16th Edition

HARRISON'S
PRINCIPLES OF
Internal
Medicine

EDITORS OF PREVIOUS EDITIONS

T. R. HARRISON
Editor-in-Chief, Editions 1, 2, 3, 4, 5

W. R. RESNICK
Editor, Editions 1, 2, 3, 4, 5

M. M. WINTROBE
Editor, Editions 1, 2, 3, 4, 5
Editor-in-Chief, Editions 6, 7

G. W. THORN
Editor, Editions 1, 2, 3, 4, 5, 6, 7
Editor-in-Chief, Edition 8

R. D. ADAMS
Editor, Editions 2, 3, 4, 5, 6, 7, 8, 9, 10

P. B. BEESON
Editor, Editions 1, 2

I. L. BENNETT, JR.
Editor, Editions 3, 4, 5, 6

E. BRAUNWALD
Editor, Editions 6, 7, 8, 9, 10, 12, 13, 14
Editor-in-Chief, Edition 11, 15

K. J. ISSELBACHER
Editor, Editions 6, 7, 8, 10, 11, 12, 14
Editor-in-Chief, Editions 9, 13

R. G. PETERSDORF
Editor, Editions 6, 7, 8, 9, 11, 12, 13
Editor-in-Chief, Edition 10

J. D. WILSON
Editor, Editions 9, 10, 11, 13, 14
Editor-in-Chief, Edition 12

J. B. MARTIN
Editor, Editions 10, 11, 12, 13, 14

A. S. FAUCI
Editor, Editions 11, 12, 13, 15
Editor-in-Chief, Edition 14

R. ROOT
Editor, Edition 12

D. L. KASPER
Editor, Editions 13, 14, 15

S. L. HAUSER
Editor, Edition 14, 15

D. L. LONGO
Editor, Edition 14, 15

J. L. JAMESON
Editor, Edition 15

16th Edition

HARRISON'S
PRINCIPLES OF
Internal
Medicine

Editors

DENNIS L. KASPER, MD
William Ellery Channing Professor of Medicine,
Professor of Microbiology and Molecular Genetics,
Harvard Medical School; Director, Channing
Laboratory, Department of Medicine, Brigham and
Women's Hospital, Boston

ANTHONY S. FAUCI, MD
Chief, Laboratory of Immunoregulation; Director,
National Institute of Allergy and Infectious Diseases,
National Institutes of Health, Bethesda

DAN L. LONGO, MD
Scientific Director, National Institute on Aging,
National Institutes of Health,
Bethesda and Baltimore

EUGENE BRAUNWALD, MD
Distinguished Hersey Professor of Medicine,
Harvard Medical School; Chairman, TIMI Study Group,
Brigham and Women's Hospital, Boston

STEPHEN L. HAUSER, MD
Robert A. Fishman Distinguished Professor and Chairman,
Department of Neurology,
University of California San Francisco, San Francisco

J. LARRY JAMESON, MD, PhD
Irving S. Cutter Professor and Chairman,
Department of Medicine,
Northwestern University Feinberg School of Medicine;
Physician-in-Chief, Northwestern
Memorial Hospital, Chicago

McGraw-Hill
MEDICAL PUBLISHING DIVISION

New York   Chicago   San Francisco   Lisbon   London   Madrid
Mexico City   Milan   New Delhi   San Juan   Seoul   Singapore   Sydney   Toronto

Harrison's
PRINCIPLES OF INTERNAL MEDICINE
Sixteenth Edition

1234567890 DOWDOW 0987654

ISBN 0-07-140235-7 (Combo)

ISBN 0-07-139140-1 (Set)
ISBN 0-07-139141-X (Vol. I)
ISBN 0-07-139142-8 (Vol. II)

FOREIGN LANGUAGE EDITIONS

Arabic (13e): McGraw-Hill Libri Italia srl (est. 1996)

Chinese Long Form (15e): McGraw-Hill International Enterprises, Inc., Taiwan

Chinese Short Form (15e): McGraw-Hill Education (Asia), Singapore

Croatian (13e): Placebo, Split, Croatia

French (15e): Medecine-Sciences Flammarion, Paris, France

German (15e): ABW Wissenschaftsverlagsgesellschaft mbH, Berlin, Germany

Greek (15e): Parissianos, S.A., Athens, Greece

Italian (15e): The McGraw-Hill Companies, Srl, Milan, Italy

Japanese (15e): MEDSI-Medical Sciences International Ltd, Tokyo, Japan

Korean (15e): McGraw-Hill Korea, Inc., Seoul, Korea

Polish (14e): Czelej Publishing Company, Lubin, Poland (est. 2000)

Portuguese (15e): McGraw-Hill Interamericana do Brazil, Rio de Janeiro, Brazil

Romanian (14e): Teora Publishers, Bucharest, Romania (est. 2000)

Serbian (15e): Publishing House Romanov, Bosnia & Herzegovina, Republic of Serbska

Spanish (15e): McGraw-Hill Interamericana de Espana S.A., Madrid, Spain

Turkish (15e): Nobel Tip Kitabevleri, Ltd., Istanbul, Turkey

Vietnamese (15e): McGraw-Hill Education (Asia), Singapore

This book was set in Times Roman by Progressive Information Technologies. The editors were Martin Wonsiewicz and Mariapaz Ramos Englis. The production director was Robert Laffler. The index was prepared by Barbara Littlewood. The text designer was Marsha Cohen/Parallelogram Graphics. Art director: Libby Pisacreta; cover design by Janice Bielawa. Medical illustrator: Jay McElroy, MAMS.

R. R. Donnelley and Sons, Inc., was the printer and binder.

Cover illustrations courtesy of Raymond J. Gibbons, MD; George V. Kelvin; Robert S. Hillman, MD; and Marilu Gorno-Tempini, MD.

Library of Congress Cataloging-in-Publication Data

Harrison's principles of internal medicine—16th ed./editors, Dennis L. Kasper . . . [et al.].   p. cm.
   Includes bibliographical references and index.
   ISBN 0-07-139140-1 (set)—ISBN 0-07-139141-X (v. 1)—ISBN 0-07-139142-8 (v. 2)—ISBN 0-07-140235-7 (combo)
     1. Internal medicine. I. Title: Principles of internal medicine. II. Kasper, Dennis L. III. Harrison, Tinsley Randolph, 1900– Principles of internal medicine.
   [DNLM: 1. Internal Medicine. WB 115 H322 2005]
RC46.H333 2005
616—dc21

2004044931

Tinsley R. Harrison

The 16th Edition of Harrison's Principles of Internal Medicine is dedicated to Tinsley R. Harrison, the founding editor and Editor-in-Chief for the first five editions.

From time to time a personality scintillates across the medical firmament who dazzles all beholders. Tinsley Harrison was such a person. A delightful, vivacious, passionate physician, he stimulated everyone with whom he came into contact, and he placed an indelible stamp on the medical events of his day.

Tinsley Randolph Harrison was born in Talladega, Alabama, on March 18, 1900. His father, Groce Harrison, was a sixth-generation physician, a student of William Osler who inculcated Osler's values into his son from an early age. Tinsley earned his undergraduate degree from the University of Michigan and his M.D. from Johns Hopkins School of Medicine. After a medical residency at the Peter Bent Brigham Hospital in Boston, where he developed his life-long interest in cardiovascular science and medicine, and additional training at Hopkins, Dr. Harrison served as chief medical resident and then joined the faculty of Vanderbilt University School of Medicine. His Chief of Medicine there, Canby Robinson, described him as "a human dynamo with unbounded energy." After a brief period of private practice, which Harrison later described as "perhaps the greatest educational experience of my entire life," he served successively as chair of medicine at Bowman-Gray School of Medicine, Winston-Salem, North Carolina; the Southwestern Medical School in Dallas, Texas; and the University of Alabama, Birmingham. He played a key role in organizing the Bowman-Gray and Southwestern medical schools. He also served as Dean of Southwestern and the University of Alabama and as Chief of Cardiology at the latter. Dr. Harrison died in Birmingham, on August 4, 1978.

For decades he was an active experimentalist, and his important contributions to the understanding of the pathophysiology of heart failure were all the more remarkable because they were obtained before the availability of measurements of intracardiac pressures, cardiac output, and regional blood flow. Harrison's research involved both basic studies in cardiovascular physiology as well as clinical research and were summarized in a classic text *Failure of the Circulation*. He was a founding member of the Council of the National Heart Institute and served as president of the American Society for Clinical Investigation and of the American Heart Association. Tinsley Harrison received the Gold Heart Award from the latter, the Kober Medal of the Association of American Physicians, and the Distinguished Teacher Award of the American College of Physicians. Few people of his generation surpassed him as a bedside teacher.

In 1945, stimulated by the publisher Blakiston, Harrison conceived of a new type of textbook of internal medicine, in which both of his interests—clinical medicine and the pathophysiologic mechanisms of disease—would be as closely interwoven as they were in his mind. He immediately recruited an editorial team; Harrison authored or co-authored almost the entire cardiovascular section. By 1950, the first edition of *Principles of Internal Medicine* was published.

Although Harrison was a distinguished investigator, teacher, academic leader, and editor, he was first and foremost a masterful physician who excelled in the care of the sick. The individual patient was always in the center of the stage. To put the disease first, to refer to the patient as "a case," would arouse Harrison's wrath. The words that he penned for the first edition of this book reflect the importance he attached to his role as a physician.

> *No greater opportunity or obligation can fall the lot of a human being than to be a physician. In the care of the suffering he needs technical skill, scientific knowledge, and human understanding. He who uses these with courage, humility, and wisdom will provide a unique service for his fellow man and will build an enduring edifice of character within himself. The physician should ask of his destiny no more than this, and he should be content with no less.*

These words express the philosophy of the original editors and of all those who have followed.

It is to the memory of this great physician, teacher, investigator, and editor, whose life and works have so inspired us, that this sixteenth edition of *Harrison's Principles of Internal Medicine* is dedicated.

THE EDITORS

CONTENTS

Part Ten
CRITICAL CARE MEDICINE

Part Eleven
DISORDERS OF THE KIDNEY AND URINARY TRACT

Part Twelve
DISORDERS OF THE GASTROINTESTINAL SYSTEM

Part Thirteen
DISORDERS OF THE IMMUNE SYSTEM, CONNECTIVE TISSUE, AND JOINTS

Part Fourteen
ENDOCRINOLOGY AND METABOLISM

Part Fifteen
NEUROLOGIC DISORDERS

SECTION 1
DIAGNOSIS OF NEUROLOGIC DISORDERS

SECTION 2
DISEASES OF THE CENTRAL NERVOUS SYSTEM

SECTION 3
NERVE AND MUSCLE DISORDERS

SECTION 4
CHRONIC FATIGUE SYNDROME

SECTION 5
PSYCHIATRIC DISORDERS

SECTION 6
ALCOHOLISM AND DRUG DEPENDENCY

Part Sixteen
POISONING, DRUG OVERDOSE, AND ENVENOMATION

APPENDICES

INDEX

Numbers in brackets refer to chapters written or co-written by the contributor.

ELIAS ABRUTYN, MD
Professor of Medicine and Public Health, Associate Provost and Associate Dean for Faculty Affairs; Interim Chief, Infectious Diseases, Drexel University College of Medicine, Philadelphia [124,125]

JOHN C. ACHERMANN, MRCP, MRCPCH, MD
Wellcome Trust Clinician Scientist, Department of Medicine and Institute of Child Health, University College London, London, UK [328]

JOHN W. ADAMSON, MD
Executive Vice President for Research, Director, Blood Research Institute, Blood Center of Southeastern Wisconsin, Milwaukee [52, 90]

DAVID A. AHLQUIST, MD
Professor of Medicine, Mayo Clinic College of Medicine; Consultant in Gastroenterology, Division of Gastroenterology and Hepatology, Mayo Clinic, Rochester [35]

LEENA ALA-KOKKO, MD, PhD
Professor of Medicine, Center for Gene Therapy, Tulane University Health Sciences Center, New Orleans [342]

KENNETH C. ANDERSON, MD
Chief, Division of Hematologic Neoplasia; Director, Jerome Lipper Multiple Myeloma Center, Dana-Farber Cancer Institute; Kraft Family Professor of Medicine, Harvard Medical School, Boston [98, 99]

ELLIOTT M. ANTMAN, MD
Professor of Medicine, Harvard Medical School; Director, Samuel A. Levine Cardiac Unit, Brigham and Women's Hospital, Boston [228]

FREDERICK R. APPELBAUM, MD
Member and Director, Clinical Research Division, Fred Hutchinson Cancer Research Center; Professor and Head, Division of Medical Oncology, University of Washington School of Medicine, Seattle [100]

GORDON L. ARCHER, MD
Professor of Medicine and Microbiology/Immunology; Chair, Division of Infectious Diseases, Department of Medicine, Virginia Commonwealth University Medical Center, Richmond [118]

JAMES O. ARMITAGE, MD
Joe Shapiro Professor of Medicine, University of Nebraska, Omaha [97]

ARTHUR K. ASBURY, MD
Van Meter Professor of Neurology Emeritus, University of Pennsylvania School of Medicine, Philadelphia [22, 363, 365]

JOHN R. ASPLIN, MD
Assistant Professor of Medicine, Section of Nephrology, University of Chicago Pritzker School of Medicine, Chicago [265, 268]

JOHN C. ATHERTON, MD
Professor of Gastroenterology, Wolfson Digestive Diseases Centre and Institute of Infections, Immunity and Inflammation, University of Nottingham, Nottingham, England [135]

PAUL S. AUERBACH, MD, MS
Clinical Professor of Surgery, Department of Surgery, Division of Emergency Medicine, Stanford University School of Medicine, Los Altos [378]

K. FRANK AUSTEN, MD
AstraZeneca Professor of Respiratory and Inflammatory Diseases, Harvard Medical School; Director, Inflammation and Allergic Diseases Research Section, Division of Rheumatology, Immunology, and Allergy, Department of Medicine, Brigham and Women's Hospital, Boston [298]

BERNARD M. BABIOR, MD, PhD
Professor and Head, Division of Biochemistry, Department of Molecular and Experimental Medicine, The Scripps Research Institute, La Jolla [92]

LINDSEY R. BADEN, MD
Assistant Professor of Medicine, Harvard Medical School; Division of Infectious Diseases, Brigham and Women's Hospital, Boston [162]

KAMAL F. BADR, MD
Professor and Chair, Department of Internal Medicine, American University of Beirut (Lebanon); Attending Physician, American University of Beirut Medical Center, Beirut, Lebanon [267]

DONALD S. BAIM, MD
Professor of Medicine, Harvard Medical School; Director, Center for Integration of Medicine and Innovative Technology, Brigham and Women's Hospital, Boston [212, 229]

ROBERT L. BARBIERI, MD
Kate Macy Ladd Professor of Obstetrics, Gynecology, and Reproductive Biology, Harvard Medical School; Chairman, Obstetrics and Gynecology, Brigham and Women's Hospital, Boston [6]

TAMAR F. BARLAM, MD
Associate Professor of Medicine, Boston University School of Medicine, Boston [106, 131]

KENNETH J. BART, MD
Director, Graduate School of Public Health, Professor of Epidemiology and Biostatistics, San Diego State University, San Diego [107]

SHARI S. BASSUK, ScD
Epidemiologist, Division of Preventive Medicine, Brigham and Women's Hospital, Boston [327]

M. FLINT BEAL, MD
Anne Parrish Titzel Professor and Chair, Department of Neurology and Neuroscience, Weill Medical College of Cornell University; Neurologist-in-Chief, New York Presbyterian Hospital, New York [345, 355]

NICHOLAS J. BEECHING, FRCP, FRACP, DCH, DTM&H
Senior Lecturer in Infectious Diseases, Liverpool School of Tropical Medicine; Clinical Lead, Tropical and Infectious Disease Unit, Royal Liverpool University Hospital, Liverpool, United Kingdom [141]

ROBERT S. BENJAMIN, MD
Professor of Medicine, Chairman, Department of Sarcoma Medical Oncology, The University of Texas MD Anderson, Houston [84]

JOHN E. BENNETT, MD
Head, Clinical Mycology Section, Laboratory of Clinical Investigation, National Institute of Allergy and Infectious Diseases, National Institutes of Health, Potomac [182–190]

EDWARD J. BENZ, JR., MD
Richard and Susan Smith Professor of Medicine, Professor of Pediatrics, Professor of Pathology, Harvard Medical School; President and CEO, Dana-Farber Cancer Institute; Director, Dana-Farber/Harvard Cancer Center, Boston [91]

SHALENDAR BHASIN, MD
Professor of Medicine, University of California Los Angeles School of Medicine; Chief, Division of Endocrinology, Charles R. Drew University, Los Angeles [325]

DAVID R. BICKERS, MD
Carl Truman Nelson Professor and Chair, Department of Dermatology, College of Physicians and Surgeons, Columbia University Medical Center, New York [51]

HENRY J. BINDER, MD
Professor of Medicine, Professor of Cellular and Molecular Physiology, Yale University, New Haven [275]

THOMAS D. BIRD, MD
Professor of Neurology and Medicine, University of Washington; Veterans Affairs Puget Sound Medical Center, Seattle [350, 364]

NEIL R. BLACKLOW, MD
Chairman Emeritus, Department of Medicine, Professor of Medicine, University of Massachusetts Medical School, Worcester; Visiting Professor of Medicine, Harvard Medical School, Boston [168]

MARTIN J. BLASER, MD
Chairman, Department of Medicine, Frederick H. King Professor of Internal Medicine; Professor of Microbiology, New York University School of Medicine, New York [135, 139]

CLARA D. BLOOMFIELD, MD
William G. Pace III Professor of Cancer Research, Cancer Scholar and Senior Advisor, The Ohio State University Comprehensive Cancer and The Arthur G. James Cancer Hospital and Richard J. Solove Research Institute, Columbus [96]

RICHARD S. BLUMBERG, MD
Chief, Division of Gastroenterology, Hepatology, and Endoscopy, Brigham and Women's Hospital, Boston [276]

DAVID M. BODINE, PhD
Chief, Hematopoiesis Section, Genetics and Molecular Biology Branch, National Human Genome Research Institute, Bethesda [59]

JEAN L. BOLOGNIA, MD
Professor of Dermatology, Yale University School of Medicine, New Haven [48]

GEORGE J. BOSL, MD
Chairman, Department of Medicine, Memorial Sloan-Kettering Cancer Center; Professor of Medicine, Weill Medical College of Cornell University, New York [82]

RICHARD C. BOUCHER JR., MD
William Rand Kenan Professor of Medicine, University of North Carolina at Chapel Hill; Director, University of North Carolina Cystic Fibrosis Center, Chapel Hill [241]

KAREN D. BRADSHAW, MD
Professor of Obstetrics/Gynecology and Surgery, Helen J. and Robert S. Strauss and Diana K. and Richard C. Strauss Distinguished Professor in Women's Health, The University of Texas Southwestern Medical Center, Dallas [326]

HUGH R. BRADY, MD, PhD, FRCPI
Professor and Head, Department of Medicine and Therapeutics, University College Dublin, Dublin, Ireland [260, 264]

KENNETH D. BRANDT, MD
Professor of Medicine and Professor of Orthopaedic Surgery, Indiana University School of Medicine; Director, Indiana University Multipurpose Arthritis and Musculoskeletal Diseases Center, Indianapolis [312]

EUGENE BRAUNWALD, MD, MA(Hon), MD(Hon), ScD(Hon)
Distinguished Hersey Professor of Medicine, Harvard Medical School; Chairman, TIMI Study Group, Brigham and Women's Hospital, Boston [29, 31, 32, 208, 209, 215, 216, 219, 221, 222, 226–228]

IRWIN M. BRAVERMAN, MD
Professor of Dermatology, Yale University School of Medicine, New Haven [48]

OTIS W. BRAWLEY, MD
Professor of Hematology, Oncology, and Epidemiology, Emory University Medical School; Associate Director, Population Sciences and Cancer Control Program, Winship Cancer Institute, Atlanta [67]

JOEL G. BREMAN, MD, DTPH
Senior Scientific Advisor, Fogarty International Center, National Institutes of Health, Bethesda [195]

BARRY M. BRENNER, MD, DSc(Hon), DMSc(Hon)
Samuel A. Levine Professor of Medicine, Harvard Medical School; Director Emeritus, Renal Division, Brigham and Women's Hospital, Boston [40, 41, 259–262, 264, 266, 267, 270]

ROBERT M. BRENNER, MD
Associate Medical Director, Clinical Research, Amgen In., Thousand Oaks, California [259]

GEORGE J. BREWER, MD
Morton S. and Henrietta K. Sellner Active Emeritus Professor of Human Genetics, Active Emeritus Professor of Internal Medicine, University of Michigan Medical School, Ann Arbor [339]

F. RICHARD BRINGHURST, MD
Associate Professor of Medicine, Harvard Medical School, Boston [331]

CLAIRE V. BROOME, MD
Senior Advisor, Centers for Disease Control and Prevention, Atlanta [123]

ROBERT H. BROWN, JR., MD, DPHil
Associate Neurologist, Massachusetts General Hospital; Professor of Neurology, Harvard Medical School, Boston [353, 368]

GREGORY BULKLEY, MD
Mark M. Ravitch Professor of Surgery, The Johns Hopkins University School of Medicine, Baltimore [279]

H. FRANKLIN BUNN, MD
Professor of Medicine, Harvard Medical School, Boston [92, 93]

DAVID M. BURNS, MD
Professor of Family and Preventive Medicine, Professor of Medicine, University of California San Diego, San Diego [375]

MICHAEL J. BURNS, MD
Assistant Professor of Medicine, Harvard Medical School, Boston [377]

JOAN R. BUTTERTON, MD, DTM&H
Assistant Professor of Medicine, Harvard Medical School; Assistant in Medicine, Infectious Disease Division, Massachusetts General Hospital, Boston [113]

JOHN C. BYRD, MD
D. Warren Brown Professor of Leukemia Research, Associate Professor of Medicine and Medical Chemistry, The Ohio State University; Director of Hematologic Malignancies, Division of Hematology and Oncology, James Cancer Hospital and Solove Research Institute, Columbus [96]

STEPHEN B. CALDERWOOD, MD
Chief, Division of Infectious Diseases, Massachusetts General Hospital; Professor of Medicine (Microbiology and Molecular Genetics), Harvard Medical School, Boston [113]

MICHAEL V. CALLAHAN, MD, MSPH, DTM&H
Program Leader, Biological Threat Defense, Center for Integration of Medicine and Innovative Technologies, Massachusetts General Hospital, Boston [18]

MICHAEL CAMILLERI, MD
Atherton and Winifred W. Bean Professor, Professor of Medicine and Physiology, Mayo Clinic College of Medicine; Consultant in Gastroenterology, Mayo Clinic, Rochester [35]

G. DOUGLAS CAMPBELL, MD
Professor of Medicine, Director, Division of Pulmonary, Critical Care, and Sleep Medicine, University of Mississippi School of Medicine, Jackson [239]

GRANT L. CAMPBELL, MD, PhD
Chief, Epidemiology Activity, Arbovirus Diseases Branch, Division of Vector-Borne Infectious Diseases, National Center for Infectious Diseases, Centers for Disease Control and Prevention, Fort Collins [143]

CHRISTOPHER P. CANNON, MD
Associate Professor of Medicine, Harvard Medical School; Senior Investigator, TIMI Study Group, Cardiovascular Division, Brigham and Women's Hospital, Boston [227]

MARK D. CARLSON, MD
Professor of Medicine, Associate Vice President for Government Relations, Case Western Reserve University; Associate Dean, Case School of Medicine, Cleveland [20]

CHARLES B. CARPENTER, MD
Professor of Medicine, Harvard Medical School; Senior Physician, Brigham and Women's Hospital, Boston [263]

BRUCE R. CARR, MD
Professor and Director, Division of Reproductive Endocrinology and Infertility; Holder, Paul C. MacDonald Distinguished Chair in Obstetrics and Gynecology, The University of Texas Southwestern Medical Center, Dallas [326]

AGUSTIN CASTELLANOS, MD
Professor of Medicine; Director, Clinical Electrophysiology, University of Miami School of Medicine, Miami [256]

PHILIP F. CHANCE, MD
Professor of Pediatrics and Neurology, University of Washington School of Medicine; Chief, Division of Genetics and Development, Children's Hospital and Regional Medical Center, Seattle [364]

FENG-YEE CHANG, MD
Professor, Department of Medicine, National Defense Medical Center; Chief, Division of Infectious Diseases and Tropical Medicine, Department of Internal Medicine, Tri-Service General Hospital, Taipei, Taiwan [132]

YUAN-TSONG CHEN, MD, PhD
Professor and Chief, Division of Medical Genetics, Duke University Medical Center; Director, Institute of Biomedical Sciences, Durham [341]

JOHN S. CHILD, MD
Streisand Professor of Medicine/Cardiology; Co-Chief, Division of Cardiology, David Geffen School of Medicine at UCLA; Director, Ahmanson/UCLA Adult Congenital Heart Disease Center, UCLA Medical Center, Los Angeles [218]

KATARINA G. CHILLER, MD
Assistant Professor, Department of Dermatology, Emory University, Atlanta [73]

OLIVIER M. CHOSIDOW, MD, PhD
Department of Internal Medicine, Hôpital Pitié-Salpêtrière, Paris, France [50]

RAYMOND T. CHUNG, MD
Assistant Professor of Medicine, Harvard Medical School; Director, Hepatology Source, Medical Director, Lung Transplant Program, Associate Physician, Massachusetts General Hospital, Boston [289]

FREDRIC L. COE, MD
Professor of Medicine and Physiology, University of Chicago Pritzker School of Medicine, Chicago [265, 268]

ALAN S. COHEN, MD
Distinguished Professor of Medicine in Rheumatology, Emeritus, Boston University School of Medicine, Boston [310]

JEFFREY I. COHEN, MD
Head, Medical Virology Section, Laboratory of Infectious Diseases, National Institute of Allergy and Infectious Diseases, National Institutes of Health, Bethesda [165, 175]

FRANCIS S. COLLINS, MD, PhD
Director, National Human Genome Research Institute, National Institutes of Health, Bethesda [68]

WILSON S. COLUCCI, MD, FACC, FAHA
Thomas J. Ryan Professor of Medicine, Boston University School of Medicine; Chief, Cardiovascular Medicine, Boston University Medical Center, Boston [223]

JOEL D. COOPER, MD
Evarts A. Graham Professor of Surgery, Department of Surgery, Division of Cardiothoracic Surgery, Washington University School of Medicine, St. Louis [248]

MAX D. COOPER, MD
Professor of Medicine, Pediatrics, and Microbiology; Howard Hughes Medical Institute Investigator, University of Alabama at Birmingham, Birmingham [297]

MICHAEL J. CORBEL, PhD, DSc(Med), FIBiol, FRCPath
Head, Division of Bacteriology, National Institute for Biological Standards and Control, Potters Bar, United Kingdom [141]

LAWRENCE COREY, MD
Professor, Medicine and Laboratory Medicine; Head, Virology Division, University of Washington; Head, Program in Infectious Diseases, Fred Hutchinson Cancer Research Center, Seattle [163, 179]

FELICIA COSMAN, MD
Associate Professor of Clinical Medicine, Columbia University College of Physicians and Surgeons; Medical Director, Clinical Research Center, Helen Hayes Hospital, West Haverstraw, New York [333]

MARK A. CREAGER, MD
Professor of Medicine, Harvard Medical School; Physician, Brigham and Women's Hospital, Boston [231, 232]

PHILIP E. CRYER, MD
Irene E. and Michael M. Karl Professor of Endocrinology and Metabolism in Medicine, Washington University School of Medicine, St. Louis [324]

RONALD G. CRYSTAL, MD
Professor and Chair, Department of Genetic Medicine, Weill Medical College of Cornell University; Chief, Division of Pulmonary and Critical Care Medicine, New York Presbyterian Hospital-Weill Cornell Medical Center, New York [309]

JOHN J. CUSH, MD
Medical Director, Arthritis Center, Presbyterian Hospital of Dallas, Dallas [311]

CHARLES A. CZEISLER, MD, PhD
Professor of Medicine, Harvard Medical School; Chief, Division of Sleep Medicine; Director, Sleep Disorders and Circadian Medicine, Brigham and Women's Hospital, Boston [24]

MARINOS C. DALAKAS, MD
Professor of Neurology; Chief, Neuromuscular Diseases Section, National Institute of Neurological Disorders and Stroke, National Institutes of Health, Bethesda [369]

JOSEP DALMAU, MD, PhD
Associate Professor of Neurology, Department of Neurology, University of Pennsylvania, Philadelphia [87]

DANIEL F. DANZL, MD
Professor and Chair, Department of Emergency Medicine, University of Louisville School of Medicine, Louisville [19]

ROBERT B. DAROFF, MD
Professor of Neurology and Associate Dean, Case Western Reserve University School of Medicine, Cleveland [20]

CHARLES E. DAVIS, MD
Professor of Pathology and Medicine Emeritus, University of California San Diego School of Medicine; Director Emeritus, Microbiology Laboratory, University of California San Diego Medical Center, San Diego [192]

STEVEN R. DEITCHER, MD
Head, Section of Hematology and Coagulation Medicine, Department of Hematology-Medical Oncology, The Cleveland Clinic Foundation, Cleveland [103]

JOHN DEL VALLE, MD
Professor and Senior Associate Chair of Medicine, Graduate Medical Education, Department of Internal Medicine, University of Michigan Health System, Ann Arbor [274]

MAHLON R. DELONG, MD
Timmie Professor of Neurology; Director of Neuroscience, Emory University School of Medicine, Atlanta [351]

MARIE B. DEMAY, MD
Associate Professor of Medicine, Harvard Medical School, Boston [331]

BRADLEY M. DENKER, MD
Assistant Professor of Medicine, Harvard Medical School; Associate Physician, Brigham and Women's Hospital, Boston [40]

DAVID T. DENNIS, MD, MPH
Faculty Affiliate, Department of Microbiology, Colorado State University; Medical Epidemiologist, Division of Vector-Borne Infectious Diseases, Centers for Disease Control and Prevention, Fort Collins [143, 156]

ROBERT J. DESNICK, MD, PhD
Professor and Chair, Department of Human Genetics, Mount Sinai School of Medicine of New York University, New York [337]

BETTY DIAMOND, MD
Chief, Division of Rheumatology, Department of Microbiology and Immunology, Albert Einstein College of Medicine, New York [299]

JULES L. DIENSTAG, MD
Professor of Medicine, Harvard Medical School; Physician, Massachusetts General Hospital, Boston [78, 285–287, 291]

WILLIAM P. DILLON, MD
Professor of Radiology, Section Chief, Neuroradiology, Vice-Chair for Research Radiology, University of California San Francisco, San Francisco [347]

CHARLES A. DINARELLO, MD
Professor of Medicine, University of Colorado Health Sciences Center, Denver [16]

ROBERT G. DLUHY, MD
Professor of Medicine, Harvard Medical School, Brigham and Women's Hospital, Boston [321]

RAPHAEL DOLIN, MD
Maxwell Finland Professor of Medicine (Microbiology and Molecular Genetics); Dean for Academic and Clinical Programs, Harvard Medical School, Boston [162, 170, 171]

DAVID M. DOSA, MD, MPH
Assistant Professor of Medicine, Brown Medical School; Division of Geriatrics, Rhode Island Hospital, Providence [8]

DANIEL B. DRACHMAN, MD
Professor of Neurology and Neuroscience; WW Smith Charitable Foundation Professor of Neuroimmunology; Director, Neuromuscular Unit, The Johns Hopkins University School of Medicine, Baltimore [366]

JEFFREY M. DRAZEN, MD
Professor of Medicine, Harvard Medical School, Boston [233–235, 252]

THOMAS D. DuBOSE, JR., MD
Professor and Chair, Department of Internal Medicine, Professor, Department of Physiology and Pharmacology, Wake Forest University School of Medicine, Winston-Salem [42]

J. STEPHEN DUMLER, MD
Professor, Division of Medical Microbiology, Department of Pathology and the Program in Cellular and Molecular Medicine, The Johns Hopkins University School of Medicine; Department of Molecular Microbiology and Immunology, The Johns Hopkins University Bloomberg School of Public Health, Baltimore [158]

ANDREA E. DUNAIF, MD
Charles F. Kettering Professor of Medicine, Northwestern University Feinberg School of Medicine; Chief, Division of Endocrinology, Metabolism and Molecular Medicine, Northwestern University, Chicago [5]

SAMUEL C. DURSO, MD
Associate Professor of Medicine, Division of Geriatric Medicine and Gerontology, The Johns Hopkins University School of Medicine; Deputy Director of Education, Co-Director Fellowship Training Program, Director of Ambulatory Clinical Services, Baltimore [28]

JANICE P. DUTCHER, MD
Professor of Medicine, New York Medical College; Associate Director, Clinical Affairs, Our Lady of Mercy Cancer Center, Bronx [88]

JOHANNA T. DWYER, DSc
Professor of Medicine and Community Health, Tufts University School of Medicine and Friedman School of Nutrition; Director, Frances Stern Nutrition Center; Tufts-New England Medical Center Senior Scientist; Nutritional Epidemiology Program, Jean Mayer USDA Human Nutrition Center on Aging at Tufts, Boston [60]

VICTOR J. DZAU, MD
Hershey Professor of Medicine, Harvard Medical School; Chairman, Department of Medicine and Director of Research, Brigham and Women's Hospital, Boston [231, 232]

JEFFERY S. DZIECZKOWSKI, MD
Physician, New Britain General Hospital, New Britain [99]

J. DONALD EASTON, MD
Professor and Chair, Department of Clinical Neurosciences, Brown Medical School and Rhode Island Hospital, Providence [349]

DAVID A. EHRMANN, MD
Associate Professor, Section of Endocrinology, Department of Medicine, University of Chicago Pritzker School of Medicine, Chicago [44]

EZEKIEL J. EMANUEL, MD, PhD
Chief, Department of Clinical Bioethics, Warren G. Magnuson Clinical Center, National Institutes of Health, Bethesda [9]

LINDA L. EMANUEL, MD
Buehler Professor of Geriatric Medicine, Director, Buehler Center on Aging, Northwestern University School of Medicine, Chicago [9]

JOHN W. ENGSTROM, MD
Professor of Neurology; Vice Chairman, Residency Program Director, University of California San Francisco, San Francisco [15, 354]

ANTHONY S. FAUCI, MD
Chief, Laboratory of Immunoregulation; Director, National Institute of Allergy and Infectious Diseases, National Institutes of Health, Bethesda [172, 173, 205, 295, 306]

MURRAY J. FAVUS, MD
Professor of Medicine, University of Chicago Pritzker School of Medicine, Division of Biological Sciences, Chicago [268, 334]

ROBERT G. FENTON, MD, PhD
Associate Professor of Medicine, University of Maryland Greenebaum Cancer Center, Baltimore [69]

HOWARD L. FIELDS, MD, PhD
Professor of Neurology and Physiology, University of California San Francisco, San Francisco [11]

GREGORY A. FILICE, MD
Chief, Infectious Disease Section, Veterans Affairs Medical Center; Associate Professor, Department of Medicine, University of Minnesota, Minneapolis [146]

ROBERT W. FINBERG, MD
Professor and Chair, Department of Medicine, University of Massachusetts Medical School, Worcester [72, 117]

JOYCE D. FINGEROTH, MD
Assistant Professor of Medicine, Harvard Medical School; Division of Infectious Diseases, Beth Israel Deaconess Medical Center, Boston [117]

NAOMI D.L. FISHER, MD
Assistant Professor, Harvard Medical School; Director, Hypertension Service, Brigham and Women's Hospital, Boston [230]

JEFFREY S. FLIER, MD
Chief Academic Officer, Beth Israel Deaconess Medical Center; George C. Reisman Professor of Medicine, Harvard Medical School, Boston [64]

SONIA FRIEDMAN, MD
Instructor of Medicine, Harvard Medical School; Associate Physician, Brigham and Women's Hospital, Boston [276]

WILLIAM F. FRIEDMAN, MD
JH Nicholson Professor of Pediatrics (Cardiology); Senior Associate Dean for Academic Affairs, David Geffen School of Medicine at UCLA, Los Angeles [218]

ROBERT F. GAGEL, MD
Professor of Medicine and Head, Division of Internal Medicine, University of Texas MD Anderson Cancer Center, Houston [330]

JOHN I. GALLIN, MD
Director, NIH Warren Grant G. Magnuson Clinical Center; NIH Associate Director for Clinical Research; Chief Laboratory of Host Defenses, National Institute of Allergy and Infectious Diseases, National Institutes of Health, Bethesda [55]

SUSAN L. GEARHART, MD
Assistant Professor of Surgery, The Johns Hopkins University School of Medicine, Baltimore [279]

ROBERT H. GELBER, MD
Leonard Wood Memorial Scientific Director, American Leprosy Foundation; Clinical Professor of Medicine and Dermatology, University of California San Francisco, San Francisco [151]

JEFFREY A. GELFAND, MD
Visiting Professor of Medicine, Harvard Medical School; Professor of Medicine, Tufts University School of Medicine; Physician, Infectious Diseases Unit, Department of Medicine, Massachusetts General Hospital, Boston [16, 18]

DALE N. GERDING, MD
Chief, Medical Service, VA Chicago Health Care System—Lakeside Division; Professor and Associate Chairman, Department of Medicine, The Feinberg School of Medicine, Northwestern University, Chicago [114]

ANNE A. GERSHON, MD
Professor of Pediatrics; Director, Division of Pediatric Infectious Diseases, Columbia University Medical Center, New York [176–178]

MARC GHANY, MD
Medical Staff Fellow, Liver Diseases Section, Digestive Diseases Branch, National Institute of Diabetes and Digestive and Kidney Diseases, National Institutes of Health, Bethesda [282]

RAYMOND J. GIBBONS, MD
Arthur M. and Gladys D. Gray Professor of Medicine, Mayo Clinic College of Medicine, Rochester [211]

BRUCE C. GILLILAND, MD
Professor of Medicine and Laboratory Medicine, University of Washington School of Medicine, Seattle [303, 308, 315, 316]

ROGER I. GLASS, MD, PhD
Viral Gastroenteritis Section, Centers for Disease Control and Prevention, Atlanta [174]

ELI GLATSTEIN, MD
Morton M. Kligerman Professor and Vice Chairman, Clinical Director, Department of Radiation Oncology, University of Pennsylvania Medical Center, Philadelphia [71, 207]

ROBERT M. GLICKMAN, MD
Professor of Medicine and Dean, New York University School of Medicine; CEO New York University Hospitals Center, New York [39]

JAMES F. GLOCKNER, MD
Assistant Professor of Radiology, Mayo Clinic College of Medicine; Consultant, Department of Radiology, Mayo Clinic, Rochester [211]

ARY L. GOLDBERGER, MD
Associate Professor of Medicine, Harvard Medical School; Director, Margret and H.A. Rey Institute for Nonlinear Dynamics in Medicine, Beth Israel Deaconess Medical Center, Boston [210]

SAMUEL Z. GOLDHABER, MD
Associate Professor of Medicine, Harvard Medical School; Director, Venous Thromboembolism Research Group, Director, Anticoagulation Service and Staff Cardiologist, Brigham and Women's Hospital, Boston [244]

RALPH GONZALES, MD, MSPH
Associate Professor of Medicine, Epidemiology and Biostatistics, University of California San Francisco, San Francisco [27]

DOUGLAS S. GOODIN, MD
Professor of Neurology, University of California San Francisco, San Francisco [359]

RAJ K. GOYAL, MD
Mallinckrodt Professor of Medicine, Harvard Medical School, Boston [33, 273]

GREGORY A. GRABOWSKI, MD
Director, Division and Program in Human Genetics, Cincinnati Children's Hospital Research Foundation; Professor, Department of Pediatrics, and Molecular Genetics and Biochemistry, University of Cincinnati College of Medicine, Cincinnati [340]

JACOB GREEN, MD
Associate Professor of Medicine, Department of Nephrology, Technion Faculty of Medicine, Haifa, Israel [261]

NORTON J. GREENBERGER, MD
Professor of Medicine, Harvard Medical School; Senior Physician, Brigham and Women's Hospital, Boston [292–294]

DAVID E. GRIFFITH, MD
Director of Tuberculosis Services and Professor of Medicine, University of Texas Health Center, Tyler [149]

WILLIAM GROSSMAN, MD
Myer Friedman Distinguished Professor of Medicine, University of California San Francisco; Chief of Cardiology, University of California San Francisco Medical Center, San Francisco [212]

RASIM GUCALP, MD
Associate Professor of Medicine, Department of Oncology, Montefiore Medical Center, Albert Einstein College of Medicine, New York [88]

BEVRA HANNAHS HAHN, MD
Professor of Medicine, David Geffen School of Medicine at the University of California Los Angeles, Los Angeles [300]

STEPHEN M. HAHN, MD
Associate Professor, Department of Radiation Oncology, Division of Hematology Oncology, University of Pennsylvania, Philadelphia [71]

JANET E. HALL, MD
Associate Professor of Medicine, Harvard Medical School; Assistant Physician, Massachusetts General Hospital, Boston [45]

JESSE B. HALL, MD
Section Chief, Pulmonary and Critical Care Medicine; Professor of Medicine, Anesthesia and Critical Care, University of Chicago, Chicago [249]

SCOTT A. HALPERIN, MD
Professor of Pediatrics; Associate Professor of Microbiology and Immunology, Dalhousie University, Halifax, Nova Scotia, Canada [133]

CHARLES H. HALSTED, MD
Professor of Internal Medicine and Nutrition, University of California-Davis School of Medicine, Davis [62]

ROBERT I. HANDIN, MD
Professor of Medicine, Harvard Medical School, Boston [53, 101, 102]

CATHLEEN A. HANLON, VMD, PhD
Veterinary Medical Officer, Rabies Section, Centers for Disease Control and Prevention, Atlanta [179]

GAVIN HART, MD, MPH
Director, STD Services, Royal Adelaide Hospital; Clinical Associate Professor, School of Medicine, Flinders University, Adelaide, South Australia, Australia [145]

WILLIAM L. HASLER, MD
Associate Professor of Internal Medicine, Division of Gastroenterology, University of Michigan Medical Center, Ann Arbor [34, 271]

TERRY J. HASSOLD, PhD
Professor of Genetics, Case Western Reserve University School of Medicine, Cleveland [57]

STEPHEN L. HAUSER, MD
Robert A. Fishman Distinguished Professor and Chairman, Department of Neurology, University of California San Francisco, San Francisco [345, 346, 355, 356, 365]

EDWARD B. HAYES, MD
Medical Epidemiologist, Division of Vector-Borne Infectious Diseases, Centers for Disease Control and Prevention, Fort Collins [156]

BARTON F. HAYNES, MD
Frederic M. Hanes Professor of Medicine, Professor of Immunology, Duke University School of Medicine, Durham [295]

J. CLAUDE HEMPHILL III, MD
Assistant Professor of Neurology, University of California San Francisco; Director, Neurovascular and Neurocritical Care Program, San Francisco General Hospital, San Francisco [258]

PATRICK H. HENRY, MD
Principal Investigator, St. Louis-Cape Girardeau Community Clinical Oncology Program, St. Louis [54]

BARBARA L. HERWALDT, MD, MPH
Medical Epidemiologist, Division of Parasitic Diseases, Centers for Disease Control and Prevention, Atlanta [196]

MARTIN S. HIRSCH, MD
Professor of Medicine, Harvard Medical School; Professor of Immunology and Infectious Diseases, Harvard School of Public Health; Director of Clinical AIDS Research, Massachusetts General Hospital, Boston [166]

HELEN HASKELL HOBBS, MD
Investigator, Howard Hughes Medical Institute; Professor of Internal Medicine and Molecular Genetics, University of Texas Southwestern Medical Center, Dallas [335]

JUDITH S. HOCHMAN, MD, FACC
Harold Snyder Family Professor of Cardiology; Clinical Chief, Division of Cardiology; Director, Cardiovascular Clinical Research, New York University School of Medicine, New York [255]

STEVEN M. HOLLAND, MD
Senior Investigator and Head, Immunopathogenesis Unit, Clinical Pathophysiology Section, Laboratory of Host Defenses, National Institute of Allergy and Infectious Diseases, National Institute of Health, Bethesda [55]

KING K. HOLMES, MD, PhD
Professor of Medicine; Director, Center for AIDS and Sexually Transmitted Diseases, University of Washington, Seattle [115]

RANDALL K. HOLMES, MD, PhD
Professor and Chair, Department of Microbiology, University of Colorado Health Sciences Center, Denver [122]

JAY H. HOOFNAGLE, MD
Director, Liver Disease Research Branch, Division of Digestive Diseases and Nutrition, National Institute of Diabetes and Digestive and Kidney Diseases, National Institutes of Health, Bethesda [282]

ROBERT J. HOPKIN, MD
Assistant Professor of Clinical Pediatrics, The University of Cincinnati College of Medicine; Division and Program in Human Genetics, Cincinnati Children's Hospital Research Foundation, Cincinnati [340]

JONATHAN C. HORTON, MD, PhD
William F. Hoyt Professor of Neuro-Ophthalmology, Departments of Ophthalmology, Neurology, and Physiology, University of California San Francisco, San Francisco [25]

LYN HOWARD, MB, FRCP
Emeritus Professor of Medicine, Associate Professor of Pediatrics, Albany Medical College, Albany [63]

HOWARD HU, MD, MPH, ScD
Professor of Occupational and Environmental Medicine, Department of Environmental Health, Harvard School of Public Health; Associate Physician Channing Laboratory, Department of Medicine, Brigham and Women's Hospital; Associate Professor of Medicine, Harvard Medical School, Boston [376]

GARY W. HUNNINGHAKE, MD
Sterba Professor of Medicine, Director, Division of Pulmonary Critical Care and Occupational Medicine; Director, Graduate Program in Translational Biomedical Research, University of Iowa College of Medicine, Iowa City [237]

SHARON A. HUNT, MD
Professor, Division of Cardiovascular Medicine, Stanford University, Stanford [217]

CHARLES G. HURST, MD
Chief, Chemical Casualty Care Division, US Army Medical Research Institute of Chemical Defense, Maryland [206]

DAVID H. INGBAR, MD
Professor, Medicine Physiology and Pediatrics; Director, Pulmonary Allergy and Critical Care Division, University of Minnesota, Minneapolis [255]

EDWARD P. INGENITO, MD, PhD
Associate Physician, Brigham and Women's Hospital; Adjunct Assistant Professor, Harvard Medical School, Boston [250, 252]

ROLAND H. INGRAM, JR., MD
Martha West Looney Professor Emeritus, Emory University School of Medicine, Atlanta [29]

MARK A. ISRAEL, MD
Professor of Pediatrics and Genetics, Dartmouth Medical School; Director, Norris Cotton Cancer Center, Dartmouth–Hitchcock Medical Center, Lebanon [358]

KURT J. ISSELBACHER, MD
Distinguished Mallinckrodt Professor of Medicine, Harvard Medical School; Physician and Director, Massachusetts General Hospital Cancer Center, Boston [78, 285–287]

RICHARD F. JACOBS, MD
Horace C. Cabe Professor of Pediatrics, University of Arkansas for Medical Sciences College of Medicine; Chief, Pediatric Infectious Diseases, Arkansas Children's Hospital, Little Rock [142]

J. LARRY JAMESON, MD, PhD
Irving S. Cutter Professor and Chair, Department of Medicine, Northwestern University Feinberg School of Medicine; Physician-in-Chief, Northwestern Memorial Hospital, Chicago [56, 58, 59, 86, 317, 318, 320, 325, 328]

JAMES L. JANUZZI, JR., MD
Assistant Professor of Medicine, Harvard Medical School; Assistant Physician, Division of Cardiology and Department of Medicine, Massachusetts General Hospital, Boston [Appendices]

ROBERT T. JENSEN, MD
Chief, Digestive Diseases Branch, National Institute of Diabetes and Digestive and Kidney Diseases, National Institutes of Health, Bethesda [329]

BRUCE E. JOHNSON, MD
Associate Professor of Medicine, Brigham and Women's Hospital and Harvard Medical School; Program Director, Lowe Center for Thoracic Oncology, Dana-Farber Cancer Institute, Boston [86]

STUART JOHNSON, MD
Attending Physician, Hines VA Hospital; Associate Professor, Department of Medicine, Stritch School of Medicine, Loyola University, Maywood, IL [114]

S. CLAIBORNE JOHNSTON, MD, PhD
Associate Professor of Neurology and Epidemiology; Director, Stroke Service, University of California San Francisco, San Francisco [349]

MARK E. JOSEPHSON, MD
Professor of Medicine, Harvard Medical School; Chief, Cardiovascular Division, Beth Israel Deaconess Medical Center; Director, Harvard-Thorndike Electrophysiology Institute and Arrhythmia Service, Boston [213, 214]

JORGE L. JUNCOS, MD
Associate Professor of Neurology, Emory University School of Medicine; Director of Neurology, Wesley Woods Hospital, Atlanta [351]

EDWARD L. KAPLAN, MD
Professor of Pediatrics, University of Minnesota Medical School, Minneapolis [302]

MARSHALL M. KAPLAN, MD
Professor of Medicine, Tufts University School of Medicine, Boston [38, 283]

ADOLF W. KARCHMER, MD
Professor of Medicine, Harvard Medical School; Chief, Division of Infectious Diseases, Beth Israel Deaconess Medical Center, Boston [109]

DENNIS L. KASPER, MD, MA(Hon)
William Ellery Channing Professor of Medicine, Professor of Microbiology and Molecular Genetics, Harvard Medical School; Director, Channing Laboratory, Department of Medicine, Brigham and Women's Hospital, Boston [104, 106, 112, 126, 131, 148]

LLOYD H. KASPER, MD
Professor of Medicine (Neurology) and Microbiology/Immunology; Director, Multiple Sclerosis Center, Dartmouth Medical School, Lebanon [198]

DANIEL L. KASTNER, MD, PhD
Chief, Genetics and Genomics Branch, National Institute of Arthritis and Musculoskeletal and Skin Diseases, National Institutes of Health, Bethesda [278]

ELAINE T. KAYE, MD
Clinical Instructor in Dermatology, Harvard Medical School; Assistant in Medicine, Department of Medicine, Children's Hospital Medical Center, Boston [17]

KENNETH M. KAYE, MD
Assistant Professor of Medicine, Harvard Medical School; Associate Physician, Division of Infectious Diseases, Brigham and Women's Hospital, Boston [17]

GERALD T. KEUSCH, MD
Assistant Provost and Associate Dean for Global Health; Professor of Medicine and International Health, Boston University Medical Campus and School of Public Health, Boston [107, 138, 140]

JAY S. KEYSTONE, MD, MSC(CTM), FRCPC
Professor of Medicine, University of Toronto; Tropical Disease Unit, Division of Infectious Disease, Toronto General Hospital, University Health Network, Toronto, Ontario, Canada [108]

ELLIOTT KIEFF, MD, PhD
Harriet Ryan Albee Professor of Medicine and Microbiology and Molecular Genetics, Harvard Medical School; Senior Physician, Brigham and Women's Hospital, Boston [161]

TALMADGE E. KING, JR., MD
The Constance B. Wofsy Distinguished Professor and Vice Chairman, Department of Medicine, University of California San Francisco; Chief, Medical Services, San Francisco General Hospital, San Francisco [243]

LOUIS V. KIRCHHOFF, MD, MPH
Professor, Departments of Internal Medicine and Epidemiology, University of Iowa; Staff Physician, Department of Veterans Affairs Medical Center, Iowa City [197]

JOEL N. KLINE, MD, MS
Professor, Director, University of Iowa Adult Asthma Center, University of Iowa College of Medicine, Iowa City [237]

HOWARD K. KOH, MD, PhD
Professor and Associate Dean, Harvard School of Public Health, Boston [73]

DENNIS J. KOPECKO, PhD
Chief, Laboratory of Enteric and Sexually Transmitted Diseases, Center for Biologics Evaluation and Research, National Institutes of Health, Bethesda [138]

PETER KOPP, MD
Associate Professor, Division of Endocrinology, Metabolism, and Molecular Medicine, Northwestern University Feinberg School of Medicine, Chicago [56]

WALTER J. KOROSHETZ, MD
Vice Chair, Neurology Service, Massachusetts General Hospital, Associate Professor of Neurology, Harvard Medical School, Boston [361]

PHYLLIS E. KOZARSKY, MD
Professor of Medicine/Infectious Diseases, Emory University School of Medicine; Chief, Traveler's Health, Division of Global Migration and Quarantine, Centers for Disease Control and Prevention, Atlanta [108]

BARNETT S. KRAMER, MD, MPH
Associate Director for Disease Prevention, National Institutes of Health; Clinical Professor of Medicine, Uniformed Services University of the Health Sciences, Bethesda [67]

STEPHEN M. KRANE, MD
Persis, Cyrus, and Marlow B. Harrison Professor of Medicine, Harvard Medical School; Physician and Chief, Arthritis Unit, Massachusetts General Hospital, Boston [331]

ALEXANDER KRATZ, MD, PhD, MPH
Assistant Professor of Pathology, Harvard Medical School; Director, Clinical Hematology Laboratory, Massachusetts General Hospital [Appendices]

JOHN P. KRESS, MD
Assistant Professor of Medicine, University of Chicago Pritzker School of Medicine, Chicago [249]

HENRY M. KRONENBERG, MD
Professor of Medicine, Harvard Medical School; Chief, Endocrine Unit, Massachusetts General Hospital, Boston [331]

LOREN LAINE, MD
Professor of Medicine, Gastrointestinal Division, Department of Medicine, Keck School of Medicine, University of Southern California School of Medicine, Los Angeles [37]

ANIL K. LALWANI, MD
Mendik Foundation Professor and Chair, Department of Otolaryngology; Professor of Physiology and Neuroscience, New York University School of Medicine, New York [26]

LEWIS LANDSBERG, MD
Professor of Medicine, Dean and Vice President for Medical Affairs, Northwestern University Feinberg School of Medicine, Chicago [322]

H. CLIFFORD LANE, MD
Head, Clinical and Molecular Retrovirology Section, Laboratory of Immunoregulation; Clinical Director, National Institute of Allergy and Infectious Diseases, National Institutes of Health, Bethesda [173, 205]

CAROL A. LANGFORD, MD
Senior Investigator, Immunologic Diseases Section, NIAID, NIH, Bethesda [306]

THOMAS J. LAWLEY, MD
Dean, Emory University School of Medicine, Atlanta [46, 47, 49]

THOMAS H. LEE, MD
Associate Professor of Medicine, Harvard Medical School; Chief Executive Officer, Partners Community Health Care, Inc; Network President, Partners Health Care, Boston [12]

OFER LEHAVI, MD
Attending Physician, Department of Obstetrics and Gynecology, Tel-Aviv Medical Center, Israel [207]

CAMMIE F. LESSER, MD, PhD
Assistant Professor in Medicine, Harvard Medical School, Cambridge [137]

BRUCE D. LEVY, MD, FACP
Assistant Professor of Medicine, Harvard Medical School; Pulmonary and Critical Care Medicine, Brigham and Women's Hospital, Boston [251]

KENT B. LEWANDROWSKI, MD
Associate Chief of Pathology, Director, Core Laboratory, Massachusetts General Hospital; Associate Professor, Harvard Medical School, Boston [Appendices]

PETER LIBBY, MD
Mallinckrodt Professor of Medicine, Harvard Medical School; Chief, Cardiovascular Medicine, Brigham and Women's Hospital, Boston [224, 225]

RICHARD W. LIGHT, MD
Professor of Medicine, Vanderbilt University, Nashville [245]

CRAIG LILLY, MD
Associate Professor of Medicine, Harvard Medical School; Division of Pulmonary and Critical Care, Department of Medicine, Brigham and Women's Hospital, Boston [250]

CHRISTOPHER H. LINDEN, MD
Professor, Department of Emergency Medicine, Division of Medical Toxicology, University of Massachusetts Medical School, Worcester [377]

ROBERT LINDSAY, MD, PhD
Professor of Clinical Medicine, Columbia University College of Physicians and Surgeons; Chief, Internal Medicine, Helen Hayes Hospital, West Haverstraw, New York [333]

MARC E. LIPPMAN, MD
John G. Searle Professor and Chair, Department of Internal Medicine, University of Michigan Health System, Ann Arbor [76]

PETER E. LIPSKY, MD
Scientific Director, National Institute of Arthritis and Musculoskeletal and Skin Diseases, National Institutes of Health, Bethesda [299, 301, 311]

DAN L. LONGO, MD
Scientific Director, National Institute on Aging, National Institutes of Health, Bethesda and Baltimore [52, 54, 66, 69, 70, 89, 97, 98, 172]

NICOLA LONGO, MD, PhD
Professor of Pediatrics and Director, Metabolic Service, Division of Medical Genetics, Department of Pediatrics, University of Utah, Salt Lake City [343, 344]

DONALD E. LOW, MD
Chief, Department of Medicine, Toronto Medical Laboratories and Mount Sinai Hospital; Professor of Medicine and Microbiology, University of Toronto, Toronto, Ontario, Canada [239]

PHILLIP A. LOW, MD
Professor of Neurology, Mayo Medical School; Chairman, Division of Clinical Neurophysiology; Consultant in Neurology, Mayo Clinic, Rochester [354]

DANIEL H. LOWENSTEIN, MD
Professor of Neurology, Vice Chairman, Department of Neurology; Director, Physician-Scientist Education and Training Program; Director UCSF Epilepsy Center, University of California San Francisco, San Francisco [346, 348]

FRANKLIN D. LOWY, MD
Professor of Medicine and Physiology, Columbia University, New York [120]

SHEILA A. LUKEHART, PhD
Research Professor, University of Washington, Seattle [153,154]

LAWRENCE C. MADOFF, MD
Assistant Professor of Medicine, Harvard Medical School; Associate Physician, Brigham and Women's Hospital, Boston [104, 126, 314]

JAMES H. MAGUIRE, MD
Chief, Parasitic Diseases Branch, Centers for Disease Control and Prevention, Atlanta [111, 314, 379]

ADEL A. F. MAHMOUD, MD, PhD
President, Merck Vaccines, Merck & Co., Inc.; Adjunct Professor of Medicine, Case Western Reserve University, Whitehouse Station [203]

RONALD V. MAIER, MD
Professor and Vice Chair, Surgery, University of Washington; Surgeon-in-Chief, Harborview Medical Center, Seattle [253]

MARK E. MAILLIARD, MD
Associate Professor, Department of Internal Medicine, University of Nebraska College of Medicine; Chief, Section of Gastroenterology, Omaha Veterans Affairs Medical Center, Omaha [288]

JoANN E. MANSON, MD, DRPH
Professor of Medicine and the Elizabeth F. Brigham Professor of Women's Health, Harvard Medical School; Chief, Division of Preventive Medicine, Brigham and Women's Hospital, Boston [327]

ELEFTHERIA MARATOS-FLIER, MD
Associate Professor of Medicine, Harvard Medical School; Chief, Obesity Section, Joslin Diabetes Center, Boston [64]

DANIEL B. MARK, MD, MPH
Professor of Medicine, Duke University Medical Center; Director, Outcomes Research, Duke Clinical Research Institute, Durham [2]

THOMAS J. MARRIE, MD, FRCPC
Professor, Department of Medicine, Dean Faculty of Medicine and Dentistry, University of Alberta, Edmonton, Alberta, Canada [158, 239]

GARY J. MARTIN, MD
Raymond J. Lagenback, MD, Professor of Medicine, Vice Chairman, Department of Medicine, Northwestern University Feinberg School of Medicine, Chicago [4]

JOSEPH B. MARTIN, MD, PhD, MA(Hon)
Dean of the Faculty of Medicine; Caroline Shields Walker Professor of Neurobiology and Clinical Neuroscience, Harvard Medical School, Boston [11, 346]

ROBERT J. MAYER, MD
Vice Chair for Academic Affairs; Director, Center for Gastrointestinal Oncology, Dana-Farber Cancer Institute; Professor of Medicine, Harvard Medical School, Boston [77, 79]

CALVIN O. McCALL, MD
Assistant Professor of Dermatology, Department of Dermatology, Emory University School of Medicine, Atlanta [47]

WILLIAM M. McCORMACK, MD
Professor of Medicine; Chief, Infectious Diseases Division, State University of New York Downstate Medical Center, New York [159]

E. REGIS McFADDEN, JR., MD
Argyl J. Beams Professor of Medicine, MetroHealth Medical Center, Cleveland [236]

RONALD D.G. McKAY, PhD
Chief, Laboratory of Molecular Biology, National Institute of Neurologic Disorders and Stroke, NIH, Bethesda [59]

KEVIN T. McVARY, MD
Associate Professor of Urology, Northwestern University Feinberg School of Medicine, Chicago [43]

NANCY K. MELLO, PhD
Professor of Psychology, Harvard Medical School, Boston [374]

SHLOMO MELMED, MD
Professor and Associate Dean, David Geffen School of Medicine at University of California Los Angeles; Senior Vice President and Chief Academic Officer at Cedars-Sinai Medical Center, Los Angeles [318]

JERRY R. MENDELL, MD
Helen C. Kurtz Professor and Chairman of Neurology, Ohio State University, Columbus [367, 368]

JACK H. MENDELSON, MD
Professor of Psychiatry (Neuroscience), Harvard Medical School, Belmont [374]

M. -MARSEL MESULAM, MD
Ruth and Evelyn Dunbar Professor of Neurology and Psychiatry; Director, Center for Behavioral and Cognitive Neurology; Director, Alzheimer's Program, Northwestern University Feinberg School of Medicine, Chicago [23]

SUSAN MIESFELDT, MD
Maine Center for Cancer Medicine and Blood Disorders, Scarborough [58]

EDGAR L. MILFORD MD
Associate Professor of Medicine, Harvard Medical School; Brigham and Women's Hospital, Boston [263]

BRUCE L. MILLER, MD
AW and Mary Margaret Clausen Distinguished Chair, Professor of Neurology, University of California San Francisco, San Francisco [350, 362]

MARK MILLER, MD
Associate Director for Research; Director, Division of International Epidemiology and Population Studies, Fogarty International Center, National Institutes of Health, Bethesda [107]

SAMUEL I. MILLER, MD
Professor of Medicine, Microbiology, and Genome Sciences, University of Washington, Seattle [137]

JOHN D. MINNA, MD
Professor of Internal Medicine and Pharmacology; Director, Hamon Center for Therapeutic Oncology Research, University of Texas Southwestern Medical Center, Dallas [75]

THOMAS A. MOORE, MD, FACP
Clinical Associate Professor of Medicine, University of Kansas School of Medicine, Wichita [193]

PAT J. MORIN, PhD
Investigator, National Institute on Aging, National Institutes of Health; Assistant Professor, Department of Pathology, The Johns Hopkins School of Medicine, Baltimore [68]

ROBERT J. MOTZER, MD
Attending Physician, Memorial Sloan-Kettering Cancer Center; Professor of Medicine, Weill Medical College of Cornell University, New York [80, 82]

HARALAMPOS M. MOUTSOPOULOS, MD
Professor and Director, Department of Pathophysiology, National University School of Medicine; President of the National Organization for Medicines, Athens, Greece [304, 307]

ROBERT S. MUNFORD, MD
Jan and Henri Bromberg Professor of Internal Medicine, University of Texas Southwestern Medical Center, Dallas [127, 254]

TIMOTHY F. MURPHY, MD
Distinguished Professor of Medicine; Chief, Division of Infectious Diseases, State University of New York at Buffalo, Buffalo [130]

DANIEL M. MUSHER, MD
Chief, Infectious Diseases Section, Veterans Affairs Medical Center; Professor of Medicine, Professor of Molecular Virology and Immunology, Baylor College of Medicine, Houston [119, 129]

ROBERT J. MYERBURG, MD
Lemberg Professor of Medicine and Physiology, Director, Division of Cardiology, University of Miami School of Medicine; American Heart Association Chair in Cardiovascular Research, Miami [256]

GERALD T. NEPOM, MD, PhD
Director, Benaroya Research Institute at Virginia Mason; Professor (Affiliate), Department of Immunology, University of Washington School of Medicine, Seattle [296]

JONATHAN NEWMARK, MD
Chief, Operations, Chemical Casualty Care, US Army Medical Research Institute of Chemical Defense, Maryland [206]

RICHARD A. NISHIMURA, MD
Judd and Mary Morris Leighton Professor of Cardiovascular Diseases, Mayo Clinic College of Medicine, Rochester [211]

ROBERT L. NORRIS, MD
Associate Professor of Surgery, Department of Surgery, Division of Emergency Medicine, Stanford University School of Medicine, Stanford [378]

THOMAS B. NUTMAN, MD
Head, Helminth Immunology Section, and Head, Clinical Parasitology Unit, Laboratory of Parasitic Diseases, National Institute of Allergy and Infectious Diseases, National Institutes of Health, Bethesda [201, 202]

RICHARD J. O'BRIEN, MD
Head of Scientific Evaluation, Foundation for Innovative New Diagnostics, Geneva, Switzerland [150]

CHRISTOPHER A. OHL, MD
Associate Professor of Medicine, Section of Infectious Diseases, Wake Forest University School of Medicine; Director, Center for Antimicrobial Utilization, Stewardship, and Epidemiology, Baptist Medical Center, Winston-Salem [136]

RICHARD K. OLNEY, MD
Professor of Neurology, University of California San Francisco, San Francisco [21]

YVONNE M. O'MEARA, MD, FRCPI
Senior Lecturer in Medicine, University College Dublin; Consultant Nephrologist, Mater Misericordiae Hospital, Dublin, Ireland [264]

ROBERT A. O'ROURKE, MD
Charles Conrad Brown Distinguished Professor of Cardiovascular Science, University of Texas Health Science Center at San Antonio, San Antonio [209]

CHUNG OWYANG, MD
Professor of Internal Medicine, H. Marvin Pollard Collegiate Professor and Chief, Division of Gastroenterology, Department of Internal Medicine, University of Michigan Medical Center, Ann Arbor [271, 277]

UMESH D. PARASHAR, MBBS, MPH
Medical Epidemiologist, Respiratory and Enteric Viruses Branch, Centers for Disease Control and Prevention, Atlanta [174]

JEFFREY PARSONNET, MD
Associate Professor of Medicine and of Microbiology, Dartmouth Medical School; Staff Physician, Infectious Diseases Section, Dartmouth-Hitchcock Medical Center, Lebanon [111]

SHREYASKUMAR R. PATEL, MD
Associate Professor of Medicine, Deputy Chairman, Department of Sarcoma Medical Oncology, University of Texas, MD Anderson Cancer Center, Houston [84]

G. ALEXANDER PATTERSON, MD
Joseph C. Bancroft Professor of Surgery, Department of Surgery, Division of Cardiothoracic Surgery, Washington University School of Medicine, St. Louis [248]

GUSTAV PAUMGARTNER, MD
Professor of Medicine, Ludwig Maximiliam University of Munich, Durchwal, Germany [292]

MICHAEL C. PERRY, MD, FACP
Professor of Internal Medicine, Director, Division of Hematology/ Oncology, Nellie B. Smith Chair of Oncology, University of Missouri/ Ellis Fischer Cancer Center, Columbia [89]

CLARENCE J. PETERS, MD
John Sealy Distinguished University Chair in Tropical and Emerging Virology, Director for Biodefense, Center for Biodefense and Emerging Infectious Diseases, University of Texas Medical Branch in Galveston, Galveston [180, 181]

ELIOT A. PHILLIPSON, MD
Sir John and Lady Eaton Professor and Chair, Department of Medicine, University of Toronto, Toronto, Ontario, Canada [246, 247]

GERALD B. PIER, PhD
Professor of Medicine (Microbiology and Molecular Genetics), Harvard School of Medicine, Boston [105]

DANIEL K. PODOLSKY, MD
Mallinckrodt Professor of Medicine, Harvard Medical School; Chief, Gastroenterology, Massachusetts General Hospital, Boston [289, 290]

RONALD E. POLK, Pharm. D.
Professor of Pharmacy and Medicine, Chair, Department of Pharmacy, School of Pharmacy, Virginia Commonwealth University, Richmond [118]

MATTHEW POLLACK, MD
Professor of Medicine, Uniformed Services University; F. Edward Hébert School of Medicine; Attending Staff Physician, Internal Medicine and Infectious Diseases, National Naval Medical Center, Bethesda [136]

RICHARD J. POLLACK, PhD
Instructor of Tropical Public Health, Department of Immunology and Infectious Diseases, Harvard School of Public Health, Boston [379]

JOHN T. POTTS, JR., MD
Jackson Distinguished Professor of Clinical Medicine, Harvard Medical School, Boston [332]

LAWRIE W. POWELL, MD, PhD
Professor of Medicine, The University of Queensland and The Royal Brisbane and Women's Hospital, Brisbane, Queensland, Australia [336]

ALVIN C. POWERS, MD
Ruth K. Scoville Professor of Medicine, Division of Diabetes, Endocrinology, and Metabolism, Vanderbilt University Medical Center; Chief, Diabetes and Endocrinology Section, VA Tennessee Valley Healthcare System, Nashville [323]

DANIEL S. PRATT, MD
Assistant Professor of Medicine, Tufts University School of Medicine; Medical Director of Liver Transplantation, New England Medical Center, Boston [38, 283]

DANIEL T. PRICE, MD
Assistant Professor of Medicine, Boston University School of Medicine; Staff Physician, Boston Veterans Affairs Medical Center, West Roxbury [223]

DARWIN J. PROCKOP, MD, PhD
Director of Center for Gene Therapy and Professor of Biochemistry, Tulane Health Sciences Center, New Orleans [342]

STANLEY B. PRUSINER, MD
Director, Institute for Neurodegenerative Diseases; Professor, Departments of Neurology, Biochemistry and Biophysics, University of California San Francisco, San Francisco [362]

DANIEL J. RADER, MD
Associate Professor, Department of Medicine, University of Pennsylvania School of Medicine, Philadelphia [335]

SANJAY RAM, MD
Assistant Professor of Medicine, Section of Infectious Diseases, Boston University School of Medicine and Boston Medical Center, Boston [128]

DIDIER RAOULT, MD
Professor of Medicine, Unité des Rickettsies, School of Medicine, University of Aux-Marseille, Marseille, France [158]

NEIL H. RASKIN, MD
Professor of Neurology, University of California San Francisco, San Francisco [14]

MARIO C. RAVIGLIONE, MD
Director, Stop TB Department, World Health Organization, Geneva, Switzerland [150]

SHARON L. REED, MD
Professor of Pathology and Medicine, Director, Microbiology and Virology Laboratories, University of California Medical Center, San Diego [194]

ANTONIO J. REGINATO, MD
Professor of Medicine; Head, Division of Rheumatology, Cooper University Medical Center, Robert Wood Johnson Medical School at Camden, Camden [313]

RICHARD C. REICHMAN, MD
Professor of Medicine, Microbiology and Immunology; Head, Infectious Diseases Unit, Senior Associate Dean for Clinical Research, University of Rochester School of Medicine and Dentistry, Rochester [169]

CAROL M. REIFE, MD
Assistant Professor of Medicine, Jefferson Medical College of Thomas Jefferson University, Philadelphia [36]

JOHN J. REILLY, MD
Associate Professor of Medicine, Harvard Medical School; Clinical Director, Pulmonary and Critical Care Medicine, Brigham and Women's Hospital, Boston [242]

JOHN T. REPKE, MD, FACOG
Professor and Chair, Department of Obstetrics and Gynecology, Pennsylvania State University College of Medicine; Obstetrician-Gynecologist In-Chief, The Milton S. Hershey Medical Center, Hershey [6]

NEIL M. RESNICK, MD
Professor of Medicine, University of Pittsburgh School of Medicine; Chief, Division of Geriatric Medicine, University of Pittsburgh Institute on Aging, Pittsburgh [8]

VICTOR I. REUS, MD
Professor of Psychiatry, University of California San Francisco; Medical Director, Langley Porter Hospital, San Francisco [371]

C. FORDHAM VON REYN, MD
Professor of Medicine, Chief, Infectious Diseases and International Health, Dartmouth Medical School, Lebanon [152]

PETER A. RICE, MD
Professor of Medicine and Chief, Section of Infectious Diseases, Boston University Medical Center, Boston [128]

STUART RICH, MD
Professor of Medicine, Rush University Medical, Chicago [220]

GARY S. RICHARDSON, MD
Assistant Professor of Psychiatry, Case Western Reserve University, Cleveland; Senior Research Scientist, Sleep Disorders and Research Center, Henry Ford Hospital, Detroit [24]

GARY L. ROBERTSON, MD
Professor of Medicine and Neurology, Northwestern University Feinberg School of Medicine, Chicago [319]

DAN M. RODEN, MD
Professor of Medicine and Pharmacology; Chief, Division of Clinical Pharmacology, Vanderbilt University School of Medicine, Nashville [3]

JAMES A. ROMANO, JR., PhD
Commander, US Army Medical Research Institute of Chemical Defense, Maryland [206]

KAREN L. ROOS, MD
John and Nancy Nelson Professor of Neurology, Indiana University School of Medicine, Indianapolis [360]

ALLAN H. ROPPER, MD
Professor and Chairman of Neurology, Tufts University School of Medicine; Chief, Department of Neurology, St. Elizabeth's Medical Center, Boston [257, 356, 357]

ROGER N. ROSENBERG, MD
Zale Distinguished Chair and Professor of Neurology, University of Texas Southwestern Medical Center at Dallas; Attending Neurologist, Parkland Memorial Hospital and Zale-Lipsky University Hospital, Dallas [352]

MYRNA R. ROSENFELD, MD, PhD
Associate Professor of Neurology, Department of Neurology, University of Pennsylvania, Philadelphia [87]

WENDELL ROSSE, MD
Florence Reynaud McAlister Professor of Medicine and Medical Research, Department of Medicine, Duke University Medical School, Durham [93]

MICHAEL A. RUBIN, MD, PhD
Assistant Professor, Internal Medicine, Division of Infectious Diseases, Division of Clinical Epidemiology, Salt Lake City [27]

ROBERT M. RUSSELL, MD
Professor, Friedman School of Nutrition Science and Policy; Director and Scientist, Jean Mayer USDA Human Nutrition Center on Aging at Tufts, Boston [61]

THOMAS A. RUSSO, MD, CM
Assistant Professor of Medicine, Division of Infectious Diseases, Department of Medicine, State University of New York at Buffalo; Veterans Affairs Medical Center, Buffalo [134, 147]

STEPHEN M. SAGAR, MD
Professor of Neurology, Case Western Reserve School of Medicine; Director of Neuro-Oncology, Ireland Cancer Center, University Hospitals of Cleveland, Cleveland [358]

MERLE A. SANDE, MD
Professor of Medicine, University of Utah School of Medicine; President, Academic Alliance for AIDS Care and Prevention in Africa Foundation, Salt Lake City [27]

EDWARD A. SAUSVILLE, MD, PhD
Associate Director for Clinical Research, Greenebaum Cancer Center, University of Maryland, Baltimore [70]

MOHAMED H. SAYEGH, MD
Associate Professor of Medicine, Harvard Medical School; Director, Transplantation Research Center, Brigham and Women's Hospital and Children's Hospital, Boston [263]

HOWARD I. SCHER, MD
D. Wayne Calloway Chair in Urologic Oncology, Attending Physician and Chief, Genitourinary Oncology Service, Department of Medicine, Memorial Sloan-Kettering Cancer Center; Professor of Medicine, Weill Medical College of Cornell University, New York [80, 81]

HARRY W. SCHROEDER, JR., MD, PhD
Professor of Medicine and Microbiology, University of Alabama at Birmingham, Birmingham [297]

ANNE SCHUCHAT, MD
Chief, Respiratory Diseases Branch, National Center for Infectious Diseases, Centers for Disease Control and Prevention, Atlanta [123]

MARC A. SCHUCKIT, MD
Professor of Psychiatry, University of California, San Diego; Director, Alcohol Research Center; Director, Alcohol and Drug Treatment Program, Veterans Affairs San Diego Healthcare System, San Diego [372, 373]

STUART SCHWARTZ, PhD
Professor of Genetics and Oncology, Center for Human Genetics Laboratory, Cleveland [57]

DAVID S. SEGAL, PhD
Professor of Psychiatry, University of California San Diego, La Jolla [373]

JULIAN L. SEIFTER, MD
Associate Professor of Medicine, Harvard Medical School, Physician, Brigham and Women's Hospital, Boston [270]

ANDREW P. SELWYN, MD
Professor of Medicine, Harvard Medical School; Physician, Brigham and Women's Hospital, Boston [226]

STEVEN D. SHAPIRO, MD
Parker B. Francis Professor of Medicine, Harvard Medical School and Brigham and Women's Hospital, Boston [242, 250, 251]

STEVEN I. SHERMAN, MD
Associate Professor, University of Texas M.D. Anderson Cancer Center; Adjunct Associate Professor, Baylor College of Medicine, Houston [330]

WILLIAM SILEN, MD
Johnson and Johnson Distinguished Professor of Surgery, Emeritus, Harvard Medical School, Boston [13, 280, 281]

EDWIN K. SILVERMAN, MD, PhD
Assistant Professor of Medicine, Harvard Medical School; Brigham and Women's Hospital, Boston [242]

GARY G. SINGER, MD
Assistant Professor of Medicine, Washington University School of Medicine; Associate Director, Transplant Nephrology, Barnes Jewish Hospital, St. Louis [41]

AJAY K. SINGH, MD
Associate Professor of Medicine, Harvard Medical School; Director of Clinical Nephrology, Brigham and Women's Hospital, Boston [262]

JEAN DOW SIPE, PhD
Professor Emeritus, Boston University School of Medicine; Scientific Review Administrator, National Institutes of Health, Bethesda [310]

KARL SKORECKI, MD
Annie Chutick Professor of Medicine, Bruce Rappaport Faculty of Medicine, Technion-Israel Institute of Technology; Director, Department of Nephrology and Molecular Medicine, Rambam Medical Center, Haifa, Israel [261]

GERALD W. SMETANA, MD
Associate Professor of Medicine, Harvard Medical School; Division of General Medicine and Primary Care, Beth Israel Deaconess Medical Center, Boston [7]

PATRICK M. SLUSS, PhD
Director, Immunodiagnostics Laboratory, Department of Pathology, Massachusetts General Hospital; Assistant Professor, Harvard Medical School, Boston [Appendices]

WADE S. SMITH, MD
Associates Professor of Neurology; Director, Neurointensive Care Service, University of California San Francisco, San Francisco [349]

MICHAEL C. SNELLER, MD
Chief of Immunologic Diseases Section, NIAID, NIH, Bethesda [306]

JAMES B. SNOW, JR., MD
Professor Emeritus, Department of Otorhinolaryngology, University of Pennsylvania; former Director, National Institute on Deafness and Other Communication Disorders, National Institutes of Health, Bethesda [26]

ARTHUR J. SOBER, MD
Professor of Dermatology, Harvard Medical School; Associate Chief of Dermatology, Massachusetts General Hospital, Boston [73]

MICHAEL F. SORRELL, MD
Robert L. Grissom Professor of Medicine; Chief, Section of Gastroenterology and Hepatology, and Medical Director, Liver Transplantation, University of Nebraska Medical Center, Omaha [288]

PETER SPEELMAN, MD, PhD
Professor of Internal Medicine, Division of Infectious Diseases, Tropical Medicine and AIDS, Department of Internal Medicine, Academic Medical Center, University of Amsterdam, Amsterdam, The Netherlands [155]

FRANK E. SPEIZER, MD
Edward H. Kass Professor of Medicine, Harvard Medical School; Co-Director, Channing Laboratory, Brigham and Women's Hospital; Professor of Environmental Science, Harvard School of Public Health, Boston [238]

ANDREW SPIELMAN, ScD
Professor of Tropical Public Health, Harvard School of Public Health, Boston [379]

JERRY L. SPIVAK, MD
Professor of Medicine and Oncology, Johns Hopkins University School of Medicine, Baltimore [95]

WALTER E. STAMM, MD
Professor of Medicine and Head, Division of Allergy and Infectious Diseases, University of Washington School of Medicine, Seattle [160, 269]

ALLEN C. STEERE, MD
Professor of Medicine, Harvard Medical School; Director of Rheumatology, Massachusetts General Hospital, Boston [157]

DAVID S. STEPHENS, MD
Director, Division of Infectious Diseases, Emory University Hospital; Stephen W. Schwarzmann Professor and Executive Vice Chair, Department of Medicine, Emory University School of Medicine, Atlanta [127]

ROBERT S. STERN, MD
Carl J. Herzog Professor of Dermatology, Harvard Medical, Boston [50]

DENNIS L. STEVENS, MD, PhD
Professor of Medicine, University of Washington School of Medicine, Seattle; Chief, Infectious Diseases, VA Medical Center, Boise [110]

RICHARD M. STONE, MD
Clinical Director, Adult Leukemia Program, Dana-Farber Cancer Institute/Brigham and Women's Hospital; Associate Professor of Medicine, Harvard Medical School, Boston [85]

STEPHEN E. STRAUS, MD
Senior Investigator, Laboratory of Clinical Investigation, National Institute of Allergy and Infectious Diseases; Director, National Center for Complementary and Alternative Medicine, National Institutes of Health, Bethesda [10, 370]

MORTON N. SWARTZ, MD
Professor, Department of Medicine, Harvard Medical School; Chief Emeritus, Infectious Disease, Chief, James Jackson Firm Medical Services, Massachusetts General Hospital, Boston [361]

A. JAMIL TAJIK, MD
Thomas J. Watson, Jr., Professor; Professor of Medicine and Pediatrics, Mayo Clinic College of Medicine Chair (Emeritus); Division of Cardiovascular Diseases and Internal Medicine; Consultant, Section of Pediatric Cardiology, Mayo Clinic, Minnesota [211]

JOEL D. TAUROG, MD
Professor of Internal Medicine, and William M. and Gatha Burnett Professor for Arthritis Research, University of Texas Southwestern Medical Center, Dallas [296, 305]

SCOTT J. THALER, MD
Chief Medical Officer, AERAS Global TB Vaccine Foundation, Bethesda [314]

ZELIG A. TOCHNER, MD
Associate Professor, Department of Radiation Oncology, University of Pennsylvania Medical Center, Philadelphia [207]

LUCY STUART TOMPKINS, MD
Professor of Medicine (Infectious Diseases and Geographic Medicine), Professor of Microbiology, Immunology and Pathology, Stanford University School of Medicine, Stanford [144]

MARK TOPAZIAN, MD
Associate Professor of Medicine, Yale University School of Medicine; Assistant Director, Gastrointestinal Procedure Center, Yale New Haven Hospital, New Haven [272]

PHILLIP P. TOSKES, MD
Professor of Medicine and Director, Division of Gastroenterology, Hepatology and Nutrition; Associate Chairman for Clinical Affairs, Department of Medicine, University of Florida, Gainesville [293, 294]

JEFFREY M. TRENT, PhD
President and Scientific Director; Senior Investigator, Molecular Diagnostics and Target Validation Division, T-Gen, Phoenix [68]

ELBERT P. TRULOCK, MD
Rosemary and I. Jerome Flance Professor of Pulmonary Medicine, Washington University School of Medicine; Medical Director, Lung Transplantation Program, Barnes-Jewish Hospital, St. Louis [248]

KENNETH L. TYLER, MD
Reuler-Lewin Family Professor of Neurology; Professor of Medicine, Microbiology and Immunology, University of Colorado Health Sciences Center; Chief, Neurology Service, Denver VA Medical Center, Denver [360]

BERT VOGELSTEIN, MD
Professor of Oncology and Pathology, Howard Hughes Investigator, The Sidney Kimmel Comprehensive Cancer Center, The Johns Hopkins University School of Medicine, Baltimore [68]

EVERETT E. VOKES, MD
Director, Section of Hematology/Oncology; John E. Ultmann Professor of Medicine and Radiation Oncology, University of Chicago, Chicago [74]

TAMARA J. VOKES, MD
Assistant Professor of Clinical Medicine, University of Chicago Pritzker School of Medicine, Chicago [334]

MATTHEW K. WALDOR, MD, PhD
Associate Professor of Medicine and Microbiology, Tufts University School of Medicine, Boston [140]

DAVID H. WALKER, MD
Professor and Chairman, Department of Pathology; Director, WHO Collaborating Center for Tropical Diseases, University of Texas Medical Branch, Galveston [158, 239]

RICHARD J. WALLACE, JR., MD
Chairman, Department of Microbiology, John Chapman Professorship in Microbiology, Professor of Medicine, University of Texas Health Center, Tyler [149]

B. TIMOTHY WALSH, MD
Ruane Professor of Psychiatry, College of Physicians and Surgeons, Columbia University; Director, Eating Disorders Research Unit, New York State Psychiatric Institute, New York [65]

PETER D. WALZER, MD
Associate Chief of Staff for Research, Cincinnati VA Medical Center; Professor of Medicine, University of Cincinnati, Cincinnati [191]

FREDERICK C.S. WANG, MD
Associate Professor of Medicine, Harvard Medical School; Medical Director, Clinical Virology Laboratory, Brigham and Women's Hospital, Boston [161,167]

CARL V. WASHINGTON, JR., MD
Assistant Professor of Dermatology, Emory University School of Medicine; Director, Mohs Surgery Unit, The Emory Clinic, Atlanta [73]

ANTHONY P. WEETMAN, MD, DSc
Professor of Medicine and Dean, University of Sheffield Medical School; Consultant Physician, Northern General Hospital, Sheffield, UK [320]

STEVEN E. WEINBERGER, MD
Professor of Medicine, Harvard Medical School; Senior Vice President, Medical Knowledge and Education Division, American College of Physicians, Philadelphia [30, 233–235, 240]

ROBERT A. WEINSTEIN, MD
Professor of Medicine, Rush Medical College; Chair, Infectious Diseases, Cook County Hospital; Chief Operating Officer, The CORE Center, Chicago [116]

PETER F. WELLER, MD, FACP
Professor of Medicine, Harvard Medical School; Co-Chief, Infectious Diseases Division; Chief, Allergy and Inflammation Division; Senior Vice Chair of Research, Department of Medicine, Beth Israel Deaconess Medical Center, Boston [199–202, 204]

MICHAEL R. WESSELS, MD
Professor of Pediatrics and Medicine (Microbiology and Molecular Genetics), Harvard Medical School; Chief, Division of Infectious Diseases, Children's Hospital, Boston [121]

LEE M. WETZLER, MD
Associate Professor of Medicine and Microbiology, Boston University School of Medicine, Boston [127]

MEIR WETZLER, MD
Associate Professor of Medicine, Roswell Park Cancer Institute, Buffalo [96]

A. CLINTON WHITE, JR., MD
Professor, Infectious Diseases Section, Department of Medicine, Baylor College of Medicine, Houston [204]

NICHOLAS J. WHITE, MD, DSc
Professor of Tropical Medicine, Mahidol University, Bangkok, Thailand; and Oxford University, Oxford, UK [195]

RICHARD J. WHITLEY, MD
Loeb Eminent Scholar in Pediatrics; Professor of Pediatrics, Microbiology, Medicine, and Neurosurgery, University of Alabama at Birmingham, Birmingham [164]

GORDON H. WILLIAMS, MD
Professor of Medicine, Harvard Medical School; Chief, Cardiovascular Endocrinology Section, Brigham and Women's Hospital, Boston [230, 321]

JOHN W. WINKELMAN, MD, PhD
Assistant Professor of Psychiatry, Harvard Medical School; Medical Director, Sleep Health Center, Brigham and Women's Hospital, Boston [24]

BRUCE U. WINTROUB, MD
Professor and Chair of Dermatology, Associate Dean, School of Medicine, University of California San Francisco, San Francisco [50]

ALLAN W. WOLKOFF, MD
Professor of Medicine and Anatomy and Structural Biology, Albert Einstein College of Medicine, New York [284]

ROBERT L. WORTMANN, MD
Professor and Chair, Department of Internal Medicine, University of Oklahoma College of Medicine, Tulsa [338]

JOSHUA WYNNE, MD, MBA, MPH
Professor of Medicine, Wayne State University; Attending Physician, Detroit Medical Center, Detroit [221]

KIM B. YANCEY, MD
Professor and Chair, Department of Dermatology, Medical College of Wisconsin, Milwaukee [46, 49]

JAMES B. YOUNG, MD
Professor of Medicine, Executive Associate Dean for Faculty Affairs, Northwestern University Feinberg School of Medicine, Chicago [322]

NEAL S. YOUNG, MD
Chief, Hematology Branch, National Heart, Lung and Blood Institute, National Institutes of Health, Bethesda [94]

ROBERT C. YOUNG, MD
President, Fox Chase Cancer Center, Philadelphia [83]

ALAN S.L. YU, MD, BChir
Assistant Professor of Medicine, University of Southern California Keck School of Medicine, Los Angeles [266]

VICTOR L. YU, MD
Professor of Medicine, University of Pittsburgh; Chief, Infectious Disease Section, VA Medical Center, Pittsburgh [132]

DORI F. ZALEZNIK, MD
Associate Clinical Professor of Medicine, Harvard Medical School; Senior Physician, Beth Israel Deaconess Medical Center, Boston [112]

PETER J. ZIMETBAUM, MD
Assistant Professor of Medicine, Harvard Medical School; Beth Israel Deaconess Medical Center, Boston [213, 214]

The first edition of *Harrison's Principles of Internal Medicine* was published more than half a century ago. Over the decades, this textbook has evolved to reflect the continuing advances in the field of internal medicine and to meet the growing information base required of medical students and clinical practitioners. The users of this sixteenth edition of *Harrison's* will not even have to open the volume to see that it marks a transition point in the book's history. The new cover is only the most obvious indication of a new direction for *Harrison's*.

In shaping and revising this new version, the Editors have committed themselves to making the textbook as useful as possible to students and practitioners coping with the demands of modern medicine. The growth of evidence-based medicine, the prominence of managed care, and the explosion of information in fundamental areas such as the genetics of disease are only three of the many factors that make these demands different from those faced by physicians only a decade ago. Just as the cover retains key elements of the classic book, the content of the sixteenth edition retains the essential facts that remain clinically useful and important. However, through modifications in both its format and its content, the new *Harrison's* addresses the changing needs of its readers.

The sixteenth edition of *Harrison's* has a full-color format that facilitates quick reference and allows the inclusion of hundreds more high-quality illustrations than in previous editions. We expect that the reader's convenience will be well served by the placement of color illustrations within the chapters rather than in the separate color atlas used in earlier editions. While providing the basic-science information that is critical to an understanding of biology and pathophysiology, this edition focuses more directly and extensively than ever on crucial aspects of clinical practice. Areas of emphasis include the approach to the patient, differential diagnosis, state-of-the-art treatment options, and disease prevention. Key topics, such as the immune system and HIV infection/AIDS, are covered in chapters amounting to "mini-textbooks." New sections offer information on the formidable challenges posed by critical care medicine and by the threat of bioterrorism. New chapters provide coverage of highly relevant clinical topics such as disease screening, perimenopausal management and hormone replacement therapy, and end-of-life care. Virtually every chapter in this edition has been substantially rewritten, and 46 chapters either are entirely new or have new authors.

These are only highlights of the changes that the Editors hope will make the new *Harrison's* a helpful tool—not only for the student who needs an expert source of basic knowledge in internal medicine, but also for the pressured practitioner who needs a clear, concise, and balanced distillation of the best information on which to base daily clinical decisions.

Part One, "Introduction to Clinical Medicine," contains a new chapter that provides practical information about the screening approaches that every internist should consider for routine health maintenance. This chapter discusses the principles and guidelines used in screening for common conditions such as cancer, hypertension, lipid disorders, and osteoporosis. Another new chapter offers a pragmatic approach to the medical evaluation of patients who are about to undergo surgical procedures. In light of the growth of the hospice movement and the increased awareness of the sensitive issues—physical, mental, social, and existential—that surround end-of-life care, a new chapter on this complex topic provides insights, information, and guidance to practitioners dealing with dying patients and their families. The chapter on women's health has been entirely revised and offers a broad overview of the approach to disorders that affect women disproportionately.

Part Two, "Cardinal Manifestations and Presentation of Diseases,"

serves as a comprehensive introduction to clinical medicine as well as a practical guide to the care of patients with these manifestations. Each section focuses on a particular group of disorders, examining the concepts of pathophysiology and differential diagnosis that must be considered in caring for patients with these common clinical presentations. Major symptoms are reviewed and correlated with specific disease states, and clinical approaches to patients presenting with these symptoms are summarized. Every chapter has been updated, and three chapters have new authors. The chapter on sexual dysfunction now addresses disorders in both men and women.

Given the rapid advances in human genetics over the past several years, Part Three, "Genetics and Disease," has once again been completely updated. The material included in this edition is strongly geared toward clinical practice, in which genetic information increasingly comes into play. The new chapter on stem cell and gene transfer in clinical medicine addresses a timely and controversial topic, defining different types of stem cells and discussing their potential clinical applications.

Part Four, "Nutrition," covers nutritional considerations related to clinical medicine. Areas of focus include nutritional and dietary assessment, nutritional requirements, protein-energy malnutrition, eating disorders, obesity, and enteral and parenteral nutrition therapy.

The core of *Harrison's* continues to encompass the disorders of the organ systems and is contained in Parts Five through Sixteen. These sections include succinct accounts of the pathophysiology of diseases involving the major organ systems as well as infectious diseases, with an emphasis on clinical manifestations, diagnostic procedures, differential diagnosis, and treatment strategies and guidelines.

Part Five, "Oncology and Hematology," includes four chapters by new authors. An increasing proportion of patients who develop cancer are being cured. It is important to detect late consequences as early as possible in their natural history to optimize outcome. The chapter on the late consequences of cancer and its treatment helps physicians following such patients to know what to look for in addition to a recurrence of the cancer. Advances in the management of many cancers are highlighted—for example, the dramatic impact of imatinib mesylate (Gleevec) on chronic myeloid leukemia and gastrointestinal stromal cell tumors and the role of rituximab in the management of lymphoma and autoimmune diseases. The chapter delineating the principles of radiation therapy has been entirely rewritten by Eli Glatstein and is a companion piece to this author's chapter on radiation bioterrorism in Part Seven (see below). The hematology section features the World Health Organization's new classification of lymphoid and myeloid neoplasms. One of the most rapidly expanding areas of medicine is the development of novel agents to interfere with blood coagulation. With a new author who is an expert in this field, the chapter on anticoagulant, fibrinolytic, and antiplatelet therapy reviews all these new products and their indications.

Part Six, "Infectious Diseases," summarizes the latest information on pathology, genetics, and epidemiology while focusing sharply on the needs of clinicians who must accurately diagnose and treat infections under time pressure and cost constraints. In particular, the inclusion of dozens more illustrations in full color provides easily accessible information to assist clinicians with these challenges. Specific recommendations are provided for therapeutic regimens, including the drug of choice, dose, duration, and alternatives. Current trends in antimicrobial resistance are presented and considered in light of their impact on therapeutic choices. A new chapter offers key information on the management of the complex clinical issues raised by *Clostridium difficile*–associated disease, including pseudomembranous colitis. New authors cover the latest advances in the management of diseases caused by staphylococci and nontuberculous mycobacteria, viral gastroenteritis, and brucellosis. The superb chapter by Raphael Dolin on common viral respiratory infections has been expanded to include thorough coverage of severe acute respiratory syndrome (SARS). Now placed in a separate section with the overview of the human retroviruses, the chapter on HIV infection and AIDS by Anthony S. Fauci and H. Clifford Lane has been completely revised and updated, with an emphasis on therapeutic strategies. This chapter is widely considered to be a classic in the field; its clinically pragmatic focus in combination with its comprehensive and analytical approach to the pathogenesis of HIV disease has allowed its use as the sole complete reference on HIV/AIDS in medical schools.

In recent years, physicians have found themselves on the front line of response to bioterrorist attacks around the world. Since the attacks on the United States on September 11, 2001, and the subsequent anthrax attacks, the nation has been preparing for the further attacks that will inevitably come. Part Seven, "Bioterrorism and Clinical Medicine," consists of entirely new material written by authorities in three areas of bioterrorism: microbial, chemical, and radiation. Edited by *Harrison's* editor Anthony S. Fauci, these chapters are written succinctly and include easily readable charts, tables, and algorithms; their goal is to confer an understanding of the pathogenesis, diagnosis, treatment, and prognosis of the diseases in question.

Part Eight, "Disorders of the Cardiovascular System," is once again edited by the preeminent expert in the field, Eugene Braunwald. A new chapter covers the clinically important topics of unstable angina and non-ST-segment elevation myocardial infarction; three other chapters have new authors; and every chapter has been revised to reflect the latest trends and strategies for management. These include primary percutaneous coronary intervention for ST-segment elevation myocardial infarction as well as new drugs and devices for the treatment of heart failure.

Enormous strides have been made in the use of lung transplantation for selected patients with end-stage, irreversible, pulmonary parenchymal and vascular disease. Part Nine, "Disorders of the Respiratory System," includes a chapter by a new author that focuses on the selection of patients for this intervention. New authors have also taken on the broad topic of pneumonia and lung abscess, providing focus and a clinical perspective to help the reader grasp the central issues involved in the diagnosis and management of both community-acquired and nosocomial disease.

With advances in health care delivery and pressures aimed at cost containment, critical care units account for a growing percentage of hospital beds. Part Ten, "Critical Care Medicine," is a new section of *Harrison's* that is devoted to the provision of optimal care in this medical setting of growing importance. Incorporating both new chapters and refocused chapters on topics covered in previous editions, this part deals with three main areas: respiratory critical care, shock and cardiac arrest, and neurologic critical care. The approach to the patient and the central tenets underlying critical care are at the heart of this part of the sixteenth edition.

Part Eleven, "Disorders of the Kidney and Urinary Tract," includes contributions from several new authors and, as in previous editions, provides a thorough overview of the urinary-tract disorders encountered in internal medicine.

Part Twelve, "Disorders of the Gastrointestinal System," includes a new chapter on familial Mediterranean fever. The chapter on the approach to the patient with gastrointestinal disease has been completely reworked by a new author, as has the chapter on diverticular and vascular disease of the bowel. The chapters on the various categories of viral hepatitis have been extensively revised and updated to reflect breakthrough advances in treatment.

The first chapter in Part Thirteen, "Disorders of the Immune System, Connective Tissue, and Joints," provides an introduction to the immune system that has become a classic in its field and is often used as the textbook of immunology in postgraduate and medical school

courses. This chapter combines an in-depth description and analysis of the principles of basic immunology with an easy flow into the application of these principles to clinical disease states. Its description of the relationship of innate to adaptive immunity is a model for understanding the intricacies of the human immune system. Once again, the authors have extensively revised this chapter to bring it up to date with regard to recent rapid advances in both basic and clinical immunology. In the section on disorders of immune-mediated injury, the spondyloarthropathies have been grouped together in one chapter that clearly and comprehensively discusses the similarities and dissimilarities among the various diseases in this category. The breakthrough advances in immunomodulatory therapy that have been realized in rheumatology over the past few years are captured in the spondyloarthropathy chapters and in the extensively revised chapters on rheumatoid arthritis and systemic lupus erythematosus. A new chapter covers fibromyalgia, arthritis associated with systemic disease, and other arthritides.

Part Fourteen, "Endocrinology and Metabolism," includes six chapters with new authors as well as a timely new chapter on the perimenopause transition and hormone replacement therapy. The writing of the latter chapter coincided with publication of results from the Women's Health Initiative that unexpectedly showed an increased risk of cardiovascular disease among women who received estrogen treatment. The author reviews the literature in this area and provides practical algorithms for the management of patients during this transition. The new authors of the chapter on disorders of sexual differentiation highlight novel insights derived from elucidation of the genetic basis of sex determination. The outstanding new review of bone and mineral metabolism lays a superb foundation for an understanding of the pathophysiology and treatment of various metabolic bone diseases. The newly authored version of the chapter on disorders of lipoprotein metabolism offers a much sharper focus on the classification, diagnosis, and treatment of disorders of cholesterol and triglyceride metabolism, emphasizing the use of statins for the reduction of cardiovascular risk. The new chapter on Wilson disease reports on the substantially modified treatment recommendations for this entity.

Part Fifteen, "Neurologic Disorders," has been extensively updated. A comprehensive new chapter on Alzheimer's disease and related dementias summarizes the recent explosion of knowledge on this topic, highlighting the new understanding of the genetics of these dementias and the molecules that trigger them as well as providing a clinical guide to diagnosis, differential diagnosis, and the latest treatments. The new chapter on Parkinson's disease reviews the recent genetic findings and provides an authoritative approach to therapy, including surgical options. The chapter on cerebrovascular diseases has been extensively rewritten, offering an evidence-based approach to the treatment and prevention of stroke, the third leading killer in the Western world. The updated chapter on multiple sclerosis presents the most recent advances in therapy and a practical approach to management of different stages of the disease. Finally, the recognition of bovine spongiform encephalopathy in many regions of the world has focused the global health care community on the biology and clinical manifestations of prion diseases; the sixteenth edition of *Harrison's* includes a comprehensive review of this subject by Nobel Laureate Stanley Prusiner.

Part Sixteen, "Poisoning, Drug Overdose, and Envenomation," has been thoroughly revised and streamlined to focus on the topics most relevant to internal medicine.

In view of the requirements for continuing education for licensure and relicensure as well as the emphasis on certification and recertification, a revision of the PreTest Self-Assessment and Review will again be published with this edition. This volume is in the capable hands of a new author, Dr. Charles Wiener from Johns Hopkins. It consists of several hundred questions based on the sixteenth edition of *Harrison's*, along with answers and explanations for the answers. The *Companion Handbook*, which was pioneered as a supplement to the eleventh edition of *Harrison's*, has been reworked as a concise quick-reference clinical manual; the *Manual of Medicine* will appear shortly after the publication of this edition, along with a PDA version, *Harrison's OnHand*. In 1998, *Harrison's* went online to provide a "living" textbook of internal medicine. In addition to permitting full search capabilities of the text, *Harrison's Online* offers frequent updates, reports of clinical trials, practice guidelines, online lectures, and concise reviews of timely topics as well as additional and updated references (with links to MEDLINE abstracts) and illustrations.

We wish to express our appreciation to our many associates and colleagues, who, as experts in their fields, have offered us constructive criticism and helpful suggestions. We acknowledge especially the contributions of the following individuals: Joseph Alpert, Michael Bray, Mark D. Carlson, Daniel H. Lowenstein, Lawrence C. Madoff, Thomas R. Martin, Chung Owyang, Alice Pau, and Mary Wright.

We thank in particular Kenneth and Elaine Kaye and Lindsey Baden, who gathered many high-quality illustrations of infectious disease manifestations. We also express our gratitude to Eileen J. Scott, who has applied her editorial expertise to the past six editions of *Harrison's*, and Marsha Cohen, who has been the text and cover designer for the past five editions.

This book could not have been edited without the dedicated help of our co-workers in the editorial offices of the individual editors. We are especially indebted to Patricia L. Duffey, Gregory K. Folkers, Sarah Matero, Julie B. McCoy, Jaylyn Olivo, Elizabeth Robbins, Leslie Runnels, Kathryn Saxon, Marie Scurti, and Sue Anne Tae.

Finally, we continue to be highly indebted to three outstanding members of the McGraw-Hill organization: Mariapaz Ramos Englis, Senior Managing Editor; Robert Laffler, Production Director; and Martin J. Wonsiewicz, Publisher. They are an effective team who have given the Editors constant encouragement and sage advice. They have been instrumental in guiding the many changes instituted with this edition of *Harrison's* and in bringing this volume to fruition in a timely manner.

THE EDITORS

1 | THE PRACTICE OF MEDICINE
The Editors

WHAT IS EXPECTED OF THE PHYSICIAN The accelerating pace of change in medicine stems from an explosion of scientific information and the need to blend this information into the art and practice of medicine.

The role of *science in medicine* is clear. Science-based technology and deductive reasoning form the foundation for the solution to many clinical problems. Spectacular advances in genetics, biochemistry, and imaging techniques allow access to the innermost parts of the cell and the most remote recesses of the body. Revelations about the nature of genes and single cells have opened the portal for formulating a new molecular basis for the physiology of systems. These physiologic insights will undoubtedly result in a better understanding of complex disease processes and new approaches to disease treatment and prevention. Highly advanced therapeutic maneuvers are increasingly a major part of medical practice. Yet skill in the most sophisticated application of laboratory technology and in the use of the latest therapeutic modality alone does not make a good physician.

The editors of the first edition of this book articulated well the responsibility of the physician in interacting with the patient:

> No greater opportunity, responsibility, or obligation can fall to the lot of a human being than to become a physician. In the care of the suffering, [the physician] needs technical skill, scientific knowledge, and human understanding. . . . Tact, sympathy, and understanding are expected of the physician, for the patient is no mere collection of symptoms, signs, disordered functions, damaged organs, and disturbed emotions. [The patient] is human, fearful, and hopeful, seeking relief, help, and reassurance.

When a patient poses challenging clinical problems, an effective physician must be able to identify the crucial elements in a complex history and physical examination and to extract the key laboratory results from the crowded computer printouts of data in order to determine whether to "treat" or to "watch." Deciding whether a clinical clue is worth pursuing or should be dismissed as a "red herring" and weighing whether a proposed treatment entails a greater risk than the disease itself are essential judgments that the skilled clinician must make many times each day. This combination of medical knowledge, intuition, experience, and judgment defines the *art of medicine*, which is as necessary to the practice of medicine as is a sound scientific base.

THE PATIENT-PHYSICIAN RELATIONSHIP: A HUMANE APPROACH IN THE FACE OF CHANGE In this era of "techno-medicine," physicians need to approach patients not as "cases" or "diseases" but as individuals whose problems all too often transcend their physical complaints. Most patients are anxious and fearful. Physicians should instill confidence and should be reassuring (as depicted humorously in Fig. 1-1) but should never be arrogant. A professional attitude, coupled with warmth and openness, can do much to alleviate anxiety and to encourage patients to share all aspects of their medical history. Whatever the patient's attitude, the physician needs to consider the setting in which an illness occurs—in terms not only of the patients themselves but also of their familial, social, and cultural backgrounds. The ideal patient-physician relationship is based on thorough knowledge of the patient, on mutual trust, and on the ability to communicate.

Technological Complexity and Managed Care The one-to-one patient-physician relationship, which has traditionally characterized the practice of medicine, is increasingly in jeopardy because of the growing complexity of medicine and the changes in health care delivery systems. Often the management of an individual patient is a team effort involving a number of physicians and other professional personnel. Increasingly, hospitalists assume the responsibility for patient management in the inpatient setting. The patient can benefit greatly from effective collaboration among health care professionals, but *it is the duty of the patient's principal physician to provide guidance through an illness*. To carry out this difficult task, this physician must be familiar with the techniques, skills, and objectives of specialist physicians and of colleagues in the fields allied to medicine. In giving the patient an opportunity to benefit from scientific advances, the primary physician must retain responsibility for the major decisions concerning diagnosis and treatment.

The practice of medicine in a managed-care setting puts additional stress on the patient-physician relationship. Whatever the potential advantages of organized medical groups such as health maintenance organizations (HMOs), there are also drawbacks, including the loss of the clear identification of the physician who is primarily and continuously responsible for the patient. Even under these circumstances, it is essential for each patient to have a physician who has an overview of the problems and who is familiar with the patient's reaction to the illness, the drugs the patient is given, and the challenges the patient faces. Moreover, in managed-care settings, many physicians must treat patients within a restricted time frame, with limited access to specialists, and under organizational guidelines that may compromise their ability to exercise their individual clinical judgment. As difficult as these restrictions may be, it is the ultimate responsibility of the physician, in close consultation with the patient, to determine what is best for the patient. This responsibility cannot be relinquished in the name of compliance with organizational guidelines.

The Modern Hospital Environment The physician must be aware that the hospital is an intimidating environment for most individuals. Hospitalized patients find themselves surrounded by air jets, buttons, and lights; invaded by tubes and wires; and beset by the numerous members of the health care team—nurses, nurses' aides, physicians' assistants, social workers, technologists, physical therapists, medical students, house officers, attending and consulting physicians, and many others. They may be transported to special laboratories and imaging facilities replete with blinking lights, strange sounds, and unfamiliar personnel; they may be obliged to share a room with other patients who have their own health problems. It is little wonder that

SIPRESS

"Let the healing begin!"

FIGURE 1-1 Although physicians must be confident and reassuring, it may be possible to go too far. (*The New Yorker Collection 2000, David Sipress, from cartoonbank.com. All Rights Reserved.*)

patients may lose their sense of reality. A strong personal relationship with the physician helps to sustain the patient in such a stressful situation.

Societal Trends   Many trends in contemporary society tend to make medical care impersonal. These trends, some of which have been mentioned already, include (1) vigorous efforts to reduce the escalating costs of health care; (2) the growing number of managed-care programs, which are intended to reduce costs but in which the patient may have little choice in selecting a physician or in seeing that physician consistently; (3) increasing reliance on technological advances and computerization for many aspects of diagnosis and treatment; (4) increased geographic mobility of both patients and physicians; (5) the need for numerous physicians to be involved in the care of most patients who are seriously ill; and (6) an increasing tendency on the part of patients to express their frustrations with the health care system through malpractice suits.

Given these changes in the medical care system, it is a major challenge for physicians to maintain the *humane* aspects of medical care. The American Board of Internal Medicine, working together with the American College of Physicians–American Society of Internal Medicine and the European Federation of Internal Medicine, has published a *Charter on Medical Professionalism* that underscores three main principles in physicians' contract with society: (1) the primacy of patient welfare, (2) patient autonomy, and (3) social justice. The humanistic qualities of a physician must encompass integrity, respect, and compassion. Availability, the expression of sincere concern, the willingness to take the time to explain all aspects of the illness, and a nonjudgmental attitude when dealing with patients whose cultures, lifestyles, attitudes, and values differ from those of the physician are just a few of the characteristics of the humane physician. Every physician will, at times, be challenged by patients who evoke strongly negative or positive emotional responses. Physicians should be alert to their own reactions to such patients and situations and should consciously monitor and control their behavior so that the patient's best interest remains the principal motivation for their actions at all times.

An important aspect of patient care involves an appreciation of the "quality of life," a subjective assessment of what each patient values most. Such an assessment requires detailed, sometimes intimate knowledge of the patient, which can usually be obtained only through deliberate, unhurried, and often repeated conversations. It is in these situations that the time constraints of a managed-care setting may prove particularly problematic. Time pressures will always threaten these interactions but do not diminish the importance of understanding patients' priorities from their point of view.

The famous statement of Dr. Francis Peabody is even more relevant today than when delivered more than three-quarters of a century ago:

*The significance of the intimate personal relationship between physician and patient cannot be too strongly emphasized, for in an extraordinarily large number of cases both the diagnosis and treatment are directly dependent on it. One of the essential qualities of the clinician is interest in humanity, **for the secret of the care of the patient is in caring for the patient**.*

CLINICAL SKILLS ■ History-Taking   The written history of an illness should embody all the facts of medical significance in the life of the patient. Recent events should be given the most attention. The patient should, at some early point, have the opportunity to tell his or her own story of the illness without frequent interruption and, when appropriate, receive expressions of interest, encouragement, and empathy from the physician. Any event related by the patient, however trivial or apparently remote, may be the key to the solution of the medical problem. In general, only patients who feel comfortable will provide the physician with complete information.

An informative history is more than an orderly listing of symptoms; something is always gained by listening to patients and noting the way in which they describe their symptoms. Inflections of voice, facial expression, gestures, and attitude may reveal important clues to the meaning of the symptoms to the patient. Because patients vary in their medical sophistication and ability to recall facts, the reported medical history should be corroborated whenever possible. The family and social history can also provide important insights into the types of diseases that should be considered. In listening to the history, the physician discovers not only something about the disease but also something about the patient. The process of history-taking provides an opportunity to observe the patient's behavior and to watch for features to be pursued more thoroughly during the physical examination.

The very act of eliciting the history provides the physician with the opportunity to establish or enhance the unique bond that is the basis for the ideal patient-physician relationship. It is helpful to develop an appreciation of the patient's perception of the illness, the patient's expectations of the physician and the medical care system, and the financial and social implications of the illness to the patient. The confidentiality of the patient-physician relationship should be emphasized, and the patient should be given the opportunity to identify any aspects of the history that should not be disclosed to others.

Physical Examination   Physical signs are objective indications of disease whose significance is enhanced when they confirm a functional or structural change already suggested by the patient's history. At times, however, the physical signs may be the only evidence of disease.

The physical examination should be performed methodically and thoroughly, with consideration for the patient's comfort and modesty. Although attention is often directed by the history to the diseased organ or part of the body, the examination of a new patient must extend from head to toe in an objective search for abnormalities. Unless the physical examination is systematic, important segments may be omitted. The results of the examination, like the details of the history, should be recorded at the time they are elicited, not hours later when they are subject to the distortions of memory. Skill in physical diagnosis is acquired with experience, but it is not merely technique that determines success in eliciting signs. The detection of a few scattered petechiae, a faint diastolic murmur, or a small mass in the abdomen is not a question of keener eyes and ears or more sensitive fingers but of a mind alert to these findings. Since physical findings are subject to changes, the physical examination should be repeated as frequently as the clinical situation warrants.

Laboratory Tests and Imaging Studies   The availability of a wide array of laboratory tests has increased our reliance on these studies for the solution of clinical problems. The accumulation of laboratory data does not relieve the physician from the responsibility of careful observation, examination, and study of the patient. It is also essential to bear in mind the limitations of such tests. By virtue of their impersonal quality, complexity, and apparent precision, they often gain an aura of authority regardless of the fallibility of the tests themselves, the instruments used in the tests, and the individuals performing or interpreting them. Physicians must weigh the expense involved in the laboratory procedures they order relative to the value of the information they are likely to provide.

Single laboratory tests are rarely ordered. Rather, physicians generally request "batteries" of multiple tests, which are often useful. For example, abnormalities of hepatic function may provide the clue to such nonspecific symptoms as generalized weakness and increased fatigability, suggesting the diagnosis of chronic liver disease. Sometimes a single abnormality, such as an elevated serum calcium level, points to particular diseases, such as hyperparathyroidism or underlying malignancy.

The thoughtful use of screening tests should not be confused with indiscriminate laboratory testing. The use of screening tests is based on the fact that a group of laboratory determinations can be carried out conveniently on a single specimen at relatively low cost. Screening tests are most useful when they are directed toward common diseases or disorders and when their results indicate other useful tests or interventions that may be costly to perform. Biochemical measurements, together with simple laboratory examinations such as blood count, urinalysis, and sedimentation rate, often provide the major clue to the presence of a pathologic process. At the same time, the physician must learn to evaluate occasional abnormalities among the screening tests that may not necessarily connote significant disease. An in-depth workup following a report of an isolated laboratory abnormality in a person who is otherwise well is almost invariably wasteful and unproductive. Among the more than 40 tests that are routinely performed, one or two are often slightly abnormal. If there is no suspicion of an underlying illness, these tests are ordinarily repeated to ensure that the abnormality does not represent a laboratory error. If an abnormality is confirmed, it is important to consider its potential significance in the context of the patient's condition and other test results.

The technical capability of imaging studies is one of the most rapidly advancing areas of medicine. These tests provide remarkably detailed anatomical information that can be a pivotal factor in medical decision-making. Ultrasonography, a variety of isotopic scans, computed tomography, magnetic resonance imaging, and positron emission tomography have benefited patients by opening new diagnostic vistas and by largely supplanting older, more invasive approaches. In our effort to make diagnoses quickly, it is tempting to order a battery of imaging studies. All physicians have had cases in which imaging studies turned up findings leading to an unexpected diagnosis. Nonetheless, patients must endure each of these tests, and the added cost of unnecessary testing is substantial. A skilled physician must learn to use these powerful diagnostic tools judiciously, always asking whether the results will alter management and benefit the patient.

PRINCIPLES OF PATIENT CARE ■ Evidence-Based Medicine Sackett has defined evidence-based medicine as "the conscientious, explicit and judicious use of current best evidence in making decisions about the care of individual patients." Rigorously obtained evidence is contrasted with anecdotal experience, which is often biased. Even the most experienced physicians can be influenced by recent experiences with selected patients, unless they are attuned to the importance of using larger, more objective studies for making decisions. The prospectively designed, double-blind, randomized clinical trial represents the "gold standard" for providing evidence regarding therapeutic decisions. →*For a more complete discussion of evidence-based medicine, see Chap. 2.*

Practice Guidelines The intelligent and cost-effective practice of medicine consists of making diagnostic and therapeutic choices that are most appropriate to a particular patient and clinical situation. Professional organizations and government agencies are developing formal clinical-practice guidelines in an effort to aid physicians and other caregivers in this endeavor. As the evidence base of medicine increases, guidelines can provide a useful framework for managing patients with particular diagnoses or symptoms. They can protect patients—particularly those with inadequate health care benefits—from receiving substandard care. Guidelines can also protect conscientious caregivers from inappropriate charges of malpractice and society from the excessive costs associated with the overuse of medical resources. On the other hand, clinical guidelines tend to oversimplify the complexities of medicine. Groups with differing perspectives may develop divergent recommendations regarding issues as basic as the need for periodic sigmoidoscopy in middle-aged persons. Furthermore, guidelines do not—and cannot be expected to—take into account the uniqueness of each individual and of his or her illness. The challenge for the physician is to integrate into clinical practice the useful recommendations offered by the experts who prepare clinical practice guidelines without accepting them blindly or being inappropriately constrained by them.

Medical Decision-Making Medical decision-making occurs throughout the diagnostic and treatment process. It involves the ordering of additional tests, requests for consults, and decisions regarding prognosis and treatment. This process requires an in-depth understanding of the pathophysiology and natural history of disease. It is for this reason that these topics are strongly emphasized in this textbook. As described above, medical decision-making should be evidence-based so that patients derive the full benefit of the scientific knowledge available to physicians. Formulating a differential diagnosis requires not only a broad knowledge base but also the ability to assess the relative probabilities of various diseases and to understand the significance of missing diagnoses that may be less likely. Arriving at a diagnosis requires the application of the scientific method. Hypotheses are formed, data are collected, and objective conclusions are reached concerning whether to accept or reject a particular diagnosis. Analysis of the differential diagnosis is an iterative process. As new information or test results are acquired, the group of disease processes being considered can be contracted or expanded appropriately.

Despite the importance of evidence-based medicine, much of medical decision-making relies on judgment—a process that is difficult to quantify or even to assess qualitatively. Especially when a relevant evidence base is unavailable, physicians must use their knowledge and experience as a basis for weighing known factors along with the inevitable uncertainties and then making a sound judgment. Several quantitative tools may be invaluable in synthesizing the available information, including diagnostic tests, Bayes' theorem, and multivariate statistical models. *Diagnostic tests* serve to reduce uncertainty about a diagnosis or prognosis in a particular individual and to help the physician decide how best to manage that individual's condition. Not only laboratory tests and procedures but also the history and the physical examination can be considered part of the battery of diagnostic tests. The accuracy of a given test is ascertained by determining its sensitivity (true positive rate) and specificity (true negative rate) as well as the predictive value of a positive and negative result. *Bayes' theorem* uses information on a test's sensitivity and specificity, in conjunction with the pretest probability of a diagnosis, to determine mathematically the posttest probability of the diagnosis. More complex clinical problems can be approached with *multivariate statistical models*, which generate highly accurate information even when multiple factors are acting individually or together to affect disease risk, progression, or response to treatment. Studies comparing the performance of statistical models with that of expert clinicians have documented equivalent accuracy, although the models tend to be more consistent. Thus multivariate statistical models may be particularly helpful to less experienced clinicians.

Information technology is playing an ever-increasing role in medicine. Laboratory data are accessed almost universally through computers. Many medical centers now have electronic medical records, computerized order entry, and bar-coded tracking of medications. Some of these systems are interactive and provide reminders or warn of potential medical errors. Nonetheless, at this point, clinical decisions are still best made by the physician. Many decisions are not easily compacted into practice guidelines or computerized approaches. Clinical knowledge and an understanding of the patient's needs, supplemented by quantitative tools, still seem to represent the best approach to practicing medicine.

Assessing the Outcome of Treatment Clinicians generally use *objective* and readily measurable parameters to judge the outcome of a therapeutic intervention. For example, findings on physical or laboratory examination—such as the level of blood pressure, the patency of a coronary artery on an angiogram, or the size of a mass on a radiologic examination—can provide information of critical importance. However, patients usually seek medical attention for *subjective* reasons; they wish to obtain relief from pain, to preserve or regain function, and to enjoy life. The components of a patient's health status or quality of life can include bodily comfort, capacity for physical activity, personal and professional function, sexual function, cognitive function, and overall perception of health. Each of these important areas can be assessed by means of structured interviews or specially designed questionnaires. Such assessments also provide useful parameters by which the physician can judge the patient's subjective view of his or her disability and the response to treatment, particularly in chronic illness.

The practice of medicine requires consideration and integration of both objective and subjective outcomes.

Care of the Elderly   Over the next several decades, the practice of medicine will be greatly influenced by the health care needs of the growing elderly population. In the United States the population over age 65 will almost triple over the next 30 years. The physician must understand and appreciate the decline in physiologic reserve associated with aging; the different responses of the elderly to common diseases; and disorders that occur commonly with aging, such as depression, dementia, frailty, urinary incontinence, and fractures. →*For a more complete discussion of medical care for the elderly, see Chap. 8.*

Diseases in Women versus Men   In the past, many epidemiologic studies and clinical trials focused on men. More recently, studies have included representative numbers of women, and some, like the Women's Health Initiative, have specifically addressed women's health issues. Significant sex differences exist in diseases that afflict both men and women. Ongoing study should enhance our understanding of the mechanisms of sex differences in the course and outcome of certain diseases. →*For a more complete discussion of women's health, see Chap. 5.*

Medical Errors   A report from the Institute of Medicine concluded that "to err is human" but called for an ambitious agenda to reduce medical-error rates and improve patient safety by designing and implementing fundamental changes in health care systems. Adverse drug reactions occur in at least 5% of hospitalized patients, and the incidence increases with use of a large number of drugs. No matter what the clinical situation, it is the responsibility of the physician to use powerful therapeutic measures wisely, with due regard for their beneficial action, potential dangers, and cost. It is also the responsibility of hospitals and health care organizations to develop systems to reduce risk and ensure patient safety. Medication errors can be reduced through the use of ordering systems that eliminate misreading of handwriting and through vigilance regarding dilution errors. Implementation of infection-control systems, enforcement of hand-washing protocols, and careful oversight of antibiotic use can minimize complications of nosocomial infections. The harm that a physician can do is not limited to the imprudent use of medication or procedures. Equally important are ill-considered or unjustified remarks. Many a patient has developed a cardiac neurosis because the physician ventured a grave prognosis on the basis of a misinterpreted finding of a heart murmur.

Informed Consent and Respect for the Patient's Autonomy   The fundamental principles of medical ethics are to act in the patient's best interest and to respect the patient's autonomy. Most patients possess only limited medical knowledge and must rely on their physicians for advice. Confusion or even disagreement about approaches to disease management may arise (see also "Medicine on the Internet," below), and—in the end—the patient's informed choices must prevail. Physicians must respect their patients' autonomy, fully discussing the alternatives for care and the risks, benefits, and likely consequences of each alternative.

When patients require diagnostic and therapeutic procedures that are painful and that pose some risk, they are generally required to sign a consent form. In such cases, it is particularly important for the patient to understand clearly the risks entailed in these procedures; this is the definition of *informed consent*. It is incumbent on the physician to explain the procedures in a clear and understandable manner and to ascertain that the patient comprehends both the nature of the procedure and the attendant risks. The dread of the unknown that is inherent in hospitalization can be mitigated by such explanations.

Incurable Disorders and Death   No problem is more distressing than that presented by the patient with an incurable disease, particularly when premature death is inevitable. What should the patient and family be told? What measures should be taken to maintain life? What can be done to maintain the quality of life? How is death to be defined?

Although some would argue otherwise, there is no ironclad rule that the patient must immediately be told "everything," even if the patient is an adult with substantial family responsibilities. How much is told should depend on the individual's ability to deal with the possibility of imminent death; often this capacity grows with time, and, whenever possible, gradual rather than abrupt disclosure is the best strategy. A wise and insightful physician is often guided by an understanding of what a patient wants to know and when he or she wants to know it. The patient's religious beliefs may also be taken into consideration. The patient must be given an opportunity to talk with the physician and ask questions. Patients may find it easier to share their feelings about death with their physician, who is likely to be more objective and less emotional, than with family members. As William Osler wrote: "One thing is certain; it is not for you to don the black cap and, assuming the judicial function, take hope away from any patient." Even when the patient directly inquires, "Am I dying?" the physician must attempt to determine whether this is a request for information or a demand for reassurance. Only open communication between the patient and the physician can resolve this question and guide the physician in what to say and how to say it.

The physician should provide or arrange for emotional, physical, and spiritual support and must be compassionate, unhurried, and open. There is much to be gained by the laying on of hands. Pain should be adequately controlled, human dignity maintained, and isolation from the family avoided. These aspects of care tend to be overlooked in hospitals, where the intrusion of life-sustaining apparatus can so easily detract from attention to the whole person and encourage concentration instead on the life-threatening disease, against which the battle will ultimately be lost in any case. In the face of terminal illness, the goal of medicine must shift from *cure* to *care*, in the broadest sense of the term. In offering care to the dying patient, the physician must be prepared to provide information to family members and to deal with their guilt and grief. It is important for the doctor to assure the family that everything possible has been done. →*For a more complete discussion of end-of-life care, see Chap. 9.*

THE EXPANDING ROLE OF THE PHYSICIAN ■ Genetics and Medicine   The genomic era is leading to a revolution in the practice of medicine. The sequencing of the entire human genome has set researchers on the path to elucidating the genetic components of common chronic diseases—hypertension, diabetes, atherosclerosis, many cancers, autoimmune disorders, dementias, and behavioral disorders. Forthcoming information should make it possible to determine individual susceptibility to these conditions early in life and to implement individualized prevention programs. Subclassification of many diseases on a genetic basis may allow the selection of appropriate therapy for each patient. As the response to drugs becomes more predictable, pharmacotherapy should become more rational.

Patients will be best served if physicians play an active role in applying this powerful, sensitive new information rather than being passive bystanders who are intimidated by the new technology. This is a rapidly evolving field, and physicians and other health care professionals must continue to educate themselves so that they can apply this new knowledge to the benefit of their patients' health and well-being. Genetic testing requires wise counsel based on an understanding of the value and limitations of the tests as well as the implications of their results for specific individuals. →*For a more complete discussion of the use of genetic testing, see Chap. 58.*

Medicine on the Internet   The explosion in use of the Internet through personal computers is having an important influence on health care. The Internet makes a wide range of information available to physicians and patients almost instantaneously at any time of the day or night and from anywhere in the world. This medium holds enormous potential for delivering up-to-date information, practice guidelines, state-of-the-art conferences, journal contents, textbooks (including this text), and direct communications with other physicians and specialists, thereby expanding the depth and breadth of information available to the physician about the diagnosis and care of patients. Most medical journals are now accessible online, providing rapid and comprehensive sources of information.

Patients, too, are turning to the Internet in increasing numbers to derive information about their illnesses and therapies and to join Internet-based support groups. Physicians are increasingly challenged by dealing with patients who arrive with sophisticated information about their illness. It is difficult, however, for patients to put this sometimes-alarming information into context, and the physician plays an invaluable role by encouraging patient education but helping the patient to assimilate new information and apply it to a particular circumstance.

A critically important caveat is that virtually anything can be published on the Internet, with easy circumvention of the peer-review process that is an essential feature of quality publications. Physicians or patients who search the Internet for medical information must be aware of this danger. Notwithstanding this limitation, appropriate use of the Internet is revolutionizing information access for physicians and patients and is a positive force in the practice of medicine.

Delivering Cost-Effective Medical Care   As the cost of medical care has risen, it has become necessary to establish priorities in the expenditure of resources. In some instances, preventive measures offer the greatest return for the expenditure; outstanding examples include vaccination, improved sanitation, reduction in accidents and occupational hazards, and biochemical- and DNA-based screening of newborns. As one more specific example, the detection of phenylketonuria by newborn screening may result in a net saving of many thousands of dollars.

As resources become increasingly constrained, society must weigh the benefits of performing costly procedures that provide only a limited increase in life expectancy against the pressing need for more primary care for those persons who do not have adequate access to medical services. For the individual patient, it is important to reduce costly hospital admissions as much as possible if total health care is to be affordable. This policy, of course, depends on close cooperation among patients, their physicians, employers, payers, and government. It is equally important for physicians to know the cost of the diagnostic procedures they order and the drugs and other therapies they prescribe and to monitor both costs and effectiveness. The medical profession should provide leadership and guidance to the public in matters of cost control, and physicians must take this responsibility seriously without being or seeming to be self-serving. However, the economic aspects of health care delivery must not interfere with the welfare of patients. The patient must be able to rely on the individual physician as his or her principal advocate in matters of health care.

Accountability   As the public has become more educated and more sophisticated regarding health-related issues, expectations of the health care system in general and of physicians in particular have risen. Physicians are expected to maintain mastery of rapidly advancing fields (the *science* of medicine) while considering their patients' unique needs (the *art* of medicine). Thus, physicians are held accountable not only for the technical aspects of the care that they provide but also for their patients' satisfaction with the delivery and costs of care.

In the United States, there are increasing demands for physicians to account for the way in which they practice medicine by meeting certain standards prescribed by federal and state governments. The hospitalization of patients whose health care costs are reimbursed by the government and other third parties is subjected to utilization review. Thus the physician must defend the cause for and duration of a patient's hospitalization if it falls outside certain "average" standards. Authorization for reimbursement is increasingly based on documentation of the nature and complexity of an illness, as reflected by recorded elements of the history and physical examination. The purpose of these regulations is both to improve standards of health care and to contain spiraling health care costs. This type of review is being extended to all phases of medical practice and is profoundly altering the practice of medicine. Physicians are also expected to give evidence of their continuing competence through mandatory continuing education, patient-record audits, recertification by examination, or relicensing.

Continued Learning   The conscientious physician must be a perpetual student because the body of medical knowledge is constantly expanding and being refined. The profession of medicine should be inherently linked to a career-long thirst for new information that can be used for the good of the patient. It is the responsibility of a physician to pursue new knowledge continually by reading, attending conferences and courses, and consulting colleagues and the Internet. This is often a difficult task for a busy practitioner; however, such a commitment to continued learning is an integral part of being a physician and must be given the highest priority.

Research and Teaching   The title *doctor* is derived from the Latin *docere*, "to teach," and physicians should share information and medical knowledge with colleagues, with students of medicine and related professions, and with their patients (Fig. 1-2). The practice of medicine is dependent on the sum total of medical knowledge, which in turn is based on an unending chain of scientific discovery, clinical observation, analysis, and interpretation. Advances in medicine depend on the acquisition of new information, i.e., on research, which often involves patients; improved medical care requires the transmission of this information. As part of broader societal responsibilities, the physician should encourage patients to participate in ethical and properly approved clinical investigations if they do not impose undue hazard, discomfort, or inconvenience. On the other hand, physicians engaged in clinical research must be alert to potential conflicts of interest between their research goals and their obligations to individual patients; the best interests of the patient must always take priority. To quote William Osler:

> To wrest from nature the secrets which have perplexed philosophers in all ages, to track to their sources the causes of disease, to correlate the vast stores of knowledge, that they may be quickly

FIGURE 1-2   Dr. Tinsley R. Harrison instructing students at a patient's bedside. Dr. Harrison was the editor-in-chief of the first five editions of this textbook. (*Photo reprinted with permission from the UAB Archives, University of Alabama at Birmingham.*)

available for the prevention and cure of disease—these are our ambitions.

FURTHER READING

COLLINS FS: Shattuck Lecture: Medical and societal consequences of the Human Genome Project. N Engl J Med 341:28, 1999

COUNCIL ON GRADUATE MEDICAL EDUCATION: *Thirteenth Report: Physician Education for a Changing Health Care Environment*. US Department of Health and Human Services, March 1999

LUDMERER KM: *Time to Heal: American Medical Education from the Turn of the Century to the Era of Managed Care*. New York, Oxford, 1999

PROJECT OF THE ABIM FOUNDATION, ACP-ASIM FOUNDATION, AND EUROPEAN FEDERATION OF INTERNAL MEDICINE: Medical professionalism in the new millennium: A physician charter. Ann Intern Med 136:243, 2002

SACKETT DL et al: *Evidence Based Medicine: How to Practise and Teach EBM*. London, Churchill Livingstone, 1997

2 | DECISION-MAKING IN CLINICAL MEDICINE
Daniel B. Mark

To the medical student who requires 2 h to collect a patient's history and perform a physical examination, and several additional hours to organize them into a coherent presentation, the experienced clinician's ability to reach a diagnosis and decide on a management plan in a fraction of the time seems extraordinary. While medical knowledge and experience play a significant role in the senior clinician's ability to arrive at a differential diagnosis and plan quickly, much of the process involves skill in clinical decision-making. The first goal of this chapter is to provide an introduction to the study of clinical reasoning.

Equally bewildering to the student are the proper use of diagnostic tests and the integration of the results into the clinical assessment. The novice medical practitioner typically uses a "shotgun" approach to testing, hoping to a hit a target without knowing exactly what that target is. The expert, on the other hand, usually has a specific target in mind and efficiently adjusts the testing strategy to it. The second goal of this chapter is to review briefly some of the crucial basic statistical concepts that govern the proper interpretation and use of diagnostic tests; quantitative tools available to assist in clinical decision-making will also be discussed.

Evidence-based medicine is the term used to describe the integration of the best available research evidence with clinical judgment and experience in the care of patients. The third goal of this chapter is to provide a brief overview of some of the tools of evidence-based medicine.

CLINICAL DECISION-MAKING

CLINICAL REASONING The most important clinical actions are not procedures or prescriptions but the judgments from which all other aspects of clinical medicine flow. In the modern era of large randomized trials and evidence-based medicine, it is easy to overlook the importance of this elusive mental activity and focus instead on the algorithmic practice guidelines constructed to improve care. One reason for this apparent neglect is that much more research has been done on how doctors *should* make decisions (e.g., using a Bayesian model discussed below) than on how they actually *do*. Thus, much of what we know about clinical reasoning comes from empirical studies of nonmedical problem-solving behavior.

Despite the great technological advances of the twentieth century, uncertainty still plays a pivotal role in all aspects of medical decision-making. We may know that a patient does not have long to live, but we cannot be certain how long. We may prescribe a potent new receptor blocker to reverse the course of a patient's illness, but we cannot be certain that the therapy will achieve the desired result and that result alone. Uncertainty in medical outcomes creates the need for probabilities and other mathematical/statistical tools to help guide decision-making. (These tools are reviewed later in the chapter.)

Uncertainty is compounded by the information overload that characterizes modern medicine. Today's experienced clinician needs close to 2 million pieces of information to practice medicine. Doctors subscribe to an average of 7 journals, representing over 2500 new articles each year. Computers offer the obvious solution both for management of information and for better quantitation and management of the daily uncertainties of medical care. While the technology to computerize medical practice is available, many practical problems remain to be solved before patient information can be standardized and integrated with medical evidence on a single electronic platform.

The following three examples introduce the subject of clinical reasoning:

- A 46-year-old man presents to his internist with a chief complaint of hemoptysis. The physician knows that the differential diagnosis of hemoptysis includes over 100 different conditions, including cancer and tuberculosis (Chap. 30). The examination begins with some general background questions, and the patient is asked to describe his symptoms and their chronology. By the time the examination is completed, and even before any tests are run, the physician has formulated a working diagnostic hypothesis and planned a series of steps to test it. In an otherwise healthy and nonsmoking patient recovering from a viral bronchitis, the doctor's hypothesis would be that the acute bronchitis is responsible for the small amount of blood-streaked sputum the patient observed. In this case, a chest x-ray may provide sufficient reassurance that a more serious disorder is not present.

- A second 46-year-old patient with the same chief complaint who has a 100-pack-year smoking history, a productive morning cough, and episodes of blood-streaked sputum may generate the principal diagnostic hypothesis of carcinoma of the lung. Consequently, along with the chest x-ray, the physician obtains a sputum cytology examination and refers this patient for fiberoptic bronchoscopy.

- A third 46-year-old patient with hemoptysis who is from a developing country is evaluated with an echocardiogram as well, because the physician thinks she hears a soft diastolic rumble at the apex on cardiac auscultation, suggesting rheumatic mitral stenosis.

These three simple vignettes illustrate two aspects of expert clinical reasoning: (1) the use of cognitive shortcuts as a way to organize the complex unstructured material that is collected in the clinical evaluation, and (2) the use of diagnostic hypotheses to consolidate the information and indicate appropriate management steps.

THE USE OF COGNITIVE SHORTCUTS Cognitive shortcuts or rules of thumb, sometimes referred to as *heuristics*, can help solve complex problems, of the sort encountered daily in clinical medicine, with great efficiency. Clinicians rely on three basic types of heuristics. When assessing a patient, clinicians often weigh the probability that this patient's clinical features match those of the class of patients with the leading diagnostic hypotheses being considered. In other words, the clinician is searching for the diagnosis for which the patient appears to be a representative example; this cognitive shortcut is called the *representativeness heuristic*.

It may take only a few characteristics from the history for an expert clinician using the representativeness heuristic to arrive at a sound diagnostic hypothesis. For example, an elderly patient with new-onset fever, cough productive of copious sputum, unilateral pleuritic chest pain, and dyspnea is readily identified as fitting the pattern for acute pneumonia, probably of bacterial origin. Evidence of focal pulmonary consolidation on the physical examination will increase the clinician's confidence in the diagnosis because it fits the expected pattern of acute bacterial pneumonia. Knowing this allows the experienced clinician to conduct an efficient, directed, and therapeutically productive patient evaluation although there may be little else in the history or physical examination of direct relevance. The inexperienced medical student or resident, who has not yet learned the patterns most prevalent in clinical medicine, must work much harder to achieve the same result and is often at risk of missing the important clinical problem in a sea of compulsively collected but unhelpful data.

However, physicians using the representativeness heuristic can reach erroneous conclusions if they fail to consider the underlying prevalence of two competing diagnoses (i.e., the prior, or pretest, probabilities). Consider a patient with pleuritic chest pain, dyspnea, and a low-grade fever. A clinician might consider acute pneumonia and acute pulmonary embolism to be the two leading diagnostic alternatives. Using the representativeness heuristic, the clinician might judge both diagnostic candidates to be equally likely, although to do so would be wrong if pneumonia was much more prevalent in the underlying population. Mistakes may also result from a failure to consider that a pattern based on a small number of prior observations will likely be less reliable than one based on larger samples.

A second commonly used cognitive shortcut, the *availability heuristic*, involves judgments made on the basis of how easily prior similar cases or outcomes can be brought to mind. For example, the experienced clinician may recall 20 elderly patients seen over the past few years who presented with painless dyspnea of acute onset and were found to have acute myocardial infarction. The novice clinician may spend valuable time seeking a pulmonary cause for the symptoms before considering and discovering the cardiac diagnosis. In this situation, the patient's clinical pattern does not fit the expected pattern of acute myocardial infarction, but experience with this atypical presentation, and the ability to recall it, can help direct the physician to the diagnosis.

Errors with the availability heuristic can come from several sources of recall bias. For example, rare catastrophes are likely to be remembered with a clarity and force out of proportion to their value, and recent experience is, of course, easier to recall and therefore more influential on clinical judgments.

The third commonly used cognitive shortcut, the *anchoring heuristic*, involves estimating a probability by starting from a familiar point (the anchor) and adjusting to the new case from there. Anchoring can be a powerful tool for diagnosis but is often used incorrectly. For example, a clinician may judge the probability of coronary artery disease (CAD) to be very high after a positive exercise thallium test, because the prediction has been anchored to the test result ("positive test = high probability of CAD"). Yet, as discussed below, this prediction would be inaccurate if the clinical (pretest) picture of the patient being tested indicates a low probability of disease (e.g., a 30-year-old woman with no risk factors). As illustrated in this example, anchors are not necessarily the same as the pretest probability (see "Measures of Disease Probability and Bayes' Theorem," below).

DIAGNOSTIC HYPOTHESIS GENERATION   Cognitive scientists studying the thought processes of expert clinicians have observed that clinicians group data into packets, or "chunks," which are stored in their memories and manipulated to generate diagnostic hypotheses. Because short-term memory can typically hold only 7 to 10 items at a time, the number of packets that can be actively integrated into hypothesis-generating activities is similarly limited. The cognitive shortcuts discussed above play a key role in the generation of diagnostic hypotheses, many of which are discarded as rapidly as they are formed.

A diagnostic hypothesis sets a context for diagnostic steps to follow and provides testable predictions. For example, if the enlarged and quite tender liver felt on physical examination is due to acute hepatitis (the hypothesis), certain specific liver function tests should be mark-edly elevated (the prediction). If the tests come back normal, the hypothesis may need to be discarded or substantially modified.

One of the factors that makes teaching diagnostic reasoning so difficult is that expert clinicians do not follow a fixed pattern in patient examinations. From the outset, they are generating, refining, and discarding diagnostic hypotheses. The questions they ask in the history are driven by the hypotheses they are working with at the moment. Even the physical examination is driven by specific questions rather than a preordained checklist. While the student is palpating the abdomen of the alcoholic patient, waiting for a finding to strike him, the expert clinician is on a focused search mission. Is the spleen enlarged? How big is the liver? Is it tender? Are there any palpable masses or nodules? Each question focuses the attention of the examiner to the exclusion of all other inputs until answered, allowing the examiner to move on to the next specific question.

Negative findings are often as important as positive ones in establishing and refining diagnostic hypotheses. Chest discomfort that is not provoked or worsened by exertion in an active patient reduces the likelihood that chronic ischemic heart disease is the underlying cause. The absence of a resting tachycardia and thyroid gland enlargement reduces the likelihood of hyperthyroidism in a patient with paroxysmal atrial fibrillation.

The acuity of a patient's illness can play an important role in overriding considerations of prevalence and other issues described above. For example, clinicians are taught to consider aortic dissection routinely as a possible cause of acute severe chest discomfort along with myocardial infarction, even though the typical history of dissection is different from myocardial infarction and dissection is far less prevalent (Chap. 231). This recommendation is based on the recognition that a relatively rare but catastrophic diagnosis like aortic dissection is very difficult to make unless it is explicitly considered. If the clinician fails to elicit any of the characteristic features of dissection by history and finds equivalent blood pressures in both arms and no pulse deficits, he or she may feel comfortable in discarding the aortic dissection hypothesis. If, however, the chest x-ray shows a widened mediastinum, the hypothesis may be reinstated and a diagnostic test ordered [e.g., thoracic computed tomography (CT) scan, transesophageal echocardiogram] to evaluate it more fully. In nonacute situations, the prevalence of potential alternative diagnoses should play a much more prominent role in diagnostic hypothesis generation.

Generation of Diagnostic Hypotheses   Because the generation and evaluation of appropriate diagnostic hypotheses is a skill that not all clinicians possess to an equal degree, errors in this process can occur; in the patient with serious acute illness these may lead to tragic consequences. Consider the following hypothetical example. A 45-year-old male patient with a 3-week history of a "flulike" upper respiratory infection (URI) presented to his physician with symptoms of dyspnea and a productive cough. Based on the presenting complaint, the clinician pulled out a "URI Assessment Form" to improve quality and efficiency of care. The physician quickly completed the examination components outlined on this structured form, noting in particular the absence of fever and a clear chest examination. He then prescribed an antibiotic for presumed bronchitis, showed the patient how to breathe into a paper bag to relieve his "hyperventilation," and sent him home with the reassurance that his illness was not serious. After a sleepless night with significant dyspnea unrelieved by rebreathing into a bag, the patient developed nausea and vomiting and collapsed. He was brought into the Emergency Department in cardiac arrest and could not be resuscitated. Autopsy showed a posterior wall myocardial infarction and a fresh thrombus in an atherosclerotic right coronary artery. What went wrong? The clinician decided, even before starting the history, that the patient's complaints were not serious. He therefore felt confident that he could perform an abbreviated and focused examination using the URI assessment protocol rather than considering the full range of possibilities and performing appropriate tests to confirm or refute his initial hypotheses. In particular, by concentrating on the "URI," the clinician failed to elicit the full dyspnea history, which would have suggested a far more serious disorder, and neglected to search for other symptoms that could have directed him to the correct diagnosis.

This example illustrates how patients can diverge from textbook symptoms and the potential consequences of being unable to adapt the diagnostic process to real-world challenges. The expert, while recognizing that common things occur commonly, approaches each evaluation on high alert for clues that the initial diagnosis may be wrong. Patients often provide information that "does not fit" with any of the leading diagnostic hypotheses being considered. Distinguishing real clues from false trails can only be achieved by practice and experience. A less experienced clinician who tries to be too efficient (as in the above example) can make serious judgment errors. Furthermore, the value of conducting a rapid systematic clinical survey of symptoms and organ systems to avoid missing important but inapparent clues cannot be overstated.

MAJOR INFLUENCES ON CLINICAL DECISION-MAKING   More than a decade of research on variations in clinician practice patterns has shed much light on forces that shape clinical decisions. The use of heuristic "shortcuts," as detailed above, provides a partial explanation, but several other key factors play an important role in shaping diagnostic hypotheses and management decisions. These factors can be grouped conceptually into three overlapping categories: (1) factors related to physician personal characteristics and practice style, (2) factors related to the practice setting, and (3) economic incentive factors.

Practice Style Factors   One of the key roles of the physician in medical care is to serve as the patient's agent to ensure that necessary care is provided at a high level of quality. Factors that influence this role include the physician's knowledge, training, and experience. It is obvious that physicians cannot practice evidence-based medicine (EBM; described later in the chapter) if they are unfamiliar with the evidence. As would be expected, specialists generally know the evidence in their field better than do generalists. Surgeons may be more enthusiastic about recommending surgery than medical doctors because their belief in the beneficial effects of surgery is stronger. For the same reason, invasive cardiologists are much more likely to refer chest pain patients for diagnostic catheterization than are noninvasive cardiologists or generalists. The physician beliefs that drive these different practice styles are based on personal experience, recollection, and interpretation of the available medical evidence. For example, heart failure specialists are much more likely than generalists to achieve target angiotensin-converting enzyme (ACE) inhibitor therapy in their heart failure patients because they are more familiar with what the targets are (as defined by large clinical trials), have more familiarity with the specific drugs (including dosages and side effects), and are less likely to overreact to foreseeable problems in therapy such as a rise in creatinine levels or symptomatic hypotension. Other intriguing research has shown a wide distribution of acceptance times of antibiotic therapy for peptic ulcer disease following widespread dissemination of the "evidence" in the medical literature. Some gastroenterologists accepted this new therapy before the evidence was clear (reflecting, perhaps, an aggressive practice style), and some gastroenterologists lagged behind (a conservative practice style, associated in this case with older physicians). As a group, internists lagged several years behind gastroenterologists.

The opinion of influential leaders can also have an important effect on practice patterns. Such influence can occur at both the national level (e.g., expert physicians teaching at national meetings) and the local level (e.g., local educational programs, "curbside consultants"). Opinion leaders do not have to be physicians. When conducting rounds with clinical pharmacists, physicians are less likely to make medication errors and more likely to use target levels of evidence-based therapies.

The patient's welfare is not the only concern that drives clinical decisions. The physician's perception about the risk of a malpractice suit resulting from either an erroneous decision or a bad outcome creates a style of practice referred to as *defensive medicine*. This practice involves using tests and therapies with very small marginal returns to preclude future criticism in the event of an adverse outcome. For example, a 40-year-old woman who presents with a long-standing history of intermittent headache and a new severe headache along with a normal neurologic examination has a very low likelihood of structural intracranial pathology. Performance of a head CT or magnetic resonance imaging (MRI) scan in this situation would constitute defensive medicine. On the other hand, the results of the test could provide reassurance to an anxious patient.

Practice Setting Factors   Factors in this category relate to the physical resources available to the physician's practice and the practice environment. *Physician-induced demand* is a term that refers to the repeated observation that physicians have a remarkable ability to accommodate to and employ the medical facilities available to them. A classic early study in this area showed that physicians in Boston had an almost 50% higher hospital admission rate than did physicians in New Haven, despite there being no obvious differences in the health of the cities' inhabitants. The physicians in New Haven were not aware of using fewer hospital beds for their patients, nor were the Boston physicians aware of using less stringent criteria to admit patients. In both cities, physicians unconsciously adopted their practice styles to the available level of hospital beds.

Other environmental factors that can influence decision-making include the local availability of specialists for consultations and procedures, "high tech" facilities such as angiography suites, a heart surgery program, and MRI machines.

Economic Incentives   Economic incentives are closely related to the other two categories of practice-modifying factors. Financial issues can exert both stimulatory and inhibitory influences on clinical practice. In general, physicians are paid on a fee-for-service, capitation, or salary basis. In fee-for-service, the more the physician does, the more the physician gets paid. The incentive in this case is to do more. When fees are reduced (discounted fee-for-service), doctors tend to increase the number of services billed for. Capitation, in contrast, provides a fixed payment per patient per year, encouraging physicians to take on more patients but to provide each patient with fewer services. Expensive services are more likely to be affected by this type of incentive than inexpensive preventive services. Salary compensation plans pay physicians the same regardless of the amount of clinical work performed. The incentive here is to see fewer patients.

In summary, expert clinical decision-making can be appreciated as a complex interplay between cognitive devices used to simplify large amounts of complex information interacting with physician biases reflecting education, training, and experience, all of which are shaped by powerful, sometimes perverse, external forces. In the next section, a set of statistical tools and concepts that can assist in making clinical decisions under uncertainty are reviewed.

QUANTITATIVE METHODS TO AID CLINICAL DECISION-MAKING

The process of medical decision-making can be divided into two parts: (1) defining the available courses of action and estimating the likely outcomes with each, and (2) assessing the desirability of the outcomes. The former task involves integrating key information about the patient along with relevant evidence from the medical literature to create the structure of a decision problem. The remainder of this chapter will review some quantitative tools available to assist the clinician in these activities. These tools can be divided into those that assist the clinician in making better outcome predictions, which are then used to make decisions, and those that support the decision process directly. While these tools are not yet used routinely in daily clinical practice, the computerization of medicine is creating the required platform for their future widespread dissemination.

The purpose of performing a test on a patient is to reduce uncertainty about the patient's diagnosis or prognosis and to aid the clinician in making management decisions. Although diagnostic tests are commonly thought of as laboratory tests (e.g., measurement of serum amylase level) or procedures (e.g., colonoscopy or bronchoscopy), any technology that changes our understanding of the patient's problem qualifies as a diagnostic test. Thus, even the history and physical examination can be considered a form of diagnostic test. In clinical medicine, it is common to reduce the results of a test to a dichotomous outcome, such as positive or negative, normal or abnormal. In many cases, this simplification results in the waste of useful information. However, such simplification makes it easier to demonstrate some of the quantitative ways in which test data can be used.

To characterize the accuracy of diagnostic tests, four terms are routinely used (Table 2-1). The *true-positive rate*, i.e., the *sensitivity*, provides a measure of how well the test correctly identifies patients with disease. The *false-negative rate* is calculated as (1 − sensitivity). The *true-negative rate*, i.e., the *specificity*, reflects how well the test correctly identifies patients without disease. The *false-positive rate* is (1 − specificity). A perfect test would have a sensitivity of 100% and a specificity of 100% and would completely separate patients with disease from those without it.

Calculating sensitivity and specificity require selection of a cutpoint value for the test, called the *positivity criterion*, to define the threshold value at or above which the test is considered "positive." As the cutpoint is moved to improve sensitivity, specificity typically falls and vice versa. This dynamic tradeoff between more accurate identification of subjects with disease versus those without disease is often displayed graphically as a receiver operating characteristic (ROC) curve (Fig. 2-1). An ROC curve plots sensitivity (*y*-axis) versus 1 − specificity (*x*-axis). Each point on the curve represents a potential cutpoint with an associated sensitivity and specificity value. The area under the ROC curve is often used as a quantitative measure of the information content of a test. Values range from 0.5 (no diagnostic information at all, test is equivalent to flipping a coin) to 1.0 (perfect test).

In the testing literature, ROC areas are often used to compare alternative tests that can be used for a particular diagnostic problem. The test with the highest area (i.e., closest to 1.0) is presumed to be the most accurate. However, ROC curves are not a panacea for evaluation of diagnostic test utility. Like Bayes' theorem (discussed below), they are typically focused on only one possible test parameter (e.g., ST-segment response in a treadmill exercise test) to the exclusion of other potentially relevant data. In addition, ROC area comparisons do not simulate the way test information is actually used in clinical practice. Finally, biases in the underlying population used to generate the ROC curves (e.g., related to an unrepresentative test sample) can bias the ROC area and the validity of a comparison among tests.

Measures of Disease Probability and Bayes' Theorem Unfortunately, there are no perfect tests; after every test is completed the true disease state of the patient remains uncertain. Quantitating this residual uncertainty

FIGURE 2-1 The receiver operating characteristic (ROC) curves for a hypothetical diagnostic test. The ROC curve illustrates the trade off that occurs between improved test sensitivity (accurate detection of patients with disease) and improved test specificity (accurate detection of patients without disease), as the test value defining when the test turns from "negative" to "positive" is varied. The 45° line indicates a test with no information (sensitivity = specificity at every test value). Point A indicates a test positivity criterion that has good specificity (90%) but poor sensitivity (60%). Point C indicates a test positivity criterion with the reverse problem: good sensitivity (90%) but poor specificity (30%). Point B may therefore represent the best compromise for clinical use.

can be done with Bayes' theorem. This theorem provides a simple mathematical way to calculate the posttest probability of disease from three parameters: the pretest probability of disease, the test sensitivity, and the test specificity (Table 2-2). The pretest probability is a quantitative expression of the confidence in a diagnosis before the test is performed. In the absence of more relevant information it is usually estimated from the prevalence of the disease in the underlying population. For some common conditions, such as CAD, nomograms and statistical models have been created to generate better estimates of pretest probability from elements of the history and physical examination. The posttest probability, then, is a revised statement of the confidence in the diagnosis, taking into account what was known both before and after the test.

To understand conceptually how Bayes' theorem creates this revised confidence statement, it is useful to examine a nomogram version of Bayes' theorem that uses the same three parameters to predict the posttest probability of disease (Fig. 2-2). In this nomogram, the accuracy of the diagnostic test in question is summarized by the likelihood ratio for a positive test, which is the ratio of the true-positive rate to the false-positive rate [or sensitivity/(1 − specificity)]. For example, a test with a sensitivity of 0.90 and a specificity of 0.90 has a likelihood ratio of 0.90/(1 − 0.90), or 9. Thus, for this hypothetical test, a "positive" result is 9 times more likely in a patient with the disease than in a patient without it. The more accurate the test, the higher the likelihood ratio. However, if sensitivity is excellent but specificity is less so, the likelihood ratio will be substantially reduced (e.g., with a 90% sensitivity but a 60% specificity, the likelihood ratio is 2.25). Most tests in medicine have likelihood ratios for a positive result between 1.5 and 20.

Applications to Diagnostic Testing in CAD Consider two tests commonly used in the diagnosis of CAD, an exercise treadmill and an exercise thallium-201 single photon emission CT (SPECT) test (Chap. 226). Meta-analysis has shown the treadmill to have an average sensitivity of 66% and an average specificity of 84%, yielding a likelihood ratio of 4.1 [0.66/(1 − 0.84)]. If we use this test on a patient with a pretest probability of CAD of 10%, the posttest probability of disease following a positive result rises only to about 30%. If a patient with a pretest probability of CAD of 80% has a positive test result, the posttest probability of disease is about 95%.

TABLE 2-1 *Measures of Diagnostic Test Accuracy*

Test Result	Disease Status	
	Present	*Absent*
Positive	True-positive (*TP*)	False-positive (*FP*)
Negative	False-negative (*FN*)	True-negative (*TN*)

IDENTIFICATION OF PATIENTS WITH DISEASE

True-positive rate (sensitivity) = *TP*/(*TP* + *FN*)
False-negative rate = *FN*/(*TP* + *FN*)
True-positive rate = 1 − false-negative rate

IDENTIFICATION OF PATIENTS WITHOUT DISEASE

True-negative rate (specificity) = *TN*/(*TN* + *FP*)
False-positive rate = *FP*/(*TN* + *FP*)
True-negative rate = 1 − false-positive rate

TABLE 2-2   *Measures of Disease Probability*

Pretest probability of disease = probability of disease before test is done. May use population prevalence of disease or more patient-specific data to generate this probability estimate.

Posttest probability of disease = probability of disease accounting for both pretest probability and test results. Also called predictive value of the test.

Bayes' theorem

  Computational version:

    Posttest probability =

$$\frac{\text{Pretest probability} \times \text{test sensitivity}}{\begin{array}{c}\text{Pretest probability} \times \text{test sensitivity} + \\ (1 - \text{disease prevalence}) \times \text{test false-positive rate}\end{array}}$$

  Example [with a pretest probability of 0.50 and a "positive" diagnostic test result (test sensitivity = 0.90, test specificity = 0.90)]:

$$\begin{aligned}\text{Posttest probability} &= \frac{(0.50)(0.90)}{(0.50)(0.90) + (0.50)(0.10)} \\ &= 0.90\end{aligned}$$

The exercise thallium SPECT test is a more accurate test for the diagnosis of CAD. For our purposes, assume that it has both a sensitivity and specificity of 90%, yielding a likelihood ratio of 9.0 [0.90/(1 − 0.90)]. If we again test our low pretest probability patient and he has a positive test, using Fig. 2-2 we can demonstrate that the posttest probability of CAD rises from 10 to 50%. However, from a decision-making point of view, the more accurate test has not been able to improve diagnostic confidence enough to change management. In fact, the test has moved us from being fairly certain that the patient did not have CAD to being completely undecided (a 50:50 chance of disease). In a patient with a pretest probability of 80%, using the more accurate thallium SPECT test raises the posttest probability to 97% (compared with 95% for the exercise treadmill). Again, the more accurate test does not provide enough improvement in posttest confidence to alter management, and neither test has improved much upon what was known from clinical data alone.

If the pretest probability is low (e.g., 20%), even a positive result on a very accurate test will not move the posttest probability to a range high enough to rule in disease (e.g., 80%). Conversely, with a high pretest probability, a negative test will not adequately rule out disease. Thus, the largest gain in diagnostic confidence from a test occurs when the clinician is most uncertain before performing it (e.g., pretest probability between 30 and 70%). For example, if a patient has a pretest probability for CAD of 50%, a positive exercise treadmill test will move the posttest probability to 80% and a positive exercise thallium SPECT test will move it to 90% (Fig. 2-2).

Bayes' theorem, as presented above, employs a number of important simplifications that should be considered. First, few tests have only two useful outcomes, positive or negative, and many tests provide numerous pieces of data about the patient. Even if these can be integrated into a summary result, multiple levels of useful information may be present (e.g., strongly positive, positive, indeterminate, negative, strongly negative). While Bayes' theorem can be adapted to this more detailed test result format, it is computationally complex to do so. Second, Bayes' theorem assumes that the information from the test is completely unique and nonoverlapping with information used to estimate the pretest probability. This independence assumption, however, is often wrong. In many cases, test results are correlated with patient characteristics. For example, the findings of cardiomegaly and pulmonary edema on chest x-ray are correlated with the historic features of heart failure and with the physical findings of a displaced left ventricular apical impulse, an S_3 gallop, and rales. The unique predictive information contributed by the test in this case (the chest x-ray) is only a fraction of its total information because much had already been learned about the probability of heart failure before the test was done.

Finally, it has long been thought that sensitivity and specificity are

prevalence-independent parameters of test accuracy, and many texts still make this assertion. This statistically useful assumption, however, is clinically wrong. For example, a treadmill exercise test has a sensitivity in a population of patients with one-vessel CAD of around 30%, whereas the sensitivity in severe three-vessel CAD approaches 80%. Thus, the best estimate of sensitivity to use in a particular decision will often vary depending on the distribution of disease stages present in the tested population. A hospitalized population typically has a higher prevalence of disease and in particular a higher prevalence of more advanced disease stages than an outpatient population. As a consequence, test sensitivity will tend to be higher in hospitalized patients, whereas test specificity will be higher in outpatients.

Statistical Prediction Models   Bayes' theorem, as presented above, deals with a clinical prediction problem that is unrealistically simple relative to most problems a clinician faces. Prediction models, based on multivariable statistical models, can handle much more complex problems and substantially enhance predictive accuracy for specific situations. Their particular advantage is the ability to take into account many overlapping pieces of information and assign a relative weight to each based on its unique contribution to the prediction in question. For example, a logistic regression model to predict the probability of CAD takes into account all of the relevant independent factors from the clinical examination and diagnostic testing instead of the small handful of data that clinicians can manage in their heads or with Bayes' theorem. However, despite this strength, the models are too complex computationally to use without a calculator or computer (although this limit may be overcome when medicine is practiced from a fully computerized platform). To date, only a handful of prediction models have been developed and properly validated. The importance of independent validation in a population separate from the one used to develop the model cannot be overstated. Unfortunately, most published models have not been properly validated, making their utility in clinical practice uncertain at best.

FIGURE 2-2   Nomogram version of Bayes' Theorem used to predict the posttest probability of disease (left-hand scale) using the pretest probability of disease (right-hand scale) and the likelihood ratio for a positive test (middle scale). The likelihood ratio is calculated as the sensitivity/(1 − specificity). To use, place a straightedge connecting the pretest probability and the likelihood ratio, and read off the posttest probability. This figure illustrates the value of a positive exercise treadmill test (likelihood ratio 4) and a positive exercise thallium SPECT study (likelihood ratio 9) in the patient with a pretest probability of coronary artery disease of 50%. Treadmill results shown in solid line; thallium results in dashed line. (*Adapted from Fagan TJ: N Engl J Med 293:257, 1975.*)

When statistical models have been compared directly with expert clinicians, they have been found to be more consistent, as would be expected, but not significantly more accurate. Their biggest promise, then, would seem to be to make less-experienced clinicians more accurate predictors of outcome.

DECISION SUPPORT TOOLS

DECISION SUPPORT SYSTEMS   Over the past 30 years, many attempts have been made to develop computer systems to help clinicians make decisions and manage patients. Conceptually, computers offer a very attractive way to handle the vast information load that today's physicians face. The computer can help by making accurate predictions of outcome, simulating the whole decision process, or providing algorithmic guidance. Computer-based predictions using Bayesian or statistical regression models inform a clinical decision but do not actually reach a "conclusion" or "recommendation." Artificial intelligence systems attempt to simulate or replace human reasoning with a computer-based analogue. To date, such approaches have achieved only limited success. Reminder or protocol-directed systems do not make predictions but use existing algorithms, such as practice guidelines, to guide clinical practice. In general, however, decision support systems have shown little impact on practice. Reminder systems, although not yet in widespread use, have shown the most promise, particularly in correcting drug dosing and in promoting guideline adherence. The full potential of these approaches will only be achieved when computers are fully integrated into medical practice.

DECISION ANALYSIS   Compared with the methods discussed above, decision analysis represents a completely different approach to decision support. Its principal application is in decision problems that are complex and involve a substantial risk, a high degree of uncertainty in some key area, or an idiosyncratic feature that does not "fit" the available evidence. Three general steps are involved. First, the decision problem must be clearly defined. Second, the elements of the decision must be made explicit. This involves specifying the alternatives being considered, their relevant outcomes, the probabilities attached to each outcome, and the relative desirability (called "utility") of each outcome. Cost can also be assigned to each branch of the decision tree, allowing calculation of cost effectiveness. Finally, the decision tree must be "analyzed" to find the strategy with the best expected outcome.

An example of a decision tree used to evaluate strategies for management of the risk of infective endocarditis after catheter-associated *Staphylococcus aureus* bacteremia is shown in Fig. 2-3. Approximately 35,000 cases of *S. aureus* bacteremia occur each year in the United States. The development of complicating endocarditis, which occurs in about 6% of cases, is associated with high morbidity (31% mortality, 21% stroke rate) and medical costs. The three choices for management of the bacteremia are (1) transesophageal echocardiography (TEE), (2) a 4-week course of intravenous antibiotics (long-course), or (3) a 2-week course of intravenous antibiotics (short-course). In the TEE strategy, a 4-week course of antibiotics is given if endocarditis is evident and a 2-week course is given if it is not. With each strategy, there is a risk that the patient will develop endocarditis with or without major complications. In this analysis, the longest quality-adjusted survival (5.47 quality-adjusted life-years) was associated with the 4-week antibiotic course strategy, which also had the highest costs ($14,136 per patient), whereas the lowest costs ($9830 per patient) and worst outcomes (5.42 quality-adjusted life-years) were associated with the 2-week antibiotic course strategy. From a clinical

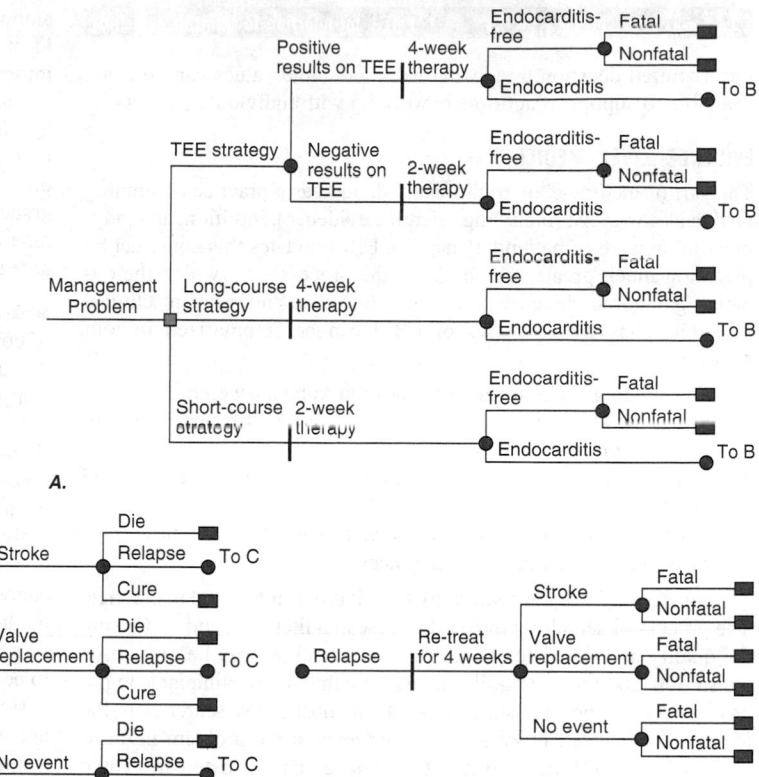

FIGURE 2-3   Decision model used to evaluate strategies for management of the risk of infective endocarditis after catheter-associated *Staphylococcus aureus* bacteremia. The square node indicates a decision between possible management strategies. Round nodes represent chance events, and rectangular (or terminal) nodes indicate the outcomes of interest. All nonterminal chance nodes in the main tree (structure *A*) enter substructure *B*. All nonterminal chance nodes in substructure *B* enter substructure *C*. TEE, transesophageal echocardiography. *(From Rosen AB et al: Ann Intern Med 130:810, 1999, with permission.)*

point of view (ignoring costs), the 4-week antibiotic course was best. From a cost-effectiveness point of view, the TEE strategy (5.46 quality-adjusted life-years and $10,051 per patient costs) provided the best balance of added benefits and costs. Thus, decision analysis can be extremely helpful in clarifying tradeoffs in outcomes and costs in difficult management areas where it is highly unlikely that an adequate randomized trial will ever be done, such as the above.

Filling in the Decision Tree   The data needed to fill in a decision tree (Fig. 2-3) are typically cobbled together from a variety of sources, including the literature (randomized trials, meta-analyses, observational studies) and expert opinion. Once the decision tree is finished, the decision is "analyzed" by calculating the average value of each limb of the tree. The decision arm with the highest net value (or expected utility) is the preferred choice. The value of this exercise, however, is not so much in developing a prescription for action as it is in exploring the key elements and pressure points of a complex or difficult decision. The process of building the decision tree forces the analyst to be explicit about the choices being considered and all their relevant outcomes. Areas of high uncertainty are readily identified. Sensitivity analyses are an integral part of decision analysis and involve systematically varying the value of each key parameter in the model alone (one-way sensitivity analysis), in pairs (two-way), or in higher combinations (multivariable) to assess the impact on choice of preferred management strategy. In the above example, varying the incidence of endocarditis resulting from *S. aureus* bacteremia from 3% to >50% had no impact on the choice of TEE as the preferred strategy.

User-friendly personal computer–based software packages now make the creation and analysis of decision trees much more straightforward than in the past. However, the process is still far too cumbersome and time-consuming to be used on a routine basis. When medicine is practiced from a fully computerized platform, a library of prestructured decision trees with user-modifiable values can be made available to support practitioners working with individual patients.

EVIDENCE-BASED MEDICINE

The "art of medicine" is traditionally defined as a practice combining medical knowledge (including scientific evidence), intuition, and judgment in the care of patients (Chap. 1). EBM updates this construct by placing a much greater emphasis on the processes by which the clinician gains knowledge of the most up-to-date and relevant clinical research. The key processes of EBM can be summarized in four steps:

1. Formulating the management question to be answered
2. Searching the literature and on-line databases for applicable research data
3. Appraising the evidence gathered with regard to its validity and relevance
4. Integrating this appraisal with knowledge about the unique aspects of the patient (including preferences).

Steps 2 and 3 are the heart of EBM as it is currently used in practice. The process of searching the world's research literature and appraising the quality and relevance of studies thus identified can be quite time consuming and requires skills and training that many clinicians do not possess. Thus, the best starting point for most EBM searches is the identification of recent systematic overviews of the problem in question. Selected resources to assist in this search are listed in (Table 2-3).

Generally, the EBM tools listed in Table 2-3 provide access to research information in one of two forms. The first, primary research reports, is the original peer-reviewed research work that is published in medical journals. Initial access to this information in an EBM search may be gained through MEDLINE, which provides access to a huge amount of data in abstract form. The difficulty with MEDLINE is locating reports that are on point in a sea of irrelevant or unhelpful information and being reasonably certain that important reports have not been overlooked. The second form, systematic reviews, comprehensively summarizes the available evidence on a particular topic up to a certain date and provides the interpretation of the reviewer. Explicit criteria are used to find all the relevant scientific research and grade its quality. The prototype for this kind of resource is the Cochrane Database of Systematic Reviews. One of the key components of a systematic review is a meta-analysis.

Meta-analysis   This is research done on research data for the purpose of combining and summarizing the available evidence quantitatively. Although it can be used to combine nonrandomized studies, meta-analysis is most valuable when used to summarize all the randomized trials on a particular therapeutic problem. Ideally, unpublished trials should be identified and included to avoid publication bias (i.e., only "positive" trials tend to get published). Furthermore, some of the best meta-analyses obtain and analyze the raw patient-level data from the individual trials rather than working only with what is available in the published reports of each trial. Importantly, not all published meta-analyses are reliable sources of evidence on a particular problem. Their methodology must be carefully scrutinized to ensure proper study design and analysis. The results of a well done meta-analysis are likely to be most persuasive if it includes at least several large-scale, properly performed randomized trials. In many cases, where the available trials are small or poorly done, the best that may be concluded is that substantial additional trials are required to reach a reliable conclusion about a particular therapy.

Meta-analyses typically focus on summary measures of relative treatment benefit, such as odds ratios or relative risks. Clinicians should also examine what absolute risk reduction (ARR) can be expected from the therapy. A useful summary metric of absolute treatment benefit is the number needed to treat (NNT) to prevent one adverse outcome event (e.g., death, stroke). NNT is simply 1/ARR. For example, if a hypothetical therapy reduced mortality over a 5-year follow-up by 33% (the relative treatment benefit) from 12% (control arm) to 8% (treatment arm), the absolute risk reduction would be 12% − 8% = 4% and the NNT = ¼ or 25. Thus, we would need to treat 25 patients for 5 years to prevent 1 death. If we applied our hypothetical treatment to a lower risk population, say with a 6% 5-year mortality, the 33% relative treatment benefit would reduce absolute mortality by 2% (from 6% to 4%) and the NNT for the same therapy in this different group of patients would be 50.

CONCLUSIONS

In this era of evidence-based medicine, it is tempting to think that all the difficult decisions practitioners face have been or soon will be solved and digested into practice guidelines and computerized reminders. However, EBM provides practitioners with an ideal rather than a finished set of tools with which to manage patients. The significant contribution of EBM has been to promote the development of more powerful and user-friendly EBM tools that can be accessed by the busy practitioners. This is an enormously important contribution that is slowly changing the way medi-

---

TABLE 2-3   *Selected Tools for Finding the Evidence in Evidence-Based Medicine*

Name	Description	Web Address	Availability
Evidence-Based Medicine Reviews	Comprehensive electronic database that combines and integrates: 1. The Cochrane Database of Systematic Reviews 2. ACP Journal Club 3. The Database of Abstracts of Reviews of Effectiveness	*www.ovid.com*	Subscription required; available through medical center libraries and other institutions
Cochrane Library	Collection of EBM databases including The Cochrane Database of Systematic Reviews—full text articles reviewing specific health care topics	*www.cochrane.org*	Subscription required; abstracts of systematic reviews available free online; some countries have funding to provide free access to all residents
ACP Journal Club	Collection of summaries of original studies and systematic reviews; published bimonthly; all data since 1991 available on Web site, updated yearly	*www.acpic.org*	Subscription required
Clinical Evidence	Monthly updated directory of concise overviews of common clinical interventions	*www.clinicalevidence.com*	Subscription required; free access for UK and for developing countries
MEDLINE	National Library of Medicine database with citations back to 1966	*www.nlm.nih.gov*	Free via Internet

Note: ACP, American College of Physicians; EBM, evidence-based medicine.

cine is practiced. One of the repeated admonitions of EBM pioneers has been to replace reliance on the local "gray-haired expert" (who may be often wrong but rarely in doubt) with a systematic search for and evaluation of the evidence. But EBM has not eliminated the need for subjective judgments; each systematic review presents the interpretation of an "expert," whose biases remain largely invisible to the consumer of the review. In addition, meta-analyses cannot generate evidence where there are no adequate randomized trials, and most of what clinicians face will never be thoroughly tested in a randomized trial. For the foreseeable future, excellent clinical reasoning skills and experience supplemented by well-designed quantitative tools and a keen appreciation for individual patient preferences will continue to be of paramount importance in the professional life of medical practitioners.

FURTHER READING

BALK EM et al: Correlation of quality measures with estimates of treatment effect in meta-analyses of randomized controlled trials. JAMA 287:2973, 2002

NAYLOR CD: Gray zones of clinical practice: Some limits to evidence-based medicine. Lancet 345:840, 1995

POYNARD T et al: Truth survival in clinical research: An evidence-based requiem? Ann Intern Med 136:888; 2002

SACKETT DL et al: *Evidence-Based Medicine: How to Practice and Teach EBM*. 2d ed. London, Churchill Livingstone, 2000

SCHULMAN KA et al: The effect of race and sex on physicians' recommendations for cardiac catheterization. N Engl J Med 340:618, 1999

3 PRINCIPLES OF CLINICAL PHARMACOLOGY
Dan M. Roden

Drugs are the cornerstone of modern therapeutics. Nevertheless, it is well recognized among physicians and among the lay community that the outcome of drug therapy varies widely among individuals. While this variability has been perceived as an unpredictable, and therefore inevitable, accompaniment of drug therapy, this is not the case. The goal of this chapter is to describe the principles of clinical pharmacology that can be used for the safe and optimal use of available and new drugs.

Drugs interact with specific target molecules to produce their beneficial and adverse effects. The chain of events between administration of a drug and production of these effects in the body can be divided into two important components, both of which contribute to variability in drug actions. The first component comprises the processes that determine drug delivery to, and removal from, molecular targets. The resultant description of the relationship between drug concentration and time is termed *pharmacokinetics*. The second component of variability in drug action comprises the processes that determine variability in drug actions despite equivalent drug delivery to effector drug sites. This description of the relationship between drug concentration and effect is termed *pharmacodynamics*. As discussed further below, pharmacodynamic variability can arise as a result of variability in function of the target molecule itself or of variability in the broad biologic context in which the drug-target interaction occurs to achieve drug effects.

Two important goals of the discipline of clinical pharmacology are (1) to provide a description of conditions under which drug actions vary among human subjects; and (2) to determine mechanisms underlying this variability, with the goal of improving therapy with available drugs as well as pointing to new drug mechanisms that may be effective in the treatment of human disease. The first steps in the discipline were empirical descriptions of the influence of disease X on drug action Y or of individuals or families with unusual sensitivities to adverse drug effects. These important descriptive findings are now being replaced by an understanding of the molecular mechanisms underlying variability in drug actions. Thus, the effects of disease, drug coadministration, or familial factors in modulating drug action can now be reinterpreted as variability in expression or function of specific genes whose products determine pharmacokinetics and pharmacodynamics. Nevertheless, it is the personal interaction of the patient with the physician or other health care provider that first identifies unusual variability in drug actions; maintained alertness to unusual drug responses continues to be a key component of improving drug safety.

Unusual drug responses, segregating in families, have been recognized for decades and initially defined the field of *pharmacogenetics*. Now, with an increasing appreciation of common polymorphisms across the human genome, comes the opportunity to reinterpret descriptive mechanisms of variability in drug action as a consequence of specific DNA polymorphisms, or sets of DNA polymorphisms, among individuals. This approach defines the nascent field of *pharmacogenomics*, which may hold the opportunity of allowing practitioners to integrate a molecular understanding of the basis of disease with an individual's genomic makeup to prescribe personalized, highly effective, and safe therapies.

INDICATIONS FOR DRUG THERAPY It is self-evident that the benefits of drug therapy should outweigh the risks. Benefits fall into two broad categories: those designed to alleviate a symptom, and those designed to prolong useful life. An increasing emphasis on the principles of evidence-based medicine and techniques such as large clinical trials and meta-analyses have defined benefits of drug therapy in specific patient subgroups. Establishing the balance between risk and benefit is not always simple: for example, therapies that provide symptomatic benefits but shorten life may be entertained in patients with serious and highly symptomatic diseases such as heart failure or cancer. These decisions illustrate the continuing highly personal nature of the relationship between the prescriber and the patient.

Some adverse effects are so common, and so readily associated with drug therapy, that they are identified very early during clinical use of a drug. On the other hand, serious adverse effects may be sufficiently uncommon that they escape detection for many years after a drug begins to be widely used. The issue of how to identify rare but serious adverse effects (that can profoundly affect the benefit-risk perception in an individual patient) has not been satisfactorily resolved. Potential approaches range from an increased understanding of the molecular and genetic basis of variability in drug actions to expanded postmarketing surveillance mechanisms. None of these have been completely effective, so practitioners must be continuously vigilant to the possibility that unusual symptoms may be related to specific drugs, or combinations of drugs, that their patients receive.

Beneficial and adverse reactions to drug therapy can be described by a series of dose-response relations (Fig. 3-1). Well-tolerated drugs demonstrate a wide margin, termed the *therapeutic ratio, therapeutic index*, or *therapeutic window*, between the doses required to produce a therapeutic effect and those producing toxicity. In cases where there is a similar relationship between plasma drug concentration and effects, monitoring plasma concentrations can be a highly effective aid in managing drug therapy, by enabling concentrations to be maintained above the minimum required to produce an effect and below the concentration range likely to produce toxicity. Such monitoring has been most widely used to guide therapy with specific agents, such as certain antiarrhythmics, anticonvulsants, and antibiotics. Many of the principles in clinical pharmacology and examples outlined below—that can

FIGURE 3-1 The concept of a therapeutic ratio. Each panel illustrates the relationship between increasing dose and cumulative probability of a desired or adverse drug effect. *Top.* A drug with a wide therapeutic ratio, i.e., a wide separation of the two curves. *Bottom* A drug with a narrow therapeutic ratio; here, the likelihood of adverse effects at therapeutic doses is increased because the curves are not well separated. Further, a steep dose-response curve for adverse effects is especially undesirable, as it implies that even small dosage increments may sharply increase the likelihood of toxicity. When there is a definable relationship between drug concentration (usually measured in plasma) and desirable and adverse effect curves, concentration may be substituted on the abscissa. Note that not all patients necessarily demonstrate a therapeutic response (or adverse effect) at any dose, and that some effects (notably some adverse effects) may occur in a dose-independent fashion.

be applied broadly to therapeutics—have been developed in these arenas.

PRINCIPLES OF PHARMACOKINETICS

The processes of absorption, distribution, metabolism, and elimination—collectively termed *drug disposition*—determine the concentration of drug delivered to target effector molecules. Mathematical analysis of these processes can define specific, and clinically useful, parameters that describe drug disposition. This approach allows prediction of how factors such as disease, concomitant drug therapy, or genetic variants affect these parameters, and how dosages therefore should be adjusted. In this way, the chances of undertreatment due to low drug concentrations or adverse effects due to high drug concentrations can be minimized.

BIOAVAILABILITY When a drug is administered intravenously, each drug molecule is by definition available to the systemic circulation. However, drugs are often administered by other routes, such as orally, subcutaneously, intramuscularly, rectally, sublingually, or directly into desired sites of action. With these other routes, the amount of drug actually entering the systemic circulation may be less than with the intravenous route. The fraction of drug available to the systemic circulation by other routes is termed *bioavailability*. Bioavailability may be <100% for two reasons: (1) absorption is reduced, or (2) the drug undergoes metabolism or elimination prior to entering the systemic circulation. Bioavailability (*F*) is defined as the area under the time-concentration curve (*AUC*) after a drug dose, divided by *AUC* after the same dose intravenously (Fig. 3-2*A*).

Absorption Drug administration by nonintravenous routes often involves an absorption process characterized by the plasma level increasing to a maximum value at some time after administration and then declining as the rate of drug elimination exceeds the rate of absorption (Fig. 3-2*A*). Thus, the peak concentration is lower and occurs later than after the same dose given by rapid intravenous injection. The extent of absorption may be reduced because a drug is incompletely released from its dosage form, undergoes destruction at its site of administration, or has physicochemical properties such as insolubility that prevent complete absorption from its site of administration.

The rate of absorption can be an important consideration for determining a dosage regimen, especially for drugs with a narrow therapeutic ratio. If absorption is too rapid, then the resulting high concentration may cause adverse effects not observed with a more slowly absorbed formulation. At the other extreme, slow absorption is

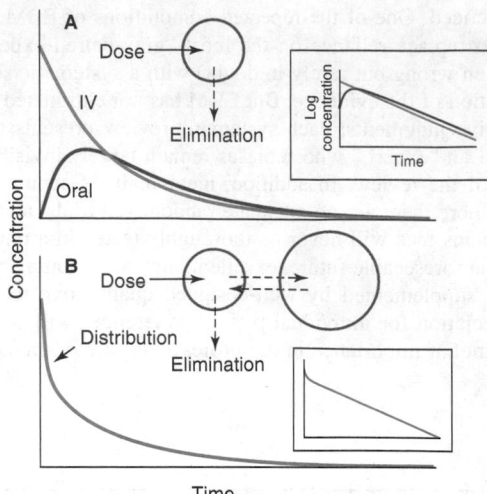

FIGURE 3-2 Idealized time-plasma concentration curves after a single dose of drug. *A.* The time course of drug concentration after an instantaneous intravenous (IV) bolus or an oral dose in the one-compartment model shown. The area under the time concentration curve is clearly less with the oral drug than the IV, indicating incomplete bioavailability. Note that despite this incomplete bioavailability, concentration after the oral dose can be higher than after the IV dose at some time points. The inset shows that the decline of concentrations over time is linear on a log-linear plot, characteristic of first-order elimination, and that oral and IV drug have the same elimination (parallel) time course. *B.* The decline of central compartment concentration when drug is both distributed to and from a peripheral compartment and eliminated from the central compartment. The rapid initial decline of concentration reflects not drug elimination but distribution.

deliberately designed into "slow-release" or "sustained-release" drug formulations in order to minimize variation in plasma concentrations during the interval between doses, because the drug's rate of elimination is offset by an equivalent rate of absorption controlled by formulation factors (Fig. 3-3).

Presystemic Metabolism or Elimination When a drug is administered orally, it must transverse the intestinal epithelium, the portal venous system, and the liver prior to entering the systemic circulation (Fig. 3-4). At each of these sites, drug availability may be reduced; this mechanism of reduction of systemic availability is termed *presystemic elimination*, or *first-pass elimination*, and its efficiency assessed as extraction ratio. Uptake into the enterocyte is a combination of passive and active processes, the latter mediated by specific drug uptake transport molecules. Once a drug enters the enterocyte, it may undergo metabolism, be transported into the portal vein, or undergo excretion back into the intestinal lumen. Both excretion into the intestinal lumen and metabolism decrease systemic bioavailability. Once a drug passes this enterocyte barrier, it may also undergo uptake (again often by specific uptake transporters such as the organic cation transporter or organic anion transporter) into the hepatocyte, where bioavailability can be further limited by metabolism or excretion into the bile.

The drug transport molecule that has been most widely studied is

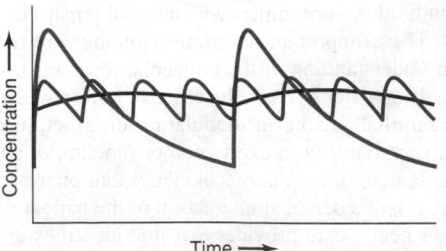

FIGURE 3-3 Concentration excursions between doses at steady state as a function of dosing frequency. With less frequent dosing (blue), excursions are larger; this is acceptable for a wide therapeutic ratio drug (Fig. 3-1). For narrower therapeutic ratio drugs, more frequent dosing (red) may be necessary to avoid toxicity and maintain efficacy. Another approach is use of a sustained-release formulation (black) that in theory results in very small excursions even with infrequent dosing.

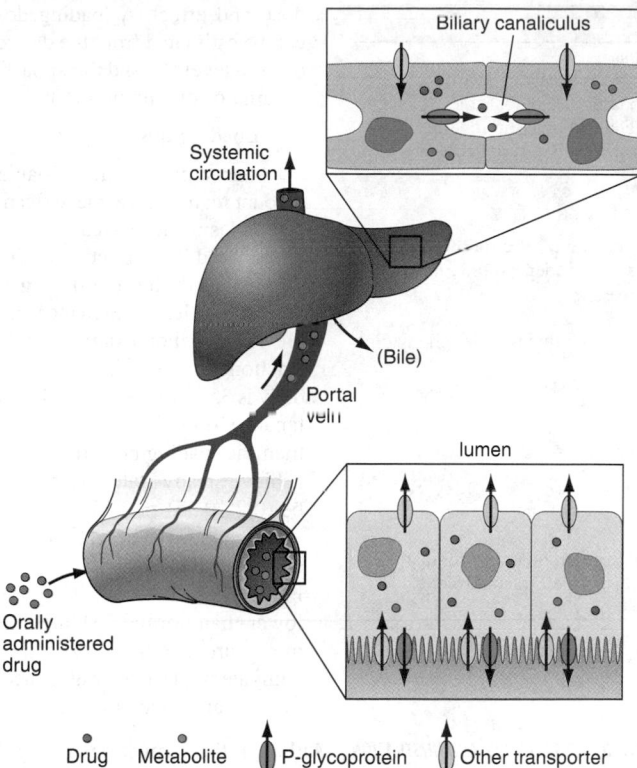

Biliary canaliculus

Systemic
circulation

(Bile)

Portal
vein

lumen

Orally
administered
drug

• Drug   ● Metabolite   ⬮ P-glycoprotein   ⬮ Other transporter

FIGURE 3-4 Mechanism of presystemic clearance. After drug enters the enterocyte, it can undergo metabolism, excretion into the intestinal lumen, or transport into the portal vein. Similarly, the hepatocyte may accomplish metabolism and biliary excretion prior to the entry of drug and metabolites to the systemic circulation. *[Adapted by permission from DM Roden, in DP Zipes, J Jalife (eds): Cardiac Electrophysiology: From Cell to Bedside, 4th ed. Philadelphia, Saunders, 2003. Copyright 2003 with permission from Elsevier.]*

P-glycoprotein, the product of the normal expression of the *MDR1* gene. P-glycoprotein is expressed on the apical aspect of the enterocyte and on the canalicular aspect of the hepatocyte (Fig. 3-4); in both locations, it serves as an efflux pump, thus limiting availability of drug to the systemic circulation.

Most drug metabolism takes place in the liver, although the enzymes accomplishing drug metabolism may be expressed, and hence drug metabolism may take place, in multiple other sites, including kidney, intestinal epithelium, lung, and plasma. Drug metabolism is generally conceptualized as "phase I," which generally results in more polar metabolites that are more readily excreted, and "phase II," during which specific endogenous compounds are conjugated to the drugs or their metabolites, again to enhance polarity and thus excretion. The major process during phase I is drug oxidation, generally accomplished by members of the cytochrome P450 (CYP) monooxygenase superfamily. CYPs that are especially important for drug metabolism (Table 3-1) include CYP3A4, CYP3A5, CYP2D6, CYP2C9, CYP2C19, CYP1A2, and CYP2E1, and each drug may be a substrate for one or more of these enzymes. The enzymes that accomplish phase II reactions include glucuronyl-, acetyl-, sulfo- and methyltransferases. Drug metabolites may exert important pharmacologic activity, as discussed further below.

Clinical Implications of Altered Bioavailability Some drugs undergo near-complete presystemic metabolism and thus cannot be administered orally. Lidocaine is an example; the drug is well absorbed but undergoes near-complete extraction in the liver, so only lidocaine metabolites (which may be toxic) appear in the systemic circulation following administration of the parent drug. Similarly, nitroglycerin cannot be used orally because it is completely extracted prior to reaching the systemic circulation. The drug is therefore used by the sublingual or transdermal routes, which bypass presystemic metabolism.

Other drugs undergo very extensive presystemic metabolism but can still be administered by the oral route, using much higher doses

than those required intravenously. Thus, a typical intravenous dose of verapamil would be 1 to 5 mg, compared to the usual single oral dose of 40 to 120 mg. Even small variations in the presystemic elimination of very highly extracted drugs such as propranolol or verapamil can cause large interindividual variations in systemic availability and effect. Oral amiodarone is 35 to 50% bioavailable because of poor solubility. Therefore, prolonged administration of usual oral doses by the intravenous route would be inappropriate. Administration of low-dose aspirin can result in exposure of cyclooxygenase in platelets in the portal vein to the drug, but systemic sparing because of first-pass de-acylation in the liver. This is an example of presystemic metabolism being exploited to therapeutic advantage.

FIRST-ORDER DISTRIBUTION AND ELIMINATION Most pharmacokinetic processes are first order; i.e., the rate of the process depends on the amount of drug present. In the simplest pharmacokinetic model (Fig. 3-2A), a drug bolus is administered instantaneously to a central compartment, from which drug elimination occurs as a first-order process. The first-order (concentration-dependent) nature of drug elimination leads directly to the relationship describing drug concentration (C) at any time (t) following the bolus:

$$C = (\text{dose}/V_c) \cdot e^{(-0.69t/t_{1/2})}$$

where V_c is the volume of the compartment into which drug is delivered and $t_{1/2}$ is elimination half-life. As a consequence of this relationship, a plot of the logarithm of concentration vs time is a straight line (Fig. 3-2A, inset). *Half-life* is the time required for 50% of a first-order process to be complete. Thus, 50% of drug elimination is accomplished after one drug elimination half-life; 75% after two; 87.5% after three, etc. In practice, first-order processes such as elimination are near-complete after four to five half-lives.

In some cases, drug is removed from the central compartment not only by elimination but also by distribution into peripheral compartments. In this case, the plot of plasma concentration vs time after a bolus demonstrates two (or more) exponential components (Fig. 3-2B). In general, the initial rapid drop in drug concentration represents not elimination but drug distribution into and out of peripheral tissues (also first-order processes), while the slower component represents drug elimination; the initial precipitous decline is usually evident with administration by intravenous but not other routes. Drug concentrations at peripheral sites are determined by a balance between drug distribution to and redistribution from peripheral sites, as well as by elimination. Once the distribution process is near-complete (four to five distribution half-lives), plasma and tissue concentrations decline in parallel.

Clinical Implications of Half-Life Measurements The elimination half-life not only determines the time required for drug concentrations to fall to near-immeasurable levels after a single bolus, but it is the key determinant of the time required for steady-state plasma concentrations to be achieved after any change in drug dosing (Fig. 3-5). This applies to the initiation of chronic drug therapy (whether by multiple oral doses or by continuous intravenous infusion), a change in chronic drug dose or dosing interval, or discontinuation of drug. When drug effect parallels drug concentrations, the time required for a change in drug dosing to achieve a new level of effect is therefore determined by the elimination half-life.

During chronic drug administration, a point is reached at which the amount of drug administered per unit time equals drug eliminated per unit time, defining the *steady state*. With a continuous intravenous infusion, plasma concentrations at steady state are stable, while with chronic oral drug administration, plasma concentrations vary during the dosing interval but the time-concentration profile between dosing intervals is stable (Fig. 3-5).

DRUG DISTRIBUTION Distribution from central to peripheral sites, or from extracellular to intracellular sites, can be accomplished by passive mechanisms such as diffusion or by specific drug transport mech-

TABLE 3-1 *Molecular Pathways Mediating Drug Disposition*[a]

Molecule	Substrates[c]	Inhibitors[c]
CYP3A	Calcium channel blockers; antiarrhythmics (lidocaine, quinidine, mexiletine); HMG-CoA reductase inhibitors ("statins"; see text); cyclosporine, tacrolimus; indinavir, saquinavir, ritonavir	Amiodarone; ketoconazole; itraconazole; erythromycin, clarithromycin; ritonavir
CYP2D6[b]	Timolol, metoprolol, carvedilol; phenformin; codeine; propafenone, flecainide; tricyclic antidepressants; fluoxetine, paroxetine	Quinidine (even at ultralow doses); tricyclic antidepressants; fluoxetine, paroxetine
CYP2C9[b]	Warfarin; phenytoin; glipizide; losartan	Amiodarone; fluconazole; phenytoin
CYP2C19[b]	Omeprazole; mephenytoin	
Thiopurine *S*-methyltransferase[b]	6-Mercaptopurine, azathioprine	
N-acetyl transferase[b]	Isoniazid; procainamide; hydralazine; some sulfonamides	
UGT1A1[b]	Irinotecan	
Pseudocholinesterase[b]	Succinylcholine	
P-glycoprotein	Digoxin; HIV protease inhibitors; many CYP3A substrates	Quinidine; amiodarone; verapamil; cyclosporine; itraconazole; erythromycin

[a] A listing of CYP substrates, inhibitors, and inducers is maintained at *http://medicine.iupui.edu/flockhart/clinlist.html*.
[b] Clinically important genetics variants described.
[c] Inhibitors affect the molecular pathway and thus may affect substrate.

anisms that are only now being defined at the molecular level. Models such as those shown in Fig. 3-2 allow derivation of a volume term for each compartment. These volumes rarely have any correspondence to actual physiologic volumes, such as plasma volume or total-body water volume. For many drugs the central volume may be viewed conveniently as a site in rapid equilibrium with plasma. Central volumes and volume of distribution at steady state can be used to estimate tissue drug uptake and, in some cases, to adjust drug dosage in disease. In a typical 70-kg human, plasma volume is ~3 L, blood volume is ~5.5 L, and extracellular water outside the vasculature is ~42 L. The volume of distribution of drugs extensively bound to plasma proteins but not to tissue components approaches plasma volume; warfarin is an example. However, for most drugs, the volume of distribution is far greater than any physiologic space. For example, the volume of distribution of digoxin and tricyclic antidepressants is hundreds of liters, obviously exceeding total-body volume. This indicates that these drugs are largely distributed outside the vascular system, and the proportion of the drug present in the plasma compartment is low. As a consequence, such drugs are not readily removed by dialysis, an important consideration in overdose.

Clinical Implications of Drug Distribution Digoxin accesses its cardiac site of action slowly, over a distribution phase of several hours. Thus after an intravenous dose, plasma levels fall but those at the site of action increase over hours. Only when distribution is near-complete does the concentration of digoxin in plasma reflect pharmacologic effect. For this reason, there should be a 6- to 8-h wait after administration before plasma levels of digoxin are measured as a guide to therapy.

Animal models have suggested, and clinical studies are confirming, that limited drug penetration into the brain, the "blood-brain barrier," often represents a robust P-glycoprotein-mediated efflux process from capillary endothelial cells in the cerebral circulation. Thus drug distribution into the brain may be modulated by changes in P-glycoprotein function.

LOADING DOSES For some drugs, the indication may be so urgent that the time required to achieve steady-state concentrations may be too long. Under these conditions, administration of "loading" dosages may result in more rapid elevations of drug concentration to achieve therapeutic effects earlier than with chronic maintenance therapy (Fig. 3-5). Nevertheless, the time required for true steady state to be achieved is still determined only by elimination half-life. This strategy is only appropriate for drugs exhibiting a defined relationship between drug

dose and effect. A loading dose can be estimated from the desired plasma level (*C*) and the apparent volume of distribution (*V*):

$$\text{Loading dose} = C \times V$$

Alternatively, the loading amount required to achieve steady-state plasma levels can also be determined if the fraction of drug eliminated during the dosing interval and the maintenance dose are known. For example, if the fraction of digoxin eliminated daily is 35% and the planned maintenance dose is 0.25 mg daily, then the loading dose required to achieve steady-state levels would be $(0.25/0.35) \approx 0.75$ mg.

In congestive heart failure, the central volume of distribution of lidocaine is reduced. Therefore, lower-than-normal loading regimens are required to achieve equivalent plasma drug concentrations and to avoid toxicity.

RATE OF INTRAVENOUS ADMINISTRATION Although the simulations in Fig. 3-2 use a single intravenous bolus, this is very rarely appropriate in practice because side effects related to transiently very high concentrations can result. Rather, drugs are more usually administered orally or as a slower intravenous infusion. Thus, administration of a full loading dose of lidocaine (3 to 4 mg/kg) as a single bolus often results transiently in very high concentrations, with a risk of adverse effects such as seizures. Since the distribution half-life of the drug is 8 min, a more appropriate loading regimen is the same dose, administered as two to four divided boluses every 8 min, or a rapid infusion (e.g., 10 mg/min for 20 min).

Some drugs are so predictably lethal when infused too rapidly that special precautions should be taken to prevent accidental boluses. For example, solutions of potassium for intravenous administration >20

FIGURE 3-5 Drug accumulation to steady state. In this simulation, drug was administered (arrows) at intervals = 50% of the elimination half-life. Steady state is achieved during initiation of therapy after ~5 elimination half-lives, or 10 doses. A loading dose did not alter the eventual steady state achieved. A doubling of the dose resulted in a doubling of the steady state but the same time course of accumulation. Once steady state is achieved, a change in dose (increase, decrease, or drug discontinuation) results in a new steady state in ~5 elimination half-lives. [*Adapted by permission from DM Roden, in DP Zipes, J Jalife (eds): Cardiac Electrophysiology: From Cell to Bedside, 4th ed. Philadelphia, Saunders, 2003. Copyright 2003 with permission from Elsevier.*]

meq/L should be avoided in all but the most exceptional and carefully monitored circumstances. This minimizes the possibility of cardiac arrest, which can occur as a result of accidental increases in infusion rates of more concentrated solutions.

Procainamide, which is almost totally absorbed after oral administration, can be given orally as a single 1000-mg loading dose with little risk of hypotension. However, administration by the intravenous route is more safely accomplished by giving the dose in fractions of about 100 mg at 5-min intervals or, more conveniently, as a 20-mg/min infusion over 50 min to avoid hypotension during the distribution phase.

As these examples illustrate, excessively rapid administration of many drugs can lead to catastrophic consequences that result from high concentrations in the blood during the distribution phase. In contrast, for some centrally active drugs, the higher concentration of drug during the distribution phase after intravenous administration is used to advantage. The use of midazolam for intravenous sedation, for example, depends upon its rapid uptake by the brain during the distribution phase to produce sedation quickly, with subsequent egress from the brain during the redistribution of the drug as equilibrium is achieved.

Similarly, adenosine must be administered as a rapid bolus in the treatment of reentrant supraventricular tachycardias (Chap. 214), to prevent elimination by very rapid ($t_{1/2}$ of seconds) uptake into erythrocytes and endothelial cells before the drug can reach its clinical site of action, the atrioventricular node.

PLASMA PROTEIN BINDING Many drugs circulate in the plasma partly bound to plasma proteins. Since only unbound (free) drug can distribute to sites of pharmacologic action, drug response is related to the free rather than the total circulating plasma drug concentration. In most cases, the degree of binding is fairly constant across the therapeutic concentration range; in this case, when plasma drug concentration is used to adjust doses, total levels in plasma can be used without resulting in significant error.

Clinical Implications of Altered Protein Binding For drugs that are normally highly bound to plasma proteins (>90%), small changes in the extent of binding (e.g., due to disease) produce a large change in the amount of unbound drug, and hence drug effect. The acute-phase reactant α_1-acid glycoprotein binds to basic drugs, such as lidocaine or quinidine, and is increased in a range of common conditions, including myocardial infarction, surgery, neoplastic disease, rheumatoid arthritis, and burns. This increased binding can lead to reduced pharmacologic effects at therapeutic concentrations of total drug. Conversely, conditions such as hypoalbuminemia, liver disease, and renal disease can decrease the extent of drug binding, particularly of acidic and neutral drugs, such as phenytoin. Here, plasma concentration of free drug is increased, so drug efficacy and toxicity are enhanced if total (free + bound) drug is used to monitor therapy.

CLEARANCE When drug is eliminated from the body, the amount of drug in the body declines over time. An important concept in quantifying this reduction is to consider that drug concentration at the beginning and end of a time period are unchanged, and that a specific volume of the body has been "cleared" of the drug during that time period. This defines clearance as volume/time. Clearance is a measure of the efficiency of drug removal that encompasses both drug metabolism as well as drug excretion.

Clinical Implications of Altered Clearance ■ ADJUSTING DRUG DOSAGES While elimination half-life determines the time required to achieve steady-state plasma concentrations (C_{ss}), the *magnitude* of that steady state is determined by clearance (Cl) and dose alone. For a drug administered as an intravenous infusion, this relationship is

$$C_{ss} = \text{dosing rate}/Cl \quad \text{or} \quad \text{dosing rate} = Cl \times C_{ss}$$

When drug is administered orally, the average plasma concentration within a dosing interval ($C_{avg,ss}$) replaces C_{ss}, and bioavailability (F) must be included:

$$F \times \text{dosing rate} = Cl \times C_{avg,ss}$$

Genetic variants, drug interactions, or diseases that reduce the activity of drug-metabolizing enzymes or excretory mechanisms may lead to decreased clearance and hence a requirement for downward dose adjustment to avoid toxicity. Genetic variants may reduce expression of CYPs (or other drug-metabolizing enzymes) or may result in normal expression of enzymes that have reduced function; in either case, dose requirements may need to be reduced. Conversely, some drug interactions and genetic variants increase CYP expression, and hence increased drug dosage may be necessary to maintain a therapeutic effect.

Clearance varies among drugs but is constant for most drugs over the therapeutic range of concentrations. In some cases, elimination becomes saturated at high doses, and the process then occurs at a fixed amount per unit time (zero order). With such nonlinear elimination kinetics, an increase in drug dosage is followed by a disproportionate rise in drug concentration, which can carry a risk of toxicity. Drugs that undergo zero-order elimination at therapeutic dosages include phenytoin, theophylline, and ethanol. Monitoring plasma concentrations of these agents is an indispensable guide to adjusting dose.

THE CONCEPT OF HIGH-RISK PHARMACOKINETICS Many drugs undergo elimination by multiple drug-metabolizing or excretory pathways. In this case, absence of one pathway (due to a genetic variant or drug interaction) may not have a large impact on drug concentrations or drug actions. However, other drugs utilize a single pathway exclusively for drug elimination. Under this scenario, any condition that inhibits that pathway (be it disease-related, genetic, or due to a drug interaction) can lead to dramatic changes in drug concentrations and hence effect. Examples of this phenomenon are discussed further below and include digoxin toxicity when P-glycoprotein, the major route of digoxin elimination, is inhibited and potentially fatal bone marrow aplasia due to azathioprine or 6-mercaptopurine in patients with genetically determined absence of function of thiopurine *S*-methyltransferase (TPMT). A dual-pathway example is the antiarrhythmic flecainide, which is eliminated by both renal excretion and CYP2D6-mediated metabolism. Rare patients with both renal dysfunction and absent CYP2D6 activity (on a genetic basis or because of drug interactions) may develop severe adverse reactions related to high plasma concentrations.

ACTIVE DRUG METABOLITES A major role of drug metabolism is generation of more polar compounds that then readily undergo renal or biliary excretion. From an evolutionary point of view, drug metabolism probably developed as a defense against noxious xenobiotics (foreign substances, e.g., from plants) to which our ancestors inadvertently exposed themselves. The organization of the drug uptake and efflux pumps, and the location of drug metabolism in the intestine and liver prior to drug entry to the systemic circulation (Fig. 3-4), support this idea of a primitive protective function.

However, drug metabolites are not necessarily pharmacologically inactive. Metabolites may produce effects similar to, overlapping with, or distinct from those of the parent drug. For example, *N*-acetyl-procainamide (NAPA) is a major metabolite of the antiarrhythmic procainamide. While it exerts antiarrhythmic effects, its electrophysiologic properties differ from those of the parent drug. Indeed, NAPA accumulation is the usual explanation for marked QT prolongation and torsades de pointes ventricular tachycardia (Chap. 214) during therapy with procainamide. Thus, the common laboratory practice of adding procainamide to NAPA concentrations to estimate a total therapeutic effect is inappropriate.

Some drugs are administered in an inactive form and require metabolism to generate active metabolites that mediate the drug effects. Examples include many angiotensin-converting enzyme (ACE) inhibitors and the analgesic codeine (whose active metabolite morphine probably underlies the opioid effect during codeine administration). Codeine and procainamide metabolism are also variable on a genetic basis, further contributing to variability in drug effects. Drug metabolism has also been implicated in bioactivation of procarcinogens and in generation of reactive metabolites that mediate certain adverse drug effects (e.g., acetaminophen hepatotoxicity, discussed below).

PRINCIPLES OF PHARMACODYNAMICS

Once a drug accesses a molecular site of action, it alters the function of that molecular target, with the ultimate result of a drug effect that the patient or physician can perceive. For drugs used in the urgent treatment of acute symptoms, little or no delay is anticipated (or desired) between the drug-target interaction and the development of a clinical effect. Examples include vascular thrombosis, shock, malignant hypertension, status epilepticus, or arrhythmias. For many conditions, however, the indication for therapy is less urgent, and in fact a delay between the interaction of a drug with its pharmacologic target(s) and a clinical effect is common. Pharmacokinetic mechanisms that can contribute to such a delay include uptake into peripheral compartments or generation and accumulation of active metabolites. A common pharmacodynamic mechanism is that the clinical effect develops as a downstream consequence of the initial molecular effect the drug produces. Thus, administration of a proton-pump inhibitor or an H_2-receptor blocker produces an immediate increase in gastric pH but ulcer healing that is delayed. Cancer chemotherapy inevitably produces delayed therapeutic effects, often long after drug is undetectable in plasma and tissue. Translation of a molecular drug action to a clinical effect can thus be highly complex and dependent on the details of the pathologic state being treated. These complexities have made pharmacodynamics and its variability less amenable than pharmacokinetics to rigorous mathematical analysis. Nevertheless, some clinically important principles can be elucidated.

A therapeutic drug effect assumes the presence of underlying pathophysiology. Thus, a drug may produce no action, or a different spectrum of actions, in unaffected individuals compared to patients. Further, concomitant disease can complicate interpretation of response to drug therapy, especially adverse effects. For example, increasing dyspnea in a patient with chronic lung disease receiving amiodarone therapy could be due to drug, underlying disease, or an intercurrent cardiopulmonary problem. Thus the presence of chronic lung disease, and interpretation of the symptom of increasing dyspnea, is one factor that should be considered in selection of antiarrhythmic therapies. Similarly, high doses of anticonvulsants such as phenytoin may cause neurologic symptoms, which may be confused with the underlying neurologic disease.

The concept that a drug interacts with a specific molecular receptor does not imply that the drug effect will be constant over time, even if stable drug and metabolite concentrations are maintained. The drug-receptor interaction occurs in a complex biologic milieu that itself can vary to modulate the drug effect. For example, ion channel blockade by drugs, an important anticonvulsant and antiarrhythmic effect, is often modulated by membrane potential, itself a function of factors such as extracellular potassium or ischemia. Thus, the effects of these drugs may vary depending on the external milieu. Receptors may be up- or downregulated by disease or by the drug itself. For example, β-adrenergic blockers upregulate β-receptor density during chronic therapy. While this effect does not usually result in resistance to the therapeutic effect of the drugs, it may produce severe β agonist–mediated effects (such as hypertension or tachycardia) if the blocking drug is abruptly withdrawn.

PRINCIPLES OF DOSE SELECTION

The desired goal of therapy with any drug is to maximize the likelihood of a beneficial effect while minimizing the risk of adverse effects. Previous experience with the drug, in controlled clinical trials or in postmarketing use, defines the relationships between dose (or plasma concentration) and these dual effects and provides a starting point for initiation of drug therapy.

Figure 3-1 illustrates the relationships among dose, plasma concentrations, efficacy, and adverse effects and carries with it several important implications:

1. *The target drug effect should be defined when drug treatment is started.* With some drugs, the desired effect may be difficult to measure objectively, and the onset of efficacy can be delayed for weeks or months; drugs used in the treatment of cancer and psychiatric disease are examples. Sometimes, a drug is used to treat a symptom, such as pain or palpitations, and here it is the patient who will report whether the selected dose is effective. In yet other settings, such as anticoagulation or hypertension, the desired response is readily measurable.

2. *The nature of anticipated toxicity often dictates the starting dose.* If side effects are minor, it may be acceptable to start at a dose highly likely to achieve efficacy and downtitrate if side effects occur. However, this approach is rarely if ever justified if the anticipated toxicity is serious or life-threatening; in this circumstance, it is more appropriate to initiate therapy with the lowest dose that may produce a desired effect.

3. *The above considerations do not apply if these relationships between dose and effects cannot be defined.* This is especially relevant to some adverse drug effects (discussed in further detail below) whose development is not readily related to drug dose.

4. *If a drug dose does not achieve its desired effect, a dosage increase is justified only if toxicity is absent and the likelihood of serious toxicity is small.* For example, a small percentage of patients with strong seizure foci require plasma levels of phenytoin >20 μg/mL to control seizures. Dosages to achieve this effect may be appropriate, if tolerated. Conversely, clinical experience with flecainide suggests that levels >1000 ng/mL, or dosages >400 mg/d, may be associated with an increased risk of sudden death; thus dosage increases beyond these limits are ordinarily not appropriate, even if the higher dosage appears tolerated.

Other mechanisms that can lead to failure of drug effect should also be considered; drug interactions and noncompliance are common examples. This is one situation in which measurement of plasma drug concentrations, if available, can be especially useful. Noncompliance is an especially frequent problem in the long-term treatment of diseases such as hypertension and epilepsy, occurring in $\geq 25\%$ of patients in therapeutic environments in which no special effort is made to involve patients in the responsibility for their own health. Multidrug regimens with multiple doses per day are especially prone to noncompliance.

Monitoring response to therapy, by physiologic measures or by plasma concentration measurements, requires an understanding of the relationships between plasma concentration and anticipated effects. For example, measurement of QT interval is used during treatment with sotalol or dofetilide to avoid marked QT prolongation that can herald serious arrhythmias. In this setting, evaluating the electrocardiogram at the time of anticipated peak plasma concentration and effect (e.g., 1 to 2 h postdose at steady state) is most appropriate. Maintained high aminoglycoside levels carry a risk of nephrotoxicity, so dosages should be adjusted on the basis of plasma concentrations measured at trough (predose). On the other hand, ensuring aminoglycoside efficacy is accomplished by adjusting dosage so that peak drug concentrations are above a minimal antibacterial concentration. For dose adjustment of other drugs (e.g., anticonvulsants, antiarrhythmics), concentration should be measured at its lowest during the dosing interval, just prior to a dose at steady state (Fig. 3-5), to ensure a maintained therapeutic effect.

CONCENTRATION OF DRUGS IN PLASMA AS A GUIDE TO THERAPY Factors such as interactions with other drugs, disease-induced alterations in elimination and distribution, and genetic variation in drug disposition combine to yield a wide range of plasma levels in patients given the same dose. Hence, if a predictable relationship can be established between plasma drug concentration and beneficial or adverse drug effect, measurement of plasma levels can provide a valuable tool to guide selection of an optimal dose. This is particularly true when there is a narrow range between the plasma levels yielding therapeutic and adverse effects, as with digoxin, theophylline, some antiarrhythmics, aminogly-cosides, cyclosporine, and anticonvulsants. The common situation of first-order elimination implies that average, maximum, and minimum steady-state concentrations are related linearly to the dosing rate. Accordingly, the maintenance dose may be adjusted on the basis of the ratio between the desired and measured concentrations *at steady state*; for example if a doubling of the steady-state plasma concentration is desired, the dose should be doubled.

For drugs that have zero-order kinetics (e.g., phenytoin and theophylline), plasma concentrations change disproportionately more than the alteration in the dosing rate. In this situation, changes in dose should be small to minimize the degree of unpredictability, and plasma concentration monitoring should be used to ensure that dose modification achieves the desired level.

DETERMINATION OF MAINTENANCE DOSE   An increase in dosage is usually best achieved by changing the drug dose but not the dosing interval, e.g., by giving 200 mg every 8 h instead of 100 mg every 8 h. However, this approach is acceptable only if the resulting maximum concentration is not toxic and the trough value does not fall below the minimum effective concentration for an undesirable period of time. Alternatively, the steady state may be changed by altering the frequency of intermittent dosing but not the size of each dose. In this case, the magnitude of the fluctuations around the average steady-state level will change—the shorter the dosing interval, the smaller the difference between peak and trough levels (Fig. 3-3).

Fluctuation within a dosing interval is determined by the relationship between the dosing interval and the drug's half-life. If the dosing interval is equal to the drug's half-life, fluctuation is about twofold, which is usually acceptable. With drugs that have a low therapeutic ratio, dosage changes should be conservative (<50% dose change) and not more frequent than every three to four half-lives. Other drugs, such as many antihypertensives, have little dose-related toxicity so the therapeutic ratio is large. Even if drug is eliminated rapidly, it can be given infrequently. Thus, 75 mg of captopril will result in reduced blood pressure for up to 12 h, even though captopril elimination half-life is about 2 h; this is because the dose raises the concentration of drug in plasma many times higher than the threshold for its pharmacologic effect.

EFFECTS OF DISEASE ON DRUG CONCENTRATION AND RESPONSE

RENAL DISEASE   Renal excretion of parent drug and metabolites is generally accomplished by glomerular filtration and by specific drug transporters, only now being identified. If a drug or its metabolites are primarily excreted through the kidneys and increased drug levels are associated with adverse effects, drug dosages must be reduced in patients with renal dysfunction to avoid toxicity. The antiarrhythmics dofetilide and sotalol undergo predominant renal excretion and carry a risk of QT prolongation and arrhythmias if doses are not reduced in renal disease. Thus, in end-stage renal disease, sotalol can be given as 40 mg after dialysis (every second day), compared to the usual daily dose, 80 to 120 mg every 12 h. The narcotic analgesic meperidine undergoes extensive hepatic metabolism, so that renal failure has little effect on its plasma concentration. However, its metabolite, normeperidine, does undergo renal excretion, accumulates in renal failure, and probably accounts for the signs of central nervous system excitation, such as irritability, twitching, and seizures, that appear when multiple doses of meperidine are administered to patients with renal disease. Protein binding of some drugs (e.g., phenytoin) may be altered in uremia, so measuring free drug concentration may be desirable.

In non-end-stage renal disease, changes in renal drug clearance are generally proportional to those in creatinine clearance, which may be measured directly or estimated from the serum creatinine (Chap. 259). This estimate, coupled with the knowledge of how much drug is normally excreted renally vs nonrenally, allows an estimate of the dose adjustment required. In practice, most decisions involving dosing adjustment in patients with renal failure use published recommended adjustments in dosage or dosing interval based on the severity of renal

dysfunction indicated by creatinine clearance. Any such modification of dose is a first approximation and should be followed by plasma concentration data (if available) and clinical observation to further optimize therapy for the individual patient.

LIVER DISEASE   In contrast to the predictable decline in renal clearance of drugs in renal insufficiency, the effects of hepatitis or cirrhosis on drug disposition range from impaired to increased drug clearance, in an unpredictable fashion. Standard tests of liver function are not useful in adjusting doses. First-pass metabolism may decrease, and thus oral bioavailability increase, as a consequence of disrupted hepatocyte function, altered liver architecture, and portacaval shunts. The oral availability for high-first-pass drugs such as morphine, meperidine, midazolam, and nifedipine is almost doubled in patients with cirrhosis, compared to those with normal liver function. Therefore, the size of the oral dose of such drugs should be reduced in this setting.

HEART FAILURE AND SHOCK   Under conditions of decreased tissue perfusion, the cardiac output is redistributed to preserve blood flow to the heart and brain at the expense of other tissues (Chap. 216). As a result, drugs may be distributed into a smaller volume of distribution, higher drug concentrations will be present in the plasma, and the tissues that are best perfused (the brain and heart) will be exposed to these higher concentrations. If either the brain or heart is sensitive to the drug, an alteration in response will occur. As well, decreased perfusion of the kidney and liver may impair drug clearance. Thus, in severe congestive heart failure, in hemorrhagic shock, and in cardiogenic shock, response to usual drug doses may be excessive, and dosage reduction may be necessary. For example, the clearance of lidocaine is reduced by about 50% in heart failure, and therapeutic plasma levels are achieved at infusion rates only about half those usually required. The volume of distribution of lidocaine is also reduced, so loading regimens should be reduced.

DRUG USE IN THE ELDERLY   Aging results in changes in organ function, especially of the organs involved in drug disposition. Therefore, pharmacokinetics are often different in elderly individuals than in younger adults. In the elderly, multiple pathologies and medications used to treat them result in more drug interactions and adverse effects.

Even in the absence of kidney disease, renal clearance may be reduced by 35 to 50% in elderly patients. Dosage adjustments are therefore necessary for drugs that are eliminated mainly by the kidneys. Because muscle mass and therefore creatinine production are reduced in older individuals, a normal serum creatinine concentration can be present even though creatinine clearance is impaired; dosages should be adjusted on the basis of creatinine clearance, as discussed above. Aging also results in a decrease in the size of and blood flow to the liver and possibly in the activity of hepatic drug-metabolizing enzymes; accordingly, the hepatic clearance of some drugs is impaired in the elderly. As with liver disease, these changes are not readily predicted.

Elderly patients may display altered drug sensitivity. Examples include increased analgesic effects of opioids, increased sedation from benzodiazepines and other CNS depressants, and increased risk of bleeding while receiving anticoagulant therapy, even when clotting parameters are well controlled. Exaggerated responses to cardiovascular drugs are also common because of the impaired responsiveness of normal homeostatic mechanisms. Conversely, the elderly display decreased sensitivity to β-adrenergic receptor blockers.

Adverse drug reactions are especially common in the elderly, because of altered pharmacokinetics and pharmacodynamics, the frequent use of multidrug regimens, and concomitant disease. For example, use of long half-life benzodiazepines is linked to the occurrence of hip fractures in elderly patients, perhaps reflecting both a risk of falls from these drugs (due to increased sedation) and the increased incidence of osteoporosis in elderly patients. In population surveys of the noninstitutionalized elderly, as many as 10% had at least one adverse drug reaction in the previous year.

Accordingly, optimization of drug therapy in the elderly, particularly in frail patients, is often difficult, as these multiple factors accentuate interindividual variability in drug response. Initial doses should be less than the usual adult dosage and should be increased slowly. The number of medications, and doses per day, should be kept as low as possible.

GENETIC DETERMINANTS OF THE RESPONSE TO DRUGS

PRINCIPLES OF GENETIC VARIATION AND HUMAN TRAITS (See also Chap. 58) Variants in the human genome resulting in variation in level of expression or function of molecules important for pharmacokinetics and pharmacodynamics are increasingly recognized. These may be mutations (very rare variants, often associated with disease) or polymorphisms, variants that are much more common in a population. Variants may occur at a single nucleotide or involve insertion or deletion of one or more nucleotides. They may be in the exons (coding regions) or introns. Exonic polymorphisms may or may not alter the encoded protein, and variant proteins may or may not display altered function. Similarly, polymorphisms in intronic regions (including those that regulate gene expression) may or may not alter protein level.

As variation in the human genome is increasingly well documented, associations are being described between polymorphisms and various traits (including response to drug therapy). Some of these rely on well-developed chains of evidence, including in vitro studies demonstrating variant protein function, familial aggregation of variant allele with the trait, and association studies in large populations. In other cases, the associations are less compelling. Identifying "real" associations is one challenge that must be overcome before genomics, and in particular the concept of genotyping to identify optimal drugs (or dosages) in individual patients prior to prescribing, can be considered for widespread clinical practice. Nevertheless, the appeal of this approach is considerable.

Rates of drug efficacy and adverse effects often vary among ethnic groups. Many explanations for such differences are plausible; genomic approaches have now established that functionally important variants determining differences in drug response often display differing distributions among ethnic groups. This finding may have importance for drug use among ethnic groups, as well as in drug development.

GENETICALLY DETERMINED DRUG DISPOSITION AND VARIABLE EFFECTS The concept that genetically determined variations in drug metabolism might be associated with variant drug levels, and hence effect, was advanced at the end of the nineteenth century, and the first examples of familial clustering of unusual drug responses due to this mechanism were noted in the mid-twentieth century. Clinically important genetic variants have been described in multiple molecular pathways of drug disposition (Table 3-1). These variants are identified either by directly establishing DNA sequence (genotyping) or by phenotyping: exposing a large group of otherwise healthy subjects to a specific probe substrate for the metabolizing enzyme under study and observing the distribution of activity (Fig. 3-6). A distinct multimodal distribution argues for a predominant effect of variants in a single gene in the metabolism of that substrate. Individuals with two alleles (variants) encoding for nonfunctional protein make up one group, often termed *poor metabolizers* (PM phenotype); many variants can produce such a loss of function, complicating the use of genotyping in clinical practice. Individuals with one functional allele make up a second (*intermediate metabolizers*), and those with two functional alleles a third (*extensive metabolizers*, EMs). On the other hand, a unimodal distribution of activity argues against the presence of important single loss-of-function alleles in the population under study.

Transferase Variants Of the variants in genes encoding drug-metabolizing enzymes that have been described to date, one, in the *TPMT* gene, has been adopted as routine clinical practice in some specialized centers. TPMT bioinactivates the antileukemic drug 6-mercaptopurine. Further, 6-mercaptopurine is itself an active metabolite of the immu-

FIGURE 3-6 CYP2D6 metabolic activity was assessed in 290 subjects by administration of a test dose of a probe substrate and measurement of urinary formation of the CYP2D6-generated metabolite. The heavy arrow indicates a clear antimode, separating poor metabolizer subjects (black), with two loss-of-function CYP2D6 alleles. Individuals with one or two functional alleles are grouped together as extensive metabolizers (blue). Also shown are ultrarapid metabolizers, with 2 to 11 functional copies of the gene (red) and 12 functional copies (green), displaying the greatest enzyme activity. *(Adapted by permission from M-L Dahl et al: J Pharmacol Exp Ther 274:516, 1995.)*

nosuppressive azathioprine. Homozygotes for alleles encoding the inactive TPMT (1 in 300 individuals) predictably exhibit severe and potentially fatal pancytopenia on standard doses of azathioprine or 6-mercaptopurine. On the other hand, homozygotes for fully functional alleles may display less anti-inflammatory or antileukemic effect with the drugs. These data illustrate the potential power of a genomic approach to optimize therapy, especially in the setting of high-risk pharmacokinetics.

N-acetylation is catalyzed by hepatic *N*-acetyl transferase (NAT), which actually represents the activity of two genes, *NAT-1* and *NAT-2*. Both enzymes transfer an acetyl group from acetyl coenzyme A to the drug; NAT-1 activity is generally constant, while polymorphisms in *NAT-2* result in individual differences in the rate at which drugs are acetylated and thus define "rapid acetylators" and "slow acetylators." Slow acetylators make up ~50% of European- and African-derived populations but are less common among Asians.

Slow acetylators have an increased incidence of the drug-induced lupus syndrome during procainamide and hydralazine therapy and of hepatitis with isoniazid. Induction of CYPs (e.g., by rifampin) also increases the risk of isoniazid-related hepatitis, likely reflecting generation of reactive metabolites of acetylhydrazine, itself an isoniazid metabolite.

Polymorphisms that reduce transcription of uridine diphosphate glucuronosyltransferase (*UGT1A1*) cause benign hyperbilirubinemia (Gilbert's disease; Chap. 284). These have also been associated with diarrhea and increased bone marrow depression with the antineoplastic irinotecan, whose active metabolite is normally detoxified by this pathway.

CYP Variants CYP3A4 is the most abundant hepatic and intestinal CYP and is also the enzyme responsible for metabolism of the greatest number of drugs in therapeutic use. CYP3A4 activity is highly variable (up to an order of magnitude) among individuals, but the distribution is unimodal, suggesting that the variability does not arise from variants in the *CYP3A4* gene. The mechanisms underlying this variability are not yet well understood. A closely related gene, encoding CYP3A5 (which shares substrates with CYP3A4), does display loss-of-function variants, especially in African-derived populations. CYP3A refers to both enzymes.

CYP2D6 accounts for very little total hepatic CYP by weight but is second to CYP3A4 in the number of commonly used drugs that it metabolizes. CYP2D6 is polymorphically distributed, with about 7% of European- and African-derived populations (but very few Asians) displaying the PM phenotype (Fig. 3-6). Over 70 loss-of-function variants in the CYP2D6 gene have been described; the PM phenotype arises in individuals with two such alleles. In addition, individuals with multiple functional copies of the CYP2D6 gene (ultrarapid metabolizers) have been identified, particularly among northern Africans. CYP2D6 represents the main metabolic pathway for a number of drugs

(Table 3-1). Codeine is biotransformed by CYP2D6 to the potent active metabolite morphine, so its effects are blunted in PMs and exaggerated in ultrarapid metabolizers. With beta blockers metabolized by CYP2D6 (including ophthalmic timolol and the antiarrhythmic propafenone), PM subjects display greater signs of beta blockade (including bradycardia and bronchospasm) than EMs. Further, in EM subjects, propafenone elimination becomes nonlinear at higher doses so, for example, a tripling of the dose may lead to a tenfold increase in drug concentration. The oral hypoglycemic agent phenformin was withdrawn because it occasionally caused profound lactic acidosis; this likely arose as a result of high concentrations in CYP2D6 PMs. Ultrarapid metabolizers may require very high dosages of tricyclic antidepressants to achieve a therapeutic effect, and with codeine may display transient euphoria and nausea due to very rapid generation of morphine.

The PM phenotype for CYP2C19 is common (20%) among Asians, and rarer (3 to 5%) in European-derived populations. The impact of polymorphic CYP2C19-mediated metabolism has been demonstrated with the proton pump inhibitor omeprazole, where ulcer cure rates with "standard" dosages were markedly lower in EM patients (29%) than in PMs (100%). Thus, understanding the importance of this polymorphism would have been important in developing the drug, and knowing a patient's CYP2C19 genotype should improve therapy.

There are common allelic variants of *CYP2C9* that encode proteins with loss of catalytic function. These variant alleles are associated with a requirement for lower maintenance dose of warfarin. In rarer (<2%) individuals homozygous for these variant alleles, maintenance warfarin dosages may be difficult to establish, and the risk of bleeding complications appears increased. Similarly, patients with loss-of-function CYP2C9 alleles display increased rates of neurologic complications with phenytoin and of hypoglycemia with glipizide.

VARIABILITY IN THE MOLECULAR TARGETS WITH WHICH DRUGS INTERACT As molecular approaches identify specific gene products as targets of drug action, polymorphisms that alter the expression or function of these drug targets—and thus modulate their actions in patients—are also being recognized. For example, genome-wide searches in families with premature Alzheimer's disease have associated variants in the *APOE* locus with the disease (Chap. 350). The *E4* allele of the gene has been associated with a worse prognosis, a finding that has been attributed to reduced expression of choline acetyltransferase. Further, this polymorphism is also linked to response to the acetylcholinesterase inhibitor tacrine; a beneficial response appears to be more common in patients with the prognostically more benign *APOE2* or *APOE3* alleles (in which the target molecule is expressed more abundantly).

Multiple polymorphisms identified in the β_2-adrenergic receptor appear to be linked to specific phenotypes in asthma and congestive heart failure, diseases in which β_2-receptor function might be expected to determine prognosis. Polymorphisms in the β_2-receptor gene have also been associated with response to inhaled β_2-receptor agonists, while those in the β_1-adrenergic receptor gene have been associated with variability in heart rate slowing and blood pressure lowering. Similarly, response to the 5-lipoxygenase inhibitor zileuton in asthma has been linked to polymorphisms that determine the expression level of the 5-lipoxygenase gene. Herceptin, which potentiates anthracycline-related cardiotoxicity, is ineffective in breast cancers that do not express the herceptin receptor; thus, "genotyping" the tumor is a mechanism to avoid potentially toxic therapy in patients who would derive no benefit.

Drugs may also interact with genetic pathways of disease, to elicit or exacerbate symptoms of the underlying conditions. In the porphyrias, CYP inducers are thought to increase the activity of enzymes proximal to the deficient enzyme, exacerbating or triggering attacks (Chap. 337). Deficiency of glucose-6-phosphate dehydrogenase (G6PD), most often in individuals of African or Mediterranean descent, increases risk of hemolytic anemia in response to primaquine and a number of other drugs that do not cause hemolysis in patients with adequate quantities of this enzyme (Chap. 93). Patients with mutations in the ryanodine receptor that controls intracellular calcium in skeletal muscle and other tissues may be asymptomatic until exposed to certain general anesthetics, which trigger the syndrome of malignant hyperthermia. Certain antiarrhythmics and other drugs can produce marked QT prolongation and torsades de pointes (Chap. 214), and in some patients this adverse effect represents unmasking of previously subclinical congenital long QT syndrome.

POLYMORPHISMS THAT MODULATE THE BIOLOGIC CONTEXT WITHIN WHICH THE DRUG-TARGET INTERACTIONS OCCUR The interaction of a drug with its molecular target is translated into a clinical action in a complex biologic milieu that is itself often perturbed by disease. Thus, polymorphisms that determine variability in this biology may profoundly influence drug response, although the genes involved are not themselves directly targets of drug action. The common insertion/deletion (I/D) polymorphism in the ACE gene determines prognosis in many types of heart disease, including heart failure. In patients with heart failure treated with β-adrenergic blockers, the best response to therapy has been associated with the DD genotype, the group with the worst prognosis. The mechanism underlying this outcome is uncertain, but a direct effect of beta blockers on ACE seems unlikely; rather the I/D genotype likely affects the biology of heart failure to allow an improved response to beta blockers. Similarly, polymorphisms in genes important for lipid homeostasis (such as the ABCA1 transporter and the cholesterol ester transport protein) modulate response to HMG-CoA reductase inhibitors. In one large study, the combination of diuretic use combined with a variant in the adducin gene (encoding a cytoskeletal protein important for renal tubular sodium absorption) decreased stroke or myocardial infarction risk, while neither factor alone has an effect. Common polymorphisms in ion channel genes that are not themselves the target of QT-prolonging drugs may nevertheless influence the extent to which those drugs affect the electrocardiogram and produce arrhythmias.

PROSPECTS FOR INCORPORATING GENETIC INFORMATION INTO CLINICAL PRACTICE These and many other examples of associations between specific genotypes and drug responses raise the tantalizing prospect that patients will undergo routine genotyping for loci known to modulate drug levels or response prior to receiving a prescription. The twin goals are to identify patients likely to exhibit adverse effects and those most likely to respond well. Obstacles that must be overcome before this vision becomes a reality include replication of even the most compelling associations, demonstrations of cost-effectiveness, development of readily useable genotyping technologies, and ethical issues involved in genotyping. While these barriers seem daunting, the field is very young and evolving rapidly. Indeed, one major result of understanding of the role of genetics in drug action has been improved screening of drugs during the development process to reduce the likelihood of highly variable metabolism or unanticipated toxicity (such as torsades de pointes).

INTERACTIONS BETWEEN DRUGS

Drug interactions can complicate therapy by adversely increasing or decreasing the action of a drug; interactions may be based on changes in drug disposition or in drug response in the absence of changes in drug levels. *Interactions must be considered in the differential diagnosis of any unusual response occurring during drug therapy.* Prescribers should recognize that patients often come to them with a legacy of drugs acquired during previous medical experiences, often with multiple physicians who may not be aware of all the patient's medications. A meticulous drug history should include examination of the patient's medications and, if necessary, calls to the pharmacist to identify prescriptions. It should also address the use of agents not often volunteered during questioning, such as over-the-counter (OTC) drugs, health food supplements, and topical agents such as eye drops. Lists of interactions are available from a number of electronic sources. The practicing physician cannot be expected to memorize these. How-

TABLE 3-2 *Drugs with a High Risk of Generating Pharmacokinetic Interactions*

Drug	Mechanism	Examples
Antacids; bile acid sequestrants	Reduced absorption	Antacids/tetracyclines; cholestryamine/digoxin
Proton pump inhibitors; H$_2$-receptor blockers	Altered gastric pH	Ketoconazole absorption decreased
Rifampin; carbamazepine; barbiturates; phenytoin; St. John's wort; glutethimide	Induction of hepatic metabolism	Decreased concentration and effects of: warfarin; quinidine; cyclosporine; losartan
Tricyclic antidepressants; fluoxetine; quinidine	Inhibitors of CYP2D6	Increased beta blockade; decreased codeine effect
Cimetidine	Inhibitor of multiple CYPs	Increased concentration and effects of: warfarin; theophylline; phenytoin
Ketoconazole, itraconazole; erythromycin, clarithromycin; calcium channel blockers; ritonavir	Inhibitor of CYP3A	Increased concentration and toxicity of: some HMG-CoA reductase inhibitors; cyclosporine; cisapride, terfenadine (now withdrawn) Increased concentration and effects of: indinavir (with ritonavir); Decreased clearance and dose requirement for: cyclosporine (with calcium channel blockers)
Allopurinol	Xanthine oxidase inhibitor	Azathioprine and 6-mercaptopurine toxicity
Amiodarone	Inhibitor of many CYPs and of P-glycoprotein	Decreased clearance (risk of toxicity) for: warfarin; digoxin; quinidine
Gemfibrazol (and other fibrates)	CYP3A inhibition	Rhabdomyolysis when co-prescribed with some HMG-CoA reductase inhibitors
Quinidine; amiodarone; verapamil; cyclosporine; itraconazole; erythromycin	P-glycoprotein inhibition	Risk of digoxin toxicity
Phenylbutazone, probenecid; salicylates	Inhibition of renal tubular transport	Salicylates $\rightarrow$ increased risk of methotrexate toxicity

ever, certain drugs consistently run the risk of generating interactions, through mechanisms that are well understood; examples (not an exhaustive listing) are presented below and in Table 3-2. When such drugs are started or stopped, prescribers must be especially alert to the possibility of interactions.

PHARMACOKINETIC INTERACTIONS CAUSING DIMINISHED DRUG DELIVERY TO TARGET SITES ■ Impaired Gastrointestinal Absorption Aluminum ions, present in antacids, can form insoluble chelates with the tetracyclines, preventing their absorption. Kaolin-pectin suspensions bind digoxin, and when the substances are administered together, digoxin absorption is reduced by about one-half. Resins that sequester bile acids in the gut can bind other drugs, such as digoxin. Ketoconazole is a weak base that dissolves well only at acidic pH. Histamine H$_2$ receptor antagonists and proton pump inhibitors reduce gastric acidity and thus impair the dissolution and absorption of ketoconazole.

Induction of CYP or Transporter Activity Expression of some genes responsible for drug elimination, notably *CYP3A* and *MDR1*, can be markedly increased by "inducing" drugs, such as rifampin, carbamazepine, phenytoin, St. John's wort, and glutethimide and by smoking, exposure to chlorinated insecticides such as DDT (CYP1A2), and chronic alcohol ingestion. One mechanism for this coordinate induction of multiple pathways is increased expression of common transcription factors (e.g., hepatocyte nuclear factor 4α). Administration of inducing agents lowers plasma levels over 2 to 3 weeks as gene expression is increased. This alters the effects of many drugs, including warfarin, quinidine, mexiletine, verapamil, ketoconazole, itraconazole, cyclosporine, dexamethasone, methylprednisolone, prednisolone (the active metabolite of prednisone), oral contraceptive steroids, methadone, and metronidazole. These interactions all have obvious clinical significance. Further, if a drug dose is stabilized in the presence of an inducer which is subsequently stopped, major toxicity can occur as clearance returns to preinduction levels and drug concentrations rise. This is a particular problem with narrow-therapeutic-ratio drugs such

as warfarin and some antiarrhythmics. Individuals vary in the extent to which drug metabolism can be induced, likely through genetic mechanisms.

Inhibition of Cellular Uptake or Binding Tricyclic antidepressants, doxepin, and chlorpromazine are potent inhibitors of norepinephrine uptake into adrenergic neurons and prevent the uptake of the guanidinium antihypertensive agents (such as guanethidine and guanadrel), thereby abolishing their antihypertensive effects. Similarly, the antihypertensive effect of clonidine is partially antagonized by tricyclic antidepressants.

PHARMACOKINETIC INTERACTIONS CAUSING INCREASED DRUG DELIVERY TO TARGET SITES ■ Inhibition of Drug Metabolism Inhibition of drug metabolism can lead to reduced clearance, prolonged half-life, accumulation of drug during maintenance therapy, and thus adverse effects. In contrast to induction, new protein synthesis is not involved, and the effect develops as drug and any inhibitor metabolites accumulate (a function of their elimination half-lives). Since shared substrates of a single enzyme can compete for access to the active site of the protein, many CYP substrates can also be considered inhibitors. However, some drugs are especially potent as inhibitors (and occasionally may not even be substrates); it is in the use of agents of the latter type that clinicians must be most alert to the potential for interactions.

Cimetidine (but not other H$_2$-receptor blockers) is a potent inhibitor of the oxidative metabolism of many drugs, including warfarin, quinidine, nifedipine, lidocaine, theophylline, and phenytoin. Severe adverse reactions can develop as a consequence.

The antifungal agents ketoconazole and itraconazole are potent inhibitors of enzymes in the CYP3A family. When fluconazole levels are elevated as a result of higher doses and/or renal insufficiency, this drug can also inhibit CYP3A. The macrolide antibiotics erythromycin and clarithromycin inhibit CYP3A4 to a clinically significant extent, but azithromycin does not. Some of the calcium channel blockers, including diltiazem, nicardipine, and verapamil can also inhibit CYP3A, as can some of the enzyme's substrates, such as cyclosporine. Examples of CYP3A substrates also include quinidine, lovastatin, simvastatin, atorvastatin, nifedipine, lidocaine, erythromycin, methylprednisolone, carbamazepine, midazolam, and triazolam.

Phenytoin, an inducer of many systems including CYP3A, inhibits CYP2C9. CYP2C9 metabolism of losartan to its active metabolite is inhibited by phenytoin, with potential loss of antihypertensive effect.

Accumulation of the prokinetic drug cisapride and the antihistamine terfenadine due to CYP3A inhibition led to QT prolongation and torsades de pointes. Measures to prevent co-prescription of these agents with CYP3A inhibitors were unsuccessful, and alternative safer agents were developed, so these drugs were eventually withdrawn.

Cyclosporine can cause serious toxicity when its metabolism via CYP3A4 is inhibited by erythromycin, ketoconazole, diltiazem, nicardipine, or verapamil. The risk of myopathy with some HMG-CoA reductase inhibitors (lovastatin, simvastatin, atorvastatin) is thought to be increased by CYP3A4 inhibition. One agent in this class, cerivastatin, was withdrawn because of an especially high incidence of this adverse effect, although cellular studies suggest inhibition of other pathways may have also contributed in this case. The antiviral ritonavir is a very potent CYP3A4 inhibitor that is often added to anti-HIV regimens not because of its antiviral effects but because it decreases clearance, and hence increases efficacy, of other anti-HIV agents. Grapefruit (but not orange) juice inhibits CYP3A, especially at high doses; patients receiving drugs where even modest CYP3A inhibition may increase the risk of adverse effects (e.g., cyclosporine, some HMG-CoA reductase inhibitors) should therefore avoid grapefruit juice.

CYP2D6 is markedly inhibited by quinidine and is also blocked by a number of neuroleptic drugs, such as chlorpromazine and haloperidol, and by fluoxetine. The analgesic effect of codeine depends on its metabolism to morphine via CYP2D6. Thus, quinidine reduces the analgesic efficacy of codeine in EMs. Since desipramine is cleared largely by metabolism via CYP2D6 in EMs, its levels are increased substantially by concurrent administration of quinidine, fluoxetine, or the neuroleptic drugs that inhibit CYP2D6. Clinical consequences of fluoxetine's interaction with CYP2D6 substrates may not be apparent for weeks after the drug is started, because of its very long half-life and slow generation of a CYP2D6-inhibiting metabolite.

6-Mercaptopurine, the active metabolite of azathioprine, is metabolized not only by TPMT but also by xanthine oxidase. When allopurinol, a potent inhibitor of xanthine oxidase, is administered with standard doses of azathioprine or 6-mercaptopurine, life-threatening toxicity (bone marrow suppression) can result.

Inhibition of Drug Transport The best studied example is P-glycoprotein (Fig. 3-4). Quinidine inhibits P-glycoprotein function in vitro, and it now appears that the long-recognized doubling of plasma digoxin when quinidine is coadministered reflects this action in vivo, particularly since the effects of quinidine (increased digoxin bioavailability and reduced renal and hepatic secretion) occur at the sites of P-glycoprotein expression. Many other drugs also elevate digoxin concentrations (e.g., amiodarone, verapamil, cyclosporine, itraconazole, and erythromycin), and a similar mechanism seems likely. Reduced CNS penetration of multiple HIV protease inhibitors (with the attendant risk of facilitating viral replication in a sanctuary site) appears attributable to P-glycoprotein-mediated exclusion of the drug from the CNS; thus inhibition of P-glycoprotein has been proposed as a therapeutic approach to enhance drug entry to the CNS.

A number of drugs are secreted by the renal tubular transport systems for organic anions. Inhibition of these systems can cause excessive drug accumulation. Salicylate, for example, reduces the renal clearance of methotrexate, an interaction that may lead to methotrexate toxicity. Renal tubular secretion contributes substantially to the elimination of penicillin, which can be inhibited (to increase its therapeutic effect) by probenecid.

Inhibition of the tubular cation transport system by cimetidine decreases the renal clearance of dofetilide and of procainamide and its active metabolite NAPA.

DRUG INTERACTIONS NOT MEDIATED BY CHANGES IN DRUG DISPOSITION Drugs may act on separate components of a common process to generate effects greater than either has alone. For example, although small doses of aspirin (<1 g daily) do not alter the prothrombin time appreciably in patients who are receiving warfarin therapy, aspirin nevertheless increases the risk of bleeding in these patients because it inhibits platelet aggregation. Thus the combination of impaired functions of platelets and of the clotting system, while useful in some patients, also increases the potential for hemorrhagic complications. Similarly, the use of other anticlotting agents (heparin, glycoprotein IIb/IIIa inhibitors, clopidogrel) with aspirin improves outcomes in acute coronary syndromes, while exacerbating this bleeding tendency.

Nonsteroidal anti-inflammatory drugs (NSAIDs) cause gastric ulcers, and, in patients treated with warfarin, the risk of bleeding from a peptic ulcer is increased almost threefold by concomitant use of a NSAID.

Indomethacin, piroxicam, and probably other NSAIDs antagonize the antihypertensive effects of β-adrenergic receptor blockers, diuretics, ACE inhibitors, and other drugs. The resulting elevation in blood pressure ranges from trivial to severe. This effect is not seen with aspirin and sulindac but has been found with cyclooxygenase-2 inhibitors (celecoxib, rofecoxib).

Torsades de pointes during administration of QT-prolonging antiarrhythmics (quinidine, sotalol, dofetilide) occur much more frequently in those patients receiving diuretics, probably reflecting hypokalemia. In vitro, hypokalemia not only prolongs the QT interval in the absence of drug but also potentiates drug block of ion channels that results in QT prolongation. Also, some diuretics have direct electrophysiologic actions that prolong QT.

The administration of supplemental potassium leads to more frequent and more severe hyperkalemia when potassium elimination is reduced by concurrent treatment with ACE inhibitors, spironolactone, amiloride, or triamterene.

The pharmacologic effects of sildenafil result from inhibition of the phosphodiesterase type 5 isoform that inactivates cyclic GMP in the vasculature. Nitroglycerin and related nitrates used to treat angina produce vasodilation by elevating cyclic GMP. Thus, coadministration of these nitrates with sildenafil can cause profound hypotension, which can be catastrophic in patients with coronary disease.

Sometimes, combining drugs can increase overall efficacy and/or reduce drug-specific toxicity. Such therapeutically useful interactions are described in chapters dealing with specific disease entities, elsewhere in this text.

ADVERSE REACTIONS TO DRUGS

The beneficial effects of drugs are coupled with the inescapable risk of untoward effects. The morbidity and mortality from these untoward effects often present diagnostic problems because they can involve every organ and system of the body and are frequently mistaken for signs of underlying disease. Major advances in the investigation, development, and regulation of drugs ensure in most instances that drugs are uniform, effective, and relatively safe and that their recognized hazards are publicized. However, prior to regulatory approval and marketing, new drugs are tested in relatively few patients who tend to be less sick and to have fewer concomitant diseases than those patients who subsequently receive the drug therapeutically. Because of the relatively small number of patients studied in clinical trials, and the selected nature of these patients, rare adverse effects may not be detected prior to a drug's approval, and physicians therefore need to be cautious in the prescription of new drugs and alert for the appearance of previously unrecognized adverse events. Often, these adverse reactions are rare, such as hematologic abnormalities, arrhythmias, hepatitis, or renal dysfunction. In these cases, often (but inappropriately) labeled "idiosyncratic," elucidating underlying mechanisms can assist development of safer compounds or allow a patient subset at especially high risk to be excluded from drug exposure. National adverse reaction reporting systems, such as those operated by the U.S. Food and Drug Administration (suspected adverse reactions can be reported online at *http://www.fda.gov/medwatch/report/hcp.htm*) and the Committee on Safety of Medicines in Great Britain, can prove useful. The publication or reporting of a newly recognized adverse reaction can in a short time stimulate many similar such reports of reactions that previously had gone unrecognized.

Occasionally, "adverse" effects may be exploited to develop an entirely new indication for a drug. Unwanted hair growth during minoxidil treatment of severely hypertensive patients led to development of the drug for hair growth. Sildenafil was initially developed as an antianginal, but its effects to alleviate erectile dysfunction not only led to a new drug indication but also to increased understanding of the role of type 5 phosphodiesterase in erectile tissue. These examples further reinforce the concept that prescribers must remain vigilant to the possibility that unusual symptoms may reflect unappreciated drug effects.

The large number and variety of drugs and herbal remedies available OTC as well as by prescription make it impossible for patient or physician to obtain or retain the knowledge necessary to use all drugs well. It is understandable, therefore, that many OTC drugs are used unwisely by the public and that restricted drugs may be prescribed incorrectly by physicians.

Some 25 to 50% of patients make errors in self-administration of prescribed medicines, and these errors can be responsible for adverse drug effects. Elderly patients are the group most likely to commit such errors, perhaps in part because they consume more medicines. One-third or more of patients also may not take their prescribed medications. Similarly, patients commit errors in taking OTC drugs by not reading or following the directions on the containers. Physicians must recognize that providing directions with prescriptions does not always guarantee compliance.

In hospital, drugs are administered in a controlled setting, and patient compliance is, in general, ensured. Errors may occur nevertheless—the wrong drug or dose may be given or the drug may be given to the wrong patient—and improved drug distribution and administration systems are addressing this problem. On the other hand, there are no easy means for controlling how ambulatory patients take prescription or OTC drugs.

EPIDEMIOLOGY Patients receive, on average, 10 different drugs during each hospitalization. The sicker the patient, the more drugs are given, and there is a corresponding increase in the likelihood of adverse drug reactions. When <6 different drugs are given to hospitalized patients the probability of an adverse reaction is ~5%, but if >15 drugs are given, the probability is >40%. Retrospective analyses of ambulatory patients have revealed adverse drug effects in 20%. Serious adverse reactions are also well recognized with "herbal" remedies and OTC compounds: examples include kava-associated hepatotoxicity, L-tryptophan-associated eosinophilia-myalgia, and phenylpropanolamine-associated stroke, each of which has caused fatalities.

A 2000 Institute of Medicine report indicated that 7000 Americans die annually because of medication errors, that 2 to 3% of hospital admissions are for illnesses attributed to drugs, that the in-hospital cost was >$2 billion, and that this represents a tiny fraction of the overall problem of medication errors and its costs. A small group of widely used drugs accounts for a disproportionate number of reactions. Aspirin and other NSAIDs, analgesics, digoxin, anticoagulants, diuretics, antimicrobials, glucocorticoids, antineoplastics, and hypoglycemic agents account for 90% of reactions, although the drugs involved differ between ambulatory and hospitalized patients.

ETIOLOGY Most adverse drug reactions are preventable, and recent studies using a systems analysis approach suggest that the most common system failure associated with an adverse drug reaction is the failure to disseminate knowledge about drugs to individuals who prescribe and administer them. Most adverse reactions may be classified in two groups. The most frequent ones result from exaggeration of an intended pharmacologic action of the drug, and the underlying mechanisms have been discussed above. Other adverse reactions ensue from toxic effects unrelated to the intended pharmacologic actions. The latter effects are often unpredictable and frequently severe, and result from recognized as well as undiscovered mechanisms.

TOXICITY UNRELATED TO A DRUG'S PRIMARY PHARMACOLOGIC ACTIVITY ■ Cytotoxic Reactions Drug or more commonly reactive metabolites generated by CYPs can covalently bind to tissue macromolecules (such as proteins or DNA) to cause tissue toxicity. Because of the reactive nature of these metabolites covalent binding often occurs close to the site of production; this is typically the liver, although CYPs are found in other tissues as well.

The most common cause of drug-induced hepatotoxicity is acetaminophen overdosage. Normally, reactive metabolites are detoxified by combining with hepatic glutathione. When glutathione becomes exhausted, the metabolites bind instead to hepatic protein, with resultant hepatocyte damage. The hepatic necrosis produced by the ingestion of acetaminophen can be prevented, or at least attenuated, by the administration of substances such as N-acetylcysteine that reduce the binding of electrophilic metabolites to hepatic proteins. The risk of hepatic necrosis is increased in patients receiving drugs such as phenobarbital or phenytoin that increase the rate of drug metabolism or ethanol that exhaust glutathione stores. Such toxicity has even occurred with therapeutic dosages, so patients at risk through these mechanisms should be warned.

Immunologic Mechanisms Most pharmacologic agents are small molecules with low molecular weights (<2000) and thus are poor immunogens. Generation of an immune response to a drug therefore usually requires in vivo activation and covalent linkage to protein, carbohydrate, or nucleic acid.

Drug stimulation of antibody production may mediate tissue injury by several mechanisms. The antibody may attack the drug when the drug is covalently attached to a cell, and thereby destroy the cell. This occurs in penicillin-induced hemolytic anemia. Antibody-drug-antigen complexes may be passively adsorbed by a bystander cell, which is then destroyed by activation of complement; this occurs in quinine- and quinidine-induced thrombocytopenia. Heparin-induced thrombocytopenia arises when antibodies against complexes of platelet factor 4 peptide and heparin generate immune complexes that activate platelets; thus the thrombocytopenia is accompanied by "paradoxical" thrombosis and is treated with thrombin inhibitors. Drugs or their reactive metabolites may alter a host tissue, rendering it antigenic and eliciting autoantibodies. For example, hydralazine and procainamide (or their reactive metabolites) can chemically alter nuclear material, stimulating the formation of antinuclear antibodies and occasionally causing lupus erythematosus. Autoantibodies can be elicited by drugs that neither interact with the host antigen nor have any chemical similarity to the host tissue; for example, the antihypertensive α-methyldopa frequently stimulates the formation of antibodies to host erythrocytes, yet the drug neither attaches to the erythrocyte nor shares any chemical similarities with the antigenic determinants on the erythrocyte. Drug-induced pure red cell aplasia (Chap. 94) is due to an immune-based drug reaction. Red cell formation in bone marrow cultures can be inhibited by phenytoin and purified IgG obtained from a patient with pure red cell aplasia associated with phenytoin.

Serum sickness (Chap. 298) results from the deposition of circulating drug-antibody complexes on endothelial surfaces. Complement activation occurs, chemotactic factors are generated locally, and an inflammatory response develops at the site of complex entrapment. Arthralgias, urticaria, lymphadenopathy, glomerulonephritis, or cerebritis may result. Foreign proteins (vaccines, streptokinase, therapeutic antibodies) and antibiotics are common causes. Many drugs, particularly antimicrobial agents, ACE inhibitors, and aspirin, can elicit anaphylaxis, with production of IgE, which binds to mast cell membranes. Contact with a drug antigen initiates a series of biochemical events in the mast cell and results in the release of mediators that can produce the characteristic urticaria, wheezing, flushing, rhinorrhea, and (occasionally) hypotension.

Drugs may also elicit cell-mediated immune responses. Topically administered substances may interact with sulfhydryl or amino groups in the skin and react with sensitized lymphocytes to produce the rash characteristic of contact dermatitis. Other types of rashes may also result from the interaction of serum factors, drugs, and sensitized lymphocytes.

DIAGNOSIS AND TREATMENT OF ADVERSE DRUG REACTIONS The manifestations of drug-induced diseases frequently resemble those of other diseases, and a given set of manifestations may be produced by different and dissimilar drugs. Recognition of the role of a drug or drugs in an illness depends on appreciation of the possible adverse reactions to drugs in any disease, on identification of the temporal relationship between drug administration and development of the illness, and on familiarity with the common manifestations of the drugs. Many associations between particular drugs and specific reactions have been described, but there is always a "first time" for a novel association, and any drug should be suspected of causing an adverse effect if the clinical setting is appropriate.

Illness related to a drug's intended pharmacologic action is often more easily recognized than illness attributable to immune or other mechanisms. For example, side effects such as cardiac arrhythmias in patients receiving digitalis, hypoglycemia in patients given insulin, and bleeding in patients receiving anticoagulants are more readily related to a specific drug than are symptoms such as fever or rash, which may be caused by many drugs or by other factors.

Electronic sources of adverse drug reactions can be useful (e.g., *http://www.hc-sc.gc.ca/hpb-dgps/therapeut/htmleng/cadrnwsletter.html*). However, exhaustive compilations often provide little sense of perspective in terms of frequency and seriousness, which can vary considerably among patients.

Eliciting a drug history from patients is important for diagnosis. Attention must be directed to OTC drugs and herbal preparations as well as to prescription drugs. Each type can be responsible for adverse drug effects, and adverse interactions may occur between OTC drugs and prescribed drugs. Loss of efficacy of oral contraceptives or cyclosporine by concurrent use of St. John's wort are examples. In addition, it is common for patients to be cared for by several physicians, and duplicative, additive, counteractive, or synergistic drug combinations may therefore be administered if the physicians are not aware of the patients' drug histories. Every physician should determine what drugs a patient has been taking, at least during the preceding 30 days, before prescribing any medications. A frequently overlooked source of additional drug exposure is topical therapy; for example, a patient complaining of bronchospasm may not mention that an ophthalmic beta blocker is being used unless specifically asked. A history of previous adverse drug effects in patients is common. Since these patients have shown a predisposition to drug-induced illnesses, such a history should dictate added caution in prescribing drugs.

Laboratory studies may include demonstration of serum antibody in some persons with drug allergies involving cellular blood elements, as in agranulocytosis, hemolytic anemia, and thrombocytopenia. For example, both quinine and quinidine can produce platelet agglutination in vitro in the presence of complement and the serum from a patient who has developed thrombocytopenia following use of this drug. Biochemical abnormalities such as G6PD deficiency, serum pseudocholinesterase level, or genotyping may also be useful in diagnosis, often after an adverse effect has occurred in the patient or a family member.

Once an adverse reaction is suspected, discontinuation of the suspected drug followed by disappearance of the reaction is presumptive evidence of a drug-induced illness. Confirming evidence may be sought by cautiously reintroducing the drug and seeing if the reaction reappears. However, that should be done only if confirmation would be useful in the future management of the patient and if the attempt would not entail undue risk. With concentration-dependent adverse reactions, lowering the dosage may cause the reaction to disappear, and raising it may cause the reaction to reappear. When the reaction is thought to be allergic, however, readministration of the drug may be hazardous, since anaphylaxis may develop. Readministration is unwise under these conditions unless no alternative drugs are available and treatment is necessary.

If the patient is receiving many drugs when an adverse reaction is suspected, the drugs likeliest to be responsible can usually be identified. All drugs may be discontinued at once or, if this is not practical, they should be discontinued one at a time, starting with the one that is most suspect, and the patient observed for signs of improvement.

The time needed for a concentration-dependent adverse effect to disappear depends on the time required for the concentration to fall below the range associated with the adverse effect; that, in turn, depends on the initial blood level and on the rate of elimination or metabolism of the drug. Adverse effects of drugs with long half-lives take a considerable time to disappear.

SUMMARY

Modern clinical pharmacology aims to replace empiricism in the use of drugs with therapy based on in-depth understanding of factor(s) that determine an individual's response to drug treatment. Molecular pharmacology, pharmacokinetics, genetics, clinical trials, and the educated prescriber all contribute to this process. No drug response should ever be termed "idiosyncratic"; all responses have a mechanism whose understanding will help guide further therapy with that drug or successors. This rapidly expanding understanding of variability in drug actions makes the process of prescribing drugs increasingly daunting for the practitioner. However, fundamental principles should guide this process:

- The benefits of drug therapy, however defined, should always outweigh the risk.
- The smallest dosage necessary to produce the desired effect should be used.
- The number of medications and doses per day should be minimized.
- Although the literature is rapidly expanding, accessing it is becoming easier; tools such as computers and hand-held devices to search databases of literature and unbiased opinion will become increasingly commonplace.
- Genetics play a role in determining variability in drug response and may become a part of clinical practice
- Prescribers should be particularly wary when adding or stopping specific drugs that are especially liable to provoke interactions and adverse reactions.
- Prescribers should use only a limited number of drugs, with which they are thoroughly familiar.

ACKNOWLEDGMENT
The author acknowledges John A. Oates, Grant Wilkinson, and Alastair Wood who wrote chapters on this material for previous editions; some of their text have been retained.

FURTHER READING

EVANS WE, JOHNSON JA: Pharmacogenomics: The inherited basis for interindividual differences in drug response. Annu Rev Genom Hum Genet 2: 9, 2001

HIGASHI MK et al: Association between CYP2C9 genetic variants and anticoagulation-related outcomes during warfarin therapy. JAMA 287:1690, 2002

MCLEOD HL, EVANS WE: Pharmacogenomics: Unlocking the human genome for better drug therapy. Annu Rev Pharmacol Toxicol 41:101, 2001

PSATY BM et al: Diuretic therapy, the alpha-adducin gene variant, and the risk of myocardial infarction or stroke in persons with treated hypertension. JAMA 287:1680, 2002

WILKINSON GR: Pharmacokinetics: The dynamics of drug absorption, distribution, and elimination, in JG Hardman, LE Limbird (eds). *Goodman and Gilman's The Pharmacological Basis of Therapeutics*, 9th ed, New York, McGraw-Hill, 2001, pp 3–30

WOOD AJ et al: Making medicines safer: The need for an independent drug safety board. N Engl J Med 339:1851, 1998

A primary goal of health care is to prevent disease or to detect it early enough that interventions will be more effective. Strategies for disease screening and prevention are driven by evidence that testing and interventions are practical and effective. Most screening tests are currently based on readily available and inexpensive biochemical (e.g., cholesterol), physiologic (e.g., blood pressure), radiologic (e.g., mammogram), or tissue specimens (e.g., Pap smear). In the future, it is anticipated that genetic testing will play an increasingly important role for predicting disease risk (Chap. 58). However, such tests are not widely used except for individuals at risk for high-penetrance genes based on family or ethnic history (e.g., *BRCA1*, *BRCA2*). The identification of low-penetrance but high-frequency genes that cause common disorders such as diabetes or hypertension offers the possibility of new genetic tests. However, any new screening test, whether based on genetic or other methods, must be subjected to rigorous evaluation of its sensitivity, specificity, impact on disease, and cost effectiveness. Physicians and patients are continuously introduced to new screening tests, often in advance of complete evaluation. For example, the use of whole-body computed tomography imaging has been advocated as a means to screen for a variety of disorders. Though appealing in concept, there is currently no evidence to justify this approach, which is associated with high cost and a substantial risk of false-positive results.

This chapter will review the basic principles of screening and strategies for measuring the impact of screening and prevention and will provide a summary of recommendations for screening and prevention in the primary care setting. Recommendations for specific disorders, such as cardiovascular disease, diabetes, or cancer, are provided in the chapters dedicated to these topics.

BASIC PRINCIPLES OF SCREENING In general, screening is most effective when applied to relatively common disorders that carry a large disease burden (Table 4-1). The five leading causes of mortality in the United States are heart diseases, malignant neoplasms, accidents, cerebrovascular diseases, and chronic obstructive pulmonary disease. Thus, many prevention strategies are targeted at these conditions.

A primary goal of screening is the early detection of a risk factor or disease at a stage when it can be corrected or cured. For example, most cancers have a better prognosis when identified as premalignant lesions or when they are still resectable. Similarly, early identification of hypertension or hyperlipidemia allows therapeutic interventions that reduce the risk of cardiovascular or cerebrovascular events. However, early detection does not necessarily influence survival. For example, in some studies of lung cancer screening, tumors are identified at an earlier stage, but overall mortality does not differ between screened and unscreened populations. The apparent improvement in 5-year survival rates can be attributed to the detection of smaller tumors rather than a real change in clinical course after diagnosis. Similarly, the detection of prostate cancer may not lead to a mortality difference because the disease is often indolent and competing morbidities, such as coronary artery disease, may ultimately cause mortality (Chap. 67).

Disorders with a long latency period increase the potential gains associated with detection. For example, cancer of the cervix has a long latency between dysplasia and invasive carcinoma, providing an opportunity for detection by routine screening. Similarly, an adenomatous polyp progresses to invasive colon cancer over 4 to 12 years, allowing an opportunity to detect early lesions by fecal occult blood testing or endoscopy. On the other hand, breast cancer screening in premenopausal women is more challenging because of the relatively short interval between development of a localized breast cancer and metastasis to regional nodes (estimated to be ~12 months).

METHODS OF MEASURING HEALTH BENEFITS It is not practical to perform all possible screening procedures. For example, screening for laryngeal cancer in smokers is not currently recommended. It is necessary to examine the strength of evidence in favor of screening measures relative to the cost and risk of false-positive tests. For example, should ultrasound be used to screen for ovarian cancer in average-risk women? It is currently estimated that the unnecessary laparotomies triggered by finding benign ovarian masses would actually cause more harm than the benefit derived from detecting the occasional curable ovarian cancer.

A variety of end points are used to assess the potential gain from screening and prevention interventions:

1. *The number of subjects screened to alter the outcome in one individual.* It is estimated, for example, that 731 women aged 65 to 69 would need to be screened by dual-energy x-ray absorptiometry (DEXA) and then treated appropriately to prevent one hip fracture from osteoporosis.

2. *The absolute and relative impact of screening on disease outcome.* A meta-analysis of Swedish mammography trials (ages 40 to 70) found that ~1.2 fewer women per thousand would die from breast cancer if they were screened over a 12-year period. By comparison, ~3 lives per 1000 might be saved from colon cancer in a population (ages 50 to 75) screened with annual fecal occult blood testing (FOBT) over a 13-year period. Based on this analysis, colon cancer screening may actually save more women's lives than mammography. The impact of FOBT (8.8/1000 versus 5.9/1000) might be stated as either 3 lives per 1000, or as a 30% reduction in colon cancer death; thus, it is important to consider both the relative and absolute impact on numbers of lives saved.

3. *The cost per year of life saved.* This is used to assess the effectiveness of many screening and prevention strategies. Typically, strategies that cost <$30,000 to $50,000 per year of life saved are considered "cost effective" (Chap. 2). For example, using alendronate to treat 65-year-old women with osteoporosis approaches this threshold of approximately $30,000 per year of life saved.

4. *Increase in average life expectancy for a population.*

Predicted increases in life expectancy for various screening procedures are listed in Table 4-2. It should be noted, however, that the life expectancy increase is an average that applies to a population and not to an individual. In reality, the vast majority of the screened population does not derive any benefit and possibly incurs a slight risk

TABLE 4-1 *Lifetime Cumulative Risk*

Breast cancer for women	10%
Colon cancer	6%
Cancer of the cervix for women[a]	2%
Domestic violence for women	Up to 15%
Hip fracture for Caucasian women	16%

[a] Assuming an unscreened population.

TABLE 4-2 *Estimated Average Increase in Life Expectancy for a Population*

Screening Procedure	Average Increase
Mammography:	
Women, 40–50 years	0–5 days
Women, 50–70 years	1 month
Pap smears, age 18–65	2–3 months
Screening treadmill for a 50-year-old (asymptomatic) man	8 days
PSA and digital rectal exam for a man >50 years	Up to 2 weeks
Getting a 35-year-old smoker to quit	3–5 years
Beginning regular exercise for a 40-year-old man (30 min 3 times a week)	9 months to 2 years

Note: PSA, prostate-specific antigen.

from false-positive results. A small subset of patients, however, will benefit greatly from being screened. For example, Pap smears do not benefit the 98% of women who never develop cancer of the cervix. However, for the 2% who would develop localized cervical cancer, Pap smears may add as much as 25 years to their lives. Some studies suggest that a 1-month gain of life expectancy is a reasonable goal for a population-based preventive strategy.

The U.S. Preventive Services Task Force provides recommendations for evidence-based screening (Table 4-3). In addition to these population-based guidelines, it is reasonable to consider family and social history to identify individuals with special risk (*www.ahrq.gov/clinic/uspstfix.htm*). For example, when there is a significant family history of breast, colon, or prostate cancer, it is prudent to initiate screening about 10 years before the age when the youngest family member developed cancer. Screening should also be considered for many other common disorders pending the development of further evidence. Three examples are screening for diabetes (using fasting blood glucose), domestic violence, and features of depression.

Cost-Effectiveness Screening techniques must be cost effective, if they are to be applied to large populations. Costs include not only the expense of testing but also time away from work and potential risks. When the risk-to-benefit ratio is less favorable, it is useful to provide information to patients and factor their perspectives into the decision-making process. For example, many expert groups, including the U.S. Preventive Services Task Force, recommend an individualized discussion about prostate cancer screening, as the decision-making process is complex and relies heavily on personal issues. Although the early detection of prostate cancer may intuitively seem desirable, risks include false-positive results that can lead to anxiety and unnecessary surgery. Potential complications from surgery and radiation treatment include erectile dysfunction, urinary incontinence, and bowel dysfunction. Some men may decline screening, while others may be more willing to accept the risks of an early detection strategy. Another example of shared decision-making is the choice of colon cancer screening techniques (Chap. 67). In controlled studies, the use of annual FOBT reduces colon cancer deaths by 15 to 30%. Flexible sigmoidoscopy reduces colon cancer deaths by ~60%. Colonoscopy offers the same, or greater, benefit than flexible sigmoidoscopy, but its use incurs additional costs and risks. These screening procedures have not been directly compared in the same population, but the estimated cost to society is similar—$10,000 to $25,000 per year of life saved. Thus, while one patient may prefer the ease of preparation, less time disruption, and the lower risk of flexible sigmoidoscopy, others may prefer the sedation and thoroughness of colonoscopy.

When considering the impact of screening tests, it is important to recognize that tobacco and alcohol use, diet, and exercise represent the vast majority of factors that influence preventable deaths. Perhaps the single greatest preventive health care measure is to help patients quit smoking (Chap. 375).

COMMONLY ENCOUNTERED ISSUES Despite compelling evidence that prevention strategies can have major health care benefits, implementation of these services is challenging because of competing demands on physician and patient time and because of gaps in health care reimbursement. Moreover, efforts to reduce disease risk frequently involve behavior changes (e.g., weight loss, exercise, seatbelts) or managing addictive conditions (e.g., tobacco and alcohol use) that are often recalcitrant to intervention. Public education and economic incentives are often useful, in addition to counseling by health care providers (Table 4-4).

A number of techniques can assist the physician with the growing number of recommended screening tests. An appropriately configured electronic medical record can provide reminder systems that make it easier for physicians to track and meet guidelines. Some systems pro-

TABLE 4-3 *Clinical Preventive Services for Normal-Risk Adults Recommended by the U.S. Preventive Services Task Force*

Test or Disorder	Population,[a] Years	Frequency	Chapter Reference
Blood pressure, height and weight	>18	Periodically	64
Cholesterol	Men > 35	Every 5 years	225
	Women > 45	Every 5 years	
Diabetes	>45 or earlier, if there are additional risk factors	Every 3 years	323
Pap smear	Within 3 years of onset of sexual activity or 21–65	Every 1–3 years	67
Chlamydia	Women 18–25	Every 1–2 years	160
Mammography[a]	Women > 40	Every 1–2 years	67, 76
Colorectal cancer[a]	>50		67, 77
fecal occult blood and/or		Every year	
sigmoidoscopy or		Every 5 years	
colonoscopy		Every 10 years	
Osteoporosis	Women > 65; >60 at risk	Periodically	333
Alcohol use	>18	Periodically	372
Vision, hearing	>65	Periodically	25, 26
Adult immunization			107, 108
Tetanus-diptheria (Td)	>18	Every 10 years	
Varicella (VZV)	Susceptibles only, >18	Two doses	
Measles, mumps, rubella (MMR)	Women, childbearing age	One dose	
Pneumococcal	>65	One dose	
Influenza	>50	Yearly	

[a] Screening is performed earlier and more frequently when there is a strong family history. Randomized, controlled trials have documented that fecal occult blood testing (FOBT) confers a 15 to 30% reduction in colon cancer mortality. Although randomized trials have not been performed for sigmoidoscopy or colonoscopy, well-designed case-control studies suggest similar or greater efficacy relative to FOBT.

Note: Prostate-specific antigen (PSA) testing is capable of enhancing the detection of early-stage prostate cancer, but evidence is inconclusive that it improves health outcomes. PSA testing is recommended by several professional organizations and is widely used in clinical practice, but it is not currently recommended by the U.S. Preventive Services Task Force (Chap. 81).

Source: Adapted from the U.S. Preventive Services Task Force, 1996. *Guide to Clinical Prevention Services*, 3d ed (*www.ahrq.gov/clinic/uspstfix.htm*)

TABLE 4-4 *Counseling to Prevent Disease*

Topic	Chapter Reference
Tobacco cessation	375
Drug and alcohol use	372, 373
Nutrition to maintain caloric balance and vitamin intake	60
Calcium intake in women > 18 years	333
Folic acid: Women of childbearing age	61
Oral health	28
Aspirin use to prevent cardiovascular disease in selected men >40 years and women >50 years	225
Chemoprevention of breast cancer in women at high risk	76
STDs and HIV prevention	115, 173
Physical activity	
Sun exposure	51
Injury prevention (loaded handgun, seat belts, bicycle helmet)	
Issues in the elderly	8
Polypharmacy	
Fall prevention	
Hot water heater <120°	
Vision, hearing, dental evaluations	
Immunizations (pneumococcal, influenza)	

Note: STDs, sexually transmitted diseases.

vide patients with secure access to their medical records, providing an additional means to ensure compliance with routine screening. Systems that provide nurses and other staff with standing orders are effective for smoking prevention and immunizations. The Agency for Healthcare Research and Quality and the Centers for Disease Control and Prevention have developed flow sheets as part of their "Put Prevention into Practice" program (*http://www.ahcpr.gov/clinic/ppipix.htm*).

A routine health care examination should be performed every 1 to 3 years before age 50 and every year thereafter. History should include medication use (prescription and nonprescription), allergies, dietary history, use of alcohol and tobacco, sexual practices, and a thorough family history, if not obtained previously. Routine measurements should include assessments of height, weight (body mass index, BMI), and blood pressure, in addition to the relevant physical examination. The increasing incidence of skin cancer underscores the importance of screening for suspicious skin lesions. Hearing and vision should be tested after age 65, or earlier if the patient describes difficulties. Other gender- and age-specific examinations are listed in Table 4-3. Counseling and instruction about self-examination (e.g., skin, breast) can be provided during the routine examination.

Many patients see a physician for ongoing care of chronic illnesses, and this visit provides an opportunity to include a "measure of prevention" for other health problems. For example, the patient seen for management of hypertension or diabetes can have breast cancer screening incorporated into one visit and a discussion about colon cancer screening at the next visit. Other patients may respond more favorably to a clearly defined visit that addresses all relevant screening and prevention interventions. In some patients, because of age or co-morbidities, it may be appropriate to abandon certain screening and prevention activities, although there are fewer data about when to "sunset" these services. The risk of certain cancers, like cancer of the cervix, ultimately declines, and it is reasonable to cease Pap smears after about age 65, if previous recent Pap smears have been negative. For breast, colon, and prostate cancer, it is reasonable to reevaluate the need for screening after about age 75. For some older patients with advanced diseases such as severe chronic obstructive pulmonary disease or congestive heart failure or who are immobile, the benefit of some screening procedures is low, and other priorities emerge when life expectancy is <10 years. This shift in focus needs to be done tactfully and allows greater focus on the conditions likely to impact quality and length of life.

FURTHER READING

BLUMENTHAL RS et al: Detecting occult coronary artery disease in a high-risk asymptomatic population. Circulation 107:702, 2003

CLINICAL PREVENTIVE SERVICES FOR NORMAL-RISK ADULTS RECOMMENDED BY THE U.S. PREVENTIVE SERVICES TASK FORCE. Put Prevention into Practice, January 2003. Agency for Healthcare Research and Quality, Rockville, MD. *www.ahrq.gov/ppip/adulttm.htm*

RANSOHOFF DF, SANDLER RS: Clinical practice: Screening for colorectal cancer. N Engl J Med 346:40, 2002

U.S. PREVENTIVE SERVICES TASK FORCE: *Guide to Clinical Preventive Services*, 3d ed. Baltimore, Williams & Wilkins, 1996

WRIGHT JC, WEINSTEIN MC: Gains in life expectancy from medical interventions—standardizing data on outcomes. N Engl J Med 339:380, 1998

---

5 WOMEN'S HEALTH
Andrea Dunaif

The study of biologic differences between sexes has emerged as a distinct scientific discipline in the United States. A report from the Institute of Medicine (IOM) found that sex has a broad impact on biologic and disease processes and succinctly concluded—sex matters. The National Institutes of Health established the Office of Research on Women's Health in 1990 to develop an agenda for future research in the field. In parallel, women's health is developing as a new clinical discipline with a focus on disorders that are disproportionately represented in women. The integration of women's health into internal medicine and other specialties has been accompanied by novel approaches to health care delivery, including greater attention to patient education and involvement in disease prevention and medical decision-making.

The IOM report recommended the terms *sex difference* to describe biologic processes that differ between males and females and *gender difference* for features related to social influences. This chapter highlights representative examples of sex differences in selected medical areas. Disorders discussed in this section are reviewed in detail in other chapters.

DISEASE RISK: REALITY AND PERCEPTION   The leading causes of death are the same in women and men: (1) heart disease, (2) cancer, and (3) cerebrovascular disease (Table 5-1; Fig. 5-1). The leading cause of cancer death, lung cancer, is the same in both sexes. Breast cancer is the second leading cause of cancer death in women but with rates that are 35% lower than those for lung cancer. Men are substantially more likely to die from suicide, homicide, and accidents than women.

Women's risk for many diseases increases at menopause, which occurs at a median age of 51.4 years. In the industrialized world, women spend one-third of their lives in the postmenopausal period. Estrogen levels fall abruptly at menopause, inducing a variety of physiologic and metabolic responses. Rates of cardiovascular disease increase and bone density begins to decrease after menopause. Nevertheless, in the United States women live on average 5.7 years longer than men, with a life expectancy of 79.5 years compared to 73.8 years in men. Elderly women outnumber elderly men, so that age-related conditions, such as hypertension, have a female preponderance.

Women's perception of disease risk is often inaccurate; <10% know that cardiovascular disease is the leading cause of death in women. The condition that they fear most is breast cancer, despite the fact that death rates from breast cancer have been falling since the 1990s. In any given decade of life, a woman's risk for breast cancer never exceeds 1 in 34. Although a woman's lifetime risk of developing breast cancer if she lives past 85 years is about 1 in 9, it is much more likely that she will die from cardiovascular disease than from breast cancer. In other words, many elderly women have breast cancer but die from other causes. Similarly, only 26% of women are aware that lung cancer is the leading cause of cancer death in women. These misconceptions are unfortunate as they perpetuate inadequate attention to modifiable risk factors, such as dyslipidemia, hypertension, and cigarette smoking. Physicians are also less likely to recognize women's risk for cardiovascular disease. When presented with actors portraying patients with chest pain, physicians' estimates for probability of coronary heart disease (CHD) were significantly lower for women than for men and were lower for black women than for white women. These perceptions on the part of both the patient and her physician lead to important differences in cardiac care that are discussed below.

SEX DIFFERENCES IN HEALTH AND DISEASE ■ Alzheimer's Disease (See also Chap. 350)   Alzheimer's disease (AD) affects approximately twice as many women as men. Because the risk for AD increases with age, part of this sex difference is accounted for by the fact that women live longer than men. However, additional factors likely contribute to the increased risk for AD in women. There are sex differences in brain size, structure, and functional organization. There is emerging evidence for sex-specific differences in gene expression, not only for genes on the X and Y chromosomes but also for some autosomal genes. Estrogens have pleiotropic genomic and nongenomic effects on the central nervous system, including neurotrophic actions in key areas involved in cognition and memory. Women with AD have lower endogenous estrogen levels compared to women without AD. These observations have led to the hypothesis that estrogen is neuroprotective.

Some studies have suggested that estrogen administration improves cognitive function in nondemented postmenopausal women as well as in women with AD, and several observational studies have suggested that postmenopausal hormone therapy (PHT) may decrease the risk of AD. However, recent placebo-controlled trials have found no improvement in disease progression or cognitive function after up to 15 months

TABLE 5-1 *Deaths and Percent of Total Deaths for the Ten Leading Causes of Death by Sex in the United States, 2000*

Cause of Death	Women			Men		
	Rank	Deaths	Percent of Total Deaths	Rank	Deaths	Percent of Total Deaths
Diseases of heart	1	365,953	29.9	1	344,807	29.3
Malignant neoplasms	2	267,009	21.8	2	286,082	24.3
Cerebrovascular diseases	3	102,892	8.4	3	64,769	5.5
Chronic lower respiratory diseases	4	62,005	5.1	5	60,004	5.1
Diabetes mellitus	5	37,699	3.1	6	31,602	2.7
Influenza and pneumonia	6	36,655	3.0	7	28,658	2.4
Alzheimer's disease	7	35,120	2.9	—	14,438	1.2
Accidents	8	34,083	2.8	4	63,817	5.4
Nephritis, nephrotic syndrome, and nephrosis	9	19,440	1.6	9	17,811	1.5
Septicemia	10	17,687	1.4	—	13,537	1.1
Intentional self-harm	—	5732	0.5	8	23,618	2.0
Chronic liver disease and cirrhosis		9338	0.8	10	17,214	1.5

Source: Data from National Vital Statistics Report, Vol. 50, No. 16, September 16, 2002, *www.cdc.gov/nchs/data/nvsr/nvsr50/nvsr50_16.pdf*

of PHT in women with AD. The findings in these observational studies may be confounded by the fact that PHT users are better educated and have higher socioeconomic status, both of which are associated with a decreased risk of AD. An ancillary study of the Women's Health Initiative (WHI) randomized clinical trial, the WHI Memory Study, is prospectively evaluating the impact of PHT on cognitive function and the development of AD in women 65 to 79 years of age at the time of enrollment. The results of this study should be available in 2007.

Coronary Heart Disease (See also Chap. 226) There are major sex differences in CHD, the leading cause of death in men and women in the United States. CHD death rates have been falling in men over the past 30 years but they have been increasing in women.

CHD presents differently in women, who are usually 10 to 15 years older than their male counterparts and are more likely to have comorbidities, such as hypertension, congestive heart failure, and diabetes. In the Framingham study, angina was the most frequent initial symptom of CHD in women, whereas myocardial infarction was the most frequent initial presentation in men. Women more often have atypical symptoms, such as nausea, vomiting, indigestion, and upper back pain.

Women with myocardial infarction are more likely to present with cardiac arrest or cardiogenic shock, whereas men are more likely to present with ventricular tachycardia. Further, younger women with myocardial infarction are more likely to die than men of similar age, with women under <50 experiencing twice the mortality rate of men, even after adjustment for differences in disease severity and management. Indeed, the younger the woman, the greater the risk of death from myocardial infarction compared to men (Fig. 5-2).

Physicians are less likely to suspect heart disease in women with chest pain and are less likely to perform diagnostic and therapeutic cardiac procedures in women. In addition, there are sex differences in the accuracy of certain diagnostic procedures. The exercise electrocardiogram has substantial false-positive as well as false-negative rates in women compared to men. Women are less likely to receive therapies such as angioplasty, thrombolytic therapy, coronary artery bypass grafts, beta-blockers, or aspirin. There are also sex differences in outcomes when women with CHD do receive therapeutic interventions. Women undergoing coronary artery bypass graft surgery have more advanced disease, a higher periop-

erative mortality rate, less relief of angina, and less graft patency; however, 5- and 10-year survival rates are similar. Women undergoing percutaneous transluminal coronary angioplasty have lower rates of initial angiographic and clinical success than men, but they also have a lower rate of restenosis and a better long-term outcome. Women may benefit less and have more frequent serious bleeding complications from thrombolytic therapy than do men. Factors such as older age, more comorbid conditions, and more severe CHD in women at the time of events or procedures appear to account in part for the observed sex differences.

Elevated cholesterol levels, hypertension, smoking, obesity, low high-density lipoprotein (HDL) cholesterol levels, diabetes, and lack of physical activity are important risk factors for CHD in both men and women. Total triglyceride levels are an independent risk factor for CHD in women but not in men. Low HDL-cholesterol and diabetes are more important risk factors for CHD in women than in men. Smoking is an important risk factor for CHD in women—it accelerates atherosclerosis, exerts direct negative effects on cardiac function, and is associated with an earlier age of menopause. Cholesterol-lowering drugs are equally effective in men and women for primary and sec-

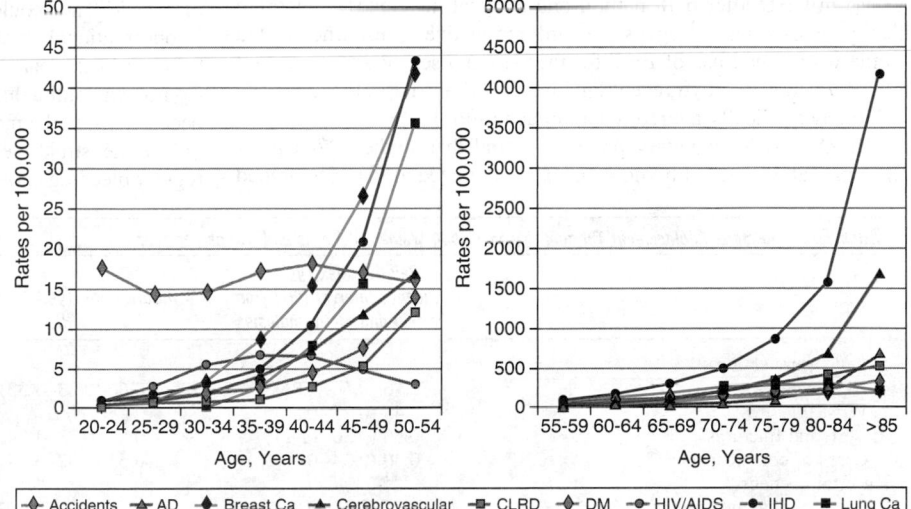

FIGURE 5-1 Death rates per 100,000 population for 1999 by 5-year age groups in U.S. women; note that the scale of the y-axis is increased by tenfold in the graph on the right compared to that on the left. Accidents and HIV/AIDS are the leading causes of death in young women 20 to 34 years of age. Accidents, breast cancer, and ischemic heart disease (IHD) are the leading causes of death in women 35 to 44 years of age. Breast cancer is the leading cause of death in women 45 to 49 years of age, and IHD becomes the leading cause of death in women beginning at 50 years of age. In older women, IHD remains the leading cause of death, cerebrovascular disease becomes the second leading cause of death, and lung cancer is the leading cause of cancer-related deaths. AD, Alzheimer's disease; Ca, cancer; CLRD, chronic lower respiratory disease; DM, diabetes mellitus; IHD, ischemic heart disease. (*Data adapted from www.cdc.gov/nchs/data/sttab/vs00199_tabl21or.pdf.*) (Writing Group for the Women's Health Initiative Investigation, JAMA 288:321, 2002. Copyright © 2002, American Medical Association.)

FIGURE 5-2 Rates of death during hospitalization for myocardial infarction among women and men according to age. The overall mortality rate during hospitalization was 16.7% among women and 11.5% among men but was twice the rate in women <50 years compared to men in the same age range. The interaction between sex and age was significant (p < .001). (*From V Vaccarino et al: N Engl J Med 341:217, 1999; with permission.*)

ondary prevention of CHD. However, because of perceptions that women are at lower risk for CHD, they receive fewer interventions for modifiable risk factors than do men. Secondary prevention in women with known CHD is also suboptimal. At baseline, only about 30% of women enrolled in the Heart and Estrogen/progestin Replacement Study (HERS), a secondary prevention trial in women with established CHD, were taking beta blockers, and only 45% received lipid-lowering medications.

Effect of Hormone Replacement Therapy on Cardiovascular Disease (See also Chap. 327) Until recently, it was widely believed that the sex-specific effects of gonadal steroids on the cardiovascular system and lipid metabolism accounted for the different rates of CHD in women compared to men. Estrogen increases HDL and lowers low-density lipoprotein (LDL), whereas androgens have the opposite effect. Estrogen has direct vasodilatory effects on the vascular endothelium, enhances insulin sensitivity, and has antioxidant properties. The striking increase in CHD after both natural and surgical menopause supported the hypothesis that estrogens are cardioprotective. These findings led to the widespread use of PHT for primary and secondary prevention of CHD. However, two recent landmark clinical trials, HERS and the WHI, have radically altered the approach to PHT.

HERS was a secondary prevention trial that studied 2763 postmenopausal women with known CHD randomized to PHT (combined

continuous conjugated equine estrogen, 0.625 mg qd, and medroxyprogesterone acetate, 2.5 mg qd) or to placebo for an average of 4.1 years. Unexpectedly, there was a 50% increase in CHD events in the first year of the trial in the PHT group. The lack of a beneficial effect on CHD events occurred in the face of a significant increase in HDL-cholesterol and fall in LDL-cholesterol levels in the PHT group. The HERS II data show no difference in CHD events after an additional 2.7 years of follow-up.

The WHI trial randomized 16,608 women 50 to 79 years of age: 8506 to estrogen plus progestin and 8102 to placebo. It was halted in May 2002 after an average follow-up of 5.2 years because women receiving PHT had an increased risk of invasive breast cancer, and an overall assessment of outcomes showed more risk than benefit. Compared to women in the placebo group, women in the PHT group had a 26% higher rate of breast cancer, a 29% higher rate of CHD, a 41% higher rate of stroke, and a greater than twofold increase in pulmonary embolism (Table 5-2). There was no difference in the rate of endometrial cancer in the PHT group compared to the placebo group. There was a 33% reduction in the rate of hip fractures and a 37% reduction in the rate of colon cancer in the PHT group. Despite these beneficial effects, the global index of outcomes showed that the PHT group had a 15% higher rate of adverse events compared to the placebo group. Nevertheless, the absolute risk of PHT is relatively small. In 10,000 women receiving PHT compared to those receiving placebo, one would predict that over 1 year there might be eight more invasive breast cancers, seven more CHD events, eight more strokes, eight more pulmonary embolic events, but six fewer colon cancers and five fewer hip fractures. An estrogen-only arm of this study is ongoing.

Why did the results of these randomized clinical trials differ so markedly from those of observational studies of PHT? Women placed on PHT tend to have higher socioeconomic status, more education, lower body weight and blood pressure, and more favorable lipid profiles than nonusers—all factors that independently decrease the risk of CHD. This phenomenon has been called the *healthy user effect*. Physicians may also choose to prescribe PHT to women they deem to be healthier. Women at risk for certain conditions, such as breast cancer, may not be placed on PHT, which could decrease the number of PHT-associated cases of breast cancer in observational studies. In addition, individuals who continue to take medication, including placebo, have decreased overall mortality. This phenomenon is known as *compliance bias* and could contribute to the better outcomes for PHT users in observational studies. It is also possible that the type of PHT was a factor in the paradoxical results of the randomized clinical trials. Combined continuous estrogen plus progestin was used in both trials, because it was the most widely prescribed preparation and it does not induce menstrual bleeding (although many women do experience irregular bleeding early in therapy), permitting blinding of the trial. The progestin used was medroxyprogesterone acetate, which has been shown to have a number of adverse metabolic effects, such as antagonizing the beneficial effects of estrogen on lipids and insulin sensitivity. Progestins may also abolish the beneficial direct vascular actions of estrogen and increase the risk for breast cancer. The estrogen-alone component of the WHI will determine whether the progestin accounted for the increased risk of PHT. The oral route of administration results in first-pass hepatic metabolism that induces the production of several clotting factors. It remains possible that more physiologic PHT, such as transdermal estradiol, may not have the adverse effects of other forms of PHT. This hypothesis needs to be tested in randomized clinical trials.

TABLE 5-2 *Hormone Replacement Therapy Use in 10,000 Women: Benefits and Harms per Year*

	Relative Risk [95% Confidence Interval (CI)] from Review and Meta-analysis	Hazard Ratio (95% CI) from WHI
Benefits (prevention)		
Hip fractures	0.76 (0.56–1.01)	0.66 (0.33–1.33)
Wrist fractures	0.44 (0.23–0.84)	NA
Vertebral fractures	0.60 (0.36–0.99)	0.66 (0.32–1.34)
Cases of colon cancer	0.80 (0.74–0.86)	0.63 (0.32–1.24)
Uncertain benefits		
Cases of dementia prevented	0.66 (0.53–0.82)	NA
Harms (caused)		
Coronary heart disease	0.91 (0.67–1.33)	1.29 (1.02–1.63)
Strokes	1.12 (1.01–1.23)	1.41 (0.86–2.31)
Thromboembolic events	2.14 (1.64–2.81)	2.11 (1.26–3.55)
Thromboembolic events during first year	3.49 (2.33–5.59)	NA
Breast cancer cases (<5 years' use)	1.0 to 1.14	NA
Breast cancer cases (5 years' use)	1.23 to 1.35	1.26 (1.00–1.59)
Cholecystitis cases (<5 years' use)	1.8 (1.6–2.0)	NA
Cholecystitis cases (5 years' use)	2.5 (2.0–2.9)	NA

Note: WHI, Women's Health Initiative; NA, not applicable.   *Source*: From Nelson, with permission.

Diabetes Mellitus (See also Chap. 323) Women are more sensitive to insulin than men. Despite this, the prevalence of type 2 diabetes mellitus (DM) is higher in women, in part related to the higher prevalence of obesity among women. Polycystic ovary syndrome and gestational diabetes mellitus—common conditions in premenopausal women—are associated with a significantly increased risk for type 2 DM. Premenopausal women with DM lose the cardioprotective effect of female sex and have identical rates of CHD to those in males. This finding is partially explained by the coexistence of several CHD risk factors: obesity, hypertension, and dyslipidemia. Premenopausal women with DM also have impaired endothelial function and reduced coronary vasodilatory responses, which may predispose to cardiovascular complications.

Hypertension (See also Chap. 230) After age 60 years, hypertension is more common in U.S. women than in men, largely because of the high prevalence of hypertension in older age groups and the longer survival of women. Isolated systolic hypertension is present in 30% of women >60 years. Sex hormones affect blood pressure. Both normotensive and hypertensive women have higher blood pressure levels during the follicular than during the luteal phase. In the Nurses Health Study, the relative risk of hypertension was 1.8 in current users of oral contraceptives, but this risk is lower with the newer low-dose contraceptive preparations. PHT is not associated with hypertension. Among secondary causes of hypertension, there is a female preponderance of renal artery fibromuscular dysplasia.

The benefits of treatment for hypertension have been dramatic in both women and men. In a meta-analysis of the effects of hypertension treatment, the Individual Data Analysis of Antihypertensive Intervention Trial found a reduction of risk for stroke and for major cardiovascular events in women. The effectiveness of various antihypertensive drugs appears to be comparable in women and men; however, women may experience more side effects. For example, women are more likely to develop cough with angiotensin-converting enzyme inhibitors.

Autoimmune Disorders (See also Chap. 299) Most autoimmune disorders occur more commonly in women than in men; these include autoimmune thyroid and liver diseases, lupus, rheumatoid arthritis, scleroderma, multiple sclerosis, and idiopathic thrombocytopenic purpura. However, there is no sex difference in the incidence of type 1 DM, and ankylosing spondylitis occurs more commonly in men. There are relatively few differences in bacterial disease infection rates in men and women. In general, sex differences in viral diseases can be accounted for by differences in behaviors, such as exposures or rates of immunization. There are, however, sex differences in HIV infection (see below). Sex differences in both immune responses and adverse reactions to vaccines have been reported. For example, there is a female preponderance of postvaccination arthritis.

The mechanisms for these sex differences remain obscure. Adaptive immune responses are more robust in women than in men, which may be explained by the stimulatory actions of estrogens and the inhibitory actions of androgens on the cellular mediators of immunity. Consistent with an important role for gonadal hormones, there is variation in immune responses during the menstrual cycle, and the activity of certain autoimmune disorders is altered by castration or pregnancy (e.g., rheumatoid arthritis and multiple sclerosis may remit during pregnancy). Nevertheless, the majority of studies show that exogenous estrogens and progestins in the form of PHT or oral contraceptives do not alter autoimmune disease incidence or activity. Exposure to fetal antigens, including circulating fetal cells that persist in certain tissues, has been speculated to increase the risk of autoimmune responses. There is clearly an important genetic component to autoimmunity, as indicated by the familial clustering and HLA association of many such disorders. However, HLA types are not sexually dimorphic.

HIV Infection (See also Chap. 173) AIDS is an important cause of death in younger women (Fig. 5-1). Heterosexual contact with an at-risk partner is the fastest-growing transmission category, and women are twice as likely as men to be infected by a partner. Women are also more likely to be infected by multiple variants of the virus than men. Women with HIV have more rapid decreases in their CD4 cell counts than men. Compared with men, HIV-infected women more frequently develop candidiasis, but Kaposi's sarcoma is less common than in men.

Other sexually transmitted diseases, such as chlamydial infection and gonorrhea, are important causes of infertility in women, and papilloma virus infection predisposes to cervical cancer.

Osteoporosis (See also Chap. 333) Osteoporosis is much more prevalent in postmenopausal women than in age-matched men, and osteoporotic hip fractures are a major cause of morbidity in elderly women. Men accumulate more bone mass, and lose bone more slowly, than women. Sex differences in bone mass are found as early as infancy. Calcium intake, vitamin D, and estrogen all play important roles in bone formation and bone loss. Particularly during adolescence, calcium intake is an important determinant of peak bone mass. Vitamin D deficiency is surprisingly common in elderly women, occurring in >40% of women living in northern latitudes. Receptors for estrogens and androgens have been identified in bone. Estrogen deficiency is associated with increased osteoclast activity and a decreased number of bone-forming units, leading to net bone loss. The aromatase enzyme, which converts androgens to estrogens, is also present in bone. Recent studies show that estrogen is an important determinant of bone mass in men (derived from the aromatization of androgens) as well as in women.

Pharmacology On average, women have lower body weights, smaller organs, higher percent body fat, and lower total body water than men. There are also important sex differences in drug action and metabolism that are not accounted for by these differences in body size and composition. Gonadal steroids alter the binding and metabolism of a number of drugs. Further, menstrual cycle phase and pregnancy can alter drug action. Women require lower doses of neuroleptics to control schizophrenia. Women awaken from anesthesia faster than men given the same doses of anesthetics. Women also take more medications than men, including over-the-counter formulations and supplements. The greater use of medications combined with these biologic differences may account for the reported higher frequency of adverse drug reactions in women than in men.

Psychological Disorders (See also Chap. 371) Depression, anxiety, and affective and eating disorders (bulimia and anorexia nervosa) are more common in women than in men. Epidemiologic studies from both developed and developing nations consistently find major depression to be twice as common in women as in men, with the sex difference becoming evident in early adolescence. Depression occurs in 10% of women during pregnancy and in 10 to 15% of women during the postpartum period. There is a high likelihood of recurrence of postpartum depression with subsequent pregnancies. The incidence of major depression diminishes after age 45 years and does not increase with the onset of menopause. Depression in women appears to have a worse prognosis than in men; episodes last longer and there is a lower rate of spontaneous remission. Schizophrenia and bipolar disorders occur at equal rates in men and women, although there may be sex differences in symptoms.

Both biologic and social factors account for the greater prevalence depressive disorders in women. Men have higher levels of the neurotransmitter serotonin. Gonadal steroids also affect mood, and fluctuations during the menstrual cycle have been linked to symptoms of premenstrual syndrome.

Substance Abuse and Tobacco (See also Chaps. 372 and 375) Substance abuse is more common in men than women. However, one-third of Americans who suffer from alcoholism are women. Women alcoholics are less likely to be diagnosed than men. A greater proportion of men than women seek help for alcohol and drug abuse. Men are more likely to go to an alcohol or drug treatment facility, while women tend to approach a primary care physician or mental health professional for help under the guise of a psychosocial problem. Late-life alcoholism is more common in women than men. On average, alcoholic women drink less than alcoholic men but exhibit the same degree of impairment. Blood alcohol levels are higher in women than in men after drinking equivalent amounts of alcohol, adjusted for body weight. This greater bioavailability of alcohol in women is due both to the smaller volume of distribution and the slower gastric metabolism of alcohol secondary to lower activity of gastric alcohol dehydrogenase than in men. In addition, alcoholic women are more likely to abuse tranquilizers, sedatives, and amphetamines. Women alcoholics have a higher mortality rate than do nonalcoholic women and alcoholic men. Women also appear to develop alcoholic liver disease and other alcohol-related diseases with shorter drinking histories and lower levels of alcohol consumption. Alcohol abuse also poses special risks to a woman, adversely affecting fertility and the health of the baby (fetal alcohol syndrome). Even moderate alcohol use increases the risk of breast cancer, hypertension, and stroke in women.

More men than women smoke tobacco, but the prevalence of smoking is declining faster in men than women. Smoking markedly increases the risk of cardiovascular disease in premenopausal women and is also associated with a decrease in the age of menopause. Women who smoke are more likely to develop chronic obstructive pulmonary disease and lung cancer than men and at lower levels of tobacco exposure.

Violence Against Women (See also Chap. 371)   Domestic violence is the most common cause of physical injury in women, exceeding the combined incidence of all other types of injury (such as from rape, mugging, and auto accidents). Sexual assault is one of the most common crimes against women. One in five adult women in the United States reports having experienced sexual assault during her lifetime. Adult women are much more likely to be raped by a spouse, ex-spouse, or acquaintance than by a stranger. Domestic violence may be an unrecognized feature of certain clinical presentations such as chronic abdominal pain, headaches, substance abuse, and eating disorders, in addition to more obvious manifestations such as trauma.

SUMMARY   Women's health has become a mature discipline over the past decade. The importance of sex differences in biologic processes is now recognized. It is clear that understanding the mechanisms of these differences will have an impact not only on women's but also on men's health. For example, estrogen is now recognized as an important regulator of bone density in men as well as in women. Elucidating the biology of sex hormone action has resulted in the design of drugs with tissue-specific hormone agonist and antagonist effects. These discoveries will make it feasible to selectively modulate the actions of sex hormones in both women and men to prevent and treat disease.

ACKNOWLEDGMENT
The author wishes to acknowledge the contributions of Dr. Anthony Komaroff and Dr. Celeste Robb-Nicholson to this chapter in previous editions of the text.

FURTHER READING

HASELTINE FP, JACOBSON BG (eds): Women's health research: An introduction, in *Women's Health Research: A Medical and Policy Primer*. Washington, DC, American Psychiatric Press, 1997, pp 1–26

HULLEY SH et al: Randomized trial of estrogen plus progestin for secondary prevention of coronary heart disease in postmenopausal women. JAMA 280:605, 1998

NELSON HD et al: Postmenopausal hormone replacement therapy (scientific review). JAMA 288:872, 2002

WIZEMANN TM, PARDUE M-L (eds): *Exploring the Biological Contributions to Human Health: Does Sex Matter?* Washington, DC, National Academy of Sciences, 2001

WRITING GROUP FOR THE WOMEN'S HEALTH INITIATIVE INVESTIGATORS: Risk and benefits of estrogen plus progestin in healthy postmenopausal women: Principal results from the women's health initiative randomized controlled trial. JAMA 288:321, 2002

---

6   MEDICAL DISORDERS DURING PREGNANCY
Robert L. Barbieri, John T. Repke

Approximately 4 million births occur in the United States each year. A significant proportion of these are complicated by one or more medical disorders. Two decades ago, many medical disorders were contraindications to pregnancy. Advances in obstetrics, neonatology, obstetric anesthesiology, and medicine have increased the expectation that pregnancy will result in an excellent outcome for both mother and fetus despite most of these conditions. Successful pregnancy requires important physiologic adaptations, such as a marked increase in cardiac output. Medical problems that interfere with the physiologic adaptations of pregnancy increase the risk for poor pregnancy outcome; conversely, in some instances pregnancy may adversely impact an underlying medical disorder.

HYPERTENSION (See also Chap. 230)   In pregnancy, cardiac output increases by 40%, most of which is due to an increase in stroke volume. Heart rate increases by approximately 10 beats per minute during the third trimester. In the second trimester of pregnancy, systemic vascular resistance decreases and this is associated with a fall in blood pressure. During pregnancy, a blood pressure of 140/90 mmHg is considered to be abnormally elevated and is associated with a marked increase in perinatal morbidity and mortality. In all pregnant women, the measurement of blood pressure should be performed in the sitting position, because for many the lateral recumbent position is associated with a blood pressure lower than that recorded in the sitting position. The diagnosis of hypertension requires the measurement of two elevated blood pressures, at least 6 h apart. Hypertension during pregnancy is usually caused by preeclampsia, chronic hypertension, gestational hypertension, or renal disease.

Preeclampsia   Approximately 5 to 7% of all pregnant women develop *preeclampsia*, the new onset of hypertension (blood pressure > 140/90 mmHg), proteinuria (>300 mg/24 h), and pathologic edema during gestation. Although the precise placental factors that cause preeclampsia are unknown, the end result is vasospasm and endothelial injury in multiple organs. Excessive placental secretion of an fms-like tyrosine kinase 1 may contribute to the endothelial dysfunction, hypertension, and proteinuria observed in preeclampsia. Glomerular endothelial cells demonstrate swelling and encroach on the vascular lumen. Preeclampsia is associated with abnormalities of cerebral circulatory autoregulation, which increase the risk of stroke at near-normal blood pressures. Risk factors for the development of preeclampsia include nulliparity, diabetes mellitus, a history of renal disease or chronic hypertension, a prior history of preeclampsia, extremes of maternal age (>35 years or <15 years), obesity, factor V Leiden mutation, angiotensinogen gene T235, antiphospholipid antibody syndrome, and multiple gestation.

There are no well-established strategies for the prevention of preeclampsia. Clinical trials have demonstrated that low-dose aspirin treatment does *not* prevent preeclampsia in either low- or high-risk women. Two meta-analyses reported that dietary calcium supplementation appeared to be effective in reducing the risk of developing preeclampsia. Subsequently, however, a large randomized clinical trial in low-risk women did not demonstrate a protective effect of calcium supplementation. Therefore, calcium supplementation *may* be considered in women at high risk for preeclampsia (see above). The observation that dietary intervention may reduce the risk of hypertension in men and nonpregnant women raises the possibility that dietary manipulations will be discovered that reduce the risk of preeclampsia.

Severe preeclampsia is the presence of new-onset hypertension and proteinuria accompanied by central nervous system dysfunction (headaches, blurred vision, seizures, coma), marked elevations of blood pressure (>160/110 mmHg), severe proteinuria (>5 g/24 h), oliguria or renal failure, pulmonary edema, hepatocellular injury (ALT > 2 × the upper limits of normal), thrombocytopenia (platelet count < 100,000/μL), or disseminated intravascular coagulation. Women with *mild preeclampsia* are those with the diagnosis of new-onset hypertension, proteinuria, and edema without evidence of severe preeclampsia. The HELLP (*h*emolysis, *e*levated *l*iver enzymes, *l*ow *p*latelets) syndrome is a special subgroup of severe preeclampsia and is a major cause of morbidity and mortality in this disease. The presence of platelet dysfunction and coagulation disorders further increases the risk of stroke.

℞ TREATMENT

Preeclampsia resolves within a few weeks after delivery. For pregnant women with preeclampsia prior to 37 weeks' gestation, delivery reduces the mother's morbidity but exposes the fetus to the risk of premature delivery. The management of preeclampsia is challenging because it requires the clinician to balance the health of both mother and fetus simultaneously and to make management decisions that afford both the best opportunities for infant survival. In general, prior to term, women with *mild* preeclampsia can be managed conservatively with bed rest, close monitoring of blood pressure and renal function, and careful fetal surveillance. For women with *severe* preeclampsia, delivery is recommended after 32 weeks' gestation. This reduces maternal morbidity and slightly increases the risks associated with prematurity for the newborn. Prior to 32 weeks' gestation, the risks of prematurity for the fetus are great, and some authorities recommend conservative management to allow for continued fetal maturation. Expectant management of severe preeclampsia remote from term affords some benefits for the fetus with significant risks for the mother. Such management should be restricted to tertiary care centers where maternal-fetal medicine, neonatal medicine, and critical care medicine expertise are available.

The definitive treatment of preeclampsia is delivery of the fetus and placenta. For women with severe preeclampsia, aggressive management of blood pressures > 160/110 mmHg reduces the risk of cerebrovascular accidents.

Intravenous labetalol or hydralazine are the drugs most commonly used to manage preeclampsia. Alternative agents such as calcium channel blockers may be used. Elevated arterial pressure should be reduced slowly to avoid hypotension and a decrease in blood flow to the fetus. *Angiotensin-converting enzyme (ACE) inhibitors as well as angiotensin-receptor blockers should be avoided in the second and third trimesters of pregnancy because of their adverse effects on fetal development.* Pregnant women treated with ACE inhibitors often develop oligohydramnios, which may be caused by decreased fetal renal function.

Magnesium sulfate is the treatment of choice for the prevention and treatment of eclamptic seizures. Two large randomized clinical trials have demonstrated the superiority of magnesium sulfate over phenytoin and diazepam, and a recent large randomized clinical trial has demonstrated the efficacy of magnesium sulphate in reducing the risk of seizure and possible reducing the risk of maternal death. Magnesium may prevent seizures by interacting with *N*-methyl-D-aspartate (NMDA) receptors in the central nervous system. Given the difficulty of predicting eclamptic seizures on the basis of disease severity, it is recommended that once the decision to proceed with delivery is made, all patients carrying a diagnosis of preeclampsia be treated with magnesium sulfate (see Guideline).

REGIMENS FOR THE ADMINISTRATION OF MAGNESIUM SULFATE FOR SEIZURE PROPHYLAXIS IN WOMEN IN LABOR WITH PREECLAMPSIA

Intramuscular	Intravenous
10 g (5 g IM deep in each buttock)[a]	6-g bolus over 15 min
5 g IM deep q4h, alternating sides	1–3 g/h by continuous infusion pump
	May be mixed in 100 mL crystalloid; if given by intravenous push, make up as 20% solution; push at maximum rate of 1g/min
	40-g MgSO$_4$·7H$_2$O in 1000 mL Ringers lactate, run at 25–75 mL/h (1–3 g/h)[a]

[a] Made up as 50% solution

Chronic Essential Hypertension Pregnancy complicated by chronic essential hypertension is associated with intrauterine growth restriction and increased perinatal mortality. Pregnant women with chronic hypertension are at increased risk for superimposed preeclampsia and abruptio placenta. Women with chronic hypertension should have a thorough prepregnancy evaluation, both to identify remediable causes of hypertension and to ensure that the prescribed antihypertensive agents are not associated with an adverse outcome of pregnancy (e.g., ACE inhibitors, angiotensin-receptor blockers). α-Methyldopa and labetalol are the most commonly used medications for the treatment of chronic hypertension in pregnancy. Baseline evaluation of renal function is necessary to help differentiate the effects of chronic hypertension versus superimposed preeclampsia should the hypertension worsen during pregnancy. There are no convincing data that demonstrate that treatment of mild chronic hypertension improves perinatal outcome.

Gestational Hypertension This is the development of elevated blood pressure during pregnancy or in the first 24 h post partum in the absence of preexisting chronic hypertension and other signs of preeclampsia. Uncomplicated gestational hypertension that does not progress to preeclampsia has not been associated with adverse pregnancy outcome or adverse long-term prognosis.

RENAL DISEASE (See also Chaps. 259 and 267) Normal pregnancy is characterized by an increase in glomerular filtration rate and creatinine clearance. This occurs secondary to a rise in renal plasma flow and increased glomerular filtration pressures. Patients with underlying renal disease and hypertension may expect a worsening of hypertension during pregnancy. If superimposed preeclampsia develops, the additional endothelial injury results in a capillary leak syndrome that may make the management of these patients challenging. In general, patients with underlying renal disease and hypertension benefit from more aggressive management of blood pressure than do those with gestational hypertension. Preconception counseling is also essential for these patients so that accurate risk assessment can occur prior to the establishment of pregnancy and important medication changes and adjustments can be made. In general, a prepregnancy serum creatinine level <133 μmol/L (<1.5 mg/dL) is associated with a favorable prognosis. When renal disease worsens during pregnancy, close collaboration between the nephrologist and the maternal-fetal medicine specialist is essential so that decisions regarding delivery can be weighed in the context of sequelae of prematurity for the neonate versus long-term sequelae for the mother with respect to future renal function.

Post-Renal Transplant Successful pregnancy after renal transplantation has been reported increasingly. Predictors for success include a normally functioning transplanted kidney, absence of rejection for at least 2 years prior to the pregnancy, absence of hypertension, and preferably minimal doses of immunosuppressant medications. Pregnancies in women using cyclosporine are more likely to be complicated by renal insufficiency and/or the development of hypertension. Such patients require very careful maternal and fetal surveillance. Nearly half of these pregnancies deliver preterm, and 20% of neonates are small for their gestational age. Rejection occurs in ~10% of pregnancies, and ~15% of patients will have deterioration in their renal function that persists after delivery. While pregnancy is generally well tolerated in renal transplant recipients, controversy remains as to whether or not deterioration of graft function is accelerated by pregnancy. More aggressive management of blood pressure has been suggested in this group of patients in an effort to protect the grafted kidney.

Systemic Lupus Erythematosus (SLE)   Another subset of patients with chronic renal disease and hypertension are those patients whose pregnancies are complicated by SLE (Chap. 300). In the past, SLE was considered to be a contraindication to pregnancy. With improved understanding of the effects of SLE on pregnancy, and vice versa, and with improved pharmacologic methods for managing SLE, successful pregnancy outcome is likely. Good prognostic factors for establishment of pregnancy in the presence of SLE are as follows:

1. Disease quiescence > 6 months
2. Normal blood pressure (with or without medication)
3. Normal renal function [creatinine < 133 μmol/L (< 1.5 mg/dL)]
4. Absence of antiphospholipid antibodies
5. Minimal or no need for immunosuppressive drugs
6. Absence of prior adverse reproductive outcome

Previously a point of controversy, there is now increasing consensus that pregnancy and the postpartum period are times of increased lupus activity. In severe flares early in gestation, pregnancy termination is often recommended. If pregnancy termination is not an option, then medical therapy to manage the lupus flare should not be influenced by the pregnancy, provided informed consent for treatment is obtained from the patient. Pulsed glucocorticoid therapy, azathioprine, hydroxychloroquine, and cyclophosphamide have all been used successfully in pregnancy.

CARDIAC DISEASE ■ **Valvular Heart Disease** (See also Chap. 219)   This is the most common cardiac problem complicating pregnancy.

MITRAL STENOSIS   This is the valvular disease most likely to cause death during pregnancy. The pregnancy-induced increase in blood volume, cardiac output, and tachycardia can cause pulmonary edema in women with mitral stenosis. Pregnancy associated with long-standing mitral stenosis may result in pulmonary hypertension. Sudden death has been reported when hypovolemia has been allowed to occur in this condition. Careful control of heart rate, especially during labor and delivery, minimizes the impact of tachycardia and reduced ventricular filling times on cardiac function. Pregnant women with mitral stenosis are at increased risk for the development of atrial fibrillation and other tachyarrythmias. Medical management of severe mitral stenosis and atrial fibrillation with digoxin and beta blockers is recommended. Balloon valvulotomy can be carried out during pregnancy.

MITRAL REGURGITATION AND AORTIC REGURGITATION   These are both generally well tolerated during pregnancy. The pregnancy-induced decrease in systemic vascular resistance reduces the risk of cardiac failure with these conditions. As a rule, mitral valve prolapse does not present problems for the pregnant patient, and aortic stenosis, unless very severe, is well tolerated. In the most severe cases of aortic stenosis, limitation of activity or balloon valvuloplasty may be indicated.

For women with artificial valves contemplating pregnancy, it is important that warfarin be stopped and heparin initiated prior to conception. Warfarin therapy during the first trimester of pregnancy has been associated with fetal chondrodysplasia punctata. In the second and third trimester of pregnancy, warfarin may cause fetal optic atrophy and mental retardation. For women with prosthetic heart valves, prophylaxis against thrombosis with low-molecular-weight heparin (LMWH) is not recommended due to reports of valvular thrombosis

despite adequate anticoagulation. Prophylaxis with unfractionated heparin is recommended for this group of women.

Congenital Heart Disease (See also Chap. 218)   The presence of a congenital cardiac lesion in the mother increases the risk of congenital cardiac disease in the newborn. Prenatal screening of the fetus for congenital cardiac disease with ultrasound is recommended. Atrial or ventricular septal defect is usually well tolerated during pregnancy in the absence of pulmonary hypertension, provided that the woman's prepregnancy cardiac status is favorable. Use of air filters on intravenous sets during labor and delivery in patients with intracardiac shunts is generally recommended.

Other Cardiac Disorders   Supraventricular tachycardia (Chap. 214) is a common cardiac complication of pregnancy. Treatment is the same as in the nonpregnant patient, and fetal tolerance of medications such as adenosine and calcium channel blockers is acceptable. When necessary, electrocardioversion may be performed and is generally well tolerated by mother and fetus.

Peripartum cardiomyopathy (Chap. 221) is a rare disorder of pregnancy associated with myocarditis, and its etiology remains unknown. Treatment is directed toward symptomatic relief and improvement of cardiac function. Many patients recover completely; others are left with a progressive dilated cardiomyopathy. Recurrence in a subsequent pregnancy has been reported, and women should be counseled to avoid pregnancy after a diagnosis of peripartum cardiomyopathy.

Specific High-Risk Cardiac Lesions ■ *MARFAN SYNDROME* (See also Chap. 342) This is an autosomal dominant disease, associated with a high risk of maternal morbidity. Approximately 15% of pregnant women with Marfan syndrome develop a major cardiovascular manifestation during pregnancy, with almost all women surviving. An aortic root diameter <40 mm is considered to be associated with a favorable outcome of pregnancy. Prophylactic therapy with beta blockers has been advocated, although large-scale clinical trials in pregnancy have not been performed.

PULMONARY HYPERTENSION (See also Chap. 220)   Maternal mortality in the setting of severe pulmonary hypertension is high, and primary pulmonary hypertension is a contraindication to pregnancy. Termination of pregnancy may be advisable in these circumstances to preserve the life of the mother. In the Eisenmenger syndrome, i.e., the combination of pulmonary hypertension with right-to-left shunting due to congenital abnormalities (Chap. 218), maternal and fetal death occur frequently. Systemic hypotension may occur after blood loss, prolonged Valsalva maneuver, or regional anesthesia; sudden death secondary to hypotension is a dreaded complication. Management of these patients is challenging, and invasive hemodynamic monitoring during labor and delivery is generally recommended.

In patients with pulmonary hypertension, vaginal delivery is less stressful hemodynamically than Cesarean section, which should be reserved for accepted obstetric indications.

DEEP VENOUS THROMBOSIS AND PULMONARY EMBOLISM (See also Chaps. 232 and 244)   A hypercoagulable state is characteristic of pregnancy, and deep venous thrombosis (DVT) is a common complication. Indeed, pulmonary embolism is the most common cause of maternal death in the United States. In pregnant women, DVT occurs much more commonly in the left leg than in the right leg, due to the compression of the left iliac vein by the right iliac artery and the uterus. Activated protein C resistance caused by the factor V Leiden mutation increases the risk for DVT and pulmonary embolism during pregnancy. Approximately 25% of women with DVT during pregnancy carry the factor V Leiden allele. The presence of the factor V Leiden mutation also increases the risk for severe preeclampsia. If the fetus carries a factor V Leiden mutation, the risk of extensive placental infarction is very high. Additional genetic mutations associated with DVT during pregnancy include the prothrombin G20210A mutation (heterozygotes and homozygotes) and the methylenetetrahydrofolate reductase C677T mutation (homozygotes).

℞ TREATMENT

Aggressive diagnosis and management of DVT and suspected pulmonary embolism optimize the outcome for mother and fetus. In general, all diagnostic and therapeutic modalities afforded the nonpregnant patient should be utilized in pregnancy. Anticoagulant therapy with LMWH or unfractionated heparin is indicated in pregnant women with DVT. LMWH may be associated with an increased risk of epidural hematoma in women receiving an epidural anesthetic in labor. One approach to this problem is to switch from LMWH heparin to unfractionated heparin about 2 weeks before the anticipated delivery date. Warfarin therapy is contraindicated in the first trimester due to its association with fetal chondrodysplasia punctata. In the second and third trimesters, warfarin may cause fetal optic atrophy and mental retardation. When DVT occurs in the postpartum period, LMWH therapy for 7 to 10 days may be followed by warfarin therapy for 3 to 6 months. Warfarin is not contraindicated in breast-feeding women.

ENDOCRINE DISORDERS ■ Diabetes Mellitus (See also Chap. 323)   In pregnancy, the fetoplacental unit induces major metabolic changes, the purpose of which is to shunt glucose and amino acids to the fetus while the mother uses ketones and triglycerides to fuel her metabolic needs. These metabolic changes are accompanied by maternal insulin resistance, caused in part by placental production of steroids, a growth hormone variant, and placental lactogen. Although pregnancy has been referred to as a state of accelerated starvation, it is better characterized as accelerated ketosis. In pregnancy, after an overnight fast, plasma glucose is lower by 0.8 to 1.1 mmol/L (15 to 20 mg/dL) than in the nonpregnant state. This is due to the use of glucose by the fetus. In early pregnancy, fasting may result in circulating glucose concentrations in the range of 2.2 mmol/L (40 mg/dL) and may be associated with symptoms of hypoglycemia. In contrast to the decrease in maternal glucose concentration, plasma hydroxybutyrate and acetoacetate levels rise to two to four times normal after a fast.

℞ TREATMENT

Pregnancy complicated by diabetes mellitus is associated with higher maternal and perinatal morbidity and mortality rates. Preconception counseling and treatment are important for the diabetic patient contemplating pregnancy. Optimizing preconception glucose control and attention to other dietary needs such as appropriate levels of folate can significantly reduce the risk of congenital fetal malformations. Folate supplementation reduces the incidence of fetal neural tube defects, which occur with greater frequency in fetuses of diabetic mothers. In addition, optimizing glucose control during key periods of organogenesis reduces other congenital anomalies including sacral agenesis, caudal dysplasia, renal agenesis, and ventricular septal defect.

Once pregnancy is established, glucose control should be managed more aggressively than in the nonpregnant state. In addition to dietary changes, this requires more frequent blood glucose monitoring and often involves additional injections of insulin or conversion to an insulin pump. Fasting blood glucose levels should be maintained at <5.8 mmol/L (<105 mg/dL) with no values exceeding 7.8 mmol/L (140 mg/dL). Commencing in the third trimester, regular surveillance of maternal glucose control as well as assessment of fetal growth (obstetric sonography) and fetoplacental oxygenation (fetal heart rate monitoring or biophysical profile) optimize pregnancy outcome. Pregnant diabetic patients without vascular disease are at greater risk for delivering a macrosomic fetus, and attention to fetal growth via clinical and ultrasound examinations is important. Fetal macrosomia is associated with an increased risk of maternal and fetal birth trauma. Pregnant women with diabetes have an increased risk of developing preeclampsia, and those with vascular disease are at greater risk for developing intrauterine growth restriction, which is associated with an increased risk of fetal and neonatal death. Excellent pregnancy outcomes in patients with diabetic nephropathy and proliferative retinopathy have been reported with aggressive glucose control and intensive maternal and fetal surveillance.

Glycemic control may become more difficult to achieve as pregnancy progresses. Because of delayed pulmonary maturation of the fetuses of diabetic mothers, early delivery should be avoided unless there is biochemical evidence of fetal lung maturity. In general, efforts to control glucose and maintain the pregnancy until the estimated date of delivery result in the best overall outcome for both mother and newborn.

Gestational Diabetes   All pregnant women should be screened for gestational diabetes unless they are in a low-risk group. Women at low risk for gestational diabetes are those <25 years of age; those with a body mass index <25 kg/m², no maternal history of macrosomia or gestational diabetes, and no diabetes in a first-degree relative; and those not members of a high-risk ethnic group (African American, Hispanic, Native American). A typical two-step strategy for establishing the diagnosis of gestational diabetes involves administration of a 50-g oral glucose challenge with a single serum glucose measurement at 60 min. If the plasma glucose is < 7.8 mmol/L (<140 mg/dL), the test is considered normal. Serum glucose > 7.8 mmol/L (>140 mg/dL) warrants administration of a 100-g oral glucose challenge with serum glucose measurements obtained in the fasting state, and at 1, 2, and 3 h. Normal values are plasma glucose concentrations <5.8 mmol/L (<105 mg/dL), 10.5 mmol/L (190 mg/dL), 9.1 mmol/L (165 mg/dL), and 8.0 mmol/L (145 mg/dL), respectively.

Pregnant women with gestational diabetes are at increased risk of preeclampsia, delivering infants who are large for their gestational age, and birth lacerations. Their fetuses are at risk of hypoglycemia and birth trauma (brachial plexus) injury.

℞ TREATMENT

Gestational diabetes is first treated with dietary measures. Inability to maintain fasting glucose concentrations <5.8 mmol/L (<105 mg/dL) or 2-h postprandial glucose concentrations <6.7 mmol/L (<120 mg/dL) should prompt initiation of insulin therapy. Patients with a diagnosis of gestational diabetes will benefit from postpartum follow-up as they are at increased risk for developing type 2 diabetes.

Thyroid Disease (See also Chap. 320)   In pregnancy, the estrogen-induced increase in thyroxine-binding globulin causes an increase in circulating levels of total T_3 and total T_4. The normal range of circulating levels of free T_4, free T_3, and thyroid stimulating hormone (TSH) remain unaltered by pregnancy.

The thyroid gland normally enlarges during pregnancy. Maternal hyperthyroidism occurs at a rate of approximately 2 per 1000 pregnancies and is generally well tolerated by pregnant women. Clinical signs and symptoms should alert the physician to the occurrence of this disease. Many of the physiologic adaptations to pregnancy may mimic subtle signs of hyperthyroidism. Although pregnant women are able to tolerate mild hyperthyroidism without adverse sequelae, more severe hyperthyroidism can cause spontaneous abortion or premature labor, and thyroid storm is associated with a significant risk of maternal mortality.

℞ TREATMENT

Hyperthyroidism in pregnancy should be aggressively evaluated and treated. The treatment of choice is propylthiouracil. Because it crosses the placenta, the minimum effective dose should be used to maintain free T_4 in the upper normal range. Methimazole crosses the placenta to a greater degree than propylthiouracil and has been associated with fetal aplasia cutis. Radioiodine should not be used during pregnancy, either for scanning or treatment, because of effects on the fetal thyroid. In emergent circumstances, additional treatment with beta blockers and a saturated solution of potassium iodide may be necessary. Hyperthyroidism is most difficult to control in the first trimester of pregnancy and easiest to control in the third trimester.

The goal of therapy for *hypothyroidism* is to maintain the serum

TSH in the normal range, and thyroxine is the drug of choice. Children born to women with an elevated serum TSH (and a normal total thyroxine) during pregnancy have impaired performance on neuropsychologic tests. During pregnancy, the dose of thyroxine required to keep the TSH in the normal range rises. In one study, the mean replacement dose of thyroxine required to maintain the TSH in the normal range was 0.1 mg daily before pregnancy, and it increased to 0.15 mg daily during pregnancy.

HEMATOLOGIC DISORDERS Pregnancy has been described as a state of physiologic anemia. Part of the reduction in hemoglobin concentration is dilutional, but iron and folate deficiencies are the major causes of correctable anemia during pregnancy. Folic acid food supplementation implemented in 1998 has reduced the risk of fetal neural tube defects.

In populations at high risk for hemoglobinopathies (Chap. 91), hemoglobin electrophoresis should be performed as part of the prenatal screen. Hemoglobinopathies can be associated with increased maternal and fetal morbidity and mortality. Management is tailored to the specific hemoglobinopathy and is generally the same for both pregnant and nonpregnant women. Prenatal diagnosis of hemoglobinopathies in the fetus is readily available and should be discussed with prospective parents either prior to or early in pregnancy.

Thrombocytopenia occurs commonly during pregnancy. The majority of cases are benign gestational thrombocytopenias, but the differential diagnosis should include immune thrombocytopenia (Chap. 101) and preeclampsia. Maternal thrombocytopenia may also be caused by catastrophic obstetric events such as retention of a dead fetus, sepsis, abruptio placenta, and amniotic fluid embolism.

NEUROLOGIC DISORDERS Headache appearing during pregnancy is usually due to migraine (Chap. 14), a condition that may worsen, improve, or be unaffected by pregnancy. A new or worsening headache, particularly if associated with visual blurring, may signal eclampsia (above) or pseudotumor cerebri (benign intracranial hypertension; Chap. 25); diplopia due to a sixth nerve palsy suggests pseudotumor cerebri. The risk of seizures in patients with epilepsy increases in the postpartum period but not consistently during pregnancy; management is discussed in Chap. 348. The risk of stroke is generally thought to increase during pregnancy because of a hypercoagulable state; however, studies suggest that the period of risk occurs primarily in the postpartum period and that both ischemic and hemorrhagic strokes may occur at this time. Guidelines for use of heparin therapy are summarized above (see "Deep Venous Thrombosis and Pulmonary Embolism"); warfarin is teratogenic and should be avoided. The onset of a new movement disorder during pregnancy suggests chorea gravidarum, a variant of Sydenham's chorea associated with rheumatic fever and streptococcal infection (Chap. 121); the chorea may recur with subsequent pregnancies. Patients with preexisting multiple sclerosis (Chap. 359) experience a gradual decrease in the risk of relapses as pregnancy progresses and, conversely, an increase in attack risk during the postpartum period. Beta interferons should *not* be administered to pregnant MS patients, but moderate or severe relapses can be safely treated with pulse glucocorticoid therapy. Finally, certain tumors, particularly pituitary adenoma and meningioma (Chap. 358), may manifest during pregnancy because of accelerated growth, possibly driven by hormonal factors.

Peripheral nerve disorders associated with pregnancy include Bell's palsy (idiopathic facial paralysis, Chap. 363), which is approximately threefold more likely to occur during the third trimester and immediate postpartum period than in the general population. Therapy with glucocorticoids should follow the guidelines established for nonpregnant patients; however, acyclovir should probably be avoided, particularly during the first two trimesters. Entrapment neuropathies (Chap. 363) are common in the later stages of pregnancy, presumably as a result of fluid retention. Carpal tunnel syndrome (median nerve) presents as pain and paresthesia in the hand, often worse at night, and later with weakness in the thenar muscles. Treatment is generally conservative;

wrist splints may be helpful, and glucocorticoid injections or surgical section of the carpal tunnel can usually be postponed. Meralgia paresthetica (lateral femoral cutaneous nerve) consists of pain and numbness in the lateral aspect of the thigh without weakness. Patients are usually reassured to learn that these symptoms are benign and can be expected to remit spontaneously after the pregnancy has been completed.

Judicious use of neuroimaging procedures is reasonable during pregnancy. Some centers require that formal consent be obtained from pregnant patients before magnetic resonance imaging (MRI) scans are administered. Experimental data indicate that high-field-strength MRI may be teratogenic to rodents; however, studies in pregnant MRI technicians have failed to show any risk to the fetus, even with chronic exposure. The paramagnetic MRI contrast agent gadolinium is usually not administered, particularly during the first trimester, because it crosses the blood-brain barrier. Computed tomography scanning of the brain is also considered safe, particularly as the procedure is fast, little radioactive scatter is produced, and pelvic contents are easily shielded; iodinated contrast media should be avoided whenever possible.

GASTROINTESTINAL AND LIVER DISEASE Up to 90% of pregnant women experience nausea and vomiting during the first trimester of pregnancy. Occasionally, hyperemesis gravidarum requires hospitalization to prevent dehydration, and sometimes parenteral nutrition is required.

Crohn's disease may be associated with exacerbations in the second and third trimesters. Ulcerative colitis is associated with disease exacerbations in the first trimester and during the early postpartum period. Medical management of these diseases during pregnancy is identical to the management in the nonpregnant state (Chap. 276).

Exacerbation of gall bladder disease is commonly observed during pregnancy. In part this may be due to pregnancy-induced alteration in the metabolism of bile and fatty acids. Intrahepatic cholestasis of pregnancy is generally a third-trimester event. Profound pruritus may accompany this condition, and it may be associated with increased fetal mortality. It has been suggested that placental bile salt deposition may contribute to progressive uteroplacental insufficiency. Therefore, regular fetal surveillance should be undertaken once the diagnosis of intrahepatic cholestasis is made. Favorable results with ursodiol have been reported.

Acute fatty liver is a rare complication of pregnancy. Frequently confused with the HELLP syndrome (see "Preeclampsia," above) and severe preeclampsia, the diagnosis of acute fatty liver of pregnancy may be facilitated by imaging studies and laboratory evaluation. Acute fatty liver of pregnancy is generally characterized by markedly increased levels of bilirubin and ammonia and by hypoglycemia. Management of acute fatty liver of pregnancy is supportive; recurrence in subsequent pregnancies has been reported.

All pregnant women should be screened for hepatitis B. This information is important for pediatricians after delivery of the infant. All infants receive hepatitis B vaccine. Infants born to mothers who are carriers of hepatitis B surface antigen should also receive hepatitis B immune globulin as soon after birth as possible and preferably within the first 72 h.

INFECTIONS ■ **Bacterial Infections** Other than bacterial vaginosis, the most common bacterial infections during pregnancy involve the urinary tract (Chap. 269). Many pregnant women have asymptomatic bacteriuria, most likely due to stasis caused by progestational effects on ureteral and bladder smooth muscle and to compression effects of the enlarging uterus. In itself, this condition is not associated with an adverse outcome of pregnancy. However, if asymptomatic bacteriuria is left untreated, symptomatic pyelonephritis may occur. Indeed, ~75% of cases of pregnancy-associated pyelonephritis are the result of untreated asymptomatic bacteriuria. All pregnant women should be screened with a urine culture for asymptomatic bacteriuria at the first prenatal visit. Subsequent screening with nitrite/leukocyte esterase strips is indicated for high-risk women, such as those with sickle cell trait or a history of urinary tract infections. All women with positive screens should be treated.

Because of the association between bacterial vaginosis and preterm delivery, screening for bacterial vaginosis has been used in an effort to reduce risk. However, standard treatment for bacterial vaginosis does not reduce the risk of preterm delivery.

Abdominal pain and fever during pregnancy create a clinical dilemma. The diagnosis of greatest concern is intrauterine amniotic infection. While amniotic infection most commonly follows rupture of the membranes, this is not always the case. In general, antibiotic therapy is not recommended as a temporizing measure in these circumstances. If intrauterine infection is suspected, induced delivery with concomitant antibiotic therapy is generally indicated. Intrauterine amniotic infection is most often caused by pathogens such as *Escherichia coli* and group B streptococcus. In high-risk patients at term or in preterm patients, routine intrapartum prophylaxis of group B streptococcal (GBS) disease is recommended. Penicillin G and ampicillin are the drugs of choice. In penicillin-allergic patients, clindamycin is recommended. Recently, it has been reported that universal screening of pregnant women for GBS disease may be superior to treatment based on presence of risk factors alone.

Postpartum infection is a significant cause of maternal morbidity and mortality. While rare after vaginal delivery, postpartum endomyometritis develops in 5% of patients having elective repeat cesarean section and in 25% of patients after emergency cesarean section following prolonged labor. Prophylactic antibiotics should be given to all patients undergoing cesarean section. As most cases of postpartum endomyometritis are polymicrobial, broad-spectrum antibiotic coverage with a penicillin, aminoglycoside, and metronidazole is recommended (Chap. 148). Most cases resolve within 72 h. Women who do not respond to antibiotic treatment for postpartum endomyometritis should be evaluated for septic pelvic thrombophlebitis. Imaging studies may be helpful in establishing the diagnosis, which is primarily a clinical diagnosis of exclusion. Patients with septic pelvic thrombophlebitis generally have tachycardia out of proportion to their fever and respond rapidly to intravenous administration of heparin.

All patients are screened prenatally for gonorrhea and chlamydial infections, and the detection of either should result in prompt treatment. Ceftriaxone and azithromycin are the agents of choice (Chaps. 128 and 160).

Viral Infections ■ *CYTOMEGALOVIRUS INFECTION* Viral infection in pregnancy presents a significant challenge. The most common cause of congenital viral infection in the United States is cytomegalovirus (CMV) (Chap. 166). As many as 50 to 90% of women of childbearing age have antibodies to CMV, but only rarely does CMV reactivation result in neonatal infection. More commonly, primary CMV infection during pregnancy creates a risk of congenital CMV. No currently accepted treatment of CMV during pregnancy has been demonstrated to protect the fetus effectively. Moreover, it is impossible to predict which fetus will sustain life-threatening CMV infection. Severe CMV disease in the newborn is characterized most often by petechiae, hepatosplenomegaly, and jaundice. Chorioretinitis, microcephaly, intracranial calcifications, hepatitis, hemolytic anemia, and purpura may also develop. Central nervous system involvement, resulting in the development of psychomotor, ocular, auditory, and dental abnormalities over time, has been described.

RUBELLA (See also Chap. 177) Rubella virus is a known teratogen; first-trimester rubella carries a high risk of fetal anomalies, though the risk decreases significantly later in pregnancy. Congenital rubella may be diagnosed by percutaneous umbilical blood sampling with the detection of IgM antibodies in fetal blood. All pregnant women should be screened for their immune status to rubella. Indeed, all women of childbearing age, regardless of pregnancy status, should have their immune status for rubella verified and be immunized if necessary. The incidence of congenital rubella in the United States is extremely low.

HERPESVIRUS (See also Chap. 163) The acquisition of genital herpes during pregnancy is associated with spontaneous abortion, prematurity, and congenital and neonatal herpes. A recent cohort study of

pregnant women without evidence of previous herpes infection demonstrated that ~2% of the women acquired a new herpes infection during the pregnancy. Approximately 60% of the newly infected women had no clinical symptoms. Infection occurred equally in all three trimesters. If herpes seroconversion occurred early in pregnancy, the risk of transmission to the newborn was very low. In women who acquired genital herpes shortly before delivery, the risk of transmission was high. The risk of active genital herpes lesions at term can be reduced by prescribing acyclovir for the last 4 weeks of pregnancy to women who have had their first episode of genital herpes during the pregnancy. However, whether or not this strategy results in less viral shedding or enhanced fetal protection at delivery remains to be determined.

Herpesvirus infection in the newborn can be devastating. Disseminated neonatal herpes carries with it high mortality and morbidity rates from central nervous system involvement. It is recommended that pregnant women with active genital herpes lesions at the time of presentation in labor be delivered by cesarean section.

PARVOVIRUS (See also Chap. 168) Parvovirus infection (human parvovirus B19) may occur during pregnancy. It rarely causes sequelae, but susceptible women infected during pregnancy may be at risk for fetal hydrops secondary to erythroid aplasia and profound anemia.

TOXOPLASMOSIS (See also Chap. 198) In the United States, approximately 70% of women of childbearing age are susceptible to *Toxoplasma*. Most primary infections of toxoplasmosis in the United States come from eating undercooked meat. The diagnosis of congenital toxoplasmosis is possible through sampling of fetal umbilical blood. If there is no evidence of placental/fetal infection, single-drug treatment with spiramycin is recommended. Triple-drug therapy with spiramycin, pyrimethamine, and sulfa is recommended if there is evidence of fetal infection and the woman does not wish to terminate the pregnancy or cannot terminate it because of advanced gestational age. Prenatal treatment has been shown to reduce the number of infants with severe infection.

HUMAN IMMUNODEFICIENCY VIRUS (HIV) (See also Chap. 173) The predominant cause of HIV infection in children is transmission of the virus from the mother to the newborn during the perinatal period. Exposures, which increase the risk of mother-to-child transmission, include vaginal delivery, preterm delivery, trauma to the fetal skin, and maternal bleeding. Additionally, recent infection with high maternal viral load, low maternal CD4+T cell count, prolonged labor, prolonged length of membrane rupture, and the presence of other genital tract infections, such as syphilis or herpes, increase the risk of transmission. Breast feeding may also transmit HIV to the newborn and is therefore contraindicated in most developed countries for HIV-infected mothers. There is no clear evidence to suggest that the course of HIV disease is altered by pregnancy. There is also no clear evidence to suggest that uncomplicated HIV disease adversely impacts pregnancy other than by its inherent infection risk.

℞ TREATMENT

The majority of cases of mother-to-child (vertical) transmission of HIV-1 occur during the intrapartum period. Mechanisms of vertical transmission include infection after rupture of the membranes and direct contact of the fetus with infected secretions or blood from the maternal genital tract. In women with HIV infection who are not receiving antiretroviral therapy, the rate of vertical transmission is approximately 25%. Cesarean section and treatment with zidovudine, administered both before and during delivery, decrease the rate of vertical transmission. In a meta-analysis, zidovudine treatment of both the mother during the prenatal and intrapartum periods and the neonate at birth reduced the risk of vertical transmission to 7.3%. The combination of elective cesarean section plus zidovudine treatment reduced the risk of vertical transmission to 2%. The role of multiple drug therapy during pregnancy has not yet been established, pending safety data for the neonate.

SUMMARY Maternal mortality has decreased steadily during the past 60 years. The maternal death rate has decreased from nearly 600/100,000 live births in 1935 to 8.5/100,000 live births in 1996. The most common causes of maternal death in the United States today are, in decreasing order of frequency, thromboembolic disease, hypertension, ectopic pregnancy, and hemorrhage. With improved diagnostic and therapeutic modalities as well as with advances in the treatment of infertility, more patients with medical complications will be seeking, and be in need of, complex obstetric care. Improving outcome of pregnancy in these women will be best obtained by assembling a team of internists and specialists in maternal-fetal medicine (high-risk obstetrics) to counsel these patients about the risks of pregnancy and to plan their treatment prior to conception. The importance of preconception counseling cannot be overstated. It is the responsibility of all physicians caring for women in the reproductive age group to assess their patient's reproductive plans as part of their overall health evaluation.

FURTHER READING

HADDOW JE et al: Maternal thyroid deficiency during pregnancy and subsequent neuropsychological development of the child. N Engl J Med 41:549, 1999

HIRSCH DR et al: Pulmonary embolism and deep venous thrombosis during pregnancy or oral contraceptive use: Prevalence of factor V Leiden. Am Heart J 131:1145, 1996

INTERNATIONAL PERINATAL HIV GROUP: The mode of delivery and the risk of vertical transmission of human immunodeficiency virus type 1—a meta-analysis of 15 prospective cohort studies. N Engl J Med 340:977, 1999

MAYNARD SE: Excess placental soluble fms-like tyrosine kinase 1 (sFlt1) may contribute to endothelial dysfunction, hypertension, and proteinuria in pre-eclampsia. J Clin Invest 111:649, 2003

RIDKER PM et al: Factor V Leiden mutation as a risk factor for recurrent pregnancy loss. Ann Intern Med 128:1000, 1998

SCHRAG SJ et al: A population-based comparison of strategies to prevent early-onset group B streptococcal disease in neonates. N Engl J Med 347:233, 2002

SCOTT LL et al: Acyclovir suppression to prevent cesarean delivery after first episode genital herpes. Obstet Gynecol 87:69, 1996

SIBAI BM: Chronic hypertension in pregnancy. Obstet Gynecol 100:369, 2002

THE MAGPIE TRIAL COLLABORATIVE GROUP: Do women with pre-eclampsia, and their babies, benefit from magnesium sulfate? The Magpie Trial: A randomised placebo-controlled trial. Lancet 359:1877, 2002

7 MEDICAL EVALUATION OF THE SURGICAL PATIENT
Gerald W. Smetana

Most individuals will require surgery at some point in their lifetimes. In the United States, surgeons performed 18 million inpatient operations in 2000; ambulatory surgery accounted for a substantial number of additional procedures. Preoperative medical consultation is, therefore, a common activity for practicing internists. However, many internists may be uncomfortable in this role as the process of preoperative risk stratification is not intuitive and relies heavily on a highly specialized literature that is not common knowledge among practicing clinicians.

The role of the medical consultant is to determine the presence of known or unrecognized comorbid disease or other factors that may increase risk of morbidity or mortality from baseline and to recommend strategies to reduce the risk and optimize the patient's condition before operation. This knowledge informs the discussion of risks and benefits for the patient and surgeon. Such consultations may range from the routine evaluation of a healthy patient before minor surgery to confirmation of high risk in a moribund patient undergoing emergency surgery for a life-threatening illness. Overall morbidity and mortality from surgery is low. Studies have demonstrated surgical mortality rates of 1% across all procedures for unselected patients. Mortality for the subset of patients undergoing ambulatory surgery is substantially lower. Surgeons select patients for ambulatory surgery when the combination of a lower risk procedure and few patient-related comorbidities suggests a low risk of adverse outcomes. Mortality in this group of patients is approximately 0.01%.

The most important contributions to postoperative morbidity and mortality are cardiac and pulmonary complications; each occurs in approximately 5% of all patients undergoing an operation. This chapter will review preoperative risk assessment and risk-reduction strategies for healthy patients and for the major categories of adverse outcomes and medical comorbidities—cardiac complications, pulmonary complications, and diabetes mellitus. Two other important perioperative considerations, venous thromboembolism prophylaxis (Chaps. 232 and 244) and endocarditis prophylaxis (Chap. 109), are discussed elsewhere in this text.

ANESTHETIC PHYSIOLOGY Modern anesthesia is extremely safe. Mortality among healthy patients undergoing surgery is low; estimates range from 0.01 to 0.03%. Patient- and procedure-related factors are more important contributors to perioperative morbidity than is anesthesia itself. Inhalational anesthetic agents have predictable physiologic effects. All inhalational anesthetic agents are myocardial depressants. While not clinically significant in healthy patients, this effect leads to a dependence on cardiac preload that may cause an accentuated response to the induction of anesthesia in patients who are volume-depleted due to illness or overdiuresis or who have left ventricular dysfunction. Anesthesia leads to a decrease in lung volumes. Both vital capacity and functional residual capacity decrease by one-third in abdominal surgery. This results from diaphragmatic dysfunction, decreased mucociliary clearance, loss of sighing breaths, and depression of the ventilatory response to hypoxemia and hypercarbia. This decrease in lung volumes may lead to atelectasis and is a principal factor leading to the development of postoperative pulmonary complications.

Controversy has long existed regarding the relative safety of general versus spinal or epidural anesthesia in patients at risk for postoperative cardiac or pulmonary complications. In a recent large meta-analysis of randomized controlled trials of anesthetic technique, patients who were randomized to spinal or epidural anesthesia as a component of their anesthesia had significantly lower rates of venous thromboembolism, pneumonia, respiratory depression, myocardial infarction, or death than patients receiving general anesthesia exclusively; relative risk reductions ranged from 30 to 55%. Clinicians should recommend spinal or epidural anesthesia, when possible, for patients at high risk for postoperative medical complications.

EVALUATION OF THE HEALTHY PATIENT Given the very low risk of complications among healthy patients undergoing surgery, additional clinical evaluation only rarely identifies patients at higher than average risk. Furthermore, due to the low prior probability of adverse events, most abnormal results from potential preoperative tests are false-positive tests. These results often contribute little to the estimation of risk, may increase patient and physician anxiety, lead to additional invasive tests that carry risk, and may increase medicolegal liability due to the possibility of abnormal test results that are ignored. A careful screening history and physical examination are the most important parts of the preoperative assessment of patients who report that they are healthy.

The history should focus on symptoms that suggest the possibility of occult cardiac or pulmonary disease. Many institutions have developed simple preoperative screening questionnaires for this purpose;

several of these instruments have been validated and shown to correctly identify most patients at higher than average risk. For example, in one study of a screening questionnaire, clinical evaluation by an anesthesiologist determined that only 2% of patients had negative responses to the questionnaire yet would have benefited from a more detailed clinical evaluation. Table 7-1 lists the questions on this validated questionnaire.

It is particularly important to query the patient about exercise capacity and to determine the reason for exercise intolerance, if present. For example, one report confirmed that a patient's self-report of the inability to walk at least four blocks on level ground or to climb at least two flights of stairs predicts a twofold increase in cardiac and all serious postoperative complications. One should inquire specifically about chest pain or shortness of breath with activity and about chronic cough. The history should also include a review of medications (both prescription and over the counter), any previous operations

TABLE 7-1 Suggested Preoperative Screening Questionnaire[a]	
1. Have you ever had a heart attack?	19. Do you have a history of thyroid problems?
2. Have you ever had heart trouble?	20. Do you have diabetes?
3. Have you ever had heart failure?	21. Do you have a kidney problem?
4. Have you ever had fluid in your lungs?	22. Do you have numbness or weakness of your arms or legs?
5. Do you have a heart murmur?	23. Do you have epilepsy, blackouts, or seizures?
6. Did you have rheumatic fever as a child?	24. Have you had problems with blood clots, or excessive bleeding?
7. Do you ever have chest pain, angina, or chest tightness?	25. Do you have any other important medical problems? Please list.
8. Have you ever been treated for an irregular heartbeat?	26. Have you ever had an anesthetic? If yes, when was your last one?
9. Do you have high blood pressure?	27. Have you or any member of your family had a reaction to an anesthetic?
10. Do you ever have difficulty with your breathing?	28. Do you have arthritis or pain in your neck or jaw?
11. Do you have asthma, bronchitis, or emphysema?	29. Do you have dentures, capped or loose teeth?
12. Do you cough frequently?	30. Do you think you may be pregnant?
13. Does climbing one flight of stairs make you short of breath?	31. Have you taken prednisone, steroid medications, or cortisone-like drugs in the past year?
14. Does walking one city block make you short of breath?	32. Please list any food or medications allergies that you have.
15. Do you now or have you recently smoked cigarettes? If yes, how many packs per day? For how many years?	33. Please list any medications you are currently taking.
16. Do you have liver disease, or a history of jaundice or hepatitis?	34. Please list any operations you have had in the past.
17. Do you drink more than three drinks of alcohol per day? If yes, how many per week?	35. If this is the day of your surgery, when did you last eat or drink?
18. Do you have indigestion, heartburn, or a hiatus hernia?	36. Age: Weight: Height:

[a] Patients who answer yes to any of questions #1–8, 10–14, 16, 19–25, or 30 should receive a complete history and physical examination as part of the preoperative evaluation.
Source: From NH Badner et al: Can J Anaesth 45:87, 1998, with permission.

or important medical problems, alcohol use, the possibility of pregnancy in reproductive-age women, previous adverse responses to anesthesia or surgery, and a family history of anesthetic reactions (that might suggest malignant hyperthermia).

Age appears to be a minor risk factor for both pulmonary and cardiac complications. Most of the risk attributed to age can be explained by medical comorbidities that are more common with advancing age. In the few studies that have looked at this question, younger and older patients with a similar burden of medical comorbidities appear to have a similar risk of postoperative complications. While counterintuitive, obesity does *not* appear to be a risk factor for cardiac or pulmonary complications or perioperative mortality.

Clinicians should not routinely obtain laboratory testing before surgery. Rather, tests should be requested selectively based on patient- or procedure-related factors that predict a higher likelihood of an abnormal result that may potentially influence perioperative management. Many studies have shown the very limited value of preoperative testing (laboratory testing, urinalysis, electrocardiogram, and chest radiograph) of healthy patients. In most reports, <1% of all routine preoperative tests are abnormal and could potentially influence management; most of these can be predicted by clinical evaluation. Among patients undergoing low-risk surgery, such as cataract surgery, there is no difference in morbidity or mortality between patients who undergo routine preoperative testing and those who do not undergo such testing. When clinicians do choose to obtain preoperative tests, tests obtained within the previous 4 months may be safely used as preoperative tests, assuming there has been no change in the patient's clinical condition. Table 7-2 lists recommendations for specific tests in healthy patients based on the incidence of abnormalities that influence management and the predictive value of an abnormal test. The positive and negative likelihood ratios refer to the change in the odds of an adverse postoperative event if the test result is abnormal or normal, respectively.

CARDIAC RISK ASSESSMENT

Cardiac complications are the most important source of perioperative morbidity and may occur even in patients previously unknown to have heart disease. Therefore, an assessment of cardiac risk must be part of every preoperative medical evaluation. In general, low-risk patients may proceed without further evaluation; high-risk patients will require treatment to reduce the risk of complications regardless of the results of preoperative cardiac testing; and intermediate-risk patients will benefit most from additional testing to stratify risk before surgery.

CARDIAC RISK INDICES In most cases, one can confidently estimate risk through a careful history and physical examination and application of a cardiac risk index. The science of cardiac risk stratification began with the landmark study of Goldman and colleagues in 1977 that identified risk factors among the history, physical examination, electrocardiogram, general medical status, and type of surgical procedure. More recently, the revised cardiac risk index of Lee and colleagues has been shown to outperform the original index and other available risk-stratification tools and is now the preferred tool for initial risk stratification before noncardiac surgery (Table 7-3). This index resulted from a multivariate analysis of patients undergoing elective noncardiac surgery and includes six independent factors that predict risk of postoperative cardiac complications. As all of these factors were associated with a similar odds ratio for complications (range, 1.9 to 3.2), each factor is assigned one point in the revised cardiac risk index. Predictive factors include high-risk surgery (intraperitoneal, intrathoracic, or suprainguinal vascular procedures), ischemic heart disease, a history of congestive heart failure, a history of symptomatic cerebrovascular disease, insulin therapy for diabetes mellitus, or a preoperative serum creatinine >177 μmol/L (>2.0 mg/dL). Risk classes result from the total number of points (of six possible points). Risk increases substantially when two points exist; the greatest risk is for patients with three or more points.

Several factors that increase the likelihood of coronary artery disease (CAD) nonetheless do not increase the risk of postoperative cardiac complications. Factors that do *not* appear to increase risk include obesity, stable hypertension with a diastolic blood pressure of <110 mmHg, elevated cholesterol, bundle branch block, and cigarette smoking.

After application of the revised cardiac risk index (Table 7-3) to

TABLE 7-2 *Recommendations for Preoperative Laboratory Testing for Healthy Patients*

Test	Incidence of Abnormalities That Influence Management, %	Likelihood Ratio [+]	Likelihood Ratio [−]	Indications
Hemoglobin	0.1	3.3	0.9	Anticipated major blood loss or symptoms of anemia
White blood cell count	0.0	0	1	Symptoms suggest infection, myeloproliferative disorder, or myelotoxic medications
Platelet count	0.0	0	1	History of bleeding diathesis, myeloproliferative disorder, or myelotoxic medications
Prothrombin time (PT)	0.0	0	1.01	History of bleeding diathesis, chronic liver disease, malnutrition, recent or long-term antibiotic use
Partial thromboplastin time (PTT)	0.1	1.7	0.86	History of bleeding diathesis
Electrolytes	1.8	4.3	0.8	Known renal insufficiency, congestive heart failure, medications that affect electrolytes
Renal function	2.6	3.3	0.81	Age > 50 years, hypertension, cardiac disease, major surgery, medications that may affect renal function
Glucose	0.5	1.6	0.85	Obesity or known diabetes
Liver function tests	0.1			No indication; consider albumin measurement for major surgery or chronic illness
Urinalysis	1.4	1.7	0.97	No indication
Electrocardiogram	2.6	1.6	0.96	Men > 40 years, women > 50 years, known CAD, diabetes, or hypertension
Chest radiograph	3.0	2.5	0.72	Age > 50 years, known cardiac or pulmonary disease, symptoms or exam suggest cardiac or pulmonary disease

Note: CAD, coronary artery disease.
Source: Reprinted from Smetana and Macpherson, with permission from Elsevier Science.

stratify risk, clinicians should apply one of the established cardiac risk guidelines to determine the optimal strategy for additional testing and risk reduction strategies. Both the American College of Physicians (ACP) and the American Heart Association/American College of Cardiology (AHA/ACC) have published guidelines that suggest criteria for additional cardiac testing for selected patients before surgery and treatment strategies to reduce risk in high-risk patients. The ACP guideline is more clinically based and easier to use but does not incorporate the revised cardiac risk index, which was published after its

TABLE 7-3 *The Revised Cardiac Risk Index*

Factor	Adjusted Odds Ratio (OR) for Cardiac Complications in Derivation Cohort
1. High-risk surgery	2.8
2. Ischemic heart disease	2.4
3. History of congestive heart failure	1.9
4. History of cerebrovascular disease	3.2
5. Insulin therapy for diabetes mellitus	3.0
6. Preoperative serum creatinine > 2.0 mg/dL	3.0

Class	Number of Factors	Cardiac Complication Rates, % Derivation Cohort	Cardiac Complication Rates, % Validation Cohort
I	0	0.5	0.4
II	1	1.3	0.9
III	2	3.6	6.6
IV	3–6	9.1	11.0

Source: Adapted from Lee et al, with permission.

release (Fig. 7-1). One can use elements of the ACP guideline along with more recent data to suggest that the first step would be to apply the revised cardiac risk index. Low-risk patients (class I) undergoing nonvascular surgery may proceed without additional evaluation. Additional noninvasive cardiac testing is appropriate for intermediate-risk patients (class II) undergoing vascular surgery. All high-risk patients (classes III and IV) should receive treatment to reduce risk (discussed below).

The AHA/ACC guideline is more complicated and relies on three separate factors: (1) clinical predictors (such as those in the revised cardiac risk index; Table 7-3), (2) functional capacity, and (3) procedure-specific risks. Examples of major clinical predictors include unstable coronary syndromes, recent myocardial infarction with evidence of ischemic risk, and decompensated congestive heart failure. Functional capacity is considered poor if patients are unable to perform activities requiring expenditure of at least four metabolic equivalents (METs). Examples in daily life include climbing one flight of stairs, doing light housework, or walking at least two blocks on level ground. Procedure-specific risks go beyond the high-risk categories defined in the revised cardiac risk index to identify low- and intermediate-risk procedures. This guideline recommends noninvasive cardiac testing for any patient with at least two of the following: (1) intermediate clinical predictors, (2) poor functional capacity, and (3) high-risk surgery.

EVALUATION BEFORE VASCULAR SURGERY Cardiac risk indices are unable to identify a subset of patients at low risk for cardiac complications after vascular surgery. This is due to the observation that the risk factors for peripheral vascular disease and CAD are the same. Therefore, patients undergoing arterial surgery are much more likely to have CAD than are patients undergoing general surgical procedures such as cholecystectomy, for example. As the prior probability of CAD is higher among such patients (92% in one angiographic study), even patients with low scores on cardiac risk indices have substantial risk for postoperative cardiac complications. Additional testing is necessary to estimate risk in these patients. Pharmacologic stress tests have been used widely to estimate cardiac risk before vascular surgery. Dipyridamole-thallium testing and dobutamine stress echocardiography have been studied most extensively. The test characteristics of the two tests are similar. Each has a negative predictive value of 95 to 100% but a positive predictive value for postoperative cardiac complications of only 10 to 20% for patients undergoing major vascular operations. As the predictive performances of these two tests are similar, clinicians may consider them to be interchangeable, and the selection of one test over the other depends on local availability and expertise.

Given the low predictive value when used in unselected patients before vascular surgery, clinicians may incorporate clinical factors to identify an intermediate probability group that will benefit most from noninvasive testing. Several strategies exist; the most widely used are the "Eagle" criteria that include Q waves on the electrocardiogram, age > 70 years, angina, ventricular ectopy requiring treatment, and diabetes requiring treatment. Patients who have none of these factors have a low risk of adverse events and can proceed without further evaluation. Those with three to five factors are at high risk and need no risk refinement by further study. Those with one to two factors benefit the most from noninvasive testing.

A.

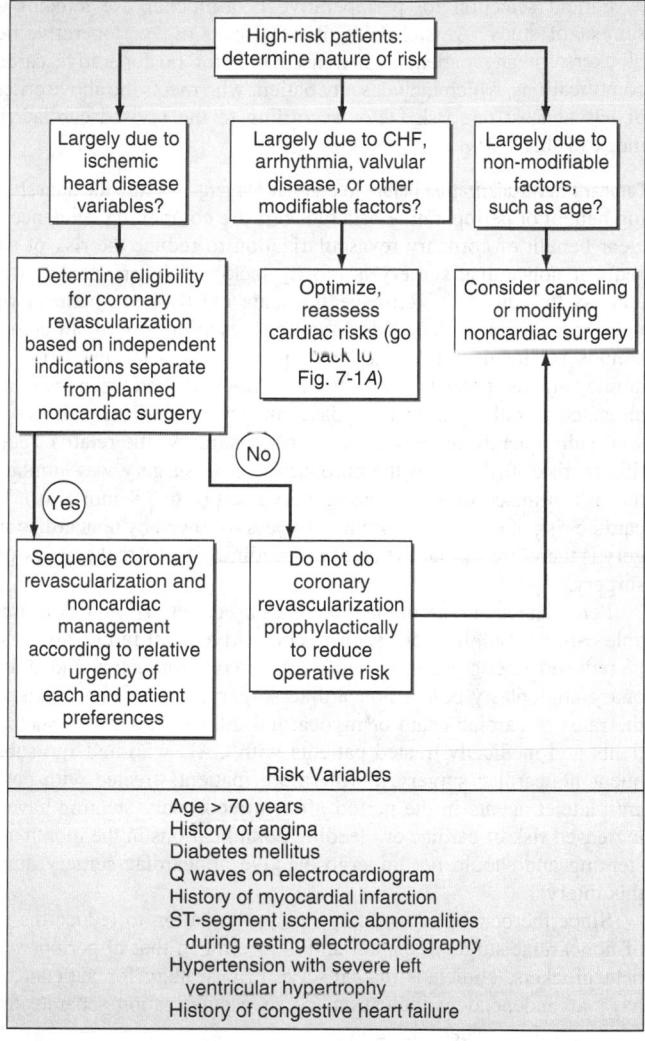

B.

FIGURE 7-1 American College of Physicians' guidelines for cardiac evaluation before noncardiac surgery. A. Guidelines for all adults facing surgery. B. Guidelines for high-risk patients. *Clinicians may use the revised cardiac risk index (Table 7-3) in place of the modified cardiac risk index for this guideline, which has been shown since the 1997 publication of the ACP guideline to be a superior tool for risk stratification. In addition, broader use of perioperative beta blockers is supported by recent studies, as described in the text. ACP, American College of Physicians; CHF, congestive heart failure; DSE, dobutamine stress echocardiography; DTI, dipyridamole-thallium imaging. (*Reprinted with permission from American College of Physicians: Ann Intern Med 127: 309, 1997.*)

STRATEGIES TO REDUCE CARDIAC RISK After identifying patients whose risk of postoperative cardiac complications is above average, one must identify interventions and strategies to reduce risk, assuming that the risk is not so high that one would consider cancelation of surgery. As a recent myocardial infarction increases the risk of adverse events, one should delay elective surgery until at least 6 months after myocardial infarction. If an operation is necessary during this interval, a functional test such as an exercise test may stratify risk and identify a subset of patients with good exercise capacity and no inducible ischemia who may consider proceeding to surgery. Active congestive heart failure increases risk, and appropriate treatment of pulmonary congestion, including diuretic therapy, will reduce this risk. One should not diurese to the point of orthostatic hypotension as this may increase the risk of hypotension with anesthetic induction.

The risk attributed to aortic stenosis is controversial. While this was an important factor in the original Goldman cardiac risk index, recent retrospective uncontrolled studies suggest that even patients with critical aortic stenosis may undergo noncardiac surgery with an acceptable degree of risk. One should evaluate the severity of aortic stenosis in all patients suspected of having symptoms caused by their valvular disease. The indication for surgical treatment of aortic ste-

nosis is the same as for patients who are not contemplating noncardiac surgery.

When risk is due to a high-risk operation, and few opportunities exist to otherwise reduce risk, clinicians may consider the possibility of an alternate lower risk procedure, if such a procedure exists.

Perioperative Beta Blockers The most important recent observation in the field of perioperative cardiac risk is that perioperative beta blockers markedly reduce the risk of cardiac complications in selected patients. Four separate large-scale randomized trials have now addressed the benefit of this intervention. In two of the trials, all patients had either known CAD or at least two of the following risk factors: age ≥ 65 years, hypertension, current cigarettes use, total cholesterol ≥ 6.2 mmol/L (≥ 240 mg/dL), and diabetes mellitus. Many patients in clinical practice would meet these broad inclusion criteria. The other trials evaluated patients undergoing vascular surgery with at least one additional risk factor or preoperative ischemia demonstrated by Holter monitoring. The results of these trials show reductions in the rate of postoperative myocardial infarction and cardiac death from 55 to 93%. The number of such patients needed to treat to prevent one event range from 2.5 to 8.3, indicating a strong effect on reducing risk.

Patient selection for perioperative beta-blocker use remains the subject of study. At this point, it is wise to use perioperative beta blockers for any patient at increased risk for postoperative cardiac complications, which includes any patient who meets the above criteria or has at least one risk factor according to the revised cardiac risk index (Table 7-3).

Coronary Revascularization Before Noncardiac Surgery

While the data showing benefit of perioperative beta blockers are compelling, evidence for clear benefit of coronary revascularization to reduce the risk of subsequent noncardiac surgery is mostly lacking. No prospective trials address this question. Retrospective data exist among patients who were recruited and studied for another reason and in whom complications for incidental noncardiac surgery were determined. For example, among patients with stable CAD who had been randomly allocated to either coronary bypass surgery or medical therapy, and who subsequently underwent noncardiac surgery, the relative reduction in risk attributed to the coronary bypass surgery was similar to the risk of the coronary bypass surgery itself (2 to 3% mortality). The cardiac risk of sequential coronary bypass followed by noncardiac surgery is therefore similar to that of proceeding directly to the noncardiac surgery.

Percutaneous revascularization fares no better. While risk of treatable cardiac complications such as congestive heart failure appears to be reduced among patients with CAD who undergo percutaneous coronary angioplasty before noncardiac surgery, no difference exists in the rates of cardiac death or myocardial infarction between such patients and medically treated patients with CAD who undergo subsequent noncardiac surgery. Furthermore, patients treated with potent antiplatelet agents in the period after intracoronary stenting have an increased risk of cardiac or bleeding complications in the month after stenting and should not undergo elective noncardiac surgery during this interval.

Since the benefit of coronary revascularization to reduce the risk of noncardiac surgery is small and is inferior to that of perioperative beta blockers, clinicians may reserve this strategy for patients who have an independent indication for revascularization separate from their need for noncardiac surgery.

PREOPERATIVE PULMONARY EVALUATION

While estimation of cardiac risk is rightfully a major focus of the preoperative evaluation, clinicians may be surprised to learn that postoperative pulmonary complications are as prevalent as cardiac complications and contribute equally to morbidity, mortality, and length of hospital stay. Therefore, estimation of the risk of pulmonary complications is a necessary part of the preoperative evaluation. Important postoperative pulmonary complications include pneumonia, respiratory failure with prolonged mechanical ventilation, atelectasis, bronchospasm, and exacerbation of underlying chronic obstructive pulmonary disease.

PATIENT-RELATED RISK FACTORS One may group risk factors for pulmonary complications into patient- and procedure-related (Table 7-4). The most important patient-related factor is chronic obstructive pulmonary disease, which increases the risk of pulmonary complications fourfold. The risk varies according to the severity of the underlying lung disease. On physical examination, decreased breath sounds, prolonged expiration, rales, wheezes, and rhonchi each predict a sixfold increase in the risk of postoperative pulmonary complications. In contrast, well-controlled asthma does not appear to increase the risk of pulmonary complications. Smoking is a risk factor even for patients with no resulting chronic lung disease; the reported relative risks for complications range from 1.5 to 4. However, patients who have reduced their cigarette use or stopped completely in the 2 months before surgery have a higher risk than current smokers. This may relate to an increase in cough and sputum production that is common in the first weeks to months after cigarette cessation.

The risk of viral respiratory infections is unknown but probably small. Bacterial lower respiratory infections, including bronchitis and pneumonia, do increase the risk of pulmonary complications. In these settings, clinicians should delay elective surgery and treat the underlying infection.

Metabolic factors shown to increase risk include renal insufficiency [BUN > 10.7 mmol/L (>30 mg/dL)] and albumin < 30 g/L (<3.0 g/dL). Poor functional capacity, known to increase risk for cardiac complications, is also a risk factor for postoperative pulmonary complications. Advanced age is a modest risk factor of approximately twofold; other patient- and procedure-related risk factors are more important than age. Surprisingly, obesity, even morbid obesity, does not increase the risk for pulmonary complications. However, obstructive sleep apnea, which is more common among obese patients, does increase the risk for airway management problems in the immediate postoperative period (such as hypoxemia and reintubation) and may increase the risk of pulmonary complications, though this latter observation is not well established.

PROCEDURE-RELATED RISK FACTORS In contrast to cardiac complications, procedure-related factors are more important than patient-related factors in predicting the risk of pulmonary complications. The most important factor is the surgical site. Risk increases as the incision approaches the diaphragm. The highest risk is for upper abdominal, thoracic, and abdominal aortic aneurysm surgery. Depending on the series, studies have shown complication of rates of 20 to 40% for these procedures. There is lower risk for lower abdominal surgery and peripheral vascular surgery. Laparoscopic abdominal surgeries carry a much lower risk of pulmonary complications (1%). Pulmonary complications are rare for surgeries outside of the chest and abdomen. Other procedure-related factors include prolonged surgical duration (>3 h), general anesthesia, emergency surgery, and the use of long-acting neuromuscular blockers such as pancuronium during anesthesia.

PREOPERATIVE PULMONARY FUNCTION TESTING (See also Chap. 234) The role of preoperative pulmonary function testing is debated. While such testing is necessary before planned lung resection (this is not the subject of this chapter), its value before other high-risk surgeries is less clear. The most commonly performed tests in this setting are simple spirometry including forced expiratory capacity in 1 s (FEV_1) and forced vital capacity (FVC). Advocates of testing suggest that clinical decision-making and patient selection for surgery may be influenced by such test results. However, most reports demonstrate that clinical factors (as described above in patient- and procedure-related risk factor sections) are as or more helpful in the estimation of risk than spirometry. Preoperative spirometry could be potentially useful were it to identify either high-risk patients who would escape clinical detection or those patients whose risk of proceeding to surgery would be prohibitive. Neither of these criteria is met.

Several reports have shown that clinical factors correctly identify

---

TABLE 7-4 *Risk Factors for Postoperative Pulmonary Complications*

Patient-Related Risk Factors	*Procedure-Related Risk Factors*
Chronic obstructive pulmonary disease	Surgical site:
	Thoracic surgery
Cigarette use < 8 weeks before surgery	Abdominal aortic aneurysm surgery
ASA class > 2	Upper abdominal surgery
Goldman class 2–4[a]	Neurosurgery
Age > 60	Peripheral vascular surgery
Dependent functional status	General anesthesia
Albumin < 3.0 g/dL	Pancuronium use
Blood urea nitrogen > 30 mg/dL	Emergency surgery
Abnormal chest radiograph	Surgery lasting > 3 hours

[a] Goldman cardiac risk index. Of four classes possible; class 4 represents the highest risk.
Note: ASA, American Society of Anesthesiologists.
Source: Reprinted from GW Smetana: Clin Geriatr Med 19:35, 2003, with permission from Elsevier Science.

patients at high risk for postoperative pulmonary complications and that there is no substantial incremental value of preoperative spirometry as a risk-stratification tool. While abnormal spirometry, in some studies, does predict risk, these patients would have been identified based on clinical criteria alone. As to prohibitive risk, it is now clear that even patients with spirometric values previously thought to represent an absolute contraindication to surgery (e.g., $FEV_1 < 1$ L or 50% predicted) can proceed to surgery with an acceptable degree of risk if the indication for surgery is compelling and if every effort is made to reduce postoperative pulmonary complications (see below). Evidence for the benefit of preoperative arterial blood gas analysis is even weaker and is based on small case series. No reports have shown that such studies are superior to clinical evaluation before high-risk nonpulmonary surgery. There is, therefore, no role for routine preoperative arterial blood gas analysis in high-risk patients.

STRATEGIES TO REDUCE POSTOPERATIVE PULMONARY COMPLICATIONS Most risk-reduction strategies follow logically from the above risk factors. One should recommend cigarette cessation for at least 8 weeks before elective surgery. Cessation for briefer periods may increase risk. Clinicians should treat patients with chronic obstructive pulmonary disease or asthma in the usual fashion so as to maximally reduce airflow obstruction. The treatment strategies are identical to those used in patients who are not preparing for surgery. Patients with asthma should be free of wheezes and have a peak flow of at least 80% of the predicted value or of personal best. Antibiotics should be reserved for patients with bacterial lower respiratory tract infection, as their indiscriminate use does not reduce risk. Intraoperative strategies include epidural or spinal anesthesia when feasible, the avoidance of pancuronium as a neuromuscular blocker in high-risk patients, and the use of shorter duration or laparoscopic procedures.

Postoperative strategies include lung expansion maneuvers and pain control. Lung expansion maneuvers reduce risk by minimizing the expected fall in lung volumes (particularly for thoracic and upper abdominal surgery) that contribute importantly to the risk of complications. These strategies include deep breathing exercises (a component of chest physical therapy) and incentive spirometry and effort-independent strategies such as continuous positive airway pressure (CPAP) (Chap. 252). Deep breathing exercises and incentive spirometry are equally effective; each reduces risk by one half. CPAP should be reserved for patients who cannot cooperate with the other maneuvers as it is more costly and carries some risk of barotrauma.

Pain control strategies decrease splinting and improve the ability to take deep breaths; they reduce pulmonary complications by these mechanisms. Epidural analgesia with local anesthetics reduces complication rates in patients undergoing abdominal, thoracic, and aortic surgery. Intercostal nerve blocks may also be beneficial, but the effect did not reach statistical significance in a large well-designed meta-analysis.

DIABETES MELLITUS (See also Chap. 323)

The most important perioperative risk attributable to diabetes mellitus is that of cardiac complications. This is due to the higher prevalence of CAD, both known and clinically inapparent, among patients with diabetes than among the general population. Therefore, the principal goal of the preparation of patients with diabetes before surgery is a careful assessment of cardiac risk, as described above. Diabetes also increases the risk of surgical wound infections. For the subset of patients with diabetic neuropathy, there is additional risk for aspiration of gastric contents during anesthesia if gastroparesis is present, and for blood pressure lability during surgery if autonomic neuropathy exists.

Strategies to control blood sugar in the perioperative period must balance the risk of hyperglycemia due to the stress of surgery and anesthesia and the need for patients to fast before surgery that may increase the risk of hypoglycemia. One achieves this balance through frequent monitoring and the use of short-acting insulin as needed to achieve blood sugar goals. Optimal perioperative blood sugars are between 120 and 200 mg/dL. Patients who are diet-controlled may proceed to surgery without additional treatment of blood sugar other than careful perioperative monitoring of blood sugar by fingerstick. Those who receive oral hypoglycemic agents should hold their medication on the morning of surgery (with the exception of metformin, which should be stopped the day before to minimize the risk of lactic acidosis). One treats these patients as needed with short-acting insulin on a sliding scale based on frequent monitoring. Intravenous fluids for oral agent– and insulin-treated patients should include glucose to decrease the risk for lipolysis and ketone production.

Controversy exists as to whether patients with insulin-requiring diabetes should be treated with a continuous insulin infusion in the perioperative period versus the conventional use of one-half of the patient's usual morning long-acting insulin dose on the morning of surgery followed by a sliding scale of regular insulin based on frequent monitoring. Patients undergoing coronary bypass grafting have a lower incidence of sternal wound infections when managed with continuous infusion insulin to achieve tight perioperative blood sugar control. Among seriously ill patients who require prolonged mechanical ventilation after surgery, intensive continuous infusion insulin to achieve near-normal blood sugars reduces overall mortality when compared to a less intensive continuous infusion insulin strategy. Until further data are available, it is reasonable to recommend continuous infusion insulin in the perioperative period for patients undergoing prolonged major surgery, cardiac surgery, or emergent surgery with metabolic abnormalities or who will require prolonged mechanical ventilation after surgery.

FURTHER READING

AUERBACH AD, GOLDMAN L: Beta-blockers and reduction of cardiac events in noncardiac surgery: Scientific review. JAMA 1987:1435, 2002

EAGLE KA et al: ACC/AHA guideline update for perioperative cardiovascular evaluation for noncardiac surgery. Executive summary: A report of the American College of Cardiology/American Heart Association Task Force on Practice Guidelines (Committee to Update the 1996 Guidelines on Perioperative Cardiovascular Evaluation for Noncardiac Surgery). Circulation 105:1257, 2002

LEE TH et al: Derivation and prospective validation of a simple index for prediction of cardiac risk of major noncardiac surgery. Circulation 100:1043, 1999

PALDA VA, DETSKY AS: Perioperative assessment and management of risk from coronary artery disease. Ann Intern Med 127:313, 1997

SMETANA GW: Preoperative pulmonary evaluation. N Engl J Med 340:937, 1999

———, MACPHERSON DS: The case against routine preoperative laboratory testing. Med Clin North Am 87:7, 2003

---

8 GERIATRIC MEDICINE
Neil M. Resnick, David Dosa

Of all the people who have ever lived to age 65, more than half are now alive. This statistic has important demographic and economic implications, and its impact on medical care is also substantial.

BIOLOGY OF AGING

Numerous molecular concomitants of aging have been described. For instance, there is an increase in chromosome structural abnormalities, DNA cross-linking, and frequency of single-strand breaks; a decline in DNA methylation; and loss of DNA telomeric sequences. The primary structure of proteins is unaltered, but there is an increase in posttranslational changes, deamidation, oxidation, cross-linking, and nonenzymatic glycation. Mitochondrial structure deteriorates, albeit not universally.

However, the biologic changes are clearer than the mechanisms that mediate them. In fact, although the senescent phenotype appears to be ubiquitous, biologists disagree about whether senescence even exists beyond zoos and civilized societies and whether it occurs at all in many species. There is little evolutionary rationale for a process that happens after reproduction is complete, particularly one associated with such a long and complex course. In nature, senescence is most notable for its absence; nearly all animals die of predation, disease, or environmental hazards rather than aging. The argument that different species have different maximum life spans can be explained without invoking a specific aging process: while growth and development are based on a genetic template, aging may reflect merely the accumulation of random damage rather than a specific mechanism.

If aging exists as a distinct process, there is consensus that the mechanisms are likely multifactorial, environmentally influenced, and species-specific, if not organ- and cell-specific, making the paucity of available human data particularly problematic. As a result, there are nearly as many theories of aging as investigators. Most theories overlap or are not mutually exclusive, and none is completely compatible with the dearth of data. As a group, the theories can be divided into two broad categories, based on whether they attribute aging to a genetic program or to progressive and random damage to homeostatic systems.

GENETIC THEORIES OF AGING   Enthusiasm for genetic theories of aging is fueled by several observations, including the dramatic species-specific differences in maximal life span, the strong correlation with survival among monozygotic compared to dizygotic twins, and the fact that single mutations can prolong life span by >50% in some nematodes, flies, and mice. However, all genetic theories must account for the fact that evolutionary selection pressure is minimal following completion of reproduction. Three genetic theories have recently been advanced, but few relevant data have yet been accrued. The first theory suggests that, since animals usually succumb to natural forces long before reaching their maximal life span, aging might reflect mutations that impair long-term survival. These mutations would accumulate in the genome because there is no selection pressure to delete them. A second theory, "pleiotropic antagonism," proposes that aging may be caused by the late and deleterious effects of genes that are conserved because of the survival advantages they confer prior to reproduction. The third theory applies to ecological niches where extrinsic hazards are relatively low. In such an environment, evolution might select for mutations that retard the aging process since these might allow an animal to produce and protect many more litters. In support of this theory, the rate of aging in an isolated clan of Virginia opossums was calculated to be roughly half of that seen in their less fortunate cousins.

The Random Damage Theories   These are based on the possibility that the balance between ongoing damage and repair is disrupted. The theories differ in the emphasis placed on increased damage (e.g., by free radicals, oxidation, or glycation) versus deficient repair, as well as in the mechanisms that might mediate each. However, all share the observation that cell and organ repair capacity declines with age. Some 40 years ago, Hayflick and Moorehead observed that the number of replications among cultured cells is finite. Subsequent research revealed that this replicative senescence was due to arrest of the cell cycle at the G_1/S phase, the point at which DNA synthesis begins. Recently, cell replication has also been linked to the length of telomeric DNA. Present at the termini of chromosomes, telomeric DNA prevents chromosomal instability, fragmentation, and rearrangement; anchors chromosomes to nuclear matrix; and provides a buffer between coding regions of DNA and the ends of the chromosomes. In addition, telomeric DNA is necessary for cell division. With each cell division, however, roughly 50 of the total 2000 base pairs of the telomere are lost. Telomeric shortening might thus result in loss of gene accessibility,

which is necessary to repair ongoing cell damage caused by metabolism. Together with cytoplasmic factors mediating arrest of DNA synthesis, telomeric shortening could also limit the cell's ability to divide and thereby replace cells lost to apoptosis.

Many mechanisms previously postulated to mediate aging have not been borne out, including the somatic mutation theory (in which aging would result from cumulative spontaneous mutations), the error catastrophe theory (in which aging would result from errors in the synthesis of proteins critical to the synthesis of genetic material or protein-synthesizing machinery), and the intrinsic mutagenesis theory (in which aging is the result of ongoing intrinsic DNA rearrangements).

To date, the only intervention known to delay aging is caloric restriction. The salutary effect of restricting caloric intake by 30 to 40% has been documented in multiple species, from single-cell organisms to rodents. In rodents, it not only increases average life expectancy and maximum life span but also delays the onset of some typical age-associated diseases as well as deterioration of physiologic systems (e.g., immune responsiveness, glucose metabolism, muscle atrophy). Moreover, its impact is evident in both mitotic and postmitotic cells, in gene expression, and in protein turnover and cross-linking. Although the mechanism is still not determined, it is specific to caloric restriction rather than to reduction of any dietary component (e.g., fat intake) or supplements with vitamins or antioxidants. Unfortunately, adequate data from primates are still limited, and the effect of caloric restriction in humans is still unknown.

PRINCIPLES OF GERIATRIC MEDICINE

Despite the biologic controversy, from a physiologic standpoint human aging is characterized by progressive constriction of the homeostatic reserve of every organ system. This decline, often referred to as *homeostenosis*, is evident by the third decade and is gradual and progressive, although the rate and extent of decline vary. The decline of each organ system (Table 8-1) appears to occur independently of changes in other organ systems and is influenced by diet, environment, and personal habits as well as by genetic factors.

Several important principles follow from these facts: (1) Individuals become more dissimilar as they age, belying any stereotype of aging; (2) an *abrupt* decline in any system or function is always due to disease and not to "normal aging"; (3) "normal aging" can be attenuated by modification of risk factors (e.g., increased blood pressure, smoking, sedentary lifestyle); and (4) "healthy old age" is not an oxymoron. In fact, *in the absence of disease, the decline in homeostatic reserve causes no symptoms and imposes few restrictions on activities of daily living regardless of age.*

Appreciation of these facts may make it easier to understand the striking increases that have occurred in life expectancy. Average life expectancy is now 18 years at age 65, 11 years at age 75, 6 years at age 85, 4 years at age 90, and 2 years at age 100. Moreover, the bulk of these years is characterized by a lack of significant impairment (Table 8-2). Even beyond age 85, only 30% of people are impaired in any activity required for daily living and only 20% reside in a nursing home. Yet, as individuals age they are more likely to suffer from disease, disability, and the side effects of drugs, all of which, when combined with the decrease in physiologic reserve, make the older person more vulnerable to environmental, pathologic, and pharmacologic challenges.

The following concepts underlie the remainder of the chapter:

1.   Disease presentation is often atypical in the elderly, especially in those >75 to 80 years old. Homeostatic strain caused by onset of a new disease often leads to symptoms associated with a different organ system, particularly one compromised by preexisting disease. For example, fewer than one-fourth of older patients with hyperthyroidism present with goiter, tremor, and exophthalmos; more likely are atrial fibrillation, confusion, depression, syncope, and weakness. Significantly, because the "weakest link" is so often the brain, the lower urinary tract, or the cardiovascular or musculoskeletal system, a limited number of presenting symptoms predominate—acute confusion, depression, incontinence, falling, and syncope—no matter

TABLE 8-1 Selected Age-Related Changes and Their Consequences

Organ/System	Age-Related Physiologic Change[a]	Consequences of Age-Related Physiologic Change	Consequences of Disease, not Age
General	↑Body fat	↑Volume of distribution for fat-soluble drugs	Obesity
	↓Total body water	↓Volume of distribution for water-soluble drugs	Anorexia
Eyes/ears	Presbyopia	↓Accommodation	
	Lens opacification	↑Susceptibility to glare	Blindness
		Need for increased illumination	
	↓High-frequency acuity	Difficulty discriminating words if background noise is present	Deafness
Endocrine	Impaired glucose homeostasis	↑Glucose level in response to acute illness	Diabetes mellitus
	↓Thyroxine clearance (and production)	↓T_4 dose required in hypothyroidism	Thyroid dysfunction
	↑ADH, ↓renin, and ↓aldosterone		↓Na^+, ↑K^+
	↓Testosterone		Impotence
	↓Vitamin D absorption and activation	Osteopenia	Osteomalacia, fracture
Respiratory	Decreased cough reflex	Microaspiration	Aspiration pneumonia
	↓Lung elasticity and ↑chest wall stiffness	Ventilation/perfusion mismatch and ↓P_{O_2}	Dyspnea, hypoxia
	Decreased DL_{CO}	Decreased resting P_{O_2}	Dyspnea
Cardiovascular	↓Arterial compliance and ↑ systolic BP →LVH	Hypotensive response to ↑HR, volume depletion, or loss of atrial contraction	Syncope
	↓β-adrenergic responsiveness	↓Cardiac output and HR response to stress	Heart failure
	↓Baroreceptor sensitivity and ↓SA node automaticity	Impaired blood pressure response to standing, volume depletion	Heart block
Gastrointestinal	↓Hepatic function	Delayed metabolism of some drugs	Cirrhosis
	↓Gastric acidity	↓Ca^{2+} absorption on empty stomach	Osteoporosis, B_{12} deficiency
	↓Colonic motility	Constipation	Fecal impaction
	↓Anorectal function		Fecal incontinence
Hematologic/immune system	↓Bone marrow reserve(?)		Anemia
	↓T cell function	False-negative PPD response	
	↑Autoantibodies	False-positive rheumatoid factor, antinuclear antibody	Autoimmune disease
Renal	↓GFR	Impaired excretion of some drugs	↑Serum creatinine
	↓Urine concentration/dilution (see also "Endocrine")	Delayed response to salt or fluid restriction/ overload; nocturia	↓↑Na^+
Genitourinary	Vaginal/urethral mucosal atrophy	Dyspareunia, bacteriuria	Symptomatic UTI
	Prostate enlargement	↑Residual urine volume	Urinary incontinence; urinary retention
Musculoskeletal	↓Lean body mass, muscle		Functional impairment
	↓Bone density	Osteopenia	Hip fracture
Nervous system	Brain atrophy	Benign senescent forgetfulness	Dementia, delirium
	↓Brain catechol synthesis		Depression
	↓Brain dopaminergic synthesis	Stiffer gait	Parkinson's disease
	↓Righting reflexes	↑Body sway	Falls
	↓Stage 4 sleep	Early wakening, insomnia	Sleep apnea
	Impaired thermal regulation	Lower resting temperature	Hypothermia, hyperthermia

[a] Changes generally observed in healthy elderly subjects free of symptoms and detectable disease in the organ system studied. The changes are usually important only when the system is stressed or other factors are added (e.g., drugs, disease, or environmental challenge); they rarely result in symptoms otherwise.

Abbreviations: T_4, thyroxine; BP, blood pressure; HR, heart rate; ADH, antidiuretic hormone; GFR, glomerular filtration rate; LVH, left ventricular hypertrophy; PPD, purified protein derivative; UTI, urinary tract infection.

what the underlying disease. Thus for the most common geriatric syndromes, regardless of the presenting symptom, the differential diagnosis is often largely similar. The corollary is equally important: The organ system usually associated with a particular symptom is less likely to be the source of that symptom in older individuals than in younger ones. Compared with middle-aged individuals, for example, acute confusion in older patients is less often due to a new brain lesion, depression to a psychiatric disorder, incontinence to bladder dysfunction, falling to a neuropathy, or syncope to heart disease.

2. Because of decreased physiologic reserve, older patients often develop symptoms at an earlier stage of their disease (Fig. 8-1). For example, heart failure may be precipitated by mild hyperthyroidism, cognitive dysfunction by mild hyperparathyroidism, urinary retention by mild prostatic enlargement, and nonketotic hyperosmolar coma by

TABLE 8-2 Life Expectancy and Number of Remaining Years Free of Dependency in Activities of Daily Living

Age	Life Expectancy[a], av		Disability-Free Years Remaining	
	Men	Women	Men	Women
65–69	13	20	9	11
70–74	12	16	8	8
75–79	10	13	7	7
80–84	7	10	5	5
≥85	7	8	3	3

[a] For independent noninstitutionalized elderly men and women in Massachusetts. Longevity and disability-free longevity are surprisingly long and must be incorporated into treatment decisions. All figures rounded to nearest year. See text for more recent data on longevity alone.
Source: S Katz et al: N Engl J Med 309:1218, 1983.

Disease severity		Compensatory mechanisms

Symptomatic		Asymptomatic

FIGURE 8-1 Even mild organ system dysfunction may cause symptoms if compensatory mechanisms are impaired. (From NM Resnick: JAMA 276:1832, 1996.)

mild glucose intolerance. Paradoxically, therefore, treatment of the underlying disease may be easier because it is frequently less advanced at the time of presentation. A corollary is that drug side effects can occur with drugs and drug doses unlikely to produce side effects in younger people. For instance, a sedating antihistamine (e.g., diphenhydramine) may cause confusion, loop diuretics may precipitate urinary incontinence, digoxin may induce depression even with normal serum levels, and over-the-counter sympathomimetics may precipitate urinary retention in men with mild prostatic obstruction.

Unfortunately, the predisposition to develop symptoms at an earlier stage of disease is often offset by two factors. First, symptoms may present later if there is functional limitation in another system. Coronary artery disease or aortic stenosis may not cause symptoms as early in patients whose mobility is compromised by arthritis. Second, a change in illness behavior occurs with age. Raised at a time when symptoms and debility were accepted as normal consequences of aging, the elderly are less likely to seek attention until symptoms become disabling. Thus, any symptom, particularly those associated with a change in functional status, must be taken seriously and evaluated promptly.

3. Since many homeostatic mechanisms may be compromised concurrently, there are usually multiple abnormalities amenable to treatment, and small improvements in each may yield dramatic benefits overall. For instance, cognitive impairment in patients with Alzheimer's disease may respond much better to interventions that alleviate comorbidity than to prescription of a cholinesterase inhibitor (Fig. 8-2). Similar approaches apply to most other geriatric syndromes, including falls, incontinence, depression, delirium, syncope, and fracture. In each case, substantial functional improvement can result from treating the contributing factors even if—as in Alzheimer's disease—the disease itself is largely untreatable.

4. Many findings that are abnormal in younger patients are relatively common in older people—e.g., bacteriuria, premature ventricular contractions, low bone mineral density, impaired glucose tolerance, and uninhibited bladder contractions. However, they may not be responsible for a particular symptom but only be incidental findings that result in missed diagnoses and misdirected therapy. For instance, the finding of bacteriuria should not end the search for a source of fever in an acutely ill older patient, nor should an elevated random blood sugar—especially in an acutely ill patient—be incriminated as the cause of neuropathy. On the other hand, certain other abnormalities must not be dismissed as due to old age—e.g., there is no anemia, impotence, depression, or confusion of old age.

5. Because symptoms in older people are often due to multiple causes, the diagnostic "law of parsimony" often does not apply. For instance, fever, anemia, retinal embolus, and a heart murmur prompt almost a reflex diagnosis of infective endocarditis in a younger patient but may reflect aspirin-induced blood loss, a cholesterol embolus, insignificant aortic sclerosis, and a viral illness in an older patient. Moreover, even when the diagnosis is correct, treatment of a single disease in an older patient is unlikely to result in cure. For instance, in a younger patient, incontinence due to involuntary bladder contractions is treated effectively with a bladder relaxant medication. However, in an older patient with the same condition but who also has fecal impaction, takes medications that cloud the sensorium, and suffers from arthritis-associated impairments of mobility and manual dexterity, treatment of the bladder spasms alone is unlikely to restore continence. On the other hand, disimpaction, discontinuation of the offending medications, and treatment of the arthritis are likely to restore continence without the need for a bladder relaxant. Failure to recognize these principles often leads to prescribing "ineffective" therapy and to unjustified therapeutic nihilism toward older patients.

6. Because the older patient is more likely to suffer the adverse consequences of disease, treatment—and even prevention—may be equally or even more effective. For instance, the survival benefits of exercise, as well as thrombolysis and beta-blocker therapy after a myocardial infarction, are as impressive in older patients as in younger ones; and treatment of hypertension and transient ischemic attacks, as well as immunization against influenza and pneumococcal pneumonia, are more effective in older patients. A proactive approach is even more effective in acute care, in which it decreases the risk of delirium by 30 to 60%. In the outpatient setting, such an approach can delay functional decline and institutionalization. In addition, prevention in older patients must often be seen in a broader context. For instance, although interventions to increase bone density may be limited in older patients, fracture may still be prevented by efforts to improve balance, strengthen legs, reduce peripheral edema, treat other contributing medical conditions, replete nutritional deficits, eliminate environmental hazards, and remove adverse medications—not so much those that affect bone metabolism, but rather those that induce orthostasis, confusion, and extrapyramidal stiffness.

In summary, optimal treatment of the older patient generally requires treating much more than the organ system usually associated with the disease or symptom, and often permits ignoring that system entirely.

EVALUATION   Evaluation of the older patient can be time-consuming, even when it is tailored to the problem. Yet, such initial investment can reduce subsequent morbidity and resource utilization and enhance patient and physician satisfaction. Additionally, the assessment can often be accomplished over several visits. Moreover, much can be gleaned from questionnaires filled out by the patient or caregiver in advance as well as from observation. For instance, greeting the patient in the waiting room allows the physician to note affective and cognitive response, the strength of the handshake, the ease of rising from a chair without using the arms, the length and steadiness of the stride, and the ability to follow directions to the examining room and to sit down safely in the examining room chair. Observing the patient dress or undress can also enhance detection of impaired cognition, fine motor skills, balance, and judgment. Such observations often provide more information than standard examinations and can shorten the clinical evaluation.

HISTORY-TAKING IN ELDERLY PATIENTS   Most older patients are able to provide a reliable medical history; however, a multitude of complaints may make obtaining a history more difficult. If the patient is unable to comprehend or communicate, data should be sought from family, friends, and caregivers. The history should also include drug and alcohol ingestion, dietary patterns, falling, incontinence, sexual dysfunction, depression, and anxiety.

FIGURE 8-2 Although young and old patients may appear to suffer equally from Alzheimer's disease, its extent in older patients is often magnified by comorbidity and drug use. Identification and treatment of these contributing factors will improve the older patient's function even though the Alzheimer's disease is inadequately treatable. CHF, congestive heart failure; COPD, chronic obstructive pulmonary disease. (*From NM Resnick, ER Marcantonio: Lancet 350:1175, 1997.*)

Advance Directives All older patients should be asked whether they have drafted advance health care directives, and, if they have, a copy should be placed in the record. Such directives may consist of a health care proxy or durable power of attorney for health care, in which patients designate a surrogate decision-maker who makes health care decisions if the patient cannot, and/or a living will or medical directive, in which patients specify their desires for treatment in specific situations if they cannot communicate at the critical time.

Whether or not the patient has formally drafted these directives, it is useful to indicate in the record who should make health care decisions if the patient is no longer able to do so. Patients should then be encouraged to discuss their thoughts with the physician as well as the designated proxy. It is not feasible to cover all possible future complications in such discussions. Ascertaining patients' perspectives on specific interventions, such as resuscitation or intubation, is also difficult because preferences will likely differ depending on prognosis. For instance, a patient may not be interested in feeding tube placement following a massive stroke with little chance of recovery but would prefer the same intervention if it is short-term and helps ensure more rapid and complete recovery from an intercurrent illness such as pneumonia. More useful is a discussion that uses open-ended questions and empathic comments to elicit the patient's values and goals. Moreover, for any given condition, preferences may differ depending on baseline clinical status. For robust elderly individuals, recovery is a realistic goal, albeit the odds of complications are higher than for younger individuals. For the frail elderly patient with comorbidity that impairs functional status, reduction or alleviation of symptoms may be the goal. For patients with advanced dementia or terminal illness, maximizing comfort may be the most appropriate strategy. In each situation, however, early elicitation of a patient's preferences and values—when the patient can still state them—can often help both physicians and families in subsequent difficult decisions by giving surrogate decision-makers the sense that they are doing as the patient would have wanted.

PHYSICAL EXAMINATION Certain features of the examination should receive special attention, depending in part on clues from the history. Weight and postural blood pressure should be measured at most visits. Vision and hearing should be checked; if hearing is impaired, excess cerumen should be removed from the external auditory canals prior to audiologic referral. Denture fit should be assessed, and the oral cavity should be inspected with the dentures removed. Although thyroid disease becomes more common with age, the sensitivity and specificity of related findings are substantially lower than in younger individuals; consequently, the physical examination can rarely corroborate or exclude thyroid dysfunction in older patients. The breasts should not be overlooked, since older women are more likely to have breast cancer and less likely to do breast self-examination. The systolic murmur of aortic sclerosis is common and may be difficult to differentiate from aortic stenosis, especially since the presence of a fourth heart sound in an elderly person does not imply significant cardiac disease, and the carotid upstroke normally increases owing to age-related arterial stiffening.

In inactive patients and those with fecal or urinary incontinence, one should check for fecal impaction. In patients with urinary incontinence—especially men—a distended bladder must be looked for, since it may be the only finding in urinary retention; perineal sensation and the bulbocavernosus reflex should also be tested. Patients who fall should be observed standing up from a chair, bending down, reaching up, walking 3 m (10 ft), turning, returning, and sitting again; abnormalities of gait and balance should be evaluated with the patient's eyes open and closed and in response to a sternal push. It should be appreciated that "frontal release signs" (e.g., "snout," "glabellar," or palmomental reflexes) and absent ankle jerks and vibratory sense in the feet may be normal in the elderly.

MENTAL STATUS EXAMINATION In addition to evaluating mood and affect, some form of cognitive testing is essential in all elderly patients, even if it involves only checking different components of the history for consistency. People with mild degrees of dementia usually retain their social graces and may mask intellectual impairment by a cheerful and cooperative manner. Thus, the examiner should always probe for content. For patients who follow the news, one can ask what stories they are particularly interested in and why; the same applies to reading, social events—even the soap operas on television.

If there is any suspicion of a cognitive deficit after this kind of conversational probing, further questioning is indicated. An examination that tests only orientation as to person, place, and time is insufficient to detect mild or moderate intellectual impairment. As a quick screen, simply assessing orientation and asking the patient to draw a clock with the hands at a set time (e.g., 10 min before 2:00) can be very informative regarding cognitive status, visuospatial deficits, ability to comprehend and execute instructions in logical sequence, and presence or absence of perseveration. For slightly more detailed examinations, many practical mental status tests are available. The most widely used is the Mini-Mental Status Examination of Folstein (Chap. 257), which provides a numerical score that can be obtained in 5 to 10 min. Regardless of the test employed, the total score is less useful diagnostically than is knowledge of the specific domain of the deficit. As a general rule, disproportionate difficulty with immediate recall (e.g., of a list of three items) suggests depression, while predominant difficulty with recalling the items 5 min later suggests dementia. For patients with deficits of attention—recognized by inability to spell simple words backwards, repeat five digits, or recite the months of the year backwards—delirium is probably present, and the accuracy of the remainder of the test is dubious. However, the test can be interpreted accurately only in the context of a comprehensive evaluation.

EVALUATION OF FUNCTIONAL CAPACITY Medical problem lists, a standard tool for assessing and following younger patients, often prove inadequate for older patients. Heart failure, stroke, and prostate cancer can describe a bedbound institutionalized person as well as a Supreme Court justice. Thus, it is essential to ascertain the patient's degree of functional incapacity owing to both medical and psychosocial problems. The functional assessment includes determination of the patient's ability to perform basic activities of daily life (ADL), which are those needed for personal self-care, as well as the ability to perform more complex tasks required for independent living, the instrumental activities of daily living (IADL). ADLs include bathing, dressing, toileting, feeding, getting in and out of chairs and bed, and walking. IADLs include shopping, cooking, money management, housework, using a telephone, and traveling outside the home. For frail patients, an assessment in the home by a trained observer may be required, but for most patients a questionnaire dealing with these activities can be completed by the family or patient. In either case, the physician must determine the cause of any impairment and whether it can be treated. Assessment should conclude with determination of the socioeconomic circumstances and social support systems.

MANAGEMENT OF COMMON GERIATRIC CONDITIONS

Diseases more common in the elderly are covered elsewhere in the text. The medical problems discussed below do not usually present as clear-cut organ-specific diagnoses and are most common in the frail elderly, especially those over 80 years of age.

INTELLECTUAL IMPAIRMENT The predominant causes of impaired mentation in older patients are delirium, dementia, and depression. Each condition is covered elsewhere in the text in detail (Chaps. 257 and 350), but their management in the elderly is discussed here.

Differentiating the causes of impaired mentation is important, but in older patients they frequently coexist. Thus, the most important first step is to search for and correct all factors that may contribute to cognitive impairment, even in patients with dementia (Fig. 8-2). Evidence of dangerous behavior should also be sought (e.g., leaving the stove on, wandering, and getting lost), and plans should be devised to deal with it. Although there is no definitive treatment for Alzheimer's disease, it is important to detect. Such knowledge allows the physician to discontinue all unnecessary medications, identify and treat new intercurrent illness, and search for alternative ways to obtain the interval history and to ensure that the patient's medications are taken correctly. In addition, the physician should help the family and patient predict and deal with the disease; indeed, the family often needs the physician's support more than the patient does.

℞ TREATMENT

Community services should be suggested as needed, including a visiting nurse, a home health aide to assist with personal hygiene, a homemaker to assist with housework, meal delivery, transportation services, day health centers, and respite care to ease the burden on family members. Support groups such as the Alzheimer's Association are often of value to the family and help them to anticipate problems. Signs of patient abuse by an overstressed caregiver should be watched for. Legal counsel should be recommended to help the patient and family devise plans for ongoing management and ultimate disposition of assets. Assessment of driving safety may be warranted and can often be completed at a driving school or rehabilitation center. Advance directives should be sought as soon as possible while the patient can still participate.

Cholinesterase inhibitors (e.g., donepezil, galantamine, and rivastigmine) can slow clinical progression and ameliorate behavior. However, they are expensive, their efficacy is modest, their utility for more than a year is largely unstudied, and their side effects (nausea, diarrhea, insomnia, dizziness, and confusion) are common, particularly at the higher dosages often needed. Thus, goals should be agreed upon prior to therapy. If they are not met within 3 to 6 months at maximum dosage, consideration may be given to discontinuing therapy. Patients should be monitored for decline when cholinesterase inhibitors are stopped, since this may point to a previously unrecognized therapeutic benefit.

Finally, abrupt worsening of mentation or the onset of disruptive behavior should always prompt a search for new illness or medication. Exacerbation of cognitive dysfunction may occur with mild infections (e.g., subungual toe abscess, vaginitis, or pressure ulcer); with "therapeutic" levels of many drugs; with use of nonprescribed drugs or alcohol; with modest abnormalities of serum sodium, calcium, glucose, or thyroxine; with mild hypoxia; with borderline nutritional deficiencies; with subdural hematoma or "minor" stroke; and with the development of fecal impaction, urinary retention, pain, or change in environment, particularly in frail older patients. However, if a cause is not found and behavior does not respond to environmental manipulation (e.g., ignoring the behavior, distracting the patient, addressing situational "triggers," and providing a calm environment), low doses of an antipsychotic medication may be helpful (e.g., haloperidol, 0.25 to 2 mg/d orally; see below). Of note, feeding tubes inserted into patients with advanced dementia do not prolong life, prevent aspiration, or promote healing of pressure ulcers.

DEPRESSION Depression of significant degree occurs in 5 to 10% of community-dwelling elderly but is often overlooked. At highest risk are individuals with recent medical illness (e.g., stroke or fracture), bereavement, lack of social supports, recent nursing home admission, or psychiatric history (including alcohol abuse). The diagnosis requires the presence of a depressed mood for at least two consecutive weeks plus at least four of the following eight symptoms: sleep disturbance, lack of interest, feelings of guilt, decreased energy, decreased concentration, decreased appetite, psychomotor agitation/retardation, and suicidal ideation. Also helpful diagnostically are a personal or family history of depression, anhedonia (loss of pleasure), and past response to an antidepressant. It is essential to bear in mind that depression in older patients is often caused or contributed to by drugs or a systemic illness. It is also important to recognize that the risk of suicide is highest in older adults. Although "subsyndromal" depression (fewer than four of the above symptoms) also causes substantial morbidity and health resource utilization, it appears to be less responsive than major depression to therapy.

℞ TREATMENT

For the hospitalized patient in whom acute depression delays recovery or rehabilitation—when correction of medical and pharmacologic contributing factors is ineffective and there is no prior history of mania or major depression—methylphenidate, 5 to 10 mg at 8 A.M. and noon (to avoid insomnia) is often very effective, with benefits discernible within a few days. For patients with major depression, there is no ideal antidepressant drug. All are about equally effective, but the side effects differ (see below and Chap. 371). Consequently, one should become familiar with more than one agent with proven efficacy in older adults (e.g., sertraline, citalopram, bupropion, venlafaxine, mirtazapine, and nortriptyline). Because of its potent anticholinergic and orthostatic side effects, amitriptyline should be avoided whenever possible in older patients. Initial low dosages should be increased slowly to avoid serious side effects; low doses of each medication (e.g., nortriptyline, 10 to 50 mg daily; desipramine, 25 to 75 mg daily; or sertraline 50 to 150 mg daily) are often effective in the elderly, especially when combined with psychotherapy. All of the selective serotonin reuptake inhibitors (SSRIs) and venlafaxine may cause hyponatremia due to the syndrome of inappropriate diuretic hormone (SIADH), and all, like the tricyclic antidepressants, may cause falls. Adverse drug reactions should not be assumed to be due to the aging process.

Treatment should be continued for up to a year after remission of the first episode of depression because relapse rates are higher in the elderly. Consideration for indefinite antidepressant therapy should be given to patients with two or more relapses. For those with psychotic depression, refractory depression, or depression where a definitive, rapid response is required (e.g., extreme frailty, actively suicidal), electroconvulsive therapy is usually well tolerated and highly effective in elderly patients.

URINARY INCONTINENCE ■ **Transient Incontinence** (Table 8-3) Because urinary continence requires adequate mobility, mentation, motivation, and manual dexterity—in addition to integrated control of the lower urinary tract—problems outside the bladder can result in incontinence.

1. *Delirium*. A clouded sensorium impedes recognition of both the need to void and the location of the nearest toilet; once delirium clears, incontinence resolves.
2. *Infection*. Symptomatic urinary tract infection commonly causes or contributes to incontinence; asymptomatic infection does not.
3. *Atrophic urethritis/vaginitis*. Atrophic urethritis/vaginitis, characterized by the presence of vaginal telangiectasia, petechiae, erythema, or friability, commonly contributes to incontinence in women and responds to a several-month course of low-dose estrogen or vaginal estrogen creams.

TABLE 8-3 Classification of Incontinence

TRANSIENT

Delirium/confusional state
Infection—urinary (symptomatic)
Atrophic urethritis/vaginitis
Pharmaceuticals
Psychological, especially depression
Excessive urine output (e.g., CHF, hyperglycemia)
Restricted mobility
Stool impaction

ESTABLISHED

Detrusor overactivity
Detrusor underactivity
Urethral obstruction
Urethral incompetence

Note: CHF, congestive heart failure.
Source: Adapted from NM Resnick: Medical Grand Rounds 3:281, 1984.

4. *Pharmaceutical*. The drugs most commonly causing transient incontinence are listed in Table 8-4.

5. *Psychological*. Depression and psychosis are uncommon but treatable causes.

6. *Excess urine output*. Excess urine output may overwhelm the ability to reach a toilet in time. Causes include diuretics, alcohol, excess fluid intake, and metabolic abnormalities (e.g., hyperglycemia, hypercalcemia, diabetes insipidus); nocturnal incontinence may also result from mobilization of peripheral edema.

7. *Restricted mobility*. If mobility cannot be improved, access to a urinal or commode may restore continence. (See "Immobility," below.)

8. *Stool impaction*. This is a common cause of urinary incontinence, especially in hospitalized or immobile patients. Although the mechanism is unknown, a clue to its presence is the coexistence of both urinary and fecal incontinence. Disimpaction restores continence.

Established Incontinence (Table 8-3) The causes of established incontinence include irreversible functional deficits, such as *end-stage* Alzheimer's disease, and intrinsic lower urinary tract dysfunction. Lower urinary tract dysfunction should be sought after transient causes have been excluded.

DETRUSOR OVERACTIVITY This disorder (involuntary bladder contraction) accounts for two-thirds of geriatric incontinence in both sexes, regardless of whether patients are demented. Detrusor overactivity can be diagnosed presumptively in a woman when leakage occurs in the absence of stress maneuvers or urinary retention and is preceded by the abrupt onset of an intense urge to urinate that cannot be forestalled. In men, the symptoms are similar, but since detrusor overactivity often coexists with urethral obstruction, urodynamic testing should be done if prescription of a bladder relaxant is planned. Because detrusor overactivity may also be due to bladder stones or tumor, the abrupt onset of otherwise unexplained urge incontinence—especially if accompanied by perineal/suprapubic discomfort or sterile hematuria—should prompt cystoscopy and cytologic examination.

℞ TREATMENT

The cornerstone of treatment is behavioral therapy with or without biofeedback. Patients without dementia are instructed to void every 1 to 2 h (while awake only) and to suppress urgency in between; once daytime continence is restored, the interval between voiding can be progressively increased. Demented patients are "prompted" to void at similar intervals. When drugs are necessary, they should be added to these regimens and monitored to avoid inducing urinary retention. Effective drugs include oxybutynin (2.5 to 5 mg three or four times daily, or sustained release, 5 to 20 mg once daily) and tolterodine (1 to 2 mg twice daily or 2 to 4 mg once daily). If prescribed for older patients, desmopressin should be used cautiously—especially in the setting of renal insufficiency or heart failure—and it probably should not be given to patients with hyponatremia or urine output >2500 mL/d. Alternative treatments, such as neuromodulation, botulinum toxin injections, and stem cell therapy, are under investigation.

Indwelling catheterization is rarely indicated for detrusor overactivity. If all measures fail, an external collection device or protective pad or undergarment may be required.

STRESS INCONTINENCE This disorder, the second most common cause of established incontinence in older women (it is rare in men), is characterized by symptoms and evidence of *instantaneous* leakage of urine in response to stress. Leakage is worse or occurs only during the day unless another abnormality (e.g., detrusor overactivity) is also present. On examination, with the bladder full and the perineum relaxed, instantaneous leakage upon coughing strongly suggests stress incontinence, especially if it reproduces symptoms and if urinary retention has been excluded by a postvoiding residual determination; a several-second delay suggests that leakage is instead caused by an involuntary bladder contraction induced by coughing.

℞ TREATMENT

Surgery is the most effective treatment. For women who can comply indefinitely, pelvic muscle exercises are an option for mild to moderate stress incontinence, but they often require specialized training using vaginal cones or biofeedback. Occasionally, a pessary or even a tampon (for women with vaginal stenosis) provides some relief.

URETHRAL OBSTRUCTION Rarely present in women, urethral obstruction (due to prostatic enlargement, urethral stricture, bladder neck contracture, or prostate cancer) is the second most common cause of established incontinence in older men. It can present as dribbling incontinence after voiding, urge incontinence due to detrusor overactivity (which coexists in two-thirds of cases), or overflow incontinence due to urinary retention. Renal ultrasound is recommended to exclude hydronephrosis in men whose postvoiding residual volume exceeds 100 to 200 mL; in older men for whom surgery is planned, urodynamic confirmation of obstruction is strongly advised.

TABLE 8-4 *Commonly Used Medications That May Affect Continence*

Type of Medication	Examples	Potential Effects on Continence
Sedatives/hypnotics	Long-acting benzodiazepines (e.g., diazepam, flurazepam)	Sedation, delirium, immobility
Alcohol		Polyuria, frequency, urgency, sedation, delirium, immobility
Anticholinergics	Dicyclomine, disopyramide, sedating antihistamines	Urinary retention, overflow incontinence, delirium, impaction
Antipsychotics	Thioridazine, haloperidol	Anticholinergic actions, sedation, rigidity, immobility
Tricyclic antidepressants	Amitriptyline, desipramine	Anticholinergic actions, sedation
Antiparkinsonians	Trihexyphenidyl, benztropine mesylate (not L-dopa/selegiline)	Anticholinergic actions, sedation
Narcotic analgesics	Opiates	Urinary retention, fecal impaction, sedation, delirium
α-Adrenergic antagonists	Prazosin, terazosin, doxazosin	Urethral relaxation may precipitate stress incontinence in women
α-Adrenergic agonists	Nasal decongestants	Urinary retention in men
Calcium channel blockers	All dihydropyridines[a]	Urinary retention; nocturnal diuresis due to fluid retention
Potent diuretics	Furosemide, bumetanide	Polyuria, frequency, urgency
Angiotensin-converting enzyme inhibitors	Captopril, enalapril, lisinopril	Drug-induced cough can precipitate stress incontinence in women and in some men with prior prostatectomy
Thiazolidinediones	Rosiglitazone	Nocturnal diuresis due to fluid retention
Cyclooxygenase 2 selective NSAIDs	Rofecoxib, celecoxib	Nocturnal diuresis due to fluid retention
Vincristine		Urinary retention

[a] Examples include nifedipine, nicardipine, israpidine, felodipine, nimodipine.
Source: Adapted from NM Resnick, in *Current Medical Diagnosis and Treatment*, LT Tierney et al (eds), Norwalk, Appleton & Lange, 1993.

TABLE 8-5 *Intrinsic Risk Factors for Falling, and Possible Interventions*

Risk Factor	Interventions	
	Medical	*Rehabilitative or Environmental*
Reduced visual acuity, dark adaptation, and perception	Refraction; cataract extraction	Home safety assessment
Reduced hearing	Removal of cerumen; audiologic evaluation	Hearing aid if appropriate (with training); reduction in background noise
Vestibular dysfunction	Avoidance of drugs affecting the vestibular system; neurologic or ear, nose, and throat evaluation, if indicated	Habituation exercises
Proprioceptive dysfunction, cervical degenerative disorders, and peripheral neuropathy	Screening for vitamin B_{12} deficiency and cervical spondylosis	Balance exercises; appropriate walking aid; correctly sized footwear with firm soles; home safety assessment
Dementia	Detection of reversible causes; avoidance of sedative or centrally acting drugs	Supervised exercise and ambulation; home safety assessment
Musculoskeletal disorders	Appropriate diagnostic evaluation	Balance-and-gait training; muscle-strengthening exercises; appropriate walking aid; home safety assessment
Foot disorders (calluses, bunions, deformities, edema)	Shaving of calluses; bunionectomy; treatment of edema	Trimming of nails; appropriate footwear
Postural hypotension	Assessment of medications; rehydration; possible alteration in situational factors (e.g., meals, change of position)	Dorsiflexion exercises; pressure-graded stockings; elevation of head of bed; use of tilt table if condition is severe
Use of medications (sedatives: benzodiazepines, phenothiazines, antidepressants; antihypertensives; others: antiarrhythmics, anticonvulsants, diuretics, alcohol)	Steps to be taken: 1. Attempted reduction in the total number of medications taken 2. Assessment of risks and benefits of each medication 3. Selection of medication, if needed, that is least centrally acting, least associated with postural hypotension, and has shortest action 4. Prescription of lowest effective dose 5. Frequent reassessment of risks and benefits	

Source: After ME Tinetti and M Speechley, N Engl J Med 320:1055, 1989.

℞ TREATMENT

Surgical decompression is the most effective treatment for obstruction, especially if there is urinary retention. For a nonoperative candidate, intermittent or indwelling catheterization is used; a condom catheter is contraindicated when urinary retention is present. For a man with prostatic obstruction who is not in retention, treatment with an α-adrenergic antagonist (e.g., terazosin, 5 to 10 mg daily, or tamsulosin, 0.4 to 0.8 mg daily) may lessen symptoms in a few weeks. The 5α-reductase inhibitor finasteride may ameliorate symptoms in a third or more of patients, but its impact is less and not apparent for many months. Combined treatment with finasteride and either terazosin or tamsulosin has proved no better than treatment with an alpha blocker alone in most men.

DETRUSOR UNDERACTIVITY Whether idiopathic or due to sacral lower motor nerve dysfunction, this is the least common cause of incontinence (<10% of cases). When it causes incontinence, detrusor underactivity is associated with urinary frequency, nocturia, and frequent leakage of small amounts. The elevated postvoiding residual volume (generally >450 mL) distinguishes it from detrusor overactivity and stress incontinence, but only urodynamic testing (rather than cystoscopy or intravenous urography) differentiates it from urethral obstruction in

℞ TREATMENT

For the patient with a poorly contractile bladder, augmented voiding techniques (e.g., double voiding or applying suprapubic pressure) are often effective; pharmacologic agents (e.g., bethanechol) are rarely effective. If further emptying is needed or for the patient with an acontractile bladder, intermittent or indwelling catheterization is the only option. Antibiotics should be used for symptomatic upper tract infection, or as prophylaxis for recurrent symptomatic infections only in a patient using intermittent catheterization; they should not be used as prophylaxis with an indwelling catheter.

FALLS Falls are a major problem for elderly people, especially women. Some 30% of community-dwelling elderly individuals fall each year, and the proportion increases with age. Nonetheless, falling must *not* be viewed as accidental, inevitable, or untreatable.

Causes of Falls Balance and ambulation require a complex interplay of cognitive, sensory, neuromuscular, and cardiovascular function and the ability to adapt rapidly to an environmental challenge. With age, balance becomes impaired and sway increases. The resulting vulnerability predisposes the older person to fall when challenged by an additional insult to *any* of these systems. Thus, a seemingly minor fall may be due to a serious problem, such as pneumonia or a myocardial infarction.

Much more commonly, however, falls are due to the complex interaction between a variably impaired patient and an environmental challenge. While a warped floorboard may pose little problem for a vigorous, unmedicated, alert person, it may be sufficient to precipitate a fall and hip fracture in the patient with impaired vision, strength, balance, or cognition. Thus, falls in older people are rarely due to a single cause, and effective prevention entails a comprehensive assessment of the patient's intrinsic deficits (usually diseases and medications), the routine activities, and the environmental obstacles.

Intrinsic deficits are those that impair sensory input, judgment, blood pressure regulation, reaction time, and balance and gait (Table 8-5). Medications and alcohol use are among the most common, significant, and reversible causes of falling. Other treatable contributors include postprandial hypotension (which peaks 30 to 60 min after a meal), insomnia, urinary urgency, foot problems, and peripheral edema [which can burden impaired leg strength and gait with an additional 2 to 5 kg (5 to 10 lb)].

Environmental obstacles are listed in Table 8-6. Since most falls occur in or around the home, a visit by a visiting nurse, physical therapist, or physician often reaps substantial dividends.

Complications of Falls and Treatment One out of four people who fall suffers serious injury. About 5% of falls result in fractures, and an equal proportion cause serious soft tissue damage. Falls are the sixth leading cause of death for older people and a contributing factor in

Environmental Area or Factor	Objective and Recommendations
All areas	
Lighting	Adequacy of illumination (older people need twice as much as younger people); absence of glare and shadows; accessible switches at room entrances; night light in bedroom, hall, bathroom
Floors	Nonskid backing for throw rugs; carpet edges tacked down; carpets with shallow pile; nonskid wax on floors; cords out of walking path; small objects (e.g., clothes, shoes) off floor
Stairs	Lighting sufficient, with switches at top and bottom of stairs; securely fastened bilateral handrails that stand out from wall; top and bottom steps marked with bright, contrasting tape; stair rises of no more than 6 in; steps in good repair; no objects stored on steps
Kitchen	Items stored so that reaching up and bending over are not necessary; secure step stool available if climbing is necessary; firm, nonmovable table
Bathroom	Grab bars for tub, shower, and toilet; nonskid decals or rubber mat in tub or shower; shower chair with handheld shower; nonskid rugs; raised toilet seat; door locks removed to ensure access in an emergency
Yard and entrances	Repair of cracks in pavement, holes in lawn; removal of rocks, tools, and other tripping hazards; well-lit walkways, free of ice and wet leaves; stairs and steps as above
Institutions	All the above; bed at proper height (not too high or low); spills on floor cleaned up promptly; appropriate use of walking aids and wheelchairs
Footwear	Shoes with firm, nonskid, nonfriction soles; low heels (unless person is accustomed to high heels); avoidance of walking in stocking feet or loose slippers

Source: After ME Tinetti and M Speechley, N Engl J Med 320:1055, 1989.

40% of admissions to nursing homes. Resultant hip problems and fear of falls are major causes of loss of independence.

Subdural hematoma is a treatable but easily overlooked complication of falls that must be considered in any elderly patient presenting with new neurologic signs, including confusion alone, even in the absence of a headache. Dehydration, electrolyte imbalance, pressure sores, rhabdomyolysis, and hypothermia may also occur and endanger the patient's life following a fall.

The risk of falling is related to the number of contributory conditions. Because the relationship is multiplicative rather than additive, however, even minor improvement in a number of these factors will reduce the risk substantially. In addition, gait training by a physical therapist often alleviates fear of falling. For those willing to wear them, hip pads have proved effective in two European trials, but the efficacy and acceptability of pads available in the United States are not yet established. Ensuring the availability of phones at floor level, a portable phone, or a lightweight radio call system is also important, as is detection and treatment of osteoporosis.

IMMOBILITY The main causes of immobility are weakness, stiffness, pain, imbalance, and psychological problems. Weakness may result from disuse of muscles, malnutrition, electrolyte disturbances, anemia, neurologic disorders, or myopathies. The most common cause of stiffness in the elderly is osteoarthritis; however, Parkinson's disease, rheumatoid arthritis, gout, pseudogout, and antipsychotic drugs such as haloperidol may also contribute. Pain, whether from bone (e.g., osteoporosis, osteomalacia, Paget's disease, metastatic bone cancer, trauma), joints (e.g., osteoarthritis, rheumatoid arthritis, gout), bursa (e.g., polymyalgia rheumatica, intermittent claudication, or "pseudoclaudication"), or foot problems may immobilize the patient.

Imbalance and fear of falling are major causes of immobilization. Imbalance may result from general debility, neurologic causes (e.g., stroke; loss of postural reflexes; peripheral neuropathy due to diabetes mellitus, alcohol, or malnutrition; and vestibulocerebellar abnormalities), orthostatic or postprandial hypotension, or drugs (e.g., diuretics, antihypertensives, neuroleptics, and antidepressants) or may occur following prolonged bed rest. Psychological conditions such as severe anxiety or depression may also contribute to immobilization.

Consequences In addition to thrombophlebitis and pulmonary embolus, there are multiple hazards of bed rest in the elderly. Deconditioning of the cardiovascular system occurs within days and involves fluid shifts, fluid loss, decreased cardiac output, decreased peak oxygen uptake, and increased resting heart rate. Striking changes also occur in skeletal muscle. At the cellular level, intracellular ATP and glycogen concentrations decrease, rates of protein degradation increase, and contractile velocity and strength decline, while at the whole-muscle level, atrophy, weakness, and shortening are seen. Pressure sores are another serious complication; mechanical pressure, moisture, friction, and shearing forces all predispose to their development. As a result, within days of being confined to bed, the risk of postural hypotension, falls, and skin breakdown rises. Moreover, these changes usually take weeks to months to reverse.

℞ TREATMENT

The most important step is preventive—to avoid bedrest whenever possible. When it cannot be avoided, several measures can be employed to minimize its consequences. Patients should be positioned as close to the upright position as possible several times daily. Range-of-motion exercises should begin immediately, and the skin over pressure points should be inspected frequently. Isometric and isotonic exercises should be performed while the patient is in bed, and whenever possible patients should assist their own positioning, transferring, and self-care. As mobility becomes feasible, graduated ambulation should begin. For individuals confined to a wheelchair, ring-shaped devices ("donuts") should not be used to prevent pressure ulcers since they cause venous congestion and edema and actually increase the risk.

If a pressure ulcer develops, therapy depends on its stage. Stage 1 ulcers are characterized by nonblanchable erythema of intact skin; stage 2 lesions involve an ulcer of the epidermis, dermis, or both; stage 3 ulcers extend to the subcutaneous tissue; and stage 4 lesions involve muscle, bone, and/or the supporting tissues. For stage 1 lesions, eliminating excess pressure and ensuring adequate nutrition and hygiene are sufficient. For the remaining types, the caregiver must also ensure that the wound stays clean and moist; thus, if saline dressings are used they should be changed when they are damp rather than dry. Synthetic dressings are more expensive than saline but are more effective because they require fewer changes (with less disruption of reepithelialization) and protect against contamination. Because bacterial colonization of pressure ulcers is universal, swab cultures should not be performed and topical treatment should be considered only for patients whose ulcers have not healed after 2 weeks of therapy. By contrast, associated cellulitis, osteomyelitis, or sepsis requires systemic therapy after cultures of blood and the wound border (by needle aspiration or biopsy) have been obtained. Surgical or enzymatic debridement is required for stage 3 and 4 lesions. In addition to a daily multivitamin, prescribing vitamin C (500 mg twice daily) is also useful. For debilitated patients, special mattresses are beneficial, including those that reduce pressure (e.g., static air mattress or foam) and those that relieve it (e.g., dynamic units that sequentially inflate and deflate).

In addition to treating all identified factors that contribute to immobility, consultation with a physical therapist should be sought. Installing handrails, lowering the bed, and providing chairs of proper height with arms and rubber skid guards may allow the patient to be safely mobile in the home. A properly fitted cane or walker may be helpful.

IATROGENIC DRUG REACTIONS   For several reasons, older patients are two or three times more likely to have adverse drug reactions (Chap. 3). Drug clearance is often markedly reduced. This is due to a decrease in renal plasma flow and glomerular filtration rate and a reduced hepatic clearance. The last is due to a decrease in activity of the drug-metabolizing microsomal enzymes and an overall decline in blood flow to the liver with aging. The volume of distribution of drugs is also affected, since the elderly have a decrease in total-body water and a relative increase in body fat. Thus, water-soluble drugs become more concentrated, and fat-soluble drugs have longer half-lives. In addition, serum albumin levels decline, particularly in sick patients, so that there is a decrease in protein binding of some drugs (e.g., warfarin, phenytoin), leaving more free (active) drug available. Thus, a lower/total serum drug level, as assessed by routine assays, may be an appropriate level in older patients.

In addition to impaired drug clearance, which alters pharmacokinetics, older patients have altered responses to similar serum drug levels, a phenomenon known as *altered pharmacodynamics*. They are more sensitive to some drugs (e.g., opiates, anticoagulants) and less sensitive to others (e.g., β-adrenergic agents). Finally, the older patient with multiple chronic conditions is likely to be taking several drugs, including nonprescribed agents. Thus, adverse drug reactions and dosage errors are more likely to occur, especially if the patient has visual, hearing, or memory deficits. Nonetheless, because undertreatment of older patients is as problematic as overtreatment, these caveats should not deter prescription of appropriate therapy.

Precautions to Avoid Drug Toxicity   ■   *DRUG SELECTION AND ADMINISTRATION*
Before initiating treatment, the physician should first ensure that the symptom requiring treatment is not itself due to another drug. For example, antipsychotic agents can cause symptoms that mimic depression (flat affect, restlessness, and pacing); such symptoms should prompt lowering of the dose rather than initiation of an antidepressant. In addition, drug therapy should be employed only after nonpharmacologic means have been considered or tried and only when the benefit clearly outweighs the risk.

Once pharmacotherapy has been decided upon, it should begin at less than the usual adult dosage and the dose should be increased slowly. However, given the marked variability in pharmacokinetics and pharmacodynamics in the elderly, dose escalation should continue until either a successful endpoint is reached or an intolerable side effect is encountered. The final dosage schedule should be kept as simple as possible, and the number of pills should be kept as low as possible. Serum drug levels are often useful in older patients, especially for monitoring drugs with narrow therapeutic indices such as phenytoin, theophylline, quinidine, aminoglycosides, lithium, and psychotropic agents such as nortriptyline. However, toxicity can occur even with "normal" therapeutic levels of some drugs (e.g., digoxin, phenytoin). Potential drug interactions should be searched for at every visit.

Over-the-Counter Agents   Nearly three-quarters of the elderly regularly use nonprescribed drugs, many of which cause significant symptoms and/or interact with other medications. Frequent offenders include nonprescribed agents for insomnia (most of which are anticholinergics), and nonsteroidal anti-inflammatory drugs (NSAIDs), which can hamper control of hypertension in addition to causing renal dysfunction and gastrointestinal bleeding. Gingko biloba, increasingly used as a "memory booster," may interfere with previously stable anticoagulation regimens. Because older patients often consider such agents "nostrums" rather than drugs, the physician must ask about them directly.

Sedative-Hypnotics   If nonpharmacologic treatment of insomnia is unsuccessful, low-dose and short-term or intermittent use of an intermediate-acting agent whose metabolism is not affected by age (e.g., oxazepam, 10 to 30 mg/d) may be useful. Because of the increased risk of confusion and other adverse effects, benzodiazepines with either short (e.g., triazolam) or long duration of action (e.g., flurazepam

and diazepam) should be avoided. Barbiturates should be avoided for the same reasons. A tricyclic antidepressant should not be prescribed for insomnia unless the patient is depressed.

Antibiotics   Serum creatinine is not a good index of renal function in old people; however, when it is elevated, special care must be taken with the administration of drugs normally excreted by the kidneys. Concentrations of relevant antibiotics should be measured directly.

Cardiac Drugs   In older patients, digitalis, procainamide, and quinidine have prolonged half-lives and narrow therapeutic windows; toxicity is common at the usual dosages. For example, digoxin toxicity—especially anorexia, confusion, or depression—can occur even with therapeutic digoxin levels.

H$_2$ Receptor Antagonists   Most of these agents interfere with hepatic metabolism of other drugs, and all can produce confusion in the elderly. Because they are renally excreted, lower doses should be used to minimize the risk of toxicity in older individuals.

Antipsychotics and Tricyclic Antidepressants   These drugs can produce anticholinergic side effects in old people (e.g., confusion, urinary retention, constipation, dry mouth). These can be minimized by switching to a nonanticholinergic agent (e.g., sertraline or citalopram) or one with less anticholinergic effect (e.g., olanzapine, nortriptyline). In general, the least potent agents for psychosis (e.g., chlorpromazine) have the most sedating and anticholinergic effects and are the most likely to induce postural hypotension. By contrast, the most potent antipsychotic agents (e.g., haloperidol) have the least sedating, anticholinergic, and hypotensive side effects but cause extrapyramidal side effects, including dystonia, akathisia, rigidity, and tardive dyskinesia. The newer potent antipsychotics (e.g., risperidone, olanzapine, quetiapine, and clozapine) are relative exceptions to this rule. More specific for serotonin than dopamine D$_2$ receptors, these medications may be safer for older demented patients, especially those with hallucinations associated with Lewy body dementia or in those receiving therapy for Parkinson's disease. Unfortunately, even these newer drugs lose their specificity at the higher doses that are commonly required in clinical practice. Thus all of these agents are potentially toxic. Moreover, since both depression and agitation often remit spontaneously, cautious discontinuation of these drugs should be considered periodically.

Glaucoma Medications   Both topical beta blockers and carbonic anhydrase inhibitors can cause systemic side effects. The latter can cause malaise and anorexia independent of the induced metabolic acidosis.

Anticoagulants   Elderly patients benefit from anticoagulation as much as do younger individuals but are more vulnerable to serious bleeding and drug interactions. Hence, more careful monitoring and aiming for the lower boundary of the therapeutic window are advisable.

Analgesics   Both propoxyphene and meperidine are associated with a disproportionate risk of delirium, and propoxyphene also increases the risk of hip fracture. Of the NSAIDs, indomethacin is most likely to induce confusion, fluid retention, and gastrointestinal bleeding. Each of these agents should be avoided in the elderly. Cyclooxygenase 2 (COX-2) inhibitors are safer than nonselective NSAIDs for older adults. However, they are more expensive and can cause fluid retention with consequent worsening of hypertension and nocturnal incontinence.

Avoidance of Overtreatment   Drugs are frequently not indicated in some common clinical situations. For instance, antibiotics need not be given for asymptomatic bacteriuria unless obstructive uropathy, other anatomic abnormalities, or stones are also present. Ankle edema is often due to venous insufficiency, drugs such as NSAIDs or some calcium antagonists, or even inactivity or malnutrition in chairbound patients. Diuretics are usually not indicated unless edema is associated with heart failure. Fitted, pressure gradient stockings are often helpful. For claudication, regular exercise should be prescribed before cilostazol. Finally, since older patients generally tolerate aspirin and other NSAIDs less well than do younger patients, localized pain should be treated when possible with local measures such as injection, physical therapy, heat, ultrasound, or transcutaneous electrical stimulation (Chap. 11).

PREVENTION

Much can be done to prevent the progression and even the onset of disease in older persons. Even when the relative benefit of an intervention is less than in younger adults, its absolute impact is often greater in the elderly because their baseline risk is higher. However, while reductions of mortality and morbidity are valuable goals for older adults, prevention must also encompass preservation of function and quality of life. Moreover, because preventive interventions are often associated with discomfort, risk, and expense, it is important to ensure that the patient believes the benefit is worth the effort.

Certain recommendations are straightforward. Dietary inadequacies should be corrected. Daily calcium intake should approximate 1500 mg, and most elderly people should take 400 to 800 IU of vitamin D daily (contained in one to two multivitamin tablets). Tobacco and alcohol use should be minimized, since the benefits of discontinuing these accrue even to individuals over age 65. Because of the prevalence, functional impact, and ease of treatment, glaucoma should be screened for, and visual and auditory impairment should be corrected. Dentures should be assessed for their fit, and oral lesions beneath them should be detected. Because thyroid dysfunction is more prevalent in the elderly, difficult to detect clinically, and treatable, serum levels of thyroid-stimulating hormone should be measured at least once in asymptomatic older people and probably every 3 to 5 years thereafter. All older women should be screened for osteoporosis. The importance of reviewing all of a patient's medications and discontinuing them whenever feasible cannot be overemphasized.

Exercise should be encouraged not only because of its beneficial effects of blood pressure, cardiovascular conditioning, glucose homeostasis, bone density, insomnia, functional status, and even longevity, but also because it may improve mood and social interaction, reduce constipation, and prevent falls. Resistance training should be encouraged as much as a walking program. Sophisticated screening tests are generally not required. Spinal flexion exercises should be avoided in patients with osteopenia.

Immunizations for influenza, pneumococcal pneumonia, and tetanus should be current. Purified protein derivative (PPD) testing should be done on residents of chronic care facilities and on others at high risk of tuberculosis; those who have recently converted probably should be treated. Since responsiveness wanes with age, the test, if negative, should be repeated in a week.

Hypertension, whether isolated systolic hypertension or combined systolic and diastolic hypertension, should be treated as outlined in Chap. 230.

Serum cholesterol should be measured in patients with established coronary heart disease. Older adults with cardiovascular risk factors experience a similar benefit from statin therapy as younger adults (Chap. 225). Low-dose aspirin is likely useful for primary prevention among those at highest risk for coronary and cerebrovascular disease, but the relative risks and benefits must be considered on an individual basis.

Cancer screening is warranted. A Papanicolaou test should be done in women who have not had one before, since the incidence of cervical carcinoma and associated death increases with age; it should be repeated triennially in all older women unless two previous tests have been normal. Screening for colon cancer is warranted until a minimum age of 80 to 85, at least in community-dwelling elderly, although the optimal method is unclear. Because older women with breast cancer are more likely to die of *of* it than *with* it, screening mammography is indicated every 1 to 2 years, at least until age 75, and thereafter if a positive finding would result in therapeutic intervention.

Perhaps the most valuable preventive measure in the elderly is to take a careful history, focusing not only on the "chief complaint" but also on common and often hidden conditions such as falls, confusion, depression, alcohol abuse, sexual dysfunction, and incontinence. In addition, one should always anticipate the complications for which the specific patient is at risk and take steps to avert them. For instance, a patient with cognitive impairment who smokes is at risk not only for lung cancer but also for starting a fire, and a patient who requires narcotics is at risk for fecal impaction, delirium, urinary retention, and confusion. Community-dwelling patients who are at highest risk of rapid deterioration and institutionalization and who should be monitored more closely include those over age 80, those who live alone, those who are bereaved or depressed, and those who are intellectually impaired.

FURTHER READING

BLAZER DG: Depression in late life: Review and commentary. J Gerontol A Biol Sci Med Sci 58A:249, 2003

BURGIO KL et al: Behavioral training with and without biofeedback in the treatment of urge incontinence in older women. A randomized controlled trial. JAMA 288:2293, 2002

CUMMINGS JL, COLE G: Alzheimer's disease. JAMA 287:2335, 2002

DUBINSKI RM et al: Practice parameter: Risk of driving and Alzheimer's disease (an evidence-based review): Report of the Quality Standards Subcommittee of the American Academy of Neurology. Neurology 54:2205, 2000

GILLICK MR: Choosing appropriate medical care for the elderly. J Am Med Dir Assoc 2:305, 2001

KANNUS P et al: Prevention of hip fracture in elderly people with the use of a hip protector. N Engl J Med 343:1506, 2000

KIRKLAND JL: The biology of senescence: Potential for prevention of disease. Clin Geriatr Med 18:383, 2002

MARCANTONIO ER et al: Reducing delirium after hip fracture. A randomized trial. J Am Geriatr Soc 49:516, 2001

SCIENTIFIC COMMITTEE OF THE FIRST INTERNATIONAL CONSULTATION ON INCONTINENCY: Assessment and treatment of urinary incontinence. Lancet 355:2153, 2000

SHEPHERD J et al: Pravastatin in elderly individuals at risk of vascular disease (PROSPER): A randomised controlled trial. Lancet 360:1623, 2002

TINETTI MP: Preventing falls in elderly persons. N Engl J Med 348:42, 2003

TRINH N-H et al: Efficacy of cholinesterase inhibitors in the treatment of neuropsychiatric symptoms and functional impairment in Alzheimer disease: A meta-analysis. JAMA 289:210, 2003

US PREVENTIVE SERVICES TASK FORCE: Screening for osteoporosis in postmenopausal women: Recommendations and rationale. Ann Intern Med 137:526, 2002

WALTER LC, COVINSKY KE: Cancer screening in elderly patients. A framework for individualized decision making. JAMA 285:2750, 2001

9 PALLIATIVE AND END-OF-LIFE CARE
Ezekiel J. Emanuel, Linda L. Emanuel

EPIDEMIOLOGY

In 2000, 2,403,351 people died in the United States (Table 9-1). Over 70% of all deaths occur in people >65 years of age. The epidemiology of mortality is similar in most developed countries; cardiovascular diseases and cancer are the predominant killers, a marked change since 1900, when heart disease caused ~8% of all deaths and cancer accounted for <4% of all deaths. In 2000, AIDS accounted for <1% of all deaths, although among those aged 35 to 44, it remains a leading cause of death.

While precise statistics are not available, it is estimated that in developed countries ~70% of all deaths are preceded by a disease or condition such that it is reasonable to plan for dying in the foreseeable future. Cancer has served as the paradigm for terminal care, but it is not the only type of illness with a recognizable and predictable terminal phase. Since congestive heart failure, chronic obstructive pul-

TABLE 9-1 *Ten Leading Causes of Death in the United States and Britain*

| | United States | | | | Britain | |
Cause of Death	Number of Deaths	Percent or Total	Number of Deaths Among People ≥65 Years of Age		Number of Deaths	Percent of Total
All deaths	2,403,351	100	1,799,825		535,664	100
Heart disease	710,760	29.6	593,707		108,418	20.2
Cancer	553,091	23.0	392,366		132,793	24.8
Stroke	167,661	7.0	148,045		52,516	9.8
Chronic obstructive pulmonary disease	122,009	5.1	106,375		23,538	4.4
Accidents	97,900	4.1	31,051		10,733	2.0
Diabetes	69,301	2.9	52,414		5,773	1.1
Pneumonia/influenza	65,313	2.7	58,557		56,329	10.5
Alzheimer's disease	49,558	2.1	48,993		14,082	2.6
Nephritis, nephritic syndrome, nephrosis	37,251	1.5	31,225		7,270	1.4
Septicemia	31,224	1.4	24,786		3,410	0.6

Source: National Center for Health Statistics (2000) *www.cdc.gov/nchs*; National Statistics (Great Britain) www.statistics.gov.uk.

monary disease (COPD), chronic liver failure, and many other conditions have recognizable terminal phases, a systematic approach to end-of-life care should be part of all medical specialties. Many patients with advanced illness can also benefit from palliative care long before the terminal phases of their illnesses.

Over the past few decades in the United States, a significant change in the site of death has occurred that coincides with patient and family preferences. Nearly 60% of Americans died as inpatients in hospitals in 1980. By 2000, the trend was reversing, with ~40% of Americans dying as hospital inpatients (Fig. 9-1). This shift has been most dramatic for people dying from cancer and COPD and for younger and very old individuals. In the past decade, it is associated with the increased use of hospice care; in 2000, ~20% of all decedents in the United States received such care. Cancer patients currently constitute >70% of hospice users, with 33 to 50% of all terminal cancer patients receiving hospice care. About 90% of patients receiving hospice care die out of the hospital. Consequently, providing optimal palliative and end-of-life care requires ensuring appropriate services in a variety of settings, including noninstitutional settings.

HOSPICE AND THE PALLIATIVE CARE FRAMEWORK

Central to this type of care is an interdisciplinary team approach that typically encompasses pain and symptom management, spiritual and psychological care for the patient, and support for family caregivers.

Terminally ill patients have a wide variety of advanced diseases, often with multiple symptoms demanding relief, and require noninvasive therapeutic regimens to be delivered in a commodious care setting. Fundamental to ensuring quality palliative and end-of-life care

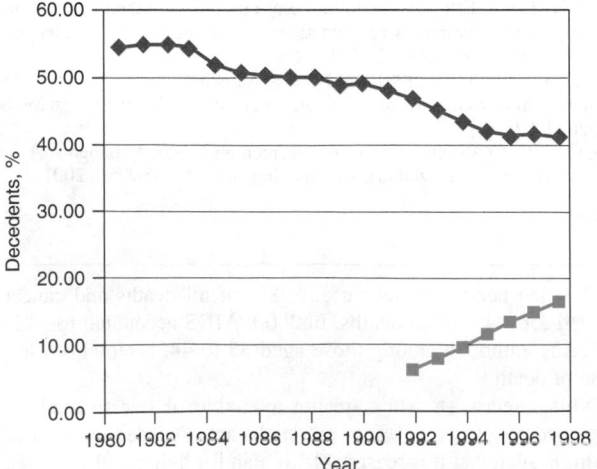

FIGURE 9-1 Graph showing trends in the site of death in the past two decades. ♦, percentage of hospital inpatient deaths; ■, percentage of decedents enrolled in a hospice.

is a focus on four broad domains: (1) physical symptoms; (2) mental or psychological symptoms; (3) social needs that include interpersonal relationships, caregiving, and economic concerns; and (4) existential or spiritual needs.

A whole-person assessment screens for and evaluates needs in each of these four domains. Goals for care are established in discussion with the patient and/or family based on the assessment in each of these domains. Interventions are aimed at improving or managing symptoms and needs. While physicians are responsible for certain especially technical interventions, and for coordinating the interventions, they cannot be responsible for providing all of them. Since failing to address any one of the domains is likely to preclude a good death, a well coordinated, effectively communicating interdisciplinary team takes on special importance in end-of-life care.

ASSESSMENT AND CARE PLANNING ■ Whole-Person Assessment Standardized methods for conducting a whole-person assessment focus on evaluating the patient's condition in all four domains affected by illness: physical, mental, social, and spiritual. The assessment of physical and mental symptoms should follow a modified version of the traditional medical history and physical examination that emphasizes symptoms. Questions should aim at elucidating symptoms but also discerning sources of suffering and how much these symptoms interfere with the patient's life. Standardized assessment questions are available from scales such as the Memorial Symptom Assessment Scale. Using such scales ensures that the assessment is comprehensive and does not just focus on pain and a few other physical symptoms. Invasive tests are best avoided in end-of-life care, and even minimally invasive tests should be carefully evaluated for their benefit-to-burden ratio for the patient. Aspects of the physical examination that are uncomfortable and unlikely to yield useful information can also be omitted.

Regarding social needs, health care providers should assess the status of important relationships, financial burdens, care-giving needs, and access to medical care. Relevant questions will include: *How often is there someone to feel close to? How much help do you need with things like getting meals or getting around? How much trouble do you have getting the medical care you need?* In the area of existential needs, providers should assess distress and the patient's sense of being emotionally and existentially settled and of finding purpose or meaning. Helpful assessment questions can include: *How much are you able to find meaning since your illness began?* In addition, it can be helpful to ask about how well the patient perceives his or her care to be: *How much do you feel your doctors and nurses respect you? How clear is the information from us about what to expect regarding your illness? How much do you feel that the medical care you are getting fits with your goals?* If concern is detected in any of these areas, deeper evaluative questions are warranted.

Communication Foremost is to ensure empathetic and effective communication. When an illness is life-threatening, there are many emotionally charged and potentially conflict-creating moments, collectively called "bad news" situations, in which good communication skills are essential. These moments include communicating to the patient and/or family about a terminal diagnosis, the patient's prognosis, any treatment failures, deemphasizing efforts to cure and prolong life while focusing more on symptom management and palliation, advance care planning, and the patient's actual death.

Just as surgeons plan and prepare for major operations or investigators rehearse a presentation of research results, physicians and health care providers caring for patients with advanced illness must develop a practiced approach to sharing important information and planning interventions. In addition, families identify as important not only how well the physician was prepared to deliver bad news but also the setting in which it was delivered. For instance, 27% of families making critical decisions for patients in the intensive care unit (ICU) desired better and more private physical space to communicate with physicians, and 48% found having clergy present reassuring.

An organized and effective procedure for communicating bad news with seven steps goes by the acronym P-SPIKES: (1) prepare for the discussion, (2) set up a suitable environment, (3) begin the discussion by finding out what the patient and/or family understand, (4) determine how they will comprehend new information best and how much they want to know, (5) provide needed new knowledge accordingly, (6) allow for emotional responses; and (7) share plans for the next steps in care. Table 9-2 provides a summary of these steps along with suggested phrases and underlying rationales for each.

Continuous Goal Assessment   Major barriers to ensuring quality palliative and end-of-life care include difficulty in providing an accurate prognosis and emotional resistance of patients and their families to accepting the implications of a poor prognosis. A practical solution to these barriers is to integrate palliative care with curative care regardless of prognosis. With this approach, palliative care no longer conveys the message of failure, having no more treatments, or "giving up hope." Fundamental to integrating palliative care with curative therapy is to include continuous goal assessment as part of the routine patient reassessment that occurs at most patient-physician encounters.

Goals for care are numerous, ranging from cure of a specific dis-

---

TABLE 9-2   Elements of Communicating Bad News—the P-SPIKES Approach

Acronym	Steps	Aim of the Interaction	Preparations, Questions, or Phrases
P	Preparation	Mentally prepare for the interaction with the patient and/or family.	Review what information needs to be communicated. Plan how you will provide emotional support. Rehearse key steps and phrases in the interaction.
S	Setting of the interaction	Ensure the appropriate setting for a serious and emotionally charged discussion.	Ensure patient, family, and appropriate social supports are present. Devote sufficient time—do not squeeze in a discussion. Ensure privacy and prevent interruptions by people or beeper. Bring a box of tissues.
P	Patient's perception and preparation	Begin the discussion by establishing the baseline and whether the patient and family can grasp the information. Ease tension by having the patient and family contribute.	Start with open-ended questions to encourage participation. Possible phrases to use: *What do you understand about your illness? When you first had symptom X, what did you think it might be? What did Dr. X tell you when he sent you here? What do you think is going to happen?*
I	Invitation and information needs	Discover what information needs the patient and/or family have and what limits they want regarding the bad information.	Possible phrases to use: *If this condition turns out to be something serious, do you want to know? Would you like me to tell you the full details of your condition? If not, then who would you like me to talk to?*
K	Knowledge of the condition	Provide the bad news or other information to the patient and/or family sensitively.	Do not just dump the information on the patient and family. Interrupt and check that the patient and family are understanding. Possible phrases to use: *I feel badly to have to tell you this, but . . . Unfortunately, the tests showed . . . I'm afraid the news is not good . . .*
E	Empathy and exploration	Identify the cause of the emotions—e.g., poor prognosis. Empathize with the patient and/or family's feeling. Explore by asking open-ended questions.	Strong feelings in reaction to bad news are normal. Acknowledge what the patient and family are feeling. Remind them such feelings are normal, even if frightening. Give them time to respond. Remind patient and family you won't abandon them. Possible phrases to use: *I imagine this is very hard for you. You look very upset. Tell me how you are feeling. I wish the news were different. I'll do whatever I can to help you.*
S	Summary and strategic planning	Delineate for the patient and the family the next steps, including additional tests or interventions.	It is the unknown and uncertain that increase anxiety. Recommend a schedule with goals and landmarks. Provide your rationale for the patient and/or family to accept (or reject). If the patient and/or family are not ready to discuss the next steps, schedule a follow-up visit.

Source: Adapted from Buckman.

ease, to relief of a symptom, to delaying the course of an incurable disease, to adapting to progressive disability without disrupting the family, to finding peace of mind or personal meaning, to dying in a manner that leaves loved ones with a positive "departure memory." Discernment of goals for care can be approached through a seven-step protocol: (1) ensure that information is as complete as reasonably possible and understood by all relevant parties (see above); (2) explore what the patient and/or family are hoping for while identifying relevant and realistic goals; (3) share all the options with the patient and family; (4) respond with empathy as they adjust to declining expectations; (5) make a plan, emphasizing what can be done toward the realistic goals; (6) follow through with the plan; and (7) review and revise this plan periodically, considering at every encounter whether the goals of care should be reviewed with the patient and/or family. If a patient or family member has difficulty letting go of an unrealistic goal, suggest that, while hoping for the best, it is still prudent to have a plan for other outcomes as well.

Advance Care Planning ■ *PRACTICES*   Advance care planning is a process of planning for future medical care in case the patient becomes incapable of making medical decisions. Ideally, such planning would occur before a health care crisis or the terminal phase of an illness. Unfortunately, diverse barriers prevent this. While 80% of Americans endorse advance care planning and completing living wills, only 20% have actually done so. Most patients expect physicians to initiate advance care planning and will wait for physicians to broach the subject. Patients also wish to discuss advance care planning with their family.

Yet patients with unrealistic expectations are significantly more likely to prefer aggressive treatments. Fewer than one-third of health care providers have completed advance care planning for themselves. Hence, a good first step is for health care providers to complete advance care planning for themselves. This makes providers aware of the critical choices in the process and the issues that are especially charged and allows them to tell their patients truthfully that they have done this themselves.

Steps in effective advance care planning center on (1) introducing the topic, (2) structuring a discussion, (3) reviewing plans that have been discussed by the patient and family, (4) documenting the plans, (5) updating them periodically, and (6) implementing the advance care directive (Table 9-3). The main barriers to advance care planning are problems in raising the topic and structuring a succinct discussion. Raising the topic can be done efficiently as a routine matter that is recommended for all patients, analogous to purchasing insurance or estate planning. It can be reassuring and effective if the physician has completed his or her own advance care directive.

Structuring a focused discussion is the central skill. Identify the health care proxy and recommend his or her involvement in the advance care planning process. Select a worksheet, preferably one that has been evaluated and demonstrated to produce reliable and valid expressions of patient preferences, and orient the patient and proxy to it. Such worksheets exist both for general and disease-specific situations. Discuss with the patient and proxy one scenario as an example to demonstrate how to think about the issues. It is often helpful to begin with a scenario in which the patient is likely to have settled preferences, such as being in a persistent vegetative state. Once the

TABLE 9-3   *Steps in Advance Care Planning*

Step	Goals to be Achieved and Measures to Cover	Useful Phrases or Points to Make
Introducing advance care planning	Ask the patient what he or she knows about advance care planning and if he or she has already completed an advanced care directive. Indicate that you as a physician have completed advance care planning. Indicate that you try to perform advance care planning with all patients regardless of prognosis. Explain the goals of the process as empowering the patient and ensuring you and the proxy understand the patient's preferences. Provide the patient relevant literature including the advance care directive that you prefer to use. Recommend the patient identify a proxy decision-maker who should attend the next meeting.	*I'd like to talk with you about something I try to discuss with all my patients. It's called advance care planning. In fact, I feel that this is such an important topic that I have done this myself. Are you familiar with advance care planning or living wills?* *Have you thought about the type of care you would want if you ever became too sick to speak for yourself? That is the purpose of advance care planning.* *There is no change in health that we have not discussed. I am bringing this up now because it is sensible for everyone, no matter how well or ill, old or young.* Have many copies of advance care directives available, including in the waiting room, for patients and families.
Structured discussion of scenarios and patient	Affirm that the goal of the process is to follow the patient's wishes if the patient looses decision-making capacity. Elicit the patient's overall goals related to health care. Elicit the patient's preferences for specific interventions in a few salient and common scenarios. Help the patient define the threshold for withdrawing and withholding interventions. Define the patient's preference for the role of the proxy.	Use a structure worksheet with typical scenarios. Begin the discussion with persistent vegetative state and consider other scenarios, such as recovery from and acute event with serious disability, asking the patient about his or her preferences regarding specific interventions, such as ventilators, nasogastric feedings, and CPR proceeding to less-invasive interventions, such as blood transfusions and antibiotics.
Review the patient's preferences	After the patient has made choices of interventions, review them to ensure they are consistent and the proxy is aware of them.	
Document the patient's preferences	Formally complete the advance care directive and have witness sign it. Provide a copy for the patient and the proxy. Insert a copy into the patient's medical record.	
Update the directive	Periodically, and with major changes in health status, review with the patient the existing choice made and make any modifications.	
Apply the directive	The directive goes into effect only when the patient becomes unable to make medical decisions for him- or herself Re-read the directive to be sure about its content. Discuss your proposed actions based on the directive with the proxy.	

Note: CPR, cardiopulmonary resuscitation.

patient's preferences for interventions in this scenario are determined, suggest that the patient and proxy discuss and complete the worksheet for the others. If appropriate, suggest they involve family members in the discussion. On a return visit, go over the patient's preferences, checking and resolving any inconsistencies. After having the patient and proxy sign the document, place it in the medical chart and be sure that copies are provided to relevant family members and care sites. Since patients' preferences can change, these documents need to be reviewed periodically or after an illness episode or personal experience.

TYPES OF DOCUMENTS Advance care planning documents are of two broad types. The first includes living wills or instructional directives; these are advisory documents that describe the types of decisions that should direct care. Some are more specific, delineating different scenarios and interventions for the patient to choose from. Among these, some are for general use and others are designed for use by patients with a specific type of disease, such as cancer or HIV. Less specific directives can be general statements of not wanting life sustaining interventions or forms that describe the values that should guide specific terminal care decisions. Health care proxy designation directives appoint an individual to make decisions. The choice is not either-or; a combined directive that both directs care and designates a proxy is often utilized, and the directive should clearly indicate whether the specified patient preferences or the proxy's choice should take precedence if they conflict.

A potentially misleading distinction relates to statutory as opposed to advisory documents. Statutory documents are drafted to fulfill relevant state laws. They tend to be written with the goal of protecting the clinician from legal action if they follow the patient's stated wishes. Advisory documents are drafted to reflect the patient's wishes. Both are legal, the first under state law, and the latter under common or constitutional law.

LEGAL ASPECTS As of 2003, 47 states and the District of Columbia had enacted living will legislation. Many states have their own statutory forms. Massachusetts, Michigan, and New York do not have living will laws. However, like all other states except Alaska, these states have enacted durable power of attorney for health care laws that permit patients to designate a proxy decision maker with authority to terminate life-sustaining treatments. Only in Alaska does the law prohibit proxies from terminating life-sustaining treatments.

The U.S. Supreme Court has ruled that patients have a constitutional right to decide about refusing and terminating medical interventions, including life-sustaining interventions, and that mentally incompetent patients can exercise this right by providing "clear and convincing evidence" of their preferences. Since advance care directives permit patients to provide such evidence, commentators agree that they are constitutionally protected. Most commentators believe that a state is required to honor any clear advance care directive. Many states explicitly honor out-of-state directives. If a patient is not using a statutory form, then a statutory form should be attached to the advance care directive being used.

INTERVENTIONS

PHYSICAL SYMPTOMS AND THEIR MANAGEMENT Great emphasis has been placed on addressing dying patients' pain. Some institutions have made it a fifth vital sign. While good end-of-life care requires good pain management, it also requires more. The frequency of symptoms varies by disease and other factors. The most common physical and psychological symptoms among all terminally ill patients include pain, fatigue, insomnia, anorexia, dyspnea, depression, anxiety, and nausea and vomiting. In the last days of life, terminal delirium is also common. Assessments of patients with advanced cancer have shown that patients experienced an average of 11.5 different physical and psychological symptoms (Table 9-4).

Evaluations to determine the etiology of these symptoms should be limited to the history and physical examination. Only in rare cases will radiologic or other diagnostic examinations provide sufficient ben-

TABLE 9-4 *Common Physical and Psychological Symptoms of Terminally Ill Patients*

Physical Symptoms	Psychological Symptoms
Pain	Anxiety
Fatigue and weakness	Depression
Dyspnea	Hopelessness
Insomnia	Meaninglessness
Dry mouth	Irritability
Anorexia	Impaired concentration
Nausea and vomiting	Confusion
Constipation	Delirium
Cough	
Swelling of arms or legs	
Itching	
Diarrhea	
Dysphagia	
Dizziness	
Loss of libido	
Fecal and urinary incontinence	
Numbness/tingling in hands/feet	

efit in directing optimal palliative care to warrant the risks, discomfort, and inconvenience to the seriously ill patient. Only a few of the common symptoms presenting difficult management issues will be addressed in this chapter. →*Management of other symptoms, such as nausea and vomiting, insomnia, and diarrhea can be found in Chaps. 34 and 66, Chap. 24, and Chap. 35, respectively.*

Pain ■ *FREQUENCY* The frequency of pain among terminally ill patients varies widely. The proportion of advanced cancer patients experiencing substantial pain is reported to range from 36 to 90%. In the SUPPORT study of hospitalized patients with diverse conditions and an estimated survival of ≤6 months, 22% reported moderate to severe pain, and caregivers of these patients reported that 50% had similar levels of pain during the last few days of life.

ETIOLOGY *Nociceptive pain* is the result of direct mechanical or chemical stimulation of nociceptors and normal neural signaling to the brain. It tends to be localized, aching, throbbing, and cramping. The classic example is bone metastases. *Visceral pain* is caused by nociceptors in gastrointestinal, respiratory, and other organ systems. It is a deep or colicky type of pain classically associated with pancreatitis, myocardial infarction, or tumor invasion of viscera. *Neuropathic pain* arises from disordered, ectopic nerve signals. It is burning or shocklike pain. Classic cases are post-stroke pain and tumor invasion of the brachial plexus. Well-recognized pain syndromes are associated with peripheral neuropathy after chemotherapy or surgery.

ASSESSMENT Pain is a subjective experience. Depending upon the patient's circumstances, perspective, and physiologic condition, the same insult can produce different levels of reported pain and need for pain relief. Systematic assessment includes eliciting the following: (1) periodicity—continuous, with or without exacerbations, or incident; (2) location; (3) intensity; (4) modifying factors; (5) effects of treatments; (6) functional impact; and (7) impact on patient. Several validated pain assessment measures may be used, such as the Visual Analogue Scale, the Brief Pain Inventory, and the pain component of the Memorial Symptom Assessment Scale. Frequent reassessments are essential to assess the effects of interventions.

INTERVENTIONS Interventions for pain must be tailored to each individual with the goal of preempting chronic pain and relieving breakthrough pain. At the end of life, there is no reason to doubt the patient's report of pain. Pain medications are the cornerstone of management. If these are failing and nonpharmacologic interventions—including radiotherapy, anesthetic or neurosurgical procedures, such as peripheral nerve blocks or epidural morphine—are required, a pain consultation is appropriate.

Pharmacologic interventions follow the World Health Organization three-step approach involving nonopioid analgesics, mild opioids, and strong opioids, with or without adjuvants (Chap. 11). Nonopioid analgesics, especially nonsteroidal anti-inflammatory drugs, are the initial treatments for mild pain. They work primarily by inhibiting peripheral prostaglandins, reducing inflammation, but may also have central nervous system (CNS) effects. They have a ceiling effect. Ibuprofen, up to 1600 mg/d, has a minimal risk of bleeding and renal impairment and is a good initial choice.

If nonopioid analgesics are insufficient, then opioids should be introduced. They work by interacting with mu opioid receptors in the CNS to activate pain-inhibitory neurons; most are receptor antagonists. The mixed agonist/antagonist opioids useful for post-acute pain should not be used for the chronic pain in end-of-life care. Weak opioids, such as codeine, should be used initially. However, if the weak opioids are escalated and also fail to relieve pain sufficiently, then strong opioids, such as morphine 5 to 10 mg every 4 h, should be used. Nonopioid analgesics should be combined with opioids because they potentiate the effect of opioids.

For continuous pain, the opioids should be administered on a regular, around-the-clock basis consistent with their duration of analgesia. They should not be provided only when the patient experiences pain; the goal is to prevent patients from experiencing pain. Patients should also be provided rescue medication, such as liquid morphine, for breakthrough pain and should be instructed to take one-half of the standing opioid dose. Patients should be informed that using the rescue medication does not obviate their taking the next standard dose of pain medication. If after 24 h the patient's pain remains uncontrolled and recurs before the next dose, requiring the patient to utilize the rescue medication, increase the daily opioid dose by the total dose of rescue medications used by the patient, or by 50% for moderate pain and 100% for severe pain of the standing opioid daily dose.

It is inappropriate to start with extended-release preparations. Once pain relief is obtained, then switch to extended-release preparations. Even with a stable extended-release preparation regimen, the patient may have incident pain, such as pain during dressing changes. Short-acting preparations should be used to cover such predictable episodes.

Because of differences in opioid receptors, cross-tolerance among opioids is incomplete and patients may experience different side effects with different opioids. Therefore, if a patient is not experiencing pain relief or is experiencing too many side effects, change to another opioid preparation. When switching, begin with ≥50% of the published equianalgesic dose of the new opioid. (Starting at 25% of the equianalgesic dose is inadequate for terminally ill patients.) Opioids have no ceiling effect; therefore, there is no maximum dose no matter how many milligrams the patient is receiving. The appropriate dose is the dose needed to achieve pain relief. Addiction or excessive respiratory depression is extremely unlikely in the terminally ill; fear of these side effects should neither prevent escalating opioid medications when the patient is experiencing insufficient pain relief nor justify using opioid antagonists, such as naloxone.

Opioid side effects should be anticipated and treated preemptively. Nearly all patients experience constipation that can be quite debilitating (see below). Failure to prevent constipation often results in noncompliance with narcotic therapy. About a third of patients experience nausea and vomiting, but tolerance develops, usually within a week. Therefore, when beginning opioids, an antiemetic, such as metoclopramide or a serotonin antagonist, should be prescribed prophylactically and stopped after 1 week. Drowsiness, a common side effect of opioids, also abates within a week. During this period, drowsiness can be treated with psychostimulants, such as dextroamphetamine or methylphenidate. Anecdotal reports suggest that donepezil may also be helpful for opiate-induced drowsiness. Metabolites of morphine and most opioids are cleared renally; doses may need to be adjusted for renal failure.

Patients and families may withhold the prescribed opioids for fear of addiction or dependence. Physicians and health care providers must reassure patients and families that the patient will not become addicted or dependent upon the opioids if used as prescribed for pain relief; this fear should not prevent the patient from taking the medications around the clock.

Seriously ill patients with chronic pain relief rarely if ever become addicted. Suspicion of addiction should not be a reason to withhold pain medications from terminally ill patients. However, diversion of drugs for use by other family members or illicit sale may occur. If this occurs, it should be managed in a way that does not inflict unnecessary pain on the dying patient. Contract writing with the patient and family can help. If that fails, transfer to a safe facility may be necessary.

Tolerance is the need for increasing medication dosage for the same pain relief without a change in disease. In the case of patients with advanced disease, the need for increasing opioid dosage for pain relief is usually caused by disease progression rather than tolerance. Physical dependence is indicated by symptoms from the abrupt withdrawal of opioids and should not be confused with addiction.

Adjuvant analgesic medications are nonopioids that potentiate the analgesic effects of opioids. In the management of neuropathic pain, tricyclic antidepressants, such as desipramine, which has fewer side effects than other tricyclic antidepressants, can begin to work in a few days at doses of 10 to 25 mg before bedtime. Similarly, anticonvulsants, especially gabapentin (begun at 100 mg tid and titrated up by 100 mg tid until relief, with usual doses between 300 mg and 1200 mg tid) or carbamazepine, have shown effectiveness in relief of neuropathic pain. Glucocorticoids, preferably dexamethasone provided once a day, can be useful in reducing inflammation that causes pain while elevating mood, energy, and appetite. Other drugs, including clonidine and baclofen, can be effective in pain relief. These drugs are adjuvants and should all be used in conjunction with—not instead of—opioids. Methadone, carefully dosed, has activity at the N-methyl D-aspartamate (NMDA) receptor and is useful for complex pain syndromes and neuropathic pain.

Radiation therapy can treat bone pain from single metastatic lesions. Bone pain from multiple metastases can be amenable to radiopharmaceuticals, such as strontium 89 and samarium 153. Pamidronate (90 mg every 4 weeks) and calcitonin (200 IU intranasally once or twice a day) can also provide relief from bone pain.

Constipation ■ *FREQUENCY*   Constipation is reported in up to 90% of terminally ill patients.

ETIOLOGY   While hypercalcemia and other factors can cause constipation, it is a predictable consequence of the use of opioids for the relief of pain and dyspnea and of tricyclic antidepressants, from their anticholinergic effects, as well as of the inactivity and poor diet that are common among seriously ill patients. If untreated, constipation can cause substantial pain, vomiting, impaction, and mental confusion. Whenever opioids, tricyclic antidepressants, and other medications known to cause constipation are used, preemptive cathartic treatment should be instituted.

ASSESSMENT   Establish the patient's previous bowel habits, including the frequency, consistency, and volume. Abdominal and rectal examinations should be performed to exclude impaction or acute abdomen. Radiographic assessments beyond a simple flat plate of the abdomen are rarely necessary except when obstruction cannot be definitively excluded.

INTERVENTION   While physical activity, adequate hydration, and dietary treatments with fiber and roughage can be helpful, each is limited in its effectiveness for most seriously ill patients, and roughage may exacerbate problems if impaired motility is the etiology. Fiber is contraindicated in the presence of opioid use. Stimulant and osmotic laxatives, stool softeners, fluids, and enemas are the mainstay of therapy (Table 9-5). When preventing constipation from opioids and other medications, a combination of a laxative and stool softener should be utilized. If after several days of treatment a bowel movement has not occurred, a rectal examination to remove impacted stool and to place a suppository is necessary. For patients with impending bowel obstruction or gastric stasis, octreotide to reduce secretions can be helpful.

Dyspnea ■ *FREQUENCY* Dyspnea is a subjective experience of being short of breath. Nearly 75% of dying patients experience dyspnea. Dyspnea is among the most distressing of physical symptoms, even more distressing than pain.

ASSESSMENT As with pain, dyspnea is a subjective experience that may not correlate with objective measures of P_{O_2}, P_{CO_2}, or respiratory rate. Consequently, measurements, much less repeated measurements, of oxygen saturation through pulse oximetry or blood gases are rarely helpful. Reversible or treatable causes of dyspnea include infection, pleural effusions, pulmonary emboli, or lung tumor encroachment on the airway. However, the risk-benefit ratio of the diagnostic and therapeutic interventions for patients with little time left to live must be carefully considered before undertaking diagnostic steps. Frequently, secondary etiologies cannot be identified, and dyspnea is the consequence of progression of the underlying disease that cannot be treated. The anxiety caused by dyspnea and the choking sensation can significantly exacerbate the underlying dyspnea in a negative reinforcing cycle.

INTERVENTIONS When reversible or treatable etiologies are diagnosed, they should be treated as long as the side effects of treatment, such as repeated drainage of effusions or anticoagulants, are less bothersome than the dyspnea itself. Usually, treatment will be symptomatic (Table 9-6). Low-dose opioids reduce the sensitivity of the central respiratory center and the sensation of dyspnea. If patients are not receiving opioids, weak opioids can be initiated; if patients are already receiving opioids, then morphine should be used. Benzodiazepines are helpful if anxiety is present. If the patient has a history of COPD, bronchodilators may also be helpful, as may glucocorticoids. Secretions can be dried with scopolamine. Oxygen can be used, although it may only be an expensive placebo. Medical staff should sit the patient upright, remove smoke or other irritants such as perfume, ensure a supply of fresh air with sufficient humidity, and minimize other factors that can increase anxiety.

Fatigue ■ *FREQUENCY* Fatigue and weakness are the most common symptoms of terminally ill patients. More than 90% of the terminally ill experience fatigue and/or weakness. Fatigue is frequently cited as among the most distressing of symptoms.

ETIOLOGY The multiple causes of fatigue in the terminally ill can be categorized as resulting from the underlying disease; from disease-induced factors, such as tumor necrosis factor and other cytokines; and from secondary factors such as cachexia, dehydration, anemia, infection, hypothyroidism, and drug side effects. Apart from low caloric intake, loss of muscle mass and changes in muscle enzymes may play an important role in fatigue of terminal illness. The importance of changes in the CNS, especially the reticular activating system, have been hypothesized based on reports of fatigue in patients receiving cranial radiation, experiencing depression, or with chronic pain in the absence of cachexia or other physiologic changes. Finally, depression and other causes of psychological distress can contribute to fatigue.

ASSESSMENT Fatigue is subjective; objective changes, even in body weight, may be absent. Consequently, assessment must rely on patient self-reporting. Scales used to measure fatigue, such as the Edmonton Functional Assessment Tool, the Fatigue Self-Report scales, or the Rhoten Fatigue scale, are usually appropriate for research rather than clinical purposes. In clinical practice, a simple performance assessment such as the Karnofsky Performance Status or the Eastern Cooperative Oncology Group's question "How much of the day does the patient spend in bed?" may be the best measure. In this 0 to 4 performance status assessment, a 0 = normal activity, 1 = symptomatic without being bedridden, 2 = requiring some, but <50%, bed time, 3 = bedbound more than half the day, and 4 = bedbound all the time. Such a scale allows for assessment over time and by third parties.

INTERVENTION At the end of life, fatigue will not be "cured." The goal is the ameliorate it and adjust expectations. Behavioral interventions should be utilized to avoid blaming the patient for inactivity, and to educate both the family and patient that the underlying disease causes physiologic changes producing low energy levels. Understanding that the problem is physiologic not psychological can help to alter expectations regarding the patient's level of physical activity. Practically, this may mean reducing routine activities, such as housework and cooking, or social events outside the house, and making it acceptable to receive guests lying on a couch. At the same time, institution of exercise regimens that are possible can raise endorphins, reduce muscle wasting, and reduce the risk of depression. In addition, ensuring good hydration without worsening edema may help reduce fatigue. Discontinuing medications that worsen fatigue, such as cardiac medications or even opioids, if pain is well controlled, may help.

TABLE 9-5 *Medications for the Management of Constipation*

Intervention	Dose	Comment
Stimulant laxatives		These agents directly stimulate peristalsis and may reduce colonic absorption of water.
Prune juice	120–240 mL/d	
Senna (Senokot)	2–4 tablets PO per day	Work in 6 to 12 h.
Bisacodyl	5–15 mg/d PO, PR	
Osmotic laxatives		These agents are not absorbed. They attract and retain water in the gastrointestinal tract.
Lactulose	15–30 mL PO q4–8h	
Magnesium hydroxide (Milk of Magnesia)	15–30 mL/d PO	Lactulose may cause flatulence and bloating. Lactulose works in 1 day;
Magnesium citrate	125–250 mL/d PO	Magnesium products in 6 h.
Stool softeners		These agents work by increasing water secretion and as detergents increasing water penetration in to the stool.
Sodium docusate (Colace)	300–600 mg/d PO	
Calcium docusate	300–600 mg/d PO	Work in 1 to 3 days.

TABLE 9-6 *Medications for the Management of Dyspnea*

Intervention	Dose	Comments
Weak opioids		For patients with mild dyspnea
Codeine (or codeine with 325 mg acetaminophen)	30 mg PO q4h	For opioid-naïve patient
Hydrocodone	5 mg PO q4h	
Strong opioids		For opioid-naïve patients with moderate to severe dyspnea
Morphine	5–10 mg PO q4h	
	30–50% of baseline opioid dose q4h	For patients already taking opioids for pain or other symptoms
Oxycodone	5–10 mg PO q4h	
Hydromorphone	1–2 mg PO q4h	
Anxiolytics		Give a dose every hour until the patient is relaxed, then provide a dose for maintenance
Lorazepam	0.5–2.0 mg PO/SL/IV qh then q4–6h	
Diazepam	5–10 mg PO or IV qh then q6–18h	
Clonazepam	0.25–2.0 mg PO q12h	
Midazolam	0.5 mg IV q15min	

Only a few pharmacologic interventions target fatigue and weakness. Glucocorticoids can increase energy and enhance mood. Dexamethasone is preferred for its once-a-day dosing and minimal mineralocorticoid activity. However, use for >1 month tends to diminish the positive effects. Psychostimulants, such as dextroamphetamine (5 to 10 mg orally) and methylphenidate (2.5 to 5 mg orally), can also enhance energy levels. Dosages should be given in the morning and at noon, otherwise they can cause counterproductive insomnia. Modafinil, developed for narcolepsy, has shown some promise in the treatment of fatigue. Its precise role in the fatigue at the end of life is yet to be determined.

MENTAL SYMPTOMS AND THEIR MANAGEMENT ■ Depression ■ *FREQUENCY*
Depression at the end of life presents an apparently paradoxical situation. Many people believe that depression is normal among seriously ill patients because they are dying. People frequently say "wouldn't you be depressed?" Depression is not a necessary part of terminal illness and constitutes needless suffering. While sadness, anxiety, anger, and irritability are normal responses to a serious condition, they are typically of modest intensity and transient. Persistent sadness and anxiety are abnormal and suggestive of major depression. While as many as 75% of terminally ill patients experience depressive symptoms, <25% of terminally ill patients have major depression.

ETIOLOGY Previous history of depression, family history of depression or manic-depression, and prior suicide attempts are associated with increased risk for depression among terminally ill patients. Other symptoms, such as pain and fatigue, are associated with higher rates of depression; uncontrolled pain can exacerbate depression, and depression can cause patients to be more distressed by pain. Many medications used in the terminal stages, including glucocorticoids, and some anticancer agents, such as tamoxifen, interleukin 2, interferon α, and vincristine, are also associated with depression. Some terminal conditions, such as pancreatic cancer and certain strokes, have been reported to be associated with higher rates of depression, although this is controversial. Finally, depression may be attributable to grief over the loss of a role or function, social isolation, or loneliness.

ASSESSMENT Diagnosing depression among patients at the end of life is complicated because many of the vegetative symptoms contained in the DSM IV criteria—insomnia, anorexia and weight loss, fatigue, decreased libido, and difficulty concentrating—are associated with the dying process itself. The assessment of depression in seriously ill patients must focus on the dysphoric mood, helplessness, hopelessness, and lack of interest and enjoyment. The single questions "how often do you feel downhearted and blue?" (more than a good bit of the time or similar responses) or "do you feel depressed most of the time?" are appropriate for screening.

Certain conditions may be confused with depression. Endocrinopathies, such as hypothyroidism or Cushing's syndrome, electrolyte abnormalities such as hypercalcemia, and akathisia, especially from dopamine blocking antiemetics such as metoclopramide and prochlorperazine, can mimic depression and should be excluded.

INTERVENTIONS Physicians must treat any physical symptom, such as pain, that may be causing or exacerbating depression. Nonpharmacologic interventions, including group or individual psychological counseling, and behavioral therapies, such as relaxation or imagery, can be helpful, especially in combination with drug therapy.

Pharmacologic interventions remain the core of therapy. The same medications are used to treat depression in terminally ill as in nonterminally ill patients. Psychostimulants may be preferred for patients with a poor prognosis or for those with fatigue or opioid-induced somnolence. Psychostimulants are comparatively fast acting, working within a few days. Dextroamphetamine or methylphenidate should be started at 2.5 to 5.0 mg in the morning and at noon, the same starting dosages used for treating fatigue. The dose can be escalated up to 15 mg twice a day; higher doses are only rarely necessary. Pemoline

is a nonamphetamine psychostimulant with minimal abuse potential. It is also effective as an antidepressant beginning at 18.75 mg in the morning and at noon. Because it can be absorbed through the buccal mucosa, it is preferred for patients with intestinal obstruction or dysphagia. If used for prolonged periods, liver function must be monitored. The psychostimulants can also be combined with more traditional antidepressants, while waiting for the latter to become effective, and then tapered after a few weeks if necessary. Psychostimulants have side effects, particularly initial anxiety, insomnia, and rarely paranoia, which may necessitate lowering the dose or discontinuing treatment. A newer, promising agent is mirtazepine starting at 7.5 mg before bed. It is sedating and has antiemetic and anxiolytic properties with few drug interactions. Its side effect of weight gain may also be beneficial for seriously ill patients, and it is available in orally disintegrating tablets.

For patients with a prognosis of several months or longer, selective serotonin reuptake inhibitors, including fluoxetine, sertraline, and citalopram, and serotonin-noradrenaline reuptake inhibitors, such as venlafaxine, are the preferred treatment because of their efficacy and comparatively few side effects. Because low doses of these medications may be effective for seriously ill patients, use half the usual starting dose for healthy adults. The starting dose for fluoxetine is 10 mg once a day. In most cases, once-a-day dosing is possible.

Atypical antidepressants are recommended only in selected circumstances, usually with the assistance of a specialty consultation. Trazadone can be an effective antidepressant but is sedating and can cause orthostatic hypotension and priapism. Therefore, it should be used only when a sedating effect is desired. In addition to its antidepressant effects, bupropion is energizing, making it useful for depressed patients suffering from fatigue. However, it can cause seizures, preventing its use for patients with a risk of CNS neoplasms or terminal delirium. Finally, alprazolam, a benzodiazepine, starting at 0.25 to 1.0 mg three times a day, can be effective in seriously ill patients suffering from a combination of anxiety and depression. While it is potent and works quickly, it has many drug interactions and may cause delirium, especially among very ill patients, because of its strong binding to the benzodiazepine-GABA receptor complex.

Unless used as adjuvants for the treatment of pain, tricyclic antidepressants are not recommended. Similarly the monoamine oxidase inhibitors are not recommended because of their side effects and dangerous drug interactions.

Delirium ■ *FREQUENCY*
In the weeks or months before death, delirium is uncommon, although it may be significantly underdiagnosed. However, delirium becomes relatively common in the hours and days immediately before death. As many as 85% of patients in the active stages of dying from cancer may experience terminal delirium.

ETIOLOGY Delirium is a global cerebral dysfunction characterized by alterations in cognition and consciousness. It is frequently preceded by anxiety, changes in sleep patterns (especially reversal of day and night), and decreased attention. In contrast to dementia, delirium has an acute onset and is reversible, although reversibility may be more theoretical than real for patients near death. It is possible to have delirium in a patient with dementia.

Causes of delirium include metabolic encephalopathy arising from liver failure, hypoxemia, or sepsis; electrolyte imbalances such as hypercalcemia; nutritional deficiencies such as vitamin B_{12} deficiency; paraneoplastic syndromes; and primary brain tumors or brain metastases. Commonly, among dying patients, delirium can be caused by side effects of treatments, including radiation for brain metastases, and medications, including opioids, glucocorticoids, anticholinergic drugs, antihistamines, antiemetics, and many chemotherapeutic agents. In many terminally ill patients, the etiology will be multifactorial; e.g., dehydration may exacerbate opioid-induced delirium.

ASSESSMENT Delirium should be recognized in any terminally ill patient with new onset of disorientation, impaired cognition, somnolence, fluctuating levels of consciousness, or delusions, with or without agitation. Delirium must be distinguished from acute anxiety and depression, as well as dementia. In some cases, use of formal assessment tools such as the Mini-Mental Status Examination (which does not distinguish delirium from dementia) or the Delirium Rating Scale (which does distinguish delirium from dementia) may be helpful in distinguishing delirium from other processes. The patient's list of medications must be carefully evaluated. Nonetheless, a reversible etiologic factor for delirium is found in fewer than half of terminally ill patients. Because most terminally ill patients experiencing delirium will be very close to death and may be at home, extensive diagnostic evaluations, such as lumbar punctures or neuroradiologic examinations, are usually inappropriate.

INTERVENTIONS   One of the most important objectives of terminal care is to provide terminally ill patients the lucidity to say goodbye to the people they love. Delirium, especially with agitation during the final days, is distressing to family and caregivers. A strong determinant of bereavement difficulties is witnessing a difficult death. Thus, terminal delirium should be treated aggressively.

At the first sign of delirium, such as day-night reversal with slight changes in mentation, let the family know that it is time to be sure that everything they want to have said has been said. The family should be informed that delirium is common just before death.

If medications such as opioids are suspected of being a cause of the delirium, then unnecessary agents should be discontinued. Other reversible causes such as constipation, urinary retention, and metabolic abnormalities should be treated. Supportive measures aimed at providing a familiar environment should be instituted, including restricting visits only to individuals with whom the patient is familiar and eliminating new experiences; orienting the patient, if possible, by providing a clock and calendar; and gently correcting the patient's hallucinations or cognitive mistakes.

Pharmacologic management focuses on the use of neuroleptics and, in the extreme, anesthetics (Table 9-7). Haloperidol remains first-line therapy. Usually, patients can be controlled with a low dose (1 to 3 mg/d), although some may require as much as 20 mg/d. It can be administered orally, subcutaneously, or intravenously. Intramuscular injections should not be used, except when it is the only way to get a patient under control. Chlorpromazine (10 to 25 mg every 4 to 6 h) can be useful if sedation is desired. Dystonic reactions resulting from dopamine blockade are a side effect of neuroleptics, although they are reported to be rare when used to treat terminal delirium. The new atypical neuroleptics—risperidone and olanzapine—have also been used successfully and are especially helpful for patients with longer anticipated life spans since they are less likely to cause dysphoria and have a lower risk of dystonic reactions. If patients develop dystonic reactions, benztropine should be administered. Neuroleptics may be combined with lorazepam to reduce agitation when the delirium is the result of alcohol or sedative withdrawal.

If no response to first-line therapy is seen, a specialty consultation should be obtained with a change to a different medication. If patients fail to improve after a second neuroleptic, then sedation with an anesthetic such as propofol or continuous-infusion midazolam may be

TABLE 9-7 *Medications for the Management of Delirium*

Interventions	Dose
Neuroleptics	
Haloperidol	0.5–5 mg q2–12h, PO/IV/SC/IM
Thioridazine	10–75 mg q4–8h, PO
Chlorpromazine	12.5–50 mg q4–12h, PO/IV/IM
Molindone	10–50 mg q8–12h, PO
Atypical neuroleptics	
Olanzapine	2.5–5 mg qd, PO
Risperidone	1–3 mg q12h, PO
Anxiolytics	
Lorazepam	0.5–2 mg q1–4h, PO/IV/IM
Midazolam	1–5 mg/h continuous infusion, IV/SC
Anesthetics	
Propofol	0.3–2.0 mg/h continuous infusion, IV

necessary. By some estimates, at the very end of life as many as 25% of patients experiencing delirium, especially restless delirium with myoclonus or convulsions, may require sedation.

Physical restraints should be used with great reluctance only when the patient's violence is threatening to self or others. If used, their appropriateness should be reevaluated frequently.

SOCIAL NEEDS AND THEIR MANAGEMENT ■ **Financial Burdens** ■ *FREQUENCY*
Dying can impose substantial economic strains on patients and families, causing distress. In the United States, with one of the least comprehensive health insurance systems among the developed countries, about 20% of terminally ill patients and their families spend >10% of family income on health care costs over and above health insurance premiums. Between 10 and 30% of families sell assets, use savings, or take out a mortgage to pay for the patient's health care costs. Nearly 40% of terminally ill patients in the United States report that the cost of their illness is a moderate or great economic hardship for their family.

The patient is likely to reduce and stop working. In 20% of cases, a family member of the terminally ill patient stops working to provide care. The major underlying causes of economic burden are related to poor physical functioning and care needs, such as the need for housekeeping, nursing, and personal care. More debilitated patients and poor patients experience greater economic burdens.

INTERVENTION   The economic burden should not be ignored as a private matter. It has been associated with a number of adverse health outcomes, including preferring comfort care over life-prolonging care as well as consideration of euthanasia or physician-assisted suicide. Economic burdens tend to increase the psychological distress of families and caregivers of terminally ill patients. Assistance from a social worker, early on if possible, to ensure access to all available benefits may be helpful. Many people and health care providers are unaware of options for long-term care insurance, respite care, the Family Medical Leave Act, and other sources of assistance.

Relationships ■ *FREQUENCY*   Settling personal issues and closing the narrative of lived relationships are universal needs. When asked if sudden death or death after an illness is preferable, respondents often initially select the former but soon change to the latter as they reflect on the importance of saying goodbye. Bereaved family members who have not had the chance to say goodbye often have a more difficult grief process.

INTERVENTION   Care of seriously ill patients requires efforts to facilitate the types of encounters and time spent with family and friends that are necessary to meet these needs. Family and close friends may need to be accommodated with unrestricted visiting hours, which perhaps may include sleeping near the patient even in otherwise regimented institutional settings. Physicians and health care providers may facilitate and resolve strained interactions between the patient and other family members. Assistance for patients and family members who are unsure about how to create or help preserve memories, whether by providing raw materials such as a scrap book or memory box or by offering them suggestions and informational resources, can be deeply appreciated. Taking photographs and creating videos can be especially helpful to terminally ill patients who have younger children or grandchildren.

Family Caregivers ■ *FREQUENCY*   Caring for seriously ill patients places a heavy burden on families. Families are frequently required to provide transportation and homemaking as well as other services. Typically, paid professionals such as home health nurses and hospice workers supplement family care; only about a quarter of all care giving is exclusively paid professional assistance. The trend toward more out-of-hospital deaths will increase reliance on families for end-of-life care.

Three-quarters of the caregivers of terminally ill patients are women—wives, daughters, and even sisters. Since many are widowed, women themselves tend to be able to rely less on family for caregiving assistance and may need more paid assistance. About 20% of terminally ill patients report substantial unmet needs for nursing and personal care.

INTERVENTION It is imperative to inquire about unmet needs and to try to ensure those needs are met either through the family or paid professional services when possible. Community assistance through houses of worship or other community groups can often be mobilized by one or two phone calls from the medical team to someone the patient or family identifies.

EXISTENTIAL NEEDS AND THEIR MANAGEMENT ■ *FREQUENCY* Religion and spirituality are often important to dying patients. Nearly 70% of patients report becoming more religious or spiritual when they became terminally ill, and many find comfort in various religious or spiritual practices such as prayer. However, ~20% of terminally ill patients become less religious, frequently feeling somehow cheated or betrayed by becoming terminally ill. For other patients, the need is for existential meaning and purpose that is distinct from and maybe even antithetical to religion or spirituality.

ASSESSMENT Health care providers are often hesitant about involving themselves in the religious, spiritual, and existential experiences of their patients, because it may seem private, related to alternative lifestyles, or "soft." But physicians and other members of the interdisciplinary team should be able to at least detect spiritual and existential needs. Screening questions have been developed for a physician's spiritual history taking. Spiritual distress can amplify other types of suffering and even masquerade as intractable physical pain, anxiety, or depression, for instance. The screening questions in the whole-person assessment are usually sufficient. Deeper evaluation and intervention are rarely appropriate for the physician unless no other member of an interdisciplinary team is available or suitable. Pastoral care providers may be helpful, whether from the medical institution or the patient's community.

INTERVENTION Precisely how religious practices, spirituality, and existential explorations can be facilitated and improve end-of-life care is not well established. In one study, only 36% of respondents indicated that a clergy member would be comforting. Nevertheless, this increase in religious and spiritual interest among a substantial fraction of dying patients suggests inquiring of individual patients how this need can be addressed.

MANAGING THE LAST STAGES

WITHDRAWING AND WITHHOLDING LIFE-SUSTAINING TREATMENT ■ *LEGAL ASPECTS* For centuries, it has been deemed ethical to withhold or withdraw life-sustaining interventions. The current legal consensus is that patients have a constitutional and common law right to refuse medical interventions (Table 9-8). Courts have held that incompetent patients have a right to refuse medical interventions. For patients who are incompetent and terminally ill and who have not completed an advance care directive, next of kin can exercise this right, although this may be restricted in some states depending how clear and convincing the evidence is of the patient's preferences. Courts are limiting families' ability to terminate life-sustaining treatments from patients who are conscious, incompetent, but not terminally ill. In theory, patients' right to refuse medical therapy can be limited by four countervailing interests: (1) preservation of life, (2) prevention of suicide, (3) protection of third parties such as children, and (4) preserving the integrity of the medical profession. In practice, these interests almost never override the right of competent patients and incompetent patients who have left explicit and advance care directives.

Regarding incompetent patients who either appointed a proxy without specific indications of their wishes or who never completed an advance care directive, three criteria have been suggested to guide the decision to terminate medical interventions. Some commentators suggest that ordinary care should be administered but extraordinary care could be terminated. Because the ordinary/extraordinary distinction is too vague, courts and commentators widely agree that it should not be used to justify decisions about stopping treatment. Many courts have advocated use of the substituted-judgment criterion, which holds that the proxy decision-makers should try to imagine what the incompetent patient would do if he or she were competent. However, most proxies, even close family members, cannot accurately predict what the patient would have wanted. Therefore, substituted judgment becomes more of a guessing game than a way of fulfilling the patient's wishes. Finally, the best-interests criterion holds that proxies should evaluate treatments by balancing their benefits and risks and select those treatments in which the benefits maximally outweigh the burdens of treatment. Yet, as many family conflicts reveal, different individuals can have very different views of what is in the patient's best interests. Indeed, this criterion has been criticized because no objective way exists of determining the balance between benefits and burdens; it depends on a patient's personal values. As a matter of practice, physicians rely on family members to make decisions that they feel are best and object only if these decisions seem to demand treatments that the physicians consider not beneficial.

PRACTICES Withholding and withdrawing acutely life-sustaining medical interventions from terminally ill patients are now standard practice. More than 90% of American patients die without cardiopulmonary resuscitation (CPR), and just as many forgo other potentially life-sustaining interventions. For instance, during 1987 to 1988 in ICUs, CPR was performed 49% of the time, but only 10% of the time in 1992 to 1993. On average, 3.8 interventions, such as vasopressors and transfusions, were stopped from each dying ICU patient.

Mechanical ventilation may be the most challenging intervention to withdraw. The two approaches are *terminal extubation*, which is the removal of the endotracheal tube, and *terminal wean*, which is the gradual reduction of the F_{IO_2} or ventilator rate. One-third of ICU physicians prefer to use the terminal wean technique, while 13% extubate; the majority of physicians utilize both techniques. Some recommend the terminal wean because patients do not develop upper airway obstruction and the distress caused by secretions or stridor; however, terminal weaning can prolong the dying process. To ensure comfort for conscious or semiconscious patients before withdrawal of the ventilator, neuromuscular blocking agents should be terminated and sedatives and analgesics administered. Removing the neuromuscular blocking agents permits patients to show discomfort, facilitating the titration of sedatives and analgesics; it also permits interactions between patients and their families. A common practice is to inject a bolus of midazolam (2 to 4 mg) before withdrawal followed by 5 to 10 mg of morphine and continuous infusion of morphine (50% of the bolus dose per hour) during weaning. Additional boluses of morphine or increases in the infusion rate should be administered for any distress. Higher doses will be needed for patients already receiving anxiolytics and opioids. Families need to be warned that up to 10% of patients unexpectedly survive for 1 day or more after mechanical ventilation is stopped.

FUTILE CARE Beginning in late 1980s, some commentators argued that physicians could terminate futile treatments demanded by families of terminally ill patients. No objective definition or standard of futility exists. Physiologic futility means that an intervention will have no physiologic effect. Some have defined qualitative futile treatments as those that "fail to end a patient's total dependence on intensive medical care." Quantitative futility occurs "when physicians conclude (either through personal experience, experiences shared with colleagues, or consideration of reported empiric data) that in the last 100 cases, a medical treatment has been useless." The term conceals subjective value judgments about when a treatment is "not beneficial." Deciding whether a treatment that obtains an additional 6 weeks of life or a 1% survival advantage confers benefit depends upon patients' preferences and goals. Furthermore, physicians' predictions of when treatments were futile deviated markedly from the quantitative definition. When residents thought CPR was quantitatively futile, more than one in five

TABLE 9-8 *Major Legal Cases Regarding the Withholding or Withdrawing of Medical Interventions*

Case and Citation	Year	State	Facts	Decision
In re Quinlan 70 N.J. 10	1976	NJ	21-year-old woman in a persistent vegetative state dependent on a respirator, artificial nutrition, and hydration.	The right to privacy includes a right to refuse medical care and extends to incompetent patients. Patient's guardian can withdraw her respirator. No need for judicial review in most cases.
Superintendent of Belchertown v Saikewicz 373 Mass 728	1977	MA	67-year-old retarded man with a mental age of 2 years 8 months who had always lived in a state institution develops acute myelomonocytic leukemia. Does he have to receive chemotherapy?	All persons including incompetent persons have the right to refuse medical treatment. Using substituted judgment, the court determined that the patient would not want chemotherapy.
In re Eichner (Brother Fox) 52 NY 2d 262	1981	NY	83-year-old priest was in a persistent vegetative state after a cardiac arrest. Prior to the event, he had publicly stated that he would not want to be respirator-dependent if he were vegetative.	Patients have the right to determine the course of their own medical care. Patient's wishes were known, even if not expressed in writing. Respirator should be withdrawn.
In re Conroy 98 N.J. 321	1985	NJ	84-year-old bedridden, totally impaired woman with organic brain syndrome fed by a nasogastric tube. Her nephew requests removal of the tube.	Nasogastric tube feedings are medical interventions that can be withdrawn.
Brophy v New England Sinai Hospital 398 Mass 417	1986	MA	49-year-old man in persistent vegetative state after a ruptured aneurysm; maintained by gastric tube feedings. He had no written living will, but he had explicitly stated that he would never want to live on life support systems.	Common law and the constitutional right of privacy given a person the right to refuse medical treatment. The patient's wishes are clearly known from explicit conversations. The gastric tube can be withdrawn.
Bouvia v Superior Court 225 Cal Rptr 297	1986	CA	29-year-old mentally competent woman with cerebral palsy that left her almost completely immobile and totally unable to care for herself. She requests a nasogastric tube to supplement her inadequate oral intake be withdrawn.	The patient has the "right to refuse any medical treatment even that which may save or prolong her life."
In re Jobes 108 N.J. 394	1987	NJ	32-year-old woman in a permanent vegetative state, receiving J-tube feedings. Her husband and parents request withdrawal of the feedings. She left no clear written or verbal indication of her wishes.	Incompetent patients have the right to refuse medical care even if they have left no clear indication of their wishes. Using substituted judgment the family can exercise her right to withdraw the J-tube feedings.
Cruzan v Director of Missouri Department of Health 110 S. Ct. 2841	1990	U.S.	33-year-old woman in a persistent vegetative state maintained by gastric tube nutrition and hydration. Her parents requested that these tube feedings be terminated.	By 8 to 1, the Supreme Court ruled that patients have a constitutional right to refuse medical care and that this applies to artificial nutrition and hydration. If there was no clear and convincing written or verbal statement of the patient's wishes, states could regulate how families exercise the right.
In re Helga Wanglie Fourth judicial district PX-91-283. Minnesota (Hennepin County)	1991	MN	85-year-old woman in a persistent vegetative state. After months, physicians suggested withdrawal of life-sustaining treatment because the patient was receiving no benefit. The family refused withdrawal.	The husband should represent the patient's interests, and his refusal to discontinue the respirator is binding.
Wendland v. Wendland 110 Cal Rptr 2d. 412	2001	CA	42-year-old conscious man with severe cognitive impairments, hemiparesis, and limited communication who was not terminally ill required feeding tube. The feeding tube fell out and needed to be replaced. After authorizing replacement of the feeling tube 3 times, wife refused replacement.	Patients have a right to refuse all medical treatments including life-sustaining treatments. This right can be exercised for mentally incompetent patients through advance care directives. For patients who are terminally ill, in persistent vegetative state, or comatose who have not completed an advance care directive, proxies who have not been formally appointed can terminate interventions. However, for mentally incompetent but conscious patients "clear and convincing" evidence is needed of the patient's wishes before life-sustaining treatment can be stopped.

patients had a >10% chance of survival to hospital discharge. Quantitative futility rarely applies in ICU settings. Most commentators reject using futility as a criterion of withdrawing care.

EUTHANASIA AND PHYSICIAN-ASSISTED SUICIDE Euthanasia and physician-assisted suicide are defined in Table 9-9. Terminating life-sustaining care and providing opioid medications to manage symptoms have long been considered ethical by the medical profession and legal by courts and should not be confused with euthanasia or physician-assisted suicide.

LEGAL ASPECTS Euthanasia is legal in the Netherlands and Belgium. Euthanasia was legalized in the Northern Territory of Australia but then repealed. Euthanasia is not legal in any state in the United States. Physician-assisted suicide is legal in Oregon but only if multiple criteria are met and then only after a process that includes a 15-day waiting period. In Switzerland, a layperson can legally assist suicide.

In all other countries and all other states in the United States, physician-assisted suicide and euthanasia are illegal explicitly or by common law.

PRACTICES Fewer than 10 to 20% of terminally ill patients actually consider euthanasia and/or physician-assisted suicide for themselves. In the Netherlands and Oregon, >70% of patients utilizing these interventions are dying of cancer; <5% of deaths by euthanasia or physician-assisted suicide involve patients with AIDS or amyotrophic lateral sclerosis. In the Netherlands, if all legal and illegal acts are grouped, euthanasia and physician-assisted suicide account for <3.5% of all deaths. In Oregon, ~0.1% of patients die by physician-assisted suicide, although many commentators suspect this is an undercount of actual cases.

Pain is not a primary motivator for patients' requests for or interest in euthanasia and/or physician-assisted suicide. Among the first patients to receive physician-assisted suicide in Oregon, only 1 patient

TABLE 9-9 *Definitions of Assisted Suicide and Euthanasia*

Term	Definition	Legal Status
Voluntary active euthanasia	Intentionally administering medications or other interventions to cause the patient's death with the patient's informed consent	Netherlands Belgium
Involuntary active euthanasia	Intentionally administering medications or other interventions to cause the patient's death when the patient was competent to consent but did not—e.g., the patient may not have been asked	Nowhere
Nonvoluntary active euthanasia	Intentionally administering medications or other interventions to cause the patient's death when the patient was incompetent and was mentally incapable of consenting—e.g., the patient might have been in a coma	Nowhere
Passive euthanasia	Withholding or withdrawing life-sustaining medical treatments from a patient to let him or her die (terminating life-sustaining treatments)	Everywhere
Indirect euthanasia	Administering opioids or other medications to relieve pain, dyspnea, or other symptoms with the incidental consequence of causing sufficient respiratory depression to result in the patient's death	Everywhere
Physician-assisted suicide	A physician provides medications or other interventions to a patient with the understanding that the patient can use them to commit suicide	Oregon Netherlands Belgium Switzerland

of 15 had inadequate pain control compared to 15 of 43 patients in a control group experiencing inadequate pain relief. Depression, hopelessness, and, more vaguely, worries about loss of dignity or autonomy appear to be the primary factors motivating a desire for euthanasia or physician-assisted suicide.

Euthanasia and physician-assisted suicide are no guarantee of a painless, quick death. Data from the Netherlands indicate that in as many as 20% of cases technical and other problems arose, including patients waking from coma, not becoming comatose, regurgitating medications, and a prolonged time to death. Problems were significantly more common in physician-assisted suicide, sometimes requiring the physician to intervene and provide euthanasia.

After receiving a request for euthanasia and/or physician-assisted suicide, health care providers should carefully clarify the request with empathic, open-ended questions to help elucidate the underlying cause for the request such as: "What makes you want to consider this option?" Endorsing either moral opposition or moral support for the act tends to be counterproductive, either lending an impression of being judgmental or of endorsing the idea that the patient's life is worthless. Health care providers must reassure the patient of continued care and commitment. The patient should be educated about alternative, less controversial options, such as symptom management and withdrawing any unwanted treatments; the reality of euthanasia and/or physician-assisted suicide, since the patient is likely to have misconceptions about its effectiveness; and also the legal implications of the choice. Depression, hopelessness, and other symptoms of psychological distress as well as physical suffering and economic burdens are likely factors motivating the request, and such factors should be assessed and treated aggressively. After these interventions and clarification of options, most patients proceed with a less controversial approach of declining life-sustaining interventions, possibly including refusal of nutrition and hydration.

CARE DURING THE LAST HOURS Most laypersons have limited experiences with the actual dying process and death. They frequently do not know what to expect of the final hours, and afterwards. Therefore, the family and other caregivers must be prepared, especially if the plan is for the patient to die at home.

Patients in the last days of life experience extreme weakness and fatigue and become bedbound; this can lead to bedsores. They stop eating and drinking with drying of mucosal membranes and dysphagia. Careful attention to oral swabbing, lubricants for lips, and use of artificial tears can provide a form of care to substitute for attempts at feeding the patient. With loss of the gag reflex and dysphagia, patients may also experience accumulation of oral secretions, producing noises during respiration sometimes called "the death rattle." Scopolamine can reduce the secretions. Patients also experience changes in respiration with periods of apnea or Cheyne-Stokes breathing. Decreased intravascular volume and cardiac output causes tachycardia, hypotension, peripheral coolness, and livedo reticularis (skin mottling). Patients can also have urinary and, less frequently, fecal incontinence. Changes in consciousness and neurologic function generally lead to two different paths to death (Fig. 9-2).

Each of these terminal changes can cause patients and families distress, requiring reassurance and targeted interventions (Table 9-10). Informing families that these changes might occur, and even providing them an information sheet, can help to preempt problems and minimize distress. Understanding that patients stop eating because they are dying, not dying because they have stopped eating, can reduce family and caregiver anxiety. Similarly, informing the family and caregivers that the "death rattle" may occur and that it is not indicative of suffocation or choking can reduce their preoccupation with the breathing sounds.

Families and caregivers can also feel guilty about stopping treatments, fearing that they are "killing" the patient. This may lead to demands for interventions that may be ineffective. In such cases, the

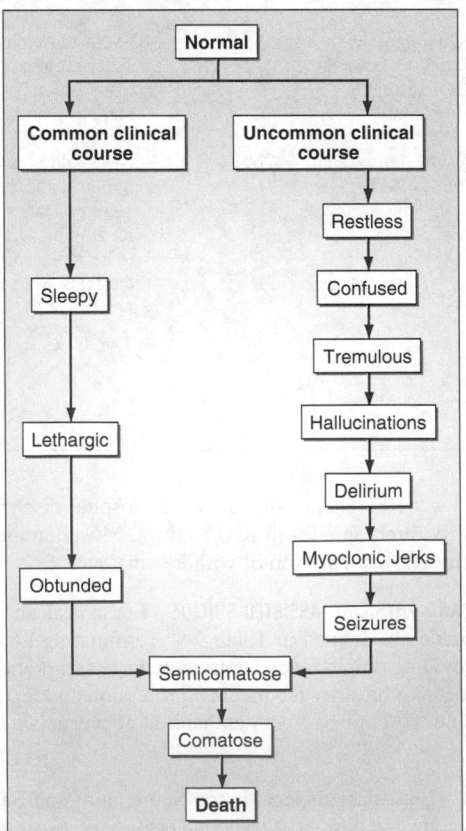

FIGURE 9-2 Common and uncommon clinical courses in the last days of terminally ill patients. (*Adapted from FD Ferris et al: Module 4: Palliative care, in Comprehensive Guide for the Care of Persons with HIV Disease. Toronto: Mt. Sinai Hospital and Casey Hospice, 1995, at www.cpsonline.info/content/resources/hivmodule4.html*)

TABLE 9-10 *Managing Changes in the Patient's Condition during the Final Days and Hours*

Changes in the Patient's Condition	Potential Complication	Family's Possible Reaction and Concern	Advice and Intervention
Profound fatigue	Bedbound with development of pressure ulcers that are prone to infection, malodor, and pain, and joint pain	Patient is lazy and giving up.	Reassure family and caregivers that terminal fatigue will not respond to interventions and should not be resisted. Use an air mattress if necessary.
Anorexia	None	Patient is giving up; patient will suffer from hunger and will starve to death.	Reassure family and caregivers that the patient is not eating because he or she is dying; not eating at the end of life does not cause suffering or death. Forced feeding, whether oral, parenteral, or enteral, does not reduce symptoms or prolong life.
Dehydration	Dry mucosal membranes (see below)	Patient will suffer from thirst and die of dehydration.	Reassure family and caregivers that terminal dehydration does not cause suffering because patients lose consciousness before any symptom distress. Intravenous hydration can worsen symptoms of dyspnea by pulmonary edema and peripheral edema as well as prolong dying process.
Dysphagia	Inability to swallow oral medications needed for palliative care		Do not force oral intake. Discontinue unnecessary medications that may have been continued including antibiotics, diuretics, anti-depressants, and laxatives. If swallowing pills is difficult, convert essential medications (analgesics, antiemetics, anxiolytics, and psychotropics) to oral solutions, buccal, sublingual, or rectal administration.
"Death rattle"—noisy breathing		Patient is choking and suffocating.	Reassure the family and caregivers that this is caused by secretions in the oropharynx and the patient is not choking. Reduce secretions with scopolamine (0.2–0.4 mg SC q4h or 1–3 patches q3d) Reposition patient to permit drainage of secretions. Do not suction. Suction can cause patient and family discomfort, and is usually ineffective.
Apnea, Cheyne-Stokes respirations, dyspnea		Patient is suffocating.	Reassure family and caregivers that unconscious patients do not experience suffocation or air hunger. Apneic episodes are frequently a premorbid change. Opioids or anxiolytics may be used for dyspnea. Oxygen is unlikely to relieve dyspneic symptoms and may prolong the dying process.
Urinary or fecal incontinence	Skin breakdown if days until death Potential transmission of infectious agents to caregivers	Patient is dirty, malodorous, and physically repellent.	Remind family and caregivers to use universal precautions. Frequent changes of bedclothes and bedding. Use diapers, urinary catheter, or rectal tube if diarrhea or high urine flow occur.
Agitation or delirium	Day/night reversal Hurt self or caregivers	Patient is in horrible pain and going to have a horrible death.	Reassure family and caregivers that agitation and delirium do not necessarily connote physical pain. Depending upon the prognosis and goals of treatment, consider evaluating for causes of delirium and modify medications. Manage symptoms with haloperidol, chlorpromazine, diazepam, or midazolam.
Dry mucosal membranes	Cracked lips, mouth sores, and candidiasis can also cause pain. Malodor	Patient may be malodorous, physically repellent.	Use baking soda mouthwash or saliva preparation q15–30min. Use topical nystatin for candidiasis. Coat lips and nasal mucosa with petroleum jelly q60–90min. Use ophthalmic lubricants q4h or artificial tears q30min.

physician should remind the family and caregivers about the inevitability of events, the palliative goals, and that interventions may prolong the dying process and cause discomfort. Physicians should also emphasize that withholding treatments is both legal and ethical, and that they are not the cause of the patient's death. This reassurance may need to be provided multiple times.

Hearing and touch are said to be the last senses to stop functioning. Therefore, families and caregivers should be permitted to communicate with the dying patient. Encouraging them to talk directly to the patient, even if he or she is unconscious, and hold the patient's hand or demonstrate affection in other ways can be an effective way to channel their urge "to do something" for the patient.

When the plan is for the patient to die at home, the physician must inform the family and caregivers how to determine that the patient has died. The cardinal signs are cessation of cardiac function and respiration; the pupils become fixed; the body becomes cool, ashen white, and waxy; muscles relax; and incontinence may occur. Remind the family and caregivers that the eyes may remain open even when the patient has died because the retroorbital fat pad may be depleted permitting the orbit to fall posteriorly, which makes it difficult for the eyelids to cover the eyeball.

The physician should establish a plan of who the family or caregivers will contact when the patient is dying and has died. Without a plan, they may panic and call 911, unleashing a cascade of unwanted events from arrival of emergency personal and resuscitation to hospital admission. The family and caregivers should be instructed to contact the hospice (if one is involved), the covering physician, or the on-call member of the palliative care team. They should also be told that the coroner need not be called, unless the state requires it for all deaths. Unless foul play is suspected, the health care team need not contact the coroner either.

Just after the patient dies, even the best-prepared family may experience shock and loss and be emotionally distraught. They need time to assimilate the event and be comforted. Health care providers should write a bereavement card or letter to the family. The purpose is to communicate about the patient, perhaps emphasizing the patient's virtues, the honor it was to care for the patient, and express concern for the family's hardship. Many physicians attend the funerals of their patients. While this is beyond any medical obligation, the presence of the physician can be a source of support to the grieving family, and the funeral provides an opportunity for closure for the physician.

Death is a strong predictor of poor health, and even mortality, for the surviving spouse. It may be important to alert the spouse's physician about the death to be aware of symptoms that might require professional attention.

PALLIATIVE CARE SERVICES: HOW AND WHERE

Determining the best approach to providing palliative care to patients will depend upon patient preferences, the availability of caregivers and specialized services in close proximity, institutional resources, and reimbursement. A hospice is a leading, but not the only, model of palliative care services. In the United States, Medicare pays for hospice services under Part A, the hospital insurance part of reimbursement. Two physicians must certify that the patient has a prognosis of ≤6 months, if the disease runs its usual course. Prognoses are probabilistic by their nature; patients are not required to die within 6 months but rather to have a condition from which half the individuals with it would be dead within 6 months. Patients sign a hospice enrollment form that states their intent to forgo curative services related to their terminal illness, but they can still receive medical services for other comorbid conditions. Patients can also un-enroll and re-enroll later; the hospice Medicare benefit can be revoked later to secure traditional Medicare benefits. Payments to the hospice are per diem, not fee-for-service. Payments are intended to cover physician services for the medical direction of the care team; regular home care visits by registered nurses and licensed practical nurses; home health aid and homemaker services; dietary counseling; chaplain services; social work services; bereavement counseling; and medical equipment, supplies, and medications. Additional clinical care, including services of the primary physician, is covered by Medicare Part B even while the hospice Medicare benefit is in place.

By 1996, the mean length of enrollment in a hospice was 65 days, with the median being <24 days. Since then, it appears the length of enrollment is declining. Such short stays create barriers to establishing high-quality palliative services in patients' homes and also place financial strains on hospice providers since the initial assessments and institution of care plans are resource intensive. Physicians should initiate early referrals to the hospice to allow more time for patients to receive palliative care.

Hospice care has been the main way of securing palliative services for terminally ill patients. However, efforts are now being made to ensure continuity of palliative care across settings and through time. Palliative care services are becoming available as consultative services in hospitals, in day care and other outpatient settings, and in nursing homes. In the United States, while the vast majority of hospice care is provided in residential homes, just over 10% now occurs in nursing homes. Palliative care consultations for non-hospice patients can be billed as for other consultations under Medicare Part B, the physician reimbursement part. Many believe palliative care should be offered to patients regardless of their prognosis. A patient and his or her family should not have to make a "curative vs. palliative care" decision because it is rarely psychologically possible to make such a decisive switch to embracing mortality.

FUTURE DIRECTIONS

OUTCOME MEASURES Care near the end of life cannot be measured by most of the available validated outcome measures since palliative care does not consider death a bad outcome. Similarly, the family and patients receiving end-of-life care may not desire the elements elicited in current quality-of-life measurements. Symptom control, enhanced family relationships, and quality of bereavement are difficult to measure and are rarely the primary focus of carefully developed or widely used outcome measures. Nevertheless, outcomes are as important in end-of-life care as in any other field of medical care. Specific end-of-life care instruments are being developed both for assessment, such as The Brief Hospice Inventory and NEST (needs near the end of life screening tool), and for outcome measures, such as the Palliative Care Outcomes Scale. The field of end-of-life care is ready to enter an era of evidence-based practice and continuous improvement through clinical trials.

FURTHER READING

AMERICAN SOCIETY OF CLINICAL ONCOLOGY: *Optimizing Cancer Care— The Importance of Symptom Management*, vols 1 and 2. Alexandria, Virginia, ASCO, 2001

BUCKMAN R: *How to Break Bad News: A Guide for Health Care Professionals.* Baltimore, Johns Hopkins University Press, 1992

LEVY MH: Pharmacologic treatment of cancer pain. N Engl J Med 335:1124, 1996

NCCN: The National Comprehensive Cancer Network (NCCN) palliative care guidelines. 2002: *www.nccn.org*

THE PALLIATIVE CARE GUIDELINES GROUP OF THE AMERICAN HOSPICE FOUNDATION: *Integrating Palliative Care into Disease Management Guidelines.* American Hospice Foundation, Washington, DC, 2003

www.epec.net

www.eperc.mcw.edu

www.partnershipforcaring.org

10 COMPLEMENTARY AND ALTERNATIVE MEDICINE
Stephen E. Straus

BACKGROUND Medicine, not long ago the domain of solitary generalists and their nurse assistants, now engages scores of specialists and allied professionals—radiation physicists, cytologists, nurse practitioners, psychiatric social workers, dental hygienists, and many more—who wield tools of unprecedented ability to extend life and sustain its quality. This evolution of the health care system has been achieved, in part, by a formidable enterprise of critical observation and formal investigation that disproves some once-accepted practices and stimulates emergence of new approaches that compete for acceptance. One need only peruse the serial editions of this textbook to comprehend the scope of these changes.

Other factors have also affected evolutionary changes in medicine. Immigration and related demographic changes yield increasingly diverse populations who value their own traditions. People's expecta-

tions of health and the nature of the health care system itself have been altered by unprecedented access to sources of information, goods, and services; the disposable income to afford them, and a patchwork quilt of regulations and laws that constrain medical practice on the one hand and facilitate increased choice in health care on the other. The emergence of complementary and alternative medicine is one manifestation of these changes in health care.

DEFINITIONS In every generation, medical practices exist that are not accepted by the mainstream: they are viewed with suspicion and dismissed as implausible or irrational. For a time, approaches that evoked some appeal, but which had not been thoroughly tested, were deemed *unconventional*. Over the past decade or so, they have been called complementary or alternative medicine (CAM), to reflect their use as adjuncts to, or as substitutes for, more generally accepted practices, respectively. CAM does not encompass practices that have yet to be translated fully from the laboratory into the clinic, nor practices that were well studied and disproved, but which manage to persist in some fashion nonetheless. Rather, CAM entails approaches with surprising pervasiveness, many of which can claim at least some evidentiary support. Until recently, CAM could also be defined as practices that are not widely taught in medical schools or reimbursed. However, medical students increasingly seek and receive some instruction about CAM, while third-party payers have identified in CAM a marketing tool to attract new, well-heeled clients. In the past few years, another term has been coined—*integrative medicine*—to suggest encouragingly that some CAM approaches, and the practitioners who deliver them, will be shown worthy of being added to the health care repertoire.

SCOPE The myriad practices and products that encompass CAM (Table 10-1) can be organized into five somewhat overlapping domains. Special diets, high doses of vitamins and minerals, and extracts of animal or botanical products are grouped together as *biologically based* CAM approaches. Massage, osteopathic and chiropractic manipulation, and cranial-sacral therapies are grouped as *manipulative and body-based* CAM approaches. Diverse forms of meditation, various uses of biofeedback, and hypnosis are considered *mind-body* approaches. All three of these CAM domains have well-accepted analogues in conventional medicine—low-fat, low-cholesterol diets; physical therapy; psychotherapy; to name but a few.

The fourth domain is known as *energy medicine*, to reflect its exploitation of veritable or putative energy fields. Today, magnets are increasingly popular health products. Over 2000 years ago, however, while Greek physicians believed that health requires a balance of vital humors, Asian practitioners postulated the flow and balance of vital energies and described tools to restore them. Acupuncture aims to correct energies that flow through special meridians, or channels. Reiki, a Japanese approach, and healing touch, a modern variant, purport to diagnose and correct one's energy by passing the hands of an adept therapist over the patient.

The fifth domain, termed *alternative systems of medicine*, combines elements of the four other domains and aims to provide primary approaches to all health needs, rather than just adjunctive solutions to them. Western variants include practices developed by Native Americans, homeopathy, and naturopathic medicine. Eastern variants such as Ayurvedic medicine of India, traditional Chinese medicine, and Tibetan medicine are rich in their use of meditative exercises and herbal products.

PATTERNS OF USE Despite its enormous success, contemporary western biomedicine has features that can discourage patients: many diseases, especially chronic ones, are not cured or even adequately ameliorated; existing treatments can impose serious adverse reactions; and the care is fragmented and impersonal. CAM, despite its lack of proof, appeals to many because its practitioners are optimistic. They spend a lot of time talking with and touching their patients. CAM empowers patients to make their own health choices, its natural products are believed to be inherently healthier and safer than synthetic ones, and care is pro-

TABLE 10-1	*Some Complementary and Alternative Medical Practices*
Type	**Description**
Acupuncture	A Chinese medical practice that involves the insertion of hair-thin needles into nonanatomic energy channels, called meridians
Alexander technique	A movement therapy that emphasizes efficient use of muscles to relieve pain, decrease skeletal strain, and improve posture
Anthroposophic medicine	A spiritually based system of medicine that incorporates herbs, homeopathy, diet, and a movement therapy called eurythmy
Aromatherapy	The use of essential plant oils (distilled concentrates) in massage, baths, or inhalation
Ayurvedic medicine	The major East Indian traditional medicine system, utilizing pulse and tongue diagnosis; treatment includes diet, exercise, herbs, oil massages, and elimination regimens (utilizing emetics, diarrheals, etc.)
Bach flower remedies	Dilute flower infusions used to treat emotional conditions
Biofeedback	The use of machinery that translates physiologic processes into audio or visual signals
Chiropractic	Adjustments of spinal vertebrae in an effort to affect neuromuscular function
Cranial-sacral therapy	Gentle manipulation of the cranium and spine
Curanderismo	A spiritual healing tradition common in Mexican-American communities that utilizes ritual cleansing, herbs and incantations
Dance therapy	Therapeutic method that uses movement to facilitate emotional expression and release
Feldenkrais bodywork	Highly structured movement sequences that emphasize proper head positioning
Guided imagery	The use of imagination to invoke specific images that are hoped to affect physiologic function
Hydropathy	Treatment utilizing water at various temperatures, sometimes aerated or under pressure, sometimes with added salts or other substances
Hypnosis	The induction of an altered of mind within which a subject becomes receptive to specific suggestions
Massage	The use of specific gliding and kneading strokes and friction to achieve muscle relaxation
Meditation	A process by which one tries to achieve awareness without thought
Music therapy	Singing, playing instruments, or listening to music
Naturopathy	A mixture of modalities that may include herbs, homeopathy, acupuncture, hydropathy, diet, and exercise
Native American medicine	Diverse systems, many of which incorporate prayer, chant, music, healing ceremonies, counseling, herbs, laying on of hands, and smudging (ritual cleansing with smoke from sacred plants)
Osteopathy	A medical field incorporating manipulative techniques for correcting abnormalities of the musculoskeletal system
Reflexology/zone therapy	Manual stimulation of points on the hands or feet, believed to affect distant organs
Rolfing/structural integration	A manual therapy that attempts to realign the body by deep tissue manipulation of fasciae
Shiatsu/acupressure	Finger pressure at points along nonanatomic meridians
Siddha medicine	An East Indian medical system (prevalent among Tamil-speaking people) utilizing breathing techniques, incantations, herbs, and muppu (a tri-salt preparation)
T'ai chi ch'aun	Chinese dancelike exercises described as a "moving meditation"
Therapeutic touch	Secular version of the laying on of hands, described as a "healing meditation" (a tri-salt preparation)
Tibetan medicine	A medical system that utilizes diagnosis by pulse and urine examination; therapies include herbs, diet, and massage
Traditional Chinese medicine	A medical system that utilizes examination of the tongue and pulses for diagnosis and acupuncture, herbal mixtures, massage, exercise, and diet
Trager bodywork	Light massage combined with gentle passive movements to help patients maximize freedom of movement
Unani medicine	An East Indian medial system, derived from Persian medicine, practiced primarily in the Muslim community
Yoga	An Indian practice that includes postures (asanas), breathing exercises (pranayama), and cleansing practices (kriyas)

vided in a "holistic" fashion, meaning that the broader medical, social, and emotional contexts of illness are considered in designing the treatment plan.

The very first large survey by Eisenberg in 1993 surprised the medical community by showing that >30% of Americans use CAM approaches. Countless studies since then have extended these conclusions by surveying specific demographic groups and patient populations. The Centers for Disease Control and Prevention (CDC) study of nearly 31,000 American adults revealed that in 1999 29% had used one or more modalities, with spiritual approaches, herbal medicine, chiropractic, and massage being the most prevalent. Over 1% underwent acupuncture treatment that year. Surveys among patients with cancer showed that 30 to 86% used CAM, with highest rates in those with more advanced disease and undergoing aggressive treatments. Similarly, among AIDS patients, 36 to 91% are reported to use CAM. In devastating chronic illnesses like these, CAM is called upon to provide hope of cures when conventional medicine cannot, to extend life, to ameliorate treatment side effects, and to provide emotional and physical comfort. While somewhat subject to vagaries of definition as to what counts as a CAM treatment, surveys have shown that Americans are willing to pay for these services out of pocket, with an estimated $7 billion each year on vitamins and mineral supplements, $4 billion on herbals and other natural products, and nearly $4 billion more on sports supplements. Eisenberg reported that total CAM expenditures in 1997 approached $30 billion, with more visits to practitioners for CAM services than to physicians in general.

FIELDS OF PRACTICE ■ Osteopathic Medicine Founded in 1892 in the American heartland by the physician Andrew Taylor Still, osteopathic medicine was based originally on the belief that manipulation of soft tissue and bone can correct a wide range of diseases of the musculoskeletal and other organ systems. Over the ensuing century, osteopathy evolved progressively towards conventional (allopathic) medicine. Today, the training, practice, credentialing, licensure, and reimbursement of osteopathic physicians is virtually indistinguishable from those of allopathic physicians, with 4 years of osteopathic medical school followed by specialty and subspecialty training and certification by organizations such as the American Board of Internal Medicine. Some osteopathic physicians continue to practice spinal manipulation, primarily as a tool to address specific musculoskeletal complaints.

Chiropractic Medicine In 1895, Daniel David Palmer founded in Missouri the first school of chiropractic medicine to teach manipulation of the spine. Palmer believed that subluxations, or partial dislocations of vertebrae, cause disease by impinging on key nerve roots. Today, chiropractors undertake 5 years of training in basic and relevant clinical sciences. Increasingly, they complete additional postgraduate training in radiology and outpatient therapeutics, primarily of musculoskeletal conditions, although within the discipline there are factions that continue to perform manipulation for many other pathologic entities. Chiropractors also advise on nutrition, exercise, and other health maintenance approaches. Over 70,000 doctors of chiropractic medicine are licensed to practice in all states and the District of Columbia.

Acupuncture A venerable component of traditional Chinese medicine, acupuncture has emerged in recent decades as a free-standing clinical discipline. Over 3000 American physicians have acquired targeted postgraduate training that permits them to practice acupuncture in over 40 states and the District of Columbia. Over 4000 non-MDs have taken far more extended training, leading to licensure to practice independently or under the supervision of a physician.

Massage Therapy Drawing upon millennia of empirical knowledge, some 80 American schools instruct students in an array of the soft tissue manipulative approaches that constitute massage. Thirty-one states and the District of Columbia license trainees to perform therapeutic massage.

Naturopathic Medicine Eleven states license practitioners of naturopathy, a discipline that emerged in central Europe in the late eighteenth century. That conventional treatments of the day were usually ineffective, if not overtly harmful, stimulated the search for safer and more "natural" approaches—naturopathy is one of them. The concept underlying this discipline is that the body possesses powerful mechanisms for self-healing that a properly instructed practitioner could harness. About 1400 naturopathic physicians have completed 4 years of education in basic and clinical sciences and are licensed to manage a predominantly outpatient population. Conventional and unconventional diagnostic tests and medications are prescribed with an emphasis on relatively low doses of drugs, herbal medicines, special diets, and exercises.

Homeopathic Medicine The late eighteenth century also witnessed the emergence of homeopathy, another discipline that reacted to toxicity of the allopathic approaches of the day. It was developed by Samuel Hahnemann, a German physician, who postulated that substances that cause particular side effects in a well person may be used to treat or prevent such symptoms in an ill person if administered in miniscule amounts—what is known as "the doctrine of similars." For example, contact with poison ivy (*Rhus toxicodendron*) causes an itchy, blistering rash. Highly diluted extracts of poison ivy are recommended to treat chickenpox. The nascent field of homeopathy used blinded tests on volunteers, presaging to some extent the use of placebo-controlled trials, to prove which materials were the most able to induce or relieve symptoms. By the mid-nineteenth century homeopathy had gained considerable presence in the American medical establishment and may, in fact, have facilitated the development of immunization and allergen desensitization, both of which utilize very small quantities of materials to elicit measurable biologic outcomes. Today, however, homeopathy is accepted less fully in the United States than in some other countries: it is the largest of all CAM practices in the United Kingdom, Germany, and France and is widely used in India. Only three states license the practice of homeopathy. The relative decline of homeopathy relates, at least in part, to the field's inability to articulate a rational mechanism as to why products that are diluted more than 10^{60}-fold, vastly greater than Avogadro's number, could incite biologic effects. Nonetheless, homeopathic remedies are readily available and commonly recommended by naturopathic physicians and other licensed and unlicensed practitioners.

Other Disciplines There are numerous other CAM practices, among which some involve formal training, such as that leading to a Doctorate of Oriental Medicine, or extended apprenticeships, as in learning herbal medicine. Unfortunately, most of the other fields have no agreed upon practice standards, credentialing processes, requirements for continuing education, or accountability.

REGULATION As indicated above, some CAM disciplines are carefully regulated. CAM products, however, are not strongly regulated. Herbal medicines, and dietary supplements more generally, occupy a unique regulatory status that affords the public remarkable freedom of choice but also many undesired challenges, summarized below. Elements of virtually all traditional healing approaches, herbal medicines were presumed safe long before the implementation of stringent drug regulations by the U.S. Food and Drug Administration (FDA). In 1994, the United States Congress passed the Dietary Supplements Health and Education Act (DSHEA) that permits sale of dietary supplements "over-the-counter," as it were, but without the requirement imposed on manufacturers of prescription or classic over-the-counter drugs to prove their products to be safe and effective before marketing. Supplements can be removed by the FDA from the market only if they are proven to be hazardous. Dietary supplements, however, cannot legally claim to prevent or treat any disease. They can, however, claim to maintain "normal structure and function" of body systems. For example, a product cannot claim to treat arthritis, but it can claim to maintain "normal joint health."

Homeopathic products predate FDA drug regulations and are sold with no requirement that they be proven effective. It would be reasonable to assume, however, given the extent to which homeopathic products are diluted, that most of them are safe.

SAFETY Despite their lack of apparent toxicities, homeopathic products, like all other CAM products and practices, do convey one type of risk, namely, that people will pursue them in lieu of more conventional modalities that are proven to be beneficial. Members of the public have considerable freedom to determine what is in their own best interest, even if those decisions deny them effective treatment, although the courts have found the rights of parents to withhold treatment of their children to be limited in instances of life-threatening illnesses. Investigators, however, have a broad ethical obligation to not withhold proven treatments for serious illnesses for the sake of testing unproven ones.

Additional risks are imposed by the use of other CAM approaches: injuries inflicted by a practice, inherent toxicities of the modality, and interference by the modality with more conventional treatments.

Injury Physical and manipulative interventions can harm patients. In past decades, reused acupuncture needles transmitted hepatitis B virus infection; today, the standard of care requires disposable needles. Aggressive massage can cause soft tissue injuries. Spinal manipulation of patients with unrecognized vertebral lesions has been associated with cord injuries, and cervical manipulation has been associated with stroke. These appear to be rare events.

Inherent Toxicity While the public may believe that "natural" equates with "safe," it is abundantly clear that natural products can be toxic. Misidentification of medicinal mushrooms has led to liver failure. Contamination of tryptophan supplements caused the eosinophilia-myalgia syndrome. Herbal products containing particular species of *Aristolochia* were associated with genitourinary malignancies. In 2001, extracts of kava, long used by Pacific Islanders for its mild anxiolytic and sedative properties, were associated with fulminant liver failure. A number of products, including the popular *Ginkgo biloba*, are known to prolong bleeding times and have been associated with postoperative hemorrhage. Among the most controversial is *Ephedra sinica*, or ma huang, a product used in traditional Chinese medicine for short-term treatment of asthma and bronchial congestion. The scientific basis for these indications was revealed when ephedra was shown to contain the ephedrine alkaloids, especially ephedrine and pseudoephedrine. With the promulgation of the DSHEA regulations, supplements containing ephedra and herbs rich in caffeine flooded the U.S. marketplace, claiming to promote weight loss and to enhance athletic performance. Reports of severe and fatal adverse events in young and, in some cases, well-known Americans led to calls for removal of ephedra-containing supplements.

Herbal-Drug Interactions The constituents of natural products may not only be toxic but may also interfere with the metabolism of life-saving drugs. This effect was illustrated most profoundly with the demonstration in 2000 that consumption of St.-John's-wort interferes with the bioavilability of the HIV protease inhibitor indinavir. Later studies showed its similar interference with metabolism of topoisomerase inhibitors such as irinotecan, with cyclosporine, and with many other drugs. The breadth of interference stems from the ability of hyperforin in St.-John's-wort to upregulate expression of the pregnane X receptor, a promiscuous nuclear regulatory factor that promotes the expression of many hepatic oxidative, conjugative, and efflux enzymes engaged in drug and food metabolism.

ACQUIRING EVIDENCE CAM evolved through an entirely different epistemologic framework than contemporary biomedicine. Empirical observations of individual patients constitute the primary evidentiary base on which CAM practices are guided and taught. Nonetheless, over the past few decades, thousands of studies have been performed of various CAM approaches, including hundreds of trials involving herbals, acupuncture, or homeopathy. To date, however, no single approach has been proven effective in a convincing way. (If they had, the practice would no longer be considered CAM!) Several factors contribute to this lack of convincing evidence. The vast majority of

CAM studies have been seriously flawed by lack of appropriate controls, bias on the part of the investigators, small sample sizes, reliance on highly subjective and nonvalidated measures of benefit, and by inappropriate statistical tests.

There are in addition, a series of methodologic issues that challenge even the better-designed CAM studies. No uniform practice guidelines exist, and the herbal products marketed in the United States are highly variable in quality and composition. Some CAM practices are not amenable to blinding. For example, both the patient and the practitioner would know if spinal manipulation had been performed. These problems are not unique to CAM, however, as they also complicate attempts to study conventional practices such as psychotherapy or surgery. Efforts are now being made to randomize patients to other equally demanding control interventions, and acupuncture at traditional needling points is being compared to needling at what are arguably irrelevant points.

Even with ongoing improvements in study design and conduct, issues of belief stand in the way of comprehending and accepting the results of some CAM studies. Many physicians are reluctant to believe positive outcomes of exotic approaches that have not emerged through the classic experimental paradigm by which drugs and biological agents are now developed, namely, the orderly progression from preclinical testing through three phases of clinical trials. More importantly, it is difficult to accept results that are counterintuitive or whose mechanism cannot be rationally explained. A powerful example of this dilemma involves studies of homeopathy. Some clinical trials of homeopathy for asthma, infantile diarrhea, and other common conditions reported positive results. Two systematic reviews of homeopathy trials gleaned an overall favorable impression of the clinical trials data, concluding that the treatments were more beneficial than placebo. Even the best trials and these reviews have been criticized on methodologic grounds. It remains unclear what evidence could compel a tidal change in belief about the benefits of homeopathy when there remain no cogent explanations for how substances diluted to the point at which only solute remains could exert physiologic effects.

By contrast, while methodologic problems continue to plague acupuncture trials, belief has been growing even in academic centers that acupuncture may be effective. The emerging acceptance of acupuncture may result, in part, from its widespread availability and use in the United States today: the CDC estimated that >1% of adult Americans received acupuncture treatments in 1999. Acupuncturists are now practicing within major medical centers, providing an ancillary approach to pain management. Yet, its acceptance may stem from more than just its communal appeal. Since the mid-1970s, studies have revealed palatable explanations for how needling may moderate pain and, not just by rephrasing the traditional explanation that acupuncture restores the flow of vital energies along meridians, for which there remain no known anatomic correlates. Rather, biochemical and imaging studies have shown that needling triggers the release of endogenous opioids that bind to specific receptors in the very brain regions that mediate the beneficial effects of narcotic analgesics.

EXISTING EVIDENCE Numerous CAM approaches lack coherent explanations and any credible body of data regarding their safety and effectiveness. And, while it is difficult to conclude decisively that an approach lacks any merit, it is quite feasible to discern that its effect size, or degree of benefit, is too small to be worth pursuing further. Over the past century, many approaches failed—one need only think back to the exotic electrical devices, procedures, and tonics that fell out of fashion. Two questions are often asked: (1) Whether any of the more contemporary CAM modalities deserve to be rejected? (2) Whether data showing it to be ineffective would change anyone's mind about using it? The case of laetrile is instructive in this regard. This extract of apricot seeds was touted in the 1970s as a cure for solid tumors. Thousands crossed the Mexican border to be treated. The lack of any positive preclinical data discouraged oncologists from agreeing to study laetrile, until public pressure required that an answer be obtained. Two studies in the 1980s showed no benefit of laetrile treatment. Today, some continue to seek the product, but the numbers are vastly smaller than before meaningful data were obtained. A similar fate befell a cocktail of drugs used for cancer patients through the 1970s and 1980s by Dr. Luigi DiBella in Italy, once large studies revealed it to have no detectable impact on the course of a variety of advanced cancers.

In contrast, modalities that have been well tested and found ineffective are still in fairly common practice. For example, the renowned biochemist and peace activist Linus Pauling proclaimed vitamin C to be the answer to the common cold. Numerous, high-quality studies failed to demonstrate clinically important effects of vitamin C in preventing or treating viral colds. The early studies were criticized for using too little of the vitamin, yet doses that well exceeded its bioavailability also proved negative. Nonetheless, ingestion of extra vitamin C remains a common habit in individuals who perceive the onset of cold symptoms. For most people, this practice is wasteful but not harmful; however, people with iron overload (either hemochromatosis or chronic transfusion requirement) can be damaged by vitamin C, which generates free radicals in the setting of iron excess.

Despite the failure of some CAM approaches, early studies have yielded positive or at least encouraging data for a number of them. Good sources of information include the Natural Medicines Comprehensive Database (www.NaturalDatabase.com) and National Institutes of Health (NIH) websites such as http://ods.od.nih.gov; http://nccam.nih.gov/health/ and http://www3.cancer.gov/occam/information.html.

Vitamins/Minerals

- *Vitamin A:* Massive studies in a number of developing nations proved that vitamin A deficiency is prevalent and associated with increased risks of mortality in young children. Prospective trials showed that 100,000 to 200,000 IU of vitamin A twice a year can reduce the overall death rate significantly.
- *Folic Acid:* Rates of neural tube defects are significantly diminished if the diet is supplemented with folic acid during pregnancy.
- *Folic acid, vitamin B_6, and vitamin B_{12}:* Randomized, double-blind, controlled trials suggest that this vitamin combination lowers serum homocysteine levels and the risk of myocardial infarction.
- *Vitamins C and E, β-carotene, and zinc:* A large, randomized controlled trial showed that these supplements combined reduce the progression of age-related macular degeneration.

Even vitamins and minerals, which are presumed safe in moderate doses, can have unexpected adverse effects. Two large controlled trials of β-carotene for prevention of cancer or retinal diseases found increased rates of lung cancer in those randomized to the supplement. Ongoing are large prospective trials seeking benefits from ingestion of supplements on rates of prostate cancer (vitamin E and selenium) and Alzheimer's disease (vitamin E).

Herbals and Other Natural Products

- *Glucosamine and/or chondroitin sulfate:* Systematic surveys of controlled trials concluded that these products of animal joints are superior to placebo in improving performance and slowing the narrowing of the joint space in patients with osteoarthritis of the knee.
- *Ginkgo biloba:* Americans consumed nearly $250 million of this herbal product in 2000. The literature shows no evidence that it improves cognition, but it may decrease the risk of dementia.

- *Saw palmetto (Serenoa repens) and African plum (Pygeum africanum):* Each of these botanicals is likely effective for the symptomatic treatment of benign prostatic hyperplasia. Sales of saw palmetto are growing, with an estimated $131 million of the product consumed by Americans in 2000.
- *St.-John's-wort (Hypericum perforatum):* Among the most popular herbal product worldwide, numerous small studies and systematic reviews suggested it to benefit patients with a wide range of depressive syndromes. High-quality, randomized, placebo-controlled trials, found St.-John's-wort to not be superior to placebo for treatment of major depression of moderate severity, a spectrum of illness that clearly warrants professional evaluation and treatment.
- *Echinacea species: Echinacea* roots are widely used to treat or prevent respiratory infections, with over $200 million in sales in 2000. Although in vitro studies have shown that *Echinacea* constituents stimulate humoral and cellular immune responses, systematic reviews of the clinical trials have not concluded that they are beneficial.

Other Modalities

- *Acupuncture:* A frequently cited NIH-led consensus development conference in 1997 concluded that evidence exists that acupuncture relieves nausea from chemotherapy and pain following extraction of molars. Some subsequent studies have confirmed these earlier impressions regarding acute nausea and vomiting, but the data regarding pain management have been mixed, with little evidence that it benefits neuropathic pain.
- *Mind-body medicine:* Clinical trials support the use of biofeedback for incontinence, headache, and stroke rehabilitation. Hypnosis may be beneficial in relieving pain due to minor surgical interventions, chemotherapy-associated nausea, and irritable bowel syndrome.
- *Spinal manipulation:* Systematic reviews of fairly well designed trials concluded that chiropractic or osteopathic manipulation provides significant improvement for patients with uncomplicated acute back pain. No proof exists that they are superior to, or more cost-effective than, other conventional approaches, nor do they alter the long-term outcome.

SUMMARY An array of unproven modalities will always be used by the patients under our care. Physicians must approach each encounter as an opportunity to better understand patients, their beliefs, and their expectations and as an opportunity to help guide their choices in a constructive way. Many of these choices are entirely innocuous and can be accommodated in the context of the larger diagnostic and therapeutic intervention. Some should be actively discouraged. Along the way, scientific evidence will drive many CAM approaches out of favor. Some modalities will garner sufficient support to become part of mainstream care: the next generation of physicians will never know they were once controversial.

FURTHER READING

DE SMET PA: Herbal remedies. N Engl J Med 347:2046, 2002

EISENBERG DM et al: Trends in alternative medicine use in the United States, 1990–1997: Results of a follow-up national survey. JAMA 280:1569, 1998

ENGEL L, STRAUS SE: Development of therapeutics: Opportunities within complementary and alternative medicine. Nat Rev Drug Discov 1:229, 2002

KAPTCHUK TJ: Acupuncture: Theory, efficacy and practice. Ann Intern Med 136:374, 2002

KINSEL JF, STRAUS SE: Complementary and alternative therapeutics: rigorous research is needed to support claims. Annu Rev Pharmacol Toxicol 43:463, 2003

RICHARDSON MA, STRAUS SE: Complementary and alternative medicine: Opportunities and challenges for cancer management and research. Semin Oncol 29:531, 2002

11 | PAIN: PATHOPHYSIOLOGY AND MANAGEMENT
Howard L. Fields, Joseph B. Martin

The task of medicine is to preserve and restore health and to relieve suffering. Understanding pain is essential to both these goals. Because pain is universally understood as a signal of disease, it is the most common symptom that brings a patient to a physician's attention. The function of the pain sensory system is to protect the body and maintain homeostasis. It does this by detecting, localizing, and identifying tissue-damaging processes. Since different diseases produce characteristic patterns of tissue damage, the quality, time course, and location of a patient's pain complaint and the location of tenderness provide important diagnostic clues and are used to evaluate the response to treatment. Once this information is obtained, it is the obligation of the physician to provide rapid and effective pain relief.

THE PAIN SENSORY SYSTEM

Pain is an unpleasant sensation localized to a part of the body. It is often described in terms of a penetrating or tissue-destructive process (e.g., stabbing, burning, twisting, tearing, squeezing) and/or of a bodily or emotional reaction (e.g., terrifying, nauseating, sickening). Furthermore, any pain of moderate or higher intensity is accompanied by anxiety and the urge to escape or terminate the feeling. These properties illustrate the duality of pain: it is both sensation and emotion. When acute, pain is characteristically associated with behavioral arousal and a stress response consisting of increased blood pressure, heart rate, pupil diameter, and plasma cortisol levels. In addition, local muscle contraction (e.g., limb flexion, abdominal wall rigidity) is often present.

PERIPHERAL MECHANISMS ■ The Primary Afferent Nociceptor A peripheral nerve consists of the axons of three different types of neurons: primary sensory afferents, motor neurons, and sympathetic postganglionic neurons (Fig. 11-1). The cell bodies of primary afferents are located in the dorsal root ganglia in the vertebral foramina. The primary afferent axon bifurcates to send one process into the spinal cord and the other to innervate tissues. Primary afferents are classified by their diameter, degree of myelination, and conduction velocity. The largest-diameter fibers, A-beta (Aβ), respond maximally to light touch and/or moving stimuli; they are present primarily in nerves that innervate the skin. In normal individuals, the activity of these fibers does not produce pain. There are two other classes of primary afferents: the small-diameter myelinated A-delta (Aδ) and the unmyelinated (C fiber) axons (Fig. 11-1). These fibers are present in nerves to the skin and to deep somatic and visceral structures. Some tissues, such as the cornea, are innervated only by Aδ and C afferents. Most Aδ and C afferents respond maximally only to intense (painful) stimuli and produce the subjective experience of pain when they are electrically stimulated; this defines them as *primary afferent nociceptors* (*pain receptors*). The ability to detect painful stimuli is completely abolished when Aδ and C axons are blocked.

Individual primary afferent nociceptors can respond to several different types of noxious stimuli. For example, most nociceptors respond to heating, intense mechanical stimuli such as a pinch, and application of irritating chemicals.

Sensitization When intense, repeated, or prolonged stimuli are applied to damaged or inflamed tissues the threshold for activating primary afferent nociceptors is lowered and the frequency of firing is higher for all stimulus intensities. Inflammatory mediators such as bradykinin, some prostaglandins, and leukotrienes contribute to this process, which is called *sensitization*. In sensitized tissues normally innocuous stimuli can produce pain. Sensitization is a clinically important process that contributes to tenderness, soreness, and hyperalgesia. A striking example of sensitization is sunburned skin, in which severe pain can be produced by a gentle slap on the back or a warm shower.

Sensitization is of particular importance for pain and tenderness in deep tissues. Viscera are normally relatively insensitive to noxious mechanical and thermal stimuli, although hollow viscera do generate significant discomfort when distended. In contrast, when affected by a disease process with an inflammatory component, deep structures such as joints or hollow viscera characteristically become exquisitely sensitive to mechanical stimulation.

A large proportion of Aδ and C afferents innervating viscera are completely insensitive in normal noninjured, noninflamed tissue. That is, they cannot be activated by known mechanical or thermal stimuli and are not spontaneously active. However, in the presence of inflammatory mediators, these afferents become sensitive to mechanical stimuli. Such afferents have been termed *silent nociceptors*, and their characteristic properties may explain how under pathologic conditions the relatively insensitive deep structures can become the source of severe and debilitating pain and tenderness. Low pH, prostaglandins, leukotrienes, and other inflammatory mediators such as bradykinin play a significant role in sensitization.

Nociceptor-Induced Inflammation One important concept to emerge in recent years is that afferent nociceptors also have a neuroeffector func-

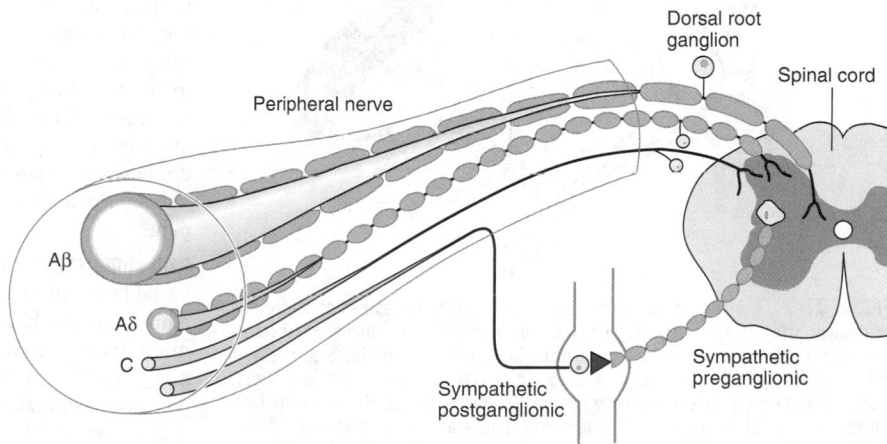

FIGURE 11-1 Components of a typical cutaneous nerve. There are two distinct functional categories of axons: primary afferents with cell bodies in the dorsal root ganglion, and sympathetic postganglionic fibers with cell bodies in the sympathetic ganglion. Primary afferents include those with large-diameter myelinated (Aβ), small-diameter myelinated (Aδ), and unmyelinated (C) axons. All sympathetic postganglionic fibers are unmyelinated.

tion. Most nociceptors contain polypeptide mediators that are released from their peripheral terminals when they are activated (Fig. 11-2). An example is substance P, an 11-amino-acid peptide. Substance P is released from primary afferent nociceptors and has multiple biologic activities. It is a potent vasodilator, degranulates mast cells, is a chemoattractant for leukocytes, and increases the production and release of inflammatory mediators. Interestingly, depletion of substance P from joints reduces the severity of experimental arthritis. Primary afferent nociceptors are not simply passive messengers of threats to tissue injury but also play an active role in tissue protection through these neuroeffector functions.

CENTRAL MECHANISMS ■ The Spinal Cord and Referred Pain The axons of primary afferent nociceptors enter the spinal cord via the dorsal root. They terminate in the dorsal horn of the spinal gray matter (Fig. 11-3). The terminals of primary afferent axons contact spinal neurons that transmit the pain signal to brain sites involved in pain perception. The axon of each primary afferent contacts many spinal neurons, and each spinal neuron receives convergent inputs from many primary afferents.

The convergence of sensory inputs to a single spinal pain-transmission neuron is of great importance because it underlies the phenomenon of referred pain. All spinal neurons that receive input from

FIGURE 11-2 Events leading to activation, sensitization, and spread of sensitization of primary afferent nociceptor terminals. *A.* Direct activation by intense pressure and consequent cell damage. Cell damage induces lower pH (H+) and leads to release of potassium (K+) and to synthesis of prostaglandins (PG) and bradykinin (BK). Prostaglandins increase the sensitivity of the terminal to bradykinin and other pain-producing substances. *B.* Secondary activation. Impulses generated in the stimulated terminal propagate not only to the spinal cord but also into other terminal branches where they induce the release of peptides, including substance P (SP). Substance P causes vasodilation and neurogenic edema with further accumulation of bradykinin. Substance P also causes the release of histamine (H) from mast cells and serotonin (5HT) from platelets.

FIGURE 11-3 The convergence-projection hypothesis of referred pain. According to this hypothesis, visceral afferent nociceptors converge on the same pain-projection neurons as the afferents from the somatic structures in which the pain is perceived. The brain has no way of knowing the actual source of input and mistakenly "projects" the sensation to the somatic structure.

the viscera and deep musculoskeletal structures also receive input from the skin. The convergence patterns are determined by the spinal segment of the dorsal root ganglion that supplies the afferent innervation of a structure. For example, the afferents that supply the central diaphragm are derived from the third and fourth cervical dorsal root ganglia. Primary afferents with cell bodies in these same ganglia supply the skin of the shoulder and lower neck. Thus sensory inputs from both the shoulder skin and the central diaphragm converge on pain-transmission neurons in the third and fourth cervical spinal segments. *Because of this convergence and the fact that the spinal neurons are most often activated by inputs from the skin, activity evoked in spinal neurons by input from deep structures is mislocalized by the patient to a place that is roughly coextensive with the region of skin innervated by the same spinal segment.* Thus inflammation near the central diaphragm is usually reported as discomfort near the shoulder. This spatial displacement of pain sensation from the site of the injury that produces it is known as *referred pain.*

Ascending Pathways for Pain A majority of spinal neurons contacted by primary afferent nociceptors send their axons to the contralateral thalamus. These axons form the contralateral spinothalamic tract, which lies in the anterolateral white matter of the spinal cord, the lateral edge of the medulla, and the lateral pons and midbrain. The spinothalamic pathway is crucial for pain sensation in humans. Interruption of this pathway produces permanent deficits in pain and temperature discrimination.

Spinothalamic tract axons ascend to several regions of the thalamus. There is tremendous divergence of the pain signal from these thalamic sites to broad areas of the cerebral cortex that subserve different aspects of the pain experience (Fig. 11-4). One of the thalamic projections is to the somatosensory cortex. This projection mediates the purely sensory aspects of pain, i.e., its location, intensity, and quality. Other thalamic neurons project to cortical regions that are linked to emotional responses, such as the cingulate gyrus and other areas of the frontal lobes. These pathways to the frontal cortex subserve the affective or unpleasant emotional dimension of pain. This affective dimension of pain produces suffering and exerts potent control of behavior. Because of this dimension, fear is a constant companion of pain.

PAIN MODULATION The pain produced by similar injuries is remarkably variable in different situations and in different individuals. For example, athletes have been known to sustain serious fractures with only minor pain, and Beecher's classic World War II survey revealed that many soldiers in battle were unbothered by injuries that would have produced agonizing pain in civilian patients. Furthermore, even the suggestion of relief can have a significant analgesic effect (placebo). On the other hand, many patients find even minor injuries (such as venipuncture) frightening and unbearable, and the expectation of pain has been demonstrated to induce pain without a noxious stimulus.

The powerful effect of expectation and other psychological varia-

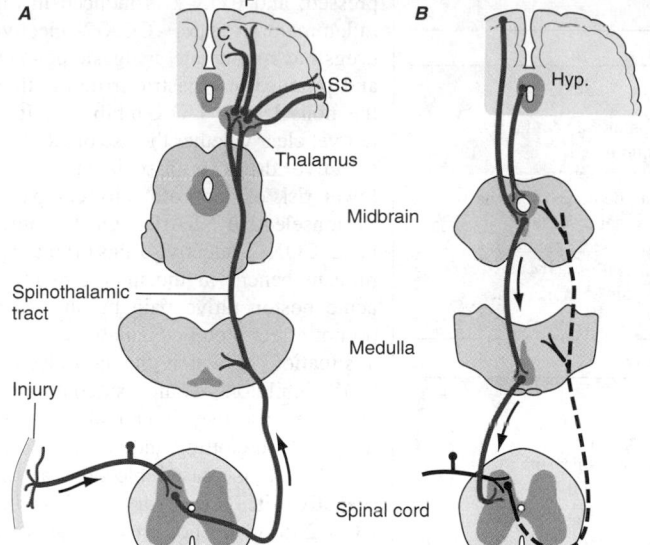

FIGURE 11-4 *A.* Transmission system for nociceptive messages. Noxious stimuli activate the sensitive peripheral ending of the primary afferent nociceptor by the process of transduction. The message is then transmitted over the peripheral nerve to the spinal cord, where it synapses with cells of origin of the major ascending pain pathway, the spinothalamic tract. The message is relayed in the thalamus to the anterior cingulate (C), frontal insular (F), and somatosensory cortex (SS). *B.* Pain-modulation network. Inputs from frontal cortex and hypothalamus (Hyp.) activate cells in the midbrain that control spinal pain-transmission cells via cells in the medulla.

bles on the perceived intensity of pain implies the existence of brain circuits that can modulate the activity of the pain-transmission pathways. One of these circuits has links in the hypothalamus, midbrain, and medulla, and it selectively controls spinal pain-transmission neurons through a descending pathway (Fig. 11-4).

Human brain imaging studies have implicated this pain-modulating circuit in the pain-relieving effect of attention, suggestion, and opioid analgesic medications. Furthermore, each of the component structures of the pathway contains opioid receptors and is sensitive to the direct application of opioid drugs. In animals, lesions of the system reduce the analgesic effect of systemically administered opioids such as morphine. Along with the opioid receptor, the component nuclei of this pain-modulating circuit contain endogenous opioid peptides such as the enkephalins and β-endorphin.

The most reliable way to activate this endogenous opioid-mediated modulating system is by prolonged pain and/or fear. There is evidence that pain-relieving endogenous opioids are released following surgical procedures and in patients given a placebo for pain relief.

Pain-modulating circuits can enhance as well as suppress pain. Both pain-inhibiting and pain-facilitating neurons in the medulla project to and control spinal pain-transmission neurons. Since pain-transmission neurons can be activated by modulatory neurons, it is theoretically possible to generate a pain signal with no peripheral noxious stimulus. In fact, functional imaging studies have demonstrated increased activity in this circuit during migraine headache. A central circuit that facilitates pain could account for the finding that pain can be induced by suggestion and could provide a framework for understanding how psychological factors can contribute to chronic pain.

NEUROPATHIC PAIN Lesions of the peripheral or central nervous pathways for pain typically result in a loss or impairment of pain sensation. Paradoxically, damage or dysfunction of these pathways can produce pain. For example, damage to peripheral nerves, as occurs in diabetic neuropathy, or to primary afferents, as in herpes zoster, can result in pain that is referred to the body region innervated by the damaged nerves. Though rare, pain may also be produced by damage to the central nervous system, particularly the spinothalamic pathway or thalamus. Such neuropathic pains are often severe and are notoriously intractable to standard treatments for pain.

Neuropathic pains typically have an unusual burning, tingling, or electric shock–like quality and may be triggered by very light touch. These features are rare in other types of pain. On examination, a sensory deficit is characteristically present in the area of the patient's pain. Hyperpathia is also characteristic of neuropathic pain; patients often complain that the very lightest moving stimuli evoke exquisite pain (allodynia). In this regard it is of clinical interest that a topical preparation of 5% lidocaine in patch form is effective for patients with postherpetic neuralgia who have prominent allodynia.

A variety of mechanisms contribute to neuropathic pain. As with sensitized primary afferent nociceptors, damaged primary afferents, including nociceptors, become highly sensitive to mechanical stimulation and begin to generate impulses in the absence of stimulation. There is evidence that this increased sensitivity and spontaneous activity is due to an increased concentration of sodium channels. Damaged primary afferents may also develop sensitivity to norepinephrine. Interestingly, spinal cord pain-transmission neurons cut off from their normal input may also become spontaneously active. Thus both central and peripheral nervous system hyperactivity contribute to neuropathic pain.

Sympathetically Maintained Pain Patients with peripheral nerve injury can develop a severe burning pain (causalgia) in the region innervated by the nerve. The pain typically begins after a delay of hours to days or even weeks. The pain is accompanied by swelling of the extremity, periarticular osteoporosis, and arthritic changes in the distal joints. The pain is dramatically and immediately relieved by blocking the sympathetic innervation of the affected extremity. Damaged primary afferent nociceptors acquire adrenergic sensitivity and can be activated by stimulation of the sympathetic outflow. A similar syndrome called *reflex sympathetic dystrophy* can be produced without obvious nerve damage by a variety of injuries, including fractures of bone, soft tissue trauma, myocardial infarction, and stroke (Chap. 354). Although the pathophysiology of this condition is poorly understood, the pain and the signs of inflammation are rapidly relieved by blocking the sympathetic nervous system. This implies that sympathetic activity can activate undamaged nociceptors when inflammation is present. Signs of sympathetic hyperactivity should be sought in patients with post-traumatic pain and inflammation and no other obvious explanation.

℞ TREATMENT

ACUTE PAIN The ideal treatment for any pain is to remove the cause; thus diagnosis should always precede treatment planning. Sometimes treating the underlying condition does not immediately relieve pain. Furthermore, some conditions are so painful that rapid and effective analgesia is essential (e.g., the postoperative state, burns, trauma, cancer, sickle cell crisis). Analgesic medications are a first line of treatment in these cases, and all practitioners should be familiar with their use.

Aspirin, Acetaminophen, and Nonsteroidal Anti-Inflammatory Agents (NSAIDS) These drugs are considered together because they are used for similar problems and may have a similar mechanism of action (Table 11-1). All these compounds inhibit cyclooxygenase (COX), and, except for acetaminophen, all have anti-inflammatory actions, especially at higher dosages. They are particularly effective for mild to moderate headache and for pain of musculoskeletal origin.

Since they are effective for these common types of pain and are available without prescription, COX inhibitors are by far the most commonly used analgesics. They are absorbed well from the gastrointestinal tract and, with occasional use, side effects are minimal. With chronic use, gastric irritation is a common side effect of aspirin and NSAIDs and is the problem that most frequently limits the dose that can be given. Gastric irritation is most severe with aspirin, which may cause erosion of the gastric mucosa, and because aspirin irreversibly acetylates platelets and thereby interferes with coagulation of the blood, gastrointestinal bleeding is a risk. The NSAIDs are less prob-

TABLE 11-1 *Drugs for Relief of Pain*

Generic Name	Dose, mg	Interval	Comments
NONNARCOTIC ANALGESICS: USUAL DOSES AND INTERVALS			
Acetylsalicylic acid	650 PO	q 4 h	Enteric-coated preparations available
Acetaminophen	650 PO	q 4 h	Side effects uncommon
Ibuprofen	400 PO	q 4–6 h	Available without prescription
Naproxen	250–500 PO	q 12 h	Delayed effects may be due to long half-life
Fenoprofen	200 PO	q 4–6 h	Contraindicated in renal disease
Indomethacin	25–50 PO	q 8 h	Gastrointestinal side effects common
Ketorolac	15–60 IM	q 4–6 h	Available for parenteral use (IM)
Rofecoxib	12.5–25 PO	q 24 h	FDA approved for pain management
Celecoxib	100–200 PO	q 12–24 h	Useful for arthritis

Generic Name	Parenteral Dose, mg	PO Dose, mg	Comments
NARCOTIC ANALGESICS: USUAL DOSES AND INTERVALS			
Codeine	30–60 q 4 h	30–60 q 4 h	Nausea common
Oxycodone	—	5–10 q 4–6 h	Usually available with acetaminophen or aspirin
Morphine	10 q 4 h	60 q 4 h	
Morphine sustained release	—	30–200 bid to tid	Oral slow-release preparation
Hydromorphone	1–2 q 4 h	2–4 q 4 h	Shorter acting than morphine sulfate
Levorphanol	2 q 6–8 h	4 q 6–8 h	Longer acting than morphine sulfate; absorbed well PO
Methadone	10 q 6–8 h	20 q 6–8 h	Delayed sedation due to long half-life
Meperidine	75–100 q 3–4 h	300 q 4 h	Poorly absorbed PO; normeperidine a toxic metabolite
Butorphanol	—	1–2 q 4 h	Intranasal spray
Fentanyl	25–100 μg/h	—	72 h Transdermal patch
Tramadol	—	50–100 q 4–6 h	Mixed opioid/adrenergic action

Generic Name	Uptake Blockade 5-HT	Uptake Blockade NE	Sedative Potency	Anticholinergic Potency	Orthostatic Hypotension	Cardiac Arrhythmia	Ave. Dose, mg/d	Range, mg/d
ANTIDEPRESSANTS[a]								
Doxepin	++	+	High	Moderate	Moderate	Less	200	75–400
Amitriptyline	++++	++	High	Highest	Moderate	Yes	150	25–300
Imipramine	++++	++	Moderate	Moderate	High	Yes	200	75–400
Nortriptyline	+++	++	Moderate	Moderate	Low	Yes	100	40–150
Desipramine	+++	++++	Low	Low	Low	Yes	150	50–300
Venlafaxine	+++	++	Low	None	None	No	150	75–400

Generic Name	PO Dose, mg	Interval	Generic Name	PO Dose, mg	Interval
ANTICONVULSANTS AND ANTIARRHYTHMICS[a]					
Phenytoin	300	daily/qhs	Clonazepam	1	q 6 h
Carbamazepine	200–300	q 6 h	Mexiletine	150–300	q 6–12 h
Oxcarbazine	300	bid	Gabapentin[b]	600–1200	q 8 h

[a] Antidepressants, anticonvulsants, and antiarrhythmics have not been approved by the U.S. Food and Drug Administration (FDA) for the treatment of pain.

[b] Gabapentin in doses up to 1800 mg/d is FDA approved for postherpetic neuralgia.

Note: 5-HT, serotonin; NE, norepinephrine.

pressed, and COX-2 is induced in the inflammatory state. COX-2-selective drugs have moderate analgesic potency and produce less gastric irritation than the nonselective COX inhibitors. It is not yet clear whether the use of COX-2-selective drugs is associated with a lower risk of nephrotoxicity compared to nonselective NSAIDs. On the other hand, COX-2-selective drugs offer a significant benefit in the management of acute postoperative pain because they do not affect blood coagulation. This is a situation in which the nonselective COX inhibitors would be contraindicated because they impair platelet-mediated blood clotting and are thus associated with increased bleeding at the operative site. A corollary of this is that COX-2 drugs do not provide the same degree of protection from thromboembolic cardiovascular adverse events such as myocardial infarction. In fact, in patients treated for arthritis, those treated with naproxen had significantly fewer adverse thromboembolic events than those treated with rofecoxib, a selective COX-2 inhibitor.

Opioid Analgesics Opioids are the most potent pain-relieving drugs currently available. Furthermore, of all analgesics, they have the broadest range of efficacy, providing the most reliable and effective method for rapid pain relief. Although side effects are common, they are usually not serious except for respiratory depression and can be reversed rapidly with the narcotic antagonist naloxone. The physician should not hesitate to use opioid analgesics in patients with acute severe pain. Table 11-1 lists the most commonly used opioid analgesics.

Opioids produce analgesia by actions in the central nervous system. They activate pain-inhibitory neurons and directly inhibit pain-transmission neurons. Most of the commercially available opioid analgesics act at the same opioid receptor (mu receptor), differing mainly in potency, speed of onset, duration of action, and optimal route of administration. Although the dose-related side effects (sedation, respiratory depression, pruritus, constipation) are similar among the different opioids, some side effects are due to accumulation of nonopioid metabolites that are unique to individual drugs. One striking example of this is normeperidine, a metabolite of meperidine. Normeperidine produces hyperexcitability and seizures that are not reversible with naloxone. Normeperidine accumulation is increased in patients with renal failure.

The most rapid relief with opioids is obtained by intravenous administration; relief with oral administration is significantly slower. Common acute side effects include nausea, vomiting, and sedation. The most serious side effect is respiratory depression. Patients with any form of respiratory compromise must be kept under close observation following opioid administration; an oxygen saturation monitor may be useful. The opioid antagonist, naloxone, should be readily

lematic, but their risk in this regard is still significant. In addition to their well known gastrointestinal toxicity, nephrotoxicity is a significant problem for patients using NSAIDs on a chronic basis, and patients at risk for renal insufficiency should be monitored closely. NSAIDs also cause an increase in blood pressure in a significant number of individuals. Long-term treatment with NSAIDs requires regular blood pressure monitoring and treatment if necessary. Although toxic to the liver when taken in a high dose, acetaminophen rarely produces gastric irritation and does not interfere with platelet function.

The introduction of a parenteral form of NSAID, ketorolac, extends the usefulness of this class of compounds in the management of acute severe pain. Ketorolac is sufficiently potent and rapid in onset to supplant opioids for many patients with acute severe headache and musculoskeletal pain.

There are two major classes of COX: COX-1 is constitutively ex-available. Opioid effects are dose-related, and there is great variability among patients in the doses that relieve pain and produce side effects. Because of this, initiation of therapy requires titration to optimal dose and interval. The most important principle is to provide adequate pain relief. This requires determining whether the drug has adequately relieved the pain and the duration of the relief. *The most common error made by physicians in managing severe pain with opioids is to prescribe an inadequate dose. Since many patients are reluctant to complain, this practice leads to needless suffering.* In the absence of sedation at the expected time of peak effect, a physician should not hesitate to repeat the initial dose to achieve satisfactory pain relief.

An innovative approach to the problem of achieving adequate pain relief is the use of patient-controlled analgesia (PCA). PCA requires a device that delivers a baseline continuous dose of an opioid drug, and preprogrammed additional doses whenever the patient pushes a button. The device can be programmed to limit the total hourly dose so that overdosing is impossible. The patient can then titrate the dose to the optimal level. This approach is used most extensively for the management of postoperative pain, but there is no reason why it should not be used for any hospitalized patient with persistent severe pain. PCA is also used for short-term home care of patients with intractable pain, such as is caused by metastatic cancer.

Many physicians, nurses, and patients have a certain trepidation about using opioids that is based on an exaggerated fear of addiction. In fact, there is a vanishingly small chance of patients becoming addicted to narcotics as a result of their appropriate medical use.

The availability of new routes of administration has extended the usefulness of opioid analgesics. Most important is the availability of spinal administration. Opioids can be infused through a spinal catheter placed either intrathecally or epidurally. By applying opioids directly to the spinal cord, regional analgesia can be obtained using a relatively low total dose. In this way, such side effects as sedation, nausea, and respiratory depression can be minimized. This approach has been used extensively in obstetric procedures and for lower-body postoperative pain. Opioids can also be given intranasally (butorphanol), rectally, and transdermally (fentanyl), thus avoiding the discomfort of frequent injections in patients who cannot be given oral medication. The fentanyl transdermal patch has the advantage of providing fairly steady plasma levels, which maximizes patient comfort.

OPIOID AND CYCLOOXYGENASE INHIBITOR COMBINATIONS When used in combination, opioids and COX inhibitors have additive effects. Because a lower dose of each can be used to achieve the same degree of pain relief and their side effects are nonadditive, such combinations can be used to lower the severity of dose-related side effects. Fixed-ratio combinations of an opioid with acetaminophen carry a special risk. Dose escalation as a result of increased severity of pain or decreased opioid effect as a result of tolerance may lead to levels of acetaminophen that are toxic to the liver.

CHRONIC PAIN

Managing patients with chronic pain is intellectually and emotionally challenging. The patient's problem is often difficult to diagnose; such patients are demanding of the physician's time and often appear emotionally distraught. The traditional medical approach of seeking an obscure organic pathology is usually unhelpful. On the other hand, psychological evaluation and behaviorally based treatment paradigms are frequently helpful, particularly in the setting of a multidisciplinary pain-management center.

There are several factors that can cause, perpetuate, or exacerbate chronic pain. First, of course, the patient may simply have a disease that is characteristically painful for which there is presently no cure. Arthritis, cancer, migraine headaches, fibromyalgia, and diabetic neuropathy are examples of this. Second, there may be secondary perpetuating factors that are initiated by disease and persist after that disease has resolved. Examples include damaged sensory nerves, sympathetic efferent activity, and painful reflex muscle contraction. Finally, a variety of psychological conditions can exacerbate or even cause pain.

There are certain areas to which special attention should be paid in the medical history. Because depression is the most common emotional disturbance in patients with chronic pain, patients should be questioned about their mood, appetite, sleep patterns, and daily activity. A simple standardized questionnaire, such as the Beck Depression Inventory, can be a useful screening device. It is important to remember that major depression is a common, treatable, and potentially fatal illness.

Other clues that a significant emotional disturbance is contributing to a patient's chronic pain complaint include: pain that occurs in multiple unrelated sites; a pattern of recurrent, but separate, pain problems beginning in childhood or adolescence; pain beginning at a time of emotional trauma, such as the loss of a parent or spouse; a history of physical or sexual abuse; and past or present substance abuse.

On examination, special attention should be paid to whether the patient guards the painful area and whether certain movements or postures are avoided because of pain. Discovering a mechanical component to the pain can be useful both diagnostically and therapeutically. Painful areas should be examined for deep tenderness, noting whether this is localized to muscle, ligamentous structures, or joints. Chronic myofascial pain is very common, and in these patients deep palpation may reveal highly localized trigger points that are firm bands or knots in muscle. Relief of the pain following injection of local anesthetic into these trigger points supports the diagnosis. A neuropathic component to the pain is indicated by evidence of nerve damage, such as sensory impairment, exquisitely sensitive skin, weakness and muscle atrophy, or loss of deep tendon reflexes. Evidence suggesting sympathetic nervous system involvement includes the presence of diffuse swelling, changes in skin color and temperature, and hypersensitive skin and joint tenderness compared with the normal side. Relief of the pain with a sympathetic block is diagnostic.

A guiding principle in evaluating patients with chronic pain is to assess both emotional and organic factors before initiating therapy. Addressing these issues together, rather than waiting to address emotional issues after organic causes of pain have been ruled out, improves compliance in part because it assures patients that a psychological evaluation does not mean that the physician is questioning the validity of their complaint. Even when an organic cause for a patient's pain can be found, it is still wise to look for other factors. For example, a cancer patient with painful bony metastases may have additional pain due to nerve damage and may also be depressed. Optimal therapy requires that each of these factors be looked for and treated.

℞ TREATMENT

Once the evaluation process has been completed and the likely causative and exacerbating factors identified, an explicit treatment plan should be developed. An important part of this process is to identify specific and realistic functional goals for therapy, such as getting a good night's sleep, being able to go shopping, or returning to work. A multidisciplinary approach that utilizes medications, counseling, physical therapy, nerve blocks, and even surgery may be required to improve the patient's quality of life. There are also some newer, relatively invasive procedures that can be helpful for some patients with intractable pain. These procedures include implanting intraspinal cannulae to deliver morphine or intraspinal electrodes for spinal stimulation. There are no set criteria for predicting which patients will respond to these procedures. They are generally reserved for patients who have not responded to conventional pharmacologic approaches. Referral to a multidisciplinary pain clinic for a full evaluation should precede any of these procedures. Such referrals are clearly not necessary for all chronic pain patients. For some, pharmacologic management alone can often provide adequate relief.

ANTIDEPRESSANT MEDICATIONS The tricyclic antidepressants (TCAs; Table 11-1) are extremely useful for the management of patients with chronic pain. Although developed for the treatment of depression, the tricyclics have a spectrum of dose-related biologic activities that include the production of analgesia in a variety of clinical conditions. Although the mechanism is unknown, the analgesic effect of TCAs has a more rapid onset and occurs at a lower dose than is typically required for the treatment of depression. Furthermore, patients with chronic pain who are not depressed obtain pain relief with antidepressants. There is evidence that tricyclic drugs potentiate opioid analgesia, so they are useful adjuncts for the treatment of severe persistent pain such as occurs with malignant tumors. Table 11-2 lists some of the painful conditions that respond to tricyclics. TCAs are of particular value in the management of neuropathic pain such as occurs in diabetic neuropathy and postherpetic neuralgia, for which there are few other therapeutic options.

The TCAs that have been shown to relieve pain have significant side effects (Table 11-1; Chap. 371). Some of these side effects, such as orthostatic hypotension, cardiac conduction delay, memory impairment, constipation, and urinary retention, are particularly problematic in elderly patients, and several are additive to the side effects of opioid analgesics. The serotonin-selective reuptake inhibitors such as fluoxetine (Prozac) have fewer and less serious side effects than TCAs, but they are much less effective for relieving pain. It is of interest that venlafaxine (Effexor), a nontricyclic antidepressant that blocks both serotonin and norepinephrine reuptake, appears to retain most of the pain-relieving effect of TCAs with a side-effect profile more like that of the serotonin-selective reuptake inhibitors. The drug may be particularly useful in patients who cannot tolerate the side effects of tricyclics.

ANTICONVULSANTS AND ANTIARRHYTHMICS (Table 11-1) These drugs are useful primarily for patients with neuropathic pain. Phenytoin (Dilantin) and carbamazepine (Tegretol) were first shown to relieve the pain of trigeminal neuralgia. This pain has a characteristic brief, shooting, electric shock–like quality. In fact, anticonvulsants seem to be helpful largely for pains that have such a lancinating quality. A new-generation anticonvulsant, gabapentin (Neurontin), is effective for a broad range of neuropathic pains.

Antiarrhythmic drugs such as low-dose lidocaine and mexiletine (Mexitil) can also be effective for neuropathic pain. These drugs block the spontaneous activity of damaged primary afferent nociceptors.

CHRONIC OPIOID MEDICATION The long-term use of opioids is accepted for patients with pain due to malignant disease. Although opioid use for chronic pain of nonmalignant origin is controversial, it is clear that for many such patients opioid analgesics are the best available option. This is understandable since opioids are the most potent and have the broadest range of efficacy of any analgesic medications. Although addiction is rare in patients who first use opioids for pain relief, some degree of tolerance and physical dependence are likely with long-term use. Therefore, before embarking on opioid therapy, other options should be explored, and the limitations and risks of opioids should be explained to the patient. It is also important to point out that some opioid analgesic medications have mixed agonist-antagonist properties (e.g., pentazocine and butorphanol). From a practical standpoint, this means that they may worsen pain by inducing an abstinence syndrome in patients who are physically dependent on other opioid analgesics.

With long-term outpatient use of orally administered opioids, it is desirable to use long-acting compounds such as levorphanol, methadone, or sustained-release morphine (Table 11-1). Transdermal fentanyl is another excellent option. The pharmacokinetic profile of these drug preparations enables prolonged pain relief, minimizes side effects such as sedation that are associated with high peak plasma levels, and reduces the likelihood of rebound pain associated with a rapid fall in plasma opioid concentration. Constipation is a virtually universal side effect of opioid use and should be treated expectantly.

It is worth emphasizing that many patients, especially those with chronic pain, seek medical attention primarily because they are suffering and because only physicians can provide the medications required for their relief. A primary responsibility of all physicians is to minimize the physical and emotional discomfort of their patients. Familiarity with pain mechanisms and analgesic medications is an important step toward accomplishing this aim.

FURTHER READING

CRAIG AD: How do you feel? Interoception: The sense of the physiological condition of the body. Nat Rev Neurosci:655, 2002

PETROVIC P et al: Placebo and opioid analgesia—imaging a shared neuronal network. Science:1737, 2002

TABLE 11-2 *Painful Conditions that Respond to Tricyclic Antidepressants*

Postherpetic neuralgia[a]	Rheumatoid arthritis[a,b]
Diabetic neuropathy[a]	Chronic low back pain[b]
Tension headache[a]	Cancer
Migraine headache[a]	Central post-stroke pain

[a] Controlled trials demonstrate analgesia.
[b] Controlled studies indicate benefit but not analgesia.

---

12 CHEST DISCOMFORT AND PALPITATIONS
Thomas H. Lee

CHEST DISCOMFORT

Chest discomfort is one of the most common challenges for clinicians in the office or emergency department. The differential diagnosis includes conditions affecting organs throughout the thorax and abdomen, with prognostic implications that vary from benign to life-threatening (Table 12-1). Failure to recognize potentially serious conditions such as acute ischemic heart disease, aortic dissection, tension pneumothorax, or pulmonary embolism can lead to serious complications, including death. Conversely, overly conservative management of low-risk patients leads to unnecessary hospital admissions, tests, procedures, and anxiety.

CAUSES OF CHEST DISCOMFORT

MYOCARDIAL ISCHEMIA AND INJURY (See also Chap. 226) Myocardial ischemia occurs when the oxygen supply to the heart is not sufficient

---

TABLE 12-1 *Differential Diagnoses of Patients Admitted to Hospital with Acute Chest Pain Ruled Not Myocardial Infarction*

Diagnosis	Percent
Gastroesophageal disease[a]	42
Gastroesophageal reflux	
Esophageal motility disorders	
Peptic ulcer	
Gallstones	
Ischemic heart disease	31
Chest wall syndromes	28
Pericarditis	4
Pleuritis/pneumonia	2
Pulmonary embolism	2
Lung cancer	1.5
Aortic aneurysm	1
Aortic stenosis	1
Herpes zoster	1

[a] In order of frequency.
Source: Fruergaard P et al: Eur Heart J 17:1028, 1996.

to meet metabolic needs. This mismatch can result from a decrease in oxygen supply, a rise in demand, or both. The most common underlying cause of myocardial ischemia is obstruction of coronary arteries by atherosclerosis; in the presence of such obstruction, transient ischemic episodes are usually precipitated by an increase in oxygen demand as a result of physical exertion. However, ischemia can also result from psychological stress, fever, or large meals or from compromised oxygen delivery due to anemia, hypoxia, or hypotension. Ventricular hypertrophy due to valvular heart disease, hypertrophic cardiomyopathy, or hypertension can predispose the myocardium to ischemia because of impaired penetration of blood flow from epicardial coronary arteries to the endocardium.

Angina Pectoris   The chest discomfort of myocardial ischemia is a visceral discomfort that is usually described as a heaviness, pressure, or squeezing (Table 12-2). Other common adjectives for anginal pain are burning and aching. Some patients deny any "pain" but may admit to dyspnea or a vague sense of anxiety. The word "sharp" is sometimes used by patients to describe intensity rather than quality.

The location of angina pectoris is usually retrosternal; most patients do not localize the pain to any small area. The discomfort may radiate to the neck, jaw, teeth, arms, or shoulders, reflecting the common origin in the posterior horn of the spinal cord of sensory neurons supplying the heart and these areas. Some patients present with aching in sites of radiated pain as their only symptoms of ischemia. Occasional patients report epigastric distress with ischemic episodes. Less common is radiation to below the umbilicus or to the back.

Stable angina pectoris usually develops gradually with exertion, emotional excitement, or after heavy meals. Rest or treatment with sublingual nitroglycerin typically leads to relief within several minutes. In contrast, pain that is fleeting (lasting only a few seconds) is rarely ischemic in origin. Similarly, pain that lasts for several hours is unlikely to represent angina, particularly if the patient's electrocardiogram does not show evidence of ischemia.

Anginal episodes can be precipitated by any physiologic or psychological stress that induces tachycardia. Most myocardial perfusion occurs during diastole, when there is minimal pressure opposing coronary artery flow from within the left ventricle. Since tachycardia decreases the percentage of the time in which the heart is in diastole, it decreases myocardial perfusion.

TABLE 12-2   *Typical Clinical Features of Major Causes of Acute Chest Discomfort*

Condition	Duration	Quality	Location	Associated Features
Angina	More than 2 and less than 10 min	Pressure, tightness, squeezing, heaviness, burning	Retrosternal, often with radiation to or isolated discomfort in neck, jaw, shoulders, or arms—frequently on left	Precipitated by exertion, exposure to cold, psychologic stress S4 gallop or mitral regurgitation murmur during pain
Unstable angina	10–20 min	Similar to angina but often more severe	Similar to angina	Similar to angina, but occurs with low levels of exertion or even at rest
Acute myocardial infarction	Variable; often more than 30 min	Similar to angina but often more severe	Similar to angina	Unrelieved by nitroglycerin May be associated with evidence of heart failure or arrhythmia
Aortic stenosis	Recurrent episodes as described for angina	As described for angina	As described for angina	Late-peaking systolic murmur radiating to carotid arteries
Pericarditis	Hours to days; may be episodic	Sharp	Retrosternal or toward cardiac apex; may radiate to left shoulder	May be relieved by sitting up and leaning forward Pericardial friction rub
Aortic dissection	Abrupt onset of unrelenting pain	Tearing or ripping sensation; knifelike	Anterior chest, often radiating to back, between shoulder blades	Associated with hypertension and/or underlying connective tissue disorder, e.g., Marfan syndrome Murmur of aortic insufficiency, pericardial rub, pericardial tamponade, or loss of peripheral pulses
Pulmonary embolism	Abrupt onset; several minutes to a few hours	Pleuritic	Often lateral, on the side of the embolism	Dyspnea, tachypnea, tachycardia, and hypotension
Pulmonary hypertension	Variable	Pressure	Substernal	Dyspnea, signs of increased venous pressure including edema and jugular venous distention
Pneumonia or pleuritis	Variable	Pleuritic	Unilateral, often localized	Dyspnea, cough, fever, rales, occasional rub
Spontaneous pneumothorax	Sudden onset; several hours	Pleuritic	Lateral to side of pneumothorax	Dyspnea, decreased breath sounds on side of pneumothorax
Esophageal reflux	10–60 min	Burning	Substernal, epigastric	Worsened by postprandial recumbency Relieved by antacids
Esophageal spasm	2–30 min	Pressure, tightness, burning	Retrosternal	Can closely mimic angina
Peptic ulcer	Prolonged	Burning	Epigastric, substernal	Relieved with food or antacids
Gallbladder disease	Prolonged	Burning, pressure	Epigastric, right upper quadrant, substernal	May follow meal
Musculoskeletal disease	Variable	Aching	Variable	Aggravated by movement May be reproduced by localized pressure on examination
Herpes zoster	Variable	Sharp or burning	Dermatomal distribution	Vesicular rash in area of discomfort
Emotional and psychiatric conditions	Variable; may be fleeting	Variable	Variable, may be retrosternal	Situational factors may precipitate symptoms Anxiety or depression often detectable with careful history

Unstable Angina and Myocardial Infarction (See also Chaps. 227 and 228) Patients with these acute ischemic syndromes usually complain of symptoms similar in quality to angina pectoris, but more prolonged and severe. The onset of these syndromes may occur with the patient at rest, or awakened from sleep, and sublingual nitroglycerin may lead to transient or no relief. Accompanying symptoms may include diaphoresis, dyspnea, nausea, and light-headedness.

The physical examination may be completely normal in patients with chest discomfort due to ischemic heart disease. Careful auscultation during ischemic episodes may reveal a third or fourth heart sound, reflecting myocardial systolic or diastolic dysfunction. A transient murmur of mitral regurgitation suggests ischemic papillary muscle dysfunction. Severe episodes of ischemia can lead to pulmonary congestion and even pulmonary edema.

Other Cardiac Causes Myocardial ischemia caused by hypertrophic cardiomyopathy, aortic stenosis, or other conditions leads to angina pectoris similar to that caused by coronary atherosclerosis. In such cases, a systolic murmur or other findings usually suggest the abnormalities other than coronary atherosclerosis that may be contributing to the patient's symptoms. Some patients with chest pain and normal coronary angiograms have functional abnormalities of the coronary circulation, ranging from coronary spasm visible on coronary angiography to abnormal vasodilator responses and heightened vasoconstrictor responses. The term "Syndrome X" is used to describe patients with angina-like chest pain and ischemic-appearing ST segment depression during stress despite normal coronary arteriograms. Some data indicate that many such patients have limited changes in coronary flow in response to pacing stress or coronary vasodilators. Despite the possibility that chest pain may be due to myocardial ischemia in such patients, their prognosis is excellent.

PERICARDITIS (See also Chap. 222) The pain in pericarditis is believed to be due to inflammation of the adjacent parietal pleura, since most of the pericardium is believed to be insensitive to pain. Thus, infectious pericarditis, which usually involves adjoining pleura surfaces, tends to be associated with pain, while conditions that cause only local inflammation (e.g., myocardial infarction or uremia) and cardiac tamponade tend to result in mild or no chest pain.

The adjacent parietal pleura receives its sensory supply from several sources, so the pain of pericarditis can be experienced in areas ranging from the shoulder and neck to the abdomen and back. Most typically, the pain is retrosternal and is aggravated by coughing, deep breaths, or changes in position—all of which lead to movements of pleural surfaces. The pain is often worse in the supine position and relieved by sitting upright and leaning forward. Less common is a steady aching discomfort that mimics acute myocardial infarction.

DISEASES OF THE AORTA (See also Chap. 231) *Aortic dissection* is a potentially catastrophic condition that is due to spread within the wall of the aorta of a subintimal hematoma. The hematoma may begin with a tear in the intima of the aorta or with rupture of the vasa vasorum within the aortic media. This syndrome can occur with trauma to the aorta, including motor vehicle accidents or medical procedures in which catheters or intraaortic balloon pumps damage the intima of the aorta. Nontraumatic aortic dissections are rare in the absence of hypertension and/or conditions associated with deterioration of the elastic or muscular components of the media within the aorta's wall. Cystic medial degeneration is a feature of several inherited connective tissue diseases, including Marfan and Ehlers-Danlos syndromes. About half of all aortic dissections in women under 40 years of age occur during pregnancy.

Almost all patients with acute dissections present with severe chest pain, although some patients with chronic dissections are identified without associated symptoms. Unlike the pain of ischemic heart disease, symptoms of aortic dissection tend to reach peak severity immediately, often causing the patient to collapse from its intensity. The adjectives used to describe the pain reflect the process occurring within the wall of the aorta—"ripping" and "tearing"—and the location usually correlates with the site and extent of the dissection. Thus, dissections that begin in the ascending aorta and extend to the descending aorta tend to cause pain in the front of the chest that extends into the back, between the shoulder blades.

Physical findings may also reflect extension of the aortic dissection that compromises flow into arteries branching off the aorta. Thus, loss of a pulse in one or both arms, cerebrovascular accident, or paraplegia can all be catastrophic consequences of aortic dissection. Hematomas that extend proximally and undermine the coronary arteries or aortic valve apparatus may lead to acute myocardial infarction or acute aortic insufficiency. Rupture of the hematoma into the pericardial space leads to pericardial tamponade.

Another abnormality of the aorta that can cause chest pain is a *thoracic aortic aneurysm*. Aortic aneurysms are frequently asymptomatic but can cause chest pain and other symptoms by compressing adjacent structures. This pain tends to be steady, deep, and sometimes severe.

PULMONARY EMBOLISM (See also Chap. 244) Chest pain due to pulmonary embolism is believed to be due to distention of the pulmonary artery or infarction of a segment of the lung adjacent to the pleura. Massive pulmonary emboli may lead to substernal pain that is suggestive of acute myocardial infarction. More commonly, smaller emboli lead to focal pulmonary infarctions that cause pain that is lateral and pleuritic. Associated symptoms include dyspnea and, occasionally, hemoptysis. Tachycardia is usually present. Although not always present, certain characteristic ECG changes can support the diagnosis.

PNEUMOTHORAX (See also Chap. 245) Sudden onset of pleuritic chest pain and respiratory distress should lead to consideration of spontaneous pneumothorax, as well as pulmonary embolism. Such events may occur without a precipitating event in people without lung disease, or as a consequence of underlying lung disorders.

PNEUMONIA OR PLEURITIS (See also Chaps. 239 and 245) Lung diseases that damage and cause inflammation of the pleura of the lung usually cause a sharp, knifelike pain that is aggravated by inspiration or coughing.

GASTROINTESTINAL CONDITIONS (See also Chap. 273) Esophageal pain from acid reflux from the stomach, spasm, obstruction, or injury can be difficult to discern from myocardial syndromes. Acid reflux typically causes a deep burning discomfort that may be exacerbated by alcohol, aspirin, or some foods; this discomfort is often relieved by antacid or other acid-reducing therapies. Acid reflux tends to be exacerbated by lying down and may be worse in early morning when the stomach is empty of food that might otherwise absorb gastric acid.

Esophageal spasm may occur in the presence or absence of acid reflux, and leads to a squeezing pain indistinguishable from angina. Prompt relief of esophageal spasm is often provided by antianginal therapies such as sublingual nifedipine, further promoting confusion between these syndromes. Chest pain can also result from injury to the esophagus, such as a Mallory-Weiss tear caused by severe vomiting.

Chest pain can result from diseases of the gastrointestinal tract below the diaphragm, including *peptic ulcer disease*, *biliary disease*, and *pancreatitis*. These conditions usually cause abdominal pain as well as chest discomfort; symptoms are not likely to be associated with exertion. The pain of ulcer disease typically occurs 60 to 90 min after meals, when postprandial acid production is no longer neutralized by food in the stomach. Cholecystitis usually causes a pain that is described as aching, occurring an hour or more after meals.

NEUROMUSCULOSKELETAL CONDITIONS *Cervical disk disease* can cause chest pain by compression of nerve roots. Pain in a dermatomal distribution can also be caused by *intercostal muscle cramps* or by *herpes zoster*. Chest pain symptoms due to herpes zoster may occur before skin lesions are apparent.

Costochondral and *chondrosternal syndromes* are the most common causes of anterior chest musculoskeletal pain. Only occasionally are physical signs of costochondritis such as swelling, redness, and warmth (Tietze's syndrome) present. The pain of such syndromes is usually fleeting and sharp, but some patients experience a dull ache that lasts for hours. Direct pressure on the chondrosternal and costochondral junctions may reproduce the pain from these and other musculoskeletal syndromes. Arthritis of the shoulder and spine and bursitis may also cause chest pain. Some patients who have these conditions and myocardial ischemia blur and confuse symptoms of these syndromes.

EMOTIONAL AND PSYCHIATRIC CONDITIONS As many as 10% of patients who present to emergency departments with acute chest pain have panic disorder or other emotional conditions. The symptoms in these populations are highly variable, but frequently the discomfort is described as visceral tightness or aching that lasts more than 30 min. Some patients offer other atypical descriptions, such as pain that is fleeting, sharp, and/or localized to a small region. The electrocardiogram in patients with emotional conditions may be difficult to interpret if hyperventilation causes ST-T-wave abnormalities. A careful history may elicit clues of depression, prior panic attacks, somatization, agoraphobia, or other phobias.

APPROACH TO THE PATIENT

The evaluation of the patient with chest discomfort must accommodate two goals—determining the diagnosis and assessing the safety of the immediate management plan. The latter issue is often dominant when the patient has acute chest discomfort, such as patients seen in the emergency department. In such settings, the clinician must focus first on identifying patients who require aggressive interventions to diagnose or manage potentially life-threatening conditions, including acute ischemic heart disease, acute aortic dissection, pulmonary embolism, and tension pneumothorax. If such conditions are unlikely, the clinician must address questions such as the safety of discharge to home, admission to a non-coronary care unit facility, or immediate exercise testing. Table 12-3 displays a sequence of questions that can be used in the evaluation of the patient with chest discomfort, with the diagnostic entities that are most important for consideration at each stage of the evaluation.

ACUTE CHEST DISCOMFORT In patients with acute chest discomfort, the clinician must first assess the patient's respiratory and hemodynamic status. If either is compromised, initial management should focus on stabilizing the patient before the diagnostic evaluation is pursued. If, however, the patient does not require emergent interventions, then a focused history, physical examination,

and laboratory evaluation should be performed to assess the patient's risk of life-threatening conditions.

The *history* should include questions about the quality and location of the chest discomfort (Table 12-2). The patient should also be asked about the nature of onset of the pain and its duration. Myocardial ischemia is usually associated with a gradual intensification of symptoms over a period of minutes. Pain that is fleeting or that lasts hours without being associated with electrocardiographic changes is not likely to be ischemic in origin. Although the presence of risk factors for coronary artery disease may heighten concern for this diagnosis, the absence of such risk factors does not lower the risk for myocardial ischemia enough to be used to justify a decision to discharge a patient.

Wide radiation of chest pain increases probability that pain is due to myocardial infarction. Radiation of chest pain to the left arm is common with acute ischemic heart disease, but radiation to the right arm is also consistent with this diagnosis. Right shoulder pain is common with acute cholecystitis, but this syndrome is usually accompanied by pain that is located in the abdomen rather than chest. Chest pain that radiates between the scapulae raises the question of aortic dissection.

The *physical examination* should include evaluation of blood pressure in both arms and of pulses in both legs. Poor perfusion of a limb may be due to an aortic dissection that has compromised flow to an artery branching from the aorta. Chest auscultation may reveal diminished breath sounds; a pleural rub; or evidence of pneumothorax, pulmonary embolism, pneumonia, or pleurisy. Tension pneumothorax may lead to a shift in the trachea from the midline, away from the side of the pneumothorax. The cardiac examination should seek pericardial rubs, systolic and diastolic murmurs, and third or fourth heart sounds. Pressure on the chest wall may reproduce symptoms in patients with musculoskeletal causes of chest pain; it is important that the clinician ask the patient if the chest pain syndrome is being completely reproduced before drawing too much reassurance that more serious underlying conditions are not present.

An *electrocardiogram* is an essential test for adults with chest discomfort that is not due to an obvious traumatic cause. In such patients, the presence of electrocardiographic changes consistent with ischemia or infarction (Chap. 210) is associated with high risks of acute myocardial infarction or unstable angina (Table 12-4); such patients should be admitted to a unit with electrocardiographic monitoring and the capacity to respond to a cardiac arrest. The absence of such changes does not exclude acute ischemic heart

---

TABLE 12-3   *Considerations in the Assessment of the Patient with Chest Pain*

1. Could the chest discomfort be due to an acute, potentially life-threatening condition that warrants immediate hospitalization and aggressive evaluation?

Acute ischemic heart disease	Pulmonary embolism
Aortic dissection	Spontaneous pneumothorax

2. If not, could the discomfort be due to a chronic condition likely to lead to serious complications?

   Stable angina
   Aortic stenosis
   Pulmonary hypertension

3. If not, could the discomfort be due to an acute condition that warrants specific treatment?

   Pericarditis
   Pneumonia/pleuritis
   Herpes zoster

4. If not, could the discomfort be due to another treatable chronic condition?

Esophageal reflux	Cervical disk disease
Esophageal spasm	Arthritis of the shoulder or spine
Peptic ulcer disease	Costochondritis
Gallbladder disease	Other musculoskeletal disorders
Other gastrointestinal conditions	Anxiety state

TABLE 12-4   *Prevalence of Myocardial Infarction and Unstable Angina Among Subsets of Patients with Acute Chest Pain in the Emergency Department*

	Prevalence	
Finding	Myocardial Infarction, %	Unstable Angina, %
ST elevation (≥ 1 mm) or Q waves on ECG not known to be old	79	12
Ischemia or strain on ECG not known to be old (ST depression ≥ 1 mm or ischemic T waves)	20	41
None of the preceding ECG changes but a prior history of angina or myocardial infarction (history of heart attack or nitroglycerin use)	4	51
None of the preceding ECG changes and no prior history of angina or myocardial infarction (history of heart attack or nitroglycerin use)	2	14

Note: ECG, electrocardiogram.
Source: Unpublished data from Brigham and Women's Hospital Chest Pain Study, 1997–1999.

disease, but the risk of life-threatening complications is low for patients with normal electrocardiograms or only nonspecific ST-T-wave changes. If these patients are not considered appropriate for immediate discharge, they are often candidates for early or immediate exercise testing.

Markers of myocardial injury are often obtained in the emergency department evaluation of acute chest discomfort. The most commonly used markers are creatine kinase (CK), CK-MB, and the cardiac troponins (I and T). Rapid bedside assays of the cardiac troponins have been developed and shown to be sufficiently accurate to predict prognosis and guide management. Some data support the use of other markers, such as serum myoglobin, C-reactive protein (CRP), and B-type natriuretic peptide (BNP); their roles are the subject of ongoing research. Single values of any of these markers do not have high sensitivity for acute myocardial infarction or for prediction of complications. Hence, decisions to discharge patients home should not be made on the basis of single negative values of these tests.

Provocative tests for coronary artery disease are not appropriate for patients with ongoing chest pain. In such patients, rest myocardial perfusion scans can be considered; a normal scan reduces the likelihood of coronary artery disease, and can help avoid admission of low-risk patients to the hospital. Clinicians frequently employ therapeutic trials with sublingual nitroglycerin or antacids or, in the stable patient seen in the office setting, a proton pump inhibitor. A common error is to assume that a response to any of these interventions clarifies the diagnosis. While such information is often helpful, the patient's response may be due to the placebo effect. Hence, myocardial ischemia should never be considered excluded solely because of a response to antacid therapy. Similarly, failure of nitroglycerin to relieve pain does not exclude the diagnosis of coronary disease.

If the patient's history or examination is consistent with aortic dissection, imaging studies to evaluate the aorta must be pursued promptly because of the high risk of catastrophic complications with this condition. A chest x-ray is not sufficient to exclude this diagnosis. Appropriate tests include a chest computed tomography scan with contrast or a magnetic resonance imaging scan in patients who are hemodynamically stable, or a transesophageal echocardiogram in patients who are less stable. Aortic angiography is no longer a first test at most institutions.

Acute pulmonary embolism should be considered in patients with respiratory symptoms, pleuritic chest pain, hemoptysis, or a history of venous thromboembolism or coagulation abnormalities. Initial tests usually include a lung scan and/or pulmonary arteriography.

If patients with acute chest discomfort show no evidence of life-threatening conditions, the clinician should then focus on serious chronic conditions with the potential to cause major complications, the most common of which is stable angina. Early use of exercise electrocardiography, stress echocardiography, or stress perfusion imaging for such patients, whether in the office or the emergency department, is now an accepted management strategy for low-risk patients. Exercise testing is not appropriate, however, for patients who (1) report pain that is believed to be ischemic occurring at rest or (2) have electrocardiographic changes not known to be old that are consistent with ischemia.

Patients with sustained chest discomfort who do not have evidence for life-threatening conditions should be evaluated for evidence of conditions likely to benefit from acute treatment (Table 12-3). Pericarditis may be suggested by the history, physical examination, and electrocardiogram (Table 12-2). Clinicians should carefully assess blood pressure patterns and consider echocardiography in such patients to detect evidence of impending pericardial tamponade. Chest x-rays can be used to evaluate the possibility of pulmonary disease.

GUIDELINES AND CRITICAL PATHWAYS FOR ACUTE CHEST PAIN

Guidelines for the initial evaluation for patients with acute chest pain have been developed by the American College of Cardiology, American Heart Association, and other organizations. These guidelines recommend performance of an electrocardiogram for virtually all patients with chest pain who do not have an obvious noncardiac cause of their pain, and performance of a chest x-ray for patients with signs or symptoms consistent with congestive heart failure, valvular heart disease, pericarditial disease, or aortic dissection or aneurysm.

Other organizations, including the Agency for Health Care Policy and Research (AHCPR) and the National Heart Attack Alert Program, have also issued guidelines for management of patients with a high probability of acute ischemic heart disease. In these and other guidelines, patients with possible or probable acute myocardial infarction as suggested by the description of their pain or ECG findings are expected to be admitted to the hospital. The AHCPR guidelines for unstable angina note that not all patients with that syndrome require admission but recommend that patients with unstable angina be monitored electrocardiographically during their evaluation; that those with ongoing rest pain should be placed at bed rest during the initial phase of stabilization.

The American Heart Association has published guidelines for the use of exercise testing in the emergency department. These recommendations include having two sets of cardiac enzymes or troponins at 4-h intervals that are normal; an ECG at presentation and preexercise ECG that shows no significant change; absence of rest ECG abnormalities that preclude accurate interpretation of an exercise ECG; and absence of ischemic chest pain at the time of exercise testing or during the observation period after admission to the emergency department.

Many medical centers have adopted critical pathways and other forms of guidelines to increase efficiency and to expedite the treatment of patients with high-risk acute ischemic heart disease syndromes. These guidelines emphasize the following strategies:

- Rapid identification and treatment of patients for whom emergent reperfusion therapy, either via percutaneous coronary interventions or thrombolytic agents, is likely to lead to improved outcomes.
- Triage to non-coronary care unit monitored facilities such as intermediate care units or chest pain units of patients with a low risk for complications, such as patients without new ischemic changes on their electrocardiograms and without ongoing chest pain. Such patients can usually be safely observed in non-coronary care unit settings, undergo early exercise testing, or be discharged home. Risk stratification can be assisted through use of prospectively validated multivariate algorithms that have been published for acute ischemic heart disease and its complications.
- Shortening lengths of stay in the coronary care unit and hospital. Recommendations regarding the minimum length of stay in a monitored bed for a patient who has no further symptoms have decreased in recent years to 12 h or less if exercise testing or other risk stratification technologies are available.

NONACUTE CHEST DISCOMFORT

The management of patients who do not require admission to the hospital or who no longer require inpatient observation should seek to identify the cause of the symptoms and the likelihood of major complications. Cost-effectiveness analyses support use of noninvasive testing for coronary disease, such as exercise electrocardiography and stress echocardiography. These tests serve both to diagnose coronary disease and to identify patients with high-risk forms of coronary disease who may benefit from revascularization. Gastrointestinal causes of chest pain can be evaluated via endoscopy or radiology studies, or with trials of medical therapy. Emotional and psychiatric conditions warrant appropriate evaluation and treatment; randomized trial data indicate that cognitive therapy and group interventions lead to decreases in symptoms for such patients.

Palpitations are characterized by an awareness of the beating of the heart. Patients commonly describe "pounding" or "fluttering" heart beats or report a sensation that the heart is stopping or skipping beats. These symptoms may be caused by a change in the heart's rhythm or rate or by an increase in the force of its contractions. In many cases, this awareness reflects lack of competing sensory stimuli, such as when a person is lying in bed, unable to sleep.

Palpitations are often manifestations of psychiatric conditions, the most common of which are depression and panic disorder. For example, in one study of outpatients referred for ambulatory electrocardiographic monitoring to evaluate palpitations, 19% were found to have a psychiatric disorder. Patients with psychiatric disorders were more likely than other patients to report that their palpitations lasted longer than 15 min or were accompanied by ancillary symptoms. In this study, physicians usually recognized the emotional basis of the patients' symptoms but frequently did not refer the patient for specific therapy.

Palpitations can also be caused by virtually any cardiac arrhythmia as well as by other cardiac and noncardiac conditions. A markedly enlarged left ventricle can cause awareness of the heart beat by contact with the chest wall. Any condition associated with increased catecholamine levels can lead to palpitations both by increasing the forcefulness of cardiac contractions and by increasing the rate of premature beats.

Palpitations can be intermittent or sustained and regular or irregular. Patients with this complaint should be asked to describe their palpitations' onset, duration, associated symptoms, and the circumstances in which they occur. Abrupt onset and termination after several minutes may reflect a sustained ventricular or supraventricular tachyarrhythmia. Gradual onset and termination of a pounding heart beat is more consistent with sinus tachycardia. Patients should try to replicate the rhythm of their palpitations by tapping on a table. This maneuver can help the physician determine the nature of any cardiac arrhythmia. Patients should also be taught to take their pulse so that they can more accurately report their approximate heart rate and whether the rhythm was regular.

DIFFERENTIAL DIAGNOSIS

Patients who report "skipped" beats or a "flopping" sensation often have atrial or ventricular extrasystoles (Chap. 214). These premature beats are followed by a compensatory pause, and the first heart beat after the pause may be unusually strong due to increased left ventricular volume and enhanced contractility (a phenomenon called *postextrasystolic potentiation*). Sustained bursts of rapid heart beats may be due to ventricular or supraventricular tachyarrhythmias. A sustained irregular rhythm suggests atrial fibrillation.

Conditions that cause marked left ventricular enlargement such as aortic regurgitation can cause an awareness of the heart beat that is sometimes positional. Presumably because of associated arrhythmias, hypertrophic cardiomyopathy, mitral valve prolapse, and other cardiac structural abnormalities are also associated with palpitations.

Palpitations can also be a prominent symptom in noncardiac conditions, including thyrotoxicosis, hypoglycemia, pheochromocytoma, and fever. The physiologic basis of palpitations with these conditions is either arrhythmia or increased catecholamine levels leading to greater myocardial contractility. Drugs that can precipitate arrhythmias and palpitations include tobacco, coffee, tea, alcohol, epinephrine, ephedrine, aminophylline, and atropine.

APPROACH TO THE PATIENT

The first goal in the evaluation of patients with palpitations is to exclude the possibility of life-threatening arrhythmias. The risk for such arrhythmias is highest in patients with coronary artery disease, congestive heart failure, or other structural cardiac abnormalities. The history, physical examination, and electrocardiogram should therefore be focused on stratifying patients according to the risk of such conditions. Palpitations are also more likely to reflect serious arrhythmias if they are associated with symptoms that suggest hemodynamic compromise, such as syncope, light-headedness, dizziness, or shortness of breath.

The most common first test after the initial evaluation of palpitations is continuous electrocardiographic (Holter) monitoring. This test is especially useful if patients have unexplained palpitations that recur frequently. For patients with more sporadic palpitations, a variety of new technologies have become available to allow capture of ECG tracings at the time of their symptoms. These technologies include loop recorders, that can freeze the last several minutes of data when the patient presses a button, and telephonic monitors, which can be used to "call in" tracings when symptoms occur. For patients who require very long-term monitoring, implantable loop recorders are available. If episodes are associated with physical stress, exercise electrocardiography can be used in an attempt to elicit an arrhythmia.

Most patients with palpitations do not have evidence of major arrhythmias or abnormal physiologic conditions associated with increased catecholamine levels. Patients with emotional or psychological causes of palpitations should be evaluated for possible cognitive and pharmaceutical therapy. Drugs and medications that may precipitate palpitations should be eliminated or reduced. A trial of beta blockers is often successful in reducing premature beats and symptoms. Regardless of the cause and treatment, the clinician should remain aware that palpitations are extremely bothersome symptoms for patients. Reassurance that a comprehensive evaluation has been performed and that the palpitations do not adversely affect the patient's prognosis is a critical part of the patient's care.

FURTHER READING

Barsky AJ et al: Somatized psychiatric disorder presenting as palpitations. Arch Intern Med 156:1102, 1996

Braunwald E et al: ACC/AHA guideline update for the management of patients with unstable angina and non-ST-segment elevation myocardial infarction, 2002: Summary article. J Am Coll Cardiol 40:1366, 2002

Cannon CP et al: National Heart Attack Alert Program (NHAAP) Coordinating Committee Critical Pathways Writing Group. Critical pathways for management of patients with acute coronary syndromes: An assessment by the National Heart Attack Alert Program. Am Heart J 143:777, 2002

Gibson PB, et al: Low event rate for stress-only perfusion imaging in patients evaluated for chest pain. J Am Coll Cardiol 39:999, 2002

Hamm CW: Cardiac biomarkers for rapid evaluation of chest pain. Circulation 104:1454, 2001

Martinez E, et al: The observation unit: A new interface between inpatient and outpatient care. Am J Med 110:274:2001

Ng SM, et al: Ninety-minute accelerated critical pathway for chest pain evaluation. Am J Cardiol 88:611:2001

Pope JH, et al: Missed diagnoses of acute cardiac ischemia in the emergency department. N Engl J Med 342:1163, 2000

Stein RA, et al: Safety and utility of exercise testing in emergency room chest pain centers: An advisory from the Committee on Exercise, Rehabilitation, and Prevention Council on Clinical Cardiology, American Heart Association. Circulation 102:1463, 2000

Van Peski-Oosterbaan AS et al: Cognitive-behavioral therapy for noncardiac chest pain: A randomized trial. Am J Med 106:424, 1999

Weber BE, Kapoor WN: Evaluation and outcomes of patients with palpitations. Am J Med 100:138, 1996

The correct interpretation of acute abdominal pain is challenging. Since proper therapy may require urgent action, the unhurried approach suitable for the study of other conditions is sometimes denied. Few other clinical situations demand greater judgment, because the most catastrophic of events may be forecast by the subtlest of symptoms and signs. A meticulously executed, detailed history and physical examination are of great importance. The etiologic classification in Table 13-1, although not complete, forms a useful basis for the evaluation of patients with abdominal pain.

The diagnosis of "acute or surgical abdomen" is not an acceptable one because of its often misleading and erroneous connotation. The most obvious of "acute abdomens" may not require operative intervention, and the mildest of abdominal pains may herald an urgently correctable lesion. Any patient with abdominal pain of recent onset requires early and thorough evaluation and accurate diagnosis.

SOME MECHANISMS OF PAIN ORIGINATING IN THE ABDOMEN ■ Inflammation of the Parietal Peritoneum The pain of parietal peritoneal inflammation is steady and aching in character and is located directly over the inflamed area, its exact reference being possible because it is transmitted by somatic nerves supplying the parietal peritoneum. The intensity of the pain is dependent on the type and amount of material to which the peritoneal surfaces are exposed in a given time period. For example, the sudden release into the peritoneal cavity of a small quantity of *sterile* acid gastric juice causes much more pain than the same amount

---

TABLE 13-1   Some Important Causes of Abdominal Pain

PAIN ORIGINATING IN THE ABDOMEN

1. Parietal peritoneal inflammation
   a. Bacterial contamination, e.g., perforated appendix, pelvic inflammatory disease
   b. Chemical irritation, e.g., perforated ulcer, pancreatitis, mittelschmerz
2. Mechanical obstruction of hollow viscera
   a. Obstruction of the small or large intestine
   b. Obstruction of the biliary tree
   c. Obstruction of the ureter
3. Vascular disturbances
   a. Embolism or thrombosis
   b. Vascular rupture
   c. Pressure or torsional occlusion
   d. Sickle cell anemia
4. Abdominal wall
   a. Distortion or traction of mesentery
   b. Trauma or infection of muscles
5. Distention of visceral surfaces, e.g., hepatic or renal capsules

PAIN REFERRED FROM EXTRAABDOMINAL SOURCE

1. Thorax, e.g., pneumonia, referred pain from coronary occlusion
2. Spine, e.g., radiculitis from arthritis, herpes zoster
3. Genitalia, e.g., torsion of the testicle

METABOLIC CAUSES

1. Exogenous
   a. Black widow spider bite
   b. Lead poisoning and others
2. Endogenous
   a. Uremia
   b. Diabetic ketoacidosis
   c. Porphyria
   d. Allergic factors (C′1 esterase inhibitor deficiency)

NEUROGENIC CAUSES

1. Organic
   a. Tabes dorsalis
   b. Herpes zoster
   c. Causalgia and others
2. Functional

---

of grossly contaminated neutral feces. Enzymatically active pancreatic juice incites more pain and inflammation than does the same amount of sterile bile containing no potent enzymes. Blood and urine are often so bland as to go undetected if their contact with the peritoneum has not been sudden and massive. In the case of bacterial contamination, such as in pelvic inflammatory disease, the pain is frequently of low intensity early in the illness until bacterial multiplication has caused the elaboration of irritating substances.

The rate at which the irritating material is applied to the peritoneum is important. Perforated peptic ulcer may be associated with entirely different clinical pictures dependent only on the rapidity with which the gastric juice enters the peritoneal cavity.

The pain of peritoneal inflammation is invariably accentuated by pressure or changes in tension of the peritoneum, whether produced by palpation or by movement, as in coughing or sneezing. The patient with peritonitis lies quietly in bed, preferring to avoid motion, in contrast to the patient with colic, who may writhe incessantly.

Another characteristic feature of peritoneal irritation is tonic reflex spasm of the abdominal musculature, localized to the involved body segment. The intensity of the tonic muscle spasm accompanying peritoneal inflammation is dependent on the location of the inflammatory process, the rate at which it develops, and the integrity of the nervous system. Spasm over a perforated retrocecal appendix or perforated ulcer into the lesser peritoneal sac may be minimal or absent because of the protective effect of overlying viscera. A slowly developing process often greatly attenuates the degree of muscle spasm. Catastrophic abdominal emergencies such as a perforated ulcer may be associated with minimal or no detectable pain or muscle spasm in obtunded, seriously ill, debilitated elderly patients or in psychotic patients.

Obstruction of Hollow Viscera The pain of obstruction of hollow abdominal viscera is classically described as intermittent, or colicky. Yet the lack of a truly cramping character should not be misleading, because distention of a hollow viscus may produce steady pain with only very occasional exacerbations. It is not nearly as well localized as the pain of parietal peritoneal inflammation.

The colicky pain of obstruction of the small intestine is usually periumbilical or supraumbilical and is poorly localized. As the intestine becomes progressively dilated with loss of muscular tone, the colicky nature of the pain may diminish. With superimposed strangulating obstruction, pain may spread to the lower lumbar region if there is traction on the root of the mesentery. The colicky pain of colonic obstruction is of lesser intensity than that of the small intestine and is often located in the infraumbilical area. Lumbar radiation of pain is common in colonic obstruction.

Sudden distention of the biliary tree produces a steady rather than colicky type of pain; hence the term *biliary colic* is misleading. Acute distention of the gallbladder usually causes pain in the right upper quadrant with radiation to the right posterior region of the thorax or to the tip of the right scapula, and distention of the common bile duct is often associated with pain in the epigastrium radiating to the upper part of the lumbar region. Considerable variation is common, however, so that differentiation between these may be impossible. The typical subscapular pain or lumbar radiation is frequently absent. Gradual dilatation of the biliary tree, as in carcinoma of the head of the pancreas, may cause no pain or only a mild aching sensation in the epigastrium or right upper quadrant. The pain of distention of the pancreatic ducts is similar to that described for distention of the common bile duct but, in addition, is very frequently accentuated by recumbency and relieved by the upright position.

Obstruction of the urinary bladder results in dull suprapubic pain, usually low in intensity. Restlessness without specific complaint of pain may be the only sign of a distended bladder in an obtunded patient. In contrast, acute obstruction of the intravesicular portion of the ureter is characterized by severe suprapubic and flank pain that radiates to the penis, scrotum, or inner aspect of the upper thigh. Obstruction of the ureteropelvic junction is felt as pain in the costovertebral angle, whereas obstruction of the remainder of the ureter is associated with flank pain that often extends into the same side of the abdomen.

Vascular Disturbances A frequent misconception, despite abundant experience to the contrary, is that pain associated with intraabdominal vascular disturbances is sudden and catastrophic in nature. The pain of embolism or thrombosis of the superior mesenteric artery or that of impending rupture of an abdominal aortic aneurysm certainly may be severe and diffuse. Yet, just as frequently, the patient with occlusion of the superior mesenteric artery has only mild continuous diffuse pain for 2 or 3 days before vascular collapse or findings of peritoneal inflammation appear. The early, seemingly insignificant discomfort is caused by hyperperistalsis rather than peritoneal inflammation. Indeed, absence of tenderness and rigidity in the presence of continuous, diffuse pain in a patient likely to have vascular disease is quite characteristic of occlusion of the superior mesenteric artery. Abdominal pain with radiation to the sacral region, flank, or genitalia should always signal the possible presence of a rupturing abdominal aortic aneurysm. This pain may persist over a period of several days before rupture and collapse occur.

Abdominal Wall Pain arising from the abdominal wall is usually constant and aching. Movement, prolonged standing, and pressure accentuate the discomfort and muscle spasm. In the case of hematoma of the rectus sheath, now most frequently encountered in association with anticoagulant therapy, a mass may be present in the lower quadrants of the abdomen. Simultaneous involvement of muscles in other parts of the body usually serves to differentiate myositis of the abdominal wall from an intraabdominal process that might cause pain in the same region.

REFERRED PAIN IN ABDOMINAL DISEASES Pain referred to the abdomen from the thorax, spine, or genitalia may prove a vexing diagnostic problem, because diseases of the upper part of the abdominal cavity such as acute cholecystitis or perforated ulcer are frequently associated with intrathoracic complications. A most important, yet often forgotten, dictum is that the possibility of intrathoracic disease must be considered in every patient with abdominal pain, especially if the pain is in the upper part of the abdomen. Systematic questioning and examination directed toward detecting myocardial or pulmonary infarction, pneumonia, pericarditis, or esophageal disease (the intrathoracic diseases that most often masquerade as abdominal emergencies) will often provide sufficient clues to establish the proper diagnosis. Diaphragmatic pleuritis resulting from pneumonia or pulmonary infarction may cause pain in the right upper quadrant and pain in the supraclavicular area, the latter radiation to be distinguished from the referred subscapular pain caused by acute distention of the extrahepatic biliary tree. The ultimate decision as to the origin of abdominal pain may require deliberate and planned observation over a period of several hours, during which repeated questioning and examination will provide the diagnosis or suggest the appropriate studies.

Referred pain of thoracic origin is often accompanied by splinting of the involved hemithorax with respiratory lag and decrease in excursion more marked than that seen in the presence of intraabdominal disease. In addition, apparent abdominal muscle spasm caused by referred pain will diminish during the inspiratory phase of respiration, whereas it is persistent throughout both respiratory phases if it is of abdominal origin. Palpation over the area of referred pain in the abdomen also does not usually accentuate the pain and in many instances actually seems to relieve it. Thoracic and abdominal disease frequently coexist and may be difficult or impossible to differentiate. For example, the patient with known biliary tract disease often has epigastric pain during myocardial infarction, or biliary colic may be referred to the precordium or left shoulder in a patient who has suffered previously from angina pectoris. →*For an explanation of the radiation of pain to a previously diseased area, see Chap. 11.*

Referred pain from the spine, which usually involves compression or irritation of nerve roots, is characteristically intensified by certain motions such as cough, sneeze, or strain and is associated with hyperesthesia over the involved dermatomes. Pain referred to the abdo-

men from the testicles or seminal vesicles is generally accentuated by the slightest pressure on either of these organs. The abdominal discomfort is of dull aching character and is poorly localized.

METABOLIC ABDOMINAL CRISES Pain of metabolic origin may simulate almost any other type of intraabdominal disease. Several mechanisms may be at work. In certain instances, such as hyperlipidemia, the metabolic disease itself may be accompanied by an intraabdominal process such as pancreatitis, which can lead to unnecessary laparotomy unless recognized. C′1 esterase deficiency associated with angioneurotic edema is often associated with episodes of severe abdominal pain. Whenever the cause of abdominal pain is obscure, a metabolic origin always must be considered. Abdominal pain is also the hallmark of familial Mediterranean fever (Chap. 278).

The problem of differential diagnosis is often not readily resolved. The pain of porphyria and of lead colic is usually difficult to distinguish from that of intestinal obstruction, because severe hyperperistalsis is a prominent feature of both. The pain of uremia or diabetes is nonspecific, and the pain and tenderness frequently shift in location and intensity. Diabetic acidosis may be precipitated by acute appendicitis or intestinal obstruction, so if prompt resolution of the abdominal pain does not result from correction of the metabolic abnormalities, an underlying organic problem should be suspected. Black widow spider bites produce intense pain and rigidity of the abdominal muscles and back, an area infrequently involved in intraabdominal disease.

NEUROGENIC CAUSES Causalgic pain may occur in diseases that injure sensory nerves. It has a burning character and is usually limited to the distribution of a given peripheral nerve. Normal stimuli such as touch or change in temperature may be transformed into this type of pain, which is frequently present in a patient at rest. The demonstration of irregularly spaced cutaneous pain spots may be the only indication of an old nerve lesion underlying causalgic pain. Even though the pain may be precipitated by gentle palpation, rigidity of the abdominal muscles is absent, and the respirations are not disturbed. Distention of the abdomen is uncommon, and the pain has no relationship to the intake of food.

Pain arising from spinal nerves or roots comes and goes suddenly and is of a lancinating type (Chap. 15). It may be caused by herpes zoster, impingement by arthritis, tumors, herniated nucleus pulposus, diabetes, or syphilis. It is not associated with food intake, abdominal distention, or changes in respiration. Severe muscle spasm, as in the gastric crises of tabes dorsalis, is common but is either relieved or is not accentuated by abdominal palpation. The pain is made worse by movement of the spine and is usually confined to a few dermatomes. Hyperesthesia is very common.

Pain due to functional causes conforms to none of the aforementioned patterns. Mechanism is hard to define. Irritable bowel syndrome (IBS) is a functional gastrointestinal disorder characterized by abdominal pain and altered bowel habits. The diagnosis is made on the basis of clinical criteria (Chap. 277) and after exclusion of demonstrable structural abnormalities. The episodes of abdominal pain are often brought on by stress, and the pain varies considerably in type and location. Nausea and vomiting are rare. Localized tenderness and muscle spasm are inconsistent or absent. The causes of IBS or related functional disorders are not known.

APPROACH TO THE PATIENT

Few abdominal conditions require such urgent operative intervention that an orderly approach need be abandoned, no matter how ill the patient. Only those patients with exsanguinating intraabdominal hemorrhage (e.g., ruptured aneurysm) must be rushed to the operating room immediately, but in such instances, only a few minutes are required to assess the critical nature of the problem. Under these circumstances, all obstacles must be swept aside, adequate venous access for fluid replacement obtained, and the operation begun. Many patients of this type have died in the radiology department or the emergency room while awaiting such unnecessary examinations as electrocardiograms or abdominal films. *There are no contraindications to operation when massive intraabdominal hemorrhage is present.* This situation fortunately is relatively rare. These comments do not pertain to gastrointestinal hemorrhage, which can often be managed by other means (Chap. 37).

Nothing will supplant an orderly, painstakingly *detailed history*, which is far more valuable than any laboratory or radiographic examination. This kind of history is laborious and time-consuming, making it not especially popular, even though a reasonably accurate diagnosis can be made on the basis of the history alone in the majority of cases. Computer-aided diagnosis of abdominal pain provides no advantage over clinical assessment alone. In cases of *acute* abdominal pain, a diagnosis is readily established in most instances, whereas success is not so frequent in patients with *chronic* pain. IBS is one of the most common causes of abdominal pain and must always be kept in mind (Chap. 277). The *chronological sequence of events* in the patient's history is often more important than emphasis on the location of pain. If the examiner is sufficiently open-minded and unhurried, asks the proper questions, and listens, the patient will usually provide the diagnosis. Careful attention should be paid to the extraabdominal regions that may be responsible for abdominal pain. An accurate menstrual history in a female patient is essential. Narcotics or analgesics should *not* be withheld until a definitive diagnosis or a definitive plan has been formulated; obfuscation of the diagnosis by adequate analgesia is unlikely.

In the examination, simple critical inspection of the patient, e.g., of facies, position in bed, and respiratory activity, may provide valuable clues. The amount of information to be gleaned is directly proportional to the *gentleness* and thoroughness of the examiner. Once a patient with peritoneal inflammation has been examined brusquely, accurate assessment by the next examiner becomes almost impossible. Eliciting rebound tenderness by sudden release of a deeply palpating hand in a patient with suspected peritonitis is cruel and unnecessary. The same information can be obtained by gentle percussion of the abdomen (rebound tenderness on a miniature scale), a maneuver that can be far more precise and localizing. Asking the patient to cough will elicit true rebound tenderness without the need for placing a hand on the abdomen. Furthermore, the forceful demonstration of rebound tenderness will startle and induce protective spasm in a nervous or worried patient in whom true rebound tenderness is not present. A palpable gallbladder will be missed if palpation is so brusque that voluntary muscle spasm becomes superimposed on involuntary muscular rigidity.

As in history taking, there is no substitute for sufficient time spent in the examination. Abdominal signs may be minimal but nevertheless, if accompanied by consistent symptoms, may be exceptionally meaningful. Abdominal signs may be virtually or totally absent in cases of pelvic peritonitis, so careful *pelvic and rectal examinations are mandatory in every patient with abdominal pain.* Tenderness on pelvic or rectal examination in the absence of other abdominal signs can be caused by operative indications such as perforated appendicitis, diverticulitis, twisted ovarian cyst, and many others.

Much attention has been paid to the presence or absence of peristaltic sounds, their quality, and their frequency. Auscultation of the abdomen is one of the least revealing aspects of the physical examination of a patient with abdominal pain. Catastrophes such as strangulating small intestinal obstruction or perforated appendicitis may occur in the presence of normal peristaltic sounds. Conversely, when the proximal part of the intestine above an obstruction becomes markedly distended and edematous, peristaltic sounds may lose the characteristics of borborygmi and become weak or absent, even when peritonitis is not present. It is usually the severe chemical peritonitis of sudden onset that is associated with the truly silent abdomen. Assessment of the patient's state of hydration is important.

Laboratory examinations may be of great value in assessment of the patient with abdominal pain, yet with few exceptions they rarely establish a diagnosis. Leukocytosis should never be the single deciding factor as to whether or not operation is indicated. A white blood cell count $>20,000/\mu L$ may be observed with perforation of a viscus, but pancreatitis, acute cholecystitis, pelvic inflammatory disease, and intestinal infarction may be associated with marked leukocytosis. A normal white blood cell count is not rare in cases of perforation of abdominal viscera. The diagnosis of anemia may be more helpful than the white blood cell count, especially when combined with the history.

The urinalysis may reveal the state of hydration or rule out severe renal disease, diabetes, or urinary infection. Blood urea nitrogen, glucose, and serum bilirubin levels may be helpful. Serum amylase levels may be increased by many diseases other than pancreatitis, e.g., perforated ulcer, strangulating intestinal obstruction, and acute cholecystitis; thus, elevations of serum amylase do not rule out the need for an operation. The determination of the serum lipase may have greater accuracy than that of the serum amylase.

Plain and upright or lateral decubitus radiographs of the abdomen may be of value in cases of intestinal obstruction, perforated ulcer, and a variety of other conditions. They are usually unnecessary in patients with acute appendicitis or strangulated external hernias. In rare instances, barium or water-soluble contrast study of the upper part of the gastrointestinal tract may demonstrate partial intestinal obstruction that may elude diagnosis by other means. If there is any question of obstruction of the colon, oral administration of barium sulfate should be avoided. On the other hand, in cases of suspected colonic obstruction (without perforation), contrast enema may be diagnostic.

In the absence of trauma, peritoneal lavage has been replaced as a diagnostic tool by ultrasound, computed tomography (CT), and laparoscopy. Ultrasonography has proved to be useful in detecting an enlarged gallbladder or pancreas, the presence of gallstones, an enlarged ovary, or a tubal pregnancy. Laparoscopy is especially helpful in diagnosing pelvic conditions, such as ovarian cysts, tubal pregnancies, salpingitis, and acute appendicitis. Radioisotopic scans (HIDA) may help differentiate acute cholecystitis from acute pancreatitis. A CT scan may demonstrate an enlarged pancreas, ruptured spleen, or thickened colonic or appendiceal wall and streaking of the mesocolon or mesoappendix characteristic of diverticulitis or appendicitis.

Sometimes, even under the best circumstances with all available aids and with the greatest of clinical skill, a definitive diagnosis cannot be established at the time of the initial examination. Nevertheless, despite lack of a clear anatomic diagnosis, it may be abundantly clear to an experienced and thoughtful physician and surgeon that on clinical grounds alone operation is indicated. Should that decision be questionable, watchful waiting with repeated questioning and examination will often elucidate the true nature of the illness and indicate the proper course of action.

FURTHER READING

CERVERO F, LAIRD JM: Visceral pain. Lancet 353:2145, 1999

JONES PF: Suspected acute appendicitis: Trends in management over 30 years. Br J Surg 88:1570, 2001

MARCO CA et al: Abdominal pain in geriatric emergency patients: Variables associated with adverse outcome. Acad Emerg Med 5:1163, 1998

TAIT IS et al: Do patients with abdominal pain wait unduly long for analgesia? J R Coll Surg Edinb 44:181, 1999

TAOUREL P et al: Acute abdomen of unknown origin: Impact of CT on diagnosis and management. Gastrointest Radiol 17:287, 1992

14 HEADACHE
Neil H. Raskin

Few of us are spared the experience of head pain. As many as 90% of individuals have at least one headache per year. Severe, disabling headache is reported to occur at least annually by 40% of individuals worldwide. A useful classification of the many causes of headache is shown in Table 14-1. Headache is usually a benign symptom, but occasionally it is the manifestation of a serious illness such as brain tumor, subarachnoid hemorrhage, meningitis, or giant cell arteritis. In emergency settings, approximately 5% of patients with headache are found to have a serious underlying neurologic disorder. Therefore, it is imperative that the serious causes of headache be diagnosed rapidly and accurately.

PAIN-SENSITIVE STRUCTURES OF THE HEAD

Pain usually occurs when peripheral nociceptors are stimulated in response to tissue injury, visceral distension, or other factors (Chap. 11). In such situations, pain perception is a normal physiologic response mediated by a healthy nervous system. Pain can also result when pain-sensitive pathways of the peripheral or central nervous system are damaged or activated inappropriately. Headache may originate from either or both mechanisms. Relatively few cranial structures are pain-sensitive: the scalp, middle meningeal artery, dural sinuses, falx cerebri, and the proximal segments of the large pial arteries. The ventricular ependyma, choroid plexus, pial veins, and much of the brain parenchyma are pain-insensitive. Electrical stimulation of the midbrain

in the region of the dorsal raphe has resulted in migraine-like headaches. Thus, whereas most of the brain is insensitive to electrode probing, a site in the midbrain represents a possible source of headache generation. Sensory stimuli from the head are conveyed to the central nervous system via the trigeminal nerves for structures above the tentorium in the anterior and middle fossae of the skull, and via the first three cervical nerves for those in the posterior fossa and the inferior surface of the tentorium.

Headache can occur as the result of (1) distention, traction, or dilation of intracranial or extracranial arteries; (2) traction or displacement of large intracranial veins or their dural envelope; (3) compression, traction, or inflammation of cranial and spinal nerves; (4) spasm, inflammation, or trauma to cranial and cervical muscles; (5) meningeal irritation and raised intracranial pressure; or (6) other possible mechanisms such as activation of brainstem structures.

GENERAL CLINICAL CONSIDERATIONS

The quality, location, duration, and time course of the headache and the conditions that produce, exacerbate, or relieve it should be carefully reviewed. Ascertaining the *quality* of cephalic pain is occasionally helpful for diagnosis. Most tension-type headaches are described as tight "bandlike" pain or as dull, deeply located, and aching pain. Jabbing, brief, sharp cephalic pain, often occurring multifocally (ice pick–like pain), is usually benign. A throbbing quality and tight muscles about the head, neck, and shoulder girdle are common nonspecific accompaniments of migraine headaches.

Pain *intensity* rarely has diagnostic value, although from the patient's perspective, it is the single aspect of pain that is most important.

TABLE 14-1 *International Headache Society Classification of Headache*

1. **Migraine**	7. **Headache associated with nonvascular intracranial disorder (cont.)**
Migraine without aura	Sarcoidosis and other noninfectious inflammatory diseases
Migraine with aura	Related to intrathecal injections
Ophthalmoplegic migraine	Intracranial neoplasm
Retinal migraine	Associated with other intracranial disorder
Childhood periodic syndromes that may be precursors to or	8. **Headache associated with substances or their withdrawal**
associated with migraine	Headache induced by acute substance use or exposure
Migrainous disorder not fulfilling above criteria	Headache induced by chronic substance use or exposure
2. **Tension-type headache**	Headache from substance withdrawal (acute use)
Episodic tension-type headache	Headache from substance withdrawal (chronic use)
Chronic tension-type headache	9. **Headache associated with noncephalic infection**
3. **Cluster headache and chronic paroxysmal hemicrania**	Viral infection
Cluster headache	Bacterial infection
Chronic paroxysmal hemicrania	Other infection
4. **Miscellaneous headaches not associated with structural lesion**	10. **Headache associated with metabolic disorder**
Idiopathic stabbing headache	Hypoxia
External compression headache	Hypercapnia
Cold stimulus headache	Mixed hypoxia and hypercapnia
Benign cough headache	Hypoglycemia
Benign exertional headache	Dialysis
Headache associated with sexual activity	Other metabolic abnormality
5. **Headache associated with head trauma**	11. **Headache or facial pain associated with disorder of facial or cranial structures**
Acute posttraumatic headache	Cranial bone
Chronic posttraumatic headache	Eyes
6. **Headache associated with vascular disorders**	Ears
Acute ischemic cerebrovascular disorder	Nose and sinuses
Intracranial hematoma	Teeth, jaws, and related structures
Subarachnoid hemorrhage	Temporomandibular joint disease
Unruptured vascular malformation	12. **Cranial neuralgias, nerve trunk pain, and deafferentation pain**
Arteritis	Persistent (in contrast to ticlike) pain of cranial nerve origin
Carotid or vertebral artery pain	Trigeminal neuralgia
Venous thrombosis	Glossopharyngeal neuralgia
Arterial hypertension	Nervus intermedius neuralgia
Other vascular disorder	Superior laryngeal neuralgia
7. **Headache associated with nonvascular intracranial disorder**	Occipital neuralgia
High CSF pressure	Central causes of head and facial pain other than tic douloureux
Low CSF pressure	13. **Headache not classifiable**
Intracranial infection	

Note: CSF, cerebrospinal fluid.
Source: After J Olesen: Cephalalgia 8(Suppl 7):1, 1988.

Although meningitis, subarachnoid hemorrhage, and cluster headache produce intense cranial pain, most patients entering emergency departments with the most severe headache of their lives usually have migraine. Contrary to common belief, the headache produced by a brain tumor is not usually distinctive or severe.

Data regarding *location* of headache may be informative. If the source is an extracranial structure, as in giant cell arteritis, the correspondence with the site of pain is fairly precise. Inflammation of an extracranial artery causes pain and exquisite tenderness localized to the site of the vessel. Lesions of paranasal sinuses, teeth, eyes, and upper cervical vertebrae induce less sharply localized pain, but pain that is still referred in a regional distribution. Intracranial lesions in the posterior fossa cause pain that is usually occipitonuchal, and supratentorial lesions most often induce frontotemporal pain.

Duration and *time-intensity* curves of headaches are diagnostically useful. A ruptured aneurysm results in head pain that peaks in an instant, thunderclap-like; much less often, unruptured aneurysms may signal their presence in the same way. Cluster headache attacks reach their peak over 3 to 5 min, remain at maximal levels for about 45 min, and then taper off. Migraine attacks build up over hours, are maintained for several hours to days, and are characteristically relieved by sleep. Sleep disruption and early morning headaches that improve during the day are characteristics of headaches produced by brain tumors or other disorders that produce increased intracranial pressure.

Facial pain must be distinguished from headache. Trigeminal and, less commonly, glossopharyngeal neuralgia are frequent causes of facial pain (Chap. 355). *Neuralgias* are painful disorders characterized by paroxysmal, fleeting, often electric shock–like episodes that are frequently caused by demyelinating lesions of nerves (the trigeminal or glossopharyngeal nerves in cranial neuralgias). Certain maneuvers characteristically trigger paroxysms of pain. However, the most common cause of facial pain by far is dental; provocation by hot, cold, or sweet foods is typical. The application of a cold stimulus will repeatedly induce dental pain, whereas in neuralgic disorders, a refractory period usually occurs after the initial response so that pain cannot be repeatedly induced.

The effect of eating on facial pain may provide insight into its cause. Is it the chewing, swallowing, or taste of the food that elicits pain? Chewing suggests trigeminal neuralgia, temporomandibular joint dysfunction, or giant cell arteritis ("jaw claudication"), whereas swallowing *and* taste provocation suggest glossopharyngeal neuralgia. Pain with swallowing is common in patients with carotidynia (see below) because the inflamed, tender carotid artery abuts the esophagus during deglutition.

Many patients with facial pain do not experience stereotypic neuralgias; the term *atypical facial pain* has been used in this setting. Vague, poorly localized, continuous facial pain is characteristic of nasopharyngeal carcinoma; a burning pain often develops as deafferentation occurs and evidence of cranial neuropathy appears. Burning facial pain may also occur with tumors of the fifth cranial nerve (meningioma or schwannoma) or with lesions of the pons that interrupt the dorsal root entry zone of the nerve (multiple sclerosis). In patients with facial pain, the finding of objective sensory loss is an important clue to a serious underlying disorder. Occasionally, the cause of a pain problem cannot be resolved promptly, necessitating periodic follow-up until further signs appear.

CLINICAL EVALUATION OF ACUTE, NEW-ONSET HEADACHE

Patients who present with their first severe headache raise entirely different diagnostic possibilities than those with recurrent headaches over many years. In new-onset and severe headaches, the probability of finding a potentially serious cause is considerably greater than in recurrent headache. When a patient complains of an acute, new-onset headache, a number of causes should be considered including meningitis, subarachnoid hemorrhage, epidural or subdural hematoma, glaucoma, and purulent sinusitis. Clinical features of acute, new-onset

TABLE 14-2   Headache Symptoms That Suggest a Serious Underlying Disorder

"Worst" headache ever
First severe headache
Subacute worsening over days or weeks
Abnormal neurologic examination
Fever or unexplained systemic signs
Vomiting precedes headache
Induced by bending, lifting, cough
Disturbs sleep or presents immediately upon awakening
Known systemic illness
Onset after age 55

headache caused by serious underlying conditions are summarized in Table 14-2.

A complete neurologic examination is an essential first step in the evaluation. In most cases, an abnormal examination should be followed by a computed tomography (CT) or a magnetic resonance imaging (MRI) study. As a screening procedure for intracranial pathology in this setting, CT and MRI methods appear to be equally sensitive. A general evaluation of acute headache might include the investigation of cardiovascular and renal status by blood pressure monitoring and urine examination; eyes by fundoscopy, intraocular pressure measurement, and refraction; cranial arteries by palpation; and cervical spine by the effect of passive movement of the head and imaging.

The psychological state of the patient should also be evaluated since a relationship exists between head pain and depression. Many patients in chronic daily pain cycles become depressed; moreover, there is a greater-than-chance coincidence of migraine with both bipolar (manic-depressive) and unipolar major depressive disorders. Drugs with antidepressant actions are also effective in the prophylactic treatment of both tension-type headache and migraine.

Underlying recurrent headache disorders may be activated by pain that follows otologic or endodontic surgical procedures. Thus, pain about the head as the result of diseased tissue or trauma may reawaken an otherwise quiescent migrainous syndrome. Treatment of the headache is largely ineffective until the cause of the primary problem is addressed.

Serious underlying conditions that are associated with headache are described below and in Table 14-3.

MENINGITIS   In general, acute, severe headache with stiff neck and fever suggests meningitis. Lumbar puncture is mandatory. Often there is striking accentuation of pain with eye movement. Meningitis is par-

TABLE 14-3   Symptoms of Serious Underlying Causes of Headache

Cause	Symptoms
Meningitis	Nuchal rigidity, headache, photophobia, and prostration; may not be febrile. Lumbar puncture is diagnostic.
Intracranial hemorrhage	Nuchal rigidity and headache; may not have clouded consciousness or seizures. Hemorrhage may not be seen on CT scan. Lumbar puncture shows "bloody tap" that does not clear by the last tube. A fresh hemorrhage may not be xanthochromic.
Brain tumor	May present with prostrating pounding headaches that are associated with nausea and vomiting. Should be suspected in progressively severe new "migraine" that is invariably unilateral.
Temporal arteritis	May present with a unilateral pounding headache. Onset generally in older patients (>50 years) and frequently associated with visual changes. The erythrocyte sedimentation rate is the best screening test and is usually markedly elevated (i.e., >50). Definitive diagnosis can be made by arterial biopsy.
Glaucoma	Usually consists of severe eye pain. May have nausea and vomiting. The eye is usually painful and red. The pupil may be partially dilated.

Note: CT, computed tomography.

ticularly easy to mistake for migraine in that the cardinal symptoms of pounding headache, photophobia, nausea, and vomiting are present. →*A detailed discussion of meningitis can be found in Chaps. 360 and 361.*

INTRACRANIAL HEMORRHAGE In general, acute, severe headache with stiff neck but without fever suggests subarachnoid hemorrhage. A ruptured aneurysm, arteriovenous malformation, or intraparenchymal hemorrhage may also present with headache alone. Rarely, if the hemorrhage is small or below the foramen magnum, the head CT scan can be normal. Therefore, a lumbar puncture may be required to make the definitive diagnosis of a subarachnoid hemorrhage. →*A detailed discussion of intracranial hemorrhage can be found in Chap. 349.*

BRAIN TUMOR Approximately 30% of patients with brain tumors consider headache to be their chief complaint. The head pain is usually nondescript—an intermittent deep, dull aching of moderate intensity, which may worsen with exertion or change in position and may be associated with nausea and vomiting. This pattern of symptoms results from migraine far more often than from brain tumor. Headache of brain tumor disturbs sleep in about 10% of patients. Vomiting that precedes the appearance of headache by weeks is highly characteristic of posterior fossa brain tumors. A history of amenorrhea or galactorrhea should lead one to question whether a prolactin-secreting pituitary adenoma (or the polycystic ovary syndrome) is the source of headache. Headache arising de novo in a patient with known malignancy suggests either cerebral metastases and/or carcinomatous meningitis. Head pain appearing abruptly after bending, lifting, or coughing can be due to a posterior fossa mass (or a Chiari malformation). →*A detailed discussion of brain tumors can be found in Chap. 358.*

TEMPORAL ARTERITIS (See also Chaps. 25 and 306) Temporal (giant cell) arteritis is an inflammatory disorder of arteries that frequently involves the extracranial carotid circulation. This is a common disorder of the elderly; its annual incidence is 77:100,000 in individuals aged 50 and older. The average age of onset is 70 years, and women account for 65% of cases. About half of patients with untreated temporal arteritis develop blindness due to involvement of the ophthalmic artery and its branches; indeed, the ischemic optic neuropathy induced by giant cell arteritis is the major cause of rapidly developing bilateral blindness in patients >60 years. Because treatment with glucocorticoids is effective in preventing this complication, prompt recognition of this disorder is important.

Typical presenting symptoms include headache, polymyalgia rheumatica (Chap. 306), jaw claudication, fever, and weight loss. Headache is the dominant symptom and often appears in association with malaise and muscle aches. Head pain may be unilateral or bilateral and is located temporally in 50% of patients but may involve any and all aspects of the cranium. Pain usually appears gradually over a few hours before peak intensity is reached; occasionally, it is explosive in onset. The quality of pain is only seldom throbbing; it is almost invariably described as dull and boring with superimposed episodic ice pick–like lancinating pains similar to the sharp pains that appear in migraine. Most patients can recognize that the origin of their head pain is superficial, external to the skull, rather than originating deep within the cranium (the pain site for migraineurs). Scalp tenderness is present, often to a marked degree; brushing the hair or resting the head on a pillow may be impossible because of pain. Headache is usually worse at night and is often aggravated by exposure to cold. Reddened, tender nodules or red streaking of the skin overlying the temporal arteries may be found in patients with headache, as is tenderness of the temporal or, less commonly, the occipital arteries.

The erythrocyte sedimentation rate (ESR) is often, though not always, elevated; a normal ESR does not exclude giant cell arteritis. A temporal artery biopsy and treatment with prednisone at 80 mg daily for the first 4 to 6 weeks should be initiated when clinical suspicion is high. The prevalence of migraine among the elderly is substantial, considerably higher than that of giant cell arteritis. Migraineurs often report amelioration of their headaches with prednisone, so that one must be cautious about interpreting the therapeutic response.

GLAUCOMA Glaucoma may present with a prostrating headache associated with nausea and vomiting. The history will usually reveal that the headache started with severe eye pain. On physical examination, the eye is often red with a fixed, moderately dilated pupil. →*A discussion of glaucoma can be found in Chap. 25.*

OTHER CAUSES OF HEADACHE ■ Systemic Illness There is hardly any illness that is never manifested by headache; however, some illnesses are frequently associated with headache. These include infectious mononucleosis, systemic lupus erythematosus, chronic pulmonary failure with hypercapnia (early morning headaches), Hashimoto's thyroiditis, inflammatory bowel disease, many of the illnesses associated with HIV, and the acute blood pressure elevations that occur in pheochromocytoma and in malignant hypertension. The last two examples are the exceptions to the generalization that hypertension per se is a very uncommon cause of headache; diastolic pressures of at least 120 mmHg are requisite for hypertension to cause headache. Persistent headache and fever are often the manifestations of an acute systemic viral infection; if the neck is supple in such a patient, lumbar puncture may be deferred. Some drugs and drug-withdrawal states, e.g., oral contraceptives, ovulation-promoting medications, and glucocorticoid withdrawal, are also associated with headache in some individuals.

Idiopathic Intracranial Hypertension (Pseudotumor Cerebri) Headache, clinically resembling that of brain tumor, is a common presenting symptom of pseudotumor cerebri, a disorder of raised intracranial pressure probably resulting from impaired cerebrospinal fluid (CSF) absorption by the arachnoid villi. Morning headaches that are worsened by coughing and straining are typical. The pain is sometimes retroocular and worsened by eye movements. Transient visual obscurations and papilledema with enlarged blind spots and loss of peripheral visual fields are additional manifestations. Most patients are young, female, and obese. They often have a history of exposure to provoking agents such as vitamin A and glucocorticoids. →*Treatment of idiopathic intracranial hypertension is discussed in Chap. 25.*

Cough A male-dominated (4:1) syndrome, cough headache is characterized by transient, severe head pain upon coughing, bending, lifting, sneezing, or stooping. Head pain persists for seconds to a few minutes. Many patients date the origins of the syndrome to a lower respiratory infection accompanied by severe coughing or to strenuous weight-lifting programs. Headache is usually diffuse but is lateralized in about one-third of patients. The incidence of serious intracranial structural anomalies causing this condition is about 25%; the Chiari malformation (Chap. 356) is a common cause. Thus, MRI is indicated for most patients with cough headache. The benign disorder may persist for a few years; it responds dramatically to indomethacin at doses ranging from 50 to 200 mg daily. Approximately half of patients will also show a response to therapeutic lumbar puncture with removal of 40 mL of CSF.

Many patients with migraine note that attacks of headache may be provoked by *sustained* physical exertion, such as during the third mile of a 5-mile run. Such headaches build up over hours, in contrast to cough headache. The term *effort migraine* has been used for this syndrome to avoid the ambiguous term *exertional headache*.

Lumbar Puncture Headache following lumbar puncture usually begins within 48 h but may be delayed for up to 12 days. Its incidence is between 10 and 30%. Head pain is dramatically positional; it begins when the patient sits or stands upright; there is relief upon reclining or with abdominal compression. The longer the patient is upright, the longer the latency before head pain subsides. It is worsened by head shaking and jugular vein compression. The pain is usually a dull ache but may be throbbing; its location is occipitofrontal. Nausea and stiff neck often accompany headache, and occasional patients report blurred vision, photophobia, tinnitus, and vertigo. The symptoms resolve over a few days but may on occasion persist for weeks to months.

Loss of CSF volume decreases the brain's supportive cushion, so

TABLE 14-4 Drugs Effective in the Treatment of Tension-Type Headache

Drug	Trade Name	Dosage
NONSTEROIDAL ANTI-INFLAMMATORY AGENTS		
Acetaminophen	Tylenol, generic	650 mg PO q4–6h
Aspirin	Generic	650 mg PO q4–6h
Diclofenac	Cataflam, generic	50–100 mg q4–6h (max 200 mg/d)
Ibuprofen	Advil, Motrin, Nuprin, generic	400 mg PO q3–4h
Naproxen sodium	Aleve, Anaprox, generic	220–550 mg bid
COMBINATION ANALGESICS		
Acetaminophen, 325 mg, *plus* butalbital, 50 mg	Phrenilin, generic	1–2 tablets; max 6 per day
Acetaminophen, 650 mg, *plus* butalbital, 50 mg	Phrenilin Forte	1 tablet; max 6 per day
Acetaminophen, 325 mg, *plus* butalbital, 50 mg, *plus* caffeine, 40 mg	Fioricet; Esgic, generic	1–2 tablets; max 6 per day
Acetaminophen, 500 mg, *plus* butalbital, 50 mg, *plus* caffeine, 40 mg	Esgicplus	1–2 tablets; max 6 per day
Aspirin, 325 mg, *plus* butalbital, 50 mg, *plus* caffeine, 40 mg	Fiorinal	1–2 tablets; max 6 per day
Aspirin, 650 mg, *plus* butalbital, 50 mg	Axotal	1 tablet q4h; max 6 per day
PROPHYLACTIC MEDICATIONS		
Amitriptyline	Elavil, generic	10–50 mg at bedtime
Doxepin	Sinequan, generic	10–75 mg at bedtime
Nortriptyline	Pamelor, generic	25–75 mg at bedtime

that when a patient is upright there is probably dilation and tension placed on the brain's anchoring structures, the pain-sensitive dural sinuses, resulting in pain. Intracranial hypotension often occurs, but severe lumbar puncture headache may be present even in patients who have normal CSF pressure.

Treatment with intravenous caffeine sodium benzoate given over a few minutes as a 500-mg dose will promptly terminate headache in 75% of patients; a second dose given in 1 h brings the total success rate to 85%. An epidural blood patch accomplished by injection of 15 mL of autologous whole blood rarely fails for those who do not respond to caffeine. The mechanism for these treatment effects is not straightforward. The blood patch has an *immediate* effect, making it unlikely that sealing off a dural hole with blood clot is its mechanism of action.

Postconcussion Following seemingly trivial head injuries and particularly after rear-end motor vehicle collisions, many patients report varying combinations of headache, dizziness, vertigo, and impaired memory. Anxiety, irritability, and difficulty with concentration are other hallmarks of this syndrome. Symptoms may remit after several weeks or persist for months and even years after the injury. Postconcussion headaches may occur whether or not a person was rendered unconscious by head trauma. Typically, the neurologic examination is normal with the exception of the behavioral abnormalities, and CT or MRI studies are unrevealing. Chronic subdural hematoma may on occasion mimic this disorder. Although the cause of postconcussive headache disorder is not known, it should not in general be viewed as a primary psychological disturbance. It often persists long after the settlement of pending lawsuits. The treatment is symptomatic support. Repeated encouragement that the syndrome eventually remits is important.

Coital Headache This is another male-dominated (4:1) syndrome. Attacks occur periorgasmically, are very abrupt in onset, and subside in a few minutes if coitus is interrupted. These are nearly always benign events and usually occur sporadically; if they persist for hours or are accompanied by vomiting, subarachnoid hemorrhage must be excluded (Chap. 349).

PRINCIPAL CLINICAL VARIETIES OF RECURRENT HEADACHE

There is usually little difficulty in diagnosing the serious types of headaches listed above because of the clues provided by the associated symptoms and signs. It is when headache is chronic, recurrent, and unattended by other important signs of disease that the physician faces a challenging and unique medical problem. The following sections describe a variety of headache types, ranging from the most common (e.g., migraine) to rare causes of recurrent headache.

TENSION-TYPE HEADACHE The term *tension-type headache* is still commonly used to describe a chronic head pain syndrome characterized by bilateral tight, bandlike discomfort. Patients may report that the head feels as if it is in a vise or that the posterior neck muscles are tight. The pain typically builds slowly, fluctuates in severity, and may persist more or less continuously for many days. Exertion does not usually worsen the headache. The headache may be episodic or chronic (i.e., present >15 days per month). Tension-type headache is common in all age groups, and females tend to predominate. In some patients, anxiety or depression coexist with tension headache.

The pathophysiologic basis of tension-type headache remains unknown. Many investigators believe that periodic tension headache is biologically indistinguishable from migraine, whereas others believe that tension-type headache and migraine are two distinct clinical entities. Abnormalities of cervical and temporal muscle contraction are likely to exist, but the exact nature of the dysfunction has not yet been elucidated.

Relaxation almost always relieves tension-type headaches. Patients should be encouraged to find a means of relaxation, which, for a given individual, could include bed rest, massage, and/or formal biofeedback training. Pharmacologic treatment consists of either simple analgesics and/or muscle relaxants. Ibuprofen and naproxen sodium are useful treatments for most individuals. When simple over-the-counter analgesics such as acetaminophen, aspirin, ibuprofen, and/or other nonsteroidal anti-inflammatory drugs (NSAIDs) alone fail, the addition of butalbital and caffeine (in a combination compound such as Fiorinal, Fioricet) to these analgesics may be effective. A list of commonly used analgesics for tension-type headaches is presented in Table 14-4. For chronic tension-type headache, prophylactic therapy is recommended. Low doses of amitriptyline (10 to 50 mg at bedtime) can provide effective prophylaxis.

MIGRAINE Migraine, the most common cause of headache, afflicts approximately 15% of women and 6% of men. A useful definition of migraine is a benign and recurring syndrome of headache, nausea, vomiting, and/or other symptoms of neurologic dysfunction in varying admixtures (Table 14-5). Migraine can often be recognized by its activators (red wine, menses, hunger, lack of sleep, glare, estrogen, worry, perfumes, let-down periods) and its deactivators (sleep, pregnancy, exhilaration, triptans). A classification of the many subtypes of migraine, as defined by the International Headache Society, is shown in Table 14-1.

Severe headache attacks, regardless of cause, are more likely to be described as throbbing and associated with vomiting and scalp tenderness. Milder headaches tend to be nondescript—tight, bandlike discomfort often involving the entire head—the profile of tension-type headache.

Pathogenesis ■ GENETIC BASIS OF MIGRAINE Migraine has a definite genetic predisposition. Specific mutations leading to *rare* causes of vascular headache have been identified (Table 14-6). For example, the MELAS syndrome consists of a *m*itochondrial *e*ncephalomyopathy, *l*actic *a*cidosis, and *s*troke-like episodes and is caused by an A → G point mutation in the mitochondrial gene encoding for tRNA$^{Leu(UUR)}$ at nucleotide position 3243. Episodic migraine-like headaches are another

TABLE 14-5 *Symptoms Accompanying Severe Migraine Attacks in 500 Patients*

Symptom	Patients Affected, %
Nausea	87
Photophobia	82
Lightheadedness	72
Scalp tenderness	65
Vomiting	56
Visual disturbances	36
Photopsia	26
Fortification spectra	10
Paresthesias	33
Vertigo	33
Alteration of consciousness	18
Syncope	10
Seizure	4
Confusional state	4
Diarrhea	16

Source: From NH Raskin, *Headache*, 2d ed. New York, Churchill Livingston, 1998; with permission.

common clinical feature of this syndrome, especially early in the course of the disease. The genetic pattern of mitochondrial disorders is unique, since only mothers transmit mitochondrial DNA. Thus, all children of mothers with MELAS syndrome are affected with the disorder.

Familial hemiplegic migraine (FHM) is characterized by episodes of recurrent hemiparesis or hemiplegia during the aura phase of a migraine headache. Other associated symptoms may include hemianesthesia or paresthesias; hemianopic visual field disturbances; dysphasia; and variable degrees of drowsiness, confusion, and/or coma. In severe attacks, these symptoms can be quite prolonged and persist for days or weeks, but characteristically they last for only 30 to 60 min and are followed by a unilateral throbbing headache.

Approximately 50% of cases of FHM appear to be caused by mutations within the CACNL1A4 gene on chromosome 19, which encodes a P/Q type calcium channel subunit expressed only in the central nervous system. The gene is very large ($>$300 kb in length) and consists of 47 exons. Four distinct point mutations have been identified within the gene (in five different families) that cosegregate with the clinical diagnosis of FHM. Analysis of haplotypes in the two families with the same mutation suggest that each mutation arose independently rather than representing a founder effect. CACNL1A4 is likely to play a role in calcium-induced neurotransmitter release and/or contraction of smooth muscle. Different mutations within this gene are the cause of two other neurogenetic disorders, spinocerebellar ataxia type 6 and episodic ataxia type 2 (Chap. 352).

In a genetic association study, a *Nco*I polymorphism in the gene encoding the D_2 dopamine receptor (DRD2) was overrepresented in a population of patients with migraine with aura compared to a control group of nonmigraineurs, suggesting that susceptibility to migraine with aura is modified by certain DRD2 alleles. In a Sardinian population, an association between different DRD2 alleles and migraine has also been demonstrated. These initial studies suggest that variations in dopamine receptor regulation and/or function may alter susceptibility to migraine since molecular variations within the DRD2 gene have been associated with variations in dopaminergic function. However, since not all individuals with the implicated DRD2 genotypes suffer from migraine with aura, additional genes or factors must also be involved. Migraine is likely to be a complex disorder with polygenic inheritance and a strong environmental component.

THE VASCULAR THEORY OF MIGRAINE It was widely held for many years that the headache phase of migrainous attacks was caused by extracranial vasodilatation and that the neurologic symptoms were produced by intracranial vasoconstriction (i.e., the "vascular" hypothesis of mi-

graine). Regional cerebral blood flow studies have shown that in patients with classic migraine there is, during attacks, a modest cortical hypoperfusion that begins in the visual cortex and spreads forward at a rate of 2 to 3 mm/min. The decrease in blood flow averages 25 to 30% (insufficient to explain symptoms on the basis of ischemia) and progresses anteriorly in a wavelike fashion independent of the topography of cerebral arteries. The wave of hypoperfusion persists for 4 to 6 h, appears to follow the convolutions of the cortex, and does not cross the central or lateral sulcus, progressing to the frontal lobe via the insula. Perfusion of subcortical structures is normal. Contralateral neurologic symptoms appear during temporoparietal hypoperfusion; at times, hypoperfusion persists in these regions after symptoms cease. More often, frontal spread continues as the headache phase begins. A few patients with classic migraine show no flow abnormalities; an occasional patient has developed focal ischemia sufficient to cause symptoms. However, focal ischemia does not appear to be *necessary* for focal symptoms to occur.

The ability of these changes to induce the symptoms of migraine has been questioned. Specifically, the decrease in blood flow that is observed does not appear to be significant enough to cause focal neurologic symptoms. Second, the increase in blood flow per se is not painful, and vasodilatation alone cannot account for the local edema and focal tenderness often observed in migraineurs. Moreover, in migraine without aura, no flow abnormalities are usually seen. Thus, it is unlikely that simple vasoconstriction and vasodilatation are the fundamental pathophysiologic abnormalities in migraine. However, it is clear that cerebral blood flow is altered during certain migraine attacks, and these changes may explain some, but clearly not all, of the clinical syndrome of migraine.

THE NEURONAL THEORY OF MIGRAINE *Fortification spectrum* is a migraine aura characterized by a slowly enlarging visual scotoma with luminous edges (see below). It is believed to result from *spreading depression*, a slowly moving (2 to 3 mm/min), potassium-liberating depression of cortical activity, preceded by a wavefront of increased metabolic activity. Spreading depression can be produced by a variety of experimental stimuli, including hypoxia, mechanical trauma, and the topical application of potassium. These observations suggest that neuronal abnormalities could be the cause of a migraine attack.

Physiologically, electrical stimulation near dorsal raphe neurons in the upper brainstem can result in migraine-like headaches. Blood flow in the pons and midbrain increases focally during migraine headache episodes; this alteration probably results from increased activity of cells in the dorsal raphe and locus coeruleus. There are projections from the dorsal raphe that terminate on cerebral arteries and alter cerebral blood flow. There are also major projections from the dorsal raphe to important visual centers, including the lateral geniculate body, superior colliculus, retina, and visual cortex. These various serotonergic projections may represent the neural substrate for the circulatory and visual characteristics of migraine. The dorsal raphe cells stop firing during deep sleep, and sleep is known to ameliorate migraine; the antimigraine prophylactic drugs also inhibit activity of the dorsal raphe cells through a direct or indirect agonist effect.

Positron emission tomography (PET) scan studies have demon-

TABLE 14-6 *Migraine Genetics*

Gene (Locus)	Function of Gene	Clinical Syndrome	Comment
tRNA^Leu(UUR) (mitochondrial)	Unknown	MELAS syndrome	Extremely rare syndrome
CACNL1A4 (19p13)	P/Q calcium channel regulating neurotransmitter release	Familial hemiplegic migraine (FHM)	Mutations account for approximately 50% of FHM cases
DRD2 (11q23)	G protein coupled D_2 receptor for dopamine	Migraine	Positive association reported in two independent laboratories

Note: MELAS, mitochondrial encephalomyopathy, lactic acidosis, and stroke-like episodes.

strated that midbrain structures near the dorsal raphe are activated during a migraine attack. In one study of acute migraine, an injection of sumatriptan relieved the headache but did not alter the brainstem changes noted on the PET scan. These data suggest that a "brainstem generator" may be the cause of migraine and that certain antimigraine medications may not interfere with the underlying pathologic process in migraine.

THE TRIGEMINOVASCULAR SYSTEM IN MIGRAINE   Activation of cells in the trigeminal nucleus caudalis in the medulla (a pain-processing center for the head and face region) results in the release of vasoactive neuropeptides, including substance P and calcitonin gene–related peptide, at vascular terminations of the trigeminal nerve. These peptide neurotransmitters have been proposed to induce a sterile inflammation that activates trigeminal nociceptive afferents originating on the vessel wall, further contributing to the production of pain. This provides a potential mechanism for the soft tissue swelling and tenderness of blood vessels that accompany migraine attacks. However, numerous pharmacologic agents that are effective in preventing or reducing inflammation in this animal model (e.g., selective 5-HT_{1D} agonists, NK-1 antagonists, endothelin antagonists) have failed to demonstrate any clinical efficacy in migraine trials.

5-HYDROXYTRYPTAMINE IN MIGRAINE   Pharmacologic and other data point to the involvement of the neurotransmitter 5-hydroxytryptamine (5-HT; also known as serotonin) in migraine. Approximately 40 years ago, methysergide was found to antagonize certain peripheral actions of 5-HT and was introduced as the first drug capable of preventing migraine attacks. Subsequently, it was found that platelet levels of 5-HT fall consistently at the onset of headache and that drugs that cause 5-HT to be released may trigger migrainous episodes. Such changes in circulating 5-HT levels proved to be pharmacologically trivial, however, and interest in the humoral role of 5-HT in migraine declined.

More recently, interest in the role of 5-HT in migraine has been renewed due to the introduction of the triptan class of antimigraine drugs. The triptans are designed to stimulate selectively a particular subpopulation of 5-HT receptors. At least 14 specific 5-HT receptors exist in humans. The triptans (e.g., naratriptan, rizatriptan, sumatriptan, and zolmitriptan) are potent agonists of 5-HT_{1B}, 5-HT_{1D}, and 5-HT_{1F} receptors and are less potent at 5-HT_{1A} and 5-HT_{1E} receptors. A growing body of data indicates that the antimigraine efficacy of the triptans relates to their ability to stimulate 5-HT_{1B} receptors, which are located on both blood vessels and nerve terminals. Selective 5-HT_{1D} receptor agonists have, thus far, failed to demonstrate clinical efficacy in migraine. Triptans that are weak 5-HT_{1F} agonists are also effective in migraine; however, only 5-HT_{1B} efficacy is currently thought to be essential for antimigraine efficacy.

DOPAMINE IN MIGRAINE   A growing body of biologic, pharmacologic, and genetic data supports a role for dopamine in the pathophysiology of certain subtypes of migraine. Most migraine symptoms can be induced by dopaminergic stimulation. Moreover, there is dopamine receptor hypersensitivity in migraineurs, as demonstrated by the induction of yawning, nausea, vomiting, hypotension, and other symptoms of a migraine attack by dopaminergic agonists at doses that do not affect nonmigraineurs. Conversely, dopamine receptor antagonists are effective therapeutic agents in migraine, especially when given parenterally or concurrently with other antimigraine agents. As noted above, genetic data also suggest that molecular variations within dopamine receptor genes play a modifying role in the pathophysiology of migraine with aura. Therefore, modulation of dopaminergic neurotransmission should be considered in the therapeutic management of migraine.

THE SYMPATHETIC NERVOUS SYSTEM IN MIGRAINE   Alterations occur within the sympathetic nervous system (SNS) of migraineurs before, during, and between migraine attacks. Factors that activate the SNS are all triggers for migraine. Specific examples include environmental changes (e.g., stress, sleep patterns, hormonal shifts, hypoglycemia) and agents that

cause release and a secondary depletion of peripheral catecholamines (e.g., tyramine, phenylethylamine, fenfluramine, m-chlorophenylpiperazine, and reserpine). By contrast, effective therapeutic approaches to migraine share an ability to mimic and/or enhance the effects of norepinephrine in the peripheral SNS. For example, norepinephrine itself, sympathomimetics (e.g., isometheptene), monoamine oxidase inhibitors (MAOIs), and reuptake blockers alleviate migraine. Dopamine antagonists, prostaglandin synthesis inhibitors, and adenosine antagonists are pharmacologic agents effective in the acute treatment of migraine. These drugs block the negative feedback inhibition or norepinephrine release induced by endogenous dopamine, prostaglandins, and adenosine. Therefore, migraine susceptibility may relate to genetically based variations in the ability to maintain adequate concentrations of certain neurotransmitters within postganglionic sympathetic nerve terminals. This hypothesis has been called the *empty neuron theory* of migraine.

Clinical Features ■ *MIGRAINE WITHOUT AURA (COMMON MIGRAINE)*   In this syndrome no focal neurologic disturbance precedes the recurrent headaches. Migraine without aura is by far the more frequent type of vascular headache. The International Headache Society criteria for migraine include moderate to severe head pain, pulsating quality, unilateral location, aggravation by walking stairs or similar routine activity, attendant nausea and/or vomiting, photophobia and phonophobia, and multiple attacks, each lasting 4 to 72 h.

MIGRAINE WITH AURA (CLASSIC MIGRAINE)   In this syndrome headache is associated with characteristic premonitory sensory, motor, or visual symptoms. Focal neurologic disturbances are more common during headache attacks than as prodromal symptoms. Focal neurologic disturbances without headache or vomiting have come to be known as *migraine equivalents* or *migraine accompaniments* and appear to occur more commonly in patients between the ages of 40 and 70 years. The term *complicated migraine* has generally been used to describe migraine with dramatic transient focal neurologic features or a migraine attack that leaves a persisting residual neurologic deficit.

The most common premonitory symptoms reported by migraineurs are visual, arising from dysfunction of occipital lobe neurons. Scotomas and/or hallucinations occur in about one-third of migraineurs and usually appear in the central portions of the visual fields. A highly characteristic syndrome occurs in about 10% of patients; it usually begins as a small paracentral scotoma, which slowly expands into a "C" shape. Luminous angles appear at the enlarging outer edge, becoming colored as the scintillating scotoma expands and moves toward the periphery of the involved half of the visual field, eventually disappearing over the horizon of peripheral vision. The entire process lasts 20 to 25 min. This phenomenon is pathognomonic for migraine and has never been described in association with a cerebral structural anomaly. It is commonly referred to as a *fortification spectrum* because the serrated edges of the hallucinated "C" seemed to resemble a fortified town with bastions around it; spectrum is used in the sense of an apparition or specter.

BASILAR MIGRAINE   Symptoms referable to a disturbance in brainstem function, such as vertigo, dysarthria, or diplopia, occur as the only neurologic symptoms of the attack in about 25% of patients. A dramatic form of basilar migraine (Bickerstaff's migraine) occurs primarily in adolescent females. Episodes begin with total blindness accompanied or followed by admixtures of vertigo, ataxia, dysarthria, tinnitus, and distal and perioral paresthesias. In about one-quarter of patients, a confusional state supervenes. The neurologic symptoms usually persist for 20 to 30 min and are generally followed by a throbbing occipital headache. This basilar migraine syndrome is now known also to occur in children and in adults over age 50. An altered sensorium may persist for as long as 5 days and may take the form of confusional states superficially resembling psychotic reactions. Full recovery after the episode is the rule.

CAROTIDYNIA   The carotidynia syndrome, sometimes called *lower-half headache* or *facial migraine*, is most common among older patients, with the incidence peaking in the fourth through sixth decades. Pain is usually located at the jaw or neck, although sometimes periorbital or maxillary pain occurs; it may be continuous, deep, dull, and aching, and it becomes pounding or throbbing episodically. There are often superimposed sharp, ice pick–like jabs. Attacks occur one to several times per week, each lasting several minutes to hours. Tenderness and prominent pulsations of the cervical carotid artery and soft tissue swelling overlying the carotid are usually present ipsilateral to the pain; many patients also report throbbing ipsilateral headache concurrent with carotidynia attacks as well as between attacks. Dental trauma is a common precipitant of this syndrome. Carotid artery involvement also appears to be common in the more traditional forms of migraine; over 50% of patients with frequent migraine attacks are found to have carotid tenderness at several points on the side most often involved during hemicranial migraine attacks.

℞ TREATMENT

Nonpharmacologic Approaches for All Migraineurs Migraine can often be managed to some degree by a variety of nonpharmacologic approaches (Table 14-7). The measures that apply to a given individual should be used routinely since they provide a simple, cost-effective approach to migraine management. Patients with migraine do not encounter more stress than headache-free individuals; overresponsiveness to stress appears to be the issue. Since the stresses of everyday living cannot be eliminated, lessening one's response to stress by various techniques is helpful for many patients. These include yoga, transcendental meditation, hypnosis, and conditioning techniques such as biofeedback. For most patients, this approach is, at best, an adjunct to pharmacotherapy. Avoidance of migraine trigger factors may also provide significant prophylactic benefits. Unfortunately, these measures are unlikely to prevent all migraine attacks. When these measures fail to prevent an attack, pharmacologic approaches are then needed to abort an attack.

Pharmacologic Treatment of Acute Migraine The mainstay of pharmacologic therapy is the judicious use of one or more of the many drugs that are effective in migraine. The selection of the optimal regimen for a given patient depends on a number of factors, the most important of which is the severity of the attack (Table 14-8). Mild migraine attacks can usually be managed by oral agents; the average efficacy rate is 50 to 70%. Severe migraine attacks may require parenteral therapy. Most drugs effective in the treatment of migraine are members of one of three major pharmacologic classes: anti-inflammatory agents, 5-HT$_1$ agonists, and dopamine antagonists.

Table 14-9 lists specific drugs effective in migraine. In general, an adequate dose of whichever agent is chosen should be used as soon as possible after the onset of an attack. If additional medication is required within 60 min because symptoms return or have not abated, the initial dose should be increased for subsequent attacks. Migraine therapy must be individualized for each patient; a standard approach for all patients is not possible. A therapeutic regimen may need to be

---

TABLE 14-7 Nonpharmacologic Approaches to Migraine

Identify and then avoid trigger factors such as:
  Alcohol (e.g., red wine)
  Foods (e.g., chocolate, certain cheeses, monosodium glutamate, nitrate-containing foods)
  Hunger (avoid missing meals)
  Irregular sleep patterns (both lack of sleep and excessive sleep)
  Organic odors
  Sustained exertion
  Acute changes in stress levels
  Miscellaneous (glare, flashing lights)
Attempt to manage environmental shifts such as:
  Time zone shifts
  High altitude
  Barometric pressure changes
  Weather changes
Assess menstrual cycle relationship

TABLE 14-8 A Staged Approach to Migraine Pharmacotherapy

Stage	Diagnosis	Therapies
Mild migraine	Occasional throbbing headaches	NSAIDs
	No major impairment of functioning	Combination analgesics
		Oral 5-HT$_1$ agonists
Moderate migraine	Moderate or severe headaches	Oral, nasal, or SC 5-HT$_1$ agonists
	Nausea common	Oral dopamine antagonists
	Some impairment of functioning	
Severe migraine	Severe headaches >3 times per month	SC, IM, or IV 5-HT$_1$ agonists
	Significant functional impairment	IM or IV dopamine antagonists
	Marked nausea and/or vomiting	Prophylactic medications

Note: NSAIDs, nonsteroidal anti-inflammatory drugs; 5-HT, 5-hydroxytryptamine.

constantly refined and personalized until one is identified that provides the patient with rapid, complete, and consistent relief with minimal side effects.

NONSTEROIDAL ANTI-INFLAMMATORY AGENTS Both the severity and duration of a migraine attack can be reduced significantly by anti-inflammatory agents. Indeed, many undiagnosed migraineurs are self-treated with nonprescription anti-inflammatory agents (Table 14-4). A general consensus is that NSAIDs are most effective when taken early in the migraine attack. However, the effectiveness of anti-inflammatory agents in migraine is usually less than optimal in moderate or severe migraine attacks. The combination of acetaminophen, aspirin, and caffeine (Excedrin Migraine) has been approved for use by the U.S. Food and Drug Administration (FDA) for the treatment of mild to moderate migraine. The combination of aspirin and metoclopramide has been shown to be equivalent to a single dose of sumatriptan. Major side effects of NSAIDs include dyspepsia and gastrointestinal irritation.

5-HT$_1$ AGONISTS ▪ Oral Stimulation of 5-HT$_1$ receptors can stop an acute migraine attack. Ergotamine and dihydroergotamine are nonselective receptor agonists, while the series of drugs known as triptans are selective 5-HT$_1$ receptor agonists. A variety of triptans (e.g., naratriptan, rizatriptan, sumatriptan, zolmitriptan, almotriptan, frovatriptan) are now available for the treatment of migraine (Table 14-9).

Each of the triptan class of drugs has similar pharmacologic properties but varies slightly in terms of clinical efficacy. Rizatriptan and almotriptan are the fastest acting and most efficacious of the triptans currently available in the United States. Sumatriptan and zolmitriptan have similar rates of efficacy as well as time to onset, whereas naratriptan and frovatriptan are the slowest acting and the least efficacious. Clinical efficacy appears to be related more to the t_{max} (time to peak plasma level) than to the potency, half-life, or bioavailability (Table 14-10). This observation is in keeping with a significant body of data indicating that faster-acting analgesics are more efficacious than slower-acting agents.

Unfortunately, monotherapy with a selective oral 5-HT$_1$ agonist does not result in rapid, consistent, and complete relief of migraine in all patients. Triptans are not effective in migraine with aura unless given after the aura is completed and the headache initiated. Side effects, although often mild and transient, occur in up to 89% of patients. Moreover, 5-HT$_1$ agonists are contraindicated in individuals with a history of cardiovascular disease. Recurrence of headache is a major limitation of triptan use, and occurs at least occasionally in 40 to 78% of patients.

Ergotamine preparations offer a nonselective means of stimulating 5-HT$_1$ receptors. A nonnauseating dose of ergotamine should be sought since a dose that provokes nausea is too high and may intensify head pain. Except for a sublingual formulation of ergotamine (Ergo-

TABLE 14-9 *Treatment of Acute Migraine*

Drug	Trade Name	Dosage
NSAIDS		
Acetaminophen, aspirin, caffeine	Excedrin Migraine	Two tablets or caplets q6h (max 8 per day)
5-HT₁ AGONISTS		
Oral		
Ergotamine	Ergomar	One 2 mg sublingual tablet at onset and q1/2h (max 3 per day, 5 per week)
Ergotamine 1 mg, caffeine 100 mg	Ercaf, Wigraine	One or two tablets at onset, then one tablet q1/2h (max 6 per day, 10 per week)
Naratriptan	Amerge	2.5 mg tablet at onset; may repeat once after 4 h
Rizatriptan	Maxalt Maxalt-MLT	5 to 10 mg tablet at onset; may repeat after 2 h (max 30 mg/d)
Sumatriptan	Imitrex	50 to 100 mg tablet at onset; may repeat after 2 h (max 200 mg/d)
Zolmitriptan	Zomig Zomig Rapimelt	2.5 mg tablet at onset; may repeat after 2 h (max 10 mg/d)
Nasal		
Dihydroergotamine	Migranal Nasal Spray	Prior to nasal spray, the pump must be primed 4 times; one spray (0.5 mg) is administered followed, in 15 min, by a second spray
Sumatriptan	Imitrex Nasal Spray	5 to 20 mg intranasal spray as 4 sprays of 5 mg or a single 20 mg spray (may repeat once after 2 h, not to exceed a dose of 40 mg/d)
Parenteral		
Dihydroergotamine	DHE-45	1 mg IV, IM, or SC at onset and q1h (max 3 mg/d, 6 mg per week)
Sumatriptan	Imitrex Injection	6 mg SC at onset (may repeat once after 1 h for max of two doses in 24 h)
DOPAMINE ANTAGONISTS		
Oral		
Metoclopramide	Reglan,[a] generic[a]	5–10 mg/d
Prochlorperazine	Compazine,[a] generic[a]	1–25 mg/d
Parenteral		
Chlorpromazine	Generic[a]	0.1 mg/kg IV at 2 mg/min; max 35 mg/d
Metoclopramide	Reglan,[a] generic	10 mg IV
Prochlorperazine	Compazine,[a] generic[a]	10 mg IV
OTHER		
Oral		
Acetaminophen, 325 mg, *plus* dichloralphenazone, 100 mg, *plus* isometheptene, 65 mg	Midrin, Duradrin, generic	Two capsules at onset followed by 1 capsule q1h (max 5 capsules)
Nasal		
Butorphanol	Stadol[a]	1 mg (1 spray in 1 nostril), may repeat if necessary in 1–2 h
Parenteral		
Narcotics	Generic[a]	Multiple preparations and dosages; see Table 11-1.

[a] Not specifically indicated by the U.S. Food and Drug Administration for migraine.
Note: NSAIDs, nonsteroidal anti-inflammatory drugs; 5-HT, 5-hydroxytryptamine.

mar), oral formulations of ergotamine also contain 100 mg caffeine (theoretically to enhance ergotamine absorption and possibly to add additional vasoconstrictor activity). The average oral ergotamine dose for a migraine attack is 2 mg. Since the clinical studies demonstrating the efficacy of ergotamine in migraine predated the clinical trial methodologies used with the triptans, it is difficult to assess the clinical efficacy of ergotamine versus the triptans. In general, ergotamine appears to have a much higher incidence of nausea than triptans, but less headache recurrence.

Nasal The fastest acting nonparenteral antimigraine therapies that can be self-administered include nasal formulations of dihydroergotamine (Migranal) or sumatriptan (Imitrex Nasal). The nasal sprays result in substantial blood levels within 30 to 60 min. However, the nasal formulations suffer from inconsistent dosing, poor taste, and variable efficacy. Although in theory the nasal sprays might provide faster and more effective relief of a migraine attack than oral formulations, their reported efficacy is only approximately 50 to 60%.

Parenteral Parenteral administration of drugs such as dihydroergotamine (DHE-45 Injectable) and sumatriptan (Imitrex SC) is approved by the FDA for the rapid relief of a migraine attack. Peak plasma levels of dihydroergotamine are achieved 3 min after intravenous dosing, 30 min after intramuscular dosing, and 45 min after subcutaneous dosing. If an attack has not already peaked, subcutaneous or intramuscular administration of 1 mg dihydroergotamine suffices for about 80 to 90% of patients. Sumatriptan, 6 mg subcutaneously, is effective in approximately 70 to 80% of patients.

DOPAMINE ANTAGONISTS ■ *Oral* Oral dopamine antagonists should be considered as adjunctive therapy in migraine. Drug absorption is impaired during migrainous attacks because of reduced gastrointestinal motility. Delayed absorption occurs in the absence of nausea and is related to the severity of the attack and not its duration. Therefore, when oral NSAIDs and/or triptan agents fail, the addition of a dopamine antagonist such as metoclopramide, 10 mg, should be considered to enhance gastric absorption. In addition, dopamine antagonists decrease nausea/vomiting and restore normal gastric motility.

Parenteral Parenteral dopamine antagonists (e.g., chlorpromazine, prochlorperazine, metoclopramide) can also provide significant acute relief of migraine; they can be used in combination with parenteral 5-HT₁ agonists. A common intravenous protocol used for the treatment of severe migraine is the administration over 2 min of a mixture of 5 mg of prochlorperazine and 0.5 mg of dihydroergotamine.

OTHER MEDICATIONS FOR ACUTE MIGRAINE ■ *Oral* The combination of acetaminophen, dichloralphenazone, and isometheptene (i.e., Midrin, Duradrin, generic), one to two capsules, has been classified by the FDA as "possibly" effective in the treatment of migraine. Since the clinical studies demonstrating the efficacy of this combination analgesic in migraine predated the clinical trial methodologies used with

TABLE 14-10 *Comparative Pharmacology of Oral Triptans[a]*

Drug and Dose, mg	t_{max}, h	$t_{1/2}$, h	Oral Bioavailability, %	Clinical Efficacy at 2 h, %
Rizatriptan, 10	1–2	2–3	45	71
Zolmitriptan, 2.5	2	2.5–3	44	65
Sumatriptan, 50	2–3	2	14	61
Naratriptan, 2.5	2–4	5–6	68	45
Frovatriptan, 2.5	2–3	26	25	43
Almotriptan, 12.5	2–3	3	70	58

[a] Data adapted from package inserts approved by the U.S. Food and Drug Administration.

the triptans, it is difficult to assess the clinical efficacy of this sympathomimetic compound in comparison to other agents.

Nasal A nasal preparation of butorphanol is available for the treatment of acute pain. As with all narcotics, the use of nasal butorphanol should be limited to a select group of migraineurs, as described below.

Parenteral Narcotics are effective in the acute treatment of migraine. For example, intravenous meperidine (Demerol), 50 to 100 mg, is given frequently in the emergency room. This regimen "works" in the sense that the pain of migraine is eliminated. However, this regimen is clearly suboptimal in patients with recurrent headache for two major reasons. First, narcotics do not treat the underlying headache mechanism; rather, they act at the thalamic level to alter pain sensation. Second, the recurrent use of narcotics can lead to significant problems. In patients taking oral narcotics such as oxycodone (Percodan) or hydrocodone (Vicodin), narcotic addiction can greatly confuse the treatment of migraine. The headache that results from narcotic craving and/or withdrawal can be difficult to distinguish from chronic migraine. Therefore, it is recommended that narcotic use in migraine be limited to patients with severe, but infrequent, headaches that are unresponsive to other pharmacologic approaches.

Prophylactic Treatment of Migraine A substantial number of drugs are now available that have the capacity to stabilize migraine (Table 14-11). The decision of whether to use this approach depends on the frequency of attacks and on how well acute treatment is working. The occurrence of at least three attacks per month could be an indication for this approach. Drugs must be taken daily, and there is usually a lag of at least 2 to 6 weeks before an effect is seen. The drugs that have been approved by the FDA for the prophylactic treatment of migraine include propranolol, timolol, sodium valproate, and methysergide. In addition, a number of other drugs appear to display prophylactic efficacy. This group of drugs includes amitriptyline, nortriptyline, verapamil, phenelzine, gabapentin, and cyproheptadine. Phenelzine and methysergide are usually reserved for recalcitrant cases because of their serious potential side effects. Phenelzine is an MAOI; therefore, tyramine-containing foods, decongestants, and meperidine are contraindicated. Methysergide may cause retroperitoneal or cardiac valvular fibrosis when it is used for >8 months, thus monitoring is required for patients using this drug; the risk of the fibrotic complication is about 1:1500 and is likely to reverse after the drug is stopped.

The probability of success with any one of the antimigraine drugs is 50 to 75%; thus, if one drug is assessed each month, there is a good chance that effective stabilization will be achieved within a few months. Many patients are managed adequately with low-dose amitriptyline, propranolol, or valproate. If these agents fail or lead to un-

acceptable side effects, then methysergide or phenelzine can be used. Once effective stabilization is achieved, the drug is continued for 5 to 6 months and then slowly tapered to assess the continued need. Many patients are able to discontinue medication and experience fewer and milder attacks for long periods, suggesting that these drugs may alter the natural history of migraine.

CLUSTER HEADACHE A variety of names have been used for this condition, including *Raeder's syndrome, histamine cephalalgia,* and *sphenopalatine neuralgia. Cluster headache* is a distinctive and treatable vascular headache syndrome. The episodic type is most common and is characterized by one to three short-lived attacks of periorbital pain per day over a 4- to 8-week period, followed by a pain-free interval that averages 1 year. The chronic form, which may begin de novo or several years after an episodic pattern has become established, is characterized by the absence of sustained periods of remission. Each type may transform into the other. Men are affected seven to eight times more often than women; hereditary factors are usually absent. Although the onset is generally between ages 20 and 50, it may occur as early as the first decade of life. Propranolol and amitriptyline are largely ineffective. Lithium is beneficial for cluster headache and ineffective in migraine. The cluster syndrome is thus clinically, genetically, and therapeutically different from migraine. Nevertheless, mixed features of the two disorders are occasionally present, suggesting some common elements to their pathogenesis.

Clinical Features Periorbital or, less commonly, temporal pain begins without warning and reaches a crescendo within 5 min. It is often excruciating in intensity and is deep, nonfluctuating, and explosive in quality; only rarely is it pulsatile. Pain is strictly unilateral and usually affects the same side in subsequent months. Attacks last from 30 min to 2 h; there are often associated symptoms of homolateral lacrimation, reddening of the eye, nasal stuffiness, lid ptosis, and nausea. Alcohol provokes attacks in about 70% of patients but ceases to be provocative when the bout remits; this on-off vulnerability to alcohol is pathognomonic of cluster headache. Only rarely do foods or emotional factors precipitate pain, in contrast to migraine.

There is a striking periodicity of attacks in at least 85% of patients. At least one of the daily attacks of pain recurs at about the same hour each day for the duration of a cluster bout. Onset is nocturnal in about 50% of the cases, and then the pain usually awakens the patient within 2 h of falling asleep.

Pathogenesis No consistent cerebral blood flow changes accompany attacks of pain. Perhaps the strongest evidence for a central mechanism is the periodicity of attacks; the existence of a central mechanism is also suggested by the observation that autonomic symptoms that accompany the pain are bilateral and are more severe on the painful side. The hypothalamus is probably the site of activation in this disorder. The posterior hypothalamus contains cells that regulate autonomic functions, and the anterior hypothalamus contains cells (in the suprachiasmatic nuclei) that constitute the principal circadian pacemaker in mammals. Activation of both is necessary to explain the symptoms of cluster headache. The pacemaker is modulated via serotonergic dorsal raphe projections. It can be concluded tentatively that both migraine and cluster headache result from abnormal serotonergic neurotransmission, albeit at different loci.

℞ TREATMENT

The most satisfactory treatment is the administration of drugs to prevent cluster attacks until the bout is over. Effective prophylactic drugs are prednisone, lithium, methysergide, ergotamine, sodium valproate, and verapamil. Lithium (600 to 900 mg daily) appears to be particularly useful for the chronic form of the disorder. A 10-day course of prednisone, beginning at 60 mg daily for 7 days followed by a rapid taper, may interrupt the pain bout for many patients. When ergotamine is used, it is most effective when given 1 to 2 h before an expected

TABLE 14-11 *Drugs Effective in the Prophylactic Treatment of Migraine*

Drug	Trade Name	Dosage
β-Adrenergic agents		
Propranolol	Inderal	80–320 mg qd
	Inderal LA	
Timolol	Blocadren	20–60 mg qd
Anticonvulsants		
Sodium valproate	Depakote	250 mg bid (max 1000 mg/d)
Tricyclic antidepressants		
Amitriptyline	Elavil,[a] generic	10–50 mg qhs
Nortriptyline	Pamelor,[a] generic	25–75 mg qhs
Monoamine oxidase inhibitors		
Phenelzine	Nardil[a]	15 mg tid
Serotonergic drugs		
Methysergide	Sansert	4–8 mg qd
Cyproheptadine	Periactin[a]	4–16 mg qd
Other		
Verapamil	Calan[a]	80–480 mg qd
	Isoptin[a]	

[a] Not specifically indicated for migraine by the U.S. Food and Drug Administration.

attack. Patients who use ergotamine daily must be educated regarding the early symptoms of ergotism, which may include vomiting, numbness, tingling, pain, and cyanosis of the limbs; a weekly limit of 14 mg should be adhered to.

For the attacks themselves, oxygen inhalation (9 L/min via a loose mask) is the most effective modality; 15 min of inhalation of 100% oxygen is often necessary. Sumatriptan, 6 mg subcutaneously, will usually shorten an attack to 10 to 15 min.

FURTHER READING

FERRARI MD et al: Oral triptans in acute migraine treatment: A meta-analysis of 53 trials. Lancet 358:1668, 2001

GOADSBY PJ: Serotonin 5-HT 1B/1D receptor agonists in migraine. CNS Drugs 10:271, 1998

LODER E: Safety of sumatriptan in pregnancy. CNS Drugs 17:1, 2003

---

15 BACK AND NECK PAIN
John W. Engstrom

The importance of back and neck pain in our society is underscored by the following: (1) the cost of back pain in the United States is between $20 and $50 billion annually, (2) back symptoms are the most common cause of disability in patients under 45 years of age, (3) low back pain is the second most common reason for visiting a physician in the United States, and (4) approximately 1% of the U.S. population is chronically disabled because of back pain.

ANATOMY OF THE SPINE

The anterior portion of the spine consists of cylindrical vertebral bodies separated by intervertebral disks and held together by the anterior and posterior longitudinal ligaments. The intervertebral disks are composed of a central gelatinous nucleus pulposus surrounded by a tough cartilagenous ring, the annulus fibrosis; disks are responsible for 25% of spinal column length (Figs. 15-1 and 15-2). The disks are largest in the cervical and lumbar regions where movements of the spine are greatest. The disks are elastic in youth and allow the bony vertebrae to move easily upon each other. Elasticity is lost with age. The function of the anterior spine is to absorb the shock of body movements such as walking and running.

The posterior portion of the spine consists of the vertebral arches and seven processes. Each arch consists of paired cylindrical pedicles anteriorly and paired laminae posteriorly. The vertebral arch gives rise to two transverse processes laterally, one spinous process posteriorly, plus two superior and two inferior articular facets. The functions of the posterior spine are to protect the spinal cord and nerves within the spinal canal and to stabilize the spine by providing sites for the attachment of muscles and ligaments. The contraction of muscles attached to the spinous and transverse processes produces a system of pulleys and levers that results in flexion, extension, and lateral bending movements of the spine.

Nerve root injury (*radiculopathy*) is a common cause of neck, arm, low back, and leg pain. The nerve roots exit at a level above their respective vertebral bodies in the cervical region (the C7 nerve root exits at the C6-C7 level) and below their respective vertebral bodies in the thoracic and lumbar regions (the T1 nerve root exits at the T1-T2 level). The cervical nerve roots follow a relatively short intraspinal course before exiting. By contrast, because the spinal cord ends at the vertebral L1 or L2 level, the lumbar nerve roots follow a long intraspinal course and can be injured anywhere from the upper lumbar spine to their exit at the intervertebral foramen. For example, it is common for disk herniation at the L4-L5 level to produce compression of the S1 nerve root (Fig. 15-3).

Pain-sensitive structures in the spine include the periosteum of the vertebrae, dura, facet joints, annulus fibrosus of the intervertebral disk, epidural veins, and the posterior longitudinal ligament. The nucleus pulposus of the intervertebral disk is not pain-sensitive under normal circumstances. Pain sensation is conveyed by the sinuvertebral nerve that arises from the spinal nerve at each spine segment and reenters the spinal canal through the intervertebral foramen at the same level. Disease of these diverse pain-sensitive spine structures may explain many cases of back pain without nerve root compression. The lumbar and cervical spine possess the greatest potential for movement and injury.

APPROACH TO THE PATIENT

Types of Back Pain   Understanding the type of pain experienced by the patient is the essential first step. Attention is also focused on identification of risk factors for serious underlying diseases.

Local pain is caused by stretching of pain-sensitive structures that compress or irritate sensory nerve endings. The site of the pain is near the affected part of the back.

Pain referred to the back may arise from abdominal or pelvic viscera. The pain is usually described as primarily abdominal or pelvic but is accompanied by back pain and usually unaffected by posture. The patient may occasionally complain of back pain only.

Pain of spine origin may be located in the back or referred to the buttocks or legs. Diseases affecting the upper lumbar spine tend to refer pain to the lumbar region, groin, or anterior thighs. Diseases affecting the lower lumbar spine tend to produce pain referred to the buttocks, posterior thighs, or rarely the calves or feet. Provocative injections into the pain-sensitive structures of the spine may produce leg pain that does not follow a dermatomal distribution. This "sclerotomal" pain may explain instances in which back and leg pain is unaccompanied by evidence of nerve root compression.

Radicular back pain is typically sharp and radiates from the spine to the leg within the territory of a nerve root (see "Lumbar Disk Disease," below). Coughing, sneezing, or voluntary contraction of abdominal muscles (lifting heavy objects or

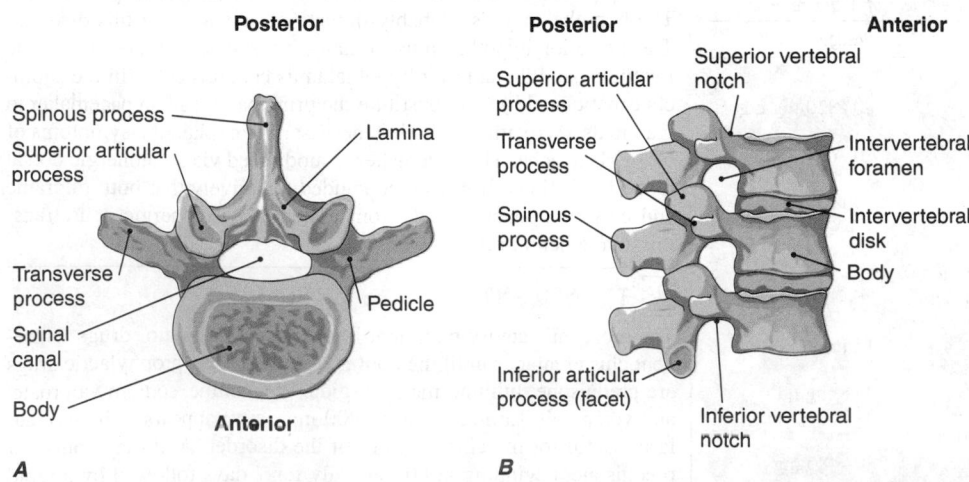

FIGURE 15-1   Vertebral anatomy. (*From A Gauthier Cornuelle, DH Gronefeld: Radiographic Anatomy Positioning. New York, McGraw-Hill, 1998, with permission.*)

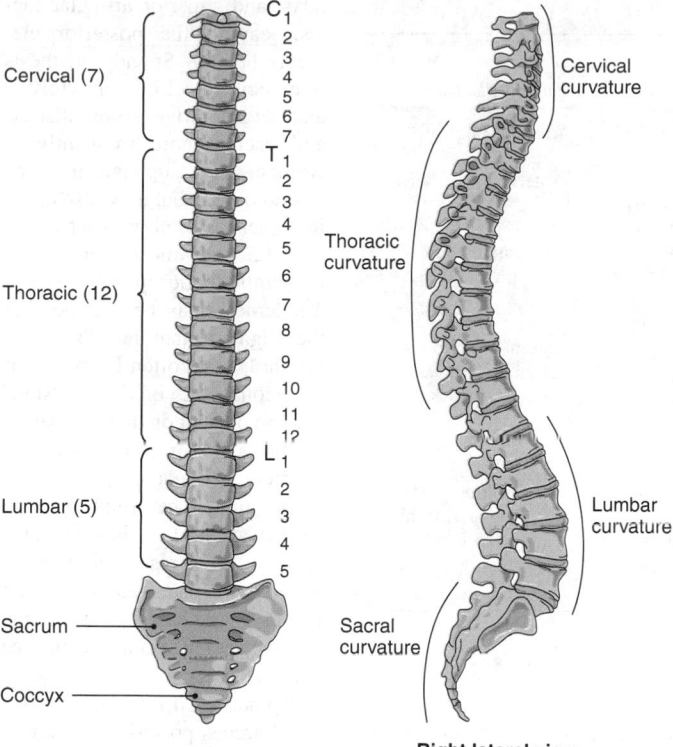

Cervical (7)

C
1
2
3
4
5
6
7

Cervical curvature

T
1
2
3
4
5
6
7
8
9
10
11
12

Thoracic (12)

Thoracic curvature

L
1
2
3
4
5

Lumbar (5)

Lumbar curvature

Sacrum

Sacral curvature

Coccyx

Right lateral view

FIGURE 15-2 Spinal column. (*From A Gauthier Cornuelle, DH Gronefeld: Radiographic Anatomy Positioning. New York, McGraw-Hill, 1998, with permission.*)

straining at stool) may elicit the radiating pain. The pain may increase in postures that stretch the nerves and nerve roots. Sitting stretches the sciatic nerve (L5 and S1 roots) because the nerve passes posterior to the hip. The femoral nerve (L2, L3, and L4 roots) passes anterior to the hip and is not stretched by sitting. The description of the pain alone often fails to distinguish clearly between sclerotomal pain and radiculopathy.

Pain associated with muscle spasm, although of obscure origin, is commonly associated with many spine disorders. The spasms are accompanied by abnormal posture, taut paraspinal muscles, and dull pain.

Back pain at rest or unassociated with specific postures should raise the index of suspicion for an underlying serious cause (e.g., spine tumor, fracture, infection, or referred pain from visceral struc-

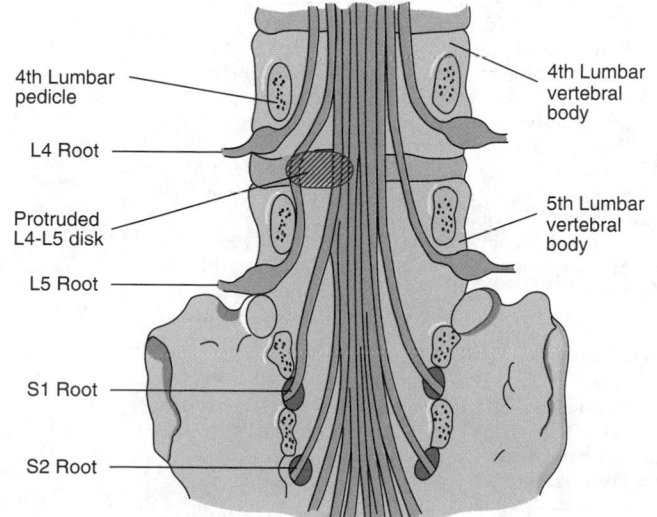

4th Lumbar pedicle

4th Lumbar vertebral body

L4 Root

Protruded L4-L5 disk

5th Lumbar vertebral body

L5 Root

S1 Root

S2 Root

FIGURE 15-3 Compression of L5 and S1 roots by herniated disk. (*From RD Adams et al: Principles of Neurology, 7th ed. New York, McGraw-Hill, 1997, with permission.*)

tures). Knowledge of the circumstances associated with the onset of back pain is important when weighing possible serious underlying causes for the pain. Some patients involved in accidents or work-related injuries may exaggerate their pain for the purpose of compensation or for psychological reasons.

Examination of the Back   A physical examination that includes the abdomen and rectum is advisable. Back pain referred from visceral organs may be reproduced during palpation of the abdomen [pancreatitis, abdominal aortic aneurysm (AAA)] or percussion over the costovertebral angles (pyelonephritis, adrenal disease).

The normal spine has a thoracic kyphosis, lumbar lordosis, and cervical lordosis. Exaggeration of these normal alignments may result in hyperkyphosis (lameback) of the thoracic spine or hyperlordosis (swayback) of the lumbar spine. Spasm of lumbar paraspinal muscles results in flattening of the usual lumbar lordosis. Inspection may reveal lateral curvature of the spine (scoliosis) or an asymmetry in the paraspinal muscles, suggesting muscle spasm. Taut paraspinal muscles limit motion of the lumbar spine. Back pain of bony spine origin is often reproduced by palpation or percussion over the spinous process of the affected vertebrae.

Forward bending is frequently limited by paraspinal muscle spasm. Flexion of the hips is normal in patients with lumbar spine disease, but flexion of the lumbar spine is limited and sometimes painful. Lateral bending to the side opposite the injured spinal element may stretch the damaged tissues, worsen pain, and limit motion. Hyperextension of the spine (with the patient prone or standing) is limited when nerve root compression or bony spine disease is present.

Pain from hip disease may resemble the pain of lumbar spine disease. Hip pain can be reproduced by internal and external rotation at the hip with the knee and hip in flexion (Patrick sign) and by tapping the heel with the examiner's palm while the leg is extended.

With the patient lying flat, passive flexion of the extended leg at the hip stretches the L5 and S1 nerve roots and the sciatic nerve. Passive dorsiflexion of the foot during the maneuver adds to the stretch. While flexion to at least 80° is normally possible without causing pain, tight hamstrings may be a source of pain in some patients. The *straight leg–raising (SLR)* test is positive if the maneuver reproduces the patient's usual back or limb pain. Eliciting the SLR sign in the sitting position may help determine if the finding is reproducible. The patient may describe pain in the low back, buttocks, posterior thigh, or lower leg, but the key feature is reproduction of the patient's usual pain. The *crossed SLR sign* is positive when flexion of one leg reproduces the pain in the opposite leg or buttocks. The crossed SLR sign is less sensitive but more specific for disk herniation than the SLR sign. The nerve or nerve root lesion is always on the side of the pain. The *reverse SLR sign* is elicited by standing the patient next to the examination table and passively extending each leg. This maneuver, which stretches the L2-L4 nerve roots and the femoral nerve, is considered positive if the patient's usual back or limb pain is reproduced.

The neurologic examination includes a search for weakness, muscle atrophy, focal reflex changes, diminished sensation in the legs, and signs of spinal cord injury. The examiner should be alert to the possibility of breakaway weakness, defined as fluctuating levels of strength in one or more muscle groups on examination. The weakness may be due to pain or a combination of pain and underlying true weakness. Breakaway weakness without pain is due to lack of effort. In uncertain cases, electromyography (EMG) can determine whether or not true weakness is present. Findings with specific nerve root lesions are shown in Table 15-1 and are discussed below.

Laboratory, Imaging, and EMG Studies   Routine laboratory studies such as a complete blood count, erythrocyte sedimentation rate, chem-

TABLE 15-1 Lumbosacral Radiculopathy—Neurologic Features

Lumbosacral Nerve Roots	Examination Findings			Pain Distribution
	Reflex	Sensory	Motor	
L2[a]	—	Upper anterior thigh	Psoas (hip flexion)	Anterior thigh
L3[a]	—	Lower anterior thigh Anterior knee	Psoas (hip flexion) Quadriceps (knee extension) Thigh adduction	Anterior thigh, knee
L4[a]	Quadriceps (knee)	Medial calf	Quadriceps (knee extension)[b] Thigh adduction Tibialis anterior (foot dorsiflexion)	Knee, medial calf Anterolateral thigh
L5[c]	—	Dorsal surface—foot Lateral calf	Peroneii (foot eversion)[b] Tibialis anterior (foot dorsiflexion) Gluteus medius (hip abduction) Toe dorsiflexors	Lateral calf, dorsal foot, posterolateral thigh, buttocks
S1[c]	Gastrocnemius/soleus (ankle)	Plantar surface—foot Lateral aspect—foot	Gastrocnemius/soleus (foot plantar flexion)[b] Abductor hallucis (toe flexors)[b] Gluteus maximus (hip extension)	Bottom foot, posterior calf, posterior thigh, buttocks

[a] Reverse straight leg–raising sign present—see "Examination of the Back."
[b] These muscles receive the majority of innervation from this root.
[c] Straight leg–raising sign present—see "Examination of the Back."

istry panel, and urinalysis are rarely needed for the initial evaluation of nonspecific ALBP (3 months). If risk factors for a serious underlying disease are present, then laboratory studies (guided by the history and examination) are indicated.

Plain films of the lumbar or cervical spine are helpful when risk factors for vertebral fracture (trauma, chronic steroid use) are present. In the absence of risk factors, routine x-rays of the lumbar spine in nonspecific ALBP are expensive and rarely helpful. Magnetic resonance imaging (MRI) and computed tomography (CT)–myelography are the radiologic tests of choice for evaluation of most serious diseases involving the spine. MRI is superior for the definition of soft tissue structures, whereas CT-myelography provides optimal imaging of bony lesions and is tolerated by claustrophobic patients. With rare exceptions, conventional myelography and bone scan are inferior to MRI and CT-myelography.

EMG can be used to assess the functional integrity of the peripheral nervous system (Chap. 363). Sensory nerve conduction studies are normal when focal sensory loss is due to nerve root damage because the nerve roots are proximal to the nerve cell bodies in the dorsal root ganglia. The diagnostic yield of needle EMG is higher than that of nerve conduction studies for radiculopathy. Denervation changes in a myotomal (segmental) distribution are detected by sampling multiple muscles supplied by different nerve roots and nerves; the pattern of muscle involvement indicates the nerve root(s) responsible for the injury. Needle EMG provides objective information about motor nerve fiber injury when the clinical evaluation of weakness is limited by pain or poor effort. EMG and nerve conduction studies will be normal when only limb pain or sensory nerve root injury or irritation is present. Mixed nerve somatosensory evoked potentials and F-wave studies are of uncertain value in the evaluation of radiculopathy.

CAUSES OF BACK PAIN (Table 15-2)

CONGENITAL ANOMALIES OF THE LUMBAR SPINE *Spondylolysis* is a bony defect in the pars interarticularis (a segment near the junction of the pedicle with the lamina) of the vertebra; the etiology may be a stress fracture in a congenitally abnormal segment. The defect (usually bilateral) is best visualized on oblique projections in plain x-rays or by CT scan and occurs in the setting of a single injury, repeated minor injuries, or growth.

Spondylolisthesis is the anterior slippage of the vertebral body, ped-

icles, and superior articular facets, leaving the posterior elements behind. Spondylolisthesis is associated with spondylolysis and degenerative spine disease and occurs more frequently in women. The slippage may be asymptomatic but may also cause low back pain, nerve root injury (the L5 root most frequently), or symptomatic spinal stenosis. Tenderness may be elicited near the segment that has "slipped" forward (most often L4 on L5 or occasionally L5 on S1). A "step" may be present on deep palpation of the posterior elements of the segment above the spondylolisthetic joint. The trunk may be shortened and the abdomen protuberant as a result of extreme forward displacement of L4 on L5; in severe cases cauda equina syndrome (CES) may occur (see below).

Spina bifida occulta is a failure of closure of one or several vertebral arches posteriorly; the meninges and spinal cord are normal. A dimple or small lipoma may overlie the defect. Most cases are asymptomatic and discovered incidentally during evaluation for back pain.

Tethered cord syndrome usually presents as a progressive cauda

TABLE 15-2 Causes of Low Back and Neck Pain

Congenital/developmental
  Spondylolysis and spondylolisthesis[a]
  Kyphoscoliosis[a]
  Spina bifida occulta[a]
  Tethered spinal cord[a]
Minor trauma
  Strain or sprain
  Whiplash injury[b]
Fractures
  Traumatic—falls, motor vehicle accidents
  Atraumatic—osteoporosis, neoplastic infiltration, exogenous steroids
Intervertebral disk herniation
Degenerative
  Disk-osteophyte complex
  Internal disk disruption
  Spinal stenosis with neurogenic claudication[a]
  Uncovertebral joint disease[b]
  Atlantoaxial joint disease (e.g., rheumatoid arthritis)[a]
Arthritis
  Spondylosis
  Facet or sacroiliac arthropathy
  Autoimmune (e.g., anklyosing spondylitis, Reiter's syndrome)
Neoplasms—metastatic, hematologic, primary bone tumors
Infection/inflammation
  Vertebral osteomyelitis
  Spinal epidural abscess
  Septic disk
  Meningitis
  Lumbar arachnoiditis[a]
Metabolic
  Osteoporosis—hyperparathyroidism, immobility
  Osteosclerosis (e.g., Paget's disease)
Other
  Referred pain from visceral disease
  Postural
  Psychiatric, malingering, chronic pain syndromes
  Vertebral artery dissection[a]

[a] Low back pain only.
[b] Neck pain only.

equina disorder (see below), although myelopathy may also be the initial manifestation. The patient is often a young adult who complains of perineal or perianal pain, sometimes following minor trauma. Neuroimaging studies reveal a low-lying conus (below L1-L2) and a short and thickened filum terminale.

TRAUMA A patient complaining of back pain and inability to move the legs may have a spinal fracture or dislocation and, with fractures above L1, spinal cord compression. Care must be taken to avoid further damage to the spinal cord or nerve roots by immobilizing the back pending results of x-rays.

Sprains and Strains The terms *low back sprain*, *strain*, or *mechanically induced muscle spasm* refer to minor, self-limited injuries associated with lifting a heavy object, a fall, or a sudden deceleration such as in an automobile accident. These terms are used loosely and do not clearly describe a specific anatomic lesion. The pain is usually confined to the lower back, and there is no radiation to the buttocks or legs. Patients with paraspinal muscle spasm often assume unusual postures.

Traumatic Vertebral Fractures Most traumatic fractures of the lumbar vertebral bodies result from injuries producing anterior wedging or compression. With severe trauma, the patient may sustain a fracture-dislocation or a "burst" fracture involving the vertebral body and posterior elements. Traumatic vertebral fractures are caused by falls from a height (a pars interarticularis fracture of the L5 vertebra is common), sudden deceleration in an automobile accident, or direct injury. Neurologic impairment is common, and early surgical treatment is indicated.

LUMBAR DISK DISEASE This is a common cause of chronic or recurrent low back and leg pain (Fig. 15-4). Disk disease is most likely to occur at the L4-L5 and L5-S1 levels, but upper lumbar levels are involved occasionally. The cause is often unknown; the risk is increased in overweight individuals. Disk herniation is unusual prior to age 20 and is rare in the fibrotic disks of the elderly. Degeneration of the nucleus pulposus and the annulus fibrosus increases with age and may be asymptomatic or painful. The pain may be located in the low back only or referred to the leg, buttock, or hip. A sneeze, cough, or trivial movement may cause the nucleus pulposus to prolapse, pushing the frayed and weakened annulus posteriorly. With severe disk disease, the nucleus may protrude through the annulus (herniation) or become extruded to lie as a free fragment in the spinal canal.

The mechanism by which intervertebral disk injury causes back

FIGURE 15-4 MRI of lumbar herniated disk; left S1 radiculopathy. Sagittal T1-weighted image on the left with arrows outlining disk margins. Sagittal T2 image on the right reveals a protruding disk at the L5-S1 level (*arrows*), which displaces the central thecal sac.

pain is controversial. The inner annulus fibrosus and nucleus pulposus are normally devoid of innervation. Inflammation and production of proinflammatory cytokines within the protruding or ruptured disk may trigger or perpetuate back pain. Ingrowth of nociceptive (pain) nerve fibers into inner portions of a diseased disk may be responsible for chronic "diskogenic" pain. Nerve root injury (radiculopathy) from disk herniation may be due to compression, inflammation, or both; pathologically, demyelination and axonal loss are usually present.

Symptoms of a ruptured disk include back pain, abnormal posture, limitation of spine motion (particularly flexion), or radicular pain. A dermatomal pattern of sensory loss or a reduced or absent deep tendon reflex is more suggestive of a specific root lesion than the pattern of pain. Motor findings (focal weakness, muscle atrophy, or fasciculations) occur less frequently than sensory or reflex changes. Symptoms and signs are usually unilateral, but bilateral involvement does occur with large central disk herniations that compress several nerve roots at the same level. Clinical manifestations of specific nerve root lesions are summarized in Table 15-1. There is evidence to suggest that lumbar disk herniation with a nonprogressive nerve root deficit can be managed nonsurgically. The size of the disk protrusion may naturally decrease over time.

The differential diagnosis includes a variety of serious and treatable conditions, including epidural abscess, hematoma, or tumor. Fever, constant pain uninfluenced by position, sphincter abnormalities, or signs of spinal cord disease suggest an etiology other than lumbar disk disease. Bilateral absence of ankle reflexes can be a normal finding in old age or a sign of bilateral S1 radiculopathy. An absent deep tendon reflex or focal sensory loss may reflect injury to a nerve root, but other sites of injury along the nerve must also be considered. For example, an absent knee reflex may be due to a femoral neuropathy rather than an L4 nerve root injury. A loss of sensation over the foot and distal lateral calf may result from a peroneal or lateral sciatic neuropathy rather than an L5 nerve root injury. Focal muscle atrophy may reflect a nerve root or peripheral nerve injury, an anterior horn cell disease, or disuse.

An MRI scan or CT-myelogram is necessary to establish the location and type of pathology. Simple MRI yields exquisite views of intraspinal and adjacent soft tissue anatomy. Bony lesions of the lateral recess or intervertebral foramen may be seen with optimal clarity on CT-myelographic studies. The correlation of neuroradiologic findings to symptoms, particularly pain, is not simple. Contrast-enhancing tears in the annulus fibrosus or disk protrusions are widely accepted as common sources of back pain; however, one study found that over half of asymptomatic adults have similar findings. Asymptomatic disk protrusions are also common, and these abnormalities may enhance with contrast. Furthermore, in patients with known disk herniation treated either medically or surgically, persistence of the herniation 10 years later had no relationship to the clinical outcome. MRI findings of disk protrusion, tears in the annulus fibrosus, or contrast enhancement are common incidental findings that by themselves should not dictate management decisions for patients with back pain.

There are four indications for intervertebral disk surgery: (1) progressive motor weakness from nerve root injury demonstrated on clinical examination or EMG, (2) bowel or bladder disturbance or other signs of spinal cord compression, (3) incapacitating nerve root pain despite conservative treatment for at least 4 weeks, and (4) recurrent incapacitating pain despite conservative treatment. The latter two criteria are more subjective and less well established than the others. Surgical treatment should also be considered if the pain and/or neurologic findings do not substantially improve over 4 to 12 weeks.

The usual surgical procedure is a partial hemilaminectomy with excision of the prolapsed disk. Fusion of the involved lumbar segments is considered only if significant spinal instability is present (i.e., degenerative spondylolisthesis or isthmic spondylolysis).

CES is an injury of multiple lumbosacral nerve roots within the spinal canal. Low back pain, weakness and areflexia in the lower extremities, saddle anesthesia, and loss of bladder function may occur. The problem must be distinguished from disorders of the lower spinal cord (conus medullaris syndrome), acute transverse myelitis (Chap. 356), and Guillain-Barré syndrome (Chap. 365). Combined involvement of the conus medullaris and cauda equina can occur. CES is commonly due to a ruptured lumbosacral intervertebral disk, lumbosacral spine fracture, hematoma within the spinal canal (e.g., following lumbar puncture in patients with coagulopathy), compressive tumors, or other mass lesions. Treatment options include surgical decompression, sometimes urgently in an attempt to restore or preserve motor or sphincter function, or palliative radiotherapy or chemotherapy for metastatic tumors.

DEGENERATIVE CONDITIONS   *Lumbar spinal stenosis* describes a narrowed lumbar spinal canal. When severe, neurogenic claudication, consisting of back and buttock or leg pain induced by walking or standing and relieved by sitting, can occur. Symptoms in the legs are usually bilateral. Unlike vascular claudication, symptoms are often provoked by standing without walking. Unlike lumbar disk disease, symptoms are usually relieved by sitting. Focal weakness, sensory loss, or reflex changes may occur when spinal stenosis is associated with radiculopathy. Severe neurologic deficits, including paralysis and urinary incontinence, occur rarely. Spinal stenosis can be acquired (75%), congenital, or due to a combination of the two causes. Congenital forms (achondroplasia, idiopathic) are characterized by short, thick pedicles that produce both spinal canal and lateral recess stenosis. Acquired factors that may contribute to spinal stenosis include degenerative diseases (spondylosis, spondylolisthesis, scoliosis), trauma, spine surgery (postlaminectomy, fusion), metabolic or endocrine disorders (epidural lipomatosis, osteoporosis, acromegaly, renal osteodystrophy, hypoparathyroidism), and Paget's disease. MRI or CT-myelography provide the best definition of the abnormal anatomy (Fig. 15-5).

Conservative treatment of symptomatic spinal stenosis includes nonsteroidal anti-inflammatory drugs (NSAIDs), exercise programs, and symptomatic treatment of acute pain exacerbations. Surgical therapy is considered when medical therapy does not relieve pain sufficiently to allow for activities of daily living or when significant focal neurologic signs are present. Between 65 and 80% of properly selected patients treated surgically experience 75% relief of back and leg pain. Up to 25% develop recurrent stenosis at the same spinal level or an adjacent level 5 years after the initial surgery; recurrent symptoms usually respond to a second surgical decompression.

Facet joint hypertrophy can produce unilateral radicular symptoms or signs due to bony compression, that are indistinguishable from disk-related radiculopathy. Patients may exhibit stretch signs, focal motor weakness, hyporeflexia, or dermatomal sensory loss. Hypertrophic superior or inferior facets can often be visualized radiologically. Foraminotomy results in long-term relief of leg and back pain in 80 to 90% of patients.

ARTHRITIS   *Spondylosis,* or osteoarthritic spine disease, typically occurs in later life and primarily involves the cervical and lumbosacral spine. Patients often complain of back pain that is increased by motion and associated with stiffness or limitation of motion. The relationship between clinical symptoms and radiologic findings is usually not straightforward. Pain may be prominent when x-ray findings are minimal; alternatively, large osteophytes can be seen in asymptomatic patients in middle and later life. Hypertrophied facets and osteophytes may compress nerve roots in the lateral recess or intervertebral foramen. Osteophytes arising from the vertebral body may cause or contribute to central spinal canal stenosis. Loss of intervertebral disk height reduces the vertical dimensions of the intervertebral foramen; the descending pedicle may compress the nerve root exiting at that level. Rarely, osteoarthritic changes in the lumbar spine compress the cauda equina.

Ankylosing Spondylitis (See also Chap. 305)   This distinctive arthritic spine disease typically presents with the insidious onset of low back and buttock pain. Patients are often males below age 40. Associated features include morning back stiffness, nocturnal pain, pain unrelieved by rest, an elevated sedimentation rate, and the histocompatibility antigen HLA-B27. Onset at a young age and back pain improving with exercise is characteristic. Loss of the normal lumbar lordosis and exaggeration of thoracic kyphosis are seen as the disease progresses. Inflammation and erosion of the outer fibers of the annulus fibrosus at the point of contact with the vertebral body are followed by ossification and bony growth that bridges adjacent vertebral bodies and reduces spine mobility in all planes. Radiologic hallmarks are periarticular destructive changes, sclerosis of the sacroiliac joints, and bridging of vertebral bodies to produce the fused "bamboo spine." Similar restricted movements may accompany Reiter's syndrome, psoriatic arthritis, and chronic inflammatory bowel disease. Stress fractures through the spontaneously ankylosed posterior bony elements of the rigid, osteoporotic spine may produce focal pain, spinal cord compression, or CES. Atlantoaxial subluxation with spinal cord compression occasionally occurs. Ankylosis of the ribs to the spine and a decrease in the height of the thoracic spine may compromise respiratory function.

NEOPLASMS (See also Chap. 358)   Back pain is the most common neurologic symptom in patients with systemic cancer and is usually due to vertebral metastases. Metastatic carcinoma (breast, lung, prostate, thyroid, kidney, gastrointestinal tract), multiple myeloma, and non-Hodgkin's and Hodgkin's lymphomas frequently involve the spine. Back pain may be the presenting symptom. The pain tends to be constant, dull, unrelieved by rest, and worse at night. In contrast, mechanical low back pain usually improves with rest. Plain x-rays usually, but not always, show destructive lesions in one or several vertebral bodies without disk space involvement. MRI or CT-myelography are the studies of choice when spinal metastasis is suspected. MRI is usually preferred, but the procedure of choice is the study most rapidly available because the patient's condition may worsen quickly.

INFECTIONS/INFLAMMATION   *Vertebral osteomyelitis* is usually caused by staphylococci, but other bacteria or the tubercle bacillus (Pott's disease) may be responsible. A primary source of infection, most often the urinary tract, skin, or lungs, can be identified in 40% of patients. Intravenous drug use is a well-recognized risk factor. Back pain exacerbated by motion and unrelieved by rest, spine tenderness over the involved spine segment, and an elevated erythrocyte sedimentation rate are the most common findings. Fever or an elevated white blood cell count are found in a minority of patients. Plain radiographs may show a narrowed disk space with erosion of adjacent vertebrae; however, these diagnostic changes may take weeks or months to appear. MRI and CT are sensitive and specific for osteomyelitis; CT may be

FIGURE 15-5   Spinal stenosis. Sagittal T2 fast spin echo magnetic resonance imaging of a normal (*left*) and stenotic (*right*) lumbar spine, revealing multifocal narrowing (*arrows*) of the cerebrospinal fluid spaces surrounding the nerve roots within the thecal sac.

more readily available in emergency settings and better tolerated by some patients with severe back pain.

Spinal epidural abscess (Chap. 356) presents with back pain (aggravated by movement or palpation) and fever. Signs of nerve root injury or spinal cord compression may be present. The abscess may track over multiple spinal levels and is best delineated by spine MRI.

Lumbar adhesive arachnoiditis with radiculopathy is due to fibrosis following inflammation within the subarachnoid space. The fibrosis results in nerve root adhesions, producing back and leg pain associated with motor, sensory, or reflex changes. Myelography-induced arachnoiditis has become rare with the abandonment of oil-based contrast. Other causes of arachnoiditis include multiple lumbar operations, chronic spinal infections, spinal cord injury, intrathecal hemorrhage, intrathecal injection of glucocorticoids or anesthetics, and foreign bodies. The MRI may show nerve roots that clump together centrally and adhere to the dura peripherally, or loculations of cerebrospinal fluid within the thecal sac. Treatment is often unsatisfactory. Microsurgical lysis of adhesions, dorsal rhizotomy, and dorsal root ganglionectomy have resulted in poor outcomes. Dorsal column stimulation for pain relief has produced varying results. Epidural injections of glucocorticoids have been of limited value.

METABOLIC CAUSES ▪ Osteoporosis and Osteosclerosis Immobilization or underlying systemic disorders such as osteomalacia, hyperparathyroidism, hyperthyroidism, multiple myeloma, metastatic carcinoma, or glucocorticoid use may accelerate osteoporosis and weaken the vertebral body. The most common causes of atraumatic vertebral body fractures are postmenopausal (type 1) or senile (type 2) osteoporosis (Chap. 333). Compression fractures occur in up to half of patients with severe osteoporosis, and those who sustain a fracture have a 4.5-fold increased risk for recurrence. The sole manifestation of a compression fracture may be localized aching (often after a trivial injury) that is exacerbated by movement. Other patients experience radicular pain only. Focal tenderness to palpation is common. The clinical context, neurologic signs, and x-ray appearance of the spine establish the diagnosis. When compression fractures are found, treatable risk factors should be sought. Antiresorptive drugs including bisphosphonates (e.g., alendronate), transdermal estrogen, and tamoxifen have been shown to reduce the risk of osteoporotic fractures. Compression fractures above the midthoracic region suggest malignancy; if tumor is suspected, a bone biopsy or diagnostic search for a primary tumor is indicated.

Interventions [percutaneous vertebroplasty (PVP), kyphoplasty] exist for osteoporotic compression fractures associated with debilitating pain. Candidates for PVP should have midline pain, focal tenderness over the spinous process of the affected vertebral body, <80% loss of vertebral body height, and onset of symptoms within the prior 4 months. The technique consists of injection of polymethylmethacrylate, under fluoroscopic guidance, into the affected vertebral body. Rare major complications include extravasation of cement into the epidural space (resulting in myelopathy) or fatal pulmonary embolism from migration of cement into paraspinal veins. Approximately three-quarters of patients who meet selection criteria have reported enhanced quality of life. Relief of pain following PVP has also been reported in patients with vertebral metastases, myeloma, or hemangiomas.

Osteosclerosis (abnormally increased bone density) is readily identifiable on routine x-ray studies (e.g., Paget's disease) and may or may not produce back pain. Spinal cord or nerve root compression may result from bony encroachment on the spinal canal or intervertebral foramina. Single dual-beam photon absorptiometry or quantitative CT can be used to detect small changes in bone mineral density. →*For further discussion of these bone disorders, see Chaps. 332–334.*

REFERRED PAIN FROM VISCERAL DISEASE Diseases of the thorax, abdomen, or pelvis may refer pain to the posterior portion of the spinal segment that innervates the diseased organ. Occasionally, back pain may be the first and only sign. Upper abdominal diseases generally refer pain to the lower thoracic or upper lumbar region (eighth thoracic to the first and second lumbar vertebrae), lower abdominal diseases to

the lumbar region (second to fourth lumbar vertebrae), and pelvic diseases to the sacral region. Local signs (pain with spine palpation, paraspinal muscle spasm) are absent, and minimal or no pain accompanies normal spine movements.

Low Thoracic or Lumbar Pain with Abdominal Disease Peptic ulcers or tumors of the posterior wall of the stomach or duodenum typically produce epigastric pain (Chaps. 77 and 274), but midline back or paraspinal pain may occur if retroperitoneal extension is present. Back pain due to peptic ulcer may be precipitated by ingestion of an orange, alcohol, or coffee and relieved by food or antacids. Fatty foods are more likely to induce back pain associated with biliary disease. Diseases of the pancreas produce back pain to the right of the spine (head of the pancreas involved) or to the left (body or tail involved). Pathology in retroperitoneal structures (hemorrhage, tumors, pyelonephritis) produces paraspinal pain that radiates to the lower abdomen, groin, or anterior thighs. A mass in the iliopsoas region often produces unilateral lumbar pain with radiation toward the groin, labia, or testicles. The sudden appearance of lumbar pain in a patient receiving anticoagulants suggests retroperitoneal hemorrhage.

Isolated low back pain occurs in 15 to 20% of patients with a contained rupture of an abdominal aortic aneurysm (AAA). The classic clinical triad of abdominal pain, shock, and back pain in an elderly man occurs in <20% of patients. Two of these three features are present in two-thirds of patients, and hypotension is present in half. The typical patient is an elderly male smoker with back pain. The diagnosis is initially missed in at least one-third of patients because the symptoms and signs can be nonspecific. Common misdiagnoses include nonspecific back pain, diverticulitis, renal colic, sepsis, and myocardial infarction. A careful abdominal examination revealing a pulsatile mass (present in 50 to 75% of patients) is an important physical finding. Patients with suspected AAA should be evaluated with ultrasound, CT, or MRI (Chap. 231).

Inflammatory bowel disorders (colitis, diverticulitis) or cancers of the colon may produce lower abdominal pain, midlumbar back pain, or both. The pain may have a beltlike distribution around the body. A lesion in the transverse or proximal descending colon may refer pain to the middle or left back at the L2-L3 level. Lesions of the sigmoid colon may refer pain to the upper sacral or midline suprapubic regions or left lower quadrant of the abdomen.

Sacral Pain with Gynecologic and Urologic Disease Pelvic organs rarely cause low back pain, except for gynecologic disorders involving the uterosacral ligaments. The pain is referred to the sacral region. Endometriosis or cancers of the uterus may invade the uterosacral ligaments; malposition of the uterus may cause uterosacral ligament traction. Pain associated with endometriosis is typically premenstrual and often continues until it merges with menstrual pain. Malposition of the uterus (retroversion, descensus, and prolapse) may produce sacral pain after prolonged standing.

Menstrual pain may be felt in the sacral region. The poorly localized, cramping pain can radiate down the legs. Pain due to neoplastic infiltration of nerves is typically continuous, progressive in severity, and unrelieved by rest at night. Less commonly, radiation therapy of pelvic tumors may produce sacral pain from late radiation necrosis of tissue or nerves. Low back pain that radiates into one or both thighs is common in the last weeks of pregnancy.

Urologic sources of lumbosacral back pain include chronic prostatitis, prostate cancer with spinal metastasis, and diseases of the kidney and ureter. Lesions of the bladder and testes do not usually produce back pain. The diagnosis of metastatic prostate carcinoma is established by rectal examination, spine imaging studies (MRI or CT), and measurement of prostate specific antigen (Chap. 81). Infectious, inflammatory, or neoplastic renal diseases may produce ipsilateral lumbosacral pain, as can renal artery or vein thrombosis. Paraspinal lumbar pain may be a symptom of ureteral obstruction due to nephrolithiasis.

OTHER CAUSES OF BACK PAIN ■ Postural Back Pain There is a group of patients with nonspecific CLBP in whom no anatomic or pathologic lesion can be found despite exhaustive investigation. These individuals complain of vague, diffuse back pain with prolonged sitting or standing that is relieved by rest. The physical examination is unrevealing except for "poor posture." Imaging studies and laboratory evaluations are normal. Exercises to strengthen the paraspinal and abdominal muscles are sometimes therapeutic.

Psychiatric Disease CLBP may be encountered in patients who seek financial compensation, in malingerers, or in those with concurrent substance abuse, chronic anxiety states, or depression. Many patients with CLBP have a history of psychiatric illness (depression, anxiety, substance abuse) or childhood trauma (physical or sexual abuse) that antedates the onset of back pain. Preoperative psychological assessment has been used to exclude patients with marked psychological impairments; these patients are likely to have a poor surgical outcome.

Unidentified The cause of low back pain occasionally remains unclear. Some patients have had multiple operations for disk disease but have persistent pain and disability. The original indications for surgery may have been questionable, with back pain only, no definite neurologic signs, or a minor disk bulge noted on CT or MRI. Scoring systems based upon neurologic signs, psychological factors, physiologic studies, and imaging studies have been devised to minimize the likelihood of unsuccessful surgical explorations.

℞ **TREATMENT**

Acute Low Back Pain A practical approach to the management of low back pain is to consider acute and chronic presentations separately. ALBP is defined as pain of <3 months duration. Full recovery can be expected in 85% of adults with ALBP unaccompanied by leg pain. Most have purely "mechanical" symptoms—i.e., pain that is aggravated by motion and relieved by rest.

Observational studies have been used to justify a minimalist approach to this problem. These studies share a number of limitations: (1) a true placebo control group is often lacking; (2) patients who consult different provider groups (generalists, orthopedists, neurologists) are assumed to have similar etiologies for their back pain; (3) no information is provided about the details of treatment; and (4) no attempt to tabulate serious causes of ALBP is made.

The algorithms for the treatment of back pain (Fig. 15-6) draw from published guidelines. However, since CPGs are based on incomplete evidence, guidelines should not substitute for clinical judgment.

The initial assessment excludes serious causes of spine pathology that require urgent intervention, including infection, cancer, and trauma. Risks factors for a possible serious underlying cause of back pain include: age >50 years, prior diagnosis of cancer or other serious medical illness, bed rest without relief, duration of pain >1 month, urinary incontinence or recent nocturia, focal leg weakness or numbness, pain radiating into the leg(s) from the back, intravenous drug use, chronic infection (pulmonary or urinary), pain increasing with standing and relieved by sitting, history of spine trauma, and glucocorticoid use. Worrisome signs include unexplained fever, unexplained weight loss, positive SLR sign or reverse SLR sign, crossed SLR sign, percussion tenderness over the spine or costovertebral angle, an abdominal mass (pulsatile or nonpulsatile), a rectal mass, focal sensory loss (saddle anesthesia or focal limb sensory loss), leg weakness, spasticity, or reflex asymmetry. Laboratory studies are unnecessary unless a serious underlying cause is suspected. Plain spine films are rarely indicated in the first month of symptoms unless a spine fracture is suspected.

Clinical trials have shown no benefit of prolonged (>2 days) bed rest for uncomplicated ALBP. There is evidence that bed rest is also ineffective for patients with sciatica or for acute back pain with findings of nerve root injury. Theoretical advantages of early ambulation for ALBP include maintenance of cardiovascular conditioning, improved disk and cartilage nutrition, improved bone and muscle strength, and increased endorphin levels. A trial examining the effects of a program of early vigorous exercise was negative, but the benefits of less vigorous exercise or other exercise programs are unknown. The early resumption of normal physical activity (without heavy manual labor) is likely to be beneficial. Traction for ALBP is not effective, as shown in well-designed clinical trials that include a "sham" traction control group. Despite this knowledge, in one survey physicians identified strict bed rest for 3 days, trigger point injections (see below), and physical therapy (PT) as beneficial for ALBP. In many instances, the behavior of treating physicians does not reflect the current medical literature.

Proof is lacking to support the treatment of acute back and neck pain with acupuncture, transcutaneous electrical nerve stimulation, massage, ultrasound, diathermy, or electrical stimulation. Cervical collars can be modestly helpful by limiting spontaneous and reflex neck movements that exacerbate pain. Evidence regarding the efficacy of ice or heat is lacking, but these interventions are optional given the lack of negative evidence, low cost, and low risk. Biofeedback has not been studied rigorously. Facet joint, trigger point, and ligament injections are not recommended.

A role for modification of posture has not been validated by rigorous clinical studies. As a practical matter, temporary suspension of activity known to increase mechanical stress on the spine (heavy lifting, prolonged sitting, bending or twisting, straining at stool) may be helpful.

Education is an important part of treatment. Satisfaction and the likelihood of follow-up increase when patients are educated about prognosis, treatment methods, activity modifications, and strategies to prevent future exacerbations. In one study, patients who felt they did not receive an adequate explanation for their symptoms wanted further diagnostic tests. Evidence for the efficacy of structured education programs ("back school") is inconclusive; in one study, patients attending back school had a shorter duration of sick leave during the initial episode but not during subsequent episodes. Randomized studies of back school for primary prevention of low back injury and pain have failed to demonstrate any benefit.

NSAIDs and acetaminophen are effective over-the-counter agents for ALBP. Muscle relaxants (cyclobenzaprine, methocarbamol) provide short-term (4 to 7 days) benefit, but drowsiness limits daytime use. Opioid analgesics are no more effective than NSAIDs or acetaminophen for initial treatment of ALBP, nor do they increase the likelihood of return to work. Short-term use of opioids in patients unresponsive to or intolerant of acetaminophen or NSAIDs may be helpful. There is no evidence to support the use of oral glucocorticoids or tricyclic antidepressants for ALBP.

Epidural glucocorticoids may occasionally produce short-term pain relief in ALBP and radiculopathy, but proof is lacking for pain relief beyond 1 month. Epidural anesthetics, glucocorticoids, or opioids are not indicated in the initial treatment of ALBP without radiculopathy. Diagnostic nerve root blocks have been advocated to determine if pain originates from a specific nerve root. However, improvement may result even when the nerve root is not responsible for the pain syndrome; this may occur with placebo effects, painful lesions located distally along the peripheral nerve, or anesthesia of the sinuvertebral nerve. Therapeutic nerve root blocks with injection of glucocorticoids and a local anesthetic is an option after conservative measures fail, particularly when temporary relief of pain is necessary.

A short course of spinal manipulation or PT for symptomatic relief of uncomplicated ALBP is an option. A prospective, randomized study comparing PT, chiropractic manipulation, and education interventions for patients with ALBP found modest trends toward benefit with both PT and chiropractic manipulation at 1 year. Costs per year were equivalent in the PT/chiropractic group and ~$280 less for the group treated with the education booklet alone. The value of such treatment beyond 1 year is unknown. Similarly, the specific PT or chiropractic protocols that may provide benefit have not been fully defined.

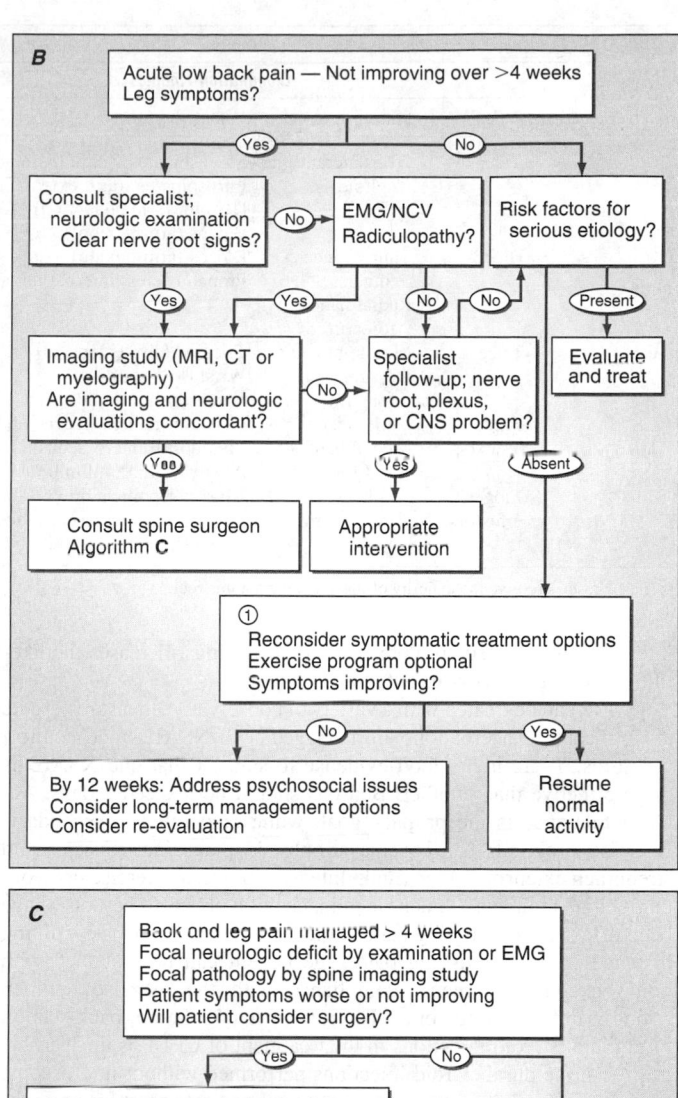

FIGURE 15-6 Algorithms for management of acute low back pain, age ≥ 18 years. *A.* Symptoms <3 months, first 4 weeks. *B.* Management weeks 4–12. ①, entry point from Algorithm *C* postoperatively or if patient declines surgery. *C.* Surgical options. (NSAIDs, nonsteroidal anti-inflammatory drugs; CBC, complete blood count; ESR, erythrocyte sedimentation rate; UA, urinalysis; EMG, electromyography; NCV, nerve conduction velocity studies; MRI, magnetic resonance imaging; CT, computed tomography; CNS, central nervous system.)

Chronic Low Back Pain CLBP, defined as pain lasting >12 weeks, accounts for 50% of total back pain costs. Overweight individuals appear to be at particular risk. Other risk factors include: female gender, older age, prior history of back pain, restricted spinal mobility, pain radiating into a leg, high levels of psychological distress, poor self-rated health, minimal physical activity, smoking, job dissatisfaction, and widespread pain. Combinations of these premorbid factors have been used to predict which individuals with ALBP are likely to develop CLBP. The initial approach to these patients is similar to that for ALBP, and the differential diagnosis is similar. Treatment of this heterogeneous group of patients is directed toward the underlying cause when known; the ultimate goal is to restore function to the greatest extent possible.

Many conditions that produce CLBP can be identified by a combination of neuroimaging and electrophysiologic studies. Spine MRI or CT-myelography are the techniques of choice but are generally not indicated within the first month after initial evaluation in the absence of risk factors for a serious underlying cause. Imaging studies should be performed only in circumstances where the results are likely to influence surgical or medical treatment.

Diskography provides no additional anatomic information beyond what is available by MRI. Reproduction of the patient's typical pain with the injection is often used as evidence that a specific disk is the pain generator, but it is not known whether this information has any value in selecting candidates for surgery. There is no proven role for thermography in the assessment of radiculopathy.

The diagnosis of nerve root injury is most secure when the history, examination, results of imaging studies, and the EMG are concordant. The correlation between CT and EMG for localization of nerve root injury is between 65 and 73%. Up to one-third of asymptomatic adults have a disk protrusion detected by CT or MRI scans. Thus, surgical

TABLE 15-3 *Cervical Radiculopathy—Neurologic Features*

Cervical Nerve Roots	Examination Findings			Pain Distribution
	Reflex	Sensory	Motor	
C5	Biceps	Over lateral deltoid	Supraspinatus[a] (initial arm abduction) Infraspinatus[a] (arm external rotation) Deltoid[a] (arm abduction) Biceps (arm flexion)	Lateral arm, medial scapula
C6	Biceps	Thumb, index fingers Radial hand/ forearm	Biceps (arm flexion) Pronator teres (internal forearm rotation)	Lateral forearm, thumb, index finger
C7	Triceps	Middle fingers Dorsum forearm	Triceps[a] (arm extension) Wrist extensors[a] Extensor digitorum[a] (finger extension)	Posterior arm, dorsal forearm, lateral hand
C8	Finger flexors	Little finger Medial hand and forearm	Abductor pollicis brevis (abduction D1) First dorsal interosseous (abduction D2) Abductor digiti minimi (abduction D5)	4th and 5th fingers, medial forearm
T1	Finger flexors	Axilla and medial arm	Abductor pollicis brevis (abduction D1) First dorsal interosseous (abduction D2) Abductor digiti minimi (abduction D5)	Medial arm, axilla

[a] These muscles receive the majority of innervation from this root.

intervention based solely upon radiologic findings increases the likelihood of an unsuccessful outcome.

CLBP can be treated with a variety of conservative measures. Acute and subacute exacerbations are managed with NSAIDs and comfort measures. There is no good evidence to suggest that one NSAID is more effective than another. Bed rest should not exceed 2 days. Activity tolerance is the primary goal, while pain relief is secondary. Exercise programs can reverse atrophy in paraspinal muscles and strengthen extensors of the trunk. Intensive physical exercise or "work hardening" regimens (under the guidance of a physical therapist) have been effective in returning some patients to work, improving walking distances, and diminishing pain. The benefit can be sustained with home exercise regimens; compliance with the exercise regimen strongly influences outcome. The role of manipulation, back school, or epidural steroid injections in the treatment of CLBP is unclear. Up to 30% of epidural steroid injections performed without fluoroscopic guidance miss the epidural space even when performed by an experienced anesthesiologist. There is no strong evidence to support the use of acupuncture or traction. A reduction in sick leave days, long-term health care utilization, and pension expenditures may offset the initial expense of multidisciplinary treatment programs. In one study comparing 3 weeks of hydrotherapy versus routine ambulatory care, hydrotherapy reduced the duration and intensity of back pain, reduced analgesic drug consumption, improved spine mobility, and improved function. Function returned to baseline at the 9-month follow-up, but all other beneficial effects were sustained. Percutaneous electrical nerve stimulation (PENS) has been shown to provide significant short-term relief of CLBP, but additional studies regarding its long-term efficacy and cost are needed.

PAIN IN THE NECK AND SHOULDER (Table 15-2)

Neck pain, which usually arises from diseases of the cervical spine and soft tissues of the neck, is common (4.6% of adults in one study). Neck pain arising from the cervical spine is typically precipitated by movements and may be accompanied by focal tenderness and limitation of motion. Pain arising from the brachial plexus, shoulder, or peripheral nerves can be confused with cervical spine disease, but the history and examination usually identify a more distal origin for the pain. Cervical spine trauma, disk disease, or spondylosis may be asymptomatic or painful and can produce a myelopathy, radiculopathy, or both. The nerve roots most commonly affected are C7 and C6.

TRAUMA TO THE CERVICAL SPINE Trauma to the cervical spine (fractures, subluxation) places the spinal cord at risk for compression. Motor vehicle accidents, violent crimes, or falls account for 87% of spinal cord injuries (Chap. 356). Immediate immobilization of the neck is essential to minimize further spinal cord injury from movement of unstable cervical spine segments.

Whiplash injury is due to trauma (usually automobile accidents) causing cervical musculoligamental sprain or strain due to hyperflexion or hyperextension. This diagnosis should not be applied to patients with fractures, disk herniation, head injury, or altered consciousness. One prospective study found that 18% of patients with whiplash injury had persistent injury-related symptoms 2 years after the car accident. These patients were older, had a higher incidence of inclined or rotated head position at impact, greater intensity of initial neck and head pain, greater number of initial symptoms, and more osteoarthritic changes on cervical spine x-rays at baseline compared to patients who ultimately recovered. Severe initial symptoms are associated with a poor long-term outcome.

CERVICAL DISK DISEASE Herniation of a lower cervical disk is a common cause of neck, shoulder, arm, or hand pain. Neck pain (worse with movement), stiffness, and a limited range of motion are the usual manifestations. With nerve root compression, pain may radiate into a shoulder or arm. Extension and lateral rotation of the neck narrows the intervertebral foramen and may reproduce radicular symptoms (Spurling's sign). In young individuals, acute nerve root compression from a ruptured cervical disk is often due to trauma. Subacute radiculopathy is less likely to be related to a specific traumatic incident and is usually due to a combination of disk disease and spondylosis. Cervical disk herniations are usually posterolateral near the lateral recess and intervertebral foramen. Typical patterns of reflex, sensory, and motor changes that accompany specific cervical nerve root lesions are summarized in Table 15-3; however, (1) overlap in function between adjacent nerve roots is common, (2) symptoms and signs may be evident in only part of the injured nerve root territory, and (3) the location of pain is the most variable of the clinical features.

CERVICAL SPONDYLOSIS Osteoarthritis of the cervical spine may produce neck pain that radiates into the back of the head, shoulders, or arms, or may be the source of headaches in the posterior occipital region (supplied by the C2-C4 nerve roots). Osteophyte formation in the lateral recess or hypertrophic facet joints may produce a monoradiculopathy (Fig. 15-7). Narrowing of the spinal canal by osteophytes, ossification of the posterior longitudinal ligament, or a large central disk may compress the cervical spinal cord. Combinations of radiculopathy and myelopathy also occur. An electrical sensation elicited by neck flexion and radiating down the spine from the neck (Lhermitte's symptom) usually indicates involvement of the cervical or upper thoracic (T1-T2) spine. When little or no neck pain accompanies the cord compression, the diagnosis may be confused with amyotrophic lateral sclerosis (Chap. 353), multiple sclerosis (Chap. 359), spinal cord tumors, or syringomyelia (Chap. 356). The possibility of treatable cervical spondylosis must be considered even when the patient presents with leg complaints only. In other cases, an unrelated lumbar radiculopathy or polyneuropathy may mask signs of an associated cervical myelopathy. MRI or CT-myelography can define the anatomic abnormalities, and EMG and nerve conduction studies can localize and assess the severity of the nerve root injury.

OTHER CAUSES OF NECK PAIN *Rheumatoid arthritis* (RA) (Chap. 301) of the cervical apophyseal joints produces neck pain, stiffness, and limitation of motion. In typical cases with symmetric inflammatory polyarthritis, the diagnosis of RA is straightforward. In advanced RA, synovitis of the atlantoaxial joint (C1-C2; Fig. 15-2) may damage the transverse ligament of the atlas, producing forward displacement of the atlas on the axis (atlantoaxial subluxation). Radiologic evidence of atlantoaxial subluxation occurs in 30% of patients with RA. Not surprisingly, the degree of subluxation correlates with the severity of erosive disease. When subluxation is present, careful neurologic assessment is important to identify early signs of myelopathy. Occasional patients develop high spinal cord compression leading to quadriparesis, respiratory insufficiency, and death. Low back pain is common in RA; however, the frequency of facet disease, fracture, and spondylolisthesis is no greater than in controls with mechanical low back pain.

Ankylosing spondylitis can cause neck pain and on occasion atlantoaxial subluxation; when spinal cord compression is present or threatened, surgical intervention is indicated. *Herpes zoster* produces acute posterior occipital or neck pain prior to the outbreak of vesicles. *Neoplasms* metastatic to the cervical spine, *infections* (osteomyelitis and epidural abscess), and *metabolic bone diseases* may also be the cause of neck pain. Neck pain may also be referred from the heart with coronary artery ischemia (cervical angina syndrome).

THORACIC OUTLET The thoracic outlet contains the first rib, the subclavian artery and vein, the brachial plexus, the clavicle, and the lung apex. Injury to these structures may result in postural or movement-induced pain around the shoulder and supraclavicular region. *True neurogenic thoracic outlet syndrome* (TOS) results from compression of the lower trunk of the brachial plexus or ventral rami of the C8 or T1 nerve roots by an anomalous band of tissue connecting an elongate transverse process at C7 with the first rib. Signs include weakness of intrinsic muscles of the hand and diminished sensation on the palmar aspect of the fourth and fifth digits. EMG and nerve conduction studies confirm the diagnosis. Treatment consists of surgical division of the anomalous band. The weakness and wasting of intrinsic hand muscles typically does not improve, but surgery halts the insidious progression of weakness. *Arterial TOS* results from compression of the subclavian artery by a cervical rib; the compression results in poststenotic dilatation of the artery and thrombus formation. Blood pressure is reduced in the affected limb, and signs of emboli may be present in the hand; neurologic signs are absent. Ultrasound can confirm the diagnosis noninvasively. Treatment is with thrombolysis or anticoagulation (with or without embolectomy) and surgical excision of the cervical rib compressing the subclavian artery or vein. *Disputed TOS* includes a large number of patients with chronic arm and shoulder pain of unclear cause. The lack of sensitive and specific findings on physical examination or laboratory markers for this condition frequently results in diagnostic uncertainty. The role of surgery in disputed TOS is controversial. Multidisciplinary pain management is a conservative approach, although treatment is often unsuccessful.

BRACHIAL PLEXUS AND NERVES Pain from injury to the brachial plexus or peripheral nerves of the arm can occasionally mimic pain of cervical spine origin. Neoplastic infiltration of the lower trunk of the brachial plexus may produce shoulder pain radiating down the arm, numbness of the fourth and fifth fingers, and weakness of intrinsic hand muscles innervated by the ulnar and median nerves. Postradiation fibrosis (breast carcinoma is the most common setting) may produce similar findings, although pain is less often present. A Pancoast tumor of the

A

B

FIGURE 15-7 Cervical spondylosis; left C6 radiculopathy. *A.* Sagittal T2 fast spin echo magnetic resonance imaging reveals a hypointense osteophyte that protrudes from the C5-C6 level into the thecal sac, displacing the spinal cord posteriorly (*white arrow*). *B.* Axial 2-mm section from a 3-D volume gradient echo sequence of the cervical spine. The high signal of the right C5-C6 intervertebral foramen contrasts with the narrow high signal of the left C5-C6 intervertebral foramen produced by osteophytic spurring (*arrows*).

lung (Chap. 75) is another cause and should be considered, especially when a Horner's syndrome is present. *Suprascapular neuropathy* may produce severe shoulder pain, weakness, and wasting of the supraspinatous and infraspinatous muscles. *Acute brachial neuritis* is often confused with radiculopathy. It consists of the acute onset of severe shoulder or scapular pain followed over days to weeks by weakness of the proximal arm and shoulder girdle muscles innervated by the upper brachial plexus. The onset is often preceeded by an infection or immunization. Complete recovery occurs in 75% of patients after 2 years and in 89% after 3 years. Occasional cases of carpal tunnel syndrome produce pain and paresthesias extending into the forearm, arm, and shoulder resembling a C5 or C6 root lesion. Lesions of the radial or ulnar nerve can mimic a radiculopathy at C7 or C8, respectively. EMG and nerve conduction studies can accurately localize lesions to the nerve roots, brachial plexus, or peripheral nerves. →*For further discussion of peripheral nerve disorders, see Chap. 363.*

SHOULDER Pain from the shoulder can be difficult to distinguish from neck pain. If symptoms and signs of radiculopathy are absent, then the differential diagnosis includes mechanical shoulder pain (tendonitis, bursitis, rotator cuff tear, dislocation, adhesive capsulitis, and cuff impingement under the acromion) and referred pain (subdiaphragmatic irritation, angina, Pancoast tumor). Mechanical pain is often worse at night, associated with local shoulder tenderness and aggravated by abduction, internal rotation, or extension of the arm. Pain from shoulder disease may on occasion radiate into the arm or hand, but sensory, motor, and reflex changes are absent.

℞ TREATMENT

There are few well-designed clinical trials that address optimal treatment of neck pain. Symptomatic treatment can include the use of analgesic medications and/or a soft cervical collar. Current indications for cervical disk surgery are similar to those for lumbar disk surgery; because of the risk of spinal cord injury with cervical spine disease, an aggressive approach is generally indicated whenever spinal cord injury is threatened. Surgical management of cervical herniated disks usually consists of an anterior approach with diskectomy followed by anterior interbody fusion. A simple posterior partial laminectomy with diskectomy is an acceptable alternative approach. The risk of subsequent radiculopathy or myelopathy at cervical segments adjacent to the fusion is ~3% per year and 26% per decade. Although this risk is sometimes portrayed as a late complication of surgery, it may also reflect the natural history of degenerative cervical spine disease. Nonprogressive cervical radiculopathy (associated with a focal neurologic deficit) due to a herniated cervical disk may be treated conservatively with a high rate of success. Cervical spondylosis with bony, compressive cervical radiculopathy is generally treated with surgical decompression to forstall the progression of neurologic signs. Cervical spondylotic myelopathy is typically managed with either anterior decompression and fusion or laminectomy. Outcomes in both surgical groups vary, but late functional deterioration occurs in 20 to 30% of patients; a prospective, controlled study comparing different surgical interventions is needed.

FURTHER READING

ATLAS SJ, NARDIN RA: Evaluation and treatment of low back pain: An evidence-based approach to clinical care. Muscle and Nerve 27:265, 2003

CASSIDY JD et al: Effect of eliminating compensation for pain and suffering on the outcome of insurance claims for whiplash injury. N Engl J Med 342:1179, 2000

HASSETT G et al: Risk factors for progression of lumbar spine disc degeneration. Arthritis Rheum 48:3112, 2003

Section 2   Alterations in Body Temperature

16   FEVER AND HYPERTHERMIA
Charles A. Dinarello, Jeffrey A. Gelfand

Body temperature is controlled by the hypothalamus. Neurons in both the preoptic anterior hypothalamus and the posterior hypothalamus receive two kinds of signals: one from peripheral nerves that reflect warmth/cold receptors and the other from the temperature of the blood bathing the region. These two types of signals are integrated by the thermoregulatory center of the hypothalamus to maintain normal temperature. In a neutral environment, the metabolic rate of humans consistently produces more heat than is necessary to maintain the core body temperature at 37°C.

A normal body temperature is ordinarily maintained, despite environmental variations, because the hypothalamic thermoregulatory center balances the excess heat production derived from metabolic activity in muscle and the liver with heat dissipation from the skin and lungs. According to studies of healthy individuals 18 to 40 years of age, the mean oral temperature is 36.8° ± 0.4°C (98.2° ± 0.7°F), with low levels at 6 A.M. and higher levels at 4 to 6 P.M. The maximum normal oral temperature is 37.2°C (98.9°F) at 6 A.M. and 37.7°C (99.9°F) at 4 P.M.; these values define the 99th percentile for healthy individuals. In light of these studies, an *A.M.* temperature of >37.2°C (>98.9°F) or a *P.M.* temperature of >37.7°C (>99.9°F) would define a fever. The normal daily temperature variation is typically 0.5°C (0.9°F). However, in some individuals recovering from a febrile illness, this daily variation can be as great as 1.0°C. During a febrile illness, diurnal variations are usually maintained but at higher levels. Daily temperature swings do not occur in patients with hyperthermia (see below). Rectal temperatures are generally 0.4°C (0.7°F) higher than oral readings. The lower oral readings are probably attributable to mouth breathing, which is a particularly important factor in patients with respiratory infections and rapid breathing. Lower esophageal temperatures closely reflect core temperature. Tympanic membrane (TM) thermometers measure radiant heat energy from the tympanic membrane and nearby ear canal and display that absolute value (unadjusted mode) or a value automatically calculated from the absolute reading on the basis of nomograms relating the radiant temperature measured to actual core temperatures obtained in clinical studies (adjusted mode). These measurements, although convenient, may be more variable than directly determined oral or rectal values. Studies in adults show that readings are lower with unadjusted-mode than with adjusted-mode TM thermometers and that unadjusted-mode TM values are 0.8°C (1.6°F) lower than rectal temperatures.

In women who menstruate, the A.M. temperature is generally lower in the 2 weeks before ovulation; it then rises by about 0.6°C (1°F) with ovulation and remains at that level until menses occur. Seasonal variation in body temperature has been described but may reflect a metabolic change and is not common. Body temperature is elevated in the postprandial state. Pregnancy and endocrinologic dysfunction also affect body temperature. The daily temperature variation appears to be fixed in early childhood; in contrast, elderly individuals can exhibit a reduced ability to develop fever, with only a modest fever even in severe infections.

FEVER VERSUS HYPERTHERMIA

FEVER   Fever is an elevation of body temperature that exceeds the normal daily variation and occurs *in conjunction with an increase in the hypothalamic set point*—for example, from 37°C to 39°C. This shift of the set point from "normothermic" to febrile levels very much resembles the resetting of the home thermostat to a higher level in order to raise the ambient temperature in a room. Once the hypothalamic set point is raised, neurons in the vasomotor center are activated and vasoconstriction commences. The individual first notices vasoconstriction in the hands and feet. Shunting of blood away from the periphery to the internal organs essentially decreases heat loss from the skin, and the person feels cold. For most fevers, body temperature increases by 1° to 2°C. Shivering, which increases heat production from the muscles, may begin at this time; however, shivering is not required if heat conservation mechanisms raise blood temperature sufficiently. Heat production from the liver also increases. In humans, behavior (e.g., putting on more clothing or bedding) helps raise body temperature.

The processes of heat conservation (vasoconstriction) and heat production (shivering and increased metabolic activity) continue until the temperature of the blood bathing the hypothalamic neurons matches the new thermostat setting. Once that point is reached, the hypothalamus maintains the temperature at the febrile level by the same mechanisms of heat balance that are operative in the afebrile state. When the hypothalamic set point is again reset downward (due to either a reduction in the concentration of pyrogens or the use of antipyretics), the processes of heat loss through vasodilation and sweating are initiated. Loss of heat by sweating and vasodilation continues until the blood temperature at the hypothalamic level matches the lower setting.

A fever of >41.5°C (>106.7°F) is called *hyperpyrexia*. This extraordinarily high fever can develop in patients with severe infections but most commonly occurs in patients with central nervous system (CNS) hemorrhages. In the preantibiotic era, fever due to a variety of infectious diseases rarely exceeded 106°F, and there has been speculation that this natural "thermal ceiling" is mediated by neuropeptides functioning as central antipyretics.

In some rare cases, the hypothalamic set point is elevated as a result of local trauma, hemorrhage, tumor, or intrinsic hypothalamic malfunction. The term *hypothalamic fever* is sometimes used to describe elevated temperature caused by abnormal hypothalamic function. However, most patients with hypothalamic damage have *sub*normal, not *supra*normal, body temperatures.

HYPERTHERMIA Hyperthermia is characterized by *an unchanged (normothermic) setting of the thermoregulatory center* in conjunction with an uncontrolled increase in body temperature that exceeds the body's ability to lose heat. Exogenous heat exposure and endogenous heat production are two mechanisms by which hyperthermia can result in dangerously high internal temperatures. Excessive heat production can easily cause hyperthermia despite physiologic and behavioral control of body temperature. For example, work or exercise in hot environments can produce heat faster than peripheral mechanisms can lose it.

Although most patients with elevated body temperature have fever, there are a few circumstances in which elevated temperature represents not fever but hyperthermia (Table 16-1). *Heat stroke*, caused by thermoregulatory failure in association with a warm environment, may be categorized as exertional or nonexertional. *Exertional heat stroke* typically occurs in younger individuals exercising at ambient temperatures and/or humidities that are higher than normal. In a dry environment and at maximal efficiency, sweating can dissipate ~600 kcal/h, requiring the production of >1 L of sweat. Even in normal individuals, dehydration or the use of common medications (e.g., over the counter antihistamines with anticholinergic side effects) may help to precipitate exertional heat stroke. *Nonexertional* or *classic heat stroke* typically occurs in either very young or elderly individuals, particularly during heat waves. According to the Centers for Disease Control and Prevention (CDC), there were 7000 deaths attributed to heat injury in the United States from 1979 to 1997. The elderly, the bedridden, persons taking anticholinergic or antiparkinsonian drugs or diuretics, and individuals confined to poorly ventilated and non-air-conditioned environments are most susceptible.

Drug-induced hyperthermia has become increasingly common as a result of the increased use of prescription psychotropic drugs and illicit drugs. Drug-induced hyperthermia may be caused by monoamine oxidase inhibitors (MAOIs), tricyclic antidepressants, and amphetamines and by the illicit use of phencyclidine (PCP), lysergic acid diethylamide (LSD), methylenedioxymethamphetamine (MDMA, "ecstasy"), or cocaine.

Malignant hyperthermia occurs in individuals with an inherited abnormality of skeletal-muscle sarcoplasmic reticulum that causes a rapid increase in intracellular calcium levels in response to halothane

---

and other inhalational anesthetics or to succinylcholine. Elevated temperature, increased muscle metabolism, muscle rigidity, rhabdomyolysis, acidosis, and cardiovascular instability develop rapidly. This condition is often fatal. The *neuroleptic malignant syndrome* (NMS) occurs in the setting of neuroleptic agent use (antipsychotic phenothiazines, haloperidol, prochlorperazine, metoclopramide) or the withdrawal of dopaminergic drugs and is characterized by "lead-pipe" muscle rigidity, extrapyramidal side effects, autonomic dysregulation, and hyperthermia. This disorder appears to be caused by the inhibition of central dopamine receptors in the hypothalamus, which results in increased heat generation and decreased heat dissipation. The *serotonin syndrome*, seen with selective serotonin uptake inhibitors (SSRIs), MAOIs, and other serotonergic medications, has many overlapping features, including hyperthermia, but may be distinguished by the presence of diarrhea, tremor, and myoclonus rather than the lead-pipe rigidity of NMS. Thyrotoxicosis and pheochromocytoma can also cause increased thermogenesis.

It is important to distinguish between fever and hyperthermia since hyperthermia can be rapidly fatal and characteristically does not respond to antipyretics. However, there is no rapid way to make this distinction. Hyperthermia is often diagnosed on the basis of the events immediately preceding the elevation of core temperature—e.g., heat exposure or treatment with drugs that interfere with thermoregulation. However, in addition to the clinical history of the patient, the physical aspects of some forms of hyperthermia may alert the clinician. For example, in patients with heat stroke syndromes and in those taking drugs that block sweating, the skin is hot but dry. Moreover, antipyretics do not reduce the elevated temperature in hyperthermia, whereas in fever—and even in hyperpyrexia—adequate doses of either aspirin or acetaminophen usually result in some decrease in body temperature.

PATHOGENESIS OF FEVER

PYROGENS The term *pyrogen* is used to describe any substance that causes fever. *Exogenous* pyrogens are derived from outside the patient; most are microbial products, microbial toxins, or whole microorganisms. The classic example of an exogenous pyrogen is the lipopolysaccharide endotoxin produced by all gram-negative bacteria. Endotoxins are potent not only as pyrogens but also as inducers of various pathologic changes in gram-negative infections. Another group of potent bacterial pyrogens is produced by gram-positive organisms and includes the enterotoxins of *Staphylococcus aureus* and the group A and B streptococcal toxins, also called *superantigens*. One staphylococcal toxin of clinical importance is the toxic shock syndrome toxin associated with isolates of *S. aureus* from patients with toxic shock syndrome. Like the endotoxins of gram-negative bacteria, the toxins produced by staphylococci and streptococci cause fever in experimental animals when injected intravenously at concentrations of <1 μg/kg of body weight. Endotoxin is a highly pyrogenic molecule in humans: a dose of 2 to 3 ng/kg produces fever and generalized symptoms of malaise in volunteers.

PYROGENIC CYTOKINES Cytokines are small proteins (molecular mass, 10,000 to 20,000 Da) that regulate immune, inflammatory, and hematopoietic processes. For example, stimulation of lymphocyte proliferation during an immune response to vaccination is the result of the cytokines interleukin (IL) 2, IL-4, and IL-6. Another cytokine, granulocyte colony-stimulating factor, stimulates granulocytopoiesis in the bone marrow. Some cytokines cause fever and hence are called *pyrogenic cytokines*. From a historic point of view, the field of cytokine biology began in the 1940s with laboratory investigations into fever induction by products of activated leukocytes. These fever-producing molecules were called *endogenous pyrogens*.

The known pyrogenic cytokines include IL-1, IL-6, tumor necrosis factor (TNF), ciliary neurotropic factor (CNTF), and interferon (IFN) α. Others probably exist, although IL-18—a member of the IL-1 family—does not appear to be a pyrogenic cytokine. Each cytokine is

---

TABLE 16-1 *Causes of Hyperthermia Syndromes*

HEAT STROKE

Exertional: Exercise in higher-than-normal heat and/or humidity
Nonexertional: Anticholinergics, including antihistamines; antiparkinsonian drugs; diuretics; phenothiazines

DRUG-INDUCED HYPERTHERMIA

Amphetamines, cocaine, phencyclidine (PCP), methylenedioxymethamphetamine (MDMA; "ecstasy"), lysergic acid diethylamide (LSD), salicylates, lithium, anticholinergics, sympathomimetics

NEUROLEPTIC MALIGNANT SYNDROME

Phenothiazines; butyrophenones, including haloperidol and bromperidol; fluoxetine; loxapine; tricyclic dibenzodiazepines; metoclopramide; domperidone; thiothixene; molindone; withdrawal of dopaminergic agents

SEROTONIN SYNDROME

Selective serotonin reuptake inhibitors (SSRIs), monoamine oxidase inhibitors (MAOIs), tricyclic antidepressants

MALIGNANT HYPERTHERMIA

Inhalational anesthetics, succinylcholine

ENDOCRINOPATHY

Thyrotoxicosis, pheochromocytoma

CENTRAL NERVOUS SYSTEM DAMAGE

Cerebral hemorrhage, status epilepticus, hypothalamic injury

Source: After FJ Curley, RS Irwin, JM Rippe et al (eds): *Intensive Care Medicine*, 3d ed. Boston, Little, Brown, 1996.

encoded by a separate gene, and each pyrogenic cytokine has been shown to cause fever in laboratory animals and in humans. When injected into humans, IL-1, IL-6, and TNF produce fever at low doses (10 to 100 ng/kg).

The synthesis and release of endogenous pyrogenic cytokines are induced by a wide spectrum of exogenous pyrogens, most of which have recognizable bacterial or fungal sources. Viruses also induce pyrogenic cytokines by infecting cells. However, in the absence of microbial infection, inflammation, trauma, tissue necrosis, or antigen-antibody complexes can induce the production of IL-1, TNF, and/or IL-6, which—individually or in combination—trigger the hypothalamus to raise the set point to febrile levels. The cellular sources of pyrogenic cytokines are primarily monocytes, neutrophils, and lymphocytes, although many other types of cells can synthesize these molecules when stimulated.

ELEVATION OF THE HYPOTHALAMIC SET POINT BY CYTOKINES During fever, levels of prostaglandin E_2 (PGE_2) are elevated in hypothalamic tissue and the third cerebral ventricle. The concentrations of PGE_2 are highest near the circumventricular vascular organs (organum vasculosum of lamina terminalis)—networks of enlarged capillaries surrounding the hypothalamic regulatory centers. Destruction of these organs reduces the ability of pyrogens to produce fever. Most studies in animals have failed to show, however, that pyrogenic cytokines pass from the circulation into the brain itself. Thus, it appears that both exogenous and endogenous pyrogens interact with the endothelium of these capillaries and that this interaction is the first step in initiating fever—i.e., in raising the set point to febrile levels.

The key events in the production of fever are illustrated in Fig. 16-1. As has been mentioned, several cell types can produce pyrogenic cytokines. Pyrogenic cytokines such as IL-1, IL-6, and TNF are released from the cells and enter the systemic circulation. Although the systemic effects of these circulating cytokines lead to fever by inducing the synthesis of PGE_2, they also induce PGE_2 in peripheral tissues. The increase in PGE_2 in the periphery accounts for the nonspecific myalgias and arthralgias that often accompany fever. However, it is the induction of PGE_2 in the brain that starts the process of raising the hypothalamic set point for core temperature.

There are four receptors for PGE_2, and each signals the cell in different ways. Of the four receptors, the third (EP-3) is essential for fever: when the gene for this receptor is deleted in mice, no fever follows the injection of IL-1 or endotoxin. Deletion of the other PGE_2 receptor genes leaves the fever mechanism intact. Although PGE_2 is essential for fever, it is not a neurotransmitter. Rather, the release of

PGE_2 from the brain side of the hypothalamic endothelium triggers the PGE_2 receptor on glial cells, and this stimulation results in the rapid release of cyclic adenosine 5′-monophosphate (cyclic AMP), which is a neurotransmitter. As shown in Fig. 16-1, the release of cyclic AMP from the glial cells activates neuronal endings from the thermoregulatory center that extend into the area. The elevation of cyclic AMP is thought to account for changes in the hypothalamic set point either directly or indirectly by inducing the release of neurotransmitters. Distinct receptors for microbial products (such as endotoxins) from gram-negative bacteria and for teichoic acids from gram-positive bacteria are located on the hypothalamic endothelium. These receptors are called *Toll-like receptors* and are similar in many ways to IL-1 receptors. The direct activation of Toll-like receptors also results in PGE_2 production and fever.

PRODUCTION OF CYTOKINES IN THE CNS Several viral diseases produce active infection in the brain. Glial and possibly neuronal cells synthesize IL-1, TNF, and IL-6. CNTF is also synthesized by neural as well as neuronal cells. What role in the production of fever is played by these cytokines produced in the brain itself? In experimental animals, the concentrations of cytokine required to cause fever are several orders of magnitude lower with direct injection into the brain than with intravenous injection. Therefore, CNS production of these cytokines apparently can raise the hypothalamic set point, bypassing the circumventricular organs involved in fever caused by circulating cytokines. CNS cytokines may account for the hyperpyrexia of CNS hemorrhage, trauma, or infection.

APPROACH TO THE PATIENT

History It is in the diagnosis of a febrile illness that the science and art of medicine come together (see also Chaps. 1, 18, and 106). In no other clinical situation is a meticulous history more important. Painstaking attention must be paid to the chronology of symptoms in relation to the use of prescription drugs (including drugs, supplements, or herbs taken without a physician's supervision) or treatments such as surgical or dental procedures. The exact nature of any prosthetic materials and/or implanted devices should be ascertained. A careful occupational history should include exposures to animals; toxic fumes; potential infectious agents; possible antigens; or other febrile or infected individuals in the home, workplace, or school. A history of the geographic areas in which the patient has lived and a travel history should include locations during military service. Information on unusual hobbies, dietary proclivities (such as raw or poorly cooked meat, raw fish, and unpasteurized milk or cheeses), and household pets should be elicited, as should that on sexual orientation and practices, including precautions taken or omitted. Attention should be directed to the use of tobacco, marijuana, intravenous drugs, or alcohol; trauma; animal bites; tick or other insect bites; and prior transfusions, immunizations, drug allergies, or hypersensitivities. A careful family history should include information on family members with tuberculosis, other febrile or infectious diseases, arthritis or collagen vascular disease, or unusual familial symptomatology such as deafness, urticaria, fevers and polyserositis, bone pain, or anemia. Ethnic origin may be critical. For example, blacks are more likely than persons in other groups to have hemoglobinopathies. Turks, Arabs, Armenians, and Sephardic Jews are especially likely to have familial Mediterranean fever (Chap. 278).

Physical Examination A meticulous physical examination should be repeated on a regular basis. All the vital signs are relevant. The temperature may be taken orally or rectally, but the site used should be consistent. Axillary temperatures are notoriously unreliable. Special attention should be paid to the skin, lymph nodes, eyes, nail beds, cardiovascular system, chest, abdomen, musculoskeletal system, and nervous system. Rectal examination is imperative. The penis, prostate, scrotum, and testes should be examined carefully and the foreskin, if present, retracted. Pelvic examination must be part of every complete physical examination of a woman, with a

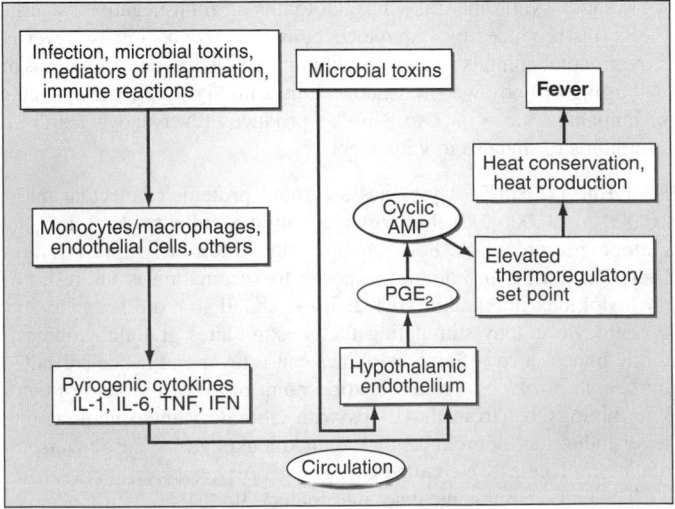

FIGURE 16-1 Chronology of events required for the induction of fever. Abbreviations: AMP, adenosine 5′-monophosphate; IFN, interferon; IL, interleukin; PGE_2, prostaglandin E_2; TNF, tumor necrosis factor.

search for such causes of fever as pelvic inflammatory disease and tubo-ovarian abscess.

Laboratory Tests   Few signs and symptoms in medicine have as many diagnostic possibilities as fever. If the history, epidemiologic situation, or physical examination suggests more than a simple viral illness or streptococcal pharyngitis, then laboratory testing is indicated. The tempo and complexity of the workup will depend on the pace of the illness, diagnostic considerations, and the immune status of the host. If findings are focal or if the history, epidemiologic setting, or physical examination suggests certain diagnoses, the laboratory examination can be focused. If fever is undifferentiated, the diagnostic nets must be cast farther, and certain guidelines are indicated, as follows.

CLINICAL PATHOLOGY   The workup should include a complete blood count; a differential count should be performed manually or with an instrument sensitive to the identification of eosinophils, juvenile or band forms, toxic granulations, and Döhle bodies, the last three of which are suggestive of bacterial infection. Neutropenia may be present with some viral infections, particularly parvovirus B19 infection; drug reactions; systemic lupus erythematosus; typhoid; brucellosis; and infiltrative diseases of the bone marrow, including lymphoma, leukemia, tuberculosis, and histoplasmosis. Lymphocytosis may occur with typhoid, brucellosis, tuberculosis, and viral disease. Atypical lymphocytes are documented in many viral diseases, including infection with Epstein-Barr virus, cytomegalovirus, or HIV; dengue; rubella; varicella; measles; and viral hepatitis. This abnormality also occurs in serum sickness and toxoplasmosis. Monocytosis is a feature of typhoid, tuberculosis, brucellosis, and lymphoma. Eosinophilia may be associated with hypersensitivity drug reactions, Hodgkin's disease, adrenal insufficiency, and certain metazoan infections. If the febrile illness appears to be severe or is prolonged, the smear should be examined carefully for malarial or babesial pathogens (where appropriate) as well as for classic morphologic features, and the erythrocyte sedimentation rate should be determined. Urinalysis, with examination of urinary sediment, is indicated. It is axiomatic that any abnormal fluid accumulation (pleural, peritoneal, joint), even if previously sampled, merits reexamination in the presence of undiagnosed fever. Joint fluids should be examined for bacteria as well as crystals. Bone marrow biopsy (not simple aspiration) for histopathologic studies (as well as culture) is indicated when marrow infiltration by pathogens or tumor cells is possible. Stool should be inspected for occult blood; an inspection for fecal leukocytes, ova, or parasites also may be indicated.

CHEMISTRY   Electrolyte, glucose, blood urea nitrogen, and creatinine levels should be measured. Liver function tests are usually indicated if efforts to identify the cause of fever do not point to the involvement of another organ. Additional assessments (e.g., measurement of creatinine phosphokinase or amylase) can be added as the workup progresses.

MICROBIOLOGY   Smears and cultures of specimens from the throat, urethra, anus, cervix, and vagina should be assessed when there are no localizing findings or when findings suggest the involvement of the pelvis or the gastrointestinal tract. If respiratory tract infection is suspected, sputum evaluation (Gram's staining, staining for acid-fast bacilli, culture) is indicated. Cultures of blood, abnormal fluid collections, and urine are indicated when fever is thought to reflect more than uncomplicated viral illness. Cerebrospinal fluid should be examined and cultured if meningismus, severe headache, or a change in mental status is noted.

RADIOLOGY   A chest x-ray is usually part of the evaluation for any significant febrile illness.

Outcome of Diagnostic Efforts   In most cases of fever, either the patient recovers spontaneously or the history, physical examination, and initial screening laboratory studies lead to a diagnosis. When

fever continues for 2 to 3 weeks, during which time repeat physical examinations and laboratory tests are unrevealing, the patient is provisionally diagnosed as having fever of unknown origin (Chap. 18).

℞ TREATMENT

The Decision to Treat Fever   Most fevers are associated with self-limited infections, most commonly of viral origin. In these cases, the general cause of the fever is easily identified. The routine use of antipyretics given automatically as "standing," "routine," or "prn" orders to treat low-grade fevers in adult patients on hospital wards is entirely unacceptable. This practice masks not only fever but also other important clinical indicators of a patient's course. For example, the daily highs and lows of normal temperature are exaggerated in most fevers, but the usual times of peak and trough temperatures may be reversed in typhoid fever and disseminated tuberculosis. Temperature-pulse dissociation (relative bradycardia) occurs in typhoid fever, brucellosis, leptospirosis, some drug-induced fevers, and factitious fever. In newborns, the elderly, patients with chronic renal failure, and patients taking glucocorticoids, fever may not be present despite infection, or core temperature may be hypothermic. Hypothermia is observed in patients with septic shock.

Some febrile diseases have characteristic patterns. With *relapsing* fevers, febrile episodes are separated by intervals of normal temperature; when paroxysms occur on the first and third days, the fever is called *tertian*. *Plasmodium vivax* causes tertian fevers. *Quartan* fevers are associated with paroxysms on the first and fourth days and are seen with *P. malariae*. Other relapsing fevers are related to *Borrelia* infections and rat-bite fever, which are both associated with days of fever followed by a several-day afebrile period and then a relapse of days of fever. Pel-Ebstein fever, with fevers lasting 3 to 10 days followed by afebrile periods of 3 to 10 days, is classic for Hodgkin's disease and other lymphomas. Another characteristic fever is that of cyclic neutropenia, in which fevers occur every 21 days and accompany the neutropenia. There is no periodicity of fever in patients with familial Mediterranean fever (Chap. 278).

Mechanisms of Antipyretic Agents   The synthesis of PGE_2 depends on the constitutively expressed enzyme cyclooxygenase. The substrate for cyclooxygenase is arachidonic acid released from the cell membrane, and this release is the rate-limiting step in the synthesis of PGE_2. Inhibitors of cyclooxygenase are potent antipyretics. The antipyretic potency of various drugs is directly correlated with the inhibition of brain cyclooxygenase. Acetaminophen is a poor cyclooxygenase inhibitor in peripheral tissue and is without noteworthy anti-inflammatory activity; in the brain, however, acetaminophen is oxidized by the p450 cytochrome system, and the oxidized form inhibits cyclooxygenase activity. Moreover, in the brain, the inhibition of another enzyme, COX-3, by acetaminophen may account for the antipyretic effect of this agent. However, COX-3 is not found outside the CNS.

Oral aspirin and acetaminophen are equally effective in reducing fever in humans. Nonsteroidal anti-inflammatory agents (NSAIDs) such as indomethacin and ibuprofen are also excellent antipyretics. Chronic high-dose therapy with antipyretics such as aspirin or the NSAIDs used in arthritis does not reduce normal core body temperature. Thus, PGE_2 appears to play no role in normal thermoregulation.

As effective antipyretics, glucocorticoids act at two levels. First, similar to the cyclooxygenase inhibitors, glucocorticoids reduce PGE_2 synthesis by inhibiting the activity of phospholipase A_2, which is needed to release arachidonic acid from the cell membrane. Second, glucocorticoids block the transcription of the mRNA for the pyrogenic cytokines.

Indications and Regimens for the Treatment of Fever   The objectives in treating fever are first to reduce the elevated hypothalamic set point and second to facilitate heat loss. There is no evidence that fever itself facilitates the recovery from infection or acts as an adjuvant to the immune system. In fact, peripheral PGE_2 production is a potent immunosuppressant. Hence, treating fever and its symptoms does no harm and does not slow the resolution of common viral and bacterial infections. Reducing fever with antipyretics also reduces systemic symptoms of headache, myalgias, and arthralgias.

Oral aspirin and NSAIDs effectively reduce fever but can adversely affect platelets and the gastrointestinal tract. Therefore, acetaminophen is preferred to all of these agents as an antipyretic. In children, acetaminophen must be used because aspirin increases the risk of Reye's syndrome. If the patient cannot take oral antipyretics, parenteral preparations of NSAIDs and rectal suppository preparations of various antipyretics can be used.

Treatment of fever in some groups of patients is recommended. Fever increases the demand for oxygen (i.e., for every increase of 1°C over 37°C, there is a 13% increase in oxygen consumption) and can aggravate preexisting cardiac, cerebrovascular, or pulmonary insufficiency. Elevated temperature can induce mental changes in patients with organic brain disease. Children with a history of febrile or nonfebrile seizure should be aggressively treated to reduce fever, although it is unclear what triggers the febrile seizure and there is no correlation between absolute temperature elevation and onset of a febrile seizure in susceptible children.

In hyperpyrexia, the use of cooling blankets facilitates the reduction of temperature; however, cooling blankets should not be used without oral antipyretics. In hyperpyretic patients with CNS disease or trauma, reducing core temperature mitigates the ill effects of high temperature on the brain.

Treating Hyperthermia   A high core temperature in a patient with an appropriate history (e.g., environmental heat exposure or treatment with anticholinergic or neuroleptic drugs, tricyclic antidepressants, succinylcholine, or halothane) along with appropriate clinical findings (dry skin, hallucinations, delirium, pupil dilation, muscle rigidity, and/or elevated levels of creatine phosphokinase) suggests hyperthermia.

The attempt to lower the already normal hypothalamic set point is of little use. Physical cooling with sponging, fans, cooling blankets, and even ice baths should be initiated immediately in conjunction with the administration of intravenous fluids and appropriate pharmacologic agents (see below). If insufficient cooling is achieved by external means, internal cooling can be achieved by gastric or peritoneal lavage with iced saline. In extreme circumstances, hemodialysis or even cardiopulmonary bypass with cooling of blood may be performed.

Malignant hyperthermia should be treated immediately with cessation of anesthesia and intravenous administration of dantrolene sodium. The recommended dose of dantrolene is 1 to 2.5 mg/kg of body weight given intravenously every 6 h for at least 24 to 48 h—until oral dantrolene can be administered, if needed. Procainamide should also be administered to patients with malignant hyperthermia because of the likelihood of ventricular fibrillation in this syndrome. Dantrolene at similar doses is indicated in NMS and in drug-induced hyperthermia and may even be useful in the hyperthermia of the serotonin syndrome and thyrotoxicosis. NMS may also be treated with bromocriptine, levodopa, amantadine, or nifedipine or by induction of muscle paralysis with curare and pancuronium. Tricyclic antidepressant overdose may be treated with physostigmine.

FURTHER READING

BOUCHAMA A, KNOCHEL JP: Heat stroke. N Engl J Med 346:1978, 2002

CHANDRASEKHARAN NV et al: COX-3, a cyclooxygenase-1 variant inhibited by acetaminophen and other analgesic/antipyretic drugs: Cloning, structure, and expression. Proc Natl Acad Sci USA 99:13926, 2002

DINARELLO CA: Proinflammatory cytokines. Chest 118:503, 2000

NETEA MG et al: Circulating cytokines as mediators of fever. Clin Infect Dis 31:178, 2000

USHIKUBI F et al: Impaired febrile response in mice lacking the prostaglandin E receptor subtype EP3. Nature 395:281, 1998

YANG RB et al: Toll-like receptor-2 mediates lipopolysaccharide-induced cellular signaling. Nature 395:284, 1998

17 FEVER AND RASH
Elaine T. Kaye, Kenneth M. Kaye

The acutely ill patient with fever and rash often presents a diagnostic challenge for physicians. The distinctive appearance of an eruption in concert with a clinical syndrome may facilitate a prompt diagnosis and the institution of life-saving therapy or critical infection-control interventions.

APPROACH TO THE PATIENT

A thorough history of patients with fever and rash includes the following relevant information: immune status, medications taken within the previous month, specific travel history, immunization status, exposure to domestic pets and other animals, history of animal or arthropod bites, existence of cardiac abnormalities, presence of prosthetic material, recent exposure to ill individuals, and exposure to sexually transmitted diseases. The history should also include the site of onset of the rash and its direction and rate of spread.

A thorough physical examination entails close attention to the rash, with an assessment and precise definition of its salient features. First, it is critical to determine the *type* of lesions that make up the eruption. *Macules* are flat lesions defined by an area of changed color (i.e., a blanchable erythema). *Papules* are raised, solid lesions <5 mm in diameter; *plaques* are lesions >5 mm in diameter with a flat, plateau-like surface; and *nodules* are lesions >5 mm in diameter with a more rounded configuration. *Wheals* (urticaria, hives) are papules or plaques that are pale pink and may appear annular (ringlike) as they enlarge; classic (nonvasculitic) wheals are transient, lasting only 24 to 48 h in any defined area.

Vesicles (<5 mm) and *bullae* (>5 mm) are circumscribed, elevated lesions containing fluid. *Pustules* are raised lesions containing purulent exudate; vesicular processes such as varicella or herpes simplex may evolve to pustules. *Nonpalpable purpura* is a flat lesion that is due to bleeding into the skin; if <3 mm in diameter, the purpuric lesions are termed *petechiae*; if >3 mm, they are termed *ecchymoses*. *Palpable purpura* is a raised lesion that is due to inflammation of the vessel wall (vasculitis) with subsequent hemorrhage. An *ulcer* is a defect in the skin extending at least into the upper layer of the dermis, and an *eschar* (tâche noire) is a necrotic lesion covered with a black crust.

Other pertinent features of rashes include their *configuration* (i.e., annular or target), the *arrangement* of their lesions, and their *distribution* (i.e., central or peripheral). →*For further discussion, see Chaps. 46 and 48.*

CLASSIFICATION OF RASH

This chapter reviews rashes that reflect systemic disease, but it does not include localized skin eruptions (i.e., cellulitis, impetigo) that may also be associated with fever (Chap. 110). Rashes are classified herein on the basis of the morphology and distribution of lesions. For practical purposes, this classification system is based on the most typical disease presentations. However, morphology may vary as rashes evolve, and the presentation of diseases with rashes is subject to many variations (Chap. 48). For instance, the classic petechial rash of Rocky Mountain spotted fever (RMSF; Chap. 158) may initially consist of blanchable erythematous macules distributed peripherally; at times, the rash associated with RMSF may not be predominantly acral, or a rash may not develop at all.

Diseases with fever and rash may be classified by type of eruption: centrally distributed maculopapular, peripheral, confluent desquamative erythematous, vesiculobullous, urticarial, nodular, purpuric, ulcerated, or eschars (Table 17-1). For a more detailed discussion of each disease associated with a rash, the reader is referred to the chapter dealing with that specific disease. (Reference chapters are cited in the text and listed in Table 17-1.)

CENTRALLY DISTRIBUTED MACULOPAPULAR ERUPTIONS Centrally distributed rashes, in which lesions are primarily truncal, are the most common type of eruption. The rash of *measles* (rubeola) starts at the hairline 2 to 3 days into the illness and moves down the body, sparing the palms and soles (Chap. 176). It begins as discrete erythematous lesions, which become confluent as the rash spreads. Koplik's spots (1- to 2-mm white or bluish lesions with an erythematous halo on the buccal mucosa) are pathognomonic for measles and are generally seen during the first 2 days of symptoms. They should not be confused with Fordyce's spots (ectopic sebaceous glands), which have no erythematous halos and are found in the mouth of healthy individuals. Koplik's spots may briefly overlap with the measles exanthem.

German measles (rubella) also spreads from the hairline downward; unlike that of measles, however, the rash of rubella tends to clear from originally affected areas as it migrates and may be pruritic (Chap. 177). Forchheimer spots (palatal petechiae) may develop but are nonspecific since they also develop in mononucleosis (Chap. 165) and scarlet fever (Chap. 121). Postauricular and suboccipital adenopathy and arthritis are common among adults with German measles. Exposure of pregnant women to ill individuals should be avoided, as rubella causes severe congenital abnormalities. Numerous strains of enteroviruses (Chap. 175), primarily echoviruses and coxsackieviruses, cause nonspecific syndromes of fever and eruptions that may mimic rubella or measles. Patients with infectious mononucleosis caused by Epstein-Barr virus (Chap. 165) or with primary infection caused by HIV (Chap. 173) may exhibit pharyngitis, lymphadenopathy, and a nonspecific maculopapular exanthem.

The rash of *erythema infectiosum* (fifth disease), which is caused by human parvovirus B19, primarily affects children 3 to 12 years old; it develops after fever has resolved as a bright blanchable erythema on the cheeks ("slapped cheeks") with perioral pallor (Chap. 168). A more diffuse rash (often pruritic) appears the next day on the trunk and extremities and then rapidly develops into a lacy reticular eruption that may wax and wane (especially with temperature change) over 3 weeks. Adults with fifth disease often have arthritis, and fetal hydrops can develop in association with this condition in pregnant women.

Exanthem subitum (roseola) is caused by human herpesvirus 6 and is most common among children <3 years of age (Chap. 166). As in erythema infectiosum, the rash usually appears after fever has subsided. It consists of 2- to 3-mm rose-pink macules and papules that rarely coalesce, occur initially on the trunk and sometimes on the extremities (sparing the face), and fade within 2 days.

Although drug reactions have many manifestations, including urticaria, exanthematous *drug-induced eruptions* (Chap. 50) are most common and are often difficult to distinguish from viral exanthems. Eruptions elicited by drugs are usually more intensely erythematous and pruritic than viral exanthems, but this distinction is not reliable. A history of new medications and an absence of prostration may help to distinguish a drug-related rash from an eruption of another etiology. Rashes may persist for up to 2 weeks after administration of the offending agent is discontinued. Certain populations are more prone than others to drug rashes. Of HIV-infected patients, 50 to 60% develop a rash in response to sulfa drugs; 50 to 100% of patients with mononucleosis due to Epstein-Barr virus develop a rash when given ampicillin.

Rickettsial illnesses (Chap. 158) should be considered in the evaluation of individuals with centrally distributed maculopapular eruptions. The usual setting for *epidemic typhus* is a site of war or natural disaster in which people are exposed to body lice. A diagnosis of recrudescent typhus should be considered in European immigrants to the United States. However, an indigenous form of typhus, presumably transmitted by flying squirrels, has been reported in the southeastern United States. *Endemic typhus* or *leptospirosis* (the latter caused by a spirochete; Chap. 155) may be seen in urban environments where rodents proliferate. Outside the United States, other rickettsial diseases cause a spotted-fever syndrome and should be considered in residents of or travelers to endemic areas. Similarly, *typhoid fever*, a nonrickettsial disease caused by *Salmonella typhi* (Chap. 137), is usually acquired during travel outside the United States. Dengue fever, caused by a mosquito-transmitted flavivirus, occurs in tropical and subtropical regions of the world (Chap. 180).

Some centrally distributed maculopapular eruptions have distinctive features. Erythema chronicum migrans (ECM), the rash of Lyme disease (Chap. 157), typically manifests as singular or multiple annular plaques. Untreated ECM lesions usually fade within a month but may persist for more than a year. *Erythema marginatum*, the rash of acute rheumatic fever (Chap. 302), has a distinctive pattern of enlarging and shifting transient annular lesions.

Collagen vascular diseases may cause fever and rash. Patients with *systemic lupus erythematosus* (Chap. 300) typically develop a sharply defined, erythematous eruption in a butterfly distribution on the cheeks (malar rash) as well as many other skin manifestations. *Still's disease* (Chap. 316) manifests as an evanescent salmon-colored rash on the trunk and proximal extremities that coincides with fever spikes.

PERIPHERAL ERUPTIONS These rashes are alike in that they are most prominent peripherally or begin in peripheral (acral) areas before spreading centripetally. Early diagnosis and therapy are critical in RMSF (Chap. 158) because of its grave prognosis if untreated. Lesions evolve from macular to petechial, start on the wrists and ankles, spread centripetally, and appear on the palms and soles only later in the disease. The rash of *secondary syphilis* (Chap. 153), which may be generalized but is prominent on the palms and soles, should be considered in the differential diagnosis of pityriasis rosea, especially in sexually active patients. *Atypical measles* (Chap. 176) is seen in individuals contracting measles who received the killed measles vaccine between 1963 and 1967 in the United States and who were not subsequently protected with the live vaccine. *Hand-foot-and-mouth disease* (Chap. 175), most commonly caused by coxsackievirus A16, is distinguished by tender vesicles distributed peripherally and in the mouth; outbreaks commonly occur within families. The classic target lesions of *erythema multiforme* appear symmetrically on the elbows, knees, palms, and soles. In relatively severe cases, these lesions may spread diffusely and involve mucosal surfaces (Stevens-Johnson syndrome). Lesions may develop on the hands and feet in *endocarditis* (Chap. 109).

CONFLUENT DESQUAMATIVE ERYTHEMAS These eruptions consist of diffuse erythema frequently followed by desquamation. The eruptions caused by group A *Streptococcus* or *Staphylococcus aureus* are toxin mediated. Certain disease features may provide diagnostic clues. *Scarlet fever* (Chap. 121) usually follows pharyngitis; patients have a facial flush, a "strawberry" tongue, and accentuated petechiae in body folds (Pastia's lines). *Kawasaki disease* (Chaps. 48 and 306) presents in the pediatric population as fissuring of the lips, a strawberry tongue, conjunctivitis, adenopathy, and sometimes cardiac abnormalities. *Streptococcal toxic shock syndrome* (Chap. 121) manifests with hypotension, multiorgan failure, and often a severe group A streptococcal infection (e.g., necrotizing fasciitis). *Staphylococcal toxic shock syndrome* (Chap. 120) also presents with hypotension and multiorgan failure, but usually only *S. aureus* colonization—not a severe *S. aureus* infection—is documented. *Staphylococcal scalded-skin syndrome* (Chap. 120) is seen primarily in children and in immunocompromised adults. Generalized erythema is often evident during the prodrome of fever and malaise; profound tenderness of the skin is distinctive. In the exfoliative stage, the skin can be induced to form bullae with light lateral pressure (Nikolsky's sign). In a mild form, a scarlatiniform eruption mimics scarlet fever, but the patient does not exhibit a straw-

TABLE 17-1 *Diseases Associated with Fever and Rash*

Disease	Etiology	Description	Group Affected/ Epidemiologic Factors	Clinical Syndrome	Chapter
CENTRALLY DISTRIBUTED MACULOPAPULAR ERUPTIONS					
Measles (rubeola, first disease)	Paramyxovirus	Discrete lesions that become confluent as rash spreads from hairline downward, sparing palms and soles; lasts ≥3 days; Koplik's spots	Nonimmune individuals	Cough, conjunctivitis, coryza, severe prostration	176
German measles (rubella, third disease)	Togavirus	Spreads from hairline downward, clearing as it spreads; Forchheimer spots	Nonimmune individuals	Adenopathy, arthritis	177
Erythema infectiosum (fifth disease)	Human parvovirus B19	Bright-red "slapped-cheek" appearance followed by lacy reticular rash that waxes and wanes over 3 weeks	Most common in children aged 3–12 years; occurs in winter and spring	Mild fever; arthritis in adults; rash follows resolution of fever	168
Exanthem subitum (roseola, sixth disease)	Human herpesvirus 6	Diffuse maculopapular eruption (sparing face); resolves within 2 days	Usually affects children <3 years old	Rash following resolution of fever; similar to Boston exanthem (echovirus 16)	166
Primary HIV infection	HIV	Nonspecific diffuse macules and papules; may be urticarial; oral or genital ulcers in some cases	Individuals recently infected with HIV	Pharyngitis, adenopathy, arthralgias	173
Infectious mononucleosis	Epstein-Barr virus	Diffuse maculopapular eruption (10–15% of cases; 90% if ampicillin is given); urticaria in some cases; periorbital edema (50%); palatal petechiae (25%)	Adolescents, young adults	Hepatosplenomegaly, pharyngitis, cervical lymphadenopathy, atypical lymphocytosis, heterophile antibody	165
Other viral exanthems	Echoviruses 2, 4, 9, 11, 16, 19, and 25; coxsackieviruses A9, B1, and B5; etc.	Skin findings mimicking rubella or measles	Affect children more commonly than adults	Nonspecific viral syndromes	175
Exanthematous drug-induced eruption	Drugs (antibiotics, anticonvulsants, diuretics, etc.)	Intensely pruritic, bright-red macules and papules, symmetric on trunk and extremities; may become confluent	Occurs 2–3 d after exposure in previously sensitized individuals; otherwise, after 2–3 weeks (but can occur anytime, even shortly after drug is discontinued)	Variable findings: fever and eosinophilia	50
Epidemic typhus	*Rickettsia prowazekii*	Maculopapular eruption appearing in axillae, spreading to trunk and later to extremities; usually spares face, palms, soles; evolves from blanchable macules to confluent eruption with petechiae; rash evanescent in recrudescent typhus (Brill-Zinsser disease)	Exposure to body lice; occurrence of recrudescent typhus as relapse after 30–50 years	Headache, myalgias; 10–40% mortality if untreated; milder clinical presentation in recrudescent form	158
Endemic (murine) typhus	*Rickettsia typhi*	Maculopapular eruption, usually sparing palms, soles	Exposure to rat or cat fleas	Headache, myalgias	158
Scrub typhus	*Orientia tsutsugamushi*	Diffuse macular rash starting on trunk; eschar at site of mite bite	Endemic in South Pacific, Australia, Asia; transmitted by mites	Headache, myalgias, regional adenopathy; mortality up to 30% if untreated	158
Rickettsial spotted fevers	*Rickettsia conorii* (boutonneuse fever), *Rickettsia australis* (North Queensland tick typhus), *Rickettsia sibirica* (Siberian tick typhus), and others	Eschar common at bite site; maculopapular (rarely, vesicular and petechial) eruption on proximal extremities, spreading to trunk and face	Exposure to ticks; *R. conorii* in Mediterranean region, India, Africa; *R. australis* in Australia; *R. sibirica* in Siberia, Mongolia	Headache, myalgias, regional adenopathy	158
Human monocytotropic ehrlichiosis[a]	*Ehrlichia chaffeensis*	Maculopapular eruption (40% of cases), involves trunk and extremities; may be petechial	Tick-borne; most common in U.S. Southeast, southern Midwest, and mid-Atlantic regions	Headache, myalgias, leukopenia	158
Leptospirosis	*Leptospira interrogans*	Maculopapular eruption; conjunctivitis; scleral hemorrhage in some cases	Exposure to water contaminated with animal urine	Myalgias; aseptic meningitis; *fulminant form*: icterohemorrhagic fever (Weil's disease)	155

(continued)

TABLE 17-1—(Continued)

Disease	Etiology	Description	Group Affected/ Epidemiologic Factors	Clinical Syndrome	Chapter
Lyme disease	*Borrelia burgdorferi*	Papule expanding to erythematous annular lesion with central clearing (erythema chronicum migrans or ECM; average diameter, 15 cm), sometimes with concentric rings, sometimes with indurated or vesicular center; multiple secondary ECM lesions in some cases	Bite of tick vector	Headache, myalgias, chills, photophobia occurring acutely; CNS disease, myocardial disease, arthritis weeks to months later in some cases	157
Typhoid fever	*Salmonella typhi*	Transient, blanchable erythematous macules and papules, 2–4 mm, usually on trunk (rose spots)	Ingestion of contaminated food or water (rare in U.S.)	Variable abdominal pain and diarrhea; headache, myalgias, hepatosplenomegaly	137
Dengue fever[b]	Dengue virus (4 serotypes; flaviviruses)	Rash in 50% of cases, initially diffuse flushing; midway through illness, onset of maculopapular rash, which begins on trunk and spreads centrifugally to extremities and face; pruritus, hyperesthesia in some cases; after defervescence, petechiae on extremities in some cases	Occurs in tropics and subtropics; transmitted by mosquito	Headache, musculoskeletal pain ("breakbone fever"); leukopenia; occasionally biphasic ("saddleback") fever	180
Rat-bite fever (sodoku)	*Spirillum minus*	Eschar at bite site; then blotchy violaceous or red-brown rash involving trunk and extremities	Rat bite; primarily found in Asia; rare in U.S.	Regional adenopathy, recurrent fevers if untreated	. . .
Relapsing fever	*Borrelia* species	Central rash at end of febrile episode; petechiae in some cases	Exposure to ticks or body lice	Recurrent fever, headache, myalgias, hepatosplenomegaly	156
Erythema marginatum (rheumatic fever)	Group A *Streptococcus*	Erythematous annular papules and plaques occurring as polycyclic lesions in waves over trunk, proximal extremities; evolving and resolving within hours	Patients with rheumatic fever	Pharyngitis preceding polyarthritis, carditis, subcutaneous nodules, chorea	302
Systemic lupus erythematosus	Autoimmune disease	Macular and papular erythema, often in sun-exposed areas; discoid lupus lesions (local atrophy, scale, pigmentary changes); periungual telangiectasis; malar rash; vasculitis sometimes causing urticaria, palpable purpura; oral erosions in some cases	Most common in young to middle-aged women; flares precipitated by sun exposure	Arthritis; cardiac, pulmonary, renal, hematologic, and vasculitic disease	300
Still's disease	Autoimmune disease	Transient 2- to 5-mm erythematous papules appearing at height of fever on trunk, proximal extremities; lesions evanescent	Children and young adults	High spiking fever, polyarthritis, splenomegaly; erythrocyte sedimentation rate, >100 mm/h	316
Arcanobacterial pharyngitis	*Arcanobacterium (Corynebacterium) haemolyticum*	Diffuse, erythematous, maculopapular eruption involving trunk and proximal extremities; may desquamate	Children and young adults	Exudative pharyngitis, lymphadenopathy	122

PERIPHERAL ERUPTIONS

Disease	Etiology	Description	Group Affected/ Epidemiologic Factors	Clinical Syndrome	Chapter
Chronic meningococcemia, disseminated gonococcal infection[c]	—	—	—	—	127, 128
Rocky Mountain spotted fever	*Rickettsia rickettsii*	Rash beginning on wrists and ankles and spreading centripetally; appears on palms and soles later in disease; lesion evolution from blanchable macules to petechiae	Tick vector; widespread but more common in southeastern and southwest-central U.S.	Headache, myalgias, abdominal pain; mortality up to 40% if untreated	158
Secondary syphilis	*Treponema pallidum*	Coincident primary chancre in 10% of cases; copper-colored, scaly papular eruption, diffuse but prominent on palms and soles; rash never vesicular in adults; condyloma latum, mucous patches, and alopecia in some cases	Sexually transmitted	Fever, constitutional symptoms	153

(continued)

TABLE 17-1   Diseases Associated with Fever and Rash—(continued)

Disease	Etiology	Description	Group Affected/ Epidemiologic Factors	Clinical Syndrome	Chapter
Atypical measles	Paramyxovirus	Maculopapular eruption beginning on distal extremities and spreading centripetally; may evolve into vesicles or petechiae; edema of extremities; Koplik's spots absent	Individuals contracting measles who received killed measles vaccine in 1963–1967 in U.S. without subsequent live vaccine	Headache, nodular pneumonia	176
Hand-foot-and-mouth disease	Coxsackievirus A16 most common cause	Tender vesicles, erosions in mouth; 0.25-cm papules on hands and feet with rim of erythema evolving into tender vesicles	Summer and fall; primarily children <10 years old; multiple family members	Transient fever	175
Erythema multiforme	Drugs, infection, idiopathic causes	Target lesions (central erythema surrounded by area of clearing and another rim of erythema) up to 2 cm; symmetric on knees, elbows, palms, soles; may become diffuse; may involve mucosal surfaces (Stevens-Johnson syndrome if 2 or more mucosal sites involved)	Drug intake (i.e., sulfa, phenytoin, penicillin); herpes simplex virus or *Mycoplasma pneumoniae* infection	Varies with predisposing factor	—[d]
Rat-bite fever (Haverhill fever)	*Streptobacillus moniliformis*	Maculopapular eruption over palms, soles, and extremities, tends to be more severe at joints; eruption sometimes becoming generalized; may be purpuric; may desquamate	Rat bite, ingestion of contaminated food	Myalgias; arthritis (50%); fever recurrence in some cases	. . .
Bacterial endocarditis	*Streptococcus*, *Staphylococcus*, etc.	*Subacute course*: Osler's nodes (tender pink nodules on finger or toe pads); petechiae on skin and mucosa; splinter hemorrhages. *Acute course* (*S. aureus*): Janeway lesions (painless erythematous or hemorrhagic macules, usually on palms and soles)	Abnormal heart valve, intravenous drug use	New heart murmur	109

CONFLUENT DESQUAMATIVE ERYTHEMAS

Disease	Etiology	Description	Group Affected/ Epidemiologic Factors	Clinical Syndrome	Chapter
Scarlet fever (second disease)	Group A *Streptococcus* (pyrogenic exotoxins A, B, C)	Diffuse blanchable erythema beginning on face and spreading to trunk and extremities; circumoral pallor; "sandpaper" texture to skin; accentuation of linear erythema in skin folds (Pastia's lines); enanthem of white evolving into red "strawberry" tongue; desquamation in second week	Most common in children aged 2–10 years; usually follows group A streptococcal pharyngitis	Fever, pharyngitis, headache	121
Kawasaki disease	Idiopathic causes	Rash similar to scarlet fever (scarlatiniform) or erythema multiforme; fissuring of lips, strawberry tongue; conjunctivitis; edema of hands, feet; desquamation later in disease	Children <8 years	Cervical adenopathy, pharyngitis, coronary artery vasculitis	48, 306
Streptococcal toxic shock syndrome	Group A *Streptococcus* (associated with pyrogenic exotoxin A and/or B or certain M types)	When present, rash often scarlatiniform	May occur in setting of severe group A streptococcal infections, such as necrotizing fasciitis, bacteremia, pneumonia	Multiorgan failure, hypotension; 30% mortality rate	121
Staphylococcal toxic shock syndrome	*S. aureus* (toxic shock syndrome toxin 1, enterotoxin B or C)	Diffuse erythema involving palms; pronounced erythema of mucosal surfaces, conjunctivitis; desquamation 7–10 days into illness	Colonization with toxin-producing *S. aureus*	Fever >39°C (102°F), hypotension, multiorgan dysfunction	120
Staphylococcal scalded-skin syndrome	*S. aureus*, phage group II	Diffuse tender erythema, often with bullae and desquamation; Nikolsky's sign	Colonization with toxin-producing *S. aureus*; occurs in children <10 years old (termed "Ritter's disease" in neonates) or adults with renal dysfunction	Irritability; nasal or conjunctival secretions	120

(continued)

TABLE 17-1—(Continued)

Disease	Etiology	Description	Group Affected/ Epidemiologic Factors	Clinical Syndrome	Chapter
Exfoliative erythroderma syndrome	Underlying psoriasis, eczema, drug eruption, mycosis fungoides	Diffuse erythema (often scaling) interspersed with lesions of underlying condition	Usually occurs in adults over age 50; more common in men	Fever, chills (i.e., difficulty with thermoregulation); lymphadenopathy	47, 50
Toxic epidermal necrolysis	Drugs, other causes (infection, neoplasm, graft-vs.-host disease)	Diffuse erythema or target-like lesions progressing to bullae, with sloughing and necrosis of entire epidermis; Nikolsky's sign	Uncommon in children; more common in patients with HIV infection or graft-vs.-host disease	Dehydration, sepsis sometimes resulting from lack of normal skin integrity; 25% mortality	50

VESICULOBULLOUS ERUPTIONS

Disease	Etiology	Description	Group Affected/ Epidemiologic Factors	Clinical Syndrome	Chapter
Hand-foot-and-mouth syndrome[e]; staphylococcal scalded-skin syndrome, toxic epidermal necrolysis[f]	—	—	—	—	—[d]
Varicella (chickenpox)	Varicella-zoster virus	Macules (2–3 mm) evolving into papules, then vesicles (sometimes umbilicated), on an erythematous base ("dewdrops on a rose petal"); pustules then forming and crusting; lesions appearing in crops; may involve scalp, mouth; intensely pruritic	Usually affects children; 10% of adults susceptible; most common in late winter and spring	Malaise; mild disease in healthy children; more severe disease with complications in adults and immunocompromised children	164
Variola (smallpox)	Variola major virus	Red macules on tongue, palate evolving to papules and vesicles; skin macules evolving to papules, then vesicles, then pustules over 1 week, with subsequent lesion crusting; lesions initially appearing on face and spreading centrifugally from trunk to extremities; differs from varicella in that (1) skin lesions in any given area are at same stage of development and (2) there is a prominent distribution of lesions on face and extremities (including palms, soles) as opposed to prominent rash on trunk	Nonimmune individuals exposed to smallpox	Prodrome of fever, headache, backache, myalgias; vomiting in 50% of cases	205
Disseminated herpesvirus infection	Varicella-zoster virus or herpes simplex virus (HSV)	Individual lesions similar for varicella-zoster and HSV; *zoster cutaneous dissemination*: >25 lesions extending outside involved dermatome; *HSV*: extensive, progressive mucocutaneous lesions in some cases; HSV lesions sometimes disseminate in eczematous skin (eczema herpeticum); HSV visceral dissemination may occur with only limited skin lesions	Immunosuppressed individuals, eczema	Visceral organ involvement (especially liver) in some cases	163, 164, 360
Rickettsialpox	*Rickettsia akari*	Eschar found at site of mite bite; generalized rash involving face, trunk, extremities; may involve palms and soles; <100 papules and plaques (2–10 mm); tops of lesions develop vesicles that may evolve into pustules	Seen in urban settings; transmitted by mouse mites	Headache, myalgias, regional adenopathy; mild disease	158
Disseminated *Vibrio vulnificus* infection	*V. vulnificus*	Erythematous lesions evolving into hemorrhagic bullae and then into necrotic ulcers	Patients with cirrhosis, diabetes, renal failure; exposure by ingestion of contaminated saltwater seafood	Hypotension; 50% mortality	140
Ecthyma gangrenosum	*Pseudomonas aeruginosa*, other gram-negative rods, fungi	Indurated plaque evolving into hemorrhagic bulla or pustule that sloughs, resulting in eschar formation; erythematous halo; most common in axillary, groin, perianal regions	Usually affects neutropenic patients; occurs in up to 28% of individuals with *Pseudomonas* bacteremia	Clinical signs of sepsis	136

(continued)

TABLE 17-1   Diseases Associated with Fever and Rash—(continued)

Disease	Etiology	Description	Group Affected/ Epidemiologic Factors	Clinical Syndrome	Chapter
URTICARIAL ERUPTIONS					
Urticarial vasculitis	Serum sickness, often due to infection (including hepatitis B viral, enteroviral, parasitic), drugs (including penicillins, sulfonamides, salicylates, barbiturates); connective tissue disease; idiopathic causes	Erythematous, circumscribed areas of edema; occasionally indurated; pruritic or burning; lesions sometimes purpuric; individual lesions lasting up to 5 days	In serum sickness, occurs 8–14 days after antigen exposure in nonsensitized individuals; may occur within 36 h in sensitized individuals	Malaise, lymphadenopathy, myalgias, arthralgias	306[d]
NODULAR ERUPTIONS					
Disseminated infection	Fungi (e.g., candidiasis, histoplasmosis, cryptococcosis, sporotrichosis, coccidioidomycosis); mycobacteria	Subcutaneous nodules (up to 3 cm); fluctuance, draining common with mycobacteria; necrotic nodules (extremities, periorbital or nasal regions) common with *Aspergillus*, *Mucor*	Immunocompromised hosts (i.e., bone marrow transplant recipients, patients undergoing chemotherapy, HIV-infected patients, alcoholics)	Features vary with organism	—[d]
Erythema nodosum (septal panniculitis)	Infections (e.g., streptococcal, fungal, mycobacterial, yersinial); drugs (e.g., sulfas, penicillins, oral contraceptives); sarcoidosis; idiopathic causes	Large, violaceous, nonulcerative, subcutaneous nodules; exquisitely tender; usually on lower legs but also on upper extremities	More common in females 15–30 years old	Arthralgias (50%); features vary with associated condition	—[d]
Sweet's syndrome (acute febrile neutrophilic dermatosis)	Yersinial infection; lymphoproliferative disorders; idiopathic causes	Tender red or blue edematous nodules giving impression of vesiculation; usually on face, neck, upper extremities; when on lower extremities, may mimic erythema nodosum	More common in women and in persons 30–60 years old; 20% of cases associated with malignancy (men and women equally affected in this group)	Headache, arthralgias, leukocytosis	48
Bacillary angiomatosis	*Bartonella henselae* or *Bartonella quintana*	Many forms, including erythematous, smooth vascular nodules; friable, exophytic lesions; erythematous plaques (may be dry, scaly); subcutaneous nodules (may be erythematous)	Usually in HIV infection	Peliosis of liver and spleen in some cases; lesions may involve multiple organs; bacteremia	144
PURPURIC ERUPTIONS					
Rocky Mountain spotted fever, rat-bite fever, endocarditis[e]; epidemic typhus[g]; dengue fever	—	—	—	—	—[d]
Acute meningococcemia	*Neisseria meningitidis*	Petechiae rapidly becoming numerous, sometimes enlarging and becoming vesicular; trunk, extremities most commonly involved; may appear on face, hands, feet; may include purpura fulminans reflecting disseminated intravascular coagulation (see below)	Most common in children, individuals with asplenia or terminal complement component deficiency (C5-C8)	Hypotension, meningitis (sometimes preceded by upper respiratory infection)	127

(continued)

TABLE 17-1—(Continued)

Disease	Etiology	Description	Group Affected/ Epidemiologic Factors	Clinical Syndrome	Chapter
Purpura fulminans	Severe disseminated intravascular coagulation	Large ecchymoses with sharply irregular shapes evolving into hemorrhagic bullae and then into black necrotic lesions	Individuals with sepsis (e.g., involving *N. meningitidis*), malignancy, or massive trauma; asplenic patients at high risk for sepsis	Hypotension	127, 254
Chronic meningococcemia	*N. meningitidis*	Variety of recurrent eruptions, including pink maculopapular; nodular (usually on lower extremities); petechial (sometimes developing vesicular centers); purpuric areas with pale blue-gray centers	Individuals with complement deficiencies	Fevers, sometimes intermittent; arthritis, myalgias, headache	127
Disseminated gonococcal infection	*Neisseria gonorrhoeae*	Papules (1–5 mm) evolving over 1–2 days into hemorrhagic pustules with gray necrotic centers; hemorrhagic bullae occurring rarely; lesions (usually fewer than 40) distributed peripherally near joints (more commonly on upper extremities)	Sexually active individuals (more often females), some with complement deficiency	Low-grade fever, tenosynovitis, arthritis	128
Enteroviral petechial rash	Usually echovirus 9 or coxsackievirus A9	Disseminated petechial lesions (may also be maculopapular, vesicular, or urticarial)	Often occurs in outbreaks	Pharyngitis, headache; aseptic meningitis with echovirus 9	175
Viral hemorrhagic fever	Arboviruses and arenaviruses	Petechial rash	Residence in or travel to endemic areas or other virus exposure	Triad of fever, shock, hemorrhage from mucosa or gastrointestinal tract	180, 181
Thrombotic thrombocytopenic purpura/hemolytic-uremic syndrome	Idiopathic, *Escherichia coli* O157:H7 (Shiga toxin), drugs	Petechiae	Individuals with *E. coli* O157:H7 gastroenteritis (especially children), cancer chemotherapy, HIV infection, autoimmune diseases; pregnant/ postpartum women	Fever (not always present), hemolytic anemia, thrombocytopenia, renal dysfunction, neurologic dysfunction; coagulation studies normal	48, 93, 101, 134, 138
Cutaneous small-vessel vasculitis (leukocytoclastic vasculitis)	Infections (including group A *Streptococcus*, viral hepatitis), drugs, chemicals, food allergens, idiopathic causes	Palpable purpuric lesions appearing in crops on legs or other dependent areas; may become vesicular or ulcerative; usually resolve over 3–4 weeks	Occurs in a wide spectrum of diseases, including connective tissue disease, cryoglobulinemia, malignancy, Henoch-Schönlein purpura (HSP); more common in children	Fever, malaise, arthralgias, myalgias; systemic vasculitis in some cases; renal, joint, and gastrointestinal involvement commonly seen in HSP	48

ERUPTIONS WITH ULCERS AND/OR ESCHARS

Disease	Etiology	Description	Group Affected/ Epidemiologic Factors	Clinical Syndrome	Chapter
Scrub typhus, rickettsial spotted fevers, rat-bite fever[g]; rickettsialpox, ecthyma gangrenosum[h]	—	—	—	—	—[d]
Tularemia	*Francisella tularensis*	Ulceroglandular form: erythematous, tender papule evolves into necrotic, tender ulcer with raised borders; in 35% of cases, eruptions (maculopapular, vesiculopapular, acneiform, urticarial, erythema nodosum, or erythema multiforme) may occur	Exposure to ticks, biting flies, infected animals	Fever, headache, lymphadenopathy	142
Anthrax	*Bacillus anthracis*	Pruritic papule enlarging and evolving into a 1- by 3-cm painless ulcer surrounded by vesicles and then developing a central eschar with edema; residual scar	Exposure to infected animals or animal products or other exposure to anthrax spores	Lymphadenopathy, headache	205

[a] In human granulocytotropic ehrlichiosis, or anaplasmosis (caused by *Anaplasma phagocytophila*; most common in the upper midwestern and northeastern regions of the United States), rash is rare.

[b] See "Viral hemorrhagic fever" under "Purpuric eruptions" for dengue hemorrhagic fever/ dengue shock syndrome.

[c] See "Purpuric eruptions."

[d] See etiology-specific chapters.

[e] See "Peripheral eruptions."

[f] See "Confluent desquamative erythemas."

[g] See "Centrally distributed maculopapular eruptions."

[h] See "Vesiculobullous eruptions."

berry tongue or circumoral pallor. In contrast to the staphylococcal scalded-skin syndrome, in which the cleavage plane is superficial in the epidermis, *toxic epidermal necrolysis* (Chap. 50) involves sloughing of the entire epidermis, resulting in severe disease. *Exfoliative erythroderma syndrome* (Chaps. 47 and 50) is a serious reaction associated with systemic toxicity that is often due to eczema, psoriasis, mycosis fungoides, or a severe drug reaction.

VESICULOBULLOUS ERUPTIONS *Varicella* (Chap. 164) is highly contagious, often occurring in winter or spring. At a given time within a given region of the body, varicella lesions are in different stages of development. In immunocompromised hosts, varicella vesicles may lack the characteristic erythematous base or may appear hemorrhagic. Lesions of *variola* (smallpox; Chap. 205) appear similar to those of varicella but are all at the same stage of development in a given region of the body. Variola lesions are most prominent on the face and extremities, while varicella lesions are most prominent on the trunk. *Rickettsialpox* (Chap. 158) is often documented in urban settings and is characterized by vesicles. It can be distinguished from varicella by an eschar at the site of the mouse-mite bite and the papule/plaque base of each vesicle. Disseminated *Vibrio vulnificus* infection (Chap. 140) or *ecthyma gangrenosum* due to *Pseudomonas aeruginosa* (Chap. 136) should be considered in immunosuppressed individuals with sepsis and hemorrhagic bullae.

URTICARIAL ERUPTIONS Individuals with classic urticaria ("hives") usually have a hypersensitivity reaction without associated fever. In the presence of fever, urticarial eruptions are usually due to *urticarial vasculitis* (Chap. 306). Unlike individual lesions of classic urticaria, which last up to 48 h, these lesions may last up to 5 days. Etiologies include serum sickness (often induced by drugs such as penicillins, sulfas, salicylates, or barbiturates), connective-tissue disease (e.g., systemic lupus erythematosus or Sjögren's syndrome), and infection (e.g., with hepatitis B virus, enteroviruses, or parasites). Malignancy may be associated with fever and chronic urticaria (Chap. 48).

NODULAR ERUPTIONS In immunocompromised hosts, nodular lesions often represent disseminated infection. Patients with disseminated *candidiasis* (often due to *Candida tropicalis*) may have a triad of fever, myalgias, and eruptive nodules (Chap. 187). Disseminated *cryptococcosis* lesions (Chap. 186) may resemble molluscum contagiosum. Necrosis of nodules should raise the suspicion of *aspergillosis* (Chap. 188) or *mucormycosis* (Chap. 189). *Erythema nodosum* presents with exquisitely tender nodules on the lower extremities. *Sweet's syndrome* (Chap. 48) should be considered in individuals with multiple nodules and plaques, often so edematous that they give the appearance of vesicles or bullae. Sweet's syndrome may affect either healthy individuals or persons with lymphoproliferative disease.

PURPURIC ERUPTIONS *Acute meningococcemia* (Chap. 127) classically presents in children as a petechial eruption, but initial lesions may appear as blanchable macules or urticaria. RMSF should be considered in the differential diagnosis of acute meningococcemia. *Echovirus 9 infection* (Chap. 175) may mimic acute meningococcemia; patients should be treated as if they have bacterial sepsis since prompt differentiation of these conditions may be impossible. Large ecchymotic areas of *purpura fulminans* (Chaps. 127 and 254) reflect severe underlying disseminated intravascular coagulation, which may be due to infectious or noninfectious causes. The lesions of *chronic meningococcemia* (Chap. 127) may have a variety of morphologies, including petechial. Purpuric nodules may develop on the legs and resemble erythema nodosum but lack its exquisite tenderness. Lesions of *disseminated gonococcemia* (Chap. 128) are distinctive, sparse, countable hemorrhagic pustules, usually located near joints. The lesions of chronic meningococcemia and those of gonococcemia may be indistinguishable in terms of appearance and distribution. *Viral hemorrhagic fever* (Chaps. 180 and 181) should be considered in patients with an appropriate travel history and a petechial rash. *Thrombotic thrombocytopenic purpura* (Chaps. 48, 93, and 101) and *hemolytic-uremic syndrome* (Chaps. 101, 134, and 138) are closely related and are noninfectious causes of fever and petechiae. *Cutaneous small-vessel vasculitis* (*leukocytoclastic vasculitis*) typically manifests as palpable purpura and has a wide variety of causes (Chap. 48).

ERUPTIONS WITH ULCERS OR ESCHARS The presence of an ulcer or eschar in the setting of a more widespread eruption can provide an important diagnostic clue. For example, the presence of an eschar may suggest the diagnosis of scrub typhus or rickettsialpox (Chap. 158) in the appropriate setting. In other illnesses (e.g., anthrax; Chap. 205), an ulcer or eschar may be the only skin manifestation.

FURTHER READING

CHERRY JD: Contemporary infectious exanthems. Clin Infect Dis 16:199, 1993
————: Cutaneous manifestations of systemic infections, in *Textbook of Pediatric Infectious Diseases*, vol. 1, 3d ed, RD Feigin and JD Cherry (eds). Philadelphia, Saunders, 1992, pp 755–782
EICHENFIELD LF et al (eds): *Textbook of Neonatal Dermatology*, Philadelphia, Saunders, 2001
FREEDBERG IM et al (eds): *Fitzpatrick's Dermatology in General Medicine*, 6th ed. New York, McGraw-Hill, 2003
LEVIN S, GOODMAN LJ: An approach to acute fever and rash (AFR) in the adult. Curr Clin Top Infect Dis 15:19, 1995
SCHLOSSBERG D: Fever and rash. Infect Dis Clin North Am 10:101, 1996
WEBER DJ et al: The acutely ill patient with fever and rash, in *Principles and Practice of Infectious Diseases*, vol 1, 5th ed, GL Mandell et al (eds). Philadelphia, Churchill Livingstone, 2000, pp 633–50

18 FEVER OF UNKNOWN ORIGIN
Jeffrey A. Gelfand, Michael V. Callahan

DEFINITION AND CLASSIFICATION *Fever of unknown origin* (FUO) was defined by Petersdorf and Beeson in 1961 as (1) temperatures of >38.3°C (>101°F) on several occasions; (2) a duration of fever of >3 weeks; and (3) failure to reach a diagnosis despite 1 week of inpatient investigation. While this classification has stood for more than 30 years, Durack and Street have proposed a new system for classification of FUO: (1) classic FUO; (2) nosocomial FUO; (3) neutropenic FUO; and (4) FUO associated with HIV infection (Table 18-1).

Classic FUO corresponds closely to the earlier definition of FUO, differing only with regard to the prior requirement for 1 week's study in the hospital. The new definition is broader, stipulating three outpatient visits or 3 days in the hospital without elucidation of a cause or 1 week of "intelligent and invasive" ambulatory investigation. In *nosocomial FUO*, a temperature of ≥38.3°C (≥101°F) develops on several occasions in a hospitalized patient who is receiving acute care and in whom infection was not manifest or incubating on admission. Three days of investigation, including at least 2 days' incubation of cultures, is the minimum requirement for this diagnosis. *Neutropenic FUO* is defined as a temperature of ≥38.3°C (≥101°F) on several occasions in a patient whose neutrophil count is <500/μL or is expected to fall to that level in 1 to 2 days. The diagnosis of neutropenic FUO is invoked if a specific cause is not identified after 3 days of investigation, including at least 2 days' incubation of cultures. *HIV-associated FUO* is defined by a temperature of ≥38.3°C (≥101°F) on several occasions over a period of >4 weeks for outpatients or >3 days for hospitalized patients with HIV infection. This diagnosis is invoked if appropriate investigation over 3 days, including 2 days' incubation of cultures, reveals no source.

Adoption of these categories of FUO on a wide scale in the literature would allow a more rational compilation of data regarding these

TABLE 18-1 Categories of FUO[a]

Feature	Category of FUO			
	Nosocomial	Neutropenic	HIV-Associated	Classic
Patient's situation	Hospitalized, acute care, no infection when admitted	Neutrophil count either <500/μL or expected to reach that level in 1–2 days	Confirmed HIV-positive	All others with fevers for ≥3 weeks
Duration of illness while under investigation	3 days[b]	3 days[b]	3 days[b] (or 4 weeks as outpatient)	3 days[b] or three outpatient visits
Examples of cause	Septic thrombophlebitis, sinusitis, *Clostridium difficile* colitis, drug fever	Perianal infection, aspergillosis, candidemia	MAI[c] infection, tuberculosis, non-Hodgkin's lymphoma, drug fever	Infections, malignancy, inflammatory diseases, drug fever

[a] All require temperatures of ≥38.3°C (≥101°F) on several occasions.
[b] Includes at least 2 days' incubation of microbiology cultures.
[c] *M. avium/M. intracellulare.*

Source: Modified from DT Durack, AC Street, in JS Remington, MN Swartz (eds): *Current Clinical Topics in Infectious Diseases.* Cambridge, MA, Blackwell, 1991.

disparate groups. In the remainder of this chapter, the discussion will focus on classic FUO unless otherwise specified.

CAUSES OF CLASSIC FUO Table 18-2 summarizes the findings of several large studies of FUO carried out since the advent of the antibiotic era, including a prospective study of 167 adult patients with FUO encompassing all 8 university hospitals in the Netherlands and using a standardized protocol in which the first author reviewed every patient. Coincident with the widespread use of antibiotics, increasingly useful diagnostic technologies—both noninvasive and invasive—have been developed. Newer studies reflect not only changing patterns of disease but also the impact of diagnostic techniques that make it possible to eliminate many patients with specific illness from the FUO category. The ubiquitous use of potent broad-spectrum antibiotics may have decreased the number of infections causing FUO. The wide availability of ultrasonography, computed tomography (CT), magnetic resonance imaging (MRI), radionuclide scanning, and positron emission tomography (PET) scanning has enhanced the detection of occult neoplasms and lymphomas in patients previously thought to have FUO. Likewise, the widespread availability of highly specific and sensitive immunologic testing has reduced the number of undetected cases of systemic lupus erythematosus and other autoimmune diseases.

Infections, especially extrapulmonary tuberculosis, remain the leading diagnosable cause of FUO. Prolonged mononucleosis syndromes caused by Epstein-Barr virus, cytomegalovirus (CMV), or HIV are conditions whose consideration as a cause of FUO is sometimes confounded by delayed antibody responses. Intraabdominal abscesses (sometimes poorly localized) and renal, retroperitoneal, and paraspinal abscesses continue to be difficult to diagnose. Renal malacoplakia, with submucosal plaques or nodules involving the urinary tract, may cause FUO and is often fatal if untreated. It is associated with coliform infection, is seen most often in patients with defects of intracellular bacterial killing, and is treated with fluoroquinolones or trimethoprim-sulfamethoxazole. Occasionally, other organs may be involved. Osteomyelitis, especially where prosthetic devices have been implanted, and infective endocarditis must be considered. Although true culture-negative infective endocarditis is rare, one may be misled by slow-growing organisms of the HACEK group (*Haemophilus aphrophilus*, *Actinobacillus actinomycetemcomitans*, *Cardiobacterium hominis*, Ei-

kenella corrodens, and *Kingella kingae*; Chap. 131), *Bartonella* spp. (previously *Rochalimaea*), *Legionella* spp., *Coxiella burnetii*, *Chlamydia psittaci*, and fungi. Prostatitis, dental abscesses, sinusitis, and cholangitis continue to be sources of occult fever.

Fungal disease, most notably histoplasmosis involving the reticuloendothelial system, may cause FUO. FUO with headache should prompt examination of spinal fluid for *Cryptococcus neoformans*. Malaria (which may result from transfusion, the failure to take a prescribed prophylactic agent, or infection with a drug-resistant strain) continues to be a cause, particularly of asynchronous FUO. A related protozoan species, *Babesia*, may cause FUO and is increasing in geographic distribution and in incidence, especially among the elderly and immunosuppressed.

In most earlier series, neoplasms were the next most common cause of FUO after infections (Table 18-2). In the two most recent series, a decrease in the percentage of FUO cases due to malignancy was attributed to improvement in diagnostic technologies—in particular, high-resolution tomography and tumor antigen assays. This observation does not diminish the importance of considering neoplasia in the initial diagnostic evaluation of a patient with fever. A number of patients in these series had temporal arteritis, adult Still's disease, drug-related fever, and factitious fever. In recent series, ~25 to 30% of cases of FUO have remained undiagnosed. The general term *noninfectious inflammatory diseases* applies to systemic rheumatologic or vasculitic diseases such as polymyalgia rheumatica, lupus, and adult Still's disease as well as to granulomatous diseases such as sarcoidosis and Crohn's and granulomatous hepatitis. Table 18-3 shows the 10 leading causes of FUO identified in an investigation at several U.S. community hospitals; the method of classification—i.e., "lumping or splitting" of specific entities—can skew rank.

In the elderly, multisystem disease is the most frequent cause of FUO, giant cell arteritis being the leading etiologic entity in this category. Tuberculosis is the most common infection causing FUO in the elderly, and colon cancer is an important cause of FUO with malignancy in this age group.

Many diseases have been grouped in the various studies as "miscellaneous." On this list are drug fever, pulmonary embolism, factitious fever, the hereditary periodic fever syndromes (familial

TABLE 18-2 Classic FUO in Adults

Authors (Year of Publication)	Years of Study	No. of Cases	Infections (%)	Neoplasms (%)	Noninfectious Inflammatory Diseases (%)	Miscellaneous Causes (%)	Undiagnosed Causes (%)
Petersdorf and Beeson (1961)	1952–1957	100	36	19	19[a]	19[a]	7
Larson and Featherstone (1982)	1970–1980	105	32	20	16[a]	11[a]	7
Knockaert and Vanneste (1992)	1980–1989	199	22.5	7	23[a]	21.5[a]	25.5
DeKleijn et al. (1997, Part I)	1992–1994	167	26	12.5	24	8	30

[a] Authors' raw data retabulated to conform to altered diagnostic categories.

Source: Modified from DeKleijn et al., 1997 (Part I).

TABLE 18-3 *Ten Leading Causes of Classic FUO among Adults at Community Hospitals in the United States*

Cause	% of Total
Lymphoma	16
Collagen vascular disease	16
Abscess	13
Undiagnosed cause	9
Solid tumor	8
Thrombosis or hematoma	7
Granulomatous disease, nonmycobacterial	5
Endocarditis	5
Mycobacterial disease	5
Viral disease	5
Remaining causes	11
	100

Source: Adapted from Kazanjian, 1992.

Mediterranean fever, hyper-IgD syndrome, tumor necrosis factor receptor–associated periodic syndrome), familial cold urticarla, the Muckle-Wells syndrome, and Fabry's disease.

A drug-related etiology must be considered in any case of prolonged fever. Any febrile pattern may be elicited by a drug, and both relative bradycardia and hypotension are uncommon. Eosinophilia and/or rash is found in only one-fifth of patients with drug fever, which usually begins 1 to 3 weeks after the start of therapy and remits 2 to 3 days after therapy is stopped. Virtually all classes of drugs cause fever, but antimicrobial agents (especially β-lactam antibiotics), cardiovascular drugs (e.g., quinidine), antineoplastic drugs, and drugs acting on the central nervous system (e.g., phenytoin) are particularly common causes.

It is axiomatic that, as the duration of fever increases, the likelihood of an infectious cause decreases, even for the more indolent infectious etiologies (e.g., brucellosis, paracoccidioidomycosis, *Plasmodium malariae*) (Table 18-4). In a series of 347 patients referred to the National Institutes of Health from 1961 to 1977, only 6% had an infection. A significant proportion (9%) had factitious fevers—i.e., fevers due either to false elevations of temperature or to self-induced disease. A substantial number of these factitious cases were in young women in the health professions. It is worth noting that 8% of the patients with prolonged fevers (some of whom had completely normal liver function studies) had granulomatous hepatitis, and 6% had adult Still's disease. After prolonged investigation, 19% of cases still had no specific diagnosis. A total of 27% of patients had no actual fever during inpatient observation or had an exaggerated circadian temperature rhythm without chills, elevated pulse, or other abnormalities.

The conditions that may be considered in a differential diagnosis of classic FUO in adults are listed in Table 18-5. This list applies strictly to the United States; the frequency of global travel underscores the need for a detailed travel history, and the continuing emergence of new infectious diseases makes this listing potentially incomplete. Increased international and domestic terrorist activity involving the intentional release of infectious agents, many of which cause illnesses presenting with prolonged fever, further underscores the need for obtaining an insightful environmental, occupational, and professional history, with early notification of public health authorities in cases of suspicious etiology (Chap. 205).

SPECIALIZED DIAGNOSTIC STUDIES ■ Classic FUO A stepwise flow chart depicting the diagnostic workup and therapeutic management of FUO is provided in Fig. 18-1. In this flow chart, reference is made to "potentially diagnostic clues," as outlined by DeKleijn and colleagues; these clues may be key findings in the history (e.g., travel), localizing signs, or key symptoms. Certain specific diagnostic maneuvers become critical in dealing with prolonged fevers. If factitious fever is suspected, electronic thermometers should be used, temperature-taking should be supervised, and simultaneous urine and body temperatures

should be measured. Thick blood smears should be examined for *Plasmodium*; thin blood smears, prepared with proper technique and quality stains and subjected to expert microscopy, should be used to speciate *Plasmodium* and to identify *Babesia*, *Trypanosoma*, *Leishmania*, *Rickettsia*, and *Borrelia*. Any tissue removed during prior relevant surgery should be reexamined; slides should be requested, and, if need be, paraffin blocks of fixed pathologic material should be reexamined and additional special studies performed. Relevant x-rays should be reexamined; reviewing of prior radiologic reports may be insufficient. Serum should be set aside in the laboratory as soon as possible and retained for future examination for rising antibody titers. *Febrile agglutinins* is a vague term that in most laboratories refers to serologic studies for salmonellosis, brucellosis, and rickettsial diseases. These studies are seldom useful, having low sensitivity and variable specificity. Multiple blood samples (no fewer than three and rarely more than six, including samples for anaerobic culture) should be cultured in the laboratory for at least 2 weeks to ensure that any HACEK group organisms that may be present have ample time to grow (Chap. 131). Lysis-centrifugation blood culture techniques should be employed in cases where prior antimicrobial therapy or fungal or atypical mycobacterial infection is suspected. Blood culture media should be supplemented with L-cysteine or pyridoxal to assist in the isolation of nutritionally variant streptococci. It should be noted that sequential cultures positive for multiple organisms may reflect self-injection of contaminated substances. Urine cultures, including cultures for mycobacteria, fungi, and CMV, are indicated. In the setting of recurrent fevers with lymphocytic meningitis (Mollaret's meningitis), cerebrospinal fluid can be tested for herpesvirus, with use of polymerase chain reaction (PCR) to amplify and detect viral nucleic acid (Chap. 163).

In any FUO workup, the erythrocyte sedimentation rate (ESR) should be determined. Striking elevation of the ESR and anemia of chronic disease are frequently seen in association with giant cell arteritis or polymyalgia rheumatica, common causes of FUO in patients >50 years of age. Still's disease is also suggested by elevations of ESR, leukocytosis, and anemia and is often accompanied by arthralgias, polyserositis (pleuritis, pericarditis), lymphadenopathy, splenomegaly, and rash. C-reactive protein may be a useful cross-reference for the ESR and is a more sensitive and specific indicator of an "acute-phase" inflammatory metabolic response. Antinuclear antibody, antineutrophil cytoplasmic antibody, rheumatoid factor, and serum cryoglobulins should be measured to rule out other collagen vascular diseases and vasculitis. Elevated levels of angiotensin-converting enzyme in serum may point to sarcoidosis. With rare exceptions, the intermediate-strength purified protein derivative (PPD) skin test should be used to screen for tuberculosis in patients with classic FUO. Concurrent control tests, such as the mumps skin test antigen (Aventis-Pasteur, Swiftwater, PA), should be employed. It should be kept in mind that both the PPD skin test and control tests may yield negative results in miliary tuberculosis, sarcoidosis, Hodgkin's disease, malnutrition, or AIDS. Noninvasive procedures should include an upper

TABLE 18-4 *Causes of FUO Lasting >6 Months*

Cause	Cases, %
None identified	19
Miscellaneous causes	13
Factitious causes	9
Granulomatous hepatitis	8
Neoplasm	7
Still's disease	6
Infection	6
Collagen vascular disease	4
Familial Mediterranean fever	3
No fever[a]	27

[a] No actual fever observed during 2 to 3 weeks of inpatient observation. Includes patients with exaggerated circadian rhythm.

Source: From a study of 347 patients referred to the National Institutes of Health from 1961 to 1977 with a presumptive diagnosis of FUO of >6 months' duration (Aduan et al.)

TABLE 18-5 Causes of FUO in Adults in the United States

INFECTIONS

Localized pyogenic infections
  Appendicitis
  Cat-scratch disease
  Cholangitis
  Cholecystitis
  Dental abscess
  Diverticulitis/abscess
  Lesser sac abscess
  Liver abscess
  Mesenteric lymphadenitis
  Osteomyelitis
  Pancreatic abscess
  Pelvic inflammatory disease
  Perinephric/intrarenal abscess
  Prostatic abscess
  Renal malacoplakia
  Sinusitis
  Subphrenic abscess
  Suppurative thrombophlebitis
  Tuboovarian abscess
Intravascular infections
  Bacterial aortitis
  Bacterial endocarditis
  Vascular catheter infection
Systemic bacterial infections
  Bartonellosis
  Brucellosis
  Campylobacter infection
  Cat-scratch disease/bacillary
    angiomatosis (*B. henselae*)
  Gonococcemia
  Legionnaires' disease
  Leptospirosis
  Listeriosis
  Lyme disease
  Melioidosis
  Meningococcemia
  Rat-bite fever
  Relapsing fever
  Salmonellosis
  Syphilis
  Tularemia
  Typhoid fever
  Vibriosis
  Yersinia infection
Mycobacterial infections
  M. avium/*M. intracellulare* infections
  Other atypical mycobacterial infections
  Tuberculosis
Fungal infections
  Aspergillosis
  Blastomycosis
  Candidiasis
  Coccidioidomycosis
  Cryptococcosis
  Histoplasmosis
  Mucormycosis
  Paracoccidioidomycosis
  Sporotrichosis

Other bacterial infections
  Actinomycosis
  Bacillary angiomatosis
  Nocardiosis
  Whipple's disease
Rickettsial infections
  Anaplasmosis
  Ehrlichiosis
  Murine typhus
  Q fever
  Rickettsialpox
  Rocky Mountain spotted fever
Mycoplasmal infections
Chlamydial infections
  Lymphogranuloma venereum
  Psittacosis
  TWAR (*C. pneumoniae*) infection
Viral infections
  Colorado tick fever
  Coxsackievirus group B infection
  Cytomegalovirus infection
  Dengue
  Epstein-Barr virus infection
  Hepatitis A, B, C, D, and E
  Human herpesvirus 6 infection
  Human immunodeficiency virus infection
  Lymphocytic choriomeningitis
  Parvovirus B19 infection
Parasitic infections
  Amebiasis
  Babesiosis
  Chagas' disease
  Leishmaniasis
  Malaria
  Pneumocystis infection
  Strongyloidiasis
  Toxocariasis
  Toxoplasmosis
  Trichinosis
Presumed infections, agent undetermined
  Kawasaki's disease (mucocutaneous lymph
    node syndrome)
  Kikuchi's necrotizing lymphadenitis

NEOPLASMS

Malignant
  Colon cancer
  Gall bladder carcinoma
  Hepatoma
  Hodgkin's lymphoma
  Immunoblastic T-cell lymphoma
  Leukemia
  Lymphomatoid granulomatosis
  Malignant histiocytosis
  Non-Hodgkin's lymphoma
  Pancreatic cancer
  Renal cell carcinoma
  Sarcoma
Benign
  Atrial myxoma
  Castleman's disease
  Renal angiomyolipoma

HABITUAL HYPERTHERMIA

(Exaggerated circadian rhythm)

COLLAGEN VASCULAR/HYPERSENSITIVITY DISEASES

Adult Still's disease
Behçet's disease
Erythema multiforme
Erythema nodosum
Giant cell arteritis/polymyalgia
  rheumatica
Hypersensitivity pneumonitis
Hypersensitivity vasculitis
Mixed connective-tissue disease
Polyarteritis nodosa
Relapsing polychondritis
Rheumatic fever
Rheumatoid arthritis
Schnitzler's syndrome
Systemic lupus erythematosus
Takayasu's aortitis
Weber-Christian disease
Wegener's granulomatosis

GRANULOMATOUS DISEASES

Crohn's disease
Granulomatous hepatitis
Midline granuloma
Sarcoidosis

MISCELLANEOUS CONDITIONS

Aortic dissection
Drug fever
Gout
Hematomas
Hemoglobinopathies
Laennec's cirrhosis
PFPA syndrome: periodic fever, adenitis,
  pharyngitis, aphthae
Postmyocardial infarction syndrome
Recurrent pulmonary emboli
Subacute thyroiditis (de Quervain's)
Tissue infarction/necrosis

INHERITED AND METABOLIC DISEASES

Adrenal insufficiency
Cyclic neutropenia
Deafness, urticaria, and amyloidosis
Fabry's disease
Familial cold urticaria
Familial Mediterranean fever
Hyperimmunoglobulinemia D and
  periodic fever
Muckle-Wells syndrome
Tumor necrosis factor receptor–
  associated periodic syndrome
Type V hypertriglyceridemia

THERMOREGULATORY DISORDERS

Central
  Brain tumor
  Cerebrovascular accident
  Encephalitis
  Hypothalamic dysfunction
Peripheral
  Hyperthyroidism
  Pheochromocytoma

FACTITIOUS FEVERS

"AFEBRILE" FUO (<38.3°C)

Source: Modified from RK Root, RG Petersdorf, in JD Wilson et al (eds): *Harrison's Principles of Internal Medicine,* 12th ed. New York, McGraw-Hill, 1991.

gastrointestinal contrast study with small-bowel follow-through and colonoscopy to examine the terminal ileum and cecum. Chest x-rays should be repeated if new symptoms arise. Sputum should be induced with an ultrasonic nebulizer for cultures and cytology. If there are pulmonary signs or symptoms, bronchoscopy with bronchoalveolar lavage for cultures and cytology should be considered. High-resolution spiral CT of the chest and abdomen should be performed with both intravenous and oral contrast. If a spinal or paraspinal lesion is sus-

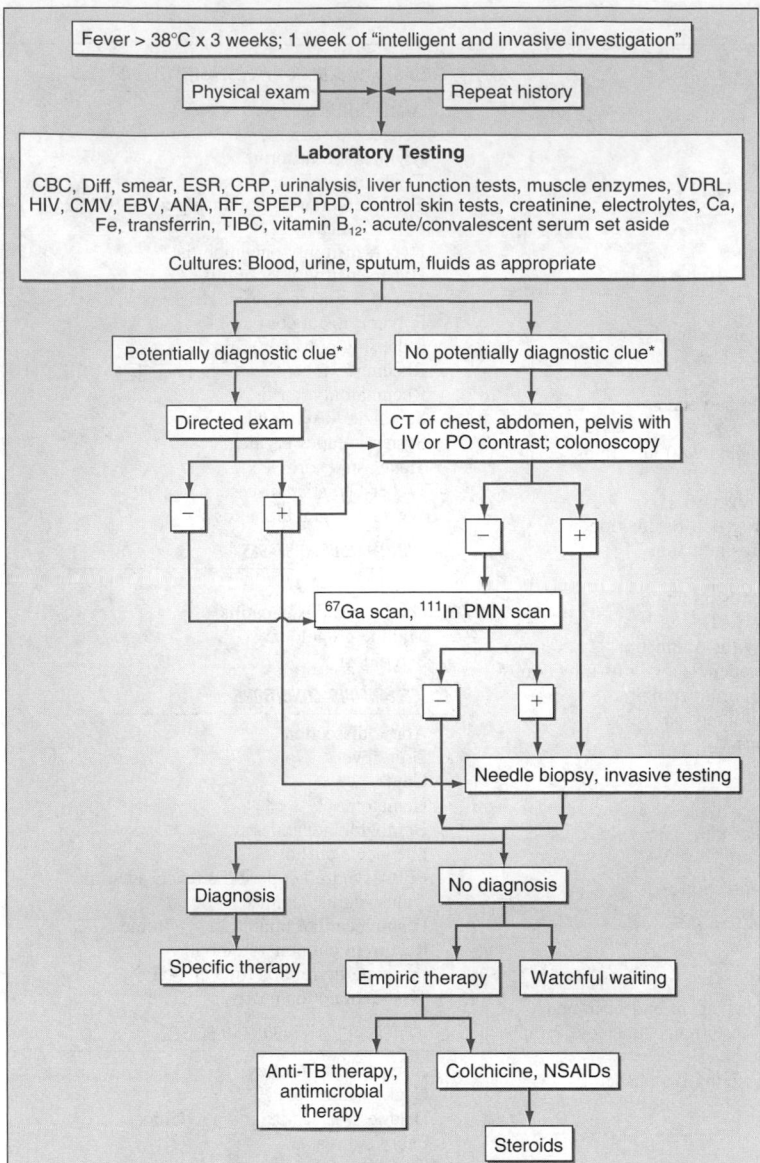

FIGURE 18-1 Approach to the patient with classic FUO. *"Potentially diagnostic clues," as outlined by DeKleijn and colleagues (1997, Part II), may be key findings in the history, localizing signs, or key symptoms. Abbreviations: ANA, antinuclear antibody; CBC, complete blood count; CMV, cytomegalovirus; CRP, C-reactive protein; CT, computed tomography; Diff, differential; EBV, Epstein-Barr virus; ESR, erythrocyte sedimentation rate; NSAIDs, nonsteroidal anti-inflammatory drugs; PMN, polymorphonuclear leukocyte; PPD, purified protein derivative; RF, rheumatoid factor; SPEP, serum protein electrophoresis; TB, tuberculosis; TIBC, total iron-binding capacity; VDRL, Venereal Disease Research Laboratory test.

- Fever > 38°C x 3 weeks; 1 week of "intelligent and invasive investigation"
- Physical exam → ← Repeat history
- **Laboratory Testing**
- CBC, Diff, smear, ESR, CRP, urinalysis, liver function tests, muscle enzymes, VDRL, HIV, CMV, EBV, ANA, RF, SPEP, PPD, control skin tests, creatinine, electrolytes, Ca, Fe, transferrin, TIBC, vitamin B$_{12}$; acute/convalescent serum set aside
- Cultures: Blood, urine, sputum, fluids as appropriate
- Potentially diagnostic clue*
- No potentially diagnostic clue*
- Directed exam
- CT of chest, abdomen, pelvis with IV or PO contrast; colonoscopy
- − +
- − +
- ^{67}Ga scan, ^{111}In PMN scan
- − +
- Needle biopsy, invasive testing
- Diagnosis
- No diagnosis
- Specific therapy
- Empiric therapy
- Watchful waiting
- Anti-TB therapy, antimicrobial therapy
- Colchicine, NSAIDs
- Steroids

pected, however, MRI is preferred. MRI may be superior to CT in demonstrating intraabdominal abscesses and aortic dissection, but the relative utility of MRI and CT in the diagnosis of FUO is unknown. At present, abdominal CT with contrast should be used unless MRI is specifically indicated. Arteriography may be useful for patients in whom systemic necrotizing vasculitis is suspected. Saccular aneurysms may be seen, most commonly in renal or hepatic vessels, and may permit diagnosis of arteritis when biopsy is difficult. Ultrasonography of the abdomen is useful for investigation of the hepatobiliary tract, kidneys, spleen, and pelvis. Echocardiography may be helpful in an evaluation for bacterial endocarditis, pericarditis, nonbacterial thrombotic endocarditis, and atrial myxomas. Transesophageal echocardiography is especially sensitive for these lesions.

Radionuclide scanning procedures using technetium (Tc) 99m sulfur colloid, gallium (Ga) 67 citrate, or indium (In) 111–labeled leukocytes may be useful in identifying and/or localizing inflammatory processes. In one study, Ga scintigraphy yielded useful diagnostic in-

formation in almost one-third of cases, and it was suggested that this procedure might actually be used before other imaging techniques if no specific organ is suspected of being abnormal. It is likely that PET scanning, which provides quicker results (hours vs days), will prove even more sensitive and specific than ^{67}Ga scanning in FUO. ^{99m}Tc bone scan should be undertaken to look for osteomyelitis or bony metastases; ^{67}Ga scan may be used to identify sarcoidosis (Chap. 309) or *Pneumocystis* (Chap. 191) in the lungs or Crohn's disease (Chap. 276) in the abdomen. ^{111}In-labeled white blood cell (WBC) scan may be used to locate abscesses. With these scans, false-positive and false-negative findings are common.

Biopsy of the liver and bone marrow should be considered in the workup of FUO if the studies mentioned above are unrevealing and if fever is prolonged. Granulomatous hepatitis has been diagnosed by liver biopsy, even when liver enzymes are normal and no other diagnostic clues point to liver disease. All biopsy specimens should be cultured for bacteria, mycobacteria, and fungi. Likewise, in the absence of clues pointing to the bone marrow, bone marrow biopsy (not simple aspiration) for histology and culture has yielded diagnoses late in the workup. When possible, a section of the tissue block should be retained for further sections or stains. PCR technology makes it potentially possible to identify and speciate mycobacterial DNA in paraffin-embedded, fixed tissues at some research centers. Thus, in some cases, a retrospective diagnosis can be made on the basis of studies of long-fixed pathologic tissues. In a patient over age 50 (or occasionally in a younger patient) with the appropriate symptoms and laboratory findings, "blind biopsy" of one or both temporal arteries may yield a diagnosis of arteritis. Tenderness or decreased pulsation, if noted, should guide the selection of a site for biopsy. Lymph node biopsy may be helpful if nodes are enlarged, but inguinal nodes are often palpable and are seldom diagnostically useful.

Exploratory laparotomy has been performed when all other diagnostic procedures fail but has largely been replaced by imaging and guided-biopsy techniques. Laparoscopic biopsy may provide more adequate guided sampling of lymph nodes or liver.

Nosocomial FUO (See also Chap. 116) The primary considerations in diagnosing nosocomial FUO are the underlying susceptibility of the patient coupled with the potential complications of hospitalization. The original surgical or procedural field is the place to begin a directed physical and laboratory examination for abscesses, hematomas, or infected foreign bodies. More than 50% of patients with nosocomial FUO are infected, and intravascular lines, septic phlebitis, and prostheses are all suspect. In this setting, the approach is to focus on sites where occult infections may be sequestered, such as the sinuses of intubated patients or a prostatic abscess in a man with a urinary catheter. *Clostridium difficile* colitis may be associated with fever and leukocytosis before the onset of diarrhea. In ~25% of patients with nosocomial FUO, the fever has a noninfectious cause. Among these causes are acalculous cholecystitis, deep-vein thrombophlebitis, and pulmonary embolism. Drug fever, transfusion reactions, alcohol/drug withdrawal, adrenal insufficiency, thyroiditis, pancreatitis, gout, and pseudogout are among the many possible causes to consider. As in classic FUO, repeated meticulous physical examinations, coupled with focused diagnostic techniques, are imperative. Multiple blood, wound, and fluid cultures are mandatory. The pace of diagnostic tests is accelerated, and the threshold for procedures—CT scans, ultrasonography, ^{111}In-WBC scans, noninvasive venous studies—is low. Even so, 20% of cases of nosocomial FUO may go undiagnosed.

Like diagnostic measures, therapeutic maneuvers must be swift and decisive, as many patients are already critically ill. Intravenous lines must be changed (and cultured), drugs stopped for 72 h, and empirical therapy started if bacteremia is a threat. In many hospital settings, empirical antibiotic coverage for nosocomial FUO now includes vancomycin for coverage of methicillin-resistant *Staphylococcus aureus* as well as broad-spectrum gram-negative coverage with piperacillin/tazobactam, ticarcillin/clavulanate, imipenem, or meropenem. Practice guidelines covering many of these issues have been published jointly by the Infectious Diseases Society of America (IDSA) and the Society for Critical Care Medicine and can be accessed on the IDSA website (www.journals.uchicago.edu/IDSA/guidelines).

Neutropenic FUO (See also Chap. 72) Neutropenic patients are susceptible to focal bacterial and fungal infections, to bacteremic infections, to infections involving catheters (including septic thrombophlebitis), and to perianal infections. *Candida* and *Aspergillus* infections are common. Infections due to herpes simplex virus or CMV are sometimes causes of FUO in this group. While the duration of illness may be short in these patients, the consequences of untreated infection may be catastrophic; 50 to 60% of febrile neutropenic patients are infected, and 20% are bacteremic. The IDSA has published extensive practice guidelines covering these critically ill neutropenic patients; these guidelines appear on the website cited in the previous section. In these patients, severe mucositis, quinolone prophylaxis, colonization with methicillin-resistant *S. aureus*, obvious catheter-related infection, or hypotension dictates the use of vancomycin plus ceftazidime, cefepime, or a carbapenem with or without an aminoglycoside to provide empirical coverage for bacterial sepsis.

HIV-Associated FUO HIV infection alone may be a cause of fever. Infection due to *Mycobacterium avium* or *Mycobacterium intracellulare*, tuberculosis, toxoplasmosis, CMV infection, *Pneumocystis* infection, salmonellosis, cryptococcosis, histoplasmosis, non-Hodgkin's lymphoma, and (of particular importance) drug fever are all possible causes of FUO. Mycobacterial infection can be diagnosed by blood cultures and by liver, bone marrow, and lymph node biopsies. Chest CT should be performed to identify enlarged mediastinal nodes. Serologic studies may reveal cryptococcal antigen, and ^{67}Ga scan may help identify *Pneumocystis* pulmonary infection. More than 80% of HIV patients with FUO are infected, but drug fever and lymphoma remain important considerations. →*Treatment of HIV-associated FUO depends on many factors and is discussed in Chap. 173.*

℞ TREATMENT

The focus here is on classic FUO. Other modifiers of FUO—neutropenia, HIV infection, a nosocomial setting—all vastly modify the risk equation and dictate therapy based on the probability of various causes of fever and on the calculated risks and benefits of a guided empirical approach. The age and physical state of the patient are factors as well: the frail elderly patient may merit a trial of empirical therapy earlier than the robust young adult.

The emphasis in patients with classic FUO is on continued observation and examination, with the avoidance of "shotgun" empirical therapy. Antibiotic therapy (even that for tuberculosis) may irrevocably alter the ability to culture fastidious bacteria or mycobacteria and delineate ultimate cause. However, vital-sign instability or neutropenia is an indication for empirical therapy with a fluoroquinolone plus piperacillin or the regimen mentioned above, for example. Cirrhosis, asplenia, intercurrent immunosuppressive drug use, or recent exotic travel may all tip the balance toward earlier empirical anti-infective therapy. If the PPD skin test is positive or if granulomatous hepatitis or other granulomatous disease is present with anergy (and sarcoid seems unlikely), then a therapeutic trial with isoniazid and rifampin (and possibly a third drug) should be undertaken, with treatment usually continued for up to 6 weeks. A failure of the fever to respond over this period suggests an alternative diagnosis.

The response of rheumatic fever and Still's disease to aspirin and nonsteroidal anti-inflammatory agents (NSAIDs) may be dramatic. The effects of glucocorticoids on temporal arteritis, polymyalgia rheumatica, and granulomatous hepatitis are equally dramatic. Colchicine is highly effective in preventing attacks of familial Mediterranean fever but is of little use once an attack is well under way. The ability of glucocorticoids and NSAIDs to mask fever while permitting the spread of infection dictates that their use be avoided unless infection has been largely ruled out and unless inflammatory disease is both probable and debilitating or threatening.

When no underlying source of FUO is identified after prolonged observation (>6 months), the prognosis is generally good, however vexing the fever may be to the patient. Under such circumstances, debilitating symptoms are treated with NSAIDs, and glucocorticoids are the last resort. The initiation of empirical therapy does not mark the end of the diagnostic workup; rather, it commits the physician to continued thoughtful reexamination and evaluation. Patience, compassion, equanimity, and intellectual flexibility are indispensable attributes for the clinician in dealing successfully with FUO.

ACKNOWLEDGMENT
Sheldon M. Wolff, MD, now deceased, was an author of a previous version of this chapter. It is to his memory that the chapter is dedicated.

FURTHER READING

ADUAN R et al: Prolonged fever of unknown origin. Clin Res 26:558A, 1978

DEKLEIJN EMHA et al: Fever of unknown origin (FUO): I. A prospective multicenter study of 167 patients with FUO, using fixed epidemiologic entry criteria. Medicine 76:392, 1997

——— et al: Fever of unknown origin (FUO): II. Diagnostic procedures in a prospective multicenter study of 167 patients. Medicine 76:401, 1997

HIRSCHMANN JV: Fever of unknown origin in adults. Clin Infect Dis 24:291, 1997

HOEN B et al: The Duke criteria for diagnosing infective endocarditis are specific: Analysis of 100 patients with acute fever or fever of unknown origin. Clin Infect Dis 23:298, 1996

HUGHES WT et al: 2002 guidelines for the use of antimicrobial agents in neutropenic patients with cancer. Clin Infect Dis 34:730, 2002

KAZANJIAN PH: Fever of unknown origin: Review of 86 patients treated in community hospitals. Clin Infect Dis 15:968, 1992

KNOCKAERT DC et al: Long-term follow-up of patients with undiagnosed fever of unknown origin. Arch Intern Med 156:618, 1996

O'GRADY NP et al: Practice guidelines for evaluating new fever in critically ill adult patients. Clin Infect Dis 26:1042, 1998

PETERSDORF RC, BEESON PB: Fever of unexplained origin. Medicine 40:1, 1961

19 HYPOTHERMIA AND FROSTBITE
Daniel F. Danzl

HYPOTHERMIA

Accidental hypothermia occurs when there is an unintentional drop in the body's core temperature below 35°C (95°F). At this temperature, many of the compensatory physiologic mechanisms to conserve heat begin to fail. *Primary accidental hypothermia* is a result of the direct exposure of a previously healthy individual to the cold. The mortality rate is much higher for those patients who develop *secondary hypothermia* as a complication of a serious systemic disorder.

CAUSES

Primary accidental hypothermia is geographically and seasonally pervasive. Although most cases occur in the winter months and in colder climates, it is surprisingly common in warmer regions as well. Multiple variables make individuals at the extremes of age, the elderly and neonates, particularly vulnerable to hypothermia (Table 19-1). The

TABLE 19-1   *Risk Factors for Hypothermia*

Age extremes	Endocrine-related
Elderly	Hypoglycemia
Neonates	Hypothyroidism
Outdoor exposure	Adrenal insufficiency
Occupational	Hypopituitarism
Sports-related	Neurologic-related
Inadequate clothing	Stroke
Drugs and intoxicants	Hypothalamic disorders
Ethanol	Parkinson's disease
Phenothiazines	Spinal cord injury
Barbiturates	Multisystem
Anesthetics	Malnutrition
Neuromuscular blockers	Sepsis
Others	Shock
	Hepatic or renal failure
	Burns and exfoliative dermatologic
	disorders
	Immobility or debilitation

elderly have diminished thermal perception and are more susceptible to immobility, malnutrition, and systemic illnesses that interfere with heat generation or conservation. Dementia, psychiatric illness, and socioeconomic factors often compound these problems by impeding adequate measures to prevent hypothermia. Neonates have high rates of heat loss because of their increased surface-to-mass ratio and their lack of effective shivering and adaptive behavioral responses. In addition, malnutrition can contribute to heat loss because of diminished subcutaneous fat and because of its association with depleted energy stores used for thermogenesis.

Individuals whose occupations or hobbies entail extensive exposure to cold weather are clearly at increased risk for hypothermia. Military history is replete with hypothermic tragedies. Hunters, sailors, skiers, and climbers also are at great risk of exposure, whether it involves injury, changes in weather, or lack of preparedness.

Ethanol causes vasodilatation (which increases heat loss), reduces thermogenesis and gluconeogenesis, and may impair judgment or lead to obtundation. Phenothiazines, barbiturates, benzodiazepines, cyclic antidepressants, and many other medications reduce centrally mediated vasoconstriction. Up to one-quarter of patients admitted to an intensive care unit because of drug overdose are hypothermic. Anesthetics can block the shivering responses; their effects may be compounded when patients are not covered adequately in the operating or recovery rooms.

Several types of endocrine dysfunction can lead to hypothermia. Hypothyroidism—particularly when extreme, as in myxedema coma—reduces the metabolic rate and impairs thermogenesis and behavioral responses. Adrenal insufficiency and hypopituitarism can also increase susceptibility to hypothermia. Hypoglycemia, most commonly caused by insulin or oral hypoglycemic drugs, is associated with hypothermia, in part the result of neuroglycopenic effects on hypothalamic function. Increased osmolality and metabolic derangements associated with uremia, diabetic ketoacidosis, and lactic acidosis can lead to altered hypothalamic thermoregulation.

Neurologic injury from trauma, cerebrovascular accident, subarachnoid hemorrhage, or hypothalamic lesions increases susceptibility to hypothermia. Agenesis of the corpus callosum, or Shapiro syndrome, is one cause of episodic hypothermia, characterized by profuse perspiration followed by a rapid fall in temperature. Acute spinal cord injury disrupts the autonomic pathways that lead to shivering and prevents cold-induced reflex vasoconstrictive responses.

Hypothermia associated with sepsis is a poor prognostic sign. Hepatic failure causes decreased glycogen stores and gluconeogenesis, as well as a diminished shivering response. In acute myocardial infarction associated with low cardiac output, hypothermia may be reversed after adequate resuscitation. With extensive burns, psoriasis, erythrodermas,

and other skin diseases, increased peripheral blood flow leads to excessive heat loss.

THERMOREGULATION

Heat loss occurs through five mechanisms: radiation (55 to 65% of heat loss), conduction (10 to 15% of heat loss, but much greater in cold water), convection (increased in the wind), respiration, and evaporation (which are affected by the ambient temperature and the relative humidity).

The preoptic anterior hypothalamus normally orchestrates thermoregulation (Chap. 16). The immediate defense of thermoneutrality is via the autonomic nervous system, whereas delayed control is mediated by the endocrine system. Autonomic nervous system responses include the release of norepinephrine, increased muscle tone, and shivering, leading to thermogenesis and an increase in the basal metabolic rate. Cutaneous cold thermoreception causes direct reflex vasoconstriction to conserve heat. Prolonged exposure to cold also stimulates the thyroid axis, leading to an increased metabolic rate.

CLINICAL PRESENTATION

In most cases of hypothermia, the history of exposure to environmental factors, such as prolonged exposure to the outdoors without adequate clothing, makes the diagnosis straightforward. In urban settings, however, the presentation is often more subtle and other disease processes, toxin exposures, or psychiatric diagnoses should be considered.

After initial stimulation by hypothermia, there is progressive depression of all organ systems. The timing of the appearance of these clinical manifestations varies widely (Table 19-2). Without knowing the core temperature, it can be difficult to interpret other vital signs. For example, a tachycardia disproportionate to the core temperature suggests secondary hypothermia resulting from hypoglycemia, hypovolemia, or a toxin overdose. Because carbon dioxide production declines progressively, the respiratory rate should be low; persistent hyperventilation suggests a central nervous system (CNS) lesion or one of the organic acidoses. A markedly depressed level of consciousness in a patient with mild hypothermia should raise suspicion of an overdose or CNS dysfunction due to infection or trauma.

Physical examination findings can also be altered by hypothermia. For instance, the assumption that areflexia is solely attributable to hypothermia can obscure and delay the diagnosis of a spinal cord lesion. Patients with hypothermia may be confused or combative; these symptoms abate more rapidly with rewarming than with the use of restraints. A classic example of maladaptive behavior in patients with hypothermia is paradoxical undressing, which involves the inappropriate removal of clothing in response to a cold stress. The cold-induced ileus and abdominal rectus spasm can mimic, or mask, the presentation of an acute abdomen (Chap. 13).

When a patient in hypothermic cardiac arrest is first discovered, cardiopulmonary resuscitation is indicated, unless (1) a do-not-resuscitate status is verified, (2) obviously lethal injuries are identified, or (3) the depression of a frozen chest wall is not possible. As the resuscitation proceeds, the prognosis is grave if there is evidence of widespread cell lysis, as reflected by potassium levels exceeding 10 meq/L. Other findings that may preclude continuing resuscitation include a core temperature <12°C, a pH <6.5, or evidence of intravascular thrombosis with a fibrinogen value <50 mg/dL. The decision to terminate resuscitation before rewarming the patient past 33°C is extremely difficult. There are no validated prognostic indicators for recovery from hypothermia. A history of asphyxia with secondary cooling is the most important negative predictor of survival.

DIAGNOSIS AND STABILIZATION

Hypothermia is confirmed by measuring the core temperature, preferably at two sites. Rectal probes should be placed to a depth of 15 cm and not adjacent to cold feces. A simultaneous esophageal probe should be placed 24 cm below the larynx; it may read falsely high during heated inhalation therapy. Relying solely on infrared tympanic thermography is not advisable.

TABLE 19-2 Physiologic Changes Associated with Hypothermia

Severity	Body Temperature	Central Nervous System	Cardiovascular	Respiratory	Renal and Endocrine	Neuromuscular
Mild	35°C (95°F)–32.2°C (90°F)	Linear depression of cerebral metabolism; amnesia; apathy; dysarthria; impaired judgment; maladaptive behavior	Tachycardia, then progressive bradycardia; cardiac-cycle prolongation; vasoconstriction; increase in cardiac output and blood pressure	Tachypnea, then progressive decrease in respiratory minute volume; declining oxygen consumption; bronchorrhea; bronchospasm	Diuresis; increase in catecholamines, adrenal steroids, triiodothyronine and thyroxine; increase in metabolism with shivering	Increased preshivering muscle tone, then fatiguing, shivering-induced thermogenesis; ataxia
Moderate	<32.2°C (90°F)–28°C (82.4°F)	EEG abnormalities; progressive depression of level of consciousness; pupillary dilatation; paradoxical undressing; hallucinations	Progressive decrease in pulse and cardiac output; increased atrial and ventricular arrhythmias; nonspecific and suggestive (J-wave) ECG changes; prolonged systole	Hypoventilation; 50% decrease in carbon dioxide production per 8°C drop in temperature; absence of protective airway reflexes; 50% decrease in oxygen consumption	50% increase in renal blood flow; renal autoregulation intact; impaired insulin action	Hyporeflexia; diminishing shivering-induced thermogenesis, rigidity
Severe	<28°C (82.4°F)	Loss of cerebrovascular autoregulation; decline in cerebral blood flow; coma; loss of ocular reflexes; progressive decrease in EEG	Progressive decreases in blood pressure, heart rate, and cardiac output; reentrant dysrhythmias; decreased ventricular arrhythmia threshold; asystole	Pulmonic congestion and edema; 75% decrease in oxygen consumption; apnea	Decrease in renal blood flow parallels decrease in cardiac output; extreme oliguria; poikilothermia; 80% decrease in basal metabolism	No motion; decreased nerve-conduction velocity; peripheral areflexia

Source: From DF Danzl, RS Pozos: N Engl J Med 331:1756, 1994.

After a diagnosis of hypothermia is established, cardiac monitoring should be instituted, along with attempts to limit further heat loss. If the patient is in ventricular fibrillation, one sequence of 3 defibrillation attempts (2 J/kg) should be administered. Supplemental oxygenation is always warranted, since tissue oxygenation is adversely affected by the leftward shift of the oxyhemoglobin dissociation curve. Pulse oximetry may be unreliable in patients with vasoconstriction. If protective airway reflexes are absent, gentle endotracheal intubation should be performed. Adequate pre-oxygenation will prevent ventricular arrhythmias. Although cardiac pacing for hypothermic bradydysrhythmias is rarely indicated, the transthoracic technique appears preferable to the transvenous.

Insertion of a gastric tube prevents dilatation secondary to decreased bowel motility. Indwelling bladder catheters facilitate monitoring of cold-induced diuresis. Dehydration is commonly encountered with chronic hypothermia, and most patients benefit from a bolus of crystalloid. Normal saline is preferable to lactated Ringer's solution, as the liver in hypothermic patients inefficiently metabolizes lactate. The placement of a pulmonary artery catheter, although of potential value, risks perforation of the less compliant pulmonary artery. Insertion of a central venous catheter into the cold right atrium should be avoided, since this can precipitate arrhythmias.

Arterial blood gases should not be corrected for temperature (Chap. 42). An uncorrected pH of 7.42 and a P_{CO_2} of 40 mmHg reflects appropriate alveolar ventilation and acid-base balance at any core temperature. Acid-base imbalances should be corrected gradually, since the bicarbonate buffering system is inefficient. A common error is overzealous hyperventilation in the setting of depressed CO_2 production. When the P_{CO_2} decreases 10 mmHg at 28°C, it doubles the pH increase of 0.08 that occurs at 37°C.

The severity of anemia may be underestimated because the hematocrit increases 2% for each 1°C drop in temperature. White blood cell sequestration and bone marrow suppression are common, potentially masking an infection. Although hypokalemia is more common in chronic hypothermia, hyperkalemia also occurs; the expected electrocardiographic changes can be obscured by hypothermia. Patients with renal insufficiency, metabolic acidoses, or rhabdomyolysis are at greatest risk for electrolyte disturbances.

Coagulopathies are common because cold inhibits the enzymatic reactions required for activation of the intrinsic cascade. In addition, the production of thromboxane B_2 by platelets is temperature-dependent, and platelet function is impaired. The administration of platelets and fresh frozen plasma is, therefore, not effective. The prothrombin or partial thromboplastin times reported by the laboratory appear deceptively normal and contrast with the observed in vivo coagulopathy. This contradiction appears because all coagulation tests are routinely performed at 37°C, and the enzymes are thus rewarmed.

REWARMING STRATEGIES

The key initial decision is whether to rewarm the patient passively or actively. *Passive external rewarming* simply involves covering and insulating the patient in a warm environment. With the head also covered, the rate of rewarming is usually 0.5° to 2.0°C per hour. This technique is ideal for previously healthy patients who develop acute, mild primary accidental hypothermia. The patient must have sufficient glycogen to support endogenous thermogenesis.

There are reservations about the application of heat directly to the extremities of patients with chronic severe hypothermia. Extinguishing peripheral vasoconstriction in the dehydrated patient may precipitate core temperature "afterdrop"—the continual decline in the core temperature after removal of the patient from the cold. Truncal heat application may minimize the risk of afterdrop.

Active rewarming is necessary under the following circumstances: core temperature <32°C (poikilothermia), cardiovascular instability, age extremes, CNS dysfunction, endocrine insufficiency, or any suspicion of secondary hypothermia. *Active external rewarming* is best accomplished with forced-air heating blankets. Other options include radiant heat sources and hot packs. Monitoring a patient with hypothermia in a heated tub is extremely difficult. Electric blankets should be avoided because vasoconstricted skin is easily burned.

There are numerous widely available *active core rewarming* options. Airway rewarming with heated humidified oxygen (40° to 45°C) is a convenient option via mask or endotracheal tube. Although airway rewarming provides less heat than some other forms of active core rewarming, it eliminates respiratory heat loss and adds 1° to 2°C to the overall rewarming rate. Crystalloids should be heated to 40° to 42°C. The quantity of heat provided is significant only during massive volume resuscitation. The most efficient method for heating and delivering fluid or blood is with a countercurrent in-line heat exchanger. Heated irrigation of the gastrointestinal tract or bladder transfers minimal heat because of the limited available surface area. These methods should be reserved for patients in cardiac arrest and then used in combination with all available active rewarming techniques. Closed thoracic lavage is far more efficient in severely hypothermic patients with cardiac arrest. The hemithoraces are irrigated through two large bore thoracostomy tubes that are inserted into the left or both of the hemithoraces. Thoracostomy tubes should not be placed in the left chest of a spontaneously perfusing patient for purposes of rewarming. Peritoneal lavage with the dialysate at 40° to 45°C efficiently transfers heat when delivered through two catheters with outflow suction. Like peritoneal dialysis, standard hemodialysis is especially useful for patients with electrolyte abnormalities, rhabdomyolysis, or toxin ingestions. The efficacy of arteriovenous anastomoses rewarming, which provides exogenous heat by immersion of the hands, forearms, feet, and calves in 44° to 45°C water, is unclear.

There are four extracorporeal blood rewarming options, which should be considered in severely hypothermic patients, especially those with *primary accidental hypothermia* (Table 19-3). Cardiopulmonary bypass should be considered in nonperfusing patients without documented contraindications to resuscitation. Circulatory support may also be the only effective option in patients with completely frozen extremities, or those with significant tissue destruction coupled with rhabdomyolysis. There is no evidence that extremely rapid rewarming improves survival in perfusing patients. The best strategy is usually a combination of passive, truncal active, and active core rewarming techniques.

DRUG THERAPY

When a patient is hypothermic, target organs and the cardiovascular system respond minimally to most medications. Moreover, cumulative doses can cause toxicity during rewarming because of increased binding of drugs to proteins, and impaired metabolism and excretion. As an example, the administration of repeated doses of digoxin or insulin would be ineffective while the patient is hypothermic, and the residual drugs are potentially toxic during rewarming.

Achieving a mean arterial pressure of at least 60 mmHg should be an early objective. If the hypotension does not respond to crystalloid/colloid infusion and rewarming, low-dose dopamine (2 to 5 μg/kg per min) support should be considered. Perfusion of the vasoconstricted cardiovascular system may also be improved with low-dose IV nitroglycerin.

Atrial arrhythmias should initially be monitored without intervention, as the ventricular response will be slow, and most will convert spontaneously during rewarming. The role of prophylaxis and treatment of ventricular arrhythmias is problematic. Preexisting ventricular ectopy may be suppressed by hypothermia, and reappear during rewarming. None of the class I agents has proved to be safe and efficacious. When available, bretylium tosylate was the class III ventricular antiarrhythmic of choice. Although class III agents such as bretylium possess direct antifibrillatory action, there is no evidence that amiodarone is safe.

Initiating empirical therapy for adrenal insufficiency is usually not

TABLE 19-3 *Options for Extracorporeal Rewarming*

Extracorporeal Rewarming (ECR) Technique	Considerations
Venovenous (VV)	Circuit—CV catheter to CV or peripheral catheter
	No oxygenator/circulatory support
	Flow rates 150–400 mL/min
	ROR 2°–3°C/h
Hemodialysis (HD)	Circuit—single-or dual-vessel cannulation
	Stabilizes electrolyte or toxicologic abnormalities
	Exchange cycle volumes 200–500 mL/min
	ROR 2°–3°C/h
Continuous arteriovenous rewarming (CAVR)	Circuit—percutaneous 8.5 Fr femoral catheters
	Requires BP 60 mmHg systolic
	No perfusionist/pump/anticoagulation
	Flow rates 225–375 mL/min
	ROR 3°–4°C/h
Cardiopulmonary bypass (CPB)	Circuit—full circulatory support with pump and oxygenator
	Perfusate-temperature gradient (5°–10°C)
	Flow rates 2–7 L/min (ave. 3–4)
	ROR up to 9.5°C/h

Note: BP, blood pressure; CV, central venous; ROR, rate of rewarming.

warranted unless there is a history suggesting steroid dependence, hypoadrenalism, or a failure to rewarm with standard therapy. However, the administration of parenteral levothyroxine to euthyroid patients with hypothermia is potentially hazardous. Because laboratory results can be delayed and confounded by the presence of the sick euthyroid syndrome (Chap. 320), historic clues or physical findings suggestive of hypothyroidism should be sought. When myxedema is the cause of hypothermia, the relaxation phase of the Achilles reflex is prolonged more than the contraction phase.

Hypothermia obscures most of the symptoms and signs of infection, notably fever and leukocytosis. Shaking rigors from infection may be mistaken for shivering. Except in mild cases, extensive cultures and repeated physical examinations are essential. Unless an infectious source is identified, empirical antibiotic prophylaxis is most warranted in the elderly, neonates, and immunocompromised patients.

Preventive measures should be discussed with high-risk individuals, such as the elderly or people whose work frequently exposes them to extreme cold. The importance of layered clothing and headgear, adequate shelter, increased caloric intake, and the avoidance of ethanol should be emphasized, along with access to rescue services.

FROSTBITE

Peripheral cold injuries include both freezing and nonfreezing injuries to tissue. Tissue freezes quickly when in contact with thermal conductors such as metal or volatile solutions. Other predisposing factors include constrictive clothing or boots, immobility, or vasoconstrictive medications. Frostbite occurs when the tissue temperature drops below 0°C. Ice crystal formation subsequently distorts and destroys the cellular architecture. Once the vascular endothelium is damaged, stasis progresses rapidly to microvascular thrombosis. After the tissue thaws, there is progressive dermal ischemia. The microvasculature begins to collapse, arteriovenous shunting increases tissue pressures, and edema forms. Finally, thrombosis, ischemia, and superficial necrosis appear. The development of mummification and demarcation may take weeks to months.

CLINICAL PRESENTATION

The initial presentation of frostbite can be deceptively benign. The symptoms always include a sensory deficiency affecting light touch, pain, and temperature perception. The acral areas and distal extremities are the most common insensate areas. Some patients complain of a clumsy or "chunk of wood" sensation in the extremity.

Deep frostbitten tissue can appear waxy, mottled, yellow, or violaceous-white. Favorable presenting signs include some warmth or sensation with normal color. The injury is often superficial if the subcutaneous tissue is pliable or if the dermis can be rolled over boney prominences.

Clinically, it is most practical to classify frostbite as superficial or deep. Superficial does not entail tissue loss. Classically, frostbite is retrospectively graded like a burn once the resultant pathology is demarcated over time. First-degree frostbite causes only anesthesia and erythema. The appearance of superficial vesiculation surrounded by edema and erythema is considered second degree (Fig. 19-1). Hemorrhagic vesicles reflect a serious injury to the microvasculature, and indicate third-degree frostbite. Fourth-degree injuries damage subcuticular, muscular, and osseous tissues.

The two most common nonfreezing peripheral cold injuries are *chilblain (pernio)* and *immersion (trench) foot*. Chilblain results from neuronal and endothelial damage induced by repetitive exposure to dry cold. Young females, particularly those with a history of Raynaud's phenomenon, are at greatest risk. Persistent vasospasticity and vasculitis can cause erythema, mild edema, and pruritus. Eventually plaques, blue nodules, and ulcerations develop. These lesions typically involve the dorsa of the hands and feet. In contrast, immersion (trench) foot results from repetitive exposure to wet cold above the freezing point. The feet initially appear cyanotic, cold, and edematous. The subsequent development of bullae is often indistinguishable from frostbite. This vesiculation rapidly progresses to ulceration and liquefaction gangrene. Patients with milder cases complain of hyperhidrosis, cold sensitivity, and painful ambulation for many years.

TABLE 19-4 Treatment for Frostbite

Before Thawing	During Thawing	After Thawing
Remove from environment	Consider parenteral analgesia and ketorolac	Gently dry and protect part; elevate; pledgets between toes, if macerated
Prevent partial thawing and refreezing	Administer ibuprofen, 400 mg PO	If clear vesicles are intact, aspirate or the fluid will reabsorb in days; if broken, debride and dress with antibiotic or sterile aloe vera ointment
Stabilize core temperature and treat hypothermia	Immerse part in 37°–40°C (thermometer-monitored) circulating water containing an antiseptic soap until distal flush (10–45 min)	Leave hemorrhagic vesicles intact to prevent dessication and infection
Protect frozen part — no friction or massage	Encourage patient to gently move part	Continue ibuprofen 400 mg PO (12 mg/kg per day) q8–12h
Address medical or surgical conditions	If pain is refractory, reduce water temperature to 33°–37°C and administer parenteral narcotics	Consider tetanus and streptococcal prophylaxis; elevate part Hydrotherapy at 37°C

℞ TREATMENT

Frozen tissue should be rapidly and completely thawed by immersion in circulating water at 37° to 40°C. Rapid rewarming often produces an initial hyperemia. The early formation of clear distal large blebs is more favorable than smaller proximal dark hemorrhagic blebs. A common error is the premature termination of thawing, since the reestablishment of perfusion is intensely painful. Parenteral narcotics will be necessary with deep frostbite. If cyanosis persists after rewarming, the tissue compartment pressures should be monitored carefully.

Numerous experimental antithrombotic and vasodilatory treatment regimens have been evaluated. There is no conclusive evidence that dextran, heparin, steroids, calcium channel blockers, or hyperbaric oxygen salvage tissue. A treatment protocol for frostbite is summarized in Table 19-4.

Unless infection develops, any decision regarding debridement or amputation should be deferred until there is clear evidence of demarcation, mummification, and sloughing. The most common symptomatic sequelae reflect neuronal injury and the persistently abnormal sympathetic tone, including paresthesias, thermal misperception, and hyperhidrosis. Delayed findings include nail deformities, cutaneous carcinomas, and epiphyseal damage in children.

FIGURE 19-1 Frostbite with vesiculation, surrounded by edema and erythema.

FURTHER READING

CAUCHY E et al: Retrospective study of 70 cases of severe frostbite lesions: A proposed new classification scheme. Wilderness Environ Med 12:248, 2001

DANZL DF: Hypothermia. Semin Respir Crit Care Med 23:57, 2002

GIESBRECHT GG: Cold stress, near drowning and accidental hypothermia: A review. Aviat Space Environ Med 71:733, 2000

VASSAL T et al: Severe accidental hypothermia treated in an ICU: Prognosis and outcome. Chest 120:1998, 2001

20 | SYNCOPE, FAINTNESS, DIZZINESS, AND VERTIGO
Robert B. Daroff, Mark D. Carlson

SYNCOPE

Syncope is defined as transient loss of consciousness due to reduced cerebral blood flow. Syncope is associated with postural collapse and spontaneous recovery. It may occur suddenly, without warning, or may be preceded by symptoms of faintness ("presyncope"). These include lightheadedness, "dizziness" without true vertigo, a feeling of warmth, diaphoresis, nausea, and visual blurring occasionally proceeding to blindness. Presyncopal symptoms vary in duration and may increase in severity until loss of consciousness occurs or may resolve prior to loss of consciousness if the cerebral ischemia is corrected. The differentiation of syncope from seizure is an important, sometimes difficult, diagnostic problem.

Syncope may be benign when it occurs as a result of normal cardiovascular reflex effects on heart rate and vascular tone, or serious when due to a life-threatening arrhythmia. Syncope may occur as a single event or may be recurrent. Recurrent, unexplained syncope, particularly in an individual with structural heart disease, is associated with a high risk of death (40% mortality within 2 years).

PATHOPHYSIOLOGY Syncope results from a sudden impairment of brain metabolism, usually brought about by hypotension with reduction of cerebral blood flow. Several mechanisms subserve circulatory adjustments to the upright posture. Approximately three-fourths of the systemic blood volume is contained in the venous bed, and any interference in venous return may lead to a reduction in cardiac output. Cerebral blood flow may still be maintained as long as systemic arterial vasoconstriction occurs, but when this adjustment fails, serious hypotension, with resultant cerebral underperfusion to less than half of normal, results in syncope. Normally, the pooling of blood in the lower parts of the body is prevented by (1) pressor reflexes that induce constriction of peripheral arterioles and venules, (2) reflex acceleration of the heart by means of aortic and carotid reflexes, and (3) improvement of venous return to the heart by activity of the muscles of the limbs. Tilting a normal person upright on a tilt table causes some blood to accumulate in the lower limbs and diminishes cardiac output slightly; this may be followed by a slight transitory fall in systolic blood pressure. In a patient with defective vasomotor reflexes, however, tilt table testing may produce an abrupt and sustained fall in blood pressure, precipitating a faint.

CAUSES OF SYNCOPE Transiently decreased cerebral blood flow is usually due to one of three general mechanisms: disorders of vascular tone or blood volume, cardiovascular disorders including cardiac arrhythmias, or cerebrovascular disease (Table 20-1). Not infrequently, however, the cause of syncope is multifactorial.

Disorders of Vascular Tone or Blood Volume Disorders of autonomic control of the heart and circulation share common pathophysiologic mechanisms: a cardioinhibitory component (e.g., bradycardia due to increased vagal activity), a vasodepressor component (e.g., inappropriate vasodilatation due to sympathetic withdrawal), or both.

NEUROCARDIOGENIC (VASOVAGAL AND VASODEPRESSOR) SYNCOPE The term *neurocardiogenic* is generally used to encompass both vasovagal and vasodepressor syncope. Strictly speaking, vasovagal syncope is associated with both sympathetic withdrawal (vasodilatation) and increased parasympathetic activity (bradycardia), whereas vasodepressor syncope is associated with sympathetic withdrawal alone.

These forms of syncope are the common faint that may be experienced by normal persons and account for approximately half of all episodes of syncope. Neurocardiogenic syncope is frequently recurrent and commonly precipitated by a hot or crowded environment, alcohol,

extreme fatigue, severe pain, hunger, prolonged standing, and emotional or stressful situations. Episodes are often preceded by a presyncopal prodrome lasting seconds to minutes, and rarely occur in the supine position. The individual is usually sitting or standing and experiences weakness, nausea, diaphoresis, lightheadedness, blurred vision, and often a forceful heart beat with tachycardia followed by cardiac slowing and decreasing blood pressure prior to loss of consciousness. The individual appears pale or ashen; in dark-skinned individuals, the pallor may only be notable in the conjunctivae and lips. Patients with a gradual onset of presyncopal symptoms have time to

---

TABLE 20-1 *Causes of Syncope*

I. Disorders of vascular tone or blood volume
  A. Vasovagal (vasodepressor, neurocardiogenic)
  B. Postural (orthostatic) hypotension
    1. Drug induced (especially antihypertensive or vasodilator drugs)
    2. Peripheral neuropathy (diabetic, alcoholic, nutritional, amyloid)
    3. Idiopathic postural hypotension
    4. Multisystem atrophies
    5. Physical deconditioning
    6. Sympathectomy
    7. Acute dysautonomia (Guillain-Barré syndrome variant)
    8. Decreased blood volume (adrenal insufficiency, acute blood loss, etc.)
  C. Carotid sinus hypersensitivity
  D. Situational
    1. Cough
    2. Micturition
    3. Defecation
    4. Valsalva
    5. Deglutition
  E. Glossopharyngeal neuralgia
II. Cardiovascular disorders
  A. Cardiac arrhythmias (Chaps. 213 and 214)
    1. Bradyarrhythmias
      a. Sinus bradycardia, sinoatrial block, sinus arrest, sick-sinus syndrome
        Atrioventricular block
    2. Tachyarrhythmias
      a. Supraventricular tachycardia with structural cardiac disease
      b. Atrial fibrillation associated with the Wolff-Parkinson-White syndrome
      c. Atrial flutter with 1:1 atrioventricular conduction
      d. Ventricular tachycardia
  B. Other cardiopulmonary etiologies
    1. Pulmonary embolism
    2. Pulmonary hypertension
    3. Atrial myxoma
    4. Myocardial disease (massive myocardial infarction)
    5. Left ventricular myocardial restriction or constriction
    6. Pericardial constriction or tamponade
    7. Aortic outflow tract obstruction
    8. Aortic valvular stenosis
    9. Hypertrophic obstructive cardiomyopathy
III. Cerebrovascular disease (Chap. 349)
  A. Vertebrobasilar insufficiency
  B. Basilar artery migraine
IV. Other disorders that may resemble syncope
  A. Metabolic
    1. Hypoxia
    2. Anemia
    3. Diminished carbon dioxide due to hyperventilation
    4. Hypoglycemia
  B. Psychogenic
    1. Anxiety attacks
    2. Hysterical fainting
  C. Seizures

protect themselves against injury; in others, syncope occurs suddenly, without warning.

The depth and duration of unconsciousness vary. Sometimes the patient remains partly aware of the surroundings, or there may be complete unresponsiveness. The unconscious patient usually lies motionless with skeletal muscles relaxed, but a few clonic jerks of the limbs and face may occur. Sphincter control is usually maintained, in contrast to a seizure. The pulse may be feeble or apparently absent, the blood pressure low or undetectable, and breathing may be almost imperceptible. The duration of unconsciousness is rarely longer than a few minutes if the conditions that provoke the episode are reversed. Once the patient is placed in a horizontal position, the strength of the pulse improves, color begins to return to the face, breathing becomes quicker and deeper, and consciousness is restored. Some patients may experience a sense of residual weakness after regaining consciousness, and rising too soon may precipitate another faint. Unconsciousness may be prolonged if an individual remains upright, thus it is essential that individuals with vasovagal syncope assume a recumbant position as soon as possible. Although commonly benign, neurocardiogenic syncope can be associated with prolonged asystole and hypotension, resulting in injury.

The syncope often occurs in this setting of increased peripheral sympathetic activity and venous pooling. Under these conditions, vigorous myocardial contraction of a relatively empty left ventricle activates myocardial mechanoreceptors and vagal afferent nerve fibers that inhibit sympathetic activity and increase parasympathetic activity. The resultant vasodilatation and bradycardia induce hypotension and syncope. Although the reflex involving myocardial mechanoreceptors is the mechanism usually accepted as responsible for neurocardiogenic syncope, other reflexes may also be operative. Patients with transplanted (denervated) hearts have experienced cardiovascular responses identical to those present during neurocardiogenic syncope. This should not be possible if the response depends solely on the reflex mechanisms described above, unless the transplanted heart has become reinnervated. Moreover, neurocardiogenic syncope often occurs in response to stimuli (fear, emotional stress, or pain) that may not be associated with venous pooling in the lower extremities, which suggests a cortical component to the reflex. Thus, a variety of afferent and efferent responses may cause neurocardiogenic syncope.

As distinct from the peripheral mechanisms, the central nervous system (CNS) mechanisms responsible for neurocardiogenic syncope are uncertain, but a sudden surge in central serotonin levels may contribute to the sympathetic withdrawal. Endogenous opiates (endorphins) and adenosine are also putative participants in the pathogenesis.

POSTURAL (ORTHOSTATIC) HYPOTENSION   This occurs in patients who have a chronic defect in, or variable instability of, vasomotor reflexes. Systemic arterial blood pressure falls on assumption of upright posture due to loss of vasoconstriction reflexes in resistance and capacitance vessels of the lower extremities. Although the syncopal attack differs little from vasodepressor syncope, the effect of posture is critical. Sudden rising from a recumbent position or standing quietly are precipitating circumstances. *Orthostatic hypotension may be the cause of syncope in up to 30% of the elderly; polypharmacy with antihypertensive or antidepressant drugs is often a contributor in these patients.*

Postural syncope may occur in otherwise normal persons with defective postural reflexes. Patients with *idiopathic postural hypotension* may be identified by a characteristic response to upright tilt on a table. Initially, the blood pressure diminishes slightly before stabilizing at a lower level. Shortly thereafter, the compensatory reflexes fail and the arterial pressure falls precipitously. The condition is often familial.

Orthostatic hypotension, often accompanied by disturbances in sweating, impotence, and sphincter difficulties, is also a primary feature of autonomic nervous system disorders (Chap. 354). The most common causes of neurogenic orthostatic hypotension are chronic diseases of the peripheral nervous system that involve postganglionic unmyelinated fibers (e.g., diabetic, nutritional, and amyloid polyneuropathy). Much less common are the multiple system atrophies; these

are CNS disorders in which orthostatic hypotension is associated with (1) parkinsonism (Shy-Drager syndrome), (2) progressive cerebellar degeneration, or (3) a more variable parkinsonian and cerebellar syndrome (striatonigral degeneration) (Chap. 351). A rare, acute postganglionic dysautonomia may represent a variant of Guillain-Barré syndrome (Chap. 365).

There are several additional causes of postural syncope: (1) After physical deconditioning (such as after prolonged illness with recumbency, especially in elderly individuals with reduced muscle tone) or after prolonged weightlessness, as in space flight; (2) after sympathectomy that has abolished vasopressor reflexes; and (3) in patients receiving antihypertensive or vasodilator drugs and those who are hypovolemic because of diuretics, excessive sweating, diarrhea, vomiting, hemorrhage, or adrenal insufficiency.

CAROTID SINUS HYPERSENSITIVITY   Syncope due to carotid sinus hypersensitivity is precipitated by pressure on the carotid sinus baroreceptors, which are located just cephalad to the bifurcation of the common carotid artery. This typically occurs in the setting of shaving, a tight collar, or turning the head to one side. Carotid sinus hypersensitivity occurs predominantly in men ≥50 years old. Activation of carotid sinus baroreceptors gives rise to impulses carried via the nerve of Hering, a branch of the glossopharyngeal nerve, to the medulla oblongata. These afferent impulses activate efferent sympathetic nerve fibers to the heart and blood vessels, cardiac vagal efferent nerve fibers, or both. In patients with carotid sinus hypersensitivity, these responses may cause sinus arrest or atrioventricular (AV) block (a cardioinhibitory response), vasodilatation (a vasodepressor response), or both (a mixed response). The mechanisms responsible for the syndrome are not clear, and validated diagnostic criteria do not exist; some authorities have questioned its very existence.

SITUATIONAL SYNCOPE   A variety of activities, including cough, deglutition, micturition, and defecation, are associated with syncope in susceptible individuals. These syndromes are caused, at least in part, by abnormal autonomic control and may involve a cardioinhibitory response, a vasodepressor response, or both. Cough, micturition, and defecation are associated with maneuvers (such as Valsalva, straining, and coughing) that may contribute to hypotension and syncope by decreasing venous return. Increased intracranial pressure secondary to the increased intrathoracic pressure may also contribute by decreasing cerebral blood flow.

Cough syncope typically occurs in men with chronic bronchitis or chronic obstructive lung disease during or after prolonged coughing fits. Micturition syncope occurs predominantly in middle-aged and older men, particularly those with prostatic hypertrophy and obstruction of the bladder neck; loss of consciousness usually occurs at night during or immediately after voiding. Deglutition syncope and defecation syncope occur in men and women. Deglutition syncope may be associated with esophageal disorders, particularly esophageal spasm. In some individuals, particular foods and carbonated or cold beverages initiate episodes by activating esophageal sensory receptors that trigger reflex sinus bradycardia or AV block. Defecation syncope is probably secondary to a Valsalva maneuver in older individuals with constipation.

GLOSSOPHARYNGEAL NEURALGIA   Syncope due to glossopharyngeal neuralgia (Chap. 355) is preceded by pain in the oropharynx, tonsillar fossa, or tongue. Loss of consciousness is usually associated with asystole rather than vasodilatation. The mechanism is thought to involve activation of afferent impulses in the glossopharyngeal nerve that terminate in the nucleus solitarius of the medulla and, via collaterals, activate the dorsal motor nucleus of the vagus nerve.

CARDIOVASCULAR DISORDERS   Cardiac syncope results from a sudden reduction in cardiac output, caused most commonly by a cardiac arrhythmia. In normal individuals, heart rates between 30 and 180 beats/min do not reduce cerebral blood flow, especially if the person is in the supine position. As the heart rate decreases, ventricular filling time and stroke volume increase to maintain normal cardiac output. At rates <30 beats/min, stroke volume can no longer increase to compensate adequately for the decreased heart rate. At rates greater than ~180 beats/min, ventricular filling time is inadequate to maintain adequate stroke volume. In either case, cerebral hypoperfusion and syncope may occur. Upright posture; cerebrovascular disease; anemia; loss of atrioventricular synchrony; and coronary, myocardial, or valvular disease all reduce the tolerance to alterations in rate.

Bradyarrhythmias (Chap. 213) may occur as a result of an abnormality of impulse generation (e.g., sinoatrial arrest) or impulse conduction (e.g., AV block). Either may cause syncope if the escape pacemaker rate is insufficient to maintain cardiac output. Syncope due to bradyarrhythmias may occur abruptly, without presyncopal symptoms, and recur several times daily. Patients with *sick sinus syndrome* may have sinus pauses (>3 s), and those with syncope due to high-degree AV block (*Stokes-Adams-Morgagni syndrome*) may have evidence of conduction system disease (e.g., prolonged PR interval, bundle branch block). However, the arrhythmia is often transitory, and the surface electrocardiogram or continuous electrocardiographic monitor (Holter monitor) taken later may not reveal the abnormality. The *bradycardia-tachycardia syndrome* is a common form of sinus node dysfunction in which syncope generally occurs as a result of marked sinus pauses, some following termination of paroxysms of atrial tachyarrhythmias. Drugs are a common cause for bradyarrhythmias, particularly in patients with underlying structural heart disease. Digoxin, β-adrenergic receptor antagonists, calcium channel blockers, and many antiarrhythmic drugs may suppress sinoatrial node impulse generation or slow AV nodal conduction.

Syncope due to a *tachyarrhythmia* (Chap. 214) is usually preceded by palpitation or lightheadedness but may occur abruptly with no warning symptoms. *Supraventricular tachyarrhythmias* are unlikely to cause syncope in individuals with structurally normal hearts but may if they occur in patients with (1) heart disease that also compromises cardiac output, (2) cerebrovascular disease, (3) a disorder of vascular tone or blood volume, or (4) a rapid ventricular rate. These tachycardias result most commonly from paroxysmal atrial flutter, atrial fibrillation, or reentry involving the AV node or accessory pathways that bypass part or all of the AV conduction system. Patients with the *Wolff-Parkinson-White syndrome* may experience syncope when a very rapid ventricular rate occurs due to reentry across an accessory AV connection.

In patients with structural heart disease, ventricular tachycardia is a common cause of syncope, particularly in patients with a prior myocardial infarction. Patients with aortic valvular stenosis and hypertrophic obstructive cardiomyopathy are also at risk for ventricular tachycardia. Individuals with abnormalities of ventricular repolarization (prolongation of the QT interval) are at risk to develop polymorphic ventricular tachycardia (*torsades de pointes*). Those with the inherited form of this syndrome often have a family history of sudden death in young individuals. Genetic markers can identify some patients with familial long-QT syndrome, but the clinical utility of these markers remains unproven. Drugs (i.e., certain antiarrhythmics and erythromycin) and electrolyte disorders (i.e., hypokalemia, hypocalcemia, hypomagnesemia) can prolong the QT interval and predispose to torsades de pointes. Antiarrhythmic medications may precipitate ventricular tachycardia, particularly in patients with structural heart disease.

In addition to arrhythmias, syncope may also occur with a variety of structural cardiovascular disorders. Episodes are usually precipitated when the cardiac output cannot increase to compensate adequately for peripheral vasodilatation. Peripheral vasodilatation may be appropriate, such as following exercise, or may occur due to inappropriate activation of left ventricular mechanoreceptor reflexes, as occurs in aortic outflow tract obstruction (aortic valvular stenosis or hypertrophic obstructive cardiomyopathy). Obstruction to forward flow is the most common reason that cardiac output cannot increase. Pericar-

dial tamponade is a rare cause of syncope. Syncope occurs in up to 10% of patients with massive pulmonary embolism and may occur with exertion in patients with severe primary pulmonary hypertension. The cause is an inability of the right ventricle to provide appropriate cardiac output in the presence of obstruction or increased pulmonary vascular resistance. Loss of consciousness is usually accompanied by other symptoms such as chest pain and dyspnea. Atrial myxoma, a prosthetic valve thrombus, and, rarely, mitral stenosis may impair left ventricular filling, decrease cardiac output, and cause syncope.

Cerebrovascular Disease   Cerebrovascular disease alone rarely causes syncope but may lower the threshold for syncope in patients with other causes. The vertebrobasilar arteries, which supply brainstem structures responsible for maintaining consciousness, are usually involved when cerebrovascular disease causes or contributes to syncope. An exception is the rare patient with tight bilateral carotid stenosis and recurrent syncope, often precipitated by standing or walking. Most patients who experience lightheadedness or syncope due to cerebrovascular disease also have symptoms of focal neurologic ischemia, such as arm or leg weakness, diplopia, ataxia, dysarthria, or sensory disturbances. Basilar artery migraine is a rare disorder that causes syncope in adolescents.

DIFFERENTIAL DIAGNOSIS ■ **Anxiety Attacks and the Hyperventilation Syndrome**
Anxiety, such as occurs in panic attacks, is frequently interpreted as a feeling of faintness or dizziness resembling presyncope. The symptoms are not accompanied by facial pallor and are not relieved by recumbency. The diagnosis is made on the basis of the associated symptoms such as a feeling of impending doom, air hunger, palpitations, and tingling of the fingers and perioral region. Attacks can often be reproduced by hyperventilation, resulting in hypocapnia, alkalosis, increased cerebrovascular resistance, and decreased cerebral blood flow. The release of epinephrine also contributes to the symptoms.

Seizures   A seizure may be heralded by an aura, which is caused by a focal seizure discharge and hence has localizing significance (Chap. 348). The aura is usually followed by a rapid return to normal or by a loss of consciousness. Injury from falling is frequent in a seizure and rare in syncope, since only in generalized seizures are protective reflexes abolished instantaneously. Sustained tonic-clonic movements are characteristic of convulsive seizures but brief clonic, or tonic-clonic, seizure-like activity can accompany fainting episodes. The period of unconsciousness tends to be longer in seizures than in syncope. Urinary incontinence is frequent in seizures and rare in syncope. The return of consciousness is prompt in syncope, slow after a seizure. Mental confusion, headache, and drowsiness are common sequelae of seizures, whereas physical weakness with a clear sensorium characterizes the postsyncopal state. Repeated spells of unconsciousness in a young person at a rate of several per day or month are more suggestive of epilepsy than syncope. See Table 348-7 for a comparison of seizures and syncope.

Hypoglycemia   Severe hypoglycemia is usually due to a serious disease such as a tumor of the islets of Langerhans; advanced adrenal, pituitary, or hepatic disease; or to excessive administration of insulin.

Acute Hemorrhage   Hemorrhage, usually within the gastrointestinal tract, is an occasional cause of syncope. In the absence of pain and hematemesis, the cause of the weakness, faintness, or even unconsciousness may remain obscure until the passage of a black stool.

Hysterical Fainting   The attack is usually unattended by an outward display of anxiety. Lack of change in pulse and blood pressure or color of the skin and mucous membranes distinguish it from the vasodepressor faint.

APPROACH TO THE PATIENT

The diagnosis of syncope is often challenging. The cause may only be apparent at the time of the event, leaving few, if any, clues when the patient is seen later by the physician. The physician should think first of those causes that constitute a therapeutic emergency. Among them are massive internal hemorrhage or myocardial infarction, which may be painless, and cardiac arrhythmias. In elderly persons, a sudden faint, without obvious cause, should arouse the suspicion of complete heart block or a tachyarrhythmia, even though all findings are negative when the patient is seen.

Figure 20-1 depicts an algorithmic approach to syncope. A careful history is the most important diagnostic tool, both to suggest the correct cause and to exclude important potential causes (Table 20-1). The nature of the events and their time course immediately prior to, during, and after an episode of syncope often provide valuable etiologic clues. Loss of consciousness in particular situations, such as during venipuncture, micturition, or with volume depletion, suggests an abnormality of vascular tone. The position of the patient at the time of the syncopal episode is important; syncope in the supine position is unlikely to be vasovagal and suggests an arrhythmia or a seizure. Syncope due to carotid sinus syndrome may occur when the individual is wearing a shirt with a tight collar, turning the head (turning to look while driving in reverse), or manipulating the neck (as in shaving). The patient's medications must be noted, including nonprescription drugs or health store supplements, with particular attention to recent changes.

The physical examination should include evaluation of heart rate and blood pressure in the supine, sitting, and standing positions. In patients with unexplained recurrent syncope, an attempt to reproduce an attack may assist in diagnosis. Anxiety attacks induced by hyperventilation can be reproduced readily by having the patient breathe rapidly and deeply for 2 to 3 min. Cough syncope may be reproduced by inducing the Valsalva maneuver. Carotid sinus massage should generally be avoided, even in patients with suspected carotid sinus hypersensitivity; it is a risky procedure that can cause a transient ischemic attack (TIA) or stroke in individuals with carotid atheromas.

Diagnostic Tests The choice of diagnostic tests should be guided by the history and the physical examination. Measurements of serum electrolytes, glucose, and the hematocrit are usually indicated. Cardiac enzymes should be evaluated if myocardial ischemia is suspected. Blood and urine toxicology screens may reveal the presence of alcohol or other drugs. In patients with possible adrenocortical insufficiency, plasma aldosterone and mineralocorticoid levels should be obtained.

Although the surface electrocardiogram is unlikely to provide a definitive diagnosis, it may provide clues to the cause of syncope *and should be performed in almost all patients*. The presence of conduction abnormalities (PR prolongation and bundle branch block) suggests a bradyarrhythmia, whereas pathologic Q waves or prolongation of the QT interval suggests a ventricular tachyarrhythmia. Inpatients should undergo continuous electrocardiographic monitoring; outpatients should wear a Holter monitor for 24 to 48 h. Whenever possible, symptoms should be correlated with the occurrence of arrhythmias. Continuous electrocardiographic monitoring may establish the cause of syncope in as many as 15% of patients. Cardiac event monitors may be useful in patients with infrequent symptoms, particularly in patients with presyncope. The presence of a late potential on a signal-averaged electrocardiogram is associated with increased risk for ventricular tacharrhythmias in patients with a prior myocardial infarction. Low-voltage (visually inapparent) T wave alternans is also associated with development of sustained ventricular arrhythmias.

Invasive cardiac electrophysiologic testing provides diagnostic and prognostic information regarding sinus node function, AV conduction, and supraventricular and ventricular arrhythmias (Chaps. 213 and 214). Prolongation of the sinus node recovery time (>1500 ms) is a specific finding (85 to 100%) for diagnosis of sinus node dysfunction but has a low sensitivity; continuous electrocardiographic monitoring is usually more effective for diagnosing this abnormality. Prolongation of the HV interval and conduction block below the His bundle indicate that His-Purkinje disease may be responsible for syncope. Programmed stimulation for ventricular arrhythmias is most useful in patients who have experienced a myocardial infarction; the sensitivity and specificity of this technique is lower in patients with normal hearts or those with heart disease other than coronary artery disease.

Upright tilt table testing is indicated for recurrent syncope, a single syncopal episode that caused injury, or a single syncopal event in a "high-risk" setting (pilot, commercial vehicle driver, etc.), whether or not there is a history of preexisting heart disease or prior vasovagal episodes. In susceptible patients, upright tilt at an angle between 60 and 80° for 30 to 60 min induces a vasovagal episode. The protocol can be shortened if upright tilt is combined with administration of drugs that cause venous pooling or increase adrenergic stimulation (isoproterenol, nitroglycerin, edrophonium, or adenosine). The sensitivity and specificity of tilt table testing is difficult to ascertain because of the lack of validated criteria. Moreover, the reflexes responsible for vasovagal syncope can be elicited in most, if not all, individuals given the appropriate stimulus. The reported accuracy of the test ranges from 30 to 80%, depending on the population studied and the techniques used. Whereas the reproducibility of a negative test is 85 to 100%, the reproducibility of a positive tilt table test is only between 62 and 88%.

A variety of other tests may be useful to determine the presence of structural heart disease that may cause syncope. The echocardiogram with Doppler examination detects valvular, myocardial, and pericardial abnormalities. The echocardiogram is the "gold standard" for the diagnosis of hypertrophic cardiomyopathy and atrial myxoma. Cardiac cine magnetic resonance (MR) imaging provides an alternative noninvasive modality that may be useful for patients in whom diagnostic-quality echocardiographic images cannot be obtained. This test is also indicated for patients suspected of having arrhythmogenic right ventricular dysplasia or right ventricular outflow tract ventricular tachycardia. Both are associated

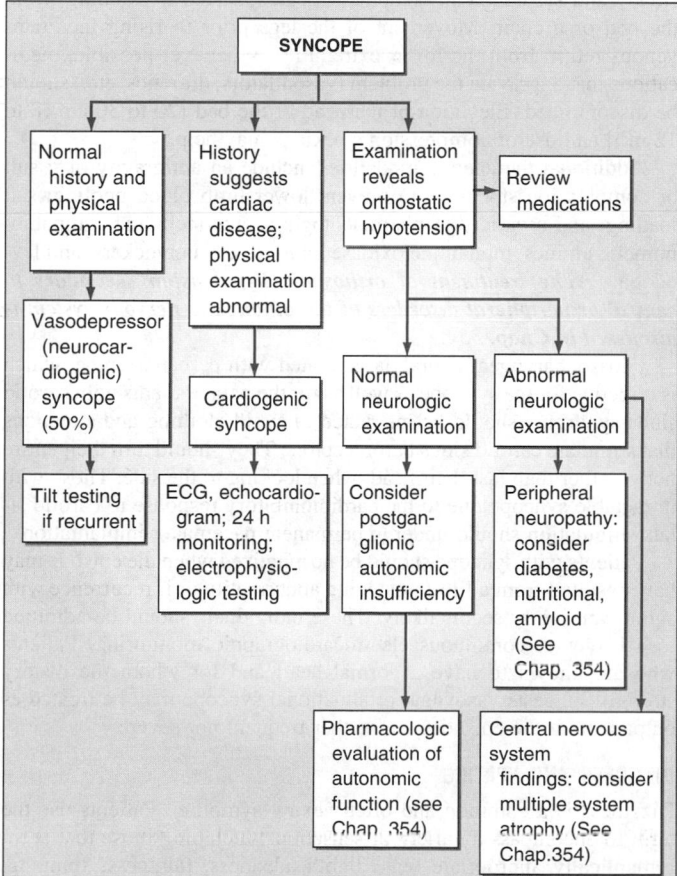

FIGURE 20-1 Approach to the patient with syncope.

with right ventricular structural abnormalities that are better visualized on MR imaging than by echocardiogram. Exercise testing may detect ischemia or exercise-induced arrhythmias. In some patients, cardiac catheterization may be necessary to diagnose the presence or severity of coronary artery disease or valvular abnormalities. Ultrafast computed tomographic scan, ventilation-perfusion scan, or pulmonary angiography is indicated in patients in whom syncope may be due to pulmonary embolus.

In possible cases of cerebrovascular syncope neuroimaging tests may be indicated, including Doppler ultrasound studies of the carotid and vertebrobasilar systems, MR imaging, MR angiography, and x-ray angiography of the cerebral vasculature (Chap. 349). Electroencephalography is indicated if seizures are suspected.

R̲x̲ TREATMENT

The treatment of syncope is directed toward the underlying cause. This discussion will focus on disorders of autonomic control. →*Arrhythmias are discussed in Chaps. 213 and 214, valvular heart diseases in Chap. 219, and cerebrovascular disorders in Chap. 349.*

Certain precautions should be taken regardless of the cause of syncope. At the first sign of symptoms, patients should make every effort to avoid injury should they lose consciousness. Patients with frequent episodes, or those who have experienced syncope without warning symptoms, should avoid situations in which sudden loss of consciousness might result in injury (e.g., climbing ladders, swimming alone, operating heavy machinery, driving). Patients should lower their head to the extent possible and preferably should lie down. Lowering the head by bending at the waist should be avoided because it may further compromise venous return to the heart. When appropriate, family members or other close contacts should be educated as to the problem. This will ensure appropriate therapy and may prevent delivery of inappropriate therapy (chest compressions associated with cardiopulmonary resuscitation) that may inflict trauma.

Patients who have lost consciousness should be placed in a position that maximizes cerebral blood flow, offers protection from trauma, and secures the airway. Whenever possible, the patient should be placed supine with the head turned to the side to prevent aspiration and the tongue from blocking the airway. Assessment of the pulse and direct cardiac auscultation may assist in determining if the episode is associated with a bradyarrhythmia or tachyarrhythmia. Clothing that fits tightly around the neck or waist should be loosened. Peripheral stimulation, such as by sprinkling cold water on the face, may be helpful. Patients should not be given anything by mouth or be permitted to rise until the sense of physical weakness has passed.

Patients with vasovagal syncope should be instructed to avoid situations or stimuli that have caused them to lose consciousness and to assume a recumbent position when premonitory symptoms occur. These behavioral modifications alone may be sufficient for patients with infrequent and relatively benign episodes of vasovagal syncope, particularly when loss of consciousness occurs in response to a specific stimulus. Tilt training (standing and leaning against a wall for progressively longer periods each day) has been used with limited success, particularly for those patients who have profound orthostatic intolerance. Episodes associated with intravascular volume depletion may be prevented by salt and fluid loading prior to provocative events.

Prescription drug therapy may be necessary when vasovagal syncope is resistant to these measures, when episodes occur frequently, or when syncope is associated with a significant risk for injury. β-Adrenergic receptor antagonists (metoprolol, 25 to 50 mg bid; atenolol, 25 to 50 mg qd; or nadolol, 10 to 20 mg bid; all starting doses), the most widely used agents, mitigate the increase in myocardial contractility that stimulates left ventricular mechanoreceptors and also block central serotonin receptors. Serotonin reuptake inhibitors (paroxetine, 20 to 40 mg qd; or sertraline, 25 to 50 mg qd), appear to be

effective for some patients. Bupropion SR (150 mg qd), another antidepressant, has also been used with success. β-Adrenergic receptor antagonists and serotonin reuptake inhibitors are well tolerated and are often used as first-line agents for younger patients. Hydrofludrocortisone (0.1 to 0.2 mg qd), a mineralocorticoid, promotes sodium retention, volume expansion, and peripheral vasoconstriction by increasing β-receptor sensitivity to endogenous catecholamines. Hydrofludrocortisone is useful for patients with intravascular volume depletion and those who also have postural hypotension. Proamatine (2.5 to 10 mg bid or tid), an α-agonist, has been used as a first-line agent for some patients. In a recent randomized controlled trial, proamatine was more effective than placebo in preventing syncope during an upright tilt-test. However, in some patients, proamatine and hydrofludrocortisone may increase resting supine systemic blood pressure, a property that may be problematic for those with hypertension.

Disopyramide (150 mg bid), a vagolytic antiarrhythmic drug with negative inotropic properties, and another vagolytic, transdermal scopolamine, have been used to treat vasovagal syncope, as have theophylline and ephedrine. Side effects associated with these drugs have limited their use for this indication. Disopyramide is a type 1A antiarrhythmic drug and should be used with great caution, if at all, in patients who are at risk for ventricular arrhythmias. Although several clinical trials have suggested that pharmacologic therapy for vasovagal syncope is effective, long-term prospective randomized controlled trials have yet to be completed.

Permanent dual-chamber cardiac pacing is effective for patients with frequent episodes of vasovagal syncope and is indicated for those with prolonged asystole associated with vasovagal episodes. Patients in whom vasodilatation contributes to loss of consciousness may also experience symptomatic benefit from permanent pacing. Pacemakers that can be programmed to transiently pace at a high rate (90 to 100 beats/min) after a profound drop in the patient's intrinsic heart rate are most effective.

Patients with orthostatic hypotension should be instructed to rise slowly and systematically (supine to seated, seated to standing) from the bed or a chair. Movement of the legs prior to rising facilitates venous return from the lower extremities. Whenever possible, medications that aggravate the problem (vasodilators, diuretics, etc.) should be discontinued. Elevation of the head of the bed [20 to 30 cm (8 to 12 in.)] and use of compression stockings may help.

Additional therapeutic modalities include an antigravity or g suit or compression stockings to prevent lower limb blood pooling; salt loading; and a variety of pharmacologic agents including sympathomimetic amines, monamine oxidase inhibitors, beta blockers, and levodopa. →*The treatment of orthostatic hypotension secondary to central or peripheral disorders of the autonomic nervous system is discussed in Chap. 354.*

Glossopharyngeal neuralgia is treated with carbamazepine, which is effective for the syncope as well as for the pain. Patients with carotid sinus syndrome should be instructed to avoid clothing and situations that stimulate carotid sinus baroreceptors. They should turn their entire body, rather than just their head, when looking to the side. Those with intractable syncope due to the cardioinhibitory response to carotid sinus stimulation should undergo permanent pacemaker implantation.

Patients with syncope should be hospitalized when the episode may have resulted from a life-threatening abnormality or if recurrence with significant injury seems likely. These individuals should be admitted to a bed with continuous electrocardiographic monitoring. Patients who are known to have a normal heart and for whom the history strongly suggests vasovagal or situational syncope may be treated as outpatients if the episodes are neither frequent nor severe.

DIZZINESS AND VERTIGO

Dizziness is a common and often vexing symptom. Patients use the term to encompass a variety of sensations, including those that seem semantically appropriate (e.g., lightheadedness, faintness, spinning, giddiness) and those that are misleadingly inappropriate, such as mental confusion, blurred vision, headache, or tingling. Moreover, some individuals with gait disorders caused by peripheral neuropathy, myelopathy, spasticity, parkinsonism, or cerebellar ataxia complain of "dizziness" despite the absence of vertigo or other abnormal cephalic sensations. In this context, the term *dizziness* is being used to describe disturbed ambulation. There may be mild associated lightheadedness, particularly with impaired sensation from the feet or poor vision; this is known as *multiple-sensory-defect dizziness* and occurs in elderly individuals who complain of dizziness only when walking. Decreased position sense (secondary to neuropathy or myelopathy) and poor vision (from cataracts or retinal degeneration) create an overreliance on the aging vestibular apparatus. A less precise but sometimes comforting designation to patients is *benign dysequilibrium of aging*. Thus, a careful history is necessary to determine exactly what a patient who states, "Doctor, I'm dizzy," is experiencing. After eliminating the misleading symptoms or gait disturbance, "dizziness" usually means either *faintness* (presyncope) or *vertigo* (an illusory or hallucinatory sense of movement of the body or environment, most often a feeling of spinning). Operationally, after obtaining the history, dizziness may be classified into three categories: (1) faintness, (2) vertigo, and (3) miscellaneous head sensations.

FAINTNESS   Prior to an actual faint (syncope), there are often prodromal presyncopal symptoms (faintness) reflecting ischemia to a degree insufficient to impair consciousness (see above).

VERTIGO   Vertigo is usually due to a disturbance in the vestibular system. The end organs of this system, situated in the bony labyrinths of the inner ears, consist of the three semicircular canals and the otolithic apparatus (utricle and saccule) on each side. The canals transduce angular acceleration, while the otoliths transduce linear acceleration and the static gravitational forces that provide a sense of head position in space. The neural output of the end organs is conveyed to the vestibular nuclei in the brainstem via the eighth cranial nerves. The principal projections from the vestibular nuclei are to the nuclei of cranial nerves III, IV, and VI; spinal cord; cerebral cortex; and cerebellum. The vestibulooocular reflex (VOR) serves to maintain visual stability during head movement and depends on direct projections from the vestibular nuclei to the sixth cranial nerve (abducens) nuclei in the pons and, via the medial longitudinal fasciculus, to the third (oculomotor) and fourth (trochlear) cranial nerve nuclei in the midbrain. These connections account for the nystagmus (to-and-fro oscillation of the eyes) that is an almost invariable accompaniment of vestibular dysfunction. The vestibular nerves and nuclei project to areas of the cerebellum (primarily the flocculus and nodulus) that modulate the VOR. The vestibulospinal pathways assist in the maintenance of postural stability. Projections to the cerebral cortex, via the thalamus, provide conscious awareness of head position and movement.

The vestibular system is one of three sensory systems subserving spatial orientation and posture; the other two are the visual system (retina to occipital cortex) and the somatosensory system that conveys peripheral information from skin, joint, and muscle receptors. The three stabilizing systems overlap sufficiently to compensate (partially or completely) for each other's deficiencies. Vertigo may represent either physiologic stimulation or pathologic dysfunction in any of the three systems.

Physiologic Vertigo   This occurs in normal individuals when (1) the brain is confronted with a mismatch among the three stabilizing sensory systems; (2) the vestibular system is subjected to unfamiliar head movements to which it is unadapted, such as in seasickness; (3) unusual head/neck positions, such as the extreme extension when painting a ceiling; or (4) following a spin. Intersensory mismatch explains carsickness, height vertigo, and the visual vertigo most commonly experienced during motion picture chase scenes; in the latter, the visual sensation of environmental movement is unaccompanied by concomitant vestibular and somatosensory movement cues. *Space sickness*, a frequent transient effect of active head movement in the weightless zero-gravity environment, is another example of physiologic vertigo.

Pathologic Vertigo   This results from lesions of the visual, somatosensory, or vestibular systems. Visual vertigo is caused by new or incorrect spectacles or by the sudden onset of an extraocular muscle paresis with diplopia; in either instance, CNS compensation rapidly counteracts the vertigo. Somatosensory vertigo, rare in isolation, is usually due to a peripheral neuropathy or myelopathy that reduces the sensory input necessary for central compensation when there is dysfunction of the vestibular or visual systems.

The most common cause of pathologic vertigo is vestibular dysfunction involving either its end organ (labyrinth), nerve, or central connections. The vertigo is frequently accompanied by nausea, jerk nystagmus, postural unsteadiness, and gait ataxia. Since vertigo increases with rapid head movements, patients tend to hold their heads still.

LABYRINTHINE DYSFUNCTION   This causes severe rotational or linear vertigo. When rotational, the hallucination of movement, whether of environment or self, is directed away from the side of the lesion. The fast phases of nystagmus beat away from the lesion side, and the tendency to fall is toward the side of the lesion, particularly in darkness or with the eyes closed.

Under normal circumstances, when the head is straight and immobile, the vestibular end organs generate a tonic resting firing frequency that is equal from the two sides. With any rotational acceleration, the anatomic positions of the semicircular canals on each side necessitate an increased firing rate from one and a commensurate decrease from the other. This change in neural activity is ultimately projected to the cerebral cortex, where it is summed with inputs from the visual and somatosensory systems to produce the appropriate conscious sense of rotational movement. After cessation of movement, the firing frequencies of the two end organs reverse; the side with the initially increased rate decreases, and the other side increases. A sense of rotation in the opposite direction is experienced; since there is no actual head movement, this hallucinatory sensation is *physiologic postrotational vertigo*.

Any disease state that changes the firing frequency of an end organ, producing unequal neural input to the brainstem and ultimately the cerebral cortex, causes vertigo. The symptom can be conceptualized as the cortex inappropriately interpreting the abnormal neural input as indicating actual head rotation. Transient abnormalities produce short-lived symptoms. With a fixed unilateral deficit, central compensatory mechanisms ultimately diminish the vertigo. Since compensation depends on the plasticity of connections between the vestibular nuclei and the cerebellum, patients with brainstem or cerebellar disease have diminished adaptive capacity, and symptoms may persist indefinitely. Compensation is always inadequate for severe fixed bilateral lesions despite normal cerebellar connections: these patients are permanently symptomatic.

Acute unilateral labyrinthine dysfunction is caused by infection, trauma, and ischemia. Often, no specific etiology is uncovered, and the nonspecific terms *acute labyrinthitis*, *acute peripheral vestibulopathy*, or *vestibular neuritis* are used to describe the event. The vertiginous attacks are brief and leave the patient with mild vertigo for several days. Infection with herpes simplex virus type 1 has been implicated. It is impossible to predict whether a patient recovering from the first bout of vertigo will have recurrent episodes.

Labyrinthine ischemia, presumably due to occlusion of the labyrinthine branch of the internal auditory artery, may be the sole manifestation of vertebrobasilar insufficiency (Chap. 349); patients with this syndrome present with the abrupt onset of severe vertigo, nausea, and vomiting, but without tinnitus or hearing loss.

Acute bilateral labyrinthine dysfunction is usually the result of toxins such as drugs or alcohol. The most common offending drugs are the aminoglycoside antibiotics that damage the hair cells of the vestibular end organs and may cause a permanent disorder of equilibrium.

Recurrent unilateral labyrinthine dysfunction, in association with signs and symptoms of cochlear disease (progressive hearing loss and tinnitus), is usually due to Ménière's disease (Chap. 26). When auditory manifestations are absent, the term *vestibular neuronitis* denotes recurrent monosymptomatic vertigo. TIAs of the posterior cerebral circulation (vertebrobasilar insufficiency) only infrequently cause recurrent vertigo without concomitant motor, sensory, visual, cranial nerve, or cerebellar signs (Chap. 349).

Positional vertigo is precipitated by a recumbent head position, either to the right or to the left. Benign paroxysmal positional (or positioning) vertigo (BPPV) of the posterior semicircular canal is particularly common. Although the condition may be due to head trauma, usually no precipitating factors are identified. It generally abates spontaneously after weeks or months. The vertigo and accompanying nystagmus have a distinct pattern of latency, fatigability, and habituation that differs from the less common central positional vertigo (Table 20-2) due to lesions in and around the fourth ventricle. Moreover, the pattern of nystagmus in posterior canal BPPV is distinctive. When supine, with the head turned to the side of the offending ear (bad ear down), the lower eye displays a large-amplitude torsional nystagmus, and the upper eye has a lesser degree of torsion combined with upbeating nystagmus. If the eyes are directed to the upper ear, the vertical nystagmus in the upper eye increases in amplitude. Mild dysequilibrium when upright may also be present.

A *perilymphatic fistula* should be suspected when episodic vertigo is precipitated by Valsalva or exertion, particularly upon a background of a stepwise progressive sensory-neural hearing loss. The condition is usually caused by head trauma or barotrauma or occurs after middle ear surgery.

VERTIGO OF VESTIBULAR NERVE ORIGIN This occurs with diseases that involve the nerve in the petrous bone or the cerebellopontine angle. Although less severe and less frequently paroxysmal, it has many of the characteristics of labyrinthine vertigo. The adjacent auditory division of the eighth cranial nerve is usually affected, which explains the frequent association of vertigo with unilateral tinnitus and hearing loss. The most common cause of eighth cranial nerve dysfunction is a tumor, usually a schwannoma (*acoustic neuroma*) or a meningioma. These tumors grow slowly and produce such a gradual reduction of labyrinthine output that central compensatory mechanisms can prevent or minimize the vertigo; auditory symptoms of hearing loss and tinnitus are the most common manifestations.

CENTRAL VERTIGO Lesions of the brainstem or cerebellum can cause acute vertigo, but associated signs and symptoms usually permit distinction from a labyrinthine etiology (Table 20-3). Occasionally, an acute lesion of the vestibulocerebellum may present with monosymptomatic vertigo indistinguishable from a labyrinthopathy.

Vertigo may be a manifestation of a migraine aura (Chap. 14), but some patients with migraine have episodes of vertigo unassociated with their headaches. Antimigrainous treatment should be considered in such patients with otherwise enigmatic vertiginous episodes.

Vestibular epilepsy, vertigo secondary to temporal lobe epileptic activity, is rare and almost always intermixed with other epileptic manifestations.

TABLE 20-2 *Benign Paroxysmal Positional Vertigo and Central Positional Vertigo*

Features	BPPV	Central
Latency[a]	3–40 s	None: immediate vertigo and nystagmus
Fatigability[b]	Yes	No
Habituation[c]	Yes	No
Intensity of vertigo	Severe	Mild
Reproducibility[d]	Variable	Good

[a] Time between attaining head position and onset of symptoms.
[b] Disappearance of symptoms with maintenance of offending position.
[c] Lessening of symptoms with repeated trials.
[d] Likelihood of symptom production during any examination session.

TABLE 20-3 *Differentiation of Peripheral and Central Vertigo*

Sign or Symptom	Peripheral (Labyrinth)	Central (Brainstem or Cerebellum)
Direction of associated nystagmus	Unidirectional; fast phase opposite lesion[a]	Bidirectional or unidirectional
Purely horizontal nystagmus without torsional component	Uncommon	Common
Vertical or purely torsional nystagmus	Never present	May be present
Visual fixation	Inhibits nystagmus and vertigo	No inhibition
Severity of vertigo	Marked	Often mild
Direction of spin	Toward fast phase	Variable
Direction of fall	Toward slow phase	Variable
Duration of symptoms	Finite (minutes, days, weeks) but recurrent	May be chronic
Tinnitus and/or deafness	Often present	Usually absent
Associated central abnormalities	None	Extremely common
Common causes	Infection (labyrinthitis), Ménière's, neuronitis, ischemia, trauma, toxin	Vascular, demyelinating, neoplasm

[a] In Ménière's disease, the direction of the fast phase is variable.

PSYCHOGENIC VERTIGO This is usually a concomitant of panic attacks (Chap. 371) or agoraphobia (fear of large open spaces, crowds, or leaving the safety of home) and should be suspected in patients so "incapacitated" by their symptoms that they adopt a prolonged housebound status. Most patients with organic vertigo attempt to function despite their discomfort. Organic vertigo is accompanied by nystagmus; a psychogenic etiology is almost certain when nystagmus is absent during a vertiginous episode.

Miscellaneous Head Sensations This designation is used, primarily for purposes of initial classification, to describe dizziness that is neither faintness nor vertigo. Cephalic ischemia or vestibular dysfunction may be of such low intensity that the usual symptomatology is not clearly identified. For example, a small decrease in blood pressure or a slight vestibular imbalance may cause sensations different from distinct faintness or vertigo but that may be identified properly during provocative testing techniques (see below). Other causes of dizziness in this category are hyperventilation syndrome, hypoglycemia, and the somatic symptoms of a clinical depression; these patients should all have normal neurologic examinations and vestibular function tests. Depressed patients often insist that the depression is "secondary" to the dizziness.

APPROACH TO THE PATIENT

The most important diagnostic tool is a detailed history focused on the meaning of "dizziness" to the patient. Is it faintness (presyncope)? Is there a sensation of spinning? If either of these is affirmed and the neurologic examination is normal, appropriate investigations for the multiple causes of cephalic ischemia or vestibular dysfunction are undertaken.

When the meaning of "dizziness" is uncertain, provocative tests may be helpful. These office procedures simulate either cephalic ischemia or vestibular dysfunction. Cephalic ischemia is obvious if the dizziness is duplicated during maneuvers that produce orthostatic hypotension. Further provocation involves the Valsalva maneuver, which decreases cerebral blood flow and should reproduce ischemic symptoms.

Hyperventilation is the cause of dizziness in many anxious individuals; tingling of the hands and face may be absent. Forced hyperventilation for 1 min is indicated for patients with enigmatic dizziness and normal neurologic examinations.

The simplest provocative test for vestibular dysfunction is rapid rotation and abrupt cessation of movement in a swivel chair. This always induces vertigo that the patients can compare with their symptomatic dizziness. The intense induced vertigo may be unlike the spontaneous symptoms, but shortly thereafter, when the vertigo has all but subsided, a lightheadedness supervenes that may be identified as "my dizziness." When this occurs, the dizzy patient, originally classified as suffering from "miscellaneous head sensations," is now properly diagnosed as having mild vertigo secondary to a vestibulopathy.

Patients with symptoms of positional vertigo should be appropriately tested (Table 20-2). A final provocative and diagnostic vestibular test, requiring the use of Frenzel eyeglasses (self-illuminated goggles with convex lenses that blur out the patient's vision, but allow the examiner to see the eyes greatly magnified), is vigorous head shaking in the horizontal plane for about 10 s. If nystagmus develops after the shaking stops, even in the absence of vertigo, vestibular dysfunction is demonstrated. The maneuver can then be repeated in the vertical plane. If the provocative tests establish the dizziness as a vestibular symptom, an evaluation of vestibular vertigo is undertaken.

Evaluation of Patients with Pathologic Vestibular Vertigo The evaluation depends on whether a central etiology is suspected (Table 20-3). If so, MR imaging of the head is mandatory. Such an examination is rarely helpful in cases of recurrent monosymptomatic vertigo with a normal neurologic examination. Typical BPPV requires no investigation after the diagnosis is made (Table 20-2).

Vestibular function tests serve to (1) demonstrate an abnormality when the distinction between organic and psychogenic is uncertain, (2) establish the side of the abnormality, and (3) distinguish between peripheral and central etiologies. The standard test is electronystagmography (calorics), where warm and cold water (or air) are applied, in a prescribed fashion, to the tympanic membranes, and the slow-phase velocities of the resultant nystagmus from the two are compared. A velocity decrease from one side indicates hypofunction ("canal paresis"). An inability to induce nystagmus with ice water denotes a "dead labyrinth." Some institutions have the capability of quantitatively determining various aspects of the VOR using computer-driven rotational chairs and precise oculographic recording of the eye movements.

CNS disease can produce dizzy sensations of all types. Consequently, a neurologic examination is always required even if the history or provocative tests suggest a cardiac, peripheral vestibular, or psychogenic etiology. Any abnormality on the neurologic examination should prompt appropriate neurodiagnostic studies.

℞ TREATMENT

Treatment of acute vertigo consists of bed rest (1 to 2 days maximum) and vestibular suppressant drugs such as antihistaminics (meclizine, dimenhydrinate, promethazine), tranquilizers with GABA-ergic effects (diazepam, clonazepam), phenothiazines (prochlorperazine), or glucocorticoids (Table 20-4). If the vertigo persists beyond a few days, most authorities advise ambulation in an attempt to induce central compensatory mechanisms, despite the short-term discomfort to the patient. Chronic vertigo of labyrinthine origin may be treated with a systematized vestibular rehabilitation program to facilitate central compensation.

BPPV is often self-limited but, when persistent, may respond dramatically to specific repositioning exercise programs designed to empty particulate debris from the posterior semicircular canal. One of

TABLE 20-4 *Treatment of Vertigo*

Agent[a]	Dose[b]
Antihistamines	
Meclizine	25–50 mg 3 times/day
Dimenhydrinate	50 mg 1–2 times/day
Promethazine[c]	25–50-mg suppository or IM
Benzodiazepines	
Diazepam	2.5 mg 1–3 times/day
Clonazepam	0.25 mg 1–3 times/day
Phenothiazines	
Prochlorperazine[c]	5 mg IM or 25-mg suppository
Anticholinergic[d]	
Scopolamine transdermal	Patch
Sympathomimetics[d]	
Ephedrine	25 mg/d
Combination preparations[d]	
Ephedrine and promethazine	25 mg/d of each
Exercise therapy	
Repositioning maneuvers[e]	
Vestibular rehabilitation[f]	
Other	
Diuretics or low-salt (1 g/d) diet[g]	
Antimigrainous drugs[h]	
Inner ear surgery[i]	
Glucocorticoids[c]	

[a] All listed drugs are U.S. Food and Drug Administration approved, but most are not approved for the treatment of vertigo.
[b] Usual oral (unless otherwise stated) starting dose in adults; maintenance dose can be reached by a gradual increase.
[c] For acute vertigo only.
[d] For motion sickness only.
[e] For benign paroxysmal positional vertigo.
[f] For vertigo other than Ménière's and positional.
[g] For Ménière's disease.
[h] For migraine-associated vertigo (see Chap. 14 for a listing of prophylactic antimigrainous drugs).
[i] For perilymphatic fistula and refractory cases of Ménière's disease.

these exercises, the Epley procedure, is graphically demonstrated, in four languages, on a website for use in both physician's offices and self-treatment (*www.charite.de/ch/neuro/vertigo.html*).

Prophylactic measures to prevent recurrent vertigo are variably effective. Antihistamines are commonly utilized but are of limited value. Ménière's disease may respond to a diuretic or, more effectively, to a very low salt diet (1 g/d). Recurrent episodes of migraine-associated vertigo should be treated with antimigrainous therapy (Chap. 14). There are a variety of inner ear surgical procedures for refractory Ménière's disease, but these are only rarely necessary.

Helpful websites for both physicians and vertigo patients are: *www.iVertigo.net* and *www.tchain.com*.

FURTHER READING

KAPOOR WN: Current evaluation in management of syncope. Circulation 106: 1606, 2002

KAUFMAN H et al: Midodrine in neurally mediated syncope: A double-blind, randomized, crossover study. Ann Neurol 52:342, 2002

KAUFMAN NH, BHATTACHARYA K: Diagnosis and treatment of neurally mediated syncope. The Neurologist 8:175, 2002

MAISEL W, STEBENSON W: Syncope—getting to the heart of the matter. N Engl J Med 347:931, 2002

SOTERIADES E et al: Incidence and prognosis of syncope. N Engl J Med 347: 878, 2002

Normal motor function requires integrated muscle activity with appropriate modulation by neuronal activity in the cerebral cortex, basal ganglia, cerebellum, and spinal cord. Symptoms and signs of motor system dysfunction may include weakness, fatigue, myalgias, spasms, cramps, dyskinetic movement, ataxia, imbalance, or disorders in the initiation or planning of movement.

WEAKNESS

Weakness is a reduction in normal power of one or more muscles. Limitation in rising from a seated position or combing hair suggests proximal weakness, whereas slapping of the feet while walking or limitation in opening jars suggests distal weakness. Increased fatigability or limitation in function due to pain is often confused with weakness by patients. *Increased fatigability* is the inability to sustain the performance of an activity that should be normal for a person of the same age, gender, and size.

Paralysis and the suffix "-plegia" indicate weakness that is so severe that it is complete or nearly complete. "Paresis" refers to weakness that is mild or moderate. The prefix "hemi-" refers to one half of the body, "para-" to both legs, and "quadri-" to all four limbs.

Tone is the resistance of a muscle to passive stretch. Central nervous system (CNS) abnormalities that cause weakness generally produce *spasticity*, an increase in tone due to upper motor neuron disease. Spasticity is velocity-dependent, has a sudden release after reaching a maximum (the "clasp-knife" phenomenon), and predominantly affects antigravity muscles (i.e., upper limb flexors and lower limb extensors). Spasticity is distinct from rigidity and paratonia, two other types of increased tone. *Rigidity* is increased tone that is present throughout the range of motion (a "lead pipe" or "plastic" stiffness) and affects flexors and extensors equally. In some patients, rigidity has a cogwheel quality that is enhanced by voluntary movement of the contralateral limb (reinforcement). Rigidity occurs with certain extrapyramidal disorders such as Parkinson's disease. *Paratonia*, also referred to as *gegenhalten*, is increased tone that varies irregularly in a manner that may seem related to the degree of relaxation, is present throughout the range of motion, and affects flexors and extensors equally. Paratonia usually results from disease of the frontal lobes. Weakness with decreased tone (flaccidity) or normal tone occurs with disorders of the *motor unit*, that is, a single lower motor neuron and all of the muscle fibers it innervates.

Three basic patterns of weakness can usually be recognized based on the signs summarized in Table 21-1. One results from upper motor neuron pathology, and the other two from disorders of the motor unit (lower motor neuron and myopathic weakness). Fasciculations and early atrophy help to distinguish lower motor neuron (neurogenic) weakness from myopathic weakness. A *fasciculation* is a visible or palpable twitch within a single muscle due to the spontaneous discharge of one motor unit. Lower motor neuron weakness also produces more prominent hypotonia and greater depression of tendon reflexes than does myopathic weakness.

PATHOGENESIS ■ Upper Motor Neuron Weakness This pattern of weakness results from disorders that affect the upper motor neurons or their axons in the cerebral cortex, subcortical white matter, internal capsule, brainstem, or spinal cord (Fig. 21-1). Upper motor neuron lesions produce weakness through decreased activation of the lower motor neurons. In general, distal muscle groups are affected more severely than proximal ones, and axial movements are spared unless the lesion is severe and bilateral. With corticobulbar involvement, weakness is usually observed only in the lower face and tongue; extraocular, upper facial, pharyngeal, and jaw muscles are almost always spared. With bilateral corticobulbar lesions, *pseudobulbar palsy* often develops, in which dysarthria, dysphagia, dysphonia, and emotional lability accompany bilateral facial weakness. Spasticity accompanies upper motor neuron weakness but may not be present in the acute phase. Upper motor neuron lesions also affect the ability to perform rapid repetitive movements. Such movements are slow and coarse, but normal rhythmicity is maintained. Finger-nose-finger and heel-knee-shin are performed slowly but adequately.

Lower Motor Neuron Weakness This pattern results from disorders of cell bodies of lower motor neurons in the brainstem motor nuclei and the anterior horn of the spinal cord, or from dysfunction of the axons of these neurons as they pass to skeletal muscle (Fig. 21-2). Weakness is due to a decrease in the number of motor units that can be activated, through a loss of the α motor neurons or disruption of their connections to muscle. With a decreased number of motor units, fewer muscle fibers are activated with full effort and maximum power is reduced. Loss of γ motor neurons does not cause weakness but decreases tension on the muscle spindles, which decreases muscular tone and contributes to less active tendon reflexes on examination. An absent tendon stretch reflex suggests involvement of the spindle afferent fibers.

When a motor unit becomes diseased, especially in anterior horn cell diseases, it may spontaneously discharge, producing a *fasciculation*. These isolated small twitches may be seen or felt clinically or recorded by electromyography (EMG). When α motor neurons or their axons degenerate, the denervated muscle fibers spontaneously discharge in a manner that cannot be seen or felt but can be recorded with EMG. These small single muscle fiber discharges are called *fibrillation potentials*. If lower motor neuron weakness is present, recruitment of motor units is delayed or reduced, with fewer than normal activated at a given discharge frequency. This contrasts with upper motor neuron weakness, in which a normal number of motor units are activated at a given frequency but in which the maximum discharge frequency is decreased.

Myopathic Weakness This pattern of weakness is produced by disorders within the motor unit that affect the muscle fibers or the neuromuscular junctions.

Two types of muscle fibers exist. Type I muscle fibers are rich in mitochondria and oxidative enzymes, produce relatively low force, but have low energy demands that can be supplied by ongoing aerobic metabolism. They produce sustained postural and nonforceful movements. Type II muscle fibers are rich in glycolytic enzymes, can produce relatively high force, but have high energy demands that cannot be supplied for long by ongoing aerobic metabolism. Thus, these units can be activated maximally for only brief periods of time to produce high-force movements.

For graded voluntary movements, type I muscle fibers are activated earlier in recruitment. For each muscle fiber, if the nerve terminal releases a normal number of acetylcholine molecules presynaptically and a sufficient number of postsynaptic acetylcholine receptors are opened, the end plate reaches threshold and thereby generates an action potential that spreads across the muscle fiber membrane and into the transverse tubular system. This electrical excitation activates intracel-

TABLE 21-1	Signs That Distinguish Patterns of Weakness		
Sign	**Upper Motor Neuron**	**Lower Motor Neuron**	**Myopathic**
Atrophy	None	Severe	Mild
Fasciculations	None	Common	None
Tone	Spastic	Decreased	Normal/decreased
Distribution of weakness	Pyramidal/regional	Distal/segmental	Proximal
Tendon reflexes	Hyperactive	Hypoactive/absent	Normal/hypoactive
Babinski's sign	Present	Absent	Absent

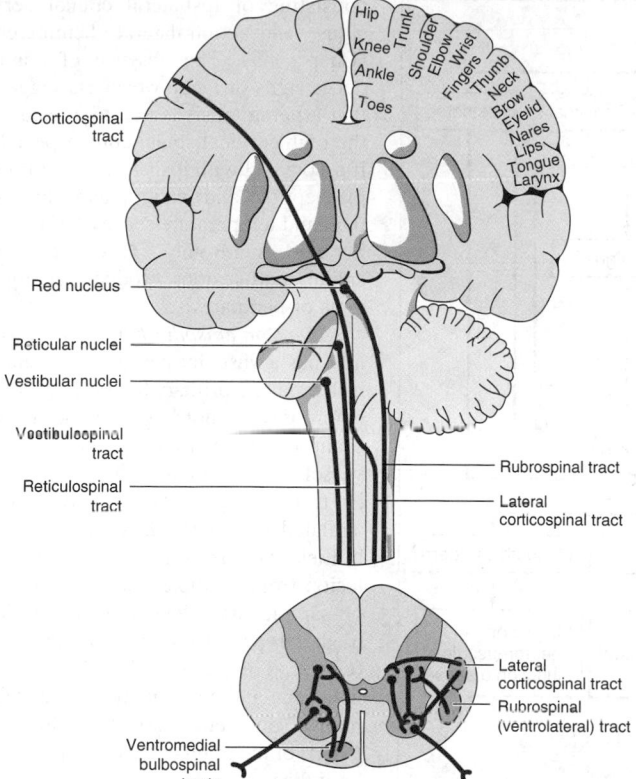

FIGURE 21-1 The corticospinal and bulbospinal upper motor neuron pathways. Upper motor neurons have their cell bodies in layer V of the primary motor cortex (the precentral gyrus, or Brodmann's area 4) and in the premotor and supplemental motor cortex (area 6). The upper motor neurons in the primary motor cortex are somatotopically organized as illustrated on the right side of the figure.

Axons of the upper motor neurons descend through the subcortical white matter and the posterior limb of the internal capsule. Axons of the *pyramidal* or *corticospinal system* descend through the brainstem in the cerebral peduncle of the midbrain, the basis pontis, and the medullary pyramids. At the cervicomedullary junction, most pyramidal axons decussate into the contralateral corticospinal tract of the lateral spinal cord, but 10 to 30% remain ipsilateral in the anterior spinal cord. Pyramidal neurons make direct monosynaptic connections with lower motor neurons. They innervate most densely the lower motor neurons of hand muscles and are involved in the execution of learned, fine movements. Corticobulbar neurons are similar to corticospinal neurons but innervate brainstem motor nuclei.

Bulbospinal upper motor neurons influence strength and tone but are not part of the pyramidal system. The descending *ventromedial bulbospinal pathways* originate in the tectum of the midbrain (tectospinal pathway), the vestibular nuclei (vestibulospinal pathway), and the reticular formation (reticulospinal pathway). These pathways influence axial and proximal muscles and are involved in the maintenance of posture and integrated movements of the limbs and trunk. The descending *ventrolateral bulbospinal pathways*, which originate predominantly in the red nucleus (rubrospinal pathway), facilitate distal limb muscles. The bulbospinal system is sometimes referred to as the *extrapyramidal upper motor neuron system*. In all figures, nerve cell bodies and axon terminals are shown, respectively, as closed circles and forks.

lular events that produce an energy-dependent contraction of the muscle fiber (excitation-contraction coupling).

Myopathic weakness is produced by a decrease in the number or contractile force of muscle fibers activated within the motor unit. With muscular dystrophies, inflammatory myopathies, or myopathies with muscle fiber necrosis, decreased numbers of muscle fibers survive within many motor units. As demonstrated with EMG, the size of each motor unit action potential is decreased so that motor units must be recruited more rapidly than normal to produce the power necessary for a certain movement. Neuromuscular junction diseases such as myasthenia gravis produce weakness in a similar manner, although the loss of muscle fibers within the motor unit is functional rather than actual. Furthermore, the number of muscle fibers activated can vary over time, depending on the state of rest of the neuromuscular junctions. Thus, fatigable weakness is suggestive of myasthenia gravis or another neuromuscular junction disease. Some myopathies produce weakness

through loss of contractile force of muscle fibers or through relatively selective involvement of the type II muscle fibers. These may not affect the size of individual motor unit action potentials observed with EMG and are detected by a discrepancy between the electrical activity and force of a muscle.

Integrated Movements Most purposeful movements require the integrated coordination of many muscle groups. Consider a simple movement, such as grasping a ball. The primary movement is a flexion of the thumb and fingers of one hand, with opposition of the thumb and little finger. This requires the contraction of several muscles, including flexor digitorum superficialis, flexor digitorum profundus, flexor pollicis longus, flexor pollicis brevis, opponens pollicis, and opponens digiti minimi. The prime movers for this action are called *agonists*. In order for the grasping to be smooth and forceful, the thumb and finger extensors need to relax at the same rate as the flexors contract. The muscles that act in a directly opposing manner to the agonists are *antagonists*. A secondary action of the thumb and finger flexors is to flex the wrist; because wrist flexion tends to weaken finger flexion if both occur, activation of wrist extensors assists the grasping movement. Muscles that produce such complementary movements are *synergists*. Finally, the arm needs to be held in a stable position as the grasp occurs, so that the ball is not knocked away before it is secured. Muscles that stabilize the arm position are *fixators*.

The coordination of activity by agonists, antagonists, synergists, and fixators is regulated by a three-level hierarchy of motor control. The lowest level of control is mediated through segmental reflexes in the spinal cord. These reflexes facilitate agonists and reciprocally inhibit the antagonists. Spinal segments also control rhythmic patterns of movement that involve more than a single pair of agonists and antagonists. For example, the lumbosacral spinal cord contains the basic programming for cyclical stepping movements that involve the synergistic activation of different muscle groups over time. The intermediate level of control is mediated through the descending bulbo-

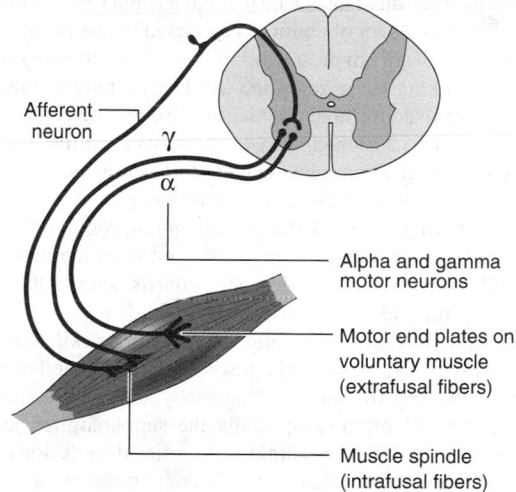

FIGURE 21-2 Lower motor neurons are divided into α and γ types. The larger α motor neurons are more numerous and innervate the extrafusal muscle fibers of the motor unit. Loss of α motor neurons or disruption of their axons produces lower motor neuron weakness. The smaller, less numerous γ motor neurons innervate the intrafusal muscle fibers of the muscle spindle and contribute to normal tone and stretch reflexes. The α motor neuron receives direct excitatory input from corticomotoneurons and primary muscle spindle afferents. The α and γ motor neurons also receive excitatory input from other descending upper motor neuron pathways, segmental sensory inputs, and interneurons. The α motor neurons receive direct inhibition from Renshaw cell interneurons, and other interneurons indirectly inhibit the α and γ motor neurons.

A tendon reflex requires the function of all illustrated structures. A tap on a tendon stretches muscle spindles (which are tonically activated by γ motor neurons) and activates the primary spindle afferent neurons. These stimulate the α motor neurons in the spinal cord, producing a brief muscle contraction, which is the familiar tendon reflex.

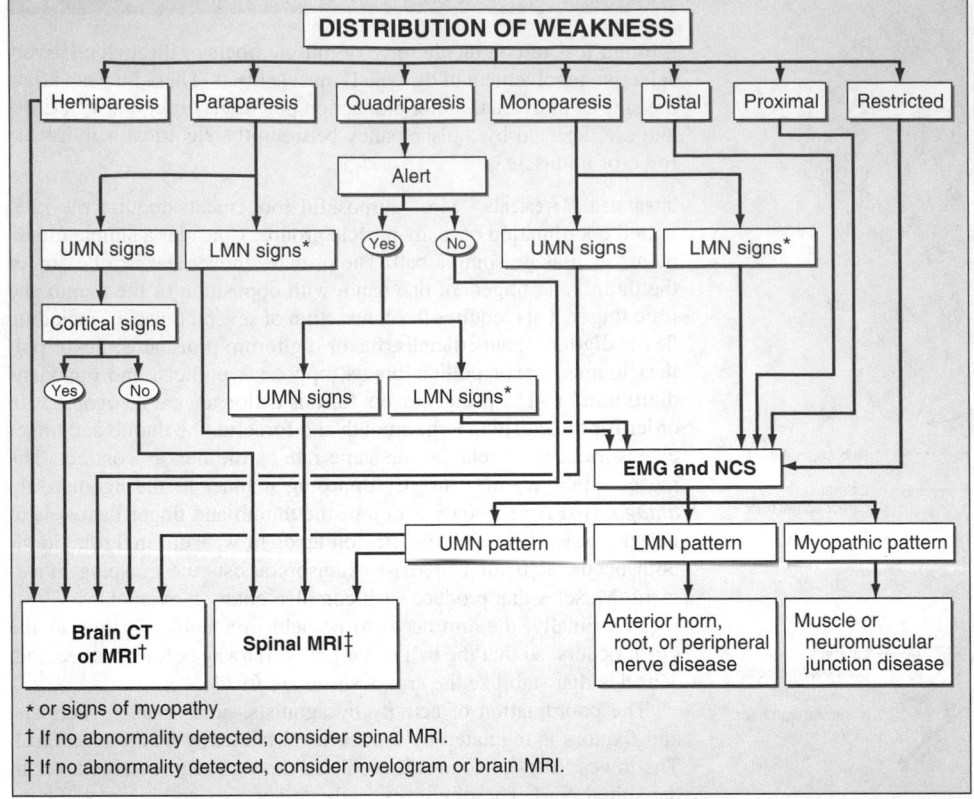

FIGURE 21-3 An algorithm for the initial workup of a patient with weakness. CT, computed tomography; EMG, electromyography; LMN, lower motor neuron; MRI, magnetic resonance imaging; NCS, nerve conduction studies; UMN, upper motor neuron.

spinal pathways, which integrate visual, proprioceptive, and vestibular feedback into the execution of an action. For example, the locomotor center in the midbrain is required to modify the cyclical stepping movements in order that balance be maintained and forward movement occurs. The highest level of control is mediated by the cerebral cortex. Superimposition of this highest level of control is necessary for activities such as walking to be goal-directed. Precise movements that are learned and improved through practice are also initiated and controlled by the motor cortex. Although only the agonists are directly activated, during the course of a complex sequence of actions such as playing the piano, the sequential activation of different groups of agonists for each note or chord is a part of the learned motor program. Further, the execution of these actions also involves input from the basal ganglia and cerebellar hemispheres to facilitate agonists, synergists, and fixators and to inhibit undesired antagonists.

Apraxia is a disorder of planning and initiating a skilled or learned movement (Chap. 23). Unilateral apraxia of the right hand may be due to a lesion of the left frontal lobe (especially anterior or inferior), the left temporoparietal region (especially the supramarginal gyrus), or their connections. Left body apraxia is produced by lesions of these regions in the right hemisphere or by lesions in the corpus callosum that disconnect the right temporoparietal or frontal regions from those on the left. Bilateral apraxia is often due to bilateral frontal lobe lesions or diffuse bilateral hemispheric disease.

Hemiparesis Hemiparesis results from an upper motor neuron lesion above the midcervical spinal cord; most lesions that produce hemiparesis are located above the foramen magnum. The presence of language disorders, cortical sensory disturbances, cognitive abnormalities, disorders of visual-spatial integration, apraxia, or seizures indicates a cortical lesion. Homonymous visual field defects reflect either a cortical or a subcortical hemispheric lesion. A "pure motor" hemiparesis of the face, arm, and/or leg is due to a small, discrete lesion in the posterior limb of the internal capsule, cerebral peduncle, or upper pons. Some brainstem lesions produce "crossed paralyses,"

consisting of ipsilateral cranial nerve signs and contralateral hemiparesis (Chap. 349). The absence of cranial nerve signs or facial weakness suggests that a hemiparesis is due to a lesion in the high cervical spinal cord, especially if associated with ipsilateral loss of proprioception and contralateral loss of pain and temperature sense (the Brown-Séquard syndrome). However, most spinal cord lesions produce quadriparesis or paraparesis.

Acute or episodic hemiparesis usually has a vascular pathogenesis, either ischemia or a primary hemorrhage. Less commonly, hemorrhage may occur into brain tumors or from rupture of normal vessels due to trauma; the trauma may be trivial in patients who are anticoagulated or elderly. Less likely possibilities include a focal inflammatory lesion from multiple sclerosis, abscess, or sarcoidosis. Evaluation begins immediately with a computed tomography (CT) scan of the brain (Fig. 21-3). If CT is normal and an ischemic stroke is unlikely, magnetic resonance imaging (MRI) of the brain or cervical spine may be indicated.

Subacute hemiparesis that evolves over days or weeks has an extensive differential diagnosis. A common cause is subdural hematoma; this readily treatable condition must always be considered, especially in elderly or anticoagulated patients, even in the absence of a history of trauma. Infectious possibilities include cerebral bacterial abscess, fungal granuloma or meningitis, and parasitic infection. Weakness from primary and metastatic neoplasms may evolve over days to weeks. AIDS may present with subacute hemiparesis due to toxoplasmosis or primary CNS lymphoma. Noninfectious inflammatory processes, such as multiple sclerosis or, less commonly, sarcoidosis, are further considerations. If the brain MRI is normal and if cortical and hemispheric signs are not present, MRI of the cervical spine may be required.

Chronic hemiparesis that evolves over months is usually due to a neoplasm, an unruptured arteriovenous malformation, a chronic subdural hematoma, or a degenerative disease. The initial diagnostic test is often an MRI of the brain, especially if the clinical findings suggest brainstem pathology. If MRI of the brain is normal, the possibility of a foramen magnum or high cervical spinal cord lesion should be considered.

Paraparesis An intraspinal lesion at or below the upper thoracic spinal cord level is most commonly responsible. A sensory level over the trunk identifies the approximate level of the cord lesion. Paraparesis can also result from lesions at other locations that disturb upper motor neurons (especially parasagittal lesions and hydrocephalus) and lower motor neurons (anterior horn cell disorders, cauda equina syndromes, and occasionally peripheral neuropathies).

Acute or episodic paraparesis due to spinal cord disease may be difficult to distinguish from disorders affecting lower motor neurons or cerebral hemispheres. Recurrent episodes of paraparesis are often due to multiple sclerosis or to vascular malformations of the spinal cord. With acute spinal cord disease, the upper motor neuron deficit is usually associated with incontinence and a sensory disturbance of the lower limbs that extends rostrally to a level on the trunk; tone is typically flaccid, and tendon reflexes absent. In such cases, the diagnostic approach begins with an imaging study of the spinal cord (Fig. 21-3). Compressive lesions (particularly epidural tumor, abscess, or hematoma), spinal cord infarction (proprioception is usually spared), an arteriovenous fistula or other vascular anomaly, and transverse myelitis, among other causes, may be responsible (Chap. 356). Diseases of the cerebral hemispheres that produce acute paraparesis include anterior cerebral artery ischemia (shoulder shrug also affected), superior sagittal sinus or cortical venous thrombosis, and acute hydrocephalus. If upper motor neuron signs are associated with drowsiness, confusion, seizures, or other hemispheric signs but not a sensory level over the trunk, the diagnostic approach starts with an MRI of the brain. Paraparesis is part of the cauda equina syndrome, which may result from trauma to the low back, a midline disk herniation, or intraspinal tumor; although sphincters are affected, hip flexion is often spared, as is sensation over the anterolateral thighs. Rarely, paraparesis is caused by a rapidly evolving peripheral neuropathy such as Guillain-Barré syndrome (Chap. 365) or by a myopathy (Chap. 368). In such cases, electrophysiologic studies are diagnostically helpful and refocus the subsequent evaluation.

Subacute or chronic paraparesis with spasticity is caused by upper motor neuron disease. When there is associated lower limb sensory loss and sphincter involvement, a chronic spinal cord disorder is likely; these are discussed in Chap. 356. The clinical approach begins with an MRI of the spinal cord. If the imaging study is normal and spasticity is present, MRI of the brain may be indicated. If hemispheric signs are present, parasagittal meningioma or chronic hydrocephalus is likely and MRI of the brain is the initial test. In the rare situation when chronic paraparesis is due to lower motor neuron or myopathic etiology, the localization is usually suspected on clinical grounds by the absence of spasticity and confirmed by EMG and nerve conduction tests.

Quadriparesis or Generalized Weakness Generalized weakness may be due to disorders of the CNS or of the motor unit. Although the terms *quadriparesis* and *generalized weakness* are often used interchangeably, quadriparesis is more often chosen when an upper motor neuron cause is suspected and generalized weakness when a disease of the motor unit is likely. Weakness from CNS disorders is usually associated with changes in consciousness or cognition, with increased muscle tone and muscle stretch reflexes, and with alterations of sensation. Most neuromuscular causes of generalized weakness are associated with normal mental function, diminished muscle tone, and hypoactive muscle stretch reflexes. Exceptions are some causes of acute quadriparesis due to upper motor neuron disorders in which transient hypotonia is present. The major causes of intermittent weakness are listed in Table 21-2. A patient with generalized fatigability without objective weakness may have the chronic fatigue syndrome (Chap. 370).

ACUTE QUADRIPARESIS Acute quadriparesis with onset over minutes may result from disorders of upper motor neurons (e.g., anoxia, hypotension, brainstem or cervical cord ischemia, trauma, and systemic metabolic abnormalities) or muscle (electrolyte disturbances, certain inborn errors of muscle energy metabolism, toxins, or periodic paralyses). Onset over hours to weeks may, in addition to the above, be due to lower motor neuron disorders. Guillain-Barré syndrome (Chap. 365)

TABLE 21-2 *Causes of Episodic Generalized Weakness*

1. Electrolyte disturbances, e.g., hypokalemia, hyperkalemia, hypercalcemia, hypernatremia, hyponatremia, hypophosphatemia, hypermagnesemia
2. Muscle disorders
   a. Channelopathies (periodic paralyses)
   b. Metabolic defects of muscle (impaired carbohydrate or fatty acid utilization; abnormal mitochondrial function)
3. Neuromuscular junction disorders
   a. Myasthenia gravis
   b. Lambert-Eaton myasthenic syndrome
4. Central nervous system disorders
   a. Transient ischemic attacks of the brainstem
   b. Transient global cerebral ischemia
   c. Multiple sclerosis

---

is the most common lower motor neuron weakness that progresses over days to 4 weeks; the finding of an elevated protein level in the cerebrospinal fluid is helpful but may be absent early in the course. If stupor or coma is present, the evaluation begins with a CT scan of the brain. If upper motor neuron signs are present but the patient is alert, the initial test is usually an MRI of the cervical cord. If weakness is lower motor neuron, myopathic, or uncertain in origin, the clinical approach begins with blood studies for muscle enzymes and electrolytes and an EMG and nerve conduction study.

SUBACUTE OR CHRONIC QUADRIPARESIS When quadriparesis due to upper motor neuron disease develops over weeks, months, or years, the distinction among disorders of the cerebral hemispheres, brainstem, and cervical spinal cord is usually possible by clinical criteria alone. The diagnostic approach begins with an MRI of the clinically suspected site of pathology. Lower motor neuron disease usually presents with weakness that is most profound distally, whereas myopathic weakness is typically proximal; the evaluation then begins with EMG and nerve conduction studies.

Monoparesis This is usually due to lower motor neuron disease, with or without associated sensory involvement. Upper motor neuron weakness occasionally presents with a monoparesis of distal and nonantigravity muscles. Myopathic weakness is rarely limited to one limb.

ACUTE MONOPARESIS Distinguishing between upper and lower motor neuron disorders may be difficult clinically because tone and reflexes are frequently decreased in both at presentation. If the weakness is predominantly in distal and nonantigravity muscles and not associated with sensory impairment or pain, focal cortical ischemia is likely (Chap. 349); in this setting, diagnostic possibilities are similar to those for acute hemiparesis. Sensory loss and pain usually accompany acute lower motor neuron weakness. The distribution of weakness is commonly localized to a single nerve root or peripheral nerve within one limb but occasionally reflects involvement of the brachial or lumbosacral plexus. If lower motor neuron weakness is suspected, or if the pattern of weakness is uncertain, the clinical approach begins with an EMG and nerve conduction study.

SUBACUTE OR CHRONIC MONOPARESIS Weakness with atrophy of one limb that develops over weeks or months is almost always lower motor neuron in origin. If the weakness is associated with numbness, a peripheral nerve or spinal root origin is likely; uncommonly, the brachial or lumbosacral plexus is affected. If numbness is absent, anterior horn cell disease is likely. In either case, an electrodiagnostic study is indicated. If upper rather than lower motor neuron signs are present, a tumor, vascular malformation, or other cortical lesion affecting the precentral gyrus may be responsible. Alternatively, if the leg is affected, a small thoracic cord lesion, often a tumor or multiple sclerosis, may be present. In these situations, the approach begins with an imaging study of the suspicious area.

Distal Weakness Involvement of two or four limbs distally suggests lower motor neuron or peripheral nerve disease. Acute distal lower limb weakness occurs occasionally from an acute toxic polyneuropathy or cauda equina syndrome. Distal symmetric weakness usually develops over weeks, months, or years and is due to metabolic, toxic, hereditary, degenerative, or inflammatory diseases of peripheral nerves (Chap. 363). With peripheral nerve disease, weakness is usually less severe than numbness. Anterior horn cell disease may begin distally but is typically asymmetric and is not associated with numbness (Chap. 353). Rarely, myopathies also present with distal weakness (Chap. 368). The first step in evaluation is an electrophysiologic study (Fig. 21-3).

Proximal Weakness Proximal weakness of two or four limbs suggests a disorder of muscle or, less commonly, neuromuscular junction or anterior horn cell. Myopathy often produces symmetric weakness of the pelvic or shoulder girdle muscles (Chap. 368). Diseases of the neuromuscular junction (such as myasthenia gravis) may present with symmetric proximal weakness (Chap. 366), often associated with ptosis, diplopia, or bulbar weakness and fluctuating in severity during the day. Extreme fatigability present in some cases of myasthenia gravis may even suggest episodic weakness, but strength rarely returns fully to normal. The proximal weakness of anterior horn cell disease is most often asymmetric, but may be symmetric if familial (Chap. 353). Numbness does not occur with any of these diseases. The evaluation usually begins with determination of the serum creatine kinase level and electrophysiologic studies.

Weakness in a Restricted Distribution   In some patients, weakness does not fit any of the above patterns. Examples include weakness limited to the extraocular, hemifacial, bulbar, or respiratory muscles. If unilateral, restricted weakness is usually due to lower motor neuron or peripheral nerve disease, such as in a facial palsy (Chap. 355) or an isolated superior oblique muscle paresis (Chap. 25). Relatively symmetric weakness of extraocular or bulbar muscles is usually due to a myopathy (Chap. 367) or neuromuscular junction disorder (Chap. 366). Bilateral facial palsy with areflexia suggests Guillain-Barré syndrome (Chap. 365). Worsening of relatively symmetric weakness with fatigue is characteristic of neuromuscular junction disorders. Asymmetric bulbar weakness is usually due to motor neuron disease. Weakness limited to respiratory muscles is uncommon and is usually due to motor neuron disease, myasthenia gravis, or polymyositis/dermatomyositis (Chap. 369).

SPASMS AND CRAMPS

Spontaneous or exercise-related discomfort from muscles is usually benign. However, a number of disorders of the motor system are characteristically painful. *Myalgias* (Chap. 367) are pains that are felt in muscle; the term does not imply an involuntary contraction. *Spasms* and *cramps* refer to episodes of involuntary contraction of one or more muscles. Cramps are usually painful, whereas spasms are not necessarily uncomfortable.

Involuntary contraction of muscle may occur with disorders of the CNS, lower motor neuron, or muscle. Contractions that originate within the CNS and are associated with upper motor neuron signs are usually referred to as spasms and generally affect the flexors or extensors of one or more limbs. Those that originate within the CNS and are not associated with upper motor neuron signs include movement disorders discussed below, as well as the rare stiff-person syndrome and tetanus. Muscle rigidity from active muscle contraction can occur in the malignant hyperthermia syndrome, usually associated with general anesthesia. In the neuroleptic malignant syndrome, muscle rigidity arises from CNS overactivity. Involuntary contractions that originate in the lower motor neurons are usually cramps, occasionally tetany, or rarely neuromyotonia. Spasms that originate in muscle or muscle membrane generally manifest as delayed relaxation after voluntary contraction (myotonia or rarely a contracture). These conditions may be difficult to distinguish clinically but are often well characterized by EMG.

Stiff-Person Syndrome   This rare syndrome is characterized by slowly progressive muscle stiffness and superimposed spasms. The stiffness commonly begins in the low back and spreads over months up the spine and into the limbs but not into the jaw. The gait becomes stiff, and there is hyperlordosis of the lumbar spine. Spasms are often produced by startle. Emotional stress tends to worsen the stiffness as well as the frequency and severity of spasms. The spontaneous motor activity disappears during sleep. The syndrome is often associated with diabetes mellitus and can be paraneoplastic, accompanying Hodgkin's lymphoma, small cell cancer of the lung, and breast cancer. Most patients have a serum antibody against glutamic acid decarboxylase, an enzyme responsible for synthesis of the inhibitory neurotransmitter γ-aminobutyric acid (GABA). Stiffness results from loss of descending brainstem or segmental spinal inhibitory influences on the lower motor

neurons. EMG studies reveal continuous motor unit activity that is similar to voluntary effort with preservation of the silent period to muscle stretch. Stiffness and spasms typically respond partially to treatment with baclofen or benzodiazepines.

Tetanus   This rare hyperexcitable state results from exposure to tetanus toxin in patients infected with *Clostridium tetani* (Chap. 124). Painful spasms typically begin with jaw closure (trismus) and soon become generalized. EMG studies reveal continuous motor unit activity that is similar to voluntary effort except for loss of the silent period to muscle stretch.

Cramps   These are the most common type of involuntary muscle contraction. Cramps are a painful contraction of a single muscle that produces a palpable knot within the muscle for seconds to minutes and is relieved by passive stretch of the muscle or spontaneously. EMG studies reveal motor unit activity that has too high a discharge frequency to be voluntary. If cramps are associated with weakness, the weakness is almost always lower motor neuron in origin. When strength is normal, no definable condition is usually found, although dehydration, hypothyroidism, or uremia is occasionally present. If prominent, membrane stabilizing drugs, such as carbamazepine, may provide symptomatic benefit.

Tetany   Tetany is characterized by contraction of distal muscles of the hands (carpal spasm with extension of interphalangeal joints and adduction and flexion of the metacarpophalangeal joints) and feet (pedal spasm) and is associated with tingling around the mouth and distally in the limbs. Tetany with carpopedal spasms is a common manifestation of hypocalcemia or respiratory alkalosis (even from hyperventilation). EMG studies reveal single or more often grouped motor unit discharges at low discharge frequency.

Neuromyotonia (Isaac's Syndrome)   Neuromyotonia is characterized by muscle stiffness at rest that persists during sleep and by delayed relaxation after voluntary effort. Distal limb muscles are usually affected most severely, but all skeletal muscle may be involved. Gait may be stiff, and close inspection of the muscle reveals undulation of the overlying skin due to continuous muscle fiber contractions (myokymia). The continuous muscle fiber activity generates heat, and excessive sweating is common. EMG studies commonly reveal myokymic discharges, especially in familial cases. Rarely, EMGs record high-frequency neuromyotonic discharges. Autoantibodies against voltage-gated potassium channels have been demonstrated in some cases, and plasma exchange may be effective.

Myotonia   This is a nonpainful delay in the relaxation of muscle after voluntary activity. Delay in opening the hand after a forceful grip (grip myotonia) is common. These disorders are usually familial and worsen in cold weather. EMG demonstrates a waxing and waning discharge of individual muscle fibers.

Contracture   A painful inability to relax a muscle after voluntary activity due to energy depletion characterizes certain metabolic disorders with failure of energy production, such as myophosphorylase deficiency (McArdle's disease). EMG studies reveal electrical silence.

MOVEMENT DISORDERS

In these disorders, abnormal movements (or *dyskinesias*) occur due to a disturbance of fluency and speed of voluntary movement or the presence of unintended extra movements. Because they are so distinct from the pyramidal disorders that cause upper motor neuron weakness, movement disorders are often referred to as *extrapyramidal diseases*. *Hyperkinetic movement disorders* are those in which an excessive amount of spontaneous motor activity is seen or in which abnormal involuntary movements occur. *Hypokinetic movement disorders* are characterized by *akinesia* or *bradykinesia*, in which purposeful motor activity is absent or reduced ("poverty of movement").

PATHOGENESIS   Movement disorders result from disease of the basal ganglia, paired subcortical gray matter structures consisting of the caudate and the putamen (which together are called the striatum), the internal and external segments of the globus pallidus, the subthalamic nucleus, and the substantia nigra (see Chap. 351).

Parkinson's disease the prototypic hypokinetic movement disorder, results from a loss of dopaminergic neurons in the substantia nigra pars compacta. This leads to less excitation of striatal neurons that express the D_1 type of dopamine receptors and less inhibition of D_2 striatal neurons, both contributing to reduced facilitation of cortically initiated movement. The resting tremor of Parkinson's disease is less readily explained by this model but may result from effects on cholinergic interneurons in the striatum. *Huntington's disease* (Chap. 350), a hyperkinetic movement disorder, may be explained by selective loss of D_2 striatal neurons, resulting in disinhibition of cortically initiated movements without normal feedback control. The pathogenesis of hemiballismus is similar—a direct lesion of the glutamatergic neurons in the subthalamic nucleus (usually from a stroke) leads to disinhibition of thalamocortical projections.

Hyperkinetic Movement Disorders Abnormal involuntary movements may be rhythmical or irregular. Those that are rhythmical are termed *tremors*, with the uncommon exception of *palatal and segmental myoclonus*. Tremors are divided into three types: rest, postural, and intention tremor. A *rest tremor* is maximal at rest and becomes less prominent with activity. A gradual onset is characteristic of parkinsonism and is commonly associated with bradykinesia and cogwheel rigidity (Chap. 351). A rest tremor that develops acutely is usually due to toxins [such as exposure to 1-methyl-4-phenyl-1,2,3,6-tetrahydropyridine (MPTP)] or dopamine blocking drugs (such as phenothiazines). A *postural tremor* is maximal while limb posture is actively maintained against gravity; it is lessened by rest and is not markedly enhanced during voluntary movement toward a target. A postural tremor that develops acutely is usually due to toxic or metabolic factors (for example, hyperthyroidism) or stress. The insidious onset of a postural tremor suggests a benign or familial essential tremor. An *intention tremor* is most prominent during voluntary movement toward a target and is not present during postural maintenance or at rest. It is a sign of cerebellar disease (Chap. 352). *Asterixis*, which may superficially resemble a tremor, is an intermittent inhibition of muscle contraction that occurs with metabolic encephalopathy (Chap. 257). This leads, for example, to a momentary and repetitive partial flexion of the wrists during attempted sustained wrist extension.

Irregular involuntary movements are characterized by their speed and location, and by whether they can be suppressed voluntarily. The slowest are athetosis and dystonia. *Athetosis* is a slow, writhing, sinuous movement that occurs nearly continuously in distal muscles. *Dystonia* is a slowly varying but nearly continuous deviation of posture about one or more joints; it may occur in a proximal or distal limb or in axial structures. Dystonia is a more sustained deviation of posture than athetosis, although these two phenomena overlap considerably. →*The further evaluation of athetosis and dystonia is discussed in Chap. 351.*

Among the rapid irregular movements, *tics* are controlled with voluntary effort, while the others are not. Tics often occur repetitively in a single location but are sometimes multifocal.

Chorea, hemiballismus, and myoclonus are rapid, irregular jerks that cannot be voluntarily suppressed. *Hemiballismus* manifests as a sudden and often violent flinging movement of a proximal limb, usually an arm. Hemiballismus usually develops acutely due to infarction of the contralateral subthalamic nucleus but occasionally develops subacutely or chronically due to other lesions of this nucleus.

Chorea is a rapid, jerky, irregular movement that tends to occur in the distal limbs or face but may also occur in proximal limbs and trunk. Acute or subacute onset is usually due to toxins including excess levodopa or dopamine-agonist therapy or, less often, neuroleptics, birth control pills, pregnancy (chorea gravidarum), hyperthyroidism, or the antiphospholipid syndrome. In children, it may be associated with rheumatic fever and, in such cases, is referred to as *Sydenham's chorea*. The gradual onset of chorea is typical of degenerative neurologic diseases, such as Huntington's disease.

Myoclonus is a rapid, brief, irregular movement that is usually multifocal. Myoclonus can occur spontaneously at rest, in response to sensory stimuli, or with voluntary movements. It is a symptom that occurs in a wide variety of metabolic and neurologic disorders. Posthypoxic intention myoclonus is a special myoclonic syndrome that occurs as a sequel to transient cerebral anoxia. Myoclonus may result from lipid storage disease, encephalitis, prion diseases, or metabolic encephalopathies due to respiratory failure, chronic renal failure, hepatic failure, or electrolyte imbalance. Myoclonus is also a feature of certain types of epilepsy (Chap. 348). *Palatal and segmental myoclonus* are uncommon rhythmic forms of myoclonus that may resemble tremor; they are caused by structural disease of the brainstem or spinal cord at the level of the abnormal movement.

Hypokinetic Movement Disorders These manifest as bradykinesia, with a masked, expressionless facial appearance, loss of associated limb movements during walking, and rigid en bloc turning. If bradykinesia is associated only with a rest tremor, cogwheel rigidity, or impairment of postural reflexes (especially with a tendency to fall backwards), Parkinson's disease is likely. If cognitive, language, upper motor neuron, sensory, or autonomic signs are also present, a *multisystem degenerative neurologic disease* is present. →*These disorders are discussed in Chaps. 351, 352, and 354.*

IMBALANCE AND DISORDERS OF GAIT

Imbalance is the impaired ability to maintain the intended orientation of the body in space. It is generally manifest as difficulty in maintaining an upright posture while standing or walking; a severe imbalance may also affect the ability to maintain posture while seated. Patients with imbalance commonly complain of a feeling of unsteadiness or dysequilibrium. Whereas imbalance and unsteadiness are synonymous, *dysequilibrium* implies the additional component of impaired spatial orientation even while lying down. Patients with dysequilibrium commonly also experience *vertigo*, defined as an hallucination of rotatory movement.

PATHOGENESIS ■ **Imbalance and Limb Ataxia** Imbalance results from disorders of the vestibular, sensory, or cerebellar systems, whereas limb ataxia is produced by disorders of the sensory or cerebellar systems. Asymmetric vestibular sensory input to the brainstem and cerebellum produces asymmetric imbalance, but not limb ataxia. Sensory ataxia is caused by lesions that affect the peripheral sensory fibers; dorsal root ganglia cells; posterior columns of the spinal cord; or lemniscal system in the brainstem, thalamus, or parietal cortex (Chap. 22). Impairment of the proprioceptive sensory feedback to the cerebellum, basal ganglia, and cortex produces sensory ataxia. Sensory ataxia results in imbalance and disturbs the fluency and integration of limb movements that can be partially alleviated by visual feedback. Imbalance with cerebellar ataxia results from disorders of proprioceptive, spinocerebellar, or vestibular sensory input; the integration of these inputs in the brainstem or midline cerebellar vermis or flocculonodular lobe; or the motor output to the spinal neurons that control muscles of the proximal limbs and trunk. Cerebellar limb ataxia results from disorders of the spinocerebellar and corticopontocerebellar inputs, the integration of these inputs in the intermediate and lateral cerebellum, or the output to the spinal neurons (via the red nucleus and rubrospinal tract) or to the cortex. These pathways ensure adequate speed, fluency, and integration of limb movements. The lateral cerebellar hemispheres coordinate a polysynaptic feedback circuit that modulates cortically initiated limb movement.

Disorders of Gait Walking is one of the most complicated motor activities. Cyclical stepping movements produced by the lumbosacral spinal cord centers are modified by cortical, basal ganglionic, brainstem, and cerebellar influences based on proprioceptive, vestibular, and visual feedback.

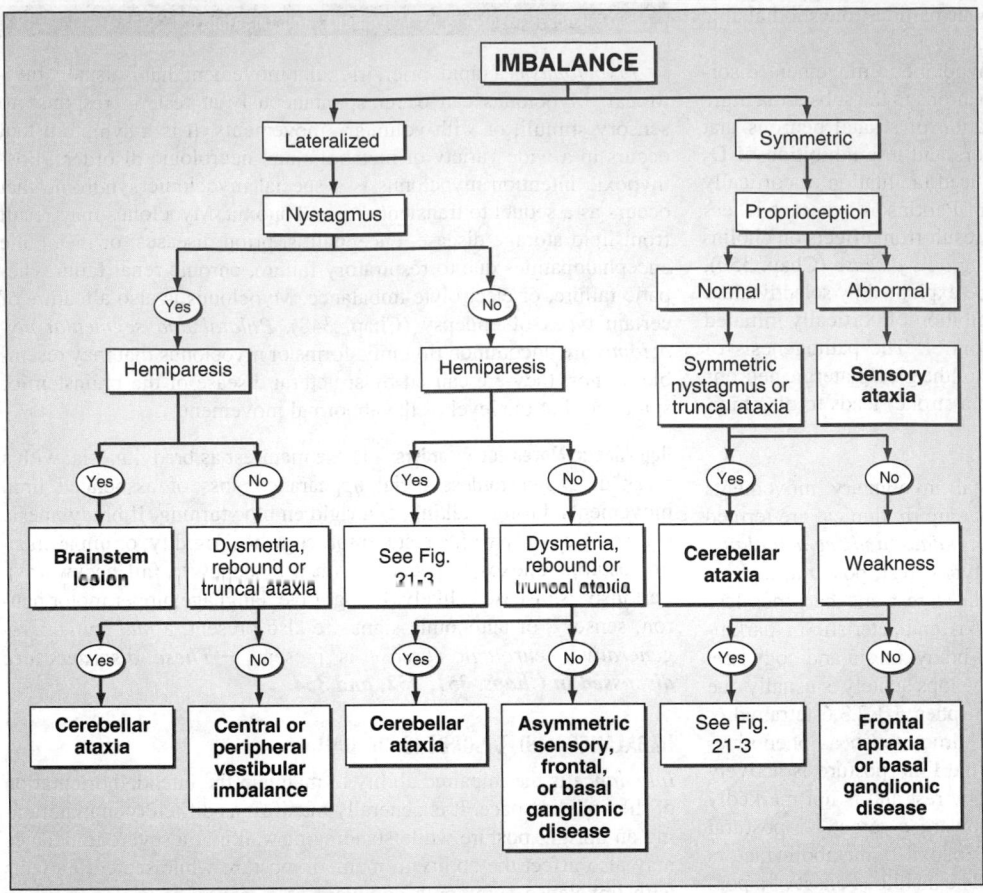

FIGURE 21-4 An algorithm for evaluation of imbalance without weakness; if weakness is present, see Fig. 21-3.

Imbalance flowchart text:

IMBALANCE
- Lateralized → Nystagmus
  - Yes → Hemiparesis
    - Yes → **Brainstem lesion**
    - No → Dysmetria, rebound or truncal ataxia
      - Yes → **Cerebellar ataxia**
      - No → **Central or peripheral vestibular imbalance**
  - No → Hemiparesis
    - Yes → See Fig. 21-3
      - Yes → **Cerebellar ataxia**
      - No → **Asymmetric sensory, frontal, or basal ganglionic disease**
    - No → Dysmetria, rebound or truncal ataxia
- Symmetric → Proprioception
  - Normal → Symmetric nystagmus or truncal ataxia
    - Yes → **Cerebellar ataxia**
      - Yes → See Fig. 21-3
      - No → **Frontal apraxia or basal ganglionic disease**
    - No → Weakness
  - Abnormal → **Sensory ataxia**

Imbalance A guide to interpretation of imbalance without weakness is presented in Fig. 21-4.

Imbalance with cerebellar ataxia typically produces truncal ataxia, which is usually revealed during the process of rising from a chair, assuming the upright stance with the feet together, or performing some other activity while standing. Once a desired position is reached, imbalance may be surprisingly mild. As walking begins, the imbalance recurs. Patients usually learn to lessen the imbalance by walking with the legs widely separated. The imbalance is usually not lateralized; may be accompanied by symmetric nystagmus; and is caused by toxic, metabolic, inflammatory, or neurodegenerative diseases. Asymmetric cerebellar ataxia suggests structural disease from ischemia, tumor, or other mass lesion.

Cerebellar limb ataxia is characterized by dysmetria (irregular errors in amplitude and force of movements); intention tremor (accentuation as the target is approached); dysdiadochokinesia (errors in rythm, velocity or force); and excessive rebound of outstretched arms against a resistance that is suddenly removed. Muscle tone is often modestly reduced; this contributes to the abnormal rebound due to decreased activation of segmental spinal cord reflexes and also to pendular reflexes, i.e., a tendency for a tendon reflex to produce multiple swings to and fro after a single tap. If involvement is asymmetric, lateralized imbalance is common and usually associated with asymmetric nystagmus. →*For further discussion of cerebellar diseases, see Chap. 352.*

Imbalance with vestibular dysfunction is characterized by a consistent tendency to fall to one side. The patient commonly complains of vertigo rather than imbalance, especially if the onset is acute. Acute vertigo associated with lateralized imbalance but no other neurologic signs is often due to disorders of the semicircular canal (Chap. 20); the presence of other neurologic signs suggests brainstem ischemia (Chap. 349) or multiple sclerosis (Chap. 359). When the vestibular dysfunction is peripheral, positional nystagmus and vertigo tend to

resolve if a provocative position is maintained (extinction) or repeated (habituation). Lateralized imbalance of gradual onset or persisting for >2 weeks, accompanied by nystagmus, may result from lesions of the semicircular canal or vestibular nerve, brainstem, or cerebellum.

Imbalance with sensory ataxia is characterized by marked worsening when visual feedback is removed. The patient can often assume the upright stance with feet together cautiously with eyes open. With eye closure, balance is rapidly lost (positive Romberg sign) in various directions at random. Sensory examination reveals impairment of proprioception at the toes and ankles, usually associated with an even more prominent abnormality of vibratory perception. Prompt evaluation for vitamin B_{12} deficiency is important, as this disorder is reversible if recognized early. Depression or absence of reflexes points to peripheral nerve disorders. Spasticity with extensor plantar responses suggests posterior column and spinal cord disorders. Rarely, sensory ataxia produces lateralized imbalance. In these cases, the disorder is usually in the parietal lobe or thalamus, but may also be due to an asymmetric sensory neuropathy or posterior column disease.

Sensory limb ataxia is similar to cerebellar limb ataxia but is markedly worse when the eyes are closed. Examination also reveals abnormal proprioception and vibratory perception. The approach focuses on localizing the proprioceptive impairment to the peripheral nerves, the posterior columns of the spinal cord, or rarely the parietal lobe.

Other forms of imbalance occur, but the fundamental problem is usually a primary disorder of strength, extrapyramidal function, or cortical initiation of movement, as indicated in Fig. 21-4.

Abnormal Gait Each of the disorders discussed in this chapter produces a characteristic gait disturbance. If the neurologic examination is normal except for an abnormal gait, diagnosis may be difficult even for the experienced clinician.

Hemiparetic gait characterizes spastic hemiparesis. In its most severe form, an abnormal posture of the limbs is produced by spasticity. The arm is adducted and internally rotated, with flexion of the elbow, wrist, and fingers and with extension of the hip, knee, and ankle. Forward swing of the spastic leg during walking requires abduction and circumduction at the hip, often with contralateral tilt of the trunk to prevent the toes catching on the floor as the leg is advanced. In its mildest form, the affected arm is held in a normal position, but swings less than the normal arm. The affected leg is flexed less than the normal leg during its forward swing and is more externally rotated. A hemiparetic gait is a common residual sign of a stroke.

Paraparetic gait is a walking pattern in which both legs are moved in a slow, stiff manner with circumduction, similar to the leg movement in a hemiparetic gait. In many patients, the legs tend to cross with each forward swing ("scissoring"). A paraparetic gait is a common sign of spinal cord disease and also occurs in cerebral palsy.

Steppage gait is produced by weakness of ankle dorsiflexion. Because of the partial or complete foot drop, the leg must be lifted higher than usual to avoid catching the toe on the floor during the forward swing of the leg. If unilateral, steppage gait is usually due to L5 radiculopathy, sciatic neuropathy, or peroneal neuropathy. If bilateral, it is the common result of a distal polyneuropathy or lumbosacral polyradiculopathy.

Waddling gait results from proximal lower limb weakness, most often from myopathy but occasionally from neuromuscular junction disease or a proximal symmetric spinal muscular atrophy. With weakness of hip flexion, the trunk is tilted away from the leg that is being moved to lift the hip and provide extra distance between the foot and the floor, and the pelvis is rotated forward to assist with forward motion of the leg. Because pelvic girdle weakness is customarily bilateral, the pelvic lift and rotation alternate from side to side, giving the waddling appearance to the gait.

Parkinsonian gait is characterized by a forward stoop, with modest flexion at the hips and knees. The arms are flexed at the elbows and adducted at the shoulders, often with a 4- to 6-Hz resting pronation-supination tremor but little other movement, even during walking. Walking is initiated slowly by leaning forward and maintained with short rapid steps, during which the feet shuffle along the floor. The pace tends to accelerate (festination) as the upper body gradually leans further ahead of the feet, whether movement is forward (propulsion) or backward (retropulsion). The postural instability leads to falls (Chap. 351).

Apraxic gait results from bilateral frontal lobe disease with impaired ability to plan and execute sequential movements. This gait superficially resembles that of parkinsonism, in that the posture is stooped and any steps taken are short and shuffling. However, initiation and maintenance of walking are impaired in a different manner. Each movement that is required for walking can usually be performed, if tested in isolation while sitting or lying. However, when asked to step forward while standing, a long pause often occurs before any attempt is made to flex at the hip and advance, as if the patient is "glued to the ground." Once walking is initiated, it is not maintained, even in an abnormal festinating manner. Rather, after one or several steps are taken, walking is stopped for several seconds or longer. The process is then repeated. Dementia and incontinence may coexist.

Choreoathetotic gait is characterized by an intermittent, irregular movement that disrupts the smooth flow of a normal gait. Flexion or extension movements at the hip are common and unpredictable but readily observed as a pelvic lurch.

Cerebellar ataxic gait is a broad-based gait disorder in which the speed and length of stride varies irregularly from step to step. With midline cerebellar disease, as in alcoholics, posture is erect but the feet are separated; lower limb ataxia is commonly present as well. With disease of the cerebellar hemispheres, limb ataxia and nystagmus are commonly present as well.

Sensory ataxic gait may resemble a cerebellar gait, with its broad-based stance and difficulty with change in position. However, although balance may be maintained with the eyes open, loss of visual input through eye closure results in rapid loss of balance with a fall (positive Romberg sign), unless the physician assists the patient.

Vestibular gait is one in which the patient consistently tends to fall to one side, whether walking or standing. Cranial nerve examination usually demonstrates an asymmetric nystagmus. The possibilities of unilateral sensory ataxia and hemiparesis are excluded by the findings of normal proprioception and strength.

Astasia-abasia is a typical hysterical gait disorder. Although the patient usually has normal coordination of leg movements in bed or while sitting, the patient is unable to stand or walk without assistance. If distracted, stationary balance is sometimes maintained and several steps are taken normally, followed by a dramatic demonstration of imbalance with a lunge toward the examiner's arms or a nearby bed.

FURTHER READING

CAPADAY C: The special nature of human walking and its neural control. Trends Neurosci 25:370, 2002

DIETZ V: Proprioception and locomotor disorders. Nat Rev Neurosci 3:781, 2002

22 NUMBNESS, TINGLING, AND SENSORY LOSS
Arthur K. Asbury

NORMAL SENSATION

Normal somatic sensation reflects a continuous day and night monitoring process that occupies considerable moment-to-moment nervous system capacity. Little of this activity reaches consciousness under ordinary conditions. In contrast, disordered sensation, particularly if experienced as painful, is alarming and dominates the sufferer's attention. Abnormalities of sensation, especially if painful, tend to make those suffering seek medical help. The physician must be able to recognize abnormal sensations by how they are described, know their type and likely site of origin, and understand their implications. →*For a consideration of pain, see Chap. 11.*

POSITIVE AND NEGATIVE PHENOMENA Abnormal sensory phenomena may be divided into two categories, positive and negative. The prototypical positive phenomenon is tingling (pins-and-needles), and the principal negative phenomenon is numbness. In addition to tingling, positive sensory phenomena include other altered sensations that are described as pricking, bandlike, lightning-like shooting feelings (lancinations), aching, knifelike, twisting, drawing, pulling, tightening, burning, searing, electrical, or raw feelings. These descriptors are frequently the actual words used by patients. Such sensations are usually experienced as painful, but not necessarily.

Positive phenomena usually result from trains of impulses generated at a site or sites of lowered threshold or heightened excitability along a sensory pathway, either peripheral or central. The nature and severity of an abnormal sensation depend on the number, rate, timing, and distribution of ectopic impulses and the type and function of nervous tissue in which they arise. Because positive phenomena represent excessive activity in sensory pathways, they are not necessarily associated with sensory deficit (loss) upon examination.

Negative phenomena represent loss of sensory function and are characterized by diminished or absent feeling, often experienced as numbness. In contrast to positive phenomena, negative phenomena are accompanied by abnormal findings on sensory examination. In disorders affecting peripheral sensation, it is estimated that at least half the afferent axons innervating a given site are lost or functionless before sensory deficit can be demonstrated by clinical examination. This threshold varies according to how rapidly sensory nerve fibers have lost function. If the rate of loss is slow and chronic, lack of cutaneous feeling may be unnoticed by the patient and difficult to demonstrate on examination, even though few sensory fibers are functioning. Rapidly evolving sensory abnormality usually evokes both positive and negative phenomena that are readily noticed. Subclinical degrees of sensory dysfunction not demonstrable on clinical sensory examination may be revealed by sensory nerve conduction studies or somatosensory evoked potentials (Chap. 359). Sensory symptoms may be either positive or negative, but sensory signs on examination are always a measure of negative phenomena.

TERMINOLOGY Words used to characterize sensory disturbance are descriptive and have been arrived at mainly by convention. Paresthesia and dysesthesia are general terms used to denote sensory symptoms (positive phenomena) and are usually stated in the plural form. *Paresthesias* usually refer to tingling or pins-and-needles sensations but may also include a wide variety of other abnormal sensations, excepting pain. Sometimes "paresthesias" carry the implication that the abnormal sensations are perceived without an apparent stimulus. *Dysesthesia* is a more general term denoting all types of abnormal sensations, even painful ones, whether a stimulus is evident or not.

While paresthesias and dysesthesias refer to sensations described by patients, another set of terms refers to sensory abnormalities found on examination. These include *hypesthesia* or *hypoesthesia* (reduction of cutaneous sensation to a specific type of testing such as pressure, light touch, and warm or cold stimuli); *anesthesia* (complete absence of skin sensation to the same stimuli plus pinprick); and *hypalgesia* (referring to reduced pain perception, i.e., nociception, such as the pricking quality elicited by a pin). *Hyperesthesia* means pain in response to touch. Similarly, *allodynia* describes the situation in which a nonpainful stimulus, once perceived, is experienced as painful, even excruciating. An example is elicitation of a painful sensation by application of a vibrating tuning fork. *Hyperalgesia* denotes severe pain in response to a mildly noxious stimulus, and *hyperpathia*, a broad term, encompasses all the phenomena described by hyperesthesia, allodynia, and hyperalgesia. With hyperpathia, the threshold for a sensory stimulus is increased and the perception is delayed, but once felt, is unduly painful.

Disorders of deep sensation, arising from muscle spindles, tendons, and joints, affect proprioception (position sense). Manifestations include imbalance (particularly with eyes closed or in the dark), clumsiness of precision movements, and unsteadiness of gait, which are referred to collectively as *sensory ataxia* (Chap. 21). Other findings on examination usually, but not invariably, include reduced or absent joint position and vibratory sensibility and absent deep tendon reflexes in the affected limbs. Romberg's sign is positive, which means that the patient sways or topples when asked to stand with feet close together and eyes closed. In severe states of deafferentation involving deep sensation, the patient cannot walk or stand unaided or even sit unsupported. Continuous, sometimes wormlike involuntary movements, called *pseudoathetosis*, of the outstretched hands and fingers occur, particularly with eyes closed. Such patients are severely disabled.

ANATOMY OF SENSATION   Cutaneous afferent innervation is conveyed by a rich variety of receptors, both naked nerve endings (nociceptors and thermoreceptors) and encapsulated terminals (mechanoreceptors). Each type of receptor has its own set of sensitivities to specific stimuli, size and distinctness of receptive fields, and adaptational qualities. Much of the knowledge about these receptors has come from the development of techniques to study single intact nerve fibers intraneurally in awake, unanesthetized human subjects. It is possible not only to record from single nerve fibers, large or small, but also to stimulate single fibers in isolation. A single impulse, whether elicited by a natural stimulus or evoked by electrical microstimulation, in a large myelinated afferent fiber may be both perceived and localized.

Afferent fibers of all sizes in peripheral nerve trunks traverse the dorsal roots and enter the dorsal horn of the spinal cord (Fig. 22-1). From there the smaller fibers take a different route to the parietal cortex than the larger fibers. The polysynaptic projections of the smaller fibers (unmyelinated and small myelinated), which subserve mainly nociception, temperature sensibility, and touch, cross and ascend in the opposite anterior and lateral columns of the spinal cord, through the brainstem, to the ventral posterolateral (VPL) nucleus of the thalamus, and ultimately project to the postcentral gyrus of the parietal cortex (Chap. 11). This is referred to as the *spinothalamic pathway*, or *anterolateral system*. The larger fibers, which subserve tactile and position sense and kinesthesia, project rostrally in the posterior column on the same side of the spinal cord and make their first synapse in the gracile or cuneate nuclei of the lower medulla. The second-order neuron decussates and ascends in the medial lemniscus located medially in the medulla and in the tegmentum of the pons and midbrain and synapses in the VPL nucleus. The third-order neuron projects to pa-

FIGURE 22-1   Schematic diagram of lemniscal and spinothalamic pathways. Note that the large fibers that subserve proprioception and discriminative touch ascend ipsilaterally as the lemniscal pathway in the posterior column of the spinal cord, and that the small fibers that subserve pain, thermal sensation, and crude touch ascend contralaterally as the spinothalamic pathway in the anterior and lateral columns of the spinal cord (insert). SS CTX, somatosensory cortex; Thal, thalamus; VPL, ventral posterolateral nucleus.

rietal cortex; this large fiber system is referred to as the *posterior column–medial lemniscal pathway* (lemniscal, for short). Note that although the lemniscal and the anterolateral pathways both project up the spinal cord to the thalamus, it is the (crossed) anterolateral pathway that is referred to as the *spinothalamic tract*, by convention.

Although the fiber types and functions that make up the spinothalamic and lemniscal systems are relatively well known, it has been found that many other fibers, particularly those associated with touch, pressure, and position sense, ascend in a diffusely distributed pattern both ipsilaterally and contralaterally in the anterolateral quadrants of the spinal cord. This explains why an individual with a complete lesion of the posterior columns of the spinal cord may have little sensory deficit on examination.

EXAMINATION OF SENSATION

The main components of the sensory examination are tests of primary sensation. These include the sense of pain, touch, vibration, joint position, and thermal sensation, both hot and cold (Table 22-1). Detailed descriptions of how to perform the various tests of the sensory examination can be found in standard texts (see "Bibliography").

Some general principles pertain. The examiner must depend on patient responses, particularly when testing cutaneous sensation (pin, touch, warm or cold). This subjective element complicates the interpretation of the sensory examination. Further, some patients are only partially examinable. In a stuporous patient, sensory examination is reduced to observing the briskness of withdrawal in response to a pinch or other noxious stimulus. Comparison of response on one side of the body to the other is essential. In the alert but uncooperative patient, cutaneous sensation may be unexaminable. However, it is usually possible to get some idea of proprioceptive function by noting the patient's best performance of movements requiring balance and precision. Frequently, patients present with sensory symptoms that do not fit an anatomic localization and that are accompanied by either no abnormalities or gross inconsistencies on examination. The examiner should then consider whether the sensory symptoms are a disguised request for help with psychological or situational problems. Discretion must be used in pursuing this possibility. Finally, sensory examination of a patient who has no neurologic complaints can be brief and consist of pin, touch, and vibration testing in the hands and feet plus evaluation of stance and gait, including the Romberg maneuver. Evaluation of stance and gait also tests the integrity of motor and cerebellar systems.

PRIMARY SENSATION (See Table 22-1)

The sense of pain is usually tested with a clean pin, asking the patient to focus on the pricking or unpleasant quality of the stimulus and not just the pressure or touch sensation elicited. Areas of hypalgesia should be mapped by proceeding radially from the most hypalgesic site (Figs. 22-2 and 22-3).

Sense	Test Device	Endings Activated	Fiber Size Mediating	Central Pathway
Pain	Pinprick	Cutaneous nociceptors	Small	SpTh, also D
Temperature, heat	Warm metal object	Cutaneous thermoreceptors for hot	Small	SpTh
Temperature, cold	Cold metal object	Cutaneous thermoreceptors for cold	Small	SpTh
Touch	Cotton wisp, fine brush	Cutaneous mechanoreceptors, also naked endings	Large and small	Lem, also D and SpTh
Vibration	Tuning fork, 128 Hz	Mechanoreceptors, especially pacinian corpuscles	Large	Lem, also D
Joint position	Passive movement of specific joints	Joint capsule and tendon endings, muscle spindles	Large	Lem, also D

TABLE 22-1 *Testing Primary Sensation*

Note: D, diffuse ascending projections in ipsilateral and contralateral anterolateral columns; SpTh, spinothalamic projection, contralateral; Lem, posterior column and lemniscal projection, ipsilateral.

Temperature sensation, to both hot and cold, is probably best tested with water flasks filled with water of the desired temperature, using a thermometer to verify the temperature. This is impractical in most settings. An alternative way to test cold sensation is to touch a metal object, such as a tuning fork at room temperature, to the skin. For testing warm temperatures, the tuning fork or other metal object may be held under warm water of the desired temperature and then used. Both cold and warm should be tested because different receptors respond to each.

Touch is usually tested with a wisp of cotton or a fine camelhair brush. In general, it is better to avoid testing touch on hairy skin because of the profusion of sensory endings that surround each hair follicle.

Joint position testing is a measure of proprioception, one of the most important functions of the sensory system. With the patient keeping eyes closed, joint position is tested in the great toe and in the fingers. If errors are made in recognizing the direction of passive movements of the toe or the finger, more proximal joints should be tested. A test of proximal joint position sense, primarily at the shoulder, is performed by asking the patient to bring the two index fingers together with arms extended and eyes closed. Normal individuals can do this accurately, with errors of a centimeter or less.

The sense of vibration is tested with a tuning fork, preferably a large one that vibrates at 128 Hz. Vibration is usually tested at bony prominences, beginning distally at the malleoli of the ankles, and at the knuckles. If abnormalities are found, more proximal sites can be examined. Vibratory thesholds at the same site in the patient and the examiner may be compared for control purposes.

QUANTITATIVE SENSORY TESTING

Effective sensory testing devices have been developed over the past two decades. Quantitative sensory testing is particularly useful for serial evaluation of cutaneous sensation in clinical trials. Threshold testing for touch and vibratory and thermal sensation is the most widely used application.

CORTICAL SENSATION

The most commonly used tests of cortical function are two-point discrimination, touch localization, and bilateral simultaneous stimulation and tests for graphesthesia and stereognosis. Abnormalities of these sensory tests, in the presence of normal primary sensation in an alert cooperative patient, signify a lesion of the parietal cortex or thalamocortical projections to the parietal lobe. If primary sensation is altered, these cortical discriminative functions will usually be abnormal, too. Comparisons should always be made between analogous sites on the two sides of the body because the deficit with a specific parietal lesion is likely to be hemilateral. Side-to-side comparisons hold true for all cortical sensory testing.

Two-point discrimination is tested by special calipers, the points of which may be set from 2 mm to several centimeters apart and then applied simultaneously to the site to be tested. The pulp of the finger tips is a common site to test; a normal individual can distinguish about 3-mm separation of points there.

Touch localization is usually carried out by light pressure for an instant with the examiner's fingertip, asking the patient, whose eyes are closed, to identify the site of touch with his or her fingertip. *Bilateral simultaneous stimulation* at analogous sites (e.g., the dorsa of both hands) can be carried out to determine whether the perception of touch is extinguished consistently on one side or the other. The phenomenon is referred to as *extinction*. *Graphesthesia* means the capacity to recognize with eyes closed letters or numbers drawn by the examiner's fingertip on the palm of the hand. Once again, the comparison of one side with the other is of prime importance. Inability to recognize numbers or letters is termed *agraphesthesia*.

Stereognosis refers to the ability to identify common objects by palpation, recognizing their shape, texture, and size. Common standard objects are the best test objects, such as a marble, a paper clip, or coins. Patients with normal stereognosis should be able to distinguish a dime from a penny and a nickel from a quarter without looking. Patients should only be allowed to feel the object with one hand at a time. If they are unable to identify it in one hand, it should be placed in the other for comparison. Individuals unable to identify common objects and coins in one hand who can do so in the other are said to have *astereognosis* of the abnormal hand.

LOCALIZATION OF SENSORY ABNORMALITIES

Sensory symptoms and signs can result from lesions at almost any level of the nervous system, including parietal cortex, deep white matter, thalamus, brainstem, spinal cord, spinal root, peripheral nerve, and sensory receptor. Noting the distribution and nature of sensory symptoms and signs is the most important way to localize their source. The extent, configuration, symmetry, quality, and severity are the key observations.

Dysesthesias without sensory findings by examination can be difficult to interpret. To illustrate, tingling dysesthesias in an acral distribution (hands and feet) can be systemic in origin, e.g., secondary to hyperventilation, or can be induced by a medication, such as the diuretic acetazolamide. Distal dysesthesias can also be an early event in an evolving polyneuropathy or can herald a myelopathy, such as with vitamin B_{12} deficiency. Sometimes distal dysesthesias have no definable basis. In contrast, dysesthesias that correspond to a particular peripheral nerve territory denote a lesion of that nerve trunk. For instance, dysesthesias restricted to the fifth digit and the adjacent one-half of the fourth finger on one hand reliably point to disorder of the ulnar nerve, most commonly at the elbow.

NERVE AND ROOT

In focal nerve trunk lesions severe enough to cause a deficit, sensory abnormalities are readily mapped and generally have discrete boundaries (Figs. 22-2 and 22-3). Root lesions, referred to as radicular, are frequently accompanied by deep, aching pain along the

FIGURE 22-2   Anterior view of dermatomes *(left)* and cutaneous areas *(right)* supplied by individual peripheral nerves. *(Modified from MB Carpenter and J Sutin, in Human Neuroanatomy, 8th ed, Baltimore, Williams & Wilkins, 1983.)*

FIGURE 22-3   Posterior view of dermatomes *(left)* and cutaneous areas *(right)* supplied by individual peripheral nerves. *(Modified from MB Carpenter and J Sutin, in Human Neuroanatomy, 8th ed, Baltimore, Williams & Wilkins, 1983.)*

course of the related nerve trunk. With compression of a fifth lumbar (L5) or first sacral (S1) root, as may occur with a ruptured intervertebral disc, sciatica (radicular pain relating to the sciatic nerve trunk) is a frequent manifestation (Chap. 15). With a lesion affecting a single root, sensory deficit in the distribution of that root is often minimal or not demonstrable at all. This is because adjacent root territories overlap extensively.

Polyneuropathies are generally graded, distal, and symmetric in distribution of deficit (Chap. 363). Dysesthesias begin in the toes and ascend symmetrically, followed by numbness. When dysesthesias reach the knees, they have usually also appeared in the fingertips. The process appears to be nerve length–dependent, and the deficit is often described as "stocking-glove" in type. Although most polyneuropathies are pansensory and affect all modalities of sensation, selective sensory dysfunction according to nerve fiber size may occur. In polyneuropathies that affect small nerve fibers selectively, the hallmark is burning, painful dysesthesias with reduced pinprick and thermal sensation but with sparing of proprioception, motor function, and even deep tendon jerks. Touch is variably involved, but when spared, the sensory pattern is referred to as *sensory dissociation.* Sensory dissociation patterns can be seen with spinal cord lesions (see below) as well as with small fiber neuropathies. In contrast to small fiber polyneuropathies, large fiber polyneuropathies are characterized by position sense deficit, imbalance, absent tendon jerks, and variable motor dysfunction but preservation of most cutaneous sensation. Dysesthesias, if present at all, tend to be tingling or bandlike.

SPINAL CORD (See also Chap. 356)   If the spinal cord is transected, all sensation is lost below the level of transection. Bladder and bowel function are also lost, as is motor function. Hemisection of the spinal cord produces the Brown-Séquard syndrome, which involves absent pain and temperature sensation on the opposite side below the lesion, and loss of proprioceptive sensation and loss of motor power on the same side below the lesion (see Figs. 22-1 and 356-1). Dissociated sensory deficit patterns (see above) are also a sign of spinothalamic tract involvement in the spinal cord, especially if the deficit is unilateral and has an upper level on the torso. Bilateral spinothalamic tract involvement occurs with lesions affecting the center of the spinal cord, such as happens with expansion of the central canal in syringomyelia. Sensory dissociation is characteristic of syringomyelia.

BRAINSTEM   Harlequin patterns of sensory disturbance, in which one side of the face and the opposite side of the body are affected, localize to the lateral medulla. Here a small lesion may damage both the ipsilateral descending trigeminal tract and ascending spinothalamic fibers subserving the opposite arm, leg, and hemitorso (see "Lateral medullary syndrome" in Fig. 349-8). In the tegmentum of the pons and midbrain, where the lemniscal and spinothalamic tracts merge, a lesion here causes pansensory loss on the contralateral side.

THALAMUS   Hemisensory disturbance with tingling numbness from head to foot is often thalamic in origin but can also be anterior parietal. If abrupt in onset, the lesion is likely to be due to a small stroke (lacunar infarction), particularly if localized to the thalamus. Occasionally, with lesions affecting the VPL nucleus or adjacent white matter, a syndrome of thalamic pain, also called *Déjerine-Roussy syndrome,* may ensue. This persistent, unrelenting hemipainful state is often described in dramatic terms such as "like the flesh is being torn from my limbs" or "as though that side is bathed in acid."

CORTEX With lesions of the parietal lobe involving either the cortex or subjacent white matter, the most prominent symptoms are contralateral hemineglect, hemi-inattention, and a tendency not to use the affected hand and arm. On cortical sensory testing (two-point discrimination, graphesthesia, etc.), abnormalities are often found, but primary sensation is usually intact. Anterior parietal infarction may present as a pseudothalamic syndrome with crossed hemilateral loss of primary sensation from head to toe. Dysesthesias or a sense of numbness may also occur, and rarely, a painful state.

FOCAL SENSORY SEIZURES These are generally due to lesions in the area of the postcentral and/or precentral gyrus. The principal symptoms of

focal sensory seizures are tingling or numbness or both, but additional, more complex sensations may occur, such as a rushing feeling, a sense of warmth, or a sense of movement without detectable motion. Likely sites of unilateral symptom origin are in the arm or hand, face, leg, or foot, and symptoms often spread as in a Jacksonian march. Duration of seizures is variable; they may be transient, lasting only seconds, or they may persist for an hour or more. Focal motor features, like clonic jerking, can supervene, and seizures often become generalized with loss of consciousness and tonic-clonic jerking. On occasion, symptoms occur in a symmetric bilateral fashion, for instance, in both hands, as a result of involvement of the second sensory area (unilaterally) located in the rolandic area at and just above the Sylvian fissure.

23 | APHASIA, MEMORY LOSS, AND OTHER FOCAL CEREBRAL DISORDERS
M.-Marsel Mesulam

The cerebral cortex of the human brain contains approximately 20 billion neurons spread over an area of 2.5 m². The *primary sensory* areas provide an obligatory portal for the entry of sensory information into cortical circuitry, whereas the *primary motor* areas provide a final common pathway for coordinating complex motor acts. The primary sensory and motor areas constitute 10% of the cerebral cortex. The rest is subsumed by unimodal, heteromodal, paralimbic, and limbic areas, collectively known as the *association cortex* (Fig. 23-1). The association cortex mediates the integrative processes that subserve cognition, emotion, and behavior. A systematic testing of these mental functions is necessary for the effective clinical assessment of the association cortex and its diseases.

According to current thinking, there are no centers for "hearing words," "perceiving space," or "storing memories." Cognitive and behavioral functions (domains) are coordinated by intersecting *large-scale neural networks* that contain interconnected cortical and subcortical components. The network approach to higher cerebral function has at least four implications of clinical relevance: (1) a single domain such as language or memory can be disrupted by damage to any one of several areas, as long as these areas belong to the same network; (2) damage confined to a single area can give rise to multiple deficits, involving the functions of all networks that intersect in that region; (3) damage to a network component may give rise to minimal or transient deficits if other parts of the network undergo compensatory reorganization; and (4) individual anatomic sites within a network display a relative (but not absolute) specialization for different behavioral aspects of the relevant function. Five anatomically defined large-scale networks are most relevant to clinical practice: a perisylvian network for language; a parietofrontal network for spatial cognition; an occipitotemporal network for face and object recognition; a limbic network for retentive memory; and a prefrontal network for attention and behavior.

THE LEFT PERISYLVIAN NETWORK FOR LANGUAGE: APHASIAS AND RELATED CONDITIONS

Language allows the communication and elaboration of thoughts and experiences by linking them to arbitrary symbols known as words. The neural substrate of language is composed of a distributed network centered in the perisylvian region of the *left* hemisphere. The posterior pole of this network is known as *Wernicke's area* and includes the posterior third of the superior temporal gyrus and a surrounding rim of inferior parietal and midtemporal cortex. An essential function of Wernicke's area is to transform sensory inputs into their neural word representations so that these can establish the distributed associations that give the word its meaning. The anterior pole of the language network, known as *Broca's area*, includes the posterior part of the inferior frontal gyrus and a surrounding rim of prefrontal heteromodal

FIGURE 23-1 Lateral (*top*) and medial (*bottom*) views of the cerebral hemispheres. The numbers refer to the Brodmann cytoarchitectonic designations. Area 17 corresponds to primary visual cortex, 41–42 to primary auditory cortex, 1–3 to primary somatosensory cortex, and 4 to primary motor cortex. The rest of the cerebral cortex contains association areas. AG, angular gyrus; B, Broca's area; CC, corpus callosum; CG, cingulate cortex; DLPFC, dorsolateral prefrontal cortex; FEF, frontal eye fields (premotor cortex); FG, fusiform gyrus; IPL, inferior parietal lobule; ITG, inferior temporal gyrus; LG, lingual gyrus; MPFC, medial prefrontal cortex; MTG, middle temporal gyrus; OFC, orbitofrontal cortex; PHG, parahippocampal gyrus; PPC, posterior parietal cortex; PSC, peristriate cortex; SC, striate cortex; SMG, supramarginal gyrus; SPL, superior parietal lobule; STG, superior temporal gyrus; STS, superior temporal sulcus; TP, temporopolar cortex; W, Wernicke's area.

TABLE 23-1 *Clinical Features of Aphasias and Related Conditions*

	Comprehension	Repetition of Spoken Language	Naming	Fluency
Wernicke's	Impaired	Impaired	Impaired	Preserved or increased
Broca's	Preserved (except grammar)	Impaired	Impaired	Decreased
Global	Impaired	Impaired	Impaired	Decreased
Conduction	Preserved	Impaired	Impaired	Preserved
Nonfluent (motor) transcortical	Preserved	Preserved	Impaired	Impaired
Fluent (sensory) transcortical	Impaired	Preserved	Impaired	Preserved
Isolation	Impaired	Echolalia	Impaired	No purposeful speech
Anomic	Preserved	Preserved	Impaired	Preserved except for word-finding pauses
Pure word deafness	Impaired only for spoken language	Impaired	Preserved	Preserved
Pure alexia	Impaired only for reading	Preserved	Preserved	Preserved

cortex. An essential function of this area is to transform neural word representations into their articulatory sequences so that the words can be uttered in the form of spoken language. The sequencing function of Broca's area also appears to involve the ordering of words into sentences that contain a meaning-appropriate *syntax* (grammar). Wernicke's and Broca's areas are interconnected with each other and with additional perisylvian, temporal, prefrontal, and posterior parietal regions, making up a neural network subserving the various aspects of language function. Damage to any one of these components or to their interconnections can give rise to language disturbances (*aphasia*). Aphasia should be diagnosed only when there are deficits in the formal aspects of language such as naming, word choice, comprehension, spelling, and syntax. Dysarthria and mutism do not, by themselves, lead to a diagnosis of aphasia. The language network shows a left hemisphere dominance pattern in the vast majority of the population. In approximately 90% of right handers and 60% of left handers, aphasia occurs only after lesions of the left hemisphere. In some individuals no hemispheric dominance for language can be discerned, and in some others (including a small minority of right handers) there is a right hemisphere dominance for language. A language disturbance occurring after a right hemisphere lesion in a right hander is called *crossed aphasia*.

CLINICAL EXAMINATION The clinical examination of language should include the assessment of naming, spontaneous speech, comprehension, repetition, reading, and writing. A deficit of naming (*anomia*) is the single most common finding in aphasic patients. When asked to name common objects (pencil or wristwatch), the patient may fail to come up with the appropriate word, may provide a circumlocutious description of the object ("the thing for writing"), or may come up with the wrong word (*paraphasia*). If the patient offers an incorrect but legitimate word ("pen" for "pencil"), the naming error is known as a *semantic paraphasia*; if the word approximates the correct answer but is phonetically inaccurate ("plentil" for "pencil"), it is known as a *phonemic paraphasia*. Asking the patient to name body parts, geometric shapes, and component parts of objects (lapel of coat, cap of pen) can elicit mild forms of anomia in patients who can otherwise name common objects. In most anomias, the patient cannot retrieve the appropriate name when shown an object but can point to the appropriate object when the name is provided by the examiner. This is known as a one-way (or retrieval-based) naming deficit. A two-way naming deficit exists if the patient can neither provide nor recognize the correct name, indicating the presence of a language comprehension impairment. *Spontaneous speech* is described as "fluent" if it maintains appropriate output volume, phrase length, and melody or as "nonfluent" if it is sparse, halting, and average utterance length is below

four words. The examiner should also note if the speech is paraphasic or circumlocutious; if it shows a relative paucity of substantive nouns and action verbs versus function words (prepositions, conjunctions); and if word order, tenses, suffixes, prefixes, plurals, and possessives are appropriate. *Comprehension* can be tested by assessing the patient's ability to follow conversation, by asking yes-no questions ("Can a dog fly?", "Does it snow in summer?") or asking the patient to point to appropriate objects ("Where is the source of illumination in this room?"). Statements with embedded clauses or passive voice construction ("If a tiger is eaten by a lion, which animal stays alive?") help to assess the ability to comprehend complex syntactic structure. Commands to close or open the eyes, stand up, sit down, or roll over should not be used to assess overall comprehension since appropriate responses aimed at such axial movements can be preserved in patients who otherwise have profound comprehension deficits.

Repetition is assessed by asking the patient to repeat single words, short sentences, or strings of words such as "No ifs, ands, or buts." The testing of repetition with tongue-twisters such as "hippopotamus" or "Irish constabulary" provides a better assessment of dysarthria and pallilalia than aphasia. Aphasic patients may have little difficulty with tongue-twisters but have a particularly hard time repeating a string of function words. It is important to make sure that the number of words does not exceed the patient's attention span. Otherwise, the failure of repetition becomes a reflection of the narrowed attention span rather than an indication of an aphasic deficit. *Reading* should be assessed for deficits in reading aloud as well as comprehension. *Writing* is assessed for spelling errors, word order, and grammar. *Alexia* describes an inability to either read aloud or comprehend single words and simple sentences; *agraphia* (or *dysgraphia*) is used to describe an acquired deficit in the spelling or grammar of written language.

The correspondence between individual deficits of language function and lesion location does not display a rigid one-to-one relationship and should be conceptualized within the context of the distributed network model. Nonetheless, the classification of aphasic patients into specific clinical syndromes helps to determine the most likely anatomic distribution of the underlying neurologic disease and has implications for etiology and prognosis (Table 23-1). Aphasic syndromes can be divided into "central" syndromes, which result from damage to the two epicenters of the language network (Broca's and Wernicke's areas), and "disconnection" syndromes, which arise from lesions that interrupt the functional connectivity of these centers with each other and with the other components of the language network. The syndromes outlined below are idealizations; pure syndromes occur rarely.

Wernicke's Aphasia Comprehension is impaired for spoken and written language. Language output is fluent but is highly paraphasic and circumlocutious. The tendency for paraphasic errors may be so pronounced that it leads to strings of neologisms, which form the basis of what is known as "jargon aphasia." Speech contains large numbers of function words (e.g., prepositions, conjunctions) but few substantive nouns or verbs that refer to specific actions. The output is therefore voluminous but uninformative. For example, a patient attempts to describe how his wife accidentally threw away something important, perhaps his dentures: "We don't need it anymore, she says. And with it when that was downstairs was my teeth-tick . . . a . . . den . . . dentith . . . my dentist. And they happened to be in that bag . . . see? How could this have happened? How could a thing like this happen . . . So she says we won't need it anymore . . . I didn't think we'd use it. And now if I have any problems anybody coming a month from now, 4 months from now, or 6 months from now, I have a new dentist. Where my two . . . two little pieces of dentist that I use . . . that I . . . all gone. If she throws the whole thing away . . . visit some friends of hers and she can't throw them away."

Gestures and pantomime do not improve communication. The patient does not seem to realize that his or her language is incomprehensible and may appear angry and impatient when the examiner fails to decipher the meaning of a severely paraphasic statement. In some patients this type of aphasia can be associated with severe agitation and paranoid behaviors. One area of comprehension that may be preserved is the ability to follow commands aimed at axial musculature. The dissociation between the failure to understand simple questions ("What is your name") in a patient who rapidly closes his or her eyes, sits up, or rolls over when asked to do so is characteristic of Wernicke's aphasia and helps to differentiate it from deafness, psychiatric disease, or malingering. Patients with Wernicke's aphasia cannot express their thoughts in meaning-appropriate words and cannot decode the meaning of words in any modality of input. This aphasia therefore has expressive as well as receptive components. Repetition, naming, reading, and writing are also impaired.

The lesion site most commonly associated with Wernicke's aphasia is the posterior portion of the language network and tends to involve at least parts of Wernicke's area. An embolus to the inferior division of the middle cerebral artery, and to the posterior temporal or angular branches in particular, is the most common etiology (Chap. 349). Intracerebral hemorrhage, severe head trauma, or neoplasm are other causes. A coexisting right hemi- or superior quadrantanopia is common, and mild right nasolabial flattening may be found, but otherwise the examination is often unrevealing. The paraphasic, neologistic speech in an agitated patient with an otherwise unremarkable neurologic examination may lead to the suspicion of a primary psychiatric disorder such as schizophrenia or mania, but the other components characteristic of acquired aphasia and the absence of prior psychiatric disease usually settle the issue. Some patients with Wernicke's aphasia due to intracerebral hemorrhage or head trauma may improve as the hemorrhage or the injury heals. In most other patients, prognosis for recovery is guarded.

Broca's Aphasia Speech is nonfluent, labored, interrupted by many word-finding pauses, and usually dysarthric. It is impoverished in function words but enriched in meaning-appropriate nouns and verbs. Abnormal word order and the inappropriate deployment of *bound morphemes* (word endings used to denote tenses, possessives, or plurals) lead to a characteristic agrammatism. Speech is telegraphic and pithy but quite informative. In the following passage, a patient with Broca's aphasia describes his medical history: "I see . . . the dotor, dotor sent me . . . Bosson. Go to hospital. Dotor . . . kept me beside. Two, tee days, doctor send me home."

Output may be reduced to a grunt or single word ("yes" or "no"), which is emitted with different intonations in an attempt to express approval or disapproval. In addition to fluency, naming and repetition are also impaired. Comprehension of spoken language is intact, except for syntactically difficult sentences with passive voice structure or embedded clauses. Reading comprehension is also preserved, with the occasional exception of a specific inability to read small grammatical words such as conjunctions and pronouns. The last two features indicate that Broca's aphasia is not just an "expressive" or "motor" disorder and that it may also involve a comprehension deficit for function words and syntax. Patients with Broca's aphasia can be tearful, easily frustrated, and profoundly depressed. Insight into their condition is preserved, in contrast to Wernicke's aphasia. Even when spontaneous speech is severely dysarthric, the patient may be able to display a relatively normal articulation of words when singing. This dissociation has been used to develop specific therapeutic approaches (melodic intonation therapy) for Broca's aphasia. Additional neurologic deficits usually include right facial weakness, hemiparesis or hemiplegia, and a buccofacial apraxia characterized by an inability to carry out motor commands involving oropharyngeal and facial musculature (e.g., pa-

tients are unable to demonstrate how to blow out a match or suck through a straw). Visual fields are intact. The cause is most often infarction of Broca's area (the inferior frontal convolution; "B" in Fig. 23-1) and surrounding anterior perisylvian and insular cortex, due to occlusion of the superior division of the middle cerebral artery (Chap. 349). Mass lesions including tumor, intracerebral hemorrhage, or abscess may also be responsible. Small lesions confined to the posterior part of Broca's area may lead to a nonaphasic and often reversible deficit of speech articulation, usually accompanied by mild right facial weakness. When the cause of Broca's aphasia is stroke, recovery of language function generally peaks within 2 to 6 months, after which time further progress is limited.

Global Aphasia Speech output is nonfluent, and comprehension of spoken language is severely impaired. Naming, repetition, reading, and writing are also impaired. This syndrome represents the combined dysfunction of Broca's and Wernicke's areas and usually results from strokes that involve the entire middle cerebral artery distribution in the left hemisphere. Most patients are initially mute or say a few words, such as "hi" or "yes." Related signs include right hemiplegia, hemisensory loss, and homonymous hemianopia. Occasionally, a patient with a lesion in Wernicke's area will present with a global aphasia that soon resolves into Wernicke's aphasia.

Conduction Aphasia Speech output is fluent but paraphasic, comprehension of spoken language is intact, and repetition is severely impaired. Naming and writing are also impaired. Reading aloud is impaired, but reading comprehension is preserved. The lesion sites spare Broca's and Wernicke's areas but may induce a functional disconnection between the two so that neural word representations formed in Wernicke's area and adjacent regions cannot be conveyed to Broca's area for assembly into corresponding articulatory patterns. Occasionally, a Wernicke's area lesion gives rise to a transient Wernicke's aphasia that rapidly resolves into a conduction aphasia. The paraphasic output in conduction aphasia interferes with the ability to express meaning, but this deficit is not nearly as severe as the one displayed by patients with Wernicke's aphasia. Associated neurologic signs in conduction aphasia vary according to the primary lesion site.

Nonfluent Transcortical Aphasia (Transcortical Motor Aphasia) The features are similar to Broca's aphasia, but repetition is intact and agrammatism may be less pronounced. The neurologic examination may be otherwise intact, but a right hemiparesis can also exist. The lesion site disconnects the intact language network from prefrontal areas of the brain and usually involves the anterior watershed zone between anterior and middle cerebral artery territories or the supplementary motor cortex in the territory of the anterior cerebral artery.

Fluent Transcortical Aphasia (Transcortical Sensory Aphasia) Clinical features are similar to those of Wernicke's aphasia, but repetition is intact. The lesion site disconnects the intact core of the language network from other temporoparietal association areas. Associated neurologic findings may include hemianopia. Cerebrovascular lesions (e.g., infarctions in the posterior watershed zone) or neoplasms that involve the temporoparietal cortex posterior to Wernicke's area are the most common causes.

Isolation Aphasia This rare syndrome represents a combination of the two transcortical aphasias. Comprehension is severely impaired, and there is no purposeful speech output. The patient may parrot fragments of heard conversations (*echolalia*), indicating that the neural mechanisms for repetition are at least partially intact. This condition represents the pathologic function of the language network when it is isolated from other regions of the brain. Broca's and Wernicke's areas tend to be spared, but there is damage to the surrounding frontal, parietal, and temporal cortex. Lesions are patchy and can be associated with anoxia, carbon monoxide poisoning, or complete watershed zone infarctions.

Anomic Aphasia   This form of aphasia may be considered the "minimal dysfunction" syndrome of the language network. Articulation, comprehension, and repetition are intact, but confrontation naming, word finding, and spelling are impaired. Speech is enriched in function words but impoverished in substantive nouns and verbs denoting specific actions. Language output is fluent but paraphasic, circumlocutious, and uninformative. The lesion sites can be anywhere within the left hemisphere language network, including the middle and inferior temporal gyri. *Anomic aphasia is the single most common language disturbance seen in head trauma, metabolic encephalopathy, and Alzheimer's disease.* The language impairment of Alzheimer's disease almost always leads to fluent aphasias (e.g., anomic, Wernicke's, conduction, or fluent transcortical aphasia). The insidious onset and relentless progression of nonfluent language disturbances (Broca's or nonfluent transcortical aphasia) can be seen in *primary progressive aphasia*, a degenerative syndrome most commonly associated with focal nonspecific neuronal loss or Pick's disease.

Pure Word Deafness   This is not a true aphasic syndrome because the language deficit is modality-specific. The most common lesions are either bilateral or left-sided in the superior temporal gyrus. The net effect of the underlying lesion is to interrupt the flow of information from the unimodal auditory association cortex to Wernicke's area. Patients have no difficulty understanding written language and can express themselves well in spoken or written language. They have no difficulty interpreting and reacting to environmental sounds since primary auditory cortex and subcortical auditory relays are intact. Since auditory information cannot be conveyed to the language network, however, it cannot be decoded into neural word representations and the patient reacts to speech as if it were in an alien tongue that cannot be deciphered. Patients cannot repeat spoken language but have no difficulty naming objects. In time, patients with pure word deafness teach themselves lip reading and may appear to have improved. There may be no additional neurologic findings, but agitated paranoid reactions are frequent in the acute stages. Cerebrovascular lesions are the most frequent cause.

Pure Alexia without Agraphia   This is the visual equivalent of pure word deafness. The lesions (usually a combination of damage to the left occipital cortex and to a posterior sector of the corpus callosum—the splenium) interrupt the flow of visual input into the language network. There is usually a right hemianopia, but the core language network remains unaffected. The patient can understand and produce spoken language, name objects in the left visual hemifield, repeat, and write. However, the patient acts as if illiterate when asked to read even the simplest sentence because the visual information from the written words (presented to the intact left visual hemifield) cannot reach the language network. Objects in the left hemifield may be named accurately because they activate nonvisual associations in the right hemisphere, which, in turn, can access the language network through transcallosal pathways anterior to the splenium. Patients with this syndrome may also lose the ability to name colors, although they can match colors. This is known as a *color anomia*. The most common etiology of pure alexia is a vascular lesion in the territory of the posterior cerebral artery or an infiltrating neoplasm in the left occipital cortex that involves the optic radiations as well as the crossing fibers of the splenium. Since the posterior cerebral artery also supplies medial temporal components of the limbic system, the patient with pure alexia may also experience an amnesia, but this is usually transient because the limbic lesion is unilateral.

Aphemia   There is an acute onset of severely impaired fluency (often mutism), which cannot be accounted for by corticobulbar, cerebellar, or extrapyramidal dysfunction. Recovery is the rule and involves an intermediate stage of hoarse whispering. Writing, reading, and comprehension are intact, so this is not a true aphasic syndrome. Partial lesions of Broca's area or subcortical lesions that undercut its connections with other parts of the brain may be present. Occasionally, the lesion site is on the medial aspects of the frontal lobes and may involve the supplementary motor cortex of the left hemisphere.

Apraxia   This generic term designates a complex motor deficit that cannot be attributed to pyramidal, extrapyramidal, cerebellar, or sensory dysfunction and that does not arise from the patient's failure to understand the nature of the task. The form that is most frequently encountered in clinical practice is known as *ideomotor apraxia*. Commands to perform a specific motor act ("cough," "blow out a match") or to pantomime the use of a common tool (a comb, hammer, straw, or toothbrush) in the absence of the real object cannot be followed. The patient's ability to comprehend the command is ascertained by demonstrating multiple movements and establishing that the correct one can be recognized. Some patients with this type of apraxia can imitate the appropriate movement (when it is demonstrated by the examiner) and show no impairment when handed the real object, indicating that the sensorimotor mechanisms necessary for the movement are intact. Some forms of ideomotor apraxia represent a disconnection of the language network from pyramidal motor systems: commands to execute complex movements are understood but cannot be conveyed to the appropriate motor areas, even though the relevant motor mechanisms are intact. *Buccofacial apraxia* involves apraxic deficits in movements of the face and mouth. *Limb apraxia* encompasses apraxic deficits in movements of the arms and legs. Ideomotor apraxia is almost always caused by lesions in the left hemisphere and is commonly associated with aphasic syndromes, especially Broca's aphasia and conduction aphasia. Its presence cannot be ascertained in patients with language comprehension deficits. The ability to follow commands aimed at axial musculature ("close the eyes," "stand up") is subserved by different pathways and may be intact in otherwise severely aphasic and apraxic patients. Patients with lesions of the anterior corpus callosum can display a special type of ideomotor apraxia confined to the left side of the body. Since the handling of real objects is not impaired, ideomotor apraxia, by itself, causes no major limitation of daily living activities.

Ideational apraxia refers to a deficit in the execution of a goal-directed sequence of movements in patients who have no difficulty executing the individual components of the sequence. For example, when asked to pick up a pen and write, the sequence of uncapping the pen, placing the cap at the opposite end, turning the point towards the writing surface, and writing may be disrupted, and the patient may be seen trying to write with the wrong end of the pen or even with the removed cap. These motor sequencing problems are usually seen in the context of confusional states and dementias rather than focal lesions associated with aphasic conditions. *Limb-kinetic apraxia* involves a clumsiness in the actual use of tools that cannot be attributed to sensory, pyramidal, extrapyramidal, or cerebellar dysfunction. This condition can emerge in the context of focal premotor cortex lesions or *corticobasal ganglionic degeneration*.

Gerstmann's Syndrome   The combination of *acalculia* (impairment of simple arithmetic), *dysgraphia* (impaired writing), *finger anomia* (an inability to name individual fingers such as the index or thumb), and *right-left confusion* (an inability to tell whether a hand, foot, or arm of the patient or examiner is on the right or left side of the body) is known as Gerstmann's syndrome. In making this diagnosis it is important to establish that the finger and left-right naming deficits are not part of a more generalized anomia and that the patient is not otherwise aphasic. When Gerstmann's syndrome is seen in isolation, it is commonly associated with damage to the inferior parietal lobule (especially the angular gyrus) in the left hemisphere.

Aprosodia   Variations of melodic stress and intonation influence the meaning and impact of spoken language. For example, the two statements "He *is* clever." and "He is *clever*?" contain an identical word choice and syntax but convey vastly different messages because of differences in the intonation and stress with which the statements are uttered. This aspect of language is known as *prosody*. Damage to perisylvian areas in the right hemisphere can interfere with speech prosody and can lead to syndromes of aprosodia. Damage to right hemisphere regions corresponding to Wernicke's area can selectively impair decoding of speech prosody, whereas damage to right hemisphere regions corresponding to Broca's area yields a greater impairment in the ability to introduce meaning-appropriate prosody into spoken language. The latter deficit is the most common type of aprosodia identified in clinical practice—the patient produces grammatically correct language with accurate word choice but the statements are uttered in a monotone that interferes with the ability to convey the intended stress and affect. Patients with this type of aprosodia give the mistaken impression of being depressed or indifferent.

Subcortical Aphasia Damage to subcortical components of the language network (e.g., the striatum and thalamus of the left hemisphere) can also lead to aphasia. The resulting syndromes contain combinations of deficits in the various aspects of language but rarely fit the specific patterns described in Table 23-1. An anomic aphasia accompanied by dysarthria or a fluent aphasia with hemiparesis should raise the suspicion of a subcortical lesion site.

THE PARIETOFRONTAL NETWORK FOR SPATIAL ORIENTATION: NEGLECT AND RELATED CONDITIONS

HEMISPATIAL NEGLECT Adaptive orientation to significant events within the extrapersonal space is subserved by a large-scale network containing three major cortical components. The *cingulate cortex* provides access to a limbic-motivational mapping of the extrapersonal space, the *posterior parietal cortex* to a sensorimotor representation of salient extrapersonal events, and the *frontal eye fields* to motor strategies for attentional behaviors (Fig. 23-2). Subcortical components of this network include the striatum and the thalamus. Contralesional hemispatial neglect represents one outcome of damage to any of the cortical or subcortical components of this network. *The traditional view that hemispatial neglect always denotes a parietal lobe lesion is inaccurate.* In keeping with this anatomic organization, the clinical manifestations of neglect display three behavioral components: sensory events

FIGURE 23-2 Functional magnetic resonance imaging of language and spatial attention in neurologically intact subjects. The dark areas show regions of task-related significant activation. (*Top*) The subjects were asked to determine if two words were synonymous. This language task led to the simultaneous activation of the two epicenters of the language network, Broca's area (B) and Wernicke's area (W). The activations are exclusively in the left hemisphere. (*Bottom*) The subjects were asked to shift spatial attention to a peripheral target. This task led to the simultaneous activation of the three epicenters of the attentional network, the posterior parietal cortex (P), the frontal eye fields (F), and the cingulate gyrus (CG). The activations are predominantly in the right hemisphere. (*Courtesy of Darren Gitelman, MD.*)

(or their mental representations) within the neglected hemispace have a lesser impact on overall awareness; there is a paucity of exploratory and orienting acts directed toward the neglected hemispace; and the patient behaves as if the neglected hemispace was motivationally devalued.

According to one model of spatial cognition, the right hemisphere directs attention within the *entire* extrapersonal space, whereas the left hemisphere directs attention mostly within the contralateral right hemispace. Consequently, unilateral left hemisphere lesions do not give rise to much contralesional neglect since the ipsilateral attentional mechanisms of the right hemisphere can compensate for the loss of the *contralaterally* directed attentional functions of the left hemisphere. Unilateral right hemisphere lesions, however, give rise to severe contralesional left hemispatial neglect because the unaffected left hemisphere does not contain ipsilateral attentional mechanisms. This model is consistent with clinical experience, which shows that contralesional neglect is more common, severe, and lasting after damage to the right hemisphere than after damage to the left hemisphere. Severe neglect for the right hemispace is rare, even in left handers with left hemisphere lesions.

Patients with severe neglect may fail to dress, shave, or groom the left side of the body; may fail to eat food placed on the left side of the tray; and may fail to read the left half of sentences. When the examiner draws a large circle [12 to 15 cm (5 to 6 in.) in diameter] and asks the patient to place the numbers 1 to 12 as if the circle represented the face of a clock, there is a tendency to crowd the numbers on the right side and leave the left side empty. When asked to copy a simple line drawing, the patient fails to copy detail on the left; and when asked to write, there is a tendency to leave an unusually wide margin on the left.

Two bedside tests that are useful in assessing neglect are *simultaneous bilateral stimulation* and *visual target cancellation*. In the former, the examiner provides either unilateral or simultaneous bilateral stimulation in the visual, auditory, and tactile modalities. Following right hemisphere injury, patients who have no difficulty detecting unilateral stimuli on either side experience the bilaterally presented stimulus as coming only from the right. This phenomenon is known as *extinction* and is a manifestation of the sensory-representational aspect of hemispatial neglect. In the target detection task, targets (e.g., As) are interspersed with foils (e.g., other letters of the alphabet) on a 21.5 to 28.0 cm (8.5 to 11 in.) sheet of paper and the patient is asked to circle all the targets. A failure to detect targets on the left is a manifestation of the exploratory deficit in hemispatial neglect (Fig. 23-3A). Hemianopia, by itself, does not interfere with performance in this task since the patient is free to turn the head and eyes to the left. The normal tendency in target detection tasks is to start from the left upper quadrant and move systematically in horizontal or vertical sweeps. Some patients show a tendency to start the process from the right and proceed in a haphazard fashion. This represents a subtle manifestation of left neglect, even if the patient eventually manages to detect all the appropriate targets. Some patients with neglect may also deny the existence of hemiparesis and may even deny ownership of the paralyzed limb, a condition known as *anosognosia*.

Cerebrovascular lesions and neoplasms in the right hemisphere are the most common causes of hemispatial neglect. Depending on the site of the lesion, the patient with neglect may also have hemiparesis, hemihypesthesia, and hemianopia on the left, but these are not invariant findings. The majority of patients display considerable improvement of hemispatial neglect, usually within the first several weeks.

BÁLINT'S SYNDROME, SIMULTANAGNOSIA, DRESSING APRAXIA, AND CONSTRUCTION APRAXIA Bilateral involvement of the network for spatial attention, especially its parietal components, leads to a state of severe spatial disorientation known as *Bálint's syndrome*. Bálint's syndrome involves deficits in the orderly visuomotor scanning of the environment (*oculomotor apraxia*) and in accurate manual reaching toward visual targets (*optic ataxia*). The third and most dramatic component of Bálint's syndrome is known as *simultanagnosia* and reflects an

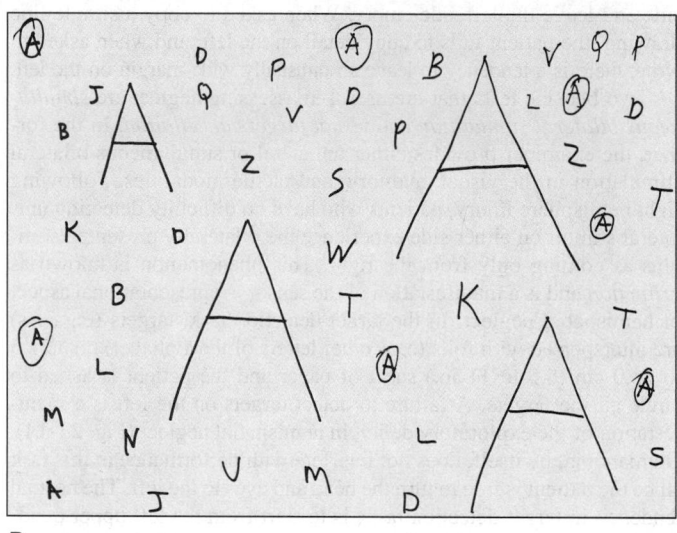

FIGURE 23-3 *A.* A 47-year-old man with a large frontoparietal lesion in the right hemisphere was asked to circle all the As. Only targets on the right are circled. This is a manifestation of left hemispatial neglect. *B.* A 70-year-old woman with a 2-year history of degenerative dementia was able to circle most of the small targets but ignored the larger ones. This is a manifestation of simultanagnosia.

be used for the bedside diagnosis of simultanagnosia. In this modification, some of the targets (e.g., As) are made to be much larger than the others [7.5 to 10 cm vs 2.5 cm (3 to 4 in. vs 1 in.) in height], and all targets are embedded among foils. Patients with simultanagnosia display a counterintuitive but characteristic tendency to miss the larger targets (Fig. 23-3*B*). This occurs because the information needed for the identification of the larger targets cannot be confined to the immediate line of gaze and requires the integration of visual information across a more extensive field of view. The greater difficulty in the detection of the larger targets also indicates that poor acuity is not responsible for the impairment of visual function and that the problem is central rather than peripheral. Bálint's syndrome results from bilateral dorsal parietal lesions; common settings include watershed infarction between the middle and posterior cerebral artery territories, hypoglycemia, sagittal sinus thrombosis, or atypical forms of Alzheimer's disease. In patients with Bálint's syndrome due to stroke, bilateral visual field defects (usually inferior quadrantanopias) are common.

Another manifestation of bilateral (or right-sided) dorsal parietal lobe lesions is *dressing apraxia*. The patient with this condition is unable to align the body axis with the axis of the garment and can be seen struggling as he or she holds a coat from its bottom or extends his or her arm into a fold of the garment rather than into its sleeve. Lesions that involve the posterior parietal cortex also lead to severe difficulties in copying simple line drawings. This is known as a *construction apraxia* and is much more severe if the lesion is in the right hemisphere. In some patients with right hemisphere lesions, the drawing difficulties are confined to the left side of the figure and represent a manifestation of hemispatial neglect; in others, there is a more universal deficit in reproducing contours and three-dimensional perspective. Dressing apraxia and construction apraxia represent special instances of a more general disturbance in spatial orientation.

THE OCCIPITOTEMPORAL NETWORK FOR FACE AND OBJECT RECOGNITION: PROSOPAGNOSIA AND OBJECT AGNOSIA

Perceptual information about faces and objects is initially encoded in primary (striate) visual cortex and adjacent (upstream) peristriate visual association areas. This information is subsequently relayed first to the downstream visual association areas of occipitotemporal cortex and then to other heteromodal and paralimbic areas of the cerebral cortex. Bilateral lesions in the fusiform and lingual gyri of occipitotemporal cortex disrupt this process and interfere with the ability of otherwise intact perceptual information to activate the distributed multimodal associations that lead to the recognition of faces and objects. The resultant face and object recognition deficits are known as *prosopagnosia* and *visual object agnosia*.

The patient with prosopagnosia cannot recognize familiar faces, including, sometimes, the reflection of his or her own face in the mirror. This is not a perceptual deficit since prosopagnosic patients can easily tell if two faces are identical or not. Furthermore, a prosopagnosic patient who cannot recognize a familiar face by visual inspection alone can use auditory cues to reach appropriate recognition if allowed to listen to the person's voice. The deficit in prosopagnosia is therefore modality-specific and reflects the existence of a lesion that prevents the activation of otherwise intact multimodal templates by relevant visual input. Damasio has pointed out that the deficit in prosopagnosia

inability to integrate visual information in the center of gaze with more peripheral information. The patient gets stuck on the detail that falls in the center of gaze without attempting to scan the visual environment for additional information. The patient with simultanagnosia "misses the forest for the trees." Complex visual scenes cannot be grasped in their entirety, leading to severe limitations in the visual identification of objects and scenes. For example, a patient who is shown a table lamp and asked to name the object may look at its circular base and call it an ash tray. Some patients with simultanagnosia report that objects they look at may suddenly vanish, probably indicating an inability to look back at the original point of gaze after brief saccadic displacements. Movement and distracting stimuli greatly exacerbate the difficulties of visual perception. Simultanagnosia can sometimes occur without the other two components of Bálint's syndrome.

A modification of the letter cancellation task described above canis not limited to the recognition of faces but that it can also extend to the recognition of individual members of larger generic object groups. For example, prosopagnosic patients characteristically have no difficulty with the generic identification of a face as a face or of a car as a car, but they cannot recognize the identity of an individual face or the make of an individual car. This reflects a visual recognition deficit for proprietary features that characterize individual members of an object class. When recognition problems become more generalized and extend to the generic identification of common objects, the condition is known as visual object agnosia. In contrast to prosopagnosic patients, those with object agnosia cannot recognize a face as a face or a car as a car.

It is important to distinguish visual object agnosia from anomia. The patient with anomia cannot name the object but can describe its use. In contrast, the patient with visual agnosia is unable either to name a visually presented object or to describe its use. The characteristic lesions in prosopagnosia and visual object agnosia consist of bilateral infarctions in the territory of the posterior cerebral arteries. Associated deficits can include visual field defects (especially superior quadrantanopias) or a centrally based color blindness known as achromatopsia. Rarely, the responsible lesion is unilateral. In such cases, prosopagnosia is associated with lesions in the right hemisphere and object agnosia with lesions in the left.

THE LIMBIC NETWORK FOR MEMORY: AMNESIAS

Limbic and paralimbic areas (such as the hippocampus, amygdala, and entorhinal cortex), the anterior and medial nuclei of the thalamus, the medial and basal parts of the striatum, and the hypothalamus collectively constitute a distributed network known as the *limbic system* (see Fig. 350-1). The behavioral affiliations of this network include the coordination of emotion, motivation, autonomic tone, and endocrine function. An additional area of specialization for the limbic network, and the one which is of most relevance to clinical practice, is that of declarative (conscious) memory for recent episodes and experiences. A disturbance in this function is known as an *amnestic state*. In the absence of deficits in motivation, attention, language, or visuospatial function, the clinical diagnosis of a persistent global amnestic state is always associated with bilateral damage to the limbic network, usually within the hippocampo-entorhinal complex or the thalamus.

Although the limbic network is the site of damage for amnestic states, it is almost certainly not the storage site for memories. Memories are stored in widely distributed form throughout the cerebral cortex. The role attributed to the limbic network is to bind these distributed fragments into coherent events and experiences that can sustain conscious recall. Damage to the limbic network does not necessarily destroy memories but interferes with their conscious (declarative) recall in coherent form. The individual fragments of information remain preserved despite the limbic lesions and can sustain what is known as *implicit memory*. For example, patients with amnestic states can acquire new motor or perceptual skills, even though they may have no conscious knowledge of the experiences that led to the acquisition of these skills.

The memory disturbance in the amnestic state is multimodal and includes retrograde and anterograde components. The *retrograde amnesia* involves an inability to recall experiences that occurred before the onset of the amnestic state. Relatively recent events are more vulnerable to retrograde amnesia than more remote and more extensively consolidated events. A patient who comes to the emergency room complaining that he cannot remember his identity but who can remember the events of the previous day is almost certainly not suffering from a neurologic cause of memory disturbance. The second and most important component of the amnestic state is the *anterograde amnesia*, which indicates an inability to store, retain, and recall new knowledge. Patients with amnestic states cannot remember what they ate a few minutes ago or the details of an important event they may have experienced a few hours ago. In the acute stages, there may also be a tendency to fill in memory gaps with inaccurate, fabricated, and often implausible information. This is known as *confabulation*. Patients with the amnestic syndrome forget that they forget and tend to deny the existence of a memory problem when questioned.

The patient with an amnestic state is almost always disoriented, especially to time. Accurate temporal orientation and accurate knowledge of current news rule out a major amnestic state. The anterograde component of an amnestic state can be tested with a list of four to five words read aloud by the examiner up to five times or until the patient can immediately repeat the entire list without intervening delay. In the next phase of testing, the patient is allowed to concentrate on the words and to rehearse them internally for 1 min before being asked to recall them. Accurate performance in this phase indicates that the patient is motivated and sufficiently attentive to hold the words online for at least 1 min. The final phase of the testing involves a retention period of 5 to 10 min, during which the patient is engaged in other tasks. Adequate recall at the end of this interval requires offline storage, retention, and retrieval. Amnestic patients fail this phase of the task and may even forget that they were given a list of words to remember. Accurate recognition of the words by multiple choice in a patient who cannot recall them indicates a less severe memory disturbance that affects mostly the retrieval stage of memory. The retrograde component of an amnesia can be assessed with questions related to autobiographical or historical events. The anterograde component of amnestic states is usually much more prominent than the retrograde component. In rare instances, usually associated with temporal lobe epilepsy or benzodiazepine intake, the retrograde component may dominate.

The assessment of memory can be quite challenging. Bedside evaluations may only detect the most severe impairments. Less severe memory impairments, as in the case of patients with temporal lobe epilepsy, mild head injury or early dementia, require quantitative evaluations by neuropsychologists. Confusional states caused by toxic metabolic encephalopathies and some types of frontal lobe damage interfere with attentional capacity and lead to secondary memory impairments, even in the absence of any limbic lesions. This sort of memory impairment can be differentiated from the amnestic state by the presence of additional impairments in the attention-related tasks described below in the section on the frontal lobes.

Many neurologic diseases can give rise to an amnestic state. These include tumors (of the sphenoid wing, posterior corpus callosum, thalamus, or medial temporal lobe), infarctions (in the territories of the anterior or posterior cerebral arteries), head trauma, herpes simplex encephalitis, Wernicke-Korsakoff encephalopathy, paraneoplastic limbic encephalitis, and degenerative dementias such as Alzheimer's or Pick's disease. The one common denominator of all these diseases is that they lead to the bilateral lesions within one or more components in the limbic network, most commonly the hippocampus, entorhinal cortex, the mammillary bodies of the hypothalamus, and the limbic thalamus. Occasionally, unilateral left-sided lesions can give rise to an amnestic state, but the memory disorder tends to be transient. Depending on the nature and distribution of the underlying neurologic disease, the patient may also have visual field deficits, eye movement limitations, or cerebellar findings.

Transient global amnesia is a distinctive syndrome usually seen in late middle age. Patients become acutely disoriented and repeatedly ask who they are, where they are, what they are doing. The spell is characterized by anterograde amnesia (inability to retain new information) and a retrograde amnesia for relatively recent events that occurred before the onset. The syndrome usually resolves within 24 to 48 h and is followed by the filling-in of the period affected by the retrograde amnesia, although there is persistent loss of memory for the events that occurred during the ictus. Recurrences are noted in approximately 20% of patients. Migraine, temporal lobe seizures, and transient ischemic events in the posterior cerebral territory have been postulated as causes of transient global amnesia. The absence of associated neurologic findings may occasionally lead to the incorrect diagnosis of a psychiatric disorder.

THE PREFRONTAL NETWORK FOR ATTENTION AND BEHAVIOR

Approximately one-third of all the cerebral cortex in the human brain is located in the frontal lobes. The frontal lobes can be subdivided into motor-premotor, dorsolateral prefrontal, medial prefrontal, and orbitofrontal components. The terms *frontal lobe syndrome* and *prefrontal cortex* refer only to the last three of these four components. These are the parts of the cerebral cortex that show the greatest phylogenetic expansion in primates and especially in humans. The dorsolateral prefrontal, medial prefrontal, and orbitofrontal areas, and the subcortical structures with which they are interconnected (i.e., the head of the caudate and the dorsomedial nucleus of the thalamus), collectively make up a large-scale network that coordinates exceedingly complex aspects of human cognition and behavior.

The prefrontal network plays an important role in behaviors that require an integration of thought with emotion and motivation. There is no simple formula for summarizing the diverse functional affiliations of the prefrontal network. Its integrity appears important for the simultaneous awareness of context, options, consequences, relevance, and emotional impact so as to allow the formulation of adaptive inferences, decisions, and actions. Damage to this part of the brain impairs mental flexibility, reasoning, hypothesis formation, abstract thinking, foresight, judgment, the online (attentive) holding of information, and the ability to inhibit inappropriate responses. Behaviors impaired by prefrontal cortex lesions, especially those related to the manipulation of mental content, are often referred to as "executive functions."

Even very large bilateral prefrontal lesions may leave all sensory, motor, and basic cognitive functions intact while leading to isolated but dramatic alterations of personality and behavior. The most common clinical manifestations of damage to the prefrontal network take the form of two relatively distinct syndromes. In the *frontal abulic syndrome*, the patient shows a loss of initiative, creativity, and curiosity and displays a pervasive emotional blandness and apathy. In the *frontal disinhibition syndrome*, the patient becomes socially disinhibited and shows severe impairments of judgment, insight, and foresight. The dissociation between intact intellectual function and a total lack of even rudimentary common sense is striking. Despite the preservation of all essential memory functions, the patient cannot learn from experience and continues to display inappropriate behaviors without appearing to feel emotional pain, guilt, or regret when such behaviors repeatedly lead to disastrous consequences. The impairments may emerge only in real-life situations when behavior is under minimal external control and may not be apparent within the structured environment of the medical office. Testing judgment by asking patients what they would do if they detected a fire in a theater or found a stamped and addressed envelope on the road is not very informative since patients who answer these questions wisely in the office may still act very foolishly in the more complex real-life setting. The physician must therefore be prepared to make a diagnosis of frontal lobe disease on the basis of historic information alone even when the office examination of mental state may be quite intact.

The abulic syndrome tends to be associated with damage to the dorsolateral prefrontal cortex, and the disinhibition syndrome with the medial prefrontal or orbitofrontal cortex. These syndromes tend to arise almost exclusively after bilateral lesions, most frequently in the setting of head trauma, stroke, ruptured aneurysms, hydrocephalus, tumors (including metastases, glioblastoma, and falx or olfactory groove meningiomas), or focal degenerative diseases. Unilateral lesions confined to the prefrontal cortex may remain silent until the pathology spreads to the other side. The emergence of developmentally primitive reflexes, also known as frontal release signs, such as grasping (elicited by stroking the palm) and sucking (elicited by stroking the lips) are seen primarily in patients with large structural lesions that extend into the premotor components of the frontal lobes or in the context of metabolic encephalopathies. The vast majority of patients with prefrontal lesions and frontal lobe behavioral syndromes do not display these reflexes.

Damage to the frontal lobe disrupts a variety of attention-related functions including working memory (the transient online holding of information), concentration span, the scanning and retrieval of stored information, the inhibition of immediate but inappropriate responses, and mental flexibility. The capacity for focusing on a trend of thought and the ability to voluntarily shift the focus of attention from one thought or stimulus to another can become impaired. Digit span (which should be seven forward and five reverse) is decreased; the recitation of the months of the year in reverse order (which should take less than 15 s) is slowed; and the fluency in producing words starting with a, f, or s that can be generated in 1 min (normally 12 or more per letter) is diminished even in nonaphasic patients. Characteristically, there is a progressive slowing of performance as the task proceeds; e.g., the patient asked to count backwards by 3s may say "100, 97, 94, . . 91, ... 88," etc., and may not complete the task. In "go–no-go" tasks (where the instruction is to raise the finger upon hearing one tap but to keep it still upon hearing two taps), the patient shows a characteristic inability to keep still in response to the "no go" stimulus; mental flexibility (tested by the ability to shift from one criterion to another in sorting or matching tasks) is impoverished; distractibility by irrelevant stimuli is increased; and there is a pronounced tendency for impersistence and perseveration.

These attentional deficits disrupt the orderly registration and retrieval of new information and lead to *secondary* memory deficits. Such memory deficits can be differentiated from the *primary* memory impairments of the amnestic state by showing that they improve when the attentional load of the task is decreased. Working memory (also known as immediate memory) is an attentional function based on the temporary online holding of information. It is closely associated with the integrity of the prefrontal network and the ascending reticular activating system. Retentive memory, on the other hand, depends on the stable (offline) storage of information and is associated with the integrity of the limbic network. The distinction of the underlying neural mechanisms is illustrated by the observation that severely amnestic patients who cannot remember events that occurred a few minutes ago may have intact if not superior working memory capacity as shown in tests of digit span.

Lesions in the caudate nucleus or in the dorsomedial nucleus of the thalamus (subcortical components of the prefrontal network) can also produce a frontal lobe syndrome. This is one reason why the mental state changes associated with degenerative basal ganglia diseases, such as Parkinson's or Huntington's disease, may take the form of a frontal lobe syndrome. Because of its widespread connections with other regions of association cortex, one essential computational role of the prefrontal network is to function as an integrator, or "orchestrator," for other networks. Bilateral multifocal lesions of the cerebral hemispheres, none of which are individually large enough to cause specific cognitive deficits such as aphasia or neglect, can collectively interfere with the connectivity and integrating function of prefrontal cortex. A frontal lobe syndrome is the single most common behavioral profile associated with a variety of bilateral multifocal brain diseases including metabolic encephalopathy, multiple sclerosis, vitamin B_{12} deficiency, and others. In fact, the vast majority of patients with the clinical diagnosis of a frontal lobe syndrome tend to have lesions that do not involve prefrontal cortex but involve either the subcortical components of the prefrontal network or its connections with other parts of the brain. In order to avoid making a diagnosis of "frontal lobe syndrome" in a patient with no evidence of frontal cortex disease, it is advisable to use the diagnostic term *frontal network syndrome*, with the understanding that the responsible lesions can lie anywhere within this distributed network.

The patient with frontal lobe disease raises potential dilemmas in differential diagnosis: the abulia and blandness may be misinterpreted as depression, and the disinhibition as idiopathic mania or acting-out. Appropriate intervention may be delayed while a treatable tumor keeps expanding. An informed approach to frontal lobe disease and its behavioral manifestations may help to avoid such errors.

CARING FOR THE PATIENT WITH DEFICITS OF HIGHER CEREBRAL FUNCTION

Some of the deficits described in this chapter are so complex that they may bewilder not only the patient and family but also the physician. It is imperative to carry out a systematic clinical evaluation in order to characterize the nature of the deficits and explain them in lay terms to the patient and family. Such an explanation can allay at least some of the anxieties, address the mistaken impression that the deficit (e.g., social disinhibition or inability to recognize family members) is psychologically motivated, and lead to practical suggestions for daily living activities. The consultation of a skilled neuropsychologist may aid in the formulation of diagnosis and management. Patients with simultanagnosia, for example, may benefit from the counterintuitive instruction to stand back when they cannot find an item so that a greater search area falls within the immediate field of gaze. Some patients with frontal lobe disease can be extremely irritable and abusive to spouses and yet display all the appropriate social graces during the visit to the medical office. In such cases, the history may be more important than the bedside examination in charting a course of treatment.

Reactive depression is common in patients with higher cerebral dysfunction and should be treated. These patients may be sensitive to the usual doses of antidepressants or anxiolytics and deserve a careful titration of dosage. Brain damage may cause a dissociation between feeling states and their expression, so that a patient who may superficially appear jocular could still be suffering from an underlying depression that deserves to be treated. In many cases, agitation may be controlled with reassurance. In other cases, treatment with benzodiazepines or sedating antidepressants may become necessary. The use of neuroleptics for the control of agitation should be reserved for refractory cases since extrapyramidal side effects are frequent in patients with coexisting brain damage.

Spontaneous improvement of cognitive deficits due to acute neurologic lesions is common. It is most rapid in the first few weeks but may continue for up to 2 years, especially in young individuals with single brain lesions. The mechanisms for this recovery are incompletely understood. Some of the initial deficits appear to arise from remote dysfunction (diaschisis) in parts of the brain that are interconnected with the site of initial injury. Improvement in these patients may reflect, at least in part, a normalization of the remote dysfunction. Other mechanisms may involve functional reorganization in surviving neurons adjacent to the injury or the compensatory use of homologous structures, e.g., the right superior temporal gyrus with recovery from Wernicke's aphasia. In some patients with large lesions involving Broca's and Wernicke's areas, only Wernicke's area may show contralateral compensatory reorganization (or bilateral functionality), giving rise to a situation where a lesion that should have caused a global aphasia becomes associated with a residual Broca's aphasia. Prognosis

for recovery from aphasia is best when Wernicke's area is spared. Cognitive rehabilitation procedures have been used in the treatment of higher cortical deficits. There are few controlled studies, but some do show a benefit of rehabilitation in the recovery from hemispatial neglect and aphasia. Some types of deficits may be more prone to recovery than others. For example, patients with nonfluent aphasias are more likely to benefit from speech therapy than patients with fluent aphasias and comprehension deficits. In general, lesions that lead to a denial of illness (e.g., anosognosia) are associated with cognitive deficits that are more resistant to rehabilitation. The recovery of higher cortical dysfunction is rarely complete. Periodic neuropsychological assessment is necessary for quantifying the pace of the improvement and for generating specific recommendations for cognitive rehabilitation, modifications in the home environment, and the timetable for returning to school or work.

In general medical practice, most patients with deficits in higher cognitive functions will be suffering from dementia. There is a mistaken belief that dementias are anatomically diffuse and that they cause global cognitive impairments. This is only true at the terminal stages. During most of the clinical course, dementias are exquisitely selective with respect to anatomy and cognitive pattern. Alzheimer's disease, for example, causes the greatest destruction in medial temporal areas belonging to the memory network and is clinically characterized by a correspondingly severe amnesia. There are other dementias where memory is intact. Frontal lobe dementia results from a selective degeneration of the frontal lobe and leads to a gradual dissolution of behavior and complex attention. Primary progressive aphasia is characterized by a gradual atrophy of the left perisylvian language network and leads to a progressive dissolution of language that can remain isolated for up to 10 years. An enlightened approach to the differential diagnosis and treatment of these patients requires an understanding of the principles that link neural networks to higher cerebral functions.

FURTHER READING

DAMASIO AR, DAMASIO H: Aphasia and the neural basis of language, in *Principles of Behavioral and Cognitive Neurology*, 2d ed, M-M Mesulam (ed). New York, Oxford University Press, 2000

GITELMAN DR et al: A large-scale distributed network for covert spatial attention. Further anatomical delineation based on stringent behavioral and cognitive controls. Brain 122:1093, 1999

HEISS W-D et al: Differential capacity of left and right hemispheric areas for compensation of poststroke aphasia. Ann Neurol 45:430, 1999

LEIGUARDA RC, MARSDEN CD: Limb apraxias. Higher-order disorders of sensorimotor integration. Brain 123:860, 2000

MESULAM M-M: Behavioral neuroanatomy: Large-scale networks, association cortex, frontal syndromes, the limbic system and hemispheric specializations, in *Principles of Behavioral and Cognitive Neurology*, 2d ed, M-M Mesulam (ed). New York, Oxford University Press, 2000

———: The human frontal lobes: Transcending the default mode through contingent encoding, in *Principles of Frontal Lobe Function*, DT Stuss, RT Knight (eds). New York, Oxford University Press, 2002

---

24 | SLEEP DISORDERS
Charles A. Czeisler, John W. Winkelman, Gary S. Richardson

Disturbed sleep is among the most frequent health complaints physicians encounter. More than one-half of adults in the United States experience at least intermittent sleep disturbances. For most, it is an occasional night of poor sleep or daytime sleepiness. However, at least 15 to 20% of adults report chronic sleep disturbance or misalignment of circadian timing, which can lead to serious impairment of daytime functioning. In addition, such problems may contribute to or exacerbate medical or psychiatric conditions. Thirty years ago, many such complaints were treated with hypnotic medications without further di-

agnostic evaluation. Since then, a distinct class of sleep and arousal disorders has been identified.

PHYSIOLOGY OF SLEEP AND WAKEFULNESS

Most adults sleep 7 to 8 h per night, although the timing, duration, and internal structure of sleep vary among healthy individuals and as a function of age. At the extremes, infants and the elderly have frequent interruptions of sleep. In the United States, adults of intermediate age tend to have one consolidated sleep episode per day, although in some cultures sleep may be divided into a midafternoon nap and a shortened night sleep. Two principal systems govern the sleep-wake cycle: one actively generates sleep and sleep-related processes and another times sleep within the 24-h day. Either intrinsic abnormalities in these sys-

FIGURE 24-1 Stages of REM sleep (solid bars), the four stages of NREM sleep, and wakefulness over the course of the entire night for representative young and older adult men. Characteristic features of sleep in older people include reduction of slow-wave sleep, frequent spontaneous awakenings, early sleep onset, and early morning awakening. *(From the Division of Sleep Medicine, Brigham and Women's Hospital.)*

tems or extrinsic disturbances (environmental, drug- or illness-related) can lead to sleep or circadian rhythm disorders.

STATES AND STAGES OF SLEEP States and stages of human sleep are defined on the basis of characteristic patterns in the electroencephalogram (EEG), the electrooculogram (EOG—a measure of eye-movement activity), and the surface electromyogram (EMG) measured on the chin and neck. The continuous recording of this array of electrophysiologic parameters to define sleep and wakefulness is termed *polysomnography.*

Polysomnographic profiles define two states of sleep: (1) rapid-eye-movement (REM) sleep, and (2) non-rapid-eye-movement (NREM) sleep. NREM sleep is further subdivided into four stages, characterized by increasing arousal threshold and slowing of the cortical EEG. REM sleep is characterized by a low-amplitude, mixed-frequency EEG similar to that of NREM stage 1 sleep. The EOG shows bursts of REM similar to those seen during eyes-open wakefulness. Chin EMG activity is absent, reflecting the brainstem-mediated muscle atonia that is characteristic of that state.

ORGANIZATION OF HUMAN SLEEP Normal nocturnal sleep in adults displays a consistent organization from night to night (Fig. 24-1). After sleep onset, sleep usually progresses through NREM stages 1 to 4 within 45 to 60 min. Slow-wave sleep (NREM stages 3 and 4) predominates in the first third of the night and comprises 15 to 25% of total nocturnal sleep time in young adults. The percentage of slow-wave sleep is influenced by several factors, most notably age (see below). Prior sleep deprivation increases the rapidity of sleep onset and both the intensity and amount of slow-wave sleep.

The first REM sleep episode usually occurs in the second hour of sleep. More rapid onset of REM sleep in a young adult (particularly if <30 min) may suggest pathology such as endogenous depression, narcolepsy, circadian rhythm disorders, or drug withdrawal. NREM and REM alternate through the night with an average period of 90 to 110 min (the "ultradian" sleep cycle). Overall, REM sleep constitutes 20 to 25% of total sleep, and NREM stages 1 and 2 are 50 to 60%.

Age has a profound impact on sleep state organization (Fig. 24-1). Slow-wave sleep is most intense and prominent during childhood, decreasing sharply at puberty and across the second and third decades of life. After age 30, there is a progressive decline in the amount of slow-wave sleep, and the amplitude of delta EEG activity comprising slow-wave sleep is profoundly reduced. The depth of slow-wave sleep, as measured by the arousal threshold to auditory stimulation, also decreases with age. In the otherwise healthy older person, slow-wave sleep may be completely absent, particularly in males.

A different age profile exists for REM sleep than for slow-wave sleep. In infancy, REM sleep may comprise 50% of total sleep time, and the percentage is inversely proportional to developmental age. The amount of REM sleep falls off sharply over the first postnatal year as

a mature REM-NREM cycle develops; thereafter, REM sleep occupies a relatively constant percentage of total sleep time.

NEUROANATOMY OF SLEEP Experimental studies in animals have variously implicated the medullary reticular formation, the thalamus, and the basal forebrain in the generation of sleep, while the brainstem reticular formation, the midbrain, the subthalamus, the thalamus, and the basal forebrain have all been suggested to play a role in the generation of wakefulness or EEG arousal.

Current hypotheses suggest that the capacity for sleep and wakefulness generation is distributed along an axial "core" of neurons extending from the brainstem rostrally to the basal forebrain. Complex commingling of neuronal groups occurs at many points along this brainstem-forebrain axis. A cluster of γ-aminobutyric acid (GABA) and galaninergic neurons in the ventrolateral preoptic (VLPO) hypothalamus is selectively activated coincident with sleep onset. These neurons project to and inhibit histaminergic cell groups in the tuberomammilary nucleus that are important to the ascending arousal system, suggesting that the hypothalamic VLPO neurons may play a key executive role in sleep regulation.

Specific regions in the pons are associated with the neurophysiologic correlates of REM sleep. Small lesions in the dorsal pons result in the loss of the descending muscle inhibition normally associated with REM sleep; microinjections of the cholinergic agonist carbachol into the pontine reticular formation appear to produce a state with all of the features of REM sleep. These experimental manipulations are mimicked by pathologic conditions in humans and animals. In narcolepsy, for example, abrupt, complete, or partial paralysis (cataplexy) occurs in response to a variety of stimuli. In dogs with this condition, physostigmine, a central cholinesterase inhibitor, increases the frequency of cataplectic attacks, while atropine decreases their frequency. Conversely, in REM sleep behavior disorder (see below), patients suffer from incomplete motor inhibition during REM sleep, resulting in involuntary, occasionally violent movement during REM sleep.

NEUROCHEMISTRY OF SLEEP Early experimental studies that focused on the raphe nuclei of the brainstem appeared to implicate serotonin as the primary sleep-promoting neurotransmitter, while catecholamines were considered to be responsible for wakefulness. Subsequent work has demonstrated that the raphe-serotonin system may facilitate sleep but is not necessary for its expression. Pharmacologic studies of sleep and wakefulness suggest roles for other neurotransmitters as well. Pontine cholinergic neurotransmission is known to play a role in REM sleep generation. The alerting influence of caffeine implicates adenosine, whereas the hypnotic effect of benzodiazepines and barbiturates suggests a role for endogenous ligands of the $GABA_A$ receptor complex. A newly characterized neuropeptide, hypocretin (orexin), has recently been implicated in the pathophysiology of narcolepsy (see below), but its role in normal sleep regulation remains to be defined.

A variety of sleep-promoting substances have been identified, although it is not known whether or not they are involved in the endogenous sleep-wake regulatory process. These include prostaglandin D_2, delta sleep–inducing peptide, muramyl dipeptide, interleukin 1, fatty acid primary amides, and melatonin. The hypnotic effect of these substances is commonly limited to NREM or slow-wave sleep, although peptides that increase REM sleep have also been reported. Many putative "sleep factors," including interleukin 1 and prostaglandin D_2, are immunologically active as well, suggesting a link between immune function and sleep-wake states.

PHYSIOLOGY OF CIRCADIAN RHYTHMICITY The sleep-wake cycle is the most evident of the many 24-h rhythms in humans. Prominent daily variations also occur in endocrine, thermoregulatory, cardiac, pulmonary, renal, gastrointestinal, and neurobehavioral functions. At the molecular level, endogenous circadian rhythmicity is driven by self-sustaining transcriptional/translational feedback loops (Fig. 24-2). In evaluating a daily variation in humans, it is important to distinguish between those rhythmic components passively evoked by periodic environmental or behavioral changes (e.g., the increase in blood pressure and heart rate upon assumption of the upright posture) and those actively driven by an endogenous oscillatory process (e.g., the circadian variation in plasma cortisol that persists under a variety of environmental and behavioral conditions).

While it is now recognized that many peripheral tissues in mammals have circadian clocks that regulate diverse physiologic processes, these independent tissue-specific oscillations are coordinated by a central neural pacemaker located in the suprachiasmatic nuclei (SCN) of the hypothalamus. Bilateral destruction of these nuclei results in a loss of the endogenous circadian rhythm of locomotor activity, which can be restored only by transplantation of the same structure from a donor animal. The genetically determined period of this endogenous neural oscillator, which averages ~24.2 h in humans, is normally synchronized to the 24-h period of the environmental light-dark cycle. Small differences in circadian period underlie variations in diurnal preference, with the circadian period shorter in morning than in evening types. Entrainment of mammalian circadian rhythms by the light-dark cycle is mediated via the retinohypothalamic tract, a monosynaptic pathway that links specialized, photoreceptive retinal ganglion cells directly to the SCN. Humans are exquisitely sensitive to the resetting effects of light, particularly at the blue end (~460 to 480 nm) of the visible spectrum.

The timing and internal architecture of sleep are directly coupled to the output of the endogenous circadian pacemaker. Paradoxically, the endogenous circadian rhythms of sleep tendency, sleepiness, and REM sleep propensity all peak near the habitual wake time, just after the nadir of the endogenous circadian temperature cycle, whereas the circadian wake propensity rhythm peaks 1 to 3 h before the habitual bedtime. These rhythms are thus timed to oppose the homeostatic decline of sleep tendency during the habitual sleep episode and the rise of sleep tendency throughout the usual waking day, respectively. Misalignment of the output of the endogenous circadian pacemaker with the desired sleep-wake cycle can, therefore, induce insomnia, decreased alertness, and impaired performance evident in night-shift workers and airline travelers.

BEHAVIORAL CORRELATES OF SLEEP STATES AND STAGES Polysomnographic staging of sleep correlates with behavioral changes during specific states and stages. During the transitional state between wakefulness and sleep (stage 1 sleep), subjects may respond to faint auditory or visual signals without "awakening." Memory incorporation is inhibited at the onset of NREM stage 1 sleep, which may explain why individuals aroused from that transitional sleep stage frequently deny having been asleep. Such transitions may intrude upon behavioral wakefulness after sleep deprivation, notwithstanding attempts to remain continuously awake (see "Shift-Work Sleep Disorder," below).

Awakenings from REM sleep are associated with recall of vivid dream imagery >80% of the time. The reliability of dream recall increases with REM sleep episodes occurring later in the night. Imagery may also be reported after NREM sleep interruptions, though these typically lack the detail and vividness of REM sleep dreams. The incidence of NREM sleep dream recall can be increased by selective REM sleep deprivation, suggesting that REM sleep and dreaming per se are not inexorably linked.

PHYSIOLOGIC CORRELATES OF SLEEP STATES AND STAGES All major physiologic systems are influenced by sleep. Changes in cardiovascular function include a decrease in blood pressure and heart rate during NREM and particularly during slow-wave sleep. During REM sleep, phasic activity (bursts of eye movements) is associated with variability in both blood pressure and heart rate mediated principally by the vagus. Cardiac dysrhythmias may occur selectively during REM sleep. Respiratory function also changes. In comparison to relaxed wakefulness, respiratory rate becomes more regular during NREM sleep (especially slow-wave sleep) and tonic REM sleep and becomes very irregular during phasic REM sleep. Minute ventilation decreases in NREM sleep out of proportion to the decrease in metabolic rate at sleep onset, resulting in a higher P_{CO_2}.

Endocrine function also varies with sleep. Slow-wave sleep is associated with secretion of growth hormone, while sleep in general is associated with augmented secretion of prolactin. Sleep has a complex effect on the secretion of luteinizing hormone (LH): during puberty, sleep is associated with increased LH secretion, whereas sleep in the mature woman inhibits LH secretion in the early follicular phase of the menstrual cycle. Sleep onset (and probably slow-wave sleep) is associated with inhibition of thyroid-stimulating hormone and of the adrenocorticotropic hormone–cortisol axis, an effect that is superimposed on the prominent circadian rhythms in the two systems.

The pineal hormone melatonin is secreted predominantly at night in both day- and night-active species, reflecting the direct modulation of pineal activity by the circadian pacemaker through a circuitous neural pathway from the SCN to the pineal gland. Melatonin secretion is not dependent upon the occurrence of sleep, persisting in individuals kept awake at night. In addition, exogenous melatonin increases sleepiness and may potentiate sleep when administered to good sleepers attempting to sleep during daylight hours at a time when endogenous melatonin levels are low. The efficacy of melatonin as a sleep-promoting therapy for patients with insomnia is currently not known.

Sleep is also accompanied by alterations of thermoregulatory function. NREM sleep is associated with an attenuation of thermoregulatory responses to either heat or cold stress, and animal studies of thermosensitive neurons in the hypothalamus document an NREM-sleep-dependent reduction of the thermoregulatory set-point. REM sleep is associated with complete absence of thermoregulatory responsiveness, effectively resulting in functional poikilothermy. However, the potential adverse impact of this failure of thermoregulation is blunted by inhibition of REM sleep by extreme ambient temperatures.

FIGURE 24-2 Model of the molecular feedback loop at the core of the mammalian circadian clock. The positive element of the feedback loop (+) is the transcriptional activation of the *Per1* gene (and probably other clock genes) by a heterodimer of the transcription factors CLOCK and BMAL1 (also called MOP3) bound to an E-box DNA regulatory element. The *Per1* transcript and its product, the clock component PER1 protein, accumulate in the cell cytoplasm. As it accumulates, the PER1 protein is recruited into a multiprotein complex thought to contain other circadian clock component proteins such as cryptochromes (CRYs), Period proteins (PERs), and others. This complex is then transported into the cell nucleus (across the dotted line), where it functions as the negative element in the feedback loop (−) by inhibiting the activity of the CLOCK-BMAL1 transcription factor heterodimer. As a consequence of this action, the concentration of PER1 and other clock proteins in the inhibitory complex falls, allowing CLOCK-BMAL1 to activate transcription of *Per1* and other genes and begin another cycle. The dynamics of the 24-h molecular cycle are controlled at several levels, including regulation of the rate of PER protein degradation by casein kinase-1 epsilon (CK1E). Additional limbs of this genetic regulatory network, omitted for the sake of clarity, are thought to contribute stability. Question marks denote putative clock proteins, such as Timeless (TIM), as yet lacking genetic proof of a role in the mammalian clock mechanism. *(Copyright © Charles J. Weitz, Ph.D., Department of Neurobiology, Harvard Medical School.)*

TABLE 24-1 *Evaluation of the Patient with the Complaint of Excessive Daytime Somnolence*

Findings on History and Physical Examination	Diagnostic Evaluation	Diagnosis	Therapy
Obesity, snoring, hypertension	Polysomnography with respiratory monitoring	Obstructive sleep apnea	Continuous positive airway pressure; ENT surgery (e.g., uvulopalatopharyngoplasty); dental appliance; pharmacologic therapy (e.g., protriptyline); weight loss
Cataplexy, hypnogogic hallucinations, sleep paralysis, family history	Polysomnography with multiple sleep latency testing	Narcolepsy-cataplexy syndrome	Stimulants (e.g., modafinil, methylphenidate); REM-suppressant antidepressants (e.g., protriptyline); genetic counseling
Restless legs syndrome, disturbed sleep, predisposing medical condition (e.g., anemia or renal failure)	Polysomnography with bilateral anterior tibialis EMG monitoring	Periodic limb movements of sleep	Treatment of predisposing condition, if possible; dopamine agonists (e.g., pramipexole); benzodiazepines (e.g., clonazepam)
Disturbed sleep, predisposing medical conditions (e.g., asthma) and/or predisposing medical therapies (e.g., theophylline)	Sleep-wake diary recording	Insomnias (see text)	Treatment of predisposing condition and/or change in therapy, if possible; behavioral therapy; short-acting benzodiazepine receptor agonist (e.g., zolpidem)

Note: ENT, ears, nose, throat; REM, rapid eye movement; EMG, electromyogram.

DISORDERS OF SLEEP AND WAKEFULNESS

APPROACH TO THE PATIENT

Patients may seek help from a physician because of one of several symptoms: (1) an acute or chronic inability to sleep adequately at night (insomnia); (2) chronic fatigue, sleepiness, or tiredness during the day; or (3) a behavioral manifestation associated with sleep itself. Complaints of insomnia or excessive daytime sleepiness should be viewed as symptoms (much like fever or pain) of underlying disorders. Knowledge of the differential diagnosis of these presenting complaints is essential to identify the underlying medical disorder. Only then can appropriate treatment, rather than nonspecific approaches (e.g., over-the-counter sleeping aids), be applied. Diagnoses of exclusion, such as primary insomnia, should be made only after other diagnoses have been ruled out. Table 24-1 outlines the diagnostic and therapeutic approach to the patient with a complaint of excessive daytime sleepiness.

A careful history is essential. In particular, the duration, severity, and consistency of the symptoms are important, along with the patient's estimate of the consequences of reported sleep loss on waking function. Information from a friend or family member can be invaluable; some patients may be unaware of, or will underreport, such potentially embarrassing symptoms as heavy snoring or falling asleep while driving.

Completion by the patient of a day-by-day sleep-work-drug log for at least 2 weeks can help the physician better understand the nature of the complaint. Work times and sleep times (including daytime naps and nocturnal awakenings) as well as drug and alcohol use, including caffeine and hypnotics, should be noted each day. In addition, the sleep times should be recorded.

Polysomnography is necessary for the diagnosis of specific disorders such as narcolepsy and sleep apnea and may be of utility in other settings as well. In addition to the three electrophysiologic variables used to define sleep states and stages, the standard clinical polysomnogram includes measures of respiration (respiratory effort, air flow, and oxygen saturation), anterior tibialis EMG, and electrocardiogram. Evaluation of penile tumescence during nocturnal sleep can also help determine whether the cause of erectile dysfunction in a patient is psychogenic or organic (Chap. 43).

EVALUATION OF INSOMNIA Insomnia is the complaint of inadequate sleep; it can be classified according to the nature of sleep disruption and the duration of the complaint. Insomnia is subdivided into difficulty falling asleep (*sleep onset insomnia*), frequent or sustained awakenings (*sleep maintenance insomnia*), early morning awakenings (*sleep offset insomnia*), or persistent sleepiness despite sleep of adequate duration (*nonrestorative sleep*). Similarly, the duration of the symptom influences diagnostic and therapeutic considerations. An insomnia complaint lasting one to several nights (within a single episode) is termed *transient insomnia* and is typically the result of situational stress or a change in sleep schedule or environment (e.g., jet lag). *Short-term insomnia* lasts from a few days to 3 weeks. Disruption of this duration is usually associated with more protracted stress, such as recovery from surgery or short-term illness. *Long-term insomnia*, or *chronic insomnia*, lasts for months or years and, in contrast with short-term insomnia, requires a thorough evaluation of underlying causes (see below). Chronic insomnia is often a waxing and waning disorder, with spontaneous or stressor-induced exacerbations.

An occasional night of poor sleep, typically in the setting of stress or excitement about external events, is both common and without lasting consequences. However, persistent insomnia can lead to impaired daytime function, injury due to accidents, and the development of major depression. In addition, there is emerging evidence that individuals with chronic insomnia have increased utilization of health care resources, even after controlling for co-morbid medical and psychiatric disorders.

All insomnias can be exacerbated and perpetuated by behaviors that are not conducive to initiating or maintaining sleep. *Inadequate sleep hygiene* is characterized by a behavior pattern prior to sleep or a bedroom environment that is not conducive to sleep. Noise or light in the bedroom can interfere with sleep, as can a bed partner with periodic limb movements during sleep or one who snores loudly. Clocks can heighten the anxiety about the time it has taken to fall asleep. Drugs that act on the central nervous system, large meals, vigorous exercise, or hot showers just before sleep may interfere with sleep onset. Many individuals participate in stressful work-related activities in the evening, producing a state incompatible with sleep onset. In preference to hypnotic medications, patients should be counseled to avoid stressful activities before bed, develop a soporific bedtime ritual, and to prepare and reserve the bedroom environment for sleeping. Consistent, regular rising times should be maintained daily, including weekends.

PRIMARY INSOMNIA ■ **Insomnia without Identifiable Cause** Many patients with chronic insomnia have no clear, single identifiable underlying cause for their difficulties with sleep. Rather, such patients often have multiple etiologies for their insomnia, which may evolve over the years. Primary insomnia is thus a diagnosis of exclusion, often without a clear underlying single cause. In addition, the chief sleep complaint may change over time, with initial insomnia predominating at one point, and multiple awakenings or nonrestorative sleep occurring at other times. Subsyndromal psychiatric disorders (e.g., anxiety and mood complaints), negative conditioning to the sleep environment (psychophysiologic insomnia, see below), amplification of the time spent awake (sleep-state misperception), physiologic hyperarousal, and poor sleep hygiene (see above) may all be present. As these processes may be both causes and consequences of chronic insomnia, many individuals will have a progressive course to their symptoms in which the severity is proportional to the chronicity, and much of the complaint may persist even after effective treatment of the initial inciting etiology. Treatment of primary insomnia is often directed to each of the putative contributing factors: behavior therapies for anxiety and negative conditioning (see below), pharmacotherapy for mood/anxiety disorders, an emphasis on maintenance of good sleep hygiene, and intermittent hypnotics for exacerbations of the insomnia.

If insomnia persists after treatment of these contributing factors, empirical pharmacotherapy is often used on a nightly or intermittent basis. A variety of sedative compounds are used for this purpose. Alcohol and antihistamines are the most commonly used nonprescription sleep aids. The former may help with sleep onset, but is associated with sleep disruption during the night and can escalate into abuse, dependence, and withdrawal in the predisposed individual. Antihistamines may be of benefit when used intermittently, but produce rapid tolerance and have multiple side effects (especially anticholinergic), which limit their use. Benzodiazepine receptor agonists are the most effective and well-tolerated class of medications for insomnia. The broad range of half-lives allows flexibility in the duration of sedative action. Zaleplon (5 to 20 mg), with a half-life of 1 to 2 h, zolpidem (5 to 10 mg) and triazolam (0.125 to 0.25 mg), with half-lives of 2 to 3 h, and temazepam (15 to 30 mg) and lorazepam (0.5 to 2 mg), with half-lives of 6 to 12 h, are the most commonly prescribed agents in this family. Generally, side effects are minimal if the dose is kept low and the serum concentration is minimized during the waking hours (by using the shortest-acting, effective agent). However, with even brief continuous use, rebound insomnia can occur upon discontinuation. There are only limited data supporting sustained efficacy of benzodiazepine receptor agonists; caution should be exercised in long-term use. The likelihood of rebound insomnia and tolerance can be minimized by short durations of treatment, intermittent use, or gradual tapering of the dose. For acute insomnia, nightly use of a benzodiazepine receptor agonist for a maximum of 2 to 4 weeks is advisable. For chronic insomnia, intermittent use is recommended. Benzodiazepine receptor agonists should be avoided, or used very judiciously, in patients with a history of substance abuse. The heterocyclic antidepressants (trazodone, amitriptyline, and doxepin) are the most commonly prescribed alternatives to benzodiazepine receptor agonists due to their lack of abuse potential and lower cost. Trazodone (25 to 100 mg) is used more commonly than the tricyclic antidepressants as it has a much shorter half-life (5 to 9 h), has much less anticholinergic activity (sparing patients, particularly the elderly, constipation, urinary retention, and tachycardia), is associated with less weight gain, and is much safer in overdose. The risk of priapism is small (~1 in 10,000).

Psychophysiologic Insomnia Persistent *psychophysiologic insomnia* is a behavioral disorder in which patients are preoccupied with a perceived inability to sleep adequately at night. The sleep disturbance is often triggered by an emotionally stressful event; however, the poor sleep habits and beliefs about sleep acquired during the stressful period persist long after the initial incident. Such patients become hyperaroused by their own persistent efforts to sleep or the sleep environment, and the insomnia is a conditioned or learned response. They may be able to fall asleep more easily at unscheduled times (when not trying) or outside the home environment. Polysomnographic recording in patients with psychophysiologic insomnia reveals an objective sleep disturbance, often with an abnormally long sleep latency; frequent nocturnal awakenings; and an increased amount of stage 1 transitional sleep. Rigorous attention should be paid to sleep hygiene and correction of counterproductive, arousing behaviors before bedtime. Behavioral therapies are the treatment modality of choice, with only intermittent use of medications. When patients are awake for >20 min, they should read or perform other relaxing activities to distract themselves from insomnia-related anxiety. In addition, bedtime and waketime should be scheduled to restrict time in bed to be equal to their perceived total sleep time. This will generally produce sleep deprivation, greater sleep drive, and, eventually, better sleep. Time in bed can then be gradually expanded.

SECONDARY INSOMNIA ■ **Transient Situational Insomnia** This typically develops after a change in the sleeping environment (e.g., in an unfamiliar hotel or hospital bed) or before or after a significant life event, such as a change of occupation, loss of a loved one, illness, or anxiety over a deadline or examination. Increased sleep latency, frequent awakenings from sleep, and early morning awakening can all occur. Recovery is generally rapid, usually within a few weeks. Treatment is symptomatic, with intermittent use of hypnotics and resolution of the underlying stress. *Altitude insomnia* describes a sleep disturbance that is a common consequence of exposure to high altitude. Periodic breathing of the Cheyne-Stokes type occurs during NREM sleep about half the time at high altitude, with restoration of a regular breathing pattern during REM sleep. Both hypoxia and hypocapnia are thought to be involved in the development of periodic breathing. Frequent awakenings and poor quality sleep characterize altitude insomnia, which is generally worst on the first few nights at high altitude but may persist. Treatment with acetazolamide can decrease time spent in periodic breathing and substantially reduce hypoxia during sleep.

Insomnia Associated with Mental Disorders Approximately 80% of patients with psychiatric disorders describe sleep complaints. There is considerable heterogeneity, however, in the nature of the sleep disturbance both between conditions and among patients with the same condition. *Depression* can be associated with sleep onset insomnia, sleep maintenance insomnia, or early morning wakefulness. However, hypersomnia occurs in some depressed patients, especially adolescents and those with either bipolar or seasonal (fall/winter) depression (Chap. 371). Indeed, sleep disturbance is an important vegetative sign of depression and may commence before any mood changes are perceived by the patient. Consistent polysomnographic findings in depression include decreased REM sleep latency, lengthened first REM sleep episode, and shortened first NREM sleep episode; however, these findings are not specific for depression, and the extent of these changes varies with age and symptomatology. Depressed patients also show decreased slow-wave sleep and reduced sleep continuity.

In *mania* and *hypomania*, sleep latency is increased and total sleep time can be reduced. Patients with *anxiety disorders* tend not to show the changes in REM sleep and slow-wave sleep seen in endogenously depressed patients. *Chronic alcoholics* lack slow-wave sleep, have decreased amounts of REM sleep (as an acute response to alcohol), and have frequent arousals throughout the night. This is associated with impaired daytime alertness. The sleep of chronic alcoholics may remain disturbed for years after discontinuance of alcohol usage. Sleep architecture and physiology are disturbed in *schizophrenia* (with a decreased amount of stage 4 sleep and a lack of augmentation of REM sleep following REM sleep deprivation); chronic schizophrenics often show day-night reversal, sleep fragmentation, and insomnia.

Insomnia Associated with Neurologic Disorders A variety of neurologic diseases result in sleep disruption through both indirect, nonspecific mechanisms (e.g., pain in cervical spondylosis or low back pain) or by impairment of central neural structures involved in the generation and control of sleep itself. For example, *dementia* from any cause has long been associated with disturbances in the timing of the sleep-wake cycle, often characterized by nocturnal wandering and an exacerbation of symptomatology at night (so-called sundowning).

Epilepsy may rarely present as a sleep complaint (Chap. 348). Often the history is of abnormal behavior, at times with convulsive movements during sleep, and the differential diagnosis includes REM sleep behavior disorder, sleep apnea syndrome, and periodic movements of sleep (see above). Diagnosis requires nocturnal EEG recording. Other neurologic diseases associated with abnormal movements, such as

FIGURE 24-3 Polysomnographic recordings of (*A*) obstructive sleep apnea and (*B*) periodic limb movement of sleep. Note the snoring and reduction in air flow in the presence of continued respiratory effort, associated with the subsequent oxygen desaturation (upper panel). Periodic limb movements occur with a relatively constant intermovement interval and are associated with changes in the EEG and heart rates acceleration (lower panel). Abbreviations: R.A.T., right anterior tibialis; L.A.T., left anterior tibialis. (*From the Division of Sleep Medicine, Brigham and Women's Hospital.*)

Parkinson's disease, hemiballismus, Huntington's chorea, and *Gilles de la Tourette syndrome* (Chap. 351), are also associated with disrupted sleep, presumably through secondary mechanisms. However, the abnormal movements themselves are greatly reduced during sleep. Headache syndromes (*migraine* or *cluster headache*) may show sleep-associated exacerbations (Chap. 14) by unknown mechanisms.

Fatal familial insomnia is a rare hereditary disorder caused by degeneration of anterior and dorsomedial nuclei of the thalamus. Insomnia is a prominent early symptom. Progressively, the syndrome produces autonomic dysfunction, dysarthria, myoclonus, coma, and death. The pathogenesis is a mutation in the prion gene (Chap. 362).

Insomnia Associated with Other Medical Disorders   A number of medical conditions are associated with disruptions of sleep. The association is frequently nonspecific, e.g., that between sleep disruption and chronic pain from rheumatologic disorders. Attention to this association is important in that sleep-associated symptoms are often the presenting complaint. Treatment of the underlying medical disorder or symptom is the most useful approach. Sleep disruption can also result from the appropriate use of drugs such as glucocorticoids (see below).

One prominent association is between sleep disruption and *asthma*. In many asthmatics there is a prominent daily variation in airway resistance that results in marked increases in asthmatic symptoms at night, especially during sleep. In addition, treatment of asthma with theophylline-based compounds, adrenergic agonists, or glucocorticoids can independently disrupt sleep. When sleep disruption is a side effect of asthma treatment, inhaled glucocorticoids (e.g., beclomethasone) that do not disrupt sleep may provide a useful alternative.

Cardiac ischemia may also be associated with sleep disruption. The ischemia itself may result from increases in sympathetic tone as a result of sleep apnea. Patients may present with complaints of nightmares or vivid, disturbing dreams, with or without awareness of the more classic symptoms of angina or of the sleep disordered breathing. Treatment of the sleep apnea may substantially improve the angina and the nocturnal sleep quality. *Paroxysmal nocturnal dyspnea* can also occur as a consequence of sleep-associated cardiac ischemia that causes pulmonary congestion exacerbated by the recumbent posture.

Chronic obstructive pulmonary disease is also associated with sleep disruption, as is *cystic fibrosis, menopause, hyperthyroidism, gastroesophageal reflux, chronic renal failure,* and *liver failure.*

Medication-, Drug-, or Alcohol-Dependent Insomnia   Disturbed sleep can result from ingestion of a wide variety of agents. Caffeine is perhaps the most common pharmacologic cause of insomnia. It produces increased latency to sleep onset, more frequent arousals during sleep, and a reduction in total sleep time for up to 8 to 14 h after ingestion. As few as three to five cups of coffee can significantly disturb sleep in some patients; therefore, a 1- to 2-month trial without caffeine should be attempted in patients with these symptoms. Similarly, alcohol and nicotine can interfere with sleep, despite the fact that many patients use them to relax and promote sleep. Although alcohol can increase drowsiness and shorten sleep latency, even moderate amounts of alcohol increase awakenings in the second half of the night. In addition, alcohol ingestion prior to sleep is contraindicated in patients with sleep apnea because of the inhibitory effects of alcohol on upper airway muscle tone. Acutely, amphetamines and cocaine suppress both REM sleep and total sleep time, which return to normal with chronic use. Withdrawal leads to a REM sleep rebound. A number of prescribed medications can produce insomnia. Antidepressants, sympathomimetics, and glucocorticoids are common causes. In addition, severe rebound insomnia can result from the acute withdrawal of hypnotics, especially following the use of high doses of benzodiazepines with a short half-life. For this reason, hypnotic doses should be low to moderate, the total duration of hypnotic therapy should usually be limited to 2 to 3 weeks, and prolonged drug tapering is encouraged.

RESTLESS LEGS SYNDROME (RLS)   Patients with this sensory-motor disorder report a creeping or crawling dysesthesia deep within the calves or feet, or sometimes even in the upper extemities, that is associated with an irresistible urge to move the affected limbs. For most patients with RLS, the dysesthesias and restlessness are much worse in the evening or night compared to the daytime and frequently interfere with the ability to fall asleep. The disorder is exacerbated by inactivity and temporarily relieved by movement. In contrast, paresthesias secondary to peripheral neuropathy persists with activity. The severity of this chronic disorder may wax and wane with time and can be exacerbated by sleep deprivation, caffeine, and pregnancy. The prevalence is 1 to 5% of young to middle-age adults and increases to 10 to 20% in those >60 years. There appear to be important differences in RLS prevalence among racial groups, with higher prevalence in those of Northern European ancestry. Roughly one-third of patients (particularly those with an early age of onset) will have multiple affected family members, possibly with an autosomal dominant pattern. Iron deficiency and renal failure may cause RLS, which is then considered secondary RLS. The symptoms of RLS are exquisitely sensitive to dopaminergic drugs (e.g., pramipexole 0.25 to 1.0 mg q8pm or ropinirole 0.5 to 4.0 mg q8pm), which are the treatment of choice. Narcotics, benzodiazepines, and certain anticonvulsants may also be of therapeutic value. Most patients with restless legs also experience periodic limb movements of sleep, although the reverse is not the case.

PERIODIC LIMB MOVEMENT DISORDER   *Periodic limb movement disorder*, previously known as *nocturnal myoclonus*, is the principal objective polysomnographic finding in 17% of patients with insomnia and 11% of those with excessive daytime somnolence (Fig. 24-3). It is often unclear whether it is an incidental finding or the cause of disturbed sleep. Stereotyped, 0.5- to 5.0-s extensions of the great toe and dorsiflexion of the foot recur every 20 to 40 s during NREM sleep, in episodes lasting from minutes to hours. Most such episodes occur during the first half of the night. The disorder occurs in a wide variety of sleep disorders (including narcolepsy, sleep apnea, REM sleep behavior disorder, and various forms of insomnia) and may be associated with frequent arousals and an increased number of sleep-stage transitions. The incidence increases with age: 44% of people over age 65 without a sleep complaint have more than five periodic leg movements per hour of sleep. The pathophysiology is not well understood, though individuals with high spinal transections can exhibit periodic leg movements during sleep, suggesting the existence of a spinal generator. Polysomnography with bilateral surface EMG recording of the anterior tibialis is used to establish the diagnosis. Treatment options include dopaminergic medications or benzodiazepines.

EVALUATION OF DAYTIME SLEEPINESS Daytime impairment due to sleep loss may be difficult to quantify for several reasons. First, sleepiness is not necessarily proportional to subjectively assessed sleep deprivation. In obstructive sleep apnea, for example, the repeated brief interruptions of sleep associated with resumption of respiration at the end of apneic episodes result in daytime sleepiness, despite the fact that the patient may be unaware of the sleep fragmentation. Second, subjective descriptions of waking impairment vary from patient to patient. Patients may describe themselves as "sleepy," "fatigued," or "tired" and may have a clear sense of the meaning of those terms, while others may use the same terms to describe a completely different condition. Third, sleepiness, particularly when profound, may affect judgment in a manner analogous to ethanol, such that subjective awareness of the condition and the consequent cognitive and motor impairment is reduced. Finally, patients may be reluctant to admit that sleepiness is a problem, both because they are generally unaware of what constitutes normal alertness and because sleepiness is generally viewed pejoratively, ascribed more often to a deficit in motivation than to an inadequately addressed physiologic sleep need.

Specific questioning about the occurrence of sleep episodes during normal waking hours, both intentional and unintentional, can overcome the inconsistencies among subjective characterizations and help to interpret the adverse impact of sleepiness on daytime function. Specific areas to be addressed include the occurrence of inadvertent sleep episodes while driving or in other safety-related settings, sleepiness while at work or school (and the relationship of sleepiness to work and school performance), and the effect of sleepiness on social and family life. Evidence for significant daytime impairment [in association either with the diagnosis of a primary sleep disorder, such as narcolepsy or sleep apnea, or with imposed or self-selected sleep-wake schedules (see "Shift-Work Sleep Disorder," below)] raises the question of the physician's responsibility to notify motor vehicle licensing authorities of the increased risk of sleepiness-related vehicle accidents. As with epilepsy, legal requirements vary from state to state, and existing legal precedents do not provide a consistent interpretation of the balance between the physician's responsibility and the patient's right to privacy. At a minimum, physicians should document discussions with the patient regarding the increased risk of operating a vehicle, as well as a recommendation that driving be suspended until successful treatment or schedule modification can be instituted.

The distinction between fatigue and sleepiness can be useful in the differentiation of patients with complaints of fatigue or tiredness in the setting of disorders such as fibromyalgia (Chap. 315), chronic fatigue syndrome (Chap. 370), or endocrine deficiencies such as hypothyroidism (Chap. 320) or Addison's disease (Chap. 321). While patients with these disorders can typically distinguish their daytime symptoms from the sleepiness that occurs with sleep deprivation, substantial overlap can occur. This is particularly true when the primary disorder also results in chronic sleep disruption (e.g., sleep apnea in hypothyroidism) or in abnormal sleep (e.g., fibromyalgia).

While clinical evaluation of the complaint of excessive sleepiness is usually adequate, objective quantification is sometimes necessary. Assessment of daytime functioning as an index of the adequacy of sleep can be made with the multiple sleep latency test (MSLT), which involves repeated measurement of sleep latency (time to onset of sleep) under standardized conditions during a day following quantified nocturnal sleep. The average latency across four to six tests (administered every 2 h across the waking day) provides an objective measure of daytime sleep tendency. Disorders of sleep that result in pathologic daytime somnolence can be reliably distinguished with the MSLT. In addition, the multiple measurements of sleep onset may identify direct transitions from wakefulness to REM sleep that are suggestive of specific pathologic conditions (e.g., narcolepsy).

NARCOLEPSY Narcolepsy is both a disorder of the ability to sustain wakefulness voluntarily and a disorder of REM sleep regulation (Table 24-2). The classic "narcolepsy tetrad" consists of excessive daytime somnolence plus three specific symptoms related to an intrusion of REM sleep characteristics (e.g., muscle atonia, vivid dream imagery) into the transition between wakefulness and sleep: (1) sudden weakness or loss of muscle tone without loss of consciousness, often elicited by emotion (cataplexy); (2) hallucinations at sleep onset (hypnogogic hallucinations) or upon awakening (hypnopompic hallucinations); and (3) muscular paralysis upon awakening (sleep paralysis). The severity of cataplexy varies, as patients may have two to three attacks per day or per decade. Some patients with objectively confirmed narcolepsy (see below) may show no evidence of cataplexy. In those with cataplexy, the extent and duration of an attack may also vary, from a transient sagging of the jaw lasting a few seconds to rare cases of flaccid paralysis of the entire voluntary musculature for up to 20 to 30 min. Symptoms of narcolepsy typically begin in the second decade, although the onset ranges from ages 5 to 50. Once established, the disease is chronic without remissions. Secondary forms of narcolepsy have been described (e.g., after head trauma).

Narcolepsy affects about 1 in 4000 people in the United States and appears to have a genetic basis. Recently, several convergent lines of evidence suggests that the hypothalamic neuropeptide hypocretin (orexin) is involved in the pathogenesis of narcolepsy: (1) a mutation in the hypocretin receptor 2 gene has been associated with canine narcolepsy; (2) hypocretin "knockout" mice that are genetically unable to produce this neuropeptide exhibit a phenotype, as assessed by behavioral and electrophysiologic criteria, that is similar to human narcolepsy; and (3) cerebrospinal fluid levels of hypocretin are reduced in most patients who have narcolepsy with cataplexy. The inheritance pattern of narcolepsy in humans is more complex than in the canine model. However, almost all narcoleptics with cataplexy are positive for HLA DQB1*0602 (Chap. 296), suggesting that an autoimmune process may be responsible.

Diagnosis The diagnostic criteria continue to be a matter of debate. Certainly, objective verification of excessive daytime somnolence, typically with MSLT mean sleep latencies <8 min, is an essential if nonspecific diagnostic feature. Other conditions that cause excessive sleepiness, such as sleep apnea or chronic sleep restriction, must be rigorously excluded. The other objective diagnostic feature of narcolepsy is the presence of REM sleep in at least two of the naps during the MSLT. Abnormal regulation of REM sleep is also manifested by

TABLE 24-2 *Prevalence of Symptoms in Narcolepsy*

Symptom	Prevalence, %
Excessive daytime somnolence	100
Disturbed sleep	87
Cataplexy	76
Hypnagogic hallucinations	68
Sleep paralysis	64
Memory problems	50

Source: Modified from TA Roth, L Merlotti in SA Burton et al (eds), *Narcolepsy 3rd International Symposium: Selected Symposium Proceedings*, Chicago, Matrix Communications, 1989.

the appearance of REM sleep immediately or within minutes after sleep onset in 50% of narcoleptic patients, a rarity in unaffected individuals maintaining a conventional sleep-wake schedule. The REM-related symptoms of the classic narcolepsy tetrad are variably present. There is increasing evidence that narcoleptics with cataplexy (one-half to two-thirds of patients) may represent a more homogeneous group than those without this symptom. However, a history of cataplexy can be difficult to establish reliably. Hypnogogic and hypnopompic hallucinations and sleep paralysis are often found in nonnarcoleptic individuals and may be present in only one-half of narcoleptics. Nocturnal sleep disruption is commonly observed in narcolepsy but is also a nonspecific symptom. Similarly, a history of "automatic behavior" during wakefulness (a trancelike state during which simple motor behaviors persist) is not specific for narcolepsy and serves principally to corroborate the presence of daytime somnolence.

℞ TREATMENT

The treatment of narcolepsy is symptomatic. Somnolence is treated with wake-promoting therapeutics. Modafinil is now the drug of choice, principally because it is associated with fewer side effects than older stimulants and has a long half-life; 200 to 400 mg is given as a single daily dose. Older drugs such as methylphenidate (10 mg bid to 20 mg qid or dextroamphetamine (10 mg bid) are still used as alternatives, particularly in refractory patients.

Treatment of the REM-related phenomena cataplexy, hypnogogic hallucinations, and sleep paralysis requires the potent REM sleep suppression produced by antidepressant medications. The tricyclic antidepressants [e.g., protriptyline (10 to 40 mg/d) and clomipramine (25–50 mg/d)] and the selective serotonin reuptake inhibitors (SSRIs) [e.g., fluoxetine (10 to 20 mg/d)] are commonly used for this purpose. Efficacy of the antidepressants is limited largely by anticholinergic side effects (tricyclics) and by sleep disturbance and sexual dysfunction (SSRIs). Adequate nocturnal sleep time and planned daytime naps (when possible) are important preventative measures.

SLEEP APNEA SYNDROMES   Respiratory dysfunction during sleep is a common, serious cause of excessive daytime somnolence as well as of disturbed nocturnal sleep. An estimated 2 to 5 million people in the United States have a reduction or cessation of breathing for 10 to 150 s, from thirty to several hundred times every night during sleep. These episodes may be due to either an occlusion of the airway (*obstructive sleep apnea*), absence of respiratory effort (*central sleep apnea*), or a combination of these factors (*mixed sleep apnea*) (Fig. 24-3). Failure to recognize and treat these conditions appropriately may lead to impairment of daytime alertness; increased risk of sleep-related motor vehicle accidents; hypertension and other serious cardiovascular complications; and increased mortality. Sleep apnea is particularly prevalent in overweight men and in the elderly, yet it is estimated to remain undiagnosed in 80 to 90% of affected individuals. This is unfortunate since effective treatments are available. →*Readers are referred to Chap. 247 for a comprehensive review of the diagnosis and treatment of patients with these conditions.*

PARASOMNIAS   The term *parasomnia* refers to abnormal behaviors that arise from or occur during sleep. A continuum of parasomnias arise from NREM sleep, from brief confusional arousals to sleepwalking and night terrors. The presenting complaint is usually related to the behavior itself, but the parasomnias can disturb sleep continuity or lead to mild impairments in daytime alertness. Only one parasomnia is known to occur in REM sleep, i.e., REM sleep behavior disorder (RBD; see below).

Sleepwalking (Somnambulism)   Patients affected by this disorder carry out automatic motor activities that range from simple to complex. Individuals may leave the bed, walk, urinate inappropriately, eat, or exit from the house while remaining only partially aware. Full arousal may be difficult, and some patients may respond to attempted awakening

with agitation or even violence. Sleepwalking arises from stage 3 or 4 NREM sleep and is most common in children and adolescents, when these sleep stages are most robust. Episodes are usually isolated but may be recurrent in 1 to 6% of patients. The cause is unknown, though it has a familial basis in roughly one-third of cases.

Sleep Terrors   This disorder, also called *pavor nocturnus*, occurs primarily in young children during the first several hours after sleep onset, in stages 3 and 4 of NREM sleep. The child suddenly screams, exhibiting autonomic arousal with sweating, tachycardia, and hyperventilation. The individual may be difficult to arouse and rarely recalls the episode on awakening in the morning. Recurrent attacks are rare. Parents are usually reassured to learn that the condition is self-limited and benign, and that no specific therapy is indicated. Both sleep terrors and sleepwalking represent abnormalities of arousal. In contrast, *nightmares* (dream anxiety attacks) occur during REM sleep and cause full arousal, with intact memory for the unpleasant episode.

REM Sleep Behavior Disorder   RBD is a rare condition that is distinct from other parasomnias in that it occurs during REM sleep. It primarily afflicts men of middle age or older, many of whom have a history of prior neurologic disease. In fact, over one-third of patients will go on to develop Parkinson's disease (Chap. 351) within 10 to 20 years. Presenting symptoms consist of agitated or violent behavior during sleep, reported by a bed partner. In contrast to typical somnambulism, injury to patient or bed partner is not uncommon, and, upon awakening, the patient reports vivid, often unpleasant, dream imagery. The principal differential diagnosis is that of nocturnal seizures, which can be excluded with polysomnography. In RBD, seizure activity is absent on the EEG, and disinhibition of the usual motor atonia is observed in the EMG during REM sleep, at times associated with complex motor behaviors. The pathogenesis is unclear, but damage to brainstem areas mediating descending motor inhibition during REM sleep may be responsible. In support of this hypothesis are the remarkable similarities between RBD and the sleep of animals with bilateral lesions of the pontine tegmentum in areas controlling REM sleep motor inhibition. Treatment with clonazepam (0.5 to 1.0 mg qhs) provides sustained improvement in almost all reported cases.

Sleep Bruxism   Bruxism is an involuntary, forceful grinding of teeth during sleep that affects 10 to 20% of the population. The patient is usually unaware of the problem. The typical age of onset is 17 to 20 years, and spontaneous remission usually occurs by age 40. Sex distribution appears to be equal. In many cases, the diagnosis is made during dental examination, damage is minor, and no treatment is indicated. In more severe cases, treatment with a rubber tooth guard is necessary to prevent disfiguring tooth injury. Stress management or, in some cases, biofeedback can be useful when bruxism is a manifestation of psychological stress. There are anecdotal reports of benefit using benzodiazepines.

Sleep Enuresis   Bedwetting, like sleepwalking and night terrors, is another parasomnia that occurs during sleep in the young. Before age 5 or 6, nocturnal enuresis should probably be considered a normal feature of development. The condition usually improves spontaneously at puberty, has a prevalence in late adolescence of 1 to 3%, and is rare in adulthood. In older patients with enuresis a distinction must be made between primary and secondary enuresis, the latter being defined as bedwetting in patients who have been fully continent for 6 to 12 months. Treatment of primary enuresis is reserved for patients of appropriate age (>5 or 6 years) and consists of bladder training exercises and behavioral therapy. Urologic abnormalities are more common in primary enuresis and must be assessed by urologic examination. Important causes of secondary enuresis include emotional disturbances, urinary tract infections or malformations, cauda equina lesions, epilepsy, sleep apnea, and certain medications. Symptomatic pharmacotherapy is usually accomplished with desmopressin (0.2 mg qhs), oxybutynin chloride (5 to 10 mg qhs) or imipramine (10 to 50 mg qhs).

Miscellaneous Parasomnias   Other clinical entities fulfill the definition of a parasomnia in that they occur selectively during sleep and are associated with some degree of sleep disruption. Examples include *jactatio capitis nocturna* (nocturnal headbanging), sleep talking, nocturnal paroxysmal dystonia, and nocturnal leg cramps.

CIRCADIAN RHYTHM SLEEP DISORDERS

A subset of patients presenting with either insomnia or hypersomnia may have a disorder of sleep *timing* rather than sleep *generation*. Disorders of sleep timing can be either organic (i.e., due to an intrinsic defect in the circadian pacemaker or its input from entraining stimuli) or environmental (i.e., due to a disruption of exposure to entraining stimuli from the environment). Regardless of etiology, the symptoms reflect the influence of the underlying circadian pacemaker on sleep-wake function. Thus, effective therapeutic approaches should aim to entrain the oscillator at an appropriate phase.

Rapid Time-Zone Change (Jet Lag) Syndrome More than 60 million people experience transmeridian air travel annually, which is often associated with excessive daytime sleepiness, sleep onset insomnia, and frequent arousals from sleep, particularly in the latter half of the night. Gastrointestinal discomfort is common. The syndrome is transient, typically lasting 2 to 14 d depending on the number of time zones crossed, the direction of travel, and the traveler's age and phase-shifting capacity. Travelers who spend more time outdoors reportedly adapt more quickly than those who remain in hotel rooms, presumably due to bright (outdoor) light exposure. Avoidance of antecedent sleep loss and obtaining nap sleep on the afternoon prior to overnight travel greatly reduces the difficulty of extended wakefulness. Laboratory studies suggest that submilligram doses of the pineal hormone melatonin can enhance sleep efficiency, but only if taken when endogenous melatonin concentrations are low (i.e., during biologic daytime), and furthermore that melatonin may induce phase shifts in human rhythms. A large-scale clinical trial evaluating the safety and efficacy of melatonin as a treatment for jet lag and other circadian sleep disorders is needed.

Shift-Work Sleep Disorder More than 7 million workers in the United States regularly work at night, either on a permanent or rotating schedule. In addition, each week millions elect to remain awake at night to meet deadlines, drive long distances, or participate in recreational activities, leading to both sleep loss and misalignment of their circadian rhythms with respect to their sleep-wake cycle. Chronic shift workers have higher rates of cardiac, gastrointestinal, and reproductive disorders. Studies of regular night-shift workers indicate that the circadian timing system usually fails to adapt successfully to such inverted schedules. This leads to a misalignment between the desired work-rest schedule and the output of the pacemaker and in disturbed daytime sleep. Sleep deprivation, increased length of time awake prior to work, and misalignment of circadian phase produce decreased alertness and performance, increased reaction time, and increased risk of performance lapses, thereby resulting in greater safety hazards among night workers and other sleep-deprived individuals. Sleep disturbance nearly doubles the risk of a fatal work accident.

Sleep onset is associated with marked attenuation in perception of both auditory and visual stimuli and lapses of consciousness. The sleepy individual may thus attempt to perform routine and familiar motor tasks during the transition state between wakefulness and sleep (stage 1 sleep) in the absence of adequate sensory input from the environment. Motor vehicle operators are especially vulnerable to sleep-related accidents since the sleep-deprived driver or operator often fails to heed the warning signs of fatigue. Such attempts to override the powerful biologic drive for sleep by the sheer force of will can yield a catastrophic outcome when sleep processes intrude involuntarily upon the waking brain. Such intrusions typically last only seconds but are known on occasion to persist for longer durations. These frequent brief intrusions of stage 1 sleep into behavioral wakefulness are a major component of the impaired psychomotor performance seen with sleepiness. There is a significant increase in the risk of sleep-related, fatal-to-the-driver highway crashes in the early morning and late af-

ternoon hours, coincident with bimodal peaks in the daily rhythm of sleep tendency.

Safety programs should promote education about sleep and increase awareness of the hazards associated with night work and should be aimed at minimizing both circadian disruption and sleep deprivation. The work schedule should minimize: (1) exposure to night work, (2) the frequency of shift rotation so that shifts do not rotate more than once every 2 to 3 weeks, (3) the number of consecutive night shifts, and (4) the duration of night shifts. In fact, shift durations of >18 h should be universally recognized as increasing the risk of sleep-related errors and performance lapses. Caffeine is undoubtedly the most widely used wake-promoting drug, but it cannot forestall sleep indefinitely and does not shield users from sleep-related performance lapses. Postural changes, exercise, and strategic placement of nap opportunities can sometimes temporarily reduce the risk of fatigue-related performance lapses. Properly timed exposure to bright light can facilitate rapid adaptation to night-shift work. An adequate number of safe highway rest areas, shoulder rumble strips, and strict enforcement and compliance monitoring of hours-of-service policies are needed to reduce the risk of sleep-related transportation crashes.

Delayed Sleep Phase Syndrome Delayed sleep phase syndrome is characterized by: (1) reported sleep onset and wake times intractably later than desired, (2) actual sleep times at nearly the same clock hours daily, and (3) essentially normal all-night polysomnography except for delayed sleep onset. Patients exhibit an abnormally delayed endogenous circadian phase, with the temperature minimum during the constant routine occurring later than normal. This delayed phase could be due to: (1) an abnormally long, genetically determined intrinsic period of the endogenous circadian pacemaker; (2) an abnormally reduced phase-advancing capacity of the pacemaker; or (3) an irregular prior sleep-wake schedule, characterized by frequent nights when the patient chooses to remain awake well past midnight (for social, school, or work reasons). In most cases, it is difficult to distinguish among these factors, since patients with an abnormally long intrinsic period are more likely to "choose" such late-night activities because they are unable to sleep at that time. Patients tend to be young adults. This self-perpetuating condition can persist for years and does not usually respond to attempts to reestablish normal bedtime hours. Treatment methods involving bright-light phototherapy during the morning hours or melatonin administration in the evening hours show promise in these patients, although the relapse rate is high.

Advanced Sleep Phase Syndrome Advanced sleep phase syndrome (ASPS) is the converse of the delayed sleep phase syndrome. Most commonly, this syndrome occurs in older people, 15% of whom report that they cannot sleep past 5 A.M., with twice that number complaining that they wake up too early at least several times per week. Patients with ASPS experience excessive daytime sleepiness during the evening hours, when they have great difficulty remaining awake, even in social settings. Typically, patients awaken from 3 to 5 A.M. each day, often several hours before their desired wake times. In addition to age-related ASPS, an early-onset familial variant of this condition has also been reported. In one such family, autosomal dominant ASPS was due to a missense mutation in a circadian clock component (PER2, as shown in Fig. 24-2) that altered the circardian period. Patients with ASPS may benefit from bright-light phototherapy during the evening hours, designed to reset the circadian pacemaker to a later hour.

Non-24-Hour Sleep-Wake Disorder This condition can occur when the maximal phase-advancing capacity of the circadian pacemaker is not adequate to accommodate the difference between the 24-h geophysical day and the intrinsic period of the pacemaker in the patient. Alternatively, patients' self-selected exposure to artificial light may drive the circadian pacemaker to a >24-h schedule. Affected patients are not able to maintain a stable phase relationship between the output of the pacemaker and the 24-h day. Such patients typically present with an incremental pattern of successive delays in sleep onsets and wake times, progressing in and out of phase with local time. When the patient's endogenous rhythms are out of phase with the local environment, insomnia coexists with excessive daytime sleepiness. Conversely, when the endogenous rhythms are in phase with the local environment, symptoms remit. The intervals between symptomatic periods may last several weeks to several months. Blind individuals unable to perceive light are particularly susceptible to this disorder. Nightly low-dose (0.5 mg) melatonin administration has been reported to improve sleep and, in some cases, even to induce synchronization of the circadian pacemaker.

MEDICAL IMPLICATIONS OF CIRCADIAN RHYTHMICITY Prominent circadian variations have been reported in the incidence of acute myocardial infarction, sudden cardiac death, and stroke, the leading causes of death in the United States. Platelet aggregability is increased after arising in the early morning hours, coincident with the peak incidence of these cardiovascular events. A better understanding of the possible role of circadian rhythmicity in the acute destabilization of a chronic condition such as atherosclerotic disease could improve the understanding of the pathophysiology.

Diagnostic and therapeutic procedures may also be affected by the time of day at which data are collected. Examples include blood pressure, body temperature, the dexamethasone suppression test, and plasma cortisol levels. The timing of chemotherapy administration has been reported to have an effect on the outcome of treatment. Few physicians realize the extent to which routine measures are affected by the time (or sleep/wake state) when the measurement is made.

In addition, both the toxicity and effectiveness of drugs can vary during the day. For example, more than a fivefold difference has been observed in mortality rates following administration of toxic agents to experimental animals at different times of day. Anesthetic agents are particularly sensitive to time-of-day effects. Finally, the physician must be increasingly aware of the public health risks associated with the ever-increasing demands made by the duty-rest-recreation schedules in our round-the-clock society.

FURTHER READING

FLEMONS WW: Clinical practice. Obstructive sleep apnea. N Engl J Med 347: 498, 2002

SCAMMELL TE: The neurobiology, diagnosis, and treatment of narcolepsy. Ann Neurol 53:154, 2003

SMITH MT: Comparative meta-analysis of pharmacotherapy and behavior therapy for persistent insomnia. Am J Psychiatry 159:5, 2002

Section 4   Disorders of the Eyes, Ears, Nose, and Throat

25 | DISORDERS OF THE EYE
Jonathan C. Horton

THE HUMAN VISUAL SYSTEM

The visual system provides a supremely efficient means for the rapid assimilation of information from the environment to aid in the guidance of behavior. The act of seeing begins with the capture of images focused by the cornea and lens upon a light-sensitive membrane in the back of the eye, called the *retina*. The retina is actually part of the brain, banished to the periphery to serve as a transducer for the conversion of patterns of light energy into neuronal signals. Light is absorbed by photopigment in two types of receptors: rods and cones. In the human retina there are 100 million rods and 5 million cones. The rods operate in dim (scotopic) illumination. The cones function under daylight (photopic) conditions. The cone system is specialized for color perception and high spatial resolution. The majority of cones are located within the macula, the portion of the retina serving the central 10° of vision. In the middle of the macula a small pit termed the *fovea*, packed exclusively with cones, provides best visual acuity.

Photoreceptors hyperpolarize in response to light, activating bipolar, amacrine, and horizontal cells in the inner nuclear layer. After processing of photoreceptor responses by this complex retinal circuit, the flow of sensory information ultimately converges upon a final common pathway: the ganglion cells. These cells translate the visual image impinging upon the retina into a continuously varying barrage of action potentials that propagates along the primary optic pathway to visual centers within the brain. There are a million ganglion cells in each retina, and hence a million fibers in each optic nerve.

Ganglion cell axons sweep along the inner surface of the retina in the nerve fiber layer, exit the eye at the optic disc, and travel through the optic nerve, optic chiasm, and optic tract to reach targets in the brain. The majority of fibers synapse upon cells in the lateral geniculate body, a thalamic relay station. Cells in the lateral geniculate body project in turn to the primary visual cortex. This massive afferent retinogeniculocortical sensory pathway provides the neural substrate for visual perception. Although the lateral geniculate body is the main target of the retina, separate classes of ganglion cells project to other subcortical visual nuclei involved in different functions. Ganglion cells

that mediate pupillary constriction and circadian rhythms are light-sensitive, owing to a novel visual pigment, melanopsin. Pupil responses are mediated by input to the pretectal olivary nuclei in the midbrain. The pretectal nuclei send their output to the Edinger-Westphal nuclei, which in turn provide parasympathetic innervation to the iris sphincter via an interneuron in the ciliary ganglion. Circadian rhythms are timed by a retinal projection to the suprachiasmatic nucleus. Visual orientation and eye movements are served by retinal input to the superior colliculus. Gaze stabilization and optokinetic reflexes are governed by a group of small retinal targets known collectively as the *brainstem accessory optic system*.

The eyes must be rotated constantly within their orbits to place and maintain targets of visual interest upon the fovea. This activity, called *foveation*, or looking, is governed by an elaborate efferent motor system. Each eye is moved by six extraocular muscles, supplied by cranial nerves from the oculomotor (III), trochlear (IV), and abducens (VI) nuclei. Activity in these ocular motor nuclei is coordinated by pontine and midbrain mechanisms for smooth pursuit, saccades, and gaze stabilization during head and body movements. Large regions of the frontal and parietooccipital cortex control these brainstem eye movement centers by providing descending supranuclear input.

CLINICAL ASSESSMENT OF VISUAL FUNCTION

REFRACTIVE STATE In approaching the patient with reduced vision, the first step is to decide whether refractive error is responsible. In *emmetropia*, parallel rays from infinity are focused perfectly upon the retina. Sadly, this condition is enjoyed by only a minority of the population. In *myopia*, the globe is too long, and light rays come to a focal point in front of the retina. Near objects can be seen clearly, but distant objects require a diverging lens in front of the eye. In *hyperopia*, the globe is too short, and hence a converging lens is used to supplement the refractive power of the eye. In *astigmatism*, the corneal surface is not perfectly spherical, necessitating a cylindrical corrective lens. In recent years it has become possible to correct refractive error with the excimer laser by performing LASIK (laser in situ keratomileusis) to alter the curvature of the cornea.

With the onset of middle age, *presbyopia* develops as the lens within the eye becomes unable to increase its refractive power to accommodate upon near objects. To compensate for presbyopia, the emmetropic patient must use reading glasses. The patient already wearing glasses for distance correction usually switches to bifocals. The only exception is the myopic patient, who may achieve clear vision at near simply by removing glasses containing the distance prescription.

Refractive errors usually develop slowly and remain stable after adolescence, except in unusual circumstances. For example, the acute onset of diabetes mellitus can produce sudden myopia because of lens edema induced by hyperglycemia. Testing vision through a pinhole aperture is a useful way to screen quickly for refractive error. If the visual acuity is better through a pinhole than with the unaided eye, the patient needs a refraction to obtain best corrected visual acuity.

VISUAL ACUITY The Snellen chart is used to test acuity at a distance of 6 m (20 ft). For convenience, a scale version of the Snellen chart, called the Rosenbaum card, is held at 36 cm (14 in) from the patient (Fig. 25-1). All subjects should be able to read the 6/6 m (20/20 ft) line with each eye using their refractive correction, if any. Patients who need reading glasses because of presbyopia must wear them for accurate testing with the Rosenbaum card. If 6/6 (20/20) acuity is not present in each eye, the deficiency in vision must be explained. If

FIGURE 25-1 The Rosenbaum card is a miniature, scale version of the Snellen chart for testing visual acuity at near. When the visual acuity is recorded, the Snellen distance equivalent should bear a notation indicating that vision was tested at near, not at 6 m (20 ft), or else the Jaeger number system should be used to report the acuity.

worse than 6/240 (20/800), acuity should be recorded in terms of counting fingers, hand motions, light perception, or no light perception. Legal blindness is defined by the Internal Revenue Service as a best corrected acuity of 6/60 (20/200) or less in the better eye, or a binocular visual field subtending 20° or less. For driving the laws vary by state, but most require a corrected acuity of 6/12 (20/40) in at least one eye. Patients with a homonymous hemianopia should not drive.

PUPILS The pupils should be tested individually in dim light with the patient fixating on a distant target. If they respond briskly to light, there is no need to check the near response, because isolated loss of constriction (miosis) to accommodation does not occur. For this reason, the ubiquitous abbreviation PERRLA (pupils equal, round, and reactive to light and accommodation) implies a wasted effort with the last step. However, it is important to test the near response if the light response is poor or absent. Light-near dissociation occurs with neurosyphilis (Argyll Robertson pupil), lesions of the dorsal midbrain (obstructive hydrocephalus, pineal region tumors), and after aberrant regeneration (oculomotor nerve palsy, Adie's tonic pupil).

An eye with no light perception has no pupillary response to direct light stimulation. If the retina or optic nerve is only partially injured, the direct pupillary response will be weaker than the consensual pupillary response evoked by shining a light into the other eye. This *relative afferent pupillary defect* (Marcus Gunn pupil) can be elicited with the swinging flashlight test. It is an extremely useful sign in retrobulbar optic neuritis and other optic nerve diseases, where it may be the sole objective evidence for disease.

Subtle inequality in pupil size, up to 0.5 mm, is a fairly common finding in normal persons. The diagnosis of essential or physiologic anisocoria is secure as long as the relative pupil asymmetry remains constant as ambient lighting varies. Anisocoria that increases in dim light indicates a sympathetic paresis of the iris dilator muscle. The triad of miosis with ipsilateral ptosis and anhidrosis constitutes Horner's syndrome, although anhidrosis is an inconstant feature. Brainstem stroke, carotid dissection, or neoplasm impinging upon the sympathetic chain are occasionally identified as the cause of Horner's syndrome, but most cases are idiopathic.

Anisocoria that increases in bright light suggests a parasympathetic palsy. The first concern is an oculomotor nerve paresis. This possibility is excluded if the eye movements are full and the patient has no ptosis or diplopia. Acute pupillary dilation (mydriasis) can occur from damage to the ciliary ganglion in the orbit. Common mechanisms are infection (herpes zoster, influenza), trauma (blunt, penetrating, surgical), or ischemia (diabetes, temporal arteritis). After denervation of the iris sphincter the pupil does not respond well to light, but the response to near is often relatively intact. When the near stimulus is removed, the pupil redilates very slowly compared with the normal pupil, hence the term *tonic pupil*. In Adie's syndrome, a tonic pupil occurs in conjunction with weak or absent tendon reflexes in the lower extremities. This benign disorder, which occurs predominantly in healthy young women, is assumed to represent a mild dysautonomia. Tonic pupils are also associated with Shy-Drager syndrome, segmental hypohidrosis, diabetes, and amyloidosis. Occasionally, a tonic pupil is discovered incidentally in an otherwise completely normal, asymptomatic individual. The diagnosis is confirmed by placing a drop of dilute (0.125%) pilocarpine into each eye. Denervation hypersensitivity produces pupillary constriction in a tonic pupil, whereas the normal pupil shows no response. Pharmacologic dilation from accidental or deliberate instillation of anticholinergic agents (atropine, scopolamine drops) into the eye can also produce pupillary mydriasis. In this situation, normal strength (1%) pilocarpine causes no constriction.

Both pupils are affected equally by systemic medications. They are small with narcotic use (morphine, heroin) and large with anticholinergics (scopolamine). Parasympathetic agents (pilocarpine, demecarium bromide) used to treat glaucoma produce miosis. In any patient with an unexplained pupillary abnormality, a slit-lamp examination is helpful to exclude surgical trauma to the iris, an occult foreign body, perforating injury, intraocular inflammation, adhesions (synechia), angle-closure glaucoma, and iris sphincter rupture from blunt trauma.

EYE MOVEMENTS AND ALIGNMENT Eye movements are tested by asking the patient with both eyes open to pursue a small target such as a penlight into the cardinal fields of gaze. Normal ocular versions are smooth, symmetric, full, and maintained in all directions without nystagmus. Saccades, or quick refixation eye movements, are assessed by having the patient look back and forth between two stationary targets. The eyes should move rapidly and accurately in a single jump to their target. Ocular alignment can be judged by holding a penlight directly in front of the patient at about 1 m. If the eyes are straight, the corneal light reflex will be centered in the middle of each pupil. To test eye alignment more precisely, the cover test is useful. The patient is instructed to gaze upon a small fixation target in the distance. One eye is covered suddenly while observing the second eye. If the second eye shifts to fixate upon the target, it was misaligned. If it does not move, the first eye is uncovered and the test is repeated on the second eye. If neither eye moves, the eyes are aligned orthotropically. If the eyes are orthotropic in primary gaze but the patient complains of diplopia, the cover test should be performed with the head tilted or turned in whatever direction elicits diplopia. With practice the examiner can detect an ocular deviation (heterotropia) as small as 1 to 2° with the cover test. Deviations can be measured by placing prisms in front of the misaligned eye to determine the power required to neutralize the fixation shift evoked by covering the other eye.

STEREOPSIS Stereoacuity is determined by presenting targets with retinal disparity separately to each eye using polarized images. The most popular office tests measure a range of thresholds from 800 to 40 seconds of arc. Normal stereoacuity is 40 seconds of arc. If a patient achieves this level of stereoacuity, one is assured that the eyes are aligned orthotropically and that vision is intact in each eye. Random dot stereograms have no monocular depth cues and provide an excellent screening test for strabismus and amblyopia in children.

COLOR VISION The retina contains three classes of cones, with visual pigments of differing peak spectral sensitivity: red (560 nm), green (530 nm), and blue (430 nm). The red and green cone pigments are encoded on the X chromosome; the blue cone pigment on chromosome 7. Mutations of the blue cone pigment are exceedingly rare. Mutations of the red and green pigments cause congenital X-linked color blindness in 8% of males. Affected individuals are not truly color blind; rather, they differ from normal subjects in how they perceive color and how they combine primary monochromatic lights to match a given color. Anomalous trichromats have three cone types, but a mutation in one cone pigment (usually red or green) causes a shift in peak spectral sensitivity, altering the proportion of primary colors required to achieve a color match. Dichromats have only two cone types and will therefore accept a color match based upon only two primary colors. Anomalous trichromats and dichromats have 6/6 (20/20) visual acuity, but their hue discrimination is impaired. Ishihara color plates can be used to detect red-green color blindness. The test plates contain a hidden number, visible only to subjects with color confusion from red-green color blindness. Because color blindness is almost exclusively X-linked, it is worth screening only male children.

The Ishihara plates are often used to detect acquired defects in color vision, although they are intended as a screening test for congenital color blindness. Acquired defects in color vision frequently result from disease of the macula or optic nerve. For example, patients with a history of optic neuritis often complain of color desaturation long after their visual acuity has returned to normal. Color blindness can also occur from bilateral strokes involving the ventral portion of the occipital lobe (cerebral achromatopsia). Such patients can perceive only shades of gray and may also have difficulty recognizing faces (prosopagnosia). Infarcts of the dominant occipital lobe sometimes give rise to color anomia. Affected patients can discriminate colors, but they cannot name them.

VISUAL FIELDS Vision can be impaired by damage to the visual system anywhere from the eyes to the occipital lobes. One can localize the site of the lesion with considerable accuracy by mapping the visual field deficit by finger confrontation and then correlating it with the topographic anatomy of the visual pathway (Fig. 25-2). Quantitative visual field mapping is performed by computer-driven perimeters (Humphrey, Octopus) that present a target of variable intensity at fixed positions in the visual field (Fig. 25-2A). By generating an automated printout of light thresholds, these static perimeters provide a sensitive means of detecting scotomas in the visual field. They are exceedingly useful for serial assessment of visual function in chronic diseases such as glaucoma or pseudotumor cerebri.

The crux of visual field analysis is to decide whether a lesion is before, at, or behind the optic chiasm. If a scotoma is confined to one eye, it must be due to a lesion anterior to the chiasm, involving either the optic nerve or retina. Retinal lesions produce scotomas that correspond optically to their location in the fundus. For example, a superior-nasal retinal detachment results in an inferior-temporal field cut. Damage to the macula causes a central scotoma (Fig. 25-2B).

Optic nerve disease produces characteristic patterns of visual field loss. Glaucoma selectively destroys axons that enter the superotemporal or inferotemporal poles of the optic disc, resulting in arcuate scotomas shaped like a Turkish scimitar, which emanate from the blind spot and curve around fixation to end flat against the horizontal meridian (Fig. 25-2C). This type of field defect mirrors the arrangement of the nerve fiber layer in the temporal retina. Arcuate or nerve fiber layer scotomas also occur from optic neuritis, ischemic optic neuropathy, optic disc drusen, and branch retinal artery or vein occlusion.

Damage to the entire upper or lower pole of the optic disc causes an altitudinal field cut that follows the horizontal meridian (Fig. 25-2D). This pattern of visual field loss is typical of ischemic optic neuropathy but also occurs from retinal vascular occlusion, advanced glaucoma, and optic neuritis.

About half the fibers in the optic nerve originate from ganglion cells serving the macula. Damage to papillomacular fibers causes a cecocentral scotoma encompassing the blind spot and macula (Fig. 25-2E). If the damage is irreversible, pallor eventually appears in the temporal portion of the optic disc. Temporal pallor from a cecocentral scotoma may develop in optic neuritis, nutritional optic neuropathy, toxic optic neuropathy, Leber's hereditary optic neuropathy, and compressive optic neuropathy. It is worth mentioning that the temporal side of the optic disc is slightly more pale than the nasal side in most normal individuals. Therefore, it can sometimes be difficult to decide whether the temporal pallor visible on fundus examination represents a pathologic change. Pallor of the nasal rim of the optic disc is a less equivocal sign of optic atrophy.

At the optic chiasm, fibers from nasal ganglion cells decussate into the contralateral optic tract. Crossed fibers are damaged more by compression than uncrossed fibers. As a result, mass lesions of the sellar region cause a temporal hemianopia in each eye. Tumors anterior to the optic chiasm, such as meningiomas of the tuberculum sella, produce a junctional scotoma characterized by an optic neuropathy in one eye and a superior temporal field cut in the other eye (Fig. 25-2G). More symmetric compression of the optic chiasm by a pituitary adenoma (Fig. 318-4), meningioma, craniopharyngioma, glioma, or aneurysm results in a bitemporal hemianopia (Fig. 25-2H). The insidious development of a bitemporal hemianopia often goes unnoticed by the patient and will escape detection by the physician unless each eye is tested separately.

It is difficult to localize a postchiasmal lesion accurately, because injury anywhere in the optic tract, lateral geniculate body, optic radiations, or visual cortex can produce a homonymous hemianopia, i.e., a temporal hemifield defect in the contralateral eye and a matching nasal hemifield defect in the ipsilateral eye (Fig. 25-2I). A unilateral postchiasmal lesion leaves the visual acuity in each eye unaffected, although the patient may read the letters on only the left or right half of the eye chart. Lesions of the optic radiations tend to cause poorly matched or incongruous field defects in each eye. Damage to the optic radiations in the temporal lobe (Meyer's loop) produces a superior quadrantic homonymous hemianopia (Fig. 25-2*J*), whereas injury to the optic radiations in the parietal lobe results in an inferior quadrantic homonymous hemianopia (Fig. 25-2*K*). Lesions of the primary visual cortex give rise to dense, congruous hemianopic field defects. Occlusion of the posterior cerebral artery supplying the occipital lobe is a frequent cause of total homonymous hemianopia. Some patients with hemianopia after occipital stroke have macular sparing, because the macular representation at the tip of the occipital lobe is supplied by collaterals from the middle cerebral artery (Fig. 25-2*L*). Destruction of both occipital lobes produces cortical blindness. This condition can be distinguished from bilateral prechiasmal visual loss by noting that the pupil responses and optic fundi remain normal.

RED OR PAINFUL EYE

Corneal Abrasions These are seen best by placing a drop of fluorescein in the eye and looking with the slit lamp using a cobalt-blue light. A penlight with a blue filter will suffice if no slit lamp is available. Damage to the corneal epithelium is revealed by yellow fluorescence of the exposed basement membrane underlying the epithelium. It is important to check for foreign bodies. To search the conjunctival fornices, the lower lid should be pulled down and the upper lid everted. A foreign body can be removed with a moistened cotton-tipped applicator after placing a drop of topical anesthetic, such as proparacaine, in the eye. Alternatively, it may be possible to flush the foreign body from the eye by irrigating copiously with saline or artificial tears. If the corneal epithelium has been abraded, antibiotic ointment and a patch should be applied to the eye. A drop of an intermediate-acting cycloplegic, such as cyclopentolate hydrochloride 1%, helps to reduce pain by relaxing the ciliary body. The eye should be reexamined the next day. Minor abrasions may not require patching and cycloplegia.

Subconjunctival Hemorrhage This results from rupture of small vessels bridging the potential space between the episclera and conjunctiva. Blood dissecting into this space can produce a spectacular red eye, but vision is not affected and the hemorrhage resolves without treatment. Subconjunctival hemorrhage is usually spontaneous but can occur from blunt trauma, eye rubbing, or vigorous coughing. Occasionally it is a clue to an underlying bleeding disorder.

Pinguecula This is a small, raised conjunctival nodule at the temporal or nasal limbus. In adults such lesions are extremely common and have little significance, unless they become inflamed (pingueculitis). A *pte-*

Monocular Prechiasmal Field Defects:

A Normal Field Right Eye (blind spot) 30°   B Central Scotoma 30°   C Nerve-Fiber Bundle (Arcuate) Scotoma 30°   D Altitudinal Scotoma 30°   E Ceco-central Scotoma 30°   F Enlarged Blind-Spot with Peripheral Constriction 30°

Binocular Chiasmal or Postchiasmal Field Defects:

(Left eye) (Right eye)

G Junctional Scotoma 30°

H Bitemporal Hemianopia 30°

I Homonymous Hemianopia 30°

J Superior Quadrantanopia 30°

K Inferior Quadrantanopia 30°

L Homonymous Hemianopia with Macular Sparing 30°

Right   Left

Optic Nerve

Optic Chiasm

Optic Tract

Lateral Geniculate Body

Optic Radiations

Primary Visual Cortex

FIGURE 25-2 Ventral view of the brain, correlating patterns of visual field loss with the sites of lesions in the visual pathway. The visual fields overlap partially, creating 120° of central binocular field flanked by a 40° monocular crescent on either side. The visual field maps in this figure were done with a computer-driven perimeter (Humphrey Instruments, Carl Zeiss, Inc.). It plots the retinal sensitivity to light in the central 30° using a gray scale format. Areas of visual field loss are shown in black. The examples of common monocular, prechiasmal field defects are all shown for the right eye. By convention, the visual fields are always recorded with the left eye's field on the left, and the right eye's field on the right, just as the patient sees the world.

rygium resembles a pinguecula but has crossed the limbus to encroach upon the corneal surface. Removal is justified when symptoms of irritation or blurring develop, but recurrence is a common problem.

Blepharitis This refers to inflammation of the eyelids. The most common form occurs in association with acne rosacea or seborrheic dermatitis. The eyelid margins are usually colonized heavily by staphylococci. Upon close inspection, they appear greasy, ulcerated, and crusted with scaling debris that clings to the lashes. Treatment consists of warm compresses, strict eyelid hygiene, and topical antibiotics such as *erythromycin*. An external *hordeolum* (sty) is caused by staphylococcal infection of the superficial accessory glands of Zeis or Moll located in the eyelid margins. An internal hordeolum occurs after suppurative infection of the oil-secreting meibomian glands within the tarsal plate of the eyelid. Systemic antibiotics, usually tetracyclines, are sometimes necessary for treatment of meibomian gland inflammation (meibomitis) or chronic, severe blepharitis. A *chalazion* is a painless, granulomatous inflammation of a meibomian gland that produces a pealike nodule within the eyelid. It can be incised and drained, or injected with glucocorticoids. Basal cell, squamous cell, or meibomian gland carcinoma should be suspected for any nonhealing, ulcerative lesion of the eyelids.

Dacrocystitis An inflammation of the lacrimal drainage system, this can produce epiphora (tearing) and ocular injection. Gentle pressure over the lacrimal sac evokes pain and reflux of mucus or pus from the tear puncta. Dacrocystitis usually occurs after obstruction of the lacrimal system. It is treated with topical and systemic antibiotics, followed by probing or surgery to reestablish patency. *Entropion* (inversion of the eyelid) or *ectropion* (sagging or eversion of the eyelid) can also lead to epiphora and ocular irritation.

Conjunctivitis This is the most common cause of a red, irritated eye. Pain is minimal, and the visual acuity is reduced only slightly. The most common viral etiology is adenovirus infection. It causes a watery discharge, mild foreign-body sensation, and photophobia. Bacterial infection tends to produce a more mucopurulent exudate. Mild cases of infectious conjunctivitis are usually treated empirically with broad-spectrum topical ocular antibiotics, such as sulfacetamide 10%, polymixin-bacitracin-neomycin, or trimethoprim-polymixin combination. Smears and cultures are usually reserved for severe, resistant, or recurrent cases of conjunctivitis. To prevent contagion, patients should be admonished to wash their hands frequently, not to touch their eyes, and to avoid direct contact with others.

Allergic Conjunctivitis This condition is extremely common and often mistaken for infectious conjunctivitis. Itching, redness, and epiphora are typical. The palpebral conjunctiva may become hypertropic with giant excrescences called cobblestone papillae. Irritation from contact lenses or any chronic foreign body can also induce formation of cobblestone papillae. *Atopic conjunctivitis* occurs in subjects with atopic dermatitis or asthma. Symptoms caused by allergic conjunctivitis can be alleviated with cold compresses, topical vasoconstrictors, antihistamines, and mast-cell stabilizers such as cromolyn sodium. Topical glucocorticoid solutions provide dramatic relief of immune-mediated forms of conjunctivitis, but their long-term use is ill-advised because of the complications of glaucoma, cataract, and secondary infection. Topical nonsteroidal anti-inflammatory agents (NSAIDs) such as ketorolac tromethamine are a better alternative.

Keratoconjunctivitis Sicca Also known as dry eye, it produces a burning, foreign-body sensation, injection, and photophobia. In mild cases the eye appears surprisingly normal, but tear production measured by wetting of a filter paper (Schirmer strip) is deficient. A variety of systemic drugs, including antihistaminic, anticholinergic, and psychotropic medications, result in dry eye by reducing lacrimal secretion. Disorders that involve the lacrimal gland directly, such as sarcoidosis or Sjögren's syndrome, also cause dry eye. Patients may develop dry eye after radiation therapy if the treatment field includes the orbits. Problems with ocular drying are also common after lesions affecting cranial nerves V or VII. Corneal anesthesia is particularly dangerous, because the absence of a normal blink reflex exposes the cornea to injury without pain to warn the patient. Dry eye is managed by frequent and liberal application of artificial tears and ocular lubricants. In severe cases the tear puncta can be plugged or cauterized to reduce lacrimal outflow.

Keratitis This is a threat to vision because of the risk of corneal clouding, scarring, and perforation. Worldwide, the two leading causes of blindness from keratitis are trachoma from chlamydial infection and vitamin A deficiency related to malnutrition. In the United States, contact lenses play a major role in corneal infection and ulceration. They should not be worn by anyone with an active eye infection. In evaluating the cornea, it is important to differentiate between a superficial infection (*keratoconjunctivitis*) and a deeper, more serious ulcerative process. The latter is accompanied by greater visual loss, pain, photophobia, redness, and discharge. Slit-lamp examination shows disruption of the corneal epithelium, a cloudy infiltrate or abscess in the

stroma, and an inflammatory cellular reaction in the anterior chamber. In severe cases, pus settles at the bottom of the anterior chamber, giving rise to a hypopyon. Immediate empirical antibiotic therapy should be initiated after corneal scrapings are obtained for Gram's stain, Giemsa stain, and cultures. Fortified topical antibiotics are most effective, supplemented with subconjunctival antibiotics as required. A fungal etiology should always be considered in the patient with keratitis. Fungal infection is common in warm humid climates, especially after penetration of the cornea by plant or vegetable material.

Herpes Simplex The *herpes viruses* are a major cause of blindness from keratitis. Most adults in the United States have serum antibodies to herpes simplex, indicating prior viral infection (Chap. 163). Primary ocular infection is generally caused by herpes simplex type 1, rather than type 2. It manifests as a unilateral follicular blepharoconjunctivitis, easily confused with adenoviral conjunctivitis unless telltale vesicles appear on the periocular skin or conjunctiva. A dendritic pattern of corneal epithelial ulceration revealed by fluorescein staining is pathognomonic for herpes infection but is seen in only a minority of primary infections. Recurrent ocular infection arises from reactivation of the latent herpes virus. Viral eruption in the corneal epithelium may result in the characteristic herpes dendrite. Involvement of the corneal stroma produces edema, vascularization, and iridocyclitis. Herpes keratitis is treated with topical antiviral agents, cycloplegics, and oral acyclovir. Topical glucocorticoids are effective in mitigating corneal scarring but must be used with extreme caution because of the danger of corneal melting and perforation. Topical glucocorticoids also carry the risk of prolonging infection and inducing glaucoma.

Herpes Zoster Herpes zoster from reactivation of latent varicella (chickenpox) virus causes a dermatomal pattern of painful vesicular dermatitis. Ocular symptoms can occur after zoster eruption in any branch of the trigeminal nerve but are particularly common when vesicles form on the nose, reflecting nasociliary (V1) nerve involvement (Hutchinson's sign). Herpes zoster ophthalmicus produces corneal dendrites, which can be difficult to distinguish from those seen in herpes simplex. Stromal keratitis, anterior uveitis, raised intraocular pressure, ocular motor nerve palsies, acute retinal necrosis, and postherpetic scarring and neuralgia are other common sequelae. Herpes zoster ophthalmicus is treated with antiviral agents and cycloplegics. In severe cases, glucocorticoids may be added to prevent permanent visual loss from corneal scarring.

Episcleritis This is an inflammation of the episclera, a thin layer of connective tissue between the conjunctiva and sclera. Episcleritis resembles conjunctivitis but is a more localized process and discharge is absent. Most cases of episcleritis are idiopathic, but some occur in the setting of an autoimmune disease. *Scleritis* refers to a deeper, more severe inflammatory process, frequently associated with a connective tissue disease such as rheumatoid arthritis, lupus erythematosus, polyarteritis nodosa, Wegener's granulomatosis, or relapsing polychondritis. The inflammation and thickening of the sclera can be diffuse or nodular. In anterior forms of scleritis, the globe assumes a violet hue and the patient complains of severe ocular tenderness and pain. With posterior scleritis the pain and redness may be less marked, but there is often proptosis, choroidal effusion, reduced motility, and visual loss. Episcleritis and scleritis should be treated with NSAIDs. If these agents fail, topical or even systemic glucocorticoid therapy may be necessary, especially if an underlying autoimmune process is active.

Uveitis Involving the anterior structures of the eye, this is also called *iritis* or *iridocyclitis*. The diagnosis requires slit-lamp examination to identify inflammatory cells floating in the aqueous humor or deposited upon the corneal endothelium (keratic precipitates). Anterior uveitis develops in sarcoidosis, ankylosing spondylitis, juvenile rheumatoid arthritis, inflammatory bowel disease, psoriasis, Reiter's syndrome, and Behçet's disease. It is also associated with herpes infections, syphilis, Lyme disease, onchocerciasis, tuberculosis, and leprosy. Although anterior uveitis can occur in conjunction with many diseases, no cause is found to explain the majority of cases. For this reason, laboratory evaluation is usually reserved for patients with recurrent or severe anterior uveitis. Treatment is aimed at reducing inflammation and scarring by judicious use of topical glucocorticoids. Dilation of the pupil reduces pain and prevents the formation of synechiae.

Posterior Uveitis This is diagnosed by observing inflammation of the vitreous, retina, or choroid on fundus examination. It is more likely than anterior uveitis to be associated with an identifiable systemic disease. Some patients have panuveitis, or inflammation of both the anterior and posterior segments of the eye. Posterior uveitis is a manifestation of autoimmune diseases such as sarcoidosis, Behçet's disease, Vogt-Koyanagi-Harada syndrome, and inflammatory bowel disease (Fig. 25-3). It also accompanies diseases such as toxoplasmosis, onchocerciasis, cysticercosis, coccidioidomycosis, toxocariasis, and histoplasmosis; infections caused by organisms such as *Candida*, *Pneumocystis carinii*, *Cryptococcus*, *Aspergillus*, herpes, and cytomegalovirus (see Fig. 166-1); and other diseases such as syphilis, Lyme disease, tuberculosis, cat-scratch disease, Whipple's disease, and brucellosis. In multiple sclerosis, chronic inflammatory changes can develop in the extreme periphery of the retina (pars planitis or intermediate uveitis).

Acute Angle-Closure Glaucoma This is a rare and frequently misdiagnosed cause of a red, painful eye. Susceptible eyes have a shallow anterior chamber, either because the eye has a short axial length (hyperopia) or a lens enlarged by the gradual development of cataract. When the pupil becomes mid-dilated, the peripheral iris blocks aqueous outflow via the anterior chamber angle and the intraocular pressure rises abruptly, producing pain, injection, corneal edema, obscurations, and blurred vision. In some patients, ocular symptoms are overshadowed by nausea, vomiting, or headache, prompting a fruitless workup for abdominal or neurologic disease. The diagnosis is made by measuring the intraocular pressure during an acute attack or by observing a narrow chamber angle by means of a specially mirrored contact lens. Acute angle closure is treated with oral or intravenous acetazolamide, topical beta blockers, prostaglandin analogues, α_2-adrenergic agonists, and pilocarpine to induce miosis. If these measures fail, a laser can be used to create a hole in the peripheral iris to relieve pupillary block. Many physicians are reluctant to dilate patients routinely for fundus examination because they fear precipitating an angle-closure glaucoma. The risk is actually remote and more than outweighed by the potential benefit to patients of discovering a hidden fundus lesion visible only through a fully dilated pupil. Moreover, a single attack of angle closure after pharmacologic dilation rarely causes any permanent damage to the eye and serves as an inadvertent provocative test to identify patients with narrow angles who would benefit from prophylactic laser iridectomy.

Endophthalmitis This occurs from bacterial, viral, fungal, or parasitic infection of the internal structures of the eye. It is usually acquired by hematogenous seeding from a remote site. Chronically ill, diabetic, or immunosuppressed patients, especially those with a history of indwelling intravenous catheters or positive blood cultures, are at greatest risk for endogenous endophthalmitis. Although most patients have ocular pain and injection, visual loss is sometimes the only symptom. Septic emboli, from a diseased heart valve or a dental abscess, that lodge in the retinal circulation can give rise to endophthalmitis. White-centered retinal hemorrhages (Roth's spots) are considered pathognomonic for subacute bacterial endocarditis, but they also appear in leukemia, diabetes, and many other conditions. Endophthalmitis also occurs as a complication of ocular surgery, occasionally months or even years after the operation. An occult penetrating foreign body or unrecognized trauma to the globe should be considered in any patient with unexplained intraocular infection or inflammation.

TRANSIENT OR SUDDEN VISUAL LOSS

Amaurosis Fugax This term refers to a transient ischemic attack of the retina (Chap. 349). Because neural tissue has a high rate of metabolism, interruption of blood flow to the retina for more than a few seconds results in *transient monocular blindness*, a term used interchangeably with amaurosis fugax. Patients describe a rapid fading of vision like a curtain descending, sometimes affecting only a portion of the visual field. Amaurosis fugax usually occurs from an embolus that becomes stuck within a retinal arteriole (Fig. 25-4). If the embolus breaks up or passes, flow is restored and vision returns quickly to normal without permanent damage. With prolonged interruption of blood flow, the inner retina suffers infarction. Ophthalmoscopy reveals zones of whitened, edematous retina following the distribution of branch retinal arterioles. Complete occlusion of the central retinal artery produces arrest of blood flow and a milky retina with a cherry-red fovea (Fig. 25-5). Emboli are composed of either cholesterol (Hollenhorst plaque), calcium, or platelet-fibrin debris. The most common source is an atherosclerotic plaque in the carotid artery or aorta, although emboli can also arise from the heart, especially in patients with diseased valves, atrial fibrillation, or wall motion abnormalities.

In rare instances, amaurosis fugax occurs from low central retinal artery perfusion pressure in a patient with a critical stenosis of the ipsilateral carotid artery and poor collateral flow via the circle of Willis. In this situation, amaurosis fugax develops when there is a dip in systemic blood pressure or a slight worsening of the carotid stenosis. Sometimes there is contralateral motor or sensory loss, indicating concomitant hemispheric cerebral ischemia.

Retinal arterial occlusion also occurs rarely in association with retinal migraine, lupus erythematosus, anticardiolipin antibodies (Fig. 25-5), anticoagulant deficiency states (protein S, protein C, and antithrombin III deficiency), pregnancy, intravenous drug abuse, blood dyscrasias, dysproteinemias, and temporal arteritis.

FIGURE 25-3 Retinal vasculitis, uveitis, and hemorrhage in a 32-year-old woman with Crohn's disease. Note that the veins are frosted with a white exudate. Visual acuity improved from 20/400 to 20/20 following treatment with intravenous methylprednisolone.

FIGURE 25-4 Hollenhorst plaque lodged at the bifurcation of a retinal arteriole proves that a patient is shedding emboli from either the carotid artery, great vessels, or heart.

FIGURE 25-5 Central retinal artery occlusion combined with ischemic optic neuropathy in a 19-year-old woman with an elevated titer of anticardiolipin antibodies. Note the orange dot (rather than cherry red) corresponding to the fovea and the spared patch of retina just temporal to the optic disc.

Marked *systemic hypertension* causes sclerosis of retinal arterioles, splinter hemorrhages, focal infarcts of the nerve fiber layer (cotton-wool spots), and leakage of lipid and fluid (hard exudate) into the macula (Fig. 25-6). In hypertensive crisis, sudden visual loss can result from vasospasm of retinal arterioles and retinal ischemia. In addition, acute hypertension may produce visual loss from ischemic swelling of the optic disc. Patients with acute hypertensive retinopathy should be treated by lowering the blood pressure. However, the blood pressure should not be reduced precipitously, because there is a danger of optic disc infarction from sudden hypoperfusion.

Impending *branch* or *central retinal vein occlusion* can produce prolonged visual obscurations that resemble those described by patients with amaurosis fugax. The veins appear engorged and phlebitic, with numerous retinal hemorrhages (Fig. 25-7). In some patients, venous blood flow recovers spontaneously, while others evolve a frank obstruction with extensive retinal bleeding ("blood and thunder" appearance), infarction, and visual loss. Venous occlusion of the retina is often idiopathic, but hypertension, diabetes, and glaucoma are prominent risk factors. Polycythemia, thrombocythemia, or other factors leading to an underlying hypercoagulable state should be corrected; aspirin treatment may be beneficial.

Anterior Ischemic Optic Neuropathy (AION)   This is caused by insufficient blood flow through the posterior ciliary arteries supplying the optic disc. It produces painless, monocular visual loss that is usually sudden, although some patients have progressive worsening. The optic disc appears swollen and surrounded by nerve fiber layer splinter hemor-

FIGURE 25-7 Central retinal vein occlusion can produce massive retinal hemorrhage ("blood and thunder"), ischemia, and vision loss.

rhages (Fig. 25-8). AION is divided into two forms: arteritic and nonarteritic. The nonarteritic form of AION is most common. No specific cause can be identified, although diabetes and hypertension are frequent risk factors. No treatment is available. About 5% of patients, especially those over age 60, develop the arteritic form of AION in conjunction with giant cell (temporal) arteritis (Chap. 306). It is urgent to recognize arteritic AION so that high doses of glucocorticoids can be instituted immediately to prevent blindness in the second eye. Symptoms of polymyalgia rheumatica may be present; the sedimentation rate and C-reactive protein level are usually elevated. In a patient with visual loss from suspected arteritic AION, temporal artery biopsy is mandatory to confirm the diagnosis. Glucocorticoids should be started immediately, without waiting for the biopsy to be completed. The diagnosis of arteritic AION is difficult to sustain in the face of a negative temporal artery biopsy, but such cases do occur.

Posterior Ischemic Optic Neuropathy   This is an infrequent cause of acute visual loss, induced by the combination of severe anemia and hypotension. Cases have been reported after major blood loss during surgery, exsanguinating trauma, gastrointestinal bleeding, and renal dialysis. The fundus usually appears normal, although optic disc swelling develops if the process extends far enough anteriorly. Vision can be salvaged in some patients by prompt blood transfusion and reversal of hypotension.

Optic Neuritis   This is a common inflammatory disease of the optic nerve. In the Optic Neuritis Treatment Trial (ONTT), the mean age of patients was 32 years, 77% were female, 92% had ocular pain (especially with eye movements), and 35% had optic disc swelling. In most patients, the demyelinating event was retrobulbar and the ocular fun-

FIGURE 25-6 Hypertensive retinopathy with scattered flame (splinter) hemorrhages and cotton wool spots (nerve fiber layer infarcts) in a patient with headache and a blood pressure of 234/120.

FIGURE 25-8 Anterior ischemic optic neuropathy from temporal arteritis in a 78-year-old woman with pallid disc swelling, hemorrhage, visual loss, myalgia, and an erythrocyte sedimentation rate of 86 mm/h.

disc pallor slowly developed over subsequent months.

Virtually all patients experience a gradual recovery of vision after a single episode of optic neuritis, even without treatment. This rule is so reliable that failure of vision to improve after a first attack of optic neuritis casts doubt upon the original diagnosis. Treatment with high-dose intravenous methylprednisolone (250 mg every 6 h for 3 days) followed by oral prednisone (1 mg/kg per day for 11 days) makes no difference in final acuity (measured 6 months after the attack), but the recovery of visual function occurs more rapidly.

For some patients, optic neuritis remains an isolated event. However, the ONTT showed that the 5-year cumulative probability of developing clinically definite multiple sclerosis following optic neuritis is 30%. In patients with two or more demyelinating plaques on brain magnetic resonance (MR) imaging, treatment with interferon beta-1a can retard the development of more lesions. In summary, an MR scan is recommended in every patient with a first attack of optic neuritis. When visual loss is severe (worse than 20/100), treatment with intravenous followed by oral glucocorticoids hastens recovery. If multiple lesions are present on the MR scan, treatment with interferon beta-1a should be broached with the patient.

Leber's Hereditary Optic Neuropathy This is a disease of young men, characterized by gradual painless, severe, central visual loss in one eye, followed weeks or months later by the same process in the other eye. Acutely, the optic disc appears mildly plethoric with surface capillary telangiectases, but no vascular leakage on fluorescein angiography. Eventually optic atrophy ensues. Leber's optic neuropathy is caused by a point mutation at codon 11778 in the mitochondrial gene encoding nicotinamide adenine dinucleotide dehydrogenase (NADH) subunit 4. Additional mutations responsible for the disease have been identified, most in mitochondrial genes encoding proteins involved in electron transport. Mitochondrial mutations causing Leber's neuropathy are inherited from the mother by all her children, but usually only sons develop symptoms. There is no treatment.

Toxic Optic Neuropathy This can result in acute visual loss with bilateral optic disc swelling and central or cecocentral scotomas. Such cases have been reported to result from exposure to ethambutol, methyl alcohol (moonshine), ethylene glycol (antifreeze), or carbon monoxide. In toxic optic neuropathy, visual loss can also develop gradually and produce optic atrophy (Fig. 25-10) without a phase of acute optic disc edema. Many agents have been implicated as a cause of toxic optic neuropathy, but the evidence supporting the association for many is weak. The following is a partial list of potential offending drugs or toxins: disulfiram, ethchlorvynol, chloramphenicol, amiodarone, monoclonal anti-CD3 antibody, ciprofloxacin, digitalis, streptomycin, lead, arsenic, thallium, D-penicillamine, isoniazid, emetine, and sulfonamides. Deficiency states, induced either by starvation, malabsorption, or alcoholism, can lead to insidious visual loss. Thiamine, vitamin B_{12}, and folate levels should be checked in any patient with unexplained, bilateral central scotomas and optic pallor.

Papilledema This connotes bilateral optic disc swelling from raised intracranial pressure (Fig. 25-11). Headache is a frequent, but not in-

FIGURE 25-10 Optic atrophy is not a specific diagnosis, but refers to the combination of optic disc pallor, arteriolar narrowing, and nerve fiber layer destruction produced by a host of eye diseases, especially optic neuropathies.

variable, accompaniment. All other forms of optic disc swelling, e.g., from optic neuritis or ischemic optic neuropathy, should be called "optic disc edema." This convention is arbitrary but serves to avoid confusion. Often it is difficult to differentiate papilledema from other forms of optic disc edema by fundus examination alone. Transient visual obscurations are a classic symptom of papilledema. They can occur in only one eye or simultaneously in both eyes. They usually last seconds but can persist longer if the papilledema is fulminant. Obscurations follow abrupt shifts in posture or happen spontaneously. When obscurations are prolonged or spontaneous, the papilledema is more threatening. Visual acuity is not affected by papilledema unless the papilledema is severe, long-standing, or accompanied by macular edema and hemorrhage. Visual field testing shows enlarged blind spots and peripheral constriction (Fig. 25-2F). With unremitting papilledema, peripheral visual field loss progresses in an insidious fashion while the optic nerve develops atrophy. In this setting, reduction of optic disc swelling is an ominous sign of a dying nerve rather than an encouraging indication of resolving papilledema.

Evaluation of papilledema requires neuroimaging to exclude an intracranial lesion. MR angiography is appropriate in selected cases to search for a dural venous sinus occlusion or an arteriovenous shunt. If neuroradiologic studies are negative, the subarachnoid opening pressure should be measured by lumbar puncture. An elevated pressure, with normal cerebrospinal fluid, points by exclusion to the diagnosis of *pseudotumor cerebri* (idiopathic intracranial hypertension). The majority of patients are young, female, and obese. Treatment with a carbonic anhydrase inhibitor such as acetazolamide lowers intracranial pressure by reducing the production of cerebrospinal fluid. Weight reduction is vital but often unsuccessful. If acetazolamide and weight loss fail, and visual field loss is progressive, a shunt should be performed without delay to prevent blindness. Occasionally, emergency

FIGURE 25-9 Retrobulbar optic neuritis is characterized by a normal fundus examination initially, hence the rubric, "the doctor sees nothing, and the patient sees nothing." Optic atrophy develops after severe or repeated attacks.

FIGURE 25-11 Papilledema means optic disc edema from raised intracranial pressure. This obese young women with pseudotumor cerebri was misdiagnosed as a migraineur until fundus examination was performed, showing optic disc elevation, hemorrhages, and cotton wool spots.

surgery is required for sudden blindness caused by fulminant papilledema.

Optic Disc Drusen   These are refractile deposits within the substance of the optic nerve head (Fig. 25-12). They are unrelated to drusen of the retina, which occur in age-related macular degeneration. Optic disc drusen are most common in people of northern European descent. Their diagnosis is obvious when they are visible as glittering particles upon the surface of the optic disc. However, in many patients they are hidden beneath the surface, producing pseudo-papilledema. It is important to recognize optic disc drusen to avoid an unneccessary evaluation for papilledema. Ultrasound or computed tomography (CT) scanning is sensitive for detection of buried optic disc drusen because they contain calcium. In most patients, optic disc drusen are an incidental, innocuous finding, but they can produce visual obscurations. On perimetry they give rise to enlarged blind spots and arcuate scotomas from damage to the optic disc. With increasing age, drusen tend to become more exposed on the disc surface as optic atrophy develops. Hemorrhage, choroidal neovascular membrane, and AION are more likely to occur in patients with optic disc drusen. No treatment is available.

Vitreous Degeneration   This occurs in all individuals with advancing age, leading to visual symptoms. Opacities develop in the vitreous, casting annoying shadows upon the retina. As the eye moves, these distracting "floaters" move synchronously, with a slight lag caused by inertia of the vitreous gel. Vitreous traction upon the retina causes mechanical stimulation, resulting in perception of flashing lights. This photopsia is brief and confined to one eye, in contrast to the bilateral, prolonged scintillations of cortical migraine. Contraction of the vitreous can result in sudden separation from the retina, heralded by an alarming shower of floaters and photopsia. This process, known as *vitreous detachment*, is a frequent involutional event in the elderly. It is not harmful unless it damages the retina. A careful examination of the dilated fundus is important in any patient complaining of floaters or photopsia to search for peripheral tears or holes. If such a lesion is found, laser application or cryotherapy can forestall a retinal detachment. Occasionally a tear ruptures a retinal blood vessel, causing vitreous hemorrhage and sudden loss of vision. On attempted ophthalmoscopy the fundus is hidden by a dark red haze of blood. Ultrasound is required to examine the interior of the eye for a retinal tear or detachment. If the hemorrhage does not resolve spontaneously, the vitreous can be removed surgically. Vitreous hemorrhage also occurs from the fragile neovascular vessels that proliferate on the surface of the retina in diabetes, sickle cell anemia, and other ischemic ocular diseases.

Retinal Detachment   This produces symptoms of floaters, flashing lights, and a scotoma in the peripheral visual field corresponding to the detachment (Fig. 25-13). If the detachment includes the fovea, there is an afferent pupil defect and the visual acuity is reduced. In most eyes, retinal detachment starts with a hole, flap, or tear in the peripheral retina (rhegmatogenous retinal detachment). Patients with peripheral retinal thinning (lattice degeneration) are particularly vulnerable to this process. Once a break has developed in the retina, liquified vitreous is free to enter the subretinal space, separating the retina from the pigment epithelium. The combination of vitreous traction upon the retinal surface and passage of fluid behind the retina leads inexorably to detachment. Patients with a history of myopia, trauma, or prior cataract extraction are at greatest risk for retinal detachment. The diagnosis is confirmed by ophthalmoscopic examination of the dilated eye.

Classic Migraine (See also Chap. 14)   This usually occurs with a visual aura lasting about 20 min. In a typical attack, a small central disturbance in the field of vision marches toward the periphery, leaving a transient scotoma in its wake. The expanding border of migraine scotoma has a scintillating, dancing, or zig-zag edge, resembling the bastions of a fortified city, hence the term *fortification spectra*. Patients' descriptions of fortification spectra vary widely and can be confused with amaurosis fugax. Migraine patterns usually last longer and are perceived in both eyes, whereas amaurosis fugax is briefer and occurs in only one eye. Migraine phenomena also remain visible in the dark or with the eyes closed. Generally they are confined to either the right or left visual hemifield, but sometimes both fields are involved simultaneously. Patients often have a long history of stereotypic attacks. After the visual symptoms recede, headache develops in most patients.

Transient Ischemic Attacks   Vertebrobasilar insufficiency may result in acute homonymous visual symptoms. Many patients mistakenly describe symptoms in their left or right eye, when in fact they are occurring in the left or right hemifield of both eyes. Interruption of blood supply to the visual cortex causes a sudden fogging or graying of vision, occasionally with flashing lights or other positive phenomena that mimic migraine. Cortical ischemic attacks are briefer in duration than migraine, occur in older patients, and are not followed by headache. There may be associated signs of brainstem ischemia, such as diplopia, vertigo, numbness, weakness, or dysarthria.

Stroke   This occurs when interruption of blood supply from the posterior cerebral artery to the visual cortex is prolonged. The only finding on examination is a homonymous visual field defect that stops abruptly at the vertical meridian. Occipital lobe stroke is usually due to thrombotic occlusion of the vertebrobasilar system, embolus, or dissection. Lobar hemorrhage, tumor, abscess, and arteriovenous malformation are other common causes of hemianopic cortical visual loss.

Factitious (Functional, Nonorganic) Visual Loss   This is claimed by hysterics or malingerers. The latter comprise the vast majority, seeking sym-

FIGURE 25-12   Optic disc drusen are calcified deposits of unknown etiology within the optic disc. They are sometimes confused with papilledema.

FIGURE 25-13   Retinal detachment appears as an elevated sheet of retinal tissue with folds. In this patient the fovea was spared, so acuity was normal, but a superior detachment produced an inferior scotoma.

pathy, special treatment, or financial gain by feigning loss of sight. The diagnosis is suspected when the history is atypical, physical findings are lacking or contradictory, inconsistencies emerge on testing, and a secondary motive can be identified. In our litigious society, the fraudulent pursuit of recompense has spawned an epidemic of factitious visual loss.

CHRONIC VISUAL LOSS

Cataract This is a clouding of the lens sufficient to reduce vision. Most cataracts develop slowly as a result of aging, leading to gradual impairment of vision. The formation of cataract occurs more rapidly in patients with a history of ocular trauma, uveitis, or diabetes mellitus. Cataracts are acquired in a variety of genetic diseases, such as myotonic dystrophy, neurofibromatosis type 2, and galactosemia. Radiation therapy and glucocorticoid treatment can induce cataract as a side effect. The cataracts associated with radiation or glucocorticoids have a typical posterior subcapsular location. Cataract can be detected by noting an impaired red reflex when viewing light reflected from the fundus with an ophthalmoscope or by examining the dilated eye using the slit lamp.

The only treatment for cataract is surgical extraction of the opacified lens. Over a million cataract operations are performed each year in the United States. The operation is generally done under local anesthesia on an outpatient basis. A plastic or silicone intraocular lens is placed within the empty lens capsule in the posterior chamber, substituting for the natural lens and leading to rapid recovery of sight. More than 95% of patients who undergo cataract extraction can expect an improvement in vision. In many patients, the lens capsule remaining in the eye after cataract extraction eventually turns cloudy, causing a secondary loss of vision. A small opening is made in the lens capsule with a laser to restore clarity.

Glaucoma This is a slowly progressive, insidious optic neuropathy, usually associated with chronic elevation of intraocular pressure. In Americans of African descent it is the leading cause of blindness. The mechanism whereby raised intraocular pressure injures the optic nerve is not understood. Axons entering the inferotemporal and superotemporal aspects of the optic disc are damaged first, producing typical nerve fiber bundle or arcuate scotomas on perimetric testing. As fibers are destroyed, the neural rim of the optic disc shrinks and the physiologic cup within the optic disc enlarges (Fig. 25-14). This process is referred to as pathologic "cupping." The cup-to-disc diameter is expressed as a ratio, e.g., 0.2/1. The cup-to-disc ratio ranges widely in normal individuals, making it difficult to diagnose glaucoma reliably simply by observing an unusually large or deep optic cup. Careful documentation of serial examinations is helpful. In the patient with physiologic cupping, the large cup remains stable, whereas in the patient with glaucoma it expands relentlessly over the years. Detection of visual field loss by computerized perimetry also contributes to the diagnosis. Finally, most patients with glaucoma have raised intraocular pressure. However, many patients with typical glaucomatous cupping and visual field loss have intraocular pressures that apparently never exceed the normal limit of 20 mmHg (so-called low-tension glaucoma).

In acute angle-closure glaucoma, the eye is red and painful due to abrupt, severe elevation of intraocular pressure. Such cases account for only a handful of patients with glaucoma. Most patients with glaucoma have open, anterior chamber angles. The cause of raised intraocular pressure in open angle glaucoma is unknown but is associated with gene mutations in the heritable forms.

Glaucoma is usually painless (except in angle-closure glaucoma). Foveal acuity is spared until end-stage disease is reached. For these reasons, severe and irreversible damage can occur before either the patient or physician recognizes the diagnosis. Screening of patients for glaucoma by noting the cup-to-disc ratio on ophthalmoscopy and by measuring intraocular pressure is vital. Glaucoma is treated with topical adrenergic agonists, cholinergic agonists, beta blockers, and prostaglandin analogues. Occasionally, systemic absorption of beta blocker

FIGURE 25-14 Glaucoma results in "cupping" as the neural rim is destroyed and the central cup becomes enlarged and excavated. The cup-to-disc ratio is about 0.7/1.0 in this patient.

from eye drops can be sufficient to cause side effects of bradycardia, hypotension, heart block, bronchospasm, or depression. Topical or oral carbonic anhydrase inhibitors are used to lower intraocular pressure by reducing aqueous production. Laser treatment of the trabecular meshwork in the anterior chamber angle improves aqueous outflow from the eye. If medical or laser treatments fail to halt optic nerve damage from glaucoma, a filter must be constructed surgically (trabeculectomy) to release aqueous from the eye in a controlled fashion.

Macular Degeneration This is a major cause of gradual, painless, bilateral central visual loss in the elderly. The old term, "senile macular degeneration," misinterpreted by many patients as an unflattering reference, has been replaced with "age-related macular degeneration." It occurs in a nonexudative (dry) form and an exudative (wet) form. The nonexudative process begins with the accumulation of extracellular deposits, called drusen, underneath the retinal pigment epithelium. On ophthalmoscopy, they are pleomorphic but generally appear as small discrete yellow lesions clustered in the macula (Fig. 25-15). With time they become larger, more numerous, and confluent. The retinal pigment epithelium becomes focally detached and atrophic, causing visual loss by interfering with photoreceptor function. Treatment with vitamins C and E, beta carotene, and zinc may retard dry macular degeneration.

Exudative macular degeneration, which develops in only a minority of patients, occurs when neovascular vessels from the choroid grow through defects in Bruch's membrane into the potential space beneath the retinal pigment epithelium. Leakage from these vessels produces elevation of the retina and pigment epithelium, with distortion (metamorphopsia) and blurring of vision. Although onset of these symptoms is usually gradual, bleeding from subretinal choroidal neovascular membranes sometimes causes acute visual loss. The neovascular membranes can be difficult to see on fundus examination because they are beneath the retina. Fluorescein or indocyanine green angiography is extremely useful for their detection. In some patients, prompt laser ablation of choroidal neovascular membranes seen on fluorescein angiography can halt the exudative process. However, the neovascular membranes frequently recur, requiring constant vigilance and repeated photocoagulation.

FIGURE 25-15 Age-related macular degeneration begins with the accumulation of drusen within the macula. They appear as scattered yellow subretinal deposits.

Major or repeated hemorrhage under the retina from neovascular membranes results in fibrosis, development of a round (disciform) macular scar, and permanent loss of central vision. Surgical attempts to remove subretinal membranes in age-related macular degeneration have not improved vision in most patients. However, outcomes have been more encouraging for patients with choroidal neovascular membranes from ocular histoplasmosis syndrome.

Central Serous Chorioretinopathy This primarily affects males between the ages of 20 and 50. Leakage of serous fluid from the choroid causes small, localized detachment of the retinal pigment epithelium and the neurosensory retina. These detachments produce acute or chronic symptoms of metamorphopsia and blurred vision when the macula is involved. They are difficult to visualize with a direct ophthalmoscope because the detached retina is transparent and only slightly elevated. Diagnosis of central serous chorioretinopathy is made easily by fluorescein angiography, which shows dye streaming into the subretinal space. The cause of central serous chorioretinopathy is unknown. Symptoms may resolve spontaneously if the retina reattaches, but recurrent detachment is common. Laser photocoagulation has benefited some patients with this condition.

Diabetic Retinopathy A rare disease until 1921, when the discovery of insulin resulted in a dramatic improvement in life expectancy for patients with diabetes mellitus, it is now a leading cause of blindness in the United States. The retinopathy of diabetes takes years to develop but eventually appears in nearly all cases. Regular surveillance of the dilated fundus is crucial for any patient with diabetes. In advanced diabetic retinopathy, the proliferation of neovascular vessels leads to blindness from vitreous hemorrhage, retinal detachment, and glaucoma (see Fig. 323-9). These complications can be avoided in most patients by administration of panretinal laser photocoagulation at the appropriate point in the evolution of the disease. →*For further discussion of the manifestations and management of diabetic retinopathy, see Chap. 323.*

Retinitis Pigmentosa This is a general term for a disparate group of rod and cone dystrophies characterized by progressive night blindness, visual field constriction with a ring scotoma, loss of acuity, and an abnormal electroretinogram (ERG). It occurs sporadically or in an autosomal recessive, dominant, or X-linked pattern. Irregular black deposits of clumped pigment in the peripheral retina, called *bone spicules* because of their vague resemblance to the spicules of cancellous bone, give the disease its name (Fig. 25-16). The name is actually a misnomer because retinitis pigmentosa is not an inflammatory process. Most cases are due to a mutation in the gene for rhodopsin, the rod photopigment, or in the gene for peripherin, a glycoprotein located in photoreceptor outer segments. Vitamin A (15,000 IU/day) slightly retards the deterioration of the ERG in patients with retinitis pigmentosa but has no beneficial effect on visual acuity or fields. Some forms of retinitis pigmentosa occur in association with rare, hereditary systemic diseases (olivopontocerebellar degeneration, Bassen-Kornzweig disease, Kearns-Sayre syndrome, Refsum's disease). Chronic treatment with chloroquine, hydroxychloroquine, and phenothiazines (especially thioridazine) can produce visual loss from a toxic retinopathy that resembles retinitis pigmentosa.

Epiretinal Membrane This is a fibrocellular tissue that grows across the inner surface of the retina, causing metamorphopsia and reduced visual acuity from distortion of the macula. A crinkled, cellophane-like membrane is visible on the retinal examination. Epiretinal membrane is most common in patients over 50 years of age and is usually unilateral. Most cases are idiopathic, but some occur as a result of hypertensive retinopathy, diabetes, retinal detachment, or trauma. When visual acuity is reduced to the level of about 6/24 (20/80), vitrectomy and surgical peeling of the membrane to relieve macular puckering are recommended. Contraction of an epiretinal membrane sometimes gives rise to a *macular hole*. Most macular holes, however, are caused by

FIGURE 25-16 Retinitis pigmentosa with black clumps of pigment in the retinal periphery known as "bone spicules." There is also atrophy of the retinal pigment epithelium, making the vasculature of the choroid easily visible.

local vitreous traction within the fovea. Vitrectomy can improve acuity in selected cases.

Melanoma and Other Tumors Melanoma is the most common primary tumor of the eye (Fig. 25-17). It causes photopsia, an enlarging scotoma, and loss of vision. A small melanoma is often difficult to differentiate from a benign choroidal nevus. Serial examinations are required to document a malignant pattern of growth. Treatment of melanoma is controversial. Options include enucleation, local resection, and irradiation. *Metastatic tumors* to the eye outnumber primary tumors. Breast and lung carcinoma have a special propensity to spread to the choroid or iris. Leukemia and lymphoma also commonly invade ocular tissues. Sometimes their only sign on eye examination is cellular debris in the vitreous, which can masquerade as a chronic posterior uveitis. *Retrobulbar tumor* of the optic nerve (meningioma, glioma) or *chiasmal tumor* (pituitary adenoma, meningioma) produces gradual visual loss with few objective findings, except for optic disc pallor. Rarely, sudden expansion of a pituitary adenoma from infarction and bleeding (*pituitary apoplexy*) causes acute retrobulbar visual loss, with headache, nausea, and ocular motor nerve palsies. In any patient with visual field loss or optic atrophy, CT or MR scanning should be considered if the cause remains unknown after careful review of the history and thorough examination of the eye.

PROPTOSIS

When the globes appear asymmetric, the clinician must first decide which eye is abnormal. Is one eye recessed within the orbit (*enophthalmos*) or is the other eye protuberant (*exophthalmos*, or *proptosis*)? A small globe or a Horner's syndrome can give the appearance of enophthalmos. True enophthalmos occurs commonly after trauma, from atrophy of retrobulbar fat, or fracture of the orbital floor. The position of the eyes within the orbits is measured using a Hertel exophthalmometer, a hand-held instrument that records the position of the anterior corneal surface relative to the lateral orbital rim. If this instrument is not available, relative eye position can be judged by

FIGURE 25-17 Melanoma of the choroid, appearing as an elevated dark mass in the inferior temporal fundus, just encroaching upon the fovea.

bending the patient's head forward and looking down upon the orbits. A proptosis of only 2 mm in one eye is detectable from this perspective. The development of proptosis implies a space-occupying lesion in the orbit, and usually warrants CT or MR imaging.

Graves' Ophthalmopathy This is the leading cause of proptosis in adults (Chap. 320). The proptosis is often asymmetric and can even appear to be unilateral. Orbital inflammation and engorgement of the extraocular muscles, particularly the medial rectus and the inferior rectus, account for the protrusion of the globe. Corneal exposure, lid retraction, conjunctival injection, restriction of gaze, diplopia, and visual loss from optic nerve compression are cardinal symptoms. Graves' ophthalmopathy is treated with oral prednisone (60 mg/d) for 1 month, followed by a taper over several months, topical lubricants, eyelid surgery, eye muscle surgery, or orbital decompression. Radiation therapy is not effective.

Orbital Pseudotumor This is an idiopathic, inflammatory orbital syndrome, frequently confused with Graves' ophthalmopathy. Symptoms are pain, limited eye movements, proptosis, and congestion. Evaluation for sarcoidosis, Wegener's granulomatosis, and other types of orbital vasculitis or collagen-vascular disease is negative. Imaging often shows swollen eye muscles (orbital myositis) with enlarged tendons. By contrast, in Graves' ophthalmopathy the tendons of the eye muscles are usually spared. The Tolosa-Hunt syndrome may be regarded as an extension of orbital pseudotumor through the superior orbital fissure into the cavernous sinus. The diagnosis of orbital pseudotumor is difficult. Biopsy of the orbit frequently yields nonspecific evidence of fat infiltration by lymphocytes, plasma cells, and eosinophils. A dramatic response to a therapeutic trial of systemic glucocorticoids indirectly provides the best confirmation of the diagnosis.

Orbital Cellulitis This causes pain, lid erythema, proptosis, conjunctival chemosis, restricted motility, decreased acuity, afferent pupillary defect, fever, and leukocytosis. It often arises from the paranasal sinuses, especially by contiguous spread of infection from the ethmoid sinus through the lamina papyracea of the medial orbit. A history of recent upper respiratory tract infection, chronic sinusitis, thick mucous secretions, or dental disease is significant in any patient with suspected orbital cellulitis. Blood cultures should be obtained, but they are usually negative. Most patients respond to empirical therapy with broad-spectrum intravenous antibiotics. Occasionally, orbital cellulitis follows an overwhelming course, with massive proptosis, blindness, septic cavernous sinus thrombosis, and meningitis. To avert this disaster, orbital cellulitis should be managed aggressively in the early stages, with immediate antibiotic therapy and imaging of the orbits. Prompt surgical drainage of an orbital abscess or paranasal sinusitis is indicated if optic nerve function deteriorates despite antibiotics.

Tumors Tumors of the orbit cause painless, progressive proptosis. The most common primary tumors are hemangioma, lymphangioma, neurofibroma, dermoid cyst, adenoid cystic carcinoma, optic nerve glioma, optic nerve meningioma, and benign mixed tumor of the lacrimal gland. Metastatic tumor to the orbit occurs frequently in breast carcinoma, lung carcinoma, and lymphoma. Diagnosis by fine-needle aspiration followed by urgent radiation therapy can sometimes preserve vision.

Carotid Cavernous Fistulas With anterior drainage through the orbit these produce proptosis, diplopia, glaucoma, and corkscrew, arterialized conjunctival vessels. Direct fistulas usually result from trauma. They are easily diagnosed because of the prominent signs produced by high-flow, high-pressure shunting. Indirect fistulas, or dural arteriovenous malformations, are more likely to occur spontaneously, especially in older women. The signs are more subtle and the diagnosis is frequently missed. The combination of slight proptosis, diplopia, enlarged muscles, and an injected eye is often mistaken for thyroid ophthalmopathy. A bruit heard upon auscultation of the head, or reported by the patient, is a valuable diagnostic clue. Imaging shows an enlarged superior ophthalmic vein in the orbits. Carotid cavernous shunts can be eliminated by intravascular embolization.

PTOSIS

Blepharoptosis This is an abnormal drooping of the eyelid. Unilateral or bilateral ptosis can be congenital, from dysgenesis of the levator palpebrae superioris, or from abnormal insertion of its aponeurosis into the eyelid. Acquired ptosis can develop so gradually that the patient is unaware of the problem. Inspection of old photographs is helpful in dating the onset. A history of prior trauma, eye surgery, contact lens use, diplopia, systemic symptoms (e.g., dysphagia or peripheral muscle weakness), or a family history of ptosis should be sought. Fluctuating ptosis that worsens late in the day is typical of myasthenia gravis. Examination should focus upon evidence for proptosis, eyelid masses or deformities, inflammation, pupil inequality, or limitation of motility. The width of the palpebral fissures is measured in primary gaze to quantitate the degree of ptosis. The ptosis will be underestimated if the patient compensates by lifting the brow with the frontalis muscle.

Mechanical Ptosis This occurs in many elderly patients from stretching and redundancy of eyelid skin and subcutaneous fat (dermatochalasis). The extra weight of these sagging tissues causes the lid to droop. Enlargement or deformation of the eyelid from infection, tumor, trauma, or inflammation also results in ptosis on a purely mechanical basis.

Aponeurotic Ptosis This is an acquired dehiscence or stretching of the aponeurotic tendon, which connects the levator muscle to the tarsal plate of the eyelid. It occurs commonly in older patients, presumably from loss of connective tissue elasticity. Aponeurotic ptosis is also a frequent sequela of eyelid swelling from infection or blunt trauma to the orbit, cataract surgery, or hard contact lens usage.

Myogenic Ptosis The causes of *myogenic ptosis* include myasthenia gravis (Chap. 366) and a number of rare myopathies that manifest with ptosis. The term *chronic progressive external ophthalmoplegia* refers to a spectrum of systemic diseases caused by mutations of mitochondrial DNA. As the name implies, the most prominent findings are symmetric, slowly progressive ptosis and limitation of eye movements. In general, diplopia is a late symptom because all eye movements are reduced equally. In the *Kearns-Sayre* variant, retinal pigmentary changes and abnormalities of cardiac conduction develop. Peripheral muscle biopsy shows characteristic "ragged-red fibers." *Oculopharyngeal dystrophy* is a distinct autosomal dominant disease with onset in middle age, characterized by ptosis, limited eye movements, and trouble swallowing. *Myotonic dystrophy*, another autosomal dominant disorder, causes ptosis, ophthalmoparesis, cataract, and pigmentary retinopathy. Patients have muscle wasting, myotonia, frontal balding, and cardiac abnormalities.

Neurogenic Ptosis This results from a lesion affecting the innervation to either of the two muscles that open the eyelid: Müller's muscle or the levator palpebrae superioris. Examination of the pupil helps to distinguish between these two possibilities. In Horner's syndrome, the eye with ptosis has a smaller pupil and the eye movements are full. In an oculomotor nerve palsy, the eye with the ptosis has a larger, or a normal, pupil. If the pupil is normal but there is limitation of adduction, elevation, and depression, a pupil-sparing oculomotor nerve palsy is likely (see next section). Rarely, a lesion affecting the small, central subnucleus of the oculomotor complex will cause bilateral ptosis with normal eye movements and pupils.

DOUBLE VISION

The first point to clarify is whether diplopia persists in either eye after covering the fellow eye. If it does, the diagnosis is monocular diplopia. The cause is usually intrinsic to the eye and therefore has no dire implications for the patient. Corneal aberrations (e.g., keratoconus, pterygium), uncorrected refractive error, cataract, or foveal traction may give rise to monocular diplopia. Occasionally it is a symptom of malingering or psychiatric disease. Diplopia alleviated by covering one eye is binocular diplopia and is caused by disruption of ocular alignment. Inquiry should be made into the nature of the double vision (purely side-by-side versus partial vertical displacement of images), mode of onset, duration, intermittency, diurnal variation, and associated neurologic or systemic symptoms. If the patient has diplopia while being examined, motility testing should reveal a deficiency corresponding to the patient's symptoms. However, subtle limitation of ocular excursions is often difficult to detect. For example, a patient with a slight left abducens nerve paresis may appear to have full eye movements, despite a complaint of horizontal diplopia upon looking to the left. In this situation, the cover test provides a more sensitive method for demonstrating the ocular misalignment. It should be conducted in primary gaze, and then with the head turned and tilted in each direction. In the above example, a cover test with the head turned to the right will maximize the fixation shift evoked by the cover test.

Occasionally, a cover test performed in an asymptomatic patient during a routine examination will reveal an ocular deviation. If the eye movements are full and the ocular misalignment is equal in all directions of gaze (concomitant deviation), the diagnosis is strabismus. In this condition, which affects about 1% of the population, fusion is disrupted in infancy or early childhood. To avoid diplopia, vision is suppressed from the nonfixating eye. In some children, this leads to impaired vision (amblyopia, or "lazy" eye) in the deviated eye.

Binocular diplopia occurs from a wide range of processes: infectious, neoplastic, metabolic, degenerative, inflammatory, and vascular. One must decide if the diplopia is neurogenic in origin or due to restriction of globe rotation by local disease in the orbit. Orbital pseudotumor, myositis, infection, tumor, thyroid disease, and muscle entrapment (e.g., from a blowout fracture) cause restrictive diplopia. The diagnosis of restriction is usually made by recognizing other associated signs and symptoms of local orbital disease in conjunction with imaging.

Myasthenia Gravis (See also Chap. 366)   This is a major cause of diplopia. The diplopia is often intermittent, variable, and not confined to any single ocular motor nerve distribution. The pupils are always normal. Fluctuating ptosis may be present. Many patients have a purely ocular form of the disease, with no evidence of systemic muscular weakness. The diagnosis can be confirmed by an intravenous edrophonium injection or by an assay for antiacetylcholine receptor antibodies. Negative results from these tests do not exclude the diagnosis. *Botulism* from food or wound poisoning can mimic ocular myasthenia.

After restrictive orbital disease and myasthenia gravis are excluded, a lesion of a cranial nerve supplying innervation to the extraocular muscles is the most likely cause of binocular diplopia.

Oculomotor Nerve   The third cranial nerve innervates the medial, inferior, and superior recti; inferior oblique; levator palpebrae superioris; and the iris sphincter. Total palsy of the oculomotor nerve causes ptosis, a dilated pupil, and leaves the eye "down and out" because of the unopposed action of the lateral rectus and superior oblique. This combination of findings is obvious. More challenging is the diagnosis of an early or partial oculomotor nerve palsy. In this setting, any combination of ptosis, pupil dilation, and weakness of the eye muscles supplied by the oculomotor nerve may be encountered. Frequent serial examinations during the evolving phase of the palsy and a high index of suspicion help ensure that the diagnosis is not missed. The advent of an oculomotor nerve palsy with any degree of pupil involvement in an otherwise healthy patient, especially when accompanied by pain, raises the specter of a circle of Willis aneurysm. If an MR imaging shows no compressive lesion, an arteriogram must be considered to rule out an aneurysm of either the posterior communicating artery or the basilar artery. If the pupil is entirely normal, with all other components of an oculomotor palsy present, aneurysm is so rare that an angiogram is seldom indicated.

A lesion of the oculomotor nucleus in the rostral midbrain produces signs that differ from those caused by a lesion of the nerve itself. There is bilateral ptosis because the levator muscle is innervated by a single central subnucleus. There is also weakness of the contralateral superior rectus, because it is supplied by the oculomotor nucleus on the other side. Occasionally both superior recti are weak. Isolated nuclear oculomotor palsy is rare. Usually neurologic examination reveals additional signs to suggest brainstem damage from infarction, hemorrhage, tumor, or infection.

Injury to structures surrounding fascicles of the oculomotor nerve descending through the midbrain has given rise to a number of classic eponymic designations. In *Nothnagel's syndrome*, injury to the superior cerebellar peduncle causes ipsilateral oculomotor palsy and contralateral cerebellar ataxia. In *Benedikt's syndrome*, injury to the red nucleus results in ipsilateral oculomotor palsy and contralateral tremor, chorea, and athetosis. *Claude's syndrome* incorporates features of both the aforementioned syndromes, by injury to both the red nucleus and the superior cerebellar peduncle. Finally, in *Weber's syndrome*, injury to the cerebral peduncle causes ipsilateral oculomotor palsy with contralateral hemiparesis.

In the subarachnoid space the oculomotor nerve is vulnerable to aneurysm, meningitis, tumor, infarction, and compression. In cerebral herniation the nerve becomes trapped between the edge of the tentorium and the uncus of the temporal lobe. Oculomotor palsy can also occur from midbrain torsion and hemorrhages during herniation. In the cavernous sinus, oculomotor palsy arises from carotid aneurysm, carotid cavernous fistula, cavernous sinus thrombosis, tumor (pituitary adenoma, meningioma, metastasis), herpes zoster infection, and the Tolosa-Hunt syndrome.

The etiology of an isolated, pupil-sparing oculomotor palsy often remains an enigma, even after neuroimaging and extensive laboratory testing. Most cases are thought to result from microvascular infarction of the nerve, somewhere along its course from the brainstem to the orbit. Usually the patient complains of pain. Diabetes, hypertension, and vascular disease are major risk factors. Spontaneous recovery over a period of months is the rule. If this fails to occur, or if new findings develop, the diagnosis of microvascular oculomotor nerve palsy should be reconsidered. Aberrant regeneration is common when the oculomotor nerve is injured by trauma or compression (tumor, aneurysm). Miswiring of sprouting fibers to the levator muscle and the rectus muscles results in elevation of the eyelid upon downgaze or adduction. The pupil also constricts upon attempted adduction, elevation, or depression of the globe. Aberrant regeneration is not seen after oculomotor palsy from microvascular infarct and hence vitiates that diagnosis.

Trochlear Nerve   The fourth cranial nerve originates in the midbrain, just caudal to the oculomotor nerve complex. Fibers exit the brainstem dorsally and cross to innervate the contralateral superior oblique. The principal actions of this muscle are to depress and to intort the globe. A palsy therefore results in hypertropia and excyclotorsion. The cyclotorsion is seldom noticed by patients. Instead, they complain of vertical diplopia, especially upon reading or looking down. The vertical diplopia is also exacerbated by tilting the head toward the side with the muscle palsy, and alleviated by tilting it away. This "head tilt test" is a cardinal diagnostic feature.

Isolated trochlear nerve palsy occurs from all the causes listed above for the oculomotor nerve, except aneurysm. The trochlear nerve is particularly apt to suffer injury after closed head trauma. The free edge of the tentorium is thought to impinge upon the nerve during a concussive blow. Most isolated trochlear nerve palsies are idiopathic and hence diagnosed by exclusion as "microvascular." Spontaneous improvement occurs over a period of months in most patients. A base-down prism (conveniently applied to the patient's glasses as a stick-on Fresnel lens) may serve as a temporary measure to alleviate diplopia. If the palsy does not resolve, the eyes can be realigned by weakening the inferior oblique muscle.

Abducens Nerve   The sixth cranial nerve innervates the lateral rectus muscle. A palsy produces horizontal diplopia, worse on gaze to the side of the lesion. A nuclear lesion has different consequences, because the abducens nucleus contains interneurons that project via the medial longitudinal fasciculus to the medial rectus subnucleus of the contralateral oculomotor complex. Therefore, an abducens nuclear lesion produces a complete lateral gaze palsy, from weakness of both the ipsilateral lateral rectus and the contralateral medial rectus. *Foville's syndrome* following dorsal pontine injury includes lateral gaze palsy, ipsilateral facial palsy, and contralateral hemiparesis incurred by damage to descending corticospinal fibers. *Millard-Gubler syndrome* from ventral pontine injury is similar, except for the eye findings. There is lateral rectus weakness only, instead of gaze palsy, because the abducens fascicle is injured rather than the nucleus. Infarct, tumor, hemorrhage, vascular malformation, and multiple sclerosis are the most common etiologies of brainstem abducens palsy.

After leaving the ventral pons, the abducens nerve runs forward along the clivus to pierce the dura at the petrous apex, where it enters the cavernous sinus. Along its subarachnoid course it is susceptible to meningitis, tumor (meningioma, chordoma, carcinomatous meningitis), subarachnoid hemorrhage, trauma, and compression by aneurysm or dolichoectatic vessels. At the petrous apex, mastoiditis can produce deafness, pain, and ipsilateral abducens palsy (*Gradenigo's syndrome*). In the cavernous sinus, the nerve can be affected by carotid aneurysm, carotid cavernous fistula, tumor (pituitary adenoma, meningioma, nasopharyngeal carcinoma), herpes infection, and Tolosa-Hunt syndrome.

Unilateral or bilateral abducens palsy is a classic sign of raised intracranial pressure. The diagnosis can be confirmed if papilledema is observed on fundus examination. The mechanism is still debated but is probably related to rostral-caudal displacement of the brainstem. The same phenomenon accounts for abducens palsy from low intracranial pressure (e.g., after lumbar puncture, spinal anesthesia, or spontaneous dural cerebrospinal fluid leak).

Treatment of abducens palsy is aimed at prompt correction of the underlying cause. However, the cause remains obscure in many instances, despite diligent evaluation. As mentioned above for isolated trochlear or oculomotor palsy, most cases are assumed to represent microvascular infarcts because they often occur in the setting of diabetes or other vascular risk factors. Some cases may develop as a postinfectious mononeuritis (e.g., following a viral flu). Patching one eye or applying a temporary prism will provide relief of diplopia until the palsy resolves. If recovery is incomplete, eye muscle surgery can nearly always realign the eyes, at least in primary position. A patient with an abducens palsy that fails to improve should be reevaluated for an occult etiology (e.g., chordoma, carcinomatous meningitis, carotid cavernous fistula, myasthenia gravis).

Multiple Ocular Motor Nerve Palsies These should not be attributed to spontaneous microvascular events affecting more than one cranial nerve at a time. This remarkable coincidence does occur, especially in diabetic patients, but the diagnosis is made only in retrospect after exhausting all other diagnostic alternatives. Neuroimaging should focus on the cavernous sinus, superior orbital fissure, and orbital apex, where all three ocular motor nerves are in close proximity. In the diabetic or compromised host, fungal infection (*Aspergillus*, Mucorales, *Cryptococcus*) is a frequent cause of multiple nerve palsies. In the patient with systemic malignancy, carcinomatous meningitis is a likely diagnosis. Cytologic examination may be negative despite repeated sampling of the cerebrospinal fluid. The cancer-associated Lambert-Eaton myasthenic syndrome can also produce ophthalmoplegia. Giant cell (temporal) arteritis occasionally manifests as diplopia from ischemic palsies of extraocular muscles. Fisher syndrome, an ocular variant of Guillain-Barré, can produce ophthalmoplegia with areflexia and ataxia. Often the ataxia is mild, and the areflexia is overlooked because the physician's attention is focused upon the eyes. Antiganglioside antibodies (GQ1b) can be detected in about 50% of cases.

Supranuclear Disorders of Gaze These are often mistaken for multiple ocular motor nerve palsies. For example, Wernicke's encephalopathy can produce nystagmus and a partial deficit of horizontal and vertical gaze that mimics a combined abducens and oculomotor nerve palsy. The disorder occurs in malnourished or alcoholic patients and can be reversed by thiamine. Infarct, hemorrhage, tumor, multiple sclerosis, encephalitis, vasculitis, and Whipple's disease are other important causes of supranuclear gaze palsy. Disorders of vertical gaze, especially downwards saccades, are an early feature of progressive supranuclear palsy. Smooth pursuit is affected later in the course of the disease. Parkinson's disease, Huntington's chorea, and olivopontocerebellar degeneration can also affect vertical gaze.

The *frontal eye field* of the cerebral cortex is involved in generation of saccades to the contralateral side. After hemispheric stroke, the eyes usually deviate towards the lesioned side, because of the unopposed action of the frontal eye field in the normal hemisphere. With time, this deficit resolves. Seizures generally have the opposite effect: the eyes deviate conjugately away from the irritative focus. *Parietal lesions* disrupt smooth pursuit of targets moving toward the side of the lesion. Bilateral parietal lesions produce *Balint's syndrome*, characterized by impaired eye-hand coordination (optic ataxia), difficulty initiating voluntary eye movements (ocular apraxia), and visuospatial disorientation (simultanagnosia).

Horizontal Gaze Descending cortical inputs mediating horizontal gaze ultimately converge at the level of the pons. Neurons in the paramedian pontine reticular formation are responsible for controlling conjugate gaze toward the same side. They project directly to the ipsilateral abducens nucleus. A lesion of either the paramedian pontine reticular formation or the abducens nucleus causes an ipsilateral conjugate gaze palsy. Lesions at either locus produce nearly identical clinical syndromes, with the following exception: vestibular stimulation (oculocephalic maneuver or caloric irrigation) will succeed in driving the eyes conjugately to the side in a patient with a lesion of the paramedian pontine reticular formation, but not in a patient with a lesion of the abducens nucleus.

INTERNUCLEAR OPHTHALMOPLEGIA This results from damage to the medial longitudinal fasciculus ascending from the abducens nucleus in the pons to the oculomotor nucleus in the midbrain (hence, "internuclear"). Damage to fibers carrying the conjugate signal from abducens interneurons to the contralateral medial rectus motoneurons results in a failure of adduction on attempted lateral gaze. For example, a patient with a left internuclear ophthalmoplegia will have slowed or absent adducting movements of the left eye. A patient with bilateral injury to the medial longitudinal fasciculus will have bilateral internuclear ophthalmoplegia. Multiple sclerosis is the most common cause, although tumor, stroke, trauma, or any brainstem process may be responsible. *One-and-a-half syndrome* is due to a combined lesion of the medial longitudinal fasciculus and the abducens nucleus on the same side. The patient's only horizontal eye movement is abduction of the eye on the other side.

Vertical Gaze This is controlled at the level of the midbrain. The neuronal circuits affected in disorders of vertical gaze are not fully elucidated, but lesions of the rostral interstitial nucleus of the medial longitudinal fasciculus and the interstitial nucleus of Cajal cause supranuclear paresis of upgaze, downgaze, or all vertical eye movements. Distal basilar artery ischemia is the most common etiology. *Skew deviation* refers to a vertical misalignment of the eyes, usually constant in all positions of gaze. The finding has poor localizing value because skew deviation has been reported after lesions in widespread regions of the brainstem and cerebellum.

PARINAUD'S SYNDROME Also known as dorsal midbrain syndrome, this is a distinct supranuclear vertical gaze disorder from damage to the posterior commissure. It is a classic sign of hydrocephalus from aqueductal stenosis. Pineal region tumors, cysticercosis, and stroke also cause Parinaud's syndrome. Features include loss of upgaze (and sometimes downgaze), convergence-retraction nystagmus on attempted upgaze, downwards ocular deviation ("setting sun" sign), lid retraction (Collier's sign), skew deviation, pseudoabducens palsy, and light-near dissociation of the pupils.

Nystagmus   This is a rhythmical oscillation of the eyes, occurring physiologically from vestibular and optokinetic stimulation or pathologically in a wide variety of diseases (Chap. 20). Abnormalities of the eyes or optic nerves, present at birth or acquired in childhood, can produce a complex, searching nystagmus with irregular pendular (sinusoidal) and jerk features. This nystagmus is commonly referred to as *congenital sensory nystagmus*. It is a poor term, because even in children with congenital lesions, the nystagmus does not appear until several months of age. *Congenital motor nystagmus*, which looks similar to congenital sensory nystagmus, develops in the absence of any abnormality of the sensory visual system. Visual acuity is also reduced in congenital motor nystagmus, probably by the nystagmus itself, but seldom below a level of 20/200.

JERK NYSTAGMUS   This is characterized by a slow drift off the target, followed by a fast corrective saccade. By convention, the nystagmus is named after the quick phase. Jerk nystagmus can be downbeat, upbeat, horizontal (left or right), and torsional. The pattern of nystagmus may vary with gaze position. Some patients will be oblivious to their nystagmus. Others will complain of blurred vision, or a subjective, to-and-fro movement of the environment (oscillopsia) corresponding to their nystagmus. Fine nystagmus may be difficult to see upon gross examination of the eyes. Observation of nystagmoid movements of the optic disc on ophthalmoscopy is a sensitive way to detect subtle nystagmus.

GAZE-EVOKED NYSTAGMUS   This is the most common form of jerk nystagmus. When the eyes are held eccentrically in the orbits, they have a natural tendency to drift back to primary position. The subject compensates by making a corrective saccade to maintain the deviated eye position. Many normal patients have mild gaze-evoked nystagmus. Exaggerated gaze-evoked nystagmus can be induced by drugs (seda-

tives, anticonvulsants, alcohol); muscle paresis; myasthenia gravis; demyelinating disease; and cerebellopontine angle, brainstem, and cerebellar lesions.

VESTIBULAR NYSTAGMUS   *Vestibular nystagmus* results from dysfunction of the labyrinth (Ménière's disease), vestibular nerve, or vestibular nucleus in the brainstem. Peripheral vestibular nystagmus often occurs in discrete attacks, with symptoms of nausea and vertigo. There may be associated tinnitus and hearing loss. Sudden shifts in head position may provoke or exacerbate symptoms.

DOWNBEAT NYSTAGMUS   *Downbeat nystagmus* occurs from lesions near the craniocervical junction (Chiari malformation, basilar invagination). It has also been reported in brainstem or cerebellar stroke, lithium or anticonvulsant intoxication, alcoholism, and multiple sclerosis. *Upbeat nystagmus* is associated with damage to the pontine tegmentum, from stroke, demyelination, or tumor.

Opsoclonus   This rare, dramatic disorder of eye movements consists of bursts of consecutive saccades (saccadomania). When the saccades are confined to the horizontal plane, the term *ocular flutter* is preferred. It can occur from viral encephalitis, trauma, or a paraneoplastic effect of neuroblastoma, breast carcinoma, and other malignancies. It has also been reported as a benign, transient phenomenon in otherwise healthy patients.

FURTHER READING

AREDS REPORT NO. 8: A randomized, placebo-controlled, clinical trial of high-dose supplementation with vitamins C and E, beta carotene, and zinc for age-related macular degeneration and vision loss. Arch Ophthalmol 119: 1417, 2001

BECK RW et al: Interferon beta-1a for early multiple sclerosis: CHAMPS trial subgroup analyses. Ann Neurol 51:481, 2002

BENAVENTE O et al: Prognosis after transient monocular blindness associated with carotid artery stenosis. N Engl J Med 345:1084, 2001

NEGI A, VERNON SA: An overview of the eye in diabetes. JR Soc Med 96: 266, 2003

SOLOMON R, DONNENFELD ED: Recent advances and future frontiers in treating age-related cataracts. JAMA 290:248, 2003

26   DISORDERS OF SMELL, TASTE, AND HEARING
Anil K. Lalwani, James B. Snow, Jr.

SMELL

The sense of smell determines the flavor and palatability of food and drink. It serves, along with the trigeminal system, as a monitor of inhaled chemicals, including dangerous substances such as natural gas, smoke, and air pollutants. Olfactory dysfunction affects ~1% of people under age 60 and more than half of the population beyond this age.

DEFINITIONS   *Smell* is the perception of odor by the nose. *Taste* is the perception of salty, sweet, sour, or bitter by the tongue. Related sensations during eating such as somatic sensations of coolness, warmth, and irritation are mediated through the trigeminal, glossopharyngeal, and vagal afferents in the nose, oral cavity, tongue, pharynx, and larynx. *Flavor* is the complex interaction of taste, smell, and somatic sensation. Terms relating to disorders of smell include *anosmia*, an absence of the ability to smell; *hyposmia*, a decreased ability to smell; *hyperosmia*, an increased sensitivity to an odorant; *dysosmia*, distortion in the perception of an odor; *phantosmia*, perception of an odorant where none is present; and *agnosia*, inability to classify, contrast, or identify odor sensations verbally, even though the ability to distinguish between odorants or to recognize them may be normal. An odor stimulus is referred to as an *odorant*. Each category of smell dysfunction can be further subclassified as total (applying to all odorants) or partial (dysfunction of only select odorants).

PHYSIOLOGY OF SMELL   The *olfactory neuroepithelium* is located in the superior part of the nasal cavities. It contains an orderly arrangement

of bipolar olfactory receptor cells, microvillar cells, sustentacular cells, and basal cells. The dendritic process of the bipolar cell has a bulb-shaped vesicle that projects into the mucous layer and bears six to eight cilia containing the odorant. Each bipolar cell contains 56 cm^2 (9 in.^{2}) of surface area to receive olfactory stimuli.

Microvillar cells are located adjacent to the receptor cells on the surface of the neuroepithelium. Sustentacular cells, unlike their counterparts in the respiratory epithelium, are not specialized to secrete mucus. Although they form a tight barrier separating neurons from the outside environment, their complete function is unknown. The basal cells are progenitors of other cell types in the olfactory neuroepithelium, including the bipolar receptor cells. There is a regular turnover of bipolar receptor cells, which function as the primary sensory neurons. In addition, with injury to the cell body or its axon, the receptor cell is replaced by a differentiated basal cell, which reestablishes a central neural connection. These primary sensory neurons are unique among sensory systems in that they are regularly replaced and regenerate after injury.

The unmyelinated axons of receptor cells form the fila of the olfactory nerve, pass through the cribriform plate, and terminate within spherical masses of neuropil, termed *glomeruli*, in the olfactory bulb. The glomeruli are the focus of a high degree of convergence of information, since many more fibers enter than leave them. The main second-order neurons are mitral cells. The primary dendrite of each mitral cell extends into a single glomerulus. Axons of the mitral cells project along with the axons of adjacent tufted cells to the limbic system, including the anterior olfactory nucleus and the amygdala. Cognitive awareness of smell requires stimulation of the prepiriform cortex or amygdaloid nuclei.

A secondary site of olfactory chemosensation is located in the epithelium of the vomeronasal organ, a tubular structure that opens on the ventral aspect of the nasal septum. Sensory neurons located in the vomeronasal organ detect pheromones, nonvolatile chemical signals that in lower mammals trigger innate and stereotyped reproductive and social behaviors, as well as neuroendocrine changes. Neurons from the organ project to the accessory olfactory bulbs and not the main olfactory bulb, as does the olfactory neuroepithelium. Whether humans use the vomeronasal organ to detect and respond to chemical signals from others remains controversial. Development of the olfactory and vomeronasal system appears to be required for normal sexual maturation.

The sensation of smell begins with introduction of an odorant to the cilia of the bipolar neuron. Most odorants are hydrophobic; as they move from the air phase of the nasal cavity to the aqueous phase of the olfactory mucous, they are transported toward the cilia by small water-soluble proteins called *odorant-binding proteins* and reversibly bind to receptors on the cilia surface. Binding leads to conformational changes in the receptor protein, activation of G protein–coupled second messengers, and generation of action potentials in the primary neurons. Intensity appears to be coded by the amount of firing in the afferent neurons.

Olfactory receptor proteins belong to the large family of G protein–coupled receptors that also includes rhodopsins; α- and β-adrenergic receptors; muscarinic acetylcholine receptors; and neurotransmitter receptors for dopamine, serotonin, and substance P. In humans, there are 300 to 1000 olfactory receptor genes belonging to 20 different families located in clusters at more than 25 different chromosomal locations. Each olfactory neuron seems to express only one or, at most, a few receptor genes, thus providing the molecular basis of odor discrimination. Bipolar cells that express similar receptors appear to be scattered across discrete spatial zones. These similar cells converge on a select few glomeruli in the olfactory bulb. The result is a potential spatial map of how we receive odor stimului, much like the tonotopic organization of how we perceive sound.

DISORDERS OF THE SENSE OF SMELL These are caused by conditions that interfere with the access of the odorant to the olfactory neuroepithelium (transport loss), injure the receptor region (sensory loss), or damage central olfactory pathways (neural loss). Currently no clinical tests exist to differentiate these different types of olfactory losses. Fortunately, the history of the disease provides important clues to the cause. The leading causes of olfactory disorders are summarized in Table 26-1; the most common etiologies are head trauma in children and young adults, and viral infections in older adults.

Head trauma is followed by unilateral or bilateral impairment of smell in up to 15% of cases; anosmia is more common than hyposmia. Olfactory dysfunction is more common when trauma is associated with loss of consciousness, moderately severe head injury (grades II to V), and skull fracture. Frontal injuries and fractures disrupt the cribriform plate and olfactory axons that perforate it. Sometimes there is an associated cerebrospinal fluid (CSF) rhinorrhea resulting from a tearing of the dura overlying the cribriform plate and paranasal sinuses. Anosmia may also follow blows to the occiput. Once traumatic anosmia develops, it is usually permanent; only 10% of patients ever improve or recover. Perversion of the sense of smell may occur as a transient phase in the recovery process.

Viral infections destroy the olfactory neuroepithelium, which is replaced by respiratory epithelium. Parainfluenza virus type 3 appears to be especially detrimental to human olfaction. HIV infection is associated with subjective distortion of taste and smell, which may become more severe as the disease progresses. The loss of taste and smell may play an important role in the development and progression of HIV-associated wasting. Congenital anosmias are rare but important. Kallmann syndrome is an X-linked disorder characterized by congen-

TABLE 26-1 *Causes of Olfactory Dysfunction*

Transport Losses	Neural Losses
Allergic rhinitis	AIDS
Bacterial rhinitis and sinusitis	Alcoholism
Congenital abnormalities	Alzheimer's disease
Nasal neoplasms	Cigarette smoke
Nasal polyps	Depression
Nasal septal deviation	Diabetes mellitus
Nasal surgery	Drugs/Toxins
Viral infections	Huntington's chorea
Sensory Losses	Hypothyroidism
Drugs	Kallmann syndrome
Neoplasms	Malnutrition
Radiation therapy	Neoplasms
Toxin exposure	Neurosurgery
Viral infections	Parkinson's disease
	Trauma
	Vitamin B_{12} deficiency
	Zinc deficiency

ital anosmia and hypogonadotropic hypogonadism resulting from a failure of migration from the olfactory placode of olfactory receptor neurons and neurons synthesizing gonadotropin-releasing hormone (Chap. 325). Anosmia can also occur in albinos. The receptor cells are present but are hypoplastic, lack cilia, and do not project above the surrounding supporting cells.

Meningiomas of the inferior frontal region are the most frequent neoplastic cause of anosmia; loss of smell may be the only neurologic abnormality. Rarely, anosmia can occur with gliomas of the frontal lobe. Occasionally, pituitary adenomas, craniopharyngiomas, suprasellar meningiomas, and aneurysms of the anterior part of the circle of Willis extend forward and damage olfactory structures. These tumors and hamartomas may also induce seizures with olfactory hallucinations, indicating involvement of the uncus of the temporal lobe.

Dysosmia, subjective distortions of olfactory perception, may occur with intranasal diseases that partially impair smell or may represent a phase in the recovery from a neurogenic anosmia. Most dysosmic disorders consist of disagreeable odors, sometimes accompanied by distortions of taste. Dysosmia also can occur with depression.

APPROACH TO THE PATIENT

Unilateral anosmia is rarely a complaint and is only recognized by separate testing of smell in each nasal cavity. Bilateral anosmia, on the other hand, brings patients to medical attention. Anosmic patients usually complain of a loss of the sense of taste even though their taste thresholds may be within normal limits. In actuality, they are complaining of a loss of flavor detection, which is mainly an olfactory function. The physical examination should include a thorough inspection of the ears, upper respiratory tract, and head and neck. A neurologic examination emphasizing the cranial nerves and cerebellar and sensorimotor function is essential. Any signs of depression should be noted.

Sensory olfactory function can be assessed by any of several methods. The Odor Stix test uses a commercially available odor-producing magic marker–like pen held approximately 8 to 15 cm (3 to 6 in.) from the patient's nose. The 30-cm alcohol test uses a freshly opened isopropyl alcohol packet held approximately 30 cm (12 in.) from the patient's nose. There is a commercially available scratch-and-sniff card containing three odors available for testing olfaction grossly. A superior test is the University of Pennsylvania Smell Identification Test (UPSIT). This consists of a 40-item, forced choice, microencapsulated odor, scratch-and-sniff paradigm. For example, one of the items reads, "This odor smells most like (a) chocolate, (b) banana, (c) onion, or (d) fruit punch." The test is highly reliable, is sensitive to age and sex differences, and provides an accurate quantitative determination of the olfactory deficit. The average score for total anosmics is slightly higher than that expected on the basis of chance because of the inclusion of some odorants that act by trigeminal stimulation.

Following assessment of sensory olfactory function, the detection threshold for the odorant phenyl ethyl alcohol should be established using a graduated stimulus. Sensitivity for each side of the nose is determined with a detection threshold for phenyl ethyl methyl ethyl carbinol. Nasal resistance can also be measured with anterior rhinomanometry for each side of the nose.

Computed tomography (CT) or magnetic resonance imaging (MRI) of the head is required to rule out paranasal sinusitis; neoplasms of the anterior cranial fossa, nasal cavity, or paranasal sinuses; or unsuspected fractures of the anterior cranial fossa. Bone abnormalities are best seen with CT. MRI is useful in evaluating olfactory bulbs, ventricles, and other soft tissue of the brain. Coronal CT is optimal for assessing cribriform plate, anterior cranial fossa, and sinus anatomy.

Techniques have been developed to biopsy the olfactory neuroepithelium, but in view of the widespread degeneration of the olfactory neuroepithelium and intercalation of respiratory epithelium in the olfactory area of adults with no apparent olfactory dysfunction, biopsy material must be interpreted cautiously.

℞ TREATMENT

Therapy for patients with transport olfactory losses due to allergic rhinitis, bacterial rhinitis and sinusitis, polyps, neoplasms, and structural abnormalities of the nasal cavities can be undertaken with a high likelihood for improvement. Allergy management; antibiotic therapy; topical and systemic glucocorticoid therapy; and surgery for nasal polyps, deviation of the nasal septum, and chronic hyperplastic sinusitis are frequently effective in restoring the sense of smell.

There is no proven treatment for sensorineural olfactory losses. Fortunately, spontaneous recovery often occurs. Zinc and vitamin therapy (especially with vitamin A) are advocated by some. Profound zinc deficiency can produce loss and distortion of the sense of smell but is not a clinically important problem except in very limited geographic areas (Chap. 61). The epithelial degeneration associated with vitamin A deficiency can cause anosmia, but in western societies the prevalence of vitamin A deficiency is low. Exposure to cigarette smoke and other airborne toxic chemicals can cause metaplasia of the olfactory epithelium. Spontaneous recovery can occur if the insult is discontinued. Counseling of patients is therefore helpful in these cases.

More than half of people over age 60 suffer from olfactory dysfunction. No effective treatment exists for presbyosmia, but patients are often reassured to learn that this problem is common in their age group. In addition, early recognition and counseling can help patients to compensate for the loss of smell. The incidence of natural gas–related accidents is disproportionately high in the elderly, perhaps due in part to the gradual loss of smell. Mercaptan, the pungent odor in natural gas, is an olfactory stimulant and does not activate taste receptors. Many elderly with olfactory dysfunction experience a decrease in flavor sensation and find it necessary to hyperflavor food, usually by increasing the amount of salt in their diet.

TASTE

Compared with disorders of smell, gustatory disorders are uncommon. Loss of olfactory sensitivity is often accompanied by complaints of loss of the sense of taste, usually with normal detection thresholds for taste.

DEFINITIONS Disturbances of the sense of taste may be categorized as *total ageusia*, total absence of gustatory function or inability to detect the qualities of sweet, salt, bitter, or sour; *partial ageusia*, ability to detect some of but not all the qualitative gustatory sensations; *specific ageusia*, inability to detect the taste quality of certain substances; *total hypogeusia*, decreased sensitivity to all tastants; *partial hypogeusia*, decreased sensitivity to some tastants; and *dysgeusia* or *phantogeusia*, distortion in the perception of a tastant, i.e., the perception of the wrong quality when a tastant is presented or the perception of a taste when there has been no tastant ingested. Confusions between sour and bitter, and less commonly between salty and bitter, may represent semantic misunderstandings or have true pathophysiologic bases. It may be possible to differentiate between the loss of flavor recognition in patients with olfactory losses who complain of a loss of taste as well as smell by asking if they are able to taste sweetness in sodas, saltiness in potato chips, etc.

PHYSIOLOGY OF TASTE The taste receptor cells are located in the taste buds, spherical groups of cells arranged in a pattern resembling the segments of a citrus fruit. At the surface, the taste bud has a pore into which microvilli of the receptor cells project. Unlike the olfactory system, the receptor cell is not the primary neuron. Instead, gustatory afferent nerve fibers contact individual taste receptor cells. There are at least five receptor populations. Taste buds are located in the papillae along the lateral margin and dorsum of the tongue; at the junction of the dorsum and the base of the tongue; and in the palate, epiglottis, larynx, and esophagus.

The sense of taste is mediated through the facial, glossopharyngeal, and vagal nerves. The chorda tympani branch of the facial nerve subserves taste from the anterior two-thirds of the tongue. The posterior third of the tongue is supplied by the lingual branch of the glossopharyngeal nerve. Afferents from the palate travel with the greater superficial petrosal nerve to the geniculate ganglion and then via the facial nerve to the brainstem. The internal branch of the superior laryngeal nerve of the vagus nerve contains the taste afferents from the larynx, including the epiglottis and esophagus.

The central connections of the nerves terminate in the brainstem in the nucleus of the tractus solitarius. The central pathway from the nucleus of the tractus solitarius projects to the ipsilateral parabrachial nuclei of the pons. Two divergent pathways project from the parabrachial nuclei. One ascends to the gustatory relay in the dorsal thalamus, synapses, and continues to the cortex of the insula. There is also evidence for a direct pathway from the parabrachial nuclei to the cortex. (Olfaction and gustation appear to be unique among sensory systems in that at least some fibers bypass the thalamus.) The other pathway from the parabrachial nuclei goes to the ventral forebrain, including the lateral hypothalamus, substantia innominata, central nucleus of the amygdala, and the stria terminalis.

Tastants gain access to the receptor cells through the taste pore. Four classes of taste are recognized: sweet, salt, sour, and bitter. Individual gustatory afferent fibers almost always respond to a number of different chemicals. Response patterns of gustatory afferent axons can be grouped into classes based on the stimulus chemical that produces the largest response. For example, for sucrose-best response neurons, the second-best stimulus is almost always sodium chloride. The fact that individual gustatory afferent fibers respond to a large number of different chemicals led to the *across-fiber-pattern* theory of gustatory coding, while the best-stimulus analysis led to the concept of *labeled* afferents. It appears that labeled fibers are important for establishing gross quality, but the across-fiber pattern within a best-stimulus category, and perhaps among categories, is needed for discriminating chemicals within qualities. For example, sweetness may be carried by sucrose-best neurons, but the differentiation of sucrose and fructose may require a comparison of the relative activity among sucrose-best, salt-best, and quinine-best neurons. As with olfaction and other sensory systems, intensity appears to be encoded by the quantity of neural activity.

DISORDERS OF THE SENSE OF TASTE Disorders of the sense of taste are caused by conditions that interfere with the access of the tastant to the receptor cells in the taste bud (transport loss), injure receptor cells (sensory loss), or damage gustatory afferent nerves and central gustatory pathways (neural loss) (Table 26-2). *Transport gustatory losses* result from xerostomia due to many causes, including Sjögren's syndrome, radiation therapy, heavy-metal intoxication, and bacterial col-

TABLE 26-2 Causes of Gustatory Dysfunction

Transport Gustatory Losses	Neural Gustatory Losses
Drugs	Diabetes mellitus
Heavy-metal intoxication	Hypothyroidism
Radiation therapy	Oral neoplasms
Sjögren's syndrome	Oral surgery
Xerostomia	Radiation therapy
Sensory Gustatory Losses	Renal disease
Aging	Stroke and other CNS disorders
Candidiasis	Trauma
Drugs (antithyroid and	Upper respiratory tract infections
antineoplastic)	
Endocrine disorders	
Oral neoplasms	
Pemphigus	
Radiation therapy	
Viral infections (especially with	
herpes viruses)	

more receptor fields as a result of a peripheral or central lesion. The history of the disease and localization studies provide important clues to the reason for taste disturbance. For example, absence of taste on the anterior two-thirds of the tongue associated with a facial paralysis indicates that the lesion is proximal to the juncture of the chorda tympani branch with the facial nerve in the mastoid.

℞ TREATMENT

Treatment of gustatory disorders is limited. No effective therapies exist for the sensorineural disorders of taste. Altered taste due to surgical stretch injury of chorda tympani nerve usually improves within 3 to 4 months, while dysfunction is usually permanent with transection of the nerve. Taste dysfunction following trauma may resolve spontaneously without intervention and is more likely to do so than post-traumatic smell dysfunction. Idiopathic alterations of taste sensitivity usually remain stable or worsen; zinc and vitamin therapy are of unproven value. Directed therapy to address factors that affect taste perception can be of value. Xerostomia can be treated with artificial saliva, providing some benefits to patients with a disturbed salivary milieu. Oral pilocarpine may be beneficial for a variety of forms of xerostomia. Appropriate treatment of bacterial and fungal infections of the oral cavity can be of great help in improving taste function. Taste disturbance related to drugs can often be resolved by changing the prescribed medication.

HEARING

Hearing loss is one of the most common sensory disorders in humans and can present at any age. Nearly 10% of the adult population has some hearing loss, and one-third of individuals over the age of 65 have a hearing loss of sufficient magnitude to require a hearing aid.

PHYSIOLOGY OF HEARING (Fig. 26-1)   The function of the external and middle ear is to amplify sound to facilitate mechanotransduction by hair cells in the inner ear. Sound waves enter the external auditory canal and set the tympanic membrane in motion, which in turn moves the malleus, incus, and stapes of the middle ear. Movement of the footplate of the stapes causes pressure changes in the fluid-filled inner ear eliciting a traveling wave in the basilar membrane of the cochlea. The tympanic membrane and the ossicular chain in the middle ear serve as an impedence-matching mechanism, improving the efficiency of energy transfer from air to the fluid-filled inner ear.

Stereocilia of the hair cells of the organ of Corti, which rests on the basilar membrane, are in contact with the tectorial membrane and are deformed by the traveling wave. A point of maximal displacement of the basilar membrane is determined by the frequency of the stimulating tone. High-frequency tones cause maximal displacement of the basilar membrane near the base of the cochlea. As the frequency of the stimulating tone decreases, the point of maximal displacement moves toward the apex of the cochlea.

The inner and outer hair cells of the organ of Corti have different innervation patterns, but both are mechanoreceptors. The afferent innervation relates principally to the inner hair cells, and the efferent innervation relates principally to outer hair cells. The motility of the outer hair cells alters the micromechanics of the inner hair cells creating a cochlear amplifier, which explains the exquisite sensitivity and frequency selectivity of the cochlea.

The current concept of cochlear transduction is that displacement of the tips of the stereocilia allows potassium to flow into the cell, resulting in its depolarization. The potassium influx opens calcium channels near the base of the cell, stimulating transmitter release. The neurotransmitter at the hair cell and cochlear nerve dendrite interface is thought to be glutamate. Each of the cochlear nerve neurons can be activated at a frequency and intensity specific for that cell. This specificity is maintained at each point of the central auditory pathway: dorsal and ventral cochlear nuclei, trapezoid body, superior olivary

onization of the taste pore. *Sensory gustatory losses* are caused by inflammatory and degenerative diseases in the oral cavity; a vast number of drugs, particularly those that interfere with cell turnover such as antithyroid and antineoplastic agents; radiation therapy to the oral cavity and pharynx; viral infections; endocrine disorders; neoplasms; and aging. *Neural gustatory losses* occur with neoplasms, trauma, and surgical procedures in which the gustatory afferents are injured. Taste buds degenerate when their gustatory afferents are transected but remain when their somatosensory afferents are severed. Patients with renal disease have increased thresholds for sweet and sour tastes, which resolves with dialysis.

A side effect of medication is the single most common cause of taste dysfunction in clinical practice. Xerostomia, regardless of the etiology, can be associated with taste dysfunction. It is associated with poor oral clearance and poor dental hygeine, and can adversely affect the oral mucosa, all leading to dysgeusia. However, severe salivary gland failure does not necessarily lead to taste complaints. Xerostomia, the use of antibiotics or glucocorticoids, or immunodeficiency can lead to overgrowth of *Candida*; overgrowth alone, without thrush or overt signs of infection, can be associated with bad taste or hypogeusia. When taste dysfunction occurs in a patient at risk for fungal overgrowth, a trial of nystatin or other antifungal medication is warranted.

Upper respiratory infections and head trauma can lead to both smell and taste dysfunction; taste is more likely to improve than smell. The mechanism of taste disturbance in these situations is not well understood. Trauma to the chorda tympani branch of the facial nerve during middle ear surgery or third molar extractions is relatively common and can cause dysgeusia. Bilateral chorda tympani injuries are usually associated with hypogeusia, whereas unilateral lesions produce only limited symptoms.

Finally, aging itself may be associated with reduced taste sensitivity. The taste dysfunction may be limited to a single compound and may be mild.

APPROACH TO THE PATIENT

Patients who complain of loss of taste should be evaluated for both gustatory and olfactory function. Clinical assessment of taste is not as well developed or standardized as that of smell. The first step is to perform suprathreshold whole-mouth taste testing for quality, intensity, and pleasantness perception of four taste qualities: sweet, salty, sour, and bitter. Most commonly used reagents for taste testing are sucrose, citric acid or hydrochloric acid, caffeine or quinine (sulfate or hydrochloride), and sodium chloride. The taste stimuli should be freshly prepared. For quantification, detection thresholds are obtained by applying graduated dilutions to the tongue quadrants or by whole mouth sips. Electric taste testing (*electrogustometry*) is used clinically to identify taste deficits in specific quadrants of the tongue. Regional gustatory testing may also be performed to assess for the possibility of loss localized to one or

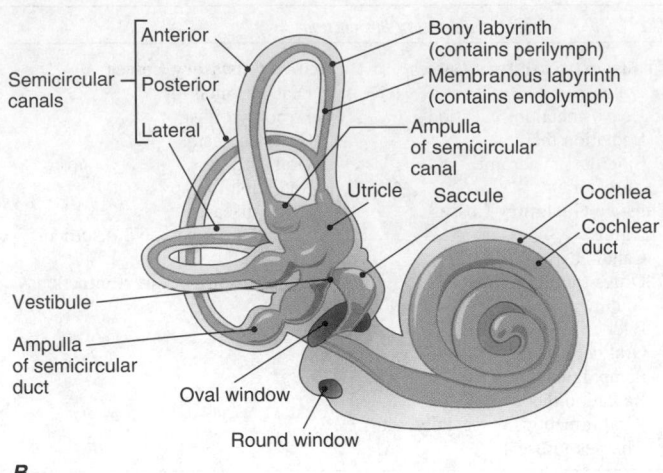

FIGURE 26-1 *A.* Drawing of modified coronal section through external ear and temporal bone, with structures of the middle and inner ear demonstrated.

B. High-resolution view of inner ear.

complex, lateral lemniscus, inferior colliculus, medial geniculate body, and auditory cortex. At low frequencies, individual auditory nerve fibers can respond more or less synchronously with the stimulating tone. At higher frequencies, phase-locking occurs so that neurons alternate in response to particular phases of the cycle of the sound wave. Intensity is encoded by the amount of neural activity in individual neurons, the number of neurons that are active, and the specific neurons that are activated.

GENETIC CAUSES OF HEARING LOSS More than half of childhood hearing impairment is thought to be hereditary; hereditary hearing impairment (HHI) can also manifest later in life. HHI may be classified as either nonsyndromic, when hearing loss is the only clinical abnormality, or syndromic, when hearing loss is associated with anomalies in other organ systems. Nearly two-thirds of HHIs are nonsyndromic, and the remaining one-third are syndromic. Between 70 and 80% of nonsyndromic HHI is inherited in an autosomal recessive manner; another 15 to 20% is autosomal dominant. Less than 5% is X-linked or maternally inherited via the mitochondria.

Over 60 loci harboring genes for nonsyndromic HHI have been mapped, with equal numbers of dominant and recessive modes of inheritance; numerous genes have now been cloned (Table 26-3). The hearing genes fall into the categories of structural proteins (MYO7A, MYO15, TECTA, DIAPH1), transcription factors (POU3F4, POU4F3), ion channels (KCNQ4, PDS), and gap junction proteins (Cx26, Cx30, Cx31). Several of these genes, including connexin 26 (Cx26), TECTA, and MYO7A, cause both autosomal dominant and recessive forms of nonsyndromic HHI. In general, the hearing loss associated with dominant genes has its onset in adolescence or adulthood and varies in severity, whereas the hearing loss associated with recessive inheritance is congenital and profound. Connexin 26 is particularly important because it is associated with nearly 20% of cases of childhood deafness; in heterozygotes the onset of hearing loss may be in adolescence or adulthood. Two frame-shift mutations, 30delG and 167delT, account for >50% of the cases, making population screening feasible. The 167delT mutation is highly prevalent in Ashkenazi Jews; it is predicted that 1 in 1765 individuals in this population will be homozygous and affected. The hearing loss can also vary among the members of the same family, suggesting that other genes or factors likely influence the auditory phenotype.

The contribution of genetics to presbycusis (see below) is also becoming better understood. In addition to connexin 26, several other nonsyndromic genes are associated with hear-

TABLE 26-3 *Nonsyndromic Genes and Loci*

Locus	Gene	Function	Inheritance
DFNB1	GBJ2 (Cx26)	Forms gap junctions, or plasma membrane channels, with connexins	AR
DFNB2	MYO7A	Moves different macromolecular structures relative to actin filaments	AR
DFNB3	MYO15	Organizes actin in hair cells	AR
DFNB4	PDS	Encodes highly hydrophobic proteins containing the sulphate transporter signature	AR
DFNB9	OTOF	Involved in trafficking of membrane vesicles	AR
DFNB21	TECTA	Includes an amino-terminal hydrophobic signal sequence for translocation across the membrane and a carboxy-terminal hydrophobic region characteristic of precursors of glycosylphosphatidylinositol-linked membrane-bound proteins	AR
DFNA1	DIAPH1	Involved in cytokinesis and establishment of cell polarity	AD
DFNA2	GJB3 (Cx31)	Forms gap junction protein	AD
	KCNQ4	Forms potassium channel	
DFNA3	GJB2 (Cx26)	Forms gap junctions, or plasma membrane channels, with connexins	AD
	GBJ6 (Cx30)		
DFNA5	DFNA5	Unknown; related to a gene that is upregulated in estrogen receptor–negative breast carcinomas	AD
DFNA8/12	TECTA	Includes an amino-terminal hydrophobic signal sequence for translocation across the membrane and a carboxy-terminal hydrophobic region characteristic of precursors of glycosylphosphatidylinositol-linked membrane-bound proteins	AD
DFNA9	COCH	Involved in hemostasis, complement system, immune system, and extracellular matrix assembly	AD
DFNA11	MYO7A	Moves different macromolecular structures relative to actin filaments	AD
DFNA15	POU4F3	Serves as a critical developmental regulator for the determination of cellular phenotypes	AD
DFN3	POU3F4	Serves as a critical developmental regulator for the determination of cellular phenotypes	X-linked

Note: AD, autosomal dominant; AR, autosomal recessive.

ing loss that progresses with age. Sensitivity to aminoglycoside ototoxicity can be maternally transmitted through a mitochondrial mutation. Susceptibility to noise-induced hearing loss may also be genetically determined.

There are over 200 syndromic forms of hearing loss. These include Usher syndrome (retinitis pigmentosa and hearing loss), Waardenburg syndrome (pigmentary abnormality and hearing loss), Pendred syndrome (thyroid organification defect and hearing loss), Alport syndrome (renal disease and hearing loss), Jervell and Lange-Nielsen syndrome (prolonged QT interval and hearing loss), neurofibromatosis type 2 (bilateral acoustic schwannoma), and mitochondrial disorders [mitochondrial encephalopathy, lactic acidosis, and stroke-like episodes (MELAS); myoclonic epilepsy and ragged red fibers (MERRF); progressive external ophthalmoplegia (PEO)].

DISORDERS OF THE SENSE OF HEARING   Hearing loss can result from disorders of the auricle, external auditory canal, middle ear, inner ear, or central auditory pathways (Fig. 26-2). *In general, lesions in the auricle, external auditory canal, or middle ear cause conductive hearing losses, whereas lesions in the inner ear or eighth nerve cause sensorineural hearing losses.*

Conductive Hearing Loss   This results from obstruction of the external auditory canal by cerumen, debris, and foreign bodies; swelling of the lining of the canal; atresia or neoplasms of the canal; perforations of the tympanic membrane; disruption of the ossicular chain, as occurs with necrosis of the long process of the incus in trauma or infection; otosclerosis; or fluid, scarring, or neoplasms in the middle ear.

Cholesteatoma, stratified squamous epithelium in the middle ear or mastoid, occurs frequently in adults. This is a benign, slowly growing lesion that destroys bone and normal ear tissue. Theories of pathogen

esis include traumatic implantation and invasion, immigration and invasion through a perforation, and metaplasia following chronic infection and irritation. On examination, there is often a perforation of the tympanic membrane filled with cheesy white squamous debris. A chronically draining ear that fails to respond to appropriate antibiotic therapy should raise suspicion of a cholesteatoma. Conductive hearing loss secondary to ossicular erosion is common. Surgery is required to remove this destructive process.

Conductive hearing loss with a normal ear canal and intact tympanic membrane suggests ossicular pathology. Fixation of the stapes from *otosclerosis* is a common cause of low-frequency conductive hearing loss. It occurs equally in men and women and has a simple autosomal dominant inheritance with incomplete penetrance. Hearing impairment usually presents between the late teens to the forties. In women, the hearing loss is often first noticeable during pregnancy, as the otosclerotic process is accelerated during pregnancy. A hearing aid or a simple outpatient surgical procedure (stapedectomy) can provide adequate auditory rehabilitation. Extension of otosclerosis beyond the stapes footplate to involve the cochlea (cochlear otosclerosis) can lead to mixed or sensorineural hearing loss. Fluoride therapy to prevent hearing loss associated with cochlear otosclerosis is of uncertain value.

Eustachian tube dysfunction is extremely common in adults and may predispose to acute otitis media (AOM) or serous otitis media (SOM). Trauma, AOM, or chronic otitis media are the usual factors responsible for tympanic membrane perforation. While small perforations often heal spontaneously, larger defects usually require surgical intervention. Tympanoplasty is highly effective (>90%) in the repair of tympanic membrane perforations. Otoscopy is usually sufficient to

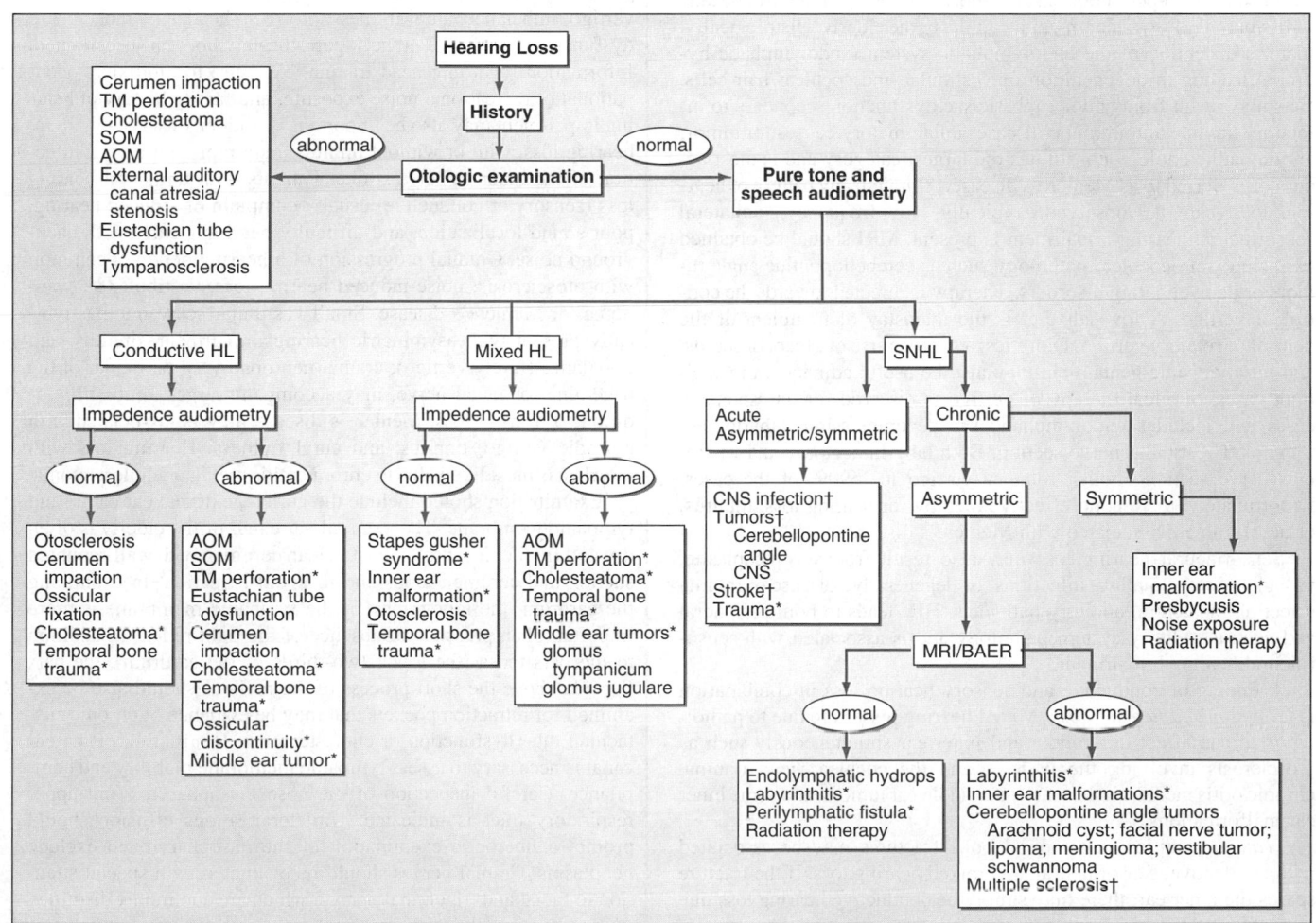

FIGURE 26-2   An algorithm for the approach to hearing loss. HL, hearing loss; SNHL, sensorineural hearing loss; TM, tympanic membrane; SOM, serous otitis media; AOM, acute otitis media; *, CT scan of temporal bone; †, MRI scan.

diagnose AOM, SOM, chronic otitis media, cerumen impaction, tympanic membrane perforation, and eustachian tube dysfunction.

Sensorineural Hearing Loss   Damage to the hair cells of the organ of Corti may be caused by intense noise, viral infections, ototoxic drugs (e.g., salicylates, quinine and its synthetic analogues, aminoglycoside antibiotics, loop diuretics such as furosemide and ethacrynic acid, and cancer chemotherapeutic agents such as cisplatin), fractures of the temporal bone, meningitis, cochlear otosclerosis (see above), Ménière's disease, and aging. Congenital malformations of the inner ear may be the cause of hearing loss in some adults. Genetic predisposition alone or in concert with environmental influences may also be responsible.

Presbycusis (age-associated hearing loss) is the most common cause of sensorineural hearing loss in adults. In the early stages, it is characterized by symmetric, gentle to sharply sloping high-frequency hearing loss. With progression, the hearing loss involves all frequencies. More importantly, the hearing impairment is associated with significant loss in clarity. There is a loss of discrimination for phonemes, recruitment (abnormal growth of loudness), and particular difficulty in understanding speech in noisy environments. Hearing aids may provide limited rehabilitation once the word recognition score deteriorates below 50%. Improvements in cochlear implants have made them the treatment of choice when hearing aids prove inadequate.

Ménière's disease is characterized by episodic vertigo, fluctuating sensorineural hearing loss, tinnitus, and aural fullness. Tinnitus and/or deafness may be absent during the initial attacks of vertigo, but they invariably appear as the disease progresses and are increased in severity during an acute attack. The annual incidence of Ménière's disease is 0.5 to 7.5 per 1000; onset is most frequently in the fifth decade of life but may also occur in young adults or the elderly. Histologically, there is distention of the endolymphatic system (endolymphatic hydrops) leading to degeneration of vestibular and cochlear hair cells. This may result from endolymphatic sac dysfunction secondary to infection, trauma, autoimmune disease, inflammatory causes, or tumor; an idiopathic etiology constitutes the largest category and is most accurately referred to as Ménière's disease. Although any pattern of hearing loss can be observed, typically, low-frequency, unilateral sensorineural hearing impairment is present. MRI should be obtained to exclude retrocochlear pathology such as cerebellopontine angle tumors or demyelinating disorders. Therapy is directed towards the control of vertigo. A low-salt diet is the mainstay of treatment of the control of rotatory vertigo. Diuretics, a short course of glucocorticoids, and intratympanic gentamicin may also be useful adjuncts in recalcitrant cases. Surgical therapy of vertigo is reserved for unresponsive cases and includes endolymphatic sac decompression, labyrinthectomy, and vestibular nerve section. Both labyrinthectomy and vestibular nerve section abolish rotatory vertigo in >90% of the cases. Unfortunately, there is no effective therapy for hearing loss, tinnitus, or aural fullness associated with Ménière's disease.

Sensorineural hearing loss may also result from any neoplastic, vascular, demyelinating, infectious, or degenerative disease or trauma affecting the central auditory pathways. HIV leads to both peripheral and central auditory system pathology and is associated with sensorineural hearing impairment.

A finding of conductive and sensory hearing loss in combination is termed *mixed hearing loss*. Mixed hearing losses are due to pathology that can affect the middle and inner ear simultaneously such as otosclerosis involving the ossicles and the cochlea, head trauma, chronic otitis media, cholesteatoma, middle ear tumors, and some inner ear malformations.

Trauma resulting in temporal bone fractures may be associated with conductive, sensorineural, and mixed hearing loss. If the fracture spares the inner ear, there may simply be conductive hearing loss due to rupture of the tympanic membrane or disruption of the ossicular chain. These abnormalities are amenable to surgical correction. Profound hearing loss and severe vertigo are associated with temporal

bone fractures involving the inner ear. A perilymphatic fistula associated with leakage of inner-ear fluid into the middle ear can occur and may require surgical repair. An associated facial nerve injury is not uncommon. CT is best suited to assess fracture of the traumatized temporal bone, evaluate the ear canal, and determine the integrity of the ossicular chain and the involvement of the inner ear. CSF leaks that accompany temporal bone fractures are usually self-limited; the use of prophylactic antibiotics is controversial.

Tinnitus is defined as the perception of a sound when there is no sound in the environment. It may have a buzzing, roaring, or ringing quality and may be pulsatile (synchronous with the heartbeat). Tinnitus is often associated with either a conductive or sensorineural hearing loss. The pathophysiology of tinnitus is not well understood. The cause of the tinnitus can usually be determined by finding the cause of the associated hearing loss. Tinnitus may be the first symptom of a serious condition such as a vestibular schwannoma. Pulsatile tinnitus requires evaluation of the vascular system of the head to exclude vascular tumors such as glomus jugulare tumors, aneurysms, and stenotic arterial lesions; it may also occur with SOM.

APPROACH TO THE PATIENT

The goal in the evaluation of a patient with auditory complaints is to determine (1) the nature of the hearing impairment (conductive vs. sensorineural), (2) the severity of the impairment (mild, moderate, severe, profound), (3) the anatomy of the impairment (external ear, middle ear, inner ear, or central auditory pathway), and (4) the etiology. The history should elicit characteristics of the hearing loss, including the duration of deafness, unilateral vs. bilateral involvement, nature of onset (sudden vs. insidious), and rate of progression (rapid vs. slow). The presence or absence of tinnitus, vertigo, imbalance, aural fullness, otorrhea, headache, facial nerve dysfunction, and head and neck paresthesias should be ascertained. Information regarding head trauma, exposure to ototoxins, occupational or recreational noise exposure, and family history of hearing impairment may also be important. A sudden onset of unilateral hearing loss, with or without tinnitus, may represent a viral infection of the inner ear or a stroke. Patients with unilateral hearing loss (sensory or conductive) usually complain of reduced hearing, poor sound localization, and difficulty hearing clearly with background noise. Gradual progression of a hearing deficit is common with otosclerosis, noise-induced hearing loss, vestibular schwannoma, or Ménière's disease. Small vestibular schwannomas typically present with asymmetric hearing impairment, tinnitus, and imbalance (rarely vertigo); cranial neuropathy, in particular of the trigeminal or facial nerve, may accompany larger tumors. In addition to hearing loss, Ménière's disease may be associated with episodic vertigo, tinnitus, and aural fullness. Hearing loss with otorrhea is most likely due to chronic otitis media or cholesteatoma.

Examination should include the auricle, external ear canal, and tympanic membrane. The external ear canal of the elderly is often dry and fragile; it is preferable to clean cerumen with wall-mounted suction and cerumen loops and to avoid irrigation. In examining the eardrum, the topography of the tympanic membrane is more important than presence or absence of the light reflex. In addition to the pars tensa (the lower two-thirds of the eardrum), the pars flaccida above the short process of the malleus should also be examined for retraction pockets that may be evidence of chronic eustachian tube dysfunction or cholesteatoma. Insufflation of the ear canal is necessary to assess tympanic membrane mobility and compliance. Careful inspection of the nose, nasopharynx, and upper respiratory tract is indicated. Unilateral serous effusion should prompt a fiberoptic examination of the nasopharynx to exclude neoplasms. Cranial nerves should be evaluated with special attention to facial and trigeminal nerves, which are commonly disturbed with tumors involving the cerebellopontine angle.

The Rinne and Weber tuning fork tests, with a 256- or 512-Hz tuning fork, are used to screen for hearing loss, differentiate conductive from sensorineural hearing losses, and to confirm the findings of audiologic evaluation. Rinne's test compares the ability to hear by air conduction with the ability to hear by bone conduction. The tines of a vibrating tuning fork are held near the opening of the external auditory canal, and then the stem is placed on the mastoid process; for direct contact, it may be placed on teeth or dentures. The patient is asked to indicate whether the tone is louder by air conduction or bone conduction. Normally, and in the presence of sensorineural hearing loss, a tone is heard louder by air conduction than by bone conduction; however, with conductive hearing loss of ≥30 dB (see "Audiologic Assessment," below), the bone-conduction stimulus is perceived as louder than the air-conduction stimulus. For the Weber test, the stem of a vibrating tuning fork is placed on the head in the midline and the patient asked whether the tone is heard in both ears or better in one ear than in the other. With a unilateral conductive hearing loss, the tone is perceived in the affected ear. With a unilateral sensorineural hearing loss, the tone is perceived in the unaffected ear. A 5-dB difference in hearing between the two ears is required for lateralization.

LABORATORY ASSESSMENT OF HEARING ■ **Audiologic Assessment** The minimum audiologic assessment for hearing loss should include the measurement of pure tone air-conduction and bone-conduction thresholds, speech reception threshold, discrimination score, tympanometry, acoustic reflexes, and acoustic-reflex decay. This test battery provides a comprehensive screening evaluation of the whole auditory system and allows one to determine whether further differentiation of a sensory (cochlear) from a neural (retrocochlear) hearing loss is indicated.

Pure tone audiometry assesses hearing acuity for pure tones. The test is administered by an audiologist and is performed in a sound-attenuated chamber. The pure tone stimulus is delivered with an audiometer, an electronic device that allows the presentation of specific frequencies (generally between 250 and 8000 Hz) at specific intensities. Air and bone conduction thresholds are established for each ear. Air conduction thresholds are established by presenting the stimulus in air with the use of headphones. Bone conduction thresholds are accomplished by placing the stem of a vibrating tuning fork or an oscillator of an audiometer in contact with the head. In the presence of a hearing loss, broad-spectrum noise is presented to the nontest ear for *masking* purposes so that responses are based on perception from the ear under test.

The responses are measured in decibels. An *audiogram* is a plot of intensity in decibels of hearing threshold versus frequency. A decibel (dB) is equal to 20 times the logarithm of the ratio of the sound pressure required to achieve threshold in the patient to the sound pressure required to achieve threshold in a normal hearing person. Therefore, a change of 6 dB represents doubling of sound pressure, and a change of 20 dB represents a tenfold change in sound pressure. Loudness, which depends on the frequency, intensity, and duration of a sound, doubles with approximately each 10-dB increase in sound pressure level. Pitch, on the other hand, does not directly correlate with frequency. The perception of pitch changes slowly in the low and high frequencies. In the middle tones, which are important for human speech, pitch varies more rapidly with changes in frequency.

Pure tone audiometry establishes the presence and severity of hearing impairment, unilateral vs. bilateral involvement, and the type of hearing loss. Conductive hearing losses with a large mass component, as is often seen in middle-ear effusions, produce elevation of thresholds that predominate in the higher frequencies. Conductive hearing losses with a large stiffness component, as in fixation of the footplate of the stapes in early otosclerosis, produce threshold elevations in the lower frequencies. Often, the conductive hearing loss involves all frequencies, suggesting involvement of both stiffness and mass. In general, sensorineural hearing losses such as presbycusis affect higher frequencies more than lower frequencies. An exception is Ménière's disease, which is characteristically associated with low-frequency sen-

sorineural hearing loss. Noise-induced hearing loss has an unusual pattern of hearing impairment in which the loss at 4000 Hz is greater than at higher frequencies. Vestibular schwannomas characteristically affect the higher frequencies, but any pattern of hearing loss can be observed.

Speech recognition requires greater synchronous neural firing than is necessary for appreciation of pure tones. *Speech audiometry* tests the clarity with which one hears. The *speech reception threshold* (SRT) is defined as the intensity at which speech is recognized as a meaningful symbol and is obtained by presenting two-syllable words with an equal accent on each syllable. The intensity at which the patient can repeat 50% of the words correctly is the SRT. Once the SRT is determined, discrimination or word recognition ability is tested by presenting one-syllable words at 25 to 40 dB above the speech reception threshold. The words are phonetically balanced in that the phonemes (speech sounds) occur in the list of words at the same frequency that they occur in ordinary conversational English. An individual with normal hearing or conductive hearing loss can repeat 88 to 100% of the phonetically balanced words correctly. Patients with a sensorineural hearing loss have variable loss of discrimination. As a general rule, neural lesions are associated with more deterioration in discrimination ability than are lesions in the inner ear. For example, in a patient with mild asymmetric sensorineural hearing loss, a clue to the diagnosis of vestibular schwannoma is the presence of greater than expected deterioration in discrimination ability. Deterioration in discrimination ability at higher intensities above the SRT also suggests a lesion in the eighth nerve or central auditory pathways.

Tympanometry measures the impedance of the middle ear to sound and is useful in diagnosis of middle-ear effusions. A *tympanogram* is the graphic representation of change in impedance or compliance as the pressure in the ear canal is changed. Normally, the middle ear is most compliant at atmospheric pressure, and the compliance decreases as the pressure is increased or decreased; this pattern is seen with normal hearing or in the presence of sensorineural hearing loss. Compliance that does not change with change in pressure suggests middle-ear effusion. With a negative pressure in the middle ear, as with eustachian tube obstruction, the point of maximal compliance occurs with negative pressure in the ear canal. A tympanogram in which no point of maximal compliance can be obtained is most commonly seen with discontinuity of the ossicular chain. A reduction in the maximal compliance peak can be seen in otosclerosis.

During tympanometry, an intense tone elicits contraction of the stapedius muscle. The change in compliance of the middle ear with contraction of the stapedius muscle can be detected. The presence or absence of this *acoustic reflex* is important in the anatomic localization of facial nerve paralysis as well as hearing loss. Normal or elevated acoustic reflex thresholds in an individual with sensorineural hearing impairment suggests a cochlear hearing loss. Assessment of *acoustic reflex decay* helps differentiate sensory from neural hearing losses. In neural hearing loss, the reflex adapts or decays with time.

Otoacoustic emissions (OAE) can be measured with microphones inserted into the external auditory canal. The emissions may be spontaneous or evoked with sound stimulation. The presence of OAEs indicates that the outer hair cells of the organ of Corti are intact and can be used to assess auditory thresholds and to distinguish sensory from neural hearing losses.

Evoked Responses *Electrocochleography* measures the earliest evoked potentials generated in the cochlea and the auditory nerve. Receptor potentials recorded include the cochlear microphonic, generated by the outer hair cells of the organ of Corti, and the summating potential, generated by the inner hair cells in response to sound. The whole nerve action potential representing the composite firing of the first-order neurons can also be recorded during electrocochleography. Clinically, the test is useful in the diagnosis of Ménière's disease, where an elevation of the ratio of summating potential to action potential is seen.

Brainstem auditory evoked responses (BAERs) are useful in differentiating the site of sensorineural hearing loss. In response to sound, five distinct electrical potentials arising from different stations along the peripheral and central auditory pathway can be identified using computer averaging from scalp surface electrodes. BAERs are valuable in situations in which patients cannot or will not give reliable voluntary thresholds. They are also used to assess the integrity of the auditory nerve and brainstem in various clinical situations, including intraoperative monitoring and in determination of brain death.

Imaging Studies The choice of radiologic tests is largely determined by whether the goal is to evaluate the bony anatomy of the external, middle, and inner ear or to image the auditory nerve and brain. Axial and coronal CT of the temporal bone with fine 1-mm cuts is ideal for determining the caliber of the external auditory canal, integrity of the ossicular chain, and presence of middle-ear or mastoid disease; it can also detect inner-ear malformations. CT is also ideal for the detection of bone erosion often seen in the presence of chronic otitis media and cholesteatoma. MRI is superior to CT for imaging of retrocochlear pathology such as vestibular schwannoma, meningioma, other lesions of the cerebellopontine angle, demyelinating lesions of the brainstem, and brain tumors. Recent experience suggests that both CT and MRI are equally capable of identifying inner-ear malformations and assessing cochlear patency for preoperative evaluation of patients for cochlear implantation.

℞ TREATMENT

In general, conductive hearing losses are amenable to surgical intervention and correction, while sensorineural hearing losses are permanent. Atresia of the ear canal can be surgically repaired, often with significant improvement in hearing. Tympanic membrane perforations due to chronic otitis media or trauma can be repaired with an outpatient tympanoplasty. Likewise, conductive hearing loss associated with otosclerosis can be treated by stapedectomy, which is successful in 90 to 95% of cases. Tympanostomy tubes allow the prompt return of normal hearing in individuals with middle-ear effusions. Hearing aids are effective and well-tolerated in patients with conductive hearing losses.

Patients with mild, moderate, and severe sensorineural hearing losses are regularly rehabilitated with hearing aids of varying configuration and strength. Hearing aids have been improved to provide greater fidelity and have been miniaturized. The current generation of hearing aids can be placed entirely within the ear canal, thus reducing the stigma associated with their use. In general, the more severe the hearing impairment, the larger the hearing aid required for auditory rehabilitation. Digital hearing aids lend themselves to individual programming, and multiple and directional microphones at the ear level may be helpful in noisy surroundings. Since all hearing aids amplify noise as well as speech, the only absolute solution to the problem found thus far is to place the microphone closer to the speaker than the noise source. This arrangement is not possible with a self-contained, cosmetically acceptable device. It is cumbersome and requires a user-friendly environment.

In many situations, including lectures and the theater, hearing-impaired persons benefit from assistive devices that are based on the principle of having the speaker closer to the microphone than any source of noise. Assistive devices include infrared and frequency modulated (FM) transmission as well as an electromagnetic loop around the room for transmission to the individual's hearing aid. Hearing aids with telecoils can also be used with properly equipped telephones in the same way.

In the event that the hearing aid provides inadequate rehabilitation, cochlear implants may be appropriate. Criteria for implantation include severe to profound hearing loss with word recognition score ≤30% under best aided conditions. Worldwide, more than 20,000 deaf individuals (including 4000 children) have received cochlear implants. Cochlear implants are neural prostheses that convert sound energy to electrical energy and can be used to stimulate the auditory division of the eighth nerve directly. In most cases of profound hearing impairment, the auditory hair cells are lost but the ganglionic cells of the auditory division of the eighth nerve are preserved. Cochlear implants consist of electrodes that are inserted into the cochlea through the round window, speech processors that extract acoustical elements of speech for conversion to electrical currents, and a means of transmitting the electrical energy through the skin. Patients with implants experience sound that helps with speech reading, allows open-set word recognition, and helps in modulating the person's own voice. Usually, within 3 months after implantation, adult patients can understand speech without visual cues. With the current generation of multichannel cochlear implants, nearly 75% of patients are able to converse on the telephone. It is anticipated that improvements in the electrode design and speech processors will permit further enhancement in understanding speech, especially in the presence of background noise.

For individuals who have had both eighth nerves destroyed by trauma or bilateral vestibular schwannomas (e.g., neurofibromatosis type 2), brainstem auditory implants placed near the cochlear nucleus may provide auditory rehabilitation. It is hoped that additional advances may provide benefits similar to those with the cochlear implant.

Tinnitus often accompanies hearing loss. Tinnitus and background noise can significantly affect understanding of speech in individuals with hearing impairment. Therapy for tinnitus is usually directed towards minimizing the appreciation of tinnitus. Relief of the tinnitus may be obtained by masking it with background music. Hearing aids are also helpful in tinnitus suppression, as are tinnitus maskers, devices that present a sound to the affected ear that is more pleasant to listen to than the tinnitus. The use of a tinnitus masker is often followed by several hours of inhibition of the tinnitus. Antidepressants have also shown beneficial effect in helping patients deal with tinnitus.

Tinnitus and background noise can significantly affect understanding of speech in individuals with hearing impairment. Hard-of-hearing individuals often benefit from a reduction in unnecessary noise (e.g., radio or television) to enhance the signal-to-noise ratio. Speech comprehension is aided by lip reading; therefore the impaired listener should be seated so that the face of the speaker is well-illuminated and easily seen. Speaking directly into the ear is occasionally helpful, but usually more is lost than gained because the speaker's face can no longer be seen. Speech should be slow enough to make each word distinct, but overly slow speech is distracting and loses contextual and speech-reading benefits. Although speech should be in a loud, clear voice, one should be aware that in sensorineural hearing losses in general and in elderly hard-of-hearing persons in particular, recruitment (abnormal perception of loud sounds) may be troublesome. Above all, optimal communication cannot take place without both parties giving it their full and undivided attention.

PREVENTION Conductive hearing losses may be prevented by prompt antibiotic therapy of adequate duration for AOM and by ventilation of the middle ear with tympanostomy tubes in middle-ear effusions lasting ≥12 weeks. Loss of vestibular function and deafness due to aminoglycoside antibiotics can largely be prevented by careful monitoring of serum peak and trough levels.

Some 10 million Americans have noise-induced hearing loss, and 20 million are exposed to hazardous noise in their employment. Noise-induced hearing loss can be prevented by avoidance of exposure to loud noise or by regular use of ear plugs or fluid-filled ear muffs to attenuate intense sound. Noise-induced hearing loss results from recreational as well as occupational activities and begins in adolescence. High-risk activities for noise-induced hearing loss include wood and metal working with electrical equipment and target practice and hunting with small firearms. All internal-combustion and electric engines, including snow and leaf blowers, snowmobiles, outboard motors, and chain saws, require protection of the user with hearing protectors. Virtually all noise-induced hearing loss is preventable through education, which should begin before the teenage years. Programs of industrial conservation of hearing are required when the exposure over an 8-h period averages 85 dB. Workers in such noisy environments can be protected with preemployment audiologic assessment, the mandatory use of hearing protectors, and annual audiologic assessments.

FURTHER READING

BALLENGER JJ, SNOW JB (eds): *Ballenger's Otorhinolaryngology Head and Neck Surgery*, 16th ed. Baltimore, BC Decker, 2002

GURTLER N, LALWANI AK: Etiology of syndromic and nonsyndromic sensorineural hearing loss. Otolaryngol Clin North Am 35:891, 2002

ZADEH MH et al: Diagnosis and treatment of sudden-onset sensorineural hearing loss: A study of 51 patients. Otolaryngol Head Neck Surg 128:92, 2003

27 | INFECTIONS OF THE UPPER RESPIRATORY TRACT
Michael A. Rubin, Ralph Gonzales, Merle A. Sande

Infections of the upper respiratory tract (URIs) have a tremendous impact on public health. They are among the most common reasons for visits to primary care providers, and, although the illnesses are typically mild, their high incidence and transmission rates place them among the leading causes of time lost from work or school. Even though the minority (~25%) of cases are caused by bacteria, URIs are the leading diagnoses for which antibiotics are prescribed on an outpatient basis in the United States. The enormous consumption of antibiotics for these illnesses has contributed to the rise in antibiotic resistance among common community-acquired pathogens such as *Streptococcus pneumoniae*—a trend that in itself has had a tremendous impact on public health.

Although most URIs are caused by viruses, distinguishing patients with primary viral infection from those with primary bacterial infection is difficult. Signs and symptoms of bacterial and viral URIs are, in fact, indistinguishable. Because routine, rapid testing is neither available nor practical for most syndromes, acute infections are diagnosed largely on clinical grounds. This situation makes the judicious use of antibiotics in this setting challenging.

NONSPECIFIC INFECTIONS OF THE UPPER RESPIRATORY TRACT

Nonspecific URIs are a broadly defined group of disorders that collectively constitute the leading cause of ambulatory care visits in the United States. Nonspecific URIs, by definition, have no prominent localizing features. They are identified by a variety of descriptive names, including *acute infective rhinitis*, *acute rhinopharyngitis/nasopharyngitis*, *acute coryza*, and *acute nasal catarrh*, as well as by the inclusive label *common cold*.

Etiology The large assortment of URI classifications reflects the wide variety of causative infectious agents and the varied manifestations of common pathogens. Nearly all nonspecific URIs are caused by viruses spanning multiple virus families and large numbers of antigenic types. For instance, rhinoviruses (Chap. 170), the most common cause (~30 to 40% of cases), consist of at least 100 immunotypes; other causes include influenza virus (3 immunotypes; Chap. 171) as well as parainfluenza virus (4 immunotypes), coronavirus (at least 3 immunotypes), and adenovirus (47 immunotypes) (Chap. 170). Respiratory syncytial virus (RSV) also accounts for a small percentage of cases each year, as do some viruses not typically associated with URIs (e.g., enteroviruses, rubella virus, and varicella-zoster virus). Even with sophisticated diagnostic and culture techniques, a substantial proportion (25 to 30%) of cases have no assigned pathogen.

Manifestations The signs and symptoms of nonspecific URI are similar to those of other URIs but lack a pronounced localization to one particular anatomic location, such as the sinuses, pharynx, or lower airway. Nonspecific URI is commonly described as an acute, mild, and self-limited catarrhal syndrome, with a median duration of ~1 week. Signs and symptoms are diverse and frequently variable across patients. The principal signs and symptoms of nonspecific URI include rhinorrhea (with or without purulence), nasal congestion, cough, and sore throat; other manifestations, such as fever, malaise, sneezing, and hoarseness, are more variable, with fever more common among infants and young children. Occasionally, clinical features reflect the underlying viral pathogen; myalgias and fatigue, for example, are sometimes seen with influenza and parainfluenza infections, while conjunctivitis may suggest infection with adenovirus or enterovirus. Findings on physical examination are frequently nonspecific and unimpressive. Between 0.5 and 2% of colds are complicated by secondary bacterial infections (e.g., rhinosinusitis, otitis media, and pneumonia), particularly in high-risk populations such as infants, elderly persons, and chronically ill patients. Secondary bacterial infections are usually associated with a prolonged course of illness, worsening of illness severity, and localization of signs and symptoms. The presence of purulent secretions from the nares or throat has often been used as an indication of sinusitis or pharyngitis. However, these secretions are also seen in nonspecific URI and, in the absence of other clinical features, are poor predictors of bacterial infection.

℞ TREATMENT

Antibiotics have no role in the treatment of uncomplicated nonspecific URI. In the absence of clinical evidence of bacterial infection, treatment remains entirely symptom-based, with use of decongestants and nonsteroidal anti-inflammatory drugs. Other therapies directed at specific symptoms are often useful, including dextromethorphan for cough and lozenges with topical anesthetic for sore throat. Clinical trials of zinc, vitamin C, echinacea, and other alternative remedies have revealed no consistent benefit for the treatment of nonspecific URI.

INFECTIONS OF THE SINUS

Sinusitis refers to an inflammatory condition involving the four paired structures surrounding the nasal cavities. Although most cases of sinusitis involve more than one sinus, the maxillary sinus is most commonly involved, followed in frequency by the ethmoid, frontal, and sphenoid sinuses. Each sinus is lined with a respiratory epithelium that produces mucus, which is transported out by ciliary action through the sinus ostium and into the nasal cavity. Normally, mucus does not accumulate in the sinuses, which remain sterile despite their adjacency to the bacterium-filled nasal passages. When the sinus ostia are obstructed, however, or when ciliary clearance is impaired or absent, the secretions can be retained, producing the typical signs and symptoms of sinusitis. The retained secretions may become infected with a variety of pathogens, including viruses, bacteria, and fungi. Sinusitis affects a tremendous proportion of the population, accounts for millions of visits to primary care physicians each year, and is the fifth leading diagnosis for which antibiotics are prescribed. It is typically classified by duration of illness (acute vs. chronic); by etiology (infectious vs. noninfectious); and, when infectious, by the offending pathogen type (viral, bacterial, or fungal).

ACUTE SINUSITIS   Acute sinusitis—defined as sinusitis of <4 weeks' duration—constitutes the vast majority of sinusitis cases. Most cases are diagnosed in the ambulatory care setting and occur primarily as a consequence of a preceding viral URI. Differentiating acute bacterial and viral sinusitis on clinical grounds is difficult. Therefore, it is perhaps unsurprising that antibiotics are prescribed frequently (in 85 to 98% of all cases) for this condition.

Etiology   A number of infectious and noninfectious factors can contribute to acute obstruction of the sinus ostia or impairment of ciliary clearance, with consequent sinusitis. Noninfectious causes include allergic rhinitis (with either mucosal edema or polyp obstruction), barotrauma (e.g., from deep-sea diving or air travel), or chemical irritants. Illnesses such as nasal and sinus tumors (e.g., squamous cell carcinoma) or granulomatous diseases (e.g., Wegener's granulomatosis or rhinoscleroma) can also produce obstruction of the sinus ostia, while conditions leading to altered mucus content (e.g., cystic fibrosis) can cause sinusitis through impaired mucus clearance. In the hospital setting, nasotracheal intubation is a major risk factor for nosocomial sinusitis in intensive care units.

Acute infectious sinusitis can be caused by a variety of organisms, including viruses, bacteria, and fungi. Viral rhinosinusitis is far more common than bacterial sinusitis, although relatively few studies have sampled sinus aspirates for the presence of different viruses. In those studies that have done so, the viruses most commonly isolated—both alone and with bacteria—have been rhinovirus, parainfluenza virus, and influenza virus. Bacterial causes of sinusitis have been better described. Among community-acquired cases, *S. pneumoniae* and nontypable *Haemophilus influenzae* are the most common pathogens, accounting for 50 to 60% of cases. *Moraxella catarrhalis* causes disease in a significant percentage (20%) of children but less often in adults. Other streptococcal species and *Staphylococcus aureus* cause a small percentage of cases. Anaerobes are occasionally found in association with infections of the roots of premolar teeth that spread into the adjacent maxillary sinuses. The role of *Chlamydia pneumoniae* and *Mycoplasma pneumoniae* in the pathogenesis of acute sinusitis is still unclear. Nosocomial cases are commonly associated with bacteria found in the hospital environment, including *S. aureus*, *Pseudomonas aeruginosa*, *Serratia marcescens*, *Klebsiella pneumoniae*, and *Enterobacter* species. Often, these infections are polymicrobial and involve organisms that are highly resistant to numerous antibiotics. Fungi are also established causes of sinusitis, although most acute cases are in immunocompromised patients and represent invasive, life-threatening infections. The best-known example is rhinocerebral mucormycosis caused by fungi of the order Mucorales, which includes *Rhizopus*, *Rhizomucor*, *Mucor*, *Absidia*, and *Cunninghamella*. These infections usually occur in diabetic patients with ketoacidosis but also develop in transplant recipients, patients with hematologic malignancies, and patients receiving chronic glucocorticoid or deferoxamine therapy. Other hyaline molds, such as *Aspergillus* and *Fusarium* species, are also occasional causes of this disease.

Manifestations   Most cases of acute sinusitis present after or in conjunction with a viral URI, and it can be difficult to discriminate the clinical features of one from the other. A large proportion of patients with colds have sinus inflammation, although bacterial sinusitis complicates only 0.2 to 2% of these viral infections. Common presenting symptoms of sinusitis include nasal drainage and congestion, facial pain or pressure, and headache. Thick, purulent or discolored nasal discharge is often thought to indicate bacterial sinusitis, but it also occurs early in viral infections such as the common cold and is not specific to bacterial infection. Other nonspecific symptoms include cough, sneezing, and fever. Tooth pain, most often involving the upper molars, is associated with bacterial sinusitis, as is halitosis.

In acute sinusitis, sinus pain or pressure often localizes to the involved sinus (particularly the maxillary sinus) and can be worse when the patient bends over or is supine. Although rare, symptoms of advanced sphenoid or ethmoid sinus infection can be profound, including severe frontal or retroorbital pain radiating to the occiput, thrombosis of the cavernous sinus, and signs of orbital cellulitis. Acute focal sinusitis is uncommon but should be considered in the patient with severe symptoms over the maxillary sinus and fever, regardless of illness duration. Similarly, advanced frontal sinusitis can present with a condition known as *Pott's puffy tumor*, with soft tissue swelling and pitting edema over the frontal bone from a communicating subperiosteal abscess. Life-threatening complications include meningitis, epidural abscess, and cerebral abscess.

Patients with acute fungal sinusitis (such as mucormycosis) often present with symptoms related to pressure effects, particularly when the infection has spread to the orbits and cavernous sinus. Signs such as orbital swelling and cellulitis, proptosis, ptosis, and decreased extraocular movement are common, as is retroorbital or periorbital pain. Nasopharyngeal ulcerations, epistaxis, and headaches are also frequent, and involvement of cranial nerves V and VII has been described in more advanced cases. Bony erosion may be evident on examination. Oftentimes, the patient does not appear seriously ill despite the rapidly progressive nature of these infections.

Patients with acute nosocomial sinusitis are often critically ill and thus do not manifest the typical clinical features of sinus disease. This diagnosis should be suspected, however, when hospitalized patients who have appropriate risk factors (e.g., nasotracheal intubation) develop fever of uncertain origin.

Diagnosis   Distinguishing viral from bacterial sinusitis in the ambulatory setting is usually difficult, given the relatively low sensitivity and specificity of the common clinical features. One clinical feature that has been used to help guide diagnostic and therapeutic decision-making is illness duration. Because acute bacterial sinusitis is uncommon in patients whose symptoms have lasted <7 days, several authorities now recommend reserving this diagnosis for patients with appropriate symptoms (e.g., facial or tooth pain in combination with purulent nasal discharge) that have persisted for >7 days (Table 27-1). Nonetheless, of the patients who meet these criteria, only 40 to 50% have true bacterial sinusitis. The use of computed tomography (CT) or sinus radiography is not recommended for routine cases, particularly early in the course of illness (i.e., at <7 days), given the high prevalence of similar abnormalities among cases of acute viral rhinosinusitis. In the evaluation of persistent, recurrent, or chronic sinusitis, CT of the sinuses is the radiographic study of choice.

The clinical history and/or setting can often identify cases of acute anaerobic bacterial sinusitis, acute fungal sinusitis, or sinusitis from noninfectious causes, such as allergic rhinosinusitis. In the case of an immunocompromised patient with acute fungal sinus infection, immediate examination by an otolaryngologist is required. Biopsies of involved areas should be examined by a pathologist for evidence of fungal hyphal elements and tissue invasion. Cases of suspected acute nosocomial sinusitis should be confirmed by a sinus CT scan. Because therapy should target the offending organism, a sinus aspirate should be obtained, if possible, for culture and susceptibility testing.

℞ **TREATMENT**

Most patients with a diagnosis of acute rhinosinusitis based on clinical grounds improve without antibiotic therapy. The preferred initial approach in adult patients with mild to moderate symptoms of <7 days' duration are therapies aimed at facilitating sinus drainage, such as oral and topical decongestants, nasal saline lavage, and—in patients with a history of chronic sinusitis or allergies—nasal glucocorticoids. Adult patients fulfilling the above criteria who do not improve after 7 days and those with more severe symptoms (regardless of duration) should be treated with antibiotics (Table 27-1). Empirical therapy should consist of the most narrow-spectrum agent active against the most common bacterial pathogens, including *S. pneumoniae* and *H. influenzae*—e.g., amoxicillin. No clinical trials support the use of broad-spectrum agents for routine cases of bacterial sinusitis, even in the current era of drug-resistant *S. pneumoniae*. Up to 10% of patients do not respond

Syndrome, Age Group	Diagnostic Criteria	Treatment Recommendations
ACUTE SINUSITIS		

Adults	Moderate symptoms (e.g., nasal purulence/congestion or cough) for >7 d or
	Severe symptoms (any duration), including unilateral/focal facial swelling or tooth pain
		Initial therapy:
		   Amoxicillin, 875 mg PO bid for 10 d or
		   TMP-SMX, 1 DS tablet PO bid for 10 d
		Exposure to antibiotics within 30 d:
		   Amoxicillin, 1000 mg PO bid for 10 d or
		   Amoxicillin/clavulanate, 875 mg PO bid for 10 d or
		   Antipneumococcal fluoroquinolone (e.g., levofloxacin, 500 mg PO qd) for 7 d
		Recent treatment failure:
		   Amoxicillin (1500 mg) *plus* clavulanate (125 mg) PO bid for 10 d or
		   Amoxicillin (1500 mg) *plus* clindamycin (300 mg qid) PO for 10 d or
		   Antipneumococcal fluoroquinolone (e.g., levofloxacin, 500 mg PO qd) for 7 d

Children	Moderate symptoms (e.g., nasal purulence/congestion or cough) for 10–14 d or longer or
	Severe symptoms (any duration), including fever (>102°F), unilateral/focal facial swelling or pain
		Initial therapy: 10-d course of oral treatment with:
		   Amoxicillin, 45–90 mg/kg per day (up to 2 g) in divided doses (bid or tid) or
		   Cefuroxime axetil, 30 mg/kg per day in divided doses (bid) or Cefdinir, 14 mg/kg qd
		Exposure to antibiotics within 30 d or recent treatment failure: 10-d course of oral treatment with:
		   Amoxicillin, 90 mg/kg per day (up to 2 g), *plus* clavulanate, 6.4 mg/kg per day; both in divided doses (bid) or
		   Cefuroxime axetil, 30 mg/kg per day in divided doses (bid) or Cefdinir, 14 mg/kg qd

ACUTE PHARYNGITIS		
Adults	Clinical suspicion of streptococcal pharyngitis (e.g., fever, tonsillar swelling, exudate, enlarged/tender anterior cervical lymph nodes, absence of cough or coryza)[a] *with* History of rheumatic fever or Documented household exposure or Positive rapid strep screen	Penicillin V, 500 mg PO bid for 10 d or Cephalexin, 250 mg PO qid for 10 d or Erythromycin, 250 mg PO qid for 10 d or Benzathine penicillin G, single dose of 1.2 million units IM
Children	Clinical suspicion of streptococcal pharyngitis (e.g., tonsillar swelling, exudate, enlarged/tender anterior cervical lymph nodes, absence of coryza) *with* History of rheumatic fever or Documented household exposure or Positive rapid strep screen or Positive throat culture (for those with negative rapid strep screen)	Amoxicillin, 45 mg/kg per day PO in divided doses (bid or tid) for 10 d or Penicillin VK, 50 mg/kg per day PO in divided doses (bid) for 10 d Cephalexin, 50 mg/kg per day PO in divided doses (qid) for 10 d Benzathine penicillin G, single dose of 25,000 units/kg IM
ACUTE OTITIS MEDIA		

Adults and children	Fluid in middle ear, evidenced by decreased tympanic membrane mobility, air/fluid level behind tympanic membrane, bulging tympanic membrane, purulent otorrhea *and*
	Signs and symptoms of middle-ear disease, including fever, irritability, otalgia, decreased hearing, tinnitus, vertigo
		Initial therapy[b]:
		   Amoxicillin, 90 mg/kg per day (up to 2 g) PO in divided doses (bid or tid) or
		   Amoxicillin, 90 mg/kg per day (up to 2 g), *plus* clavulanate, 6.4 mg/kg per day; both PO in divided doses (bid) or
		   Cefdinir, 14 mg/kg PO qd or
		   Clindamycin, 20 mg/kg per day PO in divided doses (tid), *plus* TMP-SMX, 10 mg/kg per day PO in divided doses (bid)
		Exposure to antibiotics within 30 d or recent treatment failure:
		   Amoxicillin, 90 mg/kg per day (up to 2 g), *plus* clavulanate, 6.4 mg/kg per day; both PO in divided doses (bid) for 10 d or
		   Cefdinir, 14 mg/kg PO qd for 10 d or
		   Ceftriaxone, 50 mg/kg IM qd for 3 d or
		   Consider myringotomy

[a] Some organizations support treating adults with these symptoms and signs without the need for rapid streptococcal antigen testing.

[b] Duration: 10 d for patients <2 years old, 5–7 d for patients 2–5 years old, and 5–7 d (with consideration of observation only in previously healthy individuals with mild disease) for patients >5 years old.

Note: DS, double-strength; TMP-SMX, trimethoprim-sulfamethoxazole.
Source: Cooper et al; Hickner et al; O'Brien et al; SF Dowell et al: Pediatrics 101:165, 1998; B Schwartz et al: Pediatrics 101:171, 1998.

to initial antimicrobial therapy, and these patients should be considered for sinus aspiration and/or lavage by an otolaryngologist. The use of prophylactic antibiotics to prevent episodes of recurrent acute bacterial sinusitis is not recommended.

Surgical intervention and intravenous antibiotics are usually reserved for patients with severe disease or those with intracranial complications, such as abscess or orbital involvement. Immunocompromised patients with acute invasive fungal sinusitis usually require extensive surgical debridement and treatment with intravenous antifungal agents active against fungal hyphal forms, such as amphotericin B. Specific therapy should be individualized according to the fungal species and the patient's attributes.

Treatment of nosocomial sinusitis should begin with broad-spectrum antibiotics to cover common pathogens such as *S. aureus* and gram-negative bacilli. Therapy should then be tailored to the results of culture and susceptibility testing of sinus aspirates.

CHRONIC SINUSITIS Chronic sinusitis is characterized by symptoms of sinus inflammation lasting >12 weeks. This illness is most commonly associated with either bacteria or fungi, and clinical cure in most cases is very difficult. Many patients have undergone treatment with repeated courses of antibacterial agents and multiple sinus surgeries, increasing their risk of colonization with antibiotic-resistant pathogens and of surgical complications. Patients often suffer significant morbidity, sometimes over many years.

In *chronic bacterial sinusitis*, infection is thought to be due to the impairment of mucociliary clearance from repeated infections rather than to persistent bacterial infection. However, the pathogenesis of this condition is poorly understood. Although certain conditions (e.g., cystic fibrosis) can predispose patients to chronic bacterial sinusitis, most patients with this infection do not have obvious underlying conditions that result in the obstruction of sinus drainage, the impairment of ciliary action, or immune dysfunction. Patients experience constant nasal congestion and sinus pressure, with intermittent periods of greater severity, which may persist for years. CT can be helpful in defining the extent of disease and the response to therapy. The management team should include an otolaryngologist to conduct endoscopic examinations and obtain tissue samples for histologic examination and culture.

Chronic fungal sinusitis is a disease of immunocompetent hosts and is usually noninvasive, although slowly progressive invasive disease is sometimes seen. Noninvasive disease, which is typically associated with hyaline molds such as *Aspergillus* species and dematiaceous molds such as *Curvularia* or *Bipolaris* species, can present as a number of different scenarios. In mild, indolent disease, which usually occurs in the setting of repeated failures of antibacterial therapy, only nonspecific mucosal changes may be seen on sinus CT. Endoscopic surgery is usually curative in these patients, with no need for antifungal therapy. Another form of disease presents with longstanding, often unilateral symptoms and opacification of a single sinus on imaging studies as a result of a mycetoma (fungus ball) within the sinus. Treatment for this condition is also surgical, although systemic antifungal therapy may be warranted in the rare case where bony erosion occurs. A third form of disease, known as *allergic fungal sinusitis*, is seen in patients with a history of nasal polyposis and asthma, who often have had multiple sinus surgeries. Patients with this condition produce a thick, eosinophilic mucus with the consistency of peanut butter that contains sparse fungal hyphae on histologic examination. Patients often present with pansinusitis.

℞ TREATMENT

Treatment of chronic bacterial sinusitis can be challenging and consists primarily of repeated culture-guided courses of antibiotics, sometimes for 3 to 4 weeks at a time; administration of intranasal glucocorticoids; and mechanical irrigation of the sinus with sterile saline solution. When this management approach fails, sinus surgery may be indicated and sometimes provides significant, albeit short-term, alleviation. Treatment of chronic fungal sinusitis consists of surgical removal of impacted mucus. Recurrence, unfortunately, is common.

INFECTIONS OF THE EAR AND MASTOID

Infections of the ear and associated structures can involve both the middle and external ear, including the skin, cartilage, periosteum, ear canal, and tympanic and mastoid cavities. Both viruses and bacteria are known causes of these infections, some of which result in significant morbidity if not treated appropriately.

INFECTIONS OF THE EXTERNAL EAR STRUCTURES ■ **Auricular Cellulitis** Auricular cellulitis is an infection of the skin overlying the external ear and typically follows minor local trauma. It presents with the typical signs and symptoms of a skin/soft tissue infection, with tenderness, ery-

thema, swelling, and warmth of the external ear (particularly the lobule) but without apparent involvement of the ear canal or inner structures. Treatment consists of warm compresses and oral antibiotics such as dicloxacillin that are active against typical skin and soft tissue pathogens (specifically, *S. aureus* and streptococci). Intravenous antibiotics, such as a first-generation cephalosporin (e.g., cefazolin) or a penicillinase-resistant penicillin (e.g., nafcillin) are occasionally needed for more severe cases.

Perichondritis Perichondritis, an infection of the perichondrium of the auricular cartilage, typically follows local trauma (e.g., ear piercing, burns, or lacerations). Occasionally, when the infection spreads down to the cartilage of the pinna itself, patients may also have chondritis. The infection may closely resemble auricular cellulitis, with erythema, swelling, and extreme tenderness of the pinna, although the lobule is less often involved in perichondritis. The most common pathogens are *P. aeruginosa* and *S. aureus*, although other gram-negative and gram-positive organisms are occasionally involved. Treatment consists of systemic antibiotics active against both *P. aeruginosa* and *S. aureus*. An antipseudomonal penicillin (e.g., piperacillin) or a combination of a penicillinase-resistant penicillin plus an antipseudomonal quinolone (e.g., nafcillin plus ciprofloxacin) is typically used. Incision and drainage may be helpful for culture and for resolution of infection, which often takes weeks.

Otitis Externa The term *otitis externa* refers to a collection of diseases involving primarily the auditory meatus. Otitis externa usually results from a combination of heat, retained moisture, and desquamation and maceration of the outer canal epithelium. The disease exists in a number of forms, which are identified as localized, diffuse, chronic, or invasive. They are all predominantly bacterial in origin, with *P. aeruginosa* and *S. aureus* the most common pathogens.

Acute localized otitis externa (furunculosis) can develop in the outer third of the ear canal, where skin overlies cartilage and hair follicles are numerous. As with furunculosis elsewhere on the body, *S. aureus* is the usual pathogen, and treatment typically consists of an oral antistaphylococcal penicillin (e.g., dicloxacillin), with incision and drainage in cases of abscess formation.

Acute diffuse otitis externa is also known as "swimmer's ear," although it can develop in the absence of swimming. Heat, humidity, and the loss of protective cerumen lead to excessive moisture and elevation of the pH in the ear canal, which in turn lead to skin maceration and irritation. Infection may then occur; the predominant pathogen is *P. aeruginosa*, although other gram-negative and gram-positive organisms have been recovered from patients with this condition. The illness often starts with itching and progresses to severe pain, which is usually triggered by manipulation of the pinna or tragus. The onset of pain is usually accompanied by the development of an erythematous, swollen ear canal, often with scant white, clumpy discharge. Treatment consists of cleansing the canal to remove debris and to enhance the activity of topical therapies—usually hypertonic saline or mixtures of alcohol and acetic acid. Inflammation can also be decreased by adding glucocorticoids to the treatment regimen or by using Burow's solution (aluminum acetate in water). Antibiotics are most effective when given topically. Otic mixtures provide adequate pathogen coverage; these preparations usually combine neomycin with polymyxin, with or without glucocorticoids.

Chronic otitis externa is caused primarily by repeated local irritation, most commonly arising from persistent drainage from a chronic middle-ear infection. Other causes of repeated irritation, such as cotton swabs or other foreign objects inserted into the ear canal, can lead to this condition, as can rare chronic infections such as syphilis, tuberculosis, or leprosy. Chronic otitis externa typically presents as erythematous, scaling dermatitis in which the predominant symptom is pruritus rather than pain; this condition must be differentiated from several others that produce a similar clinical picture, such as atopic dermatitis, seborrheic dermatitis, psoriasis, and dermatomycosis. Therapy consists of identifying and treating or removing the offending process, although successful resolution is frequently difficult.

Invasive otitis externa, also known as "malignant" or "necrotizing" otitis externa, is an aggressive and potentially life-threatening disease that occurs predominantly in elderly diabetics and other immunocompromised patients. The disease begins in the external canal, progresses slowly over weeks to months, and often is difficult to distinguish from a severe case of chronic otitis externa because of the presence of purulent otorrhea and an erythematous swollen ear and external canal. Severe, deep-seated otalgia is often noted and can help differentiate invasive from chronic otitis externa. The characteristic finding on examination is granulation tissue in the posteroinferior wall of the external canal, near the junction of bone and cartilage. If left unchecked, the infection can migrate to the base of the skull (resulting in skull-base osteomyelitis) and on to the meninges and brain, with a high associated mortality rate. Cranial nerve involvement is occasionally seen, with the facial nerve usually affected first and most often. Thrombosis of the sigmoid sinus can occur if the infection extends to that area. CT, which can reveal osseous erosion of the temporal bone and skull base, can be used to help determine the extent of disease, as can gallium and technetium-99 scintigraphy studies. *P. aeruginosa* is by far the most common pathogen involved, although *S. aureus*, *Staphylococcus epidermidis*, *Aspergillus*, *Actinomyces*, and some gram-negative bacteria have been associated with this disease. Cleansing of the external canal and biopsy of the granulation tissue within the canal (or of deeper tissues) should be performed in all cases to isolate the offending organism in culture. Intravenous antibiotic therapy is directed specifically toward the recovered pathogen. For *P. aeruginosa*, the regimen typically includes an antipseudomonal penicillin or cephalosporin (e.g., piperacillin or ceftazidime) with an aminoglycoside. A fluoroquinolone antibiotic is frequently used in place of the aminoglycoside and can even be administered orally, given its excellent bioavailability. Antibiotic drops containing an agent active against *Pseudomonas* (e.g., ciprofloxacin) are also usually prescribed and are combined with glucocorticoids to reduce inflammation. Cases of invasive *Pseudomonas* otitis externa recognized in the early stages can sometimes be treated with oral and otic fluoroquinolones alone, albeit with close follow-up. Extensive surgical debridement, once an important component of the treatment approach, is now rarely indicated.

INFECTIONS OF MIDDLE-EAR STRUCTURES *Otitis media* is an inflammatory condition of the middle ear that results from dysfunction of the eustachian tube in association with a number of illnesses, including URIs and chronic rhinosinusitis. The inflammatory response to these conditions leads to the development of a sterile transudate within the middle-ear and mastoid cavities. Infection may occur if bacteria or viruses from the nasopharynx contaminate this fluid, producing an acute (or sometimes chronic) illness.

Acute Otitis Media Acute otitis media results when pathogens from the nasopharynx are introduced into the inflammatory fluid collected in the middle ear—e.g., by nose blowing during a URI. The proliferation of these pathogens in this space leads to the development of the typical signs and symptoms of acute middle-ear infection. The diagnosis of acute otitis media requires the demonstration of fluid in the middle ear (with tympanic membrane immobility) and the accompanying signs or symptoms of local or systemic illness (Table 27-1).

ETIOLOGY Acute otitis media typically follows a viral URI. The causative viruses (most commonly RSV, influenza virus, rhinovirus, and enterovirus) can themselves cause subsequent acute otitis media; more often, they predispose the patient to bacterial otitis media. Studies using tympanocentesis have consistently found *S. pneumoniae* to be the most important bacterial cause, isolated in up to 35% of cases. *H. influenzae* (nontypable strains) and *M. catarrhalis* are also common bacterial causes of acute otitis media. Viruses, such as those mentioned above, have been recovered either alone or with bacteria in 17 to 40% of cases.

MANIFESTATIONS Fluid in the middle ear is typically demonstrated or confirmed with pneumatic otoscopy. In the absence of fluid, the tympanic membrane moves visibly with the application of positive and

negative pressure, but this movement is dampened when fluid is present. With bacterial infection, the tympanic membrane can also be erythematous, bulging, or retracted and occasionally can spontaneously perforate. The signs and symptoms accompanying infection can be local or systemic, including otalgia, otorrhea, diminished hearing, fever, or irritability. Erythema of the tympanic membrane is often evident but is nonspecific as it is frequently seen in association with inflammation of the upper respiratory mucosa (e.g., during examination of young children). Other signs and symptoms occasionally reported include vertigo, nystagmus, and tinnitus.

℞ TREATMENT

There has been considerable debate on the usefulness of antibiotics for the treatment of acute otitis media. Although most cases resolve clinically 1 week after the onset of illness, there appears to be some benefit to the use of antibiotics, with a higher proportion of treated than of untreated patients free of illness 3 to 5 days after diagnosis. The difficulty of predicting which patients will benefit from antibiotic therapy has led to different approaches. In the Netherlands, for instance, physicians typically manage acute otitis media with initial observation and aggressive pain management with anti-inflammatory therapy, reserving antibiotics for high-risk patients, patients with complicated disease, or patients who do not improve after 48 to 72 h. In contrast, many experts in the United States continue to recommend antibiotic therapy for children <2 years old in light of the higher frequency of secondary complications in this young and functionally immunocompromised population.

Given that most studies of the etiologic agents of acute otitis media consistently document similar pathogen profiles, therapy is generally empirical except in those few cases where tympanocentesis is warranted—e.g., cases in newborns, cases refractory to therapy, or cases in patients who are severely ill or who have an immune deficiency. Despite resistance to penicillin and amoxicillin in roughly one-quarter of *S. pneumoniae* isolates, one-third of *H. influenzae* isolates, and nearly all *M. catarrhalis* isolates, outcome studies continue to find that amoxicillin is as successful as any other agent, and it remains the drug of first choice in recommendations from the Centers for Disease Control and Prevention (CDC; Table 27-1). Therapy is typically administered for 5 to 7 days for uncomplicated acute otitis media; longer courses (e.g., 10 days) have traditionally been prescribed, but evidence suggests that this duration should be reserved for complicated cases or for children <2 years old, in whom short-course therapy may be inadequate.

A switch in regimen is recommended if there is no clinical improvement by the third day of therapy, given the possibility of infection with a β-lactamase-producing strain of *H. influenzae* or *M. catarrhalis* or with a strain of penicillin-resistant *S. pneumoniae*. Decongestants and antihistamines are frequently used as adjunctive therapy to reduce congestion and relieve obstruction of the eustachian tube, but clinical trials have yielded no significant evidence of benefit with either class of agents.

Recurrent Acute Otitis Media Recurrent acute otitis media (more than three episodes within 6 months or four episodes within 12 months) is generally due to relapse or reinfection, although data indicate that the majority of early recurrences are new infections. In general, the same pathogens responsible for acute otitis media cause recurrent disease; even so, the recommended treatment consists of antibiotics active against β-lactamase-producing organisms. Antibiotic prophylaxis for patients with recurrent acute otitis media [e.g., with trimethoprim-sulfamethoxazole (TMP-SMX) or amoxicillin] can reduce recurrences by an average of one episode per year, but this benefit is small compared with the cost of the drug and the high likelihood of colonization with antibiotic-resistant pathogens. Other approaches, including placement of tympanostomy tubes, adenoidectomy, and tonsillectomy plus adenoidectomy, are of questionable overall value, given the relatively small benefit compared with the potential for complications.

Serous Otitis Media   Serous otitis media, or otitis media with effusion, exists when fluid is present in the middle ear for an extended period and in the absence of signs and symptoms of infection. In general, acute effusions are self-limited; most resolve in 2 to 4 weeks. In some cases, however (in particular after an episode of acute otitis media), effusions can persist for months. These chronic effusions are often associated with a significant hearing loss in the affected ear. In younger children, persistent effusions and decreased hearing can be associated with impairment of language acquisition skills. The great majority of cases of otitis media with effusion resolve spontaneously within 3 months without antibiotic therapy. Antibiotic therapy or myringotomy with insertion of tympanostomy tubes is typically reserved for patients in whom bilateral effusion (1) has persisted for at least 3 months and (2) is associated with significant bilateral hearing loss. With this conservative approach and the application of strict diagnostic criteria for acute otitis media and otitis media with effusion, it is estimated that 6 to 8 million courses of antibiotics could be avoided each year.

Chronic Otitis Media   Chronic suppurative otitis media is characterized by persistent or recurrent purulent otorrhea in the setting of tympanic membrane perforation. Usually, there is also some degree of conductive hearing loss. This condition is sometimes divided into two subcategories: active and inactive. Inactive disease is characterized by a central perforation of the tympanic membrane, which allows drainage of purulent fluid from the middle ear. When the perforation is more peripheral, squamous epithelium from the auditory canal may invade the middle ear through the perforation, forming a mass of keratinaceous debris (*cholesteatoma*) at the site of invasion. This mass can enlarge and has the potential to erode bone and promote further infection, which can lead to meningitis, brain abscess, or paralysis of cranial nerve VII. Treatment of chronic active otitis media is surgical; mastoidectomy, myringoplasty, and tympanoplasty can be performed as outpatient surgical procedures, with an overall success rate of ~80%. Chronic inactive otitis media is more difficult to cure, usually requiring repeated courses of topical antibiotic drops during periods of drainage. Systemic antibiotics may offer better cure rates, but their role in the treatment of this condition remains unclear.

Mastoiditis   Acute mastoiditis was a relatively common condition in children before the introduction of antibiotics. Because the mastoid air cells connect with the middle ear, the process of fluid collection and infection in the mastoid is usually the same as in the middle ear. Early and frequent treatment of acute otitis media is most likely the reason that the incidence of acute mastoiditis has declined to only 1.2 to 2.0 cases per 100,000 person-years in countries with high prescribing rates for acute otitis media. In countries like the Netherlands, where antibiotics are used sparingly for acute otitis media, the incidence rate of acute mastoiditis is roughly twice that seen in countries like the United States. However, neighboring Denmark has a rate of acute mastoiditis similar to that in the Netherlands but an antibiotic-prescribing rate for acute otitis media more similar to that in the United States.

In typical acute mastoiditis, purulent exudate collects in the mastoid air cells, producing pressure that may result in erosion of the surrounding bone and the formation of abscess-like cavities that are usually evident on CT. Patients typically present with pain, erythema, and swelling of the mastoid process along with displacement of the pinna, usually in conjunction with the typical signs and symptoms of acute middle-ear infection. Rarely, patients can develop severe complications if the infection tracks under the periosteum of the temporal bone to cause a subperiosteal abscess, erodes through the mastoid tip to cause a deep neck abscess, or extends posteriorly to cause septic thrombosis of the lateral sinus.

Cultures of purulent fluid should be performed whenever possible to help guide antimicrobial therapy. Initial empirical therapy is usually directed against the typical organisms associated with acute otitis me-

dia, such as *S. pneumoniae*, *H. influenzae*, and *M. catarrhalis*. Some patients with more severe or prolonged courses of illness should be treated for infection with *S. aureus* and gram-negative bacilli (including *Pseudomonas*). Broad empirical therapy is usually narrowed once culture results become available. Most patients can be treated conservatively with intravenous antibiotics; surgery (cortical mastoidectomy) can be reserved for complicated cases and those in which conservative treatment has failed.

INFECTIONS OF THE PHARYNX AND ORAL CAVITY

Oropharyngeal infections range from mild, self-limited viral illnesses to serious, life-threatening bacterial infections. The most common presenting symptom is sore throat—one of the most frequent reasons for ambulatory care visits among adults and children. Although sore throat is a symptom in many noninfectious illnesses as well, the overwhelming majority of patients with a new sore throat have acute pharyngitis of viral or bacterial etiology.

ACUTE PHARYNGITIS   Millions of visits to primary care providers each year are for sore throat; the majority of cases of acute pharyngitis are caused by typical respiratory viruses. The most important source of concern is infection with group A β-hemolytic *Streptococcus* (*S. pyogenes*), which can progress to acute rheumatic fever and acute glomerulonephritis, the risk for both of which can be reduced by timely penicillin therapy.

Etiology   A wide variety of organisms cause acute pharyngitis. The relative importance of the different pathogens can only be estimated, since a significant proportion of cases (~30%) have no identified cause. Respiratory viruses are the most common identifiable cause of acute pharyngitis, with rhinoviruses (~20% of cases) and coronaviruses (at least 5%) accounting for a large proportion. Influenza virus, parainfluenza virus, and adenovirus also account for a measurable share of cases, the latter as part of the more clinically severe syndrome of pharyngoconjunctival fever. Other important but less common viral causes include herpes simplex virus (HSV) types 1 and 2, coxsackievirus A, cytomegalovirus (CMV), and Epstein-Barr virus (EBV). Acute HIV infection can present as acute pharyngitis and should be considered in high-risk populations.

Acute bacterial pharyngitis is typically caused by *S. pyogenes*, which accounts for ~5 to 15% of all cases of acute pharyngitis in adults; rates vary depending on the season and on health care system utilization. Group A streptococcal pharyngitis is primarily a disease of children 5 to 15 years of age; it is uncommon among children <3 years old, as is rheumatic fever. Streptococci of groups C and G account for a minority of cases, although these serogroups are nonrheumatogenic. The remaining bacterial causes of the acute pharyngitis are seen infrequently (<1% each) but should be considered in appropriate exposure groups because of the severity of illness if left untreated; these etiologic agents include *Neisseria gonorrhoeae*, *Corynebacterium diphtheriae*, *Corynebacterium ulcerans*, *Yersinia enterocolitica*, and *Treponema pallidum* (in secondary syphilis). Anaerobic bacteria can also cause acute pharyngitis (*Vincent's angina*) and can contribute to more serious polymicrobial infections, such as peritonsillar or retropharyngeal abscess (see below). Atypical organisms such as *M. pneumoniae* and *C. pneumoniae* have been recovered from patients with acute pharyngitis; whether these agents are commensals or causes of acute infection is debatable.

Manifestations   Although the signs and symptoms accompanying acute pharyngitis are not reliable predictors of the etiologic agent, the clinical presentation occasionally suggests that one etiology is more likely than another. Acute pharyngitis due to respiratory viruses such as rhinovirus or coronavirus is usually not severe and is typically associated with a constellation of coryzal symptoms better characterized as nonspecific URI. Findings on physical examination are uncommon; fever is rare, and tender cervical adenopathy and pharyngeal exudates are not seen. In contrast, acute pharyngitis from influenza virus can be severe and is much more likely to be associated with fever as well as with myalgias, headache, and cough. The presentation of pharyngo-conjunctival fever due to adenovirus infection is similar. Since pharyngeal exudate may be present on examination, this condition can be difficult to differentiate from streptococcal pharyngitis. However, adenoviral pharyngitis is distinguished by the presence of conjunctivitis in one-third to one-half of patients. Acute pharyngitis from primary HSV infection can also mimic streptococcal pharyngitis in some cases, with pharyngeal inflammation and exudate, but the presence of vesicles and shallow ulcers on the palate can help differentiate the two diseases. This HSV syndrome is distinct from pharyngitis caused by coxsackievirus (*herpangina*), which is associated with small vesicles that develop on the soft palate and uvula and then rupture to form shallow white ulcers. Acute exudative pharyngitis coupled with fever, fatigue, generalized lymphadenopathy, and (on occasion) splenomegaly is characteristic of infectious mononucleosis due to EBV or CMV. Acute primary infection with HIV is frequently associated with fever and acute pharyngitis as well as with myalgias, arthralgias, malaise, and occasionally a nonpruritic maculopapular rash, which later may be followed by lymphadenopathy and mucosal ulcerations without exudate.

The clinical features of acute pharyngitis caused by streptococci of groups A, C, and G are all similar, ranging from a relatively mild illness without many accompanying symptoms to clinically severe cases with profound pharyngeal pain, fever, chills, and abdominal pain. A hyperemic pharyngeal membrane with tonsillar hypertrophy and exudate is usually seen, along with tender anterior cervical adenopathy. Coryzal manifestations, including cough, are typically absent; when present, they suggest a viral etiology. Strains of *S. pyogenes* that generate erythrogenic toxin can also produce scarlet fever, characterized by an erythematous rash and strawberry tongue. The other types of acute bacterial pharyngitis (e.g., gonococcal, diphtherial, and yersinial) often present as exudative pharyngitis with or without other clinical features. Their etiologies are often suggested only by the clinical history.

Diagnosis The primary goal of diagnostic testing is to separate acute streptococcal pharyngitis from pharyngitis of other etiologies (particularly viral) so that antibiotics can be prescribed more efficiently for patients to whom they may be beneficial. The most appropriate standard for the diagnosis of streptococcal pharyngitis, however, has not been definitively established. Throat swab culture is generally regarded as such. However, this method cannot distinguish between infection and colonization, and it takes 24 to 48 h to yield results that vary according to technique and culture conditions. Rapid antigen-detection tests offer good specificity (>90%) but lower sensitivity that varies across the clinical spectrum of disease (65 to 90%). Several clinical prediction systems (see Table 27-1) can increase the sensitivity of rapid antigen-detection tests to >90% in controlled settings. Since the sensitivities achieved in routine clinical practice are often lower, several medical and professional societies continue to recommend that all negative rapid antigen-detection tests in children be confirmed by a throat culture to limit transmission and complications of illness caused by group A streptococci. The CDC, the Infectious Diseases Society of America, the American College of Physicians, and the American Academy of Family Physicians do not recommend backup culture when adults have a negative rapid antigen-detection test, however, given the lower prevalence and smaller benefit in this age group.

Cultures and rapid diagnostic tests for other causes of acute pharyngitis, such as influenza virus, adenovirus, HSV, EBV, CMV, and *M. pneumoniae*, are available in some locations and can be used when these infections are suspected. In general, the monospot test for EBV is preferable to an assay for EBV antibodies, since the latter does not distinguish antecedent from current infection. Testing is also available for HIV RNA or antigen (p24) when acute primary HIV infection is suspected. If other bacterial causes are suspected (particularly *N. gonorrhoeae*, *C. diphtheriae*, or *Y. enterocolitica*), specific cultures should be requested since these organisms may be missed on routine throat swab culture.

℞ TREATMENT

Antibiotic treatment of pharyngitis due to *S. pyogenes* confers numerous benefits, including a decrease in the risk of rheumatic fever. The magnitude of this benefit is fairly small, however, since rheumatic fever is now a rare disease, even in untreated patients. When therapy is started within 48 h of illness onset, however, symptom duration is also decreased. An additional benefit of therapy is the potential to reduce the spread of streptococcal pharyngitis, particularly in areas of overcrowding or close contact. Antibiotic therapy for acute pharyngitis is therefore recommended in cases where *S. pyogenes* is confirmed as the etiologic agent by rapid antigen-detection test or throat swab culture. Otherwise, antibiotics should be given in routine cases only when another bacterial cause has been identified. Effective therapy for streptococcal pharyngitis consists of either a single dose of intramuscular benzathine penicillin or a full 10-day course of oral penicillin (Table 27-1). Erythromycin can be used in place of penicillin, although erythromycin resistance among *S. pyogenes* strains in some parts of the world (particularly Europe) can prohibit the use of this drug. Newer (and more expensive) antibiotics are also active against streptococci but offer no greater efficacy than the above agents. Testing for cure is unnecessary and may reveal only chronic colonization. There is no evidence to support antibiotic treatment of group C or G streptococcal pharyngitis or of pharyngitis in which *Mycoplasma* or *Chlamydia* has been recovered. Penicillin prophylaxis (benzathine penicillin G, 1.2 million units intramuscularly every 3 to 4 weeks) is indicated for patients at risk of recurrent rheumatic fever.

Treatment of viral pharyngitis is entirely symptom-based except in infection with influenza virus or HSV. For influenza, a number of therapeutic agents exist, including amantadine, rimantadine, and the two newer agents oseltamivir and zanamivir. All of these agents need to be started within 36 to 48 h of symptom onset to reduce illness duration meaningfully. Of these agents, only oseltamivir and zanamivir are active against both influenza A and influenza B and therefore can be used when local infection patterns are unknown. Oropharyngeal HSV infection sometimes responds to treatment with antiviral agents such as acyclovir, although these drugs are often reserved for patients who are immunosuppressed.

Complications Although rheumatic fever is the best-known complication of acute streptococcal pharyngitis, its risk following acute infection remains quite low. Other complications include acute glomerulonephritis and numerous suppurative conditions, such as peritonsillar abscess (*quinsy*), otitis media, mastoiditis, sinusitis, bacteremia, and pneumonia—all of which occur at extremely low rates. Although antibiotic treatment of acute streptococcal pharyngitis can prevent the development of rheumatic fever, there is no evidence that it can prevent acute glomerulonephritis. Some evidence supports antibiotic use to prevent the suppurative complications of streptococcal pharyngitis, particularly peritonsillar abscess, which can also involve oral anaerobes. Abscesses are usually accompanied by severe pharyngeal pain, dysphagia, and fever, often with medial displacement of the tonsil on examination. Oral penicillin remains the recommended therapy for peritonsillar abscess, with clindamycin as an alternative. Early use of antibiotics in these cases has substantially reduced the need for surgical drainage.

ORAL INFECTIONS Aside from periodontal disease such as gingivitis, infections of the oral cavity most commonly involve HSV or *Candida* species. In addition to causing painful cold sores on the lips, HSV can infect the tongue and buccal mucosa, causing the formation of irritating vesicles. Although topical antiviral agents (such as acyclovir or penciclovir) can be used externally for cold sores, oral or intravenous acyclovir is often needed for primary infections, extensive oral infections, and infections in immunocompromised patients. Oropharyngeal candidiasis (*thrush*) is caused by a variety of *Candida* species, most often *C. albicans*. Thrush occurs predominantly in neonates, immunocompromised patients (especially those with AIDS), and patients who have received prolonged antibiotic or glucocorticoid therapy. In addition to sore throat, patients often complain of a burning tongue, and physical examination reveals friable white or gray plaques on the gingiva, tongue, and oral mucosa. Treatment usually consists of an oral antifungal suspension (nystatin or clotrimazole) or oral fluconazole. In the cases of fluconazole-refractory thrush seen occasionally in patients with AIDS, the limited therapeutic options include oral suspensions of either itraconazole or amphotericin B.

Vincent's angina, also known as *acute necrotizing ulcerative gingivitis* or *trench mouth*, is a unique and dramatic form of gingivitis characterized by painful, inflamed gingiva with ulcerations of the interdental papillae that bleed easily. Since oral anaerobes are the cause, patients typically have halitosis and frequently present with fever, malaise, and lymphadenopathy. Treatment consists of debridement and oral administration of penicillin plus metronidazole, with clindamycin alone as an alternative.

Ludwig's angina is a rapidly progressive, potentially fulminant cellulitis involving the sublingual and submandibular spaces that typically originates from an infected or recently extracted tooth, most commonly the lower second and third molars. Improved dental care has substantially reduced the incidence of this disorder. Infection in these areas leads to dysphagia, odynophagia, and "woody" edema in the sublingual region, forcing the tongue up and back with the potential for airway obstruction. Fever, dysarthria, and drooling may also be noted, and patients may speak in a "hot potato" voice. Intubation or tracheostomy may be necessary to secure the airway, as asphyxiation is the most common cause of death. Patients should be monitored closely and treated promptly with intravenous antibiotics directed against streptococci and oral anaerobes. Recommended agents include ampicillin/sulbactam and high-dose penicillin plus metronidazole.

Postanginal septicemia (Lemierre's disease) is a rare anaerobic oropharyngeal infection caused predominantly by *Fusobacterium necrophorum*. The illness typically starts as a sore throat (most commonly in adolescents and young adults), which may present as exudative tonsillitis or peritonsillar abscess. Infection of the deep pharyngeal tissue allows organisms to drain into the lateral pharyngeal space, which contains the carotid artery and internal jugular vein. Septic thrombophlebitis of the internal jugular vein can result, with associated pain, dysphagia, and neck swelling and stiffness. Sepsis usually occurs 3 to 10 days after the onset of sore throat and is often coupled with metastatic infection to the lung and other distant sites. Occasionally, the infection can extend along the carotid sheath and into the posterior mediastinum, resulting in mediastinitis, or it can erode into the carotid artery, with the early sign of repeated small bleeds into the mouth. The mortality rate from these invasive infections can be as high as 50%. Treatment consists of intravenous antibiotics (penicillin G or clindamycin) and surgical drainage of any purulent collections. The concomitant use of anticoagulants to prevent embolization remains controversial but is often advised.

INFECTIONS OF THE LARYNX AND EPIGLOTTIS

LARYNGITIS *Laryngitis* is defined as any inflammatory process involving the larynx and can be caused by a variety of infectious and noninfectious processes. The vast majority of laryngitis cases seen in clinical practice in developed countries are acute. Acute laryngitis is a common syndrome caused predominantly by the same viruses responsible for many other URIs. In fact, most cases of acute laryngitis occur in the setting of a viral URI.

Etiology Nearly all major respiratory viruses have been implicated in acute viral laryngitis, including rhinovirus, influenza virus, parainfluenza virus, adenovirus, coxsackievirus, coronavirus, and RSV. Acute laryngitis can also be associated with acute bacterial respiratory infections, such as those caused by group A *Streptococcus* or *C. diphtheriae* (although diphtheria has been all but eliminated in the United States).

Another bacterial pathogen thought to play a role (albeit unclear) in the pathogenesis of acute laryngitis is *M. catarrhalis*, which has been recovered on nasopharyngeal culture from a significant percentage of people with acute laryngitis. Chronic laryngitis of infectious etiology is much less common in developed than in developing countries. Laryngitis due to *Mycobacterium tuberculosis* is often difficult to distinguish from laryngeal cancer, in part because of the frequent absence of signs, symptoms, and radiographic findings typical of pulmonary disease. *Histoplasma* and *Blastomyces* may cause laryngitis, often as a complication of systemic infection. *Candida* species can cause laryngitis as well, often in association with thrush or esophagitis and particularly in immunosuppressed patients. Rare cases of chronic laryngitis are due to *Coccidioides* and *Cryptococcus*.

Manifestations Laryngitis is characterized by hoarseness and can also be associated with reduced vocal pitch or aphonia. As acute laryngitis is caused predominantly by respiratory viruses, these symptoms usually occur in association with other symptoms and signs of URI, including rhinorrhea, nasal congestion, cough, and sore throat. Direct laryngoscopy often reveals diffuse laryngeal erythema and edema, along with vascular engorgement of the vocal folds. Chronic disease (e.g., tuberculous laryngitis), in addition, often includes mucosal nodules and ulcerations visible on laryngoscopy; these lesions are sometimes mistaken for laryngeal cancer.

℞ TREATMENT

Acute laryngitis is usually treated with humidification and voice rest alone. Antibiotics are not recommended except when group A *Streptococcus* is cultured, in which case penicillin is the drug of choice. The choice of therapy for chronic laryngitis depends on the pathogen, whose identification usually requires biopsy with culture. Patients with laryngeal tuberculosis are highly contagious because of the large number of organisms that are easily aerosolized. These patients should be managed in the same way as patients with active pulmonary disease.

CROUP The term *croup* actually denotes a group of diseases collectively referred to as "croup syndrome," all of which are acute and predominantly viral respiratory illnesses characterized by marked swelling of the subglottic region of the larynx. Croup primarily affects children <6 years old. For a detailed discussion of this entity, the reader is referred to a text of pediatric medicine.

EPIGLOTTITIS *Acute epiglottitis* (supraglottitis) is an acute, rapidly progressive cellulitis of the epiglottis and adjacent structures that can result in complete—and potentially fatal—airway obstruction in both children and adults. Before the widespread use of *H. influenzae* type b (Hib) vaccine, this entity was much more common among children, with a peak incidence at ~3.5 years of age. In some countries, mass vaccination against Hib has reduced the annual incidence of acute epiglottitis in children by >90%; over the same period, the annual incidence in adults has changed little. Because of the danger of airway obstruction, acute epiglottitis constitutes a medical emergency, particularly in children, and prompt diagnosis and airway protection are of utmost importance.

Etiology After the introduction of the Hib vaccine, disease incidence among children in the United States declined dramatically. Nevertheless, lack of vaccination or vaccine failure have meant that many pediatric cases seen today are still due to Hib. In adults and (more recently) in children, a variety of other bacterial pathogens have been associated with epiglottitis, the most common being group A *Streptococcus*. Other pathogens seen less frequently include *S. pneumoniae*, *Haemophilus parainfluenzae*, and *S. aureus*. Viruses have not yet been established as a cause of acute epiglottitis.

Manifestations and Diagnosis Epiglottitis typically presents more acutely in young children than in adolescents or adults. On presentation, most children have had symptoms for <24 h, including high fever, severe sore throat, tachycardia, systemic toxicity, and (in many cases) drooling while sitting forward. Symptoms and signs of respiratory obstruction may also be present and may progress rapidly. The somewhat milder illness in adolescents and adults often follows 1 or 2 days of severe sore throat and is commonly accompanied by dyspnea, drooling, and stridor. Physical examination of patients with acute epiglottitis may reveal moderate or severe respiratory distress, with inspiratory stridor and retractions of the chest wall. These findings *diminish* as the disease progresses and the patient tires. Conversely, oropharyngeal examination reveals injection that is much less severe than would be predicted from the symptoms—a finding that should alert the clinician to a cause of symptoms and obstruction that lies beyond the tonsils. The diagnosis is often made on clinical grounds, although direct fiberoptic laryngoscopy is frequently performed in a controlled environment (e.g., an operating room) in order to visualize and culture the typical edematous "cherry-red" epiglottis and to facilitate placement of an endotracheal tube. Direct visualization in an examination room (e.g., with a tongue blade and indirect laryngoscopy) is not recommended because of the risk of immediate laryngospasm and complete airway obstruction. Lateral neck radiographs and laboratory tests can assist in the diagnosis but may delay the critical securing of the airway and cause the patient to be excessively moved or repositioned, risking further airway compromise. Neck radiographs typically show an enlarged edematous epiglottis (the "thumbprint sign"), usually with a dilated hypopharynx and normal subglottic structures. Laboratory tests typically show mild to moderate leukocytosis with a predominance of neutrophils. Blood cultures are positive in a significant proportion of cases.

℞ TREATMENT

Security of the airway is always of primary concern in acute epiglottitis, even if the diagnosis is only suspected. Mere observation for signs of impending airway obstruction is not routinely recommended, particularly in children. Many adults have been managed in this way since the illness is perceived to be milder in this age group, but some data suggest that this approach may be risky and probably should be reserved only for adult patients who have yet to develop dyspnea or stridor. Once the airway has been secured and blood and epiglottis specimens have been obtained for culture, treatment with intravenous antibiotics should be given to cover the most likely organisms, particularly *H. influenzae*. Because rates of ampicillin resistance in this organism have risen significantly in recent years, therapy with a β-lactam/β-lactamase inhibitor combination or a second- or third-generation cephalosporin is recommended. Typically, ampicillin/sulbactam, cefuroxime, cefotaxime, or ceftriaxone is given, with clindamycin and TMP-SMX reserved for patients allergic to β-lactams. Antibiotic therapy should be continued for 7 to 10 days and should be tailored, if necessary, to the organism recovered in culture. If the household contacts of a patient with *H. influenzae* epiglottitis include an unvaccinated child under the age of 4, all members of the household (including the patient) should receive prophylactic rifampin for 4 days to eradicate *H. influenzae* carriage.

INFECTIONS OF THE DEEP NECK STRUCTURES

Deep neck infections are usually extensions of infection from other primary sites, most often within the pharynx or oral cavity. Many of these infections are life-threatening but are difficult to detect at early stages when they may be more easily managed. Three of the most clinically relevant spaces in the neck are the submandibular (and sublingual) space, the lateral pharyngeal (or parapharyngeal) space, and the retropharyngeal space. These spaces communicate with one another and with other important structures in the head, neck, and thorax, providing infections with easy access to areas including the mediastinum, carotid sheath, skull base, and meninges. Once infection reaches these sensitive areas, mortality rates can be as high as 20 to 50%.

Infection of the submandibular and/or sublingual space typically originates from an infected or recently extracted lower tooth. The result is the severe, life-threatening infection referred to as Ludwig's angina

(see under "Oral Infections," above). Lateral pharyngeal (or parapharyngeal) space infection is most often a complication of common infections of the oral cavity and upper respiratory tract, including tonsillitis, peritonsillar abscess, pharyngitis, mastoiditis, or periodontal infection. This space, located deep to the lateral wall of the pharynx, contains a number of sensitive structures, including the carotid artery, internal jugular vein, cervical sympathetic chain, and portions of cranial nerves IX through XII; at its distal end, it opens into the posterior mediastinum. Involvement of this space with infection can therefore be rapidly fatal. Examination may reveal some tonsillar displacement, trismus, and neck rigidity, but lateral pharyngeal wall swelling can easily be missed. The diagnosis can be confirmed by CT. Treatment consists of airway management, operative drainage of fluid collections, and at least a 10-day course of intravenous therapy with an antibiotic active against streptococci and oral anaerobes (e.g., ampicillin/sulbactam). A particularly severe form of this infection involving the components of the carotid sheath, called postanginal septicemia (or Lemierre's disease), is described above ("Oral Infections"). Infection of the retropharyngeal space can also be extremely dangerous, as this space runs posterior to the pharynx from the skull base to the superior mediastinum. Infections in this space are more common in children <5 years old because of the presence of several small retropharyngeal lymph nodes that typically atrophy by the age of 4 years. Infection is usually a consequence of extension from another site of infection, most commonly acute pharyngitis. Other sources include otitis media, tonsillitis, dental infections, Ludwig's angina, and anterior extension of vertebral osteomyelitis. Retropharyngeal space infection can also follow penetrating trauma to the posterior pharynx (e.g., from an endoscopic procedure). Infections are commonly polymicrobial, with a mixture of aerobes and anaerobes; group A β-hemolytic streptococci and *S. aureus* are the most common pathogens. Tuberculosis was a frequent cause in the past but now is rarely seen in the United States.

Patients with retropharyngeal abscess typically present with sore throat, fever, dysphagia, and neck pain and are often drooling because of difficulty and pain with swallowing. Examination may reveal tender cervical adenopathy, neck swelling, and diffuse erythema and edema of the posterior pharynx as well as a bulge in the posterior pharyngeal wall, although the latter may not be obvious on routine inspection. A soft tissue mass is usually demonstrable by lateral neck radiography or CT. Because of the risk of airway obstruction, treatment begins with securing of the airway, which is followed by a combination of surgical drainage and intravenous antibiotic administration. Initial empirical therapy should cover streptococci, oral anaerobes, and *S. aureus*; ampicillin/sulbactam, clindamycin alone, or clindamycin plus ceftriaxone is usually effective. Complications occur primarily as a result of extension to other areas, including rupture into the posterior pharynx, which may lead to aspiration pneumonia and empyema. Extension may also occur to the lateral pharyngeal space and mediastinum, resulting in mediastinitis and pericarditis, or into nearby major blood vessels. All these events are associated with a high mortality rate.

FURTHER READING

Bisno AL: Acute pharyngitis. N Engl J Med 344:205, 2001

Cooper RJ et al: Principles of appropriate antibiotic use for acute pharyngitis in adults: Background. Ann Intern Med 134:509, 2001

Gonzales R et al: Principles of appropriate antibiotic use for treatment of nonspecific upper respiratory tract infections in adults: Background. Ann Intern Med 134:490, 2001

——— et al: Principles of appropriate antibiotic use for treatment of uncomplicated acute bronchitis: Background. Ann Intern Med 134:521, 2001

Hickner JM et al: Principles of appropriate antibiotic use for acute rhinosinusitis in adults: Background. Ann Intern Med 2001; 134:498, 2001

O'Brien KL et al: Acute sinusitis—principles of judicious use of antimicrobial agents. Pediatrics 101:174, 1998

Van Zuijlen DA et al: National differences in incidence of acute mastoiditis: Relationship to prescribing patterns of antibiotics for acute otitis media? Pediatr Infect Dis J 20:140, 2001

As primary care physicians and consultants, internists are often asked to evaluate patients with disease of the oral soft tissues, teeth, and pharynx. Knowledge of the oral milieu and its unique structures is necessary to guide preventive services and recognize oral manifestations of local or systemic disease. Furthermore, internists frequently collaborate with dentists in the care of patients with a variety of medical conditions that impact oral health or who undergo dental procedures that increase the patient's risk of medical complications.

DISEASES OF THE TEETH AND PERIODONTAL STRUCTURES ■ **Tooth and Periodontal Structure** Tooth formation begins during the sixth week of embryonic life and continues through the first 17 years of age. Tooth development begins in utero and continues until after the tooth erupts. Normally all 20 deciduous teeth have erupted by age 3 and have been shed by age 13. Permanent teeth, eventually totaling 32, begin to erupt by age 6 and have completely erupted by age 14, though third molars (wisdom teeth) may erupt later.

The erupted tooth consists of the visible crown covered with enamel and the root submerged below the gum line and covered with bonelike cementum. *Dentin*, a material that is denser than bone and exquisitely sensitive to pain, forms the majority of the tooth substance. Dentin surrounds a core of myxomatous *pulp* containing the vascular and nerve supply. The tooth is held firmly in the alveolar socket by the *periodontium*, supporting structures that consist of the gingivae, alveolar bone, cementum, and periodontal ligament. The periodontal ligament tenaciously binds the tooth's cementum to the alveolar bone. Above this ligament is a collar of attached gingiva just below the crown. A few millimeters of unattached or free gingiva (1 to 3 mm) overlaps the base of the crown, forming a shallow sulcus along the gum-tooth margin.

Dental Caries, Pulpal and Periapical Disease, and Complications Dental caries begin asymptomatically as a destructive process of the hard surface of the tooth. *Streptococcus mutans*, principally, along with other bacteria colonize the organic buffering film on the tooth surface to produce *plaque*. If not removed by brushing or the natural cleaning action of saliva and oral soft tissues, bacterial acids demineralize the enamel. Fissures and pits on the occlusion surfaces are the most frequent sites of decay. Surfaces adjacent to tooth restorations and exposed roots are also vulnerable, particularly as teeth are retained in an aging population. Over time dental caries extend to the underlying dentin, leading to cavitation of the enamel and ultimately penetration to the tooth pulp, producing *acute pulpitis*. At this early stage when the pulp infection is limited, the tooth becomes sensitive to percussion and hot or cold, and pain resolves immediately when the irritating stimulus is removed. Should the infection spread throughout the pulp, *irreversible pulpitis* occurs leading to pulp necrosis. At this late stage pain is severe and has a sharp or throbbing visceral quality that may be worse when the patient lies down. Once pulp necrosis is complete, pain may be constant or intermittent, but cold sensitivity is lost.

Treatment of caries involves removal of the softened and infected hard tissue; sealing the exposed dentin; and restoration of the tooth structure with silver amalgam, composite plastic, gold, or porcelain. Once irreversible pulpitis occurs, root canal therapy is necessary and the contents of the pulp chamber and root canals are removed, followed by thorough cleaning, antisepsis, and filling with an inert material. Alternatively, the tooth may be extracted.

Pulpal infection, if it does not egress through the decayed enamel, leads to *periapical abscess* formation, which produces pain on chewing. If the infection is mild and chronic, a *periapical granuloma* or eventually a *periapical cyst* forms, either of which produces radiolucency at the root apex. When unchecked, a periapical abscess can erode into the alveolar bone producing osteomyelitis, penetrate and drain through the gingivae (*parulis* or *gumboil*), or track along deep fascial planes producing a virulent cellulitis (*Ludwig's angina*) involving the submandibular space and floor of the mouth (Chap. 148). Elderly patients, those with diabetes mellitus, and patients taking glucocorticoids may experience little or no pain and fever as these complications develop.

Periodontal Disease Periodontal disease accounts for more tooth loss than caries, particularly in the elderly. Like dental caries, chronic infection of the gingiva and anchoring structures of the tooth begins with formation of bacterial plaque. The process begins invisibly above the gum line and in the gingival sulcus. Plaque, including mineralized plaque (*calculus*), is preventable by appropriate dental hygiene, including periodic professional cleaning. Left undisturbed, chronic inflammation ensues and produces a painless hyperemia of the free and attached gingivae (*gingivitis*) that typically bleeds with brushing. If ignored, severe *periodontitis* occurs, leading to deepening of the physiologic sulcus and destruction of the periodontal ligament. Pockets develop around the teeth that become filled with pus and debris. As the periodontium is destroyed, teeth loosen and exfoliate. Eventually there is resorption of the alveolar bone.

Acute and aggressive forms of periodontal disease are seen less commonly than the chronic forms described above. However, if the host is stressed or exposed to a new pathogen, rapidly progressive and destructive disease of the periodontal tissue can occur. A virulent example is *acute necrotizing ulcerative gingivitis* (ANUG), or *Vincent's infection*, characterized as "trench mouth" during World War I. Stress, poor oral hygiene, and tobacco and alcohol use are risk factors. The presentation includes sudden gingival inflammation, ulceration, bleeding, interdental gingival necrosis, and fetid halitosis. *Localized juvenile periodontitis*, seen in adolescents, is particularly destructive and appears to be associated with impaired neutrophil chemotaxis. *AIDS-related periodontitis* resembles ANUG in some patients or a more destructive form of adult chronic periodontitis in others. It may also produce a gangrene-like destructive process of the oral soft tissues and bone that resembles *noma*, seen in severely malnourished children in developing nations.

Prevention of Tooth Decay and Periodontal Infection Despite the reduced prevalence of dental caries and periodontal disease in the United States due in large part to water fluoridation and improved dental care, respectively, both diseases constitute a major public health problem worldwide and for certain groups. The internist can promote prevention by including questions about dental care and hygiene as part of health maintenance. Special populations at high risk for dental caries and periodontal disease include those with xerostomia (Sjögren's syndrome, drug-induced, postirradiation head and neck), diabetics, alcoholics, tobacco users, those with Down's syndrome, and those with gingival hyperplasia. Furthermore, patients lacking dental care access (low socioeconomic status) and those with reduced ability to provide self-care (e.g., nursing-home residents, those with dementia or upper extremity disability) suffer at a disproportionate rate. It is important to provide counseling regarding regular dental hygiene and professional cleaning, use of fluoride-containing toothpaste, professional fluoride treatments, and use of electric toothbrushes for patients with limited dexterity and to give instruction to caregivers for those unable to perform self-care.

Developmental and Systemic Disease Affecting the Teeth and Periodontium Malocclusion is the most common developmental problem, which in addition to a problem with cosmesis, can interfere with mastication unless corrected through orthodontic techniques. Impacted third molars are common and occasionally become infected. Acquired prognathism due to *acromegaly* may also lead to malocclusion, as may deformity of the maxilla and mandible due to *Paget's disease* of the bone. Delayed tooth eruption, receding chin, and a protruding tongue are occasional features of *cretinism* and *hypopituitarism*. Congenital syphilis produces tapering, notched (*Hutchinson's*) incisors and finely nodular (*mulberry*) molar crowns.

Enamel hypoplasia results in crown defects ranging from pits to deep fissures of primary or permanent teeth. Intrauterine infection (syphilis, rubella), vitamin deficiency (A, C, or D), disorders of calcium metabolism (malabsorption, vitamin D–resistant rickets, hypoparathyroidism), prematurity, high fever, or rare inherited defects (*amelogenesis imperfecta*) are all causes. Tetracycline, given in sufficiently high doses during the first 8 years, may produce enamel hypoplasia and discoloration. Exposure to endogenous pigments can discolor developing teeth: *erythroblastosis fetalis* (green or bluish-black), congenital liver disease (green or yellow-brown), and porphyria (red or brown that fluoresces with ultraviolet light). *Mottled enamel* occurs if excessive fluoride is ingested during development. Worn enamel is seen with age, bruxism, or excessive acid exposure (e.g., chronic gastric reflux or bulimia).

Premature tooth loss resulting from periodontitis is seen with cyclic neutropenia, Papillon-Lefèvre syndrome, Chédiak-Higashi syndrome, and leukemia. Rapid focal tooth loosening is most often due to infection, but rarer causes include histiocytosis X, Ewing's sarcoma, osteosarcoma, or Burkitt's lymphoma. Early loss of primary teeth is a feature of *hypophosphatasia*, a rare inborn error of metabolism.

Pregnancy may produce severe gingivitis and localized *pyogenic granulomas*. Severe periodontal disease occurs with *Down's syndrome* and *diabetes mellitus*. *Gingival hyperplasia* may be caused by phenytoin, calcium channel blockers (e.g., nifedipine), and cyclosporine. *Idiopathic familial gingival fibromatosis* and several syndrome-related disorders appear similar. Removal of the medication often reverses the drug-induced form, though surgery may be needed to control both. *Linear gingival erythema* is variably seen in patients with advanced HIV infection and probably represents immune deficiency and decreased polymorphonuclear activity. Diffuse or focal gingival swelling may be a feature of early or late *acute myelomonocytic leukemia* as well as of other lymphoproliferative disorders. A rare, but pathognomonic, sign of Wegener's granulomatosis is a red-purplish, granular gingivitis (*strawberry gums*).

DISEASES OF THE ORAL MUCOSA ■ **Infection**   Most oral mucosal diseases involve microorganisms (Table 28-1).

Pigmented Lesions   See Table 28-2

Dermatologic Diseases   See Tables 28-1, 28-2, and 28-3 and Chaps. 46 to 51

Diseases of the Tongue   See Table 28-4

HIV Disease and AIDS   See Tables 28-1, 28-2, 28-3, and 28-5; Chaps. 172 and 173; and see Figs. 165-1 and 187-1.

Ulcers   Ulceration is the most common oral mucosal lesion encountered. Although there are many possible causes, the host and pattern of lesions, including the presence of systemic features, narrow the differential diagnosis (Table 28-1). Most acute ulcers are painful and self-limited. Recurrent *aphthous ulcers* and herpes simplex infection constitute the majority. Persistent and deep aphthous ulcers can be idiopathic or seen with HIV/AIDS. Aphthous lesions are often the presenting symptom in *Behçet's disease*. Similar appearing, though less painful, lesions may occur with *Reiter's syndrome*, and aphthous ulcers are occasionally present during phases of discoid or *systemic lupus erythematosus*. Aphthous-like ulcers are seen in *Crohn's disease*, but unlike the common aphthous variety, they may exhibit granulomatous inflammation histologically. Recurrent aphthae in some patients with *celiac disease* have been reported to remit with elimination of gluten.

Of major concern are chronic, relatively painless ulcers and mixed red/white patches (*erythroplakia* and *leukoplakia*) of more than 2 weeks' duration. *Squamous cell carcinoma* and *premalignant dysplasia* should be considered early and a diagnostic biopsy obtained. The importance is underscored because early-stage malignancy is vastly more treatable than late-stage disease. High risk sites include the lower lip, floor of the mouth, ventral and lateral tongue, and soft palate–tonsillar pillar complex. Significant risk factors for oral cancer in western countries includes sun-exposure (lower lip) and tobacco and al-

cohol use. In India and some other Asian countries, smokeless tobacco mixed with betel nut, slaked lime, and spices is a common cause of oral cancer. Less common etiologies include syphilis and Plummer-Vinson syndrome.

Rarer causes of chronic ulcer such as tuberculosis, fungal infection, Wegener's granulomatosis, and midline granuloma may look identical to carcinoma. Making the correct diagnosis depends on recognizing other clinical features and biopsy of the lesion. The syphilitic *chancre* is typically painless and therefore easily missed. Regional lymphadenopathy is invariably present. Confirmation is achieved using appropriate bacterial and serologic tests.

Disorders of mucosal fragility often produce painful oral ulcers that fail to heal within 2 weeks. *Mucous membrane pemphigoid* and *pemphigus vulgaris* are the major acquired disorders. While clinical features are often distinctive, immunohistochemical examination should be performed for diagnosis and to distinguish these entities from *lichen planus* and drug reactions.

Hematologic and Nutritional Disease   Internists are more likely to encounter patients with acquired, rather than congenital, bleeding disorders. Bleeding after minor trauma should stop after 15 min and within an hour of tooth extraction if local pressure is applied. Bleeding in excess of this, if not due to continued injury or rupture of a large vessel, should lead to investigation for a clotting abnormality. In addition to bleeding, petechiae and ecchymoses are prone to occur at the line of vibration between the soft and hard palates in patients with platelet dysfunction or thrombocytopenia.

All forms of leukemia, but particularly *acute myelomonocytic leukemia*, can produce gingival bleeding, ulcers, and gingival enlargement. Oral ulcers are a feature of *agranulocytosis*, and ulcers and mucositis are often severe complications of chemotherapy and radiation therapy for hematologic and other malignancies. *Plummer-Vinson syndrome* (iron deficiency, angular stomatitis, glossitis, and dysphagia) raises the risk of oral squamous cell cancer and esophageal cancer at the postcricoidal tissue web. Atrophic papillae and a red, burning tongue may occur with *pernicious anemia*. *B group vitamin deficiencies* produce many of these same symptoms as well as oral ulceration and cheilosis. Swollen, bleeding gums, ulcers, and loosening of the teeth are a consequence of *scurvy*.

NONDENTAL CAUSES OF ORAL PAIN   Most oral pain emanates from inflamed or injured tooth pulp or periodontal tissues, and this fact often leads clinicians to overlook nonodontogenic causes. In most instances toothache is predictable and proportional to the stimulus applied and an identifiable condition (e.g., caries, abscess) is found. Local anesthesia eliminates pain originating from dental or periodontal structures, but not referred pains. The most common nondental origin is myofascial pain referred from muscles of mastication. The masticatory muscles are tender and ache with increased use. Many sufferers exhibit bruxism that is secondary to stress and anxiety. *Temporomandibular disorder* is closely related. It predominantly affects females between ages 15 and 45. Features include pain, limited mandibular movement, and temporomandibular joint sounds. The etiologies are complex, and malocclusion does not play the primary role once attributed to it. *Osteoarthritis* is a common cause of masticatory pain. Anti-inflammatory medication, jaw rest, soft foods, and heat provide relief. With treatment complete, remission of pain is the rule. The temporomandibular joint is involved in 50% of patients with *rheumatoid arthritis* and is usually a late feature of severe disease. Bilateral preauricular pain, particularly in the morning, limits range of motion.

Migrainous neuralgia is sometimes so localized to the mouth as to present a diagnostic challenge. Episodes of pain and remission without identifiable cause and absence of relief with local anesthesia are important clues. *Trigeminal neuralgia* (*tic douloureux*) may involve the entire branch or part of the mandibular or maxillary branches of the fifth cranial nerve and produce pain in one or a few teeth. Pain may occur spontaneously or may be triggered by touching the lip or gin-

Condition	Usual Location	Clinical Features	Course
VIRAL DISEASES			
Primary acute herpetic gingivostomatitis [herpes simplex virus (HSV) type 1, rarely type 2]	Lip and oral mucosa (buccal, gingival, lingual mucosa)	Labial vesicles that rupture and crust, and intraoral vesicles that quickly ulcerate; extremely painful; acute gingivitis, fever, malaise, foul odor, and cervical lymphadenopathy; occurs primarily in infants, children, and young adults	Heals spontaneously in 10–14 days. Unless secondarily infected, lesions lasting >3 weeks are not due to primary HSV infection.
Recurrent herpes labialis	Mucocutaneous junction of lip, perioral skin	Eruption of groups of vesicles that may coalesce, then rupture and crust; painful to pressure or spicy foods	Lasts about 1 week, but condition may be prolonged if secondarily infected. If severe, topical or oral antiviral may reduce healing time.
Recurrent intraoral herpes simplex	Palate and gingiva	Small vesicles on keratinized epithelium that rupture and coalesce; painful	Heals spontaneously in about 1 week. If severe, topical or oral antiviral may reduce healing time.
Chickenpox (varicella-zoster virus)	Gingiva and oral mucosa	Skin lesions may be accompanied by small vesicles on oral mucosa that rupture to form shallow ulcers; may coalesce to form large bullous lesions that ulcerate; mucosa may have generalized erythema	Lesions heal spontaneously within 2 weeks.
Herpes zoster (reactivation of varicella-zoster virus)	Cheek, tongue, gingiva, or palate	Unilateral vesicular eruptions and ulceration in linear pattern following sensory distribution of trigeminal nerve or one of its branches	Gradual healing without scarring unless secondarily infected; postherpetic neuralgia is common. Oral acyclovir, famcyclovir, or valacylovir reduce healing time and postherpetic neuralgia
Infectious mononucleosis (Epstein-Barr virus)	Oral mucosa	Fatigue, sore throat, malaise, fever, and cervical lymphadenopathy; numerous small ulcers usually appear several days before lymphadenopathy; gingival bleeding and multiple petechiae at junction of hard and soft palates	Oral lesions disappear during convalescence; no treatment though glucocorticoids indicated if tonsillar swelling compromises airway
Herpangina (coxsackievirus A; also possibly coxsackie B and echovirus)	Oral mucosa, pharynx, tongue	Sudden onset of fever, sore throat, and oropharyngeal vesicles, usually in children under 4 years, during summer months; diffuse pharyngeal congestion and vesicles (1–2 mm), grayish-white surrounded by red areola; vesicles enlarge and ulcerate	Incubation period 2–9 days; fever for 1–4 days; recovery uneventful
Hand, foot, and mouth disease (coxsackievirus A16 most common)	Oral mucosa, pharynx, palms, and soles	Fever, malaise, headache with oropharyngeal vesicles that become painful, shallow ulcers; highly infectious; usually affects children under age 10	Incubation period 2–18 days; lesions heal spontaneously in 2–4 weeks
Primary HIV infection	Gingiva, palate, and pharynx	Acute gingivitis and oropharyngeal ulceration, associated with febrile illness resembling mononucleosis and including lymphadenopathy	Followed by HIV seroconversion, asymptomatic HIV infection, and usually ultimately by HIV disease
BACTERIAL OR FUNGAL DISEASES			
Acute necrotizing ulcerative gingivitis ("trench mouth," Vincent's infection)	Gingiva	Painful, bleeding gingiva characterized by necrosis and ulceration of gingival papillae and margins plus lymphadenopathy and foul odor	Debridement and diluted (1:3) peroxide lavage provide relief within 24 h; antibiotics in acutely ill patients; relapse may occur
Prenatal (congenital) syphilis	Palate, jaws, tongue, and teeth	Gummatous involvement of palate, jaws, and facial bones; Hutchinson's incisors, mulberry molars, glossitis, mucous patches, and fissures on corner of mouth	Tooth deformities in permanent dentition irreversible
Primary syphilis (chancre)	Lesion appears where organism enters body; may occur on lips, tongue, or tonsillar area	Small papule developing rapidly into a large, painless ulcer with indurated border; unilateral lymphadenopathy; chancre and lymph nodes containing spirochetes; serologic tests positive by third to fourth weeks	Healing of chancre in 1–2 months, followed by secondary syphilis in 6–8 weeks
Secondary syphilis	Oral mucosa frequently involved with mucous patches, primarily on palate, also at commissures of mouth	Maculopapular lesions of oral mucosa, 5–10 mm in diameter with central ulceration covered by grayish membrane; eruptions occurring on various mucosal surfaces and skin accompanied by fever, malaise, and sore throat	Lesions may persist from several weeks to a year
Tertiary syphilis	Palate and tongue	Gummatous infiltration of palate or tongue followed by ulceration and fibrosis; atrophy of tongue papillae produces characteristic bald tongue and glossitis	Gumma may destroy palate, causing complete perforation

(continued)

TABLE 28-1—(Continued)

Condition	Usual Location	Clinical Features	Course
Gonorrhea	Lesions may occur in mouth at site of inoculation or secondarily by hematogenous spread from a primary focus elsewhere	Most pharyngeal infection is asymptomatic; may produce burning or itching sensation; oropharynx and tonsils may be ulcerated and erythematous; saliva viscous and fetid	More difficult to eradicate than urogenital infection, though pharyngitis usually resolves with appropriate antimicrobial treatment
Tuberculosis	Tongue, tonsillar area, soft palate	A painless, solitary, 1–5 cm, irregular ulcer covered with a persistent exudate; ulcer has a firm undermined border	Autoinoculation from pulmonary infection usual; lesions resolve with appropriate antimicrobial therapy
Cervicofacial actinomycosis	Swellings in region of face, neck, and floor of mouth	Infection may be associated with an extraction, jaw fracture, or eruption of molar tooth; in acute form resembles an acute pyogenic abscess, but contains yellow "sulfur granules" (gram-positive mycelia and their hyphae)	Typically swelling is hard and grows painlessly; multiple abscesses with draining tracks develop; penicillin first choice; surgery usually necessary
Histoplasmosis	Any area of the mouth particularly tongue, gingiva, or palate	Nodular, verrucous, or granulomatous lesions; ulcers are indurated and painful; usual source hematogenous or pulmonary source, but may be primary	Systemic antifungal therapy necessary to treat
Candidiasis (Table 28-3)			

DERMATOLOGIC DISEASES

Condition	Usual Location	Clinical Features	Course
Mucous membrane pemphigoid	Typically produces marked gingival erythema and ulceration; other areas of oral cavity, esophagus, and vagina may be affected	Painful, grayish-white collapsed vesicles or bullae of full-thickness epithelium with peripheral erythematous zone; gingival lesions desquamate, leaving ulcerated area	Protracted course with remissions and exacerbations; involvement of different sites occurs slowly; glucocorticoids may temporarily reduce symptoms but do not control the disease
Erythema multiforme minor and major (Stevens-Johnson syndrome)	Primarily the oral mucosa and the skin of hands and feet	Intraoral ruptured bullae surrounded by an inflammatory area; lips may show hemorrhagic crusts; the "iris," or "target," lesion on the skin is pathognomonic; patient may have severe signs of toxicity	Onset very rapid; usually idiopathic, but may by associated with trigger such as drug reaction; condition may last 3–6 weeks; mortality with EM major 5–15% if untreated
Pemphigus vulgaris	Oral mucosa and skin; sites of mechanical trauma (soft/hard palate, frenulum, lips buccal mucosa)	Usually (>70%) presents with oral lesions; fragile, ruptured bullae and ulcerated oral areas; mostly in older adults	With repeated occurrence of bullae, toxicity may lead to cachexia, infection, and death within 2 years; often controllable with oral glucocorticoids
Lichen planus	Oral mucosa and skin	White striae in mouth; purplish nodules on skin at sites of friction; occasionally causes oral mucosal ulcers and erosive gingivitis	White striae alone usually asymptomatic; erosive lesions often difficult to treat, but may respond to glucocorticoids

OTHER CONDITIONS

Condition	Usual Location	Clinical Features	Course
Recurrent aphthous ulcers	Usually on nonkeratinized oral mucosa (buccal and labial mucosa, floor of mouth, soft palate, lateral and ventral tongue)	Single or clusters of painful ulcers with surrounding erythematous border; lesions may be 1–2 mm in diameter in crops (herpetiform), 1–5 mm (minor), or 5–15 mm (major)	Lesions heal in 1–2 weeks but may recur monthly or several times a year; protective barrier with orabase and topical steroids give symptomatic relief; systemic glucocorticoids may be needed in severe cases
Behçet's syndrome	Oral mucosa, eyes, genitalia, gut, and CNS	Multiple aphthous ulcers in mouth; inflammatory ocular changes, ulcerative lesions on genitalia; inflammatory bowel disease and CNS disease	Oral lesions often first manifestation; persist several weeks and heal without scarring
Traumatic ulcers	Anywhere on oral mucosa; dentures frequently responsible for ulcers in vestibule	Localized, discrete ulcerated lesions with red border; produced by accidental biting of mucosa, penetration by a foreign object, or chronic irritation by a denture	Lesions usually heal in 7–10 days when irritant is removed, unless secondarily infected
Squamous cell carcinoma	Any area in the mouth, most commonly on lower lip, tongue, and floor of mouth	Ulcer with elevated, indurated border; failure to heal, pain not prominent; lesions tend to arise in areas of erythro/leukoplakia or in smooth atrophic tongue	Invades and destroys underlying tissues; frequently metastasizes to regional lymph nodes
Acute myeloid leukemia (usually monocytic)	Gingiva	Gingival swelling and superficial ulceration followed by hyperplasia of gingiva with extensive necrosis and hemorrhage; deep ulcers may occur elsewhere on the mucosa complicated by secondary infection	Usually responds to systemic treatment of leukemia; occasionally requires local radiation therapy
Lymphoma	Gingiva, tongue, palate and tonsillar area	Elevated, ulcerated area that may proliferate rapidly, giving the appearance of traumatic inflammation	Fatal if untreated; may indicate underlying HIV infection
Chemical or thermal burns	Any area in mouth	White slough due to contact with corrosive agents (e.g., aspirin, hot cheese) applied locally; removal of slough leaves raw, painful surface	Lesion heals in several weeks if not secondarily infected

Note: CNS, central nervous system.

TABLE 28-2 *Pigmented Lesions of the Oral Mucosa*

Condition	Usual Location	Clinical Features	Course
Oral melanotic macule	Any area of the mouth	Discrete or diffuse localized, brown to black macule	Remains indefinitely; no growth
Diffuse melanin pigmentation	Any area of the mouth	Diffuse pale to dark-brown pigmentation; may be physiologic ("racial") or due to smoking	Remains indefinitely
Nevi	Any area of the mouth	Discrete, localized, brown to black pigmentation	Remains indefinitely
Malignant melanoma	Any area of the mouth	Can be flat and diffuse, painless, brown to black, or can be raised and nodular	Expands and invades early; metastasis leads to death
Addison's disease	Any area of the mouth but mostly buccal mucosa	Blotches or spots of bluish-black to dark-brown pigmentation occurring early in the disease, accompanied by diffuse pigmentation of skin; other symptoms of adrenal insufficiency	Condition controlled by steroid replacement
Peutz-Jeghers syndrome	Any area of the mouth	Dark-brown spots on lips, buccal mucosa, with characteristic distribution of pigment around lips, nose, eyes, and on hands; concomitant intestinal polyposis	Oral pigmented lesions remain indefinitely; gastrointestinal polyps may become malignant
Drug ingestion (neuroleptics, oral contraceptives, minocycline, zidovudine, quinine derivatives)	Any area of the mouth	Brown, black, or gray areas of pigmentation	Gradually disappears following cessation of drug
Amalgam tattoo	Gingiva and alveolar mucosa	Small blue-black pigmented areas associated with embedded amalgam particles in soft tissues; these may show up on radiographs as radiopaque particles in some cases	Remains indefinitely
Heavy metal pigmentation (bismuth, mercury, lead)	Gingival margin	Thin blue-black pigmented line along gingival margin; rarely seen except for children exposed to lead-based paint	Indicative of systemic absorption; no significance for oral health
Black hairy tongue	Dorsum of tongue	Elongation of filiform papillae of tongue, which become stained by coffee, tea, tobacco, or pigmented bacteria	Improves within 1–2 weeks with gentle brushing of tongue or discontinuation of antibiotic if due to bacterial overgrowth
Fordyce "spots"	Buccal and labial mucosa	Numerous small yellowish spots just beneath mucosal surface; no symptoms; due to hyperplasia of sebaceous glands	Benign; remains without apparent change
Kaposi's sarcoma	Palate most common, but may occur in any other site	Red or blue plaques of variable size and shape; often enlarge, become nodular and may ulcerate	Usually indicative of HIV infection or non-Hodgkin's lymphoma; rarely fatal, but may require treatment for comfort or cosmesis
Mucous retention cysts	Buccal and labial mucosa	Bluish-clear fluid filled cyst due to extravasated mucous from injured minor salivary gland	Benign; painless unless traumatized; may be removed surgically

giva, brushing the teeth, or chewing. *Glossopharyngeal neuralgia* produces similar acute neuropathic symptoms in the distribution of the ninth cranial nerve. Swallowing, sneezing, coughing, or pressure on the tragus of the ear triggers pain that is felt in the base of the tongue, pharynx, and soft palate and may be referred to the temporomandibular joint. *Neuritis* involving the maxillary and mandibular divisions of the trigeminal nerve (e.g., maxillary sinusitis, neuroma, and leukemic infiltrate) is distinguished from ordinary toothache by the neuropathic quality of the pain. Occasionally *phantom pain* follows tooth extraction. Often the earliest symptom of *Bell's palsy* in the day or so before facial weakness develops is pain and hyperalgesia behind the ear and side of the face. Likewise, similar symptoms may precede visible lesions of herpes zoster infecting the seventh nerve (*Ramsey-Hunt syndrome*) or trigeminal nerve. Either condition may leave *postherpetic neuralgia* in its wake. *Coronary ischemia* may produce pain exclusively in the face and jaw. Like typical angina pectoris, it is usually reproducible with increased myocardial demand. Aching in several upper molar or premolar teeth may point to *maxillary sinusitis*. Failure to relieve by anesthetizing the teeth and confirmation with appropriate radiographs support the clinical diagnosis.

Giant cell arteritis is notorious for producing headache, but it may also produce facial pain or sore throat that is mistaken for other causes. Jaw and tongue claudication with prolonged chewing or talking is relatively common. Tongue infarction is rare. Patients with *subacute thyroiditis* often experience pain referred to the face or jaw. Oral and pharyngeal causes may be sought before the tender thyroid gland and transient hyperthyroidism are appreciated.

Burning mouth syndrome (*glossodynia*) is present in the absence of mucosal lesions and predominantly affects women over 50. Poorly fitting dentures, anxiety, and depression are common and treatable causes. Tongue-thrusting habit is a cause in some elderly sufferers. The symptom occasionally leads to the discovery of vitamin B_{12} deficiency, iron deficiency, *Plummer-Vinson syndrome*, diabetes mellitus, low-grade *Candida* infection, food sensitivity (e.g., cinnamon), or subtle xerostomia.

DISEASES OF THE SALIVARY GLANDS Saliva is essential to oral health. Its major components, water and mucin, serve as a cleansing solvent and lubricating fluid. In addition it contains antimicrobial factors (e.g., lysozyme, lactoperoxidase, secretory IgA), epidermal growth factor, minerals, and buffering systems. The major salivary glands secrete intermittently in response to autonomic stimulation, which is high during a meal but low otherwise. The parotid secretion is serous or watery, the sublingual is mostly mucus, and the submandibular is a balance of the two elements. Hundreds of minor glands in the lips and cheeks secrete mucus continuously. It is easy to appreciate how oral function becomes impaired when salivary function is reduced. Dry mouth (*xerostomia*) is perceived when salivary flow is reduced by 50%. The most common etiology is medication, especially drugs with anticholinergic properties, but also alpha and beta blockers, calcium channel blockers, and diuretics. Other causes of chronic dryness include Sjögren's syndrome, chronic parotitis, salivary duct obstruction, diabetes mellitus, HIV/AIDS, and irradiation for head and neck cancer. Management involves eliminating or limiting drying medications, preventive dental care, and supplementing oral liquid. Sugarless mints or chewing gum may stimulate salivary secretion if dysfunction is mild. When sufficient exocrine tissue remains, pilocarpine or cevimeline has been shown to increase secretions and reduce symptoms. Commercial

TABLE 28-3   White Lesions of Oral Mucosa

Condition	Usual Location	Clinical Features	Course
Lichen planus	Buccal mucosa, tongue, gingiva, and lips; skin	Striae, white plaques, red areas, ulcers in mouth; purplish papules on skin; may be asymptomatic, sore, or painful; lichenoid drug reactions may look similar	Protracted; responds to topical steroids
White sponge nevus	Oral mucosa, vagina, anal mucosa	Painless white thickening of epithelium; adolescent/early adult onset; familial	Benign and permanent
Smoker's leukoplakia and smokeless tobacco lesions	Any area of oral mucosa, sometimes related to location of habit	White patch that may become firm, rough, or red-fissured and ulcerated; may become sore and painful but usually painless	May or may not resolve with cessation of habit; 2% develop squamous cell carcinoma; early biopsy essential
Erythroplakia with or without white patches	Floor of mouth common in men; tongue and buccal mucosa in women	Velvety, reddish plaque; occasionally mixed with white patches or smooth red areas	High risk of squamous cell cancer; early biopsy essential
Candidiasis	Any area mouth	*Pseudomembranous type* ("thrush"): creamy white curdlike patches that reveal a raw, bleeding surface when scraped; found in sick infants, debilitated elderly patients receiving high doses of glucocorticoids or broad-spectrum antibiotics, or in patients with AIDS	Responds favorably to antifungal therapy and correction of predisposing causes where possible
		Erythematous type: flat, red, sometimes sore areas in same groups of patients	Course same as for pseudomembranous type
		Candidal leukoplakia: nonremovable white thickening of epithelium due to *Candida*	Responds to prolonged antifungal therapy
		Angular cheilitis: sore fissures at corner of mouth	Responds to topical antifungal therapy
Hairy leukoplakia	Usually lateral tongue, rarely elsewhere on oral mucosa	White areas ranging from small and flat to extensive accentuation of vertical folds; found in HIV carriers in all risk groups for AIDS	Due to EBV; responds to high dose acyclovir but recurs; rarely causes discomfort unless secondarily infected with *Candida*
Warts (papillomavirus)	Anywhere on skin and oral mucosa	Single or multiple papillary lesions, with thick, white keratinized surfaces containing many pointed projections; cauliflower lesions covered with normal-colored mucosa or multiple pink or pale bumps (focal epithelial hyperplasia)	Lesions grow rapidly and spread; consider squamous cell carcinoma and rule out with biopsy; excision or laser therapy; may regress in HIV infected patients on antiretroviral therapy

Note: EBV, Epstein-Barr virus.

saliva substitutes or gels relieve dryness but must be supplemented with fluoride applications to prevent caries.

Sialolithiasis presents most often as painful swelling but in some instances as just swelling or pain. The obstructing stone produces spasm upon eating. Conservative therapy consists of local heat, massage, and hydration. Promotion of salivary secretion with mints or lemon drops may flush out small stones. Antibiotic treatment is necessary when bacterial infection in suspected. In adults *acute bacterial parotitis* is typically unilateral and most commonly affects postoperative patients within the first 2 weeks of surgery. *Staphylococcus aureus* is the most common bacterial agent. Dehydration is a major risk for parotitis, as is advanced age and chronic debilitating disease. *Chronic bacterial sialadenitis* is a consequence of lowered salivary secretion and recurrent bacterial infection. When suspected bacterial infection is not responsive to therapy, the differential diagnosis should be expanded to include benign and malignant neoplasms, lymphoproliferative disorders, Sjögren's syndrome, sarcoidosis, tuberculosis, lymphadenitis, actinomycosis, and Wegener's granulomatosis. Bilateral nontender parotid enlargement occurs with diabetes mellitus, cirrhosis, bulimia, HIV/AIDS, and drugs (e.g., iodide, propylthiouracil).

TABLE 28-4 Alterations of the Tongue	
Type of Change	**Clinical Features**
SIZE OR MORPHOLOGY CHANGES	
Macroglossia	Enlarged tongue that may be part of a syndrome found in developmental conditions such as Down's syndrome; may be due to tumor (hemangioma or lymphangioma), metabolic disease (such as primary amyloidosis), or endocrine disturbance (such as acromegaly or cretinism)
Fissured ("scrotal") tongue	Dorsal surface and sides of tongue covered by painless shallow or deep fissures that may collect debris and become irritated
Median rhomboid glossitis	Congenital abnormality of tongue with ovoid, denuded area in median posterior portion of the tongue; may be associated with candidiasis and may respond to antifungals
COLOR CHANGES	
"Geographic" tongue (benign migratory glossitis)	Asymptomatic inflammatory condition of the tongue, with rapid loss and regrowth of filiform papillae, leading to appearance of denuded red patches "wandering" across the surface of the tongue
Hairy tongue	Elongation of filiform papillae of the medial dorsal surface area due to failure of keratin layer of the papillae to desquamate normally; brownish-black coloration may be due to staining by tobacco, food, or chromogenic organisms
"Strawberry" and "raspberry" tongue	Appearance of tongue during scarlet fever due to the hypertrophy of fungiform papillae plus changes in the filiform papillae
"Bald" tongue	Atrophy may be associated with xerostomia, pernicious anemia, iron-deficiency anemia, pellagra, or syphilis; may be accompanied by painful burning sensation; may be an expression of erythematous candidiasis and respond to antifungals

TABLE 28-5 Oral Lesions Associated with HIV Infection

Lesion Morphology	Etiologies
Papules, nodules, plaques	Candidiasis (hyperplastic and pseudomembranous)[a]
	Condyloma acuminatum (human papillomavirus infection)
	Squamous cell carcinoma (preinvasive and invasive)
	Non-Hodgkin's lymphoma[a]
	Hairy leukoplakia[a]
Ulcers	Recurrent aphthous ulcers[a]
	Angular cheilitis
	Squamous cell carcinoma
	Acute necrotizing ulcerative gingivitis[a]
	Necrotizing ulcerative periodontitis[a]
	Necrotizing ulcerative stomatitis
	Non-Hodgkin's lymphoma[a]
	Viral infection (herpes simplex, herpes zoster, cytomegalovirus)
	Mycobacterium tuberculosis, mycobacterium avium-intracellulare
	Fungal infection (histoplasmosis, cryptococcosis, candidiasis, geotrichosis, aspergillosis)
	Bacterial infection (*Escherichia coli, Enterobacter cloacae, Klebsiella pneumoniae, Pseudomonas aeruginosa*)
	Drug reactions (single or multiple ulcers)
Pigmented lesions	Kaposi's sarcoma[a]
	Bacillary angiomatosis (skin and visceral lesions more common than oral)
	Zidovudine pigmentation (skin, nails, and occasionally oral mucosa)
	Addison's disease
Miscellaneous	Linear gingival erythema[a]

[a] Strongly associated with HIV infection.

Pleomorphic adenoma comprises two-thirds of all salivary neoplasms. The parotid is the principle salivary gland affected, and the tumor presents as a firm, slow-growing mass. Though benign, recurrence is common if not completely resected. Malignant tumors such as *mucoepidermoid carcinoma, adenoid cystic carcinoma,* and *adenocarcinoma* tend to grow relatively fast, depending upon grade. They may ulcerate and invade nerves, producing numbness and facial paralysis and correspondingly worsen overall prognosis; 5-year survival is about 68% for malignant salivary gland cancers.

DENTAL CARE OF MEDICALLY COMPLEX PATIENTS Procedures performed in the course of routine dental care (e.g., extraction, scaling and cleaning, tooth restoration, and root canal) are remarkably safe. The most common concerns that arise in the care of dental patients with medical disease are fear of excessive bleeding for patients on anticoagulants, infection of the heart valves and prosthetic devices from hematogenous seeding of oral flora, and cardiovascular complication resulting from vasopressors used with local anesthetic during dental treatment. Experience has confirmed that the risks of any of these complications are very low—far lower than many physicians or dentists imagine.

Patients undergoing tooth extraction or alveolar and gingival surgery rarely experience uncontrolled bleeding when warfarin anticoagulation is maintained within the therapeutic range currently recommended for prevention of venous thrombosis, atrial fibrillation, or mechanical heart valve. While the risk of bleeding is low, embolic complications and death have been reported during subtherapeutic anticoagulation. Therapeutic anticoagulation should be confirmed before and continued through the procedure. Likewise, low-dose aspirin (e.g., 81 to 325 mg) can be safely continued. Bleeding is controlled with local pressure (e.g., gauze), suturing, topical thrombin, or tranexamic acid mouthwash.

Patients at high or moderate risk for bacterial endocarditis (Chap. 109) should maintain optimal oral hygiene, including flossing, and have regular professional cleaning. Prophylactic antibiotics are recommended for all at-risk patients who undergo dental and oral procedures likely to cause significant bleeding and therefore bacteremia. Should unexpected bleeding occur, antibiotics given within 2 h following the procedure will provide effective prophylaxis.

Hematogenous bacterial seeding from oral infection can undoubtedly produce late prosthetic joint infection and therefore requires removal of the infected tissue (e.g., drainage, extraction, root canal) and appropriate antibiotic therapy. However, scientific evidence that late prosthetic joint infection occurs following routine dental procedures is lacking. For this reason, antibiotic prophylaxis is not recommended before dental surgery in patients with orthopedic pins, screws, and plates. It is, however, advised within the first 2 years after joint replacement and for patients with prosthetic joints who have inflammatory arthropathies, immunosuppression (e.g., drug-, radiation-, or disease-induced), type 1 diabetes mellitus, previous prosthetic joint infection, hemophilia, or malnourishment.

Concern often arises regarding the use of vasoconstrictors in patients with hypertension and heart disease. Vasoconstrictors enhance the depth and duration of local anesthesia, thus reducing the anesthetic dose and potential toxicity. If caution is used to avoid intravascular injection, 2% lidocaine with 1:100,000 epinephrine (limited to a total of 0.036 mg epinephrine) can be used safely in those with controlled hypertension and stable coronary heart disease, arrhythmia, or congestive heart failure. Precaution should be taken with patients taking tricyclic antidepressants and nonselective beta blockers since these drugs may potentiate the effect of epinephrine.

Elective dental treatments should be postponed for at least 1 month after myocardial infarction. After this time the risk of reinfarction is low provided the patient is medically stable (e.g., stable rhythm, stable angina, and free of heart failure). Patients who have suffered a stroke should have elective dental care deferred until 6 months after the cerebrovascular accident. In both situations, effective stress reduction requires good pain control. This includes using the minimal amount of vasoconstrictor necessary to provide good hemostasis and local anesthesia.

HALITOSIS Halitosis, or "bad breath," typically emanates from the oral cavity or nasal passages. Volatile sulfur compounds resulting from bacterial decay of food and cellular debris account for the malodor. Periodontal disease, caries and acute forms of gingivitis, poorly fitting dentures, oral abscess, and tongue coating are usual causes. Treatment includes correcting poor hygiene, treating infection, and tongue brushing. Any cause for xerostomia can produce and exacerbate halitosis. Temporary odor due to diet (e.g., garlic) should be self-evident. Pockets of decay in the tonsillar crypts, esophageal diverticulum, esophageal stasis (e.g., achalasia, stricture), sinusitis, and lung abscess account for some instances. A few systemic diseases produce distinctive odors: renal failure (ammoniacal, urinary), hepatic (fishy), and ketoacidosis (sweet, fruity). *Helicobacter pylori* gastritis can also be associated with ammoniacal breath. Distinguishing an oral from a nasal source is accomplished by pinching the nose while exhaling through the mouth and closing the mouth while exhaling through the nose. If no odor is objectively detectable, then pseudo-halitosis or even halitophobia must be considered. These conditions represent varying degrees of psychiatric illness.

AGING AND ORAL HEALTH While tooth loss and dental disease are not normal consequences of aging, a complex array of structural and functional changes occurs with age that can impact oral heath. Subtle changes in tooth structure (e.g., diminished pulp space and volume, sclerosis of dentinal tubules, altered proportions of nerve and vascular pulp content) result in diminished or altered pain sensitivity, reduced reparative capacity, and increased tooth brittleness. In addition age-associated fatty replacement of salivary acini may reduce physiologic reserve, thus increasing the risk of xerostomia due to medication and disease.

Poor oral hygiene often results when vision fails or when patients lose manual dexterity and upper extremity flexibility. This is particularly common for nursing home residents and must be emphasized since regular oral cleaning and dental care has been shown to reduce the incidence of pneumonia. Other risks for dental decay include limited lifetime fluoride exposure and preference by some older adults for intensely sweet foods when taste and olfaction wane. These factors occur in an increasing proportion of persons over age 75 who retain teeth that have extensive restorations and exposed roots. Without assiduous personal and professional care, decay can become quite advanced, yet remain asymptomatic. The result is that much of a tooth or the entire tooth can become destroyed before the process is detected.

Periodontal disease, a leading cause of tooth loss, is indicated by loss of alveolar bone height. Over 90% of Americans have some degree of periodontal disease by age 50. Healthy adults who have not experienced significant alveolar bone loss by the sixth decade do not typically develop significant worsening with advancing age.

Complete edentulousness with advanced age is less common than in previous decades. Nevertheless, it is still present in approximately 50% of Americans age ≥85. Speech, mastication, and facial contours are dramatically affected. Dentures can improve speech articulation and restore diminished facial contours. Mastication is restored less predictably and improves chewing to no more than 15% of natural ability. Those expecting dentures to improve oral intake are often disappointed. On the other hand, more acceptable cosmetic appearance, clearer speech, and modestly improved chewing are attainable goals. Dentures require periodic adjustment to accommodate inevitable remodeling that leads to a diminished volume of the alveolar ridge. Pain can result from friction or traumatic lesions produced by loose dentures. Poor fit and poor oral hygiene may create an environment that allows candidiasis to develop. This may be asymptomatic or painful and is indicated by erythematous smooth or granular tissue conforming to an area covered by the appliance.

ACKNOWLEDGMENT

The author acknowledges the contribution to this chapter by the previous author, Dr. John S. Greenspan.

FURTHER READING

LITTLE JW et al (eds): *Dental Management of the Medically Compromised Patient*, 6th ed. St. Louis, Mosby, 2002

REGEZI JA, SCIUBBA JJ: *Oral Pathology: Clinical Pathologic Correlations*. 4th ed. Philadelphia, Saunders, 2002

SHIP JA et al: Xerostomia and the geriatric patient. J Am Geriatr Soc 50:535, 2002

SILVERMAN S et al (eds): *Essentials of Oral Medicine*. Ontario, BC Decker, 2002

TAKEYOSHI Y et al: Oral care reduces pneumonia in older patients in nursing homes. J Am Geriatr Soc 50:430, 2002

Section 5   Alterations in Circulatory and Respiratory Functions

29 DYSPNEA AND PULMONARY EDEMA
Roland H. Ingram, Jr., Eugene Braunwald

DYSPNEA

Breathing is controlled by central and peripheral mechanisms that adjust ventilation appropriate to increased metabolic demands during physical activity and increase ventilation in excess of metabolic demands in conditions such as anxiety and fear. A normal resting person is unaware of the act of breathing, and while he or she may become conscious of breathing during mild to moderate exertion, no discomfort is experienced. However, during and following exhausting exertion, an individual may become unpleasantly aware of breathing yet feel reasonably assured that the sensation will be transitory and is appropriate to the level of exercise. Therefore, as a cardinal symptom of diseases affecting the cardiorespiratory system, *dyspnea* is defined as an *abnormally uncomfortable awareness of breathing*.

Although dyspnea is not painful in the usual sense of the word, it is, like pain, involved with both the perception of a sensation and the reaction to that perception. Patients experience a number of uncomfortable sensations related to breathing and use an even larger number of verbal expressions to describe these sensations, such as "cannot get enough air," "air does not go all the way down," "smothering feeling or tightness or tiredness in the chest," and a "choking sensation." It may be necessary, therefore, to review the patient's history meticulously in order to ascertain whether the more abstruse descriptions do, in fact, represent dyspnea. Once it is established that a patient has dyspnea, it is of paramount importance to define the circumstances in which it occurs and to assess associated symptoms. There are situations in which breathing appears labored but in which dyspnea does not occur. For example, the hyperventilation associated with metabolic acidemia is rarely accompanied by dyspnea. On the other hand, patients with apparently normal breathing patterns may complain of shortness of breath.

QUANTITATION OF DYSPNEA   The gradation of dyspnea is based on the amount of physical exertion required to produce the sensation. In assessing the severity of dyspnea, it is important to obtain a clear understanding of the patient's general physical condition, work history, and recreational habits. For example, the development of dyspnea in a trained runner upon running 2 mi may signify a much more serious disturbance than a similar degree of breathlessness in a sedentary person upon running a fraction of this distance. Interindividual variation in perception must also be considered. Some patients with severe disease may complain of only mild dyspnea; others with mild disease may experience more severe shortness of breath. Some patients with lung or heart disease may have such reduced capabilities due to other disease (e.g., peripheral vascular insufficiency or severe osteoarthritis of the hips or knees) that exertional dyspnea is precluded despite serious impairment of pulmonary or cardiac function.

Some patterns of dyspnea are not directly related to physical exertion. Sudden and unexpected dyspneic episodes at rest can be associated with pulmonary emboli, spontaneous pneumothorax, hypercapnea secondary to breath holding, or anxiety. Nocturnal episodes of severe paroxysmal dyspnea are characteristic of left ventricular failure. Dyspnea upon assuming the supine posture, *orthopnea* (see below and Chap. 216), thought to be mainly characteristic of congestive heart failure, may also occur in some patients with asthma and chronic obstruction of the airways and is a regular finding in the rare occurrence of bilateral diaphragmatic paralysis. *Trepopnea* is used to describe the unusual circumstance in which dyspnea occurs only in a lateral decubitus position, most often in patients with heart disease, while *platypnea* is dyspnea that occurs only in the upright position. Positional alterations in ventilation-perfusion relationships (Chap. 234) have been invoked to explain these patterns.

MECHANISMS OF DYSPNEA (See Fig. 29-1)   Dyspnea occurs whenever the work of breathing is excessive. Increased force generation is required of the respiratory muscles to produce a given volume change if the chest wall or lungs are less compliant or if resistance to airflow is increased. Increased work of breathing also occurs when the venti-

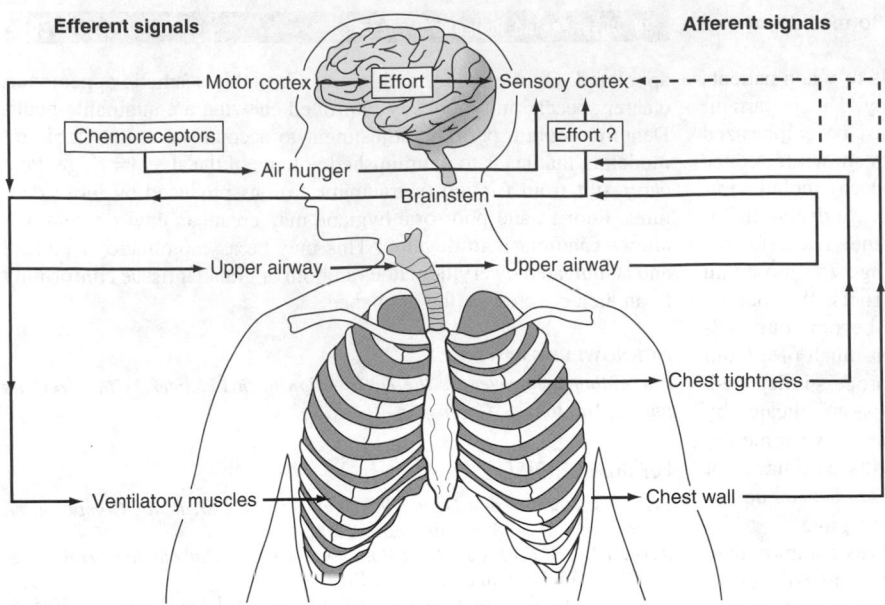

Efferent signals

Motor cortex — Effort — Sensory cortex

Chemoreceptors

Air hunger

Effort ?

Brainstem

Upper airway — Upper airway

Chest tightness

Ventilatory muscles — Chest wall

Afferent signals

FIGURE 29-1 Efferent and afferent signals that contribute to the sensation of dyspnea. There is evidence that the sense of respiratory effort arises from a signal transmitted from the motor cortex to the sensory cortex simultaneously with the outgoing motor command to the ventilatory muscles. The motor output of the brainstem may also contribute to the sense of effort, as shown in the arrow from the brainstem to the sensory cortex. The sense of air hunger arises, in part, from increased respiratory activity within the brainstem, and the sensation of chest tightness probably results from stimulation of vagal-irritant receptors. While afferent information from airway, lung, and chest wall receptors probably passes through the brainstem before reaching the sensory cortex, the dashed lines indicate uncertainty about whether some afferents bypass the brainstem and project directly to the sensory cortex. *(From HL Manning, RM Schwartzstein, Pathophysiology of dyspnea. N Engl J Med 333:1547, 1995, with permission.)*

lation is excessive for the level of activity. Although an individual is more apt to become dyspneic when the work of breathing is increased, the work theory does not account for the perceptual difference between a deep breath with a normal mechanical load and a normal-sized breath with an increased mechanical load. The work might be the same with both breaths, but the normal one with the increased load will be associated with discomfort. In fact, with respiratory loading, such as adding a resistance at the mouth, there is an increase in respiratory center output that is disproportionate to the increase in the work of breathing. It has been postulated that whenever the force that muscles actually generate during breathing approaches some fraction of their maximal force-generating ability, which may vary among individuals, dyspnea ensues due to transduction of mechanical to neural stimuli.

In all likelihood, several different mechanisms operate to different degrees in the various clinical situations in which dyspnea occurs. In some circumstances, dyspnea is evoked by stimulation of receptors in the upper respiratory tract; in others it may originate from receptors in the lungs, airways, respiratory muscles, chest wall, or some combination of these structures. In any event, dyspnea is characterized by an excessive or abnormal activation of the respiratory centers in the brainstem. This activation comes about from stimuli transmitted from or through a variety of structures and pathways, including (1) intrathoracic receptors via the vagal nerves; (2) afferent somatic nerves, particularly from the respiratory muscles and chest wall, but also from other skeletal muscles and joints; (3) chemoreceptors in the brain, aortic, and carotid bodies, and elsewhere in the circulation; (4) higher (cortical) centers; and perhaps (5) afferent fibers in the phrenic nerves. In general, despite the interindividual variations described above, there is a reasonable correlation between the severity of dyspnea and the magnitude of disturbances of pulmonary or cardiac function that are responsible.

The mechanisms responsible for dyspnea may vary in different conditions (Table 29-1).

DIFFERENTIAL DIAGNOSIS ■ Obstructive Disease of Airways (See also Chaps. 236 and 242) Obstruction to airflow can be present anywhere from the extrathoracic airways out to the small airways in the periphery of

the lung. Large extrathoracic airway obstruction can occur acutely, as with aspiration of food or a foreign body, or with angioedema of the glottis. An allergic history together with a few scattered hives should raise the possibility of glottic edema. Acute upper airway obstruction is a medical emergency. More chronic forms can occur with tumors or with fibrotic stenosis following tracheostomy or prolonged endotracheal intubation. Whether acute or chronic, the cardinal symptom is dyspnea, and the characteristic signs are stridor and retraction of the supraclavicular fossae with *inspiration*.

Obstruction of intrathoracic airways can occur acutely and intermittently or can be present chronically with worsening during respiratory infections. Acute intermittent obstruction with wheezing is typical of *asthma* (Chap. 236). Chronic cough with expectoration is typical of *chronic bronchitis* (Chap. 242) and *bronchiectasis* (Chap. 240). Most often there are prolongation of expiration and coarse rhonchi that are generalized in chronic bronchitis and may be localized in the case of bronchiectasis. Intercurrent infection results in worsening of the cough, increased expectoration of purulent sputum, and more severe dyspnea. During such episodes, the patient may complain of nocturnal paroxysms of dyspnea with wheezing relieved by cough and expectoration of sputum. Despite the fact that severe limitation of expiratory flow and hyperinflation of the lung are characteristic of these diseases, the sensory experience is often that of an inability to take in a sufficiently deep breath rather than difficulty in exhaling.

The patient with predominant *emphysema* is characterized by many years of exertional dyspnea progressing to dyspnea at rest (Chap. 242). Although a parenchymal disease by definition, emphysema is invariably accompanied by obstruction of airways.

Diffuse Parenchymal Lung Diseases (See also Chap. 243) This category includes a large number of diseases ranging from acute pneumonia to chronic disorders such as sarcoidosis and the various forms of *pneumoconiosis* (Chap. 238). History, physical findings, and radiographic abnormalities often provide clues to the diagnosis. The patients are often tachypneic with arterial P_{CO_2} and P_{O_2} values below normal. Exertion often further reduces the arterial P_{O_2}. Lung volumes are decreased, and the lungs are stiffer, i.e., less compliant, than normal.

Pulmonary Vascular Occlusive Diseases (See also Chap. 244) Repeated episodes of dyspnea at rest often occur with recurrent pulmonary em-

TABLE 29-1 *Likely Mechanisms of Dyspnea in Selected Conditions*

Condition	Mechanism
Asthma	Increased sense of effort
	Stimulation of irritant receptors in airways
Neuromuscular disease	Increased sense of effort
COPD	Increased sense of effort
	Hypoxia
	Hypercapnia
	Dynamic airway compression
Mechanical ventilation	Afferent mismatch
	Factors associated with the underlying condition
Pulmonary embolism	Stimulation of pressure receptors in pulmonary vasculature or right atrium (possible)

Note: COPD, chronic obstructive pulmonary disease.
Source: From HL Manning, RM Schwartzstein, Pathophysiology of dyspnea. N Engl J Med 333:1547, 1995, with permission.

boli. Near syncope on exertion is another suggestive symptom. Evidence of a source for emboli, such as phlebitis of a lower extremity or the pelvis, is quite helpful in leading the physician to suspect the diagnosis. Arterial blood gases are most often abnormal, but lung volumes are frequently normal or only minimally abnormal.

Diseases of the Chest Wall or Respiratory Muscles (See also Chap. 246) The physical examination establishes the presence of a chest wall disease such as severe kyphoscoliosis, pectus excavatum, or ankylosing spondylitis. Although all three of these deformities may be associated with dyspnea, only severe kyphoscoliosis regularly interferes with ventilation sufficiently to produce chronic cor pulmonale and respiratory failure.

Both weakness and paralysis of respiratory muscles can lead to respiratory failure and dyspnea (Chap. 246), but most often the signs and symptoms of the neurologic or muscular disorder are more prominently manifested in other systems.

Heart Disease In patients with cardiac disease, exertional dyspnea occurs most commonly as a consequence of an elevated pulmonary capillary pressure, which in turn may be due to left ventricular dysfunction (Chaps. 215 and 216), reduced left ventricular compliance, and mitral stenosis. The elevation of hydrostatic pressure in the pulmonary vascular bed tends to upset the Starling equilibrium (see "Pulmonary Edema," below) with resulting transudation of liquid into the interstitial space, reducing the compliance of the lungs and stimulating J (juxtacapillary) receptors in the alveolar interstitial space. When it is prolonged, pulmonary venous hypertension results in thickening of the walls of small pulmonary vessels and an increase in perivascular cells and fibrous tissue, causing a further reduction in compliance. The competition for space among vessels, airways, and increased fluid within the interstitial space compromises the lumina of small airways, increasing the airways' resistance. Diminution in compliance and an increase in the airways' resistance increase the work of breathing. In advanced congestive heart failure, usually involving elevation of both pulmonary and systemic venous pressures, hydrothorax may develop, interfering further with pulmonary function and intensifying dyspnea.

Orthopnea, i.e., dyspnea in the supine position, is the result of the alteration of gravitational forces when this position is assumed, which elevates pulmonary venous and capillary pressures. These, in turn, increase the pulmonary closing volume (Chap. 234) and reduce the vital capacity.

PAROXYSMAL NOCTURNAL DYSPNEA Also known as *cardiac asthma*, this condition is characterized by attacks of severe shortness of breath that generally occur at night and usually awaken the patient from sleep. The attack is precipitated by stimuli that aggravate previously existing pulmonary congestion; frequently, the total blood volume is augmented at night because of the reabsorption of edema from dependent portions of the body during recumbency. A sleeping patient can tolerate relatively severe pulmonary engorgement and may awaken only when actual pulmonary edema and bronchospasm have developed, with the feeling of suffocation and with wheezing respirations.

Two other forms of nocturnal dyspnea must be distinguished from that due to heart failure. Chronic bronchitis is characterized by mucus hypersecretion and, after a few hours sleep, secretions can accumulate and produce dyspnea and wheezing, both of which are relieved by cough and expectoration of sputum. Asthma patients have circadian variations in their degree of airway obstruction. The obstruction becomes most severe between 2 A.M. and 4 A.M. and can be sufficiently severe that the patient awakens with a sense of suffocation, extreme dyspnea, and wheezing. Although there is a prominent inflammatory component to nocturnal asthma, inhaled bronchodilators usually improve symptoms quickly.

CHEYNE-STOKES RESPIRATION See Chap. 216 ■ *Diagnosis* The diagnosis of cardiac dyspnea depends on the recognition of heart disease on the basis of the clinical examination supplemented by noninvasive testing. There may be a history of antecedent myocardial infarction; third and fourth heart sounds may be audible; and/or there may be evidence of

left ventricular enlargement, jugular neck vein distention, and/or peripheral edema. Often there are radiographic signs of heart failure, with evidence of interstitial edema, pulmonary vascular redistribution, and accumulation of liquid in the septal planes and pleural cavity. Transthoracic echocardiography is particularly useful in establishing the diagnosis of structural heart disease, which can be responsible for dyspnea. Specifically, left atrial and/or left ventricular dilatation, left ventricular hypertrophy, a reduced left ventricular ejection fraction, and disorders of left ventricular wall motion may be clues to the presence of a cardiac etiology of otherwise unexplained dyspnea.

DIFFERENTIATION BETWEEN CARDIAC AND PULMONARY DYSPNEA In most patients with dyspnea there is obvious clinical evidence of disease of the heart and/or lungs. Like patients with cardiac dyspnea, patients with chronic obstructive lung disease may also waken at night with dyspnea, but, as pointed out above, this is usually associated with sputum production; the dyspnea is relieved after these patients rid themselves of secretions. The difficulty in the distinction between cardiac and pulmonary dyspnea may be compounded by the coexistence of diseases involving both organ systems.

In patients in whom the etiology of dyspnea is not clear, it is desirable to carry out pulmonary function testing, for these tests may be helpful in determining whether dyspnea is produced by heart disease, lung disease, abnormalities of the chest wall, or anxiety (Chap. 235). In addition to the usual means of assessing patients for heart disease, determination of the ejection fraction at rest and during exercise by echocardiography or radionuclide ventriculography is helpful in the differential diagnosis of dyspnea. The left ventricular ejection fraction is depressed in left ventricular failure, while the right ventricular ejection fraction may be low at rest or may decline during exercise in patients with severe lung disease. Both left and right ventricular ejection fractions are normal at rest and during exercise in dyspnea due to anxiety or malingering. Careful observation during the performance of an exercise treadmill test will often help in the identification of the patient who is malingering or whose dyspnea is secondary to anxiety. Under these circumstances, the patient usually complains of severe shortness of breath but appears to be breathing either effortlessly or totally irregularly. Cardiopulmonary testing, in which the patient's maximal functional exercise capacity is assessed while measurements of the electrocardiogram, blood pressure, oxygen consumption, arterial saturation (oximetry), and ventilation are carried out, is useful in the differentiation between cardiac and pulmonary dyspnea (Table 29-2).

ANXIETY STATES Dyspnea experienced by a patient with anxiety alone is difficult to evaluate. The signs and symptoms of acute and chronic

TABLE 29-2 *Patterns of Abnormality in Cardiopulmonary Exercise Testing*[a]

Cardiovascular limitation
Heart rate ≥85% of predicted maximum
Low anaerobic threshold
Reduced maximal oxygen consumption
Drop in blood pressure with exercise
Arrhythmias or ischemic changes on ECG
Does not achieve maximal predicted ventilation
Does not have significant desaturation
Respiratory limitation
Achieves or exceeds maximal predicted ventilation
Significant desaturation (<90%)
Stable or increase dead space–to–tidal volume ratio
Development or bronchospasm with falling FEV_1
Does not achieve 85% of predicted maximal heart rate
No ischemic ECG changes

[a] All features will not be present in a particular case, and there may be elements of both cardiovascular and respiratory causes of shortness of breath. One looks for the predominant pattern in assessing the etiology of the patient's exercise limitation.
Note: ECG, electrocardiogram; FEV_1, forced expiratory volume in 1 s.
Source: From RM Schwartzstein, D Feller-Kopman, in E Braunwald, L Goldman (eds): *Primary Cardiology*, 2d ed. Philadelphia, Saunders, 2003

hyperventilation do not serve to distinguish between anxiety states and other processes, such as recurrent pulmonary emboli. Another potentially confusing situation is seen when chest pain and electrocardiographic changes accompany the hyperventilation syndrome. When present and attributable to this condition, also referred to as *neurocirculatory asthenia*, the chest pain is often sharp, fleeting, and in various loci, and the electrocardiographic changes are most often seen during repolarization. Frequent sighing respirations and an irregular breathing pattern point to a psychogenic origin of the dyspnea. Anxiety and depression in association with heart or lung disease can serve to intensify dyspnea symptoms beyond what would be expected for a given degree of dysfunction.

PULMONARY EDEMA

CARDIOGENIC PULMONARY EDEMA (See Table 29-3, IA)   An increase in pulmonary venous pressure, which results initially in engorgement of the pulmonary vasculature, is common in most instances of dyspnea in association with congestive heart failure. The lungs become less compliant, the resistance of small airways increases, and there is an increase in lymphatic flow that apparently serves to maintain a constant pulmonary extravascular liquid volume. Mild tachypnea is present. If

---

TABLE 29-3 Classification of Pulmonary Edema Based on Initiating Mechanism

I. Imbalance of Starling forces
  A. Increased pulmonary capillary pressure
    1. Increased pulmonary venous pressure without left ventricular failure (e.g., mitral stenosis)
    2. Increased pulmonary venous pressure secondary to left ventricular failure
    3. Increased pulmonary capillary pressure secondary to increased pulmonary arterial pressure (so-called overperfusion pulmonary edema)
  B. Decreased plasma oncotic pressure
    1. Hypoalbuminemia
  C. Increased negativity of interstitial pressure
    1. Rapid removal of pneumothorax with large applied negative pressures (unilateral)
    2. Large negative pleural pressures due to acute airway obstruction alone with increased end-expiratory volumes (asthma)
II. Altered alveolar-capillary membrane permeability (acute respiratory distress syndrome)
  A. Infectious pneumonia—bacterial, viral, parasitic
  B. Inhaled toxins (e.g., phosgene, ozone, chlorine, Teflon fumes, nitrogen dioxide, smoke)
  C. Circulating foreign substances (e.g., snake venom, bacterial endotoxins)
  D. Aspiration of acidic gastric contents
  E. Acute radiation pneumonitis
  F. Endogenous vasoactive substances (e.g., histamine, kinins)
  G. Disseminated intravascular coagulation
  H. Immunologic—hypersensitivity pneumonitis, drugs (nitrofurantoin), leukoagglutinins
  I. Shock lung in association with nonthoracic trauma
  J. Acute hemorrhagic pancreatitis
III. Lymphatic insufficiency
  A. After lung transplant
  B. Lymphangitic carcinomatosis
  C. Fibrosing lymphangitis (e.g., silicosis)
IV. Unknown or incompletely understood
  A. High-altitude pulmonary edema
  B. Neurogenic pulmonary edema
  C. Narcotic overdose
  D. Pulmonary embolism
  E. Eclampsia
  F. After cardioversion
  G. After anesthesia
  H. After cardiopulmonary bypass

Source: From Braunwald et al., with permission.

---

the increase in intravascular pressure is sufficient both in magnitude and duration, there is a net gain of liquid in the extravascular space, i.e., *interstitial* edema. At this point symptoms worsen, tachypnea increases, gas exchange deteriorates further, and radiographic changes, such as Kerley B lines and loss of distinct vascular margins, are seen. At this stage, the capillary endothelial intercellular junctions widen and allow passage of macromolecules into the interstices.

Further elevations in intravascular pressure disrupt the tight junctions between alveolar lining cells, and *alveolar* edema ensues, with outpouring of liquid that contains both red blood cells and macromolecules. With yet more severe disruption of the alveolar-capillary membrane, edematous liquid floods the alveoli and airways. At this point, full-blown clinical pulmonary edema with bilateral wet rales and rhonchi occurs, and the chest radiograph may show diffuse haziness of the lung fields with greater density in the more proximal hilar regions. Typically, the patient is anxious and perspires freely, and the sputum is frothy and bloodtinged. Gas exchange is more severely compromised with worsening hypoxia. Without effective treatment (Chap. 255), progressive acidemia, hypercapnia, and respiratory arrest ensue.

The sequence of liquid accumulation described above follows the Starling law of capillary-interstitial liquid exchange:

$$\text{Liquid accumulation} = K[(P_c - P_{IF}) - \sigma(\pi_{pl} - \pi_{IF})] - Q_{lymph}$$

where K, hydraulic conductance (directly proportional to membrane surface area and inversely proportional to membrane thickness); P_c, mean intracapillary pressure; π_{IF}, oncotic pressure of interstitial liquid; σ, reflection coefficient of macromolecules; P_{IF}, mean interstitial liquid pressure; π_{pl}, oncotic pressure of the plasma; Q_{lymph}, lymphatic flow.

The pressures tending to move liquid out of the vessel are P_c and π_{IF}, which are normally more than offset by pressures tending to move liquid back into the vasculature, i.e., the algebraic sum of P_{IF} and π_{pl}. Implicit in the preceding equation is that lymphatic flow can increase in the case of imbalance of forces and result in no net accumulation of interstitial liquid. Further elevations in P_c not only increase the outward movement of liquid in each capillary region but also recruit more of the capillary bed, which increases K. These two effects lead to liquid filtration that exceeds clearance capability by the lymphatics, and liquid accumulates in the loose interstitial spaces of the lung. Even greater increases in P_c open first the loose endothelial intercellular junctions and later the tight alveolar intercellular junctions with an increase in permeability to macromolecules. This secondary disruption of both the function and structure of the alveolar-capillary membrane leads to alveolar flooding.

NONCARDIOGENIC PULMONARY EDEMA (See Table 29-3, IB, IC, II, III, and IV)   Several clinical conditions are associated with pulmonary edema based on an imbalance of Starling forces other than through primary elevations of pulmonary capillary pressure. Although diminished plasma oncotic pressure in hypoalbuminemic states (e.g., severe liver disease, nephrotic syndrome, protein-losing enteropathy) might be expected to lead to pulmonary edema, the balance of forces normally so strongly favors resorption that even in these conditions some elevation of capillary pressure is usually necessary before interstitial edema develops. Increased negativity of interstitial pressure has been implicated in the genesis of unilateral pulmonary edema following rapid evacuation of a large pneumothorax. In this situation, the findings may be apparent only by radiography, but occasionally the patient experiences dyspnea with physical findings localized to the edematous lung. It has been proposed that large negative intrapleural pressures during acute severe asthma may be associated with the development of interstitial edema. Lymphatic blockade secondary to fibrotic and inflammatory diseases or lymphangitic carcinomatosis may lead to interstitial edema. In such instances, both clinical and radiographic manifestations are dominated by the underlying disease process.

Other conditions characterized by increases in the interstitial liquid content of the lungs appear to be associated primarily with disruption of the alveolar-capillary membranes. Any number of spontaneously occurring or environmental toxic insults, including diffuse pulmonary infections, aspiration, and shock (particularly due to sepsis, hemorrhagic pancreatitis, and following cardiopulmonary bypass), are associated with diffuse pulmonary edema that clearly does not have a hemodynamic origin. →*These conditions, which may lead to the acute respiratory distress syndrome, are discussed in Chap. 251.*

Other Forms of Pulmonary Edema There are three forms of pulmonary edema whose precise mechanism remains unexplained. *Narcotic overdose* is a well-recognized antecedent to pulmonary edema. Although illicit use of parenteral heroin is the most frequent cause, parenteral and oral overdoses of legitimate preparations of morphine, methadone, and dextropropoxyphene have also been associated with pulmonary edema. The earlier idea that injected impurities lead to the disorder is untenable. Available evidence suggests that there are alterations in the permeability of alveolar and capillary membranes rather than an elevation of pulmonary capillary pressure.

Exposure to high altitude in association with severe physical exertion is a well-recognized setting for pulmonary edema in unacclimatized yet otherwise healthy persons. Acclimatized high-altitude natives also develop this syndrome upon return to high altitude after a relatively brief sojourn at low altitudes. The syndrome is far more common in persons under the age of 25 years. The mechanism for high-altitude pulmonary edema (HAPE) remains obscure, and studies have been conflicting, some suggesting pulmonary venous constriction and others indicating pulmonary arteriolar constriction as the prime mechanisms. A role for hypoxia at high altitude is suggested by the fact that patients respond to the administration of oxygen and/or return to lower altitudes. Hypoxia per se does not alter permeability of the alveolar-capillary membrane. Hence increased cardiac output and pulmonary arterial pressures with exercise combined with hypoxic pulmonary arteriolar constriction, which is more prominent in young persons, may combine to make this an example of prearteriolar, high-pressure pulmonary edema. HAPE has also been attributed to a defect in the absorption of liquid driven by active alveolar transepithelial sodium transport. Prophylactic inhalation of the β_2 agonist salmeterol has been shown to reduce the incidence of this condition.

Neurogenic pulmonary edema has been described in patients with central nervous system disorders and without apparent preexisting left ventricular dysfunction. Although most experimental studies have implicated sympathetic nervous system activity, the mechanism whereby sympathetic efferent activity leads to pulmonary edema is a matter of speculation. It is known that a massive adrenergic nerve discharge leads to peripheral vasoconstriction with elevation of blood pressure and shifts of blood to the central circulation. In addition, it is probable that a reduction in left ventricular compliance also occurs, and both factors serve to increase left atrial pressures sufficiently to induce pulmonary edema on a hemodynamic basis. Some experimental evidence suggests that stimulation of adrenergic receptors increases capillary permeability directly, but this effect is relatively minor as compared with the imbalance of Starling forces.

TREATMENT OF PULMONARY EDEMA See Chap. 255

FURTHER READING

GIVERTZ ME et al: Clinical aspects of heart failure; high-output heart failure; pulmonary edema, in D Zipes et al (eds), *Braunwald's Heart Disease*, 7th ed, Philadelphia, Saunders, 2005

MANNING HL, SCHWARTZSTEIN RM: Respiratory symptoms in asthma: Physiological and clinical implications. J Asthma 38:447, 2001

MANNING HL, MAHLER DA: Pathophysiology of dyspnea. Monaldi Arch Chest Dis 56:325, 2001

SCHWARTZSTEIN RM, FELLER-KOPMAN D: Approach to the patient with dyspnea, in E Braunwald, L Goldman (eds), *Primary Cardiology*, 2d ed, Philadelphia, Elsevier, 2003

30 COUGH AND HEMOPTYSIS
Steven E. Weinberger

COUGH

Cough is an explosive expiration that provides a normal protective mechanism for clearing the tracheobronchial tree of secretions and foreign material. When excessive or bothersome, it is also one of the most common symptoms for which medical attention is sought. Reasons for the latter include discomfort from the cough itself, interference with normal lifestyle, and concern for the cause of the cough, especially fear of cancer.

MECHANISM

Coughing may be initiated either voluntarily or reflexively. As a defensive reflex it has both afferent and efferent pathways. The *afferent limb* includes receptors within the sensory distribution of the trigeminal, glossopharyngeal, superior laryngeal, and vagus nerves. The *efferent limb* includes the recurrent laryngeal nerve and the spinal nerves. The cough starts with a deep inspiration followed by glottic closure, relaxation of the diaphragm, and muscle contraction against a closed glottis. The resulting markedly positive intrathoracic pressure causes narrowing of the trachea. Once the glottis opens, the large pressure differential between the airways and the atmosphere coupled with tracheal narrowing produces rapid flow rates through the trachea. The shearing forces that develop aid in the elimination of mucus and foreign materials.

ETIOLOGY

Cough can be initiated by a variety of irritant triggers either from an exogenous source (smoke, dust, fumes, foreign bodies) or from an endogenous origin (upper airway secretions, gastric contents). These stimuli may affect receptors in the upper airway (especially the pharynx and larynx) or in the lower respiratory tract, following access to the tracheobronchial tree by inhalation or by aspiration. When cough is triggered by upper airway secretions (as with postnasal drip) or gastric contents (as with gastroesophageal reflux), the initiating factor may go unrecognized and the cough can be persistent. Additionally, prolonged exposure to such irritants may initiate airway inflammation, which can itself precipitate cough and sensitize the airway to other irritants. Cough associated with gastroesophageal reflux is due only in part to irritation of upper airway receptors or to aspiration of gastric contents, as a vagally mediated reflex mechanism secondary to acid in the distal esophagus may also contribute.

Any disorder resulting in inflammation, constriction, infiltration, or compression of airways can be associated with cough. Inflammation commonly results from airway infections, ranging from viral or bacterial bronchitis to bronchiectasis. In viral bronchitis, airway inflammation sometimes persists long after resolution of the typical acute symptoms, thereby producing a prolonged cough, lasting for weeks. Pertussis infection is also a possible cause of persistent cough in adults; however, diagnosis is generally made on clinical grounds (Chap. 133). Asthma is a common cause of cough. Although the clinical setting commonly suggests when a cough is secondary to asthma, some patients present with cough in the absence of wheezing or dyspnea, thus making the diagnosis more subtle ("cough variant asthma"). A neoplasm infiltrating the airway wall, such as bronchogenic carcinoma or a carcinoid tumor, is commonly associated with cough. Airway infiltration with granulomas may also trigger a cough, as seen with endobronchial sarcoidosis or tuberculosis. Compression of airways results from extrinsic masses, including lymph nodes, mediastinal tumors, and aortic aneurysms.

Examples of parenchymal lung disease potentially producing cough include interstitial lung disease, pneumonia, and lung abscess.

Congestive heart failure may be associated with cough, probably as a consequence of interstitial as well as peribronchial edema. A nonproductive cough complicates the use of angiotensin-converting enzyme (ACE) inhibitors in 5 to 20% of patients taking these agents. Onset is usually within 1 week of starting the drug but can be delayed up to 6 months. Although the mechanism is not known with certainty, it may relate to accumulation of bradykinin or substance P, both of which are degraded by ACE.

The most common causes of cough can be categorized according to the duration of the cough. Acute cough (<3 weeks) is most often due to upper respiratory infection (especially the common cold, acute bacterial sinusitis, and pertussis), but more serious disorders, such as pneumonia, pulmonary embolus, and congestive heart failure, can also present in this fashion. Chronic cough (>3 weeks) in a smoker raises the possibilities of chronic obstructive lung disease or bronchogenic carcinoma. In a nonsmoker who has a normal chest radiograph and is not taking an ACE inhibitor, the most common causes of chronic cough are postnasal drip, asthma, and gastroesophageal reflux. Eosinophilic bronchitis in the absence of asthma has also been recognized as a potential cause of chronic cough.

APPROACH TO THE PATIENT

A detailed *history* frequently provides the most valuable clues for etiology of the cough. Particularly important questions include:

1. Is the cough acute or chronic?
2. At its onset, were there associated symptoms suggestive of a respiratory infection?
3. Is it seasonal or associated with wheezing?
4. Is it associated with symptoms suggestive of postnasal drip (nasal discharge, frequent throat clearing, a "tickle in the throat") or gastroesophageal reflux (heartburn or sensation of regurgitation)? (The absence of such suggestive symptoms does not exclude either of these diagnoses, particularly in the case of gastroesophageal reflux.)
5. Is it associated with fever or sputum? If sputum is present, what is its character?
6. Does the patient have any associated diseases or risk factors for disease (e.g., cigarette smoking, risk factors for infection with HIV, environmental exposures)?
7. Is the patient taking an ACE inhibitor?

The general *physical examination* may point to a systemic or nonpulmonary cause of cough, such as heart failure, primary nonpulmonary neoplasm, or AIDS. Examination of the oropharynx may provide suggestive evidence for postnasal drip, including oropharyngeal mucus or erythema, or a "cobblestone" appearance to the mucosa. Auscultation of the chest may demonstrate inspiratory stridor (indicative of upper airway disease), rhonchi or expiratory wheezing (indicative of lower airway disease), or inspiratory crackles (suggestive of a process involving the pulmonary parenchyma, such as interstitial lung disease, pneumonia, or pulmonary edema).

Chest radiography may be particularly helpful in suggesting or confirming the cause of the cough. Important potential findings include the presence of an intrathoracic mass lesion, a localized pulmonary parenchymal infiltrate, or diffuse interstitial or alveolar disease. An area of honeycombing or cyst formation may suggest bronchiectasis, while symmetric bilateral hilar adenopathy may suggest sarcoidosis.

Pulmonary function testing (Chap. 234) is useful for assessing the functional abnormalities that accompany certain disorders producing cough. Measurement of forced expiratory flow rates can demonstrate reversible airflow obstruction characteristic of asthma. When asthma is considered but flow rates are normal, bronchoprovocation testing with methacholine or cold-air inhalation can demonstrate hyperreactivity of the airways to a bronchoconstrictive

stimulus. Measurement of lung volumes and diffusing capacity is useful primarily for demonstration of a restrictive pattern, often seen with any of the diffuse interstitial lung diseases.

If *sputum* is produced, gross and microscopic examination may provide useful information. Purulent sputum suggests chronic bronchitis, bronchiectasis, pneumonia, or lung abscess. Blood in the sputum may be seen in the same disorders, but its presence also raises the question of an endobronchial tumor. Greater than 3% eosinophils seen on staining of induced sputum in a patient without asthma suggests the possibility of eosinophilic bronchitis. Gram and acid-fast stains and cultures may demonstrate a particular infectious pathogen, while sputum cytology may provide a diagnosis of a pulmonary malignancy.

More specialized studies are helpful in specific circumstances. *Fiberoptic bronchoscopy* is the procedure of choice for visualizing an endobronchial tumor and collecting cytologic and histologic specimens. Inspection of the tracheobronchial mucosa can demonstrate endobronchial granulomas often seen in sarcoidosis, and endobronchial biopsy of such lesions or transbronchial biopsy of the lung interstitium can confirm the diagnosis. Inspection of the airway mucosa by bronchoscopy can also demonstrate the characteristic appearance of endobronchial Kaposi's sarcoma in patients with AIDS. *High-resolution computed tomography* (HRCT) can confirm the presence of interstitial disease and frequently suggests a diagnosis based on the pattern of disease. It is the procedure of choice for demonstrating dilated airways and confirming the diagnosis of bronchiectasis.

A diagnostic algorithm for evaluation of chronic cough is presented in Fig. 30-1.

COMPLICATIONS

Common complications of coughing include chest and abdominal wall soreness, urinary incontinence, and exhaustion. On occasion, paroxysms of coughing may precipitate syncope (cough syncope; Chap. 20), consequent to markedly positive intrathoracic and alveolar pressures, diminished venous return, and decreased cardiac output. Although cough fractures of the ribs may occur in otherwise normal patients, their occurrence should at least raise the possibility of pathologic fractures, which are seen with multiple myeloma, osteoporosis, and osteolytic metastases.

℞ TREATMENT

Definitive treatment of cough depends on determining the underlying cause and then initiating specific therapy. Elimination of an exogenous inciting agent (cigarette smoke, ACE inhibitors) or an endogenous trigger (postnasal drip, gastroesophageal reflux) is usually effective when such a precipitant can be identified. Other important management considerations are treatment of specific respiratory tract infections, bronchodilators for potentially reversible airflow obstruction, inhaled glucocorticoids for eosinophilic bronchitis, chest physiotherapy and other methods to enhance clearance of secretions in patients with bronchiectasis, and treatment of endobronchial tumors or interstitial lung disease when such therapy is available and appropriate. In patients with chronic, unexplained cough, an empirical approach to treatment is often used for both diagnostic and therapeutic purposes, starting with an antihistamine-decongestant combination or nasal ipratropium spray to treat unrecognized postnasal drip. If ineffective, this may be followed sequentially by treatment for asthma and for gastroesophageal reflux.

Symptomatic or nonspecific therapy of cough should be considered when: (1) the cause of the cough is not known or specific treatment is not possible, and (2) the cough performs no useful function or causes marked discomfort. An irritative, nonproductive cough may be suppressed by an antitussive agent, which increases the latency or threshold of the cough center. Such agents include codeine (15 mg qid) or nonnarcotics such as dextromethorphan (15 mg qid). These drugs provide symptomatic relief by interrupting prolonged, self-perpetuating paroxysms. However, a cough productive of significant quantities of sputum should usually not be suppressed, since retention of sputum in the tracheobronchial tree may interfere with the distribution of ventilation, alveolar aeration, and the ability of the lung to resist infection.

Other agents working by a variety of mechanisms have also been used to control cough, but objective information assessing their benefit is meager. For example, the inhaled anticholinergic agent, ipratropium bromide (2 to 4 puffs qid), has been used with the rationale of inhibiting the efferent limb of the cough reflex.

HEMOPTYSIS

Hemoptysis is defined as the expectoration of blood from the respiratory tract, a spectrum that varies from blood-streaking of sputum to coughing up large amounts of pure blood. *Massive hemoptysis* is variably defined as the expectoration of >100 to >600 mL over a 24-h period, although the patient's estimation of the amount of blood is notoriously unreliable. Expectoration of even relatively small amounts of blood is a frightening symptom and can be a marker for potentially serious disease, such as bronchogenic carcinoma. Massive hemoptysis, on the other hand, can represent an acutely life-threatening problem. Large amounts of blood can fill the airways and the alveolar spaces, not only seriously disturbing gas exchange but potentially causing the patient to suffocate.

ETIOLOGY

Because blood originating from the nasopharynx or the gastrointestinal tract can mimic blood coming from the lower respiratory tract, it is important to determine initially that the blood is not coming from one of these alternative sites. Clues that the blood is originating from the gastrointestinal tract include a dark red appearance and an acidic pH, in contrast to the typical bright red appearance and alkaline pH of true hemoptysis.

An etiologic classification of hemoptysis can be based on the site of origin within the lungs (Table 30-1). The most common site of bleeding is the airways, i.e., the tracheobronchial tree, which can be affected by inflammation (acute or chronic bronchitis, bronchiectasis) or by neoplasm (bronchogenic carcinoma, endobronchial metastatic carcinoma, or bronchial carcinoid tumor). The bronchial arteries, which originate either from the aorta or from intercostal arteries and are therefore part of the high-pressure systemic circulation, are the source of bleeding in bronchitis or bronchiectasis or with endobronchial tumors. Blood originating from the pulmonary parenchyma can be either from a localized source, such as an infection (pneumonia, lung abscess, tuberculosis), or from a process diffusely affecting the parenchyma (as with a coagulopathy or with an autoimmune process such as Goodpasture's syndrome). Disorders primarily affecting the pulmonary vasculature include pulmonary embolic disease and those conditions associated with elevated pulmonary venous and capillary pressures, such as mitral stenosis or left ventricular failure.

Although the relative frequency of the different etiologies of hemoptysis varies from series to series, most recent studies indicate that bronchitis and bronchogenic carcinoma are the two most common causes. Despite the lower frequency of tuberculosis and bronchiectasis seen in recent compared to older series, these two disorders still represent the most common causes of massive hemoptysis in several series. Even after extensive evaluation, a sizable proportion of patients (up to 30% in some series) have no identifiable etiology for their hemoptysis. These patients are classified as having idiopathic or cryptogenic hemoptysis, and subtle airway or parenchymal disease is presumably responsible for the bleeding.

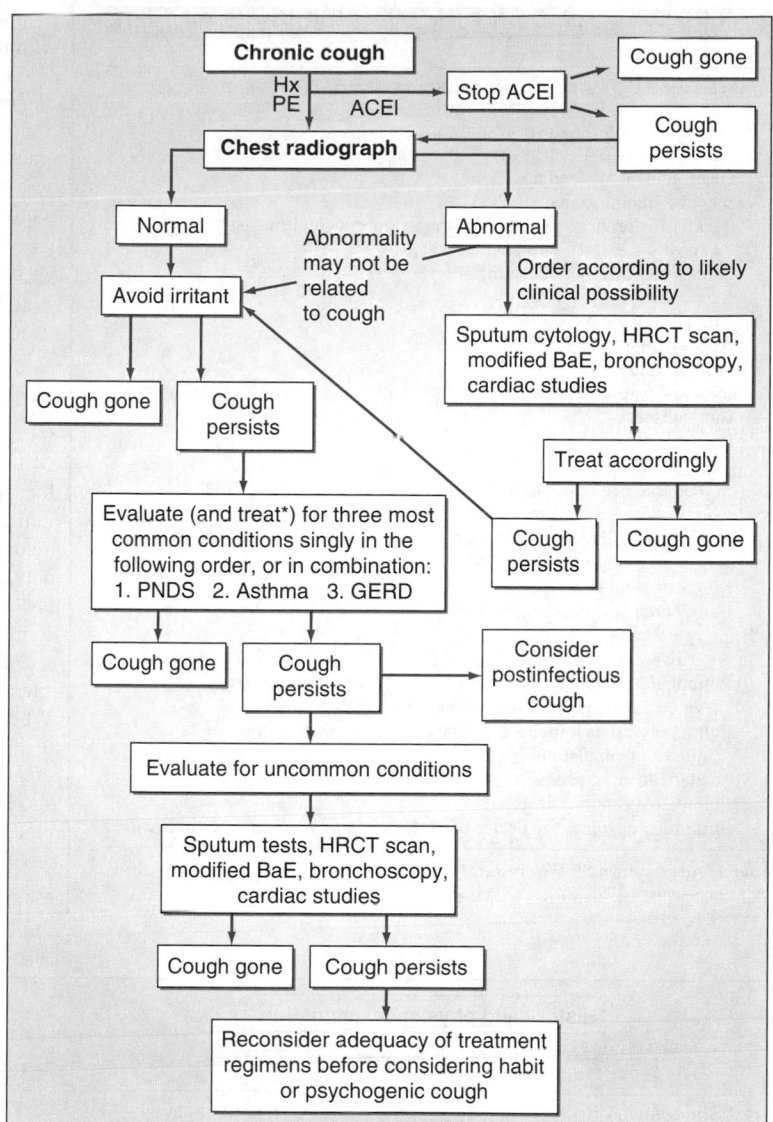

FIGURE 30-1 An algorithm for the evaluation of chronic cough. ACEI, angiotensin-converting enzyme inhibitor; BaE, barium esophagography; GERD, gastroesophageal reflux disease; HRCT, high-resolution computed tomography; Hx, history; PE, physical examination; PNDS, postnasal drip syndrome. *Treatment is either targeted to a presumptive diagnosis or given empirically. [Adapted from RS Irwin: Chest 114(Suppl):133S, 1998, with permission.]

APPROACH TO THE PATIENT

The *history* is extremely valuable. Hemoptysis that is described as blood-streaking of mucopurulent or purulent sputum often suggests bronchitis. Chronic production of sputum with a recent change in quantity or appearance favors an acute exacerbation of chronic bronchitis. Fever or chills accompanying blood-streaked purulent sputum suggests pneumonia, whereas a putrid smell to the sputum raises the possibility of lung abscess. When sputum production has been chronic and copious, the diagnosis of bronchiectasis should be considered. Hemoptysis following the acute onset of pleuritic chest pain and dyspnea is suggestive of pulmonary embolism.

A history of previous or coexisting disorders should be sought, such as renal disease (seen with Goodpasture's syndrome or Wegener's granulomatosis), lupus erythematosus (with associated pulmonary hemorrhage from lupus pneumonitis), or a previous malignancy (either recurrent lung cancer or endobronchial metastasis from a nonpulmonary primary tumor). In a patient with AIDS, endobronchial or pulmonary parenchymal Kaposi's sarcoma should be considered. Risk factors for bronchogenic carcinoma, particularly smoking and asbestos exposure, should be sought. Patients should be questioned about previous bleeding disorders,

TABLE 30-1 *Differential Diagnosis of Hemoptysis*

Source other than the lower respiratory tract
    Upper airway (nasopharyngeal) bleeding
    Gastrointestinal bleeding
Tracheobronchial source
    Neoplasm (bronchogenic carcinoma, endobronchial metastatic tumor,
     Kaposi's sarcoma, bronchial carcinoid)
    Bronchitis (acute or chronic)
    Bronchiectasis
    Broncholithiasis
    Airway trauma
    Foreign body
Pulmonary parenchymal source
    Lung abscess
    Pneumonia
    Tuberculosis
    Mycetoma ("fungus ball")
    Goodpasture's syndrome
    Idiopathic pulmonary hemosiderosis
    Wegener's granulomatosis
    Lupus pneumonitis
    Lung contusion
Primary vascular source
    Arteriovenous malformation
    Pulmonary embolism
    Elevated pulmonary venous pressure (esp. mitral stenosis)
    Pulmonary artery rupture secondary to balloon-tip pulmonary artery
     catheter manipulation
Miscellaneous/rare causes
    Pulmonary endometriosis
    Systemic coagulopathy or use of anticoagulants or thrombolytic agents

Source: Adapted from SE Weinberger, *Principles of Pulmonary Medicine*, 3d ed, Philadelphia, Saunders, 1998.

treatment with anticoagulants, or use of drugs that can be associated with thrombocytopenia.

The *physical examination* may also provide helpful clues to the diagnosis. For example, examination of the lungs may demonstrate a pleural friction rub (pulmonary embolism), localized or diffuse crackles (parenchymal bleeding or an underlying parenchymal process associated with bleeding), evidence of airflow obstruction (chronic bronchitis), or prominent rhonchi, with or without wheezing or crackles (bronchiectasis). Cardiac examination may demonstrate findings of pulmonary arterial hypertension, mitral stenosis, or heart failure. Skin examination may reveal Kaposi's sarcoma, arteriovenous malformations of Osler-Rendu-Weber disease, or lesions suggestive of systemic lupus erythematosus.

Diagnostic evaluation of hemoptysis starts with a chest radiograph (often followed by a computed tomographic scan) to look for a mass lesion, findings suggestive of bronchiectasis (Chap. 240), or focal or diffuse parenchymal disease (representing either focal or diffuse bleeding or a focal area of pneumonitis). Additional initial screening evaluation often includes a complete blood count, a coagulation profile, and assessment for renal disease with a urinalysis and measurement of blood urea nitrogen and creatinine levels. When sputum is present, examination by Gram and acid-fast stains (along with the corresponding cultures) is indicated.

Fiberoptic bronchoscopy is particularly useful for localizing the site of bleeding and for visualization of endobronchial lesions. When bleeding is massive, rigid bronchoscopy is often preferable to fiberoptic bronchoscopy because of better airway control and greater suction capability. In patients with suspected bronchiectasis, HRCT is now the diagnostic procedure of choice, having replaced bronchography.

A diagnostic algorithm for evaluation of nonmassive hemoptysis is presented in Fig. 30-2.

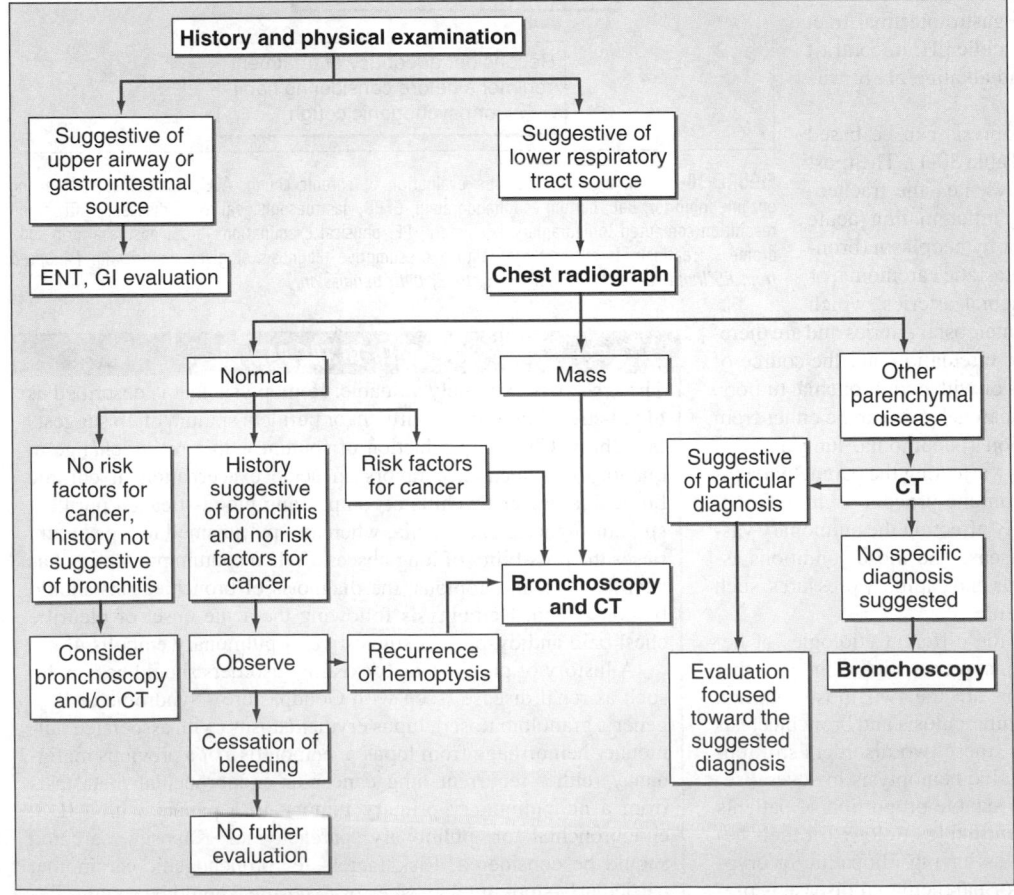

FIGURE 30-2   An algorithm for the evaluation of non-massive hemoptysis. CT, computed tomography.

TREATMENT

The rapidity of bleeding and its effect on gas exchange determine the urgency of management. When the bleeding is confined to either blood-streaking of sputum or production of small amounts of pure blood, gas exchange is usually preserved; establishing a diagnosis is the first priority. When hemoptysis is massive, maintaining adequate gas exchange, preventing blood from spilling into unaffected areas of lung, and avoiding asphyxiation are the highest priorities. Keeping the patient at rest and partially suppressing cough may help the bleeding to subside. If the origin of the blood is known and is limited to one lung, the bleeding lung should be placed in the dependent position, so that blood is not aspirated into the unaffected lung.

With massive bleeding, the need to control the airway and maintain adequate gas exchange may necessitate endotracheal intubation and mechanical ventilation. In patients in danger of flooding the lung contralateral to the side of hemorrhage despite proper positioning, isolation of the right and left mainstem bronchi from each other can be achieved by selectively intubating the nonbleeding lung (often with bronchoscopic guidance) or by using specially designed double-lumen endotracheal tubes. Another option involves inserting a balloon catheter through a bronchoscope by direct visualization and inflating the balloon to occlude the bronchus leading to the bleeding site. This technique not only prevents aspiration of blood into unaffected areas but also may promote tamponade of the bleeding site and cessation of bleeding.

Other available techniques for control of significant bleeding include laser phototherapy, electrocautery, embolotherapy, and surgical resection of the involved area of lung. With bleeding from an endobronchial tumor, the neodymium:yttrium-aluminum-garnet (Nd:YAG) laser can often achieve at least temporary hemostasis by coagulating the bleeding site. Electrocautery, which uses an electric current for thermal destruction of tissue, can be used similarly for management of bleeding from an endobronchial tumor. Embolotherapy involves an arteriographic procedure in which a vessel proximal to the bleeding site is cannulated, and a material such as Gelfoam is injected to occlude the bleeding vessel. Surgical resection is a therapeutic option either for the emergent therapy of life-threatening hemoptysis that fails to respond to other measures or for the elective but definitive management of localized disease subject to recurrent bleeding.

FURTHER READING

GIBSON PG et al: Eosinophilic bronchitis: Clinical manifestations and implications for treatment. Thorax 57:178, 2002

HIRSHBERG B et al: Hemoptysis: Etiology, evaluation, and outcome in a tertiary referral hospital. Chest 112:440, 1997

IRWIN RS, MADISON JM: The diagnosis and treatment of cough. N Engl J Med 343:1715, 2000

————, WIDDICOMBE J: Cough, in *Textbook of Respiratory Medicine*, 3d ed JF Murray, JA Nadel (eds). Philadelphia, Saunders, 2000, pp 553–566

ISRAILI ZH, HALL WD: Cough and angioneurotic edema associated with angiotensin-converting enzyme inhibitor therapy. Ann Intern Med 117:234, 1992

JEAN-BAPTISTE E: Clinical assessment and management of massive hemoptysis. Crit Care Med 28:1642, 2000

31 HYPOXIA AND CYANOSIS
Eugene Braunwald

HYPOXIA

The fundamental purpose of the cardiorespiratory system is to deliver O_2 (and substrates) to the cells and to remove CO_2 (and other metabolic products) from them. Proper maintenance of this function depends on intact cardiovascular and respiratory systems and a supply of inspired gas containing adequate O_2. When hypoxia occurs consequent to respiratory failure, Pa_{O_2} declines, Pa_{CO_2} usually rises (Chap. 234), and the hemoglobin-oxygen (Hb-O_2) dissociation curve (see Fig. 91-2) is displaced to the right, with greater quantities of O_2 released at any level of tissue P_{O_2}. Arterial hypoxemia, i.e., a reduction of O_2 saturation of arterial blood (Sa_{O_2}), and consequent cyanosis are likely to be more marked when such depression of Pa_{O_2} results from pulmonary disease than when the depression occurs as the result of a decline in the fraction of oxygen in inspired air (FI_{O_2}). In this situation Pa_{CO_2} falls secondary to anoxia-induced hyperventilation and the Hb-O_2 dissociation curve is displaced to the left, limiting the decline in Sa_{O_2} at any level of Pa_{O_2}.

CAUSES OF HYPOXIA

ANEMIC HYPOXIA A reduction in the hemoglobin concentration of the blood is attended by a corresponding decline in the O_2-carrying capacity of the blood. In anemic hypoxia, the Pa_{O_2} is normal; but as a consequence of the reduction of the hemoglobin concentration, the absolute quantity of O_2 transported per unit volume of blood is diminished. As the anemic blood passes through the capillaries and the usual quantity of O_2 is removed from it, the P_{O_2} in the venous blood declines to a greater degree than would normally be the case.

CARBON MONOXIDE INTOXICATION (See also Chap. 377) Hemoglobin that is combined with carbon monoxide (carboxyhemoglobin, COHb) is unavailable for O_2 transport. In addition, the presence of COHb shifts the Hb-O_2 dissociation curve to the left (see Fig. 91-2) so that O_2 is unloaded only at lower tensions. By such formation of COHb, a given degree of reduction in O_2-carrying power produces a far greater degree of tissue hypoxia than the equivalent reduction in hemoglobin due to simple anemia.

RESPIRATORY HYPOXIA Arterial unsaturation is a common finding in advanced pulmonary disease. The most common cause of respiratory hypoxia is ventilation-perfusion mismatch, which results from perfusion of poorly ventilated alveoli. As discussed in Chap. 234, it may also be caused by hypoventilation, and it is then associated with an elevation of Pa_{CO_2}. These two forms of respiratory hypoxia may be recognized because they are usually correctable by inspiring 100% O_2 for several minutes. A third cause is shunting of blood across the lung from right to left by perfusion of nonventilated portions of the lung, as in pulmonary atelectasis or through arteriovenous connections in the lung. The low Pa_{O_2} in this situation is correctable only in part by an FI_{O_2} of 100%.

HYPOXIA SECONDARY TO HIGH ALTITUDE As one ascends rapidly to 3000 m (approximately 10,000 ft), the alveolar P_{O_2} declines to about 60 mmHg, and impaired memory and other cerebral symptoms of hypoxia may develop. At higher altitudes, arterial saturation declines rapidly and symptoms become more serious; and at 5000 m (approximately 15,000 ft) unacclimatized individuals usually cease to be able to function normally.

HYPOXIA SECONDARY TO RIGHT-TO-LEFT EXTRAPULMONARY SHUNTING From a physiologic viewpoint, this cause of hypoxia resembles intrapulmonary right-to-left shunting but is caused by congenital cardiac malformations such as tetralogy of Fallot, transposition of the great arteries, and Eisenmenger's syndrome (Chap. 218). As in pulmonary right-to-left shunting, the Pa_{O_2} cannot be restored to normal with inspiration of 100% O_2.

CIRCULATORY HYPOXIA As in anemic hypoxia, the Pa_{O_2} is usually normal, but venous and tissue P_{O_2} values are reduced as a consequence of reduced tissue perfusion and greater tissue O_2 extraction. Generalized circulatory hypoxia occurs in heart failure (Chap. 216) and in most forms of shock (Chap. 253).

SPECIFIC ORGAN HYPOXIA Decreased perfusion of any organ resulting in localized circulatory hypoxia may occur secondary to organic arterial obstruction, as in atherosclerosis, or as a consequence of vasoconstriction (Chap. 232), as observed in Raynaud's phenomenon. Localized hypoxia may also result from venous obstruction and the resultant congestion and reduced arterial inflow. Edema, which increases the distance through which O_2 diffuses before it reaches cells, also can cause localized hypoxia. In an attempt to maintain adequate perfusion to more vital organs, vasoconstriction may reduce perfusion in the limbs and skin, causing hypoxia of these regions in patients with heart failure or hypovolemic shock.

INCREASED O_2 REQUIREMENTS If the O_2 consumption of the tissues is elevated without a corresponding increase in perfusion, tissue hypoxia ensues and the P_{O_2} in venous blood becomes reduced. Ordinarily, the clinical picture of patients with hypoxia due to an elevated metabolic rate is quite different from that in other types of hypoxia; the skin is warm and flushed, owing to increased cutaneous blood flow that dissipates the excessive heat produced, and cyanosis is usually absent.

Exercise is a classic example of increased tissue O_2 requirements. These increased demands are normally met by several mechanisms operating simultaneously: (1) increasing the cardiac output and ventilation and thus O_2 delivery to the tissues; (2) preferentially directing the blood to the exercising muscles by changing vascular resistances in various circulatory beds, directly and/or reflexly; (3) increasing O_2 extraction from the delivered blood and widening the arteriovenous O_2 difference; and (4) reducing the pH of the tissues and capillary blood, shifting the Hb-O_2 curve to the right and unloading more O_2 from hemoglobin. If the capacity of these mechanisms is exceeded, then hypoxia, especially of the exercising muscles, will result.

IMPROPER OXYGEN UTILIZATION   Cyanide (Chap. 377) and several other similarly acting poisons cause cellular hypoxia. The tissues are unable to utilize O_2, and as a consequence, the venous blood tends to have a high O_2 tension. This condition has been termed *histotoxic hypoxia.*

EFFECTS OF HYPOXIA

Changes in the central nervous system, particularly the higher centers, are especially important consequences of hypoxia. Acute hypoxia causes impaired judgment, motor incoordination, and a clinical picture closely resembling that of acute alcoholism. When hypoxia is long-standing, fatigue, drowsiness, apathy, inattentiveness, delayed reaction time, and reduced work capacity occur. As hypoxia becomes more severe, the centers of the brainstem are affected, and death usually results from respiratory failure. With the reduction of Pa_{O_2}, cerebrovascular resistance decreases and cerebral blood flow increases, in an attempt to maintain O_2 delivery to the brain. However, when the reduction of Pa_{O_2} is accompanied by hyperventilation and a reduction of Pa_{CO_2}, cerebrovascular resistance rises, cerebral blood flow falls, and hypoxia is intensified. Hypoxia also causes pulmonary arterial constriction, which shunts blood away from poorly ventilated toward better-ventilated portions of the lung. However, it also increases pulmonary vascular resistance and right ventricular afterload.

Glucose is normally broken down to pyruvic acid. However, the further breakdown of pyruvate and the generation of adenosine triphosphate (ATP) consequent to it require O_2, and in the presence of hypoxia increasing proportions of pyruvate are reduced to lactic acid, which cannot be broken down further, causing metabolic acidosis. Under these circumstances, the total energy obtained from the breakdown of carbohydrate is greatly reduced, and the quantity of energy available for the production of ATP becomes inadequate.

An important component of the respiratory response to hypoxia originates in special chemosensitive cells in the carotid and aortic bodies and in the respiratory center in the brainstem. The stimulation of these cells by hypoxia increases ventilation, with a loss of CO_2, and leads to respiratory alkalosis. When combined with the metabolic acidosis resulting from the production of lactic acid, the serum bicarbonate level declines (Chap. 42).

Diminished P_{O_2} in any tissue results in local vasodilatation, and the diffuse vasodilatation that occurs in generalized hypoxia raises the cardiac output. In patients with underlying heart disease, the requirements of the peripheral tissues for an increase of cardiac output with hypoxia may precipitate congestive heart failure. In patients with ischemic heart disease, a reduced Pa_{O_2} may intensify myocardial ischemia and further impair left ventricular function.

One of the important mechanisms of compensation for chronic hypoxia is an increase in the hemoglobin concentration and in the number of red blood cells in the circulating blood, i.e., the development of polycythemia secondary to erythropoietin production (Chap. 95). →*The approach to the patient with hypoxia is presented in Chap. 234.*

CYANOSIS

Cyanosis refers to a bluish color of the skin and mucous membranes resulting from an increased quantity of reduced hemoglobin, or of hemoglobin derivatives, in the small blood vessels of those areas. It is usually most marked in the lips, nail beds, ears, and malar eminences. Cyanosis, especially if developed recently, is more commonly detected by a family member than the patient. The florid skin characteristic of polycythemia vera (Chap. 95) must be distinguished from the true cyanosis discussed here. A cherry-colored flush, rather than cyanosis, is caused by COHb (Chap. 377). The degree of cyanosis is modified by the color of the cutaneous pigment and the thickness of the skin, as well as by the state of the cutaneous capillaries. The accurate clinical detection of the presence and degree of cyanosis is difficult, as proved by oximetric studies. In some instances, central cyanosis can be detected reliably when the Sa_{O_2} has fallen to 85%; in others, particularly in dark-skinned persons, it may not be detected until it has declined to 75%. In the latter case, examination of the mucous membranes in the oral cavity and the conjunctivae rather than examination of the skin is more helpful in the detection of cyanosis.

The increase in the quantity of reduced hemoglobin in the mucocutaneous vessels that produces cyanosis may be brought about either by an increase in the quantity of venous blood as the result of dilatation of the venules and venous ends of the capillaries or by a reduction in the Sa_{O_2} in the capillary blood. In general, cyanosis becomes apparent when the mean capillary concentration of reduced hemoglobin exceeds 40 g/L (4 g/dL). It is the *absolute* rather than the *relative* quantity of reduced hemoglobin that is important in producing cyanosis. Thus, in a patient with severe anemia, the relative amount of reduced hemoglobin in the venous blood may be very large when considered in relation to the total amount of hemoglobin in the blood. However, since the concentration of the latter is markedly reduced, the *absolute* quantity of reduced hemoglobin may still be small, and therefore patients with severe anemia and even *marked* arterial desaturation may not display cyanosis. Conversely, the higher the total hemoglobin content, the greater is the tendency toward cyanosis; thus, patients with marked polycythemia tend to be cyanotic at higher levels of Sa_{O_2} than patients with normal hematocrit values. Likewise, local passive congestion, which causes an increase in the total amount of reduced hemoglobin in the vessels in a given area, may cause cyanosis. Cyanosis is also observed when nonfunctional hemoglobin such as methemoglobin or sulfhemoglobin (Chap. 91) is present in blood.

Cyanosis may be subdivided into central and peripheral types. In the *central* type, the Sa_{O_2} is reduced or an abnormal hemoglobin derivative is present, and the mucous membranes and skin are both affected. *Peripheral* cyanosis is due to a slowing of blood flow and abnormally great extraction of O_2 from normally saturated arterial blood. It results from vasoconstriction and diminished peripheral blood flow, such as occurs in cold exposure, shock, congestive failure, and peripheral vascular disease. Often in these conditions the mucous membranes of the oral cavity or those beneath the tongue may be spared. Clinical differentiation between central and peripheral cyanosis may not always be simple, and in conditions such as cardiogenic shock with pulmonary edema there may be a mixture of both types.

DIFFERENTIAL DIAGNOSIS

CENTRAL CYANOSIS (Table 31-1)   Decreased Sa_{O_2} results from a marked reduction in the Pa_{O_2}. This reduction may be brought about by a decline in the FI_{O_2} without sufficient compensatory alveolar hyperventilation to maintain alveolar P_{O_2}. Cyanosis does not occur to a significant degree in an ascent to an altitude of 2500 m (8000 ft) but is marked in a further ascent to 5000 m (16,000 ft). The reason for this difference becomes clear on studying the *S* shape of the Hb-O_2 dissociation curve (see Fig. 91-2). At 2500 m (8000 ft) the FI_{O_2} is about 120 mmHg, the alveolar P_{O_2} is approximately 80 mmHg, and the Sa_{O_2} is nearly normal. However, at 5000 m (16,000 ft) the FI_{O_2} and alveolar P_{O_2} are about 85 and 50 mmHg, respectively, and the Sa_{O_2} is only about 75%. This leaves 25% of the hemoglobin in the arterial blood in the reduced form, an amount likely to be associated with cyanosis in the absence of anemia. Similarly, a mutant hemoglobin with a low affinity for O_2 (e.g., Hb Kansas) causes lowered Sa_{O_2} saturation and resultant central cyanosis (Chap. 91).

TABLE 31-1   Causes of Cyanosis

CENTRAL CYANOSIS

Decreased arterial oxygen saturation
    Decreased atmospheric pressure—high altitude
    Impaired pulmonary function
        Alveolar hypoventilation
        Uneven relationships between pulmonary ventilation and perfusion
            (perfusion of hypoventilated alveoli)
        Impaired oxygen diffusion
    Anatomic shunts
        Certain types of congenital heart disease
        Pulmonary arteriovenous fistulas
        Multiple small intrapulmonary shunts
    Hemoglobin with low affinity for oxygen
Hemoglobin abnormalities
    Methemoglobinemia—hereditary, acquired
    Sulfhemoglobinemia—acquired
    Carboxyhemoglobinemia (not true cyanosis)

PERIPHERAL CYANOSIS

Reduced cardiac output
Cold exposure
Redistribution of blood flow from extremities
Arterial obstruction
Venous obstruction

sides of the heart. Secondary polycythemia occurs frequently in patients with arterial O_2 unsaturation and contributes to the cyanosis.

Cyanosis can be caused by small amounts of circulating methemoglobin and by even smaller amounts of sulfhemoglobin (Chap. 91). Although they are uncommon causes of cyanosis, these abnormal hemoglobin pigments should be sought by spectroscopy when cyanosis is not readily explained by malfunction of the circulatory or respiratory systems. Generally, digital clubbing does not occur with them. The diagnosis of methemoglobinemia can be suspected if the patient's blood remains brown after being mixed in a test tube and exposed to air.

PERIPHERAL CYANOSIS   Probably the most common cause of peripheral cyanosis is the normal vasoconstriction resulting from exposure to cold air or water. When cardiac output is reduced, cutaneous vasoconstriction occurs as a compensatory mechanism so that blood is diverted from the skin to more vital areas such as the central nervous system and heart, and cyanosis of the extremities may result, even though the arterial blood is normally saturated.

Arterial obstruction to an extremity, as with an embolus, or arteriolar constriction, as in cold-induced vasospasm (Raynaud's phenomenon, Chap. 232), generally results in pallor and coldness, but there may be associated cyanosis. Venous obstruction, as in thrombophlebitis, dilates the subpapillary venous plexuses and thereby intensifies cyanosis.

APPROACH TO THE PATIENT

Certain features are important in arriving at the cause of cyanosis:

1.   A careful history must be obtained, particularly timing of the onset of cyanosis. Cyanosis present since birth or infancy is usually due to congenital heart disease.

2.   Central and peripheral cyanosis must be differentiated. Evidence of disorders of the respiratory or cardiovascular systems are helpful. Massage or gentle warming of a cyanotic extremity will increase peripheral blood flow and abolish peripheral but not central cyanosis.

3.   The presence or absence of clubbing of the digits (see below) should be ascertained. Clubbing *without* cyanosis is frequent in patients with infective endocarditis and inflammatory bowel disease; it may occasionally occur in healthy persons, and in some instances it may be occupational, e.g., in jackhammer operators. The combination of cyanosis and clubbing is frequent in patients with congenital heart disease and right-to-left shunting and is seen occasionally in patients with pulmonary disease such as lung abscess or pulmonary arteriovenous fistulae. In contrast, peripheral cyanosis or acutely developing central cyanosis is *not* associated with clubbed digits.

4. Pa_{O_2} and Sa_{O_2} should be ascertained and in patients in whom the mechanism of cyanosis is obscure spectroscopic and other examinations of the blood performed to look for abnormal types of hemoglobin (critical in the differential diagnosis of cyanosis).

Seriously *impaired pulmonary function*, through perfusion of unventilated or poorly ventilated areas of the lung or alveolar hypoventilation, is a common cause of central cyanosis (Chap. 234). This condition may occur acutely, as in extensive pneumonia or pulmonary edema, or chronically with chronic pulmonary diseases (e.g., emphysema). In the latter situation, secondary polycythemia is generally present and clubbing of the fingers may occur. However, in many types of chronic pulmonary disease with fibrosis and obliteration of the capillary vascular bed, cyanosis does not occur because there is relatively little perfusion of underventilated areas.

Another cause of reduced Sa_{O_2} is *shunting of systemic venous blood into the arterial circuit*. Certain forms of congenital heart disease are associated with cyanosis (Chap. 218). Since blood flows from a higher-pressure to a lower-pressure region, for a cardiac defect to result in a right-to-left shunt, it must ordinarily be combined with an obstructive lesion distal (downstream) to the defect or with elevated pulmonary vascular resistance. The most common congenital cardiac lesion associated with cyanosis in the adult is the combination of ventricular septal defect and pulmonary outflow tract obstruction (*tetralogy of Fallot*). The more severe the obstruction, the greater the degree of right-to-left shunting and resultant cyanosis. In patients with patent ductus arteriosus, pulmonary hypertension, and right-to-left shunt, *differential cyanosis* results; that is, cyanosis occurs in the lower but not in the upper extremities. →*The mechanisms for the elevated pulmonary vascular resistance that may produce cyanosis in the presence of intra- and extracardiac communications without pulmonic stenosis (Eisenmenger syndrome) are discussed in Chap. 218.*

Pulmonary arteriovenous fistulae (Chap. 48) may be congenital or acquired, solitary or multiple, microscopic or massive. The severity of cyanosis produced by these fistulae depends on their size and number. They occur with some frequency in hereditary hemorrhagic telangiectasia. Sa_{O_2} reduction and cyanosis may also occur in some patients with cirrhosis, presumably as a consequence of pulmonary arteriovenous fistulas or portal vein–pulmonary vein anastomoses.

In patients with cardiac or pulmonary right-to-left shunts, the presence and severity of cyanosis depend on the size of the shunt relative to the systemic flow as well as on the Hb-O_2 saturation of the venous blood. With increased extraction of O_2 from the blood by the exercising muscles, the venous blood returning to the right side of the heart is more unsaturated than at rest, and shunting of this blood intensifies the cyanosis. Also, since the systemic vascular resistance falls with exercise, the right-to-left shunt is augmented by exercise in patients with congenital heart disease and communications between the two

CLUBBING

The selective bullous enlargement of the distal segments of the fingers and toes due to proliferation of connective tissue, particularly on the dorsal surface, is termed *clubbing*; there is increased sponginess of the soft tissue at the base of the nail. Clubbing may be hereditary, idiopathic, or acquired and associated with a variety of disorders, including cyanotic congenital heart disease, infective endocarditis, and a variety of pulmonary conditions (among them primary and metastatic lung cancer, bronchiectasis, lung abscess, cystic fibrosis, and mesothelioma), as well as with some gastrointestinal diseases (including inflammatory bowel disease and hepatic cirrhosis).

Clubbing in patients with primary and metastatic lung cancer, mesothelioma, bronchiectasis, and hepatic cirrhosis may be associated with *hypertrophic osteoarthropathy*. In this condition, the subperiosteal formation of new bone in the distal diaphyses of the long bones of the extremities causes pain and symmetric arthritis-like changes in the shoulders, knees, ankles, wrists, and elbows. The diagnosis of hypertrophic osteoarthropathy may be confirmed by bone radiographs. Although the mechanism of clubbing is unclear, it appears to be secondary to a humoral substance that causes dilation of the vessels of the fingertip.

FURTHER READING

BEALL CM: Tibetan and Andean patterns of adaptation to high-altitude hypoxia. Hum Biol 72:201, 2000

FISHMAN AP: Approach to the patient with respiratory symptoms: Cyanosis and clubbing, in *Fishman's Pulmonary Diseases and Disorders*, 3d ed, Fishman AP et al (eds). Philadelphia, Saunders, 1998, pp 382–383

GRIFFEY RT et al: Cyanosis. J Emerg Med 18:369, 2000

GRIFKA RG: Cyanotic congenital heart disease with increased pulmonary blood flow. Pediatr Clin North Am 46:405, 1999

HACKETT PH, ROACH RC: Current concepts: High altitude illness. N Engl J Med 345:107, 2001

MYERS KA, FARQUHAR DR: The rational clinical examination. Does the patient have clubbing? JAMA 286:341, 2001

WALDMAN JD, WERNLY JA. Cyanotic congenital heart disease with decreased pulmonary blood flow in children. Pediatr Clin North Am 46:385, 1999

32 EDEMA
Eugene Braunwald

Edema is defined as a clinically apparent increase in the interstitial fluid volume, which may expand by several liters before the abnormality is evident. Therefore, a weight gain of several kilograms usually precedes overt manifestations of edema, and a similar weight loss from diuresis can be induced in a slightly edematous patient before "dry weight" is achieved. *Anasarca* refers to gross, generalized edema. *Ascites* (Chap. 39) and *hydrothorax* refer to accumulation of excess fluid in the peritoneal and pleural cavities, respectively, and are considered to be special forms of edema.

Depending on its cause and mechanism, edema may be localized or have a generalized distribution; it is recognized in its generalized form by puffiness of the face, which is most readily apparent in the periorbital areas, and by the persistence of an indentation of the skin following pressure; this is known as "pitting" edema. In its more subtle form, edema may be detected by noting that after the stethoscope is removed from the chest wall, the rim of the bell leaves an indentation on the skin of the chest for a few minutes. When the ring on a finger fits more snugly than in the past or when a patient complains of difficulty in putting on shoes, particularly in the evening, edema may be present.

PATHOGENESIS

About one-third of the total-body water is confined to the extracellular space. Approximately 25% of the latter, in turn, is composed of the plasma volume, and the remainder is interstitial fluid.

STARLING FORCES The forces that regulate the disposition of fluid between these two components of the extracellular compartment are frequently referred to as the *Starling forces* (see p. 204). The hydrostatic pressure within the vascular system and the colloid oncotic pressure in the interstitial fluid tend to promote movement of fluid from the vascular to the extravascular space. On the other hand, the colloid oncotic pressure contributed by the plasma proteins and the hydrostatic pressure within the interstitial fluid, referred to as the *tissue tension*, promote the movement of fluid into the vascular compartment. Consequently there is a movement of water and diffusible solutes from the vascular space at the arteriolar end of the capillaries. Fluid is returned from the interstitial space into the vascular system at the venous end of the capillary and by way of the lymphatics. Unless these channels are obstructed, lymph flow rises with increases in net movement of fluid from the vascular compartment to the interstitium. These flows are usually balanced so that a steady state exists in the sizes of the intravascular and interstitial compartments, and yet a large exchange between them occurs. However, should any one of the hydrostatic or oncotic pressure gradients be altered significantly, a further net movement of fluid between the two components of the extracellular space will take place. The development of edema then depends on one or more alterations in the Starling forces so that there is increased flow of fluid from the vascular system into the interstitium or into a body cavity.

Edema due to increase in capillary pressure may result from an elevation of venous pressure due to obstruction in venous drainage. This increase in capillary pressure may be generalized, as occurs in congestive heart failure. The Starling forces may be imbalanced when the colloid oncotic pressure of the plasma is reduced, owing to any factor that may induce hypoalbuminemia, such as saline expansion, malnutrition, liver disease, loss of protein into the urine or into the gastrointestinal tract, or a severe catabolic state.

CAPILLARY DAMAGE Edema may also result from damage to the capillary endothelium, which increases its permeability and permits the transfer of protein into the interstitial compartment. Injury to the capillary wall can result from drugs, viral or bacterial agents, and thermal or mechanical trauma. Increased capillary permeability may also be a consequence of a hypersensitivity reaction and is characteristic of immune injury. Damage to the capillary endothelium is presumably responsible for inflammatory edema, which is usually nonpitting, localized, and accompanied by other signs of inflammation—redness, heat, and tenderness.

REDUCTION OF EFFECTIVE ARTERIAL VOLUME In many forms of edema the *effective arterial blood volume*, an as yet poorly defined parameter of the filling of the arterial tree, is reduced, and as a consequence a series of physiologic responses designed to restore it to normal are set into motion. A key element of these responses is the retention of salt and therefore of water, principally by the renal proximal tubule, ultimately leading to edema.

REDUCED CARDIAC OUTPUT A reduction of cardiac output, whatever the cause, is associated with a lowering of the effective arterial blood volume as well as of renal blood flow, constriction of the efferent renal arterioles, and an elevation of the filtration fraction, i.e., the ratio of glomerular filtration rate to renal plasma flow. In severe heart failure there is a reduction in the glomerular filtration rate. Activation of the sympathetic nervous system and of the renin-angiotensin systems is responsible for renal vasoconstriction. The finding that α-adrenergic blocking agents and/or angiotensin-converting enzyme (ACE) inhibitors augment renal blood flow and induce diuresis supports the role of these two systems in elevating renal vascular resistance and salt and water retention when cardiac output is reduced.

RENAL FACTORS Heart failure and other conditions, such as nephrotic syndrome and cirrhosis that reduce effective arterial blood volume, cause renal efferent arteriolar constriction. This, in turn, reduces the hydrostatic pressure while the increased filtration fraction raises the colloid osmotic pressure in the peritubular capillaries, thus enhancing salt and water reabsorption in the proximal tubule as well as in the ascending limb of the loop of Henle.

In addition, the diminished renal blood flow characteristic of states in which the effective arterial blood volume is reduced is translated by the renal juxtaglomerular cells into a signal for increased renin release (Chap. 321). The mechanisms responsible for this release include: (1) a baroreceptor response in which reduced renal perfusion results in incomplete filling of the renal arterioles and diminished stretch of the juxtaglomerular cells, a signal that provides for the elaboration and/or release of renin (see below); (2) reduced glomerular filtration which lowers the sodium chloride load reaching the distal renal tubules; this is sensed by the macula densa, which signals the neighboring juxtaglomerular cells to secrete renin; (3) activation of the β-adrenergic receptors in the juxtaglomerular cells by the sympathetic nervous system and circulating catecholamines stimulates renin release. These three mechanisms generally act in concert.

THE RENIN-ANGIOTENSIN-ALDOSTERONE (RAA) SYSTEM (See also Chap. 321) Renin, an enzyme with a molecular weight of about 40,000, acts on its substrate, angiotensinogen, an α_2 globulin synthesized by the liver, to release angiotensin I, a decapeptide, which is broken down to angiotensin II (AII), an octapeptide. AII has generalized vasoconstrictor properties; it is especially active on the efferent arterioles and independently increases Na^+ reabsorption in the proximal tubule. The RAA system has long been recognized as a hormone system. However, it also operates locally. Both circulating and intrarenally produced AII contribute to renal vasoconstriction and to salt and water retention. These renal effects of AII are mediated by activation of AII type 1 receptors, which can be blocked by specific antagonists (angiotensin receptor blockers) such as losartan. AII also enters the circulation and stimulates the production of aldosterone by the zona glomerulosa of the adrenal cortex. In patients with heart failure, not only is aldosterone secretion elevated but the biologic half-life of aldosterone is prolonged, which further increases the plasma level of the hormone. A depression of hepatic blood flow, particularly during exercise, secondary to a reduction in cardiac output, is responsible for the reduced hepatic catabolism of aldosterone. Aldosterone, in turn, enhances Na^+ reabsorption (and K^+ excretion) by the collecting tubule. The activation of the RAA system is most striking in the early phase of acute, severe heart failure and is less intense in patients with chronic, stable, compensated heart failure.

Although increased quantities of aldosterone are secreted in heart failure and in other edematous states and although blockade of the action of aldosterone by spironolactone (an aldosterone antagonist) or amiloride (a blocker of epithelial Na^+ channels) often induces a moderate diuresis in edematous states, persistent augmented levels of aldosterone (or other mineralocorticoids) alone do not always promote accumulation of edema, as witnessed by the lack of striking fluid retention in most instances of primary aldosteronism (Chap. 321). Furthermore, although normal individuals retain some salt and water with the administration of potent mineralocorticoids, such as deoxycorticosterone acetate or fludrocortisone, this accumulation is self-limiting, despite continued exposure to the steroid, a phenomenon known as *mineralocorticoid escape*. The failure of normal individuals who receive large doses of mineralocorticoids to accumulate large quantities of extracellular fluid and to develop edema is probably a consequence of an increase in glomerular filtration rate (pressure natriuresis) and through the action of natriuretic substance(s) (see below). The continued secretion of aldosterone may be more important in the accumulation of fluid in edematous states because patients with edema secondary to heart failure, nephrotic syndrome, and cirrhosis are generally unable to repair the deficit in effective arterial blood volume. As a consequence they do not develop pressure natriuresis.

ARGININE VASOPRESSIN (AVP) (See also Chap. 319) The secretion of AVP occurs in response to increased intracellular osmolar concentration and by stimulating V_2 receptors increases the reabsorption of free water in the renal distal tubule and collecting duct, thereby increasing total-body water. Circulating AVP is elevated in many patients with heart failure secondary to a nonosmotic stimulus associated with decreased effective arterial volume. Such patients fail to show the normal reduction of AVP with a reduction of osmolality, contributing to hyponatremia and edema formation.

ENDOTHELIN This is a potent peptide vasoconstrictor released by endothelial cells; its concentration is elevated in heart failure and contributes to renal vasoconstriction, Na^+ retention, and edema in heart failure.

NATRIURETIC PEPTIDES (See also Chap. 215) Atrial distention and/or a sodium load cause release into the circulation of atrial natriuretic peptide (ANP), a polypeptide; a high-molecular-weight precursor of ANP is stored in secretory granules within atrial myocytes. Release of ANP causes (1) excretion of sodium and water by augmenting glomerular filtration rate, inhibiting sodium reabsorption in the proximal tubule, and inhibiting release of renin and aldosterone; and (2) arteriolar and venous dilatation by antagonizing the vasoconstrictor actions of AII, AVP, and sympathetic stimulation. Thus, ANP has the capacity to oppose sodium retention and arterial pressure elevation in hypervolemic states.

The closely related brain natriuretic peptide (BNP) is stored primarily in cardiac ventricular myocardium and is released when ventricular diastolic pressure rises. Its actions are similar to those of ANP. Circulating levels of ANP and BNP are elevated in congestive heart failure but obviously not sufficiently to prevent edema formation. In addition, in edematous states (particularly heart failure), there is abnormal resistance to the actions of natriuretic peptides.

CLINICAL CAUSES OF EDEMA

OBSTRUCTION OF VENOUS (AND LYMPHATIC) DRAINAGE OF A LIMB In this condition the hydrostatic pressure in the capillary bed upstream (proximal) to the obstruction increases so that an abnormal quantity of fluid is transferred from the vascular to the interstitial space. Since the alternative route (i.e., the lymphatic channels) may also be obstructed, an increased volume of interstitial fluid in the limb develops, i.e., there is trapping of fluid in the extremity, causing local edema at the expense of the blood volume in the remainder of the body, thereby reducing effective arterial blood volume and leading to the retention of salt and water until the deficit in plasma volume has been corrected. Tissue tension rises in the affected limb until it counterbalances the primary alterations in the Starling forces, at which time no further fluid accumulates. The net effect is a local increase in the volume of interstitial fluid. This same sequence occurs in ascites and hydrothorax, in which fluid is trapped or accumulates in the cavitary space, depleting the intravascular volume and leading to secondary salt and fluid retention, as already described.

CONGESTIVE HEART FAILURE (See also Chap. 216) In this disorder, the impaired systolic emptying of the ventricle(s) and/or the impairment of ventricular relaxation promotes an accumulation of blood in the venous circulation at the expense of the effective arterial volume, and the aforementioned sequence of events (Fig. 32-1) is initiated. In mild heart failure, a small increment of total blood volume may repair the deficit of arterial volume and establish a new steady state. Through the operation of Starling's law of the heart, an increase in ventricular diastolic volume promotes a more forceful contraction and may thereby restore the cardiac output (Fig. 216-1). However, if the cardiac disorder is more severe, fluid retention continues, and the increment in blood volume accumulates in the venous circulation. With reduction in cardiac output, a decrease in baroreflex-mediated inhibition of the vasomotor center activates renal vasoconstrictor nerves and the RAA system, causing sodium and water retention.

Incomplete ventricular emptying (systolic heart failure) and/or inadequate ventricular relaxation (diastolic heart failure) both lead to an elevation of ventricular diastolic pressure. If the impairment of cardiac function primarily involves the right ventricle, pressures in the systemic veins and capillaries rise, augmenting the transudation of fluid into the interstitial space and enhancing the likelihood of peripheral edema. The elevated systemic venous pressure is transmitted to the thoracic duct with consequent reduction of lymph drainage, further increasing the accumulation of edema.

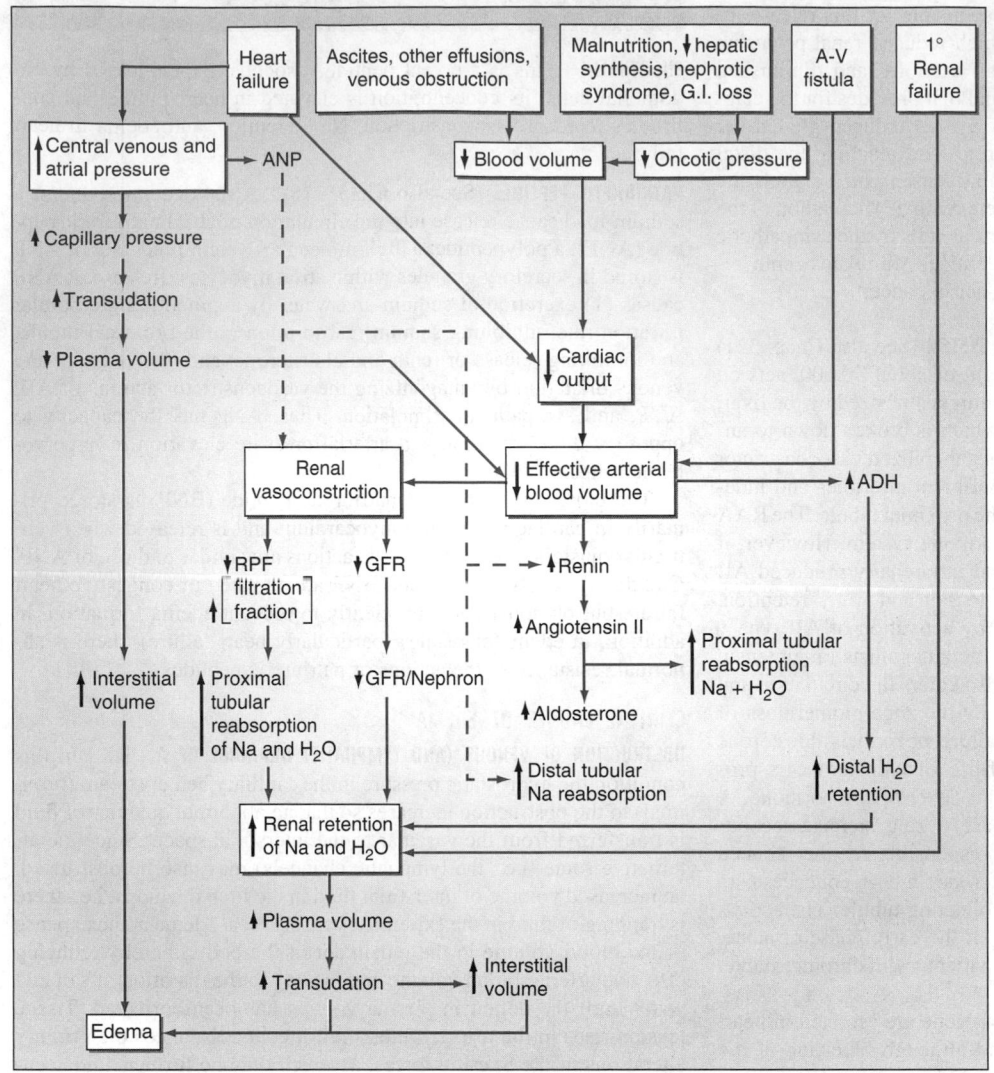

FIGURE 32-1 Sequence of events leading to the formation and retention of salt and water and the development of edema. ANP, atrial natriuretic peptide; RPF, renal plasma flow; GFR, glomerular filtration rate. Inhibitory influences are shown by broken lines. ADH, antidiuretic hormone.

CIRRHOSIS (See also Chap. 39 and Chap. 289) This condition is characterized by hepatic venous outflow blockade, which in turn expands the splanchnic blood volume and increases hepatic lymph formation. Intrahepatic hypertension acts as a potent stimulus for renal Na^+ retention and a reduction of effective arterial blood volume. These alterations are frequently complicated by hypoalbuminemia secondary to reduced hepatic synthesis, which reduce the effective arterial blood volume further, leading to activation of the RAA system, of renal sympathetic nerves, and other salt- and water-retaining mechanisms. The concentration of circulating aldosterone is elevated by the liver's failure to metabolize this hormone. Initially, the excess interstitial fluid is localized preferentially proximal (upstream) to the congested portal venous system and obstructed hepatic lymphatics, i.e., in the peritoneal cavity. In later stages, particularly when there is severe hypoalbuminemia, peripheral edema may develop. The excess production of prostaglandins (PGE_2 and PGI_2) in cirrhosis attenuates renal Na^+ retention. When the synthesis of these substances is inhibited by nonsteroidal anti-inflammatory agents, renal function deteriorates and Na^+ retention increases.

DRUG-INDUCED EDEMA A large number of widely used drugs can cause edema (Table 32-1). Mechanisms include renal vasoconstriction (nonsteroidal anti-inflammatory agents and cyclosporine), arteriolar dilatation (vasodilators), augmented renal sodium reabsorption (steroid hormones), and capillary damage (interleukin 2).

IDIOPATHIC EDEMA This syndrome, which occurs almost exclusively in women, is characterized by periodic episodes of edema (unrelated to

If the impairment of cardiac function (incomplete ventricular emptying and/or inadequate relaxation) involves the left ventricle primarily, then pulmonary venous and capillary pressures rise. Pulmonary artery pressure rises and this in turn interferes with the emptying of the right ventricle, leading to an elevation of right ventricular diastolic and of central and systemic venous pressures, thereby enhancing the likelihood of the formation of peripheral edema. The elevation of pulmonary capillary pressure may cause pulmonary edema, which impairs gas exchange. The resultant hypoxemia may impair cardiac function further, sometimes causing a vicious circle.

NEPHROTIC SYNDROME AND OTHER HYPOALBUMINEMIC STATES (See also Chap. 264) The primary alteration in this disorder is a diminished colloid oncotic pressure due to losses of large quantities of protein into the urine. This promotes a net movement of fluid into the interstitium, causes hypovolemia, and initiates the edema-forming sequence of events described above, including activation of the RAA system. With severe hypoalbuminemia and the consequent reduced colloid osmotic pressure, the salt and water that are retained cannot be restrained within the vascular compartment, total and effective arterial blood volumes decline, and hence the stimuli to retain salt and water are not abated. A similar sequence of events occurs in other conditions that lead to *severe* hypoalbuminemia, including severe nutritional deficiency states, severe, chronic liver disease, and protein-losing enteropathy. In the nephrotic syndrome, impaired renal Na^+ excretion contributes to edema, even in the absence of severe hypoalbuminemia.

TABLE 32-1 *Drugs Associated with Edema Formation*

Nonsteroidal anti-inflammatory drugs
Antihypertensive agents
   Direct arterial/arteriolar vasodilators
      Minoxidil
      Hydralazine
      Clonidine
      Methyldopa
      Guanethidine
   Calcium channel antagonists
   α-Adrenergic antagonists
Steroid hormones
   Glucocorticoids
   Anabolic steroids
   Estrogens
   Progestins
Cyclosporine
Growth hormone
Immunotherapies
   Interleukin 2
   OKT3 monoclonal antibody

Source: From Chertow.

the menstrual cycle), frequently accompanied by abdominal distention. Diurnal alterations in weight occur with orthostatic retention of sodium and water, so that the patient may weigh several pounds more after having been in the upright posture for several hours. Such large diurnal weight changes suggest an increase in capillary permeability that appears to fluctuate in severity and to be aggravated by hot weather. There is some evidence that a reduction in plasma volume occurs in this condition with secondary activation of the RAA system and impaired suppression of AVP release. Idiopathic edema should be distinguished from cyclical or premenstrual edema, in which the sodium and water retention may be secondary to excessive estrogen stimulation. There are also some cases in which the edema appears to be diuretic-induced. It has been postulated that in these patients, chronic diuretic administration leads to mild blood volume depletion, which causes chronic hyperreninemia and juxtaglomerular hyperplasia. Salt-retaining mechanisms appear to overcompensate for the direct effects of the diuretics. *Acute* withdrawal of diuretics can then leave the sodium-retaining forces unopposed, leading to fluid retention and edema. Decreased dopaminergic activity and reduced urinary kallikrein and kinin excretion have been reported in this condition and may also be of pathogenetic importance.

℞ TREATMENT

The treatment of idiopathic cyclic edema includes a reduction in salt intake, rest in the supine position for several hours each day, the wearing of elastic stockings (which should be put on before arising in the morning), and an attempt to understand any underlying emotional problems. A variety of pharmacologic agents including ACE inhibitors, progesterone, the dopamine receptor agonist bromocriptine, and the sympathomimetic amine dextroamphetamine have all been reported to be useful when administered to patients who do not respond to simpler measures. Diuretics may be helpful initially but may lose their effectiveness with continuous administration; accordingly, they should be employed sparingly, if at all. Discontinuation of diuretics paradoxically leads to diuresis in diuretic-induced edema, described above.

DIFFERENTIAL DIAGNOSIS

LOCALIZED EDEMA (See also Chap. 232)

Edema originating from inflammation or hypersensitivity is usually readily identified. Localized edema due to venous or lymphatic obstruction may be caused by thrombophlebitis, chronic lymphangitis, resection of regional lymph nodes, filariasis, etc. Lymphedema is particularly intractable because restriction of lymphatic flow results in increased protein concentration in the interstitial fluid, a circumstance that aggravates retention of fluid.

GENERALIZED EDEMA

The differences between the three major causes of generalized edema are shown in Table 32-2.

The great majority of patients with generalized edema suffer from advanced cardiac, renal, hepatic, or nutritional disorders. Consequently, the differential diagnosis of generalized edema should be directed toward identifying or excluding these several conditions.

EDEMA OF HEART FAILURE (See also Chap. 216)
The presence of heart disease, as manifested by cardiac enlargement and gallop rhythm, together with evidence of cardiac failure, such as dyspnea, basilar rales, venous distention, and hepatomegaly, usually indicate that edema results from heart failure. Noninvasive tests such as echocardiography and radionuclide angiography may be helpful in establishing the diagnosis of heart failure.

EDEMA OF THE NEPHROTIC SYNDROME (See also Chap. 264)
Marked proteinuria (>3.5 g/d), hypoalbuminemia (<35 g/L), and in some instances hypercholesterolemia are present. This syndrome may occur during the course of a variety of kidney diseases, which include glomerulonephritis, diabetic glomerulosclerosis, and hypersensitivity reactions. A history of previous renal disease may or may not be elicited.

EDEMA OF ACUTE GLOMERULONEPHRITIS AND OTHER FORMS OF RENAL FAILURE
The edema occurring during the acute phases of glomerulonephritis is characteristically associated with hematuria, proteinuria, and hypertension. Although some evidence supports the view that the fluid retention is due to increased capillary permeability, in most instances the edema results from primary retention of sodium and water by the kidneys owing to renal insufficiency. This state differs from congestive heart failure in that it is characterized by a normal (or sometimes even increased) cardiac output and a normal arterial–mixed venous oxygen difference. Patients with edema due to renal failure commonly have evidence of pulmonary congestion on chest roentgenograms before cardiac enlargement is significant, but they may not develop orthopnea. Patients with *chronic* renal failure may also develop edema due to primary renal retention of sodium and water.

TABLE 32-2 *Principal Causes of Generalized Edema: History, Physical Examination, and Laboratory Findings*

Organ System	History	Physical Examination	Laboratory Findings
Cardiac	Dyspnea with exertion prominent—often associated with orthopnea—or paroxysmal nocturnal dyspnea	Elevated jugular venous pressure, ventricular (S_3) gallop; occasionally with displaced or dyskinetic apical pulse; peripheral cyanosis, cool extremities, small pulse pressure when severe	Elevated urea nitrogen-to-creatinine ratio common; elevated uric acid; serum sodium often diminished; liver enzymes occasionally elevated with hepatic congestion
Hepatic	Dyspnea infrequent, except if associated with significant degree of ascites; most often a history of ethanol abuse	Frequently associated with ascites; jugular venous pressure normal or low; blood pressure lower than in renal or cardiac disease; one or more additional signs of chronic liver disease (jaundice, palmar erythema, Dupuytren's contracture, spider angiomata, male gynecomastia; asterixis and other signs of encephalopathy) may be present	If severe, reductions in serum albumin, cholesterol, other hepatic proteins (transferrin, fibrinogen); liver enzymes elevated, depending on the cause and acuity of liver injury; tendency toward hypokalemia, respiratory alkalosis; macrocytosis from folate deficiency
Renal	Usually chronic: may be associated with uremic signs and symptoms, including decreased appetite, altered (metallic or fishy) taste, altered sleep pattern, difficulty concentrating, restless legs or myoclonus: dyspnea can be present, but generally less prominent than in heart failure	Blood pressure may be elevated; hypertensive or diabetic retinopathy in selected cases; nitrogenous fetor; periorbital edema may predominate; pericardial friction rub in advanced cases with uremia	Albuminuria, hypoalbuminemia; sometimes, elevation of serum creatinine and urea nitrogen; hyperkalemia, metabolic acidosis, hyperphosphatemia, hypocalcemia, anemia (usually normocytic)

Source: From Chertow.
Note: S_3, third heart sound.

EDEMA OF CIRRHOSIS (See also Chap. 289) Ascites and biochemical and clinical evidence of hepatic disease (collateral venous channels, jaundice, and spider angiomas) characterize edema of hepatic origin. The ascites (Chap. 39) is frequently refractory to treatment because it collects as a result of a combination of obstruction of hepatic lymphatic drainage, portal hypertension, and hypoalbuminemia. Edema may also occur in other parts of the body in these patients as a result of hypoalbuminemia. Furthermore, a sizable accumulation of ascitic fluid may increase intraabdominal pressure and impede venous return from the lower extremities; hence, it tends to promote accumulation of edema in this region as well.

EDEMA OF NUTRITIONAL ORIGIN A diet grossly deficient in protein over a prolonged period may produce hypoproteinemia and edema. The latter may be intensified by the development of beriberi heart disease (Chap. 223), also of nutritional origin, in which multiple peripheral arteriovenous fistulae result in reduced effective systemic perfusion and effective arterial blood volume, thereby enhancing edema formation (Chap. 61). Edema may actually become intensified when famished subjects are first provided with an adequate diet. The ingestion of more food may increase the quantity of NaCl ingested, which is then retained along with water. So-called refeeding edema may also be linked to increased release of insulin, which directly increases tubular sodium reabsorption. In addition to hypoalbuminemia, hypokalemia and caloric deficits may be involved in the edema of starvation.

OTHER CAUSES OF EDEMA These include hypothyroidism, in which the edema (myxedema) is located typically in the pretibial region and which may also be associated with periorbital puffiness. Exogenous hyperadrenocortism, pregnancy, and administration of estrogens and vasodilators, particularly dihydropyridines such as nifedipine, may also all cause edema.

DISTRIBUTION OF EDEMA

The distribution of edema is an important guide to the cause. Thus, edema limited to one leg or to one or both arms is usually the result of venous and/or lymphatic obstruction. Edema resulting from hypoproteinemia characteristically is generalized, but it is especially evident in the very soft tissues of the eyelids and face and tends to be most pronounced in the morning because of the recumbent posture assumed during the night. Less common causes of facial edema include trichinosis, allergic reactions, and myxedema. Edema associated with heart failure, on the other hand, tends to be more extensive in the legs and to be accentuated in the evening, a feature also determined largely by posture. When patients with heart failure have been confined to bed, edema may be most prominent in the presacral region. Paralysis reduces lymphatic and venous drainage on the affected side and may be responsible for unilateral edema.

ADDITIONAL FACTORS IN DIAGNOSIS

The color, thickness, and sensitivity of the skin are significant. Local tenderness and warmth suggest inflammation. Local cyanosis may signify a venous obstruction. In individuals who have had repeated episodes of prolonged edema, the skin over the involved areas may be thickened, indurated, and often red.

Measurement or estimation of the venous pressure is of importance in evaluating edema. Elevation in an isolated part of the body usually reflects localized venous obstruction. Generalized elevation of systemic venous pressure usually indicates the presence of congestive heart failure. Ordinarily, a significant generalized increase in venous pressure can be recognized by the level at which cervical veins collapse (Chap. 209). In patients with obstruction of the superior vena cava, edema is confined to the face, neck, and upper extremities, where the venous pressure is elevated compared with that in the lower extremities. Measurement of venous pressure in the upper extremities is also useful in patients with massive edema of the lower extremities and ascites; it is elevated in the upper extremities when the edema is on a cardiac basis (e.g., advanced heart failure, constrictive pericarditis, or tricuspid stenosis) but is normal when it is secondary to cirrhosis. Severe heart failure may cause ascites that may be distinguished from the ascites caused by hepatic cirrhosis by the jugular venous pressure, which usually is elevated in heart failure and normal in cirrhosis.

Determination of the concentration of serum albumin aids importantly in identifying those patients in whom edema is due, at least in part, to diminished intravascular colloid oncotic pressure. The presence of proteinuria also affords useful clues. The absence of proteinuria excludes nephrotic syndrome but cannot exclude nonproteinuric causes of renal failure. Slight to moderate proteinuria is the rule in patients with heart failure.

APPROACH TO THE PATIENT

An important first question is whether the edema is localized or generalized. If it is localized, those phenomena that may be responsible should be concentrated upon. If the edema is generalized, it should be determined, first, if there is serious hypoalbuminemia, e.g., serum albumin <25 g/L. If so, the history, physical examination, urinalysis, and other laboratory data will help evaluate the question of cirrhosis, severe malnutrition, protein-losing gastroenteropathy, or the nephrotic syndrome as the underlying disorder. If hypoalbuminemia is not present, it should be determined if there is evidence of congestive heart failure of a severity to promote generalized edema. Finally, it should be determined whether the patient has an adequate urine output, or if there is significant oliguria or even anuria. →*These abnormalities are discussed in Chaps. 40, 260, and 261.*

FURTHER READING

ABASSI ZA et al: Control of extracellular fluid volume and the pathophysiology of edema formation, in *The Kidney*, 7th ed, BM Brenner (ed). Philadelphia, Saunders, 2004, pp 777–856

CHERTOW GM: Approach to the patient with edema, in E Braunwald, L Goldman (eds): *Cardiology for the Primary Care Physician,* 2nd ed, Philadelphia, Saunders, 2003, p 117–128

DISKIN CJ et al: Edema, oncotic pressure, and free entropy: Novel considerations for treatment of edema through attention to thermodynamics. Nephron 78:131, 1998

MCCULLOUGH JC: Renal disorders and heart disease, in Zipes D et al (eds): *Braunwald's Heart Disease,* 7th ed, Philadelphia, Saunders, 2005

SCHRIER RW, FASSETT RG: A critique of the overfill hypothesis of sodium and water retention in the nephrotic syndrome. Kidney Int 53:1111, 1998

33 | DYSPHAGIA
Raj K. Goyal

Dysphagia is defined as a sensation of "sticking" or obstruction of the passage of food through the mouth, pharynx, or esophagus. It should be distinguished from other symptoms related to swallowing. *Aphagia* signifies complete esophageal obstruction, which is usually due to bolus impaction and represents a medical emergency. *Difficulty in initiating a swallow* occurs in disorders of the voluntary phase of swallowing. However, once initiated, swallowing is completed normally. *Odynophagia* means painful swallowing. Frequently, odynophagia and dysphagia occur together. *Globus pharyngeous* is the sensation of a lump lodged in the throat. However, no difficulty is encountered when swallowing is performed. *Misdirection of food*, resulting in nasal regurgitation and laryngeal and pulmonary aspiration of food during swallowing, is characteristic of oropharyngeal dysphagia. *Phagophobia*, meaning fear of swallowing, and *refusal to swallow* may occur in hysteria, rabies, tetanus, and pharyngeal paralysis due to fear of aspiration. Painful inflammatory lesions that cause odynophagia may also cause refusal to swallow. Some patients may feel the food as it goes down the esophagus. This esophageal sensitivity is not associated with either food sticking or obstruction, however. Similarly, the *feeling of fullness in the epigastrium* that occurs after a meal or after swallowing air should not be confused with dysphagia.

PHYSIOLOGY OF SWALLOWING The process of swallowing begins with a voluntary (oral) phase during which a bolus of food is pushed into the pharynx by the contraction of the tongue. The bolus then activates oropharyngeal sensory receptors that initiate the involuntary (pharyngeal and esophageal) phase, or deglutition reflex. The deglutition reflex is a complex series of events and serves both to propel food through the pharynx and the esophagus and to prevent its entry into the airway. When the bolus is propelled backward by the tongue, the larynx moves forward and the upper esophageal sphincter opens. As the bolus moves into the pharynx, contraction of the superior pharyngeal constrictor against the contracted soft palate initiates a peristaltic contraction that proceeds rapidly downward to move the bolus through the pharynx and the esophagus. The lower esophageal sphincter opens as the food enters the esophagus and remains open until the peristaltic contraction has swept the bolus into the stomach. Peristaltic contraction in response to a swallow is called *primary peristalsis*. It involves inhibition followed by sequential contraction of muscles along the entire swallowing passage. The inhibition that precedes the peristaltic contraction is called *deglutitive inhibition*. Local distention of the esophagus from food activates intramural reflexes in the smooth muscle and results in *secondary peristalsis*, which is limited to the thoracic esophagus. *Tertiary contractions* are nonperistaltic because they occur simultaneously over a long segment of the esophagus. Tertiary contractions may occur in response to a swallow or esophageal distention, or they may occur spontaneously.

PATHOPHYSIOLOGY OF DYSPHAGIA The normal transport of an ingested bolus through the swallowing passage depends on the size of the ingested bolus; the luminal diameter of the swallowing passage; the force of peristaltic contraction; and deglutitive inhibition, including normal relaxation of upper and lower esophageal sphincters during swallowing. Dysphagia caused by a large bolus or luminal narrowing is called *mechanical dysphagia*, whereas dysphagia due to weakness of peristaltic contractions or to impaired deglutitive inhibition causing nonperistaltic contractions and impaired sphincter relaxation is called *motor dysphagia*.

Mechanical Dysphagia Mechanical dysphagia can be caused by a very large food bolus, intrinsic narrowing, or extrinsic compression of the lumen. In an adult, the esophageal lumen can distend up to 4 cm in diameter. When the esophagus cannot dilate beyond 2.5 cm in diameter, dysphagia to normal solid food can occur. Dysphagia is always present when the esophagus cannot distend beyond 1.3 cm. Circumferential lesions produce dysphagia more consistently than do lesions that involve only a portion of circumferences of the esophageal wall, as uninvolved segments retain their distensibility. The causes of mechanical dysphagia are listed in Table 33-1. Common causes include carcinoma, peptic and other benign strictures, and lower esophageal ring.

Motor Dysphagia Motor dysphagia may result from difficulty in initiating a swallow or from abnormalities in peristalsis and deglutitive inhibition due to diseases of the esophageal striated or smooth muscle.

Diseases of the striated muscle involve the pharynx, upper esophageal sphincter, and cervical esophagus. The striated muscle is innervated by a somatic component of the vagus with cell bodies of the lower motor neurons located in the nucleus ambiguus. These neurons are cholinergic and excitatory and are the sole determinant of the muscle activity. Peristalsis in the striated muscle segment is due to sequential central activation of neurons innervating muscles at different levels along the esophagus. Motor dysphagia of the pharynx results from neuromuscular disorders causing muscle paralysis, simultaneous nonperistaltic contraction, or loss of opening of the upper esophageal sphincter. Loss of opening of the upper sphincter is caused by paralysis of geniohyoid and other suprahyoid muscles or loss of deglutitive inhibition of the cricopharyngeus muscle. Because each side of the pharynx is innervated by ipsilateral nerves, a unilateral lesion of motor neurons leads to unilateral pharyngeal paralysis. Although lesions of striated muscle also involve the cervical part of the esophagus, the clinical manifestations of pharyngeal dysfunction usually overshadow those due to esophageal involvement.

Diseases of the smooth-muscle segment involve the thoracic part of the esophagus and the lower esophageal sphincter. The smooth muscle is innervated by the parasympathetic component of the vagal preganglionic fibers and postganglionic neurons in the myenteric ganglia. The vagal pathway consists of parallel excitatory and inhibitory pathways that use acetylcholine and nitric oxide as neurotransmitters, respectively. The activation of inhibitory nerves causes inhibition that is followed by rebound contraction. These pathways are involved in the resting tone of the lower esophageal sphincter, swallow-induced lower esophageal sphincter opening, and inhibition followed by peristaltic contractions in the esophageal body. Dysphagia results when the peristaltic contractions are weak or nonperistaltic or when the lower sphincter fails to relax normally. Loss of contractile power occurs due to muscle weakness, as in scleroderma. The nonperistaltic contractions and impaired relaxation of the lower esophageal sphincter result from a defect in inhibitory vagal innervation and account for dysphagia in achalasia.

The causes of motor dysphagia are also listed in Table 33-1. Important causes are pharyngeal paralysis, cricopharyngeal achalasia, scleroderma of the esophagus, achalasia, and diffuse esophageal spasm and related motor disorders.

APPROACH TO THE PATIENT

History The history can provide a presumptive diagnosis in >80% of patients. The type of food causing dysphagia provides useful information. Difficulty only with solids implies mechanical dysphagia with a lumen that is not severely narrowed. In advanced obstruction, dysphagia occurs with liquids as well as solids. In contrast, motor dysphagia due to achalasia and diffuse esophageal spasm is equally affected by solids and liquids from the very onset. Patients with scleroderma have dysphagia to solids that is unrelated to posture and to liquids while recumbent but not upright. When peptic stricture develops in patients with scleroderma, dysphagia becomes more persistent.

The duration and course of dysphagia are helpful in diagnosis. Transient dysphagia may be due to an inflammatory process. Pro-

TABLE 33-1 Causes of Dysphagia

MECHANICAL DYSPHAGIA

I. Luminal
  A. Large bolus
  B. Foreign body
II. Intrinsic narrowing
  A. Inflammatory condition causing edema and swelling
    1. Stomatitis
    2. Pharyngitis, epiglottitis
    3. Esophagitis
      a. Viral (herpes simplex, varicella-zoster, cytomegalovirus)
      b. Bacterial
      c. Fungal (candidal)
      d. Mucocutaneous bullous diseases
      e. Caustic, chemical, thermal injury
  B. Webs and rings
    1. Pharyngeal (Plummer-Vinson syndrome)
    2. Esophageal (congenital, inflammatory)
    3. Lower esophageal mucosal ring (Schatzki ring)
  C. Benign strictures
    1. Peptic
    2. Caustic and pill-induced
    3. Inflammatory (Crohn's disease, candidal, mucocutaneous lesions)
    4. Ischemic
    5. Postoperative, postirradiation
    6. Congenital
  D. Malignant tumors
    1. Primary carcinoma
      a. Squamous cell carcinoma
      b. Adenocarcinoma
      c. Carcinosarcoma
      d. Pseudosarcoma
      e. Lymphoma
      f. Melanoma
      g. Kaposi's sarcoma
    2. Metastatic carcinoma
  E. Benign tumors
    1. Leiomyoma
    2. Lipoma
    3. Angioma
    4. Inflammatory fibroid polyp
    5. Epithelial papilloma
III. Extrinsic compression
  A. Cervical spondylitis
  B. Vertebral osteophytes
  C. Retropharyngeal abscess and masses
  D. Enlarged thyroid gland
  E. Zenker's diverticulum
  F. Vascular compression
    1. Aberrant right subclavian artery
    2. Right-sided aorta
    3. Left atrial enlargement
    4. Aortic aneurysm
  G. Posterior mediastinal masses
  H. Pancreatic tumor, pancreatitis
  I. Postvagotomy hematoma and fibrosis

MOTOR (NEUROMUSCULAR) DYSPHAGIA

I. Difficulty in initiating swallowing reflex
  A. Paralysis of the tongue
  B. Oropharyngeal anesthesia
  C. Lack of saliva (e.g., Sjögren's syndrome)
  D. Lesions of sensory components of vagus and glossopharyngeal nerves
  E. Lesions of swallowing center
II. Disorders of pharyngeal and esophageal striated muscle
  A. Muscle weakness
    1. Lower motor neuron lesion (bulbar paralysis)
      a. Cerebrovascular accident
      b. Motor neuron disease
      c. Poliomyelitis, postpolio syndrome
      d. Polyneuritis
      e. Amyotrophic lateral sclerosis
      f. Familial dysautonomia
    2. Neuromuscular
      a. Myasthenia gravis
    3. Muscle disorders
      a. Polymyositis
      b. Dermatomyositis
      c. Myopathies (myotonic dystrophy, oculopharyngeal myopathy)
  B. Nonperistaltic contractions or impaired deglutitive inhibition
    1. Pharynx and upper esophagus
      a. Rabies
      b. Tetanus
      c. Extrapyramidal tract disease
      d. Upper motor neuron lesions (pseudobulbar paralysis)
    2. Upper esophageal sphincter (UES)
      a. Paralysis of suprahyoid muscles (causes same as paralysis of pharyngeal musculature)
      b. Cricopharyngeal achalasia
III. Disorders of esophageal smooth muscle
  A. Paralysis of esophageal body causing weak contractions
    1. Scleroderma and related collagen vascular diseases
    2. Hollow visceral myopathy
    3. Myotonic dystrophy
    4. Metabolic neuromyopathy (amyloid, alcohol?, diabetes?)
    5. Achalasia (classical)
  B. Nonperistaltic contractions or impaired deglutitive inhibition
    1. Esophageal body
      a. Diffuse esophageal spasm
      b. Achalasia (vigorous)
      c. Variants of diffuse esophageal spasm
    2. Lower esophageal sphincter
      a. Achalasia
        (1) Primary
        (2) Secondary
          (a) Chagas' disease
          (b) Carcinoma
          (c) Lymphoma
          (d) Neuropathic intestinal pseudoobstruction syndrome
          (e) Toxins and drugs
      b. Lower esophageal muscular (contractile) ring

---

gressive dysphagia lasting a few weeks to a few months is suggestive of carcinoma of the esophagus. Episodic dysphagia to solids lasting several years indicates a benign disease characteristic of a lower esophageal ring.

The site of dysphagia described by the patient helps to determine the site of esophageal obstruction; the lesion is at or below the perceived location of dysphagia.

Associated symptoms provide important diagnostic clues. Nasal regurgitation and tracheobronchial aspiration with swallowing are hallmarks of pharyngeal paralysis or a tracheoesophageal fistula. Tracheobronchial aspiration unrelated to swallowing may be secondary to achalasia, Zenker's diverticulum, or gastroesophageal reflux.

Severe weight loss that is out of proportion to the degree of dysphagia is highly suggestive of carcinoma. When hoarseness precedes dysphagia, the primary lesion is usually in the larynx. Hoarseness following dysphagia may suggest involvement of the recurrent laryngeal nerve by extension of esophageal carcinoma. Sometimes hoarseness may be due to laryngitis secondary to gastroesophageal reflux. Association of laryngeal symptoms and dysphagia also occurs in various neuromuscular disorders. Hiccups may rarely occur with a lesion in the distal portion of the esophagus. Unilateral wheezing with dysphagia indicates a mediastinal mass involving the esophagus and a large bronchus.

Chest pain with dysphagia occurs in diffuse esophageal spasm and related motor disorders. Chest pain resembling diffuse esophageal spasms may occur in esophageal obstruction due to a large bolus. A prolonged history of heartburn and reflux preceding dysphagia indicates peptic stricture. A history of prolonged nasogastric intubation, ingestion of caustic agents, ingestion of pills without water, previous radiation therapy, or associated mucocutaneous diseases may provide the cause of esophageal stricture. If odynophagia is present, candidal or herpes esophagitis or pill-induced esophagitis should be suspected.

In patients with AIDS or other immunodeficiency states, esophagitis due to opportunistic infections such as *Candida*, herpes simplex virus, or cytomegalovirus and tumors such as Kaposi's sarcoma and lymphoma should be suspected.

Physical Examination   Physical examination is important in motor dysphagia due to skeletal muscle, neurologic, and oropharyngeal diseases. Signs of bulbar or pseudobulbar palsy, including dysarthria, dysphonia, ptosis, tongue atrophy, and hyperactive jaw jerk, in addition to evidence of generalized neuromuscular disease, should be sought. The neck should be examined for thyromegaly or a spinal abnormality. A careful inspection of the mouth and pharynx should disclose lesions that may interfere with passage of food because of pain or obstruction. Changes in the skin and extremities may suggest a diagnosis of scleroderma and other collagen vascular diseases or mucocutaneous diseases such as pemphigoid or epidermolysis bullosa, which may involve the esophagus. Cancer spread to lymph nodes and liver may be evident. Pulmonary complications of acute aspiration pneumonia or chronic aspiration may be present.

Diagnostic Procedures   Dysphagia is nearly always a symptom of organic disease rather than a functional complaint. If oropharyngeal dysphagia is suspected, videofluoroscopy of oropharyngeal swallowing should be obtained. If mechanical dysphagia is suspected on clinical history, barium swallow, esophagogastroscopy and endoscopic biopsies are the diagnostic procedures of choice. Barium swallow and esophageal motility studies are diagnostic tests for motor dysphagia. Esophagogastroscopy may be needed in patients with motor dysphagia to exclude an associated structural abnormality (Chap. 273).

FURTHER READING

GOYAL RK, HIRANO I: Mechanisms of disease: The enteric nervous system. N Engl J Med 334:110, 1996

HENDRIX TR: Art and science of history taking in the patient with difficulty swallowing. Dysphagia 8:69, 1993

KOCH WM: Swallowing disorders. Diagnosis and therapy. Med Clin North Am 77:571, 1993

MORTON RE et al: Videofluoroscopy in the assessment of feeding disorders of children with neurological problems. J Dev Med Child Neurol 35:388, 1993

SPIEKER MR: Evaluating dysphagia. Am Fam Physician 61:3639, 2000

34   NAUSEA, VOMITING, AND INDIGESTION
William L. Hasler

Nausea is the subjective feeling of a need to vomit. *Vomiting* (emesis) is the oral expulsion of upper gastrointestinal contents resulting from contractions of gut and thoracoabdominal wall musculature. Vomiting is contrasted with *regurgitation*, the effortless passage of gastric contents into the mouth. *Rumination* is the repeated regurgitation of stomach contents, which are often rechewed and then reswallowed. In contrast to vomiting, these phenomena often exhibit some volitional control. *Indigestion* is a nonspecific term that encompasses a variety of upper abdominal complaints including nausea, vomiting, heartburn, regurgitation, and dyspepsia (upper abdominal discomfort or pain). Some individuals with dyspepsia report ulcer-like symptoms such as epigastric burning or gnawing discomfort. Others experience symptoms of gastric dysmotility such as postprandial fullness, bloating, eructation (belching), anorexia (loss of appetite), and early satiety (an inability to complete a meal due to premature fullness).

NAUSEA AND VOMITING

MECHANISMS   Vomiting is coordinated by the brainstem and is effected by neuromuscular responses in the gut, pharynx, and thoracoabdominal wall. The mechanisms underlying nausea are poorly understood but likely involve the cerebral cortex, as nausea requires conscious perception. Electroencephalographic studies show activation of temporofrontal cortical regions with induction of nausea.

Coordination of Emesis   Several brainstem nuclei initiate emesis, including the nucleus tractus solitarius, the dorsal vagal and phrenic nuclei, and medullary nuclei that regulate respiration; nuclei that control pharyngeal, facial, and tongue movements coordinate the initiation of emesis. The neurotransmitters involved in this coordination are uncertain; however, roles for neurokinin NK_1, serotonin, and vasopressin pathways are postulated.

Somatic and visceral muscles exhibit stereotypic responses during emesis. Inspiratory thoracic and abdominal wall muscles contract, producing high intrathoracic and intraabdominal pressures that facilitate expulsion of gastric contents. The gastric cardia herniates across the diaphragm, and the larynx moves upward to promote oral propulsion of the vomitus. Under normal conditions, distally migrating gut contractions are regulated by an electrical phenomenon, the slow wave, which cycles at 3 cycles/min in the stomach and 11 cycles/min in the duodenum. With emesis, slow waves are replaced by orally propagating spike activity, which induces retrograde contractions that assist in the oral expulsion of small-intestinal contents.

Activators of Emesis   Emetic stimuli act at several anatomic sites. Emesis provoked by noxious thoughts or smells originates in the cerebral cortex, whereas cranial nerves mediate vomiting after gag reflex activation. Motion sickness and inner ear disorders act on the labyrinthine apparatus, while gastric irritants and emetogenic anticancer agents such as cisplatin stimulate gastroduodenal vagal afferent nerves. Nongastric visceral afferents are activated by small intestinal and colonic obstruction and mesenteric ischemia. The area postrema, a medullary nucleus, responds to bloodborne emetic stimuli and is termed the *chemoreceptor trigger zone*. Many emetic drugs act on the area postrema as do bacterial toxins and metabolic disorders such as uremia, hypoxia, and ketoacidosis.

Neurotransmitters that mediate induction of vomiting are selective for these anatomic sites. Labyrinthine disorders stimulate vestibular cholinergic muscarinic M_1 and histaminergic H_1 receptors, whereas gastroduodenal vagal afferent stimuli activate serotonin 5-HT_3 receptors. The area postrema is richly served by nerve fibers acting on 5-HT_3, M_1, H_1, and dopamine D_2 receptor subtypes. Optimal pharmacologic management requires an understanding of these pathways.

DIFFERENTIAL DIAGNOSIS   Nausea and vomiting are caused by conditions within and outside the gut as well as by drugs and circulating toxins (Table 34-1).

Intraperitoneal Disorders   Visceral obstruction and inflammation of hollow and solid viscera may produce vomiting as the main symptom. Gastric obstruction results from ulcer disease and malignancy, whereas small-bowel and colonic obstructions occur as a consequence of adhesions, benign or malignant tumors, volvulus, intussusception, or inflammatory diseases such as Crohn's disease. The superior mesenteric artery syndrome, occurring after weight loss or prolonged bed rest, results when the duodenum is compressed by the overlying superior mesenteric artery. Abdominal irradiation impairs intestinal contractile function and induces strictures. Biliary colic causes nausea by action

TABLE 34-1 *Causes of Nausea and Vomiting*

Intraperitoneal	Extraperitoneal	Medications/Metabolic Disorders
Obstructing disorders	Cardiopulmonary disease	Drugs
Pyloric obstruction	Cardiomyopathy	Cancer chemotherapy
Small bowel obstruction	Myocardial infarction	Antibiotics
Colonic obstruction	Labyrinthine disease	Cardiac antiarrhythmics
Superior mesenteric artery	Motion sickness	Digoxin
syndrome	Labyrinthitis	Oral hypoglycemics
Enteric infections	Malignancy	Oral contraceptives
Viral	Intracerebral disorders	Endocrine/metabolic disease
Bacterial	Malignancy	Pregnancy
Inflammatory diseases	Hemorrhage	Uremia
Cholecystitis	Abscess	Ketoacidosis
Pancreatitis	Hydrocephalus	Thyroid and parathyroid disease
Appendicitis	Psychiatric illness	Adrenal insufficiency
Hepatitis	Anorexia and bulimia nervosa	Toxins
Impaired motor function	Depression	Liver failure
Gastroparesis	Psychogenic vomiting	Ethanol
Intestinal	Postoperative vomiting	
pseudoobstruction	Cyclic vomiting syndrome	
Functional dyspepsia		
Gastroesophageal reflux		
Biliary colic		
Abdominal irradiation		

on visceral afferent nerves. Vomiting with pancreatitis, cholecystitis, and appendicitis is due to localized visceral irritation and induction of ileus. Enteric infections with viruses or bacteria such as *Staphylococcus aureus* and *Bacillus cereus* are among the most common causes of acute vomiting, especially in children. Opportunistic infections such as cytomegalovirus or herpes simplex induce emesis in immunocompromised individuals.

Disordered gut motor function also commonly causes nausea and vomiting. *Gastroparesis* is defined as a delay in emptying of food from the stomach and occurs after vagotomy for peptic ulcer; with pancreatic adenocarcinoma; with mesenteric vascular insufficiency; or in systemic diseases such as diabetes, scleroderma, and amyloidosis. Idiopathic gastroparesis occurring in the absence of systemic illness may follow a viral prodrome suggesting an infectious etiology. *Intestinal pseudoobstruction* is characterized by disrupted intestinal and colonic motor activity and leads to intestinal retention of food residue and secretions; bacterial overgrowth; nutrient malabsorption; and symptoms of nausea, vomiting, bloating, pain, and altered defecation. Intestinal pseudoobstruction may be idiopathic, inherited as a familial visceral myopathy or neuropathy, or result from systemic disease or as a paraneoplastic consequence of malignancy (especially small-cell lung carcinoma). Patients with functional dyspepsia and irritable bowel syndrome may report prominent nausea and vomiting, as do some individuals with gastroesophageal reflux.

Extraperitoneal Disorders Myocardial infarction and congestive heart failure are cardiac causes of nausea and vomiting. Emesis occurs after 25% of surgical operations, most commonly laparotomy and orthopedic surgery, and is more prevalent in women. Increased intracranial pressure from tumors, bleeding, abscess, or obstruction to cerebrospinal fluid outflow produces prominent vomiting with or without nausea. Motion sickness, labyrinthitis, and Ménière's disease evoke symptoms via labyrinthine pathways. Cyclic vomiting syndrome is a rare disorder of unknown etiology that produces episodes of intractable nausea and vomiting, usually in children. The syndrome shows a strong association with migraine headaches, suggesting that some cases may be migraine variants. Patients with psychiatric illnesses, including anorexia nervosa, bulimia, anxiety, and depression, may report significant nausea. Psychogenic vomiting occurs most commonly in women with other emotional problems.

Medications and Metabolic Disorders Drugs evoke vomiting by action on the stomach (analgesics, erythromycin) or area postrema (digoxin, opiates, anti-parkinsonian drugs). Emetogenic agents include antibiotics, antiarrhythmics, antihypertensives, oral hypoglycemics, and contra-ceptives. Cancer chemotherapy causes vomiting that is acute (within hours of administration), delayed (after 1 or more days), or anticipatory. Acute emesis resulting from highly emetogenic agents such as cisplatin is mediated by 5-HT$_3$ pathways, whereas delayed emesis is 5-HT$_3$ independent. Anticipatory nausea often responds better to anxiolytic therapy than to antiemetics.

Metabolic disorders elicit nausea and vomiting in certain settings. Pregnancy is the most prevalent endocrinologic cause of nausea, occurring in 70% of women in the first trimester. Hyperemesis gravidarum is a severe form of nausea of pregnancy that can produce significant fluid loss and electrolyte disturbances. Uremia, ketoacidosis, adrenal insufficiency, as well as parathyroid and thyroid disease are other metabolic causes of emesis.

Circulating toxins evoke symptoms through effects on the area postrema. Endogenous toxins are generated in fulminant liver failure, whereas exogenous enterotoxins may be produced by enteric bacterial infection. Ethanol intoxication is a common toxic cause of nausea and vomiting.

APPROACH TO THE PATIENT

History and Physical Examination The history helps define the etiology of unexplained nausea and vomiting. Drugs, toxins, and gastrointestinal infections often cause acute symptoms, while established illnesses evoke chronic complaints. Pyloric obstruction and gastroparesis produce vomiting within 1 h of eating, whereas emesis from intestinal obstruction occurs later. In severe cases of gastroparesis, the vomitus may contain food residue ingested hours or days previously. Hematemesis raises suspicion of an ulcer or malignancy or a Mallory-Weiss tear, whereas feculent emesis is noted with distal intestinal or colonic obstruction. Bilious vomiting excludes gastric obstruction, whereas emesis of undigested food is consistent with a Zenker's diverticulum or achalasia. Relief of abdominal pain by emesis characterizes small-bowel obstruction, but vomiting has no effect on pancreatitis or cholecystitis pain. Pronounced weight loss raises concern about malignancy or obstruction. Fevers suggest inflammation, while an intracranial source is considered if there are headaches or visual field changes. Vertigo or tinnitus indicates labyrinthine disease.

The physical examination complements the history. Orthostatic hypotension and poor skin turgor indicate intravascular fluid depletion. Pulmonary abnormalities raise concern that vomitus was aspirated. Abdominal auscultation may reveal absent bowel sounds with ileus. High-pitched rushes suggest bowel obstruction, while a succession splash on abrupt lateral movement of the patient is found with gastroparesis or pyloric obstruction. Tenderness or involuntary guarding raises suspicion of inflammation, whereas fecal blood suggests mucosal injury from ulcer, ischemia, or tumor. Neurologic etiologies present with papilledema, visual field loss, or focal neural abnormalities. Neoplasm is suggested by palpable masses or adenopathy.

Diagnostic Testing With intractable symptoms or an elusive diagnosis, selected diagnostic tests can direct clinical management. Electrolyte replenishment is indicated for hypokalemia or metabolic alkalosis. Detection of iron-deficiency anemia mandates a search for mucosal injury. Pancreaticobiliary disease is suggested by abnormal pancreatic enzymes or liver biochemistries, whereas endocrinologic, rheumatologic, or paraneoplastic etiologies are diagnosed by specific hormone or serologic testing. If luminal obstruction is suspected, supine and upright abdominal radiographs may show intestinal air-fluid levels with reduced colonic air. Ileus is characterized by diffusely dilated air-filled bowel loops.

Anatomic studies may be indicated if initial testing is nondiagnostic. Upper endoscopy detects ulcer or malignancy, and small-bowel barium radiography diagnoses partial small-bowel obstruction. Colonoscopy or contrast barium enema can detect colonic obstruction. Abdominal ultrasound or computed tomography (CT) defines intraperitoneal inflammatory processes, while CT or magnetic resonance imaging (MRI) of the head can delineate intracranial sources of nausea and vomiting. Mesenteric angiography or MRI is useful when ischemia is considered.

TABLE 34-2 *Treatment of Nausea and Vomiting*

Treatment	Mechanism	Examples	Clinical Indications
Antiemetic agents	Antihistaminergic	Dimenhydrate, meclizine	Motion sickness, inner ear disease
	Anticholinergic	Scopolamine	Motion sickness, inner ear disease
	Antidopaminergic	Prochlorperazine, droperidol	Medication-, toxin-, or metabolic-induced emesis
	5-HT$_3$ antagonist	Ondansetron, granisetron	Chemotherapy- and radiation-induced emesis, postoperative emesis
	Tricyclic antidepressant	Amitriptyline, nortriptyline	Functional nausea
Prokinetic agents	5-HT$_4$ agonist	Cisapride	Gastroparesis, functional dyspepsia, gastroesophageal reflux disease, intestinal pseudoobstruction
	5 HT$_4$ agonist and antidopaminergic	Metoclopramide	Gastroparesis, functional dyspepsia
	Motilin agonist	Erythromycin	Gastroparesis, ?Intestinal pseudoobstruction
	Peripheral antidopaminergic	Domperidone	Gastroparesis, functional dyspepsia
	Somatostatin analogue	Octreotide	Intestinal pseudoobstruction
Special settings	Benzodiazepines	Lorazepam	Anticipatory nausea and vomiting with chemotherapy
	Glucocorticoids	Methylprednisolone, dexamethasone	Chemotherapy-induced emesis
	Cannabinoids	Tetrahydrocannabinol	?Chemotherapy-induced emesis

Gastrointestinal motility testing may detect a motor disorder that contributes to symptoms when anatomic abnormalities are absent. Gastroparesis is most commonly diagnosed with gastric scintigraphy, by which emptying of a radiolabeled meal is measured. Electrogastrography, a noninvasive method to test gastric slow-wave activity using cutaneous electrodes placed over the stomach, has been proposed as an alternative means of diagnosing gastroparesis. The diagnosis of intestinal pseudoobstruction is suggested by abnormal barium transit on small-bowel contrast radiography. Small-intestinal manometry may provide confirmation of the diagnosis and further characterize the motor abnormality as neuropathic or myopathic based on contractile patterns. Such investigation can obviate the need for open intestinal biopsy to evaluate for smooth-muscle or neuronal degeneration.

℞ TREATMENT

General Principles Therapy of vomiting is tailored to correction of medically or surgically remediable abnormalities, if possible. Hospitalization is considered for severe dehydration, especially if oral fluid replenishment cannot be sustained. Once oral intake is tolerated, nutrients are restarted with liquids that are low in fat, as lipids delay gastric emptying. Foods high in indigestible residues are avoided because these also prolong gastric retention.

Antiemetic Medications The most commonly used antiemetic agents act on the central nervous system (Table 34-2). Antihistamines such as meclizine and dimenhydrinate and anticholinergic drugs such as scopolamine act on labyrinthine-activated pathways and are useful in motion sickness and inner ear disorders. Phenothiazine and butyrophenone dopamine D$_2$ antagonists are used to treat emesis evoked by area postrema stimuli and are effective for medication, toxic, and metabolic etiologies. Dopamine antagonists freely cross the blood-brain barrier and may cause anxiety, dystonic reactions, hyperprolactinemic effects (galactorrhea and sexual dysfunction), and irreversible tardive dyskinesia.

Other drug classes have antiemetic properties. Serotonin 5-HT$_3$ antagonists such as ondansetron and granisetron are useful in the treatment of postoperative vomiting, after radiation therapy, and in the prevention of cancer chemotherapy–induced emesis. The usefulness of 5-HT$_3$ antagonists for other causes of emesis is less well established. Low-dose tricyclic antidepressants provide symptomatic benefit in patients with unexplained nausea of a functional nature, as well as in diabetic patients with nausea and vomiting whose disease is of long standing.

Gastrointestinal Motor Stimulants Drugs that stimulate gastric emptying are indicated for gastroparesis (Table 34-2). Metoclopramide, a combined 5-HT$_4$ agonist and D$_2$ antagonist, is effective in gastroparesis, but antidopaminergic side effects limit its use in 20% of patients. Erythromycin, a macrolide antibiotic, potently increases gastroduodenal motility by action on receptors for motilin, an endogenous stimulant of fasting motor activity. Intravenous erythromycin is useful in patients with refractory gastroparesis; however, oral forms of the drug also have some effect. Domperidone, a D$_2$ antagonist not available in the United States, has prokinetic and antiemetic effects but does not cross into most other brain regions; thus, anxiety and dystonic reactions are rare. The main side effects of domperidone are induction of hyperprolactinemia through effects on pituitary regions served by a porous blood-brain barrier.

Patients with refractory upper gut motility disorders pose significant challenges. Liquid suspensions of prokinetic drugs may be beneficial as liquids empty from the stomach more rapidly than pills. Metoclopramide can be administered subcutaneously in patients who do not respond to oral drugs. Intestinal pseudoobstruction may respond to the somatostatin analogue octreotide, which induces propagative small-intestinal motor complexes. Pyloric injections of botulinum toxin are reported in uncontrolled studies to benefit patients with idiopathic or diabetic gastroparesis. Placement of a feeding jejunostomy reduces hospitalizations and improves overall health in some patients with gastroparesis who do not respond to drug therapy. Surgical options are limited for refractory cases, but postvagotomy gastroparesis may improve with near-total resection of the stomach. Implanted gastric electrical pacemakers and neurostimulators may reduce symptoms, improve quality-of-life, and decrease health care expenditures in patients with medication-refractory gastroparesis.

Selected Clinical Settings Cancer chemotherapeutic agents such as cisplatin are intensely emetogenic. Given prophylactically, 5-HT$_3$ antag-

221

onists prevent chemotherapy-induced acute vomiting in most cases (Table 34-2). Optimal antiemetic effects are often obtained with a 5-HT$_3$ antagonist in combination with a glucocorticoid. High-dose metoclopramide is also effective in chemotherapy-evoked emesis, whereas benzodiazepines such as lorazepam are useful in reducing anticipatory nausea and vomiting. Delayed emesis 1 to 5 days after chemotherapy is more refractory to treatment. Novel neurokinin NK$_1$ antagonists may be potent antiemetic and antinausea drugs during both the acute and the delayed periods after chemotherapy. Cannabinoids such as tetrahydrocannabinol, long advocated for cancer-associated emesis, produce significant side effects and are no more effective than antidopaminergic agents. Most current drug regimens are more effective at controlling emesis than nausea.

The clinician should exercise caution in managing the pregnant patient with nausea. Studies of the teratogenic effects of available antiemetic agents provide conflicting results. Few controlled trials have been performed in the nausea of pregnancy, although antihistamines such as meclizine and antidopaminergics such as prochlorperazine are more effective than placebo. Alternative therapies such as pyridoxine, acupressure, or ginger are being tested.

Controlling emesis in children with cyclic vomiting syndrome is a challenge. 5-HT$_3$ antagonists are a mainstay of treatment. Considering the possible link to migraine headaches, anti-migraine therapy with antidepressants and the serotonin 5-HT$_1$ agonist, sumatriptan, may be tried.

INDIGESTION

MECHANISMS The most common causes of indigestion are gastroesophageal acid reflux and functional dyspepsia. Other cases are a consequence of a more serious organic illness.

Gastroesophageal Acid Reflux Acid reflux can result from a variety of physiologic defects. Reduced lower esophageal sphincter (LES) tone is an important cause of reflux in scleroderma and pregnancy and may also be a factor in patients without other systemic conditions. Many individuals show frequent transient LES relaxations, during which acid bathes the esophagus. Overeating and aerophagia can transiently override the barrier function of the LES, whereas impaired esophageal body motility and reduced salivary secretion prolong acid exposure. The role of hiatal hernias is controversial—although most reflux patients exhibit hiatal hernias, most individuals with hiatal hernias do not have excess heartburn.

Gastric Motor Dysfunction Disturbed gastric motility is purported to cause acid reflux in some cases of indigestion. Delayed gastric emptying also is found in 25 to 50% of functional dyspeptics. The relation of these defects to symptom induction is uncertain; many studies show poor correlation between symptom severity and the degree of motor dysfunction. Abnormal gastric fundic relaxation after eating may cause selected dyspeptic symptoms such as bloating, fullness, nausea, and early satiety. A current focus of investigation is developing drugs that enhance fundic relaxation.

Visceral Afferent Hypersensitivity Disturbed gastric sensory function may also cause functional dyspepsia. Visceral afferent hypersensitivity was first demonstrated in patients with irritable bowel syndrome who had heightened perception of rectal balloon inflation without changes in rectal compliance. Patients with dyspepsia may experience discomfort with fundic distention to lower pressures than healthy control subjects.

Other Factors *Helicobacter pylori* has a clear etiologic role in peptic ulcer disease, but ulcers cause only a minority of cases of dyspepsia. The importance of *H. pylori* in the genesis of functional dyspepsia is controversial, but most investigators believe it is of minor importance. In contrast, functional dyspepsia is associated with a reduced sense of physical and mental well-being and is exacerbated by stress, suggesting an important role for psychological factors. Analgesics cause dys-

pepsia; nitrates, calcium channel blockers, theophylline, and progesterone promote acid reflux. Other exogenous factors that induce acid reflux include ethanol, tobacco, and caffeine via LES relaxation. Genetic factors may contribute to development of acid reflux.

DIFFERENTIAL DIAGNOSIS ■ Gastroesophageal Reflux Disease Gastroesophageal reflux disease (GERD) is prevalent in Western society. Heartburn is reported once monthly by 40% of Americans and daily by 7 to 10%. Most cases of heartburn occur because of excess acid reflux; however, some patients exhibit heightened sensitivity to normal amounts of acid exposure.

Functional Dyspepsia Functional dyspepsia, defined as ≥ 3 months of dyspepsia without an organic cause, is also common. Nearly 25% of the populace has abdominal discomfort at least six times yearly, but only 10 to 20% consult physicians. Functional dyspepsia accounts for 60% of cases of dyspepsia. Most patients with functional dyspepsia follow a benign course, but a small number with *H. pylori* infection or on nonsteroidal anti-inflammatory drugs (NSAIDs) progress to ulcer formation. As with idiopathic gastroparesis, some cases of functional dyspepsia appear to result from prior gastrointestinal infection.

Ulcer Disease In most cases of GERD, the esophagus is not damaged. However, 5% of patients develop esophageal ulcers, and some form strictures. Symptoms do not reliably distinguish nonerosive from erosive or ulcerative esophagitis. From 15 to 25% of cases of dyspepsia stem from ulcers of the stomach or duodenum. The most common causes of ulcer disease are gastric infection with *H. pylori* and use of NSAIDs. Other rare causes of gastroduodenal ulcer include Crohn's disease and Zollinger-Ellison syndrome, a condition resulting from gastrin overproduction by an endocrine tumor (Chap. 274).

Malignancy Dyspeptic patients often seek care because of fear of cancer. However, <2% of cases result from gastroesophageal malignancy. Esophageal squamous cell carcinoma occurs most often in those patients with histories of tobacco or ethanol intake. Other risk factors include prior caustic ingestion, achalasia, and the hereditary disorder tylosis. Esophageal adenocarcinoma usually complicates long-standing acid reflux. Between 8 and 20% of GERD patients exhibit glandular mucosal (intestinal) metaplasia of the squamous epithelium in the lower esophagus, termed *Barrett's metaplasia*. This condition predisposes to esophageal adenocarcinoma. Gastric malignancies include adenocarcinoma, which is more prevalent in certain Asian societies, and lymphoma (Chap. 77).

Other Causes Alkaline reflux esophagitis produces GERD-like symptoms in patients who have had surgery for peptic ulcer disease. Opportunistic fungal or viral esophageal infections may produce heartburn or chest discomfort but more often cause odynophagia. Biliary colic is in the differential diagnosis of dyspepsia, but most patients with true biliary colic report discrete episodes of right upper quadrant or epigastric pain rather than chronic burning discomfort, nausea, and bloating. Intestinal lactase deficiency produces gas, bloating, discomfort, and diarrhea after lactose ingestion; it occurs in 15% of Caucasians of northern European descent but is more common in African Americans and Asians. Other carbohydrate intolerance syndromes (e.g., fructose, sorbitol) produce similar symptoms. Pancreatic disease (chronic pancreatitis and malignancy), hepatocellular carcinoma, celiac sprue, Ménétrier's disease, infiltrative diseases (sarcoidosis and eosinophilic gastroenteritis), mesenteric ischemia, thyroid and parathyroid disease, and abdominal wall strain cause dyspepsia. Extraperitoneal etiologies of indigestion include congestive heart failure and tuberculosis.

APPROACH TO THE PATIENT

History and Physical Examination GERD classically produces heartburn, a substernal warmth beginning in the epigastrium that moves toward the neck. Heartburn is often exacerbated by meals and may awaken the patient. Associated symptoms include regurgitation of acid and water brash, the reflex release of salty salivary secretions into the mouth. Atypical symptoms include pharyngitis, asthma, cough, bronchitis, hoarseness, and chest pain that mimics angina. Some patients with acid reflux on esophageal pH testing do not report heartburn and instead note abdominal pain or other symptoms.

Some individuals with dyspepsia report ulcer-like symptoms including epigastric gnawing or burning that is relieved by meals or acid suppression. Others experience dysmotility-like fullness or pain that is aggravated by eating and associated with nausea, eructation, and early satiety. There is overlap of functional dyspepsia with other functional disorders such as irritable bowel syndrome.

The physical examination of individuals with GERD and functional dyspepsia is usually normal. In atypical GERD, pharyngeal erythema and wheezing may be present. Poor dentition may occur with prolonged acid regurgitation. Patients with functional dyspepsia may have epigastric tenderness or abdominal distention.

Discrimination between functional and organic causes of indigestion mandates exclusion of selected historic and examination features. Odynophagia suggests esophageal infection; dysphagia promotes concern about a benign or malignant esophageal blockage. Other features that raise alarm include unexplained weight loss, recurrent vomiting, occult or gross gastrointestinal bleeding, jaundice, and a palpable mass or adenopathy.

Diagnostic Testing Because indigestion is prevalent and because most cases result from GERD or functional dyspepsia, a general principle of diagnostic testing is to perform only limited and directed testing of selected individuals.

Once alarm factors are excluded, patients with typical GERD do not need further evaluation and are treated empirically. Upper endoscopy is indicated to exclude mucosal injury in patients with atypical symptoms, symptoms unresponsive to acid-suppressing drugs, or alarm factors. For heartburn >5 years in duration, especially in patients >50 years old, endoscopy is recommended by some experts to screen for Barrett's metaplasia. However, the benefits of this approach have not been validated in controlled studies. Ambulatory esophageal pH testing is considered for drug-refractory symptoms and atypical symptoms such as unexplained chest pain. Esophageal manometry is most commonly ordered when surgical treatment of GERD is considered. A low LES pressure may predict failure with drug therapy and identify patients who may require surgery. Demonstration of disordered esophageal body peristalsis may affect the decision to operate or modify the type of operation chosen. Manometry with provocative testing may clarify the diagnosis in patients with atypical symptoms. Blinded perfusion of saline then acid into the esophagus, known as the *Bernstein test*, can delineate whether unexplained chest discomfort results from acid reflux.

Upper endoscopy is performed as the initial diagnostic test in patients with unexplained dyspepsia who are >45 years old, have alarm factors, or are on NSAIDs because of the elevated risk of malignancy and ulcer in these groups. For younger patients without alarm factors not on NSAIDs, the "test and treat" approach is commonly applied. Determination of *H. pylori* status is made with urea breath testing, stool antigen measurement, or blood serology testing. Those who are *H. pylori* positive are treated to eradicate the infection. For those with negative tests, an acid suppressive regimen is offered empirically. If symptoms resolve on these regimens, no further intervention is required. Endoscopy is reserved for those who fail to respond to treatment of *H. pylori*–positive or –negative dyspepsia. Some clinicians advocate an alternative approach in which those with *H. pylori* undergo endoscopy before treatment. Eradication therapy is then offered only to those with proven ulcer disease. This approach may be preferred where gastric cancer is prevalent and endoscopy less costly.

Further testing is indicated if other factors are present. If bleeding is reported, a blood count is obtained to exclude anemia. Thyroid chemistries or calcium levels are done to screen for metabolic disease. For suspected pancreaticobiliary causes, pancreatic and liver chemistry are obtained. If abnormalities are found, abdominal ultrasound or CT may give important information. Gastric emptying scintigraphy is considered for patients with dysmotility-like dyspepsia when drug treatment fails. Hydrogen breath testing after lactose ingestion may be performed for suspected lactase deficiency.

General Principles In mild indigestion, reassurance that a careful evaluation revealed no serious organic disease may be the only intervention required. Drugs that cause acid reflux or dyspepsia should be stopped if possible. Patients with GERD should limit ethanol, caffeine, chocolate, and tobacco use because of their effects on the LES. Other measures in GERD include ingestion of a low-fat diet, avoidance of snacks before bedtime, and elevation of the head of the bed.

Specific therapies for organic disease should be offered when possible. Surgery is appropriate in biliary colic, while diet changes are indicated for lactase deficiency and celiac sprue. Some illnesses such as peptic ulcer disease may be cured by specific medical regimens. However, as most indigestion is caused by GERD or functional dyspepsia, medications that reduce gastric acid, stimulate motility, or blunt gastric sensitivity are indicated.

Acid Suppressing or Neutralizing Medications Drugs that reduce or neutralize gastric acid are the most prescribed agents for GERD. Histamine H_2 receptor antagonists such as cimetidine, ranitidine, famotidine, and nizatidine are useful in mild to moderate GERD. For uncomplicated heartburn, H_2 receptor antagonists are given for 4 weeks before considering endoscopy. For severe symptoms or for many cases of erosive or ulcerative esophagitis, proton pump inhibitors such as omeprazole, lansoprazole, rabeparzole, pantoprazole, or esomeprazole are needed. These drugs, which inhibit gastric H^+, K^+-ATPase, are more potent than H_2 receptor antagonists. Acid suppressants may be taken continuously or as needed, depending on symptom severity. Many patients initially started on a proton pump inhibitor can be stepped down to an H_2 antagonist. The role of combined therapy with a proton pump inhibitor and an H_2 antagonist is undefined. Liquid antacids are useful for short-term control of mild GERD but are less effective for severe disease unless given at high doses that produce side effects (diarrhea with magnesium-containing agents and constipation with aluminum-containing agents). Sucralfate is a salt of aluminum hydroxide and sucrose octasulfate and buffers acid and binds pepsin and bile salts. Its efficacy in GERD and functional dyspepsia is unproven.

Acid-suppressing drugs are advocated for first-line therapy of *H. pylori*–negative dyspepsia, especially with ulcer-like symptoms. Ranitidine is of benefit in the treatment of functional dyspepsia versus placebo. In young patients without alarm symptoms, a 4-week trial of an H_2 receptor antagonist or proton pump inhibitor is given. Endoscopy is performed only if symptoms do not improve.

***Helicobacter pylori* Eradication** *H. pylori* eradication is indicated only for peptic ulcer and gastric mucosa–associated lymphoid tissue lymphoma. The usefulness of *H. pylori* eradication in patients with functional dyspepsia is unproven, but evidence suggests that <15% of cases relate to *H. pylori*. Patients with ulcer-like symptoms may respond. *H. pylori* eradication is not useful in the treatment of GERD; some reports suggest that elimination of the organism increases the risk of developing GERD and others show no effect. Several drug combinations show efficacy; most include 10 to 14 days of a proton pump inhibitor or bismuth subsalicylate in concert with two antibiotics.

Gastrointestinal Motor Stimulants Motor stimulants such as metoclopramide, erythromycin, and domperidone have limited utility in GERD.

The γ-aminobutyric acid B (GABA-B) agonist baclofen reduces esophageal acid exposure by inhibiting transient LES relaxations; the clinical role of the drug is being studied. Domperidone may be useful in functional dyspepsia and may be given instead of acid suppressants as initial empirical therapy of young patients without alarm symptoms and without *H. pylori* infection. Patients with dysmotility-like dyspepsia may respond preferentially to motor-stimulating drugs.

Other Options Antireflux surgery may be offered to GERD patients with poorly controlled symptoms, disease complications, or unbearable life-style impairments. Fundoplication can be performed laparoscopically; the Nissen and Toupet procedures involve wrapping the proximal stomach around the LES to increase LES pressure. Dysphagia may be a long-term complication of these procedures. Endoscopic interventions at the gastroesophageal junction including radiofrequency energy delivery, suturing, biopolymer implantation, and gastroplication have been used in refractory GERD; their efficacy is being assessed.

Some patients with functional dyspepsia are refractory to acid suppressants or prokinetic drugs but may respond to low-dose tricyclic antidepressant therapy. The mechanism of action in functional dyspepsia is unknown but may involve blunting of visceral pain processing in the brain. Gas and bloating may be the most troubling symptoms in some patients with indigestion and can be difficult to treat. Dietary exclusion of gas-producing foods such as legumes and use of simethicone or activated charcoal benefit some patients. Psychological treatments may be offered for refractory functional dyspepsia, but no convincing data suggest efficacy.

FURTHER READING

HAUG TT et al: The prevalence of nausea in the community: Psychological, social and somatic factors. Gen Hosp Psych 24:81, 2002

HESKETH PJ: Potential role of the NK₁ receptor antagonists in chemotherapy-induced nausea and vomiting. Support Care Cancer 9:350, 2001

MCCOLL KE et al: Randomised trial of endoscopy with testing for *Helicobacter pylori* compared with non-invasive *H. pylori* testing alone in the management of dyspepsia. BMJ 324:999, 2002

RABENECK L et al: A double blind, randomized, placebo-controlled trial of proton pump inhibitor therapy in patients with uninvestigated dyspepsia. Am J Gastroenterol 97:3045, 2002

TACK J et al: Clinical and pathophysiological characteristics of acute-onset functional dyspepsia. Gastroenterology 122:1738, 2002

TALLEY NJ: Dyspepsia: Management guidelines for the millennium. Gut 50 (Suppl 4):iv72, 2002

35 DIARRHEA AND CONSTIPATION
David A. Ahlquist, Michael Camilleri

Diarrhea and constipation are exceedingly common and together exact an enormous toll in terms of morbidity, loss of work productivity, and consumption of medical resources. Worldwide, more than 1 billion people suffer one or more episodes of acute diarrhea each year. Among the 100 million persons affected annually by acute diarrhea in the United States, nearly half must restrict activities, 10% consult physicians, 250,000 require hospitalization, and roughly 3000 die (primarily the elderly). The annual economic burden to society is estimated at >$20 billion. Because of poor sanitation and more limited access to health care, acute infectious diarrhea remains one of the most common causes of mortality in developing countries, particularly among children, accounting for 5 to 8 million deaths per year. Population statistics on chronic diarrhea and constipation are more uncertain, perhaps due to variable definitions and reporting, but the frequency of these conditions is also high. Based on United States population surveys, prevalence rates for chronic diarrhea range from 2 to 7% and for chronic constipation from 3 to 17%. Diarrhea and constipation are among the most common patient complaints faced by internists and primary care physicians, and they account for nearly 50% of referrals to gastroenterologists.

Although diarrhea and constipation may present as mere nuisance symptoms at one extreme, they can be severe or life-threatening at the other. Even mild symptoms may signal a serious underlying gastrointestinal lesion, such as colorectal cancer, or systemic disorder, such as thyroid disease. Given the heterogeneous causes and potential severity of these common complaints, it is imperative for clinicians to appreciate the pathophysiology, etiologic classification, diagnostic strategies, and therapeutic principles of diarrhea and constipation so that rational and cost-effective care can be delivered.

NORMAL PHYSIOLOGY

The human small intestine and colon perform important functions including the secretion and absorption of water and electrolytes, the storage and subsequent transport of intraluminal contents aborally, and the salvage of some nutrients after bacterial metabolism of carbohydrate that are not absorbed in the small intestine. The main motor functions are summarized in Table 35-1. Alterations in fluid and electrolyte handling contribute significantly to diarrhea. Alterations in motor and sensory functions of the human colon result in highly prevalent syndromes such as irritable bowel syndrome, chronic diarrhea, and chronic constipation.

NEURAL CONTROL The small intestine and colon have intrinsic and extrinsic innervation. The *intrinsic innervation*, also called the enteric nervous system, comprises myenteric, submucosal, and mucosal neuronal layers. The function of these layers is modulated by interneurons through the actions of neurotransmitter amines or peptides, including acetylcholine, opioids, norepinephrine, serotonin, ATP, and nitric oxide. The myenteric plexus regulates smooth-muscle function, and the submucosal plexus affects secretion and absorption.

The *extrinsic innervations* of the small intestine and colon are part of the autonomic nervous system and also modulate both motor and secretory functions. The parasympathetic nerve supply conveys both visceral sensory as well as excitatory pathways to the motor components of the colon. Parasympathetic fibers via the vagus nerve reach the small intestine and proximal colon along the branches of the superior mesenteric artery. The distal colon is supplied by sacral parasympathetic nerves (S₂₋₄) via the pelvic plexus; these fibers course through the wall of the colon as ascending intracolonic fibers as far as, and in some instances including, the proximal colon. The chief excitatory neurotransmitters controlling motor function are acetylcholine and the tachykinins, such as substance P. The sympathetic nerve supply modulates motor functions and reaches the small intestine and colon alongside the arterial arcades of the superior and inferior mesenteric vessels. Sympathetic input to the gut is generally excitatory to sphincters and inhibitory to nonsphincteric muscle. Visceral afferents convey sensation from the gut to the central nervous system; initially, they course along sympathetic fibers, but as they approach the spinal cord they separate, have cell bodies in the dorsal root ganglion, and enter the dorsal horn of the spinal cord. Afferent signals are conveyed

TABLE 35-1 *Normal Gastrointestinal Motility: Functions at Different Anatomic Levels*

Stomach and small bowel	Colon: Irregular mixing, absorption,
Synchronized MMCs in fasting	transit
Accommodation, trituration,	Ascending, transverse: reservoirs
mixing, transit	Descending: conduit
Stomach, ~3 h	Sigmoid/rectum: volitional reservoir
Small bowel, ~3 h	
Ileal reservoir empties boluses	

Note: MMC, migrating motor complex.

to the brain along the lateral spinothalamic tract and the nociceptive dorsal column pathway and are then perceived. Other afferent fibers synapse in the prevertebral ganglia and reflexly modulate intestinal motility.

INTESTINAL FLUID ABSORPTION AND SECRETION   On an average day, 9 L of fluid enters the gastrointestinal tract; approximately 1 L of residual fluid reaches the colon; the stool excretion of fluid constitutes about 0.2 L/d. The colon has a large capacitance and functional reserve and may recover up to four times its usual volume of 0.8 L/d, provided the rate of flow permits reabsorption to occur. Thus, the colon can partially compensate for intestinal absorptive or secretory disorders.

In the colon, sodium absorption is predominantly electrogenic, and uptake takes place at the apical membrane; it is compensated for by the export functions of the basolateral sodium pump. A variety of neural and non-neural mediators regulate colonic fluid and electrolyte balance, including cholinergic, adrenergic, and serotonergic mediators. Angiotensin and aldosterone also influence colonic absorption, reflecting the common embryologic development of the distal colonic epithelium and the renal tubules.

SMALL INTESTINAL MOTILITY   During fasting, the motility of the small intestine is characterized by a cyclical event called the migrating motor complex (MMC), which serves to clear nondigestible residue from the small intestine. This organized, propagated series of contractions lasts on average 4 min, occurs every 60 to 90 min, and usually involves the entire small intestine. After food ingestion, the small intestine produces irregular, mixing contractions of relatively low amplitude, except in the distal ileum where more powerful contractions occur intermittently and empty the ileum by bolus transfers.

ILEOCOLONIC STORAGE AND SALVAGE   The distal ileum acts as a reservoir, emptying intermittently by bolus movements. This action allows time for salvage of fluids, electrolytes, and nutrients. Segmentation by haustra compartmentalizes the colon and facilitates mixing, retention of residue, and formation of solid stools. In health, the ascending and transverse regions of colon function as reservoirs (average transit, 15 h), and the descending colon acts as a conduit (average transit, 3 h). The colon is efficient at conserving sodium and water, a function that is particularly important in sodium-depleted patients in whom the small intestine alone is unable to maintain sodium balance. Diarrhea or constipation may result from alteration in the reservoir function of the proximal colon or the propulsive function of the left colon. Constipation may also result from disturbances of the rectal or sigmoid reservoir, typically as a result of dysfunction of the pelvic floor or the coordination of defecation.

COLONIC MOTILITY AND TONE   The small intestinal MMC only rarely continues into the colon. However, short duration or phasic contractions mix colonic contents, and high-amplitude propagated contractions (HAPCs) are sometimes associated with mass movements through the colon and occur approximately five times per day, usually on awakening in the morning and postprandially. Increased frequency of HAPCs may result in diarrhea. The predominant phasic contractions are irregular and nonpropagated and serve as a "mixing" function.

Colonic tone refers to the background contractility upon which phasic contractile activity (typically contractions lasting <15 s) is superimposed. It is an important cofactor in the colon's capacitance (volume accommodation) and sensation.

COLONIC MOTILITY AFTER MEAL INGESTION   After meal ingestion, colonic phasic and tonic contractility increase for a period of approximately 2 h. The initial phase (about 10 min) is mediated by the vagus nerve in response to mechanical distention of the stomach. The subsequent response of the colon requires caloric stimulation and is at least in part mediated by hormones, e.g., gastrin and serotonin.

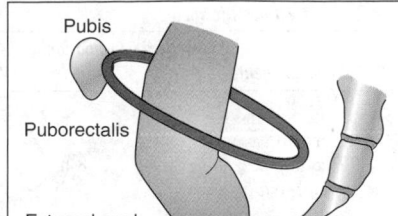

FIGURE 35-1   Mechanisms involved in continence and defecation. Note the importance of pelvic floor and anal sphincter functions. Continence requires: contraction of puborectalis, maintenance of anorectal angle, normal rectal sensation, and contraction of sphincter. Defecation requires: relaxation of puborectalis, straightening of anorectal angle, and relaxation of sphincter.

DEFECATION   Tonic contraction of the puborectalis muscle, which forms a sling around the rectoanal junction, is important to maintain continence; during defecation, sacral parasympathetic nerves relax this muscle, facilitating the straightening of the rectoanal angle (Fig. 35-1). Distention of the rectum results in transient relaxation of the internal anal sphincter via intrinsic and reflex sympathetic innervation. As sigmoid and rectal contractions increase the pressure within the rectum, the rectosigmoid angle opens by >15°. Voluntary relaxation of the external anal sphincter (striated muscle innervated by the pudendal nerve) permits the evacuation of feces; this evacuation process can be augmented by an increase in intraabdominal pressure created by the Valsalva maneuver.

DIARRHEA

DEFINITION   Diarrhea is loosely defined as passage of abnormally liquid or unformed stools at an increased frequency. For adults on a typical Western diet, stool weight >200 g/d can generally be considered diarrheal. Because of the fundamental importance of duration to diagnostic considerations, diarrhea may be further defined as *acute* if <2 weeks, *persistent* if 2 to 4 weeks, and *chronic* if >4 weeks in duration.

Two common conditions, usually associated with the passage of stool totaling <200 g/d, must be distinguished from diarrhea, as diagnostic and therapeutic algorithms differ. *Pseudodiarrhea*, or the frequent passage of small volumes of stool, is often associated with rectal urgency and accompanies the irritable bowel syndrome or anorectal disorders such as proctitis. *Fecal incontinence* is the involuntary discharge of rectal contents and is most often caused by neuromuscular disorders or structural anorectal problems. Diarrhea and urgency, especially if severe, may aggravate or cause incontinence. Pseudodiarrhea and fecal incontinence occur at prevalence rates comparable to or higher than that of chronic diarrhea and should always be considered in patients complaining of "diarrhea." A careful history and physical examination generally allow these conditions to be discriminated from true diarrhea.

ACUTE DIARRHEA   More than 90% of cases of acute diarrhea are caused by infectious agents; these cases are often accompanied by vomiting, fever, and abdominal pain. The remaining 10% or so are caused by medications, toxic ingestions, ischemia, and other conditions.

Infectious Agents   Most infectious diarrheas are acquired by fecal-oral transmission via direct personal contact or, more commonly, via ingestion of food or water contaminated with pathogens from human or animal feces. In the immunologically competent person, the resident fecal microflora, containing >500 taxonomically distinct species, are rarely the source of diarrhea and may actually play a role in suppressing the growth of ingested pathogens. Acute infection or injury occurs when the ingested agent overwhelms the host's mucosal immune and nonimmune (gastric acid, digestive enzymes, mucus secretion, peristalsis, and suppressive resident flora) defenses. Established clinical associations with specific enteropathogens may offer diagnostic clues.

Pathobiology/Agents	Incubation Period	Vomiting	Abdominal Pain	Fever	Diarrhea
Toxin producers					
Preformed toxin					
Bacillus cereus, *Staphylococcus aureus*, *Clostridium perfringens*	1–8 h 8–24 h	3–4+	1–2+	0–1+	3–4+, watery
Enterotoxin					
Vibrio cholerae, enterotoxigenic *Escherichia coli*, *Klebsiella pneumoniae*, *Aeromonas* species	8–72 h	2–4+	1–2+	0–1+	3–4+, watery
Enteroadherent					
Enteropathogenic and enteroadherent *E. coli*, *Giardia* organisms, cryptosporidiosis, helminths	1–8 d	0–1+	1–3+	1–2+	1–2+, watery
Cytotoxin-producers					
Clostridium difficile	1–3 d	0–1+	3–4+	1–2+	1–3+, usually watery, occasionally bloody
Hemorrhagic *E. coli*	12–72 h	0–1+	3–4+	1–2+	1–3+, initially watery, quickly bloody
Invasive organisms					
Minimal inflammation					
Rotavirus and Norwalk agent	1–3 d	1–2+	2–3+	3–4+	1–3+, watery
Variable inflammation					
Salmonella, *Campylobacter*, and *Aeromonas* species, *Vibrio parahaemolyticus*, *Yersinia*	12 h–11 d	0–3+	2–4+	3–4+	1–4+, watery or bloody
Severe inflammation					
Shigella species, enteroinvasive *E. coli*, *Entamoeba histolytica*	12 h–8 d	0–1+	3–4+	3–4+	1–2+, bloody

Source: Adapted from DW Powell, in T Yamada (ed): *Textbook of Gastroenterology and Hepatology*, 4th ed. Philadelphia, Lippincott, Williams & Wilkins, 2003; and DR Syndman, in SL Gorbach (ed): *Infectious Diarrhea*. London, Blackwell, 1986.

protracted diarrheal illness, and, particularly in persons with AIDS, opportunistic infections, such as by *Mycobacterium* species, certain viruses (cytomegalovirus, adenovirus, and herpes simplex), and protozoa (*Cryptosporidium*, *Isospora belli*, Microsporidia, and *Blastocystis hominis*) may also play a role (Chap. 173). In patients with AIDS, agents transmitted venereally per rectum (e.g., *Neisseria gonorrhoeae*, *Treponema pallidum*, *Chlamydia*) may contribute to proctocolitis.

4. *Daycare participants and their family members.* Infections with *Shigella*, *Giardia*, *Cryptosporidium*, rotavirus, and other agents are very common and should be considered.

5. *Institutionalized persons.* Infectious diarrhea is one of the most frequent categories of nosocomial infections in many hospitals and long-term care facilities; the causes are a variety of microorganisms but most commonly *Clostridium difficile*.

The pathophysiology underlying acute diarrhea by infectious agents produces specific clinical features that may also be helpful in diagnosis (Table 35-2). Profuse watery diarrhea secondary to small bowel hypersecretion occurs with ingestion of preformed bacterial toxins, enterotoxin-producing bacteria, and enteroadherent pathogens. Diarrhea associated with marked vomiting and minimal or no fever may occur abruptly within a few hours after ingestion of the former two types; vomiting is usually less, and abdominal cramping or bloating is greater; fever is higher with the latter. Cytotoxin-producing and invasive microorganisms all cause high fever and abdominal pain. Invasive bacteria and *Entamoeba histolytica* often cause bloody diarrhea (referred to as *dysentery*). *Yersinia* invades the terminal ileal and proximal colon mucosa and may cause especially severe abdominal pain with tenderness mimicking acute appendicitis.

Finally, infectious diarrhea may be associated with systemic manifestations. Reiter's syndrome (arthritis, urethritis, and conjunctivitis) may accompany or follow infections by *Salmonella*, *Campylobacter*, *Shigella*, and *Yersinia*. Yersiniosis may also lead to an autoimmune-type thyroiditis, pericarditis, and glomerulonephritis. Both enterohemorrhagic *E. coli* (O157:H7) and *Shigella* can lead to the *hemolytic-uremic syndrome* with an attendant high mortality rate. Acute diarrhea can also be a major symptom of several systemic infections including *viral hepatitis, listeriosis, legionellosis*, and *toxic shock syndrome*.

Other Causes Side effects from medications are probably the most common noninfectious cause of acute diarrhea, and etiology may be suggested by a temporal association between use and symptom onset. Although innumerable medications may produce diarrhea, some of the more frequently incriminated include antibiotics, cardiac antidysrhythmics, antihypertensives, nonsteroidal anti-inflammatory drugs (NSAIDs), certain antidepressants, chemotherapeutic agents, bronchodilators, antacids, and laxatives. Occlusive or nonocclusive *ischemic colitis* typically occurs in persons >50 years, often presents as

In the United States, high risk groups are recognized:

1. *Travelers.* Nearly 40% of tourists to endemic regions of Latin America, Africa, and Asia develop so-called traveler's diarrhea, most commonly due to enterotoxigenic *Escherichia coli* as well as to *Campylobacter*, *Shigella*, and *Salmonella*. Visitors to Russia (especially St. Petersburg) may have increased risk of *Giardia*-associated diarrhea; visitors to Nepal may acquire *Cyclospora*. Campers, backpackers, and swimmers in wilderness areas may become infected with *Giardia*.

2. *Consumers of certain foods.* Diarrhea closely following food consumption at a picnic, banquet, or restaurant may suggest infection with *Salmonella*, *Campylobacter*, or *Shigella* from chicken; enterohemorrhagic *E. coli* (O157:H7) from undercooked hamburger; *Bacillus aureus* from fried rice; *Staphylococcus aureus* or *Salmonella* from mayonnaise or creams; *Salmonella* from eggs; and *Vibrio* species, *Salmonella*, or acute hepatitis A or B from seafood, especially if raw.

3. *Immunodeficient persons.* Individuals at risk for diarrhea include those with either primary immunodeficiency (e.g., IgA deficiency, common variable hypogammaglobulinemia, chronic granulomatous disease) or the much more common secondary immunodeficiency states (e.g., AIDS, senescence, pharmacologic suppression). Common enteropathogens often cause a more severe and

acute lower abdominal pain preceding watery, then bloody diarrhea, and generally results in acute inflammatory changes in the sigmoid or left colon while sparing the rectum. Acute diarrhea may accompany colonic *diverticulitis* and *graft-versus-host disease*. Acute diarrhea, often associated with systemic compromise, can follow ingestion of toxins including organophosphate insecticides, amanita and other mushrooms, arsenic, and preformed environmental toxins in seafoods, such as ciguatera and scombroid. The conditions causing chronic diarrhea can also be confused with acute diarrhea early in their course. This confusion may occur with inflammatory bowel disease and some of the other inflammatory chronic diarrheas that may have an abrupt rather than insidious onset and exhibit features that mimic infection.

APPROACH TO THE PATIENT

The decision to evaluate acute diarrhea depends on its severity and duration and on various host factors (Fig. 35-2). Most episodes of acute diarrhea are mild and self-limited and do not justify the cost and potential morbidity of diagnostic or pharmacologic interventions. Indications for evaluation include profuse diarrhea with dehydration, grossly bloody stools, fever ≥38.5° C, duration >48 h without improvement, new community outbreaks, associated severe abdominal pain in patients >50 years, and elderly (≥70 years) or immunocompromised patients. In some cases of moderately severe febrile diarrhea associated with fecal leukocytes (or increased fecal levels of the leukocyte proteins) or with gross blood, a diagnostic evaluation might be avoided in favor of an empirical antibiotic trial (see below).

The cornerstone of diagnosis in those suspected of severe acute infectious diarrhea is microbiologic analysis of the stool. Workup includes cultures for bacterial and viral pathogens, direct inspection for ova and parasites, and immunoassays for certain bacterial toxins (*C. difficile*), viral antigens (rotavirus), and protozoal antigens (*Giardia, E. histolytica*). The aforementioned clinical and epidemiologic associations may assist in focusing the evaluation. If a particular pathogen or set of possible pathogens is so implicated, then either the whole panel of routine studies may not be necessary or, in some instances, special cultures may be appropriate as for enterohemorrhagic and other types of *E. coli*, *Vibrio* species, and *Yersinia*. Molecular diagnosis of pathogens in stool can be made by identification of unique DNA sequences; and evolving microarray technologies could lead to a more rapid, sensitive, specific, and cost-effective diagnostic approach in the future.

Persistent diarrhea is commonly due to *Giardia*, but additional causative organisms that should be considered include *C. difficile* (especially if antibiotics had been administered), *E. histolytica*, *Cryptosporidium*, *Campylobacter*, and others. If stool studies are unrevealing, then flexible sigmoidoscopy with biopsies and upper endoscopy with duodenal aspirates and biopsies may be indicated.

Structural examination by sigmoidoscopy, colonoscopy, or abdominal computed tomographic scanning (or other imaging approaches) may be appropriate in patients with uncharacterized persistent diarrhea to exclude inflammatory bowel disease, or as an initial approach in patients with suspected noninfectious acute diarrhea such as might be caused by ischemic colitis, diverticulitis, or partial bowel obstruction.

℞ TREATMENT

Fluid and electrolyte replacement are of central importance to all forms of acute diarrhea. Fluid replacement alone may suffice for mild cases. Oral sugar-electrolyte solutions (sport drinks or designed formulations) should be instituted promptly with severe diarrhea to limit dehydration, which is the major cause of death. Profoundly dehydrated patients, especially infants and the elderly, require intravenous rehydration.

In moderately severe nonfebrile and nonbloody diarrhea, antimotility antisecretory agents such as loperamide can be useful adjuncts to control symptoms. Such agents should be avoided with febrile dysentery, which may be exacerbated or prolonged by them. Bismuth subsalicylate may reduce symptoms of vomiting and diarrhea but should not be used to treat immunocompromised patients because of the risk of bismuth encephalopathy.

Judicious use of antibiotics is appropriate in selected instances of acute diarrhea and may reduce its severity and duration (Fig. 35-2). Many physicians treat moderately to severely ill patients with febrile dysentery empirically without diagnostic evaluation using a quinolone, such as ciprofloxacin (500 mg bid for 3 to 5 d). Empirical treatment can also be considered for suspected giardiasis with metronidazole (250 mg qid for 7 d). Selection of antibiotics and dosage regimens are otherwise dictated by specific pathogens and conditions found (Chaps. 113, 134, 137–143). Antibiotic coverage is indicated whether or not a causative organism is discovered in patients who are immunocompromised, have mechanical heart valves or recent vascular grafts, or are elderly. Antibiotic prophylaxis is indicated for certain patients traveling to high-risk countries in whom the likelihood or seriousness of acquired diarrhea would be especially high, including those with immunocompromise, inflammatory bowel disease, or gastric achlorhydria. Use of trimethoprim/sulfamethoxazole or ciprofloxacin may reduce bacterial diarrhea in such travelers by 90%.

CHRONIC DIARRHEA Diarrhea lasting >4 weeks warrants evaluation to exclude serious underlying pathology. In contrast to acute diarrhea, most of the many causes of chronic diarrhea are noninfectious. The classification of chronic diarrhea by pathophysiologic mechanism facilitates a rational approach to management (Table 35-3).

Secretory Causes Secretory diarrheas are due to derangements in fluid and electrolyte transport across the enterocolic mucosa. They are char-

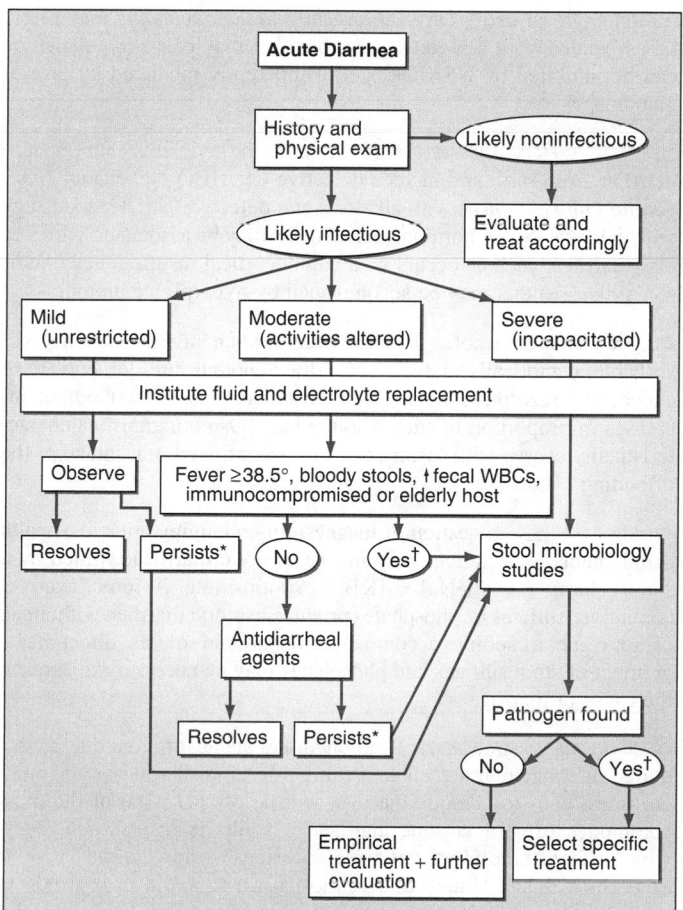

FIGURE 35-2 Algorithm for the management of acute diarrhea. Consider empirical Rx before evaluation with (*) metronidazole and (†) with quinolone.

TABLE 35-3 *Major Causes of Chronic Diarrhea According to Predominant Pathophysiologic Mechanism*

Secretory causes	Inflammatory causes
Exogenous stimulant laxatives	Idiopathic inflammatory bowel
Chronic ethanol ingestion	disease (Crohn's chronic
Other drugs and toxins	ulcerative colitis)
Endogenous laxatives (dihydroxy bile acids)	Microscopic and collagenous colitis
Idiopathic secretory diarrhea	Immune-related mucosal disease
Certain bacterial infections	(1° or 2° immunodeficiencies,
Bowel resection, disease, or fistula (↓ absorption)	food allergy, eosinophilic gastroenteritis, graft-vs-host
Partial bowel obstruction or fecal impaction	disease) Infections (invasive bacteria,
Hormone-producing tumors	viruses, and parasites)
(carcinoid, VIPoma, medullary	Radiation injury
cancer of thyroid, mastocytosis,	Gastrointestinal malignancies
gastrinoma, colorectal villous	Dysmotile causes
adenoma)	Visceral neuromyopathies
Addison's disease	Hyperthyroidism
Congenital electrolyte absorption	Drugs (prokinetic agents)
defects	Factitial causes
Osmotic causes	Munchausen
Osmotic laxatives (Mg^{2+}, PO_4^{3-}, SO_4^{2-})	Bulimia
Lactase and other disaccharide deficiencies	
Nonabsorbable carbohydrates (sorbitol, lactulose, polyethylene glycol)	
Steatorrheal causes	
Intraluminal maldigestion (pancreatic exocrine insufficiency, bacterial overgrowth, liver disease)	
Mucosal malabsorption (celiac sprue, Whipple's disease, infections, abetalipoproteinemia, ischemia)	
Postmucosal obstruction (1° or 2° lymphatic obstruction)	

acterized clinically by watery, large-volume fecal outputs that are typically painless and persist with fasting. Because there is no malabsorbed solute, stool osmolality is accounted for by normal endogenous electrolytes with no fecal osmotic gap.

MEDICATIONS Side effects from regular ingestion of drugs and toxins are the most common secretory causes of chronic diarrhea. Hundreds of prescription and over-the-counter medications (see "Other Causes of Acute Diarrhea," above) may produce unwanted diarrhea. Surreptitious or habitual use of stimulant laxatives [e.g., senna, cascara, bisacodyl, ricinoleic acid (castor oil)] must also be considered. Chronic ethanol consumption may cause a secretory-type diarrhea due to enterocyte injury with impaired sodium and water absorption as well as to rapid transit and other alterations. Inadvertent ingestion of certain environmental toxins (e.g., arsenic) may lead to chronic rather than acute forms of diarrhea. Certain bacterial infections may occasionally persist and be associated with a secretory-type diarrhea.

BOWEL RESECTION, MUCOSAL DISEASE, OR ENTEROCOLIC FISTULA These conditions may result in a secretory-type diarrhea because of inadequate surface for resorption of secreted fluids and electrolytes. Unlike other secretory diarrheas, this subset of conditions tends to worsen with eating. With disease (e.g., Crohn's ileitis) or resection of <100 cm of terminal ileum, dihydroxy bile acids may escape absorption and stimulate colonic secretion (cholorrheic diarrhea). This mechanism may contribute to so-called *idiopathic secretory diarrhea*, in which bile acids are functionally malabsorbed from a normal-appearing terminal ileum. Partial bowel obstruction, ostomy stricture, or fecal impaction may paradoxically lead to increased fecal output due to hypersecretion.

HORMONES Although uncommon, the classic examples of secretory diarrhea are those mediated by hormones. *Metastatic gastrointestinal carcinoid tumors* or, rarely, *primary bronchial carcinoids* may produce watery diarrhea alone or as part of the carcinoid syndrome that comprises episodic flushing, wheezing, dyspnea, and right-sided valvular heart disease. Diarrhea is due to the release into the circulation of potent intestinal secretagogues including serotonin, histamine, prostaglandins, and various kinins. Pellagra-like skin lesions may rarely occur as the result of serotonin overproduction with niacin depletion. *Gastrinoma*, one of the most common neuroendocrine tumors, most typically presents with refractory peptic ulcers, but diarrhea occurs in up to one-third of cases and may be the only clinical manifestation in 10%. While various secretagogues released with gastrin may play a role, the diarrhea most often results from fat maldigestion owing to pancreatic enzyme inactivation by low intraduodenal pH. The watery diarrhea hypokalemia achlorhydria syndrome, also called *pancreatic cholera*, is due to a non-β cell pancreatic adenoma, referred to as a *VIPoma*, that secretes vasoactive intestinal peptide (VIP) and a host of other peptide hormones including pancreatic polypeptide, secretin, gastrin, gastrin-inhibitory polypeptide, neurotensin, calcitonin, and prostaglandins. The secretory diarrhea is often massive with stool volumes >3 L/d; daily volumes as high as 20 L have been reported. Life-threatening dehydration; neuromuscular dysfunction from associated hypokalemia, hypomagnesemia, or hypercalcemia; flushing; and hyperglycemia may accompany a VIPoma. *Medullary carcinoma of the thyroid* may present with watery diarrhea caused by calcitonin, other secretory peptides, or prostaglandins. This tumor occurs sporadically or, in 25 to 50% of cases, as a feature of multiple endocrine neoplasia type IIa with pheochromocytomas and hyperparathyroidism. Prominent diarrhea is often associated with metastatic disease and poor prognosis. *Systemic mastocytosis*, which may be associated with the skin lesion urticaria pigmentosa, may cause diarrhea that is either secretory and mediated by histamine or inflammatory and due to intestinal filtration by mast cells. Large *colorectal villous adenomas* may rarely be associated with a secretory diarrhea that may cause hypokalemia, can be inhibited by NSAIDs, and is apparently mediated by prostaglandins.

CONGENITAL DEFECTS IN ION ABSORPTION Rarely, these defects cause watery diarrhea from birth and include defective Cl^-/HCO_3^- exchange (*congenital chloridorrhea*) with alkalosis and defective Na^+/H^+ exchange with acidosis. Some hormone deficiencies may be associated with watery diarrhea, such as occurs with adrenocortical insufficiency (Addison's disease) that may be accompanied by hyperpigmentation.

Osmotic Causes Osmotic diarrhea occurs when ingested, poorly absorbable, osmotically active solutes draw enough fluid lumenward to exceed the resorptive capacity of the colon. Fecal water output increases in proportion to such a solute load. Osmotic diarrhea characteristically ceases with fasting or with discontinued oral intake of the offending agent.

OSMOTIC LAXATIVES Ingestion of magnesium-containing antacids, health supplements, or laxatives may induce osmotic diarrhea typified by a stool osmotic gap: $2([Na] + [K]) <290$ mosm/kg. Anionic laxatives containing sulfates or phosphates produce osmotic diarrhea without an osmotic gap, as sodium accompanies the anionic solutes; direct measurement of stool sulfates and phosphates may be necessary to confirm the cause of diarrhea.

CARBOHYDRATE MALABSORPTION Carbohydrate malabsorption due to acquired or congenital defects in brush-border disaccharidases and other enzymes leads to osmotic diarrhea with a low pH. One of the most common causes of chronic diarrhea in adults is *lactase deficiency*, which affects three-fourths of non-Caucasians worldwide and 5 to 30% of persons in the United States; most learn to avoid milk products without an intervention. Some sugars, such as sorbitol, are universally malabsorbed, and diarrhea ensues with ingestion of ample medications, gum, or candies sweetened with these nonabsorbable sugars.

Lactulose, used to acidify stools in patients with hepatic failure, also causes diarrhea on this basis.

Steatorrheal Causes Fat malabsorption may lead to greasy, foul-smelling, difficult-to-flush diarrhea often associated with weight loss and nutritional deficiencies due to concomitant malabsorption of amino acids and vitamins. Increased fecal output is caused by the osmotic effects of fatty acids, especially after bacterial hydroxylation, and, to a lesser extent, by the burden of neutral fat. Quantitatively, steatorrhea is defined as stool fat exceeding the normal 7 g/d; daily fecal fat averages 15 to 25 g with small intestinal diseases and is often >40 g with pancreatic exocrine insufficiency. Intraluminal maldigestion, mucosal malabsorption, or lymphatic obstruction may produce steatorrhea.

INTRALUMINAL MALDIGESTION This condition most commonly results from pancreatic exocrine insufficiency, which occurs when >90% of pancreatic secretory function is lost. *Chronic pancreatitis*, usually a sequela of ethanol abuse, most frequently causes pancreatic insufficiency. Other causes include *cystic fibrosis*, *pancreatic duct obstruction*, and rarely, *somatostatinoma*. Bacterial overgrowth in the small intestine may deconjugate bile acids and alter micelle formation that impairs fat digestion; it occurs with stasis from a blind-loop, small bowel diverticulum or dysmotility and is especially likely in the elderly. Finally, cirrhosis or biliary obstruction may lead to mild steatorrhea due to deficient intraluminal bile acid concentration.

MUCOSAL MALABSORPTION Mucosal malabsorption occurs from a variety of enteropathies but most prototypically and perhaps most commonly from *celiac sprue*. This gluten-sensitive enteropathy characterized by villous atrophy and crypt hyperplasia in the proximal small bowel often presents with fatty diarrhea associated with multiple nutritional deficiencies of varying severity and affects all ages. *Tropical sprue* may produce a similar histologic and clinical syndrome but occurs in residents of or travelers to tropical climates; its often abrupt onset and response to antibiotics suggest an infectious etiology. *Whipple's disease*, due to the actinomycete *Treponema whippleii* and histiocytic infiltration of the small bowel mucosa, is a less common cause of steatorrhea that most typically occurs in young or middle-aged men; it is frequently associated with arthralgias, fever, lymphadenopathy, and extreme fatigue and may affect the central nervous system and endocardium. A similar clinical and histologic picture results from *Mycobacterium avium-intracellulare* infection in patients with AIDS. *Abetalipoproteinemia* is a rare defect of chylomicron formation and fat malabsorption in children associated with acanthocytic erythrocytes, ataxia, and retinitis pigmentosa. Several other conditions may cause mucosal malabsorption including infections, especially with protozoa such as *Giardia*, numerous medications (e.g., colchicine, cholestyramine, neomycin), and chronic ischemia.

POSTMUCOSAL LYMPHATIC OBSTRUCTION The pathophysiology of this condition, which is due to the rare *congenital intestinal lymphangiectasia* or to *acquired lymphatic obstruction* secondary to trauma, tumor, or infection, leads to the unique constellation of fat malabsorption with enteric losses of protein (often causing edema) and lymphocytes (with resultant lymphocytopenia) that enter the portal circulation directly. Carbohydrate and amino acid absorption are preserved.

Inflammatory Causes Inflammatory diarrheas are generally accompanied by pain, fever, bleeding, or other manifestations of inflammation. The mechanism of diarrhea may not only be exudation but, depending on lesion site, may include fat malabsorption, disrupted fluid/electrolyte absorption, and hypersecretion or hypermotility from release of cytokines and other inflammatory mediators. The unifying feature on stool analysis is the presence of leukocytes or leukocyte-derived proteins such as calprotectin. With severe inflammation, exudative protein loss can lead to anasarca (generalized edema). Any middle-aged or older person with chronic inflammatory-type diarrhea, especially with blood, should be carefully evaluated to exclude a colorectal or large enteric tumor.

IDIOPATHIC INFLAMMATORY BOWEL DISEASE The illnesses in this category, which include *Crohn's disease* and *chronic ulcerative colitis*, are among the most common organic causes of chronic diarrhea in adults and range in severity from mild to fulminant and life-threatening. They may be associated with uveitis, polyarthralgias, cholestatic liver disease (primary sclerosing cholangitis), and various skin lesions (erythema nodosum, pyoderma gangrenosum). *Microscopic colitis*, including *collagenous colitis*, is an increasingly recognized cause of chronic watery diarrhea; biopsy of a normal appearing colorectum is required for histologic diagnosis.

PRIMARY OR SECONDARY FORMS OF IMMUNODEFICIENCY Immunodeficiency may lead to prolonged infectious diarrhea. With common, variable *hypogammaglobulinemia*, diarrhea is particularly prevalent and often the result of giardiasis.

EOSINOPHILIC GASTROENTERITIS Eosinophil infiltration of the mucosa, muscularis, or serosa at any level of the gastrointestinal tract may cause diarrhea, pain, vomiting, or ascites. Affected patients often have an atopic history, Charcot-Leyden crystals due to extruded eosinophil contents may be seen on microscopic inspection of stool, and peripheral eosinophilia is present in 50 to 75% of patients. While hypersensitivity to certain foods occurs in adults, true food allergy causing chronic diarrhea is rare.

OTHER CAUSES Chronic inflammatory diarrhea may be caused by *radiation enterocolitis, chronic graft-versus-host disease, Behçet's syndrome*, and *Cronkite-Canada syndrome*, among others.

Dysmotile Causes Rapid transit may accompany many diarrheas as a secondary or contributing phenomenon, but primary dysmotility is an unusual etiology of true diarrhea. Stool features often suggest a secretory diarrhea, but mild steatorrhea of up to 14 g of fat per day can be produced by maldigestion from rapid transit alone. *Hyperthyroidism, carcinoid syndrome*, and certain drugs (e.g., prostaglandins, prokinetic agents) may produce hypermotility with resultant diarrhea. Primary visceral neuromyopathies or idiopathic acquired intestinal pseudo-obstruction may lead to stasis with secondary bacterial overgrowth causing diarrhea. *Diabetic diarrhea*, often accompanied by peripheral and generalized autonomic neuropathies, may occur in part because of intestinal dysmotility.

The exceedingly common *irritable bowel syndrome* (10% point prevalence, 1 to 2% per year incidence) is characterized by disturbed intestinal and colonic motor and sensory responses to various stimuli. Symptoms of stool frequency typically cease at night, alternate with periods of constipation, are accompanied by abdominal pain relieved with defecation, and rarely result in weight loss or true diarrhea.

Factitial Causes Factitial diarrhea accounts for up to 15% of unexplained diarrheas referred to tertiary care centers. Either as a form of *Munchausen syndrome* (deception or self-injury for secondary gain) or *bulimia*, some patients covertly self-administer laxatives alone or in combination with other medications (e.g., diuretics) or surreptitiously add water or urine to stool sent for analysis. Such patients are typically women, often with histories of psychiatric illness, and disproportionately from careers in health care. Hypotension and hypokalemia are common co-presenting features. Such patients often deny this possibility when confronted, but they do benefit from psychiatric counseling when they acknowledge their behavior.

APPROACH TO THE PATIENT

The laboratory tools available to evaluate the very common problem of chronic diarrhea are extensive, and many are costly and invasive. As such, the diagnostic evaluation must be rationally directed by a careful history and physical examination, and simple triage tests are often warranted before complex investigations are launched (Fig. 35-3). The history, physical examination, and routine blood studies should attempt to characterize the mechanism of diarrhea, identify diagnostically helpful associations, and assess the

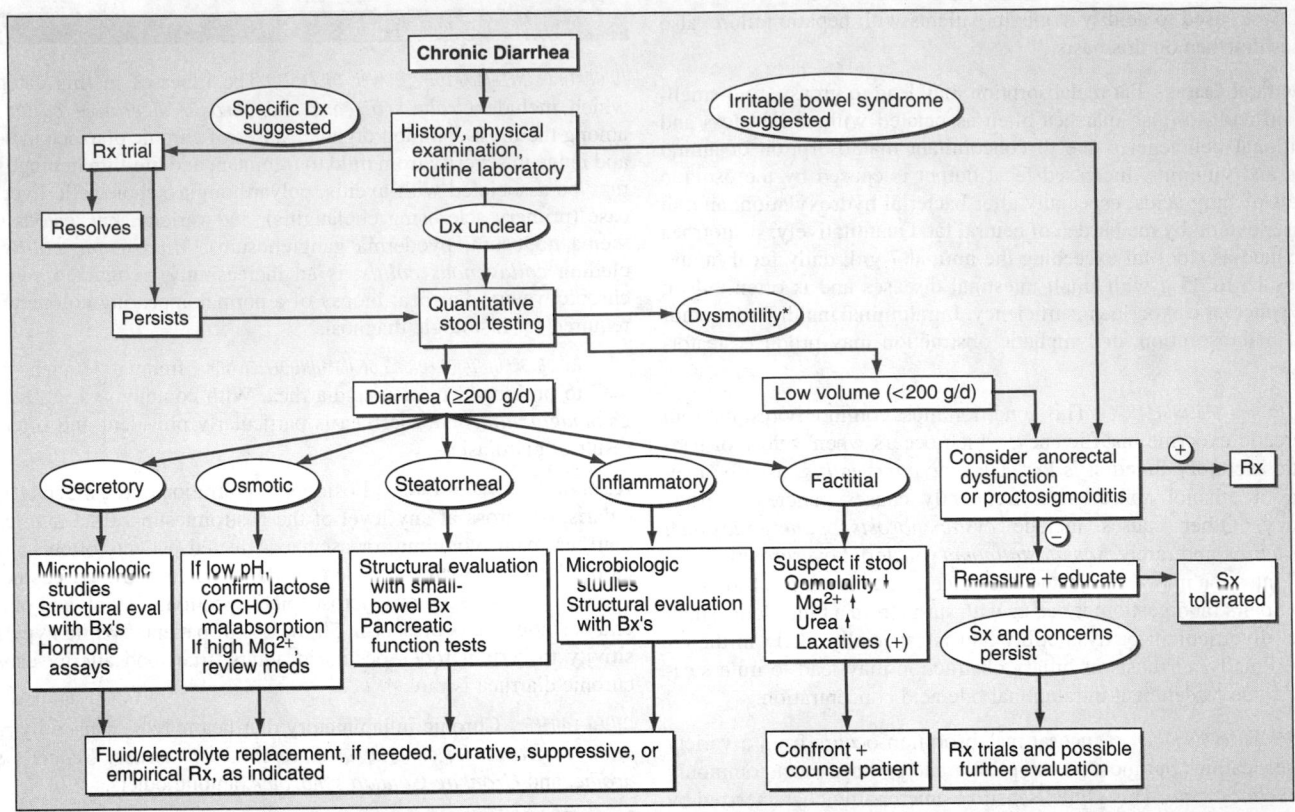

FIGURE 35-3 Algorithm for the management of chronic diarrhea.* Dysmotility presents variable stool profile.

patient's fluid/electrolyte and nutritional status. Patients should be questioned about the onset, duration, pattern, aggravating (especially diet) and relieving factors, and stool characteristics of their diarrhea. The presence or absence of fecal incontinence, fever, weight loss, pain, certain exposures (travel, medications, contacts with diarrhea), and common extraintestinal manifestations (skin changes, arthralgias, oral aphtha) should be noted. Physical findings may offer clues such as a thyroid mass, wheezing, heart murmurs, edema, hepatomegaly, abdominal masses, lymphadenopathy, mucocutaneous abnormalities, perianal fistulae, or anal sphincter laxity. Peripheral blood counts may reveal leukocytosis that suggests inflammation; anemia that reflects blood loss or nutritional deficiencies; or eosinophilia that may occur with parasitoses, neoplasia, collagen-vascular disease, allergy, or eosinophilic gastroenteritis. Blood chemistries may demonstrate electrolyte, hepatic, or other metabolic disturbances.

A therapeutic trial is often appropriate, definitive, and highly cost effective when a specific diagnosis is suggested on the initial physician encounter. For example, chronic watery diarrhea, which ceases with fasting in an otherwise healthy young adult, may justify a trial of a lactose-restricted diet; bloating and diarrhea persisting since a mountain backpacking trip may warrant a trial of metronidazole for likely giardiasis; and postprandial diarrhea persisting since an ileal resection might be due to bile acid malabsorption and be treated with cholestyramine before further evaluation. Persistent symptoms require additional investigation.

Certain diagnoses may be suggested on the initial encounter, e.g., idiopathic inflammatory bowel disease; however, additional focused evaluations may be necessary to confirm the diagnosis and characterize the severity or extent of disease so that treatment can be best guided. Patients suspected of having irritable bowel syndrome should be initially evaluated with proctosigmoidoscopy and mucosal biopsies; those with normal findings might be reassured and, as indicated, treated empirically with antispasmodics, antidiarrheals, bulk agents, anxiolytics, or antidepressants. Any patient who presents with chronic diarrhea and hematochezia should be evaluated with stool microbiologic studies and colonoscopy.

In an estimated two-thirds of cases, the cause for chronic diarrhea remains unclear after the initial encounter, and further testing is required. Quantitative stool collection and analyses can yield important objective data that may establish a diagnosis or characterize the type of diarrhea as a triage for focused additional studies (Fig. 35-3). If stool weight is >200 g/d, additional stool analyses should be performed that might include electrolyte concentration, pH, occult blood testing, leukocyte inspection (or leukocyte protein assay), fat quantitation, and laxative screens.

For secretory diarrheas (watery, normal osmotic gap), possible medication-related side effects or surreptitious laxative use should be reconsidered. Microbiologic studies should be done including fecal bacterial cultures (including media for *Aeromonas* and *Pleisiomonas*), inspection for ova and parasites, and *Giardia* antigen assay (the most sensitive test for giardiasis). Small bowel bacterial overgrowth can be excluded by intestinal aspirates with quantitative cultures or with glucose or xylose breath tests involving measurement of breath hydrogen or other metabolite (e.g., $^{14}CO_2$). However, interpretation of these breath tests may be confounded by disturbances of intestinal transit. When suggested by history or other findings, screens for peptide hormones should be pursued (e.g., serum gastrin, VIP, calcitonin, and thyroid hormone/thyroid stimulating hormone, or urinary 5-hydroxyindolacetic acid and histamine). Upper endoscopy and colonoscopy with biopsies and small-bowel barium x-rays are helpful to rule out structural or occult inflammatory disease.

Further evaluation of osmotic diarrhea should include tests for lactose intolerance and magnesium ingestion, the two most common causes. Low fecal pH suggests carbohydrate malabsorption; lactose malabsorption can be confirmed by lactose breath testing or by a therapeutic trial with lactose exclusion and observation of the effect of lactose challenge (e.g., a quart of milk). Lactase determination on small-bowel biopsy is generally not available. If fecal Mg^{2+} or laxative levels are elevated, then inadvertent or surreptitious ingestion should be considered and psychiatric help should be sought.

For those with proven fatty diarrhea, endoscopy with small-bowel biopsy (including aspiration for *Giardia* and quantitative cultures) should be performed; if this procedure is unrevealing, a small-bowel radiograph is often an appropriate next step. If small-bowel studies are negative or if pancreatic disease is suspected, pancreatic exocrine insufficiency should be excluded with direct tests, such as the secretin-cholecystokinin stimulation test, or by indirect tests, such as assay of fecal chymotrypsin activity or a bentiromide test.

Chronic inflammatory-type diarrheas should be suspected by the presence of blood or leukocytes in the stool. Such findings warrant stool cultures, inspection for ova and parasites, *C. difficile* toxin assay, colonoscopy with biopsies, and, if indicated, small-bowel oral contrast studies.

℞ TREATMENT

Treatment of chronic diarrhea depends on the specific etiology and may be curative, suppressive, or empirical. If the cause can be eradicated, treatment is curative as with resection of a colorectal cancer, antibiotic administration for Whipple's disease, or discontinuation of an offending drug. For many chronic conditions, diarrhea can be controlled by suppression of the underlying mechanism. Examples include elimination of dietary lactose for lactase deficiency or gluten for celiac sprue, use of glucocorticoids or other anti-inflammatory agents for idiopathic inflammatory bowel diseases, adsorptive agents such as cholestyramine for ileal bile acid malabsorption, proton pump inhibitors such as omeprazole for the gastric hypersecretion of gastrinomas, somatostatin analogues such as octreotide for malignant carcinoid, prostaglandin inhibitors such as indomethacin for medullary carcinoma of the thyroid, and pancreatic enzyme replacement for pancreatic insufficiency. When the specific cause or mechanism of chronic diarrhea evades diagnosis, empirical therapy may be beneficial. Mild opiates such as diphenoxylate or loperamide are often helpful in mild or moderate watery diarrhea. For those with more severe diarrhea, codeine or tincture of opium may be beneficial. Such antimotility agents should be avoided with inflammatory bowel disease, as toxic megacolon may be precipitated. Clonidine, an α_2-adrenergic agonist, may allow control of diabetic diarrhea. For all patients with chronic diarrhea, fluid and electrolyte repletion is an important component of management (see "Acute Diarrhea," above). Replacement of fat-soluble vitamins may also be necessary in patients with chronic steatorrhea.

CONSTIPATION

DEFINITION Constipation is a common complaint in clinical practice and usually refers to persistent, difficult, infrequent, or seemingly incomplete defecation. Because of the wide range of normal bowel habits, constipation is difficult to define precisely. Most persons have at least three bowel movements per week; however, stool frequency alone is not a sufficient criterion for the diagnosis of constipation because many constipated patients describe a normal frequency of defecation but subjective complaints of excessive straining, hard stools, lower abdominal fullness, and a sense of incomplete evacuation. The individual patient's symptoms must be analyzed in detail to ascertain what is meant by "constipation" or "difficulty" with defecation.

Stool form and consistency are well correlated with the time elapsed from the preceding defecation. Hard, pellety stools occur with slow transit, while loose watery stools are associated with rapid transit. Small, pellety stools are more difficult to expel than large ones.

The perception of hard stools or excessive straining is more difficult to assess objectively, and the need for enemas or digital disimpaction is a clinically useful way to corroborate the patient's perceptions of difficult defecation.

Psychosocial factors may also be important. A person whose parents attached great importance to daily defecation will become greatly concerned when he or she misses a daily bowel movement; some children withhold stool to gain attention; and some adults are simply too busy or too embarrassed to interrupt their work when the call to have a bowel movement is sensed.

CAUSES Pathophysiologically, chronic constipation generally results from inadequate fiber intake or from disordered colonic transit or anorectal function as a result of a neurogastroenterologic disturbance, certain drugs, or in association with a large number of systemic diseases that affect the gastroinestinal tract (Table 35-4). Constipation of recent onset may be a symptom of significant organic disease such as tumor or stricture. In *idiopathic constipation*, a subset of patients exhibit delayed emptying of the ascending and transverse colon with prolongation of transit (often in the proximal colon) and a reduced frequency of propulsive colonic contractions (HAPCs). *Outlet obstruction to defecation* (also called *evacuation disorders*) may cause delayed colonic transit, which is usually corrected by biofeedback retraining of the disordered defecation. Constipation of any cause may be exacerbated by chronic illnesses that lead to physical or mental impairment and result in inactivity or physical immobility.

APPROACH TO THE PATIENT

A careful history should explore the patient's symptoms and confirm whether he or she is indeed constipated based on frequency (e.g., fewer than three bowel movements per week), consistency (lumpy/hard), excessive straining, prolonged defecation time, or need to support the perineum or digitate the anorectum. In the vast majority of cases (probably >90%), there is no underlying cause (e.g., cancer, depression, or hypothyroidism), and constipation responds to ample hydration, exercise, and supplementation of dietary fiber (15 to 25 g/d). A good diet and medication history and attention to psychosocial issues are key. Physical examination and, particularly, a rectal examination should exclude most of the important diseases that present with constipation and possibly indicate features suggesting an evacuation disorder (e.g., high anal sphincter tone).

There is broad consensus on the selection of patients for further investigation. The presence of weight loss, rectal bleeding, or anemia with constipation mandates either sigmoidoscopy plus barium enema or colonoscopy alone, particularly in patients >40 years, to exclude structural diseases such as cancer or strictures. Colonoscopy alone is most cost effective in this setting since it provides an opportunity to biopsy mucosal lesions, perform polypectomy, or dilate strictures. Barium enema has advantages over colonoscopy in the patient with isolated constipation, since it is less costly and identifies colonic dilatation and all significant mucosal lesions or strictures that are likely to present with constipation. Melanosis coli, or pigmentation of the colon mucosa, indicates the use of

TABLE 35-4 *Causes of Constipation in Adults*

Types of Constipation and Causes	Examples
Recent onset	
Colonic obstruction	Neoplasm: stricture: ischemic, diverticular, inflammatory
Anal sphincter spasm	Anal fissure, painful hemorrhoids
Medications	
Chronic	
Irritable bowel syndrome	Constipation–predominant, alternating
Medications	Ca²⁺ blockers, antidepressants
Colonic pseudo-obstruction	Slow transit constipation, megacolon (rare Hirschsprung's, Chagas)
Disorders of rectal evacuation	Pelvic floor dysfunction, anismus, descending perineum syndrome, rectal mucosal prolapse, rectocele
Endocrinopathies	Hypothyroidism, hypercalcemia, pregnancy
Psychiatric disorders	Depression, eating disorders, drugs
Neurologic disease	Parkinsonism, multiple sclerosis, spinal cord injury
Generalized muscle disease	Progressive systemic sclerosis

anthraquinone laxatives such as cascara or senna; however, this is usually apparent from a careful history. An unexpected disorder such as megacolon or cathartic colon may also be detected by colonic radiographs. Measurement of serum calcium and thyroid stimulating hormone levels will identify rare patients with metabolic disorders.

Patients with more troublesome constipation may not respond to fiber alone and may be helped by a bowel training regimen: taking an osmotic laxative and evacuating with enema or glycerine suppository as needed. After breakfast, a distraction-free 15 to 20 min on the toilet without straining is encouraged. Excessive straining may lead to development of hemorrhoids, and, if there is weakness of the pelvic floor or injury to the pudendal nerve, may result in obstructed defecation from descending perineum syndrome several years later. Those few who do not benefit from the simple measures delineated above or require long-term treatment with stimulant laxatives with the attendant risk of developing laxative abuse syndrome are assumed to have severe or intractable constipation and should have further investigation (Fig. 35-4)

INVESTIGATION OF SEVERE CONSTIPATION A small minority (probably <5%) of all patients with constipation have cases that are considered severe or "intractable"; these are the patients most likely to be seen by gastroenterologists or in referral centers. Further observation of the patient may occasionally reveal a previously unrecognized cause, such as an evacuation disorder, laxative abuse, malingering, or psychiatric disorder. In these patients, recent studies suggest that evaluations of the physiologic function of the colon and pelvic floor and of psychological status aid in the rational choice of treatment. Even among these highly selected patients with severe constipation, a cause can be identified in only about 30% (see below).

Measurement of Colonic Transit Radiopaque marker transit tests are easy, repeatable, generally safe, inexpensive, reliable, and highly applicable in evaluating constipated patients in clinical practice. There are several validated methods that are very simple. For example, radiopaque

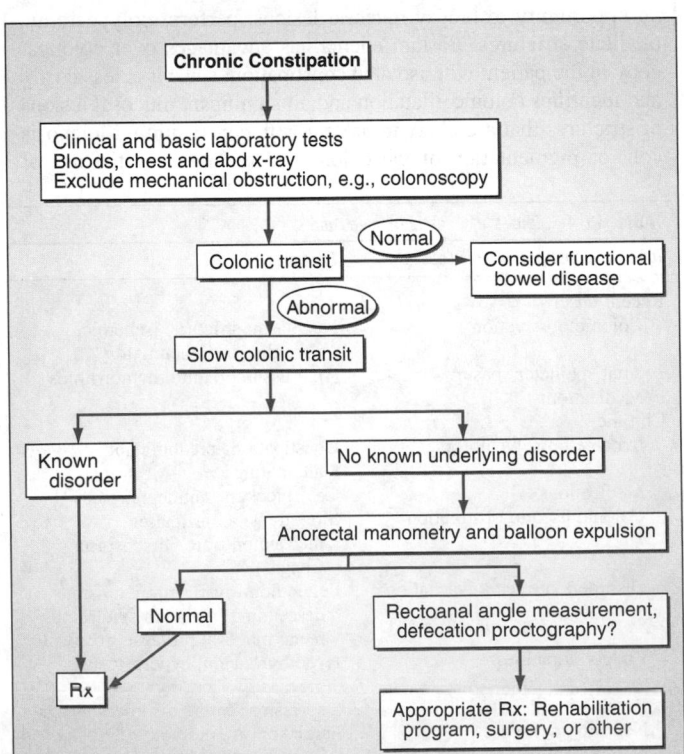

FIGURE 35-4 Algorithm for the management of constipation.

markers are ingested, and an abdominal flat film taken 5 d later should indicate passage of 80% of the markers out of the colon. This test does not provide useful information about the transit profile of the stomach and small bowel, and avoidance of laxatives or enemas during the testing period is essential.

Radioscintigraphy with a delayed-release capsule containing radiolabeled particles has been used to noninvasively characterize normal, accelerated, or delayed colonic function over 24 to 48 h with low radiation exposure. This approach simultaneously assesses gastric, small-bowel, and colonic transit. The disadvantages are the greater cost and the need for specific materials prepared in a nuclear medicine laboratory.

Anorectal and Pelvic Floor Tests Pelvic floor dysfunction is suggested by the inability to evacuate the rectum, a feeling of persistent rectal fullness, rectal pain, the need to extract stool from the rectum digitally, application of pressure on the posterior wall of the vagina, support of the perineum during straining, and excessive straining. These significant symptoms should be contrasted with the sense of incomplete rectal evacuation, which is common in irritable bowel syndrome.

Patients with clinically suspected obstruction of defecation should also be evaluated by a psychologist to identify eating disorders or a "need to control," to provide stress management or relaxation training, and to identify depression.

A simple clinical test in the office to document a nonrelaxing puborectalis muscle is to have the patient strain to expel the index finger during a digital rectal examination. Motion of the puborectalis posteriorly during straining indicates proper coordination of the pelvic floor muscles.

Measurement of perineal descent is relatively easy to gauge clinically by placing the patient in the left decubitus position and watching the perineum to assess either paucity or lack of descent (<1.5 cm, a sign of pelvic floor dysfunction) or perineal ballooning during straining relative to bony landmarks (>4 cm, suggesting excessive perineal descent).

A useful overall test of evacuation is the balloon expulsion test. A urinary catheter is placed in the rectum, the balloon is inflated to 50 mL with water, and a determination is made about whether the patient can expel it while seated on a toilet or in the left lateral decubitus position. In the lateral position, the weight needed to facilitate expulsion of the balloon (normal, 0 to 200 g) is determined.

Anorectal manometry is not often contributory in the evaluation of patients presenting with severe constipation, except when an excessively high resting or squeeze anal sphincter tone suggests anismus (anal sphincter spasm). This test also identifies rare syndromes, such as adult Hirschsprung's disease, by the absence of the rectoanal inhibitory reflex or the presence of occult incontinence.

Defecography (a dynamic barium enema including lateral views obtained during barium expulsion) reveals "soft abnormalities" in many patients; the most relevant findings are the measured changes in rectoanal angle, anatomic defects of the rectum, and enteroceles or rectoceles. In a very small proportion of patients, significant anatomic defects associated with intractable constipation respond best to surgical treatment. These defects include severe intussusception with complete outlet obstruction due to funnel-shaped plugging at the anal canal or an extremely large rectocele that is preferentially filled during attempts at defecation instead of expulsion of the barium through the anus. In summary, defecography requires an interested and experienced radiologist, and abnormalities are not pathognomonic for pelvic floor dysfunction. More commonly, outlet obstruction results from a nonrelaxing puborectalis muscle, which impedes rectal emptying, rather than from defects identified by defecography.

Dynamic imaging studies such as proctography during defecation or scintigraphic expulsion of artificial stool help measure perineal descent and the rectoanal angle during rest, squeezing, and straining, and scintigraphic expulsion quantitates the amount of "artificial stool" emptied. Failure of the rectoanal angle to increase significantly (~15°) during straining confirms pelvic floor dysfunction.

Neurologic testing (electromyography) is more helpful in the evaluation of patients with incontinence than of those with symptoms suggesting obstructed defecation. The absence of neurologic signs in the lower extremities suggests that any documented denervation of the puborectalis results from pelvic (e.g., obstetric) injury or from stretching of the pudendal nerve by chronic, long-standing straining.

Ultrasonography identifies sphincter or rectal wall defects and may help select patients for surgical correction. Spinal-evoked responses during electrical rectal stimulation or stimulation of external anal sphincter contraction by applying magnetic stimulation over the lumbosacral cord identify patients with limited sacral neuropathies with sufficient residual nerve conduction to attempt biofeedback training.

In summary, a balloon expulsion test is an important screening test for anorectal dysfunction. If positive, an anatomic evaluation of the rectum or anal sphincters and an assessment of pelvic floor relaxation are the tools for evaluating patients in whom obstructed defecation is suspected.

℞ TREATMENT

After the cause of constipation is characterized, a treatment decision can be made. Slow transit constipation requires aggressive medical or surgical treatment; anismus or pelvic floor dysfunction usually responds to biofeedback management (Fig. 35-4). However, only about 30% of patients with severe constipation are found to have such a physiologic disorder.

Patients with slow transit constipation are treated with bulk, osmotic, and stimulant laxatives, including fiber, psyllium, milk of magnesia, lactulose, polyethylene glycol (colonic lavage solution), and bisacodyl. If a 2- to 3-month trial of medical therapy fails and patients continue to have documented slow transit constipation unassociated with obstructed defecation, colectomy with ileorectostomy is indicated. The decision to resort to surgery is facilitated in the presence

of megacolon and megarectum. The complications after surgery include small-bowel obstruction (11%) and fecal soiling, particularly at night during the first postoperative year.

Patients who have a combined disorder should pursue pelvic floor retraining (biofeedback and muscle relaxation), psychological counseling, and dietetic advice first, followed by colectomy and ileorectosomy if colonic transit studies do not normalize with biofeedback alone. In patients with pelvic floor dysfunction alone, biofeedback training has a 70 to 80% success rate, measured by the acquisition of comfortable stool habits. Attempts to manage pelvic floor dysfunction with operations (internal anal sphincter or puborectalis muscle division) have achieved only mediocre success and have been largely abandoned.

FURTHER READING

AMERICAN GASTROENTEROLOGICAL ASSOCIATION: Medical Position Statement: Guidelines for the evaluation and management of chronic diarrhea. Gastroenterology 116:1461, 1991

BRANDT LJ et al: Systematic review on the management of irritable bowel syndrome in North America. Am J Gastroenterol 97 (Suppl):S1, 2002

CAMILLERI M et al: Clinical management of intractable constipation. Ann Intern Med 121:520, 1994

DUPONT HL and Practice Parameters Committee of the American College of Gastroenterology: Guidelines on acute infectious diarrhea in adults. Am J Gastroenterol 92:1962, 1997

FINE KD, SCHILLER LR: AGA technical review on the evaluation and management of chronic diarrhea. Gastroenterology 116:1461, 1999

LOCKE GR et al: AGA Medical Position Statement: Guidelines on constipation. Gastroenterology 119:1761, 2000

ROHNER P et al: Etiological agents of infectious diarrhea: Implications for requests for microbial culture. J Clin Microbiol 35:1427, 1997

36 | WEIGHT LOSS
Carol M. Reife

Significant unintentional weight loss in a previously healthy individual is often a harbinger of underlying systemic disease. During the routine medical history, inquiry should always be made about changes in weight; loss of 5% of body weight over 6 to 12 months should prompt further evaluation.

PHYSIOLOGY OF WEIGHT REGULATION

The normal individual maintains body weight at a remarkably stable "set point," given the wide variation in daily caloric intake and level of activity. Because of the physiologic importance of maintaining energy stores, voluntary weight loss is difficult to achieve and sustain.

Appetite and metabolism are regulated by an intricate network of neural and hormonal factors. The hypothalamic feeding and satiety centers play a central role in these processes (Chap. 64). Neuropeptides such as corticotropin-releasing hormone (CRH), α-melanocyte stimulating hormone (α-MSH), and cocaine- and amphetamine-related transcript (CART) induce anorexia by acting centrally on satiety centers. The gastrointestinal peptides ghrelin, glucagon, somatostatin, and cholecystokinin signal satiety and thus decrease food intake. Hypoglycemia suppresses insulin, reducing glucose utilization and inhibiting the satiety center.

Leptin is produced by adipose tissue, and it plays a central role in the long-term maintenance of weight homeostasis by acting on the hypothalamus to decrease food intake and increase energy expenditure (Chap. 64). Leptin suppresses expression of hypothalamic neuropeptide Y, a potent appetite stimulatory peptide, and it increases the expression of α-MSH, which acts through the MC4R melanocortin receptor to decrease appetite. Thus, leptin activates a series of downstream neural pathways that alter food-seeking behavior and metabolism.

However, leptin deficiency, which occurs in conjunction with the loss of adipose tissue, stimulates appetite and induces adaptive responses including inhibition of hypothalamic thyrotropin-releasing hormone (TRH) and gonadotropin-releasing hormone (GnRH).

A variety of cytokines, including tumor necrosis factor α (TNF-α), interleukin (IL) 6 (IL-6), IL-1, interferon γ (IFN-γ), ciliary neurotrophic factor (CNTF), and leukemia inhibitory factor (LIF), can induce cachexia (Chap. 16). In addition to causing anorexia, these factors may stimulate fever, depress myocardial function, modulate immune and inflammatory responses, and induce a variety of specific metabolic alterations. TNF-α, for example, preferentially mobilizes fat but spares skeletal muscle. Levels of one or more of these cytokines may be increased in patients with cancer, sepsis, chronic inflammatory conditions, AIDS, and congestive heart failure.

Weight loss occurs when energy expenditure exceeds calories available for energy utilization (Chap. 62). In most individuals, approximately half of food energy is utilized for basal processes such as maintenance of body temperature. In a 70-kg person, basal activity consumes about 1800 kcal/d. About 40% of caloric intake is used for physical activity, although athletes may use more than 50% during vigorous exercise. About 10% of caloric intake is used for dietary thermogenesis, the energy expended for digestion, absorption, and metabolism of food.

Mechanisms of weight loss include decreased food intake, malabsorption, loss of calories, and increased energy requirements (Fig. 36-1). Changes in weight may involve loss of tissue mass or body fluid content. A deficit of 3500 kcal generally correlates with the loss of 0.45 kg (1 lb) of body fat, but one must also consider water weight [1 kg/L (2.2 lb/L)] gained or lost. Weight loss that persists over weeks to months reflects the loss of tissue mass.

Food intake may be influenced by a wide variety of visual, olfactory, and gustatory stimuli as well as by genetic, psychological, and social factors. Absorption may be impaired because of pancreatic in-

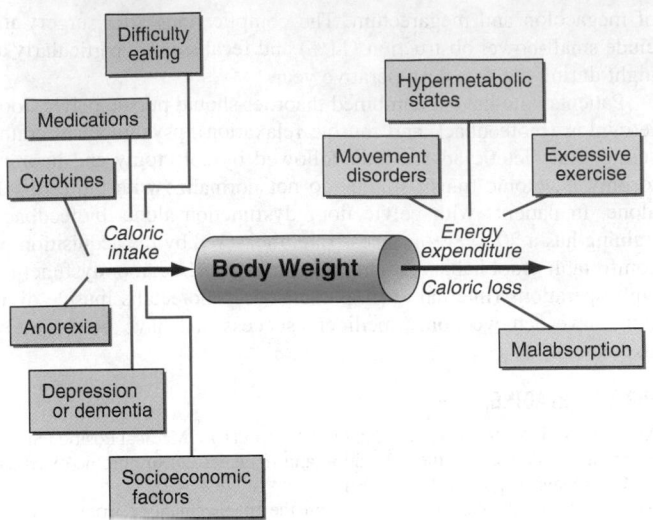

FIGURE 36-1 Energy balance and pathophysiology of weight loss.

TABLE 36-1	Causes of Weight Loss
Cancer	Medications
Endocrine and metabolic	Antibiotics
Hyperthyroidism	Nonsteroidal anti-inflammatory drugs
Diabetes mellitus	Serotonin reuptake inhibitors
Pheochromocytoma	Metformin
Adrenal insufficiency	Levodopa
Gastrointestinal disorders	ACE inhibitors
Malabsorption	Other drugs
Obstruction	Disorders of the mouth and teeth
Pernicious anemia	Age-related factors
Cardiac disorders	Physiologic changes
Chronic ischemia	Decreased taste and smell
Chronic congestive heart	Functional disabilities
failure	Neurologic
Respiratory disorders	Stroke
Emphysema	Parkinson's disease
Chronic obstructive	Neuromuscular disorders
pulmonary disease	Dementia
Renal insufficiency	Social
Rheumatologic disease	Isolation
Infections	Economic hardship
HIV	Psychiatric and behavioral
Tuberculosis	Depression
Parasitic infection	Anxiety
Subacute bacterial	Bereavement
endocarditis	Alcoholism
	Eating disorders
	Increased activity or exercise
	Idiopathic

sufficiency, cholestasis, celiac sprue, intestinal tumors, radiation injury, inflammatory bowel disease, infection, or medication effect. These disease processes may be manifest as changes in stool frequency and consistency. Calories may also be lost due to vomiting or diarrhea, glucosuria in diabetes mellitus, or fistulous drainage. Resting energy expenditure decreases with age and can be affected by thyroid status. Beginning at about age 60, body weight declines by an average of 0.5% per year. Body composition is also affected by aging; adipose tissue increases and lean muscle mass decreases with age.

SIGNIFICANCE OF WEIGHT LOSS

Unintentional weight loss, especially in the elderly, is not uncommon and is associated with increased morbidity and mortality rates, even after comorbid conditions have been taken into account. Prospective studies indicate that significant involuntary weight loss is associated with a mortality rate of 25% over the next 18 months. Retrospective studies of significant weight loss in the elderly document mortality rates of 9 to 38% over a 2- to 3-year period.

Cancer patients with weight loss have decreased performance status, impaired responses to chemotherapy, and reduced median survival (Chap. 66). Marked weight loss also predisposes to infection. Patients undergoing elective surgery, who have lost >4.5 kg (>10 lb) in 6 months, have higher surgical mortality rates. Vitamin and nutrient deficiencies also can accompany significant weight loss (Chap. 61).

CAUSES OF WEIGHT LOSS

The list of possible causes of weight loss is extensive (Table 36-1). In the elderly, the most common causes of weight loss are depression, cancer, and benign gastrointestinal disease. Lung and gastrointestinal cancer are the most common malignancies in patients presenting with weight loss. In younger individuals, diabetes mellitus, hyperthyroidism, psychiatric disturbances including eating disorders, and infection, especially with HIV, should be considered.

The cause of involuntary weight loss is rarely occult. Careful history and physical examination, in association with directed diagnostic testing, will identify the cause of weight loss in 75% of patients. The etiology of weight loss may not be found in the remaining patients, despite extensive testing. Patients with negative evaluations tend to have lower mortality rates than those found to have organic disease.

Patients with medical causes of weight loss usually have signs or symptoms that suggest involvement of a particular organ system. Gastrointestinal tumors, including those of the pancreas and liver, may affect food intake early in the course of illness, causing weight loss before other symptoms are apparent. Lung cancer may present with post-obstructive pneumonia, dyspnea, or cough and hemoptysis; how-

ever, it may be silent and should be considered even in those without a history of cigarette smoking. Depression and isolation can cause profound weight loss, especially in the elderly. Chronic pulmonary disease and congestive heart failure can produce anorexia, and they also increase resting energy expenditure. Weight loss may be the presenting sign of infectious diseases such as HIV infection, tuberculosis, endocarditis, and fungal or parasitic infections. Hyperthyroidism or pheochromocytoma increases metabolism. Elderly patients with apathetic hyperthyroidism may present with weight loss and weakness, with few other manifestations of thyrotoxicosis. New-onset diabetes mellitus is often accompanied by weight loss, reflecting glucosuria and loss of the anabolic actions of insulin. Adrenal insufficiency may be suggested by increased pigmentation, hyponatremia, and hyperkalemia.

APPROACH TO THE PATIENT

Before extensive evaluation is undertaken, it is important to confirm weight loss and to determine the time interval over which it has occurred. Almost half of patients who claim significant weight loss have no actual change when body weight is measured objectively. In the absence of documentation, changes in belt notch size or the fit of clothing may be confirmatory. Not infrequently, patients who have actually sustained significant weight loss are unaware that it has occurred. Routine documentation of weight during office visits is therefore important.

The review of systems should focus on signs or symptoms that are associated with disorders that commonly cause weight loss. These include fever, pain, shortness of breath or cough, palpitations, and evidence of neurologic disease. Gastrointestinal disturbances, including difficulty eating, dysphagia, anorexia, nausea, and change in bowel habits, should be sought. Travel history, use of cigarettes and alcohol, and all medications should be reviewed, and patients should be questioned about previous illness or surgery as well as diseases in family members. Risk factors for HIV infection should be assessed. Signs of depression, evidence of dementia, and social factors, including financial issues that might affect food intake, should be considered.

Physical examination should begin with weight determination and documentation of vital signs. The skin should be examined for

TABLE 36-2 *Screening Tests for Evaluation of Involuntary Weight Loss*

Initial testing	Additional testing
CBC	HIV test
Electrolytes, calcium, glucose	Upper and/or lower gastrointestinal endoscopy
Renal and liver function tests	Abdominal CT scan or MRI
Urinalysis	Chest CT scan
TSH	
Chest x-ray	
Recommended cancer screening	

pallor, jaundice, turgor, scars from prior surgery, and stigmata of systemic disease. The search for oral thrush or dental disease, thyroid gland enlargement, adenopathy, and respiratory or cardiac abnormalities and a detailed examination of the abdomen often lead to clues for further evaluation. Rectal examination, including prostate examination and testing of stool for occult blood, should be performed in men; and all women should have a pelvic examination, even if they have had a hysterectomy. Neurologic examination should include mental status assessment and screening for depression.

Laboratory testing should confirm or exclude possible diagnoses elicited from the history and physical examination (Table 36-2). An initial phase of testing should include a complete blood count with differential, serum chemistry tests including glucose, electrolytes, renal and liver tests, calcium, thyroid-stimulating hormone (TSH), urinalysis, and chest x-ray. Patients at risk for HIV infection should have HIV antibody testing. In all cases, recommended cancer screening tests appropriate for the gender and age group, such as mammograms and Pap smears, should be updated (Chap. 67). If gastrointestinal signs or symptoms are present, upper and/or lower endoscopy and abdominal imaging with either computed tomography (CT) or magnetic resonance imaging (MRI) have a relatively high yield, consistent with the high prevalence of gastrointestinal disorders in patients with weight loss. If an etiology of weight loss is not found, careful clinical follow-up, rather than persistent undirected testing, is reasonable.

FURTHER READING

BOURAS EP, LANGE SM: Rational approach to patients with unintentional weight loss. Mayo Clinic Proc 76:923, 2001

INUI A: Cancer anorexia-cachexia syndrome: Current issues in research and management. Cancer J Clinicians 52:72, 2002

REIFE CM: Involuntary weight loss. Med Clin North Am 79:299, 1995

SCHWARTZ MW: Brain pathways controlling food intake and body weight. Exp Biol Med 226:978, 2001

WALLACE JI: Involuntary weight loss in elderly outpatients: Recognition, etiologies, and treatment. Clin Geriatr Med 13:717, 1997

37 GASTROINTESTINAL BLEEDING
Loren Laine

Bleeding from the gastrointestinal (GI) tract may present in five ways. *Hematemesis* is vomitus of red blood or "coffee-grounds" material. *Melena* is black, tarry, foul-smelling stool. *Hematochezia* is the passage of bright red or maroon blood from the rectum. *Occult GI bleeding* (GIB) may be identified in the absence of overt bleeding by special examination of the stool (e.g., guaiac testing). Finally, patients may present only with *symptoms of blood loss or anemia* such as lightheadedness, syncope, angina, or dyspnea.

SOURCES OF GASTROINTESTINAL BLEEDING

UPPER GASTROINTESTINAL SOURCES OF BLEEDING (Table 37-1) The annual incidence of hospital admissions for upper GIB (UGIB) in the United States and Europe is approximately 0.1%, with a mortality rate of ~5 to 10%. Patients rarely die from exsanguination; rather, they die due to decompensation from other underlying illnesses. The mortality rate for patients under 60 years of age in the absence of malignancy or organ failure is <1%. The three independent clinical predictors of death in patients hospitalized with UGIB are increasing age, comorbidities, and hemodynamic compromise (tachycardia or hypotension).

Peptic ulcers are the most common cause of UGIB, accounting for about 50% of cases. Mallory-Weiss tears account for 5 to 15% of cases. The proportion of patients bleeding from varices varies widely from ~5 to 30%, depending on the population. Hemorrhagic or erosive gastropathy [e.g., due to nonsteroidal anti-inflammatory drugs (NSAIDs) or alcohol] and erosive esophagitis often cause mild UGIB, but major bleeding is rare.

Peptic Ulcers In addition to clinical features, characteristics of an ulcer at endoscopy provide important prognostic information. One-third of patients with active bleeding or a nonbleeding visible vessel have further bleeding that requires urgent surgery if they are treated conservatively. These patients clearly benefit from endoscopic therapy with bipolar electrocoagulation, heater probe, or injection therapy (e.g., absolute alcohol, 1:10,000 epinephrine), with reductions in bleeding, hospital stay, mortality rate, and costs. In contrast, patients with clean-based ulcers have rates of recurrent bleeding approaching zero. If there is no other reason for hospitalization, such patients may be discharged on the first hospital day, following stabilization. Patients without clean-based ulcers should usually remain in the hospital for 3 days, since most episodes of recurrent bleeding occur within 3 days.

Randomized controlled trials document that high-dose constant infusion intravenous omeprazole (80-mg bolus and 8-mg/h infusion), used to raise intragastric pH to between 6 and 7 and enhance clot stability, decreases further bleeding (but not mortality), even after the use of appropriate endoscopic therapy in patients with high-risk ulcers (active bleeding, nonbleeding visible vessel, and perhaps adherent clot). In the United States, the same dose of the only available intravenous proton pump inhibitor, pantoprazole, is used after endoscopic confirmation of an ulcer with high-risk findings.

Approximately one-third of patients with a bleeding ulcer will rebleed within the next 1 to 2 years. Prevention of recurrent bleeding focuses on the three main factors in ulcer pathogenesis, *Helicobacter pylori*, NSAIDs, and acid. Eradication of *H. pylori* in patients with bleeding ulcers decreases rates of rebleeding to <5%. If a bleeding ulcer develops in a patient taking NSAIDs, the NSAIDs should be discontinued if possible. If NSAIDs must be continued, initial treatment should be with a proton pump inhibitor. Subsequently patients should either switch from a nonselective NSAID to a cyclooxygenase 2 (COX-2) specific inhibitor or add GI co-therapy. Proton pump inhibitors and misoprostol are effective co-therapies, but proton pump inhibitors are preferred due to less frequent dosing (once daily) and fewer side effects (e.g., diarrhea). Patients at very high risk (e.g., el-

TABLE 37-1 *Sources of Bleeding in Patients Hospitalized for Acute UGIB*

Sources of Bleeding	Proportion of Patients (%)
Ulcers	35–62
Varices	4–31
Mallory-Weiss tears	4–13
Gastroduodenal erosions	3–11
Erosive esophagitis	2–8
Malignancy	1–4
No source identified	7–25

Source: Data from Rockall et al; GF Longstreth: Am J Gastroenterol 90:206, 1995; EM Vreeburg et al: Am J Gastroenterol 92:236, 1997; and L Laine: West J Med 155:274, 1991.

derly with prior bleeding ulcer) should probably take a COX-2 specific inhibitor and a proton pump inhibitor. Patients with bleeding ulcers unrelated to *H. pylori* or NSAIDs should remain on full-dose antisecretory therapy indefinitely. →*Peptic ulcers are discussed in Chap. 274.*

Mallory-Weiss Tears   The classic history is vomiting, retching, or coughing preceding hematemesis, especially in an alcoholic patient. Bleeding from these tears, which are usually on the gastric side of the gastroesophageal junction, stops spontaneously in 80 to 90% of patients and recurs in only 0 to 5%. Endoscopic therapy is indicated for actively bleeding Mallory-Weiss tears. Angiographic therapy with intraarterial infusion of vasopressin or embolization and operative therapy with oversewing of the tear are rarely required. →*Mallory-Weiss tears are discussed in Chap. 273.*

Esophageal Varices   Patients with variceal hemorrhage have poorer outcomes than patients with other sources of UGIB. Endoscopic therapy for acute bleeding and repeated sessions of endoscopic therapy to eradicate esophageal varices significantly reduces rebleeding and mortality. Ligation is the endoscopic therapy of choice for esophageal varices because it has less rebleeding, a lower mortality rate, fewer local complications, and requires fewer treatment sessions to achieve variceal eradication as compared to sclerotherapy.

Acute treatment with octreotide (50-μg bolus and 50-μg/h intravenous infusion for 2 to 5 days) may help in the control of acute bleeding, and this has replaced vasopressin as the medical therapy of choice for acute variceal bleeding in the United States. Agents such as somatostatin and terlipressin, available outside the United States, are also effective. Over the long term, treatment with nonselective beta blockers decreases recurrent bleeding from esophageal varices. Beta blockers are commonly given along with chronic endoscopic therapy.

In patients who have persistent or recurrent bleeding despite endoscopic and medical therapy, more invasive therapy is warranted. Transjugular intrahepatic portosystemic shunt (TIPS) decreases rebleeding more effectively than endoscopic therapy, although hepatic encephalopathy is more common and the mortality rates are comparable. Most patients with TIPS have shunt stenosis within 1 to 2 years and require reinstrumentation. Therefore, TIPS is most appropriate for patients with more severe liver disease and those in whom transplant is anticipated. Patients with milder, well-compensated cirrhosis should probably undergo decompressive surgery (e.g., distal splenorenal shunt).

Portal hypertension is also responsible for bleeding from gastric varices, varices in the small and large intestine, and portal hypertensive gastropathy and enterocolopathy.

Hemorrhagic and Erosive Gastropathy ("Gastritis")   Hemorrhagic and erosive gastropathy, or gastritis, refers to endoscopically visualized subepithelial hemorrhages and erosions. These are mucosal lesions and thus do not cause major bleeding. They develop in various clinical settings, the most important of which are NSAID use, alcohol intake, and stress. Half of patients who chronically ingest NSAIDs have erosions (15 to 30% have ulcers), while up to 20% of actively drinking alcoholic patients with symptoms of UGIB have evidence of subepithelial hemorrhages or erosions.

Stress-related gastric mucosal injury occurs only in extremely sick patients: those who have experienced serious trauma, major surgery, burns covering more than one-third of the body surface area, major intracranial disease, and severe medical illness (i.e., ventilator dependence, coagulopathy). Significant bleeding probably does not develop unless ulceration occurs. The mortality rate in these patients is quite high because of their serious underlying illnesses.

The incidence of bleeding from stress-related gastric mucosal injury or ulceration has decreased dramatically in recent years, most likely due to better care of critically ill patients. Pharmacologic prophylaxis for bleeding may be considered in the high-risk patients mentioned above. The best data suggest that intravenous H$_2$-receptor antagonist therapy is the treatment of choice, although sucralfate is also effective. Prophylactic therapy decreases bleeding but does not lower the mortality rate.

Other Causes   Other, less frequent causes of UGIB include erosive duodenitis, neoplasms, aortoenteric fistulas, vascular lesions [including hereditary hemorrhagic telengectasias (Osler-Weber-Rendu) and gastric antral vascular ectasia ("watermelon stomach")], Dieulafoy's lesion (in which an aberrant vessel in the mucosa bleeds from a pinpoint mucosal defect), prolapse gastropathy (prolapse of proximal stomach into esophagus with retching, especially in alcoholics), and hemobilia and hemosuccus pancreaticus (bleeding from the bile duct or pancreatic duct).

SMALL-INTESTINAL SOURCES OF BLEEDING   Small-intestinal sources of bleeding (bleeding from sites beyond the reach of the standard upper endoscope) are difficult to diagnose and are responsible for the majority of cases of obscure GIB. Fortunately, small-intestinal bleeding is uncommon. The most common causes are vascular ectasias and tumors (e.g., adenocarcinoma, leiomyoma, lymphoma, benign polyps, carcinoid, metastases, and lipoma). Other less common causes include Crohn's disease, infection, ischemia, vasculitis, small-bowel varices, diverticula, Meckel's diverticulum, duplication cysts, and intussusception. NSAIDs induce small-intestinal erosions and ulcers and may be a relatively common cause of chronic, obscure GIB.

Meckel's diverticulum is the most common cause of significant lower GIB (LGIB) in children, decreasing in frequency as a cause of bleeding with age. In adults <40 to 50 years, small-bowel tumors often account for obscure GIB; in patients >50 to 60 years, vascular ectasias are usually responsible.

Vascular ectasias should be treated with endoscopic therapy if possible. Surgical therapy can be used for vascular ectasias isolated to a segment of the small intestine when endoscopic therapy is unsuccessful. Although estrogen/progesterone compounds have been used for vascular ectasias, a double-blind trial found no benefit in prevention of recurrent bleeding. Isolated lesions, such as tumors, diverticula, or duplications, are generally treated with surgical resection.

COLONIC SOURCES OF BLEEDING   The incidence of hospitalizations for LGIB is about one-fifth that for UGIB. Hemorrhoids are probably the most common cause of LGIB; anal fissures also cause minor bleeding and pain. If these local anal processes, which rarely require hospitalization, are excluded, the most common causes of LGIB in adults are diverticula, vascular ectasias (especially in the proximal colon of patients >70 years), neoplasms (primarily adenocarcinoma), and colitis—most commonly infectious or idiopathic inflammatory bowel disease, but occasionally ischemic or radiation-induced. Uncommon causes include post-polypectomy bleeding, solitary rectal ulcer syndrome, NSAID-induced ulcers or colitis, trauma, varices (most commonly rectal), lymphoid nodular hyperplasia, vasculitis, and aortocolic fistulas. In children and adolescents, the most common colonic causes of significant GIB are inflammatory bowel disease and juvenile polyps.

Diverticular bleeding is abrupt in onset, usually painless, sometimes massive, and often from the right colon; minor and occult bleeding is not characteristic. Clinical reports suggest that bleeding colonic diverticula stop bleeding spontaneously in approximately 80% of patients and rebleed in about 20 to 25% of patients. Intraarterial vasopressin may halt the bleeding, at least temporarily. If bleeding persists or recurs, segmental surgical resection is indicated.

Bleeding from right colonic vascular ectasias in the elderly may be overt or occult; it tends to be chronic and only occasionally is hemodynamically significant. Endoscopic hemostatic therapy may be useful in the treatment of vascular ectasias, as well as discrete bleeding ulcers and post-polypectomy bleeding, while endoscopic polypectomy, if possible, is used for bleeding colonic polyps. Surgical therapy is generally required for major, persistent, or recurrent bleeding from the wide variety of colonic sources of GIB that cannot be treated medically or endoscopically.

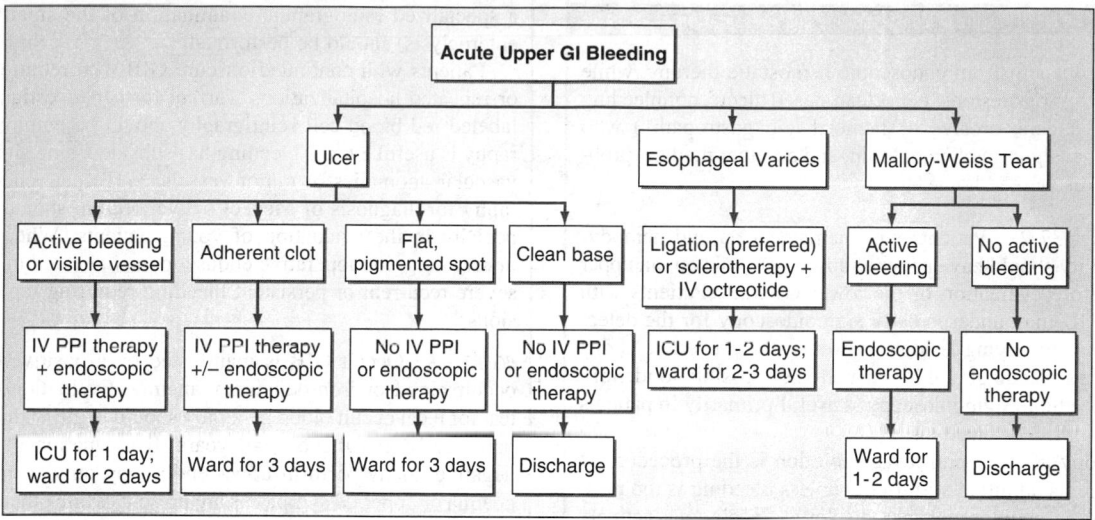

FIGURE 37-1 Suggested algorithm for patients with acute upper gastrointestinal bleeding. Recommendations on level of care and time of discharge assume patient is stabilized without further bleeding or other concomitant medical problems. PPI, proton pump inhibitor; ICU, intensive care unit.

APPROACH TO THE PATIENT

Measurement of the heart rate and blood pressure is the best way to assess a patient with GIB. Clinically significant bleeding leads to postural changes in heart rate or blood pressure, tachycardia, and, finally, recumbent hypotension. In contrast, the hemoglobin does not fall immediately with acute GIB, due to proportionate reductions in plasma and red cell volumes (i.e., "people bleed whole blood"). Thus, hemoglobin may be normal or only minimally decreased at the initial presentation of a severe bleeding episode. As extravascular fluid enters the vascular space to restore volume, the hemoglobin falls, but this process may take up to 72 h. Patients with slow, chronic GIB may have very low hemoglobin values despite normal blood pressure and heart rate. With the development of iron-deficiency anemia, the mean corpuscular volume will be low and red blood cell distribution width will be increased.

Differentiation of Upper from Lower GIB Hematemesis indicates an upper GI source of bleeding (above the ligament of Treitz). Melena indicates that blood has been present in the GI tract for at least 14 h. Thus, the more proximal the bleeding site, the more likely melena will occur. Hematochezia usually represents a lower GI source of bleeding, although an upper GI lesion may bleed so briskly that blood does not remain in the bowel long enough for melena to develop. When hematochezia is the presenting symptom of UGIB, it is associated with hemodynamic instability and dropping hemoglobin. Bleeding lesions of the small bowel may present as melena or hematochezia. Other clues to UGIB include hyperactive bowel sounds and an elevated blood urea nitrogen level (due to volume depletion and blood proteins absorbed in the small intestine).

A nonbloody nasogastric aspirate may be seen in up to 16% of patients with UGIB—usually from a duodenal source. Even a bile-stained appearance does not exclude a bleeding postpyloric lesion since reports of bile in the aspirate are incorrect in about 50% of cases. Testing of aspirates that are not grossly bloody for occult blood is not useful.

Diagnostic Evaluation of the Patient with GIB ■ *UPPER GIB* (Fig. 37-1) History and physical examination are

not usually diagnostic of the source of GIB. Upper endoscopy is the test of choice in patients with UGIB and should be performed urgently in patients with hemodynamic instability (hypotension, tachycardia, or postural changes in heart rate or blood pressure). Early endoscopy is also beneficial in cases of milder bleeding for management decisions. Patients with major bleeding and high-risk endoscopic findings (e.g., varices, ulcers with active bleeding or a

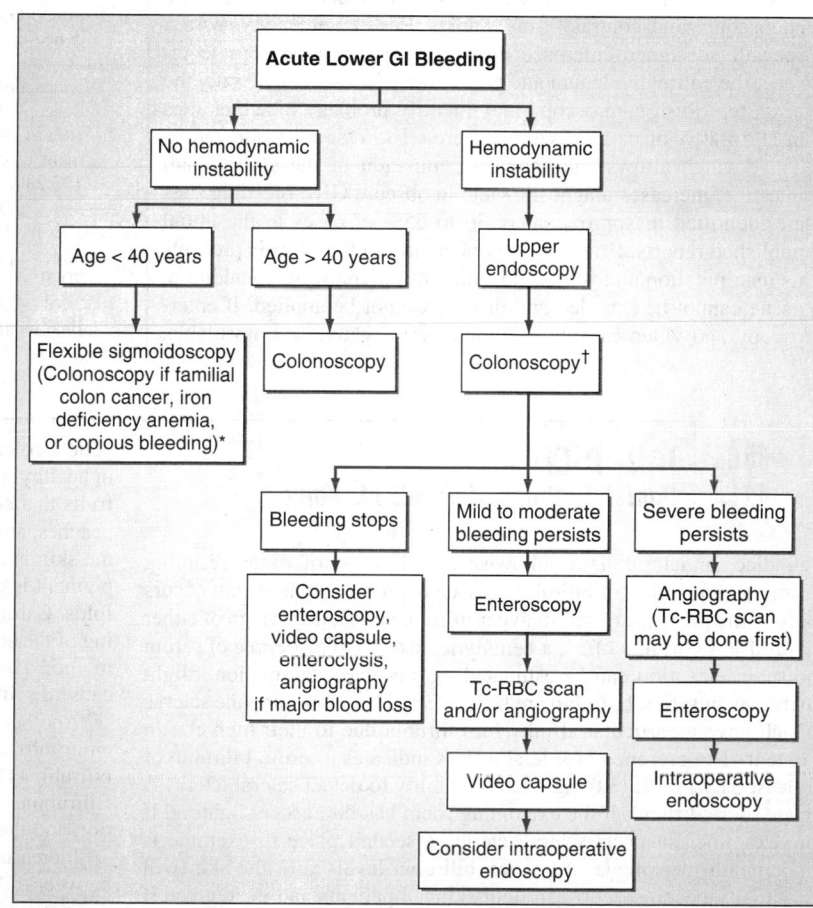

FIGURE 37-2 Suggested algorithm for patients with acute lower gastrointestinal bleeding. Sequential recommendations under "Hemodynamic instability" assume a test is found to be nondiagnostic before next test is performed. *Some suggest colonoscopy for any degree of rectal bleeding in patients <40 years old as well. †If massive bleeding does not allow time for colonic lavage, proceed to angiography. Tc-RBC, 99mtechnetium-labeled red blood cell.

visible vessel) benefit from endoscopic hemostatic therapy, while patients with low-risk lesions (e.g., clean-based ulcers, nonbleeding Mallory-Weiss tears, erosive or hemorrhagic gastropathy) who have stable vital signs and hemoglobin, and no other medical problems, can be discharged home.

LOWER GIB (Fig. 37-2) Patients with hematochezia and hemodynamic instability should have upper endoscopy to rule out an upper GI source before evaluation of the lower GI tract. Patients with presumed LGIB may undergo early sigmoidoscopy for the detection of obvious, low-lying lesions. However, the procedure is difficult with brisk bleeding, and it is usually not possible to identify the area of bleeding. Sigmoidoscopy is useful primarily in patients <40 years with minor bleeding.

Colonoscopy after an oral lavage solution is the procedure of choice in patients admitted with LGIB unless bleeding is too massive or unless sigmoidoscopy has disclosed an obvious actively bleeding lesion. ^{99M}Tc-labeled red cell scan allows repeated imaging for up to 24 h and may identify the general location of bleeding. However, radionuclide scans should be interpreted with caution because results, especially from later images, are highly variable. In active LGIB, angiography can detect the site of bleeding (extravasation of contrast into the gut) and permits treatment with intraarterial infusion of vasopressin or embolization. Even after bleeding has stopped, angiography may identify lesions with abnormal vasculature, such as vascular ectasias or tumors.

GIB OF OBSCURE ORIGIN Obscure GIB is defined as recurrent acute or chronic bleeding for which no source has been identified by routine endoscopic and contrast x-ray studies. Push enteroscopy, with a specially designed enteroscope or a pediatric colonoscope to inspect the entire duodenum and part of the jejunum, is generally the next step. Push enteroscopy may identify probable bleeding sites in 20 to 40% of patients with obscure GIB. Video capsule endoscopy, which allows endoscopic examination of the entire small intestine, increases diagnostic yield in obscure GIB: bleeding sites are identified in approximately 30 to 65% of cases in the initial published reports. However, lack of control of the capsule prevents its manipulation and full visualization of the intestine; in addition, tissue cannot be sampled and therapy cannot be applied. If enteroscopy and video capsule endoscopy are negative or unavailable,

a specialized radiographic examination of the small bowel (e.g., enteroclysis) should be performed.

Patients with continued obscure GIB who require transfusions or repeated hospitalizations warrant further investigations. ^{99M}Tc-labeled red blood cell scintigraphy should be employed. Angiography is useful even if bleeding has subsided, since it may disclose vascular anomalies or tumor vessels. ^{99M}Tc-pertechnetate scintigraphy for diagnosis of Meckel's diverticulum should be done, especially in the evaluation of young patients. When all tests are unrevealing, intraoperative endoscopy is indicated in patients with severe recurrent or persistent bleeding requiring repeated transfusions.

OCCULT GIB Occult GIB is manifested by a positive test for fecal occult blood or iron-deficiency anemia. Evaluation of a positive test for fecal occult blood generally should begin with colonoscopy, particularly in patients >40 years. If evaluation of the colon is negative, many perform upper endoscopy only if iron-deficiency anemia or upper GI symptoms are present, while others recommend upper endoscopy in all patients since up to 25 to 40% of these patients may have some abnormality noted on upper endoscopy. If standard endoscopic tests are unrevealing, enteroscopy, video capsule endoscopy, and/or enteroclysis may be considered in patients with iron-deficiency anemia.

FURTHER READING

CHAN FK et al: Celecoxib versus diclofenac and omeprazole in reducing the risk of recurrent ulcer bleeding in patients with arthritis. N Engl J Med 347: 2104, 2002

CIPOLLETTA L et al: Outpatient management for low-risk nonvariceal upper GI bleeding: A randomized controlled trial. Gastrointest Endosc 55:1, 2002

D'AMICO G et al: Pharmacological treatment of portal hypertension: An evidence-based approach. Semin Liver Dis 19:475, 1999

ELL C et al: The first prospective controlled trial comparing wireless capsule endoscopy with push enteroscopy in chronic gastrointestinal bleeding. Endoscopy 34:685, 2002

LAINE L, COOK D: Endoscopic ligation compared with sclerotherapy for treatment of esophageal variceal bleeding: A meta-analysis. Ann Intern Med 123:280, 1995

———, PETERSON WL: Bleeding peptic ulcer. N Engl J Med 331:717, 1994

LAU JYW et al: Effect of intravenous omeprazole on recurrent bleeding after endoscopic treatment of bleeding peptic ulcers. N Engl J Med 343:310, 2000

ROCKALL TA et al: Incidence of and mortality from acute upper gastrointestinal haemorrhage in the United Kingdom. BMJ 311:222, 1995

38 | JAUNDICE
Daniel S. Pratt, Marshall M. Kaplan

Jaundice, or icterus, is a yellowish discoloration of tissue resulting from the deposition of bilirubin. Tissue deposition of bilirubin occurs only in the presence of serum hyperbilirubinemia and is a sign of either liver disease or, less often, a hemolytic disorder. The degree of serum bilirubin elevation can be estimated by physical examination. Slight increases in serum bilirubin are best detected by examining the sclerae which have a particular affinity for bilirubin due to their high elastin content. The presence of scleral icterus indicates a serum bilirubin of at least 51 μmol/L (3.0 mg/dL). The ability to detect scleral icterus is made more difficult if the examining room has fluorescent lighting. If the examiner suspects scleral icterus, a second place to examine is underneath the tongue. As serum bilirubin levels rise, the skin will eventually become yellow in light-skinned patients and even green if the process is long-standing; the green color is produced by oxidation of bilirubin to biliverdin.

The differential diagnosis for yellowing of the skin is limited. In addition to jaundice, it includes carotenoderma, the use of the drug quinacrine, and excessive exposure to phenols. Carotenoderma is the

yellow color imparted to the skin by the presence of carotene; it occurs in healthy individuals who ingest excessive amounts of vegetables and fruits that contain carotene, such as carrots, leafy vegetables, squash, peaches, and oranges. Unlike jaundice, where the yellow coloration of the skin is uniformly distributed over the body, in carotenoderma the pigment is concentrated on the palms, soles, forehead, and nasolabial folds. Carotenoderma can be distinguished from jaundice by the sparing of the sclerae. Quinacrine causes a yellow discoloration of the skin in 4 to 37% of patients treated with it. Unlike carotene, quinacrine can cause discoloration of the sclerae.

Another sensitive indicator of increased serum bilirubin is darkening of the urine, which is due to the renal excretion of conjugated bilirubin. Patients often describe their urine as tea or cola colored. Bilirubinuria indicates an elevation of the direct serum bilirubin fraction and therefore the presence of liver disease.

Increased serum bilirubin levels occur when an imbalance exists between bilirubin production and clearance. A logical evaluation of the patient who is jaundiced requires an understanding of bilirubin production and metabolism.

PRODUCTION AND METABOLISM OF BILIRUBIN (See also Chap. 284) Bilirubin, a tetrapyrrole pigment, is a breakdown product of heme (ferroprotoporphyrin IX). About 70 to 80% of the 250 to 300 mg of bilirubin produced each day is derived from the breakdown of hemoglobin in senescent red blood cells. The remainder comes from prematurely destroyed erythroid cells in bone marrow and from the turnover of hemoproteins such as myoglobin and cytochromes found in tissues throughout the body.

The formation of bilirubin occurs in reticuloendothelial cells, primarily in the spleen and liver. The first reaction, catalyzed by the microsomal enzyme heme oxygenase, oxidatively cleaves the α bridge of the porphyrin group and opens the heme ring. The end products of this reaction are biliverdin, carbon monoxide, and iron. The second reaction, catalyzed by the cytosolic enzyme biliverdin reductase, reduces the central methylene bridge of biliverdin and converts it to bilirubin. Bilirubin formed in the reticuloendothelial cells is virtually insoluble in water. This is due to tight internal hydrogen bonding between the water-soluble moieties of bilirubin, proprionic acid carboxyl groups of one dipyrrolic half of the molecule with the imino and lactam groups of the opposite half. This configuration blocks solvent access to the polar residues of bilirubin and places the hydrophobic residues on the outside. To be transported in blood, bilirubin must be solubilized. This is accomplished by its reversible, noncovalent binding to albumin. Unconjugated bilirubin bound to albumin is transported to the liver, where it, but not the albumin, is taken up by hepatocytes via a process that at least partly involves carrier-mediated membrane transport. No specific bilirubin transporter has yet been identified (Chap. 284, Fig. 284-1).

After entering the hepatocyte, unconjugated bilirubin is bound to the cytosolic protein ligandin, or glutathione S-transferase B. Whereas ligandin was initially thought to be a transport protein, responsible for delivering unconjugated bilirubin from the plasma membrane to the endoplasmic reticulum, it now appears that its role may in fact be to reduce bilirubin efflux back into the plasma. Studies suggest that unconjugated bilirubin may well rapidly diffuse unaided through the aqueous cytosol between membranes. In the endoplasmic reticulum, bilirubin is solubilized by conjugation to glucuronic acid, a process that disrupts the internal hydrogen bonds and yields bilirubin monoglucuronide and diglucuronide. The conjugation of glucuronic acid to bilirubin is catalyzed by bilirubin uridine-diphosphate (UDP) glucuronosyltransferase. The now hydrophilic bilirubin conjugates diffuse from the endoplasmic reticulum to the canalicular membrane, where bilirubin monoglucuronide and diglucuronide are actively transported into canalicular bile by an energy-dependent mechanism involving the multiple drug resistance protein 2.

The conjugated bilirubin excreted into bile drains into the duodenum and passes unchanged through the proximal small bowel. Conjugated bilirubin is not taken up by the intestinal mucosa. When the conjugated bilirubin reaches the distal ileum and colon, it is hydrolyzed to unconjugated bilirubin by bacterial β-glucuronidases. The unconjugated bilirubin is reduced by normal gut bacteria to form a group of colorless tetrapyrroles called urobilinogens. About 80 to 90% of these products are excreted in feces, either unchanged or oxidized to orange derivatives called urobilins. The remaining 10 to 20% of the urobilinogens are passively absorbed, enter the portal venous blood, and are reexcreted by the liver. A small fraction (usually <3 mg/dL) escapes hepatic uptake, filters across the renal glomerulus, and is excreted in urine.

MEASUREMENT OF SERUM BILIRUBIN The terms direct- and indirect-reacting bilirubin are based on the original van den Bergh reaction. This assay, or a variation of it, is still used in most clinical chemistry laboratories to determine the serum bilirubin level. In this assay, bilirubin is exposed to diazotized sulfanilic acid, splitting into two relatively stable dipyrrylmethene azopigments that absorb maximally at 540 nm, allowing for photometric analysis. The direct fraction is that which reacts with diazotized sulfanilic acid in the absence of an accelerator substance such as alcohol. The direct fraction provides an approximate determination of the conjugated bilirubin in serum. The total serum bilirubin is the amount that reacts after the addition of alcohol. The indirect fraction is the difference between the total and the direct

bilirubin and provides an estimate of the unconjugated bilirubin in serum.

With the van den Bergh method, the normal serum bilirubin concentration usually is 17 μmol/L (<1 mg/dL). Up to 30%, or 5.1 μmol/L (0.3 mg/dL), of the total may be direct-reacting (conjugated) bilirubin. Total serum bilirubin concentrations are between 3.4 and 15.4 μmol/L (0.2 and 0.9 mg/dL) in 95% of a normal population.

Several new techniques, although less convenient to perform, have added considerably to our understanding of bilirubin metabolism. First, they demonstrate that in normal persons or those with Gilbert's syndrome, almost 100% of the serum bilirubin is unconjugated; <3% is monoconjugated bilirubin. Second, in jaundiced patients with hepatobiliary disease, the total serum bilirubin concentration measured by these new, more accurate methods is lower than the values found with diazo methods. This suggests that there are diazo-positive compounds distinct from bilirubin in the serum of patients with hepatobiliary disease. Third, these studies indicate that in jaundiced patients with hepatobiliary disease, monoglucuronides of bilirubin predominate over the diglucuronides. Fourth, part of the direct-reacting bilirubin fraction includes conjugated bilirubin that is covalently linked to albumin. This albumin-linked bilirubin fraction (*delta fraction* or *biliprotein*) represents an important fraction of total serum bilirubin in patients with cholestasis and hepatobiliary disorders. Albumin-bound conjugated bilirubin is formed in serum when hepatic excretion of bilirubin glucuronides is impaired and the glucuronides are present in serum in increasing amounts. By virtue of its tight binding to albumin, the clearance rate of albumin-bound bilirubin from serum approximates the half-life of albumin, 12 to 14 days, rather than the short half-life of bilirubin, about 4 h.

The prolonged half-life of albumin-bound conjugated bilirubin explains two previously unexplained enigmas in jaundiced patients with liver disease: (1) that some patients with conjugated hyperbilirubinemia do not exhibit bilirubinuria during the recovery phase of their disease because the bilirubin is bound to albumin and therefore not filtered by the renal glomeruli and (2) that the elevated serum bilirubin level declines more slowly than expected in some patients who otherwise appear to be recovering satisfactorily. Late in the recovery phase of hepatobiliary disorders, all the conjugated bilirubin may be in the albumin-linked form. Its value in serum falls slowly because of the long half-life of albumin.

MEASUREMENT OF URINE BILIRUBIN Unconjugated bilirubin is always bound to albumin in the serum, is not filtered by the kidney, and is not found in the urine. Conjugated bilirubin is filtered at the glomerulus and the majority is reabsorbed by the proximal tubules; a small fraction is excreted in the urine. Any bilirubin found in the urine is conjugated bilirubin. The presence of bilirubinuria implies the presence of liver disease. A urine dipstick test (Ictotest) gives the same information as fractionation of the serum bilirubin. This test is very accurate. A false-negative test is possible in patients with prolonged cholestasis due to the predominance of conjugated bilirubin covalently bound to albumin.

APPROACH TO THE PATIENT

The bilirubin present in serum represents a balance between input from production of bilirubin and hepatic/biliary removal of the pigment. Hyperbilirubinemia may result from (1) overproduction of bilirubin; (2) impaired uptake, conjugation, or excretion of bilirubin; or (3) regurgitation of unconjugated or conjugated bilirubin from damaged hepatocytes or bile ducts. An increase in unconjugated bilirubin in serum results from either overproduction, impairment of uptake, or conjugation of bilirubin. An increase in conjugated bilirubin is due to decreased excretion into the bile ductules or backward leakage of the pigment. The initial steps in evaluating the patient with jaundice are to determine (1) whether the hyperbilirubinemia is predominantly conjugated or unconjugated in na-

FIGURE 38-1 Evaluation of the patient with jaundice. ERCP, endoscopic retrograde cholangiopancreatography; CT, computed tomography; ALT, alanine aminotransferase; AST, aspartate aminotransferase; SMA, smooth-muscle antibody; AMA, antimitochondrial antibody; LKM, liver-kidney microsomal antibody; SPEP, serum protein electrophoresis; CMV, cytomegalovirus; EBV, Epstein-Barr virus.

Acquired hemolytic disorders include microangiopathic hemolytic anemia (e.g., hemolytic-uremic syndrome), paroxysmal nocturnal hemoglobinuria, and immune hemolysis. Ineffective erythropoiesis occurs in cobalamin, folate, and iron deficiencies.

In the absence of hemolysis, the physician should consider a problem with the hepatic uptake or conjugation of bilirubin. Certain drugs, including rifampicin and probenecid, may cause unconjugated hyperbilirubinemia by diminishing hepatic uptake of bilirubin. Impaired bilirubin conjugation occurs in three genetic conditions: Crigler-Najjar syndrome, types I and II, and Gilbert's syndrome. *Crigler-Najjar type I* is an exceptionally rare condition found in neonates and characterized by severe jaundice [bilirubin >342 μmol/L (> 20 mg/dL)] and neurologic impairment due to kernicterus, frequently leading to death in infancy or childhood. These patients have a complete absence of bilirubin UDP glucuronosyltransferase activity, usually due to mutations in the critical 3' domain of the UDP glucuronosyltransferase gene, and are totally unable to conjugate, hence cannot excrete bilirubin. The only effective treatment is orthotopic liver transplantation. Use of gene therapy and allogeneic hepatocyte infusion are experimental approaches of future promise for this devastating disease.

Crigler-Najjar type II is somewhat more common than type I. Patients live into adulthood with serum bilirubin levels that range from 103 to 428 μmol/L (6 to 25 mg/dL). In these patients, mutations in the bili-

ture, and (2) whether other biochemical liver tests are abnormal. The thoughtful interpretation of limited data will allow for a rational evaluation of the patient (Fig. 38-1). This discussion will focus solely on the evaluation of the adult patient with jaundice.

Isolated Elevation of Serum Bilirubin ■ *UNCONJUGATED HYPERBILIRUBINEMIA* The differential diagnosis of an isolated unconjugated hyperbilirubinemia is limited (Table 38-1). The critical determination is whether the patient is suffering from a hemolytic process resulting in an overproduction of bilirubin (hemolytic disorders and ineffective erythropoiesis) or from impaired hepatic uptake/conjugation of bilirubin (drug effect or genetic disorders).

Hemolytic disorders that cause excessive heme production may be either inherited or acquired. Inherited disorders include spherocytosis, sickle cell anemia, and deficiency of red cell enzymes such as pyruvate kinase and glucose-6-phosphate dehydrogenase. In these conditions, the serum bilirubin rarely exceeds 86 μmol/L (5 mg/dL). Higher levels may occur when there is coexistent renal or hepatocellular dysfunction, or in acute hemolysis such as a sickle cell crisis. In evaluating jaundice in patients with chronic hemolysis, it is important to remember the high incidence of pigmented (calcium bilirubinate) gallstones found in these patients, which increases the likelihood of choledocholithiasis as an alternative explanation for hyperbilirubinemia.

TABLE 38-1 *Causes of Isolated Hyperbilirubinemia*

I. Indirect hyperbilirubinemia
  A. Hemolytic disorders
    1. Inherited
      a. Spherocytosis, elliptocytosis
         Glucose-6-phosphate dehydrogenase and pyruvate kinase deficiencies
      b. Sickle cell anemia
    2. Acquired
      a. Microangiopathic hemolytic anemias
      b. Paroxysmal nocturnal hemoglobinuria
      c. Immune hemolysis
  B. Ineffective erythropoiesis
    1. Cobalamin, folate, thalassemia, and severe iron deficiencies
  C. Drugs
    1. Rifampicin, probenecid, ribavirin
  D. Inherited conditions
    1. Crigler-Najjar types I and II
    2. Gilbert's syndrome
II. Direct hyperbilirubinemia
  A. Inherited conditions
    1. Dubin-Johnson syndrome
    2. Rotor's syndrome

rubin UDP glucuronosyltransferase gene cause reduced but not completely absent activity of the enzyme. Bilirubin UDP glucuronosyltransferase activity can be induced by the administration of phenobarbital, which can reduce serum bilirubin levels in these patients. Despite marked jaundice, these patients usually survive into adulthood, although they may be susceptible to kernicterus under the stress of intercurrent illness or surgery.

Gilbert's syndrome is also marked by the impaired conjugation of bilirubin due to reduced bilirubin UDP glucuronosyltransferase activity. Patients with Gilbert's syndrome have a mild unconjugated hyperbilirubinemia with serum levels almost always <103 μmol/L (6 mg/dL). The serum levels may fluctuate, and jaundice is often identified only during periods of fasting. One molecular defect that has been identified in patients with Gilbert's syndrome is in the TATAA element in the 5′ promoter region of the bilirubin UDP glucuronosyltransferase gene upstream of exon 1. This defect alone is not necessarily sufficient for producing the clinical syndrome of Gilbert's as there are patients who are homozygous for this defect yet do not have the levels of hyperbilirubinemia typically seen in Gilbert's syndrome. Unlike both Crigler-Najjar syndromes, Gilbert's syndrome is very common. The reported incidence is 3 to 7% of the population with males predominating over females by a ratio of 2–7:1.

CONJUGATED HYPERBILIRUBINEMIA Elevated conjugated hyperbilirubinemia is found in two rare inherited conditions: *Dubin-Johnson syndrome* and *Rotor's syndrome* (Table 38-1). Patients with both conditions present with asymptomatic jaundice, typically in the second generation of life. The defect in Dubin-Johnson syndrome is mutations in the gene for multiple drug resistance protein 2. These patients have altered excretion of bilirubin into the bile ducts. Rotor's syndrome seems to be a problem with the hepatic storage of bilirubin. Differentiating between these syndromes is possible, but clinically unnecessary, due to their benign nature.

Elevation of Serum Bilirubin with Other Liver Test Abnormalities The remainder of this chapter will focus on the evaluation of the patient with a conjugated hyperbilirubinemia in the setting of other liver test abnormalities. This group of patients can be divided into those with a primary hepatocellular process and those with intra- or extrahepatic cholestasis. Being able to make this differentiation will guide the physician's evaluation (Fig. 38-1). This differentiation is made on the basis of the history and physical examination as well as the pattern of liver test abnormalities.

HISTORY A complete medical history is perhaps the single most important part of the evaluation of the patient with unexplained jaundice. Important considerations include the use of or exposure to any chemical or medication, either physician-prescribed or over-the-counter, such as herbal and vitamin preparations and other drugs such as anabolic steroids. The patient should be carefully questioned about possible parenteral exposures, including transfusions, intravenous and intranasal drug use, tattoos, and sexual activity. Other important questions include recent travel history, exposure to people with jaundice, exposure to possibly contaminated foods, occupational exposure to hepatotoxins, alcohol consumption, the duration of jaundice, and the presence of any accompanying symptoms such as arthralgias, myalgias, rash, anorexia, weight loss, abdominal pain, fever, pruritus, and changes in the urine and stool. While none of these latter symptoms are specific for any one condition, they can suggest a particular diagnosis. A history of arthralgias and myalgias predating jaundice suggests hepatitis, either viral or drug-related. Jaundice associated with the sudden onset of severe right upper quadrant pain and shaking chills suggests choledocholithiasis and ascending cholangitis.

PHYSICAL EXAMINATION The general assessment should include assessment of the patient's nutritional status. Temporal and proximal muscle wasting suggests long-standing diseases such as pancreatic cancer or cirrhosis. Stigmata of chronic liver disease, including spider nevi, palmar erythema, gynecomastia, caput medusae, Dupuytren's contractures, parotid gland enlargement, and testicular atrophy are commonly seen in advanced alcoholic (Laennec's) cirrhosis and occasionally in other types of cirrhosis. An enlarged left supraclavicular node (Virchow's node) or periumbilical nodule (Sister Mary Joseph's nodule) suggests an abdominal malignancy. Jugular venous distention, a sign of right-sided heart failure, suggests hepatic congestion. Right pleural effusion, in the absence of clinically apparent ascites, may be seen in advanced cirrhosis.

The abdominal examination should focus on the size and consistency of the liver, whether the spleen is palpable and hence enlarged, and whether there is ascites present. Patients with cirrhosis may have an enlarged left lobe of the liver which is felt below the xiphoid and an enlarged spleen. A grossly enlarged nodular liver or an obvious abdominal mass suggests malignancy. An enlarged tender liver could be viral or alcoholic hepatitis or, less often, an acutely congested liver secondary to right-sided heart failure. Severe right upper quadrant tenderness with respiratory arrest on inspiration (Murphy's sign) suggests cholecystitis or, occasionally, ascending cholangitis. Ascites in the presence of jaundice suggests either cirrhosis or malignancy with peritoneal spread.

LABORATORY TESTS When the physician encounters a patient with unexplained jaundice, there are a battery of tests that are helpful in the initial evaluation. These include total and direct serum bilirubin with fractionation, aminotransferases, alkaline phosphatase, albumin, and prothrombin time tests. Enzyme tests [alanine aminotransferase (ALT), aspartate aminotransferase (AST), and alkaline phosphatase] are helpful in differentiating between a hepatocellular process and a cholestatic process (Table 283-1; Fig. 38-1), a critical step in determining what additional workup is indicated. Patients with a hepatocellular process generally have a disproportionate rise in the aminotransferases compared to the alkaline phosphatase. Patients with a cholestatic process have a disproportionate rise in the alkaline phosphatase compared to the aminotransferases. The bilirubin can be prominently elevated in both hepatocellular and cholestatic conditions and therefore is not necessarily helpful in differentiating between the two.

In addition to the enzyme tests, all jaundiced patients should have additional blood tests, specifically an albumin level and a prothrombin time, to assess liver function. A low albumin suggests a chronic process such as cirrhosis or cancer. A normal albumin is suggestive of a more acute process such as viral hepatitis or choledocholithiasis. An elevated prothrombin time indicates either vitamin K deficiency due to prolonged jaundice and malabsorption of vitamin K or significant hepatocellular dysfunction. The failure of the prothrombin time to correct with parenteral administration of vitamin K indicates severe hepatocellular injury.

The results of the bilirubin, enzyme, albumin, and prothrombin time tests will usually indicate whether a jaundiced patient has a hepatocellular or a cholestatic disease. The causes and evaluation of each of these are quite different.

HEPATOCELLULAR CONDITIONS Hepatocellular diseases that can cause jaundice include viral hepatitis, drug or environmental toxicity, alcohol, and end-stage cirrhosis from any cause (Table 38-2). Wilson's disease should be considered in young adults. Autoimmune hepatitis is typically seen in young to middle-aged women but may affect men and women of any age. Alcoholic hepatitis can be differentiated from viral and toxin-related hepatitis by the pattern of the aminotransferases. Patients with alcoholic hepatitis typically have an AST:ALT ratio of at least 2:1. The AST rarely exceeds 300 U/L. Patients with acute viral hepatitis and toxin-related injury severe enough to produce jaundice typically have aminotransferases greater than 500 U/L, with the ALT greater than or equal to the AST. The degree of aminotransferase elevation can occasionally help in differentiating between hepatocellular and cholestatic

TABLE 38-2   Hepatocellular Conditions That May Produce Jaundice

Viral hepatitis
  Hepatitis A, B, C, D, and E
  Epstein-Barr virus
  Cytomegalovirus
  Herpes simplex
Alcohol
Drug toxicity
  Predictable, dose-dependent, e.g., acetaminophen
  Unpredictable, idosyncratic, e.g., isoniazid
Environmental toxins
  Vinyl chloride
  Jamaica bush tea—pyrrolizidine alkaloids
  Kava Kava
  Wild mushrooms—*Amanita phalloides* or *A. verna*
Wilson's disease
Autoimmune hepatitis

processes. While ALT and AST values less than 8 times normal may be seen in either hepatocellular or cholestatic liver disease, values 25 times normal or higher are seen primarily in acute hepatocellular diseases. Patients with jaundice from cirrhosis can have normal or only slight elevations of the aminotransferases.

When the physician determines that the patient has a hepatocellular disease, appropriate testing for acute viral hepatitis includes a hepatitis A IgM antibody, a hepatitis B surface antigen and core IgM antibody, and a hepatitis C viral RNA test. It can take many weeks for the hepatitis C antibody to become detectable, making it an unreliable test if acute hepatitis C is suspected. Depending on circumstances, studies for hepatitis D, E, Epstein-Barr virus (EBV), and cytomegalovirus (CMV) may be indicated. Ceruloplasmin is the initial screening test for Wilson's disease. Testing for autoimmune hepatitis usually includes an antinuclear antibody and measurement of specific immunoglobulins.

Drug-induced hepatocellular injury can be classified either as predictable or unpredictable. Predictable drug reactions are dose-dependent and affect all patients who ingest a toxic dose of the drug in question. The classic example is acetaminophen hepatotoxicity. Unpredictable or idiosyncratic drug reactions are not dose-dependent and occur in a minority of patients. A great number of drugs can cause idiosyncratic hepatic injury. Environmental toxins are also an important cause of hepatocellular injury. Examples include industrial chemicals such as vinyl chloride, herbal preparations containing pyrrolizidine alkaloids (Jamaica bush tea) and Kava Kava, and the mushrooms *Amanita phalloides* or *A. verna* that contain highly hepatotoxic amatoxins.

CHOLESTATIC CONDITIONS   When the pattern of the liver tests suggests a cholestatic disorder, the next step is to determine whether it is intra- or extrahepatic cholestasis (Fig. 38-1). Distinguishing intrahepatic from extrahepatic cholestasis may be difficult. History, physical examination, and laboratory tests are often not helpful. The next appropriate test is an ultrasound. The ultrasound is inexpensive, does not expose the patient to ionizing radiation, and can detect dilation of the intra- and extrahepatic biliary tree with a high degree of sensitivity and specificity. The absence of biliary dilatation suggests intrahepatic cholestasis, while the presence of biliary dilatation indicates extrahepatic cholestasis. False-negative results occur in patients with partial obstruction of the common bile duct or in patients with cirrhosis or primary sclerosing cholangitis (PSC) where scarring prevents the intrahepatic ducts from dilating.

Although ultrasonography may indicate extrahepatic cholestasis, it rarely identifies the site or cause of obstruction. The distal common bile duct is a particularly difficult area to visualize by ultrasound because of overlying bowel gas. Appropriate next tests include computed tomography (CT) and endoscopic retrograde

cholangiopancreatography (ERCP). CT scanning is better than ultrasonography for assessing the head of the pancreas and for identifying choledocholithiasis in the distal common bile duct, particularly when the ducts are not dilated. ERCP is the "gold standard" for identifying choledocholithiasis. It is performed by introducing a side-viewing endoscope perorally into the duodenum. The ampulla of Vater is visualized and a catheter is advanced through the ampulla. Injection of dye allows for the visualization of the common bile duct and the pancreatic duct. The success rate for cannulation of the common bile duct ranges from 80 to 95%, depending on the operator's experience. Beyond its diagnostic capabilities, ERCP allows for therapeutic interventions, including the removal of common bile duct stones and the placement of stents. In patients in whom ERCP is unsuccessful, transhepatic cholangiography can provide the same information. Magnetic resonance cholangiopancreatography is a rapidly developing, noninvasive technique for imaging the bile and pancreatic ducts; this may replace ERCP as the initial diagnostic test in cases where the need for intervention is felt to be small.

In patients with apparent *intrahepatic cholestasis*, the diagnosis is often made by serologic testing in combination with percutaneous liver biopsy. The list of possible causes of intrahepatic cholestasis is long and varied (Table 38-3). A number of conditions that typically cause a hepatocellular pattern of injury can also present as a cholestatic variant. Both hepatitis B and C can cause a cholestatic hepatitis (fibrosing cholestatic hepatitis) that has histologic features that mimic large duct obstruction. This disease variant has been reported in patients who have undergone solid organ transplantation. Hepatitis A, alcoholic hepatitis, EBV, and CMV may also present as cholestatic liver disease.

Drugs may cause intrahepatic cholestasis, a variant of drug-induced hepatitis. Drug-induced cholestasis is usually reversible after eliminating the offending drug, although it may take many

TABLE 38-3   Cholestatic Conditions That May Produce Jaundice

I. Intrahepatic
  A. Viral hepatitis
    1. Fibrosing cholestatic hepatitis—hepatitis B and C
    2. Hepatitis A, Epstein-Barr virus, cytomegalovirus
  B. Alcoholic hepatitis
  C. Drug toxicity
    1. Pure cholestasis—anabolic and contraceptive steroids
    2. Cholestatic hepatitis—chlorpromazine, erythromycin estolate
    3. Chronic cholestasis—chlorpromazine and prochlorperazine
  D. Primary biliary cirrhosis
  E. Primary sclerosing cholangitis
  F. Vanishing bile duct syndrome
    1. Chronic rejection of liver transplants
    2. Sarcoidosis
    3. Drugs
  G. Inherited
    1. Benign recurrent cholestasis
  H. Cholestasis of pregnancy
  I. Total parenteral nutrition
  J. Nonhepatobiliary sepsis
  K. Benign postoperative cholestasis
  L. Paraneoplastic syndrome
  M. Venoocclusive disease
  N. Graft-versus-host disease
II. Extrahepatic
  A. Malignant
    1. Cholangiocarcinoma
    2. Pancreatic cancer
    3. Gallbladder cancer
    4. Ampullary cancer
    5. Malignant involvement of the porta hepatis lymph nodes
  B. Benign
    1. Choledocholithiasis
    2. Primary sclerosing cholangitis
    3. Chronic pancreatitis
    4. AIDS cholangiopathy

months for cholestasis to resolve. Drugs most commonly associated with cholestasis are the anabolic and contraceptive steroids. Cholestatic hepatitis has been reported with chlorpromazine, imipramine, tolbutamide, sulindac, cimetidine, and erythromycin estolate. It also occurs in patients taking trimethoprim, sulfamethoxazole, and penicillin-based antibiotics such as ampicillin, dicloxacillin, and clavulinic acid. Rarely, cholestasis may be chronic and associated with progressive fibrosis despite early discontinuation of the drug. Chronic cholestasis has been associated with chlorpromazine and prochlorperazine.

Primary biliary cirrhosis is a disease predominantly of middle-aged women in which there is a progressive destruction of interlobular bile ducts. The diagnosis is made by the presence of the antimitochondrial antibody that is found in 95% of patients. *Primary sclerosing cholangitis* is characterized by the destruction and fibrosis of larger bile ducts. The disease may involve only the intrahepatic ducts and present as intrahepatic cholestasis. However, in 95% of patients with PSC, both intra- and extrahepatic ducts are involved. The diagnosis of PSC is made by ERCP. The pathognomonic findings are multiple strictures of bile ducts with dilatations proximal to the strictures. Approximately 75% of patients with PSC have inflammatory bowel disease.

The *vanishing bile duct syndrome* and *adult bile ductopenia* are rare conditions in which there are a decreased number of bile ducts seen in liver biopsy specimens. The histologic picture is similar to that found in primary biliary cirrhosis. This picture is seen in patients who develop chronic rejection after liver transplantation and in those who develop graft-versus-host disease after bone marrow transplantation. Vanishing bile duct syndrome also occurs in rare cases of sarcoidosis, in patients taking certain drugs including chlorpromazine, and idiopathically. There are also familial forms of intrahepatic cholestasis, including the *familial intrahepatic cholestatic syndromes, I–III*. Benign recurrent cholestasis is an autosomal recessive disease that appears to be due to mutations in a P type ATPase, which probably acts as a bile acid transporter. The disease is marked by recurrent episodes of jaundice and pruritus; the episodes are self-limited but can be debilitating. *Cholestasis of pregnancy* occurs in the second and third trimesters and resolves after delivery. Its cause is unknown, but the condition is probably inherited and cholestasis can be triggered by estrogen administration.

Other causes of intrahepatic cholestasis include total parenteral nutrition (TPN), nonhepatobiliary sepsis, benign postoperative cholestasis, and a paraneoplastic syndrome associated with a number of different malignancies, including Hodgkin's disease, medullary thyroid cancer, hypernephroma, renal sarcoma, T cell lymphoma, prostate cancer, and several gastrointestinal malignancies. In patients developing cholestasis in the intensive care unit, the major considerations should be sepsis, shock liver, and TPN jaundice. Jaundice occurring after bone marrow transplantation is most likely due to venoocclusive disease or graft-versus-host disease.

Causes of *extrahepatic cholestasis* can be split into malignant and benign (Table 38-3). Malignant causes include pancreatic, gallbladder, ampullary, and cholangiocarcinoma. The latter is most commonly associated with PSC and is exceptionally difficult to diagnose because its appearance is often identical to PSC. Pancreatic and gallbladder tumors, as well as cholangiocarcinoma, are rarely resectable and have poor prognoses. Ampullary carcinoma has the highest surgical cure rate of all the tumors that present as painless jaundice. Hilar lymphadenopathy due to metastases from other cancers may cause obstruction of the extrahepatic biliary tree.

Choledocholithiasis is the most common cause of extrahepatic cholestasis. The clinical presentation can range from mild right upper quadrant discomfort with only minimal elevations of the enzyme tests to ascending cholangitis with jaundice, sepsis, and circulatory collapse. PSC may occur with clinically important strictures limited to the extrahepatic biliary tree. In cases where there is a dominant stricture, patients can be effectively managed with serial endoscopic dilatations. Chronic pancreatitis rarely causes strictures of the distal common bile duct, where it passes through the head of the pancreas. AIDS cholangiopathy is a condition, usually due to infection of the bile duct epithelium with CMV or cryptosporidia, which has a cholangiographic appearance similar to that of PSC. These patients usually present with greatly elevated serum alkaline phosphatase levels, mean of 800 IU/L, but the bilirubin is often near normal. These patients do not typically present with jaundice.

SUMMARY The goal of this chapter is not to provide an encyclopedic review of all of the conditions that can cause jaundice. Rather, it is intended to provide a framework that helps a physician to evaluate the patient with jaundice in a logical way (Fig. 38-1).

Simply stated, the initial step is to obtain appropriate blood tests to determine if the patient has an isolated elevation of serum bilirubin. If so, is the bilirubin elevation due to an increased unconjugated or conjugated fraction? If the hyperbilirubinemia is accompanied by other liver test abnormalities, is the disorder hepatocellular or cholestatic? If cholestatic, is it intra- or extrahepatic? All of these questions can be answered with a thoughtful history, physical examination, and interpretation of laboratory and radiologic tests and procedures.

FURTHER READING

BERG CL et al: Bilirubin metabolism and the pathophysiology of jaundice, in *Schiff's Diseases of the Liver*, 8th ed, ER Schiff et al (eds). Philadelphia, Lippincott Williams & Wilkins, 1999

FOX IJ et al: Treatment of the Crigler-Najjar syndrome type I with hepatocyte transplantation. N Engl J Med 338:1422, 1998

GLASOVA H, BEUERS U: Extrahepatic manifestations of cholestasis. J Gastroenterol Hepatol 9:938, 2002

PRATT DS, KAPLAN MM: Laboratory tests, in *Schiff's Diseases of the Liver*, 8th ed, ER Schiff et al (eds). Philadelphia, Lippincott Williams & Wilkins, 1999

TRAUNER M et al: Molecular pathogenesis of cholestasis. N Engl J Med 339:1217, 1998

39 ABDOMINAL SWELLING AND ASCITES
Robert M. Glickman

ABDOMINAL SWELLING

Abdominal swelling or distention is a common problem in clinical medicine and may be the initial manifestation of a systemic disease or of otherwise unsuspected abdominal disease. *Subjective* abdominal enlargement, often described as a sensation of fullness or bloating, is usually transient and is often related to a functional gastrointestinal disorder when it is not accompanied by objective physical findings of increased abdominal girth or local swelling. *Obesity* and lumbar lordosis, which may be associated with prominence of the abdomen, may usually be distinguished from true increases in the volume of the peritoneal cavity by history and careful physical examination.

CLINICAL HISTORY Abdominal swelling may first be noticed by the patient because of a progressive increase in belt or clothing size, the appearance of abdominal or inguinal hernias, or the development of a localized swelling. Often, considerable abdominal enlargement has gone unnoticed for weeks or months, either because of coexistent obesity or because the ascites formation has been insidious, without pain or localizing symptoms. Progressive abdominal distention may be associated with a sensation of "pulling" or "stretching" of the flanks or groins and vague low back pain. Localized pain usually results from involvement of an abdominal organ (e.g., a passively congested liver, large spleen, or colonic tumor). Pain is uncommon in cirrhosis with ascites, and when it is present, pancreatitis, hepatocellular carcinoma, or peritonitis should be considered. Tense ascites or abdominal tumors may produce increased intraabdominal pressure, resulting in indigestion and heartburn due to gastroesophageal reflux or dyspnea, abdominal wall hernias (inguinal and umbilical) orthopnea, and tachypnea from elevation of the diaphragm. A coexistent pleural effusion, more commonly on the right, presumably due to leakage of ascitic fluid through lymphatic channels in the diaphragm, may also contribute to respiratory embarrassment. A large pleural effusion, obscuring most of the lung is known as a *hepatic hydrothorax*. The patient with diffuse abdominal swelling should be questioned about increased alcohol intake, a prior episode of jaundice or hematuria, or a change in bowel habits. Such historic information may provide the clues that will lead one to suspect an occult cirrhosis, a colonic tumor with peritoneal seeding, congestive heart failure, or nephrosis.

PHYSICAL EXAMINATION   A carefully executed general physical examination can yield valuable clues concerning the etiology of abdominal swelling. Thus palmar erythema and spider angiomas suggest an underlying cirrhosis, while supraclavicular adenopathy (Virchow's node) should raise the question of an underlying gastrointestinal malignancy.

Inspection of the abdomen is important. By noting the abdominal contour, one may be able to distinguish localized from generalized swelling. The tensely distended abdomen with tightly stretched skin, bulging flanks, and everted umbilicus is characteristic of ascites. A prominent abdominal venous pattern with the direction of flow away from the umbilicus is often a reflection of portal hypertension; venous collaterals with flow from the lower part of the abdomen toward the umbilicus suggest obstruction of the inferior vena cava; flow downward toward the umbilicus suggests superior vena cava obstruction. "Doming" of the abdomen with visible ridges from underlying intestinal loops is usually due to intestinal obstruction or distention. An epigastric mass, with evident peristalsis proceeding from left to right, usually indicates underlying pyloric obstruction. A liver with metastatic deposits may be visible as a nodular right upper quadrant mass moving with respiration.

Auscultation may reveal the high-pitched, rushing sounds of early intestinal obstruction or a succussion sound due to increased fluid and gas in a dilated hollow viscus. Careful auscultation over an enlarged liver occasionally reveals the harsh bruit of a vascular tumor, especially a hepatocellular carcinoma, or the leathery friction rub of a surface nodule. A venous hum at the umbilicus may signify portal hypertension and an increased collateral blood flow around the liver. A fluid wave and flank dullness that shifts with change in position of the patient are important signs that indicate the presence of peritoneal fluid. In obese patients, small amounts of fluid may be difficult to demonstrate; on occasion, the fluid may be detected by abdominal percussion with patients on their hands and knees. Small amounts of ascites often can only be detected by ultrasound examination of the abdomen, which can detect as little as 100 mL of fluid. Careful percussion should serve to distinguish generalized abdominal enlargement from localized swelling due to an enlarged uterus, ovarian cyst, or distended bladder. Percussion can also outline an abnormally small or large liver. Loss of normal liver dullness may result from massive hepatic necrosis; it also may be a clue to free gas in the peritoneal cavity, as from perforation of a hollow viscus.

Palpation is often difficult with massive ascites, and ballottement of overlying fluid may be the only method of palpating the liver or spleen. A slightly enlarged spleen in association with ascites may be the only evidence of an occult cirrhosis. When there is evidence of portal hypertension, a soft liver suggests that obstruction to portal flow is extrahepatic; a firm liver suggests cirrhosis as the likely cause of

the portal hypertension. A very hard or nodular liver is a clue that the liver is infiltrated with tumor, and when accompanied by ascites, it suggests that the latter is due to peritoneal seeding. The presence of a hard periumbilical nodule (Sister Mary Joseph's nodule) suggests metastatic disease from a pelvic or gastrointestinal primary tumor. A pulsatile liver and ascites may be found in tricuspid insufficiency.

An attempt should be made to determine whether a mass is solid or cystic, smooth or irregular, and whether it moves with respiration. The liver, spleen, and gallbladder should descend with respiration unless they are fixed by adhesions or extension of tumor beyond the organ. A fixed mass not descending with respiration may indicate that it is retroperitoneal. Tenderness, especially if localized, may indicate an inflammatory process such as an abscess; it also may be due to stretching of the visceral peritoneum or tumor necrosis. Rectal and pelvic examinations are mandatory; they may reveal otherwise undetected masses due to tumor or infection.

Radiographic and laboratory examinations are essential for confirming or extending the impressions gained on physical examination. Upright and recumbent films of the abdomen may demonstrate the dilated loops of intestine with fluid levels characteristic of intestinal obstruction or the diffuse abdominal haziness and loss of psoas margins suggestive of ascites. Ultrasonography is often of value in detecting ascites, determining the presence of a mass, or evaluating the size of the liver and spleen. Computed tomography (CT) scanning provides similar information. CT scanning is often necessary to visualize the retroperitoneum, pancreas, and lymph nodes. A plain film of the abdomen may reveal the distended colon of otherwise unsuspected ulcerative colitis and give valuable information as to the size of the liver and spleen. An irregular and elevated right side of the diaphragm may be a clue to a liver abscess or hepatocellular carcinoma. Studies of the gastrointestinal tract with barium or other contrast media are usually necessary in the search for a primary tumor.

ASCITES

The evaluation of a patient with ascites requires that the cause of the ascites be established. In most cases ascites appears as part of a well-recognized illness, that is, cirrhosis, congestive heart failure, nephrosis, or disseminated carcinomatosis. In these situations, the physician should determine that the development of ascites is indeed a consequence of the basic underlying disease and not due to the presence of a separate or related disease process. This distinction is necessary even when the cause of ascites seems obvious. For example, when the patient with compensated cirrhosis and minimal ascites develops progressive ascites that is increasingly difficult to control with sodium restriction or diuretics, the temptation is to attribute the worsening of the clinical picture to progressive liver disease. However, an occult hepatocellular carcinoma, portal vein thrombosis, spontaneous bacterial peritonitis, or even tuberculosis may be responsible for the decompensation. The disappointingly low success in diagnosing tuberculous peritonitis or hepatocullar carcinoma in the patient with cirrhosis and ascites reflects the too-low index of suspicion for the development of such superimposed conditions. Similarly, the patient with congestive heart failure may develop ascites from a disseminated carcinoma with peritoneal seeding.

Diagnostic paracentesis (50 to 100 mL) should be part of the routine evaluation of the patient with ascites. The fluid should be examined for its gross appearance; protein content, cell count, and differential cell count should be determined; and Gram's and acid-fast stains and culture should be performed. Cytologic and cell-block examination may disclose an otherwise unsuspected carcinoma. Table 39-1 presents some of the features of ascitic fluid typically found in various disease states. In some disorders, such as cirrhosis, the fluid has the characteristics of a transudate (<25 g protein per liter and a specific gravity of <1.016); in others, such as peritonitis, the features are those of an exudate. Rather than the total protein content of ascites, many authors prefer the use of a *serum-ascites albumin gradient* (SAG) to characterize ascites. The gradient correlates directly with portal pressure. A gradient >1.1 g/dL (high gradient) is characteristic

TABLE 39-1 *Characteristics of Ascitic Fluid in Various Disease States*

Condition	Gross Appearance	Protein, g/dL	Serum-Ascites Albumin Gradient, g/dL	Cell Count Red Blood Cells, >10,000/μL	Cell Count White Blood Cells, per μL	Other Tests
Cirrhosis	Straw-colored or bile-stained	<25 (95%)	>1.1	1%	<250 (90%);[a] predominantly mesothelial	
Neoplasm	Straw-colored, hemorrhagic, mucinous, or chylous	>25 (75%)	<1.1	20%	>1000 (50%); variable cell types	Cytology, cell block, peritoneal biopsy
Tuberculous peritonitis	Clear, turbid, hemorrhagic, chylous	>25 (50%)	<1.1	7%	>1000 (70%); usually >70% lymphocytes	Peritoneal biopsy, stain and culture for acid-fast bacilli
Pyogenic peritonitis	Turbid or purulent	If purulent, >25	<1.1	Unusual	Predominantly polymorphonuclear leukocytes	Positive Gram's stain, culture
Congestive heart failure	Straw-colored	Variable, 15–53	>1.1	10%	<1000 (90%); usually mesothelial, mononuclear	
Nephrosis	Straw-colored or chylous	<25 (100%)	<1.1	Unusual	<250; mesothelial, mononuclear	If chylous, ether extraction, Sudan staining
Pancreatic ascites (pancreatitis, pseudocyst)	Turbid, hemorrhagic, or chylous	Variable, often >25	<1.1	Variable, may be blood-stained	Variable	Increased amylase in ascitic fluid and serum

[a] Because the conditions of examining fluid and selecting patients were not identical in each series, the percentage figures (in parentheses) should be taken as an indication of the order of magnitude rather than as the precise incidence of any abnormal finding.

of uncomplicated cirrhotic ascites and differentiates ascites due to portal hypertension from ascites not due to portal hypertension >95% of the time. A gradient <1.1 g/dL (low gradient) suggests that the ascites is not due to portal hypertension with >95% accuracy and mandates a search for other causes (Table 39-1). Although there is variability of the ascitic fluid in any given disease state, some features are sufficiently characteristic to suggest certain diagnostic possibilities. For example, blood-stained fluid with >25 g protein per liter is unusual in uncomplicated cirrhosis but is consistent with tuberculous peritonitis or neoplasm. Cloudy fluid with a predominance of polymorphonuclear cells and a positive Gram's stain are characteristic of bacterial peritonitis; if most cells are lymphocytes, tuberculosis should be suspected. The complete examination of each fluid is most important, for occasionally only one finding may be abnormal. For example, if the fluid is a typical transudate but contains >250 white blood cells per microliter, the finding should be recognized as atypical for cirrhosis and should warrant a search for tumor or infection. This is especially true in the evaluation of cirrhotic ascites where occult peritoneal infection may be present with only minor elevations in the white blood cell count of the peritoneal fluid (300 to 500 cells/μL). Since Gram's stain of the fluid may be negative in a high proportion of such cases, careful culture of the peritoneal fluid is mandatory. Bedside innoculation of blood culture flasks with ascitic fluid results in a dramatically increased incidence of positive cultures when bacterial infection is present (90 versus 40% positivity with conventional cultures done by the laboratory). Direct visualization of the peritoneum (laparoscopy) may disclose peritoneal deposits of tumor, tuberculosis, or metastatic disease of the liver. Biopsies are taken under direct vision, often adding to the diagnostic accuracy of the procedure.

Chylous ascites refers to a turbid, milky, or creamy peritoneal fluid due to the presence of thoracic or intestinal lymph. Such a fluid shows Sudan-staining fat globules microscopically and an increased triglyceride content by chemical examination. Opaque milky fluid usually has a triglyceride concentration of >11.3 μmol/L (>1000 mg/dL). A turbid fluid due to leukocytes or tumor cells may be confused with chylous fluid (pseudochylous), and it is often helpful to carry out alkalinization and ether extraction of the specimen. Alkali tend to dissolve cellular proteins and thereby reduce turbidity; ether extraction leads to clearing if the turbidity of the fluid is due to lipid. Chylous ascites is most often the result of lymphatic obstruction from trauma, tumor, tuberculosis, filariasis (Chap. 202), or congenital abnormalities. It may also be seen in the nephrotic syndrome.

Rarely, ascitic fluid may be *mucinous* in character, suggesting either pseudomyxoma peritonei (Chap. 279) or rarely a colloid carcinoma of the stomach or colon with peritoneal implants.

On occasion, ascites may develop as a seemingly isolated finding in the absence of a clinically evident underlying disease. Then, a careful analysis of ascitic fluid may indicate the direction the evaluation should take. A useful framework for the workup starts with an analysis of whether the fluid is classified as a high (transudate) or low (exudate) gradient fluid. *High gradient (transudative) ascites* of unclear etiology is most often due to occult cirrhosis, right-sided venous hypertension raising hepatic sinusoidal pressure, or hypoalbuminemic states such as nephrosis or protein-losing enteropathy. Cirrhosis with well-preserved liver function (normal albumin) resulting in ascites is invariably associated with significant portal hypertension (Chap. 288). Evaluation should include liver function tests, liver-spleen scan, or other hepatic imaging procedure (i.e., CT or ultrasound) to detect nodular changes in the liver or a colloid shift of isotope to suggest portal hypertension. On occasion, a wedged hepatic venous pressure can be useful to document portal hypertension. Finally, if clinically indicated, a liver biopsy will confirm the diagnosis of cirrhosis and perhaps suggest its etiology. Other etiologies may result in hepatic venous congestion and resultant ascites. Right-sided cardiac valvular disease and particularly constrictive pericarditis should raise a high index of suspicion and may require cardiac imaging and cardiac catheterization for definitive diagnosis. Hepatic vein thrombosis is evaluated by visualizing the hepatic veins with imaging techniques (Doppler ultrasound, angiography, CT scans, magnetic resonance imaging) to demonstrate obliteration, thrombosis, or obstruction by tumor. Uncommonly, transudative ascites may be associated with benign tumors of the ovary, particularly fibroma (Meigs' syndrome) with ascites and hydrothorax.

Low gradient (exudative) ascites should initiate an evaluation for primary peritoneal processes, most importantly infection and tumor. Routine bacteriologic culture of ascitic fluid often yields a specific organism causing infectious peritonitis. Tuberculous peritonitis (Table 39-1) is best diagnosed by peritoneal biopsy, either percutaneously or via laparoscopy. Histologic examination invariably shows granulomata that may contain acid-fast bacilli. Since cultures of peritoneal fluid and biopsies for tuberculosis may require 6 weeks, characteristic histology with appropriate stains allows antituberculosis therapy to be started promptly. Similarly, the diagnosis of peritoneal seeding by tumor can usually be made by cytologic analysis of peritoneal fluid or by peritoneal biopsy if cytology is negative. Appropriate diagnostic studies can then be undertaken to determine the nature and site of the primary tumor. Pancreatic ascites (Table 39-1) is invariably associated with an extravasation of pancreatic fluid from the pancreatic ductal system, most commonly from a leaking pseudocyst. Ultrasound or CT examination of the pancreas followed by visualization of the pancreatic

duct by direct cannulation [viz., endoscopic retrograde cholangiopancreatography (ERCP)] usually discloses the site of leakage and permits resective surgery to be carried out.

An analysis of the physiologic and metabolic factors involved in the production of ascites (detailed in Chap. 288), coupled with a complete evaluation of the nature of the ascitic fluid, invariably discloses the etiology of the ascites and permits appropriate therapy to be instituted.

ACKNOWLEDGMENT
Dr. Kurt J. Isselbacher was the co-author of this chapter in previous editions.

FURTHER READING

LIPSKY MS, STERNBACH MR: Evaluation and initial management of patients with ascites. Am Fam Physician 54:1327, 1996

MCHUTCHISON JG: Differential diagnosis of ascites. Semin Liver Dis 17:191, 1997

PARSONS SL et al: Malignant ascites. Br J Surg 83:6, 1996

PINTO PC et al: Large volume paracentesis in nonedematous patients with tense ascites: Its effect on intravascular volume. Hepatology 8:207, 1988

RUNYON BA: Management of adult patients with ascites caused by cirrhosis. Hepatology 27:264, 1998

——— et al: The serum-ascites albumin gradient in the differential diagnosis of ascites. Ann Intern Med 117:215, 1992

Section 7   *Alterations in Renal and Urinary Tract Function*

40 | AZOTEMIA AND URINARY ABNORMALITIES
Bradley M. Denker, Barry M. Brenner

Body homeostasis is maintained predominantly through the cellular processes that together comprise normal kidney function. Disturbances to any of these functions can lead to a constellation of abnormalities that may be detrimental to survival. The clinical manifestations of these diseases will depend upon the pathophysiology of the renal injury and will often be initially identified as a complex of symptoms, abnormal physical findings, and laboratory changes that will allow the identification of specific syndromes. These renal syndromes (summarized in Table 40-1) may arise as the consequence of a systemic illness or can occur as a primary renal disease. Nephrologic syndromes usually consist of several elements that reflect the underlying pathologic processes and the duration of the disease and typically include one or more of the following features: (1) disturbances in urine volume (oliguria, anuria, polyuria); (2) abnormalities of urine sediment [red blood cells (RBC); white blood cells, casts, and crystals]; (3) abnormal excretion of serum proteins (proteinuria); (4) reduction in glomerular filtration rate (GFR) (azotemia); (5) presence of hypertension and/or expanded total body volume (edema); (6) electrolyte abnormalities; or (7) in some syndromes, fever/pain. The combination of these findings should permit identification of one of the major nephrologic syndromes (Table 40-1) and will allow the differential diagnoses to be narrowed and the appropriate diagnostic evaluation and therapeutic course to be determined. Each of these syndromes and their associated diseases are discussed in more detail in subsequent chapters. This chapter will focus on several aspects of renal abnormalities that are critically important to distinguishing these processes: (1) reduction in GFR leading to azotemia, (2) alterations of the urinary sediment and/or protein excretion, and (3) abnormalities of urinary volume.

AZOTEMIA

ASSESSMENT OF GLOMERULAR FILTRATION RATE

Monitoring the GFR is important in both the hospital and outpatient settings, and several different methodologies are available (discussed below). In most acute clinical circumstances a measured GFR is not available, and it is necessary to estimate the GFR from the serum

creatinine level in order to provide appropriate doses of drugs that are excreted into the urine. Serum creatinine is the most widely used marker for GFR, and the GFR is related directly to the urine creatinine excretion and inversely to the serum creatinine (U_{Cr}/P_{Cr}). Based upon this relationship and some important caveats (discussed below), the GFR will fall proportionately with the increase in P_{Cr}. Failure to account for GFR reductions in drug dosing can lead to significant morbidity and mortality from drug toxicities (e.g., digoxin, aminoglycosides). In the outpatient setting, the serum creatinine is often used as a surrogate for GFR (although much less accurate; see below). In patients with chronic progressive renal failure there is an approximately linear relationship between $1/P_{Cr}$ and time. The slope of this line will remain constant for an individual patient, and when values are obtained that do not fall on this line, an investigation for a superimposed acute process (e.g., volume depletion, drug reaction) should be initiated. It should be emphasized that the signs and symptoms of uremia will develop at significantly different levels of serum creatinine depending upon the patient (size, age, and sex), the underlying renal disease, existence of concurrent diseases, and true GFR. In general, patients do not develop symptomatic uremia until renal insufficiency is usually quite severe (GFR < 15 mL/min).

A reduced GFR leads to retention of nitrogenous waste products (azotemia) such as serum urea nitrogen and creatinine. Azotemia may result from reduced renal perfusion, intrinsic renal disease, or postrenal processes (ureteral obstruction; see below and Fig. 40-1). Precise determination of GFR is problematic as both commonly used markers (urea and creatinine) have characteristics that affect their accuracy as markers of clearance. Urea clearance is generally an underestimate of GFR because of tubule urea reabsorption and may be as low as one-half of GFR measured by other techniques.

Creatinine is a small, freely filtered solute that varies little from day to day (since it is derived from muscle metabolism of creatine). However, serum creatinine can increase acutely from dietary ingestion of cooked meat. Creatinine can be secreted by the proximal tubule through an organic cation pathway. There are many clinical settings where a creatinine clearance is not available, and decisions concerning

TABLE 40-1 *Initial Clinical and Laboratory Data Base for Defining Major Syndromes in Nephrology*

Syndromes	Important Clues to Diagnosis	Findings That Are Common	Location of Discussion of Diseases-Causing Syndrome
Acute or rapidly progressive renal failure	Anuria Oliguria Documented recent decline in GFR	Hypertension, hematuria Proteinuria, pyuria Casts, edema	Chaps. 260, 264, 266, 270
Acute nephritis	Hematuria, RBC casts Azotemia, oliguria Edema, hypertension	Proteinuria Pyuria Circulatory congestion	Chap. 264
Chronic renal failure	Azotemia for >3 months Prolonged symptoms or signs of uremia Symptoms or signs of renal osteodystrophy Kidneys reduced in size bilaterally Broad casts in urinary sediment	Hematuria, proteinuria Casts, oliguria Polyuria, nocturia Edema, hypertension Electrolyte disorders	Chaps. 259, 261
Nephrotic syndrome	Proteinuria >3.5 g per 1.73 m² per 24 h Hypoalbuminemia Hyperlipidemia Lipiduria	Casts Edema	Chap. 264
Asymptomatic urinary abnormalities	Hematuria Proteinuria (below nephrotic range) Sterile pyuria, casts		Chap. 264
Urinary tract infection	Bacteriuria >10⁵ colonies per milliliter Other infectious agent documented in urine Pyuria, leukocyte casts Frequency, urgency Bladder tenderness, flank tenderness	Hematuria Mild azotemia Mild proteinuria Fever	Chap. 269
Renal tubule defects	Electrolyte disorders Polyuria, nocturia Symptoms or signs of renal osteodystrophy Large kidneys Renal transport defects	Hematuria "Tubular" proteinuria Enuresis	Chaps. 265, 266
Hypertension	Systolic/diastolic hypertension	Proteinuria Casts Azotemia	Chaps. 230, 267
Nephrolithiasis	Previous history of stone passage or removal Previous history of stone seen by x ray Renal colic	Hematuria Pyuria Frequency, urgency	Chap. 268
Urinary tract obstruction	Azotemia, oliguria, anuria Polyuria, nocturia, urinary retention Slowing of urinary stream Large prostate, large kidneys Flank tenderness, full bladder after voiding	Hematuria Pyuria Enuresis, dysuria	Chap. 270

Note: GFR; glomerular filtration rate; RBC, red blood cell.

drug dosing must be made based on the serum creatinine. A formula that allows an estimate of creatinine clearance in men that accounts for age-related decreases in GFR, body weight, and sex has been derived by Cockcroft-Gault:

$$\text{Creatinine clearance (mL/min)}$$
$$= \frac{(140 - \text{age}) \times \text{lean body weight (kg)}}{\text{plasma creatinine (mg/dL)} \times 72}$$

This value should be multiplied 0.85 for women, since a lower fraction of the body weight is composed of muscle. The gradual loss of muscle from chronic illness, chronic use of glucocorticoids, or malnutrition can mask significant changes in GFR with small or imperceptible changes in serum creatinine. More accurate determinations of GFR are available using inulin clearance or radionuclide-labeled markers such as ¹²⁵I-iothalamate or EDTA. These methods are highly accurate due to precise quantitation and the absence of any renal reabsorption/secretion and should be used to follow GFR in patients in whom creatinine is not likely to be a reliable indicator (patients with decreased muscle mass secondary to age, malnutrition, concurrent illnesses). (See also Table 261-2.)

APPROACH TO THE PATIENT

Once it has been established that GFR is reduced, the physician must decide if this represents acute or chronic renal failure. The clinical situation, history, and laboratory data often make this an easy distinction. However, the laboratory abnormalities characteristic of chronic renal failure, including anemia, hypocalcemia, and hyperphosphatemia, are often also present in patients presenting with acute renal failure. Radiographic evidence of renal osteodystrophy (Chap. 261) would be seen only in chronic renal failure but is a very late finding, and these patients are usually on dialysis. The urinalysis and renal ultrasound can occasionally facilitate distinguishing acute from chronic renal failure. An approach to the evaluation of azotemic patients is shown in Fig. 40-1. Patients with advanced chronic renal insufficiency often have some proteinuria, nonconcentrated urine (isosthenuria), and small kidneys on ultrasound characterized by increased echogenicity and cortical thinning. Treatment should be directed toward slowing the progression of renal disease and providing symptomatic relief for edema, acidosis, anemia, and hyperphosphatemia, as discussed in Chap. 261. Acute renal failure (Chap. 260) can result from processes affecting renal blood flow (prerenal azotemia), intrinsic renal diseases (affecting vessels, glomeruli, or tubules), or postrenal processes (obstruction to urine flow in ureters, bladder, or urethra) (Chap. 270).

PRERENAL FAILURE Decreased renal perfusion accounts for 40 to 80% of acute renal failure and, if appropriately treated, is readily reversible. The etiologies of prerenal azotemia include any cause of decreased circulating blood volume such as volume loss (gastrointestinal hemorrhage, burns, diarrhea, diuretics), volume sequestration (pancreatitis, peritonitis, rhabdomyolysis), or decreased effective circulating volume (cardiogenic shock, sepsis). Renal perfusion can also be affected by reductions in cardiac output from peripheral vasodilatation (sepsis, drugs) or profound renal vasoconstriction [severe heart failure, hepatorenal syndrome, drugs such as nonsteroidal anti-inflammatory drugs (NSAIDs)]. True, or "ef-

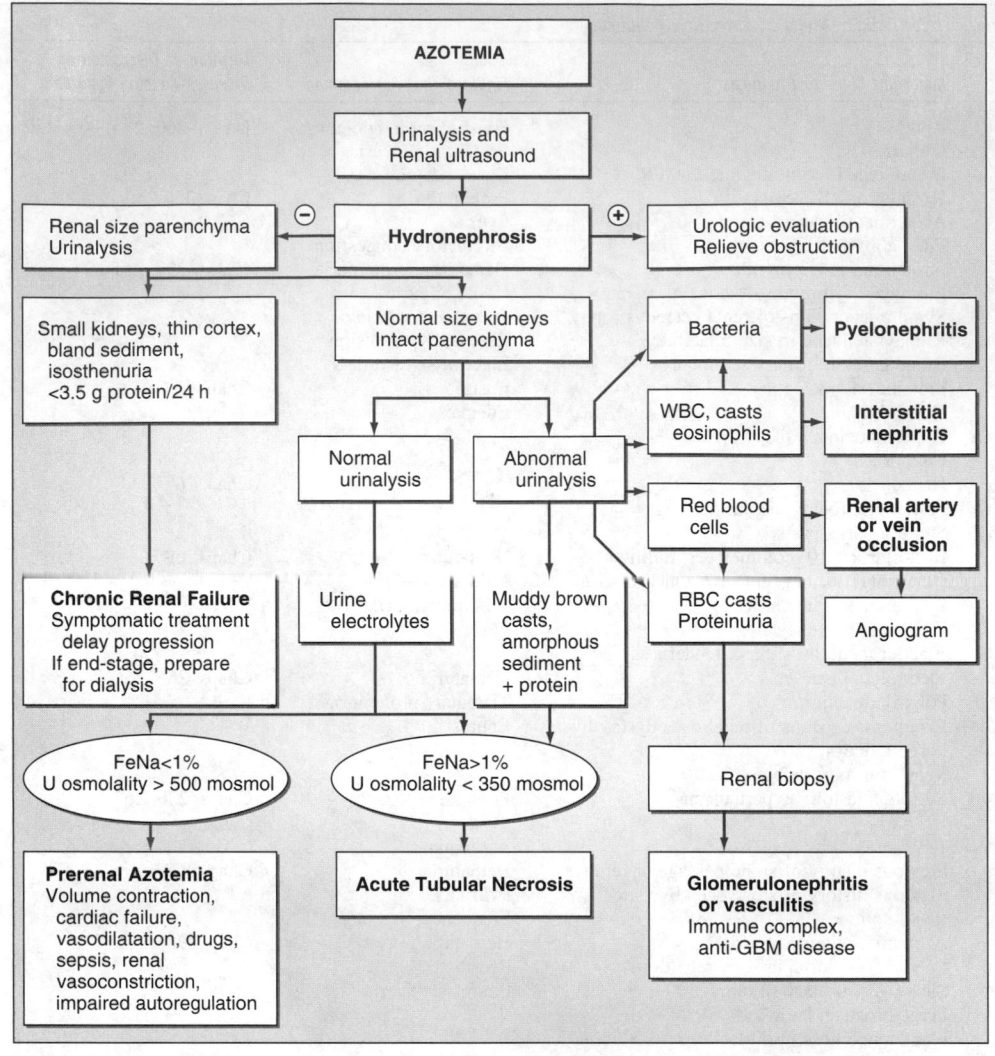

FIGURE 40-1 Approach to the patient with azotemia. WBC, white blood cell; RBC, red blood cell; GBM, glomerular basement membrane.

tention (urine Na concentration <20 mM/L; fractional excretion of Na <1%), and U_{Cr}/P_{Cr} > 40 (Table 40-2). The prerenal urine sediment is usually normal or has occasional hyaline and granular casts, while the sediment of ATN is usually filled with cellular debris and muddy brown granular casts.

INTRINSIC RENAL DISEASE When prerenal and postrenal azotemia have been excluded as etiologies of renal failure, an intrinsic parenchymal renal disease is present. Intrinsic renal disease can arise from processes involving large renal vessels, microvasculature and glomeruli, or tubulointerstitium. Ischemic and toxic ATN account for about 90% of acute intrinsic renal failure. As outlined in Fig. 40-1, the clinical setting and urinalysis are helpful in separating the possible etiologies of acute intrinsic renal failure. Prerenal azotemia and ATN are part of a spectrum of renal hypoperfusion; evidence of structural tubule injury is present in ATN, whereas prompt reversibility occurs with prerenal azotemia upon restoration of adequate renal perfusion. Thus, ATN can often be distinguished from prerenal azotemia by urinalysis and urine electrolyte composition (Table 40-2 and Fig. 40-1). Ischemic ATN is observed most frequently in patients who have undergone major surgery, trauma, severe hypovolemia, overwhelming sepsis, or extensive burns. Nephrotoxic ATN complicates the administration of many common medications, usually by inducing a combination of intrarenal vasoconstriction, direct tubule toxicity, and/or tubular obstruction. The kidney is vulnerable to toxic injury by virtue of its rich blood supply (25% of cardiac output) and its ability to concentrate and metabolize toxins. A diligent search for hypotension and nephrotoxins will usually uncover the specific etiology of ATN. Discontinuation of nephrotoxins and stabilizing blood pressure will often suffice without the need for dialysis while the tubules recover. →*An extensive list of potential drugs and toxins implicated in ATN can be found in Chap. 260.*

Processes that involve the tubules and interstitium can lead to acute renal failure. These include drug-induced interstitial nephritis

fective," hypovolemia leads to a fall in mean arterial pressure, which in turn triggers a series of neural and humoral responses that include activation of the sympathetic nervous and renin-angiotensin-aldosterone systems and ADH release. GFR is maintained by prostaglandin-mediated relaxation of afferent arterioles and angiotensin II–mediated constriction of efferent arterioles. Once the mean arterial pressure falls below 80 mmHg, there is a steep decline in GFR.

Blockade of prostaglandin production by NSAIDs can result in severe vasoconstriction and acute renal failure under these circumstances. Angiotensin-converting enzyme (ACE) inhibitors decrease efferent arteriolar tone and can decrease glomerular capillary perfusion pressure. Patients on NSAIDs and/or ACE inhibitors are most susceptible to hemodynamically mediated acute renal failure when blood volume is reduced for any reason. Patients with renal artery stenosis are dependent upon efferent arteriolar vasoconstriction for maintenance of glomerular filtration pressure and are particularly susceptible to precipitous decline in GFR when given ACE inhibitors.

Prolonged renal hypoperfusion can lead to acute tubular necrosis (ATN; an intrinsic renal disease discussed below). The urinalysis and urinary electrolytes can be useful in distinguishing prerenal azotemia from ATN (Table 40-2). The urine of patients with prerenal azotemia can be predicted from the stimulatory actions of norepinephrine, angiotensin II, ADH, and low tubule fluid flow on salt and water reabsorption. In prerenal conditions the tubules are intact, leading to a concentrated urine (>500 mosm) and avid Na re-

TABLE 40-2 *Laboratory Findings in Acute Renal Failure*

Index	Prerenal Azotemia	Oliguric Acute Renal Failure
BUN/P_{Cr} Ratio	>20:1	10–15:1
Urine sodium (U_{Na}), meq/L	<20	>40
Urine osmolality, mosmol/L H_2O	>500	<350
Fractional excretion of sodium	<1%	>2%
$FE_{Na} = \dfrac{U_{Na} \times P_{Cr} \times 100}{P_{Na} \times U_{Cr}}$		
Urine/plasma creatinine (U_{Cr}/P_{Cr})	>40	<20

Note: BUN, Blood urea nitrogen; P_{Cr}, plasma creatinine; U_{Na}, urine sodium concentration; P_{Na}, plasma sodium concentration; U_{Cr}, urine creatinine concentration.

(especially antibiotics, NSAIDs, and diuretics), severe infections (both bacterial and viral), systemic diseases (e.g., systemic lupus erythematosus), or infiltrative disorders (e.g., sarcoid, lymphoma, or leukemia). A list of drugs associated with allergic interstitial nephritis can be found in Chap. 266. The urinalysis usually shows mild to moderate proteinuria, hematuria, and pyuria (approximately 75% of cases) and occasionally white blood cell casts. The finding of RBC casts in interstitial nephritis has been reported but should prompt a search for glomerular diseases. Occasionally renal biopsy will be needed to distinguish among these possibilities. The finding of eosinophils in the urine is suggestive of allergic interstitial nephritis and is optimally observed by using a Hansel stain. The absence of eosinophiluria, however, does not exclude the possibility of acute interstitial nephritis.

Occlusion of large renal vessels including arteries and veins is an uncommon cause of acute renal failure. A significant reduction in GFR by this mechanism suggests bilateral processes or a unilateral process in a patient with a single functioning kidney. Renal arteries can be occluded with atheroemboli, thromboemboli, in situ thrombosis, aortic dissection, or vasculitis. Atheroembolic renal failure can occur spontaneously but is most often associated with recent aortic instrumentation. The emboli are cholesterol-rich and lodge in medium and small renal arteries, leading to an eosinophil-rich inflammatory reaction. Patients with atheroembolic acute renal failure often have a normal urinalysis, but the urine may contain eosinophils and casts. The diagnosis can be confirmed by renal biopsy, but this is often unnecessary when other stigmata of atheroemboli are present (livedo reticularis, distal peripheral infarcts, eosinophilia). Renal artery thrombosis may lead to mild proteinuria and hematuria, whereas renal vein thrombosis typically induces heavy proteinuria and hematuria. →*These vascular complications often require angiography for confirmation and are discussed in Chap. 267.*

Diseases of glomeruli (glomerulonephritis or vasculitis) and the renal microvasculature (hemolytic uremic syndromes, thrombotic thrombocytopenic purpura, or malignant hypertension) usually present with various combinations of glomerular injury: proteinuria, hematuria, reduced GFR, and alterations of Na excretion leading to hypertension, edema, and circulatory congestion (acute nephritic syndrome). These findings may occur as primary renal diseases or as renal manifestations of systemic diseases. The clinical setting and other laboratory data will help distinguish primary renal from systemic diseases. The finding of RBC casts in the urine is an indication for early renal biopsy (Fig. 40-1) as the pathologic pattern has important implications for diagnosis, prognosis, and treatment. Hematuria without RBC casts can also be an indication of glomerular disease, and this evaluation is summarized in Fig. 40-2. →*A detailed discussion of glomerulonephritis and diseases of the microvasculature can be found in Chap. 264.*

POSTRENAL AZOTEMIA Urinary tract obstruction accounts for fewer than 5% of cases of acute renal failure, but it is usually reversible and must be ruled out early in the evaluation (Fig. 40-1). Since a single kidney is capable of adequate clearance, acute renal failure from obstruction requires obstruction at the urethra or bladder outlet, bilateral ureteral obstruction, or unilateral obstruction in a patient with a single functioning kidney. Obstruction is usually diagnosed by the presence of ureteral dilatation on renal ultrasound. However, early in the course of obstruction or if the ureters are unable to dilate (such as encasement by pelvic tumors), the ultrasound examination may be negative. →*The specific urologic conditions that cause obstruction are discussed in Chap. 270.*

OLIGURIA AND ANURIA *Oliguria* refers to a 24-h urine output of <500 mL, and *anuria* is the complete absence of urine formation. Anuria can be caused by total urinary tract obstruction, total renal artery or vein occlusion, and shock (manifested by severe hypotension and intense renal vasoconstriction). Cortical necrosis, ATN, and rapidly progressive glomerulonephritis can occasionally cause

anuria. Oliguria can accompany any cause of acute renal failure and carries a more serious prognosis for renal recovery in all conditions except prerenal azotemia. *Nonoliguria* refers to urine output in excess of 500 mL/day in patients with acute or chronic azotemia. With nonoliguric ATN, disturbances of potassium and hydrogen balance are less severe than in oliguric patients and recovery to normal renal function is usually more rapid.

ABNORMALITIES OF THE URINE

PROTEINURIA

The evaluation of proteinuria is shown schematically in Fig. 40-3 and is typically initiated after colorimetric detection of proteinuria by dipstick examination. The dipstick measurement detects mostly albumin and gives false-positive results when pH > 7.0 and the urine is very concentrated or contaminated with blood. A very dilute urine may obscure significant proteinuria on dipstick examination, and proteinuria that is not predominantly albumin will be missed. This is particularly important for the detection of Bence Jones proteins in the urine of patients with multiple myeloma. Tests to measure total urine concentration accurately rely on precipitation with sulfosalicylic or trichloracetic acids. Currently, ultrasensitive dipsticks are available to measure microalbuminuria (30 to 300 mg/d), an early marker of glomerular disease that has been shown to predict glomerular injury in early diabetic nephropathy (Fig. 40-3).

The magnitude of proteinuria and the protein composition in the urine depend upon the mechanism of renal injury leading to protein losses. Both charge and size selectivity normally prevent virtually all

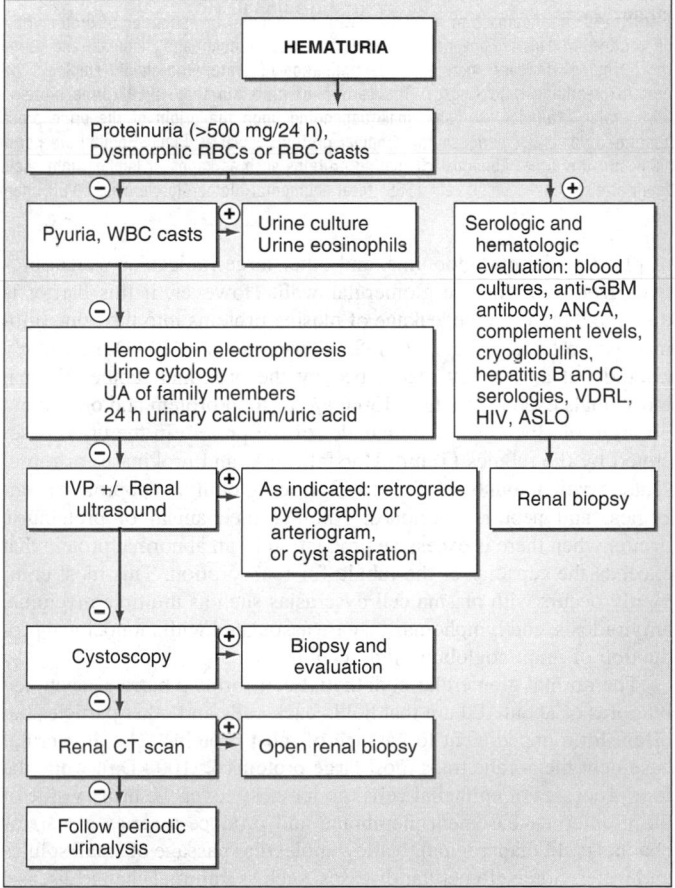

FIGURE 40-2 Approach to the patient with hematuria. RBC, red blood cell; WBC, white blood cell; GBM, glomerular basement membrane; ANCA, antineutrophil cytoplasmic antibody; VDRL, venereal disease research laboratory; ASLO, antistreptolysin O; UA, urinalysis; IVP, intravenous pyelography; CT, computed tomography.

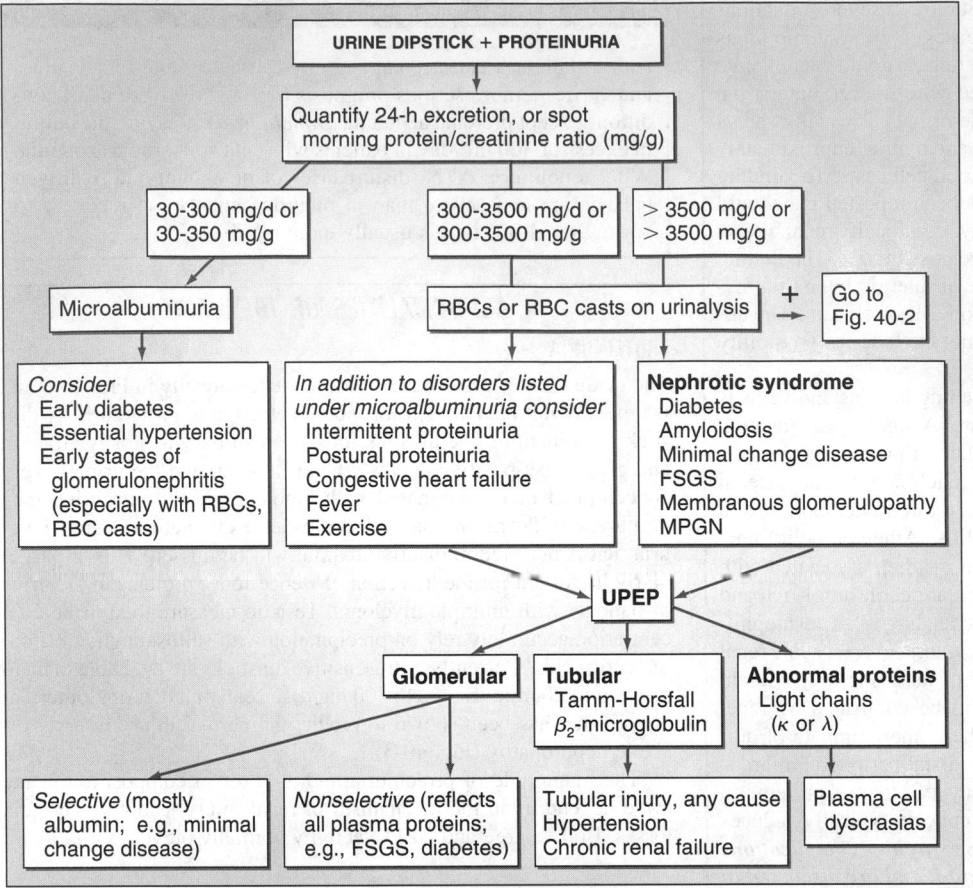

FIGURE 40-3 Approach to the patient with proteinuria. Investigation of proteinuria is often initiated by a positive dipstick on routine urinalysis. Conventional dipsticks detect predominantly albumin and cannot detect urinary albumin levels of 30 to 300 mg/d. However, more exact determination of proteinuria should employ a 24-h urine collection or a spot morning protein/creatinine ratio (mg/g). The pattern of proteinuria on UPEP (urine protein electrophoresis) can be classified as "glomerular," "tubular," or "abnormal" depending upon the origin of the urine proteins. Glomerular proteinuria is due to abnormal glomerular permeability. "Tubular proteins" such as Tamm-Horsfall are normally produced by the renal tubule and shed into the urine. Abnormal circulating proteins such as kappa or lambda light chains are readily filtered because of their small size. RBC, red blood cell; FSGS, focal segmental glomerulosclerosis; MPGN, membranoproliferative glomerulonephritis.

of plasma albumin, globulins, and other large-molecular-weight proteins from crossing the glomerular wall. However, if this barrier is disrupted, there can be leakage of plasma proteins into the urine (glomerular proteinuria; Fig. 40-3). Smaller proteins (<20 kDa) are freely filtered but are readily reabsorbed by the proximal tubule. Normal individuals excrete less than 150 mg/d of total protein and only about 30 mg/d of albumin. The remainder of the protein in the urine is secreted by the tubules (Tamm-Horsfall, IgA, and urokinase) or represents small amounts of filtered β_2-microglobulin, apoproteins, enzymes, and peptide hormones. Another mechanism of proteinuria occurs when there is excessive production of an abnormal protein that exceeds the capacity of the tubule for reabsorption. This most commonly occurs with plasma cell dyscrasias such as multiple myeloma, amyloidosis, and lymphomas that are associated with monoclonal production of immunoglobulin light chains.

The normal glomerular endothelial cell forms a barrier penetrated by pores of about 100 nm that holds back cells and other particles but offers little impediment to passage of most proteins. The glomerular basement membrane traps most large proteins (>100 kDa), while the foot processes of epithelial cells (podocytes) cover the urinary side of the glomerular basement membrane and produce a series of narrow channels (slit diaphragms) to allow molecular passage of small solutes and water. Some glomerular diseases, such as minimal change disease, cause fusion of glomerular epithelial cell foot processes, resulting in predominantly "selective" (Fig. 40-3) loss of albumin. Other glomerular diseases can present with disruption of the basement membrane and slit diaphragms (e.g., by immune complex deposition), resulting

in large amounts of protein losses that include albumin and other plasma proteins. The fusion of foot processes causes increased pressure across the capillary basement membrane, resulting in areas with larger pore sizes. The combination of increased pressure and larger pores results in significant proteinuria ("nonselective"; Fig. 40-3).

When the total daily excretion of protein exceeds 3.5 g, there is often associated hypoalbuminemia, hyperlipidemia, and edema (nephrotic syndrome; Table 40-1). However, total daily urinary protein excretion greater than 3.5 g can occur without the other features of the nephrotic syndrome in a variety of other renal diseases (Fig. 40-3). Plasma cell dyscrasias (multiple myeloma) can be associated with large amounts of excreted light chains in the urine, which may not be detected by dipstick (which detects mostly albumin). The light chains produced from these disorders are filtered by the glomerulus and overwhelm the reabsorptive capacity of the proximal tubule. A sulfosalicylic acid precipitate that is out of proportion to the dipstick estimate is suggestive of light chains (Bence Jones protein), and light chains typically redissolve upon warming of the precipitate. Renal failure from these disorders occurs through a variety of mechanisms including tubule obstruction (cast nephropathy) and light chain deposition.

Hypoalbuminemia in nephrotic syndrome occurs through excessive urinary losses, and increased proximal tubule catabolism of filtered albumin. Hepatic rates of albumin synthesis are increased. Edema forms from primary renal sodium retention and from reduced plasma oncotic pressure, which favors fluid movement from capillaries to interstitium. The mechanisms designed to correct the decrease in effective intravascular volume contribute to edema formation in some patients. These mechanisms include activation of the renin-angiotensin system, antidiuretic hormone, and the sympathetic nervous system, which contribute to excessive renal salt and water reabsorption.

The severity of edema correlates with the degree of hypoalbuminemia and is modified by other factors such as heart disease or peripheral vascular disease. The diminished plasma oncotic pressure and urinary losses of regulatory proteins appear to stimulate hepatic lipoprotein synthesis. The resulting hyperlipidemia results in lipid bodies (fatty casts, oval fat bodies) in the urine. Other proteins are lost in the urine, leading to a variety of metabolic disturbances. These include thyroxine-binding globulin, cholecalciferol-binding protein, transferrin, and metal-binding proteins. A hypercoagulable state frequently accompanies severe nephrotic syndrome due to urinary losses of antithrombin III, reduced serum levels of proteins S and C, hyperfibrinogenemia, and enhanced platelet aggregation. Some patients develop severe IgG deficiency with resulting defects in immunity. Many diseases (some listed in Fig. 40-3) and drugs can cause the nephrotic syndrome, and a complete list can be found in Chap. 264.

HEMATURIA, PYURIA, AND CASTS

Isolated hematuria without proteinuria, other cells, or casts is often indicative of bleeding from the urinary tract. Normal red blood cell excretion is up to 2 million RBCs per day. Hematuria is defined as two to five RBCs per high-power field (HPF) and can be detected by dipstick. Common causes of isolated hematuria include stones, neoplasms, tuberculosis, trauma, and prostatitis. Gross hematuria with blood clots is almost never indicative of glomerular bleeding; rather, it suggests a postrenal source in the urinary collecting system. Evaluation of patients presenting with microscopic hematuria is outlined in Fig. 40-2. A single urinalysis with hematuria is common and can result from menstruation, viral illness, allergy, exercise, or mild trauma. Annual urinalysis of servicemen over a 10-year period showed an incidence of 38%. However, persistent or significant hematuria (>three RBCs/HPF on three urinalyses, or a single urinalysis with >100 RBCs, or gross hematuria) identified significant renal or urologic lesions in 9.1% of over 1000 patients. Even patients who are chronically anticoagulated should be investigated as outlined in Fig. 40-2. The suspicion for urogenital neoplasms in patients with isolated painless hematuria (nondysmorphic RBCs) increases with age. Neoplasms are rare in the pediatric population, and isolated hematuria is more likely to be "idiopathic" or associated with a congenital anomaly. Hematuria with pyuria and bacteriuria is typical of infection and should be treated with antibiotics after appropriate cultures. Acute cystitis or urethritis in women can cause gross hematuria. Hypercalciuria and hyperuricosuria are also risk factors for unexplained isolated hematuria in both children and adults. In some of these patients (50 to 60%), reducing calcium and uric acid excretion through dietary interventions can eliminate the microscopic hematuria.

Isolated microscopic hematuria can be a manifestation of glomerular diseases. The RBCs of glomerular origin are often dysmorphic when examined by phase-contrast microscopy. Irregular shapes of RBCs may also occur due to pH and osmolarity changes found in the distal tubule. There is, however, significant observer variability in detecting dysmorphic RBCs, especially if a phase-contrast microscope is not available. The most common etiologies of isolated glomerular hematuria are IgA nephropathy, hereditary nephritis, and thin basement membrane disease. IgA nephropathy and hereditary nephritis can have episodic gross hematuria. A family history of renal failure is often present in patients with hereditary nephritis, and patients with thin basement membrane disease often have other family members with microscopic hematuria. A renal biopsy is needed for the definitive diagnosis of these disorders, which are discussed in more detail in Chap. 264. Hematuria with dysmorphic RBCs, RBC casts, and protein excretion >500 mg/d is virtually diagnostic of glomerulonephritis. RBC casts form as RBCs that enter the tubular fluid become trapped in a cylindrical mold of gelled Tamm-Horsfall protein. Even in the absence of azotemia, these patients should undergo serologic evaluation and renal biopsy as outlined in Fig. 40-2.

Isolated pyuria is unusual since inflammatory reactions in the kidney or collecting system are also associated with hematuria. The presence of bacteria suggests infection, and white blood cell casts with bacteria are indicative of pyelonephritis. White blood cells and/or white blood cell casts may also be seen in tubulointerstitial processes such as interstitial nephritis, systemic lupus erythematosus, and transplant rejection. In chronic renal diseases, degenerated cellular casts called *waxy casts* can be seen in the urine. *Broad casts* are thought to arise in the dilated tubules of enlarged nephrons that have undergone compensatory hypertrophy in response to reduced renal mass (i.e., chronic renal failure). A mixture of broad casts typically seen with chronic renal failure together with cellular casts and RBCs may be seen in smoldering processes such as chronic glomerulonephritis with active glomerulitis.

ABNORMALITIES OF URINE VOLUME

The volume of urine produced varies depending upon the fluid intake, renal function, and physiologic demands of the individual. See "Azotemia," above, for discussion of decreased (oliguria) or absent urine production (anuria). →*The physiology of water formation and renal water conservation are discussed in Chap. 259.*

POLYURIA

By history, it is often difficult for patients to distinguish urinary frequency (often of small volumes) from polyuria, and a 24-h urine collection is needed for evaluation (Fig. 40-4). It is necessary to determine if the polyuria represents a solute or water diuresis and if the diuresis is appropriate for the clinical circumstances. The average person excretes between 600 and 800 mosmol of solutes per day, primarily as urea and electrolytes. The urine osmolality can help distinguish a solute from water diuresis. If the urine output is >3 L/d (arbitrarily defined as polyuria) and the urine is dilute (<250 mosmol/L), then total mosmol excretion is normal and a water diuresis is present. This circumstance could arise from polydipsia, inadequate secretion of vasopressin (central diabetes insipidus), or failure of renal tubules to respond to vasopressin (nephrogenic diabetes insipidus). If the urine volume is >3 L/d and urine osmolality is >300 mosmol/L, then a solute diuresis is clearly present and a search for the responsible solute(s) is mandatory.

Excessive filtration of a poorly reabsorbed solute such as glucose, mannitol, or urea can depress reabsorption of NaCl and water in the proximal tubule and lead to enhanced excretion in the urine. Poorly controlled diabetes mellitus is the most common cause of a solute diuresis, leading to volume depletion and serum hypertonicity. Since the urine Na concentration is less than that of blood, more water than Na is lost, causing hypernatremia and hypertonicity. Common iatrogenic solute diuresis occurs from mannitol administration, radiocontrast media, and high-protein feedings (enterally or parenterally), leading to increased urea production and excretion. Less commonly, excessive Na loss may occur from cystic renal diseases, Bartter's syndrome, or during the course of a tubulointerstitial process (such as

FIGURE 40-4 Approach to the patient with polyuria. ATN, acute tubular necrosis; ADH, antidiuretic hormone.

resolving ATN). In these so-called salt-wasting disorders, the tubule damage results in direct impairment of Na reabsorption and indirectly reduces the responsiveness of the tubule to aldosterone. Usually, the Na losses are mild, and the obligatory urine output is less than 2 L/d (resolving ATN and postobstructive diuresis are exceptions and may be associated with significant natriuresis and polyuria.)

Formation of large volumes of dilute urine represent polydipsic states or diabetes insipidus. Primary polydipsia can result from habit, psychiatric disorders, neurologic lesions, or medications. During deliberate polydipsia, extracellular fluid volume is normal or expanded and vasopressin levels are reduced because serum osmolality tends to be near the lower limits of normal.

Central diabetes insipidus may be idiopathic in origin or secondary to a variety of hypothalamic conditions including posthypophysectomy or trauma or neoplastic, inflammatory, vascular, or infectious hypothalamic diseases. Idiopathic central diabetes insipidus is associated with selective destruction of the vasopressin-secreting neurons in the supraoptic and paraventricular nuclei and can be inherited as an autosomal dominant trait or occur spontaneously. Nephrogenic diabetes insipidus can occur in a variety of clinical situations as summarized in Fig. 40-4.

A plasma vasopressin level is recommended as the best method for distinguishing between central and nephrogenic diabetes insipidus. Alternatively, a water deprivation test plus exogenous vasopressin may also distinguish primary polydipsia from central and nephrogenic diabetes insipidus. →*For a detailed discussion, see Chap. 319.*

FURTHER READING

ANDERSON S et al: Renal and systemic manifestations of glomerular disease, in BM Brenner (ed): *Brenner & Rector's The Kidney*, 7th ed. Philadelphia, Saunders, 2004, pp 1927–1954

BERL T, VERBALIS J: Pathophysiology of water metabolism, in BM Brenner (ed): *Brenner & Rector's The Kidney*, 7th ed. Philadelphia, Saunders, 2004, pp 857–920

BICHET DG: Nephrogenic diabetes insipidus. Am J Med 105(5):431, 1998

BOUTE N et al: NPHS2, encoding the glomerular protein podocin, is mutated in autosomal recessive steroid-resistant nephrotic syndrome. Nat Genet 24: 349, 2000

GROSSFELD GD, CARROLL PR: Evaluation of asymptomatic microscopic hematuria. Urol Clin North Am 25:661, 1998

LAMIERE N, VANHOLDER R: Pathophysiologic features and prevention of human and experimental acute tubulonecrosis. J Am Soc Nephrol 12:S20, 2001

MARIANI AJ et al: The significance of adult hematuria: 1000 hematuria evaluations including a risk-benefit and cost-effectiveness analysis. J Urol 141. 350, 1989

---

41 FLUID AND ELECTROLYTE DISTURBANCES
Gary G. Singer, Barry M. Brenner

SODIUM AND WATER

COMPOSITION OF BODY FLUIDS Water is the most abundant constituent in the body, comprising approximately 50% of body weight in women and 60% in men. This difference is attributable to differences in the relative proportions of adipose tissue in men and women. Total body water is distributed in two major compartments—55 to 75% is intracellular [intracellular fluid (ICF)], and 25 to 45% is extracellular [extracellular fluid (ECF)]. The ECF is further subdivided into intravascular (plasma water) and extravascular (interstitial) spaces in a ratio of 1:3.

The solute or particle concentration of a fluid is known as its *osmolality* and is expressed as milliosmoles per kilogram of water (mosmol/kg). Water crosses cell membranes to achieve osmotic equilibrium (ECF osmolality = ICF osmolality). The extracellular and intracellular solutes or osmoles are markedly different due to disparities in permeability and the presence of transporters and active pumps. The major ECF particles are Na^+ and its accompanying anions Cl^- and HCO_3^-, whereas K^+ and organic phosphate esters (ATP, creatine phosphate, and phospholipids) are the predominant ICF osmoles. Solutes that are restricted to the ECF or the ICF determine the *effective osmolality* (or *tonicity*) of that compartment. Since Na^+ is largely restricted to the extracellular compartment, total body Na^+ content is a reflection of ECF volume. Likewise, K^+ and its attendant anions are predominantly limited to the ICF and are necessary for normal cell function. Therefore, the number of intracellular particles is relatively constant, and a change in ICF osmolality is usually due to a change in ICF water content. However, in certain situations, brain cells can vary the number of intracellular solutes in order to defend against large water shifts. This process of *osmotic adaptation* is important in the defense of cell volume and occurs in chronic hyponatremia and hypernatremia. This response is mediated initially by transcellular shifts of K^+ and Na^+, followed by synthesis, import, or export of organic solutes (so-called osmolytes) such as inositol, betaine, and glutamine. During chronic hyponatremia, brain cells lose solutes, thereby defending cell volume and diminishing neurologic symptoms. The converse occurs during chronic hypernatremia. Certain solutes, such as urea, do not contribute to water shift across cell membranes and are known as *ineffective osmoles.*

Fluid movement between the intravascular and interstitial spaces occurs across the capillary wall and is determined by the Starling forces—capillary hydraulic pressure and colloid osmotic pressure. The transcapillary hydraulic pressure gradient exceeds the corresponding oncotic pressure gradient, thereby favoring the movement of plasma ultrafiltrate into the extravascular space. The return of fluid into the intravascular compartment occurs via lymphatic flow.

WATER BALANCE (See also Chap. 259) The normal plasma osmolality is 275 to 290 mosmol/kg and is kept within a narrow range by mechanisms capable of sensing a 1 to 2% change in tonicity. To maintain a steady state, water intake must equal water excretion. Disorders of water homeostasis result in hypo- or hypernatremia. Normal individuals have an obligate water loss consisting of urine, stool, and evaporation from the skin and respiratory tract. Gastrointestinal excretion is usually a minor component of total water output, except in patients with vomiting, diarrhea, or high enterostomy output states. Evaporative or insensitive water losses are important in the regulation of core body temperature. Obligatory renal water loss is mandated by the minimum solute excretion required to maintain a steady state. Normally, about 600 mosmols must be excreted per day, and since the maximal urine osmolality is 1200 mosmol/kg a minimum urine output of 500 mL/d is required for neutral solute balance.

Water Intake The primary stimulus for water ingestion is *thirst*, mediated either by an increase in effective osmolality or a decrease in ECF volume or blood pressure. *Osmoreceptors*, located in the anterolateral hypothalamus, are stimulated by a rise in tonicity. Ineffective osmoles, such as urea and glucose, do not play a role in stimulating thirst. The average osmotic threshold for thirst is approximately 295 mosmol/kg and varies among individuals. Under normal circumstances, daily water intake exceeds physiologic requirements.

Water Excretion In contrast to the ingestion of water, its excretion is tightly regulated by physiologic factors. The principal determinant of renal water excretion is *arginine vasopressin* (AVP; formerly antidiuretic hormone), a polypeptide synthesized in the supraoptic and paraventricular nuclei of the hypothalamus and secreted by the posterior pituitary gland. The binding of AVP to V_2 receptors on the basolateral membrane of principal cells in the collecting duct activates adenylyl cyclase and initiates a sequence of events that leads to the insertion of water channels into the luminal membrane. These water channels that are specifically activated by AVP are encoded by the *aquaporin-2* gene (Chap. 319). The net effect is passive water reabsorption along an osmotic gradient from the lumen of the collecting duct to the hypertonic medullary interstitium. The major stimulus for AVP secretion is hypertonicity. Since the major ECF solutes are Na^+ salts, effective osmolality is primarily determined by the plasma Na^+ concentration. An increase or decrease in tonicity is sensed by hypothalamic osmoreceptors as a decrease or increase in cell volume, respectively, leading to enhancement or suppression of AVP secretion. The osmotic threshold for AVP release is 280 to 290 mosmol/kg, and the system is sufficiently sensitive that plasma osmolality varies by no more than 1 to 2%.

Nonosmotic factors that regulate AVP secretion include *effective circulating (arterial) volume*, nausea, pain, stress, hypoglycemia, pregnancy, and numerous drugs. The hemodynamic response is mediated by baroreceptors in the carotid sinus. The sensitivity of these receptors is significantly lower than that of the osmoreceptors. In fact, depletion of blood volume sufficient to result in a decreased mean arterial pressure is necessary to stimulate AVP release, whereas small changes in effective circulating volume have little effect.

To maintain homeostasis and a normal plasma Na^+ concentration, the ingestion of solute-free water must eventually lead to the loss of the same volume of electrolyte-free water. Three steps are required for the kidney to excrete a water load: (1) filtration and delivery of water (and electrolytes) to the diluting sites of the nephron; (2) active reabsorption of Na^+ and Cl^- without water in the thick ascending limb of the loop of Henle and, to a lesser extent, in the distal nephron; and (3) maintenance of a dilute urine due to impermeability of the collecting duct to water in the absence of AVP. Abnormalities of any of these steps can result in impaired free water excretion, and eventual hyponatremia.

SODIUM BALANCE   Sodium is actively pumped out of cells by the Na^+, K^+-ATPase pump. As a result, 85 to 90% of all Na^+ is extracellular, and the ECF volume is a reflection of total body Na^+ content. Normal volume regulatory mechanisms ensure that Na^+ loss balances Na^+ gain. If this does not occur, conditions of Na^+ excess or deficit ensue and are manifest as edematous or hypovolemic states, respectively. It is important to distinguish between disorders of osmoregulation and disorders of volume regulation since water and Na^+ balance are regulated independently. Changes in Na^+ concentration generally reflect disturbed water homeostasis, whereas alterations in Na^+ content are manifest as ECF volume contraction or expansion and imply abnormal Na^+ balance.

Sodium Intake   Individuals eating a typical western diet consume approximately 150 mmol of NaCl daily. This normally exceeds basal requirements. As noted above, sodium is the principal extracellular cation. Therefore, dietary intake of Na^+ results in ECF volume expansion, which in turn promotes enhanced renal Na^+ excretion to maintain steady state Na^+ balance.

Sodium Excretion (See also Chap. 259)   The regulation of Na^+ excretion is multifactorial and is the major determinant of Na^+ balance. A Na^+ deficit or excess is manifest as a decreased or increased effective circulating volume, respectively. Changes in effective circulating volume tend to lead to parallel changes in glomerular filtration rate (GFR). However, tubule Na^+ reabsorption, and not GFR, is the major regulatory mechanism controlling Na^+ excretion. Almost two-thirds of filtered Na^+ is reabsorbed in the proximal convoluted tubule—this process is electroneutral and isoosmotic. Further reabsorption (25 to 30%) occurs in the thick ascending limb of the loop of Henle via the apical *Na^+-K^+-$2Cl^-$ cotransporter*—this is an active process and is also electroneutral. Distal convoluted tubule reabsorption of Na^+ (5%) is mediated by the *thiazide-sensitive Na^+-Cl^- cotransporter*. Final Na^+

reabsorption occurs in the cortical and medullary collecting ducts, the amount excreted being reasonably equivalent to the amount ingested per day.

HYPOVOLEMIA

ETIOLOGY   True volume depletion, or hypovolemia, generally refers to a state of combined salt and water loss exceeding intake, leading to ECF volume contraction. The loss of Na^+ may be renal or extrarenal (Table 41-1).

Renal   Many conditions are associated with excessive urinary NaCl and water losses, including diuretics. Pharmacologic diuretics inhibit specific pathways of Na^+ reabsorption along the nephron with a consequent increase in urinary Na^+ excretion. Enhanced filtration of non-reabsorbed solutes, such as glucose or urea, can also impair tubular reabsorption of Na^+ and water, leading to an osmotic or solute diuresis. This often occurs in poorly controlled diabetes mellitus and in patients receiving high-protein hyperalimentation. Mannitol is a diuretic that produces an osmotic diuresis because the renal tubule is impermeable to mannitol. Many tubule and interstitial renal disorders are associated with Na^+ wasting. Excessive renal losses of Na^+ and water may also occur during the diuretic phase of acute tubular necrosis (Chap. 260) and following the relief of bilateral urinary tract obstruction. Finally, mineralocorticoid deficiency (hypoaldosteronism) causes salt wasting in the presence of normal intrinsic renal function.

Massive renal water excretion can also lead to hypovolemia. The ECF volume contraction is usually less severe since two-thirds of the volume lost is intracellular. Conditions associated with excessive urinary water loss include *central diabetes insipidus* (CDI) and *nephrogenic diabetes insipidus* (NDI). These two disorders are due to impaired secretion of and renal unresponsiveness to AVP, respectively, and are discussed below.

Extrarenal   Nonrenal causes of hypovolemia include fluid loss from the gastrointestinal tract, skin, and respiratory system and third-space accumulations (burns, pancreatitis, peritonitis). Approximately 9 L of fluid enters the gastrointestinal tract daily, 2 L by ingestion and 7 L by secretion. Almost 98% of this volume is reabsorbed so that fecal fluid loss is only 100 to 200 mL/d. Impaired gastrointestinal reabsorption or enhanced secretion leads to volume depletion. Since gastric secretions have a low pH (high H^+ concentration) and biliary, pancreatic, and intestinal secretions are alkaline (high HCO_3^- concentration),

TABLE 41-1   *Causes of Hypovolemia*

I. ECF volume contracted
   A. Extrarenal Na^+ loss
      1. Gastrointestinal
        (vomiting, nasogastric suction, drainage, fistula, diarrhea)
      2. Skin/respiratory
        (insensible losses, sweat, burns)
      3. Hemorrhage
   B. Renal Na^+ and water loss
      1. Diuretics
      2. Osmotic diuresis
      3. Hypoaldosteronism
      4. Salt-wasting nephropathies
   C. Renal water loss
      1. Diabetes insipidus (central or nephrogenic)
II. ECF volume normal or expanded
   A. Decreased cardiac output
      1. Myocardial, valvular, or pericardial disease
   B. Redistribution
      1. Hypoalbuminemia
        (hepatic cirrhosis, nephrotic syndrome)
      2. Capillary leak
        (acute pancreatitis, ischemic bowel, rhabdomyolysis)
   C. Increased venous capacitance
      1. Sepsis

Note: ECF, extracellular fluid.

vomiting and diarrhea are often accompanied by metabolic alkalosis and acidosis, respectively.

Water evaporation from the skin and respiratory tract contributes to thermoregulation. These *insensible losses* amount to 500 mL/d. During febrile illnesses, prolonged heat exposure, exercise, or increased salt and water loss from skin, in the form of sweat, can be significant and lead to volume depletion. The Na^+ concentration of sweat is normally 20 to 50 mmol/L and decreases with profuse sweating due to the action of aldosterone. Since sweat is hypotonic, the loss of water exceeds that of Na^+. The water deficit is minimized by enhanced thirst. Nevertheless, ongoing Na^+ loss is manifest as hypovolemia. Enhanced evaporative water loss from the respiratory tract may be associated with hyperventilation, especially in mechanically ventilated febrile patients.

Certain conditions lead to fluid sequestration in a *third space*. This compartment is extracellular but is not in equilibrium with either the ECF or the ICF. The fluid is effectively lost from the ECF and can result in hypovolemia. Examples include the bowel lumen in gastrointestinal obstruction, subcutaneous tissues in severe burns, retroperitoneal space in acute pancreatitis, and peritoneal cavity in peritonitis. Finally, severe hemorrhage from any source can result in volume depletion.

PATHOPHYSIOLOGY   ECF volume contraction is manifest as a decreased plasma volume and hypotension. Hypotension is due to decreased venous return (preload) and diminished cardiac output; it triggers baroreceptors in the carotid sinus and aortic arch and leads to activation of the sympathetic nervous system and the renin-angiotensin system. The net effect is to maintain mean arterial pressure and cerebral and coronary perfusion. In contrast to the cardiovascular response, the renal response is aimed at restoring the ECF volume by decreasing the GFR and filtered load of Na^+ and, most importantly, by promoting tubular reabsorption of Na^+. Increased sympathetic tone increases proximal tubular Na^+ reabsorption and decreases GFR by causing preferential afferent arteriolar vasoconstriction. Sodium is also reabsorbed in the proximal convoluted tubule in response to increased angiotensin II and altered peritubular capillary hemodynamics (decreased hydraulic and increased oncotic pressure). Enhanced reabsorption of Na^+ by the collecting duct is an important component of the renal adaptation to ECF volume contraction. This occurs in response to increased *aldosterone* and AVP secretion, and suppressed *atrial natriuretic peptide* secretion.

CLINICAL FEATURES   A careful history is often helpful in determining the etiology of ECF volume contraction (e.g., vomiting, diarrhea, polyuria, diaphoresis). Most symptoms are nonspecific and secondary to electrolyte imbalances and tissue hypoperfusion and include fatigue, weakness, muscle cramps, thirst, and postural dizziness. More severe degrees of volume contraction can lead to end-organ ischemia manifest as oliguria, cyanosis, abdominal and chest pain, and confusion or obtundation. Diminished skin turgor and dry oral mucous membranes are poor markers of decreased interstitial fluid. Signs of intravascular volume contraction include decreased jugular venous pressure, postural hypotension, and postural tachycardia. Larger and more acute fluid losses lead to hypovolemic shock, manifest as hypotension, tachycardia, peripheral vasoconstriction, and hypoperfusion—cyanosis, cold and clammy extremities, oliguria, and altered mental status.

DIAGNOSIS   A thorough history and physical examination are generally sufficient to diagnose the etiology of hypovolemia. Laboratory data usually confirm and support the clinical diagnosis. The blood urea nitrogen (BUN) and plasma creatinine concentrations tend to be elevated, reflecting a decreased GFR. Normally, the BUN:creatinine ratio is about 10:1. However, in *prerenal azotemia*, hypovolemia leads to increased urea reabsorption and a proportionately greater elevation in BUN than plasma creatinine, and a BUN:creatinine ratio of 20:1 or higher. An increased BUN (relative to creatinine) may also be due to increased urea production that occurs with hyperalimentation (high-protein), glucocorticoid therapy, and gastrointestinal bleeding.

The appropriate response to hypovolemia is enhanced renal Na^+ and water reabsorption, which is reflected in the urine composition. Therefore, the urine Na^+ concentration should usually be <20 mmol/L except in conditions associated with impaired Na^+ reabsorption, as in acute tubular necrosis (Chap. 260). Another exception is hypovolemia due to vomiting, since the associated metabolic alkalosis and increased filtered HCO_3^- impair proximal Na^+ reabsorption. In this case, the urine Cl^- is low (<20 mmol/L). The urine osmolality and specific gravity in hypovolemic subjects are generally >450 mosmol/kg and 1.015, respectively, reflecting the presence of enhanced AVP secretion. However, in hypovolemia due to diabetes insipidus, urine osmolality and specific gravity are indicative of inappropriately dilute urine.

℞ TREATMENT

The therapeutic goals are to restore normovolemia with fluid similar in composition to that lost and to replace ongoing losses. Symptoms and signs, including weight loss, can help estimate the degree of volume contraction and should also be monitored to assess response to treatment. Mild volume contraction can usually be corrected via the oral route. More severe hypovolemia requires intravenous therapy. Isotonic or normal saline (0.9% NaCl or 154 mmol/L Na^+) is the solution of choice in normonatremic and mildly hyponatremic individuals and should be administered initially in patients with hypotension or shock. Severe hyponatremia may require hypertonic saline (3.0% NaCl or 513 mmol/L Na^+). Hypernatremia reflects a proportionally greater deficit of water than Na^+, and its correction will therefore require a hypotonic solution such as half-normal saline (0.45% NaCl or 77 mmol/L Na^+) or 5% dextrose in water. Patients with significant hemorrhage, anemia, or intravascular volume depletion may require blood transfusion or colloid-containing solutions (albumin, dextran). Hypokalemia may be present initially or may ensue as a result of increased urinary K^+ excretion; it should be corrected by adding appropriate amounts of KCl to replacement solutions.

HYPONATREMIA

ETIOLOGY   A plasma Na^+ concentration less than 135 mmol/L usually reflects a hypotonic state. However, plasma osmolality may be normal or increased in some cases of hyponatremia. Isotonic or slightly hypotonic hyponatremia may complicate transurethral resection of the prostate or bladder because large volumes of isoosmotic (mannitol) or hypoosmotic (sorbital or glycine) bladder irrigation solution can be absorbed and result in a dilutional hyponatremia. The metabolism of sorbitol and glycine to CO_2 and water may lead to hypotonicity if the accumulated fluid and solutes are not rapidly excreted. Hypertonic hyponatremia is usually due to hyperglycemia or, occasionally, intravenous administration of mannitol. Relative insulin deficiency causes myocytes to become impermeable to glucose. Therefore, during poorly controlled diabetes mellitus, glucose is an effective osmole and draws water from muscle cells, resulting in hyponatremia. Plasma Na^+ concentration falls by 1.4 mmol/L for every 100 mg/dL rise in the plasma glucose concentration.

Most causes of hyponatremia are associated with a low plasma osmolality (Table 41-2). In general, hypotonic hyponatremia is due either to a primary water gain (and secondary Na^+ loss) or a primary Na^+ loss (and secondary water gain). In the absence of water intake or hypotonic fluid replacement, hyponatremia is usually associated with hypovolemic shock due to a profound sodium deficit and transcellular water shift. Contraction of the ECF volume stimulates thirst and AVP secretion. The increased water ingestion and impaired renal excretion result in hyponatremia. It is important to note that *diuretic-induced hyponatremia* is almost always due to thiazide diuretics. Loop diuretics decrease the tonicity of the medullary interstitium and impair maximal urinary concentrating capacity. This limits the ability of AVP to promote water retention. In contrast, thiazide diuretics lead to Na^+ and K^+ depletion and AVP-mediated water retention. Hyponatremia can also occur by a process of *desalination*. This occurs when the urine

TABLE 41-2 Causes of Hyponatremia

I. Pseudohyponatremia
   A. Normal plasma osmolality
      1. Hyperlipidemia
      2. Hyperproteinemia
      3. Posttransurethral resection of prostate/bladder tumor
   B. Increased plasma osmolality
      1. Hyperglycemia
      2. Mannitol
II. Hypoosmolal hyponatremia
   A. Primary Na^+ loss (secondary water gain)
      1. Integumentary loss: sweating, burns
      2. Gastrointestinal loss: vomiting, tube drainage, fistula, obstruction, diarrhea
      3. Renal loss: diuretics, osmotic diuresis, hypoaldosteronism, salt-wasting nephropathy, postobstructive diuresis, nonoliguric acute tubular necrosis
   B. Primary water gain (secondary Na^+ loss)
      1. Primary polydipsia
      2. Decreased solute intake (e.g., beer potomania)
      3. AVP release due to pain, nausea, drugs
      4. Syndrome of inappropriate AVP secretion
      5. Glucocorticoid deficiency
      6. Hypothyroidism
      7. Chronic renal insufficiency
   C. Primary Na^+ gain (exceeded by secondary water gain)
      1. Heart failure
      2. Hepatic cirrhosis
      3. Nephrotic syndrome

tonicity (the sum of the concentrations of Na^+ and K^+) exceeds that of administered intravenous fluids (including isotonic saline). This accounts for some cases of acute postoperative hyponatremia and cerebral salt wasting after neurosurgery.

Hyponatremia in the setting of ECF volume expansion is usually associated with edematous states, such as congestive heart failure, hepatic cirrhosis, and the nephrotic syndrome. These disorders all have in common a decreased effective circulating arterial volume, leading to increased thirst and increased AVP levels. Additional factors impairing the excretion of solute-free water include a reduced GFR, decreased delivery of ultrafiltrate to the diluting site (due to increased proximal fractional reabsorption of Na^+ and water), and diuretic therapy. The degree of hyponatremia often correlates with the severity of the underlying condition and is an important prognostic factor. Oliguric acute and chronic renal failure may be associated with hyponatremia if water intake exceeds the ability to excrete equivalent volumes.

Hyponatremia in the absence of ECF volume contraction, decreased effective circulating arterial volume, or renal insufficiency is usually due to increased AVP secretion resulting in impaired water excretion. Ingestion or administration of water is also required since high levels of AVP alone are usually insufficient to produce hyponatremia. This disorder, commonly termed the *syndrome of inappropriate antidiuretic hormone secretion* (SIADH), is the most common cause of normovolemic hyponatremia and is due to the nonphysiologic release of AVP from the posterior pituitary or an ectopic source (Chap. 319). Renal free water excretion is impaired while the regulation of Na^+ balance is unaffected. The most common causes of SIADH include neuropsychiatric and pulmonary diseases, malignant tumors, major surgery (postoperative pain), and pharmacologic agents. Severe pain and nausea are physiologic stimuli of AVP secretion; these stimuli are inappropriate in the absence of hypovolemia or hyperosmolality. The pattern of AVP secretion can be used to classify SIADH into four subtypes: (1) erratic autonomous AVP secretion (ectopic production); (2) normal regulation of AVP release around a lower osmolality set point or *reset osmostat* (cachexia, malnutrition); (3) normal AVP response to hypertonicity with failure to suppress completely at low osmolality (incomplete pituitary stalk section); and (4) normal AVP secretion with increased sensitivity to its actions or secretion of some other antidiuretic factor (rare).

Hormonal excess or deficiency may cause hyponatremia. Adrenal insufficiency (Chap. 321) and hypothyroidism (Chap. 320) may present with hyponatremia and should not be confused with SIADH. Although decreased mineralocorticoids may contribute to the hyponatremia of adrenal insufficiency, it is the cortisol deficiency that leads to hypersecretion of AVP both indirectly (secondary to volume depletion) and directly (cosecreted with corticotropin-releasing factor). The mechanisms by which hypothyroidism leads to hyponatremia include decreased cardiac output and GFR and increased AVP secretion in response to hemodynamic stimuli.

Finally, hyponatremia may occur in the absence of AVP or renal failure if the kidney is unable to excrete the dietary water load. In psychogenic or primary polydipsia, compulsive water consumption may overwhelm the normally large renal excretory capacity of 12 L/d (Chap. 319). These patients often have psychiatric illnesses and may be taking medications, such as phenothiazines, that enhance the sensation of thirst by causing a dry mouth. The maximal urine output is a function of the minimum urine osmolality achievable and the mandatory solute excretion. Metabolism of a normal diet generates about 600 mosmol/d, and the minimum urine osmolality in humans is 50 mosmol/kg. Therefore, the maximum daily urine output will be about 12 L (600 ÷ 50 = 12). A solute excretion rate of greater than ~750 mosmol/d is, by definition, an *osmotic diuresis*. A low-protein diet may yield as few as 250 mosmol/d, which translates into a maximal urine output of 5 L/d at a minimum urine tonicity of 50 mosmol/kg. Beer drinkers typically have a poor dietary intake of protein and electrolytes and consume large volumes (of beer), which may exceed the renal excretory capacity and result in hyponatremia. This phenomenon is referred to as *beer potomania*.

CLINICAL FEATURES The clinical manifestations of hyponatremia are related to osmotic water shift leading to increased ICF volume, specifically brain cell swelling or cerebral edema. Therefore, the symptoms are primarily neurologic, and their severity is dependent on the rapidity of onset and absolute decrease in plasma Na^+ concentration. Patients may be asymptomatic or complain of nausea and malaise. As the plasma Na^+ concentration falls, the symptoms progress to include headache, lethargy, confusion, and obtundation. Stupor, seizures, and coma do not usually occur unless the plasma Na^+ concentration falls acutely below 120 mmol/L or decreases rapidly. As described above, adaptive mechanisms designed to protect cell volume occur in chronic hyponatremia. Loss of Na^+ and K^+, followed by organic osmolytes, from brain cells decreases brain swelling due to secondary transcellular water shifts (from ICF to ECF). The net effect is to minimize cerebral edema and its symptoms.

DIAGNOSIS (Fig. 41-1) Hyponatremia is not a disease but a manifestation of a variety of disorders. The underlying cause can often be ascertained from an accurate history and physical examination, including an assessment of ECF volume status and effective circulating arterial volume. The differential diagnosis of hyponatremia, an expanded ECF volume, and decreased effective circulating volume includes congestive heart failure, hepatic cirrhosis, and the nephrotic syndrome. Hypothyroidism and adrenal insufficiency tend to present with a near-normal ECF volume and decreased effective circulating arterial volume. All of these diseases have characteristic signs and symptoms. Patients with SIADH are usually euvolemic.

Four laboratory findings often provide useful information and can narrow the differential diagnosis of hyponatremia: (1) the plasma osmolality, (2) the urine osmolality, (3) the urine Na^+ concentration, and (4) the urine K^+ concentration. Since ECF tonicity is determined primarily by the Na^+ concentration, most patients with hyponatremia have a decreased plasma osmolality. The appropriate renal response to hypoosmolality is to excrete the maximum volume of dilute urine, i.e., urine osmolality and specific gravity of less than 100 mosmol/kg and 1.003, respectively. This occurs in patients with primary polydipsia. If this is not present, it suggests impaired free water excretion due

FIGURE 41-1 Algorithm depicting clinical approach to hyponatremia. ECF, extracellular fluid; SIADH, syndrome of inappropriate antidiuretic hormone secretion.

to the action of AVP on the kidney. The secretion of AVP may be a physiologic response to hemodynamic stimuli or it may be inappropriate in the presence of hyponatremia and euvolemia. Since Na+ is the major ECF cation and is largely restricted to this compartment, ECF volume contraction represents a deficit in total body Na+ content. Therefore, volume depletion in patients with normal underlying renal function results in enhanced tubule Na+ reabsorption and a urine Na+ concentration less than 20 mmol/L. The finding of a urine Na+ concentration greater than 20 mmol/L in hypovolemic hyponatremia implies a salt-wasting nephropathy, diuretic therapy, hypoaldosteronism, or occasionally vomiting. Both the urine osmolality and the urine Na+ concentration can be followed serially when assessing response to therapy.

SIADH is characterized by hypoosmotic hyponatremia in the setting of an inappropriately concentrated urine (urine osmolality greater than 100 mosmol/kg). Patients are typically normovolemic and have normal Na+ balance. They tend to be mildly volume expanded secondary to water retention and have a urine Na+ excretion rate equal to intake (urine Na+ concentration usually greater than 40 mmol/L). By definition, they have normal renal, adrenal, and thyroid function and usually have normal K+ and acid-base balance. SIADH is often associated with hypouricemia due to the uricosuric state induced by volume expansion. In contrast, hypovolemic patients tend to be hyperuricemic secondary to increased proximal urate reabsorption.

℞ TREATMENT

The goals of therapy are twofold: (1) to raise the plasma Na+ concentration by restricting water intake and promoting water loss; and (2) to correct the underlying disorder. Mild asymptomatic hyponatremia is generally of little clinical significance and requires no treatment. The management of asymptomatic hyponatremia associated with ECF volume contraction should include Na+ repletion, generally in the form

of isotonic saline. The direct effect of the administered NaCl on the plasma Na+ concentration is trivial. However, restoration of euvolemia removes the hemodynamic stimulus for AVP release, allowing the excess free water to be excreted. The hyponatremia associated with edematous states tends to reflect the severity of the underlying disease and is usually asymptomatic. These patients have increased total body water that exceeds the increase in total body Na+ content. Treatment should include restriction of Na+ and water intake, correction of hypokalemia, and promotion of water loss in excess of Na+. The latter may require the use of loop diuretics with replacement of a proportion of the urinary Na+ loss to ensure net free water excretion. Dietary water restriction should be less than the urine output. Correction of the K+ deficit may raise the plasma Na+ concentration by favoring a shift of Na+ out of cells as K+ moves in. Water restriction is also a component of the therapeutic approach to hyponatremia associated with primary polydipsia, renal failure, and SIADH (Chap. 319).

The rate of correction of hyponatremia depends on the absence or presence of neurologic dysfunction. This, in turn, is related to the rapidity of onset and magnitude of the fall in plasma Na+ concentration. In asymptomatic patients, the plasma Na+ concentration should be raised by no more than 0.5 to 1.0 mmol/L per h and by less than 10 to 12 mmol/L over the first 24 h. Acute or severe hyponatremia (plasma Na+ concentration <110 to 115 mmol/L) tends to present with altered mental status and/or seizures and requires more rapid correction. Severe symptomatic hyponatremia should be treated with hypertonic saline, and the plasma Na+ concentration should be raised by 1 to 2 mmol/L per hour for the first 3 to 4 h or until the seizures subside. Once again, the plasma Na+ concentration should probably be raised by no more than 12 mmol/L during the first 24 h. The quantity of Na+ required to increase the plasma Na+ concentration by a given amount can be estimated by multiplying the deficit in plasma Na+ concentration by the total body water.

Under normal conditions, total body water is 50 or 60% of lean body weight in women or men, respectively. Therefore, to raise the plasma Na+ concentration from 105 to 115 mmol/L in a 70-kg man requires 420 mmol [(115 − 105) × 70 × 0.6] of Na+. The risk of correcting hyponatremia too rapidly is the development of the *osmotic demyelination syndrome* (ODS). This is a neurologic disorder characterized by flaccid paralysis, dysarthria, and dysphagia. The diagnosis is usually suspected clinically and can be confirmed by appropriate neuroimaging studies. There is no specific treatment for the disorder, which is associated with significant morbidity and mortality. Patients with chronic hyponatremia are most susceptible to the development of ODS, since their brain cell volume has returned to near normal as a result of the osmotic adaptive mechanisms described above. Therefore, administration of hypertonic saline to these individuals can cause sudden osmotic shrinkage of brain cells. In addition to rapid or overcorrection of hyponatremia, risk factors for ODS include prior cerebral anoxic injury, hypokalemia, and malnutrition, especially secondary to alcoholism. Water restriction in primary polydipsia and intravenous saline therapy in ECF volume–contracted patients may also lead to overly rapid correction of hyponatremia as a result of AVP suppression and a brisk water diuresis. This can be prevented by administration of water or use of an AVP analogue to slow down the rate of free water excretion. →*For further discussion, see Chap. 319.*

HYPERNATREMIA

ETIOLOGY Hypernatremia is defined as a plasma Na+ concentration greater than 145 mmol/L. Since Na+ and its accompanying anions are the major effective ECF osmoles, hypernatremia is a state of hyperosmolality. As a result of the fixed number of ICF particles, maintenance of osmotic equilibrium in hypernatremia results in ICF volume contraction. Hypernatremia may be due to primary Na+ gain or water deficit. The two components of an appropriate response to hypernatremia are increased water intake stimulated by thirst and the excretion of the minimum volume of maximally concentrated urine reflecting AVP secretion in response to an osmotic stimulus.

In practice, the majority of cases of hypernatremia result from the loss of water. Since water is distributed between the ICF and the ECF in a 2:1 ratio, a given amount of solute-free water loss will result in a twofold greater reduction in the ICF compartment than the ECF compartment. For example, consider three scenarios: the loss of 1 L of water, isotonic NaCl, or half-isotonic NaCl. If 1 L of water is lost, the ICF volume will decrease by 667 mL, whereas the ECF volume will fall by only 333 mL. Due to the fact that Na^+ is largely restricted to the ECF, this compartment will decrease by 1 L if the fluid lost is isoosmotic. One liter of half-isotonic NaCl is equivalent to 500 mL of water (one-third ECF, two-thirds ICF) plus 500 mL of isotonic saline (all ECF). Therefore, the loss of 1 L of half-isotonic saline decreases the ECF and ICF volumes by 667 mL and 333 mL, respectively.

The degree of hyperosmolality is typically mild unless the thirst mechanism is abnormal or access to water is limited. The latter occurs in infants, the physically handicapped, patients with impaired mental status, in the postoperative state, and in intubated patients in the intensive care unit. On rare occasions, impaired thirst may be due to *primary hypodipsia*. This usually occurs as a result of damage to the hypothalamic osmoreceptors that control thirst and tends to be associated with abnormal osmotic regulation of AVP secretion. Primary hypodipsia may be due to a variety of pathologic changes including granulomatous disease, vascular occlusion, and tumors. A subset of hypodipsic hypernatremia, referred to as *essential hypernatremia*, does not respond to forced water intake. This appears to be due to a specific osmoreceptor defect resulting in nonosmotic regulation of AVP release. Thus, the hemodynamic effects of water loading lead to AVP suppression and excretion of dilute urine.

The source of free water loss is either renal or extrarenal. Nonrenal loss of water may be due to evaporation from the skin and respiratory tract (insensible losses) or loss from the gastrointestinal tract. Insensible losses are increased with fever, exercise, heat exposure, and severe burns and in mechanically ventilated patients. Furthermore, the Na^+ concentration of sweat decreases with profuse perspiration, thereby increasing solute-free water loss. Diarrhea is the most common gastrointestinal cause of hypernatremia. Specifically, osmotic diarrheas (induced by lactulose, sorbitol, or malabsorption of carbohydrate) and viral gastroenteritides result in water loss exceeding that of Na^+ and K^+. In contrast, secretory diarrheas (e.g., cholera, carcinoid, VIPoma) have a fecal osmolality (twice the sum of the concentrations of Na^+ and K^+) similar to that of plasma and present with ECF volume contraction and a normal plasma Na^+ concentration or hyponatremia.

Renal water loss is the most common cause of hypernatremia and is due to drug-induced or osmotic diuresis or diabetes insipidus (Chap. 319). Loop diuretics interfere with the countercurrent mechanism and produce an isoosmotic solute diuresis. This results in a decreased medullary interstitial tonicity and impaired renal concentrating ability. The presence of non-reabsorbed organic solutes in the tubule lumen impairs the osmotic reabsorption of water. This leads to water loss in excess of Na^+ and K^+, known as an osmotic diuresis. The most frequent cause of an osmotic diuresis is hyperglycemia and glucosuria in poorly controlled diabetes mellitus. Intravenous administration of mannitol and increased endogenous production of urea (high-protein diet) can also result in an osmotic diuresis.

Hypernatremia secondary to nonosmotic urinary water loss is usually due to: (1) Central diabetes insipidus (CDI) characterized by impaired AVP secretion, or (2) NDI resulting from end-organ (renal) resistance to the actions of AVP. The most common cause of CDI is destruction of the neurohypophysis. This may occur as a result of trauma, neurosurgery, granulomatous disease, neoplasms, vascular accidents, or infection. In many cases, CDI is idiopathic and may occasionally be hereditary. The familial form of the disease is inherited in an autosomal dominant fashion and has been attributed to mutations in the propressophysin (AVP precursor) gene. Nephrogenic diabetes insipidus (NDI) may be either inherited or acquired. Congenital NDI is an X-linked recessive trait due to mutations in the V_2 receptor gene. Mutations in the autosomal *aquaporin-2* gene may also result in NDI. The *aquaporin-2* gene encodes the water channel protein whose membrane insertion is stimulated by AVP. The causes of sporadic NDI are numerous and include drugs (especially lithium), hypercalcemia, hypokalemia, and conditions that impair medullary hypertonicity (e.g., papillary necrosis or osmotic diuresis). Pregnant women, in the second or third trimester, may develop NDI as a result of excessive elaboration of vasopressinase by the placenta.

Finally, although infrequent, a primary Na^+ gain may cause hypernatremia. For example, inadvertent administration of hypertonic NaCl or NaHCO₃ or replacing sugar with salt in infant formula can produce this complication.

CLINICAL FEATURES As a consequence of hypertonicity, water shifts out of cells, leading to a contracted ICF volume. A decreased brain cell volume is associated with an increased risk of subarachnoid or intracerebral hemorrhage. Hence, the major symptoms of hypernatremia are neurologic and include altered mental status, weakness, neuromuscular irritability, focal neurologic deficits, and occasionally coma or seizures. Patients may also complain of polyuria or thirst. For unknown reasons, patients with polydipsia from CDI tend to prefer ice-cold water. The signs and symptoms of volume depletion are often present in patients with a history of excessive sweating, diarrhea, or an osmotic diuresis. As with hyponatremia, the severity of the clinical manifestations is related to the acuity and magnitude of the rise in plasma Na^+ concentration. Chronic hypernatremia is generally less symptomatic as a result of adaptive mechanisms designed to defend cell volume. Brain cells initially take up Na^+ and K^+ salts, later followed by accumulation of organic osmolytes such as inositol. This serves to restore the brain ICF volume towards normal.

DIAGNOSIS (Fig. 41-2) A complete history and physical examination will often provide clues as to the underlying cause of hypernatremia. Relevant symptoms and signs include the absence or presence of thirst, diaphoresis, diarrhea, polyuria, and the features of ECF volume contraction. The history should include a list of current and recent medications, and the physical examination is incomplete without a thorough mental status and neurologic assessment. Measurement of urine volume and osmolality are essential in the evaluation of hyperosmolality. The appropriate renal response to hypernatremia is the excretion of the minimum volume (500 mL/d) of maximally concentrated urine (urine osmolality >800 mosmol/kg). These findings suggest extrarenal

FIGURE 41-2 Algorithm depicting clinical approach to hypernatremia.

or remote renal water loss or administration of hypertonic Na$^+$ salt solutions. The presence of a primary Na$^+$ excess can be confirmed by the presence of ECF volume expansion and natriuresis (urine Na$^+$ concentration usually >100 mmol/L).

Many causes of hypernatremia are associated with polyuria and a submaximal urine osmolality. The product of the urine volume and osmolality, i.e., the solute excretion rate, is helpful in determining the basis of the polyuria (see above). To maintain a steady state, total solute excretion must equal solute production. As stated above, individuals eating a normal diet generate ~600 mosmol/d. Therefore, daily solute excretion in excess of 750 mosmol defines an osmotic diuresis. This can be confirmed by measuring the urine glucose and urea. In general, both CDI and NDI present with polyuria and hypotonic urine (urine osmolality <250 mosmol/kg). The degree of hypernatremia is usually mild unless there is an associated thirst abnormality. The clinical history, physical examination, and pertinent laboratory data can often rule out causes of acquired NDI. CDI and NDI can generally be distinguished by administering the AVP analogue desmopressin (10 μg intranasally) after careful water restriction. The urine osmolality should increase by at least 50% in CDI and will not change in NDI. Unfortunately, the diagnosis may sometimes be difficult due to partial defects in AVP secretion and action.

℞ TREATMENT

The therapeutic goals are to stop ongoing water loss by treating the underlying cause and to correct the water deficit. The ECF volume should be restored in hypovolemic patients. The quantity of water required to correct the deficit can be calculated from the following equation:

$$\text{Water deficit} = \frac{\text{Plasma Na}^+ \text{ concentration} - 140}{140} \times \text{Total body water}$$

In hypernatremia due to water loss, total body water is approximately 50 and 40% of lean body weight in men and women, respectively. For example, a 50-kg woman with a plasma Na$^+$ concentration of 160 mmol/L has an estimated free water deficit of 2.9 L {[(160 − 140) ÷ 140] × (0.4 × 50)}. As in hyponatremia, rapid correction of hypernatremia is potentially dangerous. In this case, a sudden decrease in osmolality could potentially cause a rapid shift of water into cells that have undergone osmotic adaptation. This would result in swollen brain cells and increase the risk of seizures or permanent neurologic damage. Therefore, the water deficit should be corrected slowly over at least 48 to 72 h. When calculating the rate of water replacement, ongoing losses should be taken into account, and the plasma Na$^+$ concentration should be lowered by 0.5 mmol/L per h and by no more than 12 mmol/L over the first 24 h.

The safest route of administration of water is by mouth or via a nasogastric tube (or other feeding tube). Alternatively, 5% dextrose in water or half-isotonic saline can be given intravenously. The appropriate treatment of CDI consists of administering desmopressin intranasally (Chap. 319). Other options for decreasing urine output include a low-salt diet in combination with low-dose thiazide diuretic therapy. In some patients with partial CDI, drugs that either stimulate AVP secretion or enhance its action on the kidney have been useful. These include chlorpropamide, clofibrate, carbamazepine, and nonsteroidal anti-inflammatory drugs (NSAIDs). The concentrating defect in NDI may be reversible by treating the underlying disorder or eliminating the offending drug. Symptomatic polyuria due to NDI can be treated with a low-Na$^+$ diet and thiazide diuretics as described above. This induces mild volume depletion, which leads to enhanced proximal reabsorption of salt and water and decreased delivery to the site of action of AVP, the collecting duct. By impairing renal prostaglandin synthesis, NSAIDs potentiate AVP action and thereby increase urine osmolality and decrease urine volume. Amiloride may be useful in patients with NDI who need to be on lithium. The nephrotoxicity of lithium requires the drug to be taken up into collecting duct cells via the amiloride-sensitive Na$^+$ channel.

POTASSIUM

POTASSIUM BALANCE Potassium is the major intracellular cation. The normal plasma K$^+$ concentration is 3.5 to 5.0 mmol/L, whereas that inside cells is about 150 mmol/L. Therefore, the amount of K$^+$ in the ECF (30 to 70 mmol) constitutes less than 2% of the total body K$^+$ content (2500 to 4500 mmol). The ratio of ICF to ECF K$^+$ concentration (normally 38:1) is the principal result of the resting membrane potential and is crucial for normal neuromuscular function. The basolateral Na$^+$, K$^+$-ATPase pump actively transports K$^+$ in and Na$^+$ out of the cell in a 2:3 ratio, and the passive outward diffusion of K$^+$ is quantitatively the most important factor that generates the resting membrane potential. The activity of the electrogenic Na$^+$, K$^+$-ATPase pump may be stimulated as a result of an increased intracellular Na$^+$ concentration and inhibited in the setting of digoxin toxicity or chronic illness such as heart failure or renal failure.

The K$^+$ intake of individuals on an average western diet is 40 to 120 mmol/d or approximately 1 mmol/kg per day, 90% of which is absorbed by the gastrointestinal tract. Maintenance of the steady state necessitates matching K$^+$ ingestion with excretion. Initially, extrarenal adaptive mechanisms, followed later by urinary excretion, prevent a doubling of the plasma K$^+$ concentration that would occur if the dietary K$^+$ load remained in the ECF compartment. Immediately following a meal, most of the absorbed K$^+$ enters cells as a result of the initial elevation in the plasma K$^+$ concentration and facilitated by insulin release and basal catecholamine levels. Eventually, however, the excess K$^+$ is excreted in the urine (see below). The regulation of gastrointestinal K$^+$ handling is not well understood. The amount of K$^+$ lost in the stool can increase from 10 to 50 or 60% (of dietary intake) in chronic renal insufficiency. In addition, colonic secretion of K$^+$ is stimulated in patients with large volumes of diarrhea, resulting in potentially severe K$^+$ depletion.

POTASSIUM EXCRETION (See also Chap. 259) Renal excretion is the major route of elimination of dietary and other sources of excess K$^+$. The filtered load of K$^+$ (GFR × plasma K$^+$ concentration = 180 L/d × 4 mmol/L = 720 mmol/d) is 10- to 20-fold greater than the ECF K$^+$ content. Some 90% of filtered K$^+$ is reabsorbed by the proximal convoluted tubule and loop of Henle. Proximally, K$^+$ is reabsorbed passively with Na$^+$ and water, whereas the luminal Na$^+$-K$^+$-2Cl$^-$ cotransporter mediates K$^+$ uptake in the thick ascending limb of the loop of Henle. Therefore, K$^+$ delivery to the distal nephron [distal convoluted tubule and cortical collecting duct (CCD)] approximates dietary intake. Net distal K$^+$ secretion or reabsorption occurs in the setting of K$^+$ excess or depletion, respectively. The cell responsible for K$^+$ secretion in the late distal convoluted tubule (or connecting tubule) and CCD is the principal cell. Virtually all regulation of renal K$^+$ excretion and total body K$^+$ balance occurs in the distal nephron. Potassium secretion is regulated by two physiologic stimuli—aldosterone and hyperkalemia. Aldosterone is secreted by the zona glomerulosa cells of the adrenal cortex in response to high renin and angiotensin II or hyperkalemia. The plasma K$^+$ concentration, independent of aldosterone, can directly affect K$^+$ secretion. In addition to the K$^+$ concentration in the lumen of the CCD, renal K$^+$ loss depends on the urine flow rate, a function of daily solute excretion (see above). Since excretion is equal to the product of concentration and volume, increased distal flow rate can significantly enhance urinary K$^+$ output. Finally, in severe K$^+$ depletion, secretion of K$^+$ is reduced and reabsorption in the cortical and medullary collecting ducts is upregulated.

HYPOKALEMIA

ETIOLOGY (See Table 41-3) Hypokalemia, defined as a plasma K$^+$ concentration <3.5 mmol/L, may result from one (or more) of the following: decreased net intake, shift into cells, or increased net loss. Diminished intake is seldom the sole cause of K$^+$ depletion since urinary excretion can be effectively decreased to less than 15 mmol/d as a

I. Decreased intake
  A. Starvation
  B. Clay ingestion
II. Redistribution into cells
  A. Acid-base
    1. Metabolic alkalosis
  B. Hormonal
    1. Insulin
    2. β_2-Adrenergic agonists (endogenous or exogenous)
    3. α-Adrenergic antagonists
  C. Anabolic state
    1. Vitamin B_{12} or folic acid (red blood cell production)
    2. Granulocyte-macrophage colony stimulating factor (white blood cell production)
    3. Total parenteral nutrition
  D. Other
    1. Pseudohypokalemia
    2. Hypothermia
    3. Hypokalemic periodic paralysis
    4. Barium toxicity
III. Increased loss
  A. Nonrenal
    1. Gastrointestinal loss (diarrhea)
    2. Integumentary loss (sweat)
  B. Renal
    1. Increased distal flow: diuretics, osmotic diuresis, salt-wasting nephropathies
    2. Increased secretion of potassium
      a. Mineralocorticoid excess: primary hyperaldosteronism, secondary hyperaldosteronism (malignant hypertension, renin-secreting tumors, renal artery stenosis, hypovolemia), apparent mineralocorticoid excess (licorice, chewing tobacco, carbenoxolone), congenital adrenal hyperplasia, Cushing's syndrome, Bartter's syndrome
      b. Distal delivery of non-reabsorbed anions: vomiting, nasogastric suction, proximal (type 2) renal tubular acidosis, diabetic ketoacidosis, glue-sniffing (toluene abuse), penicillin derivatives
      c. Other: amphotericin B, Liddle's syndrome, hypomagnesemia

result of net K^+ reabsorption in the distal nephron. With the exception of the urban poor and certain cultural groups, the amount of K^+ in the diet almost always exceeds that excreted in the urine. However, dietary K^+ restriction may exacerbate the hypokalemia secondary to increased gastrointestinal or renal loss. An unusual cause of decreased K^+ intake is ingestion of clay (geophagia), which binds dietary K^+ and iron. This custom was previously common among African Americans in the American South.

Redistribution into Cells Movement of K^+ into cells may transiently decrease the plasma K^+ concentration without altering total body K^+ content. For any given cause, the magnitude of the change is relatively small, often less than 1 mmol/L. However, a combination of factors may lead to a significant fall in the plasma K^+ concentration and may amplify the hypokalemia due to K^+ wasting. Metabolic alkalosis is often associated with hypokalemia. This occurs as a result of K^+ redistribution as well as excessive renal K^+ loss. Treatment of diabetic ketoacidosis with insulin may lead to hypokalemia due to stimulation of the Na^+-H^+ antiporter and (secondarily) the Na^+, K^+-ATPase pump. Furthermore, uncontrolled hyperglycemia often leads to K^+ depletion from an osmotic diuresis (see below). Stress-induced catecholamine release and administration of β_2-adrenergic agonists directly induce cellular uptake of K^+ and promote insulin secretion by pancreatic islet β cells. *Hypokalemic periodic paralysis* is a rare condition characterized by recurrent episodic weakness or paralysis (Chap. 367). Since K^+ is the major ICF cation, anabolic states can potentially result in hypokalemia due to a K^+ shift into cells. This may occur following rapid cell growth seen in patients with pernicious anemia treated with vitamin B_{12} or with neutropenia after treatment with granulocyte-macrophage colony stimulating factor. Massive transfusion with thawed washed red blood cells (RBCs) could cause hypokalemia since frozen RBCs lose up to half of their K^+ during storage.

Nonrenal Loss of Potassium Excessive sweating may result in K^+ depletion from increased integumentary and renal K^+ loss. Hyperaldosteronism, secondary to ECF volume contraction, enhances K^+ excretion in the urine (Chap. 321). Normally, K^+ lost in the stool amounts to 5 to 10 mmol/d in a volume of 100 to 200 mL. Hypokalemia subsequent to increased gastrointestinal loss can occur in patients with profuse diarrhea (usually secretory), villous adenomas, VIPomas, or laxative abuse. However, the loss of gastric secretions does not account for the moderate to severe K^+ depletion often associated with vomiting or nasogastric suction. Since the K^+ concentration of gastric fluid is 5 to 10 mmol/L, it would take 30 to 80 L of vomitus to achieve a K^+ deficit of 300 to 400 mmol typically seen in these patients. In fact, the hypokalemia is primarily due to increased renal K^+ excretion. Loss of gastric contents results in volume depletion and metabolic alkalosis, both of which promote kaliuresis. Hypovolemia stimulates aldosterone release, which augments K^+ secretion by the principal cells. In addition, the filtered load of HCO_3^- exceeds the reabsorptive capacity of the proximal convoluted tubule, thereby increasing distal delivery of $NaHCO_3$, which enhances the electrochemical gradient favoring K^+ loss in the urine.

Renal Loss of Potassium (See also Chap. 321) In general, most cases of chronic hypokalemia are due to renal K^+ wasting. This may be due to factors that increase the K^+ concentration in the lumen of the CCD or augment distal flow rate. Mineralocorticoid excess commonly results in hypokalemia. *Primary hyperaldosteronism* is due to dysregulated aldosterone secretion by an adrenal adenoma (Conn's syndrome) or carcinoma or to adrenocortical hyperplasia. In a rare subset of patients, the disorder is familial (autosomal dominant) and aldosterone levels can be suppressed by administering low doses of exogenous glucocorticoid. The molecular defect responsible for *glucocorticoid-remediable hyperaldosteronism* is a rearranged gene (due to a chromosomal crossover), containing the 5′-regulatory region of the 11β-hydroxylase gene and the coding sequence of the aldosterone synthase gene. Consequently, mineralocorticoid is synthesized in the zona fasciculata and regulated by corticotropin. A number of conditions associated with hyperreninemia result in secondary hyperaldosteronism and renal K^+ wasting. High renin levels are commonly seen in both renovascular and malignant hypertension. Renin-secreting tumors of the juxtaglomerular apparatus are a rare cause of hypokalemia. Other tumors that have been reported to produce renin include renal cell carcinoma, ovarian carcinoma, and Wilms' tumor. Hyperreninemia may also occur secondary to decreased effective circulating arterial volume.

In the absence of elevated renin or aldosterone levels, enhanced distal nephron secretion of K^+ may result from increased production of non-aldosterone mineralocorticoids in *congenital adrenal hyperplasia*. Glucocorticoid-stimulated kaliuresis does not normally occur due to the conversion of cortisol to cortisone by 11β-hydroxysteroid dehydrogenase (11β-HSDH). Therefore, 11β-HSDH deficiency or suppression allows cortisol to bind to the aldosterone receptor and leads to the *syndrome of apparent mineralocorticoid excess*. Drugs that inhibit the activity of 11β-HSDH include glycyrrhetinic acid, present in licorice, chewing tobacco, and carbenoxolone. The presentation of Cushing's syndrome may include hypokalemia if the capacity of 11β-HSDH to inactivate cortisol is overwhelmed by persistently elevated glucocorticoid levels.

Liddle's syndrome is a rare familial (autosomal dominant) disease characterized by hypertension, hypokalemic metabolic alkalosis, renal K^+ wasting, and suppressed renin and aldosterone secretion. Increased distal delivery of Na^+ with a non-reabsorbable anion (not Cl^-) enhances K^+ secretion. Classically, this is seen with *proximal (type 2) renal tubular acidosis* (RTA) and vomiting, associated with bicarbonaturia. Diabetic ketoacidosis and toluene abuse (glue-sniffing) can lead to increased delivery of β-hydroxybutyrate and hippurate, respectively, to the CCD and to renal K^+ loss. High doses of penicillin derivatives administered to volume-depleted patients may likewise promote renal K⁺ secretion as well as an osmotic diuresis. *Classic distal (type 1) RTA* is associated with hypokalemia due to increased renal K⁺ loss, the mechanism of which is uncertain. Amphotericin B causes hypokalemia due to increased distal nephron permeability to Na⁺ and K⁺ and to renal K⁺ wasting.

Bartter's syndrome is a disorder characterized by hypokalemia, metabolic alkalosis, hyperreninemic hyperaldosteronism secondary to ECF volume contraction, and juxtaglomerular apparatus hyperplasia. Finally, diuretic use and abuse are common causes of K⁺ depletion. Carbonic anhydrase inhibitors, loop diuretics, and thiazides are all kaliuretic. The degree of hypokalemia tends to be greater with long-acting agents and is dose-dependent. Increased renal K⁺ excretion is due primarily to increased distal solute delivery and secondary hyperaldosteronism (due to volume depletion).

CLINICAL FEATURES The clinical manifestations of K⁺ depletion vary greatly between individual patients, and their severity depends on the degree of hypokalemia. Symptoms seldom occur unless the plasma K⁺ concentration is less than 3 mmol/L. Fatigue, myalgia, and muscular weakness of the lower extremities are common complaints and are due to a lower (more negative) resting membrane potential. More severe hypokalemia may lead to progressive weakness, hypoventilation (due to respiratory muscle involvement), and eventually complete paralysis. Impaired muscle metabolism and the blunted hyperemic response to exercise associated with profound K⁺ depletion increase the risk of rhabdomyolysis. Smooth-muscle function may also be affected and manifest as paralytic ileus.

The electrocardiographic changes of hypokalemia (Fig. 210-17) are due to delayed ventricular repolarization and do not correlate well with the plasma K⁺ concentration. Early changes include flattening or inversion of the T wave, a prominent U wave, ST-segment depression, and a prolonged QU interval. Severe K⁺ depletion may result in a prolonged PR interval, decreased voltage and widening of the QRS complex, and an increased risk of ventricular arrhythmias, especially in patients with myocardial ischemia or left ventricular hypertrophy. Hypokalemia may also predispose to digitalis toxicity. Hypokalemia is often associated with acid-base disturbances related to the underlying disorder. In addition, K⁺ depletion results in intracellular acidification and an increase in net acid excretion or new HCO_3^- production. This is a consequence of enhanced proximal HCO_3^- reabsorption, increased renal ammoniagenesis, and increased distal H⁺ secretion. This contributes to the generation of metabolic alkalosis frequently present in hypokalemic patients. NDI (see above) is not uncommonly seen in K⁺ depletion and is manifest as polydipsia and polyuria. Glucose intolerance may also occur with hypokalemia and has been attributed to either impaired insulin secretion or peripheral insulin resistance.

DIAGNOSIS (Fig. 41-3) In most cases, the etiology of K⁺ depletion can be determined by a careful history. Diuretic and laxative abuse as well as surreptitious vomiting may be difficult to identify but should be excluded. Rarely, patients with a marked leukocytosis (e.g., acute myeloid leukemia) and normokalemia may have a low measured plasma K⁺ concentration due to white blood cell uptake of K⁺ at room temperature. This *pseudohypokalemia* can be avoided by storing the blood sample on ice or rapidly separating the plasma (or serum) from the cells.

After eliminating decreased intake and intracellular shift as potential causes of hypokalemia, examination of the renal response can help to clarify the source of K⁺ loss. The appropriate response to K⁺ depletion is to excrete less than 15 mmol/d of K⁺ in the urine, due to increased reabsorption and decreased distal secretion. Hypokalemia with minimal renal K⁺ excretion suggests that K⁺ was lost via the skin or gastrointestinal tract or that there is a remote history of vomiting or diuretic use. As described above, renal K⁺ wasting may be due to factors that either increase the K⁺ concentration in the CCD or increase the distal flow rate (or both). The ECF volume status, blood pressure,

FIGURE 41-3 Algorithm depicting clinical approach to hypokalemia. TTKG, transtubular K⁺ concentration gradient; RTA, renal tubular acidosis.

and associated acid-base disorder may help to differentiate the causes of excessive renal K⁺ loss. A rapid and simple test designed to evaluate the driving force for net K⁺ secretion is the *transtubular K⁺ concentration gradient* (TTKG). The TTKG is the ratio of the K⁺ concentration in the lumen of the CCD ($[K^+]_{CCD}$) to that in peritubular capillaries or plasma ($[K^+]_P$). The validity of this measurement depends on three assumptions: (1) few solutes are reabsorbed in the medullary collecting duct (MCD), (2) K⁺ is neither secreted nor reabsorbed in the MCD, and (3) the osmolality of the fluid in the terminal CCD is known. Significant reabsorption or secretion of K⁺ in the MCD seldom occurs, except in profound K⁺ depletion or excess, respectively. When AVP is acting ($OSM_U \geq OSM_P$), the osmolality in the terminal CCD is the same as that of plasma, and the K⁺ concentration in the lumen of the distal nephron can be estimated by dividing the urine K⁺ concentration ($[K^+]_U$) by the ratio of the urine to plasma osmolality (OSM_U/OSM_P):

$$[K^+]_{CCD} = [K^+]_U \div (OSM_U/OSM_P)$$

$$TTKG = \frac{[K^+]_{CCD}}{[K^+]_P} = \frac{[K^+]_U \div (OSM_U/OSM_P)}{[K^+]_P}$$

Hypokalemia with a TTKG greater than 4 suggests renal K⁺ loss due to increased distal K⁺ secretion. Plasma renin and aldosterone levels are often helpful in differentiating the various causes of hyperaldosteronism. Bicarbonaturia and the presence of other non-reabsorbed anions also increase the TTKG and lead to renal K⁺-wasting.

℞ **TREATMENT**

The therapeutic goals are to correct the K⁺ deficit and to minimize ongoing losses. With the exception of periodic paralysis, hypokalemia resulting from transcellular shifts rarely requires intravenous K⁺ supplementation, which can lead to rebound hyperkalemia. It is generally safer to correct hypokalemia via the oral route. The degree of K⁺ depletion does not correlate well with the plasma K⁺ concentration. A decrement of 1 mmol/L in the plasma K$^+$ concentration (from 4.0 to 3.0 mmol/L) may represent a total body K$^+$ deficit of 200 to 400 mmol, and patients with plasma levels under 3.0 mmol/L often require in excess of 600 mmol of K$^+$ to correct the deficit. Furthermore, factors promoting K$^+$ shift out of cells (e.g., insulin deficiency in diabetic ketoacidosis) may result in underestimation of the K$^+$ deficit. There- fore, the plasma K$^+$ concentration should be monitored frequently when assessing the response to treatment. Potassium chloride is usu- ally the preparation of choice and will promote more rapid correction of hypokalemia and metabolic alkalosis. Potassium bicarbonate and citrate (metabolized to HCO$_3^-$) tend to alkalinize the patient and would be more appropriate for hypokalemia associated with chronic diarrhea or RTA.

Patients with severe hypokalemia or those unable to take anything by mouth require intravenous replacement therapy with KCl. The max- imum concentration of administered K$^+$ should be no more than 40 mmol/L via a peripheral vein or 60 mmol/L via a central vein. The rate of infusion should not exceed 20 mmol/h unless paralysis or ma- lignant ventricular arrhythmias are present. Ideally, KCl should be mixed in normal saline since dextrose solutions may initially exacer- bate hypokalemia due to insulin-mediated movement of K$^+$ into cells. Rapid intravenous administration of K$^+$ should be used judiciously and requires close observation of the clinical manifestations of hypo- kalemia (electrocardiogram and neuromuscular examination).

HYPERKALEMIA

ETIOLOGY Hyperkalemia, defined as a plasma K$^+$ concentration >5.0 mmol/L, occurs as a result of either K$^+$ release from cells or decreased renal loss. Increased K$^+$ intake is rarely the sole cause of hyperkalemia since the phenomenon of *potassium adaptation* ensures rapid K$^+$ ex- cretion in response to increases in dietary consumption. Iatrogenic hyperkalemia may result from overzealous parenteral K$^+$ replacement or in patients with renal insufficiency. *Pseudohyperkalemia* represents an artificially elevated plasma K$^+$ concentration due to K$^+$ movement out of cells immediately prior to or following venipuncture. Contrib- uting factors include prolonged use of a tourniquet with or without repeated fist clenching, hemolysis, and marked leukocytosis or throm- bocytosis. The latter two result in an elevated serum K$^+$ concentration due to release of intracellular K$^+$ following clot formation. Pseudo- hyperkalemia should be suspected in an otherwise asymptomatic pa- tient with no obvious underlying cause. If proper venipuncture tech- nique is used and a plasma (not serum) K$^+$ concentration is measured, it should be normal. Intravascular hemolysis, tumor lysis syndrome, and rhabdomyolysis all lead to K$^+$ release from cells as a result of tissue breakdown.

Metabolic acidoses, with the exception of those due to the accu- mulation of organic anions, can be associated with mild hyperkalemia resulting from intracellular buffering of H$^+$ (see above). Insulin defi- ciency and hypertonicity (e.g., hyperglycemia) promote K$^+$ shift from the ICF to the ECF. The severity of exercise-induced hyperkalemia is related to the degree of exertion. It is due to release of K$^+$ from muscles and is usually rapidly reversible, often associated with rebound hy- pokalemia. Treatment with beta blockers rarely causes hyperkalemia but may contribute to the elevation in plasma K$^+$ concentration seen with other conditions. *Hyperkalemic periodic paralysis* (Chap. 367) is a rare autosomal dominant disorder characterized by episodic weak- ness or paralysis, precipitated by stimuli that normally lead to mild hyperkalemia (e.g., exercise). The genetic defect appears to be a single amino acid substitution due to a mutation in the gene for the skeletal muscle Na$^+$ channel. Hyperkalemia may occur with severe digitalis toxicity due to inhibition of the Na$^+$,K$^+$-ATPase pump. Depolarizing muscle relaxants such as succinylcholine can increase the plasma K$^+$ concentration, especially in patients with massive trauma, burns, or neuromuscular disease.

Chronic hyperkalemia is virtually always associated with decreased renal K$^+$ excretion due to either impaired secretion or diminished distal solute delivery (Table 41-4). The latter is seldom the only cause of impaired K$^+$ excretion but may significantly contribute to hyperkale-

TABLE 41-4 *Causes of Hyperkalemia*

I. Renal failure
II. Decreased distal flow (i.e., decreased effective circulating arterial volume)
III. Decreased K$^+$ secretion
  A. Impaired Na$^+$ reabsorption
    1. Primary hypoaldosteronism: adrenal insufficiency, adrenal enzyme deficiency (21-hydroxylase, 3β-hydroxysteroid dehydrogenase, corticosterone methyl oxidase)
    2. Secondary hypoaldosteronism: hyporeninemia, drugs (ACE inhibitors, NSAIDs, heparin)
    3. Resistance to aldosterone: pseudohypoaldosteronism, tubulointerstitial disease, drugs (K$^+$-sparing diuretics, trimethoprim, pentamidine)
  B. Enhanced Cl$^-$ reabsorption (chloride shunt)
    1. Gordon's syndrome
    2. Cyclosporine

Note: ACE, angiotensin-converting enzyme; NSAIDs, nonsteroidal anti-inflammatory drugs.

mia in protein-malnourished (low urea excretion) and ECF volume– contracted (decreased distal NaCl delivery) patients. Decreased K$^+$ secretion by the principal cells results from either impaired Na$^+$ reab- sorption or increased Cl$^-$ reabsorption.

Hyporeninemic hypoaldosteronism is a syndrome characterized by euvolemia or ECF volume expansion and suppressed renin and aldos- terone levels (Chaps. 321 and 323). This disorder is commonly seen in mild renal insufficiency, diabetic nephropathy, or chronic tubuloin- terstitial disease. Patients frequently have an impaired kaliuretic re- sponse to exogenous mineralocorticoid administration, suggesting that enhanced distal Cl$^-$ reabsorption (electroneutral Na$^+$ reabsorption) may account for many of the findings of hyporeninemic hypoaldo- steronism. NSAIDs inhibit renin secretion and the synthesis of vaso- dilatory renal prostaglandins. The resultant decrease in GFR and K$^+$ secretion is often manifest as hyperkalemia. As a rule, the degree of hyperkalemia due to hypoaldosteronism is mild in the absence of in- creased K$^+$ intake or renal dysfunction.

Angiotensin-converting enzyme (ACE) inhibitors block the con- version of angiotensin I to angiotensin II. Angiotensin receptor antag- onists directly inhibit the actions of angiotensin II on AT1 angiotensin II receptors. The actions of both of these classes of drugs result in impaired aldosterone release. Patients at increased risk of ACE inhib- itor or angiotensin receptor antagonist–induced hyperkalemia include those with diabetes mellitus, renal insufficiency, decreased effective circulating arterial volume, bilateral renal artery stenosis, or concurrent use of K$^+$-sparing diuretics or NSAIDs.

Decreased aldosterone synthesis may be due to *primary adrenal in- sufficiency* (Addison's disease) or congenital adrenal enzyme deficiency (Chap. 321). Heparin (including low-molecular-weight heparin) inhibits production of aldosterone by the cells of the zona glomerulosa and can lead to severe hyperkalemia in a subset of patients with underlying renal disease, diabetes mellitus, or those receiving K$^+$-sparing diuretics, ACE inhibitors, or NSAIDs. *Pseudohypoaldosteronism* is a rare familial dis- order characterized by hyperkalemia, metabolic acidosis, renal Na$^+$ wasting, hypotension, high renin and aldosterone levels, and end-organ resistance to aldosterone. The gene encoding the mineralocorticoid re- ceptor is normal in these patients, and the electrolyte abnormalities can be reversed with suprapharmacologic doses of an exogenous mineral- ocorticoid (e.g., 9α-fludrocortisone) or an inhibitor of 11β-HSDH (e.g., carbenoxolone). The kaliuretic response to aldosterone is impaired by K$^+$-sparing diuretics. Spironolactone is a competitive mineralocorticoid antagonist, whereas amiloride and triamterene block the apical Na$^+$ channel of the principal cell. Two other drugs that impair K$^+$ secretion by blocking distal nephron Na$^+$ reabsorption are trimethoprim and pen- tamidine. These antimicrobial agents may contribute to the hyperkale- mia often seen in patients infected with HIV who are being treated for *Pneumocystis carinii* pneumonia.

Hyperkalemia frequently complicates acute oliguric renal failure due to increased K^+ release from cells (acidosis, catabolism) and decreased excretion. Increased distal flow rate and K^+ secretion per nephron compensate for decreased renal mass in chronic renal insufficiency. However, these adaptive mechanisms eventually fail to maintain K^+ balance when the GFR falls below 10 to 15 mL/min or oliguria ensues. Otherwise asymptomatic urinary tract obstruction is an often overlooked cause of hyperkalemia. Other nephropathies associated with impaired K^+ excretion include drug-induced interstitial nephritis, lupus nephritis, sickle cell disease, and diabetic nephropathy.

Gordon's syndrome is a rare condition characterized by hyperkalemia, metabolic acidosis, and a normal GFR. These patients are usually volume-expanded with suppressed renin and aldosterone levels as well as refractory to the kaliuretic effect of exogenous mineralocorticoids. It has been suggested that these findings could all be accounted for by increased distal Cl^- reabsorption (electroneutral Na^+ reabsorption), also referred to as a *Cl^- shunt*. A similar mechanism may be partially responsible for the hyperkalemia associated with cyclosporine nephrotoxicity. *Hyperkalemic distal (type 4) RTA* may be due to either hypoaldosteronism or a Cl^- shunt (aldosterone-resistant).

CLINICAL FEATURES   Since the resting membrane potential is related to the ratio of the ICF to ECF K^+ concentration, hyperkalemia partially depolarizes the cell membrane. Prolonged depolarization impairs membrane excitability and is manifest as weakness, which may progress to flaccid paralysis and hypoventilation if the respiratory muscles are involved. Hyperkalemia also inhibits renal ammoniagenesis and reabsorption of NH_4^+ in the thick ascending limb of the loop of Henle. Thus, net acid excretion is impaired and results in metabolic acidosis, which may further exacerbate the hyperkalemia due to K^+ movement out of cells.

The most serious effect of hyperkalemia is cardiac toxicity, which does not correlate well with the plasma K^+ concentration. The earliest electrocardiographic changes include increased T-wave amplitude, or peaked T waves. More severe degrees of hyperkalemia result in a prolonged PR interval and QRS duration, atrioventricular conduction delay, and loss of P waves. Progressive widening of the QRS complex and merging with the T wave produces a sine wave pattern. The terminal event is usually ventricular fibrillation or asystole.

DIAGNOSIS (Fig. 41-4)   With rare exceptions, chronic hyperkalemia is always due to impaired K^+ excretion. If the etiology is not readily apparent and the patient is asymptomatic, pseudohyperkalemia should be excluded, as described above. Oliguric acute renal failure and severe chronic renal insufficiency should also be ruled out. The history should focus on medications that impair K^+ handling and potential sources of K^+ intake. Evaluation of the ECF compartment, effective circulating volume, and urine output are essential components of the physical examination. The severity of hyperkalemia is determined by the symptoms, plasma K^+ concentration, and electrocardiographic abnormalities.

The appropriate renal response to hyperkalemia is to excrete at least 200 mmol of K^+ daily. In most cases, diminished renal K^+ loss is due to impaired K^+ secretion, which can be assessed by measuring the transtubular K^+ concentration gradient (TTKG). A TTKG <10 implies a decreased driving force for K^+ secretion due to either hypoaldosteronism or resistance to the renal effects of mineralocorticoid. This can be determined by evaluating the kaliuretic response to administration of mineralocorticoid (e.g., 9α-fludrocortisone). Primary adrenal insufficiency can be differentiated from hyporeninemic hypoaldosteronism by examining the renin-aldosterone axis. Renin and aldosterone levels should be measured in the supine and upright positions, following three days of Na^+ restriction (Na^+ intake <10 mmol/d) in combination with a loop diuretic to induce mild volume contraction. Aldosterone-resistant hyperkalemia can result from the various causes of impaired distal Na^+ reabsorption or from a Cl^- shunt. The former leads to salt wasting, ECF volume contraction, and high renin

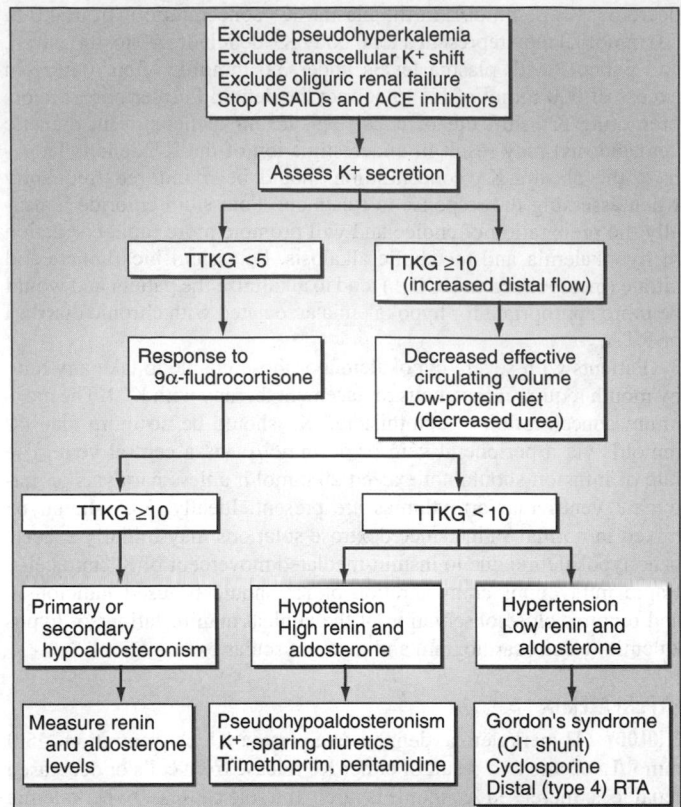

FIGURE 41-4   Algorithm depicting clinical approach to hyperkalemia. NSAID, nonsteroidal anti-inflammatory drug; ACE, angiotensin-converting enzyme; RTA, renal tubular acidosis; TTKG, transtubular K^+ concentration gradient.

and aldosterone levels. In contrast, enhanced distal Cl^- reabsorption is associated with volume expansion and suppressed renin and aldosterone secretion. As mentioned above, hypoaldosteronism seldom causes severe hypokalemia in the absence of increased dietary K^+ intake, renal insufficiency, transcellular K^+ shifts, or antikaliuretic drugs.

$\mathbb{R}$ TREATMENT

The approach to therapy depends on the degree of hyperkalemia as determined by the plasma K^+ concentration, associated muscular weakness, and changes on the electrocardiogram. Potentially fatal hyperkalemia rarely occurs unless the plasma K^+ concentration exceeds 7.5 mmol/L and is usually associated with profound weakness and absent P waves, QRS widening, or ventricular arrhythmias on the electrocardiogram.

Severe hyperkalemia requires emergent treatment directed at minimizing membrane depolarization, shifting K^+ into cells, and promoting K^+ loss. In addition, exogenous K^+ intake and antikaliuretic drugs should be discontinued. Administration of calcium gluconate decreases membrane excitability. The usual dose is 10 mL of a 10% solution infused over 2 to 3 min. The effect begins within minutes but is short-lived (30 to 60 min), and the dose can be repeated if no change in the electrocardiogram is seen after 5 to 10 min. Insulin causes K^+ to shift into cells by mechanisms described previously and will temporarily lower the plasma K^+ concentration. Although glucose alone will stimulate insulin release from normal pancreatic β cells, a more rapid response generally occurs when exogenous insulin is administered (with glucose to prevent hypoglycemia). A commonly recommended combination is 10 to 20 units of regular insulin and 25 to 50 g of glucose. Obviously, hyperglycemic patients should not be given glucose. If effective, the plasma K^+ concentration will fall by 0.5 to 1.5 mmol/L in 15 to 30 min and the effect will last for several hours. Alkali therapy with intravenous $NaHCO_3$ can also shift K^+ into cells. This is safest when administered as an isotonic solution of 3 ampules per liter (134 mmol/L NaHCO$_3$) and ideally should be reserved for severe hyperkalemia associated with metabolic acidosis. Patients with end-stage renal disease seldom respond to this intervention and may not tolerate the Na$^+$ load and resultant volume expansion. When administered parenterally or in nebulized form, β_2-adrenergic agonists promote cellular uptake of K$^+$ (see above). The onset of action is 30 min, lowering the plasma K$^+$ concentration by 0.5 to 1.5 mmol/L, and the effect lasts 2 to 4 h.

Removal of K$^+$ can be achieved using diuretics, cation-exchange resin, or dialysis. Loop and thiazide diuretics, often in combination, may enhance K$^+$ excretion if renal function is adequate. Sodium polystyrene sulfonate is a cation-exchange resin that promotes the exchange of Na$^+$ for K$^+$ in the gastrointestinal tract. Each gram binds 1 mmol of K$^+$ and releases 2 to 3 mmol of Na$^+$. When given by mouth, the usual dose is 25 to 50 g mixed with 100 mL of 20% sorbitol to prevent constipation. This will generally lower the plasma K$^+$ concentration by 0.5 to 1.0 mmol/L within 1 to 2 h and last for 4 to 6 h. Sodium polystyrene sulfonate can also be administered as a retention enema consisting of 50 g of resin and 50 mL of 70% sorbitol mixed in 150 mL of tap water. The sorbitol should be omitted from the enema in postoperative patients due to the increased incidence of sorbitol-induced colonic necrosis, especially following renal transplantation. The most rapid and effective way of lowering the plasma K$^+$ concentration is hemodialysis. This should be reserved for patients with renal failure and those with severe life-threatening hyperkalemia unresponsive to more conservative measures. Peritoneal dialysis also removes

K$^+$ but is only 15 to 20% as effective as hemodialysis. Finally, the underlying cause of the hyperkalemia should be treated. This may involve dietary modification, correction of metabolic acidosis, cautious volume expansion, and administration of exogenous mineralocorticoid.

FURTHER READING

ADROGUE HJ, MADIAS NE: Hypernatremia. N Engl J Med 342:1493, 2000

ADROGUE HJ, MADIAS NE: Hyponatremia. N Engl J Med 342:1581, 2000

BERL T, VERBALIS J: Pathophysiology of water metabolism, in BM Brenner (ed): *Brenner & Rector's The Kidney*, 7th ed. Philadelphia, Saunders, 2004, pp 857–920

COHN JN et al: New guidelines for potassium replacement in clinical practice: A contemporary review by the National Council on Potassium in Clinical Practice. Arch Intern Med 160:2429, 2000

GOLDSZMIDT MA, ILIESCU EA: DDAVP to prevent rapid correction in hyponatremia. Clin Nephrol 53:226, 2000

GROSS P: Treatment of severe hyponatremia. Kidney Int 60:2417, 2001

HARRIGAN MR: Cerebral salt wasting syndrome. Crit Care Clin 17:125, 2001

MOUNT DB: Disorders of potassium balance, in BM Brenner (ed): *Brenner & Rector's The Kidney*, 7th ed. Philadelphia, Saunders, 2004, pp 997–1040

NIELSEN S et al: Aquaporins in the kidney: From molecules to medicine. Physiol Rev 82:205, 2002

WARNOCK DG: Genetic forms of renal potassium and magnesium wasting. Am J Med 112:235, 2002

42 | ACIDOSIS AND ALKALOSIS
Thomas D. DuBose, Jr.

NORMAL ACID-BASE HOMEOSTASIS

Systemic arterial pH is maintained between 7.35 and 7.45 by extracellular and intracellular chemical buffering together with respiratory and renal regulatory mechanisms. The control of arterial CO$_2$ tension (Pa$_{CO_2}$) by the central nervous system and respiratory systems and the control of the plasma bicarbonate by the kidneys stabilize the arterial pH by excretion or retention of acid or alkali. The metabolic and respiratory components that regulate systemic pH are described by the Henderson-Hasselbalch equation:

$$pH = 6.1 + \log \frac{HCO_3^-}{Pa_{CO_2} \times 0.0301}$$

Under most circumstances, CO$_2$ production and excretion are matched, and the usual steady-state Pa$_{CO_2}$ is maintained at 40 mmHg. Underexcretion of CO$_2$ produces hypercapnia, and overexcretion causes hypocapnia. Nevertheless, production and excretion are again matched at a new steady-state Pa$_{CO_2}$. Therefore, the Pa$_{CO_2}$ is regulated primarily by neural respiratory factors (Chap. 246) and is not subject to regulation by the rate of CO$_2$ production. Hypercapnia is usually the result of hypoventilation rather than of increased CO$_2$ production. Increases or decreases in Pa$_{CO_2}$ represent derangements of neural respiratory control or are due to compensatory changes in response to a primary alteration in the plasma [HCO$_3^-$].

Primary changes in Pa$_{CO_2}$ can cause acidosis or alkalosis, depending on whether Pa$_{CO_2}$ is above or below the normal value of 40 mmHg (respiratory acidosis or alkalosis, respectively). Primary alteration of Pa$_{CO_2}$ evokes cellular buffering and renal adaptation, a slow process that becomes more efficient with time. A primary change in the plasma [HCO$_3^-$] as a result of metabolic or renal factors results in compensatory changes in ventilation that blunt the changes in blood pH that would occur otherwise. Such respiratory alterations are referred to as *secondary*, or compensatory, changes, since they occur in response to primary metabolic changes.

The kidneys regulate plasma [HCO$_3^-$] through three main processes: (1) "reabsorption" of filtered HCO$_3^-$, (2) formation of titratable

acid, and (3) excretion of NH$_4^+$ in the urine. The kidney filters approximately 4000 mmol of HCO$_3^-$ per day. To reabsorb the filtered load of HCO$_3^-$, the renal tubules must therefore secrete 4000 mmol of hydrogen ions. Between 80 and 90% of HCO$_3^-$ is reabsorbed in the proximal tubule. The distal nephron reabsorbs the remainder and secretes protons, as generated from metabolism, to defend systemic pH. While this quantity of protons, 40 to 60 mmol/d, is small, it must be secreted to prevent chronic positive H$^+$ balance and metabolic acidosis. This quantity of secreted protons is represented in the urine as titratable acid and NH$_4^+$. Metabolic acidosis in the face of normal renal function increases NH$_4^+$ production and excretion. NH$_4^+$ production and excretion are impaired in chronic renal failure, hyperkalemia, and renal tubular acidosis.

In sum, these regulatory responses, including chemical buffering, the regulation of Pa$_{CO_2}$ by the respiratory system, and the regulation of [HCO$_3^-$] by the kidneys, act in concert to maintain a systemic arterial pH between 7.35 and 7.45.

DIAGNOSIS OF GENERAL TYPES OF DISTURBANCES

The most common clinical disturbances are simple acid-base disorders, i.e., metabolic acidosis or alkalosis or respiratory acidosis or alkalosis. Since compensation is not complete, the pH is abnormal in simple disturbances. More complicated clinical situations can give rise to mixed acid-base disturbances.

SIMPLE ACID-BASE DISORDERS Primary respiratory disturbances (primary changes in Pa$_{CO_2}$) invoke compensatory metabolic responses (secondary changes in [HCO$_3^-$]), and primary metabolic disturbances elicit predictable compensatory respiratory responses. Physiologic compensation can be predicted from the relationships displayed in Table 42-1. Primary changes in Pa$_{CO_2}$ or [HCO$_3^-$] alter systemic pH and cause acidosis or alkalosis. To illustrate, metabolic acidosis due to an increase in endogenous acids (e.g., ketoacidosis) lowers extracellular fluid [HCO$_3^-$] and decreases extracellular pH. This stimulates the medullary chemoreceptors to increase ventilation and to return the ratio of [HCO$_3^-$] to Pa$_{CO_2}$, and thus pH, toward normal, although not to normal. The degree of respiratory compensation expected in a simple form of metabolic acidosis can be predicted from the relationship: Pa$_{CO_2}$ = (1.5 × [HCO$_3^-$]) + 8, i.e., the Pa$_{CO_2}$ is expected to decrease 1.25 mmHg for each mmol per liter decrease in [HCO$_3^-$]. Thus, a patient

TABLE 42-1 *Prediction of Compensatory Responses on Simple Acid-Base Disturbances*

Disorder	Prediction of Compensation
Metabolic acidosis	$Pa_{CO_2} = (1.5 \times HCO_3^-) + 8$
	or
	Pa_{CO_2} will $\downarrow$ 1.25 mmHg per mmol/L $\downarrow$ in $[HCO_3^-]$
	or
	$Pa_{CO_2} = [HCO_3^-] + 15$
Metabolic alkalosis	Pa_{CO_2} will $\uparrow$ 0.75 mmHg per mmol/L $\uparrow$ in $[HCO_3^-]$
	or
	Pa_{CO_2} will $\uparrow$ 6 mmHg per 10 mmol/L $\uparrow$ in $[HCO_3^-]$
	or
	$Pa_{CO_2} = [HCO_3^-] + 15$
Respiratory alkalosis	
Acute	$[HCO_3^-]$ will $\downarrow$ 2 mmol/L per 10 mmHg $\downarrow$ in Pa_{CO_2}
Chronic	$[HCO_3^-]$ will $\downarrow$ 4 mmol/L per 10 mmHg $\downarrow$ in Pa_{CO_2}
Respiratory acidosis	
Acute	$[HCO_3^-]$ will $\uparrow$ 1 mmol/L per 10 mmHg $\uparrow$ in Pa_{CO_2}
Chronic	$[HCO_3^-]$ will $\uparrow$ 4 mmol/L per 10 mmHg $\uparrow$ in Pa_{CO_2}

with metabolic acidosis and $[HCO_3^-]$ of 12 mmol/L would be expected to have a Pa_{CO_2} between 24 and 28 mmHg. Values for Pa_{CO_2} below 24 or greater than 28 mmHg define a mixed disturbance (metabolic acidosis and respiratory alkalosis or metabolic alkalosis and respiratory acidosis, respectively). Another way to judge the appropriateness of the response in $[HCO_3^-]$ or Pa_{CO_2} is to use an acid-base nomogram (Fig. 42-1). While the shaded areas of the nomogram show the 95% confidence limits for normal compensation in simple disturbances, finding acid-base values within the shaded area does not necessarily rule out a mixed disturbance. Imposition of one disorder over another may result in values lying within the area of a third. Thus, the nomogram, while convenient, is not a substitute for the equations in Table 42-1.

MIXED ACID-BASE DISORDERS Mixed acid-base disorders—defined as independently coexisting disorders, not merely compensatory responses—are often seen in patients in critical care units and can lead to dangerous extremes of pH. A patient with diabetic ketoacidosis (metabolic acidosis) may develop an independent respiratory problem leading to respiratory acidosis or alkalosis. Patients with underlying

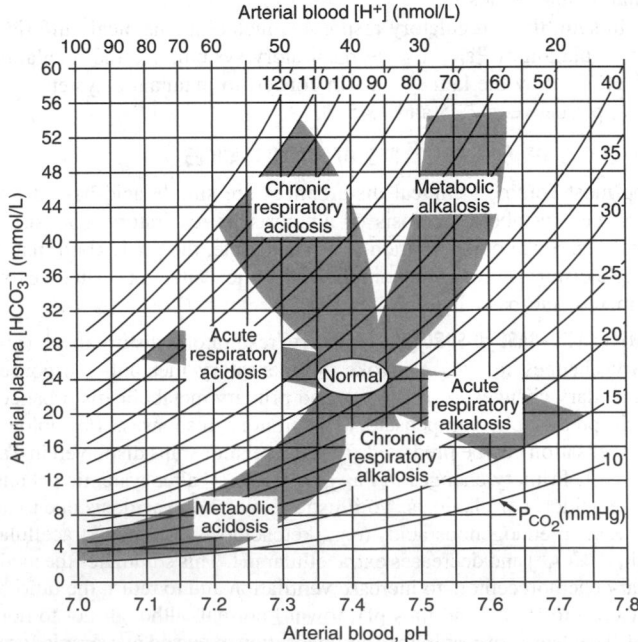

FIGURE 42-1 Acid-base nomogram. Shown are the 90% confidence limits of the normal respiratory and metabolic compensations for primary acid-base disturbances. *(From DuBose, used with permission.)*

pulmonary disease may not respond to metabolic acidosis with an appropriate ventilatory response because of insufficient respiratory reserve. Such imposition of respiratory acidosis on metabolic acidosis can lead to severe acidemia and a poor outcome. When metabolic acidosis and metabolic alkalosis coexist in the same patient, the pH may be normal or near normal. When the pH is normal, an elevated anion gap (see below) denotes the presence of a metabolic acidosis. A diabetic patient with ketoacidosis may have renal dysfunction resulting in simultaneous metabolic acidosis. Patients who have ingested an overdose of drug combinations such as sedatives and salicylates may have mixed disturbances as a result of the acid-base response to the individual drugs (metabolic acidosis mixed with respiratory acidosis or respiratory alkalosis, respectively). Even more complex are triple acid-base disturbances. For example, patients with metabolic acidosis due to alcoholic ketoacidosis may develop metabolic alkalosis due to vomiting and superimposed respiratory alkalosis due to the hyperventilation of hepatic dysfunction or alcohol withdrawal.

DIAGNOSIS OF ACID-BASE DISORDERS A stepwise approach to the diagnosis of acid-base disorders follows and is summarized in Table 42-2. Care should be taken when measuring blood gases to obtain the arterial blood sample without using excessive heparin. In the determination of arterial blood gases by the clinical laboratory, both pH and Pa_{CO_2} are measured, and the $[HCO_3^-]$ is calculated from the Henderson-Hasselbalch equation. This calculated value should be compared with the measured $[HCO_3^-]$ (total CO_2) on the electrolyte panel. These two values should agree within 2 mmol/L. If they do not, the values may not have been drawn simultaneously, a laboratory error may be present, or an error could have been made in calculating the $[HCO_3^-]$. After verifying the blood acid-base values, one can then identify the precise acid-base disorder.

The most common causes of acid-base disorders should be kept in mind while probing the history for clues about the etiology. For example, established chronic renal failure is expected to cause a metabolic acidosis, and chronic vomiting frequently causes metabolic alkalosis. Patients with pneumonia, sepsis, or cardiac failure frequently have respiratory alkalosis, and patients with chronic obstructive pulmonary disease or a sedative drug overdose often display a respiratory acidosis. The drug history is important since loop or thiazide diuretics may cause metabolic alkalosis, and the carbonic anhydrase inhibitor acetazolamide can result in metabolic acidosis.

Blood for electrolytes and arterial blood gases should be drawn simultaneously prior to therapy, since an increase in $[HCO_3^-]$ occurs with metabolic alkalosis and respiratory acidosis. Conversely, a decrease in $[HCO_3^-]$ occurs in metabolic acidosis and respiratory alkalosis.

Metabolic acidosis leads to hyperkalemia as a result of cellular shifts in which H^+ is exchanged for K^+ or Na^+. For each decrease in blood pH of 0.10, the plasma $[K^+]$ should rise by 0.6 mmol/L. This relationship is not invariable. Diabetic ketoacidosis, lactic acidosis, diarrhea, and renal tubular acidosis (RTA) are often associated with potassium depletion because of urinary K^+ wasting.

Anion Gap All evaluations of acid-base disorders should include a simple calculation of the anion gap (AG); it represents those unmeasured anions in plasma (normally 10 to 12 mmol/L) and is calculated as

TABLE 42-2 *Steps in Acid-Base Diagnosis*

1. Obtain arterial blood gases (ABGs) and electrolytes (lytes) simultaneously.
2. Compare $[HCO_3]$ on ABG and lytes to verify accuracy.
3. Calculate anion gap (AG).
4. Know four causes of high AG acidosis (ketoacidosis, lactic acid acidosis, renal failure, and toxins).
5. Know two causes of high hyperchloremic or nongap acidosis (bicarbonate loss from GI tract, renal tubular acidosis).
6. Estimate compensatory response (Table 42-1).
7. Compare ΔAG and ΔHCO_3^-.
8. Compare change in $[Cl^-]$ with change in $[Na^+]$.

follows: $AG = Na^+ - (Cl^- + HCO_3^-)$. The unmeasured anions include anionic proteins, phosphate, sulfate, and organic anions. When acid anions, such as acetoacetate and lactate, accumulate in extracellular fluid, the AG increases, causing a high-AG acidosis. An increase in the AG is most often due to an increase in unmeasured anions and less commonly is due to a decrease in unmeasured cations (calcium, magnesium, potassium). In addition, the AG may increase with an increase in anionic albumin, either because of increased albumin concentration or alkalosis, which alters albumin charge. A decrease in the AG can be due to (1) an increase in unmeasured cations; (2) the addition to the blood of abnormal cations, such as lithium (lithium intoxication) or cationic immunoglobulins (plasma cell dyscrasias); (3) a reduction in the major plasma anion albumin concentration (nephrotic syndrome); (4) a decrease in the effective anionic charge on albumin by acidosis; or (5) hyperviscosity and severe hyperlipidemia, which can lead to an underestimation of sodium and chloride concentrations. A fall in serum albumin by 1 g/dL from the normal value (4.5 g/dL) decreases the anion gap by 2.5 meq/L.

In the face of a normal serum albumin, a high AG is usually due to non-chloride-containing acids that contain inorganic (phosphate, sulfate), organic (ketoacids, lactate, uremic organic anions), exogenous (salicylate or ingested toxins with organic acid production), or unidentified anions. By definition, therefore, a high-AG acidosis has two identifying features: a low [HCO_3^-] and an elevated AG. The latter is present even if an additional acid-base disorder is superimposed to modify the [HCO_3^-] independently. Simultaneous metabolic acidosis of the high-AG variety plus either chronic respiratory acidosis or metabolic alkalosis represents such a situation in which [HCO_3^-] may be normal or even high. However, the AG is elevated, and [Cl^-] is depressed.

Similarly, normal values for [HCO_3^-], Pa_{CO_2}, and pH do not ensure the absence of an acid-base disturbance. For instance, an alcoholic who has been vomiting may develop a metabolic alkalosis with a pH of 7.55, Pa_{CO_2} of 48 mmHg, [HCO_3^-] of 40 mmol/L, [Na^+] of 135, [Cl^-] of 80, and [K^+] of 2.8. If such a patient were then to develop a superimposed alcoholic ketoacidosis with a β-hydroxybutyrate concentration of 15 mM, arterial pH would fall to 7.40, [HCO_3^-] to 25 mmol/L, and the Pa_{CO_2} to 40 mmHg. Although these blood gases are normal, the AG is elevated at 30 mmol/L, indicating a mixed metabolic alkalosis and metabolic acidosis.

METABOLIC ACIDOSIS

Metabolic acidosis can occur because of an increase in endogenous acid production (such as lactate and ketoacids), loss of bicarbonate (as in diarrhea), or accumulation of endogenous acids (as in renal failure). Metabolic acidosis has profound effects on the respiratory, cardiac, and nervous systems. The fall in blood pH is accompanied by a characteristic increase in ventilation, especially the tidal volume (Kussmaul respiration). Intrinsic cardiac contractility may be depressed, but inotropic function can be normal because of catecholamine release. Both peripheral arterial vasodilation and central venoconstriction can be present; the decrease in central and pulmonary vascular compliance predisposes to pulmonary edema with even minimal volume overload. Central nervous system function is depressed, with headache, lethargy, stupor, and, in some cases, even coma. Glucose intolerance may also occur.

There are two major categories of clinical metabolic acidosis: high-anion-gap (AG) and normal-AG, or hyperchloremic acidosis (Table 42-3 and Table 42-4).

TABLE 42-3 *Causes of High-Anion-Gap Metabolic Acidosis*

Lactic acidosis	Toxins
Ketoacidosis	Ethylene glycol
Diabetic	Methanol
Alcoholic	Salicylates
Starvation	Renal failure (acute and chronic)

TABLE 42-4 *Causes of Non-Anion-Gap Acidosis*

I. Gastrointestinal bicarbonate loss
  A. Diarrhea
  B. External pancreatic or small-bowel drainage
  C. Ureterosigmoidostomy, jejunal loop, ileal loop
  D. Drugs
    1. Calcium chloride (acidifying agent)
    2. Magnesium sulfate (diarrhea)
    3. Cholestyramine (bile acid diarrhea)
II. Renal acidosis
  A. Hypokalemia
    1. Proximal RTA (type 2)
    2. Distal (classic) RTA (type 1)
  B. Hyperkalemia
    1. Generalized distal nephron dysfunction (type 4 RTA)
      a. Mineralocorticoid deficiency
      b. Mineralocorticoid resistance
      c. $\downarrow Na^+$ delivery to distal nephron
      d. Tubulointerstitial disease
      e. Ammonium excretion defect
III. Drug-induced hyperkalemia (with renal insufficiency)
  A. Potassium-sparing diuretics (amiloride, triamterene, spironolactone)
  B. Trimethoprim
  C. Pentamidine
  D. Angiotensin-converting enzyme inhibitors and AT-II receptor blockers
  E. Nonsteroidal anti-inflammatory drugs
  F. Cyclosporine
IV. Other
  A. Acid loads (ammonium chloride, hyperalimentation)
  B. Loss of potential bicarbonate: ketosis with ketone excretion
  C. Expansion acidosis (rapid saline administration)
  D. Hippurate
  E. Cation exchange resins

Note: RTA, renal tubular acidosis; AT-II, angiotensin-II receptor blockers.

$\boxed{R_x}$ TREATMENT

Treatment of metabolic acidosis with alkali should be reserved for severe acidemia except when the patient has no "potential HCO_3^-" in plasma. Potential [HCO_3^-] can be estimated from the increment (Δ) in the AG (ΔAG = patient's AG $-$ 10). It must be determined if the acid anion in plasma is metabolizable (i.e., β-hydroxybutyrate, acetoacetate, and lactate) or nonmetabolizable (anions that accumulate in chronic renal failure and after toxin ingestion). The latter requires return of renal function to replenish the [HCO_3^-] deficit, a slow and often unpredictable process. Consequently, patients with a normal AG acidosis (hyperchloremic acidosis), a slightly elevated AG (mixed hyperchloremic and AG acidosis), or an AG attributable to a nonmetabolizable anion in the face of renal failure should receive alkali therapy, either orally ($NaHCO_3$ or Shohl's solution) or intravenously ($NaHCO_3$), in an amount necessary to slowly increase the plasma [HCO_3^-] into the 20 to 22 mmol/L range.

Controversy exists, however, in regard to the use of alkali in patients with a pure AG acidosis owing to accumulation of a metabolizable organic acid anion (ketoacidosis or lactic acidosis). In general, severe acidosis (pH <7.20) warrants the intravenous administration of 50 to 100 meq of $NaHCO_3$, over 30 to 45 min, during the initial 1 to 2 h of therapy. Provision of such modest quantities of alkali in this situation seems to provide an added measure of safety, but it is essential to monitor plasma electrolytes during the course of therapy, since the [K^+] may decline as pH rises. The goal is to increase the [HCO_3^-] to 10 meq/L and the pH to 7.15, not to increase these values to normal.

HIGH-ANION-GAP ACIDOSES There are four principal causes of a high-AG acidosis: (1) lactic acidosis, (2) ketoacidosis, (3) ingested toxins, and (4) acute and chronic renal failure (Table 42-3). Initial screening to differentiate the high-AG acidoses should include (1) a probe of the history for evidence of drug and toxin ingestion and measurement of arterial blood gas to detect coexistent respiratory alkalosis (salicylates); (2) determination of whether diabetes mellitus is present (diabetic ketoacidosis); (3) a search for evidence of alcoholism or increased levels of β-hydroxybutyrate (alcoholic ketoacidosis); (4) observation for clinical signs of uremia and determination of the blood urea nitrogen (BUN) and creatinine (uremic acidosis); (5) inspection of the urine for oxalate crystals (ethylene glycol); and (6) recognition of the numerous clinical settings in which lactate levels may be increased (hypotension, shock, cardiac failure, leukemia, cancer, and drug or toxin ingestion).

Lactic Acidosis   An increase in plasma L-lactate may be secondary to poor tissue perfusion (type A)—circulatory insufficiency (shock, circulatory failure), severe anemia, mitochondrial enzyme defects, and inhibitors (carbon monoxide, cyanide)—or to aerobic disorders (type B)—malignancies, diabetes mellitus, renal or hepatic failure, severe infections (cholera, malaria), seizures, AIDS, or drugs/toxins (biguanides, ethanol, methanol, isoniazid, AZT analogues, and fructose). Unrecognized bowel ischemia or infarction in a patient with severe atherosclerosis or cardiac decompensation receiving vasopressors is a common cause of lactic acidosis. D-Lactic acid acidosis, which may be associated with jejunoileal bypass or intestinal obstruction and is due to formation of D-lactate by gut bacteria, may cause both an increased AG and hyperchloremia.

℞ TREATMENT

The underlying condition that disrupts lactate metabolism must first be corrected; tissue perfusion must be restored when it is inadequate. Vasoconstrictors should be avoided, if possible, since they may worsen tissue perfusion. Alkali therapy is generally advocated for acute, severe acidemia (pH <7.15) to improve cardiac function and lactate utilization. However, $NaHCO_3$ therapy may paradoxically depress cardiac performance and exacerbate acidosis by enhancing lactate production (HCO_3^- stimulates phosphofructokinase). While the use of alkali in moderate lactic acidosis is controversial, it is generally agreed that attempts to return the pH or $[HCO_3^-]$ to normal by administration of exogenous $NaHCO_3$ are deleterious. A reasonable approach is to infuse sufficient $NaHCO_3$ to raise the arterial pH to no more than 7.2 over 30 to 40 min.

NaHCO3 therapy can cause fluid overload and hypertension because the amount required can be massive when accumulation of lactic acid is relentless. Fluid administration is poorly tolerated because of central venoconstriction, especially in the oliguric patient. If the underlying cause of the lactic acidosis can be remedied, blood lactate will be converted to HCO_3^- and may result in an overshoot alkalosis.

Ketoacidosis ■ *DIABETIC KETOACIDOSIS*   This condition is caused by increased fatty acid metabolism and the accumulation of ketoacids (acetoacetate and β-hydroxybutyrate). Diabetic ketoacidosis usually occurs in insulin-dependent diabetes mellitus in association with cessation of insulin or an intercurrent illness, such as an infection, gastroenteritis, pancreatitis, or myocardial infarction, which increases insulin requirements temporarily and acutely. The accumulation of ketoacids accounts for the increment in the AG and is accompanied most often by hyperglycemia [glucose >17 mmol/L (300 mg/dL)]. It should be noted that since insulin prevents production of ketones, bicarbonate therapy is rarely needed except with extreme acidemia (pH <7.1), and then in only limited amounts (see "Treatment" for lactic acidosis). →*The management of this condition is described in Chap. 323.*

ALCOHOLIC KETOACIDOSIS   Chronic alcoholics can develop ketoacidosis when alcohol consumption is abruptly curtailed; it is usually associated with binge drinking, vomiting, abdominal pain, starvation, and volume depletion. The glucose concentration is low or normal, and acidosis may be severe because of elevated ketones, predominantly β-hydrox-

ybutyrate. Mild lactic acidosis may coexist because of alteration in the redox state. The nitroprusside ketone reaction (Acetest) can detect acetoacetic acid but not β-hydroxybutyrate, so that the degree of ketosis and ketonuria can be underestimated. Typically, insulin levels are low, and concentrations of triglyceride, cortisol, glucagon, and growth hormone are increased.

℞ TREATMENT

Extracellular fluid deficits should be repleted by intravenous administration of saline and glucose (5% dextrose in 0.9% NaCl). Hypophosphatemia, hypokalemia, and hypomagnesemia may coexist and should be corrected. Hypophosphatemia usually emerges 12 to 24 h after admission, may be exacerbated by glucose infusion, and, if severe, may induce rhabdomyolysis. Upper gastrointestinal hemorrhage, pancreatitis, and pneumonia may accompany this disorder.

Drug- and Toxin-Induced Acidosis ■ *SALICYLATES* (See also Chap. 377.) Salicylate intoxication in adults usually causes respiratory alkalosis, mixed metabolic acidosis–respiratory alkalosis, or a pure high-AG metabolic acidosis. In the latter example, which is less common, only a portion of the AG is due to the salicylates. Lactic acid production is also often increased.

℞ TREATMENT

This should begin with vigorous gastric lavage with isotonic saline (not $NaHCO_3$) followed by administration of activated charcoal. In the acidotic patient, to facilitate removal of salicylate, intravenous $NaHCO_3$ is administered in amounts adequate to alkalinize the urine and to maintain urine output (urine pH >7.5). While this form of therapy is straightforward in acidotic patients, a coexisting respiratory alkalosis may make this approach hazardous. Acetazolamide may be administered when an alkaline diuresis cannot be achieved, but this drug can cause systemic metabolic acidosis if HCO_3^- is not replaced. Hypokalemia may occur with an alkaline diuresis from $NaHCO_3$ and should be treated promptly and aggressively. Glucose-containing fluids should be administered because of the danger of hypoglycemia. Excessive insensible fluid losses may cause severe volume depletion and hypernatremia. If renal failure prevents rapid clearance of salicylate, hemodialysis can be performed against a bicarbonate dialysate.

ALCOHOLS   Under most physiologic conditions, sodium, urea, and glucose generate the osmotic pressure of blood. Plasma osmolality is calculated according to the following expression: $P_{osm} = 2Na^+ + Glu + BUN$ (all in mmol/L), or, using conventional laboratory values in which glucose and BUN are expressed in milligrams per deciliter: $P_{osm} = 2Na^+ + Glu/18 + BUN/2.8$. The calculated and determined osmolality should agree within 10 to 15 mmol/kg H_2O. When the measured osmolality exceeds the calculated osmolality by more than 15 to 20 mmol/kg H_2O, one of two circumstances prevails. Either the serum sodium is spuriously low, as with hyperlipidemia or hyperproteinemia (pseudohyponatremia), or osmolytes other than sodium salts, glucose, or urea have accumulated in plasma. Examples include mannitol, radiocontrast media, isopropyl alcohol, ethylene glycol, ethanol, methanol, and acetone. In this situation, the difference between the calculated osmolality and the measured osmolality (*osmolar gap*) is proportional to the concentration of the unmeasured solute. With an appropriate clinical history and index of suspicion, identification of an osmolar gap is helpful in identifying the presence of poison-associated AG acidosis.

ETHYLENE GLYCOL (See also Chap. 377.)   Ingestion of ethylene glycol (commonly used in antifreeze) leads to a metabolic acidosis and severe damage to the central nervous system, heart, lungs, and kidneys. The increased AG and osmolar gap are attributable to ethylene glycol and its metabolites, oxalic acid, glycolic acid, and other organic acids. Lactic acid production increases secondary to inhibition of the tricarboxylic acid cycle and altered intracellular redox state. Diagnosis is facilitated by recognizing oxalate crystals in the urine, the presence of an osmolar gap in serum, and a high-AG acidosis. Treatment should not be delayed while awaiting measurement of ethylene glycol levels in this setting.

℞ TREATMENT

This includes the prompt institution of a saline or osmotic diuresis, thiamine and pyridoxine supplements, fomepizole or ethanol, and hemodialysis. The intravenous administration of the alcohol dehydrogenase inhibitor fomepizole (4-methylpyrazole; 7 mg/kg as a loading dose) or ethanol intravenously to achieve a level of 22 mmol/L (100 mg/dL) serves to lessen toxicity because they compete with ethylene glycol for metabolism by alcohol dehydrogenase. Fomepizole, although expensive, offers the advantages of a predictable decline in ethylene glycol levels without the adverse effects, such as excessive obtundation, associated with ethyl alcohol infusion.

METHANOL (See also Chap. 377.)   The ingestion of methanol (wood alcohol) causes metabolic acidosis, and its metabolites formaldehyde and formic acid cause severe optic nerve and cental nervous system damage. Lactic acid, ketoacids, and other unidentified organic acids may contribute to the acidosis. Due to its low molecular weight (32 Da), an osmolar gap is usually present.

℞ TREATMENT

This is similar to that for ethylene glycol intoxication, including general supportive measures, fomepizole or ethanol administration, and hemodialysis.

RENAL FAILURE (See also Chaps. 260 and 261)   The hyperchloremic acidosis of moderate renal insufficiency is eventually converted to the high-AG acidosis of advanced renal failure. Poor filtration and reabsorption of organic anions contribute to the pathogenesis. As renal disease progresses, the number of functioning nephrons eventually becomes insufficient to keep pace with net acid production. Uremic acidosis is characterized, therefore, by a reduced rate of NH_4^+ production and excretion, primarily due to decreased renal mass. $[HCO_3^-]$ rarely falls below 15 mmol/L, and the AG rarely exceeds 20 mmol/L. The acid retained in chronic renal disease is buffered by alkaline salts from bone. Despite significant retention of acid (up to 20 mmol/d), the serum $[HCO_3^-]$ does not decrease further, indicating participation of buffers outside the extracellular compartment. Chronic metabolic acidosis results in significant loss of bone mass due to reduction in bone calcium carbonate. Chronic acidosis also increases urinary calcium excretion, proportional to cumulative acid retention.

℞ TREATMENT

Both uremic acidosis and the hyperchloremic acidosis of renal failure require oral alkali replacement to maintain the $[HCO_3^-]$ between 20 and 24 mmol/L. This can be accomplished with relatively modest amounts of alkali (1.0 to 1.5 mmol/kg body weight per day). It is assumed that alkali replacement prevents the harmful effects of H^+ balance on bone and prevents or retards muscle catabolism. Sodium citrate (Shohl's solution) or $NaHCO_3$ tablets are equally effective alkalinizing salts. Citrate enhances the absorption of aluminum from the gastrointestinal tract and should never be given together with aluminum-containing antacids because of the risk of aluminum intoxication. When hyperkalemia is present, furosemide (60 to 80 mg/d) should be added.

HYPERCHLOREMIC (NONGAP) METABOLIC ACIDOSES   Alkali can be lost from the gastrointestinal tract in diarrhea or from the kidneys (renal tubular acidosis, RTA). In these disorders (Table 42-4), reciprocal changes in $[Cl^-]$ and $[HCO_3^-]$ result in a normal AG. In pure hyperchloremic acidosis, therefore, the increase in $[Cl^-]$ above the normal value approximates the decrease in $[HCO_3^-]$. The absence of such a relationship suggests a mixed disturbance.

In diarrhea, stools contain a higher $[HCO_3^-]$ and decomposed HCO_3^- than plasma so that metabolic acidosis develops along with

volume depletion. Instead of an acid urine pH (as anticipated with systemic acidosis), urine pH is usually around 6 because metabolic acidosis and hypokalemia increase renal synthesis and excretion of NH_4^+, thus providing a urinary buffer that increases urine pH. Metabolic acidosis due to gastrointestinal losses with a high urine pH can be differentiated from RTA (Chap. 265) because urinary NH_4^+ excretion is typically low in RTA and high with diarrhea. Urinary NH_4^+ levels can be estimated by calculating the urine anion gap (UAG): UAG = $[Na^+ + K^+]_u - [Cl^-]_u$. When $[Cl^-]_u > [Na^+ + K^+]$, and the urine gap is negative, the urine ammonium level is appropriately increased, suggesting an extrarenal cause of the acidosis. Conversely, when the urine anion gap is positive, the urine ammonium level is low, suggesting a renal cause of the acidosis.

Loss of functioning renal parenchyma by progressive renal disease leads to hyperchloremic acidosis when the glomerular filtration rate (GFR) is between 20 and 50 mL/min and to uremic acidosis with a high AG when the GFR falls to <20 mL/min. Such a progression occurs commonly with tubulointerstitial forms of renal disease, but hyperchloremic metabolic acidosis can persist with advanced glomerular disease. In advanced renal failure, ammoniagenesis is reduced in proportion to the loss of functional renal mass, and ammonium accumulation and trapping in the outer medullary collecting tubule may also be impaired. Because of adaptive increases in K^+ secretion by the collecting duct and colon, the acidosis of chronic renal insufficiency is typically normokalemic.

Proximal RTA (type 2 RTA) (Chap. 265) is most often due to generalized proximal tubular dysfunction manifested by glycosuria, generalized aminoaciduria, and phosphaturia (Fanconi syndrome). With a low plasma $[HCO_3^-]$, the urine pH is acid (pH <5.5). The fractional excretion of $[HCO_3^-]$ may exceed 10 to 15% when the serum $HCO_3^- > 20$ mmol/L. Since HCO_3^- is not reabsorbed normally in the proximal tubule, therapy with $NaHCO_3$ will enhance renal potassium wasting and hypokalemia.

The typical findings in classic distal RTA (type 1 RTA) include hypokalemia, hyperchloremic acidosis, low urinary NH_4^+ excretion (positive UAG, low urine $[NH_4^+]$), and inappropriately high urine pH (pH >5.5). Such patients are unable to acidify the urine below a pH of 5.5. Most patients have hypocitraturia and hypercalciuria, so nephrolithiasis, nephrocalcinosis, and bone disease are common. In type 4 RTA, hyperkalemia is disproportionate to the reduction in GFR because of coexisting dysfunction of potassium and acid secretion. Urinary ammonium excretion is invariably depressed, and renal function may be compromised, for example, due to diabetic nephropathy, amyloidosis, or tubulointerstital disease. →*See Chap. 265 for the pathophysiology, diagnosis, and treatment of RTA.*

Hyporeninemic Hypoaldosteronism (See also Chap. 321)   This condition typically causes hyperchloremic metabolic acidosis, most commonly in older adults with diabetes mellitus or tubulointerstitial disease and renal insufficiency. Patients usually have mild to moderate renal insufficiency and acidosis, with elevation in serum $[K^+]$ (5.2 to 6.0 mmol/L), concurrent hypertension, and congestive heart failure. Both the metabolic acidosis and the hyperkalemia are out of proportion to impairment in GFR. Nonsteroidal anti-inflammatory drugs trimethoprim, pentamidine, and angiotensin-converting enzyme (ACE) inhibitors can also cause hyperkalemia with hyperchloremic metabolic acidosis in patients with renal insufficiency (Table 42-4).

METABOLIC ALKALOSIS

Metabolic alkalosis is manifested by an elevated arterial pH, an increase in the serum $[HCO_3^-]$, and an increase in Pa_{CO_2} as a result of compensatory alveolar hypoventilation. It is often accompanied by hypochloremia and hypokalemia. The patient with a high $[HCO_3^-]$ and a low $[Cl^-]$ has either metabolic alkalosis or chronic respiratory acidosis. As shown in Table 42-1, the Pa_{CO_2} increases 6 mmHg for each 10-mmol/L increase in the $[HCO_3^-]$ above normal. Stated differently, in the range of $[HCO_3^-]$ from 10 to 40 mmol/L, the predicted Pa_{CO_2}

is approximately equal to the $[HCO_3^-] + 15$. The arterial pH establishes the diagnosis, since it is increased in metabolic alkalosis and decreased or normal in respiratory acidosis. Metabolic alkalosis frequently occurs in association with other disorders such as respiratory acidosis or alkalosis or metabolic acidosis.

PATHOGENESIS Metabolic alkalosis occurs as a result of net gain of $[HCO_3^-]$ or loss of nonvolatile acid (usually HCl by vomiting) from the extracellular fluid. Since it is unusual for alkali to be added to the body, the disorder involves a generative stage, in which the loss of acid usually causes alkalosis, and a maintenance stage, in which the kidneys fail to compensate by excreting HCO_3^- because of volume contraction, a low GFR, or depletion of Cl^- or K^+.

Under normal circumstances, the kidneys have an impressive capacity to excrete HCO_3^-. Continuation of metabolic alkalosis represents a failure of the kidneys to eliminate HCO_3^- in the usual manner. For HCO_3^- to be added to the extracellular fluid, it must be administered exogenously or synthesized endogenously, in part or entirely by the kidneys. The kidneys will retain, rather than excrete, the excess alkali and maintain the alkalosis if (1) volume deficiency, chloride deficiency, and K^+ deficiency exist in combination with a reduced GFR, which augments distal tubule H^+ secretion; or (2) hypokalemia exists because of autonomous hyperaldosteronism. In the first example, alkalosis is corrected by administration of NaCl and KCl, whereas in the latter it is necessary to repair the alkalosis by pharmacologic or surgical intervention, not with saline administration.

DIFFERENTIAL DIAGNOSIS To establish the cause of metabolic alkalosis (Table 42-5), it is necessary to assess the status of the extracellular fluid volume (ECFV), the recumbent and upright blood pressure, the serum $[K^+]$, and the renin-aldosterone system. For example, the presence of chronic hypertension and chronic hypokalemia in an alkalotic patient suggests either mineralocorticoid excess or that the hypertensive patient is receiving diuretics. Low plasma renin activity and normal urine $[Na^+]$ and $[Cl^-]$ in a patient who is not taking diuretics indicate a primary mineralocorticoid excess syndrome. The combination of hypokalemia and alkalosis in a normotensive, nonedematous patient can be due to Bartter's or Gitelman's syndrome, magnesium deficiency, vomiting, exogenous alkali, or diuretic ingestion. Determination of urine electrolytes (especially the urine $[Cl^-]$) and screening of the urine for diuretics may be helpful. If the urine is alkaline, with an elevated $[Na^+]$ and $[K^+]$ but low $[Cl^-]$, the diagnosis is usually either vomiting (overt or surreptitious) or alkali ingestion. If the urine is relatively acid and has low concentrations of Na^+, K^+, and Cl^-, the most likely possibilities are prior vomiting, the posthypercapnic state, or prior diuretic ingestion. If, on the other hand, neither the urine sodium, potassium, nor chloride concentrations are depressed, magnesium deficiency, Bartter's or Gitelman's syndrome, or current diuretic ingestion should be considered. Bartter's syndrome is distinguished from Gitelman's syndrome because of hypocalciuria and hypomagnesemia in the latter disorder. The genetic and molecular basis of these two disorders has been elucidated recently (Chap. 265).

Alkali Administration Chronic administration of alkali to individuals with normal renal function rarely, if ever causes alkalosis. However, in patients with coexistent hemodynamic disturbances, alkalosis can develop because the normal capacity to excrete HCO_3^- may be exceeded or there may be enhanced reabsorption of HCO_3^-. Such patients include those who receive oral or intravenous HCO_3^-, acetate loads (parenteral hyperalimentation solutions), citrate loads (transfusions), or antacids plus cation-exchange resins (aluminum hydroxide and sodium polystyrene sulfonate).

METABOLIC ALKALOSIS ASSOCIATED WITH ECFV CONTRACTION, K^+ DEPLETION, AND SECONDARY HYPERRENINEMIC HYPERALDOSTERONISM ■ Gastrointestinal Origin

Gastrointestinal loss of H^+ from vomiting or gastric aspiration results in retention of HCO_3^-. The loss of fluid and NaCl in vomitus or na-

TABLE 42-5 *Causes of Metabolic Alkalosis*

I. Exogenous HCO_3^- loads
   A. Acute alkali administration
   B. Milk-alkali syndrome
II. Effective ECFV contraction, normotension, K^+ deficiency, and secondary hyperreninemic hyperaldosteronism
   A. Gastrointestinal origin
      1. Vomiting
      2. Gastric aspiration
      3. Congenital chloridorrhea
      4. Villous adenoma
      5. Combined administration of sodium polystyrene sulfonate (Kayexalate) and aluminum hydroxide
   B. Renal origin
      1. Diuretics
      2. Edematous states
      3. Posthypercapnic state
      4. Hypercalcemia/hypoparathyroidism
      5. Recovery from lactic acidosis or ketoacidosis
      6. Nonreabsorbable anions including penicillin, carbenicillin
      7. Mg^{2+} deficiency
      8. K^+ depletion
      9. Bartter's syndrome (loss of function mutations in TALH)
      10. Gitelman's syndrome (loss of function mutation in Na^+-Cl^- cotransporter in DCT)
III. ECFV expansion, hypertension, K^+ deficiency, and mineralocorticoid excess
   A. High renin
      1. Renal artery stenosis
      2. Accelerated hypertension
      3. Renin-secreting tumor
      4. Estrogen therapy
   B. Low renin
      1. Primary aldosteronism
         a. Adenoma
         b. Hyperplasia
         c. Carcinoma
      2. Adrenal enzyme defects
         a. 11β-Hydroxylase deficiency
         b. 17α-Hydroxylase deficiency
      3. Cushing's syndrome or disease
      4. Other
         a. Licorice
         b. Carbenoxolone
         c. Chewer's tobacco
         d. Lydia Pinkam tablets
IV. Gain of function mutation of renal sodium channel with ECFV expansion, hypertension, K^+ deficiency, and hyporeninemic-hypoaldosteronism
   A. Liddle's syndrome

Note: ECFV, extracellular fluid volume; TALH, thick ascending limb of Henle's loop; DCT, distal convoluted tubule.

sogastric suction results in contraction of the ECFV and an increase in the secretion of renin and aldosterone. Volume contraction causes a reduction in GFR and an enhanced capacity of the renal tubule to reabsorb HCO_3^-. During active vomiting, there is continued addition of HCO_3^- to plasma in exchange for Cl^-, and the plasma $[HCO_3^-]$ exceeds the reabsorptive capacity of the proximal tubule. The excess $NaHCO_3$ reaches the distal tubule, where secretion is enhanced by an aldosterone and the delivery of the poorly reabsorbed anion, HCO_3^-. Because of contraction of the ECFV and hypochloremia, Cl^- is avidly conserved by the kidney. Correction of the contracted ECFV with NaCl and repair of K^+ deficits corrects the acid-base disorder.

Renal Origin ■ *DIURETICS* (See also Chap. 216) Drugs that induce chloruresis, such as thiazides and loop diuretics (furosemide, bumetanide, torsemide, and ethracrynic acid), acutely diminish the ECFV without altering the total body bicarbonate content. The serum $[HCO_3^-]$ increases. The chronic administration of diuretics tends to generate an alkalosis by increasing distal salt delivery, so that K^+ and H^+ secretion are stimulated. The alkalosis is maintained by persistence of the contraction of the ECFV, secondary hyperaldosteronism, K^+ deficiency, and the direct effect of the diuretic (as long as diuretic administration continues). Repair of the alkalosis is achieved by providing isotonic saline to correct the ECFV deficit.

BARTTER'S SYNDROME AND GITELMAN'S SYNDROME   See Chap. 265.

NONREABSORBABLE ANIONS AND MAGNESIUM DEFICIENCY   Administration of large quantities of nonreabsorbable anions, such as penicillin or carbenicillin, can enhance distal acidification and K^+ secretion by increasing the transepithelial potential difference (lumen negative). Mg^{2+} deficiency results in hypokalemic alkalosis by enhancing distal acidification through stimulation of renin and hence aldosterone secretion.

POTASSIUM DEPLETION   Chronic K^+ depletion may cause metabolic alkalosis by increasing urinary acid excretion. Both NH_4^+ production and absorption are enhanced and HCO_3^- reabsorption is stimulated. Chronic K^+ deficiency upregulates the renal H^+, K^+-ATPase to increase K^+ absorption at the expense of enhanced H^+ secretion. Alkalosis associated with severe K^+ depletion is resistant to salt administration, but repair of the K^+ deficiency corrects the alkalosis.

AFTER TREATMENT OF LACTIC ACIDOSIS OR KETOACIDOSIS   When an underlying stimulus for the generation of lactic acid or ketoacid is removed rapidly, as with repair of circulatory insufficiency or with insulin therapy, the lactate or ketones are metabolized to yield an equivalent amount of HCO_3^-. Other sources of new HCO_3^- are additive with the original amount generated by organic anion metabolism to create a surfeit of HCO_3^-. Such sources include (1) new HCO_3^- added to the blood by the kidneys as a result of enhanced acid excretion during the preexisting period of acidosis, and (2) alkali therapy during the treatment phase of the acidosis. Acidosis-induced contraction of the ECFV and K^+ deficiency act to sustain the alkalosis.

POSTHYPERCAPNIA   Prolonged CO_2 retention with chronic respiratory acidosis enhances renal HCO_3^- absorption and the generation of new HCO_3^- (increased net acid excretion). If the Pa_{CO_2} is returned to normal, metabolic alkalosis results from the persistently elevated $[HCO_3^-]$. Alkalosis develops if the elevated Pa_{CO_2} is abruptly returned toward normal by a change in mechanically controlled ventilation. Associated ECFV contraction does not allow complete repair of the alkalosis by correction of the Pa_{CO_2} alone, and alkalosis persists until Cl^- supplementation is provided.

METABOLIC ALKALOSIS ASSOCIATED WITH ECFV EXPANSION, HYPERTENSION, AND HYPERALDOSTERONISM   Mineralocorticoid administration or excess production [primary aldosteronism of Cushing's syndrome and adrenal cortical enzyme defects (Chap. 321)] increases net acid excretion and may result in metabolic alkalosis, which may be worsened by associated K^+ deficiency. ECFV expansion from salt retention causes hypertension and antagonizes the reduction in GFR and/or increases tubule acidification induced by aldosterone and by K^+ deficiency. The kaliuresis persists and causes continued K^+ depletion with polydipsia, inability to concentrate the urine, and polyuria. Increased aldosterone levels may be the result of autonomous primary adrenal overproduction or of secondary aldosterone release due to renal overproduction of renin. In both situations, the normal feedback of ECFV on net aldosterone production is disrupted, and hypertension from volume retention can result.

Liddle's syndrome (Chap. 265) results from increased activity of the collecting duct Na^+ channel (ENaC) and is a rare inherited disorder associated with hypertension due to volume expansion manifested as hypokalemic alkalosis and normal aldosterone levels.

Symptoms   With metabolic alkalosis, changes in central and peripheral nervous system function are similar to those of hypocalcemia (Chap. 331); symptoms include mental confusion, obtundation, and a predisposition to seizures, paresthesia, muscular cramping, tetany, aggravation of arrhythmias, and hypoxemia in chronic obstructive pulmonary disease. Related electrolyte abnormalities include hypokalemia and hypophosphatemia.

℞ TREATMENT

This is primarily directed at correcting the underlying stimulus for HCO_3^- generation. If primary aldosteronism is present, correction of the underlying cause will reverse the alkalosis. $[H^+]$ loss by the stomach or kidneys can be mitigated by the use of H_2 receptor blockers, H^+, K^+-ATPase inhibitors, or the discontinuation of diuretics. The second aspect of treatment is to remove the factors that sustain HCO_3^- reabsorption, such as ECFV contraction or K^+ deficiency. Although K^+ deficits should be repaired, NaCl therapy is usually sufficient to reverse the alkalosis if ECFV contraction is present, as indicated by a low urine $[Cl^-]$.

If associated conditions preclude infusion of saline, renal HCO_3^- loss can be accelerated by administration of acetazolamide, a carbonic anhydrase inhibitor, which is usually effective in patients with adequate renal function but can worsen K^+ losses. Dilute hydrochloric acid ($0.1\ N$ HCl) is also effective but can cause hemolysis. Alternatively, acidification can also be achieved with oral NH_4Cl, which should be avoided in the presence of liver disease. Hemodialysis against a dialysate low in $[HCO_3^-]$ and high in $[Cl^-]$ can be effective when renal function is impaired.

RESPIRATORY ACIDOSIS

Respiratory acidosis can be due to severe pulmonary disease, respiratory muscle fatigue, or abnormalities in ventilatory control and is recognized by an increase in Pa_{CO_2} and decrease in pH (Table 42-6). In acute respiratory acidosis, there is an immediate compensatory elevation (due to cellular buffering mechanisms) in HCO_3^-, which increases 1 mmol/L for every 10-mmHg increase in Pa_{CO_2}. In chronic respiratory acidosis (>24 h), renal adaptation increases the $[HCO_3^-]$ by 4 mmol/L for every 10-mmHg increase in Pa_{CO_2}. The serum HCO_3^- usually does not increase above 38 mmol/L.

The clinical features vary according to the severity and duration of the respiratory acidosis, the underlying disease, and whether there is

TABLE 42-6   *Respiratory Acid-Base Disorders*

I. Alkalosis	II. Acidosis
A. Central nervous system stimulation	A. Central
1. Pain	1. Drugs (anesthetics, morphine, sedatives)
2. Anxiety, psychosis	2. Stroke
3. Fever	3. Infection
4. Cerebrovascular accident	B. Airway
5. Meningitis, encephalitis	1. Obstruction
6. Tumor	2. Asthma
7. Trauma	C. Parenchyma
B. Hypoxemia or Tissue hypoxia	1. Emphysema
1. High altitude, $\downarrow Pa_{CO_2}$	2. Pneumoconiosis
2. Pneumonia, pulmonary edema	3. Bronchitis
	4. Adult respiratory distress syndrome
3. Aspiration	5. Barotrauma
4. Severe anemia	D. Neuromuscular
C. Drugs or hormones	1. Poliomyelitis
1. Pregnancy, progesterone	2. Kyphoscoliosis
2. Salicylates	3. Myasthenia
3. Nikethamide	4. Muscular dystrophies
D. Stimulation of chest receptors	E. Miscellaneous
1. Hemothorax	1. Obesity
2. Flail chest	2. Hypoventilation
3. Cardiac failure	3. Permissive hypercapnia
4. Pulmonary embolism	
E. Miscellaneous	
1. Septicemia	
2. Hepatic failure	
3. Mechanical hyperventilation	
4. Heat exposure	
5. Recovery from metabolic acidosis	

accompanying hypoxemia. A rapid increase in Pa_{CO_2} may cause anxiety, dyspnea, confusion, psychosis, and hallucinations and may progress to coma. Lesser degrees of dysfunction in chronic hypercapnia include sleep disturbances, loss of memory, daytime somnolence, personality changes, impairment of coordination, and motor disturbances such as tremor, myoclonic jerks, and asterixis. Headaches and other signs that mimic raised intracranial pressure, such as papilledema, abnormal reflexes, and focal muscle weakness, are due to vasoconstriction secondary to loss of the vasodilator effects of CO_2.

Depression of the respiratory center by a variety of drugs, injury, or disease can produce respiratory acidosis. This may occur acutely with general anesthetics, sedatives, and head trauma or chronically with sedatives, alcohol, intracranial tumors, and the syndromes of sleep-disordered breathing, including the primary alveolar and obesity-hypoventilation syndromes (Chaps. 246 and 247). Abnormalities or disease in the motor neurons, neuromuscular junction, and skeletal muscle can cause hypoventilation via respiratory muscle fatigue. Mechanical ventilation, when not properly adjusted and supervised, may result in respiratory acidosis, particularly if CO_2 production suddenly rises (because of fever, agitation, sepsis, or overfeeding) or alveolar ventilation falls because of worsening pulmonary function. High levels of positive end-expiratory pressure in the presence of reduced cardiac output may cause hypercapnia as a result of large increases in alveolar dead space (Chap. 234). Permissive hypercapnia is being used with increasing frequency because of studies suggesting lower mortality rates than with conventional mechanical ventilation, especially with severe central nervous system or heart disease. Although the potential beneficial effects of permissive hypercapnia may be mitigated by correction of the acidemia, it seems prudent, nevertheless, to keep the pH in the range of 7.2 to 7.3 by administration of $NaHCO_3$.

Acute hypercapnia follows sudden occlusion of the upper airway or generalized bronchospasm as in severe asthma, anaphylaxis, inhalational burn, or toxin injury. Chronic hypercapnia and respiratory acidosis occur in end-stage obstructive lung disease. Restrictive disorders involving both the chest wall and the lungs can cause respiratory acidosis because the high metabolic cost of respiration causes ventilatory muscle fatigue. Advanced stages of intrapulmonary and extrapulmonary restrictive defects present as chronic respiratory acidosis.

The diagnosis of respiratory acidosis requires, by definition, the measurement of Pa_{CO_2} and arterial pH. A detailed history and physical examination often indicate the cause. Pulmonary function studies (Chap. 234), including spirometry, diffusion capacity for carbon monoxide, lung volumes, and arterial Pa_{CO_2} and O_2 saturation, usually make it possible to determine if respiratory acidosis is secondary to lung disease. The workup for nonpulmonary causes should include a detailed drug history, measurement of hematocrit, and assessment of upper airway, chest wall, pleura, and neuromuscular function.

℞ TREATMENT

The management of respiratory acidosis depends on its severity and rate of onset. Acute respiratory acidosis can be life-threatening, and measures to reverse the underlying cause should be undertaken simultaneously with restoration of adequate alveolar ventilation. This may necessitate tracheal intubation and assisted mechanical ventilation. Oxygen administration should be titrated carefully in patients with severe obstructive pulmonary disease and chronic CO_2 retention who are breathing spontaneously (Chap. 242). When oxygen is used injudiciously, these patients may experience progression of the respiratory acidosis. Aggressive and rapid correction of hypercapnia should be avoided, because the falling Pa_{CO_2} may provoke the same complications noted with acute respiratory alkalosis (i.e., cardiac arrhythmias, reduced cerebral perfusion, and seizures). The Pa_{CO_2} should be lowered gradually in chronic respiratory acidosis, aiming to restore the Pa_{CO_2} to baseline levels and to provide sufficient Cl^- and K^+ to enhance the renal excretion of HCO_3^-.

Chronic respiratory acidosis is frequently difficult to correct, but measures aimed at improving lung function (Chap. 242) can help some patients and forestall further deterioration in most.

RESPIRATORY ALKALOSIS

Alveolar hyperventilation decreases Pa_{CO_2} and increases the HCO_3^-/Pa_{CO_2} ratio, thus increasing pH (Table 42-6). Nonbicarbonate cellular buffers respond by consuming HCO_3^-. Hypocapnia develops when a sufficiently strong ventilatory stimulus causes CO_2 output in the lungs to exceed its metabolic production by tissues. Plasma pH and $[HCO_3^-]$ appear to vary proportionately with Pa_{CO_2} over a range from 40 to 15 mmHg. The relationship between arterial $[H^+]$ concentration and Pa_{CO_2} is about 0.7 mmol/L per mmHg (or 0.01 pH unit/mmHg), and that for plasma $[HCO_3^-]$ is 0.2 mmol/L per mmHg. Hypocapnia sustained longer than 2 to 6 h is further compensated by a decrease in renal ammonium and titratable acid excretion and a reduction in filtered HCO_3^- reabsorption. Full renal adaptation to respiratory alkalosis may take several days and requires normal volume status and renal function. The kidneys appear to respond directly to the lowered Pa_{CO_2} rather than to alkalosis per se. In chronic respiratory alkalosis a 1-mmHg fall in Pa_{CO_2} causes a 0.4- to 0.5-mmol/L drop in $[HCO_3^-]$ and a 0.3-mmol/L fall (or 0.003 rise in pH) in $[H^+]$.

The effects of respiratory alkalosis vary according to duration and severity but are primarily those of the underlying disease. Reduced cerebral blood flow as a consequence of a rapid decline in Pa_{CO_2} may cause dizziness, mental confusion, and seizures, even in the absence of hypoxemia. The cardiovascular effects of acute hypocapnia in the conscious human are generally minimal, but in the anesthetized or mechanically ventilated patient, cardiac output and blood pressure may fall because of the depressant effects of anesthesia and positive-pressure ventilation on heart rate, systemic resistance, and venous return. Cardiac arrhythmias may occur in patients with heart disease as a result of changes in oxygen unloading by blood from a left shift in the hemoglobin-oxygen dissociation curve (Bohr effect). Acute respiratory alkalosis causes intracellular shifts of Na^+, K^+, and PO_4^- and reduces free $[Ca^{2+}]$ by increasing the protein-bound fraction. Hypocapnia-induced hypokalemia is usually minor.

Chronic respiratory alkalosis is the most common acid-base disturbance in critically ill patients and, when severe, portends a poor prognosis. Many cardiopulmonary disorders manifest respiratory alkalosis in their early to intermediate stages, and the finding of normocapnia and hypoxemia in a patient with hyperventilation may herald the onset of rapid respiratory failure and should prompt an assessment to determine if the patient is becoming fatigued. Respiratory alkalosis is common during mechanical ventilation.

The hyperventilation syndrome may be disabling. Paresthesia, circumoral numbness, chest wall tightness or pain, dizziness, inability to take an adequate breath, and, rarely, tetany may themselves be sufficiently stressful to perpetuate the disorder. Arterial blood-gas analysis demonstrates an acute or chronic respiratory alkalosis, often with hypocapnia in the range of 15 to 30 mmHg and no hypoxemia. Central nervous system diseases or injury can produce several patterns of hyperventilation and sustained Pa_{CO_2} levels of 20 to 30 mmHg. Hyperthyroidism, high caloric loads, and exercise raise the basal metabolic rate, but ventilation usually rises in proportion so that arterial blood gases are unchanged and respiratory alkalosis does not develop. Salicylates are the most common cause of drug-induced respiratory alkalosis as a result of direct stimulation of the medullary chemoreceptor (Chap. 377). The methylxanthines, theophylline, and aminophylline stimulate ventilation and increase the ventilatory response to CO_2. Progesterone increases ventilation and lowers arterial Pa_{CO_2} by as much as 5 to 10 mmHg. Therefore, chronic respiratory alkalosis is a common feature of pregnancy. Respiratory alkalosis is also prominent in liver failure, and the severity correlates with the degree of hepatic insufficiency. Respiratory alkalosis is often an early finding in gram-negative septicemia, before fever, hypoxemia, or hypotension develop.

The diagnosis of respiratory alkalosis depends on measurement of arterial pH and Pa_{CO_2}. The plasma $[K^+]$ is often reduced and the $[Cl^-]$ increased. In the acute phase, respiratory alkalosis is not associated with increased renal HCO_3^- excretion, but within hours net acid excretion is reduced. In general, the HCO_3^- concentration falls by 2.0 mmol/L for each 10-mmHg decrease in Pa_{CO_2}. Chronic hypocapnia reduces the serum $[HCO_3^-]$ by 5.0 mmol/L for each 10-mmHg decrease in Pa_{CO_2}. It is unusual to observe a plasma HCO_3^- <12 mmol/L as a result of a pure respiratory alkalosis.

When a diagnosis of respiratory alkalosis is made, its cause should be investigated. The diagnosis of hyperventilation syndrome is made by exclusion. In difficult cases, it may be important to rule out other conditions such as pulmonary embolism, coronary artery disease, and hyperthyroidism.

℞ TREATMENT

The management of respiratory alkalosis is directed toward alleviation of the underlying disorder. If respiratory alkalosis complicates ventilator management, changes in dead space, tidal volume, and frequency can minimize the hypocapnia. Patients with the hyperventilation syndrome may benefit from reassurance, rebreathing from a paper bag during symptomatic attacks, and attention to underlying psychological stress. Antidepressants and sedatives are not recommended. β-Adrenergic blockers may ameliorate peripheral manifestations of the hyperadrenergic state.

FURTHER READING

DuBose TD Jr: Acid-base disorders, in BM Brenner (ed): *Brenner and Rector's The Kidney*, 7th ed. Philadelphia, Saunders, 2004, pp 921–996
——, Alpern RJ: Renal tubular acidosis, in CR Scriver et al (eds): *The Metabolic and Molecular Bases of Inherited Disease*, 8th ed. New York, McGraw-Hill, 2001
Fall PJ: A stepwise approach to acid-base disorders: Practical patient evaluation for metabolic acidosis and other conditions. Postgrad Med 107:249, 253, 257, 2000
Galla JH: Metabolic alkalosis. J Am Soc Nephrol 11:369, 2000
Madias NE, Cohen JJ: Respiratory alkalosis and acidosis, in DW Seldin, G Giebisch (eds): *The Kidney: Physiology and Pathophysiology*, 2d ed. New York, Raven, 1992, pp 2733–2758
Wesson DE et al: Clinical syndromes of metabolic alkalosis, in DW Seldin, G Giebisch (eds): *The Kidney: Physiology and Pathophysiology*, 3d ed. Philadelphia: Lippincott Williams and Wilkins, 2000, pp 2055–2072

Section 8 Alterations in Sexual Function and Reproduction

43 SEXUAL DYSFUNCTION
Kevin T. McVary

Male sexual dysfunction affects 10 to 25% of middle-aged and elderly men. Female sexual dysfunction occurs with a similar frequency. Demographic changes, the popularity of newer treatments, and greater awareness of sexual dysfunction by patients and society have led to increased diagnosis and associated health care expenditures for the management of this common disorder. Because many patients are reluctant to initiate discussion of their sex lives, the physician should address this topic directly to elicit a history of sexual dysfunction.

PHYSIOLOGY OF MALE SEXUAL RESPONSE

Normal male sexual function requires (1) an intact libido; (2) the ability to achieve and maintain penile erection; (3) ejaculation; and (4) detumescence. *Libido* refers to sexual desire and is influenced by a variety of visual, olfactory, tactile, auditory, imaginative, and hormonal stimuli. Sex steroids, particularly testosterone, act to increase libido. Libido can be diminished by hormonal or psychiatric disorders or by medications.

Penile tumescence leading to erection depends on the increased flow of blood into the lacunar network after complete relaxation of the arteries and corporal smooth muscle. The microarchitecture of the corpora is composed of a mass of smooth muscle (trabecula) which contains a network of endothelial-lined vessels (lacunar spaces). Subsequent compression of the trabecular smooth muscle against the fibroelastic tunica albuginea causes a passive closure of the emissary veins and accumulation of blood in the corpora. In the presence of a full erection and a competent valve mechanism, the corpora become noncompressible cylinders from which blood does not escape.

The central nervous system exerts an important influence by either stimulating or antagonizing spinal pathways that mediate erectile function and ejaculation. The erectile response is mediated by a combination of central (psychogenic) and peripheral (reflexogenic) innervation. Sensory nerves that originate from receptors in the penile skin and glans converge to form the dorsal nerve of the penis, which travels to the S2-S4 dorsal root ganglia via the pudendal nerve. Parasympathetic nerve fibers to the penis arise from neurons in the intermediolateral columns of S2-S4 sacral spinal segments. Sympathetic innervation originates from the T-11 to the L-2 spinal segments and descends through the hypogastric plexus.

Neural input to smooth muscle tone is crucial to the initiation and maintenance of an erection. There is also an intricate interaction between the corporal smooth muscle cell and its overlying endothelial cell lining (Fig. 43-1A). Nitric oxide, which induces vascular relaxation, promotes erection and is opposed by endothelin-1 (ET-1), which mediates vascular contraction. Nitric oxide is synthesized from L-arginine by nitric oxide synthase, and is released from the nonadrenergic, noncholinergic (NANC) autonomic nerve supply to act postjunctionally on smooth muscle cells. Nitric oxide increases the production of cyclic 3',5'-guanosine monophosphate (cyclic GMP), which induces relaxation of the smooth muscle (Fig. 43-1B). Cyclic GMP is gradually broken down by phosphodiesterase type 5 (PDE-5). Inhibitors of PDE-5, such as the oral medication sildenafil, maintain erections by reducing the breakdown of cyclic GMP. However, if nitric oxide is not produced at some level, the addition of PDE-5 inhibitor is not effective, as the drug facilitates but does not initiate the initial enzyme cascade. In addition to nitric oxide, vasoactive prostaglandins (PGE_1, $PGF_{2\alpha}$) are synthesized within the cavernosal tissue and increase cyclic AMP levels, also leading to relaxation of cavernosal smooth muscle cells.

Ejaculation is stimulated by the sympathetic nervous system, which results in contraction of the epididymis, vas deferens, seminal vesicles, and prostate, causing seminal fluid to enter the urethra. Seminal fluid emission is followed by rhythmic contractions of the bulbocavernosus and ischiocavernosus muscles, leading to ejaculation. *Premature ejaculation* is usually related to anxiety or a learned behavior and is amenable to behavioral therapy or treatment with medications such as selective serotonin reuptake inhibitors (SSRIs). *Retrograde ejaculation* results when the internal urethral sphincter does not close, and it may occur in men with diabetes or after surgery involving the bladder neck.

Detumescence is mediated by released norepinephrine from the sympathetic nerves, release of endothelin from the vascular surface, and contraction of smooth muscle induced by activation of postsynaptic α-adrenergic receptors. These events increase venous outflow and restore the flaccid state. Venous leak can cause premature detumescence and is thought to be caused by insufficient relaxation of the corporal smooth muscle rather than a specific anatomic defect. *Pria-*

FIGURE 43-1 Pathways that control erection and detumescence. *A.* Erection is mediated by cholinergic parasympathetic pathways, and nonadrenergic, noncholinergic (NANC) pathways, which release nitric oxide (NO). Endothelial cells also release NO, which induces vascular smooth muscle cell relaxation, allowing enhanced blood flow, and leading to erection. Detumescence is mediated by sympathetic pathways that release norepinephrine and stimulate α-adrenergic pathways, leading to contraction of vascular smooth muscle cells. Endothelin, released from endothelial cells, also induces contraction. *B.* Biochemical pathways of NO synthesis and action. Sildenafil enhances erectile function by inhibiting phosphodiesterase type 5 (PDE-5), thereby maintaining high levels of cyclic 3′,5′-guanosine monophosphate (cyclic GMP). NOS, nitric oxide synthase; iCa²⁺, intracellular calcium.

pism refers to a persistent and painful erection and may be associated with sickle cell anemia, hypercoagulable states, spinal cord injury, or injection of vasodilator agents into the penis.

ERECTILE DYSFUNCTION

EPIDEMIOLOGY   Erectile dysfunction (ED) is not considered a normal part of the aging process. Nonetheless, it is associated with certain physiologic and psychological changes related to age. In the Massachusetts Male Aging Study (MMAS), a community-based survey of men between the ages of 40 and 70, 52% of responders reported some degree of ED. Complete ED occurred in 10% of respondents, moderate ED occurred in 25%, and minimal ED in 17%. The incidence of moderate or severe ED more than doubled between the ages of 40 and 70. In the National Health and Social Life Survey (NHSLS), which was a nationally representative sample of men and women age 18 to 59 years, 10% of men reported being unable to maintain an erection (corresponding to the proportion of men in the MMAS reporting severe ED). Incidence was highest among men in the 50 to 59 age group (21%) and among men who were poor (14%), divorced (14%), and less educated (13%).

The incidence of ED is also higher among men with certain medical disorders such as diabetes mellitus, heart disease, hypertension, and decreased HDL levels. Smoking is a significant risk factor in the development of ED. Medications used to treat diabetes or cardiovascular disease are additional risk factors (see below). There is a higher incidence of ED among men who have undergone radiation or surgery for prostate cancer and in those with a lower spinal cord injury. Psychological causes of ED include depression, anger, or stress from unemployment or other causes.

PATHOPHYSIOLOGY   ED may result from three basic mechanisms: (1) failure to initiate (psychogenic, endocrinologic, or neurogenic); (2) failure to fill (arteriogenic); or (3) failure to store (venoocclusive dysfunction) adequate blood volume within the lacunar network. These categories are not mutually exclusive, and multiple factors contribute to ED in many patients. For example, diminished filling pressure can lead secondarily to venous leak. Psychogenic factor frequently coexist with other etiologic factors and should be considered in all cases. Diabetic, atherosclerotic, and drug-related causes account for >80% of cases of ED in older men.

Vasculogenic   The most frequent organic cause of ED is a disturbance of blood flow to and from the penis. Atherosclerotic or traumatic arterial disease can decrease flow to the lacunar spaces, resulting in decreased rigidity and an increased time to full erection. Excessive outflow through the veins, despite adequate inflow, may also contribute to ED. This situation may be due to insufficient relaxation of trabecular smooth muscle and may occur in anxious individuals with excessive adrenergic tone or in those with damaged parasympathetic outflow. Structural alterations to the fibroelastic components of the corpora may cause a loss of compliance and an inability to compress the tunical veins. This condition may result from aging, increased cross-linking of collagen fibers induced by nonenzymatic glycosylation, hypoxia, or altered synthesis of collagen associated with hypercholesterolemia.

Neurogenic   Disorders that affect the sacral spinal cord or the autonomic fibers to the penis preclude nervous system relaxation of penile smooth muscle, thus leading to ED. In patients with spinal cord injury, the degree of ED depends on the completeness and level of the lesion. Patients with incomplete lesions or injuries to the upper part of the spinal cord are more likely to retain erectile capabilities than those with complete lesions or injuries to the lower part. Although 75% of patients with spinal cord injuries have some erectile capability, only 25% have erections sufficient for penetration. Other neurologic disorders commonly associated with ED include multiple sclerosis and peripheral neuropathy. The latter is often due to either diabetes or alcoholism. Pelvic surgery may cause ED through disruption of the autonomic nerve supply.

Endocrinologic   Androgens increase libido, but their exact role in erectile function remains unclear. Individuals with castrate levels of testosterone can achieve erections from visual or sexual stimuli. Nonetheless, normal levels of testosterone appear to be important for erectile function, particularly in older males. Androgen replacement therapy can improve depressed erectile function when it is secondary to hypogonadism; it is not useful for ED when endogenous testosterone levels are normal. Increased prolactin may decrease libido by suppressing gonadotropin-releasing hormone (GnRH), and it also leads to decreased testosterone levels. Treatment of hyperprolactinemia with dopamine agonists can restore libido and testosterone.

Diabetic   ED occurs in 35 to 75% of men with diabetes mellitus. Pathologic mechanisms are primarily related to diabetes-associated vascular and neurologic complications. Diabetic macrovascular complications are mainly related to age, whereas microvascular complications correlate with the duration of diabetes and the degree of glycemic control (Chap. 323). Individuals with diabetes also have reduced amounts of nitric oxide synthase in both endothelial and neural tissues.

Psychogenic   Two mechanisms contribute to the inhibition of erections in psychogenic ED. First, psychogenic stimuli to the sacral cord may inhibit reflexogenic responses, thereby blocking activation of vasodilator outflow to the penis. Second, excess sympathetic stimulation in an anxious man may increase penile smooth muscle tone. The most common causes of psychogenic ED are performance anxiety, depression, relationship conflict, loss of attraction, sexual inhibition, conflicts over sexual preference, sexual abuse in childhood, and fear of pregnancy or sexually transmitted disease. Almost all patients with ED, even when it has a clear-cut organic basis, develop a psychogenic component as a reaction to ED.

Medication-Related Medication-induced ED (Table 43-1) is estimated to occur in 25% of men seen in general medical outpatient clinics. Among the antihypertensive agents, the thiazide diuretics and beta blockers have been implicated most frequently. Calcium channel blockers and angiotensin-converting enzyme inhibitors are less frequently cited. These drugs may act directly at the corporal level (e.g., calcium channel blockers) or indirectly by reducing pelvic blood pressure, which is important in the development of penile rigidity. α Adrenergic blockers are less likely to cause ED. Estrogens, GnRH agonists, H_2 antagonists, and spironolactone cause ED by suppressing gonadotropin production or by blocking androgen action. Antidepressant and antipsychotic agents—particularly neuroleptics, tricyclics, and SSRIs—are associated with erectile, ejaculatory, orgasmic, and sexual desire difficulties.

Although many medications can cause ED, patients frequently have concomitant risk factors that confound the clinical picture. If there is a strong association between the institution of a drug and the onset of ED, alternative medications should be considered. Otherwise, it is often practical to treat the ED without attempting multiple changes in medications, as it may be difficult to establish a causal role for the drug.

CLINICAL EVALUATION A good physician-patient relationship helps to unravel the possible causes of ED, many of which require discussion of personal and sometimes embarrassing topics. For this reason, a primary care provider is often ideally suited to initiate the evaluation. A complete medical and sexual history should be taken in an effort to assess whether the cause of ED is organic, psychogenic, or multifactorial (Fig. 43-2). Initial questions should focus on the onset of symptoms, the presence and duration of partial erections, and the progression of ED. A history of nocturnal or early morning erections is useful for distinguishing physiologic from psychogenic ED. Nocturnal erections occur during rapid eye movement (REM) sleep and require intact neurologic and circulatory systems. Organic causes of ED are generally characterized by a gradual and persistent change in rigidity or the

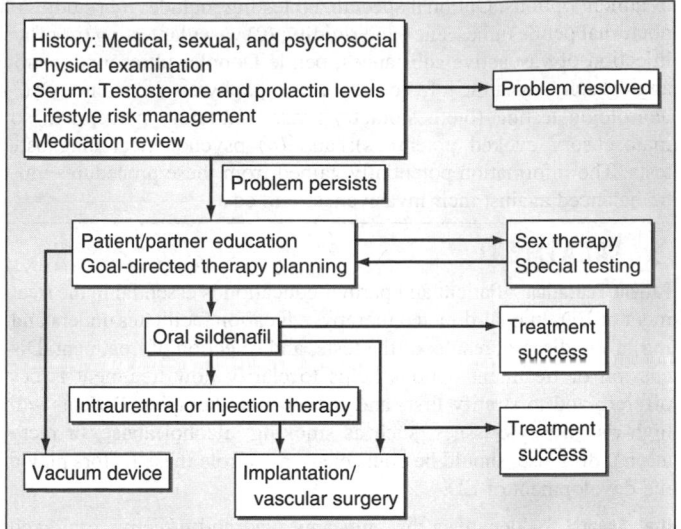

FIGURE 43-2 Algorithm for the evaluation and management of patients with ED.

inability to sustain nocturnal, coital, or self-stimulated erections. The patient should also be questioned about the presence of penile curvature or pain with coitus. It is also important to address libido, as decreased sexual drive and ED are sometimes the earliest signs of endocrine abnormalities (e.g., increased prolactin, decreased testosterone levels). It is useful to ask whether the problem is confined to coitus with one or other partners; ED arises not uncommonly in association with new or extramarital sexual relationships. Situational ED, as opposed to consistent ED, suggests psychogenic causes. Ejaculation is much less commonly affected than erection, but questions should be asked about whether ejaculation is normal, premature, delayed, or absent. Relevant risk factors should be identified, such as diabetes mellitus, coronary artery disease, lipid disorders, hypertension, peripheral vascular disease, smoking, alcoholism, and endocrine or neurologic disorders. The patient's surgical history should be explored with an emphasis on bowel, bladder, prostate, or vascular procedures. A complete drug history is also important. Social changes that may precipitate ED are also crucial to the evaluation, including health worries, spousal death, divorce, relationship difficulties, and financial concerns.

The physical examination is an essential element in the assessment of ED. Signs of hypertension as well as evidence of thyroid, hepatic, hematologic, cardiovascular, or renal diseases should be sought. An assessment should be made of the endocrine and vascular systems, the external genitalia, and the prostate gland. The penis should be carefully palpated along the corpora to detect fibrotic plaques. Reduced testicular size and loss of secondary sexual characteristics are suggestive of hypogonadism. Neurologic examination should include assessment of anal sphincter tone, the bulbocavernosus reflex, and testing for peripheral neuropathy.

Although hyperprolactinemia is uncommon, a serum prolactin level should be measured, as decreased libido and/or erectile dysfunction may be the presenting symptoms of a prolactinoma or other mass lesions of the sella (Chap. 318). The serum testosterone level should be measured and, if low, gonadotropins should be measured to determine whether hypogonadism is primary (testicular) or secondary (hypothalamic-pituitary) in origin (Chap. 325). Serum chemistries, CBC, and lipid profiles may be of value, if not performed recently, as they can yield evidence of anemia, diabetes, hyperlipidemia, or other systemic diseases associated with ED. Determination of serum PSA should be conducted according to recommended clinical guidelines (Chap. 81).

Additional diagnostic testing is rarely necessary in the evaluation of ED. However, in selected patients, specialized testing may provide insight into pathologic mechanisms of ED and aid in the selection of

TABLE 43-1 Drugs Associated with Erectile Dysfunction

Classification	Drugs
Diuretics	Thiazides
	Spironolactone
Antihypertensives	Calcium channel blockers
	Methyldopa
	Clonidine
	Reserpine
	β-Blockers
	Guanethidine
Cardiac/anti-hyperlipidemics	Digoxin
	Gemfibrozil
	Clofibrate
Antidepressants	Selective serotonin reuptake inhibitors
	Tricyclic antidepressants
	Lithium
	Monoamine oxidase inhibitors
Tranquilizers	Butyrophenones
	Phenothiazines
H_2 antagonists	Ranitidine
	Cimetidine
Hormones	Progesterone
	Estrogens
	Corticosteroids
	GnRH agonists
	5α-Reductase inhibitors
	Cyproterone acetate
Cytotoxic agents	Cyclophosphamide
	Methotrexate
	Roferon-A
Anticholinergics	Disopyramide
	Anticonvulsants
Recreational	Ethanol
	Cocaine
	Marijuana

treatment options. Optional specialized testing includes: (1) studies of nocturnal penile tumescence and rigidity; (2) vascular testing (in-office injection of vasoactive substances, penile Doppler ultrasound, penile angiography, dynamic infusion cavernosography/cavernosometry); (3) neurologic testing (biothesiometry-graded vibratory perception; somatosensory evoked potentials); and (4) psychological diagnostic tests. The information potentially gained from these procedures must be balanced against their invasiveness and cost.

℞ TREATMENT

Patient Education   Patient and partner education is essential in the treatment of ED. In goal-directed therapy, education facilitates understanding of the disease, results of the tests, and selection of treatment. Discussion of treatment options helps to clarify how treatment is best offered, and to stratify first- and second-line therapies. Patients with high-risk lifestyle issues, such as smoking, alcohol abuse, or recreational drug use, should be counseled on the role these factors play in the development of ED.

Oral Agents   Sildenafil is the only approved and effective oral agent for the treatment of ED. Sildenafil has markedly improved the management of ED because it is effective for the treatment of a broad range of causes of ED, including psychogenic, diabetic, vasculogenic, post-radical prostatectomy (nerve-sparing procedures), and spinal cord injury. Sildenafil is a selective and potent inhibitor of PDE-5, the predominant phosphodiesterase isoform found in the penis. It is administered in doses of 25, 50, or 100 mg, and enhances erections after sexual stimulation. The onset of action is approximately 60 to 90 min. Reduced initial doses should be considered for patients who are elderly, have renal insufficiency, or are taking medications that inhibit the CYP3A4 metabolic pathway in the liver (e.g., erythromycin, cimetidine, ketoconazole, and, possibly, itraconazole and mibefradil), as they may increase the serum concentration of sildenafil. The drug does not affect ejaculation, orgasm, or sexual drive. Side effects associated with sildenafil include headaches (19%), facial flushing (9%), dyspepsia (6%) and nasal congestion (4%). Approximately 7% of men may experience transient altered color vision (blue halo effect). Sildenafil is contraindicated in men receiving nitrate therapy for cardiovascular disease, including agents delivered by oral, sublingual, transnasal, or topical routes. These agents can potentiate its hypotensive effect and may result in profound shock. Likewise, amyl/butyl nitrates "poppers" may have a fatal synergistic effect on blood pressure. Sildenafil should also be avoided in patients with congestive heart failure and cardiomyopathy because of the risk of vascular collapse. Because sexual activity leads to an increase in physiologic expenditure [5 to 6 metabolic equivalents (METS)], physicians have been advised to exercise caution in prescribing any drug for sexual activity to those with active coronary disease, heart failure, borderline hypotension, hypovolemia, and to those on complex antihypertensive regimens.

Androgen Therapy   Testosterone replacement is used to treat both primary and secondary causes of hypogonadism (Chap. 325). Androgen supplementation in the setting of normal testosterone is rarely efficacious and is discouraged. Methods of androgen replacement include parenteral administration of long-acting testosterone esters (enanthate and cypionate), oral preparations (17 α-alkylated derivatives), and transdermal patches, and gels (Chap. 325). The long-acting 17 β-hydroxy esters of testosterone are the safest, most cost-effective, and practical preparations available. The administration of 200 to 300 mg intramuscularly every 2 to 3 weeks provides a practical option but is far from an ideal physiologic replacement. Oral androgen preparations have the potential for hepatotoxicity and should be avoided. Transdermal delivery of testosterone using patches or gels more closely mimics physiologic testosterone levels, but it is unclear whether this translates into improved sexual function. Testosterone therapy is contraindicated in men with androgen-sensitive cancers and may be inappropriate for men with bladder neck obstruction. It is generally advisable to measure PSA before giving androgen. Hepatic function should be tested before and during testosterone therapy.

Vacuum Constriction Devices   Vacuum constriction devices (VCD) are a well-established, noninvasive therapy. They are a reasonable treatment alternative for select patients who cannot take sildenafil or do not desire other interventions. VCD draw venous blood into the penis and use a constriction ring to restrict venous return and maintain tumescence. Adverse events with VCD include pain, numbness, bruising, and altered ejaculation. Additionally, many patients complain that the devices are cumbersome and that the induced erections have a non-physiologic appearance.

Intraurethral Alprostadil   If a patient fails to respond to oral agents, a reasonable next choice is intraurethral or self-injection of vasoactive substances. Intraurethral prostaglandin E_1 (alprostadil), in the form of a semisolid pellet (doses of 125 to 1000 μg), is delivered with an applicator. Approximately 65% of men receiving intraurethral alprostadil respond with an erection when tested in the office, but only 50% of those achieve successful coitus at home. Intraurethral insertion is associated with a markedly reduced incidence of priapism in comparison to intracavernosal injection.

Intracavernosal Self-Injection   Injection of synthetic formulations of alprostadil is effective in 70 to 80% of patients with ED, but discontinuation rates are high because of the invasive nature of administration. Doses range between 1 and 40 μg. Injection therapy is contraindicated in men with a history of hypersensitivity to the drug and in men at risk for priapism (hypercoagulable states, sickle cell disease). Side effects include local adverse events, prolonged erections, pain, and fibrosis with chronic use. Various combinations of alprostadil, phentolamine, and/or papaverine are sometimes used.

Surgery   A less frequently used form of therapy for ED involves the surgical implantation of a semi-rigid or inflatable penile prosthesis. These surgical treatments are invasive, associated with potential complications, and generally reserved for treatment of refractory ED. Despite their high cost and invasiveness, penile prostheses are associated with high rates of patient satisfaction.

SEX THERAPY   A course of sex therapy may be useful for addressing specific interpersonal factors that may affect sexual functioning. Sex therapy generally consists of in-session discussion and at-home exercises specific to the person and the relationship. It is preferable if therapy includes both partners, provided the patient is involved in an ongoing relationship.

FEMALE SEXUAL DYSFUNCTION

Female sexual dysfunction (FSD) has traditionally included disorders of desire, arousal, pain, and muted orgasm. The associated risk factors for FSD are similar to those in males: cardiovascular disease, endocrine disorders, hypertension, neurologic disorders, and smoking (Table 43-2).

TABLE 43-2   Risk Factors for Female Sexual Dysfunction

Neurologic disease: stroke, spinal cord injury, Parkinsonism
Trauma, genital surgery, radiation
Endocrinopathies: diabetes, hyperprolactinemia
Liver and/or renal failure
Cardiovascular disease
Psychological factors and interpersonal relationship disorders: sexual abuse, life stressors
Medications
   Antiandrogens: Cimetidine, spironolactone
   Antidepressants, Alcohol, hypnotics, sedatives
   Antiestrogens or GnRH antagonists
   Antihistamines, sympathomimetic amines
   Antihypertensives: Diuretics, calcium channel blockers
   Alkylating agents
   Anticholinergics

EPIDEMIOLOGY Epidemiologic data are limited but the available estimates suggest that as many as 43% of women complain of at least one sexual problem. Despite the recent interest in organic causes of FSD, desire and arousal phase disorders (including lubrication complaints) remain the most common presenting problems when surveyed in a community-based population.

PHYSIOLOGY OF THE FEMALE SEXUAL RESPONSE Although there are the obvious anatomic differences as well as variation in the density of vascular and neural beds in males and females, the primary effectors of sexual response are strikingly similar. Intact sensation is important for arousal. Thus, reduced levels of sexual functioning are more common in women with peripheral neuropathies (e.g., diabetes). Vaginal lubrication is a transudate of serum that results from the increased pelvic blood flow associated with arousal. Vascular insufficiency from a variety of causes may compromise adequate lubrication and result in dyspareunia. Similar to the male response, cavernosal and arteriole smooth muscle relaxation occurs via increased NOS activity and produces engorgement in the clitoris and surrounding vestibule. Orgasm requires an intact sympathetic outflow tract; hence, orgasmic disorders are common in female patients with spinal cord injuries.

CLINICAL EVALUATION The evaluation of FSD previously occurred mainly in a psychosocial context. However, inconsistencies between diagnostic categories based on only psychosocial considerations, and the emerging recognition of organic etiologies, has led to a new classification of FSD. This diagnostic scheme is based on four components that are not mutually exclusive: (1) *Hypoactive sexual desire*—the persistent or recurrent lack of sexual thoughts and/or receptivity to sexual activity, which causes personal distress. Hypoactive sexual desire may result from endocrine failure or may be associated with psychological or emotional disorders; (2) *Sexual arousal disorder*—the persistent or recurrent inability to attain or maintain sexual excitement, which causes personal distress; (3) *Orgasmic disorder*—the persistent or recurrent loss of orgasmic potential after sufficient sexual stimulation and arousal, which causes personal distress; (4) *Sexual pain disorder*—persistent or recurrent genital pain associated with noncoital sexual stimulation, which causes personal distress. This newer classification emphasizes "personal distress" as a requirement for dysfunction and provides clinicians an organized framework for evaluation prior to or in conjunction with more traditional counseling methods.

℞ TREATMENT

Patient Education Patient and partner education is essential in the treatment of FSD. Educating the couple about normal anatomy and physiologic responses is often necessary. Physiologic changes associated with aging and/or disease should be explained. Maximizing physical health and avoiding lifestyles (e.g., smoking, alcohol abuse) and medications likely to produce FSD are prudent (Table 43-2).

Hormonal Therapy In postmenopausal women, estrogen replacement therapy may be helpful in treating vaginal atrophy, decreasing coital pain, and improving clitoral sensitivity (Chap. 327). Estrogen replacement in the form of local cream is the preferred method, as it avoids systemic side effects. Androgen levels in women decline substantially before menopause. However, low levels of testosterone or dehydroepiandrosterone (DHEA) are not effective predictors of a positive therapeutic outcome with androgen therapy. The widespread use of exogenous androgens is not supported by the literature except in select circumstances (premature ovarian failure or menopausal states) and in secondary arousal disorders.

Oral Agents The efficacy of PDE-5 inhibitors in FDS has been a marked disappointment given the proposed role of nitric oxide-dependent physiology in the normal female sexual response. The use of sildenafil for FSD should be discouraged pending proof that it is effective.

Clitoral Vacuum Device In patients with arousal and orgasmic difficulties, the option of using a clitoral vacuum device may be explored. This handheld battery-operated device has a small soft plastic cup that applies a vacuum over the stimulated clitoris. This causes increased cavernosal blood flow, engorgement, and vaginal lubrication.

FURTHER READING

BERMAN JR et al: Female sexual dysfunction: Incidence, pathophysiology, evaluation, and treatment options. Urology 54:385–391, 1999

DAVIS SR. The clinical use of androgens in female sexual disorders. J Sex Marital Ther 24:153, 1998

FELDMAN HA et al: Impotence and its medical and psychosocial correlates: Results of the Massachusetts Male Aging Study. J Urol 151:54, 1994

LAUMANN EO et al: Sexual dysfunction in the United States. JAMA 81:553, 1999

LUE TF: Drug therapy: Erectile dysfunction. N Engl J Med 342:1802, 2000

44 HIRSUTISM AND VIRILIZATION
David A. Ehrmann

Hirsutism, defined as excessive male-pattern hair growth, affects approximately 10% of women. If often represents a variation of normal hair growth, but rarely it is a harbinger of a serious underlying condition. Hirsutism is often idiopathic but may be caused by conditions associated with androgen excess, such as polycystic ovarian syndrome (PCOS) or congenital adrenal hyperplasia (CAH) (Table 44-1). Cutaneous manifestations commonly associated with hirsutism include acne and male-pattern balding (androgenic alopecia). *Virilization* refers to the state in which androgen levels are sufficiently high to cause additional signs and symptoms such as deepening of the voice, breast atrophy, increased muscle bulk, clitoromegaly, and increased libido; virilization is an ominous sign that suggests the possibility of an ovarian or adrenal neoplasm.

HAIR FOLLICLE GROWTH AND DIFFERENTIATION

Hair can be categorized as either *vellus* (fine, soft, and not pigmented) or *terminal* (long, coarse, and pigmented). The number of hair follicles does not change over an individual's lifetime, but the follicle size and type of hair can change in response to numerous factors, particularly androgens. Androgens are necessary for terminal hair and sebaceous gland-development and mediate differentiation of pilosebaceous units (PSUs) into either a terminal hair follicle or a sebaceous gland. In the former case, androgens transform the vellus hair into a terminal hair; in the latter, the sebaceous component proliferates and the hair remains vellus.

There are three phases in the cycle of hair growth: (1) *anagen* (growth phase), (2) *catagen* (involution phase), and (3) *telogen* (rest phase). Depending on the body site, hormonal regulation may play an important role in the hair growth cycle. For example, the eyebrows, eyelashes, and vellus hairs are androgen-insensitive, whereas the axillary and pubic areas are sensitive to low levels of androgens. Hair growth on the face, chest, upper abdomen, and back requires greater levels of androgens and is therefore more characteristic of the pattern typically seen in males. Androgen excess in women leads to increased hair growth in most androgen-sensitive sites except in the scalp region, where hair loss occurs because androgens cause scalp hairs to spend less time in the anagen phase.

Although androgen excess underlies most cases of hirsutism, there is only a modest correlation between androgen levels and the quantity of hair growth. This is due to the fact that hair growth from the follicle also depends on local growth factors, and there is variability in end-

TABLE 44-1   *Causes of Hirsutism*

Gonadal hyperandrogenism
   Ovarian hyperandrogenism
   Polycystic ovary syndrome/functional ovarian hyperandrogenism
   Ovarian steroidogenic blocks
   Syndromes of extreme insulin resistance
   Ovarian neoplasms
Adrenal hyperandrogenism
   Premature adrenarche
   Functional adrenal hyperandrogenism
   Congenital adrenal hyperplasia (nonclassic and classic)
   Abnormal cortisol action/metabolism
   Adrenal neoplasms
Other endocrine disorders
   Cushing's syndrome
   Hyperprolactinemia
   Acromegaly
Peripheral androgen overproduction
   Obesity
   Idiopathic
Pregnancy related hyperandrogenism
   Hyperreactio luteinalis
   Thecoma of pregnancy
Drugs
   Androgens
   Oral contraceptives containing androgenic progestins
   Minoxidil
   Phenytoin
   Diazoxide
   Cyclosporine
True hermaphroditism

organ sensitivity. Genetic factors and ethnic background also influence hair growth. In general, dark-haired individuals tend to be more hirsute than blonde or fair individuals. Asians and Native Americans have relatively sparse hair in regions sensitive to high androgen levels, whereas people of Mediterranean descent are more hirsute.

CLINICAL ASSESSMENT

Historic elements relevant to the assessment of hirsutism include the age of onset and rate of progression of hair growth and associated symptoms or signs (e.g., acne). Depending on the cause, excess hair growth is typically first noted during the second and third decades. The growth is usually slow but progressive. Sudden development and rapid progression of hirsutism suggests the possibility of an androgen-secreting neoplasm, in which case virilization may also be present.

The age of onset of menstrual cycles (menarche) and the pattern of the menstrual cycle should be ascertained; irregular cycles from the time of menarche onward are more likely to result from ovarian rather than adrenal androgen excess. Associated symptoms such as galactorrhea should prompt evaluation for hyperprolactinemia (Chap. 318) and possibly hypothyroidism (Chap. 320). Hypertension, striae, easy bruising, centripetal weight gain, and weakness suggest hypercortisolism (Cushing's syndrome; Chap. 321). Rarely, patients with growth hormone excess (i.e., acromegaly) will present with hirsutism. Use of medications such as phenytoin, minoxidil, or cyclosporine may be associated with androgen-independent causes of excess hair growth (i.e., hypertrichosis). A family history of infertility and/or hirsutism may indicate disorders such as nonclassic CAH (Chap. 321).

Physical examination should include measurement of height, weight, and calculation of body mass index (BMI). A BMI >25 kg/m² is indicative of excess weight for height, and values >30 kg/m² are often seen in association with hirsutism. Notation should be made of blood pressure, as adrenal causes may be associated with hypertension. Cutaneous signs sometimes associated with androgen excess and insulin resistance include acanthosis nigricans and skin tags.

An objective clinical assessment of hair distribution and quantity is central to the evaluation in any woman presenting with hirsutism. This assessment permits the distinction between hirsutism and hypertrichosis and provides a baseline reference point to gauge the response to treatment. A simple and commonly used method to grade hair growth is the modified scale of Ferriman and Gallwey (Fig. 44-1), where each of nine androgen-sensitive sites is graded from 0 to 4. Approximately 95% of Caucasian women have a score below 8 on this scale; thus, it is normal for most women to have some hair growth in androgen-sensitive sites. Scores above 8 suggest excess androgen-mediated hair growth, a finding that should be assessed further by hormonal evaluation (see below). In racial/ethnic groups that are less likely to manifest hirsutism (e.g., Asian women), additional cutaneous

FIGURE 44-1   Hirsutism scoring scale of Ferriman and Gallwey. The nine body areas possessing androgen-sensitive areas are graded from 0 (no terminal hair) to 4 (frankly virile) to obtain a total score. A normal hirsutism score is less than 8. [*Reproduced from DA Ehrmann et al: Hyperandrogenism, hirsutism, and polycystic ovarian syndrome, in LJ DeGroot et al (eds), Endocrinology, 4th ed. Philadelphia, Saunders, 2000; with permission.*]

evidence of androgen excess should be sought, including pustular acne or thinning hair.

HORMONAL EVALUATION

Androgens are secreted by the ovaries and adrenal glands in response to their respective tropic hormones, luteinizing hormone (LH) and adrenocorticotropic hormone (ACTH). The principal circulating steroids involved in the etiology of hirsutism are testosterone, androstenedione, dehydroepiandrosterone (DHEA) and its sulfated form (DHEAS). The ovaries and adrenal glands normally contribute about equally to testosterone production. Approximately half of the total testosterone originates from direct glandular secretion, and the remainder is derived from the peripheral conversion of androstenedione and DHEA (Chap. 325).

Although it is the most important circulating androgen, testosterone is, in effect, the penultimate androgen in mediating hirsutism; it is converted to the more potent dihydrotestosterone (DHT) by the enzyme 5α-reductase, which is located in the PSU. DHT has a higher affinity for, and slower dissociation from, the androgen receptor. The local production of DHT allows it to serve as the primary mediator of androgen action at the level of the pilosebaceous unit. There are two isoenzymes of 5α-reductase: type 2 is found in the prostate gland and in hair follicles, whereas type 1 is found primarily in sebaceous glands.

One approach to testing for hyperandrogenemia is depicted in Fig. 44-2. In addition to measuring blood levels of testosterone and DHEAS, it is also important to measure the level of free (or unbound) testosterone. The fraction of testosterone that is not bound to its carrier protein, sex-hormone binding globulin (SHBG), is biologically available for conversion to DHT and for binding to androgen receptors. Hyperinsulinemia and/or androgen excess decrease hepatic production of SHBG, resulting in levels of total testosterone within the high-normal range, whereas the unbound hormone is more substantially elevated. Although there is a decline in ovarian testosterone production after menopause, ovarian estrogen production decreases to an even greater extent, and the concentration of SHBG is reduced. Consequently, there is an increase in the relative proportion of unbound testosterone, and it may exacerbate hirsutism after menopause.

Because adrenal androgens are readily suppressed by low doses of glucocorticoids, the dexamethasone androgen-suppression test may broadly distinguish ovarian from adrenal androgen overproduction. A blood sample is obtained before and after administering dexamethasone (0.5 mg orally every 6 h for 4 days). An adrenal source is suggested by suppression of unbound testosterone into the normal range; incomplete suppression suggests ovarian androgen excess.

A baseline plasma total testosterone level >12 nmol/L (>3.5 ng/mL) usually indicates a virilizing tumor, whereas a level >7 nmol/L (>2 ng/mL) is suggestive. A basal DHEAS level >18.5 μmol/L (>7000 μg/L) suggests an adrenal tumor. Although DHEAS has been proposed as a "marker" of predominant adrenal androgen excess, it is not unusual to find modest elevations in DHEAS among women with PCOS. Computed tomography (CT) or magnetic resonance imaging (MRI) should be used to localize an adrenal mass, and ultrasound will usually suffice to identify an ovarian mass, if clinical evaluation and hormonal levels suggest these possibilities.

PCOS is the most common cause of ovarian androgen excess (Chap. 326). However, the increased ratio of LH to follicle-stimu-

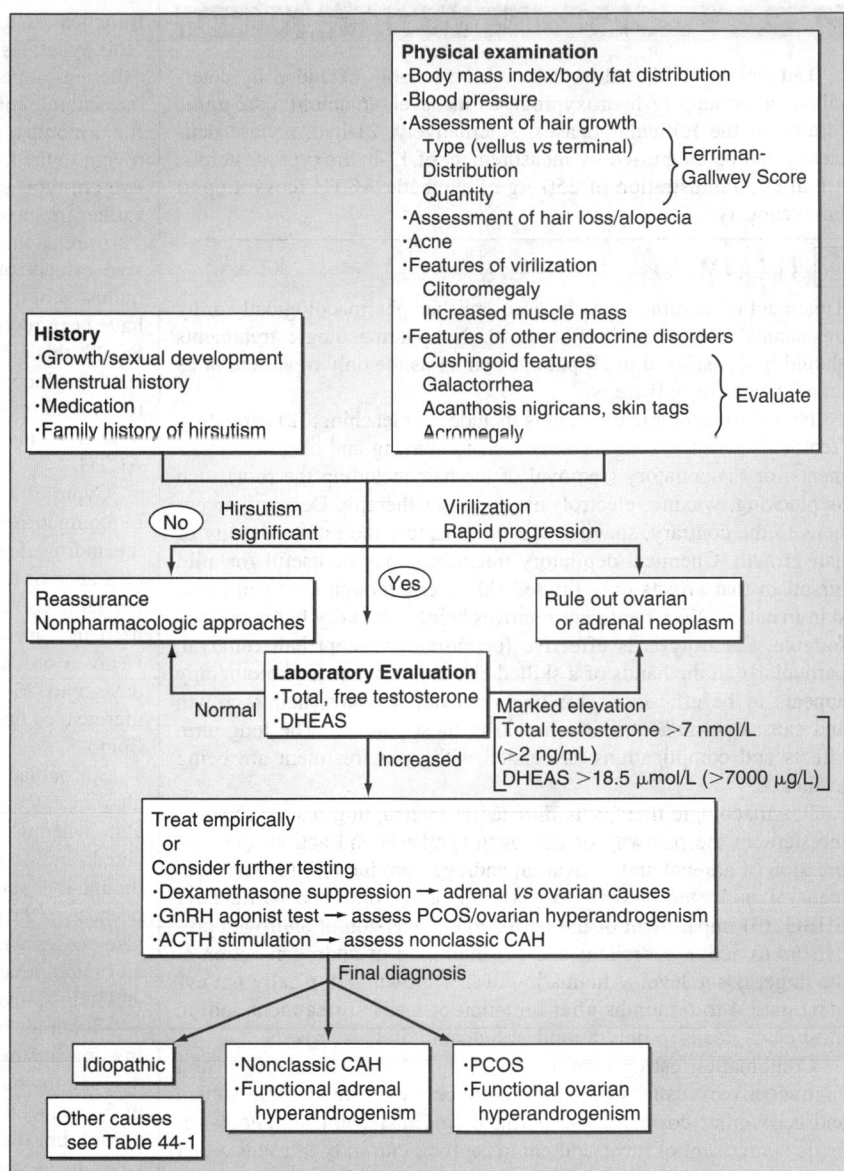

FIGURE 44-2 Algorithm for the evaluation and differential diagnosis of hirsutism. ACTH, adrenocorticotropic hormone; CAH, congenital adrenal hyperplasia; DHEAS, sulfated form of dehydroepiandrosterone; GnRH, gonadotropin-releasing hormone; PCOS, polycystic ovarian syndrome.

lating hormone that is characteristic of carefully studied patients with PCOS is not seen in up to half of these women due to the pulsatility of gonadotropins. If performed, ultrasound shows enlarged ovaries and increased stroma in many women with PCOS. However, polycystic ovaries may also be found in women without clinical or laboratory features of PCOS. Therefore, polycystic ovaries are a relatively insensitive and nonspecific finding for the diagnosis of ovarian hyperandrogenism. Gonadotropin-releasing hormone agonist testing can be used to make a specific diagnosis of ovarian hyperandrogenism. A peak 17-hydroxyprogesterone level ≥7.8 nmol/L (≥2.6 μg/L), after the administration of 100 μg nafarelin (or 10 μg/kg leuprolide) subcutaneously, is virtually diagnostic of ovarian hyperandrogenism.

Nonclassic CAH is most commonly due to 21-hydroxylase deficiency but can also be caused by autosomal recessive defects in other steroidogenic enzymes necessary for adrenal corticosteroid synthesis (Chap. 321). Because of the enzyme defect, the adrenal gland cannot secrete glucocorticoids efficiently (especially cortisol). This results in diminished negative feedback inhibition of ACTH, leading to compensatory adrenal hyperplasia and the accumulation of steroid precursors that are subsequently converted to androgen.

Deficiency of 21-hydroxylase can be reliably excluded by determining a morning 17-hydroxyprogesterone level <6 nmol/L (<2 μg/L) (drawn in the follicular phase). Alternatively, 21-hydroxylase deficiency can be diagnosed by measurement of 17-hydroxyprogesterone 1 h after administration of 250 μg of synthetic ACTH (cosyntropin) intravenously.

R̲x̲ TREATMENT

Treatment of hirsutism may be accomplished pharmacologically or by mechanical means of hair removal. Nonpharmacologic treatments should be considered in all patients, either as the only treatment or as an adjunct to drug therapy.

Nonpharmacologic treatments include (1) bleaching; (2) depilatory (removal from the skin surface) such as shaving and chemical treatments; or (3) epilatory (removal of the hair including the root) such as plucking, waxing, electrolysis, and laser therapy. Despite perceptions to the contrary, shaving does not increase the rate or density of hair growth. Chemical depilatory treatments may be useful for mild hirsutism that affects only limited skin areas, though they can cause skin irritation. Wax treatment removes hair temporarily but is uncomfortable. Electrolysis is effective for more permanent hair removal, particularly in the hands of a skilled electrologist. Laser phototherapy appears to be efficacious for hair removal. It delays hair regrowth and causes permanent hair removal in most patients. The long-term effects and complications associated with laser treatment are being evaluated.

Pharmacologic therapy is directed at interrupting one or more of the steps in the pathway of androgen synthesis and action: (1) suppression of adrenal and/or ovarian androgen production; (2) enhancement of androgen-binding to plasma-binding proteins, particularly SHBG; (3) impairment of the peripheral conversion of androgen precursors to active androgen; and (4) inhibition of androgen action at the target tissue level. Attenuation of hair growth is typically not evident until 4 to 6 months after initiation of medical treatment and, in most cases, leads to only a modest reduction in hair growth.

Combination estrogen-progestin therapy, in the form of an oral contraceptive, is usually the first-line endocrine treatment for hirsutism and acne, after cosmetic and dermatologic management. The estrogenic component of most oral contraceptives currently in use is either ethinyl estradiol or mestranol. The suppression of LH leads to reduced production of ovarian androgens. The reduced androgen levels also result in a dose-related increase in SHBG, thereby lowering the fraction of unbound plasma testosterone. Combination therapy has also been demonstrated to decrease DHEAS, perhaps by reducing ACTH levels. Estrogens also have a direct, dose-dependent suppressive effect on sebaceous cell function.

The choice of a specific oral contraceptive should be predicated on the progestational component, as progestins vary in their suppressive effect on SHBG levels and in their androgenic potential. Ethynodiol diacetate has relatively low androgenic potential, whereas progestins such as norgestrel and levonorgestrel are pargenic, as judged from their attenuation of the estrogen-induced increase in SHBG. Norgestimate exemplifies the newer generation of progestins that are virtually nonandrogenic. Drospirenone, an analogue of spironolactone that has both antiineralocorticoid and antiandrogenic activities, has been approved for use as a progestational agent in combination with ethinyl estradiol. Its properties suggest that it should be the preferred choice for the treatment of hirsutism.

Oral contraceptives are contraindicated in women with a history of thromboembolic disease or in women with increased risk of breast or other estrogen-dependent cancers (Chap. 327). There is a relative contraindication to the use of oral contraceptives in smokers or in those with hypertension or a history of migraine headaches. In most trials, estrogen-progestin therapy alone improves the extent of acne by a maximum of 50 to 70%. The effect on hair growth may not be evident for 6 months, and the maximum effect may require 9 to 12 months owing to the length of the hair growth cycle. Improvements in hirsutism are typically in the range of 20%, but there may be an arrest of further progression of hair growth.

Adrenal androgens are more sensitive than cortisol to the suppressive effects of glucocorticoids. Therefore, glucocorticoids are the mainstay of treatment in patients with CAH. Although glucocorticoids have been reported to restore ovulatory function in some women with PCOS, this effect is highly variable. Because of side effects from excessive glucocorticoids, low doses should be used. Dexamethasone (0.2 to 0.5 mg) or prednisone (5 to 10 mg) should be taken at bedtime to achieve maximal suppression by inhibiting the nocturnal surge of ACTH.

Cyproterone acetate is the prototypic antiandrogen. It acts mainly by competitive inhibition of the binding of testosterone and DHT to the androgen receptor. In addition, it may act to enhance the metabolic clearance of testosterone by inducing hepatic enzymes. Although not available for use in the United States, cyproterone acetate is widely used in Canada, Mexico, and Europe. Cyproterone (50 to 100 mg) is given on days 1 to 15 and ethinyl estradiol (50 μg) is given on days 5 to 26 of the menstrual cycle. Side effects include irregular uterine bleeding, nausea, headache, fatigue, weight gain, and decreased libido.

Spironolactone, usually used as a mineralocorticoid antagonist, is also a weak antiandrogen. It is almost as effective as cyproterone acetate when used at high enough doses (100 to 200 mg daily). Patients should be monitored intermittently for hyperkalemia or hypotension, though these side effects are uncommon. Pregnancy should be avoided because of the risk of feminization of a male fetus. Spironolactone can also cause menstrual irregularity. It is often used in combination with an oral contraceptive, which suppresses ovarian androgen production and helps prevent pregnancy.

Flutamide is a potent nonsteroidal antiandrogen that is effective in treating hirsutism, but concerns about the induction of hepatocellular dysfunction have limited its use. Finasteride is a competitive inhibitor of 5α-reductase type 2. Beneficial effects on hirsutism have been reported, but the predominance of 5α-reductase type 1 in the PSU appears to account for its limited efficacy. Finasteride would also be expected to impair sexual differentiation in a male fetus, and it should not be used in women who may become pregnant.

Eflornithine cream (Vaniqa) has been approved as a novel treatment for unwanted facial hair in women, but long-term efficacy remains to be established. It can cause skin irritation under exaggerated conditions of use. Ultimately, the choice of any specific agent(s) must be tailored to the unique needs of the patient being treated. As noted previously, pharmacologic treatments for hirsutism should be used in conjunction with nonpharmacologic approaches. It is also helpful to review the pattern of female hair distribution in the normal population to dispel unrealistic expectations.

FURTHER READING

CARMINA E: Antiandrogens for the treatment of hirsutism. Expert Opin Investig Drugs 11:357, 2002

FALSETTI L et al: Management of hirsutism. Am J Clin Dermatol 1:89, 2000

HORDINSKY M et al: Hair loss and hirsutism in the elderly. Clin Geriatr Med 18:121, 2002

LANIGAN SW: Management of unwanted hair in females. Clin Exp Dermatol 26:644, 2001

SANCHEZ LA et al: Laser hair reduction in the hirsute patient: A critical assessment. Hum Reprod Update 8:169, 2002

45 INFERTILITY AND FERTILITY CONTROL
Janet E. Hall

The concept of reproductive choice is now firmly entrenched in developed countries and has dramatically altered reproductive behavior. The availability of effective contraceptive methods prevents unintended pregnancies and has important economic and social implications. Infertility, on the other hand, can be accompanied by substantial stress and disappointment. Fortunately, the ability to diagnose and to treat various causes of infertility now provides an array of effective new approaches to this condition.

INFERTILITY

DEFINITION AND PREVALENCE *Infertility* is defined as the inability to conceive after 12 months of unprotected sexual intercourse. In a study of 5574 English and American women who ultimately conceived, pregnancy occurred in 50% within 3 months, 72% within 6 months, and 85% within 12 months. These findings are consistent with predictions based on *fecundability*, the probability of achieving pregnancy in one menstrual cycle (approximately 20 to 25% in healthy young couples). Assuming a fecundability of 0.25, 98% of couples should conceive within 13 months. Based on this definition, the National Survey of Family Growth reports a 14% rate of infertility in the United States in married women aged 15 to 44. The infertility rate has remained relatively stable over the past 30 years, although the proportion of couples without children has risen, reflecting a trend to delay childbearing. This trend has important implications because of an age-related decrease in fecundability, which begins at age 35 and is exacerbated after age 40.

CAUSES OF INFERTILITY The spectrum of infertility ranges from reduced conception rates or the need for medical intervention to irreversible causes of infertility (*sterility*). Infertility can be attributed primarily to male factors in 25%, female factors in 58%, and is unexplained in about 17% of couples (Fig. 45-1). Not uncommonly, both male and female factors contribute to infertility.

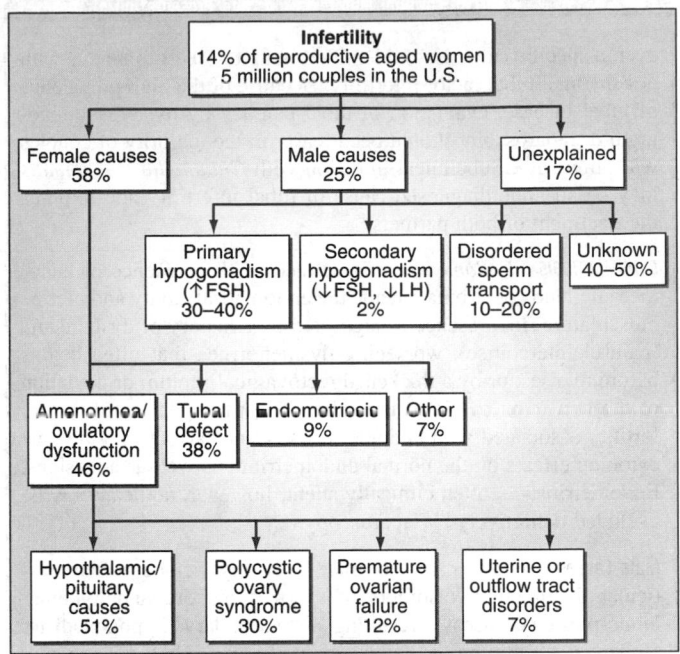

FIGURE 45-1 Causes of infertility. FSH, follicle-stimulating hormone; LH, luteinizing hormone.

APPROACH TO THE PATIENT

Initial Evaluation In all couples presenting with infertility, the initial evaluation includes discussion of the appropriate timing of intercourse and discussion of modifiable risk factors such as smoking, alcohol, caffeine, and obesity. A description of the range of investigations that may be required and a brief description of infertility treatment options, including adoption, should be reviewed. Initial investigations are focused on determining whether the primary cause of the infertility is male, female, or both. These investigations include a semen analysis in the male, confirmation of ovulation in the female, and, in the majority of situations, documentation of tubal patency in the female. Although frequently used in the past, recent studies have not supported the efficacy of postcoital testing of sperm interaction with cervical mucus as a routine component of initial testing. Strategies for further evaluation are described below and in Chaps. 325 and 326. In some cases, after an extensive evaluation has excluded identifiable male or female causes of infertility, the disorder is classified as unexplained infertility.

Psychological Aspects of Infertility Infertility is invariably associated with psychological stress. In addition to the diagnostic and therapeutic procedures, stress may result from repeated cycles of hope and loss associated with each new procedure or cycle of treatment that does not result in the birth of a child. These feelings are often combined with a sense of isolation from friends and family. Counseling and stress-management techniques should be introduced early in the evaluation of infertility. When extreme, stress can contribute to infertility; for example, stress may impair hypothalamic

control of ovulation. Infertility and its treatment do not appear to be associated with long-term psychological sequelae.

Female Causes Abnormalities in menstrual function constitute the most common cause of female infertility. These disorders, which include ovulatory dysfunction and abnormalities of the uterus or outflow tract, may present as amenorrhea (absence of menses) or as irregular or short menstrual cycles. A careful history and physical examination and a limited number of laboratory tests will help to determine whether the abnormality is (1) hypothalamic or pituitary [low follicle-stimulating hormone (FSH), luteinizing hormone (LH), and estradiol with or without an increase in prolactin]; (2) polycystic ovarian syndrome (PCOS; irregular cycles and hyperandrogenism in the absence of other causes of androgen excess); (3) ovarian (low estradiol with increased FSH); or (4) uterine or outflow tract abnormality. The frequency of these diagnoses depends on whether the amenorrhea is primary or occurs after normal puberty and menarche (Fig. 45-1). →*The approach to further evaluation of these disorders is described in detail in Chap. 326.*

OVULATORY DYSFUNCTION In women with a history of regular menstrual cycles, *evidence of ovulation* should be sought by using urinary ovulation predictor kits (they reflect the preovulatory gonadotropin surge but do not confirm ovulation), basal body temperature charts, or a mid-luteal phase progesterone level. The mid-luteal phase progesterone increase (usually >3 ng/mL) confirms ovulation and corpus luteum function and is responsible for the rise in basal body temperature [>0.3°C (>0.6°F) for 10 days]. An endometrial biopsy to exclude luteal phase insufficiency is no longer considered an essential part of the infertility workup for most patients. Even in the presence of ovulatory cycles, evaluation of *ovarian reserve* is recommended for women over 35 by measurement of FSH on day 3 of the cycle or in response to clomiphene, an estrogen antagonist (see below). An FSH level <10 IU/mL on cycle day 3 predicts adequate ovarian oocyte reserve. Inhibin B, an ovarian hormone that selectively suppresses FSH, is not of additional benefit in assessment of ovarian reserve.

TUBAL DISEASE Tubal disease may result from pelvic inflammatory disease (PID), appendicitis, endometriosis, pelvic adhesions, tubal surgery, and previous use of an intrauterine device (IUD). However, a specific cause is not identified in up to 50% of patients with documented tubal factor infertility. Because of the high prevalence of tubal disease, evaluation of tubal patency by hysterosalpingogram or laparoscopy should occur early in the majority of couples with infertility. Subclinical infection with *Chlamydia trachomatis* may be an underdiagnosed cause of tubal infertility and requires the treatment of both partners.

ENDOMETRIOSIS Endometriosis is defined as the presence of endometrial glands or stroma outside the endometrial cavity and uterine musculature. Its presence is suggested by a history of dyspareunia (painful intercourse), worsening dysmenorrhea that often begins before menses, or by a thickened rectovaginal septum or deviation of the cervix on pelvic examination. The pathogenesis of the infertility associated with endometriosis is unclear but may involve cytokine effects on the normal endometrium as well as adhesions. Endometriosis is often clinically silent, however, and can only be excluded definitively by laparoscopy.

Male Causes Known causes of male infertility include primary testicular dysfunction, disorders of sperm transport, and hypothalamic-pituitary disease resulting in secondary hypogonadism. However, the etiology is not ascertained in up to half of men with suspected male factor infertility (Fig. 45-1). The key initial diagnostic test is a *semen analysis*. Although 95% confidence limits can be used to define normal semen parameters, data relating sperm counts to fecundability are more useful. Such studies suggest that normal fertility is associated with sperm counts of >48 million/mL, with a motility of >63%, with >12% exhibiting normal morphology, whereas subfertility is seen with sperm counts of <13 million/mL, motility of <32%, and <9% normal morphology. Abnormalities of spermatogenesis may have a genetic component. Y chromosome microdeletions and *POLG* variants are increasingly recognized as a cause of *azoospermia* (absence of sperm) or *oligospermia* (low sperm count). Y chromosome microdeletions have also been identified in a subset of men with elevated FSH levels and idiopathic infertility. Testosterone levels should be measured if the sperm count is low on repeated examination or if there is clinical evidence of hypogonadism. A low testosterone level may result from *primary gonadal deficiency*; in this condition, levels of LH and FSH will be elevated. Less commonly, low testosterone and decreased spermatogenesis result from hypothalamic or pituitary disease, in which case the LH and FSH levels will be low (Chap. 325).

Acquired disorders of the testes are often associated with impaired spermatogenesis with relatively preserved Leydig cell function; thus, testosterone levels may be normal. Such abnormalities include viral orchitis (especially mumps) and other infectious causes such as tuberculosis or sexually transmitted diseases (STDs), chemotherapy (especially the alkylating agents cyclophosphamide and chlorambucil), ionizing radiation, and drugs that may impair fertility directly or through inhibition of testicular androgen production or action. Anabolic androgen abuse should be considered in a well-androgenized man with low gonadotropins and testosterone but a suppressed sperm count. Prolonged elevation of testicular temperature may impair spermatogenesis, e.g., cryptorchidism, after an acute febrile illness or in association with varicocele. A potential role for environmental toxins as a cause of impaired spermatogenesis has been suggested based on an apparent decrease in sperm counts over the past several decades, but a direct cause-and-effect relationship has not been established.

SECONDARY HYPOGONADISM Low gonadotropin levels, associated with low testosterone, may signal the presence of a pituitary macroadenoma or hypothalamic tumor (in both cases prolactin levels may be elevated; Chap. 318) or may be the first presentation of hemochromatosis (Chap. 336) or other systemic illness. Recent studies have identified several genetic causes of gonadotropin-releasing hormone (GnRH) deficiency (*KAL* and *DAX-1*), as well as mutations that lead to isolated gonadotropin deficiency (GnRH receptor, LHβ, FSHβ mutations) (Chap. 318).

DISORDERED SPERM TRANSPORT Patients with low sperm counts and normal hormonal levels may be found to have obstructive abnormalities of the vas deferens or epididymus. The most common causes of vas deferens obstruction are previous vasectomy or accidental ligation during inguinal surgery. Congenital absence of the vas deferens can be diagnosed by a deficiency of fructose in the ejaculate and is often associated with an abnormality of the cystic fibrosis transmembrane regulator (*CFTR*) gene. Young's syndrome, characterized by inspissated secretions, can also preclude normal sperm transport.

R_x TREATMENT

The treatment of infertility should be tailored to the problems unique to each couple. In many situations, including unexplained infertility, mild to moderate endometriosis, and/or borderline semen parameters, a stepwise approach to infertility is optimal, beginning with low-risk interventions and moving to more invasive, higher risk interventions only if necessary. After determination of all infertility factors and their correction, if possible, this approach might include, in increasing order of complexity: (1) expectant management, (2) clomiphene citrate (see below) with or without intrauterine insemination (IUI), (3) gonadotropins with or without IUI, and (4) in vitro fertilization (IVF). The time used to complete the evaluation, correction, and expectant management can be longer in women <30, but this process should be advanced rapidly in women >35. In some situations, expectant management will not be appropriate.

Ovulatory Dysfunction Treatment of ovulatory dysfunction should first be directed at identification of the etiology of the disorder to allow specific management when possible. Dopamine agonists, for example, may be indicated in patients with hyperprolactinemia (Chap. 318); lifestyle modification may be successful in women with low body weight or a history of intensive exercise (Chap. 65).

Medications used for ovulation induction include clomiphene citrate, gonadotropins, and pulsatile GnRH. *Clomiphene citrate* is a nonsteroidal estrogen antagonist that increases FSH and LH levels by blocking estrogen negative feedback at the hypothalamus. The efficacy of clomiphene for ovulation induction is highly dependent on patient selection. It induces ovulation in 70 to 80% of women with PCOS and is the initial treatment of choice in these patients, particularly in conjunction with the use of insulin-sensitizing agents, such as metformin. Clomiphene citrate is less successful in patients with hypogonadotropic hypogonadism.

Gonadotropins are highly effective for ovulation induction in women with hypogonadotropic hypogonadism and PCOS and are used to induce multiple follicular recruitment in unexplained infertility and in older reproductive-aged women. Disadvantages include a significant risk of multiple gestation and the risk of ovarian hyperstimulation, but careful monitoring and a conservative approach to ovarian stimulation reduce these risks. Currently available gonadotropins include urinary preparations of LH and FSH, highly purified FSH, and recombinant FSH. Though FSH is the key component, the addition of some LH (or human chorionic gonadotropin) may improve results, particularly in hypogonadotropic patients.

Pulsatile GnRH is highly effective for restoring ovulation in patients with hypothalamic amenorrhea but is not widely available in the United States. Pregnancy rates are similar to those following the use of gonadotropins, but rates of multiple gestation are lower and there is virtually no risk of ovarian hyperstimulation.

None of these methods are effective in women with premature ovarian failure in whom donor oocyte or adoption are the methods of choice.

Tubal Disease If hysterosalpingography suggests a tubal or uterine cavity abnormality, or if a patient is ≥35 at the time of initial evaluation, laparoscopy with tubal lavage is recommended, often with a hysteroscopy. Although tubal reconstruction may be attempted if tubal disease is identified, IVF is often used instead, as these patients are at increased risk of developing an ectopic pregnancy.

Endometriosis Though 60% of women with minimal or mild endometriosis may conceive within 1 year without treatment, laparoscopic resection or ablation appears to improve conception rates. Medical management of advanced stages of endometriosis is widely used for symptom control but has not been shown to enhance fertility (Chap. 326). In moderate to severe endometriosis, conservative surgery is associated with pregnancy rates of 50 and 39% respectively, compared with rates of 25 and 5% with expectant management alone. In some patients, IVF may be the treatment of choice.

Male Factor Infertility Treatment options for male factor infertility have expanded greatly in recent years. Secondary hypogonadism is highly amenable to treatment with pulsatile GnRH or gonadotropins (Chap. 325). In vitro techniques have provided new opportunities for patients with primary testicular failure and disorders of sperm transport. Choice of initial treatment options depends on sperm concentration and motility. Expectant management should be attempted initially in men with mild male factor infertility (sperm count of 15 to 20 × 10⁶/mL and normal motility). Moderate male factor infertility (10 to 15 × 10⁶/mL and 20 to 40% motility) should begin with IUI alone or in combination with treatment of the female partner with clomiphene or gonadotropins, but it may require IVF with or without intracytoplasmic sperm injection (ICSI). For men with a severe defect (sperm count of <10 × 10⁶/mL, 10% motility), IVF with ICSI or donor sperm should be used.

Assisted Reproductive Technologies The development of assisted reproductive technologies (ART) has dramatically altered the treatment of male and female infertility. IVF is indicated for patients with many causes of infertility that have not been successfully managed with more conservative approaches. IVF or ICSI is often the treatment of choice in couples with a significant male factor or tubal disease, whereas IVF using donor oocytes is used in patients with premature ovarian failure and in women of advanced reproductive age. Success rates depend on the age of the woman and the cause of the infertility and are generally 18 to 24% per cycle when initiated in women <40. In women >40, there is a marked decrease in both the number of oocytes retrieved and their ability to be fertilized. Though often effective, IVF is expensive and requires careful monitoring of ovulation induction and invasive techniques, including the aspiration of multiple follicles. IVF is associated with a significant risk of multiple gestation (31% twins, 6% triplets, and 0.2% higher order multiples).

CONTRACEPTION

Though various forms of contraception are widely available, approximately 30% of births in the United States are the result of unintended pregnancy. Teenage pregnancies continue to represent a serious public health problem in the United States, with >1 million unintended pregnancies each year—a significantly greater incidence than in other industrialized nations.

Contraceptive methods are widely used (Table 45-1). Only 15% of couples report having unprotected sexual intercourse in the past 3

TABLE 45-1 *Effectiveness of Different Forms of Contraception*

Method of Contraception	Theoretical Effectiveness, %[a]	Actual Effectiveness, %[a]	% Continuing Use at 1 Year[b]	Contraceptive Methods Used by U.S. Women[c]
Barrier methods				
Condoms	98	88	63	20
Diaphragm	94	82	58	2
Cervical cap	94	82	50	<1
Spermicides	97	79	43	1
Sterilization				
Male	99.9	99.9	100	11
Female	99.8	99.6	100	28
Intrauterine device				1
Copper T380	99	97	78	
Progestasert	98	97	81	
Mirena	99.9	99.8		
Oral contraceptive pill			72	27
Combination	99.9	97		
Progestin only	99.5	97		
Long-acting progestins				
Depo-Provera	99.7	99.7	70	<1
Norplant	99.7	99.7	85	1

[a] Adapted from Trussel J et al, Obstet Gynecol 76:558, 1990.
[b] Adapted from Contraceptive Technology Update. Contraceptive Technology, Feb. 1996, vol 17, No 1, pp 13–24.
[c] Adapted from Piccinino LJ and Mosher WD, Fam Plan Perspective 30:4, 1998.

months. A reversible form of contraception is used by >50% of couples. Sterilization (in either the male or female) has been employed as a permanent form of contraception by over a third of couples. Pregnancy termination is relatively safe when directed by health care professionals but is rarely the option of choice.

No single contraceptive method is ideal, although all are safer than carrying a pregnancy to term. The effectiveness of a given method of contraception is dependent on the efficacy of the method itself, compliance, and appropriate use. Knowledge of the advantages and disadvantages of each contraceptive is essential for counseling an individual about the methods that are safest and most consistent with his or her lifestyle. Discrepancies between theoretical and actual effectiveness emphasize the importance of patient education and compliance when considering various forms of contraception (Table 45-1).

BARRIER METHODS Barrier contraceptives (such as condoms, diaphragms, and cervical caps) and spermicides are easily available, reversible, and have fewer side effects than hormonal methods. However, their effectiveness is highly dependent on compliance and proper use (Table 45-1). A major advantage of barrier contraceptives is the protection provided against STDs (Chap. 115). Consistent use is associated with a decreased risk of gonorrhea, nongonococcal urethritis, and genital herpes, probably due in part to the concomitant use of spermicides. Condom use also reduces the transmission of HIV infection. Natural membrane condoms may be less effective than latex condoms, and petroleum-based lubricants can degrade condoms and decrease their efficacy for preventing HIV infection. A highly effective female condom, which also provides protection against STDs, was approved in 1994 but has not achieved widespread use.

STERILIZATION Sterilization is the method of birth control most frequently chosen by fertile men and multiparous women >30 (Table 45-1). Sterilization prevents fertilization by surgical interruption of the fallopian tubes in women or the vas deferens in men. Although tubal ligation and vasectomy are potentially reversible, these procedures should be considered permanent and should not be undertaken without careful patient counseling.

Several methods of *tubal ligation* have been developed, all of which are highly effective with a 10-year cumulative pregnancy rate of 1.85 per 100 women. However, when pregnancy does occur, the risk of ectopic pregnancy may be as high as 30%. In addition to prevention of pregnancy, tubal ligation reduces the risk of ovarian cancer, possibly by limiting the upward migration of potential carcinogens.

Vasectomy is an outpatient surgical procedure that has little risk and is highly effective. The development of azoospermia may be delayed for 2 to 6 months, and other forms of contraception must be used until two sperm-free ejaculations provide proof of sterility.

INTRAUTERINE DEVICES IUDs inhibit pregnancy primarily through a spermicidal effect caused by a sterile inflammatory reaction produced by the presence of a foreign body in the uterine cavity (copper IUDs) or by the release of progestins (Progestasert, Mirena). IUDs provide a high level of efficacy in the absence of systemic metabolic effects, and ongoing motivation is not required to ensure efficacy once the device has been placed. However, only 1% of women in the United States use this method compared to a utilization rate of 15 to 30% in much of Europe and Canada. This relatively low utilization rate continues despite evidence that the newer devices are not associated with increased rates of pelvic infection and infertility, as occurred with earlier devices. Screening for STDs should be performed prior to insertion, and an IUD should not be used in women at high risk for development of STDs or in women at high risk for bacterial endocarditis.

HORMONAL METHODS ■ Oral Contraceptive Pills Because of their ease of use and efficacy, oral contraceptive pills are the most widely used form of hormonal contraception. They act by suppressing ovulation, changing cervical mucus, and altering the endometrium. The current formulations are made from synthetic estrogens and progestins. The estrogen component of the pill consists of ethinyl estradiol or mestranol, which is metabolized to ethinyl estradiol. Multiple synthetic progestins are available. Norethindrone and its derivatives are used in many formulations. Low-dose norgestimate and the more recently developed progestins (desogestrel, gestodene, drospirenone) have a less androgenic profile; levonorgestrel appears to be the most androgenic of the progestins and should be avoided in patients with hyperandrogenic features. The three major formulations of oral contraceptives are: (1) fixed-dose estrogen-progestin combination, (2) phasic estrogen-progestin combination, and (3) progestin only. Combination formulations are administered daily for 3 weeks followed by a week of no medication during which menstrual bleeding generally occurs. Progestin-only pills are administered continuously. There has been recent interest in the development of extended oral contraceptives, reducing the number of episodes of withdrawal bleeding. An oral, trimonthly regimen is currently under investigation in the United States. Preliminary studies indicate that headache is reduced, although there is an early incidence of breakthrough bleeding.

Current doses of ethinyl estradiol range from 20 to 50 μg. However, indications for the 50-μg dose are rare, and the majority of formulations contain 35 μg of ethinyl estradiol. The reduced estrogen and progesterone content in the second- and third-generation pills has decreased both side effects and risks associated with oral contraceptive use (Table 45-2). At the currently used doses, patients must be cautioned not to miss pills due to the potential for ovulation. Side effects, including break-through bleeding, amenorrhea, breast tenderness, and weight gain, are often responsive to a change in formulation.

The microdose progestin-only minipill is less effective as a contraceptive, having a pregnancy rate of 2 to 7 per 100 women-years. However, it may be appropriate for women with cardiovascular disease or for women who cannot tolerate synthetic estrogens.

New Methods A *weekly contraceptive patch* (Ortho Evra) is now available. It has similar efficacy to oral contraceptives and may be associated with less breakthrough bleeding. Approximately 2% of patches fail to adhere, and a similar percentage of women have skin reactions. Efficacy is lower in women >90 kg. A *monthly contraceptive injection* (Lunelle) is also available. This estrogen/progestin combination is highly effective, with a first-year failure rate of <0.2%, but it may be less effective in obese women. Its use is associated with bleeding irregularities that diminish over time. Fertility returns rapidly after discontinuation. A *monthly vaginal ring* (NuvaRing) is now approved for contraceptive use. It is highly effective, with a 12-month failure rate of 0.7%. The device is intended to be left in place during intercourse.

TABLE 45-2 *Oral Contraceptives: Contraindications and Disease Risk*

I. Contraindications
  A. Absolute
    1. Previous thromboembolic event or stroke
    2. History of an estrogen-dependent tumor
    3. Active liver disease
    4. Pregnancy
    5. Undiagnosed abnormal uterine bleeding
    6. Hypertriglyceridemia
    7. Women over age 35 who smoke heavily (>15 cigarettes per day)
  B. Relative
    1. Hypertension
    2. Women receiving anticonvulsant drug therapy
II. Disease risks
  A. Increased
    1. Coronary heart disease—increased only in smokers > 35; no relation to progestin type
    2. Hypertension—relative risk 1.8 (current users) and 1.2 (previous users)
    3. Venous thrombosis—relative risk ~4; markedly increased with factor V Leiden or prothrombin-gene mutations
    4. Stroke—increased only in combination with hypertension; unclear relation to migraine headache
    5. Cerebral vein thrombosis—relative risk 13–15; synergistic with prothrombin-gene mutation
    6. Cervical cancer—relative risk 2–4
  B. Decreased
    1. Ovarian cancer—50% reduction in risk
    2. Endometrial cancer—40% reduction in risk
  C. No effect
    1. Breast cancer

If removed during intercourse, it must be reinserted within 3 h. Ovulation returns within the first recovery cycle after discontinuation.

Long-Term Contraceptives Long-term progestin administration in the form of Depo-Provera and Norplant (Table 45-1) act primarily by inhibiting ovulation and causing changes in the endometrium and cervical mucus that result in decreased implantation and sperm transport. Depo-Provera requires an intramuscular injection and is effective for 3 months, but return of fertility after discontinuation may be delayed for up to 12 to 18 months. Norplant requires surgical insertion but is effective for up to 5 years afer insertion; fertility is possible shortly after its removal. Amenorrhea, irregular bleeding, and weight gain are the most common adverse effects associated with both injectable forms of contraception. A major advantage of the injectable progestin-based contraceptives is the apparent lack of increased arterial and venous thromboembolic events, but increased gallbladder disease and decreased bone density may result.

POSTCOITAL CONTRACEPTION Postcoital contraceptive methods prevent implantation or cause regression of the corpus luteum and are highly efficacious if used appropriately. Unprotected intercourse without regard to the time of the month carries an 8% incidence of pregnancy, an incidence that can be reduced to 2% by the use of emergency contraceptives within 72 h of unprotected intercourse. Certain oral contraceptive pills can be used within 72 h of unprotected intercourse [Ovral (2 tablets, 12 h apart) and Lo/Ovral (4 tablets, 12 h apart)]. Preven (50 mg ethinyl estradiol and 0.25 mg levonorgestrel) and Plan B (0.75 mg levonorgestrel) are now approved for postcoital contraception. Side effects are common with these high doses of hormones and include nausea, vomiting, and breast soreness. Recent studies suggest that 600 mg mifepristone (RU486), a progesterone receptor antagonist, may be equally as effective or more effective than hormonal regimens, with fewer side effects.

MALE HORMONAL CONTRACEPTION An effective and reversible male contraceptive has long been sought, and surveys indicate that a "male pill" would be acceptable to both men and women. Complete suppression of spermatogenesis is required for acceptable contraception but is not achieved reliably with testosterone alone. However, the combination of a long-acting testosterone preparation with a GnRH antagonist or a progestin such as norgestral, desonorgestrel, or norethisterone results in effective contraception, suggesting that a male contraceptive may be forthcoming.

FURTHER READING

ABMA JC et al and the National Center for Health Statistics: Fertility, family planning, and women's health: New data from the 1995 Survey of Family Growth. Vital Health Stat 23, no. 10

ANDERSON RA et al: Male contraception. Endocr Rev 23:735, 2002

GUZIK DS et al: Sperm morphology, motility and concentration in fertile and infertile men. N Engl J Med 345:1388, 2001

KURODA-KAWAGUCHI T et al: The AZFc region of the Y chromosome features massive palindromes and uniform recurrent deletions in infertile men. Nat Genet 29:279, 2001

MARCHBANKS PA et al. Oral contraceptives and the risk of breast cancer. N Engl J Med 346:2025, 2002

TRUSSELL J, VAUGHAN B: Contraceptive failure, method-related discontinuation and resumption of use: Results from the 1995 National Survey of Family Growth. Fam Plan Perspect 31:64, 1999

Section 9   Alterations in the Skin

46 | APPROACH TO THE PATIENT WITH A SKIN DISORDER
Thomas J. Lawley, Kim B. Yancey

The challenge of examining the skin lies in distinguishing normal from abnormal, significant findings from trivial ones, and in integrating pertinent signs and symptoms into an appropriate differential diagnosis. The fact that the largest organ in the body is visible is both an advantage and a disadvantage to those who examine it. It is advantageous because no special instrumentation is necessary and because the skin can be biopsied with little morbidity. However, the casual observer can be misled by a variety of stimuli and overlook important, subtle signs of skin or systemic disease. For instance, the sometimes minor differences in color and shape that distinguish a malignant melanoma (Fig. 46-1) from a benign pigmented nevus (Fig. 46-2) can be difficult to recognize. To aid in the interpretation of skin lesions, a variety of descriptive terms have been developed to characterize cutaneous lesions (Tables 46-1 and 46-2 and Fig. 46-3) and to formulate a differential diagnosis (Table 46-3). For instance, the finding of large numbers of scaling papules, usually indicative of a primary skin disease, places the patient in a different diagnostic category than would hemorrhagic papules, which may indicate vasculitis or sepsis (Figs. 46-4 and 46-5, respectively). It is important to differentiate primary skin lesions from secondary skin changes. If the examiner focuses on linear erosions overlying an area of erythema and scaling, he or she may incorrectly assume that the erosion is the primary lesion and the redness and scale are secondary, while the correct interpretation would be that the patient has a pruritic eczematous dermatitis with erosions caused by scratching.

FIGURE 46-2   Nevi are benign proliferations of nevomelanocytes characterized by regularly shaped hyperpigmented macules or papules of a uniform color.

APPROACH TO THE PATIENT

In examining the skin it is usually advisable to assess the patient before taking an extensive history. This way, the entire cutaneous surface is sure to be evaluated, and objective findings can be integrated with relevant historic data. Four basic features of any cutaneous lesion must be noted and considered in the examination of

FIGURE 46-1   Superficial spreading melanoma is the most common type of malignant melanoma and demonstrates color variegation (black, blue, brown, pink, and white) and irregular borders.

TABLE 46-1   Descriptions of Primary Skin Lesions

Macule: A flat, colored lesion, <2 cm in diameter, not raised above the surface of the surrounding skin. A "freckle," or ephelid, is a prototype pigmented macule.

Patch: A large (>2 cm), flat lesion with a color different from the surrounding skin. This differs from a macule only in size.

Papule: A small, solid lesion, <0.5 cm in diameter, raised above the surface of the surrounding skin and hence palpable (e.g., a closed comedone, or whitehead, in acne).

Nodule: A larger (0.5–5.0 cm), firm lesion raised above the surface of the surrounding skin. This differs from a papule only in size (e.g., dermal nevus).

Tumor: A solid, raised growth >5 cm in diameter.

Plaque: A large (>1 cm), flat-topped, raised lesion; edges may either be distinct (e.g., in psoriasis) or gradually blend with surrounding skin (e.g., in eczematous dermatitis).

Vesicle: A small, fluid-filled lesion, <0.5 cm in diameter, raised above the plane of surrounding skin. Fluid is often visible, and the lesions are often translucent [e.g., vesicles in allergic contact dermatitis caused by *Toxicodendron* (poison ivy)].

Pustule: A vesicle filled with leukocytes. Note: The presence of pustules does not necessarily signify the existence of an infection.

Bulla: A fluid-filled, raised, often translucent lesion >0.5 cm in diameter.

Cyst: A soft, raised, encapsulated lesion filled with semisolid or liquid contents.

Wheal: A raised, erythematous papule or plaque, usually representing short-lived dermal edema.

Telangiectasia: Dilated, superficial blood vessels.

TABLE 46-2   *Common Dermatologic Terms*

Lichenification: A distinctive thickening of the skin that is characterized by accentuated skin-fold markings and that feels thick on palpation.

Crust: Dried exudate of body fluids that may be either yellow (serous exudate) or red (hemorrhagic exudate).

Milia: Small, firm, white papules that are filled with keratin (and may in part resemble pustules).

Erosion: Loss of epidermis without an associated loss of dermis.

Ulcer: Loss of epidermis and at least a portion of the underlying dermis.

Excoriations: Linear, angular erosions that may be covered by crust and are caused by scratching.

Atrophy: An acquired loss of substance. In the skin, this may appear as a depression with intact epidermis (i.e., loss of dermal or subcutaneous tissue) or as sites of shiny, delicate, wrinkled lesions (i.e., epidermal atrophy).

Scar: A change in the skin secondary to trauma or inflammation. Sites may be erythematous, hypopigmented, or hypertrophic depending on their age or character. Sites on hair-bearing areas may be characterized by destruction of hair follicles.

Pruritus: A sensation that elicits the desire to scratch. Pruritus is often the predominant symptom of inflammatory skin diseases (e.g., atopic dermatitis, allergic contact dermatitis); it is also commonly associated with xerosis and aged skin. Systemic conditions that can be associated with pruritus include chronic renal disease, cholestasis, pregnancy, malignancy, polycythemia vera, and delusions of parasitosis.

FIGURE 46-4   Palpable purpuric papules on the lower legs are seen in this patient with cutaneous small vessel vasculitis. *(Courtesy of Robert Swerlick, MD.)*

skin: the distribution of the eruption, the type(s) of primary lesion, the shape of individual lesions, and the arrangement of the lesions. In the initial examination it is important that the patient be disrobed as completely as possible. This will minimize chances of missing important individual skin lesions and make it possible to assess the distribution of the eruption accurately. The patient should first be viewed from a distance of about 1.5 to 2 m (4 to 6 ft) so that the general character of the skin and the distribution of lesions can be evaluated. Indeed, distribution of lesions often correlates highly with diagnosis (Fig. 46-6). For example, a hospitalized patient with a generalized erythematous exanthem is more likely to have a drug eruption than is a patient with a similar rash limited to the sun-exposed portions of the face. The presence or absence of lesions on mucosal surfaces should also be determined. Once the distribution of the lesions has been established, the nature of the primary

lesion must be determined. Thus, when lesions are distributed on elbows, knees, and scalp, the most likely possibility based solely on distribution is psoriasis or dermatitis herpetiformis (Figs. 46-7 and 46-8, respectively). The primary lesion in psoriasis is a scaly papule that soon forms erythematous plaques covered with a white scale, whereas that of dermatitis herpetiformis is an urticarial papule that quickly becomes a small vesicle. In this manner, identification of the primary lesion directs the examiner toward the proper diagnosis. Secondary changes in skin can also be quite helpful. For example, scale represents excessive epidermis, while crust is the result of a discontinuous epithelial cell layer. Palpation of skin lesions can also yield insight into the character of an eruption. Thus red papules on the lower extremities that blanch with pressure can be a manifestation of many different diseases, but hemorrhagic red papules that do not blanch with pressure indicate palpable purpura characteristic of necrotizing vasculitis (Fig. 46-4).

The shape of lesions is also an important feature. Flat, round, erythematous papules and plaques are common in many cutaneous diseases. However, target-shaped lesions that consist in part of erythematous plaques are specific for erythema multiforme (Fig. 46-9). In the same way, the arrangement of individual lesions is important. Erythematous papules and vesicles can occur in many conditions, but their arrangement in a specific linear array suggests an external etiology such as allergic contact (Fig. 46-10) or primary

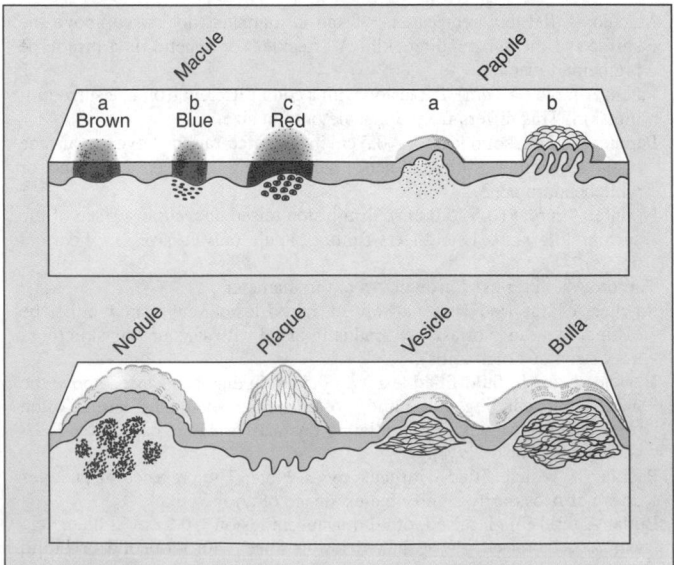

FIGURE 46-3   A schematic representation of several common primary skin lesions (see Table 46-1).

FIGURE 46-5   Fulminant meningococcemia with extensive angular purpuric patches. *(Courtesy of Stephen E. Gellis, MD.)*

TABLE 46-3 *Selected Common Dermatologic Conditions*

Diagnosis	Common Distribution	Usual Morphology	Diagnosis	Common Distribution	Usual Morphology
Acne vulgaris	Face, upper back	Open and closed comedones, erythematous papules, pustules, cysts	Seborrheic keratosis	Trunk, face	Brown plaques with adherent, greasy scale; "stuck on" appearance
Rosacea	Blush area of cheeks, nose, forehead, chin	Erythema, telangiectasias, papules, pustules	Folliculitis	Any hair-bearing area	Follicular pustules
Seborrheic dermatitis	Scalp, eyebrows, perinasal areas	Erythema with greasy yellow-brown scale	Impetigo	Anywhere	Papules, vesicles, pustules, often with honey-colored crusts
Atopic dermatitis	Antecubital and popliteal fossae; may be widespread	Patches and plaques of erythema, scaling, and lichenification; pruritus	Herpes simplex	Lips, genitalia	Grouped vesicles progressing to crusted erosions
Stasis dermatitis	Ankles, lower legs	Patches of erythema and scaling on background of hyperpigmentation associated with signs of venous insufficiency	Herpes zoster	Dermatomal, usually trunk but may be anywhere	Vesicles limited to a dermatome (often painful)
Dyshidrotic eczema	Palms, soles, sides of fingers and toes	Deep vesicles	Varicella	Face, trunk, relative sparing of extremities	Lesions arise in crops and quickly progress from erythematous macules to papules to vesicles to pustules to crusts
Allergic contact dermatitis	Anywhere	Localized erythema, vesicles, scale, and pruritus (e.g., fingers, earlobes—nickel; dorsal aspect of foot—shoe; exposed surfaces—poison ivy)	Pityriasis rosea	Trunk (Christmas tree pattern); herald patch followed by multiple smaller lesions	Symmetric erythematous patches with a collarette of scale
Psoriasis	Elbows, knees, scalp, lower back, fingernails (may be generalized)	Papules and plaques covered with silvery scale; nails have pits	Tinea versicolor	Chest, back, abdomen, proximal extremities	Scaly hyper- or hypopigmented macules
Lichen planus	Wrists, ankles, mouth (may be widespread)	Violaceous flat-topped papules and plaques	Candidiasis	Groin, beneath breasts, vagina, oral cavity	Erythematous macerated areas with satellite pustules; white, friable patches on mucous membranes
Keratosis pilaris	Extensor surfaces of arms and thighs, buttocks	Keratotic follicular papules with surrounding erythema	Dermatophytosis	Feet, groin, beard, or scalp	Varies with site, (e.g., tinea corporis—scaly annular patch)
Melasma	Forehead, cheeks, temples, upper lip	Tan to brown patches	Scabies	Groin, axillae, between fingers and toes, beneath breasts	Excoriated papules, burrows, pruritus
Vitiligo	Periorificial, trunk, extensor surfaces of extremities, flexor wrists, axillae	Chalk-white macules	Insect bites	Anywhere	Erythematous papules with central puncta
Actinic keratosis	Sun-exposed areas	Skin-colored or red-brown macule or papule with dry, rough, adherent scale	Cherry angioma	Trunk	Red, blood-filled papules
			Keloid	Anywhere (site of previous injury)	Firm tumor, pink, purple, or brown
Basal cell carcinoma	Face	Papule with pearly, telangiectatic border on sun-damaged skin	Dermatofibroma	Anywhere	Firm red to brown nodule that shows dimpling of overlying skin with lateral compression
Squamous cell carcinoma	Face, especially lower lip, ears	Indurated and possibly hyperkeratotic lesions often showing ulceration and/or crusting	Acrochordons (skin tags)	Groin, axilla, neck	Fleshy papules
			Urticaria	Anywhere	Wheals, sometimes with surrounding flare; pruritus
			Transient acantholytic dermatosis	Trunk, especially anterior chest	Erythematous papules
			Xerosis	Extensor extremities, especially legs	Dry, erythematous, scaling patches; pruritus

irritant dermatitis. In contrast, lesions with a generalized arrangement are common and suggest a systemic etiology.

As in other branches of medicine, a complete history should be obtained to emphasize the following features:

1. Evolution of lesions
   a. Site of onset
   b. Manner in which the eruption progressed or spread
   c. Duration
   d. Periods of resolution or improvement in chronic eruptions
2. Symptoms associated with the eruption
   a. Itching, burning, pain, numbness
   b. What, if anything, has relieved symptoms
   c. Time of day when symptoms are most severe

3. Current or recent medications (prescribed as well as over-the-counter)
4. Associated systemic symptoms (e.g., malaise, fever, arthralgias)
5. Ongoing or previous illnesses
6. History of allergies
7. Presence of photosensitivity
8. Review of systems

DIAGNOSTIC TECHNIQUES   Many skin diseases can be diagnosed on gross clinical appearance, but sometimes relatively simple diagnostic procedures can yield valuable information. In most instances, they can be performed at the bedside with a minimum of equipment.

A

Psoriasis
Acne vulgaris
Pityriasis rosea
Lichen planus
Perianal lesions
  Hemorrhoids
  Condyloma acuminata
  Herpes simplex
  Dermatitis
  Vitiligo

Epidermal inclusion cyst
Herpes zoster
Psoriasis
Psoriasis
Folliculitis
Dyshidrotic eczema
Hand eczema
Atopic dermatitis
Verruca plana
Tinea pedis

B

Keratosis pilaris
Verrucae vulgaris
Asteatotic eczema
Lichen simplex chronicus

Skin tags
Seborrheic keratoses
Senile angioma
Atopic dermatitis
Tinea or Candida cruris
Actinic keratoses
Psoriasis
Dermatofibroma
Stasis ulcer
Stasis dermatitis
Tinea pedis

C

Actinic keratoses
Basal cell carcinoma
Contact dermatitis
Skin tags

Seborrheic dermatitis
Melasma
Seborrheic dermatitis
Xanthelasma
Acne rosacea
Seborrheic dermatitis
Perleche
Acne vulgaris

D

Herpes labialis
Lichen planus
Aphthous stomatitis
Geographic tongue

Leukoplakia
Squamous cell carcinoma
Oral hairy leukoplakia

FIGURE 46-6 *A–D.* The distribution of some common dermatologic diseases and lesions.

Skin Biopsy   A skin biopsy is a straightforward minor surgical procedure; however, it is important to biopsy a lesion that is most likely to yield diagnostic findings. This decision may require expertise in skin diseases and knowledge of superficial anatomic structures in selected areas of the body. In this procedure, a small area of skin is anesthetized with 1% lidocaine with or without epinephrine. The skin lesion in question can be excised with a scalpel or removed by punch biopsy. In the latter technique, a punch is pressed against the surface of the skin and rotated with downward pressure until it penetrates to the subcutaneous tissue. The circular biopsy is then lifted with forceps, and the bottom is cut with iris scissors. Biopsy sites may or may not need suture closure, depending on size and location.

KOH Preparation   A potassium hydroxide (KOH) preparation is performed on scaling skin lesions where a fungal etiology is a possibility. The edge of such a lesion is scraped gently with a scalpel blade, and the removed scale is collected on a glass microscope slide and treated with 1 to 2 drops of a solution of 10 to 20% KOH. KOH dissolves keratin and allows easier visualization of fungal elements. Brief heating of the slide accelerates dissolution of keratin. When the preparation

FIGURE 46-7   Psoriasis is characterized by small and large erythematous plaques with adherent silvery scale.

FIGURE 46-8   Dermatitis herpetiformis manifested by pruritic, grouped vesicles in a typical location. The vesicles are often excoriated and may occur on knees, buttocks, and posterior scalp.

is viewed under the microscope, the refractile hyphae will be seen more easily when the light intensity is reduced and the condenser is lowered. This technique can be utilized to identify hyphae in dermatophyte infections (see Fig. 190-1), pseudohyphae and budding yeast in *Candida* infections (see Fig. 187-1), and fragmented hyphae and spores in tinea versicolor. The same sampling technique can be used to obtain scale for culture of selected pathogenic organisms.

Tzanck Smear   A Tzanck smear is a cytologic technique most often used in the diagnosis of herpesvirus infections [simplex or varicella-zoster (see Figs. 164-1 and 164-3). An early vesicle, not a pustule or crusted lesion, is unroofed, and the base of the lesion is scraped gently with a scalpel blade. The material is placed on a glass slide, air-dried, and stained with Giemsa or Wright's stain. Multinucleated epithelial giant cells suggest the presence of herpes, but culture or immunofluorescence testing must be performed to identify the specific virus.

Diascopy   Diascopy is designed to assess whether a skin lesion will blanch with pressure as, for example, in determining whether a red lesion is hemorrhagic or simply blood-filled. For instance, urticaria (Fig. 46-11) will blanch with pressure, whereas a purpuric lesion caused by necrotizing vasculitis (Fig. 46-4) will not. Diascopy is performed by pressing a microscope slide or magnifying lens against a lesion and noting the amount of blanching that occurs. Granulomas often have an "apple jelly" appearance on diascopy.

Wood's Light   A Wood's lamp generates 360-nm ultraviolet (or "black") light that can be used to aid the evaluation of certain skin

A

B

FIGURE 46-10   *A.* Allergic contact dermatitis, acute phase, with sharply demarcated, weeping, eczematous plaques in a perioral distribution. *B.* Allergic contact dermatitis to nickel, chronic phase demonstrating an erythematous, lichenified, weeping plaque on skin chronically exposed to a metal snap. (*B, Courtesy of Robert Swerlick, MD.*)

disorders. For example, a Wood's lamp will cause erythrasma (a superficial, intertriginous infection caused by *Corynebacterium minutissimum*) to show a characteristic coral red color, and wounds colonized by *Pseudomonas* to appear pale blue. Tinea capitis caused by certain dermatophytes such as *Microsporum canis* or *M. audouini* exhibits a yellow fluorescence. Pigmented lesions of the epidermis such as freckles are accentuated, while dermal pigment such as postinflammatory hyperpigmentation fades under a Wood's light. Vitiligo (Fig. 46-12)

FIGURE 46-9   Erythema multiforme is characterized by multiple erythematous plaques with a target or iris morphology and usually represents a hypersensitivity reaction to drugs or infections (especially herpes simplex virus). (*Courtesy of the Yale Resident's Slide Collection.*)

FIGURE 46-11   Urticaria showing characteristic discrete and confluent, edematous, erythematous papules and plaques.

FIGURE 46-12 Vitiligo in a typical acral distribution demonstrating striking cutaneous depigmentation, as a result of loss of melanocytes.

appears totally white under a Wood's lamp, and previously unsuspected areas of involvement often become apparent. A Wood's lamp may also aid in the demonstration of tinea versicolor and in recognition of ash leaf spots in patients with tuberous sclerosis.

Patch Tests Patch testing is designed to document sensitivity to a specific antigen. In this procedure, a battery of suspected allergens is applied to the patient's back under occlusive dressings and allowed to remain in contact with the skin for 48 h. The dressings are removed, and the area is examined for evidence of delayed hypersensitivity reactions (e.g., erythema, edema, or papulovesicles). This test is best performed by physicians with special expertise in patch testing and is often helpful in the evaluation of patients with chronic dermatitis.

FURTHER READING

ARNDT KA et al (eds): *Cutaneous Medicine and Surgery, An Integrated Program in Dermatology.* Philadelphia, Saunders, 1996

CHAMPION RH et al (eds): *Textbook of Dermatology*, 6th ed. Oxford, Blackwell Scientific, 1999

DERMATOLOGY LEXICON PROJECT: www.dermatology lexicon.org

FREEDBERG IM et al (eds): *Fitzpatrick's Dermatology in General Medicine*, 5th ed. New York, McGraw-Hill, 1999

47 ECZEMA, PSORIASIS, CUTANEOUS INFECTIONS, ACNE, AND OTHER COMMON SKIN DISORDERS
Calvin O. McCall, Thomas J. Lawley

ECZEMA AND DERMATITIS

Eczema, or dermatitis, is a reaction pattern that presents with variable clinical and histologic findings and is the final common expression for a number of disorders, including atopic dermatitis, allergic contact and irritant contact dermatitis, dyshidrotic eczema, nummular eczema, lichen simplex chronicus, asteatotic eczema, and seborrheic dermatitis. Primary lesions may include papules, erythematous macules, and vesicles, which can coalesce to form patches and plaques. In severe eczema, secondary lesions from infection or excoriation, marked by weeping and crusting, may predominate. Long-standing dermatitis is often dry and is characterized by thickened, scaling skin (*lichenification*).

ATOPIC DERMATITIS
Atopic dermatitis (AD) is the cutaneous expression of the atopic state, characterized by a family history of asthma, hay fever, or dermatitis in up to 70% of patients. Some of the features of atopic eczema are shown in Table 47-1. The prevalence of atopic dermatitis is increasing worldwide, with a point prevalence in Norwegian school children as high as 23%.

The etiology of AD is only partially defined, but there is a clear genetic predisposition. When both parents are affected by AD, over 80% of their children manifest the disease. When only one parent is affected, the prevalence drops to slightly over 50%. Patients with AD may display a variety of immunoregulatory abnormalities including increased IgE synthesis; increased serum IgE; increased specific IgE to foods, aeroallergens, bacteria, and bacterial products; increased expression of CD23 (low-affinity IgE receptor) on monocytes and B cells; and impaired delayed type hypersensitivity reactions.

The clinical presentation often varies with age. Half of patients with AD present within the first year of life, and 80% present by 5 years of age. About 80% ultimately coexpress allergic rhinitis or asthma. The infantile pattern is characterized by weeping inflammatory patches and crusted plaques that occur on the face, neck, and extensor surfaces. The childhood and adolescent pattern is marked by dermatitis of flexural skin, particularly in the antecubital and popliteal fossae (Fig. 47-1). AD may resolve spontaneously, but over half of all individuals affected as children will have dermatitis in adult life. The distribution of lesions may be similar to those seen in childhood. However, adults frequently have localized disease, manifesting as hand eczema or lichen simplex chronicus (see below). In patients with localized disease, AD may be suspected because of a typical personal history, family history, or the presence of cutaneous stigmata of AD such as perioral pallor, an extra fold of skin beneath the lower eyelid (Dennie's line), increased palmar skin markings, and an increased incidence of cutaneous infections, particularly with *Staphylococcus aureus*. Regardless of other manifestations, pruritus is a prominent characteristic of AD and is exacerbated by dry skin. Many of the cutaneous findings in affected patients, such as lichenification, are secondary to rubbing and scratching.

FIGURE 47-1 Atopic dermatitis with hyperpigmentation, lichenification, and scaling in the antecubital fossae. (Courtesy of Robert Swerlick, MD.)

TABLE 47-1 *Clinical Features of Atopic Dermatitis*

1. Pruritus and scratching
2. Course marked by exacerbations and remissions
3. Lesions typical of eczematous dermatitis
4. Personal or family history of atopy (asthma, allergic rhinitis, food allergies, or eczema)
5. Clinical course lasting longer than 6 weeks

Histologic examination of the skin affected by AD may demonstrate features of acute or chronic dermatitis. Immunopathology shows activated, memory T helper cells. AD skin lesions may also demonstrate IgE-bearing CD1a+ Langerhans cells, and these cells have been implicated in AD disease pathophysiology through mediation of hypersensitivity responses to environmental antigens.

℞ TREATMENT

Therapy of AD should include avoidance of cutaneous irritants, adequate moisturizing, judicious use of topical anti-inflammatory agents, and prompt treatment of secondary infection. Patients should be instructed to bathe using warm, but not hot, water and to limit their use of soap. Immediately after bathing while the skin is still moist, a topical anti-inflammatory agent in a cream or ointment base should be applied to areas of dermatitis, and all other skin areas should be lubricated with a moisturizer. Approximately 30 g of a topical agent is required to cover the entire body surface of an average adult.

Until recently, low- to midpotency topical glucocorticoids were employed in most treatment regimens for AD. Skin atrophy and the potential for systemic absorption, especially with more potent agents, were constant concerns. Two non-glucocorticoid anti-inflammatory agents are now available, tacrolimus ointment and pimecrolimus cream. These agents are macrolide immunosuppressants derived from soil fungi and are approved for use in AD. Reports of broader effectiveness appear in the literature. These agents do not cause skin atrophy and do not suppress the hypothalamic-pituitary-adrenal axis. They may replace topical glucocorticoids in some patients, but they are more costly than generic topical glucocorticoids. The non-steroid agents or low-potency topical glucocorticoids should be selected for use on the face or intertriginous areas to minimize the risk of skin atrophy.

Crusted and weeping skin lesions should be treated with systemic antibiotics with activity against *S. aureus* since secondary infection often exacerbates eczema. The frequency of macrolide-resistant organisms makes the use of penicillinase-resistant penicillins or cephalosporins preferable. Dicloxacillin or cephalexin (250 mg four times daily for 7 to 10 days) is generally adequate to decrease heavy colonization. As an adjunct, the use of triclosan-containing antibacterial washes and intermittent nasal mupirocin may be useful as prophylactic measures. The role of dietary allergens in atopic dermatitis is controversial, and there is little evidence that they play any role outside of infancy.

Control of pruritus is essential for treatment, since AD often represents "an itch that rashes." Antihistamines are most often used to control pruritus, and mild sedation may be responsible for their antipruritic action. Sedation may also limit their usefulness. Unlike their effects in urticaria, nonsedating antihistamines and selective H_2 blockers are of little use in controlling the pruritus of AD.

Treatment with systemic glucocorticoids should be limited to severe exacerbations unresponsive to conservative topical therapy. In the patient with chronic AD, therapy with systemic glucocorticoids will generally clear the skin only briefly, but cessation of the systemic therapy will invariably be accompanied by return, if not worsening, of the dermatitis. Patients who do not respond to conventional therapies should be considered for patch testing to rule out allergic contact dermatitis. Immunotherapy with aeroallergens has not proven useful in AD, unlike its effect in allergic rhinitis and extrinsic asthma.

CONTACT DERMATITIS Contact dermatitis is an inflammatory process in skin caused by an exogenous agent or agents that directly or indirectly injure the skin. This injury may be caused by an inherent characteristic of a compound—irritant contact dermatitis (ICD). An example of ICD would be dermatitis induced by a concentrated acid or base. Agents that cause allergic contact dermatitis (ACD) induce an antigen-specific immune response. The clinical lesions of contact dermatitis may be acute (wet and edematous) or chronic (dry, thickened, and scaly), depending on the persistence of the insult (see Fig. 46-10). The most common presentation of contact dermatitis is hand eczema, and it is frequently related to occupational exposures. Occupation-related contact dermatitis represents a significant proportion of occupation-induced injury, affecting over 60,000 persons annually.

ICD is generally strictly demarcated and often localized to areas of thin skin (eyelids, intertriginous areas) or to areas where the irritant was occluded. Lesions may range from minimal skin erythema to areas of marked edema, vesicles, and ulcers. Chronic low-grade irritant dermatitis is the most common type of ICD, and the most common area of involvement is the hands (see below). The most common irritants encountered are chronic wet work, soaps, and detergents. Treatment should be directed to avoidance of irritants and use of protective gloves or clothing.

ACD is a manifestation of delayed-type hypersensitivity mediated by memory T lymphocytes in the skin. The most common cause of ACD is exposure to plants, especially to members of the family Anacardiaceae, including the genus *Toxicodendrun*. Poison ivy, poison oak, and poison sumac are members of this genus and cause an allergic reaction marked by erythema, vesiculation, and severe pruritus. The eruption is often linear, corresponding to areas where plants have touched the skin. The sensitizing antigen common to these plants is urushiol, an oleoresin containing the active ingredient pentadecylcatechol. The oleoresin may adhere to skin, clothing, tools, and pets, and contaminated articles may cause dermatitis even after prolonged storage. Blister fluid does not contain urushiol and is not capable of inducing skin eruption in exposed subjects. Other allergens may be more difficult to identify, especially if the exposure is chronic and the skin becomes thickened and scaly.

℞ TREATMENT

If ACD is suspected and an offending agent is identified and removed, the eruption will resolve. Usually, treatment with high-potency fluorinated topical glucocorticoids is enough to relieve symptoms while the ACD runs its course. For those patients who require systemic therapy, daily oral prednisone beginning at 1 mg/kg, but usually not exceeding 60 mg/d, is sufficient. It should be tapered over 2 to 3 weeks, and each daily dose given in the morning with food.

Identification of a contact allergen can be a difficult and time-consuming task. Patients with dermatitis unresponsive to conventional therapy or with an unusual and patterned distribution should be suspected of having ACD. They should be questioned carefully regarding occupational exposures, topical medicaments, and oral medications. Common sensitizers include preservatives in topical preparations, nickel sulfate, potassium dichromate, thimerosal, neomycin sulfate, fragrances, formaldehyde, and rubber-curing agents. Patch testing is helpful in identifying these agents, but should not be attempted on patients with widespread active dermatitis or on those taking systemic glucocorticoids.

HAND ECZEMA Hand eczema is a very common, chronic skin disorder. It represents a large proportion of occupation-associated skin disease. It may be associated with other cutaneous disorders such as AD or may occur by itself. Similar to other forms of dermatitis, both exogenous and endogenous factors play important roles in the expression of hand dermatitis. Chronic, excessive exposure to water and detergents may initiate or aggravate this disorder. It may present with dryness and cracking of the skin of the hands as well as with variable amounts of erythema and edema. Often, the dermatitis will begin under rings where water and irritants are trapped. A variant of hand dermatitis, dyshidrotic eczema, presents with multiple, intensely pruritic, small papules and vesicles occurring on the thenar and hypothenar eminences and the sides of the fingers (Fig. 47-2). Lesions tend to occur in crops that slowly form crusts and heal.

The evaluation of a patient with hand eczema should include an assessment of potential occupation-associated exposures. Predominant involvement of the dorsal surface of the hands with sparing of the palmar surface suggests a possible contact dermatitis. The history

FIGURE 47-2 Dyshidrotic eczema, characterized by deep-seated vesicles and scaling on palms and lateral fingers, is often associated with an atopic diathesis.

should be directed to identifying possible irritant or allergen exposures. The use of rubber gloves to protect dermatitic skin is sometimes associated with the development of delayed-type hypersensitivity reactions to agents used for cross-linking rubber. Such reactions can be detected by patch testing. Less commonly, patients may manifest hand dermatitis as a consequence of developing immediate-type hypersensitivity reactions to latex. These are of particular concern since these patients are at risk for anaphylactic reactions. The most sensitive method of detection is the use of scratch testing with latex extract. However, this should be done with extreme caution only in a setting where an anaphylactic reaction can be treated. A latex radioallergosorbent test is available but is only about 60% sensitive.

℞ TREATMENT

Therapy of hand dermatitis is directed toward avoidance of irritants, identification of possible contact allergens, treatment of coexistent infection, and application of topical glucocorticoids. Whenever possible, the hands should be protected by gloves, preferably vinyl. Most patients can be treated with cool moist compresses (dressings) to dry and debride acute inflammatory lesions and to decrease swelling, followed by application of a mid- to high-potency topical glucocorticoid in a cream or ointment base. As with atopic dermatitis, treatment of secondary infection by staphylococci or streptococci is essential for good control. Additionally, patients with hand dermatitis should be examined for dermatophyte infection by KOH preparation and culture (see below).

NUMMULAR ECZEMA   Nummular eczema is characterized by circular or oval "coinlike" lesions. Initially, this eruption consists of small edematous papules that become crusted and scaly. The most common locations are on the trunk or the extensor surfaces of the extremities, particularly on the pretibial areas or dorsum of the hands. It occurs more frequently in men and is most commonly seen in middle age. The etiology of nummular eczema is unknown. The treatment of nummular eczema is similar to that for other forms of dermatitis.

LICHEN SIMPLEX CHRONICUS   Lichen simplex chronicus may represent the end stage of a variety of pruritic and eczematous disorders. It consists of a well-circumscribed plaque or plaques with lichenified or thickened skin due to chronic scratching or rubbing. Common areas involved include the posterior nuchal region, dorsum of the feet, or ankles. Treatment of lichen simplex chronicus centers around breaking the cycle of chronic itching and scratching, which often occur during sleep. High-potency topical glucocorticoids are helpful in alleviating pruritus in most cases, but in recalcitrant cases, application of topical glucocorticoids under occlusion or intralesional injection of glucocor-

ticoids may be required. Oral antihistamines such as hydroxyzine (10 to 25 mg every 6 h) or tricyclic antidepressants with antihistaminic activity such as doxepin (10 to 25 mg at bedtime) are useful as antipruritics primarily due to their sedating action. Higher doses of these agents may be required, but sedation can become bothersome. Patients need to be counseled regarding driving or operating heavy equipment after taking these medications due to their potentially potent sedative activity.

ASTEATOTIC ECZEMA   Asteatotic eczema, also known as *xerotic eczema* or *"winter itch,"* is a mildly inflammatory dermatitis that develops in areas of extremely dry skin, especially during the dry winter months. This form of eczema accounts for a large number of physician visits because of the associated pruritus. Fine cracks and scale, with or without erythema, characteristically develop in areas of dry skin, especially on the anterior surfaces of the lower extremities in elderly patients. Asteatotic eczema responds well to topical moisturizers and the avoidance of cutaneous irritants. Overbathing and the use of harsh soaps exacerbate asteatotic eczema. Moisturizers should be applied to dry skin areas twice daily and always applied to damp skin after bathing. Prescription emollients containing ammonium lactate or urea are useful in patients with extremely dry skin, but they may be associated with skin irritation. Emollients should be applied after leaving the bath or shower to avoid increasing the risk of falling.

STASIS DERMATITIS AND STASIS ULCERATION   Stasis dermatitis develops on the lower extremities secondary to venous incompetence and chronic edema. Early findings in stasis dermatitis consist of mild erythema and scaling associated with pruritus. The typical initial site of involvement is the medial aspect of the ankle, often over a distended vein (Fig. 47-3). As the disorder progresses, the dermatitis becomes progressively pigmented, due to chronic erythrocyte extravasation leading to cutaneous hemosiderin deposition. As with other forms of dermatitis, stasis dermatitis may become acutely inflamed, with crusting and exudate. Chronic stasis dermatitis is often associated with dermal fibrosis that is recognized clinically as brawny edema of the skin. Stasis dermatitis is often complicated by secondary infection and contact dermatitis. Severe stasis dermatitis may precede the development of stasis ulcers.

℞ TREATMENT

Patients with stasis dermatitis and stasis ulceration benefit greatly from leg elevation and the routine use of compression stockings with a gradient of at least 30 to 40 mmHg. Stockings providing less compression, such as antiembolism hose, are poor substitutes. Use of emollients and/or midpotency topical glucocorticoids and avoidance of irritants are also helpful in treating stasis dermatitis. Protecting the legs from injury, including scratching, and control of chronic edema are essential to prevent ulcers.

FIGURE 47-3 Stasis dermatitis showing erythematous, scaly, and oozing patches over the lower leg. Several stasis ulcers are also seen in this patient.

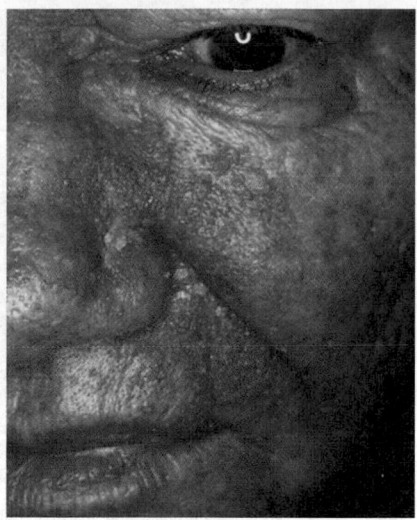

FIGURE 47-4 Seborrheic dermatitis showing central facial erythema with overlying greasy, yellowish scale. (Courtesy of Jean Bolognia, MD.)

Stasis ulcers are difficult to treat, and resolution of these lesions is slow. It is extremely important to elevate the affected limb as much as possible. The ulcer should be kept clear of necrotic material by gentle debridement and covered with a semipermeable dressing under pressure. Glucocorticoids should not be applied to ulcers, since they may retard healing. Secondarily infected lesions should be treated with appropriate oral antibiotics, but it should be noted that all ulcers will become colonized with bacteria, and the purpose of antibiotic therapy should not be to clear all bacterial growth. Care must be taken to exclude treatable causes of leg ulcers (hypercoagulation, vasculitis) before beginning the chronic management outlined above.

SEBORRHEIC DERMATITIS Seborrheic dermatitis is a common, chronic disorder, characterized by greasy scales overlying erythematous patches or plaques. The most common location is in the scalp where it may be recognized as severe dandruff. On the face, seborrheic dermatitis affects the eyebrows, eyelids, glabella, and nasolabial folds (Fig. 47-4). Scaling of the external auditory canal is common in seborrheic dermatitis and may be mistaken for a fungal infection (otomycosis). The postauricular areas often become macerated and tender. Additionally, seborrheic dermatitis may develop in the central chest, axilla, groin, submammary folds, and gluteal cleft. Rarely, it may cause a widespread generalized dermatitis.

Seborrheic dermatitis may be evident within the first few weeks of life, and within this context it occurs in the scalp ("cradle cap"), face, or groin. It is rarely seen in children beyond infancy but becomes evident again during adult life. Although it is frequently seen in patients with Parkinson's disease, in those who have had cerebrovascular accidents, and in those with HIV infection, the overwhelming majority of individuals with seborrheic dermatitis have no underlying disorder.

℞ TREATMENT

Treatment with low-potency topical glucocorticoids in conjunction with a topical antifungal agent, such as ketoconazole cream or ciclopirox cream, is often effective. The scalp and beard areas may benefit from shampoos containing coal tar and/or salicylic acid. Shampoos should be left in place 3 to 5 min before rinsing. High-potency topical glucocorticoid solutions (betamethasone or fluocinonide) are effective for control of severe scalp involvement. Fluorinated topical glucocorticoids should not be used on the face since this is often associated with the development of rebound worsening and steroid-induced rosacea or atrophy.

PAPULOSQUAMOUS DISORDERS (Table 47-2)

PSORIASIS Psoriasis is one of the most common dermatologic diseases, affecting up to 2.5% of the world's population. It is a chronic inflammatory skin disorder clinically characterized by erythematous, sharply demarcated papules and rounded plaques, covered by silvery micaceous scale. The skin lesions of psoriasis are variably pruritic. Traumatized areas often develop lesions of psoriasis (Koebner or isomorphic phenomenon). Additionally, other external factors may exacerbate psoriasis including infections, stress, and medications (lithium, beta blockers, and antimalarials).

The most common variety of psoriasis is called *plaque type*. Patients with plaque-type psoriasis will have stable, slowly enlarging plaques, which remain basically unchanged for long periods of time. The most common areas for plaque psoriasis to occur are the elbows, knees, gluteal cleft, and the scalp. Involvement tends to be symmetric. *Inverse psoriasis* affects the intertriginous regions including the axilla, groin, submammary region, and navel; it also tends to affect the scalp, palms, and soles. The individual lesions are sharply demarcated plaques (see Fig. 46-7) but may be moist due to their location. Plaque psoriasis generally develops slowly and runs an indolent course. It rarely remits spontaneously.

Eruptive psoriasis (guttate psoriasis) is most common in children and young adults. It develops acutely in individuals without psoriasis or in those with chronic plaque psoriasis. Patients present with many small erythematous, scaling papules, frequently after upper respiratory tract infection with β-hemolytic streptococci. The differential diagnosis should include pityriasis rosea and secondary syphilis. *Pustular psoriasis* is another variant. Patients may have disease localized to the palms and soles or generalized and associated with fever, malaise, diarrhea, and arthralgias.

About half of all patients with psoriasis have fingernail involvement, appearing as punctate pitting, nail thickening, or subungual hyperkeratosis. About 5 to 10% of patients with psoriasis have associated joint complaints, and these are most often found in patients with fingernail involvement. Although some have the coincident occurrence

---

TABLE 47-2 *Papulosquamous Disorders*

	Clinical Features	Other Notable Features	Histologic Features
Psoriasis	Sharply demarcated, erythematous plaques with mica-like scale; predominantly elbows, knees, and scalp; atypical forms may localize to intertriginous areas; eruptive forms may be associated with infection (Reiter's syndrome)	May be aggravated by certain drugs, infection; severe forms seen associated with HIV	Acanthosis, vascular proliferation
Lichen planus	Purple polygonal papules marked by severe pruritus; lacy white markings, especially associated with mucous membrane lesions	Certain drugs may induce: thiazides, antimalarial drugs	Interface dermatitis
Pityriasis rosea	Rash often preceded by herald patch; oval to round plaques with trailing scale; most often affects the trunk, and eruption lines up in skin folds giving a "fir tree"-like appearance; generally spares palms and soles	Variable pruritus; self-limited resolving in 2–8 weeks; may be imitated by secondary syphilis	Pathologic features often nonspecific
Dermatophytosis	Polymorphous appearance depending on dermatophyte, body site, and host response; sharply defined to ill-demarcated scaly plaques with or without inflammation; may be associated with hair loss	KOH preparation may show branching hyphae; culture helpful	Hyphae and neutrophils in stratum corneum

of classic rheumatoid arthritis (Chap. 301), many have joint disease that falls into one of three types associated with psoriasis: (1) asymmetric inflammatory arthritis most commonly involving the distal and proximal interphalangeal joints and less commonly the knees, hips, ankles, and wrists; (2) a seronegative rheumatoid arthritis–like disease; a significant portion of these patients go on to develop a severe destructive arthritis; or (3) disease limited to the spine (psoriatic spondylitis).

The etiology of psoriasis is still poorly understood, but there is clearly a genetic component to the disease. Over 50% of patients with psoriasis report a positive family history. Psoriasis has been linked to HLA-Cw6 and, to a lesser extent, to HLA-DR7. Psoriatic lesions are characterized by infiltration of skin with activated T cells, which appear to have a role in the pathophysiology of psoriasis. Presumably, cytokines from activated T cells elaborate growth factors that stimulate keratinocyte hyperproliferation. Agents that inhibit T cell activation, clonal expansion, or release of proinflammatory cytokines are often effective for the treatment of severe psoriasis.

R̲x̲ TREATMENT

Treatment of psoriasis depends on the type, location, and extent of disease. All patients should be instructed to avoid excess drying or irritation of their skin and to maintain adequate cutaneous hydration. Most patients with localized, plaque-type psoriasis can be managed with midpotency topical glucocorticoids, although their long-term use is often accompanied by loss of effectiveness (tachyphylaxis) and atrophy of the skin. A topical vitamin D analogue (calcipotriene) and a retinoid (tazarotene) are also efficacious in the treatment of psoriasis and have largely replaced other topical agents such as coal tar, salicylic acid, and anthralin.

Ultraviolet light, natural or artificial, is an effective therapy for patients with widespread psoriasis. Ultraviolet B (UV-B) light is effective alone, or may be combined with coal tar or anthralin. The combination of the ultraviolet A (UV-A) spectrum with either oral or topical psoralens (PUVA) is also extremely effective for the treatment of psoriasis, but long-term use may be associated with an increased incidence of squamous cell cancer and melanoma of the skin.

Various other agents can be used for severe, widespread psoriatic disease. Oral glucocorticoids should not be used for the treatment of psoriasis due to the potential for developing life-threatening pustular psoriasis when therapy is discontinued. Methotrexate is an effective agent, especially in patients with psoriatic arthritis; however, liver toxicity and bone marrow suppression limit its use. The synthetic retinoid, acitretin, is effective in some patients with severe psoriasis. It is a potent teratogen and should not be used in women of childbearing potential. The evidence implicating psoriasis as a T cell–mediated disorder has directed therapeutic efforts to immunoregulation. Cyclosporine is highly effective in selected patients with severe disease, but nephrotoxicity and hypertension complicate its use. Much attention is currently directed toward the development of biologic agents with more selective immunosuppressive properties and better safety profiles. Etanercept, a tumor necrosis factor α (TNF-α) inhibitor, is now approved for psoriatic arthritis and is in clinical trials for psoriasis. Other agents in clinical trials target TNF-α and other proinflammatory cytokines, T cell activation, and lymphocyte trafficking in an attempt to suppress the inflammation characteristic of psoriasis.

LICHEN PLANUS Lichen planus (LP) is a papulosquamous disorder in which the primary lesions are pruritic, polygonal, flat-topped, violaceous papules. Close examination of the surface of these papules often reveals a network of gray lines (Wickham's striae). The skin lesions may occur anywhere but have a predilection for the wrists, shins, lower back, and genitalia (Fig. 47-5). Involvement of the scalp may lead to hair loss. LP commonly involves mucous membranes, particularly the buccal mucosa, where it can present as a white netlike eruption. Its etiology is unknown, but cutaneous eruptions clinically resembling LP

FIGURE 47-5 Lichen planus showing multiple flat-topped, violaceous papules and plaques. Nail dystrophy as seen in this patient's thumbnail may also be a feature. (Courtesy of Robert Swerlick, MD.)

have been observed after administration of numerous drugs, including thiazide diuretics, gold, antimalarials, penicillamine, and phenothiazines, and in patients with skin lesions of chronic graft-versus-host disease. Additionally, LP may be associated with hepatitis C infection. The course of LP is variable, but most patients have spontaneous remissions 6 months to 2 years after the onset of disease. Topical glucocorticoids are the mainstay of therapy.

PITYRIASIS ROSEA Pityriasis rosea (PR) is a papulosquamous eruption of unknown etiology that occurs more commonly in the spring and fall. Its first manifestation is the development of a 2- to 6-cm annular lesion (the herald patch). This is followed in a few days to a few weeks by the appearance of many smaller annular or papular lesions with a predilection to occur on the trunk (Fig. 47-6). The lesions are generally oval, with their long axis parallel to the skin-fold lines. Individual lesions may range in color from red to brown and have a trailing scale. PR shares many clinical features with the eruption of secondary syphilis, but palm and sole lesions are extremely rare in PR and common in secondary syphilis. The eruption tends to be moderately pruritic and lasts 3 to 8 weeks. Treatment is generally directed at alleviating pruritus and consists of oral antihistamines, midpotency topical glucocorticoids, and, in some cases, the use of UV-B phototherapy.

CUTANEOUS INFECTIONS (Table 47-3)

IMPETIGO AND ECTHYMA Impetigo is a common superficial bacterial infection of skin caused by group A β-hemolytic streptococci (Chap.

FIGURE 47-6 Pityriasis rosea in which multiple round to oval erythematous patches with fine central scale are distributed along the skin tension lines on the trunk.

TABLE 47-3 *Common Skin Infections*

	Clinical Features	Etiologic Agent	Treatment
Impetigo	Honey-colored crusted papules, plaques, or bullae	Group A *Streptococcus* and *Staphylococcus aureus*	Systemic or topical antistaphylococcal antibiotics
Dermatophytosis	Inflammatory or noninflammatory annular scaly plaques; may have hair loss; groin involvement spares scrotum; hyphae on KOH preparation	*Trichophyton*, *Epidermophyton*, or *Microsporum* sp.	Topical azoles, systemic griseofulvin, terbinafine, or azoles
Candidiasis	Inflammatory papules and plaques with satellite pustules, frequently in intertriginous areas; may involve scrotum; pseudohyphae on KOH preparation	*Candida albicans* and other *Candida* species	Topical nystatin or azoles; systemic azoles for resistant disease
Tinea versicolor	Hyperpigmented or hypopigmented scaly patches on the trunk; characteristic mixture of hyphae and spores on KOH preparation ("spaghetti and meatballs")	*Malassezia furfur*	Topical selenium sulfide lotion or azoles

121) or *S. aureus* (Chap. 120). The primary lesion is a superficial pustule that ruptures and forms a characteristic yellow-brown honey-colored crust (see Fig. 121-1). Lesions caused by staphylococci may be tense, clear bullae, and this less common form of the disease is called *bullous impetigo*. Lesions may occur on normal skin or in areas already affected by another skin disease. Ecthyma is a variant of impetigo that generally occurs on the lower extremities and causes punched-out ulcerative lesions. Treatment of both ecthyma and impetigo involves gentle debridement of adherent crusts, which is facilitated by the use of soaks and topical antibiotics, in conjunction with appropriate oral antibiotics.

ERYSIPELAS AND CELLULITIS →*See Chap. 110*

DERMATOPHYTOSIS Dermatophytes are fungi that infect skin, hair, and nails and include members of the genera *Trichophyton*, *Microsporum*, and *Epidermophyton*. Tinea corporis, or infection of the relatively hairless skin of the body (glabrous skin), may have a variable appearance depending on the extent of the associated inflammatory reaction (see Fig. 46-11). It may have the typical annular appearance of "ringworm" or appear as deep inflammatory nodules or granulomas. Involvement of the groin (tinea cruris) is more common in males than females. It presents as a scaling, erythematous eruption that spares the scrotum. Infection of the foot (tinea pedis) is the most common dermatophyte infection and is often chronic; it is characterized by variable erythema, edema, scaling, pruritus, and occasionally vesiculation. Involvement may be widespread or localized, but almost invariably involves the web space between the fourth and fifth toes. Infection of the nails (tinea unguium or onychomycosis) occurs in many patients with tinea pedis and is characterized by opacified, thickened nails and subungual debris. Dermatophyte infection of the scalp (tinea capitis) has returned in epidemic proportions, particularly affecting inner-city children, but it also affects adults. The predominant organism is *T. tonsurans*, which can produce a relatively noninflammatory infection with mild scale and hair loss that is diffuse or localized. Localized disease may be well defined or irregular. *T. tonsurans* can also cause a markedly inflammatory dermatosis with edema and nodules. This latter presentation is a kerion.

The diagnosis of tinea can be made from skin scrapings, nail scrapings, or hair by culture or direct microscopic examination with potassium hydroxide (KOH). Hair, nail scrapings, and scrapings from markedly inflamed skin may fail to show hyphae on direct examination.

℞ TREATMENT

Both topical and systemic therapies may be used to treat dermatophyte infections. Treatment depends on the site involved and the type of infection. Topical therapy is generally effective for uncomplicated tinea corporis, tinea cruris, and limited tinea pedis. It is not effective as a monotherapy for tinea capitis or onychomycosis. Topical imidazoles, triazoles, and allylamines may all be effective topical therapies

for dermatophyte infections. Haloprogin, undecylenic acid, ciclopirox olamine, and tolnaftate are also effective, but nystatin is not active against dermatophytes. Topicals are generally applied twice daily, and treatment should continue 1 week beyond clinical resolution of the infection. Tinea pedis often requires longer treatment courses and frequently relapses. Oral antifungal agents may be required for recalcitrant tinea pedis or tinea corporis with a nodular (granulomatous) component.

Oral antifungal agents are required for dermatophyte infections involving the hair and nails and for other infections unresponsive to topical therapy. A fungal etiology should be confirmed by direct microscopic examination or by culture prior to prescribing oral antifungal agents. All of the oral agents may cause hepatotoxicity and should not be used in women who are pregnant or breast-feeding.

Griseofulvin is the only oral agent approved in the United States for dermatophyte infections involving the skin, hair, or nails. Itraconazole and terbinafine are approved for onychomycosis; however, the literature cites multiple examples of their effective use in other dermatophyte infections. When griseofulvin is used, a daily dose of 500 mg of microsized or 350 mg of ultramicrosized griseofulvin administered with a fatty meal is an adequate dose for most dermatophyte infections. Higher doses are required for tinea pedis and onychomycosis. The duration of therapy may be 2 weeks for uncomplicated tinea corporis or as long as 6 to 18 months for nail infections. Due to high relapse rates, griseofulvin is seldom used for nail infections. The usual adult dose of griseofulvin for tinea capitis is 1 g of microsized or 0.5 g of ultramicrosized given daily for 6 to 8 weeks or until cultures are negative. The adjunctive use of topical antifungal agents may be useful, but topical therapy alone is not adequate for tinea capitis. Markedly inflammatory tinea capitis may result in scarring and hair loss, and systemic or topical glucocorticoids may be helpful in preventing these sequelae. Common side effects of griseofulvin include gastrointestinal distress, headache, and urticaria.

Oral itraconazole and terbinafine are approved for onychomycosis. Itraconazole is given as either continuous daily therapy (200 mg/d) or pulses (200 mg twice daily for 1 week per month) administered with food. Fingernails require 2 months of continuous therapy or two pulses. Toenails require 3 months of continuous therapy or three pulses. Itraconazole has the potential for serious interactions with other drugs requiring the P450 enzyme system for metabolism. Terbinafine (250 mg/d) is also effective for onychomycosis. Therapy with terbinafine is continued for 6 weeks for fingernail infections and 12 weeks for toenail infections. Terbinafine has fewer drug-drug interactions, but caution should be used when patients are on multiple medications.

TINEA VERSICOLOR Tinea versicolor is caused by a non-dermatophyte, dimorphic fungus, *Malassezia furfur*, a normal inhabitant of the skin. As the yeast form, it generally does not cause disease (except for folliculitis in certain individuals). However, in some individuals, it converts to the hyphal form and causes characteristic lesions. The expression of infection is promoted by heat and humidity. The typical lesions consist of oval scaly macules, papules, and patches concentrated on the chest, shoulders, and back but only rarely on the face or distal extremities. On dark skin, they often appear as hypopigmented areas, while on light skin, they are slightly erythematous or hyperpigmented. In some darkly pigmented individuals, they may only appear as scaling patches. A KOH preparation from scaling lesions will demonstrate a confluence of short hyphae and round spores (so-called spaghetti and meatballs). Solutions containing sulfur, salicylic acid, or selenium sulfide will clear the infection if used daily for a week and then intermittently thereafter. Treatment with a single 400-mg oral dose of ketoconazole is also effective.

CANDIDIASIS Candidiasis is a fungal infection caused by a related group of yeasts, whose manifestations may be localized to the skin, or rarely, may be systemic and life-threatening. The causative organism is usually *Candida albicans*, but may also be *C. tropicalis, C. parapsilosis,* or *C. krusei*. These organisms are normal saprophytic inhabitants of the gastrointestinal tract but may overgrow (usually due to broad-spectrum antibiotic therapy) and cause disease at a number of cutaneous sites. Other predisposing factors include diabetes mellitus, chronic intertrigo, oral contraceptive use, and cellular immune deficiency. Candidiasis is a very common infection in HIV-infected individuals (Chap. 173). The oral cavity is commonly involved. Lesions may occur on the tongue or buccal mucosa (thrush) and appear as white plaques (see Fig. 46-12). Microscopic examination of scrapings demonstrate both pseudohyphae and yeast forms. Fissured, macerated lesions at the corners of the mouth (perlèche) are often seen in individuals with poorly fitting dentures and may also be associated with candidal infection. Additionally, candidal infections have an affinity for sites that are chronically wet and macerated and may occur around nails (onycholysis and paronychia) and in intertriginous areas. Intertriginous lesions are characteristically edematous, erythematous, and scaly, with scattered "satellite pustules." In males, there is often involvement of the penis and scrotum as well as the inner aspect of the thighs. In contrast to dermatophyte infections, candidal infections are frequently painful and accompanied by a marked inflammatory response. Diagnosis of candidal infection is based upon the clinical pattern and demonstration of yeast on KOH preparation or culture.

℞ TREATMENT

Treatment routinely involves removing any predisposing factors such as antibiotic therapy or chronic wetness and the use of appropriate topical or systemic antifungal therapy. Effective topical agents include nystatin or topical azoles (miconazole, clotrimazole, econazole, or ketoconazole). These agents are generally effective in clearing mucous membrane or glabrous skin involvement in nonimmunosuppressed patients. The associated inflammatory response that often accompanies candidal infection on glabrous skin can be treated with a mild glucocorticoid lotion or cream (2.5% hydrocortisone). Systemic therapy is generally reserved for immunosuppressed patients or individuals with chronic or recurrent disease who fail to respond to or tolerate appropriate topical therapy.

WARTS Warts are cutaneous neoplasms that are caused by papilloma viruses. Approximately 80 different human papilloma viruses (HPV) have been described, and this number will likely increase. Typical verruca vulgaris lesions are sessile, dome-shaped, usually about a centimeter in diameter, and their surface is hyperkeratotic consisting of many small filamentous projections. The HPV that cause typical verruca vulgaris also cause typical plantar warts, flat warts (or verruca plana), and filiform warts in intertriginous areas. Plantar warts are endophytic and are covered by thick keratin. Paring of the wart will generally demonstrate a central core of keratinized debris and punctate

bleeding points. Filiform warts are most commonly seen on the face, neck, and skin folds and present as papillomatous lesions on a narrow base. Flat warts are only slightly elevated and have a velvety, nonverrucous surface. They have a propensity for the face, arms, and legs and are often spread by shaving.

Genital warts generally begin as small papillomas that may grow to form large fungating lesions. In women, they may involve either the labia, perineum, or perianal skin. Additionally, the mucosa of the vagina, urethra, and anus can be involved, as well as the cervical epithelium. In men, the lesions often occur initially in the coronal sulcus, but may be seen on the shaft of the penis, the scrotum, perianal skin, or in the urethra.

Within the past decade, appreciable evidence has accumulated that suggests HPV plays a role in the development of neoplasia of the uterine cervix and external genitalia (Chap. 83). HPV types 16 and 18 have been most intensely studied, while recent evidence also implicates other types. Lesions may initially appear as small, flat, velvety, hyperpigmented papules occurring on the genitalia or perianal skin. Histologic examination of biopsies from affected sites may reveal changes associated with typical warts and/or features typical of intraepidermal carcinoma (Bowen's disease). Squamous cell carcinomas associated with HPV infections have also been observed in extragenital skin (Chap. 73). This is most commonly seen in patients immunosuppressed after organ transplantation.

℞ TREATMENT

There are many modalities available to treat warts, but no single therapy is universally effective. Factors that influence the choice of therapy include the location of the wart, extent of disease, the age and immunologic status of the patient, and the patient's desire for therapy. Perhaps the most useful and convenient method for treating warts in almost any location is cryotherapy with liquid nitrogen. Equally effective, but requiring much more patient compliance, is the use of keratolytic agents such as salicylic acid plasters or solutions. For genital warts, in-office application of a podophyllin solution is moderately effective but may be associated with marked local reactions. Prescription preparations of dilute, purified podophyllin are available for home use. Topical imiquimod, a potent inducer of local cytokine release, has also been approved for use in genital warts. Conventional and laser surgical procedures may be required for recalcitrant warts. Recurrence of warts appears to be common to all these modalities.

Treatment of warts, other than anogenital warts, should be tempered by the observation that a majority of warts in normal individuals resolve spontaneously within 1 to 2 years. Also, very few warts are associated with malignancy, and those are usually located in the anogenital region.

HERPES SIMPLEX →*See Chap. 163*

HERPES ZOSTER →*See Chap. 164*

ACNE

ACNE VULGARIS Acne vulgaris is a self-limited disorder primarily of teenagers and young adults, although perhaps 10 to 20% of adults may continue to experience some form of the disorder. The permissive factor for the expression of the disease in adolescence is the increase in sebum production by sebaceous glands after puberty. Small cysts, called *comedones*, form in hair follicles due to blockage of the follicular orifice by retention of sebum and keratinous material. The activity of bacteria (*Proprionobacterium acnes*) within the comedones releases free fatty acids from sebum, causes inflammation within the cyst, and results in rupture of the cyst wall. An inflammatory foreign-body reaction develops as a result of extrusion of oily and keratinous debris from the cyst.

The clinical hallmark of acne vulgaris is the comedone, which may be closed (whitehead) or open (blackhead). Closed comedones appear as 1- to 2-mm pebbly white papules, which are accentuated when the

FIGURE 47-7 Acne vulgaris with inflammatory papules, pustules, and comedones. (Courtesy of Kalman Watsky, MD.)

skin is stretched. They are the precursors of inflammatory lesions of acne vulgaris. The contents of closed comedones are not easily expressed. Open comedones, which rarely result in inflammatory acne lesions, have a large dilated follicular orifice and are filled with easily expressible oxidized, darkened, oily debris. Comedones are usually accompanied by inflammatory lesions: papules, pustules, or nodules.

The earliest lesions seen in early adolescence are generally mildly inflamed or noninflammatory comedones on the forehead. Subsequently, more typical inflammatory lesions develop on the cheeks, nose, and chin (Fig. 47-7). The most common location for acne is the face, but involvement of the chest and back is not uncommon. Most disease remains mild and does not lead to scarring. However, a small number of patients develop large inflammatory cysts and nodules, which may drain and result in significant scarring.

Exogenous and endogenous factors can alter the expression of acne vulgaris. Friction and trauma may rupture preexisting microcomedones and elicit inflammatory acne lesions. This is commonly seen with headbands or chin straps of athletic helmets. Application of comedogenic topical agents in cosmetics or hair preparations or chronic topical exposure to certain industrial compounds that are comedogenic may elicit or aggravate acne. Glucocorticoids, applied topically or administered systemically in high doses, may also elicit acne. Other systemic medications such as lithium, isoniazid, halogens, phenytoin, and phenobarbital may produce acneiform eruptions, or aggravate preexisting acne.

℞ TREATMENT

Treatment of acne vulgaris is directed toward elimination of comedones by normalization of follicular keratinization, decreasing sebaceous gland activity, decreasing the population of *P. acnes*, and decreasing inflammation. Acne vulgaris may be treated with either local or systemic medications. Minimal to moderate, pauci-inflammatory disease may respond adequately to local therapy alone. Although areas affected with acne should be kept clean, there is little evidence to suggest that removal of surface oils plays an important role in therapy. Overly vigorous scrubbing may aggravate acne due to mechanical rupture of comedones. Topical agents such as retinoic acid, benzoyl peroxide, or salicylic acid may alter the pattern of epidermal desquamation, preventing the formation of comedones and aiding in the resolution of preexisting cysts. Topical antibacterial agents such as benzoyl peroxide, azelaic acid, topical erythromycin (with or without zinc), or clindamycin are also useful adjuncts to therapy.

Patients with moderate to severe acne with a prominent inflammatory component will benefit from the addition of systemic therapy, such as tetracycline or erythromycin, in doses of 250 to 1000 mg/d. Such antibiotics appear to have an anti-inflammatory effect independent of their antibacterial effect. Female patients who do not respond to oral antibiotics may benefit from hormonal therapy. Women placed on oral contraceptives containing ethinyl estradiol and norgestimate

have demonstrated improvement in their acne when compared to a placebo control.

Patients with severe nodulocystic acne unresponsive to the therapies discussed above may benefit from treatment with the synthetic retinoid, isotretinoin. Its use is highly regulated due to its potential for severe adverse events, primarily teratogenicity. Recently there have also been concerns that it is associated with severe depression in some patients. The latter has not been proved. At present, prescribers must receive from the manufacturer training, certification, and stickers to affix to each prescription. These measures are imposed to ensure that all prescribers are familiar with the risks of isotretinoin; that all female patients have two negative pregnancy tests prior to initiating therapy and a negative pregnancy test prior to each refill; and that all patients have been warned about the risks associated with isotretinoin, including depression. Additionally, patients receiving this medication develop extremely dry skin and cheilitis and must be followed for development of hypertriglyceridemia.

ACNE ROSACEA Acne rosacea is an inflammatory disorder predominantly affecting the central face. It is seen almost exclusively in adults, only rarely affecting patients under 30 years of age. Rosacea is seen more often in women, but those most severely affected are men. It is characterized by the presence of erythema, telangiectases, and superficial pustules (Fig. 47-8), but is not associated with the presence of comedones. Rosacea only rarely involves the chest or back.

There is a relationship between the tendency for pronounced facial flushing and the subsequent development of acne rosacea. Often, individuals with rosacea initially demonstrate a pronounced flushing reaction. This may be in response to heat, emotional stimuli, alcohol, hot drinks, or spicy foods. As the disease progresses, the flush persists longer and longer and may eventually become permanent. Papules, pustules, and telangiectases can become superimposed on the persistent flush. Rosacea of very long standing may lead to connective tissue overgrowth, particularly of the nose (rhinophyma). Rosacea may also be complicated by various inflammatory disorders of the eye, including keratitis, blepharitis, iritis, and recurrent chalazion. These ocular problems are potentially sight-threatening and warrant ophthalmologic evaluation.

℞ TREATMENT

Acne rosacea can be treated topically or systemically. Mild disease often responds to topical metronidazole or sodium sulfacetamide. More severe disease requires oral tetracycline in doses ranging from 250 to 1000 mg/d. Residual telangiectasia may respond to laser therapy. Topical glucocorticoids, especially potent agents, should be avoided since chronic use of these preparations may elicit rosacea. Topical therapy of the skin is not effective treatment for ocular disease.

FIGURE 47-8 Acne rosacea with prominent facial erythema, telangiectasia, scattered papules, and small pustules. (Courtesy of Robert Swerlick, MD.)

SKIN DISEASES AND SMALLPOX VACCINATION

Given the potential threat of a bioterrorism attack with smallpox, vaccinations against smallpox are available to the general public, although they are not recommended. Because of a higher incidence of adverse events associated with smallpox vaccination in patients with a history of certain skin diseases, including atopic dermatitis, eczema, severe acne, and psoriasis, such vaccination is contraindicated in patients with these conditions in the absence of a bioterrorism attack and a real or potential exposure to smallpox. In the case of such exposure, the risk of smallpox infection outweighs the risk of adverse events from the vaccine (Chap. 205).

FURTHER READING

BOS JD, DERIE MA: The pathogenesis of psoriasis: Immunological facts and speculations. Immunol Today 20:40, 1999

COHEN DE: Occupational dermatoses, in *Handbook of Occupational Safety and Health*, 2d ed, LJ DiBerardinis (ed). New York, Wiley, 1999, p 697

FREEDBURG IM et al (eds): *Fitzpatrick's Dermatology in General Medicine*, 5th ed. New York, McGraw-Hill, 1999

HENGGE UR et al: Topical immunomodulators—progress towards treating inflammation, infection, and cancer. Lancet Infect Dis 1:189, 2001

KRUEGER JG: The immunologic basis for the treatment of psoriasis with new biologic agents. J Am Acad Dermatol 46:1, 2002

48 SKIN MANIFESTATIONS OF INTERNAL DISEASE
Jean L. Bolognia, Irwin M. Braverman

It is now a generally accepted concept in medicine that the skin can show signs of internal disease. Therefore, in textbooks of medicine one finds a chapter describing in detail the major systemic disorders that can be identified by cutaneous signs. The underlying assumption of such a chapter is that the clinician has been able to identify the disorder in the patient and needs only to read about it in the textbook. In reality, concise differential diagnoses and the identification of these disorders are actually difficult for the nondermatologist because he or she is not well versed in the recognition of cutaneous lesions or their spectrum of presentations. Therefore, the authors of this chapter have decided to cover this particular topic of cutaneous medicine not by discussing individual disorders but by describing and discussing the various presenting clinical signs and symptoms that indicate the presence of these disorders. Concise differential diagnoses will be generated in which the significant diseases will be briefly discussed and distinguished from the more common disorders that have no significance for internal diseases. The latter disorders are reviewed in table form and always need to be excluded when considering the former. For a detailed description of individual diseases, the reader should consult a dermatologic text.

PAPULOSQUAMOUS SKIN LESIONS (Table 48-1)   When an eruption is characterized by elevated lesions, papules (<1 cm), or plaques (>1 cm), in association with scale, it is referred to as a *papulosquamous lesion*. The most common papulosquamous diseases—*psoriasis*, *tinea*, *pityriasis rosea*, and *lichen planus*—are primary cutaneous disorders (Chap. 47). When psoriatic lesions are accompanied by arthritis, the possibility of psoriatic arthritis or *Reiter's disease* should be considered. A history of oral ulcers, conjunctivitis, uveitis, and/or urethritis points to the latter diagnosis. In *guttate psoriasis* there is an acute onset of small, widely scattered, uniform lesions, often in association with a streptococcal infection. Lithium, beta blockers, HIV infection, and a rapid taper of systemic glucocorticoids are also known to exacerbate psoriasis.

Whenever the diagnosis of pityriasis rosea or lichen planus is made, it is important to review the patient's medications because the eruption can be treated by simply discontinuing the offending agent. Pityriasis rosea–like drug eruptions are seen most commonly with beta blockers, angiotensin-converting enzyme (ACE) inhibitors, gold, and metronidazole, while the drugs that can produce a lichenoid eruption include gold, antimalarials, thiazides, quinidine, phenothiazines, sulfonylureas, and ACE inhibitors. Lichen planus–like lesions are also observed in chronic graft-versus-host disease.

In its early stages, *cutaneous T cell lymphoma* (CTCL) may be confused with eczema or psoriasis, but it often fails to respond to the appropriate therapy for those inflammatory diseases. CTCL can develop within lesions of large-plaque parapsoriasis and is suggested by an increase in the thickness of the lesions. The diagnosis of CTCL is established by skin biopsy in which collections of atypical T lymphocytes are found in the epidermis and dermis. As the disease progresses, cutaneous tumors and lymph node involvement may appear.

In *secondary syphilis* there are scattered red-brown papules with thin scale. The eruption often involves the palms and soles and can resemble pityriasis rosea. Associated findings are helpful in making the diagnosis and include annular plaques on the face, nonscarring alopecia, condyloma lata (broad-based and moist), and mucous patches as well as lymphadenopathy, malaise, fever, headache, and myalgias. The interval between the primary chancre and the secondary stage is usually 4 to 8 weeks, and spontaneous resolution without appropriate therapy is seen.

ERYTHRODERMA (Table 48-2)   *Erythroderma* is the term used when the majority of the skin surface is erythematous (red in color). There may be associated scale, erosions, or pustules as well as shedding of the hair and nails. Potential systemic manifestations include fever, chills, hypothermia, reactive lymphadenopathy, peripheral edema, hypoal-

---

TABLE 48-1   *Selected Causes of Papulosquamous Skin Lesions*

1. Primary cutaneous disorders
   a. Psoriasis[a]
   b. Tinea[a]
   c. Pityriasis rosea[a]
   d. Lichen planus[a]
   e. Parapsoriasis
   f. Bowen's disease (squamous cell carcinoma in situ)[b]
2. Drugs
3. Systemic diseases
   a. Lupus erythematosus[c]
   b. Cutaneous T cell lymphoma
   c. Secondary syphilis
   d. Reiter's disease
   e. Sarcoidosis[d]

[a] Discussed in detail in Chap. 47.
[b] Associated with chronic sun exposure and exposure to arsenic.
[c] See also "Red Lesions" in "Papulonodular Skin Lesions."
[d] See also "Red-Brown Lesions" in "Papulonodular Skin Lesions."

TABLE 48-2   *Causes of Erythroderma*

1. Primary cutaneous disorders
   a. Psoriasis[a]
   b. Dermatitis (atopic, stasis, contact, seborrheic)[a]
   c. Pityriasis rubra pilaris
2. Drugs
3. Systemic diseases
   a. Cutaneous T cell lymphoma
   b. Lymphoma
4. Idiopathic

[a] Discussed in detail in Chap. 47.

TABLE 48-3 *Erythroderma (Primary Cutaneous Disorders)*

	Initial Lesions	Location of Initial Lesions	Other Findings	Diagnostic Aids	Treatment
Psoriasis[a]	Pink-red, silvery scale, sharply demarcated	Elbows, knees, scalp, presacral area	Nail dystrophy, arthritis, pustules	Skin biopsy	Oral retinoid ± PUVA; UV-B; methotrexate; cyclosporine; monoclonal antibodies
Dermatitis[a] Atopic	Acute: Erythema, fine scale, crust, indistinct borders Chronic: Lichenification (increased skin markings)	Antecubital and popliteal fossae, neck, hands	Pruritus Family history of atopy, including asthma, allergic rhinitis or conjunctivitis, and atopic dermatitis Rule out secondary infection with *S. aureus* Rule out superimposed irritant contact dermatitis	Skin biopsy	Topical glucocorticoids, tacrolimus, pimecrolimus, tar, and antipruritics; oral antihistamines; open wet dressings; UV-B + UV-A; PUVA; oral/IM glucocorticoids; cyclosporine Topical or oral antibiotics
Stasis	Erythema, crusting, excoriations	Lower extremities	Pruritus, lower extremity edema History of venous ulcers, thrombophlebitis, and/or cellulitis Rule out cellulitis Rule out superimposed contact dermatitis, e.g., topical neomycin	Skin biopsy	Topical glucocorticoids; open; wet dressings; leg elevation; pressure stockings
Contact	Local: Erythema, crusting, vesicles, and bullae	Depends on offending agent	Irritant—onset often within hours Allergic—delayed-type hypersensitivity; lag time of 48 h	Patch testing	Remove irritant or allergen; topical glucocorticoids; oral antihistamines; oral/IM glucocorticoids
	Systemic: Erythema, fine scale, crust	Generalized	Patient has history of allergic contact dermatitis to topical agent and then receives systemic medication that is structurally related, e.g., ethylenediamine, (topical) aminophylline (IV)	Patch testing	Same as local
Seborrheic	Pink-red, greasy scale	Scalp, nasolabial folds, eyebrows, intertriginous zones	Flares with stress, HIV infection Associated with Parkinson's disease	Skin biopsy	Topical glucocorticoids and imidazoles
Pityriasis rubra pilaris	Orange-red, perifollicular papules	Generalized, but characteristic "skip" areas of normal skin	Wax-like keratoderma Rule out cutaneous T cell lymphoma	Skin biopsy	Isotretinoin or acitretin; methotrexate

[a] Discussed in detail in Chap. 47.

Note: PUVA, *p*soralens + *u*ltraviolet *A* irradiation; UV-B, *u*ltraviolet *B*; UV-A, *u*ltraviolet *A*; IM, intramuscular; IV, intravenous.

buminemia, and high-output cardiac failure. The major etiologies of erythroderma are (1) cutaneous diseases such as psoriasis and dermatitis (Table 48-3); (2) drugs; (3) systemic diseases, most commonly CTCL; and (4) idiopathic. In the first three groups, the location and description of the initial lesions, prior to the development of the erythroderma, aid in the diagnosis. For example, a history of red scaly plaques on the elbows and knees would point to psoriasis. It is also important to examine the skin carefully for a migration of the erythema and associated secondary changes such as pustules or erosions. Migratory waves of erythema studded with superficial pustules are seen in *pustular psoriasis*.

Drug-induced erythroderma (exfoliative dermatitis) may begin as a morbilliform eruption (Chap. 50) or may arise as diffuse erythema. Fever and peripheral eosinophilia often accompany the eruption, and occasionally there is an associated allergic interstitial nephritis. A number of drugs can produce an erythroderma, including penicillins, sulfonamides, carbamazepine, phenytoin, gold, allopurinol, and captopril. While reactions to anticonvulsants can lead to a pseudolymphoma syndrome (with adenopathy, hepatitis, and circulating atypical lymphocytes), reactions to allopurinol may be accompanied by hepatitis, gastrointestinal bleeding, and nephropathy.

The most common malignancy that is associated with erythroderma is CTCL; in some series, up to 25% of the cases of erythroderma were duc to CTCL. The patient may progress from isolated plaques and tumors, but more commonly the erythroderma is present throughout the course of the disease (Sézary syndrome). In the Sézary syndrome, there are circulating atypical T lymphocytes, pruritus, and lymphadenopathy. In cases of erythroderma where there is no apparent cause (idiopathic), longitudinal follow-up is mandatory to monitor for the possible development of CTCL. There have been isolated case reports of erythroderma secondary to some solid tumors—lung, liver, prostate, thyroid, and colon—but it is usually in a late stage of the disease.

ALOPECIA (Table 48-4) The two major forms of alopecia are scarring and nonscarring. In *scarring alopecia* there are associated fibrosis, inflammation, and loss of hair follicles. A smooth scalp with a decreased number of follicular openings is usually observed clinically, but in some cases the changes are seen only in biopsy specimens from the affected areas. In *nonscarring alopecia* the hair shafts are gone, but the hair follicles are preserved, explaining the reversible nature of nonscarring alopecia.

The most common causes of nonscarring alopecia include *telogen effluvium, androgenetic alopecia, alopecia areata, tinea capitis,* and *traumatic alopecia* (Table 48-5). In women with androgenetic alopecia, an elevation in circulating levels of androgens may be seen as a result of ovarian or adrenal gland dysfunction. When there are

TABLE 48-4   *Causes of Alopecia*

I. Nonscarring alopecia
  A. Primary cutaneous disorders
    1. Telogen effluvium
    2. Androgenetic alopecia
    3. Alopecia areata
    4. Tinea capitis
    5. Traumatic alopecia
  B. Drugs
  C. Systemic diseases
    1. Lupus erythematosus
    2. Secondary syphilis
    3. Hypothryoidism
    4. Hyperthyroidism
    5. Hypopituitarism
    6. Deficiencies of protein,
      iron, biotin, and zinc
	II. Scarring alopecia
	  A. Primary cutaneous disorders
	    1. Cutaneous lupus
	    2. Lichen planus
	    3. Folliculitis decalvans
	    4. Linear scleroderma
	      (morphea)
	    5. Traumatic alopecia[a]
	  B. Systemic diseases
	    1. Lupus erythematosus
	    2. Sarcoidosis
	    3. Cutaneous metastases

[a] Also referred to as follicular degeneration.

signs of virilization, such as a deepened voice and enlarged clitoris, the possibility of an ovarian or adrenal gland tumor should be considered.

Exposure to various drugs can also cause diffuse hair loss, usually by inducing a telogen effluvium. An exception is the anagen effluvium observed with antimitotic agents such as daunorubicin. Alopecia is a side effect of the following drugs: warfarin, heparin, propylthiouracil, carbimazole, vitamin A, isotretinoin, acitretin, lithium, beta blockers, colchicine, and amphetamines. Fortunately, spontaneous regrowth usually follows discontinuation of the offending agent.

Less commonly, nonscarring alopecia is associated with *lupus erythematosus* and *secondary syphilis*. In systemic lupus there are two forms of alopecia—one is scarring secondary to discoid lesions (see below) and the other is nonscarring. The latter form may be diffuse and involve the entire scalp, or it may be localized to the frontal scalp and result in multiple short hairs ("lupus hairs"). Scattered, poorly circumscribed patches of alopecia with a "moth-eaten" appearance are a manifestation of the secondary stage of syphilis. Diffuse thinning of the hair is also associated with hypothyroidism and hyperthyroidism (Table 48-4).

Scarring alopecia is more frequently the result of a primary cutaneous disorder such as *lichen planus*, *folliculitis decalvans*, *cutaneous lupus*, or *linear scleroderma* (*morphea*) than it is a sign of systemic disease. Although the scarring lesions of *discoid lupus* can be seen in patients with systemic lupus, in the majority of cases the disease process is limited to the skin. Less common causes of scarring alopecia include *sarcoidosis* (see "Papulonodular Skin Lesions," below) and *cutaneous metastases*.

In the early phases of discoid lupus, lichen planus, and folliculitis decalvans, there are circumscribed areas of alopecia. Fibrosis and subsequent loss of follicles are observed primarily in the center of the individual lesions, while the inflammatory process is most prominent at the periphery. The areas of active inflammation in discoid lupus are erythematous with scale, whereas the areas of previous inflammation are often hypopigmented with a rim of hyperpigmentation. In lichen planus the peripheral perifollicular macules are usually violet-colored. Complete examination of the skin and oral mucosa combined with a biopsy and direct immunofluorescence microscopy will aid in distinguishing these two entities. The peripheral active lesions in folliculitis decalvans are follicular pustules; these patients can develop a reactive arthritis.

FIGURATE SKIN LESIONS (Table 48-6) In *figurate eruptions*, the lesions form rings and arcs that are usually erythematous but can be skin-colored to brown. Most commonly, they are due to primary cutaneous diseases such as *tinea*, *urticaria*, *erythema annulare centrifugum*, and *granuloma annulare* (Chaps. 47 and 49). An underlying systemic illness is found in a second, less common group of migratory annular erythemas. It includes *erythema gyratum repens*, *erythema migrans*, *erythema marginatum*, and *necrolytic migratory erythema*.

In erythema gyratum repens, one sees hundreds of mobile concentric arcs and wavefronts that resemble the grain in wood. A search for an underlying malignancy is mandatory in a patient with this eruption. Erythema migrans is the cutaneous manifestation of Lyme disease, which is caused by the spirochete *Borrelia burgdorferi*. In the initial stage (3 to 30 days after tick bite), a single annular lesion is usually seen, which can expand to ≥10 cm in diameter. Within several days, approximately half the patients develop multiple smaller erythematous lesions at sites distant from the bite. Associated symptoms include fever, headache, photophobia, myalgias, arthralgias, and malar rash. Erythema marginatum is seen in patients with rheumatic fever, primarily on the trunk. Lesions are pink-red in color, flat to mildly elevated, and transient.

There are additional cutaneous diseases that present as annular eruptions but lack an obvious migratory component. Examples include *CTCL*, *annular cutaneous lupus* (also referred to as *subacute lupus*), *secondary syphilis*, and *sarcoidosis* (see "Papulonodular Skin Lesions," below).

ACNE (Table 48-7) In addition to *acne vulgaris* and *acne rosacea*, the two major forms of acne (Chap. 47), there are drugs and systemic diseases that can lead to acneiform eruptions (Table 48-7).

Patients with the *carcinoid syndrome* have episodes of flushing of the head, neck, and sometimes the trunk. Resultant skin changes of the face, in particular telangiectasias, may mimic the clinical appearance of acne rosacea.

PUSTULAR LESIONS *Acneiform eruptions* (see "Acne," above) and *folliculitis* represent the most common pustular dermatoses. An important consideration in the evaluation of follicular pustules is a determination of the associated pathogen, e.g., normal flora, *Staphylococcus aureus*, *Pityrosporum*. Noninfectious forms of folliculitis include HIV-associated eosinophilic folliculitis and folliculitis secondary to drugs such as glucocorticoids and lithium. Administration of high-dose oral glucocorticoids can result in a widespread eruption of follicular pustules on the trunk, characterized by lesions in the same stage of development. With regard to underlying systemic diseases, nonfollicular-based pustules are a characteristic component of pustular psoriasis and can be seen in septic emboli of bacterial or fungal origin (see "Purpura," below).

TELANGIECTASIAS (Table 48-8) In order to distinguish the various types of telangiectasias, it is important to examine the shape and configuration of the dilated blood vessels. *Linear telangiectasias* are seen on the face of patients with *actinically damaged skin* and *acne rosacea* and they are found on the legs of patients with *venous hypertension* and *essential telangiectasia*. Patients with an unusual form of *mastocytosis* (telangiectasia macularis eruptiva perstans) and the *carcinoid syndrome* (see "Acne," above) also have linear telangiectasias. Lastly, linear telangiectasias are found in areas of cutaneous inflammation. For example, lesions of discoid lupus frequently have telangiectasias within them.

Poikiloderma is a term used to describe a patch of skin with (1) reticulated hypo- and hyperpigmentation, (2) wrinkling secondary to epidermal atrophy, and (3) telangiectasias. Poikiloderma does not imply a single disease entity—although becoming less common, it is seen in skin damaged by *ionizing radiation*, as well as in patients with autoimmune connective tissue diseases, primarily *dermatomyositis* (DM).

In *scleroderma*, the dilated blood vessels have a unique configuration and are known as *mat telangiectasias*. The lesions are broad macules that usually measure 2 to 7 mm in diameter but occasionally are larger. Mats have a polygonal or oval shape, and their erythematous color may be uniform or the result of delicate telangiectasias. The most common locations for mat telangiectasias are the face, oral mucosa, and hands—peripheral sites that are prone to intermittent ischemia. The CREST (*c*alcinosis cutis, *R*aynaud's phenomenon, *e*sophageal dysmotility, *s*clerodactyly, and *t*elangiectasia) variant of scleroderma

(Chap. 303) is associated with a chronic course and anticentromere antibodies. Mat telangiectasias are an important clue to the diagnosis of the CREST syndrome as well as systemic scleroderma, for they may be the only cutaneous finding.

Periungual telangiectasias are pathognomonic signs of the three major autoimmune connective tissue diseases—*lupus erythematosus, scleroderma*, and *DM*. They are easily visualized by the naked eye and occur in at least two-thirds of these patients. In both DM and lupus there is associated nailfold erythema, and in DM the erythema is often accompanied by "ragged" cuticles and fingertip tenderness. Under $10\times$ magnification, the blood vessels in the nailfolds of lupus patients are tortuous and resemble "glomeruli," whereas in scleroderma and DM there is a loss of capillary loops and those that remain are markedly dilated.

In *hereditary hemorrhagic telangiectasia* (Osler-Rendu-Weber disease), the lesions usually appear during adulthood and are most commonly seen on the mucous membranes, face, and distal extremities, including under the nails. They represent arteriovenous (AV) malformations of the dermal microvasculature, are dark red in color, and are usually slightly elevated. When the skin is stretched over an individual lesion, an eccentric punctum with radiating legs is seen. Although the degree of systemic involvement varies in this autosomal dominant disease (due to mutations in either the endoglin or activin receptor–like kinase gene), the major symptoms are recurrent epistaxis and gastrointestinal bleeding. The fact that these mucosal telangiectasias are actually AV communications helps to explain their tendency to bleed.

TABLE 48-5 *Nonscarring Alopecia (Primary Cutaneous Disorders)*

	Clinical Characteristics	Pathogenesis	Treatment
Telogen effluvium	Diffuse shedding of normal hairs. Follows either major stress (high fever, severe infection) or change in hormones (post partum). Reversible without treatment	Stress causes the normally asynchronous growth cycles of individual hairs to become synchronous; therefore, large numbers of growing (anagen) hairs simultaneously enter the dying (telogen) phase	Observation; discontinue any drugs that have alopecia as a side effect; must exclude underlying metabolic causes, e.g., hypothyroidism, hyperthyroidism
Androgenetic alopecia	Miniaturization of hairs along the midline of the scalp. Recession of the anterior scalp line in men and some women	Increased sensitivity of affected hairs to the effects of testosterone. Increased levels of circulating androgens (ovarian or adrenal source in women)	If no evidence of hyperandrogen state, then topical minoxidil ± tretinoin; finasteride[a]; hair transplant
Alopecia areata	Well-circumscribed, circular areas of hair loss, 2–5 cm in diameter. In extensive cases, coalescence of lesions and/or involvement of other hair-bearing surfaces of the body. Pitting of the nails	The germinative zones of the hair follicles are surrounded by T lymphocytes. Occasional associated diseases: hyperthyroidism, hypothyroidism, vitiligo, Down's syndrome	Topical anthralin; intralesional glucocorticoids; topical contact sensitizers
Tinea	Varies from scaling with minimal hair loss to discrete patches with "black dots" (broken hairs) to boggy plaque with pustules (kerion)	Invasion of hairs by dermatophytes, most commonly *Trichophyton tonsurans*	Oral griseofulvin or terbinafine plus 2.5% selenium sulfide or ketoconazole shampoo; examine family members
Traumatic alopecia	Broken hairs. Irregular outline	Traction with curlers, rubber bands, braiding. Exposure to heat or chemicals. Mechanical pulling (trichotillomania)	Discontinuation of offending hair style or chemical treatments; trichotillomania may require hair clipping and observation of shaved hairs or biopsy for diagnosis, followed by psychotherapy

[a] To date, FDA-approved for men.

HYPOPIGMENTATION (Table 48-9)

Disorders of hypopigmentation are classified as either diffuse or localized. The classic example of *diffuse hypopigmentation* is *oculocutaneous albinism* (OCA). The most common forms are due to mutations in the tyrosinase gene (type I) or the *P* gene (type II); patients with type IA OCA have a total lack of enzyme activity. At birth, different forms of OCA can appear similar—white hair, gray-blue eyes, and pink-white skin. However, the patients with no tyrosinase activity maintain this phenotype, whereas those with decreased activity or *P* gene mutations will acquire some pigmentation of the eyes, hair, and skin as they age. The degree of pigment formation is also a function of racial background, and the pigmentary dilution is readily apparent when patients are compared to their first-degree relatives. The ocular findings in OCA correlate with the degree of hypopigmentation and include decreased visual acuity, nystagmus, photophobia, and monocular vision.

The differential diagnosis of *localized hypomelanosis* includes the following primary cutaneous disorders: *idiopathic guttate hypomelanosis, postinflammatory hypopigmentation, tinea (pityriasis) versicolor, vitiligo, chemical leukoderma, nevus depigmentosus* (see below), and *piebaldism* (Table 48-9). In this group of diseases, the areas of involvement are macules or patches with a decrease or absence of pigmentation. Patients with vitiligo also have an increased incidence of several autoimmune disorders, including hypothyroidism, Graves' disease, pernicious anemia, Addison's disease, uveitis, alopecia areata, chronic mucocutaneous candidiasis, and the polyglandular autoimmune syndromes (types I and II). Diseases of the thyroid gland are the most frequently associated disorders, occurring in up to 30% of patients with vitiligo. Circulating autoantibodies are often found, and the most common ones are antithyroglobulin, antimicrosomal, and antiparietal cell antibodies.

There are three systemic diseases that should be considered in a patient with skin findings suggestive of vitiligo—*Vogt-Koyanagi-Harada syndrome, scleroderma*, and *melanoma-associated leukoderma*. A history of aseptic meningitis, nontraumatic uveitis, tinnitus, hearing loss, and/or dysacousis points to the diagnosis of the Vogt-Koyanagi-Harada syndrome. In these patients, the face and scalp are the most common locations of pigment loss. The vitiligo-like leukoderma seen in patients with scleroderma has a clinical resemblance to idiopathic vitiligo that has begun to repigment as a result of treatment; that is, perifollicular macules of normal pigmentation are seen within areas of depigmentation. The basis of this leukoderma is unknown;

TABLE 48-6 *Causes of Figurate Skin Lesions*

I. Primary cutaneous disorders
  A. Tinea
  B. Urticaria (≥90%)
  C. Erythema annulare centrifugum
  D. Granuloma annulare
  E. Psoriasis
II. Systemic diseases
  A. Migratory
    1. Erythema migrans
    2. Urticaria (≤10%)
    3. Erythema gyratum repens
    4. Erythema marginatum
    5. Pustular psoriasis
    6. Necrolytic migratory erythema (glucagonoma syndrome)[a]
  B. Nonmigratory
    1. Sarcoidosis
    2. Subacute lupus erythematosus
    3. Secondary syphilis
    4. Cutaneous T cell lymphoma (e.g., mycosis fungoides)

[a] Migratory erythema with erosions; favors lower extremities and girdle area.

TABLE 48-8 *Causes of Telangiectasias*

I. Primary cutaneous disorders
  A. Linear
    1. Acne rosacea
    2. Actinically damaged skin
    3. Venous hypertension
    4. Essential telangiectasia
    5. Within basal cell carcinomas
  B. Poikiloderma
    1. Ionizing radiation[a]
    2. Poikiloderma vasculare atrophicans
  C. Spider angioma
    1. Idiopathic
    2. Pregnancy
II. Systemic diseases
  A. Linear
    1. Carcinoid
    2. Ataxia-telangiectasia
    3. Mastocytosis
  B. Poikiloderma
    1. Dermatomyositis
    2. Cutaneous T cell lymphoma
    3. Xeroderma pigmentosum
  C. Mat
    1. Scleroderma
  D. Periungual
    1. Lupus erythematosus
    2. Scleroderma
    3. Dermatomyositis
  E. Papular
    1. Hereditary hemorrhagic telangiectasia
  F. Spider angioma
    1. Cirrhosis

[a] Becoming less common.

there is no evidence of inflammation in areas of involvement, but it can resolve if the underlying connective tissue disease becomes inactive. In contrast to idiopathic vitiligo, melanoma-associated leukoderma often begins on the trunk, and its appearance should prompt a search for metastatic disease. The possibility exists that the destruction of normal melanocytes is the result of an immune response against malignant melanocytes.

There are two systemic disorders that may have the cutaneous findings of piebaldism (Table 48-10). They are *Hirschsprung's disease* and *Waardenburg's syndrome*. A possible explanation for both disorders is an abnormal embryonic migration or survival of two neural crest–derived elements, one of them being melanocytes and the other myenteric ganglion cells (Hirschsprung's disease) or auditory nerve cells (Waardenburg's syndrome). The latter syndrome is characterized by congenital sensorineural hearing loss, dystopia canthorum (lateral displacement of the inner canthi but normal interpupillary distance), heterochromic irises, and a broad nasal root, in addition to the piebaldism. Patients with Waardenburg's syndrome have been shown to have mutations in two genes that encode DNA-binding proteins, *PAX-3* and *MITF*, while patients with Hirschsprung's disease and white spotting have mutations in one of three genes—endothelin 3, endothelin B receptor, and *SOX-10*.

In *tuberous sclerosis*, the earliest cutaneous sign is an ash leaf spot. These lesions are often present at birth and are usually multiple; however, detection may require Wood's lamp examination, especially in fair-skinned individuals. The pigment within them is reduced but not absent. The average size is 1 to 3 cm, and the common shapes are polygonal and lance-ovate. Examination of the patient for additional cutaneous signs such as adenoma sebaceum (multiple angiofibromas of the face), ungual and gingival fibromas, fibrous plaques of the forehead, and connective tissue nevi (shagreen patches) is re-

commended. It is important to remember that an ash leaf spot on the scalp will result in *poliosis*, which is a circumscribed patch of gray-white hair. Internal manifestations include seizures, mental retardation, central nervous system (CNS) and retinal hamartomas, renal angiomyolipomas, and cardiac rhabdomyomas. The latter can be detected in up to 60% of children (<18 years) with tuberous sclerosis by echocardiography.

Nevus depigmentosus is a stable, well-circumscribed hypomelanosis that is present at birth. There is usually a single circular or rectangular lesion, but occasionally the nevus has a segmental or whorled pattern. It is important to distinguish this more common entity from ash leaf spots especially when there are multiple lesions. In *hypomelanosis of Ito*, swirls and streaks of hypopigmentation run parallel to one another in a pattern that resembles a marble cake. Lesions may progress or regress with time, and in up to a third of patients, associated abnormalities are found including in the musculoskeletal system (asymmetry), the CNS (seizures and mental retardation), and the eyes (strabismus and hypertelorism). Chromosomal mosaicism has been de-

TABLE 48-7 *Causes of Acneiform Eruptions*

I. Primary cutaneous disorders
  A. Acne vulgaris
  B. Acne rosacea
II. Drugs, e.g., anabolic steroids, glucocorticoids, lithium, iodides
III. Systemic diseases
  A. Increased androgen production
    1. Adrenal origin, e.g., Cushing's disease, 21-hydroxylase deficiency
    2. Ovarian origin, e.g., polycystic ovary disease
  B. Cryptococcosis, disseminated
  C. Dimorphic fungi
  D. Behçet's disease

TABLE 48-9 *Causes of Hypopigmentation*

I. Primary cutaneous disorders
  A. Diffuse
    1. Generalized vitiligo[a]
  B. Localized
    1. Idiopathic guttate hypomelanosis
    2. Postinflammatory
    3. Tinea (pityriasis) versicolor
    4. Vitiligo
    5. Chemical leukoderma
    6. Nevus depigmentosus
    7. Piebaldism
II. Systemic diseases
  A. Diffuse
    1. Oculocutaneous albinism[b]
      a. Hermansky-Pudlak syndrome[c]
      b. Chédiak-Higashi syndrome[d]
    2. Phenylketonuria
    3. Homocystinuria
  B. Localized
    1. Vogt-Koyanagi-Harada
    2. Scleroderma
    3. Melanoma-associated leukoderma
    4. Tuberous sclerosis
    5. Hypomelanosis of Ito/mosaicism
    6. Incontinentia pigmenti (stage IV)
    7. Sarcoidosis
    8. Tuberculoid and indeterminate leprosy
    9. Cutaneous T cell lymphoma

[a] Absence of melanocytes.
[b] Normal number of melanocytes.
[c] Platelet storage defect and restrictive lung disease secondary to deposits of ceroid-like material; one form due to mutations in β subunit of adaptor protein.
[d] Giant lysosomal granules and recurrent infections.

TABLE 48-10 *Hypopigmentation (Primary Cutaneous Disorders, Localized)*

	Clinical Characteristics	Wood's Lamp Examination (UV-A; Peak = 365 nm)	Skin Biopsy Specimen	Pathogenesis	Treatment
Idiopathic guttate hypomelanosis	Common; acquired; 1 to 4 mm in diameter Shins and extensor forearms	Less enhancement than vitiligo	Abrupt decrease in epidermal melanin content	Possible somatic mutations as a reflection of aging; UV exposure	None
Postinflammatory hypopigmentation	Can develop within active lesions, as in subacute lupus, or after the lesion fades, as in dermatitis	Depends on particular disease Usually less enhancement than in vitiligo	Type of inflammatory infiltrate depends on specific disease	Block in transfer of melanin from melanocytes to keratinocytes could be secondary to edema or decrease in contact time Destruction of melanocytes if inflammatory cells attack basal layer	Treat underlying inflammatory disease
Tinea (pityriasis) versicolor	Common disorder Upper trunk and neck Shawl-like distribution Young adults Macules have fine white scale when scratched	Golden fluorescence	Hyphae and budding yeast in stratum corneum	Invasion of stratum corneum by the yeast *Pityrosporum* Yeast is lipophilic and produces C_9 and C_{11} dicarboxylic acids, which in vitro inhibit tyrosinase	Selenium sulfide 2.5%; topical imidazoles; oral imidazoles or triazoles
Vitiligo	Acquired; progressive Symmetric areas of complete pigment loss Periorificial—around mouth, nose, eyes, nipples, umbilicus, anus Other areas—flexor wrists, extensor distal extremities Segmental form is less common—unilateral, dermatomal-like	More apparent Chalk-white	Absence of melanocytes Mild inflammation	Possible autoimmune phenomenon that results in destruction of melanocytes—humoral and/or cellular Alternative hypothesis is self-destruction of melanocytes and circulating antibodies or cytotoxic T cells as a secondary phenomenon	Topical glucocorticoids; UV-B; PUVA; transplants; depigmentation if widespread
Chemical leukoderma	Similar appearance to vitiligo Often begins on hands Satellite lesions in areas not exposed to chemicals	More apparent Chalk-white	Decreased number or absence of melanocytes	Exposure to chemicals that selectively destroy melanocytes, in particular phenols and catechols (germicides; adhesives) Release of cellular antigens and activation of circulating lymphocytes may explain satellite phenomenon	Avoid exposure to offending agent, then treat as vitiligo
Piebaldism	Autosomal dominant Congenital, stable White forelock Areas of hypomelanosis contain normally pigmented and hyperpigmented macules of various sizes Symmetric involvement of central forehead, ventral trunk, and mid regions of upper and lower extremities	Enhancement of leukoderma and hyperpigmented macules	Hypomelanotic areas—few to no melanocytes	Defect in migration of melanoblasts from neural crest to ventral skin or failure of melanoblasts to survive or differentiate in these areas Mutations within the c-*kit* proto-oncogene that encodes the tyrosine kinase receptor for mast/stem cell growth factor	None; occasionally transplants

Note: PUVA, psoralens + ultraviolet A irradiation; UV-B, ultraviolet B.

tected in these patients; this lends support to the hypothesis that the pattern is the result of the migration of two clones of primordial melanocytes, each with a different pigment potential.

Localized areas of decreased pigmentation are commonly seen as a result of cutaneous inflammation (Table 48-10) and have been observed in the skin overlying active lesions of sarcoidosis (see "Papulonodular Skin Lesions," below) as well as in CTCL. Cutaneous infections also present as disorders of hypopigmentation, and in *tuberculoid leprosy* there are a few asymmetric patches of hypomelanosis that have associated anesthesia, anhidrosis, and alopecia. Biopsy specimens of the palpable border show dermal granulomas that contain rare, if any, *Mycobacterium leprae* organisms.

HYPERPIGMENTATION (Table 48-11) Disorders of hyperpigmentation are also divided into two groups—localized and diffuse. The localized forms are due to an epidermal alteration, a proliferation of melanocytes, or an increase in pigment production. Both seborrheic keratoses and acanthosis nigricans belong to the first group. *Seborrheic keratoses* are common lesions, but in one clinical setting they are a sign of systemic disease, and that setting is the sudden appearance of multiple lesions, often with an inflammatory base and in association with acrochordons (skin tags) and acanthosis nigricans. This is termed the *sign of Leser-Trélat* and signifies an internal malignancy. *Acanthosis nigricans* can also be a reflection of an internal malignancy, most commonly of the gastrointestinal tract, and it appears as velvety hy-

TABLE 48-11　*Causes of Hyperpigmentation*

I. Primary cutaneous disorders
　A. Localized
　　1. Epidermal alteration
　　　a. Seborrheic keratosis
　　　b. Acanthosis nigricans (obesity)
　　　c. Pigmented actinic keratosis
　　2. Proliferation of melanocytes
　　　a. Lentigo
　　　b. Nevus
　　　c. Melanoma
　　3. Increased pigment production
　　　a. Ephelides (freckles)
　　　b. Café au lait macule
　B. Localized and diffuse
　　1. Drugs
II. Systemic diseases
　A. Localized
　　1. Epidermal alteration
　　　a. Seborrheic keratoses (sign of Leser-Trélat)
　　　b. Acanthosis nigricans (endocrine disorders, paraneoplastic)
　　2. Proliferation of melanocytes
　　　a. Lentigines (Peutz-Jeghers and LEOPARD syndromes; xeroderma pigmentosum)
　　　b. Nevi [Carney complex (LAMB and NAME syndromes)][a]
　　3. Increased pigment production
　　　a. Café au lait macules (neurofibromatosis, McCune-Albright syndrome[b])
　　　b. Urticaria pigmentosa[c]
　　4. Dermal pigmentation
　　　a. Incontinentia pigmenti (stage III)
　　　b. Dyskeratosis congenita
　B. Diffuse
　　1. Endocrinopathies
　　　a. Addison's disease
　　　b. Nelson syndrome
　　　c. Ectopic ACTH syndrome
　　2. Metabolic
　　　a. Porphyria cutanea tarda
　　　b. Hemochromatosis
　　　c. Vitamin B_{12}, folate deficiency
　　　d. Pellagra
　　　e. Malabsorption, Whipple's disease
　　3. Melanosis secondary to metastatic melanoma
　　4. Autoimmune
　　　a. Biliary cirrhosis
　　　b. Scleroderma
　　　c. POEMS syndrome
　　　d. Eosinophilia-myalgia syndrome[d]
　　5. Drugs and metals

[a] Also lentigines.
[b] Polyostotic fibrous dysplasia.
[c] See also "Papulonodular Skin Lesions."
[d] Late 1980s.

perpigmentation, primarily in flexural areas. In the majority of patients, acanthosis nigricans is associated with obesity and insulin resistance, but it may be a reflection of an endocrinopathy such as acromegaly, Cushing's syndrome, the Stein-Leventhal syndrome, or insulin-resistant diabetes mellitus (type A, type B, and lipoatrophic forms).

A proliferation of melanocytes results in the following pigmented lesions: *lentigo, melanocytic nevus,* and *melanoma* (Chap. 73). In an adult, the majority of lentigines are related to sun exposure, which explains their distribution. However, in the Peutz-Jeghers and LEOPARD [*l*entigines; *E*CG abnormalities, primarily conduction defects; *o*cular hypertelorism; *p*ulmonary stenosis and subaortic valvular stenosis; *a*bnormal genitalia (cryptorchidism, hypospadias); *r*etardation of growth; and *d*eafness (sensorineural)] syndromes, lentigines do serve as a clue to systemic disease. In *LEOPARD syndrome,* hundreds of lentigines develop during childhood and are scattered over the entire surface of the body. The lentigines in patients with *Peutz-Jeghers syndrome* are located primarily around the nose and mouth, on the hands

and feet, and within the oral cavity. While the pigmented macules on the face may fade with age, the oral lesions persist. However, similar intraoral lesions are also seen in Addison's disease and as a normal finding in darkly pigmented individuals. Patients with this autosomal dominant syndrome (due to mutations in a novel serine threonine kinase gene) have multiple benign polyps of the gastrointestinal tract, testicular tumors, and an increased risk of developing gastrointestinal (primarily colon), breast, and gynecologic cancers.

Lentigines are also seen in association with cardiac myxomas and have been described in two syndromes whose findings overlap: *LAMB* (*l*entigines, *a*trial myxomas, *m*ucocutaneous myxomas, and *b*lue nevi) *syndrome* and *NAME* [*n*evi, *a*trial myxoma, *m*yxoid neurofibroma, and *e*phelides (freckles)] *syndrome*. These patients can also have evidence of endocrine overactivity in the form of Cushing's syndrome, acromegaly, or sexual precocity (Carney complex).

The third type of localized hyperpigmentation is due to a local increase in pigment production, and it includes *ephelides* and café au lait macules (CALM). The latter are most commonly associated with two disorders—neurofibromatosis (NF) and McCune-Albright syndrome. *CALM* are flat, uniformly light brown in color, and can vary in size from 0.5 to 12 cm. Approximately 80% of adult patients with *type I NF* will have six or more CALM measuring ≥1.5 cm in diameter. Additional findings are discussed in the section on neurofibromas (see "Papulonodular Skin Lesions," below). In comparison with NF, the CALM in patients with *McCune-Albright syndrome* [polyostotic fibrous dysplasia with precocious puberty in females due to mosaicism for an activating mutation in a G protein ($G_s\alpha$) gene] are usually larger, more irregular in outline, and tend to respect the midline. CALM have also been associated with pulmonary stenosis (Watson syndrome), tuberous sclerosis, the LEOPARD syndrome, and multiple endocrine neoplasia (MEN), but a few such lesions can be found in normal individuals.

In incontinentia pigmenti, dyskeratosis congenita, and bleomycin pigmentation, the areas of localized hyperpigmentation form a pattern—swirled in the first, reticulated in the second, and flagellate in the third. In *dyskeratosis congenita*, atrophic reticulated hyperpigmentation is seen on the neck, thighs, and trunk and is accompanied by nail dystrophy, pancytopenia, and leukoplakia of the oral and anal mucosa. The latter often develops into squamous cell carcinoma. In addition to the flagellate pigmentation (linear streaks) on the trunk, patients receiving bleomycin often have hyperpigmentation on the elbows, knees, and small joints of the hand.

Localized hyperpigmentation is seen as a side effect of several other *systemic medications,* including those that produce fixed drug reactions [phenolphthalein, nonsteroidal anti-inflammatory drugs (NSAIDs), sulfonamides, and barbiturates] and those that can complex with melanin (antimalarials). Fixed drug eruptions recur in the same location as circular areas of erythema that can become bullous and then resolve as brown macules. The eruption usually appears within hours of administration of the offending agent, and common locations include the genitalia, extremities, and perioral region. Chloroquine and hydroxychloroquine produce gray-brown to blue-black discoloration of the shins, hard palate, and face, while blue macules can be seen on the lower extremities and in sites of inflammation with prolonged minocycline administration. Estrogen in oral contraceptives can induce melasma—symmetric brown patches on the face, especially the cheeks, upper lip, and forehead. Similar changes are seen in pregnancy, in patients receiving phenytoin, and in the adult form of Gaucher's disease. In the latter group there is also hyperpigmentation of the distal lower extremities.

In the diffuse forms of hyperpigmentation, the darkening of the skin may be of equal intensity over the entire body or may be accentuated in sun-exposed areas. The causes of diffuse hyperpigmentation can be divided into four groups—endocrine, metabolic, autoimmune, and drugs. The endocrinopathies that frequently have associated hyperpigmentation include *Addison's disease, Nelson syndrome,* and *ectopic ACTH syndrome.* In these diseases, the increased pigmentation is diffuse but is accentuated in the palmar creases, sites of friction, scars, and the oral mucosa. An overproduction of the pituitary hormones α-MSH (melanocyte-stimulating hormone) and ACTH can lead to an increase in melanocyte activity. These peptides are products of the proopiomelanocortin gene and exhibit homology; e.g., α-MSH and ACTH share 13 amino acids. A minority of the patients with Cushing's disease or hyperthyroidism have generalized hyperpigmentation.

The metabolic causes of hyperpigmentation include *porphyria cutanea tarda* (PCT), *hemochromatosis, vitamin B₁₂ deficiency, folic acid deficiency, pellagra, malabsorption,* and *Whipple's disease*. In patients with PCT (see "Vesicles/Bullae," below), the skin darkening is seen in sun-exposed areas and is a reflection of the photoreactive properties of porphyrins. The increased level of iron in the skin of patients with hemochromatosis stimulates melanin pigment production and leads to the classic bronze color. Patients with pellagra have a brown discoloration of the skin, especially in sun-exposed areas, as a result of nicotinic acid (niacin) deficiency. In the areas of increased pigmentation, there is a thin varnish-like scale. These changes are also seen in patients who are vitamin B₆ deficient, have functioning carcinoid tumors (increased consumption of niacin), or take isoniazid. Approximately 50% of the patients with Whipple's disease have an associated generalized hyperpigmentation in association with diarrhea, weight loss, arthritis, and lymphadenopathy. A diffuse slate-blue color is seen in patients with melanosis secondary to metastatic melanoma. Although there is a debate as to whether the color is due to single-cell metastases in the dermis or to a widespread deposition of melanin resulting from the high concentration of circulating melanin precursors, there is more evidence to support the latter.

Of the autoimmune diseases associated with diffuse hyperpigmentation, *biliary cirrhosis* and *scleroderma* are the most common, and occasionally both disorders are seen in the same patient. The skin is dark brown in color, especially in sun-exposed areas. In biliary cirrhosis the hyperpigmentation is accompanied by pruritus, jaundice, and xanthomas, whereas in scleroderma it is accompanied by sclerosis of the extremities, face, and, less commonly, the trunk. Additional clues to the diagnosis of scleroderma are telangiectasias, calcinosis cutis, Raynaud's phenomenon, and distal ulcerations (see "Telangiectasias," above). The differential diagnosis of cutaneous sclerosis with hyperpigmentation includes the POEMS [polyneuropathy; organomegaly (liver, spleen, lymph nodes); endocrinopathies (impotence, gynecomastia); M-protein; and skin changes] syndrome. The skin changes include hyperpigmentation, skin thickening, hypertrichosis, and angiomas.

Diffuse hyperpigmentation that is due to drugs or metals can result from one of several mechanisms—induction of melanin pigment formation, complexing of the drug or its metabolites to melanin, and deposits of the drug in the dermis. Busulfan; cyclophosphamide; long-term, high-dose ACTH; and inorganic arsenic induce pigment production. Complexes containing melanin or hemosiderin plus the drug or its metabolites are seen in patients receiving chlorpromazine and minocycline. The sun-exposed skin as well as the conjunctivae of patients on long-term, high-dose chlorpromazine can become blue-gray in color. Patients taking minocycline may develop a diffuse blue-gray, muddy appearance in sun-exposed areas in addition to pigmentation of the mucous membranes, teeth, nails, bones, and thyroid. Administration of amiodarone can result in both a phototoxic eruption (exaggerated sunburn) and/or a brown or blue-gray discoloration of sun-exposed skin. Biopsy specimens of the latter show yellow-brown granules in dermal macrophages, which represent intralysosomal accumulations of lipids, amiodarone, and its metabolites. Actual deposits of a particular drug or metal in the skin are seen with silver (argyria), where the skin appears blue-gray in color; gold (chrysiasis), where the skin has a brown to blue-gray color; and clofazimine, where the skin appears reddish brown. The associated hyperpigmentation is accentuated in sun-exposed areas, and discoloration of the eye is seen with gold (sclerae) and clofazimine (conjunctivae).

VESICLES/BULLAE (Table 48-12) Depending on their size, cutaneous blisters are referred to as *vesicles* (<0.5 cm) or *bullae* (>0.5 cm). The

TABLE 48-12 *Causes of Vesicles/Bullae*

I. Primary cutaneous diseases	II. Systemic diseases
A. Primary blistering diseases (autoimmune)	A. Autoimmune
1. Pemphigus[a]	1. Paraneoplastic pemphigus[a]
2. Bullous pemphigoid[b]	B. Infections
3. Gestational pemphigoid[b]	1. Cutaneous emboli[b]
4. Cicatricial pemphigoid[b]	C. Metabolic
5. Dermatitis herpetiformis[b,c]	1. Diabetic bullae[a,b]
6. Linear IgA disease[b]	2. Porphyria cutanea tarda[b]
7. Epidermolysis bullosa acquisita[b,d]	3. Porphyria variegata[b]
B. Secondary blistering diseases	4. Pseudoporphyria[b]
1. Contact dermatitis[a]	5. Bullous dermatosis of hemodialysis[b]
2. Erythema multiforme[a,b]	D. Ischemia
3. Toxic epidermal necrolysis[b]	1. Coma bullae
C. Infections	
1. Varicella/zoster virus[a,e]	
2. Herpes simplex virus[a,e]	
3. Enteroviruses, e.g., hand-foot-and-mouth disease	
4. Staphylococcal scalded-skin syndrome[a,f]	
5. Bullous impetigo[a]	

[a] Intraepidermal.
[b] Subepidermal.
[c] Associated with gluten enteropathy.
[d] Associated with inflammatory bowel disease.
[e] Also systemic.
[f] In adults, associated with renal failure and immunocompromised state.

primary blistering disorders include *pemphigus vulgaris, pemphigus foliaceus, pemphigus erythematosus, paraneoplastic pemphigus, bullous pemphigoid, gestational pemphigoid, cicatricial pemphigoid, epidermolysis bullosa acquisita, linear IgA disease,* and *dermatitis herpetiformis* (Chap. 49).

Vesicles and bullae are also seen in *contact dermatitis*, both allergic and irritant forms (Chap. 47). When there is a linear arrangement of vesicular lesions, an exogenous cause should be suspected. Bullous disease secondary to the ingestion of drugs can take one of several forms, including phototoxic eruptions, isolated bullae, toxic epidermal necrolysis (TEN), and erythema multiforme major (Chap. 50). Clinically, phototoxic eruptions resemble an exaggerated sunburn with diffuse erythema and bullae in sun-exposed areas. The most commonly associated drugs are thiazides, doxycycline, sulfonamides, NSAIDs, and psoralens. The development of a phototoxic eruption is dependent on the doses of both the drug and ultraviolet (UV)-A irradiation.

Toxic epidermal necrolysis is characterized by bullae that arise on widespread areas of erythema and then slough. This results in large areas of denuded skin. The associated morbidity, such as sepsis, and mortality are relatively high and are a function of the extent of epidermal necrosis. In addition, these patients may also have involvement of the mucous membranes and intestinal tract. Drugs are the primary cause of TEN, and the most common offenders are phenytoin, barbiturates, sulfonamides, penicillins, and NSAIDs. Severe acute graft-versus-host disease (grade 4) can also resemble TEN.

In *erythema multiforme* (EM), the primary lesions are pink-red macules and edematous papules, the centers of which may become vesicular. The clue to the diagnosis of EM, as opposed to a drug-induced morbilliform exanthem, is the development of a "dusky" violet color or petechiae in the center of the lesions. Target or iris lesions are also characteristic of EM and arise as a result of active centers and borders in combination with centrifugal spread. However, iris lesions need not be present to make the diagnosis of EM.

EM has been subdivided into two major groups: (1) herpes simplex virus (HSV)-associated and (2) EM major due to drugs or *Mycoplasma pneumoniae*. Involvement of the mucous membranes (oral, nasal, ocular, and genital) is seen more commonly in the latter form. Hemorrhagic crusts of the lips are characteristic of EM major as well as herpes simplex, pemphigus vulgaris, and paraneoplastic pemphigus. Fever, malaise, myalgias, sore throat, and cough may precede or accompany the eruption. The lesions of EM usually resolve over 3 to 6 weeks but may be recurrent, especially when due to HSV.

Induction of EM major is most often due to drugs, especially sulfonamides, phenytoin, barbiturates, penicillins, and carbamazepine. In addition to HSV (in which lesions appear 7 to 12 days after the viral eruption), EM can also follow vaccinations, radiation therapy, and exposure to environmental toxins.

In addition to primary blistering disorders and hypersensitivity reactions, bacterial and viral infections can lead to vesicles and bullae. The most common infectious agents are herpes simplex (Chap. 163), herpes varicella-zoster (Chap. 164), and staphylococci (Chap. 120).

Staphylococcal scalded-skin syndrome (SSSS) and *bullous impetigo* are two blistering disorders associated with staphylococcal (phage group II) infection. In SSSS, the initial findings are redness and tenderness of the central face, neck, trunk, and intertriginous zones. This is followed by short-lived flaccid bullae and a slough or exfoliation of the superficial epidermis. Crusted areas then develop, characteristically around the mouth. SSSS is distinguished from TEN by the following features: younger age group, more superficial site of blister formation, no oral lesions, shorter course, less morbidity and mortality, and an association with staphylococcal exfoliative toxin ("exfoliatin"), not drugs. A rapid diagnosis of SSSS versus TEN can be made by a frozen section of the blister roof or exfoliative cytology of the blister contents. In SSSS the site of staphylococcal infection is usually extracutaneous (conjunctivitis, rhinorrhea, otitis media, pharyngitis, tonsillitis), and the cutaneous lesions are sterile, whereas in bullous impetigo the skin lesions are the site of infection. Impetigo is more localized than SSSS and usually presents with honey-colored crusts. Occasionally, superficial purulent blisters also form. *Cutaneous emboli* from gram-negative infections may present as isolated bullae, but the base of the lesion is purpuric or necrotic, and it may develop into an ulcer (see "Purpura," below).

Several metabolic disorders are associated with blister formation, including diabetes mellitus, renal failure, and porphyria. Local hypoxia secondary to decreased cutaneous blood flow can also produce blisters, which explains the presence of bullae over pressure points in comatose patients (coma bullae). In *diabetes mellitus*, tense bullae with clear viscous fluid arise on normal skin. The lesions can be as large as 6 cm in diameter and are located on the distal extremities. There are several types of porphyria, but the most common form with cutaneous findings is *PCT*. In sun-exposed areas (primarily the face and hands), the skin is very fragile, and trauma leads to erosions and tense vesicles. These lesions then heal with scarring and formation of milia; the latter are firm, 1- to 2-mm white or yellow papules that represent epidermoid inclusion cysts. Associated findings can include hypertrichosis of the lateral malar region (men) or face (women) and, in sun-exposed areas, hyperpigmentation and firm sclerotic plaques. An elevated level of urinary uroporphyrins confirms the diagnosis and is due to a decrease in uroporphyrinogen decarboxylase activity. Precipitating agents include alcohol, iron, chlorinated hydrocarbons, hepatitis C infection, and hepatomas.

The differential diagnosis of PCT includes (1) *porphyria variegata*—the skin signs of PCT plus the systemic findings of acute intermittent porphyria; it has a diagnostic plasma porphyrin fluorescence emission at 626 nm; (2) *drug-induced bullous photosensitivity* (pseudoporphyria)—the clinical and histologic findings are similar to PCT, but porphyrins are normal; etiologic agents include naproxen, furosemide, tetracycline, and nalidixic acid; (3) *bullous dermatosis of hemodialysis*—the same appearance as PCT, but porphyrins are usually normal or occasionally borderline elevated; patients have chronic renal failure and are on hemodialysis; (4) PCT associated with hepatomas,

hepatic carcinomas, and hemodialysis; and (5) *epidermolysis bullosa acquisita* (Chap. 49).

EXANTHEMS (Table 48-13) Exanthems are characterized by an acute generalized eruption. The two most common presentations are erythematous macules and papules (morbilliform) and confluent blanching erythema (scarlatiniform). *Morbilliform* eruptions are usually due to either drugs or viral infections. For example, up to 5% of the patients receiving penicillins, sulfonamides, phenytoin, or gold will develop a maculopapular eruption. Accompanying signs may include pruritus, fever, eosinophilia, and transient lymphadenopathy. Similar maculopapular eruptions are seen in the classic childhood viral exanthems, including (1) *rubeola* (measles)—a prodrome of coryza, cough, and conjunctivitis followed by Koplik's spots on the buccal mucosa; the eruption begins behind the ears, at the hairline, and on the forehead and then spreads down the body, often becoming confluent; (2) *rubella*—it begins on the forehead and face and then spreads down the body; it resolves in the same order and is associated with retroauricular and suboccipital lymphadenopathy; and (3) *erythema infectiosum* (fifth disease)—erythema of the cheeks is followed by a reticulated pattern on extremities; it is secondary to a parvovirus B19 infection, and an associated arthritis is seen in adults.

Both measles and rubella are seen in unvaccinated young adults, and an atypical form of measles is seen in adults immunized with either killed measles vaccine or killed vaccine followed in time by live vaccine. In contrast to classic measles, the eruption of atypical measles begins on the palms, soles, wrists, and knuckles, and the lesions may become purpuric. The patient with atypical measles can have pulmonary involvement and be quite ill. Rubelliform and roseoliform eruptions are also associated with *Epstein-Barr virus* (5 to 15% of patients), *echovirus*, *coxsackievirus*, and *adenovirus* infections. Detection of specific IgM antibodies or fourfold elevations in IgG antibodies allows the proper diagnosis. Occasionally, a maculopapular drug eruption is a reflection of an underlying viral infection. For example, about 95% of the patients with infectious mononucleosis who are given ampicillin will develop a rash.

Of note, early in the course of infections with *Rickettsia* and meningococcus, prior to the development of purpura, the lesions may be erythematous macules and papules. This is also the case in chickenpox prior to the development of vesicles. Maculopapular eruptions are associated with early *HIV infection*, early secondary *syphilis*, *typhoid fever*, and *acute graft-versus-host disease*. In the last, lesions frequently begin on the palms and soles; the macular rose spots of typhoid fever involve primarily the anterior trunk.

The prototypic *scarlatiniform* eruption is seen in *scarlet fever* and is due to an erythrotoxin produced by group A β-hemolytic streptococcal infections, most commonly pharyngitis. This eruption is characterized by diffuse erythema, which begins on the neck and upper trunk, and red follicular puncta. Additional findings include a white

TABLE 48-13 *Causes of Exanthems*

I. Morbilliform
  A. Drugs
  B. Viral
    1. Rubeola (measles)
    2. Rubella
    3. Erythema infectiosum
    4. Epstein-Barr virus, echovirus, coxsackievirus, and adenovirus
    5. Early HIV (plus mucosal ulcerations)
  C. Bacterial
    1. Typhoid fever
    2. Early secondary syphilis
    3. Early *Rickettsia*
    4. Early meningococcemia
  D. Acute graft-versus-host disease
  E. Kawasaki's disease
II. Scarlatiniform
  A. Scarlet fever
  B. Toxic shock syndrome
  C. Kawasaki's disease

strawberry tongue (white coating with red papillae) followed by a red strawberry tongue (red tongue with red papillae); petechiae of the palate; a facial flush with circumoral pallor; linear petechiae in the antecubital fossae; and desquamation of the involved skin, palms, and soles 5 to 20 days after onset of the eruption. A similar desquamation of the palms and soles is seen in toxic shock syndrome (TSS), Kawasaki's disease, and after severe febrile illnesses. Certain strains of staphylococci also produce an erythrotoxin that leads to the same clinical findings as in streptococcal scarlet fever, except that the antistreptolysin O titers are not elevated.

In *toxic shock syndrome*, staphylococcal (phage group I) infections produce an exotoxin (TSST-1) that causes the fever and rash, as well as enterotoxins. Initially, the majority of cases were reported in menstruating women who were using tampons. However, other sites of infection, including wounds and vaginitis, can lead to TSS. The diagnosis of TSS is based on clinical criteria (Chap. 120), and three of these involve mucocutaneous sites (diffuse erythema of the skin, desquamation of the palms and soles 1 to 2 weeks after onset of illness, and involvement of the mucous membranes). The latter is characterized as hyperemia of the vagina, oropharynx, or conjunctivae. Similar systemic findings have been described in *streptococcal toxic shock–like syndrome* (Chap. 121), and although an exanthem is seen less often than in TSS due to a staphylococcal infection, the underlying infection is often in the soft tissue.

The cutaneous eruption in *Kawasaki's disease* (mucocutaneous lymph node syndrome) (Chap. 121) is polymorphous, but the two most common forms are morbilliform and scarlatiniform. Additional mucocutaneous findings include bilateral conjunctival injection; erythema and edema of the hands and feet followed by desquamation; and diffuse erythema of the oropharynx, red strawberry tongue, and erosions with crusting on the lips. This clinical picture can resemble TSS and scarlet fever, but clues to the diagnosis of Kawasaki's disease are cervical lymphadenopathy, lip erosions, and thrombocytosis. The most serious associated systemic finding in this disease is coronary aneurysm secondary to arteritis. Aneurysms may lead to sudden death, primarily within the first 30 days of the illness. Scarlatiniform eruptions are also seen in the early phase of SSSS (see "Vesicles/Bullae," above) and as reactions to drugs.

URICARIA (Table 48-14)   *Urticaria* (hives) are transient lesions that are composed of a central wheal surrounded by an erythematous halo. Individual lesions are round, oval, or figurate and are often pruritic. Acute and chronic urticaria have a wide variety of allergic etiologies and reflect edema in the dermis. Urticarial lesions can also be seen in patients with mastocytosis (urticaria pigmentosa), hyperthyroidism, and juvenile rheumatoid arthritis (JRA). In JRA, the lesions coincide with the fever spike, are transient, and are due to dermal infiltrates of neutrophils.

The common *physical urticarias* include dermographism, solar urticaria, cold urticaria, and cholinergic urticaria. Patients with *dermographism* exhibit linear wheals following minor pressure or scratching of the skin. It is a common disorder, affecting ~5% of the population.

TABLE 48-14   Causes of Urticaria

I. Primary cutaneous disorders
   A. Acute and chronic urticaria[a]
   B. Physical urticaria
      1. Dermatographism
      2. Solar urticaria[b]
      3. Cold urticaria[b]
      4. Cholinergic urticaria[b]
   C. Angioedema (hereditary and acquired)[b]
II. Systemic diseases
   A. Urticarial vasculitis
   B. Hepatitis B or C infection
   C. Serum sickness
   D. Angioedema (hereditary and acquired)

[a] A small minority develop anaphylaxis.
[b] Also systemic.

Solar urticaria characteristically occurs within minutes of sun exposure and is a skin sign of one systemic disease—erythropoietic protoporphyria. In addition to the urticaria, these patients have subtle pitted scarring of the nose and hands. *Cold urticaria* is precipitated by exposure to the cold, and therefore exposed areas are usually affected. In some cases, the disease is associated with abnormal circulating proteins—more commonly cryoglobulins and less commonly cryofibrinogens and cold agglutinins. Additional systemic symptoms include wheezing and syncope, thus explaining the need for these patients to avoid swimming in cold water. *Cholinergic urticaria* is precipitated by heat, exercise, or emotion and are characterized by small wheals with relatively large flares. They are occasionally associated with wheezing.

Whereas urticaria are the result of dermal edema, subcutaneous edema leads to the clinical picture of *angioedema*. Sites of involvement include the eyelids, lips, tongue, larynx, and gastrointestinal tract as well as the subcutaneous tissue. Angioedema occurs alone or in combination with urticaria, including urticarial vasculitis and the physical urticarias. Both acquired and hereditary (autosomal dominant) forms of angioedema occur (Chap. 298), and in the latter, urticaria is rarely, if ever, seen.

Urticarial vasculitis is an immune complex disease that may be confused with simple urticaria. In contrast to simple urticaria, individual lesions tend to last longer than 24 h and usually develop central petechiae that can be observed even after the urticarial phase has resolved. The patient may also complain of burning rather than pruritus. On biopsy, there is a leukocytoclastic vasculitis of the small blood vessels. Although many cases of urticarial vasculitis are idiopathic in origin, it can be a reflection of an underlying systemic illness such as lupus erythematosus, Sjögren's syndrome, or hereditary complement deficiency. There is a spectrum of urticarial vasculitis that ranges from purely cutaneous to multisystem involvement. The most common systemic signs and symptoms are arthralgias and/or arthritis, nephritis, and crampy abdominal pain, with asthma and chronic obstructive lung disease seen less often. Hypocomplementemia occurs in one- to two-thirds of patients, even in the idiopathic cases. Urticarial vasculitis can also be seen in patients with *hepatitis B* and *hepatitis C* infections, *serum sickness*, and *serum sickness–like illnesses*.

PAPULONODULAR SKIN LESIONS (Table 48-15)   In the *papulonodular diseases*, the lesions are elevated above the surface of the skin and may coalesce to form plaques. The location, consistency, and color of the lesions are the keys to their diagnosis; this section is organized on the basis of color.

White Lesions   In *calcinosis cutis* there are firm white to white-yellow papules with an irregular surface. When the contents are expressed, a chalky white material is seen. *Dystrophic calcification* is seen at sites of previous inflammation or damage to the skin. It develops in acne scars as well as on the distal extremities of patients with scleroderma and in the subcutaneous tissue and intermuscular fascial planes in DM. The latter is more extensive and is more commonly seen in children. An elevated calcium phosphate product, most commonly due to secondary hyperparathyroidism in the setting of renal failure, can lead to nodules of *metastatic calcinosis cutis*, which tend to be subcutaneous and periarticular. These patients can also develop calcification of muscular arteries and subsequent ischemic necrosis (calciphylaxis).

Skin-Colored Lesions   There are several types of skin-colored lesions, including epidermoid inclusion cysts, lipomas, rheumatoid nodules, neurofibromas, angiofibromas, neuromas, and adnexal tumors such as tricholemmomas. Both *epidermoid inclusion cysts* and *lipomas* are very common mobile subcutaneous nodules—the former are rubbery and compressible and drain cheeselike material (sebum and keratin) if incised. Lipomas are firm and somewhat lobulated on palpation. When extensive facial epidermoid inclusion cysts develop in childhood or there is a family history of such lesions, the patient should be examined for other signs of Gardner syndrome, including osteomas and desmoid

TABLE 48-15 Papulonodular Skin Lesions According to Color Groups

I. White
  A. Calcinosis cutis
II. Skin-colored
  A. Rheumatoid nodules
  B. Neurofibromas (von Recklinghausen's disease)
  C. Angiofibromas (tuberous sclerosis, MEN syndrome, type 1)
  D. Neuromas (MEN syndrome, type 2b)
  E. Adnexal tumors
    1. Basal cell carcinomas (nevoid basal cell carcinoma syndrome)
    2. Tricholemmomas (Cowden's disease)
  F. Osteomas (Gardner syndrome)
  G. Primary cutaneous disorders
    1. Epidermal inclusion cysts
    2. Lipomas
III. Pink/translucent[a]
  A. Amyloidosis
  B. Papular mucinosis
IV. Yellow
  A. Xanthomas
  B. Tophi
  C. Necrobiosis lipoidica
  D. Pseudoxanthoma elasticum
  E. Sebaceous adenomas (Torre syndrome)
V. Red[a]
  A. Papules
    1. Angiokeratomas (Fabry's disease)
    2. Bacillary angiomatosis (primarily in AIDS)
  B. Papules/plaques
    1. Cutaneous lupus
    2. Lymphoma cutis
    3. Leukemia cutis

  C. Nodules
    1. Panniculitis
    2. Cutaneous polyarteritis nodosa
    3. Systemic vasculitis
  D. Primary cutaneous disorders
    1. Arthropod bites
    2. Cherry hemangiomas
    3. Infections, e.g., erysipelas, sporotrichosis
    4. Polymorphous light eruption
    5. Lymphocytoma cutis (pseudolymphoma)
VI. Red-brown[a]
  A. Sarcoidosis
  B. Sweet's syndrome
  C. Urticaria pigmentosa
  D. Erythema elevatum diutinum (chronic leukocytoclastic vasculitis)
  E. Lupus vulgaris
VII. Blue[a]
  A. Venous malformations (blue rubber bleb syndrome)
  B. Primary cutaneous disorders
    1. Venous lake
    2. Blue nevus
VIII. Violaceous
  A. Lupus pernio (sarcoidosis)
  B. Lymphoma cutis
  C. Cutaneous lupus
IX. Purple
  A. Kaposi's sarcoma
  B. Angiosarcoma
  C. Palpable purpura
X. Brown-black[b]
XI. Any color
  A. Metastases

[a] May have darker hue in more darkly pigmented individuals.
[b] See also "Hyperpigmentation."
Note: MEN, multiple endocrine neoplasia.

tumors. *Rheumatoid nodules* are firm, 0.5- to 4-cm nodules that tend to localize around pressure points, especially the elbows. They are seen in approximately 20% of patients with rheumatoid arthritis and 6% of patients with Still's disease. Biopsies of the nodules show palisading granulomas. Similar lesions that are smaller and shorter-lived are seen in rheumatic fever.

Neurofibromas (benign Schwann cell tumors) are soft papules or nodules that exhibit the "button-hole" sign, that is, they invaginate into the skin with pressure in a manner similar to a hernia. Single lesions are seen in normal individuals, but multiple neurofibromas, usually in combination with six or more CALM measuring >1.5 cm (see "Hyperpigmentation," above), axillary freckling, and multiple Lisch nodules, are seen in von Recklinghausen's disease (NF type I; Chap. 359). In some patients the neurofibromas are localized and unilateral due to somatic mosaicism.

Angiofibromas are firm, pink to skin-colored papules that measure from 3 mm to several centimeters in diameter. When they are located on the central cheeks (adenoma sebaceum), the patient has tuberous sclerosis or MEN syndrome, type 1. The former is an autosomal disorder due to mutations in two different genes, and the associated findings are discussed in the section on ash leaf spots as well as in Chap. 359.

Neuromas (benign proliferations of nerve fibers) are also firm, skin-colored papules. They are more commonly found at sites of amputation and as rudimentary supernumerary digits. However, when there are multiple neuromas on the eyelids, lips, distal tongue, and/or oral mucosa, the patient should be investigated for other signs of the MEN syndrome, type 2b. Associated findings include marfanoid habitus, protuberant lips, intestinal ganglioneuromas, and medullary thyroid carcinoma (>75% of patients; Chap. 330).

Adnexal tumors are derived from pluripotential cells of the epidermis that can differentiate toward hair, sebaceous, apocrine, or eccrine glands or remain undifferentiated. *Basal cell carcinomas* (BCCs) are examples of adnexal tumors that have little or no evidence of differentiation. Clinically, they are translucent papules with rolled borders, telangiectasias, and central erosion. BCCs commonly arise in sun-damaged skin of the head and neck. When a patient has multiple BCCs, especially prior to age 30, the possibility of the nevoid basal cell carcinoma syndrome should be raised. It is inherited as an autosomal dominant trait and is associated with jaw cysts, palmar and plantar pits, frontal bossing, medulloblastomas, and calcification of the falx cerebri and diaphragma sellae. *Tricholemmomas* are also skin-colored adnexal tumors but differentiate toward hair follicles and can have a wartlike appearance. The presence of multiple tricholemmomas on the face and cobblestoning of the oral mucosa points to the diagnosis of Cowden's disease (multiple hamartoma syndrome) due to mutations in the *PTEN* gene. Internal organ involvement (in decreasing order of frequency) includes fibrocystic disease and carcinoma of the breast, adenomas and carcinomas of the thyroid, and gastrointestinal polyposis. Keratoses of the palms, soles, and dorsa of the hands are also seen.

Pink Lesions The cutaneous lesions associated with primary systemic *amyloidosis* are pink in color and translucent. Common locations are the face, especially the periorbital and perioral regions, and flexural areas. On biopsy, homogeneous deposits of amyloid are seen in the dermis and in the walls of blood vessels; the latter lead to an increase in vessel wall fragility. As a result, petechiae and purpura develop in clinically normal skin as well as in lesional skin following minor trauma, hence the term *pinch purpura*. Amyloid deposits are also seen in the striated muscle of the tongue and result in macroglossia.

Even though specific mucocutaneous lesions are rarely seen in secondary amyloidosis and are present in only about 30% of the patients with primary amyloidosis, a rapid diagnosis of systemic amyloidosis can be made by an examination of abdominal subcutaneous fat. By special staining, deposits are seen around blood vessels or individual fat cells in 40 to 50% of patients. There are also three forms of amyloidosis that are limited to the skin and that should not be construed as cutaneous lesions of systemic amyloidosis. They are macular amyloidosis (upper back), lichenoid amyloidosis (usually lower extremities), and nodular amyloidosis. In macular and lichenoid amyloidosis, the deposits are composed of altered epidermal keratin. Recently, macular and lichenoid amyloidosis have been associated with MEN syndrome, type 2a.

Patients with *multicentric reticulohistiocytosis* also have pink-colored papules and nodules on the face and mucous membranes as well as on the extensor surface of the hands and forearms. They have a polyarthritis that can mimic rheumatoid arthritis clinically. On histologic examination, the papules have characteristic giant cells that are not seen in biopsies of rheumatoid nodules. Pink to skin-colored papules that are firm, 2 to 5 mm in diameter, and often in a linear arrangement are seen in patients with *papular mucinosis*. This disease is also referred to as *lichen myxedematosus* or *scleromyxedema*. The latter name comes from the brawny induration of the face and extremities that may accompany the papular eruption. Biopsy specimens of the papules show localized mucin deposition, and serum protein electrophoresis demonstrates a monoclonal spike of IgG, usually with a λ light chain.

Yellow Lesions Several systemic disorders are characterized by yellow-colored cutaneous papules or plaques—hyperlipidemia (xanthomas), gout (tophi), diabetes (necrobiosis lipoidica), pseudoxanthoma elasticum, and Torre syndrome (sebaceous tumors). Eruptive xanthomas are the most common form of *xanthomas*, and are associated with hypertriglyceridemia (types I, III, IV, and V). Crops of yellow papules with erythematous halos occur primarily on the extensor surfaces of the extremities and the buttocks, and they spontaneously involute with a fall in serum triglycerides. Increased β-lipoproteins (primarily types II and III) result in one or more of the following types of xanthoma: xanthelasma, tendon xanthomas, and plane xanthomas. Xanthelasma are found on the eyelids, whereas tendon xanthomas are frequently associated with the Achilles and extensor finger tendons; plane xanthomas are flat and favor the palmar creases, face, upper trunk, and scars. Tuberous xanthomas are frequently associated with hypertriglyceridemia, but they are also seen in patients with hypercholesterolemia (type II) and are found most frequently over the large joints or hand. Biopsy specimens of xanthomas show collections of lipid-containing macrophages (foam cells).

Patients with several disorders, including biliary cirrhosis, can have a secondary form of hyperlipidemia with associated tuberous and planar xanthomas. However, patients with myeloma have *normolipemic flat xanthomas*. This latter form of xanthoma may be ≥12 cm in diameter and is most frequently seen on the upper trunk or side of the neck. It is important to note that the most common setting for eruptive xanthomas is uncontrolled diabetes mellitus. The least specific sign for hyperlipidemia is xanthelasma, because at least 50% of the patients with this finding have normal lipid profiles.

In *tophaceous gout* there are deposits of monosodium urate in the skin around the joints, particularly those of the hands and feet. Additional sites of *tophi* formation include the helix of the ear and the olecranon and prepatellar bursae. The lesions are firm, yellow in color, and occasionally discharge a chalky material. Their size varies from 1 mm to 7 cm, and the diagnosis can be established by polarization of the aspirated contents of a lesion. Lesions of *necrobiosis lipoidica* are found primarily on the shins (90%), and patients can have diabetes mellitus or develop it subsequently. Characteristic findings include a central yellow color, atrophy (transparency), telangiectasias, and an erythematous border. Ulcerations can also develop within the plaques. Biopsy specimens show necrobiosis of collagen, granulomatous inflammation, and obliterative endarteritis.

In *pseudoxanthoma elasticum* (PXE) there is an abnormal deposition of calcium on the elastic fibers of the skin, eye, and blood vessels. In the skin, the flexural areas such as the neck, axillae, antecubital fossae, and inguinal area are the primary sites of involvement. Yellow papules coalesce to form reticulated plaques that have an appearance similar to that of plucked chicken skin. In severely affected skin, hanging, redundant folds develop. Biopsy specimens of involved skin show swollen and irregularly clumped elastic fibers with deposits of calcium. In the eye, the calcium deposits in Bruch's membrane lead to angioid streaks and choroiditis; in the arteries of the heart, kidney, gastrointestinal tract, and extremities, the deposits lead to angina, hypertension, gastrointestinal bleeding, and claudication, respectively. Long-term administration of D-penicillamine can lead to PXE-like skin changes as well as elastic fiber alterations in internal organs.

Adnexal tumors that have differentiated toward sebaceous glands include sebaceous adenoma, sebaceous carcinoma, and sebaceous hyperplasia. Except for sebaceous hyperplasia, which is commonly seen on the face, these tumors are fairly rare. Patients with Torre syndrome have one or more *sebaceous adenoma(s)*, and they can also have sebaceous carcinomas and sebaceous hyperplasia as well as keratoacanthomas. The internal manifestations of Torre syndrome include *multiple* carcinomas of the gastrointestinal tract (primarily colon) as well as cancers of the larynx, genitourinary tract, and endometrium.

Red Lesions Cutaneous lesions that are red in color have a wide variety of etiologies; in an attempt to simplify their identification, they will be subdivided into papules, papules/plaques, and subcutaneous nodules. Common red papules include *arthropod bites* and *cherry hemangiomas*; the latter are small, bright-red, dome-shaped papules that represent benign proliferation of capillaries. In patients with AIDS, the development of multiple red hemangioma-like lesions points to bacillary angiomatosis, and biopsy specimens show clusters of bacilli that stain positive with the Warthin-Starry stain; the pathogens have been identified as *Bartonella henselae* and *B. quintana*. Disseminated visceral disease is seen primarily in immunocompromised hosts but can occur in immunocompetent individuals.

Multiple *angiokeratomas* are seen in Fabry's disease, an X-linked recessive lysosomal storage disease that is due to a deficiency of α-galactosidase A. The lesions are red to red-blue in color and can be quite small in size (1 to 3 mm), with the most common location being the lower trunk. Associated findings include chronic renal failure, peripheral neuropathy, and corneal opacities (cornea verticillata). Electron photomicrographs of angiokeratomas and clinically normal skin demonstrate lamellar lipid deposits in fibroblasts, pericytes, and endothelial cells that are diagnostic of this disease. Widespread acute eruptions of erythematous papules are discussed in the section on exanthems.

There are several infectious diseases that present as erythematous papules or nodules in a sporotrichoid pattern, that is, in a linear arrangement along the lymphatic channels. The two most common etiologies are *Sporothrix schenckii* (sporotrichosis) and *M. marinum* (atypical mycobacteria). The organisms are introduced as a result of trauma, and a primary inoculation site is often seen in addition to the lymphatic nodules. Additional causes include *Nocardia, Leishmania*, and other dimorphic fungi; culture of lesional tissue will aid in the diagnosis.

The diseases that are characterized by erythematous plaques with scale are reviewed in the papulosquamous section, and the various forms of dermatitis are discussed in the section on erythroderma. Additional disorders in the differential diagnosis of red papules/plaques include *erysipelas*, *polymorphous light eruption* (PMLE), *lymphocytoma cutis, cutaneous lupus, lymphoma cutis*, and *leukemia cutis*. The first three diseases represent primary cutaneous disorders. PMLE is characterized by erythematous papules and plaques in a primarily sun-exposed distribution—dorsum of the hand, extensor forearm, and face. Lesions follow exposure to UV-B and/or UV-A, and in northern latitudes PMLE is most severe in the late spring and early summer. A process referred to as "hardening" occurs with continued UV exposure, and the eruption fades, but in temperate climates it will recur in the spring. PMLE must be differentiated from cutaneous lupus, and this is accomplished by histologic examination and direct immunofluorescence of the lesions. Lymphocytoma cutis (pseudolymphoma) is a *benign* polyclonal proliferation of lymphocytes in the skin that presents as infiltrated pink-red to red-purple papules and plaques; it must be distinguished from lymphoma cutis.

Several types of red plaques are seen in patients with systemic *lupus*, including (1) erythematous urticarial plaques across the cheeks and nose in the classic butterfly rash; (2) erythematous discoid lesions with fine or "carpet-tack" scale, telangiectasias, central hypopigmentation, peripheral hyperpigmentation, follicular plugging, and atrophy located on the face, scalp, external ears, arms, and upper trunk; and (3) psoriasiform or annular lesions of subacute lupus with hypopigmented centers located on the face, extensor arms, and upper trunk. Additional cutaneous findings include (1) a violaceous flush on the face and V of the neck; (2) urticarial vasculitis (see "Urticaria," above); (3) lupus panniculitis (see below); (4) diffuse alopecia; (5) alopecia secondary to discoid lesions; (6) periungual telangiectasias and erythema; (7) EM-like lesions that may become bullous; and (8) distal ulcerations secondary to Raynaud's phenomenon, vasculitis, or livedoid vasculopathy. Patients with only discoid lesions usually have the form of lupus that is limited to the skin. However, 2 to 10% of these patients eventually develop systemic lupus. Direct immunofluorescence of involved skin shows deposits of IgG or IgM and C3 in a granular distribution along the dermal-epidermal junction.

In *lymphoma cutis* there is a proliferation of malignant lymphocytes or histiocytes in the skin, and the clinical appearance resembles that of lymphocytoma cutis—infiltrated pink-red to red-purple papules and plaques. Lymphoma cutis can occur anywhere on the surface of the skin, whereas the sites of predilection for lymphocytomas include the malar ridge, tip of the nose, and earlobes. Patients with non-Hodgkin's lymphomas have specific cutaneous lesions more often than those with Hodgkin's disease, and occasionally, the skin nodules precede the development of extracutaneous non-Hodgkin's lymphoma or represent the only site of involvement. Arcuate lesions are sometimes seen in lymphoma and lymphocytoma cutis as well as in CTCL. *Leukemia cutis* has the same appearance as lymphoma cutis, and specific lesions are seen more commonly in monocytic leukemias than in lymphocytic or granulocytic leukemias. Cutaneous chloromas (granulocytic sarcomas) may precede the appearance of circulating blasts in acute non lymphocytic leukemia and, as such, represent a form of aleukemic leukemia cutis.

Common causes of erythematous subcutaneous nodules include inflamed epidermoid inclusion cysts, acne cysts, and furuncles. *Panniculitis*, an inflammation of the fat, also presents as subcutaneous nodules and is frequently a sign of systemic disease. There are several forms of panniculitis, including erythema nodosum, erythema induratum/nodular vasculitis, lupus profundus, lipomembranous lipodermatosclerosis, α_1-antitrypsin deficiency, facticial, and fat necrosis secondary to pancreatic disease. Except for erythema nodosum, these lesions may break down and ulcerate or heal with a scar. The shin is the most common location for the nodules of erythema nodosum, whereas the calf is the most common location for lesions of erythema induratum. In erythema nodosum the nodules are initially red but then develop a blue color as they resolve. Patients with erythema nodosum but no underlying systemic illness can still have fever, malaise, leukocytosis, arthralgias, and/or arthritis. However, the possibility of an underlying illness should be excluded, and the most common associations are streptococcal infections, upper respiratory infections, sarcoidosis, and inflammatory bowel disease. The less common associations include tuberculosis, histoplasmosis, coccidioidomycosis, psittacosis, drugs (oral contraceptives, sulfonamides, aspartame, bromides, iodides), cat-scratch fever, and infections with *Yersinia, Salmonella*, and *Chlamydia*.

Erythema induratum and nodular vasculitis share a similar histology and were thought to represent the clinical spectrum of a single entity; subsequently they have been separated, with the latter idiopathic and the former associated with the presence of *M. tuberculosis* DNA by polymerase chain reaction (PCR) in 25 to 70% of patients. The lesions of lupus profundus are found primarily on the upper arms and buttocks (sites of abundant fat) and are seen in both the cutaneous and systemic forms of lupus. The overlying skin may be normal, erythematous, or have the changes of discoid lupus. The subcutaneous fat necrosis that is associated with pancreatic disease is presumably secondary to circulating lipases and is seen in patients with pancreatic carcinoma as well as in patients with acute and chronic pancreatitis. In this disorder there may be an associated arthritis, fever, and inflammation of visceral fat. Histologic examination of deep incisional biopsy specimens will aid in the diagnosis of the particular type of panniculitis.

Subcutaneous erythematous nodules are also seen in *cutaneous polyarteritis nodosa* (PAN) and as a manifestation of *systemic vasculitis*, e.g., systemic PAN, allergic granulomatosis, or Wegener's granulomatosis (Chap. 306). Cutaneous PAN presents with painful subcutaneous nodules and ulcers within a red-purple, netlike pattern of livedo reticularis. The latter is due to slowed blood flow through the superficial horizontal venous plexus. The majority of lesions are found on the lower extremity, and while arthralgias and myalgias may accompany cutaneous PAN, there is no evidence of systemic involvement. In both the cutaneous and systemic forms of vasculitis, skin biopsy specimens of the associated nodules will show the changes characteristic of a vasculitis; the size of the vessel involved will depend on the particular disease.

Red-Brown Lesions   The cutaneous lesions in *sarcoidosis* (Chap. 309) are classically red to red-brown in color, and with diascopy (pressure with a glass slide) a yellow-brown residual color is observed that is secondary to the granulomatous infiltrate. The waxy papules and plaques may be found anywhere on the skin, but the face is the most common location. Usually there are no surface changes, but occasionally the lesions will have scale. Biopsy specimens of the papules show "naked" granulomas in the dermis, i.e., granulomas surrounded by a minimal number of lymphocytes. Other cutaneous findings in sarcoidosis include annular lesions with an atrophic or scaly center, papules within scars, hypopigmented macules and papules, alopecia, acquired ichthyosis, erythema nodosum, and lupus pernio (see below).

The differential diagnosis of sarcoidosis includes foreign-body granulomas produced by chemicals such as beryllium and zirconium, late secondary syphilis, and *lupus vulgaris*. Lupus vulgaris is a form of cutaneous tuberculosis that is seen in previously infected and sensitized individuals. There is often underlying active tuberculosis elsewhere, usually in the lungs or lymph nodes. At least 90% of the lesions occur in the head and neck area and are red-brown plaques with a yellow-brown color on diascopy. Secondary scarring and squamous cell carcinomas can develop within the plaques. Cultures or PCR analysis of the lesions should be done because it is rare for the acid-fast stain to show bacilli within the dermal granulomas.

Sweet's syndrome is characterized by red to red-brown plaques and nodules that are frequently painful and occur primarily on the head, neck, and upper extremities. The patients also have fever, neutrophilia, and a dense dermal infiltrate of neutrophils in the lesions. In approximately 10% of the patients there is an associated malignancy, most commonly acute nonlymphocytic leukemia. Sweet's syndrome has also been reported with lymphoma, chronic leukemia, myeloma, myelodysplastic syndromes, and solid tumors (primarily of the genitourinary tract). The differential diagnosis includes neutrophilic eccrine hidradenitis and atypical forms of pyoderma gangrenosum. Extracutaneous sites of involvement include joints, muscles, eye, kidney (proteinuria, occasionally glomerulonephritis), and lung (neutrophilic infiltrates). The idiopathic form of Sweet's syndrome is seen more often in women, following a respiratory tract infection.

A generalized distribution of red-brown macules and papules is seen in the form of mastocytosis known as *urticaria pigmentosa* (Chap. 298). Each lesion represents a collection of mast cells in the dermis, with hyperpigmentation of the overlying epidermis. Stimuli such as rubbing cause these mast cells to degranulate, and this leads to the formation of localized urticaria (Darier's sign). Additional symptoms can result from mast cell degranulation and include headache, flushing, diarrhea, and pruritus. Mast cells also infiltrate various organs such as the liver, spleen, and gastrointestinal tract in up to 30 to 50% of patients with urticaria pigmentosa, and accumulations of mast cells in the bones may produce either osteosclerotic or osteolytic shadows on radiographs. In the majority of these patients, however, the internal involvement remains fairly static. A subtype of chronic leukocytoclastic vasculitis, *erythema elevatum diutinum* (EED), also presents with papules that are red-brown in color. The papules coalesce into plaques on the extensor surfaces of knees, elbows, and the small joints of the hand. Flares of EED have been associated with streptococcal infections.

Blue Lesions   Lesions that are blue in color are the result of either vascular ectasias and tumors or melanin pigment in the dermis. *Venous lakes* (ectasias) are compressible dark-blue lesions that are found commonly in the head and neck region. *Venous malformations* are also compressible blue papules and nodules that can occur anywhere on the body, including the oral mucosa. When there are multiple rather than single congenital lesions, the patient may have the blue rubber bleb syndrome or Mafucci's syndrome. Patients with the blue rubber bleb syndrome also have vascular anomalies of the gastrointestinal tract that may bleed, whereas patients with Mafucci's syndrome have associated dyschondroplasia and osteochondromas. *Blue nevi* (moles) are seen when there are collections of pigment-producing nevus cells in the dermis. These benign papular lesions are dome-shaped and occur most commonly on the dorsum of the hand or foot.

Violaceous Lesions   Violaceous papules and plaques are seen in *lupus pernio*, *lymphoma cutis*, and *cutaneous lupus*. Lupus pernio is a particular type of sarcoidosis that involves the tip of the nose and the earlobes, with lesions that are violaceous in color rather than red-brown. This form of sarcoidosis is associated with involvement of the upper respiratory tract. The plaques of lymphoma cutis and cutaneous lupus may be red or violaceous in color and were discussed above.

Purple Lesions   Purple-colored papules and plaques are seen in vascular tumors, such as *Kaposi's sarcoma* (Chap. 173) and *angiosarcoma*, and when there is extravasation of red blood cells into the skin in association with inflammation, as in *palpable purpura* (see "Purpura," below). Patients with congenital or acquired AV fistulas and venous hypertension can develop purple papules on the lower extremities that can resemble Kaposi's sarcoma clinically and histologically; this condition is referred to as pseudo-Kaposi sarcoma (acral angiodermatitis). Angiosarcoma is found most commonly on the scalp and face of elderly patients or within areas of chronic lymphedema and presents as purple papules and plaques. In the head and neck region the tumor often extends beyond the clinically defined borders and may be accompanied by facial edema.

Brown and Black Lesions   Brown- and black-colored papules are reviewed in "Hyperpigmentation," above.

Cutaneous Metastases   These are discussed last because they can have a wide range of colors. Most commonly they present as either firm, skin-colored subcutaneous nodules or firm, red to red-brown papulonodules. The lesions of lymphoma cutis range from pink-red to plum in color, whereas metastatic melanoma can be pink, blue, or black in color. Cutaneous metastases develop from hematogenous or lymphatic spread and are most often due to the following primary carcinomas: in men, lung, colon, melanoma, and oral cavity; and in women, breast, colon, and lung. These metastatic lesions may be the initial presentation of the carcinoma, especially when the primary site is the lung, kidney, or ovary.

PURPURA (Table 48-16)   *Purpura* are seen when there is an extravasation of red blood cells into the dermis and, as a result, the lesions do not blanch with pressure. This is in contrast to those erythematous or violet-colored lesions that are due to localized vasodilatation—they do blanch with pressure. Purpura ($\geq$3 mm) and petechiae ($\leq$2 mm) are divided into two major groups, palpable and nonpalpable. The most frequent causes of *nonpalpable* petechiae and purpura are primary cutaneous disorders such as *trauma*, *solar purpura*, and *capillaritis*. Less common causes are *steroid purpura* and *livedoid vasculitis* (see "Ulcers," below). Solar purpura are seen primarily on the extensor forearms, while glucocorticoid purpura secondary to potent topical steroids or endogenous or exogenous Cushing's syndrome can be more widespread. In both cases there is alteration of the supporting connective tissue that surrounds the dermal blood vessels. In contrast, the petechiae that result from capillaritis are found primarily on the lower extremities. In capillaritis there is an extravasation of erythrocytes as a result of perivascular lymphocytic inflammation. The petechiae are bright red, 1 to 2 mm in size, and scattered within annular or coin-shaped yellow-brown macules. The yellow-brown color is caused by hemosiderin deposits within the dermis.

Systemic causes of nonpalpable purpura fall into several categories, and those secondary to clotting disturbances and vascular fragility will be discussed first. The former group includes *thrombocytopenia* (Chap. 101), *abnormal platelet function* as is seen in uremia, and *clotting factor defects*. The initial site of presentation for thrombocytopenia-

TABLE 48-16   *Causes of Purpura*

I. Primary cutaneous disorders	c. Thrombotic thrombocytopenic purpura
A. Nonpalpable	d. Warfarin reaction
1. Trauma	4. Emboli
2. Solar purpura	a. Cholesterol
3. Steroid purpura	b. Fat
4. Capillaritis	5. Possible immune complex
5. Livedoid vasculitis[a]	a. Gardner-Diamond syndrome (autoerythrocyte sensitivity)
II. Systemic diseases	b. Waldenström's hypergammaglobulinemic purpura
A. Nonpalpable	B. Palpable
1. Clotting disturbances	1. Vasculitis
a. Thrombocytopenia (including ITP)	a. Leukocytoclastic vasculitis
b. Abnormal platelet function	b. Polyarteritis nodosa
c. Clotting factor defects	2. Emboli[b]
2. Vascular fragility	a. Acute meningococcemia
a. Amyloidosis	b. Disseminated gonococcal infection
b. Ehlers-Danlos syndrome	c. Rocky Mountain spotted fever
c. Scurvy	d. Ecthyma gangrenosum
3. Thrombi	
a. Disseminated intravascular coagulation	
b. Monoclonal cryoglobulinemia	

[a] Also associated with systemic diseases.
[b] Bacterial, fungal, or parasitic.
Note: ITP, idiopathic thrombocytopenic purpura.

induced petechiae is the distal lower extremity. Capillary fragility leads to nonpalpable purpura in patients with systemic *amyloidosis* (see "Papulonodular Skin Lesions," above), disorders of collagen production such as *Ehlers-Danlos syndrome*, and *scurvy*. In scurvy there are flattened corkscrew hairs with surrounding hemorrhage on the lower extremities, in addition to gingivitis. Vitamin C is a cofactor for lysyl hydroxylase, an enzyme involved in the posttranslational modification of procollagen that is necessary for cross-link formation.

In contrast to the previous group of disorders, the purpura seen in the following group of diseases are associated with thrombi formation within vessels. It is important to note that these thrombi are demonstrable in skin biopsy specimens. This group of disorders includes disseminated intravascular coagulation (DIC), monoclonal cryoglobulinemia, thrombotic thrombocytopenic purpura, and reactions to warfarin. DIC is triggered by several types of infection (gram-negative, gram-positive, viral, and rickettsial) as well as by tissue injury and neoplasms. Widespread purpura and hemorrhagic infarcts of the distal extremities are seen. Similar lesions are found in purpura fulminans, which is a form of DIC associated with fever and hypotension that occurs more commonly in children following an infectious illness such as varicella, scarlet fever, or an upper respiratory tract infection. In both disorders, hemorrhagic bullae can develop in involved skin.

Monoclonal cryoglobulinemia is associated with multiple myeloma, Waldenström's macroglobulinemia, lymphocytic leukemia, and lymphoma. Purpura, primarily of the lower extremities, and hemorrhagic infarcts of the fingers and toes are seen in these patients. Exacerbations of disease activity can follow cold exposure or an increase in serum viscosity. Biopsy specimens show precipitates of the cryoglobulin within dermal vessels. Similar deposits have been found in the lung, brain, and renal glomeruli. Patients with *thrombotic thrombocytopenic purpura* can also have hemorrhagic infarcts as a result of intravascular thromboses. Additional signs include thrombocytopenic purpura, fever, and microangiopathic hemolytic anemia (Chap. 93).

Administration of *warfarin* can result in painful areas of erythema that become purpuric and then necrotic with an adherent black eschar. This reaction is seen more often in women and in areas with abundant subcutaneous fat—breasts, abdomen, buttocks, thighs, and calves. The erythema and purpura develop between the third and tenth day of therapy, most likely as a result of a transient imbalance in the levels of anticoagulant and procoagulant vitamin K–dependent factors. Continued therapy does not exacerbate preexisting lesions, and patients with an inherited or acquired deficiency of protein C are at increased risk for this particular reaction as well as for purpura fulminans.

Purpura secondary to *cholesterol emboli* are usually seen on the lower extremities of patients with atherosclerotic vascular disease. They often follow anticoagulant therapy or an invasive vascular procedure such as an arteriogram but also occur spontaneously from disintegration of atheromatous plaques. Associated findings include livedo reticularis, gangrene, cyanosis, subcutaneous nodules, and ischemic ulcerations. Multiple step sections of the biopsy specimen may be necessary to demonstrate the cholesterol clefts with the vessels. Petechiae are also an important sign of *fat embolism* and occur primarily on the upper body 2 to 3 days after a major injury. By using special fixatives, the emboli can be demonstrated in biopsy specimens of the petechiae. Emboli of tumor or thrombus are seen in patients with atrial myxomas and marantic endocarditis.

In the *Gardner-Diamond syndrome* (autoerythrocyte sensitivity), female patients develop large ecchymoses within areas of painful, warm erythema. Intradermal injections of autologous erythrocytes or phosphatidyl serine derived from the red cell membrane can reproduce the lesions in some patients; however, there are instances where a reaction is seen at an injection site of the forearm but not in the midback region. The latter has led some observers to view Gardner-Diamond syndrome as a cutaneous manifestation of severe emotional stress. *Waldenström's hypergammaglobulinemic purpura* is a chronic disorder characterized by petechiae on the lower extremities. There are circulating complexes of IgG–anti-IgG molecules, and exacerbations are associated with prolonged standing or walking.

Palpable purpura are further subdivided into vasculitic and embolic. In the group of vasculitic disorders, *leukocytoclastic vasculitis* (LCV), also known as *allergic* or *small-vessel vasculitis*, is the one most commonly associated with palpable purpura (Chap. 306). Underlying etiologies include drugs (e.g., antibiotics), infections (e.g., hepatitis C), and connective tissue diseases. *Henoch-Schönlein purpura* is a subtype of acute LCV that is seen primarily in children and adolescents following an upper respiratory infection. The majority of lesions are found on the lower extremities and buttocks. Systemic manifestations include fever, arthralgias (primarily of the knees and ankles), abdominal pain, gastrointestinal bleeding, and nephritis. Direct immunofluorescence examination shows deposits of IgA within dermal blood vessel walls. In *polyarteritis nodosa*, specific cutaneous lesions result from a vasculitis of arterial vessels rather than postcapillary venules as in LCV. The arteritis leads to ischemia of the skin, and this explains the irregular outline of the purpura (see below).

Several types of infectious emboli can give rise to palpable purpura. These embolic lesions are usually *irregular* in outline as opposed to the lesions of LCV, which are *circular* in outline. The irregular outline is indicative of a cutaneous infarct, and the size corresponds to the area of skin that received its blood supply from that particular arteriole or artery. The palpable purpura in LCV are circular because the erythrocytes simply diffuse out evenly from the postcapillary venules as a result of inflammation. Infectious emboli are most commonly due to gram-negative cocci (meningococcus, gonococcus), gram-negative rods (Enterobacteriaceae), and gram-positive cocci (*Staphylococcus*). Additional causes include *Rickettsia* and, in immunocompromised patients, *Candida* and opportunistic fungi.

The embolic lesions in *acute meningococcemia* are found primarily on the trunk, lower extremities, and sites of pressure, and a gunmetal-gray color often develops within them. Their size varies from 1 mm to several centimeters, and the organisms can be cultured from the lesions. Associated findings include a preceding upper respiratory tract infection, fever, meningitis, DIC, and, in some patients, a deficiency of the terminal components of complement. In *disseminated gonococcal infection* (arthritis-dermatitis syndrome), a small number of papules and vesicopustules with central purpura or hemorrhagic necrosis

are found on the distal extremities. Additional symptoms include arthralgias, tenosynovitis, and fever. To establish the diagnosis, a Gram stain of these lesions should be performed. *Rocky Mountain spotted fever* is a tick-borne disease that is caused by *R. rickettsii*. A several-day history of fever, chills, severe headache, and photophobia precedes the onset of the cutaneous eruption. The initial lesions are erythematous macules and papules on the wrists, ankles, palms, and soles. With time, the lesions spread centripetally and become purpuric.

Lesions of *ecthyma gangrenosum* begin as edematous, erythematous papules or plaques and then develop central purpura and necrosis. Bullae formation also occurs in these lesions, and they are frequently found in the girdle region. The organism that is classically associated with ecthyma gangrenosum is *Pseudomonas aeruginosa*, but other gram-negative rods such as *Klebsiella*, *Escherichia coli*, and *Serratia* can produce similar lesions. In immunocompromised hosts, the list of potential pathogens is expanded to include *Candida* and opportunistic fungi.

ULCERS The approach to the patient with a cutaneous ulcer is outlined in Table 48-17. →*Peripheral vascular diseases of the extremities are reviewed in Chap. 232, as is Raynaud's phenomenon.*

Livedoid vasculitis (atrophie blanche) represents a combination of a vasculopathy with intravascular thrombosis. Purpuric lesions and livedo reticularis are found in association with painful ulcerations of the lower extremities. These ulcers are often slow to heal, but when they do, irregularly shaped white scars are formed. The majority of cases are secondary to venous hypertension, but possible underlying illnesses include cryofibrinogenemia and disorders of hypercoagulability, e.g., the antiphospholipid syndrome (Chaps. 102 and 300).

In *pyoderma gangrenosum*, the border of the ulcers has a characteristic appearance of an undermined necrotic violaceous edge and a peripheral erythematous halo. The ulcers often begin as pustules that then expand rather rapidly to a size as large as 20 cm. Although these lesions are most commonly found on the lower extremities, they can arise anywhere on the surface of the body, including sites of trauma (pathergy). An estimated 30 to 50% of cases are idiopathic, and the

---

TABLE 48-17 *Causes of Cutaneous Ulcers*

I. Primary cutaneous disorders
  A. Peripheral vascular disease (Chap. 232)
    1. Venous
    2. Arterial
  B. Livedoid vasculopathy[a]
  C. Squamous cell carcinoma, e.g., within scars
  D. Infections, e.g., ecthyma caused by *Streptococcus* (Chap. 121)
II. Systemic diseases
  A. Lower legs
    1. Leukocytoclastic vasculitis[b]
    2. Hemoglobinopathies (Chap. 91)
    3. Cryoglobulinemia,[b] cryofibrinogenemia
    4. Cholesterol emboli[b]
    5. Necrobiosis lipoidica[c]
    6. Antiphospholipid syndrome (Chap. 102)
    7. Neuropathic[d] (Chap. 323)
    8. Panniculitis
  B. Hands and feet
    1. Raynaud's phenomenon (Chap. 232)
  C. Generalized
    1. Pyoderma gangrenosum
    2. Calciphylaxis (Chap. 332)
    3. Infections, e.g., dimorphic fungi, chronic herpes varicella–zoster
    4. Lymphoma
  D. Mucosal
    1. Behçet's syndrome (Chap. 307)
    2. Erythema multiforme
    3. Primary blistering disorders (Chap. 49)
    4. Lupus erythematosus
    5. Inflammatory bowel disease

[a] Also associated with systemic diseases.
[b] Reviewed in section on "Purpura."
[c] Reviewed in section on "Papulonodular Skin Lesions."
[d] Favors plantar surface of the foot.

most common associated disorders are ulcerative colitis and Crohn's disease. Less commonly, it is associated with chronic active hepatitis, seropositive rheumatoid arthritis, acute and chronic granulocytic leukemia, polycythemia vera, and myeloma. Additional findings in these patients, even those with idiopathic disease, are cutaneous anergy and a benign monoclonal gammopathy. Because the histology of pyoderma gangrenosum is nonspecific, the diagnosis is made clinically by excluding less common causes of similar-appearing ulcers such as necrotizing vasculitis, Meleney's ulcer (synergistic infection at a site of trauma or surgery), dimorphic fungi, cutaneous amebiasis, spider bites, and facticial. In the myeloproliferative disorders, the ulcers may be more superficial with a pustulobullous border, and these lesions provide a connection between classic pyoderma gangrenosum and acute febrile neutrophilic dermatosis (Sweet's syndrome).

FEVER AND RASH   The major considerations in a patient with a fever and a rash are inflammatory diseases versus infectious diseases. In the hospital setting, the most common scenario is a patient who has a drug rash plus a fever secondary to an underlying infection. However, it should be emphasized that a drug reaction can lead to both a cutaneous eruption and a fever ("drug fever"). Additional inflammatory diseases that are often associated with a fever include pustular psoriasis, erythroderma, and Sweet's syndrome. Lyme disease, secondary syphilis, and viral and bacterial exanthems (see "Exanthems," above) are examples of infectious diseases that produce a rash and a fever. Lastly, it is important to determine whether or not the cutaneous lesions represent septic emboli (see "Purpura," above). Such lesions usually have evidence of ischemia in the form of purpura, necrosis, or impending necrosis (gunmetal-gray color). In the patient with thrombocytopenia, however, purpura can be seen in inflammatory reactions such as morbilliform drug eruptions and infectious lesions.

FURTHER READING

BOLOGNIA JL et al: *Dermatology*. Philadelphia, Mosby, 2003

BRAVERMAN IM; *Skin Signs of Systemic Disease*, 3d ed, Philadelphia, Saunders, 1998

CALLEN JP et al: *Dermatological Signs of Internal Disease*, 3d ed. Philadelphia, Saunders, 2003

SYBERT VP: *Genetic Skin Disorders*. New York, Oxford University Press, 1997

WEEDON D: *Skin Pathology*. 2d ed. London, Churchill Livingstone, 2002

49 IMMUNOLOGICALLY MEDIATED SKIN DISEASES
Kim B. Yancey, Thomas J. Lawley

A number of immunologically mediated skin diseases and immunologically mediated systemic disorders with cutaneous manifestations are now recognized as distinct entities with consistent clinical, histologic, and immunopathologic findings. Many of these disorders are due to autoimmune mechanisms. Clinically, they are characterized by morbidity (pain, pruritus, disfigurement) and in some instances by mortality (largely due to loss of epidermal barrier function and/or secondary infection). The major features of the more common immunologically mediated skin diseases are summarized in this chapter (Table 49-1).

PEMPHIGUS VULGARIS   Pemphigus vulgaris (PV) is a blistering skin disease seen predominantly in elderly patients. Patients with PV have an increased incidence of the HLA-DR4 and -DRw6 serologically defined haplotypes. This disorder is characterized by the loss of cohesion between epidermal cells (a process termed *acantholysis*) with the resultant formation of intraepidermal blisters. Clinical lesions of PV typically consist of flaccid blisters on either normal-appearing or erythematous skin. These blisters rupture easily, leaving denuded areas that may crust and enlarge peripherally (Fig. 49-1). Substantial portions of the body surface may be denuded in severe cases. Manual pressure to the skin of these patients may elicit the separation of the epidermis (Nikolsky's sign). This finding, while characteristic of PV, is not specific to this disorder and is also seen in toxic epidermal necrolysis, Stevens-Johnson syndrome, and a few other skin diseases. Lesions in PV typically present on the oral mucosa, scalp, face, neck, axilla, and trunk. In most patients, lesions begin in the mouth; involvement of other mucosal surfaces (e.g., pharyngeal, laryngeal, esophageal, conjunctival, vulval, or rectal) can occur in severe disease. Pruritus may be a feature of early pemphigus lesions; extensive denudation may be associated with severe pain. Lesions usually heal without scarring, except at sites complicated by secondary infection or mechanically induced dermal wounds. Nonetheless, postinflammatory hyperpigmentation is usually present at sites of healed lesions for some time.

Biopsies of early lesions demonstrate intraepidermal vesicle formation secondary to loss of cohesion between epidermal cells (i.e., acantholytic blisters). Blister cavities contain acantholytic epidermal cells, which appear as round homogeneous cells containing hyperchromatic nuclei. Basal keratinocytes remain attached to the epidermal basement membrane, hence blister formation is within the suprabasal portion of the epidermis. Lesional skin may contain focal collections of intraepidermal eosinophils within blister cavities; dermal alterations are slight, often limited to an eosinophil-predominant leukocytic infiltrate. Direct immunofluorescence microscopy of lesional or intact patient skin shows deposits of IgG on the surface of keratinocytes; in contrast, deposits of complement components are typically found in lesional but not uninvolved skin. Deposits of IgG on keratinocytes are derived from circulating autoantibodies directed against cell-surface antigens. Circulating autoantibodies can be demonstrated in 80 to 90% of PV patients by indirect immunofluorescence microscopy; monkey esophagus is the optimal substrate for these studies. Patients with PV have IgG autoantibodies directed against *desmogleins* (Dsgs), transmembrane desmosomal glycoproteins that belong to the cadherin supergene family of calcium-dependent adhesion molecules. Such autoantibodies can now be precisely quantitated by enzyme-linked immunosorbent assay (ELISA). Most patients with early PV (i.e., only mucosal involvement) have only anti-Dsg3 autoantibodies; most patients with advanced disease (i.e., involvement of skin and mucosa) have both anti-Dsg3 and anti-Dsg1 autoantibodies. Recent studies have shown that the anti-Dsg autoantibody profile in these patients' sera as well as the tissue distribution of Dsg3 and Dsg1 determine the site of blister formation in patients with pemphigus. Experimental studies have also shown that these autoantibodies are pathogenic (i.e., responsible for blister formation) and that their titer correlates with disease activity.

PV can be life-threatening. Prior to the availability of glucocorticoids, the mortality ranged from 60 to 90%; the current mortality is approximately 5%. Common causes of morbidity and mortality are infection and complications of treatment with glucocorticoids. Bad prognostic factors include advanced age, widespread involvement, and the requirement for high doses of glucocorticoids (with or without other immunosuppressive agents) for control of disease. The course of PV in individual patients is variable and difficult to predict. Some patients achieve remission (40% of patients in some series), but others may require long-term treatment or succumb to complications of their disease or its treatment. The mainstay of treatment is systemic glucocorticoids. Patients with moderate to severe disease are usually started on prednisone, 60 to 80 mg/d. If new lesions continue to appear

TABLE 49-1 *Immunologically Mediated Blistering Diseases*

Disease	Clinical	Histology	Immunopathology	Autoantigens[a]
Pemphigus foliaceus	Crusts and shallow erosions on scalp, central face, upper chest, and back	Acantholytic blister formed in superficial layer of epidermis	Cell surface deposits of IgG on keratinocytes	Dsg1
Pemphigus vulgaris	Flaccid blisters, denuded skin, oromucosal lesions	Acantholytic blister formed in suprabasal layer of epidermis	Cell surface deposits of IgG on keratinocytes	Dsg3 (plus Dsg1 in patients with skin involvement)
Bullous pemphigoid	Large tense blisters on flexor surfaces and trunk	Blister formed in subepidermal region; usually eosinophil-rich infiltrate	Linear band of IgG and/or C3 in epidermal BMZ[a]	BPAG1, BPAG2
Pemphigoid gestationis	Pruritic, urticarial plaques, rimmed by vesicles and bullae on the trunk and extremities	Teardrop-shaped, subepidermal blisters in dermal papillae; eosinophil-rich infiltrate	Linear band of C3 in epidermal BMZ	BPAG2 (plus BPAG1 in some patients)
Linear IgA disease	Pruritic small papules on extensor surfaces; occasionally larger, arciform blisters	Subepidermal blister with neutrophils in dermal papillae	Linear band of IgA in epidermal BMZ	BPAG2 (see text for specific details)
Cicatricial pemphigoid	Erosive and/or blistering lesions of mucous membranes and possibly the skin; scarring of some sites	Subepidermal blister that may or may not include a leukocytic infiltrate	Linear band of IgG, IgA, and/or C3 in epidermal BMZ	BPAG2, laminin 5, or others
Epidermolysis bullosa acquisita	Blisters, erosions, scars, and milia on sites exposed to trauma; widespread, inflammatory, tense blisters may be seen initially	Subepidermal blister that may or may not include a leukocytic infiltrate	Linear band of IgG and/or C3 in epidermal BMZ	Type VII collagen
Dermatitis herpetiformis	Extremely pruritic small papules and vesicles on elbows, knees, buttocks, and posterior neck	Subepidermal blister with neutrophils in dermal papillae	Granular deposits of IgA in dermal papillae	Epidermal transglutaminase

[a] Autoantigens bound by these patients' autoantibodies are defined as follows: Dsg1, desmoglein 1; Dsg3, desmoglein 3; BPAG1, bullous pemphigoid antigen 1; BPAG2, bullous pemphigoid antigen 2; BMZ, basement membrane zone.

after 1 to 2 weeks of treatment, the dose may need to be increased. Many regimens combine an immunosuppressive agent with systemic glucocorticoids for control of PV. The most frequently used are either azathioprine (1 to 2 mg/kg per day), or mycophenolate mofetil (20 to 35 mg/kg per day), cyclophosphamide (1 to 2 mg/kg per day). It is important to bring severe or progressive disease under control quickly to lessen the severity and/or duration of this disorder.

PEMPHIGUS FOLIACEUS Pemphigus foliaceus (PF) is distinguished from PV by several features. In PF, acantholytic blisters are located high within the epidermis, usually just beneath the stratum corneum. Hence PF is a more superficial blistering disease than PV. The distribution of lesions in the two disorders is much the same, except that in PF mucous membranes are almost always spared. Patients with PF rarely demonstrate intact blisters but rather exhibit shallow erosions associated with erythema, scale, and crust formation. Mild cases of PF resemble severe seborrheic dermatitis; severe PF may cause extensive exfoliation. Sun exposure (ultraviolet irradiation) may be an aggravating factor. A blistering skin disease endemic to south central Brazil known as *fogo selvagem*, or *Brazilian pemphigus*, is clinically, histologically, and immunopathologically indistinguishable from PF.

Patients with PF have immunopathologic features in common with PV. Specifically, direct immunofluorescence microscopy of perilesional skin demonstrates IgG on the surface of keratinocytes. As in PV, patients with PF frequently have circulating IgG autoantibodies against keratinocyte cell surface antigens. Guinea pig esophagus is the optimal substrate for indirect immunofluorescence microscopy studies of sera from patients with PF. In PF, autoantibodies are directed against Dsg1, a 160-kDa desmosomal cadherin. As noted for PV, the autoantibody profile in patients with PF (i.e., anti-Dsg1) and the normal tissue distribution of this autoantigen (i.e., low expression in oral mucosa) is thought to account for the distribution of lesions in this disease.

Although pemphigus has been associated with several autoimmune diseases, its association with thymoma and/or myasthenia gravis is particularly notable. To date, more than 30 cases of thymoma and/or myasthenia gravis have been reported in association with pemphigus, usually with PF. Patients may also develop pemphigus as a consequence of drug exposure. The most frequently implicated agent is penicillamine; other offenders include captopril, rifampin, piroxicam, penicillin, and phenobarbital. Drug-induced pemphigus usually resembles PF rather than PV; autoantibodies in these patients have the same antigenic specificity as they do in other pemphigus patients. In most patients, lesions resolve following discontinuation of the drug; however, some patients require treatment with systemic glucocorticoids and/or immunosuppressive agents.

PF is generally a far less severe disease than PV and carries a better prognosis. Localized disease can be treated conservatively with topical or intralesional glucocorticoids; more active cases can usually be controlled with systemic glucocorticoids.

PARANEOPLASTIC PEMPHIGUS Paraneoplastic pemphigus (PNP) is an autoimmune acantholytic mucocutaneous disease associated with an occult or confirmed neoplasm. Patients with PNP typically show painful mucosal erosive lesions in association with papulosquamous eruptions that often progress to blisters. Palm and sole involvement is common in these patients and raises the possibility that prior reports of neoplasia-associated erythema multiforme actually may have represented unrecognized cases of PNP. Biopsies of lesional skin from these patients show varying combinations of acantholysis, keratinocyte necrosis, and vacuolar-interface dermatitis. Direct immunofluorescence microscopy of patient skin shows deposits of IgG and complement on the surface

A

B

FIGURE 49-1 *A.* Pemphigus vulgaris demonstrating flaccid bullae that are easily ruptured, resulting in multiple erosions and crusted plaques. *B.* Pemphigus vulgaris almost invariably involves the oral mucosa and may present with erosions involving the gingiva, buccal mucosa, palate, posterior pharynx, or the tongue. (*B*, Courtesy of Robert Swerlick, MD.)

of keratinocytes and (variably) similar immunoreactants in the epidermal basement membrane zone. Patients with PNP have IgG autoantibodies against cytoplasmic proteins that are members of the plakin family (e.g., desmoplakins I and II, bullous pemphigoid antigen 1, envoplakin, periplakin, and plectin) and cell-surface proteins that are members of the cadherin family (e.g., Dsg3). Because immunoadsorption of anti-Dsg3 IgG is sufficient to eliminate the ability of PNP sera to induce blisters in an experimental passive transfer animal model, these particular autoantibodies are thought to play the key pathogenic role in blister formation in these patients.

Although PNP is generally resistant to conventional therapies (i.e., those used to treat PV), patients may improve (or even remit) following resection of underlying neoplasms. The predominant neoplasms associated with this disorder are non-Hodgkin's lymphoma, chronic lymphocytic leukemia, Castleman's disease, thymoma, and spindle cell tumors.

BULLOUS PEMPHIGOID Bullous pemphigoid (BP) is an autoimmune subepidermal blistering disease usually seen in the elderly. Lesions typically consist of tense blisters on either normal-appearing or erythematous skin (Fig. 49-2). The lesions are usually distributed over the lower abdomen, groin, and flexor surface of the extremities; oral mu-

cosal lesions are found in 10 to 40% of patients. Pruritus may be nonexistent or severe. As lesions evolve, tense blisters tend to rupture and be replaced by flaccid lesions or erosions with or without surmounting crust. Nontraumatized blisters heal without scarring. The major histocompatibility complex class II allele HLA-DQβ1*0301 is prevalent in patients with BP. Despite isolated reports, several studies have shown that patients with BP do not have an increased incidence of malignancy in comparison with appropriately age- and gender-matched controls.

While biopsies of early lesional skin demonstrate subepidermal blisters, the histologic features depend on the character of the particular lesion. Lesions on normal-appearing skin generally show a sparse perivascular leukocytic infiltrate with some eosinophils; conversely, biopsies of inflammatory lesions typically show an eosinophil rich infiltrate within the papillary dermis at sites of vesicle formation and in perivascular areas. In addition to eosinophils, cell-rich lesions also contain mononuclear cells and neutrophils. It is not always possible to distinguish BP from other subepidermal blistering diseases by routine histologic techniques.

Immunopathologic studies have broadened our understanding of this disease and aided its diagnosis. Direct immunofluorescence microscopy of normal-appearing perilesional skin shows linear deposits of IgG and/or C3 in the epidermal basement membrane. The sera of approximately 70% of these patients contain circulating IgG autoantibodies that bind the epidermal basement membrane of normal human skin in indirect immunofluorescence microscopy. An even higher percentage of patients shows reactivity to the epidermal side of 1 *M* NaCl split skin [an alternative immunofluorescence microscopy test substrate that is commonly used to distinguish circulating IgG anti-basement membrane autoantibodies in patients with BP from those in patients with similar, yet different, subepidermal blistering diseases (e.g., epidermolysis bullosa acquisita, see below)]. No correlation exists between the titer of these autoantibodies and disease activity. In BP, circulating autoantibodies recognize 230- and 180-kDa hemidesmosome-associated proteins in basal keratinocytes [i.e., bullous pemphigoid antigen (BPAG)1 and BPAG2, respectively]. Autoantibodies are thought to develop against these antigens (more specifically, initially against BPAG2), deposit in situ, and activate complement that subsequently produces dermal mast cell degranulation and granulocyte-rich infiltrates that cause tissue damage and blister formation.

BP may persist for months to years, with exacerbations or remissions. Although extensive involvement may result in widespread erosions and compromise cutaneous integrity, the mortality rate is rela-

FIGURE 49-2 Bullous pemphigoid with tense vesicles and bullae on erythematous, urticarial bases. (Courtesy of the Yale Resident's Slide Collection.)

tively low. Nonetheless, deaths may occur in elderly and/or debilitated patients. The mainstay of treatment is systemic glucocorticoids. Patients with local or minimal disease can sometimes be controlled with topical glucocorticoids alone; patients with more extensive lesions generally respond to systemic glucocorticoids either alone or in combination with immunosuppressive agents. Patients will usually respond to prednisone, 40 to 60 mg/d. In some instances, azathioprine (1 to 2 mg/kg per day), mycophenolate mofetil (20 to 35 mg/kg per day), or cyclophosphamide (1 to 2 mg/kg per day) are necessary adjuncts.

PEMPHIGOID GESTATIONIS Pemphigoid gestationis (PG), also known as *herpes gestationis*, is a rare, nonviral, subepidermal blistering disease of pregnancy and the puerperium. PG may begin during any trimester of pregnancy or present shortly after delivery. Lesions are usually distributed over the abdomen, trunk, and extremities; mucous membrane lesions are rare. Skin lesions in these patients may be quite polymorphic and consist of erythematous urticarial papules and plaques, vesiculopapules, and/or frank bullae. Lesions are almost always very pruritic. Severe exacerbations of PG frequently occur after delivery, typically within 24 to 48 h. PG tends to recur in subsequent pregnancies, often beginning earlier during such gestations. Brief flare-ups of disease may occur with resumption of menses and may develop in patients later exposed to oral contraceptives. Occasionally, infants of affected mothers demonstrate transient skin lesions.

Biopsies of early lesional skin show teardrop-shaped subepidermal vesicles forming in dermal papillae in association with an eosinophil-rich leukocytic infiltrate. Differentiation of PG from other subepidermal bullous diseases by light microscopy is often difficult. However, direct immunofluorescence microscopy of perilesional skin from PG patients reveals the immunopathologic hallmark of this disorder—linear deposits of C3 in the epidermal basement membrane zone. These deposits develop as a consequence of complement activation produced by low titer IgG anti-basement membrane zone autoantibodies. Recent studies have shown that the majority of PG sera contain autoantibodies that recognize BPAG2, the same 180-kDa hemidesmosome-associated protein that is targeted by autoantibodies in patients with BP—a subepidermal bullous disease that resembles PG morphologically, histologically, and immunopathologically.

The goals of therapy in patients with PG are to prevent the development of new lesions, relieve intense pruritus, and care for erosions at sites of blister formation. Most patients require treatment with moderate doses of daily glucocorticoids (i.e., 20 to 40 mg of prednisone) at some point in their course. Mild cases (or brief flare-ups) may be controlled by vigorous use of potent topical glucocorticoids. Although PG was once thought to be associated with an increased risk of fetal morbidity and mortality, the best evidence now suggests that these infants are only at increased risk of being slightly premature or "small for dates." Current evidence suggests that there is no difference in the incidence of uncomplicated live births in PG patients treated with systemic glucocorticoids and in those managed more conservatively. If systemic glucocorticoids are administered, newborns are at risk for development of reversible adrenal insufficiency.

DERMATITIS HERPETIFORMIS Dermatitis herpetiformis (DH) is an intensely pruritic, papulovesicular skin disease characterized by lesions symmetrically distributed over extensor surfaces (i.e., elbows, knees, buttocks, back, scalp, and posterior neck) (see Fig. 46-8). The primary lesion in this disorder is a papule, papulovesicle, or urticarial plaque. Because pruritus is prominent, patients may present with excoriations and crusted papules but no observable primary lesions. Patients sometimes report that their pruritus has a distinctive burning or stinging component; the onset of such local symptoms reliably heralds the development of distinct clinical lesions 12 to 24 h later. Almost all DH patients have an associated, usually subclinical, gluten-sensitive enteropathy (Chap. 275), and more than 90% express the HLA-B8/DRw3 and HLA-DQw2 haplotypes. DH may present at any age, including childhood; onset in the second to fourth decades is most common. The disease is typically chronic.

Biopsy of early lesional skin reveals neutrophil-rich infiltrates within dermal papillae. Neutrophils, fibrin, edema, and microvesicle formation at these sites are characteristic of early disease. Older lesions may demonstrate nonspecific features of a subepidermal bulla or an excoriated papule. Because the clinical and histologic features of this disease can be variable and resemble other subepidermal blistering disorders, the diagnosis is confirmed by direct immunofluorescence microscopy of normal-appearing perilesional skin. Such studies demonstrate granular deposits of IgA (with or without complement components) in the papillary dermis and along the epidermal basement membrane zone. IgA deposits in the skin are unaffected by control of disease with medication; however, these immunoreactants may diminish in intensity or disappear in patients maintained for long periods on a strict gluten-free diet (see below). Patients with DH have granular deposits of IgA in their epidermal basement membrane zone and should be distinguished from individuals with linear IgA deposits at this site (see below).

Although most DH patients do not report overt gastrointestinal symptoms or have laboratory evidence of malabsorption, biopsies of small bowel usually reveal blunting of intestinal villi and a lymphocytic infiltrate in the lamina propria. As is true for patients with celiac disease, this gastrointestinal abnormality can be reversed by a gluten-free diet. Moreover, if maintained, this diet alone may control the skin disease and eventuate in clearance of IgA deposits from these patients' epidermal basement membrane zone. Subsequent gluten exposure in such patients alters the morphology of their small bowel, elicits a flare-up of their skin disease, and is associated with the reappearance of IgA in their epidermal basement membrane zone. As in patients with celiac disease, dietary gluten sensitivity in patients with DH is associated with IgA anti-endomysial autoantibodies that target tissue transglutaminase. Recent studies suggest that patients with DH also have high-avidity IgA autoantibodies against epidermal transglutaminase and that the latter is co-localized with granular deposits of IgA in the papillary dermis of DH patients. Patients with DH also have an increased incidence of thyroid abnormalities, achlorhydria, atrophic gastritis, and antigastric parietal cell antibodies. These associations likely relate to the high frequency of the HLA-B8/DRw3 haplotype in these patients, since this marker is commonly linked to autoimmune disorders. The mainstay of treatment of DH is dapsone, a sulfone. Patients respond rapidly (24 to 48 h) to dapsone (50 to 200 mg/d) but require careful pretreatment evaluation and close follow-up to ensure that complications are avoided or controlled. All patients on more than 100 mg/d dapsone will have some hemolysis and methemoglobinemia. These are expected pharmacologic side effects of this agent. Gluten restriction can control DH and lessen dapsone requirements; this diet must rigidly exclude gluten to be of maximal benefit. Many months of dietary restriction may be necessary before a beneficial result is achieved. Good dietary counselling by a trained dietitian is essential.

LINEAR IGA DISEASE Linear IgA disease, once considered a variant form of dermatitis herpetiformis, is actually a separate and distinct entity. Clinically, these patients may resemble patients with typical cases of DH, BP, or other subepidermal blistering diseases. Lesions typically consist of papulovesicles, bullae, and/or urticarial plaques, predominantly on extensor (as seen in "classic" DH), central, or flexural sites. Oral mucosal involvement occurs in some patients. Severe pruritus resembles that in patients with DH. Patients with linear IgA disease do not have an increased frequency of the HLA-B8/DRw3 haplotype or an associated enteropathy and hence are not candidates for a gluten-free diet.

The histologic alterations in early lesions may be virtually indistinguishable from those in DH. However, direct immunofluorescence microscopy of normal-appearing perilesional skin reveals linear deposits of IgA (and often C3) in the epidermal basement membrane zone. Most patients with linear IgA disease demonstrate circulating IgA anti-basement membrane autoantibodies against epitopes in the extracellular domain of BPAG2, a transmembrane protein found in hemidesmosomes of basal keratinocytes. These patients generally respond to treatment with dapsone, 50 to 200 mg/d.

EPIDERMOLYSIS BULLOSA ACQUISITA EBA is a rare, noninherited, polymorphic, chronic, subepidermal blistering disease. (The inherited form is discussed in Chap. 342.) Patients with classic or noninflammatory EBA have blisters on noninflamed skin, atrophic scars, milia, nail dystrophy, and oral lesions. Because lesions generally occur at sites exposed to minor trauma, classic EBA is considered to be a mechanobullous disease. Other patients with EBA have widespread inflammatory, scarring, and bullous lesions that resemble severe BP. Inflammatory EBA may evolve into the classic, noninflammatory form of this disease. Rare patients present with lesions that predominate on mucous membranes. The HLA-DR2 haplotype is found with increased frequency in EBA patients. Recent studies suggest that EBA is often associated with inflammatory bowel disease (especially Crohn's disease).

The histology of lesional skin varies depending on the character of the lesion being studied. Noninflammatory bullae show subepidermal blisters with a sparse leukocytic infiltrate and resemble those in patients with porphyria cutanea tarda. Inflammatory lesions consist of a subepidermal blister and neutrophil-rich leukocytic infiltrates in the superficial dermis. EBA patients have continuous deposits of IgG (and frequently C3 as well as other complement components) in a linear pattern within the epidermal basement membrane zone. Ultrastructurally, these immunoreactants are found in the sublamina densa region in association with anchoring fibrils, wheat stack–like structures that extend from the lamina densa into the underlying papillary dermis. Approximately 50% of EBA patients have circulating IgG anti-basement membrane autoantibodies directed against type VII collagen—the collagen species that comprises anchoring fibrils. Such IgG autoantibodies bind the dermal side of 1 M NaCl split skin (in contrast to IgG autoantibodies in patients with BP that bind either epidermal or both sides of this indirect immunofluorescence microscopy test substrate).

Treatment of EBA is generally unsatisfactory. Some patients with inflammatory EBA may respond to systemic glucocorticoids, either alone or in combination with immunosuppressive agents. Other patients (especially those with neutrophil-rich inflammatory lesions) may respond to dapsone. The chronic, noninflammatory form of this disease is largely resistant to treatment, although some patients may respond to cyclosporine or intravenous immunoglobulin.

CICATRICIAL PEMPHIGOID Cicatricial pemphigoid (CP) is a rare, acquired, subepithelial blistering disease characterized by erosive lesions of mucous membranes and skin that result in scarring of at least some sites of involvement. Immunopathologically, perilesional mucosa and skin of patients with CP demonstrate in situ deposits of immunoreactants in epithelial basement membranes. Common sites of involvement include the oral mucosa (especially the gingiva) and conjunctiva; other sites that may be affected include the nasopharyngeal, laryngeal, esophageal, urogenital, and rectal mucosa. Skin lesions (present in about one-third of patients) tend to predominate on the scalp, face, and upper trunk and generally consist of a few scattered erosions or tense blisters on an erythematous or urticarial base. CP is typically a chronic and progressive disorder. Serious complications may arise as a consequence of ocular, laryngeal, esophageal, or urogenital lesions. Erosive conjunctivitis may result in shortened fornices, symblephara, ankyloblepharon, entropion, corneal opacities, and (in severe cases) blindness. Similarly, erosive lesions of the larynx may cause hoarseness, pain, and tissue loss that if unrecognized and untreated may eventuate in complete destruction of the airway. Esophageal lesions may result in stenosis and/or strictures that may place patients at risk for aspiration. Strictures may also complicate urogenital involvement.

Biopsies of lesional tissue generally demonstrate subepithelial vesiculobullae and a mononuclear leukocytic infiltrate. Neutrophils and eosinophils may be seen in biopsies of early lesions; older lesions may demonstrate a scant leukocytic infiltrate and fibrosis. Direct immu-

nofluorescence microscopy of perilesional tissue typically demonstrates deposits of IgG, IgA, and/or C3 in these patients' epithelial basement membranes. Because many of these patients show no evidence of circulating anti-basement membrane autoantibodies, testing of perilesional skin is important diagnostically. Although CP was once thought to be a single nosologic entity, it is now largely regarded as a disease phenotype that may develop as a consequence of an autoimmune reaction against a variety of different molecules in epithelial basement membranes (e.g., BPAG2, laminin 5, type VII collagen, and other antigens yet to be completely defined). Treatment of CP is largely dependent upon sites of involvement. Due to potentially severe complications, ocular, laryngeal, esophageal, and/or urogenital involvement require aggressive systemic treatment with dapsone, prednisone, or the latter in combination with another immunosuppressive agent (e.g., azathioprine, mycophenolate mofetil, or cyclophosphamide) or intravenous immunoglobulin. Less threatening forms of the disease may be managed with topical or intralesional glucocorticoids.

AUTOIMMUNE SYSTEMIC DISEASES WITH PROMINENT CUTANEOUS FEATURES

DERMATOMYOSITIS The cutaneous manifestations of dermatomyositis (Chap. 369) are often distinctive but at times may resemble those of systemic lupus erythematosus (SLE) (Chap. 300), scleroderma (Chap. 303), or other overlapping connective tissue diseases (Chap. 303). The extent and severity of cutaneous disease may or may not correlate with the extent and severity of the myositis. The cutaneous manifestations of dermatomyositis are similar whether the disease appears in childhood or old age, except that calcification of subcutaneous tissue is a common late sequela in childhood dermatomyositis.

The cutaneous signs of dermatomyositis may precede or follow the development of myositis by weeks to years. Cases lacking muscle involvement (i.e., dermatomyositis sine myositis) have also been reported. The most common manifestation is a purple-red discoloration of the upper eyelids, sometimes associated with scaling ("heliotrope" erythema; Fig. 49-3) and periorbital edema. Erythema on the cheeks and nose in a "butterfly" distribution may resemble the eruption in SLE. Erythematous or violaceous scaling patches are common on the upper anterior chest, posterior neck, scalp, and the extensor surfaces of the arms, legs, and hands. Erythema and scaling may be particularly prominent over the elbows, knees, and the dorsal interphalangeal joints. Approximately one-third of patients have violaceous, flat-topped papules over the dorsal interphalangeal joints that are pathognomonic of dermatomyositis (Gottron's sign or Gottron's papules; Fig. 49-4). These lesions can be contrasted with the erythema and scaling

FIGURE 49-3 Dermatomyositis Periorbital violaceous erythema characterizes the classic heliotrope rash. (Courtesy of James Krell, MD.)

FIGURE 49-4 Dermatomyositis often involves the hands as erythematous flat-topped papules over the knuckles (Gottron's sign) and periungual telangiectasias.

on the dorsum of the fingers in some patients with SLE, which spares the skin over the interphalangeal joints. Periungual telangiectasia may be prominent, and a lacy or reticulated erythema may be associated with fine scaling on the extensor surfaces of the thighs and upper arms. Other patients, particularly those with long-standing disease, develop areas of hypopigmentation, hyperpigmentation, mild atrophy, and telangiectasia known as *poikiloderma*. Poikiloderma is rare in both SLE and scleroderma and thus can serve as a clinical sign that distinguishes dermatomyositis from these two diseases. Cutaneous changes may be similar in scleroderma and dermatomyositis and may include thickening and binding down of the skin of the hands (sclerodactyly) as well as Raynaud's phenomenon. However, the presence of severe muscle disease, Gottron's papules, heliotrope erythema, and poikiloderma serve to distinguish patients with dermatomyositis. Skin biopsy of erythematous, scaling lesions of dermatomyositis may reveal only mild nonspecific inflammation but sometimes may show changes indistinguishable from those found in SLE, including epidermal atrophy, hydropic degeneration of basal keratinocytes, edema of the upper dermis, and a mild mononuclear cell infiltrate. Direct immunofluorescence microscopy of lesional skin is usually negative, although granular deposits of immunoglobulin(s) and complement in the epidermal basement membrane zone have been described in some patients. Treatment should be directed at the systemic disease. In the few instances where adjunctive cutaneous therapy is desirable, topical glucocorticoids are sometimes useful. These patients should avoid exposure to ultraviolet irradiation and use photoprotective measures such as sunscreens.

LUPUS ERYTHEMATOSUS The cutaneous manifestations of lupus erythematosus (LE) (Chap. 300) can be divided into acute, subacute, and chronic types. *Acute cutaneous LE* is characterized by erythema of the nose and malar eminences in a "butterfly" distribution (Fig. 49-5). The erythema is often sudden in onset, accompanied by edema and fine scale, and correlated with systemic involvement. Patients may have widespread involvement of the face as well as erythema and scaling of the extensor surfaces of the extremities and upper chest. These acute lesions, while sometimes evanescent, usually last for days and are often associated with exacerbations of systemic disease. Skin biopsy of acute lesions may show only a sparse dermal infiltrate of mononuclear cells and dermal edema. In some instances, cellular infiltrates around blood vessels and hair follicles are notable, as is hydropic degeneration of basal cells of the epidermis. Direct immunofluorescence microscopy of lesional skin frequently reveals deposits of immunoglobulin(s) and complement in the epidermal basement membrane zone. Treatment is aimed at control of systemic disease; photoprotection in this, as well as in other forms of LE, is very important.

Subacute cutaneous lupus erythematosus (SCLE) is characterized by a widespread photosensitive, nonscarring eruption. About half of these patients have SLE in which severe renal and central nervous system involvement is uncommon. SCLE may present as a papulosquamous eruption that resembles psoriasis or annular lesions that resemble those seen in erythema multiforme. In the papulosquamous form, discrete erythematous papules arise on the back, chest, shoulders, extensor surfaces of the arms, and the dorsum of the hands; lesions are uncommon on the face, flexor surfaces of the arms, and below the waist. The slightly scaling papules tend to merge into large plaques, some with a reticulate appearance. The annular form involves the same areas and presents with erythematous papules that evolve into oval, circular, or polycyclic lesions. The lesions of SCLE are more widespread but have less tendency for scarring than do lesions of discoid LE. Skin biopsy reveals a dense mononuclear cell infiltrate around hair follicles and blood vessels in the superficial dermis, combined with hydropic degeneration of basal cells in the epidermis. Direct immunofluorescence microscopy of lesional skin reveals deposits of immunoglobulin(s) in the epidermal basement membrane zone in about half these cases. A particulate pattern of IgG deposition around basal keratinocytes has recently been associated with SCLE. Most SCLE patients have anti-Ro antibodies. Local therapy is usually unsuccessful, and most patients require treatment with aminoquinoline antimalarials. Low-dose therapy with oral glucocorticoids is sometimes necessary; photoprotective measures against both ultraviolet B and A wavelengths are very important.

FIGURE 49-5 *A.* Systemic lupus erythematosus showing prominent, scaly, malar erythema. Involvement of other sun-exposed sites is also common. *B.* Acute LE on the upper chest demonstrating brightly erythematous and slightly edematous papules and plaques. (*B,* Courtesy of Robert Swerlick, MD.)

Discoid lupus erythematosus (DLE) is characterized by discrete lesions, most often on the face, scalp, or external ears. The lesions are erythematous papules or plaques with a thick, adherent scale that occludes hair follicles (follicular plugging). When the scale is removed, its underside will show small excrescences that correlate with the openings of hair follicles and is termed a "carpet tack" appearance. This finding is relatively specific for DLE. Long-standing lesions develop central atrophy, scarring, and hypopigmentation but frequently have erythematous, sometimes raised borders at the periphery (Fig. 49-6). These lesions persist for years and tend to expand slowly. Only 5 to 10% of patients with DLE meet the American Rheumatism Association criteria for SLE. However, typical discoid lesions are frequently seen in patients with SLE. Biopsy of DLE lesions shows hyperkeratosis, follicular plugging, and atrophy of the epidermis; hydropic degeneration of basal keratinocytes; and a mononuclear cell infiltrate adjacent to epidermal, adnexal, and microvascular basement membranes. Direct immunofluorescence microscopy demonstrates immunoglobulin(s) and complement deposits at the basement membrane zone in about 90% of cases. Treatment is focused on control of local cutaneous disease and consists mainly of photoprotection and topical or intralesional glucocorticoids. If local therapy is ineffective, use of aminoquinoline antimalarials may be indicated.

SCLERODERMA AND MORPHEA   The skin changes of scleroderma (Chap. 303) usually begin on the hands, feet, and face, with episodes of recurrent nonpitting edema. Sclerosis of the skin begins distally on the fingers (sclerodactyly) and spreads proximally, usually accompanied by resorption of bone of the fingertips, which may have punched out ulcers, stellate scars, or areas of hemorrhage (Fig. 49-7). The fingers may actually shrink in size and become sausage-shaped, and since the fingernails are usually unaffected, the nails may curve over the end of the fingertips. Periungual telangiectasias are usually present, but periungual erythema is rare. In advanced cases, the extremities show contractures and calcinosis cutis. Facial involvement includes a smooth, unwrinkled brow, taut skin over the nose, shrinkage of tissue around the mouth, and perioral radial furrowing (Fig. 49-8). Matlike telangiectasias are often present, particularly on the face and hands. Involved skin feels indurated, smooth, and bound to underlying structures; hyperpigmentation and hypopigmentation are also often present. Raynaud's phenomenon, i.e., cold-induced blanching, cyanosis, and reactive hyperemia, is present in almost all patients and can precede development of scleroderma by many years. The combination of calcinosis cutis, Raynaud's phenomenon, esophageal dysmotility, sclerodactyly, and telangiectasia has been termed the *CREST syndrome*. Anticentromere antibodies have been reported in a very high percentage of patients with the CREST syndrome but in only a small minority of patients with scleroderma. Skin biopsy reveals

FIGURE 49-7   Scleroderma showing acral sclerosis and focal digital ulcers.

thickening of the dermis and homogenization of collagen bundles. Direct immunofluorescence microscopy of lesional skin is usually negative.

Morphea, which has been called *localized scleroderma*, is characterized by localized thickening and sclerosis of skin, usually affecting young adults or children. Morphea begins as erythematous or flesh-colored plaques that become sclerotic, develop central hypopigmentation, and demonstrate an erythematous border. In most cases, patients have one or a few lesions, and the disease is termed *localized morphea*. In some patients, widespread cutaneous lesions may occur, without systemic involvement. This form is called *generalized morphea*. Most patients with morphea do not have autoantibodies. Skin biopsy of morphea is indistinguishable from that of scleroderma. Linear scleroderma is a limited form of disease that presents in a linear, bandlike distribution and tends to involve deep as well as superficial layers of skin. Scleroderma and morphea are usually quite resistant to therapy. For this reason, physical therapy to prevent joint contractures and to maintain function is employed and is often helpful.

Diffuse fasciitis with eosinophilia is a clinical entity that can sometimes be confused with scleroderma. There is usually the sudden onset of swelling, induration, and erythema of the extremities frequently following significant physical exertion. The proximal portions of extremities (arms, forearms, thighs, legs) are more often involved than are the hands and feet. While the skin is indurated, it is usually not bound down as in scleroderma; contractures may occur early second-

FIGURE 49-6   Violaceous, hyperpigmented, atrophic plaques, often with evidence of follicular plugging, which may result in scarring, are characteristic of discoid lupus erythematosus.

FIGURE 49-8   Scleroderma characterized by typical expressionless, mask-like facies.

ary to fascial involvement. The latter may also cause muscle groups to be separated (i.e., the "groove sign") and veins to appear depressed (i.e., sunken veins). These skin findings are accompanied by peripheral blood eosinophilia, increased erythrocyte sedimentation rate, and sometimes hypergammaglobulinemia. Deep biopsy of affected areas of skin reveals inflammation and thickening of the deep fascia overlying muscle. An inflammatory infiltrate composed of eosinophils and mononuclear cells is usually found. Patients with eosinophilic fasciitis appear to be at increased risk to develop bone marrow failure or other hematologic abnormalities. While the ultimate course of eosinophilic fasciitis is uncertain, many patients respond favorably to treatment with prednisone in doses ranging from 40 to 60 mg/d.

The *eosinophilia-myalgia syndrome*, a disorder reported in epidemic numbers in 1989 and linked to ingestion of L-tryptophan manufactured by a single company in Japan, is a multisystem disorder characterized by debilitating myalgias and absolute eosinophilia in association with varying combinations of arthralgias, pulmonary symptoms, and peripheral edema. In a later phase (i.e., 3 to 6 months after initial symptoms), these patients often develop localized sclerodermatous skin changes, weight loss, and/or neuropathy (Chap. 303). The precise cause of this syndrome, which may resemble other sclerotic skin conditions, is unknown. However, the implicated lots of L-tryptophan contained the contaminant 1,1-ethylidene bis[tryptophan]. This contaminant may be pathogenic or a marker for another substance that provokes the disorder.

FURTHER READING

AMAGAI M: Pemphigus: Autoimmunity to epidermal cell adhesion molecules. Adv Dermatol 11:319, 1996

ANHALT GJ et al: Paraneoplastic pemphigus. Adv Dermatol 12:77, 1997

SCHMIDT E, ZILLIKENS D: Autoimmune and inherited subepidermal blistering diseases: Advances in the clinic and the laboratory. Adv Dermatol 16:113, 2000

UDEY MC, STANLEY JR: Pemphigus—diseases of antidesmosomal autoimmunity. JAMA 282:572, 1999

YANCEY KB, EGAN CA: Pemphigoid: Clinical, histologic, immunopathologic, and therapeutic considerations. JAMA 284:350, 2000

50 CUTANEOUS DRUG REACTIONS
Olivier M. Chosidow, Robert S. Stern, Bruce U. Wintroub

Cutaneous reactions are among the most frequent adverse reactions to drugs. Prompt recognition of these reactions, drug withdrawal, and appropriate therapeutic interventions can minimize toxicity. This chapter focuses on adverse cutaneous reactions to drugs other than topical agents and reviews the incidence, patterns, and pathogenesis of cutaneous reactions to drugs and other therapeutic agents.

USE OF PRESCRIPTION DRUGS IN THE UNITED STATES More than 1.5 billion prescriptions for 60,000 drug products, which include over 2000 different active agents, are dispensed each year in the United States. Hospital inpatients alone annually receive about 120 million courses of drug therapy, and half of adult Americans receive prescription drugs on a regular outpatient basis. Many additional patients use over-the-counter medicines that may cause adverse cutaneous reactions.

INCIDENCE OF CUTANEOUS REACTIONS Although adverse drug reactions are common, it is difficult to ascertain their incidence, seriousness, and ultimate health effects. Available information comes from evaluations of hospitalized patients, epidemiologic surveys, premarketing studies, and voluntary reporting, most notably to the U.S. Food and Drug Administration's Medwatch System. In a systematic literature review of cutaneous reactions to drugs, the reaction rates varied from 0 to 8% and were highest for antibiotics (Table 50-1). In a series of 48,005 inpatients over a 20-year period, morbilliform rash (91%) and urticaria (6%) were the most frequent skin reactions.

The relative risk of Stevens-Johnson syndrome (SJS) and toxic epidermal necrolysis (TEN), perhaps the most important severe cutaneous reactions, has been quantified in an international case control study and case series. Sulfonamide antibiotics, allopurinol, amine antiepileptic drugs (phenytoin and carbamazepine), lamotrigine, and the oxicam nonsteroidal anti-inflammatory drugs (NSAIDs) are associated with the highest risk of these reactions.

PATHOGENESIS OF DRUG REACTIONS

Untoward cutaneous responses to drugs can arise as a result of immunologic or nonimmunologic mechanisms. Immunologic reactions require activation of host immunologic pathways and are designated *drug allergy*. Drug reactions occurring through nonimmunologic mechanisms may be due to activation of effector pathways, overdosage, cumulative toxicity, side effects, ecologic disturbance, interactions between drugs, metabolic alterations, exacerbation of preexisting dermatologic conditions, or inherited protein or enzyme deficiencies. It is often not possible to specify the responsible drug or pathogenic mechanism because the skin responds to a variety of stimuli through a limited number of reaction patterns. The mechanism of many drug reactions is unknown.

IMMUNOLOGIC DRUG REACTIONS Drugs frequently elicit an immune response, but only a small number of individuals experience clinical hypersensitivity reactions. For example, most patients exposed to penicillin develop demonstrable antibodies to penicillin but do not manifest drug reactions when exposed to penicillin. Multiple factors determine the capacity of a drug to elicit an immune response, including the molecular characteristics of the drug and host effects.

Increases in *molecular* size and complexity are associated with increased immunogenicity, and macromolecular drugs such as protein or peptide hormones are highly antigenic. Most drugs are small organic molecules <1000 Da in size, and the capacity of such small molecules to elicit an immune response depends on their ability to act as haptens, i.e., to form stable, usually covalent, bonds with tissue macromolecules, an extremely rare event.

Route of administration of a drug or simple chemical can influence the nature of the *host* immune response. For example, topical application of antigens tends to induce delayed hypersensitivity, and exposure to antigens via oral or nasal cavities stimulates production of secretory immunoglobins, IgA and IgE, and occasionally IgM. Frequency of sensitization through intravenous administration of drugs varies, but anaphylaxis is a more likely consequence with this route of exposure than following oral administration.

The degree of drug exposure and individual variability in absorption and metabolism of a given agent may alter immunogenic load. The variable degree of in vivo acetylation of hydralazine provides a

TABLE 50-1 *Cutaneous Reactions to Drugs Received by at Least 1000 Patients (BCDSP)[a]*

Drug	Reactions, No.	Recipients, No.	Rate, %	95% Confidence Interval
Amoxicillin	63	1225	5.1	3.9–6.4
Ampicillin	215	4763	4.5	3.9–5.1
Co-trimoxazole	46	1235	3.7	2.7–4.8
Semisynthetic penicillins	41	1436	2.9	2.0–3.7
Red blood cells	67	3386	2.0	1.5–2.4
Penicillin G	68	4204	1.6	1.2–2.0
Cephalosporins	27	1781	1.5	0.9–2.1
Gentamicin	13	1277	1.0	0.5–1.6

[a] BCDSP, Boston Collaborative Drug Surveillance Program.
Source: Adapted from Bigby.

clinical example of this phenomenon. Hydralazine produces a lupus-like syndrome associated with antinuclear antibody formation more frequently in patients who acetylate the drug slowly. Frequent high-dose and interrupted courses of therapy are also important risk factors for development of drug allergy.

Pathogenesis of Allergic Drug Reactions ■ *IGE-DEPENDENT REACTIONS* IgE-dependent drug reactions are usually manifest in the skin and gastrointestinal, respiratory, and cardiovascular systems (Chap. 298). Primary symptoms and signs include pruritus, urticaria, nausea, vomiting, cramps, bronchospasm, and laryngeal edema and, on occasion, anaphylactic shock with hypotension and death. Immediate reactions may occur within minutes of drug exposure, and accelerated reactions occur hours or days after drug administration. Accelerated reactions are usually urticarial and may include laryngeal edema. Penicillin and related drugs are the most frequent causes of IgE-dependent reactions. Release of chemical mediators such as histamine, adenosine, leukotrienes, prostaglandins, platelet-activating factor, enzymes, and proteoglycans from sensitized tissue, mast cells, or circulating basophilic leukocytes results in vasodilation and edema. Release is triggered when polyvalent drug protein conjugates cross-link IgE molecules fixed to sensitized cells. The clinical manifestations are determined by interaction of the released chemical mediator with its target organ, i.e., skin, respiratory, gastrointestinal, and/or cardiovascular systems. Certain routes of administration favor different clinical patterns (i.e., oral route: gastrointestinal effects; intravenous route: circulatory effects).

IMMUNE-COMPLEX–DEPENDENT REACTIONS Serum sickness is produced by circulating immune complexes and is characterized by fever, arthritis, nephritis, neuritis, edema, and an urticarial, papular, or purpuric rash (Chap. 306). The syndrome requires an antigen that remains in the circulation for prolonged periods so that when antibody is synthesized, circulating antigen-antibody complexes are formed. Serum sickness was first described following administration of foreign sera, but drugs are now the usual cause. Drugs that produce serum sickness include the penicillins, sulfonamides, thiouracils, cholecystographic dyes, phenytoin, aminosalicylic acid, heparin, and antilymphocyte globulin. Cephalosporin administration in febrile children is associated with a high risk of a clinically similar reaction, but the mechanism of this reaction is unknown. In classic serum sickness, symptoms develop 6 days or more after exposure to a drug, the latent period representing the time needed to synthesize antibody. The antibodies responsible for immune-complex–dependent drug reactions are largely of the IgG or IgM class. Vasculitis, a relatively rare cutaneous complication of drugs, may also be a result of immune complex deposition (Chap. 306).

CYTOTOXICITY AND DELAYED HYPERSENSITIVITY Cytotoxicity and delayed hypersensitivity mechanisms may be important in the etiology of morbilliform exanthema, hypersensitivity syndrome, SJS, or TEN, but this is not proven. Systemic manifestations occur frequently. The antigen may be the drug or its metabolites, and it is likely that different T lymphocyte populations are activated. T_H1 type cells will lead to the production of interleukin (IL)-2 and interferon (IFN)-γ and subsequent activation of cytotoxic T cells. In early lesions of morbilliform exanthema or TEN, histopathologic studies have shown expression of HLA-DR and intercellular adhesion molecule (ICAM)-1 by keratinocytes, CD4 cells (in the dermis), and CD8 T cells (in the epidermis) and apoptosis of keratinocytes (facilitated by tumor necrosis factor α, perforin, and granzyme secretion, and *fas*-ligand expression). T_H2 type cells produce cytokines such as IL-5 and eotaxin, which may be involved in hypersensitivity syndrome (see below).

NONIMMUNOLOGIC DRUG REACTIONS Nonimmunologic mechanisms are responsible for the majority of drug reactions; however, only the most important mechanisms will be discussed.

Nonimmunologic Activation of Effector Pathways Drug reactions may result from nonimmunologic activation of effector pathways by three mechanisms: First, drugs may release mediators directly from mast cells and basophils and present as anaphylaxis, urticaria, and/or angio-

edema. Urticarial anaphylactic reactions induced by opiates, polymyxin B, tubocurarine, radiocontrast media, and dextrans may occur by this mechanism. Second, drugs may activate complement in the absence of antibody. This is an additional mechanism through which radiocontrast media may act. Third, drugs such as aspirin and other NSAIDs may alter pathways of arachidonic acid metabolism and induce urticaria.

Phototoxicity Phototoxic reactions may be drug-induced or may occur in metabolic disorders in which a photosensitizing chemical is overproduced. A phototoxic reaction occurs when enough chromophore (drug or metabolic product) absorbs sufficient radiation to cause a reaction or interaction with target tissue. Drug-induced phototoxic reactions can occur on first exposure. Phototoxic injury is usually manifest as a photodistributed dermatitis.

Exacerbation of Preexisting Diseases A variety of agents can exacerbate preexisting diseases. For example, lithium can exacerbate acne and psoriasis in a dose-dependent manner. Beta-blocking agents and IFN-α may induce psoriasis. Withdrawal of glucocorticoids can exacerbate psoriasis or atopic dermatitis.

Inherited Enzyme or Protein Deficiencies Specific genetically determined defects in the ability of an individual to detoxify toxic reactive drug metabolites may predispose such individuals to the development of severe drug reactions, especially hypersensitivity syndrome, and perhaps TEN associated with use of sulfonamides and anticonvulsants. However, in a prospective cohort of 136 HIV-infected patients treated with sulfonamides, no association of drug eruption with acetylation genotype or glutathione levels was found.

Alterations of Immunologic Status Alterations in patients' immunologic status may also modify the risk of cutaneous reactions. Bone marrow transplant patients, HIV-infected persons, and persons with Epstein-Barr virus infection are at higher risk of developing cutaneous reactions to drugs. Skin reactions to trimethoprim-sulfamethoxazole are seen in about a third of HIV-infected users of this drug, but desensitization can be accomplished. Dapsone, trimethoprim alone, and amoxicillin-clavulanate are also frequent causes of drug eruptions in HIV-infected patients. The advent of highly active antiretroviral therapy (HAART) may have decreased the risk of cutaneous reactions in HIV patients (Chap. 173).

A CLINICAL CLASSIFICATION OF CUTANEOUS DRUG REACTIONS

URTICARIA/ANGIOEDEMA *Urticaria* is a skin reaction characterized by pruritic, red wheals. Lesions may vary from a small point to a large area. Individual lesions rarely last more than 24 h. When deep dermal and subcutaneous tissues are also swollen, this reaction is known as *angioedema*. Angioedema may involve mucous membranes and may be part of a life-threatening anaphylactic reaction. Urticarial lesions, along with pruritus and morbilliform (or maculopapular) eruptions, are among the most frequent types of cutaneous reactions to drugs.

Drug-induced urticaria may be caused by three mechanisms: an IgE-dependent mechanism, circulating immune complexes (serum sickness), and nonimmunologic activation of effector pathways. IgE-dependent urticarial reactions usually occur within 36 h but can occur within minutes. Reactions occurring within minutes to hours of drug exposure are termed *immediate reactions*, whereas those that occur 12 to 36 h after drug exposure are designated *accelerated reactions*. Immune-complex–induced urticaria associated with serum sickness usually occurs from 6 to 12 days after first exposure. In this syndrome, the urticarial eruption may be accompanied by fever, hematuria, arthralgias, hepatic dysfunction, and neurologic symptoms.

Certain drugs, such as NSAIDs, angiotensin-converting enzyme (ACE) inhibitors, and radiographic dyes, may induce urticarial reactions, angioedema, and anaphylaxis in the absence of drug-specific antibody. Although ACE inhibitors, aspirin, penicillin, and blood products are the most frequent causes of urticarial eruptions, urticaria has been observed in association with nearly all drugs. Drugs may also cause chronic urticaria, which lasts more than 6 weeks. Aspirin frequently exacerbates this problem.

The treatment of urticaria or angioedema depends on the severity of the reaction and the rate at which it is evolving. In severe cases, especially with respiratory or cardiovascular compromise, epinephrine is the mainstay of therapy, but its effect is reduced in patients using beta blockers. For more seriously affected patients, treatment with systemic glucocorticoids, sometimes intravenously administered, are helpful. In addition to drug withdrawal, for patients with only cutaneous symptoms and without symptoms of angioedema or anaphylaxis, oral antihistamines are usually sufficient.

PHOTOSENSITIVITY ERUPTIONS Photosensitivity eruptions are usually most marked in sun-exposed areas but may extend to sun-protected areas. The mechanism of photosensitivity eruptions is almost always phototoxicity. Phototoxic reactions are also most marked in sun-exposed areas, resemble sunburn, and can occur with first exposure to a drug. Their severity depends on the tissue level of the drug, the extent of exposure to light, and the efficiency of the photosensitizer (Chap. 51).

Common orally administered photosensitizing drugs include many fluoroquinolones and doxycycline. Other drugs less frequently encountered are chlorpromazine, other tetracyclines, thiazides, and at least two NSAIDs (ibuprofen and naproxen). The majority of the common photosensitizing drugs have action spectrums in the long-wave ultraviolet A (UV-A) range. Photosensitive reactions abate with removal of either the drug or ultraviolet radiation. Because UV-A and visible light, which trigger these reactions, are not easily absorbed by nonopaque sunscreens and are transmitted through window glass, these reactions may be difficult to block.

Photosensitivity reactions are treated by avoiding exposure to ultraviolet light (sunlight), use of high-potency sunscreens which block UV-A light, and treating the reaction as one would a sunburn. Rarely, individuals develop persistent reactivity to light, necessitating long-term avoidance of sun exposure.

PIGMENTATION CHANGES Drugs, either systemic or topical, may cause a variety of pigmentary changes in the skin. Oral contraceptives may induce melasma. Long-term minocycline or perfloxacin may cause blue-gray pigmentation, while amiodarone causes a more purple coloration. Long-term high-dose phenothiazine results in gray-brown pigmentation of sun-exposed areas. Numerous cancer chemotherapeutic agents may be associated with pigmentation. Bleomycin, busulphan, daunorubicin, cyclophosphamide, hydroxyurea, and methotrexate pigmentation changes may also occur in mucous membranes (busulphan), nails (zidovudine), hair, and teeth. Gold may cause blue-gray pigmentation in light-exposed areas.

VASCULITIS Cutaneous necrotizing vasculitis often presents as palpable purpuric lesions that may be generalized or limited to the lower extremities or other dependent areas (Chap. 306). Urticarial lesions, ulcers, and hemorrhagic blisters also occur. Vasculitis may involve other organs, including the liver, kidney, brain, and joints. Drugs are only one cause of vasculitis, with infection and collagen vascular disease responsible for the majority of cases.

Propylthiouracil induces a cutaneous vasculitis that is accompanied by leukopenia and splenomegaly. Direct immunofluorescent changes in these lesions suggest immune-complex deposition. Drugs implicated in vasculitic eruptions include allopurinol, thiazides, sulfonamides, penicillin, and some NSAIDs.

HYPERSENSITIVITY SYNDROME Initially described with phenytoin, hypersensitivity syndrome presents as an erythematous eruption that may become purpuric or lichenoid and is accompanied by many of the following features: fever, facial and periorbital edema, tender generalized lymphadenopathy, leukocytosis (often with atypical lymphocytes and eosinophils), hepatitis, and sometimes nephritis or pneu-

monitis. The cutaneous reaction usually begins 2 to 8 weeks after the drug is begun and may resolve with drug cessation. However, symptoms may persist for several weeks, especially hepatitis. With phenytoin, an increased risk of this syndrome is associated with an inherited deficiency of epoxide hydrolase, an enzyme required for metabolism of a toxic intermediate arene oxide that is formed during metabolism of phenytoin by the cytochrome P450 system. This explains why the eruption recurs with rechallenge, and cross-reactions among aromatic anticonvulsants, including phenytoin, carbamazepine, and barbiturates, are frequent. The role of human herpes virus (HHV)-6 infection is still unclear. Other drugs causing this syndrome include lamotrigine, minocycline, dapsone, allopurinol, sulfonamides, and abacavir and zalcitabine in HIV-infected patients. Mortality as high as 10% has been reported. In life-threatening situations such as hepatitis, systemic glucocorticoids (prednisone, 0.5 to 1.0 mg/kg) seems to reduce symptoms. Topical high-potency glucocorticoids may be helpful too. In all cases, urgent withdrawal of the suspected drug is required.

WARFARIN NECROSIS OF THE SKIN This rare reaction occurs usually between the third and tenth days of therapy with warfarin derivatives, usually in women. Lesions are sharply demarcated, erythematous, indurated, and purpuric and may resolve or progress to form large, irregular, hemorrhagic bullae with eventual necrosis and slow-healing eschar formation.

Development of the syndrome is unrelated to drug dose or underlying condition. Favored sites are breasts, thighs, and buttocks. The course is not altered by discontinuation of the drug after onset of the eruption. Similar reactions have been associated with heparin. Warfarin reactions are associated with protein C deficiency. Protein C is a vitamin K–dependent protein with a shorter half-life than other clotting proteins and is in part responsible for control of fibrinolysis. Since warfarin inhibits synthesis of vitamin K–dependent coagulation factors, warfarin anticoagulation in heterozygotes for protein C deficiency causes a precipitous fall in circulating levels of protein C, permitting hypercoagulability and thrombosis in the cutaneous microvasculature, with consequent areas of necrosis. Heparin-induced necrosis may have clinically similar features but is probably due to heparin-induced platelet aggregation with subsequent occlusion of blood vessels.

Warfarin-induced cutaneous necrosis is treated with vitamin K and heparin. Vitamin K reverses the effects of warfarin, and heparin acts as an anticoagulant. Treatment with protein C concentrates may also be helpful in individuals with deficiencies of protein C, the predisposing factor for development of these reactions.

MORBILLIFORM REACTIONS Morbilliform or maculopapular eruptions are the most common of all drug-induced reactions, often start on the trunk or areas of pressure or trauma, and consist of erythematous macules and papules that are frequently symmetric and may become confluent. Involvement of mucous membranes, palms, and soles is variable; the eruption may be associated with moderate to severe pruritus and fever.

The pathogenesis is unclear. A hypersensitivity mechanism has been suggested, although these reactions do not always recur following drug rechallenge. Diagnosis is rarely assisted by laboratory or patch testing; differentiation from viral exanthem is the principal differential diagnostic consideration. Unless the suspect drug is essential it should be discontinued. Occasionally these eruptions may decrease or fade with continued use of the responsible drug.

Morbilliform reactions usually develop within 1 week of initiation of therapy and last 1 to 2 weeks; however, reactions to some drugs, especially penicillin and drugs with long half-lives, may begin more than 2 weeks after therapy has begun and last as long as 2 weeks after therapy has ceased.

Morbilliform eruptions are usually treated by discontinuing the suspect medications symptomatically. Oral antihistamines, emollients, and soothing baths are useful for treatment of pruritus. Short courses of potent topical glucocorticoids can reduce inflammation and symptoms and are probably helpful. Systemic glucocorticoid treatment is rarely indicated.

FIXED DRUG REACTIONS These reactions are characterized by one or more sharply demarcated, erythematous lesions in which hyperpigmentation results after resolution of the acute inflammation; with rechallenge, the lesion recurs in the same (i.e., "fixed") location. Lesions often involve the lips, hands, legs, face, genitalia, and oral mucosa and cause burning. Most patients have multiple lesions. Patch testing is useful to establish the etiology. Fixed drug eruptions have been associated with phenolphthalein, sulfonamides, tetracyclines, phenylbutazone, NSAIDs, and barbiturates. Although cross-sensitivity appears to occur between different tetracycline compounds, cross-sensitivity was not elicited when different sulfonamide compounds were administered to patients as part of provocation testing.

LICHENOID DRUG ERUPTIONS A lichenoid cutaneous reaction, clinically and morphologically indistinguishable from lichen planus, is associated with a variety of drugs and chemicals. Eosinophils are more common when the reaction is drug-induced. Gold and antimalarials are most often associated with this eruption. Sulfomamides, thiazides, and antihypertensive agents, including beta blockers and captopril, have also been reported to cause lichenoid reactions.

PUSTULAR ERUPTIONS Acute generalized exanthematous pustulosis (AGEP) is often associated with exposure to drugs, most notably antibiotics. Usually beginning on the face or intertriginous areas, small nonfollicular pustules overlying erythematous and edematous skin may coalesce and lead to superficial ulceration. Fever is present, and differentiating this eruption from TEN in its initial stages may be difficult. AGEP often begins within a few days of initiating drug treatment.

STEVENS-JOHNSON SYNDROME AND TOXIC EPIDERMAL NECROLYSIS SJS and TEN are terms that, most believe, describe the same drug-induced disorder, which is characterized by blisters and epidermal detachment resulting from epidermal necrosis in the absence of substantial dermal inflammation. The term *SJS* is now used to describe patients with blisters developing on dusky or purpuric macules in which total percent body surface area blistering and eventual detachment is <10%. The term *SJS/TEN* is used to describe patients with 10 to 30% detachment, and *TEN* is used to describe patients with >30% detachment. Erythema multiforme (EM) is a third term which, in the past, was used to describe patients now designated as having SJS. EM is now used by most to describe patients with typical "target" lesions resulting as a reaction to infection, most commonly from herpes simplex virus.

SJS, SJS/TEN, and TEN patients initially present with acute symptoms, painful skin lesions, fever >39°C (102.2°F), sore throat, and visual impairment resulting from mucous membrane and ocular lesions. Intestinal and pulmonary involvement are associated with a poor prognosis, as are a greater extent of epidermal detachment and older age. About 5% of SJS and 30% of TEN affected persons die from their disease. Drugs that most commonly cause SJS, SJS/TEN, or TEN are sulfonamides, lamotrigine, aromatic anticonvulsants, and oxicam NSAIDs. Many treatments affecting immune responses or cytokines have been advocated, but none have been shown to be efficacious in well-controlled trials. Because drug-induced epidermal apoptosis has been proposed as a possible pathogenesis, intravenous immunoglobulin (IVIG) has been used recently by some with success in the absence of side effects or additional toxicity. At this time, the best results come from early diagnosis, immediate discontinuation of any suspected drug, and supportive therapy, paying close attention to ocular complications, often in burn units or intensive care units.

DRUGS OF SPECIAL INTEREST

PENICILLIN The incidence of cutaneous reactions to penicillin is about 1%. About 85% of cutaneous reactions to penicillin are morbilliform, and about 10% are urticaria or angioedema.

IgG, IgM, and IgE antibodies can be produced; IgG and IgM antipenicillin antibodies play a role in the development of hemolytic anemia, whereas anaphylaxis and serum sickness appear to be due to IgE antibodies in serum.

In patients with suspected IgE-mediated reactions to penicillin for whom future treatment is anticipated, accurate tests for sensitization are available. Current practice is to perform skin testing with a commercially available penicilloyl determinant preparation (Pre-pen, Kremers-Urban) and with fresh penicillin and, if possible, with another source of minor (nonpenicilloyl) determinants such as aged or base-treated penicillin. Antibodies to minor determinants are common in patients experiencing anaphylaxis, but testing with major determinants alone detects most patients at risk for anaphylaxis.

About one-fourth of patients with positive history of penicillin allergy have a positive skin test, while 6% (3 to 10%) with no history of penicillin sensitivity demonstrate a positive skin response to penicillin. Administering penicillin to those patients with a positive skin test produces reactions in a high proportion (50 to 100%); conversely, only a few patients (0.5%) with a negative skin test react to the drug, and reactions tend to be mild and to occur late. Since a false-negative skin test may occur during or just after an acute reaction, testing should be performed either prospectively or several months after a suspected reaction. As many as 80% of patients lose anaphylactic sensitivity and IgE antibody after several years. Radioallergosorbent tests and other in vitro tests offer no advantage over properly performed skin testing. Some cross-reactivity between penicillin and nonpenicillin β-lactam antibiotics (e.g., cephalosporins) occurs, but the majority of penicillin-allergic patients will tolerate cephalosporins. Persons who have negative skin tests to penicillin rarely develop reactions to cephalosporins.

In the face of a positive clinical history of penicillin reaction, another drug should be chosen. If this is not feasible or prudent (e.g., in a pregnant patient with syphilis or with enterococcal endocarditis), skin testing with penicillin is warranted. If skin tests are negative, cautious administration of penicillin is acceptable, although some recommend desensitization of such patients if the reaction was likely to be IgE-mediated. In those with positive skin tests, desensitization is mandatory if therapeutic use of β-lactam antibiotics is to be undertaken. Various protocols are available, including oral and parenteral approaches. Oral desensitization appears to have lower risk of serious anaphylactic reactions during desensitization. However, desensitization carries the risk of anaphylaxis regardless of how it is performed. After desensitization, many patients experience non-life-threatening IgE-mediated untoward reactions to penicillin during their course of therapy. Desensitization is not effective in those with exfoliative dermatitis or morbilliform reactions due to penicillin.

NONSTEROIDAL ANTI-INFLAMMATORY DRUGS NSAIDs, including aspirin and indomethacin (indometacin), cause two broad categories of allergic-like symptoms in susceptible individuals: (1) approximately 1% of persons experience urticaria or angioedema, and (2) about half as many (0.5%) experience rhinosinusitis and asthma; however, about 10% of adults with asthma and one-third of individuals with nasal polyposis and sinusitis may respond adversely to aspirin.

Urticaria/angioedema may be delayed up to 24 h and may occur at any age. The rhinosinusitis-asthma syndrome generally develops within 1 h of drug administration. In young patients, the reaction pattern often begins as watery rhinorrhea, which can be complicated by nasal and sinus infection, and polyposis, bloody discharge, and nasal eosinophilia. In many individuals with this syndrome, asthma that can be life-threatening eventually ensues whenever NSAIDs are subsequently ingested, and symptoms may persist despite avoidance of these drugs. Proof of the association of symptoms and NSAID use requires either clear-cut history of symptoms following drug ingestion or an oral challenge. For the latter to be performed with relative safety, (1) asthma must be under good control, (2) the procedure must be conducted in a hospital setting by experienced personnel capable of recognizing and treating acute respiratory responses, and (3) the challenge should begin with very low doses (i.e., not >30 mg) of aspirin and increase every 1 to 2 h in doubling doses as tolerated to 650 mg.

While cross-reactivity between NSAIDs is common, it is not immunologic, and patients who are sensitive to NSAIDs cannot be identified by assessment of IgE antibody to aspirin, lymphocyte sensitization, or in vitro immunologic testing.

RADIOCONTRAST MEDIA   Large numbers of patients are exposed to radiocontrast agents. High-osmolality radiocontrast media are about five times more likely to induce urticaria (1%) or anaphylaxis than newer low-osmolality media. Severe reactions are rare with either type of contrast media. About one-third of those with mild reactions to previous exposure rereact on reexposure. In most cases, these reactions are probably not immunologic. Pretreatment with prednisone and diphenhydramine reduces reaction rates. Persons with a reaction to a high-osmolality contrast media should be given low-osmolality media if later contrast studies are required.

ANTICONVULSANTS   Of the anticonvulsants, the single orally administered agent with the highest risk of severe adverse cutaneous reactions is the antiseizure medicine lamotrigine. Older anticonvulsants, including phenytoin and carbamazepine, are also associated with many types of severe reactions and a high incidence of less severe reactions, particularly in children. In addition to SJS, TEN, and the hypersensitivity syndrome discussed above, the aromatic anticonvulsants can induce a pseudolymphoma syndrome and induce gingival hyperplasia.

SULFONAMIDES   Sulfonamides have perhaps the highest risk of causing cutaneous eruptions and are the drugs most frequently implicated in SJS and TEN. The combination of sulfamethoxazole and trimethoprim frequently induces adverse cutaneous reactions in patients with AIDS (Chap. 173). Desensitization is often successful in AIDS patients with morbilliform eruptions but does not work in AIDS patients who manifest erythroderma, fever, or a bullous reaction in response to their earlier sulfonamide exposure.

VANCOMYCIN   Vancomycin causes two unusual but recognizable cutaneous reactions: Linear IgA bullous dermatosis and "red man syndrome." The first is an autoimmune disorder characterized by pruritic vesiculobullous skin lesions favoring the trunk, proximal extremities, and acral region. When the syndrome is drug-induced, most cases have been associated with vancomycin, but a variety of other drugs have been reported to cause the same clinical picture.

The red man syndrome occurs during rapid intravenous infusion of vancomycin. This is thought to be a histamine-related anaphylactoid reaction characterized by flushing, diffuse maculopapular eruption, hypotension, and, in rare cases, cardiac arrest.

AGENTS USED IN CANCER CHEMOTHERAPY   Since many agents used in cancer chemotherapy inhibit cell division, rapidly proliferating elements of the skin, including hair, mucous membranes, and appendages, are sensitive to their effects; as a result, stomatitis and alopecia are among the most frequent dose-dependent side effects of chemotherapy. Various nail abnormalities have been described: onycholysis, dystrophy, Beau's lines, white lines, and pigmentation. Sterile cellulitis and phlebitis and ulceration of pressure areas occur with many of these agents. Also reported is acral erythema, which begins with dysesthesia followed by redness and a painful edematous eruption of the palms and soles; it is caused by cytarabin, doxorubicin, methotrexate, and 5-fluorouracil. Urticaria, angioedema, and exfoliative dermatitis have also been seen, as has local and diffuse hyperpigmentation.

GLUCOCORTICOIDS   Both systemic and topical glucocorticoids cause a variety of skin changes, including acneiform eruptions, atrophy, striae, and other stigmata of Cushing's syndrome, and in sufficiently high doses can retard wound healing. Patients using glucocorticoids are at higher risk for bacterial, yeast, and fungal skin infections that may be misinterpreted as drug eruptions but are instead drug side effects.

CYTOKINE THERAPY   Alopecia is a common complication of IFN-α. Induction or exacerbation of various immune-mediated disorders (psoriasis, lichen planus, lupus erythematosus) has been also reported with this agent. IFN-β injection has been associated with local necrosis of the skin. Granulocyte colony-stimulating factor may induce various neutrophilic dermatosis, including Sweet's syndrome, pyoderma gangrenosum, neutrophilic eccrine hidradenitis, and vasculitis, and can exacerbate psoriasis.

IL-2 is associated with frequent cutaneous reactions including exanthema, facial edema, xerosis, and pruritus. Cases of pemphigus vulgaris, linear IgA disease, psoriasis, and vitiligo have also been described in association with this drug.

ANTIMALARIAL AGENTS   Antimalarial agents are used as therapy for several skin diseases, including the skin manifestations of lupus and polymorphous light eruption, but they can also induce cutaneous reactions. Although also used to treat porphyria cutanea tarda at low doses, in patients with asymptomatic porphyria cutanea tarda, higher doses of chloroquine increase porphyrin levels to such an extent that they may exacerbate the disease.

Pigmentation disturbances, including black pigmentation of the face, mucous membranes, and pretibial and subungual areas, occur with antimalarials. Quinacrine (mepacrine) causes generalized, cutaneous yellow discoloration.

GOLD   Chrysotherapy has been associated with a variety of dose-related dermatologic reactions (including maculopapular eruptions), which can develop as long as 2 years after initiation of therapy and require months to resolve. Erythema nodosum, psoriasiform dermatitis, vaginal pruritus, eruptions similar to those of pityriasis rosea, hyperpigmentation, and lichenoid eruptions resembling those seen with antimalarial agents have been reported. After a cutaneous reaction, it is sometimes possible to reinstitute gold therapy at lower doses without recurrence of the dermatitis.

DIAGNOSIS OF DRUG REACTIONS

Possible causes of an adverse reaction can be assessed as definite, probable, possible, or unlikely based on six variables: (1) previous experience with the drug in the general population, (2) alternative etiologic candidates, (3) timing of events, (4) drug levels or evidence of overdose, (5) patient reaction to drug discontinuation, and (6) patient reaction to rechallenge.

PREVIOUS EXPERIENCE   Tables of relative reaction rates are available and are useful to assess the likelihood that a given drug is responsible for a given cutaneous reaction. The specific morphologic pattern of a drug reaction, however, may modify these reaction rates by increasing or decreasing the likelihood that a given drug is responsible for a given reaction. For example, since fixed eruptions due to drugs are more often seen with barbiturates than with penicillin, a fixed drug reaction in a patient taking both types of agents is more likely to be due to the barbiturate, even though penicillins have a higher overall drug reaction rate.

ALTERNATIVE ETIOLOGIC CANDIDATES   A cutaneous eruption may be due to exacerbation of preexisting disease or to development of new disease unrelated to drugs. For example, a patient with psoriasis may have a flare-up of disease coincidental with administration of penicillin for streptococcal infection; in this case, infection is a more likely cause for the flare-up than drug reaction.

TIMING OF EVENTS   Most drug reactions of the skin occur within 1 to 2 weeks of initiation of therapy. Hypersensitivity syndrome may occur later (up to 8 weeks) after initiating drug therapy. Fixed drug reactions and generalized exanthematous pustulosis often occur earlier (within 48 h), as do reactions of all types in persons with prior sensitization to that drug or a cross-sensitizing agent.

DRUG LEVELS   Some cutaneous reactions are dependent on dosage or cumulative toxicity. For example, lichenoid dermatoses due to gold administration appear more often in patients taking high doses.

DISCONTINUATION   Most adverse cutaneous reactions to drugs remit with discontinuation of the suspected agent. A reaction is considered unlikely to be drug-related if improvement occurs while the drug is

TABLE 50-2 *Clinical and Laboratory Findings Associated with More Serious Drug-Induced Cutaneous Clinical Findings*

Cutaneous
  Confluent erythema
  Facial edema or central facial involvement
  Skin pain
  Palpable purpura
  Skin necrosis
  Blisters or epidermal detachment
  Positive Nikolsky's sign
  Mucous membrane erosions
  Urticaria
  Swelling of tongue

General
  High fever [temperature >40°C (>104°F)]
  Enlarged lymph nodes
  Arthralgias or arthritis
  Shortness of breath, wheezing, hypotension

Laboratory results
  Eosinophil count >1000/μL
  Lymphocytosis with atypical lymphocytes
  Abnormal liver function tests

Source: Adapted from Roujeau and Stern.

continued or if a patient fails to improve after stopping the drug and appropriate therapy.

RECHALLENGE Rechallenge provides the most definitive information concerning adverse cutaneous reactions to drugs, since a reaction failing to recur on rechallenge with a drug is unlikely to be due to that agent. Rechallenge is usually impractical, however, because the need to ensure patient safety and comfort outweighs the value of the possible information derived from rechallenge.

Of special importance is the rapid recognition of reactions that may become serious or life-threatening. Table 50-2 lists clinical and laboratory features that, if present, suggest the reaction may be serious. Table 50-3 provides key features of the most serious adverse cutaneous reactions.

DIAGNOSIS OF DRUG ALLERGY

Tests for IgE responses include in vivo and in vitro methods, but such tests are available for only a limited number of drugs, including penicillins and cephalosporins, some peptide and protein drugs (insulin, xenogeneic sera), and some agents used for general anesthesia. In vivo testing is accomplished by prick puncture and/or by intradermal skin testing. A wheal-and-flare response 2 × 2 mm greater than that seen with a saline control within 20 min is considered indicative of IgE-mediated mast cell degranulation, provided (1) the patient is not dermographic, (2) the drug does not nonspecifically degranulate mast cells, (3) the drug concentration is not high enough to be irritating, and (4) the buffer itself does not cause wheal-and-flare responses.

Skin testing with major and minor determinants of penicillins or cephalosporins has proved useful for identifying patients at risk of anaphylactic reactions to these agents. However, skin tests themselves carry a small risk of anaphylaxis. Negative skin tests do not rule out IgE-mediated reactivity, and the risk of anaphylaxis in response to

TABLE 50-3 *Clinical Features of Selected Severe Cutaneous Reactions Often Induced by Drugs*

Diagnosis	Mucosal Lesions	Typical Skin Lesions	Frequent Signs and Symptoms	Alternative Causes not Related to Drugs
Stevens-Johnson syndrome	Erosions usually at ≥two sites	Small blisters on dusky purpuric macules or atypical targets; rare areas of confluence; detachment ≤10% of body surface area	10–30% of cases involve fever	
Toxic epidermal necrolysis[a]	Erosions usually at ≥two sites	Individual lesions like those seen in Stevens-Johnson syndrome; confluent erythema; outer layer of epidermis separates readily from basal layer with lateral pressure; large sheet of necrotic epidermis; total detachment of >30% of body surface area	Nearly all cases involve fever, "acute skin failure," leukopenia	
Hypersensitivity syndrome	Infrequent	Severe exanthematous rash (may become purpuric), exfoliative dermatitis	30–50% of cases involve fever, lymphadenopathy, hepatitis, nephritis, carditis, eosinophilia, atypical lymphocytes	Cutaneous lymphoma
Acute generalized exanthematous pustulosis	About 50% erosions mouth, tongue	Initially nonfollicular small pustules overlying edematous erythema, sometimes leading to superficial ulcers	Fever, burning, pruritus, facial swelling, leukocytosis, hypocalcemia	Infection
Serum sickness or reactions resembling serum sickness	Absent	Morbilliform lesions, sometimes with urticaria	Fever, arthralgias	Infection
Anticoagulant-induced necrosis	Infrequent	Erythema then purpura and necrosis, especially of fatty areas	Pain in affected areas	Disseminated intravascular coagulopathy, septicemia
Angioedema	Often involved	Urticaria or swelling of central part of face	Respiratory distress, cardiovascular collapse	Insect stings, foods

[a] Overlap of Stevens-Johnson syndrome and toxic epidermal necrolysis with features of both and attachment of 10 to 30% of body surface area may occur.

Source: Adapted from Roujeau and Stern.

penicillin administration in patients with negative skin tests is about 1%; about two-thirds of patients with a positive skin test and history of a previous adverse reaction to penicillin experience an allergic response on rechallenge. Skin tests may be negative in allergic patients receiving antihistamines or in those whose allergy is to determinants not present in the test reagent. Although less well studied, similar techniques can identify patients who are sensitive to protein drugs and to agents such as gallamine and succinylcholine. Most other drugs are small molecules, and skin testing with them is unreliable.

There are no generally available and reliable tests for assessing causality of non-IgE-mediated reactions, except possibly patch tests for assessment of fixed drug reactions. Therefore, diagnosis usually relies on clinical factors rather than test results.

FURTHER READING

BIGBY M: Rates of cutaneous reactions to drugs. Arch Dermatol 137:765, 2001

BREATHNACH SM: Adverse cutaneous reactions to drugs. Clin Med 2:15, 2002

ROUJEAU JC, STERN RS: Severe adverse cutaneous reactions to drugs. N Engl J Med 331:1272, 1994

——— et al: Medication use and the risk of Stevens-Johnson syndrome or toxic epidermal necrolysis. N Engl J Med 333:1600, 1995

VAN DER LINDEN PD et al: Skin reactions to antibacterial agents in general practice. J Clin Epidemiol 51:703, 1998

WARD HA et al: Cutaneous manifestations of antiretroviral therapy. J Am Acad Dermatol 46:284, 2002

51 PHOTOSENSITIVITY AND OTHER REACTIONS TO LIGHT
David R. Bickers

SOLAR RADIATION Sunlight is the most visible and obvious source of comfort in the environment. The sun provides the beneficial effects of warmth and vitamin D synthesis; however, acute and chronic sun exposure also have pathologic consequences. Few effects of sun exposure beyond those affecting the skin have been identified, but cutaneous exposure to sunlight is the major cause of human skin cancer and can exert immunosuppressive effects as well.

The sun's energy reaching the earth's surface is limited to components of the ultraviolet (UV), the visible, and portions of the infrared spectra. The cutoff at the short end of the UV is at approximately 290 nm; this is due primarily to stratospheric ozone formed by highly energetic ionizing radiation, thereby preventing penetration to the earth's surface of the shorter, more energetic, potentially more harmful wavelengths of solar radiation. Indeed, concern about destruction of the ozone layer by chlorofluorocarbons released into the atmosphere has led to international agreements to reduce production of these chemicals.

Measurements of solar flux indicate that there is a twentyfold regional variation in the amount of energy at 300 nm that reaches the earth's surface. This variability relates to seasonal effects; the path of sunlight transmission through ozone and air; the altitude (4% increase for each 300 m of elevation); the latitude (increasing intensity with decreasing latitude); and the amount of cloud cover, fog, and pollution.

The major components of the photobiologic action spectrum capable of affecting human skin include the UV and visible wavelengths between 290 and 700 nm. In addition, the wavelengths beyond 700 nm in the infrared spectrum primarily emit heat and under certain circumstances may exacerbate the pathologic effects of energy in the UV and visible spectra.

The UV spectrum reaching the earth represents <10% of total incident solar energy and is arbitrarily divided into two major segments: UV-B, and UV-A. This includes the wavelengths between 290 and 400 nm. UV-B consists of wavelengths between 290 and 320 nm. This portion of the photobiologic action spectrum is the most efficient in producing redness or erythema in human skin and hence is sometimes known as the "sunburn spectrum." UV-A represents those wavelengths between 320 and 400 nm and is approximately 1000-fold less efficient in producing skin redness than is UV-B.

The wavelengths between 400 and 700 nm are visible to the human eye. The photon energy in the visible spectrum is not capable of damaging human skin in the absence of a photosensitizing chemical. Without the absorption of energy by a molecule there can be no photosensitivity. Thus the *absorption spectrum* of a molecule is defined as the range of wavelengths absorbed by it, whereas the *action spectrum* for an effect of incident radiation is defined as the range of wavelengths that evoke the response.

Photosensitivity occurs when a photon-absorbing chemical (chromophore) present in the skin absorbs incident energy, becomes excited, and transfers the absorbed energy to various structures or to oxygen.

UV RADIATION (UVR) AND SKIN STRUCTURE AND FUNCTION Skin consists of two major compartments: the outer epidermis, a stratified squamous epithelium, and the underlying dermis rich in matrix proteins such as collagen and elastin. Both of these compartments are susceptible to damage from sun exposure. The epidermis and the dermis contain several chromophores capable of absorbing incident solar energy including nucleic acids, proteins, and lipids. The outermost epidermal layer, the stratum corneum, is a major absorber of UV-B, and <10% of incident UV-B wavelengths penetrate through the epidermis to the dermis. Approximately 3% of radiation below 300 nm, 20% of radiation below 360 nm, and 33% of short visible radiation reaches the basal cell layer in untanned human skin. In contrast, UV-A readily penetrates to the dermis and is capable of altering structural and matrix proteins that contribute to the aged appearance of chronically sun-exposed skin, particularly in individuals of light complexion.

Epidermal DNA, predominantly in keratinocytes, absorbs UV-B and undergoes structural changes including the formation of cyclobutane dimers and 6,4-photoproducts. These structural changes are potentially mutagenic and can be repaired by mechanisms that result in their recognition and excision and the reestablishment of normal base sequences. The efficient repair of these structural aberrations is crucial, since individuals with defective DNA repair are at high risk for the development of cutaneous cancer. For example, patients with xeroderma pigmentosum (XP), an autosomal recessive disorder, are characterized by variably deficient repair of UV-induced photoproducts, and their skin phenotype often manifests the dry, leathery appearance of prematurely photoaged skin as well as basal cell and squamous cell carcinomas and melanoma in the first two decades of life. Studies in mice using knockout gene technology have verified the importance of functional genes regulating these repair pathways in preventing the development of UV-induced cancer. Furthermore, incorporation of a bacterial DNA repair enzyme, T4N5 endonuclease, into liposomes in a product applied to skin of patients with XP selectively removes cyclobutane pyrimidine dimers and reduces the degree of solar damage and skin cancer.

Cutaneous Optics and Chromophores Chromophores are endogenous or exogenous chemical components that can absorb physical energy. Endogenous chromophores are of two types: (1) chemicals that are normal components of skin, including nucleic acids, proteins, lipids, and 7-dehydrocholesterol, the precursor of vitamin D; and (2) chemicals, such as porphyrins, synthesized elsewhere in the body that circulate in the bloodstream and diffuse into the skin. Normally, only trace amounts of porphyrins are present in the skin, but in selected diseases known as the porphyrias (Chap. 337), increased amounts are released into the circulation from the bone marrow and the liver and are transported to the skin, where they absorb incident energy both in the Soret band, around 400 nm (short visible), and to a lesser extent in the red portion of the visible spectrum (580 to 660 nm). This results in the generation of reactive oxygen species that can mediate structural damage to the skin, manifest as erythema, edema, urticaria, or blister formation.

Acute Effects of Sun Exposure   The acute effects of skin exposure to sunlight include sunburn and vitamin D synthesis.

SUNBURN   This painful skin condition is caused predominantly by UV-B. Generally speaking, an individual's ability to tolerate sunlight is inversely proportional to the degree of melanin pigmentation. Melanin, a complex tyrosine polymer, is synthesized in specialized epidermal dendritic cells known as melanocytes and is packaged into *melanosomes* that are transferred via dendritic process into *keratinocytes*, thereby providing photoprotection and simultaneously darkening the skin. Sun-induced melanogenesis is a consequence of increased tyrosinase activity in melanocytes that in turn may be due to a combination of eicosanoid and endothelin-1 release. The Fitzpatrick classification of human skin is a function of the efficiency of the epidermal-melanin unit and can usually be ascertained by asking an individual two questions: (1) Do you burn after sun exposure? and (2) Do you tan after sun exposure? The answers to these questions permit division of the population into six skin types varying from type I (always burn, never tan) to type VI (never burn, always tan) (Table 51-1).

Sunburn is due to vasodilatation of dermal blood vessels. There is a lag in time between skin exposure to sunlight and the development of visible redness (usually 4 to 12 h), suggesting that an epidermal chromophore causes delayed production and/or release of vasoactive mediator(s), or cytokines, that diffuse to the dermal vasculature to evoke vasodilatation.

The action spectrum for sunburn erythema includes the UV-B and UV-A. Photons in the UV-B are at least 1000-fold more efficient than photons in the UV-A in evoking the response. However, UV-A may contribute to sunburn erythema at midday when much more UV-A than UV-B is present in the solar spectrum. UV-induced activation of nuclear factor-κB (NF-κB)-dependent gene transactivation can augment release of several proinflammatory cytokines including interleukin (IL) 1B, 1L-6, vascular endothelial growth factor, and tumor necrosis factor α. Local accumulation of these cytokines occurs in sunburned skin. It is of interest that nonsteroidal anti-inflammatory drugs can reduce sunburn erythema, perhaps by blocking I-κB kinase 2, the enzyme essential for nuclear translocation of cytosolic NF-κB.

VITAMIN D PHOTOCHEMISTRY   Cutaneous exposure to UV-B causes photolysis of epidermal 7-dehydrocholesterol converting it to pre-vitamin D$_3$, which then undergoes a temperature-dependent isomerization to form the stable hormone vitamin D$_3$. This compound then diffuses to the dermal vasculature and circulates systemically where it is converted to the functional hormone 1,25-dihydroxy vitamin D$_3$ [1,25(OH)$_2$D$_3$]. Vitamin D metabolites from the circulation or those produced in the skin itself can augment epidermal differentiation signaling. Aging substantially decreases the ability of human skin to photocatalytically produce vitamin D$_3$. This, coupled with the widespread use of sunscreens that filter out UV-B, has led to concern that vitamin D deficiency may become a significant clinical problem in the elderly. Nonetheless, at least one double-blind placebo-controlled trial has

shown that a broad-spectrum sunscreen applied topically for several months has no significant effect on measured plasma vitamin D metabolites.

Chronic Effects of Sun Exposure: Nonmalignant   The clinical features of photodamaged sun-exposed skin consist of wrinkling, blotchiness, and telangiectasia and a roughened, irregular, "weather-beaten" leathery appearance. Whether this photoaging represents accelerated chronologic aging or a separate and distinct process is not clear.

Within chronically sun-exposed epidermis, there is thickening (acanthosis) and morphologic heterogeneity within the basal cell layer. Higher but irregular melanosome content may be present in some keratinocytes, indicating prolonged residence of the cells in the basal cell layer. These structural changes may help to explain the leathery texture and the blotchy discoloration of sun-damaged skin.

The dermis and its connective tissue matrix are the major site for sun-associated chronic damage, manifest as solar elastosis, a massive increase in thickened irregular masses of abnormal elastic fibers. Collagen fibers are also abnormally clumped in the deeper dermis of sun-damaged skin. The chromophore(s), the action spectra, and the specific biochemical events orchestrating these changes are only partially understood. Chronologically aged, sun-protected skin and photoaged skin share important molecular features including connective tissue damage, elevated matrix metalloproteinase levels, and reduced collagen production.

Chronic Effects of Sun Exposure: Malignant   One of the major known consequences of chronic skin exposure to sunlight is nonmelanoma skin cancer. The two types of nonmelanoma skin cancer are *basal cell carcinoma* and *squamous cell carcinoma* (Chap. 73). There are three major steps for cancer induction: initiation, promotion, and progression. Exposure of human skin to sunlight results in *initiation*, a step whereby structural (mutagenic) changes in DNA evoke an irreversible alteration in the target cell (*keratinocyte*) that begins the tumorigenic process. Exposure to a tumor initiator such as UV-B is believed to be a necessary but not sufficient step in the malignant process, since initiated skin cells not exposed to tumor promoters do not generally develop tumors. The second stage in tumor development is *promotion*, a multistep process whereby chronic exposure to sunlight evokes epigenetic changes that culminate in the clonal expansion of initiated cells and cause the development, over many years, of premalignant growths known as *actinic keratoses*, a minority of which may progress to form skin cancer. Based on extensive studies it seems clear that UV-B is a *complete carcinogen*, meaning that it can act as both a tumor initiator and a promoter.

The third and final step in the malignant process is *malignant conversion* of benign precursors into malignant lesions, a process thought to require additional genetic alterations in already transformed cells. Skin carcinogenesis is thought to be caused by the accumulation of mutations in the tumor suppressor gene p53 as a result of UV-induced DNA damage. Indeed both human and murine UV-induced skin cancers have unique p53 mutations (C $\rightarrow$ T and CC $\rightarrow$ TT transitions) that are present in the majority of these lesions. Studies have shown that sunscreens can substantially reduce the frequency of these signature mutations in p53 and can dramatically inhibit the induction of tumors. The p53 mutations are present in normal human skin, in actinic keratoses, and in nonmelanoma skin cancers including basal cell and squamous cell carcinomas.

Basal cell carcinomas also manifest mutations in the tumor-suppressor gene known as *patched*, which results in activation of hedgehog signaling, and enhanced activity of *smoothened*, which in turn causes downstream activation of transcription factors that augment cell proliferation. Thus, these tumors can manifest mutations in both p53 and in *patched*.

Sun exposure causes nonmelanoma and melanoma cancers of the skin, although the evidence is far more direct for its role in nonmelanoma (basal cell and squamous cell carcinoma) than in melanoma.

TABLE 51-1   *Skin Type and Sunburn Sensitivity (Fitzpatrick Classification)*

Type	Description
I	Always burn, never tan
II	Always burn, sometimes tan
III	Sometimes burn, sometimes tan
IV	Sometimes burn, always tan
V	Never burn, sometimes tan
VI	Never burn, always tan

Approximately 80% of nonmelanoma skin cancers develop on exposed body area, including the face, the neck, and the hands. Major risk factors include male sex, childhood sun exposures, older age, fair skin, and residence at latitudes closer to the equator. Whites of darker complexions (e.g., Hispanics) have one-tenth the risk of developing such cancers compared to fair-skinned individuals. Blacks are at substantially reduced risk for all forms of skin cancer. One million individuals in the United States develop nonmelanoma skin cancer annually, and the lifetime risk for a fair-skinned individual to develop such a neoplasm is estimated at approximately 15%. A consensus exists that the incidence of nonmelanoma skin cancer in the population is increasing at the rate of 2 to 3% per year, for unknown reasons.

The relationship of sun exposure to melanoma development is less clear-cut, but suggestive evidence supports an association. Melanomas occasionally develop by the teenage years, indicating that the latent period for tumor growth is less than that of nonmelanoma skin cancer. Melanomas are among the most rapidly increasing of all human malignancies (Chap. 73). Epidemiologic studies of immigrant populations of similar ethnic stock indicate that individuals born in one area or who migrate to the same locale before age 10 have higher age-specific melanoma rates than individuals arriving later. It is thus reasonable to conclude that life in a sunny climate from birth or early childhood increases the risk of melanoma. In general, risk does not correlate with cumulative sun exposure but may relate to the duration and extent of exposure in childhood.

Meta-analysis of 17 case-control studies in patients with melanoma concluded that the protective effect of sunscreens against this type of tumor could not be substantiated. Since no prospective studies are available to address this issue, it seems reasonable to recommend that patients at risk for melanoma utilize photoprotection such as sun avoidance, high sun protective factor (SPF) sunscreens, and protective clothing.

Immunologic Effects Exposure to solar radiation suppresses both local and systemic immune responses. The action spectrum for UV-induced immunosuppression closely mimics the absorption spectrum of urocanic acid. UV-induced *trans-cis* isomerization of urocanic acid in the stratum corneum leads to its systemic absorption and consequent immunosuppressive effects. Furthermore administration of modest doses of UV-B to human skin reduces the degree of allergic sensitization to the potent contact allergen, dinitrochlorobenzene. This is associated with depletion of epidermal Langerhans cells.

Higher doses of UV-radiation evoke diminished immunologic responses to antigens introduced either epicutaneously or intracutaneously at sites distant from the irradiated site. These suppressed responses are also associated with the induction of antigen-specific suppressor T lymphocytes and may be mediated by as yet undefined factors that are released from epidermal cells at the irradiated site. One important consequence of chronic sun exposure and the concomitant immunosuppression is enhanced risk of skin cancer. Perhaps the most graphic demonstration of the role of immunosuppression in enhancing the risk of nonmelanoma skin cancer has come from studies of patients receiving organ transplantation who are on chronic immunosuppressive antirejection drug regimens. More than 50% of transplant patients develop basal and squamous cell carcinomas, and these cancers are the most common malignancy arising in renal transplant recipients. These patients require close periodic monitoring and rigorous photoprotection using sunscreens, protective clothing, and sun avoidance.

PHOTOSENSITIVITY DISEASES The diagnosis of photosensitivity requires a careful history to define the duration of the signs and symptoms, the length of time between exposure to sunlight and the development of subjective complaints, and visible changes in the skin. The age of onset can also be a helpful clue; for example, the acute photosensitivity of erythropoietic protoporphyria almost always begins in childhood, whereas the chronic photosensitivity of porphyria cutanea tarda (PCT) typically begins in the fourth and fifth decades. A history of exposure

to topical and systemic drugs and chemicals may provide important clues. Many classes of drugs can cause photosensitivity on the basis of either phototoxicity or photoallergy. Fragrances such as musk ambrette that were previously present in numerous cosmetic products are also potent photosensitizers.

Examination of the skin may also offer important clues. Anatomic areas that are naturally protected from direct sunlight such as the hairy scalp, the upper eyelids, the retroauricular areas, and the infranasal and submental regions may be spared, whereas exposed areas show characteristic features of the pathologic process. These anatomic localization patterns are often helpful, but not infallible, in making the diagnosis. For example, airborne contact sensitizers that are blown onto the skin may produce dermatitis that can be difficult to distinguish from photosensitivity, despite the fact that such material may trigger skin reactivity in areas shielded from direct sunlight.

Many dermatologic conditions may be caused or aggravated by sunlight (Table 51-2). The role of light in evoking these responses may be dependent on genetic abnormalities ranging from well-described defects in DNA repair that occur in XP to the inherited abnormalities in heme synthesis that characterize the porphyrias. In certain photosensitivity diseases, the chromophore has been identified, whereas in the majority, the energy-absorbing agent is unknown.

Polymorphous Light Eruption After sunburn, the most common type of photosensitivity disease is *polymorphous light eruption* (PLE), the mechanism of which is unknown. Many affected individuals never seek medical attention because the condition is often transient, becoming manifest each spring with initial sun exposure but then subsiding spontaneously with continuing exposure, a phenomenon known as "hardening." The major manifestations of PLE include pruritic (often intensely so) erythematous papules that may coalesce into plaques in

TABLE 51-2 *Classification of Photosensitivity Diseases*

Type	Disease
Genetic	Erythropoietic porphyria
	Erythropoietic protoporphyria
	Porphyria cutanea tarda—familial
	Variegate porphyria
	Hepatoerythropoietic porphyria
	Albinism
	Xeroderma pigmentosum
	Rothmund-Thompson disease
	Bloom syndrome
	Cockayne's disease
	Phenylketonuria
Metabolic	Porphyria cutanea tarda—sporadic
	Hartnup disease
	Kwashiorkor
	Pellagra
	Carcinoid syndrome
Phototoxic	
Internal	Drugs
External	Drugs, plants, food
Photoallergic	
Immediate	Solar urticaria
Delayed	Drug photoallergy
	Persistent light reaction/chronic actinic dermatitis
Neoplastic and	Photoaging
degenerative	Actinic keratosis
	Melanoma and nonmelanoma skin cancer
Idiopathic	Polymorphous light eruption
	Hydroa aestivale
	Actinic prurigo
Photoaggravated	Lupus erythematosus
	Systemic
	Subacute cutaneous
	Discoid
	Dermatomyositis
	Herpes simplex
	Lichen planus actinicus
	Acne vulgaris (aestivale)

a patchy distribution on exposed areas of the trunk and forearms. The face is usually less seriously involved.

The diagnosis can be confirmed by skin biopsy and by performing phototest procedures in which skin is exposed to multiple erythema doses of UV-A and UV-B. The action spectrum for PLE is usually within these portions of the solar spectrum.

Treatment of this PLE includes the use of sunscreens and the induction of hardening by the cautious administration of artificial UV-B and/or UV-A radiation for 2 to 3 weeks in the spring.

Phototoxicity and Photoallergy These photosensitivity disorders are related to the topical or systemic administration of drugs and other chemicals. Both reactions require the absorption of energy by a drug or chemical resulting in the production of an excited-state photosensitizer that can transfer its absorbed energy to a bystander molecule or to molecular oxygen, thereby generating tissue-destructive chemical species.

Phototoxicity is a nonimmunologic reaction caused by drugs and chemicals, a few of which are listed in Table 51-3. The usual clinical manifestations include erythema resembling a sunburn reaction that quickly desquamates, or "peels," within several days. In addition, edema, vesicles, and bullae may occur.

Photoallergy is much less common and is distinct in that the immune system participates in the pathologic process. The excited-state photosensitizer may create highly unstable haptenic free radicals that bind covalently to macromolecules to form a functional antigen capable of evoking a delayed hypersensitivity response. Some of the drugs and chemicals that produce photoallergy are listed in Table 51-4. The clinical manifestations typically differ from those of phototoxicity in that an intensely pruritic eczematous dermatitis tends to predominate and evolves into lichenified, thickened, "leathery" changes in sun-exposed areas. A small subset (perhaps 5 to 10%) of patients with photoallergy may develop a persistent exquisite hypersensitivity to light even when the offending drug or chemical is identified and eliminated, a condition known as *persistent light reaction.*

A very uncommon type of persistent photosensitivity is known as *chronic actinic dermatitis.* These patients are typically elderly men with a long history of preexisting allergic contact dermatitis or photosensitivity. They are usually exquisitely sensitive to UV-B, UV-A, and visible wavelengths.

Diagnostic confirmation of phototoxicity and photoallergy can often be obtained using phototest procedures. In patients with suspected phototoxicity, determining the minimal erythema dose (MED) while the patient is exposed to a suspected agent and then repeating the MED after discontinuation of the agent may provide a clue to the causative drug or chemical. Photopatch testing can be performed to confirm the diagnosis of photoallergy. This is a simple variant of ordinary patch testing in which a series of known photoallergens is applied to the skin in duplicate and one set is irradiated with a suberythema dose of UV-A. Development of eczematous changes at sites exposed to sensitizer and light is a positive result. The characteristic abnormality in patients with persistent light reaction is a diminished threshold to erythema evoked by UV-B. Patients with chronic actinic dermatitis usually manifest a broad spectrum of UV hyperresponsiveness and require rigorous photoprotection for relief of their symptoms.

The management of drug photosensitivity involves first and foremost the elimination of exposure to the chemical agents responsible for the reaction and minimization sun exposure. The acute symptoms of phototoxicity may be ameliorated by cool, moist compresses, topical glucocorticoids, and systemically administered NSAIDs. In severely affected individuals, a rapidly tapered course of systemic glucocorticoids may be useful. Judicious use of analgesics may be necessary.

Photoallergic reactions require a similar management approach. Furthermore, patients with persistent light reaction and chronic actinic dermatitis must be meticulously protected against light exposure. In selected patients in whom chronic systemic high-dose glucocorticoids pose unacceptable risks, it may be necessary to employ cytotoxic agents such as azathioprine or cyclophosphamide.

Porphyria The porphyrias (Chap. 337) are a group of diseases that have in common inherited or acquired derangements in the synthesis of heme. Heme is an iron-chelated tetrapyrrole or porphyrin, and the nonmetal chelated porphyrins are potent photosensitizers that absorb light intensely in both the short (400 to 410 nm) and the long (580 to 650 nm) portions of the visible spectrum.

Heme cannot be reutilized and must be continuously synthesized, and the two body compartments with the largest capacity for its production are the bone marrow and the liver. Accordingly, the porphyrias originate in one or the other of these organs, with the end result of excessive endogenous production of potent photosensitizing porphyrins. The porphyrins circulate in the bloodstream and diffuse into the skin, where they absorb solar energy, become photoexcited, generate reactive oxygen species, and evoke cutaneous photosensitivity. The mechanism of porphyrin photosensitization is known to be photodynamic, or oxygen-dependent, and is mediated by reactive oxygen species such as singlet oxygen and superoxide anions.

Porphyria cutanea tarda is the most common type of human porphyria and is associated with decreased activity of the enzyme uroporphyrinogen decarboxylase associated with a number of gene mutations. There are two basic types of PCT: (1) the sporadic or acquired type, generally seen in individuals ingesting ethanol or receiving estrogens; and (2) the inherited type, in which there is autosomal dominant transmission of deficient enzyme activity. Both forms are associated with increased hepatic iron stores.

In both types of PCT, the predominant feature is a chronic photosensitivity characterized by increased fragility of sun-exposed skin, particularly areas subject to repeated trauma such as the dorsa of the hands, the forearms, the face, and the ears. The predominant skin lesions are vesicles and bullae that rupture, producing moist erosions, often with a hemorrhagic base, that heal slowly with crusting and

TABLE 51-4 *Photoallergic Drugs*

	Topical	Systemic
6-Methylcoumarin	+	
Aminobenzoic acid and esters	+	
Bithionol	+	
Chlorpromazine		+
Diclofenac		+
Fluoroquinolones		+
Halogenated salicylanilides	+	
Hypericin (St John's Wort)	+	+
Musk ambrette	+	
Piroxicam		+
Promethazine		+
Sulfonamides		+
Sulfonylureas		+

TABLE 51-3 *Phototoxic Drugs*

	Topical	Systemic
Amiodarone		+
Dacarbazine		+
Fluoroquinolones		+
5-Fluorouracil	+	+
Furosemide		+
Nalidixic acid		+
Phenothiazines		+
Psoralens	+	+
Retinoids	+/−	+
Sulfonamides		+
Sulfonylureas		+
Tetracyclines		+
Thiazides		+
Vinblastine		+

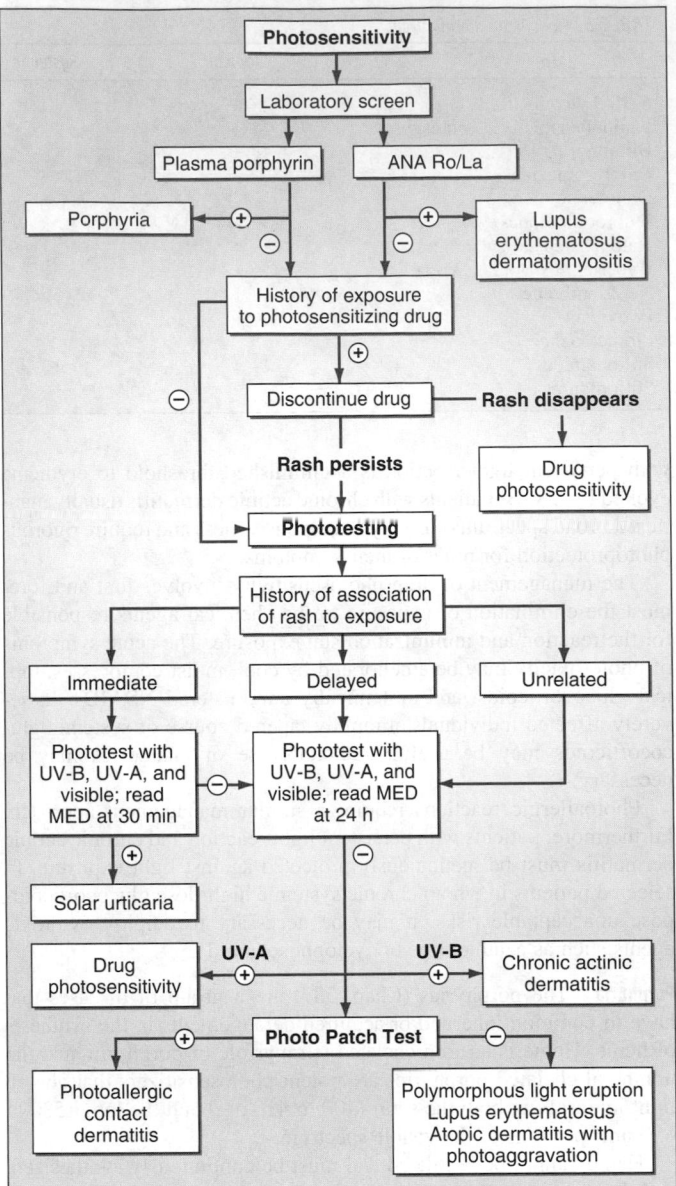

clude an acute photosensitivity characterized by subjective burning and stinging of exposed skin that often develops during or just after exposure. There may be associated skin swelling and, after repeated episodes, a waxlike scarring.

The diagnosis is confirmed by demonstration of elevated levels of free erythrocyte protoporphyrin. Detection of increased plasma protoporphyrin helps to differentiate lead poisoning and iron-deficiency anemia, in both of which elevated erythrocyte protoporphyrin levels occur in the absence of cutaneous photosensitivity and of elevated plasma protoporphyrin levels.

Treatment consists of reducing sun exposure and the oral administration of the carotenoid β-carotene, which is an effective scavenger of free radicals. This drug increases tolerance to sun exposure in many affected individuals, although it has no effect on deficient ferrochelatase.

An algorithm for managing patients with photosensitivity is illustrated in Fig. 51-1.

PHOTOPROTECTION   Since photosensitivity of the skin results from exposure to sunlight, it follows that absolute avoidance of the sun would eliminate these disorders. Unfortunately, contemporary life-styles make this an impractical alternative for most individuals, and this has led to a search for better approaches to photoprotection.

Natural photoprotection is provided by structural proteins in the epidermis, particularly keratins and melanin. The amount of melanin and its distribution in cells is genetically regulated, and individuals of darker complexion (skin types IV to VI) are at decreased risk for the development of acute sunburn and cutaneous malignancy.

Other forms of photoprotection include clothing and sunscreens. Clothing constructed of tightly woven sun-protective fabrics, irrespective of color, affords substantial protection. Wide-brimmed hats, long sleeves, and trousers all reduce direct exposure. Sunscreens are now considered to be over-the-counter drugs and category I ingredients are recognized by the U.S. Food and Drug Administration (FDA) as monographed and safe and effective. These are listed in Table 51-5. Sunscreens are rated for their photoprotective effect by their SPF. The SPF is simply a ratio of the time required to produce sunburn erythema with and without sunscreen application. The monograph stipulates that sunscreens must be rated on a scale ranging from minimal (SPF $\nleq 2$ and $\ngtr 12$) to moderate (SPF $\nleq 12$ and $\ngtr 30$) to high (SPF ≥ 30, labeled as 30+). No SPF number >30 can be placed on the label.

In addition to light absorption, a critical determinant of the sustained photoprotective effect of sunscreens is their water-resistance. The FDA monograph has also defined strict testing criteria for sunscreens making this claim.

Some degree of photoprotection can also be achieved by limiting the time of exposure during the day. Since the majority of an individual's total lifetime sun exposure may occur by the age of 18, it is important to educate parents and young children about the hazards of

purplish discoloration of the affected skin. Hypertrichosis, mottled pigmentary change, and scleroderma-like induration are associated features. Biochemical confirmation of the diagnosis can be obtained by measurement of urinary porphyrin excretion, plasma porphyrin assay, and by assay of erythrocyte and/or hepatic uroporphyrinogen decarboxylase. Multiple mutations of the uroporphyrinogen decarboxylase gene have been identified in human populations, including exon skipping and base substitutions. Some patients with PCT have associated mutations in the *HFE* gene linked to hemochromatosis. This could contribute to the iron overload seen in PCT, although iron status as measured by serum ferritin, iron levels, and transferrin saturation is no different from that in PCT patients without *HFE* mutations. Prior hepatitis C infection appears to be an independent risk factor for PCT.

Treatment of PCT consists of repeated phlebotomies to diminish the excessive hepatic iron stores and/or intermittent low doses of the antimalarial drugs chloroquine and hydroxychloroquine. Long-term remission of the disease can be achieved if the patient eliminates exposure to porphyrinogenic agents.

Erythropoietic protoporphyria originates in the bone marrow and is due to a decrease in the mitochondrial enzyme ferrochelatase secondary to numerous gene mutations. The major clinical features in-

TABLE 51-5   *FDA Category 1 Monographed Sunscreen Ingredients*[a]

Ingredients	Maximum Concentration, %
p-Aminobenzoic acid (PABA)	15
Avobenzone	3
Cinoxate	3
Dioxybenzone (benzophenone-8)	3
Homosalate	15
Menthyl anthranilate	5
Octocrylene	10
Octyl methoxycinnamate	7.5
Octyl salicylate	5
Oxybenzone (benzophenone-3)	6
Padimate (octyl dimethyl PABA)	8
Phenylbenzimidazole sulfonic acid	4
Sulisobenzone (benzophenone-4)	10
Titanium dioxide	25
Trolamine salicylate	12
Zinc oxide	25

[a] FDA, U.S. Food and Drug Administration.

sunlight. Simply eliminating exposure at midday will substantially reduce lifetime UV-B exposure.

PHOTOTHERAPY AND PHOTOCHEMOTHERAPY UV can also be used therapeutically. The administration of UV-B alone or in combination with topically applied agents can induce remissions of psoriasis and atopic dermatitis.

Photochemotherapy in which topically applied or systemically administered psoralens are combined with UV-A (PUVA) is also effective in treating psoriasis and in the early stages of cutaneous T cell lymphoma and vitiligo. Psoralens are tricyclic furocoumarins that, when intercalated into DNA and exposed to UV-A, form adducts with pyrimidine bases and eventually form DNA cross-links. These structural changes are thought to decrease DNA synthesis and relate to the improvement that occurs in psoriasis. The reason that PUVA photochemotherapy is effective in cutaneous T cell lymphoma is not clear.

In addition to its effects on DNA, PUVA photochemotherapy also stimulates melanin synthesis, and this provides the rationale for its use in the depigmenting disease vitiligo. Oral 8-methoxypsoralen and UV-A appear to be most effective in this regard, but as many as 100 treatments extending over 12 to 18 months may be required to promote satisfactory repigmentation.

Not surprisingly the major side effects of long-term UV-B phototherapy and PUVA photochemotherapy mimic those seen in individuals with chronic sun exposure and include skin dryness, actinic keratoses, and an increased risk of melanoma and nonmelanoma skin cancer. Despite these risks, the therapeutic index of these modalities continues to be excellent.

FURTHER READING

ANANTHASWAMY HN et al: Inhibition of UVB-induced p53 mutations and skin cancer by sunscreens: Implications for skin cancer prevention. Exp Dermatol 11(Suppl 1):40, 2002

DRAELOS ZD: A dermatologist's perspective on the final sunscreen monograph. J Am Acad Dermatol 44:109, 2001

MARKS R et al: The effect of regular sunscreen use on vitamin D levels in an Australian population. Results of a randomized clinical trial. Arch Dermatol 131:1337, 1995

MATSUMURA Y, ANANTHASWAMY NH: Molecular mechanisms of photocarcinogenesis. Front Biosci 7:765, 2002

ROELANDTS R: The diagnosis of photosensitivity. Arch Dermatol 136:1152, 2000

Section 10   Hematologic Alterations

52 ANEMIA AND POLYCYTHEMIA
John W. Adamson, Dan L. Longo

HEMATOPOIESIS AND THE PHYSIOLOGIC BASIS OF RED CELL PRODUCTION *Hematopoiesis* is the process by which the formed elements of the blood are produced. The process is regulated through a series of steps beginning with the pluripotent hematopoietic stem cell. Stem cells are capable of producing red cells, all classes of granulocytes, monocytes, platelets, and the cells of the immune system. Commitment of the stem cell to the specific cell lineages appears not to be regulated by known exogenous growth factors or cytokines. Rather, stem cells develop into differentiated cell types through incompletely defined molecular events that are intrinsic to the stem cell itself. Following lineage commitment (or differentiation), hematopoietic progenitor and precursor cells come increasingly under the regulatory influence of growth factors and hormones. For red cell production, erythropoietin (EPO) is the regulatory hormone. EPO is required for the maintenance of committed erythroid progenitor cells that, in the absence of the hormone, undergo programmed cell death (*apoptosis*). The regulated process of red cell production is *erythropoiesis*, and its key elements are illustrated in Fig. 52-1.

In the bone marrow, the first morphologically recognizable erythroid precursor is the pronormoblast. This cell can undergo 4 to 5 cell divisions that result in the production of 16 to 32 mature red cells. With increased EPO production, or the administration of EPO as a drug, early progenitor cell numbers are amplified and, in turn, give rise to increased numbers of erythrocytes. The regulation of EPO production itself is linked to O_2 transport.

In mammals, O_2 is transported to tissues bound to the hemoglobin contained within circulating red cells. The mature red cell is 8 μm in diameter, anucleate, discoid in shape, and extremely pliable in order to traverse the microcirculation successfully; its membrane integrity is maintained by the intracellular generation of ATP. Normal red cell production results in the daily replacement of 0.8 to 1% of all circulating red cells in the body. The average red cell lives 100 to 120 days. The machinery responsible for red cell production is called the *erythron*. The erythron is a dynamic organ made up of a rapidly proliferating pool of marrow erythroid precursor cells and a large mass of mature circulating red blood cells. The size of the red cell mass

reflects the balance of red cell production and destruction. The physiologic basis of red cell production and destruction provides an understanding of the mechanisms that can lead to anemia.

The physiologic regulator of red cell production, the glycoprotein hormone EPO, is produced and released by peritubular capillary lining cells within the kidney. These cells are highly specialized epithelial-like cells. A small amount of EPO is produced by hepatocytes. The fundamental stimulus for EPO production is the availability of O_2 for tissue metabolic needs. Impaired O_2 delivery to the kidney can result from a decreased red cell mass (*anemia*), impaired O_2 loading of the hemoglobin molecule (*hypoxemia*), or, rarely, impaired blood flow to the kidney (renal artery stenosis). EPO governs the day-to-day production of red cells, and ambient levels of the hormone can be measured in the plasma by sensitive immunoassays—the normal level being 10 to 25 U/L. When the hemoglobin concentration falls below 100 to 120 g/L (10 to 12 g/dL), plasma EPO levels increase in proportion to the severity of the anemia. In circulation, EPO has a half-clearance time of 6 to 9 h. EPO acts by binding to specific receptors on the surface of marrow erythroid precursors, inducing them to proliferate and to mature. Under the stimulus of EPO, red cell production

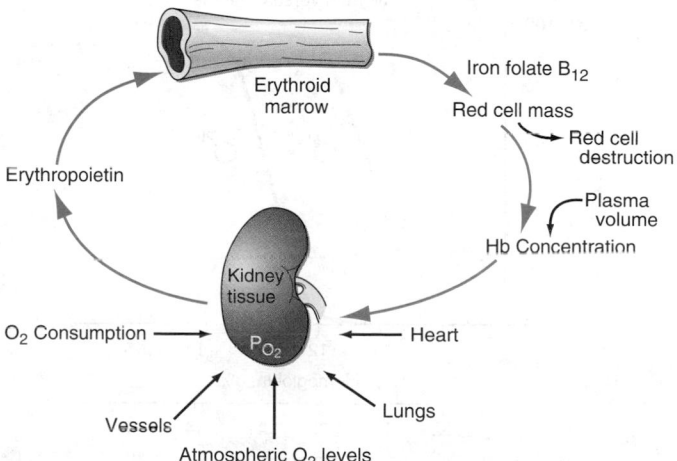

FIGURE 52-1 The physiologic regulation of red cell production by tissue oxygen tension. Hb, hemoglobin.

can increase four- to fivefold within a 1- to 2-week period but only in the presence of adequate nutrients, especially iron. The functional capacity of the erythron, therefore, requires normal renal production of EPO, a functioning erythroid marrow, and an adequate supply of substrates for hemoglobin synthesis. A defect in any of these key components can lead to anemia. Generally, anemia is recognized in the laboratory when a patient's hemoglobin level or hematocrit is reduced below an expected value (the normal range). The likelihood and severity of anemia are defined based on the deviation of the patient's hemoglobin/hematocrit from values expected for age- and sex-matched normal subjects. The lower ranges of distribution of hemoglobin/hematocrit values for adult males and females are shown in Fig. 52-2. The hemoglobin concentration in adults has a Gaussian distribution. The mean hematocrit value for adult males is 47% ($\pm$ SD 7) and that for adult females is 42% ($\pm$ 5). Any single hematocrit or hemoglobin value carries with it a likelihood of associated anemia. Thus, a hematocrit of $\leq$39% in an adult male or <35% in an adult female has only about a 25% chance of being normal. Suspected low hemoglobin or hematocrit values are more easily interpreted if there are historic values for the same patient for comparison.

The critical elements of erythropoiesis—EPO production, iron availability, the proliferative capacity of the bone marrow, and effective maturation of red cell precursors—are used for the initial classification of anemia (see below).

ANEMIA

CLINICAL PRESENTATION OF ANEMIA ■ **Signs and Symptoms**   Anemia is most often recognized by abnormal screening laboratory tests. Patients less commonly present with advanced anemia and its attendant signs and symptoms. Acute anemia is nearly always due to blood loss or hemolysis. If blood loss is mild, enhanced O_2 delivery is achieved through changes in the O_2-hemoglobin dissociation curve mediated by a decreased pH or increased CO_2 (*Bohr effect*). With acute blood loss, hypovolemia dominates the clinical picture and the hematocrit and hemoglobin levels do not reflect the volume of blood lost. Signs of vascular instability appear with acute losses of 10 to 15% of the total blood volume. In such patients, the issue is not anemia but hypotension and decreased organ perfusion. When >30% of the blood volume is lost suddenly, patients are unable to compensate with the usual mechanisms of vascular contraction and changes in regional blood flow. The patient prefers to remain supine and will show postural hypotension and tachycardia if upright. If the volume of blood lost is >40% (i.e., >2 L in the average-sized adult), signs of hypovolemic shock including confusion, dyspnea, diaphoresis, hypotension, and tachycardia appear (Chap. 93). Such patients have significant deficits in vital organ perfusion and require immediate volume replacement.

With acute hemolytic disease, the signs and symptoms depend on the mechanism that leads to red cell destruction. Intravascular hemolysis with release of free hemoglobin may be associated with acute back pain, free hemoglobin in the plasma and urine, and renal failure. Symptoms associated with more chronic or progressive anemia depend on the age of the patient and the adequacy of blood supply to critical organs. Symptoms associated with moderate anemia include fatigue, loss of stamina, breathlessness, and tachycardia (particularly with physical exertion). However, because of the intrinsic compensatory mechanisms that govern the O_2-hemoglobin dissociation curve, the gradual onset of anemia—particularly in young patients—may not be associated with signs or symptoms until the anemia is severe [hemoglobin <70 to 80 g/L (7 to 8 g/dL)]. When anemia develops over a period of days or weeks, the total blood volume is normal to slightly increased and changes in cardiac output and regional blood flow help compensate for the overall loss in O_2-carrying capacity. Changes in the position of the O_2-hemoglobin dissociation curve account for some of the compensatory response to anemia. With chronic anemia, intracellular levels of 2,3-bisphosphoglycerate rise, shifting the dissociation curve to the right and facilitating O_2 unloading. This compensatory mechanism can only maintain normal tissue O_2 delivery in the face of a 20 to 30 g/L (2 to 3 g/dL) deficit in hemoglobin concentration. Finally, further protection of O_2 delivery to vital organs is achieved by the shunting of blood away from organs that are relatively rich in blood supply, particularly the kidney, gut, and skin.

Certain disorders are commonly associated with anemia. Chronic inflammatory states (e.g., infection, rheumatoid arthritis) are associated with mild to moderate anemia, whereas lymphoproliferative disorders, such as chronic lymphocytic leukemia and certain other B cell neoplasms, may be associated with autoimmune hemolysis.

APPROACH TO THE PATIENT

The evaluation of the patient with anemia requires a careful history and physical examination. Nutritional history related to drugs or alcohol intake and family history of anemia should always be assessed. Certain geographic backgrounds and ethnic origins are associated with an increased likelihood of an inherited disorder of the hemoglobin molecule or intermediary metabolism. Glucose-6-phosphate dehydrogenase deficiency and certain hemoglobinopathies are seen more commonly in those of Middle Eastern or African origin. Other information that may be useful includes exposure to certain toxic agents or drugs and symptoms related to other disorders commonly associated with anemia. These include

FIGURE 52-2 The probability that a particular hemoglobin or hematocrit value is abnormal is different in men and women.

TABLE 52-1   *Laboratory Tests in Anemia Diagnosis*

I. Complete blood count (CBC)	II. Iron supply studies
A. Red blood cell count	A. Serum iron
1. Hemoglobin	B. Total iron-binding
2. Hematocrit	capacity
3. Reticulocyte count	C. Serum ferritin, marrow
B. Red blood cell indices	iron stain
1. Mean cell volume (MCV)	III. Marrow examination
2. Mean cell hemoglobin (MCH)	A. Aspirate
3. Mean cell hemoglobin	1. M/E ratio[a]
concentration (MCHC)	2. Cell morphology
4. Red cell distribution width	3. Iron stain
(RDW)	B. Biopsy
C. White blood cell count	1. Cellularity
1. Cell differential	2. Morphology
2. Nuclear segmentation of	
neutrophils	
D. Platelet count	
E. Cell morphology	
1. Cell size	
2. Hemoglobin content	
3. Anisocytosis	
4. Poikilocytosis	
5. Polychromasia	

[a] M/E ratio, ratio of myeloid to erythroid precursors.

TABLE 52-2 *Red Blood Cell Indices*

Index	Normal Value
Mean cell volume (MCV) = (hematocrit × 10)/(red cell count × 10^6)	90 ± 8 fL
Mean cell hemoglobin (MCH) = (hemoglobin × 10)/(red cell count × 10^6)	30 ± 3 pg
Mean cell hemoglobin concentration = (hemoglobin × 10)/hematocrit, or MCH/MCV	33 ± 2%

symptoms and signs such as bleeding, fatigue, malaise, fever, weight loss, night sweats, and other systemic symptoms. Clues to the mechanisms of anemia may be provided on physical examination by findings of infection, blood in the stool, lymphadenopathy, splenomegaly, or petechiae. Splenomegaly and lymphadenopathy suggest an underlying lymphoproliferative disease, while petechiae suggest platelet dysfunction. Past laboratory measurements may be helpful to determine a time of onset.

In the anemic patient, physical examination may demonstrate a forceful heartbeat, strong peripheral pulses, and a systolic "flow" murmur. The skin and mucous membranes may be pale if the hemoglobin is <80 to 100 g/L (8 to 10 g/dL). This part of the physical examination should focus on areas where vessels are close to the surface such as the mucous membranes, nail beds, and palmar creases. If the palmar creases are lighter in color than the surrounding skin when the hand is hyperextended, the hemoglobin level is usually <80 g/L (8 g/dL).

Laboratory Evaluation Table 52-1 lists the tests used in the initial workup of anemia. A routine complete blood count (CBC) is required as part of the evaluation and includes the hemoglobin, hematocrit, and red cell indices: the mean cell volume (MCV) in femtoliters, mean cell hemoglobin (MCH) in picograms per cell, and mean concentration of hemoglobin per volume of red cells (MCHC) in grams per liter (non-SI: grams per deciliter). The red cell indices are calculated as shown in Table 52-2, and the normal variations in the hemoglobin and hematocrit with age are shown in Table 52-3. A number of physiologic factors affect the normal CBC values including age, gender, pregnancy, smoking, and altitude. High-normal hemoglobin values may be seen in men and women who live at altitude or smoke heavily. Hemoglobin elevations due to smoking reflect normal compensation due to the displacement of O_2 by CO in hemoglobin binding. Other important information is provided by the reticulocyte count and measurements of iron supply including *serum iron*, *total iron-binding capacity* (TIBC; an indirect measure of the transferrin level), and *serum ferritin*. Marked alterations in the red cell indices usually reflect disorders of maturation or iron deficiency. Clinical laboratories also provide a description of both the red and white cells, a white cell differential count, and the platelet count. In patients with severe anemia and abnormalities in red blood cell morphology, a bone marrow aspirate or biopsy may be important to assist in the diagnosis. Other tests of value in the diagnosis of specific anemias are discussed in chapters on specific disease states.

The components of the CBC also help in the classification of anemia. *Microcytosis* is reflected by a lower than normal MCV

FIGURE 52-3 Normal blood smear (Wright's stain). High-power field showing normal red cells, a neutrophil, and a few platelets. (*From Hillman and Ault.*)

(<80), whereas high values (>100) reflect *macrocytosis*. The MCH and MCHC reflect defects in hemoglobin synthesis (*hypochromia*). Automated cell counters describe the red cell volume distribution width (RDW). The MCV (representing the peak of the distribution curve) is insensitive to the appearance of small populations of macrocytes or microcytes. An experienced laboratory technician will be able to identify minor populations of large or small cells or hypochromic cells before the red cell indices change.

PERIPHERAL BLOOD SMEAR The peripheral blood smear provides important information about defects in red cell production. As a complement to the red cell indices, the blood smear also reveals variations in cell size (*anisocytosis*) and shape (*poikilocytosis*). The degree of anisocytosis usually correlates with increases in the RDW or the range of cell sizes. Poikilocytosis suggests a defect in the maturation of red cell precursors in the bone marrow or fragmentation of circulating red cells. The blood smear may also reveal *polychromasia*—red cells that are slightly larger than normal and grayish blue in color on the Wright-Giemsa stain. These cells are reticulocytes that have been prematurely released from the bone marrow, and their color represents residual amounts of ribosomal RNA. These cells appear in circulation in response to EPO stimulation or to architectural damage of the bone marrow (fibrosis, infiltration of the marrow by malignant cells, etc.) that results in their disordered release from the marrow. The appearance of nucleated red cells, Howell-Jolly bodies, target cells, sickle cells, and others may provide clues to specific disorders (see Figs. 52-3 to 52-11).

RETICULOCYTE COUNT An accurate reticulocyte count is key to the initial classification of anemia. Normally, reticulocytes are red cells

TABLE 52-3 *Changes in Normal Hemoglobin/Hematocrit Values with Age and Pregnancy*

Age/Sex	Hemoglobin g/dL	Hematocrit %
At birth	17	52
Childhood	12	36
Adolescence	13	40
Adult man	16 (±2)	47 (±6)
Adult woman (menstruating)	13 (±2)	40 (±6)
Adult woman (postmenopausal)	14 (±2)	42 (±6)
During pregnancy	12 (±2)	37 (±6)

Source: From Hillman and Ault.

FIGURE 52-4 Severe iron-deficiency anemia. Microcytic and hypochromic red cells smaller than the nucleus of a lymphocyte associated with marked variation in size (anisocytosis) and shape (poikilocytosis). (*From Hillman and Ault.*)

FIGURE 52-5 Macrocytosis. Red cells are larger than a small lymphocyte and well hemoglobinized. Often macrocytes are oval-shaped, so-called macroovalocytes.

FIGURE 52-6 Howell-Jolly bodies. In the absence of a functional spleen, nuclear remnants are not culled from the red cells and remain as small homogeneously staining blue inclusions on Wright stain. (*From Hillman and Ault.*)

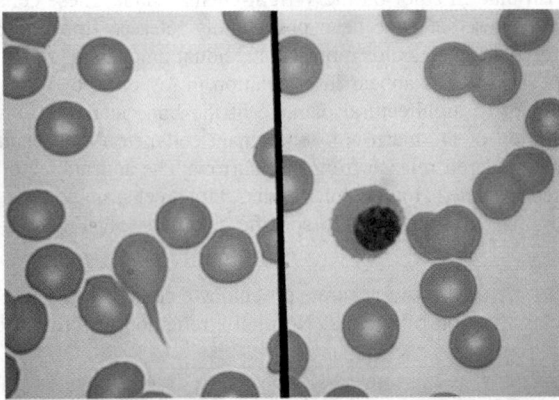

FIGURE 52-7 Red cell changes in myelofibrosis. The left panel shows a teardrop-shaped cell. The right panel shows a nucleated red cell. These forms are seen in myelofibrosis with extramedullary hematopoiesis.

FIGURE 52-8 Target cells. Target cells have a bull's-eye appearance and are seen in thalassemia and in liver disease. (*From Hillman and Ault.*)

FIGURE 52-9 Red cell fragmentation. Red cells may become fragmented in the presence of foreign bodies in the circulation such as mechanical heart valves or in the setting of thermal injury. (*From Hillman and Ault.*)

FIGURE 52-10 Uremia. The red cells in uremia may acquire numerous, regularly spaced, small spiny projections. Such cells, called burr cells or echinocytes, are readily distinguishable from irregularly spiculated acanthocytes shown in Fig. 52-11.

FIGURE 52-11 Spur cells. Spur cells are recognized as distorted red cells containing several irregularly distributed thornlike projections. Cells with this morphologic abnormality are also called acanthocytes. (*Courtesy of Elaine Jaffe, MD.*)

that have been recently released from the bone marrow. They are identified by staining with a supravital dye that precipitates the residual ribosomal RNA (Fig. 52-12). These precipitates appear as blue or black punctate spots. This residual RNA is metabolized over the first 24 to 36 h of the reticulocyte's lifespan in circulation. Normally, the reticulocyte count ranges from 1 to 2% and reflects the daily replacement of 0.8 to 1.0% of the circulating red cell population. A reticulocyte count provides a reliable measure of red cell production.

In the initial classification of anemia, the patient's reticulocyte count is compared with the expected reticulocyte response. In general, if the EPO and erythroid marrow responses to moderate ane-

mia [hemoglobin <100 g/L (10 g/dL)] are intact, the red cell production rate increases to two to three times normal within 10 days following the onset of anemia. In the face of established anemia, a reticulocyte response less than two to three times normal indicates an inadequate marrow response.

In order to use the reticulocyte count to estimate marrow response, two corrections are necessary. The first correction adjusts the reticulocyte count based on the reduced number of circulating red cells. With anemia, the percentage of reticulocytes may be increased while the absolute number is unchanged. To correct for this effect, the reticulocyte percentage is multiplied by the ratio of the patient's hemoglobin or hematocrit to the expected hemoglobin/

FIGURE 52-12 Reticulocytes. Methylene blue stain demonstrates residual RNA in newly made red cells. (*Courtesy of Elaine Jaffe, MD.*)

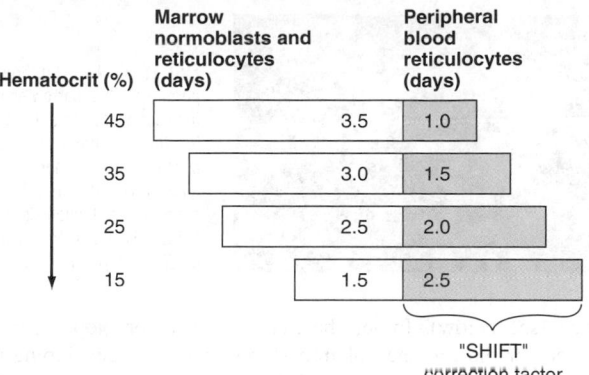

FIGURE 52-13 Correction of reticulocyte count based on level of anemia and the circulatory life span of prematurely released reticulocytes. Erythroid cells take about 4.5 days to mature. At normal hematocrit levels, they are released to the circulation with about 1 day left as reticulocytes. However, with different levels of anemia, erythroid cells are released from the marrow prematurely. Most patients come to clinical attention with hematocrits in the mid-20s and thus, a correction factor of 2 is commonly used because the observed reticulocytes will live for 2 days in the circulation before losing their RNA.

hematocrit for the age and gender of the patient (Table 52-4). This provides an estimate of the reticulocyte count corrected for anemia. In order to convert the corrected reticulocyte count to an index of marrow production, a further correction is required, depending on whether some of the reticulocytes in circulation have been released from the marrow prematurely. For this second correction, the peripheral blood smear is examined to see if there are polychromatophilic macrocytes present. These cells, representing prematurely released reticulocytes, are referred to as "shift" cells, and the relationship between the degree of shift and the necessary shift correction factor is shown in Fig. 52-13. The correction is necessary because these prematurely released cells survive as reticulocytes in circulation for >1 day, thereby providing a falsely high estimate of daily red cell production. If polychromasia is increased, the reticulocyte count, already corrected for anemia, should be divided again by a factor of 2 to account for the prolonged reticulocyte maturation time. The second correction factor varies from 1 to 3 depending on the severity of anemia. In general, a correction of 2 is commonly used. An appropriate correction is shown in Table 52-4. If polychromatophilic cells are not seen on the blood smear, the second correction is not required. The now doubly corrected reticulocyte count is the *reticulocyte production index*, and it provides an estimate of marrow production relative to normal.

Premature release of reticulocytes is normally due to increased EPO stimulation. However, if the integrity of the bone marrow release process is lost through tumor infiltration, fibrosis, or other disorders, the appearance of nucleated red cells or polychromatophilic macrocytes should still invoke the second reticulocyte correction. The shift correction should always be applied to a patient with anemia and a very high reticulocyte count to provide a true index of effective red cell production. Patients with severe chronic hemolytic anemia may increase red cell production as much as six- to sevenfold. This measure alone, therefore, confirms the fact that the patient has an appropriate EPO response, a normally functioning bone marrow, and sufficient iron available to meet the demands for new red cell formation. If the reticulocyte production index is

<2 in the face of established anemia, a defect in erythroid marrow proliferation or maturation must be present.

TESTS OF IRON SUPPLY AND STORAGE The laboratory measurements that reflect the availability of iron for hemoglobin synthesis include the serum iron, the TIBC, and the percent transferrin saturation. The percent transferrin saturation is derived by dividing the serum iron level ($\times$ 100) by the TIBC. The normal serum iron ranges from 9 to 27 μmol/L (50 to 150 μg/dL), while the normal TIBC is 54 to 64 μmol/L (300 to 360 μg/dL); the transferrin saturation ranges from 25 to 50%. A diurnal variation in the serum iron leads to a variation in the percent transferrin saturation. The serum ferritin is used to evaluate total-body iron stores. Adult males have serum ferritin levels that average about 100 μg/L, corresponding to iron stores of about 1 g. Adult females have lower serum ferritin levels averaging 30 μg/L, reflecting lower iron stores. A serum ferritin level of 10 to 15 μg/L represents depletion of body iron stores. However, ferritin is also an acute-phase reactant and, in the presence of acute or chronic inflammation, may rise severalfold above baseline levels. As a rule, a serum ferritin >200 μg/L means there is at least some iron in tissue stores.

BONE MARROW EXAMINATION A bone marrow aspirate and smear or a needle biopsy may be useful in the diagnosis of a marrow disorder such as myelofibrosis, a red cell maturation defect, or an infiltrative disease (Figs. 52-14 to 52-16). The increase or decrease of one cell lineage (myeloid vs. erythroid) compared to another is obtained by a differential count of nucleated cells in a bone marrow smear [the myeloid/erythroid (M/E) ratio]. A patient with a hypoproliferative anemia (see below) and a reticulocyte production index <2 will demonstrate an M/E ratio of 2 or 3:1. In contrast, patients with hemolytic disease and a production index >3 will have an M/E ratio of at least 1:1. Maturation disorders are identified from the discrepancy between the M/E ratio and the reticulocyte production

TABLE 52-4   Calculation of Reticulocyte Production Index

Correction #1 for anemia:
   This correction produces the corrected reticulocyte count
   In a person whose reticulocyte count is 9%, hemoglobin 7.5 g/dL, hematocrit 23%, the absolute reticulocyte count = 9 × (7.5/15)[or ×(23/45)] = 4.5%
Correction #2 for longer life of prematurely released reticulocytes in the blood:
   This correction produces the reticulocyte production index
   In a person whose reticulocyte count is 9%, hemoglobin 7.5 gm/dL, hematocrit 23%, the reticulocyte production index =

$$9 \times \frac{(7.5/15)(\text{hemoglobin correction})}{2 \text{ (maturation time correction)}} = 2.25$$

FIGURE 52-14 Normal bone marrow. This is a low-power view of a section of normal marrow stained with hematoxylin and eosin (H&E). Note that the nucleated cellular elements account for about 40 to 50% and the fat (clear areas) accounts for about 50 to 60% of the area. (*Courtesy of Elaine Jaffe, MD.*)

FIGURE 52-15 Erythroid hyperplasia. This marrow shows an increase in the fraction of cells in the erythroid lineage as might be seen when a normal marrow compensates for acute blood loss or hemolysis. The M/E ratio is about 1:1. (*Courtesy of Elaine Jaffe, MD.*)

index (see below). Either the marrow smear or biopsy can be stained for the presence of iron stores or iron in developing red cells. The storage iron is in the form of ferritin or *hemosiderin*. On carefully prepared bone marrow smears, small ferritin granules can normally be seen in 20 to 40% of developing erythroblasts. Such cells are called *sideroblasts*.

Other Laboratory Measurements   Additional laboratory tests may be of value in confirming specific diagnoses. →*For details of these tests and how they are applied in individual disorders, see Chaps. 90 to 94.*

DEFINITION AND CLASSIFICATION OF ANEMIA ■ Initial Classification of Anemia
Classifying an anemia according to the functional defect in red cell production helps organize the subsequent use of laboratory studies. The three major classes of anemia are: (1) marrow production defects (*hypoproliferation*), (2) red cell maturation defects (*ineffective erythropoiesis*), and (3) decreased red cell survival (*blood loss/hemolysis*). This functional classification of anemia then guides the selection of specific clinical and laboratory studies designed to complete the differential diagnosis and to plan appropriate therapy. The classification is shown in Fig. 52-17. A hypoproliferative anemia is typically seen with a low reticulocyte production index together with little or no change in red cell morphology (a normocytic, normochromic anemia) (Chap. 90). Maturation disorders typically have a slight to moderately elevated reticulocyte production index that is accompanied by either macrocytic (Chap. 92) or microcytic (Chaps. 90, 91) red cell indices. Increased red blood cell destruction secondary to hemolysis results in an increase in the reticulocyte production index to at least three times normal (Chap. 93), provided sufficient iron is available for hemoglobin synthesis. Hemorrhagic anemia does not typically result in production indices of more than 2.5 times normal because of the limitations placed on expansion of the erythroid marrow by iron availability.

In the first branch point of the classification of anemia, a reticulocyte production index >2.5 indicates that hemolysis is most likely. A reticulocyte production index <2 indicates either a hypoproliferative anemia or maturation disorder. The latter two possibilities can often be distinguished by the red cell indices, by examination of the peripheral blood smear, or by a marrow examination. If the red cell indices are normal, the anemia is almost certainly hypoproliferative in nature. Maturation disorders are characterized by ineffective red cell production and a low reticulocyte production index. Bizarre red cell shapes—macrocytes or hypochromic microcytes—are seen on the peripheral blood smear. With a hypoproliferative anemia, no erythroid hyperpla-

FIGURE 52-16 Myeloid hyperplasia. This marrow shows an increase in the fraction of cells in the myeloid or granulocytic lineage as might be seen in a normal marrow responding to infection. The M/E ratio is >3:1. (*Courtesy of Elaine Jaffe, MD.*)

FIGURE 52-17   The physiologic classification of anemia. CBC, complete blood count.

sia is noted in the marrow, whereas patients with ineffective red cell production have erythroid hyperplasia and an M/E ratio <1:1.

Hypoproliferative Anemias   At least 75% of all cases of anemia are hypoproliferative in nature. A hypoproliferative anemia reflects absolute or relative marrow failure in which the erythroid marrow has not proliferated appropriately for the degree of anemia. The majority of hypoproliferative anemias are due to mild to moderate iron deficiency or inflammation. A hypoproliferative anemia can result from marrow damage, iron deficiency, or inadequate EPO stimulation. The last may reflect impaired renal function, suppression of EPO production by inflammatory cytokines such as interleukin 1, or reduced tissue needs for O_2 from metabolic disease such as hypothyroidism. Only occasionally is the marrow unable to produce red cells at a normal rate, and this is most prevalent in patients with renal failure. In general, hypoproliferative anemias are characterized by normocytic, normochromic red cells, although microcytic, hypochromic cells may be observed with mild iron deficiency or long-standing chronic inflammatory disease. The key laboratory tests in distinguishing between the various forms of hypoproliferative anemia include the serum iron and iron-binding capacity, evaluation of renal and thyroid function, a marrow biopsy or aspirate to detect marrow damage or infiltrative disease, and serum ferritin to assess iron stores. Occasionally, an iron stain of the marrow will be needed to determine the pattern of iron distribution. Patients with the anemia of acute or chronic inflammation show a distinctive pattern of serum iron (low), TIBC (normal or low), percent transferrin saturation (low), and serum ferritin (normal or high). A distinct pattern of results is noted in mild to moderate iron deficiency (low serum iron, high TIBC, low percent transferrin saturation, low serum ferritin) (Chap. 90). Marrow damage by a drug, infiltrative disease such as leukemia or lymphoma, or marrow aplasia can usually be diagnosed from the peripheral blood and bone marrow morphology. With infiltrative disease or fibrosis, a marrow biopsy will likely be required.

Maturation Disorders   The presence of anemia with an inappropriately low reticulocyte production index, macro- or microcytosis on smear, and abnormal red cell indices suggests a maturation disorder. Maturation disorders are divided into two categories: nuclear maturation defects, associated with macrocytosis and abnormal marrow development, and cytoplasmic maturation defects, associated with microcytosis and hypochromia usually from defects in hemoglobin synthesis. The low reticulocyte production index is a reflection of the ineffective erythropoiesis that results from the destruction within the marrow of developing erythroblasts. Marrow morphology shows an M/E ratio of <1:1, diagnostic of erythroid hyperplasia.

Nuclear maturation defects result from vitamin B_{12} or folic acid deficiency, drug damage, or myelodysplasia. Drugs that interfere with cellular DNA metabolism, such as methotrexate or alkylating agents, can produce a nuclear maturation defect. Alcohol, alone, is also capable of producing macrocytosis and a variable degree of anemia, but this is usually associated with coincident folic acid deficiency. Measurements of folic acid and vitamin B_{12} are key not only in identifying the specific vitamin deficiency but also because they reflect different pathogenetic mechanisms.

Cytoplasmic maturation defects result from severe iron deficiency or abnormalities in globin or heme synthesis. Iron deficiency occupies an unusual position in the classification of anemia. If the iron-deficiency anemia is mild to moderate, erythroid marrow proliferation is decreased and the anemia is classified as hypoproliferative. However, if the anemia is severe and prolonged, the erythroid marrow will become hyperplastic despite the inadequate iron supply, and the anemia will be classified as ineffective erythropoiesis with a cytoplasmic maturation defect. In either case, a reduced reticulocyte production index, microcytosis, and a classic pattern of iron values make the diagnosis clear and easily distinguish iron deficiency from other cytoplasmic maturation defects such as the thalassemias. Defects in heme synthesis, in contrast to globin synthesis, are less common and may be acquired or inherited (Chap. 337). Acquired abnormalities are usually associated with myelodysplasia, may lead to either a macro- or microcytic anemia, and are frequently associated with mitochondrial iron loading. In these cases, iron is taken up by the mitochondria of the developing erythroid cell but not incorporated into heme. The iron-encrusted mitochondria surround the nucleus of the erythroid cell, forming a ring. Based on the distinctive finding of so-called ringed sideroblasts on the marrow iron stain, patients are diagnosed as having a sideroblastic anemia—almost always reflecting myelodysplasia. Again, studies of iron parameters are helpful in the differential diagnosis and management of these patients.

Blood Loss/Hemolytic Anemia   In contrast to anemias associated with an inappropriately low reticulocyte production index, blood loss or hemolysis is associated with red cell production indices ≥2.5 times normal. The stimulated erythropoiesis is reflected in the blood smear by the appearance of increased numbers of polychromatophilic macrocytes. A marrow examination is rarely indicated if the reticulocyte production index is increased appropriately. The red cell indices are typically normocytic or slightly macrocytic, reflecting the increased number of reticulocytes. Acute blood loss is not associated with an increased reticulocyte production index because of the time required to increase EPO production and, subsequently, marrow proliferation. Subacute blood loss may be associated with modest reticulocytosis. Anemia from chronic blood loss presents more often as iron deficiency than with the picture of increased red cell production.

The evaluation of blood loss anemia is usually not difficult. Most problems arise when a patient presents with an increased red cell production index from an episode of acute blood loss that went unrecognized. The cause of the anemia and increased red cell production may not be obvious. The confirmation of a recovering state may require observations over a period of 2 to 3 weeks, during which the hemoglobin concentration will be seen to rise and the reticulocyte production index fall.

Hemolytic disease, while dramatic, is among the least common forms of anemia. The ability to sustain a high reticulocyte production index reflects the ability of the erythroid marrow to compensate for hemolysis and the efficient recycling of iron from the destroyed red cells to support new hemoglobin synthesis. The level of response will depend on the severity of the anemia and the nature of the underlying disease process.

Hemoglobinopathies, such as sickle cell disease and the thalassemias, present a mixed picture. The reticulocyte index may be high but is inappropriately low for the degree of marrow erythroid hyperplasia (Chap. 91).

Hemolytic anemias present in different ways. Some appear suddenly as an acute, self-limited episode of intravascular or extravascular hemolysis, a presentation pattern often seen in patients with autoimmune hemolysis or with inherited defects of the Embden-Meyerhof pathway or the glutathione reductase pathway. Patients with inherited disorders of the hemoglobin molecule or red cell membrane generally have a lifelong clinical history typical of the disease process. Those with chronic hemolytic disease, such as hereditary spherocytosis, may actually present not with anemia but with a complication stemming from the prolonged increase in red cell destruction such as aplastic crisis, symptomatic bilirubin gallstones, or splenomegaly.

The differential diagnosis of an acute or chronic hemolytic event requires the careful integration of family history, pattern of clinical presentation, and a number of highly specific laboratory studies (Chap. 93). Some of the more common congenital hemolytic anemias may be identified from the red cell morphology, a routine laboratory test such as hemoglobin electrophoresis, or a screen for red cell enzymes. Acquired defects in red cell survival are often immunologically mediated and require a direct or indirect antiglobulin test or a cold agglutinin titer to detect the presence of hemolytic antibodies or complement-mediated red cell destruction.

R⃰ TREATMENT

An overriding principle is to initiate treatment of mild to moderate anemia only when a specific diagnosis is made. Rarely, in the acute setting, anemia may be so severe that red cell transfusions are required before a specific diagnosis is made. Whether the anemia is of acute or gradual onset, the selection of the appropriate treatment is determined by the documented cause(s) of the anemia. Often, the cause of the anemia may be multifactorial. For example, a patient with severe rheumatoid arthritis who has been taking anti-inflammatory drugs may have a hypoproliferative anemia associated with chronic inflammation as well as chronic blood loss associated with intermittent gastrointestinal bleeding. In every circumstance, it is important to evaluate the patient's iron status fully before and during the treatment of any anemia. →*Transfusion is discussed in Chap. 99; iron therapy is discussed in Chap. 90; treatment of megaloblastic anemia is discussed in Chap. 92; treatment of other entities is discussed in their respective chapters (sickle cell anemia, Chap. 91; hemolytic anemias, Chap. 93; aplastic anemia and myelodysplasia, Chap. 94).*

Therapeutic options for the treatment of anemias have expanded dramatically during the past 25 years. Blood component therapy is available and safe. Recombinant EPO as an adjunct to anemia management has transformed the lives of patients with chronic renal failure on dialysis. Improvements in the management of sickle cell crises and sickle cell anemia also have occurred. Eventually, patients with inherited disorders of globin synthesis or mutations in the globin gene, such as sickle cell disease, may benefit from the successful introduction of targeted genetic therapy (Chap. 59).

POLYCYTHEMIA

Polycythemia is defined as an increase in circulating red blood cells above normal. This increase may be real or only apparent because of a decrease in plasma volume (spurious or relative). The term *erythrocytosis* may be used interchangeably with polycythemia, but some draw a distinction between them; erythrocytosis implies documentation of increased red cell mass, whereas polycythemia refers to any increase in red cells. Often patients with polycythemia are detected through an incidental finding of elevated hemoglobin or hematocrit levels. Concern that the hemoglobin level may be abnormally high is usually triggered at 170 g/L (17 g/dL) for men and 150 g/L (15 g/dL) for women. Hematocrit levels >50% in men or >45% in women may be abnormal. Hematocrits >60% in men and >55% in women are almost invariably associated with increased red cell mass.

Historic features useful in the differential diagnosis include smoking history; living at high altitude; or a history of congenital heart disease, peptic ulcer disease, sleep apnea, chronic lung disease, or renal disease.

Patients with polycythemia may be asymptomatic or experience symptoms related to the increased red cell mass or an underlying disease process that leads to increased red cell production. The dominant symptoms from increased red cell mass are related to hyperviscosity and thrombosis (both venous and arterial), because the blood viscosity increases logarithmically at hematocrits >55%. Manifestations range from digital ischemia to Budd-Chiari syndrome with hepatic vein thrombosis. Abdominal thromboses are particularly common. Neurologic symptoms such as vertigo, tinnitus, headache, and visual disturbances may occur. Hypertension is often present. Patients with *polycythemia vera* may have aquagenic pruritus and symptoms related to hepatosplenomegaly. Patients may have easy bruising, epistaxis, or bleeding from the gastrointestinal tract. Patients with hypoxemia may develop cyanosis on minimal exertion or have headache, impaired mental acuity, and fatigue.

The physical examination usually reveals a ruddy complexion. Splenomegaly favors polycythemia vera as the diagnosis (Chap. 95). The presence of cyanosis or evidence of a right-to-left shunt suggests congenital heart disease presenting in the adult, particularly tetralogy of Fallot or Eisenmenger syndrome (Chap. 218). Increased blood viscosity raises pulmonary artery pressure; hypoxemia can lead to increased pulmonary vascular resistance. Together these factors can produce cor pulmonale.

Polycythemia can be spurious (related to a decrease in plasma volume; Gaisböck's syndrome), primary, or secondary in origin. The secondary causes are all associated with increases in EPO levels: either a physiologically adapted appropriate elevation based on tissue hypoxia (lung disease, high altitude, CO poisoning, high-affinity hemoglobinopathy) or an abnormal overproduction (renal cysts, renal artery stenosis, tumors with ectopic EPO production). A rare familial form of polycythemia is associated with normal EPO levels but hyperresponsive EPO receptors due to mutations.

APPROACH TO THE PATIENT

As shown in Fig. 52-18, the first step is to document the presence of an increased red cell mass using the principle of isotope dilution by administering ^{51}Cr-labeled autologous red blood cells to the patient and sampling blood radioactivity over a 2-h period. If the red cell mass is normal (<36 mL/kg in men, <32 mL/kg in women), the patient has spurious polycythemia. If the red cell mass is increased (>36 mL/kg in men, >32 mL/kg in women), serum EPO levels should be measured. If EPO levels are low or unmeasurable, the patient most likely has polycythemia vera. Ancillary tests that support this diagnosis include elevated white blood cell count, increased absolute basophil count, thrombocytosis, elevated leukocyte alkaline phosphatase levels, and elevated serum vitamin B_{12} and vitamin B_{12}–binding protein levels.

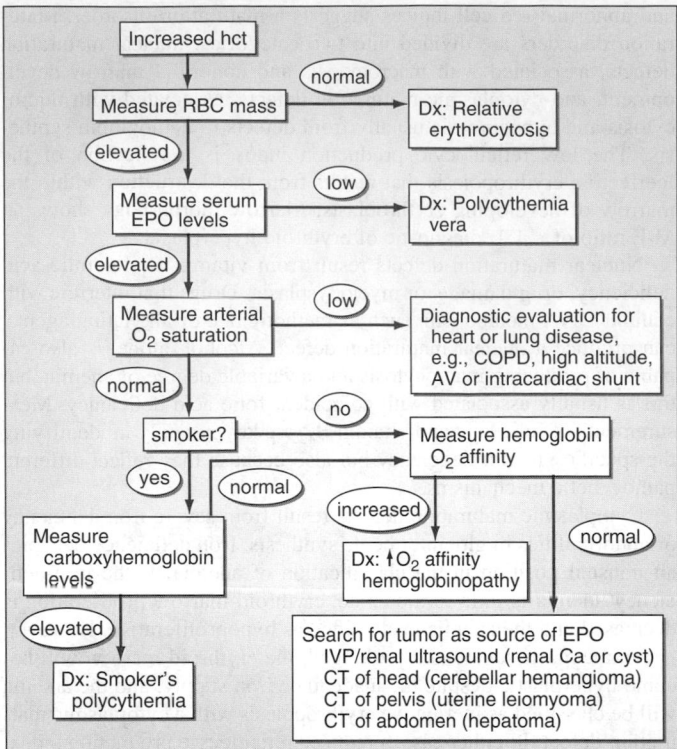

FIGURE 52-18 An approach to diagnosing patients with polycythemia. RBC, red blood cell; EPO, erythropoietin; COPD, chronic obstructive pulmonary disease; AV, atrioventricular; IVP, intravenous pyelogram; CT, computed tomography.

If serum EPO levels are elevated, one attempts to distinguish whether the elevation is a physiologic response to hypoxia or is related to autonomous production. Patients with low arterial O_2 saturation (<92%) should be further evaluated for the presence of heart or lung disease, if they are not living at high altitude. Patients with normal O_2 saturation who are smokers may have elevated EPO levels because of CO displacement of O_2. If carboxyhemoglobin (COHb) levels are high, the diagnosis is smoker's polycythemia. Such patients should be urged to stop smoking. Those who cannot stop smoking require phlebotomy to control their polycythemia. Patients with normal O_2 saturation who do not smoke either have an abnormal hemoglobin that does not deliver O_2 to the tissues (evaluated by finding elevated O_2-hemoglobin affinity) or have a source of EPO production that is not responding to the normal feedback inhibition. Further workup is dictated by the differential diagnosis of EPO-producing neoplasms. Hepatoma, uterine leiomyoma, and renal cancer or cysts are all detectable with abdominopelvic computed tomography scans. Cerebellar hemangiomas may produce EPO, but they nearly always present with localizing neurologic signs and symptoms rather than polycythemia-related symptoms.

ACKNOWLEDGMENT
Dr. Robert S. Hillman wrote this chapter in the 14th edition, and elements of his chapter were retained here.

FURTHER READING

HILLMAN RS, AULT KA: *Hematology in Clinical Practice.* New York, McGraw-Hill, 2002

Hemorrhage, intravascular thrombosis, and embolism are common clinical manifestations of many diseases. The normal hemostatic system limits blood loss by precisely regulated interactions between components of the vessel wall, blood platelets, and plasma proteins. However, when disease or trauma damages large arteries and veins, excessive bleeding may occur, despite a normal hemostatic system. Less frequently, hemorrhage is caused by an inherited or acquired disorder of the hemostatic machinery itself. A large number of bleeding disorders have been identified.

In addition, unregulated activation of the hemostatic system may cause thrombosis and embolism, which can reduce blood flow to critical organs such as the brain and myocardium. Although we understand less about the pathophysiology of thrombosis than of hemostatic failure, certain patient groups have been identified that are particularly prone to thrombosis and embolism. These include patients who (1) are immobilized after surgery, (2) have chronic congestive heart failure, (3) have atherosclerotic vascular disease, (4) have a malignancy, or (5) are pregnant. Most of these "thrombosis-prone" patients have inherited or acquired "hypercoagulable" or "prethrombotic" disorders.

Certain information in the patient's history, such as the mode of onset and sites of bleeding, a family bleeding tendency, and a record of drug ingestion, helps establish the correct diagnosis. Physical examination can identify bleeding in the skin or joint deformities due to previous hemarthroses. Ultimately, however, bleeding disorders are diagnosed by laboratory tests. General screening tests are used first, to document a systemic disorder, and are then supplemented by specific tests of coagulation protein or platelet function to arrive at an accurate diagnosis.

The hypercoagulable or prethrombotic patient can also be identified by a careful history. Three important clues to this diagnosis are: (1) repeated episodes of thromboembolism without an obvious predisposing condition, (2) a family history of thrombosis, and (3) well-documented thromboembolism in adolescents and young adults. All of the known inherited prethrombotic disorders can be diagnosed with specific immunologic, functional, or genetic tests.

NORMAL HEMOSTASIS

Accurate diagnosis and treatment of patients with either bleeding or thrombosis require knowledge of the pathophysiology of hemostasis. The process can be divided into primary and secondary components and is initiated when trauma, surgery, or disease disrupts the vascular endothelial lining and blood is exposed to subendothelial connective tissue. *Primary hemostasis* is the name given to the process of platelet plug formation at sites of injury. It occurs within seconds of injury and is of prime importance in stopping blood loss from capillaries, small arterioles, and venules (Fig. 53-1). *Secondary hemostasis* consists of the reactions of the plasma coagulation system that result in fibrin formation. It requires several minutes for completion. The fibrin strands that are produced strengthen the primary hemostatic plug. This reaction is particularly important in larger vessels and prevents bleeding from recurring hours or days after the injury. Although presented here as separate events, primary and secondary hemostasis are closely linked. For example, activated platelets accelerate plasma coagulation, and products of the plasma coagulation reaction, such as thrombin, induce platelet activation.

Effective primary hemostasis requires three critical events—platelet adhesion, granule release, and platelet aggregation. Within a few seconds of injury, platelets adhere to collagen fibrils in vascular subendothelium by at least two collagen receptors, glycoprotein (Gp) Ia/IIa, a member of the integrin family, and GpVI. GpVI binding of collagen transduces signals that activate platelets through the Fc receptor (FcRγ). As shown in Fig. 53-2, this interaction with collagen is stabilized by the von Willebrand factor (vWF), an adhesive glyco-

FIGURE 53-1 Schematic presentation of the major events in primary hemostasis. The first event is platelet adhesion, the interaction of platelets with a nonplatelet surface such as vascular subendothelium. This is followed by platelet activation and secretion. Some of the products secreted by platelets are depicted. Abbreviations: ADP, adenosine diphosphate; PDGF, platelet-derived growth factor; vWF, von Willebrand factor. The final event is the binding of activated platelets to the adherent monolayer in the process of platelet aggregation.

protein that allows platelets to remain attached to the vessel wall despite the high shear forces generated within the vascular lumen. The vWF accomplishes this task by forming a link between a platelet receptor site on Gp Ib/IX and collagen fibrils. The adherent, activated platelets then release preformed granule constituents and generate de novo mediators like those depicted in Fig. 53-1.

As in other cells, platelet activation and secretion are regulated by changes in the level of cyclic nucleotides, the influx of calcium, hydrolysis of membrane phospholipids, and phosphorylation of critical

FIGURE 53-2 The molecular basis of platelet adhesion and aggregation. Adhesion of platelets to vascular subendothelium is facilitated by the interaction of two platelet collagen receptors, GpIa/IIa ($\alpha_2\beta_1$) integrin and GpVI with collagen. The binding of collagen to GpVI causes it to interact with FcRγ, which is phosphorylated and transduces activation signals in the platelet. Adhesion is stabilized by the von Willebrand factor, which forms a bridge between collagen fibrils in the vessel wall and receptors on platelet glycoprotein Ib/IX (GpIb/IX). In a similar manner, platelet aggregation is mediated by fibrinogen, which links adjacent platelets via receptors on the platelet glycoprotein IIb/IIIa complex (GpIIb/IIIa, $\alpha_1 b/\beta_3$).

intracellular proteins. The relevant pathways are depicted in Figs. 53-3, 53-4, and 53-5. The binding of agonists such as epinephrine, collagen, or thrombin to platelet surface receptors activates two membrane enzymes—phospholipase C and phospholipase A₂. These enzymes catalyze the release of arachidonic acid from two of the major membrane phospholipids, phosphatidylinositol and phosphatidylcholine. Initially, a small quantity of the released arachidonic acid is converted to thromboxane A₂ (TXA₂), which, in turn, can activate phospholipase C. The formation of TXA₂ from arachidonic acid is mediated by the enzyme cyclooxygenase (Fig. 53-3). This enzyme is inhibited by aspirin and nonsteroidal anti-inflammatory drugs. Inhibition of TXA₂ synthesis is a cause of mild bleeding in some patients and is the same way some antithrombotic drugs work.

A finely balanced mechanism controls the rate and extent of platelet activation (Fig. 53-3). TXA₂, a platelet product of arachidonic acid, stimulates platelet activation and secretion. In contrast, prostacyclin, an endothelial cell product of arachidonic acid metabolism, inhibits platelet activation by raising intraplatelet levels of cyclic adenosine monophosphate. In addition, endothelial cells have an ecto-ADPase on their surface that hydrolyzes the platelet agonist adenosine diphosphate (ADP) and limits its effects.

Platelet signal transduction pathways are complex (Fig. 53-4). Potential platelet-activating agents bind to a surface receptor that initiates a cascade of signaling events. The four major classes of receptors are: (1) GpIb/IX complex that binds vWF; (2) integrin family receptors [GpIIB/IIIa ($\alpha IIb\beta_3$) binds fibrinogen; GpIa/IIa ($\alpha_2\beta_1$) binds collagen]; (3) seven membrane-spanning "serpentine" receptors that bind thrombin (PAR1) or TXA₂; and (4) GpVI/FcγRIIa that binds collagen. Signaling induces calcium flux and leads to remodeling of the cytoskeleton, change in shape, formation of filopodia, and granule release. These changes allow the platelet to adhere to substrata and form intravascular aggregates in concert with platelet and matrix glycoproteins such as collagen, vWF, and fibrinogen. The details of the guanine nucleotide–dependent reactions are shown in Fig. 53-5.

Following activation, platelets secrete their granule contents into plasma. Endoglycosidases and a heparin-cleaving enzyme are released from lysosomes; calcium, serotonin, and ADP are released from the dense granules; and several proteins, including vWF, fibronectin, thrombospondin, the platelet-derived growth factor (PDGF), and a heparin-neutralizing protein (platelet factor 4), are released from α granules. Released ADP binds to purinergic receptors, which, when activated, change the conformation of the GpIIb/IIIa complex so that it binds fibrinogen, linking adjacent platelets into a hemostatic plug (Fig. 53-2). The platelet-specific purinergic receptor P₂Y₁₂ is the principal activating receptor on the platelet. Released PDGF stimulates the growth and migration of fibroblasts and smooth-muscle cells within the vessel wall, an important part of the repair process.

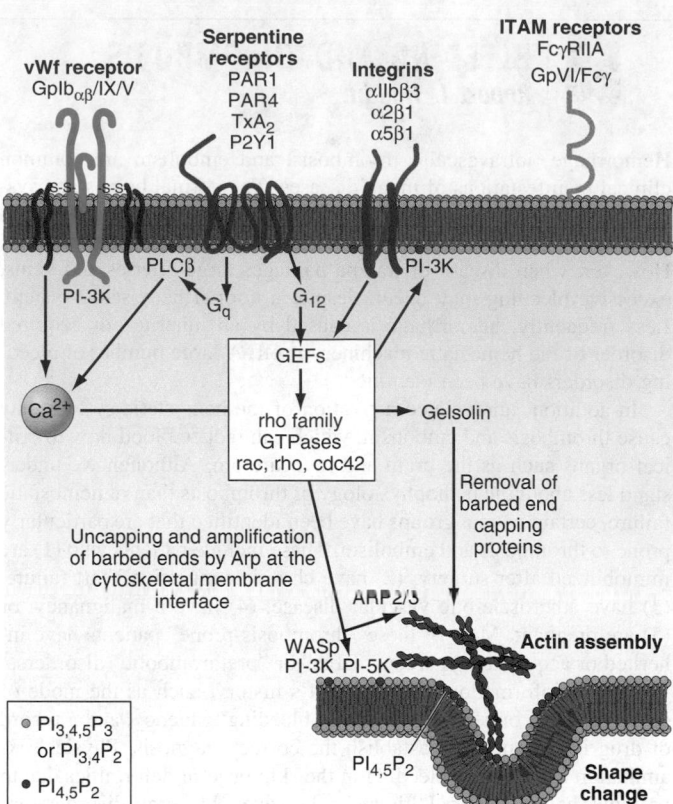

FIGURE 53-4 Platelet signal transduction overview. Actin assembly, platelet shape change, granule secretion, and the activation of some receptors are regulated by the level of intracellular calcium, the activity of guanosine triphosphatases (GTPases), and the synthesis of polyphosphoinositides. The best understood signal transduction pathway involves the multimembrane-spanning or serpentine receptors that include as agonists thrombin and thromboxane A₂. As shown, the receptors couple to downstream signaling molecules via heterotrimeric G proteins. For example, thrombin binding to PAR1 leads to the phosphorylation and dissociation of the Gq trimer complex, the activation of phospholipase Cβ (PLCβ), the hydrolysis of membrane phosphatidylinositol 4,5-bisphosphate (PI₄,₅P₂) to inositol 1,4,5-triphosphate (IP₃), and diacylglycerol (DAG). IP₃ binds to receptors on the smooth endoplasmic reticulum to release calcium into the cytosol. Calcium then activates gelsolin, which fragments actin filaments and mediates the activation of myosin II by myosin light chain kinase (MLCK). At the same time trimeric guanosine triphosphatase (GTPase) G₁₂ is activated, leading to the stimulation of guanine exchange factors (GEFs) that activate small GTPases of the rhoA family. GTP-rac activates downstream effectors including the lipid kinases phosphoinositide 5-kinase (PI-5K) and phosphoinositide 3-kinase (PI-3K). Activation of other receptors, as shown in the figure, induces other signal transduction pathways with parallel but distinct effects. Stimulation of receptors such as GpVI and FcγRIIA, which contain an immunoreceptor tyrosine-based activation motif (ITAM), increases tyrosine phosphorylation of these receptors, the tyrosine kinase Syk, the adaptor SLP76, and PLCγ. Phosphorylation activates PLCγ to hydrolyze lipids, which, in turn, promote calcium release and actin assembly. These are two of the complex signaling pathways leading to platelet activation. [From JH Hartwig, JE Italiano, Jr, in RI Handin et al (eds), Blood: Principles and Practice of Hematology, 2d ed. Philadelphia, Lippincott Williams & Wilkins, 2003, pp 1062–1079; with permission.]

As the primary hemostatic plug is being formed, plasma coagulation proteins are activated to initiate secondary hemostasis. An overall picture of the coagulation scheme, including the role of various inhibitors, is shown in Fig. 53-6. In the classic view of coagulation, four reactions have been defined (Fig. 53-7) that culminate in the production of enough thrombin to convert a small amount of plasma fibrinogen to fibrin. Each of the reactions requires the formation of a surface-bound complex and the conversion of inactive precursor proteins into active proteases by limited proteolysis, and each is regulated by both plasma and cellular cofactors and calcium.

In *reaction 1*, the intrinsic, or contact, phase of coagulation, three plasma proteins, Hageman factor (factor XII), high-molecular-weight kininogen (HMWK), and prekallikrein (PK), form a complex on vascular subendothelial collagen. After binding to HMWK, factor XII is slowly converted to an active protease (XIIa), which then activates PK to kallikrein and factor XI to XIa. Kallikrein accelerates the conversion

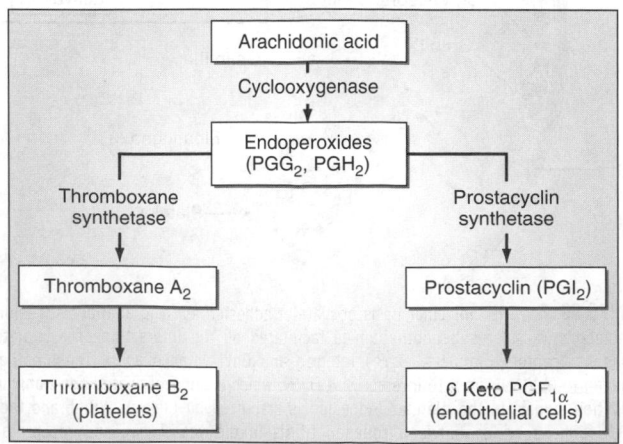

FIGURE 53-3 Generation of thromboxane A₂ in platelets and prostacyclin (PGI₂) in endothelial cells.

FIGURE 53-5 A more detailed look at G protein activation and inactivation—a key step in platelet and other cellular signal transduction pathways. G proteins exist as inactive membrane-bound heterotrimeric (α,β,γ) complexes. Binding of ligand to one of the multimembrane-spanning (usually 7 passes through the membrane) receptors leads to the conversion of the inactive guanosine diphosphate (GDP) form of the G protein complex to the active guanosine triphosphate (GTP) form that then dissociates into the GTP-α and the β,γ subunits. The dissociated subunits go on to mediate downstream events as shown in Fig. 53-4. GTP-activating proteins (GAPs) convert GTP to GDP, which then favors reassociation of the subunits to form the inactive heterotrimer. GDP dissociation inhibitors (GDI) maintain the α-GDP complex in an inactive state. The released Pi is then added to the low-molecular-weight small G proteins in the cytosol by the guanine nucleotide exchange factors (GEFs). The active forms of these low-molecular-weight G proteins also effect downstream events shown in Fig. 53-4. [From JH Hartwig, JE Italiano, Jr, in RI Handin et al (eds), Blood: Principles and Practice of Hematology, 2d ed. Philadelphia, Lippincott William & Wilkins, 2003, pp 1062–1079; with permission.]

of XII to XIIa, while XIa participates in subsequent coagulation reactions. An alternative mechanism for the activation of factor XI may exist, as patients who are deficient in either factor XII, HMWK, or PK have apparently normal hemostasis and no clinical bleeding.

Reaction 2 provides a second pathway to initiate coagulation by activating factor VII to a protease. In this extrinsic, or tissue factor–dependent, pathway, a complex is formed between factor VII, calcium, and tissue factor, a ubiquitous lipoprotein present in cellular membranes and exposed by cellular injury. The tissue factor–VII pathway

FIGURE 53-6 A schematic diagram of some of the clinically important coagulation reactions. The unactivated or precursor proteins are indicated by roman numerals, and the active form by the addition of a lowercase "a"—a standard convention. Other abbreviations: HMWK, high-molecular-weight kininogen; PK, prekallikrein; PL, phospholipid; TM, thrombomodulin; Ca²⁺, calcium. There are two independent activation pathways, the contact system and the tissue factor–mediated, or extrinsic, system. They merge at the point of factor X activation and lead to the generation of thrombin, which converts fibrinogen into fibrin. These reactions are regulated by antithrombin, which forms complexes with all of the coagulation protein serine proteases except factor VII, and by the protein C–protein S system, which inactivates factors V and VIII.

FIGURE 53-7 The major coagulation reactions are subdivided and depicted in schematic form to emphasize their similarity. They all rely on the formation of surface-bound enzyme-cofactor complexes. Abbreviations: PK, prekallikrein; K, kallikrein; HMWK, high-molecular-weight kininogen; TF, tissue factor; Ca²⁺, calcium; PT, prothrombin; Thr, thrombin. By convention, other coagulation factors are indicated by roman numerals, with a lowercase "a" appended to indicate their active form. The ^^^ is used to indicate the Gla (di-γ-carboxyglutamic acid)–containing domains of factors VII, IX, X, Xa, and PT, which bind calcium and phospholipid. Hatching is used to indicate proteins that adhere to surfaces by hydrophobic interaction.

is continuously active and makes a major contribution to basal coagulation; indeed, it seems to be the major way to initiate coagulation. Factor VII and three other coagulation proteins—factors II (prothrombin), IX, and X—require calcium and vitamin K for biologic activity. These proteins are synthesized in the liver, where a vitamin K–dependent carboxylase catalyzes a unique posttranslational modification that adds a second carboxyl group to certain glutamic acid residues. Pairs of these di-γ-carboxyglutamic acid (Gla) residues bind calcium, which alters protein comformation for binding to phospholipid surfaces and confers biologic activity. Inhibition of this modification by vitamin K antagonists (e.g., warfarin) is the basis of one of the most common forms of anticoagulant therapy.

In *reaction 3*, factor X is activated by the proteases generated in the two previous reactions. In one reaction, a calcium- and lipid-dependent complex is formed between factors VIII, IX, and X. Within this complex, factor IX is first converted to IXa by factor XIa that was generated within the intrinsic pathway (reaction 1). Factor X is then activated by factor IXa in concert with factor VIII. Alternatively, both factors IX and X can be activated more directly by factor VIIa, generated via the extrinsic pathway (reaction 2). Activation of factors IX and X provides a link between the intrinsic and extrinsic coagulation pathways (Fig. 53-6).

Reaction 4, the final step, converts prothrombin to thrombin in the presence of factor V, calcium, and phospholipid. Although prothrombin conversion can take place on various natural and artificial phospholipid-rich surfaces, it proceeds several thousand times faster on the surface of activated platelets or endothelial cells. Thrombin has multiple functions in hemostasis. Although its principal role in hemostasis is the conversion of fibrinogen to fibrin, it also activates factors V, VIII, and XIII and stimulates platelet aggregation and secretion. Following the release of fibrinopeptides A and B from the α and β chains of fibrinogen, the modified molecule, now called *fibrin monomer*, polymerizes into an insoluble gel. The fibrin polymer is then stabilized by the cross-linking of individual chains by factor XIIIa, a plasma transglutaminase (Fig. 53-6).

Although the classic view of coagulation had clinical utility, it left several important questions unanswered: (1) Why does factor XII deficiency dramatically prolong partial thromboplastin time (PTT) but not cause bleeding? (2) Why is there heterogeneity in the bleeding symptoms of patients with factor XI deficiency? (3) Why do deficiencies in factors VIII or IX produce such dramatic bleeding even though the "extrinsic" pathway remains intact? Activation of factors IX and X by the tissue factor–VIIa complex is thought to play a major role in the initiation of hemostasis. Once coagulation is initiated by this interaction, the tissue factor pathway inhibitor (TFPI) blocks the pathway, and elements of the intrinsic pathway, particularly factors VIII and IX, become the dominant regulators of thrombin generation. This step in the pathway explains why factor XII–deficient patients are asymptomatic and why factor XI–deficient patients have only a mild to moderate bleeding diathesis (Fig. 53-8).

Clot lysis and vessel repair begin immediately after the formation of the definitive hemostatic plug. Three potential activators of the fibrinolytic system are Hageman factor fragments; urinary plasminogen activator (uPA), or urokinase; and tissue plasminogen activator (tPA). The principal physiologic activators, tPA and uPA, diffuse from endothelial cells and convert plasminogen, adsorbed to the fibrin clot, into plasmin (Fig. 53-9). Plasmin then degrades fibrin polymer into small fragments, which are cleared by the monocyte-macrophage scavenger system. Although plasmin can also degrade fibrinogen, the reaction remains localized because (1) tPA and some forms of uPA activate plasminogen more effectively when it is adsorbed to fibrin clots; (2) any plasmin that enters the circulation is rapidly bound and neutralized by the α_2 plasmin inhibitor (patients who lack this factor have unchecked fibrinolysis and bleed); and (3) endothelial cells release a plasminogen activator inhibitor (PAI) 1, which blocks the action of tPA.

Only a small quantity of each coagulation enzyme is converted to its active form. As a consequence, the hemostatic plug does not propagate beyond the site of injury. Precise regulation is important, since each milliliter of blood contains enough clotting material to clot all the fibrinogen in the body in 10 to 15 s. Blood fluidity is maintained by the flow of blood, the adsorption of coagulation factors to surfaces and their trapping in the emerging clot, and by multiple inhibitors in plasma. These factors reduce the concentration of these potent enzymes and cofactors and reduce reaction rates. Antithrombin, proteins C and S, and TFPI are important inhibitors that maintain blood fluidity.

These inhibitors have distinct modes of action. Antithrombin forms complexes with all serine protease coagulation factors except factor VII (Fig. 53-6). Rates of complex formation are accelerated by heparin and heparin-like molecules on the surface of the endothelial cells. Heparin's ability to accelerate antithrombin activity is the basis for its anticoagulant action. Protein C is converted to an active protease by thrombin after it is bound to an endothelial cell protein called *thrombomodulin*. Activated protein C then inactivates the two plasma cofactors V and VIII by limited proteolysis, which slows down two critical coagulation reactions. Protein C may also stimulate the release

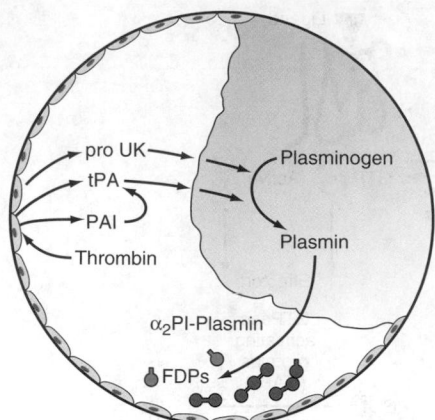

FIGURE 53-9 A schematic diagram of the fibrinolytic pathway. Tissue plasminogen activator (tPA) is released from endothelial cells, enters the fibrin clot, and activates plasminogen to plasmin. Any free plasmin is complexed with α_2 plasmin inhibitor (α_2PI). Fibrin is degraded to low-molecular-weight fragments, fibrin degradation products (FDPs).

of tPA from endothelial cells. The inhibitory function of protein C is enhanced by protein S. Reduced levels of antithrombin or proteins C and S, or dysfunctional forms of these molecules, result in a hypercoagulable or prethrombotic state. In addition, a particularly common heritable defect associated with a hypercoagulable state is the presence of a form of factor V (factor V Leiden) that is resistant to protein C inhibition. Between 20 and 50% of patients with unexplained venous thromboembolism have this defect.

Blood coagulation is not uniform throughout the body. The composition of the blood clot varies with the site of injury. Hemostatic plugs or thrombi that form in veins where blood flow is slow are rich in fibrin and trapped red blood cells and contain relatively few platelets. They are often called *red thrombi* because of their appearance in surgical and pathologic specimens. The friable ends of these red thrombi, which most often form in leg veins, can break off and embolize to the pulmonary circulation. Conversely, clots that form in arteries under conditions of high flow are predominantly composed of platelets and have little fibrin. These *white thrombi* may readily dislodge from the arterial wall and embolize to distant sites, causing temporary or permanent ischemia. These clots are a particularly common cause of embolism in the cerebral and retinal circulation, where they may lead to transient neurologic dysfunction (transient ischemic attacks), including temporary monocular blindness (amaurosis fugax), or to strokes. In addition, most episodes of myocardial infarction are due to thrombi that form after the rupture of atherosclerotic plaques within diseased coronary arteries. Hemostatic plugs, which are a physiologic response to injury, are very similar to pathologic thrombi. Thrombosis has been described as coagulation occurring in the wrong place or at the wrong time.

CLINICAL EVALUATION

HISTORY Certain elements of the history are particularly useful in determining whether bleeding is caused by an underlying hemostatic disorder or by a local anatomic defect. One clue is a history of bleeding following common hemostatic stresses such as dental extraction, childbirth, or minor surgery. Bleeding that is sufficiently severe to require a blood transfusion merits special attention. A family history of bleeding and bleeding from multiple sites that cannot be linked to trauma or surgery also suggest a systemic disorder. Since bleeding can be mild, lack of a family history of bleeding does not exclude an inherited hemostatic disorder.

Bleeding from a platelet disorder is usually localized to superficial sites such as the skin and mucous membranes, comes on immediately after trauma or surgery, and is readily controlled by local measures (Table 53-1). In contrast, bleeding from plasma coagulation defects occurs hours or days after injury and is unaffected by local therapy. Such bleeding most often occurs in deep subcutaneous tissues, muscles, joints, or body cavities. A thorough history may establish the presence of a hemostatic disorder and guide initial laboratory testing.

PHYSICAL EXAMINATION The most common site to observe bleeding is in the skin and mucous membranes. Collections of blood in the skin

FIGURE 53-8 The contribution of the tissue factor–VIIa complex (TF-VIIa) and tissue factor pathway inhibitor (TFPI) to coagulation. Initial activation of factor IX by TF-VIIa compensates for deficiencies in the early factors, e.g., factors XII and XI. The subsequent inhibition of TF-VIIa by TFPI makes sustained activation of factor X by IXa and VIIIa critical for normal hemostasis. PL, phospholipid.

TABLE 53-1 *Differences in the Clinical Manifestations of Disorders of Primary and Secondary Hemostasis*

Manifestations	Defects of Primary Hemostasis (Platelet Defects)	Defects of Secondary Hemostasis (Plasma Protein Defects)
Onset of bleeding after trauma	Immediate	Delayed—hours or days
Sites of bleeding	Superficial—skin, mucous membranes, nose, gastrointestinal and genitourinary tracts	Deep—joints, muscle, retroperitoneum
Physical findings	Petechiae, ecchymoses	Hematomas, hemarthroses
Family history	Autosomal dominant	Autosomal or X-linked recessive
Response to therapy	Immediate, local measures effective	Requires sustained systemic therapy

TABLE 53-2 *Causes of Thrombocytopenia*

Decreased marrow production of megakaryocytes
  Marrow infiltration with tumor, fibrosis
  Marrow failure—aplastic, hypoplastic anemias, drug effects
Splenic sequestration of circulating platelets
  Splenic enlargement due to tumor infiltration
  Splenic congestion due to portal hypertension
Increased destruction of circulating platelets
  Nonimmune destruction
    Vascular prostheses, cardiac valves
    Disseminated intravascular coagulation
    Sepsis
    Vasculitis
  Immune destruction
    Autoantibodies to platelet antigens
    Drug-associated antibodies
    Circulating immune complexes (systemic lupus erythematosus, viral agents, bacterial sepsis)

are called *purpura* and may be subdivided on the basis of the site of bleeding in the skin. Small pinpoint hemorrhages into the dermis due to the leakage of red cells through capillaries are called *petechiae* and are characteristic of platelet disorders—in particular, severe thrombocytopenia. Larger subcutaneous collections of blood due to leakage of blood from small arterioles and venules are called *ecchymoses* (common bruises) or, if somewhat deeper and palpable, *hematomas*. They are also common in patients with platelet defects and result from minor trauma. Dilated capillaries, or *telangiectasia*, may cause bleeding without any hemostatic defect. In addition, the loss of connective tissue support for capillaries and small veins that accompanies aging increases the fragility of superficial vessels, such as those on the dorsum of the hand, leading to extravasation of blood into subcutaneous tissue—*senile purpura*. Menorrhagia is sometimes a serious problem in women with severe thrombocytopenia or platelet dysfunction. Some patients with primary hemostatic defects, especially von Willebrand's disease, may have recurrent gastrointestinal hemorrhage, often associated with angiodysplasia, a common vascular malformation in the gastrointestinal tract.

Bleeding into body cavities, the retroperitoneum, or joints is a common manifestation of plasma coagulation defects. Repeated joint bleeding may cause synovial thickening, chronic inflammation, and fluid collections and may erode articular cartilage and lead to chronic joint deformity and limited mobility. Joint deformities are particularly common in patients with deficiencies of factors VIII and IX, the two sex-linked coagulation disorders referred to as the *hemophilias*. For unclear reasons, hemarthroses are much less common in patients with other plasma coagulation defects. Blood collections in various body cavities or soft tissues can cause secondary necrosis of tissues or nerve compression. Retroperitoneal hematomas can cause femoral nerve compression, and large collections of poorly coagulated blood in soft tissues occasionally mimic malignant growths—the *pseudotumor syndrome*. Two of the most life-threatening sites of bleeding are in the oropharynx, where bleeding can compromise the airway, and in the central nervous system. Intracerebral hemorrhage is one of the leading causes of death in patients with severe coagulation disorders. Because of their need for plasma and factor concentrates derived from multiple donors, many patients with hemophilia were infected with HIV before effective testing of donors was in place. HIV infection can induce thrombocytopenia and exacerbate bleeding in hemophilia patients.

LABORATORY TESTS The most important screening tests of the primary hemostatic system are (1) a bleeding time (a sensitive measure of platelet function), and (2) a platelet count. The latter correlates well with the propensity to bleed. The normal platelet count is 150,000 to 450,000/μL of blood. As long as the count is >100,000/μL, patients are usually asymptomatic and the bleeding time remains normal. Platelet counts of 50,000 to 100,000/μL cause mild prolongation of the bleeding time; bleeding occurs only from severe trauma or other stress. Patients with platelet counts <50,000/μL have easy bruising, mani-

fested by skin purpura after minor trauma and bleeding after mucous membrane surgery. Patients with a platelet count <20,000/μL have an appreciable incidence of spontaneous bleeding, usually have petechiae, and may have intracranial or other spontaneous internal bleeding. The major causes of thrombocytopenia are outlined in Table 53-2.

Patients with qualitative platelet abnormalities have a normal platelet count and a prolonged bleeding time (Table 53-3). The bleeding time is ascertained by making a small, superficial skin incision and timing the duration of blood flow from the wounded area. With careful standardization, bleeding time is a reliable and sensitive test of platelet function. A template or an automated scalpel controls the length and depth of the incision (usually 1 mm deep by 9 mm long), and a sphygmomanometer inflated to 40 mmHg distends the capillary bed of the forearm uniformly. The bleeding time test must be performed by an experienced technician, as small differences in technique have a big effect on outcome. Any patient with a bleeding time >10 min has an increased risk of bleeding, but the risk does not become great until the bleeding time is >15 or 20 min. As shown in Fig. 53-10, the relationship between the platelet count and the bleeding time is roughly linear. When a defect in primary hemostasis is uncovered, specialized testing is needed to determine the cause of the platelet dysfunction (Table 53-3). A precise diagnosis is important in determining the proper treatment. Occasional patients with a strong history of bleeding, particularly those with mild von Willebrand's disease, may have a normal bleeding time when initially tested, owing to cyclical variations in the level of the vWF. Repeated testing may be necessary to establish an accurate diagnosis. Bleeding time is not an effective screening test for preoperative patients.

Plasma coagulation function is readily assessed with the PTT, pro-

TABLE 53-3 *Primary Hemostatic (Platelet) Disorders*

Defects of platelet adhesion
  von Willebrand's disease
  Bernard-Soulier syndrome (absence or dysfunction of GpIb/IX)
Defects of platelet aggregation
  Glanzmann's thrombasthenia (absence or dysfunction of GpIIb/IIIa)
Defects of platelet release
  Decreased cyclooxygenase activity
    Drug-induced—aspirin, nonsteroidal anti-inflammatory agents
    Congenital
  Granule storage pool defects
    Congenital
    Acquired
  Uremia
  Platelet coating (e.g., penicillin or paraproteins)
Defect of platelet coagulant activity
  Scott's syndrome

Abbreviation: Gp, glycoprotein.

FIGURE 53-10 The relationship between the platelet count and the bleeding time. (From LA Harker, *Hemostasis Manual*, 2d ed. Philadelphia, FA Davis Company, 1974.)

thrombin time (PT), thrombin time (TT), and quantitative fibrinogen determination (Fig. 53-6, Table 53-4). The PTT screens the intrinsic limb of the coagulation system and tests for the adequacy of factors XII, HMWK, PK, XI, IX, and VIII. The PT screens the extrinsic or tissue factor–dependent pathway. Both tests also evaluate the common coagulation pathway involving all the reactions that occur after the activation of factor X. Prolongation of the PT and PTT that does not resolve after the addition of normal plasma suggests a coagulation inhibitor. A specific test for the conversion of fibrinogen to fibrin is needed when both the PTT and PT are prolonged—either a TT or a clottable fibrinogen level can be employed. When abnormalities are noted in any of the screening tests, more specific coagulation factor assays can be ordered to determine the nature of the defect.

Several rare coagulation abnormalities may be missed as they do not affect these screening tests: factor XIII deficiency, α_2 plasmin inhibitor deficiency, PAI-1 deficiency (PAI-1 is the major inhibitor of plasminogen activators), and Scott's syndrome, a platelet coagulant defect. A test for factor XIII–dependent fibrin cross-linking, like clot solubility in 5 M urea, should be ordered when the PT and PTT are both normal but the history of bleeding is strong. The fibrinolytic

system can be assessed by measuring the rate of clot lysis with the euglobulin lysis or whole blood clot lysis tests and by measuring the levels of α_2 plasmin inhibitor and PAI-1. Scott's syndrome can be detected by measuring the serum PT, which assesses the amount of residual prothrombin.

Conditions associated with thrombosis are listed in Table 53-5. Patients suspected of having a hypercoagulable or prethrombotic disorder on the basis of clinical information should be tested with specific assays to screen for the known defects. Currently available tests can identify 50 to 60% of the cases of familial or recurrent venous thrombosis.

Inhibitor syndromes or circulating anticoagulants are usually due to antibodies that impair coagulation factor activity. They are an infrequent cause of bleeding and require specialized diagnostic testing. Inhibitors are likely when screening test abnormalities cannot be reversed by adding normal plasma to patient plasma. Antibodies against specific coagulation factors may develop in: (1) postpartum women, (2) patients with autoimmune disorders such as systemic lupus erythematosus (SLE), (3) patients taking drugs such as penicillin and streptomycin, and (4) otherwise healthy elderly individuals. In addition, between 10 to 20% of patients with severe hemophilia who have received multiple plasma infusions develop inhibitory antibodies. Some patients, especially those with SLE, may also have a nonspecific form of anticoagulant antibody that interferes with phospholipid binding of coagulation factors and prolongs the PT and PTT but does not cause clinical bleeding. The presence of the lupus anticoagulant may increase the risk of thromboembolism and may cause placental infarction, recurrent midtrimester abortion, and venous and arterial thrombosis. The lupus-like anticoagulant is one manifestation of the anticardiolipin antibody syndrome. Patients may have anticardiolipin antibodies that do not prolong the PTT, but they still have an increased risk of thrombosis. Occasionally, patients develop inhibitors that are not antibodies. For example, several patients with clinical bleeding have been found to have circulating mucopolysaccharides that have heparin-like activity.

TABLE 53-4 *Relationship between Secondary Hemostatic Disorders and Coagulation Test Abnormalities*

Prolonged partial thromboplastin time (PTT)
  No clinical bleeding—factors XII, HMWK, PK
  Mild or rare bleeding—factor XI
  Frequent, severe bleeding—factors VIII and IX
Prolonged prothrombin time (PT)
  Factor VII deficiency
  Vitamin K deficiency—early
  Warfarin anticoagulant ingestion
Prolonged PTT and PT
  Factor II, V, or X deficiency
  Vitamin K deficiency—late
  Warfarin anticoagulant ingestion
Prolonged thrombin time (TT)
  Mild or rare bleeding—afibrinogenemia
  Frequent, severe bleeding—dysfibrinogenemia
  Heparin-like inhibitors or heparin administration
Prolonged PT and/or PTT not corrected with normal plasma
  Specific or nonspecific inhibitor syndromes
Clot solubility in 5 M urea
  Factor XIII deficiency
  Inhibitors or defective cross-linking
Rapid clot lysis
  α_2 plasmin inhibitor

Abbreviations: HMWK, high-molecular-weight kininogen; PK, prekallikrein.

TABLE 53-5 *Thrombotic Disorders*

Inherited
  Defective inhibition of coagulation factors
    Factor V Leiden (resistant to inhibition by activated protein C)
    Antithrombin III deficiency
    Protein C deficiency
    Protein S deficiency
    Prothrombin gene mutation (G20210A)
  Impaired clot lysis
    Dysfibrinogenemia
    Plasminogen deficiency
    tPA deficiency
    PAI-1 excess
  Uncertain mechanism
    Homocystinuria - ? endothelial damage
Acquired
  Diseases or syndromes
    Lupus anticoagulant/anticardiolipin antibody syndrome
    Malignancy
    Myeloproliferative disorder
    Thrombotic thrombocytopenic purpura
    Estrogen treatment
    Hyperlipidemia
    Diabetes mellitus
    Hyperviscosity
    Nephrotic syndrome
    Congestive heart failure
    Paroxysmal nocturnal hemoglobinuria
  Physiologic states
    Pregnancy (especially postpartum)
    Obesity
    Postoperative state
    Immobilization
    Old age

FURTHER READING

CROWTHER MA, KELTON JG: Congenital thrombophilic states associated with venous thrombosis: A qualitative overview and proposed classification. Ann Intern Med 138:128, 2003

GEORGE JN et al: Platelets: Thrombotic thrombocytopenic purpura. Hematology 2002 (American Society of Hematology Education Program book). 315:2002

HARTWIG JH, ITALIANO JE JR: Life of the blood platelet, in *Blood: Principles and Practice of Hematology*, 2nd ed, RI Handin et al (eds). Philadelpia, Lippincott Williams & Wilkins, 2003

MANN KG et al: The dynamics of thrombin formation. Arterioscler Thromb Vasc Biol 1:17, 2003

54 ENLARGEMENT OF LYMPH NODES AND SPLEEN
Patrick H. Henry, Dan L. Longo

This chapter is intended to serve as a guide to the evaluation of patients who present with enlargement of the lymph nodes (*lymphadenopathy*) or the spleen (*splenomegaly*). Lymphadenopathy is a rather common clinical finding in primary care settings, whereas palpable splenomegaly is less so.

LYMPHADENOPATHY

Lymphadenopathy may be an incidental finding in patients being examined for various reasons or it may be a presenting sign or symptom of the patient's illness. The physician must eventually decide whether the lymphadenopathy is a normal finding or one that requires further study, up to and including biopsy. Soft, flat, submandibular nodes (<1 cm) are often palpable in healthy children and young adults, and healthy adults may have palpable inguinal nodes of up to 2 cm, which are considered normal. Further evaluation of these normal nodes is not warranted. In contrast, if the physician believes the node(s) to be abnormal, then pursuit of a more precise diagnosis is needed.

APPROACH TO THE PATIENT

Lymphadenopathy may be a primary or secondary manifestation of numerous disorders, as shown in Table 54-1. Many of these disorders are infrequent causes of lymphadenopathy. Analysis of lymphadenopathy in primary care practice has shown that more than two-thirds of patients have nonspecific causes or upper respiratory illnesses (viral or bacterial), and <1% have a malignancy. In one study, researchers reported that 186 of 220 patients (84%) referred for evaluation of lymphadenopathy had a "benign" diagnosis. The remaining 34 patients (16%) had a malignancy (lymphoma or metastatic adenocarcinoma). Of the 186 patients with benign lymphadenopathy, 63% (112) had a nonspecific or reactive etiology (no causative agent found), and the remainder had a specific cause demonstrated, most commonly infectious mononucleosis, toxoplasmosis, or tuberculosis. Thus, the vast majority of patients with lymphadenopathy will have a nonspecific etiology requiring few diagnostic tests.

Clinical Assessment   The physician will be aided in the pursuit of an explanation for the lymphadenopathy by a careful medical history, physical examination, selected laboratory tests, and perhaps an excisional lymph node biopsy.

The *medical history* should reveal the setting in which lymphadenopathy is occurring. Symptoms such as sore throat, cough, fever, night sweats, fatigue, weight loss, or pain in the nodes should be sought. The patient's age, sex, occupation, exposure to pets, sexual behavior, and use of drugs such as diphenylhydantoin are other important historic points. For example, children and young adults usually have benign (i.e., nonmalignant) disorders, such as viral or bacterial upper respiratory infections, infectious mononucleosis, toxoplasmosis, and, in some countries, tuberculosis, which account for the observed lymphadenopathy. In contrast, after age 50 the incidence of malignant disorders increases and that of benign disorders decreases.

The *physical examination* can provide useful clues such as the extent of lymphadenopathy (localized or generalized), size of nodes, texture, presence or absence of nodal tenderness, signs of

inflammation over the node, skin lesions, and splenomegaly. A thorough ear, nose, and throat (ENT) examination is indicated in adult patients with cervical adenopathy and a history of tobacco use. Localized or regional adenopathy implies involvement of a single anatomic area. Generalized adenopathy has been defined as involvement of three or more noncontiguous lymph node areas. Many of the causes of lymphadenopathy (Table 54-1) can produce localized *or* generalized adenopathy, so this distinction is of limited

---

TABLE 54-1   Diseases Associated with Lymphadenopathy

1. Infectious diseases
   a. Viral—infectious mononucleosis syndromes (EBV, CMV), infectious hepatitis, herpes simplex, herpesvirus-6, varicella-zoster virus, rubella, measles, adenovirus, HIV, epidemic keratoconjunctivitis, vaccinia, herpesvirus-8
   b. Bacterial—streptococci, staphylococci, cat-scratch disease, brucellosis, tularemia, plague, chancroid, melioidosis, glanders, tuberculosis, atypical mycobacterial infection, primary and secondary syphilis, diphtheria, leprosy
   c. Fungal—histoplasmosis, coccidioidomycosis, paracoccidioidomycosis
   d. Chlamydial—lymphogranuloma venereum, trachoma
   e. Parasitic—toxoplasmosis, leishmaniasis, trypanosomiasis, filariasis
   f. Rickettsial—scrub typhus, rickettsialpox
2. Immunologic diseases
   a. Rheumatoid arthritis
   b. Juvenile rheumatoid arthritis
   c. Mixed connective tissue disease
   d. Systemic lupus erythematosus
   e. Dermatomyositis
   f. Sjögren's syndrome
   g. Serum sickness
   h. Drug hypersensitivity—diphenylhydantoin, hydralazine, allopurinol, primidone, gold, carbamazepine, etc.
   i. Angioimmunoblastic lymphadenopathy
   j. Primary biliary cirrhosis
   k. Graft-vs.-host disease
   l. Silicone-associated
3. Malignant diseases
   a. Hematologic—Hodgkin's disease, non-Hodgkin's lymphomas, acute or chronic lymphocytic leukemia, hairy cell leukemia, malignant histiocytosis, amyloidosis
   b. Metastatic—from numerous primary sites
4. Lipid storage diseases—Gaucher's, Niemann-Pick, Fabry, Tangier
5. Endocrine diseases—hyperthyroidism
6. Other disorders
   a. Castleman's disease (giant lymph node hyperplasia)
   b. Sarcoidosis
   c. Dermatopathic lymphadenitis
   d. Lymphomatoid granulomatosis
   e. Histiocytic necrotizing lymphadenitis (Kikuchi's disease)
   f. Sinus histiocytosis with massive lymphadenopathy (Rosai-Dorfman disease)
   g. Mucocutaneous lymph node syndrome (Kawasaki's disease)
   h. Histiocytosis X
   i. Familial mediterranean fever
   j. Severe hypertriglyceridemia
   k. Vascular transformation of sinuses
   l. Inflammatory pseudotumor of lymph node

Note: EBV, Epstein-Barr virus; CMV, cytomegalovirus.

utility in the differential diagnosis. Nevertheless, generalized lymphadenopathy is frequently associated with nonmalignant disorders such as infectious mononucleosis [Epstein-Barr virus (EBV) or cytomegalovirus (CMV)], toxoplasmosis, AIDS, other viral infections, systemic lupus erythematosus (SLE), and mixed connective tissue disease. Acute and chronic lymphocytic leukemias and malignant lymphomas also produce generalized adenopathy in adults.

The site of localized or regional adenopathy may provide a useful clue about the cause. Occipital adenopathy often reflects an infection of the scalp, and preauricular adenopathy accompanies conjunctival infections and cat-scratch disease. The most frequent site of regional adenopathy is the neck, and most of the causes are benign—upper respiratory infections, oral and dental lesions, infectious mononucleosis, other viral illnesses. The chief malignant causes include metastatic cancer from head and neck, breast, lung, and thyroid primaries. Enlargement of supraclavicular and scalene nodes is always abnormal. Because these nodes drain regions of the lung and retroperitoneal space, they can reflect either lymphomas, other cancers, or infectious processes arising in these areas. Virchow's node is an enlarged left supraclavicular node infiltrated with metastatic cancer from a gastrointestinal primary. Metastases to supraclavicular nodes also occur from lung, breast, testis, or ovarian cancers. Tuberculosis, sarcoidosis, and toxoplasmosis are nonneoplastic causes of supraclavicular adenopathy. Axillary adenopathy is usually due to injuries or localized infections of the ipsilateral upper extremity. Malignant causes include melanoma or lymphoma and, in women, breast cancer. Inguinal lymphadenopathy is usually secondary to infections or trauma of the lower extremities and may accompany sexually transmitted diseases such as lymphogranuloma venereum, primary syphilis, genital herpes, or chancroid. These nodes may also be involved by lymphomas and metastatic cancer from primary lesions of the rectum, genitalia, or lower extremities (melanoma).

The size and texture of the lymph node(s) and the presence of pain are useful parameters in evaluating a patient with lymphadenopathy. Nodes <1.0 cm^2 in area (1.0 × 1.0 cm or less) are almost always secondary to benign, nonspecific reactive causes. In one retrospective analysis of younger patients (9 to 25 years) who had a lymph node biopsy, a maximum diameter of >2 cm served as one discriminant for predicting that the biopsy would reveal malignant or granulomatous disease. Another study showed that a lymph node size of 2.25 cm^2 (1.5 cm × 1.5 cm) was the best discriminating limit for distinguishing malignant or granulomatous lymphadenopathy from other causes of lymphadenopathy. Patients with node(s) ≤1.0 cm^2 should be observed after excluding infectious mononucleosis and/or toxoplasmosis unless there are symptoms and signs of an underlying systemic illness.

The texture of lymph nodes may be described as soft, firm, rubbery, hard, discrete, matted, tender, movable, or fixed. Tenderness is found when the capsule is stretched during rapid enlargement, usually secondary to an inflammatory process. Some malignant diseases such as acute leukemia may produce rapid enlargement and pain in the nodes. Nodes involved by lymphoma tend to be large, discrete, symmetric, rubbery, firm, mobile, and nontender. Nodes containing metastatic cancer are often hard, nontender, and nonmovable because of fixation to surrounding tissues. The coexistence of splenomegaly in the patient with lymphadenopathy implies a systemic illness such as infectious mononucleosis, lymphoma, acute or chronic leukemia, SLE, sarcoidosis, toxoplasmosis, cat-scratch disease, or other less common hematologic disorders. The patient's story should provide helpful clues about the underlying systemic illness.

Nonsuperficial presentations (thoracic or abdominal) of adenopathy are usually detected as the result of a symptom-directed diagnostic workup. Thoracic adenopathy may be detected by routine chest roentgenography or during the workup for superficial adenopathy. It may also be found because the patient complains of a cough or wheezing from airway compression; hoarseness from recurrent laryngeal nerve involvement; dysphagia from esophageal compression; or swelling of the neck, face, or arms secondary to compression of the superior vena cava or subclavian vein. The differential diagnosis of mediastinal and hilar adenopathy includes primary lung disorders and systemic illnesses that characteristically involve mediastinal or hilar nodes. In the young, mediastinal adenopathy is associated with infectious mononucleosis and sarcoidosis. In endemic regions, histoplasmosis can cause unilateral paratracheal lymph node involvement that mimics lymphoma. Tuberculosis can also cause unilateral adenopathy. In older patients, the differential diagnosis includes primary lung cancer (especially among smokers), lymphomas, metastatic carcinoma (usually lung), tuberculosis, fungal infection, and sarcoidosis.

Enlarged intraabdominal or retroperitoneal nodes are usually malignant. Although tuberculosis may present as mesenteric lymphadenitis, these masses usually contain lymphomas or, in young men, germ cell tumors.

Laboratory Investigation   The laboratory investigation of patients with lymphadenopathy must be tailored to elucidate the etiology suspected from the patient's history and physical findings. One study from a family practice clinic evaluated 249 younger patients with "enlarged lymph nodes, not infected" or "lymphadenitis." No laboratory studies were obtained in 51%. When studies were performed, the most common were a complete blood count (33%), throat culture (16%), chest x-ray (12%), or monospot test (10%). Only eight patients (3%) had a node biopsy, and half of those were normal or reactive. The complete blood count can provide useful data for the diagnosis of acute or chronic leukemias, EBV or CMV mononucleosis, lymphoma with a leukemic component, pyogenic infections, or immune cytopenias in illnesses such as SLE. Serologic studies may demonstrate antibodies specific to components of EBV, CMV, HIV, and other viruses; *Toxoplasma gondii*; *Brucella*; etc. If SLE is suspected, then antinuclear and anti-DNA antibody studies are warranted.

The chest x-ray is usually negative, but the presence of a pulmonary infiltrate or mediastinal lymphadenopathy would suggest tuberculosis, histoplasmosis, sarcoidosis, lymphoma, primary lung cancer, or metastatic cancer and demands further investigation.

A variety of imaging techniques [computed tomography (CT), magnetic resonance imaging (MRI), ultrasound, color Doppler ultrasonography] have been employed to differentiate benign from malignant lymph nodes, especially in patients with head and neck cancer. CT and MRI are comparably accurate (65 to 90%) in the diagnosis of metastases to cervical lymph nodes. Ultrasonography has been used to determine the long (L) axis, short (S) axis, and a ratio of long to short axis in cervical nodes. An L/S ratio of <2.0 has a sensitivity and a specificity of 95% for distinguishing benign and malignant nodes in patients with head and neck cancer. This ratio has greater specificity and sensitivity than palpation or measurement of either the long or the short axis alone.

The indications for lymph node biopsy are imprecise, yet it is a valuable diagnostic tool. The decision to biopsy may be made early in a patient's evaluation or delayed for up to 2 weeks. Prompt biopsy should occur if the patient's history and physical findings suggest a malignancy; examples include a solitary, hard, nontender cervical node in an older patient who is a chronic user of tobacco; supraclavicular adenopathy; and solitary or generalized adenopathy that is firm, movable, and suggestive of lymphoma. If a primary head and neck cancer is suspected as the basis of a solitary, hard cervical node, then a careful ENT examination should be performed. Any mucosal lesion that is suspicious for a primary neoplastic process should be biopsied first. If no mucosal lesion is detected, an excisional biopsy of the largest node should be performed. Fine-needle aspiration should not be performed as the first diagnostic procedure. Most diagnoses require more tissue than such aspiration can provide, and it often delays a definitive diagnosis. Fine-needle aspiration should be reserved for thyroid nodules and for confirmation of relapse in patients whose primary diagnosis is known. If the primary physician is uncertain about whether to proceed to biopsy, consultation with a hematologist or medical oncologist should be helpful. In primary care practices, <5% of lymphadenopathy patients will require a biopsy. That percentage will be considerably larger in referral practices, i.e., hematology, oncology, or otolaryngology (ENT).

Two groups have reported algorithms that they claim will identify more precisely those lymphadenopathy patients who should have a biopsy. Both reports were retrospective analyses in referral practices. The first study involved patients 9 to 25 years of age who had a node biopsy performed. Three variables were identified that predicted those young patients with peripheral lymphadenopathy who should undergo biopsy; lymph node size >2 cm in diameter and abnormal chest x-ray had positive predictive value, whereas recent ENT symptoms had negative predictive values. The second study evaluated 220 lymphadenopathy patients in a hematology unit and identified five variables [lymph node size, location (supraclavicular or nonsupraclavicular), age (>40 years or <40 years), texture (nonhard or hard), and tenderness] that were utilized in a mathematical model to identify those patients requiring a biopsy. Positive predictive value was found for age >40 years, supraclavicular location, node size >2.25 cm², hard texture, and lack of pain or tenderness. Negative predictive value was evident for age <40 years, node size <1.0 cm², nonhard texture, and tender or painful nodes. Ninety-one percent of those who required biopsy were correctly classified by this model. Since both of these studies were retrospective analyses and one was limited to young patients, it is not known how useful these models would be if applied prospectively in a primary care setting.

Most lymphadenopathy patients do not require a biopsy, and at least half require no laboratory studies. If the patient's history and physical findings point to a benign cause for lymphadenopathy, then careful follow-up at a 2- to 4-week interval can be employed. The patient should be instructed to return for reevaluation if the node(s) increase in size. Antibiotics are not indicated for lymphadenopathy unless there is strong evidence of a bacterial infection. Glucocorticoids should not be used to treat lymphadenopathy because their lympholytic effect obscures some diagnoses (lymphoma, leukemia, Castleman's disease) and they contribute to delayed healing or activation of underlying infections. An exception to this statement is the life-threatening pharyngeal obstruction by enlarged lymphoid tissue in Waldeyer's ring that is occasionally seen in infectious mononucleosis.

SPLENOMEGALY

STRUCTURE AND FUNCTION OF THE SPLEEN The spleen is a reticuloendothelial organ that has its embryologic origin in the dorsal mesogastrium at about 5 weeks' gestation. It arises in a series of hillocks, migrates to its normal adult location in the left upper quadrant (LUQ), and is attached to the stomach via the gastrolienal ligament and to the kidney via the lienorenal ligament. When the hillocks fail to unify into a single tissue mass, accessory spleens may develop in around 20% of persons. The function of the spleen has been elusive. Galen believed it was the source of "black bile" or melancholia, and the word *hypochondria* (literally, beneath the ribs) and the idiom "to vent one's spleen" attest to the beliefs that the spleen had an important influence on the psyche and emotions. In humans, its normal physiologic roles seem to be the following:

1. Maintenance of quality control over erythrocytes in the red pulp by removal of senescent and defective red blood cells. The spleen accomplishes this function through a unique organization of its parenchyma and vasculature (Fig. 54-1).
2. Synthesis of antibodies in the white pulp.

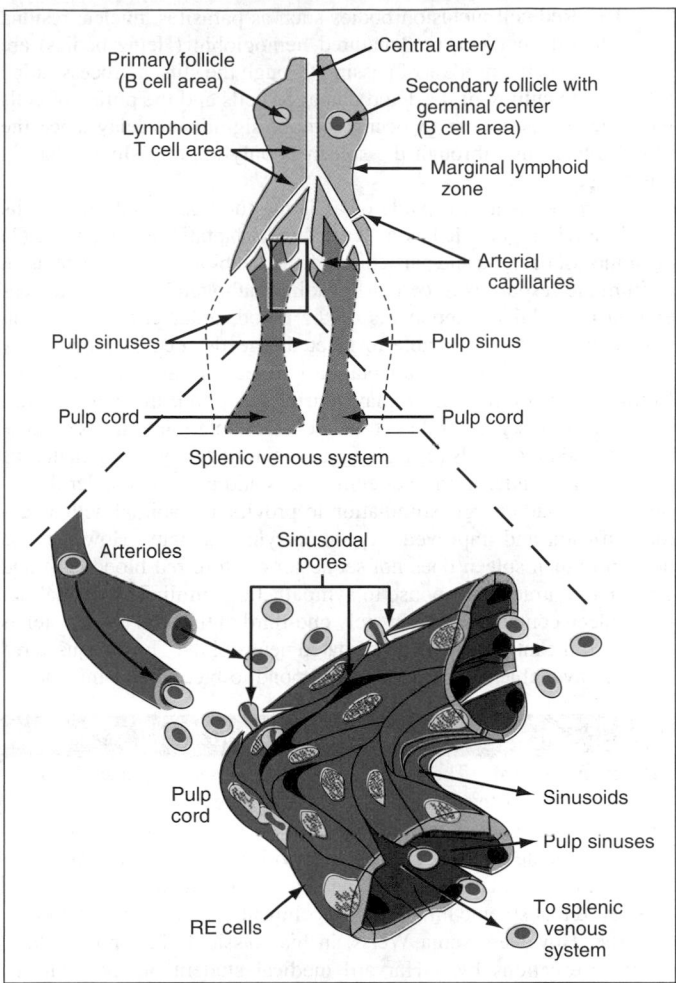

FIGURE 54-1 Schematic spleen structure. The spleen comprises many units of red and white pulp centered around small branches of the splenic artery, called central arteries. White pulp is lymphoid in nature and contains B cell follicles, a marginal zone around the follicles, and T cell–rich areas sheathing arterioles. The red pulp areas include pulp sinuses and pulp cords. The cords are dead ends. In order to regain access to the circulation, red blood cells must traverse tiny openings in the sinusoidal lining. Stiff, damaged, or old red cells cannot enter the sinuses. (*Top portion of figure from CA Janeway et al: Immunobiology, 5th edition, New York, Garland, 2001; Bottom portion of figure from RS Hillman, KA Ault: Hematology in Clinical Practice. New York, McGraw-Hill, 1995.*)

3. The removal of antibody-coated bacteria and antibody-coated blood cells from the circulation.

An increase in these normal functions may result in splenomegaly.

The spleen is composed of red pulp and white pulp, which are Malpighi's terms for the red blood–filled sinuses and reticuloendothelial cell–lined cords and the white lymphoid follicles arrayed within the red pulp matrix. The spleen is in the portal circulation. The reason for this is unknown but may relate to the fact that lower blood pressure allows less rapid flow and minimizes damage to normal erythrocytes. Blood flows into the spleen at a rate of about 150 mL/min through the splenic artery, which ultimately ramifies into central arterioles. Some blood goes from the arterioles to capillaries and then to splenic veins and out of the spleen, but the majority of blood from central arterioles flows into the macrophage-lined sinuses and cords. The blood entering the sinuses reenters the circulation through the splenic venules, but the blood entering the cords is subjected to an inspection of sorts. In order to return to the circulation, the blood cells in the cords must squeeze through slits in the cord lining to enter the sinuses that lead to the venules. Old and damaged erythrocytes are less deformable and are retained in the cords, where they are destroyed and their components recycled. Red cell inclusion bodies such as parasites, nuclear residua (Howell-Jolly bodies), or denatured hemoglobin (Heinz bodies) are pinched off in the process of passing through the slits, a process called *pitting*. The culling of dead and damaged cells and the pitting of cells with inclusions appear to occur without significant delay since the blood transit time through the spleen is only slightly slower than in other organs.

The spleen is also capable of assisting the host in adapting to its hostile environment. It has at least three adaptational functions: (1) clearance of bacteria and particulates from the blood, (2) the generation of immune responses to certain invading pathogens, and (3) the generation of cellular components of the blood under circumstances in which the marrow is unable to meet the needs (i.e., extramedullary hematopoiesis). The latter adaptation is a recapitulation of the blood-forming function the spleen plays during gestation. In some animals, the spleen also serves a role in the vascular adaptation to stress because it stores red blood cells (often hemoconcentrated to higher hematocrits than normal) under normal circumstances and contracts under the influence of β-adrenergic stimulation to provide the animal with an autotransfusion and improved oxygen-carrying capacity. However, the normal human spleen does not sequester or store red blood cells and does not contract in response to sympathetic stimuli. The normal human spleen contains approximately one-third of the total body platelets and a significant number of marginated neutrophils. These sequestered cells are available when needed to respond to bleeding or infection.

APPROACH TO THE PATIENT

Clinical Assessment   The most common *symptoms* produced by diseases involving the spleen are pain and a heavy sensation in the LUQ. Massive splenomegaly may cause early satiety.Pain may result from acute swelling of the spleen with stretching of the capsule, infarction, or inflammation of the capsule. For many years, it was believed that splenic infarction was clinically silent, which at times is true. However, Soma Weiss, in his classic 1942 report of the self-observations by a Harvard medical student on the clinical course of subacute bacterial endocarditis, documented that severe LUQ and pleuritic chest pain may accompany thromboembolic occlusion of splenic blood flow. Vascular occlusion, with infarction and pain, is commonly seen in children with sickle cell crises. Rupture of the spleen, either from trauma or infiltrative disease that breaks the capsule, may result in intraperitoneal bleeding, shock, and death. The rupture itself may be painless.

A palpable spleen is the major *physical sign* produced by diseases affecting the spleen and suggests enlargement of the organ. The normal spleen is said to weigh <250 g, decreases in size with age, normally lies entirely within the rib cage, has a maximum cephalocaudad diameter of 13 cm by ultrasonography or maximum length of 12 cm and/or width of 7 cm by radionuclide scan, and is usually not palpable. However, a palpable spleen was found in 3% of 2200 asymptomatic, male, freshman college students. Follow-up at 3 years revealed that 30% of those students still had a palpable spleen without any increase in disease prevalence. Ten-year follow-up found no evidence for lymphoid malignancies. Furthermore, in some tropical countries (e.g., New Guinea) the incidence of splenomegaly may reach 60%. Thus, the presence of a palpable spleen does not always equate with presence of disease. Even when disease is present, splenomegaly may not reflect the primary disease but rather a reaction to it. For example, in patients with Hodgkin's disease, only two-thirds of the palpable spleens show involvement by the cancer.

Physical examination of the spleen utilizes primarily the techniques of palpation and percussion. Inspection may reveal a fullness in the LUQ that descends on inspiration, a finding associated with a massively enlarged spleen. Auscultation may reveal a venous hum or a friction rub.

Palpation can be accomplished by bimanual palpation, ballot-

ment, and palpation from above (Middleton maneuver). For bimanual palpation, which is at least as reliable as the other techniques, the patient is supine with flexed knees. The examiner's left hand is placed on the lower rib cage and pulls the skin toward the costal margin, allowing the fingertips of the right hand to feel the tip of the spleen as it descends while the patient inspires slowly, smoothly, and deeply. Palpation is begun with the right hand in the left lower quadrant with gradual movement toward the left costal margin, thereby identifying the lower edge of a massively enlarged spleen. When the spleen tip is felt, the finding is recorded as centimeters below the left costal margin at some arbitrary point, i.e., 10 to 15 cm, from the midpoint of the umbilicus or the xiphisternal junction. This allows other examiners to compare findings or the initial examiner to determine changes in size over time. Bimanual palpation in the right lateral decubitus position adds nothing to the supine examination.

Percussion for splenic dullness is accomplished with any of three techniques described by Nixon, Castell, or Barkun:

1.   *Nixon's method*: The patient is placed on the right side so that the spleen lies above the colon and stomach. Percussion begins at the lower level of pulmonary resonance in the posterior axillary line and proceeds diagonally along a perpendicular line toward the lower midanterior costal margin. The upper border of dullness is normally 6 to 8 cm above the costal margin. Dullness >8 cm in an adult is presumed to indicate splenic enlargement.

2.   *Castell's method*: With the patient supine, percussion in the lowest intercostal space in the anterior axillary line (8th or 9th) produces a resonant note if the spleen is normal in size. This is true during expiration or full inspiration. A dull percussion note on full inspiration suggests splenomegaly.

3.   *Percussion of Traube's semilunar space*: The borders of Traube's space are the sixth rib superiorly, the left midaxillary line laterally, and the left costal margin inferiorly. The patient is supine with the left arm slightly abducted. During normal breathing, this space is percussed from medial to lateral margins, yielding a normal resonant sound. A dull percussion note suggests splenomegaly.

Studies comparing methods of percussion and palpation with a standard of ultrasonography or scintigraphy have revealed sensitivity of 56 to 71% for palpation and 59 to 82% for percussion. Reproducibility among examiners is better for palpation than percussion. Both techniques are less reliable in obese patients or patients who have just eaten. Thus, the physical examination techniques of palpation and percussion are imprecise at best. It has been suggested that the examiner perform percussion first and, if positive, proceed to palpation; if the spleen is palpable, then one can be reasonably confident that splenomegaly exists. However, not all LUQ masses are enlarged spleens; gastric or colon tumors and pancreatic or renal cysts or tumors can mimic splenomegaly.

The presence of an enlarged spleen can be more precisely determined, if necessary, by liver-spleen radionuclide scan, CT, MRI, or ultrasonography. The latter technique is the current procedure of choice for routine assessment of spleen size (normal = a maximum cephalocaudad diameter of 13 cm) because it has high sensitivity and specificity and is safe, noninvasive, quick, mobile, and less costly. Nuclear medicine scans are accurate, sensitive, and reliable but are costly, require greater time to generate data, and utilize immobile equipment. They have the advantage of demonstrating accessory splenic tissue. CT and MRI provide accurate determination of spleen size, but the equipment is immobile and the procedures are expensive. MRI appears to offer no advantage over CT. Changes in spleen structure such as mass lesions, infarcts, inhomogeneous infiltrates, and cysts are more readily assessed by CT, MRI, or ultrasonography. None of these techniques is very reliable in the detection of patchy infiltration (e.g., Hodgkin's disease).

Differential Diagnosis   Many of the diseases associated with splenomegaly are listed in Table 54-2. They are grouped according to the presumed basic mechanisms responsible for organ enlargement:

1. Hyperplasia or hypertrophy related to a particular splenic function such as reticuloendothelial hyperplasia (work hypertrophy) in diseases such as hereditary spherocytosis or thalassemia syndromes that require removal of large numbers of defective red blood cells; immune hyperplasia in response to systemic infection (infectious mononucleosis, subacute bacterial endocarditis) or to immunologic diseases (immune thrombocytopenia, SLE, Felty's syndrome).

2. Passive congestion due to decreased blood flow from the spleen in conditions that produce portal hypertension (cirrhosis, Budd-Chiari syndrome, congestive heart failure).

3. Infiltrative diseases of the spleen (lymphomas, metastatic cancer, amyloidosis, Gaucher's disease, myeloproliferative disorders with extramedullary hematopoiesis).

The differential diagnostic possibilities are much fewer when the spleen is "massively enlarged," that is, it is palpable more than 8 cm below the left costal margin or its drained weight is ≥1000 g (Table 54-3). The vast majority of such patients will have non-Hodgkin's lymphoma, chronic lymphocytic leukemia, hairy cell leukemia, chronic myelogenous leukemia, myelofibrosis with myeloid metaplasia, or polycythemia vera.

Laboratory Assessment The major laboratory abnormalities accompanying splenomegaly are determined by the underlying systemic illness. Erythrocyte counts may be normal, decreased (thalassemia major syndromes, SLE, cirrhosis with portal hypertension), or increased (polycythemia vera). Granulocyte counts may be normal, decreased (Felty's syndrome, congestive splenomegaly, leukemias), or increased (infections or inflammatory disease, myeloproliferative disorders). Similarly, the platelet count may be normal, decreased when there is enhanced sequestration or destruction of platelets in an enlarged spleen (congestive splenomegaly, Gaucher's disease, immune thrombocytopenia), or increased in the myeloproliferative disorders such as polycythemia vera.

The complete blood count may reveal cytopenia of one or more blood cell types, which should suggest *hypersplenism*. This condition is characterized by splenomegaly, cytopenia(s), normal or hyperplastic bone marrow, and a response to splenectomy. The latter characteristic is less precise because reversal of cytopenia, particularly granulocytopenia, is sometimes not sustained after splenectomy. The cytopenias result from increased destruction of the cellular elements secondary to reduced flow of blood through enlarged and congested cords (congestive splenomegaly) or to immune-mediated mechanisms. In hypersplenism, various cell types usually have normal morphology on the peripheral blood smear, although the red cells may be spherocytic due to loss of surface area during their longer transit through the enlarged spleen. The increased marrow production of red cells should be reflected as an increased reticulocyte production index, although the value may be less than expected due to increased sequestration of reticulocytes in the spleen.

The need for additional laboratory studies is dictated by the differential diagnosis of the underlying illness of which splenomegaly is a manifestation.

SPLENECTOMY Splenectomy is infrequently performed for diagnostic purposes, especially in the absence of clinical illness or other diagnostic tests that suggest underlying disease. More often splenectomy is performed for staging the extent of disease in patients with Hodgkin's disease, for symptom control in patients with massive splenomegaly, for disease control in patients with traumatic splenic rupture, or for correction of cytopenias in patients with hypersplenism or immune-mediated destruction of one or more cellular blood elements.

TABLE 54-2 *Diseases Associated with Splenomegaly Grouped by Pathogenic Mechanism*

ENLARGEMENT DUE TO INCREASED DEMAND FOR SPLENIC FUNCTION	ENLARGEMENT DUE TO ABNORMAL SPLENIC OR PORTAL BLOOD FLOW
Reticuloendothelial system hyperplasia (for removal of defective erythrocytes)	Cirrhosis
Spherocytosis	Hepatic vein obstruction
Early sickle cell anemia	Portal vein obstruction, intrahepatic or extrahepatic
Ovalocytosis	Cavernous transformation of the portal vein
Thalassemia major	Splenic vein obstruction
Hemoglobinopathies	Splenic artery aneurysm
Paroxysmal nocturnal hemoglobinuria	Hepatic schistosomiasis
Nutritional anemias	Congestive heart failure
Immune hyperplasia	Hepatic echinococcosis
Response to infection (viral, bacterial, fungal, parasitic)	Portal hypertension (any cause including the above): "Banti's disease"
Infectious mononucleosis	
AIDS	**INFILTRATION OF THE SPLEEN**
Viral hepatitis	
Cytomegalovirus	*Intracellular or extracellular depositions*
Subacute bacterial endocarditis	Amyloidosis
Bacterial septicemia	Gaucher's disease
Congenital syphilis	Niemann-Pick disease
Splenic abscess	Tangier disease
Tuberculosis	Hurler's syndrome and other mucopolysaccharidoses
Histoplasmosis	Hyperlipidemias
Malaria	*Benign and malignant cellular infiltrations*
Leishmaniasis	Leukemias (acute, chronic, lymphoid, myeloid, monocytic)
Trypanosomiasis	Lymphomas
Ehrlichiosis	Hodgkin's disease
Disordered immunoregulation	Myeloproliferative syndromes (e.g., polycythemia vera)
Rheumatoid arthritis (Felty's syndrome)	Angiosarcomas
Systemic lupus erythematosus	Metastatic tumors (melanoma is most common)
Collagen vascular diseases	Eosinophilic granuloma
Serum sickness	Histiocytosis X
Immune hemolytic anemias	Hamartomas
Immune thrombocytopenias	Hemangiomas, fibromas, lymphangiomas
Immune neutropenias	Splenic cysts
Drug reactions	
Angioimmunoblastic lymphadenopathy	**UNKNOWN ETIOLOGY**
Sarcoidosis	
Thyrotoxicosis (benign lymphoid hypertrophy)	Idiopathic splenomegaly
Interleukin 2 therapy	Berylliosis
Extramedullary hematopoiesis	Iron-deficiency anemia
Myelofibrosis	
Marrow damage by toxins, radiation, strontium	
Marrow infiltration by tumors, leukemias, Gaucher's disease	

TABLE 54-3 *Diseases Associated with Massive Splenomegaly*[a]

Chronic myelogenous leukemia	Gaucher's disease
Lymphomas	Chronic lymphocytic leukemia
Hairy cell leukemia	Sarcoidosis
Myelofibrosis with myeloid metaplasia	Autoimmune hemolytic anemia
Polycythemia vera	Diffuse splenic hemangiomatosis

[a] The spleen extends greater than 8 cm below left costal margin and/or weighs more than 1000 g.

Splenectomy is necessary for routine staging of patients with Hodgkin's disease only in those with clinical stage I or II disease in whom radiation therapy alone is contemplated as the treatment. Noninvasive staging of the spleen in Hodgkin's disease is not a sufficiently reliable basis for treatment decisions because one-third of normal-sized spleens will be involved with Hodgkin's disease and one-third of enlarged spleens will be tumor-free. Although splenectomy in chronic myelogenous leukemia does not affect the natural history of disease, removal of the massive spleen usually makes patients significantly more comfortable and simplifies their management by significantly reducing transfusion requirements. Splenectomy is an effective secondary or tertiary treatment for two chronic B cell leukemias, hairy cell leukemia and prolymphocytic leukemia, and for the very rare splenic mantle cell or marginal zone lymphoma. Splenectomy in these diseases may be associated with significant tumor regression in bone marrow and other sites of disease. Similar regressions of systemic disease have been noted after splenic irradiation in some types of lymphoproliferative disease, especially chronic lymphocytic leukemia and prolymphocytic leukemia. This has been termed the *abscopal effect*. Such systemic tumor responses to local therapy directed at the spleen suggest that there may be some hormone or growth factor produced by the spleen that affects tumor cell proliferation, but this conjecture is not yet substantiated. A common therapeutic indication for splenectomy is traumatic or iatrogenic splenic rupture. In a fraction of patients with splenic rupture, peritoneal seeding of splenic fragments can lead to *splenosis*—the presence of multiple rests of spleen tissue not connected to the portal circulation. This ectopic spleen tissue may cause pain or gastrointestinal obstruction, as in endometriosis. A large number of hematologic, immunologic, and congestive causes of splenomegaly can lead to destruction of one or more cellular blood elements. In the majority of such cases, splenectomy can correct the cytopenias, particularly anemia and thrombocytopenia. In a large series of patients seen in two tertiary care centers, the indication for splenectomy was diagnostic in 10% of the patients, therapeutic in 44%, staging for Hodgkin's disease in 20%, and incidental to another procedure in 26%. Perhaps the only contraindication to splenectomy is the presence of marrow failure, in which the enlarged spleen is the only source of hematopoietic tissue.

The absence of the spleen has minimal long-term effects on the hematologic profile. In the immediate postsplenectomy period, there may be some leukocytosis (up to $25,000/\mu L$) and thrombocytosis (up to $1 \times 10^6/\mu L$), but within 2 to 3 weeks, blood cell counts and survival of each cell lineage are usually normal. The chronic manifestations of splenectomy are marked variation in size and shape of erythrocytes (anisocytosis, poikilocytosis) and the presence of Howell-Jolly bodies (nuclear remnants), Heinz bodies (denatured hemoglobin), basophilic stippling, and an occasional nucleated erythrocyte in the peripheral blood. When such erythrocyte abnormalities appear in a patient whose spleen has not been removed, one should suspect splenic infiltration by tumor that has interfered with its normal culling and pitting function.

The most serious consequence of splenectomy is increased susceptibility to bacterial infections, particularly those with capsules such as *Streptococcus pneumoniae*, *Haemophilus influenzae*, and some gramnegative enteric organisms. Patients under age 20 years are particularly susceptible to overwhelming sepsis with *S. pneumoniae*, and the overall actuarial risk of sepsis in patients who have had their spleens removed is about 7% in 10 years. The case-fatality rate for pneumococcal sepsis in splenectomized patients is 50 to 80%. About 25% of patients without spleens will develop a serious infection at some time in their life. The frequency is highest within the first 3 years after splenectomy. About 15% of the infections are polymicrobial, and lung, skin, and blood are the most common sites. No increased risk of viral infection has been noted in patients who have no spleen. The susceptibility to bacterial infections relates to the inability to remove opsonized bacteria from the bloodstream and a defect in making antibodies to T cell–independent antigens such as the polysaccharide components of bacterial capsules. Pneumococcal vaccine (23-valent polysaccharide vaccine) should be administered to all patients 2 weeks before elective splenectomy. The Advisory Committee on Immunization Practices recommends that even splenectomized patients receive pneumococcal vaccine with a repeat vaccination 5 years later. Efficacy has not been proven in this setting, and the recommendation discounts the possibility that administration of the vaccine may actually lower the titer of specific pneumococcal antibodies. A more effective pneumococcal vaccine that involves T cells in the response is in development. The vaccine to *Neisseria meningitidis* should also be given to patients in whom elective splenectomy is planned. No other vaccines are routinely recommended in this setting.

Splenectomized patients should be educated to consider any unexplained fever as a medical emergency. Prompt medical attention with evaluation and treatment of suspected bacteremia may be lifesaving. Routine chemoprophylaxis with oral penicillin can result in the emergence of drug-resistant strains and is not recommended.

In addition to an increased susceptibility to bacterial infections, splenectomized patients are also more susceptible to the parasitic disease babesiosis. The splenectomized patient should avoid areas where the parasite *Babesia* is endemic (e.g., Cape Cod, MA).

Surgical removal of the spleen is an obvious cause of hyposplenism. Patients with sickle cell disease often suffer from autosplenectomy as a result of splenic destruction by the numerous infarcts associated with sickle cell crises during childhood. Indeed, the presence of a palpable spleen in a patient with sickle cell disease after age 5 suggests a coexisting hemoglobinopathy, e.g., thalassemia or hemoglobin C. In addition, patients who receive splenic irradiation for a neoplastic or autoimmune disease are also functionally hyposplenic. The term *hyposplenism* is preferred to *asplenism* in referring to the physiologic consequences of splenectomy because asplenia is a rare, specific, and fatal congenital abnormality in which there is a failure of the left side of the coelomic cavity (which includes the splenic anlagen) to develop normally. Infants with asplenia have no spleens, but that is the least of their problems. The right side of the developing embryo is duplicated on the left so there is liver where the spleen should be, there are two right lungs, and the heart comprises two right atria and two right ventricles.

FURTHER READING

BARKUN AN et al: The bedside assessment of splenic enlargement. Am J Med 91:512, 1991

GRAVES SA et al: Does this patient have splenomegaly? JAMA 270:2218, 1993

KRAUS MD et al: The spleen as a diagnostic specimen: A review of ten years' experience at two tertiary care institutions. Cancer 91:2001, 2001

MCINTYRE OR, EBAUGH FG JR: Palpable spleens: Ten year follow-up. Ann Intern Med 90:130, 1979

PANGALIS GA et al: Clinical approach to lymphadenopathy. Semin Oncol 20: 570, 1993

PREVENTION OF PNEUMOCOCCAL DISEASE: Recommendations of the Advisory Committee on Immunization Practices. MMWR 46(RR-8):1, 1997

WILLIAMSON HA JR: Lymphadenopathy in a family practice: A descriptive study of 240 cases. J Fam Pract 20:449, 1985

Leukocytes are the major cells comprising inflammatory and immune responses and include neutrophils, T and B lymphocytes, natural killer (NK) cells, monocytes, eosinophils, and basophils. These cells have specific functions, such as antibody production by B lymphocytes or destruction of bacteria by neutrophils, but in no single infectious disease is the exact role of the cell types completely established. Thus, whereas neutrophils are classically thought to be critical to host defense against bacteria, they may also play important roles in defense against viral infections.

The blood delivers leukocytes to the various tissues from the bone marrow, where they are produced. Normal blood leukocyte counts are 4.3 to 10.8 × 10⁹/L with neutrophils representing 45 to 74% of the cells, bands 0 to 4%, lymphocytes 16 to 45%, monocytes 4 to 10%, eosinophils 0 to 7%, and basophils 0 to 2%. The various leukocytes are derived from a common stem cell in the bone marrow. Three-fourths of the nucleated cells of bone marrow are committed to the production of leukocytes. Leukocyte maturation in the marrow is under the regulatory control of a number of different factors, known as colony-stimulating factors and interleukins (ILs). Because an alteration in the number and type of leukocytes is often associated with disease processes, total white blood count (WBC) (cells per microliter) and differential counts are informative. The lymphocytes and basophils are discussed in Chaps. 295 and 298, respectively. This chapter focuses on the neutrophils, monocytes, and eosinophils.

NEUTROPHILS

MATURATION Important events in neutrophil life are summarized in Fig. 55-1. In normal humans, neutrophils are produced only in the bone marrow. The minimum number of stem cells necessary to support hematopoiesis is estimated to be 400 to 500. Human blood monocytes, tissue macrophages, and stromal cells produce colony-stimulating factors, hormones required for the growth of monocytes and neutrophils in the bone marrow. The hematopoietic system not only produces enough neutrophils (~1.3 × 10¹¹ cells per 80-kg person per day) to carry out physiologic functions but also has a large reserve stored in the marrow, which can be mobilized in response to inflammation or infection. An increase in the number of blood neutrophils is called *neutrophilia*, and the presence of immature cells is termed a *shift to the left*. A decrease in the number of blood neutrophils is called *neutropenia*.

Neutrophils and monocytes evolve from pluripotent stem cells under the influence of cytokines and colony-stimulating factors (Fig. 55-2). The proliferation phase through the metamyelocyte takes about 1 week, while the maturation phase from metamyelocyte to mature neutrophil takes another week. The myeloblast is the first recognizable precursor cell and is followed by the *promyelocyte*. The promyelocyte evolves when the classic lysosomal granules, called the *primary*, or *azurophil*, *granules*, are produced. The primary granules contain hydrolases, elastase, myeloperoxidase, cathepsin G, cationic proteins, and bactericidal/permeability-increasing protein, which is important for killing gram-negative bacteria. Azurophil granules also contain *defensins*, a family of cysteine-rich polypeptides with broad antimicrobial activity against bacteria, fungi, and certain enveloped viruses. The promyelocyte divides to produce the *myelocyte*, a cell responsible for the synthesis of the spe-

cific, or *secondary, granules*, which contain unique (specific) constituents such as lactoferrin, vitamin B₁₂–binding protein, membrane components of the nicotinamide-adenine dinucleotide phosphate (NADPH) oxidase required for hydrogen peroxide production, histaminase, and receptors for certain chemoattractants and adherence-promoting factors (CR3) as well as receptors for the basement membrane component, laminin. The secondary granules do not contain acid hydrolases and therefore are not classic lysosomes. Packaging of secondary granule contents during myelopoiesis is controlled by CCAAT/enhancer binding protein-ε. Secondary granule contents are readily released extracellularly, and their mobilization is important in modulating inflammation. During the final stages of maturation no cell division occurs, and the cell passes through the metamyelocyte stage and then to the band neutrophil with a sausage-shaped nucleus (Fig. 55-3). As the band cell matures, the nucleus assumes a lobulated configuration. The nucleus of neutrophils normally contains up to four segments (Fig. 55-4). Excessive segmentation (more than five nuclear lobes) may be a manifestation of folate or vitamin B₁₂ deficiency (Fig. 92-4). The Pelger-Hüet anomaly (Fig. 55-5), an infrequent dominant benign inherited trait, results in neutrophils with distinctive bilobed nuclei that must be distinguished from band forms. The physiologic role of the multilobed nucleus of neutrophils is unknown, but it may allow great deformation of neutrophils during migration into tissues at sites of inflammation.

In severe acute bacterial infection, prominent neutrophil cytoplasmic granules, called *toxic granulations*, are occasionally seen. Toxic granulations are immature or abnormally staining azurophil granules. Cytoplasmic inclusions, also called *Döhle bodies* (Fig. 55-3), can be seen during infection and are fragments of ribosome-rich endoplasmic reticulum. Large neutrophil vacuoles are often present in acute bacterial infection and probably represent pinocytosed (internalized) membrane.

Neutrophils are heterogeneous in function. Monoclonal antibodies have been developed that recognize only a subset of mature neutrophils. The meaning of neutrophil heterogeneity is not known.

The morphology of eosinophils and basophils is shown in Fig. 55-6.

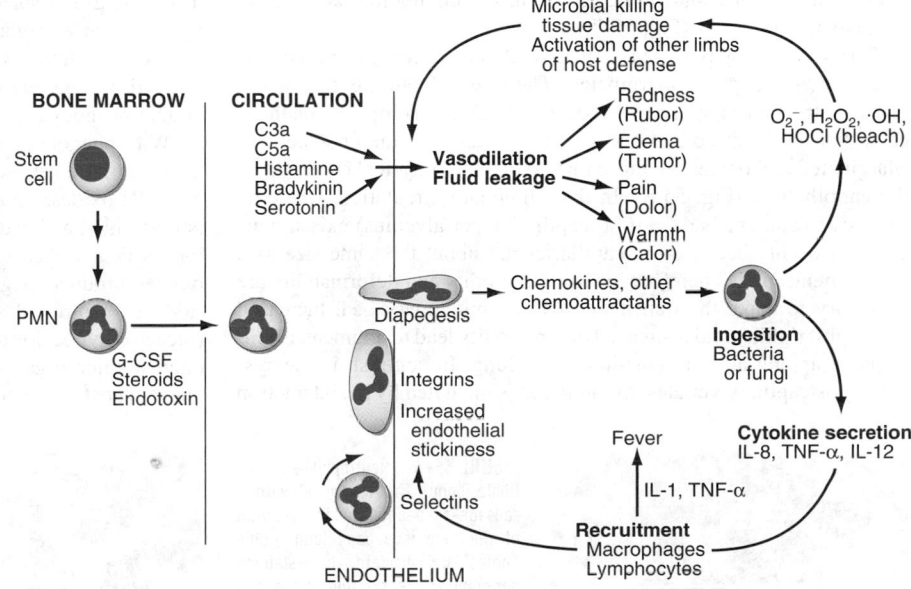

FIGURE 55-1 Schematic events in neutrophil production, recruitment, and inflammation. The four cardinal signs of inflammation (rubor, tumor, calor, dolor) are indicated, as are the interactions of neutrophils with other cells and cytokines. PMN, polymorphonuclear leukocytes; G-CSF, granulocyte colony-stimulating factor; IL, interleukin; TNF-α, tumor necrosis factor.

Cell	Stage	Surface Markers[a]	Characteristics
![myeloblast]	MYELOBLAST	CD33, CD13, CD15	Prominent nucleoli
![promyelocyte]	PROMYELOCYTE	CD33, CD13, CD15	Large cell Primary granules appear
![myelocyte]	MYELOCYTE	CD33, CD13, CD15, CD14, CD11b	Secondary granules appear
![metamyelocyte]	METAMYELOCYTE	CD33, CD13, CD15, CD14, CD11b	Kidney bean–shaped nucleus
![band form]	BAND FORM	CD33, CD13, CD15, CD14, CD11b CD10, CD16	Condensed, band–shaped nucleus
![neutrophil]	NEUTROPHIL	CD33, CD13, CD15, CD14, CD11b CD10, CD16	Condensed, multilobed nucleus

[a]CD= Cluster Determinant; ● Nucleolus; ● Primary granule; ◆Secondary granule.

FIGURE 55-2 Stages of neutrophil development are schematically shown. G-CSF and GM-CSF are critical to this process. Identifying cellular characteristics and specific cell-surface markers are listed for each maturational stage.

MARROW RELEASE AND CIRCULATING COMPARTMENTS Specific signals, including IL-1, tumor necrosis factor-α (TNF-α), the colony-stimulating factors, complement fragments, and perhaps other cytokines, mobilize leukocytes from the bone marrow and deliver them to the blood in an unstimulated state. Under normal conditions, ~90% of the neutrophil pool is in the bone marrow, 2 to 3% in the circulation, and the remainder in the tissues (Fig. 55-7).

The circulating pool exists in two dynamic compartments: one freely flowing and one marginated. The freely flowing pool is about one-half the neutrophils in the basal state and is composed of those cells that are in the blood and not in contact with the endothelium. Marginated leukocytes are those that are in close physical contact with the endothelium (Fig. 55-8). In the pulmonary circulation, where an extensive capillary bed (~1000 capillaries per alveolus) exists, margination occurs because the capillaries are about the same size as a mature neutrophil. Therefore, neutrophil fluidity and deformability are necessary to make the transit through the pulmonary bed. Increased neutrophil rigidity and decreased deformability lead to augmented neutrophil trapping and margination in the lung. In contrast, in the systemic postcapillary venules, margination is mediated by the interaction of specific cell-surface molecules. *Selectins* are glycoproteins expressed on neutrophils and endothelial cells, among others, that cause a low-affinity interaction, resulting in "rolling" of the neutrophil along the endothelial surface. On neutrophils, the molecule L-selectin [cluster determinant (CD) 62L] binds to glycosylated proteins on endothelial cells [e.g., glycosylation-dependent cell adhesion molecule (GlyCAM1) and CD34]. Glycoproteins on neutrophils, most importantly sialyl-Lewis^x (SLe^x, CD15s), are targets for binding of selectins expressed on endothelial cells [E-selectin (CD62E) and P-selectin (CD62P)] and other leukocytes. In response to chemotactic stimuli from injured tissues (e.g., complement product C5a, leukotriene B$_4$, IL-8) or bacterial products [e.g., N-formylmethionylleucylphenylalanine (f-metleuphe)], neutrophil adhesiveness increases, and the cells "stick" to the endothelium through *integrins*. The integrins are leukocyte glycoproteins that exist as complexes of a common CD18 β chain with CD11a (LFA-1), CD11b (also called either Mac-1, CR3, or the C3bi receptor), and CD11c (p150,95). CD11a/CD18 and CD11b/CD18 bind to specific endothelial receptors [intercellular adhesion molecules (ICAM) 1 and 2.]

On cell stimulation, L-selectin is shed; receptors for chemoattractants and opsonins are mobilized; and the phagocytes orient toward the chemoattractant source in the extravascular space, increase their motile activity (chemokinesis), and migrate directionally (chemotaxis) into tissues. The process of migration into tissues is called *diapedesis* and involves the crawling of neutrophils between postcapillary endothelial cells that open junctions between adjacent cells to permit leukocyte passage. Diapedesis involves platelet/endothelial cell adhesion molecule (PECAM) 1 (CD31), which is expressed on both the emigrating leukocyte and the endothelial cells. The endothelial responses (increased blood flow from increased vasodilation and permeability) are mediated by anaphylatoxins (e.g., C3a and C5a) as well as vasodilators such as histamine, bradykinin, serotonin, nitric oxide, vascular endothelial growth factor (VEGF), and prostaglandins E and I. Cytokines regulate some of these processes [e.g., TNF-α induction of VEGF, interferon (IFN) γ inhibition of prostaglandin E.

In the healthy adult, most neutrophils leave the body by migration through the mucous membrane of the gastrointestinal tract. Normally, neutrophils spend a short time in the circulation (half-life, 6 to 7 h). Senescent neutrophils are cleared from the circulation by macrophages in the lung and spleen. Once in the tissues, neutrophils release enzymes, such as collagenase and elastase, that help establish abscess cavities. Neutrophils ingest pathogenic materials that have been opsonized by IgG and C3b. Fibronectin and the tetrapeptide tuftsin facilitate phagocytosis.

With phagocytosis comes a burst of oxygen consumption and activation of the hexose-monophosphate shunt. A membrane-associated NADPH oxidase, consisting of membrane and cytosolic components, is assembled and catalyzes the reduction of oxygen to superoxide anion, which is then converted to hydrogen peroxide and other toxic oxygen products (e.g., hydroxyl radical). Hydrogen peroxide + chloride + neutrophil myeloperoxidase generate hypochlorous acid (bleach), hypochlorite, and chlorine. These products oxidize and halogenate microorganisms and tumor cells and, when uncontrolled, can damage host tissue. Strongly cationic proteins, defensins, and probably

FIGURE 55-3 Neutrophil band with Döhle body. The neutrophil with a sausage-shaped nucleus in the center of the field is a band form. Döhle bodies are discrete, blue-staining nongranular areas found in the periphery of the cytoplasm of the neutrophil in infections and other toxic states. They represent aggregates of rough endoplasmic reticulum.

FIGURE 55-4 Normal granulocyte. The normal granulocyte has a segmented nucleus with heavy, clumped chromatin; fine neutrophilic granules are dispersed throughout the cytoplasm.

FIGURE 55-5 Pelger-Hüet anomaly. In this benign disorder, the majority of granulocytes are bilobed. The nucleus frequently has a spectacle-like, or "pince-nez," configuration.

nitric oxide also participate in microbial killing. Other enzymes, such as lysozyme and acid proteases, help digest microbial debris. After 1 to 4 days in tissues neutrophils die. The apoptosis of neutrophils is also cytokine-regulated; granulocyte colony-stimulating factor (G-CSF) and IFN-γ prevent their death. Under certain conditions, such as in delayed-type hypersensitivity, monocyte accumulation occurs within 6 to 12 h of initiation of inflammation. Neutrophils, monocytes, microorganisms in various states of digestion, and altered local tissue cells make up the inflammatory exudate, pus. Myeloperoxidase confers the characteristic green color to pus and may participate in turning off the inflammatory process by inactivating chemoattractants and immobilizing phagocytic cells.

Neutrophils respond to certain cytokines [IFN-γ, granulocyte-macrophage colony-stimulating factor (GM-CSF), IL-8] and produce cytokines and chemotactic signals [TNF-α, IL-8, macrophage inflammatory protein (MIP) 1] that modulate the inflammatory response. In the presence of fibrinogen, f-metleuphe or leukotriene B_4 induces IL-8 production by neutrophils, providing autocrine amplification of inflammation. *Chemokines* (chemoattractant cytokines) are small proteins produced by many different cell types, including endothelial cells, fibroblasts, epithelial cells, neutrophils, and monocytes, that regulate neutrophil and monocyte recruitment and activation. The chemokines transduce their signals through heterotrimeric G protein–linked receptors that have seven cell membrane–spanning domains, the same type of cell-surface receptor that mediates the response to the classic chemoattractants f-metleuphe and C5a. Four major groups of chemokines are recognized based on the cysteine structure near the N terminus: C, CC, CXC, and CXXXC. The CXC cytokines such as IL-8 mainly attract neutrophils; CC chemokines such as MIP-1 attract lymphocytes, monocytes, eosinophils, and basophils; the C chemokine lymphotactin is T cell tropic; the CXXXC chemokine fractalkine attracts neutrophils, monocytes, and T cells. These molecules and their receptors not only regulate the trafficking and activation of inflammatory cells, but chemokine receptors serve as co-receptors for HIV infection (Chap. 173) and have a role in atherogenesis.

NEUTROPHIL ABNORMALITIES A defect in the neutrophil life cycle can lead to dysfunction and compromised host defenses. Inflammation is often depressed, and the clinical result is often recurrent and severe bacterial and fungal infections. Aphthous ulcers of mucous membranes (gray ulcers without pus) and gingivitis and periodontal disease suggest a phagocytic cell disorder. Patients with congenital phagocyte defects can have infections within the first few days of life. Skin, ear, upper and lower respiratory tract, and bone infections are common. Sepsis and meningitis are rare. In some disorders the frequency of infection is variable, and patients can go for months or even years without major infection. Aggressive management of these congenital diseases has extended the life span of patients well beyond 30 years.

FIGURE 55-6 Normal eosinophil and basophil. The eosinophil contains large, bright orange granules and usually a bilobed nucleus. The basophil contains large purple-black granules that fill the cell and obscure the nucleus.

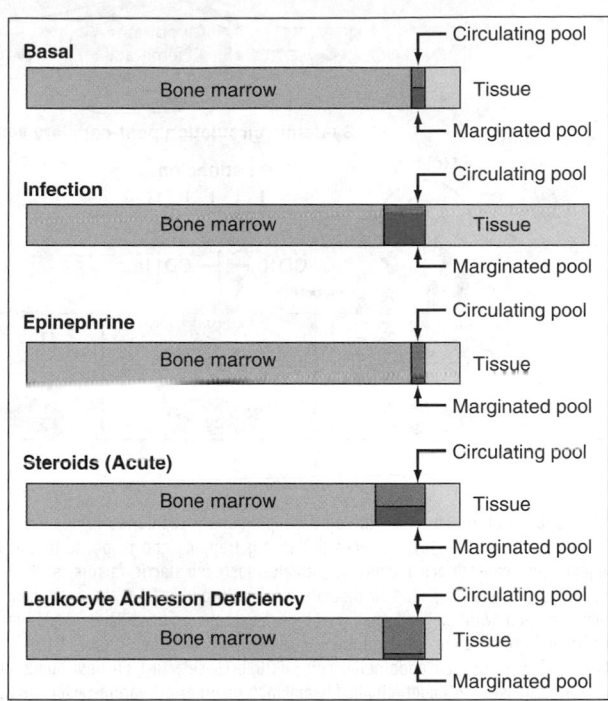

FIGURE 55-7 Schematic neutrophil distribution and kinetics between the different anatomic and functional pools.

Neutropenia The consequences of absent neutrophils are dramatic. Susceptibility to infectious diseases increases sharply when neutrophil counts fall below 1000 cells/μL. When the absolute neutrophil count (ANC; band forms and mature neutrophils combined) falls to <500 cells/μL, control of endogenous microbial flora (e.g., mouth, gut) is impaired; when the ANC is <200/μL, the inflammatory process is absent. Neutropenia can be due to depressed production, increased peripheral destruction, or excessive peripheral pooling. A falling neutrophil count or a significant decrease in the number of neutrophils below steady-state levels, together with a failure to increase neutrophil counts in the setting of infection or other challenge, requires investigation. Acute neutropenia, such as that caused by cancer chemotherapy, is more likely to be associated with increased risk of infection than neutropenia of long duration (months to years) that reverses in response to infection or carefully controlled administration of endotoxin (see "Laboratory Diagnosis," below).

Some causes of inherited and acquired neutropenia are listed in Table 55-1. The most common neutropenias are iatrogenic, resulting from the use of cytotoxic or immunosuppressive therapies for malignancy or control of autoimmune disorders. These drugs cause neutropenia because they result in decreased production of rapidly growing progenitor (stem) cells of the marrow. Certain antibiotics such as chloramphenicol, trimethoprim-sulfamethoxazole, flucytosine, vidarabine, and the antiretroviral drug zidovudine may cause neutropenia by inhibiting proliferation of myeloid precursors. The marrow suppression is generally dose-related and dependent on continued administration of the drug. Recombinant human G-CSF usually reverses this form of neutropenia.

Another important mechanism for iatrogenic neutropenia is the effect of drugs that serve as immune haptens and sensitize neutrophils or neutrophil precursors to immune-mediated peripheral destruction. This form of drug-induced neutropenia can be seen within 7 days of exposure to the drug; with previous drug exposure, resulting in pre-existing antibodies, neutropenia may occur a few hours after administration of the drug. Although any drug can cause this form of neutropenia, the most frequent causes are commonly used antibiotics, such as sulfa-containing compounds, penicillins, and cephalosporins. Fever and eosinophilia may also be associated with drug reactions, but

FIGURE 55-8 Neutrophil travel through the pulmonary capillaries is dependent on neutrophil deformability. Neutrophil rigidity (e.g., caused by C5a) enhances pulmonary trapping and response to pulmonary pathogens in a way that is not so dependent upon cell-surface receptors. Intraalveolar chemotactic factors, such as those caused by certain bacteria (e.g., *Streptococcus pneumoniae*) lead to diapedesis of neutrophils from the pulmonary capillaries into the alveolar space. Neutrophil interaction with the endothelium of the systemic postcapillary venules is dependent on molecules of attachment. The neutrophil "rolls" along the endothelium using selectins: neutrophil CD15s (sialyl-Lewis^x) binds to CD62E (E-selectin) and CD62P (P-selectin) on endothelial cells; CD62L (L-selectin) on neutrophils binds to CD34 and other molecules (e.g., GlyCAM-1) expressed on endothelium. Chemokines or other activation factors stimulate integrin-mediated "tight adhesion": CD11a/CD18 (LFA-1) and CD11b/CD18 (Mac-1, CR3) bind to CD54 (ICAM-1) and CD102(ICAM-2) on the endothelium. Diapedesis occurs between endothelial cells: CD31 (PECAM-1) expressed by the emigrating neutrophil interacts with CD31 expressed at the endothelial cell-cell junction.

often these signs are not present. Drug-induced neutropenia can be severe, but discontinuation of the sensitizing drug is sufficient for recovery, which is usually seen within 5 to 7 days and is complete by 10 days. Readministration of the sensitizing drug should be avoided, since abrupt neutropenia will often result. For this reason, diagnostic challenge should be avoided.

Autoimmune neutropenias caused by circulating antineutrophil antibodies are another form of acquired neutropenia that results in increased destruction of neutrophils. Acquired neutropenia may also be seen with viral infections, including infection with HIV. Acquired neutropenia may be cyclic in nature, occurring at intervals of several weeks. Acquired cyclic or stable neutropenia may be associated with an expansion of large granular lymphocytes (LGL), which may be T cells, NK cells, or NK-like cells. Patients with LGL lymphocytosis may have moderate blood and bone marrow lymphocytosis, neutropenia, polyclonal hypergammaglobulinemia, splenomegaly, rheumatoid arthritis, and absence of lymphadenopathy. Such patients may have a chronic and relatively stable course. Recurrent bacterial infections are frequent. Benign and malignant forms of this syndrome occur. In some patients, a spontaneous regression has occurred even after 11 years, suggesting an immunoregulatory defect as the basis for at least one form of the disorder. Glucocorticoids, cyclosporine, IFN-α, and nucleosides such as 2-chlorodeoxyadenosine each have induced remission.

Hereditary Neutropenias Hereditary neutropenias are rare and may manifest in early childhood as a profound constant neutropenia or agranulocytosis. Congenital forms of neutropenia include Kostmann's syndrome (neutrophil count < 100/μL), which is often fatal; more benign severe chronic neutropenia (neutrophil count of 300 to 1500/μL) due to mutations in neutrophil elastase; the cartilage-hair hypoplasia syndrome due to mutations in the mitochondrial RNA-processing endoribonuclease, RMRP; Shwachman-Diamond syndrome associated with pancreatic insufficiency due to mutations in the Shwachman-Bodian-Diamond syndrome gene, *SBDS*; myelokathexis, a congenital disorder characterized by neutrophil degeneration, hypersegmentation, and myeloid hyperplasia in the marrow associated with decreased expression of bcl-X$_L$ in myeloid precursors and accel-

erated apoptosis due to mutations in the chemokine receptor CXCR4; and neutropenias associated with other immune defects (X-linked agammaglobulinemia, ataxia telangiectasia, IgA deficiency). Mutations in the G-CSF receptor on chromosome 1 associated with poor response to G-CSF can develop in severe congenital neutropenia and are linked to myeloid malignancy. Hereditary cyclic neutropenia, an autosomal dominant trait, is typically diagnosed in infancy and is characterized by a remarkably regular 3-week cycle. Hereditary cyclic neutropenia actually is cyclic hematopoiesis, also due to mutations in the neutrophil elastase gene. Glucocorticoids and G-CSF blunt the cycling in some patients.

Maternal factors can be associated with neutropenia in the newborn. Transplacental transfer of IgG directed against antigens on fetal neutrophils can result in peripheral destruction. Drugs (e.g., thiazides) ingested during pregnancy can cause neutropenia in the newborn by either depressed production or peripheral destruction.

The presence of immunoglobulin directed toward neutrophils is seen in Felty's syndrome—a triad of rheumatoid arthritis, splenomegaly, and neutropenia (Chap. 301). Patients with Felty's syndrome who respond to splenectomy with an increase in their neutrophil count also have lower postoperative serum neutrophil-binding IgG. Some of these patients have neutropenia associated with an increased number of LGL. Splenomegaly with peripheral trapping and destruction of neutrophils is also seen in lysosomal storage diseases and in portal hypertension.

Neutrophilia Neutrophilia results from increased neutrophil production, increased marrow release, or defective margination (Table 55-2). The most important acute cause of neutrophilia is infection. Neutrophilia from acute infection represents both increased production and increased marrow release. Increased production is also associated with chronic inflammation and certain myeloproliferative diseases. In-

---

TABLE 55-1 *Causes of Neutropenia*

Decreased Production
Drug-induced—alkylating agents (nitrogen mustard, busulfan, chlorambucil, cyclophosphamide); antimetabolites (methotrexate, 6-mercaptopurine, 5-flucytosine); noncytotoxic agents [antibiotics (chloramphenicol, penicillins, sulfonamides), phenothiazines, tranquilizers (meprobamate), anticonvulsants (carbamazepine), antipsychotics (clozapine), certain diuretics, anti-inflammatory agents, antithyroid drugs, many others]
Hematologic diseases—idiopathic, cyclic neutropenia, Chédiak-Higashi syndrome, aplastic anemia, infantile genetic disorders (see text)
Tumor invasion, myelofibrosis
Nutritional deficiency—vitamin B$_{12}$, folate (especially alcoholics)
Infection—tuberculosis, typhoid fever, brucellosis, tularemia, measles, infectious mononucleosis, malaria, viral hepatitis, leishmaniasis, AIDS
Peripheral Destruction
Antineutrophil antibodies and/or splenic or lung trapping
Autoimmune disorders—Felty's syndrome, rheumatoid arthritis, lupus erythematosus
Drugs as haptens—aminopyrine, α-methyldopa, phenylbutazone, mercurial diuretics, some phenothiazines
Wegener's granulomatosis
Peripheral Pooling (Transient Neutropenia)
Overwhelming bacterial infection (acute endotoxemia)
Hemodialysis
Cardiopulmonary bypass

TABLE 55-2 Causes of Neutrophilia

Increased Production
  Idiopathic
  Drug-induced—glucocorticoids
  Infection—bacterial, fungal, sometimes viral
  Inflammation—thermal injury, tissue necrosis, myocardial and pulmonary
    infarction, hypersensitivity states, collagen vascular diseases
  Myeloproliferative diseases—myelocytic leukemia, myeloid
    metaplasia, polycythemia vera
Increased Marrow Release
  Glucocorticoids
  Acute infection (endotoxin)
  Inflammation—thermal injury
Decreased or Defective Margination
  Drugs—epinephrine, glucocorticoids, nonsteroidal anti-inflammatory
    agents
  Stress, excitement, vigorous exercise
  Leukocyte adhesion deficiency type 1 (integrin β chain, CD18);
    leukocyte adhesion deficiency type 2 (selectin ligand, CD15s, sialyl-
    Lewis^x)
Miscellaneous
  Metabolic disorders—ketoacidosis, acute renal failure, eclampsia,
    acute poisoning
  Drugs—lithium
  Other—metastatic carcinoma, acute hemorrhage or hemolysis

creased marrow release and mobilization of the marginated leukocyte pool are induced by glucocorticoids. Release of epinephrine, as with vigorous exercise, excitement, or stress, will demarginate neutrophils in the spleen and lungs and double the neutrophil count in minutes. Leukocytosis with cell counts of 10,000 to 25,000/μL occurs in response to infection and other forms of acute inflammation and results from both release of the marginated pool and mobilization of marrow reserves. Persistent neutrophilia with cell counts of ≥30,000 to 50,000/μL is called a *leukemoid reaction*, a term often used to distinguish this degree of neutrophilia from leukemia. In a leukemoid reaction, the circulating neutrophils are usually mature and not clonally derived.

Abnormal Neutrophil Function Inherited and acquired abnormalities of phagocyte function are listed in Table 55-3. The resulting diseases are best considered in terms of the functional defects of adherence, chemotaxis, and microbicidal activity. The distinguishing features of the important inherited disorders of phagocyte function are shown in Table 55-4.

DISORDERS OF ADHESION Two types of leukocyte adhesion deficiency (LAD) have been described. Both are autosomal recessive traits and result in the inability of neutrophils to exit the circulation to sites of

infection, leading to leukocytosis and increased susceptibility to infection (Fig. 55-8). Patients with LAD 1 have mutations in CD18, the common component of the integrins LFA-1, Mac-1, and p150,95, leading to a defect in tight adhesion between neutrophils and the endothelium. The heterodimer formed by CD18/CD11b (Mac-1) is also the receptor for the complement-derived opsonin C3bi (CR3). The CD18 gene is located on distal chromosome 21q. Variable expression of the defect determines the severity of clinical disease. Complete lack of expression of the leukocyte integrins results in severe phenotype in which inflammatory stimuli do not increase the expression of leukocyte integrins on neutrophils or activated T and B cells. Neutrophils (and monocytes) from patients with LAD 1 adhere poorly to endothelial cells and protein-coated surfaces and exhibit defective spreading, aggregation, and chemotaxis. Patients with LAD 1 have recurrent bacterial and fungal infections involving skin, oral and genital mucosa, and respiratory and intestinal tracts, persistent leukocytosis (neutrophil counts of 15,000 to 20,000/μL) because cells do not marginate; and, in severe cases, a history of delayed separation of the umbilical stump. Infections, especially of the skin, may become necrotic with progressively enlarging borders, slow healing, and development of dysplastic scars. The most common bacteria are *Staphylococcus aureus* and enteric gram-negative bacteria. LAD 2 is caused by an abnormality of fucosylation of SLe^x(CD15s), the ligand on neutrophils that interacts with selectins on endothelial cells. It is now also known as *congenital disorder of glycosylation IIc* (CDGIIc).

DISORDERS OF NEUTROPHIL GRANULES The most common neutrophil defect is myeloperoxidase deficiency, a primary granule defect inherited as an autosomal recessive trait; the incidence is ~1 in 2000 persons. Isolated myeloperoxidase deficiency is not associated with clinically compromised defenses, presumably because other defense systems such as hydrogen peroxide generation are amplified. Microbicidal activity of neutrophils is delayed but not absent. Myeloperoxidase deficiency may make other acquired host defense defects more serious. An acquired form of myeloperoxidase deficiency occurs in myelomonocytic leukemia and acute myeloid leukemia.

Chédiak-Higashi syndrome (CHS) is a rare disease with autosomal recessive inheritance due to defects in the lysosomal transport protein LYST, encoded by the gene *CHS1* at 1q42. This protein is required for normal packaging and disbursement of granules. Neutrophils (and all cells containing lysosomes) from patients with CHS characteristically have large granules (Fig. 55-9). Patients with CHS have an increased number of infections resulting from many bacterial agents. CHS neutrophils and monocytes have impaired chemotaxis and abnormal rates of microbial killing due to slow rates of fusion of the lysosomal granules with phagosomes. NK cell function is also impaired.

TABLE 55-3 Types of Granulocyte and Monocyte Disorders

Function	Cause of Indicated Dysfunction			
	Drug-Induced	Acquired	Inherited
Adherence-aggregation	Aspirin, colchicine, alcohol, glucocorticoids, ibuprofen, piroxicam	Neonatal state, hemodialysis	Leukoctye adhesion deficiency types 1 and 2
Deformability		Leukemia, neonatal state, diabetes mellitus, immature neutrophils	
Chemokinesis-chemotaxis	Glucocorticoids (high dose), auranofin, colchicine (weak effect), phenylbutazone, naproxen, indomethacin, interleukin 2	Thermal injury, malignancy, malnutrition, periodontal disease, neonatal state, systemic lupus erythematosus, rheumatoid arthritis, diabetes mellitus, sepsis, influenza virus infection, herpes simplex virus infection, acrodermatitis enteropathica, AIDS	Chédiak-Higashi syndrome, neutrophil-specific granule deficiency, hyper IgE–recurrent infection (Job's) syndrome (in some patients), Down syndrome, α-mannosidase deficiency, severe combined immunodeficiency, Wiskott-Aldrich syndrome
Microbicidal activity	Colchicine, cyclophosphamide, glucocorticoids (high dose), TNF-α blocking antibodies	Leukemia, aplastic anemia, certain neutropenias, tuftsin deficiency, thermal injury, sepsis, neonatal state, diabetes mellitus, malnutrition, AIDS	Chédiak-Higashi syndrome, neutrophil-specific granule deficiency, chronic granulomatous disease, defects in IFN-γ/IL-12 axis

Clinical Manifestations	Cellular or Molecular Defects	Diagnosis
CHRONIC GRANULOMATOUS DISEASES (70% X-LINKED, 30% AUTOSOMAL RECESSIVE)		
Severe infections of skin, ears, lungs, liver, and bone with catalase-positive microorganisms such as *S. aureus*, *Burkholderia cepacia*, *Aspergillus* spp., *Chromobacterium violaceum*; often hard to culture organism; excessive inflammation with granulomas, frequent lymph node suppuration; granulomas can obstruct GI or GU tracts; gingivitis, aphthous ulcers, seborrheic dermatitis	No respiratory burst due to the lack of one of four NADPH oxidase subunits in neutrophils, monocytes, and eosinophils	NBT or DHR test; no superoxide and H_2O_2 production by neutrophils; immunoblot for NADPH oxidase components; genetic detection
CHÉDIAK-HIGASHI SYNDROME (AUTOSOMAL RECESSIVE)		
Recurrent pyogenic infections, especially with *S. aureus*; many patients get lymphoma-like illness during adolescence; periodontal disease; partial oculocutaneous albinism, nystagmus, progressive peripheral neuropathy, mental retardation in some patients	Reduced chemotaxis and phagolysosome fusion, increased respiratory burst activity, defective egress from marrow, abnormal skin window; defect in LYST	Giant primary granules in neutrophils and other granule-bearing cells (Wright's stain); genetic detection
SPECIFIC GRANULE DEFICIENCY (AUTOSOMAL RECESSIVE?)		
Recurrent infections of skin, ears, and sinopulmonary tract; delayed wound healing; decreased inflammation; bleeding diathesis	Abnormal chemotaxis, impaired respiratory burst and bacterial killing, failure to upregulate chemotactic and adhesion receptors with stimulation, defect in transcription of granule proteins; defect in cEPB-ε	Lack of secondary (specific) granules in neutrophils (Wright's stain), no neutrophil-specific granule contents (i.e., lactoferrin), no defensins, platelet α granule abnormality; genetic detection
MYELOPEROXIDASE DEFICIENCY (AUTOSOMAL RECESSIVE)		
Clinically normal except in patients with underlying disease such as diabetes mellitus; then candidiasis or other fungal infections	No myeloperoxidase due to pre- and posttranslational defects	No peroxidase in neutrophils; genetic detection
LEUKOCYTE ADHESION DEFICIENCY (AUTOSOMAL RECESSIVE)		
Type 1: Delayed separation of umbilical cord, sustained neutrophilia, recurrent infections of skin and mucosa, gingivitis, periodontal disease	Impaired phagocyte adherence, aggregation, spreading, chemotaxis, phagocytosis of C3bi-coated particles; defective production of CD18 subunit common to leukocyte integrins	Reduced phagocyte surface expression of the CD18-containing integrins with monoclonal antibodies against LFA-1 (CD18/CD11a), Mac-1 or CR3 (CD18/CD11b), p150,95 (CD18/CD11c); genetic detection
Type 2: Mental retardation, short stature, Bombay (hh) blood phenotype, recurrent infections, neutrophilia	Impaired phagocyte rolling along endothelium	Reduced phagocyte surface expression of Sialyl-Lewis^x, with monoclonal antibodies against CD15s; genetic detection
PHACOCYTE ACTIVATION DEFECTS (X-LINKED AND AUTOSOMAL RECESSIVE)		
NEMO deficiency: mild hypohidrotic ectodermal dysplasia; broad based immune defect: pyogenic and encapsulated bacteria, viruses, *Pneumocystis*, mycobacteria; X-linked	Impaired phagocyte activiation by IL-1, IL-18, TLR, CD40, TNF-α leading to problems with inflammation and antibody production	Poor in vitro response to endotoxin; lack of NF-κB activation; genetic detection
IRAK4 deficiency: susceptibility to pyogenic bacteria such as staphylococci, streptococci, clostridia; resistant to mycobacteria; autosomal recessive	Impaired phagocyte activation by endotoxin through TLR and other pathways; TNF-α signaling preserved	Poor in vitro response to endotoxin; lack of NF-κB activation by endotoxin; genetic detection
HYPER IGE – RECURRENT INFECTION SYNDROME (AUTOSOMAL DOMINANT) (JOB'S SYNDROME)		
Eczematoid or pruritic dermatitis, "cold" skin abscesses, recurrent pneumonias with *S. aureus* with bronchopleural fistulae and cyst formation, mild eosinophilia, mucocutaneous candidiasis, characteristic facies, restrictive lung disease, scoliosis, delayed primary dental deciduation	Reduced chemotaxis in some patients, reduced suppressor T cell activity	Clinical features, involving lungs, skeleton, and immune system; serum IgE > 2000 IU/mL
MYCOBACTERIA SUSCEPTIBILITY (AUTOSOMAL DOMINANT AND RECESSIVE FORMS)		
Severe local or disseminated infections with bacille Calmette-Guérin (BCG), nontuberculous mycobacteria, salmonella, histoplasmosis, poor granuloma formation	Inability to kill intracellular organisms due to low IFN-γ production; mutations in IFN-γ receptors, IL-12 receptor, IL-12 p40, STAT-1, NEMO	Low or very high levels of IFN-γ receptor 1; functional assays of cytokine production and response; genetic detection

Abbreviations: GI, gastrointestinal; GU, genitourinary; NADPH, nicotinamide-adenine dinucleotide phosphate, NBT, nitroblue tetrazolium (dye test), DHR, dihydrorhodamine (oxidation test); LYST, lysosomal transport protein; cEBP-ε, CCAAT/enhancer binding protein-ε; NEMO, NF-κB essential modulator; TLR, Toll-like receptor; IL, interleukin; TNF, tumor necrosis factor; IRAK4, IL-1 receptor–associated kinase protein-ε, NEMO 4; IFN, interferon.

Specific granule deficiency is a rare autosomal recessive disease in which the production of secondary granules and their contents, as well as the primary granule component defensins, is defective. The defect in bacterial killing leads to severe bacterial infections. One type of specific granule deficiency is due to a mutation in the CCAAT/enhancer binding protein-ε, a regulator of expression of granule components.

CHRONIC GRANULOMATOUS DISEASE Chronic granulomatous disease (CGD) is a group of disorders of granulocyte and monocyte oxidative metab-

FIGURE 55-9 Chédiak-Higashi syndrome. In this disorder, the granulocytes contain huge cytoplasmic granules formed from aggregation and fusion of azurophilic and specific granules. Large abnormal granules are found in other granule-containing cells throughout the body.

olism. Although CGD is rare, with an incidence of 1 in 200,000 individuals, it is an important model of defective neutrophil oxidative metabolism. Most often CGD is inherited as an X-linked recessive trait; 30% of patients inherit the disease in an autosomal recessive pattern. Mutations in the genes for the four proteins that assemble at the plasma membrane account for all patients with CGD. Two proteins (a 91-kDa protein, abnormal in X-linked CGD, and a 22-kDa protein, absent in one form of autosomal recessive CGD) form the heterodimer cytochrome b-558 in the plasma membrane. Two other proteins (47 and 67 kDa, abnormal in the other autosomal recessive forms of CGD) are cytoplasmic in origin and interact with the cytochrome after cell activation to form NADPH oxidase, required for hydrogen peroxide production. Leukocytes from patients with CGD have severely diminished hydrogen peroxide production. The genes involved in each of the defects have been cloned and sequenced and the chromosome locations identified. Patients with CGD characteristically have increased numbers of infections due to catalase-positive microorganisms (organisms that destroy their own hydrogen peroxide). When patients with CGD become infected, they often have extensive inflammatory reactions, and lymph node suppuration is common despite the administration of appropriate antibiotics. Aphthous ulcers and chronic inflammation of the nares are often present. Granulomas are frequent and can obstruct the gastrointestinal or genitourinary tracts. The excessive inflammation probably reflects failure to degrade chemoattractants and antigens, leading to persistent neutrophil accumulation. Impaired killing of intracellular microorganisms by macrophages may lead to persistent cell-mediated immune activation and granuloma formation. Autoimmune complications such as immune thrombocytopenic purpura (ITP) and juvenile rheumatoid arthritis (JRA) are also increased in CGD. In addition, discoid lupus is more common in X-linked carriers.

DISORDERS OF PHAGOCYTE ACTIVATION Phagocytes depend on cell-surface stimulation to induce signals that evoke multiple levels of the inflammatory response, including cytokine synthesis, chemotaxis, and antigen presentation. Mutations affecting the major pathway that signals through NF-κB have been noted in patients with a variety of infection susceptibility syndromes. If the defects are at a very late stage of signal transduction, in the protein critical for NF-κB activation known as the NF-κB essential modulator (NEMO), then affected males develop ectodermal dysplasia and severe immune deficiency with susceptibility to bacteria, fungi, mycobacteria, and viruses. If the defect in NF-κB activation is closer to the signaling source, in the IL-1 receptor–associated kinase 4 (IRAK4), then children have a marked susceptibility to pyogenic infections early in life but develop resistance to infection later.

MONONUCLEAR PHAGOCYTES

The mononuclear phagocyte system is composed of monoblasts, promonocytes, and monocytes in addition to the structurally diverse tissue macrophages that make up what was previously referred to as the reticuloendothelial system. Macrophages are long-lived phagocytic cells capable of many of the functions of neutrophils. They are also secretory cells that participate in many immunologic and inflammatory processes distinct from neutrophils. Monocytes leave the circulation by diapedesis more slowly than neutrophils and have a half-life in the blood of 12 to 24 h.

After blood monocytes arrive in the tissues, they differentiate into

macrophages ("big eaters") with specialized functions suited for specific anatomic locations. Macrophages are particularly abundant in capillary walls of the lung, spleen, liver, and bone marrow, where they function to remove microorganisms and other noxious elements from the blood. Alveolar macrophages, liver Kupffer cells, splenic macrophages, peritoneal macrophages, bone marrow macrophages, lymphatic macrophages, brain microglial cells, and dendritic macrophages all have specialized functions. Macrophage-secreted products include lysozyme, neutral proteases, acid hydrolases, arginase, complement components, enzyme inhibitors (plasmin, α_2-macroglobulin), binding proteins (transferrin, fibronectin, transcobalamin II), nucleosides, and cytokines (TNF-α; IL-1, -8, -12, and -18). IL-1 (Chaps. 16 and 295) has many functions, including initiating fever in the hypothalamus, mobilizing leukocytes from the bone marrow, and activating lymphocytes and neutrophils. TNF-α is a pyrogen that duplicates many of the actions of IL-1 and plays an important role in the pathogenesis of gram-negative shock (Chap. 254). TNF-α stimulates production of hydrogen peroxide and related toxic oxygen species by macrophages and neutrophils. In addition, TNF-α induces catabolic changes that contribute to the profound wasting (cachexia) associated with many chronic diseases.

Other macrophage-secreted products include reactive oxygen and nitrogen metabolites, bioactive lipids (arachidonic acid metabolites and platelet-activating factors), chemokines, colony-stimulating factors, and factors stimulating fibroblast and vessel proliferation. Macrophages help regulate the replication of lymphocytes and participate in the killing of tumors, viruses, and certain bacteria (*Mycobacterium tuberculosis* and *Listeria monocytogenes*). Macrophages are key effector cells in the elimination of intracellular microorganisms. Their ability to fuse to form giant cells that coalesce into granulomas in response to some inflammatory stimuli is important in the elimination of intracellular microbes and is under the control of IFN-γ. Nitric oxide induced by IFN-γ is an important effector against intracellular parasites, including tuberculosis and *Leishmania*.

Macrophages play an important role in the immune response (Chap. 295). They process and present antigen to lymphocytes and secrete cytokines that modulate and direct lymphocyte development and function. Macrophages participate in autoimmune phenomena by removing immune complexes and other substances from the circulation. Polymorphisms in macrophage receptors for immunoglobulin (FcγRII) determine susceptibility to some infections and autoimmune diseases. In wound healing, they dispose of senescent cells, and they contribute to atheroma development. Macrophage elastase mediates development of emphysema from cigarette smoking.

DISORDERS OF THE MONONUCLEAR PHAGOCYTE SYSTEM Many disorders of neutrophils extend to mononuclear phagocytes. Thus, drugs that suppress neutrophil production in the bone marrow can cause monocytopenia. Transient monocytopenia occurs after stress or glucocorticoid administration. Monocytosis is associated with tuberculosis, brucellosis, subacute bacterial endocarditis, Rocky Mountain spotted fever, malaria, and visceral leishmaniasis (kala azar). Monocytosis also occurs with malignancies, leukemias, myeloproliferative syndromes, hemolytic anemias, chronic idiopathic neutropenias, and granulomatous diseases such as sarcoidosis, regional enteritis, and some collagen vascular diseases. Patients with LAD, hyperimmunoglobulin E–recurrent infection (Job's) syndrome, CHS, and CGD all have defects in the mononuclear phagocyte system.

Monocyte cytokine production or response is impaired in some patients with disseminated nontuberculous mycobacterial infection who are not infected with HIV. Genetic defects in the pathways regulated by IFN-γ and IL-12 lead to impaired killing of intracellular bacteria, mycobacteria, salmonellae, and certain viruses (Fig. 55-10).

Certain viral infections impair mononuclear phagocyte function. For example, influenza virus infection causes abnormal monocyte chemotaxis. Mononuclear phagocytes can be infected by HIV using

FIGURE 55-10 Lymphocyte-macrophage interactions underlying resistance to mycobacteria and other intracellular parasites such as *Salmonella*. *Mycobacteria* infect macrophages, leading to the production of IL-12, which activates T or NK cells through its receptor, leading to production of IL-2 and IFN-γ. IFN-γ acts through its receptor on macrophages to upregulate TNF-α and IL-12 and kill intracellular parasites. Mutant forms of the cytokines and receptors shown in large type have been found in severe cases of nontuberculous mycobacterial infection and salmonellosis.

CCR5, the chemokine receptor that acts as a co-receptor with CD4 for HIV. T lymphocytes produce IFN-γ, which induces FcR expression and phagocytosis and stimulates hydrogen peroxide production by mononuclear phagocytes and neutrophils. In certain diseases, such as AIDS, IFN-γ production may be deficient, while in other diseases, such as T cell lymphomas, excessive release of IFN-γ may be associated with erythrophagocytosis by splenic macrophages.

Gain-of-function mutations in the TNF-α receptor cause TNF-α receptor–associated periodic syndromes (TRAPS) that are characterized by recurrent fever in the absence of infection, due to persistent stimulation of the TNF-α receptor. Administration of the TNF-α antagonists infliximab, etanercept, and adalimumab has been associated with severe infections such as tuberculosis.

Monocytopenia occurs with acute infections, with stress, and after treatment with glucocorticoids. Monocytopenia also occurs in aplastic anemia, hairy cell leukemia, acute myeloid leukemia, and as a direct result of myelotoxic drugs.

EOSINOPHILS

Eosinophils and neutrophils share similar morphology, many lysosomal constituents, phagocytic capacity, and oxidative metabolism. Eosinophils express a specific chemoattractant receptor and respond to a specific chemokine, eotaxin. Little is known about the role of eosinophils. Eosinophils are much longer lived than neutrophils, and unlike neutrophils, tissue eosinophils can recirculate. During most infections, eosinophils are not important. However, in invasive helminthic infections, such as hookworm, schistosomiasis, strongyloidiasis, toxocariasis, trichinosis, filariasis, echinococcosis, and cysticercosis, the eosinophil plays a central role in host defense. Eosinophils are associated with bronchial asthma, cutaneous allergic reactions, and other hypersensitivity states.

The distinctive feature of the red-staining (Wright's stain) eosinophil granule is its crystalline core consisting of an arginine-rich protein (major basic protein) with histaminase activity, important in host defense against parasites. Eosinophil granules also contain a unique eosinophil peroxidase that catalyzes the oxidation of many substances by hydrogen peroxide and may facilitate killing of microorganisms.

Eosinophil peroxidase, in the presence of hydrogen peroxide and halide, initiates mast cell secretion in vitro and thereby promotes inflammation. Eosinophils contain cationic proteins, some of which bind to heparin and reduce its anticoagulant activity. Eosinophil-derived neurotoxin and eosinophil cationic protein are ribonucleases that can kill respiratory syncytial virus. Eosinophil cytoplasm contains Charcot-Leyden crystal protein, a hexagonal bipyramidal crystal first observed in a patient with leukemia and then in sputum of patients with asthma; this protein is lysophospholipase and may function to detoxify certain lysophospholipids.

Several factors enhance the eosinophil's function in host defense. T cell–derived factors enhance the ability of eosinophils to kill parasites. Mast cell–derived eosinophil chemotactic factor of anaphylaxis (ECFa) increases the number of eosinophil complement receptors and enhances eosinophil killing of parasites. Eosinophil colony-stimulating factors (e.g., IL-5) produced by macrophages increase eosinophil production in the bone marrow and activate eosinophils to kill parasites.

EOSINOPHILIA Eosinophilia is the presence of >500 eosinophils per microliter of blood and is common in many settings besides parasite infection. Significant tissue eosinophilia can occur without an elevated blood count. A common cause of eosinophilia is allergic reaction to drugs (iodides, aspirin, sulfonamides, nitrofurantoin, penicillins, and cephalosporins). Allergies such as hay fever, asthma, eczema, serum sickness, allergic vasculitis, and pemphigus are associated with eosinophilia. Eosinophilia also occurs in collagen vascular diseases (e.g., rheumatoid arthritis, eosinophilic fasciitis, allergic angiitis, and periarteritis nodosa) and malignancies (e.g., Hodgkin's disease; mycosis fungoides; chronic myelogenous leukemia; and cancer of the lung, stomach, pancreas, ovary, or uterus), as well as in Job's syndrome and CGD. Eosinophilia is commonly present in the helminthic infections. IL-5 is the dominant eosinophil growth factor. Therapeutic administration of the cytokines IL-2 and GM-CSF frequently leads to transient eosinophilia. The most dramatic hypereosinophilic syndromes are Loeffler's syndrome, tropical pulmonary eosinophilia, Loeffler's endocarditis, eosinophilic leukemia, and idiopathic hypereosinophilic syndrome (50,000 to 100,000/μL).

The idiopathic hypereosinophilic syndrome represents a heterogeneous group of disorders with the common feature of prolonged eosinophilia of unknown cause and organ system dysfunction, including the heart, central nervous system, kidneys, lungs, gastrointestinal tract, and skin. The bone marrow is involved in all affected individuals, but the most severe complications involve the heart and central nervous system. Clinical manifestations and organ dysfunction are highly variable. Eosinophils are found in the involved tissues and likely cause tissue damage by local deposition of toxic eosinophil proteins such as eosinophil cationic protein and major basic protein. In the heart, the pathologic changes lead to thrombosis, endocardial fibrosis, and restrictive endomyocardiopathy. The damage to tissues in other organ systems is similar. Some cases are due to mutations involving the platelet derived growth factor receptor and these are extremely sensitive to the tyrosine kinase inhibitor imatinib. Glucocorticoids may also induce remission. In patients who do not respond to glucocorticoids, a cytotoxic agent such as hydroxyurea has been used successfully to lower the peripheral blood eosinophil counts and to improve the prognosis markedly. IFN-α is also effective in some patients, including those unresponsive to hydroxyurea. Aggressive medical and surgical approaches are used to manage patients with cardiovascular complications.

The *eosinophilia-myalgia syndrome* is a multisystem disease with prominent cutaneous, hematologic, and visceral manifestations that frequently evolves into a chronic course and can occasionally be fatal. The syndrome is characterized by eosinophilia (eosinophil count > 1000/μL) and generalized disabling myalgias without other recognized causes. Eosinophilic fasciitis, pneumonitis, and myocarditis; neuropathy culminating in respiratory failure; and encephalopathy may occur. The disease is caused by ingesting contaminants in L-tryptophan–containing products. Eosinophils, lymphocytes, macrophages, and fibroblasts accumulate in the affected tissues, but their role in pathogenesis is unclear. Activation of eosinophils and fibroblasts and the deposition of eosinophil-derived toxic proteins in affected tissues may contribute. IL-5 and transforming growth factor β have been implicated as potential mediators. Treatment is withdrawal of products containing L-tryptophan and the administration of glucocorticoids. Most patients recover fully, remain stable, or show slow recovery, but the disease can be fatal in up to 5% of patients.

EOSINOPENIA Eosinopenia occurs with stress, such as acute bacterial infection, and after treatment with glucocorticoids. The mechanism of eosinopenia of acute bacterial infection is unknown but is independent of endogenous glucocorticoids, since it occurs in animals after total adrenalectomy. There is no known adverse effect of eosinopenia.

HYPERIMMUNOGLOBULIN E-RECURRENT INFECTION SYNDROME

The hyperimmunoglobulin E–recurrent infection (HIE) syndrome, or Job's syndrome, is a rare multisystem disease in which the immune system, bone, teeth, lung, and skin are affected. Abnormal chemotaxis is a variable feature. The molecular basis for this syndrome is not known, but some cases show autosomal dominant transmission with linkage to 4q. Patients with this syndrome have characteristic facies with broad nose, kyphoscoliosis and osteoporosis, and eczema. The primary teeth erupt normally but do not deciduate, often requiring extraction. Patients develop recurrent sinopulmonary and cutaneous infections that tend to be much less inflamed than appropriate for the degree of infection and have been referred to as "cold abscesses." A high degree of suspicion is required to diagnose infections in these patients, who may appear well despite extensive disease. The cold abscesses have been considered a reflection of too few phagocytes arriving too late, perhaps due to a lymphocyte factor inhibiting chemotaxis. However, the chemotactic defect in these patients is variable, and the fundamental basis for the impaired defenses is complex and poorly defined.

LABORATORY DIAGNOSIS AND MANAGEMENT

Initial studies of WBC and differential and often a bone marrow examination may be followed by assessment of bone marrow reserves (steroid challenge test), marginated circulating pool of cells (epinephrine challenge test), and marginating ability (endotoxin challenge test) (Fig. 55-7). In vivo assessment of inflammation is possible with a Rebuck skin window test or an in vivo blister assay, which measures the ability of leukocytes and inflammatory mediators to accumulate locally in the skin. In vitro tests of phagocyte aggregation, adherence, chemotaxis, phagocytosis, degranulation, and microbicidal activity (for *S. aureus*) may help pinpoint cellular or humoral lesions. Deficiencies of oxidative metabolism are detected with either the nitroblue tetrazolium (NBT) dye test or the dihydrorhodamine (DHR) oxidation test. These tests are based on the ability of products of oxidative metabolism to alter the oxidation states of reporter molecules so that they can be detected microscopically (NBT) or by flow cytometry (DHR). Qualitative studies of superoxide and hydrogen peroxide production may further define neutrophil oxidative function.

Patients with leukopenias or leukocyte dysfunction often have delayed inflammatory responses. Therefore, clinical manifestations may be minimal despite overwhelming infection, and unusual infections must always be suspected. Early signs of infection demand prompt, aggressive culturing for microorganisms, use of antibiotics, and surgical drainage of abscesses. Prolonged courses of antibiotics are often

required. In patients with CGD, prophylactic antibiotics (trimethoprim-sulfamethoxazole) and antifungals (itraconazole) markedly diminish the frequency of life-threatening infections. Short courses of glucocorticoids may relieve gastrointestinal or genitourinary tract obstruction by granulomas in patients with CGD. Recombinant human IFN-γ, which nonspecifically stimulates phagocytic cell function, reduces the frequency of infections in patients with CGD by 70% and reduces the severity of infection. This effect of IFN-γ in CGD is additive to the effect of prophylactic antibiotics. The recommended dose is 50 μg/m^2 subcutaneously three times weekly. IFN-γ has also been used successfully in the treatment of leprosy, nontuberculous mycobacteria, and visceral leishmaniasis.

Rigorous oral hygiene reduces but does not eliminate the discomfort of gingivitis, periodontal disease, and aphthous ulcers; chlorhexidine mouthwash and tooth brushing with a hydrogen peroxide–sodium bicarbonate paste helps many patients. Oral antifungal agents (fluconazole) have reduced mucocutaneous candidiasis in patients with Job's syndrome. Androgens, glucocorticoids, lithium, and immunosuppressive therapy have been used to restore myelopoiesis in patients with neutropenia due to impaired production. Recombinant G-CSF is useful in the management of certain forms of neutropenia due to depressed neutrophil production, especially those related to cancer chemotherapy. Patients with chronic neutropenia with evidence of a good bone marrow reserve need not receive prophylactic antibiotics. Patients with chronic or cyclic neutrophil counts < 500/μL may benefit from prophylactic antibiotics and G-CSF during periods of neutropenia. Oral trimethoprim-sulfamethoxazole (160/800 mg) twice daily can prevent infection. Increased numbers of fungal infections are not seen in patients with CGD on this regimen. Oral quinolones such as levofloxacin and ciprofloxacin are alternatives.

In the setting of cytotoxic chemotherapy with severe, persistent neutropenia, trimethoprim-sulfamethoxazole prevents *Pneumocystis carinii* pneumonia. These patients, and patients with phagocytic cell dysfunction, should avoid heavy exposure to airborne soil, dust, or decaying matter (mulch, manure), which are often rich in *Nocardia* and the spores of *Aspergillus* and other fungi. Restriction of activities or social contact has no proven role in reducing risk of infection.

Cure of some congenital phagocyte defects is possible by bone marrow transplantation (Chap. 100). However, complications of bone marrow transplantation are still serious, and with rigorous medical care many patients with phagocytic disorders can go for years without a life-threatening infection. The identification of specific gene defects in patients with LAD 1, CGD, and other immunodeficiencies has led to gene therapy trials in a number of genetic white cell disorders.

FURTHER READING

DALE DC et al: Cyclic neutropenia. Semin Hematol 39:89, 2002

LEKSTROM-HIMES JA, GALLIN JI: Immunodeficiency diseases caused by defects in phagocytes. N Engl J Med 343:1703, 2000

NATHAN C: Points of control in inflammation. Nature 420:846, 2002

PICARD C et al: Pyogenic bacterial infections in humans with IRAK-4 deficiency. Science 299:2076, 2003

ROSENBERG HF, DOMACHOWSKE JB: Eosinophils, eosinophil ribonucleases, and their role in host defense against respiratory virus pathogens. J Leukoc Biol 70:691, 2001

SEGAL BH et al: Genetic, biochemical, and clinical features of chronic granulomatous disease. Medicine (Baltimore) 79:170, 2000

56 PRINCIPLES OF HUMAN GENETICS
J. Larry Jameson, Peter Kopp

IMPACT OF GENETICS ON MEDICAL PRACTICE

The beginning of the new millennium was marked by the announcement that the vast majority of the human genome has been sequenced. This milestone in the exploration of the human genome was preceded by numerous conceptual and technological advances. They include, among others, the elucidation of the DNA double-helix structure, the discovery of restriction enzymes and the polymerase chain reaction (PCR), the development and automatization of DNA sequencing, and the generation of genetic and physical maps by the Human Genome Project (HGP). The consequences of this wealth of knowledge for the practice of medicine are profound, but the integration of genetics into the everyday practice of medicine remains challenging. To date, the most significant impact of genetics has been to enhance our understanding of disease etiology and pathogenesis. In the near term, we can expect an increasing role for genetics in the diagnosis, prevention, and treatment of disease (Chaps. 58 and 59).

Genetics has traditionally been viewed through the window of relatively rare single-gene diseases. Taken together, these rare disorders account for up to 10% of pediatric admissions and childhood mortality. It is, however, increasingly apparent that virtually every medical condition with the exception of simple trauma has a genetic component. As is often evident from a patient's family history, many common disorders such as hypertension, heart disease, asthma, diabetes mellitus, and mental illnesses are significantly influenced by the genetic background. These polygenic or multifactorial disorders involve the contributions of many different genes, as well as environmental factors, that can modify disease risk (Chap. 58). Cancer has a genetic basis since it results from acquired somatic mutations in genes controlling growth and differentiation (Chap. 68). In addition, the development of many cancers is associated with a hereditary predisposition. The prevalence of genetic diseases, combined with their severity and chronic nature, imposes a great financial, social, and emotional burden on society.

Genetics has historically focused on chromosomal and metabolic disorders, reflecting the long-standing availability of techniques to diagnose these conditions. For example, conditions such as trisomy 21 (Down syndrome) or monosomy X (Turner syndrome) can be diagnosed using cytogenetics (Chap. 57). Likewise, many metabolic disorders (e.g., phenylketonuria, familial hypercholesterolemia) are diagnosed using biochemical analyses. Recent advances in DNA diagnostics have extended the field of genetics to include virtually all medical specialties. In cardiology, for example, the molecular basis of inherited cardiomyopathies and ion channel defects that predispose to arrhythmias is being defined (Chaps. 214 and 221). In neurology, genetics has unmasked the pathophysiology of a startling number of neurodegenerative disorders (Chap. 345). Hematology has evolved dramatically, from its incipient genetic descriptions of hemoglobinopathies to the current understanding of the molecular basis of red cell membrane defects, clotting disorders, and thrombotic disorders (Chaps. 91 and 102). It is now abundantly clear that neoplasia and the acquisition of metastatic potential can be described in genetic terms (Chaps. 68 and 69).

New concepts derived from genetic studies can sometimes clarify the pathogenesis of disorders that were previously opaque. For example, although many different genetic defects can cause peripheral neuropathies, disruption of the normal folding of the myelin sheaths is frequently a common final pathway (Chap. 364). Several genetic causes of obesity appear to converge on a physiologic pathway that involves products of the proopiomelanocortin polypeptide and the MC4R receptor, thus identifying a key mechanism for appetite control (Chap. 64). A similar situation is emerging for genetically distinct forms of Alzheimer's disease, several of which lead to the formation of neurofibrillary tangles (Chap. 350). Increasingly, the identification of defective genes can pinpoint cellular pathways involved in key physiologic processes. Examples include identification of the cystic fibrosis conductance regulator (CFTR) gene, the Duchenne muscular dystrophy (DMD) gene, which encodes dystrophin, and the fibroblast growth factor receptor-3 (FGFR3) gene, which is responsible for achondroplastic dwarfism. Similarly, transgenic (over)expression, and targeted gene "knockout" and "knockin" models help to unravel the physiologic function of genes. Genetic approaches have proven invaluable for the detection of infectious pathogens and are used clinically to identify agents that are difficult to culture such as mycobacteria, viruses, and parasites. In many cases, molecular genetics has improved the feasibility and accuracy of diagnostic testing, enhanced our understanding of pathophysiology, and is beginning to open new avenues for therapy, including gene and cellular therapy (Chap. 59).

The astounding rate at which new genetic information is being generated creates a major challenge for physicians, health care providers, and basic investigators. The terminology and techniques used for discovery evolve continuously. Much genetic information presently resides in computer databases or is being published in basic science journals. Databases provide easy access to the expanding information about the human genome, genetic disease, and genetic testing (Table 56-1). For example, several thousand monogenic disorders are summarized in a large, continuously evolving compendium, referred to as the *Online Mendelian Inheritance in Man* (OMIM) catalog (Table 56-1). The ongoing refinement of bioinformatics is simplifying the access to this seemingly daunting onslaught of new information.

APPROACH TO THE PATIENT

For the practicing clinician, the family history remains an essential step in recognizing the possibility of a hereditary component. When taking the history, it is useful to draw a detailed pedigree of the first-degree relatives (e.g., parents, siblings, and children), since they share 50% of genes with the patient. Standard symbols for pedigrees are depicted in Fig. 56-1. The family history should include information about ethnic background, age, health status, and (infant) deaths. Next, the physician should explore whether there is a family history of the same or related illnesses to the current problem. An inquiry focused on commonly occurring disorders such as cancers, heart disease, and diabetes mellitus should follow. Because of the possibility of age-dependent expressivity and penetrance, the family history may need updating. If the findings suggest a genetic disorder, the clinician will have to assess whether some of the patient's relatives may be at risk of carrying or transmitting the disease. In this circumstance, it is useful to confirm and extend the pedigree based on input from several family members. This information may form the basis for carrier detection, genetic counseling, early intervention, and prevention of a disease in relatives of the index patient (Chap. 59).

In instances where a diagnosis at the molecular level may be relevant, the physician will have to identify an appropriate laboratory that can perform the test. If a disease-causing mutation is expected in all cells due to germline transmission, DNA can be collected from any tissue, most commonly nucleated blood cells. In the case of somatic mutations, which are limited to a neoplastic

TABLE 56-1 *Selected Databases Relevant for Genomics and Genetic Disorders*

Site	URL	Comment
National Center for Biotechnology Information (NCBI)	http://www.ncbi.nlm.nih.gov/	Molecular biology information, public databases, computational biology
		Software for analyzing genome data
		Extensive links to other databases, genome resources, and educational primers
National Human Genome Research Institute	http://www.genome.gov/	Web links providing information about the human genome sequence, genomes of other organisms, and genomic research
Ensembl Genome browser	http://www.ensembl.org/	Maps and sequence information of eukaryotic genomes
Online Mendelian Inheritance in Man (OMIM)	http://www.ncbi.nlm.nih.gov/omim/	Online compendium of Mendelian disorders and human genes causing genetic disorders
Office of Biotechnology Activities National Institutes of Health	www4.od.nih.gov/oba/	Information about recombinant DNA and gene transfer
		Medical, ethical, legal, and social issues raised by genetic testing
		Medical, ethical, legal, and social issues raised by xenotransplantation
American College of Medical Genetics	http://www.acmg.net/	Extensive links to other databases relevant for the diagnosis, treatment and prevention of genetic disease
Cancer Genome Anatomy Project (CGAP)	http://cgap.nci.nih.gov/	Information about gene expression profiles of normal, precancer, and cancer cells
GenLink	http://www.genlink.wustl.edu	Multimedia database resource for human genetics and telomere research
GeneTests-GeneClinics	http://www.genetests.org/	International directory of genetic testing laboratories and prenatal diagnosis clinics
		Reviews and educational materials
Dolan DNA Learning Center, Cold Spring Harbor Laboratories	http://www.dnalc.org	Educational material about selected genetic disorders, DNA, eugenics, and genetic origin
HUGO Gene Nomenclature	http://www.gene.ucl.ac.uk/nomenclature	Gene names and symbols
MITOMAP, a human mitochondrial genome database	http://www.mitomap.org	A compendium of polymorphisms and mutations of the human mitochondrial DNA
Mitochondrial disorders	http://www.neuro.wustl.edu/neuromuscular/mitosyn.html	Overview on clinical syndromes associated with mtDNA mutations
DNA repeat sequences & disease	http://www.neuro.wustl.edu/neuromuscular/mother/dnarep.htm	Overview on clinical syndromes associated with DNA repeats
Online Mendelian Inheritance in Animals (OMIA)	http://www.angis.su.oz.au/Databases/BIRX/omia	Online compendium of Mendelian disorders in animals
The Jackson Laboratory	http://www.jax.org/	Information about murine models and the mouse genome

Note: Databases are evolving constantly. Pertinent information may be found by using links listed in the few selected databases. Instructions for the use of genome-related databases have been published [Nat Genet 32 (Suppl):1–79, 2002].

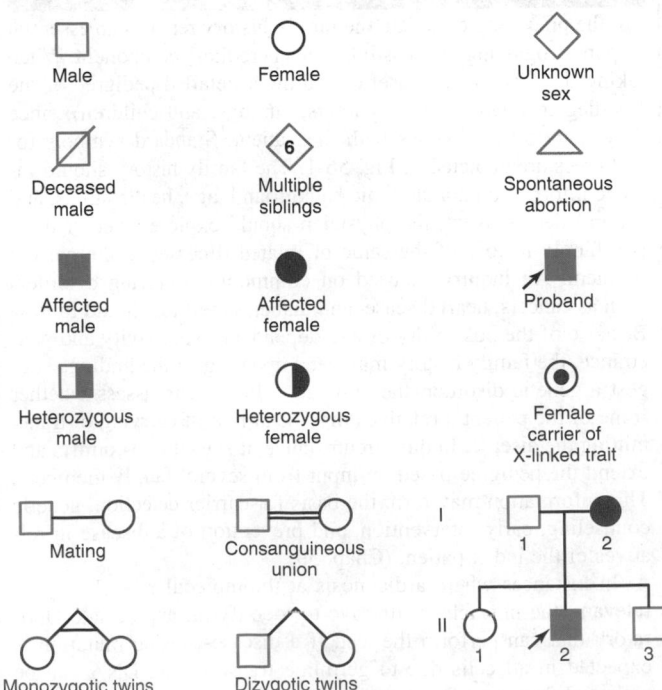

FIGURE 56-1 Standard pedigree symbols.

tissue, an adequate sample of this lesion is used for extraction of DNA or RNA. For the detection of pathogens, the material to be analyzed will vary and may include blood, cerebrospinal fluid, solid tissues, sputum, or fluid obtained through bronchioalveolar lavage.

CHROMOSOMES AND DNA REPLICATION

ORGANIZATION OF DNA INTO CHROMOSOMES ■ Size of the Human Genome

The human genome is divided into 23 different chromosomes, including 22 autosomes (numbered 1 to 22) and the X and Y sex chromosomes. Adult cells are diploid, meaning they contain two homologous sets of 22 autosomes and a pair of sex chromosomes. Females have two X chromosomes (XX), whereas males have one X and one Y chromosome (XY). As a consequence of meiosis, germ cells (sperm or oocytes) are haploid and contain one set of 22 autosomes and one of the sex chromosomes. At the time of fertilization, the diploid genome is reconstituted by pairing of the homologous chromosomes from the mother and father. With each cell division (mitosis), chromosomes are replicated, paired, segregated, and divided into two daughter cells (Chap. 57).

The human genome is estimated to contain about 30,000 to 40,000 genes, a smaller number than initially predicted, that are divided among the 23 chromosomes. A *gene* is a functional unit that is regulated by transcription (see below) and encodes a product, either RNA or protein, that exerts activity within or outside the cell. Historically, genes were identified because they conferred specific traits that are transmitted from one generation to the next. Increasingly, they are characterized based on expression in various tissues. The number of genes greatly underestimates the complexity of genetic expression, as single genes can generate multiple spliced mRNA products, which are translated into proteins that are subject to complex posttranslational modification, such as phosphorylation. *Proteomics* is an emerging field focused on protein variation and function.

Human DNA consists of about 3 billion base pairs (bp) of DNA per haploid genome. DNA length is normally measured in units of 1000 bp (kilobases, kb) or 1,000,000 bp (megabases, Mb). Not all DNA encodes genes. In fact, genes account for only about 10 to 15% of DNA. Much of the remaining DNA consists of highly repetitive sequences, the function of which is poorly understood. These repetitive DNA regions, along with nonrepetitive sequences that do not encode genes, may serve a structural role in the packaging of DNA into chromatin (DNA bound to histone proteins) and chromosomes (Fig. 56-2). If only 10% of DNA is expressed and there are 100,000 genes, the average gene would be about 3 kb in length. Although many genes are about this size, the range is quite broad. For example, some genes are only a few hundred bp, whereas others, like the *DMD* gene, are extraordinarily large (2 Mb).

Structure of DNA   Each gene is composed of a linear polymer of DNA. DNA is a double-stranded helix composed of four different bases: adenine (A), thymidine (T), guanine (G), and cytosine (C). Adenine is paired to thymidine, and guanine is paired to cytosine, by hydrogen bond interactions that span the double helix. DNA has several remarkable features that make it ideal for the transmission of genetic information. It is relatively stable, at least in comparison to RNA or proteins. The double-stranded nature of DNA and its feature of strict base-pair complementarity permit faithful replication during cell division. As described below, complementarity also allows the trans-

FIGURE 56-2   Structure of chromatin and chromosomes. Chromatin is composed of double strand DNA that is wrapped around histone and nonhistone proteins forming nucleosomes. The nucleosomes are then organized into solenoid structures. Chromosomes assume their characteristic structure, with short (p) and long (q) arms at the metaphase stage of the cell cycle.

mission of genetic information from DNA → RNA → protein (Fig. 56-3). Messenger RNA (mRNA) is encoded by the so-called sense or coding strand of the DNA double helix and is translated into proteins by ribosomes.

The presence of four different bases provides surprising genetic diversity. In the protein-coding regions of genes, the DNA bases are arranged into codons, a triplet of bases that specifies a particular amino acid. It is possible to arrange the four bases into 64 different triplet codons (4^3). Each codon specifies 1 of the 20 different amino acids, or a regulatory signal, such as initiation and stop of translation. Because there are more codons than amino acids, the genetic code is degenerate; that is, most amino acids can be specified by several different codons. By arranging the codons in different combinations and in various lengths, it is possible to generate the tremendous diversity of primary protein structure.

REPLICATION OF DNA AND MITOSIS   Genetic information in DNA is transmitted to daughter cells under two different circumstances: (1) somatic cells divide by mitosis, allowing the diploid ($2n$) genome to replicate itself completely in conjunction with cell division; and (2) germ cells (sperm and ova) undergo meiosis, a process that enables the reduction of the diploid ($2n$) set of chromosomes to the haploid state ($1n$) (Chap. 57).

Prior to mitosis, cells exit the resting, or G_0 state, and enter the cell cycle (Chap. 69). After traversing a critical checkpoint in G_1, cells undergo DNA synthesis (S phase), during which the DNA in each chromosome is replicated, yielding two pairs of sister chromatids ($2n \rightarrow 4n$). The process of DNA synthesis requires stringent fidelity in order to avoid transmitting errors to subsequent generations of cells. Genetic abnormalities of DNA mismatch/repair include xeroderma pigmentosum, Bloom syndrome, ataxia telangiectasia, and hereditary nonpolyposis colon cancer (HNPCC), among others. Many of these disorders strongly predispose to neoplasia because of the rapid acquisition of additional mutations (Chap. 68). After completion of DNA synthesis, cells enter G_2 and progress through a second checkpoint before entering mitosis. At this stage, the chromosomes condense and are aligned along the equatorial plate at metaphase. The two identical sister chromatids, held together at the centromere, divide and migrate to opposite poles of the cell (see Fig. 57-3). After formation of a nuclear membrane around the two separated sets of chromatids, the cell divides and two daughter cells are formed, thus restoring the diploid ($2n$) state.

ASSORTMENT AND SEGREGATION OF GENES DURING MEIOSIS   Meiosis occurs only in germ cells of the gonads. It shares certain features with mitosis but involves two distinct steps of cell division that reduce the chromosome number to the haploid state. In addition, there is active recombination that generates genetic diversity. During the first cell division, two sister chromatids ($2n \rightarrow 4n$) are formed for each chromosome pair and there is an exchange of DNA between homologous paternal and maternal chromosomes. This process involves the formation of *chiasmata*, structures that correspond to the DNA segments that cross over between the maternal and paternal homologues (Fig. 56-4). Usually there is at least one crossover on each chromosomal arm; recombination occurs more frequently in female meiosis than in male meiosis. Subsequently, the chromosomes segregate randomly. Because there are 23 chromosomes, there exist 2^{23} (>8 million) possible combinations of chromosomes. Together with the genetic exchanges that occur during recombination, chromosomal segregation generates tremendous diversity, and each gamete is genetically unique. The process of recombination, and the independent segregation of chromosomes, provide the foundation for performing linkage analyses, whereby one attempts to correlate the inheritance of certain chromosomal regions (or linked genes) with the presence of a disease or genetic trait (see below).

After the first meiotic division, which results in two daughter cells ($2n$), the two chromatids of each chromosome separate during a second

FIGURE 56-3 Flow of genetic information. Multiple extracellular signals activate intracellular signal cascades that result in altered regulation of gene expression through the interaction of transcription factors with regulatory regions of genes. RNA polymerase transcribes DNA into RNA that is processed to mRNA by excision of intronic sequences. The mRNA is translated into a polypeptide chain to form the mature protein after undergoing posttranslational processing. HAT, histone acetyl transferase; CBP, CREB-binding protein; CREB, cyclic AMP response element–binding protein; CRE, cyclic AMP responsive element; CoA, Co activator; TAF, TBP-associated factors; GTF, general transcription factors; TBP, TATA-binding protein; TATA, TATA box; RE, response element; NH_2, aminoterminus; COOH, carboxyterminus.

FIGURE 56-4 Crossing-over and genetic recombination. During chiasma formation, either of the two sister chromatids on one chromosome pairs with one of the chromatids of the homologous chromosome. Genetic recombination occurs through crossing-over and results in recombinant and nonrecombinant chromosome segments in the gametes. Together with the random segregation of the maternal and paternal chromosomes, recombination contributes to genetic diversity and forms the basis of the concept of linkage.

meiotic division to yield four gametes with a haploid state (1*n*). When the egg is fertilized by sperm, the two haploid sets are combined, thereby restoring the diploid state (2*n*) in the zygote.

REGULATION OF GENE EXPRESSION

Mechanisms that regulate gene expression play a critical role in the function of genes. The new field of *functional genomics* is based on the concept that understanding gene regulation and function will provide a better understanding of physiology and offer novel therapeutic opportunities. The transcription of genes is controlled primarily by *transcription factors* that bind to DNA sequences in the regulatory regions of genes. As described below, mutations in transcription factors cause a significant number of genetic disorders. Gene expression is also influenced by *epigenetic events*, such as X-inactivation and imprinting, processes in which DNA methylation is associated with the silencing (i.e., suppression) of expression. Several genetic disorders, such as Prader-Willi syndrome (neonatal hypotonia, developmental delay, obesity, short stature, and hypogonadism) and Albright hereditary osteodystrophy (resistance to parathyroid hormone, short stature, brachydactyly, resistance to other hormones in certain subtypes), exhibit the consequences of genomic imprinting. Most studies of gene expression have focused on the regulatory DNA elements of genes that control transcription. However, it should be emphasized that gene expression requires a series of steps, including mRNA processing, protein translation, and posttranslational modifications, all of which are actively regulated (Fig. 56-3).

STRUCTURE OF GENES A gene product is usually a protein but can occasionally consist of RNA that is not translated. *Exons* refer to the portion of genes that are eventually spliced together to form mRNA. *Introns* refer to the spacing regions between the exons that are spliced out of precursor RNAs during RNA processing (Fig. 56-3).

The gene locus also includes regions that are necessary to control its expression. The regulatory regions most commonly involve sequences upstream (5′) of the transcription start site, although there are also examples of control elements within introns or downstream of the coding regions of a gene. The upstream regulatory regions are also referred to as the *promoter*. The minimal promoter usually consists of a TATA box (which binds TATA-binding protein, TBP) and initiator sequences that enhance the formation of an active transcription complex. A gene may generate various transcripts through the use of alternative promoters and/or alternative splicing of exons, mechanisms that contribute to the enormous diversity of proteins and their functions. Transcriptional termination signals reside downstream, or 3′, of a gene. Specific sequences, such as the AAUAAA sequence at the 3′ end of the mRNA, designate the site for polyadenylation (poly-A tail), a process that influences mRNA transport to the cytoplasm, stability, and translation efficiency. A rigorous test of the regulatory region boundaries involves expressing a gene in a transgenic animal to determine whether the isolated DNA flanking sequences are sufficient to recapitulate the normal developmental, tissue-specific, and signal-responsive features of the endogenous gene. This has been accomplished for only a few genes; there are many examples in which large genomic fragments only partially reconstitute normal gene regulation in vivo, implying the presence of distant regulatory sequences. This approach is critical to our understanding of mechanisms that regulate genes and is also relevant for gene therapy strategies that require normal gene regulation (Chap. 59).

As genes are dissected with greater resolution, the number of DNA sequences and transcription factors that regulate transcription is much greater than originally anticipated. Most genes contain at least 15 to 20 discrete regulatory elements within 300 bp of the transcription start site. This densely packed promoter region often contains binding sites for ubiquitous transcription factors such as CAAT box/enhancer binding protein (C/EBP), cyclic AMP response element–binding (CREB) protein, selective promoter factor 1 (Sp-1), or activator protein 1 (AP-1). However, factors involved in cell-specific expression may also bind to these sequences. For example, basic helix-loop-helix (bHLH) proteins bind to E-boxes in the promoters of myogenic genes, and steroidogenic factor 1 (SF-1) binds to a specific recognition site in the regulatory region of multiple steroidogenic enzyme genes. Key regulatory elements may also reside at some distance from the proximal promoter. The globin and the immunoglobulin genes, for example, contain *locus control regions* that are several kilobases away from the structural sequences of the gene. Specific groups of transcription factors that bind to these promoter and enhancer sequences provide a combinatorial code for regulating transcription. In this manner, relatively ubiquitous factors interact with more restricted factors to allow each gene to be expressed and regulated in a unique manner that is dependent on developmental state, cell type, and numerous extracellular stimuli. As described below, the transcription factors that bind to DNA actually represent only the first level of regulatory control. Other proteins—*coactivators* and *co-repressors*—interact with the DNA-binding transcription factors to generate large regulatory complexes. These complexes are subject to control by numerous cell-signaling pathways, including phosphorylation and acetylation. Ultimately, the recruited transcription factors interact with, and stabilize, components of the basal transcription complex that assembles at the site of the TATA box and initiator region. This basal transcription factor complex consists of >30 different proteins. Gene transcription occurs when RNA polymerase begins to synthesize RNA from the DNA template.

Mutations can occur in all domains of a gene (Fig. 56-5). A point mutation occurring within the coding region leads to an amino acid substitution if the codon is altered. Point mutations that introduce a premature stop codon result in a truncated protein. Large deletions may affect a portion of a gene or an entire gene, whereas small deletions and insertions alter the reading frame if they do not represent a multiple of three bases. These "frameshift" mutations lead to an entirely altered carboxy terminus. Mutations occurring in regulatory or intronic regions may result in altered expression or splicing of genes. Examples are shown in Fig. 56-6.

TRANSCRIPTIONAL ACTIVATION AND REPRESSION Every gene is controlled uniquely, whether in its spatial or temporal pattern of expression or in its response to extracellular signals. It is estimated that transcription factors account for about 30% of expressed genes. A growing number of identified genetic diseases involve transcription factors (Table 56-2). The MODY (maturity-onset diabetes of the young) disorders are representative of this group of diseases; mutations in several different islet cell–specific transcription factors cause various forms of MODY (Chap. 323).

Transcriptional activation can be divided into three main mechanisms:

1. Events that alter chromatin structure can enhance the access of transcription factors to DNA. For example, histone acetylation opens chromatin structure and is correlated with transcriptional activation.
2. Posttranslational modifications of transcription factors, such as phosphorylation, can induce the assembly of active transcription complexes. As an example, phosphorylation of CREB protein on serine 133 induces a conformational change that allows the recruitment of CREB-binding protein (CBP), a factor that integrates the actions of many transcription factors, including proteins, with histone acetyltransferase activity.
3. Transcriptional activators can displace a repressor protein. This mechanism is particularly common during development when the pattern of transcription factor expression changes dynamically.

β-Globin Gene Cluster

FIGURE 56-5 Point mutations causing β-thalassemia as example of allelic heterogeneity. The β-globin gene is located in the globin gene cluster. Point mutations can be located in the promoter, the CAP site, the 5′-untranslated region, the initiation codon, each of the three exons, the introns, or the polyadenylation signal. Many mutations introduce missense or nonsense mutations, whereas others cause defective RNA splicing. Not shown here are deletion mutations of the β-globin gene or larger deletions of the globin locus that can also result in thalassemia. ▼, Promoter mutations; *, CAP site; •, 5′UTR; ☐1, Initiation codon; ◆, Defective RNA processing; ✦, Missense and nonsense mutations; ☐A, Poly A signal.

FIGURE 56-6 *A.* Examples of mutations. The coding strand is shown with the encoded amino acid sequence. *B.* Chromatograms of sequence analyses after amplification of genomic DNA by polymerase chain reaction.

TABLE 56-2 *Selected Examples of Diseases Caused by Mutations and Rearrangements in Transcription Factor Classes*

Transcription Factor Class	Example	Associated Disorder
Nuclear receptors	Androgen receptor	Complete or partial androgen insensitivity (recessive missense mutations)
		Spinobulbar muscular atrophy (CAG repeat expansion)
Zinc finger proteins	WT-1	WAGR syndrome: Wilm's tumor, aniridia, genitourinary malformations, mental retardation
Basic helix-loop-helix	MITF	Waardenburg syndrome type 2A
Homeobox	IPF1	Maturity onset of diabetes mellitus type 4 (heterozygous mutation/haploinsufficiency)
		Pancreatic agenesis (homozygous mutation)
Leucine zipper	Retina leucine zipper (NRL)	Autosomal dominant retinitis pigmentosa
High- mobility group (HMG) proteins	SRY	Sex-reversal
Forkhead	HNF4α, HNF1α, HNF1β	Maturity-onset of diabetes mellitus types 1, 3, 5
Paired box	PAX-3	Waardenburg syndrome types 1 and 3
T-box	TBX-5	Holt-Oram syndrome (thumb anomalies, atrial or ventricular septum defects, phocomelia)
Cell cycle control proteins	P53	Li-Fraumeni syndrome, other cancers
Coactivators	CREB binding protein (CBP)	Rubenstein-Taybi syndrome
General transcription factors	TATA-binding protein (TBP)	Spinocerebellar ataxia 17 (CAG expansion)
Transcription elongation factor	VHL	von Hippel-Lindau syndrome (renal cell carcinoma, pheochromocytoma, pancreatic tumors, hemangioblastomas)
		Autosomal dominant inheritance, somatic inactivation of second allele
Runt	CBFA2	Familial thrombocytopenia with propensity to acute myelogenous leukemia
Chimeric proteins due to translocations	PML—RAR	Acute promyelocytic leukemia t(15;17)(q22;q11.2-q12) translocation

Abbreviations: SRY, sex determining region Y; HNF, hepatocyte nuclear factor; CREB (cAMP responsive element binding) binding protein; VHL, von Hippel-Lindau; PML, promyelocytic leukemia; RAR, retinoic acid receptor.

vances and to profound insights into genetics. Examples include the discoveries of reverse transcriptase, restriction enzymes, plasmid cloning vectors, DNA sequencing, and PCR. A description of recombinant DNA techniques, the methodology used for the manipulation, analysis, and characterization of DNA segments, is beyond the scope of this chapter. As these methods are widely used in genetics and molecular diagnostics, however, it is useful to review briefly some of the fundamental principles of cloning and DNA sequencing.

CLONING OF GENES *Cloning* refers to the creation of a recombinant DNA molecule that can be propagated indefinitely. The ability to clone genes and cDNAs therefore provides a permanent and renewable source of these reagents. Cloning is essential for DNA sequencing, nucleic acid hybridization studies, expression of recombinant proteins, and other recombinant DNA procedures.

The cloning of DNA involves the insertion of a DNA fragment into a cloning vector, followed by the propagation of the recombinant DNA in a host cell. The most straightforward cloning strategy involves inserting a DNA fragment into bacterial plasmids. Plasmids are small, autonomously replicating, circular DNA molecules that propagate separately from the chromosome in bacterial cells. The process of DNA insertion relies heavily on the use of restriction enzymes, which cleave DNA at highly specific sequences (usually 4 to 6 bp in length). Restriction enzymes generate complementary, cohesive sequences at the ends of the DNA fragment, which allow them to be efficiently ligated to the plasmid vector. Because plasmids contain genes that confer resistance to antibiotics, their presence in the host cell can be used for selection and DNA amplification.

A variety of vectors (e.g., plasmids, phage, bacterial, or yeast artificial chromosomes) are used for cloning. Many of these are used for creating *libraries*, a term that refers to a collection of DNA clones. A genomic library represents an array of clones derived from genomic DNA. These overlapping DNA fragments represent the entire genome and can ultimately be arranged according to their linear order. cDNA libraries reflect clones derived from mRNA, typically from a particular tissue source. Thus, a cDNA library from the heart contains copies of mRNA expressed specifically in cardiac myocytes, in addition to those that are expressed ubiquitously. For this reason, a heart cDNA library will be enriched with cardiac-specific gene products and will differ from cDNA libraries generated from liver or pituitary mRNAs. As an example of the complexity of a genomic library, consider that the human genome contains 3×10^9 bp and the average genomic insert in a λ phage library is about 10^4 bp. Therefore, it requires at least 3×10^5 clones to represent all genomic DNA. Specific clones are isolated from the several hundred thousand clones by using DNA hybridization.

With completion of the HGP, all human genes have been cloned and sequenced. As a result, many of these cloning procedures are now unnecessary or greatly facilitated by the extensive information concerning DNA markers and the sequence of DNA (see below).

NUCLEIC ACID HYBRIDIZATION Nucleic acid *hybridization* is a fundamental principle in molecular biology that takes advantage of the fact that the two complementary strands of nucleic acids bind, or *hybridize*, to one another with very high specificity. The goal of hybridization is to

Of course, these mechanisms are not mutually exclusive, and most genes are activated by some combination of these events.

Suppression of gene expression is as important as gene activation in the control of cell differentiation and function. Some mechanisms of repression are the corollary of activation. For example, repression is often associated with histone deacetylation or protein dephosphorylation. For nuclear hormone receptors, transcriptional silencing involves the recruitment of repression complexes that contain histone deacetylase activity. Aberrant expression of repressor proteins is sometimes associated with neoplasia. The t(15;17) chromosomal translocation that occurs in promyelocytic leukemia fuses the *PML* gene to a portion of the retinoic acid receptor α (*RAR* α) gene (Table 56-2). This event causes unregulated transcriptional repression in a manner that precludes normal cellular differentiation. The addition of the RAR ligand, retinoic acid, activates the receptor, thereby relieving repression and allowing cells to differentiate and ultimately undergo apoptosis. This mechanism has therapeutic importance as the addition of retinoic acid to treatment regimens induces a higher remission rate in patients with promyelocytic leukemia (Chap. 96).

CLONING AND SEQUENCING DNA

Since the mid-1970s, eight Nobel prizes have been awarded for research that led, directly or indirectly, to major methodological ad-detect specific nucleic acid (DNA or RNA) sequences in a complex background of other sequences. This technique is used for Southern blotting, Northern blotting, and for screening libraries (see above). Further adaptation of hybridization techniques has led to the development of microarray DNA chips.

Southern Blot Southern blotting is used to analyze whether genes have been deleted or rearranged. It is also used to detect restriction fragment length polymorphisms (RFLPs). Genomic DNA is digested with restriction endonucleases and separated by gel electrophoresis. Individual fragments can then be transferred to a membrane and detected after hybridization with specific radioactive DNA probes. Because single base-pair mismatches can disrupt the hybridization of short DNA probes (oligonucleotides), a variation of the Southern blot, termed *oligonucleotide-specific hybridization* (OSH), uses short oligonucleotides to distinguish normal from mutant genes.

Northern Blot Northern blots are used to analyze patterns and levels of gene expression in different tissues. In a northern blot, mRNA is separated on a gel and transferred to a membrane, and specific transcripts are detected using radiolabeled DNA as a probe. This technique is rapidly being supplanted by more sensitive and comprehensive methods such as reverse transcriptase (RT)–PCR and gene expression arrays on DNA chips (see below).

Microarray Technology A rapidly evolving approach to genome-scale studies consists of *microarrays*, or *DNA chips*. These approaches consist of thousands of synthetic nucleic acid sequences aligned on thin glass or silicon surfaces. Fluorescently labeled test sample DNA or RNA is hybridized to the chip, and a computerized scanner detects sequence matches. Microarrays allow the detection of variations in DNA sequence and are used for mutational analysis and genotyping. Alternatively, the expression pattern of large numbers of mRNA transcripts can be determined by hybridization of RNA samples to cDNA or genomic microarrays. This method has tremendous potential in the era of functional genomics (e.g., a comprehensive analysis of gene expression profiles). As one example, microarrays can be used to develop genetic fingerprints of different types of malignancies, providing information useful for classification, pathophysiology, prognosis, and treatment.

THE POLYMERASE CHAIN REACTION The PCR, introduced in 1985, has revolutionized the way DNA analyses are performed and has become a cornerstone of molecular biology and genetic analysis. In essence, PCR provides a rapid way of cloning (amplifying) specific DNA fragments in vitro (Fig. 56-7). Exquisite specificity is conferred by the use of PCR primers, which are designed for a given DNA sequence. The geometric amplification of the DNA after multiple cycles yields remarkable sensitivity. As a result, PCR can be used to amplify DNA from very small samples, including single cells. These properties also allow DNA amplification from a variety of tissue sources including blood samples, biopsies, surgical or autopsy specimens, or cells from hair or saliva. PCR can also be used to study mRNA. In this case, the enzyme RT is first used to convert the RNA to DNA, which can then be amplified by PCR. This procedure, commonly known as *RT-PCR*, is useful as a quantitative measure of gene expression.

PCR provides a key component of molecular diagnostics. It provides a strategy for the rapid amplification of DNA (or mRNA) to search for mutations by a wide array of techniques, including DNA sequencing. PCR is also used for the amplification of highly polymorphic di- or trinucleotide repeat sequences, which allow various polymorphic alleles to be traced in genetic linkage or association studies. PCR is increasingly used to diagnose various microbial pathogens.

DNA SEQUENCING DNA sequencing is now an automated procedure. Although many protocols exist, the most commonly used strategy is based on the Sanger method in which dideoxynucleotides are used to randomly terminate DNA polymerization at each of the four bases (A,G,T,C). After separating the array of terminated DNA fragments using high-resolution gel or capillary electrophoresis, it is possible to deduce the DNA sequence by examining the progression of fragment

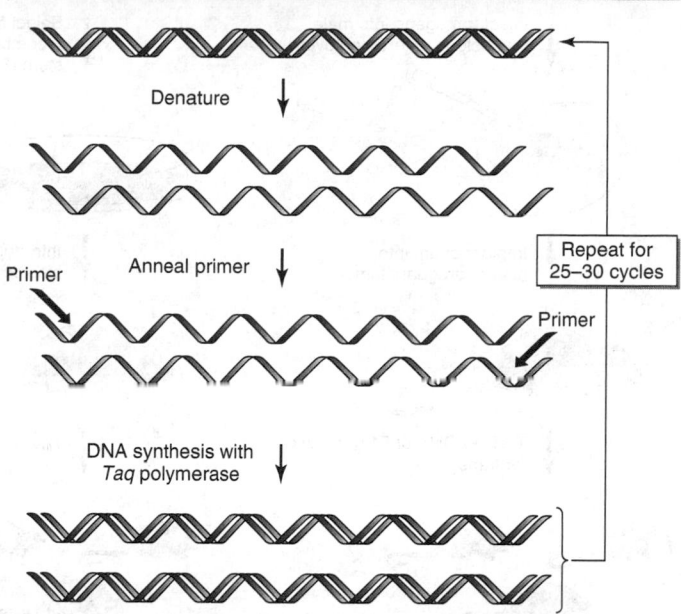

FIGURE 56-7 Polymerase chain reaction. The polymerase chain reaction (PCR) generates multiple copies of a DNA segment. After denaturing the double-stranded (ds) DNA, complementary synthetic oligonucleotide primers of about 20 bp are annealed on each side of the fragment of interest. A heat-stable polymerase then extends the oligonucleotides and synthesizes the complementary strand. This cycle is repeated 25 to 30 times. The number of DNA-amplified DNA segments is thus doubled after every PCR cycle.

lengths generated in each of the four nucleotide reactions. The use of fluorescently labeled dideoxynucleotides allows automated detection of the different bases and direct computer analysis of the DNA sequence (Fig. 56-6). Efforts are underway to develop faster, more cost-effective DNA sequencing technologies. These include the use of mass spectrometry; detection of fluorescently labeled bases in flow cytometry; direct reading of the DNA sequence by scanning, tunneling, or atomic force microscopy; and sequence analysis using DNA chips.

TRANSGENIC MICE AS MODELS OF GENETIC DISEASE

Several organisms have been studied extensively as genetic models, including *Mus musculus* (mouse), *Drosophila melanogaster* (fruit fly), *Caenorhabditis elegans* (nematode), *Saccharomyces cerevisiae* (baker's yeast), and *Escherichia coli* (colonic bacterium). The ability to use these evolutionarily distant organisms as genetic models that are relevant to human physiology reflects a surprising conservation of genetic pathways and gene function. Transgenic mouse models have been particularly valuable, because many human and mouse genes exhibit similar structure and function, and because manipulation of the mouse genome is relatively straightforward compared to those of other mammalian species.

Transgenic strategies in mice can be divided into two main approaches: (1) expression of a gene by random insertion into the genome, and (2) deletion or targeted mutagenesis of a gene by homologous recombination with the native endogenous gene (knockout, knockin) (Fig. 56-8; Table 56-3). Transgenic mice are generated by pronuclear injection of foreign DNA into fertilized mouse oocytes and subsequent transfer into the oviduct of pseudopregnant foster mothers.

Transgenic expression of genes can be useful for studying disorders that are sensitive to gene dosage. Overexpression of *PMP22*, for example, mimics a common duplication of this gene in type IA Charcot-Marie-Tooth disease (Chap. 364). Duplication of the *PMP22* gene results in high levels of expression of peripheral myelin protein 22, and this dosage effect is responsible for the demyelinating neuropathy. Expression of the Y chromosome–specific gene, *SRY*, in XX females demonstrates that *SRY* is sufficient to induce the formation of testes. This finding confirms the pathogenic role of *SRY* translocations to the

Prepare DNA transgene

Inject transgene into male pronucleus of fertilized ovum

Implant ovum into pseudopregnant female

Test tail DNA of F1 generation for transgene

Breed to homozygosity

Prepare targeting construct

Select for homologous recombination in embryonic stem (ES) cells

Introduce selected ES cells into blastocyst and implant

Mixed coat color in chimeric mice

Breed to homozygosity

FIGURE 56-8 Transgenic mouse models. *Left.* Transgenic mice are generated by pronuclear injection of foreign DNA into fertilized mouse oocytes and subsequent transfer into the oviduct of pseudopregnant foster mothers. *Right.* For targeted mutagenesis (gene knockout/knockin), embryonic stem (ES) cells are transfected with the targeted (mutagenized) transgene. The transgene undergoes homologous recombination with the wild-type gene. After selection, positive ES cells are introduced into blastocysts and implanted into foster mothers. Chimeric mice can be identified based on the mixed coat color of the offspring. Heterozygous mice are bred to obtain mice homozygous for the mutant allele.

X chromosome in sex-reversed XX females. Huntington disease is an autosomal dominant disorder caused by expansion of a CAG trinucleotide repeat that encodes a polyglutamine tract. Targeted deletion of the Huntington disease (*HD*) gene does not induce the neurologic disorder. On the other hand, transgenic expression of the entire gene or of the first exon containing the expanded polyGlu repeat is sufficient to cause many features of the neurologic disorder, indicating a gain-of-function property for the expanded polyGlu-containing protein. Transgenic strategies can also be used as a precursor to gene therapy. Expression of dystrophin, the protein that is deleted in Duchenne muscular dystrophy, partially corrects the disorder in a mouse model of Duchenne's. Targeted expression of oncogenes has been valuable to study mechanisms of neoplasia and to generate immortalized cell lines. For example, expression of the simian virus 40 (SV40) large T antigen under the direction of the insulin promoter induces the formation of islet cell tumors.

The creation of gene knockout and knockin models takes advantage of the fact that a segment of DNA can be substituted by another that is identical (homologous), or nearly identical, by recombination. This permits integration of deletions that disrupt the gene (knockout) or selected mutations (knockin) into the target gene of choice. The transgene is introduced into embryonic stem (ES) cells by transfection and, after selection of cells with an integrated transgene, the positive ES cells are introduced into blastocysts and implanted into foster mothers. Chimeric mice can be identified based on the mixed coat color of the offspring. Heterozygous mice are bred to obtain mice homozygous for the mutant allele. This is particularly useful for genes that would be lethal if deleted universally or during early development. The list of genes that have been modified by this approach is very large.

Many of these knockouts do not have an apparent phenotype, either because of redundant functions of the other genes or because the phenotype is subtle. For example, deletion of the hypoxanthine phosphoribosyltransferase (HPRT) gene (*Hprt*) does not cause characteristic features of Lesch-Nyhan syndrome in mice because of their reliance on adenine phosphoribosyltransferase (APRT) in the purine salvage pathway. Deletion of the retinoblastoma (*Rb*) gene does not lead to retinoblastoma or other tumors that characterize the human syndrome. These examples underscore the fact that the functions of genes, and their interactions with genetic background and the environment, are not necessarily identical in mice and humans. On the other hand, the deletion of many genes provides a remarkably faithful model of human disorders. In addition to clarifying pathophysiology, these models facilitate the development of therapies, both genetic and pharmaceutical.

Many variations of these basic approaches now exist that allow genes to be expressed or deleted in specific cell types, at different times during development, or at varying levels. Consequently, transgenic technology has emerged as a powerful strategy for defining the physiologic effects of deleting or overexpressing a gene, as well as providing unique genetic models for dissecting pathophysiology or testing therapies. In addition to transgenic animal models, naturally occurring mutations in mice and other species continue to provide fundamental insights into human disease. A compendium of natural and transgenic animal models is provided in continuously evolving databases (Table 56-1).

Human pluripotential *stem cells* have recently been developed, and, consistent with their potential for self-renewal, these cell lines express high levels of telomerase, an enzyme that is essential for allowing repeated replication of the ends of eukaryotic chromosomes. Although much remains to be learned about the properties of pluripotential stem cells, they may prove useful for transplantation, drug testing, or for other purposes (Chap. 59).

IMPLICATIONS OF THE HUMAN GENOME PROJECT

The HGP was initiated in the mid-1980s as an ambitious effort to characterize the human genome, culminating in a complete DNA sequence. The initial main goals were (1) creation of genetic maps, (2) development of physical maps, and (3) determination of the complete human DNA sequence. Some analogies help in appreciating the scope of the HGP. The 23 pairs of human chromosomes encode approximately 30,000 to 40,000 genes. The total length of DNA is about 3 billion bp, which is nearly 1000-fold greater than that of the *E. coli* genome. If the human DNA sequence were printed out, it would correspond to about 120 volumes of *Harrison's Principles of Internal Medicine*.

THE GENETIC MAP Given the size and complexity of the human genome, initial efforts aimed at developing genetic maps to provide orientation and to delimit where a gene of interest may be located. A *genetic map* describes the order of genes and defines the position of a gene relative to other loci on the same chromosome. It is constructed by assessing how frequently two markers are inherited together (e.g., *linked*) by association studies. Distances of the genetic map are expressed in recombination units, or centimorgans (cM). One cM corresponds to a recombination frequency of 1% between two polymorphic markers; 1 cM corresponds to approximately 1 Mb of DNA (Fig. 56-4). Any polymorphic sequence variation can be useful for mapping purposes. Examples of polymorphic markers include variable number of tandem repeats (VNTRs), RFLPs, microsatellite repeats, and single nucleotide polymorphisms (SNPs); the latter two methods are now used predominantly because of the high density of markers and because they are amenable to automated procedures. Current efforts aim at creating high quality, dense SNP maps and haplotype maps (e.g., linear arrangements of alleles) of the human genome through the identification of as many as 500,000 SNPs. These variations, which are amenable to automated analysis with DNA chips, will greatly facilitate association and linkage studies for the elucidation of the complex interactions among multiple genes and life-style factors in multifactorial disorders. SNP patterns may ultimately become useful for the prediction of disease predisposition and pharmacogenomics.

THE PHYSICAL MAP Cytogenetics and chromosomal banding techniques provide a relatively low-resolution microscopic view of genetic loci. Physical maps indicate the position of a locus or gene in absolute values. Sequence-tagged sites (STSs) are used as a standard unit for physical mapping and serve as sequence-specific landmarks for arranging overlapping cloned fragments in the same order as they occur in the genome. These overlapping clones allow the characterization of contiguous DNA sequences, commonly referred to as *contigs*. This approach led to high-resolution physical maps by cloning the whole genome into overlapping fragments and has been essential for the identification of disease-causing genes by positional cloning. The complete DNA sequence of each chromosome, now already complete for several chromosomes and as draft for the whole genome, provides the highest resolution physical map.

STATUS OF DNA SEQUENCING The primary focus of the HGP was to obtain DNA sequence for the entire human genome as well as model organisms. Although the prospect of determining the complete sequence of the human genome seemed daunting several years ago, technical advances in DNA sequencing and bioinformatics led to the completion of a draft human sequence in June 2000, well in advance of the original goal year of 2003. The whole genomes of more than 800 organisms have been sequenced partially or completely. They include, among others, eukaryotes such as man and mouse; *S. cerevisiae, C. elegans,* and *D. melanogaster*; bacteria (e.g., *E. coli*); and archeae, viruses, organelles (mitochondriae, chloroplasts), and plants (e.g., *Arabidopsis thaliana*). For the human genome, the current goal is now to achieve 99.99% (1 error in 10,000 bp) accuracy. This level of accuracy is important for many reasons, including efforts to determine the degree of DNA sequence variation in the population. Comparisons of the DNA sequence from multiple individuals or populations will allow assessments of genetic variance in the human population. Another goal is to develop a complete set of full-length human cDNAs and to define their locations on the physical map.

CURRENT DIRECTIONS ARISING FROM THE HGP The primary goals of the HGP have been achieved, but there are numerous remaining challenges, including (1) refining the sequence information and solving ambiguities, (2) establishing catalogs of sequence variations and SNPs, (3) characterizing the expression pattern of thousands of genes simultaneously in order to detect differences between various tissues in health and disease (*functional genomics*), (4) identifying the genes that play critical roles in the development of polygenic and multifactorial disorders, and (5) developing large-scale analyses of protein expression (*proteomics*).

ETHICAL ISSUES Implicit in the HGP is the idea and hope that identifying disease-causing genes can lead to improvements in diagnosis,

TABLE 56-3 Genetic Modified Animals		
Commonly Used Description	Technical Principle	Remarks
Transgenic	Pronuclear injection of transgene	Commonly used
		Genomic DNA or cDNA constructs
		Random integration of transgene
		Variable copy numbers of transgene
		Variable expression in each individual founder
		Gain of function models due to overexpression using tissue-specific promoters
		Loss of function models using anti-sense and dominant negative transgenes
		Inducible expression possible (Tetracycline, ecdysone)
		Applicable to several species
(Targeted) Knockout	Substitution of functional gene with inactive gene by homologous recombination in embryonic stem cells	Predominantly used in mice
		Tissue-specific knockout possible (Cre/lox)
		Absence of phenotype possible due to redundancy
(Targeted) Knockin	Introduction of subtle mutation(s) into gene by substitution of endogenous gene with gene carrying a specific mutation. Homologous recombination in embryonic stem cells	Predominantly used in mice
		Can accurately model human disease
Forward genetics	Mutations created randomly by ENU (N-ethyl-N-nitrourea)	Selection of phenotype followed by genetic characterization
		Useful for cloning of novel genes
Cloning	Introduction of nucleus into enucleated eggs (nuclear transfer)	Successful in several mammalian species including sheep (Dolly), mice, cows, monkeys
		Cloning of genetically identical individuals
		May affect life span
		Ethical concerns

prognosis, and treatment. It is estimated that most individuals harbor several serious recessive genes. However, completion of the human genome sequence, determination of the association of genetic defects with disease, and studies of genetic variation raise many new issues with implications for the individual and mankind. The controversies concerning the cloning of mammals and the establishment of human embryonic stem cells underscore the relevance of these questions. Moreover, the information gleaned from genotypic results can have quite different impacts, depending on the availability of strategies to modify the course of disease. For example, the identification of mutations that cause multiple endocrine neoplasia (MEN) type 2 or hemochromatosis allows specific interventions for affected family members. On the other hand, at present, the identification of an Alzheimer or Huntington disease gene does not alter therapy. Genetic test results can generate anxiety in affected individuals and family members, and there is the possibility of discrimination on the basis of the test results. Most genetic disorders are likely to fall into an intermediate category where the opportunity for prevention or treatment is significant but limited (Chap. 58). For these reasons, the scientific components of the HGP have been paralleled by efforts to examine ethical and legal implications as new issues arise. About 5% of the HGP budget had been allocated to studies addressing the ethical, legal, and social implications associated with the increasing knowledge about the human genome and the genetic basis of disease.

Many issues raised by the genome project are familiar, in principle, to medical practitioners. For example, an asymptomatic patient with increased low-density lipoprotein (LDL) cholesterol, high blood pressure, or a strong family history of early myocardial infarction is known to be at increased risk of coronary heart disease. In such cases, it is clear that the identification of risk factors and an appropriate intervention are beneficial. Likewise, patients with phenylketonuria, cystic fibrosis, or sickle cell anemia are often identified as having a genetic disease early in life. These precedents can be helpful for adapting policies that relate to genetic information. We can anticipate similar efforts, whether based on genotypes or other markers of genetic predisposition, to be applied to many disorders. One confounding aspect of the rapid expansion of information is that our ability to make clinical predictions often lags behind genetic advances. For example, when genes that predispose to breast cancer, such as *BRCA1*, are described, they generate tremendous public interest in the potential to predict disease, but many years of clinical research are still required to rigorously establish genotype and phenotype correlations.

Whether related to informed consent, participation in research, or the management of a genetic disorder that affects an individual or their families, there is a great need for more information about fundamental principles of genetics. The pervasive nature of the role of genetics in medicine makes it imperative for physicians and other health care professionals to become more informed about genetics, and to provide advice and counseling in conjunction with trained genetic counselors (Chap. 58). The application of screening and prevention strategies will therefore require intensive patient and physician education, changes in health care financing, and legislation to protect patient's rights.

TRANSMISSION OF GENETIC DISEASE

ORIGINS AND TYPES OF MUTATIONS A *mutation* can be defined as any change in the primary nucleotide sequence of DNA regardless of its functional consequences. Some mutations may be lethal, others are less deleterious, and some may confer an evolutionary advantage. Mutations can occur in the germline (sperm or oocytes); these can be transmitted to progeny. Alternatively, mutations can occur during embryogenesis or in somatic tissues. Mutations that occur during development lead to *mosaicism*, a situation in which tissues are composed of cells with different genetic constitutions. If the germline is mosaic, a mutation can be transmitted to some progeny but not others, which sometimes leads to confusion in assessing the pattern of inheritance. Somatic mutations that do not affect cell survival can sometimes be detected because of variable phenotypic effects in tissues (e.g., pigmented lesions in McCune-Albright syndrome). Other somatic mutations are associated with neoplasia because they confer a growth advantage to cells. Epigenetic events, heritable changes that do not involve changes in gene sequence (e.g., altered DNA methylation), may influence gene expression or facilitate genetic damage. With the exception of triplet nucleotide repeats, which can expand (see below), mutations are usually stable.

Mutations are structurally diverse—they can involve the entire genome, as in triploidy (one extra set of chromosomes), or gross numerical or structural alterations in chromosomes or individual genes (Chap. 57). Large deletions may affect a portion of a gene or an entire gene, or, if several genes are involved, they may lead to a *contiguous gene syndrome*. Unequal crossing-over between homologous genes can result in fusion gene mutations, as illustrated by color blindness (Chap. 25). Mutations involving single nucleotides are referred to as *point mutations* (Fig. 56-6). Substitutions are called *transitions* if a purine is replaced by another purine base (A $\leftrightarrow$ G) or if a pyrimidine is replaced by another pyrimidine (C $\leftrightarrow$ T). Changes from a purine to a pyrimidine, or vice versa, are referred to as *transversions*. If the DNA sequence change occurs in a coding region and alters an amino acid, it is called a *missense mutation*. Depending on the functional consequences of such a missense mutation, amino acid substitutions in different regions of the protein can lead to distinct phenotypes. *Polymorphisms* are sequence variations that have a frequency of at least 1%. Usually, they do not result in a perceptible phenotype. Often they consist of single base-pair substitutions that do not alter the protein coding sequence because of the degenerate nature of the genetic code, although it is possible that some might alter mRNA stability, translation, or the amino acid sequence. These types of silent base substitutions and SNPs are encountered frequently during genetic testing

and must be distinguished from true mutations that alter protein expression or function. Small nucleotide deletions or insertions cause a shift of the codon reading frame (*frameshift*). Most commonly, reading frame alterations result in an abnormal protein segment of variable length before termination of translation occurs at a stop codon (*nonsense mutation*) (Fig. 56-6). Mutations in intronic sequences or in exon junctions may destroy or create splice donor or splice acceptor sites. Mutations may also be found in the regulatory sequences of genes, resulting in reduced gene transcription.

Mutation Rates As noted before, mutations represent an important cause of genetic diversity as well as disease. Mutation rates are difficult to determine in humans because many mutations are silent and because testing is often not adequate to detect the phenotypic consequences. Mutation rates vary in different genes but are estimated to occur at a rate of about 10^{-10}/bp per cell division. Germline mutation rates (as opposed to somatic mutations) are relevant in the transmission of genetic disease. Because the population of oocytes is established very early in development, only about 20 cell divisions are required for completed oogenesis, whereas spermatogenesis involves about 30 divisions by the time of puberty and 20 cell divisions each year thereafter. Consequently, the probability of acquiring new point mutations is much greater in the male germline than the female germline, in which rates of aneuploidy are increased (Chap. 57). Thus, the incidence of new point mutations in spermatogonia increases with paternal age (e.g., achondrodysplasia, Marfan syndrome, neurofibromatosis). It is estimated that about 1 in 10 sperm carries a new deleterious mutation. The rates for new mutations are calculated most readily for autosomal dominant and X-linked disorders and are $\sim10^{-5}$ to 10^{-6}/locus per generation. Because most monogenic diseases are relatively rare, new mutations account for a significant fraction of cases. This is important in the context of genetic counseling, as a new mutation can be transmitted to the affected individual but does not necessarily imply that the parents are at risk to transmit the disease to other children. An exception to this is when the new mutation occurs early in germline development, leading to *gonadal mosaicism*.

Unequal Crossing-Over Normally, DNA recombination in germ cells occurs with remarkable fidelity to maintain the precise junction sites for the exchanged DNA sequences (Fig. 56-4). However, mispairing of homologous sequences leads to unequal crossover, with gene duplication on one of the chromosomes and gene deletion on the other chromosome. A significant fraction of growth hormone (*GH*) gene deletions, for example, involve unequal crossing-over (Chap. 318). The *GH* gene is a member of a large gene cluster that includes a growth hormone variant gene as well as several structurally related chorionic somatomammotropin genes and pseudogenes (highly homologous but functionally inactive relatives of a normal gene). Because such gene clusters contain multiple homologous DNA sequences arranged in tandem, they are particularly prone to undergo recombination and, consequently, gene duplication or deletion. On the other hand, duplication of the *PMP22* gene because of unequal crossing-over results in increased gene dosage and type IA Charcot-Marie-Tooth disease (Chap. 364). Unequal crossing-over resulting in deletion of *PMP22* causes a distinct neuropathy called *hereditary liability to pressure palsy* (Chap. 364).

Glucocorticoid-remediable aldosteronism (GRA) is caused by a rearrangement involving the genes that encode aldosterone synthase (*CYP11B2*) and steroid 11β-hydroxylase (*CYP11B1*), normally arranged in tandem on chromosome 8q. These two genes are 95% identical, predisposing to gene duplication and deletion by unequal crossing-over. The rearranged gene product contains the regulatory regions of 11β-hydroxylase fused to the coding sequence of aldosterone synthetase. Consequently, the latter enzyme is expressed in the adrenocorticotropic hormone (ACTH)-dependent zona fasciculata of the adrenal gland, resulting in overproduction of mineralocorticoids and hypertension (Chap. 321).

Gene conversion refers to a nonreciprocal exchange of homologous genetic information; it is probably more common than generally recognized. In human genetics, gene conversion has been used to explain how an internal portion of a gene is replaced by a homologous segment copied from another allele or locus; these genetic alterations may range from a few nucleotides to a few thousand nucleotides. As a result of gene conversion, it is possible for short DNA segments of two chromosomes to be identical, even though these sequences are distinct in the parents. A practical consequence of this phenomenon is that nucleotide substitutions can occur during gene conversion between related genes, often altering the function of the gene. In disease states, gene conversion often involves intergenic exchange of DNA between a gene and a related pseudogene. For example, the 21-hydroxylase gene (*CYP21A*) is adjacent to a nonfunctional pseudogene. Many of the nucleotide substitutions that are found in the *CYP21A* gene in patients with congenital adrenal hyperplasia correspond to sequences that are present in the pseudogene, suggesting gene conversion as a mechanism of mutagenesis. In addition, mitotic gene conversion has been suggested as a mechanism to explain revertant mosaicism in which an inherited mutation is "corrected" in certain cells. For example, patients with autosomal recessive generalized atrophic benign epidermolysis bullosa have acquired reverse mutations in one of the two mutated *COL17A1* alleles, leading to clinically unaffected patches of skin.

Insertions and Deletions Though many instances of insertions and deletions occur as a consequence of unequal crossing-over, there is also evidence for internal duplication, inversion, or deletion of DNA sequences. The fact that certain deletions or insertions appear to occur repeatedly as independent events suggests that specific regions within the DNA sequence predispose to these errors. For example, certain regions of the *DMD* gene appear to be hot spots for deletions.

Errors in DNA Repair Because mutations caused by defects in DNA repair accumulate as somatic cells divide, these types of mutations are particularly important in the context of neoplastic disorders (Chap. 69). Several genetic disorders involving DNA repair enzymes underscore their importance. Patients with xeroderma pigmentosum have defects in DNA damage recognition or in the nucleotide excision and repair pathway (Chap. 73). Exposed skin is dry and pigmented and is extraordinarily sensitive to the mutagenic effects of ultraviolet irradiation. More than 10 different genes have been shown to cause the different forms of xeroderma pigmentosum. This finding is consistent with the earlier classification of this disease into different complementation groups in which normal function is rescued by the fusion of cells derived from two different forms of xeroderma pigmentosum.

Ataxia telangiectasia causes large telangiectatic lesions of the face, cerebellar ataxia, immunologic defects, and hypersensitivity to ionizing radiation (Chap. 352). The discovery of the ataxia telangiectasia mutated (*ATM*) gene reveals that it is homologous to genes involved in DNA repair and control of cell cycle checkpoints. Mutations in the *ATM* gene give rise to defects in meiosis as well as increasing susceptibility to damage from ionizing radiation. Fanconi's anemia is also associated with an increased risk of multiple acquired genetic abnormalities. It is characterized by diverse congenital anomalies and a strong predisposition to develop aplastic anemia and acute myelogenous leukemia (Chap. 96). Cells from these patients are susceptible to chromosomal breaks caused by a defect in genetic recombination. At least eight different complementation groups have been identified, and several loci and genes associated with Fanconi's anemia have been mapped or cloned.

HNPCC is caused by mutations in one of several different mismatch repair (MMR) genes including MutS homologue 2 (*MSH2*) and MutL homologue 1 (*MLH1*) (Chap. 77). These enzymes are involved in the detection of nucleotide mismatches and in the recognition of slipped-strand trinucleotide repeats. Germline mutations in these genes lead to microsatellite instability and a high mutation rate in colon cancer. This syndrome is characterized by autosomal dominant transmission of colon cancer, young age (<50 years) of presentation, predisposition to lesions in the proximal large bowel, and associated malignancies such as uterine cancer and ovarian cancer. Genetic screening

tests for this disorder are now being used for families considered to be at risk (Chap. 58). Recognition of HNPCC allows early screening with colonoscopy and the implementation of prevention strategies using nonsteroidal anti-inflammatory drugs.

CpG and Dipyrimidine Sequences Certain DNA sequences are particularly susceptible to mutagenesis. Successive pyrimidine residues (e.g., T-T or C-C) are subject to the formation of ultraviolet light–induced photoadducts. If these pyrimidine dimers are not repaired by the nucleotide excision repair pathway, mutations will be introduced after DNA synthesis. The dinucleotide C-G, or CpG, is also a hot spot for a specific type of mutation. In this case, methylation of the cytosine is associated with an enhanced rate of deamination to uracil, which is then replaced with thymine. This $C \rightarrow T$ transition (or $G \rightarrow A$ on the opposite strand) accounts for at least one-third of point mutations associated with polymorphisms and mutations. Many of the *MSH2* mutations in HNPCC, for example, involve CpG sequences. In addition to the fact that certain types of mutations ($C \rightarrow T$ or $G \rightarrow A$) are relatively common, the nature of the genetic code also results in overrepresentation of certain amino acid substitutions.

Unstable DNA Sequences *Trinucleotide repeats* may be unstable and expand beyond a critical number. Mechanistically, the expansion is thought to be caused by unequal recombination and slipped mispairing. A premutation represents a small increase in trinucleotide copy number. In subsequent generations, the expanded repeat may increase further in length and result in an increasingly severe phenotype, a process called *dynamic mutation* (see below for discussion of anticipation). Trinucleotide expansion was first recognized as a cause of the fragile X syndrome, one of the most common causes of mental retardation. Other disorders arising from a similar mechanism include Huntington disease (Chap. 350), X-linked spinobulbar muscular atrophy (Chap. 353), and myotonic dystrophy (Chap. 368) (Table 56-4). Malignant cells are also characterized by genetic instability, indicating a breakdown in mechanisms that regulate DNA repair and the cell cycle.

FUNCTIONAL CONSEQUENCES OF MUTATIONS Functionally, mutations can be broadly classified as gain-of-function and loss-of-function mutations. Gain-of-function mutations are typically dominant, i.e., they result in phenotypic alterations when a single allele is affected. Inactivating mutations are usually recessive, and an affected individual is homozygous or compound heterozygous (e.g., carrying two different mutant alleles) for the disease-causing mutations. Alternatively, mutation in a single allele can result in *haploinsufficiency*, a situation in which one normal allele is not sufficient to maintain a normal phenotype. Haploinsufficiency is a commonly observed mechanism in diseases associated with mutations in transcription factors (Table 56-2). Remarkably, the clinical features among patients with an identical mutation in a transcription factor often vary significantly. One mechanism underlying this variability consists in the influence of modifying genes. Haploinsufficiency can also affect the expression of rate-limiting enzymes. For example, haploinsufficiency in enzymes involved in heme synthesis can cause porphyrias (Chap. 337).

An increase in dosage of a gene product may also result in disease, as illustrated by the duplication of the *DAX1* gene in dosage-sensitive sex-reversal (Chap. 328). Mutation in a single allele can also result in loss of function due to a dominant-negative effect. In this case, the mutated allele interferes with the function of the normal gene product by one of several different mechanisms: (1) a mutant protein may interfere with the function of a multimeric protein complex, as illustrated by mutations in type 1 collagen (*COL1A1, COL1A2*) genes in osteogenesis imperfecta (Chap. 342); (2) a mutant protein may occupy binding sites on proteins or promoter response elements, as illustrated by thyroid hormone resistance, a disorder in which inactivated thyroid hormone receptor binds to target genes and functions as an antagonist of normal receptors (Chap. 320); or (3) a mutant protein can be cytotoxic as in α_1 antitrypsin deficiency (Chap. 242) or autosomal dominant neurohypophyseal diabetes insipidus (Chap. 319), in which the

TABLE 56-4 *Selected Trinucleotide Repeat Disorders*

Disease	Locus	Repeat	Triplet Length Normal/Disease	Inheritance	Gene Product
X-Chromosomal spinobulbar muscular atrophy (SBMA)	Xq11-q12	CAG	11–34/40–62	XR	Androgen receptor
Fragile X-syndrome (FRAXA)	Xq27.3	CGG	6–50/200–300	XR	FMR-1 protein
Fragile X-syndrome (FRAXE)	Xq28	GCC	6–25/>200	XR	FMR-2 protein
Dystrophia myotonica (DM)	19q13.2-q13.3	CTG	5–30/200–1000	AD, variable penetrance	Myotonin protein kinase
Huntington disease (HD)	4p16.3	CAG	11–34/37–121	AD	Huntington
Spinocerebellar ataxia type 1 (SCA1)	6p21.3-21.2	CAG	19–36/39–83	AD	Ataxin 1
Spinocerebellar ataxia type 2 (SCA2)	12q24.1	CAG	15–31/34–400	AD	Ataxin 2
Spinocerebellar ataxia type 3 (SCA3); Machado Joseph disease (MD)	14q21	CAG	13–36/55–86	AD	SC3/MJD1
Spinocerebellar ataxia type 6 (SCA6, CACNAIA)	19p13.1-13.2	CAG	4–16/20–33	AD	Alpha 1A voltage-dependent calcium channel
Spinocerebellar ataxia type 7 (SCA7)	3p21.1-p12	CAG	4–19/37 ≥ 300	AD	Ataxin 7
Spinocerebellar ataxia type 12 (SCA12)	5q31	CAG	6–26/66–78	AD	Protein phosphatase 2A
Dentorubral pallidoluysiane atrophy (DRPLA)	12p	CAG	7–23/49–75	AD	Atrophin
Friedreich ataxia (FRDA1)	9q13-21	GAA	7–22/200–900	AR	Frataxin

Abbreviations: AD, autosomal dominant; AR, autosomal recessive; XR, X-linked recessive.

abnormally folded proteins are trapped within the endoplasmic reticulum and ultimately cause cellular damage.

GENOTYPE AND PHENOTYPE ■ Alleles, Genotypes, and Haplotypes An observed trait is referred to as a *phenotype*; the genetic information defining the phenotype is called the *genotype*. Alternative forms of a gene or a genetic marker are referred to as *alleles*. Alleles may be polymorphic variants of nucleic acids that have no apparent effect on gene expression or function. In other instances, these variants may have subtle effects on gene expression, thereby conferring the adaptive advantages associated with genetic diversity. On the other hand, allelic variants may reflect mutations in a gene that clearly alter its function. The common Glu → Val sickle cell mutation (E6V) in the *β-globin* gene and the δF508 deletion of phenylalanine (F) in the *CFTR* gene are examples of allelic variants of these genes. Because each individual has two copies of each chromosome (one inherited from the mother and one inherited from the father), he or she can have only two alleles at a given locus. However, there can be many different alleles in the population. The normal or common allele is usually referred to as *wild type*. When alleles at a given locus are identical, the individual is *homozygous*. Inheriting such identical copies of a mutant allele occurs in many autosomal recessive disorders, particularly in circumstances of consanguinity. If the alleles are different, the individual is *heterozygous* at this locus (Fig. 56-6). If two different mutant alleles are inherited at a given locus, the individual is said to be a *compound heterozygote*. *Hemizygous* is used to describe males with a mutation in an X chromosomal gene or a female with a loss of one X chromosomal locus.

Genotypes describe the specific alleles at a particular locus. For example, there are three common alleles (E2, E3, E4) of the apolipoprotein E (*APOE*) gene. The genotype of an individual can therefore be described as *APOE3/4* or *APOE4/4* or any other variant. These designations indicate which alleles are present on the two chromosomes in the *APOE* gene at locus 19q13.2. In other cases, the genotype might be assigned arbitrary numbers (e.g., 1/2) or letters (e.g., B/b) to distinguish different alleles.

A *haplotype* refers to a group of alleles that are closely linked together at a genomic locus. Haplotypes are useful for tracking the transmission of genomic segments within families and for detecting evidence of genetic recombination, if the crossover event occurs between the alleles (Fig. 56-4). As an example, various alleles at the histocompatibility locus antigen (HLA) on chromosome 6p are used to establish haplotypes associated with certain disease states. For example, 21-hydroxylase deficiency, complement deficiency, and hemochromatosis are each associated with specific HLA haplotypes. It is now recognized that these genes lie in close vicinity to the HLA locus, which explains why HLA associations were identified even before the disease genes were cloned and localized. In other cases, specific HLA associations with diseases such as ankylosing spondylitis (HLA-B27) or type 1 diabetes mellitus (HLA-DR4) reflect the role of specific HLA allelic variants in susceptibility to these autoimmune diseases.

Allelic Heterogeneity *Allelic heterogeneity* refers to the fact that different mutations in the same genetic locus can cause an identical or similar phenotype. For example, many different mutations of the *β*-globin locus can cause *β*-thalassemia (Fig. 56-5). In essence, allelic heterogeneity reflects the fact that many different mutations are capable of altering protein structure and function. For this reason, maps of inactivating mutations in genes usually show a near-random distribution. Exceptions include: (1) a founder effect, in which a particular mutation that does not affect reproductive capacity can be traced to a single individual; (2) "hot spots" for mutations, in which the nature of the DNA sequence predisposes to a recurring mutation; and (3) localization of mutations to certain domains that are particularly critical for protein function. Allelic heterogeneity creates a practical problem for genetic testing because one must often examine the entire genetic locus for mutations, as these can differ in each patient.

Phenotypic Heterogeneity *Phenotypic heterogeneity* occurs when more than one phenotype is caused by allelic mutations (e.g., different mutations in the same gene). For example, mutations in the *myosin VIIIA* gene can result in four distinct clinical disorders: (1) autosomal recessive deafness DFNB2, (2) autosomal dominant nonsyndromic deafness DFNA11, (3) Usher 1B syndrome [congenital deafness, retinitis pigmentosa (Fig. 56-9)], and (4) an atypical variant of Usher's syndrome.

FIGURE 56-9 Retinitis pigmentosa with black clumps of pigment in the retinal periphery, known as "bone spicules." There is also atrophy of the retinal pigment epithelium, making the vasculature of the choroid easily visible.

Similarly, identical mutations in the *FGFR2* gene can result in very distinct phenotypes: Crouzon syndrome (craniofacial synostosis), or Pfeiffer syndrome (acrocephalopolysyndactyly).

Locus or Nonallelic Heterogeneity and Phenocopies

Nonallelic or locus heterogeneity refers to the situation in which a similar disease phenotype results from mutations at different genetic loci (Table 56-5). This often occurs when more than one gene product produces different subunits of an interacting complex or when different genes are involved in the same genetic cascade or physiologic pathway. For example, osteogenesis imperfecta can arise from mutations in two different procollagen genes (*COL1A1* or *COL1A2*) that are located on different chromosomes (Chap. 342). The effects of inactivating mutations in these two genes are similar because the protein products comprise different subunits of the helical collagen fiber. Similarly, muscular dystrophy syndromes can be caused by mutations in various genes, consistent with the fact that it can be transmitted in an X-linked (Duchenne or Becker), autosomal dominant (limb-girdle muscular dystrophy type 1), or autosomal recessive (limb-girdle muscular dystrophy type 2) manner (Chap. 368). Mutations in the X-linked *DMD* gene, which encodes dystrophin, are the most common cause of muscular dystrophy. This feature reflects the large size of the gene as well as the fact that the phenotype is expressed in hemizygous males because they have only a single copy of the X chromosome. Dystrophin is associated with a large group of additional proteins that form the membrane-associated cytoskeleton in muscle. Mutations in several components of this protein complex can also cause muscular dystrophy syndromes. Although the phenotypic features of some of these disorders are distinct, the phenotypic spectrum caused by mutations in different genes overlaps, thereby leading to nonallelic heterogeneity. It should be noted that mutations in dystrophin also cause allelic heterogeneity. For example, mutations in the *DMD* gene can cause either Duchenne or the less severe Becker muscular dystrophy, depending on the severity of the protein defect.

Recognition of nonallelic heterogeneity is important for several reasons: (1) the ability to identify disease loci in linkage studies is reduced by including patients with similar phenotypes but different genetic disorders; (2) genetic testing is more complex because several different genes need to be considered along with the possibility of different mutations in each of the candidate genes; and (3) novel information is gained about how genes or proteins interact, providing unique insights into molecular physiology.

Phenocopies refer to circumstances in which nongenetic conditions mimic a genetic disorder. For example, features of toxin- or drug-induced neurologic syndromes can resemble those seen in Huntington disease, and vascular causes of dementia share phenotypic features with familial forms of Alzheimer dementia (Chap. 350). Children born with activating mutations of the thyroid-stimulating hormone receptor (TSH-R) exhibit goiter and thyrotoxicosis similar to that seen in neonatal Graves' disease, which is caused by the transfer of maternal autoantibodies to the fetus (Chap. 320). As in nonallelic heterogeneity, the presence of phenocopies has the potential to confound linkage studies and genetic testing. Patient history and subtle differences in phenotype can often provide clues that distinguish these disorders from related genetic conditions.

Variable Expressivity and Incomplete Penetrance

It is not uncommon for the same genetic mutation to cause a phenotypic spectrum illustrating the phenomenon of *variable expressivity*. This may include different

TABLE 56-5 *Selected Examples of Locus Heterogeneity*

Phenotype	Gene	Chromosomal Location	Protein
Familial hypertrophic cardiomyopathy			
Genes encoding for sarcomeric proteins	*MYH7*	14q12	Myosin heavy chain beta
	TNNT2	1q2	Troponin-T2
	TPM1	15q22.1	Tropomyosin α
	MYBPC3	11p11q	Myosin binding protein C
	TNN13	19q13.4	Troponin 1
	MYL3	3p	Myosin light chain 3
	MYL2	12q23-24.3	Myosin light chain 2
	TTN	2q24.3	Cardiac titin
	ACTC	15q11	Cardiac alpha actin
	MYH6	14q1	Myosin heavy chain alpha
	TNNC1	3p21.3-3p14.5	Cardiac troponin C
Nonsarcomeric proteins	*MTT1*	Mitochondrial	tRNA isoleucine and tRNA glycine
	PRKAG2	7q35-q36	AMP-activated protein kinase γ2 subunit
	DMPK	19q13	Myotonin protein kinase (myotonic dystrophy)
	FRDA	9q13	Frataxin (Friedreich ataxia)
Polycystic kidney disease			
	PKD1	16p13.3-13.12	Polycystin 1 (AD)
	PKD2	4q21.-23	Polycystin 2 (AD)
	PKHD1	6p21.1-p12	Fibrocystin (AR)
Familial breast cancer			
BRCA1	*BRCA1*	17q21	BRCA1 (RNA polymerase II component)
BRCA2	*BRCA2*	13q12.3	BRCA2

manifestations of a complex disorder (e.g., MEN), the severity of the disorder (e.g., sickle cell anemia), or the age of disease onset (e.g., Alzheimer dementia). MEN-1 illustrates several of these features. Families with this autosomal dominant disorder develop tumors of the parathyroid gland, endocrine pancreas, and the pituitary gland (Chap. 330). However, the pattern of tumors in the different glands, the age at which tumors develop, and the types of hormones produced vary among affected individuals, even within a given family. In this example, the phenotypic variability arises, in part, because of the requirement for a second mutation in the normal copy of the *MEN1* gene, as well as the large array of different cell types that are susceptible to the effects of *MEN1* gene mutations. In part, variable expression reflects the influence of modifier genes, or genetic background, on the effects of a particular mutation. Even in identical twins, in whom the genetic constitution is the same, one can occasionally see variable expression of a genetic disease.

Interactions with the environment can also influence the course of a disease. For example, the manifestations and severity of hemochromatosis can be influenced by iron intake (Chap. 336), and the course of phenylketonuria is affected by exposure to phenylalanine in the diet (Chap. 343). Other metabolic disorders, such as hyperlipidemias and porphyria, also fall into this category. Many mechanisms, including genetic effects and environmental influences, can therefore lead to variable expressivity. In genetic counseling, it is particularly important to recognize this variability, as one cannot always predict the course of disease, even when the mutation is known.

Penetrance refers to the proportion of individuals with a mutant genotype that express the phenotype. If all carriers of a mutant express the phenotype, penetrance is complete, whereas it is said to be *incomplete* or *reduced* if some individuals do not have any features of the phenotype. Dominant conditions with incomplete penetrance are characterized by skipping of generations with unaffected carriers transmitting the mutant gene. For example, hypertrophic obstructive cardiomyopathy (HCM) caused by mutations in the *myosin-binding protein C* gene is a dominant disorder with clinical features in only a subset of patients who carry the mutation (Chap. 221). Patients who have the mutation but no evidence of the disease can still transmit the disorder to subsequent generations. In many conditions with postnatal onset, the proportion of gene carriers who are affected varies with age. When describing penetrance, one has to therefore specify age. For

PCR product	Allele
120	1
123	2
126	3
129	4

FIGURE 56-10 CAG repeat length and linkage analysis in multiple endocrine neoplasia type 1. *Upper panel.* Detection of different alleles using polymorphic microsatellite markers. The example depicts a CAG trinucleotide repeat. PCR with primers flanking the polymorphic region results in products of variable length, depending on the number of CAG repeats. After characterization of the alleles in the parents, transmission of the paternal and maternal alleles can be determined. *Lower panel.* Genotype analysis using microsatellite markers in a family with multiple endocrine neoplasia type 1. Two microsatellite markers, A and B, are located in close proximity to the *MEN1* gene on chromosome 11q13. For each individual, the A and B alleles have been determined. Based on this analysis, the genotype A3,B4 is linked to the disease because it occurs in the two affected individuals I-1 and II-1 but not in unaffected siblings. Because the disease allele is linked to A3,B4 within the affected family, it is likely that the individual III-1 is a carrier of the mutated *MEN1* gene. Although III-5 also has the A3,B4 genotype, she has inherited the allele from her unaffected father (II-4), who is not related to the original family. The A3,B4 genotype is only associated with MEN-1 in the original family, but not in the general population. Therefore, individual III-5 is not at risk for developing the disease.

example, for disorders such as Huntington disease or familial amyotrophic lateral sclerosis, which present late in life, the rate of penetrance is influenced by the age at which the clinical assessment is performed. *Imprinting* can also modify the penetrance of a disease (see below). For example, in patients with Albright hereditary osteodystrophy, mutations in the Gsα subunit (*GNAS1* gene) are expressed clinically only in individuals who inherit the mutation from their mother (Chap. 334).

Sex-Influenced Phenotypes Certain mutations affect males and females quite differently. In some instances, this is because the gene resides on the X or Y sex chromosomes (X-linked disorders and Y-linked disorders). As a result, the phenotype of mutated X-linked genes will be expressed fully in males but variably in heterozygous females, depending on the degree of X-inactivation and the function of the gene. For example, most heterozygous female carriers of factor VIII deficiency (hemophilia A) are asymptomatic because sufficient factor VIII is produced to prevent a defect in coagulation (Chap. 102). On the other hand, some females heterozygous for the X-linked lipid storage

defect caused by α-galactosidase A deficiency (Fabry disease) experience mild manifestations of painful neuropathy, as well as other features of the disease (Chap. 340). Because only males have a Y chromosome, mutations in genes such as *SRY*, which causes male-to-female sex-reversal, or *DAZ* (deleted in azoospermia), which causes abnormalities of spermatogenesis, are unique to males (Chap. 328).

Other diseases are expressed in a sex-limited manner because of the differential function of the gene product in males and females. Activating mutations in the luteinizing hormone receptor cause dominant male-limited precocious puberty in boys (Chap. 325). The phenotype is unique to males because activation of the receptor induces testosterone production in the testis, whereas it is functionally silent in the immature ovary. Homozygous inactivating mutations of the follicle-stimulating hormone (FSH) receptor cause primary ovarian failure in females because the follicles do not develop in the absence of FSH action. In contrast, affected males have a more subtle phenotype, because testosterone production is preserved (allowing sexual maturation) and spermatogenesis is only partially impaired (Chap. 325). In congenital adrenal hyperplasia, most commonly caused by 21-hydroxylase deficiency, cortisol production is impaired and ACTH stimulation of the adrenal gland leads to increased production of androgenic precursors (Chap. 321). In females, the increased androgen level causes ambiguous genitalia, which can be recognized at the time of birth. In males, the diagnosis may be made on the basis of adrenal insufficiency at birth, because the increased adrenal androgen level does not alter sexual differentiation, or later in childhood, because of the development of precocious puberty. Hemochromatosis is more common in males than in females, presumably because of differences in dietary iron intake and losses associated with menstruation and pregnancy in females (Chap. 336).

GENETIC LINKAGE *Genetic linkage* refers to the fact that genes are physically connected, or linked, to one another along the chromosomes. Two fundamental principles are essential for understanding the concept of linkage: (1) when two genes are close together on a chromosome, they are usually transmitted together, unless a recombination event separates them (Fig. 56-4); and (2) the odds of a crossover, or recombination event, between two linked genes is proportional to the distance that separates them. Thus, genes that are further apart are more likely to undergo a recombination event than genes that are very close together. The detection of chromosomal loci that segregate with a disease by linkage can be used to identify the gene responsible for the disease (*positional cloning*) and to predict the odds of disease gene transmission in genetic counseling.

Polymorphisms are essential for linkage studies because they provide a means to distinguish the maternal and paternal chromosomes in an individual. On average, 1 out of every 1000 bp varies from one person to the next. Although this degree of variation seems low (99.9% identical), it means that >3 million sequence differences exist between any two unrelated individuals and the probability that the sequence at such loci will differ on the two homologous chromosomes is high (often >70 to 90%). These sequence variations include VNTRs, short tandem repeats (STRs), and SNPs. Most STRs, also called *polymorphic microsatellite markers*, consist of di-, tri-, or tetranucleotide repeats that can be measured readily using PCR (Fig. 56-10). Characterization of SNPs, using DNA chips, provides a promising means for rapid analysis of genetic variation and linkage. Although this sequence variation usually has no apparent functional consequence, it provides much of the basis for variation in genetic traits.

In order to identify a chromosomal locus that segregates with a disease, it is necessary to determine the genotype or haplotype of DNA samples from one or several pedigrees. One can then assess whether certain marker alleles cosegregate with the disease. Markers that are closest to the disease gene are less likely to undergo recombination events and therefore receive a higher linkage score. Linkage is expressed as a lod (logarithm of odds) score—the ratio of the probability that the disease and marker loci are linked rather than unlinked. Lod scores of +3 (1000:1) are generally accepted as supporting linkage, whereas a score of −2 is consistent with the absence of linkage.

An example of the use of linkage analysis is shown in Fig. 56-10. In this case, the gene for the autosomal dominant disorder, MEN-1, is known to be located on chromosome 11q13. Using positional cloning, the *MEN1* gene was identified and shown to encode menin, a tumor suppressor. Affected individuals inherit a mutant form of the *MEN1* gene, predisposing them to certain types of tumors (parathyroid, pituitary, pancreatic islet) (Chap. 330). In the tissues that develop a tumor, a "second hit" occurs in the normal copy of the *MEN1* gene. This somatic mutation may be a point mutation, a microdeletion, or loss of a chromosomal fragment (detected as loss of heterozygosity, LOH). Within a given family, linkage to the *MEN1* gene locus can be assessed without necessarily knowing the specific mutation in the *MEN1* gene. Using polymorphic STRs that are close to the *MEN1* gene, one can assess transmission of the different *MEN1* alleles and compare this pattern to development of the disorder to determine which allele is associated with risk of MEN-1. In the pedigree shown, the affected grandfather in generation I carries alleles 3 and 4 on the chromosome with the mutated *MEN1* gene and alleles 2 and 2 on his other chromosome 11. Consistent with linkage of the 3/4 genotype to the *MEN1* locus, his son in generation II is affected, whereas his daughter (who inherits the 2/2 genotype from her father) is unaffected. In the third generation, transmission of the 3/4 genotype indicates risk of developing MEN-1, assuming that no genetic recombination between the 3/4 alleles and the *MEN1* gene has occurred. After a specific mutation in the *MEN1* gene is identified within a family, it is possible to track transmission of the mutation itself, thereby eliminating uncertainty caused by recombination.

CHROMOSOMAL DISORDERS Chromosomal or cytogenetic disorders are caused by numerical or structural aberrations in chromosomes. Deviations in chromosome number are common causes of abortions, developmental disorders, and malformations. *Contiguous gene syndromes*, i.e., large deletions affecting several genes, have been useful for identifying the location of new disease-causing genes. Because of the variable size of gene deletions in different patients, a systematic comparison of phenotypes and locations of deletion breakpoints allows positions of particular genes to be mapped within the critical genomic region. →*For discussion of disorders of chromosome number and structure, see Chap. 57.*

MONOGENIC MENDELIAN DISORDERS Monogenic human diseases are frequently referred to as *Mendelian disorders* because they obey the principles of genetic transmission originally set forth in Gregor Mendel's classic work. The continuously updated OMIM catalog lists several thousand of these disorders and provides information about the clinical phenotype, molecular basis, allelic variants, and pertinent animal models (Table 56-1). The mode of inheritance for a given phenotypic trait or disease is determined by pedigree analysis. All affected and unaffected individuals in the family are recorded in a pedigree using standard symbols (Fig. 56-1). The principles of allelic segregation, and the transmission of alleles from parents to children, are illustrated in Fig. 56-11. One dominant (A) allele and one recessive (a) allele can display three Mendelian modes of inheritance: autosomal dominant, autosomal recessive, and X-chromosomal. About 65% of human monogenic disorders are autosomal dominant, 25% are autosomal recessive, and 5%

FIGURE 56-11 Segregation of alleles. Segregation of genotypes in the offspring of parents with one dominant (A) and one recessive (a) allele. The distribution of the parental alleles to their offspring depends on the combination present in the parents.

are X-linked. Genetic testing is now available for many of these disorders and plays an increasingly important role in clinical medicine (Chap. 58).

Autosomal Dominant Disorders Autosomal dominant disorders assume particular relevance because mutations in a single allele are sufficient to cause the disease. In contrast to recessive disorders, in which disease pathogenesis is relatively straightforward because there is loss of gene function, in dominant disorders there are various disease mechanisms, many of which are unique to the function of the genetic pathway involved.

In autosomal dominant disorders, individuals are affected in successive generations; the disease does not occur in the offspring of unaffected individuals. Males and females are affected with equal frequency because the defective gene resides on one of the 22 autosomes (Fig. 56-12A). Autosomal dominant mutations alter one of the two alleles at a given locus. Because the alleles segregate randomly at meiosis, the probability that an offspring will be affected is 50%. Unless there is a new germline mutation, an affected individual has an affected parent. Children with a normal genotype do not transmit the disorder. Due to differences in penetrance or expressivity (see above), the clinical manifestations of autosomal dominant disorders may be variable. Because of these variations, it is sometimes challenging to determine the pattern of inheritance.

It should be recognized, however, that some individuals acquire a mutated gene from an unaffected parent. De novo germline mutations occur more frequently during later cell divisions in gametogenesis, which explains why siblings are rarely affected. As noted before, new germline mutations occur more frequently in fathers of advanced age. For example, the average age of fathers with new germline mutations that cause Marfan's syndrome is approximately 37 years, whereas fathers who transmit the disease by inheritance have an average age of about 30 years.

Autosomal Recessive Disorders The clinical expression of autosomal recessive disorders is more uniform than in autosomal dominant disorders. Most mutated alleles lead to a complete or partial loss of function. They frequently involve enzymes in metabolic pathways, receptors, or proteins in signaling cascades. In an autosomal recessive disease, the affected individual, who can be of either sex, is a homozygote or compound heterozygote for a single-gene defect. With a few important exceptions, autosomal recessive diseases are rare and often occur in the context of parental consanguinity. The relatively high frequency of certain recessive disorders, such as sickle cell anemia, cystic fibrosis, and thalassemia, is partially explained by a selective biologic advantage for the heterozygous state (see below). Though heterozygous carriers of a defective allele are usually clinically normal, they may display subtle differences in phenotype that only become apparent with more precise testing or in the context of certain environmental influences. In sickle cell anemia, for example, heterozygotes are normally asymptomatic. However, in situations of dehydration or diminished oxygen pressure, sickle cell crises can also occur in heterozygotes (Chap. 91).

In most instances, an affected individual is the offspring of heterozygous parents. In this situation, there is a 25% chance that the off-

FIGURE 56-12 Dominant, recessive, X-linked, and mitochondrial (matrilinear) inheritance.

spring will have a normal genotype, a 50% probability of a heterozygous state, and a 25% risk of homozygosity for the recessive alleles (Fig. 56-12B). In the case of one unaffected heterozygous and one affected homozygous parent, the probability of disease increases to 50% for each child. In this instance, the pedigree analysis mimics an autosomal dominant mode of inheritance (*pseudodominance*). In contrast to autosomal dominant disorders, new mutations in recessive alleles are rarely manifest because they usually result in an asymptomatic carrier state.

X-Linked Disorders   Males have only one X chromosome; consequently, a daughter always inherits her father's X chromosome in addition to one of her mother's two X chromosomes. A son inherits the Y chromosome from his father and one maternal X chromosome. Thus, the characteristic features of X-linked inheritance are (1) the absence of father-to-son transmission, and (2) the fact that all daughters of an affected male are obligate carriers of the mutant allele (Fig. 56-12C). The risk of developing disease due to a mutant X-chromosomal gene differs in the two sexes. Because males have only one X chromosome, they are hemizygous for the mutant allele; thus, they are more likely to develop the mutant phenotype, regardless of whether the mutation is dominant or recessive. A female may be either heterozygous or homozygous for the mutant allele, which may be dominant or recessive. The terms *X-linked dominant* or *X-linked recessive* are therefore only applicable to expression of the mutant phenotype in women. In addition, the expression of X-chromosomal genes is influenced by X chromosome inactivation (see below).

Y-Linked Disorders   Only a few genes are known on the Y chromosome. One such gene, the sex-region determining Y factor (*SRY*), or testis-determining factor (*TDF*), is crucial for normal male development. Normally there is infrequent exchange of sequences on the Y chromosome with the X chromosome. Because the *SRY* region is closely adjacent to the pseudoautosomal region, a chromosomal segment on the X and Y chromosomes with a high degree of homology, a crossing-over occasionally involves the *SRY* region. Translocations can result in XY females with the Y chromosome lacking the *SRY* gene or XX males harboring the *SRY* gene on one of the X chromosomes (Chap. 328). Point mutations in the *SRY* gene may also result in individuals with an XY genotype and an incomplete female phenotype. Most of these mutations occur de novo. Men with oligospermia/azoospermia frequently have microdeletions on the long arm of the Y chromosome that involve one or more of the azoospermia factor (*AZF*) genes.

EXCEPTIONS TO SIMPLE MENDELIAN INHERITANCE PATTERNS ■ Mitochondrial Disorders   Mendelian inheritance refers to the transmission of genes encoded by DNA contained in the nuclear chromosomes. In addition, each mitochondrion contains several copies of a circular chromosome. The mitochondrial DNA (mtDNA) is small (16.5 kb) and encodes transfer and ribosomal RNAs, and 13 proteins that are components of the respiratory chain involved in oxidative phosphorylation and ATP generation. The mitochondrial genome does not recombine and is inherited through the maternal line because sperm does not contribute significant cytoplasmic components to the zygote. A noncoding region of the mitochondrial chromosome, referred to as D-loop, is highly polymorphic. This property, together with the absence of mtDNA recombination, makes it a valuable tool for studies tracing human migration and evolution, and it is also used for specific forensic applications.

Inherited mitochondrial disorders are transmitted in a matrilineal fashion; all children from an affected mother will inherit the disease, but it will not be transmitted from an affected father to his children (Fig. 56-12D). Alterations in the mtDNA affecting enzymes required for oxidative phosphorylation lead to reduction of ATP supply, generation of free radicals, and induction of apoptosis. Several syndromic disorders arising from mutations in the mitochondrial genome are known in humans and they affect both protein-coding and tRNA genes (Tables 56-1 and 56-6). The broad clinical spectrum often involves (cardio)myopathies and encephalopathies because of the high dependence of these tissues on oxidative phosphorylation. The age of onset and the clinical course are highly variable because of the unusual mechanisms of mtDNA, which replicates independently from nuclear DNA. During cell replication, the proportion of wild-type and mutant mitochondria can drift among different cells and tissues. The resulting heterogeneity in the proportion of mitochondria with and without a mutation is referred to as *heteroplasmia* and underlies the phenotypic variability that is characteristic of mitochondrial diseases.

Acquired somatic mutations in mitochondria are thought to be involved in several age-dependent degenerative disorders affecting predominantly muscle and the peripheral and central nervous system (e.g., Alzheimer's and Parkinson's disease). Establishing that a mtDNA alteration is causal for a clinical phenotype is challenging because of the high degree of polymorphism in mtDNA and the phenotypic variability characteristic of these disorders. Certain pharmacologic treatments may have an impact on mitochondria and/or their function. For

TABLE 56-6 *Selected Mitochondrial Diseases*

Disease/Syndrome	MIM #
MELAS syndrome: mitochondrial myopathy with encephalopathy, lactic acidosis, and stroke	540000 540050
Leber's optic atrophy: hereditary optical neuropathy	535000
Kearns-Sayre syndrome (KSS): ophthalmoplegia, pigmental degeneration of the retina, cardiomyopathy	530000
MERRF syndrome: myoclonic epilepsy and ragged red fibers	545030
Maternally inherited myopathy and cardiomyopathy (MMC)	590050
Neurogenic muscular weakness with ataxia and retinitis pigmentosa (NARP)	551500
Progressive external ophthalmoplegia (CEOP)	258470
Pearson syndrome (PEAR): bone marrow and pancreatic failure	557000
Autosomal dominant inherited mitochondrial myopathy with mitochondrial deletion (ADMIMY)	157640
Somatic mutations in cytochrome *b* gene: exercise intolerance, lactic acidosis, complex III deficiency, muscle pain, ragged-red fibers	

example, treatment with the antiretroviral compound azidothymidine (AZT) causes an acquired mitochondrial myopathy through depletion of muscular mtDNA.

Mosaicism Mosaicism refers to the presence of two or more genetically distinct cell lines in the tissues of an individual. It results from a mutation that occurs during embryonic, fetal, or extrauterine development. The developmental stage at which the mutation arises will determine whether germ cells and/or somatic cells are involved. Chromosomal mosaicism results from non-disjunction at an early embryonic mitotic division, leading to the persistence of more than one cell line, as exemplified by some patients with Turner syndrome (Chap. 328). Somatic mosaicism is characterized by a patchy distribution of genetically altered somatic cells. The McCune-Albright syndrome, for example, is caused by activating mutations in the stimulatory G protein α (G$_s$α) that occur early in development (Chap. 334). The clinical phenotype varies depending on the tissue distribution of the mutation; manifestations include ovarian cysts that secrete sex steroids and cause precocious puberty, polyostotic fibrous dysplasia, café-au-lait skin pigmentation, growth hormone–secreting pituitary adenomas, and hypersecreting autonomous thyroid nodules (Chap. 326).

X-Inactivation, Imprinting, and Uniparental Disomy According to traditional Mendelian principles, the parental origin of a mutant gene is irrelevant for the expression of the phenotype. Nonetheless, there are important exceptions to this rule. X-inactivation prevents the expression of most genes on one of the two X-chromosomes in every cell of a female. Gene inactivation also occurs on selected chromosomal regions of autosomes. This phenomenon, referred to as *genomic imprinting*, leads to preferential expression of an allele depending on its parental origin. It is of pathophysiologic importance in disorders where the transmission of disease is dependent on the sex of the transmitting parent and, thus, plays an important role in the expression of certain genetic disorders. Two classic examples are the Prader-Willi syndrome and Angelman syndrome (Chap. 57). Prader-Willi syndrome is characterized by diminished fetal activity, obesity, hypotonia, mental retardation, short stature, and hypogonadotropic hypogonadism. Deletions in the Prader-Willi syndrome occur exclusively on the paternal chromosome 15. In contrast, patients with Angelman syndrome, characterized by mental retardation, seizures, ataxia, and hypotonia, have deletions at the same site of chromosome 15; however, they are located on the maternal chromosome 15. These two syndromes may also result from *uniparental disomy*. In this case, the syndromes are not caused by deletions on chromosome 15 but by the inheritance of either two maternal chromosomes (Angelman syndrome) or two paternal chromosomes (Prader-Willi syndrome).

Imprinting and the related phenomenon of allelic exclusion may be more common than currently documented, as it is difficult to examine levels of mRNA expression from the maternal and paternal alleles in specific tissues or in individual cells. Genomic imprinting, or uniparental disomy, is involved in the pathogenesis of several other disorders and malignancies (Chap. 57). Hydatidiform mole contains a normal number of diploid chromosomes, but they are all of paternal origin. The opposite situation occurs in ovarian teratomata, with 46 chromosomes of maternal origin. Expression of the imprinted gene for insulin-like growth factor II (IGF-II) is involved in the pathogenesis of the cancer-predisposing Beckwith-Wiedemann syndrome (BWS) (Chap. 68). These children show somatic overgrowth with organomegalies and hemihypertrophy, and they have an increased risk of embryonal malignancies such as Wilm's tumor. Normally, only the paternally derived copy of the *IGF-II* gene is active and the maternal copy is inactive. Imprinting of the *IGF-II* gene is regulated by *H19*, which encodes an RNA transcript that is not translated into protein. Disruption or lack of *H19* methylation leads to a relaxation of *IGF-II* imprinting and expression of both alleles. Heritable changes in gene expression not associated with DNA sequence alterations are referred to as *epigenetic effects*; these changes are increasingly recognized to play a role in human diseases and possibly in aging as well.

Somatic Mutations Cancer can be defined as a genetic disease at the cellular level (Chap. 68). Cancers are monoclonal in origin, indicating that they have arisen from a single precursor cell with one or several mutations in genes controlling growth and/or differentiation. These acquired somatic mutations are restricted to the tumor and its metastases and are not found in the surrounding normal tissue. The molecular alterations include dominant gain-of-function mutations in oncogenes, recessive loss-of-function mutations in tumor supressor genes and DNA repair genes, gene amplification, and chromosome rearrangements. Rarely, a single mutation in certain genes may be sufficient to transform a normal cell into a malignant cell. In most cancers, however, the development of a malignant phenotype requires several genetic alterations for the gradual progression from a normal cell to a cancerous cell, a phenomenon termed *multistep carcinogenesis* (Chaps. 68 and 69).

In many cancer syndromes, there is an inherited *predisposition* to tumor formation. In these instances, a germline mutation is inherited in an autosomal dominant fashion. This germline alteration affects one allele of an autosomal tumor suppressor gene. If the second allele is inactivated by a somatic mutation in a given cell, this will lead to neoplastic growth (two-hit model, or Knudson hypothesis). Thus, the defective allele in the germline is transmitted in a dominant pattern, though tumorigenesis results from a recessive loss of the tumor suppressor gene in an affected tissue. The classic example to illustrate this phenomenon is retinoblastoma, which can occur as a sporadic or hereditary tumor. In sporadic retinoblastoma, both copies of the retinoblastoma (*RB*) gene are inactivated through two somatic events. In hereditary retinoblastoma, one mutated or deleted *RB* allele is inherited in an autosomal dominant manner and the second allele is inactivated by a subsequent somatic mutation. This two-hit model applies to other inherited cancer syndromes such as MEN-1 (Chap. 330) and neurofibromatosis type 2 (Chap. 358).

Nucleotide Repeat Expansion Disorders Several diseases are associated with an increase in the number of nucleotide repeats above a certain threshold (Table 56-4). The repeats are sometimes located within the coding region of the genes, as in Huntington disease or the X-linked form of spinal and bulbar muscular atrophy (SBMA, Kennedy syndrome). In other instances, the repeats probably alter gene regulatory sequences. If an expansion is present, the DNA fragment is unstable and tends to expand further during cell division. The length of the nucleotide repeat often correlates with the severity of the disease. When repeat length increases from one generation to the next, disease manifestations may worsen or be observed at an earlier age; this phenomenon is referred to as *anticipation*. In Huntington disease, for example, there is a correlation between age of onset and length of the triplet codon expansion (Chap. 350). Anticipation has also been doc-

TABLE 56-7 *Genetic Approaches for Identifying Disease Genes*

Method	Indications and Advantages	Limitations
Linkage analysis	Analysis of monogenic traits Suitable for genome scan Control population not required Useful for multifactorial disorders in isolated populations	Difficult to collect large informative pedigrees Difficult to obtain sufficient statistical power for complex traits

Allele-sharing methods
  Affected sib and relative pair analyses
 	
  Sib pair analysis
	Suitable for identification of susceptibility genes in polygenic and multifactorial disorders
	Suitable for genome scan
	Control population not required if allele frequencies are known
	Statistical power can be increased by including parents and relatives
		Difficult to collect sufficient number of subjects
		Difficult to obtain sufficient statistical power for complex traits

Association studies
  Case-control studies
  Linkage disequilibrium
  Transmission distortion test
	Suitable for identification of susceptibility genes in polygenic and multifactorial disorders
	Suitable for testing specific allelic variants of known candidate loci
	Does not necessarily need relatives
		Requires large sample size and matched control population
		False-positive results in the absence of suitable control population

umented in other diseases caused by dynamic mutations in trinucleotide repeats (Table 56-4). The repeat number may also vary in a tissue-specific manner. In myotonic dystrophy, the CTG repeat may be tenfold greater in muscle tissue than in lymphocytes (Chap. 368).

POPULATION GENETICS AND ASSOCIATION STUDIES ■ Overview of Population Genetics

In population genetics, the focus changes from alterations in an individual's genome to the distribution pattern of different genotypes of alleles in the population. In a case where there are only two alleles, A and a, the frequency of the genotypes will be $p^2 + 2pq + q^2 = 1$, with p^2 corresponding to the frequency of AA, $2pq$ to the frequency of Aa, and q^2 to aa. When the frequency of an allele is known, the frequency of the genotype can be calculated. Alternatively, one can determine an allele frequency, if the genotype frequency has been determined.

Allele frequencies vary among ethnic groups and geographical regions. For example, heterozygous mutations in the *CFTR* gene are relatively common in populations of European origin but are rare in the African population. Allele frequencies may vary because certain allelic variants confer a selective advantage. For example, heterozygotes for the sickle cell mutation, which is particularly common in West Africa, are more resistant to malarial infection because the erythrocytes of heterozygotes provide a less favorable environment for *Plasmodium* parasites. Though homozygosity for the sickle cell gene is associated with severe anemia and sickle crises (Chap. 91), heterozygotes have a higher probability of survival because of the reduced morbidity and mortality from malaria; this phenomenon has led to an increased frequency of the mutant allele. Recessive conditions are more prevalent in geographically isolated populations because of the more restricted gene pool.

Allelic Association and Linkage Disequilibrium

There are two primary strategies for mapping genes that cause or increase susceptibility to human disease: (1) classic linkage can be performed based on a known genetic model (see above) or, when the model is unknown, by studying pairs of affected relatives; or (2) disease genes can be mapped using allelic association studies (Table 56-7). *Allelic association* refers to a situation in which the frequency of an allele is significantly increased or decreased in a particular disease. Linkage and association differ in several aspects. Genetic linkage is demonstrable in families or sibships. Association studies, on the other hand, compare a population of affected individuals with a control population. Association studies can be performed as case-control studies that include unrelated affected individuals and matched controls, or as family-based studies that compare the frequencies of alleles transmitted or not transmitted to affected children.

Allelic association studies are particularly useful for identifying susceptibility genes in complex diseases. When alleles at two loci occur more frequently in combination than would be predicted (based on known allele frequencies and recombination fractions), they are said to be in *linkage disequilibrium*. In Fig. 56-13, a mutation, Z, has occurred at a susceptibility locus where the normal allele is Y. The mutation is in close proximity to a genetic polymorphism with allele A or B. With time, the chromosomes carrying the A and Z alleles accumulate and represent 10% of the chromosomes in the population. The fact that the disease susceptibility gene, Z, is found preferentially, or exclusively, in association with the A allele illustrates linkage disequilibrium. Though not all chromosomes carrying the A allele carry the disease gene, the A allele is associated with an increased risk because of its possible association with the Z allele. This model implies that it may be possible in the future to identify Z directly to provide a more accurate prediction of disease susceptibility. Evidence for linkage disequilibrium can be helpful in mapping disease genes because it suggests that the two loci, in this case A and Z, are tightly linked.

POLYGENIC DISEASE AND COMPLEX GENETIC TRAITS ■ Approach to Polygenic and Multifactorial Disease

The expression of many common diseases such as cardiovascular disease, hypertension, diabetes, asthma, psychiatric disorders, and certain cancers is determined by genetic background, environmental factors, and lifestyle (Table 56-8). A trait is called *polygenic* if multiple genes are thought to contribute to the phenotype or *multifactorial* if multiple genes are assumed to interact with environmental factors. Genetic models for complex traits need to account for genetic heterogeneity and interactions with other genes and the environment. Complex genetic traits may be influenced by modifying genes that are not linked to the main gene involved in the pathogenesis of the trait. This type of gene-gene interaction, or *epistasis*, plays an important role in polygenic traits that require the simultaneous presence of variations in multiple genes in order to result in a pathologic phenotype. Gene-environment interactions are relevant for many monogenic and polygenic disorders. In phenylketonuria, the phenotypic expression of the disease depends not only on the presence

Wild-type: Polymorphic alleles
A = 40%; B = 60%
Wild-type allele Y = 100%

Linkage disequilibrium: Allele A is associated with the mutation Z in 10%. B is never associated with the mutation Z, unless a recombination has occurred between the two loci.

Mutation Y→Z

Passage of many generations

30%   10%   60%

FIGURE 56-13   Linkage disequilibrium.

TABLE 56-8 *Genes and Loci Involved in Mono- and Polygenic Forms of Diabetes and Hypertension*

Disorder	Genes or Susceptibility Locus	Chromosomal Location	Other Factors
DIABETES MELLITUS			
Monogenic forms of diabetes			
MODY 1	HNF4α (hepatocyte nuclear factor 4α)	20q12-q13.1	
MODY 1	GCK (glucokinase)	7p15-p13	
MODY 1	HNF1α (hepatocyte nuclear factor 1α)	12q24.2	
MODY 1	IPF1 (insulin promoter factor 1)	13q12.1	
MODY 5 (Renal cysts, diabetes)	HNF1β (hepatocyte nuclear factor 1β)	17cen-q21.3	
MODY 6	NeuroD1 (neurogenic differention factor 1)	2q32	
Loci and genes associated with susceptibility for diabetes mellitus type 2	Genes and loci identified by linkage/association studies		Diet
CPN10 (Calpain-10)		2q37.3	Energy expenditure
1q, 3q, 8p, 12q, 20q		1q, 3q, 8p, 12q, 20q	Obesity
"Candidate genes" with possible contribution			
Peroxisome proliferator receptor gamma		3p25	
Insulin		11p15	
Sulfonylurea receptor		11p15.1	
IPF1 (insulin promoter factor 1)		13q12.1	
IRS-1 (insulin receptor substrate)		2q36	
KCNJ11 (ATP-sensitive K channel Kir6.2)		11p15.1	
AMP1 (adiponectin)		3q27	
PGC-1		6p21.3-p21.1	
HYPERTENSION			
Monogenic forms			
Apparent mineralocorticoid excess	11-Ketoreductase		
Glucocorticoid-remediable HTN	CYP11B1 (unequal crossover with CYP11B2)		
Glucocorticoid-remediable HTN	CYP11B2 (unequal crossover with CYP11B1)		
17-alpha hydroxylase deficiency	17α hydroxylase		
Liddle's syndrome	SCNN1B		
Liddle's syndrome	SCNN1G		
Pseudohypoaldosteronism type II	WNK1		
Pseudohypoaldosteronism type II	WNK4		
Early onset HTN (AD)	MR		
Early onset HTN (AD)	BBS2		
Bardet-Biedl syndrome type 2	BBS4		
Loci and genes associated with susceptibility for essential hypertension	Loci identified by linkage/association studies		Salt intake
1p, 2p, 2q, 3, 5p, 5q, 6p, 6q, 7q, 8q, 11q, 15q, 16q, 17, 18q, 19p, 22q, Xp			
"Candidate genes" with possible contribution			
Angiotensinogen		1q42-43	
Angiotensin converting enzyme		17q23	
Angiotensin receptor 1		3q21-25	
G-protein subunit 3		12p13	

of the mutation in the phenylalanine hydroxylase gene but also on the exposure to the amino acid phenylalanine (Chap. 343). Type 2 diabetes mellitus provides a paradigm for considering a multifactorial disorder, as genetic, nutritional, and lifestyle factors are intimately interrelated in disease pathogenesis (Chap. 323). The identification of genetic variations and environmental factors that either predispose or protect against disease is essential for predicting disease risk, designing preventive strategies, and developing novel therapeutic approaches (Chap. 58). The study of rare monogenic diseases may provide insight into genetic and molecular mechanisms that are subsequently of importance for the understanding of complex diseases. For example, the identification of the insulin promoter factor 1 in maturity-onset of diabetes type 4 defined it as a *candidate gene* in the pathogenesis of diabetes mellitus type 2 (Tables 56-2 and 56-8). Genome scans have identified various loci that may be associated with susceptibility to development of diabetes mellitus in certain populations. Efforts to identify susceptibility genes require very large sample sizes, and positive results may depend on ethnicity, ascertainment criteria, and statistical analysis. Association studies analyzing the potential influence of (biologically functional) SNPs and SNP haplotypes on a particular phenotype are a promising approach for the detection of involved genes.

APPROACH TO THE PATIENT

Identifying the Disease-Causing Gene *Genomic medicine* aims to enhance the quality of medical care through the use of genotypic analysis (DNA testing) to identify genetic predisposition to disease, to select more specific pharmacotherapy, and to design individu-

alized medical care based on genotype. Genotype can be deduced by analysis of protein (e.g., hemoglobin, apoprotein E), mRNA, or DNA. However, technological advances have made DNA analysis particularly useful because it can be readily applied to all but the largest genes (Fig. 56-14).

DNA testing is performed by mutational analysis or linkage studies in individuals at risk for a genetic disorder known to be present in a family. Mass screening programs require tests of high sensitivity and specificity to be cost-effective. Prerequisites for the success of genetic screening programs include the following: that the disorder is potentially serious; that it can be influenced at a presymptomatic stage by changes in behavior, diet, and/or pharmaceutical manipulations; and that the screening does not result in any harm or discrimination. Screening in Jewish populations for the autosomal recessive neurodegenerative storage disease Tay-Sachs has reduced the number of affected individuals. In contrast, screening for sickle cell trait/disease in African Americans has led to unanticipated problems of discrimination by health insurers and employers. Mass screening programs harbor additional potential problems. For example, screening for the most common genetic alteration in cystic fibrosis, the ΔF508 mutation with a frequency of ~70% in northern Europe, is feasible and seems to be effective. One has to keep in mind, however, that there is pronounced allelic heterogeneity and that the disease can be caused by >600 other mutations. The search for these less common mutations would substantially increase costs but not the effectiveness of the screening program as a whole. Occupational screening programs aim to detect

FIGURE 56-14 Approach to genetic disease.

individuals with increased risk for certain professional activities (e.g., α_1 antitrypsin deficiency and smoke or dust exposure).

MUTATIONAL ANALYSES DNA sequence analysis is increasingly used as a diagnostic tool and has significantly enhanced diagnostic accuracy. It is used for determining carrier status and for prenatal testing in monogenic disorders (Chap. 58). Numerous techniques are available for the detection of mutations (Table 56-9). In a very broad sense, one can distinguish between techniques that allow for screening the absence or presence of known mutations (screening mode) or techniques that definitively characterize mutations. Analyses of large alterations in the genome are possible using cytoge-

netics, fluorescent in situ hybridization (FISH), and Southern blotting (Chap. 57).

More discrete sequence alterations rely heavily on the use of the PCR, which allows rapid gene amplification and analysis. Moreover, PCR makes it possible to perform genetic testing and mutational analysis with small amounts of DNA extracted from leukocytes or even from single cells, buccal cells, or hair roots. Screening for point mutations can be performed by numerous methods (Table 56-9); most are based on the recognition of mismatches between nucleic acid duplexes, electrophoretic separation of single- or double-stranded DNA, or sequencing of DNA fragments amplified by PCR. DNA sequencing can be performed directly on PCR products or on fragments cloned into plasmid vectors amplified in bacterial host cells.

RT-PCR may be useful to detect absent or reduced levels of mRNA expression due to a mutated allele. Protein truncation tests (PTT) can be used to detect the broad array of mutations that result in premature termination of a polypeptide during its synthesis. The isolated cDNA is transcribed and translated in vitro, and the proteins are analyzed by gel electrophoresis. Comparison of electrophoretic mobility with the wild-type protein allows detection of truncated mutants.

The majority of traditional diagnostic methods are gel-based. Novel technologies for the analysis of mutations, genetic mapping, and mRNA expression profiles are in rapid development. DNA chip technologies allow hybridization of DNA or RNA to hundreds of thousands of probes simultaneously. Microarrays are being used clinically for mutational analysis of several human disease genes, as well as for the identification of viral sequence variations. Together with the knowledge gained from the HGP, these technologies provide the foundation to expand from a focus on single genes to analyses at the scale of the genome.

TABLE 56-9 *Methods Used for the Detection of Mutations*

Method	Principle	Type of Mutation Detected
COMMONLY USED TECHNIQUES		
Cytogenic analysis	Unique visual appearance of various chromosomes	Numerical or structural abnormalities in chromosomes
Fluorescent in situ hybridization (FISH)	Hybridization to chromosomes with fluorescently labeled probes	Numerical or structural abnormalities in chromosomes
Southern blot	Hybridization with genomic probe or cDNA probe after digestion of high molecular DNA	Large deletion, insertion, rearrangement, expansions of triplet repeat, amplification
Polymerase chain reaction (PCR)	Amplification of DNA segment	Expansion of triplet repeats, variable number of tandem repeats (VNTR), gene rearrangements, translocations; prepare DNA for other mutation methods
Reverse transcriptase PCR (RT-PCR)	Reverse transcription, amplification of DNA segment → absence or reduction of mRNA transcription	Analyze expressed mRNA (cDNA) sequence; detect loss of expression
DNA sequencing	Direct sequencing of PCR products. Sequencing of DNA segments cloned into plasmid vectors	Point mutations, small deletions, and insertions
Restriction fragment polymorphism (RFLP)	Detection of altered restriction pattern of genomic DNA (Southern blot) or PCR products	Point mutations, small deletions, and insertions
OTHER TECHNIQUES		
Single-strand conformational polymorphism (SSCP)	PCR of DNA segment: Mutations result in conformational change and altered mobility	Point mutations, small deletions, and insertions
Denaturing gradient gel electrophoresis (DGGE)	PCR of DNA segment: Mutations result in conformational change and altered mobility	Point mutations, small deletions, and insertions
RNAse cleavage	Cleavage of mismatch between mutated and wild type sequence	Point mutations, small deletions, and insertions
Oligonucleotide specific hybridization (OSH)	Hybridization of PCR products to wild type or mutated oligonucleotides immobilized on chips or slides	Point mutations, small deletions, and insertions
Microarrays	Hybridization of PCR products to wild type or mutated oligonucleotides	Point mutations, small deletions, and insertions
Protein truncation test (PTT)	Transcription/translation of cDNA isolated from tissue sample	Mutations leading to premature truncations

A general algorithm for the approach to mutational analysis is outlined in Fig. 56-14. The importance of a detailed clinical phenotype cannot be overemphasized. This is the step where one should also consider the possibility of genetic heterogeneity and phenocopies. If obvious candidate genes are suggested by the phenotype, they can be analyzed directly. After identification of a mutation, it is essential to demonstrate that it segregates with the phenotype. The functional characterization of novel mutations is labor intensive and may require analyses in vitro or in transgenic models in order to document the relevance of the genetic alteration.

Prenatal diagnosis of numerous genetic diseases in instances with a high risk for certain disorders is now possible by direct DNA analysis. *Amniocentesis* involves the removal of a small amount of amniotic fluid, usually at 16 weeks of gestation. Cells can be collected and submitted for karyotype analyses, FISH, and mutational analysis of selected genes. The main indications for amniocentesis include advanced maternal age above age 35, abnormal serum triple marker test (α-fetoprotein, β human chorionic gonadotropin, pregnancy-associated plasma protein A, or unconjugated estriol), a family history of chromosomal abnormalities, or a Mendelian disorder amenable to genetic testing. Prenatal diagnosis can also be performed by *chorionic villus sampling* (CVS), in which a small amount of the chorion is removed by a transcervical or transabdominal biopsy. Chromosomes and DNA obtained from these cells can be submitted for cytogenetic and mutational analyses. CVS can be performed earlier in gestation (weeks 9 to 12) than amniocentesis, an aspect that may be of relevance when termination of pregnancy is a consideration. Later in pregnancy, beginning at about 18 weeks of gestation, percutaneous umbilical blood sampling (PUBS) permits collection of fetal blood for lymphocyte culture and analysis. In combination with in vitro fertilization (IVF) techniques, it is even possible to perform genetic diagnoses in a single cell removed from the four- to eight-cell embryo or to analyze the first polar body from an oocyte. Preconceptual diagnosis thereby avoids therapeutic abortions but is extremely costly and labor intensive. Lastly, it has to be emphasized that excluding a specific disorder by any of these approaches is never equivalent to the assurance of having a normal child.

Mutations in certain cancer susceptibility genes, such as *BRCA1* and *BRCA2*, may identify individuals with an increased risk for the development of malignancies and result in risk-reducing interventions. The detection of mutations is an important diagnostic and prognostic tool in leukemias and lymphomas. The demonstration of the presence or absence of mutations and polymorphisms is also relevant for the rapidly evolving field of pharmacogenomics, including the identification of differences in drug treatment response or metabolism as a function of genetic background. For example, the thiopurine drugs 6-mercaptopurine and azathioprine are commonly used cytotoxic and immunosuppressive agents. They are metabolized by thiopurine methyltransferase (TPMT), an enzyme with variable activity associated with genetic polymorphisms in 10% of Caucasians and complete deficiency in about 1/300 individuals. Patients with intermediate or deficient TPMT activity are at risk for excessive toxicity, including fatal myelosuppression. Characterization of these polymorphisms allows mercaptopurine doses to be modified based on TPMT genotype. Pharmacogenomics may increasingly permit individualized drug therapy, improve drug effectiveness, reduce adverse side effects, and provide cost-effective pharmaceutical care.

FURTHER READING

BROWN PO, BOTSTEIN D: Exploring the new world of the genome with DNA microarrays. Nat Genet (Suppl) 21:33, 1999

COLLINS FS, MCKUSICK V: Implications of the Human Genome Project for medical science. JAMA 285:540, 2001

COTTON RGH, KAZAZIAN HH JR: The HUGO mutation database initiative: Issues, databases, and perspectives for the new millenium. Hum Mutat 15: 1, 2000

Instructions for the use of genome-related databases. Nat Genet 32 (Suppl):1, 2002

ROSES AD: Pharmacogenomics and the practice of medicine. Nature 405:857, 2000

57 CHROMOSOME DISORDERS
Terry Hassold, Stuart Schwartz

In humans, the normal diploid number of chromosomes is 46, consisting of 22 pairs of autosomal chromosomes (numbered 1 to 22 in decreasing size) and one pair of sex chromosomes (XX in females and XY in males). The genome is estimated to contain between 30,000 and 40,000 genes. Even the smallest autosome contains between 200 and 300 genes. Not surprisingly, duplications or deletions of chromosomes, or even small chromosome segments, have profound consequences on normal gene expression, leading to severe developmental and physiologic abnormalities.

Deviations in number or structure of the 46 human chromosomes are astonishingly common, despite severe deleterious consequences. Chromosomal disorders occur in an estimated 10 to 25% of all pregnancies. They are the leading cause of fetal loss and, among pregnancies surviving to term, the leading known cause of birth defects and mental retardation.

In recent years, the practice of cytogenetics has shifted from conventional cytogenetic methodology to a union of cytogenetic and molecular techniques. Formerly the province of research laboratories, fluorescence in situ hybridization (FISH) and related molecular cytogenetic technologies have been incorporated into everyday practice in clinical laboratories. As a result, there is an increased appreciation of the importance of "subtle" constitutional cytogenetic abnormalities, such as microdeletions and imprinting disorders, as well as previously recognized translocations and disorders of chromosome number.

VISUALIZING CHROMOSOMES

CONVENTIONAL CYTOGENETIC ANALYSIS In theory, chromosome preparations can be obtained from any actively dividing tissue by causing the cells to arrest in metaphase, the stage of the cell cycle when chromosomes are maximally condensed. In practice, only a small number of tissues are used for routine chromosome analysis: amniocytes or chorionic villi for prenatal testing, and blood, bone marrow, or skin fibroblasts for postnatal studies. Samples of blood, bone marrow, and chorionic villi can be processed using short-term culture techniques that yield results in 1 to 3 days. Analysis of other tissue types typically involves long-term cell culture, requiring 1 to 3 weeks of processing before cytogenetic analysis is possible.

Cells are isolated at metaphase or prometaphase, and treated chemically or enzymatically to reveal chromosome "bands" (Fig. 57-1). Analysis of the number of chromosomes in the cell, and the distribution of bands on individual chromosomes, allows the identification of numerical or structural abnormalities. This strategy is useful for characterizing the normal chromosome complement and determining the incidence and types of major chromosome abnormalities.

Each human chromosome contains two specialized structures: a centromere and two telomeres. The centromere, or primary constriction, divides the chromosome into short (p) and long (q) arms and is responsible for the segregation of chromosomes during cell division.

FIGURE 57-1 *A.* An idealized human chromosome, showing the centromere (cen), long (q) and short (p) arms, and telomeres (tel). *B.* A G-banded human karyotype from a normal (46,XX) female.

The telomeres, or chromosome ends, "cap" the p and q arms and are important for allowing DNA replication at the ends of the chromosomes. Prior to DNA replication, each chromosome consists of a single chromatid copy of the DNA double helix. After DNA replication and continuing until the time of cell division (including metaphase, when chromosomes are typically visualized), each chromosome consists of two identical sister chromatids (Fig. 57-1).

MOLECULAR CYTOGENETICS The introduction of FISH methodologies in the late 1980s revolutionized the field of cytogenetics. In principle, FISH is similar to other DNA-DNA hybridization methodologies. The probe is labeled with a hapten, such as biotin or digoxigenin, to allow detection with a fluorophore (e.g., FITC or rhodamine). After the hybridization step, the specimen is counter-stained and the preparations are visualized with a fluorescence microscope.

Types of FISH Probes A variety of probes are available for use with FISH, including chromosome-specific paints (chromosome libraries), repetitive probes, and single-copy probes (Fig. 57-2). Chromosome libraries hybridize to sequences that span the entirety of the chromosome from which they are derived and, as a result, they can be used to "paint" individual chromosomes.

Repetitive probes recognize amplified DNA sequences present in chromosomes. The most common are α-satellite DNA probes that are complementary to DNA sequences found at the centromeric regions of all human chromosomes. A vast number of *single-copy probes* are now available as a result of the human genome project. These probes can be as small as 1 kb, though normally they are much larger and are packaged into cosmids (40 kb), bacterial artificial chromosomes (BACs) or P1 clones (100 to 200 kb), or yeast artificial chromosomes (YACs) (1 to 2 Mb). Many are available commercially, including probes for a variety of microdeletion syndromes and for subtelomeric regions of individual chromosomes.

Applications of FISH The majority of FISH applications involve hybridization of one or two probes of interest as an adjunctive procedure

to conventional chromosomal banding techniques. In this regard, FISH can be utilized to identify specific chromosomes, characterize de novo duplications or deletions, and clarify subtle chromosomal rearrangements. Its greatest utilization, however, is in the detection of microdeletions (see below). Though conventional cytogenetic studies can detect some microdeletions, initial detection and/or confirmation with FISH is essential. In fact, since appropriate FISH probes have become available, detection of microdeletion syndromes has increased significantly.

In addition to metaphase FISH, cells can be analyzed at a variety of stages. Interphase analysis, for example, can be used to make a rapid diagnosis in instances when metaphase chromosome preparations are not yet available (e.g., amniotic fluid interphase analysis). Interphase analysis also increases the number of cells available for examination, allows for investigation of nuclear organization, and provides results when cells do not progress to metaphase. One specialized type of interphase analysis involves the application of FISH to paraffin-embedded sections, thereby preserving the architecture of the tissue.

The use of interphase FISH has increased recently, especially for analyses of amniocentesis samples. These studies are performed on uncultured amniotic fluid, typically using DNA probes specific for the chromosomes most commonly identified in trisomies (chromosomes 13, 18, 21, and the X and Y). These studies can be performed rapidly (24 to 72 h) and will ascertain about 60% of the abnormalities detected prenatally. Another area in which interphase analysis is routinely utilized is cancer cytogenetics (Chap. 68). Many site-specific translocations are associated with specific types of malignancies. For example, there are probes available for both the Abelson (Abl) oncogene and breakpoint cluster region (bcr) involved in chronic myelogenous leukemia (CML); these probes are labeled in red and green, respectively; the fusion of these genes in CML combines the fluorescent colors and appears as a yellow hybridization signal.

In addition to standard metaphase and interphase FISH analyses, a number of enhanced techniques have been developed for specific types of analysis, including multicolor FISH techniques, reverse painting, comparative genomic hybridization, and fiber FISH. *Spectral karyotyping* (SKY) and multicolor FISH (m-FISH) techniques use combinatorially labeled probes that create a unique color for individual chromosomes. This technology is useful in the identification of unknown chromosome material (such as markers of duplications) but is most commonly used with the complex rearrangements seen in cancer specimens.

Comparative genomic hybridization (CGH) is a method that can be used only when DNA is available from a specimen of interest. The entire DNA specimen from the sample of interest is labeled in one color (e.g., green), and the normal control DNA specimen is indicated by another color (e.g., red). These are mixed in equal amounts and hybridized to normal metaphase chromosomes. The red-to-green ratio is analyzed by a computer program, which determines where the DNA of interest may have gains or losses of material. This technique is useful in the analysis of tumors, particularly in those cases where cytogenetic analysis is not possible.

Fiber FISH is a technique in which chromosomes are mechanically stretched, using one of a variety of different methods. It provides a higher resolution of analysis than conventional FISH.

INDICATIONS FOR CYTOGENETIC ANALYSIS

Primary indications for karyotypic analysis vary according to the developmental stage/age of the conceptus/individual under investigation. One especially important application is in prenatal diagnosis (particularly for pregnancies involving older women), assaying for chromosomal abnormalities in either chorionic villi of first-trimester fetuses or amniotic fluid of second-trimester fetuses. Tissue specimens from spontaneously aborted fetuses or still-births can also be examined for chromosome abnormalities. Interphase cytogenetics (using FISH) is increasingly being used to study individual blastomeres of preimplantation embryos (with in vitro fertilization-derived pregnancies). This makes it possible to detect aneuploid or structurally unbalanced embryos or, in the case of sex-linked disorders, to identify male conceptuses; such embryos would not be used to initiate pregnancies.

Among infants and children, peripheral blood is examined, most often in individuals with specific phenotypic abnormalities. For example, karotypic analysis can be used for the confirmation or exclusion of a specific chromosomal syndrome (e.g., trisomy 21); in patients with unexplained psychomotor retardation with or without dysmorphic features; in cases of monogenic disorders associated with mental retardation and/or dysmorphic features; and with abnormalities of sexual differentiation and development.

In adults, peripheral blood can be examined in patients with infertility or recurrent miscarriages, since chromosome abnormalities can lead to meiotic arrest or to genetically unbalanced gametes. An important branch of cytogenetics is concerned with analyses of bone marrow, unstimulated peripheral blood, and lymph nodes of tumors, as chromosomal abnormalities are a common correlate of leukemia, lymphoma, and solid tumors (Chap. 68).

CYTOGENETIC TESTING IN PRENATAL DIAGNOSIS The vast majority of prenatal diagnostic studies are performed to rule out a chromosomal ab-

FIGURE 57-2 Examples of different applications of fluorescence in situ hybridization (FISH) to human metaphase and interphase preparations. Top left, chromosome-specific "paint" probes demonstrating hybridization to normal chromosomes 2 (red) and 12 (green), as well as indicating a translocation between the short arm of chromosome 12 and the long arm of chromosome 2. This hybridization also demonstrates that some of the short arm of chromosome 12 has been inserted into the short arm of chromosome 5. Top right, a repetitive DNA probe specific for centromeric α-satellite sequences on chromosome 7 (red) and chromosome 10 (green) hybridizes to the centromeric region of the appropriate chromosomes, as well as to a marker chromosome derived from chromosome 10. Bottom left, two-color FISH used to detect a microdeletion of chromosome 22 associated with velocardiofacial (VCF) syndrome. A probe for ARSA (a locus on the distal portion of chromosome 22, visualized as a green signal) is observed on both chromosomes. However, a probe for TUPLE1 (a locus within the VCF region of chromosome 22, visualized in red) hybridizes only to the normal chromosome. The arrow points to the deleted chromosome. Bottom right, interphase FISH using chromosome 13 (green) and chromosome 21 (red) unique sequence probes on interphase cells from direct amniotic fluid preparations. In each of the four interphase cells, three chromosome 21 signals are observed, indicating the presence of trisomy 21 in the fetus.

normality, but cells may also be propagated for biochemical studies or molecular analyses of DNA. Three procedures are used to obtain samples for prenatal diagnosis: amniocentesis, chorionic villus sampling (CVS), and fetal blood sampling. Amniocentesis is the most common procedure and is routinely performed at 15 to 17 weeks of gestation. On some occasions, early amniocentesis at 12 to 14 weeks is performed to expedite results, although less fluid is obtained at this time. Early amniocentesis carries a greater risk of spontaneous abortion or fetal injury but provides results at an earlier stage of pregnancy.

The vast majority of amniocenteses are performed in the context of advanced maternal age, the best-known correlate of trisomy (see below). Additional reasons for amniocentesis referral include an abnormal "triple- or quad-marker assay" and/or detection of ultrasound abnormalities. In this assay, levels of human chorionic gonadotropin, α-fetoprotein, and unconjugated estriol (and, in the quad assay, inhibin) in the maternal serum are quantified and used to adjust the maternal age-predicted risk of a trisomy 21 or trisomy 18 fetus. Specific ultrasound abnormalities, when detected at midtrimester, can also be associated with chromosomal defects. When a nonspecific ultrasound abnormality is present, the estimated risk of a chromosomal defect is approximately 16%. Associations of chromosomal abnormalities and specific types of abnormal ultrasound findings are listed in Table 57-1.

CVS is the second most common procedure for genetic prenatal diagnosis. Because this procedure is routinely performed at about 10

TABLE 57-1   *Frequency of Chromosome Abnormalities, Identified on the Basis of Abnormal Ultrasound Findings*

Ultrasound Finding	Chromosomal Abnormalities (Frequency)	
	Average, %	Range in Different Studies, %
Abnormal ultrasound (nonspecific)	16	13–35
Omphalocele	39	26–54
Cystic hygroma	68	46–78
Congenital heart disease	30	8–40
Choroid plexus cyst	5	4–10

to 12 weeks of gestation, it allows for an earlier detection of abnormalities and a safer pregnancy termination, if desired. CVS is a relatively safe procedure (spontaneous abortions, <0.5 to 1%). Because there is an increased association of limb defects when the procedure is performed earlier (<10 weeks of gestation), CVS is applicable during a narrow time frame of gestation. CVS involves the use of a catheter inserted transvaginally; approximately 25 mg of villi are aspirated from the chorion frondosum (the fetal portion of the placenta). By adding colchicine directly to the rapidly dividing cytotrophoblasts, results can be obtained within 24 to 48 h. Findings from these procedures should be confirmed by analyses of cultured mesenchymal cells, as they are more reliably derived from the fetus.

Percutaneous umbilical blood sampling (PUBS) is a method for obtaining fetal blood during the second and third trimesters of pregnancy. PUBS is usually performed when ultrasound abnormalities are detected late in the second trimester. PUBS is also used when cytogenetic results from amniocentesis need clarification, such as in the detection of mosaicism.

CHROMOSOME ABNORMALITIES

CHROMOSOMES IN CELL DIVISION   To understand the etiology of chromosome abnormalities, it is important to review the movement of chromosomes during cell division. In somatic tissues, chromosomes are replicated during the S-phase of the cell cycle, so that each replicated chromosome consists of two identical sister chromatids. When the cell enters mitosis, each of the 46 chromosomes align on the metaphase plate, with the centomeres co-oriented toward opposite spindle poles (Fig. 57-3). At anaphase the sister chromatids separate, with each of the daughter cells receiving one sister chromatid from each of the 46 chromosomes.

Chromosome segregation is more complicated in germ cell division, since the number of chromosomes must be reduced from 46 to 23 in the mature sperm and eggs. This is accomplished by two rounds of division—meiosis I and meiosis II (Fig. 57-3). In meiosis I, homologous chromosomes pair and exchange genetic material, then align on the metaphase plate, and finally separate from one another. Thus, by the end of meiosis I, only 23 of the original 46 chromosomes are represented in each of the two daughter cells. Meiosis II quickly follows meiosis I and is essentially a "haploid mitosis," involving separation of the sister chromatids in each of the 23 chromosomes.

Although the fundamentals of meiosis are the same in males and females, there are important distinctions, particularly in the timing of meiotic divisions. In males, meiosis begins with puberty and continues throughout the individual's lifetime. In females, meiosis begins prenatally, with oocytes proceeding through the first stages of meiosis I but arresting at mid-prophase. At the time of birth, the first meiotic division is suspended in oocytes. Only after ovulation many years later do oocytes complete meiosis I and proceed to the metaphase stage of meiosis II; if fertilized, the oocyte then completes the second meiotic division. Thus, in females, the first meiotic division takes at least 10 to 15 years and as many as 40 to 45 years to complete. Maternal age-related increases in the incidence of trisomy are likely the consequence of this protracted process of cell division.

INCIDENCE AND TYPES OF CHROMOSOME ABNORMALITIES   Errors in meiosis, or in early cleavage divisions, occur with extraordinary frequency. At least 10 to 25% of all pregnancies, for example, involve chromosomally abnormal conceptions. A large proportion of these terminate in the earliest stages of pregnancy, many of which go unrecognized. Nevertheless, even among clinically recognized pregnancies, nearly 10% of fetuses are chromosomally unbalanced. For the three types of clinically recognized pregnancies—spontaneous abortions, stillbirths, and livebirths—the frequencies of different chromosomal abnormalities are summarized in Table 57-2. The most common abnormalities are numerical, involving fetuses with additional (trisomy) or missing (monosomy) chromosomes, or those with one (triploidy) or two (tetraploidy) additional sets of chromosomes. Structural chromosome abnormalities are much less common, although several of the most important clinical chromosomal disorders involve structural rearrangements (see below).

By far the most common abnormality is trisomy, which is identified in approximately 25% of spontaneous abortions and 0.3% of newborns. Trisomies for all chromosomes have now been identified in embryos or fetuses, but there is considerable variation in frequency for various chromosomes. For example, trisomy 16 is extraordinarily common, accounting for about one-third of all trisomies in spontaneous abortions, whereas trisomies 1, 5, 11, and 19 have been identified less often. Available evidence suggests two reasons for this variation: (1) some chromosomes (e.g., chromosome 16) are more likely to segregate abnormally or undergo nondisjunction during meiosis than are others; and (2) the potential for development varies widely among different trisomic conditions, with some being eliminated very early in gestation, others surviving to the time of clinical pregnancy recognition, and some (e.g., trisomies 13, 18, and 21 and sex chromosome trisomies) being compatible with survival to term.

CHROMOSOMAL SYNDROMES

While most chromosomally abnormal conceptions perish in utero, several conditions are compatible with survival to term. The best-char-

FIGURE 57-3   Chromosome segregation in meiosis. *A.* In meiosis I, each of the 23 pairs of chromosomes finds its "partner," or homologue, and exchanges genetic material (recombines) with it. At metaphase, each homologous pair aligns on the equatorial plate; at anaphase, each member of the homologous pair segregates from its partner. Thus, at the end of meiosis I, each daughter cell contains 23 chromosomes, with each chromosome consisting of two sister chromatids. *B.* In meiosis II, each chromosome aligns on the metaphase plate, and at anaphase, each of the two sister chromatids divide from one another. Thus, at the end of meiosis II, each daughter cell (e.g., the oocyte or spermatocyte) contains 23 chromosomes, with each chromosome consisting of one sister chromatid. In mitosis, the chromosomes behave exactly as they do in meiosis II, except that somatically dividing cells contain 46 chromosomes, not the 23 that are present in the meiosis II cell.

acterized of these are numerical abnormalities involving loss or gain of individual chromosomes, and abnormalities resulting from unbalanced translocations. FISH and other molecular studies have led to the identification of two "new" types of chromosome abnormalities, commonly referred to as microdeletion syndromes and imprinting syndromes.

NUMERICAL ABNORMALITIES Virtually all types of numerical abnormalities are eliminated prenatally, so that only those involving small, gene-poor autosomes or the sex chromosomes are identified with any frequency among liveborns. Clinically, the most important of these is trisomy 21, the most frequent cause of Down syndrome. Depending on the maternal age structure of the population and the utilization of prenatal testing, the incidence of trisomy 21 ranges from 1/600 to 1/1000 live births, making it the most common chromosome abnormality in live-born individuals. Like most trisomies, the incidence of trisomy 21 is highly correlated with maternal age, increasing from about 1/1500 live births for women 20 years of age to 1/30 for women 45 years of age and older.

In addition to trisomy 21, only two other autosomal trisomies, 13 and 18, occur with any frequency in livebirths. Incidence rates for trisomies 13 and 18 in livebirths are 1/20,000 and 1/10,000, respectively. Unlike trisomy 21, which is associated with near-normal life expectancy, both trisomies 13 and 18 are associated with death in infancy, typically occurring during the first year of life.

Three sex chromosome trisomies—the 47,XXX, 47,XXY (Klinefelter syndrome), and 47,XYY conditions—are quite common, with each occurring in about 1/2000 newborns. Of all the trisomic conditions, these three have the fewest phenotypic complications. In fact, with the exception of infertility in Klinefelter syndrome (Chap. 328), it is likely that most individuals with such trisomic conditions would go undetected. The additional Y chromosome in the 47,XYY condition is small and contains only a few genes. Most Y-linked genes are involved in testicular development or spermatogenesis. Thus, dosage imbalance of Y-linked genes has relatively little effect on other developmental processes. The 47,XYY genotype is associated with increased height. Its role in antisocial behavior, postulated initially because of an increased prevalence among some penalized populations, is unclear.

For the 47,XXX and 47,XXY conditions, the situation is different—the X chromosome contains over 1000 genes, many of them essential for normal development. How, then, are 47,XXX and 47,XXY individuals spared from the catastrophic consequences of dosage imbalance? The answer lies in the biology of X chromosome gene expression. In normal females, one of the chromosomes undergoes *X inactivation* in somatic cells. The inactivation of the paternal or maternal X chromosome occurs randomly in each somatic cell and thereby serves as a mechanism of dosage compensation, ensuring that males and females have equal expression of most X-linked genes. The inactivation process occurs at the blastocyst stage of development; prior to this, both X chromosomes are active. In addition, not all X-linked genes are inactivated. Some genes on the X chromosome "escape" the inactivating mechanism and are expressed from both X chromosomes. In disorders such as Klinefelter syndrome, some genes may be expressed from both X chromosomes, resulting in its phenotypic features.

As a rule, monosomic conditions are incompatible with fetal development and, consequently, autosomal monosomies are only rarely identified in spontaneous abortions and are not found among live-born individuals. In fact, the only monosomy compatible with live birth is the 45,X condition, which causes Turner syndrome. The 45,X chromosome constitution occurs with surprisingly high frequency, present in at least 1 to 2% of all pregnancies. More than 99% of all 45,X conceptions are spontaneously aborted. Thus, live-born individuals with a 45,X chromosome constitution represent a rare group of survivors. The 45,X phenotype is mild, presumably because the second copy of many X chromosomal genes is normally inactivated. Nonetheless, Turner syndrome causes gonadal dysgenesis, resulting in infertility and failure to undergo secondary sexual development, along with a number of other phenotypic features (Chap. 328). Several other structural abnormalities of the X chromosome such as deletions, isochromosome X, or ring chromosomes can cause Turner syndrome. Mosaicism, including 45,X/45,XX, 45X/45,XXX, 45,X/45,XY, and others, also occurs (see below) and contributes to the phenotypic spectrum in Turner syndrome.

Because numerical abnormalities originate in meiosis (Table 57-3), affected individuals have missing or extra chromosomes in all cells. In a small proportion of cases, a mitotic nondisjunctional event occurs at an early stage in an individual with an initially normal chromosome constitution. Alternatively, a "normalizing" mitotic nondisjunctional event may result in a normal chromosome complement in some cells of an embryo. In either case, the embryo is a mosaic, with some cells bearing a normal chromosome constitution and others an aneuploid number of chromosomes. The phenotypic consequences are difficult to predict because they depend on the timing of nondisjunction and the distribution of normal and abnormal cells in different tissues. Nevertheless, mosaicism may lead to clinical abnormalities indistinguishable from those of nonmosaic individuals; for example, nearly 5% of all cases of Down syndrome involve individuals with mosaic trisomy 21, and about 15% of individuals with Turner syndrome are mosaic for various sex chromosomal constitutions as described above.

The Origin and Etiology of Numerical Abnormalities Over the past decade, a number of studies have used DNA polymorphisms to investigate the

TABLE 57-2 *Frequency and Distribution of Chromosome Abnormalities in Different Types of Clinically Recognizable Pregnancies*

Chromosome Abnormality	Frequency of Abnormality			Probability of Surviving to Term, %
	Spontaneous Abortion	Stillbirth	Livebirth	
Trisomy, all	25.1	4.0	0.3	5
+13, 18, 21	4.5	2.7	0.14	15
+16	7.5	—	—	0
Sex chromosome monosomy (45,X)	8.7	0.1	0.01	1
Triploidy	6.4	0.2	—	0
Tetraploidy	2.4	—	—	0
Structural abnormality	2.0	0.8	0.3	45
Total abnormalities	50.0	5.1	0.6	5

TABLE 57-3 *Studies of the Parent and Meiotic/Mitotic Stage of Origin of Human Trisomies and Sex Chromosome Monosomy*

	Origin, %				
	Paternal		Maternal		
	I	II	I	II	Mitotic
TRISOMY					
2	28	—	54	13	6
7	—	—	17	26	57
15	—	15	76	9	—
16	—	1	96	3	—
18	—	—	33	56	11
21	3	5	67	22	2
22	3	—	94	3	—
XXY	46	—	38	14	3
XXX	—	6	60	16	18
MONOSOMY					
X[a]		80		20	

[a] Results pertain to nonmosaic 45,X individuals.

origin of different types of chromosome abnormalities (Fig. 57-4). The most thoroughly investigated types have been numerical abnormalities (Table 57-3). Sex chromosome monosomy usually results from loss of the paternal sex chromosome, regardless of whether the conception is live-born or spontaneously aborted.

Trisomies show remarkable variation in parental origin. For example, paternal nondisjunction is responsible for nearly 50% of 47,XXY but only 5 to 10% of cases of trisomies 13, 14, 15, 21, and 22; it is rarely, if ever, the source of the additional chromosome in trisomy 16. Similarly, there is considerable variability in the meiotic stage of origin. For example, all cases of trisomy 16 may be due to meiosis I errors, whereas for trisomy 21, one-third of cases are associated with meiosis II errors, and for trisomy 18, the majority of cases are apparently due to meiosis II nondisjunction. In spite of this variation in parental and meiotic origin, nondisjunction at maternal meiosis I appears to be the most common source of trisomy.

Maternal Age and Trisomy   The association between increasing maternal age and trisomy is the most important etiologic factor in congenital chromosomal disorders. Among women under the age of 25, approximately 2% of all clinically recognized pregnancies are trisomic; by the age of 36, however, this figure increases to 10% and by the age of 42, to over 33% (Fig. 57-5). This association between maternal age and trisomy is exerted without respect to race, geography, or socioeconomic factors and likely affects segregation of all chromosomes.

Despite the importance of increasing age, little is known about the mechanism by which aging leads to abnormal chromosomal segregation. As noted above, it is thought to originate in maternal meiosis I

FIGURE 57-5   Estimated maternal age-adjusted rates of trisomy among all clinically recognized pregnancies (e.g., spontaneous abortions, stillbirths, and livebirths). Among women in their forties, over 25% of all pregnancies are estimated to involve a trisomic conception; the vast majority of these spontaneously abort, with only trisomies 13, 18, and 21 and sex chromosome trisomies surviving to term with any appreciable frequency.

owing to the protracted time to completion (often ≥40 years) in females, and recent studies suggest that it may be associated with alterations in meiotic crossing-over. In trisomy 21, for example, crossover patterns appear to be similarly abnormal in younger and older mothers of trisomic conceptions. Thus, it has been suggested that two distinct steps, or "hits," may be involved in maternal age-related nondisjunction. The first hit, which is age independent, involves the establishment of a "vulnerable" crossover configuration in the fetal oocyte; the second hit, which is age dependent, involves abnormal processing of the vulnerable bivalent structure at metaphase I. If this model is correct, it suggests that the nondisjunctional process is the same in younger and older women, but it occurs more frequently with aging, possibly because of age-dependent degradation of meiotic proteins.

STRUCTURAL CHROMOSOME ABNORMALITIES   Structural rearrangements involve breakage and reunion of chromosomes. Although less common than numerical abnormalities, they present additional challenges from a genetic counseling standpoint. This is because structural abnormalities, unlike numerical abnormalities, can be present in "balanced" form in clinically normal individuals but transmitted in "unbalanced" form to progeny, thereby resulting in a hereditary form of chromosome abnormality.

Rearrangements may involve exchanges of material between different chromosomes (translocations) or loss, gain, or rearrangements of individual chromosomes (e.g., deletions, duplications, inversions, rings, or isochromosomes). Of particular clinical importance are *translocations*, which involve two basic types: Robertsonian and reciprocal. Robertsonian rearrangements are a special class of translocation, in which the long arms of two acrocentric chromosomes (chromosomes 13, 14, 15, 21, and 22) join together, generating a fusion chromosome that contains virtually all of the genetic material of the original two chromosomes. If the Robertsonian translocation is present in unbalanced form, a monosomic or trisomic conception ensues. For example, approximately 3% of Down syndrome cases are attributable to unbalanced Robertsonian translocations, most often involving chromosomes 14 and 21. In this instance, the affected individual has 46 chromosomes, including one structurally normal chromosome 14, two structurally normal chromosomes 21, and one fusion 14/21 chromosome. This effect leads to a normal diploid dosage for chromosome 14 and to

A. Parental origin of trisomy 21   *B.* Parental origin of PWS

FIGURE 57-4   Use of DNA technology to determine the origin of chromosome abnormalities. *A.* Analysis of a chromosome 21–specific DNA polymorphism demonstrates that the trisomic individual received two chromosomes 21 from his mother and one from his father; thus, the extra chromosome 21 resulted from an error in oogenesis. *B.* Inheritance of a chromosome 15–specific DNA polymorphism in an individual with Prader-Willi syndrome (PWS). The affected individual has received two maternal, but no paternal, chromosomes 15; thus, the individual is said to have maternal uniparental disomy 15, a common cause of PWS.

a triplication of chromosome 21, thus resulting in Down syndrome. Similarly, a small proportion of individuals with trisomy 13 syndrome are clinically affected because of an unbalanced Robertsonian translocation.

Reciprocal translocations involve mutual exchanges between any two chromosomes. In this circumstance, the phenotypic consequences associated with unbalanced translocations depend on the location of the breakpoints, which dictate the amount of material that has been "exchanged" between the two chromosomes. Because most reciprocal translocations involve unique sets of breakpoints, it is difficult to predict the phenotypic consequences in any one situation. In general, severity is determined by the amount of excess or missing chromosome material in individuals with unbalanced translocations.

In addition to rearrangements between chromosomes, there are several examples of intrachromosome structural abnormalities. The most common and deleterious of these involve loss of chromosome material due to deletions. The two best-characterized deletion syndromes, Wolf-Hirschhorn syndrome and cri-du-chat syndrome, result from loss of relatively small chromosomal segments on chromosomes 4p and 5p, respectively. Nonetheless, each is associated with multiple congenital anomalies, developmental delays, profound retardation, and reduced lifespan.

Microdeletion Syndromes The term *contiguous gene syndrome* refers to genetic disorders that mimic a combination of single gene disorders. They result from the deletion of a small number of tightly clustered genes. Because some are too small to be detected cytogenetically, they are termed microdeletions. The application of molecular techniques has led to the identification of at least 18 of these microdeletion syndromes (Table 57-4). Some of the more common ones include the Wilms' tumor–aniridia complex (WAGR), Miller Dieker syndrome (MDS), and velocardiofacial (VCF) syndrome. WAGR is characterized by mental retardation and involvement of multiple organs, including kidney (Wilm's tumor), eye (aniridia), and the genitourinary system. The cytogenetic abnormality involves a deletion of a part of the short arm of chromosome 11 (11p13), which typically is detectable on well-banded chromosome preparations. In MDS, a disorder characterized by mental retardation, dysmorphic faces, and lissencephaly, the deletion involves chromosome 17 (17p13). Using FISH, 17p deletions have been detected in over 90% of patients with MDS as well as in 20% of cases of isolated lissencephaly.

Deletions involving the long arm of chromosome 22 (22q11) are the most common microdeletions identified to date, present in approximately 1/3000 newborns. VCF syndrome, the most commonly associated syndrome, consists of learning disabilities or mild mental retardation, palatal defects, a hypoplastic aloe nasi and long nose, and congenital heart defects (conotruncal defect). Some individuals with 22q11 deletion are more severely affected and present with DiGeorge syndrome, which involves abnormalities in the development of the third and fourth branchial arches leading to thymic hypoplasia, parathyroid hypoplasia, and conotruncal heart defects. In approximately 30% of these cases, a deletion at 22q11 can be detected with high-resolution banding; by combing conventional cytogenetics, FISH, and molecular detection techniques (i.e., Southern blotting or polymerase chain reaction analyses), these rates improve to over 90%. Additional studies have demonstrated a surprisingly high frequency of 22q11 deletions in individuals with nonsyndromic conotruncal defects. Approximately 10% of individuals with a 22q11 deletion inherited it from a parent with a similar deletion.

Smith-Magenis syndrome involves a microdeletion localized to the proximal region of the short arm of chromosome 17 (17p11.2). Affected individuals have mental retardation, dysmorphic facial features, delayed speech, peripheral neuropathy, and behavior abnormalities. Most of these deletions can be detected with cytogenetic analysis, although FISH is available to confirm these findings. In contrast, William syndrome, a chromosome 7 (7q11.23) microdeletion, cannot be diagnosed with standard or high-resolution analysis; it is only detectable utilizing FISH or other molecular methods. William syndrome involves a deletion of the elastin gene and is characterized by mental retardation, dysmorphic features, a gregarious personality, premature aging, and congenital heart disease (usually supravalvular aortic stenosis).

In addition to microdeletion syndromes, there is now at least one well-described microduplication syndrome, Charcot-Marie-Tooth type 1A (CMT1A). This is a nerve conduction disease previously thought to be transmitted as a simple autosomal dominant disorder. Recent molecular studies have demonstrated that affected individuals are heterozygous for duplication of a small region of chromosome 17 (17p11.2-12). Although it is not yet clear why increased gene dosage would result in CMT1A, the inheritance pattern is explained by the fact that one-half of the offspring of affected individuals inherit the duplication-carrying chromosome.

IMPRINTING DISORDERS Two other microdeletion syndromes, Prader-Willi syndrome (PWS) and Angelman syndrome (AS), exhibit parent-of-origin, or "imprinting," effects. For many years, it has been known that cytogenetically detectable deletions of chromosome 15 occur in a proportion of patients with PWS, as well as in those with AS. This

TABLE 57-4 *Some Commonly Identified Microdeletion and Microduplication Syndromes*

Syndrome	Cytogenetic Location	Principal Features	Imprinting Effects
Langer-Giedion syndrome	8q24.1 (del)	Sparse hair, bulbous nose, variable mental retardation	No
WAGR complex	11p13 (del)	Wilms' tumor, aniridia, genitourinary disorders, mental retardation	No
Beckwith-Wiedemann syndrome	11p15 (dup)	Macrosomia, macroglossia, omphalocoele	Yes, occasionally associated with "paternal uniparental disomy" (see text)
Retinoblastoma	13q14.11 (del)	Retinoblastoma due to homozygous loss of functional RB allele	No obvious effect, although abnormal RB allele more likely to be paternal
Prader-Willi syndrome	15q11-13 (del)	Obesity, hypogonadism, mental retardation	Yes; prototypic imprinting disorder (see text)
Angelman syndrome	15q11-13 (del)	Ataxic gait	With Prader-Willi syndrome, prototypic imprinting disorder (see text)
α-Thalassemia and mental retardation	16p13.3 (del)	α-thalassemia and mental retardation, due to deletion of distal 16p, including α-globin locus	No
Smith-Magenis syndrome	17p11.2 (del)	Brachycephaly, midface hypoplasia, mental retardation	No
Miller-Dieker syndrome	17p13 (del)	Dysmorphic facies, lissencephaly	No
Charcot-Marie-Tooth syndrome type 1A	17p11.2 (dup)	Progressive neuropathy due to microduplication	No
DiGeorge syndrome/ velocardiofacial syndrome	22q11 (del)	Abnormalities of third and fourth branchial arches	No

seemed curious, as the clinical manifestations of the two syndromes are very dissimilar. PWS is characterized by obesity, hypogonadism, and mild to moderate mental retardation, whereas AS is associated with microcephaly, ataxic gait, seizures, inappropriate laughter, and severe mental retardation. New insight into the pathogenesis of these disorders has been provided by the recognition that parental origin of the deletion determines which phenotype ensues: if the deletion is paternal, the result is PWS, whereas if the deletion is maternal, the result is AS (Fig. 57-2).

This scenario is complicated further by the recognition that not all individuals with PWS or AS carry the chromosome 15 deletion. For such individuals, the parental origin of the chromosome 15 region is again the important determinant. In PWS, for example, nondeletion patients invariably have two maternal and no paternal chromosomes 15 [maternal uniparental disomy (UPD)], whereas for some nondeletion AS patients the reverse is true (paternal UPD). This indicates that at least some genes on chromosome 15 are differently expressed, depending on which parent contributed the chromosome. Additionally, this means that normal fetal development requires the presence of one maternal and one paternal copy of chromosome 15.

Approximately 70% of PWS cases are due to paternal deletions of 15q11-q13, whereas 25% are due to maternal UPD, and about 5% are caused by mutations in a chromosome 15 imprinting center. In AS, 75% of cases are due to maternal deletions, and only 2% are due to paternal UPD. The remaining cases are presumably caused by imprinting mutations (5%), or mutations in the *UBE3A* gene, which is associated with AS. The UPD cases are mostly caused by meiotic nondisjunction resulting in trisomy 15, subsequently followed by a normalizing mitotic nondisjunction event ("trisomy rescue") resulting in two normal chromosomes 15, both from the same parent. *UBE3A* is the only maternally imprinted gene known in the critical region of chromosome 15. However, several paternally imprinted genes, or expressed-sequence tags (ESTs), have been identified, including *ZNF127*, *IPW*, *SNRPN*, *SNURF*, *PAR1*, and *PAR5*.

Chromosomal regions that behave in the manner observed in PWS and AS are said to be *imprinted*. This phenomenon is involved in differential expression of certain genes on different chromosomes. Chromosome 11 is one of these with an imprinted region, since it is known that a small proportion of individuals with the Beckwith-Wiedemann overgrowth syndrome have two paternal but no maternal copies of this chromosome.

ACQUIRED CHROMOSOME ABNORMALITIES IN CANCER (See also Chap. 68 for detailed discussion of cancer genetics)

In addition to the constitutional cytogenetic chromosomal abnormalities that are present at birth, somatic chromosomal changes can be acquired later in life and are often associated with malignant conditions. As with constitutional abnormalities, somatic changes can include the net loss of chromosomal material (due to a deletion or loss of a chromosome), net gain of material (duplication or gain of a chromosome), and relocation of DNA sequences (translocation). Cytogenetic changes have been particularly well studied in (1) leukemias, e.g., Philadelphia chromosome translocation in CML [t(9;22)(q34.1; q11.2)]; and (2) lymphomas, e.g., translocations of *MYC* in Burkitt's [t(8;14)(q24;q32)]. These and other translocations are useful for diagnosis, classification, and prognosis. Analyses of cytogenetic changes are also useful in certain solid tumors. For example, a complex karyotype with Wilms' tumor, diploidy in medulloblastoma, and Her-2/neu amplification in breast cancer are poor prognostic signs.

FURTHER READING

JIANG F, KATZ RL: Use of interphase fluorescence in situ hybridization as a powerful diagnostic tool in cytology. Diagn Mol Pathol 11:47, 2002

NASMYTH K: Segregating sister genomes: the molecular biology of chromosome separation. Science 297:559, 2002

NICHOLLS RD et al: Imprinting in Prader-Willi and Angelman syndromes. Trends Genet 14:194, 1998

STUMM M et al: Molecular cytogenetic techniques for the diagnosis of chromosomal abnormalities in childhood disease. Eur J Pediatr 158:531, 1999

58 THE PRACTICE OF GENETICS IN CLINICAL MEDICINE
Susan Miesfeldt, J. Larry Jameson

IMPLICATIONS OF MOLECULAR GENETICS FOR INTERNAL MEDICINE

The field of medical genetics has traditionally focused on chromosomal abnormalities (Chap. 57) and Mendelian disorders (Chap. 56). However, there is genetic susceptibility to many common adult-onset diseases including atherosclerosis, hypertension, autoimmune diseases, diabetes mellitus, Alzheimer disease, psychiatric disorders, and many forms of cancer. Genetic contributions to these common disorders involve more than the ultimate expression of an illness; these genes can also influence the severity of infirmity, response to treatment, and progression of disease.

The primary care clinician is now faced with the role of recognizing and counseling patients at risk for a number of genetically influenced illnesses. Among the greater than 30,000 genes in the human genome, it is estimated that each of us harbors several potentially deleterious mutations. Fortunately, many of these alterations are recessive and clinically silent. An even greater number, however, represent genetic variants that alter disease susceptibility or severity. Genetic medicine is changing the way diseases are classified, enhancing our understanding of pathophysiology, providing practical information concerning drug metabolism and therapeutic responses, and allowing for individualized screening and health care management programs. In view of these changes, the physician must integrate personal medical history, family history, and diagnostic molecular testing into the overall care of individual patients and their families. In addition, the internist has an important role in educating patients about the indications, benefits, risks, and limitations of genetic testing in the management of a number of diverse diseases. This is a difficult task as scientific advances in genetic medicine, and media attention to these advances, have outpaced the translation of these discoveries into standards of clinical care.

COMMON ADULT-ONSET GENETIC DISORDERS

MULTIFACTORIAL INHERITANCE The risk for many adult-onset disorders reflects the combined effects of genetic factors at multiple loci that may function independently, or in combination with other genes or environmental factors. Our understanding of the genetic basis of these disorders is incomplete, despite the clear recognition of genetic susceptibility. In type 2 diabetes mellitus, for example, the concordance rate in monozygotic twins ranges between 50 and 90%. Diabetes or impaired glucose tolerance occurs in 40% of siblings and in 30% of the offspring of an affected individual. Despite the fact that diabetes affects 5% of the population and exhibits a high degree of heritability, there are only a few examples of genetic mutations (most of which are rare) that might account for the familial nature of the disease. They include certain mitochondrial DNA disorders (Chap. 56), mutations in a cascade of genes that control pancreatic islet cell development and function (*HNF4α*, *HNF1α*, *IPF1*, *glucokinase*), insulin receptor mutations, and others (Chap. 323). Obesity and other factors that contribute to insulin resistance represent major risk factors for type 2 diabetes.

Current models for the genetic basis of type 2 diabetes propose the involvement of more than a dozen genes: some genes influence pancreatic islet cell development or function; others modulate glucose sensing; and an important group determine insulin sensitivity, either directly by affecting insulin signaling or indirectly by regulating body weight or composition. Superimposed on this genetic background are environmental influences such as diet, exercise, pregnancy, and medications.

Identifying these susceptibility genes is a formidable task. Nonetheless, a reasonable goal for this type of disease is to identify genes that increase (or decrease) disease risk by a factor of two or more. For common diseases such as diabetes or heart disease, this level of risk has important implications for health. Much the same way that cholesterol is currently used as a biochemical marker of cardiovascular risk, we can anticipate the development of genetic panels with similar predictive power. Tests for a large number of genetic disorders are available; a website (www.genetests.org) lists various laboratories that perform specific tests. The advent of DNA-sequencing chips represents an important technical advance that promises to make large-scale testing more feasible (Chap. 56). The decision whether or not to perform a genetic test for a particular inherited adult-onset disorder, such as hemochromatosis, multiple endocrine neoplasia (MEN) type 1, prolonged QT syndrome, or Huntington disease, is complex; it depends on the clinical features of the disorder, the desires of the patient and family, and whether the results of genetic testing will alter medical decision-making or treatment (see below).

THE FAMILY HISTORY Pending further advances in genetic testing, the key to assessing the inherited risk for common adult-onset diseases rests in the collection and interpretation of a detailed personal and family medical history in conjunction with a directed physical examination. For example, a history of multiple family members with early-onset coronary artery disease, glucose intolerance, and hypertension should suggest increased risk for genetic, and perhaps environmental, predisposition to insulin resistance (Chap. 323). Individual patients with this family history should be monitored for the possible development of hypertension, diabetes, and hyperlipidemia. They should be counseled about the importance of avoiding additional risk factors such as obesity and cigarette smoking.

Family history should be recorded in the form of a pedigree which greatly assists the assessment of risk in the individual patient (Chap. 56). At a minimum, pedigrees should convey health-related data on all first-degree relatives and selected second-degree relatives, including grandparents. When pedigrees appear to suggest an inherited disease, they should be extended to include additional family members. The determination of risk for an asymptomatic individual will vary depending on the size of the pedigree, the number of unaffected relatives, and the types of diagnoses within the family. For example, a woman with two first-degree relatives with breast cancer is at greater risk for a Mendelian disorder if she has a total of three female first-degree relatives than if she has a total of ten female first-degree relatives. Additional variables that should be documented in the pedigree include the age at diagnosis of each affected family member, present age of all family members, the presence or absence of nonhereditary risk factors among those affected with diseases, and the finding of multiple diseases in an individual patient. For instance, a woman with a history of both colon cancer and endometrial cancer is at risk for hereditary nonpolyposis colon cancer (HNPCC) regardless of her family history.

When assessing the personal and family history, the physician should be alert to a younger age of disease onset than is usually seen in the general population. A 30-year-old with acute myocardial infarction should be considered at risk for a hereditary trait, even if there is no family history of premature coronary artery disease (Chap. 224). The absence of the nonhereditary risk factors typically associated with a disease also raises the prospect of genetic risk factors. A personal or family history of deep-vein thrombosis, in the absence of known nongenetic risk factors, suggests a hereditary thrombotic disorder (Chap.

102). The physical examination may also provide important clues concerning the risk for a specific inherited disorder. A patient with xanthomas at a young age should prompt consideration of familial hypercholesterolemia. Some adult-onset disease-causing mutations are more prevalent in certain ethnic groups. For instance, >2% of the Ashkenazi population carry one of three specific mutations in the *BRCA1* or *BRCA2* genes. The prevalence of the factor V Leiden allele ranges from 3 to 7% in Caucasians but is much less common in Africans or Asians.

Recall of family history is sometimes inaccurate. This is especially so when the history is remote and families become more dispersed. It can be helpful to ask patients to fill out family history forms before or after their visits, as this provides them with an opportunity to contact relatives. Attempts should be made to confirm the illnesses reported in the family history before making important, and in certain circumstances, irreversible management decisions. This process is often labor intensive and ideally involves interviews of additional family members or reviewing medical records, autopsy reports, and death certificates.

Nongenetic factors associated with disease risk should also be reviewed in full, including occupation, diet, living conditions, and social habits. For example, patients at hereditary risk for heart disease should be questioned about tobacco use, diet, exercise, and lipid levels. Patients should also be asked about their health screening and prevention behaviors, as well as medication use. These nonhereditary factors contribute to the assessment of overall risk and represent an important focus for disease prevention.

Although many inherited disorders will be suggested by the clustering of relatives with the same or related conditions, it is important to note that *disease penetrance* is incomplete for most multifactorial genetic disorders. As a result, the pedigree obtained in such families may not exhibit a clear Mendelian pattern of inheritance, as not all family members carrying the disease-associated alleles will manifest a clinical disorder. Furthermore, genes associated with some of these disorders often exhibit *variable expression* of disease. For example, the breast cancer–associated gene *BRCA1* can predispose to several different malignancies in the same family, including cancers of the breast, ovary, and prostate (Chap. 68). For common diseases such as breast cancer, some family members without the disease-causing mutation may also develop breast cancer, representing another confounding variable in the pedigree analysis.

Some of the aforementioned features of the family history are illustrated in Fig. 58-1. In this example, the proband, a 36-year-old woman, has a strong history of breast and ovarian cancer on the paternal side of her family. The early age of onset, as well as the co-occurrence of breast and ovarian cancer in this family, suggests the possibility of an inherited alteration in *BRCA1* or *BRCA2*. It is unclear though—without genetic testing—whether her father inherited such a mutation and transmitted it to her. After appropriate genetic counseling of the proband and her family, one approach to DNA analysis in this family is to test the potentially affected 42-year-old living cousin for the presence of a *BRCA1* or *BRCA2* mutation. If a mutation is found, then it is possible to test for this particular alteration in the proband and other family members, if they so desire. In the example shown, if the proband's father has the *BRCA1* mutation, there is a 50:50 probability that the mutation has been transmitted to her, and genetic testing can be used to establish the absence or presence of this particular risk factor.

GENETIC TESTING FOR ADULT-ONSET DISORDERS

A critical first step before initiating genetic testing is to assure that the correct clinical diagnosis has been made, whether based on family history, characteristic physical findings, or biochemical testing. Careful clinical assessment can define the *phenotype*, thereby preventing unnecessary testing and directing testing towards the most probable candidate genes. Many disorders exhibit the feature of *locus heterogeneity*, which refers to the fact that mutations in different genes can

FIGURE 58-1 A 36-year-old woman (arrow) seeks consultation because of her family history of cancer. The patient expresses concern that the multiple cancers in her relatives imply an inherited predisposition to develop cancer. The family history is recorded and records of the patient's relatives confirm the reported diagnoses.

cause phenotypically similar disorders. For example, osteogenesis imperfecta (Chap. 342), long QT syndrome (Chap. 214), muscular dystrophy (Chap. 368), homocystinuria (Chap. 343), retinitis pigmentosa (Chap. 25) and hereditary predisposition to colon cancer (Chap. 77) or breast cancer (Chap. 76) can each be caused by mutations in distinct genes. The pattern of disease transmission, clinical course, and treatment may differ significantly, depending on which gene is affected. In these cases, the choice of which genes to test is often determined by unique clinical features, the relative prevalence of mutations in various genes, or test availability.

Like all laboratory tests, there are limitations to the accuracy and interpretation of genetic tests. In addition to technical errors, genetic tests are often designed to detect only the most common mutations. In this case, a negative result must be qualified by the possibility that the individual may have a mutation that is not included in the test.

In addition to molecular testing for established disease, genetic testing for susceptibility to chronic disease is being increasingly integrated into the practice of medicine. In most cases, however, the discovery of disease-associated genes has greatly outpaced studies that assess clinical outcomes and the impact of interventions. Until such evidence-based studies are available, predictive molecular testing must be approached with caution and should be offered only to patients who have been adequately counseled and have provided informed consent (Fig. 58-2). In the majority of cases, genetic testing should be offered only to individuals with a suggestive personal or family medical history or in the context of a clinical trial.

Predictive genetic testing falls into two distinct categories. *Presymptomatic testing* applies to diseases where a specific genetic alteration is associated with a near 100% likelihood of developing disease. In contrast, *predisposition testing* predicts a risk for disease that is less than 100%. For example, presymptomatic testing is available for those at risk for Huntington's disease, whereas predisposition testing is considered for those at risk for hereditary breast cancer. It is important to note that, for the majority of adult-onset, multifactorial genetic disorders, testing is purely predictive. Test results cannot reveal with confidence whether, when, or how the disease will manifest itself. For example, not everyone with the apolipoprotein E allele (ϵ4) will develop Alzheimer's disease, and individuals without this genetic marker can still develop the disorder (Chap. 350).

Molecular analysis is generally more informative if testing is initiated in a symptomatic family member, since the identification of a

mutation can direct the testing of other at-risk family members (whether they are symptomatic or not). In the absence of additional familial or environmental risk factors, individuals who test negative for the mutation found in the affected family member can be informed that they are at general population risk for that particular disease. Furthermore, they can be reassured that they are not at risk for passing on the mutation to their children. On the other hand, asymptomatic family members who test positive for the known mutation must be informed that they are at increased risk for disease development and for transmitting the mutation to their children.

A negative test result is interpreted differently when no genetic mutation is found in a symptomatic family member. In this difficult circumstance, the test performed on a given gene may not detect all mutations in that gene (false negative) or the individual may have a mutation in a different disease-associated gene that was not tested.

Clinicians providing pretest counseling and education should assess the patient's ability to cope with test results. Individuals who demonstrate signs and symptoms of emotional distress should have their psychosocial needs addressed before proceeding with molecular testing. Generally, genetic testing should not be offered at a time of personal crisis or acute illness within the family. Patients will derive more benefit from test results if they are emotionally able to comprehend and absorb the information. It is important to assess patients' preconceived notions of their personal likelihood of disease in preparing pretest educational strategies. Often, patients harbor unwarranted fear or denial of their likelihood of genetic risk.

Genetic testing has the potential of affecting the way individual family members relate to one another, both negatively and positively. As a result, patients addressing the option of molecular testing must consider how test results might impact their relationships with rela-

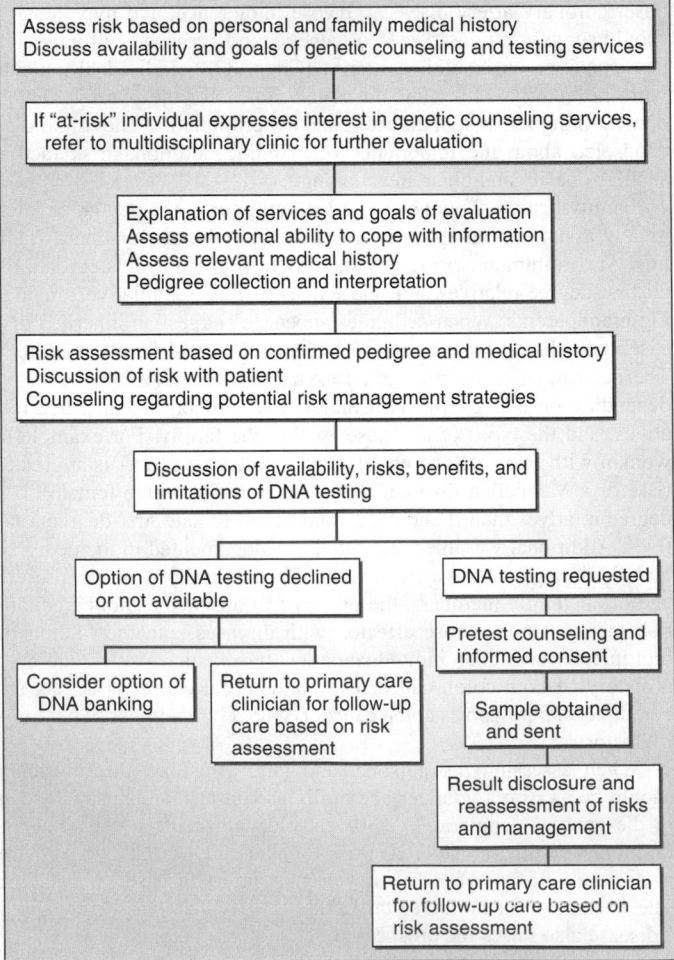

FIGURE 58-2 Algorithm for genetic counseling and testing.

tives, spouses, and friends. In families with a known genetic mutation, those who test positive must consider the impact of their carrier status on their present and future lifestyles; those who test negative may manifest *survivor guilt*. Family members are likely to differ in their emotional and social responses to the same information. Counseling should also address the potential consequences of test results on relationships with a spouse or child. Parents who are found to have a disease-associated mutation often express considerable anxiety and despair as they address the issue of risk to their children.

When a condition does not manifest until adulthood, clinicians will be faced with the question of whether at-risk children should be offered molecular testing and, if so, at what age. Although the matter is debated, several professional organizations have cautioned that genetic testing for adult-onset disorders should not be offered to children. Many of these conditions are not preventable and, consequently, such information can pose significant psychosocial risk to the child. In addition, there is concern that testing during childhood violates a child's right to make an informed decision regarding testing upon reaching adulthood. On the other hand, testing should be offered in childhood for disorders that may manifest early in life, especially when management options are available. For example, children at risk for familial adenomatous polyposis (FAP), associated with alterations in the *APC* gene, may develop polyps as early as their teens, and progression to an invasive cancer can occur by their twenties. Likewise, children at risk for MEN type 2, which is caused by mutations in the *RET* proto-oncogene, may develop medullary thyroid cancer early in childhood, and the issue of prophylactic thyroidectomy should be addressed with the parents of children with documented mutations (Chap. 330).

INFORMED CONSENT When the issue of testing is addressed, patients should be strongly encouraged to involve other relatives in the decision-making process, as molecular diagnostics will likely have an impact on the entire family. Informed consent for molecular testing begins with detailed education and counseling. The patient must fully understand the risks, benefits, and limitations of undergoing the analysis. Informed consent should include a written document, drafted clearly and concisely in a language and format that is comprehensible to the patient, who should be made aware of the disposition of test results. Informed consent should also include a discussion of the mechanics of testing. Most molecular testing for hereditary disease involves DNA-based analysis of peripheral blood. In the majority of circumstances, test results should be given only to the individual, in person, and with a support person in the room.

Because molecular testing of an asymptomatic individual often allows prediction of future risk, the patient should understand any potential long-term medical, psychological, and social implications of this decision. In the United States, legislation affecting this area is still evolving, and it is important to explore with the patient the potential impact that test results may have on employment, as well as future health, and disability and life insurance coverage.

Patients should understand that alternatives to molecular analysis remain available if they decide not to proceed with this option. They should also be notified that testing is available in the future if they are not currently prepared to undergo analysis. The option of DNA banking should be presented so that samples are readily available for future use by family members, if needed. DNA banking is a particularly valuable option for those individuals who are not expected to survive their illness and cannot immediately proceed with testing.

FOLLOW-UP CARE AFTER TESTING Depending on the nature of the genetic disorder, posttest interventions may include (1) cautious surveillance and appropriate health care screening, (2) specific medical interventions, (3) chemoprevention, (4) risk avoidance, and (5) referral to support services. For example, patients with known pathologic mutations in *BRCA1* or *BRCA2* are offered intensive screening as well as the option of prophylactic mastectomy and/or oophorectomy. In addition, such women may be eligible for preventive treatment with tamoxifen, or enrollment in a chemoprevention clinical trial. In contrast, those at known risk for Huntington's disease are offered continued follow-up

and supportive services, including physical and occupational therapy, and social services or support groups, as indicated. Specific interventions will change as translational research continues to enhance our understanding of these genetic diseases and as more is learned about the functions of the proteins involved.

Individuals who test negative for a mutation in a disease-associated gene identified in an affected family member must be reminded that they may still be at risk for the disease. This is of particular importance for common diseases such as diabetes mellitus, cancer, and coronary artery disease. For example, a woman who finds that she does not carry the disease-associated mutation in *BRCA2* previously discovered in her family must be reminded that she still requires the same breast cancer screening recommended for the general population.

GENETIC COUNSELING AND EDUCATION

Genetic counseling should be distinguished from genetic testing and screening, even though genetic counselors are often involved in issues related to testing. Genetic counseling refers to *a communication process that deals with human problems associated with the occurrence or risk of a genetic disorder in a family*. Genetic risk assessment is complex and often involves elements of uncertainty. Counseling therefore includes genetic education as well as psychosocial counseling. Genetic counselors may be called upon by other health care professionals (or by individual patients and families) to address a broad range of issues directly and indirectly involved with genetic disease (Table 58-1). The role of the genetic counselor includes the following:

- Gather and document a detailed family history
- Educate the patient about general genetic principles related to disease risk, both for themselves and others in their family
- Assess and enhance the patient's ability to cope with the genetic information offered
- Discuss how nongenetic factors may relate to the ultimate expression of disease
- Address medical management issues
- Assist in determining the role of genetic testing for the individual and family
- Ensure that the patient is aware of the risks, benefits, and limitations of the various genetic testing options
- Assist the patient, family and referring physician in the interpretation of the test results
- Refer the patient and other at-risk family members for additional medical and support services, if necessary.

The complexity of genetic counseling and the broad scope of genetic diseases have led to the development of specialized, multidisciplinary clinics designed to provide broad-based support and medical care for those at risk and their family members. Such specialty clinics are well established in the areas of cancer and neurodegenerative disorders. The multidisciplinary teams are often composed of medical geneticists, specialist physicians, genetic counselors, nurses, psychologists, social workers, and biomedical ethicists who work together to consider difficult diagnostic, treatment, and testing decisions. Such a format also provides primary care physicians with invaluable support and assistance as they follow and treat at-risk patients.

The approach to genetic counseling has important ethical, social, and financial implications. Philosophies related to genetic counseling vary widely by country and center. In North American centers, for

---

TABLE 58-1 *Indications for Genetic Counseling*

Advanced maternal (>35) or paternal (>50) age
Consanguinity
Previous history of a child with birth defects or a genetic disorder
Personal or family history suggestive of a genetic disorder
High-risk ethnic groups; known carriers of genetic alterations
Documented genetic alteration in a family member
Ultrasound or prenatal testing suggesting a genetic disorder

TABLE 58-2 *Examples of Genetic Testing and Possible Interventions*

Genetic Disorder	Inheritance	Genes	Interventions
ONCOLOGY			
Hereditary nonpolyposis colon cancer	AD	*MSH2, MLH1, MSH6, PMS1, PMS2*	Early cancer screening
Familial adenomatous polyposis	AD	*APC*	Nonsteroidal anti-inflammatory drugs
			Early endoscopic screening
			Colectomy
Familial breast and ovarian cancer	AD	*BRCA1, BRCA2*	Estrogen receptor antagonists
			Early screening by exams and mammography
			Consider prophylactic surgery
Familial melanoma	AD	*CDKN2A*	Avoid UV light
			Screening and biopsies
Basal cell nevus syndrome	AD	*PTCH*	Avoid UV light
			Screening and biopsies
HEMATOLOGY			
Factor V Leiden	AD	*F5*	Avoid thrombogenic risk factors and oral contraceptives
Hemophilia A	XL	*F8C*	Factor VIII replacement
Hemophilia B	XL	*F9*	Factor IX replacement
			Possible gene therapy
Glucose-6-PO4 dehydrogenase deficiency	XL	*G6PD*	Avoid oxidant drugs
CARDIOVASCULAR			
Hypertrophic cardiomyopathy	AD	*MYH7, MYBPC3, TNNT2, TPM1*	Echocardiographic screening
			Early pharmacologic intervention
Long QT syndrome	AD	*KCNQ1, KCNH2, SCN5A, LQT4, KCNE1, KCNE2*	Electrocardiographic screening and electrophysiologic testing
			Early pharmacologic intervention
			Possible implantable cardioverter defibrillator
Marfan syndrome	AD	*FBN1*	Echocardiographic screening
			Prophylactic beta blockers
GASTROINTESTINAL			
Familial Mediterranean fever	AR	*MEFV*	Colchicine treatment
Hemochromatosis	AR	*HFE*	Phlebotomy
PULMONARY			
α-1 Antitrypsin deficiency	AR	*PI*	Avoid smoking
			Avoid occupational and environmental toxins
Primary pulmonary hypertension	AD	*BMPR2*	Treatment with pulmonary vasodilators
RENAL			
Polycystic kidney disease	AD	*PKHD1*	Prevent hypertension
			Prevent urinary tract infections
			Kidney transplantation
Nephrogenic diabetes insipidus	XL, AR	*AVPR2, AQP2*	Fluid replacement
			Thiazides, amiloride
ENDOCRINE			
Neurohypophyseal diabetes insipidus	AD	*AVP*	Replace vasopressin
Maturity onset diabetes of the young	AD	Multiple genes	Screen and treat for diabetes
Familial hypocalciuric hypercalcemia	AD	*CASR*	Avoid parathyroidectomy
Kallmann syndrome	XL	*KAL*	Induce puberty with hormone replacement
Multiple endocrine neoplasia type 2	AD	*RET*	Prophylactic thyroidectomy
			Screen for pheochromocytoma and hyperparathyroidism
21-Hydroxylase deficiency	AR	*CYP21*	Glucocorticoid and mineralocorticoid treatment
NEUROLOGIC			
Malignant hyperthermia	AD	*RYR1*	Avoid precipitating anesthetics
Hyperkalemic periodic paralysis	AD	*SCN4A*	Acetazolamide
Adrenoleukodystrophy	XL	*ABCD1*	Possible bone marrow transplant for severe childhood CNS form
Duchenne and Becker muscular dystrophy	XL	*DMD*	Glucocorticoids
			Possible future myoblast transfer
Familial Parkinson's disease	AD	*SNCA, PARK2*	Amantadine, anticholinergics, levodopa, monoamine oxidase B inhibitors
Wilson's disease	AR	*ATP7B*	D-Penicillamine treatment

Abbreviations: AD, autosomal dominant; AR, autosomal recessive: CNS, central nervous system; XL, X-linked

example, counseling is generally offered in a nondirective manner, wherein patients learn to understand how their values factor into a particular medical decision. Nondirective counseling is particularly appropriate when there are no data demonstrating a clear benefit associated with a particular intervention or when an intervention is considered experimental. For example, nondirective genetic counseling is employed when a person is deciding whether or not to undergo genetic testing for Huntington's disease (Chap. 350). At this time, there is no clear benefit (in terms of medical outcome) to an at-risk individual undergoing genetic testing for this disease, as its course cannot be altered by therapeutic interventions. However, testing can have an important impact on this individual's perception of the future and his or her interpersonal relationships and plans for reproduction. Therefore, the decision to pursue testing rests on the individual's belief system and values. On the other hand, a more directive approach is appropriate when a condition can be treated. In a family with FAP, colon cancer screening and prophylactic colectomy should be recommended for known *APC* mutation carriers. The counselor and clinician following this family must ensure that the at-risk family members have access to the resources necessary to adhere to these recommendations.

Genetic education is central to an individual's ability to make an informed decision regarding testing options and treatment. Although genetic counselors represent one source of genetic education, other health care providers also need to contribute to patient education. Patients at risk for genetic disease should understand fundamental medical genetic principles and terminology relevant to their situation. This includes the concept of genes, how they are transmitted, and how they confer hereditary disease risk. An adequate knowledge of patterns of inheritance will allow patients to understand the probability of disease risk for themselves and other family members. It is also important to impart the concepts of disease penetrance and expression. For most complex adult-onset genetic disorders, asymptomatic patients should be advised that a positive test result does not always translate into future disease development. In addition, the role of nongenetic factors, such as environmental exposures, must be discussed in the context of multifactorial disease risk and disease prevention. Finally, patients should understand the natural history of the disease as well as the potential options for intervention, including screening, prevention, and—in certain circumstances—pharmacologic treatment or prophylactic surgery.

THERAPEUTIC INTERVENTIONS BASED ON GENETIC RISK FOR DISEASE

Specific treatments are now available for an increasing number of genetic disorders, whether identified through population-based screening or directed testing (Table 58-2). Although the strategies for therapeutic interventions are best developed for childhood hereditary metabolic diseases, these principles are making their way into the diagnosis and management of adult-onset disorders. Hereditary hemochromatosis illustrates many of the issues raised by the availability of genetic screening in the adult population. For instance, it is relatively common (approximately 1 in 200 individuals of northern European descent are homozygous), and its complications are potentially preventable through phlebotomy (Chap. 336). The identification of the *HFE* gene, mutations of which are associated with this syndrome, has sparked interest in the use of DNA-based testing for presymptomatic diagnosis of the disorder. However, up to one-third of individuals who are homozygous for the *HFE* mutation do not have evidence of iron overload. Consequently, in the absence of a positive family history, current recommendations include phenotypic screening for evidence of iron overload followed by genetic testing. Whether genetic screening for hemochromatosis will someday be coupled to assessment of phenotypic expression awaits further studies. In contrast to the issue of population screening, it is important to test and counsel other family members when the diagnosis of hemochromatosis has been made in a proband. Testing allows the physician to exclude family members who are not at risk. It also permits presymptomatic detection of iron overload and the institution of treatment (phlebotomy) before the development of organ damage.

Preventive measures and therapeutic interventions are not restricted to metabolic disorders. Identification of familial forms of long QT

syndrome, associated with ventricular arrythmias, allows early electrocardiographic testing and the use of prophylactic antiarrythmic therapy, overdrive pacemakers, or defibrillators (Chap. 214). Individuals with familial hypertrophic cardiomyopathy can be screened by ultrasound, treated with beta blockers or other drugs, and counseled about the importance of avoiding strenuous exercise and dehydration (Chap. 221). Likewise, individuals with Marfan syndrome can be treated with beta blockers and monitored for the development of aortic aneurysms (Chap. 231). Individuals with α_1 antitrypsin deficiency can be strongly counseled to avoid cigarette smoking and exposure to environmental pulmonary and hepatotoxins. Various host genes influence the pathogenesis of certain infectious diseases in humans, including HIV (Chap. 173). The factor V Leiden allele increases risk of thrombosis (Chap. 53). Approximately 3% of the worldwide population is heterozygous for this mutation. Moreover, it is found in up to 25% of patients with recurrent deep-vein thrombosis or pulmonary embolism. Women who are heterozygous or homozygous for this allele should therefore avoid the use of oral contraceptives and receive heparin prophylaxis after surgery or trauma.

The field of pharmacogenomics seeks to identify genes that alter drug metabolism or confer susceptibility to toxic drug reactions. Examples include succinylcholine sensitivity, malignant hyperthermia, dihydropyrimidine dehydrogenase deficiency, the porphyrias, and glucose-6-phosphase dehydrogenase (G6PD) deficiency.

As noted above, the identification of genes that increase the risk of specific types of neoplasia is rapidly changing the management of many cancers. Identifying family members with mutations that predispose to FAP or hereditary nonpolyposis colon cancer (HNPCC) can lead to recommendations of early cancer screening or prophylactic surgery (Chap. 77). Similar principles apply to familial forms of melanoma, basal cell carcinoma, and cancers of the breast, ovary, and thyroid gland. It should be recognized, however, that most cancers harbor several distinct genetic abnormalities by the time they acquire invasive or metastatic potential (Chaps. 68 and 69). Consequently, the major impact of genetic testing in these cases is to allow more intensive clinical screening, as it remains very challenging to predict disease penetrance, expression, or the clinical course of these diseases.

Although genetic diagnosis of these and other disorders is only beginning to be used in the clinical setting, predictive testing holds the promise of allowing earlier and more targeted interventions that can reduce the morbidity and mortality associated with these disorders. We can expect the availability of genetic tests to expand rapidly. A critical challenge for physicians and other health care providers is to keep pace with these advances in genetic medicine and to implement testing judiciously. Meeting this goal will enhance patient care through adequate counseling, directed testing, and appropriate interventions, with the ultimate objective being the reduction of morbidity and mortality from genetic diseases.

FURTHER READING

BIESECKER BB, MARTEAU TM: Future of genetic counselling: An international perspective. Nat Genet 22:133, 1999

HARPER PS: *Practical Genetic Counselling*, 5th ed. Oxford, Butterworth Heinmann, 1998

MCKINNON WC et al: Predisposition genetic testing for late-onset disorders in adults: Position paper of the National Society of Genetic Counselors. JAMA 278:1217, 1997

PATENAUDE AF et al: Genetic testing and psychology. New roles, new responsibilities. Am Psychol 57:271, 2002

THE AMERICAN COLLEGE OF MEDICAL GENETICS: Points to consider: Ethical, legal and psychosocial implications of genetic testing in children and adolescents. Am J Hum Genet 57:1233, 1995

Gene therapy uses gene replacement to repair or treat disease. *Stem cell replacement* involves the administration of pluripotent, renewable cells to organs irreversibly damaged by disease. The disciplines of gene and cell therapy are now converging, offering unique opportunities to translate new knowledge of genetics and stem cell biology into the clinical setting. The technical, safety, and ethical challenges of these new treatment approaches are substantial, but their enormous promise provides strong incentive for ongoing research.

GENE TRANSFER IN CLINICAL MEDICINE

METHODS OF GENE TRANSFER Approaches to gene transfer can be divided broadly into: (1) ex vivo, in which genes are transferred into cells that are subsequently introduced into the patient; or (2) in vivo, in which genes are introduced directly into tissues, some of which are not readily accessible for ex vivo approaches. Ex vivo approaches are amenable to combining gene transfer with stem cell replacement (see below). In vivo gene transfer approaches have found relatively few clinical applications because of problems with targeting and regulating gene expression, maintaining gene expression, and avoiding toxicity.

Techniques for transferring genes include viral vectors and non-viral methods. *Viral vectors* take advantage of the fact that viruses enter cells efficiently and already contain genes that facilitate expression in host cells. In addition, some viruses such as retroviruses, lentiviruses, and adeno-associated viruses (AAVs) integrate genes into the host genome, facilitating long-term expression. However, technical limitations with viral production, the carrying capacity for the transferred gene, and the requirement for cell replication for effective integration (e.g., retroviruses) have hampered applications using these viruses. Nonetheless, viruses currently provide the best approach for long-lasting genetic modifications, as might be applied to stem cells or somatic cells. Adenoviruses have been widely used because they are easily produced in high titer, infect both quiescent and dividing cells, and can accommodate up to 10 kb of DNA. However, DNA transferred by adenoviruses is episomal (does not integrate into the host genome), resulting in relatively short-term gene expression over several weeks. The current generation of adenoviruses induces variable cytotoxicity and elicits immune responses—features that are useful for cytotoxic gene therapy but not for gene replacement.

Nonviral gene transfer includes the use of liposomes, electroporation, particle-mediated uptake, and direct uptake of naked DNA or oligonucleotides. Although these methods are relatively simple to perform and introduce minimal toxicity, they are much less efficient than viral-mediated approaches.

CHALLENGES ASSOCIATED WITH GENE THERAPY Gene therapy can be defined as the introduction of genes into cells or tissues with the goal of modifying the function of the tissue or producing a protein product beneficial for normal physiology. Potential applications of gene therapy are summarized in Table 59-1. Progress in gene therapy has been slow, reflecting substantial hurdles as investigators move closer to clinical applications. A few examples of potential applications highlight the status of this field and illustrate the requirements for successful gene therapy.

Significant therapeutic benefit can be achieved by the delivery of a single protein—insulin—to the patient with *diabetes mellitus*. In this case, the protein is secreted and can therefore be delivered extracellularly. The ability to produce recombinant human insulin has been a major advance. However, effective intensive insulin therapy remains difficult to achieve because of the exquisite regulation needed for dynamic metabolic responses to meals, exercise, and environmental stresses (Chap. 323). Clearly, much benefit would be gained if the insulin gene could be replaced and regulated normally. Although the gene has been cloned, and its regulatory elements have been characterized, insulin regulation requires multiple features of the normal pancreatic islet beta cell, including metabolic sensing mechanisms, an array of specific transcription factors that regulate the insulin gene, specialized protein-processing enzymes and secretory granules, and various channels that depolarize in response to metabolic signals. Thus, insulin gene therapy will not be successful in the absence of critical cellular features that recapitulate the function of the beta cell.

In contrast to insulin, where the goal is to secrete the protein for actions elsewhere in the body, many proteins function within a particular cell type, significantly complicating the delivery problem. For example, patients with *sickle cell anemia* or *β-thalassemia* have mutations in their β-globin genes (Chap. 91). In this case, one must introduce the replacement genes into specific cells and ensure regulated and sustained expression. The initial delivery and the long-term expression of the introduced gene are two distinct problems. Even if β-hemoglobin is expressed and regulated successfully in a red cell, the cell itself will only last for several weeks. Successful treatment there-

TABLE 59-1 *Examples of Disorders Potentially Amenable to Gene Therapy*

Disease	Gene Therapy Strategy
Inherited disorders	**Gene addition**
Cystic fibrosis	Express CFTR in pulmonary system and/or GI tract
Familial hypercholesterolemia	Express LDL receptor in liver
Hemophilias A and B	Express factor VIII or IX and secrete in circulation
Thalassemia	Express normal globin in red blood cells
Immunodeficiencies	Express deficient genes, such as adenosine deaminase
Metabolic disorders	Express missing enzymes or transporters
Duchenne's muscular dystrophy	Express mutant dystrophin protein in muscle cells
Retinitis pigmentosa (recessive)	Express normal protein in retina
	Gene correction
Lesch-Nyhan	Modify hypoxanthine phosphoribosyl transferase locus
Retinitis pigmentosa (dominant)	Correct missense mutation
Sickle cell disease	Correct β-globin mutation
Cystic fibrosis	Correct ΔF508 mutation in pulmonary system
Cardiovascular diseases	**Modify vascular biology**
Coronary artery restenosis	Block cell proliferation in vessel wall
Peripheral vascular disease	Induce angiogenesis
Hypertension	Express genes (e.g., tissue kallikrein) to induce vasodilation
Cancer	**Multiples approaches**
Many types	Express immunostimulants in or near malignant cells
	Express toxic genes in tumor cells (e.g., HSV-TK)
	Express genes to protect from chemotherapy in normal cells
Infectious diseases	
Viral diseases	Express genes that block viral replication or function, including ribozymes, decoys, dominant negative proteins
Many	Express antigens as recombinant vaccines
Miscellaneous	
Rheumatoid arthritis	Express anti-inflammatory cytokines in joints
Parkinson's disease	Express genes required for L-dopa synthesis in striatum
Neurodegenerative disease	Express neurotrophic factors

Note: CFTR, cystic fibrous transmembrane regulator; GI, gastrointestinal; LDL, low-density lipoprotein; HSV, herpes simplex virus; TK, thymidine kinase.

fore requires that the therapeutic genes be introduced into long-lived cells that can be renewed continuously to restore normal erythrocytes. Again, it is important to combine gene replacement or correction in the context of the normal host cell, in this case, an erythroblast.

Cystic fibrosis is caused by mutations in the cystic fibrosis transmembrane regulator (CFTR), a protein that regulates epithelial cell transport of Na^+ and Cl^- in the lung, gastrointestinal tract, sweat glands, and genitourinary system (Chap. 241). Gene delivery of the CFTR is more straightforward, in principle, as regulation of its expression level is less critical. The first attempt at gene therapy for cystic fibrosis was performed in 1993 using adenovirus-mediated transfer of the CFTR. This vector provides high level expression and is particularly effective for delivery to the lung. However, adenoviral expression is transient and induces immune responses that can limit subsequent viral administration. No clinical efficacy was demonstrated in the initial trials. Other viral delivery approaches are under investigation, but the challenge remains to target expression to particular tissues and to introduce the gene into a renewable population of cells.

The delivery of toxic, or suicide, genes to cancer cells is one of the most active areas of gene therapy research. Particularly for localized tumors, such as brain tumors or endocrine tumors, it may be possible to deliver highly toxic genes such as diphtheria toxin to tumor cells. For some tumor types, specific promoters can be used to express the toxic gene selectively in the cancer cell. Viruses have also been designed to replicate selectively in cells that lack certain tumor-suppressor genes, such as p53. An advantage of gene therapy for cancer cells is that long-term expression is not required. On the other hand, like chemotherapy or radiotherapy, gene therapy approaches must kill tumor cells with high efficacy without introducing significant toxicity. One novel approach is designed to increase the immunogenicity of tumors by expressing foreign antigens or cytokines that might increase endogenous immune responses.

FACTOR IX REPLACEMENT IN HEMOPHILIA B: POTENTIAL PARADIGM FOR GENE REPLACEMENT An excellent candidate for somatic gene therapy is hemophilia B, an X-linked blood clotting disorder caused by a deficiency of factor IX (Chap. 102). Factor IX is normally produced in the liver and secreted into the circulation. Clotting times can be corrected with <5% of the normal levels of factor IX; thus, low levels of factor IX should be sufficient for clinical benefit. The factor IX gene has been inserted into AAV vectors and introduced into muscle and liver cells. AAVs can be produced at high enough titers that the factor IX gene can be transferred to relatively large numbers of cells. Wild-type AAV has no known pathology, and the AAV particle does not provoke significant inflammatory or immune responses. Studies of AAV-mediated factor IX gene transfer in canine and murine models lacking factor IX have shown efficacy, although correction of the clotting abnormality is transient because inhibitory antibodies against human factor IX are generated in these species.

In an initial human clinical trial, AAV−factor IX was injected at multiple sites in a skeletal muscle that could be excised in the event of an unanticipated adverse event. At moderate doses of vector, factor IX expression and low levels of circulating factor IX were detected. The patients had decreased need for supplemental factor IX injections, but no significant decrease in clotting time was observed.

A different strategy has been employed to express factor VIII in dermal fibroblasts of patients with hemophilia A. Factor VIII was expressed under control of the fibronectin promoter and transferred ex vivo to dermal fibroblasts. The genetically modified cells were injected into the omentum. In four of six patients, plasma levels of factor VIII increased but then declined, probably because the cells were not renewable. This ex vivo approach represents a combination of gene transfer and cellular therapy.

CHARACTERISTICS OF STEM CELLS

The use of stem cell therapy addresses several of the shortcomings of gene therapy, including the need to express genes in specific types of host cells, such as erythrocytes or neurons, and the need to regulate gene expression in response to physiologic signals. Recent advances in stem cell biology greatly enhance the prospects for applying cell therapy (Table 59-2).

Although murine embryonic stem cells (ESCs) have been studied for many years, human ESCs were successfully cultured in vitro only in 1998. *Stem cells* are the undifferentiated progenitors that can develop into highly specialized cells that form the various organs. Stem cells vary in their replicative capacity and in their differentiation potential. A convenient classification of stem cells is as follows:

1. *Totipotent stem cells* can form a placenta and can develop into a complete embryo. These features are characteristic of the cells derived from the first few divisions of the fertilized oocyte.
2. *Pluripotent stem cells* are capable of forming tissues derived from all three major germline layers—endoderm, mesoderm, and ectoderm. These features are exhibited by making chimeras in which ESCs are injected into a blastocyst to become integrated into all tissues in the animal. Cells derived from the inner cell mass of the blastocyst will divide in culture indefinitely, retain a stable genome, and maintain the potential to contribute to all tissues. Common use of the term *embryonic stem cells* refers to lines with these characteristics.
3. *Multipotent stem cells* are the progenitors of cells in particular tissues. Tissues such as bone marrow, skin, intestinal tract, and liver have tremendous regenerative potential and continuously renew their cell populations. In these cases, the multipotent stem cells give rise to multiple cell types characteristic of a particular tissue.

Embryonic germ cells (EGCs) can be derived from the precursors of the germ line. Unlike totipotent ESCs, EGCs cannot be incorporated into the inner cell mass. However, cell lines established from the developing germ cells form chimeras and, like ESCs, contribute to all tissue lines of the embryo.

Stem cells are self-renewing while at the same time generating daughter cells that are more differentiated. The expression of telomerase, an enzyme critical for maintaining the telomeres, is consistent with the self-renewing feature of stem cells. Microarray studies, which examine patterns of gene expression, have identified several hundred genes that are shared by various types of stem cells. For continuous

TABLE 59-2 *Potential Applications of Stem Cell Therapy*

Disease	Stem Cell Therapy Goal
Hematologic disorders	
Leukemias	Replace marrow; graft vs tumor
Multiple myeloma	Replace marrow; graft vs tumor
Sickle cell anemia	Replace or correct erythrocytes
Autoimmune diseases	
Systemic lupus erythematosus	Reconstitute immune system
Crohn disease	Reconstitute immune system
Immune deficiency disorders	
Severe combined immune deficiency	Gene correction in immune cells
Wiscott-Aldrich	Gene correction in immune cells
Cardiovascular diseases	
Myocardial ischemia	Replace ischemic cardiomyocytes
Hepatic disease	
Hepatic failure	Replace or regenerate hepatocytes
Metabolic disorders	
Diabetes	Replace pancreatic islets or induce beta cell differentiation
Osteoporosis	Regenerate bone
Gaucher disease	Express glucocerebrosidase in macrophages
Musculoskeletal disorders	
Duchenne muscular dystrophy	Replace myoblasts
Neurologic disorders	
Parkinson's disease	Replace dopamine-producing neurons

renewal, some daughter cells must remain undifferentiated, while others become committed and generate more differentiated cells (Fig. 59-1).

The ability of ESCs to become incorporated into the germ line has allowed the genome of mouse ESCs to be manipulated in culture before being introduced into blastocysts to form chimeric mice (Chap. 56). Because these mice contain germ cells derived from the cultured ESCs, some animals born in the second generation are derived entirely from the cultured and manipulated ESCs. The genetic manipulation of ESCs has made the mouse a very useful model organism for studying the effects of targeted mutagenesis (gene knock-out or knock-in). Access to cultured ESCs offers the potential for differentiation into multiple tissue types, including cells of the blood, brain, and other tissues.

Emerging evidence indicates that adult tissues previously thought to have little or no plasticity, such as the central nervous system (CNS) and heart, do have some regenerative potential, implying the presence of stem cells, or the ability to attract and adopt circulating stem cells (Fig. 59-2). Thus, most adult tissues appear to contain stem cells, but the characteristics of these so called adult stem cells are highly variable and appear to depend on the tissue of origin as well as on the mesenchymal niche in which the cells are located. The hematopoietic system, gastrointestinal tract, and skin exemplify highly regenerative tissues in which stem cell populations have been partially characterized.

HEMATOPOIETIC STEM CELLS (See also Chap. 100)

Hematopoietic stem cells (HSCs) provide a relatively well-studied model of adult stem cells. Although HSCs are used routinely for bone marrow transplantation, the technology is complex to implement in part because the stem cells do not grow in culture. An additional difficulty is that the stem cell property is not a stable feature but is dependent on signals derived from other cells that provide a *stem cell niche*. Adherent mesenchymal cells in the bone marrow contain a second class of stem cell, called a *stromal stem cell* or a *mesenchymal stem cell*, which is capable of generating mesodermal cells such as connective tissue or muscle. Adherent cells from the bone marrow can be expanded for long periods to generate yet another stem cell with the potential to form many other cell types, including liver, endothelial, and neural cells. This *mesenchymal adult progenitor cell* may also

have the potential to form the various cell types of the blood. The implication is that the bone marrow mesenchyme can generate a pluripotent stem cell that is similar to ESCs, at least in some ways.

All blood cells, as well as vascular endothelial cells, are derived from a common progenitor termed the *hemangioblast*. Adoptive transfer of these cells demonstrates that the myeloid and lymphoid cells of a recipient are derived from the donor. Moreover, bone marrow from primary recipients can be transplanted into secondary and tertiary recipients, demonstrating that HSCs can self-renew.

HEMATOPOIETIC STEM CELL DIFFERENTIATION Bone marrow cells cultured in semi-solid medium give rise to colonies of a specific hematopoietic lineage, such as red cells [the colony forming unit (CFU) erythroid (CFU-E)], granulocytes (CFU-G), monocytes (CFU-M), or B cells (CFU-B). Less common are cells that give rise to multiple different cell types such as the colony-forming unit granulocyte, erythroid, macrophage (CFU-GEM). Current models predict that as pluripotent stem cells proliferate, they become progressively committed to fewer hematopoietic lineages and eventually to a single lineage. The differentiation of stem cells appears to involve the ordered sequential expression of transcription factors that dictate lineage. For example, the Gata-1 transcription factor is required for the terminal differentiation of erythroid and megakaryocytic cells, whereas the Gata-2 factor is required for proliferation of the most primitive multilineage hematopoietic cells. Interleukin (IL) receptor signaling (IL-7Rα and the common chain, γc) and the JAK3 kinase are critical for the production of both T and B cells.

HEMATOPOIETIC STEM CELL ENRICHMENT Repopulation assays with limiting numbers of mouse bone marrow cells have shown that the number of HSCs is at least 100-fold lower than the frequency of colony-forming cells. Fluorescence-activated cell sorting using monoclonal antibodies against cell surface proteins has allowed the separation of HSCs from cells that cannot repopulate irradiated mice. Most methods begin with the removal of bone marrow cells expressing markers associated with a specific lineage of peripheral blood cells. Lineage negative (Lin$-$) cells, which comprise <5% of bone marrow cells, are enriched for colony-forming cells and can repopulate irradiated mice, whereas Lin$+$ cells have no colony-forming cells. HSCs among the Lin$-$ cells are positively identified by the expression of the c-*kit* receptor and the Ly-6 antigen known as Sca-1. Lin$-$ c-*kit*$+$ Sca-1$+$ cells are highly enriched for HSCs as well as for cells capable of generating T and B cells (common lymphoid progenitors). The common lymphoid progenitors express the IL-7 receptor α-chain, whereas HSCs are IL-7R$\alpha-$. Lin$-$ c-*kit*$+$ Sca-1$+$ IL-7R$\alpha-$ cells represent the most highly enriched population of mouse HSCs.

Surrogate assays have been developed for the study of human HSCs. The long term culture initiating cell assay is an in vitro system in which single human bone marrow cells are placed on a layer of bone marrow–derived fibroblasts and endothelial cells. Some of these cells can be placed onto new feeder cells where they continue to produce colony-forming cells, indicating both proliferation and self-renewal.

The most widely used in vivo surrogate assays for human HSCs involve the injection of human hematopoietic cells into genetically immune-deficient mice. The simplest model uses mice homozygous for the severe combined immune deficiency (*scid*) mutation, a deletion of the p350 DNA-dependent kinase gene that causes a failure of T and B cell development. The NOD strain of mice is deficient in natural killer cells, and NOD mice homozygous for the *scid* mutation (NOD/SCID) are good hosts for human hematopoietic cells. Human cells engraft in these animals, and their progeny can be detected in the bone marrow for ≥12 weeks after transplantation. Using these and other models, human HSCs have been shown to be Lin$-$ and express the CD34 antigen. Lin$-$ CD34$+$ cells can be further enriched for HSCs by sorting for cells that express Thy-1 and do not express CD38. Lin$-$ CD34$+$ Thy-1$+$ CD38$-$ cells are highly enriched for HSCs and are present at a frequency of <0.02% in human bone marrow.

Human and mouse HSCs share the ability to export the vital dyes

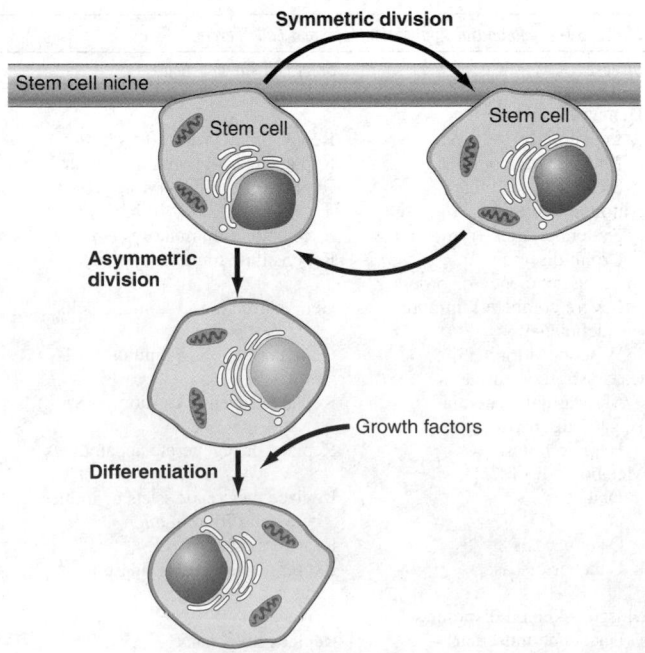

Symmetric division

Stem cell niche

Stem cell   Stem cell

Asymmetric division

Growth factors

Differentiation

FIGURE 59-1 Stem cells have the capacity for self-renewal through symmetric division or they can generate daughter cells that enter specific differentiation pathways, usually in response to extrinsic cell contacts or growth factor signals.

Hoechst 33342 and/or Rhodamine 123 efficiently. Dye export from HSCs is controlled by Bcrp, a member of the ATP-binding cassette transporter protein family that is expressed at high levels in HSCs. The ability to export Hoechst 33342 and Rhodamine 123 is shared by stem cells in other adult tissues, suggesting a common behavior of stem cells.

GENETIC MODIFICATION OF STEM CELLS

Stem cells are the ideal targets for gene therapy approaches. Because stem cells are able to self-renew, gene insertion into stem cells followed by engraftment into the patient should lead to a lifetime supply of corrected cells. In organs where cells are constantly lost and replaced, such as the hematopoietic and epithelial systems, introduction of a gene into a cell that cannot self-renew would require repeated treatments. The ability of stem cells to proliferate and differentiate into different types of mature cells ensures that the correct cell type will have the transferred gene. A problem is that most genes whose function needs to be replaced in disease states are expressed mainly in terminally differentiated cells and are not normally expressed in stem cells.

A variety of methods have been developed to transfer new genetic material into cells, including direct injection of DNA and gene transfer by viruses such as adenovirus, AAV or various RNA tumor viruses. Because RNA tumor viruses integrate into the genome of the target cell, they are currently the method of choice for stem cell gene transfer. The retroviruses have been modified such that most viral proteins are deleted, leaving only sequences important for viral integration. Recombinant virus vectors replace the protein-encoding sequences with a gene of interest. Because packaging sequences are deleted, the viruses do not replicate. The first recombinant RNA viral vectors were based on the Moloney murine leukemia viruses (MMuLV) but transduction efficiencies were very low (<1% of human cells). Although strategies to enhance MMuLV titers, attachment, and integration are ongoing, other retroviruses, such as vesicular stomatitis virus (VSV) and lentivirus, appear more promising. After the RNA virus genome enters the cell, it is converted into DNA by reverse transcriptase packaged with the RNA genome. Integration into the host genome occurs only during cell division. Thus, strategies to recruit cells into the cell cycle (e.g., transforming growth factor β antibodies) or to extend the G_1 to S-phase transition (e.g., antisense p27KIP-1 oligonucleotides) appear to enhance viral integration into stem cells.

HEMATOPOIETIC STEM CELL GENE THERAPY ■ Bone Marrow Transplantation

This is used in thousands of patients yearly and is an example of cell therapy (Chap. 100). The success of bone marrow transplantation reflects the fact that the many cell types of the blood are derived from progenitor stem cells. Bone marrow transplantation is used to treat numerous acquired (aplastic anemia, myelodysplasia, leukemia, and lymphoma) and inherited (immune deficiencies, thalassemia, and sickle cell disease) hematologic and immunologic diseases. Ongoing studies are examining its applicability in selected autoimmune disorders such as refractory systemic lupus erythematosus and Crohn disease. Genetic modification of HSCs may achieve certain therapeutic goals (e.g., resistance to chemotherapy) or allow correction of a genetic defect.

Severe Combined Immune Deficiencies (SCID)   This causes defects in both T and B lymphocyte production. Patients with SCID do not have cell-mediated or humoral immune responses and are subject to chronic life-threatening infections. The two most common forms of SCID are adenosine deaminase (ADA) deficiency (ADA-SCID) and deficiency of the X-linked IL-2 receptor γ-chain (γc, X-SCID) (Chap. 297). Bone

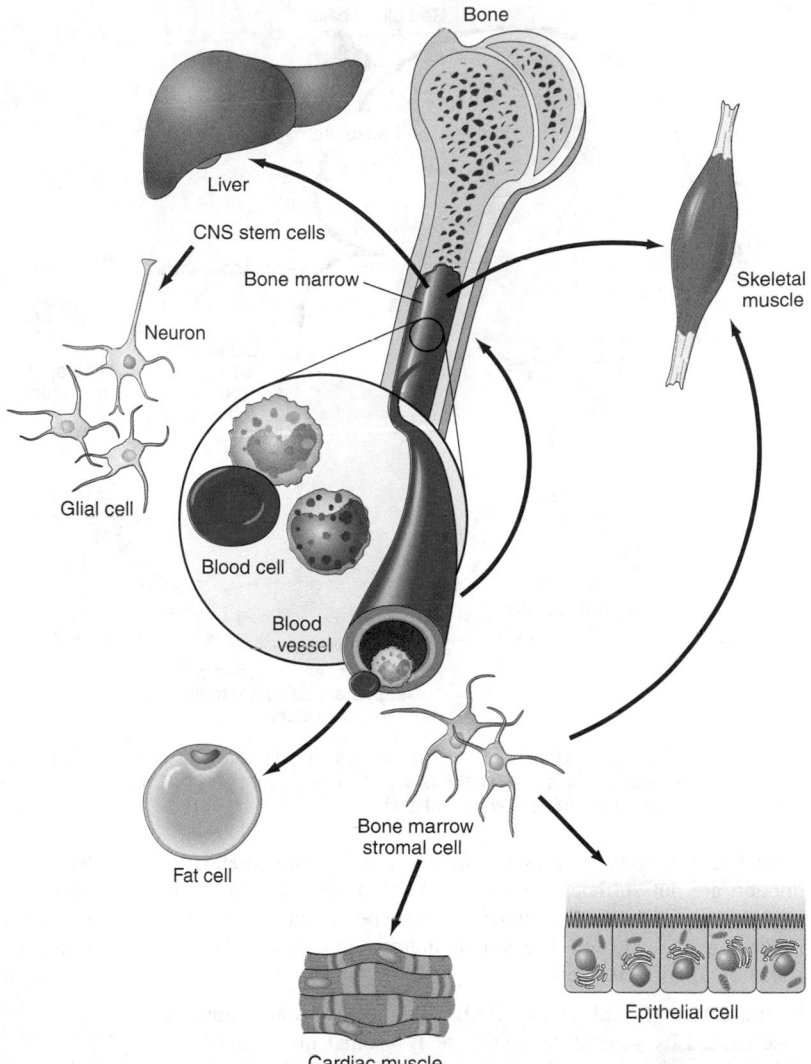

FIGURE 59-2   Plasticity of adult stem cells. CNS, central nervous system. [*Adapted from NIH Guide on Stem Cells: Scientific Promise and Future, 2001 (http://www.nih.gov/news/stemcell/scireport.htm.)*]

marrow transplantation from an MHC-matched related donor is the treatment of choice and is effective in about 70 to 80% of patients.

Because the gene defects are known, ADA-SCID and X-SCID patients without a matched donor are excellent candidates for stem cell gene therapy. The first human gene therapy trial was performed in 1991. T lymphocytes from two ADA-deficient patients receiving ADA enzyme therapy were expanded and transduced with a retrovirus vector containing the ADA gene. Between 2 and 10% of the transduced T cells expressed the transferred gene and were reinfused into the patients. Clinical improvements, including positive responses to vaccinations, were documented in both patients despite the gradual disappearance of transduced cells to background levels over the next 5 years. In 2000, the first successful stem cell gene therapy was reported. Cord blood CD34+ cells from X-SCID newborns transduced with a γc retrovirus vector were reinfused into the patients. Approximately 98% of circulating T lymphocytes and 1% of circulating B lymphocytes contained the γc vector, compared to <0.1% of myeloid cells, demonstrating in vivo selection. The patients responded to clinical vaccinations and have been living at home without supportive care. Unfortunately, two recipients of marrow transduced with a γc retrovirus vector have developed a clinical disorder that resembles leukemia, and further studies have been suspended.

Wiscott-Aldrich Syndrome (WAS)   This is an X-linked T lymphocyte disorder that can be accompanied by platelet dysfunction. Bone marrow transplantation can cure WAS, and in vivo selection for corrected cells has been demonstrated in several clinically normal WAS patients with

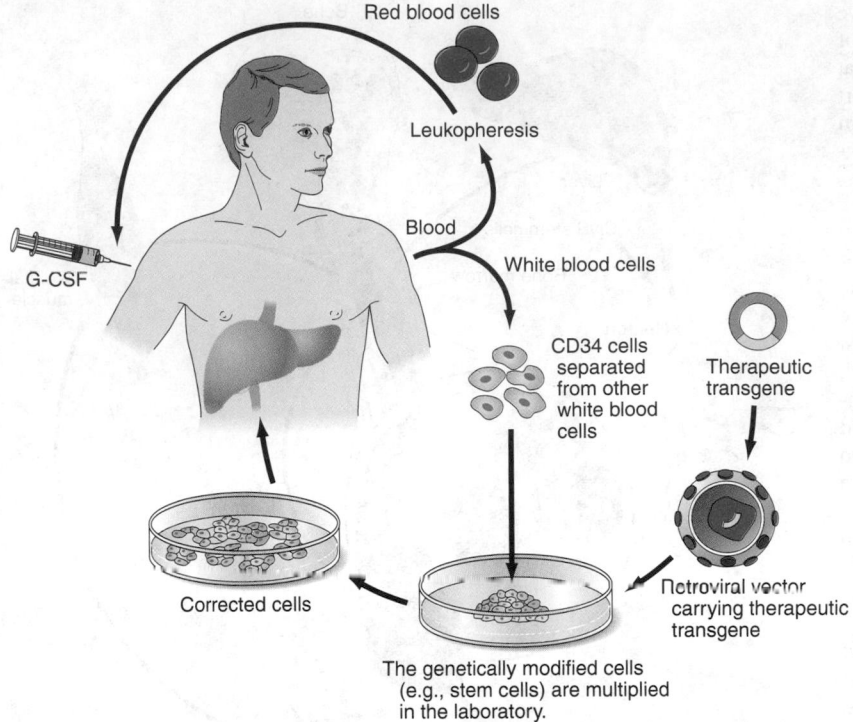

FIGURE 59-3 Strategy for introducing a therapeutic gene into hematopoietic stem cells to be used for autologous transplantation. [*Adapted from Pittsburgh Gaucher Disease Diagnosis and Treatment Program (http://gaucher.mgh.harvard.edu/centers/Pitt.html.)*]

Labels in figure: Red blood cells; Leukopheresis; Blood; White blood cells; G-CSF; CD34 cells separated from other white blood cells; Therapeutic transgene; Corrected cells; Retroviral vector carrying therapeutic transgene; The genetically modified cells (e.g., stem cells) are multiplied in the laboratory.

reversion mutations. At present, the low rates of human HSC transduction are not sufficient to treat diseases of granulocytes (chronic granulomatous disease), monocytes (Gaucher disease), or red cells (thalassemia, sickle cell disease), as there is no evidence for in vivo selection of corrected cells.

Gaucher Disease (See also Chap. 340) This is a lysosomal storage disease caused by genetic deficiency of lysosomal glucocerebrosidase. Clinical manifestations reflect the accumulation of lipid-laden macrophages, referred to as *Gaucher cells*, in bone, liver, spleen, and other viscera. Macrophage-targeted enzyme replacement therapy has proven highly effective in Gaucher disease. Trials are currently underway to harvest a patient's HSCs, insert a normal copy of the gene encoding glucocerebrosidase using retroviruses, and return the modified cells to the patient (Fig. 59-3). This strategy represents a potential paradigm for disorders in which stem cells can be modified and reconstituted into normal tissues.

EMBRYONIC AND SOMATIC STEM CELL TECHNOLOGY IN MEDICINE

CARDIOVASCULAR SYSTEM The high incidence of cardiac disease has made regeneration of damaged cardiac muscle of great interest. Skeletal myoblasts can improve function in the damaged heart, but it is not clear if these cells confer long-term benefit. Myocardium has some regenerative capacity; pluripotent cells hone into areas of damaged myocardium. In men who receive heart transplants from female donors, XY-derived host cells are found in the donor tissue, particularly in regions of injury. Stem cells with the potential to generate cardiac tissue have been isolated from the bone marrow. In mouse models, labeled ESCs are incorporated into ischemic regions of the heart and reconstitute vascular and connective tissue as well as cardiac myocytes, and they express a number of highly specific cardiac markers. These findings imply that local factors, perhaps produced in response to injury, induce specific patterns of cellular differentiation.

LIVER The liver is capable of extensive regeneration. In most cases, regeneration is not caused by rare stem cells but rather by the rapid division of differentiated hepatocytes. Hepatocytes can be transplanted serially from one animal to another, demonstrating their extensive proliferative potential in vivo. It has been difficult, however, to establish conditions for long-term growth in vitro. When hepatocytes are inadequate for regeneration, less abundant stem cells in the liver become activated. The term *oval cell* is often used to refer to stem cells in the liver, but other pluripotent cells also appear capable of liver regeneration. For example, hepatocytes may be generated from cell populations enriched for HSCs as demonstrated by engraftment into animals with an otherwise fatal deficiency in liver function. Pluripotent cells derived from the bone marrow and capable of long-term culture can differentiate into liver cells in vitro. There is also evidence that HSCs can fuse with hepatocytes to generate new liver cells. ESCs can also generate liver cells.

PANCREATIC ISLETS The liver and pancreas share a number of developmental transcription factors and growth factors but ultimately diverge into distinct organs containing highly specialized cells. The pancreas is composed of two distinct cell types, the exocrine and endocrine cells. The islets of Langerhans contain the beta cells, which secrete insulin. Improvements in islet transplantation and immunosuppression regimens have resulted in some patients being free of exogenous insulin administration. However, the number of donor islets is very limited. Expansion of the beta cell population in vivo or in vitro would be useful. Stem cells in the adult pancreas reside near the pancreatic ducts and are competent to differentiate into the endocrine cell types. Self-assembling structures similar to pancreatic islets can be derived from ESCs. These embryonic stem–derived cells secrete insulin in response to glucose. An alternative approach involves attempts to alter the differentiation program of hepatic progenitor cells by introducing pancreas-specific transcription factors, such as PDX-1, using adenoviruses. In mouse models, PDX-1 induces a small fraction of liver cells to produce insulin and some of these cells appear to cycle and maintain a beta cell–like phenotype. Although much work remains to characterize and improve these models, early findings suggest that stem cell plasticity may offer a means to increase the population of insulin-producing cells.

NERVOUS SYSTEM The peripheral nervous system (PNS) is generated by an epithelial to mesenchymal transition that occurs in the neural crest. The precursor cells of the PNS are flexible and can give rise to progeny with multiple fates. *PNS stem cells* with somewhat different properties can be found in adult as well as fetal animals.

The many complex cell types of the CNS are generated from epithelial precursors that are not committed to specific fates. *CNS stem cells* can be expanded in tissue culture and generate the three major cell types of the brain: neurons, astrocytes, and oligodendrocytes. Multipotent cells can be obtained in large numbers from both the developing and adult brain. Neurons generated by fetal and adult CNS stem cells form functional excitatory and inhibitory synapses.

Although many types of neurons exist in the brain, the idea that the brain is derived from stem cells has stimulated attempts to exploit the regenerative potential of stem cell therapy to treat neurologic disease in the adult brain.

Parkinson's Disease Transplantation of fetal brain tissue may provide benefit to patients with Parkinson's disease. Dopamine neurons that are functional and long lasting can be obtained by grafting the tissue of the ventral fetal midbrain into the dorsal striatum. Raclopride is a drug that binds to dopamine receptors and radioactive raclopride can be imaged in the human brain using position emission tomography scanning. The displacement of raclopride has been used to show that grafted midbrain neurons release dopamine. This is one of several types of data supporting the idea of transplantation in Parkinson's disease.

The current procedures also have limitations. For optimal effects, the tissue from several fetal brains must be used; as the tissue must be at a specific stage in development, the logistics are difficult. Unexplained adverse reactions have been noted, and efficacy is hard to predict. ESCs offer a potential solution to the problem of variable tissue sources as they expand for long periods in tissue culture and can differentiate through midbrain precursors into dopamine secreting neurons. *Nuclear transfer* represents another approach in which an ESC can be generated from an oocyte after replacing its nucleus with one from a host somatic cell. Preliminary studies show that these ntESCs also readily form dopamine neurons.

Both ESC-derived and normal midbrain neurons express receptors for glial derived neurotrophic factor (GDNF). Gene therapy data in monkeys suggest that GDNF delivery may provide clinical benefit in Parkinson's patients. Clinical trials with GDNF are now underway.

ESCs can also be differentiated into cells similar to motor neurons, which degenerate in amyotrophic lateral sclerosis. ESCs can also be used as a source for large numbers of oligodendrocytes, a cell type that is lost in multiple sclerosis.

New neurons are not normally produced in most regions of the adult CNS. However, large numbers of new neurons are produced in the adult dentate gyrus of the hippocampus and the olfactory bulb. Pyramidal neurons can be regenerated in the CA1 region of the hippocampus and the cerebral cortex. New neurons are also generated in the adult striatum. Thus, endogenous precursors may be capable of regenerating neurons after injury to the adult nervous system.

ETHICAL ISSUES

Gene and stem cell therapies raise ethical and socially contentious issues that must be addressed in parallel with the scientific and medical opportunities. Our society has great diversity with respect to religious beliefs, concepts of individual rights, tolerance for uncertainty and risk, and boundaries for how scientific interventions should be used to alter the outcome of disease. In the United States, the federal government has authorized research using existing human ESC lines but has restricted the use of federal funds for developing new human ESC lines. Studies of the characteristics of these existing lines, including whether they are stable over time, are ongoing.

In considering ethical issues associated with the use of stem cells, it is helpful to draw from experience with other scientific advances, such as organ transplantation, recombinant DNA technology, implantation of mechanical devices, neuroscience and cognitive research, in vitro fertilization, and prenatal genetic testing. From these and other precedents, we learn the importance of understanding and testing fundamental biology in the laboratory setting and in animal models before applying new techniques in carefully controlled clinical trials. When these trials occur, they must include full informed consent and have careful oversight by external review groups.

Ultimately, there will be medical interventions that are scientifically feasible but ethically or socially unacceptable to some members of a society. Since genetic research raises fundamentally difficult questions of identity, it has raised deep fears about our ability to assure justice, access, and safety in genetic medicine. Health care providers and experts with backgrounds in ethics, law, and sociology must help guard against the premature or inappropriate application of gene or stem cell therapies, and the inappropriate use of vulnerable population groups. On the other hand, these therapies offer important new strategies for the treatment of otherwise irreversible disorders. An open dialogue between the scientific community, physicians, patients and their advocates, lawmakers, and the lay population is critically important to raise and address important ethical issues and to balance the benefits and risks associated with gene and stem cell transfer.

FURTHER READING

BISHOP AE et al: Embryonic stem cells. J Pathol 197:424, 2002

IVANOVA NB et al: A stem cell molecular signature. Science 298:601, 2002

JIANG Y et al: Pluripotency of mesenchymal stem cells derived from adult marrow. Nature 418:41, 2002

KARBLING M, ESTROV Z: Adult stem cells for tissue repair—a new therapeutic concept? N Engl J Med 349:570, 2003

WAKAYAMA T et al: Differentiation of embryonic stem cell lines generated from adult somatic cells by nuclear transfer. Science 292:740, 2001

60 | NUTRITIONAL REQUIREMENTS AND DIETARY ASSESSMENT
Johanna Dwyer

Nutrients are substances that are not synthesized in the body in sufficient amounts and therefore must be supplied by the diet. Nutrient requirements for groups of healthy persons have been defined on the basis of experimental evidence. For good health we require energy-providing nutrients (protein, fat, and carbohydrate), vitamins, minerals, and water. Specific nutrient requirements include 9 essential amino acids, several fatty acids, 4 fat-soluble vitamins, 10 water-soluble vitamins, and choline. Several inorganic substances, including 4 minerals, 7 trace minerals, 3 electrolytes, and the ultratrace elements, must also be supplied in the diet.

The required amounts of the essential nutrients differ by age and physiologic state. Conditionally essential nutrients are not required in the diet but must be supplied to individuals who do not synthesize them in adequate amounts, such as those with genetic defects, those having pathologic states with nutritional implications, and developmentally immature infants. Many organic phytochemicals and zoochemicals present in foods have various health effects. For example, dietary fiber has beneficial effects on gastrointestinal function.

ESSENTIAL NUTRIENT REQUIREMENTS

ENERGY For weight to remain stable, energy intake must match energy output. The major components of energy output are resting energy expenditure (REE) and physical activity; minor sources include the energy cost of metabolizing food (thermic effect of food or specific dynamic action) and shivering thermogenesis (e.g., cold-induced thermogenesis). The average energy intake is about 2800 kcal/d for American men and about 1800 kcal/d for American women, though these estimates vary with body size and activity level. Formulas for estimating REE are useful for assessing the energy needs of an individual whose weight is stable. Thus, for males, REE = 900 + 10w, and for females, REE = 700 + 7w, where w is weight in kilograms. The calculated REE is then adjusted for physical activity level by multiplying by 1.2 for sedentary, 1.4 for moderately active, or 1.8 for very active individuals. The final figure provides an estimate of total caloric needs in a state of energy balance. →*For further discussion of energy balance in health and disease, see Chap. 62.*

PROTEIN Dietary protein consists of both essential and nonessential amino acids that are required for protein synthesis, whereas certain amino acids can also be used for energy and gluconeogenesis. The nine essential amino acids are histidine, isoleucine, leucine, lysine, methionine/cystine, phenylalanine/tyrosine, threonine, tryptophan, and valine. When energy intake is inadequate, protein intake must be increased, since ingested amino acids are diverted into pathways of glucose synthesis and oxidation. In extreme energy deprivation, protein-calorie malnutrition may ensue (Chap. 62).

For adults, the recommended dietary allowance (RDA) for protein is about 0.6 g/kg desirable body weight per day, assuming that energy needs are met and that the protein is of relatively high biologic value. Current recommendations for a healthy diet call for at least 10 to 14% of calories from protein. Biologic value tends to be highest for animal proteins, followed by proteins from legumes (beans), cereals (rice, wheat, corn), and roots. Combinations of plant proteins that complement one another in biologic value or combinations of animal and plant proteins can increase biologic value and lower total protein requirements.

Protein needs increase during growth, pregnancy, lactation, and rehabilitation during treatment of malnutrition. The tolerance to dietary protein is decreased in renal insufficiency and liver failure. Normal protein intake can precipitate encephalopathy in patients with cirrhosis of the liver or worsen uremia in those with renal failure.

FAT AND CARBOHYDRATE Fats are a concentrated source of energy and constitute on average 34% of calories in U.S. diets. However, for optimal health, fat intake should total no more than 30% of calories. Saturated fat and trans-fat should be limited to <10% of calories, and polyunsaturated fats to <10% of calories, with monounsaturated fats comprising the remainder of fat intake. At least 55% of total calories should be derived from carbohydrates. The brain requires about 100 g/d of glucose for fuel; other tissues use about 50 g/d. Over time, adaptations in carbohydrate needs are possible in hypocaloric states. For example, reduced insulin levels lead to adipose tissue breakdown and cause the body to burn more fatty acids. However, some tissues (e.g., brain and red blood cells) rely on glucose supplied either exogenously or from muscle proteolysis (Chap. 324).

WATER For adults, 1 to 1.5 mL water per kcal of energy expenditure is sufficient under usual conditions to allow for normal variations in physical activity, sweating, and solute load of the diet. Water losses include 50 to 100 mL/d in the feces, 500 to 1000 mL/d by evaporation or exhalation, and, depending on the renal solute load, ≥1000 mL/d in the urine. If external losses increase, intakes must increase accordingly to avoid underhydration. Fever increases water losses by approximately 200 mL/d per °C; diarrheal losses vary but may be as great as 5 L/d in severe diarrhea. Heavy sweating and vomiting also increase water losses. When renal function is normal and solute intakes are adequate, the kidneys can adjust to increased water intake by excreting up to 18 L/d of excess water (Chap. 319). However, obligatory urine outputs can compromise hydration status when there is inadequate intake or when losses increase in disease or kidney damage.

Infants have high requirements for water because of their large ratio of surface area to volume, the limited capacity of the immature kidney to handle high renal solute loads, and their inability to communicate their thirst. Increased water needs during pregnancy are low, perhaps an additional 30 mL/d. During lactation, milk production increases water requirements so that approximately 1000 mL/d of additional water is needed, or 1 mL for each mL of milk produced. Special attention must be paid to the water needs of the elderly, who have reduced total body water and blunted thirst sensation, and may be taking diuretics.

OTHER NUTRIENTS See Chap. 61 for detailed description of vitamins and trace minerals.

DIETARY REFERENCE INTAKES AND RECOMMENDED DIETARY ALLOWANCES

Fortunately, human life and well-being can be maintained within a fairly wide range for most nutrients. However, the capacity for adaptation is not infinite—too much, as well as too little, intake of a nutrient may have adverse effects or alter the health benefits conferred by another nutrient. Therefore, benchmark recommendations on nutrient intakes have been developed to guide clinical practice. These quantitative estimates of nutrient intakes are collectively referred to as the *dietary reference intakes* (DRIs). The DRIs supplant the *recommended daily allowances* (RDAs), the single reference values used in the United States since 1989. DRIs include the *estimated average requirement* (EAR) for nutrients, as well as three other reference values used for dietary planning for individuals: the RDA, the *adequate intake*

(AI), and the tolerable *upper level* (UL). The current DRIs for vitamins and elements are provided in Tables 60-1 and 60-2, respectively.

ESTIMATED AVERAGE REQUIREMENT When florid dietary deficiency diseases such as rickets, scurvy, xerophthalmia, and protein-calorie malnutrition were common, nutrient adequacy was assumed by the absence of clinical signs of a dietary deficiency disease. Later, it was determined that biochemical and other changes were evident long before the clinical deficiency became apparent. Consequently, criteria of adequacy are now based on biologic markers when they are available. Current efforts focus on the amount of a nutrient that reduces the risk of chronic degenerative diseases. Priority is given to sensitive biochemical, physiologic, or behavioral tests that reflect early changes in regulatory processes or maintenance of body stores of nutrients.

The EAR is the amount of a nutrient estimated to be adequate for half of the healthy individuals of a specific age and sex. The types of evidence and criteria used to establish nutrient requirements vary by nutrient, age, and physiologic group. The EAR is not an effective estimate of nutrient adequacy in individuals because it is a median requirement for a group; 50% of individuals in a group fall below the requirement and 50% fall above it. Thus, a person with a usual intake at the EAR has a 50% risk of an inadequate intake. For these reasons, other standards, described below, are more useful for clinical purposes.

RECOMMENDED DIETARY ALLOWANCES The RDA is the average daily dietary intake level that meets the nutrient requirements of nearly all healthy persons of a specific sex, age, life stage, or physiologic condition (such as pregnancy or lactation). The RDA is the nutrient-intake goal for planning diets of individuals.

The RDA is defined statistically as 2 standard deviations (SD) above the EAR to ensure that the needs of any given individual are met. The RDAs are used to formulate food guides such as the U.S. Department of Agriculture (USDA) Food Guide Pyramid for individuals, to create food exchange lists for therapeutic diet planning, and as a standard for describing the nutritional content of processed foods and nutrient supplements. The nutrient content in a food is stated by weight or as a percent of the daily value (DV), a variant of the RDA

TABLE 60-1   *Dietary Reference Intakes: Recommended Intakes for Individuals—Vitamins*

Life-Stage Group	Vitamin A, $\mu g/d^a$	Vitamin C, mg/d	Vitamin D, $\mu g/d^{b,c}$	Vitamin E, mg/d^d	Vitamin K, $\mu g/d$	Thiamine, mg/d	Riboflavin, mg/d	Niacin, mg/d^d	Vitamin B$_6$, mg/d	Folate, $\mu g/d^f$	Vitamin B$_{12}$, $\mu g/d$	Pantothenic Acid, mg/d	Biotin, $\mu g/d$	Choline, mg/d^g
Infants														
0–6 mo	400	40	5	4	2.0	0.2	0.3	2	0.1	65	0.4	1.7	5	125
7–12 mo	500	50	5	5	2.5	0.3	0.4	4	0.3	80	0.5	1.8	6	150
Children														
1–3 y	**300**	**15**	5	**6**	30	**0.5**	**0.5**	**6**	**0.5**	150	**0.9**	2	8	200
4–8 y	**400**	**25**	5	**7**	55	**0.6**	**0.6**	**8**	**0.6**	200	**1.2**	3	12	250
Males														
9–13 y	**600**	**45**	5	**11**	60	**0.9**	**0.9**	**12**	**1.0**	**300**	**1.8**	4	20	375
14–18 y	**900**	**75**	5	**15**	75	**1.2**	**1.3**	**16**	**1.3**	**400**	**2.4**	5	25	550
19–30 y	**900**	**90**	5	**15**	120	**1.2**	**1.3**	**16**	**1.3**	**400**	**2.4**	5	30	550
31–50 y	**900**	**90**	5	**15**	120	**1.2**	**1.3**	**16**	**1.3**	**400**	**2.4**	5	30	550
51–70 y	**900**	**90**	10	**15**	120	**1.2**	**1.3**	**16**	**1.7**	**400**	**2.4**^{h}	5	30	550
>70 y	**900**	**90**	15	**15**	120	**1.2**	**1.3**	**16**	**1.7**	**400**	**2.4**^{h}	5	30	550
Females														
9–13 y	**600**	**45**	5	**11**	60	**0.9**	**0.9**	**12**	**1.0**	**300**	**1.8**	4	20	375
14–18 y	**700**	**65**	5	**15**	75	**1.0**	**1.0**	**14**	**1.2**	**400**^{i}	**2.4**	5	25	400
19–30 y	**700**	**75**	5	**15**	90	**1.1**	**1.1**	**14**	**1.3**	**400**^{i}	**2.4**	5	30	425
31–50 y	**700**	**75**	5	**15**	90	**1.1**	**1.1**	**14**	**1.3**	**400**^{i}	**2.4**	5	30	425
51–70 y	**700**	**75**	10	**15**	90	**1.1**	**1.1**	**14**	**1.5**	**400**	**2.4**^{h}	5	30	425
>70 y	**700**	**75**	15	**15**	90	**1.1**	**1.1**	**14**	**1.5**	**400**	**2.4**^{h}	5	30	425
Pregnancy														
≤18 y	**750**	**80**	5	**15**	75	**1.4**	**1.4**	**18**	**1.6**	**600**^{j}	**2.6**	6	30	450
19–30 y	**770**	**85**	5	**15**	90	**1.4**	**1.4**	**18**	**1.9**	**600**^{j}	**2.6**	6	30	450
31–50 y	**770**	**85**	5	**15**	90	**1.4**	**1.4**	**18**	**1.9**	**600**^{j}	**2.6**	6	30	450
Lactation														
≤18 y	**1200**	**115**	5	**19**	75	**1.4**	**1.6**	**17**	**2.0**	**500**	**2.8**	7	35	550
19–30 y	**1300**	**120**	5	**19**	90	**1.4**	**1.6**	**17**	**2.0**	**500**	**2.8**	7	35	550
31–50 y	**1300**	**120**	5	**19**	90	**1.4**	**1.6**	**17**	**2.0**	**500**	**2.8**	7	35	550

Note: This table presents recommended dietary allowances (RDAs) in **bold type** and adequate intakes (AIs) in ordinary type. RDAs and AIs may both be used as goals for individual intake. RDAs are set to meet the needs of almost all individuals (97 to 98%) in a group. For healthy breastfed infants, the AI is the mean intake. The AI for other life stage and gender groups is believed to cover needs of all individuals in the group, but lack of data or uncertainty in the data prevent being able to specify with confidence the percentage of individuals covered by this intake.

^{a} As retinol activity equivalents (RAEs). 1 RAE = 1 μg retinol, 12 μg β-carotene, 24 μg α-carotene, or 24 μg β-cryptoxanthin. To calculate RAEs from retinol equivalents (REs) of provitamin A carotenoids in foods, divide the REs by 2. For preformed vitamin A in foods or supplements and for provitamin A carotenoids in supplements, 1 RE = 1 RAE.

^{b} As calciferol. 1 μg calciferol = 40 IU vitamin D.

^{c} In the absence of adequate exposure to sunlight.

^{d} As α-tocopherol. α-Tocopherol includes *RRR*-α-tocopherol, the only form of α-tocopherol that occurs naturally in foods, and the *2R*-stereoisomeric forms of α-tocopherol (*RRR*-, *RSR*-, *RRS*-, and *RSS*-α-tocopherol) that occur in fortified foods and supplements. It does not include the *2S*-stereoisomeric forms of α-tocopherol (*SRR*-, *SSR*-, *SRS*-, and *SSS*-α-tocopherol), also found in fortified foods and supplements.

^{e} As niacin equivalents (NE). 1 mg of niacin = 60 mg of tryptophan; 0–6 months = preformed niacin (not NE).

^{f} As dietary folate equivalents (DFEs). 1 DFE = 1 μg food folate = 0.6 μg of folic acid from fortified food or as a supplement consumed with food = 0.5 μg of a supplement taken on an empty stomach.

^{g} Although AIs have been set for choline, there are few data to assess whether a dietary supply of choline is needed at all stages of the life cycle, and it may be that the choline requirement can be met by endogenous synthesis at some of these stages.

^{h} Because 10 to 30% of older people may malabsorb food-bound B$_{12}$, it is advisable for those >50 years to meet their RDA mainly by consuming foods fortified with B$_{12}$ or a supplement containing B$_{12}$.

^{i} In view of evidence linking inadequate folate intake with neural tube defects in the fetus, it is recommended that all women capable of becoming pregnant consume 400 μg from supplements or fortified foods in addition to intake of food folate from a varied diet.

^{j} It is assumed that women will continue consuming 400 μg from supplements or fortified food until their pregnancy is confirmed and they enter prenatal care, which ordinarily occurs after the end of the periconceptional period—the critical time for formation of the neural tube.

Source: Food and Nutrition Board, Institute of Medicine—National Academy of Sciences Dietary Reference Intakes, 2000, 2002, reprinted with permission. Courtesy of the National Academy Press, Washington, DC. www.nap.edu

Life-Stage Group	Calcium, mg/d[a]	Chromium, μg/d	Copper, μg/d	Fluoride, mg/d	Iodine, μg/d	Iron, mg/d	Magnesium, mg/d	Manganese, mg/d	Molybdenum, μg/d	Phosphorus, mg/d	Selenium, μg/d	Zinc, mg/d
Infants												
0–6 mo	210	0.2	200	0.01	110	0.27	30	0.003	2	100	15	2
7–12 mo	270	5.5	220	0.5	130	**11**	75	0.6	3	275	20	**3**
Children												
1–3 y	500	11	**340**	0.7	**90**	**7**	**80**	1.2	**17**	**460**	**20**	**3**
4–8 y	800	15	**440**	1	**90**	**10**	**130**	1.5	**22**	**500**	**30**	**5**
Males												
9–13 y	1300	25	**700**	2	**120**	**8**	**240**	1.9	**34**	**1250**	**40**	**8**
14–18 y	1300	35	**890**	3	**150**	**11**	**410**	2.2	**43**	**1250**	**55**	**11**
19–30 y	1000	35	**900**	4	**150**	**8**	**400**	2.3	**45**	**700**	**55**	**11**
31–50 y	1000	35	**900**	4	**150**	**8**	**420**	2.3	**45**	**700**	**55**	**11**
51–70 y	1200	30	**900**	4	**150**	**8**	**420**	2.3	**45**	**700**	**55**	**11**
>70 y	1200	30	**900**	4	**150**	**8**	**420**	2.3	**45**	**700**	**55**	**11**
Females												
9–13 y	1300	21	**700**	2	**120**	**8**	**240**	1.6	**34**	**1250**	**40**	**8**
14–18 y	1300	24	**890**	3	**150**	**15**	**360**	1.6	**43**	**1250**	**55**	**9**
19–30 y	1000	25	**900**	3	**150**	**18**	**310**	1.8	**45**	**700**	**55**	**8**
31–50 y	1000	25	**900**	3	**150**	**18**	**320**	1.8	**45**	**700**	**55**	**8**
51–70 y	1200	20	**900**	3	**150**	**8**	**320**	1.8	**45**	**700**	**55**	**8**
>70 y	1200	20	**900**	3	**150**	**8**	**320**	1.8	**45**	**700**	**55**	**8**
Pregnancy												
≤18 y	1300	29	**1000**	3	**220**	**27**	**400**	2.0	**50**	**1250**	**60**	**12**
19–30 y	1000	30	**1000**	3	**220**	**27**	**350**	2.0	**50**	**700**	**60**	**11**
31–50 y	1000	30	**1000**	3	**220**	**27**	**360**	2.0	**50**	**700**	**60**	**11**
Lactation												
≤18 y	1300	44	**1300**	3	**290**	**10**	**360**	2.6	**50**	**1250**	**70**	**13**
19–30 y	1000	45	**1300**	3	**290**	**9**	**310**	2.6	**50**	**700**	**70**	**12**
31–50 y	1000	45	**1300**	3	**290**	**9**	**320**	2.6	**50**	**700**	**70**	**12**

Note: This table presents recommended dietary allowances (RDAs) in **bold type** and adequate intakes (AIs) in ordinary type. RDAs and AIs may both be used as goals for individual intake. RDAs are set to meet the needs of almost all individuals (97 to 98%) in a group. For healthy breastfed infants, the AI is the mean intake. The AI for other life stage and gender groups is believed to cover needs of all individuals in the group, but lack of data or uncertainty in the data prevent being able to specify with confidence the percentage of individuals covered by this intake.
Source: Food and Nutrition Board, Institute of Medicine—National Academy of Sciences Dietary Reference Intakes, 2000, 2002, reprinted with permission. Courtesy of the National Academy Press, Washington, DC. www.nap.edu

that, for an adult, represents the highest RDA for an adult consuming 2000 kcal/d.

The risk of dietary inadequacy increases as intake falls further below the RDA. However, the RDA is an overly generous criterion for evaluating nutrient adequacy. For example, by definition the RDA exceeds the actual requirements of all but about 2 to 3% of the population. Therefore, many people whose intake falls below the RDA may still be getting enough of the nutrient.

ADEQUATE INTAKE It is not possible to set an RDA for some nutrients that do not have an established EAR. In this circumstance, the AI is based on observed, or experimentally determined, approximations of nutrient intakes in healthy people. In the DRIs established to date, AIs rather than RDAs are proposed for infants up to age 1 year, as well as for calcium, chromium, vitamin D, fluoride, manganese, pantothenic acid, biotin, and choline for persons of all ages.

TOLERABLE UPPER LEVELS OF NUTRIENT INTAKE Excessive nutrient intake can disturb body functions and cause acute, progressive, or permanent disabilities. The tolerable UL is the highest level of chronic nutrient intake (usually daily) that is unlikely to pose a risk of adverse health effects for most of the population. Data on the adverse effects of large amounts of many nutrients are unavailable or too limited to establish a UL. Therefore, the lack of a UL does *not* mean that the risk of adverse effects from high intake is nonexistent. Healthy individuals derive no established benefit from consuming nutrient levels above the RDA or AI. Individual nutrients in foods that most people eat rarely reach levels that exceed the UL. However, nutritional supplements provide more concentrated amounts of nutrients per dose and, as a result, pose a potential risk of toxicity. Nutrient supplements are labeled with "supplement facts" that express the amount of nutrient in absolute units or as the percent of the DV provided per recommended serving size. Total nutrient consumption, including both food and supplements, should not exceed RDA levels.

FACTORS ALTERING NUTRIENT NEEDS

The DRIs are affected by age, sex, rate of growth, pregnancy, lactation, physical activity, composition of diet, concomitant diseases, and drugs. When only slight differences exist between the requirements for nutrient sufficiency and excess, dietary planning becomes more difficult.

PHYSIOLOGIC FACTORS Growth, strenuous physical activity, pregnancy, and lactation increase needs for energy and several essential nutrients. Energy needs rise during pregnancy, due to the demands of fetal growth, and during lactation, because of the increased energy required for milk production. Energy needs decrease with loss of lean body mass, the major determinant of REE. Because both health and physical activity tend to decline with age, energy needs in older persons, especially those over 70, tend to be less than those of younger persons.

DIETARY COMPOSITION Dietary composition affects the biologic availability and utilization of nutrients. For example, the absorption of iron may be impaired by high amounts of calcium or lead; non-heme iron uptake may be impaired by the lack of ascorbic acid and amino acids in the meal. Protein utilization by the body may be decreased when essential amino acids are not present in sufficient amounts. Animal foods, such as milk, eggs, and meat, have high biologic values with most of the needed amino acids present in adequate amounts. Plant proteins in corn (maize), soy, and wheat have lower biologic values and must be combined with other plant or animal proteins to achieve optimal utilization by the body.

ROUTE OF ADMINISTRATION The RDAs apply only to oral intakes. When nutrients are administered parenterally, similar values can sometimes be used for amino acids, carbohydrates, fats, sodium, chloride, potassium, and most of the vitamins, since their intestinal absorption is nearly 100%. However, the oral bioavailability of most mineral elements may be only half that obtained by parenteral administration. For

TABLE 60-3 *The USDA Food Guide Pyramid for Healthy Persons*

Servings and Examples of Standard Portion Sizes	Lower: 1600 kcal	Moderate: ~2200 kcal	Higher: ~2800 kcal

Bread group
    1 slice bread; 1 oz. ready-to-eat cereal;
    ½ cup cooked cereal, rice, or pasta
	6	9	22

Vegetable group
    1 cup raw leafy vegetables; ½ cup other vegetables, cooked
    or chopped raw; ¾ cup vegetable juice
	3	4	5

Fruit group
    1 medium banana, apple, or orange; ½ cup chopped,
    cooked, or canned fruit; ¾ cup fruit juice
	2	3	4

Milk group
    1 cup milk or yogurt, 1.5 oz natural cheese,
    1 oz processed cheese
	2–3[a]	2–3[a]	1–3[a]

Meat group
    2–3 oz cooked lean meat, poultry or fish;
    ½ cup cooked dry beans; 1 egg or 2 Tbsp.
    peanut butter count as 1 oz lean meat
	5	5	7

Total fat, g	53	73	93
Total added sugars, tsp	6	12	18

[a] Women who are pregnant or breastfeeding, teenagers, and young adults to age 24 need 3 servings.

Source: US Department of Agriculture, Human Nutrition Information Service. *The Food Guide Pyramid*, Home and Garden Bulletin Number 252, US Department of Agriculture, Washington DC, August 1992.

some nutrients that are not readily stored in the body, or cannot be stored in large amounts, timing of administration may also be important. For example, amino acids cannot be used for protein synthesis if they are not supplied together; instead they will be used for energy production.

DISEASE Specific dietary deficiency diseases include protein-calorie malnutrition; iron, iodine, and vitamin A deficiency; megaloblastic anemia due to vitamin B_{12} or folic acid deficiency; vitamin D–deficiency rickets; and scurvy, beriberi, and pellagra (Chaps. 61 and 62). Each deficiency disease is characterized by imbalances at the cellular level between the supply of nutrients or energy and the body's nutritional needs for growth, maintenance, and other functions. Imbalances in nutrient intakes are recognized as risk factors for certain chronic degenerative diseases, such as saturated fat and cholesterol in coronary artery disease; sodium in hypertension; obesity in hormone-dependent endometrial and breast cancers; and ethanol in alcoholism. Since the etiology and pathogenesis of these disorders are multifactorial, diet is only one of many risk factors. Osteoporosis, for example, is associated with calcium deficiency, as well as risk factors related to environment (e.g., smoking, sedentary lifestyle), physiology (e.g., estrogen deficiency), genetic determinants (e.g., defects in collagen metabolism), and drug use (chronic steroids) (Chap. 333).

DIETARY ASSESSMENT

In clinical situations, nutritional assessment is an iterative process that involves: (1) screening for malnutrition, (2) assessing the diet and other data to establish either the absence or presence of malnutrition and its possible causes, and (3) planning for the most appropriate nutritional therapy. Some disease states affect the bioavailability, requirements, utilization, or excretion of specific nutrients. In these circumstances, specific measurements of various nutrients may be required to ensure adequate replacement (Chap. 62).

Most health care facilities have a nutrition screening process in place for identifying possible malnutrition after hospital admission. Nutritional screening is required by the Joint Commission on Accreditation of Healthcare Organizations (JCAHO), but there are no universally recognized or validated standards. The factors that are usually assessed include abnormal weight for height or body mass index (e.g., BMI <19 or >25); reported weight change (involuntary loss or gain of >5 kg in the past 6 months) (Chap. 36); diagnoses with known nutritional implications (metabolic disease, any disease affecting the gastrointestinal tract, alcoholism, and others); present therapeutic dietary prescription; chronic poor appetite; presence of chewing and

swallowing problems or major food intolerances; need for assistance with preparing or shopping for food, eating, or other aspects of self care; and social isolation. Reassessment of nutrition status should occur periodically in hospitalized patients—at least once every week.

A more complete dietary assessment is indicated for patients who exhibit a high risk of malnutrition on nutrition screening. The type of assessment varies based on the clinical setting, severity of the patient's illness, and stability of his or her condition.

ACUTE CARE SETTINGS In acute care settings, anorexia, various diseases, test procedures, and medications can compromise dietary intake. Under such circumstances, the goal is to identify and avoid inadequate intake and assure appropriate alimentation. Dietary assessment focuses on what patients are currently eating, whether they are able and willing to eat, and whether they experience any problems with eating. Dietary intake assessment is based on information from observed intakes; medical record; history; clinical examination; and anthropometric, biochemical, and functional status. The objective is to gather enough information to establish the likelihood of malnutrition due to poor dietary intake or other causes to assess whether nutritional therapy is indicated.

Simple observations may suffice to suggest inadequate oral intake. These include dietitians' and nurses' notes, the amount of food eaten on trays, frequent tests and procedures that are likely to cause meals to be skipped, nutritionally inadequate diet orders such as clear liquids or full liquids for more than a few days, fever, gastrointestinal distress, vomiting, diarrhea, a comatose state, and diseases or treatments that involve any part of the alimentary tract. Acutely ill patients with diet-related diseases such as diabetes need assessment because an inappropriate diet may exacerbate these conditions and adversely affect other therapies. Abnormal biochemical values [serum albumin levels <35 g/L (<3.5 mg/dL); serum cholesterol levels <3.9 mmol/L (<150 mg/dL)] are nonspecific but may also indicate a need for further nutritional assessment.

Most therapeutic diets offered in hospitals are calculated to meet individual nutrient requirements and the RDA. Exceptions include clear liquids, some full liquid diets, and test diets, which are inadequate for several nutrients and should not be used, if possible, for more than 24 h. As much as half of the food served to hospitalized patients is not eaten, and so it cannot be assumed that the intakes of hospitalized patients are adequate. Dietary assessment should compare how much and what food the patient has consumed with the diet that has been provided. Major deviations in intakes of energy, protein, fluids, or other nutrients of special concern for the patient's illness should be noted and corrected.

Nutritional monitoring is especially important for patients who are very ill and who have extended lengths of stay. Patients who are fed by special enteral and parenteral routes also require special nutritional assessment and monitoring by physicians with training in nutrition support and/or dietitians with certification in nutrition support (Chap. 63).

AMBULATORY SETTINGS The aim of dietary assessment in the outpatient setting is to determine whether the patient's usual diet is a health risk in itself or if it contributes to existing chronic disease-related problems. Dietary assessment also provides the basis for planning a diet that fulfills therapeutic goals while ensuring patient adherence. The outpatient dietary assessment should review the adequacy of present and usual food intakes, including vitamin and mineral supplements, medications, and alcohol, as all of these may affect the patient's nutritional status. The assessment should focus on the dietary constituents that are most likely to be involved or compromised by a specific diagnosis, as well as any comorbidities that are present. More than one day's intake should be reviewed to provide a better representation of the usual diet.

There are many ways to assess the adequacy of the patient's habitual diet. These include a food guide, a food exchange list, a diet history, or a food frequency questionnaire. A commonly used food guide for healthy persons is the USDA's food pyramid, which is useful as a basis for identifying inadequate intakes of essential nutrients, as well as likely excesses in fat, saturated fat, sodium, sugar, and alcohol (Table 60-3). The guide can be adjusted by varying the number of servings to provide for the needs of persons of different ages and life cycle stages. Those who follow ethnic or unusual dietary patterns may need extra instruction on how foods should be categorized, as well as the appropriate portion sizes that constitute a serving. The process of reviewing the guide with patients helps them transition to healthier dietary patterns and identifies food groups eaten in excess of recommendations or in insufficient quantities. For those on therapeutic diets, assessment against food exchange lists may be useful. These include, for example, the American Diabetes Association food exchange lists for diabetes, or the American Dietetic Association food exchange lists for renal disease.

NUTRITIONAL STATUS ASSESSMENT Full nutritional status assessment is reserved for seriously ill patients and those at very high nutritional risk when the cause of malnutrition is still uncertain after initial clinical evaluation and dietary assessment. It involves multiple dimensions, including documentation of dietary intake, anthropometric measurements, biochemical measurements of blood and urine, clinical examination, health history, and functional status. →*For further discussion of nutritional assessment, see Chap. 62.*

FURTHER READING

OWEN OE et al: A reappraisal of the caloric requirements of men. Am J Clin Nutr 46:875, 1987

———: A reappraisal of caloric requirements in healthy women. Am J Clin Nutr 44:1, 1986

STANDING COMMITTEE ON THE SCIENTIFIC EVALUATION OF DIETARY REFERENCE INTAKES, FOOD AND NUTRITION BOARD, INSTITUTE OF MEDICINE: *Dietary Reference Intakes for Vitamin A, Vitamin K, Arsenic, Boron, Chromium, Copper, Iodine, Iron, Manganese, Molybdenum, Nickel, Silicon, Vanadium, and Zinc.* Washington, National Academy Press, 2001

———: *Dietary Reference Intakes: Applications in Dietary Assessment.* Washington, National Academy Press, 2000

———: *Dietary Reference Intakes for Calcium, Phosphorus, Magnesium, Vitamin D, and Fluoride.* Washington, National Academy Press, 1997

61 | VITAMIN AND TRACE MINERAL DEFICIENCY AND EXCESS
Robert M. Russell

Vitamins and trace minerals are required constituents of the human diet since they are either inadequately synthesized or not synthesized in the human body. Only small amounts of these substances are needed for carrying out essential biochemical reactions (e.g., acting as coenzymes or prosthetic groups). Overt vitamin or trace mineral deficiencies are rare in western countries due to a plentiful, varied, and inexpensive food supply; however, multiple nutrient deficiencies may appear together in persons who are ill or alcoholic. Moreover, subclinical vitamin and trace mineral deficiencies, as diagnosed by laboratory testing, are quite common in the normal population—especially in the geriatric age group.

Body stores of vitamins and minerals vary tremendously. For example, vitamin B_{12} and vitamin A stores are large, and an adult may not become deficient for 1 or more years after being on a depleted diet. However, folate and thiamine may become depleted within weeks when eating a deficient diet. Therapeutic modalities can deplete essential nutrients from the body; for example, hemodialysis removes water-soluble vitamins, which must be replaced by supplementation.

There are several roles for vitamins and trace minerals in diseases: (1) deficiencies of vitamins and minerals may be caused by disease states such as malabsorption; (2) both deficiency and excess of vitamins and minerals can cause disease in and of themselves (e.g., vitamin A intoxication and liver disease); and (3) vitamins and minerals in high doses may be used as drugs (e.g., niacin for hypercholesterolemia). The hematologic-related vitamins and minerals (Chaps. 90, 92) are considered only briefly in this chapter, as are the bone-related vitamins and minerals (vitamin D, calcium, phosphorus; Chap. 331), since they are covered elsewhere (see Tables 61-1, 61-2, and Fig. 61-1).

VITAMINS

THIAMINE (VITAMIN B₁)

Thiamine was the first B vitamin to be identified and is therefore also referred to as vitamin B_1. Thiamine functions in the decarboxylation of α-ketoacids, such as pyruvate α-ketoglutarate, and branched-chain amino acids and thus is a source of energy generation. In addition, thiamine pyrophosphate acts as a coenzyme for a transketolase reaction that mediates the conversion of hexose and pentose phosphates. It has also been postulated that thiamine plays a role in peripheral nerve conduction, although the exact chemical reactions underlying this function are unknown.

FOOD SOURCES The median intake of thiamine in the United States from food alone is 2 mg/d. Primary food sources for thiamine include yeast, pork, legumes, beef, whole grains, and nuts. Milled and polished rice contain little thiamine, if any. Thiamine deficiency is therefore more common in cultures that rely heavily on a rice-based diet. Tea, coffee (caffeinated and decaffeinated), raw fish, and shellfish contain thiamineases, which can destroy the vitamin. Thus, drinking large amounts of tea or coffee can theoretically lower thiamine body stores.

DEFICIENCY Most dietary deficiency of thiamine worldwide is the result of poor dietary intake. In western countries, the primary causes of thiamine deficiency are alcoholism and chronic illness, such as cancer. Alcohol is known to interfere directly with the absorption of thiamine and with the synthesis of thiamine pyrophosphate. Thiamine should always be replenished when refeeding a patient with alcoholism, as carbohydrate repletion without adequate thiamine can precipitate acute thiamine deficiency.

Thiamine deficiency in its early stage induces anorexia and nonspecific symptoms (e.g., irritability). Prolonged thiamine deficiency causes beriberi, which is classically categorized as wet or dry, although there is considerable overlap. In either form of beriberi, patients may complain of pain and parathesia. *Wet beriberi* presents primarily with cardiovascular symptoms, due to impaired myocardial energy metabolism and dysautonomia, and can occur after 3 months of a thiamine-deficient diet. Patients present with an enlarged heart, tachycardia, high-output congestive heart failure, peripheral edema, and peripheral neuritis. Patients with *dry beriberi* present with a symmetric peripheral neuropathy of the motor and sensory systems with diminished reflexes. The neuropathy affects the legs most markedly, and patients have difficulty rising from a squatting position.

Alcoholic patients with chronic thiamine deficiency may also have central nervous system manifestations known as *Wernicke's enceph-*

TABLE 61-1 *Principal Clinical Findings of Vitamin Malnutrition*

Nutrient	Clinical Finding	Dietary Level per Day Associated with Overt Deficiency in Adults	Contributing Factors to Deficiency
Thiamine	Beriberi: neuropathy, muscle weakness and wasting, cardiomegaly, edema, ophthalmoplegia, confabulation	<0.3 mg/1000 kcal	Alcoholism
Riboflavin	Magenta tongue, angular stomatitis, seborrhea, cheilosis	<0.6 mg	—
Niacin	Pellagra: pigmented rash of sun-exposed areas, bright red tongue, diarrhea, apathy, memory loss, disorientation	<9.0 niacin equivalents	Alcoholism, vitamin B_6 deficiency, riboflavin deficiency
Vitamin B_6	Seborrhea, glossitis convulsions, neuropathy, depression, confusion, microcytic anemia	<0.2 mg	Alcoholism, isoniazid
Folate	Megaloblastic anemia, atrophic glossitis, depression, ↑ homocysteine,	<100 µg/d	Alcoholism, sulfasalazine, pyrimethamine, triamterene
Vitamin B_{12}	Megaloblastic anemia, loss of vibratory and position sense, abnormal gait, dementia, impotence, loss of bladder and bowel control, ↑ homocysteine, ↑ methylmalonic acid	<1.0 µg/d	Gastric atrophy (pernicious anemia), terminal ileal disease, strict vegetarianism
Vitamin C	Scurvy: petechiae, ecchymosis, coiled hairs, inflamed and bleeding gums, joint effusion, poor wound healing	<10 mg/d	Smoking, alcoholism
Vitamin A	Xerophthalmia, nightblindness, Bitot spots, follicular hyperkeratosis, impaired embryonic development, immune dysfunction	<300 µg/d	Fat malabsorption, infection, measles, alcoholism, protein-energy malnutrition
Vitamin D	Rickets: skeletal deformation, rachitic rosary, bowed legs; osteomalacia	<2.0 µg/d	Aging, lack of sunlight exposure, fat malabsorption
Vitamin E	Peripheral neuropathy, spinocerebellar ataxia, skeletal muscle atrophy, retinopathy	Not described unless underlying contributing factor is present	Occurs only with fat malabsorption, or genetic abnormalities of vitamin E metabolism/transport
Vitamin K	Elevated prothrombin time, bleeding	<10 µg/d	Fat malabsorption, liver disease, antibiotic use

alopathy, consisting of horizontal nystagmus, ophthalmoplegia (due to weakness of one or more extraocular muscles), cerebellar ataxia, and mental impairment (Chap. 372). When there is an additional loss of memory and a confabulatory psychosis, the syndrome is known as *Wernicke-Korsakoff syndrome*.

The laboratory diagnosis of thiamine deficiency is usually made by a functional enzymatic assay of transketolase activity measured before and after the addition of thiamine pyrophosphate. A >25% stimulation by the addition of thiamine pyrophosphate (an activity coefficient of 1.25) is taken as abnormal. Thiamine or the phosphorylated esters of thiamine in serum or blood can also be measured by high-performance liquid chromatography (HPLC) to detect deficiency.

℞ TREATMENT

In acute thiamine deficiency with either cardiovascular or neurologic signs, 100 mg/d of thiamine should be given parenterally for 7 days, followed by 10 mg/d orally until there is complete recovery. Cardiovascular improvement occurs in ≤12 h, and ophthalmoplegic improvement occurs within 24 h. Other manifestations gradually clear, although psychosis in the Wernicke-Korsakoff syndrome may be permanent or persist for several months.

TOXICITY Although anaphylaxis has been reported after high doses of thiamine, no adverse effects have been recorded from either food or supplements at high doses. Thiamine supplements may be bought over the counter in doses of up to 50 mg/d.

RIBOFLAVIN (VITAMIN B₂)

Riboflavin is important for the metabolism of fat, carbohydrate, and protein, reflecting its role as a respiratory coenzyme and an electron donor. Enzymes that contain flavin adenine dinucleotide (FAD) or flavin-mononucleotide (FMN) as prosthetic groups are known as *flavoenzymes* (e.g., succinic acid dehydrogenase, monoamine oxidase, glutathione reductase).

Although much is known about the chemical and enzymatic reactions of riboflavin, the clinical manifestations of riboflavin deficiency are nonspecific and similar to those of other B vitamin deficiencies.

Riboflavin deficiency is manifested principally by lesions of the mucocutaneous surfaces of the mouth and skin (Table 61-1). In addition to the mucocutaneous lesions, corneal vascularization, anemia, and personality changes have been described with riboflavin deficiency.

DEFICIENCY AND EXCESS Riboflavin deficiency is almost always due to dietary deficiency. Milk, other dairy products, and enriched breads and cereals are the most important dietary sources of riboflavin in the United States, although lean meat, fish, eggs, broccoli, and legumes are also good sources. Riboflavin is extremely sensitive to light, and milk should be stored in containers that protect against photodegradation. Laboratory diagnosis of riboflavin deficiency can be made by measurement of red blood cell or urinary riboflavin concentrations or by measurement of erythrocyte glutathione reductase activity, with and without added FAD. Because the capacity of the gastrointestinal tract to absorb riboflavin is limited (~20 mg if given in one oral dose), riboflavin toxicity has not been described.

NIACIN (VITAMIN B₃)

The term *niacin* refers to nicotinic acid and nicotinamide and their biologically active derivatives. Nicotinic acid and nicotinamide serve as precursors of two coenzymes, nicotinamide adenine dinucleotide (NAD) and NAD phosphate (NADP), which are important in numerous oxidation and reduction reactions in the body. In addition, NAD and NADP are active in adenine diphosphate–ribose transfer reactions involved in DNA repair and calcium mobilization.

METABOLISM AND REQUIREMENTS Nicotinic acid and nicotinamide are absorbed well from the stomach and small intestine. Niacin bioavailability is high from beans, milk, meat, and eggs; bioavailability from cereal grains is lower. Since flour is enriched with the "free" niacin (i.e., non-coenzyme form), bioavailability is excellent. Median intakes of niacin in the United States considerably exceed the recommended dietary allowance (RDA).

The amino acid tryptophan can be converted to niacin with an efficiency of 60:1 by weight. Thus, the RDA for niacin is expressed in niacin equivalents. A lower conversion of tryptophan to niacin occurs if a patient is vitamin B_6- or riboflavin-deficient or in the presence of isoniazid. The urinary excretion products of niacin include 2-pyridone and 2-methyl nicotinamide, measurements of which are used in diagnosis of niacin deficiency.

DEFICIENCY Niacin deficiency causes *pellagra*, which is mostly found among people eating corn-based diets in parts of China, Africa, and India. Pellagra in North America is found mainly among alcoholics; in patients with congenital defects of intestinal and kidney absorption of tryptophan (Hartnup's disease; Chap. 343); and in patients with carcinoid syndrome (Chap. 329), where there is increased conversion of tryptophan to serotonin. The early symptoms of pellagra include loss of appetite, generalized weakness and irritability, abdominal pain, and vomiting. Bright-red glossitis then ensues, followed by a characteristic skin rash that is pigmented and scaling, particularly in skin areas exposed to sunlight. This rash is known as "Casal's necklace" because it forms a ring around the neck; it is seen in advanced cases. Vaginitis and esophagitis may also occur. Diarrhea (in part due to proctitis and in part due to malabsorption), depression, seizures, and dementia are also part of the pellagra syndrome—the four D's: *d*ermatitis, *d*iarrhea, and *d*ementia leading to *d*eath.

Treatment of pellagra consists of oral supplementation of 100 to 200 mg of nicotinamide or nicotinic acid three times daily for 5 days. High doses of nicotinic acid (≥3 g nicotinic acid per day) are used for the treatment of elevated cholesterol levels and in the treatment of types 2, 4, and 5 hyperlipidemias (Chap. 335).

TOXICITY Prostaglandin-mediated flushing has been observed at daily doses as low as 50 mg of niacin when taken as a supplement or as therapy for hypertriglyceridemia. There is no evidence of toxicity from niacin derived from food sources. Flushing may be accompanied by skin dryness, itching, and headache. Premedication with aspirin may alleviate these symptoms. Nausea, vomiting, and abdominal pain also occur at similar doses of niacin. Hepatic toxicity is the most serious toxic reaction due to niacin and may present as jaundice with elevated aspartate aminotransferase (AST) and alanine aminotranferase (ALT) levels. A few cases of fulminant hepatitis requiring liver transplantation have been reported at doses of 3 to 9 g/d. Other toxic reactions include glucose intolerance, macular edema, and macular cysts. The upper limit for daily niacin intake has been set at 35 mg. However, this upper limit does not pertain to the therapeutic use of niacin.

PYRIDOXINE (VITAMIN B₆)

Vitamin B_6 refers to a family of compounds including pyridoxine, pyridoxal, pyridoxamine, and their 5'-phosphate derivatives. 5'-Pyridoxal phosphate (PLP) is a cofactor for more than 100 enzymes involved in amino acid metabolism. Vitamin B_6 is also involved in heme and neurotransmitter synthesis and in the metabolism of glycogen, lipids, steroids, sphingoid bases, and several vitamins, including the conversion of tryptophan to niacin.

DIETARY SOURCES Plants contain vitamin B_6 in the form of pyridoxine, whereas animal tissues contain PLP and pyridoxamine phosphate. The

Vitamin	Active derivative or cofactor form	Principal function
Thiamine (B₁)	Thiamine pyrophosphate	Coenzyme for cleavage of carbon-carbon bonds; amino acid and carbohydrate metabolism
Riboflavin (B₂)	Flavin mononucleotide (FMN) and flavin adenine dinucleotide (FAD)	Cofactor for oxidation, reduction reactions, and covalently attached prosthetic groups for some enzymes
Niacin	Nicotinamide adenine dinucleotide phosphate (NADP) and nicotinamide adenine dinucleotide (NAD)	Coenzymes for oxidation and reduction reactions
Vitamin B₆	Pyridoxal phosphate	Cofactor for enzymes of amino acid metabolism
Folate	Polyglutamate forms of (5, 6, 7, 8) tetrahydrofolate with carbon unit attachments	Coenzyme for one carbon transfer in nucleic acid and amino acid metabolism
Vitamin B₁₂	Methylcobalamine Adenosylcobalamin	Coenzyme for methionine synthase and L-methylmalonyl-CoA mutase

FIGURE 61-1 The structures and principal functions of vitamins associated with human disorders.

Vitamin	Active derivative or cofactor form	Principal function
Vitamin C O=C—C=C—C—C—CH₂OH (OH OH O OH)	Ascorbic acid and dehydrascorbic acid	Participation as a redox ion in many biological oxidation and hydrogen transfer reactions
Vitamin A (β-Carotene) CH₂OH (Retinol)	Retinol, retinaldehyde, and retinoic acid	Formation of rhodopsin (vision) and glycoproteins (epithelial cell function); also regulates gene transcription
Vitamin D (structure, OH, CH₂, HO, OH)	1, 25-Dihyroxy vitamin	Maintenance of blood calcium and phosphorous levels; antiproliferative hormone
Vitamin E CH₃ / —CH₂[CH₂—CH₂—CH—CH₂]₃H / HO	Tocopherols and tocotrienols	Antioxidants
Vitamin K (structure, O, R, O)	Vitamin K hydroquinone	Cofactor for posttranslation carboxylation of many proteins including essential clotting factors

FIGURE 61-1—(continued)

vitamin B_6 contained in plants is less bioavailable than that from animal tissues. Rich food sources of vitamin B_6 include legumes, nuts, wheat bran, and meat, although it is present in all food groups.

DEFICIENCY Symptoms of vitamin B_6 deficiency include epithelial changes, as seen frequently with other B vitamin deficiencies. In addition, severe vitamin B_6 deficiency can lead to peripheral neuropathy, abnormal electroencephalograms, and personality changes including depression and confusion. In infants, diarrhea, seizures, and anemia have been reported. Microcytic, hypochromic anemia is due to diminished hemoglobin synthesis, since the first enzyme involved in heme biosynthesis (amino-levulinate synthase) requires PLP as a cofactor (Chap. 90). In some case reports, platelet dysfunction has also been reported. Since vitamin B_6 is necessary for the conversion of homocysteine to cystathionine, it is possible that chronic low-grade vitamin B_6 deficiency may result in hyperhomocystinemia and increased risk of cardiovascular disease (Chaps. 225 and 343).

Certain medications such as isoniazid, L-dopa, penicillamine, and cycloserine interact with PLP due to a reaction with carbonyl groups. The increased ratio of AST (or SGOT) to ALT (or SGPT) seen in alcoholic liver disease reflects the relative vitamin B_6 dependence of ALT. Vitamin B_6 dependency syndromes that require pharmacologic doses of vitamin B_6 are rare, but include cystathionine β-synthase deficiency, pyridoxine-responsive (primarily sideroblastic) anemias, and gyrate atrophy with chorioretinal degeneration due to decreased activity of the mitochondrial enzyme ornithine aminotransferase. In these situations, 100 to 200 mg/d of oral vitamin B_6 are required for treatment.

High doses of vitamin B_6 have been used to treat carpal tunnel syndrome, premenstrual syndrome, schizophrenia, autism, and diabetic neuropathy but have not been found to be effective.

The laboratory diagnosis of vitamin B_6 deficiency is generally made on the basis of low plasma PLP values (<20 nmol/L). Treatment of vitamin B_6 deficiency is 50 mg/d; higher doses of 100 to 200 mg/d are given if vitamin B_6 deficiency is related to medication use. Vitamin B_6 should not be given with L-dopa, since the vitamin interferes with the action of this drug.

TOXICITY The safe upper limit for vitamin B_6 has been set at 100 mg/d, although no adverse effects have been associated with high intakes of vitamin B_6 from food sources only. When toxicity occurs, it causes a severe sensory neuropathy, leaving patients unable to walk. Some cases of photosensitivity and dermatitis have also been reported.

FOLATE, VITAMIN B_{12} See Chap. 90.

VITAMIN C

Both ascorbic acid and its oxidized product dehydroascorbic acid are biologically active. Actions of vitamin C include antioxidant activity, promotion of nonheme iron absorption, carnitine biosynthesis, and the conversion of dopamine to norepinephrine. Vitamin C is also important for connective tissue metabolism and cross-linking, and it is a component of many drug-metabolizing enzyme systems, particularly the mixed-function oxidase systems.

ABSORPTION AND DIETARY SOURCES Almost complete absorption of vitamin C occurs if <100 mg is administered in a single dose; however, only 50% or less is absorbed at doses >1 g. Enhanced degradation and fecal and urinary excretion of vitamin C occur at higher intake levels.

Good dietary sources of vitamin C include citrus fruits, green vegetables (especially broccoli), tomatoes, and potatoes. Consumption of five servings of fruits and vegetables a day provides vitamin C in excess of the RDA, 60 mg/d for males and females. In addition, approximately 40% of the U.S. population takes vitamin C as a dietary supplement in which "natural forms" of vitamin C are no more bioavailable than synthetic forms. Smoking, hemodialysis, and stress (e.g., infection, trauma) appear to increase vitamin C requirements.

DEFICIENCY Vitamin C deficiency causes scurvy; in the United States, this is seen primarily among the poor and elderly and in alcoholics who consume <10 mg/d of vitamin C. Vitamin C deficiency has also been described among individuals consuming macrobiotic diets. Symptoms of scurvy primarily reflect impaired formation of mature connective tissue and include bleeding into skin (petechiae, ecchymoses, perifollicular hemorrhages); inflamed and bleeding gums; and manifestations of bleeding into joints, the peritoneal cavity, pericardium, and the adrenal glands. In children, vitamin C deficiency may cause impaired bone growth. Laboratory diagnosis of vitamin C deficiency is made on the basis of low plasma or leukocyte levels.

Administration of vitamin C (200 mg/d) improves the symptoms of scurvy within a matter of several days. High-dose vitamin C supplementation (e.g., 1 to 2 g/d) may slightly decrease the symptoms and duration of upper respiratory tract infections. Vitamin C supplementation has also been reported to be useful in Chédiak-Higashi syndrome (Chap. 55) and osteogenesis imperfecta (Chap. 342). Diets high in vitamin C have been claimed to lower the incidence of certain cancers, particularly esophageal and gastric cancers. If proven, this effect may be due to the fact that vitamin C can prevent the conversion of nitrites and secondary amines to carcinogenic nitrosomines. However, one intervention study from China did not show vitamin C to be protective.

TOXICITY Taking >2 g of vitamin C in a single dose may result in abdominal pain, diarrhea, and nausea; doses >3 g have been reported to elevate blood levels of ALT, lactic acid dehydrogenase, and uric acid. Since vitamin C may be metabolized to oxalate, it is feared that chronic, high-dose vitamin C supplementation could result in an increased prevalence of kidney stones. However, this has not been borne out in several trials, except in patients with preexisting renal disease. Thus, it is reasonable to advise patients with a past history of kidney stones to not take large doses of vitamin C. There is also an unproven, but possible, risk that chronic high doses of vitamin C could promote iron overload in patients taking supplemental iron. High doses of vitamin C can induce hemolysis in patients with glucose-6-phosphate dehydrogenase deficiency, and doses >1 g/d can cause false-negative guaiac reactions as well as interfere with tests for urinary glucose.

BIOTIN

Biotin is a water-soluble vitamin that plays a role in gluconeogenesis and fatty acid synthesis and serves as a CO_2 carrier on the surface of both cytosolic and mitochondrial carboxylase enzymes. The vitamin also functions in the catabolism of specific amino acids (e.g., leucine). Excellent food sources of biotin include liver, soy, beans, yeast, and egg yolks; however, egg white contains the protein avidin, which strongly binds the vitamin and reduces its bioavailability.

Biotin deficiency has been induced by experimental feeding of egg white diets and in patients with short bowels who received biotin-free parenteral nutrition. In the adult, biotin deficiency results in mental changes (depression, hallucinations), paresthesia, anorexia, and nausea. A scaling, seborrheic, and erythematous rash may occur around the eyes, nose, and mouth as well as on the extremities. In infants, biotin deficiency presents as hypotonia, lethargy, and apathy. In addition, the infant may develop alopecia and a characteristic rash that includes the ears. The laboratory diagnosis of biotin deficiency can be established based on a decreased urinary concentration. Treatment requires pharmacologic doses of biotin, using up to 10 mg/d.

PANTOTHENIC ACID

Pantothenic acid is a component of coenzyme A and phosphopantetheine, which are involved in fatty acid metabolism and the synthesis of cholesterol, steroid hormones, and all compounds formed from isoprenoid units. In addition, pantothenic acid is involved in the acetylation of proteins. The vitamin is excreted in the urine, and the laboratory diagnosis of deficiency is made on the basis of low urinary vitamin levels.

The vitamin is ubiquitous in the food supply. Liver, yeast, egg yolks, and vegetables are particularly good sources. Human pantothenic acid deficiency has only been demonstrated in experimental feeding of diets low in pantothenic acid or by giving a specific pantothenic acid antagonist. The symptoms of pantothenic acid deficiency are nonspecific and include gastrointestinal disturbance, depression, muscle cramps, paresthesia, ataxia, and hypoglycemia. Pantothenic acid deficiency is believed to have caused the burning feet syndrome seen in prisoners of war during World War II. No toxicity of this vitamin has been reported.

CHOLINE

Choline is a precursor for acetylcholine, phospholipids, and betaine. Choline is necessary for the structural integrity of cell membranes, cholinergic neurotransmission, lipid and cholesterol metabolism, and transmembrane signaling. Recently, a recommended adequate intake was set at 550 mg/d for adult males and 425 mg/d for adult females. Choline is thought to be a "conditionally essential" nutrient, in that de novo synthesis occurs in the liver and is less than the vitamin's utilization only under certain stress conditions. Choline deficiency has occurred in patients receiving parenteral nutrition devoid of choline. Deficiency results in fatty liver and elevated transaminase levels. The diagnosis of choline deficiency is made on the basis of low plasma levels.

Toxicity from choline results in hypotension, cholinergic sweating, diarrhea, salivation, and a fishy body odor. The upper limit for choline has been set at 3.5 g/d. Therapeutically, choline has been suggested for patients with dementia and for patients at high risk of cardiovascular disease, due to its ability to lower cholesterol and homocysteine levels. However, such benefits have yet to be documented.

VITAMIN A

Vitamin A, in the strictest sense, refers to retinol. However, the oxidized metabolites, retinaldehyde and retinoic acid, are also biologically active compounds. The term *retinoids* includes synthetic molecules that are chemically related to retinol. Retinaldehyde (11-*cis*) is the essential form of vitamin A that is required for normal vision, whereas retinoic acid is necessary for normal morphogenesis, growth, and cell differentiation. Retinoic acid does not function in vision and, in contrast to retinol, is not involved in reproduction. Vitamin A also plays a role in iron utilization, humoral immunity, T cell–mediated immunity, natural killer cell activity, and phagocytosis. Vitamin A is commercially available in esterified forms (e.g., acetate, palmitate) since it is more stable as an ester.

There are over 600 carotenoids in nature, and approximately 50 of these can be metabolized to vitamin A. β-Carotene is the most prevalent carotenoid in the food supply that has provitamin A activity. It is estimated that 12 μg or greater of dietary β-carotene is equivalent to 1 μg of retinol, whereas 24 μg or greater of other dietary provitamin A carotenoids (e.g., cryptoxanthin, α-carotene) is equivalent to 1 μg of retinol.

METABOLISM The liver contains approximately 90% of the vitamin A reserves and secretes vitamin A in the form of retinol, which is bound to retinol-binding protein. Once this has occurred, the retinol-binding protein complex interacts with a second protein, transthryetin. This trimolecular complex functions to prevent vitamin A from being filtered by the kidney glomerulus, to protect the body against the toxicity of retinol and to allow retinol to be taken up by specific cell-surface receptors that recognize retinol-binding protein. A certain amount of vitamin A enters peripheral cells even if it is not bound to retinol-binding protein. After retinol is internalized by the cell, it becomes bound to a series of cellular retinol-binding proteins, which function as sequestering and transporting agents as well as coligands for enzymatic reactions. Certain cells also contain retinoic acid–binding proteins, which have the same sequestering functions as well as enabling retinoic acid metabolism.

Retinoic acid is a ligand for certain nuclear receptors that act as transcription factors. Two families of receptors (RAR and RXR receptors) are active in retinoid-mediated gene transcription. Retinoid receptors regulate transcription by binding as dimeric complexes to specific DNA sites, the retinoic acid response elements, in target genes (Chap. 317). The receptors can either stimulate or repress gene expression in response to their ligands. RAR binds all-*trans* retinoic acid and 9-*cis* retinoic acid, whereas RXR binds only 9-*cis* retinoic acid.

The retinoid receptors play an important role in controlling cell proliferation and differentiation. Retinoic acid is useful in the treatment of promyeolcytic leukemia (Chap. 96) and is also used in the treatment of cystic acne because it inhibits keratinization, decreases sebum secretion, and possibly alters the inflammatory reaction (Chap. 47). RXRs dimerize with other nuclear receptors to function as co-regulators of genes responsive to retinoids, thyroid hormone, and calcitriol. RXR agonists induce insulin sensitivity experimentally, perhaps because RXR is a cofactor for the peroxisome-proliferator-activated receptors (PPARs), which are targets for the thiazolidinedione drugs such as rosiglitazone and troglitazone (Chap. 323).

DIETARY SOURCES   The retinol activity equivalent (RAE) is used to express the vitamin A value of food. One RAE is defined as 1 μg of retinol (0.003491 mmol), 12 μg of β-carotene, and 24 μg of other provitamin A carotenoids. In older literature, vitamin A was often expressed in international units (IU), with 1 RAE being equal to 3.33 IU of retinol and 20 IU of β-carotene, but these units are no longer in current scientific use.

Liver and fish are excellent food sources for preformed vitamin A; vegetable sources of provitamin A carotenoids include dark-green and -colored fruits and vegetables. Children are particularly susceptible to vitamin A deficiency because neither breast nor cow's milk supplies enough vitamin A to prevent deficiency. Areas of the world where vitamin A deficiency is particularly prevalent include parts of Africa, South America, and Southeast Asia. Vitamin A deficiency occurs in more than 250,000 children each year, resulting in blindness and a 50% mortality rate within the year. In western countries, vitamin A deficiency is seen primarily among patients with diseases associated with fat malabsorption (e.g., celiac sprue, short-bowel syndrome). Concurrent zinc deficiency can interfere with the mobilization of vitamin A from liver stores. Alcohol interferes with the conversion of retinol to retinaldehyde in the eye by competing for alcohol (retinol) dehydrogenase. Drugs that interfere with the absorption of vitamin A include mineral oil, neomycin, and cholestyramine.

DEFICIENCY   Symptoms of vitamin A deficiency include hyperkeratotic skin lesions, and xerophthalmia (e.g., Bitôt spots, which are white patches of keratinized epithelium appearing on the sclera). Aggressive xerophthalmia can result in corneal ulceration. If untreated, proteolytic destruction and rupture of the cornea ensues with permanent blindness, although vitamin A treatment of patients with corneal ulcers can also result in blindness due to permanent corneal scarring. Children with vitamin A deficiency have increased mortality, primarily from infectious diseases, measles, respiratory diseases, and diarrhea. Extremely low birth weight infants (<1000 g) should be treated parenterally with 1500 μg (or RAE) of vitamin A three times a week for 4 weeks.

There are no specific deficiency signs or symptoms that result from carotenoid deficiency. It was postulated that β-carotene would be an effective chemopreventive for cancer because numerous epidemiologic studies had shown that diets high in β-carotene were associated with lower incidences of cancers of the respiratory and digestive system. However, intervention studies using high doses of β-carotene actually resulted in more lung cancers than in placebo-treated groups. Non-provitamin A carotenoids, such as lutein and zeaxanthin, have been suggested to protect against macular degeneration. The non-provitamin A carotenoid lycopene has been proposed to protect against prostate cancer. However, the effectiveness of these agents has not been proven by intervention studies, and the mechanisms underlying these purported biologic actions are unknown.

The diagnosis of vitamin A deficiency is made by measurement of serum retinol (normal range, 30 to 65 μg/dL), tests of dark adaptation, impression cytology of the conjunctiva (decreased numbers of mucous-secreting cells), or measurement of body storage pools, either directly by liver biopsy or by isotopic dilution after administering a stable isotope of vitamin A.

Vitamin A deficiency with ocular changes should be treated by administering 30 mg of vitamin A intramuscularly, or 60 mg orally. In areas of endemic vitamin A deficiency, this is followed by 60 mg

vitamin A capsules at 6-month intervals. Vitamin A deficiency in patients with malabsorptive diseases, who have abnormal dark adaptation or symptoms of night blindness without ocular changes, should be treated for 1 month with 15 mg/d orally of a water micelle preparation of vitamin A. This is followed by lower maintenance doses with the exact amount determined by monitoring serum retinol.

TOXICITY   Acute toxicity of vitamin A was first noted in Arctic explorers who ate polar bear liver and has also been seen after administration of 150 mg in adults or 100 mg in children. Acute toxicity is manifested by increased intracranial pressure, vertigo, diplopia, bulging fontanels in children, seizures, and exfoliative dermatitis; it may result in death. Chronic vitamin A intoxication has been seen in normal adults who ingest 15 mg/d of vitamin A for a period of several months and in children who ingest 6 mg/d. Manifestations include dry skin, cheilosis, glossitis, vomiting, alopecia, bone pain, hypercalcemia, lymph node enlargement, hyperlipidemia, amenorrhea, and features of pseudotumor cerebri with increased intracranial pressure and papilledema. Liver fibrosis with portal hypertension and bone demineralization may also result from chronic vitamin A intoxication. When vitamin A is provided in excess to pregnant women, congenital malformations have included spontaneous abortions, craniofacial abnormalities, and valvular heart disease. In pregnancy, the daily dose of vitamin A should not exceed 3 mg. Commercially available retinoid derivatives are also toxic, including 13-*cis*-retinoic acid, which has been associated with birth defects. As a result, contraception should be continued for at least 1 year, and possibly longer, in women who have taken 13-*cis* retinoic acid.

High doses of carotenoids do not result in toxic symptoms. However, carotenemia, which is characterized by a yellowing of the skin (creases of the palms and soles) but not the sclerae, may be present after ingestion of >30 mg of β-carotene on a daily basis. Hypothyroid patients are particularly susceptible to the development of carotenemia due to impaired breakdown of carotene to vitamin A. Reduction of carotenes from the diet results in the disappearance of skin yellowing and carotenemia over a period of 30 to 60 days.

VITAMIN D   See Chap. 331, Fig. 61-1, and Table 61-1.

VITAMIN E

Vitamin E is a collective name for the 2R stereoisomers of α tocopherol. Vitamin E acts as a chain-breaking antioxidant and is an efficient pyroxyl radical scavenger, which protects low-density lipoproteins (LDLs) and polyunsaturated fats in membranes from oxidation. A network of other antioxidants (e.g., vitamin C, glutathione) and enzymes maintains vitamin E in a reduced state. Vitamin E also inhibits prostaglandin synthesis and the activities of protein kinase C and phospholipase A$_2$.

ABSORPTION AND METABOLISM   After absorption, vitamin E is taken up from chylomicrons by the liver, and an hepatic α tocopherol transport protein mediates intracellular vitamin E transport and incorporation into very low density lipoprotein (VLDL). The transport protein has particular affinity for the RRR isomeric form of α tocopherol; thus this natural isomer has the most biologic activity.

REQUIREMENT   Vitamin E is widely distributed in the food supply and is particularly high in sunflower oil, safflower oil, and wheat germ oil; γ tocotrionols are notably present in soybean and corn oils. Vitamin E is also found in meats, nuts, and cereal grains, and small amounts are present in fruits and vegetables. Vitamin E pills containing doses of 50 to 1000 mg are ingested by a large fraction of the U.S. population. Diets high in polyunsaturated fats may necessitate a slightly higher requirement for vitamin E.

Dietary deficiency of vitamin E does not exist. Vitamin E deficiency is seen in only severe and prolonged malabsorptive diseases, such as celiac disease, or after small-intestinal resection. Children with cystic fibrosis or prolonged cholestasis may develop vitamin E deficiency characterized by areflexia and hemolytic anemia. Children with abetalipoproteinemia cannot absorb or transport vitamin E and become deficient quite rapidly. A familial form of isolated vitamin E deficiency also exists, which is due to a defect in the α tocopherol transport protein. Vitamin E deficiency causes axonal degeneration of the large myelinated axons and results in posterior column and spinocerebellar symptoms. Peripheral neuropathy is initially characterized by areflexia, with progression to an ataxic gait, and by decreased vibration and position sensations. Ophthalmoplegia, skeletal myopathy, and pigmented retinopathy may also be features of vitamin E deficiency. The laboratory diagnosis of vitamin E deficiency is made on the basis of low blood levels of α tocopherol (<5 $\mu g/mL$, or <0.8 mg of α tocopherol per gram of total lipids).

℞ TREATMENT

Symptomatic vitamin E deficiency should be treated with 800 to 1200 mg of α tocopherol per day. Patients with abetalipoproteinemia may need as much as 5000 to 7000 mg/d. Children with symptomatic vitamin E deficiency should be treated with 400 mg/d orally of water-miscible esters; alternatively, 2 mg/kg per day may be administered intramuscularly. Vitamin E in high doses may protect against oxygen-induced retrolental fibroplasia and bronchopulmonary dysplasia, as well as intraventricular hemorrhage of prematurity. Vitamin E has been suggested to increase sexual performance, to treat intermittent claudication, and to slow the aging process, but evidence for these properties is lacking. High doses (60 to 800 mg/d) of vitamin E have been shown in controlled trials to improve parameters of immune function, but intervention studies using vitamin E to prevent cardiovascular disease have not shown efficacy.

TOXICITY High doses of vitamin E (>800 mg/d) may reduce platelet aggregation and interfere with vitamin K metabolism and are therefore contraindicated in patients taking warfarin. Nausea, flatulence, and diarrhea have been reported at doses >1 g/d.

VITAMIN K

There are two natural forms of vitamin K: vitamin K I, also known as *phylloquinone*, from vegetable and animal sources, and vitamin K II, or *menaquinone*, which is synthesized by bacterial flora and found in hepatic tissue. *Menadione*, or vitamin K III, is a chemically synthesized pro-vitamin that can be converted to menaquinone by the liver.

Vitamin K is required for the posttranslational carboxylation of glutamic acid, which is necessary for calcium binding to γ-carboxylated proteins such as prothrombin (factor II); factors VII, IX, and X; protein C; protein S; and proteins found in bone (bone gla, matrix gla protein, and osteocalcin). However, the importance of vitamin K for bone mineralization is not known. Warfarin-type drugs inhibit γ carboxylation by preventing the conversion of vitamin K to its active hydroquinone form.

DIETARY SOURCES Vitamin K is found in green leafy vegetables such as kale and spinach, but appreciable amounts are also present in butter, margarine, liver, milk, ground beef, coffee, and pears. Vitamin K is present in vegetable oils and is particularly rich in olive oil and soybean oil. The average daily intake by Americans is estimated to be approximately 100 $\mu g/d$.

DEFICIENCY The symptoms of vitamin K deficiency are due to hemorrhage, and newborns are particularly susceptible because of low fat stores, low breast milk levels of vitamin K, sterility of the infantile intestinal tract, liver immaturity, and poor placental transport. Intracranial bleeding, as well as gastrointestinal and skin bleeding, can occur in vitamin K–deficient infants 1 to 7 days after birth. Thus, vitamin K (1 mg intramuscularly) is given prophylactically at the time of delivery.

Vitamin K deficiency in adults may be seen in patients with chronic small-intestinal disease (e.g., celiac disease, Crohn's disease), obstructed biliary tracts, or after small-bowel resection. Broad-spectrum antibiotic treatment can precipitate vitamin K deficiency by reducing gut bacteria, which synthesize menaquinones, and by inhibiting the

metabolism of vitamin K. The diagnosis of vitamin K deficiency is usually made on the basis of an elevated prothrombin time or reduced clotting factors, although vitamin K may also be measured directly by HPLC. Vitamin K deficiency is treated using a parenteral dose of 10 mg. For patients with chronic malabsorption, 1 to 2 mg/d of vitamin K should be given orally, or 1 to 2 mg/week can be taken parenterally. Patients with liver disease may have an elevated prothrombin time because of liver cell destruction as well as vitamin K deficiency. If an elevated prothrombin time does not improve on vitamin K therapy, it can be deduced that it is not the result of vitamin K deficiency.

TOXICITY Parenteral doses of the water-soluble vitamin K derivative (menadione) have been reported to cause hemolytic anemia and hypobilirubinemia in infants. Toxicity from dietary phylloquinones and menaquinones has not been described. High doses of vitamin K can impair the actions of oral anticoagulants.

MINERALS See Table 61-2.

CALCIUM See Chap. 331.

ZINC

Zinc is an integral component of many metalloenzymes in the body; it is involved in the synthesis and stabilization of proteins, DNA, and RNA and plays a structural role in ribosomes and membranes. Zinc is necessary for the binding of steroid hormone receptors and several other transcription factors to DNA. Zinc is absolutely required for normal spermatogenesis, fetal growth, and embryonic development.

ABSORPTION The absorption of zinc from the diet is inhibited by dietary phytate, fiber, oxalate, iron, and copper, as well as by certain drugs including penicillamine, sodium valproate, and ethambutol. Meat, shellfish, nuts, and legumes are good sources of bioavailable zinc, whereas zinc in grains is less available for absorption.

DEFICIENCY Mild zinc deficiency has been described in many diseases including diabetes mellitus, AIDS, cirrhosis, alcoholism, inflammatory bowel disease, malabsorption syndromes, and sickle cell anemia. In these diseases, mild chronic zinc deficiency can cause stunted growth in children, decreased taste sensation (hypogusia), and impaired immune function. Severe chronic zinc deficiency has been described as a cause of hypogonadism and dwarfism in several Middle Eastern countries. In these children, hypopigmented hair is also part of the syndrome. Acrodermatitis enteropathica is a rare autosomal recessive disorder characterized by abnormalities in zinc absorption. Clinical manifestations include diarrhea, alopecia, muscle wasting, depression, irritability, and a rash involving the extremities, face, and perineum. The rash is characterized by vesicular and pustular crusting with scaling and erythema. Occasional patients with Wilson's disease have developed zinc deficiency as a consequence of penicillamine therapy (Chap. 339).

The diagnosis of zinc deficiency is usually made by a serum zinc level of <12 $\mu mol/L$ (<70 $\mu g/dL$). Pregnancy and birth control pills may cause a slight depression in serum zinc levels, and hypoalbuminemia from any cause can result in hypozincemia. In acute stress situations, zinc may be redistributed from serum into tissues. Zinc deficiency may be treated with 60 mg elemental zinc, orally twice a day. Zinc gluconate lozenges (13 mg elemental Zn every 2 h while awake) have been reported to reduce the duration and symptoms of the common cold in adults, but studies are conflicting.

TOXICITY Acute zinc toxicity after oral ingestion causes nausea, vomiting, and fever. Zinc fumes from welding may also be toxic and cause fever, respiratory distress, excessive salivation, sweating, and headache. Chronic large doses of zinc may depress immune function and cause hypochromic anemia as a result of copper deficiency.

COPPER

Copper is an integral part of numerous enzyme systems including amine oxidases, ferrooxidase (ceruloplasmin), cytochrome-c oxidase,

TABLE 61-2 *Deficiencies and Toxicities of Metals*

Element	Deficiency	Toxicity	Tolerable Upper (Dietary) Intake Level
Boron	No biologic function determined	Developmental defects, male sterility, testicular atrophy	20 mg/d (extrapolated from animal data)
Calcium	Reduced bone mass, osteoporosis	Renal insufficiency (milk-alkalai syndrome), nephrolithiasis, impaired iron absorption	2500 mg/d (milk-alkalai)
Copper	Anemia, growth retardation, defective keratinization and pigmentation of hair, hypothermia, degenerative changes in aortic elastin, osteopenia, mental deterioration	Nausea, vomiting, diarrhea, hepatic failure, tremor, mental deterioration, hemolytic anemia, renal dysfunction	10 mg/d (liver toxicity)
Chromium	Impaired glucose tolerance	Occupational: renal failure, dermatitis, pulmonary cancer	ND
Fluoride	↑ Dental caries	Dental and skeletal fluorosis, osteoscleroisis	10 mg/d (fluorosis)
Iodine	Thyroid enlargement, ↓ T_4	Thyroid dysfunction, acne-like eruptions	1100 μg/d (thyroid dysfunction)
Iron	Muscle abnormalities, kilonychia, pica, anemia, ↓ work performance, impaired cognitive development, premature labor, ↑ perinatal maternal mortality	Gastrointestinal effects (nausea, vomiting, diarrhea, constipation), iron overload with organ damage, acute systemic toxicity	45 mg/d of elemental iron (GI side effects)
Manganese	Impaired growth and skeletal development, reproduction, lipid and carbohydrate metabolism; upper body rash	General: Neurotoxicity, Parkinson-like symptoms Occupational: Encephalitis-like syndrome, Parkinson-like syndrome, psychosis, pneumoconiosis	11 mg/d (neurotoxicity)
Molybdenum	Severe neurologic abnormalities	Reproductive and fetal abnormalities	2 mg/d extrapolated from animal data
Selenium	Cardiomyopathy, heart failure, striated muscle degeneration	General: Alopecia, nausea, vomiting, abnormal nails, emotional lability, peripheral neuropathy, lassitude, garlic odor to breath, dermatitis Occupational: Lung and nasal carcinomas, liver necrosis, pulmonary inflammation	400 μg/d (hair, nail changes)
Phosphorous	Rickets (osteomalacia), proximal muscle weakness, rhabdomyolysis, paresthesia, ataxia, seizure, confusion, heart failure, hemolysis, acidosis	Hyperphosphatemia	4000 mg/d
Zinc	Growth retardation, ↓ taste and smell, alopecia, dermatitis, diarrhea, immune dysfunction, failure to thrive, gonadal atrophy, congenital malformations	General: Reduced copper absorption, gastritis, sweating, fever, nausea, vomiting. Occupational: Respiratory distress, pulmonary fibrosis	40 mg/d (impaired copper metabolism)

Note: ND, not determined; GI, gastrointestinal.

superoxide dismutase, and dopamine hydroxylase. As such, copper plays a role in iron metabolism, melanin synthesis, and central nervous system function; the synthesis and cross-linking of elastin and collagen; and the scavenging of superoxide radicals. Dietary sources of copper include shellfish, liver, nuts, legumes, bran, and organ meats.

DEFICIENCY Dietary copper deficiency is relatively rare, although it has been described in premature infants who are fed milk diets and in infants with malabsorption (Table 61-2). Copper deficiency anemia has been reported in patients with malabsorptive diseases and nephrotic syndrome and in patients treated for Wilson's disease with chronic high doses of oral zinc, which can interfere with copper absorption. Menkes kinky hair syndrome is an X-linked metabolic disturbance of copper metabolism characterized by mental retardation, hypocupremia, and decreased circulating ceruloplasmin (Chap. 342). It is caused by mutations in a copper-transporting *ATP7A* gene. Children with this disease often die within 5 years because of dissecting aneurysms or cardiac rupture.

The diagnosis of copper deficiency is usually made on the basis of low serum levels of copper (<65 μg/dL) and low ceruloplasmin levels (<18 mg/dL). Serum levels of copper may be elevated in pregnancy or stress conditions since ceruloplasmin is an acute-phase reactant and 90% of circulating copper is bound to ceruloplasmin.

TOXICITY Copper toxicity is usually accidental (Table 61-2). In severe cases, kidney failure, liver failure, and coma may ensue. In Wilson's disease, mutations in the copper-transporting *ATP7B* gene lead to accumulation of copper in the liver and brain, with low blood levels due to decreased ceruloplasmin (Chap. 339).

SELENIUM

Selenium, in the form of selenocysteine, is a component of the enzyme glutathione peroxidase, which serves to protect proteins, cell membranes, lipids, and nucleic acids from oxidant molecules. Selenocysteine is also found in the deiodinase enzymes, which mediate the deiodination of thyroxine to triiodothyronine (Chap. 320). Rich dietary sources of selenium include seafood, muscle meat, and cereals, although the selenium content of cereal is determined by the soil concentration. Countries with low soil concentrations include parts of Scandinavia, China, and New Zealand. *Keshan disease* is an endemic cardiomyopathy found in children and young women residing in regions of China where dietary intake of selenium is low (<20 μg/d). Concomitant deficiencies of iodine and selenium may worsen the clinical manifestations of cretinism.

CHROMIUM

Chromium potentiates the action of insulin in patients with impaired glucose tolerance, presumably by increasing insulin receptor–mediated signaling. In addition, in some patients, improvement in blood lipid profiles has been reported. The usefulness of chromium supplements in muscle building are not substantiated. Rich food sources of chromium include yeast, meat, and grain products. Chromium in the trivalent state is found in supplements and is largely nontoxic; however, chromium-6 is a product of stainless steel welding and is a known pulmonary carcinogen, as well as causing liver, kidney, and central nervous system damage.

MAGNESIUM See Chap. 331.

FLUORIDE, MANGANESE, AND ULTRATRACE ELEMENTS

An essential function for *fluoride* in humans has not been described, although it is useful for the maintenance of structure in teeth and bone. Adult fluorosis results in mottled and pitted defects in tooth enamel as well as brittle bone (skeletal fluorosis).

Manganese and molybdenum deficiencies have been reported in patients with rare genetic abnormalities and in a few patients receiving prolonged total parenteral nutrition. Several manganese-specific enzymes have been identified (e.g., manganese superoxide dismutase). Deficiencies of manganese have been reported to result in bone demineralization, poor growth, ataxia, and convulsions.

Ultratrace elements are defined as those needed in amounts <1 mg/d. Essentiality has not been established for most ultratrace elements, although *iodine* is clearly essential (Chap. 320). *Molybdenum* is necessary for the activity of sulfite and xanthine oxidase, and molybdenum deficiency may result in skeletal and brain lesions.

FURTHER READING

PANEL ON MICRONUTRIENTS, FOOD AND NUTRITION BOARD, INSTITUTE OF MEDICINE: *Dietary Reference Intakes for Calcium, Phosphorus, Magnesium, Vitamin D, and Fluoride: Standing Committee on the Scientific Evaluation of Dietary Reference Intakes.* Washington, DC, National Academy Press, 1997

————: *Dietary Reference Intakes for Thiamin, Riboflavin, Niacin, Vitamin B6, Folate, Vitamin B12, Pantothenic Acid, Biotin, and Choline: A Report of the Standing Committee on the Scientific Evaluation of Dietary Reference Intakes and its Panel on Folate, Other B Vitamins, and Choline and Subcommittee on Upper Reference Levels of Nutrients.* Washington, DC, National Academy Press, 2000

————: *Dietary Reference Intakes for Vitamin C, Vitamin E, Selenium, and Carotenoids: A Report of the Panel on Dietary Antioxidants and Related Compounds, Subcommittees on Upper Intakes, and the Standing Committee on the Scientific Evaluation of Dietary Reference Intakes.* Washington, DC, National Academy Press, 2000

————: *Dietary Reference Intakes for Vitamin A, Vitamin K, Arsenic, Boron, Chromium, Copper, Iodine, Iron, Manganese, Molybdenum, Nickel, Silicon, Vanadium, and Zinc: A Report of the Subcommittees on Upper Reference Levels of Nutrients and of Interpretation and Uses of Dietary Reference Intakes, and the Standing Committee on the Scientific Evaluation of Dietary Reference Intakes.* Washington, DC, National Academy Press, 2001

62 | MALNUTRITION AND NUTRITIONAL ASSESSMENT
Charles H. Halsted

Malnutrition is a frequent component of acute and chronic illness and is found in ~50% of all hospitalized adults. It contributes to increased in-hospital morbidity and mortality in both medical and surgical patients, and leads to more frequent hospital admissions among the elderly. Malnutrition results from various combinations of starvation, abnormal assimilation of the diet, the stress response of illness, and abnormal nutrient metabolism. Nutritional assessment should be considered an integral part of the clinical evaluation and used as a basis for nutritional support in the overall therapeutic plan.

Two forms of severe malnutrition are recognized under conditions of inadequate food supply or distribution: *marasmus* refers to generalized starvation with loss of body fat and protein, whereas *kwashiorkor* refers to selective protein malnutrition with edema and fatty liver. These distinctions, however, seldom apply to malnourished patients in more developed societies where features of combined protein-calorie malnutrition (PCM) are seen in acute and chronic illnesses. The potential medical consequences of unrecognized malnutrition are depicted in Fig. 62-1.

Patients lose weight when the intake or gastrointestinal assimilation of dietary calories is insufficient to meet normal energy expenditure, the expenditure of body energy stores is greater than energy assimilated by the body, or the metabolism of energy is significantly impaired by the intrinsic disease process. The etiologies of malnutrition can be categorized according to decreased intake or assimilation of diet, increased loss of nutrients from the body, and mixed mechanisms that reflect abnormal nutrient metabolism, as summarized in Table 62-1.

ENERGY BALANCE AND BODY COMPOSITION IN HEALTH AND DISEASE

Energy balance and body weight are sustained in health by the consumption of dietary energy (calories) in an amount equal to the daily expenditure of energy. Simply put, undernutrition results from the intake or absorption of fewer calories than energy spent, and overnutrition represents less expenditure of energy than calories consumed. In healthy individuals, daily total energy expenditure (TEE) is composed of basal or resting energy expenditure (REE, about 60% of total), the thermic cost of digestion (about 10% of total), and modest physical activity (about 30% of total). The REE represents the cost of all intrinsic metabolic reactions and is directly related to the fat-free mass (FFM) of the body. As depicted in Fig. 62-2, the human body stores 15 and 25% of its energy as fat (greater in women than men), which

is available for the release of stored fatty acids during starvation. The remaining FFM is composed of extracellular and intracellular water, the bony skeleton, glycogen, and skeletal and visceral protein. Aside from body fat, energy reserves are also provided by intracellular glycogen and protein, which, together with intracellular water, constitute the body cell mass (BCM). Thus, in addition to the enzymes that support the normal metabolic machinery of the body, the BCM provides reserve protein for energy production by gluconeogenesis during the stress response.

The energy stores in a healthy 70-kg man include about 15 kg as fat, 6 kg as protein, and 0.4 kg as glycogen. During a 24-h fast, energy needs are met by the consumption of liver glycogen stores and the conversion by gluconeogenesis of up to 75 g of body protein to glucose. During longer fasting, the REE decreases by as much as 25%

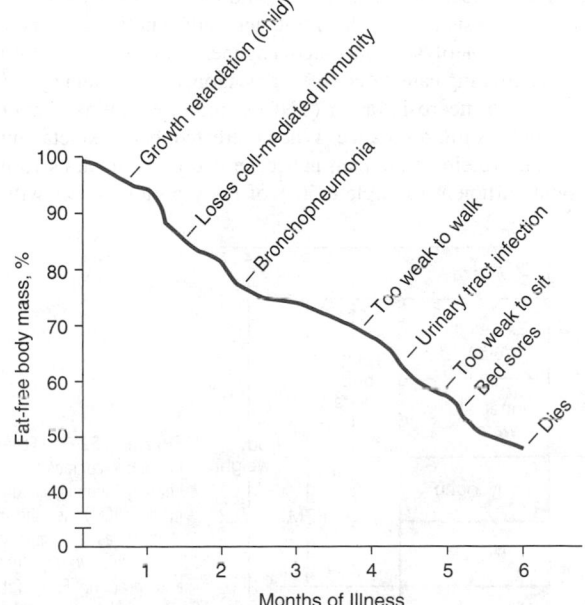

FIGURE 62-1 Hypothetical history of progressive protein-calorie malnutrition in a patient with wasting illness. *(Reproduced with permission from Heymsfield et al.)*

TABLE 62-1 *Etiologies of Protein-Calorie Malnutrition*

I. Starvation (hypometabolism with reliance on body fat stores)
  A. Decreased diet intake
    1. Social and economic: poverty, chronic alcoholism
    2. Psychiatric: anorexia nervosa, severe depression
    3. Neurodegenerative dementias of aging
    4. Anorexia associated with AIDS, disseminated cancer, renal failure
    5. Abdominal pain triggered by food intake: pancreatitis, intestinal ischemia
  B. Decreased assimilation of the diet
    1. Impaired transit of diet, e.g., benign or malignant esophageal, gastric, or intestinal obstruction
    2. Impaired digestion of diet, e.g., pancreatic insufficiency, short bowel syndrome
    3. Intestinal malabsorption of dietary constituents, e.g., celiac disease
II. Stress (hypermetabolism with reliance on protein stores for gluconeogenesis)
  A. Acute trauma, e.g., accident, burns, major surgery
  B. Acute sepsis
  C. Acute or chronic inflammation: pancreatitis, collagen diseases, chronic infectious disease, e.g., tuberculosis, AIDS opportunistic infections
III. Mixed mechanisms
  A. Futile metabolic cycles and anorexia, e.g., AIDS, disseminated cancer
  B. Increased energy demands, e.g., chronic obstructive pulmonary disease
  C. Abnormal metabolism and decreased biliary digestion, e.g., chronic liver disease
  D. Protein-losing enteropathy and chronic inflammation, e.g., Crohn's disease, ulcerative colitis

and the decreased energy needs are supplied by gluconeogenesis, derived from stores of body fat (about 150 g/d), which provides ketones, and muscle, which provides protein (about 20 g/d). While normal-weight individuals can sustain total fasting for about 2 months, obese individuals can fast for periods >12 months, depending on the size of their fat stores.

The metabolic responses to the stress of acute critical illness (e.g., following accidental or surgical trauma or sepsis) significantly modify energy balance. In contrast to the hypometabolism of starvation, the acute stress response is characterized by hypermetabolism, in which the demands of accelerated energy expenditure are met by skeletal and visceral proteolysis to provide amino acid substrate for gluconeogenesis. Muscle proteolysis and gluconeogenesis are promoted by high levels of circulating catecholamines, glucagon, cortisol, and cytokines, including tumor necrosis factor (TNF) α and interleukins 1 and 6, in the setting of insulin resistance. When untreated, body skeletal muscle and visceral protein catabolism is accelerated to as much as 150 g/d, an amount sufficient to deplete 50% of body protein stores within 3

weeks. In the malnourished patient with chronic illness in whom acute trauma or sepsis superimposes cytokine-mediated proteolysis, progressive PCM is associated with decreased cardiac and renal function, fluid retention, muscle and intestinal mucosal atrophy, loss of intracellular minerals (zinc, magnesium, and phosphorus), diminished cell-mediated immune functions, increased risk of infection, and eventual death (Fig. 62-1).

CLINICAL EVALUATION OF THE MALNOURISHED PATIENT

Both outpatients and inpatients are at risk for malnutrition if they meet one or more of the following criteria: (1) unintentional loss of ~10% of usual body weight in the preceding 3 months, (2) body weight <90% of ideal for height, or (3) body mass index [BMI; the weight (kg) divided by the height (m²)] <18.5. With regard to varying levels of severity, body weight <90% of ideal for height represents risk of malnutrition, body weight <85% of ideal constitutes *malnutrition*, <70% of ideal represents *severe malnutrition*, and <60% of ideal is usually incompatible with survival. An overview of the evaluation of malnutrition in the sick adult is depicted in Fig. 62-3.

THE PATIENT HISTORY The clinical nutritional history is based on understanding the etiologies and pathophysiology of malnutrition and should focus on changes in diet and body weight, socioeconomic conditions, and symptoms unique to each clinical setting (Table 62-2). Social and economic conditions that may lead to poverty and malnutrition include inadequate income, homelessness, drug abuse, or chronic alcoholism. During binge drinking in chronic alcoholics, ethanol typically contributes more than half of daily food calories; ethanol catabolism consumes energy and promotes unbalanced metabolism of fat and carbohydrates. Depending on the severity of injury or illness, critically ill surgical and medical patients predictably develop stress-related PCM if increased nutritional needs are not met after 5 to 10 days. The malnourished patient with digestive disease etiology may complain of dysphagia or recurrent vomiting, chronic diarrhea, or recurrent abdominal pain that is exacerbated by eating. On the general medical service, PCM may be an integral part of the clinical presentation of chronic recurrent pancreatitis, renal failure, chronic liver disease, chronic obstructive pulmonary disease, disseminated cancer, or chronic infections such as AIDS or tuberculosis.

THE PHYSICAL EXAMINATION A careful physical examination can characterize the extent of malnutrition. Measurements of unclothed weight and height are essential for establishing the severity of malnutrition in all patients but may be confounded by the effects of fluid overload as a result of edema and ascites. Normal values of weight for height are shown in Table 62-3. Without recourse to a table, a simplified approach for estimating ideal body weight is to assume 106 lb for 5 ft plus 6 lb per additional inch for men, or 105 lb for 5 ft plus 5 lb per additional inch for women, assuming a range of ±10%.

Specific Physical Findings of Malnutrition During the conventional physical examination, the observant and experienced clinician can identify multiple and specific findings of PCM and its associated micronutrient deficiencies (Chap. 61). A variety of nutritional deficiencies can be identified by examination of the patient's general appearance, including skin, hair, nails, mucus membranes, and neurologic system (Table 62-4). Initially, a pinch of the posterior upper arm may reveal loss of subcutaneous fat in the malnourished patient. Hollowing of the temporal muscles, wasting of upper arms and thigh muscles, easily plucked hair, and peripheral edema are all consistent with protein deficiency. Examination of the skin may reveal the papular keratitis ("goose bump rash") of vitamin A deficiency, perifollicular hemorrhages of vitamin C deficiency, ecchymoses of vitamin K deficiency, the "flaky paint" lower extremity rash of zinc deficiency, hyperpigmentation of skin-exposed areas from niacin deficiency, seborrhea of essential fatty acid deficiency, spooning of nails in iron deficiency, and transverse nail pigmentation in protein deficiency. The eye examination yields conjunctival pallor of anemia, pericorneal and corneal opacities of severe vitamin A deficiency ("Bitot spots"), and nystagmus

FIGURE 62-2 Schematic of body composition of a healthy subject. Body cell mass (BCM) is shown by shading as a composite of intracellular water, glycogen, and protein. FFM, fat-free mass. (*Adapted with permission from Heymsfield et al.*)

and isolated ocular muscle paresis of thiamine deficiency. The oral examination may reveal angular stomatitis and cheilosis of either riboflavin or niacin deficiency; glossitis with smooth and red tongue of riboflavin, niacin, vitamin B_{12}, or pyridoxine deficiency; and hypertrophied bleeding gums of vitamin C deficiency. Examination of the neurologic system, particularly in the setting of chronic alcohol abuse, may detect memory loss with confabulation, a wide-based gait, and past pointing, which, together with ophthalmoplegia and peripheral neuropathy, constitute the Wernicke-Korsakoff syndrome of thiamine deficiency. Other neurologic causes of dementia include pellagra due to niacin and/or tryptophan deficiency. Additional causes of peripheral neuropathy include deficiencies of pyridoxine or vitamin E; loss of distal vibratory and position sense is characteristic of the subacute combined degeneration of vitamin B_{12} deficiency.

Anthropometry Measurements of subcutaneous fat and skeletal muscle are important to determine the severity of PCM. Using specialized calipers and a tape measure, anthropometry estimates body fat from the thickness of the skin fold of the posterior mid-upper arm. Anthropometric measurements in healthy and malnourished adults are shown in Table 62-5. Mid-arm muscle circumference is estimated by using the equation:

$$Mid\text{-}arm\ muscle\ circumference = mid\text{-}upper\ circumference\ (cm)$$
$$- (\pi \times triceps\ skin\text{-}fold\ thickness)\ (cm)$$

LABORATORY ASSESSMENT Selected use of laboratory tests, most of which are widely available, is essential for characterizing and quantifying malnutrition. Laboratory findings that are often attributed to chronic disease may, in actuality, reflect the response to PCM or selected micronutrient deficiencies in the setting of chronic illness.

Serum Visceral Proteins Serum albumin, which has a 2- to 3-week half-life, is a sensitive but nonspecific measure of PCM. A normal serum albumin level in a well-hydrated patient is inconsistent with PCM. In contrast, a low serum albumin level could reflect PCM, but can also occur because of increased plasma volume in an overhydrated patient, or because of chronic liver, renal, or cardiopulmonary failure. The serum albumin level falls during the acute stress of surgery, sepsis, or other acute inflammatory illness because of a combination of increased circulating extracellular volume and TNF-α-mediated inhibition of albumin synthesis. Several shorter-lived visceral proteins can also be measured to estimate the severity of PCM. These include transferrin (1-week half-life), prealbumin or retinol-binding protein complex (2-day half-life), and fibronectin (1-day half-life).

Vitamins and Minerals Assays (see also Chap. 61) PCM is typically associated with low serum levels of vitamin A, zinc, and magnesium. Abnormal digestion and absorption of dietary fat are associated with deficiencies of fat-soluble vitamins A, D, and E, whereas intestinal mucosal malabsorption (as in celiac disease) is commonly associated with additional deficiencies of iron and folic acid. Chronic alcoholism is frequently associated with thiamine, folate, vitamin A, and zinc deficiencies. Normal ranges for vitamins are listed in the Appendix.

Assessment of Immune Function PCM is associated with atrophy of thymic-dependent lymphoid structures and reduced T cell–mediated immunity. Conversely, B cell–mediated production of immunoglobulins is usually unaffected. Total lymphocyte count (total white cell count × fraction as lymphocytes) is often <1000/μL in PCM and may be accompanied by anergy to common skin test antigens.

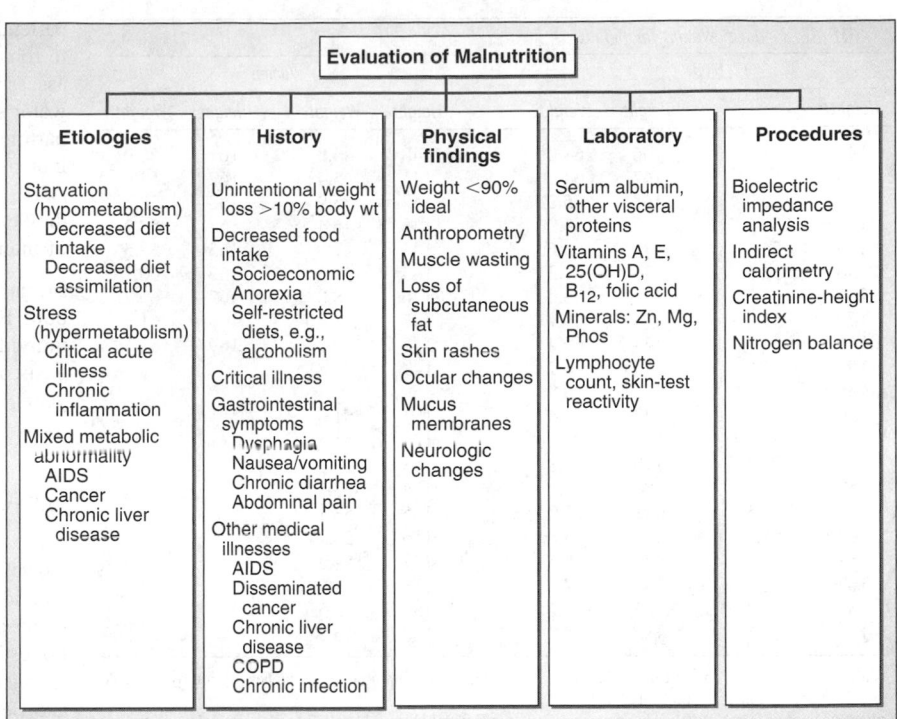

FIGURE 62-3 Conceptual framework for the nutritional assessment of sick patients. COPD, chronic obstructive pulmonary disease.

SPECIALIZED PROCEDURES FOR NUTRITIONAL ASSESSMENT Several specialized procedures are used to assess energy and protein stores and energy expenditure in malnourished patients. These procedures may be employed during the initial nutritional assessment or may serve as an index of the efficacy of nutritional support during the treatment of malnourished patients.

Bioelectric Impedance Analysis Bioelectric impedance analysis (BIA) is a simplified and portable method for measurement of body fat, FFM,

TABLE 62-2	The Patient History of Weight Loss and Malnutrition
Finding	**Example/Interpretation**
Involuntary diet restriction	Poverty due to inadequate income
Anorexia	Anorexia nervosa, severe depression, dementia, AIDS, cancer, chronic renal disease
Inadequate diet selection	Chronic alcoholism, fad diets, strict vegetarianism
Critical illness	Untreated stress response to trauma, burn, major surgery, sepsis
Gastrointestinal symptoms	
Dysphagia	Esophageal obstruction impairs diet transit
Nausea, vomiting	Gastric or intestinal obstruction impairs diet transit
Chronic diarrhea	Pancreatic, biliary, or intestinal mucosal disease impairs digestion and absorption
	Protein-losing enteropathy in inflammatory bowel disease
Chronic abdominal pain	Self-limited food intake reduces pain: e.g., pancreatitis, intestinal ischemia, inflammatory bowel disease
Other chronic medical diseases	Combinations of anorexia, increased energy demands, and abnormal nutrient metabolism: e.g., recurrent pancreatitis, AIDS, disseminated cancer, chronic liver disease, chronic obstructive pulmonary disease, chronic infectious illness

TABLE 62-3 *Ideal Weight for Height*

	Men				Women		
Height[a]	Weight[a]	Height	Weight	Height	Weight	Height	Weight
145	51.9	166	64.0	140	44.9	161	56.9
146	52.4	167	64.6	141	45.4	162	57.6
147	52.9	168	65.2	142	45.9	163	58.3
148	53.5	169	65.9	143	46.4	164	58.9
149	54.0	170	66.6	144	47.0	165	59.5
150	54.5	171	67.3	145	47.5	166	60.1
151	55.0	172	68.0	146	48.0	167	60.7
152	55.6	173	68.7	147	48.6	168	61.4
153	56.1	174	69.4	148	49.2	169	62.1
154	56.6	175	70.1	149	49.8		
155	57.2	176	70.8	150	50.4		
156	57.9	177	71.6	151	51.0		
157	58.6	178	72.4	152	51.5		
158	59.3	179	73.3	153	52.0		
159	59.9	180	74.2	154	52.5		
160	60.5	181	75.0	155	53.1		
161	61.1	182	75.8	156	53.7		
162	61.7	183	76.5	157	54.3		
163	62.3	184	77.3	158	54.9		
164	62.9	185	78.1	159	55.5		
165	63.5	186	78.9	160	56.2		

[a] Values are expressed in cm for height and kg for weight. To obtain height in inches, divide by 2.54. To obtain weight in pounds, multiply by 2.2.

Source: Adapted from GL Blackburn et al: J Parenter Enteral Nutr 1:11, 1977; with permission.

and total-body water. BIA is performed by measuring the electric conductivity of a weak current between electrodes placed on the dorsal surfaces of the hands and feet. The measurement reflects differences in the impedance to electric current, which is greatest through fat and least through water. Lean body mass can be calculated by subtracting fat mass from body weight or by dividing total-body water by 0.73.

Overall, BIA is most useful in assessing body fat and FFM in stable

TABLE 62-4 *Physical Findings of Malnutrition*

Finding	Deficiency/Interpretation
General appearance	
Weight loss	Malnutrition <90% of ideal body weight
	Severe <70% of ideal body weight
Decreased temporal and proximal extremity muscle mass	Decreased skeletal protein
Decreased skin-fold thickness by "pinch test"	Decreased body fat stores
Skin, nails, and hair	
Easily plucked hair	Protein
Easy bruising, perifollicular hemorrhages	Vitamin C
"Flaky paint" rash of lower extremities	Zinc
Coarse skin, "goose bumps"	Vitamin A
Hyperpigmentation of sun-exposed areas	Niacin, tryptophan
Spooning of nails	Iron
Eyes	
Conjunctival pallor	Anemia (nonspecific)
Bitot spot	Vitamin A
Ophthalmoplegia	Thiamine
Mouth and mucus membranes	
Nasolabial seborrhea	Essential fatty acids
Glossitis (smooth, red tongue) and/or cheilosis	Riboflavin, niacin, vitamin B_{12}, pyridoxine, folate
Diminished taste	Zinc
Neurologic system	
Disorientation	Niacin, phosphorus
Confabulation	Thiamine
Cerebellar gait, past pointing	Thiamine
Peripheral neuropathy	Thiamine, pyridoxine, vitamin E
Lost vibratory, position sense	Vitamin B_{12}

patients and in those who suffer from conditions leading to relative starvation. However, BIA can also be used to assess critically ill patients with decreased intracellular water space and BCM and expanded extracellular compartment size. Reduced BCM correlates inversely with increased metabolic rate. BIA may be confounded in AIDS patients receiving protease-inhibitor therapy, if they exhibit lipodystrophy with associated redistribution of interscapular, abdominal, and breast fat (Chap. 173).

Energy Expenditure The REE is directly proportional to both FFM and BCM and can be estimated in healthy individuals by the Harris and Benedict formula on the basis of weight in kg (W), height in cm (H), and age in years (A):

$$\text{REE (men)} = 66.473 + 13.751(W) + 5.0033\,(H) - 6.7550\,(A)\ \text{kcal/d}$$

$$\text{REE (women)} = 655.0955 + 9.4634(W) + 1.8496\,(H) - 4.6756\,(A)\ \text{kcal/d}$$

However, this equation tends to overestimate REE in obese individuals, and it is unreliable in estimating energy requirements in sick patients who may be hypo- or hypermetabolic. For estimating TEE, i.e., requirements, the REE in the non-exercising sick patient can be calculated by the Harrison and Benedict formula or estimated at 25% kcal/kg of ideal body weight for height, then modified by adding another 10% for digestion and metabolism of intravenous or enteral feeding and an additional 12.5% for each degree of fever over 37°C, as well as an additional multiplier commensurate with the severity of illness (e.g., 25% for general surgery, 50% for sepsis, and 100% for extensive third-degree burns). TEE can be measured at the bedside more precisely by the gas-exchange method of indirect calorimetry using a mobile metabolic cart. This procedure is applicable to ventilator-independent and -dependent patients whose fractional intake of oxygen is <0.45. Because the goal is to reach an accurate approximation of the 24-h energy requirement, measurements must be taken at intervals during the day and must account for several variables, including food intake and activity. To calculate the energy cost of metabolism by indirect calorimetry, the volumes (V) of oxygen consumed and carbon dioxide produced are measured over a given period of time, according to the modified Weir equation where

$$\text{REE} = 3.9\,V_{O_2} + 1.1\,V_{CO_2}$$

Indirect calorimetry also provides the respiratory quotient (RQ), which is the ratio of carbon dioxide produced to oxygen consumed during the process of gas collection. The RQ decreases when fat is the predominant substrate for metabolism (as in starvation) and increases when the contribution of carbohydrate increases (as during stress with gluconeogenesis). In healthy individuals, the RQ usually falls between 0.80 and 0.90. An RQ <0.7 is consistent with active ketogenesis from endogenous fatty acid metabolism with limited generation of carbon dioxide. An RQ >1.0 indicates net lipogenesis, or the conversion of substrate carbohydrate to fat—a situation that occurs with overfeed-

TABLE 62-5 *Anthropometric Measurements in Adults*

% Standard	Men	Women	Interpretation
TRICEPS SKIN-FOLD, MM			
100	12.5	16.5	Adequate
50	6.0	8.0	Borderline
20	2.5	3.0	Severe depletion
MID-ARM MUSCLE CIRCUMFERENCE, CM			
100	25.5	23.0	Adequate
80	20.0	18.5	Borderline
60	15.0	14.0	Depletion
40	10.0	9.0	Severe depletion

Source: Adapted from SL Morgan, Weinsier RL: *Fundamentals of Clinical Nutrition*, St. Louis, Mosby, 1998, p 167; with permission.

ing. Values that fall outside the range of 0.65 to 1.25 suggest an error in measurement technique.

Creatinine Excretion in the 24-h Urine　Creatinine, the metabolic product of skeletal muscle creatine, is produced at a constant rate and in an amount directly proportional to skeletal muscle mass. With steady-state day-to-day renal function, each gram of creatinine in the 24-h urine collection represents 18.5 g of fat-free skeletal muscle. Since skeletal muscle is the major component of FFM, measurement of creatinine in the 24-h urine collection can be used as a relative measure of this body compartment during the initial assessment or to assess the efficacy of nutritional support. The *creatinine coefficient* represents the amount of creatinine excreted per kilogram of body weight; it is equal to 23 mg/kg of ideal body weight in men and 18 mg/kg of ideal body weight in women. The *creatinine-height index* represents the ratio of the measured 24-h urine creatinine excretion to the value predicted by the creatinine coefficient for the patient's ideal body weight. These values can be calculated from estimation of the patient's ideal body weight according to height (Table 62-3). The constancy of creatinine excretion depends on steady-state renal function and the accuracy of the measurements depends on the reliability of the urine collection. Unpredictable creatinine excretion may occur through feces or skin in patients with serum creatinine levels >530 μmol/L (>6 mg/dL). The presence of ascites does not compromise the accuracy of the 24-h urine creatinine as a reflection of FFM or BCM in patients with chronic liver disease.

Urine Nitrogen Excretion and Nitrogen Balance　Nitrogen balance provides an index of protein gain or loss: 1 g nitrogen is equivalent to 6.25 g protein. Nitrogen balance can be assessed by measuring the difference between nitrogen consumed through the mouth, enteral tube, or intravenous sources and nitrogen excreted in the urine, feces, and other intestinal sources. Accurate measurement of nitrogen balance requires complete measurement of nitrogen losses from all possible excretory routes. In most cases, total urine nitrogen can be calculated by dividing 24-h urinary urea nitrogen by 0.85 and assuming approximately 2 g/d for nitrogen losses in feces and sweat. On the other hand, when the clinical condition includes extensive diarrhea and/or protein losses from pancreatic or enterocutaneous fistulas, the accuracy of nitrogen balance requires measurement of total nitrogen by the modified Kjeldahl technique in both urine and enteric sources. Total nitrogen measurements are also advisable in patients with liver failure, where urinary ammonia becomes a major and alternative source of nitrogen.

INTEGRATED BEDSIDE NUTRITIONAL ASSESSMENT　Several different approaches have been developed to simplify the process of nutritional assessment by using selective measurements that relate malnutrition to the specific medical condition and the severity of the underlying disease process.

Subjective Global Assessment　This approach incorporates historic and physical findings as a basis for nutrition assessment by the trained physician. Major components in the history include evaluation of the extent of recent weight loss, changes in dietary intake, presence of

significant gastrointestinal symptoms persisting more than 2 weeks, alterations in functional status, and the metabolic demand of the patient's underlying disease. During the physical examination, emphasis is placed on findings of depletion of subcutaneous body fat; skeletal muscle wasting; typical changes in skin, mucus membranes, and neurologic examination; as well as the presence of edema. Integration of the historic and physical data permits ranking of patients according to the following categories: adequate nutrition, moderate malnutrition, or severe malnutrition. Though the developers of the subjective global assessment have reported good sensitivity and specificity, the approach is still highly dependent on the training and experience of the clinician.

Prognostic Nutritional Assessment　Several paradigms have been developed to link different parameters of nutritional assessment with clinical prognosis. Each approach links specific features of malnutrition with certain measurements of cell-mediated immunity, since abnormal immune function is a common pathway for increased risk in the malnourished patient. A surgical prognostic nutritional index predicts morbidity based on preoperative measurements of serum albumin, transferrin, triceps skin-fold thickness, and delayed hypersensitivity to skin-test antigens. Another PCM score links survival in alcoholic liver disease to both skin-fold and mid-arm muscle measurements; the creatinine-height index; values for serum albumin, transferrin, prealbumin, and retinol-binding protein; the total lymphocyte count; and the skin-test response to a series of antigens. The Maastricht index predicts survival in patients with serious gastrointestinal diseases on the basis of factors related to serum albumin, retinol-binding protein, lymphocyte count, and deviation from the patient's ideal body weight.

FURTHER READING

BAKER JP et al: Nutritional assessment: A comparison of clinical judgment and objective measurements. N Engl J Med 306:969, 1982

GUIGOZ Y, VELLAS B: Assessing the nutritional status of the elderly: The Mini Nutritional Assessment as part of the geriatric evaluation. Nutr Rev 54:S59, 1998

HALSTED CH: Clinical nutrition education—relevance and role models. Am J Clin Nutr 67:192, 1998

HEYMSFIELD SB et al: Nutritional assessment of malnutrition by anthropomorphic methods, in *Modern Nutrition in Health and Disease*, 9th ed, ME Shils et al (eds). Philadelphia, Lea & Febiger, 1999, p 903

KLIPSTEIN-GROBUSCH K, REILLY J: Energy intake and expenditure in elderly patients admitted to the hospital with acute illness. Br J Nutr 73:323, 1995

MENDENHALL C et al: Relationship of protein calorie malnutrition to alcoholic liver disease: A reexamination of data from two Veterans Administration Cooperative Studies. Alcohol Clin Exp Res 19:635, 1995

NABER THJ et al: Prevalence of malnutrition in nonsurgical hospitalized patients and its association with disease complications. Am J Clin Nutr 66:1232, 1997

UNDERWOOD BA: Health and nutrition in women, infants, and children: Overview of the global situation and the Asian enigma. Nutr Rev 2002 60:S7, 2002

YANOVSKI SZ et al: Bioelectrical impedance analysis in body composition measurement: National Institutes of Health technology assessment conference statement. Am J Clin Nutr 64:524S, 1996

63　ENTERAL AND PARENTERAL NUTRITION THERAPY
Lyn Howard

Parenteral and enteral nutrition provide life-sustaining therapy for patients who cannot take adequate food by mouth and who consequently are at risk for malnutrition and its effects, including susceptibility to infection, weakness, and immobility; these features predispose the patient to aspiration pneumonia, pulmonary embolism, and pressure sores, all of which delay recovery from illness and increase mortality.

The term *enteral* refers to feeding via the gut and hence includes normal eating, but in the present context implies the infusion of formulas, via a tube, into the upper gastrointestinal tract. *Parenteral* refers to the infusion of nutrient solutions into the bloodstream. Although these are different approaches to nutritional support, their goals are the same.

Where feasible, enteral nutrition (EN) is the preferred route because it sustains the digestive, absorptive, and immunologic barrier functions of the gastrointestinal tract. Several developments have made tube feeding easier and more acceptable to patients. Small-bore pliable tubes have largely replaced large-bore rubber tubes, and double-lumen

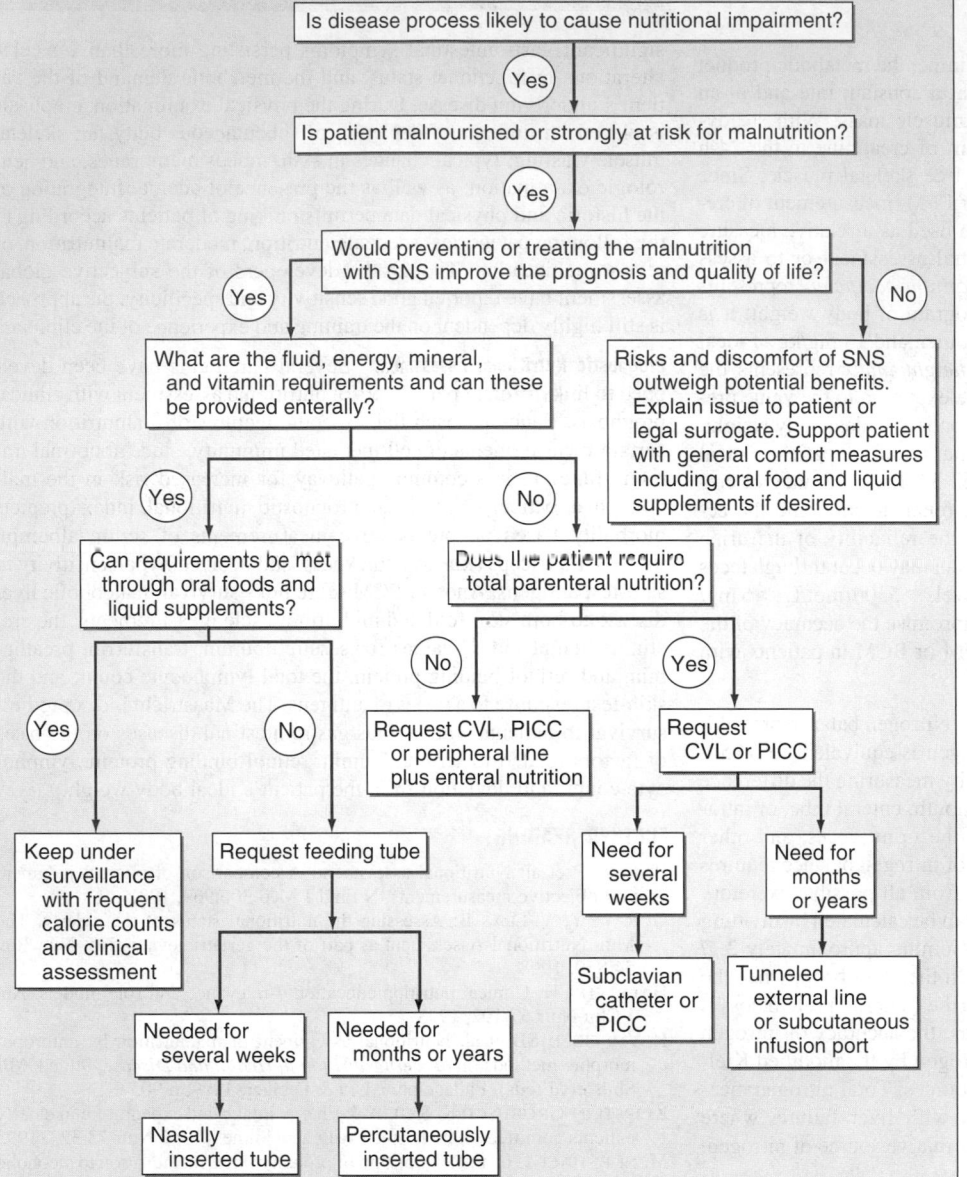

FIGURE 63-1 Should specialized nutrition support (SNS) be undertaken and, if so, how? An algorithm. PICC, peripherally inserted central catheter; CVL, central venous line.

The flow chart contains the following boxes:

- Is disease process likely to cause nutritional impairment? **Yes** →
- Is patient malnourished or strongly at risk for malnutrition? **Yes** →
- Would preventing or treating the malnutrition with SNS improve the prognosis and quality of life?
  - **Yes** → What are the fluid, energy, mineral, and vitamin requirements and can these be provided enterally?
    - **Yes** → Can requirements be met through oral foods and liquid supplements?
      - **Yes** → Keep under surveillance with frequent calorie counts and clinical assessment
      - **No** → Request feeding tube
        - Needed for several weeks → Nasally inserted tube
        - Needed for months or years → Percutaneously inserted tube
    - **No** → Does the patient require total parenteral nutrition?
      - **No** → Request CVL, PICC or peripheral line plus enteral nutrition
      - **Yes** → Request CVL or PICC
        - Need for several weeks → Subclavian catheter or PICC
        - Need for months or years → Tunneled external line or subcutaneous infusion port
  - **No** → Risks and discomfort of SNS outweigh potential benefits. Explain issue to patient or legal surrogate. Support patient with general comfort measures including oral food and liquid supplements if desired.

for others, wasting is an inevitable component of a terminal disease. A flow diagram of the steps involved in deciding whether SNS should be undertaken and, if so, how, is depicted in Fig. 63-1.

The first step requires consideration of the nutritional implications of the disease process. Is the condition or its treatment likely to impair appetite or food ingestion and absorption for a prolonged period of time? The second step is to determine whether the patient is already sufficiently malnourished that lean body mass is decreased and critical functions such as healing and ventilation are impaired. The presence or absence of metabolic stress should be noted, since injury or infection evokes the secretion of hormonal and cytokine factors that reduce the efficiency of nutrition repletion.

Weight loss without physiologic impairment is probably of no consequence. Physiologic impairment usually develops when more than 20% of body protein is lost and is more likely if key organ systems, such as the gut or liver, are directly affected by disease. Once it is recognized that the patient is malnourished or at major risk, the next question is whether SNS will impact positively on the patient's response to the disease, improving quality of life. While the provision of food and water is part of basic medical care, nutrition delivered by tube, enteral or parenteral, is associated with risk and discomfort and should be recommended only when potential benefit exceeds risk, and undertaken with the consent of the patient. Like all life support measures, these therapies are difficult to withdraw, once started.

If preventing or treating malnutrition with SNS is appropriate, then nutritional requirements must be determined and the route of nutrient delivery should be selected. The route depends primarily on the degree of gut function but somewhat on the technical resources available.

RISKS AND BENEFITS OF SPECIALIZED NUTRITION SUPPORT

The risks are determined primarily by patient factors such as state of alertness and swallowing competence, the route of delivery, and the experience of the supervising clinical team. The safest and least costly approach is to avoid SNS, if possible, by close attention to oral food intake, by adding an oral liquid supplement, or by using medications to stimulate appetite. Nutrient intake is monitored with frequent calorie counts. This more physiologic approach is the most metabolically efficient since normal eating initiates the cephalic phase of digestion. Tube-fed infants grow better if the cephalic phase is stimulated by having the infant suck on a pacifier.

Anorexia, impairment of swallowing, or bowel disease can limit intake and absorption of oral nutrients, in which case tube EN is considered next. The bowel and its associated digestive organs derive 70% of their required nutrients directly from food in the lumen. Glutamine, short-chain fatty acids, and nucleotides may have particular importance in maintaining gut integrity. Enteral feeding also supports gut function by stimulating splanchnic blood flow, neuronal activity, IgA

tubes are now available for simultaneous gastric suction and jejunal feeding when there is concern about gastric retention and aspiration. Enteral tubes can be inserted into the stomach or jejunum through the nose or, for long-term use, directly through the abdominal wall, using endoscopic, radiologic, or surgical techniques. Once the enterocutaneous tract is established, a "button" entry port can replace the protruding tube.

Complete nutrition by vein with sufficient calories, amino acids, minerals, and vitamins to permit wound healing, restoration of normal body composition of a cachectic patient, and growth in children became feasible with the development of high-flow central vein catheters. Parental nutrition (PN) is now available in all large hospitals and for some patients at home.

THE DECISION PROCESS FOR USING PARENTERAL OR ENTERAL NUTRITION

The decision to use specialized nutrition support (SNS) should be based on the likelihood that averting or redressing malnutrition will improve the quality of life, or the ability to recover from a serious illness. Approximately 15 to 20% of hospitalized patients have evidence of malnutrition. Some malnourished patients benefit from SNS;

antibody release, and secretion of gastrointestinal hormones such as epidermal growth factor that stimulate gut trophic activity. All these factors support the gut as an immunologic barrier against enteric pathogens. For these reasons, some luminal nutrition should always be provided, if possible, even when PN is required to provide most of the support. In the past, bowel rest through PN was thought to be the cornerstone of treatment for many severe gastrointestinal disorders, but the value of some EN is now widely accepted, and strict bowel rest is rarely appropriate. PN alone is necessary in severe hemorrhagic pancreatitis, necrotizing enterocolitis, prolonged ileus, and distal bowel obstruction.

SNS is expensive, accounting for >1% of all health care dollars. Consequently, in assessing effectiveness, hard clinical end points, such as mortality rate, incidence of major complications, and duration of hospital stay are required for risk-benefit studies. Better nitrogen bal-

ance, increased levels of serum albumin, and improved delayed hypersensitivity are softer end points. Table 63-1 summarizes the current evidence-based evaluation of SNS treatment in disease states. The data are strictly from randomized controlled trials, in many instances combined into meta-analyses. This analysis emphasized that SNS is beneficial primarily for conditions associated with severe protein-calorie malnutrition or when oral intake is interrupted for prolonged periods of time (e.g., >9 days).

A practical consideration is the availability of tube or line placement expertise, especially in critically ill patients. Placement of a central venous catheter is a widely available bedside technique and can be done by specially trained personnel using a peripherally inserted central catheter. While inserting a nasogastric tube is a bedside pro-

TABLE 63-1 *Evidence-Based Evaluation of SNS in Different Disease States*[a]

Disease State	Type of SNS	Comment
Perioperative		
Preoperative	PN	Only beneficial in severe PCM
		↓ Postoperative complications 10%
	EN	↓ Postoperative complications ≥25%
Postoperative	PN	↓ Complications and MR if oral intake not resumed in 9 days
	Early EN vs PN	↓ Septic complications with EN if PN calories higher
	EN with CEN	↓ Postoperative complications and hospital stay (CEN: arginine, W₃FA, nucleotides)
Critical illness	PN	Only beneficial in severe PCM
		↓ Complications if lipid not used
	Early EN vs PN	↓ Septic complications with EN if PN calories higher
	EN with CEN	Risk ≥ benefit if CEN arginine
Cancer		
Cachexia	PN	Risk ≥ benefit with CXT/RXT; beneficial in cancer surgery in severe PCM
	EN	No clear benefit
BMT	PN/EN	Better long-term survival
	PN with CEN	↓ Early MR, ↓ hospital stay (CEN: glutamine)
	Home PN vs IV hydration	Outcome same; PN associated with less weight loss but delayed oral intake
Liver failure	PN/EN with CEN	Beneficial if encephalopathy prevents adequate protein intake (CEN: ↑ BCAA, ↓ AAA)
Renal failure		
Acute	PN with AA vs PN without AA	PN with AA: ↓ septic complications; EAA or EAA and NEAA equally good
Chronic	Low-protein diet	Did not reduce rate of GFR deterioration
	IDPN	No benefit on MR shown
Pancreatitis	PN	Risk > benefit except in severe pancreatitis
Acute	Early PN vs late PN	Early PN, ↓ MR in severe pancreatitis
	EN vs PN	↓ Septic complications with EN if PN calories higher
Inflammatory bowel disease		
Crohn's	PN vs EN	No benefit from bowel rest
	EN polymeric vs elemental	No difference
	EN vs steroids	EN: slower improvement, shorter remissions
	Exclusion vs regular oral diet	Elimination of foods that induce GI distress prolongs remission
Ulcerative colitis	PN vs oral diet/steroids	No difference
Short bowel syndrome	PN with CEN	hGH and glutamine supplements did not ↑ bowel adaption
Pulmonary disease		
Acute, ventilated	PN/EN	↓ CHO, ↑ fat calories aided weaning process
	EN intermittent vs continuous	No difference in gastric colonization
Chronic	EN gastric vs jejunal	↓ Aspiration, better intake with jejunal
	EN gastric vs postpyloric	No difference in risk of aspiration
HIV disease	PN vs EN	Gain in body cell mass same but PN ↑ fat and water gain; EN led to better physical functioning
	PN vs dietary counseling	No difference in survival after 2 months, but PN led to better functioning

Note: SNS, specialized nutrition support; PN, parenteral nutrition; PCM, protein-calorie malnutrition; MR, mortality rate; Early EN, tube feeding started within 48 h of onset of acute condition; EN, tube feeding; CEN, conditionally essential nutrients; W₃FA, omega 3 fatty acids; CXT, chemotherapy; RXT, radiation therapy; BMT, bone marrow transplant; BCAA, branch chain amino acids; AAA, aromatic amino acids; EAA, essential amino acids; NEAA, nonessential amino acids; IDPN, intradialytic parenteral nutrition; GFR, glomerular filtration rate; hGH, human growth hormone; CHO, carbohydrate.

TABLE 63-2 *Summary of Outcomes for Patients on Home Parenteral and Enteral Nutrition (HPEN)*

Diagnosis	Number in Group	Age in Years	% Survival[a] on Therapy	Therapy Status, % at 1 year[b] Full Oral Nutrition	Continued on HPEN Rx	Died	Rehabilitation[c] Status, % in 1st year C	P	M	Complications[d] per Patient-Year HPEN	NonHPEN
HOME PARENTERAL NUTRITION											
Crohn's disease	562	36	96	70	25	2	60	38	2	0.9	1.1
Ischemic bowel disease	331	49	87	27	48	19	53	41	6	1.4	1.1
Motility disorder	299	45	87	31	44	21	49	39	12	1.3	1.1
Congenital bowel defect	172	5	94	42	47	9	63	27	11	2.1	1.0
Hyperemesis gravidarum	112	28	100	100	0	0	83	16	1	1.5	3.5
Chronic pancreatitis	156	42	90	82	10	5	60	38	2	1.2	2.5
Radiation enteritis	145	58	87	28	49	22	42	49	9	0.8	1.1
Chronic adhesive obstructions	120	53	83	47	34	13	23	68	10	1.7	1.4
Cystic fibrosis	51	17	50	38	13	36	24	66	16	0.8	3.7
Cancer	2122	44	20	26	8	63	29	57	14	1.1	3.3
AIDS	280	33	10	13	6	73	8	63	29	1.6	3.3
HOME ENTERAL NUTRITION											
Neurologic disorders of swallowing	1134	65	55	19	25	48	5	24	71	0.3	0.9
Cancer	1644	61	30	30	6	59	21	59	21	0.4	2.7

[a] Survival rates on therapy are values at 1 year, calculated by the life table method. This will differ from the percentage listed as died under Therapy Status, since all patients with known end points are considered in this latter measure. The ratio of observed versus expected deaths is equivalent to a Standard Mortality Ratio.

[b] Not shown are those patients who were back in hospital or who had changed therapy type by 12 months.

[c] Rehabilitation is designated complete (C), partial (P), or minimal (M), relative to the patient's ability to sustain normal age-related activity.

[d] Complications refer only to those complications that resulted in rehospitalization.

Source: Derived from North American HPEN Registry.

cedure, many sick patients have impaired gastric emptying, and intragastric feeding increases risk of aspiration pneumonia. Obtaining enteral access to the jejunum usually requires fluoroscopy in an endoscopic or radiologic unit. If a surgical laparotomy is required, a jejunal feeding tube can be placed simultaneously. Studies have shown that such tubes must be beyond the ligament of Treitz to avoid aspiration; an intraduodenal tube is no safer than an intragastric tube.

While most SNS is delivered in hospitals, some patients require SNS on a long-term basis. If they have a safe environment and a willingness to learn the self-care techniques, SNS can be administered at home. The clinical outcome of patients with severe intestinal disorders that use home PN or EN are summarized in Table 63-2. PN infused at home is usually cycled overnight to give greater daytime freedom. Cycling requires a 1-h taper up and down to avoid sudden changes in blood sugar. SNS is not usually appropriate in terminally ill patients but is an option if the patient and family request treatment and quality survival for several months is predicted.

THE DESIGN OF INDIVIDUAL REGIMENS

FLUID REQUIREMENTS   These can be determined by adding the normal daily requirement (120 mL/kg of body weight for infants, 35 mL/kg of body weight for adults) to any abnormal loss. If the patient is on PN or EN, any oral intake should be subtracted from the estimate (Table 63-3). Since abnormal loss of enteric fluid implies significant mineral losses, extra amounts of these nutrients, as well as fluid (Table 63-4), must be added to the SNS formula.

ENERGY REQUIREMENTS   (See also Chap. 62)   Ultimately, energy expenditure dictates energy requirements, but in the early phase of nutrition repletion, requirements may not reflect expenditure. For example, malnourished patients are hypometabolic and may expend only 85 kJ/kg (20 kcal/kg) per day, but more calories are needed both for tissue repletion and because the metabolic rate increases with refeeding. Conversely, a highly stressed patient (sepsis, trauma) may expend 165 kJ/kg (40 kcal/kg) per day with a significant proportion of the calories coming from protein breakdown and gluconeogenesis and

TABLE 63-3 *Estimation of Daily Fluid Requirements*

NORMAL 70-KG MAN

Intake	Output
Normal requirement: 35 × 70 = ~2500 mL/d (derived from oral liquids of 1200 mL, or 5 glasses/cups per day and solid food providing 1300 mL, 1000 mL from water in food, 300 mL from water generated by metabolism of foods)	Urine: 1600 mL/d Insensible loss: 800 mL/d Stool: 100 mL/d [sweat loss can be up to 2 L/d; each degree of fever (C) = 200 mL/d]

TUBE ENTERAL PATIENT

58-kg woman recovering from total gastrectomy for gastric cancer and supported by jejunostomy feedings, taking nothing by mouth or intravenously but experiencing 600 mL of diarrheal losses/day:
Normal requirement 35 × 58 = ~2000 mL/d
Abnormal gastrointestinal loss 600 − 100 = 500 mL/d
Total per tube requirement = 2500 mL/d

PARENTERAL PATIENT

66-kg man with a high jejunostomy following massive bowel resection for Crohn's disease with oral intake of 2000 mL/day and jejunostomy loss of 4000 mL/day:
Normal requirement 35 × 66 = 2300 mL/d
Abnormal gastrointestinal loss (4000 − 100) minus oral intake (2000) = 1900 mL/d
Total parenteral requirement = 4200 mL/d

TABLE 63-4 *Enteric Fluid Volumes and Their Sodium, Potassium, Chloride, and Bicarbonate Content[a]*

	L/d[b]	Na, mmol/L	K,[c] mmol/L	Cl, mmol/L	HCO_3,[d] mmol/L
Oral intake	2–3				
Enteric secretions					
Saliva	1–2	10	30	10	30
Gastric juice	2	60	9	90	0
Bile	2–3	150	10	90	70
Small bowel	1	100	5	100	20
Colon	Variable	40	100	15	60

[a] Enteric secretions are also rich in divalent cations (Ca, Mg, Zn, Cu), and their loss is increased by steatorrhea, a high bowel fistula, or prolonged suction.

[b] Of the 9 L/d of oral and enteric fluid presented to the upper small bowel, normally 50% is absorbed in the jejunum, 40% in the ileum, and 10% in the colon. In short bowel patients, the colon may absorb greater amounts, up to 3 L/d.

[c] Potassium losses are small except in secretions distal to the ileocecal valve. The colon ion exchange is partly controlled by aldosterone, and therefore, Na$^+$ depletion increases K$^+$ loss in the stool.

[d] Bicarbonate losses must be replaced in parenteral solutions as acetane or lactate because of potential precipitation of bicarbonate with ingredients such as calcium.

from catecholamine-induced lipolysis. Oxidation of exogenous glucose plateaus at 100 kJ/kg (25 kcal/kg) per day, and administering a higher glucose load induces hepatic steatosis. Providing such patients with additional calories as exogenous fat does not suppress endogenous lipolysis. Furthermore, lipid solutions are made from vegetable oil and egg phospholipid and lack apoproteins, which they acquire from endogenous lipoproteins. Initially, the artificial chylomicron is taken up by the reticuloendothelial system, causing potential blockade. For all these reasons, modest hypocaloric glucose feeding with minimal parenteral fat is safer in the acutely stressed subject.

Parenteral lipid solutions are available as 10 or 20% isotonic solutions and are infused separately from amino acids and glucose or as a combined "three-in-one solution," obviating the need for an extra pump. Three-in-one PN solutions are less stable, and destabilized fat particles may coalesce into larger droplets, becoming fat emboli. For this reason, three-in-one solutions have a shorter storage life and must be mixed by a pharmacist who is knowledgeable about correct mixing sequence and safe levels of electrolytes and trace elements. Iron, for example, cannot be added to this solution.

Polyunsaturated vegetable oils are used in most enteral formulas because a diseased gastrointestinal tract absorbs them better than animal fat. Median-chain triglycerides (c8–12) may be added because of their simpler absorption. Though fat must supply the long-chain essential fatty acids (1 to 4% of energy from linoleic and linolenic acid) (Table 63-5), larger amounts (30% of energy) are safe in relatively stable patients and avoid the hazard of providing large amounts of carbohydrate calories (e.g., hyperglycemia and hepatic steatosis). Substituting omega-3 polyunsaturated fish oils for polyunsaturated vegetable fats may blunt the catabolic response to burn injury, trauma, and radiation by reducing the synthesis of prostaglandins that enhance the inflammatory response. Such fats are currently available in enteral formulas and are being tested in parenteral formulas.

Carbohydrate usually provides 60 to 70% of all calories and is provided as glucose [monohydrous dextrose, 14 kJ/g (3.4 kcal/g)] in parenteral solutions and as disaccharides (sucrose) and oligosaccharides (starch fragments) in enteral formulas to maximize absorption while limiting the intraluminal osmolar load. Fructooligosaccharides have been shown to promote normal gut flora.

PROTEIN OR AMINO ACID REQUIREMENTS The recommended dietary protein allowance of 0.8 g/kg per day is adequate for nonstressed patients, such as a starved patient with a high-grade esophageal stricture. Catabolic patients, in contrast, may require up to 1.5 g/kg per day of protein to induce positive nitrogen balance and reconstitute normal lean body mass. Early studies showed that recombinant human growth hormone increases lean body mass. However, subsequent trials have

TABLE 63-6 *Central Venous Access for Parenteral Nutrition*

Type of Catheters	Advantages	Disadvantages
Peripherally inserted central catheter Single lumen Double lumen	Insertion cost low; can be done at bedside or by vascular radiology using Doppler guidance; especially advantageous for patients with neck wounds such as tracheostomies	High incidence of skin site irritation; tendency to break at hub; home patient requires assistance with weekly dressing change
Centrally inserted externalized catheter (subclavian, jugular, femoral) Single lumen Multilumen	Can be inserted at bedside; relatively low cost; can be changed over a guidewire if clinically indicated; best site subclavian > jugular > femoral vein	10% incidence of mechanical complication with insertion, higher if physician inexperienced; need dedicated nutrition line; multiple-lumen catheters have increased sepsis rate
Centrally inserted, tunneled catheter or subcutaneous port	More stable for long-term use; when needle out, patients with ports have less disturbance of body image and can shower and swim without risk	More expensive device requiring operating room insertion; ports require needle stick.

TABLE 63-5 *Daily Enteral and Parenteral Requirements of Essential Fatty Acids, Minerals, and Vitamins*

Nutrient	Daily Requirement, Adult Range	
	Enteral	Parenteral
Essential fatty acids, % kcal	1–2	2–4
Calcium, g	0.8–1.2	0.2–0.4 (10–20 mmol)
Phosphorus, g	0.8–1.2	0.4–0.8
Potassium, g	2–5	3–4 (75–100 mmol)
Sodium, g	1–3	1–3 (50–150 mmol)
Chloride, g	2.5–5	3–4^a (100–130 mmol)
Magnesium, g	0.3	0.3 (20 mmol)
Iron, mg	10	1–2
Zinc, mg	15	3–12
Copper, mg	2–3	0.3–0.5
Iodine, mg	0.15	0.15
Manganese, mg	2–5	2–5
Chromium, μg	50–200	15–30
Molybdenum, μg	150–300	20–120
Selenium, μg	50–200	50–100
Ascorbic acid, mg	60	100
Thiamine, mg	1.4	3.0
Riboflavin, mg	1.6	3.6
Niacin, mg	18	40
Biotin, μg	60	60
Pantothenic acid, mg	5	15
Pyridoxine, mg	2.0	4.0
Folic acid, μg	400	400
Cobalamin, μg	3.0	5
Vitamin A, μg	1000	1000
Vitamin D, μg	10	5–10
Vitamin E, mg	8–10	10–15
Vitamin K, μg	70–140	200

^{a} In addition to chloride anions there is a parenteral requirement for bicarbonate equivalents to protect normal acid-base balance. These are provided as 100 mmol or more per day of acetate or lactate because of potential precipitation of bicarbonate with ingredients such as calcium.

TABLE 63-7 *Monitoring the Patient on Total Parenteral Nutrition*

CLINICAL DATA MONITORED DAILY

Sense of well-being: symptoms suggesting fluid overload, high or low blood glucose, electrolyte imbalance, etc.
Strength as judged by graded activity: getting out of bed, walking, stair climbing
Vital signs: temperature, blood pressure, pulse rate, and respiratory rate
Fluid balance: weight; fluid input (intravenous +/− enteral) vs fluid output (urine, stool, gastric suction, etc.)
Delivery equipment for parenteral nutrition: tubing, pump, filter, catheter, dressing (skin checked for local infection at time of dressing change)
Composition of nutrient solution

LABORATORY DATA

Finger stick glucose	Three times daily until patient stable
Blood glucose Na, K, Cl, HCO₃ Blood urea nitrogen	Daily until glucose infusion load and patient stable, then twice weekly
Liver function studies Serum creatinine, albumin PO₄, Ca, Mg Hb/Hct, WBC	Baseline, then twice weekly
INR	Baseline, then weekly
Micronutrient tests	As indicated

Note: Hb, hemoglobin; Hct, hematocrit; WBC, white blood cell (count); INR, international normalized ratio.

TABLE 63-8 *Complications of Total Parenteral Nutrition (TPN)*

First 48 h	First 2 Weeks	3 Months Onward
MECHANICAL		

Complications from catheter insertion:
    Cephalad displacement
    Pneumothorax
    Hemothorax
Detachment of line at catheter hub with blood loss or air embolism
	Catheter coming out of vein, more common if Silastic
	Detachment of line at catheter hub with blood loss or air embolism
	Thrombosis
		Detachment of line at catheter hub with blood loss or air embolism
		Fractures or tears in catheter
		Catheter embedded in vein wall

METABOLIC		
Fluid overload Hyperglycemia Hypophosphatemia Hypokalemia	Cardiopulmonary failure Refeeding edema Hyperosmolar nonketotic hyperglycemic coma Acid-base imbalance Electrolyte imbalance	Essentially fatty acid deficiency Iron deficiency Vitamin deficiencies TPN metabolic bone disease TPN liver disease Zinc, copper, chromium, selenium, molybdenum, deficiency
INFECTIOUS		
	Catheter-induced sepsis Exit site infection	Catheter-induced sepsis Tunnel infections Exit site infection

TABLE 63-9 *Enteral Feeding Tubes*

Type/Insertion Technique	Clinical Uses	Potential Complications
NASOGASTRIC TUBE		
External measurement: nostril, ear, xiphisternum; tube stiffened by ice water or stylet; position verified by injecting air and auscultating, aspirating gastric acid, or by x-ray	Short-term clinical situation (weeks) or longer periods with intermittent insertion; bolus feeding simpler, but continuous drip with pump better tolerated	Aspiration; ulceration of nasal and esophageal tissues, leading to stricture
NASOJEJUNAL TUBE		
External measurement: nostril, ear, anterior superior iliac spine (medical malleolus in infants); tube stiffened by stylet and passed through pylorus under fluoroscopy or with endoscopic loop	Short-term clinical situations where gastric emptying impaired or proximal leak suspected; requires continuous drip with pump	Spontaneous pulling back into stomach (position verified by aspirating content, pH > 6); diarrhea common, fiber-containing formula may help
GASTROSTOMY TUBE		
Percutaneous placement endoscopically, radiologically, or surgically: after tract established, can be converted to a gastric "button"	Long-term clinical situations, swallowing disorders, or impaired small-bowel absorption requiring continuous drip	Aspiration; irritation around tube exit site; peritoneal leak; balloon migration and obstruction of pylorus
JEJUNOSTOMY TUBE		
Percutaneous placement endoscopically or radiologically via pylorus or endoscopically or surgically directly into the jejunum	Long-term clinical situations where gastric emptying impaired; requires continuous drip with pump; direct endoscopic placement (PEJ) is the most comfortable for the patient	Clogging or displacement of tube; jejunal fistula if large-bore tube used; diarrhea from dumping; irritation of surgical anchoring suture
COMBINED GASTROJEJUNOSTOMY TUBE		
Percutaneous placement endoscopically, radiologically, or surgically; intragastric arm for continuous or intermittent gastric suction; jejunal arm for enteral feeding	Used for patients with impaired gastric emptying and at high risk for aspiration or patients with acute pancreatitis or proximal leaks	Clogging: especially of small bore jejunal tube

Note: All small tubes are at risk for clogging, especially if used for crushed medications. In long-term enteral nutrition patients, gastrostomy and jejunostomy tubes can be exchanged for a low-profile "button" once the tract is established.

shown an association with increased mortality in critically ill patients.

In a stable patient the adequacy of protein support can be assessed acutely by analyzing protein balance:

Protein balance

$$= \text{protein intake} - \text{protein loss}$$

where protein loss = [(24-h urine urea nitrogen (g) + 4) × 6.25]. Over a long period, protein balance is assessed by documenting wound healing, restoration of normal body composition, or resumption of longitudinal growth. In states of disturbed protein utilization (e.g., renal and hepatic failure), azotemia and abnormal plasma amino acid patterns develop. The benefit of special enteral and parenteral solutions that correct these aberrations is only established in hepatic encephalopathy (Table 63-1).

When amino acids are infused systemically, rather than via the more physiologic portal vein, methionine, the only sulfur-containing amino acid in most parenteral solutions, is transaminated in peripheral tissues rather than transulfurated in the liver. As a result, downstream sulfur products such as carnitine, taurine, and glutathione become relatively deficient. Preliminary studies suggest that the addition of an intermediate compound, *S*-adenosyl methionine, to parenteral solutions reduces cholestasis. In enteral formulas, protein is provided either as a complete protein with high biologic value and low immunogenicity, such as egg albumin or casein, or as partially hydrolysed short oligopeptides. Studies have shown that while amino acid transport mechanisms are defective with inflamed gastrointestinal mucosa, peptide absorption remains normal.

MINERAL AND VITAMIN REQUIREMENTS

Parenteral and enteral mineral and vitamin requirements are summarized in Table 63-5. Electrolyte modifications are necessary if the patient has significant gastrointestinal losses (Table 63-4) or renal failure. Requirements of some minerals and vitamins are higher when administered parenterally rather than enterally for several reasons: (1) many micronutrients delivered into the systemic rather than the portal circulation are not captured by the liver and instead pass directly into the urine; (2) patients with bowel disease often have increased enteric loss of sodium, potassium, chloride, and bicarbonate and malabsorption of divalent cations, fat-soluble vitamins, and vitamin B_{12}; and (3) nutrients may adhere to the tubing and delivery bags, and exposure to oxygen and light may destroy vitamins (particularly vitamin A).

PARENTERAL NUTRITION

INFUSION TECHNIQUE AND PATIENT MONITORING

Partial and short-term PN can be provided via a peripheral vein if the majority of the energy is supplied by isotonic fat solutions; long-term PN using glucose as the chief energy source requires administration via a central vein catheter so the hypertonic solution is rapidly diluted in a high-flow system. The preferred site for central vein infusion is the superior vena cava. Access sites and catheter choices are summarized in Table 63-6. Peripherally inserted central catheters are the most economical option for short-term PN. Tunneled catheters and implanted subcutaneous ports require operating room insertion but are more stable for long-term use. Central catheters should be changed when clinically indicated; routine changes are costly and hazardous. Chlorhexidine solution is a more effective local antiseptic than iodophor or alcohol. Although transparent dressings are helpful in stabilizing catheters and allow easy observation of the skin site, the incidence of catheter-related sepsis is higher than with traditional dry gauze dressings; newer transparent dressings that trap less moisture are under investigation. Catheters made from Silastic material or polyurethane are associated with lower complications than polyvinylchloride catheters. Several types of needleless systems use hub valves, and while inadvertent needle sticks are prevented, contamination rates are higher with these devices used for long-term PN. Appropriate clinical and laboratory monitoring for patients on parenteral nutrition is summarized in Table 63-7.

COMPLICATIONS ■ Mechanical

The insertion of a central venous catheter should be performed only by trained personnel, using an aseptic technique. The correct catheter position must be confirmed by x-ray before hypertonic nutrient solution is infused. Insertion complications are listed in Table 63-8. Catheter thrombosis may occur, especially if the catheter is used for withdrawing blood samples, and extension of the thrombosis to the central vein is frequently coincident with infection. Thrombosed catheters can sometimes be unblocked by thrombolytic agents. The addition of heparin (1000 U/L) to the PN solution to prevent thrombosis is controversial; no randomized, controlled studies demonstrate benefit, and heparin can contribute to loss of bone mineral, which is already a problem with long-term PN. Low-dose oral warfarin (1 mg/d), which does not alter prothrombin time, has been shown to reduce catheter thrombosis.

Metabolic

Fluid overload can cause congestive heart failure, particularly in elderly and debilitated patients. Glucose overload can cause an osmotic diuresis or stimulate insulin secretion, which in turn promotes extracellular to intracellular shifts of potassium and phosphorous. Such shifts are most dangerous in cachectic patients with depletion of potassium and phosphorus stores and can cause arrhythmias, cardiopulmonary dysfunction, and neurologic symptoms. To avoid these problems, PN should be started slowly and monitored carefully. Glucose content is increased gradually as the patient demonstrates tolerance of the high glucose load. Late metabolic complications include cholestatic liver disease, with bile sludging and gallstone formation. The exact cause of the liver disease is not understood, but lack of enteral stimulation to bile flow and defective sulfur amino acid metabolism and cholesterol solubilization appear to play a role. Chole-

stasis is less likely to occur if some enteral feeding is maintained. PN induces hypercalciuria and can result in negative calcium balance and osteopenia. Once patients on long-term PN change to sustained anabolism, deficiencies of micronutrients such as essential fatty acids, trace minerals, and vitamins may develop unless they are supplied in adequate amounts (Table 63-5).

Infectious

Infection of the access line rarely occurs in the first 72 h, and fever during this period is usually due to infection elsewhere or some other cause. Infection of the access line should be suspected if the fever defervesces when the infusion of the parenteral formula is tapered.

Positive central line and peripheral blood cultures suggest catheter sepsis, if no other infectious source is identified. *Staphylococcus epidermidis* infection can often be cleared (80 to 90% of the time) without catheter removal. To improve the chances of clearing the line, the biofilm from the internal surface is removed by thrombolytic treatment and antibiotics are given through the catheter and left as a "lock" in the catheter for several hours. *S. aureus* or fungal infections require catheter removal to prevent life-threatening metastatic spread. Catheter sepsis rates are similar in single-lumen central lines dedicated to PN whether inserted peripherally, via the subclavian vein, or tunneled; multiple-lumen catheters are associated with a greater incidence of sepsis. Although there is no evidence to support the use of prophylactic antibiotics, recurrent catheter sepsis may be avoided if small amounts of an antibiotic solution are left in the line, along with a heparin lock.

ENTERAL NUTRITION

TUBE PLACEMENT AND PATIENT MONITORING

The types of enteral feeding tubes, methods of insertion, their clinical uses, and potential complications are outlined in Table 63-9. The different types of enteral formulas are listed in Table 63-10. Patients on enteral feeding are at risk for many of the same metabolic complications as those who receive PN and should be monitored in the same manner (Table 63-7). Since small-bore tubes are easily displaced, tube position should be checked

TABLE 63-10 Enteral Formulas

Composition Characteristics	Clinical Indications
STANDARD ENTERAL FORMULA	

1. Complete dietary products (+)[a]
  a. Caloric density 1 kcal/mL
  b. Protein ~14% cals, caseinates, soy, lactalbumin
  c. Fat ~30% cals, corn, soy, safflower oils
  d. CHO ~60% cals, hydrolysed corn starch, maltodextrin, sucrose
  e. Recommended daily intake of all minerals and vitamins in >1500 kcal/d
  f. Osmolality (mosmol/kg): ~300
	Suitable for most patients requiring tube feeding; flavors available for oral use

MODIFIED ENTERAL FORMULAS	
1. Caloric density 1.5–2 kcal/mL (+)	Fluid-restricted patients
2. a. High protein ~20% cals (+)	Protein malnutrition and ↓ wound healing
b. Hydrolysed protein to small peptides (++)	↓ Protein digestion/absorption or allergy
c. ↑ Glutamine, arginine, S-containing amino acids, nucleotides (+++)	Severely immunocompromised patients
d. ↑ Branch-chain amino acids, ↓ aromatic amino acids (+++)	Liver failure patients intolerant of 0.8 g/kg per day of regular protein
e. Low protein of high biologic value	Renal failure patients
3. a. Low fat, partial MCT substitution (+)	Fat malabsorption
b. ↑ Fat >40% cals (++)	Pulmonary failure with ↑ P_{CO_2} on standard formulas
c. ↑ Fat from MUFA (++)	Poorly controlled diabetes mellitus
d. Fat ↑ in w3 (fish oil) and ↓ w6 (+++)	Immunocompromised and autoimmune disorder
4. a. Fiber provided as soy polysaccharide (+)	Diarrhea/constipation
b. Fiber provided as blenderized fruits and vegetables (++)	↓ Binding of dilantin
5. ↑ Minerals (Zn) and vitamins (A and C) (++)	Decubitus ulcers

[a] Cost: + inexpensive; ++ moderately expensive; +++ very expensive.
Note: CHO, carbohydrate; MCT, medium-chain triglyceride; MUFA, monounsaturated fatty acids; w3 or w6, polyunsatuated fat with first double bond at carbon 3 (fish oils) or carbon 6 (vegetable oils).

at intervals by aspirating and measuring the pH of the gut fluid (<4 in stomach, >6 in jejunum).

COMPLICATIONS ■ Aspiration   The debilitated patient with poor gastric emptying and impairment of swallowing and cough mechanisms is at risk for aspiration; this is particularly so for those who are on respirators. Tracheal suctioning induces coughing and gastric regurgitation, and cuffs on endotracheal or tracheostomy tubes seldom protect against aspiration. Under these circumstances, it may be safer to institute jejunal feeding. A continuous gastric drip is better tolerated in sick patients than intermittent bolus feeding; a drip is essential for intrajejunal feeding.

Diarrhea   Enteral feeding often causes diarrhea, especially if bowel function is compromised by disease or drugs, particularly broadspectrum antibiotics. Diarrhea may be controlled by the use of a continuous drip, with a fiber-containing formula or by adding an anticholinergic medication to the formula. Diarrhea associated with enteral feeding does not necessarily imply inadequate absorption of nutrients, other than water and electrolytes. Since luminal nutrients exert trophic effects on the gut mucosa and enhance the enteric immunologic barrier, it is often appropriate to persist with tube feeding, despite the diarrhea, even when this necessitates supplemental parenteral fluid support.

THE SCOPE AND COST OF NUTRITION SUPPORT

As many as 25% of patients entering tertiary care hospitals have central catheters placed, and 20 to 30% of these catheters are used for parenteral nutrition. The incidence of catheter-related infection reflects the severity of the underlying medical condition and varies from 2 to 30 per thousand catheter days, depending on the type of patients involved. In critically ill patients, catheter sepsis is associated with a 35% mortality rate and a high cost per survivor. Most catheter-related complications derive from faulty insertion and management of the catheter rather than defects in the device. In large tertiary care hospitals, the insertion and management of these lines by specially trained teams can reduce complications by 80%, impacting significantly on outcome and costs. The growing shift from parenteral to enteral nutrition may produce cost savings, but the true cost of complex enteral feeding is not known. Home PN costs approximately half as much as similar treatment in the hospital, and home EN costs significantly less.

FURTHER READING

BOZZETTI F et al: Perioperative total parenteral nutrition in malnourished, gastrointestinal cancer patient, a randomized, clinical trial. JPEN 24:7, 2000

HEYLAND DK et al: Should immunonutrition become routine in critically ill patients? A systematic review of the evidence. JAMA 286(8):22, 2001

HOWARD L et al: Current use and clinical outcome of home parenteral and enteral nutrition therapies in the United States. Gastroenterology 109:335, 1995

KORETZ RL et al: AGA technical review on parenteral nutrition. Gastroenterology 121:970, 2001

WOODCOCK NP et al: Enteral versus parenteral nutrition: A pragmatic study. Nutrition 17:1, 2000

64 | OBESITY
Jeffrey S. Flier, Eleftheria Maratos-Flier

In a world where food supplies are intermittent, the ability to store energy in excess of what is required for immediate use is essential for survival. Fat cells, residing within widely distributed adipose tissue depots, are adapted to store excess energy efficiently as triglyceride and, when needed, to release stored energy as free fatty acids for use at other sites. This physiologic system, orchestrated through endocrine and neural pathways, permits humans to survive starvation for as long as several months. However, in the presence of nutritional abundance and a sedentary lifestyle, and influenced importantly by genetic endowment, this system increases adipose energy stores and produces adverse health consequences.

DEFINITION AND MEASUREMENT   *Obesity* is a state of excess adipose tissue mass. Although often viewed as equivalent to increased body weight, this need not be the case—lean but very muscular individuals may be overweight by arbitrary standards without having increased adiposity. Body weights are distributed continuously in populations, so that a medically meaningful distinction between lean and obese is somewhat arbitrary. Obesity is therefore more effectively defined by assessing its linkage to morbidity or mortality.

Although not a direct measure of adiposity, the most widely used method to gauge obesity is the *body mass index* (BMI), which is equal to weight/height^2 (in kg/m^2) (Fig. 64-1). Other approaches to quantifying obesity include anthropometry (skin-fold thickness), densitometry (underwater weighing), computed tomography (CT) or magnetic resonance imaging (MRI), and electrical impedance. Using data from the Metropolitan Life Tables, BMIs for the midpoint of all heights and frames among both men and women range from 19 to 26 kg/m^2; at a similar BMI, women have more body fat than men. Based on unequivocal data of substantial morbidity, a BMI of 30 is most commonly used as a threshold for obesity in both men and women. Large-scale epidemiologic studies suggest that all-cause, metabolic, cancer, and cardiovascular morbidity begin to rise (albeit at a slow rate) when BMIs are ≥ 25, suggesting that the cut-off for obesity should be lowered. Some authorities use the term *overweight* (rather than obese) to describe individuals with BMIs between 25 and 30. A BMI between 25 and 30 should be viewed as medically significant and worthy of therapeutic intervention, especially in the presence of risk factors that are influenced by adiposity, such as hypertension and glucose intolerance.

The distribution of adipose tissue in different anatomic depots also has substantial implications for morbidity. Specifically, intraabdominal and abdominal subcutaneous fat have more significance than subcutaneous fat present in the buttocks and lower extremities. This distinction is most easily made by determining the waist-to-hip ratio, with a ratio >0.9 in women and >1.0 in men being abnormal. Many of the most important complications of obesity, such as insulin resistance, diabetes, hypertension, and hyperlipidemia, and hyperandrogenism in women, are linked more strongly to intraabdominal and/or upper body fat than to overall adiposity. The mechanism underlying this association is unknown but may relate to the fact that intraabdominal adipocytes are more lipolytically active than those from other depots. Release of free fatty acids into the portal circulation has adverse metabolic actions, especially on the liver.

PREVALENCE   Data from the National Health and Nutrition Examination Surveys (NHANES) show that the percent of the American adult population with obesity (BMI > 30) has increased from 14.5% (between 1976 and 1980) to 30.5% (between 1999 and 2000). As many as 64% of U.S. adults ≥ 20 years of age were overweight (defined as BMI $>$ 25) between the years of 1999 and 2000. Extreme obesity (BMI ≥ 40) has also increased and affects 4.7% of the population. The increasing prevalence of medically significant obesity raises great concern. Obesity is more common among women and in the poor; the prevalence in children is also rising at a worrisome rate.

PHYSIOLOGIC REGULATION OF ENERGY BALANCE   Substantial evidence suggests that body weight is regulated by both endocrine and neural components that ultimately influence the effector arms of energy intake and expenditure. This complex regulatory system is necessary because even small imbalances between energy intake and expenditure will ultimately have large effects on body weight. For example, a 0.3%

positive imbalance over 30 years would result in a 9-kg (20-lb) weight gain. This exquisite regulation of energy balance cannot be monitored easily by calorie-counting in relation to physical activity. Rather, body weight regulation or dysregulation depends on a complex interplay of hormonal and neural signals. Alterations in stable weight by forced overfeeding or food deprivation induce physiologic changes that resist these perturbations: with weight loss, appetite increases and energy expenditure falls; with overfeeding, appetite falls and energy expenditure increases. This latter compensatory mechanism frequently fails, however, permitting obesity to develop when food is abundant and physical activity is limited. A major regulator of these adaptive responses is the adipocyte-derived hormone leptin, which acts through brain circuits (predominantly in the hypothalamus) to influence appetite, energy expenditure, and neuroendocrine function (see below).

Appetite is influenced by many factors that are integrated by the brain, most importantly within the hypothalamus (Fig. 64-2). Signals that impinge on the hypothalamic center include neural afferents, hormones, and metabolites. Vagal inputs are particularly important, bringing information from viscera, such as gut distention. Hormonal signals include leptin, insulin, cortisol, and gut peptides such as ghrelin, peptide YY (PYY), and cholecystokinin, which signal to the brain through direct action on hypothalamic control centers and/or via the vagus nerve. Metabolites, including glucose, can influence appetite, as seen by the effect of hypoglycemia to induce hunger; however, glucose is not normally a major regulator of appetite. These diverse hormonal, metabolic, and neural signals act by influencing the expression and release of various hypothalamic peptides [e.g., neuropeptide Y (NPY), Agouti-related peptide (AgRP), α melanocyte-stimulating hormone (α-MSH), and melanin-concentrating hormone (MCH)] that are integrated with serotonergic, catecholaminergic, and opioid signaling pathways (see below). Psychological and cultural factors also appear to play a role in the final expression of appetite. Apart from rare syndromes involving leptin, its receptor, and the melanocortin system, specific defects in this complex appetite control network that influence common causes of obesity are not well understood.

Energy expenditure includes the following components: (1) resting or basal metabolic rate; (2) the energy cost of metabolizing and storing food; (3) the thermic effect of exercise; and (4) adaptive thermogenesis, which varies in response to chronic caloric intake (rising with increased intake). Basal metabolic rate accounts for about 70% of daily energy expenditure, whereas active physical activity contributes 5 to 10%. Thus, a significant component of daily energy consumption is fixed.

Genetic models in mice indicate that mutations in certain genes (e.g., targeted deletion of the insulin receptor in adipose tissue) protect against obesity, apparently by increasing energy expenditure. Adaptive thermogenesis occurs in *brown adipose tissue* (BAT), which plays an important role in energy metabolism in many mammals. In contrast to white adipose tissue, which is used to store energy in the form of lipids, BAT expends stored energy as heat. A mitochondrial *uncoupling protein* (UCP-1) in BAT dissipates the hydrogen ion gradient in the oxidative respiration chain and releases energy as heat. The metabolic activity of BAT is increased by a central action of leptin, acting through the sympathetic nervous system, which heavily innervates this tissue. In rodents, BAT deficiency causes obesity and diabetes; stimulation of BAT with a specific adrenergic agonist (β_3 agonist) protects against diabetes and obesity. Although BAT exists in humans (especially neonates), its physiologic role is not yet established. Homologues of UCP-1 may mediate uncoupled mitochondrial respiration in other tissues.

THE ADIPOCYTE AND ADIPOSE TISSUE Adipose tissue is composed of the lipid-storing adipose cell and a stromal/vascular compartment in which preadipocytes reside. Adipose mass increases by enlargement of adipose cells through lipid deposition, as well as by an increase in the number of adipocytes. The process by which adipose cells are derived from a mesenchymal preadipocyte involves an orchestrated series of differentiation steps mediated by a cascade of specific transcription factors. One of the key transcription factors is *peroxisome proliferator-activated receptor* γ (PPARγ), a nuclear receptor that binds the thiazoladinedione class of insulin-sensitizing drugs used in the treatment of type 2 diabetes (Chap. 323).

Although the adipocyte has generally been regarded as a storage

FIGURE 64-1 Nomogram for determining body mass index. To use this nomogram, place a ruler or other straight edge between the body weight (without clothes) in kilograms or pounds located on the left-hand line and the height (without shoes) in centimeters or inches located on the right-hand line. The body mass index is read from the middle of the scale and is in metric units. (*Copyright 1979, George A. Bray, M.D. Used with permission.*)

FIGURE 64-2 The factors that regulate appetite through effects on central neural circuits. Some factors that increase or decrease appetite are listed. NPY, neuropeptide Y; MCH, melanin-concentrating hormone; AgRP, Agouti-related peptide; MSH, melanocyte-stimulating hormone; CART, cocaine- and amphetamine-related transcript; GLP-1, glucagon-related peptide-1; CCK, cholecystokinin.

depot for fat, it is also an endocrine cell that releases numerous molecules in a regulated fashion (Fig. 64-3). These include the energy balance-regulating hormone leptin, cytokines such as tumor necrosis factor (TNF) α, complement factors such as factor D (also known as *adipsin*), prothrombotic agents such as plasminogen activator inhibitor I, and a component of the blood pressure regulating system, angiotensinogen. Adiponectin (or ACRP30) enhances insulin sensitivity and lipid oxidation, whereas resistin may induce insulin resistance. These factors, and others not yet identified, play a role in the physiology of lipid homeostasis, insulin sensitivity, blood pressure control, and coagulation and are likely to contribute to obesity-related pathologies.

ETIOLOGY OF OBESITY Though the molecular pathways regulating energy balance are beginning to be illuminated, the causes of obesity remain elusive. In part, this reflects the fact that obesity is a heterogeneous group of disorders. At one level, the pathophysiology of obesity seems simple: a chronic excess of nutrient intake relative to the level of energy expenditure. However, due to the complexity of the neuroendocrine and metabolic systems that regulate energy intake, storage, and expenditure, it has been difficult to quantitate all the relevant parameters (e.g., food intake and energy expenditure) over time in human subjects.

Role of Genes versus Environment Obesity is commonly seen in families, and the heredibility of body weight is similar to that for height. Inheritance is usually not Mendelian, however, and it is difficult to distinguish the role of genes and environmental factors. Adoptees usually resemble their biologic rather than adoptive parents with respect to obesity, providing strong support for genetic influences. Likewise, identical twins have very similar BMIs whether reared together or apart, and their BMIs are much more strongly correlated than those of dizygotic twins. These genetic effects appear to relate to both energy intake and expenditure.

Whatever the role of genes, it is clear that the environment plays a key role in obesity, as evidenced by the fact that famine prevents obesity in even the most obesity-prone individual. In addition, the recent increase in the prevalence of obesity in the United States is too rapid to be due to changes in the gene pool. Undoubtedly, genes influence the susceptibility to obesity when confronted with specific diets and availability of nutrition. Cultural factors are also important— these relate to both availability and composition of the diet and to changes in the level of physical activity. In industrial societies, obesity is more common among poor women, whereas in underdeveloped countries, wealthier women are more often obese. In children, obesity correlates to some degree with time spent watching television. High-fat diets may promote obesity, as may diets rich in simple (as opposed to complex) carbohydrates.

Specific Genetic Syndromes For many years obesity in rodents has been known to be caused by a number of distinct mutations distributed through the genome. Most of these single-gene mutations cause both hyperphagia and diminished energy expenditure, suggesting a link between these two parameters of energy homeostasis. Identification of the *ob* gene mutation in genetically obese (ob/ob) mice represented a major breakthrough in the field. The ob/ob mouse develops severe obesity, insulin resistance, and hyperphagia, as well as efficient metabolism (e.g., it gets fat even when given the same number of calories as lean littermates). The product of the *ob* gene is the peptide leptin, a name derived from the Greek root *leptos*, meaning thin. Leptin is secreted by adipose cells and acts primarily through the hypothalamus. Its level of production provides an index of adipose energy stores (Fig. 64-4). High leptin levels decrease food intake and increase energy expenditure. Another mouse mutant, db/db, which is resistant to leptin, has a mutation in the leptin receptor and develops a similar syndrome. The *OB* gene is present in humans and expressed in fat. Several families with morbid, early-onset obesity caused by inactivating mutations in either leptin or the leptin receptor have been described, thus demonstrating the biologic relevance of leptin in humans. The obesity in these individuals begins shortly after birth, is severe, and is accompanied by neuroendocrine abnormalities. The most prominent of these is hypogonadotropic hypogonadism, which is reversed by leptin replacement. Central hypothyroidism and growth retardation are seen in the mouse model, but their occurrence in leptin-deficient humans is less clear. To date, there is no evidence to suggest that mutations or polymorphisms in the leptin or leptin receptor genes play a prominent role in common forms of obesity.

Mutations in several other genes cause severe obesity in humans (Table 64-1); each of these syndromes is rare. Mutations in the gene encoding proopiomelanocortin (POMC) cause severe obesity through failure to synthesize α-MSH, a key neuropeptide that inhibits appetite in the hypothalamus. The absence of POMC also causes secondary

FIGURE 64-3 Factors released by the adipocyte that can affect peripheral tissues. PAI, plasminogen activator inhibitor; TNF, tumor necrosis factor.

FIGURE 64-4 The physiologic system regulated by leptin. Rising or falling leptin levels act through the hypothalamus to influence appetite, energy expenditure, and neuroendocrine function and through peripheral sites to influence systems such as the immune system.

adrenal insufficiency due to absence of adrenocorticotropic hormone (ACTH), as well as pale skin and red hair due to absence of MSH. Proenzyme convertase 1 (PC-1) mutations are thought to cause obesity by preventing synthesis of α-MSH from its precursor peptide, POMC. α-MSH binds to the type 4 melanocortin receptor (MC4R), a key hypothalamic receptor that inhibits eating. Heterozygous mutations of this receptor appear to account for as much as 5% of severe obesity. These five genetic defects define a pathway through which leptin (by stimulating POMC and increasing MSH) restricts food intake and limits weight (Fig. 64-5).

In addition to these human obesity genes, studies in rodents reveal several other molecular candidates for hypothalamic mediators of human obesity or leanness. The *tub* gene encodes a hypothalamic peptide of unknown function; mutation of this gene causes late-onset obesity. The *fat* gene encodes carboxypeptidase E, a peptide-processing enzyme; muta-

TABLE 64-1	Some Obesity Genes in Humans and Mice			
Gene	Gene Product	Mechanism of Obesity	In Human	In Rodent
Lep (ob)	Leptin, a fat-derived hormone	Mutation prevents leptin from delivering satiety signal; brain perceives starvation	Yes	Yes
LepR (db)	Leptin receptor	Same as above	Yes	Yes
POMC	Proopiomelanocortin, a precursor of several hormones and neuropeptides	Mutation prevents synthesis of melanocyte-stimulating hormone (MSH), a satiety signal	Yes	Yes
MC4R	Type 4 receptor for MSH	Mutation prevents reception of satiety signal from MSH	Yes	Yes
AgRP	Agouti-related peptide, a neuropeptide expressed in the hypothalamus	Overexpression inhibits signal through MC4R	No	Yes
PC 1	Prohormone convertase 1, a processing enzyme	Mutation prevents synthesis of neuropeptide, probably MSH	Yes	No
Fat	Carboxypeptidase E, a processing enzyme	Same as above	No	Yes
Tub	Tub, a hypothalamic protein of unknown function	Hypothalamic dysfunction	No	Yes

tion of this gene is thought to cause obesity by disrupting production of one or more neuropeptides. AgRP is coexpressed with NPY in arcuate nucleus neurons. AgRP antagonizes α-MSH action at MC4 receptors, and its overexpression induces obesity. In contrast, a mouse deficient in the peptide MCH, whose administration causes feeding, is lean.

A number of complex human syndromes with defined inheritance are associated with obesity (Table 64-2). Although specific genes are undefined at present, their identification will likely enhance our understanding of more common forms of human obesity. In the Prader-Willi syndrome, obesity coexists with short stature, mental retardation, hypogonadotropic hypogonadism, hypotonia, small hands and feet, fish-shaped mouth, and hyperphagia. Most patients have a chromosome 15 deletion (Chap. 57). Laurence-Moon-Biedl syndrome is characterized by obesity, mental retardation, retinitis pigmentosa, polydactyly, and hypogonadotropic hypogonadism.

Other Specific Syndromes Associated with Obesity ■ *CUSHING'S SYNDROME* Although obese patients commonly have central obesity, hypertension, and glucose intolerance, they lack other specific stigmata of Cushing's syndrome (Chap. 321). Nonetheless, a potential diagnosis of Cushing's syndrome is often entertained. Cortisol production and urinary metabolites (17OH steroids) may be increased in simple obesity. Unlike in Cushing's syndrome, however, cortisol levels in blood and urine in the basal state and in response to corticotropin-releasing hormone (CRH) or ACTH are normal; the overnight 1-mg dexamethasone suppression test is normal in 90%, with the remainder being normal on a standard 2-day low-dose dexamethasone suppression test. Obesity may be associated with local reactivation of cortisol in fat by 11β hydroxysteroid dehydrogenase 1, an enzyme that converts cortisone to cortisol.

HYPOTHYROIDISM The possibility of hypothyroidism should be considered, but it is an uncommon cause of obesity; hypothyroidism is easily ruled out by measuring thyroid-stimulating hormone (TSH). Much of the weight gain that occurs in hypothyroidism is due to myxedema (Chap. 320).

INSULINOMA Patients with insulinoma often gain weight as a result of overeating to avoid hypoglycemia symptoms (Chap. 324). The increased substrate plus high insulin levels promote energy storage in fat. This can be marked in some individuals but is modest in most.

CRANIOPHARYNGIOMA AND OTHER DISORDERS INVOLVING THE HYPOTHALAMUS Whether through tumors, trauma, or inflammation, hypothalamic dysfunction of systems controlling satiety, hunger, and energy expenditure can cause varying degrees of obesity (Chap. 318). It is uncommon to identify a discrete anatomic basis for these disorders. Subtle hypotha-

lamic dysfunction is probably a more common cause of obesity than can be documented using currently available imaging techniques. Growth hormone (GH), which exerts lipolytic activity, is diminished in obesity and is increased with weight loss. Despite low GH levels, insulin-like growth factor (IGF) I (somatomedin) production is normal, suggesting that GH suppression is a compensatory response to increased nutritional supply.

Pathogenesis of Common Obesity Obesity can result from increased energy intake, decreased energy expenditure, or a combination of the two. Thus, identifying the etiology of obesity should involve measurements of both parameters. However, it is nearly impossible to perform direct and accurate measurements of energy intake in free-living individuals. Obese people, in particular, often underreport intake. Measurements of chronic energy expenditure have only recently become available using doubly labeled water or metabolic chamber/rooms. In subjects at stable weight and body composition, energy intake equals expenditure. Consequently, these techniques allow determination of energy intake in free-living individuals. The level of energy expenditure differs in established obesity, during periods of weight gain or loss, and in the pre- or postobese state. Studies that fail to take note of this phenomenon are not easily interpreted.

There is increased interest in the concept of a body weight "set point." This idea is supported by physiologic mechanisms centered around a sensing system in adipose tissue that reflects fat stores and a receptor, or "adipostat," that is in the hypothalamic centers. When fat

FIGURE 64-5 A central pathway through which leptin acts to regulate appetite and body weight. Leptin signals through proopiomelanocortin (POMC) neurons in the hypothalamus to induce increased production of α melanocyte-stimulating hormone (α-MSH), requiring the processing enzyme PC-1 (proenzyme convertase 1). α-MSH acts as an agonist on melanocortin-4 receptors to inhibit appetite, and the neuropeptide AgRp (Agouti-related peptide) acts as an antagonist of this receptor. Mutations that cause obesity in humans are indicated by the solid green arrows.

TABLE 64-2 *A Comparison of Syndromes of Obesity—Hypogonadism and Mental Retardation*

Feature	Prader-Willi	Laurence-Moon-Biedl	Ahlstrom	Cohen	Carpenter
			Syndrome		
Inheritance	Sporadic; two-thirds have defect	Autosomal recessive	Autosomal recessive	Probably autosomal recessive	Autosomal recessive
Stature	Short	Normal; infrequently short	Normal; infrequently short	Short or tall	Normal
Obesity	Generalized Moderate to severe Onset 1–3 yrs	Generalized Early onset, 1–2 yrs	Truncal Early onset, 2–5 yrs	Truncal Mid-childhood, age 5	Truncal, gluteal
Craniofacies	Narrow bifrontal diameter Almond-shaped eyes Strabismus V-shaped mouth High-arched palate	Not distinctive	Not distinctive	High nasal bridge Arched palate Open mouth Short philtrum	Acrocephaly Flat nasal bridge High-arched palate
Limbs	Small hands and feet Hypotonia	Polydactyly	No abnormalities	Hypotonia Narrow hands and feet	Polydactyly Syndactyly Genu valgum
Reproductive status	1° Hypogonadism	1° Hypogonadism	Hypogonadism in males but not in females	Normal gonadal function or hypogonadotrophic hypogonadism	2° Hypogonadism
Other features	Enamel hypoplasia Hyperphagia Temper tantrums Nasal speech			Dysplastic ears Delayed puberty	
Mental retardation	Mild to moderate		Normal intelligence	Mild	Slight

stores are depleted, the adipostat signal is low, and the hypothalamus responds by stimulating hunger and decreasing energy expenditure to conserve energy. Conversely, when fat stores are abundant, the signal is increased, and the hypothalamus responds by decreasing hunger and increasing energy expenditure. The recent discovery of the *ob* gene, and its product leptin, provides a molecular basis for this physiologic concept (see above).

What Is the Status of Food Intake in Obesity? (Do the Obese Eat More Than the Lean?) This question has stimulated much debate, due in part to the methodologic difficulties inherent in determining food intake. Many obese individuals believe that they eat small quantities of food, and this claim has often been supported by the results of food intake questionnaires. However, it is now established that average energy expenditure increases as people get more obese, due primarily to the fact that metabolically active lean tissue mass increases with obesity. Given the laws of thermodynamics, the obese person must therefore eat more than the average lean person to maintain their increased weight. It may be the case, however, that a subset of individuals who are predisposed to obesity have the capacity to become obese initially without an absolute increase in caloric consumption.

What Is the State of Energy Expenditure in Obesity? The average total daily energy expenditure is higher in obese than lean individuals when measured at stable weight. However, energy expenditure falls as weight is lost, due in part to loss of lean body mass and to decreased sympathetic nerve activity. When reduced to near-normal weight and maintained there for a while, (some) obese individuals have lower energy expenditure than (some) lean individuals. There is also a tendency for those who develop obesity as infants or children to have lower resting energy expenditure rates than those who remain lean.

The physiologic basis for variable rates of energy expenditure (at a given body weight and level of energy intake) is essentially unknown. A mutation in the human β_3 adrenergic receptor may be associated with increased risk of obesity and/or insulin resistance in certain (but not all) populations. Homologues of the BAT uncoupling protein, named UCP-2 and UCP 3, have been identified in both rodents and humans. UCP-2 is expressed widely, whereas UCP-3 is primarily expressed in skeletal muscle. These proteins may play a role in disordered energy balance.

One newly described component of thermogenesis, called *nonex-ercise activity thermogenesis* (NEAT), has been linked to obesity. It is the thermogenesis that accompanies physical activities other than volitional exercise, such as the activities of daily living, fidgeting, spontaneous muscle contraction, and maintaining posture. NEAT accounts for about two-thirds of the increased daily energy expenditure induced by overfeeding. The wide variation in fat storage seen in overfed individuals is predicted by the degree to which NEAT is induced. The molecular basis for NEAT and its regulation are unknown.

Leptin in Typical Obesity The vast majority of obese people have increased leptin levels but do not have mutations of either leptin or its receptor. They appear, therefore, to have a form of functional "leptin resistance." Data suggesting that some individuals produce less leptin per unit fat mass than others or have a form of relative leptin deficiency that predisposes to obesity are at present contradictory and unsettled. The mechanism for leptin resistance, and whether it can be overcome by raising leptin levels, is not yet established. Some data suggest that leptin may not effectively cross the blood-brain barrier as levels rise. It is also possible that leptin signaling inhibitors are involved in the leptin-resistant state.

PATHOLOGIC CONSEQUENCES OF OBESITY Obesity has major adverse effects on health. Morbidly obese individuals (>200% ideal body weight) have as much as a twelvefold increase in mortality. Mortality rates rise as obesity increases, particularly when obesity is associated with increased intraabdominal fat (see above). It is also apparent that the degree to which obesity affects particular organ systems is influenced by susceptibility genes that vary in the population.

Insulin Resistance and Type 2 Diabetes Mellitus Hyperinsulinemia and insulin resistance are pervasive features of obesity, increasing with weight gain and diminishing with weight loss. Insulin resistance is more strongly linked to intraabdominal fat than to fat in other depots. The molecular link between obesity and insulin resistance in tissues such as fat, muscle, and liver has been sought for many years. Major factors under investigation include: (1) insulin itself, by inducing receptor downregulation; (2) free fatty acids, known to be increased and capable of impairing insulin action; (3) intracellular lipid accumulation; and (4) various circulating peptides produced by adipocytes, including the cytokines TNF-α and interleukin (IL) 6 , and the "adipokines" adiponectin and resistin, which are produced by adipocytes, have altered expression in obese adipocytes, and are capable of modifying insulin action. Despite nearly universal insulin resistance, most obese individuals do not develop diabetes, suggesting that the onset of diabetes requires an interaction between obesity-induced insulin resistance and other factors that predispose to diabetes, such as impaired insulin secretion (Chap. 323). Obesity, however, is a major risk factor for diabetes, and as many as 80% of patients with type 2 diabetes mellitus are obese. Weight loss and exercise, even of modest degree, are associated with increased insulin sensitivity and often improve glucose control in diabetes.

Reproductive Disorders Disorders that affect the reproductive axis are associated with obesity in both men and women. Male hypogonadism is associated with increased adipose tissue, often distributed in a pattern more typical of females. In men >160% ideal body weight, plasma testosterone and sex hormone–binding globulin (SHBG) are often reduced, and estrogen levels (derived from conversion of adrenal androgens in adipose tissue) are increased (Chap. 325). Gynecomastia may be seen. However, masculinization, libido, potency, and spermatogenesis are preserved in most of these individuals. Free testosterone may be decreased in morbidly obese men whose weight exceeds 200% ideal body weight.

Obesity has long been associated with menstrual abnormalities in women, particularly in women with upper body obesity (Chap. 326). Common findings are increased androgen production, decreased SHBG, and increased peripheral conversion of androgen to estrogen. Most obese women with oligomenorrhea have the polycystic ovarian syndrome (PCOS), with its associated anovulation and ovarian hyperandrogenism; 40% of women with PCOS are obese. Most nonobese women with PCOS are also insulin-resistant, suggesting that insulin resistance, hyperinsulinemia, or the combination of the two are causative or contribute to the ovarian pathophysiology in PCOS in both obese and lean individuals. In obese women with PCOS, weight loss or treatment with insulin-sensitizing drugs often restores normal menses. The increased conversion of androstenedione to estrogen, which occurs to a greater degree in women with lower body obesity, may contribute to the increased incidence of uterine cancer in postmenopausal women with obesity.

Cardiovascular Disease The Framingham Study revealed that obesity was an independent risk factor for the 26-year incidence of cardiovascular disease in men and women [including coronary disease, stroke, and congestive heart failure (CHF)]. The waist/hip ratio may be the best predictor of these risks. When the additional effects of hypertension and glucose intolerance associated with obesity are included, the adverse impact of obesity is even more evident. The effect of obesity on cardiovascular mortality in women may be seen at BMIs as low as 25. Obesity, especially abdominal obesity, is associated with an atherogenic lipid profile, with increased low-density lipoprotein (LDL) cholesterol, very low density lipoprotein, and triglyceride, and decreased high-density lipoprotein cholesterol (Chap. 335). Obesity is also associated with hypertension. Measurement of blood pressure in the obese requires use of a larger cuff size to avoid artifactual increases. Obesity-induced hypertension is associated with increased peripheral resistance and cardiac output, increased sympathetic nervous system tone, increased salt sensitivity, and insulin-mediated salt retention; it is often responsive to modest weight loss.

Pulmonary Disease Obesity may be associated with a number of pulmonary abnormalities. These include reduced chest wall compliance, increased work of breathing, increased minute ventilation due to increased metabolic rate, and decreased total lung capacity and functional residual capacity (Chap. 234). Severe obesity may be associated with obstructive sleep apnea and the "obesity hypoventilation syndrome" (Chap. 246). Sleep apnea can be obstructive (most common), central, or mixed. Weight loss (10 to 20 kg) can bring substantial improvement, as can major weight loss following gastric bypass or restrictive surgery. Continuous positive airway pressure has been used with some success.

Gallstones Obesity is associated with enhanced biliary secretion of cholesterol, supersaturation of bile, and a higher incidence of gallstones, particularly cholesterol gallstones (Chap. 292). A person 50% above ideal body weight has about a sixfold increased incidence of symptomatic gallstones. Paradoxically, fasting increases supersaturation of bile by decreasing the phospholipid component. Fasting-induced cholecystitis is a complication of extreme diets.

Cancer Obesity in males is associated with higher mortality from cancer, including cancer of the esophagus, colon, rectum, pancreas, liver, and prostate; obesity in females is associated with higher mortality from cancer of the gallbladder, bile ducts, breasts, endometrium, cervix, and ovaries. Some of the latter may be due to increased rates of conversion of androstenedione to estrone in adipose tissue of obese individuals. It was recently estimated that obesity accounts for 14% of cancer deaths in men, and 20% in women in the United States.

Bone, Joint, and Cutaneous Disease Obesity is associated with an increased risk of osteoarthritis, no doubt partly due to the trauma of added weight bearing and joint malalignment. The prevalence of gout may also be increased (Chap. 313). Among the skin problems associated with obesity is acanthosis nigricans, manifested by darkening and thickening of the skin folds on the neck, elbows, and dorsal interphalangeal spaces. Acanthosis reflects the severity of underlying insulin resistance and diminishes with weight loss. Friability of skin may be increased, especially in skin folds, enhancing the risk of fungal and yeast infections. Finally, venous stasis is increased in the obese.

℞ TREATMENT

Obesity is a chronic medical condition. Successful treatment, defined as the sustained attainment of normal body weight without producing unacceptable treatment-induced morbidity, is rarely achieved in clinical practice. Many approaches produce short-term weight loss, and this has clear benefits for associated morbidities such as hypertension and diabetes. Although enormous resources are expended in pursuit of obesity therapies, most patients are unsuccessful at achieving and sustaining weight loss over time.

Treatment goals should be guided by the health risks of obesity in any given individual (Fig. 64-6). The clinician should always consider

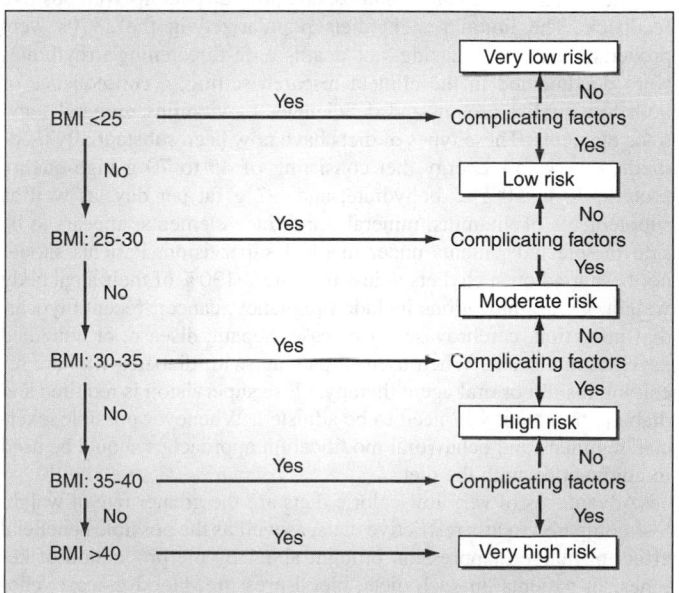

FIGURE 64-6 Risk classification algorithm. The patient is first placed into a category based on body mass index. The presence or absence of complicating factors determines the degree of health risk. Complicating factors include elevated abdominal-gluteal ratio (male: 1.0, female: 0.9), diabetes mellitus, hypertension, hyperlipidemia, male sex, and age <40. (*Copyright 1987, George A. Bray, MD. Used with permission.*)

the possibility that an individual has an identified cause of obesity, such as hypothyroidism, hypercortisolism, male hypogonadism, insulinoma, or central nervous system disease that affects hypothalamic function. Although they are infrequent causes of obesity, specific therapy may be available.

Behavior Modification The principles of behavior modification provide the underpinnings for many current programs of weight reduction. Typically, the patient is requested to monitor and record the circumstances related to eating, and rewards are designed to modify maladaptive behaviors. Patients may benefit from counseling offered in a stable group setting for extended periods of time, including after weight loss.

Diet Reduced caloric intake is the cornerstone of obesity treatment. The fundamental goal is the sustained reduction of energy intake below that of energy expenditure. The difficulty in achieving this goal has led to a wide array of suggested diets that vary in recommended calorie content (from total fasting to mild reductions), as well as specific food content and form (e.g., liquid vs. solid). There is no scientific evidence to validate the utility of specific "fad diets." The main diet regimens in use follow several general facts relevant to food intake and weight loss. First, a deficit of 7500 kcal will produce a weight loss of ~1 kg. Therefore, eating 100 kcal/d less for a year should cause a 5-kg weight loss, and a deficit of 1000 kcal/d should cause a loss of ~1 kg per week. The rate of weight loss on a given caloric intake is related to the rate of energy expenditure. Because obese individuals have a higher metabolic rate than lean individuals, and because men have a higher metabolic rate than women (due to their greater lean body mass), the rate of weight loss is greater among the more obese and among men (relative to women). With chronic caloric restriction, metabolic rate diminishes because of reduced lean body mass (along with much greater loss in fat mass) and possibly because of other adaptations. This fall in metabolic rate with food restriction slows the rate of weight loss on a constant diet. With total starvation or diets restricted to <600 kcal/d, initial weight loss over the first week results predominantly from natriuresis and the loss of fluids.

Very low energy diets (e.g., 400 to 600 kcal/d) may be appropriate for short-term treatment of obesity in selected patients. They are most commonly used for periods of 1 to 2 months to initiate more rapid weight loss, improve comorbidities, and provide patients with positive feedback. The liquid protein diets popularized in the 1970s were proved to be unsafe, causing >60 deaths. Life-threatening arrhythmias were documented in the clinical research setting, a consequence of both low-quality protein and deficiencies of vitamins, minerals, and trace elements. These types of diets have now been substantially modified. A very low energy diet consisting of 45 to 70 g high-quality protein, 30 to 50 g carbohydrate, and ~2 g fat per day, as well as supplements of vitamins, minerals, and trace elements, appears to be safe in selected patients under medical supervision. Patients should not be started on such diets unless they are >130% of their ideal body weight. Contraindications include pregnancy, cancer, recent myocardial infarction, cerebrovascular disease, hepatic disease, or untreated psychiatric disease. When used in patients with diabetes who are receiving insulin or oral agent therapy, close supervision is required and diabetic treatment will need to be adjusted. Whenever possible, exercise regimens and behavioral modification approaches should be used in conjunction with the diet.

Advantages of very low calorie diets are the greater rate of weight loss compared to less restrictive diets, as well as the possible beneficial effect of hunger suppression brought about by the production of ketones. In patients on such diets, blood pressure, blood glucose, cholesterol, and triglyceride levels fall, and pulmonary function and exercise tolerance improve. Sleep apnea may improve within a few weeks. Complications of these very low energy diets are usually minor and include fatigue, constipation or diarrhea, dry skin, hair loss, menstrual irregularities, orthostatic dizziness, and difficulty concentrating.

Cholelithiasis and pancreatitis may occur when such diets are interrupted by binge eating; gallstones have been shown to develop in as many as 25% of patients while on the diet.

Low-calorie diets, >800 kcal/d, are applicable to most patients and have fewer restrictions than the very low calorie diets. Considerable controversy has attended the question of which diet composition is most appropriate for promoting weight loss. Though commonly recommended, benefits resulting from very low fat diets are modest at best. Nonetheless, the health effects of low-fat diets—apart from curbing obesity—may be important. A diet rich in fruits, vegetables, whole grains, and other low–glycemic index carbohydrates may promote weight loss and is preferable to low-fat diets in which large amounts of simple carbohydrates are substituted for fats. The latter may actually promote obesity. Some have advocated diets with protein replacement of simple carbohydrates in an effort to minimize insulin production. The efficacy of this strategy, aside from overall calorie reduction, is unknown. Recent data suggest that very low carbohydrate "Atkins" style diets are more effective for short-term weight loss when compared to standard caloric restriction. Weight loss on such diets is not associated with adverse effects on such indices as lipid profile, glycemic control, or blood pressure. However, these diets have not been shown to be more effective in maintaining weight loss, and the possible long-term consequences of maintaining a lower body weight at the expense of consuming more saturated fat are unknown.

An important aspect of diet therapy should include education aimed at preventing weight gain. Knowledge of the caloric and nutritional content of foods is generally poor. In the absence of studies demonstrating convincingly that one type of diet is more effective and safe than another, an emphasis on helping patients understand the caloric content of specific portions is a helpful aid to weight loss and weight maintenance in many individuals.

Exercise Exercise is an important component of the overall approach to treating obesity. Increased energy expenditure is the most obvious mechanism for an effect of exercise. The impact of an exercise regimen as a sole therapy of obesity has been difficult to document. On the other hand, exercise appears to be a valuable means to sustain diet therapy (Fig. 64-7). Even if exercise had no such salutary effect, it would be valuable in the obese individual for its effects on cardiovascular tone and blood pressure. Because many obese individuals have not engaged in exercise on a regular basis and may have cardiovascular risk factors, it should be introduced gradually and under medical supervision, especially in the most obese individuals.

Drugs Despite modest short-term benefits from several agents, medication-induced weight loss is not a cure and is often associated with rebound weight gain after the cessation of drug use. Substantial side effects from several anti-obesity medications, and the potential for drug abuse, have combined to create a wariness about this approach. On the other hand, there is a great medical need for safe and effective

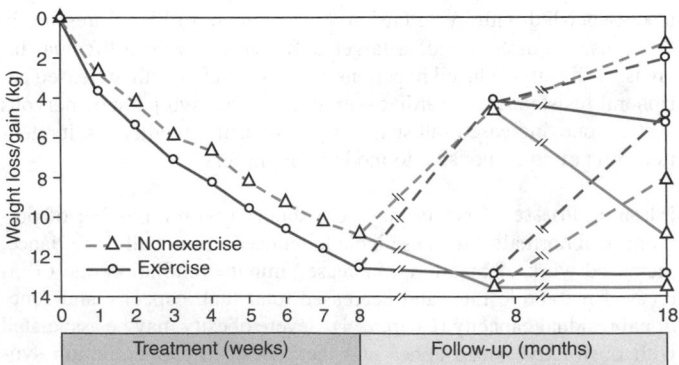

FIGURE 64-7 Weight loss and exercise. During the first 8 weeks, subjects were divided into two groups, one treated with diet and the other with diet plus exercise, with no difference in weight loss. Thereafter the subjects who exercised maintained better weight loss than those that did not. (*After KN Pavlou et al: Am J Clin Nutr 49: 1115, 1989.*)

therapies, so many possible compounds have been evaluated. On the basis of placebo-controlled trials, the U.S. Food and Drug Administration (FDA) approved several amphetamine-like agents for short-term use. Phentermine is an amphetamine-like drug with low addictive potential that showed modest efficacy (10 vs. 4.4 kg of weight loss over a 24-week period in a well-controlled study). This class of drugs is thought to act centrally by reducing appetite. The over-the-counter drug phenylpropanolamine HCl, had similar efficacy to prescription appetite suppressants in short-term studies but was withdrawn from the market in 2001 because of an association with cerebral hemorrhage. Drugs that promote serotonin release or inhibit serotonin reuptake, such as fenfluramine, have had modest efficacy as single agents. When fenfluramine was administered together with phentermine, as "fen-phen," the combination gained wide use for several years based on controlled trials that demonstrated modest but definite efficacy and reduction of comorbidities. However, the risk of primary pulmonary hypertension was increased up to 20-fold in association with this treatment. The FDA withdrew approval of the fen-phen combination in 1997 when reports demonstrated an association with right- and left-sided valvular heart disease. The histopathologic features of the valvular disease are similar to those seen in carcinoid syndrome and are thought to result from fenfluramine. The occurrence of this complication has been verified in multiple studies, and fenfluramine has been removed from the market.

Sibutramine is a central reuptake inhibitor of both norepinephrine and serotonin that was originally developed as an antidepressant. Using a once-daily dose over 24 weeks, it produced a 7% weight loss in a double-blind, placebo-controlled trial. It lowered cholesterol and triglyceride levels and exhibited similar clinical efficacy to fenfluramine. Sibutramine increases pulse by an average of 4 to 5 beats per minute and blood pressure by 1 to 3 mmHg, and this plus modest efficacy has limited its broad adoption. Orlistat is an inhibitor of intestinal lipase with no systemic availability that causes modest weight loss due to drug-induced fat malabsorption. A randomized, double-blind trial over 2 years revealed modest weight loss (8.7 kg for 120 mg orlistat versus 5.8 kg from diet alone) during the first year and better maintenance of weight loss in a second year compared to the placebo-treated group (3.2 kg regained vs. 5.6 kg regained for placebo). LDL cholesterol and insulin levels were also reduced. Gastrointestinal side effects include oily stools, flatulence, and fecal urgency and usually diminish as patients choose to limit fat intake to avoid the symptoms. Absorption of fat-soluble vitamins is decreased. In patients with obesity and type 2 diabetes mellitus, the antidiabetic medication metformin tends to decrease body weight. The mechanism appears to involve inhibition of appetite. Thyroid hormone has little place in the treatment of obesity, as the vast majority of obese individuals are euthyroid. It promotes loss of lean body mass and raises the risk of complications from the hyperthyroid state.

In the rare cases of leptin deficiency caused by mutations of the leptin gene, the administration of recombinant leptin is highly effective for regulating hunger and inducing loss of fat mass while preserving lean body mass. The response to leptin is limited or absent in common obesity, which is associated with hyperleptinemia and leptin resistance. New drugs are also being developed based on recent insights into central pathways that regulate body weight. These include antagonists for NPY receptors (subtypes Y1, Y5) and MCH receptors and agonists for melanocortin 4 receptors.

Surgery Morbid obesity, commonly defined as a BMI > 40, is estimated to increase mortality by as much as twelvefold in men between 25 and 34 years of age and sixfold between 35 and 45 years of age. Deaths from cardiovascular disease, diabetes, and accidents have been documented. In response to typically ineffective treatment using diet, exercise, and available drugs, surgical approaches are increasingly be-

FIGURE 64-8 Examples of operative interventions used for surgical manipulation of the gastrointestinal tract. *A.* Vertical banded gastroplasty; *B.* adjustable gastric banding; *C.* Roux-en-Y gastric bypass.

ing employed. The potential benefits of surgery include major weight loss and improvement in hypertension, diabetes, sleep apnea, CHF, angina, hyperlipidemia, and venous disease. Several different approaches have been used, sometimes without adequate long-term assessment of efficacy and complications. Jejunoileal bypass surgery has been abandoned because of complications, which included electrolyte disturbances, nephrolithiasis, gallstones, gastric ulcers, arthritis, and hepatic dysfunction, with cirrhosis occurring in as many as 7% of patients. Two procedures in common use today are the vertical-banded gastroplasty and the Roux-en-Y gastric bypass (Fig. 64-8). The former is a purely restrictive procedure, while the latter combines restriction with slight malabsorption and may also reduce appetite via suppression of the gastric hormone ghrelin, which stimulates appetite. Gastric bypass is most often performed by laparotomy but may be performed laparoscopically in some patients. A third procedure, laparoscopic adjustable gastric banding, is widely used in Europe and Australia and is being introduced in the United States. This procedure may be viewed as "less drastic" than gastric bypass but appears capable of producing substantial weight loss, albeit with shorter periods of follow-up.

Following the National Institutes of Health Consensus Conference on Gastrointestinal Surgery for Severe Obesity in 1991, it was recommended that suitable patients be selected using the following criteria: (1) a BMI > 35 with an associated comorbidity or a BMI > 40; (2) repeated failures of other therapeutic approaches; (3) at eligible weight for 3 to 5 years; (4) capability of tolerating surgery; (5) absence of alcoholism, other addictions, or major psychopathology; and (6) prior clearance by a psychiatrist. It is recommended that an appropriately experienced surgeon work together with nutritionists and other support personnel; evaluation and follow-up programs should be monitored closely.

ACKNOWLEDGMENT
The authors acknowledge the contributions of Dr. George A. Bray, who wrote this chapter in the 14th edition.

FURTHER READING

CROWLEY VE et al: Obesity therapy: Altering the energy intake and expenditure balance sheet. Nat Rev Drug Disc 1:276, 2002

FAROOQI IS et al: Clinical spectrum of obesity and mutations of the melanocortin 4 receptor gene. N Engl J Med 348:1160, 2003

FLEGAL KM et al: Prevalence and trends in obesity among US adults, 1999–2000. JAMA 288:1723, 2002

FLIER JS, MARATOS-FLIER E Editorial: The stomach speaks—ghrelin and weight reduction. N Engl J Med 346:1662, 2002

FONTAINE KR et al: Years of life lost due to obesity. JAMA:289, 2003

SPIEGELMAN BM, FLIER JS et al: Obesity and the regulation of energy balance. Cell 104:531, 2001

Anorexia nervosa and bulimia nervosa are characterized by severe disturbances of eating behavior. The salient feature of *anorexia nervosa* (AN) is a refusal to maintain a minimally normal body weight. *Bulimia nervosa* (BN) is characterized by recurrent episodes of binge eating followed by abnormal compensatory behaviors, such as self-induced vomiting. AN and BN are distinct clinical syndromes but share certain features in common. Both disorders occur primarily among previously healthy young women who become overly concerned with body shape and weight. Many patients with BN have past histories of anorexia nervosa, and many patients with anorexia nervosa engage in binge eating and purging behavior. In the current diagnostic system, the critical distinction between AN and BN depends on body weight: patients with AN are, by definition, significantly underweight, whereas patients with BN have body weights in the normal range or above.

Binge eating disorder (BED) is a more recently described syndrome characterized by repeated episodes of binge eating, similar to those of BN, in the absence of inappropriate compensatory behavior. Patients with BED are typically middle-aged men or women with significant obesity. They have an increased frequency of anxiety and depression compared to similarly obese patients without BED. It is not known whether patients with BED are at increased risk for medical complications or what treatment strategies are indicated.

ANOREXIA NERVOSA

EPIDEMIOLOGY Among women, the lifetime prevalence of the full syndrome of AN is approximately 0.5%. AN is much less common in males. AN is more prevalent in cultures where food is plentiful and in which being thin is associated with attractiveness. Individuals who pursue interests that place a premium on thinness, such as ballet and modeling, are at greater risk. The incidence of AN appears to have increased in recent decades.

ETIOLOGY The etiology of AN is unknown but appears to involve a combination of psychological, biologic, and cultural risk factors. Risk factors, such as sexual or physical abuse and a family history of mood disturbance, are best viewed as nonspecific risk factors that increase vulnerability to a range of psychiatric disorders, including AN.

Patients who develop AN are inclined to be more obsessional and perfectionist than their peers. The disorder often begins as a diet not distinguishable at the outset from those undertaken by many adolescents and young women. As weight loss progresses, the fear of gaining weight grows; dieting becomes stricter; and psychological, behavioral, and medical aberrations increase. Eating disorders, including AN, may develop among individuals with type 1 diabetes mellitus, and are associated with poorer glycemic control and an increased frequency of complications (Chap. 323).

Numerous physiologic disturbances, including abnormalities in a variety of neurotransmitter systems, have been described in AN (see below). It is difficult to distinguish neurochemical, metabolic, and hormonal changes that may have a role in the initiation or perpetuation of the syndrome from those that are secondary to the disorder. The resolution of most of these abnormalities with weight restoration argues against their having a critical etiologic role.

Genetic factors contribute to the risk of development of AN, as its incidence is greater in families with one affected member and the concordance in monozygotic twins is greater than in dizygotic twins. However, specific genes have not been identified.

CLINICAL FEATURES (Table 65-1) AN typically begins in mid to late adolescence, sometimes in association with a stressful life event such as leaving home for school. The disorder occasionally develops in early puberty, before menarche, but seldom begins after age 40. Despite being underweight, patients with AN are irrationally afraid of gaining weight, often out of a concern that weight gain will get "out

of control." They also exhibit a distortion of body image, which may express itself in several ways. For example, despite being emaciated, patients with AN may believe that their body as a whole, or some part of their body, is too fat. Further weight loss is viewed by the patient as a fulfilling accomplishment, while weight gain is seen as a personal failure. Patients with AN rarely complain of hunger or fatigue and often exercise extensively. Despite the denial of hunger, one-quarter to one-half of patients with AN engage in eating binges. Patients tend to become socially withdrawn and increasingly committed to work or study, dieting, and exercise. As weight loss progresses, thoughts of food dominate mental life and idiosyncratic rules develop around eating. Patients with AN may obsessively collect cookbooks and recipes and be drawn to food-related occupations.

Physical Features Patients with AN typically have few physical complaints but may note cold intolerance. Gastrointestinal motility is diminished, leading to reduced gastric emptying and constipation. Some women who develop AN after menarche report that their menses ceased before significant weight loss occurred. Weight and height should be measured to allow calculation of body mass index (BMI; kg/m²). Vital signs may reveal bradycardia, hypotension, and mild hypothermia. Soft, downy hair growth (lanugo) sometimes occurs, and alopecia may be seen. Salivary gland enlargement, which is associated with starvation as well as with binge eating and vomiting, may make the face appear surprisingly full in contrast to the marked general wasting. Acrocyanosis of the digits is common, and peripheral edema can be seen in the absence of hypoalbuminemia, particularly when the patient begins to regain weight. Some patients who consume large amounts of vegetables containing vitamin A develop a yellow tint to the skin (*hypercarotenemia*), which is especially notable on the palms.

Laboratory Abnormalities Mild normochromic, normocytic anemia is frequent, as is mild to moderate leukopenia, with a disproportionate reduction of polymorphonuclear leukocytes. Dehydration may result in slightly increased levels of blood urea nitrogen and creatinine. Serum transaminase levels may increase, especially during the early phases of refeeding. The level of serum proteins is usually normal. Blood sugar is often low and serum cholesterol may be moderately elevated. Hypokalemic alkalosis suggests self-induced vomiting or the use of diuretics. Hyponatremia is common and may result from excess fluid intake and disturbances in the secretion of antidiuretic hormone.

Endocrine Abnormalities The regulation of virtually every endocrine system is altered in AN, but the most striking changes occur in the reproductive system. Amenorrhea is hypothalamic in origin and reflects diminished production of gonadotropin-releasing hormone (GnRH). When exogenous GnRH is administered in a pulsatile manner, pituitary responses of luteinizing hormone (LH) and follicle stimulating hormone (FSH) are normalized, indicating the absence of a primary pituitary abnormality. The resulting gonadotropin deficiency causes low plasma estrogen in women and reduced testosterone in men. The hypothalamic GnRH pulse generator is exquisitely sensitive, particularly in women, to body weight, stress, and exercise, each of which may contribute to *hypothalamic amenorrhea* in AN (Chap. 326). Although the mechanisms underlying these effects are unknown, the decreased adipose tissue associated with weight loss leads to a marked reduction in leptin, a hormone that plays a permissive role in GnRH production (Chap. 64).

Serum cortisol and 24-h urine free cortisol levels are generally elevated but without characteristic clinical signs of cortisol excess. Thyroid function tests resemble the pattern seen in euthyroid sick syndrome (Chap. 320). Thyroxine (T_4) and free T_4 levels are usually in the low-normal range, triiodothyronine (T_3) levels are reduced, and reverse T_3 (rT_3) is elevated. The level of thyroid stimulating hormone (TSH) is normally or partially suppressed. Growth hormone is increased, but insulin-like growth factor 1 (IGF-1), which is produced mainly by the liver, is reduced, as in other conditions of starvation. Diminished bone density is routinely observed in AN and reflects the effects of multiple nutritional deficiencies, reduced gonadal steroids, and increased cortisol. The degree of bone density reduction is proportional to the length of the illness, and patients are at risk for the development of symptomatic fractures. The occurrence of AN during adolescence may lead to the premature cessation of linear bone growth and a failure to achieve expected adult height.

Cardiac Abnormalities Cardiac output is reduced, and congestive heart failure occurs rarely during rapid refeeding. The electrocardiogram usually shows sinus bradycardia, reduced QRS voltage, and nonspecific ST-T-wave abnormalities. Some patients develop a prolonged QT_c interval, which may predispose to serious arrhythmias, particularly when electrolyte abnormalities are also present.

DIAGNOSIS The diagnosis of AN is based on the presence of characteristic behavioral, psychological, and physical attributes (Table 65-2). Widely accepted diagnostic criteria are provided by the American Psychiatric Association's *Diagnostic and Statistical Manual of Mental Disorders* (DSM-IV). These criteria include weight <85% of that expected for age and height, which is roughly equivalent to a BMI of 18.5 kg/m² for adult women. This weight criterion is somewhat arbitrary, so that a patient who meets all other diagnostic criteria but weighs between 85 and 90% of expected would still merit the diagnosis of AN. The current diagnostic criteria require that women with AN not have spontaneous menses, but occasional patients with the characteristics and complications of AN describe regular menstruation. Two mutually exclusive subtypes of AN are specified in DSM-IV. Patients whose weight loss is maintained primarily by caloric restriction, perhaps augmented by excessive exercise, are considered to have the "restricting" subtype of AN. The "binge eating/purging" subtype is characterized by binge eating, self-induced vomiting and/or laxative abuse. Patients with the binge/purge subtype are more prone to develop electrolyte imbalances, are more emotionally labile, and are more likely to have other problems with impulse control, such as drug abuse.

The diagnosis of AN can usually be made confidently on the basis of history when significant weight loss is accomplished by restrictive dieting and excessive exercise and is accompanied by a marked reluctance to gain weight. Patients with AN often deny that they have a serious problem and may be brought to medical attention by concerned family or friends. In atypical presentations, other causes of significant weight loss in previously healthy young people should be considered, including inflammatory bowel disease, gastric outlet obstruction, diabetes mellitus, central nervous system (CNS) tumors, and neoplasm (Chap. 36).

PROGNOSIS The course and outcome of AN are highly variable. One-quarter to one-half of patients eventually recover fully, with few psychological or physical sequelae. However, many patients have persistent difficulties with weight maintenance, depression, and eating disturbances, including BN. The development of obesity following AN is rare. The long-term mortality of AN is among the highest associated with any psychiatric disorder. Approximately 5% of patients die per decade of follow-up, primarily due to the physical effects of chronic starvation or by suicide.

Virtually all of the physiologic abnormalities associated with AN are observed in other forms of starvation and markedly improve or disappear with weight gain. A worrisome exception is the reduction in bone mass, which may not recover fully, particularly when AN occurs during adolescence when peak bone mass is normally achieved.

TABLE 65-1 *Common Characteristics of Anorexia Nervosa and Bulimia Nervosa*

	Anorexia Nervosa[a]	Bulimia Nervosa
CLINICAL CHARACTERISTICS		
Onset	Mid-adolescence	Late adolescence/early adulthood
Female:male	10:1	10:1
Prevalence in women	0.5%	1–3%
Weight	Markedly decreased	Usually normal
Menstruation	Absent	Usually normal
Binge eating	25–50%	Required for diagnosis
Mortality	~5% Per decade	Low
PHYSICAL AND LABORATORY FINDINGS[a]		
Skin/extremities	Lanugo	
	Acrocyanosis	
	Edema	
Cardiovascular	Bradycardia	
	Hypotension	
Gastrointestinal	Salivary gland enlargement	Salivary gland enlargement
	Slow gastric emptying	Dental erosion
	Constipation	
	Elevated liver enzymes	
Hematopoietic	Normochromic, normocyctic anemia	
	Leukopenia	
Fluid/Electrolyte	Increased BUN, creatinine	Hypokalemia
	Hyponatremia	Hypochloremia
		Alkalosis
Endocrine	Hypoglycemia	
	Low estrogen or testosterone	
	Low LH and FSH	
	Low-normal thyroxine	
	Normal TSH	
	Increased cortisol	
Bone	Osteopenia	

[a] Patients with the binge-eating/purging subtype of anorexia nervosa may also exhibit the physical and laboratory findings associated with bulimia nervosa.
Abbreviations: BUN, blood urea nitrogen; LH, luteinizing hormone; FSH, follicle stimulating hormone; TSH, thyroid stimulating hormone.

Rx TREATMENT

Because of the profound physiologic and psychological effects of starvation, there is a broad consensus that weight restoration to 90% of predicted weight is the primary goal in the treatment of AN. Unfortunately, because most patients resist this goal, the management of AN is often accompanied by frustration for the patient, the family, and the physician. Patients typically exaggerate their food intake and minimize their symptoms. Some patients resort to subterfuge to make their weights appear higher, for example, by water-loading before they are weighed. In attempting to engage the patient in treatment, it may be useful for the physician to elicit the patient's physical concerns (e.g., about osteoporosis, weakness, or fertility) and, if possible, educate the patient regarding the importance of normalizing nutritional status in order to address those concerns. The physician should attempt to reassure the patient that weight gain will not be permitted to get "out of control" but simultaneously emphasize that weight restoration is medically and psychologically imperative.

TABLE 65-2 *Diagnostic Features of Anorexia Nervosa*

Refusal to maintain body weight at or above a minimally normal weight for age and height. (This includes a failure to achieve weight gain expected during a period of growth leading to an abnormally low body weight.)
Intense fear of weight gain or becoming fat.
Distortion of body image (e.g., feeling fat despite an objectively low weight or minimizing the seriousness of low weight).
Amenorrhea. (This criterion is met if menstrual periods occur only following hormone—e.g., estrogen—administration.)

The intensity of the initial treatment, including the need for hospitalization, is determined by the patient's current weight, the rapidity of recent weight loss, and the severity of medical and psychological complications (Fig. 65-1). Hospitalization should be strongly considered for patients weighing <75% of expected, even if the results of routine blood studies are within normal limits. Acute medical problems, such as severe electrolyte imbalances, should be identified and addressed. Nutritional restoration can almost always be successfully accomplished by oral feeding, and parenteral methods are rarely required. For severely underweight patients, sufficient calories (approximately 1500 to 1800 kcal/d) should be provided initially in divided meals as food or liquid supplements to maintain weight and to permit stabilization of fluid and electrolyte balance. Calories can then be gradually increased to achieve a weight gain of 1 to 2 kg (2 to 4 lb) per week, typically requiring an intake of 3000 to 4000 kcal/d. Meals must be supervised, ideally by personnel who are firm regarding the necessity of food consumption, empathic regarding the challenges entailed, and reassuring regarding the patient's eventual recovery. Patients have great psychological difficulty complying with the need for increased caloric consumption, and the assistance of psychiatrists or psychologists experienced in the treatment of AN is usually necessary.

Less severely affected patients may be treated in a partial hospitalization program where medical and psychiatric supervision is available and several meals can be monitored each day. Outpatient treatment may suffice for mildly ill patients. Weight must be monitored at frequent intervals, and explicit goals agreed on for weight gain, with the understanding that more intensive treatment will be required if the level of care initially employed is not successful. For younger patients, the active involvement of the family in treatment is crucial regardless of the treatment venue.

Psychiatric treatment focuses primarily on two issues. First, patients require much emotional support during the period of weight gain. Patients often intellectually agree with the need to gain weight, but strenuously resist increases in caloric intake, and often surreptitiously discard food that is provided. Second, patients must learn to base their self-esteem not on the achievement of an inappropriately low weight, but on the development of satisfying personal relationships and the attainment of reasonable academic and occupational goals. While this is often possible, some patients with AN develop other serious emotional and behavioral symptoms such as depression, self-mutilation, obsessive-compulsive behavior, and suicidal ideation. These symptoms may require additional therapeutic interventions, in the form of psychotherapy, medication, or hospitalization.

Medical complications occasionally occur during refeeding. As in other forms of malnutrition, fluid retention and peripheral edema may occur, but generally do not require specific treatment in the absence of cardiac, renal, or hepatic dysfunction. Acute gastric dilatation has been described when refeeding has been rapid. Transient modest elevations in serum levels of liver enzymes occasionally occur. Low levels of magnesium and phosphate should be repleted. Multivitamins should be given, and it is important to ensure adequate intake of vitamin D (400 IU/d) and calcium (1500 mg/d) to minimize bone loss.

No psychotropic medications are of established value in the treatment of AN; tricyclic antidepressants are contraindicated when there is prolongation of the QT_c interval. The alterations of cortisol and thyroid hormone metabolism do not require specific treatment and are corrected by weight gain. Estrogen treatment appears to have minimal impact on bone density in underweight patients but may be helpful to relieve symptoms of estrogen deficiency.

BULIMIA NERVOSA

EPIDEMIOLOGY   In women, the full syndrome of BN occurs with a lifetime prevalence of 1 to 3%. Variants of the disorder, such as occasional binge eating or purging, are much more common and occur in 5 to 10% of young women. The frequency of BN among men is less than one-tenth of that among women. The prevalence of BN increased dra-

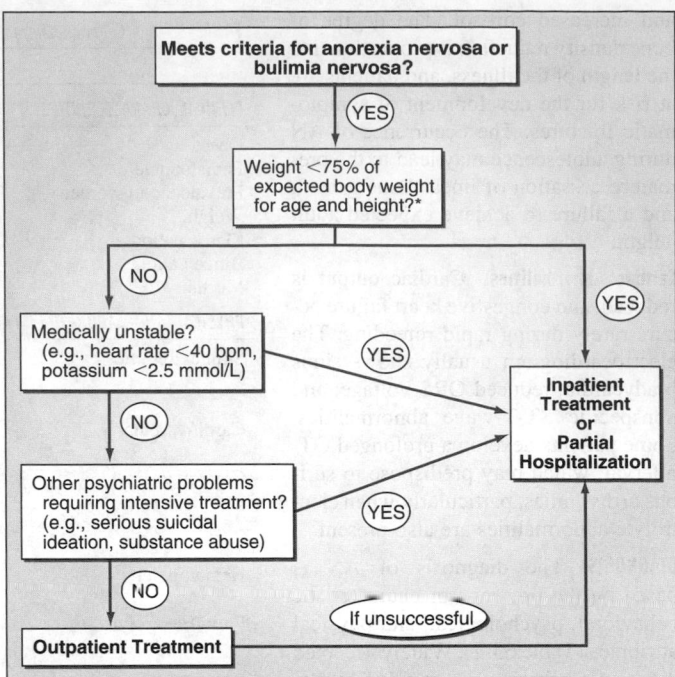

FIGURE 65-1   An algorithm for basic treatment decisions regarding patients with anorexia nervosa or bulimia nervosa. Based on the American Psychiatric Association's practice guidelines for the treatment of patients with eating disorders. *Although outpatient management may be considered for patients with anorexia nervosa weighing more than 75% of expected, there should be a low threshold for using more intensive interventions if the weight loss has been rapid or if current weight is <80% of expected.

matically in the early 1970s and 1980s but may have leveled off or declined somewhat in recent years.

ETIOLOGY   As with AN, the etiology of BN is likely to be multifactorial. Patients who develop BN describe a higher-than-expected prevalence of childhood and parental obesity, suggesting that a predisposition towards obesity may increase vulnerability to this eating disorder. The marked increase in the number of cases of BN during the past 25 years and the rarity of BN in underdeveloped countries suggest that cultural factors are important. Several biologic abnormalities in patients with BN may perpetuate this disorder once it has begun. These include abnormalities of CNS serotonergic function, which is involved in the regulation of eating behavior, and disruption of peripheral satiety mechanisms, including the release of cholecystokinin (CCK) from the small intestine.

CLINICAL FEATURES   (Table 65-3)   The typical patient presenting for treatment of BN is a woman of normal weight in her mid-twenties who reports binge eating and purging 5 to 10 times a week for 5 to 10 years. The disorder usually begins in late adolescence or early adulthood during or following a diet, often in association with depressed mood. The self-imposed caloric restriction leads to increased hunger and to overeating. In an attempt to avoid weight gain, the patient induces vomiting, takes laxatives or diuretics, or engages in some other form of compensatory behavior. During binges, patients with this dis-

TABLE 65-3   *Diagnostic Features of Bulimia Nervosa*

Recurrent episodes of binge eating, which is characterized by the consumption of a large amount of food in a short period of time and a feeling that the eating is out of control.
Recurrent inappropriate behavior to compensate for the binge eating, such as self-induced vomiting.
The occurrence of both the binge eating and the inappropriate compensatory behavior at least twice weekly, on average, for 3 months.
Overconcern with body shape and weight.

Note: If the diagnostic criteria for anorexia nervosa are simultaneously met, only the diagnosis of anorexia nervosa is given.

order tend to consume large amounts of sweet foods with a high fat content, such as dessert items. The most frequent compensatory behaviors are self-induced vomiting and laxative abuse, but a wide variety of techniques have been described, including the omission of insulin injections by individuals with type 1 diabetes mellitus. Initially, patients may experience a sense of satisfaction that appealing food can be eaten without weight gain. However, as the disorder progresses, patients perceive diminished control over eating. Binges increase in size and frequency and are provoked by a variety of stimuli, such as transient depression, anxiety, or a sense that too much food has been consumed in a normal meal. Between binges, patients attempt to restrict caloric intake, which increases hunger and sets the stage for the next binge. Typically, patients with BN are ashamed of their behavior and endeavor to keep their disorder hidden from family and friends. Like patients with AN, those with BN place an unusual emphasis on weight and shape as a basis for their self esteem. Many patients with BN have mild symptoms of depression. Some patients exhibit serious mood and behavioral disturbances, such as suicide attempts, sexual promiscuity, and drug and alcohol abuse. Although vomiting may be triggered initially by manual stimulation of the gag reflex, most patients with BN develop the ability to induce vomiting at will. Rarely, patients resort to the regular use of syrup of ipecac. Laxatives and diuretics are frequently taken in impressive quantities, such as 30 or 60 laxative pills on a single occasion. The resulting fluid loss produces dehydration and a feeling of emptiness but has little impact on caloric balance.

The physical abnormalities associated with BN primarily result from the purging behavior. Painless bilateral salivary gland hypertrophy (sialadenosis) may be noted. A scar or callus on the dorsum of the hand may develop due to repeated trauma from the teeth among patients who manually stimulate the gag reflex. Recurrent vomiting and the exposure of the lingual surfaces of the teeth to stomach acid lead to loss of dental enamel and eventually to chipping and erosion of the front teeth. Laboratory abnormalities are surprisingly infrequent, but hypokalemia, hypochloremia, and hyponatremia are observed occasionally. Repeated vomiting may lead to alkalosis, whereas repeated laxative abuse may produce a mild metabolic acidosis. Serum amylase may be mildly elevated due to an increase in the salivary isoenzyme.

Serious physical complications resulting from BN are rare. Oligomenorrhea and amenorrhea are more frequent than among women without eating disorders. Arrhythmias occasionally occur secondary to electrolyte disturbances. Tearing of the esophagus and rupture of the stomach have been reported, and constitute life-threatening events. Some patients who have chronically abused laxatives or diuretics develop transient peripheral edema when this behavior ceases, presumably due to high levels of aldosterone secondary to persistent fluid and electrolyte depletion.

DIAGNOSIS The critical diagnostic features of BN are repeated episodes of binge eating followed by inappropriate and abnormal behaviors aimed at avoiding weight gain (Table 65-3). The diagnosis of BN requires a candid history from the patient detailing frequent, large eating binges followed by the purposeful use of inappropriate mechanisms to avoid weight gain. Most patients with BN who present for

treatment are distressed by their inability to control their eating behavior but are able to provide such details if queried in a supportive and nonjudgmental fashion.

As in AN, there are two mutually exclusive subtypes of BN. Patients with the "purging" subtype utilize compensatory behaviors that directly rid the body of calories or fluids (e.g., self-induced vomiting, laxative or diuretic abuse), whereas those with the "nonpurging" subtype attempt to compensate for binges by fasting or by excessive exercise. Patients with the nonpurging subtype tend to be heavier and are less prone to fluid and electrolyte disturbances.

PROGNOSIS The prognosis of BN is much more favorable than that of AN. Mortality is low, and full recovery occurs in approximately 50% of patients within 10 years. Approximately 25% of patients have persistent symptoms of BN over many years. Few patients progress from BN to AN.

℞ TREATMENT

BN can usually be treated on an outpatient basis (Figure 65-1). Cognitive behavioral therapy (CBT) is a short-term (4 to 6 months) psychological treatment that focuses on the intense concern with shape and weight, the persistent dieting, and the binge eating and purging that characterize this disorder. Patients are directed to monitor the circumstances, thoughts, and emotions associated with binge/purge episodes, to eat regularly, and to challenge their assumptions linking weight to self-esteem. CBT produces symptomatic remission in 25 to 50% of patients.

Numerous double-bind, placebo-controlled trials have documented that antidepressant medications are useful in the treatment of BN but are probably somewhat less effective than CBT. Although efficacy has been established for virtually all chemical classes of antidepressants, only the selective serotonin reuptake inhibitor fluoxetine (Prozac) has been approved for use in BN by the U.S. Food and Drug Administration. Antidepressant medications are helpful even for patients with BN who are not depressed, and the dose of fluoxetine recommended for BN (60 mg/d) is higher than that typically used to treat depression. These observations suggest that different mechanisms may underlie the utility of these medications in BN and in depression.

A subset of patients with BN does not respond adequately to CBT, antidepressant medication, or their combination. More intensive forms of treatment, including hospitalization, may be required for such patients.

FURTHER READING

AMERICAN PSYCHIATRIC ASSOCIATION: Practice guideline for the treatment of patients with eating disorders (revision). Am J Psychiatry 157(Suppl 1): 1, 2000.

BECKER AE et al: Eating disorders. N Engl J Med 340:1092, 1999

KAYE WH et al: Anorexia and bulimia nervosa. Annu Rev Med 51:299, 2000

MEHLER PS: Diagnosis and care of patients with anorexia nervosa in primary care settings. Ann Intern Med 134:1048, 2001

WALSH BT, DEVLIN MJ: Eating disorders: Progress and problems. Science 280:1387, 1998

66 | APPROACH TO THE PATIENT WITH CANCER
Dan L. Longo

The application of current treatment techniques (surgery, radiation therapy, chemotherapy, and biological therapy) results in the cure of >50% of patients diagnosed with cancer. Nevertheless, patients experience the diagnosis of cancer as one of the most traumatic and revolutionary events that has ever happened to them. Independent of prognosis, the diagnosis brings with it a change in a person's self-image and in his or her role in the home and workplace. The prognosis of a person who has just been found to have pancreatic cancer is the same as the prognosis of the person with aortic stenosis who develops the first symptoms of congestive heart failure (median survival, about 8 months). However, the patient with heart disease may remain functional and maintain a self-image as a fully intact person with just a malfunctioning part, a diseased organ ("a bum ticker"). By contrast, the patient with pancreatic cancer has a completely altered self-image and is viewed differently by family and anyone who knows the diagnosis. He or she is being attacked and invaded by a disease that could be anywhere in the body. Every ache or pain takes on desperate significance. Cancer is an exception to the coordinated interaction among cells and organs. In general, the cells of a multicellular organism are programmed for collaboration. Many diseases occur because the specialized cells fail to perform their assigned task. Cancer takes this malfunction one step further. Not only is there a failure of the cancer cell to maintain its specialized function, but it also strikes out on its own; the cancer cell competes to survive using natural mutability and natural selection to seek advantage over normal cells in a recapitulation of evolution. One consequence of the traitorous behavior of cancer cells is that the patient feels betrayed by his or her body. The cancer patient feels that he or she, and not just a body part, is diseased.

THE MAGNITUDE OF THE PROBLEM

No nationwide cancer registry exists; therefore, the incidence of cancer is estimated on the basis of the National Cancer Institute's Surveillance, Epidemiology, and End Results (SEER) database, which tabulates cancer incidence and death figures from nine sites, accounting for about 10% of the U.S. population, and from population data from the Bureau of the Census. In 2004, 1.36 million new cases of invasive cancer (699,560 men, 668,470 women) were diagnosed and 563,700 persons (290,890 men, 272,810 women) died from cancer. The percent distribution of new cancer cases and cancer deaths by site for men and women are shown in Table 66-1. Cancer incidence has been declining by about 2% each year since 1992.

The most significant risk factor for cancer overall is age; two-thirds of all cases were in those over age 65. Cancer incidence increases as the third, fourth, or fifth power of age in different sites. For the interval between birth and age 39, 1 in 72 men and 1 in 51 women will develop cancer; for the interval between ages 40 and 59, 1 in 12 men and 1 in 11 women will develop cancer; and for the interval between ages 60 and 79, 1 in 3 men and 1 in 5 women will develop cancer.

Cancer is the second leading cause of death behind heart disease. Deaths from heart disease have declined 45% in the United States since 1950 and continue to decline. After a 70-year period of increases, cancer deaths began to decline in 1997 (Fig. 66-1). The five leading causes of cancer deaths are shown for various populations in Table 66-2. Along with the decrease in incidence has come an increase in survival for cancer patients. The 5-year survival for white patients was 39% in 1960–1963 and 64% in 1992–1998. Cancers are more often deadly in blacks; the 5-year survival was 53% for the 1992–1998

TABLE 66-1 Distribution of Cancer Incidence and Deaths for 2004[a]

Male			Female		
Sites	%	Number	Sites	%	Number
CANCER INCIDENCE					
Prostate	33	230,110	Breast	32	215,990
Lung and bronchus	13	93,110	Lung and bronchus	12	80,660
Colon and rectum	11	73,620	Colon and rectum	11	73,380
Bladder	6	44,640	Endometrium	6	40,320
Melanoma	4	29,900	Ovary	4	25,580
Lymphoma	4	28,850	Lymphoma	4	25,520
Kidney	3	22,080	Melanoma	4	25,200
Leukemia	3	19,020	Thyroid	3	17,640
Oral cavity	3	18,550	Pancreas	2	16,120
Pancreas	2	15,740	Bladder	2	15,600
All other	18	123,940	All other	20	132,460
CANCER DEATHS					
Lung and bronchus	32	91,930	Lung and bronchus	25	68,510
Prostate	10	29,900	Breast	15	40,110
Colon and rectum	10	28,320	Colon and rectum	10	28,410
Pancreas	5	15,440	Ovary	6	16,090
Leukemia	5	12,990	Pancreas	6	15,830
Lymphoma	4	11,090	Leukemia	6	10,310
Esophagus	4	10,250	Lymphoma	4	9,020
Liver and bile duct	3	9,450	Endometrium	3	7,090
			Myeloma	2	5,640
Bladder	3	8,780	Brain	2	5,490
Kidney	3	7,870	All other	24	66,310
All other	21	64,870			

[a] Data exclude basal and squamous cell skin cancers and carcinoma in situ except the bladder.
Source: From Jemal et al, with permission.

interval. Incidence and mortality vary among racial and ethnic groups (Table 66-3). The basis for these differences is unclear.

PATIENT MANAGEMENT

Important information is obtained from every portion of the routine history and physical examination. The duration of symptoms may reveal the chronicity of disease. The past medical history may alert the physician to the presence of underlying diseases that may affect the choice of therapy or the side effects of treatment. The social history may reveal occupational exposure to carcinogens or habits, such as smoking or alcohol consumption, that may influence the course of disease and its treatment. The family history may suggest an underlying familial cancer predisposition and point out the need to begin surveillance or other preventive therapy for unaffected siblings of the patient. The review of systems may suggest early symptoms of metastatic disease or a paraneoplastic syndrome.

DIAGNOSIS The diagnosis of cancer relies most heavily on invasive tissue biopsy and should never be made without obtaining tissue; no noninvasive diagnostic test is sufficient to define a disease process as cancer. Although in rare clinical settings (e.g., thyroid nodules) fine-needle aspiration is an acceptable diagnostic procedure, the diagnosis generally depends on obtaining adequate tissue to permit careful eval-

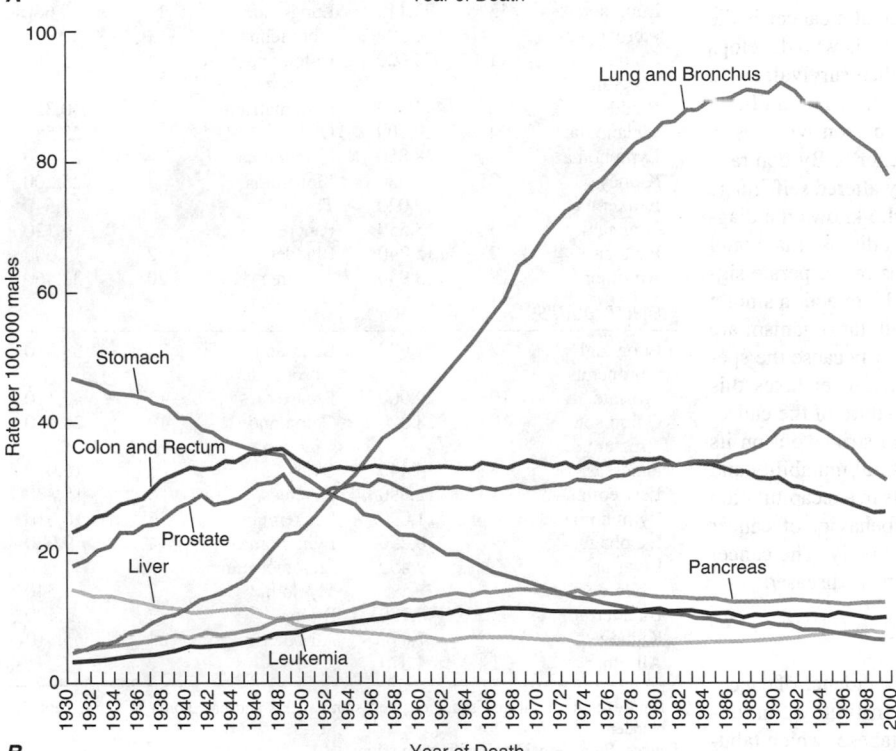

FIGURE 66-1 Sixty-year trend in cancer death rates for (*A*) women and (*B*) men, by site in the United States, 1930–1999. Rates are per 100,000 age-adjusted to the 2000 U.S. standard population. (*From Jemal et al.*)

t(8;14) translocation of Burkitt's lymphoma. Increasing evidence links the expression of certain genes with the prognosis and response to therapy (Chaps. 68, 69).

Occasionally a patient will present with a metastatic disease process that is defined as cancer on biopsy but has no apparent primary site of disease. Efforts should be made to define the primary site based on age, sex, sites of involvement, histology and tumor markers, and personal and family history. Particular attention should be focused on ruling out the most treatable causes (Chap. 85).

Once the diagnosis of cancer is made, the management of the patient is best undertaken as a multidisciplinary collaboration among the primary care physician, medical oncologists, surgical oncologists, radiation oncologists, oncology nurse specialists, pharmacists, social workers, rehabilitation medicine specialists, and a number of other consulting professionals working closely with each other and with the patient and family.

DEFINING THE EXTENT OF DISEASE AND THE PROGNOSIS The first priority in patient management after the diagnosis of cancer is established and shared with the patient is to determine the extent of disease. The curability of a tumor usually is inversely proportional to the tumor burden. Ideally, the tumor will be diagnosed before symptoms develop or as a consequence of screening efforts (Chap. 67). A very high proportion of such patients can be cured. However, most patients with cancer present with symptoms related to the cancer, caused either by mass effects of the tumor or by alterations associated with the production of cytokines or hormones by the tumor.

For most cancers, the extent of disease is evaluated by a variety of noninvasive and invasive diagnostic tests and procedures. This process is called *staging*. There are two types. *Clinical staging* is based on physical examination, radiographs, isotopic scans, computed tomography, and other imaging procedures; *pathologic staging* takes into account information obtained during a surgical procedure, which might include intraoperative palpation, resection of regional lymph nodes and/or tissue adjacent to the tumor, and inspection and biopsy of organs commonly involved in disease spread. Pathologic staging includes histologic examination of all tissues removed during the surgical procedure. Surgical procedures performed may include a simple lymph node biopsy or more extensive procedures such as thoracotomy, mediastinoscopy, or laparotomy. Surgical staging may occur in a separate procedure or may be done at the time of definitive surgical resection of the primary tumor.

Knowledge of the predilection of particular tumors for spread to adjacent or distant organs helps direct the staging evaluation.

Information obtained from staging is used to define the extent of disease either as localized, as exhibiting spread

uation of the histology of the tumor, its grade, and its invasiveness and to yield further molecular diagnostic information, such as the expression of cell-surface markers or intracellular proteins that typify a particular cancer, or the presence of a molecular marker, such as the

TABLE 66-2 *The Five Leading Primary Tumor Sites for Patients Dying of Cancer Based on Age and Sex in 2001*

			Age			
Rank	All Ages	Under 20	20–39	40–59	60–79	>80
1	M,F: lung	M,F: leukemia	M: leukemia F: breast	M: lung F: breast	M,F: lung	M,F: lung
2	M: prostate F: breast	M,F: brain	M: brain F: cervix	M: colorectal F: lung	M: colorectal F: breast	M: prostate F: colorectal
3	M,F: colorectal	M: bone sarcoma F: endocrine	M: colorectal F: leukemia	M: pancreas F: colorectal	M: prostate F: colorectal	M: colorectal F: breast
4	M,F: pancreas	M: endocrine F: bone sarcoma	M: lymphoma F: lung	M: liver F: ovary	M,F: pancreas	M: bladder F: pancreas
5	M: leukemia F: ovary	M, F: soft tissue sarcoma	M: lung F: brain	M: esophagus F: pancreas	M: leukemia F: ovary	M: leukemia F: lymphoma

Note: M, male; F, female.

outside of the organ of origin to regional but not distant sites, or as metastatic to distant sites. The most widely used system of staging is the TNM (tumor, node, metastasis) system codified by the International Union Against Cancer and the American Joint Committee on Cancer (AJCC).[1] The TNM classification is an anatomically based system that categorizes the tumor on the basis of the size of the primary tumor lesion (T1–4, where a higher number indicates a tumor of larger size), the presence of nodal involvement (usually N0 and N1 for the absence and presence, respectively, of involved nodes, although some tumors have more elaborate systems of nodal grading), and the presence of metastatic disease (M0 and M1 for the absence and presence, respectively, of metastases). The various permutations of T, N, and M scores (sometimes including tumor

TABLE 66-3	Cancer Incidence and Mortality in Racial and Ethnic Groups 1992–1999				
Site	White	Black	Asian/Pacific Islander	American Indian	Hispanic
INCIDENCE PER 100,000 POPULATION					
All	M: 568.2	M: 703.6	M: 408.9	M: 277.7	M: 393.1
	F: 424.4	F: 404.8	F: 306.5	F: 224.2	F: 290.5
Breast (F)	137	120.7	93.4	59.4	82.6
Colon/rectum	M: 64.4	M: 70.7	M: 58.7	M: 40.7	M: 43.9
	F: 46.1	F: 55.8	F: 39.5	F: 30.8	F: 29.7
Lung	M: 82.9	M: 124.1	M: 63.8	M: 51.4	M: 44.1
	F: 51.1	F: 53.2	F: 28.5	F: 23.3	F: 22.8
Prostate (M)	172.9	275.3	107.2	60.7	127.6
MORTALITY PER 100,000 POPULATION					
All	M: 258.1	M: 369	M: 160.6	M: 154.5	M: 163.7
	F: 171.2	F: 204.5	F: 104.4	F: 110.4	F: 105.7
Breast (F)	29.3	37.3	13.1	14.8	17.5
Colon	M: 26.1	M: 34.8	M: 16.5	M: 14.6	M: 16.6
	F: 18.4	F: 25.4	F: 11.6	F: 11.3	F: 10.6
Lung	M: 81.7	M: 113	M: 42.3	M: 49.3	M: 38.2
	F: 41.1	F: 39.6	F: 19.3	F: 24.9	F: 13.8
Prostate (M)	32.9	75.1	15.1	18.8	22.6

Note: M, male; F, female.

histologic grade G) are then broken into stages, usually designated by the roman numerals I through IV. Tumor burden increases and curability decreases with increasing stage. Other anatomic staging systems are used for some tumors, e.g., the Dukes classification for colorectal cancers, the International Federation of Gynecologists and Obstetricians (FIGO) classification for gynecologic cancers, and the Ann Arbor classification for Hodgkin's disease.

Certain tumors cannot be grouped on the basis of anatomic considerations. For example, hematopoietic tumors such as leukemia, myeloma, and lymphoma are often disseminated at presentation and do not spread like solid tumors. For these tumors, other prognostic factors have been identified (Chaps. 96, 97, 98).

In addition to tumor burden, a second major determinant of treatment outcome is the physiologic reserve of the patient. Patients who are bedridden before developing cancer are likely to fare worse, stage for stage, than fully active patients. Physiologic reserve is a determinant of how a patient is likely to cope with the physiologic stresses imposed by the cancer and its treatment. This factor is difficult to assess directly. Instead, surrogate markers for physiologic reserve are used, such as the patient's age or Karnofsky performance status (Table 66-4). Older patients and those with a Karnofsky performance status <70 have a poor prognosis unless the poor performance is a reversible consequence of the tumor.

Increasingly, biologic features of the tumor are being related to prognosis. The expression of particular oncogenes, drug-resistance genes, apoptosis-related genes, and genes involved in metastasis are being found to influence response to therapy and prognosis. The presence of selected cytogenetic abnormalities may influence survival. Tumors with higher growth fractions, as assessed by expression of proliferation-related markers such as proliferating cell nuclear antigen (PCNA), behave more aggressively than tumors with lower growth fractions. Information obtained from studying the tumor itself will increasingly be used to influence treatment decisions.

MAKING A TREATMENT PLAN From information on the extent of disease and the prognosis and in conjunction with the patient's wishes, it is determined whether the treatment approach should be curative or palliative in intent. Cooperation among the various professionals involved in cancer treatment is of the utmost importance in treatment planning. For some cancers, chemotherapy or chemotherapy plus radiation therapy delivered before the use of definitive surgical treatment (so-called neoadjuvant therapy) may improve the outcome, as seems to be the

case for locally advanced breast cancer and head and neck cancers. In certain settings in which combined modality therapy is intended, coordination among the medical oncologist, radiation oncologist, and surgeon is crucial to achieving optimal results. Sometimes the chemotherapy and radiation therapy need to be delivered sequentially, and other times concurrently. Surgical procedures may precede or follow other treatment approaches. It is best for the treatment plan either to follow a standard protocol precisely or else to be part of an ongoing clinical research protocol evaluating new treatments. Ad hoc modifications of standard protocols are likely to compromise treatment results.

The choice of treatment approaches was formerly dominated by the local culture in both the university and the practice settings. However, it is now possible to gain access electronically to standard treatment protocols and to every approved clinical research study in North America through a personal computer interface with the Internet.[2]

The skilled physician also has much to offer the patient for whom curative therapy is no longer an option. Often a combination of guilt and frustration over the inability to cure the patient and the pressure of a busy schedule greatly limit the time a physician spends with a patient who is receiving only palliative care. Resist these forces. In addition to the medicines administered to alleviate symptoms (see below), it is important to remember the comfort that is provided by holding the patient's hand, continuing regular examinations, and taking time to talk.

MANAGEMENT OF DISEASE AND TREATMENT COMPLICATIONS Because cancer therapies are toxic (Chaps. 70, 71), patient management involves addressing complications of both the disease and its treatment as well as the complex psychosocial problems associated with cancer. In the short term during a course of curative therapy, the patient's functional status may decline. Treatment-induced toxicity is less acceptable if the goal of therapy is palliation. The most common side effects of treatment are nausea and vomiting (see below), febrile neutropenia (Chap. 72), and myelosuppression (Chap. 70). Therapeutic tools are now available to minimize the acute toxicity of cancer treatment.

New symptoms developing in the course of cancer treatment should

---

[1]The AJCC *Manual for Staging Cancer*, 5th edition, can be obtained from the AJCC at 55 East Erie Street, Chicago, IL, 60611.

[2]The National Cancer Institute maintains a database called PDQ (Physician Data Query) that is accessible on the Internet under the name CancerNet at *wwwicic.nci.nih.gov/health.htm*. Information can be obtained through a facsimile machine using CancerFax by dialing 301 402 5874. Patient information is also provided by the National Cancer Institute in at least three formats: on the Internet via CancerNet at *wwwicic.nci.nih.gov/patient.htm*, through the CancerFax number listed above, or by calling 1-800-4-CANCER. The quality control for the information provided through these services is rigorous.

TABLE 66-4 *Karnofsky Performance Index*

Performance Status	Functional Capability of the Patient
100	Normal; no complaints; no evidence of disease
90	Able to carry on normal activity; minor signs or symptoms of disease
80	Normal activity with effort; some signs or symptoms of disease
70	Cares for self; unable to carry on normal activity or do active work
60	Requires occasional assistance but is able to care for most needs
50	Requires considerable assistance and frequent medical care
40	Disabled; requires special care and assistance
30	Severely disabled; hospitalization is indicated although death is not imminent
20	Very sick; hospitalization necessary; active supportive treatment is necessary
10	Moribund, fatal processes progressing rapidly
0	Dead

always be assumed to be reversible until proven otherwise. The fatalistic attribution of anorexia, weight loss, and jaundice to recurrent or progressive tumor could result in a patient dying from a reversible intercurrent cholecystitis. Intestinal obstruction may be due to reversible adhesions rather than progressive tumor. Systemic infections, sometimes with unusual pathogens, may be a consequence of the immunosuppression associated with cancer therapy. Some drugs used to treat cancer or its complications (e.g., nausea) may produce central nervous system symptoms that look like metastatic disease or may mimic paraneoplastic syndromes such as the syndrome of inappropriate antidiuretic hormone. A definitive diagnosis should be pursued and may even require a repeat biopsy.

A critical component of cancer management is assessing the response to treatment. In addition to a careful physical examination in which all sites of disease are physically measured and recorded in a flow chart by date, response assessment usually requires periodic repeating of imaging tests that were abnormal at the time of staging. If imaging tests have become normal, repeat biopsy of previously involved tissue is performed to document complete response by pathologic criteria. Biopsies are not usually required if there is macroscopic residual disease. A *complete response* is defined as disappearance of all evidence of disease, and a *partial response* as >50% reduction in the sum of the products of the perpendicular diameters of all measureable lesions. *Progressive disease* is defined as the appearance of any new lesion or an increase of >25% in the sum of the products of the perpendicular diameters of all measurable lesions. Tumor shrinkage or growth that does not meet any of these criteria is considered *stable disease*. Some sites of involvement (e.g., bone) or patterns of involvement (e.g., lymphangitic lung or diffuse pulmonary infiltrates) are considered unmeasurable. No response is complete without biopsy documentation of their resolution, but partial responses may exclude their assessment unless clear objective (though unmeasurable) progression has occurred.

Tumor markers may be useful in patient management in certain tumors. Response to therapy may be difficult to gauge with certainty. However, some tumors produce or elicit the production of markers that can be measured in the serum or urine and, in a particular patient, rising and falling levels of the marker are usually associated with increasing or decreasing tumor burden, respectively. Some clinically useful tumor markers are shown in Table 66-5. Tumor markers are not in themselves specific enough to permit a diagnosis of malignancy to be made, but once a malignancy has been diagnosed and shown to be associated with elevated levels of a tumor marker, the marker can be used to assess response to treatment.

The recognition and treatment of depression are important components of management. The incidence of depression in cancer patients is ~25% overall and may be greater in patients with greater debility. This diagnosis is likely in a patient with a depressed mood (dysphoria) and/or a loss of interest in pleasure (anhedonia) for at least 2 weeks. In addition, three or more of the following symptoms are usually present: appetite change, sleep problems, psychomotor retardation or agitation, fatigue, feelings of guilt or worthlessness, inability to concentrate, and suicidal ideation. Patients with these symptoms should receive therapy. Medical therapy with a serotonin reuptake inhibitor such as fluoxetine (10 to 20 mg/d), sertraline (50 to 150 mg/d), or paroxetine (10 to 20 mg/d) or a tricyclic antidepressant such as amitriptyline (50 to 100 mg/d) or desipramine (75 to 150 mg/d) should be tried, allowing 4 to 6 weeks for response. Effective therapy should be continued at least 6 months after resolution of symptoms. If therapy is unsuccessful, other classes of antidepressants may be used. In addition to medication, psychosocial interventions such as support groups, psychotherapy, and guided imagery may be of benefit.

Many patients opt for unproven or unsound approaches to treatment when it appears that conventional medicine is unlikely to be curative. Those seeking such alternatives are often well educated and may be early in the course of their disease. Unsound approaches are usually hawked on the basis of unsubstantiated anecdotes and not only cannot help the patient but may be harmful. Physicians should strive to keep communications open and nonjudgmental, so that patients are more likely to discuss with the physician what they are actually doing. The appearance of unexpected toxicity may be an indication that a supplemental therapy is being taken.[3]

LONG-TERM FOLLOW-UP/LATE COMPLICATIONS   At the completion of treatment, sites originally involved with tumor are reassessed, usually by radiography or imaging techniques, and any persistent abnormality is biopsied. If disease persists, the multidisciplinary team discusses a new salvage treatment plan. If the patient has been rendered disease-free by the original treatment, the patient is followed regularly for disease recurrence. The optimal guidelines for follow-up care are not known. For many years, a routine practice has been to follow the patient monthly for 6 to 12 months, then every other month for a year, every 3 months for a year, every 4 months for a year, every 6 months for a year, and then annually. At each visit, a battery of laboratory and radiographic and imaging tests were obtained on the assumption that it is best to detect recurrent disease before it becomes symptomatic. However, where follow-up procedures have been examined, this assumption has been found to be untrue. Studies of breast cancer, melanoma, lung cancer, colon cancer, and lymphoma have all failed to support the notion that asymptomatic relapses are more readily cured by salvage therapy than symptomatic relapses. In view of the enormous cost of a full battery of diagnostic tests and their manifest lack of impact on survival, new guidelines are emerging for less frequent follow-up visits, during which the history and physical examination are the major investigations performed.

As time passes, the likelihood of recurrence of the primary cancer diminishes. For many types of cancer, survival for 5 years without recurrence is tantamount to cure. However, important medical problems can occur in patients treated for cancer and must be examined (Chap. 89). Some problems emerge as a consequence of the disease and some as a consequence of the treatment. An understanding of these disease- and treatment-related problems may help in their detection and management.

Despite these concerns, most patients who are cured of cancer return to normal lives.

SUPPORTIVE CARE   In many ways, the success of cancer therapy depends on the success of the supportive care. Failure to control the symptoms

---

[3]Information about unsound methods may be obtained from the National Council Against Health Fraud, Box 1276, Loma Linda, CA 92354, or from the Center for Medical Consumers and Health Care Information, 237 Thompson Street, New York, NY 10012.

of cancer and its treatment may lead patients to abandon curative therapy. Of equal importance, supportive care is a major determinant of quality of life. Even when life cannot be prolonged, the physician must strive to preserve its quality. Quality-of-life measurements have become common end-points of clinical research studies. Furthermore, palliative care has been shown to be cost-effective when approached in an organized fashion. A credo for oncology could be to cure sometimes, to extend life often, and to comfort always.

Pain Pain occurs with variable frequency in the cancer patient: 25 to 50% of patients present with pain at diagnosis, 33% have pain associated with treatment, and 75% have pain with progressive disease. The pain may have several causes. In about 70% of cases, pain is caused by the tumor itself—by invasion of bone, nerves, blood vessels, or mucous membranes or obstruction of a hollow viscus or duct. In about 20% of cases, pain is related to a surgical or invasive medical procedure, to radiation injury (mucositis, enteritis, or plexus or spinal cord injury), or to chemotherapy injury (mucositis, peripheral neuropathy, phlebitis, steroid-induced aseptic necrosis of the femoral head). In 10% of cases, pain is unrelated to cancer or its treatment.

Assessment of pain requires the methodical investigation of the history of the pain, its location, character, temporal features, provocative and palliative factors, and intensity (Chap. 11); a review of the oncologic history and past medical history as well as personal and social history; and a thorough physical examination. The patient should be given a 10-division visual analogue scale on which to indicate the severity of the pain. The clinical condition is often dynamic, making it necessary to reassess the patient frequently. Pain therapy should not be withheld while the cause of pain is being sought.

A variety of tools are available with which to address cancer pain. About 85% of patients will have pain relief from pharmacologic intervention. However, other modalities, including antitumor therapy (such as surgical relief of obstruction, radiation therapy, and strontium-89 or samarium-153 treatment for bone pain), neurostimulatory techniques, regional analgesia, or neuroablative procedures are effective in an additional 12% or so. Thus, very few patients will have inadequate pain relief if appropriate measures are taken. →*A specific approach to pain relief is detailed in Chap. 9.*

Nausea Emesis in the cancer patient is usually caused by chemotherapy (Chap. 70). Its severity can be predicted from the drugs used to treat the cancer. Three forms of emesis are recognized on the basis of their timing with regard to the noxious insult. *Acute emesis*, the most common variety, occurs within 24 h of treatment. *Delayed emesis* occurs 1 to 7 days after treatment; it is rare, but, when present, usually follows cisplatin administration. *Anticipatory emesis* occurs before administration of chemotherapy and represents a conditioned response to visual and olfactory stimuli previously associated with chemotherapy delivery.

Acute emesis is the best understood form. Stimuli that activate signals in the chemoreceptor trigger zone in the medulla, the cerebral cortex, and peripherally in the intestinal tract lead to stimulation of the vomiting center in the medulla, the motor center responsible for coordinating the secretory and muscle contraction activity that leads to emesis. Diverse receptor types participate in the process, including

TABLE 66-5	Tumor Markers		
Tumor Markers	*Cancer*		*Non-Neoplastic Conditions*
HORMONES			
Human chorionic gonadotropin	Gestational trophoblastic disease, gonadal germ cell tumor		Pregnancy
Calcitonin	Medullary cancer of the thyroid		
Catecholamines	Pheochromocytoma		
ONCOFETAL ANTIGENS			
Alphafetoprotein	Hepatocellular carcinoma, gonadal germ cell tumor		Cirrhosis, hepatitis
Carcinoembryonic antigen	Adenocarcinomas of the colon, pancreas, lung, breast, ovary		Pancreatitis, hepatitis, inflammatory bowel disease, smoking
ENZYMES			
Prostatic acid phosphatase	Prostate cancer		Prostatitis, prostatic hypertrophy
Neuron-specific enolase	Small cell cancer of the lung, neuroblastoma		
Lactate dehydrogenase	Lymphoma, Ewing's sarcoma		Hepatitis, hemolytic anemia, many others
TUMOR-ASSOCIATED PROTEINS			
Prostate-specific antigen	Prostate cancer		Prostatitis, prostatic hypertrophy
Monoclonal immunoglobulin	Myeloma		Infection, MGUS[a]
CA-125	Ovarian cancer, some lymphomas		Menstruation, peritonitis, pregnancy
CA 19-9	Colon, pancreatic, breast cancer		Pancreatitis, ulcerative colitis
CD30	Hodgkin's disease, anaplastic large cell lymphoma		—
CD25	Hairy cell leukemia, adult T cell leukemia/lymphoma		—

[a] MGUS, monoclonal gammopathy of uncertain significance.

dopamine, serotonin, histamine, opioid, and acetylcholine receptors. The serotonin receptor antagonists ondansetron and granisetron are the most effective drugs against highly emetogenic agents, but they are expensive.

As with the analgesia ladder, emesis therapy should be tailored to the situation. For mildly and moderately emetogenic agents, prochlorperazine, 5 to 10 mg orally or 25 mg rectally, is effective. Its efficacy may be enhanced by administering the drug before the chemotherapy is delivered. Dexamethasone, 10 to 20 mg intravenously, is also effective and may enhance the efficacy of prochlorperazine. For highly emetogenic agents such as cisplatin, mechlorethamine, dacarbazine, and streptozocin, combinations of agents work best and administration should begin 6 to 24 h before treatment. Ondansetron, 8 mg orally every 6 h the day before therapy and intravenously on the day of therapy, plus dexamethasone, 20 mg intravenously before treatment, is an effective regimen. Addition of oral aprepitant (a substance P/neurokinin 1 receptor antagonist) to this regimen (125 mg on day 1, 80 mg on days 2 and 3) further decreases the risk of both acute and delayed vomiting. Like pain, emesis is easier to prevent than to alleviate.

Delayed emesis may be related to bowel inflammation from the therapy and can be controlled with oral dexamethasone and oral metoclopramide, a dopamine receptor antagonist that also blocks serotonin receptors at high dosages. The best strategy for preventing anticipatory emesis is to control emesis in the early cycles of therapy to prevent the conditioning from taking place. If this is unsuccessful, prophylactic antiemetics the day before treatment may help. Experimental studies are evaluating behavior modification.

Effusions Fluid may accumulate abnormally in the pleural cavity, pericardium, or peritoneum. Asymptomatic malignant effusions may not require treatment. Symptomatic effusions occurring in tumors responsive to systemic therapy usually do not require local treatment but respond to the treatment for the underlying tumor. Symptomatic effusions occurring in tumors unresponsive to systemic therapy may require local treatment in patients with a life expectancy of at least 6 months.

Pleural effusions due to tumors may or may not contain malignant cells. Lung cancer, breast cancer, and lymphomas account for about 75% of malignant pleural effusions. Their exudative nature is usually gauged by an effusion/serum protein ratio of ≥ 0.5 or an effusion/serum lactate dehydrogenase ratio of ≥ 0.6. When the condition is symptomatic, thoracentesis is usually performed first. In most cases, symptomatic improvement occurs for <1 month. Chest tube drainage is required if symptoms recur within 2 weeks. Fluid is aspirated until the flow rate is <100 mL in 24 h. Then either 60 units of bleomycin or 1 g of doxycycline is infused into the chest tube in 50 mL of 5% dextrose in water; the tube is clamped; the patient is rotated on four sides, spending 15 min in each position; and, after 1 to 2 h, the tube is again attached to suction for another 24 h. The tube is then disconnected from suction and allowed to drain by gravity. If <100 mL drains over the next 24 h, the chest tube is pulled, and a radiograph taken 24 h later. If the chest tube continues to drain fluid at an unacceptably high rate, sclerosis can be repeated. Bleomycin may be somewhat more effective than doxycycline but is very expensive. Doxycycline is usually the drug of first choice. If neither doxycycline nor bleomycin is effective, talc can be used.

Symptomatic pericardial effusions are usually treated by creating a pericardial window or by stripping the pericardium. If the patient's condition does not permit a surgical procedure, sclerosis can be attempted with doxycycline and/or bleomycin.

Malignant ascites is usually treated with repeated paracentesis of small volumes of fluid. If the underlying malignancy is unresponsive to systemic therapy, peritoneovenous shunts may be inserted. Despite the fear of disseminating tumor cells into the circulation, widespread metastases are an unusual complication. The major complications are occlusion, leakage, and fluid overload. Patients with severe liver disease may develop disseminated intravascular coagulation.

Nutrition Cancer and its treatment may lead to a decrease in nutrient intake of sufficient magnitude to cause weight loss and alteration of intermediary metabolism. The prevalence of this problem is difficult to estimate because of variations in the definition of cancer cachexia, but most patients with advanced cancer experience weight loss and decreased appetite. A variety of both tumor-derived factors (e.g., bombesin, adrenocorticotropic hormone) and host-derived factors (e.g., tumor necrosis factor, interleukins 1 and 6, growth hormone) contribute to the altered metabolism, and a vicious cycle is established in which protein catabolism, glucose intolerance, and lipolysis cannot be reversed by the provision of calories.

It remains controversial how to assess nutritional status and when and how to intervene. Efforts to make the assessment objective have included the use of a prognostic nutritional index based on albumin levels, triceps skin fold thickness, transferrin levels, and delayed-type hypersensitivity skin testing. However, a simpler approach has been to define the threshold for nutritional intervention as >10% unexplained body weight loss, serum transferrin level <1500 mg/L (150 mg/dL), and serum albumin <34 g/L (3.4 g/dL).

The decision is important, because it appears that cancer therapy is substantially more toxic and less effective in the face of malnutrition. Nevertheless, it remains unclear whether nutritional intervention can alter the natural history. Unless some pathology is affecting the absorptive function of the gastrointestinal tract, enteral nutrition provided orally or by tube feeding is preferred over parenteral supplementation. However, the risks associated with the tube may outweigh the benefits. Megestrol acetate, a progestational agent, has been advocated as a pharmacologic intervention to improve nutritional status. Research in this area may provide more tools in the future as cytokine-mediated mechanisms are further elucidated.

Psychosocial Support The psychosocial needs of patients vary with their situation. Patients undergoing treatment experience fear, anxiety, and depression. Self-image is often seriously compromised by deforming surgery and loss of hair. Women who receive cosmetic advice that enables them to look better also feel better. Loss of control over how one spends time can contribute to the sense of vulnerability. Juggling the demands of work and family with the demands of treatment may create enormous stresses. Sexual dysfunction is highly prevalent and needs to be discussed openly with the patient. An empathetic health care team is sensitive to the individual patient's needs and permits negotiation where such flexibility will not adversely affect the course of treatment.

Cancer survivors have other sets of difficulties. Patients may have fears associated with the termination of a treatment they associate with their continued survival. Adjustments are required to physical losses and handicaps, real and perceived. Patients may be preoccupied with minor physical problems. They perceive a decline in their job mobility and view themselves as less desirable workers. They may be victims of job and/or insurance discrimination. Patients may experience difficulty reentering their normal past life. They may feel guilty for having survived and may carry a sense of vulnerability to colds and other illnesses. Perhaps the most pervasive and threatening concern is the ever-present fear of relapse (the Damocles syndrome).

Patients in whom therapy has been unsuccessful have other problems related to the end of life.

Death and Dying The most common causes of death in patients with cancer are infection (leading to circulatory failure), respiratory failure, hepatic failure, and renal failure. Intestinal blockage may lead to inanition and starvation. Central nervous system disease may lead to seizures, coma, and central hypoventilation. About 70% of patients develop dyspnea preterminally. However, many months usually pass between the diagnosis of cancer and the occurrence of these complications, and during this period the patient is severely affected by the possibility of death. The path of unsuccessful cancer treatment usually occurs in three phases. First, there is optimism at the hope of cure; when the tumor recurs, there is the acknowledgment of an incurable disease, and the goal of palliative therapy is embraced in the hope of being able to live with disease; finally, at the disclosure of imminent death, another adjustment in outlook takes place. The patient imagines the worst in preparation for the end of life and may go through stages of adjustment to the diagnosis. These stages include denial, isolation, anger, bargaining, depression, acceptance, and hope. Of course, patients do not all progress through all the stages or proceed through them in the same order or at the same rate. Nevertheless, developing an understanding of how the patient has been affected by the diagnosis and is coping with it is an important goal of patient management.

It is best to speak frankly with the patient and the family regarding the likely course of disease. These discussions can be difficult for the physician as well as for the patient and family. The critical features of the interaction are to reassure the patient and family that everything that can be done to provide comfort will be done. They will not be abandoned. Many patients prefer to be cared for in their homes or in a hospice setting rather than a hospital. The American College of Physicians has published a book called *Home Care Guide for Cancer: How to Care for Family and Friends at Home* that teaches an approach to successful problem-solving in home care. With appropriate planning, it should be possible to provide the patient with the necessary medical care as well as the psychological and spiritual support that will prevent the isolation and depersonalization that can attend in-hospital death.

The care of dying patients may take a toll on the physician. A "burnout" syndrome has been described that is characterized by fatigue, disengagement from patients and colleagues, and a loss of self-fulfillment. Efforts at stress reduction, maintenance of a balanced life, and setting realistic goals may combat this disorder.

End-of-Life Decisions Unfortunately, a smooth transition in treatment goals from curative to palliative may not be possible in all cases because of the occurrence of serious treatment-related complications or rapid disease progression. Vigorous and invasive medical support for a reversible disease or treatment complication is assumed to be justified. However, if the reversibility of the condition is in doubt, the patient's wishes determine the level of medical care. These wishes should be elicited before the terminal phase of illness and reviewed periodically. Information about advance directives can be obtained from the American Association of Retired Persons, 601 E Street, NW, Washington, DC 20049, 202-434-2277 or Choice in Dying, 250 West 57th Street, New York, NY 10107, 212-366-5540. →*A full discussion of end-of-life management is in Chap. 9.*

FURTHER READING

CLINICAL PRACTICE GUIDELINE NUMBER 9, MANAGEMENT OF CANCER PAIN. U.S. Department of Health and Human Services, Agency for Health Care Policy and Research publication no. 94-0592, 1994

GRUNBERG SM, HESKETH PJ: Control of chemotherapy-induced emesis. N Engl J Med 329:1790, 1993

JEMAL A, JIWARI RC, MURRAY T et al: Cancer statistics, 2004. CA Cancer J Clin 54:8, 2004

LEVY MH: Pharmacologic treatment of cancer pain. N Engl J Med 335:1124, 1996

THERASSE P et al: New guidelines to evaluate response to treatment in solid tumors. J Natl Cancer Inst 92:205, 2000

WALSH D et al: The symptoms of advanced cancer: Relationship to age, gender, and performance status in 1000 patients. Support Care Cancer 8:175, 2000

67 PREVENTION AND EARLY DETECTION OF CANCER
Otis W. Brawley, Barnett S. Kramer

Cancer prevention and control is a burgeoning field because of advances in understanding the biology of carcinogenesis. The field has expanded beyond the identification and avoidance of carcinogens to include studies of specific interventions to lower cancer risk, as well as screening for early detection of cancer.

Central to cancer prevention and control is the concept that carcinogenesis is not an event but a process, a series of discrete cellular changes that result in progressively more autonomous cellular processes. *Primary prevention* concerns the identification and manipulation of the genetic, biologic, and environmental factors in the causal pathway. Smoking cessation, diet modification, and chemoprevention are primary prevention activities. *Secondary prevention* concerns the identification of asymptomatic neoplastic lesions combined with effective therapy. Screening is a form of secondary prevention.

EDUCATION AND HEALTHFUL HABITS Public education on the avoidance of identified risk factors for cancer and encouraging healthy habits were among early efforts in cancer prevention and control. Many educational messages have come to the public through commercials in the print and electronic media and through school health courses. The physician is a potentially powerful messenger in this education campaign about the hazards of smoking, the benefits of a healthful diet and exercise, use of proven screening methods, and sun avoidance.

Smoking Cessation Tobacco use through cigarettes and other means is the most avoidable risk factor for cardiovascular disease and cancer. The degree of smoke exposure, meaning the number of cigarettes smoked per day as well as the level of inhalation of cigarette smoke, is correlated with risk of lung cancer mortality. Light and low-tar cigarettes are not safer because smokers tend to inhale them more frequently and deeply. Those who stop smoking have a lower lung cancer mortality rate than those who continue smoking, despite the fact that some carcinogen-induced genetic mutations persist for years. In addition to lung cancer, cigarette smoking is a causative agent in cancers of the larynx, oropharynx, esophagus, bladder, and pancreas.

Smoking cessation and avoidance have the potential to save and extend more lives than any other public health activity. A smoker has a one in three lifetime risk of dying prematurely of a smoking-related cancer or cardiovascular or pulmonary disease. Indeed, more human lives are lost due to cardiovascular disease caused by smoking than from smoking-related cancer. The risk of tobacco smoke is not necessarily limited to the smoker. Epidemiologic studies suggest that environmental tobacco smoke may cause lung cancer and other pulmonary diseases in nonsmokers.

Nonsmoking persons should be encouraged not to start smoking, and persons who smoke should be encouraged to stop. Tobacco prevention is a pediatric issue. Over 80% of American smokers begin smoking before the age of 18. Nearly 20% of Americans aged 12 to 18 have smoked a cigarette in the past month. Counseling of adolescents and young adults is critical to prevent smoking. A physician's simple advice to not start smoking or to quit smoking can be of benefit. Physicians should query patients on tobacco use on every office visit, record the answer with the vital signs, and ask smokers if they would like assistance in quitting.

Current approaches to smoking cessation recognize that smoking is an addiction (Chap. 375). The smoker who is quitting goes through a process with identifiable stages that include contemplation of quitting, an action phase in which the smoker quits, and a maintenance phase. Smokers who quit completely are more likely to be successful than those who gradually reduce the number of cigarettes smoked or change to lower tar or nicotine cigarettes. More than 90% of the Americans who have successfully quit smoking did so on their own without participation in an organized cessation program, but cessation programs are helpful for some smokers. The Community Intervention Trial for Smoking Cessation (COMMIT) was a community-based 4-year program. COMMIT demonstrated that light smokers (<25 cigarettes per day) can benefit from simple cessation messages and cessation programs. The quit rate (fraction of the subjects followed who achieved and maintained cessation at the end of the trial) was 30.6% in the intervention communities and 27.5% in the control communities. This finding is statistically significant, but modest. The control communities enjoyed a substantial decrease in smoking through study participation. The COMMIT interventions were not successful for heavy smokers (>25 cigarettes per day). Heavy smokers need an intensive, broad-based cessation program that includes counseling, behavioral strategies, and pharmacologic adjuncts such as nicotine replacement and bupropion.

Cigar smoking has increased in the past 10 years, especially in younger adults. The health risks of cigars are similar to those of cigarettes. Smoking two cigars per day doubles the risk for oral and esophageal cancer; three to four cigars per day increases the risk of oral cancer eight-fold and esophageal cancer four-fold. The risks of occasional cigar smoking are unknown.

Smokeless tobacco is the fastest growing part of the tobacco industry and represents a significant health risk. Chewing tobacco is a carcinogen linked to dental caries, gingivitis, oral leukoplakia, and oral cancer. The systemic effects of smokeless tobacco may increase risks for other cancers.

Diet Modification Dietary modification may have significant potential for lowering cancer risk in western culture. Studies of international dietary patterns and animal studies suggest that diets high in fat increase the risk for cancers of the breast, colon, prostate, and endometrium. These cancers have their highest incidence and mortalities in western countries, where fat comprises an average of 40 to 45% of the total calories consumed. In populations at low risk for these cancers, fat accounts for <20% of calories.

Despite correlations, dietary fat has not been proven to cause cancer. Case-control and cohort epidemiologic studies give conflicting results. In addition, diet is a highly complex exposure to many nutrients and chemicals. Low-fat diets may render some protection through anticarcinogens found in vegetables, fruits, legumes, nuts, and grains. Protective substances found in these foods include phenols, sulfur-containing compounds, flavones, and fiber.

In observational studies, dietary fiber appears protective against colonic polyps and invasive cancer of the colon. The mechanisms involved are complex and speculative. They involve binding of oxidized bile acids and generation of soluble fiber products, such as butyrate, that may have differentiating properties. Transit time is not greatly affected. High-fiber diets may also protect against breast and prostate cancer by absorbing and inactivating dietary estrogenic and androgenic cancer promoters. Protective effects of fiber have not been proved in a prospective clinical trial.

The Polyp Prevention Trial randomly assigned 2000 elderly persons to a low-fat, high-fiber diet versus routine diet for 4 years. No differences were noted in polyp formation.

The U.S. National Institutes of Health Women's Health Initiative, launched in 1994, is a long-term clinical trial enrolling more than 100,000 women aged 45 to 69. It studies the potential cancer-preventing effects of a low-fat diet and vitamin supplementation. Results are not yet available. Scientific evidence does not currently establish the anticarcinogenic value of vitamin, mineral, or nutritional supplements in amounts greater than that provided by a good diet. However, consuming at least five servings of fruits and vegetables a day decreases dietary fat and increases fiber; such a diet may lower the risk of cardiovascular disease.

Sun Avoidance   Nonmelanoma skin cancers (basal cell and squamous cell) are induced by cumulative exposure to ultraviolet radiation. Intermittent acute sun exposure and sun damage have been linked to melanoma. Sunburns, especially in childhood and adolescence, are associated with an increased risk of melanoma in adulthood. Reduction of sun exposure through use of protective clothing and changes in the pattern of outdoor activities can reduce skin cancer risk. Sunscreens decrease the risk of actinic keratoses, the precursor to squamous cell skin cancer, but melanoma risk may be increased. Sunscreens prevent burning and may encourage more prolonged exposure to the sun; yet they may not filter out wavelengths of energy that cause melanoma.

Educational interventions to help people assess their risk of developing skin cancer accurately have some impact. Self-examination for skin pigment characteristics associated with melanoma, such as freckling, may be useful in identifying people at high risk. People who recognize themselves as being at risk tend to be more compliant with sun-avoidance recommendations. Possible risk factors for melanoma include a propensity to sunburn, a large number of benign melanocytic nevi, and atypical nevi.

CANCER CHEMOPREVENTION   Chemoprevention of cancer involves the use of specific natural or synthetic chemical agents to reverse, suppress, or prevent carcinogenesis before the development of invasive malignancy.

Cancer develops through an accumulation of genetic changes that are potential points of intervention to prevent cancer. The initial genetic changes are termed *initiation*. The alteration can be inherited or acquired through the action of physical, infectious, or chemical carcinogens. Like most human diseases, cancer arises through an interaction between genetics and environmental exposures (Table 67-1). Influences that cause the initiated cell to progress through the carcinogenic process and to change phenotypically are termed *promoters*. Promoters include hormones such as androgens, linked to prostate cancer, and estrogen, linked to breast and endometrial cancer. The distinction between an initiator and a promoter is sometimes arbitrary; some components of cigarette smoke are "complete carcinogens," acting as both initiators and promoters. Cancer can be prevented or controlled through interference with the factors that cause initiation, promotion, or progression. Compounds of interest in chemoprevention

TABLE 67-1   *Carcinogens and Associated Cancers or Neoplasms*

Carcinogens[a]	Associated Cancer or Neoplasm
Alkylating agents	Acute myelocytic leukemia, bladder cancer
Androgens	Prostate cancer
Aromatic amines (dyes)	Bladder cancer
Arsenic	Cancer of the lung, skin
Asbestos	Cancer of the lung, pleura, peritoneum
Benzene	Acute myelocytic leukemia
Chromium	Lung cancer
Diethylstilbestrol (prenatal)	Vaginal cancer (clear cell)
Epstein-Barr virus	Burkitt's lymphoma, nasal T cell lymphoma
Estrogens	Cancer of the endometrium, liver, breast
Ethyl alcohol	Cancer of the liver, esophagus, head and neck
Helicobacter pylori	Gastric cancer
Hepatitis B or C virus	Liver cancer
Human immunodeficiency virus	Non-Hodgkin's lymphoma, Kaposi's sarcoma, squamous cell carcinomas (especially of the urogenital tract)
Human papilloma virus	
Human T cell lymphotropic virus type I (HTLV-I)	Adult T cell leukemia/lymphoma
Immunosuppressive agents (azathioprine, cyclosporine, glucocorticoids)	Non-Hodgkin's lymphoma
Nitrogen mustard gas	Cancer of the lung, head and neck, nasal sinuses
Nickel dust	Cancer of the lung, nasal sinuses
Phenacetin	Cancer of the renal pelvis and bladder
Polycyclic hydrocarbons	Cancer of the lung, skin (especially squamous cell carcinoma of scrotal skin)
Schistosomiasis	Bladder cancer (squamous cell)
Sunlight (ultraviolet)	Skin cancer (squamous cell and melanoma)
Tobacco (including smokeless)	Cancer of the upper aerodigestive tract, bladder
Vinyl chloride	Liver cancer (angiosarcoma)

[a] Agents that are thought to act as cancer initiators and/or promoters.

often have antimutagenic, antioxidant, antiproliferative, or pro-apoptotic activity.

A number of chemoprevention strategies are undergoing clinical trials. However, tamoxifen is the only chemoprevention currently approved by the U.S. Food and Drug Administration; it lowers risk of breast cancer in high-risk women.

Multiple Cancer Site Prevention Trials   The Physicians' Health Trial involves 22,071 American male physicians. Participants were randomly assigned to receive β-carotene, aspirin, and/or placebo in a 2 × 2 factorial design. All major medical events were recorded. In 1988, the aspirin arm was unblinded after the trial demonstrated that aspirin therapy causes a significant reduction in cardiovascular mortality. β-Carotene was not associated with a decreased cancer risk compared to placebo.

The Women's Health Study, launched in 1992, is a 10-year trial involving 44,000 female nurses. Subjects are randomly assigned to β-carotene, α-tocopherol, aspirin, and/or placebo in a factorial design yielding eight different treatment groups. The end points are total epithelial cancers, breast cancer, lung cancer, colon cancer, and vascular disease.

The Women's Health Initiative uses a partial factorial design that places women in 22 intervention groups. Participants can receive calcium and vitamin D supplementation, hormone replacement therapy, and counseling to increase exercise and cease smoking. Prevention of a number of cancers, cardiovascular disease, osteoporosis, and other diseases will be assessed. The portion of the trial comparing combined estrogen plus progestin replacement therapy to placebo in women with an intact uterus was halted in 2002 due to an excess of cardiovascular events and breast cancer in the hormone therapy arm. Colon cancer was decreased in the hormone therapy arm. Prior epidemiologic studies had consistently shown a decrease in cardiovascular disease in women taking hormone replacement therapy. The risk of developing Alzheimer's disease was doubled in the combined hormone therapy arm, and quality of life was not improved compared to placebo. Therefore the strength of evidence from prospective randomized, controlled trials is considered to outweigh the prior evidence of benefit. At present combined estrogen plus progestin therapy is not recommended for disease prevention because of the results of this study. The estrogen-only portion of the trial (in women with prior hysterectomy) is still in progress.

Chemoprevention of Cancers of the Upper Aerodigestive Tract Smoking causes diffuse epithelial injury in the head, neck, esophagus, and lung. Patients cured of squamous cell cancers of the lung, esophagus, head, and neck are at risk (as high as 5% per year) of developing a second cancer of the upper aerodigestive tract. Cessation of cigarette smoking does not markedly decrease the cured cancer patient's risk of second malignancy, even though it does lower the cancer risk in those who have never developed a malignancy. Smoking cessation may halt the early stages of the carcinogenic process (such as metaplasia), but it may have no effect on late stages of carcinogenesis. This "field carcinogenesis" hypothesis for cancer of the upper aerodigestive tract has made "cured" patients an important population for chemoprevention of second malignancies. A randomized, placebo-controlled clinical trial has demonstrated that adjuvant isoretinoin (13-*cis*-retinoic acid) can reduce the incidence of second primary tumors in patients treated with local therapy for head and neck cancer. However, overall survival was not improved due to mortality from recurrences of the primary tumor.

Oral leukoplakia, a premalignant lesion commonly found in smokers, has been used as an intermediate marker allowing the demonstration of chemopreventive activity in smaller, shorter-duration, randomized, placebo-controlled trials. Response was associated with upregulation of retinoic acid receptor β. Therapy with isoretinoin causes regression of oral leukoplakia. However, the lesions recur when the agent is withdrawn, suggesting the need for chronic administration of retinoids. Premalignant lesions in the oropharyngeal area have also responded to β-carotene, retinol, α-tocopherol (vitamin E), and selenium. Further study to improve the definition of the activity of these drugs is ongoing. Isoretinoin was shown not to prevent second malignancies in patients cured of early-stage non-small cell lung cancer, and those who were current smokers had higher lung cancer mortality rates than those not taking isoretinoin.

Several large-scale trials have assessed agents in the chemoprevention of lung cancer in patients at high risk. In the Alpha-Tocopherol/Beta-Carotene (ATBC) Lung Cancer Prevention Trial, participants were male smokers, aged 50 to 69 at entry. At entry, participants had smoked an average of one pack of cigarettes per day for 35.9 years. Participants received α-tocopherol, β-carotene, and/or placebo in a randomized, 2 × 2 factorial design. After a median follow-up of 6.1 years, lung cancer incidence and mortality were statistically significantly *increased* in those receiving β-carotene. α-Tocopherol had no effect on lung cancer mortality, and no evidence suggested interaction between the two drugs. Patients receiving α-tocopherol had a higher incidence of hemorrhagic stroke.

The Beta-Carotene and Retinol Efficacy Trial (CARET) involved 17,000 American smokers and workers with asbestos exposure. Entrants were randomly assigned to one of four arms and received β-carotene, retinol, and/or placebo in a 2 × 2 factorial design. This trial demonstrated harm from β-carotene: a lung cancer rate of 5 per 1000 subjects per year for those taking placebo and of 6 per 1000 subjects per year for those taking β-carotene. The difference was statistically significant.

These ATBC and CARET results demonstrate the importance of testing chemoprevention hypotheses before implementing them widely, because the results stand in contrast to a number of observational epidemiologic studies. In the ATBC trial, participants taking α-tocopherol had a one-third reduction in the incidence of prostate cancer, compared to those not taking α-tocopherol. The Physicians' Health Trial showed neither an increased nor a decreased risk of lung cancer in those using β-carotene; fewer of its participants were smokers than those in the ATBC and CARET studies.

Chemoprevention of Colon Cancer Many of the current colon cancer prevention trials are based on the premise that most colorectal cancers develop from adenomatous polyps. These trials use adenoma recurrence or disappearance as a surrogate end point to assess colon cancer prevention. Early clinical trial results suggest that nonsteroidal anti-inflammatory drugs (NSAIDs), such as piroxicam, sulindac, and aspirin, may prevent adenoma formation or cause regression of adenomatous polyps. The mechanism of action of NSAIDs is unknown, but they are presumed to work through the cyclooxygenase pathway. In the Physicians' Health Trial, aspirin had no effect on colon cancer incidence, although the 6-year assessment period may not have been long enough to evaluate this end point definitively. Studies evaluating NSAIDs as colon cancer chemopreventive agents have not yet been completed.

Cyclooxygenase 2 inhibitors may be even more effective at colon cancer prevention. High-dose celecoxib reduces the number of colorectal polyps in patients with familial adenomatous polyposis and is under study for prevention of sporadic colorectal cancer.

Epidemiologic studies suggest that diets high in calcium lower colon cancer risk. Calcium binds bile and fatty acids, which cause hyperproliferation of colonic epithelium. It is hypothesized that this effect reduces intraluminal exposure to these compounds. Early data from randomized studies suggest that calcium supplementation decreases the risk of adenomatous polyp recurrence by about 20%, even though it does not decrease the proliferative rate of the colonic epithelium. Epithelial proliferative rate may not be an adequate surrogate marker in colon cancer prevention trials. Trials of calcium with cancer incidence end points are underway.

The Women's Health Initiative demonstrated a significant reduction in colon cancer among women taking combined hormone replacement therapy. However, the increased risk of cardiovascular events and breast cancer probably outweighs the benefit.

Prevention of Hormonally Driven Cancers Hormonal manipulation is being tested in the primary prevention of breast and prostate cancer. Tamoxifen is an antiestrogen with partial estrogen agonistic activity in some tissues, such as endometrium and bone. One of its actions is to upregulate transforming growth factor β, which decreases breast cell proliferation. In randomized placebo-controlled trials to assess tamoxifen as an adjuvant in breast cancer treatment, this drug reduced the number of new breast cancers in the uninvolved breast by more than a third. In a randomized placebo-controlled trial involving >13,000 women at high risk, tamoxifen decreased the risk of developing cancer by 49% compared to placebo. Tamoxifen also reduced the risk of bone fractures; a small increase in risk of endometrial cancer, stroke, pulmonary emboli, and deep vein thrombosis was noted. A trial to compare tamoxifen with another selective estrogen receptor modulator, raloxifene, is ongoing. Raloxifene may have less risk of endometrial cancer.

Finasteride is a 5α-reductase inhibitor. It inhibits the conversion of testosterone to dihydrotestosterone, a more potent stimulator of prostate cell proliferation than testosterone. In an F344 rat model of carcinogen-induced prostate cancer, finasteride decreased the incidence of cancers. Finasteride produced a 20% decrease in overall prostate cancer, but a slight increase in high-grade (Gleason score 7–10) prostate cancer in men over age 55 years.

Selenium is being tested as a prostate cancer preventive agent based on laboratory studies and a small clinical trial aimed at prevention of skin cancer. Men taking selenium to prevent skin cancer were found to have a significantly reduced incidence of prostate cancer (16 on placebo arm; 4 on selenium arm). The ATBC study cited above showed that risk of prostate cancer was reduced in those taking vitamin E (99 prostate cancers on vitamin E; 151 cases on placebo). The findings on selenium and vitamin E were serendipitous and based on secondary analysis. A prospective study is underway.

Vaccines and Cancer Prevention   A number of infectious agents have been linked to the development of cancer, leading to interest in developing vaccines to protect against these agents. The hepatitis B vaccine is quite effective in preventing hepatitis and hepatomas due to chronic hepatitis B infection. Public health officials are encouraging widespread administration of this vaccine, especially in Asia, where the disease is epidemic. Human papilloma virus (HPV) vaccines are being developed to prevent cervical cancer, and *Helicobacter pylori* vaccines are aimed at gastric cancer. Antibiotic eradication of *H. pylori* may also be a cancer prevention strategy.

SURGICAL PREVENTION OF CANCER   Some organs in some people are at such high risk of developing cancer that surgical removal of the organ at risk is recommended. Women with severe cervical dysplasia are treated with conization and occasionally even hysterectomy. Colectomy is used to prevent colon cancer in people with familial polyposis and those with ulcerative colitis. Based on a study in 139 women with *BRCA1* and *BRCA2* mutations, many women with a genetic predisposition to breast cancer opt to have bilateral mastectomy rather than close surveillance. Of the 139 women, 76 chose mastectomy and 63 chose surveillance; none of the 76 who underwent mastectomy developed breast cancer, but 8 of the 63 women under careful surveillance developed breast cancer. A randomized study is unlikely to be done, and assessment of the effects of prophylactic mastectomy on mortality is also unlikely to be done.

CANCER SCREENING   Screening is a means of detecting disease early in asymptomatic individuals, with the goal of decreasing morbidity and mortality. While screening can potentially save lives and has clearly been shown to do so in the case of cervical, colon, and probably breast cancer, it is also subject to a number of biases, which can suggest a benefit when actually there is none. Bias can even mask net harm. Early detection does not in itself confer benefit. To be of value, screening must detect disease earlier, and treatment of earlier disease must yield a better outcome than treatment at the onset of symptoms. Cause-specific mortality, rather than survival after diagnosis, is the preferred end point (see below).

Because screening is done on asymptomatic, healthy persons, it should offer substantial likelihood of benefit that outweighs harm. Screening tests and their appropriate use should be carefully evaluated before their use is widely encouraged in screening programs as a matter of public policy.

Screening examinations, tests, or procedures are usually not diagnostic of cancer but instead indicate that a cancer may be present. The diagnosis is then made following a workup that includes a biopsy and pathologic confirmation.

A number of genes have been identified that predispose for a disease, and many more will be identified in the near future. Testing for these genes can define a high-risk population. The ability to predict the development of a particular cancer may some day present therapeutic options as well as ethical dilemmas. It may eventually allow for early intervention to prevent a cancer or limit its severity. People at high risk will be ideal candidates for chemoprevention and screening; however, efficacy of these interventions in the high-risk population should be investigated. Currently, persons at high risk for a particular cancer can engage in intensive screening. While this course is clinically prudent, it is not known if it saves lives in these populations.

TABLE 67-2   Definition of Terms

Term	Definition
Sensitivity	The proportion of persons with the condition who test positive: $a/(a + c)$
Specificity	The proportion of persons without the condition who test negative: $d/(b + d)$
Positive predictive value	The proportion of persons with a positive test who have the condition: $a/(a + b)$
Negative predictive value	The proportion of persons with a negative test who do not have the condition: $d/(c + d)$

		Condition present	Condition absent
a = true positive			
b = false positive	Positive test	a	b
c = false negative			
d = true negative	Negative test	c	d

The Accuracy of Screening   A screening test's accuracy or ability to discriminate disease is described by four indices: sensitivity, specificity, positive predictive value, and negative predictive value (Table 67-2). *Sensitivity* is the proportion of persons with the disease who test positive in the screen (i.e., the ability of the test to detect disease when it is present). *Specificity* is the proportion of persons who do not have the disease and test negative in the screening test (i.e., the ability of a test to tell that the disease is not present). The *positive predictive value* is the proportion of persons who test positive who actually have the disease. Similarly, *negative predictive value* is the proportion of who test negative and do not have the disease. The sensitivity and specificity of a test are relatively independent of the underlying prevalence (or risk) of the disease in the population screened, but the predictive values depend strongly on the prevalence of the disease (Table 67-3).

Screening is most beneficial, efficient, and economical when the target disease is common in the population being screened. To be valuable, the screening test should have a high specificity; sensitivity need not be very high, as demonstrated in Table 67-3.

Potential Biases of Screening Tests   The common biases of screening are lead time, length, and selection. These biases can make a screening test seem beneficial when actually it is not (or even causes net harm). Whether beneficial or not, screening can create the false impression of an epidemic by increasing the number of cancers diagnosed. It can also produce a shift in proportion of patients diagnosed at an early stage that improves survival statistics without reducing mortality (i.e., the number of deaths from a given cancer relative to the number of people at risk for the cancer). In such a case, the *apparent* duration of

TABLE 67-3   Predictive Value Relationships[a]

Positive predictive value (PPV) is a function of sensitivity, specificity, and prevalence:

$$PPV = \frac{prevalence \times sensitivity}{(prevalence \times sensitivity) + (1 - prevalence)(1 - specificity)}$$

PPV for a prevalence of 5 per 1000:

	PPV for a Sensitivity of, %	
Specificity	0.8	0.95
0.95	7	9
0.999	80	83

PPV for a prevalence of 1 per 10,000:

	PPV for a Sensitivity of, %	
Specificity	0.8	0.95
0.95	0.2	0.2
0.999	7	9

[a] The positive predictive value is expressed as a percentage. It is influenced by the sensitivity and specificity of the screening test and the prevalence of the disease being screened for. As shown here, for relatively uncommon diseases, such as cancer, the positive predictive value is influenced particularly strongly by the specificity of the screening test at a given prevalence.

survival increases without lives being saved or life expectancy changed.

Lead-time bias occurs when a test does not influence the natural history of the disease; the patient is merely diagnosed at an earlier date. When lead-time bias occurs, survival *appears* increased, but life is not really prolonged. The screening test only prolongs the time the subject is aware of the disease and spends as a patient.

Length bias occurs when slow-growing, less aggressive cancers are detected during screening. Cancers diagnosed due to the onset of symptoms between scheduled screenings are on average more aggressive, and treatment outcomes are not as favorable. An extreme form of length bias is termed *overdiagnosis*, the detection of "pseudodisease." The reservoir of some undetected slow-growing tumors is large. Many of these tumors fulfill the histologic criteria of cancer but will never become clinically significant or cause death. This problem is compounded by the fact that the most common cancers appear most frequently at ages when competing causes of death are more frequent.

Selection bias must be considered in assessing the results of any screening effort. The population most likely to seek screening may differ from the general population to which the screening test might be applied. The individuals screened may have volunteered because of a particular risk factor not found in the general population, such as a strong family history. In general, volunteers for studies may be more health conscious and likely to have a better prognosis or lower mortality rate, irrespective of the screening result. This is termed the *healthy volunteer effect*.

Potential Drawbacks of Screening Risks associated with screening include harm caused by the screening intervention itself, harm due to the further investigation of persons with positive test results (both true and false positives), and harm from the treatment of persons with a true-positive result, even if life is extended by treatment. The diagnosis and treatment of cancers that would never have caused medical problems can lead to the harm of unnecessary treatment and give patients the anxiety of a cancer diagnosis. The psychosocial impact of cancer screening, whether the result is positive or negative, can also be substantial when applied to the entire population.

Assessment of Screening Tests Good clinical trial design can offset some biases of screening and demonstrate the relative risks and benefits of a screening test. A randomized, controlled screening trial with cause-specific mortality as the end point provides the strongest support for a screening intervention. In a randomized trial, two like populations are randomly established. One is given the medical standard of care (which may be no screening at all), and the other receives the screening intervention being assessed. The two populations are compared over time. Efficacy for the population studied is established when the group receiving the screening test has a better cause-specific mortality rate than the control group. Studies showing a reduction in the incidence of advanced-stage disease, an improved survival, or a stage shift are weaker (and possibly misleading) evidence of benefit. These latter criteria are necessary but not sufficient to establish the value of a screening test.

Although a randomized, controlled screening trial provides the strongest evidence to support the usefulness of a screening test, it is not perfect. Unless the trial is population-based, it does not remove the issue of generalizability to the target population. Screening trials generally involve thousands of persons and last for years. Less definitive study designs are therefore often used to estimate the effectiveness of screening practices. After a randomized controlled clinical trial, in descending order of strength, evidence may be derived from:

The findings of internally controlled trials using intervention allocation methods other than randomization (e.g., allocation determined by birth date, date of clinic visit);

The findings of cohort or case-control analytic observational studies;

The results of multiple time series studies with or without the intervention;

The opinions of respected authorities based on clinical experience, descriptive studies, or consensus reports of experts (the weakest evidence because even experts can be misled by the biases described above).

Screening for Specific Cancers Widespread screening for cervical, colon, and probably breast cancer is beneficial for certain age groups. Special surveillance of those at high risk for a specific cancer because of a family history or a genetic risk factor may be prudent, but few studies have been carried out to assess the impact of this practice on mortality in specific high-risk populations. A number of organizations have considered whether or not to endorse routine use of certain screening tests. Because these groups have not used the same criteria to judge whether a screening test should be endorsed, they have arrived at different recommendations. The screening guidelines of the U.S. Preventive Services Task Force, the Canadian Task Force on Preventive Health Care, and the American Cancer Society are often quoted and show a range of recommendations (Table 67-4).

BREAST CANCER Breast self-examination, clinical breast examination by a care giver, and mammography have been advocated as useful screening tools. Only breast self-examination, screening mammography alone, and screening mammography with clinical examination have been evaluated in randomized controlled trials. Magnetic resonance

TABLE 67-4 *Screening Recommendations for Asymptomatic Normal-Risk Subjects[a]*

Test or Procedure	USPSTF	ACS	CTFPHC
Sigmoidoscopy	>50, periodically <50, not recommended	≥50, every 3–5 years	Insufficient evidence
Fecal occult blood testing	≥50, every year	≥50, every year	Insufficient evidence
Digital rectal examination	No recommendation	≥40, every year	Poor evidence to include or exclude
Prostate-specific antigen	Insufficient evidence to recommend	M: ≥50, every year	Recommendation against
Pap test	F: 18–65, every 1–3 years	F with uterine cervix, beginning 3 years after first intercourse or by age 21. Yearly for standard Pap; every 2 years with liquid test.	Fair evidence to include in examination of sexually active women
Pelvic examination	Do not recommend, advise adnexal palpation during exam for other reasons	F: 18–40, every 1–3 years with Pap test; >40, every year	Not considered
Endometrial tissue sampling	Not considered	At menopause if obese or a history of unopposed estrogen use	Not considered
Breast self-examination	No recommendation	≥20, monthly	Insufficient evidence to make a recommendation
Breast clinical examination	F: >50, every year	F: 20–40, every 3 years; >40, yearly	F: >50, every year
Mammography	F: 40–75, every 1–2 years	F: ≥40, every year	F: 50–69, every year
Complete skin examination	Not recommended	20–39, every 3 years	Poor evidence to include or exclude

[a] Summary of the screening procedures recommended for the general population by U.S. Preventive Services Task Force (USPSTF), the American Cancer Society (ACS), and the Canadian Task Force on Prevention Health Care (CTFPHC). These recommendations refer to asymptomatic persons who have no risk factors, other than age or gender, for the targeted condition. *Note*: F, female; M, male.

imaging is being assessed and may be more accurate than mammography in women at high risk.

A number of trials have suggested that annual or biennial screening with mammography or mammography plus clinical breast examination in women over the age of 50 saves lives. Each trial has been criticized for design flaws. In most trials, the breast cancer mortality rate is decreased by 20 to 30%. Experts disagree on whether average-risk women aged 40 to 49 should receive regular screening (Table 67-4). The significance of the screening effect in women aged 40 to 49 depends on the statistical test used. An analysis of eight large randomized trials showed no benefit from mammographic screening for women aged 40 to 49 when assessed 5 to 7 years after trial entry. However, a small benefit emerged 10 to 12 years after study entry. What proportion of this benefit is due to screening after these women turned 50 is not known. In randomized screening studies of women aged 50 to 69, the decline in mortality begins about 5 years after initiation of screening. Nearly half of women aged 40 to 49 years screened annually will have false-positive mammograms necessitating further evaluation, often including biopsy. The risk of false-positive testing should be discussed with the patient.

While no study has shown breast self-examination to decrease mortality, it is recommended as prudent by many organizations. A substantial fraction of breast cancers are first detected by patients. Self-examination leads to increased biopsy rate without reducing breast cancer mortality.

Genetic screening for *BRCA1* and *BRCA2* mutations and other markers of breast cancer risk has identified a group of women at high risk for breast cancer. Unfortunately, when to begin and the optimal frequency of screening have not been defined. Mammography is less sensitive at detecting breast cancers in women carrying *BRCA* mutations, possibly because such cancers occur in younger women, in whom mammography is known to be less sensitive.

CERVICAL CANCER Screening with Papanicolaou smears decreases cervical cancer mortality. The cervical cancer mortality rate has fallen substantially since the widespread use of the Pap smear, although this trend actually began earlier. Most screening guidelines recommend regular Pap testing for all women who are or have been sexually active for 3 years or have reached the age of 21. With the onset of sexual activity comes the risk of sexual transmission of HPV, the most common etiologic factor for cervical cancer. The recommended interval for Pap screening varies from 1 to 3 years. At age 30, women who have had three normal test results in a row may get screened every 2 to 3 years. An upper age limit at which screening ceases to be effective is not known, but women age $\geq$70 years who have had no abnormal results in the previous 10 years may choose to stop screening.

COLORECTAL CANCER Fecal occult blood testing, digital rectal examination, rigid and flexible sigmoidoscopy, radiographic barium contrast studies, and colonoscopy have been considered for colorectal cancer screening. Annual fecal occult blood testing using hydrated specimens could reduce colorectal cancer mortality by a third. The sensitivity for fecal occult blood is increased if specimens are rehydrated before testing, but at the cost of lower specificity. The false-positive rate for rehydrated fecal occult blood testing is high; 1 to 5% of persons tested have a positive result. About 2 to 10% of those with occult blood in the stool have cancer, and 20 to 30% have adenomas. The high false-positive rate of fecal occult blood testing dramatically increases the number of colonoscopies performed.

Two case-control studies suggest that regular screening of people over 50 with sigmoidoscopy decreases mortality. These types of studies are prone to selection biases. A quarter to a third of polyps can be discovered with the rigid sigmoidoscope; half are found with a 35-cm flexible scope, and two-thirds to three-quarters are found with a 60-cm scope. Diagnosis of polyposis by sigmoidoscopy should lead to evaluation of the entire colon with colonoscopy and/or barium enema. The most efficient interval for screening sigmoidoscopy is unknown.

Case-control studies suggest that testing at intervals of up to 15 years may confer benefit.

One-time colonoscopy detects about 25% more advanced lesions (polyps > 10 mm, villous adenomas, polyps with high-grade dysplasia, invasive cancer) than does one-time fecal occult blood testing with sigmoidoscopy. Colonoscopy is well suited to screening subjects at high risk, such as those with ulcerative colitis or family predisposition. Perforation rates are 3/1000 for colonoscopy and 1/1000 for sigmoidoscopy. Debate continues on whether full colonoscopy is too expensive and invasive for widespread use as a screening tool in standard-risk populations. Data are not available on digital rectal examination or barium enema as colon cancer screening tools, but both are insensitive.

LUNG CANCER Chest radiographs and sputum cytology have been evaluated as methods for lung cancer screening. No reduction in lung cancer mortality has been found in these studies, although all the controlled trials performed have had low statistical power. Even screening of high-risk subjects (smokers) has not been proved to be beneficial. Spiral computed tomography (CT) can diagnose lung cancers at early stages; however, false-positive rates are high. Spiral CT screening increases the number of lesions detected and increases the number of diagnostic and therapeutic procedures. However, its capacity to save lives is being tested.

OVARIAN CANCER Adnexal palpation, transvaginal ultrasound, and serum CA-125 determination have been considered for ovarian cancer screening. Adnexal palpation is too insensitive to detect ovarian cancer at an early enough stage to affect mortality substantially. Neither transvaginal ultrasound nor CA-125 screening has been tested in a completed randomized prospective trial. Ovarian cancer screening can lead to an invasive diagnostic workup, which may include laparotomy. In a clinical study, 0.6% of 900 adult women had a serum CA-125 level >35 U/mL. Thus, if 100,000 adult women were screened, 600 would be identified as having a high CA-125 level. The prevalence of ovarian cancer in the female adult population is ~20 per 100,000. Thus, the screening test would identify 600 women who would undergo further evaluation to identify 20 cases of ovarian cancer. Some of these 600 would only be inconvenienced by an ultrasound examination. Others would undergo an exploratory laparotomy. A large proportion of the 20 women identified as having ovarian cancer would have advanced, incurable disease and thus not benefit from screening. A National Institutes of Health consensus conference in 1994 concluded that routine screening for ovarian cancer was not indicated for standard-risk women or those with a single affected family member, but that it might be worthwhile in families with genetic ovarian cancer syndromes.

PROSTATE CANCER The most common prostate cancer screening modalities are digital rectal examination and assays for serum prostate-specific antigen (PSA). Newer serum tests, such as measurement of the ratio of bound to free serum PSA, have yet to be fully evaluated. An emphasis on PSA screening has caused prostate cancer to become the most common non-skin cancer diagnosed in American males. Screening for this disease is very prone to lead-time bias, length bias, and overdiagnosis, and substantial debate rages among experts on whether it is effective. Some experts are concerned that prostate cancer screening, more than screening for other cancers, may cause net harm. Prostate cancer screening clearly detects many asymptomatic cancers, but the ability to distinguish tumors that are lethal but still curable from those that pose little or no threat to health is limited. Men over age 50 have a very high prevalence of indolent, clinically insignificant prostate cancers. No well-designed trial has demonstrated the benefit of prostate cancer screening and treatment.

The placebo arm of the Prostate Cancer Prevention Trial showed that rigorous screening of low-risk men for 7 years leads to the diagnosis of prostate cancer in >12% of patients. However, >12% of patients with normal annual DREs and PSAs biopsied after 7 years were found to have cancer. Thus, prostate cancer screening had moderate success in early detection, but screening missed half the prostate cancers.

The effectiveness of radical prostatectomy, radiation therapy, and other treatments for low-stage prostate cancer is also under study in randomized trials. Definitive treatment of cancers detected by screening may cause morbidity for some men, such as impotence and urinary incontinence, and carries a low but finite risk of death. Comparison of radical prostatectomy to "watchful waiting" in clinically diagnosed (not screening PSA-detected) prostate cancers showed a decreased rate of death from prostate cancer for those undergoing surgery, but overall mortality was not different in the two arms. Patients undergoing surgery had a higher rate of impotence and urinary incontinence.

Ongoing randomized trials are comparing usual care to prostate screening and comparing definitive therapy to "watchful waiting." The American Cancer Society and the American Urologic Association recommend that men be offered screening after being informed of the potential risks and benefits. A man should have a life expectancy of at least 10 years to be eligible for screening. The U.S. Preventive Services Task Force finds insufficient evidence to recommend prostate cancer screening (Table 67-4).

ENDOMETRIAL CANCER Transvaginal ultrasound and endometrial sampling have been advocated as screening tests for endometrial cancer. Benefit from routine screening has not been shown. Transvaginal ultrasound and endometrial sampling are indicated for workup of vaginal bleeding in postmenopausal women but are not considered as screening tests in symptomatic women.

SKIN CANCER Visual examination of all skin surfaces by the patient or by a health care provider is used in screening for basal and squamous cell cancers and melanoma. No prospective randomized study has been performed to look for a mortality decrease. Observational epidemiologic evidence from Scotland and Australia suggests that screening programs have caused a stage shift in melanomas diagnosed. Screening may reinforce sun avoidance and other skin cancer prevention behaviors.

FURTHER READING

THE CANADIAN TASKFORCE ON PREVENTIVE HEALTH CARE: www.ctfphc.org/
HUMPHREY LL et al: Breast cancer screening: A summary of the evidence for the U.S. Preventive Services Task Force. Ann Intern Med 137:347, 2002
KIM ES et al: Chemoprevention of aerodigestive tract cancers Annu Rev Med 53:223, 2002
THE NATIONAL CANCER INSTITUTE CANCERNET: cancernet.nci.nih.gov/
NATIONAL INSTITUTES OF HEALTH CONSENSUS DEVELOPMENT PANEL: Breast cancer screening for women ages 40–49. J Natl Cancer Inst 89: 1015, 1997
SCREENING FOR PROSTATE CANCER: Recommendation and rationale. Ann Intern Med 137:915, 2002
SMITH RA et al: American Cancer Society guidelines for the early detection of cancer, 2003. CA Cancer J Clin 53:27, 2003
STOUTJESDIJK M: Magnetic resonance imaging and mammography in women with a hereditary risk of breast cancer. J Natl Cancer Inst 93:1095, 2001

68 | CANCER GENETICS
Pat J. Morin, Jeffrey M. Trent, Francis S. Collins, Bert Vogelstein

CANCER IS A GENETIC DISEASE Cancer arises through a series of somatic alterations in DNA that results in unrestrained cellular proliferation. Most of these alterations involve actual sequence changes in DNA (i.e., mutations). They may arise as a consequence of random replication errors, exposure to carcinogens (e.g., radiation), or faulty DNA repair processes. While most cancers arise sporadically, familial clustering of cancers occurs in certain families who carry a germline mutation in a cancer gene.

HISTORIC PERSPECTIVE The concept of cancer genetics is relatively new. The idea that cancer progression is driven by sequential somatic mutations in specific genes has only gained general acceptance in the last 25 years. Before the advent of the microscope, cancer was believed to be composed of aggregates of mucus or other noncellular matter. By the middle of the nineteenth century, it became clear that tumors were masses of cells and that these cells arose from the normal cells of the tissue in which the cancer originated. However, the molecular basis for the uncontrolled proliferation of cancer cells was to remain a mystery for another century. During that time, a number of theories for the origin of cancer were postulated. The great biochemist Otto Warburg proposed the combustion theory of cancer, which stipulated that cancer was due to abnormal oxygen metabolism: while normal cells required oxygen, cancer cells could survive in its absence. In addition, some believed that all cancers were caused by viruses, and that cancer was in fact a contagious disease.

In the end, observations of cancer occurring in chimney sweeps, studies of x-rays, and the overwhelming data demonstrating cigarette smoke as a causative agent in lung cancer, together with Ames's work on chemical mutagenesis, were sufficient to convince many that cancer originated through changes in DNA. Although the viral theory of cancer did not prove to be generally accurate, the study of retroviruses led to the discovery of the first human *oncogenes* in the mid to late 1970s. Soon after, the study of families with genetic predisposition to cancer was instrumental in the discovery of *tumor suppressor genes*. The field that studies the type of mutations, as well as the consequence of these mutations in tumor cells, is now known as cancer genetics.

THE CLONAL ORIGIN AND MULTISTEP NATURE OF CANCER Nearly all cancers originate from a single cell; this clonal origin is a critical discriminating feature between neoplasia and hyperplasia. Multiple cumulative mutational events are invariably required for the progression from normal to fully malignant phenotype. The process can be seen as Darwinian microevolution in which, at each successive step, the mutated cells gain a growth advantage resulting in an increased representation relative to their neighbors (Fig. 68-1). It is believed that five to ten accumulated mutations are necessary for a cell to progress from the normal to the fully malignant phenotype.

We are beginning to understand the precise nature of the genetic alterations responsible for some malignancies and to get a sense of the order in which they occur. The best studied example is colon cancer, in which analyses of DNA from tissues extending from normal colon epithelium through adenoma to carcinoma have identified some of the genes mutated in the process (Fig. 68-2). Similar progression models are being elucidated for other malignancies.

GENERAL CLASSES OF CANCER GENES There are two major classes of cancer genes. The first class comprises genes that directly affect cell growth either positively (*oncogenes*) or negatively (*tumor suppressor*

FIGURE 68-1 Multistep clonal development of malignancy. In this diagram a series of five cumulative mutations (T1, T2, T4, T5, T6), each with a modest growth advantage acting alone, eventually results in a malignant tumor. Note that not all such alterations result in progression; for example, the T3 clone is a dead end. The actual number of cumulative mutations necessary to transform from the normal to the malignant state is unknown in most tumors. (*After P Nowell, Science 194:23, 1976, with permission.*)

FIGURE 68-2 Progressive somatic mutational steps in the development of colon carcinoma. The accumulation of alterations in a number of different genes results in the progression from normal epithelium through adenoma to full-blown carcinoma. Genetic instability (microsatellite or chromosomal) accelerates the progression by increasing the likelihood of mutation at each step. Patients with familial polyposis are already one step into this pathway, since they inherit a germline alteration of the *APC* gene. TGF, transforming growth factor.

genes). These genes exert their effects on tumor growth through their ability to control cell division (cell birth) or cell death (apoptosis). Oncogenes are tightly regulated in normal cells. In cancer cells, oncogenes acquire mutations that relieve this control and lead to increased activity of the gene product. This mutational event typically occurs in a single allele of the oncogene and acts in a dominant fashion. In contrast, the normal function of tumor suppressor genes is to restrain cell growth and this function is lost in cancer. Because of the diploid nature of mammalian cells, both alleles must be inactivated to completely lose the function of a tumor suppressor gene, leading to a recessive mechanism at the cellular level. From these ideas and studies on the inherited form of retinoblastoma, Knudson and others formulated the *two-hit hypothesis*, which in its modern version states that both copies of a tumor suppressor gene must be inactivated in cancer.

The second class of cancer genes, the *caretakers*, do not directly affect cell growth but rather affect the ability of the cell to maintain the integrity of its genome. Cells with deficiency in these genes have an increased rate of mutations in all the genes, including oncogenes and tumor suppressor genes. This "mutator" phenotype was first hypothesized by Loeb to explain how the multiple mutational events required for tumorigenesis can occur in the lifetime of an individual. A mutation phenotype has now been observed in cancer at both the nucleotide sequence and chromosomal levels.

MECHANISMS OF TUMOR SUPPRESSOR INACTIVATION The two major types of somatic lesions observed in tumor suppressor genes during tumor development are *point mutations* and *large deletions*. Point mutations in the coding region of tumor suppressor genes will frequently lead to truncated protein products or otherwise nonfunctional proteins. Similarly, deletions lead to the loss of a functional product and sometimes encompass the entire gene or even the entire chromosome arm, leading to loss of heterozygosity (LOH) in the tumor DNA compared to the corresponding normal tissue DNA (Fig. 68-3). LOH in tumor DNA is considered a hallmark for the presence of a tumor suppressor gene at a particular locus and LOH studies have been useful in the positional cloning of many tumor suppressor genes. Gene silencing, which occurs in conjunction with hypermethylation of the promoter, is another mechanism of tumor suppressor gene inactivation.

FAMILIAL CANCER SYNDROMES A small fraction of the cancers occur in patients with a genetic predisposition. In these families, the affected individuals have a predisposing loss-of-function mutation in one allele of a tumor suppressor gene or caretaker gene. The tumors in these patients show a loss of the remaining normal allele as a result of somatic events (point mutations or deletions), in agreement with the Knudson hypothesis (Fig. 68-3). Thus, most cells of an individual with an inherited loss-of-function mutation in a tumor suppressor gene are functionally normal and only the rare cells that develop a mutation in the remaining normal allele will exhibit uncontrolled growth. The normal function of tumor suppressors is to restrain growth, to promote

differentiation (gatekeeper genes), or to preserve genome integrity (caretaker genes).

Roughly 100 syndromes of familial cancer have been reported, although many are rare. The majority are inherited as autosomal dominant traits although some of those associated with DNA repair abnormalities (xeroderma pigmentosum, Fanconi's anemia, ataxia telangiectasia) are autosomal recessive. Table 68-1 shows a number of cancer predisposition syndromes and the responsible genes. The current paradigm states that the genes mutated in familial syndromes can also be targets for somatic mutations in sporadic (noninherited) tumors. The study of cancer syndromes has thus provided invaluable insights into the mechanisms of progression for many tumor types. This section examines the case of inherited colon cancer in detail, but the same general lessons can be applied to all the cancer syndromes listed in Table 68-1.

Familial adenomatous polyposis (FAP) is a dominantly inherited colon cancer syndrome due to germline mutations in the adenomatous polyposis coli (*APC*) tumor suppressor gene on chromosome 5. Patients with this syndrome develop hundreds to thousands of adenomas in the colon. Each of these adenomas has lost the normal remaining allele of *APC* but has not yet accumulated the required additional mutations to generate fully malignant cells (Fig. 68-2). However, out of these thousands of benign adenomas, several will invariably acquire further abnormalities and a subset will even develop into fully malignant cancers. *APC* is thus considered to be a gatekeeper for colon tumorigenesis; Fig. 68-4 shows germline and somatic mutations found in the *APC* gene. The function of the APC protein is still not completely understood but likely provides differentiation and apoptotic cues to colonic cells as they migrate up the crypts. Defects in this process may lead to abnormal accumulation of cells that should normally undergo apoptosis and slough off.

In contrast to FAP, patients with hereditary nonpolyposis colon cancer (HNPCC or Lynch syndrome) do not develop multiple polyposis but instead develop only one or a small number of adenomas that rapidly progress to cancer. HNPCC is commonly defined by family

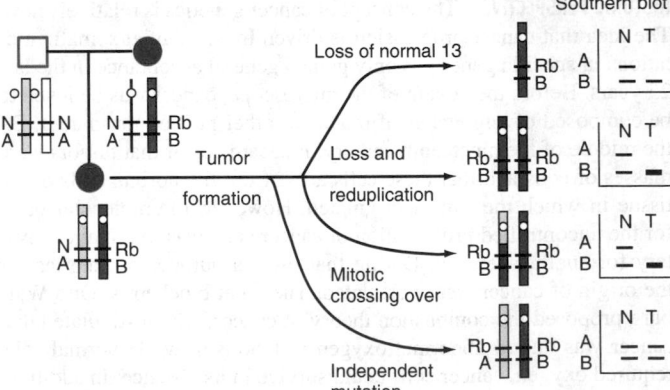

FIGURE 68-3 Diagram of possible mechanisms for tumor formation in an individual with hereditary (familial) retinoblastoma. On the left is shown the pedigree of an affected individual who has inherited the abnormal (Rb) allele from her affected mother. The four chromosomes of her two parents are drawn to indicate their origin. Just below the retinoblastoma locus a polymorphic marker is also analyzed in this family. The patient is AB at this locus, like her mother, whereas her father is AA. Thus the B allele must be on the chromosome carrying the retinoblastoma disease gene. Tumor formation results when the normal allele (N), which this patient inherited from her father, is inactivated. On the right are shown four possible ways in which this could occur. In each case, the resulting chromosome 13 arrangement is shown, as well as the results of a Southern blot comparing normal tissue with tumor tissue. Note that in the first three situations the normal allele (A) has been lost in the tumor tissue, which is referred to as loss of heterozygosity (LOH). (*From TD Gelehrter and FS Collins, in Principles of Medical Genetics, Baltimore, Williams and Wilkins, 1990, with permission.*)

history, with at least three individuals over at least two generations developing colon or endometrial cancer, and with at least one individual diagnosed before the age of 50. Most HNPCC is due to mutations in one of four DNA mismatch repair genes (Table 68-1), which are components of a repair system that is normally responsible for correcting errors in freshly replicated DNA. Germline mutations in *MSH2* and *MLH1* account for more than 60% of HNPCC cases, while mutations in *MSH6* and *PMS2* are much less frequent. When a somatic mutation inactivates the remaining wild-type allele of a mismatch repair gene, the cell develops a hypermutable phenotype characterized by profound genomic instability, especially for the short repeated sequences called *microsatellites*. This microsatellite instability (MIN) favors the development of cancer by increasing the rate of mutations in many genes, including oncogenes and tumor suppressor genes (Fig. 68-2). These genes can thus be considered caretakers. Figure 68-5 shows an example of the instability in allele sizes for dinucleotide repeats in the cancers of HNPCC patients.

While most autosomal dominant inherited cancer syndromes are due to mutations in tumor suppressor genes (Table 68-1), there are a few interesting exceptions. Multiple endocrine neoplasia type II, a dominant disorder characterized by pituitary adenomas, medullary carcinoma of the thyroid, and (in some pedigrees) pheochromocytoma, is due to gain-of-function mutations in the protooncogene *RET* on chromosome 10. Similarly, gain-of-function mutations in the tyrosine kinase domain of the *MET* oncogene lead to hereditary papillary renal carcinoma. Interestingly, loss-of-function mutations in the *RET* gene cause a completely different disease, Hirschsprung's disease [aganglionic megacolon (Chaps. 279 and 330)].

Although the Mendelian forms of cancer described above have taught us much about the mechanisms of growth control, most forms of cancer do not follow simple patterns of inheritance. In many instances (e.g., lung cancer), a strong environmental contribution is at work. Even in such circumstances, however, some individuals may be more genetically susceptible to developing cancer, given the appropriate exposure, due to the presence of modifier alleles.

GENETIC TESTING FOR FAMILIAL CANCER The discovery of cancer susceptibility genes raises the possibility of DNA testing to predict the risk of cancer in individuals of affected families. An algorithm for cancer risk assessment and decision-making in high-risk families using genetic testing is shown in Fig. 68-6. Once a mutation is discovered in a family, subsequent testing of asymptomatic family members can be crucial in patient management. A negative gene test in these individuals can prevent years of anxiety in the knowledge that their cancer risk is no higher than that of the general population. On the other hand, a positive test may lead to alteration of clinical management, such as increased frequency of cancer screening and, when feasible and appropriate, prophylactic surgery. Potential negative consequences of a positive test result include psychological distress (anxiety, depression) and discrimination (insurance, employment). Testing should therefore not be conducted without counseling before and after disclosure of the test result. In addition, the decision to test should depend on whether effective interventions exist for the particular type of cancer to be tested. Despite these caveats, genetic cancer testing for some cancer syndromes already appears to have greater benefits than risks and many companies now offer testing for various genes associated with the predisposition to breast cancer (*BRCA1* and *BRCA2*), melanoma (*p16INK4*), and colon cancer (*APC* and the HNPCC genes).

Because of the inherent problems of genetic testing such as cost,

TABLE 68-1 *Cancer Syndromes and Associated Genes*

Syndrome	Gene	Chromosome	Inheritance	Tumors
Ataxia telangiectasia	ATM	11q22-q23	AR	Breast cancer
Bloom syndrome	BLM	15q26.1	AR	Cancer of all types
Familial adenomatous polyposis	APC	5q21	AD	Intestinal adenoma, colorectal cancer
Familial melanoma	p16INK4	9p21	AD	Melanoma, pancreatic cancer
Familial Wilms' tumor	WT1	11p13	AD	Pediatric kidney cancer
Hereditary breast/ ovarian cancer	BRCA1 BRCA2	17q21 13q12.3	AD	Breast, ovarian, colon, prostate
Hereditary multiple exostoses	EXT1 EXT2	8q24 11p11-12	AD	Exostoses, chondrosarcoma
Hereditary prostate cancer	HPC1	1q24-25	AD	Prostate carcinoma
Hereditary retinobastoma	RB1	13q14.2	AD	Retinoblastoma, osteosarcoma
Hereditary nonpolyposis colon cancer (HNPCC)	MSH2 MLH1 MSH6 PMS2	2p16 3p21.3 2p16 7p22	AD	Colon, endometrial, ovarian, stomach, small bowel, ureter carcinoma
Hereditary papillary renal carcinoma	MET	7q31	AD	Papillary renal tumor
Li-Fraumeni	TP53	17p13.1	AD	Sarcoma, breast cancer
Multiple endocrine neoplasia type 1	MEN1	11q13	AD	Parathyroid, endocrine, pancreas, pituitary
Multiple endocrine neoplasia type 2a	RET	10q11.2	AD	Medullary thyroid carcinoma, pheochromocytoma
Neurofibromatosis type 1	NF1	17q11.2	AD	Neurofibroma, neurofibrosarcoma, brain tumor
Neurofibromatosis type 2	NF2	22q12.2	AD	Vestibular schwannoma, meningioma, spine
Nevoid basal cell carcinoma syndrome (Gorlin syndrome)	PTCH	9q22.3	AD	Basal cell carcinoma, medulloblastoma, jaw cysts
Tuberous sclerosis	TSC1 TSC2	9q34 16p13.3	AD	Angiofibroma, renal angiomyolipoma
Von Hippel– Lindau	VHL	3p25-26	AD	Kidney, cerebellum, pheochromocytoma

Note: AD, autosomal dominant; AR, autosomal recessive.

specificity, and sensitivity, it is not yet appropriate to offer these tests to the general population. However, testing may be appropriate in some subpopulations with a known increased risk, even without a defined family history. For example, two mutations in the breast cancer susceptibility gene *BRCA1*, 185delAG and 5382insC, exhibit a sufficiently high frequency in the Ashkenazi Jewish population that genetic testing of an individual of this ethnic group may be warranted.

It is important that genetic test results be communicated to families by trained genetic counselors. To ensure that the families clearly understand its advantages and disadvantages and the impact it may have on their management and psyche, genetic testing should never be done before counseling. Significant expertise is needed to communicate the results of genetic testing to families. For example, one common mistake is to misinterpret the result of negative genetic tests. For many cancer predisposition genes, the sensitivity of genetic testing is only 70% or less (i.e., of 100 kindreds tested, disease-causing mutations can be identified in only 70). Therefore, such testing should in general begin with an affected member of the kindred (the youngest family member still alive who has had the cancer of interest). If a mutation is not identified in this individual, then the test should be reported as noninformative (Fig. 68-6) rather than negative (because it is possible that the mutation in this individual is not detectable by standard genetic assays for purely technical reasons). On the other hand, if a mutation can be identified in this individual, then testing of other family mem-

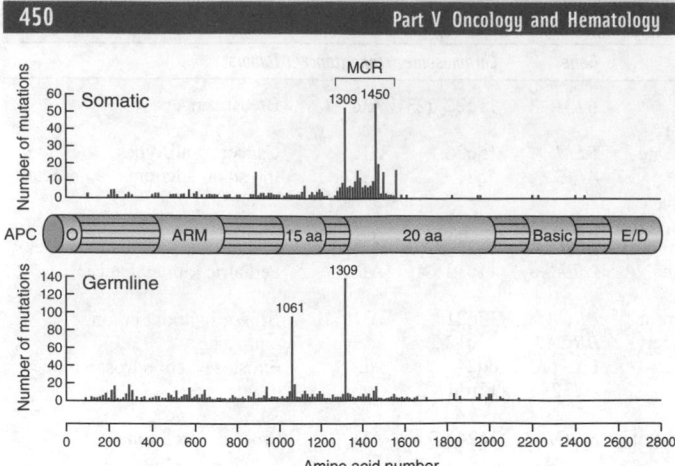

FIGURE 68-4 Germline and somatic mutations in the tumor suppressor gene *APC*. *APC* encodes a 2843-amino-acid protein with 6 major domains: an oligomerization region (O), armadillo repeats (ARM), 15-amino-acid repeats (15 AA), 20-amino-acid repeats (20 AA), a basic region, and a domain involved in binding FB1 and the *Drosophila* discs large homologue (E/D). Shown are the positions within the *APC* gene of a total of 650 somatic and 826 germline mutations (from the APC database at http://p53.curie.fr/). The vast majority of these mutations result in the truncation of the APC protein. Germline mutations are found to be relatively evenly distributed up to codon 1600 except for 2 mutation hotspots at amino acids 1061 and 1309, which together account for one-third of the mutations found in familial adenomatous polyposis (FAP) families. Somatic *APC* mutations in colon tumors cluster in an area of the gene known as the *mutation cluster region* (MCR). The location of the MCR suggests that the 20-amino-acid domain plays a crucial role in tumor suppression. Note that loss of the second functional *APC* allele in tumors from FAP families often occurs through loss of heterozygosity.

bers can be performed, and the sensitivity of such subsequent tests will be 100% (because the mutation in the family is in this case known to be detectable by the assay methods used).

ONCOGENES IN HUMAN CANCER Oncogenes of the kind found in human cancers were initially discovered through their presence in the genome of retroviruses capable of causing cancers in chickens, mice, and rats. The cellular homologues of these viral genes are often targets of mutation or aberrant regulation in human cancer. Whereas many oncogenes were discovered because of their presence in retroviruses, other oncogenes, particularly those involved in translocations characteristic of particular leukemias and lymphomas, were isolated through genomic approaches. Investigators cloned the sequences surrounding the chromosomal translocations observed cytogenetically and then de-

FIGURE 68-5 Demonstration of microsatellite instability in normal and tumor tissue from hereditary nonpolyposis colon cancer (HNPCC) patients. In each case the lane marked T contains DNA from a tumor, and the lane marked N contains DNA from normal tissue of the same patient. The marker (*D2S123*, located on chromosome 2) is a microsatellite composed of a tandem repeat of the dinucleotide CA, which varies in length from chromosome to chromosome. Normally, however, the length of the repeat is stable in somatic tissues. In this example, a polymerase chain reaction analysis has been applied to genomic DNA, and new alleles for the marker are apparent in tumors 1, 2, 5, and 7. Because the tumor tissue is defective in DNA mismatch repair, clonal abnormalities in copying of the CA repeat have arisen. Errors are also occurring in functional genes, eventually resulting in the malignant phenotype. (*From LA Aaltonen et al, Clues to the pathogenesis of familial colorectal cancer.* Science 260:812, *1993 with permission; Copyright 1993 AAAS.*)

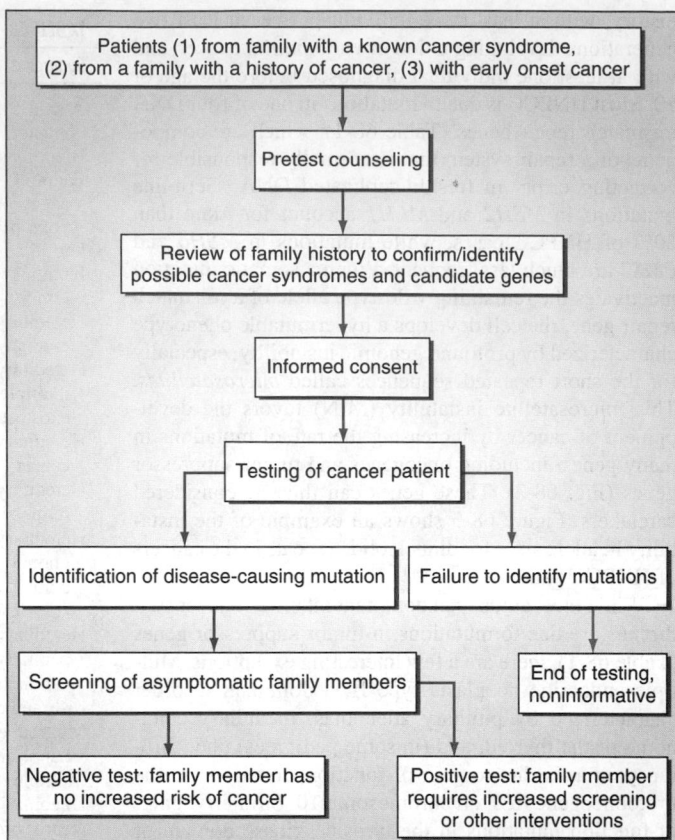

FIGURE 68-6 Algorithm for genetic testing in a family with cancer predisposition. The key step is the identification of a mutation in a cancer patient, which allows testing of asymptomatic family members. Asymptomatic family members who test positive may require increased screening or surgery, whereas others are at no greater risk for cancer than the general population.

duced the nature of the genes that were the targets of these translocations (see below). Some of these were oncogenes known from retroviruses [like *ABL*, involved in chronic myelogenous leukemia (CML)], while others were new (like *BCL2*, involved in B cell lymphoma). In the normal cellular environment, protooncogenes have crucial roles in cell proliferation and differentiation. Table 68-2 is a partial list of oncogenes known to be involved in human cancer.

The normal growth and differentiation of cells is controlled by growth factors, which bind to receptors on the surface of the cell. The signals generated by the membrane receptors are transmitted inside the cells through signaling cascades involving kinases, G proteins, and other regulatory proteins. Ultimately, these signals affect the activity of transcription factors in the nucleus, which regulate the expression of genes crucial in cell proliferation, cell differentiation, and cell death. Oncogene products have been found to function at critical steps in these pathways (Chap. 69), and inappropriate activation of these pathways can lead to tumorigenesis.

MECHANISMS OF ONCOGENE ACTIVATION Mechanisms that upregulate (or activate) cellular oncogenes fall into three broad categories: point mutation, DNA amplification, and chromosomal rearrangement.

Point Mutation Point mutation is a common mechanism of oncogene activation. For example, mutations in one of the *RAS* genes (*HRAS*, *KRAS*, or *NRAS*) are present in up to 85% of pancreatic cancers and 50% of colon cancers but are relatively uncommon in other cancer types. Remarkably—and in contrast to the diversity of mutations found in tumor suppressor genes (Fig. 68-4)—most of the activated *RAS* genes contain point mutations in codons 12, 13, or 61 (which convey resistance to GAP, a protein that interacts with RAS and inactivates it through substitution of the GTP cofactor with GDP). The restricted pattern of mutation compared to tumor suppressor genes reflects the fact that gain-of-function mutations of oncogenes are more difficult to attain than simple inactivation. Indeed, inactivation of a gene can be attained through the introduction of a stop codon anywhere in the coding sequence, whereas activations require precise substitutions at residues that normally downregulate the activity of the encoded protein. The specificity of oncogene mutations provides specific diagnostic opportunities, as it is much simpler to find mutations at specified positions than it is when mutations can be scattered throughout the gene (as in tumor suppressor genes).

DNA Amplification The second mechanism for activation of oncogenes is DNA sequence amplification, leading to overexpression of the gene product. This increase in DNA copy number may cause cytologically recognizable chromosome alterations referred to as *homogeneous staining regions* (HSRs), if integrated within chromosomes or *double minutes* (dmins), if extrachromosomal in nature. The recognition of DNA amplification is accomplished through various cytogenetic techniques such as comparative genomic hybridization (CGH) and fluorescence in situ hybridization (FISH), which allow the visualization of chromosomal aberrations using fluorescent dyes. With these techniques, the entire genome can be surveyed for gains and losses of DNA sequences, thus pinpointing chromosomal regions likely to contain genes important in the development or progression of cancer. Noncytogenetic, molecular techniques for identifying amplifications have more recently become available.

Numerous genes have been reported to be amplified in cancer. Several genes, including *NMYC* and *LMYC*, were identified through their presence within the amplified DNA sequences of a tumor and had homology to known oncogenes. Because the region amplified often extends to hundreds of thousands of base pairs, more than one oncogene may be amplified in some cancers (particularly sarcomas). Genes simultaneously amplified in many cases include *MDM2*, *GLI*, *CDK4*, and *SAS*. Demonstration of amplification of a cellular gene is often a predictor of poor prognosis. For example, *ERBB2/HER2* and *NMYC* are often amplified in aggressive breast cancers and neuroblastoma, respectively.

Chromosomal Rearrangement Chromosomal alterations provide important clues to the genetic changes in cancer. The chromosomal alterations in human solid tumors such as carcinomas are heterogeneous and complex and likely reflect selection for the loss of tumor suppressor genes on the involved chromosome. In contrast, the chromosome alterations in liquid tumors (leukemias and lymphomas) are often simple translocations, i.e., reciprocal transfers of chromosome arms from one chromosome to another. Consequently, many detailed and informative chromosome analyses have been performed on hematopoietic cancers. The breakpoints of recurring chromosome abnormalities usually occur at the site of cellular oncogenes. Table 68-3 lists representative examples of recurring chromosome alterations in malignancy and the associated gene(s) rearranged or deregulated by the chromosomal rearrangement. Translocations are particularly common in lymphoid tumors, probably because these cell types normally rearrange their DNA to generate antigen receptors. Indeed, antigen receptor genes are commonly involved in the translocations, implying that an imperfect regulation of receptor gene rearrangement may be involved in the pathogenesis. An example is Burkitt's lymphoma, a B cell tumor characterized by a reciprocal translocation between chromosomes 8 and 14. Molecular analysis of Burkitt's lymphomas demonstrated that the breakpoints occurred within or near the *MYC* locus on chromosome 8 and within the immunoglobulin heavy chain locus on chromosome 14, resulting in the transcriptional activation of *MYC*. Enhancer activation by translocation, although not universal, appears to play an important role in malignant progression. In addition to transcription factors and signal transduction molecules, translocation may result in the overexpression of cell cycle regulatory proteins such as cyclins and of proteins that regulate cell death such as bcl-2.

The first reproducible chromosome abnormality detected in human malignancy was the Philadelphia chromosome detected in CML. This cytogenetic abnormality is generated by reciprocal translocation involving the *ABL* oncogene, a tyrosine kinase on chromosome 9, being placed in proximity to the *BCR* (breakpoint cluster region) on chromosome 22. Figure 68-7 illustrates the generation of the translocation and its protein product. The consequence of expression of the *BCR-ABL* gene product is the activation of signal transduction pathways leading to cell growth independent of normal external signals. Interestingly, a compound (gleevec) that specifically blocks the activity of *BCR-ABL* was synthesized and shown to exhibit remarkable efficacy with little toxicity in patients with CML. Knowledge of genetic alterations in cancer can lead to mechanism-based design and development of a new generation of cancer drugs.

TABLE 68-2 *Common Oncogenes Altered in Human Cancers*

Oncogene	Function	Alteration in Cancer	Neoplasm
AKT1	Serine/threonine kinase	Amplification	Gastric carcinoma
AKT2	Serine/threonine kinase	Amplification	Ovarian, breast, pancreas
CTNNB1	Signal transduction	Point mutation	Colon, prostate, melanoma, skin, others
FOS	Transcription factor	Overexpression	Osteosarcomas
ERBB2	Receptor tyrosine kinase	Point mutation, amplification	Breast, ovary, stomach, neuroblastoma
JUN	Transcription factor	Overexpression	Lung
MET	Receptor tyrosine kinase	Point mutation, rearrangement	Osteocarcinoma, kidney, glioma
MYB	Transcription factor	Amplification	AML, CML, colon, melanoma
MYC	Transcription factor	Amplification	Breast, colon, gastric, lung
LMYC	Transcription factor	Amplification	Lung carcinoma, bladder
NMYC	Transcription factor	Amplification	Neuroblastoma, lung cancer
HRAS	GTPase	Point mutation	Colon, lung, pancreas
KRAS	GTPase	Point mutation	Melanoma, colorectal cancer, AML
NRAS	GTPase	Point mutation	Various carcinomas, melanoma
REL	Transcription factor	Rearrangement, amplification	Lymphomas
WNT1	Growth factor	Amplification	Retinoblastoma

Note: AML, acute myelogenous leukemia; CML, chronic myelogenous leukemia.

TABLE 68-3 *Representative Oncogenes at Chromosomal Translocations*

Gene (Chromosome)	Translocation	Malignancy
ABL (9q34.1)–BCR (22q11)	(9;22)(q34;q11)	Chronic myelogenous leukemia
ATF1 (12q13)–EWS (22q12)	(12;22)(q13;q12)	Malignant melanoma of soft parts (MMSP)
BCL1 (11q13.3)–IgH (14q32)	(11;14)(q13;q32)	Mantle cell lymphoma
BCL2 (18q21.3)–IgH (14q32)	(14;18)(q32;q21)	Follicular lymphoma
FLI1 (11q24)–EWS (22q12)	(11;22)(q24;q12)	Ewing's sarcoma
LCK (1p34)–TCRB (7q35)	(1;7)(p34;q35)	T cell acute lymphocytic leukemia (ALL)
MYC (8q24)–IgH (14q32)	(8;14)(q24;q32)	Burkitt's lymphoma, B cell ALL
WT1 (11p13)–EWS (22q12)	(11;22)(p13;q12)	Desmoplastic small round cell tumor (DSRCT)
PAX3 (2q35)–FKHR/ALV(13q14)	(2;13)(q35;q14)	Alveolar rhabdomyosarcoma
PAX7 (1p36)–KHR/ALV(13q14)	(1;13)(p36;q14)	Alveolar rhabdomyosarcoma
RET (10q11.2)	(10;17)(q11.2;q23)	Papillary thyroid carcinomas

Source: From R Hesketh: *The Oncogene and Tumour Suppressor Gene Facts Book*, 2d ed. San Diego, Academic Press, 1997; with permission.

FIGURE 68-7 Specific translocation seen in chronic myelogenous leukemia (CML). The Philadelphia chromosome (Ph) is derived from a reciprocal translocation between chromosomes 9 and 22 with the breakpoint joining the sequences of the *ABL* oncogene with the *BCR* gene. The fusion of these DNA sequences allows the generation of an entirely novel fusion protein with modified function. (*Courtesy of ER Fearon and KR Cho.*)

CHROMOSOMAL INSTABILITY IN SOLID TUMORS   Solid tumors are generally highly aneuploid, containing an abnormal number of chromosomes; these chromosomes also exhibit structural alterations such as translocations, deletions, and amplifications. Again, colon cancer has proven to be a particularly useful model for the study of chromosomal instability (CIN). As described above, some familial cases are characterized by the presence of MIN. Interestingly, MIN and CIN appear to be mutually exclusive in colon cancer, suggesting that they represent alternative mechanisms for the generation of a mutator phenotype in this cancer (Fig. 68-2). Other cancer types rarely exhibit MIN but almost always exhibit CIN. Normal cells possess several cell cycle checkpoints, often defined as quality control requirements that have to be met before subsequent events are allowed to take place. The spindle checkpoint, which ensures proper chromosome attachment to the mitotic spindle before allowing the sister chromatid to separate, has been shown to be deficient in certain cancers. The genes that, when mutated, may cause CIN have in general not yet been identified, although a few candidates mutated in a small number of tumors have been discovered. The identification of the cause of CIN in tumors will likely be a formidable task, considering that several hundred genes are thought to control the mitotic checkpoint and other cellular processes assuring proper chromosome segregation. Regardless of the mechanisms underlying CIN, the measurement of the number of chromosomal alterations present in tumors is now possible with both cytogenetic and molecular techniques, and several studies have shown that this information can be useful for prognostic purposes.

VIRUSES IN HUMAN CANCER   Certain human malignancies are associated with viruses. Examples include Burkitt's lymphoma (Epstein-Barr virus), hepatocellular carcinoma (hepatitis virus), cervical cancer [human papillomavirus (HPV)], and T cell leukemia (retroviruses). The mechanisms of action of these viruses are varied but always involve activation of growth-promoting pathways or inhibition of tumor suppressor products in the infected cells. For example, HPV proteins E6 and E7 bind and inactivate cellular tumor suppressors p53 and pRB, respectively. Viruses are not sufficient for cancer development but constitute one alteration in the multistep process of cancer.

EPIGENETIC REGULATION OF GENE EXPRESSION IN CANCER   An *epigenetic modification* refers to a change in the genome, heritable by cell progeny, that does not involve a change in the DNA sequence. The inactivation of the second X chromosome in female cells is an example of an epigenetic mechanism that prevents gene expression from the inactivated chromosome. During embryologic development, regions of chromosomes from one parent are silenced and gene expression proceeds from the chromosome of the other parent. For most genes, expression occurs from both alleles or randomly from one allele or the other. The preferential expression of a particular gene exclusively from the allele contributed by one parent is called *parental imprinting* and is thought to be regulated by covalent modifications of chromatin protein and DNA (particularly methylation) of the silenced llele.

The role of epigenetic control mechanisms in the development of human cancer is unclear. However, a general decrease in the level of DNA methylation has been noted as a common change in cancer. In addition, numerous genes, including some tumor suppressor genes, appear to become hypermethylated and silenced during tumorigenesis. *VHL* and *p16INK4* are well-studied examples of tumor suppressor genes that are silenced through methylation in human cancers. Overall, epigenetic mechanisms may be responsible for reprogramming the expression of a large number of genes in cancer and, together with the mutation of specific genes, are likely to be crucial in the development of human malignancies.

GENE EXPRESSION PROFILING IN CANCER   The tumorigenesis process, driven by alterations in tumor suppressors, oncogenes, and epigenetic regulation, is accompanied by changes in gene expression. The advent of powerful new techniques such as microarrays and serial analysis of gene expression (SAGE) has allowed the study of gene expression in neoplastic cells on a scale never before accomplished. Indeed, it is now possible to identify expression levels of thousands of genes expressed in normal and cancer tissues. Figure 68-8 shows a typical cDNA array experiment examining gene expression in cancer. This global knowledge of gene expression allows the identification of differentially expressed genes and, in principle, the understanding of the complex molecular circuitry regulating normal and neoplastic behaviors. Such studies have led to molecular profiling of tumors, which has suggested general methods for distinguishing tumors of various biologic behaviors (molecular classification), elucidating pathways relevant to the development of tumors and identifying molecular targets for the detection and therapy of cancer. The first practical applications of this technology have suggested that global gene expression profiling can provide prognostic information not evident from other clinical or

FIGURE 68-8 A cDNA array experiment. RNA is prepared from cells, reverse transcribed to cDNA, and labeled with fluorescent dyes (typically green for normal cells and red for cancer cells). The fluorescent probes are mixed and hybridized to the cDNA array. Each spot on the array is a cDNA fragment that represents a different gene. The image is then captured with a fluorescence camera; red spots indicate higher expression in tumor compared with reference while green spots represent the opposite. Yellow signals indicate equal expression levels in normal and tumor specimens. After clustering analysis of multiple arrays, the results are typically represented graphically using Treeview software, which shows, for each sample, a color-coded representation of gene expression for every gene on the array.

laboratory tests. The National Cancer Institute, in conjunction with the National Center for Biotechnology Information, has undertaken the Cancer Genome Anatomy Project (CGAP) (*www.ncbi.nlm.nih.gov/ncicgap/*) to collect data on gene expression in normal and malignant tissues and make it available on the Internet.

THE FUTURE   It is clear that there has been a revolution in cancer genetics in the past 20 years. Identification of cancer genes has led to a better understanding of the tumorigenesis process and has had important repercussions on all fields of biology. In spite of these spectacular advances, however, there has been little overall improvement in cancer death rates. It is hoped that, as the molecular mechanisms of cancer initiation and development continue to be elucidated, novel therapies based on pathophysiology rather than empiricism will emerge. Time will tell whether these strategies will rely on novel combinations or dosing schedules of conventional drugs or will be based on new approaches such as those involving gene therapy or immunotherapy. In addition, a better understanding of the molecular pathways and genetic alterations in cancer cells may lead to the development of sensitive strategies for early detection of cancer.

FURTHER READING

EMERY J: Common hereditary cancers and implications for primary care. Lancet 358:56, 2001

GOLUB TR et al: Molecular classification of cancer: Class discovery and class prediction by gene expression monitoring. Science 286:531, 1999

JALLEPALLI PV, LENGAUER C: Chromosome segregation and cancer: Cutting through the mystery. Nat Rev Cancer 1:109, 2001

LOEB LA: Mutator phenotype may be required for multistage carcinogenesis. Cancer Res 51:3075, 1991

MUNGER K: Disruption of oncogene/tumor suppressor networks during human carcinogenesis. Cancer Invest 20:71, 2002

STRAUSBERG RL et al: In silico analysis of cancer through the Cancer Genome Anatomy Project. Trends Cell Biol 11:S66, 2001

VOGELSTEIN B, KINZLER KW: The multistep nature of cancer. Trends Genet 9:138, 1993

YAN et al: Genetic testing—present and future. Science 289:1890, 2000

69   CANCER CELL BIOLOGY AND ANGIOGENESIS
Robert G. Fenton, Dan L. Longo

Two characteristic features define a cancer: unregulated cell growth and tissue invasion/metastasis. Unregulated cell growth without invasion is a feature of *benign neoplasms*, or new growths. Cancer is a synonym for *malignant neoplasm*. Cancers of epithelial tissues are called *carcinomas*; cancers of nonepithelial (mesenchymal) tissues are called *sarcomas*.

Cancer is a genetic disease. The malignant phenotype often requires mutations in several different genes. Cancer cells generally retain the capacity to proliferate by acquiring mutations in cell cycle regulatory genes (particularly those regulating the G_1 checkpoint). Often mutations activate cell pathways leading to proliferation and block pathways of differentiation. The normal cell has protective mechanisms that lead to the repair of cell damage; these repair pathways are often abnormal in cancer cells. When a normal cell has sustained too much damage to repair, the cell activates a suicide pathway to prevent damage to the organ. These cell death pathways are also commonly altered in cancer cells, leading to the survival of damaged cells that would normally die.

The accumulation of genetic lesions may lead through an identifiable progression of altered phenotypes as is noted in colon cancer: hyperplasia → adenoma → dysplasia → carcinoma in situ → invasive carcinoma. However, in many tissues, premalignant changes cannot be readily identified. Genetic changes lead to both loss and acquisition of properties: a loss of the differentiated function of the cell but the acquisition of novel characteristics that facilitate metastasis, such as the ability to break through basement membranes, migrate through the extracellular matrix and into the vascular tree, and generate new blood vessels to support colonization in remote sites.

CANCER CELL BIOLOGY

The treatment of most human cancers with conventional cytoreductive agents has been unsuccessful due to the Gompertzian-like growth kinetics of solid tumors and the genetic instability that predisposes to the development of intrinsic and acquired drug resistance. Rationally designed, target-based therapeutic agents directed against the specific molecular derangements that distinguish malignant from nonmalignant cells have become possible with advances in the understanding of oncogene and tumor-suppressor pathways. New agents can be classified by their specific molecular targets, such as tyrosine kinase inhibitors or farnesyltransferase inhibitors, or by their general mechanism of action, such as inhibition of cell cycle progression or angiogenesis. Novel therapeutics include small molecules, peptides, oligonucleotides, and monoclonal antibodies. This chapter describes the convergence of scientific, pharmacologic, and medical knowledge that has led to the targeted therapy of cancer.

THERAPEUTIC APPROACHES TO CELL CYCLE ABNORMALITIES IN CANCER   The mechanism of cell division is substantially the same in all dividing cells and has been conserved throughout evolution. The process assures that the cell accurately duplicates its contents, especially its chromosomes. The cell cycle is divided into four phases. During M-phase, the replicated chromosomes are separated and packaged into two new nuclei by mitosis and the cytoplasm is divided between the two daughter cells by cytokinesis. The other three phases of the cell cycle are called *interphase*: G_1 (gap 1), during which the cell determines its readiness to commit to DNA synthesis; S (DNA synthesis), during which the genetic material is replicated and no re-replication is permitted; and G_2 (gap 2), during which the fidelity of DNA replication is assessed and errors are corrected.

Deregulation of the molecular mechanisms controlling cell cycle progression is a hallmark of cancer. Progression from one phase of the cell cycle to the next is controlled by the orderly activation of cyclin-dependent kinases (CDKs) that are regulated by signaling events that couple a cell's physiologic response to its extracellular milieu. The transition through G_1 into S-phase is a critical regulator of cell proliferation, and the phosphorylation state of the retinoblastoma tumor-suppressor protein (pRB) at the restriction point determines whether a cell will enter S-phase (where DNA synthesis occurs). The complex of CDK4 or CDK6 with D type cyclins forms a G_1-specific kinase whose activity is regulated by growth factors, nutrients, and cell-cell and cell-matrix interactions. Subsequent formation of an active CDK2/cyclin E complex results in full phosphorylation of pRB, relieving its inhibitory effects on the S-phase-regulating transcription factor E2F/DP1, and permitting the activation of genes required for S-phase (such as dihydrofolate reductase, thymidine kinase, and DNA polymerase). The activity of CDK/cyclin complexes can be blocked by CDK-inhibitors including $p21^{Cip1/Waf1}$, $p16^{Ink4a}$, and $p27^{Kip1}$, which block S-phase progression by preventing the phosphorylation of pRB.

Genetic lesions that render the retinoblastoma pathway nonfunctional are thought to occur in almost all human cancers. The result of these lesions is loss of the function of pRB as guardian of the G_1 restriction point, enabling cancer cells to enter a mitotic cycle without the normal input from external signals. Current therapeutic efforts to reverse the derangements of the retinoblastoma pathway have taken two main approaches. All kinases require the binding of ATP (and substrate) to the enzyme active site, followed by transfer of the γ-phosphate to serine, threonine, or tyrosine residues of the substrate. One of the first kinase inhibitors to reach clinical trial was UCN-01, a staurosporine analogue, which had broad activity against many serine/threonine kinases and hence lacked specificity. Flavopiridol was the first relatively selective CDK inhibitor identified, with Ki or IC_{50}s in the 40- to 400-nM range. Although flavopiridol was initially thought to inhibit tumor cell proliferation by inhibition of cell cycle CDKs, it is now clear that non-cell cycle functions of the CDK7/cyclin H and CDK9/cyclin T1 complexes may be critical for flavopiridol's antitumor activity due to inhibition of transcription of cellular mRNA. Phase II clinical trials of flavopiridol are in progress. Laboratory efforts are focused on the development of novel classes of CDK inhibitors capable of specifically targeting individual CDK/cyclin complexes. This may prove difficult given the great structural similarity of the active sites of these kinases. A second therapeutic endeavor to regain control of pRB function involves reversing the epigenetic silencing of p16^{Ink4a} gene and is discussed below.

p53, the "guardian of the genome," is a sequence-specific transcription factor whose activity is regulated through tight control of p53 protein levels. Normally, levels of p53 are kept low by its association with the mdm2 oncogene product, which binds p53 and shuttles it out of the nucleus for proteolytic degradation. In response to noxious stimuli that induce DNA damage, such as gamma irradiation or chemotherapy, p53 is phosphorylated by several kinases that regulate the DNA damage checkpoint. This causes dissociation of p53 from mdm2, leading to increased p53 protein levels. This activates transcription of genes leading to cell cycle arrest (p21$^{Cip1/Waf1}$) or apoptosis (pro-apoptotic Bcl-2 family members, genes regulating metabolism of reactive oxygen species, and death receptors such as DR5). Inducers of p53 include hypoxia, DNA damage (caused by ultraviolet radiation, gamma irradiation, or chemotherapy), ribonucleotide depletion, and telomere shortening. Further, deregulated activity of oncogenes such as *Myc*, which promote aberrant G$_1$/S transition, results in p53-induced apoptosis. This is mediated by a second product of the Ink4a locus, p14^{ARF}, which is encoded by an *a*lternative *r*eading *f*rame from p16^{Ink4a}. Levels of ARF are upregulated by *Myc* and E2F, and ARF binds to mdm2 and rescues p53 from its inhibitory effect. This oncogene checkpoint leads to the death of renegade cells that attempt to transverse the restriction point without appropriate physiologic signals.

Acquired mutation in p53 is the most common genetic alteration found in human cancer (>50%); germline mutation in p53 is the causative genetic lesion of the Li-Fraumeni familial cancer syndrome. In many tumors, one p53 allele on chromosome 17p is deleted and the other is mutated. The mutations often abrogate the DNA binding function of p53 that is required for its transcription factor activity and tumor-suppressor functions. Inactivation of the p53 pathway compromises cell cycle arrest, attenuates apoptosis induced by DNA damage or other stimuli, and predisposes cells to chromosome instability. This genomic instability greatly increases the probability that p53 null cells will acquire additional mutations and become malignant. Almost all human cancers have genetic alterations that bypass the Rb and p53 tumor-suppressor pathways.

Therapies directed at p53 are based on the observations that tumors expressing mutant p53 are often more resistant to chemotherapy than tumors with wild-type p53, and that mutant p53 proteins accumulate to high levels in tumor cells. If the transcriptional functions of the mutant p53 could be reestablished in tumor cells, massive apoptosis might ensue, whereas normal cells would be protected because they express very low levels of wild-type 53. Investigators have screened chemical libraries for compounds that inhibit tumor cell growth in a mutant p53-dependent manner. One compound entered cells and induced mutant p53 to adopt an active conformation such that p53-de-

pendent transcriptional activation was restored and apoptosis was selectively induced. This compound also had anti-tumor activity in murine xenograft models. These experiments constitute a proof of principle for targeting mutant p53 in human cancer through the novel mechanism of restoring an active conformation to a mutant tumor-suppressor protein. Clinical development is planned.

Compounds have been identified that act through a p53-dependent mechanism to protect normal cells from genotoxic damage. Selenium has been known as a cancer preventative for many years, but its mechanism of action is unknown. Selenomethionine, the main form of selenium in our diets, participates in a redox reaction resulting in the reduction of two cysteine residues within p53, leading to an induction of p53 DNA-binding activity. However, this form of p53 activates DNA repair pathways without affecting cell growth; the repair of genetic lesions may explain the cancer-preventative activity of selenomethionine. Other investigators have identified a low-molecular-weight, cell-permeable compound that inhibits the apoptotic functions of wild-type p53. This compound protected mice from the toxic effects of radiation therapy and chemotherapy, including bone marrow suppression, gastrointestinal dysfunction, and hair loss.

Knowledge of the molecular events governing cell cycle regulation has led to the development of viruses that replicate selectively in tumor cells with defined genetic lesions. Such "oncolytic" viruses include adenoviruses designed to replicate in tumor cells that lack functional p53 or have defects in the pRB pathway, in which replication of the mutant virus is dependent on deregulated E2F transcription factor activity. The former group includes an adenovirus mutant lacking the viral p55 protein (which binds and inhibits p53 in normal cells). This virus has demonstrated efficacy in phase II clinical trials of head and neck tumors, especially when combined with 5-fluorouracil and cisplatin (50% partial or complete response). The complexities of virus-host interactions (i.e., the immune response against replicating virus) will require further refinements of this novel technology before the clinical utility of this approach can be fully realized.

TELOMERASE DNA polymerase is unable to replicate the end of chromosomes, resulting in the loss of DNA at the specialized ends of chromosomes (called *telomeres*) with each replication cycle. At birth, human telomeres are 15- to 20-kilobase pairs long and are composed of tandem repeats of a six-nucleotide sequence (TTAGGG) that associate with specialized telomere-binding proteins to form a T-loop structure that protects the ends of chromosomes from being recognized as broken or damaged DNA. The loss of telomeric repeats with each cell division cycle causes gradual telomere shortening, leading to growth arrest (called *replicative senescence*) when one or more critically short telomeres triggers a p53-regulated DNA-damage checkpoint response. Cells can bypass this growth arrest if pRB and p53 are nonfunctional, but cell death ensues when the unprotected ends of chromosomes precipitate chromosome fusions or other catastrophic DNA rearrangements (termed *crisis*). The ability to bypass telomere-based growth limitations is thought to be a critical step in the evolution of most malignancies. This occurs by the reactivation of telomerase expression in cancer cells. Telomerase is an enzyme that adds TTAGGG repeats onto the 3' ends of chromosomes. It contains a catalytic subunit with reverse transcriptase activity (hTERT) and an RNA component that provides the template for telomere extension. Most normal somatic cells do not express sufficient telomerase to prevent telomere attrition with each cell division. Exceptions include stem cells (including those found in hematopoietic tissues, gut and skin epithelium, and germ cells) that require extensive cell division to maintain tissue homeostasis. More than 90% of human cancers express high levels of telomerase that prevent telomere exhaustion and allow indefinite cell proliferation. In vitro experiments indicate that inhibition of telomerase enzymatic activity leads to tumor cell apoptosis. Major efforts are underway to develop methods to inhibit telomerase activity in cancer cells. The reverse transcriptase activity of telomerase is a prime target for small-molecule pharmaceuticals that will enter clinical trials. The protein component of telomerase (hTERT) can act as a tumor-associated antigen that could be recognized by antigen-specific cytotoxic T lymphocytes (CTL) that lyse human melanoma, prostate, lung, breast, and colon cancer cells in vitro. Phase I clinical studies of telomerase vaccines are underway.

SIGNAL TRANSDUCTION PATHWAYS AS THERAPEUTIC TARGETS IN CANCER CELLS

Since the discovery that the v-*src* oncogene has protein tyrosine kinase activity, the central role of tyrosine phosphorylation in the regulation of cell proliferation in response to growth factors has become apparent. Many tyrosine kinases act at the apex of signaling pathways and are transmembrane proteins (receptor tyrosine kinases, RTK) or are associated with structures at the plasma membrane (*Src-*, Janus-, and *Fak*-family kinases). Tyrosine kinases are normally activated by specific ligands, and their activity is short-lived and reversed by protein tyrosine phosphatases (PTP). Phosphotyrosine and adjacent amino acid residues serve as docking sites for signal transduction proteins including those with protein-kinase, lipid-kinase, nucleotide exchange, lipase, and other enzymatic activities (Fig. 69-1). The unregulated activity of specific tyrosine kinases characterizes a number of human cancers, and their important roles in cancer cell proliferation and survival has validated these enzymes as targets for drug development efforts. Tyrosine kinases become constitutively activated and lead to the development of neoplastic diseases in three ways: chromosomal translocation, overexpression, and point mutation (Table 69-1). More than 30 different tyrosine kinases have been implicated in human cancer.

TARGETING Bcr-Abl WITH IMATINIB: PROOF OF PRINCIPLE

The protein product of the Philadelphia chromosome occurs in all patients with chronic myeloid leukemia (CML) and in about 30% of patients with adult acute lymphoid leukemia (ALL) and encodes the fusion protein Bcr-Abl. Although the c-*Abl* protooncogene is a nuclear protein whose kinase activity is tightly regulated as a part of the DNA damage response pathway (and actually induces growth arrest), the Bcr-Abl fusion protein is largely cytoplasmic with a constitutively activated tyrosine kinase domain. The deregulated tyrosine kinase activity of Bcr-Abl is required for its transforming activity. The Abl tyrosine kinase inhibitor, imatinib mesylate (Gleevec), has validated the concept of a molecularly targeted approach to cancer treatment.

Imatinib is a low-molecular-weight competitive inhibitor of the ATP binding site of Bcr-Abl, c-Abl, platelet-derived growth factor receptor (PDGFR), and c-Kit; hence it is not absolutely specific for the *Bcr-Abl* oncogene product. Clinical studies have demonstrated remarkable activity of this agent in CML. In Phase II studies of 532 chronic phase CML patients in whom interferon treatment had failed, 95% obtained a hematologic complete response, with only 9% relapse after a median follow-up of 18 months. Imatinib was also active in CML blast crisis with a 52% response rate, although the responses were short lived (78% relapse within 1 year). Relapse during treatment with imatinib was associated with reactivation of the tyrosine kinase either by amplification of the *Bcr-Abl* locus leading to increased levels of Bcr-Abl protein or, more commonly, by point mutations within the Bcr-Abl kinase domain that decreased imatinib binding without loss of Bcr-Abl kinase activity. These data constitute genetic proof that the

FIGURE 69-1 Therapeutic targeting of signal transduction pathways in cancer cells. Three major signal transduction pathways are activated by receptor tyrosine kinases (RTK). 1. The protooncogene Ras is activated by the Grb2/mSOS guanine nucleotide exchange factor, which induces an association with Raf and activation of downstream kinases (MEK and ERK1/2). 2. Activated PI3K phosphorylates the membrane lipid PIP2 to generate PIP3, which acts as a membrane-docking site for a number of cellular proteins including the serine/threonine kinases PDK1 and Akt. PDK1 has numerous cellular targets including Akt and mTOR. Akt phosphorylates target proteins that promote resistance to apoptosis and cell cycle progression, while mTOR and its target p70S6K upregulate protein synthesis to potentiate cell growth. 3. Activation of PLC-γ leads the formation of diacylglycerol (DAG) and increased intracellular calcium, with activation of multiple isoforms of PKC and other enzymes regulated by the calcium/calmodulin system. Other important signaling pathways involve non-RTKs that are activated by cytokine or integrin receptors. Janus kinases (JAK) phosphorylate STAT (signal transducer and activator of transcription) transcription factors, which translocate to the nucleus and activate target genes. Integrin receptors mediate cellular interactions with the extracellular matrix (ECM), inducing activation of FAK (focal adhesion kinase) and c-Src, which activate multiple downstream pathways, including modulation of the cell cytoskeleton. Many activated kinases and transcription factors migrate into the nucleus where they regulate gene transcription, thus completing the path from extracellular signals, such as growth factors, to a change in cell phenotype, such as induction of differentiation or cell proliferation. The nuclear targets of these processes include transcription factors (e.g., Myc, AP-1, and serum response factor) and the cell cycle machinery (CDKs and cyclins). Inhibitors of many of these pathways have been developed for the treatment of human cancers. Examples of inhibitors that are currently being evaluated in clinical trials are shown in blue.

target of imatinib is the Bcr-Abl tyrosine kinase, and that Bcr-Abl kinase activity is still required by imatinib-resistant cells. Computer modeling of the x-ray crystal structure of Bcr-Abl and its mutant forms is being used to guide the synthesis of the next generation of kinase inhibitors that may be able to overcome this acquired drug resistance.

Imatinib has also demonstrated targeted activity against gastrointestinal stromal tumors (GIST), rare mesenchymal tumors of the gastrointestinal tract (stomach and small intestine). The pathogenic molecular event in this disease is mutation of the proto-oncogene c-*Kit*, leading to the constitutive activation of this receptor tyrosine kinase. This prevents the normal differentiation of gut stem cells into interstitial cells of Cajal and induces proliferation and survival of tumor cells. Imatinib, which inhibits the c-Kit kinase domain, has demonstrated significant activity (>50% partial responses, many of long duration) in this chemotherapy-refractory tumor. Patients with chronic myelomonocytic leukemia (CMML, a myeloproliferative disorder) often harbor a Tel-PDGFR translocation that results in constitutive activation of the PDGFR kinase domain exclusively in the leukemic cells. Imatinib inhibits this kinase and has demonstrated significant activity in this disease. It may have activity in glioblastomas, which often express a PDGFR/PDGF autocrine growth loop.

TABLE 69-1 *Tyrosine Kinases Are Activated by Multiple Genetic Events in Human Cancers*[a]

Mechanisms	Tyrosine Kinases	Cancers
1. Translocations generate fusion proteins with BCR, TEL, or NPM. Oligomerization leads to activation of the kinase by cross-phosphorylation.	ABL, ALK, FGFR, JAK2, PDGFR, TRKC	Acute and chronic leukemias, fibrosarcoma
2. Overexpression causing receptor dimerization in absence of ligand.	EGFR family, IGFR PDGFR, FGFR family, c-MET	Breast, ovarian, lung, gastric, prostate, glioblastoma, others
3. Gain-of-function point mutation leading to receptor dimerization and kinase activation	c-KIT c-RET	Gastrointestinal stromal tumors Medullary thyroid CA
4. Autocrine growth pathway	MET/HGF PDGF/PDGFR	Rhabdomyosarcomas Glioblastoma
5. Overexpression of ligands such as VEGF or angiopoietins by stroma or tumor cells	VEGFR TIE2	Many tumors

[a] Deregulation of protein tyrosine kinases is a common genetic event leading to the development of human neoplasia. Tumor cells are highly mutagenic and have defects in DNA-damage checkpoints. This permits the outgrowth of tumor clones with multiple genetic anomalies, some of which promote tumor progression by increasing proliferation, enhancing resistance to apoptosis, and promoting angiogenesis.
Abbreviations: BCR, breakpoint cluster region; TEL, Ets-family transcription factor; NPM, nucleophosmin; ABL, Abelson tyrosine kinase; ALK, anaplastic lymphoma kinase; FGFR, fibroblast growth factor receptor; JAK2, Janus kinase 2; PDGFR, platelet-derived growth factor receptor; TRKC, neurotropin tyrosine receptor kinase C; EGFR, epidermal growth factor receptor; IGFR, insulin-like growth factor receptor; c-MET, receptor for hepatocyte growth factor (HGF); c-KIT, receptor for stem cell factor; c-RET, receptor for glial-derived neurotrophic factors; VEGFR, vascular endothelial growth factor receptor; TIE2, angiopoietin receptor.

These examples extend the proof of principle that selective targeting of signaling pathways in cancer cells can be highly efficacious with minimal toxicity. Imatinib has become the paradigm of targeted drug development in other diseases. For instance, 30% of acute myeloid leukemias (AML) encode mutations in the Fms-like tyrosine kinase FLT-3. Internal tandem duplications of the juxtamembrane domain of this RTK, or point mutations in the activation loop of the kinase domain, lead to constitutive activation of the kinase and confer a poor prognosis. Four chemically distinct inhibitors of FLT-3 are currently in clinical trials. These differ in potency of inhibition of the FLT-3 kinase and in the spectrum of cross-reactivity against other tyrosine kinases. Differences in toxicity are expected, as is the development of drug resistance. However, if multiple clinically active inhibitors can be developed, drug resistance may be avoided by combination therapy.

RECEPTOR TYROSINE KINASES RTKs are transmembrane glycoproteins that undergo dimerization upon ligand binding, with activation of their cytoplasmic tyrosine kinase domains by proximity-induced transphosphorylation of the activation loop. Tyrosine residues of the receptor or adaptor proteins (such as IRS-1 or Shc) are phosphorylated and act as docking sites for proteins containing SH2 (Src-homology 2) or PTB (phosphotyrosine binding) domains, thus initiating multiple signal transduction pathways (Fig. 69-1). These pathways regulate the proliferation, survival, migration, and angiogenesis of many solid tumors and are therefore viewed as attractive potential targets for cancer therapy. HER2/*neu* is a target in human breast cancer.

The gene encoding HER2/*neu* [a member of the epidermal growth factor receptor (EGFR) family] is amplified in ~30% of breast cancers. Tumors that overexpress HER2/*neu* are less responsive to chemotherapy, and patients with these tumors have a reduced survival compared with patients with normal levels of HER2/*neu*. Trastuzumab (Hercep-

tin) is a humanized monoclonal antibody that binds HER2/*neu* on the surface of tumor cells and induces internalization of the receptor, thereby reducing the level of surface expression. This leads to inhibition of cell cycle progression and renders cancer cells more susceptible to the induction of apoptosis. In clinical trials, trastuzumab as a single agent induced 15% responses in previously treated metastatic breast cancer patients. In phase III studies, a statistically significant increased survival occurred when trastuzumab was combined with chemotherapy in breast cancers in which HER-2/*neu* was overexpressed.

The EGFR (ERBB1) is another member of the RTK family that includes ERBB2 (HER2/*neu*), ERBB3, and ERB4. The EGFR is broadly expressed in normal cells and is overexpressed in many human cancers including head and neck, lung, esophageal, gastric, pancreatic, colon, renal cell, breast, ovarian, cervical, and prostate cancers, and gliomas. Overexpression correlates with poor clinical outcome. Targeted approaches include the use of antibodies directed against the EGFR extracellular domain and small-molecule inhibitors of the kinase domain. Single-agent clinical trials of anti-EGFR monoclonal antibodies or tyrosine kinase inhibitors in patients with previously treated lung and colon cancer demonstrated some antitumor activity, and studies combining these agents with chemotherapy are in progress. Overall, however, the therapeutic efficacy of EGFR-targeted agents has been disappointing. Of interest is that some breast cancers overexpress both the EGFR and HER2/*neu*, and clinical trials to simultaneously target both RTKs are under consideration.

The PDGFR and its ligand platelet-derived growth factor (PDGF), are overexpressed in many glioblastomas and in subsets of melanoma, ovarian, pancreatic, gastric, lung, and prostate cancers. Overexpression of the hepatocyte growth factor receptor MET has been observed in many human cancers and correlates with a poor prognosis, perhaps due to its role in invasion and metastasis. Small-molecular inhibitors of these RTKs are being developed for clinical use. As described below, the vascular endothelial growth factor receptor (VEGFR), TIE, and EPH RTK families have been identified as important therapeutic targets for inhibition of angiogenesis.

Signaling Pathways Downstream of RTKs: Ras and PI3K Several oncogene and tumor-suppressor gene products are components of signal transduction pathways that emanate from RTK activation (Fig. 69-1). The most extensively studied are the Ras/mitogen-activated protein (MAP) kinase pathway and the phosphatidylinositol-3-kinase (PI3K) pathway, both of which regulate multiple processes in cancer cells, including cell cycle progression, resistance to apoptotic signals, and cell motility. The development of inhibitors of these pathways constitutes an important avenue of anticancer drug development.

Mutations of the *Ras* protooncogene occur in 20% of human cancers and result in loss of the response of oncogenic Ras to GTPase-activating proteins (GAPs). The constitutively activated, GTP-bound Ras activates downstream effectors including the Ras/MAP kinase and PI3K/Akt pathways. Cancers of the pancreas, colon, and lung and AML harbor frequent *Ras* mutations, with the K-*Ras* allele affected more commonly (85%) than N-*Ras* (15%); H-*Ras* mutations are uncommon in human cancers. In addition, *Ras* activity in tumor cells can be aberrantly increased by other mechanisms, including upregulation of RTK activity and mutation of GAP proteins (e.g., *NF1* mutations in type I neurofibromatosis). Ras proteins localize to the inner plasma membrane and require posttranslational modifications, including addition of a farnesyl lipid moiety to the cysteine residue of the carboxy-terminal CAAX-box motif. Inhibition of RAS farnesylation by rationally designed farnesyltransferase inhibitors (FTIs) demonstrated encouraging efficacy in preclinical models, most of which utilized oncogenic forms of H-Ras. Despite this, clinical trials of FTIs in patients whose tumors harbor *Ras* mutations have been disappointing. Lack of efficacy has been shown in pancreatic, colon, and bladder carcinomas, while some activity has been seen in AML and CML. Upon further study, it appears that in the presence of FTIs, lipid modification of the K- and N-Ras proteins occurs by addition of a distinct lipid (geranylgeranyl) by the action of geranylgeranyl transferase (GGT), which results in restoration of Ras function. Thus, while FTIs are likely to have antitumor activity in select human cancers, their mechanism of action appears to occur by inhibition of farnesylation of proteins other than Ras, perhaps RhoB.

Effector pathways downstream of Ras are also targets of anticancer drug efforts. Activation of the Raf serine/threonine kinase is induced by binding to Ras and leads to activation of the MAP kinase pathway (Fig. 69-1). Two-thirds of melanomas and 10% of colon cancers harbor activating mutations in the *BRAF* gene, leading to constitutive activation of the downstream MAP/ERK kinase (MEK) and extracellular signal-regulated kinases (ERK1/2). This results in the phosphorylation of ERK's cytoplasmic and nuclear targets and alters the pattern of normal cellular gene expression. Inhibitors of Raf kinases have entered phase I clinical trials; their activity against tumors expressing mutant *BRAF* will be of special interest. MEK inhibitors are also demonstrating activity in phase I clinical trials.

PI3K is a heterodimeric lipid kinase that catalyses the conversion of phosphatidylinositol bisphosphate (PIP$_2$) to phosphatidylinositol trisphosphate (PIP$_3$), which acts as a plasma membrane docking site for proteins that contain a pleckstrin homology (PH) domain. These include the serine/threonine kinases Akt and PDK1 that are key downstream effectors of PI3K action (Fig. 69-1). The PI3K pathway is activated in 30 to 40% of human cancers and is thought to play a critical role in tumor cell survival, as well as promoting proliferation and migration. Amplification of the gene encoding the catalytic subunit of PI3K (p110) is observed in ovarian cancer, and amplification of the *Akt2* gene occurs in breast, ovarian, and pancreatic cancers. The tumor suppressor PTEN (phosphatase with tensin homology), a lipid phosphatase that acts as an off signal for PI3K by dephosphorylating PIP$_3$, is mutated in many human cancers, leading to unchecked activity of the PI3K pathway. Akt promotes cell survival by inhibiting apoptosis-promoting proteins and through activation of the transcription factor nuclear factor of κB (NFκB); it also enhances cell cycle progression by inhibition of glycogen synthetase kinase 3 (GSK3), which prevents cyclin D1 degradation. Furthermore, the growth of cancer cells requires the activation of two downstream kinases, mammalian target of rapamycin (mTOR) and p70S6K, whose activities promote the translation of cellular mRNAs. Targeted interruption of the PI3K pathway is being attempted at multiple levels. Inhibitors of mTOR, including rapamycin and its more soluble ester derivative CCI-779, selectively kill human tumor cell lines with PTEN mutations and up-regulated PI3K pathway activity. Clinical trials of CCI-779 are under way. Because of the great sequence homology between kinase domains, it is unclear if isoform-specific drugs can be developed and whether these will enable tumor targeting without undue toxicity.

RTKs activate other signaling pathways. Activation of phospholipase C-γ(PLC) results in the hydrolysis of PIP$_2$ into diacylglycerol (DAG) and IP$_3$. DAG together with calcium ion (Ca^{2+}) activates protein kinase C (PKC), a family of serine/threonine-specific protein kinases with different activation requirements, subcellular locations, and substrates in different cell types. PKC is the target of tumor-promoting phorbol esters, and its activation can modulate cell proliferation, differentiation, and tumorigenesis. The PKC inhibitor bryostatin 1 has reached phase II clinical trials and thus far has demonstrated only minimal antitumor activity. However, an antisense oligonucleotide directed against PKC and a number of small molecule inhibitors that demonstrate greater selectivity for PKC isoforms are undergoing clinical evaluation.

FIGURE 69-2 Epigenetic regulation of gene expression in cancer cells. Tumor-suppressor genes are often epigenetically silenced in cancer cells. In the upper panel, a CpG island within the promoter and enhancer regions of the gene has been methylated, resulting in the recruitment of methyl-cytosine binding proteins and complexes with histone deacetylase (HDAC) activity. Chromatin is in a condensed, nonpermissive conformation that inhibits transcription. Clinical trials are under way utilizing the combination of demethylating agents such as 5-aza-2'-deoxycytidine plus HDAC inhibitors, which together confer an open, permissive chromatin structure (*lower panel*). Transcription factors bind to specific DNA sequences in promoter regions and, through protein-protein interactions, recruit coactivator complexes containing histone acetyl transferase (HAT) activity. This enhances transcription initiation by RNA polymerase II and associated general transcription factors. The expression of the tumor suppressor gene commences, with phenotypic changes that may include growth arrest, differentiation, or apoptosis.

ALTERATIONS IN GENE TRANSCRIPTION IN CANCER CELLS: ROLE OF EPIGENETIC CHANGES

Chromatin structure regulates the hierarchical order of sequential gene transcription that governs differentiation and tissue homeostasis. Disruption of chromatin remodeling leads to aberrant gene expression and can induce proliferation of undifferentiated cells, leading to cancer. *Epigenetics* is defined as changes that alter the pattern of gene expression that persist across at least one cell division, but are not caused by changes in the DNA code. Epigenetic changes include alterations of chromatin structure mediated by methylation of cytosine residues in CpG dinucleotides, modification of histones by acetylation or methylation, or changes in higher-order chromosome structure (Fig. 69-2). The transcriptional regulatory regions of active genes often contain a high frequency of CpG dinucleotides (referred to as *CpG islands*), which under normal circumstances remain unmethylated. Expression of these genes is regulated by transient association with repressor or activator proteins. However, hypermethylation of promoter regions is a common mechanism by which tumor-suppressor loci are epigenetically silenced in cancer cells. Thus one allele may be inactivated by mutation or deletion (as occurs in loss of heterozygosity), while expression of the other allele is epigenetically silenced. The mechanisms that target suppressor oncogenes for this form of gene silencing are unknown.

Acetylation of the amino terminus of the core histones H3 and H4 induces an open chromatin conformation that promotes transcription initiation. Histone acetylases are components of coactivator complexes recruited to promoter/enhancer regions by sequence-specific transcription factors during the activation of genes (Fig. 69-2). Histone deacetylases (HDACs; at least 17 encoded in the human genome) are recruited to genes by transcriptional repressors and prevent the initiation of gene transcription. Methylated cytosine residues in promoter regions become associated with methyl-cytosine–binding proteins that recruit protein complexes with HDAC activity. The balance between permissive and inhibitory chromatin structure is therefore largely determined by the activity of transcription factors in modulating the "histone code" and the methylation status of the genetic regulatory elements of genes.

The pattern of gene transcription is aberrant in all human cancers, and in many cases, epigenetic events are responsible. Unlike genetic events that alter DNA primary structure (e.g., deletions), epigenetic changes are potentially reversible and appear amenable to therapeutic intervention. In many human cancers, including pancreatic cancer and multiple myeloma, the p16^{Ink4a} promoter is inactivated by methylation, thus permitting the unchecked activity of CDK4/cyclin D and rendering pRB nonfunctional. In sporadic forms of renal, breast, and colon cancer, the von Hippel–Lindau (*VHL*), breast cancer 1 (*BRCA1*), and serine/threonine kinase 11 (*STK11*) genes, respectively, are epigenetically silenced. Other targeted genes include the p15^{Ink4b} CDK inhibitor, glutathione-S-transferase (which detoxifies reactive oxygen species), and the E-cadherin molecule (important for junction formation between epithelial cells). Epigenetic silencing can occur in premalignant lesions and can affect genes involved in DNA repair, thus predisposing to further genetic damage. Examples include MLH1 (mut L homologue) in hereditary nonpolyposis colon cancer (HNPCC), which is critical for repair of mismatched bases that occur during DNA synthesis, and 0^6-methylguanine-DNA methyltransferase, which removes alkylated guanine adducts from DNA and is often silenced in colon, lung, and lymphoid tumors.

Many human leukemias have chromosomal translocations that code for novel fusion proteins with enzymatic activities that alter chromatin structure. The PML-RARα fusion protein, generated by the t(15;17) observed in most cases of acute promyelocytic leukemia (APL), binds to promoters containing retinoic acid response elements and recruits HDAC to these promoters, effectively inhibiting gene expression. This arrests differentiation at the promyelocyte stage and promotes tumor cell proliferation and survival. Treatment with pharmacologic doses of all-*trans* retinoic acid (ATRA), the ligand for RARα, results in the release of HDAC activity and the recruitment of coactivators, which overcomes the differentiation block. This induced differentiation of APL cells has greatly improved treatment of these patients and has provided a treatment paradigm for the reversal of epigenetic changes in cancer. However, for other leukemia-associated fusion proteins, such as AML-ETO and the MLL fusion proteins seen in AML and ALL, no ligand is known. Therefore, efforts are ongoing to determine the structural basis for interactions between translocation fusion proteins and chromatin remodeling proteins, and to use this information to rationally design small molecules that will disrupt specific protein-protein associations. Drugs that block the enzymatic activity of HDAC are being developed. A number of different chemical classes of HDAC inhibitors have demonstrated antitumor activity in phase I studies. The next generation of such agents may have specific activity against a subset of HDAC proteins, permitting selective activation of genes in different types of cancers.

Major therapeutic efforts are also under way to reverse the hypermethylation of CpG islands that characterizes many solid tumors. Drugs that induce DNA demethylation, such as 5-aza-2'-deoxycytidine, can lead to reexpression of silenced genes in cancer cells with restoration of function. However, 5-aza-2'-deoxycytidine has limited aqueous solubility and is myelosuppressive. Other inhibitors of DNA methyltransferases are in development. In ongoing clinical trials, inhibitors of DNA methylation are being combined with HDAC inhibitors. The hope is that by reversing coexisting epigenetic changes, the deregulated patterns of gene transcription in cancer cells will be at least partially reversed.

Aberrant signal transduction pathways activate a number of transcription factors that promote tumor cell proliferation and survival. These include signal transducer and activator of transcription (STAT)-3 and STAT5, NFκB, β-catenin (a component of the APC tumor-suppressor pathway), the heterodimer of c-Jun and Fos known as AP1, and c-Myc. The ability to target these transcription factors therapeutically does not currently exist. However, structural and molecular approaches may make it possible to identify small molecules that would inhibit protein-protein interactions needed for transcription factor dimerization or interaction with coactivator proteins. A small-molecule inhibitor has been developed that blocks the association of Myc with its partner Max, thereby inhibiting Myc-induced transformation. Many transcription factors are activated by phosphorylation, which can be prevented by tyrosine- or serine/threonine kinase inhibitors. The transcription factor NFκB is a heterodimer composed of p65 and p50 subunits that associate with an inhibitor, IκB, in the cell cytoplasm. In response to growth factor or cytokine signaling, a multi-subunit kinase called IKK (IκB-kinase) phosphorylates IκB and directs its degradation by the ubiquitin/proteasome system. NFκB, free of its inhibitor, translocates to the nucleus and activates target genes, many of which promote the survival of tumor cells. Novel drugs called *proteasome inhibitors* block the proteolysis of IκB, thereby preventing NFκB activation. For unexplained reasons, this is selectively toxic to tumor cells. Further studies have indicated that the antitumor effects of proteasome inhibitors are more complicated and involve the inhibition of the degradation of multiple cellular proteins. Proteasome inhibitors [bortezomib (Velcade)] have shown very significant activity in patients with multiple myeloma, including partial and complete remissions. Inhibitors of IKK are also in development, with the hope of more selectively blocking the degradation of IκB, thus "locking" NFκB in an inhibitory complex and rendering the cancer cell more susceptible to apoptosis-inducing agents.

Estrogen receptors (ERs) and androgen receptors, members of the steroid hormone family of nuclear receptors, are targets of inhibition by drugs used to treat breast and prostate cancers, respectively. Tamoxifen, a partial agonist and antagonist of ER function, can mediate tumor regression in metastatic breast cancer and can prevent disease recurrence in the adjuvant setting, saving thousands of lives each year. Tamoxifen binds to the ER and modulates its transcriptional activity, inhibiting activity in the breast but promoting activity in bone and uterine epithelium. Selective estrogen receptor modulators (SERMs) have been developed with the hope of a more beneficial modulation of ER activity, i.e., antiestrogenic activity in the breast, uterus, and ovary, but estrogenic for bone, brain, and cardiovascular tissues. Aromatase inhibitors, which block the conversion of androgens to estrogens in breast and subcutaneous fat tissues, have significant antitumor activity in postmenopausal breast cancer patients. However, deleterious effects may occur in other tissues due to estrogen deprivation, such as loss of bone density. The development of agents that modulate the activity of transcription factors in defined ways will yield important new agents for the treatment of cancer and other diseases.

APOPTOSIS

The homeostasis of adult organisms requires a balance between the death of aged, terminally differentiated cells and their renewal by proliferation of committed stem cell progenitors. Genetic damage to growth-regulating genes of stem cells could lead to catastrophic results for the host as a whole. However, genetic events such as activation of Myc expression or loss of the Rb checkpoint, which would be predicted to lead to unregulated cell proliferation, instead lead to the death of that cell. Metazoans have evolved a genetic program that induces the programmed death of cells that lose normal growth regulation; this process is referred to as *apoptosis*. Much as a panoply of intra- and extracellular signals impinge upon the core cell cycle machinery to regulate cell division, so too these signals regulate a core enzymatic machinery that regulates cell death and survival.

Programmed cell death is induced by two main pathways (Fig. 69-3). The extrinsic pathway of apoptosis is activated by cross-linking members of the tumor necrosis factor (TNF) receptor superfamily, such as CD95 (Fas) by its ligand (CD95L), or the binding to death receptors DR4 and DR5 by their ligand TRAIL (TNF-related apoptosis-inducing ligand). This induces the association of FADD (Fas-associated death domain) and procaspase-8 to death domain motifs of the receptors. Caspase-8 is activated by proximity-induced proteolysis and then cleaves and activates effector caspases-3 and -7, which then target cellular constituents (including DNA, cytoskeletal proteins, and a variety of regulatory proteins), inducing the morphologic appearance characteristic of apoptosis. The intrinsic pathway of apoptosis is initiated by the release of cytochrome c and SMAC (second mitochondrial activator of caspases) from the mitochondrial intermembrane space in response to a variety of noxious stimuli, including DNA damage, loss of adherence to the extracellular matrix (ECM), oncogene-induced proliferation, and growth factor deprivation. Upon release into the cytoplasm, cytochrome c associates with dATP, procaspase-9, and the adaptor protein APAF-1, leading to the sequential activation of caspase-9 and effector caspases. SMAC binds to and blocks the function of inhibitor of apoptosis proteins (IAPs), negative regulators of caspase activation. The release of apoptosis-inducing proteins from the mitochondria is regulated by pro- and antiapoptotic members of the Bcl-2 family. Antiapoptotic members (e.g., Bcl-2, Bcl-XL, and Mcl-1) associate with the mitochondrial outer membrane via their carboxy termini, exposing to the cytoplasm a hydrophobic binding pocket composed of Bcl-2 homology (BH) domains 1, 2, and 3 that is crucial for their activity. Perturbations of normal physiologic processes in specific cellular compartments lead to the activation of BH3-only proapoptotic family members (such as Bad, Bik, Bid, Puma, and others) that can induce pore formation in the mitochondrial outer membrane by altering the conformation of the outer-membrane proteins Bax and Bak. If BH3-only proteins are sequestered by Bcl-2, Bcl-XL, or Mcl-1, pores do not form and apoptosis-inducing proteins are not released from the mitochondrion. The relative levels of expression of antiapoptotic Bcl-2 family members compared to the levels of proapoptotic BH3-only proteins at the mitochondrial membrane determines the activation state of the intrinsic pathway. The mitochondrion must therefore be recognized not only as an organelle with vital roles in intermediary metabolism and oxidative phosphorylation but also as a central regulatory structure of the apoptotic process.

The evolution of tumor cells to a more malignant phenotype requires the acquisition of a broad range of genetic changes that subvert apoptosis pathways and permit the cancer cells to survive. Resistance to apoptosis predisposes not only to the development of cancer but also to resistance to anticancer therapies, including radiation and chemotherapy. However, because of their deranged physiology, cancer cells may be more vulnerable than normal cells to therapeutic interventions that target apoptosis pathways. For instance, overexpression of Bcl-2 occurs in non-Hodgkin lymphoma; prostate, breast, and lung cancers; and melanoma. Genasense is phosphorothioate antisense oligonucleotide directed at the first six codons of the Bcl-2 open reading frame, which mediates the destruction of Bcl-2 mRNA and subsequent downmodulation of Bcl-2 protein levels. Genasense has demonstrated activity in phase I and phase II clinical trials. Targeting of antiapoptotic Bcl-2 family members has also been accomplished by the identification of several low-molecular-weight compounds that bind to the hydrophobic pockets of either Bcl-2 or Bcl-XL and block their ability to associate with death-inducing BH3-only proteins. These first-generation compounds inhibit the antiapoptotic activities of Bcl-2 and Bcl-XL at micromolar concentrations, and higher-affinity derivatives with better pharmacokinetic properties should soon enter clinical testing. Of note is that the chemotherapeutic drug, paclitaxel, binds to and stabilizes microtubules. This induces the

FIGURE 69-3 Therapeutic strategies to overcome aberrant survival pathways in cancer cells. 1. The extrinsic pathway of apoptosis can be selectively induced in cancer cells by TRAIL (the ligand for death receptors 4 and 5) or by agonistic monoclonal antibodies. 2. Inhibition of antiapoptotic Bcl-2 family members with antisense oligonucleotides or inhibitors of the BH3-binding pocket will promote formation of Bak- or Bax-induced pores in the mitochondrial outer membrane. 3. Epigenetic silencing of APAF-1, caspase-8, and other proteins can be overcome using demethylating agents and inhibitors of histone deacetylases. 4. Inhibitor of apoptosis proteins (IAP) block activation of caspases; small-molecule inhibitors of IAP function (mimicking SMAC action) should lower the threshold for apoptosis. 5. Signal transduction pathways originating with activation of receptor tyrosine kinase receptors (RTKs) or cytokine receptors promote survival of cancer cells by a number of mechanisms. Inhibiting receptor function with monoclonal antibodies, such as trastuzumab, or inhibition of receptor-associated tyrosine kinase activity can inhibit the pathway. 6. The Akt kinase phosphorylates many regulators of apoptosis to promote cell survival; inhibitors of Akt may render tumor cells more sensitive to apoptosis-inducing signals; however, the possibility of toxicity to normal cells may limit the therapeutic value of these agents. 7 and 8. Activation of the transcription factor NFκB (composed of p65 and p50 subunits) occurs when its inhibitor, IκB, is phosphorylated by IκB-kinase (IKK), with subsequent degradation of IκB by the proteasome. Inhibition of IKK activity should selectively block the activation of NFκB target genes, many of which promote cell survival. Inhibitors of proteasome function have entered clinical trials and may work in part by preventing destruction of IκB, thus blocking NFκB nuclear localization. NFκB is unlikely to be the only target for proteasome inhibitors.

phosphorylation and inactivation of Bcl-2, thus enhancing its activity against resistant tumor cells.

The IAP family member, survivin, is highly expressed in many human cancers but is undetectable in most adult tissues, suggesting that tumor-specific modalities can be found to inhibit its antiapoptotic functions. Small-molecule inhibitors are in development that will block the caspase-inhibitory functions of survivin and other IAP family members. Preclinical studies targeting death receptors DR4 and DR5 have demonstrated that recombinant, soluble, human TRAIL or humanized monoclonal antibodies with agonist activity against DR4 or DR5 can induce apoptosis of tumor cells while sparing normal cells. The mechanisms for this selectivity may include expression of decoy receptors or elevated levels of intracellular inhibitors (such as FLIP, which competes with caspase-8 for FADD) by normal cells but not tumor cells. Synergy has been shown between TRAIL-induced apoptosis and chemotherapeutic agents. For instance, some colon cancers encode mutated Bax protein as the result of mismatch repair (MMR) defects and are resistant to TRAIL. However, upregulation of Bak by chemotherapy restores the ability of TRAIL to activate the mitochondrial pathway of apoptosis (by death receptor–mediated cleavage of the BH3-only protein Bid, which activates Bak). Other protein-based therapeutics, including the use of monoclonal antibodies trastuzumab (see previous sections) and rituximab (directed against CD20 on B cell malignancies), may owe efficacy in part to the inhibition of survival pathways leading to apoptosis.

Many of the signal transduction pathways perturbed in cancer promote tumor cell survival. These include activation of the PI3K/Akt pathway, increased levels of the NFκB transcription factor in many cancers, and epigenetic silencing of genes such as APAF-1 and caspase-8. Each of these pathways is a target for therapeutic agents that, in addition to affecting cancer cell proliferation or gene expression, can be expected to render cancer cells more susceptible to apoptosis, thus promoting synergy when combined with other chemotherapeutic agents.

Some tumor cells resist drug-induced apoptosis by expression of one or more members of the ABC family of ATP-dependent efflux pumps that mediate the multidrug resistance (MDR) phenotype. The prototype, P-glycoprotein (PGP), spans the plasma membrane 12 times and has two ATP-binding sites. Hydrophobic drugs (e.g., anthracyclines and vinca alkaloids) are recognized by PGP as they enter the cell and are pumped out. Numerous clinical studies have failed to demonstrate that drug resistance can be overcome using inhibitors of PGP. However, ABC transporters have different substrate specificities, and inhibition of a single family member may not be sufficient to overcome the MDR phenotype. A new generation of inhibitors is under development with higher affinities for transporters and better pharmacokinetic profiles.

OTHER THERAPEUTIC TARGETS

The geldanamycin derivative 17-AAG (17-allylaminogeldanamycin) has entered clinical trials as a selective inhibitor of heat-shock protein (Hsp)90. Hsp90 functions as a chaperone by binding to and promoting the proper folding of many cellular proteins including steroid hormone receptors, HER2/*neu*, Raf, Cdk4 and -6, Bcr-Abl, and mutant forms of p53. Inhibition of Hsp90 function results in the unfolding and subsequent degradation of its target proteins, leading to an inhibition of cell proliferation. Hsp90 inhibitors have activity against CML cells that are resistant to imatinib, perhaps by destabilizing mutant Bcr-Abl proteins. The growth of a wide range of human cancer cells was inhibited by 17AAG, often with rapid decrease in the levels of Raf and loss of MAP kinase signaling activity. Promising synergy was noted with a number of chemotherapeutic agents, including paclitaxel and doxorubicin. Inhibition of Hsp90 also blocks signaling via the androgen and estrogen receptors, thus making it an attractive therapeutic target in prostate and breast cancers. The fact that tumor cells express high levels of Hsp90 supports an important role in tumor cell survival. Phase I clinical trials of 17AAG did not demonstrate dramatic single-agent activity, but studies of 17AAG in combination with other chemotherapeutic agents are planned.

Cyclooxygenase 2 (COX-2) catalyzes the rate-limiting step in prostaglandin biosynthesis. Prostaglandins bind to G protein–coupled receptors and have pleiotropic biologic effects, promoting proliferation, enhanced survival, migration, and angiogenesis. Prostaglandins are pro-inflammatory and some can directly damage DNA. Tumor cell expression of COX-2 and the synthesis of prostaglandins such as PGE$_2$ are upregulated by cytokines and growth factors and by tumor-associated inflammatory cells. Chronic inflammation is etiologic in some cases of stomach cancers (*Helicobacter pylori*), colon cancer (ulcerative colitis), hepatic cancer (chronic hepatitis), and bladder cancer (schistosomiasis). COX-2 levels are upregulated in many premalignant lesions including oral leukoplakia, actinic keratosis, and carcinoma in situ of the bladder, breast, and prostate. Its overexpression in many cancers correlates with invasiveness and decreased survival. COX-2 upregulation in HER2/*neu*-expressing breast cancer is associated with induction of aromatase expression, leading to increased production of estrogen and enhanced tumor growth. In a number of animal models, COX-2 inhibitors prevented the development of tumors, including the

Min mouse model of adenomatous polyposis. Clinical data indicate that patients taking cyclooxygenase inhibitors have decreased risk of cancer, especially colon cancers. Studies are in progress to define the cyclooxygenase products and their downstream targets that promote tumorigenesis in efforts to further enhance chemoprevention of human cancers.

METASTASIS: DETERMINING RISK AND DEVELOPING THERAPEUTIC STRATEGIES

The three major features of tissue invasion are cell adhesion to the basement membrane, local proteolysis of the membrane, and movement of the cell through the rent in the membrane and the ECM. Malignant cells that gain access to the circulation must then repeat those steps at a remote site and generate blood vessels to support local growth. There are currently few drugs that directly target the process of metastasis. Metalloproteinase inhibitors (see "Tumor Angiogenesis," below) represent an initial attempt to inhibit the migration of tumor cells into blood and lymphatic vessels. The rate-limiting step for metastasis is the ability for tumor cells to survive and expand in the novel microenvironment of the metastatic site, and multiple host-tumor interactions determine the ultimate outcome.

Analysis of gene expression patterns of primary tumors by microarray technology may predict the likelihood of metastasis. It remains unclear if the metastatic phenotype is a characteristic of most cells constituting the primary tumor, or if clonal variants with this capacity evolve during tumor progression. About eight metastasis-suppressor genes have been identified that normally suppress the growth of micrometastases in their new environment. The loss of function of these genes enhances metastasis, although the molecular mechanisms remain to be determined. It may soon be possible to predict which primary tumors are at greatest risk to metastasize and to block tumor spread using specific inhibitors of the metastatic process.

Bone metastases are extremely painful, cause fractures of weight-bearing bones, can lead to hypercalcemia, and are a major cause of morbidity for cancer patients. Osteoclasts and their bone marrow–derived precursors express the surface receptor RANK (receptor activator of NFκB), which is required for terminal differentiation and activation of osteoclasts. Osteoblasts and other stromal cells express RANK ligand, as both a membrane-bound and soluble ligand. Osteoprotegerin (OPG), a soluble receptor for RANK ligand produced by stromal cells, acts as a decoy receptor to inhibit RANK activation. The relative balance of RANK ligand and OPG determines the activation state of RANK on osteoclasts. Many tumors increase osteoclast activity by secretion of substances such as parathyroid hormone (PTH), PTH-related peptide, interleukin (IL) 1, or Mip1, that perturb the homeostatic balance of bone remodeling by increasing RANK signaling. One example is multiple myeloma, where tumor cell–stromal cell interactions activate osteoclasts and inhibit osteoblasts, leading to the development of multiple lytic lesions. Inhibition of RANK ligand by intravenous administration of recombinant OPG or the extracellular domain of RANK linked to an immunoglobulin Fc-receptor (RANK-Fc) can prevent further bone destruction. Bisphosphonates are also effective inhibitors of osteoclast function. Better understanding of signaling pathways downstream of RANK and the mechanisms that regulate the formation of blastic bone lesions should lead to novel therapies to prevent bone destruction, induce bone healing, and may even alter the bone microenvironment in ways that induce the death of metastatic tumor cells.

TUMOR ANGIOGENESIS

The growth of primary and metastatic tumors to larger than a few millimeters requires the recruitment of neighboring blood vessels and vascular endothelial cells to support their metabolic requirements. This is because the diffusion limit for oxygen in tissues is ~ 100 μM. This is true of solid tumors and hematologic malignancies such as lymphomas, acute leukemia, and multiple myeloma, where increased numbers of blood vessels are observed in the pathologic bone marrow. A critical element in the growth of primary tumors and formation of metastatic sites is the *angiogenic switch*: the ability of the tumor to promote the formation of new capillaries from preexisting host vessels. The angiogenic switch is a phase in tumor development when the dynamic balance of pro- and antiangiogenic factors is tipped in favor of vessel formation by the effects of the tumor on its immediate environment. Stimuli for tumor angiogenesis include hypoxia, inflammation, and genetic lesions in oncogenes or tumor suppressors that alter tumor cell gene expression. Angiogenesis consists of several steps, including the stimulation of endothelial cells (ECs) by growth factors, the degradation of the ECM by proteases, proliferation of ECs and migration into the tumor, and the eventual formation of new capillary tubes.

Tumor blood vessels are not normal; they have chaotic architecture and blood flow. Due to an imbalance of angiogenic regulators such as vascular endothelial growth factor (VEGF) and angiopoietins (see below), tumor vessels are tortuous and dilated with an uneven diameter, excessive branching, and shunting. Tumor blood flow is variable, with areas of hypoxia and acidosis leading to the selection of variants that are resistant to hypoxia-induced apoptosis (often due to the loss of p53 expression). Tumor vessel walls have numerous openings, widened interendothelial junctions, and discontinuous or absent basement membrane; this contributes to the high vascular permeability of these vessels and, together with lack of functional intratumoral lymphatics, causes interstitial hypertension within the tumor (which also interferes with the delivery of therapeutics to the tumor). Tumor blood vessels lack perivascular cells such as pericytes and smooth muscle cells that normally regulate vasoactive control in response to tissue metabolic needs.

Unlike normal blood vessels, the vascular lining of tumor vessels is not a homogenous layer of ECs but often consists of a mosaic of ECs and tumor cells; the concept of cancer cell–derived vascular channels, which may be lined by ECM secreted by the tumor cells, is referred to as *vascular mimickry*. It is unclear whether tumor cells actually form structural elements of vascular channels or represent tumor cells in transit into or out of the vessel. However, the former is supported by evidence that in some human colon cancers, tumor cells can comprise up to 15% of vessel walls. The ECs of angiogenic blood vessels are unlike quiescent ECs found in adult vessels, where only 0.01% of ECs are dividing. During tumor angiogenesis, ECs are highly proliferative and express a number of plasma membrane proteins that are characteristic of activated endothelium, including growth factor receptors and adhesion molecules such as integrins.

MECHANISMS OF TUMOR VESSEL FORMATION Tumors utilize a number of mechanisms to promote their vascularization, and in each case they subvert normal angiogenic processes to suit this purpose (Fig. 69-4). Primary or metastatic tumor cells sometimes arise in proximity to host blood vessels and grow around these vessels, parasitizing nutrients by coopting the local blood supply. However, most tumor blood vessels arise by the process of *sprouting*, in which tumors secrete trophic angiogenic molecules, the most potent being VEGF, that induce the proliferation and migration of host ECs into the tumor. Sprouting in normal and pathogenic angiogenesis is regulated by three families of transmembrane RTKs expressed on ECs and their ligands (VEGFs, angiopoietins, ephrins), which are produced by tumor cells, inflammatory cells, or stromal cells in the tumor microenvironment.

When tumor cells arise in or metastasize to an avascular area, they grow to a size limited by hypoxia and nutrient deprivation. Hypoxia, a key regulator of tumor angiogenesis, causes the transcriptional induction of the gene encoding VEGF by a process that involves stabilization of the transcription factor hypoxia-inducible factor (HIF)1. Under normoxic conditions, EC HIF-1 levels are maintained at a low level by proteasome-mediated destruction regulated by a ubiquitin E3-ligase encoded by the VHL tumor-suppressor locus. However, under hypoxic conditions, the HIF-1 protein is not hydroxylated and association with VHL does not occur; therefore HIF-1 levels increase, and target genes including VEGF, nitric oxide synthetase (NOS), and Ang2 are induced. Loss of the *VHL* genes, as occurs in familial and sporadic renal cell carcinomas, also results in HIF-1 stabilization and induction

FIGURE 69-4 Tumor angiogenesis is a complex process involving many different cell types that must proliferate, migrate, invade, and differentiate in response to signals from the tumor microenvironment. Endothelial cells (ECs) sprout from host vessels in response to VEGF, bFGF, Ang2, and other proangiogenic stimuli. Sprouting is stimulated by VEGF/VEGFR2, Ang2/Tie-2, and integrin/extracellular matrix (ECM) interactions. Bone marrow–derived circulating endothelial precursors (CEPs) migrate to the tumor in response to VEGF and differentiate into ECs, while hematopoietic stem cells differentiate into leukocytes, including tumor-associated macrophages that secrete angiogenic growth factors and produce MMPs that remodel the ECM and release bound growth factors. Tumor cells themselves may directly form parts of vascular channels within tumors. The pattern of vessel formation is haphazard: vessels are tortuous, dilated, leaky, and branch in random ways. This leads to uneven blood flow within the tumor, with areas of acidosis and hypoxia (which stimulate release of angiogenic factors) and high intratumoral pressures that inhibit delivery of therapeutic agents.

of VEGF. Most tumors have hypoxic regions due to poor blood flow, and tumor cells in these areas stain positive for HIF-1 expression; in renal cancers with *VHL* deletion, all of the tumor cells express high levels of HIF-1, and VEGF-induced angiogenesis leads to high microvascular density (hence the term *hypernephroma*).

VEGF and its receptors are required for *vasculogenesis* (the de novo formation of blood vessels from differentiating endothelial cells, as occurs during embryonic development) and angiogenesis under normal (wound healing, corpus luteum formation) and pathologic processes (tumor angiogenesis, inflammatory conditions such as rheumatoid arthritis). VEGF-A is a heparin-binding glycoprotein with at least four isoforms (splice variants) that regulates blood vessel formation by binding to the RTKs VEGFR1 and VEGFR2, which are expressed on all ECs in addition to a subset of hematopoietic cells (Fig. 69-5). VEGFR2 regulates EC proliferation, migration, and survival, while VEGFR1 may act as an antagonist of R1 in ECs but is probably also important for angioblast differentiation during embryogenesis. Tumor vessels appear to be more dependent on VEGFR signaling for growth and survival than normal ECs. While VEGF signaling is a critical initiator of angiogenesis, this is a complex process regulated by additional signaling pathways. The angiopoietin, Ang1,

Endothelial cell "specific" ligand/receptor complexes

Generalized growth factor receptors

PlGF VEGF-A VEGF-B VEGF-C Ang-1 Ang-2 Ephrins Extracellular matrix bFGF PDGF

Kinase domain

VEGFR1 (Endothelial cells) | VEGFR2 | VEGFR3 (Lymphatics) | Tie-2 (Blood vessel stabilization and remodeling) | EPHB4 (Artery-vein differentiation, vessel remodeling) | αvβ3 Matrix (attachment) | FGF receptor (Recruitment of smooth muscle cells and pericytes) | PDGF receptor

Downstream pathways
Ras/MAPK
PI3K/AKT
Rho/Rac/cdc42
NFκB

Endothelial cell proliferation, migration, survival

FIGURE 69-5 *Critical molecular determinants of endothelial cell biology. Angiogenic endothelium expresses a number of receptors not found on resting endothelium. These include receptor tyrosine kinases (RTK) and integrins that bind to the extracellular matrix and mediate endothelial cells adhesion, migration, and invasion. Endothelial cells (ECs) also express RTK (i.e., the FGF and PDGF receptors) that are found on many other cell types. Critical functions mediated by activated RTK include proliferation, migration, and enhanced survival of endothelial cells, as well as regulation of the recruitment of perivascular cells and bloodborne circulating endothelial precursors and hematopoietic stem cells to the tumor. Intracellular signaling via EC-specific RTK utilizes molecular pathways that may be targets for future antiangiogenic therapies.*

produced by stromal cells, binds to the EC RTK Tie-2 and promotes the interaction of ECs with the ECM and perivascular cells, such as pericytes and smooth muscle cells, to form tight, non-leaky vessels. PDGF and basic fibroblast growth factor (bFGF) help to recruit these perivascular cells. Ang1 is required for maintaining the quiescence and stability of mature blood vessels and prevents the vascular permeability normally induced by VEGF and inflammatory cytokines.

For tumor cell–derived VEGF to initiate sprouting from host vessels, the stability conferred by the Ang1/Tie2 pathway must be perturbed; this occurs by the secretion of Ang2 by ECs that are undergoing active remodeling. Ang2 binds to Tie2 and is a competitive inhibitor of Ang1 action: under the influence of Ang2, preexisting blood vessels become more responsive to remodeling signals, with less adherence of ECs to stroma and associated perivascular cells and more responsiveness to VEGF. Therefore, Ang2 is required at early stages of tumor angiogenesis for destabilizing the vasculature by making host ECs more sensitive to angiogenic signals. Since tumor ECs are blocked by Ang2, there is no stabilization by the Ang1/Tie2 interaction, and tumor blood vessels are leaky, hemorrhagic, and have poor association of ECs with underlying stroma. Sprouting tumor ECs express high levels of the transmembrane protein Ephrin-B2 and its receptor, the RTK EPH whose signaling appears to work with the angiopoietins during vessel remodeling. During embryogenesis, EPH receptors are expressed on the endothelium of primordial venous vessels while the transmembrane ligand ephrin-B2 is expressed by cells of primordial arteries; the reciprocal expression may regulate differentiation and patterning of the vasculature.

A number of ubiquitously expressed host molecules play critical roles in normal and pathologic angiogenesis. Proangiogenic cytokines, chemokines, and growth factors secreted by stromal cells or inflammatory cells make important contributions to neovascularization, including bFGF, transforming growth factor-α (TGF-α), TNF-α, and IL-8. In contrast to normal endothelium, angiogenic endothelium overexpresses specific members of the integrin family of ECM-binding

proteins that mediate EC adhesion, migration, and survival. Specifically, expression of integrins $\alpha_v\beta_3$, $\alpha_v\beta_5$, and $\alpha_5\beta_1$ mediate spreading and migration of ECs and are required for angiogenesis induced by VEGF and bFGF, which in turn can upregulate EC integrin expression. The $\alpha_v\beta_3$ integrin physically associates with VEGFR2 in the plasma membrane and promotes signal transduction from each receptor to promote EC proliferation (via focal adhesion kinase, src, PI3K, and other pathways) and survival (by inhibition of p53 and increasing the Bcl2/Bax expression ratio). In addition, $\alpha_v\beta_3$ forms cell surface complexes with matrix metalloproteinases (MMPs), zinc-requiring proteases that cleave ECM proteins, leading to enhanced EC migration and the release of heparin-binding growth factors including VEGF and bFGF. EC adhesion molecules can be upregulated (i.e., by VEGF, TNF-α) or downregulated (by TGF-β); this, together with chaotic blood flow explains poor leukocyte-endothelial interactions in tumor blood vessels and may help tumor cells avoid immune surveillance.

In addition to sprouting, the architecture of the tumor vasculature is influenced by two other mechanisms. One process, called *intussuception*, occurs when tumor cells grow into a vessel, functionally dividing it into two branches. More recently, it was discovered that cells derived from hematopoietic progenitors in the host bone marrow contribute to tumor angiogenesis in a process linked to the secretion of VEGF, and PlGF (placenta-derived growth factor) by tumor cells and their surrounding stroma. VEGF promotes the mobilization and recruitment of circulating endothelial cell precursors (CEPs) and hematopoietic stem cells (HSCs) to tumors where they colocalize and appear to cooperate in neovessel formation. CEPs express VEGFR2, while HSCs express VEGFR1, a receptor, or VEGF and PlGF. Both CEPs and HSCs are derived from a common precursor, the hemangioblast. CEPs are thought to differentiate into ECs, whereas the role of HSC-derived cells (such as tumor-associated macrophages) may be to secrete angiogenic factors required for sprouting and stabilization of ECs (VEGF, bFGF, angiopoietins) and to activate MMPs, resulting in ECM remodeling and growth factor release. In mouse tumor models and in human cancers, increased numbers of CEPs and subsets of VEGFR1+ or VEGFR-expressing HSCs can be detected in the circulation, which may correlate with increased levels of serum VEGF. It is not yet known whether levels of these cells have prognostic value or if changes during treatment correlate with inhibition of tumor angiogenesis. Whether CEPs and VEGFR1-expressing HSCs are required to maintain the long-term integrity of established tumor vessels is also unknown.

Lymphatic vessels also exist within tumors. Development of tumor lymphatics is associated with expression of VEGFR3 and its ligands VEGF-C and VEGF-D. The role of these vessels in tumor cell metastasis to regional lymph nodes remains to be determined, since, as discussed above, interstitial pressures within tumors are high and most lymphatic vessels may exit in a collapsed and nonfunctional state. However, VEGF-C levels in primary human tumors, including lung, prostate, and colorectal cancers, correlate significantly with metastasis to regional lymph nodes.

ANTIANGIOGENIC THERAPY Understanding the molecular mechanisms that regulate tumor angiogenesis may provide unique opportunities for cancer treatment. Acquired drug resistance of tumor cells due to their high intrinsic mutation rate is a major cause of treatment failure in human cancers. ECs comprising the tumor vasculature are genetically stable and do not share genetic changes with tumor cells; the EC apoptosis pathways are therefore intact. Each EC of a tumor vessel helps provide nourishment to many tumor cells, and although tumor angiogenesis can be driven by a number of exogenous proangiogenic stimuli, experimental data indicate that blockade of a single growth factor (e.g., VEGF) may inhibit tumor-induced vascular growth. Because tumor blood vessels are distinct from normal ones, they may be selectively destroyed without affecting normal vessels. Angiogenesis inhibitors function by targeting the critical molecular pathways involved in EC proliferation, migration, and/or survival, many of which are unique to the activated endothelium in tumors. Inhibition of growth factor and adhesion-dependent signaling pathways can induce EC apoptosis with concomitant inhibition of tumor growth. Different types of tumors use distinct molecular mechanisms to activate the angiogenic switch. Therefore, it is doubtful that a single antiangiogenic strategy will suffice for all human cancers; rather, a number of therapeutics will need to be developed, each responding to distinct programs of angiogenesis that have been developed by specific human cancers.

A number of strategies have been developed to selectively target tumor vasculature (Table 69-2, Fig. 69-6), and many novel antiangiogenic agents are currently in clinical trials. Inhibition of VEGF function blunts angiogenesis and tumor growth in a variety of tumor models by selectively inducing the apoptosis of immature ECs that are not associated with pericytes or smooth muscle cells, but spares normal host vessels. Humanized anti-VEGF monoclonal antibodies are active in colon cancer. A number of small, cell-permeable chemicals that inhibit the tyrosine kinase activity of VEGFR2 or VEGFR1 are being tested. The latter drugs may synergize in their antiangiogenic effects, since VEGFR2 inhibitors should block EC proliferation, migration, and survival, while VEGFR1 inhibitors are predicted to inhibit VEGF and PlGF-mediated recruitment of CEPs, HSCs, and inflammatory cells to the tumor bed. The relative efficacy of these agents may vary since some tumors may be dependent on VEGFR2-induced sprouting while others are more dependent on the bone marrow–derived EC precursors. Angiogenesis induced by bFGF can be blocked by inhibitors of the VEGF pathway, demonstrating a linkage between these pathways. Inhibitors of the Ang/Tie2 and Ephrin/EPH pathways are in development.

Blocking antibodies or antagonistic peptides to $\alpha_v\beta_3$ integrin, which interrupt the $\alpha_v\beta_3$- mediated adhesion to matrix proteins, leads to the inhibition of tumor and growth factor–induced angiogenesis in vivo by selectively inducing apoptosis of ECs in newly formed vessels. This indicates that ligation of the $\alpha_v\beta_3$ receptor is required for the survival of ECs of the angiogenic phenotype. Integrins are also required for EC migration and are important regulators of MMP activity, which modulates movement through and the release of growth factors from the ECM. Humanized monoclonal antibodies directed against $\alpha_v\beta_3$ are currently in clinical trial, as are small-molecule inhibitors of $\alpha_v\beta_3$, such as circular peptides containing the arg-gly-asp (RGD) integrin binding site. A number of clinical trials are testing the ability of MMP inhibitors to block tumor metastasis as well as angiogenesis. The discovery that ECs from various normal tissues encode unique surface markers suggests that tumors arising in different tissues may also express unique "vascular addressins," which could be targeted.

A number of endogenous, physiologic inhibitors of angiogenesis have been discovered. *Angiostatin* is a 38-kDa kringle domain–containing polypeptide fragment of plasminogen generated in the tumor microenvironment by proteases derived from tumor and stromal cells (including MMPs secreted by tumor-associated macrophages). Angiostatin inhibits in vivo tumor angiogenesis and induces tumor dormancy in murine models, and its antiangiogenic effects are mediated in part by induction of EC apoptosis. *Endostatin* is a C-terminal cleavage product of collagen XVIII generated by cathepsin or elastase-like proteolytic activities. It inhibits EC migration and promotes apoptosis by binding to $\alpha_v\beta_3$ and -β_5 integrins and downregulating expression of survival factors such as Bcl-2 and Bcl-XL. Antiangiogenic peptide domains of other normal host proteins have also been defined. Purified angiostatin and endostatin are highly specific inhibitors of activated ECs in vitro and in murine models and have entered clinical trials. Although tumor responses have been disappointingly rare, pharmacokinetic data indicate bolus administration of recombinant endostatin

TABLE 69-2 *Antiangiogenic Treatments Currently in Clinical Trials: Molecular Pathways as Targets*

I. Receptor tyrosine kinase pathways	
A. Endothelial cell (EC) specific	
1. VEGFR1 kinase inhibitors	Decreased recruitment of CEPs, HSCs to tumor vessels
2. VEGFR2 kinase inhibitors	Inhibition of EC proliferation, migration, survival
3. Anti-VEGF monoclonal antibody	Inhibition of VEGF signaling to EC, CEPs, HSCs
B. Non-EC specific	
1. FGFR, PDGF kinase inhibitors	Inhibition of EC functions; decreased recruitment of perivascular cells
2. Anti-ERB-B2 monoclonal antibody	Inhibition of tumor VEGF production; increased thrombospondin-1
II. Integrin receptors/ extracellular matrix	
A. Integrin inhibitors	
1. RGD circular pentapeptides	Inhibition of integrin-mediated attachment to ECM with induction of EC apoptosis
2. Anti-$\alpha_v\beta_3$ monoclonal antibodies	Detachment of EC from matrix with induction of apoptosis
B. Matrix metalloproteinase inhibitors	Inhibition of EC and tumor invasion; decreased release of GF from matrix binding sites
III. Endogenous angiogenesis inhibitors	
A. Peptides derived from host proteins	
1. Angiostatin (plasminogen fragment)	Mechanisms of action unclear; may inhibit EC cell surface ATP synthase activity; binds to $\alpha_v\beta_3$ and other integrins
2. Endostatin (collagen XVIII fragment)	Mechanisms unclear; binds to EC integrins; may block GF binding to heparin sulfate; inhibits EC migration and induces apoptosis
B. Hormones	Inhibits EC microtubules
1. 2-methoxy-estradiol (2-ME)	
IV. Other agents	
A. Chemokines/cytokines	
1. IL-12	Induction of IFN-γ, IP-10, and MiG
2. IFN-α	Inhibition of bFGF production by tumor
B. Synthetic compounds	
1. TNP-490 (fumagillan analogue)	Inhibition of EC methionine aminopeptidase (required for EC proliferation)
2. Thalidomide	In vitro evidence for antiangiogenic activity; proven therapeutic activity in human multiple myeloma

Abbreviations: VEGFR, vascular endothelial growth factor receptor; CEP, circulating endothelial cell precursors; HSC, hematopoietic stem cells; FGFR, fibroblast growth factor receptor; PDGF, platelet-derived growth factor; RGD, arg-gly-asp; ECM, extracellular matrix; GF, growth factor; IL, interleukin; IFN, interferon; IP-10, interferon-inducible protein-10; MiG, monokine induced by IFN-γ; bFGF, basic fibroblast growth factor.

does not maintain sufficient serum concentrations of the inhibitor for antiangiogenic activity to occur.

A number of more general signaling pathways are also important for EC function and can be targeted. Trastuzumab, a monoclonal antibody that inhibits signaling from the ERB-B2 tyrosine kinase receptor expressed by some breast and ovarian cancers, decreases expression of VEGF and upregulates expression of thrombospondin-1 (an angiogenic inhibitor), by tumor cells. Inhibition of fibroblast growth

FIGURE 69-6 *Knowledge of the molecular events governing tumor angiogenesis has led to a number of therapeutic strategies to block tumor blood vessel formation. Multiple inhibitors of the VEGF/VEGFR pathway are in clinical trial, and other endothelial cell–specific receptor tyrosine kinase pathways (e.g., angiopoietin/Tie2 and ephrin/EPH) are likely targets for the future. Inhibition of integrin binding to the ECM, and ECM breakdown by matrix-metalloproteinase inhibitors (MMPs), should lead to EC apoptosis and inhibition of EC migration and invasion. Other targets include intracellular signaling pathways, inhibition of cytoskeletal elements (i.e., by 2-methoxy estradiol, 2-ME), and compounds whose mechanisms of antiangiogenic activity are unknown, such as thalidomide and the endogenous inhibitors (endostatin, angiostatin).*

factor (FGF) and PDGF receptor signaling by kinase inhibitors may block EC proliferation and recruitment of supporting stromal cells into the tumor milieu. Signal transduction pathways downstream of RTK and integrin signaling, such as the Ras/MAP kinase, PI3K/Akt, and Src family kinase pathways, are important antitumor therapeutic targets that are also important for angiogenesis. FTIs have been shown to block VEGF expression by tumor cells. EC survival requires the activity of the serine/threonine kinase Akt, and inhibitors of this kinase may have potent antiangiogenic activity. Src kinases integrate VEGF/integrin signaling associated with focal adhesion kinase (FAK) activation and dynamic remodeling of the cell cytoskeleton; Src inhibitors should block EC motility as well as survival. Arachidonic acid metabolism may be important for $\alpha_v\beta_3$-induced proliferation and migration of EC; COX-2 inhibitors may inhibit $\alpha_v\beta_3$-mediated EC activities. Giant cell tumors of bone and angioblastomas that occur in young children, and can be severely debilitating or life-threatening, appear to depend uniquely on bFGF as their main angiogenic factor. Low daily doses of interferon block tumor cell production of bFGF and after 1 to 2 years of treatment can mediate the complete eradication of these tumors.

The conceptual design of antiangiogenic clinical trials may require a paradigm shift from conventional chemotherapy. In tumor models, the combination of low daily doses of standard chemotherapy agents combined with antiangiogenic agents can synergize to induce apoptosis of the tumor vasculature, even when the tumor cells are resistant to high doses of the same agents. The initial response to successful antiangiogenic treatment is a decrease in vascular permeability and lower intratumoral pressure; this results in an initial increase in tumor blood flow that can transiently increase tumor growth (but could also provide increased delivery of chemotherapeutic drugs to the tumor). Clinicians will need to be prepared to weather this initial "tumor flare" without stopping antiangiogenic treatment. Inhibition of new vessel formation in human cancers may induce stable disease rather than tumor regression, and progression-free survival may be a more appropriate endpoint than a reduction of tumor volume. This implies a need for chronic, daily administration to prevent regrowth of blood vessels between doses, and will require orally administered drugs that can be tolerated for prolonged times. Surrogate markers will therefore be needed to evaluate the clinical effectiveness of antiangiogenic therapies. Circulating factors may not be useful, since tumors and their stroma produce a number of positive and negative regulators of angiogenesis. The circulating levels of CEPs might be a marker of response, but this remains speculative. The promise of the antiangiogenic approach to cancer treatment depends on tumor selectivity, which may not always be predictable. Phase I clinical trial testing of a VEGFR2 kinase inhibitor demonstrated no serious toxicity. Yet when it was combined with cisplatin and gemcitibine for the treatment of solid tumors, 8 of 19 patients experienced serious thrombotic events, including pulmonary embolism and stroke. Antiangiogenic agents may sensitize normal ECs to apoptosis induction by chemotherapeutic agents, with exposure of tissue factor in subendothelial vessel wall. This underscores the potential toxicity of targeting ECs in vivo.

FURTHER READING

BYKOV VJN et al: Restoration of the tumor suppressor function of mutant p53 by a low-molecular-weight compound. Nat Med 8:282, 2002

CRISTOFANILLI M et al: Angiogenesis modulation in cancer research: Novel clinical approaches. Nat Rev Drug Discovery 1:415, 2002

DANCEY J, SAUSVILLE EA: Issues and progress with protein kinase inhibitors for cancer treatment. Nat Rev Drug Discovery 2:296, 2003

DRUKER BJ: Inhibition of the Bcr-Abl tyrosine kinase as a therapeutic strategy for CML. Oncogene 21:8541, 2002

HANAHAN D, WEINBERG RA: The hallmarks of cancer. Cell 100:57, 2000

JOHNSTONE RW: Histone-deacetylase inhibitors: Novel drugs for the treatment of cancer. Nat Rev Drug Discovery 1:287, 2002

JONES PA, BAYLIN SB: The fundamental role of epigenetic events in cancer. Nat Rev Genetics 3:415, 2002

REED JC: Apoptosis-based therapies. Nat Rev Drug Discovery 1:111, 2002

RODEN DM, GEORGE AL: The genetic basis of variability in drug responses. Nat Rev Drug Discovery 1:37, 2002

SAUSVILLE EA: Complexities in the development of cyclin-dependent kinase inhibitor drugs. Trends Mol Med 8:S32, 2002

70 PRINCIPLES OF CANCER TREATMENT: SURGERY, CHEMOTHERAPY, AND BIOLOGIC THERAPY
Edward A. Sausville, Dan L. Longo

The goal of cancer treatment is first to eradicate the cancer. If this primary goal cannot be accomplished, the goal of cancer treatment shifts to palliation, the amelioration of symptoms, and preservation of quality of life while striving to extend life. The dictum *primum non nocere* is not necessarily the guiding principle of cancer therapy. When cure of cancer is possible, cancer treatments may be undertaken despite the certainty of severe and perhaps life-threatening toxicities. Every cancer treatment has the potential to cause harm, and treatment may be given that produces toxicity with no benefit. The therapeutic index of many interventions is quite narrow, and most treatments are given to the point of toxicity. Conversely, when the clinical goal is palliation, careful attention to minimizing the toxicity of potentially toxic treatments becomes a significant goal. Irrespective of the clinical scenario, the guiding principle of cancer treatment should be *primum succerrere*, "first hasten to help." Radical surgical procedures, large-field hyperfractionated radiation therapy, high-dose chemotherapy, and maximum tolerable doses of cytokines such as interleukin (IL) 2 are all used in certain settings where 100% of the patients will experience toxicity and side effects from the intervention, and only a fraction of the patients will experience benefit. One of the challenges of cancer treatment is to use the various treatment modalities alone and together in a fashion that maximizes the chances for patient benefit.

Cancer treatments are divided into four main types: surgery, radiation therapy (including photodynamic therapy), chemotherapy (including hormonal therapy and molecularly targeted therapy), and biologic therapy (including immunotherapy and gene therapy). The modalities are often used in combination, and agents in one category can act by several mechanisms. For example, cancer chemotherapy agents can induce differentiation, and antibodies (a form of immunotherapy) can be used to deliver radiation therapy. Surgery and radiation therapy are considered local treatments, though their effects can influence the behavior of tumor at remote sites. Chemotherapy and biologic therapy are usually systemic treatments. *Oncology*, the study of tumors including treatment approaches, is a multidisciplinary effort with surgical-, radiotherapy-, and internal medicine–related areas of expertise. Treatments for patients with hematologic malignancies are often shared by hematologists and medical oncologists. →*Principles of radiation therapy are discussed in Chap. 71.*

Cancer behaves in many ways as an organ that attempts to regulate its own growth. However, cancers have not set an appropriate limit on how much growth should be permitted. Normal organs and cancers share the property of having a population of cells in cycle and actively renewing and a population of cells not in cycle. In cancers, cells that are not dividing are heterogeneous; some have sustained too much genetic damage to replicate but have defects in their death pathways that permit their survival; some are starving for nutrients and oxygen; and some are reversibly out of cycle poised to be recruited back into cycle and expand if needed. Severely damaged and starving cells are unlikely to kill the patient. The problem is that the cells that are reversibly not in cycle are capable of replenishing tumor cells physically removed or damaged by radiation and chemotherapy.

Tumors follow a Gompertzian growth curve (Fig. 70-1); the growth

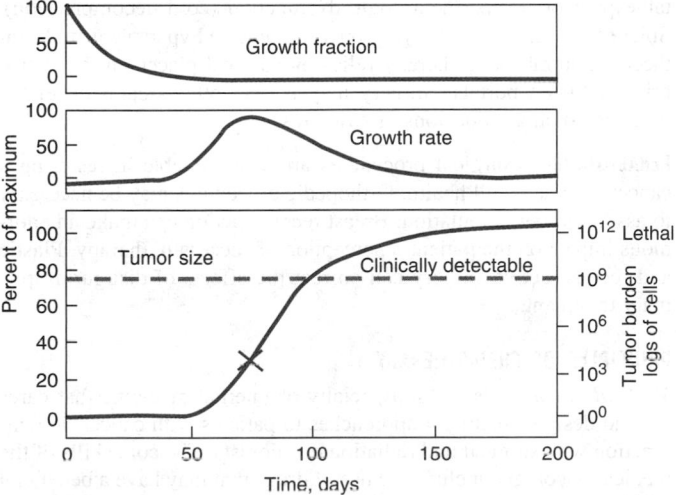

FIGURE 70-1 Gompertzian tumor growth. The growth fraction of a tumor declines exponentially over time (*top*). The growth rate of a tumor peaks before it is clinically detectable (*middle*). Tumor size increases slowly, goes through an exponential phase, and slows again as the tumor reaches the size at which limitation of nutrients or auto- or host regulatory influences can occur. The maximum growth rate occurs at 1/e, the point at which the tumor is about 37% of its maximum size (marked with an X). Tumor becomes detectable at a burden of about 10^9 (1 cm^3) and kills the patient at a tumor burden of about 10^{12} (1 kg). Efforts to treat the tumor and reduce its size can result in an increase in the growth fraction and an increase in growth rate.

fraction of a neoplasm starts at 100% with the first transformed cell and declines exponentially over time until by the time of diagnosis at a tumor burden of 1 to 5×10^9 tumor cells, the growth fraction is usually 1 to 4%. Thus, peak growth rate may actually occur before the tumor is detectable. A key aspect of a successful tumor is the ability to stimulate the development of a new supporting stroma through angiogenesis and production of proteases to allow invasion through basement membranes and normal tissue barriers (Chap. 69). Specific cellular mechanisms promote entry or withdrawal of tumor cells from the cell cycle. For example, when a tumor recurs after surgery or chemotherapy, frequently its growth is accelerated and the growth fraction of the tumor is increased. This pattern is similar to that seen in regenerating organs. Partial resection of the liver results in the recruitment of cells into the cell cycle, and the resected liver volume is replaced. Similarly, chemotherapy-damaged bone marrow increases its growth to replace cells killed by chemotherapy. However, cancers do not recognize a limit on their expansion. Monoclonal gammopathy of uncertain significance may be an example of a clonal neoplasm with intrinsic features that stop its growth before a lethal tumor burden is reached. A fraction of patients with this disorder go on to develop fatal multiple myeloma, but probably this occurs because of the accumulation of additional genetic lesions. Elucidation of the mechanisms that regulate this "organ-like" behavior of tumors may provide additional clues to cancer control and treatment.

PRINCIPLES OF CANCER SURGERY

Surgery is used in cancer prevention, diagnosis, staging, treatment (for both localized and metastatic disease), palliation, and rehabilitation.

PREVENTION Cancer can be prevented by surgery in people who have premalignant lesions resected (e.g., premalignant lesions of skin, colon, cervix) and in those who are at increased risk of cancer from either an underlying disease (colectomy in those with pancolonic involvement with ulcerative colitis), the presence of genetic lesions (colectomy for familial polyposis; thyroidectomy for multiple endocrine neoplasia type 2; bilateral mastectomy or oophorectomy for familial breast or ovarian cancer syndromes), or a developmental anomaly (orchiectomy in those with an undescended testis). In some cases, prophylactic surgery is more radical than the surgical procedures used to treat the cancer after it develops. The assessment of risk involves many factors and should be undertaken with care before advising a patient to undergo such a major procedure. For breast cancer prevention, many experts use a 20% risk of developing breast cancer over the next 5 years as a threshold. However, patient fears play a major role in defining candidates for cancer prevention surgery. Counseling and education may not be enough to allay the fears of someone who has lost close family members to a malignancy.

DIAGNOSIS The ideal diagnostic procedure varies with the type of cancer, its anatomical location, and the medical condition of the patient. However, the underlying principle is to obtain as much tissue as safely possible. Tumors may be heterogeneous in appearance. Pathologists are better able to make the diagnosis when they have more tissue to examine. In addition to light-microscopic inspection of a tumor for pattern of growth, degree of cellular atypia, invasiveness, and morphologic features that aid in the differential diagnosis, sufficient tissue is of value in searching for genetic abnormalities and protein expression patterns that may aid in differential diagnosis or to provide information about prognosis or likely response to treatment. Histologically similar tumors may have very different gene expression patterns when assessed by such techniques as microarray analysis using gene chips, with important differences in response to treatment. Such testing requires that the tissue be handled properly (e.g., immunologic detection of proteins is more effective in fresh-frozen tissue rather than in formalin-fixed tissue); thus, coordination among the surgeon, pathologist, and primary care physician is essential to ensure that the amount of information learned from the biopsy material is maximized.

These goals are best met by an *excisional biopsy* in which the entire tumor mass is removed with a small margin of normal tissue surrounding it. If an excisional biopsy cannot be performed, *incisional biopsy* is the procedure of second choice. A wedge of tissue is removed, and an effort is made to include the majority of the cross-sectional diameter of the tumor in the biopsy to minimize sampling error. When the diagnosis is being made through an endoscope or via fluoroscopy, it may be necessary to obtain a *core-needle biopsy* of the mass; considerably less tissue is obtained and the diagnosis may be less certain. However, this procedure often provides enough information to plan a definitive surgical procedure. Least reliable in diagnosis of primary cancer is *fine-needle aspiration*. This technique generally obtains only a suspension of cells from within a mass. This approach (with stereotactic guidance of the needle) is the procedure of choice in the diagnosis of brain tumors and may be useful in diagnosing thyroid nodules and in confirming persistent or recurrent disease in a patient with known cancer, but the procedure is overutilized in primary diagnosis. It would be preferable to perform a larger open operation to obtain more tissue in most sites. The biopsy techniques that involve cutting into tumor carry with them a risk of facilitating the spread of the tumor.

STAGING   As noted in Chap. 66, an important component of patient management is defining the extent of disease. Radiographic and other imaging tests can be helpful in defining the clinical stage; however, pathologic staging requires defining the extent of involvement by documenting the histologic presence of tumor in tissue biopsies obtained through a surgical procedure. Axillary lymph node sampling in breast cancer and lymph node sampling at laparotomy for lymphomas and testicular, colon, and other intraabdominal cancers provide crucial information for treatment planning and may determine the extent and nature of primary cancer treatment.

TREATMENT   Surgery is the most effective means of treating cancer. About 40% of cancer patients are cured today by surgery. Unfortunately, a large fraction of patients with solid tumors (perhaps 60%) have metastatic disease that is not accessible for removal. However, even when the disease is not curable by surgery alone, the removal of tumor can obtain important benefits, including local control of tumor, preservation of organ function, debulking that permits subsequent therapy to work better, and staging information on extent of involvement. Cancer surgery aiming for cure is usually planned to excise the tumor completely with an adequate margin of normal tissue (the margin varies with the tumor and the anatomy), touching the tumor as little as possible to prevent vascular and lymphatic spread, and minimizing operative risk. Extending the procedure to resect draining lymph nodes obtains prognostic information, but such resections alone generally do not improve survival.

Increasingly, laparoscopic approaches are being used to address primary abdominal and pelvic tumors. Lymph node spread may be assessed using the sentinel node approach, in which the first draining lymph node a spreading tumor would encounter is defined by injecting a dye at operation and then resecting the first node to turn blue. The sentinel node assessment is continuing to undergo clinical evaluation but appears to provide reliable information without the risks (lymphedema, lymphangiosarcoma) associated with resection of all the regional nodes. Advances in adjuvant chemotherapy and radiation therapy following surgery have permitted a substantial decrease in the extent of primary surgery necessary to obtain the best outcomes. Thus, lumpectomy with radiation therapy is as effective as modified radical mastectomy for breast cancer, and limb-sparing surgery followed by adjuvant radiation therapy and chemotherapy has replaced radical primary surgical procedures involving amputation and disarticulation for childhood rhabdomyosarcomas. More limited surgery is also being employed to spare organ function, as in larynx and bladder cancer. The magnitude of operations necessary to optimally control and cure cancer has also been diminished by technical advances; for example, the circular anastomotic stapler has allowed narrower (<2 cm) margins

in colon cancer without compromise of local control rates, and many patients who would have had colostomies are able to maintain normal anatomy.

In some settings, e.g., bulky testicular cancer or stage III breast cancer, surgery is not the first treatment modality employed. After an initial diagnostic biopsy, chemotherapy and/or radiation therapy are delivered to reduce the size of the tumor and control clinically undetected metastatic disease, and such therapy is followed by a surgical procedure to remove residual masses. This is called *neoadjuvant therapy*. Because the sequence of treatment is critical to success and is different from the standard surgery-first approach, coordination among the surgical oncologist, radiation oncologist, and medical oncologist is crucial.

Surgery may be curative in a subset of patients with metastatic disease. Patients with lung metastases from osteosarcoma may be cured by resection of the lung lesions. In patients with colon cancer who have fewer than five liver metastases restricted to one lobe and no extrahepatic metastases, hepatic lobectomy may produce long-term disease-free survival in 25% of selected patients. Surgery can also be associated with systemic antitumor effects. In the setting of hormonally responsive tumors, oophorectomy and/or adrenalectomy may control estrogen production and orchiectomy may reduce androgen production, both with effects on metastatic tumor growth. If resection of the primary lesion takes place in the presence of metastases, the noted change in tumor behavior is most often acceleration of growth, perhaps based on the removal of a source of angiogenesis inhibitors and mass-related growth regulators in the tumor. However, on rare occasions (certain renal cancers), primary tumor resection is accompanied by regression of metastatic lesions. Similarly, splenectomy in some cases of lymphoma may be associated with regression of disease at remote sites. This phenomenon, called the *abscopal effect*, is attributed to the removal of a source of growth or angiogenic factors upon which the remote sites depend for growth.

PALLIATION   Surgery is employed in a number of ways for supportive care: insertion of central venous catheters, diagnostic evaluation of pulmonary infiltrates, control of pleural and pericardial effusions and ascites, caval interruption for recurrent pulmonary emboli, stabilization of cancer-weakened weight-bearing bones, and control of hemorrhage, among others. Surgical bypass of gastrointestinal, urinary tract, or biliary tree obstruction can alleviate symptoms and prolong survival. Surgical procedures may provide relief of otherwise intractable pain or reverse neurologic dysfunction (cord decompression). Splenectomy may relieve symptoms and reverse hypersplenism. Intrathecal or intrahepatic therapy relies on surgical placement of appropriate infusion portals. Surgery may correct other treatment-related toxicities such as adhesions or strictures.

REHABILITATION   Surgical procedures are also valuable in restoring a cancer patient to full health. Orthopedic procedures may be necessary to assure proper ambulation. Breast reconstruction can make an enormous impact on the patient's perception of successful therapy. Plastic and reconstructive surgery can correct the effects of disfiguring primary treatment.

PRINCIPLES OF CHEMOTHERAPY

Medical oncology is the subspecialty of internal medicine that cares for and designs treatment approaches to patients with cancer, in conjunction with surgical and radiation oncologists. The core skills of the medical oncologist include the use of drugs that may have a beneficial effect on the natural history of the patient's illness or favorably influence the patient's quality of life.

HISTORIC BACKGROUND   The treatment of patients with cancer using chemicals, in the hope of causing regressions of established tumors or to slow the rate of tumor growth, arose by analogy to the proposition of Ehrlich that bacteria might be killed selectively by compounds with intrinsic affinity for bacteria, in effect acting as "magic bullets." Candidate compounds that might have selectivity for cancer cells were suggested by the marrow-toxic effects of sulfur and nitrogen mustards, first noted in their use in chemical warfare. These observations led in the 1940s to the first clinical experiments where notable regressions of hematopoietic tumors followed use of these compounds by Gilman and colleagues. As these compounds caused covalent modification of DNA, the structure of DNA was thereby identified as a potential target for drug design efforts to produce antineoplastic agents. Biochemical studies demonstrating the requirement of growing tumor cells for precursors of nucleic acids led to nearly contemporaneous studies by Farber of folate analogues. The cure of patients with advanced choriocarcinoma by methotrexate in the 1950s provided further impetus to define the value of chemotherapeutic agents in many different tumor types. This resulted in efforts to understand unique metabolic requirements for biosynthesis of nucleic acids and led to the design, rational for the time, of compounds that might selectively inhibit DNA synthesis in proliferating cancer cells. The capacity of hormonal manipulations including oophorectomy and orchiectomy to cause regressions of breast and prostate cancers, respectively, provided a rationale for efforts to interdict various aspects of hormone function in hormone-dependent tumors. The serendipitous finding that certain poisons derived from bacteria or plants could affect normal DNA or mitotic spindle function allowed completion of the classic armamentarium of drugs with proven efficacy and a relative margin of safety in the treatment of certain cancers.

END POINTS OF DRUG ACTION   Chemotherapy agents may be used for the treatment of active, clinically apparent cancer. Table 70-1,**A** lists those

tumors considered curable by conventionally available chemotherapeutic agents when used to address disseminated or metastatic cancers. If a tumor is localized to a single site, serious consideration of surgery or primary radiation therapy should be given, as these treatment modalities may be curative as local treatments. Chemotherapy may be employed after the failure of these modalities to eradicate a local tumor or as part of multimodality approaches to offer primary treatment to a clinically localized tumor. In this event, it can allow organ preservation when given with radiation, as in larynx or other upper airway sites; or sensitize tumors to radiation when given, for example, to patients concurrently receiving radiation for lung or cervix cancer (Table 70-1,**B**). Chemotherapy can be administered as an adjuvant, i.e., in addition to surgery (Table 70-1,**C**) or radiation, after all clinically apparent disease has been removed. This use of chemotherapy may have curative potential in breast and colorectal neoplasms, as it attempts to eliminate clinically unapparent tumor that may have already disseminated. As noted above, small tumors frequently have high growth fractions and therefore may be intrinsically more susceptible to the action of antiproliferative agents. Chemotherapy is routinely used in "conventional" dose regimens. In general, these doses produce reversible acute side effects primarily consisting of transient myelosuppression with or without gastrointestinal toxicity (usually nausea), which are readily managed. High-dose chemotherapy regimens are predicated on the observation that the concentration-effect curve for many anticancer agents is rather steep, and increased dose can produce markedly increased therapeutic effect, although at the cost of potentially life-threatening complications that require intensive support, usually in the form of hematopoietic stem cell support from the patient (*autologous*) or from donors matched for histocompatibility loci (*allogeneic*). High-dose regimens nonetheless have definite curative potential in defined clinical settings (Table 70-1,**D**).

Karnofsky was among the first to champion the evaluation of a chemotherapeutic agent's benefit by carefully quantitating its effect on tumor size and using these measurements to decide objectively the basis for further treatment of a particular patient or further clinical evaluation of a drug's potential. A partial response (PR) is defined conventionally as a decrease by at least 50% in a tumor's bi-dimensional area; a complete response (CR) connotes disappearance of all tumor; progression of disease signifies an increase in size of existing lesions by >25% from baseline or best response or development of new lesions; and "stable" disease fits into none of the above categories. More recently proposed evaluation systems utilize unidimensional measurement, but the intent is similar in rigorously defining evidence for the activity of the agent in assessing its value to the patient.

If cure is not possible, chemotherapy may be undertaken with the goal of palliating some aspect of the tumor's effect on the host. Common tumors that may be meaningfully addressed with palliative intent are listed in Table 70-1,**E**. Usually tumor-related symptoms may manifest as pain, weight loss, or some local symptom related to the tumor's effect on normal structures. Patients treated with palliative intent should be aware of their diagnosis and the limitations of the proposed treatments, have access to supportive care, and have suitable "performance status," according to assessment algorithms such as the one developed by Karnofsky or by the Eastern Cooperative Oncology Group (ECOG). ECOG performance status 0 (PS0) patients are without symptoms; PS1 patients have mild symptoms not requiring treatment; PS2, symptoms requiring some treatment; PS3, disabling symptoms, but allowing ambulation for >50% of the day; PS4, ambulation <50% of the day. Only PS0 to PS2 patients are generally considered suitable for palliative (noncurative) treatment. If there is curative potential, even poor performance status patients may be treated, but their prognosis is usually inferior to that of good performance patients treated with similar regimens.

PATH FOR NEW CANCER DRUG DISCOVERY AND DEVELOPMENT   The usefulness of any drug is governed by the extent to which a given dose causes a

---

TABLE 70-1   Curability of Cancers with Chemotherapy

A. Advanced cancers with possible cure
- Acute lymphoid and acute myeloid leukemia (pediatric/adult)
- Hodgkin's disease (pediatric/adult)
- Lymphomas—certain types (pediatric/adult)
- Germ cell neoplasms
  - Embryonal carcinoma
  - Teratocarcinoma
  - Seminoma or dysgerminoma
  - Choriocarcinoma
- Gestational trophoblastic neoplasia
- Pediatric neoplasms
  - Wilm's tumor
  - Embryonal rhabdomyocarcinoma
  - Ewing's sarcoma
  - Peripheral neuroepithelioma
  - Neuroblastoma
- Small-cell lung carcinoma
- Ovarian carcinoma

B. Advanced cancers possibly cured by chemotherapy and radiation
- Squamous carcinoma (head and neck)
- Squamous carcinoma (anus)
- Breast carcinoma
- Carcinoma of the uterine cervix
- Non-small cell lung carcinoma (stage III)
- Small-cell lung carcinoma

C. Cancers possibly cured with chemotherapy as adjuvant to surgery
- Breast carcinoma
- Colorectal carcinoma[a]
- Osteogenic sarcoma
- Soft tissue sarcoma

D. Cancers possibly cured with "high-dose" chemotherapy with stem cell support
- Relapsed leukemias, lymphoid and myeloid
- Relapsed lymphomas, Hodgkin's and non-Hodgkin's
- Chronic myeloid leukemia
- Multiple myeloma

E. Cancers responsive with useful palliation, but not cure, by chemotherapy
- Bladder carcinoma
- Chronic myeloid leukemia
- Hairy cell leukemia
- Chronic lymphocytic leukemia
- Lymphoma—certain types
- Multiple myeloma
- Gastric carcinoma
- Cervix carcinoma
- Endometrial carcinoma
- Soft tissue sarcoma
- Head and neck cancer
- Adrenocortical carcinoma
- Islet-cell neoplasms
- Breast carcinoma
- Colorectal carcinoma

F. Tumor poorly responsive in advanced stages to chemotherapy
- Pancreatic carcinoma
- Biliary-tract neoplasms
- Renal carcinoma
- Thyroid carcinoma
- Carcinoma of the vulva
- Non-small cell lung carcinoma
- Prostate carcinoma
- Melanoma
- Hepatocellular carcinoma

[a] Rectum also receives radiation therapy.

useful result (therapeutic effect; in the case of anticancer agents, toxicity to tumor cells) as opposed to a toxic effect, reflecting injury to the host. The *therapeutic index* is the degree of separation between toxic and therapeutic doses. Really useful drugs have large therapeutic indices, and this usually occurs when the drug target is expressed in the disease-causing compartment as opposed to the normal compartment. Classically, selective toxicity of an agent for an organ is governed by the expression of an agent's target; or differential accumulation into or elimination from compartments where toxicity is experienced or ameliorated, respectively. Current "conventional cytotoxic" antineoplastic agents have the unfortunate property that their targets are present in both normal and tumor tissues. In the main they therefore have relatively narrow therapeutic indices.

Agents with promise for the treatment of cancer have in the past been detected empirically through screening for antiproliferative effects in animal or human tumors, usually in rodent hosts or through inhibition of tumor cells growing in tissue culture. An optimal schedule for demonstrating antitumor activity in animals is defined in further preclinical studies, as is the optimal drug formulation for a given route and schedule. Safety testing in two species on an analogous schedule of administration defines the starting dose for a phase I trial in humans. This is established as a fraction, usually one-sixth to one-tenth, of the dose just causing easily reversible toxicity in the more sensitive animal species. Escalating doses of the drug are then given during the human phase I trial until reversible toxicity is observed. Dose-limiting toxicity (DLT) defines a dose that conveys greater toxicity than would be acceptable in routine practice, allowing definition of a lower maximal tolerated dose (MTD). The occurrence of toxicity is correlated if possible with plasma drug concentrations. The MTD or a dose just lower than the MTD is usually the dose suitable for phase II trials, where a fixed dose is administered to a relatively homogeneous set of patients in an effort to define whether the drug causes regression of tumors. An "active" agent conventionally has PR rates of at least 20 to 25% with reversible non-life-threatening side effects, and it may then be suitable for study in phase III trials to assess efficacy in comparison to standard or no therapy. Response is but the most immediate indicator of drug effect. To be clinically valuable, responses must translate into clinical benefit. This is conventionally established by a beneficial effect on overall survival, or at least an increased time to further progression of disease. Active efforts are being made to quantitate effects of anticancer agents on quality of life. Cancer drug clinical trials conventionally use a toxicity grading scale where grade I toxicities do not require treatment; grade II often require symptomatic treatment but are not life-threatening; grade III toxicities are potentially life-threatening if untreated; grade IV toxicities are actually life-threatening; and grade V toxicities are those that result in the patient's death.

The process of cancer drug development is likely to evolve in significant ways in the near future as (1) the molecular analysis of human tumors defines more precisely the molecular targets that can be the focus of drug discovery efforts, and (2) clinical trials are undertaken only after means of assessing the behavior of the drug in relation to its target have been developed. The basis for optimism and anticipated change in clinical trials methodology extends from emerging understanding of the basis for cancer incidence and progression. Cancer arises from genetic lesions that cause an excess of cell growth or division, with inadequate cell death (Chap. 68). In addition, failure of cellular differentiation results in altered cellular position and capacity to proliferate while cut off from normal cell regulatory signals. An overall schema for understanding cancer progression can be seen in Fig. 70-2. Normally, cells in a differentiated state are stimulated to enter the cell cycle from a quiescent state, or G_0, or continue after completion of a prior cell division cycle in response to environmental cues including growth factor and hormonal signals. Cells progress through G_1 and enter S-phase after passing through "checkpoints," which are biochemically regulated transition points, to assure that the genome is "ready" for replication. The cyclin-dependent kinases

FIGURE 70-2 Basis for neoplastic growth and progression. Normally cells are stimulated to enter a proliferating state through the action of growth factors, positional signals, or cytokines. Cells enter G_1 under the influence of normal signaling pathways including tyrosine kinase receptors coupled to ras protooncogenes or seven-transmembrane receptors coupled through heterotrimeric guanine nucleotide binding (0) proteins, especially Gq linked to calcium- and lipid-mediated signaling pathways through protein kinase C (PKC). Cells activate transcription and translation of key regulatory molecules such as the cyclins, which activate cyclin-dependent kinases (CDKs) 4 or 6. Phosphorylation of the retinoblastoma susceptibility protein (pRb) causes release of E2F transcription factors to an active state, promoting the transcription of multiple genes allowing progression through S-phase, where DNA is replicated. Tumor cells possess activated oncogenes such as *erbB*1, *erbB*2, and *sis* or mutated *ras* gene products that are tonically activated, thus driving proliferation autonomously. *Raf* and the mitogen-activated kinases, MAPKK and MAPK, amplify the growth signal in a kinase cascade. "Brakes" to cell cycle progression include the p53-mediated G_1 to S-phase checkpoint, mediated by the CDK inhibitors p16^INK4a and p21^WAF1. Progression through S-phase is also promoted by CDK2 acting in concert with cyclins E and A, and initiation of cell division is governed by the action of CDK1 acting in concert with cyclin B.

(CDKs) are enzymes that critically regulate cell cycle progression from one phase to the next. One important checkpoint is mediated by the p53 tumor-suppressor gene product, acting through its upregulation of the p21^WAF1 inhibitor of CDK function, acting on CDKs 4 or 6. These kinase molecules can also be inhibited by the p16^INK4A and p27^KIP1 CDK inhibitors, but in turn are activated by cyclins of the D family (which appear during G_1) and the proper sequence of regulatory phosphorylations. Activated CDKs 4 or 6 phosphorylate, and thus inactivate, the product of the retinoblastoma susceptibility gene, *pRb*, which in its nonphosphorylated state complexes with transcription factors of the E2F family. Phosphorylated *pRb* releases E2Fs, which activate genes important in completing DNA replication during S-phase, progression through which is promoted by CDK2 acting in concert with cylins A and E. During G_2, another checkpoint occurs, in which the cell assures the completion of correct DNA synthesis. Cells then progress into M-phase under the influence of CDK1 and cyclin B. Cells may then go on to a subsequent division cycle or enter into a quiescent, differentiated state.

Also shown in Fig. 70-2 are the sites of action of protooncogenes, regulators of cellular proliferation that, in an active state, promote cell growth, and whose deregulation produces oncogenes, originally discovered as the genes encoded by tumor-forming viruses in animals. Oncogenes can be divided into two families: (1) those that act in the cytoplasm to disrupt normal growth factor–related signaling, including *ras*, *raf*, and the tyrosine kinases of the *src* and *erb*B or *sis* families; and (2) nuclear oncogenes, including *jun*, *fos*, *myc*, and *myb*, that act to alter transcriptional control of cassettes of genes. In contrast, tumor-suppressor genes, including *p53* and *pRb*, act as cellular "brakes" whose normal function is to inhibit or prevent unregulated cellular growth. The capacity to divide indefinitely is provided by activation of telomerase, which allows continued replication of chromosomes by addressing the unique need of chromosome ends to be continually renewed to a proper length to allow normal mitosis. The capacity to invade and metastasize is conveyed by elaboration of matrix metalloproteases and plasminogen activators and the capacity to recruit host stromal cells at the site of invasion through tumor-induced angiogenesis.

Currently used drugs for the treatment of cancer focus principally on the proximate biochemistry of nucleic acid and mitotic spindle structure or function. Drugs of the future may seek to replace lost function of tumor-suppressor genes; counter the action of activated oncogenes; influence the capacity of cells to die; prevent normal chromosomal end replication; actually infect cells with viruses designed to replicate in the milieu of the cancer but not the normal cell; cause differentiation of cells with exit from the cell cycle by activating the appropriate genes; and use immunologic strategies, including antibodies and engineered cells to be directed at targets expressed on the surface of cancer cells.

BIOLOGIC BASIS FOR CANCER CHEMOTHERAPY The classic view of how cancer chemotherapeutic agents cause regressions of tumors focused on animal models such as the L1210 murine leukemia system, where cancer cells grow exponentially after inoculation into the peritoneal cavity of an isogenic mouse. The interaction of drug with its biochemical target in the cancer cell was proposed to result in "unbalanced growth" that was not sustainable and therefore resulted in cell death, directly as a result of interacting with the drug's proximal target. Agents could be categorized (Fig. 70-3) as cell cycle–active, phase-specific (e.g., antimetabolites, purines, and pyrimidines in S-phase; vinca alkaloids in M), and phase-nonspecific agents [e.g., alkylators, and antitumor antibiotics including the anthracyclines, dactinomycin (formerly actinomycin D), and mitomycin], which can injure DNA at any phase of the cell cycle but appear to then block in S-phase or G_2 at a checkpoint in the cell cycle before cell division. Cells arrested at a checkpoint may repair DNA lesions. Checkpoints have been defined at the G_1 to S transition, mediated by the tumor-suppressor gene $p53$ (giving rise to the characterization of $p53$ as a "guardian of the genome"); at the G_2 to M transition, mediated by the $chk1$ kinase and additional p53-related pathways influencing the function of CDK1; and during M-phase, to ensure the integrity of the mitotic spindle. The importance of the concept of checkpoints extends from the hypothesis that repair of chemotherapy-mediated damage can occur while cells are stopped at a checkpoint; therefore, manipulation of checkpoint function emerges as an important basis of affecting resistance to chemotherapeutic agents.

Resistance to drugs was postulated to arise either from cells not being in the appropriate phase of the cell cycle or from decreased uptake, increased efflux, metabolism of the drug, or alteration of the target, e.g., by mutation or overexpression. Indeed, p170PGP (p170 P-glycoprotein; mdr gene product) was recognized from experiments with cells growing in tissue culture as mediating the efflux of chemotherapeutic agents in resistant cells. Certain neoplasms, particularly hematopoietic tumors, have an adverse prognosis if they express high levels of p170PGP, and modulation of this protein's function has been attempted by a variety of strategies.

Combinations of agents were proposed to afford the opportunity to affect many different targets or portions of the cell cycle at once, particularly if the toxic effects for the host of the different components of the combination were distinct. Combinations of agents were actually more effective in animal model systems than single agents, particularly if the tumor cell inoculum was high. This thinking led to the design of "combination chemotherapy" regimens, where drugs acting by different mechanisms (e.g., an alkylating agent plus an antimetabolite plus a mitotic spindle blocker) were combined. Particular combinations were chosen to emphasize drugs whose individual toxicities to the host were, if possible, distinct.

This view of cancer drug action is grossly oversimplified. Most tumors do not grow in an exponential pattern but rather follow Gompertzian kinetics, where the rate of tumor growth decreases as tumor mass increases (Fig. 70-1). Thus, a tumor has quiescent, differentiated compartments; proliferating compartments; and both well-vascularized and necrotic regions. Also, cell death is itself a closely regulated process. *Necrosis* refers to cell death induced, for example, by physical damage with the hallmarks of cell swelling and membrane disruption. *Apoptosis*, or programmed cell death, refers to a highly ordered process whereby cells respond to defined stimuli by dying, and it recapitulates the necessary cell death observed during the ontogeny of the organism. *Anoikis* refers to death of epithelial cells after removal from the normal milieu of substrate, particularly from cell-to-cell contact. Cancer chemotherapeutic agents can cause both necrosis and apoptosis. Apoptosis is characterized by chromatin condensation (giving rise to "apoptotic bodies"); cell shrinkage; and, in living animals, phagocytosis by surrounding stromal cells without evidence of inflammation. This process is regulated either by signal transduction systems that promote a cell's demise after a certain level of insult is achieved, or in response to specific cell-surface receptors that mediate cell death signals. Modulation of apoptosis by manipulation of signal transduction pathways has emerged as a basis for understanding the actions of currently used drugs and designing new strategies to improve their use.

The current view envisions that the interaction of a chemotherapeutic drug with its target, e.g., of an alkylating agent with DNA, causes or is itself a signal that initiates a "cascade" of further signaling steps to trigger an "execution phase" where proteases, nucleases, and endogenous regulators of the cell death pathway are activated. Effective cancer chemotherapeutic agents are efficient activators of apoptosis through signal transduction pathways (Fig. 70-4). For example, in the cytokine-mediated pathway, exogenous ligands such as the Fas ligand (FasL) bind to cell-surface receptors (CD95; Fas), or tumor necrosis factor (TNF) or its homologue Apo2L binds to its cognate receptors and directly recruits accessory molecules to activate a protease cascade (utilizing members of the caspase family of *cy*steine *asp*artyl prote*ases*), resulting in apoptosis. In a second pathway, growth factor deprivation elicits poorly defined signals that result in protease activation. Chemotherapeutic agents create molecular lesions (in DNA or cellular membranes) as a consequence of combining with their respective molecular targets. These lesions are sensed by a cellular "damage sensor," whose molecular nature is unclear, which leads to mitochondrial damage. Release of mitochondrial factors (e.g.,

FIGURE 70-3 *Location of drug action in the cell cycle. Cancer chemotherapy agents can be broadly described as phase specific agents acting in S-(antimetabolites) and M-(spindle poisons) phase, respectively, and phase-nonspecific agents that injure their targets throughout the cycle but cause arrest of cell cycle progression at checkpoints. The G_1 checkpoint is mediated through p53 acting on CDKs 4,6, and 2, and the G_2 checkpoint is mediated in part by the $chk1$ kinase acting on CDK1.*

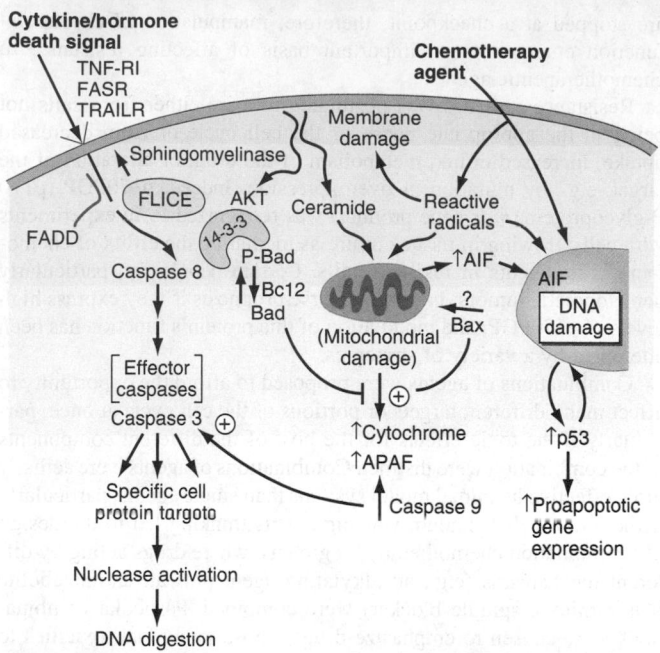

FIGURE 70-4 Integration of cell death responses. Cell death through an apoptotic mechanism requires active participation of the cell. In response to hormonal or cytokine death signals, receptors activate "upstream" cysteine aspartyl proteases (caspases), which then directly digest cytoplasmic and nuclear proteins, resulting in activation of "downstream" caspases; these cause activation of nucleases resulting in the characteristic DNA fragmentation that is a hallmark of apoptosis. Chemotherapy agents that create lesions in DNA seem to activate aspects of this process through a pathway that appears to result in damage to mitochondria, perhaps by activating the transcription of genes whose products can produce or modulate the toxicity of free radicals. In addition, membrane damage with activation of sphingomyelinases results in the production of ceramides that can have a direct action at mitochondria. The antiapoptotic protein bcl2 attenuates mitochondrial toxicity, while proapoptotic gene products such as bax antagonize the action of bcl2. Damaged mitochondria release cytochrome C and "apoptosis activating factor," which can directly activate caspase 9, resulting in propagation of a direct signal to other downstream caspases through protease activation. Apoptosis-inducing factor (AIF) is also released from the mitochondrion and then can translocate to the nucleus, bind to DNA, and generate free radicals to further damage DNA. An additional proapoptotic stimulus is the bad protein, which can heterodimerize with *bcl2* gene family members to antagonize apoptosis. Importantly, though, bad protein function can be retarded by its sequestration as phospho-bad through the 14-3-3 adapter proteins. The phosphorylation of bad is mediated by the action of the AKT kinase in a way that defines how growth factors that activate this kinase can retard apoptosis and promote cell survival.

APAF1, cytochrome c) promotes the activation of another set of caspases. Apoptosis-inducing factor (AIF) is another mitochondrial factor that upon release can translocate to the nucleus and promote DNA damage in its own right, without necessarily activating caspases. Damage to the plasma membrane, e.g., from free radicals generated by certain chemotherapeutic agents, leads to activation of acid sphingomyelinase to release lipid components including ceramides, which then promote apoptosis through a variety of pathways including direct mitochondrial damage.

While apoptotic mechanisms are important in regulating cellular proliferation and the behavior of tumor cells in vitro, in vivo it is unclear whether all of the actions of chemotherapeutic agents to cause cell death can be attributed to apoptotic mechanisms. Loss of clonogenic survival (conventionally detecting the capacity of a few cells to survive) may predict clinical value more reliably than detection of apoptotic changes in the majority of tumor cells. However, changes in molecules that regulate apoptosis are clearly correlated with clinical outcomes (e.g., *bcl2* overexpression in certain lymphomas conveys poor prognosis; proapoptotic bax expression is associated with a better outcome in ovarian carcinoma). A better understanding of the relationship of cell death and cell survival mechanisms is needed.

CHEMOTHERAPEUTIC AGENTS USED FOR CANCER TREATMENT Table 70-2 lists commonly used cancer chemotherapy agents and pertinent clinical aspects of their use. The drugs and schedules listed are examples of regimens that have proved tolerable and useful; the specific doses that may be used in a particular patient may vary somewhat with the particular treatment protocol, or plan, of treatment. Significant variation from these dose ranges should be carefully verified to avoid or anticipate toxicity. Not included in Table 70-2 are hormone receptor–directed agents, as the side effects are generally those expected from the interruption or augmentation of hormonal effect, and doses used in most cases are those that adequately saturate the intended hormone receptor. The drugs listed may be usefully grouped into three general categories: those affecting DNA, those affecting microtubules, and molecularly targeted agents.

Direct DNA-Interactive Agents ■ *FORMATION OF COVALENT DNA ADDUCTS* Alkylating agents as a class break down, either spontaneously or after normal organ or tumor cell metabolism, to reactive intermediates that covalently modify bases in DNA. This leads to cross-linkage of DNA strands or the appearance of breaks in DNA as a result of repair efforts. "Broken" or cross-linked DNA is intrinsically unable to complete normal replication or cell division; in addition, it is a potent activator of cell cycle checkpoints and signaling pathways that can activate apoptosis. As a class, alkylating agents share similar toxicities: myelosuppression, alopecia, gonadal dysfunction, mucositis, and pulmonary fibrosis. They differ greatly in a spectrum of normal organ toxicities. As a class they share the capacity to cause "second" neoplasms, particularly leukemia, many years after use, particularly when used in low doses for protracted periods.

Nitrogen mustard (mechlorethamine) is the prototypic agent of this class, decomposing rapidly in aqueous solution to yield potentially a bifunctional carbonium ion. It must be administered shortly after preparation into a rapidly flowing intravenous line. It is a powerful vesicant, and infiltration may be symptomatically ameliorated by infiltration of the affected site with $1/6$ *M* thiosulfate. Even without infiltration, aseptic thrombophlebitis is frequent. It can be used topically as a dilute solution in cutaneous lymphomas, with a notable incidence of hypersensitivity reactions. It causes moderate nausea after intravenous administration.

Cyclophosphamide is inactive unless metabolized by the liver to 4-hydroxy-cyclophosphamide, which decomposes into alkylating species, as well as to chloroacetaldehyde and acrolein. The latter causes chemical cystitis; therefore excellent hydration must be maintained while using cyclophosphamide. If severe, the cystitis may be effectively treated by mesna (2-mercaptoethanesulfonate). Liver disease impairs drug activation. Sporadic interstitial pneumonitis leading to pulmonary fibrosis can accompany the use of cyclophosphamide, and high doses used in conditioning regimens for bone marrow transplant can cause cardiac dysfunction. Ifosfamide is a cyclophosphamide analogue also activated in the liver, but more slowly, and it requires coadministration of mesna to prevent bladder injury. Central nervous system (CNS) effects, including somnolence, confusion, and psychosis, can follow ifosfamide use; the incidence appears related to low body surface area or the presence of nephrectomy.

Several alkylating agents are less commonly used. Chlorambucil causes predictable myelosuppression, azoospermia, nausea, and pulmonary side effects. Busulfan can cause profound myelosuppression, alopecia, and pulmonary toxicity but is relatively "lymphocyte sparing." Its routine use in treatment of chronic myeloid leukemia (CML) has been curtailed in favor of imatinib (Gleevec), hydroxyurea, and interferon (IFN), but it still is employed in transplant preparation regimens. Melphalan shows variable oral bioavailability and undergoes extensive binding to albumin and α_1-acidic glycoprotein. Mucositis appears more prominently.

Nitrosoureas break down to carbamoylating species that not only cause a distinct pattern of DNA base pair–directed toxicity but also can covalently modify proteins. They share the feature of causing relatively delayed bone marrow toxicity, which can be cumulative and

TABLE 70-2   *Commonly Used Cancer Chemotherapy Agents*

Drug	Examples of Usual Doses	Toxicity	Interactions, Issues
DIRECT DNA-INTERACTING AGENTS			
Alkylators			
Cyclophosphamide	400–2000 mg/m² IV 100 mg/m² PO qd	Marrow (relative platelet sparing) Cystitis Common alkylator[a] Cardiac (high dose)	Liver metabolism required to activate to phosphoramide mustard + acrolein Mesna protects against "high-dose" bladder damage
Mechlorethamine	6 mg/m² IV day 1 and day 8	Marrow Vesicant Nausea	Topical use in cutaneous lymphoma
Chlorambucil	1–3 mg/m² qd PO	Marrow Common alkylator[a]	
Melphalan	8 mg/m² qd × 5, PO	Marrow (delayed nadir) GI (high dose)	Decreased renal function delays clearance
Carmustine (BCNU)	200 mg/m² IV 150 mg/m² PO	Marrow (delayed nadir) GI, liver (high dose) Renal	
Lomustine (CCNU)	100–300 mg/m² PO	Marrow (delayed nadir)	
Ifosfamide	1.2 g/m² per day qd × 5 + mesna	Myelosuppressive Bladder Neurologic Metabolic acidosis Neuropathy	Isomeric analogue of cyclophosphamide More lipid soluble Greater activity vs testicular neoplasms and sarcomas Must use mesna
Procarbazine	100 mg/m² per day qd ×14	Marrow Nausea Neurologic Common alkylator[a]	Liver and tissue metabolism required Disulfiran-like effect with ethanol Acts as MAOI HBP after tyrosinase-rich foods
Dacarbazine (DTIC)	375 mg/m² IV day 1 & day 15	Marrow Nausea Flulike	Metabolic activation
Temozolomide	150–200 mg/m² qd × 5 q28d *or* 75 mg/m² qd × 6–7 weeks	Nausea/vomiting Headache/fatigue Constipation	Infrequent myelosuppression
Altretamine (formerly hexamethylmelamine)	260 mg/m² per day qd ×14–21 as 4 divided oral doses	Nausea Neurologic (mood swing) Neuropathy Marrow (less)	Liver activation Barbiturates enchance/cimetidine diminishes
Cisplatin	20 mg/m² qd ×5 IV 1 q3–4 weeks *or* 100–200 mg/m² per dose IV q3–4 weeks	Nausea Neuropathy Auditory Marrow platelets > WBCs Renal Mg²⁺, Ca²⁺	Maintain high urine flow; osmotic diuresis, monitor intake/output K⁺, Mg²⁺ Emetogenic—prophylaxis needed Full dose if CrCl > 60 mL/min and tolerate fluid push
Carboplatin	365 mg/m² IV q3–4 weeks as adjusted for CrCl	Marrow platelets > WBCs Nausea Renal (high dose)	Reduce dose according to CrCl: to AUC of 5–7 mg/mL per min [AUC = dose/(CrCl + 25)]
Oxaliplatin	130 mg/m² q3 weeks over 2 h *or* 85 mg/m² q2 weeks	Nausea Anemia	Acute reversible neurotoxicity; chronic sensory neurotox cumulative with dose; reversible laryngopharyngeal spasm
Antitumor antibiotics			
Bleomycin	15–25 mg/d qd ×5 IV bolus or continuous IV	Pulmonary Skin effects Raynaud's Hypersensitivity	Inactivate by bleomycin hydrolase (decreased in lung/skin) O₂ enhances pulmonary toxicity Cisplatin-induced decrease in CrCl may increase skin/lung toxicity Reduce dose if CrCl < 60 mL/min
Actinomycin D	10–15 μg/kg per day qd ×5 IV bolus	Marrow Nausea Mucositis Vesicant Alopecia	Radiation recall

(continued)

TABLE 70-2 Commonly Used Cancer Chemotherapy Agents—(Continued)

Drug	Examples of Usual Doses	Toxicity	Interactions, Issues
Mithramycin	15–20 μg/kg qd ×4–7 (hypercalcemia) or 50 μg/kg qod ×3–8 (antineoplastic)	Marrow Liver Renal Mucositis Hypocalcemia Nausea Vesicant	Acute hemorrhagic syndrome
Mitomycin C	6–10 mg/m² q6 weeks	Marrow Vesicant Hemolytic-uremic syndrome Lung CV—heart failure	Treat superficial bladder cancers by intravesical infusion Delayed marrow toxicity Cumulative marrow toxicity
Etoposide (VP16-213)	100–150 mg/m² IV qd ×3–5d or 50 mg/m² PO qd ×21d or up to 1500 mg/m² per dose (high dose with stem cell support)	Marrow (WBCs > platelet) Alopecia Hypotension Hypersensitivity (rapid IV) Nausea Mucositis (high dose)	Hepatic metabolism—renal 30% Reduce doses with renal failure Schedule-dependant (5 day better than 1 day) Late leukemogenic Accentuate antimetabolite action
Teniposide (VM-26)	150–200 mg/m² twice per week for 4 weeks	Marrow Alopecia	
Amsacrine	100–150 mg/m² IV qd ×5	Marrow Mucositis Nausea CV—arrhythmia (avoid hypokalemia)	Decrease dose by 30% if liver or renal failure
Topotecan	20 mg/m² IV q3–4 weeks over 30 min or 1.5–3 mg/m² q3–4 weeks over 24 h or 0.5 mg/m² per day over 21 days	Marrow Mucositis Nausea Mild alopecia	Reduce dose with renal failure No liver toxicity
Irinotecan (CPT II)	100–150 mg/m² IV over 90 min q3–4 weeks or 30 mg/m² per day over 120 h	Diarrhea: "early onset" with cramping, flushing, vomiting; "late onset" after several doses Marrow Alopecia Nausea Vomiting Pulmonary	Prodrug requires enzymatic clearance to active drug "SN 38" Early diarrhea likely due to biliary excretion Late diarrhea, use "high-dose" loperamide (2 mg q2–4 h)
Doxorubicin and daunorubicin	45–60 mg/m² dose q3–4 weeks or 10–30 mg/m² dose q week or continuous-infusion regimen	Marrow Mucositis Alopecia Cardiovascular acute/chronic Vesicant	Heparin aggregate; coadministration increases clearance Acetaminophen, BCNU increase liver toxicity Radiation recall
Idarubicin	10–15 mg/m² IV q 3 weeks or 10 mg/m² IV qd ×3	Marrow Cardiac (less than doxorubicin)	None established
Epirubicin	150 mg/m² IV q3 weeks	Marrow Cardiac	None established
Mitoxantrone	12 mg/m² qd ×3 or 12–14 mg/m² q3 weeks	Marrow Cardiac (less than doxorubicin) Vesicant (mild) Blue urine, sclerae, nails	Interacts with heparin Less alopecia, nausea than doxorubicin Radiation recall

INDIRECT DNA-INTERACTING AGENTS

Antimetabolites

Drug	Examples of Usual Doses	Toxicity	Interactions, Issues
Deoxycoformycin	4 mg/m² IV every other week	Nausea Immunosuppression Neurologic Renal	Excretes in urine Reduce dose for renal failure Inhibits adenosine deaminase
6-Mercaptopurine	75 mg/m² PO or up 500 mg/m² PO (high dose)	Marrow Liver Nausea	Variable bioavailability Metabolize by xanthine oxidase Decrease dose with allopurinol Increased toxicity with thiopurine methyltransferase deficiency

(continued)

TABLE 70-2—(Continued)

Drug	Examples of Usual Doses	Toxicity	Interactions, Issues
6-Thioguanine	2–3 mg/kg per day for up to 3–4 weeks	Marrow Liver Nausea	Variable bioavailability Increased toxicity with thiopurine methyltransferase deficiency
Azathioprine	1–5 mg/kg per day	Marrow Nausea Liver	Metabolizes to 6MP, therefore reduce dose with allopurinol Increased toxicity with thiopurine methyltransferase deficiency
2-Chlorodeoxyadenosine	0.09 mg/kg per day qd ×7 as continuous infusion	Marrow Renal Fever	Notable use in hairy cell leukemia
Hydroxyurea	20–50 mg/kg (lean body weight) PO qd or 1–3 g/d	Marrow Nausea Mucositis Skin changes Rare renal, liver, lung, CNS	Decrease dose with renal failure Augments antimetabolite effect
Methotrexate	15–30 mg PO or IM qd ×3–5 or 30 mg IV days 1 and 8 or 1.5–12 g/m^2 per day (with leucovorin)	Marrow Liver/lung Renal tubular Mucositis	Rescue with leucovorin Excreted in urine Decrease dose in renal failure NSAIDs increase renal toxicity
5-Fluorouracil	375 mg/m^2 IV qd ×5 or 600 mg/m^2 IV days 1 and 8	Marrow Mucositis Neurologic Skin changes	Toxicity enhanced by leucovorin Dihydropyrimidine dehydrogenase deficiency increases toxicity Metabolizes in tissues
Capecitabine	665 mg/m^2 bid continuous; 1250 mg/m^2 bid 2 weeks on/ 1 off; 829 mg/m^2 bid 2 weeks on/ 1 off + 60 mg/d leucovorin	Diarrhea Hand-foot syndrome	Prodrug of 5FU due to intratumoral metabolism
Cytosine arabinoside	100 mg/m^2 per day qd ×7 by continuous infusion or 1–3 g/m^2 dose IV bolus	Marrow Mucositis Neurologic (high dose) Conjunctivitis (high dose) Noncardiogenic pulmonary edema	Enhances activity of alkylating agents Metabolizes in tissues by deamination
Azacytidine	750 mg/m^2 per week or 150–200 mg/m^2 per day ×5–10 (bolus) or (continuous IV)	Marrow Nausea Liver Neurologic Myalgia	Use limited to leukemia Altered methylation of DNA alters gene expression
Gemcitabine	1000 mg/m^2 IV weekly ×7	Marrow Nausea Hepatic Fever/"flu syndrome"	
Fludarabine phosphate	25 mg/m^2 IV qd ×5	Marrow Neurologic Lung	Dose reduction with renal failure Metabolized to F-ara converted to F-ara ATP in cells by deoxycytidine kinase
Asparaginase	25,000 IU/m^2 q3–4 weeks or 6000 IU/m^2 per day qod for 3–4 weeks or 1000–2000 IU/m^2 for 10–20 days	Protein synthesis Clotting factors Glucose Albumin Hypersensitivity CNS Pancreatitis Hepatic	Blocks methotrexate action
Antimitotic agents Vincristine	1–1.4 mg/m^2 per week	Vesicant Marrow Neurologic GI: ileus/constipation; bladder hypotoxicity; SIADH Cardiovascular	Hepatic clearance Dose reduction for bilirubin >1.5 mg/dL Prophylactic bowel regimen

(continued)

TABLE 70-2 *Commonly Used Cancer Chemotherapy Agents—(Continued)*

Drug	Examples of Usual Doses	Toxicity	Interactions, Issues
Vinblastine	6–8 mg/m² per week	Vesicant Marrow Neurologic (less common but similar spectrum to other vincas) Hypertension Raynaud's	Hepatic clearance Dose reduction as with vincristine
Vinorelbine	15–30 mg/m² per week	Vesicant Marrow Allergic/bronchospasm (immediate) Dyspnea/cough (subacute) Neurologic (less prominent but similar spectrum to other vincas)	Hepatic clearance
Paclitaxel	135–175 mg/m² per 24-h infusion *or* 175 mg/m² per 3-h infusion *or* 140 mg/m² per 96-h infusion *or* 250 mg/m² per 24-h infusion plus G-CSF	Hypersensitivity Marrow Mucositis Alopecia Sensory neuropathy CV conduction disturbance Nausea—infrequent	Premedicate with steroids, H_1 and H_2 blockers Hepatic clearance Dose reduction as with vincas
Docetaxel	100 mg/m² per 1-h infusion q3 weeks	Hypersensitivity Fluid retention syndrome Marrow Dermatologic Sensory neuropathy Nausea infrequent Some stomatitis	Premedicate with steroids, H_1 and H_2 blockers
Estramustine phosphate	14 mg/kg per day in 3–4 divided doses with water >2 h after meals Avoid Ca^{2+}-rich foods	Nausea Vomiting Diarrhea CHF Thrombosis Gynecomastia	
MOLECULARLY TARGETED AGENTS			
Imatinib	400 mg/d, continuous	Nausea Periorbital edema	Myelosuppression not frequent in solid tumor indications
Tretinoin	45 mg/m² per day until complete response + anthrocycline-based regimen in APL	Teratogenic Cutaneous	APL differentiation syndrome: pulmonary dysfunction/infiltrate, pleural/pericardial effusion, fever
Bexarotene	300–400 mg/m² per day, continuous	Hypercholesterolemia Hypertriglyceridemia Cutaneous Teratogenic	Central hypothyroidism
Gemtuzumab ogomicin	9 mg/m² over 2 h q2 weeks, usually followed by chemotherapy or marrow transplant	Neutropenia Thrombosytopenia Hepatic	Postinfusion syndrome: fever, chills, hypotension Rare hepatic venoocclusive disease Mucositis uncommon
Denileukin deftitox	9–18 μg/kg per day × 5 d q 3 wk	Nausea/vomiting Chills/fever Asthenia Hepatic	Acute hypersensitivity: hypotension, vasodilation, rash, chest tightness Vascular leak: hypotension, edema, hypoalbuminemia, thrombotic events (MI, DVT, CVA)
MISCELLANEOUS			
Arsenic trioxide	0.16 mg/kg per day up to 50 days in APL	↑QT_c Peripheral neuropathy Musculoskeletal pain Hyperglycemia	APL differentiation syndrome (see under tretinoin)

[a] Common alkylator: alopecia, pulmonary, infertility, plus teratogenesis.
Note: APL, acute promyelocytic leukemia; AUC, area under the curve; CHF, congestive heart failure; CNS, central nervous system; CrCl, creatinine clearance; CV, cardiovascular; CVA, cerebrovascular accident; DVT, deep venous thrombosis; G-CSF, granulocyte colony-stimulating factor; GI, gastrointestinal; HBP, high blood pressure; MAOI, monoamine oxidase inhibitors; MI, myocardial infarction; 6MP, 6-mercaptopurine; NSAIDs, nonsteroidal anti-inflammatory drugs; SIADH, syndrome of inappropriate antidiuretic hormone; WBCs, white blood cells.

long-lasting. Streptozotocin is unique in that its glucose-like structure conveys specific toxicity to the islet cells of the pancreas (for whose derivative tumor types it is prominently indicated) as well as causing renal toxicity in the form of Fanconi's syndrome, including amino aciduria, glycosuria, and renal tubular acidosis. Methyl CCNU (lomustine) causes direct glomerular as well as tubular damage, cumulatively related to dose and time of exposure.

Procarbazine is metabolized in the liver and possibly in tumor cells to yield a variety of free radical and alkylating species. In addition to myelosuppression, it causes hypnotic and other CNS effects, including vivid nightmares. It can cause a disulfiram-like syndrome on ingestion of ethanol. Altretamine (formerly hexamethylmelamine) and thiotepa can chemically give rise to alkylating species, although the nature of the DNA damage has not been well characterized in either case. Thiotepa can be used for intrathecal treatment of neoplastic meningitis. Dacarbazine (DTIC) is activated in the liver to yield the highly reactive methyl diazonium cation. It causes only modest myelosuppression 21 to 25 days after a dose but causes prominent nausea on day 1. Temozolomide is structurally related to dacarbazine but was designed to be activated by nonenzymatic hydrolysis in tumors, and is orally bioavailable.

Cisplatin was discovered fortuitously by observing that bacteria present in electrolysis solutions could not divide. Only the *cis* diamine configuration is active as an antitumor agent. It is hypothesized that in the intracellular environment, a chloride is lost from each position, being replaced by a water molecule. The resulting positively charged species is an efficient bifunctional interactor with DNA, forming Pt-based cross-links. Cisplatin requires administration with adequate hydration, including forced diuresis with mannitol to prevent kidney damage; even with the use of hydration, gradual decrease in kidney function is common, along with noteworthy anemia. Hypomagnesemia frequently attends cisplatin use and can lead to hypocalcemia and tetany. Other common toxicities include neurotoxocity with stocking and glove sensorimotor neuropathy. Hearing loss occurs in 50% of patients treated with conventional doses. Cisplatin is intensely emetogenic, requiring prophylactic antiemetics. Myelosuppression is less evident than with other alkylating agents. Chronic vascular toxicity (Raynaud's syndrome, coronary artery disease) is a more unusual toxicity. Carboplatin displays less nephro-, oto-, and neurotoxicity. However, myelosuppression is more frequent, and as the drug is exclusively cleared through the kidney, adjustment of dose for creatinine clearance must be accomplished through use of various dosing nomograms. Oxaliplatin is used in colon cancers refractory to other treatments. Its place in the primary and adjuvant treatment of colon tumors is being defined, along with tests of activity in other tumors. It is prominently neurotoxic.

ANTITUMOR ANTIBIOTICS AND TOPOISOMERASE POISONS Antitumor antibiotics are substances produced by bacteria that in nature appear to provide chemical defense against other hostile microorganisms. As a class they bind to DNA directly and can frequently undergo electron transfer reactions to generate free radicals in close proximity to DNA, leading to DNA damage in the form of single strand breaks or cross-links. Topoisomerase poisons include natural products or semi-synthetic species derived ultimately from plants, and they modify enzymes that regulate the capacity of DNA to unwind to allow normal replication or transcription. DNA damage from these agents can occur in any cell cycle phase, but cells tend to arrest in S-phase or G_2 of the cell cycle in cells with p53 and Rb pathway lesions as the result of defective checkpoint mechanisms in cancer cells.

Doxorubicin is the most widely active and frequently used antineoplastic agent. It can intercalate into DNA, thereby altering DNA structure, replication, and topoisomerase function. It can also undergo redox cycling by accepting electrons into its quinone ring system. It causes predictable myelosuppression, alopecia, nausea, and mucositis. In addition, it causes acute cardiotoxicity in the form of atrial and ventricular dysrhythmias, but these are rarely of clinical significance. In contrast, cumulative doses >550 mg/m² are associated with a 10%

incidence of chronic cardiomyopathy. The incidence of cardiomyopathy appears to be related to schedule (peak serum concentration), with low dose, frequent treatment, or continuous infusions better tolerated than intermittent higher dose exposures. Its cardiotoxicity is increased when given together with trastuzumab (Herceptin), the anti-HER2/*neu* antibody. Radiation recall or interaction with concomitantly administered radiation to cause local site complications is frequent. The drug is a powerful vesicant, with necrosis of tissue apparent 4 to 7 days after an extravasation; therefore it should be administered into a rapidly flowing intravenous line. The drug is metabolized by the liver, so doses must be reduced by 50 to 75% in the presence of liver dysfunction. Daunorubicin is closely related to doxorubicin and was actually introduced first into leukemia treament, where it remains part of curative regimens and has been shown preferable to doxorubicin owing to less mucositis and colonic damage. Idarubicin is an orally acting doxorubicin analogue whose ultimate place in therapy is uncertain. Encapsulation of daunorubicin into a liposome has been accomplished, with attenuation of cardiac toxicity and noteworthy activity in Kaposi's sarcoma. Liposome-encapsulated doxorubicin may have activity in prostate cancer.

Bleomycin refers to a mixture of glycopeptides that have the unique feature of forming complexes with Fe^{2+} while also bound to DNA. Oxidation of Fe^{2+} gives rise to superoxide and hydroxyl radicals. The drug causes little, if any, myelosuppression. The drug is cleared rapidly, but augmented skin and pulmonary toxicity in the presence of renal failure has led to the recommendation that doses be reduced by 50 to 75% in the face of a creatinine clearance <25 mL/min. Bleomycin is not a vesicant and can be administered intravenously, intramuscularly, or subcutaneously. Common side effects include fever and chills, facial flush, and Raynaud's syndrome. Hypertension can follow rapid intravenous administration, and the incidence of anaphylaxis with early preparations of the drug has led to the practice of administering a test dose of 0.5 to 1 unit before the rest of the dose. The most feared complication of bleomycin treatment is pulmonary fibrosis, which increases in incidence at >300 cumulative units administered and is minimally responsive to treatment (e.g., glucocorticoids). The earliest indicator of an adverse effect is a decline in the DL_{CO}, although cessation of drug immediately upon documentation of a decrease in DL_{CO} may not prevent further decline in pulmonary function. Bleomycin is inactivated by a bleomycin hydrolase, whose concentration is diminished in skin and lung. Because bleomycin-dependent electron transport is dependent on O_2, bleomycin toxicity may become apparent after exposure to transient very high PI_{O_2}. Thus, during surgical procedures, patients with prior exposure to bleomycin should be maintained on the lowest PI_{O_2} consistent with maintaining adequate tissue oxygenation.

Dactinomycin intercalates into DNA and appears to have less, but not absent, capacity to undergo electron transfer reactions. It causes severe myelosuppression, nausea, alopecia, and mucositis. It is a notable vesicant. Mithramycin historically was used against testicular and other neoplasms; however, in addition to causing nausea, myelosuppression, and vesicant properties, it causes an acute hemorrhagic syndrome consisting of platelet function defects in association with indicators of disseminated intravascular coagulation. It is used in current practice to control hypercalcemia. In addition, renal and hepatic dysfunction may complicate its use.

Mitomycin C undergoes reduction of its quinone function to generate a bifunctional DNA alkylating agent. It is a broadly active antineoplastic agent with a number of unpredictable toxicities, including delayed bronchospasm 12 to 14 h after dosing and a chronic pulmonary fibrosis syndrome more frequent at doses of 50 to 60 mg/m². Cardiomyopathy has been described, particularly in a setting of prior radiation therapy. A hemolytic/uremic syndrome carries an ultimate mortality rate of 25 to 50% and is poorly treated by conventional component support and exchange transfusion. Mitomycin is a notable vesicant and causes substantial nausea and vomiting. It can be used for intravesical instillation for curative treatment of superficial transitional bladder carcinomas and, with radiation therapy, for curative treatment of anal carcinoma.

Mitoxantrone is a synthetic compound that was designed to recapitulate features of doxorubicin but with less cardiotoxicity. It is quantitatively less cardiotoxic (comparing the ratio of cardiotoxic to therapeutically effective doses), but its status in therapy is unclear as doses of 150 mg/m² have produced evidence of 10% incidence of cardiotoxicity; it also causes alopecia.

Etoposide was synthetically derived from the plant product podophyllotoxin; it binds directly to topoisomerase II and DNA in a reversible ternary complex. It stabilizes the covalent intermediate in the enzyme's action where the enzyme is covalently linked to DNA. This "alkali-labile" DNA bond was historically a first hint that an enzyme such as a topoisomerase might exist. The drug therefore causes a prominent G_2 arrest, reflecting the action of a DNA damage checkpoint. Prominent clinical effects include myelosuppression, nausea, and transient hypotension related to the speed of administration of the agent. Etoposide is a mild vesicant but is relatively free from other large-organ toxicities. Teniposide is a structural relative with unique activity in childhood acute lymphoid leukemia. When given at high doses or very frequently, topoisomerase inhibitors may cause acute leukemia associated with chromosome 11q23 abnormalities in up to 1% of exposed patients.

Camptothecin was isolated from extracts of a Chinese tree and had notable antileukemia activity. Early clinical studies with the sodium salt of the hydrolyzed camptothecin lactone showed evidence of toxicity with little antitumor activity. Identification of topoisomerase I as the target of camptothecins and the need to preserve lactone structure allowed additional efforts to identify active members of this series. Topoisomerase I is responsible for unwinding the DNA strand by introducing single strand breaks and allowing rotation of one strand about the other. In S-phase, topoisomerase I–induced breaks that are not promptly resealed lead to progress of the replication fork off the end of a DNA strand. The DNA damage is a potent signal for induction of apoptosis. Camptothecins promote the stabilization of the DNA linked to the enzyme in a so-called cleavable complex, analogous to the action of etoposide with topoisomerase II. Topotecan is a camptothecin derivative approved for use in ovarian tumors. Toxicity is limited to myelosuppression and mucositis. CPT-11, or irinotecan, is a camptothecin with evidence of activity in colon carcinoma. In addition to myelosuppression, it causes a secretory diarrhea, which can be treated effectively with loperamide or octreotide.

Indirect Effectors of DNA Function: Antimetabolites A broad definition of antimetabolites would include compounds with structural similarity to precursors of purines or pyrimidines or that interfere with purine or pyrimidine synthesis. Antimetabolites can cause DNA damage indirectly, through misincorporation into DNA, abnormal timing or progression through DNA synthesis, or altered function of pyrimidine and purine biosynthetic enzymes. They tend to convey greatest toxicity to cells in S-phase, and the degree of toxicity increases with duration of exposure. Common toxic manifestations include stomatitis, diarrhea, and myelosuppression. Second malignancies are not associated with their use.

Methotrexate inhibits dihydrofolate reductase, which regenerates reduced folates from the oxidized folates produced when thymidine monophosphate is formed from deoxyuridine monophosphate. Without reduced folates, cells die a "thymineless" death. N-5 tetrahydrofolate or N-5 formyltetrahydrofolate (leucovorin) can bypass this block and rescue cells from methotrexate, which is maintained in cells by polyglutamylation. The drug and other reduced folates are transported into cells by the folate carrier, and high concentrations of drug can bypass this carrier and allow diffusion of drug directly into cells. These properties have suggested the design of "high-dose" methotrexate regimens with leucovorin rescue of normal marrow and mucosa as part of curative approaches to osteosarcoma in the adjuvant setting and hematopoietic neoplasms of children and adults. Methotrexate is cleared by the kidney by both glomerular filtration and tubular secretion, and toxicity is augmented by renal dysfunction and drugs such as salicylates, probenecid, and nonsteroidal anti-inflammatory agents that undergo tubular secretion. With normal renal function, 15 mg/m² leucovorin will rescue 10^{-8} to 10^{-6} M methotrexate in three to four doses. However, with decreased creatinine clearance, doses of 50 to 100 mg/m² are continued until methotrexate levels are $<5 \times 10^{-8}$ M. In addition to bone marrow suppression and mucosal irritation, methotrexate can cause renal failure itself at high doses owing to crystallization in renal tubules; therefore high-dose regimens require alkalinization of urine with increased flow by hydration. Methotrexate can be sequestered in third space collections and leech back into the general circulation, causing prolonged myelosuppression. Less frequent adverse effects include reversible increases in transaminases and hypersensitivity-like pulmonary syndrome. Chronic low-dose methotrexate can cause hepatic fibrosis. When administered to the intrathecal space, methotrexate can cause chemical arachnoiditis and CNS dysfunction. Trimetrexate is a methotrexate derivative that is not polyglutamylated and does not use the reduced folate carrier.

5-Fluorouracil (5FU) represents an early example of "rational" drug design in that it originated from the observation that tumor cells incorporate radiolabeled uracil more efficiently into DNA than normal cells, especially gut. 5FU is metabolized in cells to 5′FdUMP, which inhibits thymidylate synthetase (TS). In addition, misincorporation can lead to single strand breaks, and RNA can aberrantly incorporate FUMP. 5FU is metabolized by dihydropyrimidine dehydrogenase, and deficiency of this enzyme can lead to excessive toxicity from 5FU. Oral bioavailability varies unreliably, but orally administered analogues of 5FU such as capecitabine have been developed that allow at least equivalent activity to many parenteral 5FU-based approaches to refractory cancers. Intravenous administration of 5FU leads to bone marrow suppression after short infusions but to stomatitis after prolonged infusions. Leucovorin augments the activity of 5FU by promoting formation of the ternary covalent complex of 5FU, the reduced folate, and TS. Less frequent toxicities include CNS dysfunction, with prominent cerebellar signs, and endothelial toxicity manifested by thrombosis, including pulmonary embolus and myocardial infarction.

Cytosine arabinoside (ara-C) is incorporated into DNA after formation of ara-CTP, resulting in S-phase-related toxicity. Continuous infusion schedules allow maximal efficiency, with uptake maximal at 5 to 7 μM. Ara-C can be administered intrathecally. Adverse effects include nausea, diarrhea, stomatitis, chemical conjunctivitis, and cerebellar ataxia. Gemcitabine is a cytosine derivative that is similar to ara-C in that it is incorporated into DNA after anabolism to the triphosphate, rendering DNA susceptible to breakage and repair synthesis, which differs from that in ara-C in that gemcitabine-induced lesions are very inefficiently removed. In contrast to ara-C, gemcitabine appears to have useful activity in a variety of solid tumors, with limited nonmyelosuppressive toxicities. 6-Thioguanine and 6-mercaptopurine (6MP) are used in the treatment of acute lymphoid leukemia. Although administered orally, they display variable bioavailability. 6MP is metabolized by xanthine oxidase and therefore requires dose reduction when used with allopurinol.

Fludarabine phosphate is a prodrug of F-adenine arabinoside (F-ara-A), which in turn was designed to diminish the susceptibility of ara-A to adenosine deaminase. F-ara-A is incorporated into DNA and can cause delayed cytotoxicity even in cells with low growth fraction, including chronic lymphocytic leukemia and follicular B cell lymphoma. CNS dysfunction and T cell depletion leading to opportunistic infections can occur in addition to myelosuppression. 2-Chlorodeoxyadenosine is a similar compound with activity in hairy cell leukemia. 2-Deoxycoformycin inhibits adenosine deaminase, with resulting increase in dATP levels. This causes inhibition of ribonucleotide reductase as well as augmented susceptibility to apoptosis, particularly in T cells. Renal failure and CNS dysfunction are notable toxicities in addition to immunosuppression.

Hydroxyurea inhibits ribonucleotide reductase, resulting in S-phase block. It is orally bioavailable and the drug of choice for the acute management of myeloproliferative states. Asparaginase is not classically considered an antimetabolite as it causes breakdown of extracellular asparagine required for protein synthesis in certain leukemic cells. However, it effectively stops DNA synthesis by preventing the requisite concurrent protein synthesis, and therefore it has a similar functional outcome as the classic antimetabolites. As asparaginase is a foreign protein, hypersensitivity reactions are common, as are effects on organs such as pancreas and liver that require continuing protein synthesis. This results in decreased insulin secretion with hyperglycemia, with or without hyperamylasemia and clotting function abnormalities. The latter may be associated with CNS and dural vein thrombosis.

Mitotic Spindle Inhibitors Microtubules are cellular structures that form the mitotic spindle and in interphase cells are responsible for the cellular "scaffolding" along which various motile and secretory processes occur. Microtubules are composed of repeating noncovalent multimers of a heterodimer of α and β subunits of the protein tubulin. Vincristine binds to the tubulin dimer with the result that microtubules are disaggregated. This results in the block of growing cells in M-phase; however, toxic effects in G_1 and S-phase are also evident. The drug is bound to blood-formed elements, leading to its occasional use as vinca-loaded platelets to treat autoimmune thrombocytopenia. The drug is metabolized by the liver, and dose adjustment in the presence of hepatic dysfunction is required. It is a powerful vesicant, and infiltration can be treated by local heat and infiltration of hyaluronidase. At clinically used intravenous doses, neurotoxicity in the form of glove-and-stocking neuropathy is frequent. Children tolerate 2 mg/m^2, but adult doses may be capped at 2 mg total to lower the incidence of disabling chronic neuropathy; whether this compromises needed dose intensity in curative regimens is uncertain. Acute neuropathic effects include jaw pain, paralytic ileus, urinary retention, and the syndrome of inappropriate antidiuretic hormone secretion. Myelosuppression is not seen. Vinblastine is similar to vincristine, except that it tends to be more myelotoxic, with more frequent thrombocytopenia and also mucositis and stomatitis. Vinorelbine is a vinca alkaloid that appears to have differences in resistance patterns in comparison to vincristine and vinblastine; it may be administered orally.

The taxanes include paclitaxel and docetaxel. These agents differ from the vinca alkaloids in that the taxanes stabilize microtubules against depolymerization. The "stabilized" microtubules function abnormally and are not able to undergo the normal dynamic changes of microtubule function necessary for cell cycle completion. Taxanes are among the most broadly active antineoplastic agents for use in solid tumors, with evidence of activity in ovarian cancer, breast cancer, Kaposi's sarcoma, and lung tumors. They are administered intravenously, and paclitaxel requires use of a cremophore-containing vehicle that can cause hypersensitivity reactions. Premedication with regimens including dexamethasone (20 mg orally or intravenously 12 and 6 h before treatment) and diphenhydramine (50 mg) and cimetidine (300 mg), both 30 min before treatment, decreases but does not eliminate the risk of hypersensitivity reactions to the paclitaxel vehicle. Docetaxel uses a polysorbate 80 formulation, which can cause fluid retention in addition to hypersensitivity reactions, and dexamethasone premedication with or without antihistamines is frequently used. Paclitaxel causes hypersensitivity reactions, myelosuppression, neurotoxicity in the form of glove-and-stocking numbness, and paresthesia. Cardiac rhythm disturbances were observed in phase I and II trials, most commonly asymptomatic bradycardia but also, much more rarely, varying degrees of heart block. These have not emerged as clinically significant in the majority of patients. Infrequently occurring evidence of myocardial ischemia during paclitaxel administration cannot yet be clearly related to the drug. Docetaxel causes comparable degrees of myelosuppression and neuropathy. Hypersensitivity reactions, including bronchospasm, dyspnea, and hypotension, are less frequent but occur to some degree in up to 25% of patients. Fluid reten-

tion appears to result from a vascular leak syndrome that can aggravate preexisting effusions. Rash can complicate docetaxel administration, appearing prominently as a pruritic maculopapular rash affecting the forearms, but it has also been associated with fingernail ridging, breakdown, and skin discoloration. Stomatitis appears to be somewhat more frequent than with paclitaxel.

Estramustine was originally synthesized as a mustard derivative that might be useful in neoplasms that possessed estrogen receptor sites. However, no evidence of interaction with DNA was observed. Surprisingly, the drug caused metaphase arrest, and subsequent study revealed that it binds to microtubule-associated proteins, resulting in abnormal microtubule function. Estramustine binds to estramustine-binding proteins (EMBP), which are notably present in prostate tumor tissue. The drug is used as an oral formulation in patients with prostate cancer. Gastrointestinal and cardiovascular adverse effects related to the estrogen moiety occur in up to 10% of patients, including worsened heart failure and thromboembolic phenomena. Gynecomastia and nipple tenderness can also occur.

Hormonal Agents The family of steroid hormone receptor–related molecules have emerged as prominent targets for small molecules useful in cancer treatment. When bound to their cognate ligands, these receptors can alter gene transcription and, in certain tissues, induce apoptosis. The pharmacologic effect is a mirror or parody of the normal effects of the agent acting in nontransformed tissue, although the effects on tumors are mediated by indirect effects in some cases.

Glucocorticoids are generally given in "pulsed" high-dose exposure in leukemias and lymphomas, where they induce apoptosis in tumor cells. Cushing's syndrome or inadvertent adrenal suppression on withdrawal from high-dose glucocorticoids can be significant complications, along with infections common in immunosuppressed patients, in particular *Pneumocystis* pneumonia, which classically appears a few days after completing a course of high-dose steroids. Tamoxifen is a partial estrogen receptor antagonist; it has a tenfold greater degree of antitumor activity in breast cancer patients whose tumors express estrogen receptors than in those who have low or no levels of expression. Side effects include a somewhat increased risk of estrogen-related cardiovascular complications, such as thromboembolic phenomena, and a small increased incidence of endometrial carcinoma, which appears after chronic use. Progestational agents including medroxyprogesterone acetate, androgens including fluoxymesterone (Halotestin), and, paradoxically, estrogens have approximately the same degeree of activity in primary hormonal treatment of breast cancers that have elevated expression of estrogen receptor protein. Estrogen is not used often owing to prominent cardiovascular and uterotropic activity.

Prostate cancer is classically treated by diethylstilbesterol (DES) acting as an estrogen at the level of the hypothalamus to downregulate hypothalamic luteinizing hormone (LH) production, resulting in decreased elaboration of testosterone by the testicle. For this reason, orchiectomy is equally as effective as moderate-dose DES, inducing responses in 80% of previously untreated patients with prostate cancer but without the prominent cardiovascular side effects of DES, including thrombosis and exacerbation of coronary artery disease. In the event that orchiectomy is not accepted by the patient, testicular androgen suppression can also be effected by luteinizing hormone–releasing hormone (LHRH) agonists such as leuprolide and goserelin. These agents cause tonic stimulation of the LHRH receptor, with the loss of its normal pulsatile activation resulting in its desensitization and decreased output of LH by the anterior pituitary. Therefore, as primary hormonal manipulation in prostate cancer one can choose orchiectomy or leuprolide, not both. The addition of actual antagonists of androgens acting at the androgen receptor, including flutamide or bicalutamide, is of uncertain additional benefit in extending overall response duration, but it clearly prevents the activation of androgen receptors by adrenal androgens, and the combined use of orchiectomy or leuprolide plus flutamide is referred to as "total androgen blockade."

Tumors that respond to a primary hormonal manipulation may frequently respond to second and third hormonal manipulations. Thus, breast tumors that had previously responded to tamoxifen have, on relapse, notable response rates to withdrawal of tamoxifen itself or to subsequent addition of a progestin. Likewise, initial treatment of prostate cancers with leuprolide plus flutamide may be followed after disease progression by response to withrawal of flutamide. These responses may result from the removal of antagonists from mutant steroid hormone receptors that have come to depend on the presence of the antagonist as a growth-promoting influence.

Additional strategies to treat refractory breast and prostate cancers that possess steroid hormone receptors may also address adrenal capacity to produce androgens and estrogens, even after orchiectomy or oophorectomy, respectively. Thus, aminoglutethimide or ketoconazole can be used to block adrenal synthesis by interfering with the enzymes of steroid hormone metabolism. Administration of these agents requires concomitant hydrocortisone replacement and additional glucocorticoid doses administered in the event of physiologic stress. Steroid hormone–inducing "aromatase" activity may be present in tumor tissue, and second- or third-line approaches to inhibition of aromatase activity may also be affected by such agents as anastrazole and letrozole. The toxicity profile and activity of the aromatase inhibitors make them candidates for first-line therapy for breast cancer.

Humoral mechanisms can also result in complications of an underlying malignancy. Adrenocortical carcinomas can cause Cushing's syndrome as well as syndromes of androgen or estrogen excess. Mitotane can counteract these by decreasing synthesis of steroid hormones. Islet cell neoplasms can cause debilitating diarrhea, treated with the somatostatin analogue octreotide. Prolactin-secreting tumors can be effectively managed by the dopaminergic agononist bromocriptine.

MOLECULARLY TARGETED THERAPIES　A better understanding of cancer cell biology has suggested many new targets for cancer drug discovery and development. These include the products of oncogenes and tumor-suppressor genes; regulators of cell death pathways; mediators of cellular immortality such as telomerase; and molecules responsible for microenvironmental molding such as proteases or angiogenic factors. The essential difference in the development of agents that would target these processes is that the basis for discovery of the candidate drug is the a priori importance of the target in the biology of the tumor, rather than the initial detection of drug candidates based on the phenomenon of tumor cell regression in tissue culture or in animals.

The most successful example of this class is imatinib mesylate (Gleevec). This protein kinase antagonist was selected as an inhibitor of the platelet-derived growth factor receptor (PDGFR) tyrosine kinase and was subsequently found to inhibit the bcr-abl kinase present in CML cells and reflecting the pathogenic t(9;22) chromosomal translocation in that tumor. It is also a potent inhibitor of the kit kinase originally defined as the stem cell factor receptor, a hematopoetic growth factor. Outstanding activity of imatinib has been noted in IFN-refractory CML with minimal toxicity, and it is also active in neoplasms driven by kit, such as gastrointestinal stromal sarcomas (GISTs), and by PDGFR, such as dermatofibrosarcoma protuberans. In each of these cases a clear link of the biology of the successfully treated neoplasm to the activity of the drug-susceptible target was a key factor in identifying patients who derived benefit from the drug.

Many classes of molecularly targeted small-molecule cancer therapeutics are under development or are in active clinical trials, including various protein kinase antagonists, farnesyltransferase antagonists originally designed to counter ras oncogene function, and protease inhibitors (Chap. 69). Many of these agents have not had evidence of frequent antitumor activity as single drugs in phase II trials. Their future use will likely depend on the evolution of more refined strategies to diagnose with accuracy the dependence of the tumor's biology on the presence of the drugs' targets. Alternatively, combinations of molecularly targeted agents with chemotherapeutic agents or with each other may evolve to address the multiplicity of genetic lesions present in solid tumors. These combinations will differ strategically from the approach used to evolve combinations of cytotoxic agents, which frequently combined agents with the same target, but which possessed differing toxicity. In contrast, combinations of molecularly targeted agents may address different pathways governing tumor biology in a manner more conceptually analogous to highly active antiretroviral therapy, where optimal disease suppression results from addressing two different gene products upon which successful viral replication depends.

An additional example related conceptually to molecularly targeted strategies is the use of retinoids, including tretinoin, the all-*trans*-isomer of retinoic acid, or isotretinoin, the 13-*cis* isomer of retinoic acid, to cause "differentiation" by acting on the retinoid receptor, a member of the steroid hormone receptor family. Leukemias and certain squamous neoplasms, including those of the skin and cervix, appear to be uniquely responsive in certain cases to retinoids. In particular, tretinoin is part of curative regimens for acute promyelocytic leukemia (APL) and appears to act by causing accelerated degradation of the fusion protein created by the t(15; 17) translocation that fuses the retinoic acid receptor α and the promyelocytic leukemia (PML) transcription factor. Acute side effects related to differentiation of promyelocytes to mature granulocytes may result in pulmonary symptoms related to granulocyte sequestration in the pulmonary vasculature; these are treated by respiratory support and glucocorticoids. This example also illustrates the important role of defining the molecular basis of empirical observations to refine a treatment strategy. Long before the definition of the t(15; 17)-derived fusion protein transcription factor now known to be the target of tretinoin, the growth and differentiation of certain leukemia cells including APL cells were known to be greatly influenced by retinoids. Empirical clinical trials of retinoids in China confirmed evidence of clinical activity of the agent before trials in the west. In this case, understanding the action of a drug led to the definition of the target. Another retinoid with activity in empirically driven clinical trials is the synthetic retinoid X receptor ligand bexarotene, which has noteworthy activity in cutaneous T cell lymphoma.

Whether derived by design a priori or through the explication of antiproliferative activity on the part of novel agents, the future will evolve additional classes of molecules whose targets are known to be causally related to neoplastic behavior. How to evaluate these agents efficiently and thoroughly is a current challenge. Empirical strategies treat a series of diseases with the novel agents without reference to the expression or activity of the target. Clinical utility dictates which agents move forward in development. While potentially inefficient, this approach has nonetheless yielded curative regimens in leukemias, lymphomas, germ cell neoplasms, and breast and colon tumors; e.g., when the latter two diseases are treated with chemotherapy after primary treatment of the local tumor with surgery and/or radiation therapy. Rigorously applied molecularly targeted development strategies, exemplified by imatinib's initial studies, would restrict drug use only to tumors with known activity or presence of the target. The former strategy risks inefficiency but is open to clinical observations that importantly influence development strategies. In all likelihood, a mix of empirical and targeted strategies will be of value in defining new, useful treatments for cancer. Examples of encouraging results of the empirical type include preliminary evidence of activity of bortezomib (Velcade), a proteosome inhibitor, in refractory multiple myeloma, and the epidermal growth factor receptor (EGFR) antagonist gefitinib (Iressa) in refractory lung cancer. Bortezomib was rationally designed to inhibit the proteosome, the multicomponent subcellular complex that degrades cell proteins as part of their normal turnover processes. The observation of activity in myeloma was an empirical outcome of a clinical trial. Likewise, simple expression of EGFR does not appear to uniquely correlate with gefitinib activity in patients with lung cancer. These examples highlight a difficulty in the more general use of molecularly targeted agents; specifically, how to select patients likely to respond to such agents. In many cases it is not obvious, as the relation of their target's action to the biologic success of the tumors in which they might be used is not clear. This is in contrast to conventional chemotherapeutic agents, where successful tumor growth obviously depends on DNA synthesis and microtubule function. These issues are very much a matter for current clinical and basic research.

An alternative way of thinking about molecularly targeted cancer therapeutics might recognize that there are actually many classes of cancer molecular targets. *Pathogenic targets* address the important events in the incidence and spread of a tumor; *differentiation-related targets* might reflect the tissue of origin; *pharmacological targets* would capitalize on intratumoral capacity to metabolize potentially active agents; *microenvironmental targets* would define processes important in molding stroma to allow successful blood supply and invasive properties. Drugs addressing all of these types of targets are in development. Certain "targeted toxins" exemplify some of these approaches. Targeted toxins utilize molecules with high affinity for defined tumor cell surface molecules, such as a leukemia differentiation antigen, to which a therapeutic antibody can deliver a covalently linked potent cytotoxin (e.g., gemtuzumab ozogamicin, a drug linked to anti-CD33), or a growth factor such as IL-2 to deliver a toxin (in the form of diphtheria toxin in denileukin diftitox) to cells bearing the IL-2 receptor. The value of such targeted approaches is that in addition to maximizing the therapeutic index by differential expression of the target in tumor (as opposed to nonrenewable normal cells), selection of patients for clinical trial and (perhaps eventually for routine clinical use) can capitalize on assessing the target in the tumor. The tools to accomplish this goal will include newer strategies to categorize tumors based on their biology rather than simply tissue of origin or histologic features.

ACUTE COMPLICATIONS OF CANCER CHEMOTHERAPY ■ Myelosuppression The
common cytotoxic chemotherapeutic agents almost invariably affect bone marrow function. Titration of this effect determines in many cases the MTD of the agent on a given schedule. The normal kinetics of blood cell turnover influence the sequence and sensitivity of each of the formed elements. Polymorphonuclear leukocytes (PMNs; $t_{1/2} =$ 6 to 8 h), platelets ($t_{1/2} = 5$ to 7 days), and red blood cells (RBCs; $t_{1/2} = 120$ days) have respectively most, less, and least susceptibility to usually administered cytotoxic agents. The nadir count of each cell type in response to classes of agents is characteristic. Maximal neutropenia occurs 6 to 14 days after conventional doses of anthracyclines, antifolates, and antimetabolites. Alkylating agents differ from each other in the timing of cytopenias. Nitrosoureas, DTIC, and procarbazine can display delayed marrow toxicity, first appearing 6 weeks after dosing.

Complications of myelosuppression result from the predictable sequelae of the missing cells' function. *Febrile neutropenia* refers to the clinical presentation of fever (one temperature $\geq 38.5°C$ or three readings $\geq 38°C$ but $\leq 38.5°C$ per 24 h) in a neutropenic patient with an uncontrolled neoplasm involving the bone marrow or, more usually, in a patient undergoing treatment with cytotoxic agents. Mortality from uncontrolled infection varies inversely with the neutrophil count. If the nadir neutrophil count is $>1000/\mu L$, there is little risk; if $<500/\mu L$, risk of death is markedly increased. Management of febrile neutropenia has conventionally included empirical coverage with antibiotics for the duration of neutropenia (Chap. 72). Selection of antibiotics is governed by the expected association of infections with certain underlying neoplasms; careful physical examination (with scrutiny of catheter sites, dentition, mucosal surfaces, and perirectal and genital orifices by gentle palpation); chest x-ray; and Gram stain and culture of blood, urine, and sputum (if any) to define a putative site of infection. In the absence of any originating site, a broadly acting β-lactam with anti-*Pseudomonas* activity, such as ceftazidime, is begun empirically. The addition of vancomycin to cover potential cutaneous sites of origin (until these are ruled out or shown to originate from methicillin-sensitive organisms) or metronidazole or imipenem for abdominal or other sites favoring anaerobes reflects modifications tailored to individual patient presentations. The coexistence of pulmo-

nary compromise raises a distinct set of potential pathogens, including *Legionella*, *Pneumocystis*, and fungal agents that may require further diagnostic evaluations such as bronchoscopy with bronchoalveolar lavage. Febrile neutropenic patients can be stratified broadly into two prognostic groups. The first, with expected short duration of neutropenia and no evidence of hypotension or abdominal or other localizing symptoms, may be expected to do well even with less complex, oral regimens, e.g., ciprofloxacin or amoxicillin and clavulinic acid. Detailed evaluation of such simple oral programs and intravenous regimens is ongoing. A less favorable prognostic group are patients with expected prolonged neutropenia, evidence of sepsis, and end-organ compromise, particularly pneumonia. These patients clearly require tailoring of their antibiotic regimen to their underlying presentation, with frequent empirical addition of antifungal agents if fever persists for 7 days without identification of an adequately treated organism or site.

Transfusion of granulocytes has no role in the management of febrile neutropenia, owing to their exceedingly short half-life, mechanical fragility, and clinical syndromes of pulmonary compromise with leukostasis after their use. Instead, colony-stimulating factors (CSFs) are used to augment bone marrow production of PMNs. These include early-acting factors such as IL-1, IL-3, and stem cell factor, which act on multiple lineages, and late-acting lineage-specific factors such as G-CSF (granulocyte colony-stimulating factor) or GM-CSF (granulocyte-macrophage colony-stimulating factor), erythropoietin, thrombopoietin, IL-6, and IL-11. CSFs are overused in oncology practice. The settings in which their use has been proved effective are limited. G-CSF, GM-CSF, erythropoietin, and IL-11 are currently approved for use. The American Society of Clinical Oncology has developed practice guidelines for the use of G-CSF and GM-CSF (Table 70-3). Primary administration (i.e., shortly after completing chemotherapy to reduce the nadir) of G-CSF to patients receiving cytotoxic regimens associated with a 40% incidence of febrile neutropenia has reduced the incidence of febrile neutropenia in several studies by about 50%. Most patients, however, receive regimens that do not have such a high risk of expected febrile neutropenia, and therefore most patients initially should not receive G-CSF or GM-CSF. Special circumstances such as a documented history of febrile neutropenia with the regimen in a particular patient; extensive compromise of marrow by prior radiation or chemotherapy; or active, open wounds or deep-seated infection may support primary treatment with G-CSF or GM-CSF. Administration of G-CSF or GM-CSF to afebrile neutropenic patients or to patients with low-risk febrile neutropenia as defined above is not recommended, although administration to high-risk patients with febrile neutropenia and evidence of organ compromise is reasonable. G-CSF or GM-CSF is conventionally started 24 to 72 h after completion of chemotherapy and continued until a PMN count of $10,000/\mu L$ is achieved. Also, patients with myeloid leukemias undergoing induction therapy may have a slight reduction in the duration of neutropenia if G-CSF (not GM-CSF) is commenced after completion of therapy and may be of particular value in elderly patients, but the influence on long-term outcome has not been defined. GM-CSF probably has a more restricted utility than G-CSF, with its use currently limited to patients after autologous bone marrow transplants, although proper head-to-head comparisons with G-CSF have not been conducted in most instances. GM-CSF may be associated with more systemic side effects.

Dangerous degrees of thrombocytopenia do not frequently complicate the management of patients with solid tumors receiving cytotoxic chemotherapy (with the possible exception of certain carboplatin-containing regimens), but they are frequent in patients with certain hematologic neoplasms where marrow is infiltrated with tumor. Severe bleeding related to thrombocytopenia occurs with increased frequency at platelet counts $<20,000/\mu L$ and is very prevalent at counts $<5000/\mu L$. Prophylactic transfusions to keep platelets $>20,000/\mu L$ are warranted in patients with leukemia (the threshold for transfusion is

TABLE 70-3 *Indications for the Clinical Use of G-CSF or GM-CSF*

Preventive Uses
With the first cycle of chemotherapy (so-called primary CSF administration)
  Not needed on a routine basis
  Use if the probability of febrile neutropenia is ≥40%
  Use if patient has preexisting neutropenia or active infection
With subsequent cycles if febrile neutropenia has previously occurred (so-called secondary CSF administration)
  Not needed after short duration neutropenia without fever
  Use if patient had febrile neutropenia in previous cycle
  Use if prolonged neutropenia (even without fever) delays therapy
Therapeutic Uses
Afebrile neutropenic patients
  No evidence of benefit
Febrile neutropenic patients
  No evidence of benefit
  May feel compelled to use in the face of clinical deterioration from sepsis, pneumonia, or fungal infection, but benefit unclear
To augment dose-intensity of chemotherapy in patients with curable malignancies
  No evidence of benefit
In bone marrow or peripheral blood stem cell transplantation
  Use to mobilize stem cells from marrow
  Use to hasten myeloid recovery
In acute myeloid leukemia
  G-CSF of minor or no benefit
  GM-CSF of no benefit and may be harmful
In myelodysplastic syndromes
  Not routinely beneficial
  Use intermittently in subset with neutropenia and recurrent infection
What Dose and Schedule Should Be Used?
G-CSF: 5 μg/kg per day subcutaneously
GM-CSF: 250 μg/m^2 per day subcutaneously
When Should Therapy Begin and End?
When indicated, start 24–72 h after chemotherapy
Continue until absolute neutrophil count is 10,000/μL
Do not use concurrently with chemotherapy or radiation therapy

Note: G-CSF, granulocyte colony-stimulating factor; GM-CSF, granulocyte-macrophage colony-stimulating factor.
Source: From the American Society of Clinical Oncology.

10,000/μL in patients with solid tumors and no other bleeding diathesis or physiologic stressors such as fever or hypotension). Careful review of medication lists to prevent exposure to nonsteroidal anti-inflammatory agents and maintenance of clotting factor levels adequate to support near-normal prothrombin and partial thromboplastin time tests are of import in minimizing the risk of bleeding in the thrombocytopenic patient. Certain cytokines in clinical investigation have shown ability to increase platelets (e.g., IL-6, IL-1, thrombopoietin), but clinical benefit and safety are not yet proven. IL-11 (oprelvekin) is approved for use in the setting of expected thrombocytopenia, but its effects on platelet counts are small and it is associated with side effects such as headache, fever, malaise, syncope, cardiac arrhythmias, and fluid retention.

Anemia associated with chemotherapy can be managed by transfusion of packed RBCs. Transfusion is not undertaken until the hemoglobin falls to <80 g/L (8 g/dL) or if compromise of end-organ function occurs or an underlying condition (e.g., coronary artery disease) calls for maintenance of hemoglobin >90 g/L (9 g/dL). Patients who are to receive therapy for >2 months on a "stable" regimen and who are likely to require continuing transfusions are also candidates for erythropoietin to maintain hemoglobin of 90 to 100 g/L (9 to 10 g/dL). In the setting of adequate iron stores and serum erythropoietin levels <100 ng/mL, erythropoietin, 150 U three times a week, can produce a slow increase in hemoglobin over about 2 months of administration. Depot formulations can be administered less frequently. It is unclear whether higher hemoglobin levels, up to 110 to 120 g/L (11 to 12 g/dL) are associated with improved quality of life to a degree that justifies the more intensive erythropoietin use. In addition, certain

treatment regimens, e.g., chemoradiation of cervix and head and neck neoplasms, may have enhanced likelihood of response in association with improved delivery of O_2. Evidence is emerging that erythropoietin may have undesirable effects in that it can rescue hypoxic cells from death. This may be a disadvantage in cancer but a great advantage in the setting of heart attacks and strokes.

Nausea and Vomiting The most common side effect of chemotherapy administration is nausea, with or without vomiting. Antineoplastic agents vary in their capacity to cause nausea and vomiting. Mechlorethamine, nitrosoureas, streptozotocin, DTIC, cisplatin, and actinomycin are highly emetogenic and produce vomiting in virtually all patients. Doxorubicin, daunorubicin, and conventional-dose cyclophosphamide are moderately emetogenic. Antimetabolites are dose- and schedule-dependent, with single doses of methotrexate and fluorouracil producing at worst anorexia; while 5-day regimens of 5FU and high-dose methotrexate produce nausea in ~50% of patients. Other agents such as chlorambucil, melphalan, and busulfan in conventional doses produce little tendency to emesis.

Emesis is a reflex caused by stimulation of the vomiting center in the medulla. Input to the vomiting center comes from the chemoreceptor trigger zone (CTZ) and afferents from the peripheral gastrointestinal tract, cerebral cortex, and heart. In addition, a conditioned reflex may contribute to anticipatory nausea arising after repeated cycles of chemotherapy. Accordingly, antiemesis agents differ in their locus of action. Combining agents from different classes or the sequential use of different classes of agent is the cornerstone of successful management of chemotherapy-induced nausea and vomiting. Of great importance are the prophylactic administration of agents and such psychological techniques as the maintenance of a supportive milieu, counseling, and relaxation to augment the action of antiemetic agents.

Antidopaminergic phenothiazines act directly at the CTZ and include prochlorperazine (Compazine), 10 mg intramuscularly or intravenously, 10 to 25 mg orally, or 25 mg per rectum every 4 to 6 h for up to four doses; and thiethylperazine (Torecan), 10 mg by potentially all the above routes every 6 h. Haloperidol (Haldol) is a butyrophenone dopamine antagonist given at 0.5 to 1.0 mg intramuscularly or orally every 8 h. Antihistamines such as diphenhydramine (Benadryl) have little intrinsic antiemetic capacity but are frequently given to prevent or treat dystonic reactions that can complicate use of the antidopaminergic agents. Lorazepam (Ativan) is a short-acting benzodiazepine that provides an anxiolytic effect to augment the effectiveness of a variety of agents when used at 1 to 2 mg intramuscularly, intravenously, or orally every 4 to 6 h. Dexamethasone (Decadron) likewise augments the action of a variety of agents when used at 4 to 40 mg intravenously or orally, given before treatment and repeated up to 10 mg orally every 6 h four times. Metoclopramide (Reglan) acts on peripheral dopamine receptors to augment gastric emptying and is used in high doses for highly emetogenic regimens (1 to 2 mg/kg intravenously 30 min before chemotherapy and every 2 h for up to three additional doses as needed); intravenous doses of 10 to 20 mg every 4 to 6 h as needed or 50 mg orally 4 h before and 8 and 12 h after chemotherapy are used for moderately emetogenic regimens. Serotonin antagonists are useful in moderately to severely emetogenic regimens; ondansetron (Zofran) is given as 0.15 mg/kg intravenously for three doses just before and at 4 and 8 h after chemotherapy, and granisetron (Kytril) is given as a single dose of 0.01 mg/kg just before chemotherapy. 5-9-Tetrahydrocannabinol (Marinol) is a rather weak antiemetic compared to other available agents, but it may be useful for persisting nausea and is used orally at 10 mg every 3 to 4 h as needed. Aprepitant is the first of a novel class of drugs, neurokinin receptor blockers; its addition to serotonin antagonists improves control of emesis against strongly emetogenic agents such as cisplatin. The usual dose is 125 mg orally on day 1, 80 mg orally on days 2 and 3.

Alopecia Chemotherapeutic agents vary widely in causing alopecia, with anthracyclines, alkylating agents, and topoisomerase inhibitors reliably causing near total alopecia when given at therapeutic doses. Antimetabolites are more variably associated with alopecia. Psychological support and the use of cosmetic resources are to be encouraged, and "chemo caps" that reduce scalp temperature to decrease the degree of alopecia should be discouraged, particularly during the treatment with curative intent of neoplasms such as leukemia, lymphoma, or in adjuvant breast cancer therapy. The richly vascularized scalp can certainly harbor micrometastatic or disseminated disease.

Gonadal Dysfunction and Pregnancy Cessation of ovulation and azoospermia reliably result from alkylating agent– and topoisomerase poison–containing regimens. The duration of these effects varies with age and sex. Males treated for Hodgkin's disease with mechlorethamine- and procarbazine-containing regimens are effectively sterile, whereas fertility usually returns after regimens including cisplatin, vinblastine, or etoposide and after bleomycin for testicular cancer. Sperm banking before treatment may be considered to support patients likely to be sterilized by treatment. Females experience amenorrhea with anovulation after alkylating agent therapy but are likely to recover normal menses if treatment is completed before age 30 and unlikely to recover menses after age 35. Even those who regain menses usually experience premature menopause. As the magnitude and extent of decreased fertility can be difficult to predict, patients should be counseled to maintain effective contraception, preferably by barrier means, during and after therapy. Resumption of efforts to conceive should be considered in the context of the likely prognosis of the patient. Hormone-replacement therapy should be undertaken in women who do not have a hormonally responsive tumor. For those patients who have had a hormone-sensitive tumor primarily treated by a local modality, conventional practice would counsel against hormone replacement, but this issue is very much a matter for current clinical investigations.

Chemotherapy agents have variable effects on the success of pregnancy (Chap. 6). All agents tend to have increased risk of adverse outcomes when administered during the first trimester, and strategies to delay chemotherapy, if possible, until after this milestone should be considered if the pregnancy is to continue to term. Patients in their second or third trimester can be treated with most regimens for the common neoplasms afflicting women in their child-bearing years with the exception of antimetabolites, particularly antifolates, which have notable teratogenic or fetotoxic effects throughout pregnancy. The need for anticancer chemotherapy per se is infrequently a clear basis to recommend termination of a concurrent pregnancy, although each treatment strategy in this circumstance must be tailored to the individual needs of the patient. →*Chronic effects of cancer treatment are reviewed in Chap. 89.*

BIOLOGIC THERAPY

No postulates resembling principles have emerged from efforts to develop biologic approaches to cancer treatment. The goal of biologic therapy is to manipulate the host-tumor interaction in favor of the host. Theoretically, biologic approaches should reflect a bell-shaped dose-response curve where the maximum biologic effect is less than the MTD. Empirical trial and error has led to the discovery that a number of biologic treatment approaches may produce antitumor effects, but nearly all of them are most active at their MTD. As a class, biologic therapies may be distinguished from molecularly targeted agents in that biologic therapies require an active response (e.g., reexpression of silenced genes) on the part of the tumor cell or on the part of the host (e.g., immunologic effects) to allow therapeutic effect. This may be contrasted with the antiproliferative or apoptotic response that is the ultimate goal of molecularly targeted agents discussed above. However, there is much commonality in the strategies to evaluate and use molecularly targeted and biologic therapies.

IMMUNE MEDIATORS OF ANTITUMOR EFFECTS The very existence of a cancer in a person is testimony to the failure of the immune system to deal effectively with the cancer. Tumors have a variety of means of avoiding the immune system: (1) they are often only subtly different from their normal counterparts; (2) they are capable of downregulating

their major histocompatibility complex antigens, effectively masking them from recognition by T cells; (3) they are inefficient at presenting antigens to the immune system; (4) they can cloak themselves in a protective shell of fibrin to minimize contact with surveillance mechanisms; and (5) they can produce a range of soluble molecules, including potential immune targets, that can distract the immune system from recognizing the tumor cell. Some of the cell products initially polarize the immune response away from cellular immunity (shifting from T_H1 to T_H2 responses; Chap. 295) and ultimately lead to defects in T cells that prevent their activation and cytotoxic activity. Cancer treatment further suppresses host immunity. A variety of strategies are being tested to overcome these barriers.

Cell-Mediated Immunity The strongest evidence that the immune system can exert clinically meaningful antitumor effects comes from allogeneic bone marrow transplantation. Adoptively transferred T cells from the donor expand in the tumor-bearing host, recognize the tumor as being foreign, and can mediate impressive antitumor effects (graft-versus-tumor effects). Three types of experimental interventions are being developed to take advantage of the ability of T cells to kill tumor cells.

1. Allogeneic T cells are being transferred to cancer-bearing hosts in three major settings: in the form of allogeneic bone marrow transplantation, as pure lymphocyte transfusions following bone marrow recovery after allogeneic bone marrow transplantation, and as pure lymphocyte transfusions following immunosuppressive (but not myeloablative) therapy (so-called minitransplants). In each of these settings, the effector cells are donor T cells that recognize the tumor as being foreign, probably through minor histocompatibility differences. The main risk of such therapy is the development of graft-versus-host disease because of the minimal difference between the cancer and the normal host cells. This approach has been highly effective in certain hematologic cancers.

2. Autologous T cells are being removed from the tumor-bearing host, manipulated in several ways in vitro, and given back to the patient. The two major classes of autologous T cell manipulation are (1) to develop tumor antigen–specific T cells and expand them to large numbers over many weeks ex vivo before administration, and (2) to activate the cells with polyclonal stimulators such as anti-CD3 and anti-CD28 after a short period ex vivo and try to expand them in the host after adoptive transfer with stimulation by IL-2, for example. Short periods removed from the patient permit the cells to overcome the tumor-induced T cell defects, and such cells traffic and home to sites of disease better than cells that have been in culture for many weeks. Individual centers have successful experiences with one or the other approach but not both, and whether one is superior to the other is not known.

3. Tumor vaccines are aimed at boosting T cell immunity. The finding that mutant oncogenes that are expressed only intracellularly can be recognized as targets of T cell killing greatly expanded the possibilities for tumor vaccine development. No longer is it difficult to find something different about tumor cells. However, major difficulties remain in getting the tumor-specific peptides presented in a fashion to prime the T cells. Tumors themselves are very poor at presenting their own antigens to T cells at the first antigen exposure (*priming*). Priming is best accomplished by professional antigen-presenting cells (dendritic cells). Thus, a number of experimental strategies are aimed at priming host T cells against tumor-associated peptides. Vaccine adjuvants such as GM-CSF appear capable of attracting antigen-presenting cells to a skin site containing a tumor antigen. Such an approach has been documented to eradicate microscopic residual disease in follicular lymphoma and give rise to tumor-specific T cells. Purified antigen-presenting cells can be pulsed with tumor, its membranes, or particular tumor antigens and delivered as a vaccine. Tumor cells can be transfected with genes that attract antigen-presenting cells. Other ideas are also being tested. In a variation on the theme of adop-

tive transfer, the tumor vaccine may be given to the normal bone marrow and lymphoid cell donor of an allogeneic transplant so that the donor immune system has more cells capable of recognizing the tumor specifically. Vaccines against viral cancers (papilloma virus in cervical cancer), lymphomas, and melanomas have had modest clinical success.

Antibodies In general, antibodies are not very effective at killing cancer cells. Because the tumor seems to influence the host toward making antibodies rather than generating cellular immunity, it is inferred that antibodies are easier for the tumor to fend off. Many patients can be shown to have serum antibodies directed at their tumors, but these do not appear to influence disease progression. However, the ability to grow very large quantities of high-affinity antibody directed at a tumor by the hybridoma technique has led to the application of antibodies to the treatment of cancer. The first study of a monoclonal antibody in cancer was published in 1980 and demonstrated many hurdles that needed to be overcome to make the approach successful. It seemed best to attack a determinant that was not shed or modulated by the tumor. A target that was involved in an important function for the tumor cells might be superior to a physiologically irrelevant target. Murine antibodies were not very effective because they did not mediate human effector mechanisms well and the host nearly always made antibodies against the therapeutic antibody that prevented it from finding the target.

The lessons were learned; humanized antibodies against the CD20 molecule expressed on B cell lymphomas (rituximab) and against the HER-2/*neu* receptor overexpressed on epithelial cancers, especially breast cancer (trastuzumab), have become reliable tools in the oncologists armamentarium. Each used alone can cause tumor regression (rituximab > trastuzumab), and both appear to potentiate the effects of combination chemotherapy given just after antibody administration. Antibodies to CD52 and vascular endothelial growth factor are active in chronic lymphoid leukemia and colon cancer, respectively. Conjugation of antibodies to drugs and toxins was discussed above, and conjugates of antibodies with isotopes, photodynamic agents, and other killing moieties may also be effective. Radioconjugates targeting CD20 on lymphomas have been approved for use [ibritumomab tiuxctan (Zevalin), using yttrium-90]. Other conjugates are associated with problems that have not yet been solved (e.g., antigenicity, instability, poor tumor penetration).

Cytokines There are >70 separate proteins and glycoproteins with biologic effects in humans: IFN-α, -β, -γ; IL-1 through -29 (so far); the TFN family [including lymphotoxin, TFN-related apoptosis-inducing ligand (TRAIL), CD40 ligand, and others]; and the chemokine family. Only a fraction of these has been tested against cancer; only IFN-α and IL-2 are in routine clinical use.

About 20 different genes encode IFN-α, and their biologic effects are indistinguishable. Interferon induces the expression of many genes, inhibits protein synthesis, and exerts a number of different effects on diverse cellular processes. Its antitumor effects appear to be antagonized in vitro by thymidine, suggesting that de novo thymidylate synthesis is also affected. The two recombinant forms that are commercially available are IFN-α2a and -α2b. In general, interferon antitumor effects are dose-related, and IFN is most effective at its MTD. Interferon is not curative for any tumor but can induce partial responses in follicular lymphoma, hairy cell leukemia, CML, melanoma, and Kaposi's sarcoma. It has been used in the adjuvant setting in stage II melanoma, multiple myeloma, and follicular lymphoma, with uncertain effects on survival. It produces fever, fatigue, a flulike syndrome, malaise, myelosuppression, and depression and can induce clinically significant autoimmune disease.

IL-2 must exert its antitumor effects indirectly through augmentation of immune function. Its biologic activity is to promote the growth and activity of T cells and natural killer (NK) cells. High doses of IL-2 can produce tumor regressions in certain patients with metastatic melanoma and renal cell cancer. About 2 to 5% of patients may experience complete remissions that are durable, unlike any other treatment for these tumors. IL-2 is associated with myriad clinical side effects: intravascular volume depletion, capillary leak syndrome, adult respiratory distress syndrome, hypotension, fever, chills, skin rash, and impaired renal and liver function. Patients may require blood pressure support and intensive care to manage the toxicity. However, once the agent is stopped, most of the toxicities reverse completely within 3 to 6 days.

GENE THERAPIES

No gene therapy has been approved for routine clinical use. Several strategies are under evaluation, including the use of viruses that cannot replicate to express genes that can allow the action of drugs or directly inhibit cancer cell growth; viruses that can actually replicate but only in the context of the tumor cell; or viruses that can express antigens in the context of the tumor and therefore provoke a host-mediated immune response. Key issues in the success of these approaches will be in defining safe viral vector systems that escape host immune function and effectively target the tumor or tumor cell milieu. Other gene therapy strategies would utilize therapeutic oligonucleoides to target the expression of genes important in the maintenance of tumor cell viability.

FURTHER READING

AMERICAN SOCIETY OF CLINICAL ONCOLOGY: Update of recommendations for use of hematopoietic colony-stimulating factors: Evidence-based clinical practice guidelines. J Clin Oncol 14:1957, 1996

CHABNER BA, LONGO DL (eds): *Cancer Chemotherapy and Biotherapy: Principles and Practice*, 3d ed. Philadelphia, Lippincott Williams & Wilkins, 2001

SAUSVILLE E et al: Signal transduction-directed cancer treatments. Annu Rev Pharmacol Toxicol 43:199, 2003

71 PRINCIPLES OF RADIATION THERAPY
Stephen M. Hahn, Eli Glatstein

All human beings are constantly exposed to ionizing radiation. Environmental sources include the cosmic radiation from space and radiation from the ground and from inhaled and ingested materials. Airline travel and mining both increase exposure to the background radiation. For example, air travel at 30,000 ft exposes individuals to a dose equivalent of 0.5 mrem/h. Radiation originating in the body comes mainly from radioactive potassium, which emits beta and gamma rays. Lungs are exposed to radiation from inhaled air, which contains small amounts of radioactive radon. Cosmic exposure contributes ~28 mrem per year. The ground and internal sources contribute ~26 and 27 mrem per year, respectively. The most prominent man-made sources of radiation include x-ray equipment, nuclear weapons, and radioactive medications.

TERMINOLOGY AND DEFINITIONS

The first major unit of radiation exposure was the roentgen (R), defined as an amount of x-rays or gamma rays that produces a specific amount of ionization in a unit of air under standard temperature and pressure (Table 71-1); this quantity can be measured directly in an ionization chamber. The rad (*radiation absorbed dose*) is defined as 100 ergs/g of tissue. Thus, the rad represents a net deposition of energy in a three-dimensional volume, because x-rays attenuate as they traverse tissue. The rad has been replaced by the Système Internationale (SI) unit of the gray (Gy), which represents 100 rad. Roentgens and rads can be

TABLE 71-1 *Units and Definitions*

Unit	Quantity Measured	Definition
Roentgen (R)	Exposure	Amount of x-rays or gamma rays that produces a specific amount of ionization in a given volume of air
Rad	Dose	100 ergs deposited per gram of tissue
Gray (Gy)	Dose	SI unit of dose; equals 100 rad
Rem	Dose equivalence	Unit that reflects the biologic response. It is used to compare various types of radiation
Sievert (Sv)	Dose equivalence	SI unit of dose equivalence; equals 100 rem

converted by means of various tables; the relation between them depends on photon energy.

The above definitions reflect physical variables. The unit that reflects the biologic response and that can be used to compare the effects of various types of radiation is the unit of dose equivalence, the rem (*r*oentgen *e*quivalent in *m*an). The rem has been replaced by the SI unit, the sievert (Sv), which equals 100 rem. These units reflect the exposure or absorption dose multiplied by a biologic factor that represents the biologic effectiveness of the specific type of radiation (see below).

TYPES OF IONIZING RADIATION

The absorption of energy from radiation in tissue often leads to excitation or ionization. Excitation involves elevation of an electron in an atom or molecule to a higher energy state without actual ejection of the electron. Ionization involves actual ejection of one or more electrons from the atom. Ionizing radiation is subclassified as electromagnetic (photon) or particulate radiation (Table 71-2). X-rays and gamma rays are examples of electromagnetic photon radiation; they differ only in their source. X-rays are produced mechanically, by making electrons strike a target, which causes the electrons to give up their kinetic energy as x-rays, while gamma rays are produced by nuclear disintegration of radioactive isotopes.

X-rays can be thought of as packets of energy, or photons. X-rays have no mass or charge, travel in straight lines, and attenuate continuously as they traverse tissue. Gamma rays have similar properties. Each photon contains an amount of energy equal to $h\nu$, where h is Planck's constant and ν is the radiation frequency. The critical difference between nonionizing and ionizing radiation is the energy of individual photons, not the energy of the total dose.

Types of *particulate radiation* include electrons, protons, alpha particles, neutrons, negative pi-mesons, and heavy charged ions; these have discrete mass and charge (except for neutrons, which lack charge;

TABLE 71-2 *Common Types of Ionizing Radiation*

Type	Mass	Charge	Comment
Electromagnetic			
X-ray	0	0	X-rays and gamma rays do not differ except in the source. Gamma rays are produced intranuclearly, and x-rays are produced extranuclearly (i.e., mechanically).
Gamma ray	0	0	
Particulate			
Electron (e)	9.1×10^{-31} kg	−1	—
Proton (p)	$2000 \times e$	+1	Exhibits a Bragg peak
Neutron (n)	$2000 \times e$	0	Cannot be accelerated by an electrical field
Alpha particle	$2p + 2n$ $\sim 8000 \times e$	+2	Helium nucleus

Table 71-2). *Electrons*, or *beta particles*, are small and negatively charged and can be accelerated to close to the speed of light. They decelerate fairly rapidly in tissue and penetrate it to only a limited depth. Thus, electron beams are often used to treat superficial problems. *Protons* are positively charged and have a mass about 2000 times that of an electron. Protons stop abruptly, depending on their energy; in the process of sudden deceleration, most of their energy is given up, which tends to cause ionization just before the proton stops. This region of enhanced ionization, sometimes called the Bragg peak, means that proton beams exert their effects in a relatively compact region. Therefore, protons may have advantages over other types of particulate radiation with respect to conforming the dose to the treatment volume. *Alpha particles* are helium nuclei, consisting of two protons and two neutrons. The mass and charge are great enough that these particles do not penetrate far through matter unless they have tremendous energy; even a piece of paper is enough to protect against most alpha particles. Because these particles are charged, they can be accelerated in electrical fields.

Neutrons are similar in mass to protons (having an atomic mass of 1), but they are not charged and therefore cannot be accelerated in an electrical field. Neutron beams are produced by colliding charged particles into a suitable target or are emitted as a fission product of heavy radioactive atoms. *Heavy charged ions* are nuclei of heavier elements that have a positive charge owing to the stripping away of some or all of the orbiting electrons.

Equal doses of different types of radiation do not necessarily produce equal biologic effects; thus 1 Gy of neutrons produces a greater biologic effect than 1 Gy of x-rays. The biologic effects produced by a given dose of radiation can be quantified by the relative biologic effectiveness (RBE) value, which relates them to the effects produced by 250-keV photon radiation as a standard. In general, the greater the RBE value for a given type of radiation, the greater the biologic effect. The RBE value will be greater for more densely ionizing radiation, such as neutrons. The RBE value depends on the linear energy transfer (see below), the dose, the dose rate, and the nature of the biologic system.

The linear energy transfer (LET) is the amount of ionization occurring per unit length of the radiation track. It is usually expressed as kilovolts per micron and increases with the square of the charge of the incident particle. High-LET radiation is biologically different from low-LET (i.e., conventional) radiation: Hypoxic and oxygenated cells respond similarly to high-LET irradiation, whereas it takes about three times as much low-LET radiation to produce a given killing effect in hypoxic cells as in oxygenated cells. It is thought that low-LET radiation must produce multiple hits on DNA to destroy a cell, whereas high-LET radiation need produce only a single hit on DNA to kill a cell. Representative values of LET and RBE are given in Table 71-3.

Radiation, especially x-rays, is absorbed and causes ionization in three major ways: the *photoelectric effect*, the *Compton effect*, and *pair production*. At low energies (30 to 100 keV), as in diagnostic radiology, the photoelectric effect is important. In this process, the incident photon interacts with an electron in one of the outer shells of an atom (typically K, L, or M). If the energy of the photon is greater than the

TABLE 71-3 *Linear Energy Transfer and Relative Biologic Effectiveness Values*

Type of Radiation	LET Values, keV/μm
Cobalt-60 gamma rays	0.2
250-keV x-rays	2.0
10 MeV protons	4.7

Type of Radiation	RBE Values (Quality Factors)
X-rays, gamma rays, and electrons	1
Neutrons	3–20
Heavy particles	1–20

FIGURE 71-1 Shape of survival curve for mammalian cells exposed to radiation. The fraction of cells surviving is plotted on a logarithmic scale against dose on a linear scale. For alpha particles or low-energy neutrons (said to be densely ionizing), the dose-response curve is a straight line from the origin (i.e., survival is an exponential function of dose). The survival curve can be described by just one parameter, the slope. For x-rays or gamma rays (said to be sparsely ionizing), the dose-response curve has an initial linear slope, followed by a shoulder; at higher doses the curve tends to become straight again. A. The experimental data are fitted to a linear-quadratic function. There are two components of cell killing: one is proportional to dose (αD), while the other is proportional to the square of the dose (βD^2). The dose at which the linear and quadratic components are equal is the ratio α/β. The linear-quadratic curve bends continuously but is a good fit to experimental data for the first few decades of survival. B. The curve is described by the initial slope (D_1), the final slope (D_0), and a parameter that represents the width of the shoulder, either n or D_q. (From Hall, with permission.)

binding energy of the electron, then the electron is expelled from the orbit with a kinetic energy that is equal to the energy of the incident photon minus the binding energy of the electron. The photoelectric effect varies as a function of the cube of the atomic number of the material exposed (Z^3); this fact explains why bone is visualized much better than soft tissue on radiographs.

At higher energies, as used in therapeutic radiology, the Compton effect dominates. In this process, the incident photon interacts with an electron in an orbital shell. Part of the incident photon energy appears as kinetic energy of electrons, and the residual energy continues as a less energetic deflected photon.

At energy levels >1.02 MeV, the photons may be absorbed through pair production. In this process, both a positron and an electron are produced in the absorbing material. A positron has the same mass as an electron but has a positive instead of a negative charge. The positron travels a very short distance in the absorbing medium before it interacts with another electron. When that happens, the entire mass of both particles is converted to energy, with the emission of two photons in exactly opposite directions.

BIOLOGIC EFFECTS OF RADIATION

Radiation must produce double-strand breaks in DNA to kill a cell, owing partly to the high capacity of mammalian cells for repairing single-strand damage. Radiation can also produce effects indirectly by interacting with water (which makes up ~80% of a cell's volume) to generate free radicals, which can damage the cell. Free radicals are highly reactive chemical entities that lack a stable number of outer-shell electrons. A free radical is not stable and has a life span of a fraction of a second. It is estimated that most x-ray-induced cell damage is due to the formation of hydroxyl radicals, as follows:

$$Ionizing\ radiation + H_2O \rightarrow H_2O^+ + e^-$$
$$H_2O^+ + H_2O \rightarrow H_3O^+ + OH\bullet$$
$$OH\bullet \rightarrow Cell\ damage$$

The usual end result of radiation damage is cell death. The biologic effects on epithelial cell reproduction are typically expressed only when the damaged cells attempt to divide. Another biologic effect is the induction of cancerous growth by mutation many years after ra-

diation exposure. Patients who receive radiation have a significant risk of neoplasm for at least two to three decades after their exposure; this risk is significantly higher than that of the population as a whole.

RADIATION-INDUCED CHROMOSOME ABERRATIONS

Chromosome breaks can occur when cells are irradiated. The broken ends of chromosomes can combine with broken ends of different chromosomes. These abnormal combinations are most readily seen during mitosis. Chromosome abnormalities typically occur in cells irradiated in the G_1 phase of the cell cycle, before the doubling of genetic material. If cells are irradiated in the G_2 phase, chromatid aberrations may result. The frequency of chromosomal aberrations in peripheral circulating lymphocytes can be used to correlate with the total body dose received. The dose can be estimated by comparing the chromosomal changes to in vitro cultures exposed to controlled doses of irradiation. The minimum dose that can be detected by peripheral lymphocyte analysis is about 0.1 to 0.2 Sv (10 to 20 rem). Lymphocyte analysis may provide evidence of recent total-body exposure.

CELL SURVIVAL CURVE The dose-response curve for all mammalian cells appears to have a linear-quadratic relationship. In simple terms, the mathematical model that explains the relationship between the dose and the fraction of surviving cells has both linear and exponential components. The linear component results from double-stranded chromosomal breaks produced by single hits. The exponential component represents breaks produced by multiple hits. Figure 71-1 shows the shape of a typical survival curve for mammalian cells exposed to radiation. The fraction of cells surviving is plotted on a semilogarithmic scale. For x-rays or gamma rays, the dose-response curve has a shoulder that is followed by a straight line curve as the dose is increased. The shoulder appears to represent the cell's ability to repair sublethal injury. For alpha particles or lower energy neutrons, the dose-response curve is a straight line from the origin. Thus, the survival rate is an exponential function of the dose.

In all mammalian cell lines studied, increases in the radiation dose decrease the survival rate of cells. However, a number of factors may contribute to a reduced sensitivity to radiation in human tumors in vivo, including extrinsic factors such as hypoxia and intrinsic factors such as expression of particular oncogenes, including *ras*. The biologic basis for this altered sensitivity to radiation has not been fully defined.

Four important processes that occur after radiation exposure can be summarized as the "four R's" of radiobiology. The first is *repair*. Repair is temperature dependent and is thought to represent the enzymatic mechanisms for healing intracellular injury. The second R is *reoxygenation*, a process whereby oxygen (and other nutrients) are actually better distributed to viable cells following radiation injury and cell killing. The third R is *repopulation*, the ability of the cell population to continue to divide and to replace dying and dead cells. The fourth R is *redistribution*, which reflects the variability of a cell's radiosensitivity over the cell cycle. Radiosensitivity can vary through the cell cycle by as much as a factor of 3. The G_1 phase has the most variable length of all the phases of the cell cycle. For most cell lines, cells that have a short G_1 period are most sensitive at the G_2/mitosis interface, less sensitive in G_1, and most resistant toward the end of the synthesis (S) period.

Radiation therapy is effective in cancer treatment when it exerts greater cytotoxic effects on tumor cells than on normal tissues (i.e., improving the therapeutic index). A major determinant of the therapeutic index is exploiting differences in the four R's between tumor cells and normal tissues. Fractionated radiation exploits differences in the four R's between tumor and normal tissues, thereby improving the therapeutic index.

NORMAL TISSUE EFFECTS OF RADIATION Therapeutic radiation leads to acute effects that typically manifest during treatment and resolve a few weeks after the completion of therapy. Late effects are also produced by radiotherapy and typically do not occur until several months or years after treatment is delivered. The clinical response to radiation may be related to the interactions of various growth factors and cytokines. For example, radiation can induce growth factors and cytokines such as tumor necrosis factor (TNF) and interleukin (IL) 1. TNF can induce proliferation of fibroblasts and enhance the inflammatory response. TNF and IL-1 have been shown to radioprotect hematopoietic cells in vitro by increasing the D_0 of the cell survival curve (Fig. 71-1). TNF also enhances killing of a human tumor cell line by irradiation. TNF may produce radioprotection or radiosensitization, depending on the cell type. Efforts to modulate radiation effects with TNF remain experimental. Other factors implicated in the radiation response are basic fibroblast growth factor and platelet-derived growth factor β, which may be associated with late effects of radiation on vessels.

The degree and the duration of functional recovery of normal tissues are related to the number of stem cells surviving after irradiation. If the stem cells are destroyed in the irradiated volume and replacement from adjacent tissues is inadequate, radiation injury will persist, causing late toxic effects. True late effects develop independent of early reactions; they may also occur despite recovery from acute radiation injury.

Table 71-4 shows the frequency of radiation tolerance seen with fractionated radiotherapy at 5 years of follow-up. These numbers are rough estimates at best. The clinical manifestations of irradiation will depend on the volume of the organ irradiated, the total dose, the dose per fraction, and the length of time taken to deliver the dose, and probably genetic/biologic factors. Dose per fraction is the most important factor determining normal tissue effects. This is why daily fractionation doses of 180 cGy to 200 cGy are used in most curative treatment situations. In addition, the cellular consequences of treatment can be progressive over time. Thus, length of follow-up is also crucial in judging late clinical sequelae from radiation.

THERAPEUTIC RADIATION Radiation therapy is a physical form of treatment that damages any tissue in its path. In the target tissue, radiation damages DNA (usually single-strand breaks) and generates free radi-

cals from cell water that are capable of damaging cell membranes, proteins, and organelles. Radiation damage is dependent on oxygen; hypoxic cells are more resistant. Augmentation of oxygen is the basis for radiation sensitization. Sulfhydryl compounds interfere with free radical generation and may act as radiation protectors. The challenge for radiation treatment planning is to deliver the radiation to the tumor volume with as little normal tissue in the field as possible.

Therapeutic radiation is delivered in three ways: *teletherapy*, with beams of radiation generated at a distance and aimed at the tumor within the patient; *brachytherapy*, with encapsulated sources of radiation implanted directly into or adjacent to tumor tissues; and *systemic therapy*, with radionuclides targeted in some fashion to a site of tumor. Teletherapy is the most commonly used form of radiation therapy.

Radiation from any source decreases in intensity as a function of the square of the distance from the source (inverse square law). Thus, if the radiation source is 5 cm above the skin surface and the tumor is 5 cm below the skin surface, the intensity of radiation in the tumor will be $5^2/10^2$, or 25% of the intensity at the skin. By contrast, if the radiation source is moved to 100 cm from the patient, the intensity of radiation in the tumor will be $100^2/105^2$, or 91% of the intensity at the skin. Teletherapy maintains intensity over a larger volume of target tissue by increasing the source-to-surface distance. In brachytherapy, the source-to-surface distance is small; thus, the effective treatment volume is small.

X-rays and gamma rays are the forms of radiation most commonly used to treat cancer. They are both electromagnetic, nonparticulate waves that cause the ejection of an orbital electron when absorbed. This orbital electron ejection is called *ionization*. X-rays are generated by linear accelerators; gamma rays are generated from decay of atomic nuclei in radioisotopes such as cobalt and radium. These waves behave biologically as packets of energy, called *photons*. Particulate forms of radiation are also used in certain circumstances. Electron beams have a very low tissue penetrance and are used to treat skin conditions such as mycosis fungoides. Neutron beams may be somewhat more effective than x-rays in treating salivary gland tumors. However, aside from these specialized uses, particulate forms of radiation such as neutrons, protons, and negative mesons, which should do more tissue damage because of their higher LET and be less dependent on oxygen, have not yet found wide applicability to cancer treatment.

A number of parameters influence the damage done to tissue by radiation. Hypoxic cells are relatively resistant. Nondividing cells are more resistant than dividing cells. In addition to these biologic parameters, physical parameters of the radiation are also crucial. The energy of the radiation determines its ability to penetrate tissue. Low-energy orthovoltage beams (150 to 400 kV) scatter when they strike the body, much like light diffuses when it strikes particles in the air. Such beams result in more damage to adjacent normal tissues and less radiation delivered to the tumor. Megavoltage radiation (>1 MeV) has very low lateral scatter; this produces a skin-sparing effect, more homogeneous distribution of the radiation energy, and greater deposit of the energy in the tumor, or *target volume*. The tissues that the beam passes through to get to the tumor are called the *transit volume*. The maximum dose in the target volume is often the cause of complications to tissues in the transit volume, and the minimum dose in the target volume influences the likelihood of tumor recurrence. Dose homogeneity in the target volume is the goal.

Radiation is quantitated on the basis of the amount of radiation absorbed in the patient, not based upon the amount of radiation generated by the machine. Radiation dose is measured by placing detectors at the body surface or calculating the dose based on radiating phantoms that resemble human form and substance. Radiation dose has three determinants: total absorbed dose, number of fractions, and time. A frequent error is to omit the number of fractions and the duration of treatment. This is analogous to saying that a runner completed a race in 20 s; without knowing how far he or she ran, the result is difficult to interpret. The time could be very good for a 200-m race or very

TABLE 71-4 *Class 1 Organs: Fatal or Severe Morbidity Following Cumulative Doses of Radiation Delivered with Standard Fractionation*

Organ	Injury	$TD_{5/5}$[a]	$TD_{50/5}$[b]	Whole or Partial Organ (Field Size or Length)
Bone marrow	Aplasia, pancytopenia	250	450	Whole
		3000	4000	Segmental
Liver	Acute and chronic hepatitis	2500	4000	Whole
		1500	2000	Whole (strip)
Stomach	Perforation, ulcer, hemorrhage	4500	5500	100 cm
Intestine	Ulcer, perforation, hemorrhage	4500	5500	400 cm
		5000	6500	100 cm
Brain	Infarction, necrosis	5000	6000	Whole
Spinal cord	Infarction, necrosis	4500	5500	10 cm
Heart	Pericarditis, pancarditis	4500	5500	60%
		7000	8000	25%
Lung	Acute and chronic pneumonitis	3000	3500	100 cm
		1500	2500	Whole
Kidney	Acute and chronic nephrosclerosis	1500	2000	Whole (strip)
		2000	2500	Whole
Fetus	Death	200	400	Whole

[a] $TD_{5/5}$ is the minimal tolerance dose—the dose that, when administered to a given patient population under a standard set of treatment conditions, results in a rate of severe complications of 5% or less within 5 years of treatment.

[b] $TD_{50/5}$ is the maximal tolerance dose—the dose that, when administered to a given population under a standard set of treatment conditions, results in a rate of severe complications of 50% within 5 years of treatment.

Source: From P Rubin et al (eds): *Radiation Biology and Radiation Pathology Syllabus*, set RT 1: *Radiation Oncology*. Chicago, American College of Radiology, 1975.

poor for a 100-m race. Thus, a typical course of radiation therapy should be described as 4500 cGy delivered to a particular target (e.g., mediastinum) over 5 weeks in 180-cGy fractions. Most curative radiation treatment programs are delivered once a day, 5 days a week in 150- to 200-cGy fractions.

Although radiation can interfere with many cellular processes, many experts feel that a cell must undergo a double-strand DNA break from radiation in order to be killed. The factors that influence tumor cell killing include the D_0 of the tumor (the dose required to deliver an average of one lethal hit to all the cells in a population), the D_q of the tumor (the threshold dose—a measure of the cell's ability to repair sublethal damage), hypoxia, tumor mass, growth fraction, and cell cycle time and phase (cells in late G_1 and S are more resistant). Rate of clinical response is not predictive; some cells do not die after radiation exposure until they attempt to replicate.

Compounds that incorporate into DNA and alter its stereochemistry (e.g., halogenated pyrimidines, cisplatin) augment radiation effects. Hydroxyurea, another DNA synthesis inhibitor, also potentiates radiation effects. Compounds that deplete thiols (e.g., buthionine sulfoximine) can also augment radiation effects. Hypoxia is a major factor that interferes with radiation effects.

APPLICATION TO PATIENTS ■ **Teletherapy** Radiation therapy can be used alone or together with chemotherapy to produce cure of localized tumors and control of the primary site of disease in tumors that have disseminated. Therapy is planned based on the use of a simulator with the treatment field or fields designed to accommodate an individual patient's anatomic features. Individualized treatment planning employs lead shielding tailored to shape the field and limit the radiation exposure of normal tissue. Often the radiation is delivered from two or three different positions. Conformal three-dimensional treatment planning permits the delivery of higher doses of radiation to the target volume without increasing complications in the transit volume.

Radiation therapy is a component of curative therapy for a number of diseases including breast cancer, Hodgkin's disease, head and neck cancer, prostate cancer, and gynecologic cancers. Radiation therapy can also palliate disease symptoms in a variety of settings: relief of bone pain from metastatic disease, control of brain metastases, reversal of spinal cord compression and superior vena caval obstruction, shrinkage of painful masses, and opening threatened airways. In high-risk settings, radiation therapy can prevent the development of leptomeningeal disease and brain metastases in acute leukemia and lung cancer.

Brachytherapy Brachytherapy involves placing a sealed source of radiation into or adjacent to the tumor and withdrawing the radiation source after a period of time precisely calculated to deliver a chosen dose of radiation to the tumor. This approach is often used to treat brain tumors and cervical cancer. The difficulty with brachytherapy is the short range of radiation effects (the inverse square law) and the inability to shape the radiation to fit the target volume. Normal tissue may receive substantial exposure to the radiation, with attendant radiation enteritis or cystitis in cervix cancer or brain injury in brain tumors.

Radionuclides and Radioimmunotherapy Nuclear medicine physicians or radiation oncologists may administer radionuclides with therapeutic effects. Iodine 131 is used to treat thyroid cancer as iodine is naturally taken up preferentially by the thyroid. It emits gamma rays that destroy the normal thyroid as well as the tumor. Strontium 89 and samarium 153 are two radionuclides that are preferentially taken up in bone, particularly sites of new bone formation. Both are capable of controlling bone metastases and the pain associated with them, but the dose-limiting toxicity is myelosuppression.

Monoclonal antibodies and other ligands can be attached to radioisotopes by conjugation (for nonmetal isotopes) or by chelation (for metal isotopes), and the targeting moiety can result in the accumulation of the radionuclide preferentially in tumor. Iodine 131–labeled anti-CD20 and yttrium 90–labeled anti-CD20 are active in B cell lymphoma, and other labeled antibodies are being evaluated. Thyroid uptake of labeled iodine is blocked by cold iodine. Dose-limiting toxicity is myelosuppression.

Photodynamic Therapy Some chemical structures (porphyrins, phthalocyanines) are selectively taken up by cancer cells by mechanisms not fully defined. When light, usually delivered by a laser, is shone on cells containing these compounds, free radicals are generated and the cells die. Hematoporphyrins and light are being used with increasing frequency to treat skin cancer; ovarian cancer; and cancers of the lung, colon, rectum, and esophagus. Palliation of recurrent locally advanced disease can sometimes be dramatic and last many months.

TOXICITY Though radiation therapy is most often administered to a local region, systemic effects, including fatigue, anorexia, nausea, and vomiting, may develop related in part to the volume of tissue irradiated, dose fractionation, radiation fields, and individual susceptibility. Bone is among the most radioresistant organs, radiation effects being manifested mainly in children through premature fusion of the epiphyseal growth plate. By contrast, the male testis, female ovary, and bone marrow are the most sensitive organs. Any bone marrow in a radiation field will be eradicated by therapeutic irradiation. Organs with less need for cell renewal, such as heart, skeletal muscle, and nerves, are more resistant to radiation effects. In radiation-resistant organs, the vascular endothelium is the most sensitive component. Organs with more self-renewal as a part of normal homeostasis, such as the hematopoietic system and mucosal lining of the intestinal tract, are more sensitive. Acute toxicities include mucositis, skin erythema (ulceration in severe cases), and bone marrow toxicity. Often these can be alleviated by interruption of treatment.

Chronic toxicities are more serious. Radiation of the head and neck region often produces thyroid failure. Cataracts and retinal damage can lead to blindness. Salivary glands stop making saliva, which leads to dental caries and poor dentition. Taste and smell can be affected. Mediastinal irradiation leads to a threefold increased risk of fatal myocardial infarction. Other late vascular effects include chronic constrictive pericarditis, lung fibrosis, viscus stricture, spinal cord transection, and radiation enteritis. A serious late toxicity is the development of second solid tumors in or adjacent to the radiation fields. Such tumors can develop in any organ or tissue and occur at a rate of about 1% per year beginning in the second decade after treatment. Some organs vary in susceptibility to radiation carcinogenesis. Women under age 30 experience a ≥100-fold increase in the incidence of breast cancer after chest or mantle-field radiation; women treated after age 30 have little or no increased risk of breast cancer. No data suggest that a threshold dose of therapeutic radiation exists below which the incidence of second cancers is decreased. High rates of second tumors have been documented in people who receive as little as 1000 cGy.

Central Nervous System Traditionally, the central nervous system (CNS) has been described as relatively resistant to radiation-induced changes. When the human brain is treated with standard fractionation (180 to 200 cGy/d), acute reactions are seldom observed.

Subacute CNS reactions to radiation treatment are more common. The clinical manifestations may include *Lhermitte's sign*, which is a self-limited paresthesia occurring with flexion of the neck. It is believed to be due to transient demyelination of the spinal cord following significant radiation exposure. It can be seen 1 to 3 months after completion of radiation treatment to the spinal cord. The frequency of Lhermitte's sign varies according to the type of radiation therapy and has been reported to be as high as 15% after mantle-field radiation. Mild encephalopathy and focal neurologic changes can also occur after irradiation limited to the cranium. If radiation treatments to the brain are given at the same time that chemotherapeutic agents are administered, the effects can be more severe, presumably reflecting altered permeability to the drugs. The effect of cranial irradiation is believed to be secondary to radiation effects on the replicating oligodendrocytes and possibly on the microvasculature. Both clinical and radiologic changes may simulate tumor progression and can often pose diagnostic and treatment dilemmas. A typical example of this kind of conundrum would be attempting to distinguish clinically between radionecrosis and recurrent tumor in patients with gliomas after radiotherapy.

Postirradiation pathology and associated clinical symptoms typically begin 6 to 36 months after radiation therapy and are related to the total dose and volume treated. Fraction size appears to be the most important variable affecting the rate of postirradiation brain necrosis. Neurocognitive changes can also be seen in children after cranial irradiation. The important pretreatment factors that predict the degree of late CNS effects include the age of the patient when cranial irradiation was given and neurocognitive functional level at the time of treatment.

A unique late effect of cranial irradiation combined with chemotherapy, known as *leukoencephalopathy*, has been described in some patients. Leukoencephalopathy is a necrotizing reaction usually noted 4 to 12 months after combined treatment with methotrexate and cranial irradiation. Dementia and dysarthria are often observed and may progress to seizures, ataxia, or death.

Transverse myelitis after radiation treatment is a spinal cord reaction similar to cerebral necrosis. This syndrome consists of progressive and irreversible leg weakness and loss of bladder function and sensation referrable to a single spinal cord level. Flaccid paralysis eventually occurs. Symptoms can occur as early as 6 months after radiation treatment, but the usual time to onset is 12 to 24 months. Lhermitte's sign does not correlate with transverse myelitis.

Skin   Skin reaction can be seen within 2 weeks of fractionated radiotherapy, a delay that correlates with the time required for cells to move from the basal to the keratinized layer of skin. The severity of the reaction depends on the skin dose per fraction and the total dose delivered to an area of skin. Erythema is observed, soon followed by dry desquamation. The skin at this time can be erythematous, warm, and sometimes edematous. The vessels in the upper dermis are dilated, and inflammatory infiltration with granulocytes, macrophages, eosinophils, plasma cells, and lymphocytes is noted.

When a severe skin reaction occurs, it is usually located where the beam strikes the skin tangentially. *Moist desquamation* consists of eruption of the epidermal layer. Healing is through reepithelialization from cells of less affected basal layers. When skin reactions are severe, treatment interruptions are needed to permit healing.

Dry desquamation is treated conservatively. Symptoms of dryness can be alleviated by advising the patient to wear only cotton fabric next to the affected skin and to refrain from the use of irritants of any kind. If treatment becomes necessary, hydrophilic agents that do not contain heavy metals are recommended. Moist desquamation is best managed by leaving the affected area dry and open to air.

A chronic reaction to radiation can be seen starting 6 to 12 months after irradiation. The epidermis may become atrophic and may be more easily injured than normal skin. Interstitial fibrosis and telangiectasia may also be increased. Hyperpigmentation of irradiated skin outlining the treatment field can be seen within a couple of months after completion of irradiation. This will fade gradually. The skin becomes thin, and hair loss may be permanent. Radiation therapy can induce second malignancies, which tend to be more aggressive than cancers arising in patients without significant radiation exposure.

Heart and Blood Vessels   When cardiac disease appears after radiation treatment, it is often difficult to tell to what extent the radiation treatment was causative. The pathogenesis of atherosclerotic heart disease is multifactorial. Exposure of a large heart volume to high-dose radiation therapy accelerates the development of coronary artery disease. Acute "pericarditis" may result from cardiac irradiation. The symptoms may include chest pain and fever, with or without pericardial effusion. This syndrome is usually self-limited and typically manifests itself a few months after treatment. Asymptomatic pericardial effusion may be the most common manifestation of radiation-induced heart

disease. It is usually detected by chest x-ray and confirmed by an echocardiogram.

Most patients with symptomatic radiation-induced constrictive pericarditis will have received >40 Gy to a large portion of the heart. The risk increases significantly with cardiac doses >50 Gy.

Chronic cardiac changes may have their onset from 6 months to several years after irradiation. The clinical symptoms may indicate chronic constrictive disease due to pericardial, myocardial, and endocardial fibrosis—a pancarditis. The clinical signs may include dyspnea, chest pain, venous distention, pleural effusion, and paradoxical pulse.

Lung   The clinical symptoms of radiation pneumonitis can be separated into early and late phases. During the early phase, clinical manifestations may include dyspnea, cough, and fever. Shortness of breath is relatively infrequent. It is more common to observe only the radiologic changes on a chest x-ray, without clinical symptoms. The clinical signs and symptoms of radiation pneumonitis may appear in 3 to 6 weeks if a large region of lung is irradiated to a dose >25 Gy. An infiltrate outlining the treatment field may become evident on the chest x-ray. Radiation changes rarely occur outside the treated field. Computed tomography can often help in distinguishing radiation pneumonitis from other causes of the infiltrate. The frequency of radiation pneumonitis can be reduced with careful treatment planning designed to lower the total dose given to the treated lung volume. Permanent scarring that results in respiratory compromise may develop if the dose and the volume of lung irradiated are excessive. Dyspnea and cough may be severe and debilitating.

Patients with symptoms of radiation pneumonitis may respond rapidly to glucocorticoids, but the medication has little effect on fibrotic changes. Glucocorticoids must be tapered very slowly to avoid rebound exacerbation of symptoms, which can prove lethal for some patients. Prophylactic administration of glucocorticoids is of no proven merit. Supportive care includes bronchodilators and oxygen at the lowest possible FI_{O_2}.

Digestive Tract   Pathologic changes of the epithelial layer occur early during radiation treatments. The underlying submucosa may become edematous, with dilation of capillaries. Recovery from radiation damage can be expected within a few weeks after completion of radiation therapy, provided that sufficient numbers of stem cells are left. The radioresponsiveness of the aerodigestive tract, like that of other structures, is not uniform but varies according to the location.

Patients often have symptoms from radiation exposure that are similar to other forms of acute gastritis. The clinical signs include epigastric pain, loss of appetite, nausea, and vomiting. Decreased gastric acidity is observed after 15 to 20 Gy of fractionated radiation therapy. The tolerance of the stomach to radiation is also aggravated by addition of systemic chemotherapy, such as 5-fluorouracil.

The germinal centers of the bowel mucosa are in the crypts of Lieberkühn. Newly formed cells move upward along the walls of the crypts as transitional cells, undergoing maturation. The epithelial lining of the small bowel is the most rapidly renewed system in the human body and is completely renewed in 3 to 6 days. Within 12 to 24 h after the first dose of radiation therapy, pathologic evidence of dead cells are seen in the mucosal lining. Complete denudation of the mucosal surface rarely occurs during a regular course of radiation treatment because of the high capacity of the mucosa for regeneration. However, a focal area of erosion may be seen. The histologic appearance may be nearly normal within 2 to 3 weeks after radiation therapy.

Clinical manifestations of acute radiation enteropathy are nausea and vomiting, diarrhea, and cramping pain. Relevant factors contributing to the pathogenesis of diarrhea include malabsorption and alterations in the intestinal bacterial flora. The severity of symptoms, as in other anatomic areas, is proportional to the irradiated volume and the total dose.

Symptoms of chronic radiation enteropathy include diarrhea, abdominal cramping, nausea, malabsorption, vomiting, and obstruction. Progressive fibrosis, perforation, fistula formation, and stenosis of the irradiated portion of the bowel can occur during the chronic phase of radiation enteropathy. Most clinical manifestations of chronic changes occur between 6 months and 5 years after radiation therapy.

Conservative noninvasive treatment can frequently control gastrointestinal symptoms. A low-residue or elemental diet may be beneficial. When nonsurgical treatment fails to relieve severe symptoms, surgical intervention is often indicated.

Bladder   Radiation injury to the bladder generally becomes symptomatic 3 to 6 weeks after the start of treatment, and symptoms usually subside 3 to 4 weeks after completion of radiation therapy. Patients often complain of increased frequency and dysuria. Cystoscopy often shows diffuse mucosal changes similar to those of acute cystitis. Sometimes desquamation and ulceration can be seen. Without infection, urinary symptoms are managed symptomatically. Concurrent chemotherapy with cytotoxic agents such as cyclophosphamide increases the severity of the acute bladder reaction.

The late effects of high radiation doses to the bladder may include contracture in size, interstitial fibrosis, telangiectasia, and ulceration. The blood vessels may be dilated and prone to rupture, resulting in painless hematuria. These changes are often difficult to distinguish from tumor recurrence and progression. A contracted bladder may result from doses >60 Gy.

Testes and Ovaries   In general, type B spermatogonia are exquisitely sensitive to the effects of radiation. The type A spermatogonia are thought to be more resistant because their longer cell cycle time allows considerable variation in radiosensitivity among different phases of the cell cycle. Sertoli cells and Leydig cells are less radiosensitive than the spermatogonia. Elevated levels of follicle-stimulating hormone (FSH) and luteinizing hormone (LH) have been observed after as little as 75 cGy. Doses as low as 10 cGy to the testicles may result in injury to the type B spermatogonia. The single dose required for permanent sterilization on normal human males is believed to be between 6 and 10 Gy. In normal human males, sperm count recovery requires 9 to 18 months after a fractionated dose of 8 to 100 cGy.

The radiation dose necessary to induce ovarian failure is age-dependent. A single dose of 3 to 4 Gy can induce amenorrhea in almost all women over 40 years of age. In young women, oogenesis is much less sensitive to radiation than is spermatogenesis in men.

ACUTE TOTAL-BODY IRRADIATION   The data regarding the acute effects of total-body irradiation on humans come primarily from Japanese survivors of the atomic bomb, Marshallese exposed to radioactive fallout in 1954, and persons exposed to radiation from the Chernobyl nuclear accident. Early symptoms of acute total-body irradiation, known as the *prodromal radiation syndrome*, may last for a limited time. Clinical manifestations depend on the total-body dose. At doses >100 Gy, death usually occurs 24 to 48 h later from neurologic and cardiovascular failure. This is known as the *cerebrovascular syndrome*. Because cerebrovascular damage causes death very quickly, the failures of other systems do not have time to develop.

At doses between 5 and 12 Gy, death may occur in a matter of days as a result of the *gastrointestinal syndrome*. The symptoms during this period may include nausea, vomiting, and prolonged diarrhea for several days leading to dehydration, sepsis, and death. A total-body dose >10 Gy is uniformly fatal unless supportive therapy (fluid, electrolytes, blood products, and antibiotics) is given. The process of intestinal denudation depends on the dose and may take between 3 and 120 days. Death from intestinal denudation usually occurs before the full effects of radiation on the blood-forming elements are seen.

At total-body doses between 2 and 8 Gy, death may occur 2 to 4 weeks after exposure from bone marrow failure, the *hematopoietic syndrome*. The full effect of radiation is not apparent until the mature hematopoietic cells are depleted. Clinical symptoms during this period

may include chills, fatigue, and petechial hemorrhage. Peripheral blood lymphopenia develops during the first 12 to 48 h after any significant exposure. Beyond 5 to 6 Gy, the rate and magnitude of the drop are not well correlated to radiation exposure. Some stem cells may survive acute exposure to ≥10 Gy. Death is from infection or bleeding and usually occurs before anemia can develop (red blood cell half-life is 100 to 120 days).

The $LD_{50/60}$ (the dose at which 50% of the population is dead by 60 days) is around 3.25 Gy if support is not given. There is considerable variability in the total-body dose tolerated. The very young and the old are more radiosensitive than middle-aged and young adults. Females in general appear to be more tolerant of radiation than males. Persons exposed to <2 Gy will require little or no therapy but should probably be observed closely with daily blood counts for a few days.

The role of bone marrow transplantation for patients exposed to acute total-body irradiation is debated. At doses <8 Gy, the patient is likely to survive with supportive care. Most people exposed to doses >10 Gy will die from the gastrointestinal syndrome. Therefore, 8 to 10 Gy may be the dose range in which bone marrow transplantation could have a role, although the Chernobyl experience did not confirm this prediction. Estimating the dose received by a given patient after radiation exposure is difficult. However, exposure estimation must be done quickly because bone marrow transplantation is most effective if it is performed within the first 3 to 5 days after exposure.

RADIATION AND CANCER INDUCTION   Some nonlethal changes in DNA sequences caused by irradiation may cause malignant transformations. Thus, it is not surprising that second neoplasms can be caused by exposure to ionizing radiation. However, paradoxically, this risk decreases with doses above a certain level. Whether there is a "safe" dose that will not induce any cancer is not likely. Estimates of the risk of developing cancer after low-level exposure to ionizing radiation are often derived by extrapolation from the risks for higher doses and acute exposures. Predicted risks of cancer are, therefore, prone to modification depending on the assumptions made about the data available for analysis.

Throughout the history of human exposure to ionizing radiation, increased rates of cancer have been noted after exposure to radiation. The populations studied include survivors of the atomic bomb during World War II; radium watch-dial painters who shaped their brush tips with their tongues; patients who underwent multiple fluoroscopic examinations for tuberculosis, received spinal irradiation for ankylosing spondylitis, and received breast irradiation for postpartum mastitis; and others. Exposure to ionizing radiation at an earlier age appears to increase the chance of developing radiation-induced carcinomas. However, the radiation-induced cancers have an age of onset similar to that of the native cancers, and the available data argue against radiation as the only cause of the increased incidence of cancers seen after exposure to radiation. Table 71-5 shows examples of cancer observed in specific situations.

Because a safe dose of radiation is unknown at present, it is prudent to avoid routine exposures to ionizing irradiation.

TABLE 71-5   *Examples of Radiation-Induced Cancers*

Types of Exposure	Types of Cancer Observed
Neck irradiation during infancy for benign conditions	Thyroid carcinoma
Radiation therapy for other malignant tumors	Thyroid carcinoma
	Breast cancer
	Gastric cancer
	Melanoma
	Lung cancer
	Sarcomas in the field
Cranial irradiation	Central nervous system tumors
Breast irradiation for postpartum mastitis	Breast cancer
Brush-licking by radium dial painters	Bone sarcomas
Uranium mining	Lung cancer
In utero exposure	Leukemia

FURTHER READING

HALL EJ: *Radiobiology for the Radiologist*, 5th ed. Philadelphia, Lippincott Williams & Wilkins, 2000

HEVEZI JM: Emerging technology in cancer treatment: Radiotherapy modalities. Oncology 17:1445, 2003

METTLER FA JR, UPTON AC: *Medical Effects of Ionizing Radiation*, 2d ed, Philadelphia, Saunders, 1995

MOSS WT, COX JD: *Moss' Radiation Oncology: Rationale, Technique, Results*, 7th ed. St. Louis, Mosby, 1994

PEREZ CP, BRADY LW: *Principles and Practice of Radiation Oncology*, 3d ed. Philadelphia, Lippincott Williams & Wilkins, 1998

RUBIN P: Late effects of normal tissues consensus conference. Int J Radiat Oncol Biol Phys 31:5, 1995

RUIFROK ACC, MCBRIDE WH: Growth factors: Biological and clinical aspects. Int J Radiat Oncol Biol Phys 43:877, 1999

72 INFECTIONS IN PATIENTS WITH CANCER
Robert Finberg

Infections are a common cause of death and an even more common cause of morbidity in patients with a wide variety of neoplasms. Autopsy studies show that most deaths from acute leukemia and half of deaths from lymphoma are caused directly by infection. With more intensive chemotherapy, patients with solid tumors have also become more likely to die of infection.

A physical predisposition to infection (Table 72-1) can be a result of the neoplasm's production of a break in the skin; for example, a squamous cell carcinoma may cause local invasion of the epidermis, which allows bacteria to gain access to the subcutaneous tissue and permits the development of cellulitis. The artificial closing of a normally patent orifice can also predispose to infection: Obstruction of a ureter by a tumor can cause urinary tract infection, and obstruction of the bile duct can cause cholangitis. Part of the host's normal defense against infection depends on the continuous emptying of a viscus; without emptying, a few bacteria present as a result of bacteremia or local transit can multiply and cause disease.

A similar problem can affect patients whose lymph node integrity has been disrupted by radical surgery, particularly patients who have had radical node dissections. A common clinical problem following radical mastectomy is the development of cellulitis (usually caused by streptococci or staphylococci) because of lymphedema and/or inadequate lymph drainage. In most cases, this problem can be addressed by local measures designed to prevent fluid accumulation and breaks in the skin, but antibiotic prophylaxis has been necessary in refractory cases.

A life-threatening problem common to many cancer patients is the loss of the reticuloendothelial capacity to clear microorganisms after splenectomy. Splenectomy may be performed as part of the management of hairy cell leukemia, chronic lymphocytic leukemia (CLL), and chronic myelocytic leukemia (CML) and in Hodgkin's disease. Even after curative therapy for the underlying disease, the lack of a spleen predisposes such patients to rapidly fatal infections. The loss of the spleen through trauma similarly predisposes the normal host to overwhelming infection for as long as 25 years after splenectomy. The splenectomized patient should be counseled about the risks of infection with certain organisms, such as the protozoan *Babesia* (Chap. 195) and *Capnocytophaga canimorsus* (formerly dysgonic fermenter 2, or DF-2), a bacterium carried in the mouths of animals (Chap. 131). Since encapsulated bacteria (*Streptococcus pneumoniae*, *Haemophilus influenzae*, and *Neisseria meningitidis*) are the organisms most commonly associated with postsplenectomy sepsis, splenectomized persons should be vaccinated (and revaccinated; Table 72-2) against the capsular polysaccharides of these organisms. Many clinicians recommend giving splenectomized patients a small supply of antibiotics effective against *S. pneumoniae*, *N. meningitidis*, and *H. influenzae* to avert rapid, overwhelming sepsis in the event that they cannot present for medical attention immediately after the onset of fever or other symptoms of bacterial infection.

The level of suspicion of infections with certain organisms should depend on the type of cancer diagnosed (Table 72-3). Diagnosis of multiple myeloma or CLL should alert the clinician to the possibility of hypogammaglobulinemia. While immunoglobulin replacement therapy can be effective, in most cases prophylactic antibiotics are a cheaper, more convenient method of eliminating bacterial infections in CLL patients with hypogammaglobulinemia. Patients with acute lymphocytic leukemia (ALL), patients with non-Hodgkin's lymphoma, and all cancer patients treated with high-dose glucocorticoids (or glucocorticoid-containing chemotherapy regimens) should receive antibiotic prophylaxis for *Pneumocystis* infection (Table 72-3) for the duration of their chemotherapy. In addition to exhibiting susceptibility to certain infectious organisms, patients with cancer are likely to manifest their infections in characteristic ways.

TABLE 72-1 *Normal Barriers to Infections*

Type of Defense	Specific Lesion	Cells Involved	Organism	Cancer Association	Disease
Physical barrier	Breaks in skin	Skin epithelial cells	Staphylococci, streptococci	Head and neck, squamous cell carcinoma	Cellulitis, extensive skin infection
Emptying of fluid collections	Occlusion of orifices: ureters, bile duct, colon	Luminal epithelial cells	Gram-negative bacilli	Renal, ovarian, biliary tree, metastatic diseases of many cancers	Rapid, overwhelming bacteremia, urinary tract infection
Lymphatic disease	Node dissection	Lymph nodes	Staphylococci, streptococci	Breast cancer surgery	Cellulitis
Splenic clearance of microorganisms	Splenectomy	Splenic reticuloendothelial cells	*Streptococcus pneumoniae*, *Haemophilus influenzae*, *Neisseria meningitidis*, *Babesia*, *Capnocytophaga canimorsus*	Hodgkin's disease, leukemia, idiopathic thrombocytopenic purpura	Rapid, overwhelming sepsis
Phagocytosis	Lack of granulocytes	Granulocytes (neutrophils)	Staphylococci, streptococci, enteric organisms, fungi	Hairy cell, acute myelocytic, and acute lymphocytic leukemias	Bacteremia
Humoral immunity	Lack of antibody	B cells	*S. pneumoniae*, *H. influenzae*, *N. meningitidis*	Chronic lymphocytic leukemia, multiple myeloma	Infections with encapsulated organisms, sinusitis, pneumonia
Cellular immunity	Lack of T cells	T cells and macrophages	*Mycobacterium tuberculosis*, *Listeria*, herpesviruses, fungi, other intracellular parasites	Hodgkin's disease, leukemia, T cell lymphoma	Infections with intracellular bacteria, fungi, parasites

TABLE 72-2 *Vaccination of Cancer Patients Receiving Chemotherapy*

Vaccine	Use in Indicated Patients		
	Intensive Chemotherapy	Hodgkin's Disease	Bone Marrow Transplantation
Diphtheria-tetanus (diphtheria, pertussis, tetanus; DPT) for children <7 years old	Primary series and boosters as necessary	No special recommendation	12, 14, and 24 months after transplantation
Poliomyelitis[a]	Complete primary series and boosters	No special recommendation	12, 14, and 24 months after transplantation
Haemophilus influenzae type b conjugate	Primary series and booster for children	Immunization before treatment and booster 3 months afterward	12, 14, and 24 months after transplantation
Hepatitis A	Not routinely recommended	Not routinely recommended	Not routinely recommended
Hepatitis B	Complete series	No special recommendation	12, 14, and 24 months after transplantation
23-Valent pneumococcal	Every 5 years	Immunization before treatment and booster 3 months afterward	12 and 24 months after transplantation
4-Valent meningococcal	Should be administered to splenectomized patients and patients living in endemic areas, including college students in dormitories	Should be administered to splenectomized patients and patients living in endemic areas, including college students in dormitories	Should be administered to splenectomized patients and patients living in endemic areas, including college students in dormitories
Influenza	Seasonal immunization	Seasonal immunization	Seasonal immunization
Measles/mumps/rubella	Contraindicated	Contraindicated	After 24 months in patients without graft versus host disease
Varicella-zoster virus	Contraindicated[b]	Contraindicated	Contraindicated

[a] Live-virus vaccine is contraindicated; inactivated vaccine should be used.
[b] Contact the manufacturer for more information on use in children with acute lymphocytic leukemia.

SYSTEM-SPECIFIC SYNDROMES

SKIN-SPECIFIC SYNDROMES Skin lesions are common in cancer patients, and their appearance may permit the diagnosis of systemic bacterial or fungal infection. While cellulitis caused by skin organisms such as *Streptococcus* or *Staphylococcus* is common, neutropenic patients [those with fewer than 500 functional polymorphonuclear leukocytes (PMNs) per microliter] and patients with impaired blood or lymphatic drainage may develop infections with unusual organisms. Innocent-looking macules or papules may be the first sign of bacterial or fungal sepsis in immunocompromised patients (Fig. 72-1). In the neutropenic host, a macule progresses rapidly to ecthyma gangrenosum, a usually painless, round, necrotic lesion consisting of a central black or gray-black eschar with surrounding erythema. Ecthyma gangrenosum is located in nonpressure areas (as distinguished from necrotic lesions associated with lack of circulation) and is often associated with *Pseudomonas aeruginosa* bacteremia (Chap. 136) but may be caused by other bacteria.

Candidemia (Chap. 187) is also associated with a variety of skin conditions and commonly presents as a maculopapular rash. Punch biopsy of the skin may be the best method for diagnosis.

Cellulitis, an acute spreading inflammation of the skin, is most often caused by infection with group A *Streptococcus* or *Staphylococcus aureus*, virulent organisms normally found on the skin (Chap. 110). Although cellulitis tends to be circumscribed in normal hosts, it may spread rapidly in neutropenic patients. A tiny break in the skin may lead to spreading cellulitis, which is characterized by pain and erythema; in such patients, signs of infection (e.g., purulence) are often lacking. What might be a furuncle in a normal host may require amputation because of uncontrolled infection in a patient presenting with leukemia. A dramatic response to an infection that might be trivial in a normal host can mark the first sign of leukemia. Fortunately, granulocytopenic patients are likely to be infected with certain types of organisms (Table 72-4); thus the selection of an antibiotic regimen is somewhat easier than it might otherwise be. (See discussion below on the selection of antibiotics for use in neutropenic patients.) It is essential to recognize cellulitis early and to treat it aggressively. Patients who are neutropenic or have previously received antibiotics for other reasons may develop cellulitis with unusual organisms (e.g., *Escherichia coli*, *Pseudomonas*, or fungi). Early treatment, even of innocent-looking lesions, is essential to prevent necrosis and loss of tissue. Debridement to prevent spread may sometimes be necessary early in the course of disease, but it can often be performed after chemotherapy, when the PMN count increases.

Sweet's syndrome, or *febrile neutrophilic dermatosis*, was originally described in women with elevated white blood cell counts. The disease is characterized by the presence of leukocytes in the lower dermis, with edema of the papillary body. Ironically, this disease now is usually seen in neutropenic patients with cancer, most often in association with acute leukemia but also in association with a variety of other malignancies. Sweet's syndrome usually presents as red or bluish-red papules or nodules that may coalesce and form sharply bordered plaques. The edema may suggest vesicles, but on palpation the lesions are solid, and vesicles probably never arise in this disease. The lesions are most common on the face, neck, and arms. On the legs, they may

TABLE 72-3 *Infections and Cancer*

Cancer	Underlying Immune Abnormality	Organisms Causing Infection
Multiple myeloma	Hypogammaglobulinemia	*Streptococcus pneumoniae, Haemophilus influenzae, Neisseria meningitidis*
Chronic lymphocytic leukemia	Hypogammaglobulinemia	*S. pneumoniae, H. influenzae, N. meningitidis*
Acute myelocytic or lymphocytic leukemia	Granulocytopenia, skin and mucous-membrane lesions	Extracellular gram-positive and gram-negative bacteria, fungi
Hodgkin's disease	Abnormal T cell function	Intracellular pathogens (*Mycobacterium tuberculosis, Listeria, Salmonella, Cryptococcus, Mycobacterium avium*)
Non-Hodgkin's lymphoma and acute lymphocytic leukemia	Glucocorticoid chemotherapy, T and B cell dysfunction	*Pneumocystis*
Colon and rectal tumors	Local abnormalities[a]	*Streptococcus bovis* (bacteremia)
Hairy cell leukemia	Abnormal T cell function	Intracellular pathogens (*M. tuberculosis, Listeria, Cryptococcus, M. avium*)

[a] The reason for this association is not well defined.

FIGURE 72-1 *A.* Papules related to *Escherichia coli* bacteremia in a neutropenic patient with acute lymphocytic leukemia. *B.* The same lesion the following day.

be confused with erythema nodosum. The development of lesions is often accompanied by high fevers and an elevated erythrocyte sedimentation rate. Both the lesions and the temperature elevation respond dramatically to glucocorticoids. Treatment begins with high doses of glucocorticoids (60 mg/d of prednisone) followed by tapered doses over the next 2 to 3 weeks.

Data indicate that *erythema multiforme* with mucous membrane involvement is often associated with herpes simplex virus (HSV) infection and is distinct from Stevens-Johnson syndrome, which is associated with drugs and tends to have a more widespread distribution. Since cancer patients are both immunosuppressed (and therefore susceptible to herpes infections) and heavily treated with drugs (and therefore subject to Stevens-Johnson syndrome), both of these conditions are common in this population.

Cytokines, which are used as adjuvants or primary treatments for cancer, can themselves cause characteristic rashes, further complicating the differential diagnosis. This phenomenon is a particular problem in bone marrow transplant recipients (Chap. 117), who, in addition to having the usual chemotherapy-, antibiotic-, and cytokine-induced rashes, are plagued by graft-versus-host disease.

CATHETER-RELATED INFECTIONS Because intravenous catheters are commonly used in cancer chemotherapy and are prone to infection (Chap. 116), they pose a major problem in the care of patients with cancer. Some catheter-associated infections can be treated with antibiotics, while in others the catheter must be removed. If the patient has a "tunneled" catheter (which consists of an entrance site, a subcutaneous tunnel, and an exit site), a red streak over the subcutaneous part of the line (the tunnel) is grounds for immediate removal of the catheter. Failure to remove catheters under these circumstances may result in extensive cellulitis and tissue necrosis.

More common than tunnel infections are exit-site infections, often with erythema around the area where the line penetrates the skin. Most

authorities (Chap. 120) recommend treatment (usually with vancomycin) for an exit-site infection caused by a coagulase-negative *Staphylococcus*. Treatment of coagulase-positive staphylococcal infection is associated with a poorer outcome, and it is advisable to remove the catheter if possible. Similarly, many clinicians remove catheters associated with infections due to *P. aeruginosa* and *Candida* species, since such infections are difficult to treat and bloodstream infections with these organisms are likely to be deadly. Catheter infections caused by *Burkholderia cepacia*, *Stenotrophomonas* spp., *Agrobacterium* spp., and *Acinetobacter baumannii* as well as *Pseudomonas* spp. other than *aeruginosa* are likely to be very difficult to eradicate with antibiotics alone. Similarly, isolation of *Bacillus*, *Corynebacterium*, and *Mycobacterium* spp. should prompt removal of the catheter.

GASTROINTESTINAL TRACT–SPECIFIC SYNDROMES ■ **Upper Gastrointestinal Tract Disease** ■ *INFECTIONS OF THE MOUTH* The oral cavity is rich in aerobic and anaerobic bacteria (Chap. 148) that normally live in a commensal relationship with the host. The antimetabolic effects of chemotherapy cause a breakdown of host defenses, leading to ulceration of the mouth and the potential for invasion by resident bacteria. Mouth ulcerations afflict most patients receiving chemotherapy and have been associated with viridans streptococcal bacteremia. A variety of topical rinses and elixirs have been proposed to treat these ulcerations. Although some may have a local anesthetic effect, the efficacy of any of these therapies in the prevention of disease is unproven. Similarly, the efficacy of mouthwashes in the prevention of esophagitis or invasive candidiasis is doubtful. Fluconazole, on the other hand, is clearly effective in the treatment of both local infections (thrush) and systemic infections (esophagitis) due to *Candida albicans*. Newer azoles (such as voriconazole) are similarly effective.

Noma (*cancrum oris*), commonly seen in malnourished children, is a penetrating disease of the soft and hard tissues of the mouth and adjacent sites, with resulting necrosis and gangrene. It has a counterpart in immunocompromised patients and is thought to be due to invasion of the tissues by *Bacteroides*, *Fusobacterium*, and other normal inhabitants of the mouth. Noma is associated with debility, poor oral hygiene, and immunosuppression.

Viruses, particularly HSV, are a prominent cause of morbidity in immunocompromised patients, in whom they are associated with severe mucositis. The use of acyclovir, either prophylactically or therapeutically, is of value.

ESOPHAGEAL INFECTIONS The differential diagnosis of esophagitis (usually presenting as substernal chest pain upon swallowing) includes herpes simplex and candidiasis, both of which are readily treatable.

Lower Gastrointestinal Tract Disease Hepatic candidiasis (Chap. 187) results from seeding of the liver (usually from a gastrointestinal source)

TABLE 72-4 *Organisms Likely to Cause Infections in Granulocytopenic Patients*

Gram-positive cocci	*Enterobacter* spp.
Staphylococcus epidermidis	*Serratia* spp.
Staphylococcus aureus	*Acinetobacter* spp.[a]
Viridans *Streptococcus*	*Citrobacter* spp.
Enterococcus faecalis	Gram-positive bacilli
Streptococcus pneumoniae	Diphtheroids
Gram-negative bacilli	JK bacillus[a]
Escherichia coli	Fungi
Klebsiella spp.	*Candida* spp.
Pseudomonas aeruginosa	*Aspergillus* spp.
Non-*aeruginosa Pseudomonas* spp.[a]	

[a] Often associated with intravenous catheters.

in neutropenic patients. It is most common in patients being treated for acute leukemia and usually presents symptomatically around the time the neutropenia resolves. The characteristic picture is that of persistent fever unresponsive to antibiotics; abdominal pain and tenderness or nausea; and elevated serum levels of alkaline phosphatase in a patient with hematologic malignancy who has recently recovered from neutropenia. The diagnosis of this disease (which may present in an indolent manner and persist for several months) is based on the finding of yeasts or pseudohyphae in granulomatous lesions. Hepatic ultrasound or computed tomography (CT) may reveal bull's-eye lesions. In some cases, magnetic resonance imaging (MRI) reveals small lesions not visible by other imaging modalities. The pathology (a granulomatous response) and the timing (with resolution of neutropenia and an elevation in granulocyte count) suggest that the host response to *Candida* is an important component of the manifestations of disease. In many cases, although organisms are visible, cultures of biopsied material may be negative. The designation *hepatosplenic candidiasis or hepatic candidiasis* is a misnomer because the disease often involves the kidneys and other tissues; the term *chronic disseminated candidiasis* may be more appropriate. Because of the risk of bleeding with liver biopsy, diagnosis is often based on imaging studies (MRI, CT). Amphotericin B is traditionally used for therapy (often for several months, until all manifestations of disease have disappeared), but fluconazole may be useful for outpatient therapy. The use of other antifungal agents and combination therapy is less well studied.

Typhlitis   *Typhlitis*, sometimes referred to as necrotizing colitis, neutropenic colitis, necrotizing enteropathy, ileocecal syndrome, or cecitis, is a clinical syndrome of fever and right-lower-quadrant tenderness in an immunosuppressed host. This syndrome is classically seen in neutropenic patients after chemotherapy with cytotoxic drugs. It may be more common among children than among adults and appears to be much more common among patients with acute myelocytic leukemia (AML) or ALL than among those with other types of cancer. Physical examination reveals right-lower-quadrant tenderness, with or without rebound tenderness. Associated diarrhea (often bloody) is common, and the diagnosis can be confirmed by the finding of a thickened cecal wall on CT or ultrasonography. Plain films may reveal a right-lower-quadrant mass, but CT with contrast or MRI is a much more sensitive means of making the diagnosis. Although surgery is sometimes attempted to avoid perforation from ischemia, most cases resolve with medical therapy alone. The disease is sometimes associated with positive blood cultures (usually for aerobic gram-negative bacilli), and therapy is recommended for a broad spectrum of bacteria (particularly gram-negative bacilli, likely bowel flora).

Clostridium difficile–Induced Diarrhea   Cancer patients are predisposed to the development of *C. difficile* diarrhea (Chap. 114) as a consequence of chemotherapy alone. Thus, they may have positive toxin tests before receiving antibiotics. Obviously, such patients are also subject to *C. difficile*–induced diarrhea as a result of antibiotic pressure. *C. difficile* should always be considered as a possible cause of diarrhea in cancer patients who have received antibiotics.

CENTRAL NERVOUS SYSTEM–SPECIFIC SYNDROMES ■ Meningitis The presentation of meningitis in patients with lymphoma or CLL, patients receiving chemotherapy (particularly with glucocorticoids) for solid tumors, and patients who have received bone marrow transplants suggests a diagnosis of cryptococcal or listerial infection. As noted previously, splenectomized patients are susceptible to rapid, overwhelming infection with encapsulated bacteria (including *S. pneumoniae, H. influenzae,* and *N. meningitidis*). Similarly, patients who are antibody-deficient (such as patients with CLL, those who have received intensive chemotherapy, or those who have undergone bone marrow transplantation) are likely to have infections caused by these bacteria. Other cancer patients, however, because of their defective cellular immunity, are likely to be infected with other pathogens (Table 72-3).

TABLE 72-5 *Differential Diagnosis of Central Nervous System Infections in Patients with Cancer*

Findings on CT or MRI	Underlying Predisposition	
	Prolonged Neutropenia	Defects in Cellular Immunity[a]
Mass lesions	*Aspergillus* brain abscess *Nocardia* brain abscess *Cryptococcus* brain abscess	Toxoplasmosis EBV-LPD
Diffuse encephalitis	PML (J-C virus)	Infection with VZV, CMV, HSV, HHV-6, J-C virus (PML), *Listeria*

[a] High-dose glucocorticoid therapy, cytotoxic chemotherapy.
Abbreviations: CMV, cytomegalovirus; CT, computed tomography; EBV-LPD, Epstein-Barr virus lymphoproliferative disease; HHV-6, human herpesvirus type 6; HSV, herpes simplex virus; PML, progressive multifocal leukoencephalopathy.

Encephalitis   The spectrum of disease resulting from viral encephalitis is expanded in immunocompromised patients. Cancer patients receiving high-dose cytotoxic chemotherapy or any chemotherapy that affects T cell function (e.g., fludarabine) or antibodies that eliminate T cells (e.g., anti-CD3) or cytokine activity are predisposed to infections with intracellular organisms similar to those encountered in patients with AIDS (Chap. 173). Infection with varicella-zoster virus (VZV) has been associated with encephalitis that may be caused by VZV-related vasculitis. Chronic viral infections may also be associated with dementia and encephalitic presentations, and a diagnosis of progressive multifocal leukoencephalopathy should be considered when a patient who has received chemotherapy presents with dementia (Table 72-5). Other abnormalities of the central nervous system (CNS) that may be confused with infection include normal-pressure hydrocephalus and vasculitis resulting from CNS irradiation. It may be possible to differentiate these conditions by MRI.

Brain Masses   Mass lesions of the brain most often present as headache with or without fever or neurologic abnormalities. Infections associated with mass lesions may be caused by bacteria (particularly *Nocardia*), fungi (particularly *Cryptococcus* or *Aspergillus*), or parasites (*Toxoplasma*). Epstein-Barr virus (EBV)–associated lymphoproliferative disease may also present as single or multiple mass lesions of the brain. A biopsy may be required for a definitive diagnosis.

PULMONARY INFECTIONS   Pneumonia (Chap. 239) in immunocompromised patients may be difficult to diagnose because conventional methods of diagnosis depend on the presence of neutrophils. Bacterial pneumonia in neutropenic patients may present without purulent sputum—or, in fact, without any sputum at all—and may not produce physical findings suggestive of chest consolidation (rales or egophony).

In granulocytopenic patients with persistent or recurrent fever, the chest x-ray pattern may help to localize an infection and thus to determine which investigative tests and procedures should be undertaken and which therapeutic options should be considered (Table 72-6). The difficulties encountered in the management of pulmonary infiltrates relate in part to the difficulties of performing diagnostic procedures on

TABLE 72-6 *Differential Diagnosis of Chest Infiltrates in Immunocompromised Patients*

Infiltrate	Cause of Pneumonia	
	Infectious	Noninfectious
Localized	Bacteria, *Legionella,* mycobacteria	Local hemorrhage or embolism, tumor
Nodular	Fungi (e.g., *Aspergillus* or *Mucor*), *Nocardia*	Recurrent tumor
Diffuse	Viruses (especially CMV), *Chlamydia, Pneumocystis, Toxoplasma gondii,* mycobacteria	Congestive heart failure, radiation pneumonitis, drug-induced lung injury, diffuse alveolar hemorrhage (described after BMT)

Abbreviations: BMT, bone marrow transplantation; CMV, cytomegalovirus.

the patients involved. When platelet counts can be increased to adequate levels by transfusion, microscopic and microbiologic evaluation of the fluid obtained by endoscopic bronchial lavage is often diagnostic. Lavage fluid should be cultured for *Mycoplasma*, *Chlamydia*, *Legionella*, *Nocardia*, fungi, and more common bacterial pathogens. In addition, the possibility of *Pneumocystis* pneumonia should be considered, especially in patients with ALL or lymphoma who have not received prophylactic trimethoprim-sulfamethoxazole (TMP-SMX). The characteristics of the infiltrate may be helpful in decisions about further diagnostic and therapeutic maneuvers. Nodular infiltrates suggest fungal pneumonia (e.g., that caused by *Aspergillus* or *Mucor*). Such lesions may best be approached by visualized biopsy procedures.

Aspergillus spp. (Chap. 188) can colonize the skin and respiratory tract or cause fatal systemic illness. Although *Aspergillus* may cause aspergillomas in a previously existing cavity or may produce allergic bronchopulmonary aspergillosis, the major problem posed by this genus in neutropenic patients is invasive disease due to *A. fumigatus* or *A. flavus*. The organisms enter the host following colonization of the respiratory tract, with subsequent invasion of the blood vessels. The disease is likely to present as a thrombotic or embolic event because of the ability of the organisms to invade blood vessels. The risk of infection with *Aspergillus* correlates directly with the duration of neutropenia. In prolonged neutropenia, positive surveillance cultures for colonization of the nasopharynx with *Aspergillus* may predict the development of disease.

Patients with *Aspergillus* infection often present with pleuritic chest pain and fever, which are sometimes accompanied by cough. Hemoptysis may be an ominous sign. Chest x-rays may reveal new focal infiltrates or nodules. Chest CT may reveal a characteristic halo consisting of a mass-like infiltrate surrounded by an area of low attenuation. The presence of a "crescent sign" on a chest x-ray or a chest CT scan, in which the mass progresses to central cavitation, is characteristic of invasive *Aspergillus* infection but may develop as the lesions are resolving.

In addition to causing pulmonary disease, *Aspergillus* may invade through the nose or palate, with deep sinus penetration. The appearance of a discolored area in the nasal passages or on the hard palate should prompt a search for invasive *Aspergillus*. This situation is likely to require surgical debridement. Treatment (Chap. 188) with high doses of amphotericin B has been successful in curing granulocytopenic patients of invasive *Aspergillus* infection after the return of granulocytes. Catheter infections with *Aspergillus* usually require both removal of the catheter and antifungal therapy.

Diffuse interstitial infiltrates suggest viral, parasitic, or *Pneumocystis* pneumonia. If the patient has a diffuse interstitial pattern on chest x-ray, it may be reasonable to institute empirical treatment with TMP-SMX (for *Pneumocystis*) and a quinolone (for *Chlamydia*, *Mycoplasma*, and *Legionella*) or an erythromycin derivative (e.g., azithromycin) while considering invasive diagnostic procedures. Noninvasive procedures, such as staining of sputum smears for *Pneumocystis*, serum cryptococcal antigen tests, and urine testing for *Legionella* only, may be helpful. In transplant recipients who are seropositive for cytomegalovirus (CMV), a determination of CMV load in the serum should be considered. The availability of viral load studies (which allow physicians to quantitate viruses) has superseded simple measurement of serum IgG, which merely documents prior exposure to virus. Infections with viruses that cause only upper respiratory symptoms in immunocompetent hosts, such as respiratory syncytial virus, influenza viruses, and parainfluenza viruses, may be associated with fatal pneumonitis in immunocompromised hosts. An attempt at early diagnosis by nasopharyngeal aspiration should be considered so that appropriate treatment can be instituted.

While bleomycin is the most common cause of chemotherapy-induced lung disease, other causes include alkylating agents (such as cyclophosphamide, chlorambucil, and melphalan), nitrosoureas [carmustine (BCNU), lomustine (CCNU), and methyl-CCNU], busulfan, procarbazine, methotrexate, and hydroxyurea. Both infectious and noninfectious (drug- and/or radiation-induced) pneumonitis can cause

fever and abnormalities on chest x-ray; thus, the differential diagnosis of an infiltrate in a patient receiving chemotherapy encompasses a broad range of conditions (Table 72-6). Since the treatment of radiation pneumonitis (which may respond dramatically to glucocorticoids) or drug-induced pneumonitis is different from that of infectious pneumonia, a biopsy may be important in the diagnosis. Unfortunately, no definitive diagnosis can be made in ~30% of cases, even after bronchoscopy.

Open-lung biopsy is the "gold standard" of diagnostic techniques. Biopsy via a visualized thoracostomy can replace an open procedure in many cases. When a biopsy cannot be performed, empirical treatment can be undertaken with a quinolone or erythromycin (or an erythromycin derivative such as azithromycin) and TMP-SMX (in the case of diffuse infiltrates) or with amphotericin B or other antifungal agents (in the case of nodular infiltrates). The risks should be weighed carefully in these cases. If inappropriate drugs are administered, empirical treatment may prove toxic or ineffective; either of these outcomes may be riskier than biopsy.

CARDIOVASCULAR INFECTIONS Patients with Hodgkin's disease are prone to persistent infections by *Salmonella*, sometimes (and particularly often in elderly patients) affecting a vascular site. The use of intravenous catheters deliberately lodged in the right atrium is associated with a high incidence of bacterial endocarditis (presumably related to valve damage followed by bacteremia). Nonbacterial thrombotic endocarditis has been described in association with a variety of malignancies (most often solid tumors) and may follow bone marrow transplantation as well. The presentation of an embolic event with a new cardiac murmur suggests this diagnosis. Blood cultures are negative in this disease of unknown pathogenesis.

ENDOCRINE SYNDROMES In addition to infections of the skin, gastrointestinal tract, and pulmonary and cardiovascular systems, infections of the endocrine system have been described in immunocompromised patients. *Candida* infection of the thyroid during neutropenia can be defined by indium-labeled white cell scans or gallium scans after neutrophil counts increase. CMV infection can cause adrenalitis with or without resulting adrenal insufficiency. The presentation of a sudden endocrine anomaly in an immunocompromised patient may be a sign of infection in the involved end organ.

MUSCULOSKELETAL INFECTIONS Infection that is a consequence of vascular compromise (resulting in gangrene) can occur when a tumor restricts the blood supply to muscles, bones, or joints. The process of diagnosis and treatment of such infection is similar to that in normal hosts, with the following caveats: (1) In terms of diagnosis, a lack of physical findings resulting from a lack of granulocytes in the granulocytopenic patient should make the clinician more aggressive in obtaining tissue rather than relying on physical signs. (2) In terms of therapy, aggressive debridement of infected tissues may be required, but it is usually difficult to operate on patients who have recently received chemotherapy, both because of a lack of platelets (which results in bleeding complications) and because of a lack of white blood cells (which may lead to secondary infection). A blood culture positive for *Clostridium perfringens* (an organism commonly associated with gas gangrene) can have a number of meanings (Chap. 126). Bloodstream infections with intestinal organisms like *Streptococcus bovis* and *C. perfringens* may arise spontaneously from lower gastrointestinal lesions (tumor or polyps); alternatively, these lesions may be harbingers of invasive disease. The clinical setting must be considered in order to define the appropriate treatment for each case.

RENAL AND URETERAL INFECTIONS Infections of the urinary tract are common among patients whose ureteral excretion is compromised (Table 72-1). *Candida*, which has a predilection for the kidney, can invade either from the bloodstream or in a retrograde manner (via the ureters or bladder) in immunocompromised patients. The presence of "fungus balls" or persistent candiduria suggests invasive disease. Persistent funguria (with *Aspergillus* as well as *Candida*) should prompt a search for a nidus of infection in the kidney.

Certain viruses are typically seen only in immunosuppressed patients. BK virus (polyomavirus hominis 1) has been documented in the urine of bone marrow transplant recipients and, like adenovirus, may be associated with hemorrhagic cystitis. BK-induced cystitis usually remits with decreasing immunosuppression. Anecdotal reports have described the treatment of infections due to adenovirus and BK virus with cidofovir (see below).

ABNORMALITIES THAT PREDISPOSE TO INFECTION

THE LYMPHOID SYSTEM   It is beyond the scope of this chapter to detail how all the immunologic abnormalities that result from cancer or from chemotherapy for cancer lead to infections. Disorders of the immune system are discussed in other sections of this book. As has been noted, patients with antibody deficiency are predisposed to overwhelming infection with encapsulated bacteria (including *S. pneumoniae*, *H. influenzae*, and *N. meningitidis*). Infections that result from the lack of a functional cellular immune system are described in Chap. 173. It is worth mentioning, however, that patients undergoing intensive chemotherapy for any form of cancer will have not only defects due to granulocytopenia but also lymphocyte dysfunction, which may be profound. Thus, these patients—especially those receiving glucocorticoid-containing regimens or drugs that inhibit T cell activation or cytokine induction—should be given prophylaxis for *Pneumocystis* pneumonia.

THE HEMATOPOIETIC SYSTEM   Initial studies in the 1960s revealed a dramatic increase in the incidence of infections (fatal and nonfatal) among cancer patients with a granulocyte count of <500/μL. Recent studies have cited a figure of 48.3 infections per 100 neutropenic patients (<1000 granulocytes per microliter) with hematologic malignancies and solid tumors, or 46.3 infections per 1000 days at risk.

Neutropenic patients are unusually susceptible to infection with a wide variety of bacteria; thus, antibiotic therapy should be initiated promptly to cover likely pathogens if infection is suspected. Indeed, early initiation of antibacterial agents is mandatory to prevent deaths. These patients are susceptible to gram-positive and gram-negative organisms found commonly on the skin and in the bowel (Table 72-4). Because treatment with narrow-spectrum agents leads to infection with organisms not covered by the antibiotics used, the initial regimen should target pathogens likely to be initial causes of bacterial infection in neutropenic hosts (Fig. 72-2).

℞ TREATMENT

Antibacterial Therapy   Hundreds of antibacterial regimens have been tested for use in patients with cancer. The major risk of infection is related to the degree of neutropenia seen as a consequence of either the disease or therapy. Many of the relevant studies involved small populations in which the outcomes were generally good, and most lacked the statistical power to detect differences among the regimens studied. Each febrile neutropenic patient should be approached as a unique problem, with particular attention given to previous infections and recent exposures to antibiotics. Several general guidelines are useful in the initial treatment of neutropenic patients with fever (Fig. 72-2):

1. It is necessary to use antibiotics active against both gram-negative and gram-positive bacteria (Table 72-4) in the initial regimen.
2. An aminoglycoside or an antibiotic without good activity against gram-positive organisms (e.g., ciprofloxacin or aztreonam) alone is not adequate in this setting.
3. The agents used should reflect both the epidemiology and the antibiotic resistance pattern of the hospital. For example, in hospitals where there is gentamicin resistance, amikacin-containing regimens should be considered; in hospitals with frequent *P. aeruginosa* infections, a regimen with the highest level of activity against

Physical examination: skin lesions, mucous membranes, IV catheter sites, perirectal area
Granulocyte count: absolute count < 500/μL; duration of expected neutropenia
Blood cultures; chest radiogram; other appropriate studies based on history (sputum, urine, skin biopsy)

Initial evaluation

Initial therapy → Treat with antibiotic(s) effective against both gram-negative and gram-positive aerobes.

Follow-up → Obvious infectious site found / No obvious infectious site

Subsequent therapy → Treat the infection with the best available antibiotics. Do not narrow the spectrum unnecessarily (continue to treat for both gram-positive and gram-negative aerobes). / Afebrile / Febrile

Continue regimen. / Add antifungal agent.

Continue treatment until neutropenia resolves (granulocyte count > 500/μL).

FIGURE 72-2   Algorithm for the diagnosis and treatment of febrile neutropenic patients.

this pathogen (such as tobramycin plus a semisynthetic penicillin) would be reasonable for initial therapy.

4. A single third-generation cephalosporin constitutes an appropriate initial regimen in many hospitals (if the pattern of resistance justifies its use).
5. Most standard regimens are designed for patients who have not previously received prophylactic antibiotics. The development of fever in a patient receiving antibiotics affects the choice of subsequent therapy (which should target resistant organisms and organisms known to cause infections in patients being treated with the antibiotics already administered).
6. Randomized trials have indicated that it is safe to use oral antibiotic regimens to treat "low-risk" patients with fever and neutropenia. Outpatients who are expected to remain neutropenic for <10 days and who have no concurrent medical problems (such as hypotension, pulmonary compromise, or abdominal pain) can be classified as low risk and treated with a broad-spectrum oral regimen. On the basis of large studies, it can be concluded that this therapy is safe and effective, at least when delivered in the inpatient setting. Outpatient treatment has been assessed in small studies, but data from large randomized trials demonstrating the safety of outpatient treatment of fever and neutropenia are not yet available.

The initial antibacterial regimen should be refined on the basis of culture results (Fig. 72-2). Blood cultures are the most relevant on which to base therapy; surface cultures of skin and mucous membranes may be misleading. In the case of gram-positive bacteremia or another gram-positive infection, it is important that the antibiotic be optimal for the organism isolated. If the infection is caused by certain gram-negative pathogens (such as *P. aeruginosa*), a synergistic combination of antibiotics (usually a semisynthetic penicillin, such as piperacillin, plus an aminoglycoside) may be appropriate. Although it is not desirable to leave the patient unprotected, the addition of more and more antibacterial agents to the regimen is not appropriate unless there is a clinical or microbiologic reason to do so. Planned progressive therapy (the serial, empirical addition of one drug after another without culture data) is not efficacious in most settings and may have unfortunate consequences. Simply adding another antibiotic for fear that a gram-negative infection is present is a dubious practice. The synergy exhibited by β-lactams and aminoglycosides against certain gram-negative organisms (especially *P. aeruginosa*) provides the rationale for using two antibiotics in this setting. Mere addition of a quinolone or another antibiotic not likely to exhibit synergy for "double coverage" has not been shown to be of benefit and may cause additional toxicities and side effects. Cephalosporins can cause bone marrow suppression, and vancomycin is associated with neutropenia in some healthy people (Chap. 118). Furthermore, the addition of multiple cephalosporins may induce β-lactamase production by some organisms; cephalosporins and double β-lactam combinations should probably be avoided altogether in *Enterobacter* infections.

Antifungal Therapy Fungal infections in cancer patients are most often associated with neutropenia. Neutropenic patients are predisposed to the development of invasive fungal infections, most commonly those due to *Candida* and *Aspergillus* species and occasionally those caused by

TABLE 72-7 *Antiviral Agents Active against Herpesviruses*

Agent	Description	Spectrum	Toxicity	Other Issues
Acyclovir	Inhibits HSV polymerase	HSV, VZV (± CMV, EBV)	Rarely has side effects; crystalluria can occur at high doses	Long history of safety; original antiviral agent
Famciclovir	Prodrug of penciclovir (a guanosine analogue)	HSV, VZV (± CMV)	Associated with cancer in rats	Longer effective half-life than acyclovir
Valacyclovir	Prodrug of acyclovir; better absorption	HSV, VZV (± CMV)	Associated with thrombotic microangiopathy in one study of immunocompromised patients	Better oral absorption and longer effective half-life than acyclovir; can be given as a single daily dose for prophylaxis
Ganciclovir	More potent polymerase inhibitor; more toxic than acyclovir	HSV, VZV, CMV, HHV-6	Bone marrow suppression	Neutropenia may respond to G-CSF or GM-CSF
Valganciclovir	Prodrug of ganciclovir; better absorption	HSV, VZV, CMV, HHV-6	Bone marrow suppression	—
Cidofovir	Nucleotide analogue of cytosine	HSV, VZV, CMV; has good in vitro activity against adenovirus and others	Nephrotoxic marrow suppression	Given IV once a week
Foscarnet	Phosphonoformic acid; inhibits viral DNA polymerase	HSV, VZV, CMV, HHV-6	Nephrotoxic; electrolyte abnormalities common	IV only

Abbreviations: ±, agent has some activity but not enough for the treatment of infections; CMV, cytomegalovirus; EBV, Epstein-Barr virus; G-CSF, granulocyte colony-stimulating factor; GM-CSF, granulocyte-macrophage colony-stimulating factor; HHV, human herpesvirus; HSV, herpes simplex virus; VZV, varicella-zoster virus.

Fusarium, *Trichosporon*, and *Bipolaris*. Cryptococcal infection, which is common among patients taking immunosuppressive agents, is uncommon among neutropenic patients receiving chemotherapy for AML. Invasive candidal disease is usually caused by *C. albicans* or *C. tropicalis* but can be caused by *C. krusei*, *C. parapsilosis*, and *C. glabrata*.

For decades it has been common clinical practice to add amphotericin B to antibacterial regimens if a neutropenic patient remains febrile despite 4 to 7 days of treatment with antibacterial agents. The rationale for the empirical addition of amphotericin B is that it is difficult to culture fungi before they cause disseminated disease and that mortality from disseminated fungal infections in granulocytopenic patients is high. Prior to the introduction of newer azoles into clinical practice, amphotericin B was the mainstay of antifungal therapy. The insolubility of amphotericin B has resulted in the marketing of several amphotericin B–lipid formulations. Lipid preparations have been shown to be less toxic than the amphotericin B deoxycholate complex. However, because of the high cost of the lipid preparations, at many centers their use is reserved for patients who fail to respond to standard amphotericin B. Since the side effects of the formulations differ, unnecessary switching from one to another is not recommended.

Although fluconazole has been demonstrated to be efficacious in the treatment of infections due to many *Candida* spp., its use against serious fungal infections in immunocompromised patients has been limited by its narrow spectrum: it has no activity against *Aspergillus* or against several non-*albicans Candida* spp. The release of newer broad-spectrum azoles (such as voriconazole) has provided another option for the treatment of *Aspergillus* infection (including CNS infection, in which amphotericin B has usually failed). In fact, experience indicates that these drugs may well supplant amphotericin B as the mainstay of treatment because of their lesser toxicity and better penetration into cerebrospinal fluid and other sites. Clinicians should be aware that the spectrum of each azole is somewhat different and that no drug can be assumed to be efficacious against all fungi. For example, while voriconazole is active against *Pseudallescheria boydii*,

amphotericin B is not; however, voriconazole has no activity against *Mucor*. →*For a full discussion of antifungal therapy, see Chap. 182.*

The introduction of new antifungal agents with different mechanisms of activity (e.g., the echinocandins) has opened the door to combination antifungal therapy. Studies in progress are assessing the use of these agents in cancer patients.

Antiviral Therapy The availability of a variety of agents with activity against herpes group viruses (and of some new agents with a broader spectrum of activity) has resulted in a greater focus on the treatment of viral infections, which pose a major problem in cancer patients. Among the viral diseases that affect cancer patients, those caused by the herpes group viruses are prominent. Serious (and sometimes fatal) infections due to HSV and CMV are well documented, and VZV infections may be fatal to patients receiving chemotherapy. The roles of human herpesvirus (HHV) 6, HHV-7, and HHV-8 (also known as Kaposi's sarcoma herpesvirus) in cancer patients are currently being defined (Chap. 166). While most clinical experience is with acyclovir, which can be used therapeutically or prophylactically, a number of derivative drugs offer advantages over this agent (Table 72-7).

In addition to the herpes group viruses, several respiratory viruses (especially respiratory syncytial virus) may cause serious disease in cancer patients. While vaccination with influenza vaccine is recommended (see below), it may be ineffective in this patient population. The availability of antiviral drugs with activity against influenza viruses gives the clinician additional options for the treatment of these patients (Table 72-8).

Other Therapeutic Modalities Another way to address the problems of the febrile neutropenic patient is to replenish the neutrophil population. Although granulocyte transfusions are efficacious in the treatment of refractory gram-negative bacteremia, they do not have a documented role in prophylaxis. Because of the expense, the risk of leukoagglutinin reactions (which has probably been decreased by improved cell-separation procedures), and the risk of transmission of CMV from unscreened donors (which has been reduced by the use of filters),

TABLE 72-8 *Other Antiviral Agents Useful in the Treatment of Infections in Cancer Patients*

Agent	Description	Spectrum	Toxicity	Other Issues
Amantadine Rimantadine	Interferes with uncoating	Influenza A only	5–10% fewer CNS effects with rimantadine	May be given prophylactically
Zanamivir	Neuraminidase inhibitor	Influenza A and B	Usually well tolerated	Inhalation only
Oseltamivir	Neuraminidase inhibitor	Influenza A and B	Usually well tolerated	PO dosing
Pleconaril	Blocks enterovirus binding and uncoating	90% of enteroviruses, 80% of rhinoviruses	Generally well tolerated	Decreases duration of meningitis; available for compassionate use only
Interferons	Cytokines with broad spectrum of activity	Used locally for warts, systemically for hepatitis	Fever, myalgias, bone marrow suppression	Not shown to be helpful in CMV infection; use limited by toxicity
Ribavirin	Purine analogue (precise mechanism of action unknown)	Broad theoretical spectrum; documented use against RSV, Lassa fever virus, and hepatitis viruses (with interferon)	IV form causes anemia	Given by aerosol for RSV infection (efficacy in doubt); approved for use in children with heart/lung disease

Abbreviations: CMV, cytomegalovirus; CNS, central nervous system; RSV, respiratory syncytial virus.

granulocyte transfusion is reserved for patients unresponsive to antibiotics. This modality is efficacious for documented gram-negative bacteremia refractory to antibiotics, particularly in situations where granulocyte numbers will be depressed for only a short period. The demonstrated usefulness of granulocyte colony-stimulating factor (G-CSF) in mobilizing neutrophils and advances in preservation techniques may make this option more useful than in the past.

A variety of cytokines, including G-CSF and granulocyte-macrophage colony-stimulating factor, enhance granulocyte recovery after chemotherapy and consequently shorten the period of maximal vulnerability to fatal infections. The role of these cytokines in routine practice is still a matter of some debate. Most authorities recommend their use only when neutropenia is both severe and prolonged. The cytokines themselves may have adverse effects, including fever, hypoxemia, and pleural effusions or serositis in other areas (Chap. 295). Since there is little evidence that their routine administration lessens the risk of death and since they are still expensive, the use of these cytokines has not become the standard of care in all centers. The role of other cytokines (such as macrophage colony-stimulating factor for monocytes or interferon-γ) in preventing or treating infections in granulocytopenic patients is under investigation.

Once neutropenia has resolved, patients are not at increased risk of infection. However, depending on what drugs they receive, patients who continue on chemotherapeutic protocols remain at high risk for certain diseases. Any patient receiving more than a maintenance dose of glucocorticoids (including many treatment regimens for diffuse lymphoma) should also receive prophylactic TMP-SMX because of the risk of *Pneumocystis* infection; those with ALL should receive such prophylaxis for the duration of chemotherapy.

PREVENTION OF INFECTION IN CANCER PATIENTS

EFFECT OF THE ENVIRONMENT Outbreaks of fatal *Aspergillus* infection have been associated with construction projects and materials in several hospitals. The association between spore counts and risk of infection suggests the need for a high-efficiency air-handling system in hospitals that care for large numbers of neutropenic patients. The use of laminar-flow rooms and prophylactic antibiotics has decreased the number of infectious episodes in severely neutropenic patients. However, because of the expense of such a program and the failure to show that it dramatically affects mortality, most centers do not routinely use laminar flow to care for neutropenic patients. Some centers use "reverse isolation," in which health care providers and visitors to a patient who is neutropenic wear gowns and gloves. Since most of the infec-

tions these patients develop are due to organisms that colonize the patients' own skin and bowel, the validity of such schemes is dubious, and limited clinical data do not support their use. Hand washing by all staff caring for neutropenic patients should be required to prevent the spread of resistant organisms.

The presence of large numbers of bacteria (particularly *P. aeruginosa*) in certain foods, especially fresh vegetables, has led some authorities to recommend a special "low-bacteria" diet. A diet consisting of cooked and canned food is satisfactory to most neutropenic patients and does not involve elaborate disinfection or sterilization protocols However, there are no studies to support even this type of dietary restriction. Counseling of patients to avoid leftovers, deli foods, and unpasteurized dairy products is recommended.

PHYSICAL MEASURES Although few studies address this issue, patients with cancer are predisposed to infections resulting from anatomic compromise (e.g., lymphedema resulting from node dissections after radical mastectomy). Surgeons who specialize in cancer surgery can provide specific guidelines for the care of such patients, and patients benefit from common-sense advice about how to prevent infections in vulnerable areas.

IMMUNOGLOBULIN REPLACEMENT Many patients with multiple myeloma or CLL have immunoglobulin deficiencies as a result of their disease, and all allogeneic bone marrow transplant recipients are hypogammaglobinemic for a period after transplantation. However, current recommendations reserve intravenous immunoglobulin (IVIg) replacement therapy for those patients with severe (<400 mg/dL), prolonged hypogammaglobulinemia. Antibiotic prophylaxis has been shown to be cheaper and efficacious in preventing infections in most CLL patients with hypogammaglobulinemia. Routine use of IVIg replacement is not recommended.

SEX The use of condoms is recommended for severely immunocompromised patients. Any sexual practice that results in oral exposure to feces is not recommended. Neutropenic patients should be advised to avoid any practice that results in trauma, as even microscopic cuts may result in bacterial invasion and fatal sepsis.

ANTIBIOTIC PROPHYLAXIS There is no consensus on the use of prophylactic antibiotics in neutropenic patients. The incidence of infection is lower among patients who receive broad-spectrum antibiotic prophylaxis than among those who do not. Because of the prolongation of neutropenia associated with the use of TMP-SMX, some clinicians use broad-spectrum agents such as quinolones (e.g., levofloxacin). Either regimen can be given orally, and both have the advantage of inactivity against anaerobic organisms; thus, neither is likely to disrupt the bowel flora and permit colonization with new aerobes or *Candida*. However, all antibiotic regimens have adverse effects and can lead to the selection of resistant organisms in a hospital. For these reasons, many clinicians reserve their use for patients with the longest periods of neutropenia (e.g., bone marrow transplant recipients). The same issues apply to the use of antifungal agents. While agents such as fluconazole may prevent infections with susceptible organisms (e.g., *C. albicans*), they can cause a concomitant increase in infections due to resistant fungi (e.g., *C. krusei*). Thus, the decision to use antifungal prophylaxis may vary with the fungi endemic in a given hospital. Prophylaxis for

Pneumocystis is mandatory for patients with ALL and for all cancer patients receiving glucocorticoid-containing chemotherapy regimens.

VACCINATION OF CANCER PATIENTS In general, patients undergoing chemotherapy respond less well to vaccines than normal hosts. Their greater need for vaccines thus leads to a dilemma in their management. Purified proteins and inactivated vaccines are almost never contraindicated and should be given to patients even during chemotherapy. For example, all adults should receive diphtheria-tetanus toxoid boosters at the indicated times as well as seasonal influenza vaccine. However, if possible, vaccination should not be undertaken concurrent with cytotoxic chemotherapy. If patients are expected to be receiving chemotherapy for several months and vaccination is indicated (for example, influenza vaccination in the fall), the vaccine should be given midcycle—as far apart in time as possible from the antimetabolic agents that will prevent an immune response. The meningococcal and pneumococcal polysaccharide vaccines should be given to patients before splenectomy, if possible. The *H. influenzae* type b conjugate vaccine should be administered to all splenectomized patients.

In general, live virus (or live bacterial) vaccines should not be given to patients during intensive chemotherapy because of the risk of disseminated infection. Recommendations on vaccination are summarized in Table 72-2.

FURTHER READING

BERGHMANS T et al: Therapeutic use of granulocyte and granulocyte-macrophage colony-stimulating factors in febrile neutropenic cancer patients. A systematic review of the literature with meta-analysis. Support Care Cancer 10:181, 2002

CENTERS FOR DISEASE CONTROL AND PREVENTION: Guidelines for preventing opportunistic infections among hematopoietic stem cell transplant recipients. MMWR Recomm Rep 49:1, 2000

HUGHES WT et al: 2002 guidelines for the use of antimicrobial agents in neutropenic patients with cancer. Clin Infect Dis 34:730, 2002

MERMEL LA et al: Guidelines for the management of intravascular catheter–related infections. Clin Infect Dis 32:1249, 2001

WALSH TJ et al: Voriconazole compared with liposomal amphotericin B for empirical antifungal therapy in patients with neutropenia and persistent fever. N Engl J Med 346:225, 2002

73 CANCER OF THE SKIN
Katarina G. Chiller, Carl Washington, Arthur J. Sober, Howard K. Koh

NONMELANOMA SKIN CANCER

Nonmelanoma skin cancer (NMSC) is the most common cancer in the United States, with an estimated annual incidence of >1.3 million cases. Basal cell carcinomas (BCCs) account for 70 to 80% of NMSCs. Squamous cell carcinomas (SCCs), while representing only ~20% of NMSC, are more significant because of their ability to metastasize; they account for most of the 2300 deaths annually. Incidence rates have risen dramatically over the past decade.

ETIOLOGY The cause of BCC and SCC is multifactorial. Cumulative exposure to sunlight, principally the ultraviolet B (UV-B) spectrum, is the most significant factor. Other factors associated with a higher incidence of skin cancer are male sex, older age, Celtic descent, a fair complexion, a tendency to sunburn easily, and an outdoor occupation. The incidence of these tumors increases with decreasing latitude. Most tumors develop on sun-exposed areas of the head and neck. Tumors are more common on the left side of the body in the United States but on the right side in England, presumably owing to asymmetric exposure during driving. As the earth's protective ozone shield continues to thin, further increases in the incidence of skin cancer can be anticipated. In certain geographic areas, exposure to arsenic in well water or from industrial sources may significantly increase the risk of BCC and SCC. Skin cancer in affected individuals may be seen with or without other cutaneous markers of chronic arsenism (e.g., arsenical keratoses). Less common is exposure to the cyclic aromatic hydrocarbons in tar, soot, or shale. The risk of lip or oral SCC is increased with cigarette smoking. Human papillomaviruses and UV radiation may act as cocarcinogens.

Host factors associated with a high risk of skin cancer include immunosuppression induced by disease or drugs. Transplant recipients receiving chronic immunosuppressive therapy are particularly prone to SCC. The frequency of skin cancer is proportional to the duration of immunosuppression and the extent of sun exposure. Skin cancer is not uncommon in patients infected with HIV, and it may be more aggressive in this setting. Other factors include ionizing radiation, thermal burn scars, and chronic ulcerations. Several heritable conditions are associated with skin cancer (e.g., albinism, xeroderma pigmentosum, and basal cell nevus syndrome). Mutations in the tumor suppressor *patch* gene have been implicated in the development of BCC.

CLINICAL PRESENTATION NMSCs are often asymptomatic, but nonhealing ulceration, bleeding, or pain can occur in advanced lesions.

Basal Cell Carcinoma BCC is a malignancy arising from epidermal basal cells. The least invasive of BCC subtypes, *superficial BCC*, classically consists of truncal erythematous, scaling plaques that slowly enlarge. This BCC subtype may be confused with benign inflammatory dermatoses, especially nummular eczema and psoriasis. BCC can also present as a small, slow growing pearly nodule, often with small telangiectatic vessels on its surface (*nodular BCC*). The occasional presence of melanin in this variant of nodular BCC (*pigmented BCC*) may lead to the erroneous diagnosis of malignant melanoma. *Morpheaform (fibrosing) BCC*, the most invasive subtype, manifests itself as a solitary, flat or slightly depressed, indurated, whitish or yellowish plaque. Borders are typically indistinct, a feature associated with a greater potential for extensive subclinical spread.

Squamous Cell Carcinoma Primary *cutaneous SCC* is a malignant neoplasm of keratinizing epidermal cells. SCC can grow rapidly and metastasize. The clinical features of SCC vary widely. Commonly, SCC appears as an ulcerated erythematous nodule or superficial erosion on the skin or lower lip, but it may present as a verrucous papule or plaque. Overlying telangiectasias are uncommon. The margins of this tumor may be ill defined, and fixation to underlying structures may occur. Cutaneous SCC may develop anywhere on the body but usually arises on sun-damaged skin. A related neoplasm, keratoacanthoma, typically appears as a dome-shaped papule with a central keratotic crater, expands rapidly, and commonly regresses without therapy. This lesion can be difficult to differentiate from SCC.

Actinic keratoses and *cheilitis*, both premalignant forms of SCC, present as hyperkeratotic papules on sun-exposed areas. The potential for malignant degeneration in untreated lesions ranges from 0.25 to 20%. *Bowen's disease*, the in situ form of SCC, presents as a scaling, erythematous plaque. Treatment of premalignant and in situ lesions reduces the subsequent risk of invasive disease.

NATURAL HISTORY ■ Basal Cell Carcinoma The natural history of BCC is that of a slowly enlarging, locally invasive neoplasm. The degree of local destruction and risk of recurrence vary with the size, duration, location, and histologic subtype of the tumor; presence of recurrent disease; and various patient characteristics. Location on the central face, ears, or the scalp may portend a higher risk. Small nodular, pigmented, cystic, or superficial BCCs respond well to most treatments. Large lesions or morpheaform subtype may be more aggressive. The metastatic potential of BCC has been estimated to be 0.0028 to 0.1%. Persons with either BCC or SCC have an increased risk of developing subsequent skin cancers, estimated to be up to 40% in 5 years.

Squamous Cell Carcinoma The natural history of SCC depends on both tumor and host characteristics. Tumors arising on actinically damaged skin have a lower metastatic potential than those on protected surfaces. The metastatic frequency of cutaneous SCC, reported at 0.3 to 5.2%, occurs most frequently in regional draining lymph nodes. Tumors occurring on the lower lip and ear have metastatic potentials approaching 13 and 11%, respectively. The metastatic potential of SCC arising in scars, chronic ulcerations, and genital or mucosal surfaces is higher. The overall metastatic rate for recurrent tumors may approach 30%. Large, poorly differentiated, deep tumors, with perineural or lymphatic invasion, often behave aggressively. Multiple tumors with rapid growth and aggressive behavior can be a therapeutic challenge in immunosuppressed patients.

℞ TREATMENT

Basal Cell Carcinoma The most frequently used treatment modalities for BCC include electrodesiccation and curettage (ED&C), excision, cryosurgery, radiation therapy, laser therapy, Mohs micrographic surgery (MMS), topical 5-fluorouracil, and topical immunomodulators. The mode of therapy chosen depends on tumor characteristics, patient age, medical status, preferences of the patient, and other factors. ED&C remains the method most commonly employed by dermatologists. This method is selected for low-risk tumors (e.g., a small primary tumor of a less aggressive subtype in a favorable location). Excision, which offers the advantage of histologic control, is usually selected for more aggressive tumors or those in high-risk locations or, in many instances, for aesthetic reasons. Cryosurgery using liquid nitrogen may be used in certain low-risk tumors, but it requires specialized equipment (cryoprobes) to be effective for advanced neoplasms. Radiation therapy, while not employed as often as surgical modalities, offers an excellent chance for cure in many cases of BCC. It is useful in patients not considered surgical candidates and as a surgical adjunct in high-risk tumors. Younger patients may not be good candidates for radiation therapy because of the risks of long-term carcinogenesis and radiodermatitis. Despite rapidly advancing technology in laser development, their long-term efficacy in treating infiltrative or recurrent lesions is still unknown. On the other hand, MMS, a specialized type of surgical excision that permits the best histologic control and preservation of uninvolved tissue, is associated with cure rates >98%. It is the preferred modality for lesions that are recurrent, in a high-risk location, or large and ill-defined and where maximal tissue conservation is critical (e.g., the eyelids). Topical 5-fluorouracil therapy should be limited to superficial BCC. New lines of topicals, the immunomodulators, show promise in their efficacy at treating superficial and even nodular BCCs. Imiquimod, a relatively well-tolerated cream, has successfully undergone phase III clinical trials. Intralesional chemotherapy (5-fluorouracil and interferon) and photodynamic therapy (which employs selective activation of a photoactive drug by visible light) have been used successfully in patients with numerous tumors.

Squamous Cell Carcinoma The therapy of cutaneous SCC should be based on an analysis of risk factors influencing the biologic behavior of the tumor. These include the size, location, and degree of histologic differentiation of the tumor as well as the age and physical condition of the patient. Surgical excision, MMS, and radiation therapy are standard methods of treatment. Cryosurgery and ED&C have been used successfully for premalignant lesions and small primary tumors. Metastases are treated with lymph node dissection, irradiation, or both. 13-*cis*-retinoic acid (1 mg orally every day) plus interferon α (3 million units subcutaneously or intramuscularly every day) may produce a partial response in most patients. Systemic chemotherapy combinations that include cisplatin may also be palliative in some patients.

PREVENTION As the vast majority of skin cancers are related to chronic UV radiation exposure, patient and physician education could dramatically reduce their incidence. Emphasis should be placed on preventive measures beginning early in life. Patients must understand that damage from UV-B begins early, despite the fact that cancers develop years later. Regular use of sunscreens and protective clothing should be encouraged. Avoidance of tanning salons and midday (10 A.M. to 2 P.M.) sun exposure is recommended. Precancerous and in situ lesions should be treated early. Early detection of small tumors affords simpler treatment modalities with higher cure rates and lower morbidity. In patients with a history of skin cancer, long-term follow-up for the detection of recurrence, metastasis, and new skin cancers should be emphasized. Chemoprophylaxis using synthetic retinoids is useful in controlling new lesions in some patients with multiple tumors.

OTHER NONMELANOMA CUTANEOUS MALIGNANCIES Neoplasms of cutaneous adnexa and sarcomas of fibrous, mesenchymal, fatty, and vascular tissues make up 1 to 2% of NMSC (Table 73-1). Some can portend a poor prognosis such as *Merkel cell carcinoma*, which is a neural crest–derived, highly aggressive malignancy that exhibits a metastatic rate of 75%, and a 5-year survival rate of 30 to 40%. Others, such as the human herpes virus 8–induced, HIV-related *Kaposi's sarcoma*, exhibit a more indolent course. The recent marked decrease in incidence of this tumor parallels the institution of the highly active antiretroviral therapy.

MELANOMA

Pigmented skin lesions are among the most common findings on physical examination. The challenge is to distinguish cutaneous melanomas, which may be lethal, from the remainder, which with rare exceptions are benign. Cutaneous neoplasms are depicted in Fig. 73-1; benign and malignant pigmented lesions are shown in Fig. 73-2.

EPIDEMIOLOGY Melanomas originate from neural crest–derived melanocytes, pigment cells present normally in the epidermis and sometimes in the dermis. This tumor will affect approximately 54,200 individuals per year in the United States, resulting in >8,200 deaths. The tumor can affect adults of all ages, even young individuals (starting in the mid-teens); it has distinct clinical features that make it detectable at a time when cure by surgical excision is possible; and it is located on the skin surface, where it is visible. The incidence has increased dramatically (a 300% increase in the past 40 years). If the incidence continues to increase at the present rate, within a decade, lifetime risk of melanoma will be ≥1%. The reason for this increase is uncertain but may involve increased recreational sun exposure, especially early in life. Individuals of similar ethnic background who immigrate after childhood to areas of high sun exposure (e.g., Israel and Australia) have lower melanoma rates than individuals of similar age who were either born in those countries or immigrated before age 10. The individuals most susceptible to development of melanoma are those with fair complexions, red or blond hair, blue eyes, and freckles and who tan poorly and sunburn easily. In one literature survey, 9 of 11 studies linked increased melanoma risk to history of sunburn. Other factors associated with increased risk include a family history of melanoma (~1 in 10 melanoma patients have a family member with mel-

TABLE 73-1 *Other Nonmelanoma Cutaneous Malignancies*

Tumor Type	Most Common Location	Recurrence Rate,[a] %	Metastatic Rate, %
Atypical fibroxanthoma	Head and neck	21	4
Merkel cell carcinoma	Head and neck	40	75
Dermatofibrosarcoma protuberans	Trunk	50	1
Sebaceous carcinoma	Eyelid	12	30
Microcystic adnexal carcinoma	Face	50	1 case
Porocarcinoma	Extremity	20	10
Eccrine carcinoma	Head and neck	36	11
Angiosarcoma	Head and neck	75	75

[a] Recurrence rates are the highest reported and were established prior to widespread use of Mohs micrographic surgery.

FIGURE 73-1   *A.* Non-Hodgkin's lymphoma involves the skin with typical violaceous, "plum-colored" nodules. *B.* Squamous cell carcinoma is seen here as a hyperkeratotic crusted and somewhat eroded plaque on the lower lip. Sun-exposed skin such as the head, neck, hands, and arms are other typical sites of involvement. *C.* Actinic keratoses consists of hyperkeratotic erythematous papules and patches on sun-exposed skin. They arise in middle-aged to older adults and have some potential for malignant transfor- mation. *D.* Metastatic carcinoma to the skin is characterized by inflammatory, often ulcerated dermal nodules. *E.* Mycosis fungoides is a cutaneous T cell lymphoma, and plaque stage lesions are seen in this patient. *F.* Keratoacanthoma is a low-grade squa- mous cell carcinoma that presents as an exophytic nodule with central keratinous debris. *G.* This basal cell carcinoma shows central ulceration and a pearly, rolled, telangiectatic tumor border.

anoma); the presence of a clinically atypical mole (dysplastic nevus), a giant congenital melanocytic nevus, or a small to medium-sized con- genital melanocytic nevus (see below); the presence of a higher than average number of ordinary melanocytic nevi; and immunosuppres- sion (Table 73-2). A 64-fold increased risk for individuals with 50 or more moles ≥2 mm in size has been reported. About 30% of mela- nomas arise in a nevus. Melanoma is relatively rare in heavily pig- mented peoples. Dark-skinned populations (such as those of India and Puerto Rico), blacks, and East Asians have rates 10 to 20 times lower than lighter-skinned whites. In keeping with the role of sun exposure, the incidence is inversely correlated with the latitude of residence; at any latitude, darker-skinned persons have the lowest incidence.

CLINICAL CHARACTERISTICS   There are four types of cutaneous melanoma (Table 73-3). In three of these—*superficial spreading melanoma*, *len- tigo maligna melanoma*, and *acral lentiginous melanoma*—the lesion has a period of superficial (so-called radial) growth during which it increases in size but does not penetrate deeply. It is during this period that the melanoma is most capable of being cured by surgical excision. The fourth type—*nodular melanoma*—does not have a recognizable radial growth phase and usually presents as a deeply invasive lesion, capable of early metastasis. When tumors begin to penetrate deeply into the skin, they are in the so-called vertical growth phase. Mela- nomas with a radial growth phase are characterized by irregular and sometimes notched borders, variation in pigment pattern, and variation

FIGURE 73-2   *A.* Acral lentiginous melanoma is more common in blacks, Asians, and Hispanics and occurs as an enlarging hyperpigmented macule or plaque on the palms and soles. Lateral pigment diffusion is present. *B.* Nodular melanoma most commonly manifests itself as a rapidly growing, often ulcerated or crusted black nodule. *C.* Lentigo maligna melanoma occurs on sun-exposed skin as a large, hyperpigmented macule or plaque with irregular borders and variable pigmentation. *D.* Dysplastic nevi are irreg- ularly pigmented and shaped nevomelanocytic lesions which may be associated with familial melanoma.

TABLE 73-2   Risk Factors for Cutaneous Melanoma

High risk (>50-fold increase in risk)
   Persistently changing mole
   Clinically atypical moles in patient with two family members with
     melanoma
   Adulthood (vs. childhood)
   >50 nevi ≥2 mm in diameter
Intermediate risk (~10-fold increase in risk)
   Family history of melanoma
   Sporadic clinically atypical moles
   Congenital nevi (?)
   White ethnicity (vs. black or East Asian ethnicity)
   Personal history of prior melanoma
Low risk (2- to 4-fold increase in risk)
   Immunosuppression
   Sun sensitivity or excess exposure to sun

Source: Adapted from AR Rhodes et al: JAMA 258:3146, 1987.

in color. An increase in size or change in color is noted by the patient in 70% of early lesions. Bleeding, ulceration, and pain are late signs and are of little help in early recognition. Nodular melanomas are dark brown-black to blue-black nodules. Melanomas occasionally are amelanotic, in which case the diagnosis is established histologically after biopsy of a new or changing skin nodule. Lentigo maligna melanoma is usually confined to chronically sun-damaged, sun-exposed sites (face, neck, back of hands) in older individuals. Acral lentiginous melanoma occurs on the palms, soles, nail beds, and mucous membranes. While this type occurs in whites, it is most frequent (along with nodular melanoma) in blacks and East Asians. Superficial spreading melanoma is most frequent in whites. Melanomas arising in dysplastic nevi (see below) are usually of this type. The back is the most common site for melanoma in men. In women, the back and the lower leg (from knee to ankle) are frequent sites.

PROGNOSTIC FACTORS   The most important prognostic factor is the stage at the time of presentation. Fortunately, most melanomas are diagnosed in clinical stages I and II. The revised staging system for melanoma is based on microscopic primary tumor depth (Breslow's thickness), presence of ulceration, evidence of nodal involvement, presence of microscopic satellites, and presence of metastatic disease (Table 73-4). Certain anatomic sites may affect the prognosis. The favorable sites appear to be the forearm and leg (excluding feet), while unfavorable sites include scalp, hands, feet, and mucous membranes. In general, women with stage I or II disease have a better survival than men, perhaps in part because of earlier diagnosis; women frequently have melanomas on the lower leg, where self-recognition is more likely and prognosis is better. Older individuals, in general, have poorer prognoses. This finding has been explained in part by a tendency toward later diagnosis (and thus thicker tumors) in men and by a higher proportion in men of acral melanomas (palmar-plantar), which have a poorer prognosis. Melanoma may recur after many years. About 10 to 15% of first-time recurrences develop >5 years after treatment of the original lesion. The time to recurrence varies inversely with tumor thickness. An alternative prognostic scheme for clinical stages I and II melanoma, proposed by Clark, is based on the anatomic level of invasion in the skin. Level I is intraepidermal (in situ); level II penetrates the papillary dermis; level III spans the papillary dermis; level IV penetrates the reticular dermis; and level V penetrates into the subcutaneous fat. The 5-year survival for these stages averages 100, 95, 82, 71, and 49%, respectively.

NATURAL HISTORY   Melanomas may spread by the lymphatic channels or the bloodstream. The earliest metastases are often to regional lymph nodes. Surgical lymphadenectomy may control early regional disease. Liver, lung, bone, and brain are common sites of hematogenous spread, but unusual sites, such as the anterior chamber of the eye, may also be involved. Once widespread metastatic disease is established, the likelihood of cure is low.

MANAGEMENT   The entire cutaneous surface, including the scalp and mucous membranes, should be examined in each patient. Bright room illumination is important, and a 7× to 10× hand lens is helpful for evaluating variation in pigment pattern. A history of relevant risk factors should be elicited. Any suspicious lesions should be biopsied, evaluated by a specialist, or recorded by chart and/or photography for follow-up. Examination of the lymph nodes and palpation of the abdominal viscera are part of the staging examination for suspected melanoma. The patient should be advised to have other family members screened if either melanoma or clinically atypical moles (dysplastic nevi) are present. The detection of early melanoma in relatives on screening has been reported. Melanoma prevention is based on protection from the sun. Routine use of a sunblock with sun protection factor ≥15, use of protective clothing, and avoiding intense midday ultraviolet exposure should be recommended. The patient should be educated in the clinical features of melanoma and advised to report any growth or other change in a pigmented lesion. Patient education brochures are available from the American Cancer Society, the American Academy of Dermatology, the National Cancer Institute, and the Skin Cancer Foundation. Self-examination at 6- to 8-week intervals may enhance the likelihood of detecting change. The importance of routine follow-up visits for melanoma patients and patients with clinically atypical moles (dysplastic nevi) should be emphasized, as these visits may facilitate early detection of new tumors.

Precursor Lesions   Clinically atypical moles, also termed *dysplastic nevi*, occur in certain families affected by melanoma. In some families, melanomas occur nearly exclusively in the individuals with dysplastic nevi. These nevi appear to be transmitted as an autosomal dominant trait that involves chromosome 9p16. In other families, the nevi may

TABLE 73-3   Clinical Features of Malignant Melanoma

Type	Site	Average Age at Diagnosis, Years	Duration of Known Existence, Years	Color
Lentigo maligna melanoma	Sun-exposed surfaces, particularly malar region of cheek and temple	70	5–20[a] or longer	In flat portions, shades of brown and tan predominant, but whitish gray occasionally present; in nodules, shades of reddish brown, bluish gray, bluish black
Superficial spreading melanoma	Any site (more common on upper back and, in women, on lower legs)	40–50	1–7	Shades of brown mixed with bluish red (violaceous), bluish black, reddish brown, and often whitish pink, and the border of lesion is at least in part visibly and/or palpably elevated
Nodular melanoma	Any site	40–50	Months to less than 5 years	Reddish blue (purple) or bluish black; either uniform in color or mixed with brown or black
Acral lentiginous melanoma	Palm, sole, nail bed, mucous membrane	60	1–10	In flat portions, dark brown predominantly; in raised lesions (plaques) brown-black or blue-black predominantly

[a] During much of this time, the precursor stage, lentigo maligna, is confined to the epidermis.

Source: Adapted from AJ Sober, in *Pathophysiology of Dermatologic Diseases*, NA Soter, HP Baden (eds). New York, McGraw-Hill, 1984.

not be present in all individuals with an increased risk of melanoma. The melanomas may arise in clinically atypical moles or in normal skin (in the latter situation the mole acts as a marker of increased risk). Individuals with clinically atypical moles and two family members with melanoma have been reported to have a >50% lifetime risk for developing melanoma. Table 73-5 lists the features that are characteristic of clinically atypical moles and that differentiate them from benign acquired nevi. The number of clinically atypical moles may vary from one to several hundred. Clinically atypical moles usually differ from each other in appearance. The borders are often hazy and indistinct, and the pigment pattern is more highly varied than that in benign acquired nevi. Of the 90% of melanoma patients whose disease is regarded as sporadic (i.e., who lack a family history of melanoma), ~40% have clinically atypical moles, as compared with an estimated 5 to 10% of the population at large. Further studies to determine the background frequency of clinically atypical moles are required, once greater unanimity exists regarding their clinical and histopathologic features. The observation that at least 20% of sporadic melanomas arise in association with a clinically atypical mole makes this the most important precursor for melanoma. Less frequent precursors include the giant congenital melanocytic nevus and the small congenital melanocytic nevus (although the latter relationship is disputed by some). Congenital melanocytic nevi are present at birth or appear in the neonatal period (tardive form). The *giant melanocytic nevus*, also called the bathing trunk, cape, or garment nevus, is a rare malformation that affects perhaps 1 in 30,000 to 1 in 100,000 individuals. These nevi are usually >20 cm in diameter and may cover more than half the body surface. Giant nevi often occur in association with multiple small congenital nevi. The borders are sharp, and hair may be present. The lesions are usually dark brown and may have darker and lighter areas. Pigment is haphazardly displayed. The surface is smooth to rugose or cerebriform and may vary from one portion of the lesion to another. A lifetime risk of melanoma development of 6% has been estimated. The risk is greatest before age 5 and next greatest between ages 5 and 10. Early detection of melanoma is difficult in these lesions because of the deep dermal or subcutaneous origin of primary melanoma and because of the large and varied surface of the nevus. Prophylactic excision early in life can be accomplished by staged removal with coverage by split-thickness skin grafts. The use of cultured keratinocytes for coverage appears promising. At present, there are no uniform management guidelines for giant congenital nevi. The *small- to medium-sized congenital melanocytic nevus*, which affects approximately 1% of persons, presents usually as a raised dark- to medium-brown lesion with a smooth or papillomatous surface. The border is sharp, and lesions may be oriented along lines of skin cleavage. Follicular hyper- and hypopigmentation may coexist in a salt-and-pepper configuration. The lesion may have an excess of thick, coarse hairs. The risk of melanoma developing in these lesions is not known; however, melanomas can arise in these lesions. Considerations of body surface area suggest that the incidence of melanomas arising in small congenital melanocytic nevi is probably higher than would be expected by chance. The remnants of a nevus with histopathologic features of a congenital nevus have been observed in 2 to 6% of melanomas. The management of small- to medium-sized congenital melanocytic nevi remains controversial; prophylactic removal under local anesthesia in the early teen years is appropriate. Melanomas in small congenital melanocytic nevi appear to occur after this period of life.

Differential Diagnosis   The aim of differential diagnosis is to distinguish benign pigmented lesions from melanoma and its precursor. If melanoma is a consideration, then biopsy is appropriate. Some benign look-alikes may be removed in the process of trying to detect authentic melanoma. Table 73-6 summarizes the distinguishing features of benign lesions that may be confused with melanoma. Early detection of melanoma may be facilitated by applying the "ABCD rules": A—asymmetry, benign lesions are usually symmetric; B—border irregularity, most nevi have clear-cut borders; C—color variegation, benign lesions usually have uniform light or dark pigment; D—diameter >6 mm (the size of a pencil eraser). Consideration may be given for ev-

TABLE 73-4   *Prognosis of Melanoma by Thickness (Breslow) and Revised AJCC Stages: 5-Year Survival Rates*

AJCC Stage	Thickness, mm	Ulceration	Nodal Disease	Distant Metastases
0	In situ	N/A	No	No
IA	<1	No	No	No
IB	<1	Yes	No	No
	1.01–2.0	No	No	No
IIA	1.01–2.0	Yes	No	No
	2.01–4.0	No	No	No
IIB	2.01–4.0	Yes	No	No
	>4.0	No	No	No
IIC	>4.0	Yes	No	No
IIIA	Any	No	Yes	
			1 node w/microscopic disease	No
			2–3 nodes w/microscopic disease	No
IIIB	Any	Yes	1 node w/microscopic disease	No
	Any	Yes	2–3 nodes w/microscopic disease	No
	Any	No	1 node w/macroscopic disease	No
	Any	No	2–3 nodes w/macroscopic disease	No
	Any	Any	In transit or satellite disease w/out nodal disease	No
	Any			
IIIC	Any	Yes	1 node w/macroscopic disease	No
		Yes	2–3 nodes w/macroscopic disease	No
		Any	≥4 metastatic or matted nodes, or in transit mets/satellites or metastatic nodes	No
IV	Any	Any	Any	Yes

Note: AJCC, American Joint Commission for Cancer.

TABLE 73-5   *Clinical Features Distinguishing Atypical Moles from Benign Acquired Nevi*

Clinical Feature	Clinically Atypical Moles	Benign Acquired Nevi
Color	Variable mixtures of tan, brown, black, or red/pink within a single nevus; nevi may look very different from each other	Uniformly tan or brown
Shape	Irregular borders; pigment may fade off into surrounding skin; macular portion at the edge of the nevus	Round; sharp, clear-cut borders between the nevus and the surrounding skin; may be flat or elevated
Size	Usually >6 mm in diameter; may be >10 mm; occasionally <6 mm	Usually <6 mm in diameter
Number	Often very many (>100), but occasionally may be only one	In a typical adult, 10 to 40 are scattered over the body; perhaps 15% of patients have no nevi
Location	Sun-exposed areas; the back is the most common site, but dysplastic nevi may also be seen on the scalp, breasts, and buttocks	Generally on the sun-exposed surfaces of the skin above the waist; the scalp, breasts, and buttocks are rarely involved

Source: Modified from RI Friedman et al (eds): *Cancer of the Skin*. Philadelphia, Saunders, 1991.

TABLE 73-6 *Pigmented Lesions that Must Be Distinguished from Cutaneous Melanoma and Its Precursors*

Blue nevus	Gunmetal or cerulean blue, blue-gray. Stable over time. One-half occur on dorsa of hands and feet. Lesions are usually single, small, 3 mm to <1 cm. Must be distinguished from nodular melanoma.
Compound nevus	Round or oval shape, well-demarcated, smooth-bordered. May be dome-shaped or papillomatous; colors range from flesh colored to very dark brown, with individual nevi being relatively homogeneous in color.
Hemangioma	Dome-shaped reddish, purple, blue nodule. Compression with a glass microscope slide may result in blanching. Must be distinguished from nodular melanoma.
Junctional nevus	Flat to barely raised brown lesion. Sharp border. Fine pigmentary stippling visible, especially upon magnification.

Lentigo
  Juvenile
  Solar
	Flat, uniformly medium or dark brown lesion with sharp border. Solar lentigines are acquired lesions on sites of chronic solar exposure (face and backs of hands). Lesions are 2 mm to ≥1 cm. Solar lentigines have reticulate pigmentation upon magnification.

Pigmented basal cell carcinoma	Papular border. May have central ulceration. Usually on a sun-exposed surface in an older patient. Patient usually has dark brown eyes and dark brown or black hair.
Pigmented dermatofibroma	Lesion is not well demarcated visually, is firm, and dimples downward when compressed laterally. Usually on extremities. Usually <6 mm.
Seborrheic keratosis	Rough, sharp-bordered lesions that feel waxy and "stuck on"; range in color from flesh to tan, to dark brown. Presence of keratin plugs in surface is helpful for discriminating especially dark lesions from melanoma.
Subungual hematoma	Maroon (red-brown) coloration. As lesion grows out from nail fold, a curving clear area is seen.
Tattoo (medical or traumatic)	In medical tattoo, lesions are small pigmentary dots, often blue or green, which make a regular pattern (rectangle). Traumatic tattoos are irregular, and pigmentation may appear black.

olution ("E"), as any of the other features become more significant as the lesion is changing.

Biopsy Any pigmented cutaneous lesion that has changed in size or shape or has other features suggestive of malignant melanoma is a candidate for biopsy. The recommended technique is a full-thickness excisional biopsy, as that facilitates pathologic assessment of the lesion, permits accurate measurement of thickness if the lesion is melanoma, and constitutes treatment if the lesion is benign. Shave biopsy or curettage of a suspected melanoma is contraindicated. For large lesions or lesions on anatomic sites where excisional biopsy may not be feasible (such as the face, hands, or feet), an incisional biopsy through the most nodular or darkest area of the lesion is acceptable; this should include the vertical growth phase of the primary tumor, if present. Data from prospective studies do not indicate that an incisional biopsy facilitates the spread of melanoma.

Staging Once the diagnosis of malignant melanoma has been confirmed, the tumor must be staged to determine prognosis and treatment. The history should probe for evidence of metastatic disease, such as malaise, weight loss, headaches, visual difficulty, or bone pain. The physical examination should be directed especially to the skin, regional draining lymph nodes, central nervous system, liver, and spleen. In the absence of signs or symptoms of metastasis, few laboratory or radiologic tests are indicated for staging purposes. Aside from a chest radiograph and, possibly, liver function tests, no other tests or scans

are routinely indicated unless the history or physical examination suggests metastasis to a specific organ. Specifically, liver-spleen scans and computed tomography have a low yield and are not cost-effective. However, once signs of metastasis exist, favored sites of spread, such as the liver, lungs, bone, and brain, should be scanned. Appropriate evaluations place patients into four clinical stages (Table 73-4).

℞ TREATMENT

Surgical Management For a newly diagnosed cutaneous melanoma, wide surgical excision of the lesion with a margin of normal skin is necessary to remove all malignant cells and minimize local recurrence. The appropriate width of the margin is a source of controversy. A World Health Organization trial prospectively randomized between 1- and 3-cm margins in 612 patients with thin malignant melanomas (≤2 mm thick) reported that the narrower margin resulted in higher rates of local recurrence but no difference in rates of nodal or distant metastases, disease-free survival, or overall survival after 7.5 years of follow-up. Another large randomized trial comparing 2- or 4-cm surgical margins for intermediate-thickness lesions (1 to 4 mm thick) also found no significant differences in overall survival. The following margins can be recommended for primary melanoma: in situ: 0.5 cm; invasive up to 1 mm thick: 1.0 cm; 1 to 4 mm thick: 2.0 cm; >4 mm thick: 2.5 to 3.0 cm. For lesions on the face, hands, and feet, strict adherence to these margins must give way to individual considerations about the constraints of surgery and minimization of morbidity. In all instances, however, inclusion of subcutaneous fat in the surgical specimen facilitates adequate thickness measurement and assessment of surgical margins by the pathologist.

ELECTIVE REGIONAL NODE DISSECTION Elective regional node dissection in the American Joint Commission for Cancer (AJCC) stage II disease (without palpable adenopathy) has been advocated, based on the hypothesis that melanoma metastasizes in an orderly fashion from the skin to regional lymph nodes and finally to distant sites. If that is the case, surgical excision of nodal micrometastasis could theoretically provide definitive treatment at a time of relatively low tumor burden and perhaps improve survival. The efficacy of this procedure remains controversial; while some retrospective series suggest a survival benefit, two randomized studies examining this question in patients with limb melanomas and clinical stage I disease showed no survival advantage for wide local excision followed by immediate elective regional node dissection compared with wide local excision followed by delayed dissection (only if nodes became palpable). Furthermore, the procedure has associated morbidity, and some lesions, especially those on the trunk, have ambiguous nodal draining sites, making it difficult to decide which area to dissect. Sentinel lymph node examination has been shown to be a valuable staging tool and, in instances of a negative sentinel lymph node, may obviate the need for elective regional nodal dissection. Patients with lesions <0.75 mm thick have an excellent prognosis and need no node dissection; at the other extreme, patients with lesions 3.5 mm thick have such a high risk for distant metastases that elective node dissection may not alter the ultimate clinical outcome. A subset of patients with AJCC stage II lesions of intermediate thickness may benefit from elective regional node dissection, but there is no consensus about which patients should undergo this procedure. An ongoing randomized surgical trial may resolve this issue.

Adjuvant Therapy For patients who are free of disease but at high risk for metastases, adjuvant therapy that complements surgery is needed to destroy occult micrometastases, prolong disease-free survival, and improve the cure rate. Many strategies have been tried unsuccessfully. However, adjuvant interferon α (either 2a or 2b) may be capable of improving disease-free and overall survival in some, particularly in patients with nodal metastases (stage III disease). The U.S. Food and Drug Administration has approved a high-dose interferon adjuvant protocol consisting of 20 million units per square meter intravenously 5 days a week for 4 weeks followed by 10 million units per square meter subcutaneously three times a week for 11 months. Ongoing studies are attempting to define the minimal effective dose, because, in nearly half of patients, these doses of interferon are associated with severe toxicity, including flulike illness and decline in performance status. The toxicity reverses promptly with lower doses and when therapy is stopped.

Treatment of Metastatic Disease Melanoma can metastasize to any organ, the brain being a particularly common site. Metastatic melanoma is generally incurable, with survival in patients with visceral metastases generally <1 year. Thus, the goal of treatment is usually palliation. Patients with soft tissue and node metastases fare better than those with liver and brain metastases. Metastases limited to regional nodes (AJCC stage III disease) warrant a therapeutic lymph node dissection. Surgical excision of a single metastasis to the lung or to a surgically accessible brain site can prolong survival. Trials of stereotactic radiosurgery will determine its future role in the treatment of brain metastases. More often, however, patients have multiple brain metastases that require radiation therapy and glucocorticoids. Radiation therapy can provide local palliation for recurrent tumors or metastases. Patients who have advanced regional disease limited to a limb may benefit from hyperthermic limb perfusion with melphalan and tumor necrosis factor. Complete response rates >90% have been reported; responses are associated with significant palliation of symptoms.

A number of drugs and biologicals have minimal antitumor activity (15 to 20% partial response rates) in metastatic melanoma, including dacarbazine (DTIC); the nitrosoureas carmustine (BCNU), lomustine (CCNU), and semustine (methyl-CCNU); platinum analogues such as cisplatin and carboplatin; vinca alkyloids such as vincristine, vinblastine, and vindesine; the taxanes paclitaxel and docetaxel; interferon α; and interleukin 2 (IL-2). Single-agent dacarbazine is considered the standard treatment. This agent has been given at a number of different doses and schedules; 250 mg/m² intravenously every day for 5 days every 3 weeks is a standard schedule. Dacarbazine-based combination regimens are probably more effective. Ongoing trials are attempting to define superior combinations. Interferon and IL-2 produce response rates similar to those seen with cytotoxic agents; however, at active doses, they usually cause greater toxicity than chemotherapy.

Melanoma can express cell surface antigens that may be recognized by host immune cells. Melanoma antigens (MAGEs)-1, -2, and -3 (endogenous proteins controlled by genes on the X chromosome; there may be up to 12 of these genes) and tyrosinase, an enzyme involved in melanin synthesis, are antigens that are processed into peptides and presented to T cells via HLA-A antigens on the tumor, particularly the HLA-A1 and A2 alleles, which are expressed in about 85% of patients with melanoma. In addition, a melanoma antigen called MART is recognized in the context of class II MHC antigens. These melanoma-associated antigens alone or in combination may make it possible to develop vaccination strategies against melanoma. Such strategies include the use of purified proteins as immunogens and the use of genetically altered tumor cells to elicit a T cell response. Alternative experimental approaches include efforts to expand tumor-specific T cells (obtained either from the tumor as tumor-infiltrating lymphocytes or harvested from the peripheral blood after vaccination) in vitro and transfer them into patients in large numbers. In addition, monoclonal antibodies to tumor antigens are being tested, with some early indication of efficacy in ~15% of patients. All of these experimental approaches will need considerable further development before being applicable on a wide scale. Advances in treating metastatic disease may be applicable in the adjuvant setting.

The absence of curative therapy for patients with metastatic melanoma underscores the importance of early detection and prevention as strategies to decrease melanoma mortality.

FURTHER READING

BALCH CM et al: Prognostic factors analysis of 17,600 melanoma patients: Validation of the AJCC staging system. J Clin Oncol 19:2001

CREAGAN ET et al: Randomized surgical adjuvant clinical trial of recombinant interferon-alfa-2a in selected patients with malignant melanoma. J Clin Oncol 13:2776, 1995

DRAKE LA et al: Guidelines of care of basal cell carcinoma. J Am Acad Dermatol 26:117, 1992

——— et al: Guidelines of care for cutaneous squamous cell carcinoma. J Am Acad Dermatol 28:628, 1993

GEISSE JK et al: Imiquimod 5% cream for the treatment of superficial basal cell carcinoma: A double-blind, randomized, vehicle-controlled study. J Am Acad Dermatol 47:390, 2002

JOHNSON TM et al: Staging workup, sentinel node biopsy, and follow-up tests for melanoma: Update of current concepts, 140:107, 2004

74 HEAD AND NECK CANCER
Everett E. Vokes

Epithelial carcinomas of the head and neck arise from the mucosal surfaces in the head and neck area and typically are squamous cell in origin. This category includes tumors of the paranasal sinuses, the oral cavity, and the nasopharynx, oropharynx, hypopharynx, and larynx. Tumors of the salivary glands differ from the more common carcinomas of the head and neck in etiology, histopathology, clinical presentation, and therapy. Thyroid malignancies are described in Chap. 320.

INCIDENCE AND EPIDEMIOLOGY The number of new cases of head and neck cancers in the United States was 38,530 in 2004, accounting for about 3% of adult malignancies. The worldwide incidence exceeds half a million cases annually. In North America and Europe, the tumors usually arise from the oral cavity, oropharynx, or larynx, whereas nasopharyngeal cancer is more common in the Mediterranean countries and in the Far East.

ETIOLOGY AND GENETICS Alcohol and tobacco use are the most common risk factors for head and neck cancer in the United States. Smokeless tobacco is an etiologic agent for oral cancers. Other potential carcinogens include marijuana and occupational exposures such as nickel refining, exposure to textile fibers, and woodworking.

Dietary factors may contribute. The incidence of head and neck cancer is highest in people with the lowest consumption of fruits and vegetables. Certain vitamins, including dietary carotenoids, may be protective; retinoids are being tested for prevention.

Some head and neck cancers may have a viral etiology. The DNA of human papillomavirus has been detected in the tissue of oral and tonsil cancers, and may predispose to oral cancer in the absence of tobacco and alcohol use. Epstein-Barr virus (EBV) infection is associated with nasopharyngeal cancer. Nasopharyngeal cancer occurs endemically in some countries of the Mediterranean and Far East, where EBV antibody titers can be measured to screen high-risk populations. Nasopharyngeal cancer has also been associated with consumption of salted fish.

No specific risk factors or environmental carcinogens have been identified for salivary gland tumors.

HISTOPATHOLOGY, CARCINOGENESIS, AND MOLECULAR BIOLOGY Squamous cell head and neck cancers can be divided into well-differentiated, moderately well-differentiated, and poorly differentiated categories. Patients with poorly differentiated tumors have a worse prognosis than those with well-differentiated tumors. For nasopharyngeal cancers, the less common differentiated squamous cell carcinoma is distinguished from nonkeratinizing and undifferentiated carcinoma (lymphoepithelioma) that contains infiltrating (bystander) lymphocytes.

Salivary gland tumors can arise from the major (parotid, submandibular, sublingual) or minor salivary glands (located in the submucosa of the upper aerodigestive tract). Most parotid tumors are benign, but half of submandibular and sublingual gland tumors and most minor salivary gland tumors are malignant. Malignant tumors include mucoepidermoid and adenoidcystic carcinomas and adenocarcinomas.

The mucosal surface of the entire pharynx is exposed to alcohol- and tobacco-related carcinogens and is at risk for the development of a premalignant or malignant lesion, such as erythroplakia or leukoplakia (hyperplasia, dysplasia), that can progress to invasive carcinoma. Alternatively, multiple synchronous or metachronous cancers can develop. In fact, patients with early-stage head and neck cancer are at greater risk of dying of a second malignancy than of dying from a recurrence of the primary disease.

Second head and neck malignancies are not therapy-induced; they reflect the exposure of the upper aerodigestive mucosa to the same carcinogens that caused the first cancer. These second primaries develop in the head and neck area, the lung, or the esophagus.

Chromosomal deletions and other alterations, most frequently involving chromosomes 3p, 9p, 17p, and 13q, have been identified in both premalignant and malignant head and neck lesions, as have mutations in tumor suppressor genes, commonly the p53 gene. Amplification of oncogenes is less common, but overexpression of PRAD-1/bcl-1 (cyclin D1), bcl-2, transforming growth factor β, and the epidermal growth factor receptor have been described. The latter finding correlates positively with tumor size and poor outcome and is a target for experimental treatments.

Resected tumor specimens with histopathologically negative margins ("complete resection") can have undetectable residual tumor cells with persistent p53 mutations at the margins. Thus, a tumor-specific p53 mutation can be detected in some phenotypically "normal" surgical margins, indicating residual disease. Patients with such submicroscopic marginal involvement may have a worse prognosis than patients with negative margins.

CLINICAL PRESENTATION AND DIFFERENTIAL DIAGNOSIS Most head and neck cancers occur after age 50, although these cancers can appear in younger patients, including those without known risk factors. The manifestations vary according to the stage and primary site of the tumor. Patients with nonspecific signs and symptoms in the head and neck area should be evaluated with a thorough otolaryngologic exam, particularly if symptoms persist longer than 2 to 4 weeks.

Cancer of the nasopharynx typically does not cause early symptoms. However, on occasion it may cause unilateral serous otitis media due to obstruction of the eustachian tube, unilateral or bilateral nasal obstruction, or epistaxis. Advanced nasopharyngeal carcinoma causes neuropathies of the cranial nerves.

Carcinomas of the oral cavity present as nonhealing ulcers, changes in the fit of dentures, or painful lesions. Tumors of the tongue base or oropharynx can cause decreased tongue mobility and alterations in speech. Cancers of the oropharynx or hypopharynx rarely cause early symptoms, but they may cause sore throat and/or otalgia.

Hoarseness may be an early symptom of laryngeal cancer, and persistent hoarseness requires referral to a specialist for indirect laryngoscopy and/or radiographic studies. If a head and neck lesion treated initially with antibiotics does not resolve in a short period, further workup is indicated; to simply continue the antibiotic treatment may be to lose the chance of early diagnosis of a malignancy.

Advanced head and neck cancers in any location can cause severe pain, otalgia, airway obstruction, cranial neuropathies, trismus, odynophagia, dysphagia, decreased tongue mobility, fistulas, skin involvement, and massive cervical lymphadenopathy, which may be unilateral or bilateral. Some patients have enlarged lymph nodes even though no primary lesion can be detected by endoscopy or biopsy; these patients are considered to have carcinoma of unknown primary (Fig. 74-1). If the enlarged nodes are located in the upper neck and the tumor cells are of squamous cell histology, the malignancy probably arose from a mucosal surface in the head or neck. Tumor cells in supraclavicular

FIGURE 74-1 Evaluation of a patient with cervical adenopathy without a primary mucosal lesion; a diagnostic workup. FNA, fine-needle aspiration.

lymph nodes may also arise from a primary site in the chest or abdomen.

The physical examination should include inspection of all visible mucosal surfaces and palpation of the floor of mouth and tongue and of the neck. In addition to tumors themselves, leukoplakia, a white mucosal patch, or erythroplakia, a red mucosal patch, may be observed; these "premalignant" lesions can represent hyperplasia, dysplasia, or carcinoma in situ. All visible or palpable lesions should be biopsied. Further examination should be performed by a specialist. Additional staging procedures include computed tomography of the head and neck to identify the extent of the disease. Patients with lymph node involvement should have chest radiography and a bone scan to screen for distant metastases. The definitive staging procedure is an endoscopic examination under anesthesia, which may include laryngoscopy, esophagoscopy, and bronchoscopy; during this procedure, multiple biopsy samples are obtained to establish a primary diagnosis, define the extent of primary disease, and identify any additional premalignant lesions or second primaries.

Head and neck tumors are classified according to the TNM system of the American Joint Committee on Cancer. This classification varies according to the specific anatomic subsite (Tables 74-1 and 74-2). Distant metastases are found in <10% of patients at initial diagnosis, but in autopsy series, microscopic involvement of the lungs, bones, or liver is more common, particularly in patients with advanced neck lymph node disease.

In patients with lymph node involvement and no visible primary, the diagnosis should be made by lymph node excision. If the results indicate squamous cell carcinoma, a panendoscopy should be performed, with biopsy of all suspicious-appearing areas and directed biopsies of common primary sites, such as the nasopharynx, tonsil, tongue base, and pyriform sinus.

Rx TREATMENT

Patients with head and neck cancer can be categorized into three clinical groups: those with localized disease, those with locally or regionally advanced disease, and those with recurrent and/or metastatic disease. Comorbidities associated with tobacco and alcohol abuse can affect treatment outcome.

Localized Disease Nearly one-third of patients have localized disease; that is, T1 or T2 (stage I or stage II) lesions without detectable lymph node involvement or distant metastases. These lesions are treated with curative intent by surgery or radiation therapy. The choice of modality differs according to institutional expertise. Radiation therapy is often preferred for laryngeal cancer to preserve voice function, and surgery is preferred for small lesions in the oral cavity to avoid the long-term complications of radiation, such as xerostomia and dental decay. Overall 5-year survival is 60 to 90%.

Locally or Regionally Advanced Disease   Locally or regionally advanced disease—disease with a large primary tumor and/or lymph node metastases—can also be treated with curative intent, but not with surgery or radiation therapy alone. Combined modality therapy including surgery, radiation therapy, and chemotherapy is most successful. Concomitant chemotherapy and radiation therapy appears to be most effective.

INDUCTION CHEMOTHERAPY   In this strategy, patients receive chemotherapy [usually cisplatin and fluorouracil (5FU)] before surgery and radiation therapy. Most patients who receive three cycles show tumor reduction, and the response is clinically "complete" in up to half. This "sequential" multimodality therapy does not cure more patients than surgery plus radiation therapy alone. However, induction chemotherapy allows for organ preservation in patients with laryngeal and hypopharyngeal cancer.

CONCOMITANT CHEMORADIOTHERAPY   With the concomitant strategy, chemotherapy and radiation therapy are given simultaneously rather than sequentially. Because most patients with head and neck cancer develop recurrent disease in the head and neck area, this approach is aimed at killing radiation-resistant cancer cells with chemotherapy. In addition, chemotherapy can enhance cell killing by radiation therapy. Toxicity (mucositis) is increased with concomitant chemoradiotherapy; however, meta-analysis of randomized trials documents an improvement in 5-year survival of 8% with concomitant 5FU and radiation therapy. Results seem even better with 5FU and cisplatin plus radiation therapy. Five-year survival is 34 to 50%. In addition, concomitant chemoradiotherapy produces better laryngectomy-free survival (organ preservation) than induction chemotherapy in patients with advanced larynx cancer. The use of radiation therapy together with cisplatin has produced markedly improved survival in patients with advanced nasopharyngeal cancer. The success of concomitant chemoradiotherapy in patients with unresectable disease has led to the testing of a similar approach in patients with resected disease as a postoperative therapy, but results to date have not convincingly shown improvement over postoperative radiation therapy alone.

Recurrent and/or Metastatic Disease
Patients with recurrent and/or

TABLE 74-1   *TNM Classification for Head and Neck Cancer (Except Nasopharyngeal)*

PRIMARY TUMOR SITE

T Grade	Oropharynx	Hypopharynx
T1	0–2 cm	0–2 cm
T2	2.1–4 cm	>1 site, 2–4 cm
T3	>4 cm	>4 cm
T4a	Larynx, muscle of tongue, medial pterygoid, hard palate, mandible invasion	Thyroid/cricoid cartilage, hyoid bone, thyroid gland, esophagus, or central compartment soft tissue invasion
T4b	Lateral pterygoid muscle, pterygoid plates, lateral nasopharynx, or skull base or encases carotid artery invasion	Invasion of prevertebral fascia, encases carotid artery, or involves mediastinal structures

REGIONAL LYMPH NODES (N)

NX	Regional lymph nodes cannot be assessed
N0	No regional lymph node metastasis
N1	Unilateral metastasis in lymph node(s), ≤6 cm in greatest dimension, above the supraclavicular fossa
N2	Bilateral metastasis in lymph node(s), ≤6 cm in greatest dimension, above the supraclavicular fossa
N3	Metastasis in a lymph node(s) >6 cm and/or to supraclavicular fossa
	N3a > 6 cm
	N3b Extension to the supraclavicular fossa
MX	Distant metastasis cannot be assessed
M0	No distant metastasis
M1	Distant metastasis

STAGE GROUPING

Stage 0	Tis	N0	M0
Stage I	T1	N0	M0
Stage II	T2	N0	M0
Stage III	T3	N0	M0
	T1	N1	M0
	T2	N1	M0
	T3	N1	M0
Stage IVA	T4a	N0	M0
	T4a	N1	M0
	T1	N2	M0
	T2	N2	M0
	T3	N2	M0
	T4a	N2	M0
Stage IVB	T4b	Any N	M0
	Any T	N3	M0
Stage IVC	Any T	Any N	M1

TABLE 74-2   *Definition of TNM—Nasopharynx*

Primary Tumor (T)		Stage Grouping			
TX	Cannot be assessed	Stage 0	Tis	N0	M0
T0	No evidence	Stage I	T1	N0	M0
Tis	Carcinoma in situ	Stage IIA	T2a	N0	M0
T1	Tumor confined to the nasopharynx	Stage IIB	T1	N1	M0
T2	Tumor extends to soft tissues		T2	N1	M0
	T2a Tumor extends to the oropharynx and/or nasal cavity w/o parapharyngeal extension		T2a	N1	M0
	T2b Any tumor with parapharyngeal extension		T2b	N1	M0
T3	Tumor involves bony structures and/or paranasal sinuses		T2b	N1	M0
T4	Tumor with intracranial extension and/or involvement of cranial nerves, infratemporal fossa, hypopharynx, orbit, or masticator space	Stage III	T1	N2	M0
			T2a	N2	M0
Regional Lymph Nodes (N)			T2b	N2	M0
The distribution and the prognostic impact of regional lymph node spread from nasopharynx cancer, particularly of the undifferentiated type, are different from those of other head and neck mucosal cancers and justify the use of a different N classification scheme.			T3	N0	M0
NX Regional lymph nodes cannot be assessed			T3	N1	M0
N0 No regional lymph node metastasis			T3	N2	M0
N1 Unilateral metastasis in lymph node(s), ≤6 cm in greatest dimension, above the supraclavicular fossa			T4	N0	M0
N2 Bilateral metastasis in lymph node(s), ≤6 cm in greatest dimension, above the supraclavicular fossa			T4	N1	M0
N3 Metastasis in lymph node(s), >6 cm and/or to supraclavicular fossa			T4	N2	M0
N3a Greater than 6 cm in dimension			Any T	N3	M0
N3b Extension to the supraclavicular fossa			Any T	Any N	M1

metastatic disease are, with few exceptions, treated with palliative intent. Some patients may require local or regional radiation therapy for pain control, but most are given chemotherapy. Response rates to chemotherapy average only 30 to 50%; the duration of response averages only 3 months, and the median survival time is 6 to 8 months. Therefore, chemotherapy provides transient symptomatic benefit. Drugs with single-agent activity in this setting include methotrexate, 5FU, cisplatin, paclitaxel, and docetaxel. Combinations of cisplatin and 5FU, carboplatin and 5FU, and cisplatin or carboplatin and paclitaxel or docetaxel are frequently used.

CHEMOPREVENTION β-Carotene and *cis*-retinoic acid can lead to the regression of leukoplakia. However, *cis*-retinoic acid does not reduce the incidence of second primaries.

TREATMENT COMPLICATIONS   Complications from treatment of head and neck cancer are usually related to the extent of surgery. Several attempts have been made to limit the extent of surgery or to replace it with chemotherapy and radiation therapy. Acute complications of radiation include mucositis and dysphagia. Long-term complications include xerostomia, loss of taste, decreased tongue mobility, second malignancies, dysphagia, and neck fibrosis. The complications of chemotherapy vary with the regimen used but usually include myelosuppression, mucositis, nausea and vomiting, and nephrotoxicity (with cisplatin).

SALIVARY GLAND TUMORS   Most benign salivary gland tumors are treated with surgical excision, and patients with invasive salivary gland tumors are treated with surgery and radiation therapy. Neutron radiation may be particularly effective. These tumors may recur regionally; adenoidcystic carcinoma has a tendency to recur along the nerve tracks. Distant metastases may occur as late as 10 to 20 years after the initial diagnosis. For metastatic disease, therapy is given with palliative intent, usually chemotherapy with doxorubicin and/or cisplatin.

FURTHER READING

CALIFANO J et al: Genetic progression model for head and neck cancer: Implications for field cancerization. Cancer Res 56:2488, 1996

FORASTIERE A et al: Head and neck cancer. N Engl J Med 345:1890, 2001

LAMONT EB, VOKES EE: Chemotherapy in the management of squamous-cell carcinoma of the head and neck. Lancet Oncol 2:261, 2001

LICITRA L, VERMORKEN JB: Is there still a role for neoadjuvant chemotherapy in head and neck cancer? Ann Oncol 15:7, 2004

RICE DH: Salivary gland disorders, Neoplastic and nonneoplastic. Med Clin North Am 83:197, 1999

VOKES E et al: Weekly carboplatin and paclitaxel followed by concomitant TFHX chemoradiotherapy: Curative and organ preserving therapy for advanced head and neck cancer. J Clin Oncol 21:320, 2003

75   NEOPLASMS OF THE LUNG
John D. Minna

Each year, primary carcinoma of the lung affects 93,000 males and 80,000 females in the United States, 86% of whom die within 5 years of diagnosis, making it the leading cause of cancer death in both men and women. The incidence of lung cancer peaks between ages 55 and 65 years. Lung cancer accounts for 28% of all cancer deaths (32% in men, 25% in women). The smoking cessation efforts begun 30 years ago have lowered the age-adjusted lung cancer death rate in males ($\sim$70 per 100,000 male population); but, unfortunately, the rate in females is still increasing ($\sim$35 per 100,000 female population). The 5-year overall lung cancer survival rate (14%) has nearly doubled in the past 30 years. The improvement is due to advances in combined-modality treatment with surgery, radiotherapy, and chemotherapy. Thus, primary carcinoma of the lung is a major health problem with a generally grim prognosis.

PATHOLOGY

The term *lung cancer* is used for tumors arising from the respiratory epithelium (bronchi, bronchioles, and alveoli). Mesotheliomas, lymphomas, and stromal tumors (sarcomas) are distinct from epithelial lung cancer. Four major cell types make up 88% of all primary lung neoplasms according to the World Health Organization classification (Table 75-1). These are *squamous* or *epidermoid carcinoma*, *small cell* (also called *oat cell*) *carcinoma*, *adenocarcinoma* (including bronchoalveolar), and *large cell* (also called *large cell anaplastic*) *carcinoma*. The remainder include undifferentiated carcinomas, carcinoids, bronchial gland tumors (including adenoid cystic carcinomas and mucoepidermoid tumors), and rarer tumor types. The various cell types have different natural histories and responses to therapy, and thus a correct histologic diagnosis by an experienced pathologist is the first step to correct treatment. In the past 25 years, for unknown reasons, adenocarcinoma has replaced squamous cell carcinoma as the most frequent histologic subtype (Table 75-1).

Major treatment decisions are made on the basis of whether a tumor is classified as a small cell carcinoma or as one of the non-small cell varieties (squamous, adenocarcinoma, large cell carcinoma, bronchoalveolar carcinoma, and mixed versions of these). Some of the distinctions are summarized in Tables 75-1 and 75-2. At presentation, small cell carcinomas usually have already spread such that surgery is unlikely to be curative, and they are managed primarily by chemotherapy with or without radiotherapy. In contrast, non-small cell cancers that are localized at the time of presentation may be cured with either surgery or radiotherapy. Non-small cell cancers do not respond as well to chemotherapy as small cell cancers.

Ninety percent of patients with lung cancer of all histologic types are current or former cigarette smokers. Of the an-

TABLE 75-1 *Frequency, Age-Adjusted Incidence, and Survival Rates for Different Histologic Types of Lung Cancer*[a]

Histologic Type of Thoracic Malignancy	Frequency, %	Age-Adjusted Rate	5-Year Survival Rate (All Stages)
Adenocarcinoma (and all subtypes)	32	17	17
Bronchioloalveolar carcinoma	3	1.4	42
Squamous cell (epidermoid) carcinoma	29	15	15
Small cell carcinoma	18	9	5
Large cell carcinoma	9	5	11
Carcinoid	1.0	0.5	83
Mucoepidermoid carcinoma	0.1	<0.1	39
Adenoid cystic carcinoma	<0.1	<0.1	48
Sarcoma and other soft tissue tumors	0.1	0.1	30
All others and unspecified carcinomas	11.0	6	NA
Total	100	52	14

[a] Data on histology frequency and age-adjusted incidence rates per 100,000 U.S. population are from 60,514 cases of invasive lung cancer involving all races and both sexes obtained from the data for 1983–1987 of the Surveillance, Epidemiology, and End Results (SEER) Program of the National Cancer Institute; 5-year relative survival rates for all stages, all races, and both sexes are from the SEER data on 87,128 carcinomas, 1978–1986. NA, not available.
Source: Summarized from Travis et al: Cancer 75:191, 1995.

nual 171,900 new cases of lung cancer, ~50% develop in former smokers. With increased success in smoking cessation efforts, the number of former smokers will grow, and these individuals will be important candidates for early detection and chemoprevention efforts. By far the most common form of lung cancer arising in lifetime nonsmokers, in women, and in young patients (<45 years) is adenocarcinoma. However, in nonsmokers with adenocarcinoma involving the lung, the possibility of other primary sites should be considered. Squamous and small cell cancers usually present as central masses with endobronchial growth, while adenocarcinomas and large cell cancers tend to present as peripheral nodules or masses, frequently with pleural involvement. Squamous and large cell cancers cavitate in ~10 to 20% of cases. Bronchoalveolar carcinoma, a form of adenocarcinoma arising from peripheral airways, can present radiographically as a single mass; as a diffuse, multinodular lesion; or as a fluffy infiltrate.

ETIOLOGY

Most lung cancers are caused by carcinogens and tumor promoters ingested via cigarette smoking. The prevalence of smoking in the United States is 28% for males and 25% for females, age 18 years or older; 38% of high school seniors smoke. The relative risk of developing lung cancer is increased about 13-fold by active smoking and about 1.5-fold by long-term passive exposure to cigarette smoke. Chronic obstructive pulmonary disease, which is also smoking-related, further increases the risk of developing lung cancer. The lung cancer death rate is related to the total amount (often expressed in "cigarette pack-years") of cigarettes smoked, such that the risk is increased 60- to 70-fold for a man smoking two packs a day for 20 years as compared with a nonsmoker. Conversely, the chance of developing lung cancer decreases with cessation of smoking but may never return to the nonsmoker level. The increase in lung cancer rate in women is also associated with a rise in cigarette smoking. Women have a higher relative risk per given exposure than men (~1.5 fold higher), and women with lung cancer are more likely than men to have never smoked. This sex difference is likely due to a higher susceptibility to tobacco carcinogens in women.

Efforts to get people to stop smoking are mandatory. However, smoking cessation is extremely difficult, because the smoking habit represents a powerful addiction to nicotine (Chap. 375). Smoking addiction is both biologic and psychosocial. Different methods are available to help motivated smokers give up the habit including counseling, behavioral therapy, nicotine replacement (gum, patch, sublingual spray, inhaler), and antidepressants (buproprion). However, these methods are successful in only 20 to 25% of individuals at 1 year. Preventing people from starting to smoke may be more effective, an effort that needs to be targeted to children.

Molecular genetic studies have shown the acquisition by lung cancer cells of a number of genetic lesions, including activation of dominant oncogenes and inactivation of tumor suppressor or recessive oncogenes (Chaps. 68 and 69). In fact, lung cancer cells may have to accumulate a large number (perhaps ≥20) of such lesions. For the

TABLE 75-2 *Comparison of Small Cell and Non-Small Cell Lung Cancers*

Feature	Small Cell	Non-Small Cell
Histology	Scant cytoplasm; small, hyperchromatic nuclei with fine chromatin pattern; nucleoli indistinct; diffuse sheets of cells	Abundant cytoplasm; pleomorphic nuclei with coarse chromatin pattern; nucleoli often prominent; glandular or squamous architecture
GENERAL NEUROENDOCRINE PROPERTIES		
Dense-core granules	Present	Absent
Chromogranin	Present	Absent
Synaptophysin	Present	Absent
CD56 and CD57 antigens	Present	Absent
PEPTIDE HORMONE PRODUCTION		
Gastrin-releasing peptide gene products	Present	Absent
Other neuropeptides	ACTH, AVP, calcitonin, ANF	PTH
Autocrine loops	GRP/GRP receptor SCF/KIT	HGF/MET NDF/ERBB2
OTHER MARKERS		
HLA, β_2-microglobulin	Absent/low	Present
Intermediate filament pattern	"SCLC"	"Non SCLC"
Neurofilaments	Present	Absent
Opioid receptors	Present	Present
Nicotine receptors	Present	Present
EGF receptors	Low or absent	Present
Mucin	Absent	Present in adenocarcinomas
Surfactant-associated proteins	Absent	Often present
Carcinoembryonic antigen	Present	Present
RECESSIVE ONCOGENE (TUMOR SUPPRESSOR GENE) AND ALLELOTYPE ABNORMALITIES		
3p allele loss	100%	>90%
RASSF1A methylation	90%	40%
rb mutations	~90%	~20%
p16/CDKN2 mutations/absent expression	~10%	~50%
p53 mutations/abnormal expression	>90%	>50%
Promoter hypermethylation overall (*p16*, DAP Kinase, GSTP1, MGMT, *FHIT*, *RARβ*, *APC*, *ECAD*, *HCAD*, *RASSF1A*)	>80%	>80%
4p, 4q, 5q, 8p, 11p and other allele losses	Present	Present
Microsatellite alterations	Present	Present
DOMINANT ONCOGENE ABNORMALITIES		
ras mutations	<1%	~30%
myc family overexpression	>50%	10–35%
bcl-2 overexpression	>75%	>50%
Her-2/neu overexpression	<10%	~30%
Telomerase overexpression	>90%	>90%
RESPONSE		
Radiotherapy	Objective shrinkage in 80–90%; often complete response	Objective shrinkage in 30–50%; response uncommonly complete
Combination chemotherapy		
Overall regression rate	90%	40–60%
Rate of complete regression	30%	5%

dominant oncogenes, these include point mutations in the coding regions of the *ras* family of oncogenes (particularly in the K-*ras* gene in adenocarcinoma of the lung); amplification, rearrangement, and/or loss of transcriptional control of *myc* family oncogenes (c-, N-, and L-*myc*; changes in c-*myc* are found in non-small cell cancers, while changes in all *myc* family members are found in small cell lung cancer); and overexpression of *bcl-2*, *Her-2/neu*, and the telomerase gene (Table 75-2). Tumor mutations in *ras* genes are associated with a poor prognosis in non-small cell lung cancer, while tumor amplification of c-*myc* is associated with a poor prognosis in small cell lung cancer.

For the recessive oncogenes (*tumor suppressor genes*), allele loss occurs at chromosome regions 1p, 1q, 3p12-13, 3p14 (*FHIT* gene), 3p21 (*RASSF1A* gene), 3p24-25 (*RARβ* gene), 4p, 4q, 5q, 8p, 9p (*p16/CDKN2*, *p15,p14ARF* gene cluster), 11p13, 11p15, 13q14 (retinoblastoma, *rb*, gene), 16q, and 17p13 (*p53* gene), as well as other sites. Several candidate recessive oncogenes on chromosome 3p appear to be involved in nearly all lung cancers and may be affected early in preneoplastic lesions. The *p53* and *rb* genes are both mutated in >90% of small cell lung cancers, while *p53* is mutated in >50% and *rb* in 20% of non-small cell lung cancers. *p16/CDKN2* is abnormal in 10% of small cell and >50% of non-small cell lung cancers. The *rb* and *p16/CDKN2* genes are part of the same G_1-to-S cell cycle regulatory pathway. Either one or the other of these elements appears to be mutated or to have its expression turned off (e.g., by hypermethylation of the promoter) in the large majority of lung cancers. Tumor acquired promoter methylation may be the most frequent method of inactivating tumor-suppressor genes in lung cancer (>10 such genes commonly affected). These methylation changes inhibit gene expression and can be detected in tumor cells, preneoplastic lesions, and DNA in the sputum; their detection may improve early diagnosis and follow-up of the disease. Preneoplastic lesions found in the respiratory epithelium of lung cancer patients and smokers include hyperplasia, dysplasia (progressively severe), and carcinoma in situ. 3p allele loss (hyperplasia) followed by 9p (*p16/CDKN2*) allele loss (hyperplasia) are the earliest events; 17p (*p53*) abnormalities and then *ras* mutations are usually found only in carcinoma in situ and invasive cancer. Thus, molecular changes can be found in the earliest preneoplastic lesions and potentially even before any histologic changes are noted. Clinical trials of early diagnosis are needed to prove the usefulness of these molecular markers in the identification of very early lung cancer and in the monitoring of treatment and chemoprevention.

The large number of genetic and epigenetic lesions shows that lung cancer, like other common epithelial malignancies, is a multistep process that is likely to involve both carcinogens and tumor promoters. Prevention can be directed at both processes. Lung cancer cells produce many peptide hormones and express receptors for these hormones, which can act to stimulate tumor cell growth in an "autocrine" fashion. Highly carcinogenic derivatives of nicotine are formed in cigarette smoke. Lung cancer cells of all histologic types (and the cells from which they are derived) express nicotinic acetylcholine receptors. Nicotine activates signaling pathways in tumor and normal cells that block apoptosis. Thus, nicotine itself could be directly involved in lung cancer pathogenesis.

While lung cancer does not have a clear pattern of Mendelian inheritance, several features suggest a potential for familial association. Inherited mutations in *rb* (patients with retinoblastomas living to adulthood) and *p53* (Li-Fraumeni syndrome) genes may develop lung cancer. First-degree relatives of lung cancer probands have a two- to threefold excess risk of lung cancer or other cancers, many of which are not smoking-related. Certain alleles of the P450 enzyme system (which metabolizes carcinogens) or chromosome fragility (*mutagen sensitivity*) genotypes are associated with the development of lung cancer. The use of these polymorphisms to identify persons at very high risk of developing lung cancer would be useful in early detection and prevention efforts.

CLINICAL MANIFESTATIONS

Lung cancer gives rise to signs and symptoms caused by local tumor growth, invasion or obstruction of adjacent structures, growth in regional nodes through lymphatic spread, growth in distant metastatic sites after hematogenous dissemination, and remote effects of tumor products (paraneoplastic syndromes) (Chaps. 86 and 87).

Although 5 to 15% of patients with lung cancer are identified while they are asymptomatic, usually as a result of a routine chest radiograph, most patients present with some sign or symptom. Central or endobronchial growth of the primary tumor may cause cough, hemoptysis, wheeze and stridor, dyspnea, and postobstructive pneumonitis (fever and productive cough). Peripheral growth of the primary tumor may cause pain from pleural or chest wall involvement, cough, dyspnea on a restrictive basis, and symptoms of lung abscess resulting from tumor cavitation. Regional spread of tumor in the thorax (by contiguous growth or by metastasis to regional lymph nodes) may cause tracheal obstruction, esophageal compression with dysphagia, recurrent laryngeal nerve paralysis with hoarseness, phrenic nerve paralysis with elevation of the hemidiaphragm and dyspnea, and sympathetic nerve paralysis with Horner's syndrome (enophthalmos, ptosis, miosis, and ipsilateral loss of sweating). Malignant pleural effusion often leads to dyspnea. *Pancoast's* (or *superior sulcus tumor*) *syndrome* results from local extension of a tumor growing in the apex of the lung with involvement of the eighth cervical and first and second thoracic nerves, with shoulder pain that characteristically radiates in the ulnar distribution of the arm, often with radiologic destruction of the first and second ribs. Often Horner's syndrome and Pancoast's syndrome coexist. Other problems of regional spread include *superior vena cava syndrome* from vascular obstruction; pericardial and cardiac extension with resultant tamponade, arrhythmia, or cardiac failure; lymphatic obstruction with resultant pleural effusion; and lymphangitic spread through the lungs with hypoxemia and dyspnea. In addition, bronchoalveolar carcinoma can spread transbronchially, producing tumor growing along multiple alveolar surfaces with impairment of gas exchange, respiratory insufficiency, dyspnea, hypoxemia, and sputum production.

Extrathoracic metastatic disease is found at autopsy in >50% of patients with squamous carcinoma, 80% of patients with adenocarcinoma and large cell carcinoma, and >95% of patients with small cell cancer. Lung cancer metastases may occur in virtually every organ system. Common clinical problems related to metastatic lung cancer include brain metastases with neurologic deficits; bone metastases with pain and pathologic fractures; bone marrow invasion with cytopenias or leukoerythroblastosis; liver metastases causing liver dysfunction, biliary obstruction, and pain; lymph node metastases in the supraclavicular region and occasionally in the axilla and groin; and spinal cord compression syndromes from epidural or bone metastases. Adrenal metastases are common but rarely cause adrenal insufficiency.

Paraneoplastic syndromes are common in patients with lung cancer and may be the presenting finding or first sign of recurrence. In addition, paraneoplastic syndromes may mimic metastatic disease and, unless detected, lead to inappropriate palliative rather than curative treatment. Often the paraneoplastic syndrome may be relieved with successful treatment of the tumor. In some cases, the pathophysiology of the paraneoplastic syndrome is known, particularly when a hormone with biologic activity is secreted by a tumor (Chap. 86). However, in many cases the pathophysiology is unknown. Systemic symptoms of anorexia, cachexia, weight loss (seen in 30% of patients), fever, and suppressed immunity are paraneoplastic syndromes of unknown etiology. *Endocrine syndromes* are seen in 12% of patients: hypercalcemia and hypophosphatemia resulting from the ectopic production by squamous tumors of parathyroid hormone (PTH) or, more commonly, PTH-related peptide; hyponatremia with the syndrome of inappropriate secretion of antidiuretic hormone or possibly atrial natriuretic factor by small cell cancer; and ectopic secretion by small cell cancer of adrenocorticotropic hormone (ACTH). ACTH secretion usually results in additional electrolyte disturbances, especially hypokalemia, rather than the changes in body habitus that occur in Cushing's syndrome from a pituitary adenoma.

Skeletal–connective tissue syndromes include clubbing in 30% of cases (usually non-small cell carcinomas) and hypertrophic pulmonary osteoarthropathy in 1 to 10% of cases (usually adenocarcinomas) with periostitis and clubbing causing pain, tenderness, and swelling over the affected bones and a positive bone scan. *Neurologic-myopathic syndromes* are seen in only 1% of patients but are dramatic and include the myasthenic *Eaton-Lambert syndrome* and retinal blindness with small cell cancer, while peripheral neuropathies, subacute cerebellar degeneration, cortical degeneration, and polymyositis are seen with all lung cancer types. Many of these are caused by autoimmune responses such as the development of anti-voltage-gated calcium channel antibodies in the Eaton-Lambert syndrome (Chap. 87). Coagulation, thrombotic, or other hematologic manifestations occur in 1 to 8% of patients and include migratory venous thrombophlebitis (*Trousseau's syndrome*), nonbacterial thrombotic (marantic) endocarditis with arterial emboli, disseminated intravascular coagulation with hemorrhage, and anemia, granulocytosis, and leukoerythroblastosis. Thrombotic disease complicating cancer is usually a poor prognostic sign. Cutaneous manifestations such as dermatomyositis and acanthosis nigricans are uncommon (≤1%), as are the renal manifestations of nephrotic syndrome or glomerulonephritis (≤1%).

DIAGNOSIS AND STAGING

EARLY DIAGNOSIS The screening of asymptomatic persons at high risk (men >45 years who smoke ≥40 cigarettes per day) by means of sputum cytology and chest radiographs has not improved the survival rate. Although 90% of patients whose lung cancer was detected by screening were asymptomatic, no difference was found in the survival rates of the screened and nonscreened groups. Women have not been studied. The use of low-dose spiral computed tomography (CT) lung scanning may be more sensitive, particularly for peripheral lesions. However, false-positive rates are high (25% have abnormal tests, only 10% of which are cancers), and survival benefit for screening has not yet been shown (Chap. 67).

ESTABLISHING A TISSUE DIAGNOSIS OF LUNG CANCER Once signs, symptoms, or screening studies suggest lung cancer, a tissue diagnosis must be established. Tumor tissue can be obtained by a bronchial or transbronchial biopsy during fiberoptic bronchoscopy; by node biopsy during mediastinoscopy; from the operative specimen at the time of definitive surgical resection; by percutaneous biopsy of an enlarged lymph node, soft tissue mass, lytic bone lesion, bone marrow, or pleural lesion; by fine-needle aspiration of thoracic or extrathoracic tumor masses using CT guidance; or from an adequate cell block obtained from a malignant pleural effusion. In most cases, the pathologist should be able to make a definite diagnosis of epithelial malignancy and distinguish small cell from non-small cell lung cancer.

STAGING PATIENTS WITH LUNG CANCER Lung cancer staging consists of two parts: first, a determination of the location of tumor (anatomic staging) and, second, an assessment of a patient's ability to withstand various antitumor treatments (physiologic staging). In a patient with non-small cell lung cancer, *resectability* (whether the tumor can be entirely removed by a standard surgical procedure such as a lobectomy or pneumonectomy), which depends on the anatomic stage of the tumor, and *operability* (whether the patient can tolerate such a surgical procedure), which depends on the cardiopulmonary function of the patient, are determined.

Non-Small Cell Lung Cancer The TNM International Staging System should be used for cases of non-small cell lung cancer, particularly in preparing patients for curative attempts with surgery or radiotherapy (Table 75-3). The various T (tumor size), N (regional node involvement), and M (presence or absence of distant metastasis) factors are combined to form different stage groups. At presentation, approximately one-third of patients have disease localized enough for a curative attempt with surgery or radiotherapy (patients with stage I or II

TABLE 75-3 *Tumor, Node, Metastasis International Staging System for Lung Cancer*

Stage	TNM Descriptors	5-Year Survival Rate, %	
		Clinical Stage	Surgical-Pathologic Stage
IA	T1 N0 M0	61	67
IB	T2 N0 M0	38	57
IIA	T1 N1 M0	34	55
IIB	T2 N1 M0	24	39
IIB	T3 N0 M0	22	38
IIIA	T3 N1 M0	9	25
	T1–2–3 N2 M0	13	23
IIIB	T4 N0–1–2 M0	7	<5
	T1–2–3–4 N3 M0	3	<3
IV	Any T any N M1	1	<1

TUMOR (T) STATUS DESCRIPTOR

T0	No evidence of a primary tumor
TX	Primary tumor cannot be assessed, or tumor proven by the presence of malignant cells in sputum or bronchial washings but not visualized by imaging or bronchoscopy
TIS	Carcinoma in situ
T1	Tumor <3 cm in greatest dimension, surrounded by lung or visceral pleura, without bronchoscopic evidence of invasion more proximal than lobar bronchus (i.e., not in main bronchus)
T2	Tumor with any of following: >3 cm in greatest dimension; involves main bronchus, ≥2 cm distal to the carcina; invades visceral pleura; associated with atelectasis or obstructive pneumonitis extending to hilum but does not involve entire lung
T3	Tumor of any size that directly invades any of the following: chest wall (including superior sulcus tumors), diaphragm, mediastinal pleura, parietal pericardium; or tumor in main bronchus <2 cm distal to carina but without involvement of carina; or associated atelectasis or obstructive pneumonitis of entire lung
T4	Tumor of any size that invades any of the following: mediastinum, heart, great vessels, trachea, esophagus, vertebral body, carina; or tumor with a malignant pleural or pericardial effusion[a], or with satellite tumor nodule(s) within the ipsilateral primary-tumor lobe of the lung.

LYMPH NODE (N) INVOLVEMENT DESCRIPTOR

NX	Regional lymph nodes cannot be assessed
N0	No regional lymph node metastasis
N1	Metastasis to ipsilateral peribronchial and/or ipsilateral hilar lymph nodes, and intrapulmonary nodes involved by direct extension of the primary tumor
N2	Metastasis to ipsilateral mediastinal and/or subcarinal lymph nodes(s)
N3	Metastasis to contralateral mediastinal, contralateral hilar, ipsilateral or contralateral scalene, or supraclavicular lymph node(s)

DISTANT METASTASIS (M) DESCRIPTOR

MX	Presence of distant metastasis cannot be assessed
M0	No distant metastasis
M1	Distant metastasis present[b]

[a] Most pleural effusions associated with lung cancer are due to tumor. However, in a few patients with multiple negative cytopathologic exams of a non-bloody, non-exudative pleural or pericardial effusion that clinical judgment dictates is not related to the tumor, the effusion should be excluded as a staging element and the patient's disease staged as T1, T2, or T3.

[b] Separate metastatic pulmonary tumor nodule(s) in the ipsilateral nonprimary tumor lobe(s) of the lung are classified as M1.

Source: Adapted from CF Mountain. Revisions in the International System for Staging of Lung Cancer. Chest 111:1710, 1997; with permission.

disease and some with stage IIIA disease), one-third have distant metastatic disease (stage IV disease), and one-third have local or regional disease that may or may not be amenable to a curative attempt (some patients with stage IIIA disease and others with stage IIIB disease) (see below). This staging system provides useful prognostic information.

Small Cell Lung Cancer   A simple two-stage system is used. In this system, limited-stage disease (seen in about 30% of all patients with small cell lung cancer) is defined as disease confined to one hemithorax and regional lymph nodes (including mediastinal, contralateral hilar, and usually ipsilateral supraclavicular nodes), while extensive-stage disease (seen in about 70% of patients) is defined as disease exceeding those boundaries. Clinical studies such as physical examination, x-rays, CT and bone scans, and bone marrow examination are used in staging. In part, the definition of limited-stage disease relates to whether the known tumor can be encompassed within a tolerable radiation therapy port. Thus, contralateral supraclavicular nodes, recurrent laryngeal nerve involvement, and superior vena caval obstruction can all be part of limited-stage disease. However, cardiac tamponade, malignant pleural effusion, and bilateral pulmonary parenchymal involvement generally qualify disease as extensive-stage because the organs within a curative radiation therapy port cannot safely tolerate curative radiation doses.

GENERAL STAGING PROCEDURES (Table 75-4)   All patients with lung cancer should have a complete history and physical examination, with evaluation of all other medical problems, determination of performance status and history of weight loss, and a CT scan of the chest and abdomen with contrast. Positron emission tomography (PET) scans are sensitive in detecting both intrathoracic and metastatic disease. PET is useful in assessing the mediastinum and solitary pulmonary nodules. A Standardized Uptake Value (SUV) of >2.5 is highly suspicious for malignancy. False negatives can be seen in diabetes, slow-growing tumors such as bronchoalveolar carcinoma, concurrent infection such as tuberculosis, and in lesions <1 cm. Fiberoptic bronchoscopy obtains material for pathologic examination and information on tumor size, location, degree of bronchial obstruction (i.e., assesses resectability), and recurrence.

Chest radiographs and CT scans are needed to evaluate tumor size and nodal involvement; old radiographs are useful for comparison. CT scans of the thorax and upper abdomen are of use in the preoperative staging of non-small cell lung cancer to detect mediastinal nodes and pleural extension and occult abdominal disease (e.g., liver, adrenal), and in planning curative radiation therapy. However, mediastinal nodal involvement should be documented histologically if the findings will influence therapeutic decisions. Thus, sampling of lymph nodes via mediastinoscopy or thoracotomy to establish the presence or absence of N2 or N3 nodal involvement is crucial in considering a curative surgical approach for patients with non-small cell lung cancer with clinical stage I, II, or III disease. A standard nomenclature for referring to the location of lymph nodes involved with cancer has evolved (Fig. 75-1). Likewise, unless the CT-detected abnormalities are unequivocal, histology of suspicious abdominal lesions should be confirmed by procedures such as fine-needle aspiration if the patient would otherwise be considered for curative treatment. In small cell lung cancer, CT scans are used in the planning of chest radiation treatment and in the assessment of the response to chemotherapy and radiation therapy. Surgery or radiotherapy can make interpretation of conventional chest x-rays difficult; after treatment, CT scans can provide good evidence of tumor recurrence.

If signs or symptoms suggest involvement by tumor, brain CT or bone scans are performed, as well as radiography of any suspicious bony lesions. Any accessible lesions suspicious for cancer should be biopsied if involvement would influence treatment.

In patients presenting with a mass lesion on chest x-ray or CT scan and no obvious contraindications to a curative approach after the initial evaluation, the mediastinum must be investigated. Approaches vary among centers and include performing chest CT scan and mediastinoscopy (for right-sided tumors) or mediastinotomy (for left-sided lesions) on all patients and proceeding directly to thoracotomy for staging of the mediastinum. In patients presenting with disease that is confined to the chest but not resectable, and who thus are candidates for neoadjuvant chemotherapy plus surgery or for curative radiother-

TABLE 75-4 *Pretreatment Staging Procedures for Patients with Lung Cancer*

ALL PATIENTS

Complete history and physical examination
  Determination of performance status and weight loss
Complete blood count with platelet determination
Measurement of serum electrolytes, glucose, calcium, and phosphorus; renal and liver function tests
Electrocardiogram
Skin test for tuberculosis
Chest x-ray
CT scan of chest and abdomen
CT scan of brain and radionuclide scan of bone if any finding suggests the presence of tumor metastasis in these organs
Fiberoptic bronchoscopy with washings, brushings, and biopsy of suspicious lesions unless medically contraindicated or if it would not alter therapy (e.g., very late stage patient)
X-rays of suspicious bony lesions detected by scan or symptom
Barium-swallow radiographic examination if esophageal symptoms exist
Pulmonary function studies and arterial blood gas measurements if signs or symptoms of respiratory insufficiency are present
Biopsy of accessible lesions suspicious for cancer if a histologic diagnosis is not yet made or if treatment or staging decisions would be based on whether or not a lesion contained cancer

PATIENTS WITH NON-SMALL CELL LUNG CANCER WHO HAVE NO CONTRAINDICATION^a TO CURATIVE SURGERY OR RADIOTHERAPY WITH OR WITHOUT CHEMOTHERAPY

All the above procedures, plus the following:
PET scan to evaluate mediastinum and detect metastatic disease
Pulmonary function tests and arterial blood gas measurements
Coagulation tests
CT scan of brain if symptoms suggestive
Cardiopulmonary excercise testing if performance status or pulmonary function tests are borderline
  If surgical resection is planned: surgical evaluation of the mediastinum at mediastinoscopy or at thoracotomy
  If the patient is a poor surgical risk or a candidate for curative radiotherapy: transthoracic fine-needle aspiration biopsy or transbronchial forceps biopsy of peripheral lesions if material from routine fiberoptic bronchoscopy is negative

PATIENTS PRESENTING WITH SMALL CELL OR ADVANCED NON-SMALL CELL LUNG CANCER

For proven small cell lung cancer, all the procedures under "All Patients," plus the following:
  CT scan of brain
  Bone marrow aspiration and biopsy (if peripheral blood counts abnormal)
For non-small cell lung cancer or cancer of unknown histology, all the procedures under "All Patients," plus the following:
  Fiberoptic bronchoscopy if indicated by hemoptysis, obstruction, pneumonitis, or no histologic diagnosis of cancer
  Biopsy of accessible lesions suspicious for tumor to obtain a histologic diagnosis or if therapy would be altered by finding of tumor
  Transthoracic fine-needle aspiration biopsy or transbronchial forceps biopsy of peripheral lesions if fiberoptic bronchoscopy is negative and no other material exists for a histologic diagnosis
  Diagnostic and therapeutic thoracentesis if a pleural effusion is present

^{a} Patients with non-small cell lung cancer and extrathoracic metastatic disease, malignant pleural effusion, or intrathoracic disease beyond the bounds of a tolerable radiotherapy port.
Note: CT, computed tomography; PET, positron emission tomography.

apy with or without chemotherapy, other tests are done as indicated to evaluate specific symptoms. In patients presenting with non-small cell cancer that is not curable, all the general staging procedures are done, plus fiberoptic bronchoscopy as indicated to evaluate hemoptysis, obstruction, or pneumonitis, as well as thoracentesis with cytologic examination (and chest tube drainage as indicated) if fluid is present. As a rule, a radiographic finding of an isolated lesion (such as an enlarged adrenal gland) should be confirmed as cancer by fine-needle aspiration before a curative attempt is rejected.

STAGING OF SMALL CELL LUNG CANCER   Pretreatment staging for patients with small cell lung cancer includes the initial general lung cancer evaluation with chest and abdominal CT scans (because of the high frequency of hepatic and adrenal involvement) as well as fiberoptic bronchoscopy with washings and biopsies to determine the tumor extent before therapy; brain CT scan (10% of patients have metastases); bone marrow biopsy and aspiration (20 to 30% of patients have tumor in the bone marrow); and radionuclide scans (bone) if symptoms or other findings suggest disease involvement in these areas. Chest and abdominal CT scans are very useful to evaluate and follow tumor response to therapy, and chest CT scans are helpful in planning chest radiotherapy ports.

If signs or symptoms of spinal cord compression or leptomeningitis develop at any time in lung cancer patients with disease of any histologic type, a spinal CT scan or magnetic resonance imaging (MRI) scan and examination of the cerebrospinal fluid cytology are performed. If malignant cells are detected, radiotherapy to the site of compression and intrathecal chemotherapy (usually with methotrexate) are given. In addition, a brain CT or MRI scan is performed to search for brain metastases, which often are associated with spinal cord or leptomeningeal metastases.

DETERMINATION OF RESECTABILITY AND OPERABILITY

In patients with non-small cell lung cancer, the following are major contraindications to curative surgery or radiotherapy alone: extrathoracic metastases; superior vena cava syndrome; vocal cord and, in most cases, phrenic nerve paralysis; malignant pleural effusion; cardiac tamponade; tumor within 2 cm of the carina (not curable by surgery but potentially curable by radiotherapy); metastasis to the contralateral lung; bilateral endobronchial tumor (potentially curable by radiotherapy); metastasis to the supraclavicular lymph nodes; contralateral mediastinal node metastases (potentially curable by radiotherapy); and involvement of the main pulmonary artery. Most patients with small cell lung cancer have unresectable disease; however, if clinical findings suggest the potential for resection (most common with peripheral lesions), that option should be considered.

PHYSIOLOGIC STAGING Patients with lung cancer often have cardiopulmonary and other problems related to chronic obstructive pulmonary disease as well as other medical problems. To improve their preoperative condition, correctable problems (e.g., anemia, electrolyte and fluid disorders, infections, and arrhythmias) should be addressed, smoking stopped, and appropriate chest therapy instituted. Since it is not always possible to predict whether a lobectomy or pneumonectomy will be required until the time of operation, a conservative approach is to restrict resectional surgery to patients who could potentially tolerate a pneumonectomy. In addition to nonambulatory performance status, a myocardial infarction within the past 3 months is a contraindication to thoracic surgery because 20% of patients will die of reinfarction, while an infarction in the past 6 months is a relative contraindication. Other major contraindications include uncontrolled major arrhythmias, an FEV_1 (forced expiratory volume in 1 s) <1 L, CO_2 retention (resting PCO_2 > 45 mmHg), D_LCO < 40%, and severe pulmonary hypertension. Recommending surgery when the FEV_1 is 1.1 to 2.0 L or <80% predicted requires careful judgment, while an FEV_1 > 2.5 L or >80% predicted usually permits a pneumonectomy. In patients with borderline lung function but a resectable tumor, cardiopulmonary exercise testing could be performed as part of the physiologic evaluation. This test allows an estimate of the maximal oxygen consumption ($\dot{V}max_{O_2}$). A $\dot{V}max_{O_2}$ < 15 mL/kg per min predicts for high risk of postoperative complications.

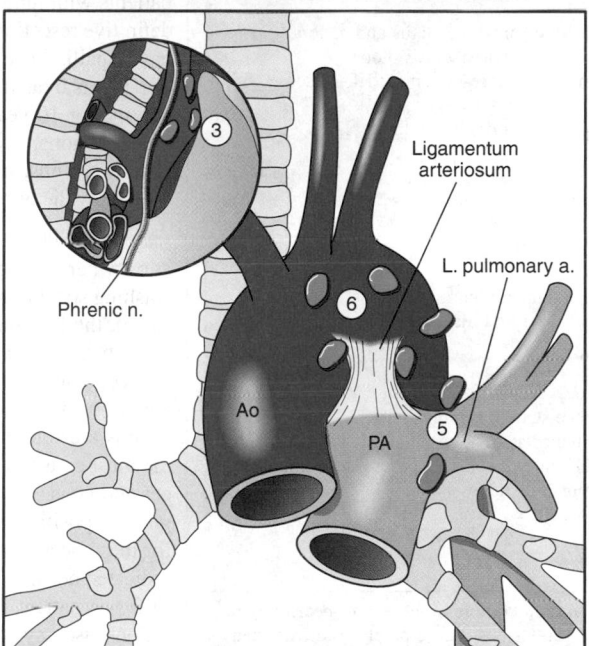

FIGURE 75-1 Regional lymph node stations for lung cancer staging. (*Used by permission from CF Mountain, C Dresler: Chest 111:1718, 1997.*)

Superior Mediastinal Nodes
1 Highest mediastinal
2 Upper paratracheal
3 Prevascular and retrotracheal
4 Lower paratracheal (including azygos nodes)
N2 = single digit, ipsilateral
N3 = single digit, contralateral or supraclavicular

Aortic Nodes
5 Subaortic (A-P window)
6 Para-aortic (ascending aorta or phrenic)

Inferior Mediastinal Nodes
7 Subcarinal
8 Paraesophageal (below carina)
9 Pulmonary ligament

N1 Nodes
10 Hilar
11 Interlobar
12 Lobar
13 Segmental
14 Subsegmental

℞ TREATMENT

The overall treatment approach to patients with lung cancer is shown in Table 75-5. Patients should be encouraged to stop smoking. Those who do fare better than those who continue to smoke.

Non-Small Cell Lung Cancer: Localized Disease ■ SURGERY In patients with non-small cell lung cancer of stages IA, IB, IIA and IIB (Table 75-3) who can tolerate operation, the treatment of choice is pulmonary resection. In stage IIIA cases where the patient's age, cardiopulmonary function, and anatomy are favorable, a team approach (involving pulmonary medicine, thoracic surgery, medical and radiation oncology) is useful. Neoadjuvant chemotherapy with or without radiotherapy

TABLE 75-5   Summary of Treatment Approach to Patients with Lung Cancer

NON-SMALL CELL LUNG CANCER

Stages IA, IB, IIA, IIB, and some IIIA:
  Surgical resection for stages IA, IB, IIA, and IIB
  Surgical resection with complete-mediastinal lymph node dissection
    and consideration of neoadjuvant CRx for stage IIIA disease with
    "minimal N2 involvement" (discovered at thoracotomy or
    mediastinoscopy)
  Postoperative RT for patients found to have N2 disease if no
    neoadjuvant CRx given
  Discussion of risks/benefits of adjuvant CRx with individual patients
  Curative potential RT for "nonoperable" patients
Stage IIIA with selected types of stage T3 tumors:
  Tumors with chest wall invasion (T3): en bloc resection of tumor with
    involved chest wall and consideration of postoperative RT
  Superior sulcus (Pancoast's) (T3) tumors: preoperative RT (30–45 Gy)
    followed by en bloc resection of involved lung and chest wall with
    consideration of postoperative RT or intraoperative brachytherapy
  Proximal airway involvement (<2 cm from carina) without
    mediastinal nodes; sleeve resection if possible preserving distal
    normal lung or pneumonectomy
Stages IIIA "advanced, bulky, clinically evident N2 disease" (discovered
  preoperatively) and IIIB disease that can be included in a tolerable RT
  port:
  Curative potential RT + CRx if performance status and general
    medical condition are reasonable; otherwise, RT alone
  Consider neoadjuvant CRx and surgical resection for IIIA disease with
    advanced N2 involvement
Stage IIIB disease with carinal invasion (T4) but without N2
  involvement:
  Consider pneumonectomy with tracheal sleeve resection with direct
    reanastomosis to contralateral mainstem bronchus
Stage IV and more advanced IIIB disease:
  RT to symptomatic local sites
  CRx for ambulatory patients
  Chest tube drainage of large malignant pleural effusions
  Consider resection of primary tumor and metastasis for isolated brain
    or adrenal metastases

SMALL CELL LUNG CANCER

  Limited stage (good performance status): combination CRx + chest RT
  Extensive stage (good performance status): combination CRx
  Complete tumor responders (all stages): consider prophylactic cranial RT
  Poor-performance-status patients (all stages):
    Modified-dose combination CRx
    Palliative RT

ALL PATIENTS

  RT for brain metastases, spinal cord compression, weight-bearing lytic
    bony lesions, symptomatic local lesions (nerve paralyses, obstructed
    airway, hemoptysis, intrathoracic large venous obstruction, in non-
    small cell lung cancer and in small cell cancer not responding to CRx)
  Appropriate diagnosis and treatment of other medical problems and
    supportive care during CRx
  Encouragement to stop smoking
  Entrance into clinical trial, if eligible

Abbreviations: CRx, chemotherapy; RT, radiotherapy.

may shrink the local tumor, treat micrometastases, and make surgical resection safer and more effective in selected patients. If a complete resection is possible, the 5-year survival rate for N1 disease is about 50%, while it is about 20% for N2 disease. However, only 20% of cases of N2 disease are technically resectable, and most of these are discovered to be N2 only at thoracotomy. Surgery for N2 disease is the most controversial area in the surgical management of lung cancer. Patients with N2 disease can be divided into "minimal" disease (involvement of only one node with microscopic foci, usually discovered at thoracotomy or mediastinoscopy) and the more common "advanced," bulky disease, clinically obvious on CT scans and discovered preoperatively. Patients with contralateral or bilateral positive mediastinal (N3) nodes, extracapsular nodal involvement, or fixed nodes are not considered candidates for resection. Approaches that may make

resection possible include chest wall resection for direct extension of tumor, tracheal sleeve pneumonectomy, and sleeve lobectomy for lesions near the carina. Neoadjuvant (preoperative) chemotherapy has response rates of 50 to 60% and causes unresectable disease to become resectable in many patients who respond (see below). Video-assisted thoracic surgery (VATS) via thoracoscopy is not usually used for curative lung cancer resection but may be useful for peripheral lesions in patients with poor lung function. VATS has been advocated to reduce postoperative impairment of lung function, pain, length of hospital stay, and recovery time. However, randomized controlled trials have not confirmed the advantages. Open thoracotomy remains the preferred surgical approach to curative resection of lung cancer. VATS can be used for diagnostic purposes to examine the pleural surface and cavity and biopsy peripheral lung nodules or accessible mediastinal nodes; its major therapeutic use is resection of peripheral lung nodules.

The extent of resection is a matter of surgical judgment based on findings at exploration. Conservative resection that encompasses all known tumor gives survival equal to that obtained with more extensive procedures. However, lobectomy is superior to wedge resection in reducing the rate of local recurrence. Thus, lobectomy is preferred to pneumonectomy and wedge resection. Wedge resection and segmentectomy (potentially by VATS) are reserved for patients with poor pulmonary reserve and small peripheral lesions. About 40% of all patients with lung cancer undergo thoracotomy. Of these, 75% have a definitive resection, 12% are explored only for disease extent, and 12% have a palliative procedure with known disease left behind. About 30% of patients treated with resection for cure survive for 5 years, and 15% survive for 10 years (Table 75-3). The 30-day hospital mortality rate after pulmonary resection is 3% for lobectomy and 6% for pneumonectomy. Thus, most patients thought to have a "curative" resection ultimately die of metastatic disease (usually within 5 years of surgery).

MANAGEMENT OF OCCULT AND STAGE 0 CARCINOMAS   In the uncommon situation where malignant cells are identified in a sputum or bronchial washing specimen but the chest radiograph appears normal (TX tumor stage), the lesion must be localized. More than 90% can be localized by meticulous examination of the bronchial tree with a fiberoptic bronchoscope under general anesthesia and collection of a series of differential brushings and biopsies. Often, carcinoma in situ or multicentric lesions are found in these patients. Current recommendations are for the most conservative surgical resection, allowing removal of the cancer and conservation of lung parenchyma, even if the bronchial margins are positive for carcinoma in situ. The 5-year overall survival rate for these occult cancers is ~60%. Close follow-up of these patients is indicated because of the high incidence of second primary lung cancers (5% per patient per year). One approach to in situ or multicentric lesions uses systemically administered hematoporphyrin (which localizes to tumors and sensitizes them to light) followed by bronchoscopic phototherapy.

SOLITARY PULMONARY NODULE   When a patient presents with an asymptomatic, solitary pulmonary nodule (defined as an x-ray density completely surrounded by normal aerated lung, with circumscribed margins, of any shape, usually 1 to 6 cm in greatest diameter), a decision to resect or follow the nodule must be made. Approximately 35% of all such lesions in adults are malignant, most being primary lung cancer, while <1% are malignant in nonsmokers under 35 years of age. A complete history, including a smoking history, physical examination, routine laboratory tests, chest CT scan, fiberoptic bronchoscopy, and old chest x-rays are obtained. PET scans are useful in detecting lung cancers >1 cm in diameter. If no diagnosis is immediately apparent, the following risk factors would all argue strongly in favor of proceeding with resection to establish a histologic diagnosis: a history of cigarette smoking; age ≥ 35 years; a relatively large lesion; lack of calcification; chest symptoms; associated atelectasis, pneumonitis, or adenopathy; growth of the lesion revealed by comparison with old x-rays; or positive PET scan. At present, only two radiographic criteria are reliable predictors of the benign nature of a solitary pulmonary nodule: lack of growth over a period >2 years and certain characteristic patterns of calcification. Calcification alone does not exclude malignancy. However, a dense central nidus, multiple punctate foci, and "bull's eye" (granuloma) and "popcorn ball" (hamartoma) calcifications are all highly suggestive of a benign lesion. An algorithm for evaluating a solitary pulmonary nodule is shown in Fig. 75-2.

When old x-rays are not available and the characteristic calcification patterns are absent, the following approach is reasonable: Nonsmoking patients <35 years can be followed with serial CT every 3 months for 1 year and then yearly. If any significant growth is found, a histologic diagnosis is needed. For patients >35 years and all patients with a smoking history, a histologic diagnosis must be made. The sample for histologic diagnosis can be obtained either at the time of nodule resection or, if the patient is a poor operative risk, via VATS or transthoracic fine-needle biopsy. Some institutions use preoperative fine-needle aspiration on all such lesions; however, all positive lesions have to be resected, and negative cytologic findings in most cases have to be confirmed by histology on a resected specimen. While much has been made of sparing patients an operation, the high probability of finding a malignancy (particularly in smokers >35 years) and the excellent chance for surgical cure when the tumor is small both suggest an aggressive approach to these lesions.

The application of low-dose spiral CT scanning to high-risk populations is under investigation. The test identifies a large number of asymptomatic pulmonary nodules that require evaluation. Approximately 23% of screened high-risk patients have an abnormality, and ~12% of the detected abnormalities are lung cancer. The American College of Radiology has developed scoring of CT-detected lesions as "benign," "indeterminate," or "abnormal." Lesions > 1 cm are usually resected; those ≤1 cm are followed for change at 3 to 6-month intervals. Although a number of early lung cancers are detected in this way, it is not yet clear that survival is improved.

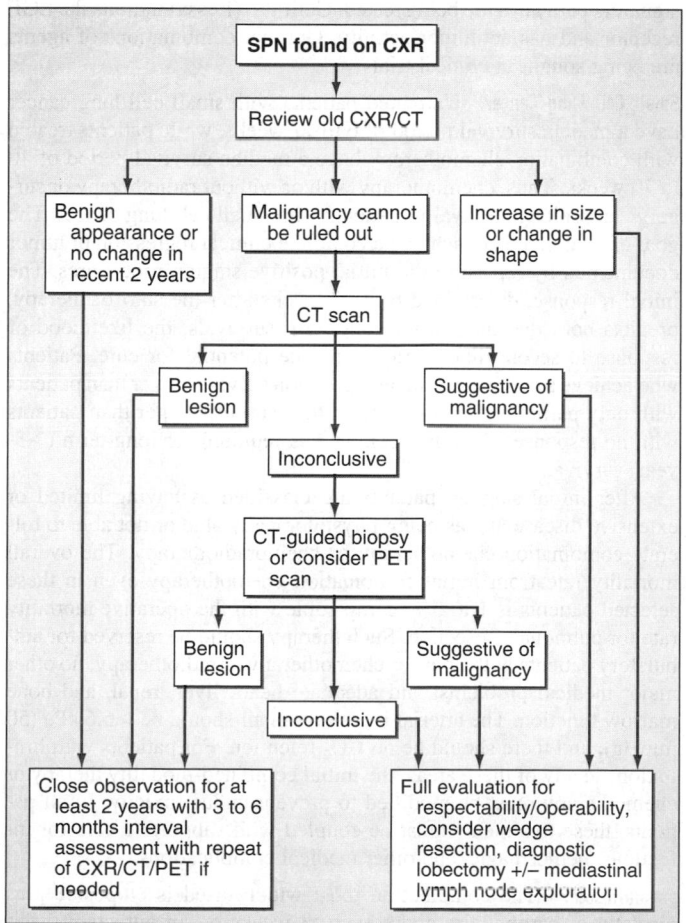

FIGURE 75-2 Algorithm for evaluation of a solitary pulmonary nodule (SPN). (CXR, chest x-ray; CT, computed tomography scan; PET, positron emission tomography.)

RADIOTHERAPY WITH CURATIVE INTENT Patients with stage III disease, as well as patients with stage I or II disease who refuse surgery or are not candidates for pulmonary resection, should be considered for radiation therapy with curative intent. The decision to administer high-dose radiotherapy is based on the extent of disease and the volume of the chest that requires irradiation. Patients with distant metastases, malignant pleural effusion, or cardiac involvement are generally not considered for curative radiation treatment. The median survival period for patients with unresectable non-small cell lung cancer localized to the chest who undergo primary radiotherapy with curative intent is <1 year. However, 6% of these patients are alive at 5 years and are cured by radiotherapy alone. In addition to being potentially curative, radiotherapy, by controlling the primary tumor, may increase the quality and length of life of noncured patients. Treatment usually involves midplane doses of 55 to 60 Gy, and the major concern is the amount of lung parenchyma and other organs in the thorax included in the treatment plan, including the spinal cord, heart, and esophagus. In patients with a major degree of underlying pulmonary disease, the treatment plan may have to be compromised because of the deleterious effect of radiation on pulmonary function. The risk of radiation pneumonitis is proportional to the radiation dose and the volume of lung in the field. The full clinical syndrome (dyspnea, fever, and radiographic infiltrate corresponding to the treatment port) occurs in 5% of cases. Acute radiation esophagitis occurs during treatment but is usually self-limited, while spinal cord injury should be avoided by careful treatment planning. Continuous hyperfractionated accelerated radiation therapy (CHART) involves delivery of 36 treatments of 1.5 Gy given 3 times a day for 12 consecutive days to a total dose of 54 Gy. The 2-year survival rate increased from 20 to 29% with CHART, although more esophagitis occurred. Brachytherapy (local radiotherapy delivered by placing radioactive "seeds" in a catheter in the tumor bed) provides a way to give a high local dose while sparing surrounding normal tissue.

COMBINED-MODALITY THERAPY WITH CURATIVE INTENT After apparently complete resection, adjuvant radiation therapy does not improve survival and may be detrimental in N0 and N1 disease.

Carcinomas of the superior pulmonary sulcus producing *Pancoast's syndrome* are usually treated with combined radiotherapy and surgery. Patients with these carcinomas should have the usual preoperative staging procedures, including mediastinoscopy and CT and PET scans, to determine tumor extent and a neurologic examination (and sometimes nerve conduction studies) to document neurologic findings. Sometimes a histologic diagnosis is not made, but the combination of tumor location and pain distribution permit a diagnostic accuracy for cancer of >90%. If mediastinoscopy is negative, curative approaches may be used in treating a Pancoast's syndrome tumor. Preoperative irradiation [30 Gy in 10 treatments] is given to the area, followed by an en bloc resection of the tumor and involved chest wall 3 to 6 weeks later. The 3-year survival rate is 40% for squamous and 20% for adeno- and large cell carcinomas. Another approach involves radiotherapy alone in curative doses and standard fractionation, which leads to survival rates similar to those from combined-modality therapy. Chemotherapy with etoposide and cisplatin plus radiotherapy to the area produces high rates of tumor resectability and >50% survival at 4 years.

A meta-analysis of chemotherapy in non-small cell lung cancer used updated data on 9387 individual patients from 52 randomized trials, both published and unpublished, with the main outcome measure being survival. Regimens containing cisplatin were significantly more effective than no treatment. Trials in early-stage disease comparing surgery with surgery plus chemotherapy gave a hazard ratio of 0.87 (13% reduction in risk of death at 5 years) in favor of chemotherapy. Confidence intervals of these data are wide. Ongoing randomized trials of adjuvant chemotherapy for stage I and II disease appear to show benefit.

The most impressive benefits were obtained when chemotherapy was added to radiotherapy for locally advanced disease (stage IIIB and some stage IIIA disease) and when chemotherapy was given preoperatively in a neoadjuvant fashion in stage IIIA disease. Preoperative neoadjuvant chemotherapy is widely used for stage IIIA disease. Preoperative combined modality therapy followed by surgical resection has given promising early results. Whether the surgery adds benefit after chemoradiotherapy has not been defined. Provided the risk/benefit ratio of using chemotherapy is discussed appropriately with patients, such therapy can be given in a noninvestigational setting. For stage IIIA disease, resection followed by postoperative radiation plus chemotherapy for N2 disease, neoadjuvant chemotherapy followed by surgical resection, or neoadjuvant chemoradiotherapy followed by resection are options. For stage IIIB and bulky IIIA disease, neoadjuvant chemotherapy (two or three cycles of a cisplatin-based combination) followed by chest radiation therapy (60 Gy) has improved median survival time from 10 to 14 months and the 5-year survival rate from 7 to 17% compared to results with radiation therapy alone. Administration of radiation and chemotherapy concurrently is being tested; myelotoxicity and esophagitis are increased, but survival improvement is not yet proven. Randomized clinical trials are also needed to evaluate the usefulness of the new agents with activity against non-small cell lung cancer, including the taxanes (paclitaxel and docetaxel), vinorelbine, gemcitabine, and the camptothecins (topotecan and irinotecan) in both adjuvant and neoadjuvant settings.

Disseminated Non-Small Cell Lung Cancer   The 70% of patients who have unresectable non-small cell cancer have a poor prognosis. Patients with performance status scores of 0 (asymptomatic), 1 (symptomatic, fully ambulatory), 2 (in bed <50% of the time), 3 (in bed >50% of the time), and 4 (bedridden) have median survival times of 34, 25, 17, 8, and 4 weeks, respectively. Standard medical management, the judicious use of pain medications, the appropriate use of radiotherapy, and outpatient chemotherapy form the cornerstone of management. Patients whose primary tumor is causing symptoms such as bronchial obstruction with pneumonitis, hemoptysis, or upper airway or superior vena cava obstruction should have radiotherapy to the primary tumor. The case for prophylactic treatment of the asymptomatic patient is to prevent major symptoms from occurring in the thorax. Usually a course of 30 to 40 Gy over 2 to 4 weeks is given to the tumor. Radiation therapy provides relief of intrathoracic symptoms with the following frequencies: hemoptysis, 84%; superior vena cava syndrome, 80%; dyspnea, 60%; cough, 60%; atelectasis, 23%; and vocal cord paralysis, 6%. Cardiac tamponade (treated with pericardiocentesis and radiation therapy to the heart), painful bony metastases (with relief in 66%), brain or spinal cord compression, and brachial plexus involvement may also be palliated with radiotherapy. Usually, with brain metastases and cord compression, dexamethasone (25 to 100 mg/d in four divided doses) is also given and then rapidly tapered to the lowest dosage that relieves symptoms.

Brain metastases are often isolated instances of relapse in patients with adenocarcinoma of the lung otherwise controlled by surgery or radiotherapy. However, there is no proven value for prophylactic cranial irradiation or for CT scans of the head in asymptomatic patients.

Pleural effusions are common and are usually treated with thoracentesis. If they recur and are symptomatic, chest tube drainage with a sclerosing agent such as intrapleural talc is used. First, the chest cavity is completely drained. Xylocaine 1% is instilled (15 mL), followed by 50 mL normal saline. Then, 10 g sterile talc is dissolved in 100 mL normal saline, and this solution is injected through the chest tube. The chest tube is clamped for 4 h if tolerated, and the patient is rotated onto different sides to distribute the sclerosing agent. The chest tube is removed 24 to 48 h later, after drainage has become slight (usually <100 mL/24 h). VATS has been used to drain and treat large malignant effusions. An indwelling pleurex catheter is equivalent to chest tube drainage and better tolerated by the patient. Symptomatic

endobronchial lesions that recur after surgery or radiotherapy or that develop in patients with severely compromised pulmonary function are difficult to treat with conventional therapy. Neodynium-YAG (yttrium-aluminum-garnet) laser therapy administered through a flexible fiberoptic bronchoscope (usually under general anesthesia) can provide palliation in 80 to 90% of patients even when the tumor has relapsed after radiotherapy. Local radiotherapy delivered by brachytherapy, photodynamic therapy using a photosensitizing agent, and endobronchial stents are other measures that can relieve airway obstruction from tumor.

CHEMOTHERAPY   The use of chemotherapy for non-small cell lung cancer requires careful judgment to balance potential benefits and toxicity. Modest survival benefits (of 1 to 2 months), symptom palliation, and improved quality of life may accrue from combination chemotherapy. Randomized trials in advanced disease comparing supportive care with supportive care plus chemotherapy gave a hazard ratio of 0.73 (27% reduction in risk of death at 1 year) in favor of including chemotherapy. Economic analysis has found chemotherapy to be cost-effective palliation. Combination chemotherapy produces an objective tumor response in ~20 to 30% of patients; the response is complete in <5%. Median survival for chemotherapy-treated patients is 9 to 10 months, and the 1-year survival rate is 40%. Thus, in patients with non-small cell lung cancer who desire chemotherapy, it is reasonable to give chemotherapy if the patient is ambulatory and is able to understand and accept the risk/benefit ratio from such therapy. The chemotherapy should be one of the published standard regimens, such as paclitaxel plus carboplatin, paclitaxel plus cisplatin, or vinorelbine plus cisplatin. Improved antiemetics have made treatment tolerable on an outpatient basis. New drugs with proven activity in non-small cell lung cancer include docetaxel, irinotecan, and gemcitabine. Docetaxel may provide a survival benefit after relapse from initial chemotherapy. Furthermore, novel agents aimed at growth factor and angiogenesis receptors and signaling pathways are being tested. Gefitinib (Iressa) inhibits the EGF receptor and has antitumor activity. Optimal combinations of agents are being sought in clinical trials.

Small Cell Lung Cancer   Untreated patients with small cell lung cancer have a median survival period of 6 to 17 weeks, while patients treated with combination chemotherapy have a median survival period of 40 to 70 weeks. Thus, chemotherapy with or without radiotherapy or surgery can prolong survival in patients with small cell lung cancer. The goal of treatment is to achieve a complete clinical regression of tumor documented by repeating the initial positive staging procedures. The initial response, determined 6 to 12 weeks after the start of therapy, predicts both the median and long-term survivals, the likelihood of response to second line therapy, and the potential for cure. Patients who achieve a complete clinical regression survive longer than patients with only partial regression, who in turn survive longer than patients with no response. Complete response is required for long-term (>3-year) survival.

After initial staging, patients are classified as having limited or extensive disease and as being physiologically able or not able to tolerate combination chemotherapy or chemoradiotherapy. The overall mortality rate from initial combination chemotherapy even in these selected patients is 1 to 5%, comparable with the operative mortality rate for pulmonary resection. Such therapy should be reserved for ambulatory patients with no prior chemotherapy or radiotherapy; no other major medical problems; and adequate heart, liver, renal, and bone marrow function. The arterial P_{O_2} on room air should be >6.6 kPa (50 mmHg), and there should be no CO_2 retention. For patients with limitations in any of these areas, the initial combined-modality therapy or chemotherapy must be modified to prevent undue toxicity. In all patients, these treatments must be coupled with supportive care for infectious, hemorrhagic, and other medical complications.

CHEMOTHERAPY   The combination most widely used is etoposide plus cisplatin or carboplatin, given every 3 weeks on an outpatient basis for 4 to 6 cycles. Other active regimens are etopside, cisplatin, and paclitaxel or the combination of irinotecan and etoposide, which conveys a longer median survival but is more toxic than etoposide plus cisplatin. Increased dose intensity of chemotherapy adds toxicity without clear survival benefit. Appropriate supportive care (antiemetic therapy, administration of fluid and saline boluses with cisplatin, monitoring of blood counts and blood chemistries, monitoring for signs of bleeding or infection, and, as required, administration of erythropoietin and granulocyte colony-stimulating factor) and adjustment of chemotherapy doses on the basis of nadir granulocyte counts are essential. The initial combination chemotherapy may result in moderate to severe granulocytopenia (e.g., granulocyte counts <500 to 1500/μL) and thrombocytopenia (platelet counts <50,000 to 100,000/μL). After the initial 4 to 6 cycles of therapy, patients should be restaged to determine if they have entered a complete clinical remission, indicated by complete disappearance of all clinically evident lesions and paraneoplastic syndromes; a partial remission; or have no response or tumor progression (seen in 10 to 20% of patients). Chemotherapy is then stopped in responding patients. More prolonged chemotherapy has not been shown to be of value. Patients whose tumors are progressing or not responding should be switched to a new, experimental chemotherapy regimen. Topotecan alone or combined with paclitaxel is active in such second-line therapy. Oral etoposide, as a single agent, has been shown to be of clinical benefit in the initial treatment of patients who are elderly or have a very poor performance status.

RADIOTHERAPY High-dose (40-Gy) radiotherapy to the whole brain should be given to patients with documented brain metastases. Prophylactic cranial irradiation (PCI) may be given to patients with complete responses, since it significantly decreases the development of brain metastases (which occur in 60 to 80% of patients living ≥2 years who do not receive PCI), but survival benefit is small (5%). Because some studies indicate possible deficits in cognitive ability that could be related to PCI, the long-term quality of life after PCI needs to be further studied. The patient needs to be informed of the risks and benefits of PCI. In the case of symptomatic, progressive lesions in the chest or at other critical sites, if radiotherapy has not yet been given to these areas, it may be administered in full doses (e.g., 40 Gy to the chest tumor mass).

COMBINED-MODALITY THERAPY Most patients with limited-stage small cell lung cancer should receive combined-modality therapy with etoposide plus cisplatin (or other platinum-containing regimen) and concurrent chest radiotherapy encompassing sites of known disease in the chest. Acute and chronic toxicities are expected with chemoradiotherapy, particularly when the chemotherapy and radiotherapy are given concurrently. However, the addition of chest radiation therapy to chemotherapy reduces the local failure rate and improves survival. Patients should be selected (limited-stage disease, a performance status of 0 to 1, and initial good pulmonary function) such that radiotherapy can be given in full doses and in a manner that does not sacrifice too much lung function. Some studies show twice-daily radiation fractions produce less toxicity and improve survival compared to once-daily treatments.

For extensive-stage disease, initial chest radiotherapy is usually not advocated. However, for favorable patients (e.g., those with a performance status of 0 to 1, good pulmonary function, and only one site of extensive disease), the addition of chest radiotherapy to chemotherapy can be considered. In patients who are in a chemotherapy-induced complete remission, radiotherapy appears to increase survival. For all patients, if chemotherapy is inadequate to relieve local tumor symptoms, a course of radiotherapy can be added.

About 20 to 30% of patients with limited-stage disease and 1 to 5% of patients with extensive-stage disease are cured. About 50% of patients with limited-stage and 30% of patients with extensive-stage disease enter complete remission, and 90 to 95% of all patients have complete or partial responses. These responses increase the median survival period to 10 to 12 months for patients with extensive-stage disease and to 14 to 18 months for patients with limited-stage disease, as compared with 2 to 4 months for untreated patients. In addition, most patients have relief of their tumor-related symptoms and im-

provement of performance status. However, the maintenance of good performance status in a patient receiving outpatient chemotherapy requires judgment and skill to avoid undue therapeutic toxicity. New treatments, such as new drug combinations, very intensive initial or "reinduction" therapy with autologous bone marrow infusion, and novel ways of combining chemotherapy, radiotherapy, and surgery should be given only in the context of an approved clinical protocol.

Although surgical resection is not routinely recommended for small cell lung cancer, occasional patients meet the usual requirements for resectability (stage I or II disease with negative mediastinal nodes). Moreover, this histologic diagnosis is made in some patients only on review of the resected surgical specimen. Such patients have been reported to have high cure rates (>25%) if adjuvant chemotherapy is used.

LUNG CANCER PREVENTION

Deterring children from taking up smoking and helping young adults stop smoking is likely to be the most effective lung cancer prevention. Smoking cessation programs are successful in 5 to 20% of volunteers; the poor efficacy is because of the nature of nicotine addiction.

Chemoprevention is an experimental approach to reduce lung cancer risk; at present, no benefit has been proven for chemoprevention intervention, and at least two putative chemoprevention agents, vitamin E and β-carotene, actually increase the risk of lung cancer in heavy smokers.

BENIGN LUNG NEOPLASMS

The benign neoplasms of the lung, representing <5% of all primary tumors, include bronchial adenomas and hamartomas (90% of such lesions) and a group of very uncommon benign neoplasms (epithelial tumors such as bronchial papillomas, fibroepithelial polyps; mesenchymal tumors such as chondromas, fibromas, lipomas, hemangiomas, leiomyomas, pseudolymphomas; tumors of mixed origin such as teratomas; and other diseases such as endometriosis). The diagnostic and primary-treatment approach (surgery) is basically the same for all these neoplasms. They can present as central masses causing airway obstruction, cough, hemoptysis, and pneumonitis. The masses may or may not be visible on radiographs but are usually accessible to fiberoptic bronchoscopy. Alternatively, they can present without symptoms as solitary pulmonary nodules and thus will be evaluated as part of a solitary pulmonary nodule workup. In all cases, the extent of surgery must be determined at operation, and a conservative procedure with appropriate reconstructions is usually performed.

BRONCHIAL ADENOMAS Bronchial adenomas (80% are central) are slow-growing, endobronchial lesions; they represent 50% of all benign pulmonary neoplasms. About 80 to 90% are carcinoids, 10 to 15% are adenocystic tumors (or cylindromas), and 2 to 3% are mucoepidermoid tumors. Adenomas present in patients 15 to 60 years old (average age, 45) as endobronchial lesions and are often symptomatic for several years. Patients may have a chronic cough, recurrent hemoptysis, or obstruction with atelectasis, lobar collapse, or pneumonitis and abscess formation. Bronchial carcinoids, which usually follow a benign course, and small cell lung cancers, which are highly malignant, both express a neuroendocrine phenotype. Carcinoids, like small cell lung cancers, may secrete other hormones, such as ACTH or arginine vasopressin, and can cause paraneoplastic syndromes that resolve on resection. Uncommonly, bronchial carcinoid metastases (usually to the liver) may produce the carcinoid syndrome, with cutaneous flush, bronchoconstriction, diarrhea, and cardiac valvular lesions (Chap. 329), which small cell lung cancer does not. Occasionally, pathologists may have difficulty distinguishing carcinoids from small cell lung cancers. Carcinoid tumors that have an unusually aggressive histologic appearance (referred to as *atypical carcinoids*) metastasize in 70% of cases to regional nodes, liver, or bone, compared with only a 5% rate of metastasis for carcinoids with typical histology.

Bronchial adenomas of all types, because of their endobronchial and often central location, are usually visible by fiberoptic bronchoscopy, and tissue for histologic diagnosis is obtained in this manner. Because they are hypervascular, they can bleed profusely after bronchoscopic biopsy, and this problem should be anticipated. Bronchial adenomas must be dealt with as potentially malignant and thus require removal not only for symptom relief but also because they can be locally invasive or recurrent, potentially can metastasize, and may produce paraneoplastic syndromes. Surgical excision is the primary treatment for all types of bronchial adenomas. The extent of surgery is determined at operation and should be as conservative as possible. Often bronchotomy with local excision, sleeve resection, segmental resection, or lobectomy is sufficient. Five-year survival rates after surgical resection are 95%, decreasing to 70% if regional nodes are involved. The treatment of metastatic pulmonary carcinoids is unclear because they can either be indolent or behave more like small cell lung carcinoma. Assessment of the tempo and histology of the disease in the individual patient is necessary to determine if and when chemotherapy or radiotherapy is indicated.

HAMARTOMAS Pulmonary hamartomas have a peak incidence at age 60 and are more frequent in men than in women. Histologically, they contain normal pulmonary tissue components (smooth muscle and collagen) in a disorganized fashion. They are usually peripheral, clinically silent, and benign in their behavior. Unless the radiographic findings are pathognomonic for hamartoma, with "popcorn" calcification, the lesions usually have to be resected for diagnosis, particularly if the patient is a smoker. VATS may minimize the surgical complications.

METASTATIC PULMONARY TUMORS

The lung is a frequent site of metastases from primary cancers outside the lung. Usually such metastatic disease is considered incurable. However, two special situations should be borne in mind. The first is the development of a solitary pulmonary shadow on a chest x-ray in a patient known to have an extrathoracic neoplasm. This shadow may represent a metastasis or a new primary lung cancer. Because the natural history of lung cancer is often worse than that of other primary tumors, a single pulmonary nodule in a patient with a known extrathoracic tumor is approached as though the nodule is a primary lung cancer, particularly if the patient is older than 35 years and a smoker. If a vigorous search for other sites of active cancer proves negative, the nodule is surgically resected. Second, in some cases, multiple pulmonary nodules can be resected with curative intent. This tactic is usually recommended if, after careful staging, it is found that (1) the patient can tolerate the contemplated pulmonary resection, (2) the primary tumor has been definitively and successfully treated (disease-free for >1 year), and (3) all known metastatic disease can be encompassed by the projected pulmonary resection. The key is selection and screening of patients to exclude those with uncontrolled primary tumors and other extrapulmonary metastases. Primary tumors whose pulmonary metastases have been successfully resected for cure include osteogenic and soft tissue sarcomas; colon, rectal, uterine, cervix, and corpus tumors; head and neck, breast, testis, and salivary gland cancer; melanoma; and bladder and kidney tumors. Five-year survival rates of 20 to 30% have been found in carefully selected patients, and dramatic results have been achieved in patients with osteogenic sarcomas, where resection of pulmonary metastases (sometimes requiring several thoracotomies) is becoming a standard curative treatment approach.

FURTHER READING

AMERICAN COLLEGE OF CHEST PHYSICIANS: Diagnosis and management of lung cancer: ACCP evidence-based guidelines. Chest, 123:1S, 2003

KARNATH B: Smoking cessation. Am J Med 112:399, 2002

MOUNTAIN CF: Revisions in the international system for staging lung cancer. Chest 111:1710, 1997

PAO W et al: Targeting the epidermal growth factor receptor tyrosine kinase with gefitinib in non-small–cell lung cancer. Semin Cancer Biol 14:33, 2004

SEKIDO Y et al: Molecular genetics of lung cancer. Annu Rev Med 54:73, 2003

SPECIAL ISSUE DEALING WITH ALL ASPECTS OF THE DIAGNOSIS AND TREATMENT OF SMALL CELL LUNG CANCER. Semin Oncol 30:3, 2003

SPIRA A, ETTINGER DS: Drug therapy: Multidisciplinary management of lung cancer. N Engl J Med 350:379, 2004

76 BREAST CANCER
Marc E. Lippman

Breast cancer is a malignant proliferation of epithelial cells lining the ducts or lobules of the breast. In the year 2004, about 216,000 cases of invasive breast cancer and 40,000 deaths occurred in the United States. Epithelial malignancies of the breast are the most common cause of cancer in women (excluding skin cancer), accounting for about one-third of all cancer in women. As a result of improved treatment and earlier detection, mortality from breast cancer has begun to decrease substantially in the United States. This chapter will not consider rare malignancies of the breast, such as sarcomas and lymphomas, but will focus on the epithelial cancers. Human breast cancer is a clonal disease; a single transformed cell—the product of a series of somatic (acquired) or germline mutations—is eventually able to express full malignant potential. Thus, breast cancer may exist for a long period as either a noninvasive disease or an invasive but nonmetastatic disease. These facts have very significant clinical ramifications.

GENETIC CONSIDERATIONS Not more than 10% of human breast cancers can be linked directly to germline mutations. Several genes have been implicated in familial cases. The Li-Fraumeni syndrome is characterized by inherited mutations in the p53 tumor-suppressor gene, which lead to an increased incidence of breast cancer, osteogenic sarcomas, and other malignancies. Inherited mutations in *PTEN* have also been reported.

Another tumor-suppressor gene, *BRCA-1*, has been identified at the chromosomal locus 17q21; this gene encodes a zinc finger protein, and the product therefore may function as a transcriptional factor. The gene appears to be involved in gene repair. Women who inherit a mutated allele of this gene from either parent have at least a 60 to 80% lifetime chance of developing breast cancer and about a 33% chance of developing ovarian cancer. The risk is higher among women born after 1940, presumably due to promotional effects of hormonal factors. Men who carry a mutant allele of the gene have an increased incidence of prostate cancer and breast cancer. A fourth gene, termed *BRCA-2*, which has been localized to chromosome 13q12, is also associated with an increased incidence of breast cancer in men and women.

BRCA-1 and *BRCA-2* can now be sequenced readily and germline mutations detected; patients with these mutations can be counseled appropriately. All women with strong family histories for breast cancer should be referred to genetic screening programs whenever possible, particularly women of Ashkenazi Jewish descent who have a high likelihood of a specific *BRCA-1* mutation (deletion of adenine and guanine at position 185).

Even more important than the role these genes play in inherited forms of breast cancer may be their role in sporadic breast cancer. The p53 mutation is present in approximately 40% of human breast cancers as an acquired defect. Acquired mutations in *PTEN* occur in about 10% of the cases. *BRCA-1* mutation in primary breast cancer has not been reported. However, decreased expression of *BRCA-1* mRNA (possibly via gene methylation) and abnormal cellular location of the *BRCA-1* protein have been found in some breast cancers. Loss of heterozygosity of *BRCA-1* and *BRCA-2* suggests that tumor-suppressor activity may be inactivated in sporadic cases of human breast cancer.

Finally, increased expression of a dominant oncogene plays a role in about a quarter of human breast cancer cases. The product of this gene, a member of the epidermal growth factor receptor superfamily, is called *erbB2* (HER-2, neu) and is overexpressed in these breast cancers due to gene amplification; this overexpression can contribute to transformation of human breast epithelium.

EPIDEMIOLOGY Breast cancer is a hormone-dependent disease. Women without functioning ovaries who never receive estrogen-replacement therapy do not develop breast cancer. The female to male ratio is about 150:1. For most epithelial malignancies, a log-log plot of incidence versus age shows a single-component straight-line increase with every year of life. A similar plot for breast cancer shows two components: a straight-line increase with age but with a decrease in slope beginning at the age of menopause. The three dates in a woman's life that have a major impact on breast cancer incidence are age at menarche, age at first full-term pregnancy, and age at menopause. Women who experience menarche at age 16 have only 50 to 60% of the breast cancer risk of a woman having menarche at age 12; the lower risk persists throughout life. Similarly, menopause occurring 10 years before the median age of menopause (52 years), whether natural or surgically induced, reduces lifetime breast cancer risk by about 35%. Women who have a first full-term pregnancy by age 18 have a 30 to 40% lower risk of breast cancer compared with nulliparous women. Thus, length of menstrual life—particularly the fraction occurring before first full-term pregnancy—is a substantial component of the total risk of breast cancer. These three factors (menarche, age of first full-term pregnancy, and menopause) can account for 70 to 80% of the variation in breast cancer frequency in different countries. A meta-analysis has shown that duration of maternal nursing correlates with substantial risk reduction independent of either parity or age at first full-term pregnancy.

International variation in incidence has provided some of the most important clues on hormonal carcinogenesis. A woman living to age 80 in North America has one chance in nine of developing invasive breast cancer. Asian women have one-fifth to one-tenth the risk of breast cancer of women in North America or Western Europe. Asian women have substantially lower concentrations of estrogens and progesterone. These differences cannot be explained on a genetic basis because Asian women living in a western environment have sex steroid hormone concentrations and risks identical to those of their western counterparts. These migrant women and more notably their daughters also differ markedly in height and weight from Asian women in Asia; height and weight are critical regulators of age of menarche and have substantial effects on plasma concentrations of estrogens.

The role of diet in breast cancer etiology is controversial. While there are associative links between total caloric and fat intake and breast cancer risk, the exact role of fat in the diet is unproven. Increased caloric intake contributes to breast cancer risk in multiple ways: earlier menarche, later age at menopause, and increased postmenopausal estrogen concentrations reflecting enhanced aromatase activities in fatty tissues. Moderate alcohol intake also increases the risk by an unknown mechanism. Recommendations favoring abstinence from alcohol must be weighed against other social pressures and the possible cardioprotective effect of moderate alcohol intake.

Understanding the potential role of exogenous hormones in breast cancer is of extraordinary importance because millions of American women regularly use oral contraceptives and postmenopausal hormone replacement therapy (HT). The most credible meta-analyses of oral contraceptive use suggest that these agents cause little if any increased risk of breast cancer. By contrast, oral contraceptives offer a substantial protective effect against ovarian epithelial tumors and endometrial cancers. Far more controversial are the data surrounding HT in postmenopausal women. Data from the Women's Health Initiative (WHI) trial showed in a prospectively randomized design that conjugated equine estrogens plus progestins increased the risk of breast cancer and adverse cardiovascular events but with decreases in bone fractures and colorectal cancer. On balance there were more negative events

with HT. A parallel WHI trial with >12,000 women enrolled testing conjugated estrogens alone (in women who have had hysterectomies) continues. A meta-analysis of nonrandomized HT studies suggests that most of the previously attributed benefit of HT can be accounted for by higher socioeconomic status among users, which is presumably associated with better access to health care and healthier behaviors. Certain potential benefits of HT, such as a putative protective effect on cognition with age, were not assessed in WHI. HT is an area of rapid reevaluation, but it would appear (at least from breast cancer and cardiovascular disease vantage points) that there are serious grounds for concern about long-term HT use.

In addition to the other factors, radiation may be a risk factor in younger women. Women who have been exposed before age 30 to radiation in the form of multiple fluoroscopies (200 to 300 cGy) or treatment for Hodgkin's disease (>3600 cGy) have a substantial increase in risk of breast cancer, whereas radiation exposure after age 30 appears to have a minimal carcinogenic effect on the breast.

EVALUATION OF BREAST MASSES IN MEN AND WOMEN Because the breasts are a common site of potentially fatal malignancy in women and because they frequently provide clues to underlying systemic diseases in both men and women, examination of the breast is an essential part of the physical examination. Unfortunately, internists frequently do not examine breasts in men, and, in women, they are apt to defer this evaluation to gynecologists. Because of the plausible association between early detection and improved outcome, it is the duty of every physician to distinguish breast abnormalities at the earliest possible stage and to institute a definite diagnostic workup. It is for this reason that all women should be trained in breast self-examination (BSE). Although breast cancer in men is unusual, unilateral lesions should be evaluated in the same manner as in women, with the recognition that gynecomastia in men can sometimes begin unilaterally and is often asymmetric.

Virtually all breast cancer is diagnosed by biopsy of a nodule detected either on a mammogram or by palpation. Algorithms have been developed to enhance the likelihood of diagnosing breast cancer and reduce the frequency of unnecessary biopsy (Fig. 76-1).

The Palpable Breast Mass Women should be strongly encouraged to examine their breasts monthly. A flawed study from China has sug-

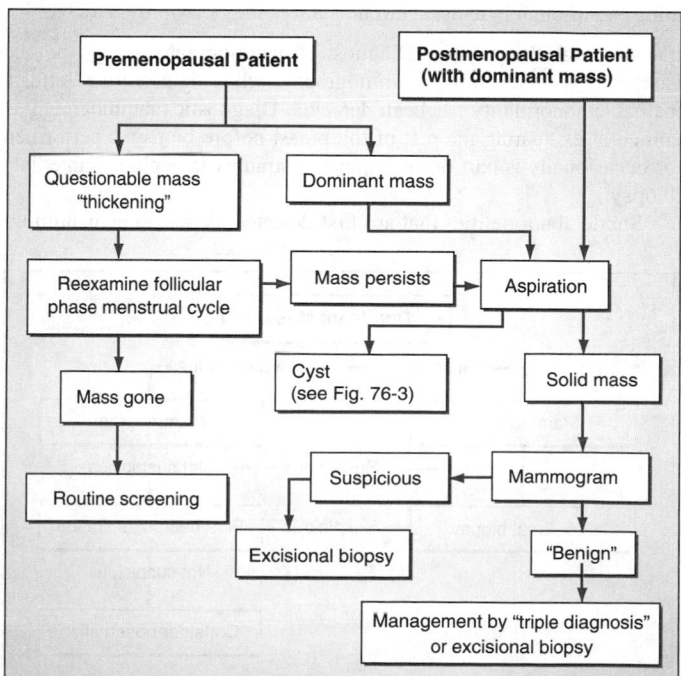

FIGURE 76-1 Approach to a palpable breast mass.

gested that BSE does not alter survival, but given its safety, the procedure should still be encouraged. The minimum benefit of this practice is the greater likelihood of detecting a mass at a smaller size when it can be treated with more limited surgery. Breast examination by the physician should be performed in good light so as to see retractions and other skin changes. The nipple and areolae should be inspected, and an attempt should be made to elicit nipple discharge. All regional lymph node groups should be examined, and any lesions should be measured. While lesions with certain features are more likely to be cancerous (hard, irregular, tethered or fixed, or painless lesions), physical examination alone cannot exclude malignancy. Furthermore, a negative mammogram in the presence of a persistent lump in the breast does not exclude malignancy.

In premenopausal women, lesions that are either equivocal or nonsuspicious on physical examination should be reexamined in 2 to 4 weeks, during the follicular phase of the menstrual cycle. Days 5 to 7 of the cycle are the best time for breast examination. A dominant mass in a postmenopausal woman or a dominant mass that persists through a menstrual cycle in a premenopausal woman should be aspirated by fine-needle biopsy or referred to a surgeon. If nonbloody fluid is aspirated and the lesion is thereby cured, the diagnosis (cyst) and therapy have been accomplished together. Solid lesions that are persistent, recurrent, complex, or bloody cysts require mammography and biopsy, although in selected patients the so-called triple diagnostic techniques (palpation, mammography, aspiration) can be used to avoid biopsy (Figs. 76-1 to 76-3). Ultrasound can be used in place of fine-needle aspiration to distinguish cysts from solid lesions. Not all solid masses are detected by ultrasound; thus, a palpable mass that is not visualized on ultrasound must be presumed to be solid.

Several points are essential in pursuing these management decision trees. First, risk factor analysis is not part of the decision structure. No constellation of risk factors, by their presence or absence, can be used to exclude biopsy. Second, fine-needle aspiration should be used only in centers that have proven skill in obtaining such specimens and analyzing them. Although the likelihood of cancer is low in the setting of a "triple negative" (benign-feeling lump, negative mammogram, and negative fine-needle aspiration), it is not zero, and the patient and physician must be aware of an 1% risk of false negativity. Third, additional technologies such as magnetic resonance imaging, ultrasound, and sestamibi imaging cannot be used to exclude the need for biopsy, although in unusual circumstances they may provoke a biopsy.

The Abnormal Mammogram   Diagnostic mammography should not be confused with screening mammography, which is performed after a palpable abnormality has been detected. Diagnostic mammography is aimed at evaluating the rest of the breast before biopsy is performed or occasionally is part of the triple-test strategy to exclude immediate biopsy.

Subtle abnormalities that are first detected by screening mammog-

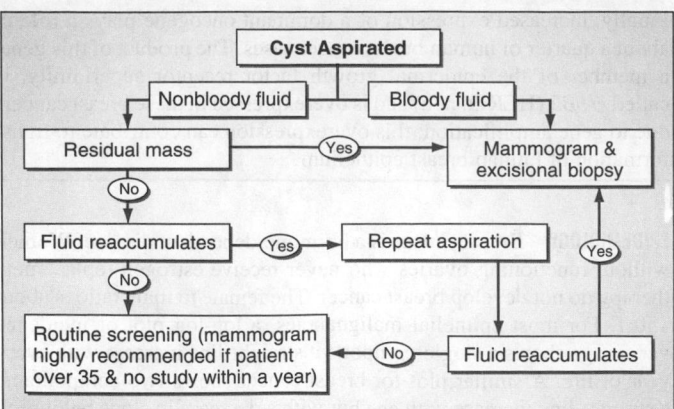

FIGURE 76-3   Management of a breast cyst.

raphy should be evaluated carefully by compression or magnified views. These abnormalities include clustered microcalcifications, densities (especially if spiculated), and new or enlarging architectural distortion. For some nonpalpable lesions ultrasound may be helpful either to identify cysts or to guide biopsy. If there is no palpable lesion and detailed mammographic studies are unequivocally benign, the patient should have routine follow-up appropriate to the patient's age.

If a nonpalpable mammographic lesion has a low index of suspicion, mammographic follow-up in 3 to 6 months is reasonable. Workup of indeterminate and suspicious lesions has been rendered more complex by the advent of stereotactic biopsies. Morrow and colleagues have suggested that these procedures are indicated for lesions that require biopsy but are likely to be benign—that is, for cases in which the procedure probably will eliminate additional surgery. When a lesion is more probably malignant, open excisional biopsy should be performed with a needle localization technique. Others have proposed more widespread use of stereotactic core biopsies for nonpalpable lesions, on economic grounds and because diagnosis leads to earlier treatment planning. However, stereotactic diagnosis of a malignant lesion does not eliminate the need for definitive surgical procedures, particularly if breast conservation is attempted. For example after a breast biopsy with needle localization (i.e., local excision) of a stereotactically diagnosed malignancy, reexcision may still be necessary to achieve negative margins. To some extent, these issues are decided on the basis of referral pattern and the availability of the resources for stereotactic core biopsies. A reasonable approach is shown in Fig. 76-4.

Breast Masses in the Pregnant or Lactating Woman   During pregnancy, the breast grows under the influence of estrogen, progesterone, prolactin, and human placental lactogen. Lactation is suppressed by progester-

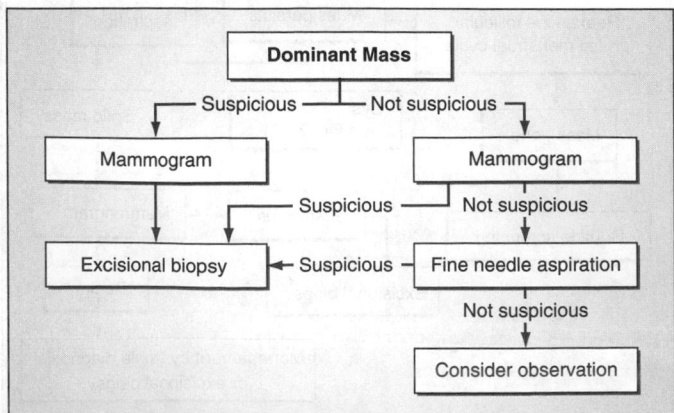

FIGURE 76-2   The "triple diagnosis" technique.

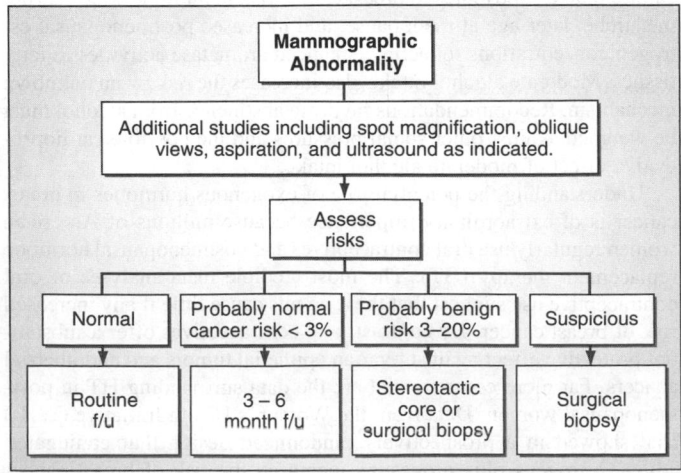

FIGURE 76-4   Approaches to abnormalities detected by mammogram. Note: f/u, follow-up; bx, biopsy.

TABLE 76-1 *Staging of Breast Cancer*

PRIMARY TUMOR (T)

T0	No evidence of primary tumor
TIS	Carcinoma in situ
T1	Tumor ≤2 cm
T2	Tumor >2 cm but ≤5 cm
T3	Tumor >5 cm
T4	Extension to chest wall, inflammation, satellite lesions, ulcerations

REGIONAL LYMPH NODES (N)

N0	No regional lymph nodes
N1	Metastasis to movable ipsilateral nodes
N2	Metastasis to matted or fixed ipsilateral nodes
N3	Metastasis to ipsilateral internal mammary nodes

DISTANT METASTASIS (M)

M0	No distant metastasis
M1	Distant metastasis (includes spread to ipsilateral supraclavicular nodes)

STAGE GROUPING

Stage 0	TIS	N0	M0
Stage I	T1	N0	M0
Stage IIA	T0	N1	M0
	T1	N1	M0
	T2	N0	M0
Stage IIB	T2	N1	M0
	T3	N0	M0
Stage IIIA	T0	N2	M0
	T1	N2	M0
	T2	N2	M0
	T3	N1, N2	M0
Stage IIIB	T4	Any N	M0
	Any T	N3	M0
Stage IV	Any T	Any N	M1

Source: Modified from the American Joint Committee on Cancer, 1992.

one, which blocks the effects of prolactin. After delivery, lactation is promoted by the fall in progesterone levels, which leaves the effects of prolactin unopposed. The development of a dominant mass during pregnancy or lactation should never be attributed to hormonal changes, and biopsy should never be performed under local anesthesia. Breast cancer develops in 1 in every 3000 to 4000 pregnancies. Stage for stage, breast cancer in pregnant patients is no different from premenopausal breast cancer in nonpregnant patients. However, pregnant women often have more advanced disease because the significance of a breast mass was not fully considered. Persistent lumps in the breast of pregnant or lactating women *can not* be attributed to benign changes based on physical findings; such patients should be promptly referred for diagnostic evaluation.

Benign Breast Masses Only about 1 in every 5 to 10 breast biopsies leads to a diagnosis of cancer, although the rate of positive biopsies varies in different countries. (These differences may be related to interpretation, medicolegal considerations, and availability of mammograms.) The vast majority of benign breast masses are due to "fibrocystic" disease, a descriptive term for small fluid-filled cysts and modest epithelial cell and fibrous tissue hyperplasia. However, fibrocystic disease is a histologic, not a clinical, diagnosis, and women who have had a biopsy with benign findings are at greater risk of developing breast cancer than those who have not had a biopsy. The subset of women with ductal or lobular cell proliferation (about 30% of patients), particularly the small fraction (3%) with atypical hyperplasia, have a fourfold greater risk of developing breast cancer than unbiopsied women, and the increase in the risk is about ninefold for women in this category who also have an affected first-degree relative. Thus, careful follow-up of these patients is required. By contrast, patients with a benign biopsy without atypical hyperplasia are at little risk and may be followed routinely.

SCREENING Breast cancer is virtually unique among the epithelial tumors in adults in that screening (in the form of annual mammography) has been proven to improve survival. Meta-analysis examining outcomes from every randomized trial of mammography conclusively shows a 25 to 30% reduction in the chance of dying from breast cancer with annual screening after age 50; the data for women between ages 40 and 50 are almost as positive. While controversy continues to surround the assessment of screening mammography, the preponderance of data as well as this author's evaluation of the literature continue to strongly support the positive benefits of screening mammography. New analyses of older randomized studies have suggested that screening may not work. While the defects in some studies cannot be corrected, most experts, including panels of the American Society of Clinical Oncology and the American Cancer Society, continue to believe that screening conveys substantial benefit. Furthermore, the profound drop in breast cancer mortality seen over the past decade is unlikely to be solely attributable to improvements in therapy. It seems prudent to recommend annual mammography for women past the age of 40. Although no randomized study of BSE has ever shown any improvement in survival, its major benefit appears to be identification of tumors appropriate for conservative local therapy. Better mammographic technology, including digitized mammography, routine use of magnified views, and greater skill in mammographic interpretation, combined with newer diagnostic techniques (magnetic resonance imaging, magnetic resonance spectroscopy, positron emission tomography, etc.) may make it possible to identify breast cancers even more reliably and earlier.

STAGING Correct staging of breast cancer patients is of extraordinary importance. Not only does it permit an accurate prognosis, but in many cases therapeutic decision-making is based largely on the TNM classification (Table 76-1). Comparison with historic series should be undertaken with caution, as the staging has changed several times in the past 20 years.

℞ TREATMENT

PRIMARY BREAST CANCER A series of randomized clinical trials both in the United States and abroad have shown that breast-conserving treatments, consisting of the removal of the primary tumor by some form of lumpectomy with or without irradiating the breast, results in a survival that is as good as that after extensive procedures, such as mastectomy or modified radical mastectomy, with or without further irradiation. Postlumpectomy breast irradiation greatly reduces the risk of recurrence in the breast. While breast conservation is associated with a possibility of recurrence in the breast, 10-year survival is at least as good as that after more radical surgery. Postoperative radiation to regional nodes following mastectomy is also associated with an improvement in survival. Since radiation therapy can also reduce the rate of local or regional recurrence, it should be strongly considered following mastectomy for women with high-risk primary tumors (i.e., T2 in size, positive margins, positive nodes). At present, approximately one-third of women in the United States are managed by lumpectomy. Breast-conserving surgery is not suitable for all patients: it is not generally suitable for tumors >5 cm (or for smaller tumors if the breast is small), for tumors involving the nipple areola complex, for tumors with extensive intraductal disease involving multiple quadrants of the breast, for women with a history of collagen-vascular disease, and for women who either do not have the motivation for breast conservation or do not have convenient access to radiation therapy. However, these groups probably do not account for more than one-third of patients who are treated with mastectomy. Thus, a great many women still undergo mastectomy who could safely avoid this procedure and probably would if appropriately counseled.

An extensive intraductal component is a predictor of recurrence in the breast, and so are several clinical variables. Both axillary lymph node involvement and involvement of vascular or lymphatic channels by metastatic tumor in the breast are associated with a higher risk of relapse in the breast but are not contraindications to breast-conserving treatment. When these patients are excluded, and when lumpectomy with negative tumor margins is achieved, breast conservation is associated with a recurrence rate in the breast of substantially <10%. The survival of patients who have recurrence in the breast is somewhat worse than that of women who do not. Thus, recurrence in the breast is a negative prognostic variable for long-term survival. However, recurrence in the breast is not the *cause* of distant metastasis. If recurrence in the breast caused metastatic disease, then women treated with lumpectomy, who have a higher rate of recurrence in the breast, should have poorer survival than women treated with mastectomy and they do not. Most patients should consult with a radiation oncologist before making a final decision concerning local therapy. However, a multi-modality clinic in which the surgeon, radiation oncologist, medical oncologist, and other caregivers cooperate to evaluate the patient and develop a treatment is usually considered a major advantage by patients.

Adjuvant Therapy   The use of systemic therapy after local management of breast cancer improves survival. More than one-third of the women who would otherwise die of metastatic breast cancer remain disease-free when treated with the appropriate systemic regimen.

PROGNOSTIC VARIABLES   The most important prognostic variables are provided by *tumor staging*. The size of the tumor and the status of the axillary lymph nodes provide reasonably accurate information on the likelihood of tumor relapse. The relation of pathologic stage to 5-year survival is shown in Table 76-2. For most women, the need for adjuvant therapy can be readily defined on this basis alone. In the absence of lymph node involvement, involvement of microvessels (either capillaries or lymphatic channels) in tumors is nearly equivalent to lymph node involvement. The greatest controversy concerns women with intermediate prognoses. *There is rarely justification for adjuvant chemotherapy in most women with tumors <1 cm in size whose axillary lymph nodes are negative.* The most exciting development in this area is the use of gene expression arrays to analyze patterns of tumor gene expression.

Other prognostic variables have been sought, and some appear to influence disease-free and overall survival. What is less clear is whether they add to the information from pathologic staging.

Estrogen and progesterone receptor status are of prognostic significance. Tumors that lack either or both of these receptors are more likely to recur than tumors that have them.

Several *measures of tumor growth rate* correlate with early relapse. S-phase analysis using flow cytometry is the most accurate measure. Indirect S-phase assessments using antigens associated with the cell cycle, such as PCNA (Ki67), are also valuable. Several studies suggest that tumors with a high proportion (more than the median) of cells in the S phase pose a greater risk of relapse and that chemotherapy offers the greatest survival benefit for these tumors. For this reason, some clinicians use S-phase assessment as a deciding factor for instituting adjuvant therapy when other pathologic features are unclear. Assessment of DNA content in the form of ploidy is of modest value, with nondiploid tumors having a somewhat worse prognosis.

TABLE 76-2   *5-Year Survival Rate for Breast Cancer by Stage*

Stage	5-Year Survival, %
0	99
I	92
IIA	82
IIB	65
IIIA	47
IIIB	44
IV	14

Source: Modified from data of the National Cancer Institute—Surveillance, Epidemiology, and End Results (SEER).

Histologic classification of the tumor has also been used as a prognostic factor. Tumors with a poor nuclear grade have a higher risk of recurrence than tumors with a good nuclear grade. Semiquantitative measures such as the Elston score improve the reproducibility of this measurement.

Molecular changes in the tumor are also useful. Tumors that overexpress *erbB2* (HER-2/neu) or have a mutated p53 gene have a worse prognosis. Particular interest has centered on *erbB2* overexpression as measured by histochemistry or by fluorescence in situ hybridization. In experienced hands either methodology is acceptable. Tumors that overexpress *erbB2* are more likely to respond to higher doses of doxorubicin-containing regimens. For this reason, *erbB2* expression is usually worth measuring as a means of deciding on therapy. Results of ongoing adjuvant therapy trials evaluating the role of monoclonal HER-2/neu antibodies (trastuzumab) are awaited with great interest.

To grow, a tumor must generate a neovasculature (Chap. 69). The presence of more microvessels, particularly when localized in so-called "hot spots," in a tumor is associated with a worse prognosis.

Other variables that have also been used to evaluate prognosis include proteins associated with invasiveness, such as type IV collagenase, cathepsin D, plasminogen activator, plasminogen activator receptor, and the metastasis-suppressor gene, *nm23*. None of these has been widely accepted as a prognostic variable for therapeutic decision-making. One problem in interpreting these prognostic variables is that most of them have not been examined in a study using a large cohort of patients.

ADJUVANT REGIMENS   Adjuvant therapy is the use of systemic therapies in patients whose known disease has received local therapy but who are at risk of relapse. Selection of appropriate adjuvant chemotherapy or hormone therapy is highly controversial in some situations. Meta-analyses have helped to define broad limits for therapy but do not help in choosing optimal regimens or in choosing a regimen for certain subgroups of patients. A summary of recommendations is shown in Table 76-3. In general, premenopausal women for whom any form of adjuvant systemic therapy is indicated should receive multidrug chemotherapy. The antiestrogen (tamoxifen) improves survival in premenopausal patients with positive estrogen receptor values and should be added following completion of chemotherapy. Prophylactic castration may also be associated with a substantial survival benefit (primarily in estrogen receptor–positive patients) but is not widely used in this country.

Data on postmenopausal women are also controversial. The impact of adjuvant chemotherapy is quantitatively less clear-cut than in premenopausal patients, although some survival advantage has been shown. The first decision is whether chemotherapy or tamoxifen should be used. While adjuvant tamoxifen improves survival regardless of axillary lymph node status, the improvement in survival is modest for patients in whom multiple lymph nodes are involved. For this reason, it has been usual to give chemotherapy to postmenopausal patients who have no medical contraindications and who have more than one positive lymph node; tamoxifen is commonly given simultaneously or subsequently. For postmenopausal women for whom systemic therapy is warranted but who have a more favorable prognosis, tamoxifen may be used as a single agent. Data from the ATAC trial in which >9000 women were randomly assigned to tamoxifen, anastrazole (an aromatase inhibitor), or the combination showed that anastrazole was superior to tamoxifen or the combination in preventing recurrence at 32 months of follow-up. Whether these observations will persist with longer follow-up and/or other effects on cardiovascular disease will become issues awaits further follow-up.

Most comparisons of adjuvant chemotherapy regimens show little difference among them, although slight advantages for doxorubicin-containing regimens are usually seen.

One approach—so-called neoadjuvant chemotherapy—involves the administration of adjuvant therapy before definitive surgery and radiation therapy. Because the objective response rates of patients with breast cancer to systemic therapy in this setting exceed 75%, many patients will be "downstaged" and may become candidates for breast-conserving therapy. At least one large randomized study has failed to show any difference in survival using this approach.

Other adjuvant treatments under investigation include the use of new drugs, such as paclitaxel and docetaxel, and therapy based on alternative kinetic and biologic models. In such approaches, high doses of single agents are used separately in relatively dose-intensive cycling regimens. One large randomized trial for node-positive patients suggests that patients treated with doxorubicin-cyclophosphamide for four cycles followed by four cycles of paclitaxel have a substantial additional gain in survival as compared with women receiving doxorubicin-cyclophosphamide alone, an outcome not validated in another large trial. Taxane use remains controversial. Very high dose therapy with stem cell transplantation in the adjuvant setting has not proved superior to standard dose therapy and should not be routinely used.

Systemic Therapy of Metastatic Disease Nearly half of patients treated for apparently localized breast cancer develop metastatic disease. Although a very small number of these patients can enjoy long remissions when treated with combinations of systemic and local therapy, most eventually succumb. Soft tissue, bony, and visceral (lung and liver) metastases each account for approximately one-third of sites of initial relapses. However, by the time of death, most patients will have bony involvement. Recurrences can appear at any time after primary therapy. Half of all initial cancer recurrences occur >5 years after initial therapy.

Because the diagnosis of metastatic disease alters the outlook for the patient so drastically, it should not be made without biopsy. Every oncologist has seen patients with tuberculosis, gallstones, primary hyperparathyroidism, or other nonmalignant diseases misdiagnosed and treated as though they had metastatic breast cancer. This is a catastrophic mistake and justifies biopsy for virtually every patient at the time of initial suspicion of metastatic disease.

The choice of therapy requires consideration of local therapy needs, the overall medical condition of the patient, and the hormone receptor status of the tumor, as well as the exercise of clinical judgment. Because therapy of systemic disease is palliative, the potential toxicities of therapies should be balanced against the response rates. Several variables influence the response to systemic therapy. For example, the presence of estrogen and progesterone receptors is a strong indication for endocrine therapy, since the response rates for tumors that express both receptors may approach 70%. On the other hand, patients with short disease-free intervals, rapidly progressive visceral disease, lymphangitic pulmonary disease, or intracranial disease are unlikely to respond to endocrine therapy.

In many cases, systemic therapy can be withheld while the patient is managed with appropriate local therapy. Radiation therapy and occasionally surgery are effective at relieving the symptoms of metastatic disease, particularly when bony sites are involved. Many patients with bone-only or bone-dominant disease have a relatively indolent course. Under such circumstances, systemic chemotherapy has a modest effect, whereas radiation therapy may be effective for long periods. Other systemic treatments, such as strontium 89 and/or bisphosphonates, may provide a palliative benefit without inducing objective responses. Most patients with metastatic disease and certainly all who have bone involvement should receive concurrent bisphosphonates. Since the goal of therapy is to maintain well-being for as long as possible, emphasis should be placed on avoiding the most hazardous complications of metastatic disease, including pathologic fracture of the axial skeleton and spinal cord compression. New back pain in patients with cancer should be explored aggressively on an emergent basis; to wait for neurologic symptoms is a potentially catastrophic error. Metastatic involvement of endocrine organs can cause profound dysfunction, including adrenal insufficiency and hypopituitarism. Similarly, obstruction of the biliary tree or other impaired organ function may be better managed with a local therapy than with a systemic approach.

Endocrine Therapy Normal breast tissue is estrogen-dependent. Both primary and metastatic breast cancer may retain this phenotype. The best means of ascertaining whether a breast cancer is hormone-dependent is through analysis of estrogen and progesterone receptor levels on the tumor. Tumors that are positive for the estrogen receptor and negative for the progesterone receptor have a response rate of ~30%. Tumors that have both receptors have a response rate approaching 70%. If neither receptor is present, the objective response rates are <10%. Receptor analyses provide information as to the correct ordering of endocrine therapies as opposed to chemotherapy. Because of their lack of toxicity and because some patients whose receptor analyses are reported as negative respond to endocrine therapy, an endocrine treatment should be attempted in virtually every patient with metastatic breast cancer. Potential endocrine therapies are summarized in Table 76-4. The choice of endocrine therapy is usually determined

TABLE 76-3 *Suggested Approaches to Adjuvant Therapy*

Age Group	Lymph Node Status[a]	Endocrine Receptor (ER) Status	Tumor	Recommendation
Premenopausal	Positive	Any	Any	Multidrug chemotherapy + tamoxifen if ER-positive
Premenopausal	Negative	Any	>2 cm, or 1–2 cm with other poor prognostic variables	Multidrug chemotherapy + tamoxifen if ER-positive
Postmenopausal	Positive	Negative	Any	Multidrug chemotherapy
Postmenopausal	Positive	Positive	Any	Tamoxifen with or without chemotherapy
Postmenopausal	Negative	Positive	>2 cm, or 1–2 cm with other poor prognostic variables	Tamoxifen
Postmenopausal	Negative	Negative	>2 cm, or 1–2 cm with other poor prognostic variables	Consider multidrug chemotherapy

[a] As determined by pathologic examination.

TABLE 76-4 *Endocrine Therapies for Breast Cancer*

Therapy	Comments
Castration Surgical LHRH agonists	For premenopausal women
Antiestrogens Tamoxifen	Useful in pre- and postmenopausal women
"Pure" antiestrogens	Promising early clinical data; responses in tamoxifen-resistant patients
Surgical adrenalectomy	Rarely employed second-line choice
Aromatase inhibitors	Low toxicity and superiority to additive hormone therapy; now first choice for metastatic disease
High-dose progestogens	Common third-line choice
Hypophysectomy	Rarely used
Additive androgens or estrogens	Plausible third-line therapies; potentially toxic

Note: LHRH, luteinizing hormone–releasing hormone.

by toxicity profile and availability. In most patients, the initial endocrine therapy should now be an aromatase inhibitor rather than tamoxifen. Newer "pure" antiestrogens that are free of agonist effects are also in clinical trial. Cases in which tumors shrink in response to tamoxifen withdrawal (as well as withdrawal of pharmacologic doses of estrogens) have been reported. Endogenous estrogen formation may be blocked by analogues of luteinizing hormone–releasing hormone in premenopausal women. Additive endocrine therapies, including treatment with progestogens, estrogens, and androgens, may also be tried in patients who respond to initial endocrine therapy; the mechanism of action of these latter therapies is unknown. Patients who respond to one endocrine therapy have at least a 50% chance of responding to a second endocrine therapy. It is not uncommon for patients to respond to two or three sequential endocrine therapies; however, combination endocrine therapies do not appear to be superior to individual agents, and combinations of chemotherapy with endocrine therapy are not useful. The median survival of patients with metastatic disease is approximately 2 years, and many patients, particularly older persons and those with hormone-dependent disease, may respond to endocrine therapy for 3 to 5 years or longer.

Chemotherapy   Unlike many other epithelial malignancies, breast cancer responds to several chemotherapeutic agents, including anthracyclines, alkylating agents, taxanes, and antimetabolites. Multiple combinations of these agents have been found to improve response rates somewhat, but they have had little effect on duration of response or survival. The choice among multidrug combinations frequently depends on whether adjuvant chemotherapy was administered and, if so, what type. While patients treated with adjuvant regimens such as cyclophosphamide, methotrexate, and fluorouracil (CMF regimens) may subsequently respond to the same combination in the metastatic disease setting, most oncologists use drugs to which the patients have not been previously exposed. Once patients have progressed after combination drug therapy, it is most common to treat them with single agents. Given the significant toxicity of most drugs, the use of a single effective agent will minimize toxicity by sparing the patient exposure to drugs that would be of little value. Unfortunately, no form of in vitro drug sensitivity testing to select the drugs most efficacious for a given patient has been demonstrated to be useful.

Most oncologists use either an anthracycline or paclitaxel following failure with the initial regimen. However, the choice has to be balanced with individual needs.

The use of a humanized antibody to *erbB2* [trastuzumab (Herceptin)] combined with paclitaxel can improve response rate and survival for women whose metastatic tumors overexpress *erbB2*. The magnitude of the survival extension is modest in patients with metastatic disease. Application to adjuvant therapy may prove even more beneficial. In the past few years a series of newer agents has emerged as useful in inducing objective responses in previously treated patients, including gemcitabine, capecitabine, navelbine, and oral etoposide.

HIGH-DOSE CHEMOTHERAPY INCLUDING AUTOLOGOUS BONE MARROW TRANSPLANTATION   Autologous bone marrow transplantation combined with high doses of single agents can produce improvement even in heavily pretreated patients. However, such responses are rarely, if ever, durable and are unlikely to substantially alter the clinical course for most patients with advanced metastatic disease. Randomized trials have not been encouraging, and these approaches cannot be recommended as part of clinical care outside of research settings.

STAGE III BREAST CANCER   Between 10 and 25% of patients present with so-called locally advanced, or stage III, breast cancer at diagnosis. Many of these cancers are technically operable, whereas others, particularly cancers with chest wall involvement, inflammatory breast cancers, or cancers with large matted axillary lymph nodes, cannot be managed with surgery initially. Although no randomized trials have proved the efficacy of induction chemotherapy, this approach has gained widespread use. More than 90% of patients with locally advanced breast cancer show a partial or better response to multidrug chemotherapy regimens that include an anthracycline. Early administration of this treatment reduces the bulk of the disease and frequently makes the patient a suitable candidate for salvage surgery and/or radiation therapy. These patients should be managed in multimodality clinics to coordinate surgery, radiation therapy, and systemic chemotherapy. Such approaches produce long-term disease-free survival in about 30 to 50% of patients.

BREAST CANCER PREVENTION   Women who have one breast cancer are at risk of developing a contralateral breast cancer at a rate of approximately 0.5% per year. When adjuvant tamoxifen is administered to these patients, the rate of development of contralateral breast cancers is reduced. In other tissues of the body, tamoxifen has estrogen-like effects that are beneficial: preservation of bone mineral density and long-term lowering of cholesterol. However, tamoxifen has estrogen-like effects on the uterus, leading to an increased risk of uterine cancer (0.75% incidence after 5 years on tamoxifen). Tamoxifen also increases the risk of cataract formation. The Breast Cancer Prevention Trial (BCPT) revealed a >49% reduction in breast cancer among women with a risk of at least 1.66% taking the drug for 5 years. Raloxifene has shown similar breast cancer prevention potency but may have different effects on bone and heart. The two agents are being compared in a prospective randomized prevention trial (the STAR trial).

NONINVASIVE BREAST CANCER   Breast cancer develops as a series of molecular changes in the epithelial cells that lead to ever more malignant behavior. Increased use of mammography has led to more frequent diagnosis of noninvasive breast cancer. These lesions fall into two groups: ductal carcinoma in situ (DCIS) and lobular carcinoma in situ (lobular neoplasia). The management of both entities is controversial.

Ductal Carcinoma in Situ   Proliferation of cytologically malignant breast epithelial cells within the ducts is termed *DCIS*. Significant disagreement can occur in differentiating atypical hyperplasia from DCIS. At least one-third of the cases of untreated DCIS progress to invasive breast cancer within 5 years. For many years, the standard treatment for this disease was mastectomy. However, since treatment of this condition by lumpectomy and radiation therapy gives survival that is as good as the survival for invasive breast cancer by mastectomy, it appears paradoxical to recommend more aggressive therapy for a "less" malignant disease. In one randomized trial, the combination of wide excision plus irradiation for DCIS caused a substantial reduction in the local recurrence rate as compared with wide excision alone with negative margins, though survival was identical in the two arms. No studies have compared either of these regimens to mastectomy. Addition of tamoxifen to any DCIS surgical/radiation therapy regimen further improves local control.

Several prognostic features may help to identify patients at high risk for local recurrence after either lumpectomy alone or lumpectomy with radiation therapy. These include extensive disease; age < 40; and cytologic features such as necrosis, poor nuclear grade, and comedo subtype with overexpression of *erbB2*. Some data suggest that adequate excision with careful determination of pathologically clear margins is associated with a low recurrence rates. When surgery is combined with radiation therapy, recurrence (which is usually in the same quadrant) occurs with a frequency of ≤10%. Given the fact that half of these recurrences will be invasive, about 5% of the initial cohort will eventually develop invasive breast cancer. A reasonable expectation of mortality for these patients is about 1%, a figure that approximates the mortality rate for DCIS managed by mastectomy. Although this train of reasoning has not formally been proved valid, it is reasonable at present to recommend that patients who desire breast preservation, and in whom DCIS appears to be reasonably localized, be managed by adequate surgery with meticulous pathologic evaluation, followed by breast irradiation and tamoxifen. For patients with localized DCIS, axillary lymph node dissection is unnecessary. More controversial is the question of what management is optimal when there is any degree of invasion. Because of a significant likelihood (10 to

TABLE 76-5 *Breast Cancer Surveillance Guidelines*

Test	Frequency
RECOMMENDED	
History; eliciting symptoms; physical examination	q3–6 months × 3 years; q6–12 months × 2 years; then annually
Breast self-examination	Monthly
Mammography	Annually
Pelvic examination	Annually
Patient education about symptoms of recurrence	Ongoing
Coordination of care	Ongoing
NOT RECOMMENDED	
Complete blood count	
Serum chemistry studies	
Chest radiographs	
Bone scans	
Ultrasound examination of the liver	
Computed tomography of chest, abdomen, or pelvis	
Tumor marker CA 15-3	
Tumor marker CEA	

Source: Recommended Breast Cancer Surveillance Guidelines, ASCO Education Book, Fall, 1997.

15%) of axillary lymph node involvement even when the primary lesion shows only microscopic invasion, it is prudent to do at least a level 1 and 2 axillary lymph node dissection for all patients with any degree of invasion; sentinel node biopsy may be substituted. Further management is dictated by the presence of nodal spread.

Lobular Neoplasia Proliferation of cytologically malignant cells within the lobules is termed *lobular neoplasia*. Nearly 30% of patients who have had adequate local excision of the lesion develop breast cancer (usually infiltrating ductal cell carcinoma) over the next 15 to 20 years. Ipsilateral and contralateral disease are equally common. Therefore, lobular neoplasia may be a premalignant lesion that suggests an elevated risk of subsequent breast cancer, rather than a form of malignancy itself, and aggressive local management seems unreasonable. Most patients should be treated with tamoxifen for 5 years and followed with careful annual mammography and semiannual physical examinations. Additional molecular analysis of these lesions may make it possible to discriminate between patients who are at risk of further progression and who require additional therapy and those in whom simple follow-up is adequate.

MALE BREAST CANCER Breast cancer is about 1/150th as frequent in men as in women. It usually presents as a unilateral lump in the breast and is frequently not diagnosed promptly. Given the small amount of soft tissue and the unexpected nature of the problem, locally advanced presentations are somewhat more common. When male breast cancer is matched to female breast cancer by age and stage, its overall prognosis is identical. Although gynecomastia may initially be unilateral or asymmetric, any unilateral mass in a man over the age of 40 should receive a careful workup all the way through biopsy. On the other hand, bilateral symmetric breast development rarely represents breast cancer and is almost invariably due to endocrine disease or a drug effect. It should be kept in mind, nevertheless, that the risk of cancer is much greater in men with gynecomastia; in such men, gross asymmetry of the breasts should arouse suspicion of cancer. Male breast cancer is best managed by mastectomy and axillary lymph node dissection (modified radical mastectomy). Patients with locally advanced disease or positive nodes should also be treated with irradiation. Approximately 90% of male breast cancers contain estrogen receptors, and approximately 60% of cases with metastatic disease respond to endocrine therapy. No randomized studies have evaluated adjuvant therapy for male breast cancer. Two historic experiences suggest that the disease responds well to adjuvant systemic therapy, and, if not medically contraindicated, the same criteria for the use of adjuvant therapy in women should be applied to men.

The sites of relapse and spectrum of response to chemotherapeutic drugs are virtually identical for breast cancers in the two sexes.

FOLLOW-UP OF BREAST CANCER PATIENTS Despite the availability of sophisticated and expensive imaging techniques and a wide range of serum tumor marker tests, no studies document that survival is influenced by early diagnosis of relapse. Surveillance guidelines are given in Table 76-5.

FURTHER READING

BENICHOU J et al: Graphs to estimate an individualized risk of breast cancer. J Clin Oncol 14:103, 1996

FISHER B et al: Twenty-year follow-up of a randomized trial comparing total mastectomy, lumpectomy, and lumpectomy plus irradiation for the treatment of invasive breast cancer. N Engl J Med 347:1233, 2002

GIORDANO S et al: Breast cancer in men. Ann Intern Med 137:678, 2002

ROUSSOUW JE et al: Risks and benefits of estrogen plus progestin in healthy postmenopausal women. JAMA 288:321, 2002

SHAPIRO CL, WINER EL (eds): Late effects of treatment and survivorship issues in early-stage breast cancer. Sem Oncol 30:729, 2003

STOCKLER M et al: Systematic reviews of chemotherapy and endocrine therapy for metastatic breast cancer. Cancer Treat Rev 26:151, 2000

VAN DE VIJVER M et al: A gene-expression signature as a predictor of survival in breast cancer. N Engl J Med 347:1999, 2002

WONG ZW, ELLIS MJ: First-line endocrine treatment of breast cancer: Aromatase inhibitor or antiestrogen? Br J Cancer 90:20, 2004

77 GASTROINTESTINAL TRACT CANCER
Robert J. Mayer

The gastrointestinal tract is the second most common noncutaneous site for cancer and the second major cause of cancer-related mortality in the United States.

ESOPHAGEAL CANCER

INCIDENCE AND ETIOLOGY Cancer of the esophagus is a relatively uncommon but extremely lethal malignancy. The diagnosis was made in 14,250 Americans in 2004 and led to 13,300 deaths. Worldwide, the incidence of esophageal cancer varies strikingly. It occurs frequently within a geographic region extending from the southern shore of the Caspian Sea on the west to northern China on the east and encompassing parts of Iran, Central Asia, Afghanistan, Siberia, and Mongolia. High-incidence "pockets" of the disease are also present in such disparate locations as Finland, Iceland, Curaçao, southeastern Africa, and northwestern France. In North America and western Europe, the disease is more common in blacks than whites and in males than females; it appears most often after age 50 and seems to be associated with a lower socioeconomic status.

A variety of causative factors have been implicated in the development of the disease (Table 77-1). In the United States, esophageal cancer cases are either squamous cell carcinomas or adenocarcinomas. The etiology of squamous cell esophageal cancer is related to excess alcohol consumption and/or cigarette smoking. The relative risk increases with the amount of tobacco smoked or alcohol consumed, with these factors acting synergistically. The consumption of whiskey is linked to a higher incidence than the consumption of wine or beer. Squamous cell esophageal carcinoma has also been associated with the ingestion of nitrites, smoked opiates, and fungal toxins in pickled vegetables, as well as mucosal damage caused by such physical insults as long-term exposure to extremely hot tea, the ingestion of lye, radiation-induced strictures, and chronic achalasia. The presence of an esophageal web in association with glossitis and iron deficiency (i.e.,

TABLE 77-1 *Some Etiologic Factors Believed to Be Associated with Esophageal Cancer*

Excess alcohol consumption
Cigarette smoking
Other ingested carcinogens
    Nitrates (converted to nitrites)
    Smoked opiates
    Fungal toxins in pickled vegetables
Mucosal damage from physical agents
    Hot tea
    Lye ingestion
    Radiation-induced strictures
    Chronic achalasia
Host susceptibility
    Esophageal web with glossitis and iron deficiency (i.e., Plummer-
        Vinson or Paterson-Kelly syndrome)
    Congenital hyperkeratosis and pitting of the palms and soles (i.e.,
        tylosis palmaris et plantaris)
? Dietary deficiencies molybdenum, zinc, vitamin A
? Celiac sprue
Chronic gastric reflux (i.e., Barrett's esophagus) for adenocarcinoma

Plummer-Vinson or Paterson-Kelly syndrome) and congenital hyperkeratosis and pitting of the palms and soles (i.e., tylosis palmaris et plantaris) have each been linked with squamous cell esophageal cancer, as have dietary deficiencies of molybdenum, zinc, and vitamin A.

For unclear reasons, the incidence of squamous cell esophageal cancer has decreased somewhat in both the black and white population in the United States over the past 25 years, while the rate of adenocarcinoma has risen dramatically, particularly in white males. Adenocarcinomas arise in the distal esophagus in the presence of chronic gastric reflux and gastric metaplasia of the epithelium (Barrett's esophagus), which is more common in obese persons. Adenocarcinomas arise within dysplastic columnar epithelium in the distal esophagus. Even before frank neoplasia is detectable, aneuploidy and p53 mutations are found in the dysplastic epithelium. These adenocarcinomas behave clinically like gastric adenocarcinoma and now account for >50% of esophageal cancers.

CLINICAL FEATURES About 15% of esophageal cancers occur in the upper third of the esophagus (cervical esophagus), 35% in the middle third, and 50% in the lower third. Squamous cell carcinomas and adenocarcinomas of the esophagus cannot be distinguished radiographically or endoscopically.

Progressive dysphagia and weight loss of short duration are the initial symptoms in the vast majority of patients. Dysphagia initially occurs with solid foods and gradually progresses to include semisolids and liquids. By the time these symptoms develop, the disease is usually incurable, since difficulty in swallowing does not occur until >60% of the esophageal circumference is infiltrated with cancer. Dysphagia may be associated with pain on swallowing (odynophagia), pain radiating to the chest and/or back, regurgitation or vomiting, and aspiration pneumonia. The disease most commonly spreads to adjacent and supraclavicular lymph nodes, liver, lungs, and pleura. Tracheoesophageal fistulas may develop as the disease advances, leading to severe suffering. As with other squamous cell carcinomas, hypercalcemia may occur in the absence of osseous metastases, probably from parathormone-related peptide secreted by tumor cells (Chap. 86).

DIAGNOSIS Attempts at endoscopic and cytologic screening for carcinoma in patients with Barrett's esophagus, while effective as a means of detecting high-grade dysplasia, have not yet been shown to improve the prognosis in individuals found to have a carcinoma. Routine contrast radiographs effectively identify esophageal lesions large enough to cause symptoms. In contrast to benign esophageal leiomyomas, which result in esophageal narrowing with preservation of a normal mucosal pattern, esophageal carcinomas characteristically cause ragged, ulcerating changes in the mucosa in association with deeper infiltration, producing a picture resembling achalasia. Smaller, potentially resectable tumors are often poorly visualized despite technically adequate esophagograms. Because of this, esophagoscopy should be performed in all patients suspected of having an esophageal abnormality, to visualize the tumor and to obtain histopathologic confirmation of the diagnosis. Because the population of persons at risk for squamous cell carcinoma of the esophagus (i.e., smokers and drinkers) also has a high rate of cancers of the lung and the head and neck region, endoscopic inspection of the larynx, trachea, and bronchi should also be done. A thorough examination of the fundus of the stomach (by retroflexing the endoscope) is imperative as well. Endoscopic biopsies of esophageal tumors fail to recover malignant tissue in one-third of cases because the biopsy forceps cannot penetrate deeply enough through normal mucosa pushed in front of the carcinoma. Cytologic examination of tumor brushings frequently complements standard biopsies and should be performed routinely. The extent of tumor spread to the mediastinum and paraaortic lymph nodes should also be assessed by computed tomography (CT) scans of the chest and abdomen and by endoscopic ultrasound. Positron emission tomography (PET) scanning may also provide useful assessment of resectability.

℞ TREATMENT

The prognosis for patients with esophageal carcinoma is poor. Fewer than 5% of patients are alive 5 years after the diagnosis; thus, management focuses on symptom control. Surgical resection of all gross tumor (i.e., total resection) is feasible in only 45% of cases, with residual tumor cells frequently present at the resection margins. Such esophagectomies have been associated with a postoperative mortality rate of 5 to 10% due to anastomotic fistulas, subphrenic abscesses, and respiratory complications. About 20% of patients who survive a total resection live 5 years. The outcome of primary radiation therapy (5500 to 6000 cGy) for squamous cell carcinomas is similar to that of radical surgery, sparing patients perioperative morbidity but often resulting in less satisfactory palliation of obstructive symptoms. The evaluation of chemotherapeutic agents in patients with esophageal carcinoma has been hampered by ambiguity in the definition of "response" (i.e., benefit) and the debilitated physical condition of many treated individuals. Nonetheless, significant reductions in the size of measurable tumor masses have been reported in 15 to 25% of patients given single-agent treatment and in 30 to 60% of patients treated with drug combinations that include cisplatin. Combination chemotherapy and radiation therapy as the initial therapeutic approach, either alone or followed by an attempt at operative resection, may be of benefit. When administered along with radiation therapy, chemotherapy produces a better survival outcome than radiation therapy alone. The use of preoperative chemotherapy and radiation therapy followed by esophageal resection appears to prolong survival as compared with historic controls, but randomized trials have produced inconsistent results.

For the incurable, surgically unresectable patient with esophageal cancer, dysphagia, malnutrition, and the management of tracheoesophageal fistulas loom as major issues. Approaches to palliation include repeated endoscopic dilatation, the surgical placement of a gastrostomy or jejunostomy for hydration and feeding, and endoscopic placement of an expansive metal stent to bypass the tumor. Endoscopic fulguration of the obstructing tumor with lasers appears to be the most promising of these techniques.

TUMORS OF THE STOMACH

GASTRIC ADENOCARCINOMA ■ **Incidence and Epidemiology** For unclear reasons, the incidence and mortality rates for gastric cancer have decreased markedly during the past 65 years. The mortality rate from gastric cancer in the United States has dropped in men from 28 to 5.0 per 100,000 population, while in women, the rate has decreased from 27 to 2.3 per 100,000. Nonetheless, 22,710 new cases of stomach cancer were diagnosed in the United States and 11,780 Americans died of the disease in 2004. Gastric cancer incidence has decreased worldwide but remains high in Japan, China, Chile, and Ireland.

The risk of gastric cancer is greater among lower socioeconomic classes. Migrants from high- to low-incidence nations maintain their susceptibility to gastric cancer, while the risk for their offspring approximates that of the new homeland. These findings suggest that an environmental exposure, probably beginning early in life, is related to the development of gastric cancer, with dietary carcinogens considered the most likely factor(s).

Pathology   About 85% of stomach cancers are adenocarcinomas, with 15% due to lymphomas and gastrointestinal stromal tumors (GIST, formerly called *leiomyosarcomas*). Gastric adenocarcinomas may be subdivided into two categories: a *diffuse type* in which cell cohesion is absent, so that individual cells infiltrate and thicken the stomach wall without forming a discrete mass; and an *intestinal type* characterized by cohesive neoplastic cells that form glandlike tubular structures. The diffuse carcinomas occur more often in younger patients, develop throughout the stomach (including the cardia), result in a loss of distensibility of the gastric wall (so-called linitis plastica or "leather bottle" appearance), and carry a poorer prognosis. Intestinal-type lesions are frequently ulcerative, more commonly appear in the antrum and lesser curvature of the stomach, and are often preceded by a prolonged precancerous process. While the incidence of diffuse carcinomas is similar in most populations, the intestinal type tends to predominate in the high-risk geographic regions and is less likely to be found in areas where the frequency of gastric cancer is declining. Thus, different etiologic factor(s) may be involved in these two subtypes. In the United States, the distal stomach is the site of origin of ~30% of gastric cancers, ~20% arise in the midportion of the stomach, and ~37% originate in the proximal third of the stomach. The remaining 13% involve the entire stomach.

Etiology   The long-term ingestion of high concentrations of nitrates in dried, smoked, and salted foods appears to be associated with a higher risk. The nitrates are thought to be converted to carcinogenic nitrites by bacteria (Table 77-2). Such bacteria may be introduced exogenously through the ingestion of partially decayed foods, which are consumed in abundance worldwide by the lower socioeconomic classes. Bacteria such as *Helicobacter pylori* may also contribute to this effect by causing chronic gastritis, loss of gastric acidity, and bacterial growth in the stomach. The effect of *H. pylori* eradication on the subsequent risk for gastric cancer in high-incidence areas is under investigation. Loss of acidity may occur when acid-producing cells of the gastric antrum have been removed surgically to control benign peptic ulcer disease or when achlorhydria, atrophic gastritis, and even pernicious anemia develop in the elderly. Serial endoscopic examinations of the stomach in patients with atrophic gastritis have documented replacement of the usual gastric mucosa by intestinal-type cells. This process of intestinal metaplasia may lead to cellular atypia and eventual neoplasia. Since the declining incidence of gastric cancer in the United States primarily reflects a decline in distal, ulcerating, intestinal-type lesions, it is conceivable that better food preservation and the availability of refrigeration to all socioeconomic classes have decreased the dietary ingestion of exogenous bacteria.

Several additional etiologic factors have been associated with gas-

tric carcinoma. Gastric ulcers and adenomatous polyps have occasionally been so linked, but data regarding a cause-and-effect relationship are unconvincing. The inadequate clinical distinction between benign gastric ulcers and small ulcerating carcinomas may, in part, account for this presumed association. The presence of extreme hypertrophy of gastric rugal folds (i.e., Ménétrier's disease), giving the impression of polypoid lesions, has been associated with a striking frequency of malignant transformation; such hypertrophy, however, does not represent the presence of true adenomatous polyps. Individuals with blood group A have a higher incidence of gastric cancer than persons with blood group O; this observation may be related to differences in the mucous secretion leading to altered mucosal protection from carcinogens. A germline mutation in the E-cadherin gene, inherited in an autosomal dominant pattern and coding for a cell adhesion protein, has been linked to a high incidence of occult gastric cancers in young asymptomatic carriers. Duodenal ulcers are not associated with gastric cancer.

Clinical Features   Gastric cancers, when superficial and surgically curable, usually produce no symptoms. As the tumor becomes more extensive, patients may complain of an insidious upper abdominal discomfort varying in intensity from a vague, postprandial fullness to a severe, steady pain. Anorexia, often with slight nausea, is very common but is not the usual presenting complaint. Weight loss may eventually be observed, and nausea and vomiting are particularly prominent with tumors of the pylorus; dysphagia may be the major symptom caused by lesions of the cardia. There are no early physical signs. A palpable abdominal mass indicates long-standing growth and predicts regional extension.

Gastric carcinomas spread by direct extension through the gastric wall to the perigastric tissues, occasionally adhering to adjacent organs such as the pancreas, colon, or liver. The disease also spreads via lymphatics or by seeding of peritoneal surfaces. Metastases to intraabdominal and supraclavicular lymph nodes occur frequently, as do metastatic nodules to the ovary (Krukenberg's tumor), periumbilical region ("Sister Mary Joseph node"), or peritoneal cul-de-sac (Blumer's shelf palpable on rectal or vaginal examination); malignant ascites may also develop. The liver is the most common site for hematogenous spread of tumor.

The presence of iron-deficiency anemia in men and of occult blood in the stool in both sexes mandates a search for an occult gastrointestinal tract lesion. A careful assessment is of particular importance in patients with atrophic gastritis or pernicious anemia. Unusual clinical features associated with gastric adenocarcinomas include migratory thrombophlebitis, microangiopathic hemolytic anemia, and acanthosis nigricans.

Diagnosis   A double-contrast radiographic examination is the simplest diagnostic procedure for the evaluation of a patient with epigastric complaints. The use of double-contrast techniques helps to detect small lesions by improving mucosal detail. The stomach should be distended at some time during every radiographic examination, since decreased distensibility may be the only indication of a diffuse infiltrative carcinoma. Although gastric ulcers can be detected fairly early, distinguishing benign from malignant lesions is difficult. The anatomic location of an ulcer is not in itself an indication of the presence or absence of a cancer.

Gastric ulcers that appear benign by radiography present special problems. Some physicians believe that gastroscopy is not mandatory if the radiographic features are typically benign, if complete healing can be visualized by x-ray within 6 weeks, and if a follow-up contrast radiograph obtained several months later shows a normal appearance. However, we recommend gastroscopic biopsy and brush cytology for all patients with a gastric ulcer in order to exclude a malignancy. Malignant gastric ulcers must be recognized before they penetrate into surrounding tissues, because the rate of cure of early lesions limited to the mucosa or submucosa is >80%. Since gastric carcinomas are

---

TABLE 77-2   *Nitrate-Converting Bacteria as a Factor in the Causation of Gastric Carcinoma[a]*

Exogenous sources of nitrate-converting bacteria:
   Bacterially contaminated food (common in lower socioeconomic classes, who have a higher incidence of the disease; diminished by improved food preservation and refrigeration)
   ? *Helicobacter pylori* infection
Endogenous factors favoring growth of nitrate-converting bacteria in the stomach:
   Decreased gastric acidity
   Prior gastric surgery (antrectomy) (15- to 20-year latency period)
   Atrophic gastritis and/or pernicious anemia
   ? Prolonged exposure to histamine H_2-receptor antagonists

[a] Hypothesis: Dietary nitrates are converted to carcinogenic nitrites by bacteria.

TABLE 77-3 *Staging System for Gastric Carcinoma*

Stage	TNM	Features	Data from ACS No. of Cases, %	Data from ACS 5-Year Survival, %
0	TisN0M0	Node negative; limited to mucosa	1	90
IA	T1N0M0	Node negative; invasion of lamina propria or submucosa	7	59
IB	T2N0M0	Node negative; invasion of muscularis propria	10	44
II	T1N2M0 T2N1M0	Node positive; invasion beyond mucosa but within wall		
		or	17	29
	T3N0M0	Node negative; extension through wall		
IIIA	T2N2M0 T3N1-2M0	Node positive; invasion of muscularis propria or through wall	21	15
IIIB	T4N0-1M0	Node negative; adherence to surrounding tissue	14	9
IV	T4N2M0	Node positive; adherence to surrounding tissue		
		or	30	3
	T1-4N0-2M1	Distant metastases		

difficult to distinguish clinically or radiographically from gastric lymphomas, endoscopic biopsies should be made as deeply as possible, due to the submucosal location of lymphoid tumors.

The staging system for gastric carcinoma is shown in Table 77-3.

℞ TREATMENT

Complete surgical removal of the tumor with resection of adjacent lymph nodes offers the only chance for cure. However, this is possible in fewer than a third of patients. A subtotal gastrectomy is the treatment of choice for patients with distal carcinomas, while total or near-total gastrectomies are required for more proximal tumors. The inclusion of extended lymph node dissection to these procedures appears to confer an added risk for complications without enhancing survival. The prognosis following complete surgical resection depends on the degree of tumor penetration into the stomach wall and is adversely influenced by regional lymph node involvement, vascular invasion, and abnormal DNA content (i.e., aneuploidy), characteristics found in the vast majority of American patients. As a result, the probability of survival after 5 years for the 25 to 30% of patients able to undergo complete resection is ~20% for distal tumors and <10% for proximal tumors, with recurrences continuing to occur for at least 8 years after surgery. In the absence of ascites or extensive hepatic or peritoneal metastases, even patients whose disease is believed to be incurable by surgery should be offered resection of the primary lesion. Reduction of tumor bulk is the best form of palliation and may enhance the probability of benefit from chemotherapy and/or radiation therapy.

Gastric adenocarcinoma is a relatively radioresistant tumor, and adequate control of the primary tumor requires doses of external beam irradiation that exceed the tolerance of surrounding structures, such as bowel mucosa and spinal cord. As a result, the major role of radiation therapy in patients has been palliation of pain. Radiation therapy alone after a complete resection does not prolong survival. In the setting of surgically unresectable disease limited to the epigastrium, patients treated with 3500 to 4000 cGy did not live longer than similar patients not receiving radiotherapy; however, survival was prolonged slightly when 5-fluorouracil (5-FU) was given in combination with radiation therapy. In this clinical setting, the 5-FU may well be functioning as a radiosensitizer.

The administration of combinations of cytotoxic drugs to patients with advanced gastric carcinoma has been associated with partial responses in 30 to 50% of cases, providing significant benefit to individuals who respond to treatment. Such drug combinations have generally included 5-FU and doxorubicin together with either mitomycin-C or cisplatin. Despite this encouraging response rate, complete remissions are uncommon, the partial responses are transient, and the overall influence of multidrug therapy on survival has been a source of debate. The use of adjuvant chemotherapy alone following the complete resection of a gastric cancer has only minimally improved sur-

vival. However, postoperative chemotherapy combined with radiation therapy has been shown to reduce the recurrence rate and prolong survival.

PRIMARY GASTRIC LYMPHOMA Primary lymphoma of the stomach is relatively uncommon, accounting for <15% of gastric malignancies and about 2% of all lymphomas. The stomach is, however, the most frequent extranodal site for lymphoma, and gastric lymphoma has increased in frequency during the past 25 years. The disease is difficult to distinguish clinically from gastric adenocarcinoma; both tumors are most often detected during the sixth decade of life; present with epigastric pain, early satiety, and generalized fatigue; and are usually characterized by ulcerations with a ragged, thickened mucosal pattern demonstrated by contrast radiographs. The diagnosis of lymphoma of the stomach may occasionally be made through cytologic brushings of the gastric mucosa but usually requires a biopsy at gastroscopy or laparotomy. Failure of gastroscopic biopsies to detect lymphoma in a given case should not be interpreted as being conclusive, since superficial biopsies may miss the deeper lymphoid infiltrate. The macroscopic pathology of gastric lymphoma may also mimic adenocarcinoma, consisting of either a bulky ulcerated lesion localized in the corpus or antrum or a diffuse process spreading throughout the entire gastric submucosa and even extending into the duodenum. Microscopically, the vast majority of gastric lymphoid tumors are non-Hodgkin's lymphomas of B cell origin; Hodgkin's disease involving the stomach is extremely uncommon. Histologically, these tumors may range from well-differentiated, superficial processes [mucosa-associated lymphoid tissue (MALT)] to high-grade, large-cell lymphomas. Infection with *H. pylori*, the same bacterium associated with the development of gastric adenocarcinoma, appears to increase the risk for gastric lymphoma in general and MALT lymphomas in particular. Gastric lymphomas spread initially to regional lymph nodes (often to Waldeyer's ring) and may then disseminate. Gastric lymphomas are staged like other lymphomas (Chap. 97).

℞ TREATMENT

Primary gastric lymphoma is a far more treatable disease than adenocarcinoma of the stomach, a fact that underscores the need for making the correct diagnosis. Antibiotic treatment to eradicate *H. pylori* infection has led to regression of about 75% of gastric MALT lymphomas and should be considered before surgery, radiation therapy, or chemotherapy are undertaken in patients having such tumors. A lack of response to such antimicrobial treatment has been linked to a specific chromosomal abnormality, i.e., t(11;18). Responding patients should undergo periodic endoscopic surveillance because it remains unclear whether the neoplastic clone is eliminated or merely suppressed. Subtotal gastrectomy, usually followed by combination chemotherapy, has led to 5-year survival rates of 40 to 60% in patients with localized high-grade lymphomas. The need for a major surgical procedure is not clear, particularly in patients with preoperative radiographic evidence of nodal involvement, for whom chemotherapy alone [CHOP (cyclophosphamide, doxorubicin, vincristine, and prednisone) plus rituximab] is effective therapy. A role for radiation therapy is not defined because most recurrences develop at sites distant from the epigastrium. If widespread disease is discovered at the time of laparotomy, combination chemotherapy should be used.

GASTRIC (NONLYMPHOID) SARCOMA Leiomyosarcomas and GISTs make up 1 to 3% of gastric neoplasms. They most frequently involve the anterior and posterior walls of the gastric fundus and often ulcerate and bleed. Even those lesions that appear benign on histologic examination may behave in a malignant fashion. These tumors rarely invade adjacent viscera and characteristically do not metastasize to lymph nodes, but they may spread to the liver and lungs. The treatment of choice is surgical resection. Combination chemotherapy should be reserved for patients with metastatic disease. All such tumors should be analyzed for a mutation in the c-*kit* receptor. GISTs are unresponsive to conventional chemotherapy; ~50% of patients with such tumors, however, experience objective response when treated with imatinib mesylate (Gleevec), a selective inhibitor of the c-*kit* tyrosine kinase.

COLORECTAL CANCER

INCIDENCE Cancer of the large bowel is second only to lung cancer as a cause of cancer death in the United States; 146,940 new cases occurred in 2004, and 56,730 deaths were due to colorectal cancer. The incidence rate has remained relatively unchanged during the past 30 years while the mortality rate has decreased, particularly in females. Colorectal cancer generally occurs in individuals ≥50 years.

POLYPS AND MOLECULAR PATHOGENESIS Most colorectal cancers, regardless of etiology, arise from adenomatous polyps. A polyp is a grossly visible protrusion from the mucosal surface and may be classified pathologically as a nonneoplastic hamartoma (*juvenile polyp*), a hyperplastic mucosal proliferation (*hyperplastic polyp*), or an adenomatous polyp. Only adenomas are clearly premalignant, and only a minority of such lesions ever develop into cancer. Population-screening studies and autopsy surveys have revealed that adenomatous polyps may be found in the colons of >30% of middle-aged or elderly people; however, <1% of polyps ever become malignant. Most polyps produce no symptoms and remain clinically undetected. Occult blood in the stool may be found in <5% of patients with such lesions.

A number of molecular changes have been described in DNA obtained from adenomatous polyps, dysplastic lesions, and polyps containing microscopic foci of tumor cells (carcinoma in situ), which are thought to represent a multistep process in the evolution of normal colonic mucosa to life-threatening invasive carcinoma. These developmental steps towards carcinogenesis include, but are not restricted to, point mutations in the K-*ras* protooncogene; hypomethylation of DNA, leading to gene activation; loss of DNA ("allelic loss") at the site of a tumor-suppressor gene [the adenomatous polyposis coli (*APC*) gene] on the long arm of chromosome 5 (5q21); allelic loss at the site of a tumor-suppressor gene located on chromosome 18q [the deleted in colorectal cancer (*DCC*) gene]; and allelic loss at chromosome 17p, associated with mutations in the p53 tumor-suppressor gene (Fig. 68-2). Thus, the altered proliferative pattern of the colonic mucosa, which results in progression to a polyp and then to carcinoma, may involve the mutational activation of an oncogene followed by and coupled with the loss of genes that normally suppress tumorigenesis. It remains uncertain whether the genetic aberrations always occur in a defined order. Based on this model, however, cancer is believed to develop only in those polyps in which all of these mutational events take place.

Clinically, the probability of an adenomatous polyp becoming a cancer depends on the gross appearance of the lesion, its histologic features, and its size. Adenomatous polyps may be pedunculated (stalked) or sessile (flat-based). Cancers develop more frequently in sessile polyps. Histologically, adenomatous polyps may be tubular, villous (i.e., papillary), or tubulovillous. Villous adenomas, most of which are sessile, become malignant more than three times as often as tubular adenomas. The likelihood that any polypoid lesion in the large bowel contains invasive cancer is related to the size of the polyp, being negligible (<2%) in lesions <1.5 cm, intermediate (2 to 10%) in lesions 1.5 to 2.5 cm in size, and substantial (10%) in lesions >2.5 cm.

Following the detection of an adenomatous polyp, the entire large bowel should be visualized endoscopically or radiographically, since synchronous lesions are present in about one-third of cases. Colonoscopy should then be repeated periodically, even in the absence of a previously documented malignancy, since such patients have a 30 to 50% probability of developing another adenoma and are at a higher-than-average risk for developing a colorectal carcinoma. Adenomatous

polyps are thought to require >5 years of growth before becoming clinically significant; colonoscopy need not be carried out more frequently than every 3 years.

ETIOLOGY AND RISK FACTORS Risk factors for the development of colorectal cancer are listed in Table 77-4.

Diet The etiology for most cases of large-bowel cancer appears to be related to environmental factors. The disease occurs more often in upper socioeconomic populations who live in urban areas. Mortality from colorectal cancer is directly correlated with per capita consumption of calories, meat protein, and dietary fat and oil as well as elevations in the serum cholesterol concentration and mortality from coronary artery disease. Geographic variations in incidence are unrelated to genetic differences, since migrant groups tend to assume the large-bowel cancer incidence rates of their adopted countries. Furthermore, population groups such as Mormons and Seventh Day Adventists, whose lifestyle and dietary habits differ somewhat from those of their neighbors, have significantly lower-than-expected incidence and mortality rates for colorectal cancer. Colorectal cancer has increased in Japan since that nation has adopted a more "western" diet. At least two hypotheses have been proposed to explain the relationship to diet, neither of which is fully satisfactory.

ANIMAL FATS One hypothesis is that the ingestion of animal fats such as are found in red meats and processed meat leads to an increased proportion of anaerobes in the gut microflora, resulting in the conversion of normal bile acids into carcinogens. This provocative hypothesis is supported by several reports of increased amounts of fecal anaerobes in the stools of patients with colorectal cancer. Diets high in animal (but not vegetable) fats are also associated with high serum cholesterol, which is also associated with enhanced risk for the development of colorectal adenomas and carcinomas.

INSULIN RESISTANCE The enhanced number of calories inherent in "western" diets coupled with physical inactivity have been associated with a higher prevalence of obesity. Persons with such excess weight gain develop insulin resistance with increased circulating levels of insulin, leading to higher circulating concentrations of insulin-like growth factor type I (IGF-I). This growth factor appears to stimulate proliferation of the intestinal mucosa.

FIBER Contrary to one hypothesis, the results of randomized trials and case-controlled studies have failed to show any value for dietary fiber or diets high in fruits and vegatables in preventing the recurrence of colorectal adenomas or the development of colorectal cancer. The weight of epidemiologic evidence, however, implicates diet as being the major etiologic factor for colorectal cancer, particularly diets high in animal fat and in calories.

HEREDITARY FACTORS AND SYNDROMES As many as 25% of patients with colorectal cancer have a family history of the disease, suggesting a hereditary predisposition. Inherited large-bowel cancers can be divided into two main groups: the well-studied but uncommon polyposis syndromes and the more common nonpolyposis syndromes (Table 77-5).

Polyposis Coli Polyposis coli (familial polyposis of the colon) is a rare condition characterized by the appearance of thousands of adenomatous polyps throughout the large bowel. It is transmitted as an autosomal dominant trait; the occasional patients with no family history

TABLE 77-4   *Risk Factors for the Development of Colorectal Cancer*

Diet: Animal fat
Hereditary syndromes (autosomal dominant inheritance)
  Polyposis coli
  Nonpolyposis syndrome (Lynch syndrome)
Inflammatory bowel disease
Streptococcus bovis bacteremia
Ureterosigmoidostomy
? Tobacco use

TABLE 77-5 *Hereditable (Autosomal Dominant) Gastrointestinal Polyposis Syndromes*

Syndrome	Distribution of Polyps	Histologic Type	Malignant Potential	Associated Lesions
Familial adenomatous polyposis	Large intestine	Adenoma	Common	None
Gardner's syndrome	Large and small intestines	Adenoma	Common	Osteomas, fibromas, lipomas, epidermoid cysts, ampullary cancers, congenital hypertrophy of retinal pigment epithelium
Turcot's syndrome	Large intestine	Adenoma	Common	Brain tumors
Nonpolyposis syndrome (Lynch syndrome)	Large intestine (often proximal)	Adenoma	Common	Endometrial and ovarian tumors
Peutz-Jeghers syndrome	Small and large intestines, stomach	Hamartoma	Rare	Mucocutaneous pigmentation; tumors of the ovary, breast, pancreas, endometrium
Juvenile polyposis	Large and small intestines, stomach	Hamartoma, rarely progressing to adenoma	Rare	Various congenital abnormalities

In contrast to polyposis coli, HNPCC is associated with an unusually high frequency of cancer arising in the proximal large bowel. The median age for the appearance of an adenocarcinoma is <50 years, 10 to 15 years younger than the median age for the general population. Despite having a poorly differentiated histologic appearance, the proximal colon tumors in HNPCC have a better prognosis than sporadic tumors from patients of similar age. Families with HNPCC often include individuals with multiple primary cancers; the association of colorectal cancer with either ovarian or endometrial carcinomas is especially strong in women. It has been recommended that members of such families undergo biennial colonoscopy beginning at age 25 years, with intermittent pelvic ultrasonography and endometrial biopsy offered for potentially afflicted women; such a screening strategy has not yet been validated. HNPCC is associated with germline mutations of several genes, particularly *hMSH2* on chromosome 2 and *hMLH1* on chromosome 3. These mutations lead to errors in DNA replication and are thought to result in DNA instability because of defective repair of DNA mismatches, resulting in abnormal cell growth and tumor development. Testing tumor cells for "microsatellite instability" (sequence changes reflecting defective mismatch repair) in patients under age 50 with colorectal cancer and a positive family history for colorectal or endometrial cancer may identify probands with HNPCC.

probably developed the condition due to a spontaneous mutation. Polyposis coli is associated with a deletion in the long arm of chromosome 5 (including the *APC* gene) in both neoplastic (somatic mutation) and normal (germline mutation) cells. The loss of this genetic material (i.e., allelic loss) results in the absence of tumor-suppressor genes whose protein products would normally inhibit neoplastic growth. The presence of soft tissue and bony tumors, congenital hypertrophy of the retinal pigment epithelium, mesenteric desmoid tumors, and of ampullary cancers in addition to the colonic polyps characterizes a subset of polyposis coli known as *Gardner's syndrome*. The appearance of malignant tumors of the central nervous system accompanying polyposis coli defines *Turcot's syndrome*. The colonic polyps in all these conditions are rarely present before puberty but are generally evident in affected individuals by age 25. If the polyposis is not treated surgically, colorectal cancer will develop in almost all patients before age 40. Polyposis coli results from a defect in the colonic mucosa leading to an abnormal proliferative pattern and an impaired DNA repair following exposure to radiation or ultraviolet light. Once the multiple polyps that constitute polyposis coli are detected, patients should undergo a total colectomy. The ileoanal anastomotic technique allows removal of the entire bowel while retaining the anal sphincter; this appears to be the best treatment. Medical therapy with nonsteroidal anti-inflammatory drugs (NSAIDs) such as sulindac and cyclooxygenase-2 inhibitors such as celecoxib can decrease the number and size of polyps in patients with polyposis coli; however, this effect on polyps is only temporary. Colectomy remains the primary therapy. The offspring of patients with polyposis coli, who often are prepubertal when the diagnosis is made in the parent, have a 50% risk for the development of this premalignant disorder and should be carefully screened by annual flexible sigmoidoscopy until age 35. Proctosigmoidoscopy is a sufficient screening procedure because polyps tend to be evenly distributed from cecum to anus, making more-invasive and expensive techniques such as colonoscopy or barium enema unnecessary. Testing for occult blood in the stool is an inadequate screening maneuver. An alternative method for identifying carriers is testing DNA from peripheral blood mononuclear cells for the presence of a mutated *APC* gene. The detection of such a germline mutation can lead to a definitive diagnosis before the development of polyps.

Hereditary Nonpolyposis Colon Cancer Hereditary nonpolyposis colon cancer (HNPCC), also known as *Lynch syndrome*, is another autosomal dominant trait. It is characterized by the presence of three or more relatives with histologically documented colorectal cancer, one of whom is a first-degree relative of the other two; one or more cases of colorectal cancer diagnosed before age 50 in the family; and colorectal

INFLAMMATORY BOWEL DISEASE (See also Chap. 276) Large-bowel cancer is increased in incidence in patients with long-standing inflammatory bowel disease (IBD). Cancers develop more commonly in patients with ulcerative colitis than in those with granulomatous colitis, but this impression may result in part from the occasional difficulty of differentiating these two conditions. The risk of colorectal cancer in a patient with IBD is relatively small during the initial 10 years of the disease, but then it appears to increase at a rate of ~0.5 to 1% per year. Cancer may develop in 8 to 30% of patients after 25 years. The risk is higher in younger patients with pancolitis.

Cancer surveillance in patients with IBD is unsatisfactory. Symptoms such as bloody diarrhea, abdominal cramping, and obstruction, which may signal the appearance of a tumor, are similar to the complaints caused by a flare-up of the underlying disease. In patients with a history of IBD lasting ≥15 years who continue to experience exacerbations, the surgical removal of the colon can significantly reduce the risk for cancer and also eliminate the target organ for the underlying chronic gastrointestinal disorder. The value of such surveillance techniques as colonoscopy with mucosal biopsies and brushings for less symptomatic individuals with chronic IBD is uncertain. The lack of uniformity regarding the pathologic criteria that characterize dysplasia and the absence of data that such surveillance reduces the development of lethal cancers have made this costly practice an area of controversy.

OTHER HIGH-RISK CONDITIONS ■ ***Streptococcus bovis* Bacteremia** For unknown reasons, individuals who develop endocarditis or septicemia from this fecal bacteria have a high incidence of occult colorectal tumors and, possibly, upper gastrointestinal cancers as well. Endoscopic or radiographic screening appears advisable.

Ureterosigmoidostomy Colon cancer develops in 5 to 10% of people 15 to 30 years after ureterosigmoidostomy to correct congenital extrophy of the bladder. Neoplasms characteristically are found at a site distal to the ureteral implant where colonic mucosa is chronically exposed to both urine and feces.

Tobacco Use Cigarette smoking is linked to the development of colorectal adenomas, particularly after >35 years of tobacco use. No biologic explanation for this association has yet been proposed.

PRIMARY PREVENTION Several orally administered compounds have been assessed as possible inhibitors of colon cancer. The most effective class of these chemopreventive agents is aspirin and other NSAIDs, which are thought to suppress cell proliferation by inhibiting prostaglandin synthesis. Regular aspirin use reduces the risk for colonic adenomas and carcinomas as well as for death from large-bowel cancer; such use also appears to diminish the likelihood for developing additional premalignant adenomas following treatment for a prior colon carcinoma. This inhibiting effect of aspirin on colon carcinogenesis appears to increase with the duration of drug use. Oral folic acid supplements and oral calcium supplements reduce the risk of adenomatous polyps and colorectal cancers in case-controlled studies. While antioxidant vitamins such as ascorbic acid, tocopherols, and β-carotene are present in diets rich in fruits and vegetables, which have been associated with lower rates of colorectal cancer, they are ineffective at reducing the incidence of subsequent adenomas in patients who have undergone the removal of a colon adenoma. Estrogen-replacement therapy has been associated with a reduction in the risk of colorectal cancer in women, conceivably by an effect on bile acid synthesis and composition or by decreasing synthesis of IGF-I. The otherwise unexplained reduction in colorectal cancer mortality in women may be a result of the widespread use of estrogen replacement in postmenopausal individuals.

SCREENING The rationale for colorectal cancer screening programs is that the earlier detection of localized, superficial cancers in asymptomatic individuals will increase the surgical cure rate. Such screening programs are important for individuals having a family history of the disease in first-degree relatives. The relative risk for developing colorectal cancer increases to 1.75 in such individuals and may be even higher if the relative was afflicted before age 60. The prior use of proctosigmoidoscopy as a screening tool was based on the observation that 60% of early lesions are located in the rectosigmoid. For unexplained reasons, however, the proportion of large-bowel cancers arising in the rectum has been decreasing during the past several decades, with a corresponding increase in the proportion of cancers in the more proximal descending colon. As such, the potential for rigid proctosigmoidoscopy to detect a sufficient number of occult neoplasms to make the procedure cost-effective has been questioned. Flexible, fiberoptic sigmoidoscopes permit trained operators to visualize the colon for up to 60 cm, which enhances the capability for cancer detection. However, this technique still leaves the proximal half of the large bowel unscreened.

Most programs directed at the early detection of colorectal cancers have focused on digital rectal examinations and fecal occult blood testing. The digital examination should be part of any routine physical evaluation in adults older than age 40, serving as a screening test for prostate cancer in men, a component of the pelvic examination in women, and an inexpensive maneuver for the detection of masses in the rectum. The development of the Hemoccult test has greatly facilitated the detection of occult fecal blood. Unfortunately, even when performed optimally, the Hemoccult test has major limitations as a screening technique. About 50% of patients with documented colorectal cancers have a negative fecal Hemoccult test, consistent with the intermittent bleeding pattern of these tumors. When random cohorts of asymptomatic persons have been tested, 2 to 4% have Hemoccult-positive stools. Colorectal cancers have been found in <10% of these "test-positive" cases, with benign polyps being detected in an additional 20 to 30%. Thus, a colorectal neoplasm will not be found in most asymptomatic individuals with occult blood in their stool. Nonetheless, persons found to have Hemoccult-positive stool routinely undergo further medical evaluation, including sigmoidoscopy, barium

enema, and/or colonoscopy—procedures that are not only uncomfortable and expensive but also associated with a small risk for significant complications. The added cost of these studies would appear justifiable if the small number of patients found to have occult neoplasms because of Hemoccult screening could be shown to have an improved prognosis and prolonged survival. Prospectively controlled trials showed a statistically significant reduction in mortality from colorectal cancer for individuals undergoing annual screening. However, this benefit only emerged after >13 years of follow-up and was extremely expensive to achieve, since all positive tests (most of which were false-positive) were followed by colonoscopy. Moreover, these colonoscopic examinations quite likely provided the opportunity for cancer prevention through the removal of potentially premalignant adenomatous polyps since the eventual development of cancer was reduced by 20% in the cohort undergoing annual screening.

Screening techniques for large-bowel cancer in asymptomatic persons remain unsatisfactory. Compliance with any screening strategy within the general population is poor. At present, the American Cancer Society suggests fecal Hemoccult screening annually and flexible sigmoidoscopy every 5 years beginning at age 50 for asymptomatic individuals having no colorectal cancer risk factors. The American Cancer Society has proposed a "total colon examination" (i.e., colonoscopy or double-contrast barium enema) every 10 years as an alternative to Hemoccult testing with periodic flexible sigmoidoscopy. Colonoscopy has been shown to be superior to double-contrast barium enema and also to have a higher sensitivity for detecting villous or dysplastic adenomas or cancers than the strategy employing occult fecal blood testing and flexible sigmoidoscopy. Whether colonoscopy performed every 10 years beginning after age 50 will prove to be cost-effective and whether it may be supplanted as a screening maneuver by sophisticated radiographic techniques ("virtual colonoscopy") remains unclear. More effective techniques for screening are needed, perhaps taking advantage of the molecular changes that have been described in these tumors. Analysis of stool for mutation in the *APC* tumor-suppressor gene is being tested.

CLINICAL FEATURES ■ Presenting Symptoms Symptoms vary with the anatomic location of the tumor. Since stool is relatively liquid as it passes through the ileocecal valve into the right colon, cancers arising in the cecum and ascending colon may become quite large without resulting in any obstructive symptoms or noticeable alterations in bowel habits. Lesions of the right colon commonly ulcerate, leading to chronic, insidious blood loss without a change in the appearance of the stool. Consequently, patients with tumors of the ascending colon often present with symptoms such as fatigue, palpitations, and even angina pectoris and are found to have a hypochromic, microcytic anemia indicative of iron deficiency. Since the cancer may bleed intermittently, a random fecal occult blood test may be negative. As a result, the unexplained presence of iron-deficiency anemia in any adult (with the possible exception of a premenopausal, multiparous woman) mandates a thorough endoscopic and/or radiographic visualization of the entire large bowel (Fig. 77-1).

Since stool becomes more concentrated as it passes into the transverse and descending colon, tumors arising there tend to impede the passage of stool, resulting in the development of abdominal cramping, occasional obstruction, and even perforation. Radiographs of the abdomen often reveal characteristic annular, constricting lesions ("apple-core" or "napkin-ring") (Fig. 77-2).

Cancers arising in the rectosigmoid are often associated with hematochezia, tenesmus, and narrowing of the caliber of stool; anemia is an infrequent finding. While these symptoms may lead patients and their physicians to suspect the presence of hemorrhoids, the development of rectal bleeding and/or altered bowel habits demands a prompt digital rectal examination and proctosigmoidoscopy.

Staging, Prognostic Factors, and Patterns of Spread The prognosis for individuals having colorectal cancer is related to the depth of tumor

FIGURE 77-1   Double-contrast air-barium enema revealing a sessile tumor of the cecum in a patient with iron-deficiency anemia and guaiac-positive stool. The lesion at surgery was a stage B adenocarcinoma.

penetration into the bowel wall and the presence of both regional lymph node involvement and distant metastases. These variables are incorporated into the staging system introduced by Dukes and applied to a TNM classification method, in which T represents the depth of tumor penetration, N the presence of lymph node involvement, and M the presence or absence of distant metastases (Table 77-6). Superficial lesions that do not penetrate into the muscularis or involve regional lymph nodes are designated as *stage A* (T1N0M0) disease; tumors that penetrate more deeply but have not spread to lymph nodes are *stage B* disease [subclassified as stage B_1 (T2N0M0) if lesions are restricted to the muscularis and as stage B_2 (T3N0M0) if lesions involve or

FIGURE 77-2   Annular, constricting adenocarcinoma of the descending colon. This radiographic appearance is referred to as an "apple-core" lesion and is always highly suggestive of malignancy.

TABLE 77-6   *Staging of and Prognosis for Colorectal Cancer*

Stage				Approximate 5-Year Survival, %
Dukes	TNM	Numerical	Pathologic Description	
A	T1N0M0	I	Cancer limited to mucosa and submucosa	>90
B_1	T2N0M0	I	Cancer extends into muscularis	85
B_2	T3N0M0	II	Cancer extends into or through serosa	70–80
C	TxN1M0	III	Cancer involves regional lymph nodes	35–65
D	TxNxM1	IV	Distant metastases (i.e., liver, lung)	5

penetrate the serosa]; regional lymph node involvement defines *stage C* (TxN1M0) disease; and metastatic spread to sites such as liver, lung, or bone indicates *stage D* (TxNxM1) disease. Unless gross evidence of metastatic disease is present, disease stage cannot be determined accurately before surgical resection and pathologic analysis of the operative specimens. It is not clear whether the detection of nodal metastases by special immunohistochemical molecular techniques has the same prognostic implications as disease detected by routine light microscopy.

Most recurrences after a surgical resection of a large-bowel cancer occur within the first 4 years, making 5-year survival a fairly reliable indicator of cure. The likelihood for 5-year survival in patients with colorectal cancer is stage-related (Table 77-6). That likelihood has improved during the past several decades when similar surgical stages have been compared. The most plausible explanation for this improvement appears to be more thorough intraoperative and pathologic staging. In particular, more exacting attention to pathologic detail has revealed that the prognosis following the resection of a colorectal cancer is not related merely to the presence or absence of regional lymph node involvement. Prognosis may be more precisely gauged by the number of involved lymph nodes (one to four lymph nodes versus five or more lymph nodes). Other predictors of a poor prognosis after a total surgical resection include tumor penetration through the bowel wall into pericolic fat, poorly differentiated histology, perforation and/or tumor adherence to adjacent organs (increasing the risk for an anatomically adjacent recurrence), and venous invasion by tumor (Table 77-7). Regardless of the clinicopathologic stage, a preoperative elevation of the plasma carcinoembryonic antigen (CEA) level predicts eventual tumor recurrence. The presence of aneuploidy and specific chromosomal deletions, such as allelic loss in chromosome 18q (involving the *DCC* gene) in tumor cells, appears to predict a higher risk for metastatic spread, particularly in patients with stage B_2 (T3N0M0) disease. Conversely, the detection of microsatellite instability in tumor tissue has been associated with a more favorable outcome. In contrast to most other cancers, the prognosis in colorectal cancer is not influenced by the size of the primary lesion when adjusted for nodal involvement and histologic differentiation.

TABLE 77-7   *Predictors of Poor Outcome Following Total Surgical Resection of Colorectal Cancer*

Tumor spread to regional lymph nodes
Number of regional lymph nodes involved
Tumor penetration through the bowel wall
Poorly differentiated histology
Perforation
Tumor adherence to adjacent organs
Venous invasion
Preoperative elevation of CEA titer (>5.0 ng/mL)
Aneuploidy
Specific chromosomal deletion (e.g., allelic loss on chromosome 18q)

Note: CEA, carcinoembryonic antigen.

Cancers of the large bowel generally spread to regional lymph nodes or to the liver via the portal venous circulation. The liver represents the most frequent visceral site of metastatic dissemination; it is the initial site of distant spread in one-third of recurring colorectal cancers and is involved in more than two-thirds of such patients at the time of death. In general, colorectal cancer rarely metastasizes to the lungs, supraclavicular lymph nodes, bone, or brain without prior spread to the liver. A major exception to this rule occurs in patients having primary tumors in the distal rectum, from which tumor cells may spread through the paravertebral venous plexus, escaping the portal venous system and thereby reaching the lungs or supraclavicular lymph nodes without hepatic involvement. The median survival after the detection of distant metastases is 6 to 9 months (hepatomegaly, abnormal liver chemistries) to 24 to 30 months (small liver nodule initially identified by elevated CEA level and subsequent CT scan).

℞ TREATMENT

Total resection of tumor is the optimal treatment when a malignant lesion is detected endoscopically or radiographically in the large bowel. An evaluation for the presence of metastatic disease, including a thorough physical examination, chest radiograph, biochemical assessment of liver function, and measurement of the plasma CEA level, should be performed before surgery. When possible, a colonoscopy of the entire large bowel should be performed to identify synchronous neoplasms and/or polyps. The detection of metastases should not preclude surgery in patients with tumor-related symptoms such as gastrointestinal bleeding or obstruction, but it often prompts the use of a less radical operative procedure. At the time of laparotomy, the entire peritoneal cavity should be examined, with thorough inspection of the liver, pelvis, and hemidiaphragm and careful palpation of the full length of the large bowel. Following recovery from a complete resection, patients should be observed carefully for 5 years by semiannual physical examinations and yearly blood chemistry measurements. If a complete colonoscopy was not performed preoperatively, it should be carried out within the first several postoperative months. Some authorities favor measuring plasma CEA levels at 3-month intervals because of the sensitivity of this test as a marker for otherwise undetectable tumor recurrence. Subsequent endoscopic or radiographic surveillance of the large bowel, probably at triennial intervals, is indicated, since patients who have been cured of one colorectal cancer have a 3 to 5% probability of developing an additional bowel cancer during their lifetime and a >15% risk for the development of adenomatous polyps. Anastomotic ("suture-line") recurrences are infrequent in colorectal cancer patients provided the surgical resection margins were adequate and free of tumor. Periodic CT screening, chest radiographs, or more frequent colonoscopic examinations do not affect prognosis and add unnecessary costs to postoperative surveillance.

Radiation therapy to the pelvis is recommended for patients with rectal cancer because it reduces the 20 to 25% probability of regional recurrences following complete surgical resection of stage B_2 or C tumors, especially if they have penetrated through the serosa. This alarmingly high rate of local disease recurrence is believed to be due to the fact that the contained anatomic space within the pelvis limits the extent of the resection and because the rich lymphatic network of the pelvic side wall immediately adjacent to the rectum facilitates the early spread of malignant cells into surgically inaccessible tissue. The use of sharp rather than blunt dissection of rectal cancers ("total mesorectal excision") appears to reduce the likelihood of local disease recurrence to ~10%. Radiation therapy, either pre- or postoperatively, reduces the likelihood of pelvic recurrences but does not appear to prolong survival. Preoperative radiotherapy is indicated for patients with large, potentially unresectable rectal cancers; such lesions may shrink enough to permit subsequent surgical removal. Radiation therapy is not effective in the primary treatment of colon cancer.

Chemotherapy in patients with advanced colorectal cancer has proven to be of only marginal benefit. 5-FU is the most effective single agent for this disease. Partial responses are obtained in 15 to 20% of patients. The probability of tumor response appears to be somewhat greater for patients with liver metastases when chemotherapy is infused directly into the hepatic artery, but intraarterial treatment is costly and toxic and does not appear to prolong survival. The concomitant administration of folinic acid (leucovorin) improves the efficacy of 5-FU in patients with advanced colorectal cancer, presumably by enhancing the binding of 5-FU to its target enzyme, thymidylate synthase. A threefold improvement in the partial response rate is noted when folinic acid is combined with 5-FU; however, the effect on survival is marginal, and the optimal dose schedule remains to be defined. 5-FU is generally administered intravenously but may also be given orally in the form of capecitabine with seemingly similar efficacy.

Irinotecan (CPT-11), a topoisomerase 1 inhibitor, prolongs survival when compared to supportive care in patients whose disease has progressed on 5-FU. Furthermore, the addition of irinotecan to 5-FU and leucovorin (LV) improves response rates and survival of patients with metastatic disease. The *FOLFIRI regimen* is as follows: irinotecan, 180 mg/m² as a 90-min infusion day 1; LV, 400 mg/m² as a 2-h infusion during irinotecan, immediately followed by 5-FU bolus, 400 mg/m² and 46-h continuous infusion of 2.4 to 3 g/m² every 2 weeks. Oxaliplatin, a platinum analogue, also improves the response rate when added to 5-FU and LV as initial treatment of patients with metastatic disease. The *FOLFOX regimen* is the following: 2-h infusion of LV (200 mg/m² per day) followed by a 5-FU bolus (400 mg/m² per day) and 22-h infusion (600 mg/m² per day) for 2 consecutive days every 2 weeks, together with oxaliplatin, 85 mg/m² as a 2-h infusion on day 1.

Patients with solitary hepatic metastases without clinical or radiographic evidence of additional tumor involvement should be considered for partial liver resection, because such procedures are associated with 5-year survival rates of 25 to 30% when performed on selected individuals by experienced surgeons.

The administration of 5-FU and LV for 6 months after resection of tumor in patients with stage C disease leads to a 40% decrease in recurrence rates and 30% improvement in survival. Patients with stage B_2 tumors do not appear to benefit from adjuvant therapy. In rectal cancer, the delivery of postoperative (and probably preoperative) combined modality therapy (5-FU plus radiation therapy) reduces the risk of recurrence and increases the chance of cure for patients with stages B_2 and C tumors. The 5-FU acts as a radiosensitizer when delivered together with radiation therapy. A surprising lack of use of life-extending adjuvant therapy has been documented in patients over age 65 years. This age bias is completely inappropriate as the benefits of adjuvant therapy have been documented in patients over age 65 years.

TUMORS OF THE SMALL INTESTINE

Small-bowel tumors comprise <5% of gastrointestinal neoplasms. Because of their rarity, a correct diagnosis is often delayed. Abdominal symptoms are usually vague and poorly defined, and conventional radiographic studies of the upper and lower intestinal tract often appear normal. Small-bowel tumors should be considered in the differential diagnosis in the following situations: (1) recurrent, unexplained episodes of crampy abdominal pain; (2) intermittent bouts of intestinal obstruction, especially in the absence of IBD or prior abdominal surgery; (3) intussusception in the adult; and (4) evidence of chronic intestinal bleeding in the presence of negative conventional contrast radiographs. A careful small-bowel barium study is the diagnostic procedure of choice; the diagnostic accuracy may be improved by infusing barium through a nasogastric tube placed into the duodenum (enteroclysis).

BENIGN TUMORS The histology of benign small-bowel tumors is difficult to predict on clinical and radiologic grounds alone. The symptomatology of benign tumors is not distinctive, with pain, obstruction, and hemorrhage being the most frequent symptoms. These tumors are usually discovered during the fifth and sixth decades of life, more often in the distal rather than the proximal small intestine. The most common benign tumors are adenomas, leiomyomas, lipomas, and angiomas.

Adenomas   These tumors include those of the islet cells and Brunner's glands as well as polypoid adenomas. *Islet cell adenomas* are occasionally located outside the pancreas; the associated syndromes are discussed in Chap. 329. *Brunner's gland adenomas* are not truly neoplastic but represent a hypertrophy or hyperplasia of submucosal duodenal glands. These appear as small nodules in the duodenal mucosa that secrete a highly viscous alkaline mucus. Most often, this is an incidental radiographic finding not associated with any specific clinical disorder.

Polypoid Adenomas   About 25% of benign small-bowel tumors are polypoid adenomas (Table 77-5). They may present as single polypoid lesions or, less commonly, as papillary villous adenomas. As in the colon, the sessile or papillary form of the tumor is sometimes associated with a coexisting carcinoma. Occasionally, patients with Gardner's syndrome develop premalignant adenomas in the small bowel; such lesions are generally in the duodenum. Multiple polypoid tumors may occur throughout the small bowel (and occasionally the stomach and colorectum) in the Peutz-Jeghers syndrome. The polyps are usually hamartomas (juvenile polyps) having a low potential for malignant degeneration. Mucocutaneous melanin deposits as well as tumors of the ovary, breast, pancreas, and endometrium are also associated with this autosomal dominant condition.

Leiomyomas   These neoplasms arise from smooth-muscle components of the intestine and are usually intramural, affecting the overlying mucosa. Ulceration of the mucosa may cause gastrointestinal hemorrhage of varying severity. Cramping, intermittent abdominal pain is frequently encountered.

Lipomas   These tumors occur with greatest frequency in the distal ileum and at the ileocecal valve. They have a characteristic radiolucent appearance, are usually intramural and asymptomatic, but on occasion cause bleeding.

Angiomas   While not true neoplasms, these lesions are important because they frequently cause intestinal bleeding. They may take the form of telangiectasia or hemangiomas. Multiple intestinal telangiectasias occur in a nonhereditary form confined to the gastrointestinal tract or as part of the hereditary Osler-Rendu-Weber syndrome. Vascular tumors may also take the form of isolated hemangiomas, most commonly in the jejunum. Angiography, especially during bleeding, is the best procedure for evaluating these lesions.

MALIGNANT TUMORS   While rare, small-bowel malignancies occur in patients with long-standing regional enteritis and celiac sprue as well as in individuals with AIDS. Malignant tumors of the small bowel are frequently associated with fever, weight loss, anorexia, bleeding, and a palpable abdominal mass. After ampullary carcinomas (many of which arise from biliary or pancreatic ducts), the most frequently occurring small-bowel malignancies are adenocarcinomas, lymphomas, carcinoid tumors, and leiomyosarcomas.

Adenocarcinomas   The most common primary cancers of the small bowel are adenocarcinomas, accounting for ~50% of malignant tumors. These cancers occur most often in the distal duodenum and proximal jejunum, where they tend to ulcerate and cause hemorrhage or obstruction. Radiologically, they may be confused with chronic duodenal ulcer disease or with Crohn's disease if the patient has long-standing regional enteritis. The diagnosis is best made by endoscopy and biopsy under direct vision. Surgical resection is the treatment of choice.

Lymphomas   Lymphoma in the small bowel may be primary or secondary. A diagnosis of a primary intestinal lymphoma requires histologic confirmation in a clinical setting in which palpable adenopathy and hepatosplenomegaly are absent and no evidence of lymphoma is seen on chest radiograph, CT scan, or peripheral blood smear or on bone marrow aspiration and biopsy. Symptoms referable to the small bowel are present, usually accompanied by an anatomically discernible lesion. Secondary lymphoma of the small bowel consists of involvement of the intestine by a lymphoid malignancy extending from involved retroperitoneal or mesenteric lymph nodes (Chap. 97).

Primary intestinal lymphoma accounts for ~20% of malignancies of the small bowel. These neoplasms are non-Hodgkin's lymphomas; they usually have a diffuse, large-cell histology and are of T cell origin. Intestinal lymphoma involves the ileum, jejunum, and duodenum, in decreasing frequency, a pattern that mirrors the relative amount of normal lymphoid cells in these anatomic areas. The risk of small-bowel lymphoma is increased in patients with a prior history of malabsorptive conditions (e.g., celiac sprue), regional enteritis, and depressed immune function due to congenital immunodeficiency syndromes, prior organ transplantation, autoimmune disorders, or AIDS.

The development of localized or nodular masses that narrow the lumen results in periumbilical pain (made worse by eating) as well as weight loss, vomiting, and occasional intestinal obstruction. The diagnosis of small-bowel lymphoma may be suspected from the appearance on contrast radiographs of patterns such as infiltration and thickening of mucosal folds, mucosal nodules, areas of irregular ulceration, or stasis of contrast material. The diagnosis can be confirmed by surgical exploration and resection of involved segments. Intestinal lymphoma can occasionally be diagnosed by peroral intestinal mucosal biopsy, but since the disease mainly involves the lamina propria, full-thickness surgical biopsies are usually required.

Resection of the tumor constitutes the initial treatment modality. While postoperative radiation therapy has been given to some patients following a total resection, most authorities favor short-term (three cycles) systemic treatment with combination chemotherapy. The frequent presence of widespread intraabdominal disease at the time of diagnosis and the occasional multicentricity of the tumor often make a total resection impossible. The probability of sustained remission or cure is ~75% in patients with localized disease but is ~25% in individuals with unresectable lymphoma. In patients whose tumors are not resected, chemotherapy may lead to bowel perforation.

A unique form of small-bowel lymphoma, diffusely involving the entire intestine, was first described in oriental Jews and Arabs and is referred to as *immunoproliferative small intestinal disease* (IPSID), *Mediterranean lymphoma,* or *α-heavy chain disease*. This is a B cell tumor. The typical presentation includes chronic diarrhea and steatorrhea associated with vomiting and abdominal cramps; clubbing of the digits may be observed. A curious feature in many patients with IPSID is the presence in the blood and intestinal secretions of an abnormal IgA that contains a shortened α-heavy chain and is devoid of light chains. It is suspected that the abnormal α chains are produced by plasma cells infiltrating the small bowel. The clinical course of patients with IPSID is generally one of exacerbations and remissions, with death frequently resulting from either progressive malnutrition and wasting or the development of an aggressive lymphoma. The use of oral antibiotics such as tetracycline appears to be beneficial in the early phases of the disorder, suggesting a possible infectious etiology. Combination chemotherapy has been administered during later stages of the disease, with variable results. Results are better when antibiotics and chemotherapy are combined.

Carcinoid Tumors   Carcinoid tumors arise from argentaffin cells of the crypts of Lieberkühn and are found from the distal duodenum to the ascending colon, areas embryologically derived from the midgut. More than 50% of intestinal carcinoids are found in the distal ileum, with most congregating close to the ileocecal valve. Most intestinal carcinoids are asymptomatic and of low malignant potential, but invasion and metastases may occur, leading to the carcinoid syndrome (Chap. 329).

Leiomyosarcomas   Leiomyosarcomas often are >5 cm in diameter and may be palpable on abdominal examination. Bleeding, obstruction, and perforation are common. Such tumors should be analyzed for the expression of mutant c-*kit* receptor (defining GIST), and in the presence of metastatic disease, justifying treatment with imatinib mesylate (Gleevec).

CANCERS OF THE ANUS

Cancers of the anus account for 1 to 2% of the malignant tumors of the large bowel. Most such lesions arise in the anal canal, the anatomic area extending from the anorectal ring to a zone approximately halfway between the pectinate (or dentate) line and the anal verge. Carcinomas arising proximal to the pectinate line (i.e., in the transitional zone between the glandular mucosa of the rectum and the squamous epithelium of the distal anus) are known as basaloid, cuboidal, or cloacogenic tumors; about one-third of anal cancers have this histologic pattern. Malignancies arising distal to the pectinate line have a squamous cell histology, ulcerate more frequently, and constitute ~55% of anal cancers. The prognosis for patients with basaloid and squamous cell cancers of the anus is identical when corrected for tumor size and the presence or absence of nodal spread.

The development of anal cancer is associated with infection by human papillomavirus, the same organism etiologically linked to cervical cancer. The virus is sexually transmitted. The infection may lead to anal warts (condyloma accuminata), which may progress to anal intraepithelial neoplasia and on to squamous cell carcinoma. The risk for anal cancer is increased among homosexual males, presumably related to anal intercourse. Anal cancer risk is increased in both men and women with AIDS, possibly because their immunosuppressed state permits more severe papillomavirus infection. Anal cancers occur most commonly in middle-aged persons and are more frequent in women than men. At diagnosis, patients may experience bleeding, pain, sensation of a perianal mass, and pruritus.

Radical surgery (abdominal-perineal resection with lymph node sampling and a permanent colostomy) used to be the treatment of choice for this tumor type. The 5-year survival rate after such a procedure was 55 to 70% in the absence of spread to regional lymph nodes and <20% if nodal involvement was present. An alternative therapeutic approach combining external beam radiation therapy with concomitant chemotherapy has resulted in biopsy-proven disappearance of all tumor in >80% of patients whose initial lesion was <3 cm in size. Tumor has recurred in <10% of these patients, and ~70% of patients with anal cancers can be cured with nonoperative treatment. Surgery should be reserved for the minority of individuals who are found to have residual tumor after being managed initially with radiation therapy combined with chemotherapy.

FURTHER READING

BARON JA et al: A randomized trial of aspirin to prevent colorectal adenomas. N Engl J Med 348:391, 2003

CRUMP W et al: Lymphoma of the gastrointestinal tract. Semin Oncol 26:324, 1999

DEMETRI GD et al: Efficacy and safety of imatinib mesylate in advanced gastrointestinal stromal tumors. N Engl J Med 347:472, 2002

ENZINGER PC, MAYER RJ: Esophageal cancer. N Engl J Med 349:2241, 2003

FUCHS CS, MAYER RJ: Gastric carcinoma. N Engl J Med 333:32, 1995

LYNCH HT, DE LA CHAPELLE A: Hereditary colorectal cancer. N Engl J Med 348:919, 2003

MACDONALD JS, ASTROW AB: Adjuvant therapy of colon cancer. Semin Oncol 28:30, 2001

RYAN DP et al: Carcinoma of the anal canal. N Engl J Med 342:792, 2000

SPECHLER SJ: Barrett's esophagus. N Engl J Med 346:836, 2002

UEMURA N et al: *Helicobacter pylori* infection and the development of gastric cancer. N Engl J Med 345:784, 2001

WALSH JME, TERDIMAN JP: Colorectal cancer screening. JAMA 289:1288, 2003

78 TUMORS OF THE LIVER AND BILIARY TRACT
Jules L. Dienstag, Kurt J. Isselbacher

BENIGN LIVER TUMORS

HEPATOCELLULAR ADENOMAS Hepatocellular adenomas are benign tumors of the liver found predominantly in women in their third and fourth decades. Their preponderance in women suggests a hormonal influence in their pathogenesis, and oral contraceptives are thought to contribute. The risk of liver adenomas is increased among those who take anabolic steroids and exogenous androgens. Multiple hepatic adenomas have been associated with glycogen storage disease type I.

Hepatic adenomas occur predominantly in the right lobe of the liver, may be multiple, and are often quite large (>10 cm). Microscopically, they consist of normal or slightly atypical hepatocytes. These cells contain increased glycogen, making them appear paler and larger than normal. Clinical features include pain and the presence of a palpable mass or features of intratumor hemorrhage (pain and circulatory collapse). The diagnosis is usually made by a combination of techniques: sonography, computed tomography (CT), magnetic resonance imaging (MRI), selective hepatic arteriography, and radionuclide scans. The angiographic appearance is typically hypervascular but often also includes hypovascular regions. Technetium 99m scans usually show a defect, because phagocytosing Kupffer cells are absent. Like hepatocellular carcinomas, adenomas have a T_1-intense MRI appearance. The risk of malignant change is small; the risk is higher for large (>10 cm) and multiple adenomas.

Management involves imaging surveillance for small tumors. If the lesion is large (8 to 10 cm), near the surface, and resectable, surgical removal is appropriate. A patient with liver adenoma should stop taking oral contraceptives. Surgical resection may be required for tumors that do not shrink after oral contraceptives are stopped. Pregnancy increases the risk of hemorrhage and should be avoided in women with large adenomas. Patients with multiple large adenomas (e.g., those with glycogen-storage disease) may benefit from liver transplantation.

FOCAL NODULAR HYPERPLASIA Focal nodular hyperplasia is a benign tumor often identified incidentally on imaging studies or at laparoscopy done for other reasons. Like hepatic adenomas, it occurs predominantly in women; however, oral contraceptives are not implicated, and hemorrhage and necrosis are rare. The risk of hemorrhage, however, appears to be higher in women taking oral contraceptives. Typically, the lesion is a solid tumor, often in the right lobe, with a fibrous core and stellate projections. The fibrous projections contain atypical hepatocytes, biliary epithelium, Kupffer cells, and inflammatory cells. A technetium scan will usually show a hot spot because of the presence of Kupffer cells. The lesion appears vascular on angiography, and septations may be detectable by angiography, helical CT scan, and, most reliably, MRI, but only rarely by ultrasound. Surgery is indicated only for symptomatic lesions.

HEMANGIOMA AND OTHER BENIGN TUMORS *Hemangiomas* are the most common benign liver tumors, occurring predominantly in women and usually detected incidentally. The prevalence in the general population is in the range of 0.5 to 7.0%. These asymptomatic vascular lesions can be identified by MRI, contrast-enhanced CT, labeled red blood cell nuclide scans, or hepatic angiography. They do not need to be removed unless they are large and are producing a mass effect. Hemorrhage is rare, and malignant change does not occur.

Nodular regenerative hyperplasia consists of multiple hepatic nodules resulting from periportal hepatocyte regeneration with surrounding atrophy. It may be associated with an underlying condition such as malignancy or connective tissue disease. Portal hypertension (in the absence of cirrhosis) is the most common clinical manifestation. Other less common benign hepatic lesions include *bile duct adenomas* and *cystadenomas*.

CARCINOMAS OF THE LIVER

HEPATOCELLULAR CARCINOMA ■ **Epidemiology and Etiology** Primary hepatocellular carcinoma (HCC) is one of the most common tumors in the world and the third most frequent cause of cancer mortality. It is especially prevalent in regions of Asia and sub-Saharan Africa, where the annual incidence is up to 500 cases per 100,000 population. In the United States and western Europe, it is much less common; however, the annual incidence in the United States has increased from 1.4 per 100,000 during 1976 to 1980 to 2.4 per 100,000 in the 1990s. HCC is up to 4 times more common in men than in women and usually arises in a cirrhotic liver. The incidence peaks in the fifth to sixth decades of life in western countries but 1 to 2 decades earlier in regions of Asia and Africa with a high prevalence of liver carcinoma.

The principal reason for the high incidence of HCC in parts of Asia and Africa is the frequency of chronic infection with *hepatitis B virus* (HBV) and *hepatitis C virus* (HCV). These chronic infections frequently lead to cirrhosis, which itself is an important risk factor for HCC (the risk of liver cancer in a cirrhotic liver is ~3% per year); 60 to 90% of these tumors occur in patients with macronodular cirrhosis. Studies in regions of Asia where HCC and HBV infection are prevalent have shown that the incidence of this cancer is about 100-fold higher in individuals with evidence of HBV infection than in noninfected controls, particularly in those with markers of high-level HBV replication, e.g., hepatitis B e antigen (HBeAg) (Chap. 285). In China, the lifetime risk of HCC in patients with chronic hepatitis B approaches 40%. In patients with HBV infection and HCC, HBV DNA may be integrated into host genomic DNA, both in the tumor cells and in adjacent, uninvolved hepatocytes. In addition, modifications of cellular gene expression occur by insertional mutagenesis, chromosomal rearrangements, or the transcriptional transactivating activity of the X and the pre-S2 regions of the HBV genome.

HCV also leads to HCC. HCV genetic material does not become integrated into host genomic DNA. Therefore, the mechanism of HCV carcinogenesis is unclear. Whether the ability of the HCV NS3 domain or the core protein to transform cells in vitro contributes to HCC in humans remains conjectural; alternatively, repeated cycles of liver regeneration and repair common in cirrhosis may permit the emergence of a malignant clone. In Europe and Japan, HCV appears to be substantially more prevalent than HBV in cases of HCC. Both HBV and HCV can be demonstrated in some patients, but the clinical course of liver malignancy in these patients does not appear to differ from that when only one virus is implicated. One distinction in high-prevalence areas between HCC associated with HBV infection and that associated with HCV infection is in the timing of onset. In Asia, HBV is acquired at birth via perinatal transmission, whereas HCV infection is acquired primarily during adulthood from transfused blood and injections. Correspondingly, the onset of HCC occurs one to two decades earlier in those with lifelong hepatitis B than in persons with adult-acquired hepatitis C. Retrospective analysis indicates that HCC occurs on average approximately 30 years after HCV infection and almost exclusively in patients with cirrhosis. The annual incidence of HCC in cirrhotic patients with chronic hepatitis C is 1.5 to 4%. Over the last decade, the frequency of HCC in Japan has increased substantially, primarily in patients with cirrhosis associated with chronic hepatitis C. The same trend is beginning to emerge in the United States and Europe; based on the known frequency of HCV-associated cirrhosis in these populations, the incidence of new HCC cases is expected to increase more than 250-fold over the next decade.

Any agent or factor that contributes to chronic, low-grade liver cell damage and mitosis makes hepatocyte DNA more susceptible to genetic alterations. Thus, as indicated above, *chronic liver disease* of any type is a risk factor and predisposes to the development of HCC. These conditions include alcoholic liver disease, α_1-antitrypsin deficiency, hemochromatosis, tyrosinemia, primary biliary cirrhosis, and even cirrhosis associated with nonalcoholic steatohepatitis. In Africa and southern China, *aflatoxin B$_1$* is an important public health hazard. This mycotoxin appears to induce a very specific G-to-T mutation at codon 249 in the tumor suppressor gene p53.

The loss, inactivation, or mutation of the p53 gene has been im-

plicated in tumorigenesis and is the most common genetic derangement present in human cancers. Thus HBV and aflatoxin B$_1$ have been implicated in the pathogenesis of HCC in regions of Africa and southern China where both agents are prevalent.

In view of the male predominance of HCC, hormonal factors may also play a role. HCC may occur with long-term androgenic steroid administration, with exposure to thorium dioxide or vinyl chloride (see below), and possibly with exposure to estrogens in the form of oral contraceptives.

Clinical and Laboratory Features   HCC initially may escape clinical recognition because it occurs in patients with underlying cirrhosis, and the symptoms and signs may suggest progression of the underlying disease. The most common presenting features are abdominal *pain* with detection of an abdominal mass in the right upper quadrant. A *friction rub* or *bruit* may be heard over the liver. Blood-tinged ascites occurs in about 20% of cases. Jaundice is rare, unless significant deterioration of liver function or mechanical obstruction of the bile ducts occurs. Serum elevations of alkaline phosphatase and α fetoprotein (AFP) are common (see below). An abnormal type of prothrombin, des-γ-carboxy prothrombin, is made and correlates with AFP elevations.

A small percentage of patients with HCC have a *paraneoplastic syndrome*; erythrocytosis may result from erythropoietin-like activity produced by the tumor; hypercalcemia may result from secretion of a parathyroid-like hormone. Other manifestations may include hypercholesterolemia, hypoglycemia, polymyositis, acquired porphyria, dysfibrinogenemia, cryofibrinogenemia, and vasoactive peptide-associated diarrhea.

Imaging procedures to detect liver tumors include ultrasound, CT, MRI, and hepatic artery angiography (Chap. 271). Ultrasound is frequently used to screen high-risk populations and should be the first test if HCC is suspected; it is less costly than scans, is relatively sensitive, and can detect most tumors >3 cm. Helical CT and MRI (hyperintense T2-weighted imaging) scans are being used with increasing frequency and have higher sensitivities.

AFP levels >500 μg/L are found in about 70 to 80% of patients with HCC. Lower levels may be found in patients with large metastases from gastric or colonic tumors and in some patients with acute or chronic hepatitis. High levels of serum AFP (>500 to 1000 μg/L) in an adult with liver disease and without an obvious gastrointestinal tumor strongly suggest HCC. A rising level suggests progression of the tumor or recurrence after hepatic resection or therapeutic approaches such as ablation or chemoembolization (see below). The presence of an arterially enhancing liver mass >2 cm documented with two imaging procedures or with one imaging technique together with an AFP >400 ng/mL is highly suggestive of HCC.

Percutaneous *liver biopsy* can be diagnostic if the sample is taken from an area localized by ultrasound or CT. Because these tumors tend to be vascular, percutaneous biopsies should be done with caution. Another possible risk of liver biopsy is seeding the needle track with tumor; however, despite anecdotal reports, the likelihood of needle-track seeding is estimated to be as low as 0.006% and as high as 1%. Cytologic examination of ascitic fluid is invariably negative for tumor cells. Occasionally, *laparoscopy* or *minilaparotomy*, to permit liver biopsy under direct vision, may be used. This approach has the additional advantage of sometimes identifying patients who have a localized resectable tumor suitable for partial hepatectomy.

R̲x̲ TREATMENT

Staging of HCC is based on four criteria: tumor size (< or > 50% of the liver), ascites (absent or present), bilirubin (< or > 3 mg/dL), and albumin (< or >3 g/dL) to establish Okuda stages I (no positive criteria), II (1or 2 positives), and III (3 or 4 positives). The Okuda system predicts clinical course better than the American Joint Cancer Commission TNM system. The natural history of each stage without treatment is as follows: stage I, 8 months; stage II, 2 months; stage III, less than 1 month. Several newly proposed staging systems take additional variables into account; however, none of the new systems has been validated. As screening for HCC has detected earlier tumors, survival has increased. Surgery alone can produce survivals of 54% at 1 year, 40% at 2 years, and 28% at 3 years when cancers are detected before symptoms appear.

The course of *clinically apparent* disease is rapid; if untreated, most patients die within 3 to 6 months of diagnosis. When HCC is detected very early by serial screening of AFP and ultrasound, survival is 1 to 2 years after resection. In selected cases, therapy may prolong life. *Surgical resection* offers a chance for cure; however, few patients have a resectable tumor at the time of presentation, because of underlying cirrhosis, involvement of both hepatic lobes, or distant metastases (common sites are lung, brain, bone, and adrenal), and the 5-year survival is low. Even after successful "curative" resection of HCC, the predisposing primary liver disorder (e.g., cirrhosis, hepatitis B) persists and new cancers can arise in the residual liver.

Screening for HCC in High-risk Patients Because 20 to 30% of patients with early HCC do not have elevated levels of circulating AFP, ultrasonographic screening is recommended along with AFP determination. In a study in the Far East, persons positive for hepatitis B surface antigen, with or without liver disease, were screened serially; a number of patients with small, subclinical tumors were identified and surgical resection was performed. Follow-up observation revealed a 5-year survival rate of 70% in this group and a 10-year survival rate of 50%. These Asian patients, however, were unusual in that they had minimal or no liver disease, and their tumors tended to be unifocal or encapsulated. In another study, AFP screening every 6 months (without ultrasound) among remote Native Alaskan populations of noncirrhotic patients with chronic hepatitis B led to improved survival rates compared with historic outcomes. These findings are in contrast with those of a study in a large population of Italian patients with cirrhosis, associated in most cases with chronic HBV and/or HCV infections. Screening every 3 to 12 months permitted the detection of a 3% annual incidence of cancer in this cohort but in most cases failed to achieve the goal of early detection of surgically treatable disease. No randomized study has yet shown a survival benefit for screening patients at high risk of HCC, but most clinicians screen high-risk patients with twice-annual AFP and ultrasound.

Liver transplantation may be considered as a therapeutic option; tumor recurrence or metastases are the major problems. Patients who have a single lesion ≤5 cm or three or fewer lesions ≤3 cm have survival after liver transplantation that is the same as survival after transplantation for nonmalignant liver disease (Chap. 291). Other approaches are primarily palliative and include (1) hepatic artery embolization and chemotherapy (chemoembolization), (2) alcohol or radiofrequency ablation via ultrasound-guided percutaneous injection, and (3) ultrasound-guided cryoablation. Radiofrequency ablation and surgical resection have been equally effective for potentially resectable HCC in some studies; 5-year survival >50% has been seen. Thus, some consider radiofrequency ablation as potentially curative. Unresectable HCC is usually managed by chemoembolization ("transcatheter arterial embolization"), but results have been mixed. Some randomized trials have shown no survival advantage. Two studies (from Hong Kong and Spain) showed >20% improvement in survival with chemoembolization compared to supportive care. The Hong Kong study mainly involved patients with hepatitis B given cisplatin chemotherapy. Survival at 1 (57%), 2 (31%), and 3 years (26%) was better than that seen in the supportive care group (32, 11, and 3%, respectively). The Spanish study mainly involved patients with hepatitis C given doxorubicin chemotherapy. Survival at 1 (82%) and 2 years (63%) in the chemoembolization group was superior to survival for supportive care (63 and 27%, respectively). Outcome is related to the experience of the treating institution; highly specialized centers obtain better results than those doing fewer procedures and those using less stringent criteria for intervention. The procedure may be complicated by a postembolization syndrome (fever, chills, abdominal pain, nausea, vomiting, leukocytosis) and transient (but occasionally irreversible) hepatic decompensation.

Treatment options for unresectable disease are limited. The liver cannot tolerate high doses of radiation and the disease is not responsive to chemotherapy. Investigative immunotherapy and gene therapy techniques have not yet been successful. Based on the presence of hormone receptors on the tumor, tamoxifen has been tested, but without success, and octreotide has shown some modest activity. In patients with resectable tumors, polyprenoic acid (a retinoic acid formulation) and intra-arterial ^{131}I-labeled lipiodol have been reported to reduce the rate of recurrence.

Prevention is the preferred strategy. Hepatitis B vaccine can prevent infection and its sequelae, and a reduction in HCC has been seen in Taiwan with the introduction of universal vaccination of children. Interferon treatment reduces the incidence of hepatic failure, death, and HCC in HBV-infected patients. Whether antiviral therapy with lamivudine, adefovir, or other agents (Chap. 287) will reduce the risk of HCC in HBV-infected cirrhotic patients is unknown. Interferon may lower the risk of HCC in patients with hepatitis C–related cirrhosis, but the evidence is mainly from retrospective studies that are confounded by lead-time bias. Prospective trials have produced conflicting results. Interferon may also reduce the risk of HCV-associated HCC recurrence after resection or percutaneous ablation.

OTHER MALIGNANT LIVER TUMORS

Fibrolamellar carcinoma differs from typical HCC in that it tends to occur in young adults without underlying cirrhosis. This tumor is non-encapsulated but well circumscribed and contains fibrous lamellae; it grows slowly and is associated with a longer survival if treated. Surgical resection has resulted in 5-year survivals >50%; if the lesion is nonresectable, liver transplantation is an option, and the outcome far exceeds that observed in the nonfibrolamellar variety of HCC. *Hepatoblastoma* is a tumor of infancy that typically is associated with very high serum AFP levels. The lesions are usually solitary, may be resectable, and have a better 5-year survival than that of HCC. *Angiosarcoma* consists of vascular spaces lined by malignant endothelial cells. Etiologic factors include prior exposure to thorium dioxide, polyvinyl chloride, arsenic, and androgenic anabolic steroids. *Epithelioid hemangioendothelioma* is of borderline malignancy; most cases are benign, but bone and lung metastases occur. This tumor occurs in early adulthood, presents with right upper quadrant pain, and is heterogeneous on sonography, hypodense on CT, and without neovascularity on angiography. Immunohistochemical staining reveals expression of factor VIII antigen. In the absence of extrahepatic metastases, these lesions can be treated by surgical resection or liver transplantation.

METASTATIC TUMORS Metastatic tumors of the liver are common, ranking second only to cirrhosis as a cause of fatal liver disease. In the United States, the incidence of metastatic carcinoma is at least 20 times greater than that of primary carcinoma. At autopsy, hepatic metastases occur in 30 to 50% of patients dying from malignant disease.

Pathogenesis The liver is uniquely vulnerable to invasion by tumor cells. Its size, high rate of blood flow, double perfusion by the hepatic artery and portal vein, and Kupffer cell filtration function combine to make it the next most common site of metastases after the lymph nodes. In addition, local tissue factors or endothelial membrane characteristics appear to enhance metastatic implants. Virtually all types of neoplasms except those primary in the brain may metastasize to the liver. The most common primary tumors are those of the gastrointestinal tract, lung, and breast, as well as melanomas. Less common are metastases from tumors of the thyroid, prostate, and skin.

Clinical Features Most patients with metastases to the liver present with symptoms referable only to the primary tumor, and the asymptomatic hepatic involvement is discovered in the course of clinical evaluation. Sometimes hepatic involvement is reflected by nonspecific symptoms of weakness, weight loss, fever, sweating, and loss of appetite. Rarely, features indicating active hepatic disease, especially abdominal pain, hepatomegaly, or ascites, are present. Patients with widespread metastatic liver involvement usually have clinical signs suggestive of cancer and hepatic enlargement. Some have localized induration or tenderness, and, occasionally, a friction rub may be found over tender areas of the liver.

Results of liver biochemical tests are often abnormal, but the elevations in marker levels are often only mild and nonspecific. These signs reflect the effects of fever and wasting as well as those of the infiltrating neoplastic process itself. An increase in serum alkaline phosphatase is the most common and frequently the only abnormality. Hypoalbuminemia, anemia, and occasionally a mild elevation of aminotransferase levels may also be found with more widespread disease. Substantially elevated serum levels of carcinoembryonic antigen are usually found when the metastases are from primary malignancies in the gastrointestinal tract, breast, or lung.

Diagnosis Evidence of metastatic invasion of the liver should be sought actively in any patient with a primary malignancy, especially of the lung, gastrointestinal tract, or breast, before resection of the primary lesion. An elevated level of alkaline phosphatase or a mass apparent on ultrasound, CT, or MRI examination of the liver may provide a presumptive diagnosis. Blind percutaneous needle biopsy of the liver will result in a positive diagnosis of metastatic disease in only 60 to 80% of cases with hepatomegaly and elevated alkaline phosphatase levels. Serial sectioning of specimens, two or three repeated biopsies, or cytologic examination of biopsy smears may increase the diagnostic yield by 10 to 15%. The yield is increased when biopsies are directed by ultrasound or CT or obtained during laparoscopy.

℞ TREATMENT

Most metastatic carcinomas respond poorly to all forms of treatment, which is usually only palliative. Rarely a single, large metastasis can be removed surgically. Systemic chemotherapy may slow tumor growth and reduce symptoms, but it does not alter the prognosis. Chemoembolization, intrahepatic chemotherapy, and alcohol or radiofrequency ablation may provide palliation.

CHOLANGIOCARCINOMA Benign tumors of the extrahepatic bile ducts are extremely rare causes of mechanical biliary obstruction. Most of these are papillomas, adenomas, or cystadenomas and present with obstructive jaundice or hemobilia. Adenocarcinoma of the extrahepatic ducts is more common. There is a slight male preponderance (60%), and the incidence peaks in the fifth to seventh decades. Apparent predisposing factors include (1) some chronic hepatobiliary parasitic infestations, (2) congenital anomalies with ectactic ducts, (3) sclerosing cholangitis and chronic ulcerative colitis, and (4) occupational exposure to possible biliary tract carcinogens (employment in rubber or automotive plants). Cholelithiasis is not clearly a predisposing factor for cholangiocarcinoma. The lesions of cholangiocarcinoma may be diffuse or nodular. Nodular lesions often arise at the bifurcation of the common bile duct (Klatskin tumors) and are usually associated with a *collapsed gallbladder*, a finding that mandates cholangiography to view proximal hepatic ducts.

Patients with cholangiocarcinoma usually present with biliary obstruction, painless jaundice, pruritus, weight loss, and acholic stools. A deep-seated, vaguely localized right upper quadrant pain may be noted. Hepatomegaly and a palpable, distended gallbladder (unless the lesion is high in the duct) are frequent accompanying signs. Fever is unusual unless associated with ascending cholangitis. Because the obstructing process is gradual, the cholangiocarcinoma is often far advanced by the time it presents clinically. The diagnosis is most frequently made by cholangiography following ultrasound demonstration of dilated intrahepatic bile ducts. Any focal strictures of the bile ducts should be considered malignant until proven otherwise. Endoscopic cholangiography permits obtaining specimens for cytology (sensitivity ~60%) and insertion of stents for biliary drainage. Survival of 1 to 2 years is possible in some cases. Perhaps 20% of patients

have surgically resectable tumors, but 5-year survival is only 10 to 30%. The high recurrence rate limits the value of liver transplantation. Photodynamic therapy (intravenous hematoporphyrin with cholangioscopically delivered light) has been used with promising early results.

CARCINOMA OF THE PAPILLA OF VATER The ampulla of Vater may be involved by extension of tumor arising elsewhere in the duodenum or may itself be the site of origin of a sarcoma, carcinoid tumor, or adenocarcinoma. Papillary adenocarcinomas are associated with slow growth and a more favorable clinical prognosis than diffuse, infiltrative cancers of the ampulla, which are more frequently widely invasive. The presenting clinical manifestation is usually obstructive jaundice. Endoscopic retrograde cannulation of the pancreatic duct is the preferred diagnostic technique when ampullary carcinoma is suspected, because it allows for direct endoscopic inspection and biopsy of the ampulla and for pancreatography to exclude a pancreatic malignancy. Cancer of the papilla is usually treated by wide surgical excision. Lymph node or other metastases are present at the time of surgery in approximately 20% of cases, and the 5-year survival rate following surgical therapy in this group is only 5 to 10%. In the absence of metastases, radical pancreaticoduodenectomy (the Whipple procedure) is associated with 5-year survival rates as high as 40%.

CANCER OF THE GALLBLADDER Most cancers of the gallbladder develop in conjunction with stones rather than polyps. In patients with gallstones, the risk for developing gallbladder cancer, while increased, is still quite low. In one study, gallbladder cancer developed in only 5 of 2583 patients with gallstones followed for a median of 13 years. In the United States, adenocarcinomas make up the vast majority of the estimated 6500 new cases of gallbladder cancer diagnosed each year. The female/male ratio is 4:1, and the mean age at diagnosis is approximately 70 years. The clinical presentation is most often one of unremitting right upper quadrant pain associated with weight loss, jaundice, and a palpable right upper quadrant mass. Cholangitis may supervene. The preoperative diagnosis of the condition has been facilitated by ultrasound and CT, which are also useful in guiding fine-needle aspiration and biopsy. The presence on imaging of a calcified ("porcelain") gallbladder can suggest gallbladder carcinoma; however, cancer is associated with <25% of patients with porcelain gallbladder.

Once symptoms have appeared, spread of the tumor outside the gallbladder by direct extension or by lymphatic or hematogenous routes is almost invariable. Over 75% of gallbladder carcinomas are unresectable at the time of surgery, the exceptions being tumors discovered incidentally at laparotomy. If the tumor is found by the pathologist, no additional therapy is required. If the tumor is noted by the surgeon on routine cholecystectomy, a second operation is generally performed to resect the adjacent liver, bile duct, and local lymph nodes. Incidental resectable gallbladder tumors have a 50% 5-year survival. The 1-year mortality rate for unresectable disease is about 95%, and <5% of patients survive 5 years. Radical operative resection does not appear to improve survival. Trials of radiation and chemotherapy in patients with gallbladder cancer have been disappointing.

FURTHER READING

BEFELER AS, DI BISCEGLIE AM: Hepatocellular carcinoma: Diagnosis and treatment. Gastroenterology 122:1609, 2002

BRUIX J, LLOVET JM: Clinical management of hepatocellular carcinoma. Conclusions of the Barcelona-2000 EASL conference. J Hepatology 35:421, 2001

CHANG MH: Decreasing incidence of hepatocellular carcinoma among children following universal hepatitis B immunization. Liver Int 23:309, 2003

HASSOUN Z, GORES GJ: Treatment of hepatocellular carcinoma. Clin Gastroenterol Hepatol 1:10, 2003

LLOVET JM et al: Hepatocellular carcinoma. Lancet 362:1907, 2003

———— et al: Arterial embolisation of chemoembolisation versus symptomatic treatment in patients with unresectable hepatocellular carcinoma. A randomised controlled trial. Lancet 359:1734, 2002

YANG H-I et al: Hepatitis B e antigen and the risk of hepatocellular carcinoma. N Engl J Med 347:168, 2002

79 PANCREATIC CANCER
Robert J. Mayer

INCIDENCE AND ETIOLOGY The incidence of pancreatic carcinoma in the United States has increased as the median life expectancy of the American population has lengthened. The tumor results in the death of >98% of afflicted patients. In 2004, 31,270 individuals died of pancreatic cancer making it the fourth most common cause of cancer-related mortality. The disease is more common in males than in females and in blacks than in whites. It rarely develops before the age of 50.

Little is known about the causes of pancreatic cancer. Cigarette smoking is the most consistent risk factor, with the disease being two to three times more common in heavy smokers than in nonsmokers. Whether this association is due to a direct carcinogenic effect of tobacco metabolites on the pancreas or an as yet undefined exposure that occurs more frequently in cigarette smokers is uncertain. Patients with chronic pancreatitis are at increased risk of pancreatic cancer, as are persons with long-standing diabetes mellitus. Obesity is a risk factor for pancreatic cancer; risk is directly related to increased calorie intake. Alcohol abuse or cholelithiasis are not risk factors for pancreatic cancer. Nor is pancreatic cancer associated with coffee consumption. Mutations in K-*ras* genes have been found in >85% of specimens of human pancreatic cancer. Pancreatic cancer has been associated with mutation of the *p16*^{INK4} gene located on chromosome 9p21, a gene also implicated in the pathogenesis of malignant melanoma, as well as mutations of the *p53*, *DPC4*, and *BRCA2* tumor suppressor genes. A series of molecular events involving a sequence of these mutations has been proposed to occur as the normal pancreatic duct progresses through dysplasia to infiltrating carcinoma.

CLINICAL FEATURES More than 90% of pancreatic cancers are ductal adenocarcinomas, with islet cell tumors constituting the remaining 5 to 10%. Pancreatic cancers occur twice as frequently in the pancreatic head (70% of cases) as in the body (20%) or tail (10%) of the gland.

With the exception of jaundice, the initial symptoms associated with pancreatic cancer are often insidious and are usually present for >2 months before the cancer is diagnosed (Table 79-1). Pain and weight loss are present in >75% of patients. The pain typically has a gnawing, visceral quality, occasionally radiating from the epigastrium to the back. Pain is often a more severe problem in lesions arising in the body or tail of the gland, as such tumors may become quite large before being detected. Characteristically, the pain improves somewhat when the patient bends forward. The development of significant pain suggests retroperitoneal invasion and infiltration of the splanchnic nerves, indicating that the primary lesion is advanced and is not surgically resectable. Rarely, such pain may be transient and associated with hyperamylasemia, indicative of acute pancreatitis caused by ductal obstruction by tumor. The weight loss observed in most patients is primarily the result of anorexia, although in the initial period of the disease, subclinical malabsorption may also be a contributing factor.

Jaundice due to biliary obstruction is found in >80% of patients having tumors in the pancreatic head and is typically accompanied by dark urine, a claylike appearance of stool, and pruritus. In contrast to the "painless jaundice" sometimes observed in patients having carcinomas of the bile ducts, duodenum, or periampullary regions, most icteric individuals with ductal carcinomas of the pancreatic head will complain of significant abdominal discomfort. Although the gallblad-

der is usually enlarged in patients with carcinoma of the head of the pancreas, it is palpable in <50% (Courvoisier's sign). However, the presence of an enlarged gallbladder in a jaundiced patient without biliary colic should suggest malignant obstruction of the extrahepatic biliary tree.

Glucose intolerance, presumably a direct consequence of the tumor, often develops within 2 years of the clinical diagnosis. Other initial manifestations include venous thrombosis and migratory thrombophlebitis (Trousseau's syndrome), gastrointestinal hemorrhage from varices due to compression of the portal venous system by tumor, and splenomegaly caused by cancerous encasement of the splenic vein.

DIAGNOSTIC PROCEDURES (Fig. 79-1) Despite the availability of serologic tests for tumor-associated antigens such as the carcinoembryonic antigen (CEA) and CA 19-9 and noninvasive imaging techniques such as computed tomography (CT) and ultrasonography, the early diagnosis of a potentially resectable pancreatic carcinoma remains extremely difficult. The nonspecificity of the initial symptoms and the poor sensitivity of both serologic assays and noninvasive techniques have frustrated the development of effective screening procedures. When the disease is clinically suspected in a patient having vague, persistent abdominal complaints, ultrasound should be performed to visualize the gallbladder and the pancreas, as should upper gastrointestinal contrast radiographs to rule out a hiatal hernia or a peptic ulcer. If these studies fail to provide an explanation for the symptoms, a CT scan should be considered. It should encompass not only the pancreas but also the liver, retroperitoneal lymph nodes, and pelvis, as pancreatic cancer frequently spreads within the abdomen. While more costly than ultrasonography, CT is technically simpler and more reproducible, provides better definition of the body and tail of the pancreas, and requires less interpretive skill. CT generally detects a malignant pancreatic lesion in >80% of cases; in 5 to 15% of patients with proven pancreatic carcinoma, the CT scan shows only generalized pancreatic enlargement suggesting pancreatitis rather than malignancy. False-positive results occur in about 5 to 10% of cases in which no tumor was found on laparotomy. Magnetic resonance imaging (MRI), while not superior to CT in the evaluation of pancreatic lesions, may occasionally distinguish benign from malignant neoplasms. The value of positron emission tomography (PET) has not been determined. When clinical circumstances dictate additional diagnostic evaluation, endoscopic retrograde cholangiopancreatography (ERCP) with endoscopic ultrasonography (EUS) may clarify the cause of ambiguous CT or ultrasound findings. The characteristic findings are stenosis or obstruction of either the pancreatic or the common bile duct; both duct systems are abnormal in over half of cases. Carcinoma and chronic pancreatitis can be difficult to distinguish by ERCP, particularly if both diseases are present. False-negative results with ERCP are infrequent (<5%) and usually occur in the setting of islet cell, rather than ductal, carcinomas.

Angiography, once a commonly utilized means of detecting carcinomas in the body and tail of the pancreas, has been largely replaced as a diagnostic and staging procedure by spiral CT scanning with contrast imaging. This high-resolution technology predicts the resectability of the tumor if no disease is found outside the pancreas, obstruction of the superior mesenteric-portal vein confluence is absent, or tumor extension to the celiac axis and superior mesenteric arteries is not found. Radiographic staging criteria are shown in Table 79-2.

Regardless of the results of the above diagnostic studies, a histologic confirmation of pancreatic cancer is mandatory; similar radiographic and endoscopic findings can result from other neoplasms such as islet cell tumor or lymphoma, for which the therapeutic approach and prognosis differ from those for ductal carcinoma. In patients with unresectable disease or medical contraindications to surgical resection, tissue may be obtained through a percutaneous needle aspiration biopsy of the pancreas with CT or ultrasonographic guidance.

Unfortunately, however, even laparotomy may not provide a definitive diagnosis, because chronic pancreatitis may also produce a hard mass in the head of the pancreas indistinguishable from carcinoma by

TABLE 79-1 *Presenting Signs and Symptoms of Pancreatic Carcinoma*	
Frequent	**Infrequent**
Abdominal pain	Glucose intolerance
Weight loss	Palpable gallbladder
Jaundice (lesions of pancreatic head only)	Migratory thrombophlebitis
	Gastrointestinal hemorrhage
	Splenomegaly

FIGURE 79-1 Carcinoma of the pancreas. *A.* Sonogram showing pancreatic carcinoma (P), dilated intrahepatic bile ducts (d), dilated portal vein (pv), and inferior vena cava (IVC). *B.* Computed tomography scan showing pancreatic carcinoma (*dark arrows*). *C.* Endoscopic retrograde showing abrupt cutoff of the duct of Wirsung (*arrow*). *D.* Arteriogram showing sheathing of splenic artery by tumor encasement (*arrow*).

palpation. Furthermore, a superficial biopsy of such a mass may not show neoplastic tissue, revealing only evidence of pancreatitis, as the cancer is often surrounded by edematous, inflamed, and fibrotic tissue (i.e., chronic pancreatitis).

℞ TREATMENT

Complete surgical resection of pancreatic tumors offers the only effective treatment for this disease. Unfortunately, such "curative" operations are only possible in 10 to 15% of patients with pancreatic cancer, usually those individuals with a tumor in the pancreatic head in whom jaundice was the initial symptom. Patients considered for such a procedure should have no evidence of metastatic spread on a chest radiograph and abdominal-pelvic CT scan and should be oper-

TABLE 79-2 *Clinical (Radiographic) Staging of Pancreatic Cancer*

Stage	Clinical/Radiographic Criteria
I	Resectable (T1–T2, selected T3,[a] NX, M0) 　No encasement of celiac axis or SMA 　Patent SMPV confluence 　No extrapancreatic disease
II	Locally advanced (T3, NX–1, M0) 　Arterial encasement (celiac axis or SMA) or venous occlusion (SMV or portal vein) 　No extrapancreatic disease
III	Metastatic (T1–3, NX–1, M1) 　Metastases typically to liver, peritoneum, and occasionally lung

[a] Resectable T3 lesions include those with isolated involvement of the SMV, portal vein, or hepatic artery without encasement of the celiac axis or SMA.

Note: T1, restricted to pancreas; T2, extension to duodenum, bile duct, or peripancreatic tissues; T3, extension to stomach, spleen, colon, or adjacent large vessels; NX, nodal status unknown; N0, regional nodes uninvolved; N1, regional nodes involved; M0, metastases absent; M1, metastases present; SMA, superior mesenteric artery; SMPV, superior mesenteric vein confluence with portal vein; SMV, superior mesenteric vein

ated on by an experienced surgeon, as mortality rates of >15% have been associated with this procedure. Curative resection is usually preceded by laparoscopic inspection of the abdomen to confirm absence of occult disease spread to the omentum, peritoneum, or liver, which would preclude curative resection. Although the potential for cure in patients with pancreatic cancer is restricted to the few who are able to undergo a complete surgical resection, the 5-year survival rate following such operations is only 10%. Nonetheless, the procedure is worth attempting, particularly for lesions in the pancreatic head, since ductal carcinomas often cannot be distinguished preoperatively from ampullary, duodenal, and distal bile duct tumors or pancreatic cyst adenocarcinomas, all of which have far higher rates of resectability and cure. Furthermore, patients who undergo resection and eventually experience disease recurrence survive three to four times longer than those whose tumor is not excised, indicating that such operations have a palliative effect. The risk for tumor recurrence is not affected by the type of operative procedure—i.e., total pancreatectomy versus pancreaticoduodenectomy ("Whipple resection")—but it is increased by the presence of lymph node metastases or tumor invasion into adjacent viscera. As a rule, pancreaticoduodenectomy or distal pancreatectomy seems preferable to total pancreatectomy because of the retention of exocrine function and avoidance of brittle diabetes.

The median survival for patients whose pancreatic cancers are surgically unresectable is 6 months. Management is directed at palliation of symptoms. Ambulatory patients having tumors in the pancreatic head should be considered for surgical diversion of the biliary system. If jaundice has already developed, therapeutic options include either nonoperative biliary decompression by endoscopic or percutaneous, transhepatic biliary drainage or surgical biliary bypass. External beam radiation in patients with unresectable tumors that have not spread beyond the pancreas does not appear to prolong survival, although a sufficient reduction in tumor size may lead to palliation of pain. However, the addition of chemotherapy with fluorouracil (5-FU) or gemcitabine to external beam irradiation has increased the survival time for these patients, presumably because the drugs act as radiosensitizing agents. In a small patient population, a combination of radiation therapy and 5-FU prolonged the survival and increased the cure rate compared to an untreated control group who had a complete surgical resection of their pancreatic cancer. Attempts at confirming this observation have resulted in controversial outcomes. The possibility of administering such chemoradiation therapy at diagnosis and before surgery (neoadjuvant treatment) to increase the potential for resectability is under investigation. Intraoperative radiation therapy has the potential to deliver higher doses of radiation to the tumor while sparing neighboring tissues but does not give better results than external beam treatment.

Chemotherapy in the management of patients with widely metastatic pancreatic cancer has been disappointing. Gemcitabine, a deoxycytidine analogue, produces improvement in the quality of life for patients with advanced pancreatic cancer. However, duration of survival is only modestly improved. Newer forms of treatment, including combining gemcitabine with other cytotoxic agents or therapies directed at specific molecular targets, such as the epidermal growth factor receptor or the vascular endothelial growth factor receptor are being evaluated. Experimental therapy should constitute the initial treatment for consenting, ambulatory patients. →*Pancreatic endocrine tumors are discussed in Chap. 329.*

FURTHER READING

ADAMEK HE et al: Pancreatic cancer detection with magnetic resonance cholangiopancreatography and endoscopic retrograde cholangiopancreatography: A prognostic controlled study. Lancet 356:190, 2000

BURRIS HA et al: Improvements in survival and clinical benefit with gemcitabine as first-line therapy for patients with advanced pancreatic cancer. A randomized trial. J Clin Oncol 15:2403, 1997

CONLON KC et al: Long-term survival after curative resection for pancreatic ductal adenocarcinoma. Clinicopathologic analysis of 5-year survivors. Ann Surg 223:273, 1996

HALLER DG: New perspectives in the management of pancreas cancer. Semin Oncol 30(suppl 11):3, 2003

HANSEL DE et al: Molecular pathogenesis of pancreatic cancer. Annu Rev Genomics Hum Genet 4:237, 2003

NEOPTOLEMOS JP et al: Adjuvant chemoradiotherapy and chemotherapy in resectable pancreatic cancer: A randomised controlled trial. Lancet 358: 1576, 2001

80 BLADDER AND RENAL CELL CARCINOMAS
Howard I. Scher, Robert J. Motzer

BLADDER CANCER

A transitional cell epithelium lines the urinary tract from the renal pelvis to the ureter, urinary bladder, and the proximal two-thirds of the urethra. Cancers can occur at any point: 90% of malignancies develop in the bladder, 8% develop in the renal pelvis, and the remaining 2% develop in the ureter or urethra. Bladder cancer is the fourth most common cancer in men and the tenth in women, with an estimated 60,240 new cases and 12,710 deaths predicted for the year 2004. The almost 5:1 ratio of incidence to mortality reflects the higher frequency of the less lethal superficial variants compared to the more lethal invasive and metastatic variants. The incidence is four times higher in men than in women, and twofold higher in whites than blacks, with a median age at diagnosis of 65 years. Once diagnosed, urothelial tumors exhibit polychronotropism—the tendency to recur over time and in new locations in the urothelial tract. As long as urothelium is present, continuous monitoring of the tract is required.

EPIDEMIOLOGY Cigarette smoking is believed to contribute to up to 50% of the diagnosed urothelial cancers in men and up to 40% in women. The risk of developing a urothelial malignancy in male smokers is increased two- to fourfold relative to nonsmokers and continues for 10 years or longer after cessation. Other implicated agents include the aniline dyes, the drugs phenacetin and chlornaphazine, and external beam radiation. Chronic cyclophosphamide exposure may also increase risk, whereas vitamin A supplements appear to be protective. Exposure to *Schistosoma haematobium*, a parasite found in many developing countries, is associated with an increase in both squamous and transitional cell carcinomas of the bladder.

PATHOLOGY More than 95% of urothelial tumors in the United States are transitional cell in origin. Pure squamous cancers with keratinization constitute 3%, adenocarcinomas 2%, and small cell tumors (with paraneoplastic syndromes) <1%. Adenocarcinomas develop primarily in the urachal remnant in the dome of the bladder or in the periurethral tissues; some assume a signet cell histology. Lymphomas or melanomas are rare. Clinical subtypes are grouped into three categories: 75% are superficial, 20% invade muscle, and 5% present with de novo metastatic disease. Of the transitional cell tumors, low-grade papillary lesions that grow on a central stalk are most common. These tumors are very friable, have a tendency to bleed, are at high risk for recurrence, and yet rarely progress to the more lethal invasive variety. About half of all invasive tumors progressed from a superficial stage. In contrast, carcinoma in situ (CIS) is a high-grade tumor that is considered a precursor of the more lethal muscle-infiltrating cancers. Tumors are rated by histologic type and grade. Grade I lesions (highly differentiated tumors) rarely progress to a higher stage, whereas grade III tumors do.

PATHOGENESIS The multicentric nature of the disease and high rate of recurrence has led to the hypothesis of a field defect in the urothelium. Molecular genetic analyses suggest that the superficial and invasive lesions develop along distinct pathways in which primary tumorigenic aberrations precede secondary changes associated with progression to a more advanced stage. Deletions of 9q are an early event; 3p and 5q deletions occur more frequently in invasive lesions. Deletions at the *TP53* locus on 17p, the *DCC* locus in 18q, and the *RB* locus on 13q24 have been seen only in invasive disease. Deletions of 3p and 11p occur in both superficial and invasive tumors. Within all clinical stages, including Tis, T1, and T2 or greater lesions, tumors with altered *TP53* have a higher risk of metastasis and death from disease.

CLINICAL PRESENTATION, DIAGNOSIS, AND STAGING Hematuria occurs in 80 to 90% of patients and often reflects exophytic tumors. Irritative symptoms are the next most common presentation and may reflect in situ disease. The bladder is the most common source of gross hematuria (40%), but benign cystitis (22%) is a more common cause than bladder cancer (15%) (Chap. 40). Microscopic hematuria is more commonly of prostate origin (25%); only 2% of bladder cancers produce microscopic hematuria. Once hematuria is documented, a urinary cytology, visualization of the urothelial tract by computed tomography (CT) or intravenous pyelogram (IVP), and cystoscopy are recommended, if no other etiology is found. Screening asymptomatic individuals for hematuria increases the diagnosis of tumors at an early stage but has not been shown to prolong life. Obstruction of the ureters may cause flank pain. Symptoms of metastatic disease are rarely the first presenting sign.

The endoscopic evaluation includes an examination under anesthesia to determine whether a palpable mass is present. A flexible endoscope is inserted into the bladder, and a bladder barbotage is performed. The visual inspection includes mapping the location, size, and number of lesions, as well as a description of the growth pattern (solid vs papillary). An intraoperative video is often recorded. All visible tumors should be resected, and a sample of the muscle underlying the tumor should be obtained to assess the depth of invasion. Normal mucosal areas are biopsied at random to ensure no field defect. A notation is made as to whether a tumor was completely or incompletely resected. Selective catheterization and visualization of the upper tracts should be performed if the cytology is positive and no disease is visible in the bladder. Ultrasonography, CT, and/or magnetic resonance imaging (MRI) may help to determine whether a tumor extends to perivesical fat (T3), and to document nodal spread. Distant metastases are assessed by CT of the chest and abdomen, MRI, or radionuclide imaging of the skeleton. Ta lesions grow as exophytic lesions; CIS lesions start on the surface and tend to invade. The revised tumor, node, metastasis (TNM) staging system is illustrated in Fig. 80-1.

℞ TREATMENT

Management depends on whether the tumor invades muscle and whether there is spread to the regional lymph nodes and beyond. The probability of spread increases with increasing T stage. At a minimum, the management of a superficial tumor is a complete endoscopic re-

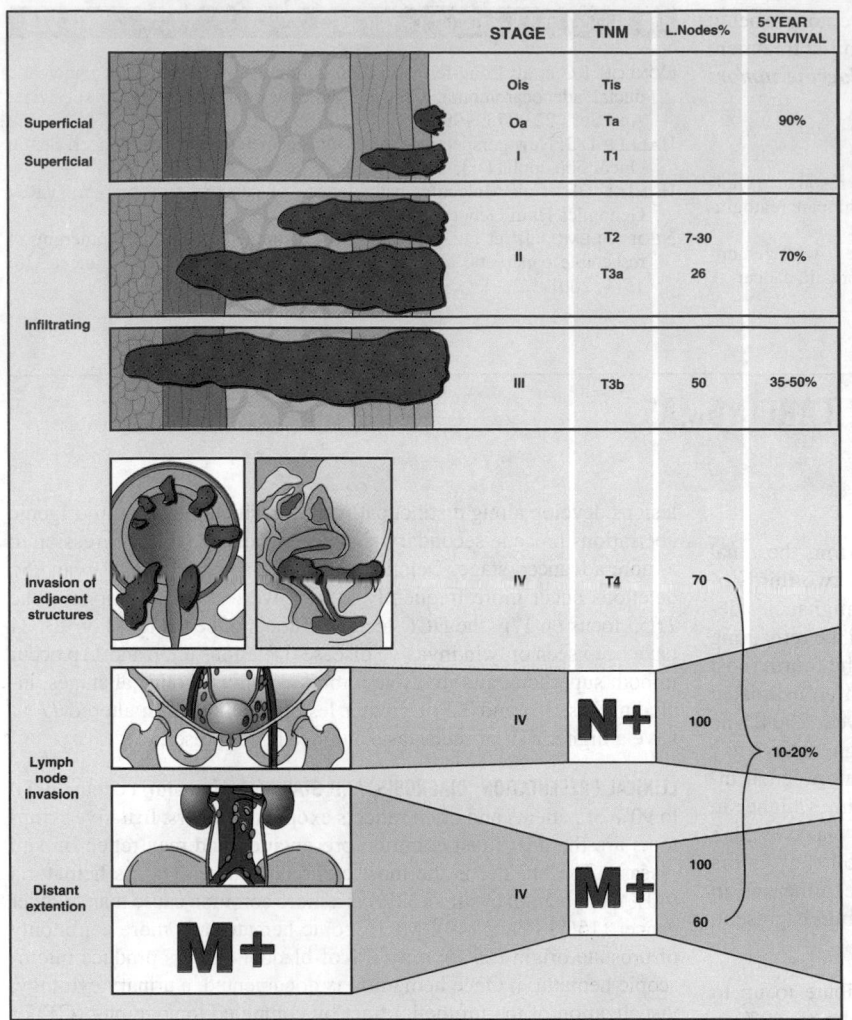

	STAGE	TNM	L.Nodes%	5-YEAR SURVIVAL
Superficial	Ois	Tis		90%
	Oa	Ta		
Superficial	I	T1		
Infiltrating	II	T2	7-30	70%
		T3a	26	
	III	T3b	50	35-50%
Invasion of adjacent structures	IV	T4	70	
Lymph node invasion	IV	N+	100	10-20%
Distant extention	IV	M+	100	
			60	

FIGURE 80-1 Bladder staging. TNM, tumor, node, metastasis.

section with or without intravesical therapy. The decision to recommend intravesical therapy depends on the histologic subtype, number of lesions, depth of invasion, and presence or absence of CIS. Recurrences develop in upwards of 50% of cases, and 5 to 20% progress to a more advanced stage. Solitary papillary lesions are generally managed by transurethral surgery alone. CIS and recurrent disease are treated by transurethral surgery followed by intravesical therapy. Radical cystectomy is the standard treatment for a tumor that has invaded muscle, either at the time of diagnosis or following treatment for superficial disease. The decision to administer systemic therapy is then based on the pathologic findings.

Superficial Disease Intravesical therapies are used in two general contexts: as an adjuvant to a complete endoscopic resection to prevent recurrence or, less commonly, to eliminate disease that cannot be controlled by endoscopic resection alone. Intravesical treatments are advised for patients with recurrent disease, >40% involvement of the bladder surface by tumor, the presence of diffuse CIS, or T1 disease. Bacillus Calmette-Guerin (BCG) in six weekly instillations, followed by maintenance, is considered standard based on randomized comparisons. Other agents with activity include mitomycin-C and interferon (IFN). The side effects include dysuria, urinary frequency, and, depending on the drug, myelosuppression or a contact dermatitis. Rarely, intravesical BCG may produce a systemic illness associated with granulomatous infections in multiple sites that requires antituberculin therapy.

Following the endoscopic resection, patients are monitored for recurrence at 3-month intervals during the first year. Those with persistent disease or new tumors are generally considered for a second course of BCG or for intravesical chemotherapy with valrubicin or

gemcitabine. In some cases cystectomy is recommended, although the specific indications vary. Recurrence may develop anywhere along the urothelial tract including the renal pelvis, ureter, or urethra. A consequence of the "successful" treatment of tumors in the bladder is an increase in the frequency of extravesical recurrences. Tumors in the ureter or renal pelvis are typically managed by resection during retrograde examination or, in some cases, by instillation through the renal pelvis. Tumors of the prostatic urethra may require cystectomy if a complete resection cannot be achieved.

Invasive Disease The treatment of a tumor that has invaded muscle can be separated into control of the primary tumor and, depending on the pathologic findings at surgery, systemic chemotherapy. Radical cystectomy is the standard, although in selected cases a bladder-sparing approach that includes a complete endoscopic resection, partial cystectomy, or a combination of resection, systemic chemotherapy, and external beam radiation therapy is used. Indications for cystectomy include muscle-invading tumors not suitable for segmental resection, low-stage tumors unsuitable for conservative management (e.g., due to multicentric and frequent recurrences resistant to intravesical instillations), high-grade tumors (T1G3) associated with CIS, and bladder symptoms such as frequency or hemorrhage that impair quality of life. In some countries, external beam radiation therapy is considered standard. In the United States, its role is limited to those patients deemed unfit for cystectomy and those with unresectable local disease, and as part of an experimental approach that seeks to spare the bladder.

Radical cystectomy is major surgery that requires appropriate preoperative evaluation and management. The procedure involves removal of the bladder and pelvic lymph nodes, and creation of a conduit or reservoir for urinary flow. Grossly abnormal lymph nodes are evaluated by frozen section. If metastases are confirmed, the procedure is often aborted. In males, radical cystectomy involves the removal of the bladder, prostate and seminal vesicles, and proximal urethra. Impotence is universal unless the nerves responsible for erectile function are preserved. In females, the procedure includes removal of the bladder, urethra, uterus, fallopian tubes, ovaries, anterior vaginal wall, and surrounding fascia. Previously, urine flow was managed by directing the ureters to the abdominal wall, where it was collected in an external appliance. Currently, most patients receive a continent cutaneous reservoir that is constituted from detubularized bowel, or an orthotopic neobladder. Some 70% of men receive a neobladder. With a continent reservoir, 65 to 85% of men will be continent at night and 85 to 90% during the day. Cutaneous reservoirs are drained by intermittent catheterization; orthotopic neobladders are drained more naturally. Contraindications to a neobladder include renal insufficiency, an inability to self-catheterize, or the presence of an exophytic tumor or CIS in the urethra. Diffuse CIS in the bladder is a relative contraindication based on the risk of a urethral recurrence. Concurrent diseases in the bowel such as ulcerative colitis or Crohn's disease may hinder the use of resected bowel.

A partial cystectomy may be considered when the disease is limited to the dome of the bladder, a minimum of a 2-cm margin can be achieved, there is no CIS in other sites, and the bladder capacity is adequate after the tumor has been removed. This occurs in 5 to 10% of cases. Carcinomas in the ureter or in the renal pelvis are treated with nephroureterectomy with a bladder cuff to remove the tumor.

The probability of recurrence following surgery is predicted on the basis of pathologic stage, presence or absence of lymphatic or vascular invasion, and nodal spread. Among those who recur, the recurrence develops in a median of 1 year (range, 0.04 to 11.1 years). Long-term outcomes vary by pathologic stage and histology (Table 80-1). The number of lymph nodes removed is also prognostic whether or not tumor was in the nodes.

Metastatic Disease The primary goal of treatment for metastatic disease is to achieve a complete remission with chemotherapy alone, or with a combined-modality approach of chemotherapy followed by surgical resection of residual disease, as is done routinely for the treatment of germ cell tumors. One can define a goal in terms of cure or palliation on the basis of the probability of achieving a complete response to chemotherapy using prognostic factors, such as Karnofsky Performance Status (<80%), and whether the pattern of spread is nodal or visceral (liver, lung, or bone). For those with zero, 1, or 2 risk factors, the probability of a complete remission is 38, 25, and 5%, respectively, and median survival is 33, 13.4, and 9.3 months, respectively. Toxicities also vary as a function of risk. Treatment-related mortality has been reported in 3 to 4% of cases using some combinations. Patients with a compromised performance status, visceral disease, or bone metastases are rarely cured with chemotherapy alone; in these cases, median survivals rarely exceed 6 months.

A number of chemotherapeutic drugs have shown activity as single agents; cisplatin, paclitaxel, and gemcitabine are considered most active. Standard therapy consists of two-, three-, or four-drug combinations. Overall response rates of >50% have been reported using combinations such as methotrexate, vinblastine, doxorubicin, and cisplatin (M-VAC); cisplatin and paclitaxel (PT); gemcitabine and cisplatin (GC); or gemcitabine, paclitaxel, and cisplatin (GTC). M-VAC was considered standard, but the toxicities of neutropenia and fever, mucositis, diminished renal and auditory function, and peripheral neuropathy led to the development of alternative regimens. A comparative trial of M-VAC versus GC showed less neutropenia and fever, less mucositis, and more anemia and thrombocytopenia with the two-drug regimen.

Chemotherapy has also been evaluated in the neoadjuvant and adjuvant settings. In a randomized trial, patients receiving three cycles of neoadjuvant M-VAC followed by cystectomy had significantly better median (6.2 years) and 5-year survival (57%) compared to cystectomy alone (median survival, 3.8 years; 5-year survival, 42%). Adjuvant therapy with cisplatin, methotrexate, and vinblastine (CMV) (three cycles) appears to reduce the risk of recurrence by 15%. Additional trials are studying taxane- and gemcitabine-based combinations.

Chemotherapy has a role in invasive disease; however, for the majority of patients, chemotherapy alone is inadequate to clear the bladder of disease. Experimental studies are evaluating combined-modality approaches using chemotherapy and radiation therapy together in patients whose tumors were endoscopically removed.

The recommendation to administer adjuvant therapy is based on the risk of recurrence following cystectomy. Indications include the presence of nodal disease, extravesical tumor extension, or vascular invasion in the resected specimen. Adjuvant therapy (four cycles of combination chemotherapy) delays recurrence, although an effect on survival is less clear.

The management of bladder cancer is summarized in Table 80-2.

RENAL CELL CARCINOMA

Renal cell carcinomas account for 90 to 95% of malignant neoplasms arising from the kidney. Notable features include refractoriness to cy-

TABLE 80-2 *Management of Bladder Cancer*

Nature of Lesion	Management Approach
Superficial	Endoscopic removal, usually with intravesical therapy
Invasive disease	Cystectomy ± systemic chemotherapy (before or after surgery)
Metastatic disease	Curative or palliative chemotherapy (based on prognostic factors) ± surgery

totoxic agents, infrequent but reproducible responses to biologic response modifiers such as IFN-α and interleukin 2 (IL-2), and a variable clinical course for patients with metastatic disease, including anecdotal reports of spontaneous regression.

EPIDEMIOLOGY AND ETIOLOGY The annual incidence of renal cell carcinoma continues to rise and now includes nearly 36,000 cases annually in the United States resulting in 12,500 deaths. The male:female ratio is 2:1. Incidence peaks between the ages of 50 to 70, although this malignancy may be diagnosed at any age. Many environmental factors have been investigated as possible contributing causes; the strongest association is with cigarette smoking (accounting for 20 to 30% of cases) and obesity. Risk is also increased for patients who have acquired cystic disease of the kidney associated with end-stage renal disease, and for those with tuberous sclerosis. Most cases are sporadic, although familial forms have been reported. One is associated with von Hippel-Lindau (VHL) syndrome, which predisposes to renal cell carcinomas, retinal hemangioma, hemangioblastoma of the spinal cord and cerebellum, and pheochromocytoma. Roughly 35% of individuals with VHL disease develop renal cell cancer. An increased incidence has also been reported for first-degree relatives. Most renal cancers arise from the epithelial cells of the proximal tubules. A number of genetic alterations have been described; 97% show allelic loss at 3p. Deletions of 3p21–26 (where the *VHL* gene maps) have been identified in familial as well as sporadic tumors.

PATHOLOGY Renal cell neoplasia represents a heterogeneous group of tumors with distinct histopathologic, genetic, and clinical features ranging from benign to high-grade malignant (Table 80-3). They are classified on the basis of morphology and histology. Categories include clear cell carcinoma (60% of cases), papillary (5 to 15%), chromophobic tumors (5 to 10%), oncocytomas (5 to 10%), and collecting or Bellini duct tumors (<1%). Clear cell tumors have clear cytoplasm and usually show chromosome 3p deletions. Papillary tumors tend to be bilateral and multifocal and show trisomy 7 or 17. Chromophobic tumors are characterized by multiple chromosomal losses but do not exhibit 3p deletions and have a more indolent clinical course. Oncocytomas have a characteristic morphology including a deeply eosinophilic cytoplasm, do not exhibit 3p deletions or trisomy 7 or 17, and are considered benign neoplasms. In contrast, Bellini duct carcinomas are very rare and are thought to arise from the collecting ducts within the renal medulla. They tend to affect younger patients and are very aggressive tumors.

TABLE 80-1 *Survival Following Surgery for Bladder Cancer*

Pathologic Stage	5-Year Survival, %	10-Year Survival, %
T2,N0	89	87
T3a,N0	78	76
T3b,N0	62	61
T4,N0	50	45
Any T,N1	35	34

TABLE 80-3 *Classification of Epithelial Neoplasms Arising from the Kidney*

Carcinoma Type	Growth Pattern	Cell of Origin	Cytogenetics
Clear cell	Acinar or sarcomatoid	Proximal tubule	3p−
Papillary	Papillary or sarcomatoid	Proximal tubule	+7, +17, −Y
Chromophobic	Solid, tubular, or sarcomatoid	Cortical collecting duct	Hypodiploid
Oncocytic	Tumor nests	Cortical collecting duct	Undetermined
Collecting duct	Papillary or sarcomatoid	Medullary collecting duct	Undetermined

CLINICAL PRESENTATION The presenting signs and symptoms include hematuria, abdominal pain, and a flank or abdominal mass. This classic triad occurs in 10 to 20% of patients. Other symptoms are fever, weight loss, anemia, and a varicocele (Table 80-4). The tumor can also be found incidentally on a radiograph. Widespread use of radiologic cross-sectional imaging procedures (CT, ultrasound, MRI) contributes to earlier detection, including incidental renal masses detected during evaluation for other medical conditions. The increasing number of incidentally discovered low-stage tumors contributes to an improved 5-year survival for patients with renal cell carcinoma and increased use of nephron-sparing surgery (partial nephrectomy).

A spectrum of paraneoplastic syndromes has been associated with these malignancies, including erythrocytosis, hypercalcemia, nonmetastatic hepatic dysfunction (Stauffer syndrome), and acquired dysfibrinogenemia. Erythrocytosis is noted at presentation in only about 3% of patients. Anemia, a sign of advanced disease, is more common.

The standard evaluation of patients with suspected renal cell tumors includes a CT scan of the abdomen and pelvis, a chest radiograph, urine analysis, and urine cytology. A CT of the chest is warranted if metastatic disease is suspected from the chest radiograph, as it will detect significantly smaller lesions, and their presence may influence the approach to the primary tumor. MRI is useful in evaluating the inferior vena cava in cases of suspected tumor involvement or invasion by thrombus, as well as for patients in whom contrast cannot be administered owing to either allergy or renal dysfunction. In clinical practice, any solid renal masses should be considered malignant until proven otherwise; a definitive diagnosis is required. If no metastases are demonstrated, surgery is indicated, even if the renal vein is invaded. The differential diagnosis of a renal mass includes cysts, benign neoplasms (adenoma, angiomyolipoma, oncocytoma), inflammatory lesions (pyelonephritis or abscesses), and other primary or metastatic malignant neoplasms. Other malignancies that may involve the kidney include transitional cell carcinoma of the renal pelvis, sarcoma, lymphoma, Wilms' tumor, and metastatic disease, especially from melanoma. All of these are less common causes of renal masses than is renal cell cancer.

STAGING AND PROGNOSIS Two staging systems used commonly are the Robson classification and the American Joint Committee on Cancer (AJCC) staging system. According to the Robson system, stage I tumors are confined to the kidney; stage II tumors extend through the renal capsule but are confined to Gerota's fascia; stage III tumors involve the renal vein or vena cava (stage III A) or the hilar lymph nodes (stage III B); and stage IV disease includes tumors that are locally invasive to adjacent organs (excluding the adrenal gland) or distant metastases. The rate of 5-year survival varies by stage: 66% for stage I, 64% for stage II, 42% for stage III, and 11% for stage IV. The prognosis for patients with stage IIIA lesions is similar to that of stage II disease; 5-year survival for patients with stage IIIB disease is only 20%, closer to that of stage IV.

TABLE 80-4 *Signs and Symptoms in Patients with Renal Cell Cancer*

Presenting Sign or Symptom	Incidence, %
Classic triad: hematuria, flank pain, flank mass	10–20
Hematuria	40
Flank pain	40
Palpable mass	25
Weight loss	33
Anemia	33
Fever	20
Hypertension	20
Abnormal liver function	15
Hypercalcemia	5
Erythrocytosis	3
Neuromyopathy	3
Amyloidosis	2
Increased erythrocyte sedimentation rate	55

℞ TREATMENT

Localized Tumors The standard management for stage I or II tumors and selected cases of stage III disease is radical nephrectomy. This procedure involves en bloc removal of Gerota's fascia and its contents including the kidney, the ipsilateral adrenal gland, and adjacent hilar lymph nodes. The role of a regional lymphadenectomy is controversial. Extension into the renal vein or inferior vena cava, stage III disease, does not preclude resection even if cardiopulmonary bypass is required. Half of these patients have prolonged survival if the tumor is resected. Stauffer syndrome describes the rare patient with no detectable metastatic disease who has hepatic dysfunction. These patients are also candidates for renal resection because the hepatopathy is often reversible after the primary is removed.

In selected patients who have only one kidney—depending on the size and location of the lesion—nephron-sparing approaches may be used via an open or laparoscopic approach. A nephron-sparing approach can also be used for patients with bilateral tumors, accompanied by a radical nephrectomy on the opposite side. Partial nephrectomy techniques are being applied electively to resect small masses for patients with a normal contralateral kidney. Adjuvant chemotherapy, immunotherapy, and radiation therapy are not useful following surgery, even in cases with a poor prognosis.

Advanced Disease Investigational therapy is first-line treatment for metastatic disease as no immune approach or chemotherapeutic agent has shown significant antitumor activity. The prognosis is highly variable; in one analysis, no prior nephrectomy, a Karnofsky performance status <80, low hemoglobin, high corrected calcium, and abnormal lactate dehydrogenase (LDH) were poor prognostic factors. Patients with zero, one or two, and three or more factors had a median survival of 24, 12, and 5 months, respectively. These tumors often follow an unpredictable and protracted clinical course. In one study, 10% of patients with established metastatic disease did not progress after 1 year of observation. It may be best to document progression before considering potentially toxic treatment approaches.

Surgery has a limited role for patients with metastatic disease. One indication for nephrectomy is to alleviate pain or hemorrhage of a primary tumor. Nephrectomy is not indicated to induce tumor regression (occurs in <1% of cases) or to increase sensitivity to cytokine therapy. However, long-term survival may occur in patients who relapse after nephrectomy in a solitary site that can be removed.

IFN-α and IL-2 produce regressions in 10 to 20% of patients but these are rarely durable. IL-2 was approved on the observation of durable complete remission in a small proportion of cases. IFN has also been evaluated as an adjuvant to cytoreductive surgery. In one study, patients were randomized to surgery plus IFN (5×10^6 IU/m², 3 times per week) versus IFN alone. The median time to progression was 5 versus 3 months, and median survival was 17 versus 7 months (hazard ratio, .54) in favor of the combined-modality approach. A second trial with a similar design showed a 3-month difference in median survival (11.1 versus 8.1 months) in favor of the combined approach. Newer cytokines and novel biologic agents are under investigation, and promising results have been reported using an inhibitor of vascular endothelial growth factor.

CARCINOMA OF THE RENAL PELVIS AND URETER

About 2500 cases of renal pelvis and ureter cancer occur each year; nearly all are transitional cell carcinomas similar to bladder cancer in biology and appearance. This tumor also is associated with chronic phenacetin abuse and with Balkan nephropathy, a chronic interstitial nephritis endemic in Bulgaria, Greece, Bosnia-Herzegovina, and Romania.

The most common symptom is painless gross hematuria, and the disease usually is detected on IVP during the workup for hematuria. Patterns of spread are like those in bladder cancer. For disease localized to the renal pelvis and ureter, nephroureterectomy (including excision of the distal ureter with a portion of the bladder) is associated with a 5-year survival of 80 to 90% for low-grade lesions. More invasive or histologically poorly differentiated tumors are more likely to recur locally and metastasize. Metastatic disease is treated with the chemotherapy used in bladder cancer, and the outcome is similar to that of metastatic transitional cell cancer of bladder origin.

FURTHER READING

ADVANCED BLADDER CANCER META-ANALYSIS COLLABORATION: Neoadjuvant chemotherapy in invasive bladder cancer: A systematic review and meta-analysis. Lancet 361:1927, 2003

BORDEN LS JR et al: Bladder cancer. Curr Opin Oncol 15:227, 2003
LINEHAN WM et al: The genetic basis of cancer of the kidney. J Urol 170: 2163, 2003
MEJEAN A et al: Prognostic factors of renal cell carcinoma. J Urol 169:821, 2003
WHANG YE, GODLEY PA: Renal cell carcinoma. Curr Opin Oncol 15:213, 2003
WINQUIST E et al: Neoadjuvant chemotherapy for transitional cell carcinoma of the bladder: A systematic review and meta-analysis. J Urol 171:561, 2004

81 HYPERPLASTIC AND MALIGNANT DISEASES OF THE PROSTATE
Howard I. Scher

The frequency of both benign and malignant changes in the prostate increase with age. Autopsies of men in the eighth decade of life show hyperplastic changes in >90% and malignant changes in >70% of individuals. The high prevalence of these diseases in an elderly population with competing causes of morbidity and mortality mandates a risk-adapted approach to diagnosis and treatment. This can be achieved by considering these diseases as a series of states. Each state represents a distinct clinical milestone for which intervention(s) may be recommended based on the presence or risk of developing symptoms or death from disease in a given time frame (Fig. 81-1). For benign proliferative disorders, symptoms of urinary frequency, infection, and potential for obstruction are weighed against the side effects and complications of medical or surgical therapy. For prostate malignancies, the risk of developing the disease, symptoms, or death from cancer are balanced against the morbidities of interventions recommended and preexisting comorbid conditions.

In 2004, around 230,000 prostate cancer cases were diagnosed, of whom 29,900 succumbed. The absolute number of prostate cancer deaths has decreased in the past 5 years; this has been attributed by some to the widespread use of detection strategies based on monitoring prostate-specific antigen (PSA). However, screening has not been proven to improve survival in prospective randomized trials. The paradox of management is that although the disease remains the second leading cause of cancer deaths in men, the almost 8:1 ratio in incidence to prostate cancer–specific mortality shows that the majority of men do not die of their disease.

ANATOMY AND PATHOLOGY

The prostate is located in the pelvis and is surrounded by the rectum, the bladder, the periprostatic and dorsal vein complexes that are responsible for erectile function, and the urinary sphincter that is responsible for passive urinary control. The prostate is composed of branching tubuloalveolar glands arranged in lobules and surrounded by a stroma. The acinal unit includes an epithelial compartment made up of epithelial, basal, and neuroendocrine cells and a stromal compartment that includes fibroblasts and smooth-muscle cells. The compartments are separated by a basement membrane. PSA and acid phosphatase (ACP) are produced in the epithelial cells. Both cell types express androgen receptors and depend on androgens for growth. Testosterone, the major circulating androgen, is converted by the enzyme 5-α reductase to dihydrotestosterone in the gland. Changes in prostate size occur during puberty and after the age of 55 in the periurethral portion of the gland. Most cancers develop in the peripheral zone, which can often be palpated by a digital rectal examination (DRE).

Nonmalignant growth occurs predominantly in the transition zone around the urethra.

EPIDEMIOLOGY

The development of a prostate cancer involves a multistep process. Hypermethylation of the GSTP1 gene promoter, leading to a loss of function of a gene that detoxifies carcinogens, is one early change. Epidemiologic studies show that the risk of being diagnosed with prostate cancer increases by a factor of 2 if one first-degree relative is affected and by 4 if two or more are affected. Current estimates are that 40% of early-onset and 5 to 10% of all cancers are hereditary and follow a Mendelian inheritance pattern. Prostate cancer affects ethnic groups differently. Matched for age, the prostates of African-American males have both a greater number of precursor prostatic intraepithelial neoplasia (PIN) lesions and larger tumors than white males, possibly related to the higher levels of testosterone seen in African-American males. These lesions are highly unstable, and typically multifocal. Polymorphic variants of the androgen receptor gene, the cytochrome P450 C17 gene, and the steroid 5α-reductase type II (*SRD5A2*) gene have also been implicated in the variations in incidence. The incidence of autopsy-detected cancers is similar around the world, while the incidence of the clinical disease varies. Thus, environmental factors may play a role. High consumption of dietary fats, such as α-linoleic acid, or polycyclic aromatic hydrocarbons that form when red meats are cooked is believed to increase risk. Similar to breast cancer in Asian women, the risk of prostate cancer in Asian males increases when they move to western environments. Protective factors include the isoflavinoid genistein (which inhibits 5α-reductase), cruciferous vegetables that contain isothiocyanate sulfuraphane, retinoids such as lycopene (in pizza and tomatoes), and inhibitors of cholesterol biosynthesis. The antioxidant α-tocopherol (vitamin E) and selenium may also reduce risk.

DIAGNOSIS AND TREATMENT BY CLINICAL STATE

The clinical states framework considers the risk of morbidity from an enlarging but nonmalignant gland; the probability that a clinically significant cancer is present in an individual with or without urinary symptoms; or, for those with a prostate cancer diagnosis, the probability of developing symptoms or dying from disease. At any point in time, a patient resides in one state and remains there until the disease has progressed to the next state. Applying this paradigm, a patient with localized prostate cancer who has had all cancer removed surgically remains in the state of localized disease as long as the PSA remains undetectable. The time within a state becomes a measure of the impact of an intervention on the natural history of disease, be it benign or malignant in etiology, recognizing that the impact may not be assessable for years. It also allows a distinction between *cure*—the elimination of all cancer cells, the primary therapeutic objective when treating most cancers—and *cancer control*, in which the tempo of the illness is modulated and symptoms controlled until the patient dies of other causes. It is the concept of cancer control that makes the man-

FIGURE 81-1 Clinical states of prostate cancer. PSA, prostate-specific antigen.

agement of prostate cancer unique. Even when a recurrence is documented, immediate therapy is not always necessary. Rather, as at the time of diagnosis, the need for intervention is based on the tempo of the illness as it unfolds in the individual, relative to the risk:reward ratio of the therapy being considered.

NO CANCER DIAGNOSIS ■ Symptoms The need to pursue a diagnosis of prostate cancer is based on symptoms, an abnormal DRE, or an elevated serum PSA. The urologic history should focus on symptoms of outlet obstruction, continence, potency, or a change in ejaculatory pattern. Benign proliferative disease may produce hesitancy, intermittent voiding, a diminished stream, incomplete emptying, and postvoid leakage. The severity of these symptoms can be quantitated with the self-administered American Urological Association (AUA) *Symptom Index* (Table 81-1) recognizing that the degree of symptoms does not always relate to gland size. Resistance to urine flow reduces bladder compliance, leading to nocturia, urgency, and, ultimately, to retention. Infection, tranquilizing drugs, antihistamines, or alcohol can precipitate urinary retention. Prostatitis often produces pain or induration. Symptoms of metastatic disease include pain secondary to osseous metastases, although many are asymptomatic despite extensive spread. Less common are symptoms related to marrow compromise (myelophthisis), a coagulopathy, or spinal cord compression.

Physical Examination The DRE focuses on the size, consistency, and abnormalities within or beyond the gland. Many cancers occur in the peripheral zone and can be palpated on DRE. Carcinomas are characteristically hard, nodular, and irregular, while induration may be due to benign prostatic hypertrophy (BPH) or to calculi or tumor. Overall, 20 to 25% of men with an abnormal DRE have cancer.

PROSTATE-SPECIFIC ANTIGEN

PSA is a kallikrein-like serine protease that causes liquefaction of seminal coagulum. It is produced by both nonmalignant and malignant epithelial cells. PSA is prostate specific, not prostate cancer specific, and increases may occur from prostatitis, nonmalignant enlargement of the gland (BPH), prostate cancer, and prostate biopsies. The level is not affected by the performance of a DRE. It circulates in the blood as an inactive complex with the protease inhibitors α-$_1$-antichymotrypsin and β_2-macroglobulin and has an estimated half-life in the serum of 2 to 3 days. Levels should be undetectable if the prostate has been removed. PSA immunostaining is used to establish a prostate cancer diagnosis.

PSA testing was approved for early detection in 1994. It is recommend on an annual basis along with a DRE for men over age 50 (with an anticipated survival of >10 years; this includes men up to age 76 years). For African Americans and men with a family history, testing is advised to begin at age 40. The normal range of PSA is 0 to 4 ng/mL. For values >4, the sensitivity for prostate cancer detection is 57 to 79%, the specificity is 59 to 68%, and the positive predictive value is 40 to 49%.

The PSA-based criteria used to recommend a diagnostic prostate biopsy have evolved over time. PSA values may fluctuate for no apparent reason; thus, an isolated abnormal value should be confirmed before proceeding with further testing. These evolving criteria aim to increase the sensitivity of the test for younger men more likely to die of the disease and to reduce the frequency of detecting cancers of low malignant potential in elderly men more likely to die of other causes. Age-specific reference ranges apply a lower "upper" limit of normal for younger males and higher "upper" limit for older individuals. Different thresholds alter sensitivity and specificity of detection. The threshold for performance of a biopsy is now 2.6 ng/mL for men under age 60. Prostate-specific antigen density (PSAD) measurements were developed to correct for the contribution of BPH to the total PSA level. PSAD is calculated by dividing the serum PSA by the estimated prostate weight calculated by transrectal ultrasound (TRUS). Values <0.10 are consistent with BPH, while those >0.15 suggest cancer. *PSA velocity* is the rate of change in PSA levels over time. It is particularly useful for men with values that are rising in the seemingly "normal" range. Rates of rise >0.75 ng/mL per year suggest cancer. As an example, an increase from 2.5 to 3.9 in a 1-year period would warrant further testing. Free and complexed PSA measurements are used when levels are between 4 and 10 ng/mL to decide who needs a biopsy. In cancer, the level of free PSA is lower. The ratios of free to total, complexed to total, and free to complexed PSA have also been used. In one series, specificity improved by 20% using a normal range of free/total >0.15; complexed/total <0.70; and free/complexed >0.25. A diagnostic algorithm based on the DRE and PSA findings is illustrated in Fig. 81-2. In general, a biopsy is recommended if the DRE or PSA are abnormal.

Prostate Biopsy A diagnosis of cancer is established by a TRUS-guided needle biopsy. Direct visualization assures that all areas of gland are sampled. A minimum of six separate cores, three from the right and three from the left, are advised, as is a separate biopsy of the transition zone, if clinically indicated. Performance of a biopsy is not advised in a patient with prostatitis until a course of antibiotics has been administered. The positive predictive value of an abnormal DRE is 21%, while 25% of men with a PSA > 4 ng/mL and an abnormal DRE, and 17% of men with a PSA of 2.5 to 4.0 ng/mL and normal DRE, have cancer. Those with an abnormal PSA and negative biopsy are advised to undergo a repeat biopsy.

TABLE 81-1   *AUA System Index*

Questions to Be Answered	Not at All	Less than 1 Time in 5	Less than Half the Time	About Half the Time	More than Half the time	Almost Always
Over the past month, how often you have had a sensation of not emptying your bladder completely after you finished urinating?	0	1	2	3	4	5
Over the past month, how often have you had to urinate again less than 2 h after you finished urinating?	0	1	2	3	4	5
Over the past month, how often have you found you stopped and started again several times when you urinated?	0	1	2	3	4	5
Over the past month, how often have you found it difficult to postpone urination?	0	1	2	3	4	5
Over the past month, how often have you had a weak urinary stream?	0	1	2	3	4	5
Over the past month, how often have you had to push or strain to begin urination?	0	1	2	3	4	5
Over the past month, how many times did you most typically get up to urinate from the time you went to bed at night until the time you got up in the morning?	(None)	(1 time)	(2 times)	(3 times)	(4 times)	(5 times)
Sum of 7 circled numbers (AUA Symptom Score): ————						

Note: AUA, American Urological Association.

Source: Barry MJ et al: J Urol 148:1549, 1992. Used with permission.

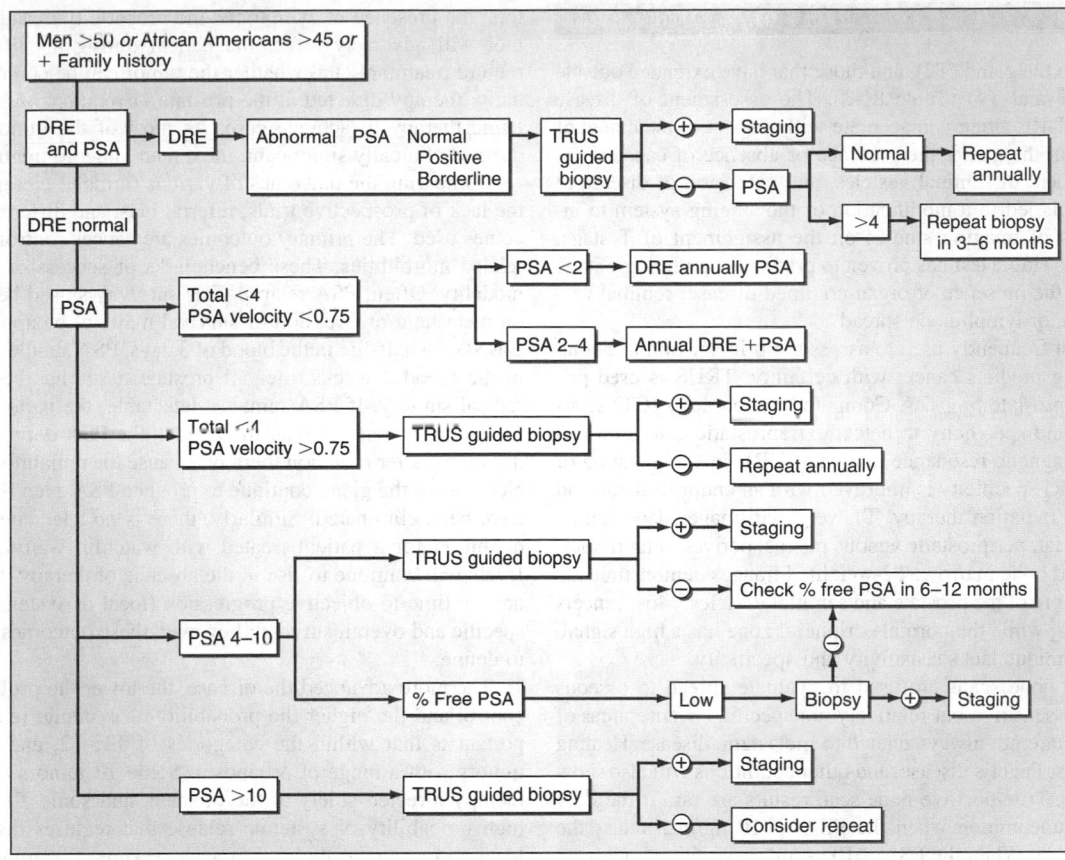

FIGURE 81-2 Algorithm for diagnostic evaluation of men based on digital rectal examination and prostate-specific antigen levels.

Pathology The noninvasive proliferation of epithelial cells within ducts is termed *prostatic intraepithelial neoplasia*. PIN is a precursor of cancer, but not all PIN lesions develop into invasive cancers. Of the cancers identified, >95% are adenocarcinomas; the remaining are squamous, transitional cell tumors, and rarely, carcinosarcomas. Metastases to the prostate are rare, but in some cases, transitional cell tumors of the bladder or colon cancers invade the gland by direct extension. Each core of the biopsy is examined for the presence of cancer, and the amount of cancer present is quantified. A measure of histologic aggressiveness is also assigned using the *Gleason grading system*, in which the dominant and secondary glandular histologic patterns are scored from 1 (well differentiated) to 5 (undifferentiated) and summed to give a total score of 2 to 10 for each tumor. The most poorly differentiated area of tumor (i.e., the area with the highest histologic grade) often determines biologic behavior. The presence or absence of perineural invasion and extracapsular spread are also recorded.

PSA-based detection strategies have changed the clinical spectrum of the disease. Now, 95 to 99% of newly diagnosed cancers are clinically localized, 40% are not palpable, and, of these, 70% are pathologically organ-confined. The downside of widespread use is the detection and treatment of cancers with such a low malignant potential that they would not have shortened survival or produced symptoms during the patient's lifetime. The side effects of treatment, including impotence, incontinence, and bowel dysfunction, are unacceptable for these cases. Formal clinical trials to assess the value of screening on prostate cancer morbidity and mortality are ongoing. Until the results of these studies are available, men are advised to make an informed decision about whether to undergo testing.

Prevention It is difficult to identify individuals who are at risk for developing a cancer that is clinically significant. The Prostate Cancer Prevention Trial is a double-blinded, randomized multicenter trial designed to investigate the ability of finasteride, a 5α-reductase inhibitor, to prevent the development of prostate cancer in men age ≥55 years.

The prostate cancer detection rate was 18.4% (803 of 4364) for finasteride and 24.4% (1147 of 4692) for placebo-treated men. However, more of the cancers detected in the finasteride group were high-grade [37% (280 of 757) vs. 22% (237 of 1068 cancers) for the placebo]. No effect on survival was detected. Vitamin E and selenium (the SELECT study) are also being tested as preventive agents.

Treatment of Benign Disease Asymptomatic patients do not require treatment regardless of the size of the gland, while those with an inability to urinate, gross hematuria, recurrent infection, or bladder stones may require surgery. Typically, obstruction does not occur and the symptoms remain stable over time. In these cases, uroflowmetry can identify patients with normal flow rates who are unlikely to benefit from treatment and those with high postvoid residuals who may need other interventions. Pressure-flow studies detect primary bladder dysfunction. Cystoscopy is recommended if hematuria is documented and to assess the urinary outflow tract before surgery. Imaging of the upper tracts is advised for patients with hematuria, a history of calculi, or prior urinary tract problems. Therapies such as finasteride, which blocks the conversion of testosterone to dihydrotestosterone, have been shown to decrease prostate size, increase urine flow rates, and improve symptoms. They will also lower baseline PSA levels by 50%, an important consideration when using PSA to guide biopsy recommendations. α-Adrenergic blockers such as terazosin act by relaxing the smooth muscle of the bladder neck and increasing peak urinary flow rates. No data show that these agents influence the progression of the disease. Surgical approaches include a transurethral resection of the prostate (TURP), transurethral incision, or removal of the gland via a retropubic, suprapubic or perineal approach. TULIP (transurethral ultrasound-guided laser-induced prostatectomy), coils, stents, and hyperthermia are also utilized.

PROSTATE CANCER STAGING The TNM staging system includes categories for cancers that are palpable on DRE, those identified solely on the basis of an abnormal PSA (T1c), those that are palpable but clinically confined to the gland (T2), and those that have extended outside of the gland (T3 and T4) (Table 81-2). The assessment of disease extent based on DRE alone is inaccurate with respect to the extent of the disease within the gland, the presence or absence of capsular invasion, involvement of seminal vesicles, and extension of disease to lymph nodes. This led to a modification of the staging system to include the results of imaging studies on the assignment of T stage. Unfortunately, no single test has proven to predict the pathologic stage accurately, be it the presence of organ-confined disease, seminal vesical involvement, or lymph node spread.

TRUS is most frequently used to assess the primary tumor, but no consistent finding predicts cancer with certainty. TRUS is used primarily to direct prostate biopsies. Computed tomography (CT) scans lack sensitivity and specificity to detect extraprostatic extension and are inferior to magnetic resonance imaging (MRI) in visualization of lymph nodes. MRI specificity is improved with an endorectal coil and aids in planning radiation therapy. T1-weighted images demonstrate the periprostatic fat, periprostatic venous plexus, perivesicular tissues, lymph nodes, and bone marrow. T2-weighted images demonstrate the internal architecture of the prostate and seminal vesicles. Most cancers have a low signal, while the normal peripheral zone has a high signal, although the technique lacks sensitivity and specificity.

Radionuclide bone scans are used to evaluate spread to osseous sites. This test is sensitive but relatively nonspecific because areas of increased uptake are not always related to metastatic disease. Healing fractures, arthritis, Paget's disease, and other conditions will also show abnormal uptake. True-positive bone scan results are rare if the PSA <8 ng/mL and uncommon when the PSA < 10 ng/mL unless the tumor is high grade. When the PSA <10 ng/mL, a positive bone scan is usually falsely positive, which in turn, leads to additional low-yield testing.

CLINICALLY LOCALIZED DISEASE   Localized prostate cancers are clinically confined to the prostate. Patients with localized disease are managed by radical surgery, radiation therapy, or watchful waiting. Data from the literature do not provide clear evidence for the superiority of any one treatment. Choice of therapy needs consideration of several factors: the presence of symptoms, the probability that the untreated tumor will adversely affect the patient during his lifetime and thus require treatment, and whether the tumor can be cured by single-modality therapy directed at the prostate or requires both local and systemic therapy to achieve cure. As most of the tumors detected are deemed clinically significant, most men undergo treatment.

Comparing the outcomes of various forms of therapy is limited by the lack of prospective trials, referral bias, and differences in the outcomes used. The primary outcomes are cancer control and treatment-related morbidities. These benchmarks of success or failure vary by modality. Often, PSA relapse–free survival is used because an effect on metastatic progression or survival may not be apparent for years. Based on a half-life in the blood of 3 days, PSA should be undetectable in the blood 4 weeks after all prostate tissue has been removed by radical surgery. If PSA remains detectable, the patient is considered to have persistent disease. In contrast, the PSA does not become undetectable after radiation therapy because the remaining nonmalignant elements of the gland continue to produce PSA even if all cancer cells have been eliminated. Similarly, there is no adequate cancer control definition for a patient treated with watchful waiting because PSA levels will continue to rise in the absence of therapy. Other outcomes are the time to objective progression (local or systemic) and cancer-specific and overall survival; however, these outcomes may take years to define.

The more advanced the disease, the lower the probability of local control and the higher the probability of systemic relapse. More important is that within the categories of T1, T2, and T3 disease are tumors with a range of prognoses. Some T3 tumors are curable with therapy directed solely at the prostate, and some T1 lesions have a high probability of systemic relapse that requires the integration of local and systemic therapy to achieve cure. T1c tumors particularly require the use of other factors to predict outcomes and select treatment. Many groups have developed prognostic models based on a combination of the initial T stage, Gleason score, and baseline PSA. Some are based on discrete cut points (PSA <10 or $\geq$ 10; Gleason score of $\leq$6, 7, or $\geq$8). Others are nomograms that use PSA and Gleason score as continuous variables. These algorithms are used to predict disease extent: organ confined vs. nonorgan confined, node negative or positive, and the probability of success using a PSA-based definition of failure specific to the local therapy under consideration. Exactly what cut-off value would lead a patient to accept one form of therapy vs. another is an area of active debate. One nomogram to predict PSA relapse–free survival following radical surgery is illustrated in Fig. 81-2. Specific nomograms have been developed for radical prostatectomy, external-beam radiation therapy, and brachytherapy (seed implantation). These are being refined continually to incorporate other clinical parameters and biologic determinants. Surgical technique, radiation therapy delivery, and criteria for watchful waiting continue to be refined and improved; the year treatment was given affects outcomes independent of other factors. The improvements make treatment decisions a dynamic process.

The frequency of adverse events for the different modalities is highly variable. Of greatest concern to patients are the effects on continence, sexual potency, and bowel function. Part of the variability relates to the definition used for a specific complication and whether the patient or physician is reporting the event. Incontinence figures range from 2% to 47% and impotence rates range from 25% to 89% following radical prostatectomy. The time of the assessment is also important. After surgery, impotence is immediate but may reverse over time, while with radiation therapy, impotence is not immediate but may develop over time.

Radical Retropubic Prostatectomy (RRP)   The goal of radical prostatectomy is to excise the cancer completely with a clear margin, to maintain continence by preserving the external sphincter, and to preserve potency by sparing the autonomic nerves in the neurovascular bundle. RRP is advised for patients with a life expectancy of >10 years and is performed using a retropubic, perineal, or laparoscopic approach.

TABLE 81-2   *Comparison of Clinical Stage by the TNM Classification System and the Whitmore-Jewett Staging System*

TNM Stage	Description	Whitmore-Jewett Stage	Description
T1a	Nonpalpable, with 5% or less of resected tissue with cancer	A1	Well differentiated tumor on few chips from 1 lobe
T1b	Nonpalpable, with >5% of resected tissue with cancer	A2	Involvement more diffuse
T1c	Nonpalpable, detected due to elevated serum PSA		
T2a	Palpable, half of one lobe or less	BIN	Palpable, < one lobe, surrounded by normal tissue
T2b	Palpable, > half of one lobe but not both lobes	B1	Palpable, < one lobe
T2c	Palpable, involves both lobes	B2	Palpable, one entire lobe or both lobes
T3a	Palpable, unilateral extracapsular extension	C1	Palpable, outside capsule, not into seminal vesicles
T3b	Palpable, bilateral extracapsular extension		
T3c	Tumor invades seminal vesicle(s)	C2	Palpable, seminal vesicle involved
MI	Distant metastases	D	Metastatic disease

Source: Adapted from FF Schroder et al: TNM classification of prostate cancer. Prostate (Suppl) 4:129, 1992; and American Joint Committee on Cancer, 1992.

Outcomes can be predicted using postoperative nomograms that consider pretreatment factors and the pathologic findings at surgery. PSA failure is defined as a detectable value of 0.2 or 0.4 ng/mL, although the exact definition varies among series. The techniques continue to improve as the ability to localize the tumor within or beyond the prostate are refined with different biopsy algorithms and with imaging. The result is better case selection and surgical planning, which in turn have led to more rapid recovery and higher rates of continence and potency. Factors associated with incontinence include older age, shorter urethra length, surgical technique, preservation of neurovascular bundles, and development of an anastomotic stricture. Surgical experience is also a factor. In one series, 6% of patients had mild stress urinary incontinence (SUI) (requiring 1 pad/day), 2% moderate SUI (>1 pad/day), and 0.3% severe SUI (requiring an artificial urinary sphincter). At 1 year, 92% were completely continent. In contrast, the results in a Medicare population treated at multiple centers showed that at 3, 12, and 24 months following surgery, 58, 35, and 42% wore pads in their underwear, and 24, 11, and 15% reported "a lot" of urine leakage. Factors associated with recovery of erectile function include younger age, quality erections before surgery, and the absence of damage to the neurovascular bundles. Erectile function returns in a median of 4 to 6 months if both bundles are preserved. Potency is reduced by half if at least one nerve bundle is sacrificed. In cases where cancer control requires the removal of both bundles, sural nerve grafts are being explored. Overall, with the availability of drugs such as sildenafil, intraurethral inserts of alprostadil, and intracavernosal injections of vasodilators, many patients recover satisfactory sexual function.

High-risk patients are those with a predicted high probability of failure with surgery alone based on pretreatment factors. In these situations, nomograms and predictive models can only go so far. Exactly what probability of success or failure would lead a physician to recommend and a patient to seek alternative approaches is controversial. For example, it may be appropriate to recommend radical surgery for a younger patient with a low probability of cure. To improve the outcomes of surgery for high-risk patients, neoadjuvant hormonal therapy has been explored. The results of several large trials testing 3 or 8 months of androgen ablation before surgery showed that serum PSA levels decreased by 96%, prostate volumes reduced by 34%, and margin positivity rates declined from 41 to 17%. Unfortunately, hormones did not produce an improvement in PSA relapse–free survival. Thus, neoadjuvant hormonal therapy is not recommended.

Radiation Therapy Radiation therapy is given by external beam, the implantation of radioactive sources into the gland, or a combination of both. Contemporary external beam radiation techniques now use three-dimensional conformal treatment plans to maximize the administered dose to the tumor and to minimize the exposure of the surrounding normal structures. The addition of intensity modulation (IMRT) has allowed further shaping of the isodose curves and the delivery of higher doses to the tumor and a further reduction in normal tissue exposure. These advances have allowed the safe administration of doses >80 Gy, higher local control rates, and fewer side effects. Overall, radiation therapy is associated with a higher frequency of bowel complications (mainly diarrhea) than surgery. Measures of cancer control include the proportion of patients who show a decline in PSA to <0.5 or 1 ng/mL, the proportion with "nonrising" PSA values, or the proportion with a negative biopsy of the prostate 2 years after completion of treatment. PSA relapse is defined as three consecutive rising PSA values from the nadir value, with the time to failure as the midpoint between the nadir and first rising value.

Radiation dose is important. A PSA nadir of <1.0 ng/mL was observed in 90% of patients receiving 75.6 or 81.0 Gy vs. 76 and 56% for those receiving 70.2 Gy and 64.8 Gy, respectively. The positive biopsy rates at 2.5 years were 4% for those treated with 81 Gy, vs. 36 and 27% for those receiving 70.2 or 75.6 Gy. The frequency of rectal complications relates directly to the volume of the anterior rectal wall receiving full-dose treatment. Grade 3 rectal or urinary toxicities were seen in 2.1% of cases at a median dose of 75.6 Gy. Grade 3 urethral strictures requiring dilatation developed in 1% of cases, all of whom had undergone a TURP. Pooled data show that the frequency of grade 3 to 4 toxicities is 6.9 and 3.5%, respectively, for patients who received >70 Gy. The frequency of erectile dysfunction is related to the quality of erections pretreatment, the dose administered, and the time of assessment. The etiology is related to a disruption of the vascular supply and not the nerve fibers.

Neoadjuvant hormone therapy has also been studied in combination with radiation therapy to increase local control rates, decrease the size of the prostate so that the exposure of normal tissues to full-dose radiation is reduced, and decrease the rate of systemic failure. Short-term hormone exposures can reduce toxicities and improve local control rates, but long-term (2 to 3 years) treatment is needed to prolong the time to PSA failure and the development of metastatic disease. The impact on survival has been less clear.

Brachytherapy involves the direct implantation of the prostate with radioactive sources. It is based on the principle that the deposition of radiation energy in tissues decreases exponentially as a function of the square of the distance from the source. The goal is to deliver intensive irradiation to the prostate, minimizing the exposure of the surrounding tissues. Techniques have evolved from intraoperative manual insertion methods to the current standard, in which customized templates based on CT and ultrasonographic assessment of the tumor are used for seed placement based on computer-optimized dosimetry to achieve more homogeneous dose distributions. The implants themselves are now performed transperineally, without an open procedure, with real-time imaging. The result is a marked reduction in local failure rates with fewer complications. In a series of 197 patients followed for a median of 3 years, 5-year actuarial PSA relapse–free survival for patients with pretherapy PSA levels of 0 to 4, 4 to 10, and >10 μg/mL were 98, 90 and 89%, respectively. In a separate report of 201 patients who underwent posttreatment biopsies, 80% were negative, 17% indeterminate, and 3% were positive. The results did not change with longer follow-up. Nevertheless, many physicians feel that implantation is best reserved for patients with good or intermediate prognostic features. The procedure is well tolerated, although most patients experience urinary frequency and urgency that can persist for several months. Incontinence has been seen in 2 to 4% of cases. Higher complication rates are observed in patients who have undergone a prior TURP or who have obstructive symptoms at baseline. Proctitis has been reported in <2% of patients.

Watchful waiting, or deferred therapy, is a policy of no therapeutic intervention(s) until the tumor progresses. Progression can be based on PSA changes, local tumor growth, the development of symptoms, or metastatic disease. The practice evolved from studies of predominantly elderly men with well-differentiated tumors in whom clinically significant progression could not be demonstrated for protracted periods, during which a significant proportion died of intercurrent disease. In a structured literature review of patients treated by radical surgery, a deferred approach, or external beam radiation, the 10-year mean survivals were 93% for radical prostatectomy, 84% for deferred treatment, and 74% for external beam radiation. Risk of progression was related to grade. Men with grade 1 or 2 tumors had a 13% risk of death and 19% risk of metastases at 10 years; those with grade 3 tumors had 63 and 74% risks, respectively.

Case selection is critical, and the criteria to select those to whom watchful waiting can be applied safely are under intense study. In a recent prostatectomy series, it was estimated that 10 to 15% of patients had "insignificant" cancers. Given the multifocality of the disease, a concern is the limited ability to predict pathologic findings on the basis of a needle biopsy, even when multiple cores are obtained. Arguing against this approach is the result of a randomized trial of radical prostatectomy vs. watchful waiting from Sweden. With a median follow-up of 6.2 years, men treated by radical surgery had a lower risk of prostate cancer death relative to watchful waiting patients (4.6 vs. 8.9%) and a lower risk of metastatic progression, hazard ratio .63.

FIGURE 81-3 Sites of action of different hormone therapies.

Nevertheless, it can be anticipated that more patients may be candidates for a deferred approach as PSA testing is applied more widely and earlier.

RISING PSA This state includes patients in whom the sole manifestation of disease is a rising PSA after surgery and/or radiation therapy. By definition, no evidence of disease is found on scan. For these patients the central issue is whether the rise in PSA is the result of persistent disease in the primary site, a systemic recurrence, or both. In theory, disease that persists or has recurred in the primary site may be curable by additional local treatment. For patients who had undergone surgery, the question is whether external beam radiation therapy to the prostate bed can eliminate the disease and lead to an undetectable PSA. For radiation therapy–treated patients, the question is whether a prostatectomy would achieve cure.

The decision to recommend radiation therapy is often made on clinical grounds, as imaging studies such as CT and bone scan are typically uninformative. Some recommend a Prostascint scan: imaging with a radiolabeled antibody to prostate-specific membrane antigen (PSMA), which is highly expressed on prostate epithelial cells. Antibody localization to the prostatic fossa suggests local recurrence; localization to extrapelvic sites predicts failure of radiation therapy. Others recommend that a biopsy of the urethrovesical anastamosis be obtained before considering radiation. Factors that predict for response to salvage radiation are a positive surgical margin, a lower Gleason grade, a long interval from surgery to PSA failure, a slow PSA doubling time, and a low (<0.5 to 1.0 ng/mL) PSA value at the time of treatment. Radiation is generally not recommended if the PSA was persistently elevated after surgery (indicating that disease-free status was not achieved).

For patients with a rising PSA after radiation therapy, a salvage prostatectomy can be considered if the disease was "curable" at the onset, persistent disease has been documented by a biopsy of the prostate, and no metastatic disease is seen on imaging studies. Unfortunately, case selection is poorly defined in most series, and morbidities are significant. As currently performed, virtually all patients are impotent, and ~45% have either total urinary incontinence or stress incontinence. Major bleeding, bladder neck contractures, and rectal injury are not uncommon.

In the majority of cases, the rise in PSA indicates systemic disease. In these cases, the need for treatment should consider the probability of developing clinically detectable disease on scan and in what time frame. That immediate therapy is not required was shown in a series where patients did not receive systemic therapy until metastatic disease was documented. Overall, the median time to metastatic progression was 8 years and 63% of the patients with rising PSA values remained free of metastases at 5 years. Factors associated with progression include Gleason grade, time to recurrence, and PSA doubling times. For those with Gleason grade ≥8 tumors, the probability of metastatic progression was 37, 51, and 71% at 3, 5, and 7 years, respectively. If the time to recurrence was <2 years and PSA doubling time was long (> 10 months), the proportion with metastatic disease was 23, 32, and 53% vs. 47, 69, and 79% if the doubling time was short (< 10 months) during the same time intervals. These models continue to be refined. A difficulty making these predictions is that most patients with a rising PSA receive some form of therapy before the development of metastases.

METASTATIC DISEASE: NONCASTRATE *Metastatic disease noncastrate* refers to patients with tumors visible on an imaging study and noncastrate levels of testosterone. The patient may be newly diagnosed or have recurrent disease after treatment for localized disease. Standard treatment is to block androgen action or decrease androgen production by medical or surgical means. Over 90% of male hormones originate in the testes; <10% are synthesized in the adrenal gland. Surgical orchiectomy is the "gold standard" approach but is least acceptable by patients. Medical therapies can be divided into those that lower testosterone levels, e.g., gonadotropin-releasing hormone (GnRH) agonists and antagonists, estrogens and progestational agents, and the antiandrogens that bind to the androgen receptor but do not signal (Fig. 81-3). Ketoconazole inhibits adrenal androgen synthesis and is used after first-line castration is no longer effective. In this setting, the adrenal glands may contribute up to 40% of the active androgens in the prostate.

GnRH analogues (leuprolide acetate and goserelin acetate) initially produce a rise in luteinizing hormone and follicle-stimulating hormone (FSH), followed by a downregulation of receptors in the pituitary gland, which effects a chemical castration. They were approved on the basis of randomized comparisons showing an improved safety profile (specifically, reduced cardiovascular toxicities) relative to diethylstilbestrol (DES), with equivalent potency. The initial rise in testosterone may result in a clinical flare of the disease. As such, these agents are contraindicated in men with significant obstructive symptoms, cancer-related pain, or spinal cord compromise. Estrogens such as DES also lower testosterone levels but have fallen out of favor due to the risk of vascular complications such as fluid retention, phlebitis, emboli, and stroke.

In contrast, nonsteroidal antiandrogens such as flutamide, bicalutamide, or nilutamide block the binding of androgens to the receptor. Given alone, testosterone levels remain the same or increase. These agents were approved initially to block the flare associated with the initial rise in testosterone that results following GnRH administration. They have also been studied as part of a combined androgen blockade (CAB) or maximal androgen blockade (MAB) and as monotherapy. The concept of CAB was developed to inhibit testicular and adrenal androgens at the outset, and it preoccupied the field for many years. It is achieved clinically by combining an antiandrogen with a GnRH agonist or surgical orchiectomy. Cumulative results of randomized comparisons involving thousands of patients showed no advantage for combining an antiandrogen with surgical orchiectomy, while separate analyses of trials combining an antiandrogen with a GnRH analogue have shown a modest (<10%) survival advantage. Meta-analysis of all combined androgen blockade trials concluded that there was no benefit to the approach. In practice, most patients treated with GnRH analogue therapy receive an antiandrogen for the first 2 to 4 weeks of treatment.

The anti–prostate cancer effects of agents that lower serum testosterone levels are similar, and the clinical course is predictable: an initial response, a period of stability in which the cells are dormant and not proliferating, followed by regrowth after a variable period of time as a hormone-independent tumor. Androgen ablation is not curative. Cells that survive castration are present when the disease is first diagnosed. Considered by disease manifestation, PSA levels return to normal in 60 to 70% of cases and measurable disease regression occurs in 50%; while improvements in bone scan occur in 25% of cases, the majority remain stable. Survival is inversely proportional to disease extent. Agents that lower testosterone are associated with an androgen-deprivation syndrome that includes hot flushes, weakness, fatigue, impotence, loss of muscle mass, changes in personality, anemia, depression, and a reduction in bone density. The bone changes can be prevented by treatment with bisphosphonates along with vitamin D and calcium supplementation.

A question often asked is whether antiandrogens, which are associated with fewer hot flashes, less of an effect on libido, less muscle wasting, fewer personality changes, and less bone loss, can be used alone without compromising outcomes. Gynecomastia remains a significant problem but can be alleviated in part with the addition of tamoxifen. Most reported randomized trials suggest that the cancer-specific outcomes are inferior. Even a comparison of bicalutamide, 150 mg (three times the recommended dose of 50 mg), versus surgical castration showed a shorter time to progression and inferior survival for patients with established metastatic disease. Nevertheless, some men may accept the trade-off of a potentially inferior cancer outcome for an improved quality of life.

Another question is whether hormones should be given early, in the adjuvant setting or at the time recurrence is first documented, or late, when metastatic disease or symptoms are manifest. Trials in support of early therapy have often been underpowered relative to the "net benefit" reported or have been criticized on methodologic grounds. In one, although a survival benefit was shown for patients treated with radiation therapy and 3 years of androgen ablation relative to radiation alone, the trial was criticized for the poor outcomes for the control group. Another showing a survival benefit for patients with positive nodes randomized to medical or surgical castration compared to observation ($p = .02$) was criticized because the confidence intervals around the 5- and 8-year survival distributions overlapped between the two groups. A large randomized study comparing early to late hormone treatment (orchiectomy or GnRH analogue) in patients with locally advanced or asymptomatic metastatic disease showed that patients treated early were less likely to progress from M0 to M1 disease, develop pain, and die of prostate cancer. This trial was criticized because therapy was delayed "too long" in the late-treatment group. When patients treated by radical surgery, radiation therapy, or watchful waiting were randomly assigned to receive bicalutamide, 150 mg, or placebo, hormone treatment produced a significant reduction in the proportion of patients who developed osseous metastases at 2 years (9% for bicalutamide; 13.8% for placebo). This result has not gained acceptance in part because too many "good-risk" patients were treated and because no effect on survival was demonstrated. These criticisms are valid; however, the net influence on survival from early hormone intervention is similar to that observed in patients with breast cancer where adjuvant hormonal therapy is routinely given.

Another way to reduce the side effects of androgen ablation is to administer hormones on an intermittent basis. This was proposed as a way to prevent the emergence of castration-resistant cells by "forcing" the cells that survive androgen ablation into a normal differentiation pathway by repleting testosterone. Theoretically, surviving cells that are allowed to proliferate in the presence of androgen will retain sensitivity to androgen ablation. The duration of treatment varies from 2 to 6 months beyond the point of maximal response. Once therapy is stopped, endogenous testosterone levels increase, and the symptoms associated with androgen ablation abate. PSA levels also begin to rise, and, at some level, androgen ablation is restarted. Using this approach, multiple cycles of regression and proliferation have been documented in individual patients. It is unknown whether the intermittent approach

increases, decreases, or does not change the overall duration of sensitivity to androgen ablation. A trial to address this question is ongoing.

METASTATIC DISEASE: CASTRATE Castration-resistant disease can be manifest in many ways. For some it is a rise in PSA with no change in radiographs and no new symptoms. In others, it is a rising PSA and progression in bone, with or without symptoms of disease. Still others will show soft tissue disease with or without osseous metastases, and others have a pattern of visceral spread. The prognosis, highly variable, can also be predicted using nomograms designed for this cohort. The important distinction is that despite the failure of first-line hormone treatment, the majority of these tumors remain sensitive to second- and third-line hormonal treatments. Castration resistance does not indicate hormonal resistance. The rising PSA is an indication of continued signaling through the androgen receptor axis.

The manifestations of disease in this patient group hinder the development of drugs and treatment standards because the traditional measures of outcome such as tumor regression do not apply. No PSA-based outcomes are true surrogates for a survival benefit, and assessing changes in osseous disease using bone scans is notoriously inaccurate. It is essential to define therapeutic objectives before initiating treatment, as standards of care have changed on the basis of randomized comparisons that provide clinical benefits without prolonging life. These endpoints include the relief of symptoms and delaying metastases or the time to the development of new symptoms of disease.

The management of these patients requires first that the castrate status be documented. Patients receiving an antiandrogen alone who have elevated levels of serum testosterone should be treated first with a GnRH analogue or orchiectomy and observed for response. Patients on an anti-androgen in combination with a GnRH analogue should have the antiandrogen discontinued, as ~30% will respond to the withdrawal of the antiandrogen. Any response occurs within weeks of stopping flutamide, but may take 8 to 12 weeks with nilutamide and bicalutamide (they have a long terminal half-life). At the time of progression, a different antiandrogen can be given as these agents are not cross-resistant. Other hormones that may be active include estrogens, progestins, ketoconazole, and glucocorticoids. Those who respond to estrogens or progestins should also be evaluated for a withdrawal response at the time of progression. Cytotoxic agents are considered when hormone responses stop.

No chemotherapy regimen has been proven to prolong life in these patients. However, responses to chemotherapy that improve symptom control are not uncommon. Drugs directed at the tumor cell cytoskeleton such estramustine (Emcyt) and a taxane such as paclitaxel or docetaxel can induce responses in ≥50% using measurable disease regression as the endpoint. Seventy percent will show a >50% decline in PSA from baseline. Studies evaluating survival effects are nearly done.

Management of pain is a critical part of therapy. Optimal palliation requires assessing whether the symptoms and metastases are focal or diffuse and whether disease threatens the spinal cord, the cauda equina, or the base of the skull. Neurologic symptoms require emergent evaluation because loss of function may be permanent if not addressed in a timely manner. Single sites of pain or areas of neurologic involvement are best treated with external beam radiation. As the disease is often diffuse, palliation at one site often leads to the emergence of symptoms at another. An important principle of management was established in two randomized trials of mitoxantrone and prednisone vs. prednisone alone. In both studies, mitoxantrone-treated patients had a greater reduction in pain, used fewer narcotics, were more mobile, and had less fatigue. No survival benefit was shown.

Given the bone-dominant nature of prostate cancer spread, bone-directed therapies may be useful in patients with diffuse disease. Two bone-seeking radioisotopes, [89]Sr (metastron) and [153]Sm-EDTMP (quadramet), are approved for palliation of pain although they have no effect on PSA or on survival. Fewer patients treated with an isotope developed new areas of pain or required additional radiation therapy compared to patients receiving external beam radiation therapy alone. Addition of zoledronate to "standard therapy" in patients with castration-resistant disease resulted in fewer skeletal events relative to placebo-treated patients. The bone events included development of new pain, need for radiation therapy, and microfractures. Finally, patients randomly assigned to a combination of ^{89}Sr and doxorubicin after induction chemotherapy had fewer skeletal events and longer survival than patients treated with doxorubicin alone. Confirmatory studies are ongoing.

FURTHER READING

GONZALGO ML, ISAACS WB: Molecular pathways to prostate cancer. J Urol 170:2444, 2003

KHAN MA, PARTIN AW: Partin tables: Past and present. BJU Int 92:7, 2003

NELSON WG et al: Prostate cancer. N Engl J Med 349:366, 2003

SCHAFFER DR, SCHER HI: Prostate cancer: A dynamic illness with shifting targets. Lancet Oncol 4:407, 2003

THOMPSON IM et al: The influence of finasteride on the development of prostate cancer. N Engl J Med 349:215, 2003

THORPE A, NEAL D: Benign prostatic hyperplasia. Lancet 366:1359, 2003

YAO SL, DIPAOLA RS: evidence-based approach to prostate cancer follow-up. Semin Oncol 30:390, 2003

82 TESTICULAR CANCER
Robert J. Motzer, George J. Bosl

Primary germ cell tumors (GCTs) of the testis, arising by the malignant transformation of primordial germ cells, constitute 95% of all testicular neoplasms. Infrequently, GCTs arise from an extragonadal site, including the mediastinum, retroperitoneum, and, very rarely, the pineal gland. This disease is notable for the young age of the afflicted patients, the totipotent capacity for differentiation of the tumor cells, and its curability; about 95% of all newly diagnosed patients will be cured. Experience in the management of GCTs leads to improved outcome.

INCIDENCE AND EPIDEMIOLOGY Nearly 9000 new cases of testicular GCT were diagnosed in the United States in 2004; the incidence of this malignancy has increased slowly over the past 40 years. The tumor occurs most frequently in men between the ages of 20 and 40. A testicular mass in a man ≥50 years should be regarded as a lymphoma until proved otherwise. GCT is at least four to five times more common in white than in African-American males, and a higher incidence has been observed in Scandinavia and New Zealand than in the United States.

ETIOLOGY AND GENETICS Cryptorchidism is associated with a severalfold higher risk of GCT. Abdominal cryptorchid testes are at a higher risk than inguinal cryptorchid testes. Orchiopexy should be performed before puberty, if possible. Early orchiopexy reduces the risk of GCT and improves the ability to save the testis. An abdominal cryptorchid testis that cannot be brought into the scrotum should be removed. About 2% of men with GCTs of one testis will develop a primary tumor in the other testis. Testicular feminization syndromes increase the risk of testicular GCT, and Klinefelter's syndrome is associated with mediastinal GCT.

An isochromosome of the short arm of chromosome 12 [i(12p)] is pathognomonic for GCT of all histologic types. Excess 12p copy number either in the form of i(12p) or as increased 12p on aberrantly banded marker chromosomes occurs in nearly all GCTs, but the gene(s) on 12p involved in the pathogenesis are not yet defined.

CLINICAL PRESENTATION A painless testicular mass is pathognomonic for a testicular malignancy. More commonly, patients present with testicular discomfort or swelling suggestive of epididymitis and/or orchitis. In this circumstance, a trial of antibiotics is reasonable. However, if symptoms persist or a residual abnormality remains, then testicular ultrasound examination is indicated.

Ultrasound of the testis is indicated whenever a testicular malignancy is considered and for persistent or painful testicular swelling. If a testicular mass is detected, a radical inguinal orchiectomy should be performed. Because the testis develops from the gonadal ridge, its blood supply and lymphatic drainage originate in the abdomen and descend with the testis into the scrotum. An inguinal approach is taken to avoid breaching anatomic barriers and permitting additional pathways of spread.

Back pain from retroperitoneal metastases is common and must be distinguished from musculoskeletal pain. Dyspnea from pulmonary metastases occurs infrequently. Patients with increased serum levels of human chorionic gonadotropin (hCG) may present with gynecomastia. A delay in diagnosis is associated with a more advanced stage and possibly worse survival.

The staging evaluation for GCT includes a determination of serum levels of α fetoprotein (AFP), hCG, and lactate dehydrogenase (LDH). After orchiectomy, a chest radiograph and a computed tomography (CT) scan of the abdomen and pelvis should be performed. A chest CT scan is required if pulmonary nodules or mediastinal or hilar disease is suspected. Stage I disease is limited to the testis, epididymis, or spermatic cord. Stage II disease is limited to retroperitoneal (regional) lymph nodes. Stage III disease is disease outside the retroperitoneum, involving supradiaphragmatic nodal sites or viscera. The staging may be "clinical"—defined solely by physical examination, blood marker evaluation, and radiographs—or "pathologic"—defined by an operative procedure.

The regional draining lymph nodes for the testis are in the retroperitoneum, and the vascular supply originates from the great vessels (for the right testis) or the renal vessels (for the left testis). As a result, the lymph nodes that are involved first by a right testicular tumor are the interaortocaval lymph nodes just below the renal vessels. For a left testicular tumor, the first involved lymph nodes are lateral to the aorta (para-aortic) and below the left renal vessels. In both cases, further nodal spread is inferior and contralateral and, less commonly, above the renal hilum. Lymphatic involvement can extend cephalad to the retrocrural, posterior mediastinal, and supraclavicular lymph nodes. Treatment is determined by tumor histology (seminoma versus nonseminoma) and clinical stage (Table 82-1).

PATHOLOGY GCTs are divided into nonseminoma and seminoma subtypes. Nonseminomatous GCTs are most frequent in the third decade of life and can display the full spectrum of embryonic and adult cellular differentiation. This entity comprises four histologies: embryonal carcinoma, teratoma, choriocarcinoma, and endodermal sinus (yolk sac) tumor. Choriocarcinoma, consisting of both cytotrophoblasts and syncytiophoblasts, represents malignant trophoblastic differentiation and is invariably associated with secretion of hCG. Endodermal sinus tumor is the malignant counterpart of the fetal yolk sac and is associated with secretion of AFP. Pure embryonal carcinoma may secrete AFP or hCG, or both; this pattern is biochemical evidence of differentiation. Teratoma is composed of somatic cell types derived from two or more germ layers (ectoderm, mesoderm, or endoderm). Each of these histologies may be present alone or in combination with others. Nonseminomatous GCTs tend to metastasize early to sites such as the retroperitoneal lymph nodes and lung parenchyma. One-third of patients present with disease limited to the testis (stage I), one-third with retroperitoneal metastases (stage II), and one-third with more extensive supradiaphragmatic nodal or visceral metastases (stage III).

Seminoma represents about 50% of all GCTs, has a median age in the fourth decade, and generally follows a more indolent clinical course. Most patients (70%) present with stage I disease, about 20% with stage II disease, and 10% with stage III disease; lung or other visceral metastases are rare. Radiation therapy is the treatment of choice in patients with stage I disease and stage II disease where the nodes are <5 cm in maximum diameter. When a tumor contains both seminoma and nonseminoma components, patient management is directed by the more aggressive nonseminoma component.

TUMOR MARKERS Careful monitoring of the serum tumor markers AFP and hCG is essential in the management of patients with GCT, as these markers are important for diagnosis, as prognostic indicators, in monitoring treatment response, and in the detection of early relapse. Approximately 70% of patients presenting with disseminated nonseminomatous GCT have increased serum concentrations of AFP and/or hCG. While hCG concentrations may be increased in patients with either nonseminoma or seminoma histology, the AFP concentration is increased only in patients with nonseminoma. The presence of an increased AFP level in a patient whose tumor showed only seminoma indicates that an occult nonseminomatous component exists and the patient should be treated for nonseminomatous GCT. LDH levels are not as specific as AFP or hCG, but are increased in 50 to 60% patients with metastatic nonseminoma and in up to 80% of patients with advanced seminoma.

AFP, hCG, and LDH levels should be determined before and after orchiectomy. Increased serum AFP and hCG concentrations decay according to first-order kinetics; the half-life is 24 to 36 h for hCG and 5 to 7 days for AFP. AFP and hCG should be assayed serially during and after treatment. The reappearance of hCG and/or AFP or the failure of these markers to decline according to the predicted half-life is an indicator of persistent or recurrent tumor.

TABLE 82-1 *Germ Cell Tumor Staging and Treatment*

Stage	Extent of Disease	Treatment	
		Seminoma	Nonseminoma
IA	Testis only, no vascular/lymphatic invasion (T1)	Radiation therapy	RPLND or observation
IB	Testis only, with vascular/lymphatic invasion (T2), or extension through tunica albuginea (T2), or involvement of spermatic cord (T3) or scrotum (T4)	Radiation therapy	RPLND
IIA	Nodes < 2 cm	Radiation therapy	RPLND or chemotherapy often followed by RPLND
IIB	Nodes 2–5 cm	Radiation therapy	RPLND +/− adjuvant chemotherapy or chemotherapy followed by RPLND
IIC	Nodes > 5 cm	Chemotherapy	Chemotherapy, often followed by RPLND
III	Distant metastases	Chemotherapy	Chemotherapy, often followed by surgery (biopsy or resection)

Note: RPLND, retroperitoneal lymph node dissection.

Rx TREATMENT

Stage I Nonseminoma If, after an orchiectomy (for clinical stage I disease), radiographs and physical examination show no evidence of disease, and serum AFP and hCG concentrations are either normal or declining to normal according to the known half-life, patients may be managed by either a nerve-sparing retroperitoneal lymph node dissection (RPLND) or surveillance. The retroperitoneal lymph nodes are involved by GCT (pathologic stage II) in 20 to 50% of these patients. The choice of surveillance or RPLND is based on the pathology of the primary tumor. If the primary tumor shows no evidence for lymphatic or vascular invasion and is limited to the testis (T1), then either option is reasonable. If lymphatic or vascular invasion is present or the tumor extends into the tunica, spermatic cord, or scrotum (T2 through T4), then surveillance should not be offered. Either approach should cure >95% of patients.

A RPLND is the standard operation for removal of the regional lymph nodes of the testis (retroperitoneal nodes). The operation removes the lymph nodes ipsilateral to the primary site and the nodal groups adjacent to the primary landing zone. The standard (modified bilateral) RPLND removes all node-bearing tissue down to the bifurcation of the great vessels, including the ipsilateral iliac nodes. The major long-term effect of this operation is retrograde ejaculation and infertility. A nerve-sparing RPLND, usually accomplished by identification and dissection of individual nerve fibers, may avoid injury to the sympathetic nerves responsible for ejaculation. Normal ejaculation is preserved in ~90% of patients. Patients with pathologic stage I disease are observed, and only the <10% who relapse require additional therapy. If retroperitoneal nodes are found to be involved at RPLND, then a decision regarding adjuvant chemotherapy is made on the basis of the extent of retroperitoneal disease (see below).

Surveillance is an option in the management of clinical stage I disease when no vascular/lymphatic invasion is found (T1). Only 20 to 30% of patients have pathologic stage II disease, implying that most

RPLNDs in this situation are not therapeutic. Although surveillance has not been compared to RPLND in a randomized trial, all large studies show that surveillance and RPLND lead to equivalent long-term survival rates. Patient compliance is essential if surveillance is to be successful. Patients must be carefully followed with periodic chest radiography, physical examination, CT scan of the abdomen, and serum tumor marker determinations. The median time to relapse is about 7 months, and late relapses (>2 years) are rare. The 70 to 80% of patients who do not relapse require no intervention after orchiectomy; treatment is reserved for those who do relapse. When the primary tumor is classified as T2 through T4 (extension beyond testis and epididymis or lymphatic/vascular invasion is identified), nerve-sparing RPLND is preferred. About 50% of these patients have pathologic stage II disease and are destined to relapse without the RPLND.

Stage II Nonseminoma Patients with limited, ipsilateral retroperitoneal adenopathy (nodes usually ≤3 cm in largest diameter) and normal levels of AFP and hCG generally undergo a modified bilateral RPLND as primary management. Increased levels of either AFP or hCG or both imply metastatic disease outside the retroperitoneum; chemotherapy is used in this setting. The local recurrence rate after a properly performed RPLND is very low. Depending on the extent of disease, the postoperative management options include either surveillance or two cycles of adjuvant chemotherapy. Surveillance is the preferred approach for patients with resected "low-volume" metastases (tumor nodes ≤2 cm in diameter *and* <6 nodes involved) because the probability of relapse is one-third or less. For those who relapse, risk-directed chemotherapy is indicated (see below). Because relapse occurs in ≥50% of patients with "high-volume" metastases (>6 nodes involved, *or* any involved node >2 cm in largest diameter, *or* extranodal tumor extension), two cycles of adjuvant chemotherapy should be considered, as it results in cure in ≥98% of patients. Regimens consisting of etoposide (100 mg/m^2 daily on days 1 through 5) plus cisplatin (20 mg/m^2 daily on days 1 through 5) with or without bleomycin (30 units per day on days 2, 9, and 16) given at 3-week intervals are effective and well tolerated.

Stages I and II Seminoma Inguinal orchiectomy followed by retroperitoneal radiation therapy cures ~98% of patients with stage I seminoma. The dose of radiation therapy (2500 to 3000 cGy) is low and well tolerated, and the in-field recurrence rate is negligible. About 2% of patients relapse with supradiaphragmatic or systemic disease. Surveillance has been proposed as an option, and studies have shown that about 15% of patients relapse. The median time to relapse is 12 to 15 months, and late relapses (>5 years) may be more frequent than with nonseminoma. The relapse is usually treated with chemotherapy. Surveillance for clinical stage I seminoma is generally not recommended.

Nonbulky retroperitoneal disease (stage IIA and IIB) is also treated with radiation therapy. Prophylactic supradiaphragmatic fields are not used. Relapses in the anterior mediastinum are unusual. Approximately 90% of patients achieve relapse-free survival with retroperitoneal masses <5 cm in diameter. Because at least one-third of patients with bulkier disease relapse, initial chemotherapy is preferred for stage IIC disease.

Chemotherapy for Advanced GCT   Regardless of histology, patients with stage IIC and stage III GCT are treated with chemotherapy. Combination chemotherapy programs based on cisplatin at doses of 100 mg/m^2 plus etoposide at doses of 500 mg/m^2 per cycle cure 70 to 80% of such patients, with or without bleomycin, depending on risk stratification (see below). A complete response (the complete disappearance of all clinical evidence of tumor on physical examination and radiography plus normal serum levels of AFP and hCG for ≥1 month) occurs after chemotherapy alone in ~60% of patients, and another 10 to 20% become disease-free with surgical resection of residual masses containing viable GCT. Lower doses of cisplatin result in inferior survival rates.

The toxicity of four cycles of the cisplatin/bleomycin/etoposide (BEP) regimen is substantial. Nausea, vomiting, and hair loss occur in most patients, although nausea and vomiting have been markedly ameliorated by modern antiemetic regimens. Myelosuppression is frequent, and symptomatic bleomycin pulmonary toxicity occurs in ~5% of patients. Treatment-induced mortality due to neutropenia with septicemia or bleomycin-induced pulmonary failure occurs in 1 to 3% of patients. Dose reductions for myelosuppression are rarely indicated. Long-term permanent toxicities include nephrotoxicity (reduced glomerular filtration and persistent magnesium wasting), ototoxicity, and peripheral neuropathy. When bleomycin is administered by weekly bolus injection, Raynaud's phenomenon appears in 5 to 10% of patients. Other evidence of small blood vessel damage is seen less often, including transient ischemic attacks and myocardial infarction.

Risk-Directed Chemotherapy   Because not all patients are cured and treatment may cause significant toxicities, patients are stratified into "good-risk" and "poor-risk" groups according to pretreatment clinical features. For good-risk patients, the goal is to achieve maximum efficacy with minimal toxicity. For poor-risk patients, the goal is to identify more effective therapy with tolerable toxicity.

The International Germ Cell Cancer Consensus Group (IGCCCG) developed criteria to assign patients to three risk groups (good, intermediate, poor) (Table 82-2). The marker cut-offs have been incorporated into the revised TNM staging of GCT. Hence, TNM stage groupings are now based on both anatomy (site and extent of disease) and biology (marker status and histology). Seminoma is either good or intermediate risk based on the absence or presence of nonpulmonary visceral metastases. No poor-risk category exists for seminoma. Marker levels play no role in defining risk for seminoma. Nonseminomas have good-, intermediate-, and poor-risk categories based on the site of the primary tumor, the presence or absence of nonpulmonary visceral metastases, and marker levels.

For ~90% of patients with good-risk GCTs, four cycles of etoposide plus cisplatin (EP) or three cycles of BEP produce durable complete responses, with minimal acute and chronic toxicity. Pulmonary toxicity is absent when bleomycin is not used and is rare when therapy is limited to 9 weeks; myelosuppression with neutropenic fever is less frequent; and the treatment mortality rate is negligible. About 75% of intermediate-risk patients and 45% of poor-risk patients achieve durable complete remission with four cycles of BEP, and no regimen has proved superior. More effective therapy is needed.

Postchemotherapy Surgery   Resection of residual metastases after the completion of chemotherapy is an integral part of therapy. If the initial histology is nonseminoma and the marker values have normalized, all

TABLE 82-2   IGCCCG Risk Classification for Advanced Germ Cell Tumors

Risk	Nonseminoma	Seminoma
Good	Gonadal or retroperitoneal primary site	Any primary site
	Absent nonpulmonary visceral metastases	Absent nonpulmonary visceral metastases
	AFP < 1000 ng/mL	Any LDH, hCG
	Beta-hCG < 5000 mIU/mL	
	LDH < 1.5 × upper limit or normal (ULN)	
Intermediate	Gonadal or retroperitoneal primary site	Any primary site
	Absent nonpulmonary visceral metastases	Presence of nonpulmonary visceral metastases
	AFP 1000–10,000 ng/mL	
	Beta-hCG 5000–50,000 mIU/mL	Any LDH, hCG
	LDH 1.5–10 × ULN	
Poor	Mediastinal primary site	No patients classified as poor prognosis
	Presence of nonpulmonary visceral metastases	
	AFP ≥ 10,000 ng/ML	
	Beta-hCG > 50,000 mIU/mL	
	LDH > 10 × ULN	

Note: AFP, α fetoprotein; hCG, human chorionic gonadotropin; LDH, lactate dehydrogenase.
Source: From International Germ Cell Cancer Consensus Group.

sites of residual disease should be resected. In general, residual retroperitoneal disease requires a modified bilateral RPLND. Thoracotomy (unilateral or bilateral) and neck dissection are less frequently required to remove residual mediastinal, pulmonary parenchymal, or cervical nodal disease. Viable tumor (seminoma, embryonal carcinoma, yolk sac tumor, or choriocarcinoma) will be present in 15%, mature teratoma in 40%, and necrotic debris and fibrosis in 45% of resected specimens. The frequency of teratoma or viable disease is highest in residual mediastinal tumors. If necrotic debris or mature teratoma is present, no further chemotherapy is necessary. If viable tumor is present but is completely excised, two additional cycles of chemotherapy are given.

If the initial histology is pure seminoma, mature teratoma is rarely present, and the most frequent finding is necrotic debris. For residual retroperitoneal disease, a complete RPLND is technically difficult owing to extensive postchemotherapy fibrosis. Observation is recommended when no radiographic abnormality exists or a residual mass <3 cm is present. Controversy exists over what to do when the residual mass exceeds 3 cm in diameter. About 25% of such masses contain viable GCT. Some investigators prefer excision or biopsy, but radiation therapy and surveillance are alternatives.

Salvage Chemotherapy   Of patients with advanced GCT, 20 to 30% fail to achieve a durable complete response to first-line chemotherapy. A combination of cisplatin, ifosfamide and vinblastine (VeIP) will cure about 25% of patients as a second-line therapy. Substitution of paclitaxel for vinblastine may be more effective in this setting. Patients are more likely to achieve a durable complete response if they had a testicular primary tumor and relapsed from a prior complete remission to first-line cisplatin-containing chemotherapy. In contrast, if the patient failed to achieve a complete response or has a primary mediastinal nonseminoma, then standard-dose salvage therapy is rarely beneficial. Treatment options for such patients include dose-intensive treatment, experimental therapies, and surgical resection.

Chemotherapy consisting of dose-intensive, high-dose carboplatin (≥1500 mg/m^2) plus etoposide (≥1200 mg/m^2), with or without cyclophosphamide or ifosfamide, with peripheral blood stem cell support induces a complete response in 25 to 40% of patients who have progressed after ifosfamide-containing salvage chemotherapy. About one-half of the complete responses will be durable. High-dose therapy is the treatment of choice and standard of care for this patient population. Paclitaxel is also active in previously treated patients and shows promise in high-dose combination programs. Cure is still possible in some relapsed patients.

EXTRAGONADAL GCT AND MIDLINE CARCINOMA OF UNCERTAIN HISTOGENESIS

The prognosis and management of patients with extragonadal GCTs depends on the tumor histology and site of origin. All patients with a diagnosis of extragonadal GCT should have a testicular ultrasound examination. Nearly all patients with retroperitoneal or mediastinal seminoma achieve a durable complete response to BEP or EP. The clinical features of patients with primary retroperitoneal nonseminoma GCT are similar to those of patients with a primary of testis origin, and careful evaluation will find evidence of a primary testicular GCT in about two-thirds of cases. In contrast, a primary mediastinal non-seminomatous GCT is associated with a poor prognosis; one-third of patients are cured with standard therapy (four cycles of BEP). Patients with newly diagnosed mediastinal nonseminoma are considered to have poor-risk disease and should be considered for clinical trials testing regimens of possibly greater efficacy. In addition, mediastinal non-seminoma is associated with hematologic disorders, including acute myelogenous leukemia, myelodysplastic syndrome, and essential thrombocytosis unrelated to previous chemotherapy. These hematologic disorders are very refractory to treatment. Nonseminoma of any primary site may change into other malignant histologies such as embryonal rhabdomyosarcoma or adenocarcinoma. This is called malignant transformation. i(12p) has been identified in the transformed cell type, indicating GCT clonal origin.

A group of patients with poorly differentiated tumors of unknown histogenesis, midline in distribution, and not associated with secretion of AFP or hCG has been described; a few (10 to 20%) are cured by standard cisplatin-containing chemotherapy. i(12p) is present in ~25% of such tumors (the fraction that are cisplatin-responsive), confirming their origin from primitive germ cells. This finding is also predictive of the response to cisplatin-based chemotherapy and resulting long-term survival. These tumors are heterogeneous; neuroepithelial tumors and lymphoma may also present in this fashion.

FERTILITY Infertility is an important consequence of the treatment of GCTs. Preexisting infertility or impaired fertility is often present. Azoospermia and/or oligospermia are present at diagnosis in at least 50% of patients with testicular GCTs. Ejaculatory dysfunction is associated with RPLND, and germ cell damage may result from cisplatin-containing chemotherapy. Nerve-sparing techniques to preserve the retroperitoneal sympathetic nerves have made retrograde ejaculation less likely in the subgroups of patients who are candidates for this operation. Spermatogenesis does recur in some patients after chemotherapy. However, because of the significant risk of impaired reproductive capacity, semen analysis and cryopreservation of sperm in a sperm bank should be recommended to all patients before treatment.

FURTHER READING

BOSL GJ et al: Testicular germ-cell cancer. N Engl J Med 337:242, 1997

CHAGANTI RSK, HOULDSWORTH J: Genetics and biology of human male germ cell tumors. Cancer Res 60:1475, 2000

INTERNATIONAL GERM CELL CANCER CONSENSUS GROUP: International Germ Cell Consensus Classification: A prognostic factor-based staging system for metastatic germ cell cancers. J Clin Oncol 15:594, 1997

KONDAGUNTA GV, MOTZER R: Adjuvant chemotherapy for stage II nonseminomatous germ cell tumors. Semin Urol 20:239, 2002

MCGLYNN KA et al: Trends in the incidence of testicular germ cell tumors in the United States. Cancer 97:63, 2003

MCGUIRE MS et al: The role of thoracotomy in managing postchemotherapy residual thoracic masses in patients with nonseminomatous germ cell tumors. BJU Int 91:469, 2003

MOTZER R et al: Sequential dose-intensive paclitaxel, ifosfamide, carboplatin, and etoposide salvage therapy for germ cell tumor patients. J Clin Oncol 18:1173, 2000

83 GYNECOLOGIC MALIGNANCIES
Robert C. Young

OVARIAN CANCER

Incidence and Epidemiology Epithelial ovarian cancer is the leading cause of death from gynecologic cancer in the United States. In 2004, 25,580 new cases were diagnosed and 16,090 women died from ovarian cancer. The disease accounts for 5% of all cancer deaths in women in the United States; more women die of this disease than from cervical and endometrial cancer combined.

The age-specific incidence of the common epithelial type of ovarian cancer increases progressively and peaks in the eighth decade. Epithelial tumors, unlike germ cell and stromal tumors, are uncommon before the age of 40. Epidemiologic studies suggest higher incidences in industrialized nations and an association with disordered ovarian function, including infertility, nulliparity, frequent miscarriages, and use of ovulation-inducing drugs such as clomiphene. Each pregnancy reduces the ovarian cancer risk by about 10%, and breast-feeding and tubal ligation also appear to reduce the risk. Oral contraceptives reduce the risk of ovarian cancer in patients with a familial history of cancer and in the general population. Many of these risk-reduction factors support the "incessant ovulation" hypothesis for ovarian cancer etiology, which implies that an aberrant repair process of the surface epithelium is central to ovarian cancer development. Estrogen replacement after menopause does not appear to increase the risk of ovarian cancer, although one study showed a modest increase in risk with >11 years of use.

Familial cases account for about 5% of all ovarian cancer, and a family history of ovarian cancer is a major risk factor. Compared to a lifetime risk of 1.6% in the general population, women with one affected first-degree relative have a 5% risk. In families with two or more affected first-degree relatives, the risk may exceed 50%. Three types of autosomal dominant familial cancer are recognized: (1) site-specific, in which only ovarian cancer is seen; (2) families with cancer of the ovary and breast; and (3) the Lynch type II cancer family syndrome with nonpolyposis colorectal cancer, endometrial cancer, and ovarian cancer.

Etiology and Genetics In women with hereditary breast/ovarian cancer, two susceptibility loci have been identified: BRCA1, located on chromosome 17q12-21, and BRCA2, on 13q12-13. Both are tumor-suppressor genes, and their protein products act as inhibitors of tumor growth. Both genes are large, and numerous mutations have been described; most are frameshift or nonsense mutations, and 86% produce truncated protein products. The implications of the many other mutations including many missense mutations are not known. The cumulative risk of ovarian cancer with critical mutations of BRCA1 or -2 is 25%, compared to the lifetime risk of 50% for breast cancer for similar mutations. Men in such families have an increased risk of prostate cancer.

Cytogenetic analysis of sporadic epithelial ovarian cancers generally reveals complex karyotypic rearrangements. Structural abnormalities frequently appear on chromosomes 1 and 11, and loss of heterozygosity is common on 3q, 6q, 11q, 13q, and 17. Abnormalities of oncogenes are frequently found in ovarian cancer and include c-myc, H-ras, K-ras, and neu.

Ovarian tumors (usually not epithelial) are sometimes components of complex genetic syndromes. Peutz-Jeghers syndrome (mucocutaneous pigmentation and intestinal polyps) is associated with ovarian sex cord stromal tumors and Sertoli cell tumors in men. Patients with gonadal dysgenesis (46XY genotype or mosaic for Y-containing cell lines) develop gonadoblastomas, and women with nevoid basal cell carcinomas have an increased risk of ovarian fibromas.

Clinical Presentation and Differential Diagnosis Most patients with ovarian cancer are first diagnosed when the disease has already spread beyond the true pelvis. The occurrence of abdominal pain, bloating, and urinary symptoms usually indicates advanced disease. Localized ovarian cancer is generally asymptomatic. However, progressive enlargement of a localized ovarian tumor can produce urinary frequency or constipation, and rarely torsion of an ovarian mass causes acute abdominal pain or a surgical abdomen. In contrast to cervical or endometrial cancer, vaginal bleeding or discharge is rarely seen with early ovarian cancer. The diagnosis of early disease usually occurs with palpation of an asymptomatic adnexal mass during routine pelvic examination. However, most ovarian enlargements discovered this way, especially in premenopausal women, are benign functional cysts that characteristically resolve over one to three menstrual cycles. Adnexal masses in premenarchal or postmenopausal women are more likely to be pathologic. A solid, irregular, fixed pelvic mass is usually ovarian cancer. Other causes of adnexal masses include pedunculated uterine fibroids, endometriosis, benign ovarian neoplasms, and inflammatory lesions of the bowel.

Evaluation of patients with suspected ovarian cancer should include measurement of serum levels of the tumor marker CA-125. CA-125 determinants are glycoproteins with molecular masses from 220 to 1000 kDa, and a radioimmunoassay is used to determine circulating CA-125 antigen levels. Between 80 and 85% of patients with epithelial ovarian cancer have levels of CA-125 $\geq$ 35 U/mL. Other malignant tumors can also elevate CA-125 levels, including cancers of the endometrium, cervix, fallopian tubes, pancreas, breast, lung, and colon. Certain nonmalignant conditions that can produce moderate elevations of CA-125 levels include pregnancy, endometriosis, pelvic inflammatory disease, and uterine fibroids. About 1% of normal females have serum CA-125 levels >35 U/mL. However, in postmenopausal women with an asymptomatic pelvic mass and CA-125 levels $\geq$65 U/mL, the test has a sensitivity of 97% and a specificity of 78%.

Screening In contrast to patients who present with advanced disease, patients with early ovarian cancers (stages I and II) are commonly curable with conventional therapy. Thus, effective screening procedures would improve the cure rate in this disease. Although pelvic examination can occasionally detect early disease, it is a relatively insensitive screening procedure. Transvaginal sonography is often useful, but significant false-positive results are noted, particularly in premenopausal women. In one study, 67 laparotomies were required to diagnose 1 primary ovarian cancer. Doppler flow imaging coupled with transvaginal ultrasound may improve accuracy and reduce the high rate of false positives.

CA-125 has been studied as a screening tool. Unfortunately, half of women with stages I and II ovarian cancer have CA-125 levels <65 U/mL. Attempts have been made to improve the sensitivity and specificity by combinations of procedures, commonly transvaginal ultrasound and CA-125 levels. In a screening study of 22,000 women, 42 had a positive screen and 11 had ovarian cancer (7 with advanced disease). In addition, eight women with a negative screen developed ovarian cancer. Thus, the false-positive rate would lead to a large number of unnecessary (i.e., negative) laparotomies if each positive screen resulted in a surgical exploration. The National Institutes of Health Consensus Conference recommended against screening for ovarian cancer among the general population without known risk factors for the disease. Although no evidence shows that screening saves lives, many physicians use annual pelvic examinations, transvaginal ultrasound, and CA-125 levels to screen women with a family history of ovarian cancer or breast/ovarian cancer syndromes.

In one study, proteomic spectra in the serum analyzed by an iterative searching algorithm were used to identify women with ovarian cancer. Preliminary studies have identified all 50 stage I patients with a sensitivity of 100%, a specificity of 95%, and a positive predictive value of 94%. The procedure can be automated, requires a pinprick of blood, and has many characteristics of an ideal screening test. However, difficulty in consistency of replicate samples, variation in spectroscopy equipment, and the tendency of the artificial intelligence algorithms to overfit the data makes conformation studies necessary before widespread application to screening is warranted.

Pathology Common epithelial tumors comprise most (85%) of the ovarian neoplasms. These may be benign (50%), frankly malignant (33%), or tumors of low malignant potential (16%) (tumors of borderline malignancy). Epithelial tumors of low malignant potential have the cytologic features of malignancy but do not invade the ovarian stroma. More than 75% of borderline malignancies present in early stage and generally occur in younger women. They have a much better natural history than their malignant counterpart.

There are five major subtypes of common epithelial tumors: serous (50%), mucinous (25%), endometroid (15%), clear cell (5%), and Brenner tumors (1%), the latter derived from the urothelium. Benign common epithelial tumors are almost always serous or mucinous and develop in women ages 20 to 60. They are frequently large (20 to 30 cm), bilateral, and cystic.

Malignant epithelial tumors are usually seen in women over 40. They present as solid masses, with areas of necrosis and hemorrhage. Masses >10 to 15 cm have usually already spread into the intraabdominal space. Spread eventually results in intraabdominal carcinomatosis, which leads to bowel and renal obstruction and cachexia.

Although most ovarian tumors are epithelial, two other important ovarian tumor types exist—stromal and germ cell tumors. These tumors are distinct in their cell of origin but also have different clinical presentations and natural histories and are often managed differently (see below).

Metastasis to the ovary can occur from breast, colon, gastric, and pancreatic cancers, and the Krukenberg tumor was classically described as bilateral ovarian masses from metastatic mucin-secreting gastrointestinal cancers.

Staging and Prognostic Factors Laparotomy is often the primary procedure used to establish the diagnosis. Less invasive studies useful in defining the extent of spread include chest x-rays, abdominal computed tomography scans, and abdominal and pelvic sonography. If the woman has specific gastrointestinal symptoms, a barium enema or gastrointestinal series can be performed. Symptoms of bladder or renal dysfunction can be evaluated by cystoscopy or intravenous pyelography.

A careful staging laparotomy will establish the stage and extent of disease and allow for the cytoreduction of tumor masses in patients with advanced disease. Proper laparotomy requires a vertical incision of sufficient length to ensure adequate examination of the abdominal contents. The presence, amount, and cytology of any ascites fluid should be noted. The primary tumor should be evaluated for rupture, excrescences, or dense adherence. Careful visual and manual inspection of the diaphragm and peritoneal surfaces is required. In addition to total abdominal hysterectomy and bilateral salpingo-oophorectomy, a partial omentectomy should be performed and the paracolic gutters inspected. Pelvic lymph nodes as well as para-aortic nodes in the region of the renal hilus should be biopsied. Since this surgical procedure defines stage, establishes prognosis, and determines the necessity for subsequent therapy, it should be performed by a surgeon with special expertise in ovarian cancer staging. Studies have shown that patients operated upon by gynecologic oncologists were properly staged 97% of the time, compared to 52% and 35% of cases staged by obstetricians/gynecologists and general surgeons, respectively. At the end of staging, 23% of women have stage I disease (cancer confined to the ovary or ovaries); 13% have stage II (disease confined to the true pelvis); 47% have stage III (disease spread into but confined to the abdomen); and 16% have stage IV disease (spread outside the pelvis and abdomen). The 5-year survival correlates with stage of disease: stage I—90%, stage II—70%, stage III—15 to 20%, and stage IV—1 to 5% (Table 83-1).

Prognosis in ovarian cancer is dependent not only upon stage but on the extent of residual disease and histologic grade. Patients presenting with advanced disease but left without significant residual disease after surgery have a median survival of 39 months, compared to 17 months for those with suboptimal tumor resection.

Prognosis of epithelial tumors is also highly influenced by histologic grade but less so by histologic type. Although grading systems differ among pathologists, all grading systems show a better prognosis for well- or moderately differentiated tumors and a poorer prognosis for poorly differentiated histologies. Typical 5-year survivals for patients with all stages of disease are: well-differentiated—88%, moderately differentiated—58%, poorly differentiated—27%.

The prognostic significance of pre- and postoperative CA-125 levels is uncertain. Serum levels generally reflect volume of disease, and high levels usually indicate unresectability and a poorer survival. Postoperative levels, if elevated, usually indicate residual disease. The rate of decline of CA-125 levels during initial therapy or the absolute level after one to three cycles of chemotherapy correlates with prognosis but is not sufficiently accurate to guide individual treatment decisions. Even when the CA-125 level falls to normal after surgery or chemotherapy, "second-look" laparotomy identifies residual disease in 60% of women.

Genetic and biologic factors may influence prognosis. Increased tumor levels of p53 are associated with a worse prognosis in advanced disease. Epidermal growth factor receptors in ovarian cancer are associated with a high risk of progression, but the increased expression of HER-2/neu has given conflicting prognostic results, and expression of Mdr-1 has not been of prognostic value. HER-2/neu is highly expressed in 20% of ovarian cancers, and responses have been seen to trastuzumab in this subset of patients.

Rx TREATMENT

The selection of therapy for patients with epithelial ovarian cancer depends upon the stage, extent of residual tumor, and histologic grade. In general, patients are considered in three separate treatment groups: (1) those with early (stages I and II) ovarian cancer and microscopic or no residual disease; (2) patients with advanced (stage III) disease but minimal residual tumor (<1 cm) after initial surgery; and (3) patients with bulky residual tumor and advanced (stage III or IV) disease.

Patients with stage I disease, no residual tumor, and well or moderately differentiated tumors need no adjuvant therapy after definitive surgery, and 5-year survival exceeds 95%. For all other patients with early disease and those stage I patients with poor prognosis histologic grade, adjuvant therapy is probably warranted, and single-agent cisplatin or platinum-containing drug combinations improve survival by 8% (82% vs 76%, $p = .08$).

For the patients with advanced (stage III) disease but with limited or no residual disease after definitive cytoreductive surgery (about half of all stage III patients), the primary therapy is platinum-based combination chemotherapy. Approximately 70% of women respond to initial combination chemotherapy, and 40 to 50% have a complete regression of disease. Only about half of these patients are free of disease if surgically restaged. Although a variety of combinations are active, a randomized prospective trial of paclitaxel and cisplatin compared to paclitaxel and carboplatin in patients with optimally resected advanced disease demonstrated equivalent results (median time to progression 20.7 months vs 19.4 months, median survival 57.4 months vs 48.7 months) but with significantly reduced toxicity using carboplatin. This regimen of paclitaxel, 175 mg/m³ by 3-h infusion, and carboplatin, dosed to an AUC (area under the curve) of 7.5 is the treatment of choice for patients with previously untreated advanced-stage disease.

TABLE 83-1 *Staging and Survival in Gynecologic Malignancies*

Stage	Ovarian	5-Year Survival, %	Endometrial	5-Year Survival, %	Cervix	5-Year Survival, %
0	—		—		Carcinoma in situ	100
I	Confined to ovary	90	Confined to corpus	89	Confined to uterus	85
II	Confined to pelvis	70	Involves corpus and cervix	80	Invades beyond uterus but not to pelvic wall	60
III	Intraabdominal spread	15–20	Extends outside the uterus but not outside the true pelvis	30	Extends to pelvic wall and/or lower third of vagina, or hydronephrosis	33
IV	Spread outside abdomen	1–5	Extends outside the true pelvis or involves the bladder or rectum	9	Invades mucosa of bladder or rectum or extends beyond the true pelvis	7

Patients with advanced disease (stages III and IV) and bulky residual tumor are generally treated with a paclitaxel-platinum combination regimen as well and, while the overall prognosis is poorer, 5-year survival may reach 10 to 15%.

Historically, patients who had an excellent initial response to chemotherapy and no clinical evidence of disease have had a second-look laparotomy. For patients with stage I ovarian cancer or for germ cell tumors, the operation rarely detects residual tumor and has been largely abandoned. Even for those with stages II and III epithelial tumors, the second-look surgical procedure itself does not prolong overall survival. Its routine use cannot be recommended. Maintenance therapy (12 cycles of paclitaxel every 28 days) may extend progression-free survival among patients who achieve a complete response; an effect on overall survival has not yet been shown.

Patients with advanced disease whose disease recurs after initial treatment are usually not curable but may benefit significantly from limited surgery to relieve intestinal obstruction, localized radiation therapy to relieve pressure or pain from mass lesions or metastasis, or palliative chemotherapy. The selection of chemotherapy for palliation depends upon the initial regimen and evidence of drug resistance. Patients who have a complete regression of disease that lasts ≥6 months often respond to reinduction with the same agents. Patients relapsing within the first 6 months of initial therapy rarely do. Chemotherapeutic agents with >15% response rates in patients relapsing after initial combination chemotherapy include gemcitabine, topotecan, liposomal doxorubicin, and vinorelbine. Intraperitoneal chemotherapy (usually cisplatin) may be used if a small residual volume (<1 cm³) of tumor exists. Progestational agents and antiestrogens produce responses in 5 to 15% of patients and have minimal side effects.

Patients with tumor of low malignant potential, even with advanced-stage disease, have longer survivals when managed with surgery alone. The added value of radiation and chemotherapy has not been shown.

OVARIAN GERM CELL TUMORS Fewer than 5% of all ovarian tumors are germ cell in origin. They include teratoma, dysgerminoma, endodermal sinus tumor, and embryonal carcinoma. Germ cell tumors of the ovary generally occur in younger women (75% of ovarian malignancies in women <30), display an unusually aggressive natural history, and are commonly cured with less extensive nonsterilizing surgery and chemotherapy. Women cured of these malignancies are able to conceive and have normal children.

These neoplasms can be divided into three major groups: (1) benign tumors (usually dermoid cysts); (2) malignant tumors that arise from dermoid cysts; and (3) primitive malignant germ cell tumors including dysgerminoma, yolk sac tumors, immature teratomas, embryonal carcinomas, and choriocarcinoma.

Dermoid cysts are teratomatous cysts usually lined by epidermis and skin appendages. They often contain hair, and calcified bone or teeth can sometimes be seen on conventional pelvic x-ray. They are almost always curable by surgical resection. Approximately 1% of these tumors have malignant elements, usually squamous cell carcinoma.

Malignant germ cell tumors are usually large (median—16 cm). Bilateral disease is rare except in dysgerminoma (10 to 15% bilaterality). Abdominal or pelvic pain in young women is the usual presenting symptom. Serum human chorionic gonadotropin (β-hCG) and α fetoprotein levels are useful in the diagnosis and management of these patients. Before the advent of chemotherapy, extensive surgery was routine, but it has now been replaced by careful evaluation of extent of spread followed by resection of bulky disease and preservation of one ovary, uterus, and cervix, if feasible. This allows many affected women to preserve fertility. After surgical staging, 60 to 75% of women have stage I disease and 25 to 30% have stage III disease. Stages II and IV are infrequent.

Most of the malignant germ cell tumors are managed with chemotherapy after surgery. Regimens used in testicular cancer such as PVB (cisplatin, vinblastine, bleomycin) and BEP (bleomycin, 30 units IV weekly; etoposide, 100 mg/m² days 1 to 5; and cisplatin, 20 mg/m² days 1 to 5), with three or four courses given at 21-day intervals, have produced 95% long-term survival in patients with stages I to III disease. This regimen is the treatment of choice for all malignant germ cell tumors except grade I, stage I immature teratoma, where surgery alone is adequate, and perhaps early-stage dysgerminoma, where surgery and radiation therapy are used.

Dysgerminoma is the ovarian counterpart of testicular seminoma. The tumor is very sensitive to radiation therapy. The 5-year disease-free survival is 100% in early-stage patients and 61% in stage III disease. Unfortunately, the use of radiation therapy makes many patients infertile. BEP chemotherapy is equally or more effective and does not cause infertility. In incompletely resected patients with dysgerminoma, the 2-year disease-free survival is 95% and infertility is not observed. Combination chemotherapy (BEP) has replaced postoperative radiation therapy as the treatment of choice in women with ovarian dysgerminoma.

OVARIAN STROMAL TUMORS   Stromal tumors make up <10% of ovarian tumors. They are named for the stromal tissue involved: granulosa, theca, Sertoli, Leydig, and collagen-producing stromal cells. The granulosa and theca cell stromal cell tumors occur most frequently in the first three decades of life. Granulosa cell tumors frequently produce estrogen and cause menstrual abnormalities, bleeding, and precocious puberty. Endometrial carcinoma can be seen in 5% of these women, perhaps related to the persistent hyperestrogenism. Sertoli and Leydig cell tumors, when functional, produce androgens with resultant virilization or hirsutism. Some 75% of these stromal cell tumors present in stage I and can be cured with total abdominal hysterectomy and bilateral salpingo-oophorectomy. Stromal tumors generally grow slowly, and recurrences can occur 5 to 10 years after initial surgery. Neither radiation therapy nor chemotherapy have been documented to be consistently effective, and surgical management remains the primary treatment.

CARCINOMA OF THE FALLOPIAN TUBE

The fallopian tube is the least common site of cancer in the female genital tract, although its epithelial surface far exceeds that of the ovary, where epithelial cancer is 20 times more common. Approximately 300 new cases occur yearly; 90% are papillary serous adenocarcinomas, with the remainder being mixed mesodermal, endometroid, and transitional cell tumors. *BRCA1* and *-2* mutations are found in 7% of cases. The gross and microscopic characteristics and the spread of the tumor are similar to those of ovarian cancer but can be distinguished if the tumor arises from the endosalpinx where the tubal epithelium shows a transition between benign and malignant, and the ovaries and endometrium are normal or minimally involved.

The differential diagnosis includes primary or metastatic ovarian cancer, chronic salpingitis, tuberculous salpingitis, salpingitis isthmica nodosa, and cautery artifact.

Unlike patients with ovarian cancer, patients often present with early symptoms, usually postmenopausal vaginal bleeding, pain, and leukorrhea. Surgical staging is similar to that used for ovarian cancer, and prognosis is related to stage and extent of residual disease. Patients with stages I and II disease are generally treated with surgery alone or with surgery and pelvic radiation therapy, although radiation therapy does not clearly improve 5-year survival (5-year survival stage I: 74 versus 75%, stage II: 43 versus 48%). Patients with stages III and IV disease are treated with the same chemotherapy regimens used in advanced ovarian carcinoma, and 5-year survival is similar (stage III—20%, stage IV—5%).

UTERINE CANCER

Carcinoma of the endometrium is the most common female pelvic malignancy. Approximately 40,300 new cases are diagnosed yearly, although in most (75%), tumor is confined to the uterine corpus at diagnosis and therefore most can be cured. The 7,000 deaths yearly make uterine cancer only the eighth leading cause of cancer death in females. It is primarily a disease of postmenopausal women, although 25% of cases occur in women <age 50 and 5% <age 40. The disease is common in Eastern Europe and the United States and uncommon in Asia.

Phenotypic characteristics and risk factors common in patients with endometrial cancer include obesity, altered menstruation, low fertility index, late menopause, anovulation, and postmenopausal bleeding. Exposure to unopposed estrogen from either endogenous or exogenous sources may play a central etiologic role. Women taking tamoxifen for breast cancer treatment or prevention have a twofold increased risk.

Endometrial carcinoma occurs most often in the sixth and seventh decades of life. Symptoms often include abnormal vaginal discharge (90%); abnormal bleeding (80%), which is usually postmenopausal; and leukorrhea (10%). Evaluation of such patients should include a history and physical and pelvic examinations followed by an endometrial biopsy or a fractional dilation and curettage. Outpatient procedures such as endometrial biopsy or aspiration curettage can be used but are definitive only when positive.

Between 75 and 80% of all endometrial carcinomas are adenocarcinomas, and the prognosis depends upon stage, histologic grade, and extent of myometrial invasion. Grade I tumors are highly differentiated adenocarcinomas, grade II contain some solid areas, and grade III tumors are largely solid or undifferentiated. Adenocarcinoma with squamous differentiation is seen in 10% of patients; the most differentiated form is known as *adenoacanthoma*, and the poorly differentiated form is called *adenosquamous carcinoma*. Other less common pathologies include mucinous carcinoma (5%) and papillary serous carcinoma (<10%). This latter type has a natural history similar to ovarian carcinoma and should be managed as an ovarian cancer. Rarer histologies include secretory (2%), ciliated, clear cell, and undifferentiated carcinomas.

The staging of endometrial cancer requires surgery to establish the extent of disease and the depth of myometrial invasion. Peritoneal fluid should be sampled; the abdomen and pelvis explored; and pelvic and para-aortic lymphadenectomy performed depending upon the histology, grade, and depth of invasion in the uterine specimen on frozen section. After evaluation and staging, 74% of patients are stage I, 13% are stage II, 9% are stage III, and 3% are stage IV. Five-year survival by stage is as follows: stage I—89%, stage II—80%, stage III—30%, and stage IV—9% (Table 83-1).

Patients with uncomplicated endometrial carcinoma are effectively managed with total abdominal hysterectomy and bilateral salpingo-oophorectomy. Pre- or postoperative irradiation has been used, and although vaginal cuff recurrence is reduced, survival is not altered. In women with poor histologic grade, deep myometrial invasion, or extensive involvement of the lower uterine segment or cervix, intracavitary or external beam irradiation is warranted.

About 15% of women have endometrial carcinoma with extension to the cervix only (stage II), and management depends upon the extent of cervical invasion. Superficial cervical invasion can be managed like stage I disease, but extensive cervical invasion requires radical hysterectomy or preoperative radiotherapy followed by extrafascial hysterectomy. Once disease is outside the uterus but still confined to the true pelvis (stage III), management generally includes surgery and irradiation. Patients who have involvement only of the ovary or fallopian tubes generally do well with such therapy (5-year survivals of 80%). Other stage III patients with disease extending beyond the adnexa or those with serous carcinomas of the endometrium have a significantly poorer prognosis (5-year survival of 15%).

Patients with stage IV disease (outside the abdomen or invading the bladder or rectum) are treated palliatively with irradiation, surgery, and/or progestational agents. Progestational agents produce responses in about 25% of patients. Well-differentiated tumors respond most frequently, and response can be correlated with the level of progesterone receptor expression in the tumor. The commonly used progestational agents hydroxyprogesterone (Dilalutin), megastrol (Megace), and deoxyprogesterone (Provera) all produce similar response rates, and the antiestrogen tamoxifen (Nolvadex) produces responses in 10 to 25% of patients in a salvage setting.

Chemotherapy is not very successful in advanced endometrial carcinoma. The most active single agents with consistent response rates of ≥20% include cisplatin, carboplatin, doxorubicin, epirubicin, and paclitaxel. Combinations of drugs with or without progestational agents have generally produced response rates similar to single agents.

CERVIX CANCER Carcinoma of the cervix was once the most common cause of cancer death in women, but over the past 30 years, the mortality rate has decreased by 50% due to widespread screening with the Pap smear. In 2004, ~10,500 new cases of invasive cervix cancer occurred, and >50,000 cases of carcinoma in situ were detected. There were 3,900 deaths from the disease, and of those patients, ~85% had never had a Pap smear. It remains the major gynecologic cancer in underdeveloped countries. It is more common in lower socioeconomic groups, in women with early initial sexual activity and/or multiple sexual partners, and in smokers. Venereal transmission of human papilloma virus (HPV) has an important etiologic role. Over 66 types of HPVs have been isolated, and many are associated with genital warts. Those types associated with cervical carcinoma are 16, 18, 31, 45, and 51 to 53. These, along with many other types, are also associated with cervical intraepithelial neoplasia (CIN). The protein product of HPV-16, the E7 protein, binds and inactivates the tumor-suppressor gene Rb, and the E6 protein of HPV-18 has sequence homology to the SV40 large T antigen and has the capacity to bind and inactivate the tumor-suppressor gene p53. E6 and E7 are both necessary and sufficient to cause cell transformation in vitro. These binding and inactivation events may explain the carcinogenic effects of the viruses (Chap. 169).

Vaccination against pathologic HPV appears quite promising as a cervix cancer prevention strategy. The administration of HPV-16 vaccine in a double-blind study of 2392 women completely prevented infection with the virus, and no cases of HPV-16-related CIN were seen in vaccinated women. Although this vaccine is promising, polyvalent vaccines incorporating the known pathologic HPV virus types may ultimately be required.

Uncomplicated HPV lower genital tract infection and condylomatous atypia of the cervix can progress to CIN. This lesion precedes invasive cervical carcinoma and is classified as low-grade squamous intraepithelial lesion (SIL), high-grade SIL, and carcinoma in situ. Carcinoma in situ demonstrates cytologic evidence of neoplasia without invasion through the basement membrane, can persist unchanged for 10 to 20 years, but eventually progresses to invasive carcinoma.

The Pap smear is 90 to 95% accurate in detecting early lesions such as CIN but is less sensitive in detecting cancer when frankly invasive cancer or fungating masses are present. Inflammation, necrosis, and hemorrhage may produce false-positive smears, and colposcopic-directed biopsy is required when any lesion is visible on the cervix, regardless of Pap smear findings. The American Cancer Society recommends that women after onset of sexual activity, or >age 20, have two consecutive yearly smears. If negative, smears should be repeated every 3 years. The American College of Obstetrics and Gynecology recommends yearly Pap smears with routine annual pelvic and breast examinations. The Pap smear can be reported as normal (includes benign, reactive, or reparative changes); atypical squamous cells of undetermined significance (ASCUS) or cannot exclude high-grade SIL (ASC-H); low- or high-grade CIN; or frankly malignant. Women with ASCUS, ASC-H, or low-grade CIN should have repeat smears in 3 to 6 months and be tested for HPV. Women with high-grade CIN or frankly malignant Pap smears should have colposcopic-directed cervical biopsy. Colposcopy is a technique using a binocular microscope and 3% acetic acid applied to the cervix in which abnormal areas appear white and can be biopsied directly. Cone biopsy is still required when endocervical tumor is suspected, colposcopy is inadequate, the biopsy shows microinvasive carcinoma, or when a discrepancy is noted between the Pap smear and the colposcopic findings. Cone biopsy alone is therapeutic for CIN in many patients, although a less radical electrocautery excision may be sufficient.

Approximately 80% of invasive cervix cancers are squamous cell tumors, 10 to 15% are adenocarcinomas, 2 to 5% are adenosquamous with epithelial and glandular structures, and 1 to 2% are clear cell mesonephric tumors.

Patients with cervix cancer generally present with abnormal bleeding or postcoital spotting that may increase to intermenstrual or prominent menstrual bleeding. Yellowish vaginal discharge, lumbosacral back pain, and urinary symptoms can also be seen.

The staging of cervical carcinoma is clinical and generally completed with a pelvic examination under anesthesia with cystoscopy and proctoscopy. Chest x-rays, intravenous pyelograms, and computed tomography are generally required, and magnetic resonance imaging (MRI) may be used to assess extracervical extension. Stage 0 is carcinoma in situ, stage I is disease confined to the cervix, stage II disease invades beyond the cervix but not to the pelvic wall or lower third of the vagina, stage III disease extends to the pelvic wall or lower third of the vagina or causes hydronephrosis, stage IV is present when the tumor invades the mucosa of bladder or rectum or extends beyond the true pelvis. Five-year survivals are as follows: stage I—85%, stage II—60%, stage III—33%, and stage IV—7% (Table 83-1).

Carcinoma in situ (stage 0) can be managed successfully by cone biopsy or by abdominal hysterectomy. For stage I disease, results appear equivalent for either radical hysterectomy or radiation therapy. Patients with stages II to IV disease are primarily managed with radical radiation therapy or combined modality therapy. Retroperitoneal lymphadenectomy has no proven therapeutic role. Pelvic exenterations, although uncommon, are performed for centrally recurrent or persistent disease. Reconstruction of the vagina, bladder, and rectum can often be done following this operation.

In women with locally advanced disease (stages IIB to IVA), platinum-based chemotherapy given concomitantly with radiation therapy improves survival compared to radiation therapy alone. Cisplatin, 75 mg/m² over 4 h, followed by 5-fluorouracil (5-FU), 4 g given by 96-h infusion on days 1 to 5 of radiation therapy, is a common regimen. Two additional cycles of chemotherapy are given at 3-week intervals. Concurrent chemoradiotherapy reduced the risk of recurrence by 30 to 50% across a wide spectrum of stages and presentations and is the treatment of choice in stages IIB to IV cervix cancer.

Chemotherapy has been used in patients with unresectable advanced disease or recurrent disease. Active agents with ≥20% response rates include cisplatin, 5-FU, ifosfamide, and irinotecan. No combination of agents has proved better than single agents. Intraarterial chemotherapy has been studied, either pre- or postoperatively, but is associated with substantial local toxicity and response rates of 20%.

GESTATIONAL TROPHOBLASTIC NEOPLASIA

Gestational trophoblastic diseases are a group of interrelated diseases that form a spectrum from benign hydatidiform mole to trophoblastic malignancy (placental-site trophoblastic tumor and choriocarcinoma). Malignant forms account for <1% of female gynecologic malignancies and can be cured with appropriate chemotherapy. Deaths from this disease have become rare in the United States.

Epidemiology The incidence is about 1 per 1500 pregnancies in the United States and is nearly tenfold higher in Asia. Maternal age >45 years is a risk factor for hydatidiform mole. A prior history of molar pregnancy is also a risk factor. Choriocarcinoma occurs in ~1 in 25,000 pregnancies or 1 in 20,000 live births. Prior history of hydatidiform mole is a risk factor for choriocarcinoma. A woman with a molar pregnancy is 1000 times more likely to develop choriocarcinoma than a woman with a prior normal-term pregnancy.

Pathology and Etiology The trophoblastic neoplasms have been divided by morphology into complete or partial hydatidiform mole, invasive mole, placental-site trophoblastomas, and choriocarcinomas. Hydatidiform moles contain clusters of villi with hydropic changes, hyperplasia of the trophoblast, and the absence of fetal vessels. Invasive moles differ only by invasion into the uterine myometrium. Placental-site trophoblastic tumors are predominately made up of cytotrophoblast cells arising from the placental implantation site. Choriocarcinomas consist of anaplastic trophoblastic tissue with both cytotrophoblastic and syncytiotrophoblastic elements and no identifiable villi.

Complete moles result from uniparental disomy in which loss of the maternal genes (23 autosomes plus X) occurs by unknown mechanisms and is followed by duplication of the paternal haploid genome (23 autosomes plus X). Uncommonly (5%), moles result from dispermic fertilization of an empty egg, resulting in either 46XY or 46XX genotype. Partial moles result from dispermic fertilization of an egg with retention of the maternal haploid set of chromosomes, resulting in diandric triploidy (Chap. 56).

Clinical Presentation Molar pregnancies are generally associated with first-trimester bleeding, ectopic pregnancies, or threatened abortions. The uterus is inappropriately large for the length of gestation, and β-hCG levels are higher than expected. Fetal parts and heart sounds are not present. The diagnosis is generally made by the passage of grape-like clusters from the uterus, but ultrasound demonstration of the hydropic mole can be diagnostic. Patients suspected of a molar pregnancy require a chest film, careful pelvic examinations, and weekly serial monitoring of β-hCG levels.

℞ TREATMENT

Patients with hydatidiform moles require suction curettage coupled with postevacuation monitoring of β-hCG levels. In most women (80%), the β-hCG titer progressively declines within 8 to 10 days of evacuation (serum half-life is 24 to 36 h). Patients should be monitored on a monthly basis and should not become pregnant for at least a year.

Patients found to have invasive mole at curettage are generally treated with hysterectomy and chemotherapy. Approximately half of patients with choriocarcinoma develop the malignancy after a molar pregnancy, and the other half develop the malignancy after abortion, ectopic pregnancy, or occasionally after a normal full-term pregnancy.

Chemotherapy is generally used for gestational trophoblastic neoplasia and is often used in hydatidiform mole if β-hCG levels rise or plateau or if metastases develop. Patients with invasive mole or choriocarcinoma require chemotherapy. Several regimens are effective, including methotrexate at 30 mg/m² intramuscularly on a weekly basis until β-hCG titers are normal. However, methotrexate (1 mg/kg) every other day for 4 days followed by leukovorin (0.1 mg/kg) intravenously 24 h after methotrexate is associated with a cure rate of ≥90% and low toxicity. Intermittent courses are continued until the β-hCG titer becomes undetectable for 3 consecutive weeks, and then patients are monitored monthly for a year.

Patients with high-risk tumors (high β-hCG levels, disease presenting ≥4 months after antecedent pregnancy, brain or liver metastasis, or failure of single-agent methotrexate) are initially treated with combination chemotherapy. EMA-CO (a cyclic non-cross-resistant combination of etoposide, methotrexate, and dactinomycin alternating with cyclophosphamide and vincristine); cisplatin, bleomycin, and vinblastine; and cisplatin, etoposide, and bleomycin are effective regimens. EMA-CO is now the regimen of choice for patients with high-risk disease because of excellent survival rates (>80%) and less toxicity. The use of etoposide carries a 1.5% lifetime risk of acute myeloid leukemia (16-fold relative risk). Because of this problem, etoposide-containing regimens should be reserved for patients with high-risk features. Patients with brain or liver metastases are usually treated with local irradiation to metastatic sites in conjunction with chemotherapy. Long-term studies of patients cured of trophoblastic disease have not demonstrated an increased risk of maternal complications or fetal abnormalities with subsequent pregnancies.

FURTHER READING

JACOBS IJ: Screening for ovarian cancer: A pilot randomized trial. Lancet 353: 1207, 1999

KOUTSKY LA: A controlled trial of a human papilloma virus type 16 vaccine. N Engl J Med 347:1645, 2002

MARKMAN M et al: Phase III randomized trial of 12 versus 3 months of maintenance paclitaxel in patients with advanced ovarian cancer after complete response to platinum and paclitaxel-based chemotherapy: A Southwest Oncology Group and Gynecologic Oncology Group Trial. J Clin Oncol 21: 2460, 2003

MORRIS M et al: Pelvic radiation with concurrent chemotherapy compared with pelvic and para-aortic radiation for high-risk cervical cancer. N Engl J Med 340:1137, 1999

PETRICOIN EF et al: Use of proteomic patterns in serum to identify ovarian cancer. Lancet 359:572, 2002

SOLOMON D et al: The 2001 Bethesda System. JAMA 287:2114, 2002

STEHMAN FB et al: Innovations in the treatment of invasive cervical cancer. Cancer 98:2052, 2003

WRIGHT JD, MUTCH DG: Treatment of high-risk gestational trophoblastic tumors. Clin Obstet Gynecol 46:593, 2003

84 SOFT TISSUE AND BONE SARCOMAS AND BONE METASTASES
Shreyaskumar R. Patel, Robert S. Benjamin

Sarcomas are rare (<1% of all malignancies) mesenchymal neoplasms that arise in bone and soft tissues. These tumors are usually of mesodermal origin, although a few are derived from neuroectoderm, and they are biologically distinct from the more common epithelial malignancies. Sarcomas affect all age groups; 15% are found in children <15 years and 40% occur after age 55. Sarcomas are one of the most common solid tumors of childhood and are the fifth most common cause of cancer deaths in children. Sarcomas may be divided into two groups, those derived from bone and those derived from soft tissues.

SOFT TISSUE SARCOMAS

Soft tissues include muscles, tendons, fat, fibrous tissue, synovial tissue, vessels, and nerves. Approximately 60% of soft tissue sarcomas arise in the extremities, with the lower extremities involved three times as often as the upper extremities. Thirty percent arise in the trunk, the retroperitoneum accounting for 40% of all trunk lesions. The remaining 10% arise in the head and neck.

INCIDENCE   Approximately 8680 new cases of soft tissue sarcomas occurred in the United States in 2004. The annual age-adjusted incidence is ~2 per 100,000 population, but the incidence varies with age. Soft tissue sarcomas constitute 0.7% of all cancers in the general population and 6.5% of all cancers in children.

EPIDEMIOLOGY   Malignant transformation of a benign soft tissue tumor is extremely rare, with the exception that malignant peripheral nerve sheath tumors (neurofibrosarcoma, malignant schwannoma) can arise from neurofibromas in patients with neurofibromatosis. Several etiologic factors have been implicated in soft tissue sarcomas.

Environmental Factors   Trauma or previous injury is rarely involved, but sarcomas can arise in scar tissue resulting from a prior operation, burn, fracture, or foreign body implantation. Chemical carcinogens such as polycyclic hydrocarbons, asbestos, and dioxin may be involved in the pathogenesis.

Iatrogenic Factors   Sarcomas in bone or soft tissues occur in patients who are treated with radiation therapy. The tumor nearly always arises in the irradiated field. The risk increases with time.

Viruses   Kaposi's sarcoma (KS) in patients with HIV type 1, classic KS, and KS in HIV-negative homosexual men is caused by human herpes virus (HHV) 8 (Chap. 166). No other sarcomas are associated with viruses.

Immunologic Factors   Congenital or acquired immunodeficiency, including therapeutic immunosuppression, increases the risk of sarcoma.

Genetic Factors   Li-Fraumeni syndrome is a familial cancer syndrome in which affected individuals have germ-line abnormalities of the tumor-suppressor gene p53 and an increased incidence of soft tissue sarcomas and other malignancies, including breast cancer, osteosarcoma, brain tumor, leukemia, and adrenal carcinoma (Chap. 68). Neurofibromatosis 1 (NF-1, peripheral form, von Recklinghausen's disease) is characterized by multiple neurofibromas and café au lait spots. Neurofibromas occasionally undergo malignant degeneration to become malignant peripheral nerve sheath tumors. The gene for NF-1 is located in the pericentromeric region of chromosome 17 and encodes neurofibromin, a tumor-suppressor protein with GTPase-activating activity that inhibits Ras function (Chap. 358). Germ-line mutation of the *Rb-1* locus (chromosome 13q14) in patients with inherited retinoblastoma is associated with the development of osteosarcoma in those who survive the retinoblastoma and of soft tissue sarcomas unrelated to radiation therapy. Other soft tissue tumors, including desmoid tumors, lipomas, leiomyomas, neuroblastomas, and paragangliomas, occasionally show a familial predisposition.

Ninety percent of synovial sarcomas contain a characteristic chromosomal translocation t(X;18) (p11;q11) involving a nuclear transcription factor on chromosome 18 called *SYT* and two breakpoints on X. Patients with translocations to the second X breakpoint (*SSX2*) may have longer survival than those with translocations involving *SSX1*.

Insulin-like growth factor (IGF) type 2 is produced by some sarcomas and may act as an autocrine growth factor and as a motility factor that promotes metastatic spread. IGF-2 stimulates growth through IGF-1 receptors but its effects on motility are through different receptors. If secreted in large amounts, IGF-2 may produce hypoglycemia (Chaps. 86 and 324).

CLASSIFICATION   Approximately 20 different groups of sarcomas are recognized on the basis of the pattern of differentiation toward normal tissue. For example, rhabdomyosarcoma shows evidence of skeletal muscle fibers with cross-striations; leiomyosarcomas contain interlacing fascicles of spindle cells resembling smooth muscle; and liposarcomas contain adipocytes. When precise characterization of the group is not possible, the tumors are called *unclassified sarcomas*. All of the primary bone sarcomas can also arise from soft tissues (e.g., extraskeletal osteosarcoma). The entity *malignant fibrous histiocytoma* includes many tumors previously classified as fibrosarcomas or as pleomorphic variants of other sarcomas and is characterized by a mixture of spindle (fibrous) cells and round (histiocytic) cells arranged in a storiform pattern with frequent giant cells and areas of pleomorphism.

For purposes of treatment, most soft tissue sarcomas can be considered together. However, some specific tumors have distinct features. For example, *liposarcoma* can have a spectrum of behaviors. Pleomorphic liposarcomas and dedifferentiated liposarcomas behave like other high-grade sarcomas; in contrast, well-differentiated liposarcomas (better termed *atypical lipomatous tumors*) lack metastatic potential, and myxoid liposarcomas metastasize infrequently but, when they do, have a predilection for unusual metastatic sites containing fat, such as the retroperitoneum, mediastinum, and subcutaneous tissue. Rhabdomyosarcomas, Ewing's sarcoma, and other small-cell sarcomas tend to be more aggressive and are more responsive to chemotherapy than other soft tissue sarcomas.

Gastrointestinal stromal cell tumors (GISTs), previously classified as gastrointestinal leiomyosarcomas, are now recognized as a distinct entity within soft tissue sarcomas. Its cell of origin resembles the interstitial cell of Cajal, which controls peristalsis. The majority of malignant GISTs have activating mutations of the c-*kit* gene that result in ligand-independent phosphorylation and activation of the KIT receptor tyrosine kinase, leading to tumorigenesis.

DIAGNOSIS   The most common presentation is an asymptomatic mass. Mechanical symptoms referable to pressure, traction, or entrapment of nerves or muscles may be present. All new and persistent or growing masses should be biopsied, either by a cutting needle (core-needle biopsy) or by a small incision, placed so that it can be encompassed in the subsequent excision without compromising a definitive resection. Lymph node metastases occur in 5%, except in synovial and epithelioid sarcomas, clear-cell sarcoma (melanoma of the soft parts), angiosarcoma, and rhabdomyosarcoma, where nodal spread may be seen in 17%. The pulmonary parenchyma is the most common site of metastases. Exceptions are GISTs, which metastasize to the liver; myxoid liposarcomas, which seek fatty tissue: and clear-cell sarcomas, which may metastasize to bones. Central nervous system metastases are rare, except in alveolar soft part sarcoma.

Radiographic Evaluation   Imaging of the primary tumor is best with plain radiographs and magnetic resonance imaging (MRI) for tumors of the extremities or head and neck and by computed tomography (CT) for tumors of the chest, abdomen, or retroperitoneal cavity. A radiograph and CT scan of the chest are important for the detection of lung metastases. Other imaging studies may be indicated, depending on the symptoms, signs, or histology.

STAGING AND PROGNOSIS   The histologic grade, relationship to fascial planes, and size of the primary tumor are the most important prognostic factors. The current American Joint Commission on Cancer (AJCC) staging system is shown in Table 84-1. Prognosis is related to the stage. Cure is common in the absence of metastatic disease, but a small number of patients with metastases can also be cured. Most patients with stage IV disease die within 12 months, but some patients may live with slowly progressive disease for many years.

Rx TREATMENT

AJCC stage I patients are adequately treated with surgery alone. Stage II patients are considered for adjuvant radiation therapy. Stage III patients may benefit from adjuvant chemotherapy. Stage IV patients are managed primarily with chemotherapy with or without other modalities.

Surgery   Soft tissue sarcomas tend to grow along fascial planes, with the surrounding soft tissues compressed to form a pseudocapsule that gives the sarcoma the appearance of a well-encapsulated lesion. This is invariably deceptive, because "shelling out" or marginal excision of

TABLE 84-1 AJCC Staging System for Sarcomas

Histologic Grade (G)	Tumor Size (T)	Node Status (N)	Metastases (M)
Well differentiated (G1)	≤5 cm (T1)	Not involved (N0)	Absent (M0)
Moderately differentiated (G2)	>5 cm (T2)	Involved (N1)	Present (M1)
Poorly differentiated (G3)	Superficial fascial involvement (Ta)		
Undifferentiated (G4)	Deep fascial involvement (Tb)		

Disease Stage	5-Year Survival, %
Stage I	98.8
A: G1,2; T1a,b; N0; M0	
B: G1,2; T2a; N0; M0	
Stage II	81.8
A: G1,2; T2b; N0; M0	
B: G3,4; T1; N0; M0	
C: G3,4; T2a; N0; M0	
Stage III G3,4; T2b; N0; M0	51.7
Stage IV	<20
A: any G; any T; N1; M0	
B: any G; any T; any N; M1	

such lesions results in a 50 to 90% probability of local recurrence. Wide excision with a negative margin, incorporating the biopsy site, is the standard surgical procedure for local disease. The adjuvant use of radiation therapy and/or chemotherapy improves the local control rate and permits the use of limb-sparing surgery with a local control rate (85 to 90%) comparable to that achieved by radical excisions and amputations. Limb-sparing approaches are indicated except when negative margins are not obtainable, when the risks of radiation are prohibitive, or when neurovascular structures are involved so that resection will result in serious functional consequences to the limb.

Radiation Therapy External beam radiation therapy is an adjuvant to limb-sparing surgery for improved local control. Preoperative radiation therapy allows the use of smaller fields and smaller doses but results in a higher rate of wound complications. Postoperative radiation therapy must be given to larger fields, as the entire surgical bed must be encompassed, and in higher doses to compensate for hypoxia in the operated field. Brachytherapy or interstitial therapy, in which the radiation source is inserted into the tumor bed, is comparable in efficacy (except in low-grade lesions), less time consuming, and less expensive.

Adjuvant Chemotherapy Chemotherapy is the mainstay of treatment for Ewing's primitive neuroectodermal tumors (PNET) and rhabdomyosarcomas. Meta-analysis of 14 randomized trials revealed a highly significant improvement in local control and disease-free survival in favor of doxorubicin-based chemotherapy. Overall survival is improved only for extremity sarcomas, however. A chemotherapy regimen including an anthracycline and ifosfamide with growth factor support improved overall survival for high-risk (high-grade, ≥5 cm primary, or locally recurrent) extremity soft tissue sarcomas.

Advanced Disease Metastatic soft tissue sarcomas are largely incurable, but up to 20% of patients who achieve a complete response become long-term survivors. The therapeutic intent, therefore, is to produce a complete remission with chemotherapy and/or surgery. Surgical resection of metastases, whenever possible, is an integral part of the management. Some patients benefit from repeated surgical excision of metastases. The two most active chemotherapeutic agents are doxorubicin and ifosfamide. These drugs show a steep dose-response relationship in sarcomas. Gemcitabine and dacarbazine also have some activity. Taxanes have selective activity in angiosarcomas, and vincristine, etoposide, and irinotecan are effective in rhabdomyosarcomas and Ewing's sarcomas. Imatinib mesylate targets the KIT tyrosine kinase activity and is standard therapy for advanced/metastatic GISTs.

BONE SARCOMAS

INCIDENCE AND EPIDEMIOLOGY Bone sarcomas are rarer than soft tissue sarcomas; they accounted for only 0.2% of all new malignancies and ~2400 new cases in the United States in 2004. Several benign bone lesions have the potential for malignant transformation. Enchondromas and osteochondromas can transform into chondrosarcoma; fibrous dysplasia, bone infarcts, and Paget's disease of bone can transform into either malignant fibrous histiocytoma or osteosarcoma.

CLASSIFICATION ■ Benign Tumors The common benign bone tumors include enchondroma, osteochondroma, chondroblastoma, and chondromyxoid fibroma, of cartilage origin; osteoid osteoma and osteoblastoma, of bone origin; fibroma and desmoplastic fibroma, of fibrous tissue origin; hemangioma, of vascular origin; and giant cell tumor, of unknown origin.

Malignant Tumors The most common malignant tumors of bone are plasma cell tumors (Chap. 98). The four most common malignant nonhematopoietic bone tumors are osteosarcoma, chondrosarcoma, Ewing's sarcoma, and malignant fibrous histiocytoma. Rare malignant tumors include chordoma (of notochordal origin), malignant giant cell tumor and adamantinoma (of unknown origin), and hemangioendothelioma (of vascular origin).

Musculoskeletal Tumor Society Staging System Sarcomas of bone are staged according to the Musculoskeletal Tumor Society staging system based on grade and compartmental localization. A Roman numeral reflects the tumor grade: stage I is low-grade, stage II is high-grade, and stage III includes tumors of any grade that have lymph node or distant metastases. In addition, the tumor is given a letter reflecting its compartmental localization. Tumors designated A are intracompartmental (i.e., confined to the same soft tissue compartment as the initial tumor), and tumors designated B are extracompartmental (i.e., extending into the adjacent soft tissue compartment or into bone). The tumor node metastasis (TNM) staging system is shown in Table 84-2.

TABLE 84-2 Staging System for Bone Sarcomas

Primary tumor (T)	TX	Primary tumor cannot be assessed
	T0	No evidence of primary tumor
	T1	Tumor ≤8 cm in greatest dimension
	T2	Tumor >8 cm in greatest dimension
	T3	Discontinuous tumors in the primary bone site
Regional lymph nodes (N)	NX	Regional lymph nodes cannot be assessed
	N0	No regional lymph node metastasis
	N1	Regional lymph node metastasis
Distant metastasis (M)	MX	Distant metastasis cannot be assessed
	M0	No distant metastasis
	M1	Distant metastasis
	M1a	Lung
	M1b	Other distant sites
Histologic grade (G)	GX	Grade cannot be assessed
	G1	Well differentiated—low grade
	G2	Moderately differentiated—low grade
	G3	Poorly differentiated—high grade
	G4	Undifferentiated—high grade (Ewing's is always classed G4)

STAGE GROUPING

Stage IA	T1	N0	M0	G1,2 low grade
Stage IB	T2	N0	M0	G1,2 low grade
Stage IIA	T1	N0	M0	G3,4 high grade
Stage IIB	T2	N0	M0	G3,4 high grade
Stage III	T3	N0	M0	Any G
Stage IVA	Any T	N0	M1a	Any G
Stage IVB	Any T	N1	Any M	Any G
	Any T	Any N	M1b	Any G

OSTEOSARCOMA Osteosarcoma, accounting for almost 45% of all bone sarcomas, is a spindle cell neoplasm that produces osteoid (unmineralized bone) or bone. About 60% of all osteosarcomas occur in children and adolescents in the second decade of life, and about 10% occur in the third decade of life. Osteosarcomas in the fifth and sixth decades of life are frequently secondary to either radiation therapy or transformation in a preexisting benign condition, such as Paget's disease. Males are affected 1.5 to 2 times as often as females. Osteosarcoma has a predilection for metaphyses of long bones; the most common sites of involvement are the distal femur, proximal tibia, and proximal humerus. The classification of osteosarcoma is complex, but 75% of osteosarcomas fall in the "classic" category, which include osteoblastic, chondroblastic, and fibroblastic osteosarcomas. The remaining 25% are classified as "variants" on the basis of (1) clinical characteristics, as in the case of osteosarcoma of the jaw, postradiation osteosarcoma, or Paget's osteosarcoma; (2) morphologic characteristics, as in the case of telangiectatic osteosarcoma, small-cell osteosarcoma, or epithelioid osteosarcoma; or (3) location, as in parosteal or periosteal osteosarcoma. Diagnosis usually requires a synthesis of clinical, radiologic, and pathologic features. Patients typically present with pain and swelling of the affected area. A plain radiograph reveals a destructive lesion with a moth-eaten appearance, a spiculated periosteal reaction (sunburst appearance), and a cuff of periosteal new bone formation at the margin of the soft tissue mass (Codman's triangle). A CT scan of the primary tumor is best for defining bone destruction and the pattern of calcification, whereas MRI is better for defining intramedullary and soft tissue extension. A chest radiograph and CT scan are used to detect lung metastases. Metastases to the bony skeleton should be imaged by a bone scan. Almost all osteosarcomas are hypervascular. Angiography is not helpful for diagnosis, but it is the most sensitive test for assessing the response to preoperative chemotherapy. Pathologic diagnosis is established either with a core-needle biopsy, where feasible, or with an open biopsy with an appropriately placed incision that does not compromise future limb-sparing resection. Most osteosarcomas are high-grade. The most important prognostic factor for long-term survival is response to chemotherapy. Preoperative chemotherapy followed by limb-sparing surgery (which can be accomplished in >80% of patients) followed by postoperative chemotherapy is standard management. The effective drugs are doxorubicin, ifosfamide, cisplatin, and high-dose methotrexate with leucovorin rescue. The various combinations of these agents that have been used have all been about equally successful. Long-term survival rates in extremity osteosarcoma range from 60 to 80%. Osteosarcoma is radioresistant; radiation therapy has no role in the routine management. Malignant fibrous histiocytoma is considered a part of the spectrum of osteosarcoma and is managed similarly.

CHONDROSARCOMA Chondrosarcoma, which constitutes ~20 to 25% of all bone sarcomas, is a tumor of adulthood and old age with a peak incidence in the fourth to sixth decades of life. It has a predilection for the flat bones, especially the shoulder and pelvic girdles, but can also affect the diaphyseal portions of long bones. Chondrosarcomas can arise de novo or as a malignant transformation of an enchondroma or, rarely, of the cartilaginous cap of an osteochondroma. Chondrosarcomas have an indolent natural history and typically present as pain and swelling. Radiographically, the lesion may have a lobular appearance with mottled or punctate or annular calcification of the cartilaginous matrix. It is difficult to distinguish low-grade chondrosarcoma from benign lesions by x-ray or histologic examination. The diagnosis is therefore influenced by clinical history and physical examination. A new onset of pain, signs of inflammation, and progressive increase in the size of the mass suggest malignancy. The histologic classification is complex, but most tumors fall within the classic category. Like other bone sarcomas, high-grade chondrosarcomas spread to the lungs. Most chondrosarcomas are resistant to chemotherapy, and surgical resection of primary or recurrent tumors, including pulmonary metastases, is the mainstay of therapy. There are two histologic variants for which this rule does not hold, however. Dedifferentiated chondrosarcoma has a

high-grade osteosarcoma or a malignant fibrous histiocytoma component that responds to chemotherapy. Mesenchymal chondrosarcoma, a rare variant composed of a small cell element, also is responsive to systemic chemotherapy and is treated like Ewing's sarcoma.

EWING'S SARCOMA Ewing's sarcoma, which constitutes ~10 to 15% of all bone sarcomas, is common in adolescence and has a peak incidence in the second decade of life. It typically involves the diaphyseal region of long bones and also has an affinity for flat bones. The plain radiograph may show a characteristic "onion peel" periosteal reaction with a generous soft tissue mass, which is better demonstrated by CT or MRI. This mass is composed of sheets of monotonous, small, round, blue cells and can be confused with lymphoma, embryonal rhabdomyosarcoma, and small-cell carcinoma. The presence of p30/32, the product of the *mic-2* gene (which maps to the pseudoautosomal region of the X and Y chromosomes) is a cell-surface marker for Ewing's sarcoma (and other members of a family of tumors called PNETs). Most PNETs arise in soft tissues; they include peripheral neuroepithelioma, Askin's tumor (chest wall), and esthesioneuroblastoma. Glycogen-filled cytoplasm detected by staining with periodic acid–Schiff is also characteristic of Ewing's sarcoma cells. The classic cytogenetic abnormality associated with this disease (and other PNETs) is a reciprocal translocation of the long arms of chromosomes 11 and 22, t(11; 22), which creates a chimeric gene product of unknown function with components from the *fli-1* gene on chromosome 11 and *ews* on 22. This disease is very aggressive, and it is therefore considered a systemic disease. Common sites of metastases are lung, bones, and bone marrow. Systemic chemotherapy is the mainstay of therapy, often being used before surgery. Doxorubicin, cyclophosphamide or ifosfamide, etoposide, vincristine, and dactinomycin are active drugs. Local treatment for the primary tumor includes surgical resection, usually with limb salvage or radiation therapy. Patients with lesions below the elbow and below the mid-calf have a 5-year survival rate of 80% with effective treatment. Ewing's sarcoma is a curable tumor, even in the presence of obvious metastatic disease, especially in children <11 years old.

TUMORS METASTATIC TO BONE

Bone is a common site of metastasis for carcinomas of the prostate, breast, lung, kidney, bladder, and thyroid and for lymphomas and sarcomas. Prostate, breast, and lung primaries account for 80% of all bone metastases. Metastatic tumors of bone are more common than primary bone tumors. Tumors usually spread to bone hematogenously, but local invasion from soft tissue masses also occurs. In descending order of frequency, the sites most often involved are the vertebrae, proximal femur, pelvis, ribs, sternum, proximal humerus, and skull. Bone metastases may be asymptomatic or may produce pain, swelling, nerve root or spinal cord compression, pathologic fracture, or myelophthisis (replacement of the marrow). Symptoms of hypercalcemia may be noted in cases of bony destruction.

Pain is the most frequent symptom. It usually develops gradually over weeks, is usually localized, and often is more severe at night. When patients with back pain develop neurologic signs or symptoms, emergency evaluation for spinal cord compression is indicated (Chap. 88). Bone metastases exert a major adverse effect on quality of life in cancer patients.

Cancer in the bone may produce osteolysis, osteogenesis, or both. Osteolytic lesions result when the tumor produces substances that can directly elicit bone resorption (vitamin D–like steroids, prostaglandins, or parathyroid hormone–related peptide) or cytokines that can induce the formation of osteoclasts (interleukin 1 and tumor necrosis factor). Osteoblastic lesions result when the tumor produces cytokines that activate osteoblasts. In general, purely osteolytic lesions are best detected by plain radiography, but they may not be apparent until they are >1 cm. These lesions are more commonly associated with hypercalcemia and with the excretion of hydroxyproline-containing peptides indicative of matrix destruction. When osteoblastic activity is prominent, the lesions may be readily detected using radionuclide bone scanning (which is sensitive to new bone formation), and the radiographic appearance may show increased bone density or sclerosis. Osteoblastic lesions are associated with higher serum levels of alkaline phosphatase, and, if extensive, may produce hypocalcemia. Although some tumors may produce mainly osteolytic lesions (e.g., kidney cancer) and others mainly osteoblastic lesions (e.g., prostate cancer), most metastatic lesions produce both types of lesion and may go through stages where one or the other predominates.

In older patients, particularly women, it may be necessary to distinguish metastatic disease of the spine from osteoporosis. In osteoporosis, the cortical bone may be preserved, whereas cortical bone destruction is usually noted with metastatic cancer.

R̽ TREATMENT

Treatment of metastatic bone disease depends on the underlying malignancy and the symptoms. Some metastatic bone tumors are curable (lymphoma, Hodgkin's disease), and others are treated with palliative intent. Pain may be relieved by local radiation therapy. Hormonally responsive tumors are responsive to hormone inhibition (antiandro-

gens for prostate cancer, antiestrogens for breast cancer). Strontium 89 and samarium 153 are bone-seeking radionuclides that can exert antitumor effects and relieve symptoms. Bisphosphonates such as pamidronate may relieve pain and inhibit bone resorption. Monthly administration prevents bone-related clinical events and may reduce the incidence of bone metastases in women with breast cancer. When the integrity of a weight-bearing bone is threatened by an expanding metastatic lesion that is refractory to radiation therapy, prophylactic internal fixation is indicated. Overall survival is related to the prognosis of the underlying tumor. Bone pain at the end of life is particularly common; an adequate pain relief regimen including sufficient amounts of narcotic analgesics is required. →*The management of hypercalcemia is discussed in Chap. 332.*

FURTHER READING

BORDEN EC et al: Soft tissue sarcomas of adults: State of the translational science. Clin Cancer Res 9:1941, 2003

DEMETRI GD et al: Efficacy and safety of imatinib mesylate in advanced gastrointestinal stromal tumors. N Engl J Med 347:472, 2002

FRUSTACI S et al: Adjuvant chemotherapy for adult soft tissue sarcomas of the extremities and girdles: Results of the Italian Randomized Cooperative Group trial. J Clin Oncol 19:1238, 2001

HELMAN LJ, MELTZER P: Mechanisms of sarcoma development. Nat Rev Cancer 3:685, 2003

WITTIG JC et al: Osteosarcoma: A multidisciplinary approach to diagnosis and treatment. Am Fam Physician 65:1123, 2002

85 METASTATIC CANCER OF UNKNOWN PRIMARY SITE
Richard M. Stone

INCIDENCE AND EPIDEMIOLOGY

The presenting findings in a patient with a newly discovered malignancy may not reveal its site of origin. Patients with cancer of unknown primary site (CUPS) present difficult diagnostic and therapeutic dilemmas. First, as additional studies may be many, costly, and/or uncomfortable for the patient, the strategy used in searching for the primary must assess what, if any, result the identification of the site of origin would have on the patient's treatment and survival. Second, while individuals with CUPS fare poorly overall (median survival is 4 to 11 months), certain subgroups of patients are more likely to benefit from treatment and, in some cases, to enjoy long disease-free survival. Population-based analysis shows that two-thirds receive only supportive treatment and that only 15% are alive 1 year after diagnosis, suggesting the selection bias inherent in the more typically reported studies from tertiary care centers.

No universally accepted definition of the CUPS syndrome exists. An occult neoplasm should fulfill all of the following criteria: (1) biopsy-proven malignancy; (2) unrevealing history, physical examination, chest film, abdominal and pelvic computed tomography (CT) scans, complete blood counts, chemistry survey, mammography (women), β human chorionic gonadotropin (βhCG) levels (men), α fetoprotein (AFP) levels (men), and prostate-specific antigen (PSA) levels (men); (3) histologic evaluation not consistent with a primary tumor at the biopsy site; and (4) failure of additional diagnostic studies (based only on findings from the laboratory and pathologic review) to identify the primary site. Such additional diagnostic tests could include, for example, colonoscopy in a patient whose rectal examination discloses guaiac-positive stool or a meticulous otolaryngologic examination in a patient who presents with squamous cell carcinoma in a cervical node. Many cases that fulfill the definition of CUPS offer clues that a given organ is the probable site of origin. Epidemiologic data suggest that the incidence of cancers for which the primary site is unknown is decreasing. CUPS accounts for about 2% of all cancer diagnoses—about 24,400 cases in the year 2000. Most patients with CUPS are over age 60.

BIOLOGIC CONSIDERATIONS The biologic behavior of CUPS is unique. In ~25% of patients, the primary site becomes apparent during the course of the illness; in about 57% of patients, the primary site can be diagnosed at autopsy; but in almost 20%, the primary site remains obscure even at autopsy. Cancers presenting as CUPS often display unusual patterns of metastatic spread (e.g., pancreatic cancer presenting with bony metastases). The fact that more tumor bulk is present at distant sites than in the tissue of origin suggests that the genetic lesions underlying cases of CUPS produce a distinctly aggressive phenotype. Microsatellite DNA analysis has shown that the same pattern of genetic alterations that appears in a cervical lymph node metastasis can be found in seemingly morphologically normal aerodigestive tissue. Such data imply that clinically evident metastases may be able to arise from microscopic primary lesions. Tumors in 11% of CUPS patients, almost all with poorly differentiated adenocarcinoma, express the HER2/neu protein. Although physiologic and genetic data that might account for the distinctive natural history of CUPS neoplasms are scant, cell lines derived from such tumors may have abnormalities of chromosome 1, a finding generally associated with advanced malignancy. In some patients, the primary tumor spontaneously regresses (perhaps under immunologic attack) or necroses. In some, a primary lesion was resected years before presentation (e.g., melanoma).

CLINICAL PRESENTATION, DIAGNOSTIC EVALUATION, AND PATHOLOGY ■ History and Physical Examination Patients present with a variety of symptoms and signs, including fatigue, weight loss, other systemic symptoms, pain, abnormal bleeding, abdominal swelling, subcutaneous masses, and lymphadenopathy. Once CUPS is considered, the physician's approach must involve reasonable efforts to identify the primary site or to determine the histology or subcategory of the metastatic tumor to decide on the optimal therapy. Though usually unrevealing, a thorough history and physical examination should be carried out to elicit easily obtainable clues regarding the primary site. The patient should be questioned concerning epigastric pain, which, if present, would mandate careful exclusion of pancreatic carcinoma as well as other gastrointestinal malignancies. Symptoms referable to a given location (e.g., new cough, hematochezia, hemoptysis, change in bowel habits, unusual vaginal bleeding, nipple discharge) should prompt an aggressive specific diagnostic approach. Occupational exposure to asbestos, for example, would raise the suspicion of mesothelioma. The absence of prior smoking reduces the likelihood of lung cancer but does not exclude it. A history of fulguration of a skin lesion, colonic polypectomy, dilatation and curettage, or prostate biopsy should prompt a review of the original histology.

Pathology Review   The most important aspect of the workup of a patient with CUPS is the thorough evaluation of the tissue obtained at biopsy by light microscopy, immunohistochemistry, ultrastructural studies, immunophenotyping, and karyotypic and molecular biologic analysis. First, if the original biopsy sample is inadequate for either confirmation of malignancy or the performance of additional specialized studies, rebiopsy is mandatory. The clinician must have a close working relationship with a pathologist skilled in the evaluation of tumor specimens, especially when the organ of origin is uncertain. Plans may be made to process the tissue for (1) routine light-microscopic, histochemical, and immunohistochemical analysis; (2) freezing for DNA and RNA isolation or for in situ genetic and immunologic evaluation; and (3) special fixation for ultrastructural analysis. Single-cell tumor suspensions in short-term culture permit cytogenetic analysis.

If routine histologic analysis fails to suggest the tissue of origin (e.g., gland formation in adenocarcinoma, psammoma bodies in ovarian or thyroid cancer, or spindle architecture in sarcomas), special histochemical studies may be helpful. For example, mucin positivity is helpful in recognizing a poorly differentiated adenocarcinoma. Light-microscopic analysis will show ~60% of CUPS tumors to be well or moderately differentiated adenocarcinomas, 30% poorly differentiated carcinomas/adenocarcinomas, and 5% poorly differentiated malignant neoplasms not further classifiable. In the poorly differentiated neoplasms, immunohistochemical, cytogenetic, and molecular biologic studies can be extremely useful in identifying sarcomas, germ cell carcinomas, lymphomas, neuroendocrine neoplasms (including melanoma), and other tumors whose diagnosis would suggest a more specific therapeutic approach.

Immunohistochemical Analysis   Antibodies to specific cell components make it possible to characterize tumors that are not identified by standard techniques. Table 85-1 provides a list of antigens that may be assessed in undifferentiated or poorly differentiated specimens. A diagnosis of lymphoma should be excluded by employing antibodies reactive to the leukocyte common antigen (LCA, CD45). LCA-positive tumors are lymphomas and have the same chances of responding to therapy as if the diagnosis were unambiguous. About half of patients with aggressive-histology lymphoma can be cured with combination chemotherapy (Chap. 97). The immunohistochemical detection of specific types of filament proteins is helpful in the identification of carcinomas and sarcomas. The presence of keratin suggests carcinoma; all epithelial tumors contain this protein. Specific types of cytokeratins (CKs) may aid in diagnosis. For example, ovarian and lung cancers are CK20−/CK7+, colorectal cancers are CK20+/CK7−, and pancreaticobiliary tumors and transitional cell cancers are CK20+/CK7+. However, certain sarcomas, mesotheliomas, and germ cell tumors are also keratin-positive. Sarcomas may react with antibodies to desmin. Coexpression of p53 and CK5/6 is suggestive of a squamous cell primary. Sarcoma subgroups may be identified by expression of myoglobin (rhabdomyosarcoma) or factor VIII (angiosarcoma or Kaposi's sarcoma). Prostate, breast, and thyroid carcinomas express, respectively, PSA, gross cystic fluid protein, or thyroglobulin. The finding of AFP, βhCG, or placental alkaline phosphatase staining is very helpful in assigning a germ cell origin. The S-100 protein is present in virtually all primary and metastatic melanomas, including the amelanotic variety. However, S-100 positivity is also found in other tumors of neuroendocrine origin (e.g., small cell lung cancer, carcinoid, neuroepithelioma); a more specific marker for melanomas is the HMB45 (human melanoma black) antigen.

TABLE 85-1   *Possible Pathologic Evaluation of Biopsy Specimens from Patients with Metastatic Cancer of Unknown Primary Site*

Evaluation/Findings	Suggested Primary Site or Neoplasm
HISTOLOGY (HEMATOXYLIN AND EOSIN STAINING)	
Psammoma bodies, papillary configuration	Ovary, thyroid
Signet ring cells	Stomach
IMMUNOHISTOLOGY	
Leukocyte common antigen (LCA, CD45)	Lymphoid neoplasm
Leu-M1	Hodgkin's disease
Epithelial membrane antigen	Carcinoma
Cytokeratin	Carcinoma[a]
CEA	Carcinoma
HMB45	Melanoma
Desmin	Sarcoma
Thyroglobulin	Thyroid carcinoma
Calcitonin	Medullary carcinoma of the thyroid
Myoglobin	Rhabdomyosarcoma
PSA/prostatic acid phosphatase	Prostate
AFP	Liver, stomach, germ cell
Placental alkaline phosphatase	Germ cell
B, T cell markers	Lymphoid neoplasm
S-100 protein	Neuroendocrine tumor, melanoma
Gross cystic fluid protein	Breast, sweat gland
Factor VIII	Kaposi's sarcoma, angiosarcoma
Thyroid transcription factor-1 (TTF-1)	Lung adenocarcinoma, thyroid
FLOW CYTOMETRY	
B, T cell markers	Lymphoid neoplasm
ULTRASTRUCTURE	
Actin-myosin filaments	Rhabdomyosarcoma
Secretory granules	Neuroendocrine tumors
Desmosomes	Carcinoma
Premelanosomes	Melanoma
CYTOGENETICS	
Isochromosome 12p; 12q(−)	Germ cell
t(11;22)	Ewing's sarcoma, primitive neuroectodermal tumor
t(8;14)[b]	Lymphoid neoplasm
3p(−)	Small cell lung carcinoma; renal cell carcinoma, mesothelioma
t(X;18)	Synovial sarcoma
t(12;16)	Myxoid liposarcoma
t(12;22)	Clear cell sarcoma (melanoma of soft parts)
t(2;13)	Alveolar rhabdomyosarcoma
1p(−)	Neuroblastoma
RECEPTOR ANALYSIS	
Estrogen/progesterone receptor	Breast
MOLECULAR BIOLOGIC STUDIES	
Immunoglobulin, *bcl*-2, T-cell receptor gene rearrangement	Lymphoid neoplasm

[a] See text for discussion of cytokeratins.
[b] Or any other rearrangement involving an antigen-receptor gene.
Note: CEA, carcinoembryonic antigen; PSA, prostate-specific antigen; AFP, α fetoprotein.

Other Diagnostic Approaches   Electron microscopy can identify cell junctions (i.e., desmosomes, typical of epithelial cancers), neuroendocrine granules, melanosomes, and muscle filaments. Cytogenetic analysis may identify tumors with specific chromosomal translocations or other genetic abnormalities (Table 85-1). Cytogenetic abnormalities can also be determined by fluorescence in situ hybridization with chromosome-specific probes, a technique that does not require cells to divide, as is the case with traditional karyotype analysis. Fresh tissue may be required for detection of estrogen or progesterone receptors (to assess breast cancer) or antigens that are sensitive to fixation. Lineage can be assigned by analysis of DNA for signature gene rearrangements, such as those of immunoglobulin (B cell) or T cell receptor (T cell). Technological advances promise to influence the diagnosis of cancer. Isolation of mRNA from tumor specimens may permit the molecular profiling of tumors by microarray analysis of gene expression. This could lead to novel classifications of tumors based on molecular characteristics that may predict clinical behavior and/or response to specific therapies.

Additional Studies If the pathologist does not identify the likely tissue of origin, it is unlikely that additional expensive diagnostic tests will benefit the patient. In females with metastatic adenocarcinoma or poorly differentiated carcinoma, mammography should be performed, although the diagnostic yield will be quite low except in patients with axillary metastases. Magnetic resonance imaging, positron-emission tomography (PET), or indium 111-pentreotide scanning can identify occult primary lesions but are expensive. The use of abdominal/pelvic CT scans leads to the identification of the primary site (often the pancreas) in up to 35% of patients but has little effect on natural history. While more sensitive than CT in detection of a primary site, the now frequently employed PET scan does not clearly lead to better outcomes. Whether to measure serum tumor markers such as AFP, βhCG, carcinoembryonic antigen (CEA), CA-125 (associated with ovarian cancer), and PSA is controversial; value has not been proved. Numerous studies have shown a lack of benefit of contrast studies (upper gastrointestinal series, barium enema, or intravenous pyelogram) in patients with CUPS who have no specific symptoms and no findings referable to the gastrointestinal or urinary tract. Moreover, autopsy series reveal that the most likely primary site of origin includes epithelial tissues such as lung, stomach, colon, and kidney, which give rise to tumors that respond poorly to chemotherapy, minimizing the therapeutic impact of such a diagnosis.

Additional invasive diagnostic studies are indicated if the presentation strongly suggests a particular primary site. For example, radiographic evidence of lung or mediastinal involvement would mandate fiberoptic bronchoscopy to exclude lung cancer. In the relatively unusual case of metastatic squamous cell cancer presenting in an inguinal lymph node, anoscopy and colposcopy should be performed to detect carcinoma of the vulva, cervix, vagina, penis, or anus, all of which may be cured even with lymph node spread. A reasonable diagnostic approach is provided in Table 85-2.

℞ TREATMENT

Prognostic Subgroups The exclusion of treatable and potentially curable neoplasms is important. Patients with squamous cell carcinoma have a somewhat longer median survival (9 months) than do those with adenocarcinoma or unclassifiable neoplasms (4 to 6 months). If laboratory studies indicate a significant likelihood that the neoplasm is a lymphoma, germ cell tumor, sarcoma, neuroendocrine tumor, or breast or prostate cancer, then disease-appropriate therapy should be administered. Patients with lymphoma or a germ cell neoplasm may be cured with combination chemotherapy. In other malignancies, effective palliative chemotherapy (for sarcoma or a breast or neuroendocrine tumor) or hormonal therapy (for breast or prostate cancer) should be strongly considered. Although often requiring electron microscopy for diagnosis, neuroendocrine tumors (especially if anaplastic) often respond to cisplatin-based chemotherapy.

Patients in whom the primary site can be identified fare somewhat better than those in whom it remains undefined. A validated prognostic model based on a multivariate analysis of clinical parameters suggested those with a good performance status without liver metastases had a median survival of 10.8 months compared with 2.4 months for patients who were more symptomatic and who had spread to the liver. Elevated serum lactate dehydrogenase alone predicted a median sur-

TABLE 85-2 *Suggested Clinical Evaluation of Patients with Metastatic Cancer of Unknown Primary Site*

History: smoking history, asbestos exposure, abdominal pain
Physical examination: lymph nodes, thyroid, skin;
   Men: prostate
   Women: breasts, pelvic examination
Laboratory evaluation: stool evaluation for occult blood; urinalysis; complete blood count; liver function tests; calcium, electrolytes, creatine; measurement of serum levels of βhCG, AFP, CEA, and CA-125 (women); chest x-ray; abdominal and pelvic CT; mammography
Pathologic evaluation: see Table 85-1

Note: PSA, prostate-specific antigen; βhCG, β-human chorionic gonadotropin; AFP, α fetoprotein; CEA, carcinoembryonic antigen; CT, computed tomography.

vival of 3.9 months (Table 85-3). Forty percent of CUPS patients may be found to have one of several clinical syndromes for which a specific therapeutic approach may be useful:

SYNDROME OF UNRECOGNIZED EXTRAGONADAL GERM CELL CANCER Some patients with poorly differentiated CUPS are responsive to chemotherapy. These patients display one or more of the following features: age <50; tumor involving midline structures, lung parenchyma, or lymph nodes; an elevated serum AFP or βhCG level; evidence of rapid tumor growth; or tumor responsiveness to previously administered radiotherapy or chemotherapy. Platinum-based chemotherapy has led to long-term survival in a fraction of patients with these features, especially those who have a favorable performance status at diagnosis, suggesting that their tumors behaved like germ cell neoplasms. If all patients with poorly differentiated carcinoma (including poorly differentiated adenocarcinoma) are treated with a chemotherapy regimen designed for germ cell cancer (e.g., cisplatin plus etoposide or vinblastine, often also with bleomycin) (Chap. 82), about 25% will respond completely and 33% will have a partial response. Patients whose disease does not respond to two cycles of therapy should not continue

TABLE 85-3 *Presentations That Dictate Specific Therapies in Patients with CUPS*

Clinicopathologic Features	Suspected Primary Site	Suggested Therapy
Squamous cell carcinoma, cervical node	Head and neck cancer	Radical neck dissection; radiotherapy ± chemotherapy
Carcinoma, axillary nodes (female)	Breast cancer	Breast radiotherapy or mastectomy, systemic adjuvant therapy
Peritoneal carcinomatosis (female)	Ovarian cancer	Debulking surgery, cisplatin-based chemotherapy
Pleural effusion, adenocarcinoma cells estrogen and/or progesterone receptor positive	Breast cancer	Systemic therapy for metastatic breast cancer
Poorly differentiated cancer, age <50, lung or retroperitoneal or mediastinal mass or lymph nodes, elevated serum βhCG or AFP levels	Germ cell tumor (extragonadal)	Cisplatin/VP-16-based chemotherapy
Bony metastases (male)	Prostate cancer	Androgen blockade (leuprolide plus flutamide)
Adenocarcinoma, liver metastases, elevated CEA level	Gastrointestinal malignancy	Surgical resection of liver lesion feasible; colonoscopy with resection (if appropriate) of tumors; 5-fluorouracil/leucovorin

Note: βhCG, β-human chorionic gonadotropin; AFP, α fetoprotein; CEA, carcinoembryonic antigen.

therapy. One in six patients survives >5 years without evidence of disease. Patients with poorly differentiated carcinoma or adenocarcinoma whose tumors have abnormalities of chromosome 12 similar to those described in patients with proven germ cell cancer are more likely to respond to platinum-based chemotherapy than are patients with a similar presentation whose tumors lack this cytogenetic abnormality.

PERITONEAL CARCINOMATOSIS IN WOMEN Women who present with increased abdominal girth and a pelvic mass or pain and who are found to have adenocarcinoma throughout the peritoneal cavity without a clear site of origin may also benefit from platinum-based chemotherapy. This syndrome has been termed *primary peritoneal papillary serous carcinoma* or *multifocal extraovarian serous carcinoma*. While breast cancer or a gastrointestinal malignancy can produce these findings, peritoneal carcinomatosis is most commonly ascribed to ovarian cancer, even in patients with apparently normal ovaries at the time of laparotomy. Especially if psammoma bodies or a papillary configuration is noted in the pathology examination or if the CA-125 level is elevated, women with adenocarcinoma of the peritoneal cavity without a defined primary should receive maximum surgical cytoreduction followed by cisplatin (or carboplatin) plus paclitaxel. The stage-specific response to such therapy appears to be comparable to that for patients with proven ovarian cancer. About 10% of patients who present in this fashion may remain free of disease 2 years after diagnosis.

CARCINOMA IN AN AXILLARY LYMPH NODE IN A FEMALE Women with adenocarcinoma or poorly differentiated carcinoma in an axillary mass should receive treatment for stage II breast cancer whether or not a careful breast examination or mammography suggests the diagnosis of primary breast cancer and whether or not estrogen or progesterone receptors are detectable in the node. Even if no lesion is found in the breast, a breast recurrence will develop in one-half of these patients if no mastectomy is performed. Modified radical mastectomy or breast irradiation may be equivalent in reducing the risk of local recurrence. In addition, adjuvant systemic therapy (chemotherapy and/or tamoxifen, depending on menopausal and estrogen receptor status) should be given to reduce the risk of developing evident metastatic breast cancer (Chap. 76). Adjuvant systemic therapy may be administered before definitive local radiation treatment. Women with axillary metastases without an obvious breast primary appear to have the same likelihood of prolonged disease-free survival as patients with typical stage II breast cancer.

BONE METASTASES IN MALES Particularly if the lesions are osteoblastic, the serum PSA level should be measured, as the probability of prostate carcinoma is high. Empirical hormonal therapy (e.g., leuprolide and flutamide) should be strongly considered.

CERVICAL LYMPH NODE METASTASES Patients who present with a neck mass should be considered to have a primary tumor of the upper aerodigestive tract (head and neck cancer) until a different source is proven. Especially if the pathologist diagnoses squamous histology and the node is located in a high or midcervical area, a careful ear, nose, and throat examination including direct laryngoscopy, nasopharyngoscopy, and random blind biopsies should be undertaken. A thyroid examination and scan should be performed to rule out a primary thyroid tumor, especially if the histology is not definitely squamous. Definitive local therapy (external beam radiation or radical neck dissection) combined with platinum-based chemotherapy may lead to prolonged survival in those with head and neck primaries (Chap. 74).

ADENOCARCINOMA AND LIVER METASTASES Liver metastases from an adenocarcinoma are not as well characterized as a syndrome as the unrecognized germ cell cancer syndrome (nor as responsive to therapy). However, such patients may have a primary stomach, biliary, or colorectal tumor. Tumors with limited hepatic involvement may be amenable to resection. A flexible sigmoidoscopy or colonoscopy may detect a potentially obstructive colon lesion. If a tumor is found, resection may be beneficial, depending on the tumor's size; even if none is found, treatment with a combination of 5-fluorouracil plus leucovorin, with or without irinotecan, is palliative for some patients with presumed metastatic gastrointestinal malignancy. Given the severe diarrhea that may be a consequence of this regimen and the relative resistance of gastrointestinal tumors to chemotherapy, patients should be informed of the risks before treatment.

Other Patients Patients not falling into one of the preceding categories should be treated palliatively. In some patients, observation is appropriate. For example, individuals without evidence of additional metastatic disease who have undergone resection of a solitary pulmonary nodule containing malignant cells may actually have undergone definitive therapy for a small primary lung tumor. Patients presenting with a solitary brain metastasis from an unknown primary source who undergo resection of the lesion followed by whole-brain radiation therapy have a median survival of 13 months, suggesting benefit for aggressive local therapy. Radiation therapy may relieve symptoms in patients with bony pain or neurologic compromise. The largest and most poorly responsive subgroup are those with moderate to well-differentiated adenocarcinomas. Combination chemotherapy is frequently employed in such patients; however, response rates to "all-purpose" regimens [e.g., FACP (5-fluorouracil, doxorubicin, cyclophosphamide, cisplatin)] or to ICE (ifosfamide, carboplatin, etoposide) are generally well under 50%, especially if patients with poorly differentiated adenocarcinoma, who have a higher response rate, are excluded; complete responses are rare. The addition of a taxane (taxotere or paclitaxel) to such regimens has been associated with a higher response rate, albeit in selected patients. High-dose chemotherapy is not beneficial. In some series, patients with a good performance status whose disease is limited to soft tissue sites or extends only above the diaphragm have shown a better rate of response to therapy. While patients whose disease responds to treatment seem to have better survival than those whose disease does not respond, the difference may be related to inherent characteristics of the tumor rather than to a beneficial effect of chemotherapy.

Before combination chemotherapy is attempted in a patient with CUPS, the potential benefits must be weighed carefully against the certainty of toxicity. While some randomized studies have reported a benefit of one form of therapy over another, these reports are generally plagued by small numbers of patients and inadequate control of potential prognostic variables. Depending on motivation, eligibility, and availability, patients with CUPS may be candidates for evaluation of new (phase I) therapies.

FURTHER READING

CULINE S et al: Development and validation of a prognostic model to predict the length of survival in patients with carcinomas of an unknown primary. J Clin Oncol 20:4679, 2002

DENNIS JL et al: Identification from public data of molecular markers of adenocarcinoma characteristic of the site of origin. Cancer Res 62:5999, 2002

ETTINGER DS et al: NCCN practice guidelines for occult primary tumors. Oncology 12:226, 1998

FOGARTY GB et al: The usefulness of fluorine 18-labelled deoxyglucose positron emission tomography in the investigation of patients with cervical lymphadenopathy from an unknown primary tumor. Head Neck 25:138, 2002

HAINSWORTH JD, GRECO FA: Management of patients with cancer of an unknown primary site. Oncology 14:563, 2000

PAVLIDIS N et al: Diagnostic and therapeutic management of cancer of an unknown primary. Eur J Cancer 39:1990, 2003

SAAD ED, ABBRUZZESE JL: Prognostic stratification in UPC: A role for assessing the value of conventional-dose and high-dose chemotherapy for unknown primary carcinoma. Crit Rev Oncol Hematol 41:205, 2002

VAN DE WOUW AJ et al: Epidemiology of unknown primary tumours: Incidence and population-based survival of 1285 patients in Southeast Netherlands, 1984–1992. Eur J Cancer 38:409, 2002

In addition to local tissue invasion and metastasis, neoplastic cells can produce a variety of peptides that exert biologic actions at local and distant sites and can elicit responses that cause a variety of hormonal, hematologic, dermatologic, and neurologic symptoms. *Paraneoplastic syndromes* refer to the disorders that accompany benign or malignant tumors but are not directly related to mass effects or invasion by the primary tumor or its metastases. Tumors of neuroendocrine origin, such as small cell lung carcinoma (SCLC) and carcinoids, produce a wide array of peptide hormones and are common causes of paraneoplastic syndromes. However, almost every type of malignancy has the potential to produce hormones or cytokines or to induce immunologic responses. Careful studies of the prevalence of paraneoplastic syndromes indicate that they are more common than is generally appreciated. The signs, symptoms, and metabolic alterations associated with paraneoplastic disorders may be overlooked in the context of a malignancy and its treatment. Consequently, atypical clinical manifestations in a patient with cancer should prompt consideration of a paraneoplastic syndrome. In this chapter, we review the most common endocrinologic, hematologic, and dermatologic syndromes associated with underlying neoplasia.

ENDOCRINE PARANEOPLASTIC SYNDROMES

ETIOLOGY Hormones can be produced from eutopic or ectopic sources. *Eutopic* refers to the expression of a hormone from its normal tissue of origin, whereas *ectopic* refers to hormone production from an atypical tissue source. For example, adrenocorticotropic hormone (ACTH) is expressed eutopically by the corticotrope cells of the anterior pituitary but it can be expressed ectopically in SCLC. As assay methodologies have become more sensitive, it is now apparent that many hormones are produced at low levels from a wide array of tissues, in addition to the classic endocrine source. Thus, ectopic expression is often a quantitative change rather than an absolute change in tissue expression. Nevertheless, the term *ectopic expression* is firmly entrenched and conveys the abnormal physiology associated with neoplastic hormone production. In addition to high levels of hormones, ectopic expression is typically characterized by abnormal regulation of hormone production (e.g., defective feedback control) and peptide processing (resulting in large, unprocessed precursors).

A diverse array of molecular mechanisms has been suggested to cause ectopic hormone production, but this process remains incompletely understood. In rare instances, genetic rearrangements explain aberrant hormone expression. For example, translocation of the *parathyroid hormone (PTH)* gene resulted in high levels of PTH expression in an ovarian carcinoma, presumably because the genetic rearrangement brings the *PTH* gene under the control of ovary-specific regulatory elements. A related phenomenon is well documented in many forms of leukemia and lymphoma, in which somatic genetic rearrangements confer a growth advantage and frequently alter cellular differentiation and function (see Chap. 97). Although genetic rearrangements may cause selected cases of ectopic hormone production, this mechanism is probably unusual, as many tumors are associated with excessive production of a wide variety of peptides. It is likely that cellular dedifferentiation underlies most cases of ectopic hormone production. In support of this idea, many cancers are poorly differentiated histologically, and certain tumor products, such as human chorionic gonadotropin (hCG), parathyroid hormone–related protein (PTHrP), and α fetoprotein, are characteristic of gene expression at earlier developmental stages. On the other hand, the propensity of certain cancers to produce particular hormones (e.g., squamous cell carcinomas produce PTHrP) suggests that dedifferentiation is partial or that selective pathways are derepressed. These expression profiles are likely to be driven by alterations in transcriptional repression, changes in DNA methylation, or other factors that govern cell differentiation. In SCLC, the pathway of differentiation has been relatively well defined. The neuroendocrine phenotype is dictated in part by the basic-helix-loop-helix (bHLH) transcription factor human achaete-scute homologue-1 (hASH1), which is expressed at abnormally high levels in SCLC associated with ectopic ACTH. The activity of hASH-1 is inhibited by hairy enhancer of split-1 (HES-1) and by Notch proteins, which are also capable of inducing growth arrest. Thus, abnormal expression of these developmental transcription factors appears to provide a link between cell proliferation and differentiation.

Ectopic hormone production would only be an epiphenomenon associated with cancer if it did not sometimes result in clinical manifestations. Excessive and unregulated production of hormones such as ACTH, PTHrP, or vasopressin can lead to substantial morbidity and can complicate the cancer treatment plan. Moreover, the paraneoplastic endocrinopathies are sometimes the presenting feature of underlying malignancy and may prompt the search for an unrecognized tumor.

A large number of paraneoplastic endocrine syndromes have been described, linking overproduction of particular hormones with specific types of tumors. However, certain recurring syndromes emerge from this large group (Table 86-1). The most common paraneoplastic endocrine syndromes include hypercalcemia from overproduction of PTHrP and other factors, hyponatremia from excess vasopressin, and Cushing's syndrome from ectopic ACTH.

SELECTED PARANEOPLASTIC ENDOCRINE SYNDROMES

HYPERCALCEMIA CAUSED BY ECTOPIC PRODUCTION OF PTHrP (See also Chap. 332) ■ **Etiology** Humoral hypercalcemia of malignancy (HHM) occurs in up to 5% of patients with cancer. HHM is most common in cancers of the lung, breast, head and neck, genitourinary tract, esophagus, and skin, and in multiple myeloma and lymphomas. There are several humoral causes of HHM but it is most often associated with overproduction of PTHrP. In addition to acting as a circulating humoral factor, many bone metastases (e.g., breast, multiple myeloma) produce PTHrP, leading to local osteolysis and hypercalcemia.

PTHrP is structurally related to PTH and it binds to the PTH receptor, explaining the similar biochemical features of HHM and hyperparathyroidism. PTHrP plays a key role in skeletal development and regulates cellular proliferation and differentiation in other tissues including skin, bone marrow, breast, and hair follicles. The mechanism of PTHrP induction in malignancy is incompletely understood but it is notable that tumor-bearing tissues commonly associated with HHM normally produce PTHrP during development or cellular renewal. Mutations in certain oncogenes, such as *Ras*, can activate PTHrP expression. In adult T cell lymphoma, the transactivating Tax protein produced by human T-cell lymphotropic virus-1 (HTLV-1) stimulates PTHrP promoter activity. Metastatic lesions to bone are more likely to produce PTHrP than are metastases in other tissues, suggesting that bone produces factors that enhance PTHrP production, or that PTHrP-producing metastases have a selective growth advantage in bone. Thus, PTHrP production can be stimulated by mutations in oncogenes, by altered expression of viral or cellular transcription factors, and by local growth factors.

Another relatively common cause of HHM is excess production of 1,25-dihydroxyvitamin D. Like granulomatous disorders associated with hypercalcemia, lymphomas can produce an enzyme that converts 25-hydroxyvitamin D to the more active 1,25-dihydroxyvitamin D, leading to enhanced gastrointestinal calcium absorption. Other causes of HHM include tumor-mediated production of osteolytic cytokines and inflammatory mediators.

Clinical Manifestations The typical presentation of HHM is a patient with a known malignancy who is found to be hypercalcemic on routine laboratory tests. Less often, hypercalcemia is the initial presenting feature of malignancy. Particularly when calcium levels are markedly increased (>14 mg/dL), patients may experience fatigue, mental status changes, dehydration, or symptoms of nephrolithiasis.

Diagnosis Features that favor HHM as opposed to primary hyperparathyroidism include known malignancy, recent onset of hypercalcemia, and very high serum calcium levels. Like hyperparathyroidism, hypercalcemia caused by PTHrP is accompanied by hypercalciuria and hypophosphatemia. Measurement of PTH is useful to exclude primary hyperparathyroidism; the PTH level should be suppressed in HHM. An elevated PTHrP level confirms the diagnosis, and it is increased in about 80% of hypercalcemic patients with cancer. 1,25-Dihydroxyvitamin D levels may be increased in patients with lymphoma.

℞ TREATMENT

The management of HHM begins with saline rehydration to dilute serum calcium and promote calciuresis. Forced diuresis with furosemide or other loop diuretics can enhance calcium excretion but provides relatively little value except in life-threatening hypercalcemia. When used, loop diuretics should be administered only after complete rehydration and with careful monitoring of fluid balance. Bisphosphonates such as pamidronate (30 to 90 mg IV) or zoledronate (4 to 8 mg IV) can reduce serum calcium within 1 to 2 days and suppress calcium release for several weeks. Oral bisphosphonates can also be used for chronic treatment. Previously used agents, such as calcitonin and mithramycin, have little utility now that bisphosphonates are available. Calcitonin (2 to 8 U/kg SC every 6 to 12 h) should be considered when rapid correction of severe hypercalcemia is needed. Hypercalcemia associated with lymphomas, multiple myeloma, or leukemia may respond to glucocorticoid treatment (e.g., prednisone 40 to 100 mg PO in four divided doses).

TABLE 86-1 *Paraneoplastic Syndromes Caused by Ectopic Hormone Production*

Paraneoplastic Syndrome	Ectopic Hormone	Typical Tumor Types[a]
COMMON		
Hypercalcemia of malignancy	Parathyroid hormone-related protein (PTHrP)	Squamous cell (head and neck, lung, skin), breast, genitourinary, gastrointestinal
	1,25 dihydroxyvitamin D	Lymphomas
	Parathyroid hormone (PTH) (rare)	Lung, ovary
	Prostaglandin E2 (PGE2) (rare)	Renal, lung
Syndrome of inappropriate antidiuretic hormone secretion (SIADH)	Vasopressin	Lung (squamous, small cell), gastrointestinal, genitourinary, ovary
Cushing's syndrome	Adrenocorticotropic hormone (ACTH)	Lung (small cell, bronchial carcinoid, adenocarcinoma, squamous), thymus, pancreatic islet, medullary thyroid carcinoma
	Corticotropin-releasing hormone (CRH) (rare)	Pancreatic islet, carcinoid, lung, prostate
	Ectopic expression of gastric inhibitory peptide (GIP), luteinizing hormone (LH)/ human chorionic gonadotropin (hCG), other G protein–coupled receptors (rare)	Macronodular adrenal hyperplasia
LESS COMMON		
Non-islet cell hypoglycemia	Insulin-like growth factor (IGF-II)	Mesenchymal tumors, sarcomas, adrenal, hepatic, gastrointestinal, kidney, prostate
	Insulin (rare)	Cervix (small cell carcinoma)
Male feminization	hCG[b]	Testis (embryonal, seminomas), germinomas, choriocarcinoma, lung, hepatic, pancreatic islet
Diarrhea or intestinal hypermotility	Calcitonin[c]	Lung, colon, breast, medullary thyroid carcinoma
	Vasoactive intestinal peptide (VIP)	Pancreas, pheochromocytoma, esophagus
RARE		
Oncogenic osteomalacia	Phosphatonin [Fibroblast growth factor 23 (FGF23)]	Hemangiopericytomas, osteoblastomas, fibromas, sarcomas, giant cell tumors, prostate, lung
Acromegaly	Growth hormone–releasing hormone (GHRH)	Pancreatic islet, bronchial and other carcinoids
	Growth hormone (GH)	Lung, pancreatic islet
Hyperthyroidism	Thyroid-stimulating hormone (TSH)	Hydatidiform mole, embryonal tumors, struma ovarii
Hypertension	Renin	Juxtaglomerula tumors, kidney, lung, pancreas, ovary

[a] Only the most common tumor types are listed. For most ectopic hormone syndromes, an extensive list of tumors has been reported to produce one or more hormones.

[b] hCG is produced eutopically by trophoblastic tumors. Certain tumors produce disproportionate amounts of the hCG α or hCG β subunits. High levels of hCG rarely cause hyperthyroidism because of weak binding to the TSH receptor.

[c] Calcitonin is produced eutopically by medullary thyroid carcinoma and is used as a tumor marker.

ECTOPIC VASOPRESSIN: TUMOR-ASSOCIATED SIADH (See also Chap. 41) ■
Etiology Vasopressin is an antidiuretic hormone normally produced by the posterior pituitary gland. Ectopic vasopressin production by tumors is a common cause of the syndrome of inappropriate antidiuretic hormone (SIADH), occurring in at least half of patients with SCLC. Compensatory mechanisms, such as decreased thirst, suppression of aldosterone, and production of atrial natriuretic peptide (ANP), may mitigate the development of hyponatremia in patients who produce excessive vasopressin. Tumors with neuroendocrine features, such as SCLC and carcinoids, are the most common sources of ectopic vasopressin production, but it also occurs in other forms of lung cancer and with CNS lesions, head and neck cancer, and genitourinary, gastrointestinal, and ovarian cancers. The mechanism of activation of the vasopressin gene in these tumors is unknown but often involves concomitant expression of the adjacent oxytocin gene, suggesting derepression of this locus.

Clinical Manifestations Most patients with ectopic vasopressin secretion are asymptomatic and are identified because of the presence of hyponatremia on routine chemistry testing. Symptoms may include weakness, lethargy, nausea, confusion, depressed mental status, and seizures. The severity of symptoms reflects the rapidity of onset as well as the extent of hyponatremia. In most cases, hyponatremia develops slowly but may be exacerbated by the administration of intravenous fluids or the institution of new medications. Thirst is typically suppressed.

Diagnosis The diagnostic features of ectopic vasopressin production are the same as those of other causes of SIADH (see Chaps. 41 and 318). Hyponatremia and reduced serum osmolality occur in the setting of an inappropriately normal or increased urine osmolality. Unless there is concomitant volume depletion, urine sodium excretion is normal or increased. Other causes of hyponatremia should be excluded, including renal, adrenal, or thyroid insufficiency. Physiologic sources of vasopressin stimulation (CNS lesions, pulmonary disease, nausea) and adaptive circulatory mechanisms (hypotension, heart failure, hepatic cirrhosis), as well as medications, including many chemotherapeutic agents, should also be considered as possible causes of hyponatremia. Measurement of vasopressin is not usually necessary to make the diagnosis.

Rx TREATMENT

Most patients with ectopic vasopressin production develop hyponatremia over several weeks or months and it is reasonable to correct the disorder gradually unless mental status is altered or there is risk of seizures. Treatment of the underlying malignancy may reduce ectopic vasopressin production but this response is slow, if it occurs at all. Fluid restriction to less than urine output, plus insensible losses, is often sufficient to partially correct hyponatremia. However, strict monitoring of the amount and types of liquids consumed or administered intravenously is required for fluid restriction to be effective. Salt tablets or saline are not helpful unless there is concomitant volume depletion. Demeclocycline (150 to 300 mg orally three to four times daily) can be used to inhibit vasopressin action on the renal distal tubule but its onset of action is relatively slow (1 to 2 weeks). Other vasopressin antagonists are under investigation. Severe hyponatremia (Na <115 mEq/L) or mental status changes may require treatment with hypertonic (3%) or normal saline infusion together with furosemide, to enhance free water clearance. The rate of sodium correction should be slow (0.5 to 1 mEq/L per h) to prevent rapid fluid shifts and the possible development of central pontine myelinolysis.

CUSHING'S SYNDROME CAUSED BY ECTOPIC ACTH PRODUCTION (See also Chap. 321) ■ **Etiology** Ectopic production of ACTH accounts for 10 to 20% of Cushing's syndrome. The syndrome is particularly common in neuroendocrine tumors. SCLC ($>50\%$) is by far the most common cause of ectopic ACTH, followed by thymic carcinoid (15%), islet cell tumors (10%), bronchial carcinoid (10%), other carcinoids (5%), and pheochromocytomas (2%). As noted above, the mechanism of ectopic ACTH production in neuroendocrine tumors appears to be linked to the expression of transcription factors that dictate pathways of cell differentiation. Ectopic ACTH production is caused by increased expression of the proopiomelanocortin (POMC) gene, which encodes ACTH, along with melanocyte-stimulating hormone (MSH), β lipotropin, and several other peptides. In many tumors, there is abundant but aberrant expression of the POMC gene from an internal promoter, proximal to the third exon, which encodes ACTH. However, because this product lacks the signal sequence necessary for protein processing, it is not secreted. Increased production of ACTH arises instead from less abundant, but unregulated, POMC expression from the same promoter site used in the pituitary. However, because the tumors lack many of the enzymes needed to process the POMC polypeptide, it is typically released as multiple large, biologically inactive fragments along with relatively small amounts of fully processed, active ACTH.

Rarely, corticotropin-releasing hormone (CRH) is produced by pancreatic islet tumors, SCLC, medullary thyroid cancer, carcinoids, or prostate cancer. When levels are high enough, CRH can cause pituitary corticotrope hyperplasia and Cushing's syndrome. Tumors that produce CRH sometimes also produce ACTH, raising the possibility of a paracrine mechanism for ACTH production.

A distinct mechanism for ACTH-independent Cushing's syndrome involves ectopic expression of various G protein–coupled receptors in the adrenal nodules. Ectopic expression of the gastric inhibitory peptide (GIP) receptor is the best-characterized example of this mechanism. In this case, meals induce GIP secretion, which inappropriately stimulates adrenal growth and glucocorticoid production.

Clinical Manifestations The clinical features of hypercortisolemia are detected in only a small fraction of patients with documented ectopic ACTH production. However, the ectopic ACTH syndrome is associated with several clinical features that distinguish it from other causes

of Cushing's syndrome (e.g., pituitary adenomas, adrenal adenomas, iatrogenic glucocorticoid excess). The metabolic manifestations of ectopic ACTH syndrome are dominated by fluid retention and hypertension, hypokalemia, metabolic alkalosis, glucose intolerance, and, often, steroid psychosis. Patients with ectopic ACTH syndrome generally exhibit less marked weight gain and centripetal fat redistribution, probably because the exposure to excess steroids is relatively short and because cachexia reduces the propensity for weight gain and fat deposition. The very high levels of ACTH often cause increased pigmentation, and melanotrope-stimulating hormone (MSH) activity derived from the POMC precursor peptide is also increased. The extraordinarily high glucocorticoid levels in patients with ectopic sources of ACTH can lead to marked skin fragility and easy bruising. In addition, the high cortisol levels often overwhelm the renal 11β-hydroxysteroid dehydrogenase type II enzyme, which normally inactivates cortisol and prevents it from binding to renal mineralocorticoid receptors. Consequently, in addition to the excess mineralocorticoids produced by ACTH stimulation of the adrenal gland, high levels of cortisol exert activity through the mineralocorticoid receptor, leading to severe hypokalemia.

Diagnosis The diagnosis of ectopic ACTH syndrome is usually not difficult in the setting of a known malignancy. Urine free cortisol levels fluctuate but are typically greater than 2 to 4 times normal and the plasma ACTH level is usually >100 pg/mL. A suppressed ACTH level excludes this diagnosis and indicates an ACTH-independent cause of Cushing's syndrome (e.g., adrenal or exogenous glucocorticoid). In contrast to pituitary sources of ACTH, most ectopic sources of ACTH do not respond to glucocorticoid suppression. Therefore, high-dose dexamethasone (8 mg PO) suppresses 8:00 A.M. serum cortisol (50% decrease from baseline) in about 80% of pituitary ACTH-producing adenomas but fails to suppress ectopic ACTH in about 90% of cases. Bronchial and other carcinoids are well-documented exceptions to these general guidelines, as these ectopic sources of ACTH may exhibit feedback regulation indistinguishable from pituitary adenomas, including suppression by high-dose dexamethasone, and ACTH responsiveness to adrenal blockade with metyrapone. If necessary, petrosal sinus catheterization can be used to evaluate a patient with ACTH-dependent Cushing's syndrome when the source of ACTH is unclear. After CRH stimulation, a 3:1 petrosal sinus:peripheral ACTH ratio strongly suggests a pituitary ACTH source. Imaging studies are also useful in the evaluation of suspected carcinoid lesions, allowing biopsy and characterization of hormone production using special stains.

Rx TREATMENT

The morbidity associated with the ectopic ACTH syndrome can be substantial. Patients may experience depression or personality changes because of extreme cortisol excess. Metabolic derangements including diabetes mellitus and hypokalemia can worsen fatigue. Poor wound healing and predisposition to infections can complicate the surgical management of tumors, and opportunistic infections, caused by organisms such as *Pneumocystis carinii* and mycoses, are often the cause of death in patients with ectopic ACTH production. Depending on prognosis and treatment plans for the underlying malignancy, measures to reduce cortisol levels are often indicated. Treatment of the underlying malignancy may reduce ACTH levels but is rarely sufficient to reduce cortisol levels to normal. Adrenalectomy is not practical for most of these patients but should be considered if the underlying tumor is not resectable and the prognosis is otherwise favorable (e.g., carcinoid). Medical therapy with ketoconazole (200 to 400 mg PO twice daily), metyrapone (250 to 500 mg PO every 6 h), mitotane (3 to 6 g PO in four divided doses, tapered to maintain low cortisol production), or other agents that block steroid synthesis or action is often the most practical strategy for managing the hypercortisolism associated with ectopic ACTH production (see Chap. 318). Glucocorticoid replacement should be provided to avoid adrenal insufficiency. Unfortunately, many patients will eventually escape from medical blockade.

TUMOR-INDUCED HYPOGLYCEMIA CAUSED BY EXCESS PRODUCTION OF IGF-II (See also Chap. 324) Mesenchymal tumors, hemangiopericytomas, hepatocellular tumors, adrenal carcinomas, and a variety of other large tumors have been reported to produce excessive amounts of insulin-like growth factor type II (IGF-II) precursor, which binds weakly to insulin receptors and strongly to IGF-I receptors, leading to insulin-like actions. The IGF-II gene resides on a locus on chromosome 11p15 that is normally imprinted (that is, expression is exclusively from a single parental allele). There is mounting evidence for biallelic expression of the IGF-II gene in a subset of tumors, suggesting loss of methylation and loss of imprinting as a mechanism for gene induction. In addition to increased IGF-II production, IGF-II bioavailability is increased due to complex alterations in circulating binding proteins. Increased IGF-II suppresses growth hormone (GH) and insulin, resulting in reduced IGF binding protein-3 (IGFBP-3), IGF-I, and acid-labile subunit (ALS). The reduction in ALS and IGFBP-3, which normally sequester IGF-II, causes it to be displaced to a small circulating complex that has greater access to insulin target tissues. For this reason, circulating IGF-II levels may not be markedly increased, despite causing hypoglycemia. In addition to IGF-II–mediated hypoglycemia, tumors may occupy enough of the liver to impair gluconeogenesis.

In most cases, the tumor causing hypoglycemia is clinically apparent and hypoglycemia develops in association with fasting. The diagnosis is made by documenting low serum glucose and suppressed insulin levels in association with symptoms of hypoglycemia. Serum IGF-II levels may not be increased (IGF-II assays may not detect IGF-II precursors). Increased IGF-II mRNA expression is found in most tumors. Any medications associated with hypoglycemia should be eliminated. Treatment of the underlying malignancy, if possible, may reduce the predisposition to hypoglycemia. Frequent meals and intravenous glucose, especially during sleep or fasting, are often necessary to prevent hypoglycemia. Glucagon, GH, and glucocorticoids have also been used to enhance glucose production.

HUMAN CHORIONIC GONADOTROPIN hCG is composed of α and β subunits and can be produced as intact hormone, which is biologically active, or as uncombined biologically inert subunits. Ectopic production of intact hCG occurs most often in association with testicular embryonal tumors, germ cell tumors, extragonadal germinomas, lung cancer, hepatoma, and pancreatic islet tumors. Eutopic production of hCG occurs with trophoblastic malignancies. Low levels of hCG or its uncombined α or β subunits have been reported in a wide range of tumors. hCG α subunit production is particularly common in lung cancer and pancreatic islet cancer. In men, high hCG levels stimulate steroidogenesis and aromatase activity in testicular Leydig cells, resulting in increased estrogen production and the development of gynecomastia. Precocious puberty in boys or gynecomastia in men should prompt measurement of hCG and consideration of a testicular tumor or another source of ectopic hCG production. Most women are asymptomatic. hCG is easily measured using sensitive immunoradiometric assays. Treatment should be directed at the underlying malignancy.

ONCOGENIC OSTEOMALACIA Hypophosphatemic oncogenic osteomalacia is characterized by markedly reduced serum phosphorus and renal phosphate wasting, leading to muscle weakness and osteomalacia. Serum calcium and PTH levels are normal and 1,25 dihydroxyvitamin D is low. Oncogenic osteomalacia is usually caused by benign mesenchymal tumors, such as hemangiopericytomas, fibromas, or giant cell tumors, often of the skeletal extremities or head. It has also been described in sarcomas and in patients with prostate and lung cancer. Resection of the tumor reverses the disorder, confirming its humoral basis. The circulating phosphaturic factor is called *phosphatonin*—a factor that inhibits renal tubular reabsorption of phosphate and renal conversion of 25-hydroxyvitamin D to 1,25-dihydroxyvitamin D. Phosphatonin has been identified as fibroblast growth factor 23 (FGF23). The disorder exhibits biochemical features similar to those seen with inactivating mutations in the *PHEX* gene, the cause of hereditary X-linked hypophosphatemia. The *PHEX* gene encodes a protease that activates FGF23. Treatment involves removal of the tumor, if possible, and supplementation with phosphate and vitamin D. Octreotide treatment reduces phosphate wasting in some patients with tumors that express somatostatin receptor subtype 2. Octreotide scans may also be useful to detect these tumors.

HEMATOLOGIC SYNDROMES

The elevation of granulocyte, platelet, and eosinophil counts in most patients with myeloproliferative disorders is caused by the proliferation of the myeloid elements due to the underlying disease rather than a paraneoplastic syndrome. The paraneoplastic hematologic syndromes in patients with solid tumors are less well characterized than the endocrine syndromes because the ectopic hormone(s) or cytokines responsible have not been identified in most of these tumors (Table 86-2). The severity of the paraneoplastic syndromes parallels the course of the cancer.

ERYTHROCYTOSIS Ectopic production of erythropoietin by cancer cells causes most paraneoplastic erythrocytosis. The ectopically produced erythropoietin stimulates the production of red blood cells in the bone marrow and raises the hematocrit. Other lymphokines and hormones produced by cancer cells may stimulate erythropoietin release but have not been proven to cause erythrocytosis.

Most patients with erythrocytosis have an elevated hematocrit (>52% in men; >48% in women) that is detected on a routine blood count. Approximately 3% of patients with renal cell cancer, 10% of patients with hepatoma, and 15% of patients with cerebellar hemangioblastomas have erythrocytosis. In most cases the erythrocytosis is asymptomatic.

Patients with erythrocytosis due to a renal cell cancer, hepatoma, or CNS cancer should have measurement of red cell mass. If the red cell mass is elevated, the serum erythropoietin level should then be measured. Patients with an appropriate cancer, elevated erythropoietin levels, and no other explanation for erythrocytosis (e.g., hemoglobinopathy that causes increased O_2 affinity; see Chap. 91) have the paraneoplastic syndrome.

℞ TREATMENT

Successful resection of the cancer usually resolves the erythrocytosis. If the tumor cannot be resected or treated effectively with radiation

---

TABLE 86-2 *Paraneoplastic Hematologic Syndromes*

Syndrome	Proteins	Cancers Typically Associated with Syndrome
Erythrocytosis	Erythropoietin	Renal cancers
		Hepatocarcinoma
		Cerebellar hemangioblastomas
Granulocytosis	G-CSF	Lung cancer
	GM-CSF	Gastrointestinal cancer
	IL-6	Ovarian cancer
		Genitourinary cancer
		Hodgkin's disease
Thrombocytosis	IL-6	Lung cancer
		Gastrointestinal cancer
		Breast cancer
		Ovarian cancer
		Lymphoma
Eosinophilia	IL-5	Lymphoma
		Leukemia
		Lung cancer
Thrombophlebitis	Unknown	Lung cancer
		Pancreatic cancer
		Gastrointestinal cancer
		Breast cancer
		Genitourinary cancer
		Ovarian cancer
		Prostate cancer
		Lymphoma

therapy or chemotherapy, phlebotomy may control any symptoms related to erythrocytosis.

GRANULOCYTOSIS   Approximately 30% of patients with solid tumors have granulocytosis (granulocyte count >8000/μL). In about half of patients with granulocytosis and cancer, the granulocytosis has an identifiable nonparaneoplastic etiology (infection, tumor necrosis, glucocorticoid administration, etc.). The other patients have proteins in urine and serum that stimulate the growth of bone marrow cells. Tumors and tumor cell lines from patients with lung, ovarian, and bladder cancers have been documented to produce granulocyte colony-stimulating factor (G-CSF), granulocyte-macrophage colony-stimulating factor (GM-CSF), and/or interleukin 6 (IL-6). However, the etiology of granulocytosis has not been characterized in most patients.

Patients with granulocytosis are nearly all asymptomatic, and the differential white blood cell count does not have a shift to immature forms of neutrophils. Granulocytosis occurs in 40% of patients with lung and gastrointestinal cancers, 20% of patients with breast cancer, 30% of patients with brain tumors and ovarian cancers, and 10% of patients with renal cell carcinoma. Patients with advanced-stage disease are more likely to have granulocytosis than those with early-stage disease.

Paraneoplastic granulocytosis does not require treatment. The granulocytosis resolves when the underlying cancer is successfully treated.

THROMBOCYTOSIS   Some 35% of patients with thrombocytosis (platelet count >400,000/μL) have an underlying diagnosis of cancer. IL-6, a candidate molecule for the etiology of paraneoplastic thrombocytosis, stimulates the production of platelets in vitro and in vivo. Some patients with cancer and thrombocytosis have elevated levels of IL-6 in plasma. Another candidate molecule is thrombopoietin, a peptide hormone that stimulates megakaryocyte proliferation and platelet production. The etiology of thrombocytosis has not been established in most cases.

Patients with thrombocytosis are nearly all asymptomatic. Thrombocytosis is not clearly linked to thrombosis in patients with cancer. Thrombocytosis is present in 40% of patients with lung and gastrointestinal cancers, 20% of patients with breast, endometrial, and ovarian cancers, and 10% of patients with lymphoma. Patients with thrombocytosis are more likely to have advanced-stage disease and have a poorer prognosis than patients without thrombocytosis. Paraneoplastic thrombocytosis does not require treatment.

EOSINOPHILIA   Eosinophilia is present in ~1% of patients with cancer. Tumors and tumor cell lines from patients with lymphomas or leukemia may produce IL-5, which stimulates eosinophil growth. Activation of IL-5 transcription in lymphomas and leukemias may involve translocation of the long arm of chromosome 5, to which the genes for IL-5 and other cytokines map.

Patients with eosinophilia are typically asymptomatic. Eosinophilia is present in 10% of patients with lymphoma, 3% of patients with lung cancer, and occasional patients with cervical, gastrointestinal, renal, and breast cancer. Patients with markedly elevated eosinophil counts (>5000/μL) can develop shortness of breath and wheezing. A chest radiograph may reveal diffuse pulmonary infiltrates from eosinophil infiltration and activation in the lungs.

℞ TREATMENT

Definitive treatment is directed at the underlying malignancy: tumors should be resected or treated with radiation or chemotherapy. In most patients who develop shortness of breath related to eosinophilia, symptoms resolve with the use of oral or inhaled glucocorticoids.

THROMBOPHLEBITIS   Deep venous thrombosis and pulmonary embolism are the most common thrombotic conditions in patients with cancer. Migratory or recurrent thrombophlebitis may be the initial manifestation of cancer. Nearly 15% of patients who develop deep venous thrombosis or pulmonary embolism have a diagnosis of cancer (Chap. 102). The coexistence of peripheral venous thrombosis with visceral carcinoma, particularly pancreatic cancer, is called *Trousseau's syndrome.*

Pathogenesis   Patients with cancer are predisposed to thromboembolism because they are often at bedrest or immobilized, and tumors may obstruct or slow blood flow. Chronic intravenous catheters also predispose to clotting. In addition, clotting may be promoted by release of procoagulants or cytokines from tumor cells or associated inflammatory cells, or by platelet adhesion or aggregation. The specific molecules that mediate the increased risk of thromboembolism have not been identified.

Clinical Manifestations   Patients with cancer who develop deep venous thrombosis usually develop swelling or pain in the leg, and physical examination reveals tenderness, warmth, and redness. Patients who present with pulmonary embolism develop dyspnea, chest pain, and syncope, and physical examination shows tachycardia, cyanosis, and hypotension. Some 5% of patients with no history of cancer who have a diagnosis of deep venous thrombosis or pulmonary embolism will have a diagnosis of cancer within 1 year. The most common cancers associated with thromboembolic episodes include lung, pancreatic, gastrointestinal, breast, ovarian, and genitourinary cancers, lymphomas, and brain tumors. Patients with cancer who undergo surgical procedures requiring general anesthesia have a 20 to 30% risk of deep venous thrombosis.

Diagnosis   The diagnosis of deep venous thrombosis in patients with cancer is made by impedance plethysmography or bilateral compression ultrasonography of the leg veins. Patients with a noncompressible venous segment have deep venous thrombosis. If compression ultrasonography is normal and a high clinical suspicion exists for deep venous thrombosis, venography should be done to look for a luminal filling defect. Elevation of D-dimer is not as predictive of deep venous thrombosis in patients with cancer as it is in patients without cancer.

Patients with symptoms and signs suggesting a pulmonary embolism should be evaluated with a chest radiograph, electrocardiogram, arterial blood gas analysis, and ventilation–perfusion scan. Patients with mismatched segmental perfusion defects have a pulmonary embolus. Patients with equivocal ventilation–perfusion findings should be evaluated as described above for deep venous thrombosis in their legs. If deep venous thrombosis is detected, they should be anticoagulated. If deep venous thrombosis is not detected, they should be considered for a pulmonary angiogram.

Patients without a diagnosis of cancer who present with an initial episode of thrombophlebitis or pulmonary embolus need no additional tests for cancer other than a careful history and physical exam. In light of the many possible primary sites, diagnostic testing in asymptomatic patients is wasteful. However, if the clot is refractory to standard treatment or is in an unusual site, or if the thrombophlebitis is migratory or recurrent, efforts to find an underlying cancer are indicated.

℞ TREATMENT

Patients with cancer and a diagnosis of deep venous thrombosis or pulmonary embolism should be treated initially with intravenous unfractionated heparin or low-molecular-weight heparin for at least 5 days and warfarin started within 1 or 2 days. The warfarin dose should be adjusted so the international normalized ratio (INR) is 2 to 3. Patients with proximal deep venous thrombosis and a relative contraindication to heparin anticoagulation (hemorrhagic brain metastases or pericardial effusion) should be considered for placement of a filter in the inferior vena cava (Greenfield filter) to prevent pulmonary embolism. Warfarin should be administered for 3 to 6 months. An alternative approach is to use low-molecular-weight heparin for 6 months. Patients with cancer who undergo a major surgical procedure should be considered for heparin prophylaxis or pneumatic boots. Breast cancer patients undergoing chemotherapy and patients with implanted catheters should be considered for prophylaxis (1 mg warfarin per day).

→*Cutaneous paraneoplastic syndromes are discussed in Chap. 48. Neurologic paraneoplastic syndromes are discussed in Chap. 87. More extensive discussion of functional endocrine tumors is given in Chap. 329.*

FURTHER READING

JONES PA, BAYLIN SB: The fundamental role of epigenetic events in cancer. Nat Rev Genet 3:415, 2002

LEE AY et al: Clinical utility of a rapid whole-blood D-dimer assay in patients with cancer who present with suspected acute deep venous thrombosis. Ann Intern Med 131:417, 1999

LEVINE MN: Can we optimise treatment of thrombosis? Cancer Treat Rev 29(Suppl 2):19, 2003

RHEE I et al: DNMT1 and DNMT3b cooperate to silence genes in human cancer cells. Nature 416:552, 2002

SEUFERT J et al: Octreotide therapy for tumor-induced osteomalacia. N Engl J Med 345:1883, 2001

STREWLER GJ: The parathyroid hormone-related protein. Endocrinol Metab Clin North Am 29:629, 2000

87 PARANEOPLASTIC NEUROLOGIC SYNDROMES
Josep Dalmau, Myrna R. Rosenfeld

Paraneoplastic neurologic disorders (PNDs) are cancer-related syndromes that can affect any part of the nervous system (Table 87-1). They are remote effects of cancer, caused by mechanisms other than metastasis or by any of the complications of cancer such as coagulopathy, stroke, metabolic and nutritional conditions, infections, and side effects of cancer therapy. In 60% of patients the neurologic symptoms precede the cancer diagnosis. Overall, clinically disabling PNDs occur in 0.5 to 1% of all cancer patients, but they occur in 2 to 3% of patients with neuroblastoma or small-cell lung cancer (SCLC), and in 30 to 50% of patients with thymoma or sclerotic myeloma.

PATHOGENESIS Most PNDs are mediated by immune responses triggered by the tumor expression of neuronal proteins (onconeuronal antigens). In PNDs of the central nervous system (CNS), many antibody-associated immune responses have been identified (Table 87-2). These antibodies usually react with the patient's tumor, and their detection in serum or cerebrospinal fluid (CSF) strongly predicts the presence

of cancer. The target antigens are usually intracellular proteins with roles in neuronal development and function. Some of the antibodies react with epitopes located in critical protein domains, disrupting protein function leading to neuronal apoptosis. In addition to onconeuronal antibodies, most PNDs of the CNS are associated with infiltrates of CD4+ and CD8+ T cells, microglial activation, gliosis, and variable neuronal loss. The infiltrating T cells are often in close contact with neurons undergoing degeneration, suggesting a primary pathogenic role. T cell–mediated cytotoxicity may contribute directly to cell death in these PNDs. Thus both humoral and cellular immune mechanisms participate in the pathogenesis of many PNDs. This complex immunopathogenesis may underlie the resistance of many of these conditions to therapy.

Only three of the antibodies listed in Table 87-2 have been shown to play a direct pathogenic role in PNDs; all produce distinctive disorders of the peripheral nervous system. These are: antibodies to P/Q-type voltage-gated calcium channels (VGCC) in patients with the Lambert-Eaton myasthenic syndrome (LEMS); antibodies to acetylcholine receptors in patients with myasthenia gravis; and antibodies to voltage-gated potassium channels (VGKC) in some patients with peripheral nerve hyperexcitability (neuromyotonia). Common features of these three antibodies are that they target cell-surface molecules and that their passive transfer to animals reproduces the disorders. Plasma exchange or immunomodulation with intravenous immunoglobulin (IVIg) usually produces neurologic improvement. Each of these disorders can occur without cancer, and therefore detection of these antibodies does not predict the presence of cancer.

Other PNDs are likely immune-mediated although their antigens are unknown. These include several syndromes of inflammatory neuropathies and myopathies. In addition, many patients with typical PND syndromes are antibody-negative.

For still other PNDs, the cause remains quite obscure. These include, among others, several neuropathies that occur in the terminal stages of cancer and a number of neuropathies associated with plasma cell dyscrasias or lymphoma without evidence of inflammatory infiltrates or deposits of immunoglobulin, cryoglobulin, or amyloid.

TABLE 87-1 *Paraneoplastic Syndromes of the Nervous System*

Syndromes of the brain, brainstem, and cerebellum
  Focal encephalitis
    Cortical encephalitis
    Limbic encephalitis
    Brainstem encephalitis
    Cerebellar dysfunction
    Autonomic dysfunction
  Paraneoplastic cerebellar degeneration
  Opsoclonus-myoclonus
Syndromes of the spinal cord
  Subacute necrotizing myelopathy
  Motor neuron dysfunction
  Myelitis
  Stiff-person syndrome
Syndromes of dorsal root ganglia
  Sensory neuronopathy
Multiple levels of involvement
  Encephalomyelitis[a], sensory neuronopathy, autonomic dysfunction
Syndromes of peripheral nerve
  Chronic and subacute sensorimotor peripheral neuropathy
  Vasculitis of nerve and muscle
  Neuropathy associated with malignant monoclonal gammopathies
  Peripheral nerve hyperexcitability
  Autonomic neuropathy
Syndromes of the neuromuscular junction
  Lambert-Eaton myasthenic syndrome
  Myasthenia gravis
Syndromes of the muscle
  Polymyositis/dermatomyositis
  Acute necrotizing myopathy
Syndromes affecting the visual system
  Cancer-associated retinopathy (CAR)
  Melanoma-associated retinopathy (MAR)
  Uveitis (usually in association with encephalomyelitis)

[a] Includes cortical, limbic, or brainstem encephalitis, cerebellar dysfunction, myelitis.

APPROACH TO THE PATIENT

The diagnosis and management of PNDs may be difficult for several reasons. First, it is common for symptoms to appear before the presence of a tumor is known. Second, the neurologic syndrome can evolve in a rapidly progressive fashion, producing a severe and usually irreversible neurologic deficit in a short period of time. There is evidence that prompt tumor control improves the course of PNDs. Therefore, the major concern of the physician is to recognize a disorder promptly as paraneoplastic in order to identify and treat the tumor.

PND of the Central Nervous System and Dorsal Root Ganglia When symptoms involve brain, spinal cord, or dorsal root ganglia, the

TABLE 87-2 *Paraneoplastic Antineuronal Antibodies, Associated Syndromes and Cancers*

Antibody	Syndrome	Associated Cancers
Anti-Hu (ANNA-1)	PEM (including cortical, limbic, brainstem encephalitis, cerebellar dysfunction, myelitis), PSN, autonomic dysfunction	SCLC, other neuroendocrine tumors
Anti-Yo (PCA-1)	PCD	Ovary and other gynecologic cancers, breast
Anti-Ri (ANNA-2)	PCD, brainstem encephalitis, opsoclonus-myoclonus	Breast, gynecological, SCLC
Anti-Tr	PCD	Hodgkin's lymphoma
Anti-Zic	PCD, encephalomyelitis	SCLC and other neuroendocrine tumors
Anti-CV$_2$/CRMP5	PEM, PCD, chorea, peripheral neuropathy, uveitis	SCLC, thymoma, other
Anti-Ma proteins[a]	Limbic, hypothalamic, brainstem encephalitis (infrequently PCD)	Germ-cell tumors of testis, lung cancer, other solid tumors
Anti-amphiphysin	Stiff-person syndrome, PEM	Breast, SCLC
Anti-VGCC[b]	LEMS, PCD	SCLC, lymphoma
Anti-AChR[b]	MG	Thymoma
Anti-VGKC[b]	Peripheral nerve hyperexcitability (neuromyotonia)	Thymoma, SCLC, others
Anti-recoverin	Cancer-associated retinopathy (CAR)	SCLC and other
Anti-bipolar cells of the retina	Melanoma-associated retinopathy (MAR)	Melanoma

[a] Patients with antibodies to Ma2 are usually men with testicular cancer. Patients with additional antibodies to other Ma proteins are men or women with a variety of solid tumors.
[b] These antibodies can occur with or without a cancer association.
Note: PEM: paraneoplastic encephalomyelitis; PCD, paraneoplastic cerebellar degeneration; PSN, paraneoplastic sensory neuronopathy; LEMS, Lambert-Eaton myasthenic syndrome; MG, myasthenia gravis; VGCC, voltage-gated calcium channel; AChR, acetylcholine receptor; VGKC, voltage-gated potassium channel; SCLC, small-cell lung cancer.

and degree of effort needed to demonstrate a neoplasm. For example, the frequent association of LEMS with SCLC should lead to a chest and abdomen computed tomography or body positron emission tomography (PET) scan and, if negative, periodic tumor screening for at least 3 years after the neurologic diagnosis. In contrast, the weak association of polymyositis with cancer calls into question the need for repeated cancer screenings in this situation. Serum and urine immunofixation studies should be considered in patients with peripheral neuropathy of unknown cause; detection of a monoclonal gammopathy suggests the need for additional studies to uncover a B cell or plasma cell malignancy. In paraneoplastic neuropathies, diagnostically useful antineuronal antibodies are limited to anti-CV$_2$/CRMP5 and anti-Hu.

For any type of PND, if antineuronal antibodies are negative, the diagnosis relies on the demonstration of cancer and the exclusion of other cancer-related or independent neurologic disorders. Body PET scans often uncover tumors undetected by other tests.

suspicion of PND is usually based on a combination of clinical, radiologic, and CSF findings. In these cases, a biopsy of the affected tissue is often difficult to obtain, and although useful to rule out other disorders (e.g., metastasis, infection), neuropathologic findings are not specific for PND. Furthermore, there are no specific radiologic or electrophysiologic tests that are diagnostic of PND. The presence of antineuronal antibodies (Table 87-2) may help in the diagnosis with the following caveats: (1) antibodies are detected in only 40 to 50% of PNDs of the CNS; (2) antibodies may be present in both the serum and CSF, but in some patients only the CSF is positive (especially with antibodies to Tr and Ma proteins); (3) antibodies (usually at low titer) are present in a variable proportion of cancer patients without PND; (4) there is an imperfect correlation between antibody titers and the course of the neurologic disorder; (5) several antibodies may associate with a similar syndrome, with the antibody specificity often correlating with the tumor type (e.g., cerebellar degeneration is associated with anti-Tr antibodies if the tumor is Hodgkin's disease but with anti-Yo antibodies if the tumor is ovarian or breast cancer); and (6) several antibodies may be present in the serum or CSF of the same patient (e.g., anti-Hu and anti-CV$_2$/CRMP5, or less frequently anti-Ri).

Magnetic resonance imaging (MRI) and CSF studies are important to rule out neurologic complications due to the direct spread of cancer, particularly metastatic and leptomeningeal disease. In most PNDs the MRI findings are nonspecific. Paraneoplastic limbic encephalitis is usually associated with characteristic MRI abnormalities in the mesial temporal lobes (see below), but similar findings can occur with other disorders [e.g., systemic lupus erythematosus, human herpesvirus (HHV) 6 encephalitis]. The CSF profile of patients with PND of the CNS or dorsal root ganglia typically consists of mild to moderate pleocytosis (<200 mononuclear cells, predominantly lymphocytes), an increase in the protein concentration, intrathecal synthesis of IgG, and a variable presence of oligoclonal bands.

PND of Nerve and Muscle If symptoms involve peripheral nerve, neuromuscular junction, or muscle, the diagnosis of a specific PND is usually established on clinical, electrophysiologic, and pathologic grounds. The clinical history, accompanying symptoms (e.g., anorexia, weight loss), and type of syndrome dictate the studies

SPECIFIC PARANEOPLASTIC NEUROLOGIC SYNDROMES (Table 87-3)
PARANEOPLASTIC ENCEPHALOMYELITIS AND FOCAL ENCEPHALITIS The term *encephalomyelitis* describes an inflammatory process with multifocal involvement of the nervous system, including brain, brainstem, cerebellum, and spinal cord. It is often associated with dorsal root ganglia and autonomic dysfunction. For any given patient, the clinical manifestations are determined by the area or areas predominantly involved, but pathology almost always reveals abnormalities (inflammatory infiltrates, neuronal loss, gliosis) beyond the symptomatic regions. Several clinicopathologic syndromes may occur alone or in combination: (1) *cortical encephalitis*, which may present as "epilepsia partialis continua"; (2) *limbic encephalitis*, characterized by confusion, depression, agitation, anxiety, severe short-term memory deficits, partial complex seizures, and dementia; the MRI usually shows unilateral or bilateral medial temporal lobe abnormalities, best seen with T2 and fluid-attenuated inversion recovery sequences, and occasionally enhancing with gadolinium; (3) *brainstem encephalitis,* resulting in eye movement disorders (nystagmus, opsoclonus, supranuclear or nuclear paresis), cranial nerve paresis, dysarthria, dysphagia, and central autonomic dysfunction; (4) *cerebellar gait and limb ataxia*; (5) *myelitis*, which may cause lower or upper motor neuron symptoms, myoclonus, muscle rigidity, and spasms; and (6) *autonomic dysfunction* as a result of involvement of the neuraxis at multiple levels, including hypothalamus, brainstem, and autonomic nerves (see autonomic neuropathy). Cardiac arrhythmias, postural hypotension, or central hypoventilation are frequent causes of death in patients with encephalomyelitis.

Paraneoplastic encephalomyelitis and focal encephalitis are usually associated with SCLC, but many other cancers have also been reported. Patients with SCLC and these syndromes usually have anti-Hu antibodies in serum and CSF. Anti-CV$_2$/CRMP5 antibodies occur less frequently; some of these patients may develop chorea or uveitis. Antibodies to Ma proteins are associated with limbic and brainstem encephalitis and occasionally with cerebellar symptoms; prominent hypothalamic dysfunction, hypersomnia, and cataplexy can also occur. MRI abnormalities are frequent, including those described with limbic

	Antibodies		
	Paraneoplastic		
Syndrome	Frequent	Infrequent	Non-Paraneoplastic
Limbic encephalitis	Ma2, Hu, CV₂/CRMP5	Tr, VGKC	VGKC
Cerebellar degeneration	Yo, Tr, P/Q VGCC, Hu, *Zic*, Ri, CV₂/CRMP5, Ma1-2	*mGluR1*; *MAZ*	Gliadin GAD
Hypothalamic, brainstem encephalitis	Ma2, Hu	CV₂/CRMP5	
Encephalomyelitis	Hu, *Zic*	CV₂/CRMP5, Ri, amphiphysin	
Chorea	CV₂/CRMP5		
Opsoclonus-myoclonus	Ri	Hu, Ma2, Yo,	*APC*
Stiff-person syndrome	Amphiphysin	*Gephyrin*, Ri	GAD
PNH (neuromyotonia)	VGKC		VGKC
Myasthenia gravis	AChR		AChR, MuSK
LEMS	P/Q-type VGCC	*MysB*	P/Q-type VGCC
Sensory neuronopathy	Hu		
Axonal sensorimotor neuropathy	Hu, CV₂/CRMP5		Monoclonal gammopathy (M protein)[b]
Autonomic neuropathy	Hu	CV₂/CRMP5, ganglionic AChR	Ganglionic AChR
Predominant sensory demyelinating neuropathy		MAG, ganglioside antibodies: often present with Waldenström's macroglobulinemia	MAG, ganglioside antibodies, often present with MGUS
Paraneoplastic retinopathy	Recoverin (CAR), anti-bipolar cell antibodies (*MAR*)	*Tubby-like protein 1, PNR*	

[a] Antibodies have been validated by more than one laboratory and/or the protein sequence of the target antigen is known.

[b] The M protein usually does not have specific antibody activity.

Note: Italics indicate that commercial testing for these antibodies is not available. PNH, peripheral nerve hyperexcitability; CAR, cancer-associated retinopathy; MAR, melanoma-associated retinopathy; PNR, photoreceptor-specific nuclear receptor; MGUS, monoclonal gammopathy of uncertain significance; VGKC, voltage-gated potassium channel; GAD, glutamic acid decarboxylase; AChR, acetylcholine receptor; LEMS, Lambert-Eaton myasthenic syndrome; VGCC, voltage-gated calcium channel; MAG, myelin-associated glycoprotein.

encephalitis and variable involvement of the hypothalamus, basal ganglia, or brainstem. The oncologic associations of these antibodies are shown in Table 87-2.

All types of paraneoplastic encephalitis and encephalomyelitis, except limbic encephalitis, respond poorly to treatment. Stabilization of symptoms or partial neurologic improvement may occasionally occur, particularly if there is a satisfactory response of the tumor to treatment. The roles of plasma exchange, IVIg, and immunosuppression have not been established. Rare patients with limbic encephalitis have shown dramatic improvement after treatment, but it is not known whether remission of the cancer, glucocorticoids, or IVIg was responsible.

PARANEOPLASTIC CEREBELLAR DEGENERATION This disorder is often preceded by a prodrome that may include dizziness, oscillopsia, blurry or double vision, nausea, and vomiting. A few days or weeks later, dysarthria, gait and limb ataxia, and variable dysphagia can appear. The examination usually shows downbeating nystagmus and, rarely, opsoclonus. Brainstem dysfunction, upgoing toes, or a mild neuropathy may occur, but more often the symptoms and signs are restricted to the cerebellum. Early in the course, MRI studies are usually normal; in some patients a transient enhancement of the cerebellar cortex has been noted. Later, the MRI typically reveals cerebellar atrophy. The disorder results from extensive degeneration of Purkinje cells, with variable involvement of other cerebellar cortical neurons, deep cerebellar nuclei, and spinocerebellar tracts. An immune-mediated pathogenesis is supported by CSF findings and biopsy studies obtained during the early stage of the disorder. The tumors more frequently involved are SCLC, cancer of the breast and ovary, and Hodgkin's lymphoma.

Anti-Yo antibodies in patients with breast and gynecologic cancers and anti-Tr antibodies in patients with Hodgkin's lymphoma are the two paraneoplastic antibodies typically associated with prominent or pure cerebellar degeneration. Antibodies to P/Q-type VGCC occur in some patients with SCLC and cerebellar dysfunction; only some of these patients develop LEMS. A subacute cerebellar ataxia can also be the presenting symptom of paraneoplastic encephalomyelitis; in this syndrome, symptoms of widespread CNS involvement eventually occur. Of note, a variable degree of cerebellar dysfunction can be associated with virtually any type of antibody-related PND of the CNS

(Table 87-2). A number of single case reports have described neurologic improvement after tumor removal, plasma exchange, IVIg, cyclophosphamide, or glucocorticoids. However, large series of patients with well-defined antibody-positive paraneoplastic cerebellar degeneration show that these disorders rarely improve with any treatment.

PARANEOPLASTIC OPSOCLONUS-MYOCLONUS SYNDROME *Opsoclonus* is a disorder of eye movement characterized by involuntary, chaotic saccades that occur in all directions of gaze; it is frequently associated with myoclonus and ataxia. Opsoclonus-myoclonus may be cancer-related or idiopathic. When the cause is paraneoplastic, the tumors involved are usually cancer of the lung and breast in adults and neuroblastoma in children. The pathologic substrate of opsoclonus-myoclonus is unclear. The majority of SCLC patients do not harbor antineuronal antibodies. A small subset of patients with ataxia, opsoclonus, and other eye movement disorders develop anti-Ri antibodies; in rare instances muscle rigidity, autonomic dysfunction, and dementia also occur. The tumor most frequently involved in anti-Ri-associated syndromes is breast cancer; however, only 50% of patients with anti-Ri antibodies develop opsoclonus.

If the tumor is not successfully treated, the paraneoplastic opsoclonus-myoclonus syndrome in adults often progresses to encephalopathy, coma, and death. In addition to treating the tumor, symptoms may respond to immunotherapy (glucocorticoids and/or IVIg).

At least 50% of children with opsoclonus-myoclonus have an underlying neuroblastoma. Hypotonia, ataxia, behavioral changes, and irritability are frequent accompanying symptoms. Although some patients harbor anti-Hu antibodies, most are antibody-negative. Neurologic symptoms often improve with treatment of the tumor (including chemotherapy) and with glucocorticoids, adrenocorticotropic hormone (ACTH), plasma exchange, and IVIg. The response to treatment varies; patients who do not improve with glucocorticoids may respond to ACTH. Neurologic relapses are frequent, and many patients are left with psychomotor retardation and behavioral and sleep problems.

PARANEOPLASTIC SYNDROMES OF THE SPINAL CORD The number of reports of paraneoplastic spinal cord syndromes, such as *subacute motor neuronopathy* and *acute necrotizing myelopathy*, has decreased in recent years. This may represent a true decrease in incidence, due to improved and prompt oncologic interventions, or may be because of the identification of nonparaneoplastic etiologies; e.g., subacute necrotizing myelopathy may occur with HSV infection, usually HSV-2.

Some patients with cancer develop *upper* or *lower motor neuron dysfunction* or both, resembling amyotrophic lateral sclerosis. Because paraneoplastic antibody markers are lacking, it is unclear whether these disorders have a paraneoplastic etiology or simply coincide with the presence of cancer. There are isolated case reports of cancer patients with motor neuron dysfunction who had neurologic improvement after tumor treatment. A more than coincidental association occurs between lymphoma and motor neuron dysfunction. A search for lymphoma should be undertaken in patients with a motor neuron syndrome who are found to have a monoclonal protein in serum or CSF or an increased protein concentration in the CSF.

Paraneoplastic myelitis may present with upper or lower motor neuron symptoms, segmental myoclonus, and rigidity. This syndrome can appear as the presenting manifestation of encephalomyelitis and may be associated with SCLC and serum anti-Hu, anti-CV$_2$/CRMP5, or anti-amphiphysin antibodies.

Paraneoplastic myelopathy can also produce several syndromes characterized by prominent muscle stiffness and rigidity. The spectrum ranges from focal symptoms in one or several extremities (*stiff-limb syndrome* or *stiff-person syndrome*) to a disorder that also affects the brainstem (known as *encephalomyelitis with rigidity*) and likely has a different pathogenesis.

PARANEOPLASTIC STIFF-PERSON SYNDROME   This disorder is characterized by progressive muscle rigidity, stiffness, and painful spasms triggered by auditory, sensory, or emotional stimuli. Rigidity mainly involves the lower trunk and legs, but it can affect the upper extremities and neck. Symptoms improve with sleep and general anesthetics. Electrophysiologic studies demonstrate continuous motor unit activity. Antibodies associated with the stiff-person syndrome target proteins [glutamic acid decarboxylase (GAD), amphiphysin] involved in the function of inhibitory synapses utilizing γ-aminobutyric acid (GABA) or glycine as neurotransmitters. Paraneoplastic stiff-person syndrome and amphiphysin antibodies are often related to breast cancer. By contrast, antibodies to GAD may occur in some cancer patients but are much more frequently present in the non-paraneoplastic disorder. Optimal treatment of stiff-person syndrome requires therapy of the underlying tumor, glucocorticoids, and symptomatic use of drugs that enhance GABA-ergic transmission (diazepam, baclofen, sodium valproate, vigabatrin). A benefit of IVIg has been demonstrated for the non-paraneoplastic disorder but remains to be established for the paraneoplastic syndrome.

PARANEOPLASTIC SENSORY NEURONOPATHY OR DORSAL ROOT GANGLIONOPATHY   This syndrome is characterized by sensory deficits that may be symmetric or asymmetric, painful dysesthesias, radicular pain, and decreased or absent reflexes. All modalities of sensation and any part of the body including face and trunk can be involved. Specialized sensations such as taste and hearing can also be affected. Electrophysiologic studies show decreased or absent sensory nerve potentials with normal or near-normal motor conduction velocities. Symptoms result from an inflammatory, likely immune-mediated, process that targets the dorsal root ganglia, causing neuronal loss, proliferation of satellite cells, and secondary degeneration of the posterior columns of the spinal cord. The dorsal nerve roots, and less frequently the anterior nerve roots and peripheral nerves, may also be involved.

This disorder often precedes or is associated with encephalomyelitis and autonomic dysfunction and has the same immunologic and oncologic associations, i.e., anti-Hu antibodies and SCLC. As with anti-Hu-associated encephalomyelitis, the therapeutic approach focuses on prompt treatment of the tumor. Glucocorticoids occasionally produce clinical stabilization or improvement. The benefit of IVIg and plasma exchange is not proved.

PARANEOPLASTIC PERIPHERAL NEUROPATHIES   These disorders may develop any time during the course of the neoplastic disease. Neuropathies occurring at late stages of cancer or lymphoma usually cause mild to moderate sensorimotor deficits due to axonal degeneration of unclear etiology. These neuropathies are often masked by concurrent neurotoxicity from chemotherapy and other cancer therapies. In contrast, the neuropathies that develop in the early stages of cancer often show a rapid progression, sometimes with a relapsing and remitting course, and evidence of inflammatory infiltrates and axonal loss or demyelination in biopsy studies. If demyelinating features predominate (Chap. 363), IVIg or glucocorticoids may improve symptoms. These neuropathies are not usually associated with antineuronal antibodies. Occasionally anti-CV$_2$/CRMP5 antibodies are present; detection of anti-Hu suggests concurrent dorsal root ganglionitis.

Guillain-Barré syndrome and *brachial plexitis* have occasionally been reported in patients with lymphoma, but there is no clear evidence of a paraneoplastic association.

Malignant monoclonal gammopathies include: (1) multiple myeloma and sclerotic myeloma associated with IgG or IgA monoclonal proteins; and (2) Waldenström's macroglobulinemia, B cell lymphoma, and chronic B cell lymphocytic leukemia associated with IgM monoclonal proteins. These disorders may cause neuropathy by a variety of mechanisms, including compression of roots and plexuses by metastasis to vertebral bodies and pelvis, deposits of amyloid in peripheral nerves, and paraneoplastic mechanisms. The paraneoplastic variety has several distinctive features. Approximately half of patients with sclerotic myeloma develop a sensorimotor neuropathy with predominantly motor deficits, resembling a chronic inflammatory demyelinating neuropathy (Chap. 365); some patients develop elements of the POEMS syndrome (*p*olyneuropathy, *o*rganomegaly, *e*ndocrinopathy, *M* protein, *s*kin changes). Treatment of the plasmacytoma or sclerotic lesions usually improves the neuropathy. In contrast, the sensorimotor or sensory neuropathy associated with multiple myeloma rarely responds to treatment. Between 5 and 10% of patients with Waldenström's macroglobulinemia develop a distal symmetric sensorimotor neuropathy with predominant involvement of large sensory fibers. These patients may have IgM antibodies in their serum against myelin-associated glycoprotein (Chap. 365). In addition to treating the Waldenström's macroglobulinemia, other therapies may improve the neuropathy, including plasma exchange, IVIg, chlorambucil, cyclophosphamide, fludarabine, or rituximab.

Vasculitis of the nerve and muscle causes a painful symmetric or asymmetric distal sensorimotor neuropathy with variable proximal weakness. It predominantly affects elderly men and is associated with an elevated erythrocyte sedimentation rate and increased CSF protein concentration. SCLC and lymphoma are the primary tumors involved. Pathology demonstrates axonal degeneration and T cell infiltrates involving the small vessels of the nerve and muscle. Immunosuppressants (glucocorticoids and cyclophosphamide) often result in neurologic improvement.

Peripheral nerve hyperexcitability (*neuromyotonia* or *Isaacs' syndrome*) is characterized by spontaneous and continuous muscle fiber activity of peripheral nerve origin. Clinical features include cramps, muscle twitching (fasciculations or myokymia), stiffness, delayed muscle relaxation (pseudomyotonia), and spontaneous or evoked carpal or pedal spasms. The involved muscles may be hypertrophic, and some patients develop paresthesias and hyperhydrosis. CNS dysfunction, including mood changes, sleep disorder, or hallucinations, may occur. The electromyogram (EMG) shows fibrillations; fasciculations; and doublet, triplet, or multiplet single unit (myokymic) discharges that have a high intraburst frequency. An immune pathogenesis is suggested by the frequent presence of serum antibodies to VGKC. The disorder often occurs without cancer; if paraneoplastic, benign and malignant thymomas and SCLC are the usual tumors. Some patients with thymoma develop acetylcholine receptor antibodies with or without myasthenia gravis. Diphenylhydantoin, carbamazepine, and plasma exchange improve symptoms.

The *cramps-fasciculation syndrome* resembles neuromyotonia, but the EMG does not show myokymic discharges. It may also occur with thymoma, lung cancer, and antibodies to VGKC.

Paraneoplastic autonomic neuropathy usually develops as a component of other disorders, such as LEMS and encephalomyelitis. It may rarely occur as a pure or predominantly autonomic neuropathy with adrenergic or cholinergic dysfunction at the pre- or postganglionic levels. Patients can develop several life-threatening complications, such as gastrointestinal paresis with pseudoobstruction, cardiac dysrhythmias, and postural hypotension. Other symptoms include dry mouth, erectile dysfunction, anhidrosis, and sphincter dysfunction. The disorder has been reported to occur in association with several tumors, including SCLC, cancer of the pancreas or testis, carcinoid tumors, and lymphoma. Because autonomic symptoms can also be the presenting feature of encephalomyelitis, serum anti-Hu and anti-CV$_2$/CRMP5 antibodies should also be sought. Serum antibodies to ganglionic acetylcholine receptors have been reported in this syndrome, but they also occur without a cancer association. (See also Table 354-6).

LAMBERT-EATON MYASTHENIC SYNDROME →*LEMS is discussed in Chap. 366.*

MYASTHENIA GRAVIS →*For discussion of myasthenia gravis, see Chap. 366.*

POLYMYOSITIS-DERMATOMYOSITIS →*Polymyositis and dermatomyositis are discussed in detail in Chap. 369.*

ACUTE NECROTIZING MYOPATHY
Patients with this syndrome develop myalgias and rapid progression of weakness involving the extremities and the pharyngeal and respiratory muscles, often resulting in death. Serum muscle enzymes are elevated, and muscle biopsy shows extensive necrosis with minimal or absent inflammation and sometimes deposits of complement. The disorder occurs as a paraneoplastic manifestation of a variety of cancers including SCLC and cancer of the gastrointestinal tract, breast, kidney, and prostate, among others. Glucocorticoids or treatment of the underlying tumor rarely control the disorder.

PARANEOPLASTIC VISUAL SYNDROMES
This group of disorders involves the retina and, less frequently, the uvea and optic nerves. The term *cancer-associated retinopathy* is used to describe paraneoplastic cone and rod dysfunction characterized by photosensitivity, progressive loss of vision and color perception, central or ring scotomas, night blindness, and attenuation of photopic and scotopic responses in the electroretinogram (ERG). The most commonly associated tumor is SCLC. Melanoma-associated retinopathy affects patients with metastatic cutaneous melanoma. Patients develop the acute onset of night blindness and shimmering, flickering, or pulsating photopsias that often progress to visual loss. The ERG demonstrates reduction in the b-wave amplitude. Paraneoplastic optic neuritis and uveitis are very uncommon and can develop in association with encephalomyelitis. Some patients with paraneoplastic uveitis harbor anti-CV$_2$/CRMP5 antibodies.

Some paraneoplastic retinopathies are associated with serum antibodies that specifically react with the subset of retinal cells undergoing degeneration, supporting an immune-mediated pathogenesis (Tables 87-2 and 87-3). Paraneoplastic retinopathies usually fail to improve with treatment, although rare responses to glucocorticoids, plasma exchange, and IVIg have been reported.

FURTHER READING

CHAN JW: Paraneoplastic retinopathies and optic neuropathies. Surv Ophthalmol 48:12, 2003

DROPCHO EJ: Remote neurologic manifestations of cancer. Neurol Clin 20:85, 2002

ROSENFELD MR, DALMAU J: Current therapy of paraneoplastic syndromes. Curr Treat Opt Neurol 5:69, 2003

88 ONCOLOGIC EMERGENCIES
Rasim Gucalp, Janice Dutcher

Emergencies in patients with cancer may be classified into three groups: pressure or obstruction caused by a space-occupying lesion, metabolic or hormonal problems (paraneoplastic syndromes, Chap. 86), and complications arising from the effects of treatment.

STRUCTURAL-OBSTRUCTIVE ONCOLOGIC EMERGENCIES

SUPERIOR VENA CAVA SYNDROME
Superior vena cava syndrome (SVCS) is the clinical manifestation of superior vena cava (SVC) obstruction, with severe reduction in venous return from the head, neck, and upper extremities. Malignant tumors, such as lung cancer, lymphoma, and metastatic tumors, are responsible for more than 90% of all SVCS cases. Lung cancer, particularly of small-cell and squamous-cell histologies, accounts for approximately 85% of all cases of malignant origin. In young adults, malignant lymphoma is a leading cause of SVCS. Hodgkin's lymphoma involves the mediastinum more commonly than other lymphomas but rarely causes SVCS. When SVCS is noted in a young man with a mediastinal mass, the differential diagnosis is lymphoma vs primary mediastinal germ cell tumor. Metastatic cancers to the mediastinum, such as testicular and breast carcinomas, account for a small proportion of cases. Other causes include benign tumors, aortic aneurysm, thyroid enlargement, thrombosis, and fibrosing mediastinitis caused by prior irradiation or histoplasmosis.

Patients with SVCS usually present with neck and facial swelling (especially around the eyes), dyspnea, and cough. Other symptoms include hoarseness, tongue swelling, headaches, nasal congestion, epistaxis, hemoptysis, dysphagia, pain, dizziness, syncope, and lethargy. Bending forward or lying down may aggravate the symptoms. The characteristic physical findings are dilated neck veins, an increased number of collateral veins covering the anterior chest wall, cyanosis, and edema of the face, arms, and chest. More severe cases include proptosis, glossal and laryngeal edema, and obtundation. The clinical picture is milder if the obstruction is located above the azygos vein.

Signs and symptoms of cerebral and/or laryngeal edema, though rare, are associated with a poorer prognosis and require urgent evaluation. Seizures may be related to brain metastases rather than cerebral edema from venous occlusion. Patients with small cell lung cancer and SVCS have a higher incidence of brain metastases than those without SVCS.

Cardiorespiratory symptoms at rest, particularly with positional changes, suggest significant airway and vascular obstruction and limited physiologic reserve. Cardiac arrest or respiratory failure can occur, particularly in patients receiving sedatives or undergoing general anesthesia.

The diagnosis of SVCS is a clinical one. The most significant chest radiographic finding is widening of the superior mediastinum, most commonly on the right side. Pleural effusion occurs in only 25% of patients, often on the right side. However, a normal chest radiograph is still compatible with the diagnosis if other characteristic findings are present. Computed tomography (CT) provides the most reliable view of the mediastinal anatomy. The diagnosis of SVCS requires diminished or absent opacification of central venous structures with prominent collateral venous circulation. Magnetic resonance imaging (MRI) has no advantages over CT. Invasive procedures, including bronchoscopy, percutaneous needle biopsy, mediastinoscopy, and even thoracotomy, can be performed by a skilled clinician without any major risk of bleeding. For patients with a known cancer, a detailed workup usually is not necessary, and appropriate treatment may be started after obtaining a CT scan of the thorax. For those with no

A

B

C

FIGURE 88-1 *A.* Chest radiographs of a 59-year-old man with recurrent SVCS caused by non-small cell lung cancer showing right paratracheal mass with right pleural effusion. *B.* Computed tomography of same patient demonstrating obstruction of SVC with thrombosis (arrow) by the lung cancer (square) and collaterals (arrowheads). *C.* Balloon angioplasty (arrowhead) with walstent (arrow) in same patient.

history of malignancy, a detailed evaluation is essential to rule out benign causes and determine a specific diagnosis to direct the appropriate therapy.

℞ TREATMENT

The one potentially life-threatening complication of a superior mediastinal mass is tracheal obstruction. Upper airway obstruction demands emergent therapy. Diuretics with a low salt diet, head elevation, and oxygen may produce temporary symptomatic relief. Glucocorticoids may be useful at shrinking lymphoma masses; they are of no benefit in patients with lung cancer.

Radiation therapy is the primary treatment for SVCS caused by non-small cell lung cancer and other metastatic solid tumors. Chemotherapy is effective when the underlying cancer is small cell carcinoma of the lung or lymphoma. Recurrent SVCS occurs in 10 to 30% of patients after initial therapy; it may be palliated with the use of intravascular self-expanding stents (Fig. 88-1). Early stenting may be necessary in patients with severe symptoms; however, the prompt increase in venous return after stenting may precipitate heart failure and pulmonary edema. Surgery may provide immediate relief for patients in whom a benign process is the cause.

Clinical improvement occurs in most patients, although this improvement may be due to the development of adequate collateral circulation. The mortality associated with SVCS does not relate to caval obstruction, but rather to the underlying cause.

SVCS and Central Venous Catheters in Adults The use of long-term central venous catheters has become common practice in patients with cancer. Major vessel thrombosis may occur. In these cases, catheter removal should be combined with anticoagulation to prevent embolization. SVCS in this setting, if detected early, can be treated by fibrinolytic therapy without sacrificing the catheter. Warfarin (1 mg/d) reduces the incidence of thrombosis without altering coagulation tests.

PERICARDIAL EFFUSION/TAMPONADE Malignant pericardial disease is found at autopsy in 5–10% of patients with cancer, most frequently with lung cancer, breast cancer, leukemias, and lymphomas. Cardiac tamponade as the initial presentation of extrathoracic malignancy is rare. The origin is not malignancy in about 50% of cancer patients with symptomatic pericardial disease, but can be related to irradiation, drug-induced pericarditis, hypothyroidism, idiopathic pericarditis, infection, or autoimmune diseases. Two types of radiation pericarditis occur: an acute inflammatory, effusive pericarditis occurring within months of irradiation, which usually resolves spontaneously, and a chronic effusive pericarditis that may appear up to 20 years after radiation therapy and is accompanied by a thickened pericardium.

Most patients with pericardial metastasis are asymptomatic. However, the common symptoms are dyspnea, cough, chest pain, orthopnea, and weakness. Pleural effusion, sinus tachycardia, jugular venous distension, hepatomegaly, peripheral edema, and cyanosis are the most frequent physical findings. Relatively specific diagnostic findings, such as paradoxical pulse, diminished heart sounds, pulsus alternans (pulse waves alternating between those of greater and lesser amplitude with successive beats), and friction rub are less common than with nonmalignant pericardial disease. Chest radiographs and ECG reveal abnormalities in 90% of patients, but half of these abnormalities are nonspecific. Echocardiography is the most helpful diagnostic test. Pericardial fluid may be serous, serosanguineous, or hemorrhagic, and cytologic examination of pericardial fluid is diagnostic in most patients. False negative cytology may occur in patients with lymphoma and mesothelioma.

℞ TREATMENT

Pericardiocentesis with or without the introduction of sclerosing agents, the creation of a pericardial window, complete pericardial stripping, cardiac irradiation, or systemic chemotherapy are effective treatments. Acute pericardial tamponade with life-threatening hemodynamic instability requires immediate drainage of fluid. This can be quickly achieved by pericardiocentesis. Alternatively, subxiphoid pericardiotomy can be performed in 45 min under local anesthesia. Thoracoscopic pericardial fenestration can be employed for benign causes; however, 60% of malignant pericardial effusions recur after this procedure.

INTESTINAL OBSTRUCTION Intestinal obstruction and reobstruction are common problems in patients with advanced cancer, particularly colorectal or ovarian carcinoma. However, other cancers, such as lung or breast cancer and melanoma, can metastasize within the abdomen, leading to intestinal obstruction. Typically, obstruction occurs at multiple sites. Melanoma has a predilection to involve the small bowel; this involvement may be isolated and resection may result in prolonged survival. Intestinal pseudoobstruction is caused by infiltration of the mesentery or bowel muscle by tumor, involvement of the celiac plexus, or paraneoplastic neuropathy in patients with small cell lung cancer. Paraneoplastic neuropathy is associated with IgG antibodies reactive to neurons of the myenteric and submucosal plexuses of the jejunum and stomach. Ovarian cancer can lead either to authentic luminal obstruction or to pseudoobstruction that results when circumferential invasion of a bowel segment arrests the forward progression of peristaltic contractions.

The onset of obstruction is usually insidious. Pain is the most common symptom and is usually colicky in nature. Pain can also be due to abdominal distention, tumor masses, or hepatomegaly. Vomiting can be intermittent or continuous. Patients with complete obstruction usually have constipation. Physical examination may reveal abdominal distention with tympany, ascites, visible peristalsis, high-pitched bowel sounds, and tumor masses. Erect plain abdominal films may reveal multiple air-fluid levels and dilation of the small or large bowel. Acute cecal dilation to more than 12 to 14 cm is considered a surgical emergency because of the high likelihood of rupture. CT is useful in differentiating benign from malignant causes of obstruction in patients who have undergone surgery for malignancy. Malignant obstruction is suggested by a mass at the site of obstruction or prior surgery, adenopathy, or an abrupt transition zone and irregular bowel thickening at the obstruction site. Benign obstruction is more likely when CT shows mesenteric vascular changes, a large volume of ascites, or a smooth transition zone and smooth bowel thickening at the obstruction site. The prognosis for the patient with cancer who develops intestinal obstruction is poor; median survival is 3 to 4 months. About 25–30% are found to have intestinal obstruction due to causes other than cancer. Adhesions from previous operations are a common benign cause. Ileus induced by vincristine is another reversible cause.

℞ TREATMENT

The management of intestinal obstruction in patients with advanced malignancy depends on the extent of the underlying malignancy and the functional status of the major organs. The initial management should include surgical evaluation. Operation is not always successful and may lead to further complications with a substantial mortality rate (10 to 20%). Self-expanding metal stents placed in the gastric outlet, duodenum, proximal jejunum, colon, or rectum may palliate obstructive symptoms at those sites without major surgery. Patients known to have advanced intraabdominal malignancy should receive a prolonged course of conservative management, including nasogastric decom-

pression. Treatment with antiemetics, antispasmodics, and analgesics may allow patients to remain outside the hospital. The somatostatin analogue octreotide may relieve obstructive symptoms through its inhibitory effect on gastrointestinal secretion.

URINARY OBSTRUCTION Urinary obstruction may occur in patients with prostatic or gynecologic malignancies, particularly cervical carcinoma, or metastatic disease from other primary sites such as carcinomas of the breast, stomach, lung, colon, and pancreas, and lymphomas. Radiation therapy to pelvic tumors may cause fibrosis and subsequent ureteral obstruction. Bladder outlet obstruction is usually due to prostate and cervical cancers and may lead to bilateral hydronephrosis and renal failure.

Flank pain is the most common symptom. Persistent urinary tract infection, persistent proteinuria, or hematuria in patients with cancer should raise suspicion of ureteral obstruction. Total anuria and/or anuria alternating with polyuria may occur. A slow, continuous rise in the serum creatinine level necessitates immediate evaluation. Renal ultrasound is the safest and cheapest way to identify hydronephrosis. The function of an obstructed kidney can be evaluated by a nuclear scan. CT can reveal the point of obstruction and identify a retroperitoneal mass or adenopathy.

℞ TREATMENT

Obstruction associated with flank pain, sepsis, or fistula formation is an indication for immediate palliative urinary diversion. Internal ureteral stents can be placed under local anesthesia. Percutaneous nephrostomy offers an alternative approach for drainage. In the case of bladder outlet obstruction due to malignancy, a suprapubic cystostomy can be used for urinary drainage.

MALIGNANT BILIARY OBSTRUCTION This common clinical problem can be caused by a primary carcinoma arising in the pancreas, ampulla of Vater, bile duct, or liver or by metastatic disease to the periductal lymph nodes or liver parenchyma. The most common metastatic tumors causing biliary obstruction are gastric, colon, breast, and lung cancers. Jaundice, light-colored stools, dark urine, pruritus, and weight loss due to malabsorption are usual symptoms. Pain and secondary infection are uncommon in malignant biliary obstruction. Ultrasound, CT, or percutaneous transhepatic or endoscopic retrograde cholangiography will identify the site and nature of the biliary obstruction.

℞ TREATMENT

Palliative intervention is indicated only in patients with disabling pruritus resistant to medical treatment, severe malabsorption, or infection. Stenting under radiographic control, surgical bypass, or radiation therapy with or without chemotherapy may alleviate the obstruction. The choice of modality should be based on the site of obstruction (proximal versus distal), the type of tumor (sensitive to radiotherapy, chemotherapy, or neither), and the general condition of the patient. In the absence of pruritus, biliary obstruction may be a largely asymptomatic cause of death.

SPINAL CORD COMPRESSION Spinal cord compression occurs in 5–10% of patients with cancer. Epidural tumor is the first manifestation of malignancy in about 10% of patients. The underlying cancer is usually identified during the initial evaluation; lung cancer is most commonly the primary malignancy.

Metastatic tumor involves the vertebral column more often than any other part of the bony skeleton. Lung, breast, and prostate cancer are the most frequent offenders. Multiple myeloma also has a high incidence of spine involvement. Lymphomas, melanoma, renal cell cancer, and genitourinary cancers also cause cord compression. The thoracic spine is the most common site (70%), followed by the lumbosacral spine (20%) and the cervical spine (10%). Involvement of multiple sites is most frequent in patients with breast and prostatic carcinoma. Cord injury develops when metastases to the vertebral body or pedicle enlarge and compress the underlying dura. Another cause of cord compression is direct extension of a paravertebral lesion through the intervertebral foramen. These cases usually involve a lymphoma, myeloma, or pediatric neoplasm. Parenchymal spinal cord metastasis due to hematogenous spread is rare.

Expanding extradural tumors induce injury through several mechanisms. Obstruction of the epidural venous plexus leads to edema. Local production of inflammatory cytokines enhances blood flow and edema formation. Compression compromises blood flow leading to ischemia.

The most common initial symptom in patients with spinal cord compression is localized back pain and tenderness due to involvement of vertebrae by tumor. Pain is usually present for days or months before other neurologic findings appear. It is exacerbated by movement and by coughing or sneezing. It can be differentiated from the pain of disk disease by the fact that it worsens when the patient is supine. Radicular pain is less common than localized back pain and usually develops later. Radicular pain in the cervical or lumbosacral areas may be unilateral or bilateral. Radicular pain from the thoracic roots is often bilateral and is described by patients as a feeling of tight, band-like constriction around the thorax and abdomen. Typical cervical radicular pain radiates down the arm; in the lumbar region, the radiation is down the legs. Lhermitte's sign, a tingling or electric sensation down the back, upper and lower limbs upon flexing or extending the neck, may be an early sign of cord compression. Loss of bowel or bladder control may be the presenting symptom, but usually occurs late in the course.

On physical examination, pain induced by straight leg raising, neck flexion, or vertebral percussion may help to determine the level of cord compression. Patients develop numbness and paresthesias in the extremities or trunk. Loss of sensibility to pinprick is as common as loss of sensibility to vibration or position. The upper limit of the zone of sensory loss is often one or two vertebrae below the site of compression. Motor findings include weakness, spasticity, and abnormal muscle stretching. An extensor plantar reflex reflects significant compression. Deep tendon reflexes may be brisk. Motor and sensory loss usually precede sphincter disturbance. Patients with autonomic dysfunction may present with decreased anal tonus, decreased perineal sensibility, and a distended bladder. The absence of the anal wink reflex or the bulbocavernosus reflex confirms cord (conus or cauda equina) involvement. In doubtful cases, evaluation of post-voiding urinary residual volume can be helpful. A residual volume of more than 150 mL suggests bladder dysfunction. Autonomic dysfunction is an unfavorable prognostic factor. Patients with progressive neurologic symptoms should have frequent neurologic examinations and rapid therapeutic intervention. Other illnesses that may mimic cord compression include osteoporotic vertebral collapse, disc disease, pyogenic abscess or vertebral tuberculosis, radiation myelopathy, neoplastic leptomeningitis, benign tumors, epidural hematoma, and spinal lipomatosis.

Patients with cancer who develop back pain should be evaluated for spinal cord compression as quickly as possible (Fig. 88-2). Treatment is more often successful in patients who are ambulatory and still have sphincter control at the time treatment is initiated. Patients should have a neurologic examination and plain films of the spine. Those whose physical examination suggests cord compression should receive dexamethasone (24 mg intravenously every 6 h), starting immediately.

Erosion of the pedicles (the "winking owl" sign) is the earliest radiologic finding of vertebral tumor. Other radiographic changes include increased intrapedicular distance, vertebral destruction, lytic or sclerotic lesions, scalloped vertebral bodies, and vertebral body collapse. Vertebral collapse is not a reliable indicator of the presence of tumor; about 20% of cases of vertebral collapse, particularly those in older patients and postmenopausal women, are due not to cancer but to osteoporosis. Also, a normal appearance on plain films of the spine does not exclude the diagnosis of cancer. The role of bone scans in

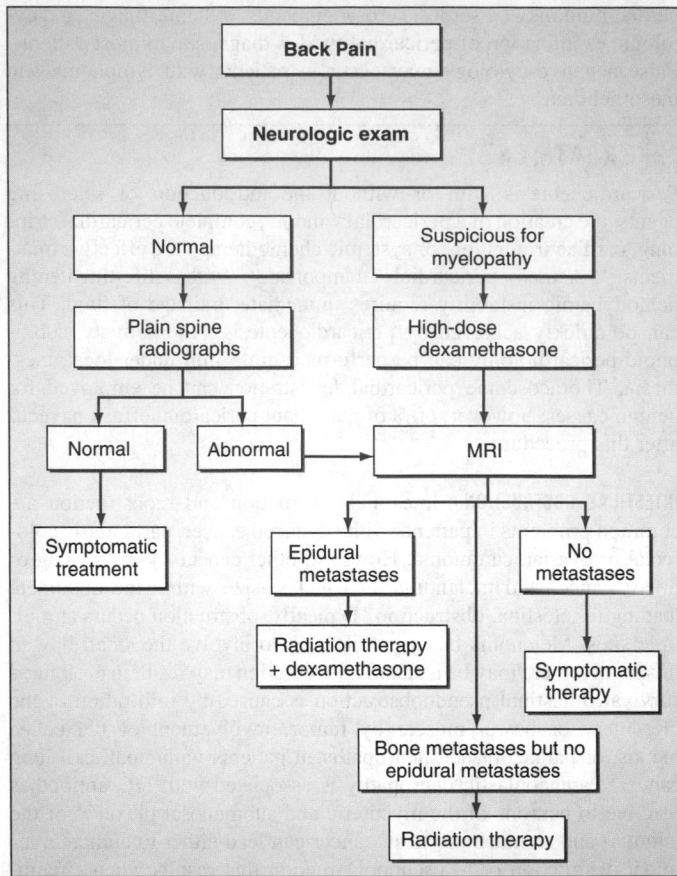

FIGURE 88-2 Management of cancer patients with back pain.

the detection of cord compression is not clear; this method is sensitive but less specific than spinal radiography.

The full-length image of the cord provided by MRI is useful. Multiple epidural metastases are noted in 25% of patients with cord compression and their presence influences treatment plans. On T1-weighted images, good contrast is noted between the cord, cerebrospinal fluid, and extradural lesions. Owing to its sensitivity in demonstrating the replacement of bone marrow by tumor, MRI can show which parts of a vertebra are involved by tumor (the body, pedicle, lamina, spinous process). MRI also visualizes intraspinal extradural masses compressing the cord. T2-weighted images are most useful for the demonstration of intramedullary pathology. Gadolinium-enhanced MRI can help to delineate intramedullary disease. MRI is as good as or better than myelography plus postmyelogram CT in detecting metastatic epidural disease with cord compression. Myelography should be reserved for patients who have poor MR images or who cannot undergo MRI promptly. CT in conjunction with myelography enhances the detection of small areas of spinal destruction.

In patients with cord compression and an unknown primary tumor, a simple workup including chest radiography, mammography, measurement of prostate-specific antigen, and abdominal CT usually reveals the underlying malignancy.

℞ TREATMENT

The treatment of patients with spinal cord compression is aimed at relief of pain and restoration of neurologic function (Fig. 88-2).

Radiation therapy plus glucocorticoids is generally the initial treatment of choice for spinal cord compression. Up to 75% of patients treated when still ambulatory remain ambulatory, but only 10% of patients with paraplegia recover walking capacity. Indications for surgical intervention include unknown etiology, failure of radiation therapy, a radioresistant tumor type (e.g., melanoma or renal cell cancer), pathologic fracture dislocation, and rapidly evolving neurologic symptoms. Until recently, laminectomy was the standard operation for metastatic spinal cord compression, although results were poor. At present, laminectomy should be used only for tissue diagnosis and for the removal of posteriorly localized epidural deposits in the absence of vertebral disease. Because most cases of epidural spinal cord compression are due to anterior or anterolateral extradural disease, resection of the anterior vertebral body along with the tumor, followed by spinal stabilization, has achieved good results and low mortality rate. Chemotherapy may have a role in patients with chemosensitive tumors who have had prior radiation therapy to the same region and who are not candidates for surgery. Most patients with prostate cancer who develop cord compression have already had hormonal therapy; however, for those who have not, androgen deprivation is combined with surgery and radiation therapy.

Patients with metastatic vertebral tumors may benefit from percutaneous vertebroplasty, the injection of acrylic cement into a collapsed vertebra to stabilize the fracture. Pain palliation is common and local antitumor effects have been noted. Cement leakage may cause symptoms in about 10% of patients.

The histology of the tumor is an important determinant of both recovery and survival. Rapid onset and quick progression are poor prognostic features.

INCREASED INTRACRANIAL PRESSURE About 25% of patients with cancer die with intracranial metastases. The cancers that most often metastasize to the brain are lung and breast cancers and melanoma. Brain metastases often occur in the presence of systemic disease, and they frequently cause major symptoms, disability, and early death.

The signs and symptoms of a metastatic brain tumor are similar to those of other intracranial expanding lesions: headache, nausea, vomiting, behavioral changes, seizures, and focal, progressive neurologic changes. Occasionally the onset is abrupt, resembling a stroke, with the sudden appearance of headache, nausea, vomiting, and neurologic deficits. This picture is usually due to hemorrhage into the metastasis. Melanoma, germ cell tumors, and renal cell cancers have a particularly high incidence of intracranial bleeding. The tumor mass and surrounding edema may cause obstruction of the circulation of cerebrospinal fluid, with resulting hydrocephalus. Patients with increased intracranial pressure may have papilledema with visual disturbances and neck stiffness. As the mass enlarges, brain tissue may be displaced through the fixed cranial openings, producing various herniation syndromes.

CT and MRI are equally effective in the diagnosis of brain metastases. CT with contrast should be used as a screening procedure. The CT scan shows brain metastases as multiple enhancing lesions of various sizes with surrounding areas of low-density edema. If a single lesion or no metastases are visualized by contrast-enhanced CT, MRI of the brain should be performed. Gadolinium-enhanced MRI is more sensitive than CT at revealing meningeal involvement and small lesions, particularly in the brainstem or cerebellum.

℞ TREATMENT

If signs and symptoms of brain herniation (particularly headache, drowsiness, and papilledema) are present, the patient should be intubated and hyperventilated to maintain P_{CO_2} between 25 and 30 mmHg and should receive infusions of mannitol (1 to 1.5 g/kg) every 6 h. Dexamethasone is the best initial treatment for all symptomatic patients with brain metastases (see above). Patients with multiple lesions should receive whole-brain radiation therapy. Patients with a single brain metastasis and with controlled extracranial disease may be treated with surgical excision followed by whole-brain radiation therapy, especially if they are younger than 60 years. Radioresistant tumors should be resected if possible. Stereotactic radiosurgery is an effective treatment for inaccessible or recurrent lesions. With a gamma knife or linear accelerator, multiple small, well-collimated beams of ionizing radiation destroy lesions seen on MRI. Some patients with increased intracranial pressure associated with hydrocephalus may benefit from shunt placement. If neurological deterioration is not reversed with

medical therapy, ventriculotomy to remove cerebrospinal fluid (CSF) or craniotomy to remove tumors or hematomas may be necessary.

NEOPLASTIC MENINGITIS Tumor involving the leptomeninges is a complication of both primary tumors of the central nervous system (CNS) and tumors that metastasize to the CNS. The incidence is estimated at 3 to 8% of patients with cancer. Melanoma, breast and lung cancer, lymphoma (including AIDS-associated), and acute leukemia are the most common causes.

Patients typically present with multifocal neurologic signs and symptoms including headache, gait abnormality, mental changes, nausea, vomiting, seizures, back or radicular pain, and limb weakness. Signs include cranial nerve palsies, extremity weakness, paresthesia, and decreased deep tendon reflexes.

Diagnosis is made by demonstrating malignant cells in the cerebrospinal fluid (CSF); however, up to 40% of patients may have false negative CSF cytology. An elevated CSF protein level is nearly always present (except in HTLV-1-associated adult T cell leukemia). Patients with neurologic signs and symptoms consistent with neoplastic meningitis who have a negative CSF cytology but an elevated CSF protein level should have the spinal tap repeated at least three times for repeated cytologic examination before the diagnosis is rejected. MRI findings suggestive of neoplastic meningitis include leptomeningeal, subependymal, dural or cranial nerve enhancement, superficial cerebral lesions, and communicating hydrocephalus. Spinal cord imaging by MRI is a necessary component of the evaluation of non-leukemia neoplastic meningitis as ~20% of patients have cord abnormalities including intradural enhancing nodules that are diagnostic for leptomeningeal involvement. Cauda equina lesions are common but lesions may be seen anywhere in the spinal canal. Radiolabeled CSF flow studies are abnormal in up to 70% of patients with neoplastic meningitis; ventricular outlet obstruction, abnormal flow in the spinal canal, or impaired flow over the cerebral convexities may affect distribution of intrathecal chemotherapy resulting in decreased efficacy or increased toxicity. Radiation therapy may correct CSF flow abnormalities before use of intrathecal chemotherapy.

The development of neoplastic meningitis usually occurs in the setting of uncontrolled cancer outside the CNS; thus, prognosis is poor (median survival 10 to 12 weeks). However, treatment of the neoplastic meningitis may successfully alleviate symptoms and control the CNS spread.

℞ TREATMENT

Intrathecal chemotherapy, usually methotrexate, cytarabine, or thiotepa, is delivered by lumbar puncture or by an intraventricular reservoir (Ommaya) three times a week until the CSF is free of malignant cells. Then injections are given twice a week for a month and then weekly for a month. An extended release preparation of cytarabine (Depocyte) has a longer half-life and is more effective than regular formulations. Among solid tumors, breast cancer responds best to therapy. Patients with neoplastic meningitis from either acute leukemia or lymphoma may be cured of their CNS disease if the systemic disease can be eliminated.

SEIZURES Seizures occurring in a patient with cancer can be caused by the tumor itself, by metabolic disturbances, by radiation injury, by cerebral infarctions, by chemotherapy-related encephalopathies, or by CNS infections. Metastatic disease to the CNS is the most common cause of seizures in patients with cancer. However, seizures occur more frequently in primary brain tumors than in metastatic brain lesions. Seizures are a presenting symptom of CNS metastasis in 6 to 29% of cases. Approximately 10% of patients with CNS metastasis eventually develop seizures. The presence of frontal lesions correlates with early seizures, and the presence of hemispheric symptoms increases the risk for late seizures. Both early and late seizures are uncommon in patients with posterior fossa lesions. Seizures are also common in patients with CNS metastases from melanoma. Very rarely, cytotoxic drugs such as etoposide, busulfan, and chlorambucil cause seizures.

℞ TREATMENT

Patients in whom seizures due to CNS metastases have been demonstrated should receive anticonvulsive treatment with diphenylhydantoin. Prophylactic anticonvulsant therapy is not recommended unless the patient is at a high risk for late seizures (melanoma primary, hemorrhagic metastases, treatment with radiosurgery). In those patients, serum diphenylhydantoin levels should be monitored closely and the dosage adjusted according to serum levels. Phenytoin induces the hepatic metabolism of dexamethasone, reducing its half-life, while dexamethasone may decrease phenytoin levels. Most anti-seizure medications alter the metabolism of antitumor agents.

PULMONARY AND INTRACEREBRAL LEUKOCYTOSTASIS Hyperleukocytosis and the leukostasis syndrome associated with it is a potentially fatal complication of acute leukemia (particularly myeloid leukemia) that can occur when the peripheral blast cell count is greater than 100,000/mL. The frequency of hyperleukocytosis is 5–13% in AML and 10–30% in acute lymphoid leukemia; however, leukostasis is rare in lymphoid leukemia. At such high blast cell counts, blood viscosity is increased, blood flow is slowed by aggregates of tumor cells, and the primitive myeloid leukemic cells are capable of invading through endothelium and causing hemorrhage. Brain and lung are most commonly affected. Patients with brain leukostasis may experience stupor, headache, dizziness, tinnitus, visual disturbances, ataxia, confusion, coma, or sudden death. Administration of 600 cGy of whole-brain irradiation can protect against this complication and can be followed by rapid institution of antileukemic therapy. Pulmonary leukostasis may present as respiratory distress, hypoxemia, and progress to respiratory failure. Chest radiographs may be normal but usually show interstitial or alveolar infiltrates. Leukapheresis may be helpful in decreasing circulating blast counts. Treatment of the leukemia can result in pulmonary hemorrhage from lysis of blasts in the lung, called "leukemic cell lysis pneumopathy." Intravascular volume depletion and unnecessary blood transfusions may increase blood viscosity and worsen leukostasis syndrome. Leukostasis is not a feature of the high white cell counts associated with chronic lymphoid or chronic myeloid leukemia.

When acute promyelocytic leukemia is treated with differentiating agents like tretinoin and arsenic trioxide, cerebral or pulmonary leukostasis may occur. This complication can be largely avoided by using cytotoxic chemotherapy together with the differentiating agents.

HEMOPTYSIS Hemoptysis may be caused by nonmalignant conditions, but lung cancer accounts for a large proportion of cases. Up to 20% of patients with lung cancer have hemoptysis some time in their course. Endobronchial metastases from carcinoid tumors, breast, colon, kidney cancer, and melanoma may also cause hemoptysis. The volume of bleeding is often difficult to gauge. Massive hemoptysis is defined as more than 600 mL of blood produced in 48 h. When respiratory difficulty occurs, hemoptysis should be treated emergently. Often patients can tell where the bleeding is occurring. They should be placed bleeding side down, given supplemental oxygen, and subjected to emergency bronchoscopy. If the site of the lesion is detected, either the patient undergoes a definitive surgical procedure or the lesion is treated with a neodymium:yttrium-aluminum-garnet (Nd:YAG) laser. The surgical option is preferred. Bronchial artery embolization may control brisk bleeding in 75 to 90% of patients, permitting the definitive surgical procedure to be done more safely. Embolization without definitive surgery is associated with rebleeding in 20 to 50% of patients. Recurrent hemoptysis usually responds to a second embolization procedure. A post-embolization syndrome characterized by pleuritic pain, fever, dysphagia, and leukocytosis may occur; it lasts 5–7 days and resolves with symptomatic treatment. Bronchial or

esophageal wall necrosis, myocardial infarction, and spinal cord infarction are rare complications.

Pulmonary hemorrhage with or without hemoptysis in hematologic malignancies is often associated with fungal infections, particularly *Aspergillus* sp. After granulocytopenia resolves, the lung infiltrates in aspergillosis may cavitate and cause massive hemoptysis. Thrombocytopenia and coagulation defects should be corrected, if possible. Surgical evaluation is recommended in patients with aspergillosis-related cavitary lesions.

AIRWAY OBSTRUCTION Generally, airway obstruction refers to a blockage at the level of the mainstem bronchi or above. It may result either from intraluminal tumor growth or from extrinsic compression of the airway. The most common cause of malignant upper airway obstruction is invasion from an adjacent primary tumor, most commonly lung cancer, followed by esophageal, thyroid, and mediastinal malignancies.Extrathoracic primary tumors such as renal cell, colon, or breast cancer can cause airway obtruction through endobronchial and/or mediastinal lymph node metastases. Patients may present with dyspnea, hemoptysis, stridor, wheezing, intractable cough, post-obstructive pneumonia, or hoarseness. Chest radiographs usually demonstrate obstructing lesions. CT scans provide more detailed information about the extent of tumor. Cool humidified oxygen, glucocorticoids, and ventilation with a mixture of helium and oxygen (Heliox) may provide temporary relief. If the obstruction is proximal to the larynx, a tracheostomy may be life-saving. For more distal obstructions, particularly intrinsic lesions incompletely obstucting the airway, bronchoscopy with laser treatment, photodynamic therapy, or stenting can produce immediate relief in most patients. However, radiation therapy (either external-beam irradiation or brachytherapy) given together with glucocorticoids may also open the airway. Symptomatic extrinsic compression may be palliated by stenting. Patients with primary airway tumors such as squamous cell carcinoma, carcinoid tumor, adenocystic carcinoma, or non-small cell lung cancer should have surgery.

METABOLIC EMERGENCIES

HYPERCALCEMIA Hypercalcemia is the most common paraneoplastic syndrome. →*Its pathogenesis and management are fully discussed in Chaps. 86 and 332.*

SYNDROME OF INAPPROPRIATE SECRETION OF ANTIDIURETIC HORMONE (SIADH) Hyponatremia is a common electrolyte abnormality in cancer patients, and SIADH is the most common cause of hyponatremia among patients with cancer. →*SIADH is discussed fully in Chaps. 86 and 319.*

LACTIC ACIDOSIS Lactic acidosis is a rare and potentially fatal metabolic complication of cancer. Lactic acidosis associated with sepsis and circulatory failure is a common preterminal event in many malignancies. Lactic acidosis in the absence of hypoxemia may occur in patients with leukemia, lymphoma, or solid tumors. Extensive involvement of the liver by tumor is present in most cases. Alteration of liver function may be responsible for the lactate accumulation. HIV-infected patients have an increased risk of aggressive lymphoma; lactic acidosis may occur in such patients either related to the rapid growth of the tumor or from toxicity of nucleoside reverse transcriptase inhibitors (components of HAART). Severe liver toxicity manifesting as acute lactic acidosis may be seen from nucleosides. Symptoms of lactic acidosis include tachypnea, tachycardia, change of mental status, and hepatomegaly. The serum level of lactic acid may reach 10 to 20 meq/L (90 to 180 mg/dL). Treatment is aimed at the underlying disease. The danger from lactic acidosis is from the acidosis, not the lactate. Sodium bicarbonate should be added if acidosis is very severe or if hydrogen ion production is very rapid and uncontrolled. The prognosis is poor.

HYPOGLYCEMIA Persistent hypoglycemia occasionally is associated with tumors other than pancreatic islet cell tumors. Usually these tumors are large, and often they are of mesenchymal origin or are hepatomas or adrenocortical tumors. Mesenchymal tumors are usually located in the retroperitoneum or thorax. In these patients, obtundation, confusion, and behavioral aberrations occur in the postabsorptive period and may precede the diagnosis of the tumor. These tumors often secrete incompletely processed insulin-like growth factor II (IGF-II), a hormone capable of activating insulin receptors and causing hypoglycemia. Rarely, hypoglycemia is due to insulin secretion by a non-islet cell carcinoma. Also, the development of hepatic dysfunction from liver metastases and increased glucose consumption by the tumor can contribute to hypoglycemia. If the tumor cannot be resected, hypoglycemia symptoms may be relieved by the administration of glucose, glucocorticoids, or glucagon.

Hypoglycemia can be artifactual; hyperleukocytosis from leukemia, myeloproliferative diseases, leukemoid reactions, or colony stimulating factor treatment can increase glucose consumption in the test tube after blood is drawn, leading to pseudohypoglycemia.

ADRENAL INSUFFICIENCY In patients with cancer, adrenal insufficiency may go unrecognized because the symptoms, such as nausea, vomiting, anorexia, and orthostatic hypotension, are nonspecific and may be mistakenly attributed to progressive cancer or to cancer therapy. Primary adrenal insufficiency may develop owing to replacement of both glands by metastases (lung, breast, colon, or kidney cancer, lymphoma), to removal of both glands, or to hemorrhagic necrosis in association with sepsis or anticoagulation. Impaired adrenal steroid synthesis occurs in patients being treated for cancer with mitotane, ketoconazole, aminoglutethimide, or the investigational agent suramin or in those undergoing rapid reduction in glucocorticoid therapy. Rarely, metastatic replacement causes primary adrenal insufficiency as the first manifestation of an occult malignancy. Metastasis to the pituitary or hypothalamus is found at autopsy in up to 5% of patients with cancer, but associated secondary adrenal insufficiency is rare. Megesterol acetate, used to manage cancer and HIV-related cachexia, may suppress plasma levels of cortisol and adrenocorticotropic hormone (ACTH). Patients taking megesterol may develop adrenal insufficiency, and even those whose adrenal dysfunction is not symptomatic may have inadequate adrenal reserve if they become seriously ill.

Acute adrenal insufficiency is potentially lethal. Treatment of suspected adrenal crisis is initiated after the sampling of serum cortisol and ACTH levels (Chap. 321).

TREATMENT-RELATED EMERGENCIES

TUMOR LYSIS SYNDROME Tumor lysis syndrome is a well-recognized clinical entity that is characterized by various combinations of hyperuricemia, hyperkalemia, hyperphosphatemia, lactic acidosis, and hypocalcemia and is caused by the destruction of a large number of rapidly proliferating neoplastic cells. Frequently, acute renal failure develops as a result of the syndrome.

Tumor lysis syndrome is most frequently associated with the treatment of Burkitt's lymphoma, acute lymphoblastic leukemia, and other high-grade lymphomas, but it also may be seen with chronic leukemias and, rarely, with solid tumors. This syndrome has been seen in patients with chronic lymphocytic leukemia after treatment with fludarabine and cladribine. Tumor lysis syndrome usually occurs during or shortly (1 to 5 days) after chemotherapy. Rarely, spontaneous necrosis of malignancies causes tumor lysis syndrome.

Hyperuricemia may be present at the time of chemotherapy. Effective treatment kills malignant cells and leads to increased serum uric acid levels from the turnover of nucleic acids. Owing to the acidic local environment, uric acid can precipitate in the tubules, medulla, and collecting ducts of the kidney, leading to renal failure. Lactic acidosis and dehydration may contribute to the precipitation of uric acid in the renal tubules. The finding of uric acid crystals in the urine is strong evidence for uric acid nephropathy. The ratio of urinary uric acid to urinary creatinine is >1 in patients with acute hyperuricemic nephropathy and <1 in patients with renal failure due to other causes.

Hyperphosphatemia, which can be caused by the release of intracellular phosphate pools by tumor cell lysis, produces a reciprocal depression in serum calcium, which causes severe neuromuscular irritability and tetany. Deposition of calcium phosphate in the kidney

and hyperphosphatemia may cause renal failure. Potassium is the principal intracellular cation, and massive destruction of malignant cells may lead to hyperkalemia. Hyperkalemia in patients with renal failure may rapidly become life-threatening. Hyperkalemia can cause ventricular arrhythmias and sudden death.

The likelihood that the tumor lysis syndrome will occur in patients with Burkitt's lymphoma is related to the tumor burden and renal function. Hyperuricemia and high serum levels of lactate dehydrogenase (LDH >1500 U/L), both of which correlate with total tumor burden, also correlate with the risk of tumor lysis syndrome. In patients at risk for tumor lysis, pretreatment evaluations should include a complete blood count, serum chemistry evaluation, and urine analysis. High leukocyte and platelet counts may artificially elevate potassium levels ("pseudohyperkalemia") due to lysis of these cells after the blood is drawn. In these cases, plasma potassium instead of serum potassium should be followed. In pseudohyperkalemia, no electrocardiographic abnormalities are present. In patients with abnormal baseline renal function, the kidneys and retroperitoneal area should be evaluated by sonography and/or CT to rule out obstructive uropathy. Urine output should be watched closely.

℞ TREATMENT

Recognition of risk and prevention are the most important steps in the management of this syndrome (Fig. 88-3). The standard preventive approach consists of allopurinol, urinary alkalinization, and aggressive hydration. Intravenous allopurinol may be given in patients who cannot tolerate oral therapy. In some cases, uric acid levels cannot be lowered sufficiently with the standard preventive approach. Rasburicase (recombinant urate oxidase) can be effective in these instances.

FIGURE 88-3 *Management of patients at high risk for the tumor lysis syndrome.*

Urate oxidase is missing from primates and catalyzes the conversion of poorly soluble uric acid to readily soluble allantoin. Rasburicase acts rapidly decreasing uric acid levels within hours; however, it may cause hypersensitivity reactions such as bronchospasm, hypoxemia, and hypotension. Rasburicase is contraindicated in patients with glucose-6-phosphate dehydrogenase deficiency who are unable to breakdown hydrogen peroxide, an end product of the urate oxidase reaction. Despite aggressive prophylaxis, tumor lysis syndrome and/or oliguric or anuric renal failure may occur. Care should be taken to prevent worsening of symptomatic hypocalcemia by induction of alkalosis during bicarbonate infusion. Administration of sodium bicarbonate may also lead to urinary precipitation of calcium phosphate, which is less soluble at alkaline pH. Dialysis is often necessary and should be considered early in the course. Hemodialysis is preferred. Hemofiltration offers a gradual, continuous method of removing cellular byproducts and fluid. The prognosis is excellent, and renal function recovers after the uric acid level is lowered to ≤ 10 mg/dL.

HUMAN ANTIBODY INFUSION REACTIONS   The initial infusion of human or humanized antibodies (e.g., rituximab, gemtuzumab, trastuzumab) is associated with fever, chills, nausea, asthenia, and headache in up to half of treated patients. Bronchospasm and hypotension occur in 1% of patients. The pathogenesis is thought to be activation of immune effector processes (cells and complement). In the presence of high levels of circulating lymphoid tumor cells, thrombocytopenia, a rapid fall in circulating tumor cells, and mild electrolyte evidence of tumor lysis syndrome may also occur. In addition, increase of liver enzymes, D-dimer, LDH, and prolongation of the prothrombin time may occur. This syndrome is related to release of inflammatory cytokines, such as tumor necrosis factor-α and IL-6. Diphenhydramine and acetaminophen can often prevent or suppress the symptoms. If they occur, the infusion should be stopped and restarted at half the initial infusion rate after the symptoms have abated.

HEMOLYTIC-UREMIC SYNDROME   Hemolytic-uremic syndrome (HUS) and, less commonly, thrombotic thrombocytopenic purpura (TTP) occurring after treatment with antineoplastic drugs have been described. Mitomycin is by far the most common agent causing this peculiar syndrome. Other chemotherapeutic agents, including cisplatin, bleomycin, and gemcitabine, have also been reported to be associated with this syndrome. It occurs most often in patients with gastric, colorectal, and breast carcinoma. In one series, 35% of patients were without evident cancer at the time this syndrome appeared. Secondary HUS/TTP has also been reported as a rare but sometimes fatal complication of bone marrow transplantation.

HUS usually has its onset 4 to 8 weeks after the last dose of chemotherapy, but it is not rare to detect it several months later. HUS is characterized by microangiopathic hemolytic anemia, thrombocytopenia, and renal failure. Dyspnea, weakness, fatigue, oliguria, and purpura are also common initial symptoms and findings. Systemic hypertension and pulmonary edema frequently occur. Severe hypertension, pulmonary edema, and rapid worsening of hemolysis and renal function may occur after a blood or blood product transfusion. Cardiac findings include atrial arrhythmias, pericardial friction rub, and pericardial effusion. Raynaud's phenomenon is part of the syndrome in patients treated with bleomycin.

Laboratory findings include severe to moderate anemia associated with red blood cell fragmentation and numerous schistocytes on peripheral smear. Reticulocytosis, decreased plasma haptoglobin, and an elevated lactic dehydrogenase (LDH) level document hemolysis. The serum bilirubin level is usually normal or slightly elevated. The Coombs test is negative. The white cell count is usually normal, and thrombocytopenia ($<100,000/\mu L$) is almost always present. Most patients have a normal coagulation profile, although some have mild elevations in thrombin time and in level of fibrin degradation products. The serum creatinine level is elevated at presentation and shows a pattern of subacute worsening within weeks of the initial azotemia.

The urinalysis reveals hematuria, proteinuria, and granular or hyaline casts; and circulating immune complexes may be present.

The basic pathologic lesion appears to be deposition of fibrin in the walls of capillaries and arterioles, and these deposits are similar to those seen in HUS due to other causes. These microvascular abnormalities involve mainly the kidneys and rarely occur in other organs. The pathogenesis of chemotherapy-related HUS is unknown. Immune complexes have been proposed but not confirmed to be etiologic.

The case fatality rate is high; most patients die within a few months. Plasmapheresis and plasma exchange may normalize the hematologic abnormalities, but renal failure is not reversed in most patients. Immunoperfusion over a staphylococcal protein A column is the most successful treatment. About half of the patients treated with immunoperfusion respond with resolution of thrombocytopenia, improvement in anemia, and stabilization of renal failure. Treatment is well tolerated. It is not clear how the treatment works.

NEUTROPENIA AND INFECTION   These remain the most common serious complications of cancer therapy. →*They are covered in detail in Chap. 72.*

PULMONARY INFILTRATES   Patients with cancer may present with dyspnea associated with diffuse interstitial infiltrates on chest radiographs. Such infiltrates may be due to progression of the underlying malignancy, treatment-related toxicities, infection, and/or unrelated diseases. The cause may be multifactorial; however, most commonly they occur as a consequence of treatment. Infiltration of the lung by malignancy has been described in patients with leukemia, lymphoma, and breast and other solid cancers. Pulmonary lymphatics may be involved diffusely by neoplasm (pulmonary lymphangitic carcinomatosis), resulting in a diffuse increase in interstitial markings on chest radiographs. The patient is often mildly dyspneic at the onset, but pulmonary failure develops over a period of weeks. In some patients, dyspnea precedes changes on the chest radiographs and is accompanied by a nonproductive cough. This syndrome is characteristic of solid tumors. In patients with leukemia, diffuse microscopic neoplastic peribronchial and peribronchiolar infiltration is frequent but may be asymptomatic. However, some patients present with diffuse interstitial infiltrates, an alveolar capillary block syndrome, and respiratory distress. In these situations, glucocorticoids can provide symptomatic relief, but specific chemotherapy should always be started promptly.

Several cytotoxic agents, such as bleomycin, methotrexate, busulfan, and the nitrosoureas, may cause pulmonary damage. The most frequent presentations are interstitial pneumonitis, alveolitis, and pulmonary fibrosis. Some cytotoxic agents, including methotrexate and procarbazine, may cause an acute hypersensitivity reaction. Cytosine arabinoside has been associated with noncardiogenic pulmonary edema. Administration of multiple cytotoxic drugs, as well as radiation therapy and preexisting lung disease, may potentiate the pulmonary toxicity. Supplemental oxygen may potentiate the effects of drugs and radiation injury. Patients should always be managed with the lowest $F_{I_{O_2}}$ that is sufficient to maintain hemoglobin saturation.

The onset of symptoms may be insidious, with symptoms including dyspnea, nonproductive cough, and tachycardia. Patients may have bibasilar crepitant rales, end-inspiratory crackles, fever, and cyanosis. The chest radiograph generally shows an interstitial and sometimes an intraalveolar pattern that is strongest at the lung bases and may be symmetric. A small effusion may occur. Hypoxemia with decreased carbon monoxide diffusing capacity is always present. Glucocorticoids may be helpful in patients in whom pulmonary toxicity is related to radiation therapy or to chemotherapy. Treatment is otherwise supportive.

Radiation pneumonitis and/or fibrosis is a relatively frequent side effect of thoracic radiation therapy when the dosage exceeds 40 Gy; it may be acute or chronic. It has its onset usually from 2 to 6 months after completion of radiation therapy. The clinical syndrome, which varies in severity, consists of dyspnea, cough with scanty sputum, low-grade fever, and an initial hazy infiltrate on chest radiographs. The infiltrate and tissue damage usually are confined to the radiation field.

The patients subsequently may develop a patchy alveolar infiltrate and air bronchograms, which may progress to acute respiratory failure that is sometimes fatal. A lung biopsy may be necessary to make the diagnosis. Asymptomatic infiltrates found incidentally after radiation therapy need not be treated. However, prednisone should be administered to patients with fever or other symptoms. The dosage should be tapered slowly after the resolution of radiation pneumonitis, as abrupt withdrawal of glucocorticoids may cause an exacerbation of pneumonia. Delayed radiation fibrosis may occur years after radiation therapy and is signaled by dyspnea on exertion. Often it is mild, but it can progress to chronic respiratory failure. Therapy is supportive.

Classical radiation pneumonitis that leads to pulmonary fibrosis is due to radiation-induced production of local cytokines such as platelet-derived growth factor β, tumor necrosis factor, and transforming growth factor β in the radiation field. An immunologically mediated sporadic radiation pneumonitis occurs in about 10% of patients; bilateral alveolitis mediated by T cells results in infiltrates outside the radiation field. This form of radiation pneumonitis usually resolves without sequelae.

Pneumonia is a common problem in patients undergoing treatment for cancer. Bacterial pneumonia typically causes a localized infiltrate on chest radiographs. Therapy is tailored to the causative organism. When diffuse interstitial infiltrates appear in a febrile patient, the differential diagnosis is extensive and includes pneumonia due to infection with *Pneumocystis carinii*, cytomegalovirus, or intracellular pathogens such as *mycoplasma* and *Legionella*; effects of drugs or radiation; tumor progression; nonspecific pneumonitis; and fungal disease. Patients with cancer who are neutropenic and have fever and local infiltrates on chest radiograph should be treated with a third generation cephalosporin perhaps together with an aminoglycoside or imipenem. A new or persistent focal infiltrate not responding to broad spectrum antibiotics argues for initiation of empiric antifungal therapy. When diffuse bilateral infiltrates develop in patients with febrile neutropenia, broad spectrum antibiotics plus trimethoprim-sulfamethoxazole with or without erythromycin should be initiated. The empiric administration of trimethoprim-sulfamethoxazole plus erythromycin to patients without neutropenia and these antibiotics plus ceftazidime to patients with neutropenia covers nearly every treatable diagnosis (except tumor progression) and gives as good overall survival as a strategy based on early invasive intervention with bronchoalveolar lavage or open lung biopsy. If the patient does not improve in 4 days, open lung biopsy is the procedure of choice. Bronchoscopy with bronchoalveolar lavage may be used in patients who are poor candidates for surgery.

In patients with pulmonary infiltrates who are afebrile, heart failure and multiple pulmonary emboli form part of the differential diagnosis.

TYPHLITIS Neutropenic enterocolitis (typhlitis) is an inflammation and necrosis of the cecum and surrounding tissues that may complicate the treatment of acute leukemia. This complication has also been seen in patients with other forms of cancer treated with taxanes and in patients receiving high-dose chemotherapy. The patient develops right lower quadrant abdominal pain, often with rebound tenderness and a tense, distended abdomen, in a setting of fever and neutropenia. Watery diarrhea (often containing sloughed mucosa) and bacteremia are common, and bleeding may occur. Plain abdominal films are generally of little value in the diagnosis; CT scan may show marked bowel wall thickening, particularly in the cecum, with bowel wall edema. Patients with bowel wall thickness >10 mm on ultrasonogram have higher mortality rates. Rapid institution of broad-spectrum antibiotic coverage and nasogastric suction may reverse the disease. Surgical intervention should be considered if there is no improvement by 24 h after the start of antibiotic treatment. If the localized abdominal findings become diffuse, the prognosis is poor.

HEMORRHAGIC CYSTITIS Hemorrhagic cystitis can develop in patients receiving cyclophosphamide or ifosfamide. Both drugs are metabolized to acrolein, which is a strong chemical irritant that is excreted in the urine. Prolonged contact or high concentrations may lead to bladder irritation and hemorrhage. Symptoms include gross hematuria, frequency, dysuria, burning, urgency, incontinence, and nocturia. The best management is prevention. Maintaining a high rate of urine flow minimizes exposure. In addition, 2-mercaptoethanesulfonate (mesna) detoxifies the metabolites and can be coadministered with the instigating drugs. Mesna usually is given three times on the day of ifosfamide administration in doses that are each 20% of the total ifosfamide dose. If hemorrhagic cystitis develops, the maintenance of a high urine flow may be sufficient supportive care. If conservative management is not effective, irrigation of the bladder with an 0.37 to 0.74% formalin solution for 10 min stops the bleeding in most cases. *N*-acetylcysteine may also be an effective irrigant. Prostaglandins (carboprost tromethamine) can inhibit the progress. In extreme cases, ligation of the hypogastric arteries, urinary diversion, or cystectomy may be necessary.

Hemorrhagic cystitis also occurs in patients who undergo bone marrow transplantation (BMT). In the BMT setting, early onset hemorrhagic cystitis is related to drugs in the treatment regimen (e.g. cyclophosphamide) and late onset hemorrhagic cystitis is usually due to the polyoma virus BKV or adenovirus type 11. Viral causes are usually detected by PCR-based diagnostic tests. Treatment of viral hemorrhagic cystitis is largely supportive with reduction in doses of immunosuppressive agents, if possible. No antiviral therapy is in use, though cidofovir is being tested.

FURTHER READING

ALBANELL J, BASELGA J: Systemic therapy emergencies. Semin Oncol 27: 347, 2000

APARICIO A et al: Neoplastic meningitis. Curr Neurol Neurosci Rep 2:225, 2002

DAVIS MP et al: Modern management of cancer-related intestinal obstruction. Curr Oncol Rep 2:343, 2000

JAECKLE KA et al: An open label trial of sustained release cytarabine (DepoCyte) for intrathecal treatment of solid tumor neoplastic meningitis. J Neuro Oncol 57:231, 2002

RIPAMONTI C et al: Respiratory problems in advanced cancer. Support Care Cancer 10:204, 2002

VAITKUS PT et al: Treatment of malignant pericardial effusion. JAMA 272: 59, 1994

YIM BT et al: Rasburicase for the treatment and prevention of hyperuricemia. Ann Pharmacother 37:1047, 2003

89 LATE CONSEQUENCES OF CANCER AND ITS TREATMENT
Michael C. Perry, Dan L. Longo

Over 9 million Americans alive today have had cancer. Virtually all of these survivors will bear some mark of their diagnosis and its therapy, and many will experience long-term complications, including medical problems, psychosocial disturbances, sexual dysfunction, and inability to find employment or insurance.

Problems may be related to the cancer itself (e.g., patients with primary cancers of the head and neck are at increased risk for subsequent lung cancer), or to the normal aging process (surviving one cancer does not necessarily alter the risk of other common tumors that increase in frequency with age). However, many of the problems affecting cured patients are related to the treatments. Individuals carefully followed for periods up to 30 years have taught us the spectrum

TABLE 89-1 *Late Effects of Cancer Therapy*

Surgical Procedure	Effect
Amputation	Functional loss
Lymph node dissection	Risk of lymphedema
Ostomy	Psychosocial impact
Splenectomy	Risk of sepsis
Adhesions	Risk of obstruction
Bowel anastomoses	Malabsorption syndromes

Radiation Therapy	Effect
Organ	
Bone	Premature termination of growth, osteonecrosis
Soft tissues	Atrophy, fibrosis
Brain	Neuropsychiatric deficits, cognitive dysfunction
Thyroid	Hypothyroidism, Graves' disease, cancer
Salivary glands	Dry mouth, caries, dysgeusia
Eyes	Cataracts
Heart	Pericarditis, myocarditis, coronary artery disease
Lung	Pulmonary fibrosis
Kidney	Decreased function, hypertension
Liver	Decreased function
Intestine	Malabsorption, stricture
Gonads	Infertility, premature menopause
Any	Secondary neoplasia

Chemotherapy		Effect
Organ	Drug	
Bone	Glucocorticoids	Osteoporosis, avascular necrosis
Brain	Methotrexate, ara-C, others	Neuropsychiatric deficits, cognitive decline?
Peripheral nerves	Vincristine, platinum	Neuropathy, hearing loss
Eyes	Glucocorticoids	Cataracts
Heart	Anthracyclines, herceptin	Cardiomyopathy
Lung	Bleomycin	Pulmonary fibrosis
	Methotrexate	Pulmonary hypersensitivity
Kidney	Platinum, others	Decreased function, hypomagnesemia
Liver	Various	Altered function
Gonads	Alkylating agents, others	Infertility, premature menopause
Bone marrow	Various	Aplasia, myelodysplasia, secondary leukemia

of problems that can be encountered. Because of heterogeneity in treatment details and in completeness of follow-up, some treatment-related problems went undetected for many years. However, studies of long-term survivors of childhood cancers, acute leukemia, Hodgkin's disease, lymphomas, testicular cancer, and localized solid tumors have identified the features of cancer treatment that are associated with later morbidity and mortality. We have been somewhat slow to act in changing those aspects of primary treatment that contribute to these late problems. This reticence is due to the uncertainty associated with changing a treatment that is known to work before having a replacement that works as well.

The first task is always to eradicate the diagnosed malignancy. Late problems occurring in cured patients reflect the success of treatment. Such problems never develop in those who do not survive the cancer. Morbidity and mortality from iatrogenic disease should be avoided, if possible. However, the risk of late complications should not lead to the failure to apply potentially curative treatment. The challenge is to preserve or augment the cure rate while decreasing the risk of serious treatment-related illness.

The mechanisms of damage vary. Surgical procedures can create abnormal physiology (such as blind loops leading to malabsorption) or interfere with normal organ function (splenectomy leading to impaired immune response). Radiation therapy can damage organ function directly (salivary gland toxicity leading to dry mouth and dental caries), act as a carcinogen (second solid tumors in radiation ports), or promote accelerated aging-associated changes (atherosclerosis). Cancer chemotherapy can produce damage to the bone marrow and immune system and induce a spectrum of organ dysfunctions. Therapy may produce subclinical damage that may only become recognized in

the presence of a second inciting factor (such as the increased incidence of melanoma in patients with dysplastic nevus syndrome treated for Hodgkin's disease with radiation therapy). Finally, although the mechanisms are not elucidated, cancer and its treatment are associated with psychosocial problems that can impair the survivor's ability to adapt to life after cancer.

Late effects by treatment modality are shown in Table 89-1. →*Drug toxicities are discussed in Chap. 70; radiation toxicity is discussed in Chap. 71.*

CONSEQUENCES BY ORGAN SYSTEM ■ Cardiovascular Dysfunction Most anthracyclines damage the heart muscle. A dose-dependent dropout of myocardial cells is seen on endomyocardial biopsy, and eventually ventricular failure ensues. About 5% of patients who receive >550 mg/m^2 of doxorubicin will develop congestive heart failure (CHF). Coexisting cardiac disease, hypertension, advanced age, and concomitant therapy with thoracic radiation therapy or mitomycin may hasten the onset of CHF. Anthracycline-induced CHF is not readily reversible; mortality is as high as 50%, thus, prevention is the best approach. Mitoxantrone is a related drug that has less cardiac toxicity. Administration of doxorubicin by continuous infusion or encapsulated in liposomes appears to decrease the risk of heart damage. Dexrazoxane, an intracellular iron chelator, may protect the heart against anthracycline toxicity by preventing iron-dependent free-radical generation.

Mediastinal radiation therapy that includes the heart can induce acute pericarditis, chronic constrictive pericarditis, myocardial fibrosis, or accelerated premature coronary atherosclerosis. The incidence of acute pericarditis is 5 to 13%; patients may be asymptomatic or have dyspnea on exertion, fever, and chest pain. Onset is insidious, with a peak about 9 months after treatment. Pericardial effusion may be present. Chronic constrictive pericarditis can develop 5 to 10 years after treatment and usually presents with dyspnea on exertion. Myocardial fibrosis may present as unexplained CHF with diagnostic evaluation showing restrictive cardiomyopathy. Patients may have aortic insufficiency from valvular thickening or mitral regurgitation from papillary muscle dysfunction. Patients who receive mantle field radiation therapy have a threefold increased risk of *fatal* myocardial infarction. Similarly, radiation of the carotids is associated with premature atherosclerosis of the carotids and can produce central nervous system embolic disease. At very high doses, cyclophosphamide can produce a hemorrhagic myocarditis. Herceptin has been associated with heart failure.

Pulmonary Dysfunction Pulmonary fibrosis from bleomycin is dose-related, with potential exacerbation by age, preexisting lung disease, thoracic radiation, high concentrations of inhaled oxygen, and the concomitant use of other chemotherapeutic agents. Several other chemotherapy agents and radiation therapy can cause pulmonary fibrosis, and at least five can cause pulmonary venoocclusive disease, especially following high-dose therapy such as that involved in stem cell/bone marrow transplantation.

Liver Dysfunction Clinically significant long-term damage to the liver from standard-dose chemotherapy is relatively infrequent and mostly confined to patients who have received chronic methotrexate for maintenance therapy of acute lymphoblastic leukemia. Radiation doses to the liver >1500 cGy can produce liver dysfunction. Although rarely seen with standard-dose chemotherapy, hepatic venoocclusive disease is more common with high-dose therapy, such as that given to prepare patients for autologous or allogeneic stem cell transplantation. Endothelial damage is probably the inciting event.

Renal/Bladder Dysfunction Reduced renal function may be produced by cisplatin; it is usually asymptomatic but may render the patient more susceptible to other renal insults. Cyclophosphamide cystitis may eventually lead to the development of bladder cancer. Ifosfamide produces cystitis and a proximal tubular defect, a Fanconi-like syndrome that is usually, but not always, reversible.

Endocrine Dysfunction Long-term survivors of childhood cancer who received cranial irradiation are shorter, more likely to be obese, and have reductions in strength, exercise tolerance, and bone mineral density. The obesity may be related to alterations in leptin biology. Growth hormone deficiency is the most common hormone deficiency.

Thyroid disease is common in patients who have received radiation therapy to the neck, such as patients with Hodgkin's disease, with an incidence of up to 62% at 26 years post-therapy. Hypothyroidism is the most common abnormality, followed by Graves' disease, thyroiditis, and cancer. Such patients should have frequent thyroid-stimulating hormone (TSH) levels to detect hypothyroidism early and suppress the TSH drive, which may contribute to thyroid cancer.

Nervous System Dysfunction Although many patients experience peripheral neuropathy during chemotherapy, only a few have chronic problems, perhaps because they have other coexisting diseases such as diabetes mellitus. High doses of cisplatin can produce severe sensorimotor neuropathy. Vincristine may produce permanent numbness and tingling in the fingers and toes.

Neurocognitive sequelae from intrathecal chemotherapy, with or without radiation therapy, are recognized complications of the successful therapy of childhood acute lymphoblastic leukemia. Cognitive decline has been attributed to radiating the brain in the treatment of a variety of tumor types. In addition, cognitive decline can follow the use of adjuvant chemotherapy in women being treated for breast cancer. Because the agents are given at modest doses and are not thought to cross the blood-brain barrier, the mechanism of the cognitive decline is not defined.

Many patients suffer intrusive thoughts about cancer recurrence for many years after successful treatment. Adjustment to normal expectations can be difficult. Cancer survivors may often have more problems holding a job, staying in a stable relationship, and coping with the usual stresses of daily life.

A dose-related hearing loss can occur with the use of cisplatin, usually with doses >400 mg/m². This is irreversible, and patients should be screened with audiometric examinations periodically during such therapy.

Eyes Cataracts may be caused by chronic glucocorticoid use, radiation therapy to the head, and, rarely, by tamoxifen.

Sexual and Reproductive Dysfunction Reversible azoospermia can be caused by many chemotherapy agents. The gonads may also be permanently damaged by radiation therapy or by chemotherapeutic agents, particularly the alkylating agents. The extent of the damage depends upon the patient's age and the total dose administered. As a woman nears menopause, smaller amounts of chemotherapy will produce ovarian failure. In men, chemotherapy may produce infertility, but hormone production is not usually affected. Women, however, commonly lose both fertility and hormone production. The premature induction of menopause in a young woman can have serious medical and psychological consequences. Hormone therapy is controversial. Paroxetine may be useful in controlling hot flashes.

Musculoskeletal Dysfunction Late consequences of radiation therapy on the musculoskeletal system occur mostly in children and are related to the radiation dose, volume of tissue irradiated, and the age of the child at the time of therapy. Damage to the microvasculature of the epiphyseal growth zone may result in leg length discrepancy, scoliosis, and short stature.

Raynaud's Phenomenon Up to 40% of patients with testicular cancer treated with bleomycin may experience Raynaud's phenomenon varying in severity from mild and transient to severe. The mechanism is unknown.

Oral Complications Radiation therapy can damage the salivary glands, producing dry mouth. Without saliva, dental caries develop, and many patients have poor dentition. In rare patients, taste can be adversely affected and appetite can be suppressed.

SECOND MALIGNANCIES Second malignancies are a major cause of death for those cured of cancer. Second malignancies can be grouped into three categories: those associated with the primary cancer, those caused by radiation therapy, and those caused by chemotherapy.

Primary cancers increase the risk of secondary cancers in a number of settings. Patients with head and neck cancers are at increased risk of developing a lung cancer, and vice versa, probably because of shared risk factors, especially tobacco abuse. Patients with breast cancer are at increased risk of a second breast cancer in the contralateral breast. Patients with Hodgkin's disease are at increased risk of non-Hodgkin's lymphoma. Patients with genetic syndromes, such as multiple endocrine neoplasia type 1 or Lynch syndrome, are at increased risk of second cancers of specific types. In none of these examples does it appear that treatment of the primary cancer is the cause of the secondary cancer, but a role for treatment is difficult to exclude. These predispositions should result in heightened surveillance in persons at risk. Patients with head and neck cancer may have a reduced risk of developing lung cancer with retinoic acid treatment. Other cancer preventions have not been proved effective.

Patients treated with radiation therapy have an increasing and apparently life-long risk of developing second solid tumors, usually in or adjacent to the radiation field. The risk is modest in the first decade after treatment but reaches 1% per year in the second decade, such that populations followed for 25 years or more have a ≥25% chance of developing a second treatment-related tumor. Some organs differ in their susceptibility to radiation carcinogenesis with age; women receiving chest radiation therapy after age 30 have a small increased risk of breast cancer, but those <30 have a 19-fold increased risk. The chances of curing the second malignancies hinge on early diagnosis. Patients who were treated with radiation therapy should be carefully examined on an annual basis and evaluated for any abnormalities in organs and tissues that were in the radiation field. Symptoms in a patient cured of cancer should not be dismissed as they may be an early sign of second cancers.

Chemotherapy produces two clinical syndromes that can be fatal: myelodysplasia and acute myeloid leukemia. Two types of acute leukemia have been described. The first occurs in patients treated with alkylating agents, especially over a protracted period. The malignant cells frequently carry genetic deletions in chromosomes 5 or 7. The lifetime risk is about 2%; the risk is increased by the addition of radiation therapy and is about three times higher in people treated over age 40. It peaks in incidence 4 to 6 years after treatment; the risk returns to baseline if no disease has developed within 10 years of treatment. The second type of acute leukemia occurs after exposure to topoisomerase II inhibitors such as doxorubicin or etoposide. It is morphologically indistinguishable from the first but contains a characteristic chromosome translocation involving 10q23. The incidence is <1%, and it usually occurs 1.5 to 3 years after treatment. Both forms of acute leukemia are highly refractory to treatment, and no preventive strategy has been developed.

Hormonal manipulations can also cause second tumors. Tamoxifen induces endometrial cancer in about 1 to 2% of women taking it for 5 years or longer. Usually these tumors are found at an early stage; mortality from endometrial cancer is very low compared to the benefit from tamoxifen use as adjuvant therapy in women with breast cancer.

CONSEQUENCES BY CANCER TYPE ■ Pediatric Cancers Quality of life is often excellent, although the majority have at least one late effect. About one-third of long-term survivors have moderate to severe problems. Cognitive function may be impaired. Late effects are worse for those with poor socioeconomic status. Functional impairments in the cardiovascular system due to radiation therapy and anthracyclines, and in the lungs due to radiation therapy, are rare. Scoliosis and/or delayed growth due to radiation of the skeleton is more common. Many survivors have psychosocial and sexual problems. Second malignant neoplasms are a significant cause of death.

Hodgkin's Disease   The patient cured of Hodgkin's disease remains subject to long-term medical problems such as thyroid dysfunction, premature coronary artery disease, gonadal dysfunction, postsplenectomy sepsis, and second malignancies. The second malignancies encountered include myelodysplasia and acute myeloid leukemia, non-Hodgkin's lymphomas, breast cancer, lung cancer, and melanoma. The major risk factor for hematologic malignancies is treatment with alkylating agents plus radiation therapy, while solid tumors are more likely to be seen with the use of radiation therapy. Patients cured of Hodgkin's disease seem to have greater fatigue, more psychosocial and sexual problems, and report a poorer quality of life than patients cured of acute leukemia.

Non-Hodgkin's Lymphomas   The patient cured of a non-Hodgkin's lymphoma may be at increased risk of myelodysplasia and acute leukemia if high doses or prolonged courses of alkylating agents were used. Chronic exposure to cyclophosphamide increases the risk of bladder cancer. Patients cured of lymphoma report a very good quality of life.

Acute Leukemia   The late effects of anti-leukemic therapy include second malignancies (hematologic and solid tumors), neuropsychiatric difficulties, subnormal growth, thyroid abnormalities, and infertility.

Head and Neck Cancer   Patients frequently have poor dentition, dry mouth, trismus, difficulty in eating, and poor nutrition. Those with nasopharyngeal cancer report the poorest long-term quality of life, possibly related to the volume of disease that is radiated.

Stem Cell Transplantation   Cured patients are at risk of second cancers, especially if radiation therapy was part of the treatment. They are also subject to gonadal damage and infertility. Graft-versus-host disease is the leading factor contributing to the morbidity and mortality from allogeneic bone marrow transplantation, with an immune-mediated attack against the skin, liver, and gut epithelium. About half of patients report psychosexual problems.

Breast Cancer   Patients treated with adjuvant chemotherapy and/or hormonal therapy for breast cancer are at risk for endometrial cancer from the use of tamoxifen. Those patients who have received chemotherapy may be at risk from doxorubicin- or radiation-induced cardiomyopathy and acute leukemia. Herceptin may contribute to heart failure. The development of premature ovarian failure from chemotherapy may cause hormone-deficient symptoms (hot flashes, decreased vaginal secretions, dyspareunia) and places women at risk for osteoporosis and cardiovascular death. Patients commonly report intrusive thoughts of cancer and psychological distress.

Testicular Cancer   Depending on the modalities used for therapy, patients cured of testicular cancer can anticipate Raynaud's phenomenon, renal and/or pulmonary damage from chemotherapy, and retrograde ejaculation from retroperitoneal lymph node dissection. Sexual dysfunction is reported by 15% of patients cured of testicular cancer.

Colon Cancer   To date the major threat to patients with colorectal cancer treated with chemotherapy and/or radiation therapy remains the risk of a second colorectal cancer. Quality of life is reported as high in long-term survivors.

Prostate Cancer   Radical surgical treatment is often accompanied by impotence, and about 10 to 15% develop some urine incontinence. Use of radiation therapy increases the risk of second cancers.

OUTLOOK   The challenge for the future is to integrate new chemotherapy and biologic agents and newer techniques of delivering radiation therapy in a fashion that increases cure rates and lowers the late effects of treatment. Additional populations at risk for late effects include those with cancers where therapy is becoming more effective, such as ovarian cancer, and cancers where chemotherapy and radiation therapy are used together in an organ-sparing approach, such as bladder, anal, and laryngeal cancers. Patients who have been cured of a cancer represent an important resource for cancer prevention studies.

FURTHER READING

AHLES T et al: Neuropsychiatric impact of standard-dose chemotherapy in long-term survivors of breast cancer and lymphoma. J Clin Oncol 20:485, 2002

BOOKMAN MA et al: Late complications of curative treatment in Hodgkin's disease. JAMA 260:680, 1988

MACKIE E et al: Adult psychosocial outcomes in long-term survivors of acute lymphoblastic leukemia and Wilms' tumor: A controlled study. Lancet 355:1310, 2000

TRAVIS LB: Therapy-associated solid tumors. Acta Oncol 41:323, 2002

Section 2   **Hematopoietic Disorders**

90 | IRON DEFICIENCY AND OTHER HYPOPROLIFERATIVE ANEMIAS
John W. Adamson

Anemias associated with normocytic and normochromic red cells and an inappropriately low reticulocyte response (reticulocyte index <2.5) are *hypoproliferative anemias*. This category includes early iron deficiency (before hypochromic microcytic red cells develop), acute and chronic inflammation (including many malignancies), renal disease, hypometabolic states such as protein malnutrition and endocrine deficiencies, and anemias from marrow damage. Marrow damage states are discussed in Chap. 94. Hypoproliferative anemias are the most common anemias and anemia associated with acute and chronic inflammation is the most common of these. The anemia of acute and chronic inflammation, like iron deficiency, is related in part to abnormal iron metabolism. The anemias associated with renal disease, inflammation, cancer, and hypometabolic states are characterized by an abnormal erythropoietin response to anemia.

IRON METABOLISM

Iron is a critical element in the function of all cells, although the amount of iron required by individual tissues varies during development. At the same time, the body must protect itself from free iron, which is highly toxic in that it participates in chemical reactions that generate free radicals such as singlet O_2 or OH^-. Consequently, elaborate mechanisms have evolved that allow iron to be made available for critical physiologic functions while at the same time conserving this element and handling it in such a way that toxicity is avoided.

The major role of iron in mammals is to carry O_2 as part of the heme protein that, in turn, is part of hemoglobin. O_2 is also bound by a heme protein in muscle, myoglobin. Iron is a critical element in iron-containing enzymes, including the cytochrome system in mitochondria; iron distribution in the body is shown in Table 90-1. Without

TABLE 90-1 *Body Iron Distribution*

	Iron Content, mg	
	Adult Male, 80 kg	Adult Female, 60 kg
Hemoglobin	2500	1700
Myoglobin/enzymes	500	300
Transferrin iron	3	3
Iron stores	600–1000	0–300

iron, cells lose their capacity for electron transport and energy metabolism; in erythroid cells hemoglobin synthesis is impaired, resulting in anemia and reduced O_2 delivery to tissue.

THE IRON CYCLE IN HUMANS Figure 90-1 outlines the major pathways of internal iron exchange in humans. Iron absorbed from the diet or released from stores circulates in the plasma bound to *transferrin*, the iron transport protein. Transferrin is a bilobed glycoprotein with two iron binding sites. Transferrin that carries iron exists in two forms—*monoferric* (one iron atom) or *diferric* (two iron atoms). The turnover (half-clearance time) of transferrin-bound iron is very rapid—typically 60 to 90 min. Because the overwhelming majority of iron transported by transferrin is delivered to the erythroid marrow, the clearance time of transferrin-bound iron from the circulation is affected most by the plasma iron level and the activity of the erythroid marrow. When erythropoiesis is markedly stimulated, the pool of erythroid cells requiring iron increases and the clearance time of iron from the circulation decreases. The half-clearance time of iron in the presence of iron deficiency is as short as 10 to 15 min; this value reflects the limits of iron delivery as a function of the cardiac output going to the bone marrow. With suppression of the erythroid marrow, the plasma iron level typically is increased and the half-clearance time is prolonged to as much as several hours. Normally, the iron bound to transferrin turns over 10 to 20 times per day. Assuming a normal plasma iron level of 80 to 100 μg/dL, the amount of iron passing through the transferrin pool is 20 to 24 mg/d.

The iron-transferrin complex circulates in the plasma until the iron-carrying transferrin interacts with specific *transferrin receptors* on the surface of marrow erythroid cells. Diferric transferrin has the highest affinity for transferrin receptors; apotransferrin (transferrin not carrying iron) has very little affinity. While transferrin receptors are found on cells in many tissues within the body—and all cells at some time

during development will display transferrin receptors—the cell having the greatest number of receptors (300,000 to 400,000/cell) is the developing erythroblast.

Once the iron-bearing transferrin interacts with its receptor, the iron-transferrin-receptor complex is internalized via clathrin-coated pits and transported to an acidic endosome, where the iron is released at the low pH. The iron is then made available for heme synthesis while the transferrin-receptor complex is recycled to the surface of the cell, where the bulk of the transferrin is released back into the circulation and the transferrin receptor reanchors into the cell membrane. At this point a certain amount of the transferrin receptor protein may be released into circulation. Within the erythroid cell, iron that is in excess of the amount needed for hemoglobin synthesis binds to a storage protein, *apoferritin*, forming *ferritin*. This mechanism of iron exchange also takes place in other cells of the body expressing transferrin receptors, especially liver parenchymal cells where the iron can be incorporated into heme-containing enzymes or stored. The iron incorporated into hemoglobin subsequently enters the circulation as new red cells are released from the bone marrow. The iron is then part of the red cell mass and will not become available for reutilization until the red cell dies.

In a normal individual, the average red cell life span is 120 days. Thus, 0.8 to 1.0% of red cells turn over each day. At the end of its life span, the red cell is recognized as senescent by the cells of the *reticuloendothelial (RE) system*, and the cell undergoes phagocytosis. Once within the RE cell, the hemoglobin from the ingested red cell is broken down, the globin and other proteins are returned to the amino acid pool, and the iron is shuttled back to the surface of the RE cell, where it is presented to circulating transferrin. The "harvesting" of iron from senescent red cells is both efficient and rapid, with newly recycled iron appearing in the circulation within 10 min of ingestion of the red cell. It is the efficient and highly conserved recycling of iron from senescent red cells that supports steady state (and even mildly accelerated) erythropoiesis.

Since each milliliter of red cells contains 1 mg of elemental iron, the amount of iron needed to replace those red cells lost through senescence amounts to 16 to 20 mg/d (assuming an adult with a red cell mass of 2 L). Any additional iron required for daily red cell production comes from the diet. Normally, an adult male will need to absorb at least 1 mg of elemental iron daily to meet needs, while females in the childbearing years will need to absorb an average of 1.4 mg/d. However, to achieve a maximum proliferative erythroid marrow response to anemia, additional iron must be available. With markedly stimulated erythropoiesis, demands for iron are increased by as much as six- to eightfold. With hemolytic anemias, the rate of red cell destruction is increased, but the iron recovered from the red cells is efficiently reutilized for hemoglobin synthesis. In contrast, with blood loss anemia the rate of red cell production is limited by the amount of iron that can be mobilized from ferritin and hemosiderin stores. Typically, the rate of mobilization under these circumstances will not support red cell production more than 2.5 to 3 times normal. If the delivery of iron to the stimulated marrow is suboptimal, the marrow's proliferative response is blunted and normal hemoglobin synthesis is impaired. The result is a hypoproliferative marrow accompanied by microcytic, hypochromic anemia.

While blood loss or hemolysis places a demand for iron to be supplied to the erythroid marrow, other conditions such as inflammation interfere with iron release from stores and can result in a rapid decrease in the serum iron (see below).

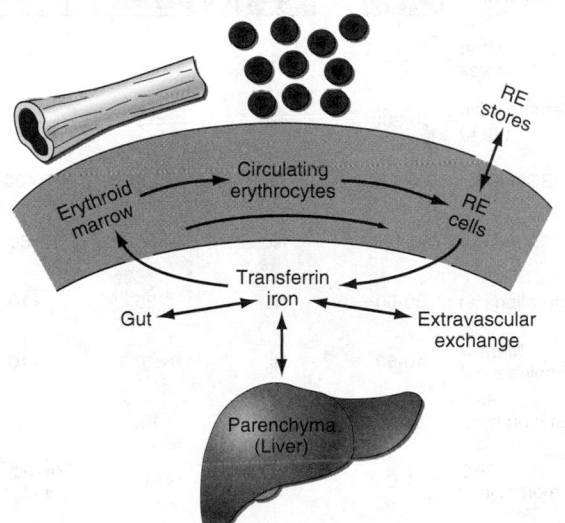

FIGURE 90-1 Internal iron exchange. Normally about 80% of iron passing through the plasma transferrin pool is recycled from broken-down red cells. Absorption of about 1 mg/d is required from the diet in men, 1.4 mg/d in women to maintain homeostasis. As long as transferrin saturation is maintained between 20 to 60% and erythropoiesis is not increased, iron stores are not required. However, in the event of blood loss, dietary iron deficiency, or inadequate iron absorption, up to 40 mg/d of iron can be mobilized from stores. RE, reticuloendothelial.

NUTRITIONAL IRON BALANCE The balance of iron metabolism in the organism is tightly controlled and designed to conserve iron for reutilization. There is no excretory pathway for iron, and the only mechanisms by which iron is lost from the body are blood loss (via gastrointestinal bleeding, menses, or other forms of bleeding) and the loss of epidermal cells from the skin and gut. Normally, the only route by which iron comes into the body is via absorption from food (dietary iron intake) or from medicinal iron taken orally. Iron may also enter the body through red cell transfusions or injection of iron complexes. The margin between the amount of iron available for absorption and the requirement for iron in growing infants and the adult female is narrow. The narrowness of this margin accounts for the great prevalence of iron deficiency worldwide—currently estimated at one-half billion people.

External iron exchange—the amount of iron required from the diet to replace losses—averages about 10% of body iron content a year in men and 15% in women of childbearing age, equivalent to 1.0 and 1.4 mg of elemental iron daily, respectively. Dietary iron content is closely related to total caloric intake (approximately 6 mg of elemental iron per 1000 calories). Iron bioavailability is affected by the nature of the foodstuff, with heme iron (e.g., red meat) being most readily absorbed. In the United States, the average iron intake in an adult male is 15 mg/d with 6% absorption; for the average female, the daily intake is 11 mg/d with 12% absorption. An individual with iron deficiency can increase iron absorption to about 20% of the iron present in a meat-containing diet but only 5 to 10% of the iron in a vegetarian diet. As a result, nearly one-third of the female population in the United States has virtually no iron stores. Vegetarians are at an additional disadvantage because certain foodstuffs that include phytates and phosphates reduce iron absorption by about 50%. When ionizable iron salts are given together with food, the amount of iron absorbed is reduced. This is particularly true with iron in the ferric state. When the percentage of iron absorbed from individual food items is compared with the percentage for an equivalent amount of ferrous salt, iron in vegetables is only about one-twentieth as available, egg iron one-eighth, liver iron one-half, and heme iron one-half to two-thirds. Therefore, liver and heme iron are absorbed nearly as well as iron salt added to food, while the iron in vegetables and eggs is much less available.

Infants, children, and adolescents may be unable to maintain normal iron balance because of the demands of body growth and lower dietary intake of iron. In pregnancy during the last two trimesters, daily iron requirements increase to 5 to 6 mg. That is the reason why iron supplements are strongly recommended for pregnant women in developed countries. Enthusiasm for supplementing foods such as bread and cereals with iron has waned in the face of concerns that the very prevalent hemochromatosis gene would result in an unacceptable risk of iron overload.

Iron absorption takes place largely in the proximal small intestine and is a carefully regulated process. For absorption, iron must be taken up by the luminal cell. That process is facilitated by the acidic contents of the stomach, which maintains the iron in solution. At the brush border of the absorptive cell, the ferric iron is converted to the ferrous form by a ferrireductase. Transport across the membrane is accomplished by divalent metal transporter 1 (DMT 1, also known as Nramp 2 or DCT 1). DMT 1 is a general cation transporter. Once iron is inside the gut cell, the iron may be stored as ferritin or transported through the cell to be released at the basolateral surface to plasma transferrin. It is likely that another transporter acts here in concert with hephaestin, another ferroxidase. Hephaestin is similar to ceruloplasmin, the copper-carrying protein.

Iron absorption is influenced by a number of physiologic states. Erythroid hyperplasia, for example, stimulates iron absorption, even in the face of normal or increased iron stores. Patients with anemias associated with high levels of ineffective erythropoiesis absorb excess amounts of dietary iron. Over time, this may lead to iron overload and tissue damage. In iron deficiency, iron is much more efficiently absorbed from a given diet; the contrary is true in the presence of iron overload. This is possibly mediated through signals that become fixed before the jejunal crypt cell migrates up the villus to become an absorptive cell. The normal individual can reduce iron absorption in situations of excessive intake or medicinal iron intake; however, while the percentage of iron absorbed goes down, the absolute amount goes

up. This accounts for the acute iron toxicity occasionally seen when children ingest large numbers of iron tablets. Under these circumstances, the amount of iron absorbed exceeds the transferrin binding capacity of the plasma, resulting in free iron that affects critical organs such as cardiac muscle cells.

IRON DEFICIENCY ANEMIA

STAGES OF IRON DEFICIENCY Iron deficiency anemia is the condition in which there is anemia and clear evidence of iron deficiency. However, iron deficiency occurs in steps (Fig. 90-2). These can be divided into three stages. The first stage is *negative iron balance*, in which the demands for (or losses of) iron exceed the body's ability to absorb iron from the diet. This stage can result from a number of physiologic mechanisms including blood loss, pregnancy (in which the demands for red cell production by the fetus outstrip the mother's ability to provide iron), rapid growth spurts in the adolescent, or inadequate dietary iron intake. Most commonly, the growth needs of the fetus or rapidly growing child exceed the individual's ability to absorb the iron necessary for hemoglobin synthesis from the diet. Blood loss in excess of 10 to 20 mL of red cells per day is greater than the amount of iron that the gut can absorb from a normal diet. Under these circumstances the iron deficit must be made up by mobilization of iron from RE storage sites. During this period measurements of iron stores—such as the serum ferritin level or the appearance of stainable iron on bone marrow aspirations—will decrease. As long as iron stores are present and can be mobilized, the serum iron, total iron-binding capacity (TIBC), and red cell protoporphyrin levels remain within normal limits. At this stage, red cell morphology and indices are normal.

When iron stores become depleted, the serum iron begins to fall. Gradually, the TIBC increases, as do red cell protoporphyrin levels. By definition, marrow iron stores are absent when the serum ferritin level is <15 μg/L. As long as the serum iron remains within the normal range, hemoglobin synthesis is unaffected despite the dwindling iron stores. Once the transferrin saturation falls to 15 to 20%, hemoglobin synthesis becomes impaired. This is a period of *iron-*

	Normal	Negative iron balance	Iron-deficient erythropoiesis	Iron-deficiency anemia
Iron stores Erythron iron				
Marrow iron stores	1-3+	0-1+	0	0
Serum ferritin (μg/L)	50-200	<20	<15	<15
TIBC (μg/dL)	300-360	>360	>380	>400
SI (μg/dL)	50-150	NL	<50	<30
Saturation (%)	30-50	NL	<20	<10
Marrow sideroblasts (%)	40-60	NL	<10	<10
RBC protoporphyrin (μg/dL)	30-50	NL	>100	>200
RBC morphology	NL	NL	NL	Microcytic/hypochromic

FIGURE 90-2 Laboratory studies in the evolution of iron deficiency. Measurements of marrow iron stores, serum ferritin, and total iron-binding capacity (TIBC) are sensitive to early iron-store depletion. Iron-deficient erythropoiesis is recognized from additional abnormalities in the serum iron (SI), percent transferrin saturation, the pattern of marrow sideroblasts, and the red cell protoporphyrin level. Patients with iron deficiency anemia demonstrate all the same abnormalities plus hypochromic microcytic anemia. (*From Hillman and Finch, with permission.*)

deficient erythropoiesis. Careful evaluation of the peripheral blood smear reveals the first appearance of microcytic cells, and if the laboratory technology is available, one finds hypochromic reticulocytes in circulation. Gradually, the hemoglobin and hematocrit begin to fall, reflecting *iron deficiency anemia*. The transferrin saturation at this point is 10 to 15%.

When moderate anemia is present (hemoglobin 10–13 g/dL), the bone marrow remains hypoproliferative. With more severe anemia (hemoglobin 7–8 g/dL), hypochromia and microcytosis become more prominent, misshapen red cells (poikilocytes) appear on the blood smear as cigar- or pencil-shaped forms and target cells, and the erythroid marrow becomes increasingly ineffective. Consequently, with severe prolonged iron deficiency anemia, erythroid hyperplasia of the marrow develops rather than hypoproliferation.

CAUSES OF IRON DEFICIENCY Conditions that increase demand for iron, increase iron loss, or decrease iron intake or absorption can produce iron deficiency (Table 90-2).

CLINICAL PRESENTATION OF IRON DEFICIENCY Certain clinical conditions carry an increased likelihood of iron deficiency. Pregnancy, adolescence, periods of rapid growth, and an intermittent history of blood loss of any kind should alert the clinician to possible iron deficiency. A cardinal rule is that the appearance of iron deficiency in an adult male means gastrointestinal blood loss until proven otherwise. Signs related to iron deficiency depend on the severity and chronicity of the anemia in addition to the usual signs of anemia—fatigue, pallor, and reduced exercise capacity. *Cheilosis* (fissures at the corners of the mouth) and *koilonychia* (spooning of the fingernails) are signs of advanced tissue iron deficiency. The diagnosis of iron deficiency is typically based on laboratory results.

LABORATORY IRON STUDIES ■ **Serum Iron and Total Iron-Binding Capacity** The serum iron level represents the amount of circulating iron bound to transferrin. The TIBC is an indirect measure of the circulating transferrin. The normal range for the serum iron is 50 to 150 μg/dL; the normal range for TIBC is 300 to 360 μg/dL. Transferrin saturation, which is normally 25 to 50%, is obtained by the following formula: serum iron × 100 ÷ TIBC. Iron deficiency states are associated with saturation levels below 18%. In evaluating the serum iron, the clinician should be aware that there is a diurnal variation in the value. A transferrin saturation of >50% indicates that a disproportionate amount of the iron bound to transferrin is being delivered to nonerythroid tissues. If this condition persists for an extended time, tissue iron overload may occur.

Serum Ferritin Free iron is toxic to cells, and the body has established an elaborate set of protective mechanisms to bind iron in various tissue compartments. Within cells, iron is stored complexed to protein as ferritin or hemosiderin. Apoferritin binds to free ferrous iron and stores it in the ferric state. As ferritin accumulates within cells of the RE system, protein aggregates are formed as hemosiderin. Iron in ferritin or hemosiderin can be extracted for release by the RE cells although hemosiderin is less readily available. Under steady state conditions,

FIGURE 90-3 Serum ferritin levels as a function of sex and age. Iron store depletion and iron deficiency are accompanied by a fall in serum ferritin level below 20 μg/L. (*From Hillman and Ault, with permission.*)

the serum ferritin level correlates with total body iron stores; thus, the serum ferritin level is the most convenient laboratory test to estimate iron stores. The normal value for ferritin varies according to the age and gender of the individual (Fig. 90-3). Adult males have serum ferritin values averaging about 100 μg/L, while adult females have levels averaging 30 μg/L. As iron stores are depleted, the serum ferritin falls to <15 μg/L. Such levels are virtually always diagnostic of absent body iron stores.

Evaluation of Bone Marrow Iron Stores Although RE cell iron stores can also be estimated from the iron stain of a bone marrow aspirate or biopsy, the measurement of serum ferritin has largely supplanted bone marrow aspirates for determination of storage iron (Table 90-3). The serum ferritin level is a better indicator of iron overload than the marrow iron stain. However, in addition to storage iron the marrow iron stain provides information about the effective delivery of iron to developing erythroblasts. Normally, 20 to 40% of developing erythroblasts—called *sideroblasts*—will have visible ferritin granules in their cytoplasm. This represents iron in excess of that needed for hemoglobin synthesis. In states in which release of iron from storage sites is blocked, RE iron will be detectable, and there will be few or no sideroblasts. In the myelodysplastic syndromes, mitochondrial dysfunction occurs, and accumulation of iron in mitochondria appears in a necklace fashion around the nucleus of the erythroblast. Such cells are referred to as *ringed sideroblasts*.

Red Cell Protoporphyrin Levels Protoporphyrin is an intermediate in the pathway to heme synthesis. Under conditions in which heme synthesis is impaired, protoporphyrin accumulates within the red cell. This can reflect an inadequate iron supply to erythroid precursors to support hemoglobin synthesis. Normal values are less than 30 μg/dL of red cells. In iron deficiency, values in excess of 100 μg/dL are seen. The most common causes of increased red cell protoporphyrin levels are absolute or relative iron deficiency and lead poisoning.

TABLE 90-2 *Causes of Iron Deficiency*

Increased demand for iron and/or hematopoiesis
   rapid growth in infancy or adolescence
   pregnancy
   erythropoietin therapy
Increased iron loss
   chronic blood loss
   menses
   acute blood loss
   blood donation
   phlebotomy as treatment for polycythemia vera
Decreased iron intake or absorption
   inadequate diet
   malabsorption from disease (sprue, Crohn's disease)
   malabsorption from surgery (post-gastrectomy)
   acute or chronic inflammation

TABLE 90-3 *Iron Store Measurements*

Iron Stores	Marrow Iron Stain, 0–4+	Serum Ferritin, μg/L
0	0	<15
1–300 mg	Trace to 1+	15–30
300–800 mg	2+	30–60
800–1000 mg	3+	60–150
1–2 g	4+	>150
Iron overload	—	>500–1000

TABLE 90-4 *Diagnosis of Microcytic Anemia*

Tests	Iron Deficiency	Inflammation	Thalassemia	Sideroblastic Anemia
Smear	Micro/hypo	Normal micro/hypo	Micro/hypo with targeting	Variable
SI	<30	<50	Normal to high	Normal to high
TIBC	>360	<300	Normal	Normal
Percent saturation	<10	10–20	30–80	30–80
Ferritin (μg/L)	<15	30–200	50–300	50–300
Hemoglobin pattern	Normal	Normal	Abnormal	Normal

Note: SI, serum iron; TIBC, total iron-binding capacity.

Serum Levels of Transferrin Receptor Protein Because erythroid cells have the highest numbers of transferrin receptors on their surface of any cell in the body, and because transferrin receptor protein (TRP) is released by cells into the circulation, serum levels of TRP reflect the total erythroid marrow mass. Another condition in which TRP levels are elevated is absolute iron deficiency. Normal values are 4 to 9 μg/L determined by immunoassay. This laboratory test is becoming increasingly available and has been proposed to measure the serial expansion of the erythroid marrow in response to recombinant erythropoietin therapy.

DIFFERENTIAL DIAGNOSIS Other than iron deficiency, only three conditions need to be considered in the differential diagnosis of a hypochromic microcytic anemia (Table 90-4). The first is inherited defects in globin chain synthesis: the thalassemias. These are differentiated from iron deficiency most readily by serum iron values, since it is characteristic to have normal or increased serum iron levels and transferrin saturation with the thalassemias.

The second condition is chronic inflammatory disease with inadequate iron supply to the erythroid marrow. The distinction between true iron deficiency anemia and the anemia associated with chronic inflammatory states is among the most common diagnostic problems encountered by clinicians (see below). Usually the anemia of chronic disease is normocytic and normochromic. Again, the iron values usually make the differential diagnosis clear, as the ferritin level is normal or increased and the TIBC is typically below normal.

Finally, the myelodysplastic syndromes represent the third and most rare condition. Occasionally, patients with myelodysplasia have impaired hemoglobin synthesis with mitochondrial dysfunction resulting in impaired iron incorporation into heme. The iron values again reveal normal stores and more than an adequate supply to the marrow, despite the microcytosis and hypochromia.

℞ TREATMENT

The severity and cause of iron deficiency anemia will determine the appropriate approach to treatment. As an example, symptomatic elderly patients with severe iron deficiency anemia and cardiovascular instability may require red cell transfusions. Younger individuals who have compensated for their anemia can be treated more conservatively with iron replacement. The foremost issue for the latter patient is the precise identification of the cause of the iron deficiency.

For the majority of cases of iron deficiency (pregnant women, growing children and adolescents, patients with infrequent episodes of bleeding, and those with inadequate dietary intake of iron), oral iron therapy will suffice. For patients with unusual blood loss or malabsorption, specific diagnostic tests and appropriate therapy take priority. Once the diagnosis of iron deficiency anemia and its cause is made, and a therapeutic approach is charted, there are three major approaches.

Red Cell Transfusion Transfusion therapy is reserved for those individuals who have symptoms of anemia, cardiovascular instability, and continued and excessive blood loss from whatever source, and those who require immediate intervention. The management of these patients is less related to the iron deficiency than it is to the consequences of the severe anemia. Not only do transfusions correct the anemia acutely, but the transfused red cells provide a source of iron for reu-

tilization, assuming they are not lost through continued bleeding. Transfusion therapy will stabilize the patient while other options are reviewed.

Oral Iron Therapy In the patient with established iron deficiency anemia who is asymptomatic, treatment with oral iron is usually adequate. Multiple preparations are available ranging from simple iron salts to complex iron compounds designed for sustained release throughout the small intestine (Table 90-5). While the various preparations contain different amounts of iron, they are generally all absorbed well and are effective in treatment. Some come with other compounds designed to enhance iron absorption, such as ascorbic acid. It is not clear whether the benefits of such compounds justify their costs. Typically, for iron replacement therapy up to 300 mg of elemental iron per day is given, usually as three or four iron tablets (each containing 50 to 65 mg elemental iron) given over the course of the day. Ideally, oral iron preparations should be taken on an empty stomach, since foods may inhibit iron absorption. Some patients with gastric disease or prior gastric surgery require special treatment with iron solutions, since the retention capacity of the stomach may be reduced. The retention capacity is necessary for dissolving the shell of the iron tablet before the release of iron. A dose of 200 to 300 mg of elemental iron per day should result in the absorption of iron up to 50 mg/d. This supports a red cell production level of two to three times normal in an individual with a normally functioning marrow and appropriate erythropoietin stimulus. However, as the hemoglobin level rises, erythropoietin stimulation decreases, and the amount of iron absorbed is reduced. The goal of therapy in individuals with iron deficiency anemia is not only to repair the anemia, but also to provide stores of at least 0.5 to 1.0 g of iron. Sustained treatment for a period of 6 to 12 months after correction of the anemia will be necessary to achieve this.

Of the complications of oral iron therapy, gastrointestinal distress is the most prominent and is seen in 15 to 20% of patients. For these patients, abdominal pain, nausea, vomiting, or constipation often lead to noncompliance. Although small doses of iron or iron preparations with delayed release may help somewhat, the gastrointestinal side effects are a major impediment to the effective treatment of a number of patients.

The response to iron therapy varies, depending on the erythropoietin stimulus and the rate of absorption. Typically, the reticulocyte count should begin to increase within 4 to 7 days after initiation of therapy and peak at 1½ weeks. The absence of a response may be due to poor adsorption, noncompliance (which is common), or a confounding diagnosis. If iron deficiency persists, it may be necessary to switch to parenteral iron therapy.

Parenteral Iron Therapy Intravenous iron can be given to patients who are unable to tolerate oral iron, whose needs are relatively acute, or who need iron on an ongoing basis, usually due to persistent gastrointestinal blood loss. Parenteral iron use has been rising rapidly in the last several years with the recognition that recombinant erythropoietin therapy induces a large demand for iron—a demand that frequently

TABLE 90-5 *Oral Iron Preparations*

Generic Name	Tablet (Iron Content), mg	Elixir (Iron Content), mg in 5 mL
Ferrous sulfate	325 (65)	300 (60)
	195 (39)	90 (18)
Extended release	525 (105)	
Ferrous fumarate	325 (107)	
	195 (64)	100 (33)
Ferrous gluconate	325 (39)	300 (35)
Polysaccharide iron	150 (150)	100 (100)
	50 (50)	

cannot be met through the physiologic release of iron from RE sources. Concern has been raised about the safety of parenteral iron—particularly iron dextran. The serious adverse reaction rate to intravenous iron dextran is 0.7%. Fortunately, newer iron complexes are available in the United States that have a much lower rate of adverse effects. The most recently approved preparations are intravenous sodium ferric gluconate (Ferrlecit) and iron sucrose (Venofer).

Parenteral iron is used in two ways: one is to administer the total dose of iron required to correct the hemoglobin deficit and provide the patient with at least 500 mg of iron stores; the second is to give repeated small doses of parenteral iron over a protracted period. The latter approach is common in dialysis centers, where it is not unusual for 100 mg of elemental iron to be given weekly for 10 weeks to augment the response to recombinant erythropoietin therapy. The amount of iron needed by an individual patient is calculated by the following formula:

$$\text{Body weight (kg)} \times 2.3 \times (15 - \text{patient's hemoglobin, g/dL}) + 500 \text{ or } 1000 \text{ mg (for stores).}$$

In administering intravenous iron dextran, anaphylaxis is a concern. Anaphylaxis is almost never seen with the newer preparations. The factors that have correlated with a serious anaphylactic-like reaction include a history of multiple allergies or a prior allergic reaction to dextran (in the case of iron dextran). Generalized symptoms appearing several days after the infusion of a large dose of iron can include arthralgias, skin rash, and low-grade fever. This may be dose-related, but it does not preclude the further use of parenteral iron in the patient. To date, patients with sensitivity to iron dextran have been safely treated with iron gluconate. If a large dose of iron dextran is to be given (>100 mg) the iron preparation should be diluted in 5% dextrose in water or 0.9% NaCl solution. The iron solution can then be infused over a 60- to 90-min period (for larger doses) or at a rate convenient for the attending nurse or physician. While a test dose (25 mg) of parenteral iron is recommended, in reality a slow infusion of a larger dose of parenteral iron solution will afford the same kind of early warning as a separately injected test dose. Early in the infusion of iron, if chest pain, wheezing, a fall in blood pressure, or other systemic manifestations occur, the infusion of iron—whether as a large solution or a test dose—should be interrupted immediately.

OTHER HYPOPROLIFERATIVE ANEMIAS

In addition to mild to moderate iron deficiency anemia, the hypoproliferative anemias can be divided into four categories: (1) chronic inflammation/infection; (2) renal disease; (3) endocrine and nutritional deficiencies (hypometabolic states); and (4) marrow damage (Chap. 94). With chronic inflammation, renal disease, or hypometabolism, endogenous erythropoietin production is inadequate for the degree of anemia observed. For the anemia of chronic inflammation (anemia of chronic disease), the erythroid marrow also responds inadequately to stimulation, due in part to defects in *iron reutilization*. As a result of the lack of adequate erythropoietin stimulation, an examination of the peripheral blood smear will disclose only an occasional polychromatophilic ("shift") reticulocyte. In the cases of iron deficiency or marrow damage, appropriate elevations in endogenous erythropoietin levels are typically found, and shift reticulocytes will be present on the blood smear.

ANEMIA OF ACUTE AND CHRONIC INFLAMMATION/INFECTION (THE ANEMIA OF CHRONIC DISEASE) The anemia of chronic disease—which encompasses inflammation, infection, tissue injury, and conditions associated with the release of proinflammatory cytokines (such as cancer)—is one of the most common forms of anemia seen clinically and is probably the most important in the differential diagnosis of iron deficiency, since many of the features of the anemia are brought about by inadequate iron delivery to the marrow, despite the presence of normal or increased iron stores. This is reflected by a low serum iron, increased red cell protoporphyrin, a hypoproliferative marrow, transferrin saturation in the range of 15 to 20%, and a normal or increased serum ferritin. The serum ferritin values are often the most distinguishing

feature between true iron deficiency anemia and the iron-deficient erythropoiesis associated with inflammation. Typically, serum ferritin values increase threefold over basal levels in the face of inflammation. All of these changes are due to the effects of inflammatory cytokines and hepcidin, the storage iron regulator, acting at several levels of erythropoiesis (Fig. 90-4). Interleukin 1 (IL-1) directly decreases erythropoietin production in response to anemia. IL-1, acting through accessory cell release of interferon γ (IFN-γ), suppresses the response of the erythroid marrow to erythropoietin—an effect that can be overcome by increased erythropoietin administration in vitro and in vivo. In addition, tumor necrosis factor (TNF), acting through the release of IFN-γ by marrow stromal cells, also suppresses the response to erythropoietin. Hepcidin, made by the liver, is increased in inflammation and acts to suppress iron absorption and iron release from storage sites. The overall result is a chronic hypoproliferative anemia with classic changes in iron metabolism. The anemia is further compounded by a mild to moderate shortening in red cell survival.

With chronic inflammation/infection, the primary disease will determine the severity and characteristics of the anemia. For instance, many patients with cancer also have anemia that is typically normocytic and normochromic. In contrast, patients with long-standing active rheumatoid arthritis or chronic infections such as tuberculosis will have a microcytic, hypochromic anemia. In both cases, the bone marrow is hypoproliferative, but the differences in red cell indices reflect differences in the availability of iron for hemoglobin synthesis. Occasionally, conditions associated with chronic inflammation are also associated with chronic blood loss. Under these circumstances, a bone marrow aspirate stained for iron may be necessary to rule out absolute iron deficiency. However, the administration of iron in this case will correct the iron deficiency component of the anemia and leave the inflammatory component unaffected.

The anemia associated with acute infection or inflammation is typically mild but becomes more pronounced over time. Acute infection can produce a fall in hemoglobin levels of 2 to 3 g/dL within 1 or 2 days; this is largely related to the hemolysis of red cells near the end of their natural life span. The fever and cytokines released exert a selective pressure against cells with more limited capacity to maintain the red cell membrane. In most individuals the mild anemia is reasonably well tolerated, and symptoms, if present, are associated with the underlying disease. Occasionally, in patients with preexisting cardiac disease, moderate anemia (hemoglobin 10–11 g/dL) may be associated with angina, exercise intolerance, and shortness of breath. The red cell indices vary from normocytic, normochromic to microcytic, hypochromic. The serum iron values tend to correlate with the red cell indices. The erythropoietic profile that distinguishes the anemia of

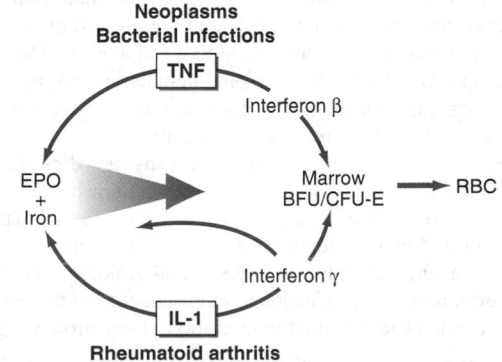

FIGURE 90-4 Suppression of erythropoiesis by inflammatory cytokines. Through the release of tumor necrosis factor (TNF) and interferon γ (IFN-γ) neoplasms and bacterial infections suppress erythropoietin (EPO) production, the release of iron from reticuloendothelial stores, and the proliferation of erythroid progenitors [erythroid burst-forming units and erythroid colony-forming units (BFU/CFU-E)]. The mediators in patients with vasculitis and rheumatoid arthritis include interleukin 1 (IL-1) and IFN-γ. The red arrows indicate sites of inflammatory cytokine inhibitory effects.

TABLE 90-6 *Diagnosis of Hypoproliferative Anemias*

Tests	Iron Deficiency	Inflammation	Renal Disease	Hypometabolic States
Anemia	Mild to severe	Mild	Mild to severe	Mild
MCV (fL)	60–90	80–90	90	90
Morphology	Normo-microcytic	Normocytic	Normocytic	Normocytic
SI	<30	<50	Normal	Normal
TIBC	>360	<300	Normal	Normal
Saturation (%)	<10	10–20	Normal	Normal
Serum ferritin (μg/L)	<15	30–200	115–150	Normal
Iron stores	0	2–4+	1–4+	Normal

Note: MCV, mean corpuscular volume; SI, serum iron; TIBC, total iron-binding capacity.

inflammation from the other causes of hypoproliferative anemias is shown in Table 90-6.

ANEMIA OF RENAL DISEASE Chronic renal failure is usually associated with a moderate to severe hypoproliferative anemia; the level of the anemia correlates with the severity of the renal failure. Red cells are typically normocytic and normochromic. Reticulocytes are decreased. The anemia is due to a failure to produce adequate amounts of erythropoietin and a reduction in red cell survival. In certain forms of acute renal failure, the correlation between the anemia and renal function is weaker. Patients with the hemolytic-uremic syndrome increase erythropoiesis in response to the hemolysis, despite renal failure requiring dialysis. Polycystic renal disease also shows a smaller degree of erythropoietin deficiency for a given level of renal failure. By contrast, patients with diabetes have more severe erythropoietin deficiency for a given level of renal failure.

Assessment of iron status provides information to distinguish the anemia of renal disease from the other forms of hypoproliferative anemia (Table 90-6) and to guide management. Patients with the anemia of renal disease usually present with normal serum iron, TIBC, and ferritin levels. However, those maintained on chronic hemodialysis may develop iron deficiency from blood loss through the dialysis procedure. Iron must be replenished in these patients to ensure an adequate response to erythropoietin therapy (see below).

ANEMIA IN HYPOMETABOLIC STATES Patients who are starving, particularly for protein, and those with a variety of endocrine disorders that produce lower metabolic rates may develop a mild to moderate hypoproliferative anemia. The release of erythropoietin from the kidney is sensitive to the need for O_2, not just O_2 levels. Thus, erythropoietin production is triggered at lower levels of O_2 tension in disease states (such as hypothyroidism and starvation) where metabolic activity, and thus O_2 demand, is decreased.

Endocrine Deficiency States The difference in the levels of hemoglobin between men and women is related to the effects of androgen and estrogen on erythropoiesis. Testosterone and anabolic steroids augment erythropoiesis; castration and estrogen administration to males decrease erythropoiesis. Patients who are hypothyroid or have deficits in pituitary hormones also may develop a mild anemia. Pathogenesis may be complicated by other nutritional deficiencies as iron and folic acid absorption can be affected by these disorders. Usually, correction of the hormone deficiency reverses the anemia.

Anemia may be more severe in Addison's disease, depending on the level of thyroid and androgen hormone dysfunction; however, anemia may be masked by decreases in plasma volume. Once such patients are given cortisol and volume replacement, the hemoglobin level may fall rapidly. Mild anemia complicating hyperparathyroidism may be due to decreased erythropoietin production as a consequence of the renal effects of hypercalcemia or to impaired proliferation of erythroid progenitors.

Protein Starvation Decreased dietary intake of protein may lead to mild to moderate hypoproliferative anemia; this form of anemia may be prevalent in the elderly. The anemia can be more severe in patients with a greater degree of starvation. In marasmus, where patients are both protein- and calorie-deficient, the release of erythropoietin is impaired in proportion to the reduction in metabolic rate; however, the degree of anemia may be masked by volume depletion and becomes

apparent after refeeding. Deficiencies in other nutrients (iron, folate) may also complicate the clinical picture but may not be apparent at diagnosis. Changes in the erythrocyte indices on refeeding should prompt evaluation of iron, folate, and B_{12} status.

Anemia in Liver Disease A mild hypoproliferative anemia may develop in patients with chronic liver disease from nearly any cause. The peripheral blood smear may show spur cells and stomatocytes from the accumulation of excess cholesterol in the membrane from a deficiency of lecithin cholesterol acyltransferase. Red cell survival is shortened, and the production of erythropoietin is inadequate to compensate. In alcoholic liver disease, nutritional deficiencies can add complexity to the management. Folate deficiency from inadequate intake, as well as iron deficiency from blood loss and inadequate intake, can alter the red cell indices.

℞ TREATMENT

Many patients with hypoproliferative anemias experience recovery of normal hemoglobin levels when the underlying disease is appropriately treated. For those in whom such reversals are not possible—such as patients with end-stage renal failure, cancer, and chronic inflammatory diseases—symptomatic anemia requires treatment. The two major forms of treatment are transfusions and erythropoietin.

Transfusions Thresholds for transfusion should be altered based on the patient's symptoms. In general, patients without serious underlying cardiovascular or pulmonary disease can tolerate hemoglobin levels above 8 g/dL and do not require intervention until the hemoglobin falls below that level. Patients with more physiologic compromise may need to have their hemoglobin levels kept above 11 g/dL. A typical unit of packed red cells increases the hemoglobin level by 1 g/dL. Transfusions are associated with certain infectious risks (Chap. 99), and chronic transfusions can produce iron overload.

Erythropoietin Erythropoietin is particularly useful in anemias in which endogenous erythropoietin levels are inappropriately low, such as the hypoproliferative anemias. Iron status must be evaluated and iron repleted to obtain optimal effects from erythropoietin. In patients with chronic renal failure, the usual dose of erythropoietin is 50 to 150 U/kg three times a week subcutaneously. Hemoglobin levels of 10 to 12 g/dL are usually reached within 4 to 6 weeks if iron levels are adequate; 90% of these patients respond. Once a target hemoglobin level is reached, the erythropoietin dose can be decreased. A fall in hemoglobin level occurring in the face of erythropoietin therapy usually signifies the development of an infection or iron depletion. Aluminum toxicity and hyperparathyroidism can also compromise the erythropoietin response. When an infection intervenes, it is best to interrupt the erythropoietin therapy and rely on transfusion to correct the anemia until the infection is adequately treated. The dose needed to correct the anemia in patients with cancer is higher, up to 300 U/kg three times a week, and only about 60% of patients respond.

ACKNOWLEDGMENT

Dr. Robert S. Hillman was the author of this chapter in the 14th edition, and material from his chapter has been retained.

FURTHER READING

BAILIE GR et al: Parenteral iron use in the management of anemia in end-stage renal disease patients. Am J Kidney Dis 35:1, 2000

BRUGNARA C: Iron deficiency and erythropoiesis: New diagnostic approaches. Clin Chem 49:1573, 2003

HILLMAN RS, AULT KA: *Hematology in Clinical Practice*, 3d ed. New York, McGraw-Hill, 2002

HILLMAN RS, FINCH CA: *Red Cell Manual*, 7th ed. Philadelphia, Davis, 1996

TSAKIRIS D: Morbidity and mortality reduction associated with the use of erythropoietin. Nephron 85(Suppl S1):2, 2000

WEINSTEIN DA et al: Inappropriate expression of hepcidin is associated with iron refractory anemia: Implications for the anemia of chronic disease. Blood 100:3776, 2002

91 HEMOGLOBINOPATHIES
Edward J. Benz

Hemoglobin is critical for normal oxygen delivery to tissues; it is also present in erythrocytes in such high concentrations that it can alter red cell shape, deformability, and viscosity. Hemoglobinopathies are disorders affecting the structure, function, or production of hemoglobin. These conditions are usually inherited and range in severity from asymptomatic laboratory abnormalities to death in utero. Different forms may present as hemolytic anemia, erythrocytosis, cyanosis, or vasoocclusive stigmata.

PROPERTIES OF THE HUMAN HEMOGLOBINS

HEMOGLOBIN STRUCTURE Different hemoglobins are produced during embryonic, fetal, and adult life (Fig. 91-1). Each consists of a tetramer of globin polypeptide chains: a pair of α-like chains 141 amino acids long and a pair of β-like chains 146 amino acids long. The major adult hemoglobin, HbA, has the structure $\alpha_2\beta_2$. HbF ($\alpha_2\gamma_2$) predominates during most of gestation, and HbA$_2$ ($\alpha_2\delta_2$) is a minor adult hemoglobin. Embryonic hemoglobins need not be considered here.

Each globin chain enfolds a single heme moiety, consisting of a protoporphyrin IX ring complexed with a single iron atom in the ferrous state (Fe^{2+}), positioned in a manner optimal for reversible binding of oxygen. Each heme moiety can bind a single oxygen molecule; every molecule of hemoglobin can thus transport up to four oxygen molecules.

The amino acid sequences of the various globins are highly homologous to one another. Each has a highly helical *secondary structure*. Their globular *tertiary structures* can cause the exterior surfaces to be rich in polar (hydrophilic) amino acids that enhance solubility and the interior to be lined with nonpolar groups, forming a hydrophobic pocket into which heme is inserted. The tetrameric *quaternary structure* of HbA contains two $\alpha\beta$ dimers. Numerous tight interactions (i.e., $\alpha_1\beta_1$ contacts) hold the α and β chains together. The complete tetramer is held together by interfaces (i.e., $\alpha_1\beta_2$ contacts) between the α-like chain of one dimer and the non-α chain of the other dimer.

The hemoglobin tetramer is highly soluble but individual globin chains are insoluble. Unpaired globin precipitates, forming inclusions that damage the cell. Normal globin chain synthesis is balanced so that each newly synthesized α or non-α globin chain will have an available partner with which to pair to form hemoglobin.

Solubility and reversible oxygen binding are the key properties deranged in hemoglobinopathies. Both depend most on the hydrophilic surface amino acids, the hydrophobic amino acids lining the heme pocket, a key histidine in the F helix, and the amino acids forming the $\alpha_1\beta_1$ and $\alpha_1\beta_2$ contact points. Mutations in these strategic regions tend to be the ones that alter clinical behavior.

FUNCTION OF HEMOGLOBIN To support oxygen transport, hemoglobin must bind O_2 efficiently at the partial pressure of oxygen (P_{O_2}) of the alveolus, retain it, and release it to tissues at the P_{O_2} of tissue capillary beds. Oxygen acquisition and delivery over a relatively narrow range of oxygen tensions depend on a property inherent in the tetrameric arrangement of heme and globin subunits within the hemoglobin molecule called *cooperativity* or *heme-heme interaction*.

At low oxygen tensions, the hemoglobin tetramer is fully deoxygenated (Fig.

FIGURE 91-1 The globin genes. The α-like genes (α, ζ) are encoded on chromosome 16; the β-like genes ($\beta, \gamma, \delta, \varepsilon$) are encoded on chromosome 11. The ζ and ε genes encode embryonic globins.

91-2). Oxygen binding begins slowly as O_2 tension rises. However, as soon as some oxygen has been bound by the tetramer, an abrupt increase occurs in the slope of the curve. Thus, hemoglobin molecules that have bound some oxygen develop a higher oxygen affinity, greatly accelerating their ability to combine with more oxygen. This S-shaped oxygen equilibrium curve (Fig. 91-2), along which substantial amounts of oxygen loading *and unloading* can occur over a narrow range of oxygen tensions, is physiologically more useful than the high-affinity hyperbolic curve of individual monomers.

Oxygen affinity is modulated by several factors. The Bohr effect arises from the stabilizing action of protons on deoxyhemoglobin, which binds protons more readily than oxyhemoglobin because it is a weaker acid (Fig. 91-2). Thus, hemoglobin has a lower oxygen affinity at low pH, facilitating delivery to tissues. The major small molecule that alters oxygen affinity in humans is 2,3-bisphosphoglycerate (2,3-BPG, formerly 2,3-DPG), which lowers oxygen affinity when bound to hemoglobin. HbA has a reasonably high affinity for 2,3-BPG. HbF does not bind 2,3-BPG, so it tends to have a higher oxygen affinity in vivo. Hemoglobin also binds nitric oxide reversibly; this interaction may influence vascular tone, but its physiologic relevance remains unclear.

To understand hemoglobinopathies, it is important to understand

FIGURE 91-2 Hemoglobin-oxygen dissociation curve. The hemoglobin tetramer can bind up to four molecules of oxygen in the iron-containing sites of the heme molecules. As oxygen is bound, 2,3-BPG and CO_2 are expelled. Salt bridges are broken, and each of the globin molecules changes its conformation to facilitate oxygen binding. Oxygen release to the tissues is the reverse process, salt bridges being formed and 2,3-BPG and CO_2 bound. Deoxyhemoglobin does not bind oxygen efficiently until the cell returns to conditions of higher pH, the most important modulator of O_2 affinity (Bohr effect). When acid is produced in the tissues, the dissociation curve shifts to the right, facilitating oxygen release and CO_2 binding. Alkalosis has the opposite effect, reducing oxygen delivery.

that proper oxygen transport depends on the tetrameric structure of the proteins, the proper arrangement of the charged amino acids, and interaction with low-molecular-weight substances such as protons or 2,3-BPG.

DEVELOPMENTAL BIOLOGY OF HUMAN HEMOGLOBINS   Red cells first appearing at about 6 weeks after conception contain the embyronic hemoglobins Hb Portland ($\zeta_2\gamma_2$), Hb Gower I ($\zeta_2\varepsilon_2$), and Hb Gower II ($\alpha_2\varepsilon_2$). At 10 to 11 weeks, fetal hemoglobin (HbF; $\alpha_2\gamma_2$) becomes predominant. The switch to nearly exclusive synthesis of adult hemoglobin (HbA; $\alpha_2\beta_2$) occurs at about 38 weeks (Fig. 91-1). Fetuses and newborns therefore require α-globin but not β-globin for normal gestation. Small amounts of HbF are produced during postnatal life. A few red cell clones called *F cells* are progeny of a small pool of immature committed erythroid precursors (BFU-e) that retain the ability to produce HbF. Profound erythroid stress, such as that seen in severe hemolytic anemias, after bone marrow transplant, or during chemotherapy, causes more of the F-potent BFU-e to be recruited. HbF levels thus tend to rise in some patients with sickle cell anemia or thalassemia. This phenomenon is also important because it probably explains the ability of hydroxyurea to increase levels of HbF in adults. Fetal globin genes can also be activated partially after birth by agents such as butyrate that inhibit histone deacetylase and modify the structure of chromatin.

GENETICS AND BIOSYNTHESIS OF HUMAN HEMOGLOBIN   The human hemoglobins are encoded in two tightly linked gene clusters; the α-like globin genes are clustered on chromosome 16, and the β-like genes on chromosome 11 (Fig. 91-1). The α-like cluster consists of two α-globin genes and a single copy of the ζ gene. The non-α gene cluster consists of a single ε gene, the Gγ and Aγ fetal globin genes, and the adult δ and β genes.

Important regulatory sequences flank each gene. Immediately upstream are typical promoter elements needed for the assembly of the transcription initiation complex. Sequences in the 5' flanking region of the γ and the β genes appear to be crucial for the correct developmental regulation of these genes, while elements that function like classic enhancers and silencers are in the 3' flanking regions. The locus control region (LCR) elements located far upstream appear to control the overall level of expression of each cluster. These elements achieve their regulatory effects by interacting with *trans*-acting transcription factors. Some of these factors are ubiquitous (e.g., Sp1 and YY1), while others are more or less limited to erythroid cells (e.g., GATA-1, NFE-2, and EKLF). The LCR controlling the α globin gene cluster is modulated by a SWI/SNF-like protein called *ATRX*; this protein appears to influence chromatin remodeling and DNA methylation. The association of α thalassemia with mental retardation and myelodysplasia in some families appears to be related to mutations in the pathway governed by ATRX. The latter also appear to modulate genes specifically expressed during erythropoiesis, such as the genes that encode the enzymes for heme biosynthesis. This is relevant since normal red blood cell (RBC) differentiation also requires the coordinated expression of the globin genes with the genes responsible for heme and iron metabolism.

CLASSIFICATION OF HEMOGLOBINOPATHIES

There are five major classes of hemoglobinopathies (Table 91-1). *Structural hemoglobinopathies* occur when mutations alter the amino acid sequence of a globin chain, altering the physiologic properties of the variant hemoglobins and producing the characteristic clinical abnormalities. The variant hemoglobins relevant to this chapter polymerize abnormally, as in sickle cell anemia, or exhibit altered solubility or oxygen-binding affinity. *Thalassemia syndromes* arise from mutations that impair production or translation of globin mRNA, leading to deficient globin chain biosynthesis. Clinical abnormalities are attributable to the inadequate supply of hemoglobin and the imbalances in the production of individual globin chains, leading to premature

TABLE 91-1   *Classification of Hemoglobinopathies*

I. Structural hemoglobinopathies—hemoglobins with altered amino acid sequences that result in deranged function or altered physical or chemical properties
   A. Abnormal hemoglobin polymerization—HbS, hemoglobin sickling
   B. Altered O$_2$ affinity
      1. High affinity—polycythemia
      2. Low affinity—cyanosis, pseudoanemia
   C. Hemoglobins that oxidize readily
      1. Unstable hemoglobins—hemolytic anemia, jaundice
      2. M hemoglobins—methemoglobinemia, cyanosis
II. Thalassemias—defective biosynthesis of globin chains
   A. α Thalassemias
   B. β Thalassemias
   C. $\delta\beta$, $\gamma\delta\beta$, $\alpha\beta$ Thalassemias
III. Thalassemic hemoglobin variants—structurally abnormal Hb associated with coinherited thalassemic phenotype
   A. HbE
   B. Hb Constant Spring
   C. Hb Lepore
IV. Hereditary persistence of fetal hemoglobin—persistence of high levels of HbF into adult life
V. Acquired hemoglobinopathies
   A. Methemoglobin due to toxic exposures
   B. Sulfhemoglobin due to toxic exposures
   C. Carboxyhemoglobin
   D. HbH in erythroleukemia
   E. Elevated HbF in states of erythroid stress and bone marrow dysplasia

destruction of erythroblasts and red cells. *Thalassemic hemoglobin variants* combine features of thalassemia (e.g., abnormal globin biosynthesis) and of structural hemoglobinopathies (e.g., an abnormal amino acid sequence). *Hereditary persistence of fetal hemoglobin* (HPFH) is characterized by synthesis of high levels of fetal hemoglobin in adult life. *Acquired hemoglobinopathies* include modifications of the hemoglobin molecule by toxins (e.g., acquired methemoglobinemia) and abnormal hemoglobin synthesis (e.g., high levels of HbF production in preleukemia and α thalassemia in myeloproliferative disorders).

EPIDEMIOLOGY   Hemoglobinopathies are especially common in areas in which malaria is endemic. This clustering of hemoglobinopathies is assumed to reflect a selective survival advantage for the abnormal red cells, which presumably provide a less hospitable environment during the obligate intraerythrocytic stages of the parasitic life cycle. Very young children with α thalassemia are *more* susceptible to infection with the nonlethal *Plasmodium vivax*. Thalassemia might then favor a natural protection against infection with the more lethal *P. falciparum*.

Thalassemias are the most common genetic disorders in the world, affecting nearly 200 million people worldwide. About 15% of American blacks are silent carriers for α thalassemia; α-thalassemia trait (minor) occurs in 3% of American blacks and in 1 to 15% of persons of Mediterranean origin. β Thalassemia has a 10 to 15% incidence in individuals from the Mediterranean and Southeast Asia and 0.8% in American blacks. The number of severe cases of thalassemia in the United States is about 1000. Sickle cell disease is the most common structural hemoglobinopathy occurring in heterozygous form in about 8% of American blacks and in homozygous form in 1 in 400. Between 2 and 3% of American blacks carry a hemoglobin C allele.

INHERITANCE AND ONTOGENY   Hemoglobinopathies are autosomal codominant traits—compound heterozygotes who inherit a different abnormal mutant allele from each parent exhibit composite features of each. For example, patients inheriting sickle β thalassemia exhibit features of β thalassemia and sickle cell anemia. The α chain is present in HbA, HbA$_2$, and HbF; α-chain mutations thus cause abnormalities in all three. The α-globin hemoglobinopathies are symptomatic in utero and after birth because normal function of the α-globin gene is required throughout gestation and adult life. In contrast, infants with β-globin hemoglobinopathies tend to be asymptomatic until 3 to 9 months of age, when HbA has largely replaced HbF.

DETECTION AND CHARACTERIZATION OF HEMOGLOBINOPATHIES—GENERAL METHODS

Of the many methods available for hemoglobin analysis, electrophoretic techniques are used for routine clinical purposes. Electrophoresis at pH 8.6 on cellulose acetate membranes is especially simple, inexpensive, and reliable for initial screening. Agar gel electrophoresis at pH 6.1 in citrate buffer is often used as a complementary method because each method detects different variants. Comparison of results obtained in each system usually allows unambiguous diagnosis, but some important variants are electrophoretically silent. These mutant hemoglobins can usually be characterized by more specialized techniques such as isoelectric focusing and/or high pressure liquid chromatography (HPLC).

Quantitation of the hemoglobin profile is often desirable. HbA_2 is frequently elevated in β-thalassemia trait and depressed in iron deficiency. HbF is elevated in HPFH, some β-thalassemia syndromes, and occasional periods of erythroid stress or marrow dysplasia. For characterization of sickle cell trait, sickle thalassemia syndromes, or HbSC disease, and for monitoring the progress of exchange transfusion therapy to lower the percentage of circulating HbS, quantitation of individual hemoglobins is also required. In most laboratories, quantitation is performed only if the test is specifically ordered.

Because some variants can comigrate with HbA or HbS (sickle hemoglobin), electrophoretic assessment should always be regarded as incomplete unless functional assays for hemoglobin sickling, solubility, or oxygen affinity are also performed, as dictated by the clinical presentation. The best sickling assays involve measurement of the degree to which the hemoglobin sample becomes insoluble, or gelated, as it is deoxygenated (i.e., sickle solubility test). Unstable hemoglobins are detected by their precipitation in isopropanol or after heating to 50°C. High-O_2 affinity and low-O_2 affinity variants are detected by quantitating the P_{50}, the partial pressure of oxygen at which the hemoglobin sample becomes 50% saturated with oxygen. Direct tests for the percent carboxyhemoglobin and methemoglobin, employing spectrophotometric techniques, can readily be obtained from most clinical laboratories on an urgent basis.

Complete characterization, including amino acid sequencing or gene cloning and sequencing, is available from several investigational laboratories around the world. The advent of the polymerase chain reaction (PCR), allele-specific oligonucleotide hybridization, and automated DNA sequencing has made it possible to identify globin gene mutations in a few days.

Laboratory evaluation remains an adjunct, rather than the primary diagnostic aid. Diagnosis is best established by recognition of a characteristic history, physical findings, peripheral blood smear morphology, and abnormalities of the complete blood cell count (e.g., profound microcytosis with minimal anemia in thalassemia trait).

STRUCTURALLY ABNORMAL HEMOGLOBINS

SICKLE CELL SYNDROMES The sickle cell syndromes are caused by a mutation in the β-globin gene that changes the sixth amino acid from glutamic acid to valine. HbS ($\alpha_2\beta_2^{6\ Glu\to Val}$) polymerizes reversibly when deoxygenated to form a gelatinous network of fibrous polymers that stiffen the erythrocyte membrane, increase viscosity, and cause dehydration due to potassium leakage and calcium influx (Fig. 91-3). These changes also produce the char-

FIGURE 91-3 Pathophysiology of sickle cell crisis.

acteristic sickle shape. Sickled cells lose the pliability needed to traverse small capillaries. They possess altered sticky membranes (especially reticulocytes) that are abnormally adherent to the endothelium of small venules. These abnormalities provoke unpredictable episodes of microvascular vasoocclusion and premature RBC destruction (hemolytic anemia). Hemolysis occurs because the abnormal erythrocytes are destroyed by the spleen. The rigid adherent cells also clog small capillaries and venules, causing tissue ischemia, acute pain, and gradual end-organ damage. This venoocclusive component usually dominates the clinical course. Prominent manifestations include episodes of ischemic pain (i.e., painful crises) and ischemic malfunction or frank infarction in the spleen, central nervous system, bones, liver, kidneys, and lungs (Fig. 91-3).

Several sickle syndromes occur as the result of inheritance of HbS from one parent and another hemoglobinopathy, such as β thalassemia or HbC ($\alpha_2\beta_2^{6\ Glu\to Lys}$), from the other parent. The prototype disease, sickle cell anemia, is the homozygous state for HbS (Table 91-2).

Clinical Manifestations of Sickle Cell Anemia Most patients with sickling syndromes suffer from hemolytic anemia, with hematocrits from 15 to 30%, and significant reticulocytosis. Anemia was once thought to exert protective effects against vasoocclusion by reducing blood viscosity. However, natural history and drug therapy trials suggest that an *increase* in the hematocrit and feedback inhibition of reticulocytosis might be beneficial, even at the expense of increased blood viscosity. The role of adhesive reticulocytes in vasoocclusion might account for these paradoxical effects.

Granulocytosis is common. The white count can fluctuate substan-

TABLE 91-2 *Clinical Features of Sickle Hemoglobinopathies*

Condition	Clinical Abnormalities	Hemoglobin Level g/L (g/dL)	MCV, fl	Hemoglobin Electrophoresis
Sickle cell trait	None; rare painless hematuria	Normal	Normal	Hb S/A:40/60
Sickle cell anemia	Vasoocclusive crises with infarction of spleen, brain, marrow, kidney, lung; aseptic necrosis of bone; gallstones; priapism; ankle ulcers	70–100 (7–10)	80–100	Hb S/A:100/0 Hb F:2–25%
S/β° thalassemia	Vasoocclusive crises; aseptic necrosis of bone	70–100 (7–10)	60–80	Hb S/A:100/0 Hb F:1–10%
S/β+ thalassemia	Rare crises and aseptic necrosis	100–140 (10–14)	70–80	Hb S/A:60/40
Hemoglobin SC	Rare crises and aseptic necrosis; painless hematuria	100–140 (10–14)	80–100	Hb S/A:50/0 Hb C:50%

tially and unpredictably during and between painful crises, infectious episodes, and other intercurrent illnesses.

Vasoocclusion causes protean manifestations. Intermittent episodes of vasoocclusion in connective and musculoskeletal structures produce painful ischemia manifested by acute pain and tenderness, fever, tachycardia, and anxiety. These recurrent episodes, called *painful crises*, are the most common clinical manifestation. Their frequency and severity vary greatly. Pain can develop almost anywhere in the body and may last from a few hours to 2 weeks. Repeated crises requiring hospitalization (>3 per year) correlate with reduced survival in adult life, suggesting that these episodes are associated with accumulation of chronic end-organ damage. Provocative factors include infection, fever, excessive exercise, anxiety, abrupt changes in temperature, hypoxia, or hypertonic dyes.

Repeated microinfarction can destroy tissues having microvascular beds that promote sickling. Thus, the spleen is frequently lost within the first 18 to 36 months of life, causing susceptibility to infection, particularly by pneumococci. Acute venous obstruction of the spleen (*splenic sequestration crisis*), a rare occurrence in early childhood, may require emergency transfusion and/or splenectomy to prevent trapping of the entire arterial output in the obstructed spleen. Occlusion of retinal vessels can produce hemorrhage, neovascularization, and eventual detachments. Renal papillary necrosis invariably produces isosthenuria. More widespread renal necrosis leads to renal failure in adults, a common late cause of death. Bone and joint ischemia can lead to aseptic necrosis, especially of the femoral or humeral heads; chronic arthropathy; and unusual susceptibility to osteomyelitis, which may be caused by organisms, such as *Salmonella*, rarely encountered in other settings. The *hand-foot syndrome* is caused by painful infarcts of the digits and dactylitis. Stroke is especially common in children, a small subset of whom tend to suffer repeated episodes; stroke is less common in adults and is often hemorrhagic. A particularly painful complication in males is priapism, due to infarction of the penile venous outflow tracts; permanent impotence is a frequent consequence. Chronic lower leg ulcers probably arise from ischemia and superinfection in the distal circulation.

Acute chest syndrome is a distinctive manifestation characterized by chest pain, tachypnea, fever, cough, and arterial oxygen desaturation. It can mimic pneumonia, pulmonary emboli, bone marrow infarction and embolism, myocardial ischemia, or in situ lung infarction. Acute chest syndrome is thought to reflect in situ sickling within the lung producing pain and temporary pulmonary dysfunction. It is frequently difficult or impossible to distinguish among other possibilities. Pulmonary infarction and pneumonia are the most frequent underlying or concomitant conditions in patients with this syndrome. Repeated episodes of acute chest pain correlate with reduced survival. Acutely, reduction in arterial oxygen saturation is especially ominous because it promotes sickling on a massive scale. Chronic acute or subacute pulmonary crises lead to pulmonary hypertension and cor pulmonale, an increasingly common cause of death as patients survive further into adult life.

Sickle cell syndromes are remarkable for their clinical heterogeneity. Some patients remain virtually asymptomatic into or even through adult life, while others suffer repeated crises requiring hospitalization from early childhood. Patients with sickle thalassemia and sickle-HbE tend to have similar, slightly milder, symptoms, perhaps because of the ameliorating effects of production of other hemoglobins within the RBC. Hemoglobin SC disease, one of the more common variants of sickle cell anemia, is frequently marked by lesser degrees of hemolytic anemia and a greater propensity for the development of retinopathy and aseptic necrosis of bones. In most respects, however, the clinical manifestations resemble sickle cell anemia. Some rare hemoglobin variants actually aggravate the sickling phenomenon.

Clinical Manifestations of Sickle Cell Trait Sickle cell trait is usually asymptomatic. Anemia and painful crises are exceedingly rare. An uncommon, but highly distinctive, symptom is painless hematuria often occurring in adolescent males, probably due to papillary necrosis. Isosthenuria is a more common manifestation of the same process. Sloughing of papillae with ureteral obstruction has been reported, as have isolated cases of massive sickling or sudden death due to exposure to high altitudes or extraordinary extremes of exercise and dehydration.

Diagnosis Sickle cell syndromes are readily suspected on the basis of characteristic hemolytic anemia, red cell morphology (Fig. 91-4), and intermittent episodes of ischemic pain. Diagnosis is confirmed by hemoglobin electrophoresis and the sickling tests already discussed. Thorough characterization of the exact hemoglobin profile of the patient is important, because sickle thalassemia and hemoglobin SC disease are correlated with alterations in prognosis or clinical features. Diagnosis is usually established in childhood, but occasional patients, often with compound heterozygous states, do not develop symptoms until the onset of puberty, pregnancy, or early adult life. Genotyping of family members and potential parental partners is critical for genetic counseling. Details of the childhood history establish prognosis and eligibility for aggressive or experimental therapies. Factors associated with increased morbidity and reduced survival are more than three crises requiring hospitalization per year, a chronic neutrophilia, a history of splenic sequestration or hand-foot syndrome, and second episodes of acute chest syndrome. Patients with a history of cerebrovascular accidents are at higher risk for repeated episodes and require especially close monitoring.

℞ TREATMENT

Patients with sickle cell syndromes require ongoing continuity of care. Familiarity with the pattern of symptoms provides the best safeguard against excessive use of the emergency room, hospitalization, and habituation to addictive narcotics. Additional preventive measures include regular slit-lamp examinations to monitor development of retinopathy; antibiotic prophylaxis appropriate for splenectomized patients during dental or other invasive procedures; and vigorous oral hydration during or in anticipation of periods of extreme exercise, exposure to heat or cold, emotional stress, or infection. Pneumococcal and *Haemophilus influenzae* vaccines are less effective in splenectomized individuals. Thus, patients with sickle cell anemia should be vaccinated early in life.

The management of acute painful crisis includes vigorous hydration, thorough evaluation for underlying causes (such as infection), and aggressive analgesia administered by a standing order and/or patient-controlled analgesia (PCA) pump. Morphine (0.1 to 0.15 mg/kg every 3 to 4 h) or meperidine (0.75 to 1.5 mg/kg every 2 to 4 h) should control severe pain. Meperidine should be used only for acute short-term pain control; as a chronic analgesic, it is unsuitable. Bone pain may respond as well to ketorolac (30 to 60 mg initial dose, then 15 to 30 mg every 6 to 8 h). Inhalation of nitrous oxide can provide short-term pain relief, but great care must be exercised to avoid hypoxia and respiratory depression. Nitrous oxide also elevates O_2 affinity, reducing O_2 delivery to tissues. Its use should be restricted to experts. Many crises can be managed at home with oral hydration and oral analgesia. Use of the emergency room should be reserved for especially severe symptoms or circumstances in which other processes, e.g., infection, are strongly suspected. Nasal oxygen should be employed as appropriate to protect arterial saturation. Most crises resolve in 1 to 7 days.

FIGURE 91-4 Sickle cell anemia. The elongated and crescent-shaped red blood cells seen on this smear represent circulating irreversibly sickled cells. Target cells and a nucleated red blood cell are also seen.

Use of blood transfusion should be reserved for extreme cases: no evidence exists for a beneficial effect in shortening the duration of the crisis.

No tests are definitive to diagnose acute painful crisis. Critical to good management is an approach that recognizes that most patients reporting crisis symptoms do indeed have crisis or another significant medical problem. Diligent diagnostic evaluation for underlying causes is imperative, even though these are found infrequently. In adults, the possibility of aseptic necrosis or sickle arthropathy must be considered, especially if pain and immobility become repeated or chronic at a single site. Nonsteroidal anti-inflammatory agents are often effective for sickle cell arthropathy.

Acute chest syndrome is a medical emergency that may require management in an intensive care unit. Hydration should be monitored carefully to avoid the development of pulmonary edema, and oxygen therapy should be especially vigorous for protection of arterial saturation. Diagnostic evaluation for pneumonia and pulmonary embolism should be especially thorough, since these may occur with atypical symptoms. Critical interventions are transfusion to maintain a hematocrit >30, and emergency exchange transfusion if arterial saturation drops to <90%. As patients with sickle cell syndrome increasingly survive into their fifth and sixth decades, end-stage renal failure and pulmonary hypertension are becoming increasingly prominent causes of end-stage morbidity. Anecdotal evidence suggests that a sickle cell cardiomyopathy and/or premature coronary artery disease may compromise cardiac function in later years. Sickle cell patients have received kidney transplants, but they often experience an increase in the frequency and severity of crises, possibly due to increased infection as a consequence of immunosuppression.

The most significant advance in the therapy of sickle cell anemia has been the introduction of hydroxyurea as a mainstay of therapy for patients with severe symptoms. Hydroxyurea (10 to 30 mg/kg per day) increases fetal hemoglobin and may also exert beneficial affects on red cell hydration, vascular wall adherence, and suppression of the granulocyte and reticulocyte counts; indeed, dosage is titrated to maintain a white count between 5000 and 8000 cells/μL. White cells and reticulocytes may play a major role in the pathogenesis of sickle cell crisis, and their suppression may be an important benefit of hydroxyurea therapy.

Hydroxyurea should be considered in patients experiencing repeated episodes of acute chest syndrome or with more than three crises per year requiring hospitalization. The utility of this agent for reducing the incidence of other complications (priapism, retinopathy) is under evaluation, as are the long-term side effects. The preponderance of evidence, however, is that hydroxyurea offers broad benefits to most patients whose disease is severe enough to impair their functional status. One long-term study suggests that hydroxyurea may improve survival. A number of experts are advocating more widespread use of this agent. HbF levels increase in most patients within a few months.

The antitumor drug, 5-azacytidine, was the first agent found to elevate HbF. It never achieved widespread use because of concerns about acute toxicity and carcinogenesis. However, low doses of the related agent, 5-deoxyazacytidine (decitabine) can elevate HbF with acceptable toxicity.

Bone marrow transplantation can provide definitive cures but is known to be effective and safe only in children. Prognostic features justifying bone marrow transplant are the presence of repeated crises early in life, a high neutrophil count, or the development of hand-foot syndrome. Children at risk for stroke can now be identified through the use of Doppler ultrasound techniques. Prophylactic exchange transfusion appears to substantially reduce the risk of stroke in this population. Children who do suffer a cerebrovascular accident should be maintained for at least 3 to 5 years on a program of vigorous exchange transfusion, since the risk of second strokes is extremely high in this population.

Gene therapy for sickle cell anemia is being intensively pursued, but no safe measures are currently available. Agents blocking RBC dehydration or vascular adhesion, such as clotrimazole or magnesium, may have value as an adjunct to hydroxyurea therapy, pending the completion of ongoing trials. Combinations of clotrimazole and magnesium are being evaluated in clinical trials.

UNSTABLE HEMOGLOBINS   Amino acid substitutions that reduce solubility or increase susceptibility to oxidation produce unstable hemoglobins that precipitate, forming inclusion bodies injurious to the red cell membrane. Representative mutations are those that interfere with contact points between the α and β subunits [e.g., Hb Philly ($\beta^{35Tyr \to Phe}$)], alter the helical segments [e.g., Hb Genova ($\beta^{28Leu \to Pro}$)], or disrupt interactions of the hydrophobic pockets of the globin subunits with heme [e.g., Hb Koln ($\beta^{98Val \to Met}$)] (Table 91-3). The inclusions, called *Heinz bodies*, are clinically detectable by staining with supravital dyes such as crystal violet (Heinz body test). Removal of these inclusions by the spleen generates pitted, rigid cells that have shortened life spans, producing hemolytic anemia of variable severity, sometimes requiring chronic transfusion support. Splenectomy may be needed to correct the anemia. Leg ulcers and premature gallbladder disease due to bilirubin turnover are frequent stigmata.

Unstable hemoglobins occur sporadically, often by spontaneous new mutations. Heterozygotes are often symptomatic because a significant Heinz body burden can develop even when the unstable variant accounts for a portion of the total hemoglobin. Symptomatic unstable hemoglobins tend to be β-globin variants, because sporadic mutations affecting only one of the four α globins would generate only 20 to 30% abnormal hemoglobin.

HEMOGLOBINS WITH ALTERED OXYGEN AFFINITY   *High-affinity hemoglobins* [e.g., Hb Yakima ($\beta^{99 Asp \to His}$)] bind oxygen more readily but deliver less O_2 to tissues at normal capillary P_{O_2} levels (Fig. 91-2). Mild tissue hypoxia ensues, stimulating RBC production and erythrocytosis (Table 91-3). In extreme cases, the hematocrits can rise to 60 to 65%, increasing blood viscosity and producing typical symptoms (headache, somnolence, or dizziness). Phlebotomy may be required. Typical mutations alter interactions within the heme pocket or disrupt the Bohr effect or salt-bond site. Mutations that impair the interaction of HbA with 2,3-BPG can increase O_2 affinity because 2,3-BPG binding lowers O_2 affinity.

Low-affinity hemoglobins [e.g., Hb Kansas ($\beta^{102Asn \to Lys}$)] bind sufficient oxygen in the lungs, despite their lower oxygen affinity, to achieve nearly full saturation. At capillary oxygen tensions, they lose sufficient amounts of oxygen to maintain homeostasis at a low hematocrit (Fig. 91-2) (*pseudoanemia*). Capillary hemoglobin desaturation can also be sufficient to produce clinically apparent cyanosis. Despite these findings, patients usually require no specific treatment.

METHEMOGLOBINEMIAS   Methemoglobin is generated by oxidation of the heme iron moieties to the ferric state, causing a characteristic bluish-brown muddy color resembling cyanosis. Methemoglobin has such

TABLE 91-3 *Representative Abnormal Hemoglobins with Altered Synthesis or Function*

Designation	Mutation	Population	Main Clinical Effects[a]
Sickle or S	$\beta^{6Glu \to Val}$	African	Anemia, ischemic infarcts
C	$\beta^{6Glu \to Lys}$	African	Mild anemia; interacts with HbS
E	$\beta^{26Glu \to Lys}$	Southeast Asian	Microcytic anemia, splenomegaly, thalassemic phenotype
Köln	$\beta^{98Val \to Met}$	Sporadic	Hemolytic anemia, Heinz bodies when splenectomized
Yakima	$\beta^{99Asp \to His}$	Sporadic	Polycythemia
Kansas	$\beta^{102Asn \to Lys}$	Sporadic	Mild anemia
M. Iwata	$\alpha^{87His \to Tyr}$	Sporadic	Methemoglobinemia

[a] See text for details.

high oxygen affinity that virtually no oxygen is delivered to tissues. Levels >50 to 60% are often fatal.

Congenital methemoglobinemia arises from globin mutations that stabilize iron in the ferric state [e.g., HbM Iwata ($\alpha^{87\ His \rightarrow Tyr}$), Table 91-3] or from mutations that impair the enzymes that reduce methemoglobin to hemoglobin (e.g., methemoglobin reductase, NADP diaphorase). Acquired methemoglobinemia is caused by toxins that oxidize heme iron, notably nitrate and nitrite-containing compounds.

DIAGNOSIS AND MANAGEMENT OF PATIENTS WITH UNSTABLE HEMOGLOBINS, HIGH-AFFINITY HEMOGLOBINS, AND METHEMOGLOBINEMIA
Unstable hemoglobin variants should be suspected in patients with nonimmune hemolytic anemia, jaundice, splenomegaly, or premature biliary tract disease. Severe hemolysis usually presents during infancy as neonatal jaundice or anemia. Milder cases may present in adult life with anemia or only as unexplained reticulocytosis, hepatosplenomegaly, premature biliary tract disease, or leg ulcers. Because spontaneous mutation is common, family history of anemia may be absent. The peripheral blood smear often shows anisocytosis, abundant cells with punctate inclusions, and irregular shapes (i.e., poikilocytosis).

The two best tests for diagnosing unstable hemoglobins are the Heinz body preparation and the isopropanol or heat stability test. Many unstable Hb variants are electrophoretically silent. A normal electrophoresis does not rule out the diagnosis.

Severely affected patients may require transfusion support for the first 3 years of life, because splenectomy before age 3 is associated with a significantly higher immune deficit. Splenectomy is usually effective thereafter, but occasional patients may require lifelong transfusion support. Even after splenectomy, patients can develop cholelithiasis and leg ulcers. Splenectomy can also be considered in patients exhibiting severe secondary complications of chronic hemolysis, even if anemia is absent. Precipitation of unstable hemoglobins is aggravated by oxidative stress, e.g., infection, antimalarial drugs.

High-O$_2$ affinity hemoglobin variants should be suspected in patients with erythrocytosis. The best test for confirmation is measurement of the P$_{50}$. A high-O$_2$ affinity Hb causes a significant left shift (i.e., lower numeric value of the P$_{50}$); confounding conditions, e.g., tobacco smoking or carbon monoxide exposure, can also lower the P$_{50}$.

High-affinity hemoglobins are often asymptomatic; rubor or plethora may be telltale signs. When the hematocrit reaches to 55 to 60%, symptoms of high blood viscosity and sluggish flow (headache, lethargy, dizziness, etc.) may be present. These persons may benefit from judicious phlebotomy. Erythrocytosis represents an appropriate attempt to compensate for the impaired oxygen delivery by the abnormal variant. Overzealous phlebotomy may stimulate increased erythropoiesis or aggravate symptoms by thwarting this compensatory mechanism. The guiding principle of phlebotomy should be to improve oxygen delivery by reducing blood viscosity and increasing blood flow rather than restoration of a normal hematocrit. Modest iron deficiency may aid in control.

Low-affinity hemoglobins should be considered in patients with cyanosis or a low hematocrit with no other reason apparent after thorough evaluation. The P$_{50}$ test confirms the diagnosis. Counseling and reassurance are the interventions of choice.

Methemoglobin should be suspected in patients with hypoxic symptoms who appear cyanotic but have a Pa$_{O_2}$ sufficiently high that hemoglobin should be fully saturated with oxygen. A history of nitrite or other oxidant ingestions may not always be available; some exposures may be unapparent to the patient, and others may result from suicide attempts. The characteristic muddy appearance of freshly drawn blood can be a critical clue. The diagnostic test of choice is measurement of the methemoglobin content, which is usually available on an emergency basis.

Methemoglobinemia often causes symptoms of cerebral ischemia at levels >15%; levels >60% are usually lethal. Intravenous injection of 1 mg/kg of methylene blue is effective emergency therapy. Milder cases and follow-up of severe cases can be treated orally with methylene blue (60 mg three to four times each day) or ascorbic acid (300 to 600 mg/d).

THALASSEMIA SYNDROMES

The thalassemia syndromes are inherited disorders of α- or β-globin biosynthesis. The reduced supply of globin diminishes production of hemoglobin tetramers, causing hypochromia and microcytosis. Unbalanced accumulation of α and β subunits occurs because the synthesis of the unaffected globins proceeds at a normal rate. Unbalanced chain accumulation dominates the clinical phenotype. Clinical severity varies widely, depending on the degree to which the synthesis of the affected globin is impaired, altered synthesis of other globin chains, and coinheritance of other abnormal globin alleles.

CLINICAL MANIFESTATIONS OF β-THALASSEMIA SYNDROMES
Mutations causing thalassemia can affect any step in the pathway of globin gene expression: transcription, processing of the mRNA precursor, translation, and posttranslational metabolism of the β-globin polypeptide chain. The most common forms arise from mutations that derange splicing of the mRNA precursor or prematurely terminate translation of the mRNA.

Hypochromia and microcytosis characterize all forms of β thalassemia because of the reduced amounts of hemoglobin tetramers (Fig. 91-5). In heterozygotes (β-thalassemia trait), this is the only abnormality seen. Anemia is minimal. In more severe homozygous states, unbalanced α- and β-globin accumulation causes accumulation of highly insoluble unpaired α chains. They form toxic inclusion bodies that kill developing erythroblasts in the marrow. Few of the proerythroblasts beginning erythroid maturation survive. The few RBCs surviving bear a burden of inclusion bodies that are detected in the spleen, shortening the RBC life span and producing severe hemolytic anemia. The resulting profound anemia stimulates erythropoietin release and compensatory erythroid hyperplasia, but the marrow response is sabotaged by ineffective erythropoiesis. Anemia persists. Erythroid hyperplasia can become exuberant and produce masses of extramedullary erythropoietic tissue in the liver and spleen.

Massive bone marrow expansion deranges growth and development. Children develop characteristic chipmunk facies due to maxillary marrow hyperplasia and frontal bossing, thinning and pathologic fracture of long bones and vertebrae due to cortical invasion by erythroid elements, and profound growth retardation. Hemolytic anemia causes hepatosplenomegaly, leg ulcers, gallstones, and high-output congestive heart failure. The conscription of caloric resources to support erythropoiesis leads to inanition, susceptibility to infection, endocrine dysfunction, and in the most severe cases, death during the first decade of life. Chronic transfusions with RBCs improves oxygen delivery, suppresses the excessive ineffective erythropoiesis, and prolongs life, but the inevitable side effects, notably iron overload, usually prove fatal by age 30.

Severity is highly variable. Known modulating factors are those that ameliorate the burden of unpaired α-globin inclusions. Alleles associated with milder synthetic defects and coinheritance of α-thalassemia trait reduce clinical severity by reducing accumulation of excess α globin. HbF persists to various degrees in β thalassemias. γ-Globin gene chains can substitute for β chains, simultaneously generating more hemoglobin and reducing the burden of α-globin inclu-

FIGURE 91-5 β-Thalassemia intermedia. Microcytic and hypochromic red blood cells are seen that resemble the red blood cells of severe iron deficiency anemia. Many elliptical and teardrop-shaped red blood cells are noted.

sions. The terms *β-thalassemia major* and *β-thalassemia intermedia* are used to reflect the clinical heterogeneity. Patients with *β*-thalassemia major require intensive transfusion support to survive. Patients with *β*-thalassemia intermedia have a somewhat milder phenotype and can survive without transfusion. The terms *β-thalassemia minor* and *β-thalassemia trait* describe asymptomatic heterozygotes for *β*-thalassemia.

α-THALASSEMIA SYNDROMES The four classic α-thalassemias, most common in Asians, are α-thalassemia-2 trait, in which one of the four α globin loci is deleted; α-thalassemia-1 trait, with two deleted loci; HbH disease, with three loci deleted; and hydrops fetalis with Hb Bart's, with all four loci deleted (Table 91-4). Nondeletion forms of α-thalassemia also exist.

α-Thalassemia-2 trait is an asymptomatic, silent carrier state. *α-Thalassemia-1 trait* resembles *β*-thalassemia minor. Offspring doubly heterozygous for α-thalassemia-2 and α-thalassemia-1 exhibit a more severe phenotype called HbH disease. Heterozygosity for a deletion that removes both genes from the same chromosome (*cis* deletion) is common in Asians and Mediterranean individuals, as is homozygosity for α-thalassemia-2 (*trans* deletion). Both produce asymptomatic hypochromia and microcytosis.

In *HbH disease,* HbA production is only 25 to 30% of normal. Fetuses accumulate some unpaired *β* chains. In adults, unpaired *β* chains accumulate and are soluble enough to form β_4 tetramers called HbH. HbH forms few inclusions in erythroblasts but does not precipitate in circulating red cells. Patients with HbH disease have thalassemia intermedia characterized by moderately severe hemolytic anemia but milder ineffective erythropoiesis. Survival into mid-adult life without transfusions is common.

The homozygous state for the α-thalassemia-1 *cis* deletion (hydrops fetalis) causes total absence of α-globin synthesis. No physiologically useful hemoglobin is produced beyond the embryonic stage. Excess γ globin forms tetramers called *Hb Barts* (γ_4), which has an extraordinarily high oxygen affinity. It delivers almost no O_2 to fetal tissues, causing tissue asphyxia, edema (hydrops fetalis), congestive heart failure, and death in utero. α-Thalassemia-2 trait is common (15 to 20%) among people of African descent. The *cis* α-thalassemia-1 deletion is almost never seen, however. Thus, α-thalassemia-2 and the *trans* form of α-thalassemia-1 are very common, but HbH disease and hydrops fetalis are almost never encountered.

It has been known for some time that some patients with myelodysplasia or erythroleukemia produce red cell clones containing HbH. It now appears that this phenomenon is due to mutations in the ATRX pathway that affect the LCR of the α-globin gene cluster.

DIAGNOSIS AND MANAGEMENT OF THALASSEMIAS The diagnosis of *β*-thalassemia major is readily made during childhood on the basis of severe anemia accompanied by the characteristic signs of massive ineffective erythropoiesis: hepatosplenomegaly, profound microcytosis, a characteristic blood smear (Fig. 91-5), and elevated levels of HbF, HbA_2, or both. Many patients require chronic hypertransfusion therapy designed to maintain a hematocrit of at least 27 to 30% so that erythropoiesis is suppressed. Splenectomy is required if the annual transfusion requirement (volume of RBCs per kilogram of body weight per year) increases by >50%. Folic acid supplements may be useful. Vaccination with Pneumovax in anticipation of eventual splenectomy is advised, as is close monitoring for infection, leg ulcers, and biliary tract disease. Early endocrine evaluation is required for glucose intolerance, thyroid dysfunction, and delayed onset of puberty or secondary sexual characteristics. Many patients develop endocrine deficiencies as a result of iron overload.

Patients with *β*-thalassemia intermedia exhibit similar stigmata but

TABLE 91-4 *The α Thalassemias*

Condition	Hemoglobin A, %	Hemoglobin H (β^4), %	Hemoglobin level, g/L (g/dL)	MCV, fL
Normal	97	0	150 (15)	90
Silent thalassemia: $-\alpha/\alpha\alpha$	98–100	0	150 (15)	90
Thalassemia trait: $-\alpha/-\alpha$ homozygous α-thal-2[a] or $--/\alpha\alpha$ heterozygous α-thal-1[a]	85–95	Rare red blood cell inclusions	120–130 (12–13)	70–80
Hemoglobin H disease: $--/-\alpha$ heterozygous α-thal-1/α-thal-2	70–95	5–30	60–100 (6–10)	60–70
Hydrops fetalis: $--/--$ homozygous α-thal-1	0	5–10[b]	Fatal in utero or at birth	

[a] When both α alleles on one chromosome are deleted, the locus is called α-thal-1; when only a single α allele on one chromosome is deleted, the locus is called α-thal-2.
[b] 90–95% of the hemoglobin is hemoglobin Barts (tetramers of γ chains).

can survive without chronic hypertransfusion. Management is particularly challenging because a number of factors can aggravate the anemia, including infection, onset of puberty, and development of splenomegaly and hypersplenism. Some patients may eventually benefit from splenectomy. The expanded erythron can cause absorption of excessive dietary iron and hemosiderosis, even without transfusion.

β-Thalassemia minor (i.e., thalassemia trait) usually presents as profound microcytosis and hypochromia with target cells, but only minimal or mild anemia. The mean corpuscular volume is rarely >75 fL; the hematocrit is rarely <30 to 33%. Hemoglobin electrophoresis classically reveals an elevated HbA_2 (3.5 to 7.5%), but some forms are associated with normal HbA_2 and/or elevated HbF. Genetic counseling and patient education are essential. Patients with *β*-thalassemia trait should be warned that their blood picture resembles iron deficiency and can be misdiagnosed. They should eschew routine use of iron but know that iron deficiency requiring supplementation can develop, as in other persons, during pregnancy or from chronic bleeding.

Persons with α-thalassemia trait may exhibit mild hypochromia and microcytosis usually without anemia. HbA_2 and HbF levels are normal. Affected individuals usually require only genetic counseling. HbH disease resembles *β*-thalassemia intermedia, with the added complication that the HbH molecule behaves like a moderately unstable hemoglobin. Patients with HbH disease should undergo splenectomy if excessive anemia or a transfusion requirement develops. Oxidative drugs should be avoided. Iron overload leading to death can occur in more severely affected patients.

PREVENTION Antenatal diagnosis of thalassemia syndromes is now widely available. DNA diagnosis is based on PCR amplification of fetal DNA, obtained by amniocentesis or chorionic villus biopsy followed by hybridization to allele-specific oligonucleotides probes. The probes can be designed to detect simultaneously the subset of mutations that account for 95 to 99% of the α- or *β*-thalassemias that occur in a particular ethnic group.

THALASSEMIC STRUCTURAL VARIANTS

Thalassemic structural variants are characterized by both defective synthesis and abnormal structure.

HEMOGLOBIN LEPORE Hb Lepore [$\alpha_2(\delta\beta)_2$] arises by an unequal crossover and recombination event that fuses the proximal end of the *δ*-gene with the distal end of the closely linked *β*-gene. The resulting chromosome contains only the fused *δβ* gene. The Lepore (*δβ*) globin is synthesized poorly because the fused gene is under the control of the weak *δ*-globin promoter. Hb Lepore alleles have a phenotype like *β*-thalassemia, except for the added presence of 2 to 20% Hb Lepore. Compound heterozygotes for Hb Lepore and a classic *β*-thalassemia allele may also have severe thalassemia.

HEMOGLOBIN E HbE (i.e., $\alpha_2\beta_2^{26Glu\rightarrow Lys}$) is extremely common in Cambodia, Thailand, and Vietnam. The gene has become far more prevalent in the United States as a result of immigration of Asian persons, especially in California, where HbE is the most common variant detected. HbE is mildly unstable but not enough to affect RBC life span significantly. The high frequency of the HbE gene may be a result of the thalassemia phenotype associated with its inheritance. Heterozygotes resemble individuals with mild β-thalassemia trait. Homozygotes have somewhat more marked abnormalities but are asymptomatic. Compound heterozygotes for HbE and a β-thalassemia gene can have β-thalassemia intermedia or β-thalassemia major, depending on the severity of the coinherited thalassemic gene.

The β^E allele contains only a single base change, in codon 26, that causes the amino acid substitution. However, this mutation activates a cryptic RNA splice site generating a structurally abnormal globin mRNA that cannot be translated from about 50% of the initial pre-mRNA molecules. The remaining 40 to 50% that are normally spliced generate functional mRNA that is translated into β^E-globin because the mature mRNA carries the base change that alters codon 26.

Genetic counseling of the persons at risk for HbE should be concerned with the interaction of HbE with β thalassemia rather than HbE homozygosity, a condition associated with asymptomatic microcytosis, hypochromia, and hemoglobin levels rarely <10 g/dL.

HEREDITARY PERSISTENCE OF FETAL HEMOGLOBIN   HPFH is characterized by continued synthesis of high levels of HbF in adult life. No deleterious effects are apparent, even when all of the hemoglobin produced is HbF. These rare patients demonstrate convincingly that prevention or reversal of the fetal to adult hemoglobin switch would provide efficacious therapy for sickle cell anemia and β thalassemia.

ACQUIRED HEMOGLOBINOPATHIES   The two most important acquired hemoglobinopathies are carbon monoxide poisoning and methemoglobinemia, which is covered elsewhere in this chapter. Carbon monoxide has a higher affinity for hemoglobin than does oxygen; it can replace oxygen and diminish O_2 delivery. Chronic elevation of carboxyhemoglobin levels to 10 or 15%, as occurs in smokers, can lead to secondary polycythemia. Carboxyhemoglobin is cherry red in color and masks the development of cyanosis usually associated with poor O_2 delivery to tissues.

Abnormalities of hemoglobin biosynthesis have also been described in blood dyscrasias. In some patients with myelodysplasia, erythroleukemia, or myeloproliferative disorders, a mild form of HbH disease may also be seen. The abnormalities are not severe enough to alter the course of the underlying disease.

MANAGEMENT OF TRANSFUSIONAL HEMOSIDEROSIS

Chronic blood transfusion can lead to bloodborne infection, alloimmunization, febrile reactions, and lethal iron overload. A unit of packed RBCs contains 250 to 300 mg iron (1 mg/mL). The iron assimilated by single transfusion of two units of packed RBCs is thus equal to a 1- to 2-year intake of iron. Iron accumulates in chronically transfused patients because no mechanisms exist for increasing iron excretion: an expanded erythron causes especially rapid development of iron overload because accelerated erythropoiesis promotes excessive absorption of dietary iron. Vitamin C should not be supplemented because it generates free radicals in iron excess states.

Patients who receive >100 units of packed RBCs usually develop hemosiderosis. The ferritin level rises, followed by early endocrine dysfunction (glucose intolerance and delayed puberty), cirrhosis, and cardiomyopathy. Liver biopsy shows both parenchymal and reticuloendothelial iron. The superconducting quantum-interference device (SQUID) is accurate at measuring hepatic iron but not widely available. Cardiac toxicity is often insidious. Early development of pericarditis is followed by dysrhythmia and pump failure. The onset of heart failure is ominous, often presaging death within a year (Chap. 336).

The decision to start long-term transfusion support should also prompt one to institute therapy with iron-chelating agents. The only approved and available iron chelator, desferoxamine (Desferal), is expensive and poorly absorbed from the gastrointestinal tract. Its iron-binding kinetics require chronic slow infusion via a metering pump.

The constant presence of the drug improves the efficiency of chelation and protects tissues from occasional releases of the most toxic fraction of iron—low-molecular-weight iron—which may not be sequestered by protective proteins. Oral iron-chelating agents such as deferiprone showed initial promise, but long-term trials have raised serious doubts about their efficacy and safety. Newer oral agents are in clinical trials.

Desferoxamine is relatively nontoxic. Occasional cataracts, deafness, and local skin reactions, including urticaria, occur. Skin reactions can usually be managed with antihistamines. Negative iron balance can be achieved, even in the face of a high transfusion requirement, but this alone does not prevent long-term morbidity and mortality in chronically transfused patients. Irreversible end-organ deterioration develops at relatively modest levels of iron overload, even if symptoms do not appear for many years thereafter. To enjoy a significant survival advantage, chelation must begin before 5 to 8 years of age in β thalassemia major.

EXPERIMENTAL THERAPIES

BONE MARROW TRANSPLANTATION, GENE THERAPY, AND MANIPULATION OF HbF
Bone marrow transplantation provides stem cells able to express normal hemoglobin; it has been used in a large number of patients with β thalassemia and a smaller number of patients with sickle cell anemia. Early in the course of disease, before end-organ damage occurs, transplantation is curative in 80 to 90% of patients. In highly experienced centers, the treatment-related mortality is <10%. Since survival into adult life is possible with conventional therapy, the decision to transplant is best made in consultation with specialized centers.

Gene therapy of thalassemia and sickle cell disease has proved to be an exceptionally elusive goal. Uptake of gene vectors into the nondividing hematopoietic stem cells has been disappointingly inefficient. Lentiviral-type vectors that can transduce nondividing cells may solve this problem.

Reestablishing high levels of fetal hemoglobin synthesis should ameliorate the symptoms of β thalassemia. Cytotoxic agents such as hydroxyurea and cytarabine promote high levels of HbF synthesis, probably by stimulating proliferation of the primitive HbF-producing progenitor cell population (i.e., F cell progenitors). Unfortunately, no regimen has yet been identified that ameliorates the clinical manifestations of β thalassemia. Butyrates stimulate HbF production, but only transiently. Pulsed or intermittent administration has recently been found to sustain HbF induction in the majority of patients with sickle cell disease. It is unclear whether butyrates will have similar activity in patients with β thalassemia.

APLASTIC AND HYPOPLASTIC CRISIS IN PATIENTS WITH HEMOGLOBINOPATHIES

Patients with hemolytic anemias sometimes exhibit an alarming decline in hematocrit during and immediately after acute illnesses. Bone marrow suppression occurs in almost everyone during acute inflammatory illnesses. In patients with short RBC life spans, suppression can affect RBC counts more dramatically. These hypoplastic crises are usually transient and self-correcting before intervention is required.

Aplastic crisis refers to a profound cessation of erythroid activity in patients with chronic hemolytic anemias. It is associated with a rapidly falling hematocrit. Episodes are usually self-limited. Aplastic crises are caused by infection with a particular strain of parvovirus, B19A. Children infected with this virus usually develop permanent immunity. Aplastic crises do not often recur and are rarely seen in adults. Management requires close monitoring of the hematocrit and reticulocyte count. If anemia becomes symptomatic, transfusion support is indicated. Most crises resolve spontaneously within 1 to 2 weeks.

FURTHER READING

ATAGA KI, ORRINGA EP: Hypercoagulability in sickle cell disease: a curious paradox. Am J. Med 115:721, 2003

BRUGNARA C et al: Therapy with oral clotrimazole induces inhibition of the Gardos channel and reduction of erythrocyte dehydration in patients with sickle cell disease. J Clin Invest 97:1227, 1996

CLASTA S, VICHINSKY EP: Managing sickle cell disease. BMJ 327:1151, 2003

DeSIMONE J et al: Maintenance of elevated fetal hemoglobin levels by decitabine during dose interval treatment of sickle cell anemia. Blood 99:3905, 2002

OLIVIERI NF: The beta-thalassemias. N Engl J Med 341:99, 1999

VICHINSKY E: New therapies in sickle cell disease. Lancet 360:629, 2002

WARE RE et al: Predictors of fetal hemoglobin response in children with sickle cell anemia receiving hydroxyurea therapy. Blood 99:10, 2002

92 | MEGALOBLASTIC ANEMIAS
Bernard M. Babior, H. Franklin Bunn

The megaloblastic anemias are disorders caused by impaired DNA synthesis. Cells primarily affected are those having relatively rapid turnover, especially hematopoietic precursors and gastrointestinal epithelial cells. Cell division is sluggish, but cytoplasmic development progresses normally, so megaloblastic cells tend to be large, with an increased ratio of RNA to DNA. Megaloblastic erythroid progenitors tend to be destroyed in the marrow. Thus, marrow cellularity is often increased but production of red blood cells (RBC) is decreased, an abnormality termed *ineffective erythropoiesis* (Chap. 52).

Most megaloblastic anemias are due to a deficiency of cobalamin (vitamin B$_{12}$) and/or folic acid. The various clinical entities associated with megaloblastic anemia are listed in Table 92-1.

PHYSIOLOGIC AND BIOCHEMICAL CONSIDERATIONS

FOLIC ACID Folic acid is the common name for pteroylmonoglutamic acid. It is synthesized by many different plants and bacteria. Fruits and vegetables constitute the primary dietary source of the vitamin. Some forms of dietary folic acid are labile and may be destroyed by cooking. The minimum daily requirement is normally about 50 μg, but this may be increased severalfold during periods of enhanced metabolic demand such as pregnancy.

The assimilation of adequate amounts of folic acid depends on the nature of the diet and its means of preparation. Folates in various foodstuffs are largely conjugated to a chain of glutamic acid residues. This highly polar side chain impairs the intestinal absorption of the vitamin. However, conjugases (γ-glutamyl carboxypeptidases) in the lumen of the gut convert polyglutamates to mono- and diglutamates, which are readily absorbed in the proximal jejunum.

Plasma folate is primarily in the form of N^5-methyltetrahydrofolate, a monoglutamate, which is transported into cells by a carrier that is specific for the tetrahydro forms of the vitamin. Once in the cell, the N^5-methyl group is removed in a cobalamin-requiring reaction (see below), and the folate is then reconverted to the polyglutamate form. Conjugation to polyglutamate may be useful for retention of folate within the cell.

A folate-binding protein occurs in plasma, milk, and other body fluids. The function of this folate binder and its membrane-bound precursor is unknown. Neither the binder nor its precursor is related to the tetrahydrofolate carrier.

Normal individuals have about 5 to 20 mg folic acid in various body stores, half in the liver. In light of the minimum daily requirement, it is not surprising that a deficiency will occur within months if dietary intake or intestinal absorption is curtailed.

The prime function of folate compounds is to transfer 1-carbon moieties such as methyl and formyl groups to various organic compounds (Fig. 92-1). The sources of these 1-carbon moieties is usually serine, which reacts with tetrahydrofolate to produce glycine and $N^{5,10}$-methylenetetrahydrofolate. An alternative source is formiminoglutamic acid, an intermediate in histidine catabolism, which gives up its formimino group to tetrahydrofolate to yield N^5-formiminotetrahydrofolate and glutamic acid. These derivatives provide entry into an interconvertible donor pool consisting of tetrahydrofolate derivatives carrying various 1-carbon moieties. The constituents of this pool can donate their 1-carbon moieties to appropriate acceptor compounds to form metabolic intermediates, which are ultimately converted to build-

TABLE 92-1 *Classification of the Megaloblastic Anemias*

COBALAMIN DEFICIENCY

I. Inadequate intake: vegans (rare)
II. Malabsorption
  A. Defective release of cobalamin from food
    1. Gastric achlorhydria
    2. Partial gastrectomy
    3. Drugs that block acid secretion
  B. Inadequate production of intrinsic factor (IF)
    1. Pernicious anemia
    2. Total gastrectomy
    3. Congenital absence or functional abnormality of IF (rare)
  C. Disorders of terminal ileum
    1. Tropical sprue
    2. Nontropical sprue
    3. Regional enteritis
    4. Intestinal resection
    5. Neoplasms and granulomatous disorders (rare)
    6. Selective cobalamin malabsorption (Imerslund's syndrome) (rare)
  D. Competition for cobalamin
    1. Fish tapeworm (*Diphyllobothrium latum*)
    2. Bacteria: "blind loop" syndrome
  E. Drugs: *p*-aminosalicylic acid, colchicine, neomycin
III. Other
  A. Nitrous oxide
  B. Transcobalamin II deficiency (rare)
  C. Congenital enzyme defects (rare)

FOLIC ACID DEFICIENCY

I. Inadequate intake: unbalanced diet (common in alcoholics, teenagers, some infants)
II. Increased requirements
  A. Pregnancy
  B. Infancy
  C. Malignancy
  D. Increased hematopoiesis (chronic hemolytic anemias)
  E. Chronic exfoliative skin disorders
  F. Hemodialysis
III. Malabsorption
  A. Tropical sprue
  B. Nontropical sprue
  C. Drugs: Phenytoin, barbiturates, (?) ethanol
IV. Impaired metabolism
  A. Inhibitors of dihydrofolate reductase: methotrexate, pyrimethamine, triamterene, pentamidine, trimethoprim
  B. Alcohol
  C. Rare enzyme deficiencies: dihydrofolate reductase, others

OTHER CAUSES

I. Drugs that impair DNA metabolism
  A. Purine antagonists: 6-mercaptopurine, azathioprine, etc.
  B. Pyrimidine antagonists: 5-fluorouracil, cytosine arabinoside, etc.
  C. Others: procarbazine, hydroxyurea, acyclovir, zidovudine
II. Metabolic disorders (rare)
  A. Hereditary orotic aciduria
  B. Lesch-Nyhan syndrome
  C. Others
III. Megaloblastic anemia of unknown etiology
  A. Refractory megaloblastic anemia
  B. Di Guglielmo's syndrome[a]
  C. Congenital dyserythropoietic anemia

[a] A form of acute myeloid leukemia with atypical, dysplastic changes in erythroid series.

FIGURE 92-1 Folate metabolism. Folate is essential for the de novo synthesis of purines, deoxythymidylate monophosphate (dTMP), and methionine, serving as an intermediate carrier of 1-carbon fragments used in the biosynthesis of these compounds. Its active form is tetrahydrofolate (THF). THF acquires the 1-carbon fragment principally from serine, which is converted to glycine in the course of the reaction. For purine synthesis, the 1-carbon fragment is first oxidized to the level of formic acid, then transferred to substrate. For methionine synthesis, a cobalamin-requiring reaction, the 1-carbon fragment is first reduced to the level of a methyl group, then transferred to homocysteine. In these reactions the cofactor is released as THF, which can immediately participate in another 1-carbon transfer cycle. During the production of dTMP from dUMP, however, the 1-carbon fragment is reduced from formaldehyde to a methyl group in the course of the transfer reaction. The hydrogen atoms used for this reduction come from the cofactor, which is therefore released, not as THF, but as dihydrofolate (DHF). To participate further in the 1-carbon transfer cycle, the DHF has to be re-reduced to THF, a reaction catalyzed by dihydrofolate reductase.

ing blocks used in the synthesis of macromolecules. The most important building blocks are (1) purines, in which the C-2 and C-8 atoms are introduced in folate-dependent reactions; (2) deoxythymidylate monophosphate (dTMP), synthesized from $N^{5,10}$-methylenetetrahydrofolate and deoxyuridylate monophosphate (dUMP); and (3) methionine, formed by the transfer of a methyl group from N^5-methyltetrahydrofolate to homocysteine (two of these three reactions are shown in Fig. 92-1).

In all but one of the 1-carbon transfer reactions, tetrahydrofolate is produced. It can immediately accept a 1-carbon moiety and reenter the donor pool. The single exception is the thymidylate synthase reaction (dUMP → dTMP), in which dihydrofolate is the product (Fig. 92-1). This must be reduced to tetrahydrofolate by the enzyme dihydrofolate reductase before it can reenter the donor pool. A number of drugs are able to inhibit dihydrofolate reductase (Table 92-1), thereby diverting folate from the donor pool and producing what amounts to a state of folate deficiency in the face of normal tissue folate concentrations.

COBALAMIN This vitamin is a complex organometallic compound in which a cobalt atom is situated within a corrin ring, a structure similar to the porphyrin from which heme is formed. Unlike heme, however, cobalamin cannot be synthesized in the human body and must be supplied in the diet. The only dietary source of cobalamin is animal products: meat and dairy foods. The minimum daily requirement for cobalamin is about 2.5 μg.

During gastric digestion, cobalamin in food is released and forms a stable complex with gastric R binder, one of a closely related group of glycoproteins of unknown function that are found in secretions (e.g., saliva, milk, gastric juice, bile), phagocytes, and plasma. On entering the duodenum, the cobalamin–R binder complex is digested, releasing the cobalamin, which then binds to intrinsic factor (IF), a 50-kDa gly-

coprotein produced by the parietal cells of the stomach. The secretion of IF generally parallels that of hydrochloric acid. The cobalamin-IF complex is resistant to proteolytic digestion and travels to the distal ileum, where specific receptors on the mucosal brush border bind and absorb the cobalamin-IF complex. Thus, IF, like iron-binding transferrin, is a cell-directed carrier protein. The receptor-bound cobalamin-IF complex is taken into the ileal mucosal cell, where the IF is destroyed and the cobalamin is transferred to another transport protein, transcobalamin (TC) II. The cobalamin–TC II complex is then secreted into the circulation, from which it is rapidly taken up by the liver, bone marrow, and other cells. The pathway of cobalamin absorption is shown in Fig. 92-2. Normally, about 2 mg cobalamin is stored in the liver, and another 2 mg is stored elsewhere in the body. In view of the minimum daily requirement, about 3 to 6 years would be required for a normal individual to become deficient in cobalamin if absorption were to cease abruptly.

Although TC II is the acceptor for newly absorbed cobalamin, most circulating cobalamin is bound to TC I, a glycoprotein closely related to gastric R binder. TC I appears to be derived in part from leukocytes. The paradox that most circulating cobalamin is bound to TC I rather than TC II, even though TC II initially carries all the cobalamin that is absorbed by the intestine, is explained by the fact that cobalamin bound to TC II is rapidly cleared from the blood ($t_{1/2}$ about 1 h), while clearance of cobalamin bound to TC I requires many days. The function of TC I is unknown.

Cobalamin is an essential cofactor for two enzymes in human cells: methionine synthase and methylmalonyl–coenzyme A (CoA) synthase. Cobalamin exists in two metabolically active forms, identified by the alkyl group attached to the sixth coordination position of the cobalt atom: methylcobalamin and adenosylcobalamin. The vitamin preparation that is used therapeutically is cyanocobalamin (also called vitamin B_{12}). Cyanocobalamin has no known physiologic role and must be converted to a biologically active form before it can be used by tissues.

Methylcobalamin is the form required for methionine synthase,

FIGURE 92-2 The assimilation of cobalamin. On entering the stomach, dietary cobalamin (Cbl) forms a complex with R binding protein. As this protein is digested in the small intestine, cobalamin is transferred to intrinsic factor (IF). This complex passes through the intestine until it reaches specific receptors on the mucosa of the distal ileum. The internalized Cbl is then transferred to transcobalamin II (TC II), which circulates in the plasma until it binds to receptors on cells throughout the body and is internalized.

which catalyzes the conversion of homocysteine to methionine (Fig. 92-1). When this reaction is impaired, folate metabolism is deranged; it is this derangement that underlies the defect in DNA synthesis and the megaloblastic maturation pattern in patients who are deficient in cobalamin. In cobalamin deficiency, the unconjugated N^5-methyltetra-hydrofolate newly taken from the bloodstream cannot be converted to other forms of tetrahydrofolate by methyl transfer. This is the so-called folate trap hypothesis. Because N^5-methyltetrahydrofolate is a poor substrate for the conjugating enzyme, it largely remains in the unconjugated form and slowly leaks from the cell. Tissue folate deficiency therefore develops, and this results in megaloblastic hematopoiesis. This hypothesis explains why tissue folate stores in cobalamin deficiency are substantially reduced, with a disproportionate reduction in conjugated, as compared with unconjugated, folates, despite normal or supranormal serum folate levels. It also explains why large doses of folate can produce a partial hematologic remission in patients with cobalamin deficiency.

Megaloblastic changes in both cobalamin and folate deficiency as well as in methotrexate treatment are related to a deficiency in production of dTMP. In addition, the excess deoxyuridylate that accumulates can be phosphorylated and mistakenly incorporated into DNA in place of thymidylate; base pairing can be affected by this U-for-T substitution.

Plasma homocysteine levels are elevated in both folate and cobalamin deficiency, and high levels of plasma homocysteine appear to be a risk factor for venous and arterial thrombosis. It is not yet known if hyperhomocysteinemia due to folate or cobalamin deficiency predisposes to thrombosis or alters its response to treatment.

Impairment in the conversion of homocysteine to methionine may also contribute to the neurologic complications of cobalamin deficiency (see below). The methionine formed in this reaction is needed for the production of choline and choline-containing phospholipids. Nervous system damage is postulated to result at least in part from interference with these processes due to decreased methionine production in cobalamin deficiency.

Adenosylcobalamin is required for the conversion of methylmalonyl CoA to succinyl CoA. Lack of this cofactor leads to large increases in the tissue levels of methylmalonyl CoA and its precursor, propionyl CoA. As a consequence, nonphysiologic fatty acids containing an odd number of carbon atoms are synthesized and incorporated into neuronal lipids. This biochemical abnormality may also contribute to the neurologic complications of cobalamin deficiency (see below).

CLINICAL DISORDERS

CLASSIFICATION OF MEGALOBLASTIC ANEMIAS (Table 92-1) The cause of megaloblastic anemia varies in different parts of the world. In temperate zones, folate deficiency in alcoholics and cobalamin deficiency due to pernicious anemia or achlorhydria are the common types of megaloblastic anemias. In certain areas close to the equator, tropical sprue is endemic and an important cause of megaloblastic anemia, while in Scandinavia, infestations by the fish tapeworm, *Diphyllobothrium latum*, may be a cause.

The dietary intake of cobalamin is more than adequate for the body's requirements, except in complete vegetarians (vegans) and their breast-fed infants. Thus deficiency of cobalamin is almost always due to malabsorption. Malabsorption can occur at several levels. In contrast, the dietary intake of folic acid is marginal in many parts of the world. Furthermore, because the body's stores of folate are relatively low, folic acid deficiency can arise rather suddenly during periods of decreased dietary intake or increased metabolic demand. Finally, folic acid deficiency may be due to malabsorption. Often two or more of these factors coexist in a given patient.

Combined deficiencies of cobalamin and folic acid are not uncommon. Patients with tropical sprue are often deficient in both vitamins. The biochemical lesion that results in megaloblastic maturation of bone marrow cells also causes structural and functional abnormalities of the rapidly proliferating epithelial cells of the intestinal mucosa.

Thus severe deficiency of one vitamin can lead to malabsorption of the other. Furthermore, as discussed above, a deficiency of cobalamin causes a secondary reduction in cellular folic acid.

Finally, megaloblastic anemias may occasionally be induced by factors unrelated to a vitamin deficiency. Most such cases are caused by drugs that interfere with DNA synthesis. Less commonly, megaloblastic maturation is a feature of certain acquired hematopoietic stem cell defects. Rarest of all are specific congenital enzyme deficiencies.

COBALAMIN DEFICIENCY The clinical features of cobalamin deficiency involve the blood, the gastrointestinal tract, and the nervous system.

The hematologic manifestations are almost entirely the result of anemia, although very rarely purpura may appear, due to thrombocytopenia. Symptoms of anemia may include weakness, light-headedness, vertigo, and tinnitus, as well as palpitations, angina, and the symptoms of congestive failure. On physical examination, the patient with florid cobalamin deficiency is pale, with slightly icteric skin and eyes. Elevated bilirubin levels are related to high erythroid cell turnover in the marrow. The pulse is rapid, and the heart may be enlarged; auscultation will usually reveal a systolic flow murmur.

The gastrointestinal manifestations reflect the effect of cobalamin deficiency on the rapidly proliferating gastrointestinal epithelium. The patient sometimes complains of a sore tongue, which on inspection will be smooth and beefy red. Anorexia with moderate weight loss may also be evident, possibly accompanied by diarrhea and other gastrointestinal symptoms. These latter manifestations may be caused in part by megaloblastosis of the small intestinal epithelium, which results in malabsorption.

The neurologic manifestations often fail to remit fully on treatment. The initial pathology is demyelination, followed by axonal degeneration and eventual neuronal death; the final stage, of course, is irreversible. Sites of involvement include peripheral nerves; the spinal cord, where the posterior and lateral columns undergo demyelination; and the cerebrum itself. Signs and symptoms include numbness and paresthesia in the extremities (the earliest neurologic manifestations), weakness, and ataxia. There may be sphincter disturbances. Reflexes may be diminished or increased. The Romberg and Babinski's signs may be positive, and position and vibration senses are usually diminished. Disturbances of mentation will vary from mild irritability and forgetfulness to severe dementia or frank psychosis. It should be emphasized that *neurologic disease may occur in a patient with a normal hematocrit* and normal RBC indices. Although it has many benefits, folate supplementation of food may increase the likelihood of neurologic presentations of cobalamin deficiency.

In the classic patient, in whom hematologic problems predominate, the blood and bone marrow show characteristic megaloblastic changes (described under "Diagnosis," below). The anemia may be very severe—hematocrits of 15 to 20 are not infrequent—but is surprisingly well tolerated by the patient because it develops slowly.

Defective Release of Cobalamin from Food Cobalamin in food is tightly bound to enzymes in meat and is split from these enzymes by hydrochloric acid and pepsin in the stomach. People >70 years commonly have achlorhydria. Therefore, they are unable to release cobalamin from food sources but retain the ability to absorb crystalline B_{12}, the form most commonly found in multivitamins. The exact incidence of the defect in cobalamin release from food has not been well defined; estimates vary from 10 to >50% of those over age 70 years. Only a minority of these persons go on to develop frank cobalamin deficiency, but many have biochemical changes, including low levels of cobalamin bound to TC II and elevated homocysteine levels, that augur cobalamin deficiency (see below).

Similarly, patients on drugs that suppress gastric acid production, such as omeprazole, may also fail to release cobalamin from food. However, the proton pump inhibitors do not inhibit IF secretion by parietal cells.

Pernicious Anemia Pernicious anemia, considered the most common cause of cobalamin deficiency, is caused by the absence of IF, due to either atrophy of the mucosa or autoimmune destruction of parietal cells. It is most frequently seen in individuals of northern European descent and African Americans and is much less common in southern Europeans and Asians. Men and women are equally affected. It is a disease of the elderly, the average patient presenting near age 60; it is rare under age 30, although typical pernicious anemia can be seen in children under age 10 (juvenile pernicious anemia). Inherited conditions in which a histologically normal stomach secretes either an abnormal IF or none at all will induce cobalamin deficiency in infancy or early childhood.

The incidence of pernicious anemia is substantially increased in patients with other diseases thought to be of immunologic origin, including Graves' disease, myxedema, thyroiditis, idiopathic adrenocortical insufficiency, vitiligo, and hypoparathyroidism. Patients with pernicious anemia also have abnormal circulating antibodies related to their disease: 90% have antiparietal cell antibody, which is directed against the H^+,K^+-ATPase, while 60% have anti-IF antibody. Antiparietal cell antibody is also found in 50% of patients with gastric atrophy without pernicious anemia, as well as in 10 to 15% of an unselected patient population, but anti-IF antibody is usually absent from these patients. Relatives of patients with pernicious anemia have an increased incidence of the disease, and even clinically unaffected relatives may have anti-IF antibody in their serum. Finally, treatment with glucocorticoids may reverse the disease.

Cytotoxic T cells may also contribute to the destruction of parietal cells in pernicious anemia. Pernicious anemia is unusually common in patients with agammaglobulinemia, supporting a role for the cellular immune system in its pathogenesis. In contrast, *Helicobacter pylori* does not cause parietal cell destruction in pernicious anemia.

The most characteristic finding in pernicious anemia is gastric atrophy affecting the acid- and pepsin-secreting portion of the stomach; the antrum is spared. Other pathologic changes are secondary to the deficiency of cobalamin; these include megaloblastic alterations in the gastric and intestinal epithelium and the neurologic changes described above. The abnormalities in the gastric epithelium appear as cellular atypia in gastric cytology specimens, a finding that must be carefully distinguished from the cytologic abnormalities seen in gastric malignancy.

The *clinical manifestations* are primarily those of cobalamin deficiency, as described above. The disease is of insidious onset and progresses slowly. Laboratory examination will reveal hypergastrinemia and pentagastrin-fast achlorhydria as well as the hematologic and other laboratory abnormalities discussed under "Diagnosis."

Through appropriate replacement therapy, patients with pernicious anemia should experience complete and lifelong correction of all abnormalities that are due to cobalamin deficiency, except to the extent that irreversible changes in the nervous system may have occurred before treatment. These patients, however, are unusually subject to gastric polyps and have about twice the normal incidence of cancer of the stomach. Thus, patients should be followed with frequent stool guaiac examinations and endoscopy when indicated.

Postgastrectomy Following total gastrectomy or extensive damage to gastric mucosa as, for example, by ingestion of corrosive agents, megaloblastic anemia will develop because the source of IF has been removed. In all such patients, the absorption of orally administered cobalamin is impaired. Megaloblastic anemia may also follow partial gastrectomy, but the incidence is lower than after total gastrectomy. The cause of cobalamin deficiency after partial gastrectomy is not clear; defective release of cobalamin from food and intestinal overgrowth of bacteria have been suggested, but response to antibiotics is not common.

Intestinal Organisms Megaloblastic anemia may occur with intestinal stasis due to anatomic lesions (strictures, diverticula, anastomoses, "blind loops") or pseudoobstruction (diabetes mellitus, scleroderma, amyloid). This anemia is caused by colonization of the small intestine by large masses of bacteria that consume intestinal cobalamin before absorption. Steatorrhea may also be seen under these circumstances because bile salt metabolism is disturbed when the intestine is heavily colonized with bacteria. Hematologic responses have been observed after administration of oral antibiotics such as tetracycline and ampicillin. Megaloblastic anemia is seen in persons harboring the fish tapeworm, *D. latum*, due to competition by the worm for cobalamin. Destruction of the worm eliminates the problem.

Ileal Abnormalities Cobalamin deficiency is common in tropical sprue, while it is an unusual complication of nontropical sprue (gluten-sensitive enteropathy; Chap. 275). Virtually any disorder that compromises the absorptive capacity of the distal ileum can result in cobalamin deficiency. Specific entities include regional enteritis, Whipple's disease, and tuberculosis. Segmental involvement of the distal ileum by disease can cause megaloblastic anemia without any other manifestations of intestinal malabsorption such as steatorrhea. Cobalamin malabsorption is also seen after ileal resection. The Zollinger-Ellison syndrome (intense gastric hyperacidity due to a gastrin-secreting tumor) may cause cobalamin malabsorption by acidifying the small intestine, retarding the transfer of the vitamin from R binder to IF and impairing the binding of the cobalamin-IF complex to the ileal receptors. Chronic pancreatitis may also cause cobalamin malabsorption by impairing the transfer of the vitamin from R binder to IF. This abnormality can be detected by tests of cobalamin absorption (see below, Schilling test), but it is invariably mild and never causes clinical cobalamin deficiency. Finally, a rare congenital disorder, Imerslund-Gräsbeck disease, involves a selective defect in cobalamin absorption accompanied by proteinuria. Affected individuals have a mutation in cubulin, a receptor that mediates intestinal absorption of the cobalamin-IF complex.

Nitrous Oxide Inhalation of nitrous oxide as an anesthetic destroys endogenous cobalamin. As ordinarily used, the magnitude of the effects are not sufficient to cause clinical cobalamin deficiency, but repeated or protracted exposure (>6 h), particularly in older patients with borderline cobalamin stores, can lead to severe megaloblastic anemia and/or acute neurologic deficits.

FOLIC ACID DEFICIENCY Since January 1998, folic acid has been added to all enriched grain products by order of the U.S. Food and Drug Administration; accordingly, the incidence of folic acid deficiency has fallen markedly. Patients with folic acid deficiency are more often malnourished than those with cobalamin deficiency. The gastrointestinal manifestations are similar to but may be more widespread and more severe than those of pernicious anemia. Diarrhea is often present, and cheilosis and glossitis are also encountered. However, in contrast to cobalamin deficiency, neurologic abnormalities do not occur.

The hematologic manifestations of folic acid deficiency are the same as those of cobalamin deficiency. Folic acid deficiency can generally be attributed to one or more of the following factors: inadequate intake, increased demand, or malabsorption.

Inadequate Intake Alcoholics may become folate deficient because their main source of caloric intake is alcoholic beverages. Distilled spirits are virtually devoid of folic acid, while beer and wine do not contain enough of the vitamin to satisfy the daily requirement. In addition, alcohol may interfere with folate metabolism. Narcotic addicts are also prone to become folate deficient because of malnutrition. Many indigent and elderly individuals who subsist primarily on canned foods or "tea and toast" and occasional teenagers whose diet consists of "junk food" develop folate deficiency.

Increased Demand Tissues with a relatively high rate of cell division such as the bone marrow or gut mucosa have a large requirement for folate. Therefore, patients with chronic hemolytic anemias or other causes of very active erythropoiesis may become deficient. Pregnant women formerly were at risk to become deficient in folic acid because of the high demand of the developing fetus. Deficiency in the first weeks of pregnancy can cause neural tube defects in newborns. Often the pregnancy was not detected until the defect had developed; thus, provision of folate supplementation to women after they learned they were pregnant was ineffective. However, folate food supplementation has decreased neural tube defects by >50%. Folate deficiency may also occur during the growth spurts of infancy and adolescence. Patients on chronic hemodialysis may require supplementary folate to replace that lost in the dialysate.

Malabsorption Folic acid deficiency is a common accompaniment of tropical sprue. Both the gastrointestinal symptoms and malabsorption are improved by the administration of either folic acid or antibiotics by mouth. Patients with nontropical sprue (gluten-sensitive enteropathy) may also develop significant folic acid deficiency that parallels other parameters of malabsorption. Similarly, folate deficiency in alcoholics may be due in part to malabsorption. In addition, other primary small-bowel disorders are sometimes associated with folate deficiency (Chap. 275).

DRUGS Next to deficiency of folate or cobalamin, the most common cause of megaloblastic anemia is drugs. Agents that cause megaloblastic anemia do so by interfering with DNA synthesis, either directly or by antagonizing the action of folate. They can be classified as follows:

1. *Direct inhibitors of DNA synthesis.* They include purine analogues (6-thioguanine, azathioprine, 6-mercaptopurine), pyrimidine analogues (5-fluorouracil, cytosine arabinoside), and other drugs that interfere with DNA synthesis by a variety of mechanisms (hydroxyurea, procarbazine). The antiviral agent zidovudine (AZT), used for treating HIV, often causes severe megaloblastic anemia.

2. *Folate antagonists.* The most toxic of these is methotrexate, a powerful inhibitor of dihydrofolate reductase, which is used in the treatment of certain malignancies and rheumatologic disorders. Much less toxic but still capable of inducing a megaloblastic anemia are several weak dihydrofolate reductase inhibitors used to treat a variety of nonmalignant conditions. These drugs include pentamidine, trimethoprim, triamterene, and pyrimethamine.

3. *Others.* A number of drugs antagonize folate by mechanisms that are poorly understood but are thought to involve an effect on absorption of the vitamin by the intestine. In this category are the anticonvulsants phenytoin, primidone, and phenobarbital. Megaloblastic anemia induced by these agents is mild.

OTHER MECHANISMS ■ **Hereditary** Megaloblastic anemia may be seen in several hereditary disorders. Orotic aciduria is a deficiency of orotidylic decarboxylase and phosphorylase, leading to a defect in pyrimidine metabolism and characterized by retarded growth and development as well as by the excretion of large amounts of orotic acid. Congenital folate malabsorption causes megaloblastic anemia, accompanied by ataxia and mental retardation. A thiamine-responsive megaloblastic anemia accompanied by nerve deafness and diabetes mellitus has been reported in several children. Megaloblastic changes as well as multinuclearity of RBC precursors are seen in the marrow of certain patients with congenital dyserythropoietic anemia, a group of inherited disorders characterized by mild to moderate anemia and a benign course.

TC II deficiency, like the congenital abnormalities in cobalamin absorption, causes pronounced deficiency in cobalamin in infancy or early childhood. Megaloblastic anemia is not seen in hereditary TC I deficiency.

Refractory Megaloblastic Anemia Megaloblastic erythropoiesis may sometimes be seen in myelodysplasia. Megaloblastic changes are restricted to the RBC series (see below). Myelodysplasia often produces a distinct morphologic picture most apparent in orthochromatic normoblasts in which a megaloblastic nucleus is associated with severely hypochromic cytoplasm. This variant has been called "megaloblastoid" and refers to the presence of both nuclear and cytoplasmic maturation defects. "Megaloblastoid" does not mean "mildly megaloblas-

tic." As with other forms of myelodysplasia, refractory megaloblastic anemia is associated with an increased incidence of acute leukemia.

Megaloblastic changes are seen in erythremic myelosis and acute erythroleukemia, where RBC precursors are prominently involved. Here, the marrow is characterized by bizarre erythroid maturation, with multinuclearity and multipolar mitotic figures in the RBC precursors (Chap. 96).

MEGALOBLASTIC DISEASE WITHOUT ANEMIA Megaloblastic disease is easily overlooked in nonanemic patients. It can present in one of two ways.

Acute Megaloblastic Disease Occasionally, a full-blown megaloblastic state can develop over the course of just a few days. This is usually seen following nitrous oxide anesthesia but may occur in any patient with a serious illness requiring intensive care, especially a patient receiving multiple transfusions, dialysis, or total parenteral nutrition. An acute megaloblastic state can also be precipitated by the administration of a weak antifolate (e.g., trimethoprim) to a patient with marginal tissue folate stores.

The condition resembles an immune cytopenia, with a rapidly developing thrombocytopenia and/or leukopenia in the absence of anemia. The blood smear may be completely normal, but the marrow is floridly megaloblastic. Acute megaloblastic anemia responds rapidly to treatment with folate plus cobalamin in the usual therapeutic doses.

Cobalamin Deficiency without Anemia Cobalamin deficiency without hematologic abnormalities is surprisingly common, especially in the elderly. The risk of a nonhematologic presentation for cobalamin deficiency is increased by the folate food fortification because folate can mask the hematologic effects of cobalamin deficiency. Between 10 and 30% of persons over age 70 years have metabolic evidence of cobalamin deficiency, either elevated homocysteine levels, low cobalamin-TC II levels, or both. Only 10% of these patients have defective production of IF, and the remainder often have atrophic gastritis and cannot release cobalamin from their food (see above). Serum cobalamin levels may be normal or low, but serum levels of methylmalonic acid are almost invariably increased due to a deficiency of cobalamin at the tissue level. The neuropsychiatric abnormalities tend to improve, and serum methylmalonic acid levels generally return to normal after treatment with cobalamin. Neurologic defects do not always reverse with cobalamin supplementation.

DIAGNOSIS The finding of significant macrocytosis [mean corpuscular volume (MCV) > 100 fL] suggests the presence of a megaloblastic anemia. Other causes of macrocytosis include hemolysis, liver disease, alcoholism, hypothyroidism, and aplastic anemia. If the macrocytosis is marked (MCV > 110 fL), the patient is much more likely to have a megaloblastic anemia. Macrocytosis is less marked with concurrent iron deficiency or thalassemia. The reticulocyte index is low, and the leukocyte and platelet count may also be decreased, particularly in severely anemic patients. The blood smear (Fig. 92-3) demonstrates marked anisocytosis and poikilocytosis, together with macroovalocytes, which are large, oval, fully hemoglobinized erythrocytes typical of megaloblastic anemias. There is some basophilic stippling, and an occasional nucleated RBC may be seen. In the white blood cell series, the neutrophils show hypersegmentation of the nucleus (Fig. 92-4). This is such a characteristic finding that a single cell with a nucleus of six lobes or more should raise the immediate suspicion of a meg-

FIGURE 92-3 Megaloblastic anemia. Oval macrocytes, well filled with hemoglobin, are admixed with lesser numbers of large red blood cells, some of which are teardrop-shaped. Note also hypersegmented granulocyte.

FIGURE 92-4 This marrow section demonstrates nuclear-cytoplasmic dissociation. Nuclei of late stage (orthochromatic) erythroblasts have loose chromatin more characteristic of more immature cells while their cytoplasms are nearly filled with hemoglobin. Slow nuclear maturation is related to a decrese in DNA synthesis related to an insufficient supply of thymidylate. An inadequate supply of reduced folate (usually folate or B12 deficiency) or drugs that inhibit DNA synthesis can produce this picture. (*From RS Hillman, MD, and KA Ault, MD, courtesy of the American Society of Hematology Slide Bank.*)

aloblastic anemia. A rare myelocyte may also be seen. Bizarre, misshapen platelets are also observed. The bone marrow is hypercellular with a decreased myeloid/erythroid ratio and abundant stainable iron. RBC precursors are abnormally large and have nuclei that appear much less mature than would be expected from the development of the cytoplasm (nuclear-cytoplasmic asynchrony). The nuclear chromatin is more dispersed than expected, and it condenses in a peculiar fenestrated pattern that is very characteristic of megaloblastic erythropoiesis. Abnormal mitoses may be seen. Granulocyte precursors are also affected, many being larger than normal, including giant bands and metamyelocytes. Megakaryocytes are decreased and show abnormal morphology.

Megaloblastic anemias are characterized by ineffective erythropoiesis (Chap. 52). In a severely megaloblastic patient, as many as 90% of the RBC precursors may be destroyed before they are released into the bloodstream, compared with 10 to 15% in normal individuals. Enhanced intramedullary destruction of erythroblasts results in an increase in unconjugated bilirubin and lactic acid dehydrogenase (isoenzyme 1) in plasma.

In evaluating a patient with megaloblastic anemia, it is important to determine whether there is a specific vitamin deficiency by measuring serum cobalamin and folate levels. The normal range of cobalamin in serum is 300 to 900 pg/mL; values <200 pg/mL indicate clinically significant deficiency. Measurements of cobalamin bound to TC II would be a more physiologic measure of cobalamin status, but such assays are not yet routinely available. The normal serum concentration of folic acid ranges from 6 to 20 ng/mL; values ≤4 ng/mL are generally considered to be diagnostic of folate deficiency. Unlike serum cobalamin, serum folate levels may reflect recent alterations in dietary intake. Measurement of RBC folate level provides useful information because it is not subject to short-term fluctuations in folate intake and is better than serum folate as an index of folate stores.

Once cobalamin deficiency has been established, its pathogenesis can be delineated by means of a Schilling test. A patient is given radioactive cobalamin by mouth, followed shortly thereafter by an intramuscular injection of unlabeled cobalamin. The proportion of the administered radioactivity excreted in the urine during the next 24 h provides an accurate measure of absorption of cobalamin, assuming that a complete urine sample has been collected. Because cobalamin deficiency is almost always due to malabsorption (Table 92-1), this first stage of the Schilling test should be abnormal (i.e., small amounts of radioactivity in the urine). The patient is then given labeled cobalamin bound to IF. Absorption of the vitamin will now approach normal if the patient has pernicious anemia or some other type of IF deficiency. If cobalamin absorption is still decreased, the patient may have bacterial overgrowth (blind loop syndrome) or ileal disease (including an ileal absorptive defect secondary to the cobalamin deficiency itself). Cobalamin malabsorption due to bacterial overgrowth can frequently

be corrected by the administration of antibiotics. The Schilling test can provide equally reliable information after the patient has had adequate therapy with parenteral cobalamin.

A normal Schilling test in a patient with documented cobalamin deficiency may indicate poor absorption of the vitamin when mixed with food. This can be established by repeating the Schilling test with radioactive cobalamin scrambled with an egg.

Serum methylmalonic acid and homocysteine levels are also useful in the diagnosis of megaloblastic anemias. Both are elevated in cobalamin deficiency, while elevated levels of homocysteine but not methylmalonic acid are seen in folate deficiency. These tests measure tissue vitamin stores and may demonstrate a deficiency even when the more traditional but less reliable folate and cobalamin levels are borderline or even normal. Patients (particularly older patients) without anemia and with normal serum cobalamin levels but elevated levels of serum methylmalonic acid may develop neuropsychiatric abnormalities. Treatment of patients with this "subtle" cobalamin deficiency will usually prevent further deterioration and may result in improvement.

℞ TREATMENT

Cobalamin Deficiency   Apart from specific therapy related to the underlying disorder (e.g., antibiotics for intestinal overgrowth with bacteria), the mainstay of treatment for cobalamin deficiency is replacement therapy. Because the defect is nearly always malabsorption, patients are generally given parenteral treatment, specifically in the form of intramuscular cyanocobalamin. Parenteral treatment begins with 1000 μg cobalamin per week for 8 weeks, followed by 1000 μg cyanocobalamin intramuscularly every month for the rest of the patient's life. Cobalamin deficiency can also be managed very effectively by oral replacement therapy with 2 mg crystalline B_{12} per day; however, compliance is a greater concern with oral than intramuscular treatment.

The response to treatment is gratifying. Shortly after treatment is begun, and several days before a hematologic response is evident in the peripheral blood, the patient will experience an increase in strength and an improved sense of well-being. Marrow morphology begins to revert toward normal within a few hours after treatment is initiated. Reticulocytosis begins 4 to 5 days after therapy is started and peaks at about day 7 (Fig. 92-5), with subsequent remission of the anemia over the next several weeks. If a reticulocytosis does not occur, or if it is less brisk than expected from the level of the hematocrit, a search should be made for other factors contributing to the anemia (e.g., infection, coexisting iron and/or folate deficiency, or hypothyroidism). Hypokalemia and salt retention may occur early in the course of therapy. Thrombocytosis may also be seen.

In most cases, replacement therapy is all that is needed for the treatment of cobalamin deficiency. Occasionally, however, a patient with a severe anemia will have such a precarious cardiovascular status that emergency transfusion is necessary. This must be done with great

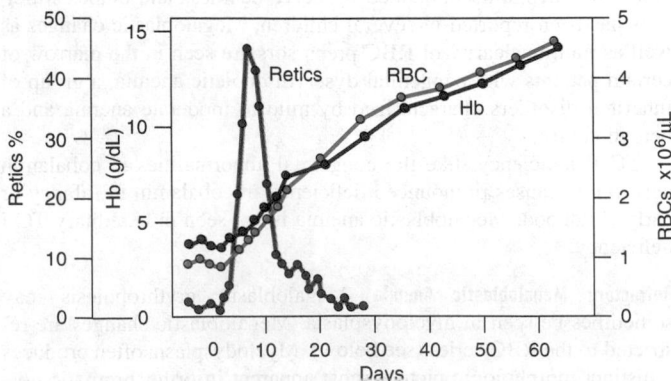

FIGURE 92-5   Hematologic response of a patient with pernicious anemia to an intramuscular injection of 100 μg cobalamin on day 0. Retics, reticulocytes; RBC, red blood cell; Hb, hemoglobin. (*From A Erslev, TG Gabuzda, Pathophysiology of Blood, Philadelphia, Saunders, 1975, with permission.*)

care, because such patients may develop heart failure from fluid overload. Blood must be administered slowly in the form of packed RBCs, with very close observation. A small volume of packed RBCs will frequently be enough to ameliorate the acute cardiovascular problems. If necessary, blood may be administered by exchanging patient blood (mostly plasma) for packed cells.

With lifelong treatment, patients should experience no further manifestations of cobalamin deficiency, although neurologic symptoms may not be fully corrected even by optimal therapy. The potential for late development of gastric carcinoma in pernicious anemia necessitates careful follow-up of the patient.

Folate, particularly in large doses, can correct the megaloblastic anemia of cobalamin deficiency without altering the neurologic abnormalities. The neurologic manifestations may even be aggravated by folate therapy. Cobalamin deficiency can thus be masked in patients who are taking large doses of folate. For this reason, a hematologic response to folate must never be used to rule out cobalamin deficiency in a given patient; cobalamin deficiency can be excluded only by appropriate laboratory evaluation.

In light of the high frequency of defective cobalamin absorption in older people and the possible increased risk that overt cobalamin deficiency will present with neurologic rather than hematologic symptoms (because of folate food fortification), some experts have recommended the use of 0.1 mg oral crystalline cobalamin prophylaxis daily in people over age 65 years.

Folate Deficiency Like cobalamin deficiency, folate deficiency is treated by replacement therapy. The usual dose of folic acid is 1 mg/d, by mouth, but higher doses (up to 5 mg/d) may be required for folate deficiency due to malabsorption. Parenteral folate is rarely necessary. The hematologic response is similar to that seen after replacement therapy for cobalamin deficiency, i.e., a brisk reticulocytosis after about 4 days, followed by correction of the anemia over the next 1 to 2 months. The duration of therapy depends on the basis of the deficiency state. Patients with a continuously increased requirement (such as patients with hemolytic anemia) or those with malabsorption or chronic malnutrition should continue to receive oral folic acid indefinitely. In addition, the patient should be encouraged to maintain an optimal diet containing adequate amounts of folate.

Other Causes of Megaloblastic Anemia Megaloblastic anemia due to drugs can be treated, if necessary, by reducing the dose of the drug or eliminating it altogether. The effects of folate antagonists that inhibit dihydrofolate reductase can be counteracted by folinic acid [5-formyl tetrahydrofolate (THF)] in a dose of 100 to 200 mg/d (Fig. 92-1), which circumvents the block in folate metabolism by providing a form of folate that can be converted to 5,10-methylene THF. For the megaloblastic forms of sideroblastic anemia, pyridoxine in pharmacologic doses (as high as 300 mg/d) should be tried. Simple supportive measures are all that appear to be in order for treatment of refractory megaloblastic anemia. Acute erythroleukemia is treated like other types of acute myeloid leukemia (Chap. 96).

FURTHER READING

CARMEL R: Current concepts in cobalamin deficiency. Annu Rev Med 51:357, 2000

D'ANGELO A, SELHUB J: Homocysteine and thrombotic disease. Blood 90:1, 1997

DHAMARAJAN TS et al: Vitamin B12 deficiency: Recognizing subtle symptoms in older adults. Geriatrics 58:30, 2003

JACQUES PF et al: The effect of folic acid fortification on plasma folate and total homocysteine concentrations. N Engl J Med 340:1449, 1999

KUZMINSKI AM et al: Effective treatment of cobalamin deficiency with oral cobalamin. Blood 92:1191, 1998

TOH BH et al: Pernicious anemia. N Engl J Med 337:1441, 1997

WICKRAMASINGHE SN: The wide spectrum and unresolved issues of megaloblastic anemia. Semin Hematol 36:3, 1999

93 HEMOLYTIC ANEMIAS AND ACUTE BLOOD LOSS
H. Franklin Bunn, Wendell Rosse

The loss of red cells either through hemorrhage or, less commonly, through premature destruction of the red cells (hemolysis) may cause anemia. Hemolysis or blood loss normally leads to an increase in red cell production, detected by an increase in reticulocyte index.

HEMOLYTIC ANEMIAS

Red blood cells (RBC) normally survive 90 to 120 days in the circulation. The life span of RBC may be shortened in a number of disorders, often resulting in anemia if the bone marrow is not able to replenish adequately the prematurely destroyed RBC.

In all patients with hemolytic anemia, a careful history and physical examination provide important clues to the diagnosis. The patient may complain of fatigue and other symptoms of anemia (Chap. 52). Less commonly, jaundice and even red-brown urine (hemoglobinuria) are reported. A complete drug and toxin exposure history and the family history often provide crucial information. The physical examination may show jaundice of skin and mucosae. Splenomegaly is encountered in a variety of hemolytic anemias. Other historic and physical findings are associated with specific hemolytic anemias (see below).

Laboratory tests may be used initially to demonstrate the presence of hemolysis (Table 93-1) and define its cause. An elevated reticulocyte count in the patient with anemia is the most useful indicator of hemolysis, reflecting erythroid hyperplasia of the bone marrow; biopsy of the bone marrow is often unnecessary. Reticulocytes are also elevated in patients with active blood loss, those with myelophthisis, and those who are recovering from suppression of erythropoiesis (Chap. 52). The morphology of the RBC may provide evidence both of hemolysis and of its cause; the characteristic abnormalities and their associated causes and syndromes are listed in Table 93-2. While the findings on the peripheral blood smear alone are rarely pathognomonic, they may provide important clues to the presence of hemolysis and to diagnosis.

Hemolysis results in increased heme catabolism and enhanced formation of unconjugated bilirubin. The plasma level of unconjugated bilirubin may be high enough to produce readily apparent jaundice (detectable usually when serum bilirubin is >34 μmol/L or 2 mg/dL).

TABLE 93-1 *Laboratory Evaluation of Hemolysis*

	Extravascular	Intravascular
HEMATOLOGIC		
Routine blood film	Polychromatophilia	Polychromatophilia
Reticulocyte count	↑	↑
Bone marrow examination	Erythroid hyperplasia	Erythroid hyperplasia
PLASMA OR SERUM		
Bilirubin	↑ Unconjugated	↑ Unconjugated
Haptoglobin	↓, Absent	Absent
Plasma hemoglobin	N–↑	↑↑
Lactate dehydrogenase	↑ (Variable)	↑↑ (Variable)
URINE		
Bilirubin	0	0
Hemosiderin	0	+
Hemoglobin	0	+ in severe cases

Note: N, normal.

TABLE 93-2   *Red Blood Cell Morphology in the Diagnosis of Hemolytic Anemia*

Morphology	Cause	Syndromes
Spherocytes	Loss of membrane	Hereditary spherocytosis, immunohemolytic anemia
Target cells	Increased ratio of RBC surface area to volume	Hemoglobin disorders: thalassemias, hemoglobin S, C, etc.; liver disease
Schistocytes	Traumatic disruption of membrane	Microangiopathy, intravascular prostheses
Sickled cells	Polymerization of hemoglobin S	Sickle cell syndromes
Acanthocytes	?Abnormal membrane lipids	Severe liver disease (spur cell anemia)
Agglutinated cells	Presence of IgM antibody	Cold agglutinin disease
Heinz bodies	Precipitated hemoglobin	Unstable hemoglobin, oxidant stress

The unconjugated (indirect) bilirubin level can be further elevated by a commonly encountered defect in conjugation of bilirubin (Gilbert's syndrome) (Chap. 284). In patients with hemolysis, the level of unconjugated bilirubin never exceeds 70 to 85 μmol/L (4 to 5 mg/dL) unless liver function is impaired.

In the absence of tissue damage in other organs, serum enzyme levels can be useful in the diagnosis and monitoring of patients with hemolysis. Lactate dehydrogenase (LDH), particularly LDH-2, is elevated by accelerated RBC destruction. Serum AST (SGOT) may be somewhat elevated, whereas ALT (SGPT) is not.

Haptoglobin is an α globulin that is present in high concentration ($\sim$1.0 g/L) in the serum. It binds specifically to the globin in hemoglobin. The hemoglobin-haptoglobin complex is cleared rapidly by the mononuclear phagocyte system. Thus patients with significant hemolysis, either intravascular or extravascular, have low or absent levels of serum haptoglobin. The fact that haptoglobin synthesis is decreased in patients with hepatocellular disease and increased in inflammatory states must be considered in the interpretation of serum haptoglobin.

Intravascular hemolysis (which is uncommon) results in the release of hemoglobin into the plasma. In these cases, plasma hemoglobin is increased in proportion to the degree of hemolysis (plasma hemoglobin may be falsely elevated due to lysis of RBC in vitro). If the haptoglobin-binding capacity of the plasma is exceeded, free hemoglobin tetramer dissociates into dimers that pass through renal glomeruli. This filtered hemoglobin is reabsorbed by the proximal tubule, where it is catabolized in situ, and the heme iron is incorporated into storage proteins (ferritin and hemosiderin). The presence of hemosiderin in the urine, detected by staining the sediment with Prussian blue, indicates that a significant amount of circulating free hemoglobin has been filtered by the kidneys. When the absorptive capacity of the tubular cells is exceeded, hemoglobinuria ensues and indicates severe intravascular hemolysis. Hemoglobinuria must be distinguished from hematuria (in which case RBC are seen on urine examination) and from myoglobinuria due to rhabdomyolysis; in all three cases, the urine is positive with the benzidine reaction, commonly used in analysis of urine. After centrifugation of an anticoagulated blood specimen, the plasma of patients with hemoglobinuria has a reddish-brown color, whereas that of patients with myoglobinuria is normal in color. Because of its higher molecular weight, hemoglobin has lower glomerular permeability than myoglobin and is less rapidly cleared by the kidneys.

CLASSIFICATION   The hemolytic anemias can be grouped into three categories (Table 93-3). Accelerated RBC destruction can be caused by (1) a molecular defect (hemoglobinopathy or enzymopathy) inside the red cell, (2) an abnormality in membrane structure and function, or (3)

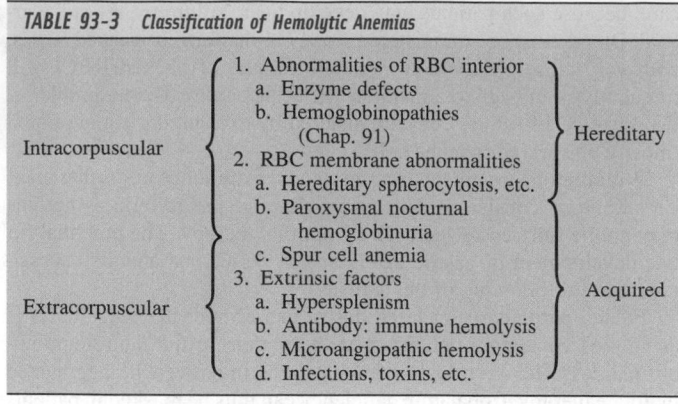

TABLE 93-3   *Classification of Hemolytic Anemias*

Intracorpuscular	1. Abnormalities of RBC interior
	  a. Enzyme defects
	  b. Hemoglobinopathies (Chap. 91)
	2. RBC membrane abnormalities
	  a. Hereditary spherocytosis, etc.
	  b. Paroxysmal nocturnal hemoglobinuria
	  c. Spur cell anemia
		Hereditary

Extracorpuscular	3. Extrinsic factors
	  a. Hypersplenism
	  b. Antibody: immune hemolysis
	  c. Microangiopathic hemolysis
	  d. Infections, toxins, etc.
		Acquired

an environmental factor such as mechanical trauma or an autoantibody. In *intracorpuscular types* of hemolysis, the patient's RBC have an abnormally short life span in a normal recipient (with a compatible blood type), while compatible normal RBC survive normally in the patient. The opposite is true in *extracorpuscular* types of hemolysis. Finally, hemolytic disorders can be either inherited or acquired.

INHERITED HEMOLYTIC ANEMIAS   The inherited hemolytic anemias are due to inborn defects in one of three main components of red cells: the membrane, enzymes, or hemoglobin. These defects are often known at the genomic level, but their identification still largely depends on their clinical and laboratory manifestations.

Red Cell Membrane Disorders   These are usually readily detected by morphologic abnormalities of the RBC on the blood film. The three inherited RBC membrane abnormalities are hereditary spherocytosis, hereditary elliptocytosis (including hereditary pyropoikilocytosis), and hereditary stomatocytosis.

HEREDITARY SPHEROCYTOSIS   Hereditary spherocytosis is characterized by spherical RBC due to a molecular defect in one of the proteins in the cytoskeleton of the RBC membrane; this leads to a loss of membrane and hence decreased ratio of surface area to volume and consequently spherocytosis. Usually an autosomal dominant trait, this disorder has an incidence of 1:1000 to 1:4500. In $\sim$20% of patients, the absence of hematologic abnormalities in family members suggests either autosomal recessive inheritance or a spontaneous mutation. The disorder is sometimes clinically apparent in early infancy but often escapes detection until adult life.

Clinical Manifestations   The major clinical features of hereditary spherocytosis are anemia, splenomegaly, and jaundice. Jaundice may be intermittent and tends to be less pronounced in early childhood. Because of the increased bile pigment production, pigmented gallstones are common, even in childhood. Compensatory erythroid hyperplasia of the bone marrow occurs, with the extension of red marrow into the midshafts of long bones and occasionally with extramedullary erythropoiesis, at times leading to the formation of paravertebral masses visible on chest x-ray. Because the bone marrow's capacity to increase erythropoiesis nearly matches the rate of hemolysis, anemia is usually mild or moderate and may even be absent in an otherwise healthy individual. Compensation may be temporarily interrupted by episodes of relative erythroid hypoplasia precipitated by infections, particularly parvovirus. Splenomegaly is very common. The hemolytic rate may increase transiently during systemic infections, which induce further splenic enlargement. Chronic leg ulcers, similar to those observed in sickle cell anemia, occur occasionally.

The characteristic erythrocyte abnormality is the spherocyte (Fig. 93-1). The mean corpuscular volume (MCV) is usually normal or slightly decreased, and the mean corpuscular hemoglobin concentration (MCHC) is increased to 350 to 400 g/L. Spheroidicity may be quantitatively assessed by measurement of the osmotic fragility of the RBC on exposure to hyposmotic solutions causing a net influx of water (Fig. 93-2). On microscopic examination, spherocytes are usually detected as small cells without central pallor.

FIGURE 93-1 *Hereditary spherocytosis* Small, densely staining red blood cells are seen that have lost their central area of pallor (microspherocytes). Microspherocytes may also be found in other hemolytic disorders (Fig. 93-5).

Pathogenesis The molecular abnormality in hereditary spherocytosis primarily involves the proteins responsible for tethering the lipid bilayer to the underlying cytoskeletal network. About 50% of patients have a defect in ankyrin, the protein that forms a bridge between protein 3 and spectrin (Fig. 93-3). Homozygotes who have a recessive inheritance pattern for ankyrin deficiency have more severe anemia than heterozygotes with the more common dominant form. About 25% of patients have a mutation of protein 3, resulting in a deficiency of that protein and mild anemia with dominant inheritance. Most of the remaining 25% have mutations of spectrin, leading to impaired synthesis or self-association. β-spectrin mutants are generally mild, with dominant inheritance, while α-spectrin deficiency is severe, with a recessive inheritance pattern. Less often, deficiency of palladin (protein 4.2) is a cause of hereditary spherocytosis. Because the lipid bilayer is not well anchored when these proteins are defective, part of it is lost by vesiculation, resulting in a more spherical and less deformable cell. Because of their shape and rigidity, spherocytes are trapped in the spleen where their increased metabolic rate cannot be sustained, causing a further loss of surface membrane. This "conditioning" produces a subpopulation of hyperspheroidal RBC in the peripheral blood.

Diagnosis Hereditary spherocytosis must be distinguished primarily from the spherocytic hemolytic anemias associated with RBC antibodies. The family history of anemia and/or splenectomy is helpful, when present. The diagnosis of immune spherocytosis is usually readily established by a positive direct Coombs test (see below). Spherocytes are also seen in association with hemolysis induced by splenomegaly in patients with cirrhosis, in clostridial infections, and in certain snake envenomations (due to the action of phospholipases on the membrane). A few spherocytes are seen in the course of a wide variety of hemolytic disorders, particularly glucose-6-phosphate dehydrogenase (G6PD) deficiency.

℞ TREATMENT

Splenectomy is recommended in patients with moderate or severe hemolysis. Although the RBC defect and its consequent morphology persist, anemia is ameliorated. The operative risk is low, particularly if performed by laparoscopy. RBC survival after splenectomy is normal or nearly so; if it is not, an accessory spleen or another diagnosis should be sought. Because of the potential for gallstones and for episodes of bone marrow hypoplasia or hemolytic crises, splenectomy should be performed in symptomatic individuals; cholecystectomy should not be performed without splenectomy, as intrahepatic gallstones may result. Splenectomy in children should be postponed until age 4, if possible, to minimize the risk of severe infections with gram-positive encapsulated organisms. Pneumococcal, meningococcal, and *Haemophilus influenzae* vaccines should be administered at least 2 weeks before splenectomy. In patients with severe hemolysis, folic acid (1 mg/d) should be administered prophylactically.

FIGURE 93-2 Osmotic fragility of RBC in hereditary spherocytosis (HS). The results from two patients are compared to those from a normal individual.

HEREDITARY ELLIPTOCYTOSIS AND HEREDITARY PYROPOIKILOCYTOSIS *Hereditary elliptocytosis* is an autosomal dominant trait and affects 1 per 4000 to 5000 people, a frequency similar to that of hereditary spherocytosis (rarely, patients with myelodysplastic disorders of the bone marrow may have acquired elliptocytosis). In most affected individuals, a structural abnormality of erythrocyte spectrin leads to impaired assembly of the cytoskeleton. In some families, affected individuals have a deficiency of erythrocyte membrane protein 4.1, which stabilizes the interaction of spectrin and actin in the cytoskeleton (Fig. 93-3). In Southeast Asia, the incidence of hereditary ovalocytosis is high; a small internal deletion of protein 3 makes the membrane rigid and confers resistance against malaria.

The great majority of patients manifest only mild hemolysis, with little or no anemia. RBC destruction occurs predominantly in an enlarged spleen. Hemolysis is corrected by splenectomy.

The blood smear reveals elongated or oval red cells (elliptocytes). Patients with marked hemolysis have microovalocytes, bizarre-shaped RBC, and RBC fragments, all of which increase in number after splenectomy. The degree of hemolysis does not correlate with the percentage of elliptocytes.

Hereditary pyropoikilocytosis is a rare disorder related to hereditary elliptocytosis and is characterized by bizarre-shaped, microcytic RBC that undergo disruption at temperatures of 44 to 45°C (in contrast,

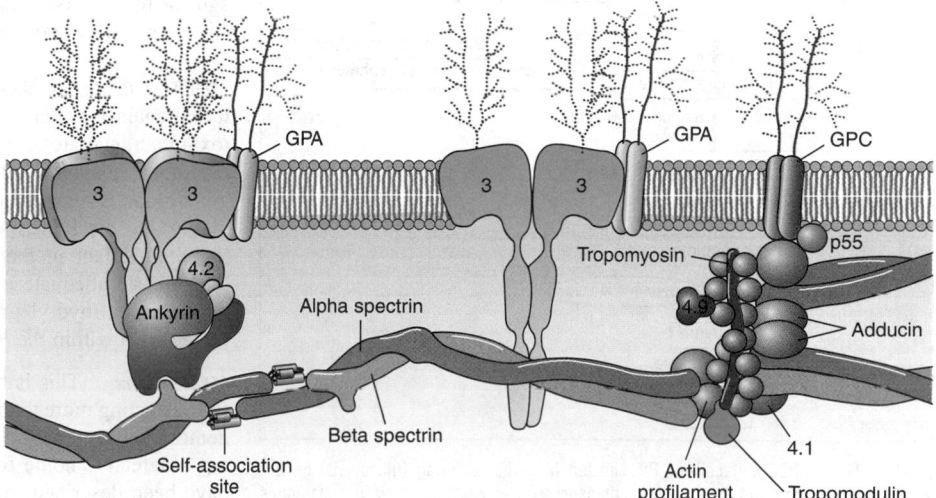

FIGURE 93-3 Diagram of a cross-section of the RBC membrane. Spectrin, actin, tropomyosin, adducin, and protein 4.1 form a meshwork that laminates the inner surface of the membrane. In contrast, other proteins such as the glycophorins (GPA and GPC) and protein 3 (anion transport channel) traverse the lipid bilayer. Long polysaccharide chains are covalently attached to these proteins on the outer surface of the cell and also to glycolipid. Ankyrin and protein 4.2 form a bridge between spectrin and a fraction of the anion transport proteins. Protein 4.1 binds to GPC. [*From Lux SE, Palek J, in Blood: Principles and Practice of Hematology, RI Handin et al (eds). Philadelphia, Lippincott, 1995.*]

normal RBC are stable up to 49°C). This condition results from a deficiency of spectrin and an abnormality of spectrin self-assembly. Hemolysis is usually severe, is recognized in childhood, and is partially responsive to splenectomy.

HEREDITARY STOMATOCYTOSIS   Stomatocytes are cup-shaped RBC that have a slitlike central zone of pallor on blood smears. The disorder is inherited in an autosomal dominant pattern. RBC have an increased permeability to sodium and potassium, which is compensated for by an increased active transport of these cations. In some patients, the RBC are swollen with an excess of ions and water and a decreased mean corpuscular hemoglobin concentration (overhydrated stomatocytes, "hydrocytosis"); many of these patients lack the RBC membrane protein 7.2 (stomatin). RBC lacking Rh proteins (Rh_{null} cells) are also stomatocytic and have a shortened life span. In other patients, the RBC are shrunken, with a decreased ion and water content, appearing as target cells on blood smears. Most patients have splenomegaly and mild anemia. Splenectomy decreases but does not totally correct the hemolytic process.

Red Cell Enzyme Defects   During its maturation, the RBC loses its nucleus, ribosomes, and mitochondria and thus its capability for protein synthesis and oxidative phosphorylation. The mature circulating RBC has a relatively simple pattern of intermediary metabolism (Fig. 93-4)

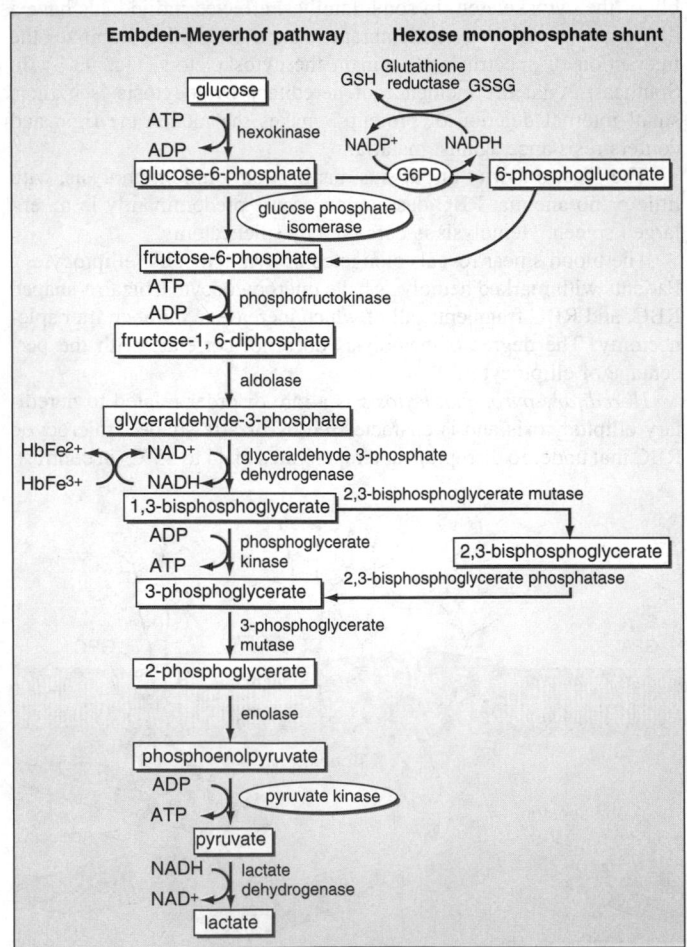

FIGURE 93-4   RBC metabolism. The Embden-Meyerhof pathway (glycolysis) generates ATP for energy and membrane maintenance. The generation of NADPH maintains hemoglobin in a reduced state. The hexose monophosphate shunt generates NADPH that is used to reduce glutathione, which protects the red cell against oxidant stress. Regulation of 2,3-bisphosphoglycerate levels is a critical determinant of oxygen affinity of hemoglobin. Enzyme deficiency states in order of prevalence: glucose-6-phosphate dehydrogenase (G6PD) ≫ pyruvate kinase > glucose-6-phosphate isomerase > rare deficiencies of other enzymes in the pathway. The more common enzyme deficiencies are encircled.

in keeping with its modest metabolic obligations. ATP must be generated from the Embden-Meyerhof pathway to drive the cation pump that maintains the ionic milieu in the RBC. Smaller amounts of energy are needed for the preservation of hemoglobin iron in the ferrous (Fe^{2+}) state and perhaps for the renewal of the lipids in the RBC membrane. About 10% of the glucose consumed by the RBC is metabolized via the hexose-monophosphate shunt (Fig. 93-4), which protects both hemoglobin and the membrane from oxidants, including certain drugs.

DEFECTS IN THE EMBDEN-MEYERHOF PATHWAY   Most of the glycolytic enzyme defects are inherited in an autosomal recessive pattern. Since the gene frequency for this group of defects is low, true heterozygotes are often the offspring of a consanguineous mating. More often, affected individuals are compound heterozygotes. Patients with severe hemolysis usually present during early childhood with anemia, jaundice, and splenomegaly. The RBC are often relatively deficient in ATP, resulting in a leak of potassium ion out of these cells. These RBC are rigid and thus more readily sequestered by the mononuclear phagocyte system.

Some of these glycolytic enzyme deficiencies such as pyruvate kinase (PK) deficiency and hexokinase deficiency are localized to the RBC, with no apparent metabolic abnormality in other cells. In other disorders, the enzyme deficiency is more widespread.

About 95% of the clinically significant defects in the glycolytic pathway are due to PK deficiency, and about 4% are due to glucose phosphate isomerase deficiency. The remainder, shown in Fig. 93-4, are extremely rare. Most have been encountered in isolated families; clinical manifestations are variable.

Laboratory Findings   Patients have a normocytic (or slightly macrocytic), normochromic anemia with reticulocytosis. In those with PK deficiency, bizarre erythrocytes, including spiculated cells, are noted on the peripheral smear, especially after splenectomy. Spherocytes are usually absent; the term *congenital nonspherocytic hemolytic anemia* has been applied to these disorders. The diagnosis of this group of anemias depends on specific enzymatic assays. Abnormalities in enzymatic properties may be useful in distinguishing among enzyme mutants. DNA sequencing is the only definitive way to identify a mutant.

℞ TREATMENT

Most patients do not require therapy. Those with severe hemolysis should be given folic acid (1 mg/d). Blood transfusions may be necessary during a hypoplastic crisis. Women with PK deficiency may become very anemic during pregnancy, sometimes leading to the diagnosis for the first time. Patients with PK or glucose phosphate isomerase deficiency may benefit from splenectomy.

DEFECTS IN THE HEXOSE-MONOPHOSPHATE SHUNT   Normal RBC are well protected against oxidant stress. When the cells are exposed to a drug or toxin that generates oxygen radicals, glucose metabolism via the hexose-monophosphate shunt is normally increased severalfold. Reduced glutathione is regenerated, protecting the sulfhydryl groups of hemoglobin and the RBC membrane from oxidation. Individuals with an inherited defect in the hexose-monophosphate shunt are unable to maintain an adequate level of reduced glutathione in their RBC, hemoglobin sulfhydryl groups become oxidized, and the hemoglobin precipitates within the RBC, forming Heinz bodies.

G6PD Deficiency   This is by far the most common congenital shunt defect, affecting more than 200 million people throughout the world; like hemoglobin S, it partially protects the patient from malaria by providing a defective home for the merozoite. Over 400 variants of G6PD have been described, resulting in considerable clinical heterogeneity among affected individuals. Most are missense mutations resulting in altered enzymatic properties.

The normal G6PD is designated as type B. About 20% of individuals of African descent have a G6PD (designated A+) that differs by a single amino acid and is electrophoretically distinguishable but functionally normal. Among the clinically significant G6PD variants, the most common, the so-called A− type, is due to two base substitutions and is encountered primarily in individuals of central African descent. The A− G6PD has the same electrophoretic mobility as the A+ type, but it is unstable and has abnormal kinetic properties. This variant is found in about 11% of African-American males. A second relatively common G6PD variant is encountered among groups of Mediterranean origin, particularly Sardinians and Sephardic Jews; this variant is more severe than the A− variant and may result in nonspherocytic hemolytic anemia in the absence of known oxidative stress. A third relatively common and slightly less severe variant occurs in southern Chinese populations.

The G6PD gene is located on the X chromosome; thus the deficiency state is a sex-linked trait. Affected males (hemizygotes) inherit the abnormal gene from their mothers who are usually carriers (heterozygotes). Because of inactivation of one of the two X chromosomes (Lyon hypothesis: Chap. 56), the heterozygote has two populations of RBC: normal and deficient in G6PD. Most female carriers have no problems. Those who happen to have a high proportion of deficient cells resemble the male hemizygotes. G6PD activity normally declines ~50% during the 120-day life span of the RBC. This decay is moderately accelerated in A− RBC and markedly so in RBC containing the Mediterranean variant. Individuals with the A− variant normally have a slightly shortened RBC survival time, but they are not anemic. Clinical problems arise only when the affected individual is subjected to some type of environmental stress. Most often, hemolytic episodes are triggered by viral and bacterial infections. The mechanism is unknown. In addition, drugs or toxins that pose an oxidant threat to the RBC (most commonly sulfa drugs, antimalarials, and nitrofurantoin) cause hemolysis in individuals deficient in G6PD (Table 93-4). Although aspirin is frequently mentioned as a likely offender, it has no deleterious effect in A− individuals. Accidental ingestion of toxic compounds such as naphthalene (moth balls) may cause severe hemolysis. Metabolic acidosis can precipitate an episode of hemolysis in individuals deficient in G6PD.

Clinical and Laboratory Features   The patient may experience an acute hemolytic crisis within hours of exposure to the oxidant stress, leading to hemoglobinuria and peripheral vascular collapse in severe cases. Since only the older population of RBC is rapidly destroyed, the hemolytic crisis is usually self-limited, even if the exposure to the oxidant continues. Among black males with the A− variant, the RBC mass decreases by a maximum of 25 to 30%. The oxidation of hemoglobin leads to the formation of Heinz bodies, visualized by means of a supravital stain such as crystal violet. However, Heinz bodies are usually not seen after the first day or so, since these inclusions are readily removed by the spleen. Their removal leads to the formation of "bite cells" (RBC that have lost a peripheral portion of the cell). Multiple bites cause the formation of fragments. A few spherocytes also may be present. Individuals with the Mediterranean type G6PD have much lower overall enzyme activity than those with the A− variant and, therefore, have more severe clinical manifestations. A minority of patients are exquisitely sensitive to fava beans and develop a fulminant hemolytic crisis after exposure. The oxidants in *Vicia fava* are two β-glycosides whose aglycones, when autooxidized, produce oxygen free radicals. The incidence of favism is highly variable due to variations in concentration, in absorption, or in metabolism of the aglycones. Favism is seldom encountered in individuals with the A− variant.

The *diagnosis* of G6PD deficiency should be considered in any individual, particularly a male of African or Mediterranean descent,

who experiences an acute hemolytic episode. The patient should be questioned about possible exposure to oxidant agents. The diagnosis can be established by a number of tests that assess either the enzyme activity or the effects of its deficiency. However, the test may yield a false-negative result during a hemolytic episode when the old RBC deficient in the enzyme have already lysed.

℞ TREATMENT

Since hemolysis in patients deficient in A− G6PD is usually self-limited, no specific treatment is necessary. Splenectomy does not benefit Mediterranean patients with chronic hemolysis. Blood transfusions are rarely indicated. Adequate urine flow should be maintained if hemoglobinuria develops during an acute hemolytic episode.

Hemolytic episodes can be prevented by warning patients about risks posed by oxidant drugs and fava beans and by prompt treatment of infections.

Other Defects of the Hexose-Monophosphate Shunt   A few kindreds have been found to have congenital deficiency in RBC glutathione due to a defect in either of the two enzymes responsible for the synthesis of this tripeptide. Affected individuals have a hemolytic anemia with Heinz bodies that is aggravated by oxidant drugs.

OTHER ENZYME DEFECTS   Hemolytic anemia may sometimes be caused by abnormalities in enzymes of nucleotide metabolism. Individuals with pyrimidine 5′-nucleotidase deficiency have marked coarse basophilic stippling in their RBC because the mRNA of the cell is not properly metabolized. Hemolytic anemia also has been noted in individuals whose RBC have supranormal levels of adenosine deaminase and relatively low levels of ATP.

Hemoglobinopathies   Hemolysis is a component of anemias related to some hemoglobinopathies (Chap. 91).

ACQUIRED HEMOLYTIC ANEMIAS   In most patients with acquired hemolytic anemia, RBC are made normally but are prematurely destroyed because of damage acquired in the circulation. (The exceptions are rare disorders characterized by acquired dysplasia of the cells of the bone marrow and the production of structurally and functionally abnormal RBC.) The damage that occurs may be mediated by antibodies or toxins or may be due to abnormalities in the circulation, including an overactive mononuclear phagocyte system or traumatic lysis by natural or artificial impediments to circulation. The acquired hemolytic anemias are classified into five categories (Table 93-5).

TABLE 93-5   *Causes of Acquired Hemolytic Anemia*
I. Entrapment
II. Immune
A. Warm-reactive (IgG) antibody
B. Cold-reactive IgM antibody (cold agglutinin disease)
C. Cold-reactive IgG antibody (paroxysmal cold hemoglobinuria)
D. Drug-dependent antibody
1. Autoimmune
2. Haptene
III. Traumatic hemolytic anemia
A. Impact hemolysis
B. Macrovascular defects—prostheses
C. Microvascular causes
1. Thrombotic thrombocytopenic purpura/hemolytic-uremic syndrome
2. Other causes of microvascular abnormalities
3. Disseminated intravascular hemolysis
IV. Hemolytic anemia due to toxic effects on the membrane
A. Spur cell anemia
B. External toxins
1. Animal or spider bites
2. Metals (e.g., copper)
3. Organic compounds
V. Paroxysmal nocturnal hemoglobinuria

TABLE 93-4   *Drugs Causing Hemolysis in Subjects Deficient in G6PD*
Antimalarials: Primaquine, pamaquine, dapsone
Sulfonamides: Sulfamethoxazole
Nitrofurantoin
Analgesics: Acetanilid
Miscellaneous: Vitamin K (water-soluble form), doxorubicin, methylene blue, nalidixic acid, furazolidone, niridazole, phenazopyridine

Hypersplenism The spleen is particularly efficient in trapping and destroying RBC that have minimal defects. This unique ability of the spleen to filter mildly damaged RBC results from its unusual vascular anatomy (Chap. 54). Almost all the blood circulating through the spleen flows rapidly from arterioles in the white pulp to sinuses in the spleen's red pulp and then into the venous system. In contrast, a small portion of splenic blood flow (normally 1 to 2%) passes into the "marginal zone" of the lymphatic white pulp. Although the cells that occupy this zone are not phagocytic, they serve as a mechanical filter that hinders the progress of severely damaged blood cells. As RBC leave this zone and enter the red pulp, they flow into narrow cords, rich in macrophages, that end blindly but communicate with sinuses through small openings between the lining cells of the sinuses. These openings, averaging 3 μm in diameter, test the ability of RBC (4.5 μm in diameter) to undergo deformation. RBC that cannot re-enter the vascular sinuses are engulfed by phagocytic cells and destroyed (see Fig. 54-1).

The normal spleen retains reticulocytes for 1 to 2 days but otherwise poses no threat to normal RBC until they become senescent. However, in the face of splenomegaly, increased destruction of the cells of the blood, including the RBC, may take place due to pooling of the blood in a relatively nutrient-poor environment full of phagocytic cells. Splenic sequestration that causes cytopenia is called hypersplenism. In infiltrative diseases of the spleen, substantial splenomegaly may exist with no apparent hemolysis; inflammatory and congestive splenomegaly is commonly associated with modest shortening of RBC survival time, along with more marked granulocytopenia and thrombocytopenia. Patients with cytopenia(s) sufficient to produce symptoms generally benefit from splenectomy.

Immunologic Causes of Hemolysis Immune hemolysis in the adult is usually induced by IgG or IgM antibodies reacting specifically with antigens associated with the patient's RBC (often called "autoantibodies") or with alloantigens on transfused RBC (alloantibodies) (Chap. 99).

The Coombs antiglobulin test is the major tool for diagnosing autoimmune hemolysis. This test relies on the ability of antibodies specific for immunoglobulins (especially IgG) or complement components (especially C3) to agglutinate RBC coated with these proteins. With specific anti-IgG and anti-C3, the *direct Coombs test* detects IgG or C3 on the patient's RBC, which indicates the presence of immune hemolysis and may help define its cause (Table 93-6). Rarely, neither IgG nor complement may be found on the RBC of the patient (Coombs-negative immune hemolytic anemia).

Antibodies in the serum of the patient that recognize RBC antigens can be detected by reacting the serum with normal RBC bearing the antigen. With the exception of cold-reacting antibodies and some drug-related antibodies (see below), this is of value primarily in compatibility testing for transfusion.

"WARM" ANTIBODIES Antibodies that react at body temperature (warm antibodies) are nearly always IgG, rarely IgM or IgA. Autologous warm antibodies cause *autoimmune hemolytic (or immunohemolytic) anemia, warm antibody type.*

Clinical Manifestations Immunohemolytic anemia of the warm antibody type occurs at all ages, but it is more common in adults, particularly women. In approximately one-fourth of patients this disorder occurs as a complication of an underlying disease affecting the immune system, especially lymphoid neoplasms (Chap. 97); collagen vascular diseases, especially systemic lupus erythematosus (SLE); and congenital immunodeficiency diseases (Table 93-7). A wide variety of drugs may stimulate antibody formation, resulting in a similar syndrome (see below).

The presentation and course of IgG immunohemolytic anemia are quite variable. In its mildest form, the only manifestation is a positive direct Coombs test. In this instance, insufficient antibody is present on the RBC surface to permit the reticuloendothelial system to recognize

TABLE 93-6 *Use of the Direct Coombs Test in Diagnosing the Cause of Autoimmune Hemolytic Anemia*

Reaction with		
Anti-IgG	Anti-C3	Causes
Yes	No	Antibodies to Rh proteins, hemolysis caused by α-methyldopa or penicillin
Yes	Yes	Antibodies to glycoprotein antigens, SLE
No	Yes	Cold-reacting antibodies (agglutinins or Donath-Landsteiner antibody), most drug-related antibodies, IgM antibodies, IgG antibodies of low affinity, activation of complement by immune complexes

the cell as abnormal. Most symptomatic patients have a moderate to severe anemia [hemoglobin levels 60 to 100 g/L and reticulocyte counts 10 to 30% (200 to 600 × 10³/μL)], spherocytosis (Fig. 93-5), and splenomegaly. Occasionally, venous thrombosis occurs.

Severe immunohemolytic anemia presents with fulminant hemolysis associated with hemoglobinemia, hemoglobinuria, and shock; this syndrome may be rapidly fatal unless aggressively treated.

The direct Coombs test is positive in 98% of patients; usually IgG is detected with or without C3. The pattern of IgG and C3 fixation on the patient's RBC may indicate the origin of the disorder.

Immune thrombocytopenia also may be present (*Evans syndrome*), a disorder in which separate antibodies are directed against platelets and RBC.

Pathogenesis IgG antibodies lyse RBC by two mechanisms: (1) immune adherence of RBC to phagocytes mediated by the antibody and by complement components that become fixed to the membrane (by far the more important mechanism of destruction), and (2) complement activation. IgG antibodies bind to Fc receptors on macrophages, activating those cells to engulf the coated RBC. If internalization is only partial, a portion of the RBC membrane is removed, resulting in the formation of spherocytes, which are destroyed in the spleen. Complement-mediated immune adherence involves the interaction of C3b and C4b with receptors on the macrophage; while much less likely to lead to RBC lysis, this mechanism markedly increases the immune adherence due to IgG. Immune adherence, particularly that due to the IgG antibody, is also enhanced by the transit of RBC into splenic cords and sinuses, which brings cells into direct contact with phagocytic cells.

℞ TREATMENT

Patients having a mild degree of hemolysis usually do not require therapy. In those with clinically significant hemolysis, initial therapy consists of glucocorticoids (e.g., prednisone, 1.0 mg/kg per day). A rise in hemoglobin is frequently noted within 3 or 4 days and occurs

TABLE 93-7 *Hemolysis due to Antibodies*

WARM-ANTIBODY IMMUNOHEMOLYTIC ANEMIA

1. Idiopathic
2. Lymphomas: Chronic lymphocytic leukemia, non-Hodgkin's lymphomas, Hodgkin's disease (infrequent)
3. SLE and other collagen-vascular diseases
4. Drugs
   a. α-Methyldopa type (autoantibody to Rh antigens)
   b. Penicillin type (stable hapten)
   c. Quinidine type (unstable hapten)
5. Postviral infections
6. Other tumors (rare)

COLD-ANTIBODY IMMUNOHEMOLYTIC ANEMIA

1. Cold agglutinin disease
   a. Acute: *Mycoplasma* infection, infectious mononucleosis
   b. Chronic: Idiopathic, lymphoma
2. Paroxysmal cold hemoglobinuria

FIGURE 93-5 *Immunohemolytic anemia* Microspherocytes are seen on this blood smear along with several macrocytes with a slight purple tinge (polychromasia). The latter represent new red blood cells released early from the bone marrow. The microspherocytes seen in immunohemolytic anemia may be indistinguishable from the microspherocytes seen in hereditary spherocytosis (Fig. 93-1).

in most patients within 1 to 2 weeks. Prednisone is continued until the hemoglobin level has risen to normal values, and thereafter it is tapered rapidly to about 20 mg/d, then slowly over the course of several months. An algorithm for this tapering process is given in Fig. 93-6. For chronic therapy with prednisone, alternate-day administration is preferred. More than 75% of patients achieve an initial significant and sustained reduction in hemolysis; however, in half these patients the disease recurs, either during glucocorticoid tapering or after its cessation. Glucocorticoids have two modes of action: an immediate effect due to inhibiting clearance of IgG-coated RBC by the mononuclear phagocyte system and a later effect due to inhibiting antibody synthesis. Splenectomy is recommended for patients who cannot tolerate or fail to respond to glucocorticoid therapy.

Patients who have been refractory to glucocorticoid therapy and to splenectomy are treated with immunosuppressive drugs. A success rate of ~50% has been reported. Intravenous gamma globulin may cause rapid cessation of hemolysis; however, it is not nearly as effective in this disorder as in immune thrombocytopenia.

Patients with severe anemia may require blood transfusions. Because the antibody in this disease is usually a "panagglutinin," reacting with nearly all normal donor cells, compatible cross-matching is impossible. The goal in selecting blood for transfusion is to avoid administering RBC with antigens to which the patient may have alloantibodies. A common procedure is to adsorb the panagglutinin

FIGURE 93-6 Algorithm for the treatment of patients with IgG-mediated immune hemolytic anemia. The patient with minimal disease may be watched carefully. The patient with very severe disease may need all modalities of treatment applied at once. The more common patient with moderate disease may be treated with prednisone at a high dose; if no response is seen, then either splenectomy is performed or an immunosuppressive agent is given. If a response is seen, the dose of prednisone is reduced over time. If relapse occurs during this process, splenectomy or chemotherapy may be needed.

present in the patient's serum with the patient's own RBC from which antibody has been previously eluted. Serum cleared of autoantibody can then be tested for the presence of alloantibody to donor blood groups. ABO-compatible RBC matched in this fashion are administered slowly, with watchfulness for signs of an immediate-type hemolytic transfusion reaction.

Prognosis Immune hemolytic anemia is often transient in children, particularly when it follows a viral infection, but is usually chronic in adults, lasting many years with exacerbations and remissions. In most patients, hemolysis is controlled by glucocorticoid therapy alone, by splenectomy, or by a combination. Fatalities occur among three rare subsets of patients: (1) those with overwhelming hemolysis who die from anemia; (2) those whose host defenses are impaired by glucocorticoids, splenectomy, and/or immunosuppressive agents; and (3) those with major thrombotic events coincident with active hemolysis.

When immunohemolysis develops as a complication of an underlying disorder, the prognosis is often determined by the primary disease.

IMMUNOHEMOLYTIC ANEMIA SECONDARY TO DRUGS Drugs cause immunohemolytic anemia by two mechanisms of action: (1) they induce a disorder identical in almost every respect to warm-antibody immunohemolytic anemia [e.g., α-methyldopa (an antihypertensive; Chap. 230)], or (2) they become associated as haptens with the RBC surface and induce the formation of an antibody directed against the RBC-drug complex (e.g., penicillin, quinidine).

A positive direct Coombs test is observed in up to 10% of patients receiving α-methyldopa therapy in doses of 2 g/d or higher. A small minority of these patients develop spherocytosis and hemolysis, which may be severe. The autoantibodies cross-react with the normal Rh protein.

In most other cases of drug-induced hemolysis, the antibody is directed against the combination of the drug and the membrane glycoprotein to which it is attached. The hemolytic reaction in vivo is dependent on the presence of the drug and usually ceases shortly after the drug has been discontinued. Penicillin and its congeners may cause this type of reaction if the drug is given in very high doses (10 million units per day or more). The direct Coombs test is positive only with anti-IgG; the indirect Coombs test is positive only when the normal cells have been coated with penicillin. Complement is not usually fixed, and the hemolysis in vivo is usually not severe. Since the antibody is usually IgG, spherocytosis and splenic destruction may occur.

Most other drugs (such as quinine, quinidine, sulfonamides, sulfonureas, phenacetin, stibophen, and dipyrone) do not adhere as tightly to their glycoproteins, and the drug-antibody complexes are removed during the washing steps of the direct and indirect Coombs reactions. These antibodies (particularly IgM) are usually able to fix complement, and C3d and C4d remain on the RBC surface; thus the direct Coombs test is positive with anti-C3 but not anti-IgG. The antibody is detected in the *indirect* Coombs test only when the drug is added to the incubation mixture. Hemolysis may be quite severe, sometimes resulting in signs of intravascular hemolysis; resolution is usually prompt after the drug is discontinued.

IMMUNE HEMOLYSIS DUE TO COLD-REACTIVE ANTIBODIES Antibodies that react with polysaccharide antigens are usually IgM and bind antigen better at temperatures lower than 37°C, hence the name *cold-reactive antibodies*. Uncommonly, the antibody is IgG (the Donath-Landsteiner antibody of paroxysmal cold hemoglobinuria).

IgM cold-reacting antibodies readily agglutinate RBC and are called *cold agglutinins*. They arise in two clinical settings: (1) monoclonal antibodies, the product of lymphocytic neoplasia or paraneoplasia; and (2) polyclonal antibodies in response to infection. In many elderly patients, the "neoplasm" is benign monoclonal gammopathy that does not progress, and the paraprotein remains its only manifestation. Occasionally, cold agglutinins are found in patients with non-lymphoid neoplasms.

Transient cold agglutinins occur commonly in two infections: *Mycoplasma pneumoniae* infection and infectious mononucleosis. In both, the titer of antibody is usually too low to cause clinical symptoms, but its presence is of diagnostic value; only occasionally is hemolysis present. Cold agglutinins are less frequently encountered in a number of other viral infections. Their manifestations are usually benign.

The specificity of the antibody may be of diagnostic value. Cold agglutinins reacting more strongly with adult RBC than fetal (cord) RBC are called *anti-I*; these antibodies are seen in benign lymphoproliferation (chronic cold agglutinin monoclonal gammopathy) and in Mycoplasma infections. Those reacting more strongly with cord RBC cells are called *anti-i*; these antibodies are seen in aggressive lymphomas and in infectious mononucleosis. Rarely, the antibody may react with other antigens that are equally expressed on adult and cord RBC. The clinical manifestations elicited by the antibody on exposure to cold are of two sorts: intravascular agglutination (acrocyanosis) and hemolysis. Acrocyanosis is the marked purpling of the extremities, ears, and nose when the blood becomes cold enough to agglutinate in the veins; it clears on warming and does not have the vasospastic characteristics of Raynaud's phenomenon (Chap. 232). Patients may also have symptoms when swallowing cold food or drinks.

The hemolysis is usually not severe and is manifested by a mild reticulocytosis, agglutination on the blood film, and agglutination during analysis of the blood by particle analysis (giving rise to a falsely high mean corpuscular volume). The degree of hemolysis depends on several variables.

1. *Antibody titer.* The titer in symptomatic patients is usually above 1:2000 dilution of serum and may range to as high as 1:50,000. When collecting samples, great care must be taken to keep the serum separated from the cells while the sample is maintained at 37°C so that the antibody will not adsorb onto the patient's own cells.
2. *Thermal amplitude of the antibody* (the highest temperature at which the antibody will react with the RBC). For most antibodies, this is 23 to 30°C. Those with a higher thermal amplitude (up to 37°C) are more hemolytic, since it is more likely that these temperatures will be encountered during RBC circulation.
3. *Environmental temperature.* Since the reaction can occur only at temperatures below body temperature, frequency and degree of exposure to cold are major determinants of the rate of hemolysis.

The hemolysis that occurs is due primarily to the hemolytic action of complement, since there are no functional Fc receptors for the IgM antibody on phagocytes. Complement is readily fixed; a single molecule of IgM is enough to effect binding of C1 and initiate the cascade. However, normal human RBC are remarkably resistant to the hemolytic action of complement because of several defense mechanisms. Therefore, severe hemolysis with hemoglobinuria occurs only with massive activation of the antibody, such as by sudden cooling. The activation of complement is always marked by the accumulation of a degradation product of C3, C3dg, on the surface; this product is what is detected with appropriate antisera in the direct Coombs test in all patients with significant cold agglutinin disease.

The cutaneous manifestations are best treated by maintaining the patient in a warm environment. Splenectomy is usually not of value in this disorder. Glucocorticoids are of limited value, although patients with the panthermal variety of cold agglutinin disease may respond. Chlorambucil and cyclophosphamide are commonly used to treat patients who have hemolysis associated with monoclonal gammopathy, but their efficacy is usually marginal. Rituximab (anti-CD20) has been effective in some cases. Successful treatment of the neoplasm responsible for the cold agglutinin often lowers the antibody titer and the severity of hemolysis.

Chronic cold agglutinin disease tends to be unremitting. The overall prognosis is dominated by the underlying lymphoma, if present. In those patients in whom cold agglutinin disease appears to arise spontaneously, malignant lymphoma may develop after several years.

PAROXYSMAL COLD HEMOGLOBINURIA (PCH) Now a rare disorder, PCH was more frequent when tertiary syphilis was prevalent; now, most cases are either secondary to a viral infection or are autoimmune. PCH results from the formation of the Donath-Landsteiner antibody, an IgG antibody that is directed against the P antigen (Chap. 99) and that can induce complement-mediated lysis. Attacks are precipitated by exposure to cold and are associated with hemoglobinemia and hemoglobinuria; chills and fever; back, leg, and abdominal pain; headache; and malaise. Recovery from the acute episode is prompt, and between episodes patients are usually asymptomatic. When this syndrome accompanies acute viral infections (e.g., measles and mumps in children), it is self-limited but may be severe. Although the direct Coombs test may show complement to be present (seldom IgG), this test may be negative. The diagnosis is made by demonstrating cold-reacting IgG antibodies either by lytic tests (when the titer is very high) or by special antiglobulin tests. When PCH is secondary to syphilis, it responds to therapy for syphilis. Chronic autoimmune PCH may respond to prednisone or cytotoxic therapy (azathioprine or cyclophosphamide) but does not respond to splenectomy. The natural history of this disease often extends over many years.

Hemolysis Due to Trauma in the Circulation RBC may be fragmented by mechanical trauma as they circulate; this circumstance leads to intravascular hemolysis and in most cases to RBC fragments called *schistocytes*. Schistocytes are identified by the sharp points that result from the faulty resealing of the fractured membrane (Fig. 93-7). Mechanical trauma leading to hemolysis occurs in three clinical settings: (1) when RBC flow through small vessels over the surface of bony prominences and are subject to external impact during various physical activities, (2) when RBC flow across a pressure gradient created by an abnormal heart valve or valve prosthesis (macrovascular), and (3) when the deposition of fibrin or small platelet thrombi in the microvasculature exposes RBC to a physical impediment that fragments them (microvascular) (Table 93-8).

EXTERNAL IMPACT Hemoglobinemia and hemoglobinuria have been observed in a small proportion of individuals who have undergone a prolonged march or a prolonged run, most typically on a hard surface and while wearing thin-soled shoes. Hemolysis can be prevented by the insertion of a soft inner sole in the runner's shoes. No abnormality of RBC has been demonstrated, even during the acute episode.

MACROVASCULAR TRAUMATIC HEMOLYSIS Hemolysis associated with fragmented RBC (Fig. 93-7) occurs in approximately 10% of patients with artificial aortic valve prostheses. In contrast, traumatic hemolysis is rare in recipients of porcine valves. Severe hemolysis may occur after repair of ostium primum or endocardial cushion defects with a prosthetic patch. Mitral valve prostheses may produce hemolysis, but since the pressure gradient across these valves is lower than across aortic prostheses, the incidence is lower. A moderately shortened RBC survival time with little or no anemia occurs in some patients with severe calcific aortic stenosis. Indeed, almost any intracardiac lesion that alters hemodynamics may lead to some shortening of RBC survival. Traumatic hemolysis has been observed in patients who have undergone aortofemoral bypass.

FIGURE 93-7 The helmet-shaped red blood cell and the small triangular-shaped red blood cells seen on this smear represent morphologic evidence of mechanical damage to red blood cells within the blood vessels.

Etiology	Fragments	Hemolysis	Thrombocytopenia
Impact: march hemoglobinuria, etc.	0	+	0
Cardiac (turbulence):			
Aortic valve prosthesis	++++	++++	0
Mitral valve prosthesis	++	++	0
Calcific aortic stenosis	+	±	0
Vessel disease[a]	+++	+	+
Thrombotic thrombocytopenic purpura	++++	++++	++++
Hemolytic-uremic syndrome	++++	++++	++++
Adenocarcinoma	++++	++++	++++
Disseminated intravascular coagulation	++	±	++++

[a] Malignant hypertension, eclampsia, renal graft rejection, hemangiomas, immune disease (scleroderma).

Clinical Manifestations In severe cases, hemoglobin levels fall to 50 to 70 g/L with reticulocytosis, fragmented RBC in the peripheral blood, depressed haptoglobin, elevated serum LDH, and hemoglobinemia and hemoglobinuria. Iron loss (as hemoglobin or hemosiderin) in the urine may lead to iron deficiency. The direct Coombs test may rarely become positive.

℞ TREATMENT

Iron deficiency should be corrected by the administration of oral iron. The elevated hemoglobin that results may permit a decrease in the cardiac output and a slowing of the hemolytic rate. Limitation in physical activity also lessens the hemolytic rate. When these measures fail, any paravalvular leak must be repaired or the prosthetic valve replaced.

MICROVASCULAR TRAUMATIC HEMOLYSIS If fibrin or platelet microthrombi are deposited in arteriolar sites, RBC may be trapped on the meshwork and fragmented by high shear forces.

Abnormalities of the Vessel Wall Disorders such as malignant hypertension, eclampsia [hemolysis, elevated liver enzymes, low platelets (HELLP) syndrome], renal allograft rejection, disseminated cancer, hemangiomas, or disseminated intravascular coagulation (DIC) may cause traumatic hemolysis (Chaps. 101, 102). The degree of hemolysis induced by this family of disorders is usually quite mild, but a large number of fragments may be seen in the peripheral blood. In some patients, thrombocytopenia may be severe. Therapy is best directed at the primary disease. Thus, reversal of renal graft rejection, treatment of malignant hypertension and eclampsia, control of cancer, and the like lead to a cessation of hemolysis. The relative importance of the primary vascular abnormality versus fibrin deposition is unclear.

THROMBOTIC THROMBOCYTOPENIA PURPURA (TTP) This disorder is characterized by arteriolar lesions in various organs that contain platelet thrombi and produce thrombocytopenia and hemolytic anemia due to fragmentation of RBC (see Chap. 101).

HEMOLYTIC-UREMIC SYNDROME This disorder is similar to TTP and is characterized by the same arteriolar lesions, which may be confined to the kidney, and by similar laboratory findings (see Chap. 101).

DISSEMINATED INTRAVASCULAR COAGULATION Inappropriate activation of the clotting system with deposition of fibrin in small vessels may lead to RBC fragmentation in the microvasculature. RBC fragmentation occurs in about one-fourth of patients with DIC (Chap. 102). The degree of hemolysis is much less in DIC than in either TTP or the hemolytic-uremic syndrome, and anemia with reticulocytosis is rare.

Environmental Alteration of the Red Cell Membrane by "Toxic" Effects A variety of infections may be associated with severe hemolysis. The microbes that cause bartonellosis (Chap. 144), as well as malaria and babesiosis (Chap. 195), directly parasitize RBC. *Clostridium welchii* (Chap. 126) produces a phospholipase that can cleave the phosphoryl bond of lecithin, thereby lysing human RBC. A mild, transient hemolysis frequently accompanies bacteremia with diverse organisms such as pneumococci, staphylococci, and *Escherichia coli*.

Hemolysis may result from the direct action of snake and spider venoms on the RBC. Although cobra venom is directly lytic in vitro, the clinical disease induced by the bite of the cobra is one of moderate hemolysis associated with spherocytosis. Spider bites, particularly the bite of the brown recluse spider, induce acute intravascular hemolysis associated with spherocytosis and fragments of complement components on the RBC. The hemolysis continues for several days up to 1 week.

Copper has a direct hemolytic effect on RBC. Hemolysis has been observed after exposure of individuals to copper salts (such as during hemodialysis). Transient episodes of hemolysis occur in patients with Wilson's disease (Chap. 339).

The RBC membrane is unstable at temperatures above 49°C due to denaturation of the cytoskeletal protein spectrin. The RBC undergoes a process of budding, cleavage, and resealing above this temperature. Patients with extensive burns have prominent spherocytosis, hemoglobinemia, and sometimes hemoglobinuria.

Spur Cell Anemia Hemolytic anemia with bizarre-shaped RBC occurs in about 5% of patients with severe hepatocellular disease, particularly advanced Laennec's cirrhosis.

Clinical Manifestations Anemia is more severe than that observed in otherwise uncomplicated cirrhosis. Splenomegaly is always present and is greater than in patients who have cirrhosis without spur cell anemia. The RBC are irregularly shaped with multiple spicules, and a small number of bizarre-shaped fragments are commonly seen on peripheral blood smears (see Fig. 98-3).

Pathogenesis The surface membrane of a spur cell contains 50 to 70% excess cholesterol, but its total phospholipid content is normal. Cholesterol out of proportion to phospholipid decreases the membrane fluidity and cell deformability. These rigid, cholesterol-laden RBC cannot pass through the filtering system of the spleen, further impeded by congestive splenomegaly in cirrhosis. In contrast, the target-shaped RBC is more common in liver disease and has an excess of both cholesterol and phospholipid.

Diagnosis Patients with spur cell anemia have severe hemolysis and characteristic RBC morphology. Spur cells or acanthocytes have irregular spikes (irregular in length of projections and their spacing) and must be distinguished from regularly spaced, crenated RBC (echinocytes). Echinocytes are a frequent artifact on portions of some blood smears, and they are uniformly present in some patients with uremia ("burr cells") (Fig. 93-8). Small, dense, crenated spheres (spheroechinocytes) are sometimes seen in congenital nonspherocytic hemolytic anemia due to enzyme deficiencies in the Embden-Meyerhof pathway (see above). RBC of similar morphology are seen in patients with abetalipoproteinemia. However, hemolysis is minimal.

℞ TREATMENT

Transfusion therapy is of limited benefit. Lipid-lowering agents have been unsuccessful. Splenectomy has been reported to prevent both the

FIGURE 93-8 The red blood cells in uremia may acquire numerous, regularly spaced, small spiny projections. Such cells, called burr cells or echinocytes, are readily distinguishable from irregularly spiculated acanthocytes or spur cells.

conditioning of RBC in the spleen and their premature destruction. However, splenectomy carries a high risk in patients with severe liver disease complicated by portal hypertension and coagulation defects. It must be reserved for patients in whom hemolysis is a major problem and who are relatively good surgical risks.

Prognosis Spur cell anemia occurs during the late stages of cirrhosis, and >90% of patients succumb to their underlying liver disease within 1 year of the diagnosis of spur cell anemia.

Paroxysmal Nocturnal Hemoglobinuria (PNH) This hemolytic disorder is distinctive because it is an intracorpuscular defect acquired at the stem cell level.

Clinical Manifestations The three common manifestations of PNH are hemolytic anemia, venous thrombosis, and deficient hematopoiesis. Anemia is highly variable, with hematocrit values ranging from ≤20% to normal. RBC are normochromic and normocytic unless iron deficiency has occurred from chronic iron loss in the urine.

Clinical hemoglobinuria is intermittent in most patients and never occurs in some, but hemosiderinuria is usually present. Since hemolysis is due to abnormalities of the RBC leading to sensitivity to the hemolytic action of complement, it is manifest when complement is activated, for example, by infection.

Granulocytopenia and thrombocytopenia are common and reflect impaired hematopoiesis. The life span of the platelet is normal. However, the activation of complement indirectly stimulates platelet aggregation and hypercoagulability; this probably accounts for the tendency toward thrombosis seen in PNH.

Venous thrombosis is a common complication of patients of European origin, affecting ~40% at one time or another; it is less common in Asian patients. It occurs primarily in intra-abdominal veins (hepatic, portal, mesenteric) and results in Budd-Chiari syndrome, congestive splenomegaly, and abdominal pain. It may occur in cerebral venous sinuses and is a common cause of death in patients with PNH.

The bone marrow may appear normocellular, but in vitro marrow progenitor assays are abnormal. In about 15 to 30% of long-term survivors of aplastic anemia, PNH cells appear in the circulation; in some patients, the manifestations of PNH become dominant. Patients with PNH may have aplastic periods lasting from weeks to years. PNH may be seen in association with other stem cell disorders, including myelofibrosis and (rarely) other myelodysplastic or myeloproliferative disorders.

Pathogenesis PNH is an acquired clonal disease, arising from an inactivating somatic mutation in a single hematopoietic stem cell of a gene on the X-chromosome (*pig-A*) necessary for the biosynthesis of the glycosylphosphatidylinositol (GPI) anchor. This anchor attaches a number of proteins to the external membrane surface, and its partial or complete absence results in the absence of those proteins; to date, about 20 proteins have been found to be missing on the blood cells of patients with PNH. Two of these are the complement defense proteins CD55 [PNH decay accelerating factor (DAF)] and CD59, which block complement activation on the cell surface. Their absence accounts for the sensitivity of RBC to complement lysis and for the tendency of platelets to abnormally initiate clotting. The normal clones of stem cells do not completely disappear, and the proportion of cells that are abnormal varies among patients and over time in a single patient.

Diagnosis PNH should be suspected in anyone with otherwise unexplained hemolytic anemia, especially with leukopenia and/or thrombocytopenia and with evidence of intravascular hemolysis (hemoglobinemia, hemoglobinuria, hemosiderinuria, elevated LDH). Anyone recovering from aplastic anemia should be examined at intervals for the appearance of the diagnostic cells. The diagnosis is often delayed because (1) it is not considered, (2) hemoglobinuria is confused with hematuria, (3) elevation of the LDH is attributed to liver disease, and (4) the diagnostic tests [the acidified serum lysis test (Ham test) and the sucrose lysis test] are not reliable.

For many years, the diagnosis of PNH depended on the demonstration of the lysis of RBC after complement activation either by acid (Ham test) or by reduction in ionic strength (sucrose lysis test). These tests are inferior to the analysis of GPI-linked proteins (e.g., CD59, DAF) on RBC and granulocytes by flow cytometry.

Rx TREATMENT

Transfusion therapy is useful in PNH not only for raising the hemoglobin level but also for suppressing the marrow production of RBC during episodes of sustained hemoglobinuria. Washed RBC are the preferred source to prevent exacerbation of hemolysis. Therapy with androgens sometimes results in a rise in hemoglobin level. Glucocorticoids reduce the rate of hemolysis in moderate doses (15 to 30 mg prednisone) on alternate days.

Iron deficiency is common. Iron replacement may exacerbate hemolysis because of the formation of many new RBC, which may be sensitive to complement. This occurrence may be minimized by giving prednisone (60 mg/d) or by suppressing the bone marrow with transfusions.

Acute thrombosis in PNH, particularly Budd-Chiari syndrome and cerebral thrombosis, should be treated with thrombolytic agents. Heparin therapy should be instituted rapidly and maintained using low-molecular-weight heparin, at least for several weeks to months and perhaps indefinitely in severe cases. Anyone who has had a major thrombosis should chronically receive at least warfarin therapy. Antithymocyte globulin (total dose, 150 mg/kg over 4 to 10 days) is often of use in treating marrow hypoplasia; prednisone counteracts the immune-complex disease that results from the administration of this foreign protein.

In patients with either hypoplasia or thrombosis who have an appropriate sibling donor, marrow transplantation should be considered early in the course of the disease. The usual conditioning programs are sufficient to eradicate the aberrant clone.

ANEMIA OF ACUTE BLOOD LOSS

The normal capacity to compensate for acute blood loss involves cardiovascular mechanisms, an adjustment in the oxygen affinity of hemoglobin, and an increase in erythropoiesis in the marrow. The signs and symptoms of blood loss relate to the volume of the blood loss and the time frame over which the hemorrhage occurs (Table 93-9). Losses of up to 20% of the blood volume are normally tolerated by redistribution of blood flow mediated by reflex venospasm, but the presence of fever or pain may interfere with this compensation. With larger losses, blood volume redistribution is not adequate to maintain normal blood pressure: initially, hypotension is only seen on standing, but with greater losses the patient has hypotension in sitting or supine positions. If the blood loss is more gradual, plasma volume increases, but albumin production usually lags behind the fluid shifts. It may take 2 to 3 days for the liver to generate the albumin lost in a 1500-mL bleed.

TABLE 93-9 *Signs and Symptoms of Acute Blood Loss*

Blood Loss			
%,[a]	Volume, mL	Symptoms	Signs
<20	<1000	Restlessness	+/− Vasovagal reaction
20–30	1000–1500	Anxiety, DOE	Orthostatic hypotension, tachycardia on exertion
30–40	1500–2000	Syncope on sitting or standing	Orthostatic hypotension, tachycardia at rest
>40	>2000	Confusion, shortness of breath	Shock, poor perfusion

[a] Based on an estimated total blood volume of 5000 mL (70-kg adult).

The most rapid hematologic adjustment to acute blood loss is an increase in oxygen delivery to the tissues. This is first mediated by the Bohr effect, in which the more acidic milieu of the hypoperfused hypoxic tissues shifts the hemoglobin-oxygen dissociation curve to the right. Over several hours the RBC increase their production of 2,3-bisphosphoglycerate, which also enhances the unloading of oxygen to tissues. These two mechanisms can substantially increase the capacity of RBC to deliver oxygen to the tissues.

The marrow response to hemorrhage is related to the erythropoietin response to decreased oxygen tension. A normal response depends on the production of erythropoietin, the presence of normal erythroid progenitors in the marrow, and an adequate supply of iron. If these three elements are normal, reticulocytes begin to increase in the first 2 days based on early release of reticulocytes from the marrow. However, it takes 3 to 6 days for erythroid hyperplasia to appear and 7 to 10 days before the erythropoietic response is maximal, producing reticulocyte counts up to 20 to 30%, a reticulocyte index of ≥ 3, and a marked increase in the marrow erythroid/granulocytic ratio.

DIAGNOSIS Usually it is clear that a patient is bleeding; however, in some cases, large volumes of blood loss can occur internally from the gastrointestinal tract (esophageal varices, cancer in the stomach or colon), a ruptured spleen, fractures and other trauma, or other lesions that can cause massive hemorrhage into the peritoneal cavity, the pleural cavity, or the retroperitoneal space. Patients who have bled sufficiently to develop hypotension generally develop anemia, which is apparent only after volume replacement. The granulocyte count may increase to $\geq 20,000$ cells/μL and include immature cell types such as

metamyelocytes and myelocytes. Epinephrine-induced demargination of peripheral granulocytes and release of cells from the marrow may account for this change. Nucleated RBC may appear in the circulation, and platelet counts may exceed $1 \times 10^6/\mu$L. The basis for the increased platelet count is unclear. Hemorrhage in an internal cavity is accompanied by a rise in unconjugated bilirubin and a fall in serum haptoglobin.

Rx TREATMENT

Treatment of the underlying cause of the hemorrhage is of paramount importance. If the patient is severely anemic or sufficiently hypovolemic, packed RBC should be transfused. In less severe cases, if the patient has normal kidneys (and presumably a normal erythropoietin response to anemia), normal bone marrow function, and an adequate supply of iron, no specific therapy for the anemia is required.

FURTHER READING

AMIDON TM et al: Mitral and aortic paravalvular leaks with hemolytic anemia. Am Heart J 125:266, 1993

GARRATY G, PETZ LD: Approaches to selecting blood for transfusion to patients with autoimmune hemolytic anemia. Transfusion 42:1390, 2002

MAURO FR et al: Autoimmune hemolytic anemia in chronic lymphocytic leukemia: Clinical, therapeutic, and prognostic features. Blood 95:2786, 2000

PRUSS A et al: Immune hemolysis-serological and clinical aspects. Clin Exp Med 3:55, 2003

ROSSE WF: Paroxysmal nocturnal hemoglobinuria as a molecular disease. Medicine 76:63, 1997

94 APLASTIC ANEMIA, MYELODYSPLASIA, AND RELATED BONE MARROW FAILURE SYNDROMES
Neal S. Young

The hypoproliferative anemias associated with marrow damage include aplastic anemia, myelodysplasia (MDS), pure red cell aplasia (PRCA), and myelophthisis. Anemia in these disorders, which is normochromic, normocytic or macrocytic, and characterized by low reticulocyte count, is not a solitary or even the major finding in these diseases, which are better described as marrow failure states. In bone marrow failure, pancytopenia—anemia, leukopenia, and thrombocytopenia (sometimes in various combinations)—results from deficient hematopoiesis, as distinguished from blood count depression due to peripheral destruction of red cells (hemolytic anemias), platelets (idiopathic thrombocytopenic purpura or due to splenomegaly), and granulocytes (as in the immune leukopenias).

Hematopoietic failure syndromes are classified by dominant morphologic features of the bone marrow (Table 94-1). While practical distinction among these syndromes usually is clear, they can occur secondary to other diseases, and some processes are so closely related that the differential diagnosis may be arbitrary. Patients may seem to suffer from two or three related diseases simultaneously, or one diagnosis may appear to evolve into another. Finally, many of these syndromes share an immune-mediated pathophysiologic mechanism of marrow destruction and some element of genomic instability resulting in a higher rate of malignant transformation.

APLASTIC ANEMIA

DEFINITION Aplastic anemia is pancytopenia with bone marrow hypocellularity. Acquired aplastic anemia is distinguished from iatrogenic marrow aplasia, the common occurrence of marrow hypocellularity after intensive cytotoxic chemotherapy for cancer. Aplastic anemia can also be constitutional: the genetic diseases Fanconi's anemia and dyskeratosis congenita, while frequently associated with typical physical anomalies and the development of pancytopenia

early in life, can also present as marrow failure in normal-appearing adults. Acquired aplastic anemia is often stereotypical in its manifestations, with the abrupt onset of low blood counts in a previously well young adult; seronegative hepatitis or a course of an incriminated medical drug may precede the onset. The diagnosis in these instances is

TABLE 94-1 *Differential Diagnosis of Pancytopenia*

PANCYTOPENIA WITH HYPOCELLULAR BONE MARROW

Acquired aplastic anemia
Constitutional aplastic anemia (Fanconi's anemia, dyskeratosis congenita)
Some myelodysplasia syndromes
Rare aleukemic leukemia (AML)
Some acute lymphoid leukemia
Some lymphomas of bone marrow

PANCYTOPENIA WITH CELLULAR BONE MARROW

Primary bone marrow diseases	Secondary to systemic diseases
Myelodysplasia syndromes	Systemic lupus erythematosus
Paroxysmal nocturnal hemoglobinuria	Hypersplenism
Myelofibrosis	B$_{12}$, folate deficiency
Some aleukemic leukemia	Overwhelming infection
Myelophthisis	Alcohol
Bone marrow lymphoma	Brucellosis
Hairy cell leukemia	Sarcoidosis
	Tuberculosis
	Leishmaniasis

HYPOCELLULAR BONE MARROW ± CYTOPENIA

Q fever
Legionnaires' disease
Anorexia nervosa, starvation
Mycobacteria

uncomplicated. Sometimes blood count depression is moderate or incomplete, resulting in anemia, leukopenia, and thrombocytopenia in some combination. Aplastic anemia is related to both paroxysmal nocturnal hemoglobinuria (PNH; Chap. 93) and to MDS, and in some cases a clear distinction among these disorders may not be possible.

EPIDEMIOLOGY   The incidence of acquired aplastic anemia in Europe and Israel is 2 cases per million persons annually. In Thailand and China, rates of 5 to 7 per million have been established. In general, men and women are affected with equal frequency, but there is a biphasic age distribution, with the major peak in the teens and twenties and a second rise in the elderly.

ETIOLOGY   The origins of aplastic anemia have been inferred from several recurring clinical associations (Table 94-2); unfortunately, these relationships are neither a reliable guide in an individual patient nor necessarily etiologic. In addition, while most cases of aplastic anemia are idiopathic, little other than history separates these cases from those with a presumed etiology such as a drug exposure.

Radiation   Marrow aplasia is a major acute sequela of radiation. Radiation damages DNA; tissues dependent on active mitosis are particularly susceptible. Nuclear accidents can involve not only power plant workers but also employees of hospitals, laboratories, and industry (food sterilization, metal radiography, etc.), as well as innocents exposed to stolen, misplaced, or misused sources. While the radiation dose can be approximated from the rate and degree of decline in blood counts, dosimetry by reconstruction of the exposure can help to estimate the patient's prognosis and also to protect medical personnel from contact with radioactive tissue and excreta. MDS and leukemia, but probably not aplastic anemia, are late effects of irradiation.

Chemicals   Benzene is a notorious cause of bone marrow failure. Vast quantities of epidemiologic, clinical, and laboratory data link benzene to aplastic anemia, acute leukemia, and blood and marrow abnormalities. The occurrence of leukemia is roughly correlated with cumulative exposure, but susceptibility must also be important, as only a minority of even heavily exposed workers develop benzene myelotoxicity. The employment history is important, especially in industries where benzene is used for a secondary purpose, usually as a solvent. Benzene-related blood diseases have declined with regulation of industrial exposure. Although benzene is no longer generally available as a household solvent, exposure to its metabolites occurs in the normal diet and in the use of lead-free gasoline. The association between marrow failure and other chemicals is much less well substantiated.

Drugs (See Table 94-3)   Many chemotherapeutic drugs have marrow suppression as a major toxicity; effects are dose-dependent and will occur in all recipients. In contrast, idiosyncratic reactions to a large and diverse group of drugs may lead to aplastic anemia without a clear dose-response relationship. These associations rested largely on accumulated case reports until a large international study in Europe in the 1980s quantitated drug relationships, especially for nonsteroidal analgesics, sulfonamides, thyrostatic drugs, some psychotropics, penicillamine, allopurinol, and gold. Not all associations necessarily reflect causation: a drug may have been used to treat the first symptoms of bone marrow failure (antibiotics for fever or the preceding viral illness) or provoked the first symptom of a preexisting disease (petechiae by nonsteroidal anti-inflammatory agents administered to the thrombocytopenic patient). In the context of total drug use, idiosyncratic reactions, while individually devastating, are rare events. Chlor-

TABLE 94-2   *Classification of Aplastic Anemia and Single Cytopenias*

Acquired	Inherited
APLASTIC ANEMIA	
Secondary	Fanconi's anemia
Radiation	Dyskeratosis congenita
Drugs and chemicals	Shwachman-Diamond syndrome
Regular effects	Reticular dysgenesis
Idiosyncratic reactions	Amegakaryocytic
	thrombocytopenia
Viruses	Familial aplastic anemias
Epstein-Barr virus (infectious	Preleukemia (monosomy 7, etc.)
mononucleosis)	Nonhematologic syndrome
Hepatitis (non-A, non-B, non-	(Down's, Dubowitz, Seckel)
C hepatitis)	
Parvovirus B19 (transient	
aplastic crisis, PRCA)	
HIV-1 (AIDS)	
Immune diseases	
Eosinophilic fasciitis	
Hypoimmunoglobulinemia	
Thymoma/thymic carcinoma	
Graft-versus-host disease in	
immunodeficiency	
Paroxysmal nocturnal	
hemoglobinuria	
Pregnancy	
Idiopathic	
CYTOPENIAS	
PRCA (see Table 94-4)	Congenital PRCA (Diamond-Blackfan anemia)
Neutropenia/Agranulocytosis	
Idiopathic	Kostmann's Syndrome
Drugs, toxins	Shwachman-Diamond syndrome
Pure white cell aplasia	Reticular dysgenesis
Thrombocytopenia	
Drugs, toxins	Amegakaryocytic
	thrombocytopenia
Idiopathic amegakaryocytic	Thrombocytopenia with absent radii

Note: PRCA, pure red cell aplasia.

TABLE 94-3   *Some Drugs and Chemicals Associated with Aplastic Anemia*

Agents that regularly produce marrow depression as major toxicity in commonly employed doses or normal exposures:
  Cytotoxic drugs used in cancer chemotherapy: *alkylating agents*, antimetabolites, antimitotics, some antibiotics

Agents that frequently but not inevitably produce marrow aplasia:
  Benzene

Agents associated with aplastic anemia but with a relatively low probability:
  Chloramphenicol
  Insecticides
  Antiprotozoals: *quinacrine* and chloroquine, mepacrine
  Nonsteroidal anti-inflammatory drugs (including *phenylbutazone*, indomethacin, ibuprofen, sulindac, aspirin)
  Anticonvulsants (*hydantoins, carbamazepine*, phenacemide, felbamate)
  Heavy metals (*gold*, arsenic, bismuth, mercury)
  Sulfonamides: some antibiotics, antithyroid drugs (methimazole, methylthiouracil, propylthiouracil), antidiabetes drugs (tolbutamide, chlorpropamide), carbonic anhydrase inhibitors (acetazolamide and methazolamide)
  Antihistamines (*cimetidine*, chlorpheniramine)
  D-Penicillamine
  Estrogens (in pregnancy and in high doses in animals)

Agents whose association with aplastic anemia is more tenuous:
  Other antibiotics (streptomycin, tetracycline, methicillin, mebendazole, trimethoprim/sulfamethoxazole, flucytosine)
  Sedatives and tranquilizers (chlorpromazine, prochlorperazine, piperacetazine, chlordiazepoxide, meprobamate, methyprylon)
  Allopurinol
  Methyldopa
  Quinidine
  Lithium
  Guanidine
  Potassium perchlorate
  Thiocyanate
  Carbimazole

Note: Terms set in italic show the most consistent association with aplastic anemia.

amphenicol, the most infamous culprit, reportedly produced aplasia in only about 1/60,000 therapy courses, and even this number is almost certainly an overestimate (risks are almost invariably exaggerated when based on collections of cases; although the introduction of chloramphenicol was perceived to have created an epidemic of aplastic anemia, its diminished use was not followed by a changed frequency of marrow failure). Risk estimates are usually lower when determined in population-based studies; furthermore, the low absolute risk is also made more obvious: even a 10- or 20-fold increase in risk translates, in a rare disease, to but a handful of drug-induced aplastic anemia cases among hundreds of thousands of exposed patients.

Infections Hepatitis is the most common preceding infection, and posthepatitis marrow failure accounts for about 5% of etiologies in most series. Patients are usually young men who have recovered from a bout of liver inflammation 1 to 2 months earlier; the subsequent pancytopenia is very severe. The hepatitis is seronegative (non-A, non-B, non-C, non-G) and presumably due to a novel, as yet undiscovered, virus. Fulminant liver failure in childhood also follows seronegative hepatitis, and marrow failure occurs at a high rate in these patients. Marrow failure can rarely follow infectious mononucleosis, and Epstein-Barr virus has been found in the marrow of a few aplastic anemia patients, some without a suggestive preceding history. Parvovirus B19, the cause of transient aplastic crisis in hemolytic anemias and of some pure red cell aplasia (see below), does not usually cause generalized bone marrow failure. Blood count depression is frequent in the course of many viral and bacterial infections but is moderate and resolves with the infection.

Immunologic Diseases Aplasia is a major consequence and the cause of death in *transfusion-associated graft-versus-host disease*, which can occur after infusion of unirradiated blood products to an immunodeficient recipient. Aplastic anemia is strongly associated with the rare collagen vascular syndrome called *eosinophilic fasciitis*, which is characterized by painful induration of subcutaneous tissues (Chap. 303). Pancytopenia with marrow hypoplasia can also occur in systemic lupus erythematosus.

Pregnancy Aplastic anemia very rarely may occur and recur during pregnancy and resolve with delivery or with spontaneous or induced abortion.

Paroxysmal Nocturnal Hemoglobinuria An acquired mutation in the *PIG-A* gene in a hematopoietic stem cell is required for the development of PNH, but *PIG-A* mutations probably occur commonly in normal individuals. If the PIG-A mutant stem cell proliferates, the result is a clone of progeny deficient in glycosylphosphatidylinositol-linked cell surface membrane proteins (Chap. 93). Such PNH cells are now most accurately enumerated using fluorescence-activated flow cytometry of CD55 or CD59 expression on granulocytes rather than Ham or sucrose lysis tests on red cells. Small clones of deficient cells can be detected in about half of patients with aplastic anemia at the time of presentation [and PNH cells are also seen in MDS (see below)]; frank hemolysis and thrombotic episodes occur in patients with PNH clones. Functional studies of bone marrow from PNH patients, even those with mainly hemolytic manifestations, show evidence of defective hematopoiesis. Patients with an initial clinical diagnosis of PNH, especially younger individuals, may later develop frank marrow aplasia and pancytopenia; patients with an initial diagnosis of aplastic anemia may suffer from hemolytic PNH years after recovery of blood counts. One explanation for the aplastic anemia/PNH syndrome is selection of the deficient clones, because they are favored for proliferation in the peculiar environment of immune-mediated marrow destruction.

Congenital Disorders Fanconi's anemia, an autosomal recessive disorder, manifests as congenital developmental anomalies, progressive pancytopenia, and an increased risk of malignancy. Chromosomes in Fanconi's anemia are peculiarly susceptible to DNA cross-linking agents, the basis for a diagnostic assay. Patients with Fanconi's anemia typically have short stature, café au lait spots, and anomalies involving the thumb, radius, and genitourinary tract. At least eight different ge-

netic defects have been defined by complementation analysis. The most common, type A Fanconi's anemia, is due to a mutation in *FANCA*. The Fanconi's anemia genes play a role in the cellular response to DNA damage, a response that includes BRCA1, ATM, and NBS1.

Dyskeratosis congenita is characterized by mucous membrane leukoplakia, dystrophic nails, reticular hyperpigmentation, and the development of aplastic anemia during childhood. The common X-linked variety is due to mutations in the *DKC1* (*dyskerin*) gene; the more unusual autosomal dominant type has been linked to *hTERC*, the RNA component of the telomerase complex. These two gene products cooperate in maintaining telomere length. In Shwachman-Diamond syndrome, marrow failure is seen with pancreatic insufficiency and malabsorption.

PATHOPHYSIOLOGY Bone marrow failure results from severe damage to the hematopoietic cell compartment. In aplastic anemia, replacement of the bone marrow by fat is apparent in the morphology of the biopsy specimen (Fig. 94-1) and magnetic resonance imaging (MRI) of the spine; cells bearing the CD34 antigen, a marker of early hematopoietic cells, are greatly diminished; and in functional studies, committed and primitive progenitor cells are virtually absent—in vitro assays have suggested that the stem cell pool is reduced to ≤1% of normal in severe disease at the time of presentation. Qualitative abnormalities, such as limited number of operating stem cell clones or shortened telomere length, may follow from the quantitative deficiency, reflecting the shrunken and stressed state of hematopoiesis. An intrinsic stem cell defect exists for constitutional aplastic anemia, as cells from patients with Fanconi's anemia exhibit chromosome damage and death on exposure to certain chemical agents. Aplastic anemia does not appear to result from defective stroma or growth factor production.

Drug Injury Extrinsic damage to the marrow follows massive physical or chemical insults such as high doses of radiation and toxic chemicals. For the more common idiosyncratic reaction to modest doses of medical drugs, altered drug metabolism has been invoked as a likely mechanism. The metabolic pathways of many drugs and chemicals, especially if they are polar and have limited water solubility, involve enzymatic degradation to highly reactive electrophilic compounds; these intermediates are toxic because of their propensity to bind to cellular macromolecules. For example, derivative hydroquinones and quinolones are responsible for benzene-induced tissue injury. Excessive generation of toxic intermediates or failure to detoxify the intermediates may be genetically determined and apparent only on specific drug challenge; the complexity and specificity of the pathways imply multiple susceptibility loci and would provide an explanation for the rarity of idiosyncratic drug reactions.

Immune-Mediated Injury The recovery of marrow function in some patients prepared for bone marrow transplantation with antilymphocyte globulin (ALG) first suggested that aplastic anemia might be immune-mediated. Consistent with this hypothesis was the frequent failure of simple bone marrow transplantation from a syngeneic twin, without conditioning cytotoxic chemotherapy, which also argued both *against* simple stem cell absence as the cause and *for* the presence of a host factor producing marrow failure. Laboratory data support an important role for the immune system in aplastic anemia. Blood and bone marrow cells of patients can suppress normal hematopoietic progenitor cell growth, and removal of T cells from aplastic anemia bone marrow improves colony formation in vitro. Increased numbers of activated cytotoxic T cells are observed in aplastic anemia patients and usually decline with successful immunosuppressive therapy; cytokine measurements show a T_H1 immune response (interferon γ, interleukin 2, and tumor necrosis factor). Interferon and tumor necrosis factor induce Fas expression on CD34 cells, leading to apoptotic cell death; localization of activated T cells to bone marrow and local production of their soluble factors are probably important in stem cell destruction.

Early immune system events in aplastic anemia are not well understood. Analysis of T cell receptor expression suggests an oligoclonal, antigen-driven cytotoxic T cell response. Many different exogenous antigens appear capable of initiating a pathologic immune response, but at least some of the T cells may recognize true self-antigens. The rarity of aplastic anemia despite common exposures (medicines, hepatitis virus) suggests that genetically determined features of the immune response can convert a normal physiologic response into a sustained abnormal autoimmune process.

CLINICAL FEATURES ■ History

Aplastic anemia can appear with seeming abruptness or have a more insidious onset. Bleeding is the most common early symptom; a complaint of days to weeks of easy bruising, oozing from the gums, nose bleeds, heavy menstrual flow, and sometimes petechiae will have been noticed. With thrombocytopenia, massive hemorrhage is unusual, but small amounts of bleeding in the central nervous system can result in catastrophic intracranial or retinal hemorrhage. Symptoms of anemia are also frequent, including lassitude, weakness, shortness of breath, and a pounding sensation in the ears. Infection is an unusual first symptom in aplastic anemia (unlike in agranulocytosis, where pharyngitis, anorectal infection, or frank sepsis occur early). A striking feature of aplastic anemia is the restriction of symptoms to the hematologic system, and patients often feel and look remarkably well despite drastically reduced blood counts. Systemic complaints and weight loss should point to other etiologies of pancytopenia. Prior drug use, chemical exposure, and preceding viral illnesses must often be elicited with repeated questioning. A family history of hematologic diseases or blood abnormalities may indicate a constitutional etiology of marrow failure.

Physical Examination

Petechiae and ecchymoses are typical, and retinal hemorrhages may be present. Pelvic and rectal examinations should be performed with great gentleness to avoid trauma; these will often show bleeding from the cervical os and blood in the stool. Pallor of the skin and mucous membranes is common except in the most acute cases or those already transfused. Infection on presentation is unusual but may occur if the patient has been symptomatic for a few weeks. Lymphadenopathy and splenomegaly are highly atypical of aplastic anemia. Café au lait spots and short stature suggest Fanconi's anemia; peculiar nails and leukoplakia suggest dyskeratosis congenita.

LABORATORY STUDIES ■ Blood

The smear shows large erythrocytes and a paucity of platelets and granulocytes. Mean corpuscular volume (MCV) is commonly increased. Reticulocytes are absent or few, and lymphocyte numbers may be normal or reduced. The presence of immature myeloid forms suggests leukemia or MDS; nucleated red blood cells suggest marrow fibrosis or tumor invasion; abnormal platelets suggest either peripheral destruction or MDS.

Bone Marrow

The bone marrow is usually readily aspirated but appears dilute on smear, and the fatty biopsy specimen may be grossly pale on withdrawal; a "dry tap" suggests fibrosis or myelophthisis. In severe aplasia the smear of the aspirated specimen shows only red cells, residual lymphocytes, and stromal cells; the biopsy, which should be >1 cm in length, is superior for determination of cellularity and shows mainly fat under the microscope, with hematopoietic cells occupying <25% of the marrow space. In the most serious cases the biopsy is virtually 100% fat. The correlation between marrow cellularity and disease severity is imperfect. Some patients with moderate disease by blood counts will have empty iliac crest biopsies, while "hot spots" of hematopoiesis may be seen in severe cases. If an iliac crest specimen is inadequate, cells may also be obtained by aspiration from the sternum. Residual hematopoietic cells should have normal morphology, except for mildly megaloblastic erythropoiesis; megakaryocytes are invariably greatly reduced and usually absent. Areas adjacent to the spicule should be searched for myeloblasts. Granulomas (in cellular specimens) may indicate an infectious etiology of the marrow failure.

Ancillary Studies

Chromosome breakage studies of peripheral blood using diepoxybutane (DEB) or mito-

A   C

B   D

FIGURE 94-1 *A.* Normal bone marrow biopsy. *B.* Normal bone marrow aspirate smear. The marrow is normally 30 to 70% cellular, and there is a heterogeneous mix of myeloid, erythroid, and lymphoid cells. *C.* Aplastic anemia biopsy. *D.* Marrow smear in aplastic anemia. The marrow shows replacement of hematopoietic tissue by fat and only residual stromal and lymphoid cells.

mycin C should be performed on children and younger adults to exclude Fanconi's anemia. Chromosome studies of bone marrow cells are often revealing in MDS and should be negative in typical aplastic anemia. Flow cytometric assays have replaced the Ham test for the diagnosis of PNH. Serologic studies may show evidence of viral infection, especially Epstein-Barr virus and HIV. Posthepatitis aplastic anemia is typically seronegative. The spleen size should be determined by scanning if the physical examination of the abdomen is unsatisfactory. MRI may be helpful to assess the fat content on a few vertebrae in order to distinguish aplasia from MDS.

DIAGNOSIS The diagnosis of aplastic anemia is usually straightforward, based on the combination of pancytopenia with a fatty, empty bone marrow. Aplastic anemia is a disease of the young and should be a leading diagnosis in the pancytopenic adolescent or young adult. When pancytopenia is secondary, the primary diagnosis is usually obvious from either history or physical examination: the massive spleen of alcoholic cirrhosis, the history of metastatic cancer or systemic lupus erythematosus, or obvious miliary tuberculosis on chest radiograph (Table 94-1).

Diagnostic problems can occur with atypical presentations and among related hematologic diseases. While pancytopenia is most common, some patients with bone marrow hypocellularity have depression of only one or two of three blood lines, sometimes showing later progression to more recognizable aplastic anemia. The bone marrow in constitutional aplastic anemia is indistinguishable morphologically from the aspirate in acquired disease. The diagnosis can be suggested by family history, abnormal blood counts since childhood, or the presence of associated physical anomalies. Aplastic anemia may be difficult to distinguish from the hypocellular variety of MDS: MDS is favored by finding morphologic abnormalities, particularly of megakaryocytes and myeloid precursor cells, and typical cytogenetic abnormalities (see below).

PROGNOSIS The natural history of severe aplastic anemia is rapid deterioration and death. Provision first of red blood cell and later platelet transfusions and effective antibiotics were of some benefit, but few patients showed spontaneous recovery. The major prognostic determinant is the blood count; severe disease is defined by the presence of two of three parameters: absolute neutrophil count $<500/\mu$L, platelet count $<20,000/\mu$L, and corrected reticulocyte count $<1\%$ (or absolute reticulocyte count $<60,000/\mu$L). Survival of patients who fulfill these criteria is about 20% at 1 year after diagnosis with only supportive care; patients with very severe disease, defined by an absolute neutrophil count $<200/\mu$L, fare even more poorly. Treatment has markedly improved survival in this disease.

℞ TREATMENT

Severe acquired aplastic anemia can be cured by replacement of the absent hematopoietic cells (and the immune system) by stem cell transplant, or it can be ameliorated by suppression of the immune system to allow recovery of the patient's residual bone marrow function. Hematopoietic growth factors have limited usefulness and glucocorticoids are of no value. Suspect exposures to drugs or chemicals should be discontinued; however, spontaneous recovery of severe blood count depression is rare, and a waiting period before beginning treatment may not be advisable unless the blood counts are only modestly depressed.

Bone Marrow Transplantation This is the best therapy for the young patient with a fully histocompatible sibling donor (Chap. 100). Human leukocyte antigen (HLA) typing should be ordered as soon as the diagnosis of aplastic anemia is established in a child or younger adult. In transplant candidates, transfusion of blood from family members should be avoided so as to prevent sensitization to histocompatibility antigens; while transfusions in general should be minimized, limited numbers of blood products probably do not seriously affect outcome.

For allogeneic transplant from fully matched siblings, long-term survival rates for children are 80% or better. Transplant morbidity and

mortality are increased among adults, due mainly to the higher risk of chronic graft-versus-host disease and serious infections. Graft rejection was historically a major determinant of outcome in bone marrow transplant for aplastic anemia; high rates of primary or secondary graft failure may be related to the pathophysiology of marrow failure as well as to alloimmunization from transfusions.

Most patients do not have a suitable sibling donor. Occasionally, a full phenotypic match can be found within the family and serve as well. Far more available are other alternative donors, either unrelated but histocompatible volunteers, or closely but not perfectly matched family members. Survival using alternative donors is about half that of conventional sibling transplants. These patients will be at risk for late complications, especially a higher rate of cancer, if radiation is used as a component of conditioning. Most older adults who undergo alternative donor transplants succumb to transplant-related complications.

Immunosuppression Used alone, ALG or antithymocyte globulin (ATG) induces hematologic recovery (independence from transfusion and a leukocyte count adequate to prevent infection) in about 50% of patients. The addition of cyclosporine to either ALG or ATG has further increased response rates to about 70% and especially improved outcomes for children and for severely neutropenic patients. Combined treatment is now standard for patients with severe disease. Hematologic response strongly correlates with survival. Improvement in granulocyte number is generally apparent within 2 months of treatment. Most recovered patients continue to have some degree of blood count depression, the MCV remains elevated, and the bone marrow cellularity returns toward normal only very slowly, if at all. Relapse (recurrent pancytopenia) is frequent, often occurring as cyclosporine is discontinued; most, but not all, patients respond to reinstitution of immunosuppression, but some responders become dependent on continued cyclosporine administration. Development of MDS, with typical marrow morphologic or cytogenetic abnormalities, occurs in about 15% of treated patients, usually but not invariably associated with a return of pancytopenia, and some patients develop leukemia. Although the laboratory diagnosis of PNH can generally be made at the time of presentation of aplastic anemia by flow cytometry, recovered patients showing frank hemolysis should be retested for PNH. Bone marrow examinations should be performed if there is an unfavorable change in blood counts.

Horse ATG is given at 40 mg/kg per day for 4 days; rabbit ALG is administered at 3.5 mg/kg per day for 5 days. For ATG, anaphylaxis is a rare but occasionally fatal complication; allergy should be tested by a skin-prick test with an undiluted solution and immediate observation; desensitization is feasible. ATG binds to peripheral blood cells; therefore, platelet and granulocyte numbers may fall further during active treatment. Serum sickness, a flulike illness with a characteristic cutaneous eruption and arthralgia, often develops about 10 days after initiating treatment. Most patients are given methylprednisolone, 1 mg/kg per day for 2 weeks, to ameliorate the immune consequences of heterologous protein infusion. Excessive or extended glucocorticoid therapy is associated with avascular joint necrosis. Cyclosporine is administered orally at an initial dose of 12 mg/kg per day in adults (15 mg/kg per day in children), with subsequent adjustment according to blood levels obtained every 2 weeks. Trough levels should be between 150 and 200 ng/mL. The most important side effects of chronic cyclosporine treatment are nephrotoxicity, hypertension, seizures, and opportunistic infections, especially *Pneumocystis carinii* (prophylactic treatment with monthly inhaled pentamidine is recommended).

Most patients with aplastic anemia lack a suitable marrow donor and immunosuppression is the treatment of choice. Long-term survival is equivalent with transplantation and immunosuppression. However, successful transplant cures marrow failure, while patients who recover adequate blood counts after immunosuppression remain at risk of relapse and malignant evolution. Because of the excellent results in children, allogeneic transplant should be performed in the pediatric population if a suitable sibling donor is available. Increasing age and the severity of neutropenia are the most important factors weighing in the decision between transplant and immunosuppression in adults who have a matched family donor: older patients do better with ATG and cyclosporine, whereas transplant is preferred if granulocytopenia is profound. Some reluctant patients may be treated by immunosuppression; transplant is used for failure to recover blood counts or occurrence of late complications.

Outcomes following both transplant and immunosuppression have improved with time. High doses of cyclophosphamide, without stem cell rescue, have been reported to produce durable hematologic recovery, without relapse or evolution to MDS, but this treatment can produce sustained severe fatal neutropenia and response is often delayed. Several new immunosuppressive drugs in clinical trial may further improve outcome.

Other Therapies   The effectiveness of androgens has not been verified in controlled trials, but occasional patients will respond or even demonstrate blood count dependence on continued therapy. For patients with moderate disease or those with severe pancytopenia in whom immunosuppression has failed, a 3- to 4-month trial is appropriate. Hematopoietic growth factors, granulocyte colony-stimulating factor (G-CSF), granulocyte-macrophage CSF (GM-CSF), and interleukin 3 are not recommended as initial therapy for severe aplastic anemia, and even their role as adjuncts to immunosuppression is not well defined. Some patients may respond to combinations of growth factors after immunosuppression has failed. Splenectomy may occasionally increase blood counts in relapsed or refractory cases.

Supportive Care   Meticulous medical attention is required so that the patient may survive to benefit from definitive therapy or, having failed treatment, to maintain a reasonable existence in the face of pancytopenia. First and most important, infection in the presence of severe neutropenia must be aggressively treated by prompt institution of parenteral, broad-spectrum antibiotics, usually ceftazidime or a combination of an aminoglycoside, cephalosporin, and semisynthetic penicillin. Therapy is empirical and must not await results of culture, although specific foci of infection such as oropharyngeal or anorectal abscesses, pneumonia, sinusitis, and typhlitis (necrotizing colitis) should be sought on physical examination and with radiographic studies. When indwelling plastic catheters become contaminated, vancomycin should be added. Persistent or recrudescent fever implies fungal disease: *Candida* or *Aspergillus* are common, especially after several courses of antibacterial antibiotics, and a progressive course may be averted by timely initiation of antifungal therapy. Granulocyte transfusions using G-CSF–mobilized peripheral blood have been effective in the treatment of overwhelming or refractory infections in a few patients. Hand washing, the single best method of preventing the spread of infection, remains a neglected practice. Nonabsorbed antibiotics for gut decontamination are poorly tolerated and not of proven value. Total reverse isolation does not reduce mortality from infections.

Both platelet and erythrocyte numbers can be maintained by transfusion. Alloimmunization limits the usefulness of platelet transfusions and can be avoided or minimized by several strategies, including use of single donors to reduce exposure and physical or chemical methods to diminish leukocytes in the product; HLA-matched platelets are often effective in patients refractory to random donor products. Inhibitors of fibrinolysis such as aminocaproic acid have not been shown to relieve mucosal oozing; the use of low-dose glucocorticoids to induce "vascular stability" is unproven. Whether platelet transfusions are better used prophylactically or only as needed remains unclear. Any rational regimen of prophylaxis requires transfusions once or twice weekly in order to maintain the platelet count >10,000/μL (oozing from the gut, and presumably also from other vascular beds, increases precipitously at counts <5000/μL). Menstruation should be suppressed either by oral estrogens or nasal follicle-stimulating hormone/luteinizing hormone (FSH/LH) antagonists. Aspirin and other nonsteroidal anti-inflammatory agents inhibit platelet function and must be avoided.

Red blood cells should be transfused to maintain a normal level of activity, usually at a hemoglobin value of 70 g/L (90 g/L if there is underlying cardiac or pulmonary disease); a regimen of 2 units every 2 weeks will replace normal losses in a patient without a functioning bone marrow. In chronic anemia, the iron chelator deferoxamine should be added at around the fiftieth transfusion in order to avoid secondary hemochromatosis.

PURE RED CELL APLASIA

Other, more restricted forms of marrow failure occur, in which only a single circulating cell type is affected and the aregenerative marrow shows corresponding absence or decreased numbers of specific precursor cells: aregenerative anemia as in PRCA (see below), thrombocytopenia with amegakaryocytosis (Chap. 101), and neutropenia without marrow myeloid cells in agranulocytosis (Chap. 55). In general, and in contrast to aplastic anemia and MDS, the unaffected lineages appear quantitatively and qualitatively normal. Agranulocytosis, the most frequent of these syndromes, is usually a complication of medical drug use (with agents similar to those related to aplastic anemia), either by a mechanism of direct chemical toxicity or by immune destruction. Agranulocytosis has an incidence similar to aplastic anemia but is especially frequent among the elderly and in women. The syndrome should resolve with discontinuation of exposure, but significant mortality is attached to neutropenia in the older and often previously unwell patient. Both pure white cell aplasia (agranulocytosis without incriminating drug exposure) and amegakaryocytic thrombocytopenia are exceedingly rare and, like PRCA, appear to be due to destructive antibodies or lymphocytes and can respond to immunosuppressive therapies. In all the single lineage failure syndromes, progression to pancytopenia or leukemia is unusual.

DEFINITION AND DIFFERENTIAL DIAGNOSIS   PRCA is characterized by anemia, reticulocytopenia, and absent or rare erythroid precursor cells in the bone marrow. The classification of PRCA is shown in Table 94-4. In adults, PRCA is acquired. An identical syndrome can occur constitutionally: Diamond-Blackfan anemia, or congenital PRCA, is diagnosed at birth or in early childhood and often responds to glucocorticoid treatment. Temporary red cell failure occurs in transient aplastic crisis of hemolytic anemias, due to acute parvovirus infection

TABLE 94-4   *Classification of Pure Red Cell Aplasia*

Self-limited
    Transient erythroblastopenia of childhood
    Transient aplastic crisis of hemolysis (acute B19 parvovirus infection)
Fetal red blood cell aplasia
    Nonimmune hydrops fetalis (in utero B19 parvovirus infection)
Hereditary pure red cell aplasia
    Congenital pure red cell aplasia (Diamond-Blackfan syndrome)
Acquired pure red cell aplasia
    Thymoma and malignancy
       Thymoma
       Lymphoid malignancies (and more rarely other hematologic diseases)
       Paraneoplastic to solid tumors
    Connective tissue disorders with immunologic abnormalities
       Systemic lupus erythematosus, juvenile rheumatoid arthritis, rheumatoid arthritis
       Multiple endocrine gland insufficiency
    Virus
       Persistent B19 parvovirus, hepatitis, adult T cell leukemia virus, Epstein-Barr virus
    Pregnancy
    Drugs
       Especially phenytoin, azathioprine, chloramphenicol, procaineamide, isoniazid
    Idiopathic

(Chap. 168), and in transient erythroblastopenia of childhood, which affects normal children.

CLINICAL ASSOCIATIONS AND ETIOLOGY PRCA has important associations with immune system diseases. A small minority of cases occur with a thymoma. More frequently, red cell aplasia can be the major manifestation of large granular lymphocytosis or may occur in chronic lymphocytic leukemia. Some patients may be hypogammaglobulinemic. As with agranulocytosis, PRCA can be due to an idiosyncratic reaction to a drug.

Like aplastic anemia, PRCA results from diverse mechanisms. Antibodies to red blood cell precursors are frequently present in the blood, but T cell inhibition is probably the more common immune mechanism. Cytotoxic lymphocyte activity restricted by histocompatibility locus or specific for human T cell leukemia/lymphoma virus I–infected cells, as well as natural killer cell activity inhibitory of erythropoiesis, have been demonstrated in particularly well-studied individual cases.

Persistent Parvovirus B19 Infection Chronic parvovirus infection is an important, treatable cause of PRCA. This common virus causes a benign exanthem of childhood (fifth disease) and a polyarthralgia syndrome in adults. In patients with underlying hemolysis (or any condition that increases demand for red blood cell production), parvovirus infection can cause a transient aplastic crisis and an abrupt but temporary worsening of the anemia due to failed erythropoiesis. In normal individuals, acute infection is resolved by production of neutralizing antibodies to the virus, but in the setting of congenital, acquired, or iatrogenic immunodeficiency, persistent viral infection may occur. The bone marrow shows red cell aplasia and the presence of giant pronormoblasts (Fig. 94-2), which is the cytopathic sign of B19 parvovirus infection. Viral tropism for human erythroid progenitor cells is due to its use of erythrocyte P antigen as a cellular receptor for entry. Direct cytotoxicity of virus causes anemia if demands on

A

B

C

D

FIGURE 94-2 Pathognomonic cells in marrow failure syndromes. *A*. Giant pronormoblast, the cytopathic effect of B19 parvovirus infection of the erythroid progenitor cell. *B*. Uninuclear megakaryocyte and microblastic erythroid precursors typical of the 5q– myelodysplasia syndrome. *C*. Ringed sideroblast showing perinuclear iron granules. *D*. Tumor cells present on a touch preparation made from the marrow biopsy of a patient with metastatic carcinoma.

erythrocyte production are high; in normal individuals, the temporary cessation of red cell production is not clinically apparent, and skin and joint symptoms are mediated by immune complex deposition.

Rx TREATMENT

History, physical examination, and routine laboratory studies may disclose an underlying disease or a suspect drug exposure. Thymoma should be sought by radiographic procedures. Tumor excision is indicated, but anemia does not necessarily improve with surgery. The diagnosis of parvovirus infection requires detection of viral DNA sequences in the blood (IgG and IgM antibodies are commonly absent). The presence of erythroid colonies has been considered predictive of response to immunosuppressive therapy in idiopathic PRCA.

Red cell aplasia is compatible with long survival with supportive care alone: a combination of erythrocyte transfusions and iron chelation. For persistent B19 parvovirus infection, almost all patients respond to intravenous immunoglobulin therapy (for example, 0.4 g/kg daily for 5 days), although relapse and retreatment may be expected, especially in patients with AIDS. The majority of patients with idiopathic PRCA respond favorably to immunosuppression. Most first receive a course of glucocorticoids, followed in the absence of a response by cyclosporine, ATG, azathioprine, or cyclophosphamide.

MYELODYSPLASIA

DEFINITION The myelodysplasias (MDS) are a heterogeneous group of hematologic disorders broadly characterized by cytopenias associated with a dysmorphic (or abnormal appearing) and usually cellular bone marrow, and consequent ineffective blood cell production. A clinically useful nosology of these entities was first developed by the French-American-British Cooperative Group in 1983. Five entities were defined: refractory anemia (RA), refractory anemia with ringed sideroblasts (RARS), refractory anemia with excess blasts (RAEB), refractory anemia with excess blasts in transformation (RAEB-t), and chronic myelomonocytic leukemia (CMML). The World Health Organization classification (2002) recognizes that the distinction between RAEB-t and acute myeloid leukemia is arbitrary and groups them together as acute leukemia, notes that CMML behaves as a myeloproliferative disease, and separates refractory anemias with dysmorphic change restricted to erythroid lineage from those with multilineage changes (Table 94-5).

EPIDEMIOLOGY Idiopathic MDS is a disease of the elderly; the mean age at onset is 68 years. There is a slight male preponderance. MDS is a relatively common form of bone marrow failure, with reported incidence rates of 35 to >100 per million persons in the general population and 120 to >500 per million in the elderly. MDS is rare in children, but monocytic leukemia can be seen. Therapy-related MDS is not age-related and may occur in as many as 15% of patients within a decade following intensive combined modality treatment for cancer. Rates of MDS have increased over time, due to the recognition of the syndrome by physicians and the aging of the population.

ETIOLOGY AND PATHOPHYSIOLOGY MDS is caused by environmental exposures such as radiation and benzene; other risk factors have been reported inconsistently. Secondary MDS occurs as a late toxicity of cancer treatment, usually with a combination of radiation and the radiomimetic alkylating agents such as busulfan, nitrosourea, or procarbazine (with a latent period of 5 to 7 years) or the DNA topoisomerase inhibitors (2 years). Both acquired aplastic anemia following immunosuppressive treatment and Fanconi's anemia can evolve into MDS.

MDS is a clonal hematopoietic stem cell disorder leading to impaired cell proliferation and differentiation. Cytogenetic abnormalities are found in about half of patients, and some of the same specific lesions are also seen in frank leukemia; aneuploidy is more frequent

TABLE 94-5 *World Health Organization Classification of Myelodysplastic Syndromes*

Disease	Frequency	Blood Findings	Bone Marrow Findings	Prognosis
Refractory anemia (RA)	5–10%	Anemia No or rare blasts	Erythroid dysplasia only <5% blasts <15% ringed sideroblasts	Protracted course Leukemic transformation in ~6%
Refractory anemia with ringed sideroblasts (RARS)	10–12%	Anemia No blasts	Erythroid dysplasia only ≥15% ringed sideroblasts <5% blasts	Protracted course Leukemia in ~1–2%
Refractory cytopenia with multilineage dysplasia (RCMD)	24%	Cytopenias (2 or 3 lineages) No or rare blasts No Auer rods <1 × 10⁹/L monocytes	Dysplasia in ≥10% of cells in ≥2 lineages <5% blasts No Auer rods <15% ringed sideroblasts	Variable clinical course Leukemia in ~11%
RCMD with ringed sideroblasts (RCMD-RS)	15%	Cytopenias (2 or 3 lineages) No or rare blasts No Auer rods <1 × 10⁹/L monocytes	Dysplasia in ≥10% of cells in ≥2 lineages ≥15% ringed sideroblasts <5% blasts No Auer rods	
Refractory anemia with excess blasts-1 (RAEB-1)	40% (RAEB-1 +2)	Cytopenias <5% blasts No Auer rods <1 × 10⁹/L monocytes	Unilineage or multilineage dysplasia 5–9% blasts No Auer rods	Progressive BM failure Leukemia in ~25%
Refractory anemia with excess blasts-2 (RAEB-2)		Cytopenias 5–19% blasts ±Auer rods <1 × 10⁹/L monocytes	Unilineage or multilineage dysplasia 10–19% blasts ±Auer rods	Progressive BM failure Leukemia in ~33%
Myelodysplastic syndrome, unclassified (MDS-U)	Unknown	Cytopenias No or rare blasts No Auer rods	Dysplasia in myeloid or platelet lineage <5% blasts No Auer rods	Unknown
MDS with isolated del(5q)	Unknown	Anemia <5% blasts Platelets nl or increased	Nl or increased megakaryocytes with hypolobated nuclei <5% blasts No Auer rods Isolated del(5q)	Long survival

Note: BM, bone marrow.
Source: Extracted from Jaffe ES et al (eds): *Pathology and Genetics of Tumors of Haematopoietic and Lymphoid Tissues*. Lyon, IARC Press, 2001

than translocations. Both presenting and evolving hematologic manifestations result from the accumulation of multiple genetic lesions, loss of tumor suppressor genes, activating oncogene mutations, or other harmful alterations. Cytogenetic abnormalities are not random (loss of all or part of 5, 7, and 20, trisomy of 8) and may be related to etiology (11q23 following topoisomerase II inhibitors); chronic myelomonocytic leukemia is often associated with t(5;12) that creates a chimeric *tel-PDGFβ* gene. The type and number of cytogenetic abnormalities strongly correlate with the probability of leukemic transformation and survival. Mutations of N *ras* (an oncogene), *p53* and *IRF-1* (tumor suppressor genes), *Bcl-2* (an antiapoptotic gene), and others have been reported in some patients but may occur relatively late in the sequence leading to leukemic transformation. Apoptosis of marrow cells is increased in MDS, presumably due to these acquired genetic alterations or possibly to an overlaid immune response. Sideroblastic anemia may be related to mutations in mitochondrial genes. Ineffective erythropoiesis and disordered iron metabolism are the functional consequences of the genetic alterations.

CLINICAL FEATURES

Anemia dominates the early course. Most symptomatic patients complain of the gradual onset of fatigue and weakness, dyspnea, and pallor, but at least half the patients are asymptomatic and their MDS is discovered only incidentally on routine blood counts. Previous chemotherapy or radiation exposure is an important historic fact. Fever and weight loss should point to a myeloproliferative rather than myelodysplastic process. Children with Down syndrome are susceptible to MDS, and a family history may indicate a hereditary form of sideroblastic anemia or Fanconi's anemia.

The physical examination is remarkable for signs of anemia; about 20% of patients have splenomegaly. Some unusual skin lesions, including Sweet's syndrome (febrile neutrophilic dermatosis), occur with MDS. Autoimmune syndromes are not infrequent.

LABORATORY STUDIES ■ Blood

Anemia is present in the majority of cases, either alone or as part of bi- or pancytopenia; isolated neutropenia or thrombocytopenia is more unusual. Macrocytosis is common, and the smear may be dimorphic with a distinctive population of large red blood cells. Platelets are also large and lack granules. In functional studies, they may show marked abnormalities, and patients may have bleeding symptoms despite seemingly adequate numbers. Neutrophils are hypogranulated; have hyposegmented, ringed, or abnormally segmented nuclei; contain Dohle bodies; and may be functionally deficient. Circulating myeloblasts usually correlate with marrow blast numbers, and their quantitation is important for classification and prognosis. The total white blood cell count is usually normal or low, except in chronic myelomonocytic leukemia. As in aplastic anemia, MDS also can be associated with a clonal population of PNH cells.

Bone Marrow

The bone marrow is usually normal or hypercellular but in 20% of cases is sufficiently hypocellular to be confused with aplasia. No single characteristic feature of marrow morphology distinguishes MDS, but the following are commonly observed: dyserythropoietic changes (especially nuclear abnormalities) and ringed sideroblasts in the erythroid lineage; hypogranulation and hyposegmentation in granulocytic precursors, with an increase in myeloblasts; and megakaryocytes showing reduced numbers of disorganized nuclei. Megaloblastic nuclei associated with defective hemoglobinization in the erythroid lineage are common. Prognosis strongly correlates with the proportion of marrow blasts. Cytogenetic analysis and fluorescent in situ hybridization can identify genetic lesions.

DIFFERENTIAL DIAGNOSIS

Deficiencies of vitamin B_{12} or folate should be excluded by appropriate blood tests; vitamin B_6 deficiency can be assessed by a therapeutic trial of pyridoxine if the bone marrow shows ringed sideroblasts. Marrow dysplasia can be observed in acute viral

TABLE 94-6 *International Prognostic Scoring System*

Prognostic Variable	Score Value				
	0	0.5	1.0	1.5	2.0
Bone marrow blasts (%)	<5%	5–10%		11–20%	21–30%
Karyotype[a]	Good	Intermediate	Poor		
Cytopenia[b] (lineages affected)	0 or 1	2 or 3			
Risk Group Scores	**Score**				
Low	0				
Intermediate-1	0.5–1.0				
Intermediate-2	1.5–2.0				
High	≥2.5				

[a] Good, normal, -Y, del(5q), del (20q); intermediate, all other abnormalities; poor, complex (≥3 abnormalities) or chromosome 7 abnormalities.

[b] Cytopenias defined as Hb <100 g/L, platelet count < 100,000/μL, absolute neutrophil count <1500/μL.

infections, drug reactions, or chemical toxicity but should be transient. More difficult are the distinctions between hypocellular MDS and aplasia or between refractory anemia with excess blasts and early acute leukemia. The World Health Organization considers the presence of 20% blasts in the marrow as the criterion that separates acute myeloid leukemia from MDS.

PROGNOSIS

The median survival varies greatly from years for patients with 5q– or sideroblastic anemia to a few months in refractory anemia with excess blasts or severe pancytopenia associated with monosomy 7; an International Prognostic Scoring System (Table 94-6) assists in making predictions. Most patients die as a result of complications of pancytopenia and not due to leukemic transformation; perhaps one-third will succumb to other diseases unrelated to their MDS. Precipitous worsening of pancytopenia, acquisition of new chromosomal abnormalities on serial cytogenetic determination, and increase in the number of blasts are all poor prognostic indicators. The outlook in therapy-related MDS, regardless of type, is poor, and most patients will progress within a few months to refractory acute myeloid leukemia.

℞ TREATMENT

The therapy of MDS is generally unsatisfactory. Only stem cell transplantation offers cure: survival rates of 50% at 3 years have been reported, but older patients are particularly prone to develop treatment-related mortality and morbidity. Results of transplant using matched unrelated donors are comparable, although most series contain younger and more highly selected cases. MDS associated with trisomy 8 may respond to cyclosporine.

MDS has been regarded as particularly refractory to cytotoxic chemotherapy regimens but is probably no more resistant to effective treatment than acute myeloid leukemia in the elderly, in whom drug toxicity is often fatal and remissions, if achieved, are brief. Low doses of cytotoxic drugs have been administered for their "differentiating" potential. 5-azacytidine inhibits DNA methylation and may induce the expression of genes; its use in MDS can improve blood counts and modestly improves survival compared to best supportive care. Amifostine, an organic thiophosphonate that blocks apoptosis, can improve blood counts but has significant toxicities. Both azacytidine and amifostine are approved by the U.S. Food and Drug Administration for use in MDS. ATG may improve blood counts in one-third of MDS patients; those who are young, HLA-D2 positive, and have a PNH clone are more likely to respond.

Hematopoietic growth factors can improve blood counts but, as in most other marrow failure states, have been most beneficial to patients with the least severe pancytopenia. G-CSF treatment alone failed to improve survival in a controlled trial. Erythropoietin alone or in combination with G-CSF can improve hemoglobin levels, especially in those with low serum erythropoietin levels who have no or only a modest need for transfusions.

The same principles of supportive care described for aplastic anemia apply to MDS. Because many patients will be anemic for years, erythrocyte transfusion support should be accompanied by iron chelation in order to prevent secondary hemochromatosis.

MYELOPHTHISIC ANEMIAS

Fibrosis of the bone marrow (see Fig. 95-2), usually accompanied by a characteristic blood smear picture called *leukoerythroblastosis*, can occur as a primary hematologic disease, called *myelofibrosis* or *myeloid metaplasia* (Chap. 95), and as a secondary process, called *myelophthisis*. Myelophthisis, or secondary myelofibrosis, is reactive. Fibrosis can be a response to invading tumor cells, usually of an epithelial cancer of breast, lung, and prostate or neuroblastoma. Marrow fibrosis may occur with infection of mycobacteria (both *Mycobacterium tuberculosis* and *M. avium*), fungi, or HIV, and in sarcoidosis. Intracellular lipid deposition in Gaucher disease and obliteration of the marrow space related to absence of osteoclast remodeling in congenital osteopetrosis also can produce fibrosis. Secondary myelofibrosis is a late consequence of radiation therapy or treatment with radiomimetic drugs. Usually, the infectious or malignant underlying processes are obvious. Marrow fibrosis can also be a feature of a variety of hematologic syndromes, especially chronic myeloid leukemia, multiple myeloma, lymphomas, myeloma, and hairy cell leukemia.

The pathophysiology has three distinct features: proliferation of fibroblasts in the marrow space (myelofibrosis); the extension of hematopoiesis into the long bones and, most particularly, into extramedullary sites usually the spleen, liver, and lymph nodes (myeloid metaplasia); and ineffective erythropoiesis. The etiology of fibrosis is unknown but most likely involves dysregulated production of growth factors: platelet-derived growth factor and transforming growth factor β have been implicated. Abnormal regulation of other hematopoietins

would lead to localization of blood-producing cells in nonhematopoietic tissues and uncoupling of the usually balanced processes of stem cell proliferation and differentiation. Myelofibrosis is remarkable for pancytopenia despite extraordinarily large numbers of circulating hematopoietic progenitor cells.

Anemia is dominant in secondary myelofibrosis, usually normocytic and normochromic. The diagnosis is suggested by the characteristic leukoerythroblastic smear (see Fig. 95-1). Erythrocyte morphology is highly abnormal, with circulating nucleated red blood cells, teardrops, and shape distortions. White blood cell numbers are often elevated, sometimes mimicking a leukemoid reaction, with circulating myelocytes, promyelocytes, and myeloblasts. Platelets may be abundant and are often giant size. Inability to aspirate the bone marrow, the characteristic "dry tap," can allow a presumptive diagnosis in the appropriate setting before the biopsy is decalcified.

The course of secondary myelofibrosis is determined by its cause, usually a metastatic tumor or an advanced hematologic malignancy. Treatable causes must be excluded, especially tuberculosis and fungus. Transfusion support can relieve symptoms.

FURTHER READING

D'ANDREA AD, GROMPE M: The Fanconi anaemia/BRCA pathway. Nat Rev Cancer 3:23, 2003

FISCH P et al: Pure red cell aplasia. Br J Haematol 111:1010, 2000

MOLLDREM JJ et al: Antithymocyte globulin for treatment of the bone marrow failure associated with myelodysplastic syndromes. Ann Intern Med 137: 156, 2002

SILVERMAN JR et al: Randomized controlled trial of azacitidine in patients with the myelodysplastic syndrome: A study of the Cancer and Leukemia Group B. J Clin Oncol 20:2429, 2002

YOUNG NS: Acquired aplastic anemia. Ann Intern Med 136:534, 2002

YOUNG NS, BROWN KE: Parvovirus B19. N Engl J Med 350:586, 2004

95 POLYCYTHEMIA VERA AND OTHER MYELOPROLIFERATIVE DISEASES
Jerry L. Spivak

Polycythemia vera, chronic idiopathic myelofibrosis, essential thrombocytosis, and chronic myeloid leukemia (CML) are commonly classified together under the rubric *the chronic myeloproliferative disorders*, because their pathophysiology involves the clonal expansion of a multipotent hematopoietic progenitor cell with the overproduction of one or more of the formed elements of the blood. These entities may transform into acute leukemia naturally or as a consequence of mutagenic treatment. However, while polycythemia vera, idiopathic myelofibrosis, essential thrombocytosis, and CML share similar phenotypic characteristics, CML is genotypically distinct from the other three disorders because it alone is associated with translocation of genetic material between the long arms of chromosomes 9 and 22, resulting in the production of the unique fusion protein, bcr-abl.

The new World Health Organization classification of myeloid neoplasms has expanded the list of chronic myeloproliferative disorders to include the exceedingly rare entities chronic neutrophilic leukemia, chronic eosinophilic leukemia, and the hypereosinophilic syndrome. In addition, a category of myelodysplastic/myeloproliferative diseases was created to encompass juvenile myelomonocytic leukemia, atypical chronic myeloid leukemia [lacking t(9;22)], and chronic myelomonocytic leukemia. The word "chronic" was also added to idiopathic myelofibrosis to distinguish this disorder from the rarer syndrome of acute panmyelosis with myelofibrosis, a rare form of acute leukemia.

These classification changes were made in recognition of the considerable overlap in clinical presentation and hematopathology that characterizes the chronic myeloproliferative disorders. Systemic mastocytosis, while having phenotypic overlap with the chronic myeloproliferative diseases, was given its own category in recognition of the many distinct clinical syndromes that characterize mast cell proliferation. In this chapter, only polycythemia vera, chronic idiopathic mye-

lofibrosis, and essential thrombocytosis will be discussed as their clinical overlap is substantial and their clinical course distinct from the other myeloproliferative disorders. →*CML is discussed in Chap. 96.*

POLYCYTHEMIA VERA

Polycythemia vera is a clonal disorder involving a multipotent hematopoietic progenitor cell in which there is accumulation of phenotypically normal red cells, granulocytes, and platelets in the absence of a recognizable physiologic stimulus. The most common of the chronic myeloproliferative disorders, polycythemia vera occurs in about 2 per 100,000 persons, sparing no adult age group. Vertical transmission has been documented, establishing a genetic basis for the disorder. A slight overall male predominance has been observed, but females predominate within the reproductive age range.

ETIOLOGY   The etiology of polycythemia vera is unknown. Although nonrandom chromosome abnormalities such as $20q-$, trisomy 8 or 9 have been documented in a small percentage of untreated polycythemia vera patients, no consistent cytogenetic abnormality has been associated with the disorder and no specific genetic defect has yet been identified. Impaired posttranslational processing of the thrombopoietin receptor, Mpl, has been noted in polycythemia vera patients; the extent of the defect correlated with disease duration and splenomegaly. While this defect is specific for polycythemia vera and is not found in secondary erythrocytosis, its role in the pathophysiology of the disorder is still undefined. Polycythemia vera leukocytes also overexpress mRNA for *PRV*-1. In contrast to normal erythroid progenitor cells, polycythemia vera erythroid progenitor cells can grow in vitro in the absence of erythropoietin due to hypersensitivity to insulin-like growth factor I. However, this phenotypic abnormality is not specific for polycythemia vera and has been documented in essential thrombocytosis and secondary erythrocytosis. Polycythemia vera erythroid progenitor cells are more resistant to apoptosis induced by erythropoietin deprivation, due to upregulation of bcl-X_L, an antiapoptotic protein. Polycythemia vera erythroid progenitors do not divide more rapidly than their normal counterparts, but they accumulate because they do not die normally. Additionally, the transformed hematopoietic progenitor cells in polycythemia vera, as in other neoplastic disorders, exhibit clonal dominance and suppress the proliferation of normal hematopoietic progenitor cells by an unknown mechanism. Consequently, the circulating formed elements of the blood represent only progeny of the transformed clone.

CLINICAL FEATURES   Although massive splenomegaly may be the initial presenting sign in polycythemia vera, most often the disorder is first recognized by the discovery of a high hemoglobin or hematocrit, but with the exception of aquagenic pruritus, no symptoms distinguish polycythemia vera from other causes of erythrocytosis.

Uncontrolled erythrocytosis can lead to neurologic symptoms such as vertigo, tinnitus, headache, and visual disturbances. Systolic hypertension also accompanies the elevated red cell mass. In some patients, venous or arterial thrombosis may be the presenting manifestation of polycythemia vera. Intraabdominal venous thrombosis is particularly common and may be catastrophic when there is sudden compromise of the hepatic vein. Polycythemia vera should be suspected in any patient who develops the Budd-Chiari syndrome. Digital ischemia may also occur. Easy bruising, epistaxis, or gastrointestinal hemorrhage may be observed, and polycythemia vera patients are frequently hypermetabolic. Hyperuricemia with secondary gout, uric acid stones, and acid-peptic disease also complicate the disorder. Because isolated erythrocytosis is a common initial presentation for polycythemia vera but no clonal marker is available for the disease, the first task of the physician is to distinguish this autonomous clonal form of erythrocytosis from the many other types of erythrocytosis, most of which are correctable (Table 95-1).

Erythropoiesis is normally regulated by the glycoprotein hormone erythropoietin. Erythropoietin, which in adults is produced primarily in the kidneys and to a small extent in the liver, promotes the proliferation of erythroid progenitor cells, maintains their survival, and facilitates their differentiation. Because erythropoietin acts as a survival factor, it is constitutively produced and, like the red cell mass, its level is constant as long as tissue oxygenation is adequate. The plasma erythropoietin level, like the red cell mass, differs among individuals but in adults is not affected by either age or gender. Erythropoietin production is regulated at the level of gene transcription. Hypoxia is the only physiologic stimulus that increases the number of cells producing erythropoietin, and thus the production of erythropoietin is independent of its plasma level. In the absence of renal or hepatic disease, plasma erythropoietin levels reflect erythropoietin production, and therefore the assay for plasma erythropoietin is a surrogate assay

for tissue hypoxia. Erythropoietin is active at the picomolar level, and its production is tightly regulated. Thus, the plasma erythropoietin level does not rise outside the normal range until the hemoglobin level falls below 105 g/L. This is not meant to imply that an increase in erythropoietin production does not occur as the hemoglobin level falls below normal, but because the normal range for plasma erythropoietin is wide (4 to 26 mU/mL), unless the patient's baseline level is known, any increase will not be recognized until the hemoglobin falls below 105 g/L. Thereafter, there is a log-linear inverse correlation between the plasma erythropoietin and hemoglobin levels. With erythrocytosis, erythropoietin production is suppressed; this suppression reflects not only the increase in tissue oxygen transport associated with the increase in red cell number but also additional negative-feedback mechanisms unrelated to oxygen transport but related to the increase in blood viscosity and an increase in red cell precursors capable of metabolizing erythropoietin. The summation of these mechanisms accounts for the paradoxical observation that many patients with hypoxic erythrocytosis due to cyanotic congenital heart disease or obstructive lung disease have a "normal" plasma erythropoietin level. The plasma erythropoietin level is a useful diagnostic test in patients with isolated erythrocytosis, because an elevated level excludes polycythemia vera as the cause for the erythrocytosis.

DIAGNOSIS   When confronted with an elevated hemoglobin or hematocrit level, it is important to obtain previous values to determine the duration of this abnormality. Because the hemoglobin or hematocrit level is affected by the plasma volume, and hematocrit and red cell mass are not linearly related, a red cell mass determination must also be performed to distinguish absolute erythrocytosis from relative erythrocytosis due to a reduction in plasma volume alone (also known as stress or spurious erythrocytosis or Geisböck's syndrome). Red cell mass determination is important because in polycythemia vera, in contrast to erythropoietin-driven erythrocytosis, the plasma volume is frequently elevated, masking not only the true extent of red cell mass expansion but often its presence. Indeed, a significant proportion of patients with polycythemia vera have a hematocrit within the normal range, particularly patients with a substantial splenomegaly. Failure to recognize this phenomenon is undoubtedly the basis for many of the reported instances of hepatic or portal vein thrombosis in patients with an "undefined" myeloproliferative disorder.

Red cell mass is reliably determined by isotope dilution using the patient's ^{51}Cr-tagged red cells; extrapolations made after determining only the plasma volume are unacceptable. Furthermore, to allow ample time for equilibration of the labeled red cells, measurements should be made over a period of ≥ 90 min.

Once the presence of absolute erythrocytosis has been established, its cause must be determined. An elevated plasma erythropoietin level suggests either an hypoxic cause for erythrocytosis or autonomous erythropoietin production, in which case assessment of pulmonary function and an abdominal computed tomography scan to evaluate renal and hepatic anatomy are appropriate. A normal erythropoietin level does not exclude an hypoxic cause for erythrocytosis. In polycythemia vera, in contrast to hypoxic erythrocytosis, the arterial oxygen saturation is normal. However, a normal oxygen saturation does not exclude a high-affinity hemoglobin as a cause for erythrocytosis, and it is here that documentation of previous hemoglobin levels and a family study become important. Because there is no clonal marker for polycythemia vera, clinical guidelines have been proposed to define the disease. A modified version is provided in Table 95-2. However, these guidelines do not establish clonality, and in some patients the underlying disorder only becomes apparent over time. Diagnostic ambiguity does not preclude the initiation of therapy.

Other laboratory studies that may aid in diagnosis include the red cell count, mean corpuscular volume, and red cell distribution width (RDW). Only three situations cause microcytic erythrocytosis: β-thalassemia trait, hypoxic erythrocytosis, and polycythemia vera. However, with β-thalassemia trait the RDW is normal, whereas with hy-

---

TABLE 95-1   Causes of Absolute Erythrocytosis

Hypoxia	Tumors
Carbon monoxide intoxication	Hypernephroma
High altitude	Hepatoma
Pulmonary disease	Cerebellar hemangioblastoma
High-affinity hemoglobin	Adrenal adenoma
Sleep-apnea syndrome	Pheochromocytoma
Respiratory center	Meningioma
dysfunction	Uterine fibromyoma
Supine hypoventilation	Familial (with normal hemoglobin
Right-to-left cardiac shunts	function)
Renal disease	VHL mutations
Renal cysts	Erythropoietin receptor mutations
Hydronephrosis	BPG mutase deficiency
Renal artery stenosis	Bartter's syndrome
Focal glomerulonephritis	Androgen therapy
Renal transplantation	Recombinant erythropoietin therapy
	Polycythemia vera

Note: BPG, bisphosphoglycerate; VHL, von Hippel–Lindau.

TABLE 95-2 *Suggested Criteria for the Clinical Diagnosis of Polycythemia Vera*[a]

Elevated red cell mass
Normal arterial oxygen saturation
Splenomegaly
In the absence of splenomegaly:
  Leukocytosis and thrombocytosis

[a] It must be emphasized that these criteria do not establish clonality.

poxic erythrocytosis and polycythemia vera, the RDW is usually elevated. A properly made blood smear from a patient with erythrocytosis will be virtually unreadable due to the marked elevation in red cell count, but no specific morphologic abnormalities are seen in the leukocytes or platelets in polycythemia vera. However, when these are also elevated the diagnosis is assured. In many patients, the leukocyte alkaline phosphatase level is also increased, as is the uric acid level. Elevated serum vitamin B_{12} or B_{12}-binding capacity may be present. In patients with associated acid-peptic disease, occult gastrointestinal bleeding may lead to presentation with hypochromic, microcytic anemia.

A bone marrow aspirate and biopsy will provide no specific diagnostic information, and unless there is a need to establish the presence of myelofibrosis or exclude some other disorder, these procedures need not be done. Although the presence of a cytogenetic abnormality such as trisomy 8 or 9 or 20q− in the setting of an expanded red cell mass supports a clonal etiology, no specific cytogenetic abnormality is associated with polycythemia vera, and the absence of a cytogenetic marker does not exclude the diagnosis.

COMPLICATIONS   The major clinical complications of polycythemia vera relate directly to the increase in blood viscosity associated with elevation of the red cell mass and indirectly to the increased turnover of red cells, leukocytes, and platelets and the attendant increase in uric acid and cytokine production. The latter appears to be responsible for the increase in peptic ulcer disease and for the pruritus associated with this disorder, although little formal proof for this has been obtained. A sudden massive increase in spleen size is another problem and can be associated with splenic infarction or progressive cachexia. Myelofibrosis and myeloid metaplasia can also develop with transfusion-dependent anemia, but the frequency is low in those not receiving chemotherapy or irradiation. Although acute nonlymphocytic leukemia is reported to be increased in polycythemia vera, the incidence of acute leukemia in patients not exposed to chemotherapy or radiation is low and the development of leukemia is not related to disease duration, suggesting that the treatment exposure may be a more important risk factor than the disease itself.

Erythromelalgia is a curious syndrome of unknown etiology primarily involving the lower extremities and manifested usually by erythema, warmth, and pain of the affected appendage and occasionally digital infarction. It occurs with a variable frequency in patients with a myeloproliferative disorder and is usually responsive to salicylates. Some of the central nervous system symptoms observed in patients with polycythemia vera may represent a variant of erythromelalgia.

If left uncontrolled, erythrocytosis can lead to intravascular thrombosis involving vital organs such as the liver, heart, brain, or lungs. Patients with massive splenomegaly are particularly prone to thrombotic events because the associated increase in plasma volume masks the true extent of the red cell mass elevation as measured by the hematocrit or hemoglobin level. A "normal" hematocrit or hemoglobin level in a polycythemia vera patient with massive splenomegaly should be considered as indicative of an elevated red cell mass until proven otherwise.

℞ TREATMENT

Polycythemia vera is generally an indolent disorder whose clinical course can run many decades, and its medical management should

reflect the tempo of the disorder. Maintenance of the hemoglobin level at ≤140 g/L in men and ≤120 g/L in women is mandatory to avoid the thrombotic complications. Thrombosis due to erythrocytosis is the most significant complication of this disorder. Phlebotomy serves initially to reduce hyperviscosity by bringing the red cell mass into the normal range. Periodic phlebotomies thereafter serve to maintain the red cell mass within the range of normal and to induce a state of iron deficiency, which prevents an accelerated reexpansion of the red cell mass. In most polycythemia vera patients, once an iron-deficient state is achieved, phlebotomy is usually required only at 3-month intervals. Although both phlebotomy and iron deficiency, in addition to the disease itself, tend to increase the platelet count, thrombocytosis is not correlated with thrombosis in polycythemia vera, in contrast to the strong correlation between erythrocytosis and thrombosis in this disease. The use of salicylates as a tonic against thrombosis in polycythemia vera patients is potentially harmful, and salicylates should be employed only to treat erythromelalgia. Anticoagulants are not routinely indicated and are difficult to monitor owing to the artifactual imbalance between the test tube anticoagulant and plasma that occurs when blood from these patients is assayed for prothrombin or partial thromboplastin activity. Asymptomatic hyperuricemia requires no therapy, but allopurinol should be administered to avoid further elevation of the uric acid when chemotherapy is employed to reduce splenomegaly, leukocytosis, or pruritus. Generalized pruritus intractable to antihistamines can be a major problem in polycythemia vera, and hydroxyurea, interferon (IFN)-α, and psoralens with ultraviolet light in the A range (PUVA) therapy are methods of palliation. Asymptomatic thrombocytosis requires no therapy. Symptomatic splenomegaly can be treated with hydroxyurea or IFN-α, although each can be associated with significant side effects. Anagrelide, a quinazolin derivative and platelet antiaggregant that also lowers the platelet count, can control thrombocytosis and is preferable to hydroxyrurea or IFN-α. A reduction in platelet number may be necessary in the treatment of erythromelalgia if salicylates are not effective or if the thrombocytosis is associated with migraine-like symptoms. Alkylating agents and sodium phosphate P32 (^{32}P) are leukemogenic in polycythemia vera, and their use should be avoided. If a cytotoxic agent must be used, hydroxyurea is preferred, but it also may be leukemogenic. Chemotherapy should be used for as short a time as possible. In some patients, massive splenomegaly unresponsive to reduction by hydroxyurea or IFN-α therapy and associated with intractable weight loss will require splenectomy. Allogeneic bone marrow transplantation may be curative in young patients.

Patients with polycythemia vera can be expected to live long and useful lives when their red cell mass is effectively managed with phlebotomy. Chemotherapy is never indicated to control the red cell mass unless venous access is impossible.

CHRONIC IDIOPATHIC MYELOFIBROSIS

Chronic idiopathic myelofibrosis (other designations include *agnogenic myeloid metaplasia* or *myelofibrosis with myeloid metaplasia*) is a clonal disorder of a multipotent hematopoietic progenitor cell of unknown etiology characterized by marrow fibrosis, myeloid metaplasia with extramedullary hematopoiesis, and splenomegaly. Chronic idiopathic myelofibrosis is uncommon; in the absence of a specific clonal marker, establishing this diagnosis is difficult because myelofibrosis and myeloid metaplasia with splenomegaly are also features of both polycythemia vera and CML. Furthermore, myelofibrosis and splenomegaly occur in a variety of benign and malignant disorders (Table 95-3), many of which are amenable to specific therapies not effective in chronic idiopathic myelofibrosis. In contrast to the other chronic myeloproliferative disorders and so-called acute or malignant myelofibrosis, which can occur at any age, chronic idiopathic myelofibrosis primarily afflicts individuals in their sixth decade or later.

ETIOLOGY   The etiology of chronic idiopathic myelofibrosis is unknown. Although nonrandom chromosome abnormalities such as 20q−, 13q−, and trisomy 1q are not uncommon, no specific cytoge-

TABLE 95-3 *Causes of Myelofibrosis*

Carcinoma metastatic to the marrow	Polycythemia vera
Infection	Chronic idiopathic myelofibrosis
Lymphoma	Systemic mastocytosis
Hodgkin's disease	Thorium dioxide (Thorotrast) exposure
Acute leukemia (lymphoid or myeloid)	Systemic lupus erythematosus
Hairy cell leukemia	Renal osteodystrophy
Multiple myeloma	HIV infection
Chronic myeloid leukemia	Hyperparathyroidism
	Gray-platelet syndrome

FIGURE 95-2 This marrow section shows the marrow cavity replaced by fibrous tissue composed of reticulin fibers and collagen. When this fibrosis is due to a primary hematologic process, it is called *myelofibrosis*. When the fibrosis is secondary to a tumor or a granulomatous process, it is called *myelophthisis*.

netic abnormality has been identified. The degree of myelofibrosis and the extent of extramedullary hematopoiesis are not related. Fibrosis in this disorder is associated with overproduction of transforming growth factor β and thrombopoietin. Importantly, fibroblasts in chronic idiopathic myelofibrosis are not part of the neoplastic clone.

CLINICAL FEATURES No specific signs or symptoms are associated with chronic idiopathic myelofibrosis. Most patients are asymptomatic at presentation and usually detected by the discovery of splenic enlargement and/or abnormal blood counts during a routine examination. A blood smear reveals the characteristic features of extramedullary hematopoiesis: teardrop-shaped red cells, nucleated red cells, myelocytes, and promyelocytes; myeloblasts may also be present but have no prognostic significance (Fig. 95-1). Anemia, usually mild initially, is the rule, while the leukocyte and platelet counts are either normal or increased but either can be depressed. Mild hepatomegaly may accompany the splenomegaly, and both the lactate dehydrogenase and serum alkaline phosphatase levels can be elevated. The level of leukocyte alkaline phosphatase can be low, normal, or elevated. Marrow may be unaspirable due to the myelofibrosis (Fig. 95-2), and bone x-rays may reveal osteosclerosis. Exuberant extramedullary hematopoiesis can cause ascites, pulmonary hypertension, intestinal or ureteral obstruction, intracranial hypertension, pericardial tamponade, spinal cord compression, or skin nodules. Splenic enlargement can be sufficiently rapid to cause splenic infarctions with fever and pleuritic chest pain. Hyperuricemia and secondary gout may ensue.

DIAGNOSIS While the clinical picture described above is characteristic of chronic idiopathic myelofibrosis, all of the clinical features described can be observed in polycythemia vera or CML. Massive splenomegaly commonly masks erythrocytosis in polycythemia vera, and reports of intraabdominal thromboses in chronic idiopathic myelofibrosis likely represent instances of unrecognized polycythemia vera. Furthermore, many other disorders have features that overlap with chronic idiopathic myelofibrosis but respond to distinctly different therapies. Therefore, the diagnosis of chronic idiopathic myelofibrosis is one of exclusion, which requires that the disorders listed in Table 95-3 be ruled out.

The presence of teardrop-shaped red cells, nucleated red cells, myelocytes, and promyelocytes establishes the presence of extramedullary hematopoiesis; the presence of leukocytosis, thrombocytosis with large and bizarre platelets, as well as circulating myeloblasts suggests

the presence of a myeloproliferative disorder as opposed to a secondary form of myelofibrosis (Table 95-3). Marrow is usually not aspirable due to increased marrow reticulin, but marrow biopsy will reveal a hypercellular marrow with trilineage hyperplasia and, in particular, increased megakaryocytes, but there are no characteristic morphologic abnormalities that distinguish idiopathic myelofibrosis from the other chronic myeloproliferative disorders. Splenomegaly due to extramedullary hematopoiesis may be sufficiently massive to cause portal hypertension and variceal formation. In some patients, exuberant extramedullary hematopoiesis can dominate the clinical picture. An intriguing feature of chronic idiopathic myelofibrosis is the occurrence of autoimmune abnormalities such as immune complexes, antinuclear antibodies, rheumatoid factor, or a positive Coombs' test. Whether these represent a host reaction to the disorder or are involved in its pathogenesis is unknown. Cytogenetic analysis of blood or marrow is useful both to exclude CML and for prognostic purposes, because complex karyotype abnormalities portend a poor prognosis in chronic idiopathic myelofibrosis. For unknown reasons, the number of circulating CD34 cells is markedly increased in chronic idiopathic myelofibrosis.

COMPLICATIONS Chronic idiopathic myelofibrosis has a median survival of only 5 years (range 1 to 15 years), a duration much shorter than for polycythemia vera or essential thrombocytosis. The natural history of chronic idiopathic myelofibrosis is one of inexorable marrow failure with transfusion-dependent anemia and increasing organomegaly. Patients are prone to deep-seated tissue infections, particularly of the lungs. As with CML, chronic idiopathic myelofibrosis can evolve from a chronic phase to an accelerated phase with constitutional symptoms and increasing marrow failure. About 10% of patients develop an aggressive form of acute leukemia for which therapy is usually ineffective. Important prognostic factors for disease acceleration include anemia; thrombocytopenia; age; the presence of complex cytogenetic abnormalities; and constitutional symptoms such as unexplained fever, night sweats, or weight loss. Any nonrandom cytogenetic abnormality is associated with a shortened life span, and the presence or development of multiple cytogenetic abnormalities is highly indicative of disease acceleration.

℞ TREATMENT

No specific therapy exists for chronic idiopathic myelofibrosis. Anemia may be exacerbated by deficiency of folic acid or iron, and in rare instances, pyridoxine therapy has been effective. However, anemia is more often due to ineffective erythropoiesis not compensated for by the extramedullary hematopoiesis in the spleen and liver; neither androgens nor erythropoietin has been consistently effective therapy. Erythropoietin may worsen splenomegaly. A red cell splenic sequestration study can establish the presence of hypersplenism, for which splenectomy is indicated. Splenectomy may also be necessary if splenomegaly impairs alimentation and should be performed before cachexia sets in. In this situation, splenectomy should not be avoided because of concern over rebound thrombocytosis, loss of hematopoietic capacity, or compensatory hepatomegaly. However, for unexplained reasons, splenectomy increases the risk of blastic transformation. Allopurinol can control significant hyperuricemia, and

FIGURE 95-1 Teardrop-shaped red blood cells indicative of membrane damage from collagen fibers, a nucleated red blood cell indicative of premature release of erythroid precursors, and immature myeloid cells indicative of extramedullary hematopoiesis are noted. This peripheral blood smear is related to marrow fibrosis, either primary myelofibrosis or secondary myelophthisis.

hydroxyurea has proved useful for controlling organomegaly. The role of IFN-α is undefined, and its side effects are more pronounced in the older individuals who are affected with this disorder, but reversal of myelofibrosis has been observed. Glucocorticoids are used to control autoimmune complications and may ameliorate anemia alone or in combination with thalidomide. Allogeneic bone marrow transplantation should be considered in younger patients.

ESSENTIAL THROMBOCYTOSIS

Essential thrombocytosis (other designations include *essential thrombocythemia*, *idiopathic thrombocytosis*, *primary thrombocytosis*, *hemorrhagic thrombocythemia*) is a clonal disorder of unknown etiology involving a multipotent hematopoietic progenitor cell and is manifested clinically by the overproduction of platelets without a definable cause. Essential thrombocytosis is an uncommon disorder, but its exact frequency is unknown. No clonal marker distinguishes it from the more common nonclonal, reactive forms of thrombocytosis (Table 95-4). Clinical recognition of thrombocytosis is unlikely in the largely asymptomatic persons affected by this disorder. As a consequence, essential thrombocytosis was formerly considered to be a disease of the elderly and to be responsible for significant morbidity due to hemorrhage or thrombosis. However, with the widespread application of platelet counting, it is now clear that essential thrombocytosis can occur at any age in adults and often occurs without symptoms or disturbances of hemostasis. There is an unexplained female predominance, in contrast to the reactive forms of thrombocytosis where no sex bias exists. Because no clonal marker is available for the disorder, clinical criteria have been proposed to distinguish it from the other chronic myeloproliferative disorders, which may also present with thrombocytosis but have differing prognoses and treatment (Table 95-5). These criteria do not establish clonality; therefore, they are truly useful only in identifying disorders such as CML, polycythemia vera, or myelodysplasia, which can masquerade as essential thrombocytosis, as opposed to establishing the presence of essential thrombocytosis. Furthermore, as with "primary" erythrocytosis, nonclonal, benign forms of thrombocytosis exist (such as hereditary overproduction of thrombopoietin) that are not widely recognized because we currently lack the diagnostic tools to do so.

ETIOLOGY   Megakaryocytopoiesis and platelet production depend upon thrombopoietin and its receptor, Mpl. As in the case of early erythroid and myeloid progenitor cells, early megakaryocytic progenitors require the presence of interleukin (IL) 3 and stem cell factor for optimal proliferation, and their subsequent development is enhanced by IL-6 and -11. However, megakaryocyte maturation and differentiation require thrombopoietin.

Megakaryocytes are unique among hematopoietic progenitor cells because they undergo endomitotic as opposed to mitotic reduplication of their genome. In the absence of thrombopoietin, endomitotic megakaryocytic reduplication and, by extension, the cytoplasmic development necessary for platelet production are impaired. Like erythropoietin, thrombopoietin is produced in both the liver and the kidneys,

TABLE 95-4   Causes of Thrombocytosis

Iron-deficiency anemia	Idiopathic myelofibrosis
Hyposplenism	Essential thrombocytosis
Postsplenectomy[a]	Chronic myeloid leukemia
Malignancy	Idiopathic sideroblastic anemia
Collagen vascular disease	Myelodysplasia (5q− syndrome)
Inflammatory bowel disease	Postsurgery
Infection	Rebound (cessation of ethanol intake,
Hemolysis	correction of vitamin B_{12} or folate
Hemorrhage	deficiency)
Polycythemia vera	

[a] If the platelet count is greater than $2 \times 10^6/\mu L$, the etiology is most likely a myeloproliferative disorder.

TABLE 95-5   Suggested Criteria for the Clinical Diagnosis of Essential Thrombocytosis[a]

Platelet count $\geq$ 500,000/μL
Absence of a known cause of reactive thrombocytosis (see Table 95-4)
Absence of the Ph chromosome and the bcr-abl gene rearrangement
Normal red cell mass
Presence of marrow iron
Absence of myelofibrosis
Absence of myelodysplasia clinically and by cytogenetic analysis
Splenomegaly

[a] The concept that a platelet count greater than $1 \times 10^6/\mu L$ distinguishes essential thrombocytosis from other causes of thrombocytosis has no clinical validity.

and an inverse correlation exists between the platelet count and plasma thrombopoietic activity. Like erythropoietin, plasma levels of thrombopoietin are controlled in part by the size of its progenitor cell pool. In contrast to erythropoietin, but like its myeloid counterparts granulocyte and granulocyte-macrophage colony-stimulating factors, thrombopoietin not only enhances the proliferation of its target cells but also enhances the reactivity of their end-stage product, the platelet. In addition to its role in thrombopoiesis, thrombopoietin enhances the survival of multipotent hematopoietic stem cells.

The clonality of essential thrombocytosis was established by the use of the isoenzymes of glucose-6-phosphate dehydrogenase in patients who are hemizygous for this gene, by the use of X-linked DNA polymorphisms, and by the identification of nonrandom, although variable, cytogenetic abnormalities. The multipotent hematopoietic progenitor cell involved in this disorder can vary; in some patients lymphocytes contained the same clonal marker as the megakaryocytes, erythrocytes, and myeloid cells, whereas in others the lymphocytes were not involved. Similar observations have been made in polycythemia vera. Furthermore, a number of families have been described in which essential thrombocytosis was inherited, in one instance as an autosomal dominant trait. In one kindred, in addition to essential thrombocytosis, idiopathic myelofibrosis and polycythemia vera were also individually documented.

CLINICAL FEATURES   Clinically, essential thrombocytosis is most often identified incidentally when a platelet count is obtained during the course of a routine evaluation. Occasionally, review of previous platelet counts will reveal that an elevation was present but overlooked. No symptoms or signs are specific for essential thrombocytosis, but patients do have hemorrhagic and thrombotic tendencies expressed as easy bruising for the former or microvascular occlusions for the latter, which may be manifested by erythromelalgia, migraine, or transient ischemic attacks. Physical examination is generally unremarkable except occasionally for mild splenomegaly. Massive splenomegaly is more characteristic of the other myeloproliferative disorders, particularly polycythemia vera or idiopathic myelofibrosis.

Anemia is unusual, but a mild neutrophilic leukocytosis is not. The blood smear, however, is most remarkable for the number of platelets present, some of which may be very large. The leukocyte alkaline phosphatase score is either normal or elevated. The large mass of circulating platelets may prevent the accurate measurement of serum potassium due to the release of platelet potassium upon blood clotting. This hyperkalemia is a laboratory artifact and is not associated with any electrocardiographic abnormalities. Similarly, arterial oxygen measurements can be inaccurate unless the blood is collected on ice. The prothrombin and partial thromboplastin times are normal, while abnormalities of platelet function such as a prolonged bleeding time and impaired platelet aggregation can be present. However, in spite of much study, characteristic platelet function abnormalities are not yet defined, and no platelet function test predicts clinically significant bleeding or thrombosis.

The elevated platelet count may hinder the collection of a marrow aspirate, but marrow biopsy usually reveals both megakaryocyte hyperplasia and hypertrophy, as well as an overall increase in marrow cellularity. A slight increase in marrow reticulin may be present, but if extensive, another diagnosis should be considered. The absence of stainable iron demands an explanation, because iron deficiency alone can cause thrombocytosis and absent marrow iron is a feature of polycythemia vera.

While nonrandom cytogenetic abnormalities have been identified in essential thrombocytosis, no consistently identifiable abnormality is notable, even involving chromosomes 3 and 1 where the genes for thrombopoietin and its receptor Mpl, respectively, are located.

DIAGNOSIS   Thrombocytosis is encountered in a variety of clinical disorders (Table 95-4) in which production of cytokines is increased. Thus, the first obligation when confronted with a high platelet count is to determine if it is a consequence of another disorder. Cytogenetic evaluation is mandatory to determine if the thrombocytosis is due to CML or a myelodysplastic disorder such as the 5q− syndrome. Because the bcr-abl translocation can be present in the absence of the Ph chromosome, fluorescence in situ hybridization (FISH) analysis for bcr-abl expression should be performed in all patients with thrombocytosis rather than a cytogenetic study. Anemia and ringed sideroblasts are not features of essential thrombocytosis, but they are features of idiopathic refractory sideroblastic anemia, in which thrombocytosis can also occur. The presence of massive splenomegaly should suggest the possibility of another myeloproliferative disorder, and in this setting a red cell mass determination is mandatory because substantial splenomegaly can mask the presence of erythrocytosis. What appears to be essential thrombocytosis can evolve into polycythemia vera, revealing the true nature of the underlying myeloproliferative disorder.

COMPLICATIONS   Perhaps no other condition in clinical medicine has caused otherwise astute physicians to intervene inappropriately more often than thrombocytosis, particularly if the platelet count is $>1 \times 10^6/\mu L$. It is commonly believed that a high platelet count must cause intravascular stasis and thrombosis; however, no controlled clinical study has ever established this association.

To the contrary, very high platelet counts are associated primarily with hemorrhage due to acquired von Willebrand disease, while platelet counts of $<1 \times 10^6/\mu L$ are more often associated with thrombosis. This is not meant to imply that an elevated platelet count cannot cause symptoms in a patient with essential thrombocytosis, but rather that the focus should be on the patient, not the platelet count. For example, some of the most dramatic neurologic problems in essential thrombocytosis are migraine-related and may respond only to lowering of the platelet count; other symptoms may be a manifestation of erythromelalgia and respond simply to platelet cyclooxygenase inhibitors such as aspirin, without a reduction in platelet number. Still others may represent an interaction between an atherosclerotic vascular system and a high platelet count, and others may have no relationship to the platelet count whatsoever. Progress in distinguishing essential thrombocytosis from polycythemia vera and in defining new causes of hypercoagulability (such as factor V Leiden) make the older literature on thrombocytosis less reliable.

R_x TREATMENT

An elevated platelet count in an asymptomatic patient requires no therapy, and before any therapy is initiated in a patient with thrombocytosis, the cause of symptoms must be clearly identified to be a consequence of the elevated platelet count. Platelet pheresis has not been proven efficacious and cannot be recommended. Furthermore, patients with essential thrombocytosis treated with ^{32}P, hydroxyurea, or alkylating agents are placed at risk of developing acute leukemia without any proof of benefit from such therapy. If platelet reduction is deemed necessary on the basis of neurologic symptoms refractory to salicylates, IFN-α or anagrelide, a quinazolin derivative, can reduce the platelet count, but neither is uniformly effective nor without significant side effects. Hydroxyurea should be considered only if these agents are not effective or tolerable. Bleeding associated with thrombocytosis usually responds to ϵ-aminocaproic acid, which can be given prophylactically before and after elective surgery. As more clinical experience is acquired, it appears that essential thrombocytosis is more benign than previously thought, and that evolution to acute leukemia is more likely to be a consequence of prior therapy than of the disease itself. In managing patients with thrombocytosis, the physician's first obligation is to do no harm.

FURTHER READING

BAROSI G: Myelofibrosis with myeloid metaplasia: Diagnostic definition and prognostic classification for clinical studies and treatment guidelines. J Clin Oncol 17:2954, 1999

BUSS DH et al: The incidence of thrombotic and hemorrhagic disorders in association with extreme thrombocytosis: An analysis of 129 cases. Am J Hematol 20:365, 1985

SPIVAK JL: Polycythemia vera: Myths, mechanisms, and management. Blood 100:4272, 2002

SPIVAK JL et al: Chronic myeloproliferative disorders. Hematology (Am Soc Hematol Educ Program):200, 2003

TEFFERI A: The forgotten myeloproliferative disorder: Myeloid metaplasia. Oncologist 8:255, 2003

VARDIMAN JW et al: The World Health Organization (WHO) classification of the myeloid neoplasms. Blood 100:2292, 2002

96 ACUTE AND CHRONIC MYELOID LEUKEMIA
Meir Wetzler, John C. Byrd, Clara D. Bloomfield

The myeloid leukemias are a heterogeneous group of diseases characterized by infiltration of the blood, bone marrow, and other tissues by neoplastic cells of the hematopoietic system. In 2004, the estimated number of new myeloid leukemia cases in the United States was 16,520. These leukemias comprise a spectrum of malignancies that, untreated, range from rapidly fatal to slowly growing. Based on their untreated course, the myeloid leukemias have traditionally been designated acute or chronic.

ACUTE MYELOID LEUKEMIA

INCIDENCE   The incidence of acute myeloid leukemia (AML) is ~3.6 per 100,000 people per year, and the age-adjusted incidence is higher in men than in women (4.4 versus 3.0). AML incidence increases with age; it is 1.7 in individuals <65 years and 16.2 in those >65. A significant increase in AML incidence has occurred over the past 10 years.

ETIOLOGY   Heredity, radiation, chemical and other occupational exposures, and drugs have been implicated in the development of AML. No direct evidence suggests a viral etiology.

Heredity   Certain syndromes with somatic cell chromosome aneuploidy, e.g., Down (chromosome 21 trisomy), Klinefelter (XXY and variants), and Patau (chromosome 13 trisomy), are associated with an increased incidence of AML. Inherited diseases with excessive chromatin fragility, e.g., Fanconi anemia, Bloom syndrome, ataxia telangiectasia, and Kostmann syndrome, are also associated with AML.

Radiation   Survivors of the atomic bomb explosions in Japan had an increased incidence of myeloid leukemias that peaked 5 to 7 years after exposure. Therapeutic radiation alone seems to add little risk of AML but can increase the risk in people exposed to alkylating agents.

Chemical and Other Exposures Exposure to benzene, which is used as a solvent in the chemical, plastic, rubber, and pharmaceutical industries, is associated with an increased incidence of AML. Smoking and exposure to petroleum products, paint, embalming fluids, ethylene oxide, herbicides, and pesticides, have also been associated with an increased risk of AML.

Drugs Anticancer drugs are the leading cause of treatment-associated AML. Alkylating agent–associated leukemias occur on average 4 to 6 years after exposure, and affected individuals have aberrations in chromosomes 5 and 7. Topoisomerase II inhibitor–associated leukemias occur 1 to 3 years after exposure, and affected individuals often have aberrations involving chromosome 11q23. Chloramphenicol, phenylbutazone, and, less commonly, chloroquine and methoxypsoralen can result in bone marrow failure that may evolve into AML.

CLASSIFICATION The categorization of acute leukemia into biologically distinct groups is based on morphology, cytochemistry, and immunophenotype as well as cytogenetic and molecular techniques.

Morphologic and Cytochemical Classification The diagnosis of AML is established by the presence of ≥20% myeloblasts in blood and/or bone marrow according to the World Health Organization (WHO) classification. Myeloblasts have nuclear chromatin that is uniformly fine or lacelike in appearance and large nucleoli (2 to 5 per cell). If specific cytoplasmic granules, Auer rods, or the nuclear folding and clefting characteristic of monocytoid cells are not present, the morphologic features observed under light microscopy may not be sufficient to clarify the diagnosis. A positive myeloperoxidase reaction in >3% of the blasts may be the only feature distinguishing AML from acute lymphoblastic leukemia (ALL).

Until 2000, the diagnosis of AML was established by the presence of ≥30% myeloblasts in the marrow and further classified based on morphology and cytochemistry according to the French, American, and British (FAB) schema, which includes eight major subtypes, M0 to M7 (Table 96-1). The WHO classification modified the FAB schema by reducing the number of blasts required for a diagnosis and incorporating molecular (including cytogenetic), morphologic (multilineage dysplasia), and clinical features (such as prior hematologic disorder) in defining disease entities (Table 96-1).

Immunophenotypic Classification The phenotype of human myeloid leukemia cells can be studied by multiparameter flow cytometry after the cells are labeled with monoclonal antibodies to cell-surface antigens. For example, M0, which is characterized by immature morphology and no lineage-specific cytochemical reactions, is diagnosed by flow cytometric demonstration of the myeloid-specific antigens cluster designation (CD) 13 or 33. Similarly, M7 can often be diagnosed only by expression of the platelet-specific antigens CD41 and/or CD61 or by electron microscopic demonstration of myeloperoxidase.

Chromosomal Classification Chromosomal analysis of the leukemic cell provides the most important pretreatment prognostic information in AML. Two cytogenetic abnormalities have been invariably associated with a specific FAB group: t(15;17)(q22;q12) with M3 and inv(16)(p13q22) with M4Eo, and many chromosomal abnormalities have been associated primarily with one FAB group, including t(8;21)(q22;q22) with M2, and t(9;11)(p22;q23), and other translocations involving 11q23, with M5. As a result of their prognostic significance and association with specific morphologic features, the WHO classification incorporates cytogenetics (Table 96-1). Many of the recurring chromosomal abnormalities in AML have been associated with specific clinical characteristics. More commonly associated with younger age are t(8;21) and t(15;17), and with older age, del(5q) and del(7q). Myeloid sarcomas (see below) are associated with t(8;21) and disseminated intravascular coagulation (DIC) with t(15;17).

Molecular Classification Molecular study of many recurring cytogenetic abnormalities has revealed genes that may be involved in leukemo-

TABLE 96-1 *Acute Myeloid Leukemia (AML) Classification Systems*

French-American-British (FAB) Classification[a]
M0: Minimally differentiated leukemia
M1: Myeloblastic leukemia without maturation
M2: Myeloblastic leukemia with maturation
M3: Hypergranular promyelocytic leukemia
M4: Myelomonocytic leukemia
M4Eo: Variant: Increase in abnormal marrow eosinophils
M5: Monocytic leukemia
M6: Erythroleukemia (DiGuglielmo's disease)
M7: Megakaryoblastic leukemia

World Health Organization Classification[b]
  I. AML with recurrent genetic abnormalities
    AML with t(8;21)(q22;q22);*AML1(CBFα)/ETO*
    AML with abnormal bone marrow eosinophils [inv(16)(p13q22) or
    t(16;16)(p13;q22);*CBFβ/MYH11*]
    Acute promyelocytic leukemia [AML with t(15;17)(q22;q12) (*PML/RARα* and variants]
    AML with 11q23 (*MLL*) abnormalities
  II. AML with multilineage dysplasia
    Following a myelodysplastic syndrome or myelodysplastic syndrome/myeloproliferative disorder
    Without antecedent myelodysplastic syndrome
  III. AML and myelodysplastic syndromes, therapy-related
    Alkylating agent–related
    Topoisomerase type II inhibitor–related
    Other types
  IV. AML not otherwise categorized
    AML minimally differentiated
    AML without maturation
    AML with maturation
    Acute myelomonocytic leukemia
    Acute monoblastic and monocytic leukemia
    Acute erythroid leukemia
    Acute megakaryoblastic leukemia
    Acute basophilic leukemia
    Acute panmyelosis with myelofibrosis
    Myeloid sarcoma

[a] JM Bennett et al: Ann Intern Med 103:620, 1985
[b] ES Jaffe et al: *World Health Organization Classification of Tumours. Pathology and Genetics of Tumours of Haematopoietic and Lymphoid Tissues.* Lyon, IARC Press, 2001.

genesis. The 15;17 translocation encodes a chimeric protein, Pml/Rarα, which is formed by the fusion of the retinoic acid receptor-α (*RARα*) gene from chromosome 17 and the promyelocytic leukemia (*PML*) gene from chromosome 15. The *RARα* gene encodes a member of the nuclear hormone receptor family of transcription factors. After binding retinoic acid, *RARα* can promote expression of a variety of genes. The 15;17 translocation juxtaposes *PML* with *RARα* in a head-to-tail configuration that is under the transcriptional control of *PML*. Three different breakpoints in the *PML* gene lead to various fusion proteins. The Pml-Rarα fusion protein tends to suppress gene transcription and blocks differentiation of the cells. Pharmacologic doses of the Rarα ligand, all-*trans*-retinoic acid (tretinoin), relieve the block and promote differentiation (see below).

The inv(16), characteristic of M4Eo or AML with abnormal bone marrow eosinophils, and the t(8;21) both involve subunits of the transcription factor complex core-binding factor (Cbf), also known as polyomavirus enhancer binding protein 2 (Pebp2). This transcription factor contains two subunits, an α subunit, the Am11 protein, and a β subunit, the Pebp2 protein, and is involved in the expression of a number of differentiation-dependent genes in myeloid cells. The inv(16) results in a fusion of the core-binding factor β (*CBFB*) gene on the q arm (encodes Pebp2 protein) and the myosin heavy chain (*MYH11*) gene on the p arm. The 8;21 translocation involves the core binding factor α (*CBFA*) gene on chromosome 21, called the *AML1* (also *RUNX1*) gene, joining the *ETO* gene on chromosome 8. Similar to the t(15;17) gene product, the Am11/Eto protein acts to block transcription of *CBFA-CBFB*-controlled genes.

Most translocations that involve 11q23 rearrange the myeloid-lymphoid [or mixed-lineage leukemia (*MLL*)] gene. The *MLL* gene has two regions that encompass multiple zinc fingers and has at least two additional potential DNA-binding motifs. Abnormalities in the *MLL* gene are relatively common in patients with AML who do not have 11q23 rearrangements cytogenetically.

The above molecular aberrations are increasingly being used for diagnosis and detection of residual disease after treatment. Molecular aberrations are also being identified that are useful for classifying risk of relapse in patients without cytogenetic abnormalities. A partial tandem duplication (PTD) of the *MLL* gene is found in 5 to 10% of patients with normal cytogenetics and results in short remission duration. Flt3 (FMS-like tyrosine kinase 3) is a tyrosine kinase receptor important in the development of myeloid and lymphoid lineages. Activating mutations of *FLT3* are present in ~30% of adult AML patients due to internal tandem duplications (ITD) in the juxtamembrane domain or mutations of the activating loop of the kinase. Continuous activation of Flt3 and downstream target kinases, including signal transducer and activator of transcription protein 5, Ras/mitogen-activated protein kinase, and phosphatidylinositol 3-kinase/Akt, provides increased proliferation and antiapoptotic signals to the myeloid progenitor cell. Several clinical studies have demonstrated that presence of *FLT3* ITD in patients with normal cytogenetics predicts for short remission duration and inferior survival.

CLINICAL PRESENTATION ■ **Symptoms** Patients with AML most often present with nonspecific symptoms that begin gradually or abruptly and are the consequence of anemia, leukocytosis, leukopenia or leukocyte dysfunction, or thrombocytopenia. Nearly half have had symptoms for ≥3 months before the leukemia was diagnosed.

Half mention fatigue as the first symptom, but most complain of fatigue or weakness at the time of diagnosis. Anorexia and weight loss are common. Fever with or without an identifiable infection is the initial symptom in ~10% of patients. Signs of abnormal hemostasis (bleeding, easy bruising) are noted first in 5% of patients. On occasion, bone pain, lymphadenopathy, nonspecific cough, headache, or diaphoresis is the presenting symptom.

Rarely patients may present with symptoms from a mass lesion located in the soft tissues, breast, uterus, ovary, cranial or spinal dura, gastrointestinal tract, lung, mediastinum, prostate, bone, or other organs. The mass lesion represents a tumor of leukemic cells and is called a *granulocytic sarcoma*, or *chloroma*. Typical AML may occur simultaneously, later, or not at all in these patients. This rare presentation is more common in patients with 8;21 translocations.

Physical Findings Fever, splenomegaly, hepatomegaly, lymphadenopathy, sternal tenderness, and evidence of infection and hemorrhage are often found at diagnosis. Significant gastrointestinal bleeding, intrapulmonary hemorrhage, or intracranial hemorrhage occur most often in acute promyelocytic leukemia (APL). Bleeding associated with coagulopathy may also occur in monocytic AML and with extreme degrees of leukocytosis or thrombocytopenia in other morphologic subtypes. Retinal hemorrhages are detected in 15% of patients. Infiltration of the gingivae, skin, soft tissues, or the meninges with leukemic blasts at diagnosis is characteristic of the monocytic subtypes (FAB M4 and M5).

Hematologic Findings Anemia is usually present at diagnosis and can be severe. The degree varies considerably irrespective of other hematologic findings, splenomegaly, or the duration of symptoms. The anemia is usually normochromic normocytic. Decreased erythropoiesis often results in a reduced reticulocyte count, and erythrocyte survival is decreased by accelerated destruction. Active blood loss also contributes to the anemia.

The median presenting leukocyte count is about 15,000/μl. Between 25 and 40% of patients have counts <5000/μl, and 20% have counts >100,000/μl. Fewer than 5% have no detectable leukemic cells in the blood. Poor neutrophil function may be noted functionally by impaired phagocytosis and migration and morphologically by abnormal lobulation and deficient granulation.

Platelet counts <100,000/μl are found at diagnosis in ~75% of patients, and about 25% have counts <25,000/μl. Both morphologic and functional platelet abnormalities can be observed, including large and bizarre shapes with abnormal granulation and inability of platelets to aggregate or adhere normally to one another.

Pretreatment Evaluation Once the diagnosis of AML is suspected, a rapid evaluation and initiation of appropriate therapy should follow (Table 96-2). In addition to clarifying the subtype of leukemia, initial studies should evaluate the overall functional integrity of the major organ systems, including the cardiovascular, pulmonary, hepatic, and renal systems. Factors that have prognostic significance, either for achieving complete remission (CR) or for predicting the duration of CR, should also be assessed before initiating treatment. Leukemic cells

TABLE 96-2 *Initial Diagnostic Evaluation and Management of Adult Patients with AML*

History
  Increasing fatigue or decreased exercise tolerance (anemia)
  Excess bleeding or bleeding from unusual sites (DIC, thrombocytopenia)
  Fevers or recurrent infections (granulocytopenia)
  Headache, vision changes, nonfocal neurologic abnormalities (CNS leukemia or bleed)
  Early satiety (splenomegaly)
  Family history of AML (Fanconi, Bloom, or Kostmann syndromes or ataxia telangiectasia)
  History of cancer (exposure to alkylating agents, radiation, topoisomerase II inhibitors)
  Occupational exposures (radiation, benzene, petroleum products, paint, smoking, pesticides)
Physical Examination
  Performance status (prognostic factor)
  Ecchymosis and oozing from IV sites (DIC, possible acute promyelocytic leukemia)
  Fever and tachycardia (signs of infection)
  Papilledema, retinal infiltrates, cranial nerve abnormalities (CNS leukemia)
  Poor dentition, dental abscesses
  Gum hypertrophy (leukemic infiltration, most common in monocytic leukemia)
  Skin infiltration or nodules (leukemia infiltration, most common in monocytic leukemia)
  Lymphadenopathy, splenomegaly, hepatomegaly
  Back pain, lower extremity weakness [spinal granulocytic sarcoma, most likely in t(8;21) patients]
Laboratory and radiologic studies
  CBC with manual differential cell count
  Chemistry tests (electrolytes, creatinine, BUN, calcium, phosphorus, uric acid, hepatic enzymes, bilirubin, LDH, amylase, lipase)
  Clotting studies (prothrombin time, partial thromboplastin time, fibrinogen, D-dimer)
  Viral serologies (CMV, HSV-1, varicella zoster)
  RBC type and screen
  HLA-typing of patient, siblings, and parents for potential allogeneic SCT
  Bone marrow aspirate and biopsy (morphology, cytochemistry, cytogenetics, flow cytometry, molecular studies)
  Cryopreservation of viable leukemia cells
  Echocardiogram
  PA and lateral chest radiograph
  Placement of central venous access device
Interventions for specific patients
  Dental evaluation (for those with poor dentition)
  Lumbar puncture (for those with symptoms of CNS involvement)
  Screening spine MRI (for patients with back pain, lower extremity weakness, paresthesias)
  Social work referral for patient and family psychosocial support
Counseling for all patients
  Provide patient with information regarding their disease, financial counseling, and support group contacts

Abbreviations: BUN, blood urea nitrogen; CBC, complete blood count; CMV, cytomegalovirus; CNS, central nervous system; DIC, disseminated intravascular coagulation; HSV, herpes simplex virus; LDH, lactate dehydrogenase; MRI, magnetic resonance imaging; PA, posteroanterior; RBC, red blood (cell) count; SCT, stem cell transplant.

should be obtained from all patients and cryopreserved for future use as new tests and therapeutics become available. All patients should be evaluated for infection.

Most patients are anemic and thrombocytopenic at presentation. Replacement of the appropriate blood components, if necessary, should begin promptly. Because qualitative platelet dysfunction or the presence of an infection may increase the likelihood of bleeding, evidence of hemorrhage justifies the immediate use of platelet transfusion, even if the platelet count is only moderately decreased.

About 50% of patients have a mild to moderate elevation of serum uric acid at presentation. Only 10% have marked elevations, but renal precipitation of uric acid and the nephropathy that may result is a serious but uncommon complication. The initiation of chemotherapy may aggravate hyperuricemia, and patients are usually started immediately on allopurinol or rasburicase (recombinant uric oxidase) and hydration at diagnosis. Finally, the presence in high concentrations of lysozyme, a marker for monocytic differentiation, may be etiologic in renal tubular dysfunction, which could worsen other renal problems that arise during the initial phases of therapy.

PROGNOSTIC FACTORS   Many factors influence the likelihood of entering CR, the length of CR, and the curability of AML. CR is defined after examination of both blood and bone marrow. The blood neutrophil count must be $\geq 1500/\mu l$ and the platelet count $\geq 100,000/\mu l$. Hemoglobin concentration or hematocrit are not considered in determining CR. Circulating blasts should be absent. While rare blasts may be detected in the blood during marrow regeneration, they should disappear on successive studies. Bone marrow cellularity should be >20% with trilineage maturation. The bone marrow should contain <5% blasts, and Auer rods should be absent. Extramedullary leukemia should not be present. For patients in CR, reverse transcriptase polymerase chain reaction (RT-PCR) to detect AML-associated molecular abnormalities and fluorescence in situ hybridization (FISH) to detect AML-associated cytogenetic aberrations are currently used to detect residual disease. Such detection of minimal residual disease may become a reliable discriminator between patients in CR who do or do not require additional and/or alternative therapies. Prognostic factors are influenced by the treatment used.

Age at diagnosis remains among the most important pretreatment risk factors, with advancing age being associated with a poorer prognosis primarily because of its influence on the patient's ability to survive induction therapy and thus achieve CR. Age may also influence outcome because AML in older patients differs biologically. The leukemic cells in elderly patients more commonly express CD34 and the multidrug resistance 1 (Mdr1) efflux pump that conveys resistance to natural product–derived agents such as the anthracyclines (see below). With each successive decade of age, a greater proportion of patients have more resistant disease. Chronic and intercurrent diseases impair tolerance to rigorous therapy; acute medical problems at diagnosis reduce the likelihood of survival. Performance status, independent of age, also influences ability to survive induction therapy and thus respond to treatment.

Chromosome findings at diagnosis are an independent prognostic factor. Patients with t(8;21), inv(16), or t(15;17) have good prognoses, while those with no cytogenetic abnormality have a moderately favorable outcome when treated with high-dose cytarabine. Patients with a complex karyotype, inv(3), or −7 have a very poor prognosis. Molecular markers such as the presence of a PTD of *MLL* or the ITD of *FLT3* may also predict poor outcome of AML patients who otherwise have an intermediate prognosis.

A prolonged symptomatic interval with cytopenias preceding diagnosis or a history of an antecedent hematologic disorder are other pretreatment clinical features that are associated with a lower CR rate and shorter survival time. The CR rate is lower in patients who have had anemia, leukopenia, and/or thrombocytopenia for >1 month before the diagnosis of AML when compared to those without such a

history. Responsiveness to chemotherapy declines as the duration of the antecedent disorder(s) increases. Secondary AML developing after treatment with cytotoxic agents for other malignancies is extremely difficult to treat successfully.

A high presenting leukocyte count is an independent prognostic factor; duration of CR is inversely related to the presenting leukocyte count or absolute circulating myeloblast count. Among patients with hyperleukocytosis ($>100,000/\mu l$), early central nervous system bleeding and pulmonary leukostasis and relapse contribute to poor outcome.

The FAB classification diagnosis has been found to be an independent prognostic factor in some series. Other characteristics of leukemic cells have been reported to have prognostic significance, including Auer rods, ultrastructural features, in vitro and in vivo growth characteristics and chemotherapeutic sensitivity, and immunophenotype. Expression of the *MDR1* gene adversely influences outcome.

In addition to pretreatment variables, several treatment factors correlate with prognosis in AML, including, most importantly, achievement of CR. Another is the rapidity with which the blast cells disappear from the blood after the institution of therapy. In addition, patients who achieve CR after one induction cycle have longer CR durations than those requiring multiple cycles.

Rx TREATMENT

Treatment of the newly diagnosed patient with AML is usually divided into two phases, induction and postremission management (Fig. 96-1). The initial goal is to quickly induce CR. Once CR is obtained, further therapy must be used to prolong survival and achieve cure. The initial induction treatment and subsequent consolidation therapy are often chosen based upon the patient's age. The influence of intensifying therapy with traditional chemotherapy agents such as cytarabine and

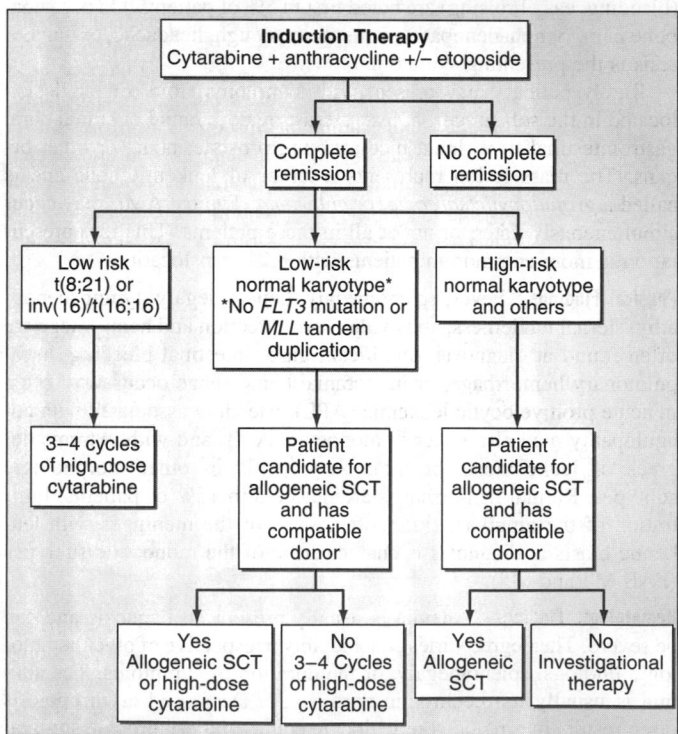

FIGURE 96-1   Flow chart for the therapy of newly diagnosed AML. For all forms of AML except APL, standard therapy includes a 7-day continuous infusion of cytarabine (100–200 mg/m² per day) and a 3-day course of daunorubicin (45–60 mg/m² per day) or idarubicin (12–13 mg/m² per day) with or without 3 days of etoposide. Patients who achieve complete remission undergo some form of consolidation therapy, including sequential courses of high-dose cytarabine, high-dose combination chemotherapy with allogeneic stem cell transplant (SCT), or novel therapies, based on their predicted risk of relapse (i.e., risk-stratified therapy). Patients with APL usually receive tretinoin together with anthracycline chemotherapy for remission induction and then receive consolidation chemotherapy (daunorubicin and cytarabine) followed by maintenance tretinoin, with or without chemotherapy.

anthracyclines in younger patients (<60 years) appears to increase the cure rate of AML. In older patients, the benefit of intensive therapy has been more difficult to document and therefore pursuit of novel therapies as consolidation for these patients has recently been actively pursued.

Induction Chemotherapy The most commonly used CR induction regimens (for patients other than those with APL) consist of combination chemotherapy with cytarabine (cytosine arabinoside) and an anthracycline. Cytarabine is a cell cycle S-phase-specific antimetabolite that becomes phosphorylated intracellularly to an active triphosphate form that interferes with DNA synthesis. Anthracyclines are DNA intercalaters. Their primary mode of action is thought to be inhibition of topoisomerase II, leading to DNA breaks. Cytarabine is usually administered as a continuous intravenous infusion at 100 to 200 mg/m² per day for 7 days. Anthracycline therapy generally consists of daunorubicin, 45 to 60 mg/m², intravenously on days 1, 2, and 3 (the 7 and 3 regimen). Treatment with idarubicin at 12 or 13 mg/m² per day for 3 days in conjunction with cytarabine by 7-day continuous infusion is at least as effective and may be superior to daunorubicin in younger patients. The addition of etoposide does not increase the CR rate but may improve the CR duration.

After induction chemotherapy, the bone marrow is examined to determine if the leukemia has been eliminated. If >5% blasts exist with ≥20% cellularity, the patient has traditionally been retreated with cytarabine and an anthracycline in doses similar to those given initially, but for 5 and 2 days, respectively. Our recommendation, however, is to change therapy in this setting. Patients who fail to attain CR after two induction courses should immediately proceed to an allogeneic stem cell transplant (SCT) if an appropriate donor exists. This approach is only applied to patients under the age of 65 to 70 with acceptable end-organ function.

With the 7 and 3 cytarabine/daunorubicin regimen outlined above, 65 to 75% of adults with de novo AML achieve CR. Two-thirds achieve CR after a single course of therapy, and one-third require two courses. About 50% of patients who do not achieve CR have a drug-resistant leukemia, and 50% do not achieve CR because of fatal complications of bone marrow aplasia or impaired recovery of normal stem cells. A higher induction treatment–related mortality and frequency of resistant disease has been observed as age increases in virtually all studies.

High-dose cytarabine-based regimens have very high CR rates after a single cycle of therapy. When given in high doses, more cytarabine may enter the cells, saturate the cytarabine-inactivating enzymes, and increase the intracellular levels of 1-β-D-arabinofuranylcytosine-triphosphate, the active metabolite incorporated into DNA. Thus, higher doses of cytarabine may increase the inhibition of DNA synthesis and thereby overcome resistance to standard-dose cytarabine. In two randomized studies, high-dose cytarabine with an anthracycline produced CR rates similar to those achieved with standard 7 and 3 regimens. However, the CR duration was longer after high-dose cytarabine than after standard-dose cytarabine.

The hematologic toxicity of high-dose cytarabine-based induction regimens has typically been greater than that associated with 7 and 3 regimens. Toxicity with high-dose cytarabine includes myelosuppression, pulmonary toxicity, and significant and occasionally irreversible cerebellar toxicity. All patients treated with high-dose cytarabine must be closely monitored for cerebellar toxicity. Full cerebellar testing should be performed before each dose, and further high-dose cytarabine should be withheld if evidence of cerebellar toxicity develops. This toxicity occurs more commonly in patients with renal impairment and in those over the age of 60. Indeed, it is the increased toxicity observed with high-dose cytarabine, as opposed to the lack of benefit of this therapy, that has limited the use of this more intensive therapy in elderly AML patients. Clinical trials in the elderly patients have therefore focused upon new agents and attenuated doses of high-dose cytarabine therapy.

Supportive Care Measures geared to supporting patients through several weeks of granulocytopenia and thrombocytopenia are critical to the success of AML therapy. Patients with AML should be treated in centers expert in providing supportive measures for their management.

Recombinant hematopoietic growth factors have been incorporated into clinical trials in AML. These trials have been designed to lower the infection rate after chemotherapy. Both granulocyte colony-stimulating factor (G-CSF) and granulocyte-macrophage colony-stimulating factor (GM-CSF) have reduced the median time to neutrophil recovery by an average of 5 to 7 days. This accelerated rate of neutrophil recovery, however, has not always translated into significant reductions in infection rates. In most randomized studies, both G-CSF and GM-CSF have failed to improve the CR rate, disease-free survival, or overall survival. Although receptors for both G-CSF and GM-CSF are present on AML blasts, therapeutic efficacy is neither enhanced nor inhibited by these agents. The use of growth factors as supportive care for AML patients is controversial. We favor their use in elderly patients, those receiving intensive regimens, patients with uncontrolled infections, or those participating in clinical trials.

Multilumen right atrial catheters should be inserted through a subcutaneous tunnel as soon as patients with newly diagnosed AML have been stabilized. They should be used thereafter for administration of intravenous medications and transfusions, as well as for blood drawing. Antibiotic-impregnated catheters should be considered if the risk or subsequent consequence of line-related infection is high. The separation between the vascular access site and the exit site and the presence of a Dacron cuff in the subcutaneous channel reduce the risk of infection. With meticulous attention to sterile technique in catheter placement and maintenance, catheters may often be left in place for months.

Adequate and prompt blood bank support is critical to therapy of AML. Platelet transfusions should be given as needed to maintain a platelet count >10,000 to 20,000/μl. We believe that the platelet count should be kept at higher levels in febrile patients and during episodes of active bleeding or DIC. Patients with poor posttransfusion platelet count increments may benefit from administration of platelets from human leukocyte antigen (HLA)-matched donors. Red blood cell transfusions should be administered to keep the hemoglobin level >80 g/L (8 g/dL) in the absence of active bleeding, DIC, or congestive heart failure. Blood products leukodepleted by filtration should be used to avert or delay alloimmunization as well as febrile reactions. Blood products should also be irradiated to prevent graft-versus-host disease (GVHD). Cytomegalovirus (CMV)-negative blood products should be used for CMV-seronegative patients who are potential candidates for allogeneic SCT. Leukodepleted products are also effective for these patients if CMV-negative products are not available.

Infectious complications remain the major cause of morbidity and death during induction and postremission chemotherapy for AML. Prophylactic administration of antibiotics in the absence of fever is controversial. Oral nystatin or clotrimazole is recommended to prevent localized candidiasis. For patients who are herpes simplex virus antibody titer–positive, acyclovir prophylaxis is effective in preventing reactivation of latent oral herpes infections.

Fever develops in most patients with AML, but infections are documented in only half of febrile patients. Early initiation of empirical broad-spectrum antibacterial and antifungal antibiotics has significantly reduced the number of patients dying of infectious complications (Chap. 72). An antibiotic regimen adequate to treat gram-negative and gram-positive organisms should be instituted at the onset of fever in a granulocytopenic patient after clinical evaluation, including a detailed physical examination with inspection of the indwelling catheter exit site and a perirectal examination, as well as procurement of cultures and radiographs aimed at documenting the source of fever. Specific antibiotic regimens should be based on antibiotic sensitivity data obtained from the institution at which the patient is being treated. Acceptable regimens include imipenem-cilastin; an antipseudomonal semisynthetic penicillin (e.g., piperacillin) combined with an aminoglycoside; a third-generation cephalosporin with antipseudomonal activity (i.e., ceftazidime or cefepime); or double β-lactam combinations (ceftazidime and piperacillin). Aminoglycosides should be avoided if possible in patients with renal insufficiency. For patients with known immediate-type hypersensitivity reactions to penicillin, aztreonam may be substituted for β-lactams. Aztreonam should be combined with an aminoglycoside or a quinolone antibiotic rather than used alone.

Empirical vancomycin is not given initially in the absence of suspected gram-positive infection or mucositis but should be initiated in neutropenic patients who remain febrile for 3 days; emperical systemic antifungal therapy is added at 7 days if fever persists. While amphotericin B has been used in the past for this, itraconazole and voriconazole have been shown to be equivalent in efficacy and less toxic. Our approach is therefore to use either itraconozole or voriconazole. Liposomal amphotericin, which has also been demonstrated to be equivalent to regular amphotericin and to have less renal toxicity, is utilized when this treatment approach fails. Antibacterial and antifungal antibiotics should be continued until patients are no longer neutropenic, regardless of whether a specific source has been found for the fever.

Treatment of Promyelocytic Leukemia Tretinoin is an oral drug that induces the differentiation of leukemic cells bearing the t(15;17); it is not effective in other forms of AML. APL is responsive to cytarabine and daunorubicin, but about 10% of patients treated with these drugs die from DIC induced by the release of granule components by dying tumor cells. Tretinoin does not produce DIC but produces another complication called the *retinoic acid syndrome*. Occurring within the first 3 weeks of treatment, it is characterized by fever, dyspnea, chest pain, pulmonary infiltrates, pleural and pericardial effusions, and hypoxia. The syndrome is related to adhesion of differentiated neoplastic cells to the pulmonary vasculature endothelium. Glucocorticoids, chemotherapy, and/or supportive measures can be effective. The mortality of this syndrome is about 10%.

Tretinoin (45 mg/m^2 per day orally until remission is documented) plus concurrent anthracycline chemotherapy appears to be the safest and most effective treatment for APL. Unlike patients with other types of AML, patients with this subtype benefit from maintenance therapy with either tretinoin or chemotherapy. The optimal regimen is being sought in clinical studies.

Arsenic trioxide produces meaningful responses in up to 85% of patients refractory to tretinoin. The use of arsenic trioxide is being explored as part of initial treatment in clinical trials of APL.

The detection of minimal residual disease by RT-PCR amplification of the t(15;17) chimeric gene product appears to predict relapse. Disappearance of the signal is associated with long-term disease-free survival; its persistence predicts relapse. With increases in the sensitivity of the assay, some patients with persistent abnormal gene product have been found who do not suffer a relapse. Studies are underway to determine whether there is a critical threshold level of transcripts that predicts for leukemia relapse.

Postremission Therapy Induction of a durable first CR is critical to long-term disease-free survival in AML. However, without further therapy virtually all patients experience relapse. Once relapse has occurred, AML is generally curable only by SCT.

Postremission therapy is designed to eradicate any residual leukemic cells; therefore, it should prevent relapse and prolong survival. Approaches to postremission therapy in AML are often based upon age (<55 to 65 and >55 to 65). For younger patients, most studies include intensive chemotherapy and allogeneic or autologous SCT. High-dose cytarabine is more effective than standard-dose cytarabine. The Cancer and Leukemia Group B (CALGB), for example, compared the duration of CR in patients randomly assigned postremission to four cycles of high (3 g/m^2, every 12 h on days 1, 3, and 5), intermediate (400 mg/m^2 for 5 days by continuous infusion), or standard (100 mg/m^2 per day for 5 days by continuous infusion) doses of cytarabine. A

dose-response effect for cytarabine in patients with AML who were ≤60 years was demonstrated. High-dose cytarabine significantly prolonged CR and increased the fraction cured in patients with favorable [t(8;21) and inv(16)] and normal cytogenetics, but it had no significant effect on patients with other abnormal karyotypes. For older patients, exploration of attenuated intensive therapy that includes either chemotherapy or nonmyeloablative allogeneic SCT has been pursued. In addition, early introduction of new agents (Table 96-3) is often pursued.

Allogeneic and autologous SCT in first CR have been studied extensively in younger patients with no major organ dysfunction. Allogeneic SCT is used in patients <65 to 70 years with an HLA-compatible donor. Relapse with this therapy occurs in only a small fraction of patients, but toxicity is relatively high from treatment; complications include venoocclusive disease, GVHD, and infections. Autologous transplantation can be administered in young and older patients and uses the same preparative regimens. Patients subsequently receive their own stem cells collected while in remission. The toxicity is lower with autologous SCT (5% mortality rate), but the relapse rate is higher than with allogeneic SCT. The increased relapse rate is due to the absence of the graft-vs-leukemia (GVL) effect seen with allogeneic SCT and possible contamination of the autologous stem cells with tumor cells. Purging the autologous stem cells does not lower the relapse rate with autologous SCT.

Randomized trials comparing intensive therapy and autologous and allogeneic SCT have shown improved duration of remission with allogeneic SCT compared to autologous SCT or chemotherapy alone. However, overall survival is generally not different; the improved disease control with allogeneic SCT is erased by the increase in fatal toxicity. While stem cells were previously harvested from the bone marrow, virtually all efforts currently collect these from the peripheral blood following mobilization regimens including growth factors with or without chemotherapy. Prognostic factors may help select patients in first CR for whom transplant is most effective.

Our approach includes strong consideration for allogeneic SCT in first CR for patients with high-risk karyotypes. Patients with normal karyotypes who have other poor risk factors (antecedent hematologic disorder, failure to attain remission with a single induction course, hyperleukocytosis, PTD of the *MLL* gene, and *FLT3* abnormalities) are also potential candidates. If a suitable HLA donor does not exist, autologous SCT or novel therapeutic approaches are considered. Other novel transplant strategies including nonmyeloblative SCT are being actively explored for consolidation of high-risk AML patients. Patients with t(8;21) and inv(16) are treated with repetitive doses of high-dose

TABLE 96-3 *Selected New Agents Under Study for Treatment of Adults with AML*

Class of Drugs	Example Agent(s)
MDR1 modulator	Cyclosporine analogues, PSC-833
Demethylating agent	Decitabine, 5-azacytidine
Histone deacetylase inhibitor	Depsipeptide, suberoylanilide hydroxamic acid (SAHA), MS275, Valproic Acid
Heavy metals	Arsenic trioxide, antimony
Farnesyl transferase inhibitors	R115777, SCH66336
FLT3 inhibitors	SU11248, PKC412, MLN518
HSP-90 antagonists	17-Allylaminogeldanamycin (17-AAG)
BCR/ABL PDGFR/c-*kit* inhibitor	Imatinib (ST1571, Gleevec)
Protein kinase C inhibitor	Bryostatin, UCN-01, CGP41251
Cell cycle inhibitor	Flavopiridol
Humanized antibodies	Anti-CD33 (HuM195), Hu1D10 (β-chain, HLA-DR)
Toxin-conjugated antibodies	Gemtuzumab ozogamicin (Mylotarg)
Radiolabeled antibodies	Yttrium-90-labeled human M195
Cytokines	Recombinant human interleukin (IL) 2 and IL-12
Anticytokines	Antivascular endothelial growth factor (Avastin)

cytarabine, which offers a high frequency of cure without the morbidity of transplant.

Relapse   Once relapse occurs after the standard induction and postremission chemotherapy approach described above and outlined in Fig. 96-1, patients are rarely cured with further standard-dose chemotherapy. Patients eligible for allogeneic SCT should receive transplants expeditiously at the first sign of relapse. Long-term disease-free survival is approximately the same (30 to 50%) with allogeneic SCT in first relapse or in second remission. Chemotherapy is administered prior to allogeneic transplant if the AML is rapidly progressing. Autologous SCT rescues about 20% of relapsed patients with AML who have chemosensitive disease. The most important factors predicting response at relapse are the length of the previous CR, whether initial CR was achieved with one or two courses of chemotherapy, and the type of postremission therapy. Because of the poor outcome of patients in early (<12 months) first relapse, it is justified (for patients without HLA-compatible donors) to explore innovative approaches, such as new drugs or immunotherapies (Table 96-3). Patients with longer (>12 months) first CR generally relapse with drug-sensitive disease and have a higher chance of attaining a CR. However, cure for these patients is uncommon, and treatment with novel approaches should be considered if SCT is not possible. New agents (Table 96-3) that may have clinical activity in AML are needed.

For elderly patients (age >60) for whom clinical trials are not available, gemtuzumab ozogamicin (Mylotarg) is another alternative. This therapy is an antibody-targeted chemotherapy consisting of the humanized anti-CD33 antibody linked to calicheamicin, a potent antitumor antibiotic. The CR rate in response to this therapy is ~30%. The effectiveness of this agent in early relapsing (<6 months) or refractory AML patients is limited, possibly due to calicheamicin being a potent Mdr1 substrate. Toxicity, including myelosuppression, infusion toxicity, and venoocclusive disease, can be observed with gemtuzumab ozogamicin. Currently, studies are examining the efficacy of this treatment in combination with chemotherapy for both young and older patients with previously untreated AML.

CHRONIC MYELOGENOUS LEUKEMIA

INCIDENCE   The incidence of chronic myelogenous leukemia (CML) is 1.5 per 100,000 people per year, and the age-adjusted incidence is higher in men than in women (2.0 versus 1.2). The incidence of CML increases slowly with age until the middle forties, when it starts to rise rapidly. CML incidence decreased slightly between 1973 and 1999 (1.9 versus 1.5).

DEFINITION   The diagnosis of CML is established by identifying a clonal expansion of a hematopoietic stem cell possessing a reciprocal translocation between chromosomes 9 and 22. This translocation results in the head-to-tail fusion of the breakpoint cluster region (*BCR*) gene on chromosome 22q11 with the *ABL* (named after the abelson murine leukemia virus) gene located on chromosome 9q34. Untreated, the disease is characterized by the inevitable transition from a chronic phase to an accelerated phase and on to blast crisis.

ETIOLOGY   No clear correlation with exposure to cytotoxic drugs, such as alkylating agents, has been found, and there is no direct evidence of a viral etiology. Cigarette smoking has been shown to accelerate the progression to blast crisis and therefore has an adverse effect on survival in CML. The effect of radiation was demonstrated in a study of the atomic bomb survivors, where it has been estimated that the development of a CML cell mass of 10,000/μl takes 6.3 years. No increase in CML incidence was found in the survivors of the Chernobyl accident, suggesting that only large doses of radiation can induce CML.

PATHOPHYSIOLOGY   The product of the fusion gene resulting from the t(9;22) plays a central role in the development of CML. This chimeric gene is transcribed into a hybrid *BCR/ABL* mRNA in which exon 1 of *ABL* is replaced by variable numbers of 5' *BCR* exons. Bcr/Abl fusion proteins, p210$^{BCR/ABL}$, are produced that contain NH$_2$-terminal domains

of Bcr and the COOH-terminal domains of Abl. A rare breakpoint, occurring within the 3' region of the *BCR* gene, yields a fusion protein of 230 kDa, p230$^{BCR/ABL}$. Bcr/Abl fusion proteins can transform hematopoietic progenitor cells *in vitro*. Furthermore, reconstituting lethally irradiated mice with bone marrow cells infected with retrovirus carrying the gene encoding the p210$^{BCR/ABL}$ leads to the development of a myeloproliferative syndrome resembling CML in 50% of the mice. Specific antisense oligomers to the *BCR/ABL* junction inhibit the growth of t(9;22)-positive leukemic cells without affecting normal colony formation.

The mechanism(s) by which p210$^{BCR/ABL}$ promotes the transition from the benign state to the fully malignant one is still unclear. Messenger RNA for *BCR/ABL* can occasionally be detected in normal individuals. However, attachment of the *BCR* sequences to *ABL* results in three critical functional changes: (1) the Abl protein becomes constitutively active as a tyrosine kinase enzyme, subsequently activating downstream kinases that prevent apoptosis; (2) the DNA-protein-binding activity of Abl is attenuated; and (3) the binding of Abl to cytoskeletal actin microfilaments is enhanced.

Disease Progression   The events associated with transition to the acute phase are poorly understood. Chromosomal instability of the malignant clone, resulting, for example, in the acquisition of an additional t(9;22), trisomy 8, or 17p- (p53 loss), is a fundamental characteristic of CML. Acquisition of these additional genetic and/or molecular abnormalities is critical to the phenotypic transformation. Large deletions adjacent to the translocation breakpoint on the derivative 9 chromosome, detected by microsatellite polymerase chain reaction (PCR) or FISH, are associated with shorter survival time. Heterogeneous structural alterations of the p53 gene, as well as structural alterations and lack of protein production of the retinoblastoma gene, have been associated with disease progression in a subset of patients. Rare patients show alterations in *RAS*. Sporadic reports also document the presence of an altered *MYC* (named after the myelocytomatosis virus) gene. Progressive de novo DNA methylation at the *BCR/ABL* locus has also been shown to herald blastic transformation. Finally, interleukin (IL)-1β may be involved in the progression of CML to the blastic phase. Multiple pathways to disease transformation exist, but the exact timing and relevance of each remain unclear.

CLINICAL PRESENTATION ■ **Symptoms**   The clinical onset of the chronic phase is generally insidious. Accordingly, some patients are diagnosed while still asymptomatic, during health screening tests; other patients present with fatigue, malaise, and weight loss or have symptoms resulting from splenic enlargement, such as early satiety and left upper quadrant pain or mass. Less common are features related to granulocyte or platelet dysfunction, such as infections, thrombosis, or bleeding. Occasionally, patients present with leukostatic manifestations due to severe leukocytosis or thrombosis such as vasoocclusive disease, cerebrovascular accidents, myocardial infarction, venous thrombosis, priapism, visual disturbances, and pulmonary insufficiency. Patients with p230$^{BCR/ABL}$-positive CML have a more indolent course.

Progression of CML is associated with worsening symptoms. Unexplained fever, significant weight loss, increasing dose requirement of the drugs controlling the disease, bone and joint pain, bleeding, thrombosis, and infections suggest transformation into accelerated or blastic phases. Fewer than 10 to 15% of newly diagnosed patients present with accelerated disease or with de novo blastic phase CML.

Physical Findings   In most patients the abnormal finding on physical examination at diagnosis is minimal to moderate splenomegaly; mild hepatomegaly is found occasionally. Persistent splenomegaly despite continued therapy is a sign of disease acceleration. Lymphadenopathy and myeloid sarcomas are unusual except late in the course of the disease; when they are present, the prognosis is poor.

Hematologic Findings   Elevated white blood cell counts, with various degrees of immaturity of the granulocytic series, are present at diagnosis. Usually <5% circulating blasts and <10% blasts and promyelocytes are noted. Cycling of the counts may be observed in patients followed without treatment. Platelet counts are almost always elevated at diagnosis, and a mild degree of normochromic normocytic anemia is present. Leukocyte alkaline phosphatase is characteristically low in CML cells. Serum levels of vitamin B_{12} and vitamin B_{12}–binding proteins are generally elevated. Phagocytic functions are usually normal at diagnosis and remain normal during the chronic phase. Histamine production secondary to basophilia is increased in later stages, causing pruritus, diarrhea, and flushing.

At diagnosis, bone marrow cellularity, primarily of the myeloid and megakaryocytic lineages, with a greatly altered myeloid to erythroid ratio, is increased in almost all patients with CML. The marrow blast percentage is generally normal or slightly elevated. Marrow or blood basophilia, eosinophilia, and monocytosis may be present. While collagen fibrosis in the marrow is unusual at presentation, significant degrees of reticulin stain–measured fibrosis are noted in about half of the patients.

Disease acceleration is defined by the development of increasing degrees of anemia unaccounted for by bleeding or chemotherapy; cytogenetic clonal evolution; or blood or marrow blasts between 10 and 20%, blood or marrow basophils ≥20%, or platelet count <100,000/ µl. *Blast crisis* is defined as acute leukemia, with blood or marrow blasts ≥ 20%. Hyposegmented neutrophils may appear (Pelger-Huet anomaly). Blast cells can be classified as myeloid, lymphoid, erythroid, or undifferentiated, based on morphologic, cytochemical, and immunologic features. About half the cases are myeloid, one-third lymphoid, 10% erythroid, and the rest are undifferentiated.

Chromosomal Findings The cytogenetic hallmark of CML, found in 90 to 95% of patients, is the t(9;22)(q34;q11.2). Originally, this was recognized by the presence of a shortened chromosome 22 (22q-), designated as the *Philadelphia chromosome*, that arises from the reciprocal 9;22 translocation. Some patients may have complex translocations (designated as *variant translocations*) involving three, four, or five chromosomes (usually including chromosomes 9 and 22). However, the molecular consequences of these changes appear similar to those resulting from the typical t(9;22). All patients should have evidence of the translocation either by cytogenetics, FISH, or molecularly to make a diagnosis of CML.

PROGNOSTIC FACTORS The clinical outcome of patients with CML is variable. Before imatinib mesylate, death was expected in 10% of patients within 2 years and in about 20% yearly thereafter and the median survival time was ~4 years. Therefore, several prognostic models that identify different risk groups in CML have been developed. The most commonly used staging systems have been derived from multivariate analyses of prognostic factors. The *Sokal index* identified percentage of circulating blasts, spleen size, platelet count, cytogenetic clonal evolution, and age as the most important prognostic indicators. This system was based on chemotherapy-treated patients. The *Hasford system* was developed on interferon α-treated patients. It identified age, spleen size, percentage of circulating blasts, platelet count, and percentage of eosinophils and basophils as the most important prognostic indicators. This system differs from the Sokal index by ignoring clonal evolution and incorporating percentage of eosinophils and basophils. When applied to a data set of 272 patients treated with interferon α (IFN-α), the Hasford system was more potent than the Sokal score for predicting survival time; it identified more low-risk patients but left only a small number of cases in the high-risk group. The Hasford system has not yet been validated in patients undergoing transplantation. However, preliminary results suggest that it is applicable to imatinib-treated patients.

℞ TREATMENT

The therapy of CML is rapidly undergoing evolution because we have a curative treatment (allogeneic transplantation) that has significant

TABLE 96-4   Response Criteria in CML

Hematologic	
Complete response[a]	White blood cell count <10,000/µl, normal morphology
	Normal hemoglobin and platelet counts
Incomplete response	White blood cell count ≥ 10,000/µl
Cytogenetic	Percentage of bone marrow metaphases with t(9;22)
Complete response	0
Partial response	≤35
Minor response	36–85[b]
No response	85–100
Molecular	Presence of *BCR/ABL* transcript by RT-PCR
Complete response	None
Incomplete response	Any

[a] Complete hematologic response requires the disappearance of splenomegaly.
[b] Up to 15% normal metaphases are occasionally seen at diagnosis (when 30 metaphases are analyzed).
Note: RT-PCR, reverse transcriptase polymerase chain reaction.

toxicity and a new targeted treatment (imatinib) without long-term follow-up data. Therefore, physician experience and patient preference must be factored into the treatment selection process. Discussion of both treatment options with a patient is indicated. The decision should focus on the outcomes, risks, and toxicities of the various approaches. Some centers would employ allogeneic SCT in patients <30 years, as the risk of transplant-related toxicity is minimal in that population.

At present, the goal of therapy in CML is to achieve prolonged, durable, nonneoplastic, nonclonal hematopoiesis, which entails the eradication of any residual cells containing the *BCR/ABL* transcript. Hence the goal is complete molecular remission and cure (Table 96-4). A proposed treatment plan for the newly diagnosed patient with CML is presented in Fig. 96-2.

Allogeneic SCT Allogeneic SCT is currently the only curative therapy for CML and, when feasible, is the treatment of choice. However, it is complicated by a high early-mortality rate owing to the transplant procedure. Outcome of SCT depends on multiple factors including: (1) the patient (e.g., age and phase of disease); (2) the type of donor [e.g., syngeneic (monozygotic twins) or HLA-compatible allogeneic, related or unrelated]; (3) the preparative regimen; (4) GVHD; and (5) posttransplantation treatment.

THE PATIENT As experience has been gained and safety and efficacy have been established, it has become clear that patients should have acceptable end-organ function, be <65 to 70 years, and have a healthy

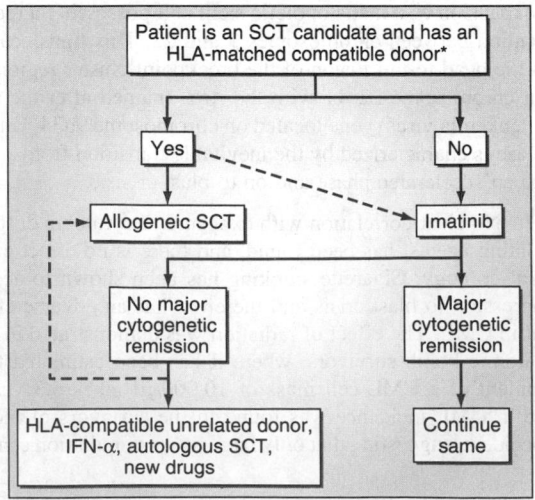

FIGURE 96-2 Flow chart for the therapy of newly diagnosed CML. Patients with an HLA-compatible donor have the possibility to undergo allogeneic stem cell transplant (SCT) as initial therapy or treatment with imatinib. The asterisk denotes that some centers employ allogeneic SCT only if imatinib fails to induce a response. Broken lines denote lack of long-term survival data. IFN, interferon.

and histocompatible donor. Furthermore, survival after SCT in the accelerated and blastic phases of the disease is significantly diminished and is associated with a very high rate of relapse. The Seattle pre-imatinib data demonstrate that bone marrow transplantation (BMT) early in the chronic phase (1 to 2 years from diagnosis) is superior to later BMT.

THE DONOR Transplantation from a family donor, who is either fully matched or mismatched at only one HLA locus, should be considered the only curative therapy for any patient with CML who is a candidate for an HLA-related sibling transplant. Syngeneic BMT in patients with chronic phase CML has been reported from the Seattle group to result in 7-year disease-free survival in 55% of the patients, with a 30% relapse rate. With HLA-identical sibling BMT in the chronic phase, many groups have reported 5-year disease-free survival in 40 to 70% of patients, with a 25% relapse rate. BMT from an HLA-matched unrelated donor in chronic phase <1 year from diagnosis and <30 years resulted in similar 5-year disease-free survival as matched sibling donor transplantation. For all other groups, patients receiving transplants from unrelated individuals have higher rates of graft failure and acute and chronic GVHD and prolonged convalescence after treatment, compared to those who receive allogeneic transplants from related individuals. Peripheral blood is now being studied as a source of hematopoietic progenitor cells; it may offer rapid engraftment and less risk for the donor. With unrelated donors, some studies demonstrated no difference in GVHD and improved disease-free survival when comparing peripheral blood to bone marrow stem cells. No such data are available using matched sibling donors to date. At the current time, some centers collect bone marrow and some peripheral blood from sibling donors for newly diagnosed CML patients. Umbilical-cord blood may permit mismatched SCT with notably less GVHD; GVL effects do not appear to be impaired. A problem with cord blood is obtaining a sufficient number of progenitor cells to reconstitute hematopoiesis in an adult.

PREPARATIVE REGIMENS These regimens have been studied by several groups. A randomized study by the Seattle group compared cyclophosphamide and total-body irradiation with busulphan and cyclophosphamide. They found no significant differences in the 3-year probabilities of survival, relapse, event-free survival, speed of engraftment, or incidence of venoocclusive disease of the liver. Significantly more patients in the total-body irradiation arm experienced major elevations of creatinine, acute GVHD, longer periods of fever, positive blood cultures, hospital admissions, and longer inpatient hospital stays. However, increased chronic GVHD, obstructive bronchiolitis, and alopecia were noted with busulphan. Measurement of busulphan levels revealed no significant association between busulphan levels and regimen-related toxicity, but low levels were associated with an increased risk of relapse. Intravenous busulphan allows better control of serum levels. We tend to favor the use of busulphan and cyclophosphamide. Nonmyeloblative transplants in which the preparative regimen is aimed at eliminating host lymphocytes rather than bone marrow are being tested. Reduced toxicity with preserved antitumor efficacy is the goal.

DEVELOPMENT AND TYPE OF GVHD Development of grade I GVHD, as compared to no GVHD, decreases the risk of relapse. A lower relapse rate was observed also in patients with grade II GVHD but was accompanied by a substantially higher transplant-related mortality rate. The decreased relapse rate may be caused by a GVL effect. Depletion of T lymphocytes from donor marrow can prevent GVHD but results in an increased risk of relapse, which exceeds the relapse rate after syngeneic SCT. Thus, T lymphocytes from the donor marrow mediate a significant antileukemic, or GVL, effect, and even syngeneic marrow may exhibit limited GVL activity in CML.

POSTTRANSPLANTATION TREATMENT Further support for the existence of an immunologically mediated GVL effect came from the observation that donor leukocyte infusions (without any preparative chemotherapy or GVHD prophylaxis) can induce hematologic and cytogenetic remissions in patients with CML who have relapsed after allogeneic SCT.

Imatinib's effect in the chronic phase of the disease prompted its study in patients who relapse after allogeneic SCT. Studies with small numbers of patients have proved that imatinib can control CML that has recurred after allogeneic SCT but is associated with myelosuppression and recurrence of severe GVHD. Imatinib studies after allogeneic SCT to prevent relapse in patients with advanced disease at the time of transplantation (patients at high risk for relapse) or patients undergoing non-myeloblative transplants are under way.

The activity of IFN-α in patients with early chronic-phase CML was the basis for the use of IFN-α after SCT, either to induce cytogenetic remissions in relapsed patients or to prevent relapse after SCT for high-risk patients. The main concern about IFN-α use after allogeneic SCT has been the development or worsening of GVHD, because IFN-α acts as an immunomodulator. IFN-α has also been combined with mononuclear cells obtained from donor blood to induce cytogenetic remissions in relapsed patients. Cytogenetic remissions have been achieved, but the exact role of IFN-α as opposed to the mononuclear cells is unclear.

Imatinib Mesylate Imatinib mesylate (Gleevec, STI571) functions through competitive inhibition at the adenosine triphosphate (ATP) binding site of the Abl kinase, which leads to inhibition of tyrosine phosphorylation of proteins involved in Bcr/Abl signal transduction. It shows a high degree of specificity for Bcr/Abl, the receptor for platelet-derived growth factor, and c-*kit* tyrosine kinases. Imatinib induces apoptosis in cells expressing Bcr/Abl. Based on its antileukemic activity in vitro it was tested in clinical trials.

Most patients with CML in chronic phase have a rapid hematologic response to imatinib therapy. In the initial studies with imatinib in patients with chronic-phase CML who were intolerant to IFN-α, 95% of patients achieved complete hematologic remission, and 60% achieved major cytogenetic remission, with a complete cytogenetic remission rate of 41%. Those who did not achieve at least a major cytogenetic remission following 3 months of therapy had a higher risk of disease progression to the accelerated/blastic phases of the disease. Patients in the accelerated/blastic phases of the disease are less sensitive to imatinib, and the treatment outcome is less favorable. In newly diagnosed CML, a recent randomized phase III study of imatinib (400 mg/d) versus IFN-α and cytarabine revealed the complete hematologic remission rate, at 18 months, of patients treated with imatinib to be 97% as compared to 69% in patients treated with IFN-α and cytarabine. Similarly, the complete cytogenetic remission rate was 76% in patients treated with imatinib as compared to 14% in patients treated with IFN-α and cytarabine. Progression to accelerated/blastic phases of the disease was noted in 3% of patients treated with imatinib as compared to 8.5% of patients treated with IFN-α and cytarabine. These results led to rapid Food and Drug Administration approval of imatinib for all stages of CML.

Imatinib is administered orally and has an acceptable toxicity profile. The main side effects are fluid retention, nausea, muscle cramps, diarrhea, and skin rashes. The management of these side effects is usually supportive. Myelosuppression is the most common hematologic side effect, and patients who received busulphan are at a greater risk than patients who were treated with IFN-α. It seems to result from the eradication of the malignant clone and delayed recovery of the normal nonclonal progenitor cells. Blood and platelet support should be provided, and therefore dose reduction is rarely recommended in the absence of infection. Doses <300 mg/d seem ineffective and may lead to development of resistance.

Four mechanisms of resistance to imatinib have been described to date. These are (1) gene amplification, (2) mutations at the kinase site, (3) enhanced expression of multidrug exporter proteins, and (4) alternative signaling pathways functionally compensating for the imatinib-sensitive mechanisms. The unfavorable prognosis associated with imatinib-resistance was shown in the accelerated and blast crisis phases of the disease. Specifically, patients who do not achieve major cytogenetic remission within 3 months of initiation of imatinib have shorter survival than patients who achieve that level of remission. Therefore, all four mechanisms are being targeted in clinical trials.

The encouraging results with imatinib have led many clinicians to offer it as a first-line therapy for newly diagnosed CML patients, including those who otherwise would have benefited from transplant (e.g., young patients with a sibling matched donor). This may be unwise since the clinical studies so far have very short follow-up, thus limiting knowledge regarding the curative potential of imatinib. Delaying transplantation until after development of imatinib resistance may worsen outcome.

Interferons   When allogeneic SCT is not feasible, IFN-α therapy used to be the treatment of choice before imatinib became available. Only longer follow-up of patients treated with imatinib will prove whether IFN-α will still have a role in the treatment of CML. The interferons are a complex group of naturally occurring proteins produced by eukaryotic cells in response to viruses, antigens, and mitogens. Three distinct groups of IFN species have been identified: IFN-α, -β and -γ. Although various interferons have become available for clinical investigation, most data have been generated with IFN-α preparations.

Interferons have potent, pleiotropic biologic effects, spanning a spectrum of antiviral, microbicidal, immunomodulatory, and antiproliferative properties. While interferons downregulate the expression of several oncogenes and cytokines, they also upregulate the expression of IFN regulatory factor-1 (a transcriptional activator with antioncogenic activity), adhesion molecules, and the histocompatibility genes. Interferons also inhibit angiogenesis and induce a cellular immune response. However, the mode(s) of action in CML is still unknown.

In randomized studies comparing IFN-α and chemotherapy, patients treated with IFN-α survived longer than patients treated with hydroxyurea or busulphan. The 5-year survival rate was 51% with IFN-α and 42% with chemotherapy. Of note, achieving complete cytogenetic or molecular response after IFN-α therapy is associated with a 10-year survival rate as high as 78%.

Patients develop both acute and chronic side effects from IFN-α therapy. Acute side effects (flulike symptoms) appear early in the course of the treatment. Most flulike symptoms respond to acetaminophen, and tachyphylaxis develops within 1 to 2 weeks. Chronic reactions, such as fatigue and lethargy, depression, weight loss, myalgias, and arthralgias, occur in about half of the patients and often require dose reduction. Patients also report cough, postnasal drip, and dryness of the skin. Infrequently, immune-mediated thrombocytopenia and anemia develop. In addition, long-term therapy has been associated with late autoimmune side effects, such as hypothyroidism and occasionally generalized autoimmune phenomena.

The most important persistent side effects in patients with CML who are treated with IFN-α are neurologic. All patients treated with IFN-α are subject to some neurologic toxicity, the most common symptom being lethargy. Up to 20% of patients have neurologic side effects that are associated with compromised quality of life and reduced ability to carry out their regular activity, such as full-time work. In addition, at the required doses, impotence in men is not infrequent. The combination of IFN-α with cytarabine has produced better results in one study but not in another.

Chemotherapy   Innovative approaches are still important in CML; the exact role of imatinib in the armamentarium of CML remains undefined. Initial management of patients with chemotherapy is currently reserved for rapid lowering of white blood cell counts, reduction of symptoms, and reversal of symptomatic splenomegaly. Hydroxyurea, a ribonucleotide reductase inhibitor, induces rapid disease control. The initial dose is 1 to 4 g/d; the dose should be halved with each 50% reduction of the leukocyte count. Unfortunately, cytogenetic remissions with hydroxyurea are uncommon. Busulphan, an alkylating agent that acts on early progenitor cells, has a more prolonged effect. However, we do not recommend its use because of its serious side effects, which include unexpected, and occasionally fatal, myelosuppression in 5 to 10% of patients; pulmonary, endocardial, and marrow fibrosis; and an Addison-like wasting syndrome.

Homoharringtonine (HHT) is a plant alkaloid derived from a tree, *Cephalotaxus fortuneii* sp. *harringtonii*. HHT blocks peptide bond formation after binding of the aminoacyl-transfer RNA to the ribosome. In patients whose disease progressed during treatment with IFN-α or who were in later chronic phase ($>$1 year from diagnosis), HHT induced 72% complete hematologic responses and 15% major cytogenetic responses. The use of HHT before IFN-α in early chronic phase resulted in a 92% complete hematologic response rate and a 27% major cytogenetic response rate. Toxicity is mainly related to myelosuppression. In vitro synergism between HHT and imatinib have led to the development of combination trials.

Arsenic trioxide gained recognition as a therapeutic agent following reports from China of a high incidence of favorable hematologic responses in patients with APL. The mechanism(s) of action of arsenic trioxide in non-APL leukemias is unknown. Initial studies of arsenic trioxide in Bcr/Abl-expressing cell lines demonstrated downregulation of Bcr/Abl expression as well as activation of apoptosis. More recent studies have demonstrated an initial effect of arsenic trioxide on Bcr/Abl expression prior to activation of the apoptotic pathway. In vitro synergism between arsenic trioxide and imatinib have led to the clinical investigation of this combination.

Intensive combination chemotherapy has also been used in chronic-phase CML, with 30 to 50% of patients achieving complete cytogenetic responses. However, these cytogenetic remissions have been short-lived. Consequently, intensive combination chemotherapy regimens are being used today only to mobilize normal progenitors in the blood in order to collect circulating stem cells for autologous transplantation.

Autologous SCT   Autologous SCT could potentially cure CML if a means to select the residual normal progenitors, which coexist with their malignant counterparts, could be developed. As a source of autologous hematopoietic stem cells for transplantation, blood offers certain advantages over marrow (e.g., faster engraftment for the patient and no general anesthesia for the donor). Normal hematopoietic stem cells appear with increased frequency in the blood of patients with CML during the recovery phase after chemotherapy and G-CSF. A role for imatinib before stem cell collection to achieve minimal residual disease and following transplantation to maintain this status is currently being investigated. However, only a few cases have been reported to successfully engraft following imatinib therapy. Therefore such approaches should be performed only in clinical trials.

Leukapheresis and Splenectomy   Intensive leukapheresis may control the blood counts in chronic-phase CML; however, it is expensive and cumbersome. It is useful in emergencies where leukostasis-related complications such as pulmonary failure or cerebrovascular accidents are likely. It may also have a role in the treatment of pregnant women in whom it is important to avoid potentially teratogenic drugs.

Splenectomy was used in CML in the past because of the suggestion that evolution to the acute phase might occur in the spleen. However, this does not appear to be the case, and splenectomy is now reserved for symptomatic relief of painful splenomegaly unresponsive to chemotherapy or for significant anemia or thrombocytopenia associated with hypersplenism. Splenic radiation is used rarely to reduce the size of the spleen.

Minimal Residual Disease   After allogeneic SCT, RT-PCR analysis may be positive for residual disease during the first 6 months in patients who subsequently achieve a long-lasting remission. However, late persistence of RT-PCR positivity appears to indicate a reduced probability of cure. RT-PCR positivity at any single time point is not predictive of imminent relapse. After allogeneic SCT, patients are often divided according to RT-PCR results into one of three groups: (1) persistently positive, (2) intermittently negative, and (3) persistently negative.

These three groups have low, intermediate, and high probability of maintaining remission and disease free-survival, respectively. Although these data suggest that patients who are persistently RT-PCR positive >6 months after allogeneic SCT need additional therapeutic interventions, this conclusion has not been rigorously established. The studies have used an assortment of techniques for measuring minimal residual disease, the level of sensitivity has been variable, and the follow-up durations of patients are short. Quantitative PCR may provide a more sensitive tool to predict relapse in CML. In patients who do not have any evidence for GVHD and are intermittently RT-PCR negative, GVL may be induced by alloreactive donor cells (without the side effects of GVHD) to suppress the proliferation of the leukemic cells. Another approach may be the use of imatinib to eradicate minimal residual disease.

Following imatinib therapy, only a minority (5 to 10%) of the patients develop molecular remission. Extrapolating from the SCT data, most patients without molecular remission are at risk of relapse. However, patients with AML with t(8;21) who are in long-term remission have persistent multipotent progenitor cells expressing *AML1/ETO* transcripts. Therefore it is unclear whether indeed achieving durable molecular remission should still be the goal of treatment in this disease. Until this issue is sorted out, approaches have been developed to try and improve the current results. Based on improved outcome with higher doses of imatinib in patients with the advanced stages of the disease, trials have been initiated that compare 400 mg to 800 mg of imatinib in newly diagnosed patients. Similarly, combination regimens have been developed; based on the effect of IFN-α in the chronic phase of the disease, imatinib with IFN-α or with its long-acting (pegylated) member are being studied. Likewise, based on the combined effect of cytarabine and IFN-α, a regimen of imatinib and cytarabine is being evaluated. The results from these trials are premature at this point. However, they will most probably lead to a randomized trial of imatinib versus imatinib with IFN-α versus imatinib with cytarabine.

After IFN α therapy, residual disease was found in all samples tested from patients with complete cytogenetic remissions. More recent studies have demonstrated the eventual elimination of the *BCR/ABL* mRNA transcript after more prolonged IFN-α treatment in some cases.

Future Directions Abrogation of DNA methylation with 5-aza-2'deoxyycytidine (decitabine) has shown clinical activity in the advanced stages of the disease. Inhibition of *Ras* with a farnesyl transferase inhibitor that blocks its insertion into the membrane may have anti-tumor activity in CML on the basis of early clinical trials. Preclinical efforts to use Bcr/Abl peptides as a tumor vaccine appear promising. The use of *BCR/ABL* antisense oligonucleotides to purge residual leukemic cells from autologous hematopoietic progenitors before reinfusion, as well as new approaches to induce GVL in the setting of minimal residual disease without inducing GVHD, are under way. All these agents and others are being or will be studied in combination with imatinib. Further, treatment with the histone deacetylase inhibitor suberoylanilide hydroxamic acid (SAHA) was shown to enhance imatinib-induced apoptosis of Bcr/Abl-positive cell lines, and the heat-shock protein 90 antagonist 17-allylaminogeldanamycin (17-AAG) inhibited cell growth of cell lines containing mutations at the kinase site.

Treatment of Blast Crisis The treatment for all forms of blast crisis is generally ineffective, including imatinib. Only 52% of patients treated with imatinib achieved hematologic remission (21% complete hematologic remission), and the median overall survival was 6.6 months. Patients who achieve complete hematologic remission or whose disease returns to a second chronic phase should be considered for allogeneic SCT. Other approaches include induction chemotherapy tailored to the phenotype of the blast cell followed by imatinib, with or without additional chemotherapy and SCT. Blast crisis following initial therapy with imatinib carries a dismal prognosis.

FURTHER READING

AML

KELLY LM, GILLILAND DG: Genetics of myeloid leukemias. Annu Rev Genomics Hum Genet 3:179, 2002

LOWENBERG B et al: Acute myeloid leukemia and acute promyelocytic leukemia. Hematology (Am Soc Hematol Educ Program):82, 2003

STONE RM: The difficult problem of acute myeloid leukemia in the older adult. CA Cancer J Clin 52:363, 2002

TALLMAN MS, NABHAN G: Management of acute promyelocytic leukemia. Curr Oncol Rep 4:381, 2002

CML

CORTES J, KANTARJIAN H: Advanced-phase chronic myeloid leukemia. Semin Hematol 40:79, 2003

DEININGER MW, DRUKER BJ: Specific targeted therapy of chronic myelogenous leukemia with imatinib. Pharmacol Rev 55:401, 2003

GOLDMAN JM, MELO JV: Chronic myeloid leukemia—advances in biology and new approaches to treatment. N Engl J Med 349:1451, 2003

97 MALIGNANCIES OF LYMPHOID CELLS
James O. Armitage, Dan L. Longo

Malignancies of lymphoid cells range from the most indolent to the most aggressive human malignancies. These cancers arise from cells of the immune system at different stages of differentiation, resulting in a wide range of morphologic, immunologic, and clinical findings. Insights on the normal immune system have allowed a better understanding of these sometimes confusing disorders.

Some malignancies of lymphoid cells almost always present as leukemia (i.e., primary involvement of bone marrow and blood), while others almost always present as lymphomas (i.e., solid tumors of the immune system). However, other malignancies of lymphoid cells can present as either leukemia or lymphoma. In addition, the clinical pattern can change over the course of the illness. This change is more often seen in a patient who seems to have a lymphoma and then develops the manifestations of leukemia over the course of the illness.

BIOLOGY OF LYMPHOID MALIGNANCIES: CONCEPTS OF THE WHO CLASSIFICATION OF LYMPHOID MALIGNANCIES

The classification of lymphoid cancers evolved steadily throughout the twentieth century. The distinction between leukemia and lymphoma was made early, and separate classification systems were developed for each. Leukemias were first divided into acute and chronic subtypes based on average survival. Chronic leukemias were easily subdivided into those of lymphoid or myeloid origin based on morphologic characteristics. However, in recent years, a spectrum of diseases that were formerly all called chronic lymphoid leukemia has become apparent (Table 97-1). The acute leukemias were usually malignancies of blast cells with few identifying characteristics. When cytochemical stains became available, it was possible to divide these objectively into myeloid malignancies and acute leukemias of lymphoid cells. Acute leu-

TABLE 97-1 *Lymphoid Disorders That Can Present as "Chronic Leukemia" and Be Confused with Typical B Cell Chronic Lymphoid Leukemia*

Follicular lymphoma	Prolymphocytic leukemia (B cell or T cell)
Splenic marginal zone lymphoma	
Nodal marginal zone lymphoma	Lymphoplasmacytic lymphoma
Mantle cell lymphoma	Sézary syndrome
Hairy cell leukemia	Smoldering adult T cell leukemia/lymphoma

TABLE 97-2 *Classification of Acute Lymphoid Leukemia (ALL)*

Immunologic Subtype	% of Cases	FAB Subtype	Cytogenetic Abnormalities
Pre-B ALL	75	L1, L2	t(9;22), t(4;11), t(1;19)
T cell ALL	20	L1, L2	14q11 or 7q34
B cell ALL	5	L3	t(8;14), t(8;22), t(2;8)

Note: FAB, French-American-British classification.

kemias of lymphoid cells have been subdivided based on morphologic characteristics by the French-American-British (FAB) group (Table 97-2). Using this system, lymphoid malignancies of small uniform blasts (e.g., typical childhood acute lymphoblastic leukemia) were called L1, lymphoid malignancies with larger and more variable size cells were called L2, and lymphoid malignancies of uniform cells with basophilic and sometimes vacuolated cytoplasm were called L3 (e.g., typical Burkitt's lymphoma cells). Acute leukemias of lymphoid cells have also been subdivided based on immunologic (i.e., T cell vs. B cell) and cytogenetic abnormalities (Table 97-2). Major cytogenetic subgroups include the t(9;22) (e.g., Philadelphia chromosome–positive acute lymphoblastic leukemia) and the t(8;14) found in the L3 or Burkitt's leukemia.

Non-Hodgkin's lymphomas were separated from Hodgkin's disease by recognition of the Sternberg-Reed cells early in the twentieth century. The histologic classification for non-Hodgkin's lymphomas was has been one of the most contentious issues in oncology. Imperfect morphologic systems were supplanted by imperfect immunologic systems, and poor reproducibility of diagnosis has hampered progress. In 1999, the World Health Organization (WHO) classification of lymphoid malignancies was devised through a process of consensus development among international leaders in hematopathology and clinical oncology. The WHO classification takes into account morphologic, clinical, immunologic, and genetic information and attempts to divide non-Hodgkin's lymphomas and other lymphoid malignancies into clinical/pathologic entities that have clinical and therapeutic relevance. This system is presented in Table 97-3. Clinical studies have shown that this new system is clinically relevant and has a higher degree of diagnostic accuracy than those used previously. The possibilities for subdividing lymphoid malignancies are extensive. However, Table 97-3 presents in bold those malignancies that occur in at least 1% of patients. Specific lymphoma subtypes will be dealt with in more detail below.

GENERAL ASPECTS OF LYMPHOID MALIGNANCIES

ETIOLOGY AND EPIDEMIOLOGY Chronic lymphoid leukemia (CLL) is the most prevalent form of leukemia in western countries. It occurs most frequently in older adults and is exceedingly rare in children. In 2004, 8190 new cases were diagnosed in the United States, but because of the prolonged survival associated with this disorder, the total prevalence is many times higher. CLL is more common in men than in women and more common in whites than in blacks. This is an uncommon malignancy in Asia. The etiologic factors for typical CLL are unknown.

In contrast to CLL, acute lymphoid leukemias (ALLs) are predominantly cancers of children and young adults. The L3 or Burkitt's leukemia occurring in children in developing countries seems to be associated with infection by the Epstein-Barr virus (EBV) in infancy. However, the explanation for the etiology of more common subtypes of ALL is much less certain. Childhood ALL occurs more often in higher socioeconomic subgroups. Children with trisomy 21 (Down's syndrome) have an increased risk for childhood acute lymphoblastic leukemia as well as acute myeloid leukemia. Exposure to high-energy radiation in early childhood increases the risk of developing T cell acute lymphoblastic leukemia.

The etiology of ALL in adults is also uncertain. ALL is unusual in middle-aged adults but increases in incidence in the elderly. However, acute myeloid leukemia is still much more common in older patients. Environmental exposures including certain industrial exposures, exposure to agricultural chemicals, and smoking might increase the risk of developing ALL as an adult.

The preponderance of evidence suggests that Hodgkin's disease is of B cell origin. The incidence of Hodgkin's disease appears fairly stable, with ~7800 new cases diagnosed in 2004 in the United States. Hodgkin's disease is more common in whites than in blacks and more common in males than in females. A bimodal distribution of age at diagnosis has been observed, with one peak incidence occurring in patients in their 20s and the other in those in their 80s.

TABLE 97-3 *WHO Classification of Lymphoid Malignancies*

B Cell	T Cell	Hodgkin's Disease
Precursor B cell neoplasm	Precursor T cell neoplasm	Nodular lymphocyte-predominant Hodgkin's disease
Precursor B lymphoblastic leukemia/lymphoma (precursor B cell acute lymphoblastic leukemia)	**Precursor T lymphoblastic lymphoma/leukemia (precursor T cell acute lymphoblastic leukemia)**	
Mature (peripheral) B cell neoplasms	Mature (peripheral) T cell neoplasms	Classic Hodgkin's disease
B cell chronic lymphocytic leukemia/small lymphocytic lymphoma	T cell prolymphocytic leukemia	Nodular sclerosis Hodgkin's disease
B cell prolymphocytic leukemia	T cell granular lymphocytic leukemia	Lymphocyte-rich classic Hodgkin's disease
Lymphoplasmacytic lymphoma	Aggressive NK cell leukemia	Mixed-cellularity Hodgkin's disease
Splenic marginal zone B cell lymphoma (± villous lymphocytes)	Adult T cell lymphoma/leukemia (HTLV-I+)	Lymphocyte-depletion Hodgkin's disease
Hairy cell leukemia	Extranodal NK/T cell lymphoma, nasal type	
Plasma cell myeloma/plasmacytoma	Enteropathy-type T cell lymphoma	
Extranodal marginal zone B cell lymphoma of MALT type	Hepatosplenic $\gamma\delta$ T cell lymphoma	
Mantle cell lymphoma	Subcutaneous panniculitis-like T cell lymphoma	
Follicular lymphoma	**Mycosis fungoides/Sézary syndrome**	
Nodal marginal zone B cell lymphoma (± monocytoid B cells)	Anaplastic large cell lymphoma, primary cutaneous type	
Diffuse large B cell lymphoma	**Peripheral T cell lymphoma, not otherwise specified (NOS)**	
Burkitt's lymphoma/Burkitt cell leukemia	Angioimmunoblastic T cell lymphoma	
	Anaplastic large cell lymphoma, primary systemic type	

Note: HTLV, human T cell lymphotropic virus; MALT, mucosa-associated lymphoid tissue; NK, natural killer; WHO, World Health Organization.
Source: Adapted from Harris et al.

Some of the late age peak may be attributed to confusion among entities with similar appearance such as anaplastic large cell lymphoma and T cell–rich B cell lymphoma. Patients in the younger age groups diagnosed in the United States largely have the nodular sclerosing subtype of Hodgkin's disease. Elderly patients, patients infected with HIV, and patients in third world countries more commonly have mixed-cellularity Hodgkin's disease or lymphocyte-depleted Hodgkin's disease. Infection by HIV is a risk factor for developing Hodgkin's disease. In addition, an association between infection by EBV and Hodgkin's disease has been demonstrated. A monoclonal or oligoclonal proliferation of EBV-infected cells in 20 to 40% of the patients with Hodgkin's disease has led to proposals for this virus having an etiologic role in Hodgkin's disease. However, the matter is not settled definitively.

For unknown reasons, non-Hodgkin's lymphomas increased in frequency in the United States at the rate of 4% per year between 1950 and the late 1990s. For uncertain reasons, the rate of increase in the past few years seems to be decreasing. About 54,000 new cases of non-Hodgkin's lymphoma were diagnosed in the United States in the year 2004. Non-Hodgkin's lymphomas are more frequent in the elderly and more frequent in men. Patients with both primary and secondary immunodeficiency states are predisposed to developing non-Hodgkin's lymphomas. These include patients with HIV infection; patients who have undergone organ transplantation; and patients with inherited immune deficiencies, the sicca syndrome, and rheumatoid arthritis.

The incidence of non-Hodgkin's lymphomas and the patterns of expression of the various subtypes differ geographically. T cell lymphomas are more common in Asia than in western countries, while certain subtypes of B cell lymphomas such as follicular lymphoma are more common in western countries. A specific subtype of non-Hodgkin's lymphoma known as the angiocentric nasal T/natural killer (NK) cell lymphoma has a striking geographic occurrence, being most frequent in Southern Asia and parts of Latin America. Another subtype of non-Hodgkin's lymphoma associated with infection by human T cell lymphotropic virus (HTLV) I is seen particularly in southern Japan and the Caribbean (Chap. 172).

A number of environmental factors have been implicated in the occurrence of non-Hodgkin's lymphoma, including infectious agents, chemical exposures, and medical treatments. Several studies have demonstrated an association between exposure to agricultural chemicals and an increased incidence in non-Hodgkin's lymphoma. Patients treated for Hodgkin's disease can develop non-Hodgkin's lymphoma; it is unclear whether this is a consequence of the Hodgkin's disease or its treatment. However, the infectious etiology of non-Hodgkin's lymphoma is the area where evidence has been expanding most rapidly in recent years. Table 97-4 illustrates those infectious agents associated with the development of non-Hodgkin's lymphoma. HTLV-I infects T cells and leads directly to the development of adult T cell lymphoma (ATL) in a small percentage of infected patients. The cumulative lifetime risk of developing lymphoma in an infected patient is 2.5%. The

virus is transmitted by infected lymphocytes ingested by nursing babies of infected mothers, blood-borne transmission, or sexually. The median age of patients with ATL is about 56 years, emphasizing the long latency. HTLV-I is also the cause of tropical spastic paraparasis—a neurologic disorder that occurs somewhat more frequently than lymphoma and with shorter latency.

EBV is associated with the development of Burkitt's lymphoma in Central Africa and the occurrence of aggressive non-Hodgkin's lymphomas in immunosuppressed patients in western countries. The majority of primary central nervous system (CNS) lymphomas are associated with EBV. EBV infection is strongly associated with the occurrence of extranodal nasal T/NK cell lymphomas in Asia and South America. Infection with HIV predisposes to the development of aggressive, B cell non-Hodgkin's lymphoma. This may be through overexpression of interleukin 6 by infected macrophages. Infection of the stomach by the bacterium *Helicobacter pylori* induces the development of gastric MALT (mucosa-associated lymphoid tissue) lymphomas. This association is supported by evidence that patients treated with antibiotics to eradicate *H. pylori* have regression of their MALT lymphoma. The bacterium does not transform lymphocytes to produce the lymphoma; instead, a vigorous immune response is made to the bacterium and the chronic antigenic stimulation leads to the neoplasia. MALT lymphomas of the skin may be related to *Borrelia* sp. infections.

Chronic hepatitis C virus infection has been associated with the development of lymphoplasmacytic lymphoma. Human herpesvirus 8 is associated with primary effusion lymphoma in HIV-infected persons and multicentric Castleman's disease, a diffuse lymphadenopathy associated with systemic symptoms of fever, malaise, and weight loss.

In addition to infectious agents, a number of other diseases or exposures may predispose to developing lymphoma (Table 97-5).

IMMUNOLOGY   All lymphoid cells are derived from a common hematopoietic progenitor that gives rise to lymphoid, myeloid, erythroid, monocyte, and megakaryocyte lineages. Through the ordered and sequential activation of a series of transcription factors, the cell first becomes committed to the lymphoid lineage and then gives rise to B and T cells. About 75% of all lymphoid leukemias and 90% of all lymphomas are of B cell origin. A cell becomes committed to B cell development when it begins to rearrange its immunoglobulin genes. The sequence of cellular changes, including changes in cell-surface phenotype, that characterizes normal B cell development is shown in Fig. 97-1. A cell becomes committed to T cell differentiation upon migration to the thymus and rearrangement of T cell antigen receptor genes. The sequence of the events that characterize T cell development is depicted in Fig. 97-2.

Although lymphoid malignancies often retain the cell-surface phenotype of lymphoid cells at particular stages of differentiation, this information is of little consequence. The so-called stage of differentiation of a malignant lymphoma does not predict its natural history. For example, the clinically most aggressive lymphoid leukemia is

TABLE 97-4   *Infectious Agents Associated with the Development of Lymphoid Malignancies*

Infectious Agent	Lymphoid Malignancy
Epstein-Barr virus	Burkitt's lymphoma
	Post–organ transplant lymphoma
	Primary CNS diffuse large B cell lymphoma
	Hodgkin's disease
	Extranodal NK/T cell lymphoma, nasal type
HTLV-I	Adult T cell leukemia/lymphoma
HIV	Diffuse large B cell lymphoma
	Burkitt's lymphoma
Hepatitis C virus	Lymphoplasmacytic lymphoma
Helicobacter pylori	Gastric MALT lymphoma
Human herpesvirus 8	Primary effusion lymphoma
	Multicentric Castleman's disease

Note: CNS, central nervous system; HTLV, human T cell lymphotropic virus; MALT, mucosa-associated lymphoid tissue; NK, natural killer.

TABLE 97-5   *Diseases or Exposures Associated with Increased Risk of Development of Malignant Lymphoma*

Inherited immunodeficiency disease	Autoimmune disease
Klinefelter's syndrome	Sjögren's syndrome
Chédiak-Higashi syndrome	Celiac sprue
Ataxia telangiectasia syndrome	Rheumatoid arthritis and systemic
Wiscott-Aldrich syndrome	lupus erythematosus
Common variable	Chemical or drug exposures
immunodeficiency disease	Phenytoin
Acquired immunodeficiency	Dioxin, phenoxyherbicides
diseases	Radiation
Iatrogenic immunosuppression	Prior chemotherapy and radiation
HIV-1 infection	therapy
Acquired	
hypogammaglobulinemia	

FIGURE 97-1 Pathway of normal B cell differentiation and relationship to B cell lymphomas. HLA-DR, CD10, CD19, CD20, CD21, CD22, CD5, and CD38 are cell markers used to distinguish stages of development. Terminal transferase (TdT) is a cellular enzyme. Immunoglobulin heavy chain gene rearrangement (HCR) and light chain gene rearrangement or deletion (κ R or D, λ R or D) occur early in B cell development. The approximate normal stage of differentiation associated with particular lymphomas is shown. ALL, acute lymphoid leukemia; CLL, chronic lymphoid leukemia; SL, small lymphocytic lymphoma.

arrangement of specific genes that may or may not be apparent from cytogenetic studies; and overexpression, underexpression, or mutation of specific oncogenes. Altered expression or mutation of specific proteins is particularly important. Many lymphomas contain balanced chromosomal translocations involving the antigen receptor genes; immunoglobulin genes on chromosomes 2, 14, and 22 in B cells; and T cell antigen receptor genes on chromosomes 7 and 14 in T cells. The rearrangement of chromosome segments to generate mature antigen receptors must create a site of vulnerability to aberrant recombination. B cells are even more susceptible to acquiring mutations during their maturation in germinal centers; the generation of antibody of higher affinity requires the introduction of mutations into the variable region genes in the germinal centers. Other nonimmunoglobulin genes, for example *bcl-6*, may acquire mutations as well.

In the case of diffuse large B cell lymphoma, the translocation t(14;18) occurs in ~30% of patients and leads to overexpression of the *bcl-2* gene found on chromosome 18. Some other patients without the translocation also overexpress the BCL-2 protein. This protein is involved in suppressing apoptosis—i.e., the mechanism of cell death most often induced by cytotoxic chemotherapeutic agents. A higher relapse rate has been observed in patients whose tumors overexpress the BCL-2 protein, but not in those patients whose lymphoma cells show only the translocation. Thus, particular genetic mechanisms have clinical ramifications.

Table 97-6 presents the best documented translocations and associated oncogenes for various subtypes of lymphoid malignancies. In some cases, such as the association of the t(14;18) in follicular lymphoma, the t(2;5) in anaplastic large T/null-cell lymphoma, the t(8;14) in Burkitt's lymphoma, and the t(11;14) in mantle cell lymphoma, the great majority of tumors in patients with these diagnoses display these abnormalities. In other types of lymphoma where a minority of the patients have tumors expressing specific genetic abnormalities, the defects may have prognostic significance. No specific genetic abnormalities have been identified in Hodgkin's disease other than aneuploidy.

In typical B cell CLL, trisomy 12 conveys a poorer prognosis. In ALL in both adults and children, genetic abnormalities have important prognostic significance. Patients whose tumor cells display the t(9;22) have a much poorer outlook than patients who do not have this translocation. Other genetic abnormalities that occur frequently in adults with ALL include the t(4;11) and the t(8;14). The t(4;11) is associated with younger age, female predominance, high white cell counts, and L1 morphology. The t(8;14) is associated with older age, male predominance, frequent CNS involvement, and L3 morphology. Both are associated with a poor prognosis. In childhood ALL, hyperdiploidy has been shown to have a favorable prognosis.

Gene profiling using array technology allows the simultaneous assessment of the expression of thousands of genes. This technology provides the possibility to identify new genes with pathologic importance in lymphomas, the identification of patterns of gene expression with diagnostic and/or prognostic significance, and the identification

Burkitt's leukemia, which has the phenotype of a mature follicle center IgM-bearing B cell. Leukemias bearing the immunologic cell-surface phenotype of more primitive cells (e.g., pre-B ALL, CD10+) are less aggressive and more amenable to curative therapy than the "more mature" appearing Burkitt's leukemia cells. Furthermore, the apparent stage of differentiation of the malignant cell does not reflect the stage at which the genetic lesions that gave rise to the malignancy developed. For example, follicular lymphoma has the cell-surface phenotype of a follicle center cell, but its characteristic chromosomal translocation, the t(14;18), which involves juxtaposition of the antiapoptotic *bcl-2* gene next to the immunoglobulin heavy chain gene (see below), had to develop early in ontogeny as an error in the process of immunoglobulin gene rearrangement. Why the subsequent steps that led to transformation became manifest in a cell of follicle center differentiation is not clear.

The major value of cell-surface phenotyping is to aid in the differential diagnosis of lymphoid tumors that appear similar by light microscopy. For example, benign follicular hyperplasia may resemble follicular lymphoma; however, the demonstration that all the cells bear the same immunoglobulin light chain isotype strongly suggests the mass is a clonal proliferation rather than a polyclonal response to an exogenous stimulus.

GENETIC CONSIDERATIONS Malignancies of lymphoid cells are associated with recurring genetic abnormalities. While specific genetic abnormalities have not been identified for all subtypes of lymphoid malignancies, it is presumed that they exist. Genetic abnormalities can be identified at a variety of levels including gross chromosomal changes (i.e., translocations, additions, or deletions); re-

| T CELL DIFFERENTIATION | THYMUS | T CELL MALIGNANCIES |

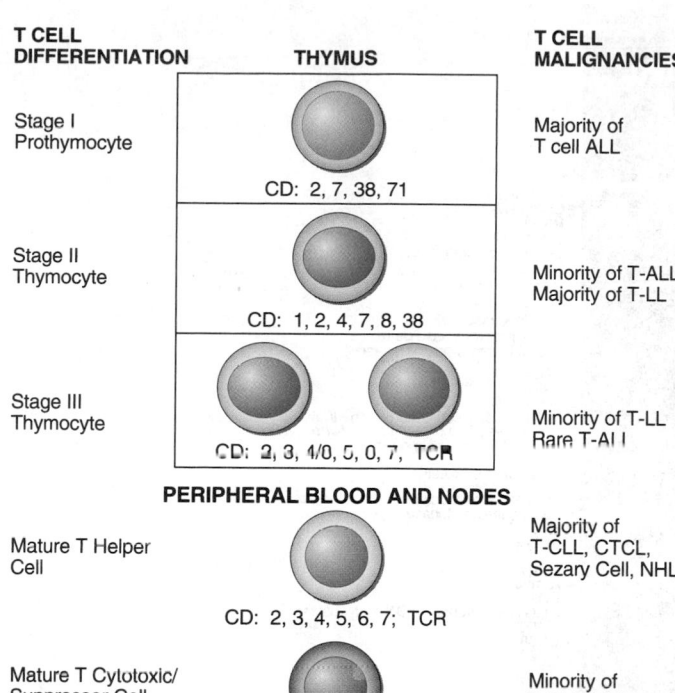

FIGURE 97-2 Pathway of normal T cell differentiation and relationship to T cell lymphomas. CD1, CD2, CD3, CD4, CD5, CD6, CD7, CD8, CD38, and CD71 are cell markers used to distinguish stages of development. T cell antigen receptors (TCR) rearrange in the thymus, and mature T cells emigrate to nodes and peripheral blood. ALL, acute lymphoid leukemia; T-ALL, T cell ALL; T-LL, T cell lymphoblastic lymphoma; T-CLL, T cell chronic lymphoid leukemia; CTCL, cutaneous T cell lymphoma; NHL, non-Hodgkin's lymphoma.

of new therapeutic targets. Recognition of patterns of gene expression is complicated and requires sophisticated mathematical techniques. Early successes using this technology in lymphoma include the identification of previously unrecognized subtypes of diffuse large B cell lymphoma whose gene expression patterns resemble either those of follicular center B cells or activated peripheral blood B cells (Fig. 97-3). Patients whose lymphomas have a germinal center B cell pattern of gene expression have a considerably better prognosis than those whose lymphomas have a pattern resembling that seen in activated

TABLE 97-6 *Cytogenetic Translocation and Associated Oncogenes Often Seen in Lymphoid Malignancies*

Disease	Cytogenetic Abnormality	Oncogene
CLL/small lymphocytic lymphoma	t(14;15)(q32;q13)	—
MALT lymphoma	t(11;18)(q21;q21)	—
Precursor B cell acute lymphoid leukemia	t(9;22)(q34;q11) or variant	BCR/ABL
	t(4;11)(q21;q23)	AF4, ALLI
Precursor acute lymphoid leukemia	t(9;22)	BCR, ABL
	t(1;19)	E2A, PBX
	t(17;19)	HLF, E2A
	t(5;14)	IL3, IGμ
Mantle cell lymphoma	t(11;14)(q13;q32)	BCL-1, IgH
Follicular lymphoma	t(14;18)(q32;q21)	BCL-2, IgH
Diffuse large-cell lymphoma	t(3;-)(q27;-)[a]	BCL-6
	t(17;-)(p13;-)	p53
Burkitt's lymphoma, Burkitt's leukemia	t(8;-)(q24;-)[a]	C-MYC
CD30+ Anaplastic large cell lymphoma	t(2;5)(p23;q35)	ALK
Lymphoplasmacytoid lymphoma	t(9;14)(p13;q32)	—

[a] Numerous sites of translocation may be involved with these genes.
Note: CLL, chronic lymphoid leukemia; MALT, mucosa-associated lymphoid tissue; IgH, immunoglobulin heavy chain.

peripheral blood B cells. This improved prognosis is independent of other known prognostic factors and provides the opportunity to identify better treatments for these subgroups of patients. Similar information is being generated in follicular lymphoma and mantle cell lymphoma. The challenge remains to provide information from such techniques in a clinically useful time frame.

APPROACH TO THE PATIENT

Regardless of the type of lymphoid malignancy, the initial evaluation of the patient should include performance of a careful history and physical examination. These will help confirm the diagnosis, identify those manifestations of the disease that might require prompt attention, and aid in the selection of further studies to optimally characterize the patient's status to allow the best choice of therapy. It is difficult to overemphasize the importance of a carefully done history and physical examination. They might provide observations that lead to reconsidering the diagnosis, provide hints at etiology, clarify the stage, and allow the physician to establish rapport with the patient that will make it possible to develop and carry out a therapeutic plan.

For patients with ALL, evaluation is usually completed after a complete blood count, chemistry studies reflecting major organ function, a bone marrow biopsy with genetic and immunologic studies, and a lumbar puncture. The latter is necessary to rule out occult CNS involvement. At this point, most patients would be ready to begin therapy. In ALL, prognosis is dependent upon the genetic characteristics of the tumor, the patient's age, the white cell count, and the patient's overall clinical status and major organ function.

In CLL, the patient evaluation should include a complete blood count, chemistry tests to measure major organ function, serum protein electrophoresis, and a bone marrow biopsy. However, some physicians believe that the diagnosis would not always require a bone marrow biopsy. Patients often have imaging studies of the chest and abdomen looking for pathologic lymphadenopathy. Patients with typical B cell CLL can be subdivided into three major prognostic groups. Those patients with only blood and bone marrow involvement by leukemia but no lymphadenopathy, organomegaly, or signs of bone marrow failure have the best prognosis. Those with lymphadenopathy and organomegaly have an intermediate prognosis, and patients with bone marrow failure, defined as hemoglobin <100 g/L (10 g/dL) or platelet count $<100,000/\mu L$, have the worst prognosis. The pathogenesis of the anemia or thrombocytopenia is important to discern. The prognosis is adversely affected when either or both of these abnormalities are due to progressive marrow infiltration and loss of productive marrow. However, either or both may be due to autoimmune phenomena or to hypersplenism that can develop during the course of the disease. These destructive mechanisms are usually completely reversible (glucocorticoids for autoimmune disease; splenectomy for hypersplenism) and do not influence disease prognosis.

Two popular staging systems have been developed to reflect these prognostic groupings (Table 97-7). Patients with typical B cell CLL can have their course complicated by immunologic abnormalities including autoimmune hemolytic anemia, autoimmune thrombocytopenia, and hypogammaglobulinemia. Patients with hypogammaglobulinemia benefit from regular (monthly) γ globulin administration. Because of expense, γ globulin is often withheld until the patient experiences a significant infection. These abnormalities do not have a clear prognostic significance and should not be used to assign a higher stage.

The initial evaluation of a patient with Hodgkin's disease or non-Hodgkin's lymphoma is similar. In both situations, the determination of an accurate anatomic stage is an important part of the evaluation. The staging system is the Ann Arbor staging system originally developed for Hodgkin's disease (Table 97-8).

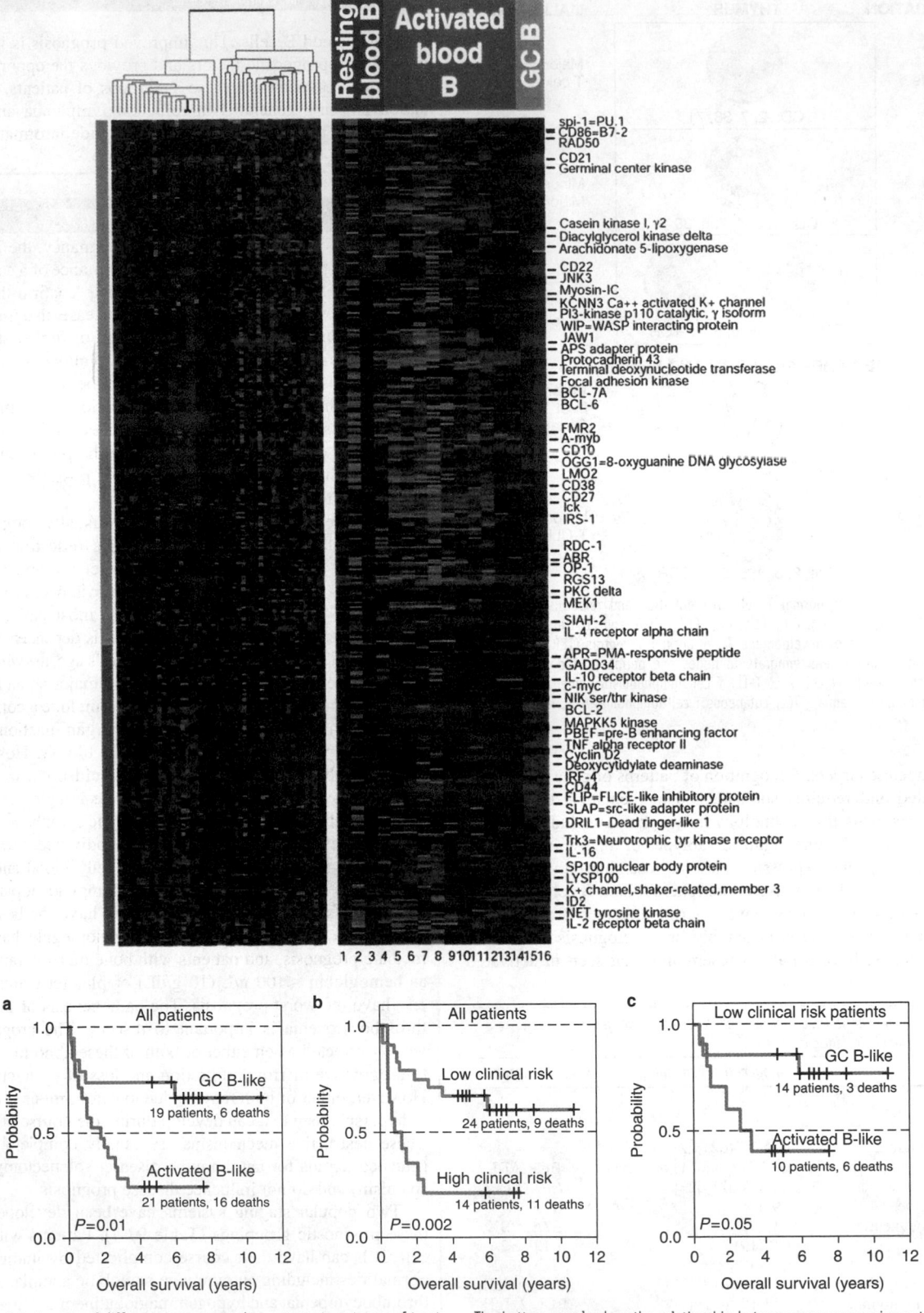

FIGURE 97-3 Relationship of different gene expression patterns to outcome of treatment for diffuse large B cell lymphoma. The top panel reveals the pattern of expression of a large number of lymphocyte-expressed genes in tumors from patients with diffuse large B cell lymphoma, a lymphoma recognized as morphologically heterogeneous but before now not classifiable reproducibly. Two dominant patterns are seen, one mimicking germinal center B cells and one mimicking activated peripheral blood B cells. The bottom panels show the relationship between gene expression pattern and clinical outcome. *A.* Kaplan-Meier survival plots of all patients according to gene profile showing significant differences between follicular center and activated B cell types. *B.* Kaplan-Meier survival of patients based upon the IPI scores. *C.* Kaplan-Meier survival plots showing that among patients with IPI low risk, the gene expression profile has prognostic significance. (IPI, International Prognostic Index.)

TABLE 97-7 *Staging of Typical B Cell Lymphoid Leukemia*

Stage	Clinical Features	Median Survival, Years
RAI SYSTEM		
0: Low risk	Lymphocytosis only in blood and marrow	>10
I: Intermediate risk	Lymphocytosis + lymphadenopathy + splenomegaly ± hepatomegaly	7
II		
III: High risk	Lymphocytosis + anemia	1.5
IV	Lymphocytosis + thrombocytopenia	
BINET SYSTEM		
A	Fewer than three areas of clinical lymphadenopathy; no anemia or thrombocytopenia	>10
B	Three or more involved node areas; no anemia or thrombocytopenia	7
C	Hemoglobin ≤10 g/dL and/or platelets <100,000/μl	2

Evaluation of patients with Hodgkin's disease will typically include a complete blood count; erythrocyte sedimentation rate; chemistry studies reflecting major organ function; computed tomography (CT) scans of the chest, abdomen, and pelvis; and a bone marrow biopsy. Neither a positron emission tomography (PET) scan nor a gallium scan is absolutely necessary for primary staging, but one performed at the completion of therapy allows evaluation of persisting radiographic abnormalities, particularly the mediastinum. Knowing that the PET scan or gallium scan is abnormal before treatment is initiated can help in this assessment. In most cases, these studies will allow assignment of anatomic stage and the development of a therapeutic plan.

In patients with non-Hodgkin's lymphoma, the same evaluation described for patients with Hodgkin's disease is usually carried out. In addition, serum levels of lactate dehydrogenase (LDH) and β_2-

TABLE 97-8 *The Ann Arbor Staging System for Hodgkin's Disease*

Stage	Definition
I	Involvement of a single lymph node region or lymphoid structure (e.g., spleen, thymus, Waldeyer's ring)
II	Involvement of two or more lymph node regions on the same side of the diaphragm (the mediastinum is a single site; hilar lymph nodes should be considered "lateralized" and, when involved on both sides, constitute stage II disease)
III	Involvement of lymph node regions or lymphoid structures on both sides of the diaphragm
III₁	Subdiaphragmatic involvement limited to spleen, splenic hilar nodes, celiac nodes, or portal nodes
III₂	Subdiaphragmatic involvement includes paraaortic, iliac, or mesenteric nodes plus structures in III₁
IV	Involvement of extranodal site(s) beyond that designated as "E" More than one extranodal deposit at any location Any involvement of liver or bone marrow
A	No symptoms
B	Unexplained weight loss of >10% of the body weight during the 6 months before staging investigation Unexplained, persistent, or recurrent fever with temperatures >38°C during the previous month Recurrent drenching night sweats during the previous month
E	Localized, solitary involvement of extralymphatic tissue, excluding liver and bone marrow

TABLE 97-9 *International Prognostic Index for NHL*

Five clinical risk factors:
  Age ≥ 60 years
  Serum lactate dehydrogenase levels elevated
  Performance status ≥ 2 (ECOG) or ≤ 70 (Karnofsky)
  Ann Arbor stage III or IV
  >1 site of extranodal involvement
Patients are assigned a number for each risk factor they have
Patients are grouped differently based upon the type of lymphoma
For diffuse large B cell lymphoma:

0,1 factor = low risk	35% of cases; 5-year survival, 73%
2 factors = low-intermediate risk	27% of cases; 5-year survival, 51%
3 factors = high intermediate risk	22% of cases; 5-year survival, 43%
4,5 factors = high risk	16% of cases; 5-year survival, 26%

microglobulin and serum protein electrophoresis are often included in the evaluation. Anatomic stage is assigned in the same manner as used for Hodgkin's disease. However, the prognosis of patients with non-Hodgkin's lymphoma is best assigned using the International Prognostic Index (IPI) (Table 97-9). This is a powerful predictor of outcome in all subtypes of non-Hodgkin's lymphoma. Patients are assigned an IPI score based on the presence or absence of five adverse prognostic factors and may have none or all five of these adverse prognostic factors. Figure 97-4 shows the prognostic significance of this score in 1300 patients with all types of non-Hodgkin's lymphoma. CT scans are routinely used in the evaluation of patients with all subtypes of non-Hodgkin's lymphoma but PET and gallium scans are much more useful in aggressive subtypes such as diffuse large B cell lymphoma than in more indolent subtypes such a follicular lymphoma or small lymphocytic lymphoma.

CLINICAL FEATURES, TREATMENT, AND PROGNOSIS OF SPECIFIC LYMPHOID MALIGNANCIES

PRECURSOR CELL B CELL NEOPLASMS ■ Precursor B Cell Lymphoblastic Leukemia/Lymphoma
The most common cancer in childhood is B cell ALL. Although this disorder can also present as a lymphoma in either adults or children, presentation as lymphoma is quite rare.

The malignant cells in patients with precursor B cell lymphoblastic leukemia are most commonly of pre-B cell origin. Patients typically present with signs of bone marrow failure such as pallor, fatigue, bleeding, fever, and infection related to peripheral blood cytopenias. Peripheral blood counts regularly show anemia and thrombocytopenia but might show leukopenia, a normal leukocyte count, or leukocytosis based largely on the number of circulating malignant cells (Fig. 97-5). Extranodal sites of disease are frequently involved in patients who

FIGURE 97-4 Relationship of International Prognostic Index (IPI) to survival. Kaplan-Meier survival curves for 1300 patients with various kinds of lymphoma stratified according to the IPI.

FIGURE 97-5 Acute lympho-blastic leukemia. The cells are heterogeneous in size, have round or convoluted nuclei, high nuclear/cytoplasmic ratio, and absence of cytoplasmic granules.

present with leukemia, which might be manifested by lymphadenopathy, hepato- or splenomegaly, CNS disease, testicular enlargement, and/or cutaneous infiltration.

The diagnosis is usually made by bone marrow biopsy, which shows infiltration by malignant lymphoblasts. Demonstration of a pre-B cell immunophenotype (Fig. 97-1) and, often, characteristic cytogenetic abnormalities (Table 97-6) confirm the diagnosis. An adverse prognosis in patients with precursor B cell ALL is predicted by a very high white cell count, the presence of symptomatic CNS disease, and unfavorable cytogenetic abnormalities. For example, t(9;22) is frequently found in adults with B cell lymphoblastic leukemia and is associated with a very poor outlook.

℞ TREATMENT

The treatment of patients with precursor B cell lymphoblastic leukemia involves remission induction with combination chemotherapy, a consolidation phase that includes administration of high-dose systemic therapy and treatment to eliminate disease in the CNS, and a period of continuing therapy to prevent relapse and effect cure. The overall cure rate in children is 85%, while about 50% of adults are long-term disease-free survivors. This reflects the high proportion of adverse cytogenetic abnormalities seen in adults with precursor B cell lymphoblastic leukemia.

Precursor B cell lymphoblastic lymphoma is a rare presentation of precursor B cell lymphoblastic malignancy. These patients often have a rapid transformation to leukemia, and similar treatment approaches as are used in patients presenting with leukemia are appropriate. In the few patients who present with the disease confined to lymph nodes, a high cure rate has been reported.

MATURE (PERIPHERAL) B CELL NEOPLASMS ■ B Cell Chronic Lymphoid Leukemia/Small Lymphocytic Lymphoma B cell CLL/small lymphocytic lymphoma represents by far the most common lymphoid leukemia, and

when presenting as a lymphoma, it accounts for ~7% of non-Hodgkin's lymphomas. As the name implies, presentation can be as either leukemia or lymphoma. The major clinical characteristics of B cell CLL/small lymphocytic lymphoma are presented in Table 97-10.

The diagnosis of typical B cell CLL is made when an increased number of circulating lymphocytes (i.e., $>4 \times 10^9$/L and usually $>10 \times 10^9$/L) is found (Fig. 97-6) that are monoclonal B cells and display the CD5 antigen. Finding bone marrow infiltration by the same cells confirms the diagnosis. The peripheral blood smear in such patients typically shows many "smudge" or "basket" cells, nuclear remnants of cells damaged by the physical shear stress of making the blood smear. If cytogenetic studies are performed, trisomy 12 is found in ~25 to 30% of patients. Abnormalities in chromosome 13 are also seen.

If the primary presentation is lymphadenopathy and a lymph node biopsy is performed, pathologists usually have little difficulty in making the diagnosis of small lymphocytic lymphoma based on morphologic findings and immunophenotype. However, even in these patients, ~70 to 75% will be found to have bone marrow involvement and the search for circulating monoclonal B lymphocytes is often positive.

The differential diagnosis of typical B cell CLL is extensive and presented in Table 97-1. Immunophenotyping will eliminate the T cell disorders and can often help sort out other B cell malignancies. For example, only mantle cell lymphoma and typical B cell CLL are usually CD5 positive. Typical B cell small lymphocytic lymphoma can be confused with other B cell disorders including lymphoplasmacytic lymphoma (i.e., the tissue manifestation of Waldenström's macroglobulinemia), nodal marginal zone B cell lymphoma, and mantle cell lymphoma. In addition, some small lymphocytic lymphomas have areas of large cells that can lead to confusion with diffuse large B cell lymphoma. An expert hematopathologist is vital for making this distinction.

Typical B cell CLL is often found incidentally when a complete blood count is done for another reason. However, complaints that might lead to the diagnosis include fatigue, frequent infections, and new lymphadenopathy. The diagnosis of typical B cell CLL should be considered in a patient presenting with an autoimmune hemolytic anemia or autoimmune thrombocytopenia. B cell CLL has also been associated with red cell aplasia. When this disorder presents as lymphoma, the most common abnormality is asymptomatic new lymphadenopathy, with or without splenomegaly. The staging systems used to predict prognosis in patients with typical B cell CLL are presented in Table 97-7. The IPI for non-Hodgkin's lymphomas, which also predicts prognosis in these patients, is presented in Table 97-9. The evaluation of a new patient with typical B cell CLL/small lym-

TABLE 97-10 Clinical Characteristics of Patients with Common Types of Non-Hodgkin's Lymphomas (NHL)

Disease	Median Age, years	Frequency in Children	% Male	Stage I/II vs III/IV, %	B Symptoms, %	Bone Marrow Involvement, %	Gastrointestinal Tract Involvement, %	% Surviving 5 years
B cell chronic lymphocytic leukemia/small lymphocytic lymphoma	65	Rare	53	9 vs 91	33	72	3	51
Mantle cell lymphoma	63	Rare	74	20 vs 80	28	64	9	27
Extranodal marginal zone B cell lymphoma of MALT type	60	Rare	48	67 vs 33	19	14	50	74
Follicular lymphoma	59	Rare	42	33 vs 67	28	42	4	72
Diffuse large B cell lymphoma	64	~25% of childhood NHL	55	54 vs 46	33	16	18	46
Burkitt's lymphoma	31	~30% of childhood NHL	89	62 vs 38	22	33	11	45
Precursor T cell lymphoblastic lymphoma	28	~40% of childhood NHL	64	11 vs 89	21	50	4	26
Anaplastic large T/null cell lymphoma	34	Common	69	51 vs 49	53	13	9	77
Peripheral T cell non-Hodgkin's lymphoma	61	~5% of childhood NHL	55	20 vs 80	50	36	15	25

Note: MALT, mucosa-associated lymphoid tissue.

FIGURE 97-6 *Chronic lymphocytic leukemia. The peripheral white blood cell count is high due to increased numbers of small, well-differentiated, normal-appearing lymphocytes. The leukemia lymphocytes are fragile, and substantial numbers of broken, smudged cells are usually also present on the blood smear.*

phocytic lymphoma will include many of the studies included in Table 97-11, which describes the initial evaluation of a new patient with non-Hodgkin's lymphoma. In addition, particular attention needs to be given to detecting immune abnormalities such as autoimmune hemolytic anemia, autoimmune thrombocytopenia, hypogammaglobulinemia, and red cell aplasia. Molecular analysis of immunoglobulin gene sequences in CLL has demonstrated that about half the patients have tumors expressing mutated immunoglobulin genes and half have tumors expressing unmutated or germ-line immunoglobulin sequences. Patients with unmutated immunoglobulins tend to have a more aggressive clinical course and are less responsive to therapy. Unfortunately, immunoglobulin gene sequencing is not routinely available. CD38 expression is said to be low in the better-prognosis patients expressing mutated immunoglobulin and high in poorer-prognosis patients expressing unmutated immunoglobulin, but this test has not been confirmed as a reliable means of distinguishing the two groups.

℞ TREATMENT

Patients whose presentation is typical B cell CLL with no manifestations of the disease other than bone marrow involvement and lymphocytosis (i.e., Rai stage O and Binet stage A; Table 97-7) can be followed without specific therapy for their malignancy. These patients have a median survival >10 years, and some will never require therapy for this disorder. If the patient has an adequate number of circulating normal blood cells and is asymptomatic, many physicians would not initiate therapy for patients in the intermediate stage of the disease manifested by lymphadenopathy and/or hepatosplenomegaly. However, the median survival for these patients is ~7 years, and most will require treatment in the first few years of follow-up. Patients who present with bone marrow failure (i.e., Rai stage III or IV or Binet stage C) will require initial therapy in almost all cases. These patients have a serious disorder with a median survival of only 1.5 years. It must be remembered that immune manifestations of typical B cell CLL should be managed independently of specific antileukemia therapy. For example, glucocorticoid therapy for autoimmune cytopenias and γ globulin replacement for patients with hypogammaglobulinanemia should be used whether or not antileukemia therapy is given.

Patients who present primarily with lymphoma and have a low IPI score have a 5-year survival of ~75%, but those with a high IPI score

TABLE 97-11   *Staging Evaluation for Non-Hodgkin's Lymphoma*

Physical examination
Documentation of B symptoms
Laboratory evaluation
   Complete blood counts
   Liver function tests
   Uric acid
   Calcium
   Serum protein electrophoresis
   Serum β_2-microglobulin
Chest radiograph
CT scan of abdomen, pelvis, and usually chest
Bone marrow biopsy
Lumbar puncture in lymphoblastic, Burkitt's, and diffuse large B cell
   lymphoma with positive marrow biopsy
Gallium scan (SPECT) or PET scan in large-cell lymphoma

Note: CT, computed tomography; SPECT, single photon emission CT; PET, position emission tomography.

have a 5-year survival of <40% and are more likely to require early therapy.

The most common treatments for patients with typical B cell CLL/small lymphocytic lymphoma have been single-agent chlorambucil or fludarabine alone or in combination. Chlorambucil can be administered orally with few immediate side effects, while fludarabine is administered intravenously and is associated with significant immune suppression. However, fludarabine is by far the more active agent and is the only drug associated with a significant incidence of complete remission. The combination of rituximab (375 to 500 mg/m² day 1), fludarabine (25 mg/m² days 2 to 4 on cycle 1 and 1 to 3 in subsequent cycles), and cyclophosphamide (250 mg/m² with fludarabine) achieves complete responses in 69% of patients and those responses are associated with molecular remissions in half of the cases. Half the patients experience grade III or IV neutropenia. For young patients presenting with leukemia requiring therapy, regimens containing fludarabine are today the treatment of choice. Because fludarabine is an effective second-line agent in patients with tumors unresponsive to chlorambucil, the latter agent is often chosen in elderly patients who require therapy. Many patients who present with lymphoma will receive a combination chemotherapy regimen used in other lymphomas such as CVP (cyclophosphamide, vincristine, and prednisone), or CHOP (cyclophosphamide, doxorubicin, vincristine, and prednisone) although fludarabine-containing regimens may be preferrable. Alemtuzimab (anti-CD52) is another antibody with activity in the disease, but it kills both B and T cells and is associated with more immune compromise that rituximab. Young patients with this disease can be candidates for bone marrow transplantation. Allogeneic bone marrow transplantation can be curative but is associated with a significant treatment-related mortality. The use of autologous transplantation in patients with this disorder has been discouraging.

Extranodal Marginal Zone B Cell Lymphoma of MALT Type   Extranodal marginal zone B cell lymphoma of MALT type makes up ~8% of non-Hodgkin's lymphomas. This small-cell lymphoma presents in extranodal sites. It was previously considered a small lymphocytic lymphoma or sometimes a pseudolymphoma. The recognition that the gastric presentation of this lymphoma was associated with *H. pylori* infection was an important step in recognizing it as a separate entity. The clinical characteristics of extranodal marginal zone B cell lymphoma of MALT type are presented in Table 97-10.

The diagnosis of extranodal marginal zone B cell lymphoma of MALT type can be made accurately by an expert hematopathologist based on a characteristic pattern of infiltration of small lymphocytes that are monoclonal B cells and CD5 negative. In some cases, transformation to diffuse large B cell lymphoma occurs, and both diagnoses may be made in the same biopsy. The differential diagnosis includes benign lymphocytic infiltration of extranodal organs and other small-cell B cell lymphomas.

Extranodal marginal zone B cell lymphoma of MALT type may occur in the stomach, orbit, intestine, lung, thyroid, salivary gland, skin, soft tissues, bladder, kidney, and CNS. It may present as a new mass, be found on routine imaging studies, or be associated with local symptoms such as upper abdominal discomfort in gastric lymphoma. Most MALT lymphomas are gastric in origin. At least two genetic forms of gastric MALT exist: one (accounting for ~50% of cases) characterized by t(11;18)(q21;q21) that juxtaposes the amino terminal of the *API2* gene with the carboxy terminal of the *MALT1* gene creating an API2/MALT1 fusion product, and the other characterized by multiple sites of genetic instability including trisomies of chromosomes 3, 7, 12, and 18. Ninety-five percent of gastric MALT lymphomas are associated with *H. pylori* infection, and those that are not usually express t(11;18). The t(11;18) usually results in activation of NF-κB, which acts a survival factor for the cells. Lymphomas with t(11;18) translocations are genetically stable and do not evolve to diffuse large B cell lymphoma. By contrast, t(11;18)-negative MALT lymphomas often acquire *BCL6* mutations and progress to aggressive histology lymphoma. MALT lymphomas are localized to the organ of origin in ~40% of cases and to the organ and regional lymph nodes in ~30% of patients. However, distant metastasis can occur—particularly with transformation to diffuse large B cell lymphoma. Many patients who develop this lymphoma will have an autoimmune or inflammatory process such as Sjögren's syndrome (salivary gland MALT), Hashimoto's thyroiditis (thyroid MALT), or *Helicobacter* gastritis (gastric MALT).

Evaluation of patients with extranodal marginal zone B cell lymphoma of MALT type follows the pattern set forth in Table 97-11 for staging a patient with non-Hodgkin's lymphoma. In particular, patients with gastric lymphoma need to have studies performed to document the presence or absence of *H. pylori* infection. Endoscopic studies including ultrasound can help define the extent of gastric involvement. Most patients with extranodal marginal zone B cell lymphoma of MALT type have a good prognosis, with a 5-year survival of ~75%. In patients with a low IPI score, the 5-year survival is ~90%, while it drops to ~40% in patients with a high IPI score.

℞ TREATMENT

Extranodal marginal zone B cell lymphoma of MALT type is curable when localized. Local therapy such as radiation or surgery can effect cure, and this is one of the few times where surgery might be a reasonable primary therapy for a patient with non-Hodgkin's lymphoma. Patients with gastric MALT lymphomas who are infected with *H. pylori* can achieve remission in the majority of cases with eradication of the infection. These remissions can be durable, but molecular evidence of persisting neoplasia is frequent and the long-term outcome is uncertain. Patients who present with more extensive disease are most often treated with single-agent chemotherapy such as chlorambucil. Coexistent diffuse large B cell lymphoma must be treated with combination chemotherapy. The additional acquired mutations that mediate the histologic progression also convey *Helicobacter* independence to the growth.

Mantle Cell Lymphoma Mantle cell lymphoma makes up ~6% of all non-Hodgkin's lymphomas. Recognized as a separate entity only in the past decade, this lymphoma was previously placed in a number of other subtypes. Its existence was confirmed by the recognition that these lymphomas have a characteristic chromosomal translocation, t(11;14), between the immunoglobulin heavy chain gene on chromosome 14 and the *bcl-1* gene on chromosome 11, and regularly overexpress the BCL-1 protein. The clinical characteristics of mantle cell lymphoma are presented in Table 97-10.

The diagnosis of mantle cell lymphoma can be made accurately by an expert hematopathologist based on morphologic findings and proof that the tumor is a B cell lymphoma. As with all subtypes of lymphoma, an adequate biopsy is important. The differential diagnosis of mantle cell lymphoma includes other small-cell B cell lymphomas. In particular, mantle cell lymphoma and small lymphocytic lymphoma share a characteristic expression of CD5. Mantle cell lymphoma usually has a slightly indented nucleus.

The most common presentation of mantle cell lymphoma is with palpable lymphadenopathy, frequently accompanied by systemic symptoms. Approximately 70% of patients will be stage IV at the time of diagnosis, with frequent bone marrow and peripheral blood involvement. Of the extranodal organs that can be involved, gastrointestinal involvement is particularly important to recognize. Patients who present with lymphomatosis polyposis in the large intestine usually have mantle cell lymphoma. The evaluation of patients with mantle cell lymphoma involves the studies presented in Table 97-11 for staging of patients with non-Hodgkin's lymphoma. Patients who present with gastrointestinal tract involvement often have Waldeyer's ring involvement, and vice versa. The 5-year survival for all patients with mantle cell lymphoma is ~25%, with only occasional patients who

present with a high IPI score surviving 5 years and ~50% of patients with a low IPI score surviving 5 years.

℞ TREATMENT

Current therapies for mantle cell lymphoma are unsatisfactory. Patients with localized disease might be treated with combination chemotherapy followed by radiotherapy; however, these patients are exceedingly rare. For the usual presentation with disseminated disease, treatments have been unsatisfactory, with the minority of patients achieving complete remission. Aggressive combination chemotherapy regimens followed by autologous or allogeneic bone marrow transplantation are frequently offered to younger patients. For the occasional elderly, asymptomatic patient, observation followed by single-agent chemotherapy might be the most practical approach. An intensive combination chemotherapy regimen originally used in the treatment of acute leukemia, HyperC-VAD (cyclophosphamide, vincristine, doxorubicin, dexamethasone, cytarabine, and methotrexate) in combination with rituximab seems to be associated with better response rates—particularly in younger patients. CHOP plus rituximab has shown better response rates than CHOP alone, but long-term follow-up is lacking.

Follicular Lymphoma Follicular lymphomas make up 22% of non-Hodgkin's lymphomas worldwide and at least 30% of non-Hodgkin's lymphomas diagnosed in the United States. This type of lymphoma can be diagnosed accurately on morphologic findings alone and has been the diagnosis in the majority of patients in therapeutic trials for "low-grade" lymphoma in the past. The clinical characteristics of follicular lymphoma are presented in Table 97-10.

Evaluation of an adequate biopsy by an expert hematopathologist is sufficient to make a diagnosis of follicular lymphoma. The tumor is composed of small cleaved and large cells in varying proportions organized in a follicular pattern of growth (Fig. 97-7). Confirmation of B cell immunophenotype and the existence of the t(14;18) and abnormal expression of BCL-2 protein are confirmatory. The major differential diagnosis is between lymphoma and reactive follicular hyperplasia. The coexistence of diffuse large B cell lymphoma must be considered. Patients with follicular lymphoma are often subclassified into those with predominantly small cells, those with a mixture of small and large cells, and those with predominantly large cells. While this distinction cannot be made simply or very accurately, these subdivisions do have prognostic significance. Patients with follicular lymphoma with predominantly large cells have a higher proliferative fraction, progress more rapidly, and have a shorter overall survival with simple chemotherapy regimens.

The most common presentation for follicular lymphoma is with new, painless lymphadenopathy. Multiple sites of lymphoid involvement are typical, and unusual sites such as epitrochlear nodes are sometimes seen. However, essentially any organ can be involved, and extranodal presentations do occur. Most patients do not have fevers, sweats, or weight loss, and an IPI score of 0 or 1 is found in ~50% of patients. Fewer than 10% of patients have a high (i.e., 4 or 5) IPI score. The staging evaluation for patients with follicular lymphoma should include the studies included in Table 97-11 for the staging of patients with non-Hodgkin's lymphoma.

℞ TREATMENT

Follicular lymphoma is one of the malignancies most responsive to chemotherapy and radiotherapy. In addition, as many as 25% of the patients undergo spontaneous regression—usually transient—when followed without therapy. In an asymptomatic patient, no initial treatment and watchful waiting can be an appropriate management strategy and is particularly likely to be adopted for older patients. For patients who do require treatment, single-agent chlorambucil or cyclophosphamide or combination chemotherapy with CVP or CHOP are most frequently used. With adequate treatment, 50 to 75% of patients will achieve a complete remission. While most patients relapse (median response duration is ~2 years), at least 20% of complete responders

FIGURE 97-7 Follicular lymphoma. The normal nodal architecture is effaced by nodular expansions of tumor cells. Nodules vary in size and contain predominantly small lymphocytes with cleaved nuclei along with variable numbers of larger cells with vesicular chromatin and prominent nucleoli.

FIGURE 97-8 Diffuse large B cell lymphoma. The neoplastic cells are heterogeneous but predominantly large cells with vesicular chromatin and prominent nucleoli.

will remain in remission for >10 years. For the rare patient with localized follicular lymphoma, involved field radiotherapy produces an excellent treatment result.

A number of new therapies have been shown to be active in the treatment of patients with follicular lymphoma. These include new cytotoxic agents such as fludarabine, and biologic agents such as interferon α, monoclonal antibodies with or without radionuclides, and lymphoma vaccines. In patients treated with a doxorubicin-containing combination chemotherapy regimen, interferon α given to patients in complete remission seems to prolong survival. The monoclonal antibody rituximab can cause objective responses in 35 to 50% of patients with relapsed follicular lymphoma, and radiolabeled antibodies appear to have response rates well in excess of 50%. Trials with tumor vaccines have been encouraging. Both autologous and allogeneic hematopoietic stem cell transplantation yield high complete response rates in patients with relapsed follicular lymphoma, and long-term remissions can occur.

Patients with follicular lymphoma with a predominance of large cells have a shorter survival when treated with single-agent chemotherapy but seem to benefit from receiving an anthracycline-containing combination chemotherapy regimen. When their disease is treated aggressively, the overall survival for such patients is no lower than for patients with other follicular lymphomas, and the failure-free survival is superior.

Patients with follicular lymphoma have a high rate of histologic transformation to diffuse large B cell lymphoma (~7% per year). This is recognized ~40% of the time during the course of the illness by repeat biopsy and is present in almost all patients at autopsy. This transformation is usually heralded by rapid growth of lymph nodes—often localized—and the development of systemic symptoms such as fevers, sweats, and weight loss. Although these patients have a poor prognosis, aggressive combination chemotherapy regimens can sometimes cause a complete remission in the diffuse large B cell lymphoma, often leaving the patient with persisting follicular lymphoma.

Diffuse Large B Cell Lymphoma Diffuse large B cell lymphoma is the most common type of non-Hodgkin's lymphoma, representing approximately one-third of all cases. This lymphoma makes up the majority of cases in previous clinical trials of "aggressive" or "intermediate-grade" lymphoma. The clinical characteristics of diffuse large B cell lymphoma are presented in Table 97-10.

The diagnosis of diffuse large B cell lymphoma can be made accurately by an expert hematopathologist when review of an adequate biopsy and proof of B cell immunophenotype are available (Fig. 97-8). Cytogenetic and molecular genetic studies are not necessary for diagnosis, but some evidence has accumulated that patients who overexpress the BCL-2 protein might be more likely to relapse than others. Patients with prominent mediastinal involvement are sometimes diagnosed as a separate subgroup having primary mediastinal diffuse large B cell lymphoma. This latter group of patients has a younger median age (i.e., 37 years) and a female predominance (66%). Subtypes of diffuse large B cell lymphoma, including those with an immunoblastic subtype and tumors with extensive fibrosis, are recognized by pathologists but do not appear to have important, independent prognostic significance.

Diffuse large B cell lymphoma can present as either primary lymph node disease or at extranodal sites. More than 50% of patients will have some site of extranodal involvement at diagnosis, with the most common sites being the gastrointestinal tract and bone marrow, each being involved in 15 to 20% of patients. Essentially any organ can be involved, making a diagnostic biopsy imperative. For example, diffuse large B cell lymphoma of the pancreas has a much better prognosis than pancreatic carcinoma but would be missed without biopsy. Primary diffuse large B cell lymphoma of the brain is being diagnosed with increasing frequency. Other unusual subtypes of diffuse large B cell lymphoma such as pleural effusion lymphoma and intravascular lymphoma have been difficult to diagnose and associated with a very poor prognosis.

The initial evaluation of patients with diffuse large B cell lymphoma involves the studies presented in Table 97-11 for staging of patients with non-Hodgkin's lymphoma. After a careful staging evaluation, ~50% of patients will be found to have stage I or II disease and ~50% will have widely disseminated lymphoma. Bone marrow biopsy shows involvement by lymphoma in about 15% of cases, with marrow involvement by small cells more frequent than with large cells.

TREATMENT

The initial treatment of all patients with diffuse large B cell lymphoma should be with a combination chemotherapy regimen. The most popular regimen in the United States is CHOP, sometimes in combination with rituximab, although a variety of other anthracycline-containing combination chemotherapy regimens appear to be equally efficacious. Patients with stage I or nonbulky stage II can be effectively treated with three to four cycles of combination chemotherapy followed by involved field radiotherapy. The results are at least equal and probably superior to six to eight cycles of combination therapy, and cure rates of 60 to 70% in stage II disease and 80 to 90% in stage I disease can be expected.

For patients with bulky stage II, stage III, or stage IV, six to eight cycles of a combination chemotherapy regimen such as CHOP, often in combination with rituximab, are usually administered. A large randomized trial showed the superiority of CHOP combined with rituximab over CHOP alone in elderly patients. A frequent approach would be to administer four cycles of therapy and then reevaluate. If the patient has achieved a complete remission after four cycles, two more cycles of treatment might be given and then therapy discontinued. Using this approach, 70% of patients can be expected to achieve a complete remission, and 50 to 70% of complete responders will be cured. The chances for a favorable response to treatment are predicted by the IPI. In fact, the IPI was developed specifically to predict outcome in patients with diffuse large B cell lymphoma. For the 35% of patients with a low IPI score of 0 to 1, the 5-year survival is >70%, while for the 20% of patients with a high IPI score of 4 to 5, the 5-year survival is ~20%. A number of other factors, including molecular features of the tumor, levels of circulating cytokines and soluble receptors, and other surrogate markers, have been shown to influence prognosis. However, they have not been validated as rigorously as the IPI and have not been uniformly applied clinically.

Because a large number of patients with diffuse large B cell lymphoma are either initially refractory to therapy or relapse after apparently effective chemotherapy, nearly half of patients will be candidates for salvage treatment at some point. Alternative combination chemotherapy regimens can induce complete remission in as many as 50% of these patients, but long-term disease-free survival is seen in ≤10%. Autologous bone marrow transplantation has been shown to be superior to salvage chemotherapy at usual doses and leads to long-term disease-free survival in ~40% of patients whose lymphomas remain chemotherapy-sensitive after relapse.

Burkitt's Lymphoma/Leukemia   Burkitt's lymphoma/leukemia is a rare disease in adults in the United States, making up <1% of non-Hodgkin's lymphomas, but it makes up ~30% of childhood non-Hodgkin's lymphoma. Burkitt's leukemia, or L3 ALL, makes up a small proportion of childhood and adult acute leukemias. The clinical features of Burkitt's lymphoma occurring in adults are presented in Table 97-10.

Burkitt's lymphoma can be diagnosed morphologically by an expert hematopathologist with a high degree of accuracy. The cells are homogeneous in size and shape (Fig. 97-9). Demonstration of a very high proliferative fraction and the presence of the t(8;14) or one of its variants, t(2;8) (c-myc and the λ light chain gene) or t(8;22) (c-myc and the κ light chain gene), can be confirmatory. Burkitt's cell leukemia is recognized by the typical monotonous mass of medium-sized cells with round nuclei, multiple nucleoli, and basophilic cytoplasm with cytoplasmic vacuoles. Demonstration of a B cell immunophenotype and one of the above-noted cytogenetic abnormalities is confirmatory.

The three distinct clinical forms of Burkitt's lymphoma that are recognized are endemic, sporadic, and immunodeficiency-associated. Endemic and sporadic Burkitt's lymphomas occur frequently in children in Africa, and the sporadic form in western countries. Immunodeficiency-associated Burkitt's lymphoma is seen in patients with HIV infection.

Pathologists sometimes have difficulty distinguishing between Burkitt's lymphoma and diffuse large B cell lymphoma. In the past, a separate subgroup of non-Hodgkin's lymphoma intermediate between the two was recognized. When tested, this subgroup could not be diagnosed accurately. Distinction between the two major types of B cell aggressive non-Hodgkin's lymphoma can sometimes be made based on the extremely high proliferative fraction seen in patients with Burkitt's lymphoma (i.e., essentially 100% of tumor cells are in cycle) caused by c-myc deregulation.

Most patients in the United States with Burkitt's lymphoma present with peripheral lymphadenopathy or an intraabdominal mass. The disease is typically rapidly progressive and has a propensity to metastasize to the CNS. Initial evaluation should always include an examination of cerebral spinal fluid to rule out metastasis in addition to the other staging evaluations noted in Table 97-11. Once the diagnosis of Burkitt's lymphoma is suspected, a diagnosis must be made promptly and staging evaluation must be accomplished expeditiously. This is the most rapidly progressive human tumor, and any delay in initiating therapy can adversely affect the patient's prognosis.

℞ TREATMENT

Treatment of Burkitt's lymphoma in both children and adults should begin within 48 h of diagnosis and involves the use of intensive combination chemotherapy regimens incorporating high doses of cyclophosphamide. Prophylactic therapy to the CNS is mandatory. Burkitt's

FIGURE 97-9 Burkitt's lymphoma. The neoplastic cells are homogenous, medium-sized B cells with frequent mitotic figures, a morphologic correlate of high growth fraction. Reactive macrophages are scattered through the tumor and their pale cytoplasm in a background of blue-staining tumor cells give the tumor a so-called starry sky appearance.

lymphoma was one of the first cancers shown to be curable by chemotherapy. Today, cure can be expected in 70 to 80% of both children and young adults when effective therapy is administered precisely. Salvage therapy has been generally ineffective in patients failing the initial treatment, emphasizing the importance of the initial treatment approach.

Other B Cell Lymphoid Malignancies   B-cell prolymphocytic leukemia involves blood and marrow infiltration by large lymphocytes with prominent nucleoli. Patients typically have a high white cell count, splenomegaly, and minimal lymphadenopathy. The chances for a complete response to therapy are poor.

Hairy cell leukemia is a rare disease that presents predominantly in older males. Typical presentation involves pancytopenia, although occasional patients will have a leukemic presentation. Splenomegaly is usual. The malignant cells appear to have "hairy" projections on light and electron microscopy and show a characteristic staining pattern with tartrate-resistant acid phosphatase. Bone marrow is typically not able to be aspirated, and biopsy shows a pattern of fibrosis with diffuse infiltration by the malignant cells. Patients with this disorder are prone to unusual infections including infection by *Mycobacterium avium intracellulare*, and vasculitic syndromes have been described. Hairy cell leukemia is responsive to chemotherapy with interferon α, pentostatin, or cladribine, with the latter being the usually preferred treatment. Clinical complete remissions with cladribine occur in the majority of patients, and long-term disease-free survival is frequent.

Splenic marginal zone lymphoma involves infiltration of the splenic white pulp by small, monoclonal B cells. This is a rare disorder that can present as leukemia as well as lymphoma. Definitive diagnosis is often made at splenectomy, which is also an effective therapy. This is an extremely indolent disorder, but when chemotherapy is required, the most usual treatment has been chlorambucil.

Lymphoplasmacytic lymphoma is the tissue manifestation of Waldenström's macroglobulinemia (Chap. 98). This type of lymphoma has been associated with chronic hepatitis C virus infection, and an etiologic association has been proposed. Patients typically present with lymphadenopathy, splenomegaly, bone marrow involvement, and occasionally peripheral blood involvement. The tumor cells do not express CD5. Patients often have a monoclonal IgM protein, high levels of which can dominate the clinical picture with the symptoms of hyperviscosity. Treatment of lymphoplasmacytic lymphoma can be aimed primarily at reducing the abnormal protein, if present, but will usually also involve chemotherapy. Chlorambucil, fludarabine, and cladribine have been utilized. The median 5-year survival for patients with this disorder is ~60%.

Nodal marginal zone lymphoma, also known as *monocytoid B cell lymphoma*, represents ~1% of non-Hodgkin's lymphomas. This lymphoma has a slight female predominance and presents with disseminated disease (i.e., stage III or IV) in 75% of patients. Approximately one-third of patients have bone marrow involvement, and a leukemic presentation occasionally occurs. The staging evaluation and therapy should use the same approach as used for patients with follicular lymphoma. Approximately 60% of the patients with nodal marginal zone lymphoma will survive 5 years after diagnosis.

PRECURSOR CELL T CELL MALIGNANCIES ■ **Precursor T Cell Lymphoblastic Leukemia/Lymphoma**   Precursor T cell malignancies can present either as ALL or as an aggressive lymphoma. These malignancies are more common in children and young adults, with males more frequently affected than females.

Precursor T cell ALL can present with bone marrow failure, although the severity of anemia, neutropenia, and thrombocytopenia is often less than in precursor B cell ALL. These patients sometimes have very high white cell counts, a mediastinal mass, lymphadenopathy, and hepatosplenomegaly. Precursor T cell lymphoblastic lymphoma is most often found in young men presenting with a large mediastinal mass and pleural effusions. Both presentations have a propensity to metastasize to the CNS, and CNS involvement is often present at diagnosis.

Children with precursor T cell ALL seem to benefit from very intensive remission induction and consolidation regimens. The majority of patients treated in this manner can be cured. Older children and young adults with precursor T cell lymphoblastic lymphoma are also often treated with "leukemia-like" regimens. Patients who present with localized disease have an excellent prognosis. However, advanced age is an adverse prognostic factor. Adults with precursor T cell lymphoblastic lymphoma who present with high LDH levels or bone marrow or CNS involvement are often offered bone marrow transplantation as part of their primary therapy.

MATURE (PERIPHERAL) T CELL DISORDERS ■ Mycosis Fungoides Mycosis fungoides is also known as *cutaneous T cell lymphoma*. This lymphoma is more often seen by dermatologists than internists. The median age of onset is in the mid-fifties, and the disease is more common in males and in blacks.

Mycosis fungoides is an indolent lymphoma with patients often having several years of eczematous or dermatitic skin lesions before the diagnosis is finally established. The skin lesions progress from patch stage to plaque stage to cutaneous tumors. Early in the disease, biopsies are often difficult to interpret, and the diagnosis may only become apparent by observing the patient over time. In advanced stages, the lymphoma can metastasize to lymph nodes and visceral organs. A particular syndrome in patients with this lymphoma involves erythroderma and circulating tumor cells. This is known as *Sézary's syndrome*.

Rare patients with localized early stage mycosis fungoides can be cured with radiotherapy, often total-skin electron beam irradiation. More advanced disease has been treated with topical glucocorticoids, topical nitrogen mustard, phototherapy, psoralen with ultraviolet A (PUVA), electron beam radiation, interferon, antibodies, fusion toxins, and systemic cytotoxic therapy. Unfortunately, these treatments are palliative.

Adult T Cell Lymphoma/Leukemia Adult T cell lymphoma/leukemia is one manifestation of infection by the HTLV-I retrovirus. Patients can be infected through transplacental transmission, blood transfusion, and by sexual transmission of the virus. Patients who acquire the virus from their mother through breast milk are most likely to develop lymphoma, but the risk is still only 2.5% and the latency averages 55 years. Nationwide testing for HTLV-I antibodies and the aggressive implementation of public health measures could theoretically lead to the disappearance of adult T cell lymphoma/leukemia. Tropical spastic paraparesis, another manifestation of HTLV-I infection (Chap. 172), occurs after a shorter latency (1 to 3 years) and is most common in people who acquire the virus during adulthood from transfusion or sex.

The diagnosis of adult T cell lymphoma/leukemia is made when an expert hematopathologist recognizes the typical morphologic picture, a T cell immunophenotype (i.e., CD4 positive) of malignant cells has been demonstrated, and the existence of antibodies to HTLV-I is proven. Examination of the peripheral blood will usually reveal characteristic, pleomorphic abnormal CD4-positive cells with indented nuclei, which have been called "flower" cells (Fig. 97-10).

A subset of patients have a smoldering clinical course and long survival, but most patients present with an aggressive disease mani-

fested by lymphadenopathy, hepatosplenomegaly, skin infiltration, hypercalcemia, lytic bone lesions, and elevated LDH levels. The skin lesions can be papules, plaques, tumors, and ulcerations. Bone marrow involvement is not usually extensive, and anemia and thrombocytopenia are not usually prominent. Although treatment by combination chemotherapy regimens can result in objective responses, true complete remissions are unusual, and the median survival of patients is about 7 months.

Anaplastic Large T/Null Cell Lymphoma Anaplastic large T/null cell lymphoma was previously usually diagnosed as undifferentiated carcinoma or malignant histiocytosis. Discovery of the CD30, or Ki-1, antigen and the recognition that some patients with previously unclassified malignancies displayed this antigen led to the identification of a new type of lymphoma. Subsequently, discovery of the t(2;5) and the resultant frequent overexpression of the anaplastic lymphoma kinase (ALK) protein confirmed the existence of this entity. This lymphoma accounts for ~2% of all non-Hodgkin's lymphomas. The clinical characteristics of patients with anaplastic large T/null cell lymphoma are presented in Table 97-10.

The diagnosis of anaplastic large T/null cell lymphoma is made when an expert hematopathologist recognizes the typical morphologic picture and a T cell or null cell immunophenotype is demonstrated along with CD30 positivity. Documentation of the t(2;5) and/or overexpression of ALK protein confirm the diagnosis. Some diffuse large B cell lymphomas can also have an anaplastic appearance but have the same clinical course or response to therapy as other diffuse large B cell lymphomas.

Patients with anaplastic large T/cell null cell lymphoma are typically young (median age, 33 years) and male (~70%). Some 50% of patients present in stage I/II, and the remainder with more extensive disease. Systemic symptoms and elevated LDH levels are seen in about one-half of patients. Bone marrow and the gastrointestinal tract are rarely involved, but skin involvement is frequent. Some patients with disease confined to the skin have a different and more indolent disorder that has been termed *cutaneous anaplastic large T/null cell lymphoma* and might be related to lymphomatoid papulosis.

Treatment regimens appropriate for other aggressive lymphomas, such as diffuse large B cell lymphoma, should be utilized in patients with anaplastic large T/null cell lymphoma. Surprisingly, given the anaplastic appearance, this disorder has the best survival rate of any aggressive lymphoma. The 5-year survival is >75%. While traditional prognostic factors such as the IPI predict treatment outcome, overexpression of the ALK protein is an important prognostic factor, with patients overexpressing this protein having a superior treatment outcome.

Peripheral T Cell Lymphoma The peripheral T cell lymphomas make up a heterogenous morphologic group of aggressive neoplasms that share a mature T cell immunophenotype. They represent ~7% of all cases of non-Hodgkin's lymphoma. A number of distinct clinical syndromes are included in this group of disorders. The clinical characteristics of patients with peripheral T cell lymphoma are presented in Table 97-10.

The diagnosis of peripheral T cell lymphoma, or any of its specific subtypes, requires an expert hematopathologist, an adequate biopsy, and immunophenotyping. Most peripheral T cell lymphomas are CD4+, but a few will be CD8+, both CD4+ and CD8+, or have an NK cell immunophenotype. No characteristic genetic abnormalities have yet been identified, but translocations involving the T cell antigen receptor genes on chromosomes 7 or 14 may be detected. The differential diagnosis of patients suspected of having peripheral T cell lymphoma includes reactive T cell infiltrative processes. In some cases,

FIGURE 97-10 Adult T cell leukemia/lymphoma. Peripheral blood smear showing leukemia cells with typical "flower-shaped" nucleus.

demonstration of a monoclonal T cell population using T cell receptor gene rearrangement studies will be required to make a diagnosis.

The initial evaluation of a patient with a peripheral T cell lymphoma should include the studies in Table 97-11 for staging patients with non-Hodgkin's lymphoma. Unfortunately, patients with peripheral T cell lymphoma usually present with adverse prognostic factors, with >80% of patients having an IPI score ≥2 and >30% having an IPI score ≥4. As this would predict, peripheral T cell lymphomas are associated with a poor outcome, and only 25% of the patients survive 5 years after diagnosis. Treatment regimens are the same as those used for diffuse large B cell lymphoma, but patients with peripheral T cell lymphoma have a poorer response to treatment. Because of this poor treatment outcome, hematopoietic stem cell transplantation is often considered early in the care of young patients.

A number of specific clinical syndromes are seen in the peripheral T cell lymphomas. *Angioimmunoblastic T cell lymphoma* is one of the more common subtypes, making up ~20% of T cell lymphomas. These patients typically present with generalized lymphadenopathy, fever, weight loss, skin rash, and polyclonal hypergammaglobulinemia. In some cases, it is difficult to separate patients with a reactive disorder from those with true lymphoma.

Extranodal T/NK cell lymphoma of nasal type has also been called *angiocentric lymphoma* and was previously termed *lethal midline granuloma*. This disorder is more frequent in Asia and South America than in the United States and Europe. Although most frequent in the upper airway, it can involve other organs. The course is aggressive, and patients frequently have the hemophagocytic syndrome. When marrow and blood involvement occur, distinction between this disease and leukemia might be difficult. Some patients will respond to aggressive combination chemotherapy regimens, but the overall outlook is poor.

Enteropathy-type intestinal T cell lymphoma is a rare disorder that occurs in patients with untreated gluten-sensitive enteropathy. Patients are frequently wasted and sometimes present with intestinal perforation. The prognosis is poor. *Hepatosplenic γδ T cell lymphoma* is a systemic illness that presents with sinusoidal infiltration of the liver, spleen, and bone marrow by malignant T cells. Tumor masses generally do not occur. The disease is associated with systemic symptoms and is often difficult to diagnosis. Treatment outcome is poor. *Subcutaneous panniculitis-like T cell lymphoma* is a rare disorder that is often confused with panniculitis. Patients present with multiple subcutaneous nodules, which progress and can ulcerate. Hemophagocytic syndrome is common. Response to therapy is poor. The development of the hemophagocytic syndrome (profound anemia, ingestion of erythrocytes by monocytes and macrophages) in the course of any peripheral T cell lymphoma is generally associated with a fatal outcome.

HODGKIN'S DISEASE ■ Classic Hodgkin's Disease

Hodgkin's disease occurs in 7600 patients in the United States each year, and the disease does not appear to be increasing in frequency. Most patients present with palpable lymphadenopathy that is nontender; in most patients, these lymph nodes are in the neck, supraclavicular area, and axilla. More than half the patients will have mediastinal adenopathy at diagnosis, and this is sometimes the initial manifestation. Subdiaphragmatic presentation of Hodgkin's disease is unusual and more common in older males. Approximately one-third of patients present with fevers, night sweats, and/or weight loss—B symptoms in the Ann Arbor staging classification (Table 97-8). Occasionally, Hodgkin's disease can present as a fever of unknown origin. This is more common in older patients who are found to have mixed-cellularity Hodgkin's disease in an abdominal site. Rarely, the fevers persist for days to weeks, followed by afebrile intervals and then recurrence of the fever. This pattern is known as *Pel-Epstein fever*. Hodgkin's disease can occasionally present with unusual manifestations. These include severe and unexplained itching, cutaneous disorders such as erythema nodosum

and ichthyosiform atrophy, paraneoplastic cerebellar degeneration and other distant effects on the CNS, nephrotic syndrome, immune hemolytic anemia and thrombocytopenia, hypercalcemia, and pain in lymph nodes on alcohol ingestion.

The diagnosis of Hodgkin's disease is established by review of an adequate biopsy specimen by an expert hematopathologist. In the United States, most patients would be classified as having nodular sclerosing Hodgkin's disease, with a minority of patients having mixed-cellularity Hodgkin's disease. Lymphocyte-predominant and lymphocyte-depleted Hodgkin's disease are rare. Mixed-cellularity Hodgkin's disease or lymphocyte-depletion Hodgkin's disease are seen more frequently in patients infected by HIV (Fig. 97-11). The differential diagnosis of a lymph node biopsy suspicious for Hodgkin's disease includes inflammatory processes, mononucleosis, non-Hodgkin's lymphoma, phenytoin-induced lymphadenopathy, and nonlymphomatous malignancies.

The staging evaluation for a patient with Hodgkin's disease would typically include a careful history and physical examination; complete blood count; erythrocyte sedimentation rate; serum chemistry studies including LDH; chest radiograph; CT scan of the chest, abdomen, and pelvis; and bone marrow biopsy. Many patients would also have a PET scan or a gallium scan. Although rarely utilized, a bipedal lymphangiogram can be helpful. PET and gallium scans are most useful at the completion of therapy to document remission. Staging laparotomies were once popular for most patients with Hodgkin's disease but are now done rarely because of an increased reliance on systemic rather than local therapy.

℞ TREATMENT

Patients with localized Hodgkin's disease are cured >90% of the time. In patients with good prognostic factors, extended field radiotherapy has a high cure rate. Increasingly, patients with all stages of Hodgkin's disease are treated initially with chemotherapy. Patients with localized or good-prognosis disease receive a brief course of chemotherapy followed by radiotherapy to sites of node involvement. Patients with more extensive disease or those with B symptoms receive a complete course of chemotherapy. The most popular chemotherapy regimens used in the treatment of Hodgkin's disease include doxorubicin, bleomycin, vinblastine, and dacarbazine (ABVD) and mechlorethamine, vincristine, procarbazine, and prednisone (MOPP), or combinations of the drugs in these two regimens. Today, most patients in the United States receive ABVD, but a weekly chemotherapy regimen administered for 12 weeks called *Stanford V* is becoming increasingly popular, but includes radiation therapy, which has been associated with life-threatening late toxicities such as premature coronary artery disease and second solid tumors. In Europe a high-dose regimen called *BEACOPP* incorporating alkylating agents has become popular and might have a better response rate in very high risk patients. Long-term disease-free survival in patients with advanced disease can be achieved in >75% of patients who lack systemic symptoms and in 50 to 70% of patients with systemic symptoms.

Patients who relapse after primary therapy of Hodgkin's disease can frequently still be cured. Patients who relapse after initial treatment only with radiotherapy have an excellent outcome when treated with chemotherapy. Patients who relapse after an effective chemotherapy regimen are usually not curable with subsequent chemotherapy administered at standard doses. However, patients with a long initial

FIGURE 97-11 Mixed cellularity Hodgkin's disease. A Reed-Sternberg cell is present near the center of the field; a large cell with a bilobed nucleus and prominent nucleoli giving an "owl's eyes" appearance. The majority of the cells are normal lymphocytes, neutrophils, and eosinophils that form a pleiomorphic cellular infiltrate.

remission can be an exception to this rule. Autologous bone marrow transplantation can cure half of patients who fail effective chemotherapy regimens.

Because of the very high cure rate in patients with Hodgkin's disease, long-term complications have become a major focus for clinical research. In fact, in some series of patients with early-stage disease, more patients died from late complications of therapy than from Hodgkin's disease itself. This is particularly true in patients with localized disease. The most serious late side effects include second malignancies and cardiac injury. Patients are at risk for the development of acute leukemia in the first 10 years after treatment with combination chemotherapy regimens that contain alkylating agents plus radiation therapy. The risk for development of acute leukemia appears to be greater after MOPP-like regimens than with ABVD. The risk of development of acute leukemia after treatment for Hodgkin's disease is also related to the number of exposures to potentially leukemogenic agents (i.e., multiple treatments after relapse) and the age of the patient being treated, with those >60 years at particularly high risk. The development of carcinomas as a complication of treatment for Hodgkin's disease has become a major problem. These tumors usually occur ≥10 years after treatment and are associated with use of radiotherapy. For this reason, young women treated with thoracic radiotherapy for Hodgkin's disease should institute screening mammograms 5 to 10 years after treatment, and all patients who receive thoracic radiotherapy for Hodgkin's disease should be discouraged from smoking. Thoracic radiation also accelerates coronary artery disease, and patients should be encouraged to minimize risk factors for coronary artery disease such as smoking and elevated cholesterol levels.

A number of other late side effects from the treatment of Hodgkin's disease are well known. Patients who receive thoracic radiotherapy are at very high risk for the eventual development of hypothyroidism and should be observed for this complication; intermittent measurement of thyrotropin should be made to identify the condition before it becomes symptomatic. Lhermitte's syndrome occurs in ~15% of patients who receive thoracic radiotherapy. This syndrome is manifested by an "electric shock" sensation into the lower extremities on flexion of the neck. Infertility is a concern for all patients undergoing treatment for Hodgkin's disease. In both women and men, the risk of permanent infertility is age-related, with younger patients more likely to recover fertility. In addition, treatment with ABVD rather than MOPP increases the chances to retain fertility.

Nodular Lymphocyte-Predominant Hodgkin's Disease Nodular lymphocyte-predominant Hodgkin's disease is now recognized as an entity distinct from classic Hodgkin's disease. Previous classification systems recognized that biopsies from a subset of patients diagnosed as having Hodgkin's disease contained a predominance of small lymphocytes and rare Reed-Sternberg cells. A subset of these patients have tumors with nodular growth pattern and a clinical course that varied from that of patients with classic Hodgkin's disease. This is an unusual clinical entity and represents <5% of cases of Hodgkin's disease.

Nodular lymphocyte-predominant Hodgkin's disease has a number of characteristics that suggest its relationship to non-Hodgkin's lymphoma. These include a clonal proliferation of B cells and a distinctive immunophenotype; tumor cells express J chain and display CD45 and epithelial membrane antigen (ema) and do not express two markers normally found on Sternberg-Reed cells, CD30 and CD15. This lymphoma tends to have a chronic, relapsing course and sometimes transforms to diffuse large B cell lymphoma.

The treatment of patients with nodular lymphocyte-predominant Hodgkin's disease is controversial. Some clinicians favor no treatment and merely close follow-up. In the United States, most physicians will treat localized disease with radiotherapy and disseminated disease with regimens utilized for patients with classic Hodgkin's disease. Regardless of the therapy utilized, most series report a long-term survival of >80%.

LYMPHOMA-LIKE DISORDERS

The most common condition that pathologists and clinicians might confuse with lymphoma is reactive, atypical lymphoid hyperplasia. Patients might have localized or disseminated lymphadenopathy and might have the systemic symptoms characteristic of lymphoma. Underlying causes include a drug reaction to phenytoin or carbamezepine. Immune disorders such as rheumatoid arthritis and lupus erythematosus, viral infections such as cytomegalovirus and EBV, and bacterial infections such as cat-scratch disease may cause adenopathy (Chap. 54). In the absence of a definitive diagnosis after initial biopsy, continued follow-up, further testing, and repeated biopsies, if necessary, are the appropriate approach rather than instituting therapy.

Specific conditions that can be confused with lymphoma include *Castleman's disease*, which can present with localized or disseminated lymphadenopathy; some patients have systemic symptoms. The disseminated form is often accompanied by anemia and polyclonal hypergammaglobulinemia, and the condition has been associated with overproduction of interleukin 6, possibly produced by human herpesvirus 8. Patients with localized disease can be treated effectively with local therapy, while the initial treatment for patients with disseminated disease is usually with systemic glucocorticoids.

Sinus histiocytosis with massive lymphadenopathy (Rosai-Dorfman's disease) usually presents with bulky lymphadenopathy in children or young adults. The disease is usually nonprogressive and self-limited, but patients can manifest autoimmune hemolytic anemia.

Lymphomatoid papulosis is a cutaneous lymphoproliferative disorder that is often confused with anaplastic large-cell lymphoma involving the skin. The cells of lymphomatoid papulosis are similar to those seen in lymphoma and stain for CD30, and T cell receptor gene rearrangements are sometimes seen. However, the condition is characterized by waxing and waning skin lesions that usually heal, leaving small scars. In the absence of effective communication between the clinician and the pathologist regarding the clinical course in the patient, this disease will be misdiagnosed. Since the clinical picture is usually benign, misdiagnosis is a serious mistake.

FURTHER READING

ARMITAGE JO et al: *Text Atlas of Lymphomas.* London, Martin Dunitz, 2002

DIEHL V et al: Hodgkin's lymphoma—diagnosis and treatment. Lancet Oncol 5:19, 2004

HARRIS NL et al: World Health Organization classification of neoplastic diseases of the hematopoietic and lymphoid tissues: Report of the Clinical Advisory Committee Meeting, Airlie House, Virginia, November, 1997. J Clin Oncol 17:3835, 1999

HAUKE RJ, ARMITAGE JO: A new approach to non-Hodgkin's lymphoma. Intern Med 39:197, 2000

ROSENWALD A et al: The use of molecular profiling to predict survival after chemotherapy for diffuse large B cell lymphoma. N Engl J Med 346:1937, 2002

URBA WJ, LONGO DL: Hodgkin's disease. N Engl J Med 326:678, 1992

YUNG L, LINCH D: Hodgkin's lymphoma. Lancet 361:943, 2003

98 PLASMA CELL DISORDERS
Dan L. Longo, Kenneth C. Anderson

GENERAL PRINCIPLES The *plasma cell disorders* are monoclonal neoplasms related to each other by virtue of their development from common progenitors in the B lymphocyte lineage. Multiple myeloma, Waldenström's macroglobulinemia, primary amyloidosis (Chap. 310), and the heavy chain diseases comprise this group and may be designated by a variety of synonyms such as *monoclonal gammopathies*, *paraproteinemias*, *plasma cell dyscrasias*, and *dysproteinemias*. Mature B lymphocytes destined to produce IgG bear surface immunoglobulin molecules of both M and G heavy chain isotypes with both isotypes having identical idiotypes (variable regions). Under normal circumstances, maturation to antibody-secreting plasma cells is stimulated by exposure to the antigen for which the surface immunoglobulin is specific; however, in the plasma cell disorders the control over this process is lost. The clinical manifestations of all the plasma cell disorders relate to the expansion of the neoplastic cells, to the secretion of cell products (immunoglobulin molecules or subunits, lymphokines), and to some extent to the host's response to the tumor. →*Normal development of B lymphocytes is discussed in Chap. 295.*

There are three categories of structural variation among immunoglobulin molecules that form antigenic determinants, and these are used to classify immunoglobulins (Chap. 295). *Isotypes* are those determinants that distinguish among the main classes of antibodies of a given species and are the same in all normal individuals of that species. Therefore, isotypic determinants are, by definition, recognized by antibodies from a distinct species (heterologous sera) but not by antibodies from the same species (homologous sera). There are five heavy chain isotypes (M, G, A, D, E) and two light chain isotypes (κ, λ). *Allotypes* are distinct determinants that reflect regular small differences between individuals of the same species in the amino acid sequences of otherwise similar immunoglobulins. These differences are determined by allelic genes; by definition, they are detected by antibodies made in the same species. *Idiotypes* are the third category of antigenic determinants. They are unique to the molecules produced by a given clone of antibody-producing cells. Idiotypes are formed by the unique structure of the antigen-binding portion of the molecule.

Antibody molecules (Fig. 295-9) are composed of two heavy chains (mol wt ~50,000) and two light chains (mol wt ~25,000). Each chain has a constant portion (limited amino acid sequence variability) and a variable region (extensive sequence variability). The light and heavy chains are linked by disulfide bonds and are aligned so that their variable regions are adjacent to one another. This variable region forms the antigen recognition site of the antibody molecule; its unique structural features form a particular set of determinants, or idiotypes, that are reliable markers for a particular clone of cells because each antibody is formed and secreted by a single clone. Each chain is specified by distinct genes, synthesized separately, and assembled into an intact antibody molecule after translation (Fig. 98-1). Because of the mechanics of the gene rearrangements necessary to specify the immunoglobulin variable regions (VDJ joining for the heavy chain, VJ joining for the light chain), a particular clone rearranges only one of the two chromosomes to produce an immunoglobulin molecule of only one light chain isotype and only one allotype (allelic exclusion). After exposure to antigen, the variable region may become associated with a new heavy chain isotype (class switch). Each clone of cells performs these sequential gene arrangements in a unique way. This results in each clone producing a unique immunoglobulin molecule. In most cells, light chains are synthesized in slight excess, are secreted as free light chains by plasma cells, and are cleared by the kidney, but <10 mg of such light chains is excreted per day.

Electrophoretic analysis of components of the serum proteins permits determination of the amount of immunoglobulin in the serum (Fig. 98-2). The variety of immunoglobulins move heterogeneously in an electric field and form a broad peak in the gamma region. The γ globulin region of the electrophoretic pattern is usually increased in the sera of patients and animals with plasma cell tumors. There is a sharp spike in this region called an *M component* (M for monoclonal). Less commonly, the M component may appear in the β_2 or α_2 globulin region. The antibody must be present at a concentration of at least 5 g/L (0.5 g/dL) to be detectable by this method. This corresponds to approximately 10^9 cells producing the antibody. Confirmation that such an M component is truly monoclonal relies on the use of immunoelectrophoresis that shows a single light and heavy chain type. Hence immunoelectrophoresis and electrophoresis provide qualitative and quantitative assessment of the M component, respectively. Once the presence of an M component has been confirmed, electrophoresis provides the more practical information for managing patients with monoclonal gammopathies. In a given patient, the amount of M component in the serum is a reliable measure of the tumor burden. This makes the M component an excellent tumor marker, yet it is not specific enough to be used to screen asymptomatic patients. In addition

CELL TYPES	GENE ORDER	GENE PRODUCT
Nonlymphoid Cells Uncommitted B Cell Precursors	V_1 V_2 V_3 V_n D_1 D_2 D_3 D_n J_1 J_2 J_3 J_4 μ δ γ_1 α_1 γ_2 γ_4 ϵ α_2	None

Rearrangements juxtapose $V_3 D_2 J_1 \mu$ and $V_3 D_2 J_1 \delta$ genes

B Lymphocytes Prior to Antigen Exposure

$V_3 D_2 J_1$ μ δ γ_3 γ_1 α_1 γ_2 γ_4 ϵ α_2

$V_3 D_2 J_1$ δ γ_3 γ_1 α_1 γ_2 γ_4 ϵ α_2

$\left. \begin{array}{c} V_3 D_2 J_1 \mu \\ V_3 D_2 J_1 \delta \end{array} \right\}$ Surface Ig

Class switch rearrangement brings $V_3 D_2 J_1 \mu$ next to another heavy chain gene

B Lymphocytes After Antigen Exposure

$V_3 D_2 J_1$ α_1 γ_2 γ_4 ϵ α_2

$V_3 D_2 J_1 \alpha_1$ Secreted Ig

FIGURE 98-1 Immunoglobulin heavy chains are encoded by four distinct genetic elements: variable (Igh-V), diversity (Igh-D), joining (Igh-J), and constant (Igh-C) genes. The variable region of the immunoglobulin heavy chain is encoded by the V, D, and J genes. The same variable region may be associated with any of the 10 heavy chain constant region genes. In the germ-line genome (all cells except B cells) the V, D, and J genes are widely separated and exist in numerous forms. Once a cell becomes committed to B cell differentiation, a single V gene and a single D gene translocate to a single J gene, and the intervening genetic material is excised (VDJ joining). The newly formed VDJ gene is transcribed into a single message along with either an M or D isotype C gene. Upon exposure to antigen, another rearrangement may occur so that the VDJ gene may be associated with a G, A, or E isotype C gene. In light chain genes there appear to be no D genes, and thus light chain variable regions are formed by VJ joining.

FIGURE 98-2 Representative patterns of serum electrophoresis. The upper panel illustrates the normal pattern of serum protein on electrophoresis. Since there are many different immunoglobulins in the serum, their differing mobilities in an electric field produce a broad peak. In conditions associated with increases in polyclonal immunoglobulin, the broad peak is more prominent (middle panel). In monoclonal gammopathies, the predominance of a product of a single cell produces a "church spire" sharp peak, usually in the γ globulin region (bottom panel).

Normal

alb α₁ α₂ β   γ

Polyclonal gammopathy

alb α₁ α₂ β   γ

Monoclonal gammopathy

alb α₁ α₂ β   γ

to the plasma cell disorders, M components may be detected in other lymphoid neoplasms such as chronic lymphocytic leukemia and lymphomas of B or T cell origin; nonlymphoid neoplasms such as chronic myeloid leukemia, breast cancer, and colon cancer; a variety of nonneoplastic conditions such as cirrhosis, sarcoidosis, parasitic diseases, Gaucher disease, and pyoderma gangrenosum; and a number of autoimmune conditions, including rheumatoid arthritis, myasthenia gravis, and cold agglutinin disease. A very rare skin disease known as lichen myxedematosus or papular mucinosis is associated with a monoclonal gammopathy. Highly cationic IgG is deposited in the dermis of patients with this disease. This organ specificity may reflect the specificity of the antibody for some antigenic component of the dermis.

The nature of the M component is variable in plasma cell disorders. It may be an intact antibody molecule of any heavy chain subclass, or it may be an altered antibody or fragment. Isolated light or heavy chains may be produced. In some plasma cell tumors such as extramedullary or solitary bone plasmacytomas, <1/3 of patients will have an M component. In about 20% of myelomas, only light chains are produced and in most cases are secreted in the urine as Bence Jones proteins. The frequency of myelomas of a particular heavy chain class is roughly proportional to the serum concentration, and therefore IgG myelomas are more common than IgA and IgD myelomas.

MULTIPLE MYELOMA ■ Definition Multiple myeloma represents a malignant proliferation of plasma cells derived from a single clone. The terms *multiple myeloma* and *myeloma* may be used interchangeably. The tumor, its products, and the host response to it result in a number of organ dysfunctions and symptoms of bone pain or fracture, renal failure, susceptibility to infection, anemia, hypercalcemia, and occasionally clotting abnormalities, neurologic symptoms, and vascular manifestations of hyperviscosity.

Etiology The cause of myeloma is not known. Myeloma occurred with increased frequency in those exposed to the radiation of nuclear warheads in World War II after a 20-year latency. A variety of chromosomal alterations have been found in patients with myeloma; 13q14 deletions, 17p13 deletions, and 11q abnormalities predominate. The most common translocation is t(11;14)(q13;q32), and evidence is strong that errors in switch recombination—the genetic mechanism to change antibody heavy chain isotype—participate in the transformation pathway. Overexpression of *myc* or *ras* genes has been noted in some cases. Mutations in p53 and Rb-1 have also been described, but no common molecular pathogenesis has yet emerged.

Myeloma has been seen more commonly than expected among farmers, wood workers, leather workers, and those exposed to petroleum products. The neoplastic event in myeloma may involve cells

earlier in B cell differentiation than the plasma cell. Circulating B cells bearing surface immunoglobulin that share the idiotype of the M component are present in myeloma patients. Interleukin (IL) 6 may play a role in driving myeloma cell proliferation; a large fraction of myeloma cells exposed to IL-6 in vitro respond by proliferating. The IL-6 dependency of myeloma is controversial. It remains difficult to distinguish benign from malignant plasma cells on the basis of morphologic criteria in all but a few cases (Fig. 98-3).

Incidence and Prevalence About 15,270 cases of myeloma were diagnosed in 2004, and 11,070 people died from the disease. Myeloma increases in incidence with age. The median age at diagnosis is 68 years; it is rare under age 40. The yearly incidence is around 4 per 100,000 and remarkably similar throughout the world. Males are slightly more commonly affected than females, and blacks have nearly twice the incidence of whites. In the age group over 25 the incidence is 30 per 100,000. Myeloma accounts for about 1% of all malignancies in whites and 2% in blacks; 13% of all hematologic cancers in whites and 33% in blacks.

Pathogenesis and Clinical Manifestations (Table 98-1) Bone pain is the most common symptom in myeloma, affecting nearly 70% of patients. The pain usually involves the back and ribs, and unlike the pain of metastatic carcinoma, which often is worse at night, the pain of myeloma is precipitated by movement. Persistent localized pain in a patient with myeloma usually signifies a pathologic fracture. The bone lesions of myeloma are caused by the proliferation of tumor cells and the activation of osteoclasts that destroy the bone. The osteoclasts respond to osteoclast activating factors (OAF) made by the myeloma cells [OAF activity can be mediated by several cytokines, including IL-1, lymphotoxin, vascular endothelial growth factor (VEGF), receptor activator of NF-κB (RANK) ligand, macrophage inhibitory factor (MIP)-1α, and tumor necrosis factor (TNF)]. However, production of these factors decreases following administration of glucocorticoids or interferon (IFN)-α. The bone lesions are lytic in nature and are rarely associated with osteoblastic new bone formation. Therefore, radioisotopic bone scanning is less useful in diagnosis than is plain radiography. The bony lysis results in substantial mobilization of calcium from bone, and serious acute and chronic complications of hypercalcemia may dominate the clinical picture (see below). Localized bone lesions may expand to the point that mass lesions may be palpated, especially on the skull (Fig. 98-4), clavicles, and sternum, and the collapse of vertebrae may lead to spinal cord compression.

The next most common clinical problem in patients with myeloma is susceptibility to bacterial infections. The most common infections are pneumonias and pyelonephritis, and the most frequent pathogens are *Streptococcus pneumoniae*, *Staphylococcus aureus*, and *Klebsiella pneumoniae* in the lungs and *Escherichia coli* and other gram-negative organisms in the urinary tract. In about 25% of patients, recurrent infections are the presenting features, and over 75% of patients will have a serious infection at some time in their course. The susceptibility to infection has several contributing causes. First, patients with myeloma have diffuse hypogammaglobulinemia if the M component is excluded. The hypogammaglobulinemia is related to both decreased production and increased destruction of normal antibodies. Moreover, some patients generate a population of circulating regulatory cells in response to their myeloma that can suppress normal antibody synthe-

FIGURE 98-3 Multiple myeloma (marrow). The cells bear characteristic morphologic features of plasma cells, round or oval cells with an eccentric nucleus composed of coarsely clumped chromatin, a densely basophilic cytoplasm, and a perinuclear clear zone (hof) containing the Golgi apparatus. Binucleate and multinucleate malignant plasma cells can be seen.

TABLE 98-1 *Pathogenesis and Clinical Manifestations of Multiple Myeloma*

Clinical Finding	Underlying Cause	Pathogenic Mechanism
Hypercalcemia, pathologic fractures, cord compression, lytic bone lesions, osteoporosis, bone pain	Skeletal destruction	Tumor expansion; production of osteoclast activating factors (OAF) by tumor cells
Renal failure	Light chain proteinuria, hypercalcemia, urate nephropathy, amyloid glomerulopathy (rare) Pyelonephritis	Toxic effects of tumor products, light chains, OAF, DNA breakdown products Hypogammaglobulinemia
Anemia	Myelophthisis, decreased production, increased destruction	Tumor expansion; production of inhibitory factors and autoantibodies by tumor cells
Infection	Hypogammaglobulinemia, decreased neutrophil migration	Decreased production due to tumor-induced suppression; increased IgG catabolism
Neurologic symptoms	Hyperviscosity, cryoglobulins, amyloid deposits Hypercalcemia, cord compression	Products of tumor; properties of M component; light chains OAF
Bleeding	Interference with clotting factors, amyloid damage of endothelium, platelet dysfunction	Products of tumor; antibodies to clotting factors; light chains; antibody coating of platelets
Mass lesions		Tumor expansion

sis. In the case of IgG myeloma, normal IgG antibodies are broken down more rapidly than normal because the catabolic rate for IgG antibodies varies directly with the serum concentration. The large M component results in fractional catabolic rates of 8 to 16% instead of the normal 2%. These patients have very poor antibody responses, especially to polysaccharide antigens such as those on bacterial cell walls. Most measures of T cell function in myeloma are normal, but

FIGURE 98-4 Bony lesions in multiple myeloma. The skull demonstrates the typical "punched out" lesions characteristic of multiple myeloma. The lesion represents a purely osteolytic lesion with little or no osteoblastic activity. (Courtesy of Dr. Geraldine Schechter.)

a subset of CD4+ cells may be decreased. Granulocyte lysozyme content is low, and granulocyte migration is not as rapid as normal in patients with myeloma, probably the result of a tumor product. There are also a variety of abnormalities in complement functions in myeloma patients. All these factors contribute to the immune deficiency of these patients.

Renal failure occurs in nearly 25% of myeloma patients, and some renal pathology is noted in over half. Many factors contribute to this. Hypercalcemia is the most common cause of renal failure. Glomerular deposits of amyloid, hyperuricemia, recurrent infections, and occasional infiltration of the kidney by myeloma cells all may contribute to renal dysfunction. However, tubular damage associated with the excretion of light chains is almost always present. Normally, light chains are filtered, reabsorbed in the tubules, and catabolized. With the increase in the amount of light chains presented to the tubule, the tubular cells become overloaded with these proteins, and tubular damage results either directly from light chain toxic effects or indirectly from the release of intracellular lysosomal enzymes. The earliest manifestation of this tubular damage is the adult Fanconi syndrome (a type 2 proximal renal tubular acidosis), with loss of glucose and amino acids, as well as defects in the ability of the kidney to acidify and concentrate the urine. The proteinuria is not accompanied by hypertension, and the protein is nearly all light chains. Generally, very little albumin is in the urine because glomerular function is usually normal. When the glomeruli are involved, the proteinuria is nonselective. Patients with myeloma also have a decreased anion gap [i.e., $Na^+ - (Cl^- + HCO_3^-)$) because the M component is cationic, resulting in retention of chloride. This is often accompanied by hyponatremia that is felt to be artificial (pseudohyponatremia) because each volume of serum has less water as a result of the increased protein. Myeloma patients are susceptible to developing acute renal failure if they become dehydrated.

Anemia occurs in about 80% of myeloma patients. It is usually normocytic and normochromic and related both to the replacement of normal marrow by expanding tumor cells and to the inhibition of hematopoiesis by factors made by the tumor. In addition, mild hemolysis may contribute to the anemia. A larger than expected fraction of patients may have megaloblastic anemia due to either folate or vitamin B_{12} deficiency. Granulocytopenia and thrombocytopenia are very rare. Clotting abnormalities may be seen due to the failure of antibody-coated platelets to function properly or to the interaction of the M component with clotting factors I, II, V, VII, or VIII. Raynaud's phenomenon and impaired circulation may result if the M component forms cryoglobulins, and hyperviscosity syndromes may develop depending on the physical properties of the M component (most common with IgM, IgG3, and IgA paraproteins). Hyperviscosity is defined on the basis of the relative viscosity of serum as compared with water. Normal relative serum viscosity is 1.8 (i.e., serum is normally almost twice as viscous as water). Symptoms of hyperviscosity occur at a level of 5 to 6, a level usually reached at paraprotein concentrations of around 40 g/L (4 g/dL) for IgM, 50 g/L (5 g/dL) for IgG3, and 70 g/L (7 g/dL) for IgA.

Although neurologic symptoms occur in a minority of patients, they may have many causes. Hypercalcemia may produce lethargy, weakness, depression, and confusion. Hyperviscosity may lead to headache, fatigue, visual disturbances, and retinopathy. Bony damage and collapse may lead to cord compression, radicular pain, and loss of bowel and bladder control. Infiltration of peripheral nerves by amyloid can be a cause of carpal tunnel syndrome and other sensorimotor mono- and polyneuropathies.

Many of the clinical features of myeloma, e.g., cord compression, pathologic fractures, hyperviscosity, sepsis, and hypercalcemia, can present as medical emergencies. Despite the widespread distribution of plasma cells in the body, tumor expansion is dominantly within bone and bone marrow and, for reasons unknown, rarely causes enlargement of spleen, lymph nodes, or gut-associated lymphatic tissue.

Diagnosis and Staging The classic triad of myeloma is marrow plasmacytosis (>10%), lytic bone lesions, and a serum and/or urine M component. The diagnosis may be made in the absence of bone lesions if the plasmacytosis is associated with a progressive increase in the M component over time or if extramedullary mass lesions develop. There are two important variants of myeloma, solitary bone plasmacytoma and extramedullary plasmacytoma. These lesions are associated with an M component in fewer than 30% of the cases, they may affect younger individuals, and both are associated with median survivals of 10 or more years. Solitary bone plasmacytoma is a single lytic bone lesion without marrow plasmacytosis. Extramedullary plasmacytomas usually involve the submucosal lymphoid tissue of the nasopharynx or paranasal sinuses without marrow plasmacytosis. Both tumors are highly responsive to local radiation therapy. If an M component is present, it should disappear after treatment. Solitary bone plasmacytomas may recur in other bony sites or evolve into myeloma. Extramedullary plasmacytomas rarely recur or progress.

The most difficult differential diagnosis in patients with myeloma involves their separation from individuals with benign monoclonal gammopathies or monoclonal gammopathies of uncertain significance (MGUS). MGUS are vastly more common than myeloma, occurring in 1% of the population over age 50 and in up to 10% over age 75. Patients with MGUS usually have <10% bone marrow plasma cells; <30 g/L (3 g/dL) of M components; no urinary Bence Jones protein; and no anemia, renal failure, lytic bone lesions, or hypercalcemia. When bone marrow cells are exposed to radioactive thymidine in order to quantitate dividing cells, patients with MGUS always have a labeling index <1%; patients with myeloma always have a labeling index >1%. With long-term follow-up, about 1% per year of patients with MGUS go on to develop myeloma. Typically, patients with MGUS require no therapy. Their survival is about 2 years shorter than age-matched controls without MGUS.

The clinical evaluation of patients with myeloma includes a careful physical examination searching for tender bones and masses. Only a small minority of patients has an enlargement of the spleen and lymph nodes, the physiologic sites of antibody production. Chest and bone radiographs may reveal lytic lesions or diffuse osteopenia. MRI offers a sensitive means to document cord or root compression in patients with pain syndromes. A complete blood count with differential may reveal anemia. Erythrocyte sedimentation rate is elevated. Rare patients (~2%) may have plasma cell leukemia with more than 2000 plasma cells/μL. This may be seen in disproportionate frequency in IgD (12%) and IgE (25%) myelomas. Serum calcium, urea nitrogen, creatinine, and uric acid levels may be elevated. Protein electrophoresis and measurement of serum immunoglobulins are useful for detecting and characterizing M spikes, supplemented by immunoelectrophoresis, which is especially sensitive for identifying low concentrations of M components not detectable by protein electrophoresis. A 24-h urine specimen is necessary to quantitate protein excretion, and a concentrated aliquot is used for electrophoresis and immunologic typing of any M component. Serum alkaline phosphatase is usually normal even with extensive bone involvement because of the absence of osteoblastic activity. It is also important to quantitate serum β_2-microglobulin (see below). Serum soluble IL-6 receptor levels and C-reactive protein may reflect physiologic IL-6 levels in the patient.

The serum M component will be IgG in 53% of patients, IgA in 25%, and IgD in 1%; 20% of patients will have only light chains in serum and urine. Dipsticks for detecting proteinuria are not reliable at identifying light chains, and the heat test for detecting Bence Jones protein is falsely negative in about 50% of patients with light chain myeloma. Fewer than 1% of patients have no identifiable M component; these patients usually have light chain myelomas in which renal catabolism has made the light chains undetectable in the urine. IgD myeloma may also present as light chain myeloma. About two-thirds of patients with serum M components also have urinary light chains. The light chain isotype may have an impact on survival. Patients secreting lambda light chains have a significantly shorter overall survival than those secreting kappa light chains. It is not clear whether this is due to some genetically important determinant of cell proliferation or

because lambda light chains are more likely to cause renal damage and form amyloid than are kappa light chains. The heavy chain isotype may have an impact on patient management as well. About half of patients with IgM paraproteins develop hyperviscosity compared with only 2 to 4% of patients with IgA and IgG M components. Among IgG myelomas, it is the IgG3 subclass that has the highest tendency to form both concentration- and temperature-dependent aggregates, leading to hyperviscosity and cold agglutination at lower serum concentrations.

The staging system for patients with myeloma is a functional system for predicting survival and is based on a variety of clinical and laboratory tests, unlike the anatomic staging systems for solid tumors. Details of the staging system are given in Table 98-2. Based on the hemoglobin, calcium, M component, and degree of skeletal involvement, the total-body tumor burden is estimated to be low (stage I, $<0.6 \times 10^{12}$ cells/m^2), intermediate (stage II, 0.6 to 1.2×10^{12} cells/m^2), or high (stage III, $>1.2 \times 10^{12}$ cells/m^2), and the stages are further subdivided on the basis of renal function [A if serum creatinine <177 mol/L (<2 mg/dL), B if >177 (>2). Patients in stage IA have a median survival of more than 5 years and those in stage IIIB about 15 months. β_2-Microglobulin is a protein of 11,000 mol wt with homologies with the constant region of immunoglobulins that is the light chain of the class I major histocompatibility antigens (HLA-A, -B, -C) on the surface of every cell. Serum β_2-microglobulin is the single most powerful predictor of survival and can substitute for staging. Patients with β_2-microglobulin levels <0.004 g/L have a median survival of 43 months and those with levels >0.004 g/L only 12 months. It is also felt that once the diagnosis of myeloma is firm, histologic features of atypia may also exert an influence on prognosis. IL-6 may be an autocrine and/or paracrine growth factor for myeloma cells; el-

TABLE 98-2 *Myeloma Staging System*

Stage	Criteria	Estimated Tumor Burden, $\times 10^{12}$ cells/m^2

I	All of the following:
	1. Hemoglobin >100 g/L (>10 g/dL)
	2. Serum calcium <3 mmol/L (<12 mg/dL)
	3. Normal bone x-ray or solitary lesion
	4. Low M-component production
	  a. IgG level <50 g/L (<5 g/dL)
	  b. IgA level <30 g/L (<3 g/dL)
	  c. Urine light chain <4 g/24 h
		<0.6 (low)

II	Fitting neither I nor III	0.6–1.20 (intermediate)

III	One or more of the following:
	1. Hemoglobin <85 g/L (<8.5 g/dL)
	2. Serum calcium >3 mmol/L (>12 mg/dL)
	3. Advanced lytic bone lesions
	4. High M-component production
	  a. IgG level >70 g/L (>7 g/dL)
	  b. IgA level >50 g/L (>5 g/dL)
	  c. Urine light chains >12 g/24 h
		>1.20 (high)

Level	Stage	Median Survival, Months
SUBCLASSIFICATION BASED ON SERUM CREATININE LEVELS		
A < 177 μmol/L (<2 mg/dL)	IA	61
B > 177 μmol/L (>2 mg/dL)	IIA,B	55
	IIIA	30
	IIIB	15
STAGING BASED ON SERUM β_2-MICROGLOBULIN LEVELS		
<0.004 g/L (<4 μg/mL)	I	43
>0.004 g/L (>4 μg/mL)	II	12

evated levels are associated with more aggressive disease. High labeling index and high levels of lactate dehydrogenase and thymidine kinase are also associated with poor prognosis.

Other factors that may influence prognosis are the number of cytogenetic abnormalities, chromosome 13q deletion, % plasma cells in the marrow, circulating plasma cells, performance status, and serum levels of IL-6, soluble IL-6 receptors, C-reactive protein, hepatocyte growth factor, C-terminal cross-linked telopeptide of collagen I, TGF-β, and syndecan-1.

℞ TREATMENT

About 10% of patients with myeloma will have an indolent course demonstrating only very slow progression of disease over many years. Such patients only require antitumor therapy when the serum myeloma protein level rises above 50 g/L (5 g/dL) or progressive bone lesions develop. Patients with solitary bone plasmacytomas and extramedullary plasmacytomas may be expected to enjoy prolonged disease-free survival after local radiation therapy to a dose of around 40 Gy. There is a low incidence of occult marrow involvement in patients with solitary bone plasmacytoma. Such patients are usually detected because their serum M component falls slowly or disappears initially only to return after a few months. These patients respond well to systemic chemotherapy.

The vast majority of patients with myeloma require therapeutic intervention. In general such therapy is of two sorts: systemic chemotherapy to control the progression of myeloma, and symptomatic supportive care to prevent serious morbidity from the complications of the disease. All patients with stage II or III disease and stage I patients exhibiting Bence Jones proteinuria, progressive lytic bone lesions, vertebral compression fractures, recurrent infections, or rising serum M component should be treated with systemic combination chemotherapy. Therapy can prolong and improve the quality of life for myeloma patients.

The standard treatment has consisted of intermittent pulses of an alkylating agent [L-phenylalanine mustard (L-PAM, melphalan), cyclophosphamide, or chlorambucil] and prednisone administered for 4 to 7 days every 4 to 6 weeks. The alkylating agents appear to be roughly equally active, but resistance to one agent is often accompanied by resistance to the others. The usual doses are as follows: melphalan, 8 mg/m^2 per day; cyclophosphamide, 200 mg/m^2 per day; chlorambucil, 8 mg/m^2 per day; prednisone, 25 to 60 mg/m^2 per day. Melphalan is used most commonly, but because of their near equivalence in antitumor efficacy, we favor cyclophosphamide as the alkylating agent because it is less toxic to the marrow stem cell compartment and results in a lower incidence of myelodysplastic syndromes than do the other alkylating agents. Doses may need adjustment based on marrow tolerance. However, there are few constraints on the dose of the steroid pulse, and it appears that more is better. Patients responding to therapy generally have a prompt and gratifying reduction in bone pain, hypercalcemia, and anemia, and often have fewer infections. The serum M component lags substantially behind the symptomatic improvement, often taking 4 to 6 weeks to fall. This fall depends on the rate of tumor kill and the fractional catabolic rate of immunoglobulin, which in turn depends on the serum concentration (for IgG). Light chain excretion, with a functional half-life of approximately 6 h, may fall within the first week of treatment. However, since urine light chain levels may relate to renal tubular function, they are not a reliable measure of tumor cell kill. Calculations of tumor cell kill are made by extrapolation of the serum M component level and rely heavily on the assumption that every tumor cell produces immunoglobulin at a constant rate. About 60% of patients will achieve at least a 75% reduction in serum M component level and tumor cell mass in response to an alkylating agent and prednisone. Although this is a tumor reduction of less than 1 log, clinical responses may last many months. The important feature of the level of the M protein is not how far or how fast it falls, but the rate of its increase after therapy. Efforts to improve the fraction of patients responding and the degree of response have involved adding other active chemotherapeutic agents to the treatment program. Patients with more advanced disease may benefit most from such an approach. High-dose therapy with hematopoietic stem cell support can modestly extend progression-free and overall survival but few, if any, patients are cured. Sequential treatment with combination chemotherapy regimens followed by two successive high-dose melphalan treatments, each supported with peripheral blood stem cell transplants, have achieved complete responses in 50% of patients treated within a year of diagnosis. Complete responses are rare (<10%) with standard therapy. Long-term follow-up is not yet available. Allogeneic transplants may also produce high response rates, but treatment-related mortality may be as high as 40%. Nonmyeloablative allogeneic transplantation is now under evaluation to reduce toxicity while permitting an immune graft-vs-tumor effect.

The ideal duration of therapy has not been determined. Most physicians treat every 4 to 6 weeks for 1 or 2 years. Cessation of therapy is followed by relapse, usually within a year. Retreatment may be associated with a second response in up to 80% of patients. Maintenance therapy (e.g., with IFN-α) may prolong the duration of response, but this therapy is toxic and has generally not prolonged survival. Oral prednisone maintenance therapy appears to improve response duration and survival. The regrowth rate of the tumor during relapse accelerates with each relapse. This observation suggests that kinetic resistance to therapy (i.e., increase in cycling cells) is perhaps more important than drug resistance controlled by mdr-1 expression. Patients often respond to treatment, but the length of the response progressively shortens. Patients primarily resistant to initial therapy have a median survival of less than a year. High-dose pulsed glucocorticoids used alone (200 mg prednisone every other day or 1 g/m^2 per day methylprednisolone for 5 days) or VAD combination chemotherapy (vincristine, 0.4 mg/d in a 4-day continuous infusion; doxorubicin, 9 mg/m^2 per day in a 4-day continuous infusion; dexamethasone, 40 mg/d for 4 days per week for 3 weeks) may offer useful palliation in patients resistant to primary therapy. High-dose melphalan has activity in patients with refractory disease. Thalidomide, which inhibits angiogenesis, also produces responses in refractory cases, but at doses that may cause somnolence. Novel agents, including immunomodulatory derivatives of thalidomide (IMIDs) and the proteasome inhibitor, PS-341, target not only the tumor cell but also the tumor cell-bone marrow interaction and production of myeloma growth, survival, drug resistance, and migration factors. These agents can achieve responses in relapsed refractory disease and are under evaluation for efficacy earlier in the disease course.

About 15% of patients die within the first 3 months after diagnosis; subsequently, the death rate is about 15% per year. The disease usually follows a chronic course for 2 to 5 years before developing an acute terminal phase, usually marked by the development of pancytopenia with a cellular marrow that is refractory to treatment. Widespread organ infiltration by myeloma cells occurs, and survival is less than 6 months. About 46% of patients die in the chronic phase of disease from progressive myeloma (16%) and renal failure (10%), sepsis (14%), or both (6%). Death in the acute terminal phase (26%) is chiefly from progressive myeloma (13%) and sepsis (9%). Five percent of patients die of acute leukemia, myeloblastic or monocytic. Although it has been debated that this is related to the primary disease, it appears more likely to be the result of chronic therapy with alkylating agents. Nearly 23% of patients die of myocardial infarction, chronic lung disease, diabetes, or stroke, all intercurrent illnesses related more to the age of the patient group than to the tumor.

Supportive care directed at the anticipated complications of the disease may be as important as primary antitumor therapy. The hypercalcemia generally responds well to bisphosphonates, glucocorticoid therapy, hydration, and natriuresis. Calcitonin may add to the inhibitory effects of steroids on bone resorption. Bisphosphonates (e.g., pamidronate 90 mg or zoledronate 4 mg once a month) reduce osteoclastic bone resorption and preserve performance status and quality of life; antitumor effects are also possible. Treatments aimed at strengthening the skeleton, such as fluorides, calcium, and vitamin D, with or without androgens, have been suggested but are not of proven efficacy. Iatrogenic worsening of renal function may be prevented by the use of allopurinol during chemotherapy to avoid urate nephropathy and by maintaining a high fluid intake to prevent dehydration and to help excrete light chains and calcium. In the event of acute renal failure, plasmapheresis is approximately 10 times more effective at clearing light chains than peritoneal dialysis, and acutely reducing the protein load may result in functional improvement. Urinary tract infections should be watched for and treated early. Chronic dialysis probably should not be initiated in patients who have failed to respond to antitumor therapy. Plasmapheresis may be the treatment of choice for hyperviscosity syndromes. Although the pneumococcus is a dreaded pathogen in myeloma patients, pneumococcal polysaccharide vaccines may not elicit an antibody response. Prophylactic administration of intravenous γ globulin preparations is used in the setting of recurrent serious infections. Chronic oral antibiotic prophylaxis is probably not warranted. Patients developing neurologic symptoms in the lower extremities, severe localized back pain, or problems with bowel and bladder control may need emergency myelography and radiation therapy for palliation. Most bone lesions respond to analgesics and chemotherapy, but certain painful lesions may respond most promptly to localized radiation. The chronic anemia may respond to hematinics (iron, folate, cobalamin), and some have responded to androgens. The pathogenesis of the anemia should be established and specific therapy instituted, where possible. In the setting of renal disease and low serum erythropoietin levels, erythropoietin is useful to increase red cell mass.

WALDENSTRÖM'S MACROGLOBULINEMIA In 1948, Waldenström described a malignancy of lymphoplasmacytoid cells that secreted IgM. In contrast to myeloma, the disease was associated with lymphadenopathy and hepatosplenomegaly, but the major clinical manifestation was the hyperviscosity syndrome. The disease resembles the related diseases chronic lymphocytic leukemia, myeloma, and lymphocytic lymphoma. Waldenström's macroglobulinemia and IgM myeloma both follow a similar clinical course. The diagnosis of IgM myeloma is usually reserved for patients with lytic bone lesions and is important only because of the hazard of pathologic fractures.

The cause of macroglobulinemia is unknown. The disease is similar to myeloma in being slightly more common in men and occurring with increased incidence with age (median 64 years). There have been reports that the IgM in some patients with macroglobulinemia may have specificity for myelin-associated glycoprotein (MAG), a protein that has been associated with demyelinating disease of the peripheral nervous system and may be lost earlier and to a greater extent than the better known myelin basic protein in patients with multiple sclerosis. Sometimes patients with macroglobulinemia develop a peripheral neuropathy before the appearance of the neoplasm. There is speculation that the whole process begins with a viral infection that may elicit an antibody response that cross-reacts with a normal tissue component.

Like myeloma, the disease involves the bone marrow, but unlike myeloma, it does not cause bone lesions or hypercalcemia. Like myeloma, a serum M component is present in the serum in excess of 30 g/L (3 g/dL), but unlike myeloma, the size of the IgM paraprotein results in little renal excretion and only around 20% of patients excrete light chains. Therefore, renal disease is not common. The light chain isotype is kappa in 80% of the cases. Patients present with weakness, fatigue, and recurrent infections, similar to myeloma patients, but epistaxis, visual disturbances, and neurologic symptoms such as peripheral neuropathy, dizziness, headache, and transient paresis are much more common in macroglobulinemia. Physical examination reveals adenopathy and hepatosplenomegaly, and ophthalmoscopic examination may reveal vascular segmentation and dilatation of the retinal veins characteristic of hyperviscosity states. Patients may have a normocytic, normochromic anemia, but rouleaux formation and a positive Coombs' test are much more common than in myeloma. Malignant

lymphocytes are usually present in the peripheral blood. About 10% of macroglobulins are cryoglobulins. These are pure M components and are not the mixed cryoglobulins seen in rheumatoid arthritis and other autoimmune diseases. Mixed cryoglobulins are composed of IgM or IgA complexed with IgG, for which they are specific. In both cases, Raynaud's phenomenon and serious vascular symptoms precipitated by the cold may occur, but mixed cryoglobulins are not commonly associated with malignancy. Patients suspected of having a cryoglobulin based on history and physical examination should have their blood drawn into a warm syringe and delivered to the laboratory in a container of warm water to avoid errors in quantitating the cryoglobulin.

℞ TREATMENT

Control of serious hyperviscosity symptoms such as an altered state of consciousness or paresis can be achieved acutely by plasmapheresis because 80% of the IgM paraprotein is intravascular. Fludarabine (25 mg/m^2 per day for 5 days every 4 weeks) or cladribine (0.1 mg/kg per day for 7 days every 4 weeks) are highly effective single agents. About 80% of patients respond to chemotherapy, and their median survival is over 3 years. Rituximab (anti-CD20) can produce responses alone or combined with chemotherapy. The absence of other serious organ toxicities results in a longer life span of patients with macroglobulinemia compared with those with myeloma.

POEMS SYNDROME The features of this syndrome are *p*olyneuropathy, *o*rganomegaly, *e*ndocrinopathy, *m*ultiple myeloma, and *s*kin changes (POEMS). Patients usually have a severe, progressive sensorimotor polyneuropathy associated with sclerotic bone lesions from myeloma. Polyneuropathy occurs in about 1.4% of myelomas, but the POEMS syndrome is only a rare subset of that group. Unlike typical myeloma, hepatomegaly and lymphadenopathy occur in about two-thirds of patients, and splenomegaly is seen in one-third. The lymphadenopathy frequently resembles Castleman's disease histologically, a condition that has been linked to IL-6 overproduction. The endocrine manifestations include amenorrhea in women and impotence and gynecomastia in men. Hyperprolactinemia due to loss of normal inhibitory control by the hypothalamus may be associated with other central nervous system manifestations such as papilledema and elevated cerebrospinal fluid pressure and protein. Type 2 diabetes mellitus occurs in about one-third of patients. Hypothyroidism and adrenal insufficiency are occasionally noted. Skin changes are diverse: hyperpigmentation, hypertrichosis, skin thickening, and digital clubbing. Other manifestations include peripheral edema, ascites, pleural effusions, fever, and thrombocytosis.

The pathogenesis of the disease is unclear, but high circulating levels of the proinflammatory cytokines IL-1, IL-6, VEGF, and TNF have been documented and levels of the inhibitory cytokine transforming growth factor (TGF-β) are lower than expected. Treatment of the myeloma may result in an improvement in the other disease manifestations.

HEAVY CHAIN DISEASES The heavy chain diseases are rare lymphoplasmacytic malignancies. Their clinical manifestations vary with the heavy chain isotype. Patients secrete a defective heavy chain that usually has an intact Fc fragment and a deletion in the Fd region. Gamma, alpha, and mu heavy chain diseases have been described, but no reports of delta or epsilon heavy chain diseases have appeared. Molecular biologic analysis of these tumors has revealed structural genetic defects that may account for the aberrant chain secreted.

Gamma Heavy Chain Disease (Franklin's Disease) This disease affects people of widely different age groups and countries of origin. It is characterized by lymphadenopathy, fever, anemia, malaise, hepatosplenomegaly, and weakness. Its most distinctive symptom is palatal edema, resulting from node involvement of Waldeyer's ring, and this may progress to produce respiratory compromise. The diagnosis depends on the demonstration of an anomalous serum M component [often <20 g/L (<2 g/dL)] that reacts with anti-IgG but not anti-light chain reagents. *The M component is typically present in both serum and urine.* Most of the paraproteins have been of the gamma₁ subclass, but other subclasses have been seen. The patients may have thrombocytopenia, eosinophilia, and nondiagnostic bone marrow. Patients usually have a rapid downhill course and die of infection; however, some patients have survived 5 years with chemotherapy.

Alpha Heavy Chain Disease (Seligmann's Disease)

This is the most common of the heavy chain diseases. It is closely related to a malignancy known as *Mediterranean lymphoma*, a disease that affects young people in parts of the world where intestinal parasites are common, such as the Mediterranean, Asia, and South America. The disease is characterized by an infiltration of the lamina propria of the small intestine with lymphoplasmacytoid cells that secrete truncated alpha chains. Demonstrating alpha heavy chains is difficult because the alpha chains tend to polymerize and appear as a smear instead of a sharp peak on electrophoretic profiles. Despite the polymerization, hyperviscosity is not a common problem in alpha heavy chain disease. Without J chain–facilitated dimerization, viscosity does not increase dramatically. Light chains are absent from serum and urine. The patients present with chronic diarrhea, weight loss, and malabsorption and have extensive mesenteric and para-aortic adenopathy. Respiratory tract involvement occurs rarely. Patients may vary widely in their clinical course. Some may develop diffuse aggressive histologies of malignant lymphoma. Chemotherapy may produce long-term remissions. Rare patients appear to have responded to antibiotic therapy, raising the question of the etiologic role of antigenic stimulation, perhaps by some chronic intestinal infection. Chemotherapy plus antibiotics may be more effective than chemotherapy alone.

Mu Heavy Chain Disease

The secretion of isolated mu heavy chains into the serum appears to occur in a very rare subset of patients with chronic lymphocytic leukemia. The only features that may distinguish patients with mu heavy chain disease are the presence of vacuoles in the malignant lymphocytes and the excretion of kappa light chains in the urine. The diagnosis requires ultracentrifugation or gel filtration to confirm the nonreactivity of the paraprotein with the light chain reagents, because some intact macroglobulins fail to interact with these serums. The tumor cells seem to have a defect in the assembly of light and heavy chains, because they appear to contain both in their cytoplasm. There is no evidence that such patients should be treated differently from other patients with chronic lymphocytic leukemia (Chap. 97).

FURTHER READING

BARLOGIE B et al: Treatment of myeloma. Blood 103:20, 2004

BERENSON JR et al: Maintenance therapy with alternate-day prednisone improves survival in multiple myeloma patients. Blood 99:3163, 2002

BERENSON JR et al: American Society of Clinical Oncology clinical practice guidelines: The role of bisphosphonates in multiple myeloma. J Clin Oncol 20:3719, 2002

GHODRIAL IM et al: Waldenstrom macroglobulinaemia. Lancet Oncol 4:679, 2003

HIDESHIMA T, ANDERSON KC: Novel therapeutic approaches for multiple myeloma. Nature Rev Cancer 2:927, 2002

KUEHL WM, BERGSAGEL PL: Multiple myeloma: Evolving genetic events and host interactions. Nature Rev Cancer 2:175, 2002

KYLE RA et al: A long-term study of prognosis in monoclonal gammopathy of undetermined significance. N Engl J Med 346:564, 2002

KYLE RA et al: Review of 1027 patients with newly diagnosed multiple myeloma. Mayo Clin Proc 78:21, 2003

WAHNER-ROEDLER DL et al: Gamma-heavy chain disease: review of 23 cases. Medicine 82:236, 2003

---

99 TRANSFUSION BIOLOGY AND THERAPY
Jeffery S. Dzieczkowski, Kenneth C. Anderson

BLOOD GROUP ANTIGENS AND ANTIBODIES

The study of red blood cell (RBC) antigens and antibodies forms the foundation of transfusion medicine. Serologic studies initially characterized these antigens, but now the molecular composition and structure of many are known. Antigens, either carbohydrate or protein, are assigned to a blood group system based upon the structure and similarity of the determinant epitopes. Other cellular blood elements and plasma proteins are also antigenic and can result in *alloimmunization*, the production of antibodies directed against the blood group antigens of another individual. These antibodies are called *alloantibodies*.

Antibodies directed against RBC antigens may result from "natural" exposure, particularly to carbohydrates that mimic some blood group antigens. Those antibodies that occur via natural stimuli are usually produced by a T cell–independent response (thus, generating no memory) and are IgM isotype. *Autoantibodies* (antibodies against autologous blood group antigens) arise spontaneously or as the result of infectious sequelae (e.g., from *Mycoplasma pneumoniae*) and are also often IgM. These antibodies are often clinically insignificant due to their low affinity for antigen at body temperature. However, IgM antibodies can activate the complement cascade and result in hemolysis. Antibodies that result from allogeneic exposure, such as transfusion or pregnancy, are usually IgG. IgG antibodies commonly bind to antigen at warmer temperatures and may hemolyze RBCs. Unlike IgM antibodies, IgG antibodies can cross the placenta and bind fetal erythrocytes bearing the corresponding antigen, resulting in hemolytic disease of the newborn, or *hydrops fetalis*.

Alloimmunization to leukocytes, platelets, and plasma proteins may also result in transfusion complications such as fevers and urticaria but generally does not cause hemolysis. Assay for these other alloantibodies is not routinely performed; however, they may be detected using special assays.

ABO ANTIGENS AND ANTIBODIES

The first blood group antigen system, recognized in 1900, was ABO, the most important in transfusion medicine. The major blood groups of this system are A, B, AB, and O. O type RBCs lack A or B antigens. These antigens are carbohydrates attached to a precursor backbone, may be found on the cellular membrane either as glycosphingolipids or glycoproteins, and are secreted into plasma and body fluids as glycoproteins. H substance is the immediate precursor upon which the A and B antigens are added. This H substance is formed by the addition of fucose to the glycolipid or glycoprotein backbone. The subsequent addition of *N*-acetylgalactosamine creates the A antigen, while the addition of galactose produces the B antigen.

The genes that determine the A and B phenotypes are found on chromosome 9p and are expressed in a Mendelian codominant manner. The gene products are glycosyl transferases, which confer the enzymatic capability of attaching the specific antigenic carbohydrate. Individuals who lack the "A" and "B" transferases are phenotypically type "O," while those who inherit both transferases are type "AB." Rare individuals lack the H gene, which codes for fucose transferase, and cannot form H substance. These individuals are homozygous for the silent h allele (hh) and have Bombay phenotype (O_h).

The ABO blood group system is important because essentially all individuals produce antibodies to the ABH carbohydrate antigen that they lack. The naturally occurring anti-A and anti-B antibodies are termed *isoagglutinins*. Thus, type A individuals produce anti-B, while type B individuals make anti-A. Neither isoagglutinin is found in type AB individuals, while type O individuals produce both anti-A and anti-B. Thus, persons with type AB are "universal recipients" because they do not have antibodies against any ABO phenotype, while persons with type O blood can donate to essentially all recipients because their cells are not recognized by any ABO isoagglutinins. The rare individuals with Bombay phenotype produce antibodies to H substance (which is present on all red cells except those of hh phenotype) as well as to both A and B antigens and are therefore compatible only with other hh donors.

In most people, A and B antigens are secreted by the cells and are present in the circulation. Nonsecretors are susceptible to a variety of infections (e.g., *Candida albicans*, *Neisseria meningitidis*, *Streptococcus pneumoniae*, *Haemophilus influenzae*) as many organisms may bind to polysaccharides on cells. Soluble blood group antigens may block this binding.

Rh SYSTEM The Rh system is the second most important blood group system in pretransfusion testing. The Rh antigens are found on a 30- to 32-kDa RBC membrane protein that has no defined function. Although >40 different antigens in the Rh system have been described, five determinants account for the vast majority of phenotypes. The presence of the D antigen confers Rh "positivity," while persons who lack the D antigen are Rh negative. Two allelic antigen pairs, E/e and C/c, are also found on the Rh protein. The three Rh genes, E/e, D, and C/c, are arranged in tandem on chromosome 1 and inherited as a haplotype, i.e., cDE or Cde. Two haplotypes can result in the phenotypic expression of two to five Rh antigens.

The D antigen is a potent alloantigen. About 15% of individuals lack this antigen. Exposure of these Rh-negative people to even small amounts of Rh-positive cells, by either transfusion or pregnancy, can result in the production of anti-D alloantibody.

OTHER BLOOD GROUP SYSTEMS AND ALLOANTIBODIES More than 100 blood group systems are recognized, composed of more than 500 antigens. The presence or absence of certain antigens has been associated with various diseases and anomalies; antigens also act as receptors for infectious agents. Alloantibodies of importance in routine clinical practice are listed in Table 99-1.

Antibodies to *Lewis system* carbohydrate antigens are the most common cause of incompatibility during pretransfusion screening. The Lewis gene product is a fucosyl transferase and maps to chromosome 19. The antigen is not an integral membrane structure but is adsorbed to the RBC membrane from the plasma. Antibodies to Lewis antigens are usually IgM and cannot cross the placenta. Lewis antigens may be adsorbed onto tumor cells and may be targets of therapy.

I system antigens are also oligosaccharides related to H, A, B, and Le. I and i are not allelic pairs but are carbohydrate antigens that differ only in the extent of branching. The i antigen is an unbranched chain that is converted by the I gene product, a glycosyltransferase, into a branched chain. The branching process affects all the ABH antigens, which become progressively more branched in the first 2 years of life. Some patients with cold agglutinin disease or lymphomas can produce anti-I autoantibodies that cause RBC destruction. Occasional patients with mononucleosis or *Mycoplasma* pneumonia may develop cold agglutinins of either anti-I or anti-i specificity. Most adults lack i expression; thus, finding a donor for patients with anti-i is not difficult.

Even though most adults express I antigen, binding is generally low at body temperature. Thus, administration of warm blood prevents isoagglutination.

The *P system* is another group of carbohydrate antigens controlled by specific glycosyltransferases. Its clinical significance is in rare cases of syphilis and viral infection that lead to paroxysmal cold hemoglobinuria. In these cases, an unusual autoantibody to P is produced that binds to RBCs in the cold and fixes complement upon warming. Antibodies with these biphasic properties are called *Donath-Landsteiner antibodies*. The P antigen is the cellular receptor of parvovirus B19 and also may be a receptor for *Escherichia coli* binding to urothelial cells.

The *MNSsU system* is regulated by genes on chromosome 4. M and N are determinants on glycophorin A, an RBC membrane protein, and S and s are determinants on glycophorin B. Anti-S and anti-s IgG antibodies may develop after pregnancy or transfusion and lead to hemolysis. Anti-U antibodies are rare but problematic; virtually every donor is incompatible because nearly all persons express U.

The *Kell* protein is very large (720 amino acids) and its secondary structure contains many different antigenic epitopes. The immunogenicity of Kell is third behind the ABO and Rh systems. The absence of the Kell precursor protein (controlled by a gene on X) is associated with acanthocytosis, shortened RBC survival, and a progressive form of muscular dystrophy that includes cardiac defects. This rare condition is called the *McLeod phenotype*. The K_x gene is linked to the 91-kDa component of the NADPH-oxidase on the X chromosome, deletion or mutation of which accounts for about 60% of cases of chronic granulomatous disease.

The *Duffy* antigens are codominant alleles, Fy^a and Fy^b, that also serve as receptors for *Plasmodium vivax*. More than 70% of persons in malaria endemic areas lack these antigens, probably from selective influences of the infection on the population.

The *Kidd* antigens, Jk^a and Jk^b, may elicit antibodies transiently. A delayed hemolytic transfusion reaction that occurs with blood tested as compatible is often related to delayed appearance of anti-Jk^a.

PRETRANSFUSION TESTING

Pretransfusion testing of a potential recipient consists of the "type and screen." The "forward type" determines the ABO and Rh phenotype of the recipient's RBC by using antisera directed against the A, B, and D antigens. The "reverse type" detects isoagglutinins in the patient's serum and should correlate with the ABO phenotype, or forward type.

The alloantibody screen identifies antibodies directed against other RBC antigens. The alloantibody screen is performed by mixing patient serum with type O RBCs that contain the major antigens of most blood group systems and whose extended phenotype is known. The specificity of the alloantibody is identified by correlating the presence or absence of antigen with the results of the agglutination.

Cross-matching is ordered when there is a high probability that the patient will require a packed RBC (PRBC) transfusion. Blood selected for cross-matching must be ABO compatible and lack antigens for which the patient has alloantibodies. Nonreactive cross-matching confirms the absence of any major incompatibility and reserves that unit for the patient.

In the case of Rh-negative patients, every attempt must be made to provide Rh-negative blood components to prevent alloimmunization to the D antigen. In an emergency, Rh-positive blood can be safely transfused to a Rh-negative patient who lacks anti-D; however, the recipient is likely to become alloimmunized and produce anti-D. Rh-negative women of childbearing age who are transfused with products containing Rh-positive RBCs should receive passive immunization with anti-D (RhoGam or WinRho) to reduce or prevent sensitization.

BLOOD COMPONENTS

Blood products intended for transfusion are routinely collected as whole blood (450 mL) in various anticoagulants. Most donated blood is processed into components: PRBCs, platelets, and fresh-frozen

TABLE 99-1 RBC Blood Group Systems and Alloantigens

Blood Group System	Antigen	Alloantibody	Clinical Significance
Rh (D, C/c, E/e)	RBC protein	IgG	HTR, HDN
Lewis (Le^a, Le^b)	Oligosaccharide	IgM/IgG	Rare HTR
Kell (K/k)	RBC protein	IgG	HTR, HDN
Duffy (Fy^a/Fy^b)	RBC protein	IgG	HTR, HDN
Kidd (Jk^a/Jk^b)	RBC protein	IgG	HTR (often delayed), HDN (mild)
I/i	Carbohydrate	IgM	None
MNSsU	RBC protein	IgM/IgG	Anti-M rare HDN, anti-S, -s, and -U HDN, HTR

Note: RBC, red blood cell; HDN, hemolytic disease of the newborn; HTR, hemolytic transfusion reaction.

TABLE 99-2 Characteristics of Selected Blood Components

Component	Volume, mL	Content	Clinical Response
PRBC	180–200	RBCs with variable leukocyte content and small amount of plasma	Increase hemoglobin 10 g/L and hematocrit 3%
Platelets	50–70	5.5×10^{10}/RD unit	Increase platelet count 5000–10,000/μL
	200–400	$\geq 3.0 \times 10^{11}$/SDAP product	CCI $\geq 10 \times 10^9$/L within 1 h and $\geq 7.5 \times 10^9$/L within 24 h posttransfusion
FFP	200–250	Plasma proteins—coagulation factors, proteins C and S, antithrombin	Increases coagulation factors about 2%
Cryoprecipitate	10–15	Cold-insoluble plasma proteins, fibrinogen, factor VIII, vWF	Topical fibrin glue, also 80 IU factor VIII

Note: PRBC, packed red blood cells; RBC, red blood cell; RD, random donor; SDAP, single-donor apheresis platelets; CCI, corrected count increment; FFP, fresh frozen plasma; vWF, von Willebrand factor.

plasma (FFP) or cryoprecipitate (Table 99-2). Whole blood is first separated into PRBCs and platelet-rich plasma by slow centrifugation. The platelet-rich plasma is then centrifuged at high speed to yield one unit of random donor (RD) platelets and one unit of FFP. Cryoprecipitate is produced by thawing FFP to precipitate the plasma proteins, then separated by centrifugation.

Apheresis technology is used for the collection of multiple units of platelets from a single donor. These single-donor apheresis platelets (SDAP) contain the equivalent of at least six units of RD platelets and have fewer contaminating leukocytes than pooled RD platelets.

Plasma may also be collected by apheresis. Plasma derivatives such as albumin, intravenous immunoglobulin, antithrombin, and coagulation factor concentrates are prepared from pooled plasma from many donors and are treated to eliminate infectious agents.

WHOLE BLOOD Whole blood provides both oxygen-carrying capacity and volume expansion. It is the ideal component for patients who have sustained acute hemorrhage of $\geq$25% total blood volume loss. Whole blood is stored at 4°C to maintain erythrocyte viability, but platelet dysfunction and degradation of some coagulation factors occurs. In addition, 2,3-bisphosphoglycerate levels fall over time, leading to an increase in the oxygen affinity of the hemoglobin and a decreased capacity to deliver oxygen to the tissues, a problem with all red cell storage. Whole blood is not readily available since it is routinely processed into components.

PACKED RED BLOOD CELLS This product increases oxygen-carrying capacity in the anemic patient. Adequate oxygenation can be maintained with a hemoglobin content of 70 g/L in the normovolemic patient without cardiac disease; however, comorbid factors often necessitate transfusion at a higher threshold. The decision to transfuse should be guided by the clinical situation and not by an arbitrary laboratory value. In the critical care setting, liberal use of transfusions to maintain near normal levels of hemoglobin may have unexpected negative effects on survival. In most patients requiring transfusion, levels of hemoglobin of 100 g/L are sufficient to keep oxygen supply from being critically low.

PRBCs may be modified to prevent certain adverse reactions. Leukocyte reduction of cellular blood products is increasingly common, and universal prestorage leukocyte reduction has been recommended. Prestorage filtration appears superior to bedside filtration as smaller amounts of cytokines are generated in the stored product. These PRBC units contain $<5 \times 10^6$ donor white blood cells (WBCs), and their use lowers the incidence of posttransfusion fever, cytomegalovirus (CMV) infections, and alloimmunization. Other theoretical benefits include less immunosuppression in the recipient and lower risk of infections. Plasma, which may cause allergic reactions, can be removed from cellular blood components by washing.

PLATELETS Thrombocytopenia is a risk factor for hemorrhage, and platelet transfusion reduces the incidence of bleeding. The threshold

for prophylactic platelet transfusion is 10,000/μL. In patients without fever or infections, a threshold of 5000/μL may be sufficient to prevent spontaneous hemorrhage. For invasive procedures, 50,000/μL platelets is the usual target level.

Platelets are given either as pools prepared from five to eight RDs or as SDAPs from a single donor. In an unsensitized patient without increased platelet consumption [splenomegaly, fever, disseminated intravascular coagulation (DIC)], six to eight units of RD platelets (about 1 unit per 10 kg body weight) are transfused, and each unit is anticipated to increase the platelet count 5000 to 10,000/μL. Patients who have received multiple transfusions may be alloimmunized to many HLA- and platelet-specific antigens and have little or no increase in their posttransfusion platelet counts. Patients who may require multiple transfusions are best served by receiving SDAP and leukocyte-reduced components to lower the risk of alloimmunization.

Refractoriness to platelet transfusion may be evaluated using the corrected count increment (CCI):

$$CCI = \frac{\text{posttransfusion count} - \text{pretransfusion count}}{\text{number of platelets transfused} \times 10^{11}} \times BSA$$

where BSA is body surface area measured in square meters. The platelet count performed 1 h after the transfusion is acceptable if the CCI is 10×10^9/mL, and after 18 to 24 h an increment of 7.5×10^9/mL is expected. Patients who have suboptimal responses are likely to have received multiple transfusions and have antibodies directed against class I HLA antigens. Refractoriness can be investigated by detecting anti-HLA antibodies in the recipient's serum. Patients who are sensitized will often react with 100% of the lymphocytes used for the HLA-antibody screen, and HLA-matched SDAPs should be considered for those patients who require transfusion. Although ABO-identical HLA-matched SDAPs provide the best chance for increasing the platelet count, locating these products is difficult. Platelet cross-matching is available in some centers. Additional clinical causes for a low platelet CCI include fever, bleeding, splenomegaly, DIC, or medications in the recipient.

FRESH-FROZEN PLASMA FFP contains stable coagulation factors and plasma proteins: fibrinogen, antithrombin, albumin, as well as proteins C and S. Indications for FFP include correction of coagulopathies, including the rapid reversal of warfarin; supplying deficient plasma proteins; and treatment of thrombotic thrombocytopenic purpura. FFP should not be routinely used to expand blood volume. FFP is an acellular component and does not transmit intracellular infections, e.g., CMV. Patients who are IgA-deficient and require plasma support should receive FFP from IgA-deficient donors to prevent anaphylaxis (see below).

CRYOPRECIPITATE Cryoprecipitate is a source of fibrinogen, factor VIII, and von Willebrand factor (vWF). It is ideal for supplying fibrinogen to the volume-sensitive patient. When factor VIII concentrates are not available, cyroprecipitate may be used since each unit contains approximately 80 units of factor VIII. Cryoprecipitate may also supply vWF to patients with dysfunctional (type II) or absent (type III) von Willebrand disease.

PLASMA DERIVATIVES Plasma from thousands of donors may be pooled to derive specific protein concentrates, including albumin, intravenous immunoglobulin, antithrombin, and coagulation factors. In addition, donors who have high-titer antibodies to specific agents or antigens provide hyperimmune globulins, such as anti-D (RhoGam, WinRho), and antisera to hepatitis B virus (HBV), varicella-zoster virus, CMV, and other infectious agents.

ADVERSE REACTIONS TO BLOOD TRANSFUSION

Adverse reactions to transfused blood components occur despite multiple tests, inspections, and checks. Fortunately, the most common reactions are not life-threatening, although serious reactions can present with mild symptoms and signs. Some reactions can be reduced or prevented by modified (filtered, washed, or irradiated) blood components. When an adverse reaction is suspected, the transfusion should be stopped and reported to the blood bank for investigation.

Transfusion reactions may result from immune and nonimmune mechanisms. Immune-mediated reactions are often due to preformed donor or recipient antibody; however, cellular elements may also cause adverse effects. Nonimmune causes of reactions are due to the chemical and physical properties of the stored blood component and its additives.

Transfusion-transmitted viral infections are increasingly rare due to improved screening and testing. As the risk of viral infection is reduced, the relative risk of other reactions increases, such as hemolytic transfusion reactions and sepsis from bacterially contaminated components. More effort is being directed at improving pretransfusion quality assurance to further increase the safety of transfusion therapy. Infections, like any adverse transfusion reaction, must be brought to the attention of the blood bank for appropriate studies (Table 99-3).

IMMUNE-MEDIATED REACTIONS ■ Acute Hemolytic Transfusion Reactions

Immune-mediated hemolysis occurs when the recipient has preformed antibodies that lyse donor erythrocytes. The ABO isoagglutinins are responsible for the majority of these reactions, although alloantibodies directed against other RBC antigens, i.e., Rh, Kell, and Duffy, may result in hemolysis.

Acute hemolytic reactions may present with hypotension, tachypnea, tachycardia, fever, chills, hemoglobinemia, hemoglobinuria, chest and/or flank pain, and discomfort at the infusion site. Monitoring the patient's vital signs before and during the transfusion is important to identify reactions promptly. When acute hemolysis is suspected, the transfusion must be stopped immediately, intravenous access maintained, and the reaction reported to the blood bank. A correctly labeled posttransfusion blood sample and any untransfused blood should be sent to the blood bank for analysis. The laboratory evaluation for hemolysis includes the measurement of serum haptoglobin, lactate dehydrogenase (LDH), and indirect bilirubin levels.

TABLE 99-3 *Risks of Transfusion Complications*

	Frequency, Episodes:Unit
Reactions	
Febrile (FNHTR)	1–4:100
Allergic	1–4:100
Delayed hemolytic	1:1,000
TRALI	1:5,000
Acute hemolytic	1:12,000
Fatal hemolytic	1:100,000
Anaphylactic	1:150,000
Infections[a]	
Hepatitis B	1:63,000
Hepatitis C	1:1,600,000
HIV-1	1:1,960,000
HIV-2	None reported
HTLV-I and -II	1:641,000
Malaria	1:4,000,000
Other complications	
RBC allosensitization	1:100
HLA allosensitization	1:10
Graft-versus-host disease	Rare

[a] Infectious agents rarely associated with transfusion, theoretically possible or of unknown risk include: Hepatitis A virus, parvovirus B-19, *Babesia microti* (babesiosis), *Borrelia burgdorferi* (Lyme disease), *Trypanosoma cruzi* (Chagas disease), and *Treponema pallidum*, human herpesvirus-8 and hepatitis G virus.
Note: FNHTR, febrile nonhemolytic transfusion reaction; TRALI, transfusion-related acute lung injury; HTLV, human T lymphotropic virus; RBC, red blood cell

The immune complexes that result in RBC lysis can cause renal dysfunction and failure. Diuresis should be induced with intravenous fluids and furosemide or mannitol. Tissue factor released from the lysed erythrocytes may initiate DIC. Coagulation studies including prothrombin time (PT), activated partial thromboplastin time (aPTT), fibrinogen, and platelet count should be monitored in patients with hemolytic reactions.

Errors at the patient's bedside, such as mislabeling the sample or transfusing the wrong patient, are responsible for the majority of these reactions. The blood bank investigation of these reactions includes examination of the pre- and posttransfusion samples for hemolysis and repeat typing of the patient samples; direct antiglobulin test (DAT), sometimes called the direct Coombs test, of the posttransfusion sample; repeating the cross-matching of the blood component; and checking all clerical records for errors. DAT detects the presence of antibody or complement bound to RBCs in vivo.

Delayed Hemolytic and Serologic Transfusion Reactions Delayed hemolytic transfusion reactions (DHTRs) are not completely preventable. These reactions occur in patients previously sensitized to RBC alloantigens who have a negative alloantibody screen due to low antibody levels. When the patient is transfused with antigen-positive blood, an anamnestic response results in the early production of alloantibody that binds donor RBCs. The alloantibody is detectable 1 to 2 weeks following the transfusion, and the posttransfusion DAT may become positive due to circulating donor RBCs coated with antibody or complement. The transfused, alloantibody-coated erythrocytes are cleared by the reticuloendothelial system. These reactions are detected most commonly in the blood bank when a subsequent patient sample reveals a positive alloantibody screen or a new alloantibody in a recently transfused recipient.

No specific therapy is usually required, although additional RBC transfusions may be necessary. Delayed serologic transfusion reactions are similar to DHTR, as the DAT is positive and alloantibody is detected; however, RBC clearance is not increased.

Febrile Nonhemolytic Transfusion Reaction The most frequent reaction associated with the transfusion of cellular blood components is a febrile nonhemolytic transfusion reaction (FNHTR). These reactions are characterized by chills and rigors and a $\geq 1°C$ rise in temperature. FNHTR is diagnosed when other causes of fever in the transfused patient are ruled out. Antibodies directed against donor leukocyte and HLA antigens may mediate these reactions; thus, multiply transfused patients and multiparous women are felt to be at increased risk. Although antibodies may be demonstrated in the recipient's serum, investigation is not routinely done because of the mild nature of most FNHTR. The use of leukocyte-reduced blood products may prevent or delay sensitization to leukocyte antigens and thereby reduce the incidence of these febrile episodes. Cytokines released from cells within stored blood components may mediate FNHTR; thus, leukoreduction before storage may prevent these reactions. The incidence and severity of these reactions can be decreased in patients with recurrent reactions by premedicating with acetaminophen or other antipyretic agents.

Allergic Reactions Urticarial reactions are related to plasma proteins found in transfused components. Mild reactions may be treated symptomatically by temporarily stopping the transfusion and administering antihistamines (diphenhydramine, 50 mg orally or intramuscularly). The transfusion may be completed after the signs and/or symptoms resolve. Patients with a history of allergic transfusion reaction should be premedicated with an antihistamine. Cellular components can be washed to remove residual plasma for the extremely sensitized patient.

Anaphylactic Reaction This severe reaction presents after transfusion of only a few milliliters of the blood component. Symptoms and signs include difficulty breathing, coughing, nausea and vomiting, hypotension, bronchospasm, loss of consciousness, respiratory arrest, and shock. Treatment includes stopping the transfusion, maintaining vascular access, and administering epinephrine (0.5 to 1.0 mL of 1:1000 dilution subcutaneously). Glucocorticoids may be required in severe cases.

Patients who are IgA-deficient may be sensitized to this Ig class and are at risk for anaphylactic reactions associated with plasma transfusion. Individuals with severe IgA deficiency should therefore receive only IgA-deficient plasma and washed cellular blood components. Patients who have anaphylactic or repeated allergic reactions to blood components should be tested for IgA deficiency.

Graft-versus-Host Disease   Graft-versus-host disease (GVHD) is a frequent complication of allogeneic stem cell transplantation, in which lymphocytes from the donor attack and cannot be eliminated by an immunodeficient host. Transfusion-related GVHD is mediated by donor T lymphocytes that recognize host HLA antigens as foreign and mount an immune response, which is manifested clinically by the development of fever, a characteristic cutaneous eruption, diarrhea, and liver function abnormalities. GVHD can also occur when blood components that contain viable T lymphocytes are transfused to immunodeficient recipients or to immunocompetent recipients who share HLA antigens with the donor (e.g., a family donor). In addition to the aforementioned clinical features of GVHD, transfusion-associated GVHD (TA-GVHD) is characterized by marrow aplasia and pancytopenia. TA-GVHD is highly resistant to treatment with immunosuppressive therapies, including glucocorticoids, cyclosporine, antithymocyte globulin, and ablative therapy followed by allogeneic bone marrow transplantation. Clinical manifestations appear at 8 to 10 days, and death occurs at 3 to 4 weeks posttransfusion.

TA-GVHD can be prevented by irradiation of cellular components (minimum of 2500 cGy) before transfusion to patients at risk. Patients at risk for TA-GVHD include fetuses receiving intrauterine transfusions, selected immunocompetent (e.g., lymphoma patients) or immunocompromised recipients, recipients of donor units known to be from a blood relative, and recipients who have undergone marrow transplantation. Directed donations by family members should be discouraged (they are not less likely to transmit infection); lacking other options, the blood products from family members should always be irradiated.

Transfusion-Related Acute Lung Injury   This uncommon reaction results from the transfusion of donor plasma that contains high-titer anti-HLA antibodies that bind recipient leukocytes. The leukocytes aggregate in the pulmonary vasculature and release mediators that increase capillary permeability. The recipient develops symptoms of respiratory compromise and signs of noncardiogenic pulmonary edema, including bilateral interstitial infiltrates on chest x-ray. Treatment is supportive, and patients usually recover without sequelae. Testing the donor's plasma for anti-HLA antibodies can support this diagnosis. The implicated donors are frequently multiparous women, and transfusion of their plasma component should be avoided.

Posttransfusion Purpura   This reaction presents as thrombocytopenia 7 to 10 days after platelet transfusion and occurs predominantly in women. Platelet-specific antibodies are found in the recipient's serum, and the most frequently recognized antigen is HPA-1a found on the platelet glycoprotein IIIa receptor. The delayed thrombocytopenia is due to the production of antibodies that react to both donor and recipient platelets. Additional platelet transfusions can worsen the thrombocytopenia and should be avoided. Treatment with intravenous immunoglobulin may neutralize the effector antibodies, or plasmapheresis can be used to remove the antibodies.

Alloimmunization   A recipient may become alloimmunized to a number of antigens on cellular blood elements and plasma proteins. Alloantibodies to RBC antigens are detected during pretransfusion testing, and their presence may delay finding antigen-negative cross-match-compatible products for transfusion. Women of childbearing age who are sensitized to certain RBC antigens (i.e., D, c, E, Kell, or Duffy) are at

risk for bearing a fetus with hemolytic disease of the newborn. Matching for D antigen is the only pretransfusion selection test to prevent RBC alloimmunization.

Alloimmunization to antigens on leukocytes and platelets can result in refractoriness to platelet transfusions. Once alloimmunization has developed, HLA-compatible platelets from donors who share similar antigens with the recipient may be difficult to find. Hence, prudent transfusion practice is directed at preventing sensitization through the use of leukocyte-reduced cellular components, as well as limiting antigenic exposure by the judicious use of transfusions and use of SDAPs.

NONIMMUNOLOGIC REACTIONS ■ Fluid Overload   Blood components are excellent volume expanders, and transfusion may quickly lead to volume overload. Monitoring the rate and volume of the transfusion, along with the use of a diuretic, can minimize this problem.

Hypothermia   Refrigerated (4°C) or frozen (−18°C or below) blood components can result in hypothermia when rapidly infused. Cardiac dysrhythmias can result from exposing the sinoatrial node to cold fluid. Use of an in-line warmer will prevent this complication.

Electrolyte Toxicity   RBC leakage during storage increases the concentration of potassium in the unit. Neonates and patients in renal failure are at risk for hyperkalemia. Preventive measures, such as using fresh or washed RBCs, are warranted for neonatal transfusions because this complication can be fatal.

Citrate, commonly used to anticoagulate blood components, chelates calcium and thereby inhibits the coagulation cascade. Hypocalcemia, manifested by circumoral numbness and/or tingling sensation of the fingers and toes, may result from multiple rapid transfusions. Because citrate is quickly metabolized to bicarbonate, calcium infusion is seldom required in this setting. If calcium or any other intravenous infusion is necessary, it must be given through a separate intravenous line.

Iron Overload   Each unit of RBCs contains 200 to 250 mg of iron. Symptoms and signs of iron overload affecting endocrine, hepatic, and cardiac function are common after 100 units of RBCs have been transfused (total body iron load of 20 g). Preventing this complication by using alternative therapies (e.g., erythropoietin) and judicious transfusion is preferable and cost effective. Deferoxamine and other chelating agents are available, but the response is often suboptimal.

Hypotensive Reactions   Transient hypotension may be noted among transfused patients who take angiotensin-converting enzyme (ACE) inhibitors. Since blood products contain bradykinin that is normally degraded by ACE, patients on ACE inhibitors may have increased bradykinin levels that cause hypotension. The blood pressure typically returns to normal without intervention.

Immunomodulation   Transfusion of allogeneic blood is immunosuppressive. Multiply transfused renal transplant recipients are less likely to reject the graft, and transfusion may result in poorer outcomes in cancer patients and increase the risk of infections. Transfused leukocytes are thought to mediate the immunosuppression. Leukocyte-depleted cellular products may cause less immunosuppression, though controlled data have not been obtained and are unlikely to be obtained as the blood supply becomes universally leukocyte-depleted.

INFECTIOUS COMPLICATIONS   Nucleic acid amplification testing (NAT) has been used since 1999 to screen donated blood for the presence of HIV and hepatitis C virus RNA.

Viral Infections ■ *HEPATITIS C VIRUS (HCV)*   Fewer than 150 donors have been found to be HCV RNA positive in the absence of HCV antibodies, and the risk of acquiring HCV through transfusion is now 1 in 1,600,000 units. Infection with HCV may be asymptomatic or lead to chronic active hepatitis, cirrhosis, and liver failure.

HUMAN IMMUNODEFICIENCY VIRUS TYPE 1   Improved donor screening and testing (NAT) have dramatically reduced the risk of HIV-1 infection by blood transfusion. Donated blood is tested for HIV-1 p24 antigen.

Only eight seronegative donors have been shown to harbor HIV RNA. The risk of HIV-1 infection per transfusion episode is 1 in 1.9 million. Antibodies to HIV-2 are also measured in donated blood. No cases of HIV-2 infection have been reported in the United States since 1992.

HEPATITIS B VIRUS Donated blood is screened for HBV using assays for hepatitis B surface antigen (HbsAg). NAT testing is not practical because of slow viral replication and lower levels of viremia. The risk of transfusion-associated HBV infection is 1 in 63,000 units, twentyfold greater than for HCV. Vaccination of individuals who require long-term transfusion therapy can prevent this complication.

OTHER HEPATITIS VIRUSES Hepatitis A virus is rarely transmitted by transfusion, and the disease is typically asymptomatic and does not lead to chronic infection. Hepatitis G virus, now called GBV-C, along with two other transfusion-transmitted viruses, TTV and SEN-V, do not cause chronic hepatitis or other disease states. Routine testing does not appear to be warranted.

CYTOMEGALOVIRUS This ubiquitous virus infects ≥50% of the general population and is transmitted by the infected "passenger" WBCs found in transfused PRBCs or platelet components. Cellular components that are leukocyte-reduced have a decreased risk of transmitting CMV, regardless of the serologic status of the donor. Groups at risk for CMV infections include immunosuppressed patients, CMV-seronegative transplant recipients, and neonates; these patients should receive leukocyte-depleted components or CMV seronegative products.

HUMAN T LYMPHOTROPIC VIRUS (HTLV) TYPE I Assays to detect HTLV-I and -II are used to screen all donated blood. HTLV-1 is associated with adult T cell leukemia/lymphoma and tropical spastic paraparesis in a small percentage of infected persons (Chap. 172). The risk of HTLV-I infection via transfusion is 1 in 641,000 transfusion episodes. HTLV-II is not clearly associated with any disease.

PARVOVIRUS B-19 Blood components and products derived from pooled plasma can transmit this virus, the etiologic agent of erythema infectiosum, or fifth disease, in children. Parvovirus B-19 shows tropism for erythroid precursors and inhibits both erythrocyte production and maturation. Pure red cell aplasia, presenting either as acute aplastic crisis or chronic anemia with shortened RBC survival, may occur in individuals with an underlying hematologic disease, such as sickle cell disease or thalassemia (Chap. 94). The fetus of a seronegative woman is at risk for developing hydrops from this virus. NAT testing has reduced the risk of transfusion transmission.

Bacterial Contamination Most bacteria do not grow well at cold temperatures; thus, PRBCs and FFP are not common sources of bacterial contamination. However, some gram-negative bacteria, notably *Yersinia* and *Pseudomonas* species, can grow at 1° to 6°C. Platelet concentrates, which are stored at room temperature, are more likely to contain skin contaminants such as gram-positive organisms, including coagulase-negative staphylococci.

Recipients of transfusions contaminated with bacteria may develop fever and chills, which can progress to septic shock and DIC. These reactions may occur abruptly, within minutes of initiating the transfusion, or after several hours. The onset of symptoms and signs is often sudden and fulminant, which distinguishes bacterial contamination from a FNHTR. The reactions, particularly those related to gram-negative contaminants, are the result of infused endotoxins formed within the contaminated stored component.

When contaminated transfusions are suspected (i.e., when there is sudden development of shock), the transfusion must be stopped immediately. Therapy is directed at supporting the recipient's blood pressure, cardiac output, oxygenation, and renal function. The laboratory investigation should include cultures of any untransfused component, along with the routine blood bank clerical checks and serologic studies. Broad-spectrum antibiotic coverage should be started immediately and may be adjusted based on culture and sensitivity.

Other Infectious Agents Various parasites including those causing malaria, babesiosis, and Chagas disease can be transmitted by blood transfusion rarely. Geographic migration and travel of donors can shift the incidence of these rare infections. West Nile virus may be transmitted by transfusion. Other agents implicated in transfusion transmission include Lyme disease and varian Creutzfeld-Jakob disease. Because these infections can prove fatal, they should be considered in the transfused patient in the appropriate clinical setting.

ALTERNATIVES TO TRANSFUSION

Alternatives to allogeneic blood transfusions that avoid homologous donor exposures with attendant immunologic and infectious risks remain attractive. Autologous blood is the best option when transfusion is anticipated. However, the cost:benefit ratio of autologous transfusion remains high. No transfusion is a zero-risk event; clerical errors and bacterial contamination remain potential complications even with autologous transfusions. Additional methods of autologous transfusion in the surgical patient include preoperative hemodilution, recovery of shed blood from sterile surgical sites, and postoperative drainage collection. Directed or designated donation from friends and family of the potential recipient has not been safer than volunteer donor component transfusions. Such directed donations may in fact place the recipient at higher risk for complications such as GVHD and alloimmunization.

Oxygen-carrying blood substitutes, such as perfluorocarbons and aggregated hemoglobin solution, are presently in various stages of clinical trials. Granulocyte and granulocyte-macrophage colony-stimulating factor are clinically useful to hasten leukocyte recovery in patients with leukopenia related to high-dose chemotherapy. Erythropoietin stimulates erythrocyte production in patients with anemia of chronic renal failure and other conditions, thus avoiding or reducing the need for transfusion. This hormone can also stimulate erythropoiesis in the autologous donor to enable additional donation. Thrombopoietin, a cytokine that promotes megakaryocyte proliferation and maturation, is being tested for its ability to reduce the need for platelet transfusion.

FURTHER READING

BARON JF et al: The effect of universal leukodepletion of packed red blood cells on postoperative infections in high-risk patients undergoing abdominal aortic surgery. Anesth Analg 94:529, 2002

BRECHER ME et al: *The Technical Manual*, 14th ed. Arlington, VA, American Association of Blood Banks, 2002

DODD RY et al: Current prevalence and incidence of infectious disease markers and estimated window-period risk in the American Red Cross blood donor population. Transfusion 42:975, 2002

DZIK WH et al: Patient safety and blood tranfusion: New solutions. Transfus Med Rev 17:169, 2003

GOODNOUGH LT: Risks of blood transfusion. Crit Care Med 31(12 Suppl): 5678, 2003

RUBELLA P et al: A multicenter randomized study of the threshold for prophylactic platelet transfusions in adults with acute myeloid leukemia. N Engl J Med 337:1870, 1997

TABOR E et al: NAT screening of blood and plasma donations: Evolution of technology and regulatory policy. Transfusion 42:1230, 2002

Bone marrow transplantation was the original term used to describe the collection and transplantation of hematopoietic stem cells, but with the recent demonstration that the peripheral blood and umbilical cord blood are also useful sources of stem cells, *hematopoietic cell transplantation* has become the preferred generic term for this process. The procedure is usually carried out for one of two purposes: (1) to replace an abnormal but nonmalignant lymphohematopoietic system with one from a normal donor, or (2) to treat malignancy by allowing the administration of higher doses of myelosuppressive therapy than would otherwise be possible. The use of bone marrow transplantation has been steadily increasing, both because of its demonstrated effectiveness in selected diseases and because of increasing availability of donors. The International Bone Marrow Transplant Registry (*http://www.ibmtr.org*) estimates that about 50,000 transplants are performed each year.

THE HEMATOPOIETIC STEM CELL

Several features of the hematopoietic stem cell make transplantation clinically feasible, including its remarkable regenerative capacity, its ability to home to the marrow space following intravenous injection, and the ability of the stem cell to be cryopreserved. Transplantation of a single stem cell can replace the entire lymphohematopoietic system of an adult mouse. In humans, transplantation of a few percent of a donor's bone marrow volume regularly results in complete and sustained replacement of the recipient's entire lymphohematopoietic system, including all red cells, granulocytes, B and T lymphocytes, and platelets, as well as cells comprising the fixed macrophage population, including Kupffer cells of the liver, pulmonary alveolar macrophages, osteoclasts, Langerhans cells of the skin, and brain microglial cells. The ability of the hematopoietic stem cell to home to the marrow following intravenous injection is mediated, at least in part, by the interaction of specific cell molecules, termed *selectins*, on bone marrow endothelial cells with their unique ligands, termed *integrins*, on early hematopoietic cells. Human hematopoietic stem cells can survive freezing and thawing with little, if any, damage, making it possible to remove and store a portion of the patient's own bone marrow for later reinfusion following treatment of the patient with high-dose myelotoxic therapy.

CATEGORIES OF HEMATOPOIETIC CELL TRANSPLANTATION

Hematopoietic cell transplantation can be described according to the relationship between the patient and the donor and by the anatomic source of stem cells. In ~1% of cases, patients have identical twins who can serve as donors. Syngeneic donors represent the best source of stem cells; unlike the use of allogeneic donors, there is no risk of graft-versus-host disease (GVHD) and, unlike the use of autologous marrow, there is no risk that the stem cells are contaminated with tumor cells.

Allogeneic transplantation involves a donor and recipient who are not immunologically identical. Following allogeneic transplantation immune cells transplanted with the marrow or developing from it can react against the patient, causing GVHD. Alternatively, if the immunosuppressive preparative regimen used to treat the patient before transplant is inadequate, immunocompetent cells of the patient can cause graft rejection. The risks of these complications are greatly influenced by the degree of matching between donor and recipient for antigens encoded by genes of the major histocompatibility complex.

The human leukocyte antigen (HLA) molecules are responsible for binding antigenic proteins and presenting them to T cells. The antigens presented by HLA molecules may derive from exogenous sources (e.g., during active infections) or may be endogenous proteins produced by the cell. If individuals are not matched for HLA, T cells from one individual will react strongly to the mismatched HLA, or "major antigens," of the second. Even if the individuals are HLA-matched, the T cells of the donor may react to differing endogenous, or "minor antigens," presented by the HLA of the recipient. Reactions to minor antigens tend to be less vigorous. The genes of major relevance to transplantation include HLA-A, -B, -C, and -D; they are closely linked and therefore tend to be inherited as haplotypes, with only rare crossovers between them. Thus, the odds that any one full sibling will match a patient are one in four, and the probability that the patient has an HLA-identical sibling is $1 - (0.75)^n$, where n equals the number of siblings.

With current techniques, the risk of graft rejection is 1 to 3%, and the risk of severe, life-threatening acute GVHD is ~15% following transplantation between HLA-identical siblings. The incidence of graft rejection and GVHD increases progressively with the use of family member donors mismatched for one, two, or three antigens. While survival following a one-antigen mismatched transplant is not markedly altered, survival following two- or three-antigen mismatched transplants is significantly impaired, and such transplants should be performed only as part of clinical trials.

The formation of the National Marrow Donor Program has allowed for the identification of HLA-matched unrelated donors for many patients. The genes encoding HLA antigens are highly polymorphic, and thus the odds of any two unrelated individuals being HLA-identical are extremely low, somewhat less than 1 in 10,000. However, by identifying and typing >7 million volunteer donors, HLA-matched donors can now be found for ~50% of patients for whom a search is initiated. It takes, on average, 3 to 4 months to complete a search and schedule and initiate an unrelated donor transplant. Results so far suggest that GVHD is somewhat increased and survival somewhat poorer with such donors than with HLA-matched siblings.

Autologous transplantation involves the removal and storage of the patient's own stem cells with subsequent reinfusion after the patient receives high-dose myeloablative therapy. Unlike allogeneic transplantation, there is no risk of GVHD or graft rejection with autologous transplantation. On the other hand, autologous transplantation lacks a graft-versus-tumor (GVT) effect, and the autologous stem cell product can be contaminated with tumor cells that could lead to relapse. A variety of techniques have been developed to "purge" autologous products of tumor cells. Some use antibodies directed at tumor-associated antigens plus complement, antibodies linked to toxins, or antibodies conjugated to immunomagnetic beads. In vitro incubation with certain chemotherapeutic agents such as 4-hydroperoxycyclophosphamide and long-term culture of bone marrow have also been shown to diminish tumor cell numbers in stem cell products. Another technique is positive selection of stem cells using antibodies to CD34, with subsequent column adherence or flow techniques to select normal stem cells while leaving tumor cells behind. All these approaches can reduce the number of tumor cells from 1000- to 10,000-fold and are clinically feasible; however, no prospective randomized trials have yet shown that any of these approaches results in a decrease in relapse rates or improvements in disease-free or overall survival.

Bone marrow aspirated from the posterior and anterior iliac crests has traditionally been the source of hematopoietic stem cells for transplantation. Typically, anywhere from 1.5 to 5×10^8 nucleated marrow cells per kilogram are collected for allogeneic transplantation. Several recent studies have found improved survival in the settings of both matched sibling and unrelated transplantation by transplanting higher numbers of bone marrow cells.

Hematopoietic stem cells circulate in the peripheral blood but in very low concentrations. Following the administration of certain hematopoietic growth factors, including granulocyte colony-stimulating factor (G-CSF) or granulocyte-macrophage colony-stimulating factor (GM-CSF), and during recovery from intensive chemotherapy, the concentration of hematopoietic progenitor cells in blood, as measured either by colony-forming units or expression of the CD34 antigen, increases markedly. This has made it possible to harvest adequate numbers of stem cells from the peripheral blood for transplantation. Donors are typically treated with 4 or 5 days of hematopoietic growth factor, following which stem cells are collected in one or two 4-h pheresis sessions. In the autologous setting, transplantation of $>2.5 \times 10^6$ CD34 cells per kilogram, a number easily collected in most circumstances, leads to rapid and sustained engraftment in virtually all cases. Compared to the use of autologous marrow, use of peripheral blood stem cells results in more rapid hematopoietic recovery, with granulocytes recovering to $500/\mu L$ by day 12 and platelets recovering to $20,000/\mu L$ by day 14. While this more rapid recovery diminishes the morbidity of transplantation, no studies show an improvement in survival.

Hesitation in studying the use of peripheral blood stem cells for allogeneic transplantation was because peripheral blood stem cell products contain as much as one log more T cells than are contained in the typical marrow harvest; in animal models, the incidence of GVHD is related to the number of T cells transplanted. Nonetheless, phase II and randomized phase III trials have shown that the use of growth factor–mobilized peripheral blood stem cells from HLA-matched family members leads to faster engraftment without an increase in acute GVHD. Chronic GVHD may be increased with peripheral blood stem cells, but in trials conducted so far, this has been more than balanced by reductions in relapse rates and nonrelapse mortality, with the use of peripheral blood stem cells resulting in improved overall survival.

Umbilical cord blood contains a high concentration of hematopoietic progenitor cells, allowing for its use as a source of stem cells for transplantation. Cord blood transplantation from family members has been explored in the setting where the immediate need for transplantation precludes waiting the 9 or so months generally required for the baby to mature to the point of donating marrow. Use of cord blood in such settings results in somewhat slower engraftment than seen with marrow but a low incidence of GVHD, perhaps reflecting the low number of T cells in cord blood. Several banks have been developed to harvest and store cord blood for possible transplantation to unrelated patients from material that would otherwise be discarded. A summary of the first 562 unrelated cord blood transplants, facilitated by the New York Blood Center, reported engraftment in ~85% of patients but at a slower pace than seen with marrow. Severe GVHD was seen in 23% of patients. The risk of graft failure was related to the dose of cord blood cells per kilogram infused. The low cell content of most cord blood collections has limited the use of this approach as a source of stem cells for adult patients.

THE TRANSPLANT PREPARATIVE REGIMEN

The treatment regimen administered to patients immediately preceding transplantation is designed to eradicate the patient's underlying disease and, in the setting of allogeneic transplantation, immunosuppress the patient adequately to prevent rejection of the transplanted marrow. The appropriate regimen, therefore, depends on the disease setting and source of marrow. For example, when transplantation is performed to treat severe combined immunodeficiency and the donor is a histocompatible sibling, no treatment is required because no host cells require eradication and the patient is already too immunoincompetent to reject the transplanted marrow. For aplastic anemia, there is no large population of cells to eradicate and high-dose cyclophosphamide plus antithymocyte globulin are sufficient to immunosuppress the patient adequately to accept the marrow graft. In the setting of thalassemia and sickle cell anemia, high-dose busulfan is frequently added to cyclophosphamide in order to eradicate the hyperplastic host hematopoiesis. A variety of different regimens have been developed to treat malignant diseases. Most of these regimens include agents that have high activity against the tumor in question at conventional doses and have myelosuppression as their predominant dose-limiting toxicity. Therefore, these regimens commonly include busulfan, cyclophospha-

mide, melphalan, thiotepa, carmustine, etoposide, and total-body irradiation in various combinations.

Although high-dose treatment regimens have typically been used in transplantation, the understanding that much of the antitumor effect of transplantation derives from an immunologically mediated GVT response has led investigators to ask if less intensive "nonmyeloablative" regimens might be effective and more tolerable. Evidence for a GVT effect comes from studies showing posttransplant relapse rates are lowest in patients who develop acute and chronic GVHD, higher in those without GVHD, and higher still in recipients of T cell–depleted allogeneic or syngeneic marrow. The demonstration that complete remissions can be obtained in many patients who have relapsed posttransplant by simply administering viable lymphocytes from the original donor further strengthens the argument for a potent GVT effect. Accordingly, a variety of less intensive nonmyeloablative regimens have been studied, ranging in intensity from the very minimum required to achieve engraftment (e.g., fludarabine plus 200 cGy total-body irradiation) to regimens of more immediate intensity (e.g., fludarabine plus melphalan). Studies to date document that engraftment can be readily achieved with less toxicity than seen with conventional transplantation. Complete sustained responses have been documented in many patients, particularly those with more indolent hematologic malignancies. The precise role of nonmyeloablative transplants in any one disease category, however, has not yet been fully defined.

THE TRANSPLANT PROCEDURE

Marrow is usually collected from the donor's posterior and sometimes anterior iliac crests with the donor under general or spinal anesthesia. Typically, 10 to 15 mL/kg of marrow is aspirated, placed in heparinized media, and filtered through 0.3- and 0.2 mm screens to remove fat and bony spicules. The collected marrow may undergo further processing depending on the clinical situation, such as the removal of red cells to prevent hemolysis in ABO-incompatible transplants, the removal of donor T cells to prevent GVHD, or attempts to remove possible contaminating tumor cells in autologous transplantation. Marrow donation is safe, with only very rare complications reported.

Peripheral blood stem cells are collected by leukopheresis after the donor has been treated with hematopoietic growth factors or, in the setting of autologous transplantation, sometimes after treatment with a combination of chemotherapy and growth factors. Stem cells for transplantation are generally infused through a large-bore central venous catheter. Such infusions are usually well tolerated, although occasionally patients develop fever, cough, or shortness of breath. These symptoms usually resolve with slowing of the infusion. When the stem cell product has been cryopreserved using dimethyl sulfoxide, patients more often experience short-lived nausea or vomiting due to the odor and taste of the cryoprotectant.

ENGRAFTMENT

Peripheral blood counts usually reach their nadir several days to a week posttransplant as a consequence of the preparative regimen, then cells produced by the transplanted stem cells begin to appear in the peripheral blood. The rate of recovery depends on the source of stem cells, the use of posttransplant growth factors, and the form of GVHD prophylaxis employed. If marrow is the source of stem cells, recovery to 100 granulocytes/μL occurs by day 16 and $500/\mu L$ by day 22. Use of G-CSF-mobilized peripheral blood stem cells speeds the rate of recovery by ~1 week when compared to marrow. Use of myeloid growth factor (G-CSF or GM-CSF) posttransplant can further accelerate recovery by 3 to 5 days, while use of methotrexate to prevent GVHD delays engraftment by a similar period. Following allogeneic transplantation, engraftment can be documented using fluorescence in situ hybridization of sex chromosomes if donor and recipient are sex-mismatched, HLA-typing if HLA-mismatched, or restriction fragment length polymorphism analysis if sex- and HLA-matched.

COMPLICATIONS FOLLOWING HEMATOPOIETIC CELL TRANSPLANT

EARLY DIRECT CHEMORADIOTOXICITIES The transplant preparative regimens commonly used cause a spectrum of acute toxicities that vary according to the specific regimen but frequently result in nausea, vomiting, and mild skin erythema (Fig. 100-1). Regimens that include high-dose cyclophosphamide can result in hemorrhagic cystitis, which can usually be prevented by bladder irrigation or with the sulfhydryl compound, mercaptoethanesulfonate (MESNA); rarely, acute hemorrhagic carditis is seen. Most preparative regimens will result in oral mucositis, which typically develops 5 to 7 days posttransplant and often requires narcotic analgesia. Use of a patient-controlled analgesic pump provides the greatest patient satisfaction and results in a lower cumulative dose of narcotic. Patients begin losing their hair 5 to 6 days posttransplant and by 1 week are usually profoundly pancytopenic.

Approximately 10% of patients will develop venoocclusive disease of the liver, a syndrome resulting from direct cytotoxic injury to hepatic-venular and sinusoidal endothelium, with subsequent deposition of fibrin and the development of a local hypercoagulable state. This chain of events results in the clinical symptoms of tender hepatomegaly, ascites, jaundice, and fluid retention. These symptoms can develop any time during the first month posttransplant, with the peak incidence at day 16. The mortality of venoocclusive disease is ~30%, with progressive hepatic failure culminating in a terminal hepatorenal syndrome. Both thrombolytic and antithrombotic agents, such as tissue plasminogen activator, heparin, and prostaglandin E, have been studied as therapy, but none has proven of consistent major benefit in controlled trials and all have significant toxicity. Early studies with defibrotide, a polydeoxyribonucleotide, seem encouraging.

Although most pneumonias developing posttransplant are caused by infectious agents, in ~5% of patients a diffuse interstitial pneumonia will develop that is thought to be the result of direct toxicity of the preparative regimen. Bronchoalveolar lavage typically shows alveolar hemorrhage, and biopsies are typically characterized by diffuse alveolar damage, although some cases may have a more clearly interstitial pattern. High-dose glucocorticoids are often used as treatment, although randomized trials testing their utility have not been reported.

LATE DIRECT CHEMORADIOTOXICITIES Late complications of the preparative regimen include decreased growth velocity in children and delayed development of secondary sex characteristics. These complications can be partly ameliorated with the use of appropriate growth and sex hormone replacement. Most men become azoospermic, and most postpubertal women will develop ovarian failure, which should be treated. Thyroid dysfunction, usually well compensated, is sometimes seen. Cataracts develop in 10 to 20% of patients and are most common in patients treated with total-body irradiation and those who receive glucocorticoid therapy posttransplant for treatment of GVHD. Aseptic necrosis of the femoral head is seen in 10% of patients and is particularly frequent in those receiving chronic glucocorticoid therapy.

GRAFT-VERSUS-HOST DISEASE GVHD is the result of allogeneic T cells that were either transferred with the donor's stem cell inoculum or develop from it, reacting with antigenic targets on host cells. GVHD developing within the first 3 months posttransplant is termed *acute GVHD*, while GVHD developing or persisting beyond 3 months posttransplant is termed *chronic GVHD*. Acute GVHD most often first becomes apparent 2 to 4 weeks posttransplant and is characterized by an erythematous maculopapular rash; persistent anorexia or diarrhea, or both; and by liver disease with increased serum levels of bilirubin, alanine and aspartate aminotransferase, and alkaline phosphatase. Since many conditions can mimic acute GVHD, diagnosis usually requires skin, liver, or endoscopic biopsy for confirmation. In all these organs, endothelial damage and lymphocytic infiltrates are seen. In skin, the epidermis and hair follicles are damaged; in liver, the small bile ducts show segmental disruption; and in intestines, destruction of the crypts and mucosal ulceration may be noted. A commonly used rating system for acute GVHD is shown in Table 100-1. Grade I acute GVHD is of little clinical significance, does not affect the likelihood of survival, and does not require treatment. In contrast, grades II to IV GVHD are associated with significant symptoms and a poorer probability of survival and require aggressive therapy. The incidence of acute GVHD is higher in recipients of stem cells from mismatched or unrelated donors, in older patients, and in patients unable to receive full doses of drugs used to prevent the disease.

One general approach to the prevention of GVHD is the administration of immunosuppressive drugs early after transplant. Combinations of methotrexate and either cyclosporine or tacrolimus are among the most effective and widely used regimens. Prednisone, anti–T cell antibodies, mycophenolate mofetil, and other immunosuppressive agents have also been or are being studied in various combinations. A second general approach to GVHD prevention is removal of T cells from the stem cell inoculum. While effective in preventing GVHD, T cell depletion is associated with an increased incidence of graft failure and of tumor recurrence posttransplant; as yet, little evidence suggests that this approach improves cure rates in any specific setting.

Despite prophylaxis, significant acute GVHD will develop in ~30% of recipients of stem cells from matched siblings and in as many as 60% of those receiving stem cells from unrelated donors. The disease is usually treated with glucocorticoids, antithymocyte globulin, or monoclonal antibodies targeted against T cells or T cell subsets.

Between 20 and 50% of patients surviving >6 months after allogeneic transplantation will develop chronic GVHD. The disease is more common in older patients, in recipients of mismatched or unrelated stem cells, and in those with a preceding episode of acute GVHD. The disease resembles an autoimmune disorder with malar rash, sicca syndrome, arthritis, obliterative bronchiolitis, and bile duct degeneration and cholestasis. Single-agent prednisone or cyclosporine is standard treatment at present, although trials of other agents, including thalidomide, are under way. In most patients, chronic GVHD resolves, but it may require 1 to 3 years of immunosuppressive treatment before these agents can be withdrawn without the disease recurring. Because patients with chronic GVHD are susceptible to significant infection, they should receive prophylactic trimethoprim-sulfamethoxazole, and all suspected infections should be investigated and treated aggressively.

GRAFT FAILURE While complete and sustained engraftment are usually seen posttransplant, occasionally marrow function either does not return or, after a brief period of engraftment, is lost. Graft failure after autologous transplantation can be the result of inadequate numbers of stem cells being transplanted, damage during ex vivo treatment or

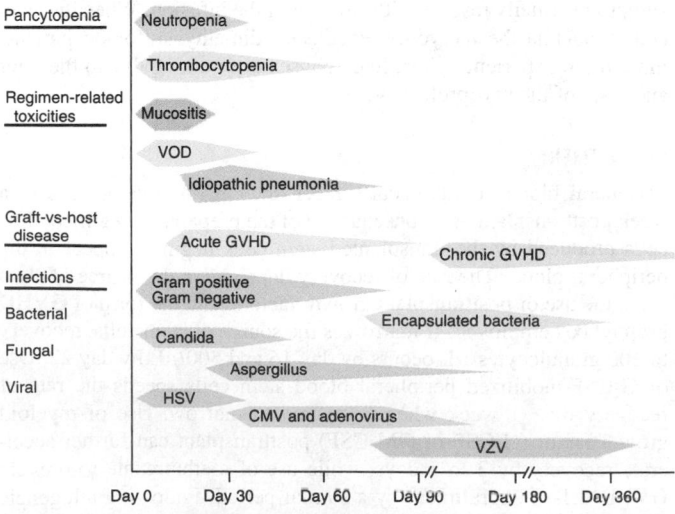

FIGURE 100-1 Major syndromes complicating marrow transplantation. VOD, venoocclusive disease; GVHD, graft-versus-host disease; HSV, herpes simplex virus; CMV, cytomegalovirus; VZV, varicella-zoster virus. The size of the shaded area roughly reflects the risk of the complication.

storage, or exposure of the patient to myelotoxic agents posttransplant. Infections with cytomegalovirus (CMV) or human herpes virus type 6 have also been associated with loss of marrow function. Graft failure after allogeneic transplantation can also be due to immunologic rejection of the graft by immunocompetent host cells. Immunologically based graft rejection is more common following use of less immunosuppressive preparative regimens, in recipients of T cell–depleted stem cell products, and in patients receiving grafts from HLA-mismatched donors.

Treatment of graft failure usually involves removing all potentially myelotoxic agents from the patient's regimen and attempting a short trial of myeloid growth factor. Persistence of lymphocytes of host origin in allogeneic transplant recipients with graft failure indicates immunologic rejection. Reinfusion of donor stem cells in such patients is usually unsuccessful unless preceded by a second immunosuppressive preparative regimen. Standard preparative regimens are generally tolerated poorly if administered within 100 days of a first transplant because of cumulative toxicities. However, use of regimens combining, for example, anti-CD3 antibodies with high-dose glucocorticoids have been successful in achieving engraftment in >50% of patients.

INFECTION Posttransplant patients, particularly recipients of allogeneic transplantation, require unique approaches to the problem of infection. Early after transplantation, patients are profoundly neutropenic, and because the risk of bacterial infection is so great, most centers initiate antibiotic treatment once the granulocyte count falls to <500/µL. Fluconazole prophylaxis at a dose of 200 to 400 mg/kg per day reduces the risk of candidal infections. Patients seropositive for herpes simplex should receive acyclovir prophylaxis. One approach to infection prophylaxis is shown in Table 100-2. Despite these prophylactic measures, most patients will develop fever and signs of infection posttransplant. The management of patients who become febrile despite bacterial and fungal prophylaxis is a difficult challenge and is guided by individual aspects of the patient and by the institution's experience. →*The general problem of infection in the immunocompromised host is discussed in Chap. 117.*

Once patients engraft, the incidence of bacterial infection diminishes; however, patients, particularly allogeneic transplant recipients, remain at significant risk of infection. During the period from engraftment until about 3 months posttransplant, the most common causes of infection are gram-positive bacteria, fungi (particularly *Aspergillus*) and viruses including CMV. CMV infection, which in the past was frequently seen and often fatal, can be prevented in seronegative patients by the use of seronegative blood products. The use of ganciclovir, either as prophylaxis beginning at the time of engraftment or initiated when CMV first reactivates as evidenced by development of antigenemia, can significantly reduce the risk of CMV disease in seropositive patients. Foscarnet is effective for some patients who develop CMV antigenemia or infection despite the use of ganciclovir or who cannot tolerate the drug.

Pneumocystis carinii pneumonia, once seen in 5 to 10% of patients, can be prevented by treating patients with oral trimethoprim-sulfamethoxazole for 1 week pretransplant and resuming the treatment once patients have engrafted.

The risk of infection diminishes considerably beyond 3 months after transplant unless chronic GVHD develops, requiring continuous immunosuppression. Most transplant centers recommend continuing trimethoprim-sulfamethoxazole prophylaxis while patients are receiving any immunosuppressive drugs and also recommend careful monitoring for late CMV reactivation. In addition, many centers recommend prophylaxis against varicella zoster, using acyclovir for 1 year posttransplant.

TABLE 100-1	Clinical Staging and Grading of Acute Graft-versus-Host Disease			
Clinical Stage	Skin	Liver— Bilirubin, µmol/L (mg/dL)	Gut	
1	Rash <25% body surface	34–51 (2–3)	Diarrhea 500–1000 mL/d	
2	Rash 25–50% body surface	51–103 (3–6)	Diarrhea 1000–1500 mL/d	
3	Generalized erythroderma	103–257 (6–15)	Diarrhea >1500 mL/d	
4	Desquamation and bullae	>257 (> 15)	Ileus	
Overall Clinical Grade		Skin Stage	Liver Stage	Gut Stage
I		1–2	0	0
II		1–3	1	1
III		1–3	2–3	2–3
IV		2–4	2–4	2–4

TREATMENT OF SPECIFIC DISEASES USING HEMATOPOIETIC CELL TRANSPLANTATION

NONMALIGNANT DISEASES ■ Immunodeficiency Disorders By replacing abnormal stem cells with cells from a normal donor, hematopoietic cell transplantation can cure patients of a variety of immunodeficiency disorders including severe combined immunodeficiency, Wiskott-Aldrich syndrome, and Chédiak-Higashi syndrome. The widest experience has been with severe combined immunodeficiency disease, where cure rates of 90% can be expected with HLA-identical donors and success rates of 50 to 70% have been reported using haplotype-mismatched parents as donors (Table 100-3).

Aplastic Anemia Transplantation from matched siblings after a preparative regimen of high-dose cyclophosphamide and antithymocyte globulin can cure up to 90% of patients <40 years with severe aplastic anemia. Results in older patients and in recipients of mismatched family member or unrelated marrow are less favorable; therefore, a trial of immunosuppressive therapy is generally recommended for such patients before considering transplantation. Transplantation is effective in all forms of aplastic anemia including, for example, the syndromes associated with paroxysmal nocturnal hemoglobinuria and Fanconi's anemia. Patients with Fanconi's anemia are abnormally sensitive to the toxic effects of alkylating agents and so less intensive preparative regimens must be used in their treatment (Chap. 94).

Hemoglobinopathies Marrow transplantation from an HLA-identical sibling following a preparative regimen of busulfan and cyclophosphamide can cure 70 to 90% of patients with thalassemia major. The best outcomes can be expected if patients are transplanted before they develop hepatomegaly or portal fibrosis and if they have been given adequate iron chelation therapy. Among such patients, the probabilities of 5-year survival and disease-free survival are 95 and 90%, respectively. Although prolonged survival can be achieved with aggressive chelation therapy, transplantation is the only curative treatment for

TABLE 100-2	Approach to Infection Prophylaxis in Allogeneic Transplant Recipients	
Organism		Approach
Bacterial	Ceftazidime	2 g IV q8h while neutropenic
Fungal	Fluconazole	400 mg PO qd to day 75 posttransplant
Pneumocystis carinii	Trimethoprim-sulfamethoxazole	1 double strength tablet PO bid 2 days/week until day 180 or off immunosuppression
Viral		
Herpes simplex	Acyclovir	800 mg PO bid to day 30
Varicella zoster	Acyclovir	800 mg PO bid to day 365
Cytomegalovirus	Ganciclovir	5 mg/kg IV bid for 7 days, then 5 (mg/kg)/d 5 days/week to day 100

TABLE 100-3 *Estimated 5-Year Survival Rates following Transplantation*[a]

Disease	Allogeneic, %	Autologous, %
Severe combined immunodeficiency	90	N/A
Aplastic anemia	90	N/A
Thalassemia	90	N/A
Acute myeloid leukemia		
First remission	55–60	50
Second remission	40	30
Acute lymphocytic leukemia		
First remission	50	40
Second remission	40	30
Chronic myeloid leukemia		
Chronic phase	70	ID
Accelerated phase	40	ID
Blast crisis	15	ID
Chronic lymphocytic leukemia	50	ID
Myelodysplasia	45	ID
Multiple myeloma	30	35
Non-Hodgkin's lymphoma		
First relapse/second remission	40	40
Hodgkin's disease		
First relapse/second remission	40	50
Breast cancer		
High-risk stage II	N/A	70
Stage IV	N/A	15

[a] These estimates are generally based on data reported by the International Bone Marrow Transplant Registry. The analysis has not been reviewed by their Advisory Committee. *Note*: N/A, not applicable; ID, insufficient data.

thalassemia. Transplantation is being studied as a curative approach to patients with sickle cell anemia. Two-year survival and disease-free survival rates of 90 and 80%, respectively, have been reported following matched sibling transplantation. Decisions about patient selection and the timing of transplantation remain difficult, but transplantation seems to represent a reasonable option for younger patients who suffer repeated crises or other significant complications and who have not responded to other interventions (Chap. 91).

Other Nonmalignant Diseases Theoretically, hematopoietic cell transplantation should be able to cure any disease that results from an inborn error of the lymphohematopoietic system. Transplantation has been used successfully to treat congenital disorders of white blood cells such as Kostmann's syndrome, chronic granulomatous disease, and leukocyte adhesion deficiency. Congenital anemias such as Black-fan-Diamond anemia can also be cured with transplantation. Infantile malignant osteopetrosis is due to an inability of the osteoclast to resorb bone, and since osteoclasts derive from the marrow, transplantation can cure this rare inherited disorder.

Hematopoietic cell transplantation has been used as treatment for a number of storage diseases caused by enzymatic deficiencies, such as Gaucher's disease, Hurler's syndrome, Hunter's syndrome, and infantile metachromatic leukodystrophy. Transplantation for these diseases has not been uniformly successful, but treatment early in the course of these diseases, before irreversible damage to extramedullary organs has occurred, increases the chance for success.

Transplantation is being explored as a treatment for severe acquired autoimmune disorders. These trials are based on studies demonstrating that transplantation can reverse autoimmune disorders in animal models and on the observation that occasional patients with coexisting autoimmune disorders and hematologic malignancies have been cured of both with transplantation.

MALIGNANT DISEASES ■ Acute Leukemia Allogeneic hematopoietic cell transplantation cures 15 to 20% of patients who do not achieve complete response from induction chemotherapy for acute myeloid leukemia (AML) and is the only form of therapy that can cure such patients. Cure rates of 30 to 35% are seen when patients are transplanted in second remission or in first relapse. The best results with allogeneic transplantation are achieved when applied during first re-

mission, with disease-free survival rates averaging 55 to 60%. Chemotherapy alone can cure a portion of AML patients, and so the relative merits of transplanting all patients during first remission versus only transplanting very high risk patients and those who relapse continue to be discussed. Autologous transplantation is also able to cure a portion of patients with AML. The rates of disease recurrence with autologous transplantation are higher than seen after allogeneic transplantation, and cure rates are generally somewhat less.

Similar to patients with AML, adults with acute lymphocytic leukemia who do not achieve a complete response to induction chemotherapy can be cured in 15 to 20% of cases with immediate transplantation. Cure rates improve to 30 to 50% in second remission, and therefore transplantation can be recommended for adults who have persistent disease after induction chemotherapy or who have subsequently relapsed. Transplantation in first remission results in cure rates around 55%. While transplantation appears to offer a clear advantage over chemotherapy for patients with high-risk disease, such as those with Philadelphia chromosome–positive disease, debate continues about whether adults with standard-risk disease should be transplanted in first remission or whether transplantation should be reserved until relapse. Autologous transplantation is associated with a higher relapse rate but a somewhat lower risk of nonrelapse mortality when compared to allogeneic transplantation. On balance, most experts recommend use of allogeneic stem cells if an appropriate donor is available.

Chronic Leukemia Allogeneic hematopoietic cell transplantation is the only therapy shown to cure a substantial portion of patients with chronic myeloid leukemia (CML). Five-year disease-free survival rates are 15 to 20% for patients transplanted for blast crisis, 25 to 50% for accelerated-phase patients, and 60 to 70% for chronic phase patients, with cure rates as high as 80% at selected centers. Time from diagnosis to transplantation influences outcome, with best results obtained among patients transplanted within 1 year of diagnosis. Use of unrelated donors results in more GVHD and slightly worse survival than seen with matched siblings, although, at some large centers, 3-year disease-free survival rates of 70% have been reported. Autologous transplantation is being studied; however, few data suggest that this approach has curative potential in this disease. The timing of transplantation in CML has become more complicated with the introduction of imatinib mesylate, a remarkably effective, relatively nontoxic oral agent. Because imatinib does not generally result in complete molecular remissions, many would argue that allogeneic transplantation remains the treatment of choice for younger patients with matched donors. For older patients and those without matched donors, an initial trial of imatinib is appropriate (Chap. 96).

Allogeneic transplantation has been used to only a limited extent for chronic lymphocytic leukemia, in large part because of the chronic nature of the disease and because of the age profile of patients. With allogeneic transplantation, complete remissions have been achieved in the majority of patients so far reported, with disease-free survival rates of ~50% at 3 years. However, treatment-related mortality has been substantial, and further follow-up is needed. There is even less experience with autologous transplantation in this disorder.

Myelodysplasia Between 40 and 50% of patients with myelodysplasia appear to be cured with allogeneic transplantation. Results are better among younger patients and those with less advanced disease. However, some patients with myelodysplasia can live for extended periods without intervention, and so transplantation is generally recommended only for patients with disease categorized as intermediate risk I or greater according to the International Prognostic Scoring System (Chap. 94).

Lymphoma Patients with disseminated intermediate- or high-grade non-Hodgkin's lymphoma who have not been cured by first-line chemotherapy and are transplanted in first relapse or second remission can still be cured in 40 to 50% of cases. This represents a clear advantage over results obtained with salvage chemotherapy. It is unsettled whether patients with high-risk disease benefit from transplantation in first remission. Most experts favor the use of autologous rather than allogeneic transplantation for patients with non-Hodgkin's lymphoma, because fewer complications occur with this approach and survival appears equivalent. The role of transplantation in patients with indolent non-Hodgkin's lymphoma is less well defined. Long-term remissions can be obtained in many patients with acceptable toxicity and results with transplantation in patients with recurrent disease generally appear better than one would expect with conventional-dose chemotherapy. However, late relapses are seen after transplantation, and no randomized study has confirmed its superiority.

The role of transplantation in Hodgkin's disease is similar to that in non-Hodgkin's lymphoma. With transplantation, 5-year disease-free survival is 20 to 30% in patients who never achieve a first remission with standard chemotherapy and up to 60% for those transplanted in second remission. Transplantation has no defined role in first remission in Hodgkin's disease.

Myeloma Patients with myeloma who have progressed on first-line therapy can sometimes benefit from allogeneic or autologous transplantation. Autologous transplantation has been studied as part of the initial therapy of patients, and in randomized trials, both disease-free survival as well as overall survival were improved with this approach. A strategy of autologous transplantation followed by nonmyeloablative allogeneic transplantation has shown encouraging results.

Solid Tumors Among women with metastatic breast cancer, 15 to 20% disease-free survival rates at 3 years have been reported, with better results seen in younger patients who have responded completely to standard-dose therapy before undergoing transplantation. Randomized trials have not shown superior survival for patients treated for metastatic disease with high-dose chemotherapy plus stem cell support. Randomized trials evaluating transplantation as treatment for primary breast cancer are being conducted, but final results are not yet available.

Patients with testicular cancer who have failed first-line chemotherapy have been treated with autologous transplantation; ~10 to 20% of such patients apparently have been cured with this approach.

The use of high-dose chemotherapy with autologous stem cell support is being studied for several other solid tumors, including ovarian cancer, small cell lung cancer, neuroblastoma, and pediatric sarcomas. As in most other settings, the best results have been obtained in patients with limited amounts of disease and where the remaining tumor retains sensitivity to conventional-dose chemotherapy. Few randomized trials of transplantation in these diseases have been completed.

Partial and complete responses have been reported following non-myeloablative allogeneic transplantation for several solid tumors, most notably renal cell carcinomas. These results suggest that the GVT effect, well documented in the treatment of hematologic malignancies, may under certain circumstances apply to selected solid tumors.

Posttransplant Relapse Patients who relapse following autologous transplantation sometimes respond to further chemotherapy, particularly if the remission following transplantation was long. More options are available for patients who relapse following allogeneic transplantation. Of particular interest are the response rates seen with infusion of unirradiated donor lymphocytes. Complete responses in as many as 75% of patients with chronic myeloid leukemia, 40% in myelodysplasia, 25% in AML, and 15% in myeloma have been reported. Major complications of donor lymphocyte infusions include transient myelosuppression and the development of GVHD. These complications appear to be dependent on the number of donor lymphocytes given and the schedule of infusions, with less GVHD seen with lower dose, fractionated schedules.

FURTHER READING

APPELBAUM FR: Haematopoietic cell transplantation as immunotherapy. Nature 411:385, 2001

BENSINGER WI et al: Transplantation of bone marrow as compared with peripheral-blood cells from HLA-identical relatives in patients with hematologic cancers. N Engl J Med 344:175, 2001

HANSEN JA et al: Bone marrow transplants from unrelated donors for patients with chronic myeloid leukemia. N Engl J Med 338:962, 1998

PHILIP T et al: Autologous bone marrow transplantation as compared with salvage chemotherapy in relapses of chemotherapy-sensitive non-Hodgkin's lymphoma. N Engl J Med 333:1540, 1995

RUBINSTEIN P et al: Outcomes among 562 recipients of placental-blood transplants from unrelated donors. N Engl J Med 339:1565, 1998

Section 3   Disorders of Hemostasis

101   DISORDERS OF THE PLATELET AND VESSEL WALL
Robert I. Handin

Patients with platelet or vessel wall disorders usually bleed into superficial sites such as the skin, mucous membranes, or genitourinary or gastrointestinal tract. Bleeding begins immediately after trauma and either responds to simple measures, such as pressure and packing, or requires systemic therapy with glucocorticoids, desmopressin, plasma fractions, or platelet concentrates. The most common platelet/vessel wall disorders are (1) various forms of thrombocytopenia, (2) von Willebrand's disease (vWD), and (3) drug-induced platelet dysfunction. This chapter reviews the diagnosis and treatment of quantitative and qualitative platelet disorders as well as vessel wall defects that cause bleeding. →*For further discussion of the physiology of normal hemostasis and the cardinal manifestations of bleeding arising from hemostatic disorders, see Chap. 53.*

PLATELET DISORDERS

Platelets arise from the fragmentation of megakaryocytes, which are very large, polyploid bone marrow cells produced by the process of endomitosis. They undergo from three to five cycles of chromosomal duplication without cytoplasmic division. After leaving the marrow space, about one-third of the platelets are sequestered in the spleen, while the other two-thirds circulate for 7 to 10 days. Normally, only a small fraction of the platelet mass is consumed in the process of hemostasis, so most platelets circulate until they become senescent and are removed by phagocytic cells. The normal blood platelet count is 150,000 to 450,000/μL. A decrease in platelet count stimulates an increase in the number, size, and ploidy of megakaryocytes, releasing additional platelets into the circulation. This process is regulated by thrombopoietin (TPO) binding to its megakaryocyte receptor, a proto-oncogene c-mpl. TPO (c-mpl ligand) is secreted continuously at a low level and binds tightly to circulating platelets. A reduction in platelet count increases the level of free TPO and thereby stimulates megakaryocyte and platelet production.

The platelet count varies during the menstrual cycle, rising following ovulation and falling at the onset of menses. It is also influenced by the patient's nutritional state and can be decreased in severe iron, folic acid, or vitamin B_{12} deficiency. Platelets are acute-phase reac-

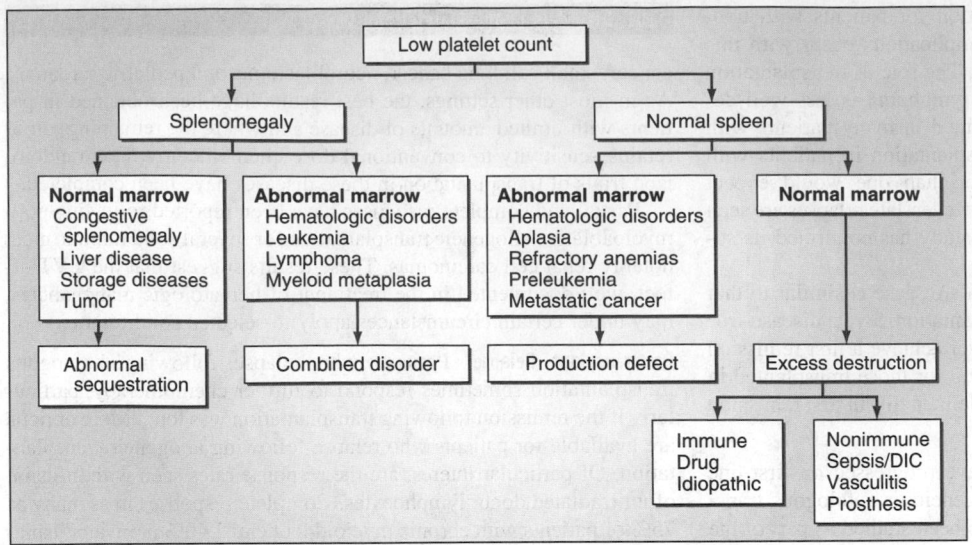

FIGURE 101-1 Clinical evaluation of patients with thrombocytopenia. [*Modified from RI Handin, in W Berk (ed), Hematology, 4th ed. Cambridge, MA, MIT Press, 1985.*]

tants, and patients with systemic inflammation, tumors, bleeding, and mild iron deficiency may have an increased platelet count, a benign condition called *secondary, or reactive, thrombocytosis.* The cytokines interleukin (IL) 3, IL-6, and IL-11 may stimulate platelet production in acute inflammation. In these conditions, the platelet count is usually < 1 million/μL. In contrast, the increase in platelet count that is characteristic of the myeloproliferative disorders such as polycythemia vera, chronic myeloid leukemia, myeloid metaplasia, and essential thrombocytosis can be much higher and cause either severe bleeding or thrombosis. In these patients, unregulated platelet production is secondary to a clonal stem cell abnormality affecting all bone marrow progenitors.

THROMBOCYTOPENIA Thrombocytopenia is caused by one of three mechanisms—decreased bone marrow production, increased splenic sequestration, or accelerated destruction of platelets. In order to determine the etiology of thrombocytopenia, each patient should have a careful examination of the peripheral blood film, an assessment of marrow morphology by examination of an aspirate or biopsy, and an estimate of splenic size by bedside palpation supplemented, if necessary, by ultrasonography or computed tomography (CT). Occasional patients have "pseudothrombocytopenia," a benign condition in which platelets agglutinate or adhere to leukocytes when blood is collected with EDTA as anticoagulant. This is a laboratory artifact, and the actual platelet count in vivo is normal. A scheme for classifying patients with thrombocytopenia based on these clinical observations and laboratory tests is outlined in Fig. 101-1.

Impaired Production Disorders that injure stem cells or prevent their proliferation frequently cause thrombocytopenia. They usually affect multiple hematopoietic cell lines so that thrombocytopenia is accompanied by varying degrees of anemia and leukopenia. Diagnosis of a platelet production defect is readily established by examination of a bone marrow aspirate or biopsy, which should show a reduced number of megakaryocytes. The most common causes of decreased platelet production are marrow aplasia, fibrosis, or infiltration with malignant cells, all of which produce highly characteristic marrow abnormalities. Occasionally, thrombocytopenia is the presenting laboratory abnormality in these disorders. Cytotoxic drugs impair megakaryocyte proliferation and maturation and frequently cause thrombocytopenia. Rare marrow disorders, such as congenital amegakaryocytic hypoplasia and thrombocytopenia with absent radii (TAR syndrome), produce a selective decrease in megakaryocyte production.

Splenic Sequestration Since one-third of the platelet mass is normally sequestered in the spleen, splenectomy will increase the platelet count by 30%. Postsplenectomy thrombocytosis is a benign self-limited con-

dition that does not require specific therapy. In contrast, when the spleen enlarges, the fraction of sequestered platelets increases, lowering the platelet count. The most common causes of splenomegaly are portal hypertension secondary to liver disease and splenic infiltration with tumor cells in myeloproliferative or lymphoproliferative disorders (Chap. 54). Isolated splenomegaly is rare, and in most patients it is accompanied by other clinical manifestations of an underlying disease. Many patients with leukemia, lymphoma, or a myeloproliferative syndrome have both marrow infiltration and splenomegaly and develop thrombocytopenia from a combination of impaired marrow production and splenic sequestration of platelets.

Accelerated Destruction Abnormal vessels, fibrin thrombi, and intravascular prostheses can all shorten platelet survival and cause nonimmunologic thrombocytopenia. Thrombocytopenia is common in patients with vasculitis, the hemolytic uremic syndrome (HUS), thrombotic thrombocytopenic purpura (TTP), or as a manifestation of disseminated intravascular coagulation (DIC). In addition, platelets coated with antibody, immune complexes, or complement are rapidly cleared by mononuclear phagocytes in the spleen or other tissues, inducing immunologic thrombocytopenia. The most common causes of immunologic thrombocytopenia are viral or bacterial infections, drugs (often heparin), and a chronic autoimmune disorder referred to as *idiopathic thrombocytopenic purpura* (ITP). Patients with immunologic thrombocytopenia do not usually have splenomegaly and have an increased number of bone marrow megakaryocytes.

DRUG-INDUCED THROMBOCYTOPENIA Many common drugs can cause thrombocytopenia (Table 101-1). Cancer chemotherapeutic agents may depress megakaryocyte production. Ingestion of large quantities of alcohol has a marrow-depressing effect leading to transient thrombocytopenia, particularly in binge drinkers. Thiazide diuretics, used to treat hypertension or congestive heart failure, impair megakaryocyte production and can produce mild thrombocytopenia (50,000 to 100,000/μL), which may persist for several months after the drug is discontinued.

Most drugs induce thrombocytopenia by eliciting an immune response in which the platelet is an innocent bystander. The platelet is damaged by complement activation following the formation of drug-antibody complexes. Current laboratory tests can identify the causative agent in 10% of patients with clinical evidence of drug-induced thrombocytopenia. The best proof of a drug-induced etiology is a prompt rise in the platelet count when the suspected drug is discontinued. Patients with drug-induced platelet destruction may also have a secondary increase in megakaryocyte number without other marrow abnormalities.

Although most patients recover within 7 to 10 days and do not require therapy, occasional patients with platelet counts <10,000 to 20,000/μL have severe hemorrhage and may require temporary support with glucocorticoids, plasmapheresis, or platelet transfusions

TABLE 101-1 Drugs That May Cause Thrombocytopenia

1. Chemotherapeutic agents—especially carboplatin, alkylating agents, anthracyclines, antimetabolites
2. Antibiotics—sulfonamides, penicillins, cephalosporins
3. Heparins—highest incidence is with unfractionated products
4. Cardiovascular agents—thiazide diuretics, rarely angiotensin converting enzyme inhibitors

while waiting for the platelet count to rise. A patient who has recovered from drug-induced immunologic thrombocytopenia should be instructed to avoid the offending drug in the future, since only minute amounts of drug are needed to set up subsequent immune reactions. Certain drugs that are cleared from body storage depots quite slowly, such as phenytoin, may induce prolonged thrombocytopenia.

Heparin is a common cause of thrombocytopenia in hospitalized patients. Between 10 and 15% of patients receiving therapeutic doses of unfractionated heparin develop thrombocytopenia (heparin-induced thrombocytopenia, HIT) and, occasionally, may have severe bleeding or intravascular platelet aggregation and paradoxical thrombosis. Heparin-induced thrombosis, sometimes called the "white clot syndrome," can be fatal unless recognized promptly. Heparin can cause mild thrombocytopenia by directly agglutinating platelets (type I HIT). The more serious form (type II HIT) results from an immune reaction. The offending antigen is a complex formed between heparin and the platelet-derived heparin-neutralizing protein, platelet factor 4. Type II HIT is particularly severe because the heparin–PF-4 antibody complexes bind the platelet Fc receptor and induce platelet activation and secretion. Prompt cessation of heparin will reverse both thrombocytopenia and heparin-induced thrombosis. Low-molecular-weight heparin products have reduced the incidence of HIT. They are effective antithrombotic agents (Chap. 103) and are less immunogenic. Unfortunately, 80 to 90% of the antibodies generated against conventional heparins cross-react with low-molecular-weight heparins, so only a minority of patients with preformed antibody can be treated with these products. Several potent thrombin inhibitors with different structures from heparin can be used to treat patients with HIT (Chap. 103). Argatroban is the current drug of choice, but pentasaccharides that mimic heparin's active site are in development.

IDIOPATHIC THROMBOCYTOPENIC PURPURA The immunologic thrombocytopenias can be classified on the basis of the pathologic mechanism, the inciting agent, or the duration of the illness. The explosive onset of severe thrombocytopenia following recovery from a viral exanthem or upper respiratory illness (*acute ITP*) is common in children and accounts for 90% of the pediatric cases of immunologic thrombocytopenia. Of these patients, 60% recover in 4 to 6 weeks and >90% recover within 3 to 6 months. Transient immunologic thrombocytopenia also complicates some cases of infectious mononucleosis, acute toxoplasmosis, or cytomegalovirus infection and can be part of the prodromal phase of viral hepatitis and initial infection with HIV. Acute ITP is rare in adults and accounts for <10% of postpubertal patients with immune thrombocytopenia. Acute ITP is caused by immune complexes containing viral antigens that bind to platelet Fc receptors or by antibodies produced against viral antigens that cross-react with the platelet. In addition to these viral disorders, the differential diagnosis includes atypical presentations of aplastic anemia, acute leukemias, or metastatic tumor. A bone marrow examination is essential to exclude these disorders, which can occasionally mimic acute ITP.

Most adults present with a more indolent form of thrombocytopenia that may persist for many years and is referred to as *chronic ITP*. Women age 20 to 40 are afflicted most commonly and outnumber men by a ratio of 3:1. They may present with an abrupt fall in platelet count and bleeding similar to patients with acute ITP. More often they have a prior history of easy bruising or menometrorrhagia. These patients have an autoimmune disorder with antibodies directed against target antigens on the glycoprotein (Gp) IIb/IIIa or, less frequently, the Gp Ib/IX complex (Fig. 53-2). Although most antibodies function as opsonins and accelerate platelet clearance by phagocytic cells, occasional antibodies bind to epitopes on critical regions of these glycoproteins and impair platelet function. Platelet-associated IgG can be measured, but specificity is a problem. High "background" level of IgG on normal platelets and elevations in plasma immunoglobulin levels or in circulating immune complexes will nonspecifically increase platelet-associated IgG. Few clinical situations require platelet-associated IgG testing.

A low platelet count may be the initial manifestation of systemic lupus erythematosus (SLE) or the first sign of a primary hematologic disorder. Thus, patients with chronic ITP should have a bone marrow examination and an antinuclear antibody determination. In addition, patients with hepatic or splenic enlargement, lymphadenopathy, or atypical lymphocytes should have serologic studies for hepatitis viruses, cytomegalovirus, Epstein-Barr virus, *Toxoplasma*, and HIV. HIV infection is a common cause of immunologic thrombocytopenia. Thrombocytopenia can be the initial symptom of HIV infection or a complication of fully developed clinical AIDS.

℞ TREATMENT

Treatment of patients with ITP must take into account the age of the patient, the severity of the illness, and the anticipated natural history. Although adults have a higher incidence of intracranial bleeding than children, specific therapy may not be necessary unless the platelet count is <20,000/μL or there is extensive bleeding. Hemorrhage in patients with either acute or chronic ITP can usually be controlled with glucocorticoids but, in rare cases, may require temporary phagocytic blockade with intravenous immunoglobulin (IVIg) or anti-RhD (WinRho). Although antibody preparations are effective, they are expensive and should be reserved for patients with severe thrombocytopenia and clinical bleeding who are refractory to other measures. Emergency splenectomy is usually reserved for patients with acute or chronic ITP who are desperately ill and have not responded to any medical measures. The treatment of symptomatic thrombocytopenia in patients with HIV infection is more complex because the administration of glucocorticoids or splenectomy may increase susceptibility to opportunistic infections. Splenectomy has been effective in the course of HIV before the onset of symptomatic AIDS. Treatment with zidovudine (AZT) and other antiviral agents that reduce viral load can improve the platelet count in patients with HIV-induced thrombocytopenia.

Symptomatic patients with chronic ITP are usually placed on prednisone, 60 mg/d for 4 to 6 weeks. The drug is then decreased slowly over another few weeks. About 50% of patients with chronic ITP will normalize their platelet count on high doses of prednisone. However, the majority will have a fall in platelet count following steroid withdrawal. Patients with chronic ITP who fail to maintain a normal platelet count after a course of prednisone are eligible for elective splenectomy. These glucocorticoid-responsive but glucocorticoid-dependent patients are very likely to respond to splenectomy, and 70% will have a normal platelet count within 1 week after surgery. Splenectomy can now often be performed by minimally invasive laparoscopic techniques that reduce morbidity and shorten hospital stay. Some patients who do not respond to glucocorticoids may still respond to splenectomy. Occasionally, patients may fail to respond to splenectomy because of the failure to remove an accessory spleen. In other patients, a small, inactive accessory spleen may grow or new splenic foci may develop from splenic cells shed at the time of surgery and cause the late onset of thrombocytopenia. In either case, the presence of splenic tissue can be diagnosed by examination of the blood smear for Howell-Jolly bodies that appear in the red cells of asplenic individuals. Persistent splenic tissue can be confirmed by a radionuclide scan.

Patients still thrombocytopenic after splenectomy or who relapse months to years after initial therapy have received a variety of immunosuppressive drugs including azathioprine, cyclophosphamide, vincristine, vinblastine, and cyclosporine. Danazol has also been used with some success. Although each of these drugs may be beneficial, they have serious side effects and should be used judiciously. IVIg and anti-RhD are only transiently effective and expensive. IVIg can cause meningismus and headache, and some lots have carried hepatitis C virus. Anti-RhD can cause hemolysis. These drugs should be used to raise the platelet count temporarily and to support patients before surgery or labor and delivery; they are not substitutes for splenectomy. If a patient is not bleeding and maintains a platelet count >20,000/

μL, consideration should be given to withholding therapy. Patients with severe chronic thrombocytopenia may live with their disease for two or three decades.

Rituximab, an anti-CD20 monoclonal antibody used to treat lymphoma, has also proven an effective approach to ITP and is probably preferable to long-term glucocorticoid therapy. Rituximab eliminates normal B cells, including those producing the antiplatelet antibody. This B cell depletion is transient (lasting 12 to 18 months, normally) and has surprisingly few side effects or toxicities.

FUNCTIONAL PLATELET DISORDERS As described in Chap. 53, normal hemostasis requires three critical platelet reactions—adhesion, aggregation, and granule release. Clinical bleeding can result from a failure of any of these important functions. Table 101-2 lists the major functional platelet disorders. Table 101-3 lists methods to assess platelet function.

von Willebrand's Disease vWD is the most common inherited bleeding disorder, occurring in 1 in 100 to 500 individuals. The von Willebrand factor (vWF) is a heterogeneous multimeric plasma glycoprotein with two major functions: (1) It facilitates platelet adhesion under conditions of high shear stress by linking platelet membrane receptors to vascular subendothelium; and (2) it serves as the plasma carrier for factor VIII, the antihemophilic factor, a critical blood coagulation protein. Discrete domains in each vWF subunit mediate each of these important functions. The normal plasma vWF level is 10 mg/L. The vWF activity is distributed among a series of plasma multimers with estimated molecular weights ranging from 400,000 to >20 million. A single large vWF precursor subunit is synthesized in endothelial cells and megakaryocytes, where it is cleaved and assembled into the disulfide-linked multimers present in plasma, platelets, and vascular subendothelium. A modest reduction in plasma vWF concentration or a selective loss in the high-molecular-weight multimers decreases platelet adhesion and causes clinical bleeding.

Although vWD is heterogeneous, certain clinical features are common to all the syndromes. With one exception (type III disease), all forms are inherited as autosomal dominant traits, and affected patients are heterozygous with one normal and one abnormal vWF allele. In mild cases, bleeding occurs only after surgery or trauma. More severely affected patients have spontaneous epistaxis or oral mucosal, gastrointestinal, or genitourinary bleeding. The laboratory findings are variable. The most diagnostic pattern is the combination of (1) a pro-

TABLE 101-2 *Classification of Functional Platelet Disorders*

I. Disorders of adhesion
  A. Inherited
    1. Bernard-Soulier syndrome
    2. von Willebrand's disease (vWD)
  B. Acquired
    1. Uremia
    2. Acquired vWD
II. Disorders of aggregation
  A. Inherited
    1. Glanzmann's thrombasthenia
    2. Afibrinogenemia
  B. Acquired
    1. Fibrin degradation product inhibition
    2. Dysproteinemias
    3. Drugs—e.g., ticlopidine, Gp IIb/IIIa inhibitors
III. Disorders of granule release
  A. Inherited
    1. Oculocutaneous albinism (Hermansky-Pudlak syndrome)
    2. Chédiak-Higashi syndrome
    3. Isolated dense (δ) granule deficiency
    4. Gray-platelet syndrome—combined α and β granule deficiency
  B. Acquired
    1. Cardiopulmonary bypass
    2. Myeloproliferative disorders
    3. Drugs—aspirin and other nonsteroidal anti-inflammatory agents

TABLE 101-3 *Evaluation of Platelet Function*

Bleeding time
  Modified Ivy method
  Skin incision—time to stop bleeding
  Global screen of platelet role in hemostasis
von Willebrand factor assays
  vWF Ag—immunoassay of total vWF protein
  vWF: RCof—bioassay of vWF that measures ability of patient plasma to support agglutination of normal platelets in the presence of ristocetin
  Factor VIII—coagulation assay of factor VIII bound and carried by plasma vWF
Platelet aggregometry
  Measures platelet aggregation in response to a panel of agonists, usually ADP, collagen, arachidonic acid, and epinephrine
Membrane glycoproteins
  Presence of glycoproteins Ib/IX and IIb/IIIa can be measured using monoclonal antibodies and flow cytometry
Platelet granule content
  Dense granules—electron microscopy or uptake and retention of radiolabeled serotonin
  Alpha granules—electron microscopy and/or immunoassays for platelet-associated proteins—vWF, fibrinogen, platelet factor 4

Note: vWF, von Willebrand factor; ADP, adenosine diphosphate; Ag, antigen, R:Cof, ristocetin cofactor.

longed bleeding time, (2) a reduction in plasma vWF concentration, (3) a parallel reduction in biologic activity as measured with the ristocetin cofactor assay, and (4) reduced factor VIII activity. The variability in laboratory tests is related to both the heterogeneous nature of the defects in vWD and the fact that plasma levels are influenced by ABO blood group type, central nervous system disorders, systemic inflammation, and pregnancy. Since vWD is an autosomal dominant disorder, some vWF is produced by the remaining normal allele. Thus patients with mild defects may have laboratory values that fluctuate over time and may occasionally be within the normal range.

There are three major types of vWD. Their mode of inheritance and laboratory findings are shown in Fig. 101-2. Patients with type I disease, the most common abnormality, have a mild to moderate decrease in plasma vWF. In the milder cases, although hemostasis is impaired, the vWF level is just below normal (50% activity, or 5 mg/L). In type I disease, vWF antigen, factor VIII activity, and ristocetin cofactor activity are decreased with a normal spectrum of multimers detected by sodium dodecyl sulfate (SDS)–agarose gel electrophoresis.

The variant forms of vWD (type II disease) are much less common and characterized by normal or near-normal levels of a dysfunctional protein. Patients with the type IIa variant of vWD have a deficiency in the high- and medium-molecular-weight forms of vWF multimer detected by SDS-agarose electrophoresis. This is due either to an inability to secrete the high-molecular-weight vWF multimers or to proteolysis of the multimers soon after they leave the endothelial cell and enter the circulation. Mutations in a localized region of the vWF A-2 domain have been identified in families with type IIa vWD (Fig. 101-3). The quantity of vWF antigen and the amount of associated factor VIII are usually normal. In the type IIb variant, high-molecular-weight multimers are also decreased; however, the decrease is due to the inappropriate binding of vWF to platelets. Intravascular platelet aggregates form that are rapidly cleared from the circulation, causing mild, variable thrombocytopenia. Mutations in a disulfide-bonded loop in the A-1 domain that binds to Gp Ib/IX are the cause of the type IIb defect (Fig. 101-3). A few patients have a platelet membrane disorder that mimics type IIb vWD—*platelet-type vWD*. It is due to mutations in the portion of Gp Ib/IX that interacts with vWF. Levels of total vWF antigen and factor VIII are normal.

Approximately 1 in 1 million individuals has a very severe form of vWD that is phenotypically recessive (type III disease). Type III patients are usually the offspring of two parents (usually asymptomatic) with mild type I disease. Type III patients may inherit a different abnormality from each parent (a doubly heterozygous or compound

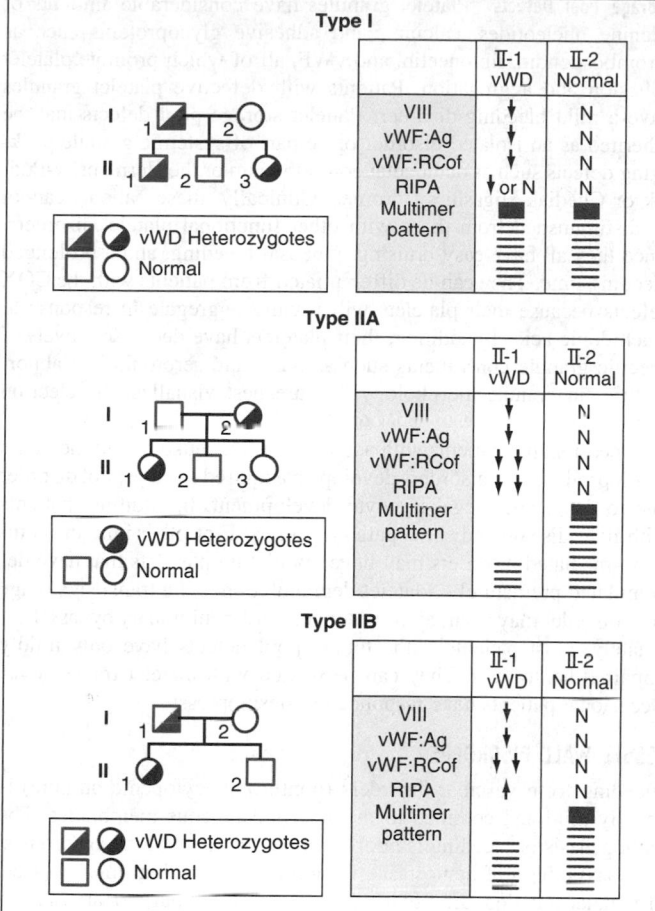

FIGURE 101-2 Pattern of inheritance and laboratory findings in von Willebrand's disease. The assays of platelet function include a coagulation assay of factor VIII bound and carried by von Willebrand factor (vWF), abbreviated as VIII; immunoassay of total vWF protein, abbreviated vWF:Ag; bioassay of the ability of patient plasma to support ristocetin-induced agglutination of normal platelets, abbreviated vWF:RCof; and ristocetin-induced aggregation of patient platelets, abbreviated RIPA. The multimer pattern illustrates the protein bonds present when plasma is electrophoresed in a polyacrylamide gel. The II-1 and II-2 columns refer to the phenotypes of the second-generation offspring.

heterozygous state) or be homozygous for a single defect. Type III patients have severe mucosal bleeding and no detectable vWF antigen or activity and, like patients with mild hemophilia, may have sufficiently low factor VIII that they have occasional hemarthroses. Major deletions in the vWF gene have been found in some type III families. Families with nonsense mutations and the combination of a deleted and nonsense mutant allele have also been described.

Type IIn disease is due to a defect in the factor VIII binding site of vWF. Patients resemble those with mild hemophilia and have low levels of factor VIII. The presence of disease in both males and females in a family is a clue to the role of vWF in this disease.

℞ TREATMENT

There are two therapeutic options. Factor VIII concentrates retain high-molecular-weight vWF multimers (Humate-P, Alfanate), are highly purified and heat-treated to destroy HIV, and are appropriate treatments for all the inherited forms of vWD. During surgery or after major trauma, patients should receive factor VIII concentrates twice daily for 2 to 3 days to assure optimal hemostasis. Minor bleeding episodes such as prolonged epistaxis or severe menorrhagia may respond to a single infusion. Recurrent menorrhagia, a major

problem for women with severe vWD, can be treated effectively with oral contraceptive agents that suppress menses.

A second therapeutic option, which avoids the use of plasma, is the use of desmopressin, a vasopressin analogue that has minimal blood pressure–elevating and fluid-retaining properties and raises the plasma vWF level in both normal individuals and patients with mild vWD. Patients with type I disease are the best candidates for desmopressin therapy. However, they must be tested for an adequate response before anticipated surgery, and vWF levels must be monitored closely during therapy, since the patient may develop tachyphylaxis when therapy is continued for >48 h. Desmopressin should not be given to patients with variant forms of vWD without prior testing, since it may not improve multimer pattern or homostasis in type IIa patients and may actually worsen the defect by depleting high-molecular-weight multimers, inducing intravascular platelet aggregation, and lowering the platelet count in type IIb patients. It is ineffective therapy for the severe (type III) form of vWD.

ACQUIRED vWD Although most cases of vWD are inherited, acquired vWD may be caused by antibodies that inhibit vWF function or by lymphoid or other tumors that selectively adsorb vWF multimers onto their surfaces. Anti-vWF antibodies have developed in patients with severe vWD following multiple transfusions, as well as in patients with autoimmune and lymphoproliferative disorders. Adsorption of vWF to tumor surfaces has been documented in patients with Waldenström's macroglobulinemia and Wilms' tumor and inferred in other patients with lymphoma. Treatment of acquired vWD should focus on the underlying disease, since plasma derivatives and desmopressin are often not effective and the disorder can be fatal.

Platelet Membrane Defects   Receptors that modulate platelet adhesion and aggregation are located on the two major platelet surface glycoproteins. vWF facilitates platelet adhesion by binding to Gp Ib/IX, while fibrinogen links platelets into aggregates via sites on the Gp IIb/IIIa complex. Two rare platelet defects are characterized by a loss of or a defect in these Gp receptors. Patients with the *Bernard-Soulier syndrome* have markedly reduced platelet adhesion and cannot bind vWF to their platelets due to deficiency or dysfunction of the Gp Ib/IX complex. They also have reduced levels of another membrane protein (GpV that associates with Gp Ib/II), mild thrombocytopenia, and extremely large, lymphocytoid platelets. Platelets from patients with *Glanzmann's disease*, or *thrombasthenia*, are deficient or defective in the Gp IIb/IIIa complex. Their platelets do not bind fibrinogen and cannot form aggregates, although the platelets undergo shape change and secretion and are of normal size.

Both these disorders are autosomal recessive traits and markedly

FIGURE 101-3 Location of mutations in types IIa and IIb von Willebrand's disease. Mutations in the region of the protein between amino acids 742 and 875 have been identified in patients with type IIa disease. These result in a deficiency in high- and medium-molecular-weight multimers due either to failure to secrete high-molecular-weight forms of von Willebrand factor (vWF) or to their proteolytic degradation in the circulation. In type IIb disease, there is also a decrease in high-molecular-weight vWF, but the defect is due to the failure of vWF with mutations in the A-1 domain of the protein (amino acids 509–695) to bind properly to platelet glycoprotein Ib/IX.

impair hemostasis, leading to recurrent episodes of severe mucosal hemorrhage. Bernard-Soulier platelets react normally to all stimuli except ristocetin. In contrast, thrombasthenic platelets adhere normally and will agglutinate with ristocetin but will not aggregate with any of the agonists that require fibrinogen binding, such as adenosine diphosphate (ADP), thrombin, or epinephrine.

The only effective therapy for hemorrhagic episodes in these two disorders is transfusion with normal platelets. Alloimmunization will eventually limit the life span of infused platelets. In addition, a few patients have developed inhibitor antibodies with specificity for the missing protein. These antibodies bind to the protein that is expressed on the transfused normal platelets and impair their function.

Platelet Release Defects   The most common mild bleeding disorders arise from the ingestion of aspirin and other nonsteroidal anti-inflammatory drugs (NSAIDs) that inhibit platelet production of thromboxane A_2, an important mediator of platelet secretion and aggregation (Figs. 53-3 and 53-4). These drugs inhibit cyclooxygenase (COX), which converts arachidonic acid to a labile endoperoxide intermediate that is critical for thromboxane formation. Aspirin is the most potent of these agents; it irreversibly acetylates the platelet enzyme so that a single dose impairs hemostasis for 5 to 7 days. The other agents are competitive and reversible inhibitors with more transient effects. Blocking thromboxane A_2 synthesis partially inhibits platelet release and aggregation with weak agonists, such as ADP and epinephrine, and produces a mild hemostatic defect. Cyclooxygenase exists in two isoforms, COX-1, which is constitutively expressed and active in the normal platelet, and COX-2, which is induced, especially in inflamed tissue. The selective COX-2 inhibitors, such as celecoxib, are increasingly being used to control arthritis pain and in other settings where NSAIDs are clinically useful. The COX-2 inhibitors are long-acting reversible inhibitors that have no adverse effects on platelet function. Their chronic use may be associated with high blood pressure and risk of thrombosis. The administration of high doses of certain antibiotics, particularly penicillin, can coat the platelet surface, block platelet release, and impair hemostasis.

Patients with release defects generally have minimal symptoms such as easy bruising, and bleeding is usually confined to the skin. Occasional patients will have prolonged oozing after surgery, particularly with procedures involving mucous membranes such as periodontal, oral, or reconstructive plastic surgery. The antiplatelet effect of drugs such as aspirin is more dramatic when they are administered to patients with underlying defects such as vWD or hemophilia. Patients with drug-induced COX deficiency often have a mildly prolonged bleeding time, and their platelets fail to aggregate when incubated with arachidonic acid, epinephrine, or low doses of ADP. Patients who have taken aspirin should be treated as if they have a mild hemostatic defect for the next 5 to 7 days. Platelet responses to collagen and thrombin are impaired at low doses but normal at higher doses. Symptomatic patients should be encouraged to use drugs such as acetaminophen that do not impair platelet function. Although most cases of COX deficiency are drug-induced, occasional patients have inherited disorders in platelet COX activity that impair thromboxane production or receptor level defects that prevent platelets from responding to thromboxane A_2.

Of the metabolic disorders that can perturb hemostasis, uremic platelet dysfunction is clinically the most important. The mechanism by which uremia impairs platelet function is not well understood, and retention of phenolic and guanidinosuccinic acids, excess prostacyclin production, or impaired vWF-platelet interactions have all been implicated. The degree of uremia correlates with bleeding symptoms and anemia. Bleeding can usually be reversed by dialysis and often improves after red cell transfusion or treatment with erythropoietin. In addition, factor VIII concentrate or desmopressin, both of which raise plasma vWF levels, can also improve hemostasis. Conjugated estrogens improve hemostasis and can be used as long-term therapy.

Storage Pool Defects   Platelet granules have considerable amounts of adenine nucleotides, calcium, and adhesive glycoproteins such as thrombospondin, fibronectin, and vWF, all of which promote platelet adhesion and aggregation. Patients with defective platelet granules have a mild bleeding disorder. Platelet storage pool defects may be inherited as an isolated disorder or be part of systemic granule packaging defects such as oculocutaneous albinism or the Hermansky-Pudlak or Chédiak-Higashi syndromes. Clinically, these patients cannot be distinguished from those with other functional platelet disorders, since they all have easy bruising, mucosal bleeding, and a prolonged bleeding time. They can be differentiated from patients with the COX defects because their platelets will usually aggregate in response to arachidonic acid. In addition, their platelets have decreased levels of specific granule constituents such as ADP and serotonin and abnormalities in granule morphology that are best visualized by electron microscopy.

Occasionally, patients with acute or chronic leukemia or one of the myeloproliferative disorders develop an acquired storage pool disorder due to dysplastic megakaryocyte development. In addition, patients with liver disease and some patients with SLE or other immune complex–mediated disorders may have circulating platelets that have degranulated prematurely. Platelet degranulation and a transient storage pool disorder may occur after prolonged cardiopulmonary bypass. Fortunately, most patients with storage pool defects have only mildly impaired hemostasis. They can be treated with platelet transfusions. Occasional patients have responded to desmopressin.

VESSEL WALL DISORDERS

Bleeding from vascular disorders (nonthrombocytopenic purpura) is usually mild and confined to the skin and mucous membranes. The pathogenesis of bleeding is poorly defined in many of the syndromes, and classic tests of hemostasis, including the bleeding time and tests of platelet function, are usually normal. Vascular purpura arises from damage to capillary endothelium, abnormalities in the vascular subendothelial matrix or extravascular connective tissues that support blood vessels, or from the formation of abnormal blood vessels. Several idiopathic disorders involve the vessel wall and can cause more severe bleeding and organ dysfunction.

THROMBOTIC THROMBOCYTOPENIC PURPURA   TTP is a fulminant, often lethal disorder that may be initiated by endothelial injury and subsequent release of vWF and other procoagulant materials from the endothelial cell. Causes include pregnancy, metastatic cancer, mitomycin C, high-dose chemotherapy, HIV infection, and certain drugs, such as the antiplatelet agent ticlopidine. Characteristic findings include the microvascular deposition of hyaline fibrin thrombi, thrombocytopenia, microangiopathic hemolytic anemia, fever, renal failure, fluctuating levels of consciousness, and evanescent focal neurologic deficits. The presence of hyaline thrombi in arterioles, capillaries, and venules without any inflammatory changes in the vessel wall is diagnostic. The presence of a severe Coombs-negative hemolytic anemia with schistocytes or fragmented red blood cells in the peripheral blood smear, coupled with thrombocytopenia, and minimal activation of the coagulation system help to confirm the clinical suspicion of TTP. This disorder should be distinguished from vasculitis and SLE, which can predispose patients to TTP. Platelet-associated IgG and complement levels are usually normal in TTP.

Clinical Manifestations   The classic pentad of TTP consists of hemolytic anemia with fragmentation of erythrocytes and signs of intravascular hemolysis, thrombocytopenia, diffuse and nonfocal neurologic findings, decreased renal function, and fever. These signs and symptoms occur variably, depending on the number and sites of the arteriolar lesions. The anemia may be very mild to very severe, and the thrombocytopenia often parallels it. The neurologic and renal symptoms are usually seen only when the platelet count is markedly diminished (<20 to $30 \times 10^3/\mu L$). Fever is not reliably present. TTP may be acute in onset, but its course spans days to weeks in most patients and occasionally continues for months. Proteinuria and a moderate elevation of blood urea nitrogen may be found on initial presentation; the latter continues to rise while urine output falls if the patient develops renal failure. Neurologic symptoms develop in >90% of patients whose disease terminates in death. Initially, changes in mental status such as confusion, delirium, or altered states of consciousness may occur. Focal findings include seizures, hemiparesis, aphasia, and visual field defects. These neurologic symptoms may fluctuate and terminate in coma. Involvement of myocardial blood vessels may be a cause of sudden death. The severity of the disorder can be estimated from the degree of anemia and thrombocytopenia and the serum lactic dehydrogenase level. Prothrombin time, partial thromboplastin time, fibrinogen concentration, and the level of fibrin split products are usually normal or only mildly abnormal. If the coagulation tests indicate a major consumption of clotting factors, the diagnosis of TTP is doubtful. A positive antinuclear antibody (ANA) determination is obtained in ~20% of patients.

Pathogenesis TTP is due to a deficiency in the activity of a specific metalloproteinase called *ADAMTS 13*, a normal plasma constituent that cleaves the ultra-high-molecular-weight (UHMW) forms of vWF secreted by endothelial cells to yield the heterogeneous set of multimers normally present in plasma (Fig. 101-4). A small number of patients have recurrent episodes of a TTP-like illness (*Upshaw-Schulman syndrome*) and are deficient in ADAMTS 13; the syndrome is inherited as an autosomal recessive trait. The more common acquired form of TTP is due to an inhibitory antibody that blocks ADAMTS 13 activity. These findings have led to more reliable diagnostic tests based on ADAMTS 13 enzyme activity and may have implications beyond TTP. Studies are underway to see if asymptomatic carriers with 50% levels of ADAMTS 13 are at increased risk of thromboembolism.

℞ TREATMENT

The treatment of acute TTP has focused on the use of exchange transfusion or intensive plasmapheresis coupled with infusion of fresh-frozen plasma. Therapy may remove abnormal forms of vWF, lower the concentration of ADAMTS 13 inhibitor, and replenish the deficient enzyme. Overall mortality has been markedly reduced, and the majority of patients with TTP recover from this formerly fatal disorder. Most patients surviving the acute illness recover completely, with no residual renal or neurologic disease. Occasional patients with a chronic, relapsing form of TTP require maintenance plasmapheresis and plasma infusion, and a few patients are controlled only with glucocorticoids. They presumably have persistence of the ADAMTS 13 inhibitor. In the future, TTP patients may be treated with some combination of enzyme replacement and immunosuppression to block inhibitor production.

HEMOLYTIC-UREMIC SYNDROME HUS is a disease of infancy and early childhood that closely resembles TTP. Patients present with fever, thrombocytopenia, microangiopathic hemolytic anemia, hypertension, and varying degrees of acute renal failure. In many cases, onset is preceded by a minor febrile or viral illness, and an infectious or immune complex–mediated cause has been proposed. Epidemics related to infection with a specific strain of *Escherichia coli* (O157:H7) have been documented. The bacteria contain a *Shigella*-like toxin that damages endothelial cells. As in TTP, DIC is not found. In contrast to TTP, the disorder remains localized to the kidney, where hyaline thrombi are seen in the afferent arterioles and glomerular capillaries. Thrombi are not present in other vessels, and neurologic symptoms, other than those associated with uremia, are uncommon. No therapy is proven effective; however, with dialysis for acute renal failure, the initial mortality is only 5% in children but may be higher in adults. Between 10 and 50% of patients have some chronic renal impairment. ADAMTS 13 levels are normal, and no inhibitors of the enzyme are present in this disorder.

HENOCH-SCHÖNLEIN PURPURA Henoch-Schönlein, or anaphylactoid, purpura is a distinct, self-limited type of vasculitis that occurs in children and young adults. Patients have an acute inflammatory reaction in capillaries, mesangial tissues, and small arterioles that leads to increased vascular permeability, exudation, and hemorrhage. Vessel lesions contain IgA and complement components. The syndrome may be preceded by an upper respiratory infection or streptococcal pharyngitis or be associated with food or drug allergies. Patients develop a purpuric or urticarial rash on the extensor surfaces of the arms and legs and on the buttocks as well as polyarthralgias or arthritis, colicky abdominal pain, and hematuria from focal glomerulonephritis. Despite the hemorrhagic features, all coagulation tests are normal. A small number of patients may develop fatal acute renal failure, and 5 to 10% develop chronic nephritis. Glucocorticoids provide symptomatic relief of the joint and abdominal pains but do not alter the course of the illness.

METABOLIC AND INFLAMMATORY DISORDERS Acute febrile illnesses may cause capillary fragility and skin bleeding. Immune complexes containing viral antigens or the viruses themselves may damage endothelial cells. In addition, certain pathogens such as the rickettsiae that cause Rocky Mountain spotted fever replicate in endothelial cells and damage them. Thrombocytopenia is also a frequent finding in acute infectious disorders and may contribute to skin bleeding. In addition, whenever the platelet count is <10,000/μL, gaps develop between endothelial cells, which allow the diapedesis of red cells into the dermis, forming petechiae. Drugs such as the sulfonamides, penicillin, and allopurinol may cause vascular inflammation, resulting in maculopapular or urticarial rashes. Some of these mechanisms are additive, and drug reactions in thrombocytopenic individuals cause an intensely hemorrhagic rash.

Occasionally, patients with diffuse polyclonal hyperglobulinemia will develop purpuric lesions on the lower limbs—a benign condition referred to as *hyperglobulinemic purpura*. Vascular purpura may occur in patients with various monoclonal gammopathies, including Waldenström's macroglobulinemia, multiple myeloma, and cryoglobuli-

vWF and Platelet Adhesion

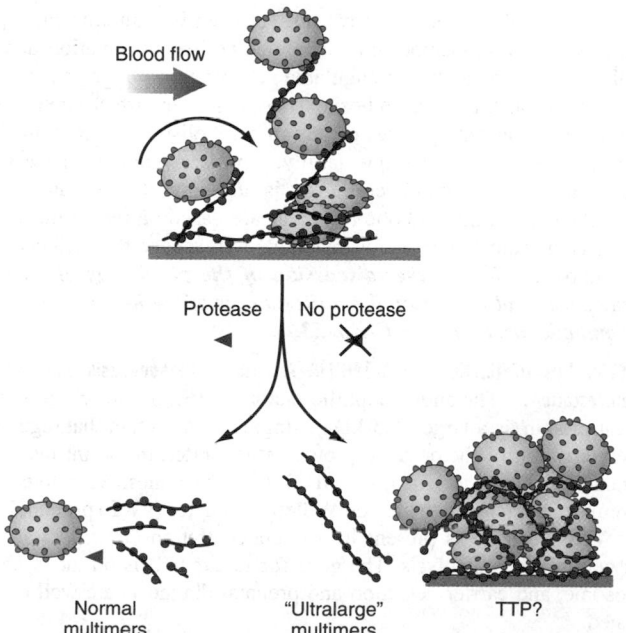

Blood flow

Protease   No protease

Normal multimers   "Ultralarge" multimers   TTP?

FIGURE 101-4 Pathogenesis of thrombotic thrombocytopenic purpura (TTP). Normally, the ultra-high-molecular-weight multimers of von Willebrand factor (vWF) produced by the endothelial cells are processed into smaller multimers by a plasma metalloproteinase called ADAMTS 13. In TTP, the activity of the protease is inhibited, and the ultra-high-molecular-weight multimers of vWF initiate platelet aggregation and thrombosis. (*From Vesely et al., Copyright American Society of Hematology.*)

nemia. These proteins markedly increase serum viscosity and may impair blood flow through capillaries and lead to retinal hemorrhage, central nervous system dysfunction, and skin necrosis. In addition, the globulins may impair platelet aggregation and adhesion and interfere with fibrin polymerization. Patients with mixed cryoglobulinemia develop a more extensive maculopapular lesion due to immune complex–mediated damage to the vessel wall. The mixed cryoglobulinemia (usually IgG and anti-IgG) may be associated with arthralgias, diffuse weakness, and unexplained nephritis. Plasmapheresis will temporarily lower the level of globulins, remove immune complexes, and improve symptoms in these patients. However, long-term management must include control of the underlying disease that produces the abnormal globulins or immune complexes.

Patients with *scurvy* (vitamin C deficiency) develop painful episodes of perifollicular skin bleeding as well as bleeding into muscles and, occasionally, into the gastrointestinal and genitourinary tracts. The diagnosis is confirmed by the presence of hyperkeratosis of skin, gum swelling, and low levels of the vitamin in leukocytes. Vitamin C is needed to synthesize hydroxyproline, an essential constituent of collagen. Thus, collagen synthesis is impaired by scurvy. Patients with *Cushing's syndrome*, an excess production of glucocorticoids, or patients on large doses of glucocorticoids develop generalized protein wasting and may show skin bleeding or easy bruising due to atrophy of the supporting connective tissue around blood vessels. Aging causes a similar atrophy of perivascular connective tissue on the extensor surfaces of the hands and arms, leading to *senile purpura*—dark purple, irregularly shaped hemorrhagic areas due to abnormal skin mobility that tears small blood vessels.

Patients with inherited disorders of the connective tissue matrix such as *Marfan's syndrome*, *Ehlers-Danlos syndrome*, and *pseudoxanthoma elasticum* also have easy bruising. In addition to having fragile skin vessels and easy bruising, patients with Ehlers-Danlos syndrome may develop aneurysms in intraabdominal vessels and apoplectic rupture and hemorrhage due to defects in the vascular collagen network. Primary vascular abnormalities can also lead to bleeding. Patients with *Osler-Rendu-Weber disease* [hereditary hemorrhagic telangiectasia (HHT)], an inherited autosomal dominant disorder, have frequent episodes of nasal and gastrointestinal bleeding from abnormal telangiectatic capillaries. They may develop pulmonary arteriovenous fistulas. Two genetic defects have been identified in these patients, both involving proteins that bind to transforming growth factor β (TGF-β); HHT-1 has mutations in endoglin, and HHT-2 has mutations in ALK-1. Patients with *angiodysplasia of the colon* have increased incidence of gastrointestinal bleeding. In the *Kasabach-Merritt syndrome*, patients may have very extensive and progressively enlarging vascular malformation that may involve large portions of their extremities. Bleeding is secondary to DIC triggered by stagnant blood flow through the tortuous vessels.

FURTHER READING

ALVING BM: How I treat heparin-induced thrombocytopenia and thrombosis. Blood 101:31, 2003

Guidelines for the investigation and management of idiopathic thrombocytopenic purpura in adults, children, and pregnancy. Br J Haematol 120:574, 2003

HANDIN RI, EWENSTEIN BM: von Willebrand's disease, in *Blood: Principles and Practice of Hematology*, 2d ed, RI Handin et al (eds). Philadelphia, Lippincott Williams & Wilkins, 2003, pp 1103–1130

VESELY SK et al: ADAMTS 13 activity in thrombotic thrombocytopenic purpura—hemolytic uremic syndrome: Relation to presenting features and clinical outcomes in a prospective cohort of 142 patients. Blood 102:60, 2003

————: Management of adult patients with persistent idiopathic thrombocytopenic purpura following splenectomy: A systematic review. Ann Intern Med 140:112, 2004

102   DISORDERS OF COAGULATION AND THROMBOSIS
Robert I. Handin

Patients with congenital plasma coagulation defects characteristically bleed into muscles, joints, and body cavities hours or days after an injury. Most of the *inherited* plasma coagulation disorders are due to defects in single coagulation proteins, with the two X-linked disorders, factors VIII and IX deficiency, accounting for the majority. These patients may have severe bleeding and chronic disability and require specialized medical therapy. With rare exceptions, the known disorders prolong either the prothrombin time (PT), partial thromboplastin time (PTT), or both. If they are abnormal, quantitative assays of specific coagulation proteins are then carried out using the PT or PTT tests with plasma from congenitally deficient individuals as substrate. The corrective effect of varying concentrations of patient plasma is measured and expressed as a percentage of a normal pooled plasma standard. The interval range for most coagulation factors is 50 to 150% of this average value, and the minimal level of most individual factors needed for adequate hemostasis is 25%.

Acquired coagulation disorders are both more frequent and more complex, arising from deficiencies of multiple coagulation proteins and simultaneously affecting both primary and secondary hemostasis. The most common acquired hemorrhagic disorders are (1) disseminated intravascular coagulation (DIC), (2) the hemorrhagic diathesis of liver disease, and (3) vitamin K deficiency and complications of anticoagulant therapy.

Although congenital and acquired bleeding disorders are relatively rare, venous and arterial thrombosis and embolism are common medical disorders that have been recognized for >100 years. Although risk factors such as atherosclerotic vascular disease, congestive heart failure, malignancy, and immobility predispose patients to thrombosis, specific coagulation defects have not yet been identified in most patients with thromboembolism. Several inherited coagulation abnormalities induce a hypercoagulable or prethrombotic state and predispose patients to thrombosis. These disorders affect young people, cause recurrent episodes of thromboembolism, and may involve multiple members of a single family. An understanding of the biochemical basis of thromboembolism is also important because anticoagulant and antithrombotic regimens are based on the premise that modifying critical coagulation reactions will reduce the incidence of thrombosis. →*For further discussion of the physiology of normal hemostasis and the cardinal manifestations of the hemorrhagic and thrombotic disorders, see Chap. 53.*

FACTOR VIII DEFICIENCY—HEMOPHILIA A   ■   **Pathogenesis and Clinical Manifestations**   The antihemophilic factor (AHF), or factor VIII coagulant protein, is a large (265-kDa), single-chain protein that regulates the activation of factor X by proteases generated in the intrinsic coagulation pathway (Figs. 53-6 and 53-7). It is synthesized in liver and circulates complexed to the von Willebrand factor (vWF) protein. Factor VIII molecule is present in low concentration (10 μg/L) and is susceptible to proteolysis. The gene for factor VIII is on the X chromosome, and carrier detection and prenatal diagnosis are well established.

One in 10,000 males is born with deficiency or dysfunction of the factor VIII molecule. The resulting disorder, *hemophilia A*, is characterized by bleeding into soft tissues, muscles, and weight-bearing joints. Symptomatic patients usually have factor VIII levels <5%, with a close correlation between the clinical severity of hemophilia and plasma AHF level. Patients with <1% factor VIII activity have *severe* disease; they bleed frequently even without discernible trauma. Patients with levels of 1 to 5% have *moderate* disease with less frequent bleeding episodes. Those with levels >5% have *mild* disease with infrequent bleeding that is usually secondary to trauma. Occasional patients with factor VIII levels as high as 25% are discovered when they bleed after major trauma or surgery. The majority of patients with hemophilia A have factor VIII levels <5%.

Hemophilic bleeding occurs hours or days after injury, can involve any organ, and, if untreated, may continue for days or weeks. This can result in large collections of partially clotted blood putting pressure on adjacent normal tissues and can cause necrosis of muscle (compartment syndromes), venous congestion (pseudophlebitis), or ischemic damage to nerves. Patients with hemophilia often develop femoral neuropathy due to pressure from an unsuspected retroperitoneal hematoma. They can also develop large calcified masses of blood and inflammatory tissue that are mistaken for cancers (pseudotumor syndrome).

Patients with severe hemophilia are usually diagnosed shortly after birth because of an extensive cephalhematoma or profuse bleeding at circumcision. However, young children with moderate disease may not bleed until they begin to walk or crawl, and individuals with mild hemophilia may not be diagnosed until they are adolescents or young adults. Typically, a hemophilia patient presents with pain followed by swelling in a weight-bearing joint, such as the hip, knee, or ankle. The presence of blood in the joint (*hemarthrosis*) causes synovial inflammation, and repetitive bleeding erodes articular cartilage and causes osteoarthritis, articular fibrosis, joint ankylosis, and eventually muscle atrophy. Bleeding may occur into any joint, but after a joint has been damaged, it may become a site for subsequent bleeding episodes.

Hematuria, without any genitourinary pathology, is also common. It is usually self-limited and may not require specific therapy. The most feared complications of hemophilia are oropharyngeal and central nervous system bleeding. Patients with oropharyngeal bleeding may require emergency intubation to maintain an adequate airway. Central nervous system bleeding can occur without antecedent trauma or without evidence of a specific lesion.

Patients suspected of having hemophilia should have a platelet count, bleeding time, PT, and PTT determination. Typically, the patient will have a prolonged PTT with all other tests normal. Because of the clinical similarity of factor VIII deficiency and factor IX deficiency, any male with an appropriate bleeding history and a prolonged PTT should have specific assays for factor VIII and factor IX.

℞ TREATMENT

Tenets regarding the treatment of bleeding in hemophilia patients include the following: (1) Symptoms often precede objective evidence of bleeding. (2) Signs of bleeding may not appear until several days after well-documented trauma. The patients can generally be relied upon to identify early symptoms, usually pain. Early treatment is more effective, less costly, and can be lifesaving. (3) Avoid the use of aspirin or aspirin-containing drugs, which impair platelet function and may cause severe hemorrhage. Cyclooxygenase inhibitors can be used, as they do not impair platelet function.

Plasma products enriched in factor VIII reduce the degree of orthopedic deformity and permit virtually any form of elective and emergency surgery. The widespread use of factor VIII concentrates has also produced serious complications, including viral hepatitis, chronic liver disease, and AIDS. *Cryoprecipitate*, which contains about half the factor VIII activity of fresh-frozen plasma in one-tenth the original volume, is simple to prepare and is produced in hospital or regional blood banks.

Three developments have increased the safety of factor VIII therapy and have changed medical practice. First, heating of lyophilized factor VIII concentrates under carefully controlled conditions can inactivate HIV without destroying factor VIII activity. Second, highly purified factor VIII can be produced by adsorbing and eluting factor VIII from monoclonal antibody columns. Third, recombinant factor

VIII is now available. Patients with hemophilia should receive either monoclonal purified or recombinant factor VIII to minimize viral infections and exposure to irrelevant proteins.

Each unit of factor VIII infused, defined as the amount present in 1 mL normal plasma, will raise the plasma level of the recipient by 2%/kg of body weight. Factor VIII has a half-life of 8 to 12 h, making it necessary to infuse it continuously or at least twice daily to sustain a chosen factor VIII level. In patients with mild hemophilia, an alternative treatment is desmopressin (DDAVP), which transiently increases the factor VIII level. Desmopressin will increase the factor level two- to threefold. Although generally safe, it occasionally causes hyponatremia or may precipitate thrombosis in elderly patients.

An uncomplicated episode of soft tissue bleeding or an early hemarthrosis can be treated with one infusion of sufficient factor VIII concentrate to raise the factor VIII level to 15 or 20%. A more extensive hemarthrosis or retroperitoneal bleeding requires twice-daily or continuous infusions in order to keep the factor VIII level at 25 to 50% for at least 72 h. Life-threatening bleeding into the central nervous system or major surgery may require therapy for 2 weeks with levels kept at a minimum of 50% normal. Patients also need skilled orthopedic care, with immobilization of inflamed joints to promote healing and to prevent contractures, and physical therapy to strengthen muscles and maintain joint mobility.

Before surgery, every hemophilia patient should be screened for the presence of an inhibitor to factor VIII. Patients with hemophilia who do not have an inhibitor should receive factor VIII infusions just before surgery and will require daily monitoring so that the factor VIII level is maintained >50% for 10 to 14 days after surgery. When patients undergo joint replacement or other major orthopedic surgery, therapy should be continued for 3 weeks to permit wound healing and the institution of physical therapy.

Hemophilia patients also require treatment before dental procedures. Filling of a carious tooth can be managed by a single infusion of factor VIII concentrate coupled with the administration of 4 to 6 g of ε-aminocaproic acid (EACA) four times daily for 3 to 4 days after the dental procedure. EACA is a potent antifibrinolytic agent that inhibits plasminogen activators present in oral secretions and stabilizes clot formation in oral tissue. Alternatives include tranexamic acid, a longer-acting antifibrinolytic. EACA is also effective when used as a mouthwash. For major oral and periodontal surgery and extractions of permanent teeth, patients should probably be hospitalized briefly and also treated with factor VIII concentrates. Therapy should begin just before surgery and continue for at least 2 to 3 days.

Many centers have organized home-care programs so that patients can administer their own factor VIII infusions with the onset of symptoms. Occasional patients with very frequent bleeding receive regularly scheduled infusions. Despite the expense and inconvenience of "prophylactic" infusions, their use in early childhood has reduced or eliminated hemarthroses. Concern about transmission of AIDS has made some patients reluctant to treat themselves, despite the fact that current blood products carry a very low or no risk of transmitting HIV.

The prospects for correcting factor VIII deficiency by gene therapy are promising; some success has been achieved in dogs. Clinical studies in humans are underway. Concerns about the side effects of current viral vectors used to deliver the factor VIII cDNA are slowing clinical trials.

Complications Most hemophilia patients have had multiple episodes of hepatitis, and a majority have elevated hepatocellular enzyme levels and abnormalities on liver biopsy. Donated blood is now being screened for various types of hepatitis, so the risk of this disease is diminishing. Between 10 and 20% of patients also have hepatosplenomegaly, and a small number develop chronic active or persistent hepatitis or cirrhosis. A few patients with hemophilia and end-stage liver disease have received liver transplants with cure of both diseases. Along with homosexuals and intravenous drug abusers, long-time hemophilia patients are at high risk for AIDS because they frequently received blood products before the era of testing them for HIV; they can also present with the full range of AIDS-related syndromes, including diffuse lymphadenopathy and immune thrombocytopenia. Although up to 50% of current multiply transfused hemophiliacs are HIV-positive and many have clinical AIDS, the advances in factor VIII concentrate production should prevent future HIV infection.

Despite frequent bleeding, severe iron-deficiency anemia is uncommon because most of the bleeding is internal and iron is effectively recycled. Mild iron deficiency from chronic epistaxis or gastrointestinal bleeding occurs in some patients. In addition, some patients have developed a mild Coombs-positive hemolytic anemia due to small amounts of anti-A and anti-B antibody that are present in intermediate purity factor VIII concentrates.

Following multiple transfusions, 10 to 20% of patients with severe hemophilia develop inhibitors to factor VIII. Inhibitors are usually IgG antibodies that rapidly neutralize factor VIII activity. Two types of inhibitors are found with different biologic characteristics and different clinical presentations. Patients with type I inhibitors have a typical anamnestic response and raise their antibody titer following exposure to factor VIII. Patients with a type II inhibitor have a low antibody titer that is not stimulated by factor VIII infusion. Patients with the type I inhibitor should not receive factor VIII. Control of bleeding may require the infusion of either porcine factor VIII concentrates, which may not be affected by inhibitors, or prothrombin complex concentrates, which contain trace quantities of activated coagulation factors and can bypass the block in coagulation produced by the inhibitor. Patients with low-titer type II antibodies may respond to higher doses of factor VIII. Another alternative is the infusion of recombinant factor VIIa; it activates factor X directly and bypasses the inhibitor-induced block.

Protocols to induce tolerance to human factor VIII use massive doses of the factor coupled with immunosuppression. Tolerance induction is expensive and not always effective; it should be reserved for severely affected patients.

Genetic Counseling and Carrier Detection   It is possible to trace the defective allele in some families by examining the inheritance of restriction fragment length polymorphisms (RFLP) linked to the factor VIII gene. In addition, in families in which a specific mutation has been defined in the factor VIII gene, it can be readily detected by gene amplification and allele-specific oligonucleotide hybridization. For example, 45% of patients with severe hemophilia A have a chromosomal inversion arising from homologous recombination between sequences in intron 22 and an upstream gene. The inversion is readily detected by polymerase chain reaction (PCR) or Southern blotting. Precise diagnosis is possible early in pregnancy from either chorionic villus biopsy or amniocentesis.

Female carriers of hemophilia, who are heterozygotes, usually produce sufficient factor VIII from the factor VIII allele on their normal X chromosome for normal hemostasis. However, occasional hemophilia carriers will have factor VIII levels far below 50% due to random inactivation of normal X chromosomes in tissue producing factor VIII. These symptomatic carriers may bleed with major surgery or bleed occasionally with menses. Rarely, true female hemophiliacs arise from consanguinity within families with hemophilia or from concomitant Turner's syndrome or XO mosaicism in a carrier female.

FACTOR IX DEFICIENCY—HEMOPHILIA B   Factor IX is a single-chain, 55-kDa proenzyme that is converted to an active protease (IXa) by factor XIa or by the tissue factor–VIIa complex. Factor IXa then activates factor X in conjunction with activated factor VIII. Factor IX is one of six proteins synthesized in the liver that require vitamin K for biologic activity. Vitamin K is a cofactor for a unique posttranslational modification that inserts a second carboxyl group onto certain glutamic acid residues on factor IX (Chap. 53). This modification permits calcium

binding and adsorption onto phospholipid surfaces. Factor IX gene is on the X chromosome.

Factor IX deficiency or dysfunction (hemophilia B, Christmas disease) occurs in 1 in 100,000 male births. Accurate laboratory diagnosis is critical, since it is indistinguishable clinically from factor VIII deficiency (hemophilia A) but requires different treatment. Either fresh-frozen plasma or a plasma fraction enriched in the prothrombin complex proteins is used. Monoclonally purified or recombinant factor IX preparations are now available. In addition to the expected complications of hepatitis, chronic liver disease, and AIDS, the therapy of factor IX deficiency has a special hazard. Trace quantities of activated coagulation factors in prothrombin complex concentrates may activate the coagulation system and cause thrombosis and embolism. This is particularly common in immobilized surgical patients and patients with liver disease. As a result, some centers have returned to fresh-frozen plasma for factor IX–deficient surgical patients, while others have recommended the addition of small doses of heparin to the concentrate to activate antithrombin III during the infusion and reduce hypercoagulability. The recombinant or monoclonally purified products are less likely to be thrombogenic.

FACTOR XI DEFICIENCY   Factor XI is a 160-kDa dimeric protein activated to an active protease (XIa) by factor XIIa, in conjunction with high-molecular-weight kininogen and kallikrein (Figs. 53-6 and 53-7). Factor XI deficiency is inherited as an autosomal recessive trait and is especially common in Ashkenazi Jews. In contrast to deficiency in factors VIII and IX, the correlation between factor level and propensity to bleed is not as precise, spontaneous bleeding is less, and hemarthroses are rare. Many patients with factor XI deficiency present with posttraumatic bleeding or with bleeding in the perioperative period, and occasional factor XI–deficient women have menorrhagia. Daily infusions of fresh-frozen plasma are sufficient, since the half-life of factor XI is approximately 24 h. The majority of defective factor XI alleles were accounted for by a limited number of mutations.

OTHER FACTOR DEFICIENCIES   Deficiencies in factors V, VII, X, and prothrombin (factor II) are exceedingly rare autosomal recessive disorders. Spontaneous or posttraumatic musculoskeletal bleeding or menorrhagia can occur with these deficiencies, but hemarthroses are uncommon. Fresh-frozen plasma is the appropriate therapy, although prothrombin concentrates may be employed for patients with severe prothrombin deficiency or decreases in factors VII and X as long as the risks of hepatitis and thrombosis are recognized.

Defects in the contact activation pathway involving Hageman factor (factor XII), high-molecular-weight kininogen, and prekallikrein cause laboratory abnormalities but no clinical bleeding. Despite dramatic prolongation of the PTT, often to greater than 100 s, deficient individuals have normal hemostasis and can undergo major surgery without plasma replacement therapy. Direct activation of factor IX by the tissue factor–VIIa complex may bypass this defective step in coagulation (Fig. 53-8). Patients with these disorders should neither be treated inappropriately with plasma nor denied indicated surgery on the basis of these laboratory abnormalities.

AFIBRINOGENEMIA AND DYSFIBRINOGENEMIA   Fibrinogen is a 340-kDa dimeric molecule made up of two sets of three covalently linked polypeptide chains. Thrombin sequentially cleaves fibrinopeptides A and B from the Aα and Bβ chains of fibrinogen to produce fibrin monomer, which then polymerizes to form a fibrin clot. Although fibrinogen is needed for platelet aggregation and fibrin formation, severe fibrinogen deficiency does not usually cause serious bleeding except after surgery. Patients with afibrinogenemia, who have no detectable fibrinogen in plasma or platelets, may have infrequent, mild bleeding episodes. Genetic analyses do not show any gross deletion or structural changes in the genes encoding the α, β, and γ chains of fibrinogen despite the total absence of plasma fibrinogen.

Fibrinogen is an abundant plasma protein (2.5 g/L). Mutations have been identified that alter the release of fibrinopeptides from the Aα and Bβ chains of fibrinogen, the rate of polymerization of fibrin monomers, and the sites for fibrin cross-linking. These dysfibrinogenemias are almost always inherited as autosomal dominant traits, so patients have nearly equal concentrations of normal and mutant fibrinogen in their plasma. Patients with dysfibrinogenemia have a slightly prolonged PT and PTT, a prolonged thrombin time, and a disparity in levels of fibrinogen measured with functional and immunologic assays. Despite these abnormalities, most patients have no symptoms or only moderate bleeding. A few dysfibrinogenemias induce a hypercoagulable state and increase the risk of thrombosis, and others have been associated with an increased incidence of abortion (Chap. 103). Some patients with liver disease, hepatomas, AIDS, and lymphoproliferative disorders develop an acquired form of dysfibrinogenemia.

FACTOR XIII DEFICIENCY AND DEFECTIVE FIBRIN CROSS-LINKING Factor XIII is a transglutaminase that stabilizes fibrin clots by forming ϵ-amino–γ-glutamyl cross-links between adjacent α and γ chains of fibrin. Factor XIII deficiency is an extremely rare inherited syndrome. Patients usually bleed in the neonatal period from their umbilical stump or circumcision. In addition to hemorrhage, these patients may have poor wound healing, a high incidence of infertility among males and abortion among affected females, and a high incidence of intracerebral hemorrhage. These observations suggest that the enzyme may be important in other physiologic processes beyond hemostasis, including placental implantation, spermatogenesis, and wound healing. Several drugs, including isoniazid, may bind to cross-linking sites on fibrinogen and mimic factor XIII deficiency by blocking enzyme activity. Normal hemostasis requires only 1% of normal enzyme activity; a single infusion of fresh-frozen plasma or a purified factor XIII–rich product derived from human placenta called Fibrogammin is effective. Factor XIII has a 14-day half-life.

VITAMIN K DEFICIENCY Vitamin K is a fat-soluble vitamin that plays a critical role in hemostasis. Dietary vitamin K is absorbed in the small intestine and stored in the liver. The vitamin is also synthesized by endogenous bacterial flora in the small intestine and colon; however, the quantity of endogenous vitamin K absorbed from the large intestine is debated. Following absorption, vitamin K is converted to an active epoxide in liver microsomes and serves as a cofactor in the enzymatic carboxylation of glutamic acid residues on prothrombin complex proteins (Fig. 102-1).

The three major causes of vitamin K deficiency are inadequate dietary intake, intestinal malabsorption, and loss of storage sites due to hepatocellular disease. Neonatal vitamin K deficiency, which causes hemorrhagic disease of the newborn, has disappeared from western countries with the routine administration of vitamin K to all newborn infants. Although a 30-day supply of vitamin K is stored in the normal liver, acutely ill patients can become deficient within 7 to 10 days. Acute vitamin K deficiency is particularly common in patients recovering from biliary tract surgery who have no dietary intake of vitamin K, have T-tube drainage of bile, and are on broad-spectrum antibiotics. Vitamin K deficiency is also seen in chronic liver disease, particularly primary biliary cirrhosis, and in some malabsorption states (Chaps. 275 and 286). The cephalosporins inhibit the reduction and recycling of vitamin K, much like warfarin.

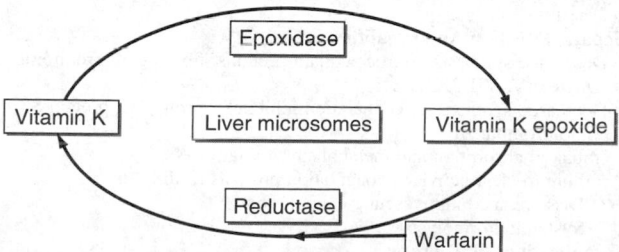

FIGURE 102-1 The mechanism of action of vitamin K, a cofactor in the formation of di-γ-carboxyglutamic acid residues on coagulation proteins, is depicted. Vitamin K is converted to an epoxide in liver microsomes. The epoxide is the active form and is reduced back to vitamin K by a liver membrane reductase. Warfarin blocks the action of the reductase and competitively inhibits the effects of vitamin K.

With vitamin K deficiency, plasma levels of all the prothrombin complex proteins (factors II, VII, IX, X; proteins C and S) decrease. Those with the shortest half-lives, factor VII and protein C, decrease first. Because of the rapid fall in factor VII, patients with mild vitamin K deficiency may have a prolonged PT and a normal PTT. Later, as the levels of the other factors fall, the PTT will also become prolonged. Parenteral administration of 10 mg vitamin K rapidly restores vitamin K levels in the liver and permits normal production of prothrombin complex proteins within 8 to 10 h. Severe hemorrhage can be treated with fresh-frozen plasma, which immediately corrects the hemostatic defect. If the cause of vitamin K deficiency cannot be eliminated, patients may need monthly injections. Purified prothrombin complex concentrates should be avoided because they contain trace quantities of activated forms of the prothrombin complex proteins and can cause thrombosis in patients with liver disease. They also carry an increased risk of hepatitis.

DISSEMINATED INTRAVASCULAR COAGULATION DIC can be either an explosive and life-threatening bleeding disorder or a relatively mild or subclinical disorder. Although a long list of diseases can be complicated by DIC, it is most frequently associated with obstetric catastrophes, metastatic malignancy, massive trauma, and bacterial sepsis (Table 102-1). Tentative triggering mechanisms have been identified. Tumors and traumatized or necrotic tissue release tissue factor into the circulation. Endotoxin from gram-negative bacteria activates several steps in the coagulation cascade. In addition to a direct effect on the activation of Hageman factor (factor XII), endotoxin induces the expression of tissue factor on the surface of monocytes and endothelial cells. These activated cell surfaces then accelerate coagulation reactions. These potent thrombogenic stimuli cause the deposition of small thrombi and emboli throughout the microvasculature. This early thrombotic phase of DIC is then followed by a phase of procoagulant consumption and secondary fibrinolysis. Continued fibrin formation and fibrinolysis lead to hemorrhage from the coagulation factor and platelet depletion and the antihemostatic effects of fibrin degradation products (Fig. 102-2).

The clinical presentation varies with the stage and severity of the

TABLE 102-1 Etiologic Factors and Disorders Causing Disseminated Intravascular Coagulation

Liberation of tissue factors	Obstetric syndromes—abruptio placentae, amniotic fluid embolism, retained dead fetus, second trimester abortion
	Hemolysis
	Neoplasms, particularly mucinous adenocarcinomas, acute promyelocytic leukemia
	Intravascular hemolysis
	Fat embolism
	Tissue damage—burns, frostbite, head injury, gunshot wounds
Endothelial damage	Aortic aneurysm
	Hemolytic uremic syndrome
	Acute glomerulonephritis
	Rocky Mountain spotted fever
Vascular malformation, decreased blood flow	Kasabach-Merritt syndrome
Infections	
	Bacterial: staphylococci, streptococci, pneumococci, meningococci, gram-negative bacilli
	Viral: arboviruses, varicella, variola, rubella
	Parasitic: malaria, kala-azar
	Rickettsial: Rocky Mountain spotted fever
	Mycotic: acute histoplasmosis

Source: Modified from RI Handin, RD Rosenberg, in *Hematology*, 4th ed, WS Beck (ed), Cambridge, MA, MIT Press, 1985.

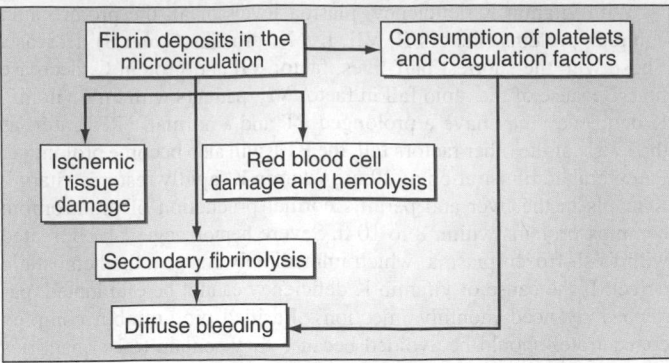

FIGURE 102-2   The pathophysiology of disseminated intravascular coagulation (DIC). Shown are the interactions between coagulation and fibrinolytic pathways that result in bleeding in patients with DIC.

syndrome. Most patients have extensive skin and mucous membrane bleeding and hemorrhage from surgical incisions or venipuncture or catheter sites. Less often, patients present with peripheral acrocyanosis, thrombosis, and pregangrenous changes in digits, genitalia, and nose—areas where blood flow is markedly reduced by vasospasm or microthrombi. Some patients, particularly those with chronic DIC and malignancy, have laboratory abnormalities without any evidence of thrombosis or hemorrhage.

The laboratory manifestations include thrombocytopenia and the presence of schistocytes or fragmented red blood cells that arise from cell trapping and damage within fibrin thrombi; prolonged PT and PTT and thrombin time and a reduced fibrinogen level from depletion of coagulation proteins; and elevated fibrin degradation products (FDP) from intense secondary fibrinolysis. The D dimer immunoassay, which measures cross-linked fibrin derivatives (i.e., those that have been in blood clots), is a more specific FDP assay. Low fibrinogen levels in DIC predict more bleeding.

Rx TREATMENT

DIC, although sometimes indolent, can cause life-threatening hemorrhage and may require emergency treatment including (1) an attempt to correct any reversible cause of DIC; (2) measures to control the major symptom, either bleeding or thrombosis; and (3) a prophylactic regimen to prevent recurrence in cases of chronic DIC. Treatment will vary with the clinical presentation. In patients with an obstetric complication such as abruptio placentae or acute bacterial sepsis, prompt delivery of the fetus and placenta or treatment with appropriate antibiotics will reverse the DIC syndrome. In patients with metastatic tumor causing DIC, control of the primary disease may not be possible, and long-term prophylaxis may be necessary.

Patients with bleeding as a major symptom should receive fresh-frozen plasma to replace depleted clotting factors and platelet concentrates to correct thrombocytopenia. Those with acrocyanosis and incipient gangrene or other thrombotic problems need immediate anticoagulation with intravenous heparin. The use of heparin in the treatment of bleeding is still controversial. Although it is a logical way to reduce thrombin generation and prevent further consumption of clotting proteins, it should be reserved for patients with thrombosis or who continue to bleed despite vigorous treatment with plasma and platelets.

Patients who initially have mild asymptomatic DIC may begin to bleed following surgery or chemotherapy. For example, mild DIC, without clinical bleeding, has been documented during saline- or prostaglandin-induced midtrimester abortions. Prophylactic treatment of patients with heparin may prevent progression of a mild DIC syndrome and has been used in the treatment of patients with acute promyelocytic leukemia and in some patients with a retained dead fetus who require surgical extraction. However, most patients with low-grade DIC can be managed with plasma and platelet replacement and do not require

heparin. Chronic DIC does not respond to oral warfarin anticoagulants, but it can be controlled with long-term heparin infusion. Occasional patients with indolent tumors and severe DIC have been maintained on heparin administered by intermittent subcutaneous injection or continuous infusion with portable pumps.

Despite our detailed understanding of the pathophysiology of DIC and a vigorous approach to therapy, treatment does not usually change the natural history of the underlying disorder. Therapy will only stabilize the patient, prevent exsanguination or massive thrombosis, and permit institution of definitive therapy.

COAGULATION DISORDERS IN LIVER DISEASE   Liver dysfunction is frequently accompanied by a hemostatic defect. The major causes of hemorrhage in patients with liver disease are shown in Table 102-2. Bleeding is usually due to an anatomic lesion that is exacerbated by a hemostatic defect. Most patients bleed from complications of portal hypertension, esophageal varices, or gastritis and peptic ulcer disease. Portal hypertension also causes splenomegaly, with splenic sequestration of platelets and thrombocytopenia, which contributes to the hemostatic defect.

Patients with hepatocellular liver disease cannot store vitamin K optimally and may have some degree of vitamin K deficiency. Cholestasis, a frequent feature of liver disease, impairs vitamin K absorption and further decreases liver vitamin K stores. Abnormalities in the γ-carboxylation of prothrombin complex proteins independent of vitamin K and the production of abnormal proteins have also been described. Patients may also have decreased production of other coagulation proteins, including fibrinogen and factor V. The liver also produces inhibitors of coagulation such as antithrombin III and proteins C and S and is the clearance site for activated coagulation factors and fibrinolytic enzymes. Thus patients with liver disease are also "hypercoagulable" and predisposed to developing DIC or systemic fibrinolysis. Coagulation defects in advanced liver failure are often difficult to distinguish from those of DIC.

Each patient with hemorrhage and liver disease should have a PT, PTT, platelet count, and fibrinogen determination, although it is not always possible to determine the major hemostatic abnormality from a single set of laboratory values. It is helpful to have previous laboratory data available for patients with chronic liver disease who develop an acute complication. The degree of prolongation of the PT predicts the risk of bleeding. Most patients present with moderate prolongation of the PT and PTT, mild thrombocytopenia, and a normal fibrinogen level. However, they may also present with a more complex defect combining defective synthesis, abnormal clearance, and active consumption of coagulation proteins. Since vitamin K deficiency is so common, a single parenteral dose of vitamin K is given after initial

---

TABLE 102-2   *Causes of Bleeding in Liver Disease*

Anatomic Factors
  Portal hypertension
    Varices
    Splenomegaly and secondary thrombocytopenia
  Peptic ulceration
  Gastritis
Hepatic Function Abnormalities
  Decreased synthesis of procoagulant proteins: fibrinogen, prothrombin,
    factors V, VII, IX, X, XI
  Decreased synthesis of coagulation inhibitors: protein C, protein S,
    antithrombin III
  Impaired absorption and metabolism of vitamin K
  Failure to clear activated coagulation proteins leading to:
    Disseminated intravascular coagulation
    Systemic fibrinolysis
Complications of Therapy
  Dilution of platelets and coagulation proteins from massive
    transfusions
  Infusion of activated coagulation proteins in prothrombin complex
    concentrates
  Bleeding from heparin; thrombosis from ε-aminocaproic acid (EACA)

laboratory studies have been obtained, even though this may only partially correct the laboratory abnormalities. The presence of severe thrombocytopenia or a low fibrinogen level suggests the additional complication of DIC and may require further studies and therapy.

The safest replacement therapy for a patient with liver disease is fresh-frozen plasma, since it supplies all known coagulation factors. However, even this form of therapy has drawbacks, since large quantities of plasma may precipitate hepatic encephalopathy and cause fluid and sodium overload. Prothrombin complex concentrates should be avoided because they replace only the vitamin K–dependent factors, may be contaminated with hepatitis and AIDS virus, and contain trace quantities of activated coagulation proteins. Similarly, fibrinogen concentrates (or cryoprecipitate), rich in factor VIII and fibrinogen, should not be used without additional fresh-frozen plasma. Anticoagulation with heparin has been advocated to control DIC, but this is particularly hazardous and not recommended in cirrhosis because heparin is metabolized erratically and may lead to severe bleeding.

FIBRINOLYTIC DEFECTS   Bleeding can also occur from defects in the fibrinolytic system. Patients with α_2 plasmin inhibitor deficiency or plasminogen activator inhibitor (PAI) 1 have rapid fibrinolysis following fibrin deposition after trauma or surgery and may experience recurrent hemorrhage. Similarly, patients with cirrhosis have an impaired clearance of tissue plasminogen activator (tPA) and systemic fibrinolysis that may contribute to their hemorrhagic defect. Rarely, patients with tumors such as metastatic prostatic cancer may develop diffuse bleeding from primary fibrinolysis rather than DIC. Clues to the diagnosis include a disproportionately low fibrinogen level with a relatively normal PT and PTT and the presence of a normal or nearly normal platelet count. With rare exceptions, patients with primary fibrinolysis should have an elevated titer of FDP but a normal D dimer level. However, it is sometimes difficult or impossible to differentiate primary fibrinolysis from the secondary fibrinolysis in DIC. Patients with clearly established primary fibrinolysis should not receive heparin; they require plasma therapy and, occasionally, fibrinolytic inhibitors such as EACA. However, EACA should not be given to patients suspected of having DIC unless they are also receiving heparin, since EACA can cause massive, often fatal, thrombosis in a patient with DIC.

CIRCULATING ANTICOAGULANTS   Circulating anticoagulants, or inhibitors, are usually IgG antibodies that interfere with coagulation reactions. Specific inhibitors inactivate individual coagulation proteins and may cause severe hemorrhage. They arise in 15 to 20% of patients with factor VIII or factor IX deficiency who have received plasma infusions. *Specific* inhibitors also occur in previously normal individuals. Although the most common target protein is factor VIII, inhibitors with specificity for each of the coagulation proteins occur. In addition to hemophiliacs, anti-factor VIII antibodies are seen in postpartum females, in patients on various drugs, as part of the spectrum of autoantibodies in systemic lupus erythematosus (SLE) patients, and in normal elderly individuals. Circulating anticoagulants also occur in patients with AIDS.

Nonspecific (lupus-like) inhibitors prolong coagulation tests by binding to phospholipids. They are assayed by their anticoagulant effect [lupus anticoagulant (LA) activity] or their ability to bind to the complex phospholipid cardiolipin [anticardiolipin antibody (ACLA) activity]. While most often encountered in patients with SLE, these nonspecific inhibitors may develop in patients with many other disorders and also in otherwise normal individuals.

The critical laboratory feature that identifies the presence of either type of inhibitor is the failure of normal plasma to correct a prolonged PT, PTT, or both. Plasma from patients with a specific inhibitor will progressively inactivate a coagulation protein and thus prolong whichever of these screening tests requires the participation of that clotting factor. This effect persists after dilution. Nonspecific inhibitors immediately prolong the PT and PTT and, at low dilution, block multiple coagulation reactions. However, these effects can be overcome by altering the quantity or type of phospholipid or by diluting the plasma.

Hemorrhage in patients with specific inhibitors may require treatment with massive plasma or concentrate infusion, the use of activated prothrombin complex concentrates to bypass the antibodies against factors VIII or IX, and plasmapheresis or exchange transfusion to lower antibody titer. Chronic immunosuppressive regimens have been particularly useful in otherwise normal individuals with an acquired factor VIII antibody. Many patients lose their antibody and recover within 6 to 12 months, although the acute mortality rate from bleeding may approach 10%.

Patients with LA activity have normal hemostasis and will not bleed unless they have concomitant thrombocytopenia or prothrombin deficiency. Both thrombocytopenia and hypoprothrombinemia are secondary to autoantibodies that bind either to platelets or the prothrombin molecule. While these antibodies have no effect on function, they accelerate clearance of the coated platelets or the antibody-prothrombin complexes.

The presence of LA activity may predispose patients to venous and arterial thromboembolism and may cause midtrimester abortions. However, the risk of thrombosis is difficult to estimate, and the appropriate therapy for individual patients difficult to choose. Tests for either LA or ACLA activity are not well standardized, and results vary among and within patients. The best predictor is a consistent prolongation of more than one coagulation test coupled with a high titer of ACLA activity. Second, the risk of thrombosis is increased in patients who have SLE compared with those with idiopathic LA or ACLA activity. Prophylactic therapy is not clearly beneficial, and treatments aimed at reducing the titer of antibody are not superior to conventional antithrombotic therapy.

Therapy should be individualized. Patients with SLE and either LA or ACLA activity who have had a thrombotic episode are at high risk for a recurrence and should receive long-term anticoagulant therapy. Women who have had more than one midtrimester abortion, especially those with SLE, should have a trial of anticoagulant therapy. Patients with a single thrombotic episode (stroke or pulmonary embolus) and no other risk factor except LA or ACLA activity should be treated. No consensus has been reached about treatment after an initial minor event [deep venous thrombosis (DVT)]. Asymptomatic patients with only laboratory abnormalities should not be treated. Glucocorticoids should be administered only in conjunction with antithrombotic agents and are not of proven efficacy.

INHERITED PROTHROMBOTIC DISORDERS   Coagulation is carefully regulated by a series of inhibitors that limit thrombin generation and fibrin formation and by the fibrinolytic system, which effectively removes fibrin thrombi (Figs. 53-6 and 53-7). Inherited defects in the natural coagulation inhibitors (i.e., antithrombin, proteins C and S), abnormalities in the fibrinolytic system, and certain dysfibrinogenemias predispose patients to thrombosis (Table 53-5). A single point mutation in the factor V gene (factor V Leiden), which converts arginine 506 to glutamine and makes the molecule resistant to degradation by activated protein C, may account for 25% of inherited prethrombotic states. Antithrombin, protein C, and protein S defects are all autosomal dominant traits, so heterozygous individuals, who have a 50% reduction in protein concentration or a mixture of mutant and normal molecules, will have an increased risk of thrombosis. The patients have similar clinical presentations with a strong family history of thrombosis, episodes of recurrent venous thromboembolism, and symptoms by their early twenties. Any patient with this distinctive history should be tested for specific abnormalities.

ANTITHROMBIN DEFICIENCY   Antithrombin complexes with activated coagulation proteins and blocks their biologic activity (Fig. 53-6). The rate of this reaction is enhanced by heparin-like molecules within the vessel wall or on endothelial cells. Plasma antithrombin III content is 5 to 15 mg/L (50 to 150%), with values only slightly below normal increasing the risk of thrombosis. For optimal screening, the antithrombin III concentration is measured by immunoassay and the plasma antithrombin and heparin cofactor activity assessed with functional assays. The most common defect (1 in 2000 indidivuals) is mild (heterozygous) antithrombin deficiency. Dysfunctional antithrombin molecules with mutations affecting either the serine protease or heparin-binding site or activation of inhibitor by heparin have also been described.

Patients with antithrombin deficiency who develop acute thrombosis or embolism can be treated with intravenous heparin, since there is usually sufficient normal antithrombin to act as a heparin cofactor. Following their first episode of thromboembolism, patients should be placed on oral anticoagulants for life to prevent recurrent thrombosis. Family studies should be conducted when an antithrombin-deficient individual is discovered, since up to half the members of a kindred may be affected. Asymptomatic individuals with antithrombin deficiency should receive prophylactic anticoagulation with heparin or plasma infusions to raise their antithrombin level before medical or surgical procedures that may increase their risk of thrombosis. Chronic oral anticoagulation is not recommended until individuals at risk have a thrombotic episode.

DEFICIENCIES OF PROTEINS C AND S   Protein C is a vitamin K–dependent hepatic protein that binds to the endothelial cell surface protein thrombomodulin and is converted to an active protease by thrombin (Fig. 53-6). Activated protein C, in conjunction with protein S, proteolyzes factors Va and VIIIa, which shuts off fibrin formation. Activated protein C may also stimulate fibrinolysis and accelerate clot lysis. Deficiencies of proteins C and S are usually autosomal dominant disorders, and deficiencies in the two proteins cause an identical syndrome of recurrent venous thrombosis and pulmonary embolism. Dysfunctional molecules have also been identified in some patients with thrombosis. Rare patients with homozygous protein C deficiency have fulminant neonatal intravascular coagulation and require prompt diagnosis and treatment.

The correlation between levels of proteins C and S and the risk of thrombosis is not as precise as for antithrombin III deficiency. In fact, some asymptomatic individuals with protein C "deficiency" have been discovered. In some well-studied protein C–deficient kindreds, asymptomatic individuals may have protein C levels as low as or lower than relatives with recurrent thrombosis. It is possible that an undiscovered cofactor is present in symptomatic patients. Finally, since a fraction of the available protein S is bound to C4b-binding protein and is unavailable for coagulation reactions, both free and total protein S levels or C4b-binding protein levels should be assessed for maximum accuracy.

Heterozygous patients with protein C or S deficiencies who develop acute thrombosis should be heparinized and then placed on oral anticoagulants. There are, however, two potential problems with the use of warfarin anticoagulants in these patients. First, these vitamin K antagonists (Fig. 102-1), which lower the level of the procoagulant factors II, VII, IX, and X, may also reduce the concentration of proteins C and S sufficiently to nullify the desired antithrombotic effect. In addition, patients who are protein C–deficient may develop warfarin-induced skin necrosis; this defect may predispose patients to a rare but serious complication. Patients with homozygous protein C deficiency require periodic plasma infusions rather than oral anticoagulants to prevent recurrent intravascular coagulation and thrombosis.

RESISTANCE TO ACTIVATED PROTEIN C AND THE FACTOR V LEIDEN MUTATION
Some patients with familial or recurrent venous thromboembolism were found not to prolong their PTT when activated protein C was added to their plasma. These patients were found to have an identical mutation in which arginine 506 in factor V is converted to glutamine. This amino acid substitution abolishes a protein C cleavage site in factor V and thus prolongs the thrombogenic effect of factor V activation. About 3% of the population worldwide is heterozygous for this mutation. The mutation is absent in certain populations, e.g., Asians,

TABLE 102-3   *Relationship between Coagulation Defect and Site of Thrombosis*

Abnormality	Arterial	Venous
Factor V Leiden R506 Q	−	+
Prothrombin G20210A	−	+
Antithrombin III	−	+
Protein C	−	+
Protein S	−	+
Homocysteinemia	+	+
Antiphospholipid antibody[a]	+	+

[a] Anticardiolipin antibody—lupus anticoagulant.

African Americans, and Native Americans. It may account for 25% of patients with recurrent DVT or pulmonary embolism.

Heterozygosity at this allele increases an individual's lifetime risk of venous thromboembolism sevenfold. The risk rises steadily with age. A homozygote has a twentyfold increased risk of thrombosis. Heterozygosity coupled with ingestion of oral contraceptives or pregnancy increases the risk at least fifteenfold. Coinheritance of factor V Leiden and another low-penetrance defect such as protein C or S deficiency is also additive. Many previous studies of risk factors predisposing patients to venous thromboembolism are being reevaluated to take into account this common mutation.

PROTHROMBIN GENE MUTATION   A specific point mutation in the prothrombin gene [conversion of G to A at position 20210 (G20210A)] also predisposes to venous thrombosis and embolism. This mutation is in the 3′-untranslated region of the gene and results in a 30% increase in plasma prothrombin levels, either through more efficient translation or greater stability of the message. Heterozygotes account for ~18% of cases with family histories of venous thrombosis and 6% of patients with first episodes of DVT.

The inheritance of multiple mutations increases the risk of thrombosis. The relationship between known mutations and the type of thrombosis is shown in Table 102-3. The fraction of patients with DVT with known mutations is shown in Table 102-4.

℞ TREATMENT

Patients who develop venous thromboembolism without a clear predisposing factor, have a strong family history, present under age 30, or have more than one episode should have assays for antithrombin III, proteins C and S, and factor V Leiden. Patients who present with DVT or pulmonary embolism during pregnancy or while using oral contraceptives have a 30% chance of having factor V Leiden.

Treatment recommendations for patients with the inherited prethrombotic disorders are still evolving. All patients should receive standard initial therapy with heparin, either conventional or low dose (Chap. 103), followed by 3 months of oral warfarin. This regimen should allow for maximal healing and reendothelialization of the thrombosed vessels and minimize recurrence in the damaged vascular beds. It is not clear which patients should go on to receive long-term (perhaps lifelong) anticoagulation, a judgment that depends on assessing the risk/benefit ratio.

Patients with antithrombin III deficiency who become symptomatic have a high likelihood of recurrent events and should be placed on lifelong anticoagulation. Patients with protein C or S deficiency or heterozygous factor V Leiden and prothrombin G20210A patients have a lower likelihood of recurrent disease. Long-term anticoagula-

TABLE 102-4   *Prevalence of Coagulation Defects in Patients with Venous Thrombosis*

Defect	Prevalence, %
Factor V Leiden (Arg506Gln) R506 Q	12–40
Hyperhomocysteinemia	10–20
Prothrombin G20210A	6–18
Deficiencies of antithrombin III, proteins C and S	5–15
Antiphospholipid antibody syndrome	10–20

tion should be reserved until their second or subsequent episode of thromboembolism. Homozygous factor V Leiden patients should be placed on long-term anticoagulation after their initial episode, and all patients should receive replacement therapy or receive heparin prophylaxis during surgery or after trauma; women with these defects should avoid the use of oral contraceptives. The asymptomatic relatives of patients shown to have these disorders should be screened to determine if they have inherited the defective gene. If so, they should receive appropriate prophylaxis but not start anticoagulation until they are symptomatic. In the absence of a congenital defect predisposing a patient to thrombosis, recurring or migratory thrombophlebitis may indicate an underlying malignancy.

DYSFIBRINOGENEMIAS AND FIBRINOLYTIC DEFECTS Recurrent venous thrombosis and embolism may be due to familial defects in fibrinogen or plasminogen or decreased synthesis or release of tPA. While most dysfibrinogenemias cause bleeding, several variants have excessively rapid release of fibrinopeptides and recurrent thromboembolism. Patients with this disorder and those with an abnormal plasminogen that resists activation by streptokinase and urokinase have been treated successfully with heparin and oral anticoagulants. Defects in tPA content or release have not been completely characterized. One group of patients with recurrent venous thrombosis and embolism failed to increase venous blood fibrinolytic activity when challenged with local ischemia or physical exercise. The other group had impaired fibrinolytic activity in extracts prepared from biopsied veins. Young patients with acute myocardial infarction may have impaired fibrinolysis due to increased plasma levels of PAI, a serine protease inhibitor that binds to tPA and is derived from endothelial cells.

Many common illnesses are associated with an increased risk of thrombosis (Table 53-5). These patients are said to have a "hypercoagulable" or "prethrombotic" state. This increased risk is seen in patients with chronic congestive heart failure and metastatic cancer and in patients undergoing major surgery. The generation of tissue factor activity in damaged or ischemic tissue or metastatic tumor, coupled with venous stasis and endothelial injury, induces the formation of venous and, more rarely, arterial thrombi. Several hematologic disorders, paroxysmal nocturnal hemoglobinuria, essential thrombocythemia, and polycythemia vera predispose patients to venous and arterial thrombosis through diverse mechanisms related to increased blood viscosity and abnormal blood cells. Diseases that affect the endothelial cell, such as Behçet's syndrome, Kawasaki's disease, and homocystinuria, or the administration of drugs such as oral contraceptives, which lower antithrombin III levels, or L-asparaginase, which inhibits production of multiple coagulation factors, may also predispose patients to thrombosis. Infusion of granulocyte-macrophage colony-stimulating factor (GM-CSF) has been associated with thrombosis. Tamoxifen, an estrogen receptor antagonist, can cause venous thrombosis. The mechanism is unclear.

Plasma homocysteine levels influence the risk of both venous and arterial thromboembolism. Individuals with the congenital homocystinuria syndrome have, in addition to their Marfanoid habitus, an increased incidence of strokes and coronary artery disease. These patients have well-recognized enzyme defects (Chap. 343), excrete homocysteine in their urine, and have very high plasma levels of the amino acid. Some patients with early-onset cerebral vascular events have mild homocystinuria that can be brought out by a methionine loading test. Epidemiologic studies show a relationship between homocysteine levels that are nearer to the normal range and coronary artery disease. Vitamin B_{12} deficiency occurs in about 30% of people over age 70, produces elevated homocysteine levels, and may be a reversible cause of thrombotic disease.

FURTHER READING

ARNOUT J, VERYLEN J: Current status and implications of autoimmune antiphospholipid antibodies in relation to thrombotic disease. J Thromb Haemost 1:931, 2003

CROWTHER MA, KELTON JG: Congenital thrombophilic states associated with venous thrombosis: A qualitative overview and proposed classification system. Ann Intern Med 138:128, 2003

HEDNER U: Recombinant factor VIIa (NovoSeven) as a hemostatic agent. Dis Mon 49:39, 2003

HIGH KA: Gene transfer as an approach to treating hemophilia. Semin Thromb Hemost 1:107, 2003

LEE C: Recombinant clotting factors in the treatment of hemophilia. Thromb Haemost 82:516, 1999

LEVI M, TEN CATE H: Current concepts: Disseminated intravascular coagulation. N Engl J Med 341:586, 1999

MANNUCCI PM: Hemophilia: Treatment options in the twenty-first century. J Thromb Haemost 1:1349, 2003

103 | ANTIPLATELET, ANTICOAGULANT, AND FIBRINOLYTIC THERAPY
Steven R. Deitcher

Arterial and venous thrombosis together with complicating embolic phenomena are major causes of mortality in the developed countries of the world. In the United States alone, myocardial infarction (MI) and thromboembolic stroke account for >800,000 deaths annually, and from one-half to 2 million venous thromboembolic events (VTE) including deep venous thrombosis (DVT) and pulmonary embolism (PE) occur annually. A common feature of the management of *all* thromboembolic vascular diseases is the use of antithrombotic agents. Antithrombotic agents, including antiplatelet drugs, anticoagulants, and fibrinolytic agents, are used to prevent thrombotic events, prevent or mitigate the complications of thrombotic events, and restore vascular patency in order to prevent loss of tissue, limb, and organ function as well as life. The pathologic basis of thrombosis in different vascular beds dictates the choice of agents: drugs that inhibit platelet activation and aggregation play a primary role in arterial disease management; drugs that inhibit thrombin and fibrin generation play a primary role in venous disease.

ANTIPLATELET DRUGS

Antiplatelet treatment reduces overall mortality from vascular disease by 15% and nonfatal vascular events by 30%. Multiple targets exist for antiplatelet therapy (Fig. 103-1), including cyclooxygenase (COX), adenosine diphosphate (ADP) receptors, the platelet adhesion glycoprotein (Gp) Ib, and the platelet agonist thrombin. Prostaglandin E_1 and stable analogues of prostacyclin inhibit platelet activation by increasing platelet cyclic AMP levels. Dipyridamole inhibits platelet activation by inhibiting phosphodiesterase to increase cyclic AMP. Because expression of functionally active GpIIb/IIIa on platelet surfaces is the final common pathway of platelet activation regardless of initial stimulus, it is a logical therapeutic target.

ASPIRIN Aspirin (acetylsalicylic acid) irreversibly inactivates by acetylation the activity of platelet prostaglandin H synthase-1 and -2 (COX-1 and -2). COX inhibition leads to the prevention of thromboxane A_2 synthesis and impairment of platelet secretion and aggregation. Non-enteric-coated aspirin is rapidly absorbed from the upper gastrointestinal tract; plasma salicylate concentrations peak within 1 h of ingestion. The effects of aspirin on platelet function occur within 1 h and last for the duration of the affected platelets' life span (1 week). Toxicities including gastrointestinal discomfort, blood loss, and systemic bleeding are dose-related. Aspirin doses as low as 30 mg/d are antithrombotic. Aspirin has been convincingly shown to be effective in treatment of stable and unstable angina, acute MI, transient ischemic

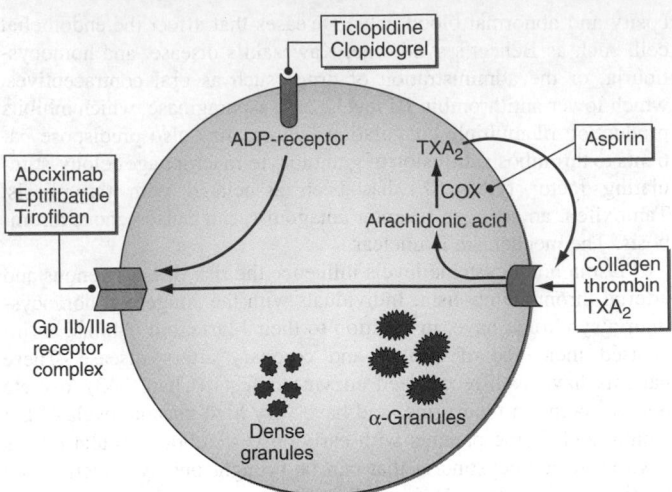

FIGURE 103-1 Antiplatelet drugs and targets for platelet function inhibition. The thienopyridines, ticlopidine and clopidogrel, inhibit the ADP-receptor of platelets. Aspirin targets platelet cyclooxygenase (COX). The disintegrins bind to and inhibit the final common pathway of platelet activation, namely the glycoprotein (Gp) IIb/IIIa complex. (TXA$_2$, thromboxane A$_2$.)

attack and incomplete stroke, stroke following carotid artery surgery, and atrial fibrillation. The minimum effective aspirin dose for these indications is 75 to 325 mg/d. Aspirin reduces mortality after coronary artery bypass surgery. In patients with acute MI or stroke, aspirin prevents 35 to 40 cardiovascular events per 1000 patients treated (secondary prevention). For primary prevention in persons >50 years of age with at least one major risk factor for coronary artery disease, aspirin prevents 4 events per 1000 patients treated. Aspirin is advisable following peripheral arterial bypass surgery and carotid endarterectomy and in patients with intermittent claudication. Though beneficial when compared to placebo, aspirin cannot be recommended as first-line VTE prophylaxis in hip fracture patients because the benefit of aspirin is less than with anticoagulants.

THIENOPYRIDINES Ticlopidine and clopidogrel are structurally related compounds that selectively inhibit ADP-induced platelet aggregation and likely ADP-mediated amplification of the platelet response to other agonists. Though more effective than aspirin in reducing vascular events in many settings, enthusiasm for ticlopidine is dampened by hematologic toxicities, including thrombotic thrombocytopenic purpura (TTP). Clopidogrel is rapidly absorbed, extensively metabolized, and inhibits ADP-induced platelet aggregation in a dose-dependent fashion with inhibition detectable 2 h after an oral dose of 400 mg. The plasma half-life of the main metabolite, SR 26334, is ~8 h. On repeated daily dosing of 50 to 100 mg, 25 to 30% inhibition of ADP-induced platelet aggregation is noted on the second day of therapy, with 50 to 60% steady-state inhibition noted after 4 to 7 days. Platelet function returns to normal about 7 days after the last dose of clopidogrel. The CAPRIE trial demonstrated a modest reduction in ischemic events in patients with recent stroke or MI and in those with symptomatic peripheral arterial disease randomly assigned to clopidogrel, 75 mg/d, compared to aspirin (5.32% vs. 5.83%). The majority of the difference in efficacy occurred in the patients who entered because of symptomatic peripheral arterial disease, with a 23.8% relative risk reduction. Another trial (PCI-CURE) demonstrated an advantage of pretreatment clopidogrel plus aspirin followed by long-term therapy over aspirin alone in patients with acute coronary syndromes. Clopidogrel rarely precipitates TTP.

GpIIb/IIIa (αIIbβ3) ANTAGONISTS GpIIb/IIIa is a member of the integrin family of receptors. These receptors recognize the amino acid sequence arginine-glycine-aspartate (Arg-Gly-Asp; RGD), which represents the cell attachment recognition sequence present in adhesive proteins such

as fibrinogen. Three potent parenteral GpIIb/IIIa inhibitors (disintegrins) have been extensively studied, primarily in the settings of percutaneous coronary intervention (PCI), unstable angina, and non-Q-wave MI. Abciximab (c7E3 Fab) is a chimeric monoclonal Fab fragment of human and murine protein that binds to GpIIb/IIIa. Eptifibatide is a synthetic cyclic heptapeptide with a KGD sequence more specific for GpIIb/IIIa than RGD. Tirofiban is a synthetic peptidomimetic based on the RGD sequence. Oral, in contrast to intravenous, GpIIb/IIIa inhibitors have been generally disappointing.

ANTICOAGULANT DRUGS

Anticoagulant drugs are used to prevent and treat thrombosis in medical and surgical patients. Narrow-spectrum (single-protein target) anticoagulants (e.g., fondaparinux and ximelagatran) are being developed to supplant more broad-spectrum anticoagulants (e.g., heparin and warfarin). The molecular targets of selected agents are shown in Fig. 103-2. Oral delivery and lack of obligatory therapeutic monitoring are desired anticoagulant characteristics.

HEPARIN Commercial unfractionated heparin (UFH), obtained from bovine lung or porcine intestinal mucosa, consists of a heterogeneous mixture of highly sulfated polysaccharides (glycosaminoglycans) with molecular masses ranging from 4 to 30 kDa, with a mean molecular mass of ~15 kDa (≈45 saccharide units). UFH molecules contain a randomly distributed unique pentasaccharide sequence that binds to antithrombin. Once bound to UFH, the natural anticoagulant effect of antithrombin is potentiated, resulting in accelerated binding and inactivation of serine proteases such as the common pathway coagulation factors, factor Xa and thrombin. Heparin is active when given intravenously or subcutaneously. Delivery systems utilizing synthetic amino acids such as sodium N-[8(2-hydroxybenzoyl)amino] caprylate (SNAC) facilitate oral heparin gut absorption. The half-life of heparin increases with increasing dosage. A 100-U/kg intravenous dose is cleared with a half-life of ~1 h. Heparin is cleared by the reticuloendothelial system and metabolized by the liver, and metabolic products are excreted in the urine. "True" heparin resistance, manifesting as inadequate anticoagulant [activated partial thromboplastin time (aPTT) prolongation] and antithrombotic (anti-factor Xa activity) responses from what would otherwise be perceived as an adequate heparin dose, likely results from the nonspecific heparin binding to white blood cells, vascular endothelial cells, and acute-phase proteins. In "apparent" heparin resistance, usually as a result of elevated factor VIII levels, the aPTT may be normal or near normal while the anti-factor Xa activity assay reveals a therapeutic heparin activity level. Simply escalating the dose of heparin to achieve the desired aPTT without checking a heparin assay may result in a pronounced bleeding

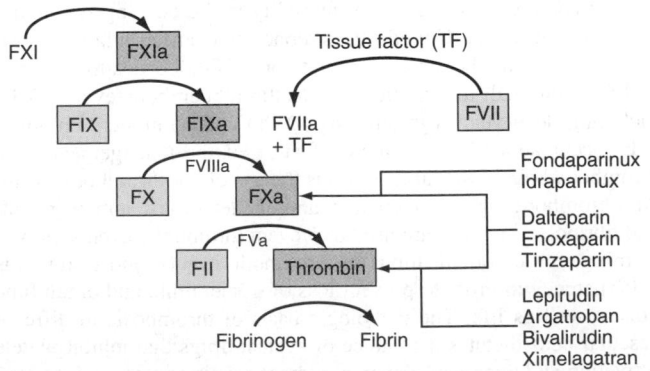

FIGURE 103-2 Anticoagulant drugs and molecular targets of anticoagulation. Unfractionated heparin targets the serine protease coagulation factors (highlighted in pale red); warfarin affects the vitamin K–dependent factors (highlighted in pale gray); pentasaccharide-based agents such as fondaparinux and idraparinux are select factor Xa inhibitors; the low-molecular-weight heparins target both factor Xa and thrombin with preference for factor Xa; and the direct thrombin inhibitors selectively target thrombin.

risk. These variables warrant close laboratory monitoring of heparin therapy.

LOW-MOLECULAR-WEIGHT HEPARINS (LMWHS) LMWHs are derived from the enzymatic or chemical cleavage of UFH into a mixture of glycosaminoglycans with a mean molecular mass of ~5 kDa (≈15 saccharide units). LMWHs bind antithrombin via the same pentasaccharide sequence as UFH. Due to the predominance of molecules <18 saccharide units in length, LMWHs have limited antithrombin activity compared to anti-factor Xa activity, and LMWH therapy is unable to be monitored by aPTT. Whereas UFH has an anti-factor Xa:antithrombin activity ratio of 1:1, LMWHs have reported ratios of 1.9:1 to 4.1:1. LMWHs differ in their degree of tissue factor pathway inhibitor release, degree of sulfation, and degree of stimulated von Willebrand factor (vWF) release. Superior bioavailability, limited nonspecific binding, and non-dose-dependent half-lives facilitate once- or twice-daily subcutaneous dosing based solely on weight and without laboratory monitoring. LMWH is cleared by renal mechanisms; therefore, multiday use in patients with severe renal insufficiency (creatinine clearance <30 mL/min) should be avoided. Reversible elevations of liver transaminases may occur during the administration of LMWH and UFH. LMWHs are associated with less heparin-induced thrombocytopenia (HIT) (Chap. 101) and osteopenia than UFH but are only partially (≈60%) neutralized by protamine sulfate.

HEPARINOIDS The heparinoid dermatan sulfate acts as an anticoagulant by activating heparin cofactor II. Danaparoid is a glycosaminoglycan mixture derived from porcine intestinal mucosa composed of heparan sulfate (84%), dermatan sulfate (12%), and chondroitin sulfate (4%). Danaparoid has an anti-factor Xa:antithrombin activity ratio of >22:1. Danaparoid's potential for heparin cross-reactivity and longer half-life (24 h) make it less desirable than a direct thrombin inhibitor for the treatment of patients with HIT, the main indication for heparinoid use.

PENTASACCHARIDES Fondaparinux is a synthetic pentasaccharide that causes selective indirect inhibition of factor Xa. Fondaparinux is administered subcutaneously and does not require therapeutic monitoring. Fondaparinux elimination is prolonged in patients with renal impairment, in those >75 years, and in those weighing <50 kg. Fondaparinux is primarily used for thromboprophylaxis in patients with hip fracture undergoing surgery and in those undergoing elective knee and hip joint replacement. Fondaparinux does not bind platelet factor 4 and may result in less HIT than UFH and LMWH. A long-acting pentasaccharide, idraparinux, has a half-life of 130 h, which may facilitate once-weekly dosing for primary and/or secondary prevention of thromboembolic events.

DIRECT THROMBIN INHIBITORS (DTI) Despite elimination of all heparin exposure and platelet count recovery, patients with isolated, serologically confirmed HIT have up to a 50% risk of developing a confirmed thrombotic event during the 30-day period following HIT diagnosis. The persistent prothrombotic tendency associated with HIT, the presence of thrombus in HIT with thrombosis, and a patient's original indication for heparin therapy all warrant use of an alternative anticoagulant agent such as DTI following heparin cessation.

Lepirudin Lepirudin is a recombinant hirudin that, unlike native hirudin in medicinal leech saliva, lacks sulfation on tyrosine 63 and has a leucine at position 1. Lepirudin is a potent, irreversible DTI that lacks any structural homology with heparin, does not cross-react with heparin, has a short half-life (1.5 h), inactivates clot-bound thrombin, and can be monitored by the aPTT assay or ecarin clotting time. The rate of death, amputation, and new thromboembolic events is reduced by >50% in HIT patients treated with lepirudin, compared with historic controls. Current lepirudin dosing recommendations for acute HIT management are 0.4 mg/kg as a bolus followed by 0.15 mg/kg per hour (up to 110 kg). The target aPTT is 1.5 to 2.5 times the median value for the normal range. The target plasma lepirudin concentration during heart bypass is 2.0 μg/mL. Outpatient subcutaneous lepirudin has been used to treat patients with HIT and patients refractory to other

anticoagulant therapy. The major challenges of lepirudin treatment are the lack of an antidote, the extreme care needed when treating patients with even mild renal insufficiency, and immunogenicity. Marked bolus and infusion rate reductions are necessary in patients with a creatinine clearance of <60 mL/min. Lepirudin should be avoided completely or administered with extreme care in the settings of hemodialysis and acute renal failure. Approximately 40% of HIT patients treated with lepirudin develop IgG anti-hirudin antibodies that decrease renal elimination of the drug rather than exerting any in vivo neutralizing effect. This enhancement of anticoagulant effect often warrants a major reduction of the infusion rate.

Argatroban Argatroban is a synthetic, small-molecule, L-arginine derivative, rapid, and reversible DTI capable of inhibiting both free and fibrin-bound thrombin. Argatroban exerts its antithrombotic effects by inhibiting thrombin-mediated fibrin formation; coagulation factor V, VII, and XIII activation; and platelet activation. Argatroban does not cross-react with heparin. Argatroban is hepatically metabolized with biliary excretion and has a half-life of 40 min. Dose reduction is required in patients with significant hepatic disease. In HIT, the combined incidence of death, amputation, and new thromboembolic events is significantly lower in argatroban recipients compared with controls. The recommended starting intravenous infusion rate is 2 μg/kg per min with a target aPTT of 1.5 to 3 times the baseline value. Prothrombin time (PT) prolongation makes an accurate International Normalized Ratio (INR) determination during conversion to oral warfarin a challenge. Argatroban [350-μg/kg bolus followed by 25 μg/kg per min titrated to achieve an activated clotting time (ACT) of 300 to 450 s] provides adequate anticoagulation with minimal bleeding risk while enabling procedural success in HIT patients undergoing a PCI.

Bivalirudin Bivalirudin is a semisynthetic, bivalent DTI consisting of a dodecapeptide analogue of the carboxyterminus of hirudin. Bivalirudin has four glycine residues that connect the thrombin exocite 1 and thrombin active-site binding moieties. Bivalirudin has a very short half-life (25 min) and is a reversible DTI. Bivalirudin is primarily used during PCI, where it is at least as effective as heparin with an improved safety profile.

Ximelagatran Ximelagatran is an oral prodrug of the DTI melagatran. Ximelagatran is administered in a fixed-dose fashion, does not require therapeutic monitoring, and has no apparent major food or drug interactions. Ximelagatran is rapidly absorbed (peak levels in 15 to 30 min) and rapidly converted to melagatran (peak levels in 1 to 2 h). Melagatran is renally eliminated. Melagatran binds to the thrombin active site resulting in inhibition of thrombin-mediated activation of coagulation factors and platelets. It is active against free and clot-bound thrombin. Ximelagatran is promising as a treatment of acute VTE, chronic management of atrial fibrillation, and prevention of VTE in high-risk settings such as following surgery and HIT. Reversible liver function abnormalities have been reported.

WARFARIN Warfarin inhibits vitamin K epoxide reductase and vitamin K reductase, thus inhibiting γ-carboxylation of select glutamic acid residues in the N-terminus of prothrombin; factors VII, IX, and X; and protein C and protein S. Inhibition of γ-carboxylation leads to synthesis of hypofunctional coagulation proteins that are unable to bind to cellular surfaces to mediate coagulation reactions. Commercially available warfarin is a racemic mixture of levo- and dextrorotatory forms of the drug. The half-life of warfarin in plasma is ~36 h. Because factor X and prothrombin have half-lives >2 days, reduction of all vitamin K−dependent coagulation proteins into the therapeutic range (~20% of normal) requires 4 to 5 days of therapy. Warfarin dosage is influenced by dietary stores of vitamin K, liver function, coexisting medical disorders, concurrent medications, and presence or absence of a common cytochrome P450 2C9 gene mutation. Warfarin metabolism is affected by other drugs metabolized by the cytochrome P450, by drugs that displace albumin-bound warfarin and impair gastrointestinal absorption, and by antibiotics that alter the natural flora of the colon (an endogenous source of vitamin K). The PT assay is useful to monitor warfarin therapy because this assay measures three vitamin K–dependent coagulation proteins—factors VII, X, and prothrombin. The PT is particularly sensitive to factor VII deficiency; with a half-life of 4 to 6 h, the factor VII level may drop rapidly after only 1 day of warfarin therapy and prolong the PT value. Large loading doses of warfarin result in a more rapid drop in factor VII levels, delay in attainment of a stable PT, a precipitous fall in protein C levels, and predisposition to warfarin-induced skin necrosis. The INR is a method that standardizes PT assays. Each new PT reagent (thromboplastin) is calibrated against the World Health Organization reference thromboplastin. A relative sensitivity of the unknown preparation compared with the reference called the International Sensitivity Index (ISI) is derived. By adjusting for the ISI of a particular thromboplastin, an INR, defined as the PT ratio (patient PT divided by the mean normal PT) that would have been obtained if the reference thromboplastin had been used, can be determined. The INR is calculated using the following formula: $INR = (PT ratio)^{ISI}$. An INR of 2.0 to 3.0 is recommended for all indications except prosthetic mechanical heart valves and prophylaxis of recurrent MI, for which higher-intensity warfarin therapy (INR 2.5 to 3.5) is suggested, and primary prophylaxis where an INR <2.0 is usually desired. In part because many patients with lupus anticoagulants have elevated baseline PTs, the INR may not be an accurate means of monitoring warfarin therapy in this setting. Factors contributing to warfarin-associated bleeding include an INR > 3.0, structural gastrointestinal lesions, concomitant antiplatelet therapy, hypertension, renal disease, and cerebrovascular disease. Visceral bleeding while on warfarin therapy often results in identification of structural lesions. In pregnant women, warfarin can cause an embryopathy consisting of nasal hypoplasia and epiphyseal stippling. The risk may be greatest between weeks 6 and 12 of gestation and may reflect the effect of warfarin on a vitamin K–dependent bone matrix protein, osteocalcin. Most practitioners avoid warfarin during pregnancy. Warfarin-induced skin necrosis is a devastating complication of warfarin therapy, occurring within the first week of therapy and associated in some with protein C deficiency. The skin lesions often begin on fatty body parts (breasts, abdomen, thighs) as erythematous patches and progress to blebs followed by demarcated skin necrosis. Skin biopsy reveals generalized thrombosis of skin vessels. The "purple-toe syndrome" is an uncommon syndrome described in patients with underlying atherosclerotic vascular disease receiving warfarin. These patients present with atheroembolic symptoms including ischemic (purple) toes, livedo reticularis, gangrene, abdominal pain, or symptoms of renal infarction. Skin biopsy reveals cholesterol emboli in the purple-toe syndrome.

FIBRINOLYTIC DRUGS

Most thrombolytic agents are recombinant forms of physiologic plasminogen activators (PAs) that differ in plasma half-life, fibrin specificity, primary clinical usage, primary infusion strategy, and immunogenicity. Therapeutic PAs are fashioned after endogenous tissue-type plasminogen activator (t-PA) or urokinase that converts plasminogen into the active enzyme plasmin. Plasmin degrades fibrinogen and fibrin into fibrin(ogen) degradation products. Major goals of new thrombolytic agent development include increasing fibrin specificity to theoretically reduce bleeding complications, prolonging initial plasma half-life to facilitate bolus administration, and reducing sensitivity to inactivation by plasminogen activator inhibitor (PAI) 1.

STREPTOKINASE Streptokinase is obtained from cultures of β-hemolytic streptococci. By itself, streptokinase has no PA activity, but when complexed with plasminogen, it can convert other plasminogen molecules to plasmin. It is not fibrin-selective in that the so-called lytic state resulting from its therapeutic use is due to lysis of fibrinogen as well as fibrin. Platelet function may be perturbed because plasmin can

proteolyze key platelet membrane receptors. The half-life of streptokinase is ~20 min. Because streptokinase is a bacterial protein, it is antigenic; allergic reactions occur in up to 6% of patients, and anaphylaxis occurs in ~0.1% of patients. Patients previously exposed to streptokinase or with previous streptococcal infections may acquire antistreptococcal antibody levels sufficient to neutralize its activity. Streptokinase has been primarily used to treat VTE and MI as well as to treat central venous line–associated thrombosis.

UROKINASE-TYPE PLASMINOGEN ACTIVATOR Native urokinase is obtained from human fetal kidney cell cultures. Recombinant high-molecular-weight urokinase is produced using nonhuman, mammalian tissue cultures. Urokinase is not fibrin-selective and thus produces a lytic state. Its half-life is ~20 min, and it is used to treat DVT, PE, MI, peripheral arterial thrombosis, and occluded catheters.

TISSUE-TYPE PLASMINOGEN ACTIVATOR Recombinant tissue-type plasminogen activator (rt-PA) produced by recombinant technology demonstrates high in vitro affinity for fibrin with which it forms a ternary complex with plasminogen. Despite reported fibrin-specificity, the lytic state is produced with dosages currently used. Bleeding complications with t-PA are similar to those of streptokinase or urokinase. The half-life of t-PA is ~5 min. t-PA is used to treat DVT, PE, acute MI, acute thrombotic stroke, and dysfunctional central venous lines.

TISSUE-TYPE PLASMINOGEN ACTIVATOR VARIANTS Recombinant PA (r-PA; reteplase) is a nonglycosylated deletion mutant of wild-type human t-PA composed of only the kringle 2 and the protease domains of the parent molecule. Lack of the finger domain imparts lower fibrin-binding affinity. Lack of glycosylation, a finger domain, and epidermal growth factor domain imparts an extended half-life (15 min versus 5 min). TNK-t-PA differs from t-PA by three sets of mutations. The $Asn^{117} \rightarrow Gln$ and $Thr^{103} \rightarrow Asn$ mutations promote a lower plasma clearance rate and greater fibrin specificity. The Lys^{296}-His^{297}-Arg^{298}-$Arg^{299} \rightarrow$ Ala-Ala-Ala-Ala mutation imparts an 80-fold increased resistance to PAI-1. The longer half-lives of r-PA and TNK-rt-PA compared with rt-PA facilitate bolus administration primarily for acute coronary thrombosis.

NEWER NON-t-PA FIBRINOLYTICS Recombinant glycosylated pro-urokinase is a rapid acting and safe fibrin-specific PA. Staphylokinase produced by *Staphylococcus aureus* possesses substantial thrombolytic activity but may be immunogenic. Vampire bat (*Desmodus rotundus*) salivary PA, possessing 85% primary structure homology to human t-PA but lacking a kringle 2 domain, holds promise as a potent thrombolytic. Alfimiprase is a novel thrombolytic based on the snake venom–derived protein fibrolase. Alfimiprase is a direct fibrinolytic (not a PA) neutralized by α_2-macroglobulin that holds promise as a rapid and safe catheter-delivered thrombolytic.

THROMBOLYTIC THERAPY–ASSOCIATED BLEEDING Bleeding associated with all PAs stems from plasmin's inability to differentiate between hemostatic and pathologic thrombi. Bleeding complications range from minor bleeding to life-threatening hemorrhage including intracranial hemorrhage. Older age, female sex, black ethnicity, systolic blood pressure $\geq$ 140 mmHg, diastolic blood pressure $\geq$ 100 mmHg, history of stroke, t-PA dose > 1.5 mg/kg, and lower body weight are all associated with increased intracranial hemorrhage risk. The ability of a thrombolytic agent (PA) to distinguish between plasminogen in the general circulation and plasminogen bound to fibrin surfaces dictates its fibrin specificity. Activation of fibrin-bound plasminogen results in the generation of fibrin-bound plasmin that is protected from inactivation by α_2-antiplasmin. Bound plasmin generates soluble fibrin degradation products, whereas circulating plasmin degrades fibrinogen into fibrinogen degradation products. High fibrin specificity is thought to be associated with lower risk for hemorrhagic complications because of the belief that plasmin born on the fibrin surface of a thrombus will restrict its activity only to that surface. This view is not supported by available data from large-scale clinical trials. Unlike in acute MI where intravenous bolus PA dosing is necessary to facilitate rapid lysis of a relatively small thrombus, lysis of larger diameter and longer peripheral thromboses is best achieved with catheter-directed infusions of PA over several hours to days. Drugs designed for bolus infusion to treat acute coronary thrombosis (e.g., r-PA and TNK-t-PA) may be associated with loss of fibrin specificity, accumulation of fragment X, and increased bleeding rates when given by extended continuous infusion.

MANAGEMENT OF VENOUS THROMBOEMBOLIC DISEASE (Fig. 103-3)

The major clinical consequences of extremity DVT include the post-thrombotic syndrome (swelling, stasis dermatitis, ulceration, and venous claudication all due to venous insufficiency), PE, and paradoxical embolism resulting in stroke. The major clinical consequences of PE include chronic dyspnea, pulmonary hypertension, pulmonary infarction, and death. Inadequately treated DVT involving the popliteal or more proximal leg veins is associated with a 20 to 50% risk of clinically relevant recurrence and is strongly associated with both symptomatic and fatal pulmonary embolism. Death from PE occurs most frequently within 2 days of presentation in untreated patients. All-cause mortality rates in treated patients with PE run as high as 11% at 2 weeks and 17% at 3 months.

CALF DEEP VENOUS THROMBOSIS While calf DVT and proximal DVT may be considered separate diseases at their outset, 15 to 25% of calf DVTs propagate and convert into proximal DVT. Symptomatic and asymptomatic calf DVT appear to propagate with equal frequency. Such "proximal conversion" renders what was initially a calf DVT just as dangerous as any proximal DVT. Proximal conversion has been shown to occur within the initial 2 weeks after diagnosis in the majority of cases and warrants treatment accordingly. The most essential goal of calf DVT treatment should be to prevent early proximal conversion. Treatment approaches for isolated calf DVT range from identical therapy as is used for proximal DVT to a complete lack of any pharmacologic therapy. Appropriate management, which falls between these extremes, includes serial duplex ultrasound surveillance (twice-weekly for 2 to 3 weeks) with therapy begun only in the event of proximal conversion and abbreviated courses of standard anticoagulation. Serial surveillance seems especially prudent in situations such as recent gastrointestinal bleeding where the risk of anticoagulation likely exceeds the benefit. Situational calf DVT (DVT with a clear precipitant) can be safely treated with anticoagulation for only 6 weeks, assuming the precipitating illness or event has resolved. Infe-

Initial-Phase Anticoagulation
4 to 14 days
Acute management usually with a parenteral agent (heparin or LMWH) intended to rapidly abrogate thrombin generation, prevent thrombus extension, and serve as a "bridge" to subacute anticoagulation

Chronic-Phase Anticoagulation
Long term
Chronic management usually with subacute-phase intensity or reduced-intensity (INR, 1.5 to 2.0) oral warfarin and perhaps in the future with oral ximelagatran or once-weekly SC idraparinux

Subacute-Phase Anticoagulation
up to 6 months
Subacute management usually with an oral agent such as warfarin (INR, 2.0 to 3.0) or SC LMWH intended to stabilize the thrombus, prevent early recurrence, and allow time for endogenous fibrinolysis-mediated recanalization

FIGURE 103-3 Phases of anticoagulation for venous thromboembolic events. Anticoagulation for a venous thromboembolic event can be divided into three distinct phases. Acute-phase anticoagulation usually consists of several days of parenteral therapy with intravenous unfractionated heparin or subcutaneous low-molecular-weight heparin (LMWH). Acute-phase therapy is usually continued for at least 4 days and until stable-dose, subacute-phase anticoagulation has been achieved. Subacute anticoagulation traditionally consists of oral warfarin for up to 6 months. Low-molecular-weight heparin therapy may offer superior and more convenient subacute anticoagulation in select populations. Long-term, chronic-phase anticoagulation consists of identical intensity therapy as is employed during subacute-phase therapy in high-risk patients and attenuated-intensity warfarin in others.

rior vena cava (IVC) filter placement is not recommended for calf DVT in most circumstances.

PROXIMAL DEEP VENOUS THROMBOSIS The goals of proximal DVT therapy include restoration of venous patency and prevention of embolization, thrombus extension, early and late recurrence, and postthrombotic syndrome. Studies done before the routine use of anticoagulant therapy demonstrated that 20% of patients with untreated DVT died of PE. Intravenous, aPTT-adjusted UFH and weight-based LMWH effectively prevent embolization, extension, and recurrence. LMWHs appear to be slightly but significantly better than standard heparin at restoring venous patency and may reduce the incidence of early postthrombotic syndrome. Placement of an IVC filter prevents PE in the short run but probably at the expense of a greater long-term DVT recurrence rate.

PULMONARY EMBOLISM In general, acute PE should be treated in the same fashion as acute proximal DVT. It is advisable to start anticoagulation at the time of suspected PE even before diagnostic testing has been performed. LMWHs have been shown to be safe and effective in patients with acute PE treated in hospital. Outpatient treatment of PE is investigational. Placement of an IVC filter at the time of PE diagnosis is usually reserved for those with an absolute contraindication to anticoagulation. Filters may be reasonable in select patients with underlying cardiac or pulmonary disease perceived as being at high risk for death in the event of even a small PE. Placement of a filter because of a "free-floating" DVT is probably not indicated.

INITIAL VTE ANTICOAGULATION Initial anticoagulation refers to the therapy begun at the time of VTE diagnosis and continued only until stable, usually oral, more long-term therapy has been achieved. Treatment with heparin or LMWH should be begun as soon as possible unless an absolute contraindication exists. A delay in achieving a therapeutic intensity of initial parenteral therapy may increase a patient's long-term VTE recurrence rate. Weight-based initial dosing of heparin (80 U/kg bolus followed by 18 U/kg per hour) with subsequent dose adjustments based on any published standardized nomogram facilitates achieving a target aPTT. An aPTT that correlates with an anti-FXa activity level of 0.3 to 0.7 IU/mL is considered therapeutic. The aPTT should be checked every 4 to 6 h until the aPTT surpasses the minimum of the target range. Fixed-dose boluses and initial infusions are preferred by some and are not necessarily inferior to weight-based dosing. Active bleeding, HIT or a history of HIT, and known sensitivity to UFH or pork products are absolute contraindications to heparin therapy. Patients with acute DVT and active bleeding require placement of an IVC filter. In patients with filters placed because of bleeding, appropriate anticoagulation should be begun as soon as the bleeding source has been properly and completely treated. Because of the risk of re-bleeding, such a patient may benefit from inpatient anticoagulation initiation. Placement and subsequent removal of a temporary (or retrievable) IVC filter once the contraindication to anticoagulation has passed seems ideal. Patients who are excessively anticoagulated with heparin without serious bleeding can be treated simply by stopping the drug; the short half-life (1 to 2 h) of heparin ensures rapid return of the aPTT to the therapeutic range. In occasional patients with thrombosis, such as those with lupus anticoagulants, the aPTT assay may not be reliable in monitoring heparin therapy. For these patients, one can follow heparin levels determined using the anti-factor Xa method or give a LMWH, with the dosage determined solely by body weight. Excessively anticoagulated and actively bleeding patients should be considered for reversal of anticoagulation with protamine sulfate. Protamine is given by slow IV infusion, with 1 mg of protamine neutralizing ~100 U of heparin. Protamine infusion may be associated with anaphylaxis, and excess protamine may lead to a paradoxical bleeding disorder. Weight-based subcutaneous LMWH is an established standard of care. Whether to use LMWH or UFH for acute anticoagulation should be determined for each patient taking into account the individual patient medical history, bleeding risk, ambulatory status, and insurance coverage. LMWHs are at least as safe and effective as UFH for the initial treatment of DVT. The major advantage of subcutaneous LMWH is its ability to be self-administered at home without the need for therapeutic monitoring. This translates into a significant reduction in mean hospital length of stay (6.5 days for UFH versus 1.1 days for LMWH in one study). Patients may be started on LMWH in the hospital and then discharged in an "accelerated" fashion to continue their conversion to oral warfarin or treated exclusively in the outpatient setting. Meta-analyses have shown a survival advantage in patients with acute DVT treated initially with LMWH versus those treated initially with UFH. This survival advantage seems primarily derived from a survival advantage in cancer patients with DVT. Enoxaparin is dosed at 1 mg/kg body weight every 12 h or 1.5 mg/kg once daily. Dalteparin is dosed at 200 IU/kg (up to 18,000 IU) once-daily. Tinzaparin is dosed at 175 IU/kg once daily. Patients at increased risk for bleeding should probably be treated initially in an inpatient setting. Such patients include those with active bleeding (including occult stool blood), a history of recent surgery, past gastrointestinal tract or neuraxial bleeding, recent trauma or stroke, concomitant regular use of nonsteroidal anti-inflammatory drugs (NSAIDs), thrombocytopenia, and renal insufficiency. Severe renal dysfunction (creatinine clearance < 30 mL/min) results in a ≥25% reduction in LMWH clearance and thus results in drug accumulation. LMWH therapy may not be suitable for the morbidly obese. Monitored heparin therapy is always a choice for the obese patient with acute DVT or PE. Therapeutic monitoring of LMWH therapy using the anti-factor Xa activity assay is not indicated in most patients. An exact therapeutic range has not been carefully determined, and adjusting the dose of LMWH based on such testing has not been shown to be superior to weight-based dosing. Fondaparinux has been shown to be equivalent to enoxaparin for the initial management of DVT and equivalent to intravenous UFH for the initial management of PE. Ximelagatran holds promise as an oral acute VTE treatment. Warfarin therapy *alone* is contraindicated as initial therapy of acute thrombosis because of the inherent delay in achieving therapeutic anticoagulation and the theoretical transient exacerbation of hypercoagulability caused by a rapid reduction in protein C functional activity. This warfarin-induced paradoxical hypercoagulability may explain warfarin-induced skin necrosis and warfarin-induced limb gangrene in patients with HIT.

SUBACUTE VTE ANTICOAGULATION *Subacute anticoagulation* refers to treatment (usually oral warfarin) that follows acute-phase therapy and continues for up to 6 months (Table 103-1). Warfarin therapy (oral or intravenous) can be started as soon as an aPTT > 1.5 times control has been achieved with heparin or an initial weight-based dose of LMWH has been given. Bolus dosing of warfarin does not help achieve a stable, target INR faster and may actually delay achievement of a stable INR and prolong hospitalization. Initial dosing with 2.5 to 7.5 mg/d (based on patient weight and nutritional status) seems prudent. Heparin and LMWH therapy must overlap oral warfarin therapy for a minimum of 4 days and ideally until a stable, target range (2.0 to 3.0) INR has been achieved. Starting warfarin therapy early after heparin therapy (day 1 or 2) facilitates earlier hospital discharge and potential reduction in the incidence of HIT. Patients with massive DVT

or PE may benefit from 7 to 10 days of initial heparin or LMWH therapy. Because of its teratogenic effects, warfarin therapy is contraindicated in pregnancy, so continued heparin or LMWH is prudent. Patients should be encouraged to consume a constant intake of dietary vitamin K and avoid large variations or fluctuations in their diet. Because of the number of pharmacologic interactions that exist between warfarin and other drugs, patients should be instructed to inform their physician of the addition or withdrawal of any medication, vitamin, and herbal preparation (Table 103-2). Recently completed studies (LITE, ONCENOX, and CLOT) provide strong evidence to support the use of LMWH as acute *plus* subacute VTE treatment. Once-daily tinzaparin (175 IU/kg) was as effective and safer than INR-adjusted oral warfarin in a mixed population of acute DVT patients. Once-daily tinzaparin, enoxaparin, and dalteparin were shown to be more effective than oral warfarin at preventing recurrent VTE in cancer patients with thrombosis. Patients with DVT secondary to a transient risk such as surgery, trauma, or pregnancy may be anticoagulated for a duration of 6 weeks to 3 months, as long as the risk factor has passed. Patients with a first idiopathic VTE should be anticoagulated for a minimum of 3 to 6 months.

CHRONIC ANTICOAGULATION FOR VTE Patients with persistent risk factors for thrombosis such as an anti-phospholipid antibody, hyperhomocysteinemia, active malignancy, or a deficiency of a natural anticoagulant (protein C, protein S, and antithrombin), homozygous factor V Leiden, and those with recurrent idiopathic VTE may benefit from long-term therapy (Table 103-1). The risk of VTE recurrence is very low as long as therapeutic anticoagulation is continued. It is the up to 3 to 4% annual risk of major hemorrhage secondary to warfarin (INR 2.0 to 3.0) that prevents physicians from prescribing long-term anticoagulation with abandon. The long-term risks and inconvenience of chronic (>6 months) therapeutic-intensity warfarin anticoagulation have led to the study of alternative approaches to chronic-phase anticoagulation following VTE. Extended secondary prevention with the oral DTI ximelagatran (24 mg bid) for 18 months after 6 months of standard anticoagulation in patients with VTE (THRIVE III) revealed recurrence rates of 2.0% and 11.6% ($p < .0001$) in the ximelagatran and placebo groups, respectively. Reported major and minor bleeding rates on therapy were not different between groups. Another successful approach

---

TABLE 103-1 *Duration of Anticoagulation for Venous Thromboembolic Events (VTE)*

Event	Duration of Anticoagulation
Situational DVT	6 weeks to 3 months
Idiopathic DVT	3 to 6 months (minimum)
Recurrent idiopathic DVT	12 months (minimum)
VTE with ongoing risk factors[a]	Long-term/indefinite
Pulmonary embolism	6 months (minimum)
Massive pulmonary embolism	Long-term/indefinite

[a] Malignancy, anti-phospholipid antibodies, homozygous factor V Leiden, natural anticoagulant deficiency, etc.

Note: DVT, deep venous thrombosis.

TABLE 103-2 *Effect of Select Drugs and Medical Conditions on Oral Warfarin Anticoagulation*

DRUGS THAT POTENTIATE WARFARIN EFFECT (INCREASE THE PROTHROMBIN TIME)

Acetaminophen	Phenylbutazone
Anabolic steroids	Phenytoin
Broad-spectrum antibiotics	Propranolol
Cimetidine	Protease inhibitors (except retinovir)
Fluconazole	Quinidine
Lovastatin	Salicylate
Metronidazole	Tamoxifen
Omeprazole	Trimethoprim-sulfamethoxazole

MEDICAL CONDITIONS THAT POTENTIATE WARFARIN EFFECT (INCREASE THE PROTHROMBIN TIME)

Advanced age	Fever
Hepatobiliary disease	Hyperthyroidism
Malabsorption	Malnutrition
Congestive heart failure	Cancer

DRUGS THAT ANTAGONIZE WARFARIN EFFECT (DECREASE THE PROTHROMBIN TIME)

Adrenal glucocorticoids	Griseofulvin
Barbiturates	Penicillin
Carbamazepine	Rifampin
Cholestyramine	Sulcrafate
Efavirenz	Trazadone

MEDICAL CONDITIONS THAT ANTAGONIZE WARFARIN EFFECT (DECREASE THE PROTHROMBIN TIME)

Excess dietary vitamin K	Hypothyroidism
Inherited warfarin resistance	Nephrotic syndrome

to chronic-phase anticoagulation involves long-term, low-intensity oral warfarin therapy with infrequent (every 8 weeks) INR monitoring (PREVENT). In this landmark study, patients with idiopathic VTE who had received standard acute- and subacute-phase anticoagulant therapy were randomly assigned to placebo or low-intensity warfarin (target INR 1.5 to 2.0). Recurrent VTE rates were 7.2 per 100 person-years and 2.6 per 100 person-years in the placebo and warfarin groups, respectively. This 64% risk reduction was accomplished in both those with and without inherited thrombophilia without any increase in major hemorrhage rates. Such safe and effective regimens have the potential to redefine the standard of care for VTE.

THROMBOLYSIS FOR VTE   Benefits of DVT thrombolysis include the ability to subsequently diagnosis and treat underlying venous stenosis, venous compression (as in May-Thurner syndrome) or venous webs. Thrombolysis results in improved venous patency and symptom resolution and in a decrease in postthrombolic syndrome symptoms, and it may improve health-related quality of life. Because of the bleeding risk, thrombolysis is best reserved to treat iliofemoral DVT in the young and those with extensive thrombosis resulting in venous limb gangrene (*phlegmasia cerulea dolens*). Intravenous thrombolysis has been demonstrated to improve survival in patients with massive PE plus shock and is probably indicated in these patients. When compared to anticoagulation alone, thrombolytic therapy results in more rapid thrombus lysis, an early improvement in pulmonary blood flow, and improvement of right ventricular function. However, these improvements in cardiopulmonary function alone have not resulted in decreased mortality in stable patients without significant hemodynamic compromise. It remains unclear whether patients with PE and evidence of right ventricular dysfunction and/or elevated cardiac troponin levels are subgroups that benefit more from thrombolysis. Major hemorrhage rates have varied between 4 and 22% when thrombolytic agents are used in studies at the currently recommended doses.

VENOUS THROMBOEMBOLIC DISEASE PREVENTION   If physicians focused more on VTE prophylaxis, much less time would need to be dedicated to emphasizing methods for VTE treatment. Fatal PE is the most common preventable cause of hospital death. A key to proper prophylaxis is the recognition of risk factors for thrombosis. Established clinical risk factors include: advanced age; prolonged immobility, stroke, or paralysis; prior VTE; active malignancy and its treatment; major surgery especially involving the abdomen, pelvis, and lower extremities; trauma, especially involving fracture of the pelvis, hip, or leg; obesity; varicose veins; depressed left ventricular ejection fraction; central venous access devices; inflammatory bowel disease; lobar pneumonia; nephrotic syndrome; pregnancy; estrogen use; and inherited and acquired hypercoagulable states. The number of risk factors, risk of DVT, risk of clinical PE, risk of fatal PE, and the required intensity of prophylactic therapy necessary to mitigate the risk all seem to increase in parallel. Medically ill patients (predominantly those immobilized with severe cardiopulmonary disease) have a 14.9% risk of developing DVT within 14 days of admission in the absence of active prophylaxis (MEDENOX). The DVT rate is reduced to 5.5% by the addition of a once-daily dose of LMWH (enoxaparin, 40 mg) without a significant increase in bleeding risk. Other studies have demonstrated equivalency between LMWH and heparin (5000 U tid) in medical patients with acute cardiac or pulmonary disease. Not all patients at risk will develop a thrombosis, and not all thromboses will result in symptoms, morbidity, or death. The benefit of pharmacologic thromboprophylaxis must always be weighed against the bleeding risk. Patients at high risk for bleeding should still receive prophylaxis in the form of intermittent pneumatic compression and/or thromboembolism-deterrence stockings.

FURTHER READING

DEITCHER SR, CARMAN TL: Heparin-induced thrombocytopenia: Natural history, diagnosis, and management. Vasc Med 6:113, 2001

———, ———: Deep venous thrombosis and pulmonary embolism. Curr Treat Options Cardiovasc Med 4:223, 2002

———: Cancer and thrombosis: Mechanisms and treatment. J Thromb Thrombolysis 16:21, 2003

GOLDHABER SZ: Thrombolysis in pulmonary embolism: A debatable indication. Thromb Haemost 86:444, 2001

HAYDEN M et al: Aspirin for the primary prevention of cardiovascular events: A summary of the evidence for the U.S. Preventive Services Task Force. Ann Intern Med 136:161, 2002

VERSTRAETE M: Third-generation thrombolytic drugs. Am J Med 109:52, 2001

104 | INTRODUCTION TO INFECTIOUS DISEASES: HOST–PATHOGEN INTERACTIONS
Lawrence C. Madoff, Dennis L. Kasper

Despite decades of dramatic progress in their treatment and prevention, infectious diseases remain a major cause of death and debility and are responsible for worsening the living conditions of many millions of people around the world. Infections frequently challenge the physician's diagnostic skill and must be considered in the differential diagnoses of syndromes affecting every organ system.

CHANGING EPIDEMIOLOGY OF INFECTIOUS DISEASES With the advent of antimicrobial agents, some medical leaders believed that infectious diseases would soon be eliminated and become of historic interest only. Indeed, the hundreds of chemotherapeutic agents developed since World War II, most of which are potent and safe, include drugs effective not only against bacteria but also against viruses, fungi, and parasites. Nevertheless, we now realize that as we developed antimicrobial agents, microbes developed the ability to elude our best weapons and to counterattack with new survival strategies. Antibiotic resistance occurs at an alarming rate among all classes of mammalian pathogens. Pneumococci resistant to penicillin and enterococci resistant to vancomycin have become commonplace. Even *Staphylococcus aureus* that is resistant to vancomycin has appeared. Such pathogens present real clinical problems in managing infections that were easily treatable just a few years ago. Diseases once thought to have been nearly eradicated from the developed world—tuberculosis, cholera, and rheumatic fever, for example—have rebounded with renewed ferocity. Newly discovered and emerging infectious agents appear to have been brought into contact with humans by changes in the environment and by movements of human and animal populations. An example of the propensity for pathogens to escape from their usual niche is the alarming 1999 outbreak in New York of encephalitis due to West Nile virus, which had never previously been isolated in the Americas. In 2003, severe acute respiratory syndrome (SARS) was first recognized. This emerging clinical entity is caused by a novel coronavirus that may have jumped from an animal niche to become a significant human pathogen. In early 2004, avian influenza spread rapidly through poultry farms in Asia and caused deaths in exposed humans, raising the specter of a new influenza pandemic.

Many infectious agents have been discovered only in recent decades (Fig. 104-1). Ebola virus, human metapneumovirus, *Anaplasma phagocytophila* (the agent of human granulocytotropic ehrlichiosis), and retroviruses such as HIV humble us despite our deepening understanding of pathogenesis at the most basic molecular level. Even in developed countries, infectious diseases have made a resurgence. Between 1980 and 1996, mortality from infectious diseases in the United States increased by 64% to levels not seen since the 1940s.

The role of infectious agents in the etiology of diseases once believed to be noninfectious is being increasingly recognized. For example, it is now widely accepted that *Helicobacter pylori* is the causative agent of peptic ulcer disease and perhaps of gastric malignancy. Human papillomavirus is likely to be the most important cause of invasive cervical cancer. Human herpesvirus type 8 is believed to be the cause of most cases of Kaposi's sarcoma. Epstein-Barr virus is a cause of certain lymphomas and may play a role in the genesis of Hodgkin's disease. The possibility certainly exists that other diseases of unknown cause, such as rheumatoid arthritis, sarcoidosis, or inflammatory bowel disease, have infectious etiologies. There is even evidence that atherosclerosis may have an infectious component. In contrast, there are data to suggest that decreased exposures to pathogens in childhood may be contributing to an increase in the observed rate of allergic diseases.

Medical advances over infectious diseases have been hindered by changes in the patient population. Immunocompromised hosts now constitute a significant proportion of the seriously infected population. Physicians immunosuppress their patients to prevent the rejection of

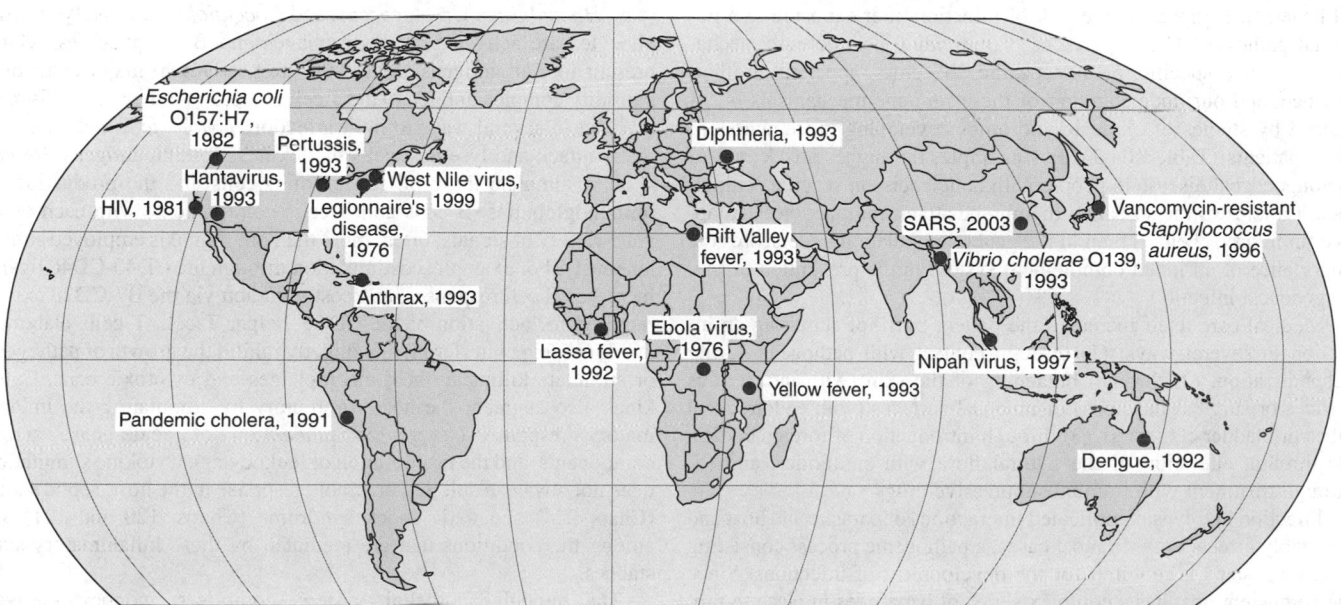

FIGURE 104-1   Map of the world showing examples of geographic locales where infectious diseases were noted to have emerged or resurged. (Adapted from *Addressing Emerging Infectious Disease Threats: A Prevention Strategy for the United States,* Department of Health and Human Services, Centers for Disease Control and Prevention, 1994.)

transplants and to treat neoplastic and inflammatory diseases. Some infections, most notably that caused by HIV, immunocompromise the host in and of themselves. Lesser degrees of immunosuppression are associated with other infections, such as influenza and syphilis. Infectious agents that coexist peacefully with immunocompetent hosts wreak havoc in those who lack a complete immune system. AIDS has brought to prominence once-obscure organisms such as *Pneumocystis*, *Cryptosporidium parvum*, and *Mycobacterium avium*.

HOST FACTORS IN INFECTION For any infectious process to occur, the pathogen and the host must first encounter each other. Factors such as geography, environment, and behavior thus influence the likelihood of infection. Although the initial encounter between a susceptible host and a virulent organism frequently results in disease, some organisms can be harbored in the host for years before disease becomes clinically evident. For a complete view, individual patients must be considered in the context of the population to which they belong. Infectious diseases do not often occur in isolation; rather, they spread through a group exposed from a point source (e.g., a contaminated water supply) or from individual to individual (e.g., via respiratory droplets). Thus, the clinician must be alert to infections prevalent in the community as a whole. A detailed history, including information on travel, behavioral factors, exposures to animals or potentially contaminated environments, and living and occupational conditions, must be elicited. For example, the likelihood of infection by *Plasmodium falciparum* can be significantly affected by altitude, climate, terrain, season, and even time of day. Antibiotic-resistant strains are localized to specific geographic regions, and a seemingly minor alteration in a travel itinerary can dramatically influence the likelihood of acquiring chloroquine-resistant malaria. If such important details in the history are overlooked, inappropriate treatment may result in the death of the patient. Likewise, the chance of acquiring a sexually transmitted disease can be greatly affected by a relatively minor variation in sexual practices, such as the method used for birth control. Knowledge of the relationship between specific risk factors and disease allows the physician to influence a patient's health even before the development of infection by modification of these risk factors and—when a vaccine is available—by immunization.

Many specific host factors influence the likelihood of acquiring an infectious disease. Age, immunization history, prior illnesses, level of nutrition, pregnancy, coexisting illness, and perhaps emotional state all have some impact on the risk of infection after exposure to a potential pathogen. The importance of individual host defense mechanisms, either specific or nonspecific, becomes apparent in their absence, and our understanding of these immune mechanisms is enhanced by studies of clinical syndromes developing in immunodeficient patients (Table 104-1). For example, the higher attack rate of meningococcal disease in people with deficiencies in specific complement proteins of the so-called membrane attack complex (see "Adaptive Immunity," below) than in the general population underscores the importance of an intact complement system in the prevention of meningococcal infection.

Medical care itself increases the patient's risk of acquiring an infection in several ways: (1) through contact with pathogens during hospitalization, (2) through breaching of the skin (with intravenous devices or surgical incisions) or mucosal surfaces (with endotracheal tubes or bladder catheters), (3) through introduction of foreign bodies, (4) through alteration of the natural flora with antibiotics, and (5) through treatment with immunosuppressive drugs.

Infection involves complicated interactions of parasite and host and inevitably affects both. In most cases, a pathogenic process consisting of several steps is required for the development of infections. Since the competent host has a complex series of barricades in place to prevent infection, the successful parasite must use specific strategies at each of these steps. The specific strategies used by bacteria, viruses, and parasites (Chap. 105) have some remarkable conceptual similarities, but the strategic details are unique not only for each class of organism but also for individual species within a class.

THE IMMUNE RESPONSE ■ Innate Immunity As they have co-evolved with microbes, higher organisms have developed mechanisms for recognizing and responding to microorganisms. Many of these mechanisms, referred to together as *innate immunity*, are evolutionarily ancient, having been conserved from insects to humans (Fig. 104-2). In general, innate immune mechanisms exploit molecular patterns found specifically in pathogenic microorganisms. These "pathogen signatures" are recognized by host molecules that either directly interfere with the pathogen or initiate a response that does so. Innate immunity serves to protect the host without prior exposure to an infectious agent—i.e., before specific or adaptive immunity has had a chance to develop. Innate immunity also functions as a warning system that activates components of adaptive immunity early in the course of infection.

Examples of innate immune effectors include defensins, simple peptides found on the skin and mucosal surfaces with activity against bacteria, fungi, and viruses. Macrophages that engulf and kill microbes (and other cells with similar function) are found even in invertebrates, such as *Drosophila*. The complement system (described below and discussed in more detail in Chap. 295) can respond to microbes without prior exposure.

The response to lipopolysaccharide (LPS), a molecule found uniquely in gram-negative bacteria, is instructive in understanding innate immunity. Even minuscule amounts of LPS are detected by LPS-binding protein, CD14, and Toll-like receptor 4 (Fig. 104-2). The interaction of LPS with these components of the innate immune system prompts macrophages, via the transcriptional activator NFκB, to produce cytokines that lead to inflammation and enzymes that enhance the clearance of microbes. These initial responses serve not only to limit infection but also to initiate specific or adaptive immune responses.

Adaptive Immunity Once in the bloodstream or a normally sterile body site, the microorganism faces the host's tightly integrated cellular and humoral immune systems. Cellular immunity (Chap. 295), comprising T lymphocytes, macrophages, and natural killer cells, primarily recognizes and combats pathogens that proliferate intracellularly. Cellular immune mechanisms are important in immunity to all classes of infectious agents, including most viruses and many bacteria (e.g., *Mycoplasma*, *Chlamydia*, *Listeria*, *Salmonella*, and *Mycobacterium*), parasites (e.g., *Trypanosoma*, *Toxoplasma*, and *Leishmania*), and fungi (e.g., *Histoplasma*, *Cryptococcus*, and *Coccidioides*). Usually, T lymphocytes are activated by macrophages and B lymphocytes, which present foreign antigens along with the host's own major histocompatibility complex antigen to the T cell receptor. Activated T cells may then act in several ways to fight infection. *Cytotoxic* T cells may directly attack and lyse host cells that express foreign antigens. *Helper* T cells stimulate the proliferation of B cells and the production of immunoglobulins. B cells and T cells communicate with each other via a variety of signals; often, more than one signal is employed simultaneously. For example, costimulation through the CD40-CD40 ligand increases B cell responses, and costimulation via the B7-CD28 axis is required for activation of the CD4+ helper T cell. T cells elaborate cytokines (e.g., interferon) that directly inhibit the growth of pathogens or stimulate killing by host macrophages and cytotoxic cells. Cytokines also augment the host's immunity by stimulating the inflammatory response (fever, the production of acute-phase serum components, and the proliferation of leukocytes). Cytokine stimulation does not always result in a favorable response in the host; septic shock (Chap. 254) and toxic shock syndrome (Chaps. 120 and 121) are among the conditions that are mediated by these inflammatory substances.

The reticuloendothelial system comprises monocyte-derived phagocytic cells that are located in the liver (Kupffer cells), lung (alveolar macrophages), spleen, kidney (mesangial cells), brain (microglia), and lymph nodes and that clear circulating microorganisms.

TABLE 104-1 Infections Associated with Selected Defects in Immunity

Host Defect	Disease or Therapy Associated with Defect	Common Etiologic Agent of Infection
NONSPECIFIC IMMUNITY		
Impaired cough	Rib fracture, neuromuscular dysfunction	Bacteria causing pneumonia, aerobic and anaerobic oral flora
Loss of gastric acidity	Achlorhydria, histamine blockade	*Salmonella* spp., enteric pathogens
Loss of cutaneous integrity	Penetrating trauma, athlete's foot	*Staphylococcus* spp., *Streptococcus* spp.
	Burn	*Pseudomonas aeruginosa*
	Intravenous catheter	*Staphylococcus* spp., *Streptococcus* spp., gram-negative rods, coagulase-negative staphylococci
Implantable device	Heart valve	*Streptococcus* spp., coagulase-negative staphylococci, *Staphylococcus aureus*
	Artificial joint	*Staphylococcus* spp., *Streptococcus* spp., gram-negative rods
Loss of normal bacterial flora	Antibiotic use	*Clostridium difficile*, *Candida* spp.
Impaired clearance		
Poor drainage	Urinary tract infection	*Escherichia coli*
Abnormal secretions	Cystic fibrosis	Chronic pulmonary infection with *P. aeruginosa*
INFLAMMATORY RESPONSE		
Neutropenia	Hematologic malignancy, cytotoxic chemotherapy, aplastic anemia, HIV infection	Gram-negative enteric bacilli, *Pseudomonas* spp., *Staphylococcus* spp., *Candida* spp.
Chemotaxis	Chédiak-Higashi syndrome, Job's syndrome, protein-calorie malnutrition	*S. aureus*, *Streptococcus pyogenes*, *Haemophilus influenzae*, gram-negative bacilli
	Leukocyte adhesion defects 1 and 2	Bacteria causing skin and systemic infections, gingivitis
Phagocytosis (cellular)	Systemic lupus erythematosus (SLE), chronic myelogenous leukemia, megaloblastic anemia	*Streptococcus pneumoniae*, *H. influenzae*
Splenectomy	—	*H. influenzae*, *S. pneumoniae*, other streptococci, *Capnocytophaga* spp., *Babesia microti*, *Salmonella* spp.
Microbicidal defect	Chronic granulomatous disease	Catalase-positive bacteria and fungi: staphylococci, *E. coli*, *Klebsiella* spp., *P. aeruginosa*, *Aspergillus* spp., *Nocardia* spp.
	Chédiak-Higashi syndrome	*S. aureus*, *S. pyogenes*
	Interferon γ receptor defect, interleukin 12 deficiency, interleukin 12 receptor defect	*Mycobacterium* spp., *Salmonella* spp.
INNATE IMMUNITY		
Complement system		
C3	Congenital liver disease, SLE, nephrotic syndrome	*S. aureus*, *S. pneumoniae*, *Pseudomonas* spp., *Proteus* spp.
C5	Congenital	*Neisseria* spp., gram-negative rods
C6, C7, C8	Congenital, SLE	*Neisseria meningitidis*, *N. gonorrhoeae*
Alternative pathway	Sickle cell disease	*S. pneumoniae*, *Salmonella* spp.
Toll-like receptor 4	Congenital	Gram-negative bacilli
Interleukin 1 receptor–associated kinase (IRAK) 4	Congenital	*S. pneumoniae*, *S. aureus*, other bacteria
Mannan-binding lectin	Congenital	*N. meningitidis*, other bacteria
ADAPTIVE IMMUNITY		
T lymphocyte deficiency/dysfunction	Thymic aplasia, thymic hypoplasia, Hodgkin's disease, sarcoidosis, lepromatous leprosy	*Listeria monocytogenes*, *Mycobacterium* spp., *Candida* spp., *Aspergillus* spp., *Cryptococcus neoformans*, herpes simplex virus, varicella-zoster virus
	AIDS	*Pneumocystis*, cytomegalovirus, herpes simplex virus, *Mycobacterium avium-intracellulare*, *C. neoformans*, *Candida* spp.
	Mucocutaneous candidiasis	*Candida* spp.
	Purine nucleoside phosphorylase deficiency	Fungi, viruses
B cell deficiency/dysfunction	Bruton's X-linked agammaglobulinemia	*S. pneumoniae*, other streptococci
	Agammaglobulinemia, chronic lymphocytic leukemia, multiple myeloma, dysglobulinemia	*H. influenzae*, *N. meningitidis*, *S. aureus*, *Klebsiella pneumoniae*, *E. coli*, *Giardia lamblia*, *Pneumocystis*, enteroviruses
	Selective IgM deficiency	*S. pneumoniae*, *H. influenzae*, *E. coli*
	Selective IgA deficiency	*G. lamblia*, hepatitis virus, *S. pneumoniae*, *H. influenzae*
Mixed T and B cell deficiency/dysfunction	Common variable hypogammaglobulinemia	*Pneumocystis*, cytomegalovirus, *S. pneumoniae*, *H. influenzae*, various other bacteria
	Ataxia-telangiectasia	*S. pneumoniae*, *H. influenzae*, *S. aureus*, rubella virus, *G. lamblia*
	Severe combined immunodeficiency	*S. aureus*, *S. pneumoniae*, *H. influenzae*, *Candida albicans*, *Pneumocystis*, varicella-zoster virus, rubella virus, cytomegalovirus
	Wiskott-Aldrich syndrome	Agents of infections associated with T and B cell abnormalities
	X-linked hyper-IgM syndrome	*Pneumocystis*, cytomegalovirus, *Cryptosporidium parvum*

FIGURE 104-2   Conserved pathways in innate immunity in *Drosophila* and mammals. Examples chosen are, left, the induction of the antifungal gene drosomycin by binding of processed Spaetzle protein to the transmembrane receptor Toll and, right, activation of costimulatory protein genes by binding of an LPS-LBP-CD14 complex to a human Toll homologue, TLR4. DD, death domain; IκB, inhibitor of κB; IKK, IκB kinase; IRAK, interleukin 1 receptor–associated kinase; KD, kinase domain; LBP, LPS-binding protein; LPS, lipopolysaccharide; LRR, leucine-rich domain; NFκB, nuclear factor κB; NIK, NFκB-inducing kinase; TIR, Toll/IL-1 receptor homology domain; TRAF6, tumor necrosis factor receptor–associated factor 6. (*Reprinted with permission from JA Hoffman et al: Science 284:1315, 1999. Copyright 1999 American Association for the Advancement of Science.*)

Although these tissue macrophages and polymorphonuclear leukocytes (PMNs) are capable of killing microorganisms without help, they function much more efficiently when pathogens are first *opsonized* (Greek, "to prepare for eating") by components of the complement system such as C3b and/or by antibodies.

Extracellular pathogens, including most encapsulated bacteria (those surrounded by a complex polysaccharide coat), are attacked by the humoral immune system, which includes antibodies, the complement cascade, and phagocytic cells. Antibodies are complex glycoproteins (also called immunoglobulins) that are produced by mature B lymphocytes, circulate in body fluids, and are secreted on mucosal surfaces. Antibodies specifically recognize and bind to foreign antigens. One of the most impressive features of the immune system is the ability to generate an incredible diversity of antibodies capable of recognizing virtually every foreign antigen yet not reacting with self. In addition to being exquisitely specific for antigens, antibodies come in different structural and functional classes: IgG predominates in the circulation and persists for many years after exposure; IgM is the earliest specific antibody to appear in response to infection; secretory IgA is important in immunity at mucosal surfaces, while monomeric IgA appears in the serum; and IgE is important in allergic and parasitic diseases. Antibodies may directly impede the function of an invading organism, neutralize secreted toxins and enzymes, or facilitate the removal of the antigen (invading organism) by phagocytic cells. Immunoglobulins participate in cell-mediated immunity by promoting the antibody-dependent cellular cytotoxicity functions of certain T lymphocytes. Antibodies also promote the deposition of complement components on the surface of the invader.

The complement system (Chap. 295) consists of a group of serum proteins functioning as a cooperative, self-regulating cascade of enzymes that adhere to—and in some cases disrupt—the surface of invading organisms. Some of these surface-adherent proteins (e.g., C3b) can then act as opsonins for destruction of microbes by phagocytes. The later, "terminal" components (C7, C8, and C9) can directly kill some bacterial invaders (notably, many of the neisseriae) by forming a membrane attack complex and disrupting the integrity of the bacterial membrane, thus causing bacteriolysis. Other complement components, such as C5a, act as chemoattractants for PMNs. Complement activation and deposition occur by either or both of two pathways: the classic pathway is activated primarily by immune complexes (i.e., antibody bound to antigen), and the alternative pathway is activated by microbial components, frequently in the absence of antibody. PMNs have receptors for both antibody and C3b, and antibody and complement function together to aid in the clearance of infectious agents.

PMNs, short-lived white blood cells that engulf and kill invading microbes, are first attracted to inflammatory sites by chemoattractants such as C5a, which is a product of complement activation at the site of infection. PMNs localize to the site of infection by adhering to cellular adhesion molecules expressed by endothelial cells. Endothelial cells express these receptors, called *selectins* (CD-62, ELAM-1), in response to inflammatory cytokines such as tumor necrosis factor (TNF) α and interleukin 1. The binding of these selectin molecules to specific receptors on PMNs results in the adherence of the PMNs to the endothelium. Cytokine-mediated upregulation and expression of intercellular adhesion molecule 1 (ICAM 1) on endothelial cells then take place, and this latter receptor binds to β_2 integrins on PMNs, thereby facilitating diapedesis into the extravascular compartment. Once the PMNs are in the extravascular compartment, various molecules such as arachidonic acids further enhance the inflammatory process.

APPROACH TO THE PATIENT

The clinical manifestations of infectious diseases at presentation are myriad, varying from fulminant life-threatening processes to brief and self-limited conditions to indolent chronic maladies. The clinician must use all the skills of medicine to diagnose the infection and prescribe appropriate treatment. First, a careful history is essential and must include details on underlying chronic diseases; medications; occupation; travel; and risk factors for exposure to certain types of pathogens, such as those associated with sexual contacts, family illnesses, illicit drug use, particular animals, blood transfusions, ingestion of contaminated liquids or foods, or bites of insect vectors. Since infectious diseases may involve many organ systems, a careful review of systems may elicit important clues as to the disease process. The physical examination must be thorough, and attention must be paid to seemingly minor details: a soft heart murmur that might indicate bacterial endocarditis; an evanescent skin rash that suggests rheumatic fever; or a retinal lesion that suggests disseminated candidiasis or cytomegalovirus (CMV) infection.

LABORATORY INVESTIGATIONS   Laboratory studies must be carefully considered and directed toward establishing an etiologic diagnosis in the shortest possible time, at the lowest possible cost, and with the least possible discomfort to the patient. Cultures must be performed in a manner that minimizes the likelihood of contamination with normal flora while maximizing the yield. A sputum sample is far more likely to be valuable when elicited with careful coaching by the clinician than when collected in a container simply left at the bedside with cursory instructions. Gram's stains of specimens should be interpreted carefully and the quality of the specimen assessed. The findings on Gram's staining should correspond to the results of culture; a discrepancy may suggest diagnostic possibilities such as infection due to fastidious or anaerobic bacteria.

The microbiology laboratory must be an ally in the diagnostic endeavor. Astute laboratory personnel will suggest optimal culture and transport conditions or alternative tests to facilitate diagnosis. If informed about specific potential pathogens, an alert laboratory staff will allow sufficient time for these organisms to become evident in culture, even when present in small numbers or when slow-growing. The parasitology technician who is attuned to the specific diagnostic considerations relevant to a particular case may be able to detect the rare, otherwise-elusive egg or cyst in a stool specimen. In cases where a diagnosis appears difficult, serum should be stored during the early acute phase of the illness so that a diagnostic rise in titer of antibody to a specific pathogen can be detected later. Bacterial and fungal antigens can sometimes be detected in body fluids, even when cultures are negative or are rendered sterile by antibiotic therapy. Techniques such as the polymerase chain reaction allow the amplification of specific DNA sequences so that minute quantities of foreign nucleic acids can be recognized in host specimens.

R̥ TREATMENT

Optimal therapy for infectious diseases requires a broad knowledge of medicine and careful clinical judgment. Life-threatening infections such as bacterial meningitis or sepsis, viral encephalitis, or falciparum malaria must be treated immediately, often before a specific causative organism is identified. Antimicrobial agents must be chosen empirically and must be active against the range of potential infectious agents consistent with the clinical scenario. In contrast, good clinical judgment sometimes dictates withholding of antimicrobials in a self-limited process or until a specific diagnosis is made. The dictum *primum non nocere* should be adhered to, and it should be remembered that all antimicrobials carry a risk (and a cost) to the patient. Direct toxicity may be encountered—e.g., ototoxicity due to aminoglycosides, lipodystrophy due to antiretroviral agents, and hepatotoxicity due to antituberculous agents such as isoniazid and rifampin. Allergic reactions are common and can be serious. Since superinfection sometimes follows the eradication of the normal flora and colonization by a resistant organism, one invariable principle is that infectious disease therapy should be directed toward as narrow a spectrum of infectious agents as possible. Treatment specific for the pathogen should result in as little perturbation as possible of the host's microflora. With few exceptions, abscesses require surgical or percutaneous drainage for cure. Foreign bodies, including medical devices, must generally be removed in order to eliminate an infection of the device or of the adjacent tissue. Other infections, such as necrotizing fasciitis, peritonitis due to a perforated organ, gas gangrene, and chronic osteomyelitis, require surgery as the primary means of cure; in these conditions, antibiotics play only an adjunctive role.

The role of immunomodulators in the management of infectious diseases has received increasing attention. Glucocorticoids have been shown to be of benefit in the treatment of *Haemophilus influenzae* meningitis in children and in therapy for *Pneumocystis* pneumonia in patients with AIDS. The use of these agents in other infectious processes remains less clear and in some cases (in cerebral malaria and septic shock, for example) is detrimental. Activated protein C is the first immunomodulatory agent widely available for the treatment of severe sepsis. Its usefulness demonstrates the interrelatedness of the clotting cascade and systemic immunity. Other agents that modulate the immune response include prostaglandin inhibitors, specific lymphokines, and TNF inhibitors. Specific antibody therapy plays a role in the treatment and prevention of many diseases. Specific immunoglobulins have long been known to prevent the development of symptomatic rabies and tetanus. More recently, CMV immune globulin has been recognized as important not only in preventing the transmission of the virus during organ transplantation but also in treating CMV pneumonia in bone marrow transplant recipients. There is a strong need for well-designed clinical trials to evaluate each new interventional modality.

PERSPECTIVE The genetic simplicity of many infectious agents allows them to undergo rapid evolution and to develop selective advantages that result in constant variation in the clinical manifestations of infection. Moreover, changes in the environment and the host can predispose new populations to a particular infection. The dramatic march of West Nile virus from a single focus in New York City in 1999 to locations across the North American continent by the summer of 2002

caused widespread alarm, illustrating the fear that new plagues induce in the human psyche. The intentional release of deadly spores of *Bacillus anthracis* awakened many from a sense of complacency regarding biological weapons.

"The terror of the unknown is seldom better displayed than by the response of a population to the appearance of an epidemic, particularly when the epidemic strikes without apparent cause." Edward Kass made this statement in 1977 in reference to the newly discovered Legionnaire's disease, but it could apply equally to SARS or to any other new and mysterious disease. The potential for infectious agents to emerge in novel and unexpected ways requires that physicians and public health officials be knowledgeable, vigilant, and open-minded in their approach to unexplained illness. The emergence of antimicrobial-resistant pathogens (e.g., enterococci that are resistant to all known antimicrobial agents and cause infections that are essentially untreatable) has led some to conclude that we are entering the "post-antibiotic era." Others have held to the perception that infectious diseases no longer represent as serious a concern to world health as they once did. The progress that science, medicine, and society as a whole have made in combating these maladies is impressive, and it is ironic that, as we stand on the threshold of an understanding of the most basic biology of the microbe, infectious diseases are posing renewed problems. We are threatened by the appearance of new diseases such as AIDS, SARS, hepatitis C, and Ebola virus infection and by the reemergence of old foes such as tuberculosis, cholera, plague, and *Streptococcus pyogenes* infection. True students of infectious diseases were perhaps less surprised than anyone else by these developments. Those who know pathogens are aware of their incredible adaptability and diversity. As ingenious and successful as therapeutic approaches may be, our ability to develop methods to counter infectious agents so far has not matched the myriad strategies employed by the sea of microbes that surrounds us. Their sheer numbers and the rate at which they can evolve are daunting. Moreover, environmental changes, rapid global travel, population movements, and medicine itself—through its use of antibiotics and immunosuppressive agents—all increase the impact of infectious diseases. Although new vaccines, new antibiotics, improved global communication, and new modalities for treating and preventing infection will be developed, pathogenic microbes will continue to develop new strategies of their own, presenting us with an unending and dynamic challenge.

FURTHER READING

ARMSTRONG G et al: Trends in infectious disease mortality in the United States during the 20th century. JAMA 281:61, 1999

BARTLETT JG: Update in infectious diseases. Ann Intern Med 133:285, 2000

BERKELMAN RL, HUGHES JM: The conquest of infectious diseases: Who are we kidding? Ann Intern Med 119:426, 1993

BUCKLEY RH: Immunodeficiency diseases. JAMA 268:2797, 1992

DE JONG R et al: Severe mycobacterial and *Salmonella* infections in interleukin-12 receptor–deficient patients. Science 280:1435, 1998

GOLD HS, EISENSTEIN BI: Introduction to bacterial diseases, in *Principles and Practice of Infectious Diseases*, 5th ed, GL Mandell et al (eds). New York, Churchill Livingstone, 2000, p 2065

HENDERSON DA: Bioterrorism as a public health threat. Emerg Infect Dis 4: 488, 1998

HOFFMAN J et al: Phylogenetic perspectives in innate immunity. Science 284: 1313, 1999

PROMED-MAIL: The Program for Monitoring Emerging Diseases. http://www.promedmail.org

PUCK JM: Primary immunodeficiency diseases. JAMA 278:1835, 1997

TYLER KL, NATHANSON N: Pathogenesis of viral infections, in *Fields Virology*, DM Knipe, PM Howley (eds). Philadelphia, Lippincott Williams & Wilkins, 2001, pp 199–244

WEISS ST: Eat dirt—the hygiene hypothesis and allergic diseases. N Engl J Med 347:930, 2002

Over the past three decades, molecular studies of the pathogenesis of microorganisms have yielded an explosion of information about the various microbial and host molecules that contribute to the processes of infection and disease. These processes can be classified into several stages: microbial encounter with and entry into the host; microbial growth after entry; avoidance of innate host defenses; tissue invasion and tropism; tissue damage; and transmission to new hosts. *Virulence* is the measure of an organism's capacity to cause disease and is a function of the pathogenic factors elaborated by microbes. These factors promote *colonization* (the simple presence of potentially pathogenic microbes in or on a host), *infection* (attachment and growth of pathogens and avoidance of host defenses), and *disease* (often, but not always, the result of activities of secreted toxins or toxic metabolites). In addition, the host's inflammatory response to infection greatly contributes to disease and its attendant clinical signs and symptoms.

MICROBIAL ENTRY AND ADHERENCE

ENTRY SITES A microbial pathogen can potentially enter any part of a host organism. In general, the type of disease produced by a particular microbe is often a direct consequence of its route of entry into the body. The most common sites of entry are mucosal surfaces (the respiratory, alimentary, and urogenital tracts) and the skin. Ingestion, inhalation, and sexual contact are typical routes of microbial entry. Other portals of entry include sites of skin injury (cuts, bites, burns, trauma) along with injection via natural (i.e., vector-borne) or artificial (i.e., needle-stick injury) routes. A few pathogens, such as *Schistosoma* spp., can penetrate unbroken skin. The conjunctiva can serve as an entry point for pathogens of the eye.

Microbial entry usually relies on the presence of specific microbial factors needed for persistence and growth in a tissue. Fecal-oral spread via the alimentary tract requires a biology consistent with survival in the varied environments of the gastrointestinal tract (including the low pH of the stomach and the high bile content of the intestine) as well as in contaminated food or water outside the host. Organisms that gain entry via the respiratory tract survive well in small moist droplets produced during sneezing and coughing. Pathogens that enter by venereal routes often survive best on the warm moist environment of the urogenital mucosa and have restricted host ranges (e.g., *Neisseria gonorrhoeae*, *Treponema pallidum*, and HIV).

The biology of microbes entering through the skin is highly varied. Some of these organisms can survive in a broad range of environments, such as the salivary glands or alimentary tracts of arthropod vectors, the mouths of larger animals, soil, and water. A complex biology allows protozoan parasites such as *Plasmodium*, *Leishmania*, and *Trypanosoma* spp. to undergo morphogenic changes that permit transmission of the organism to mammalian hosts during insect feeding for blood meals. Plasmodia are injected as infective sporozoites from the salivary glands during mosquito feeding. *Leishmania* parasites are regurgitated as promastigotes from the alimentary tract of sandflies and injected by bite into a susceptible host. Trypanosomes are first ingested from infected hosts by reduviid bugs; the pathogens then multiply in the gastrointestinal tract of the insects and are released in feces onto the host's skin during subsequent feedings. Most microbes that land directly on intact skin are destined to die, as survival on the skin or in hair follicles requires resistance to fatty acids, low pH, and other antimicrobial factors on skin. Once it is damaged (and particularly if it becomes necrotic), the skin can be a major portal of entry and growth for pathogens or their toxic products. Tetanus and burn wound infections are clear examples. After animal bites, pathogens resident in the animal's saliva gain access to the victim's tissues through the skin. Rabies is the paradigm for this pathogenic process; rabies virus grows in striated muscle cells at the site of inoculation.

MICROBIAL ADHERENCE Once in or on a host, most microbes must anchor themselves to a tissue or tissue factor; the possible exceptions are organisms that directly enter the bloodstream and multiply there. Specific ligands or adhesins for host receptors constitute a major area of study in the field of microbial pathogenesis. Adhesins comprise a wide range of surface structures, not only anchoring the microbe to a tissue and promoting cellular entry where appropriate but also eliciting host responses critical to the pathogenic process (Table 105-1). Most microbes produce multiple adhesins specific for multiple host receptors. These adhesins are often redundant, are serologically variable, and act additively or synergistically with other microbial factors to promote microbial sticking to host tissues. In addition, some microbes adsorb host proteins onto their surface and utilize the natural host protein receptor for microbial binding and entry into target cells.

TABLE 105-1 *Examples of Microbial Ligand-Receptor Interactions*

Microorganism	Type of Microbial Ligand	Host Receptor
VIRAL PATHOGENS		
Influenza virus	Hemagglutinin	Sialic acid
Measles virus		
Vaccine strain	Hemagglutinin	CD46/moesin
Wild-type strains	Hemagglutinin	Signaling lymphocytic activation molecule (SLAM)
Human herpesvirus type 6	?	CD46
Herpes simplex virus	Glycoprotein C	Heparin sulfate
HIV	Surface glycoprotein	CD4 and chemokine receptors (CCR5 and CXCR4)
Epstein-Barr virus	Envelope protein	CD21 (=CR2)
Adenovirus	Fiber protein	Coxsackie-adenovirus receptor (CAR)
Coxsackievirus	Fiber protein	CAR and major histocompatibility class I antigens
BACTERIAL PATHOGENS		
Neisseria species	Pili	Membrane cofactor protein (CD46)
Pseudomonas aeruginosa	Pili and flagella	Asialo-GM1
	Lipopolysaccharide	Cystic fibrosis transmembrane conductance regulator (CFTR)
Escherichia coli	Pili	Ceramides/mannose and digalactosyl residues
Yersinia spp.	Invasin/accessory invasin locus	β_1 Integrins
Bordetella pertussis	Filamentous hemagglutinin	CR3
Legionella pneumophila	Adsorbed C3bi	CR3
Mycobacterium tuberculosis	Adsorbed C3bi	CR3
FUNGAL PATHOGENS		
Blastomyces dermatitidis	WI-1	Possibly matrix proteins and integrins
Candida albicans	Int1p	Extracellular matrix proteins
PROTOZOAL PATHOGENS		
Plasmodium vivax	Merozoite form	Duffy Fy antigen
Plasmodium falciparum	EBA-175	Glycophorin A
Entamoeba histolytica	Surface lectin	*N*-Acetylglucosamine

Viral Adhesins All viral pathogens must bind to host cells, enter them, and replicate within them. Viral coat proteins serve as the ligands for cellular entry, and more than one ligand-receptor interaction may be needed; for example, HIV utilizes its envelope glycoprotein (gp) 120 to enter host cells by binding to both CD4 and one of two receptors for chemokines (designated CCR5 and CXCR4). Similarly, the measles virus H glycoprotein binds to both CD46 and the membrane-organizing protein moesin on host cells. The gC protein on herpes simplex virus binds to heparin sulfate; this step is followed by attachment to mammalian cells mediated by the viral gD (and possibly gH) protein. CD46 has now been shown to be the cellular receptor for human herpesvirus type 6.

Bacterial Adhesins Among the microbial adhesins studied in greatest detail are bacterial pili and flagella (Fig. 105-1). *Pili* or *fimbriae* are commonly used by gram-negative bacteria for attachment to host cells and tissues. In electron micrographs, these hairlike projections (up to several hundred per cell) may be confined to one end of the organism (polar pili) or distributed more evenly over the surface. An individual cell may have pili with a variety of functions. Most pili are made up of a major pilin protein subunit (molecular weight, 17,000 to 30,000) that polymerizes to form the pilus. Many strains of *Escherichia coli* express mannose-binding type 1 pili, whose binding to host tissues is inhibited by D-mannose. Other strains produce the Pap (pyelonephritis-associated) or P pilus adhesin that mediates binding to digalactose (gal-gal) residues on globosides of the human P blood groups. These pili have proteins located at the tips of the main pilus unit that are critical to the binding specificity of the whole pilus unit. Immunization with the mannose-binding FimH tip protein of type 1 pili prevents experimental *E. coli* bladder infections in mice and monkeys. *E. coli* cells causing diarrheal disease express pilus-like receptors for enterocytes on the small bowel, along with other receptors termed *colonization factors*.

FIGURE 105-1 Bacterial surface structures. *A and B.* Traditional electron micrographic images of fixed cells of *Pseudomonas aeruginosa.* Flagella (*A*) and pili (*B*) projecting out from the bacterial poles can be seen. *C and D.* Atomic force microscopic image of live *P. aeruginosa* freshly planted onto a smooth mica surface. This new technology reveals the fine, three-dimensional detail of the bacterial surface structures. *(Images courtesy of Dr. Martin Lee and Mr. Milan Bajmociz, Harvard Medical School.)*

A common type of pilus found in *Neisseria* spp., *Moraxella* spp., *Vibrio cholerae*, and *Pseudomonas aeruginosa* mediates adherence of these organisms to target surfaces. These pili tend to have a relatively conserved amino-terminal region and a more variable carboxyl-terminal region. For some species such as *N. gonorrhoeae* and *Neisseria meningitidis*, the pili are critical for attachment to mucosal epithelial cells. For others, such as *P. aeruginosa*, the pili only partially mediate the cells' adherence to host tissues. *V. cholerae* cells appear to use two different types of pili for intestinal colonization. Whereas interference with this stage of colonization would appear to be an effective antibacterial strategy, attempts to develop pilus-based vaccines for human diseases have not been highly successful to date.

Flagella are long appendages attached at either one or both ends of the bacterial cell (polar flagella) or distributed over the entire cell surface (peritrichous flagella). Flagella, like pili, are composed of a polymerized or aggregated basic protein. In flagella, the protein subunits form a tight helical structure and vary serologically with the species. Spirochetes such as *T. pallidum* and *Borrelia burgdorferi* have axial filaments similar to flagella running down the long axis of the center of the cell, and they "swim" by rotation around these filaments. Some bacteria can glide over a surface in the absence of obvious motility structures.

Other bacterial structures involved in adherence to host tissues include specific staphylococcal and streptococcal proteins that bind to human extracellular matrix proteins such as fibrin, fibronectin, laminin, and collagen. Fibronectin appears to be a commonly used receptor for various pathogens; a particular amino acid sequence in fibronectin, Arg-Gly-Asp or RGD, is critical for bacterial binding. The surface lipopolysaccharide (LPS) of *P. aeruginosa* mediates binding to the cystic fibrosis transmembrane conductance regulator (CFTR) on airway epithelial cells. Coagulase-negative staphylococci and *Staphylococcus aureus* readily colonize prosthetic devices and catheters commonly used in medical care; a surface polysaccharide composed of poly-N-acetyl glucosamine elaborated by these organisms promotes binding to the prosthetic material. High-powered imaging techniques such as atomic force microscopy have revealed that bacterial cells have a nonhomogeneous surface that is likely attributable to different concentrations of cell surface molecules, including microbial adhesins, at specific places on the cell surface (Fig. 105-1D).

Fungal Adhesins Several fungal adhesins have been described that mediate colonization of epithelial surfaces, particularly adherence to structures like fibronectin, laminin, and collagen. The product of the *Candida albicans INT1* gene, Int1p, bears similarity to mammalian integrins that bind to extracellular matrix proteins. Transformation of normally nonadherent *Saccharomyces cerevisiae* with this gene allows these yeast cells to adhere to human epithelial cells. Disruption of *INT1* in *C. albicans* diminishes but does not eliminate epithelial cell adhesion; this result indicates that other adhesins participate in binding of *C. albicans* to epithelial cells. Moreover, Int1p is needed for filamentous growth of *C. albicans*—a phenotype linked to virulence, and particularly to the ability to penetrate keratinized epithelium. *INT1*-deficient *C. albicans* exhibits markedly reduced virulence in a mouse model of infection.

For several fungal pathogens that initiate infections after inhalation of infectious material, the inoculum is ingested by alveolar macrophages, in which the fungal cells transform to pathogenic phenotypes. Like *C. albicans*, *Blastomyces dermatitidis* binds to CD11b/CD18 integrins as well as to CD14 on macrophages. *B. dermatitidis* produces a 120-kDa surface protein, designated WI-1, that mediates this adherence. The binding domain of WI-1 is homologous to the invasin protein of *Yersinia* that binds to the same type of host cell receptor. An unidentified factor on *Histoplasma capsulatum* also mediates binding of this fungal pathogen to the integrin surface proteins.

Eukaryotic Pathogen Adhesins Eukaryotic parasites use complicated surface glycoproteins as adhesins, some of which are lectins (proteins that bind to specific carbohydrates on host cells). For example, *Plasmodium vivax*, one of four *Plasmodium* species causing malaria, binds (via Duffy-binding protein) to the Duffy blood group carbohydrate antigen Fy on erythrocytes. *Entamoeba histolytica*, the third leading cause of death from parasitic diseases, expresses two proteins that bind to the disaccharide galactose/N-acetyl galactosamine. Reports indicate that children with mucosal IgA antibody to one of these lectins are resistant to reinfection with virulent *E. histolytica*. A major surface glycoprotein (gp63) of *Leishmania* promastigotes is needed for these parasites to enter human macrophages—the principal target cell of infection. This glycoprotein promotes complement binding but inhibits complement lytic activity, allowing the parasite to use complement receptors for entry into macrophages; gp63 also binds to fibronectin receptors on macrophages. In addition, the pathogen can express a carbohydrate that mediates binding to host cells. Evidence suggests that, as part of hepatic granuloma formation, *Schistosoma mansoni* expresses a carbohydrate epitope related to the Lewis X blood group antigen that promotes adherence of helminthic eggs to vascular endothelial cells under inflammatory conditions.

HOST RECEPTORS Host receptors are found both on target cells (such as epithelial cells lining mucosal surfaces) and within the mucus layer covering these cells. Microbial pathogens bind to a wide range of host receptors to establish infection (Table 105-1). Selective loss of host receptors for a pathogen may confer natural resistance to an otherwise susceptible population. For example, 70% of individuals in West Africa lack Fy antigens and are resistant to *P. vivax* infection. *Salmonella typhi*, the etiologic agent of typhoid fever, uses CFTR to enter the gastrointestinal submucosa after being ingested. As homozygous mutations in *CFTR* are the cause of the life-shortening disease cystic fibrosis, heterozygote carriers (e.g., 4 to 5% of individuals of European ancestry) may have had a selective advantage due to decreased susceptibility to *S. typhi* infection.

Numerous virus–target cell interactions have been described, and it is now clear that different viruses can use similar host cell receptors for entry. The list of certain and likely host receptors for viral pathogens is long. Among the host membrane components that can serve as receptors for viruses are sialic acids, gangliosides, glycosaminoglycans, integrins and other members of the immunoglobulin superfamily, histocompatibility antigens, and regulators and receptors for complement components.

MICROBIAL GROWTH AFTER ENTRY

Once established on a mucosal or skin site, pathogenic microbes must replicate before causing full-blown infection and disease. Within cells, viral particles release their nucleic acids, which may be directly translated into viral proteins (positive-strand RNA viruses), transcribed from a negative strand of RNA into a complementary mRNA (negative-strand RNA viruses), or transcribed into a complementary strand of DNA (retroviruses); for DNA viruses, mRNA may be transcribed directly from viral DNA, either in the cell nucleus or in the cytoplasm. To grow, bacteria must acquire specific nutrients or synthesize them from precursors in host tissues. Many infectious processes are usually confined to specific epithelial surfaces—influenza to the respiratory mucosa, gonorrhea to the urogenital epithelium, shigellosis to the gastrointestinal epithelium. While there are multiple reasons for this specificity, one important consideration is the ability of these pathogens to obtain from these specific environments the nutrients needed for growth and survival.

Temperature restrictions also play a role in limiting certain pathogens to specific tissues. Rhinoviruses, a cause of the common cold, grow best at 33°C and replicate in cooler nasal tissues but not in the lung. Leprosy lesions due to *Mycobacterium leprae* are found in and on relatively cool body sites. Fungal pathogens that infect the skin, hair follicles, and nails (dermatophyte infections) remain confined to the cooler, exterior, keratinous layer of the epithelium.

A topic of major interest is the ability of many bacterial, fungal, and protozoal species to grow in multicellular masses referred to as *biofilms*. These masses are biochemically and morphologically quite distinct from the free-living individual cells referred to as *planktonic cells*. Growth in biofilms leads to altered microbial metabolism, production of extracellular virulence factors, and decreased susceptibility to biocides, antimicrobial agents, and host defense molecules and cells. *P. aeruginosa* growing on the bronchial mucosa during chronic infection, staphylococci and other pathogens growing on implanted medical devices, and dental pathogens growing on tooth surfaces to form plaques represent several examples of microbial biofilm growth associated with human disease. Many other pathogens can form biofilms during in vitro growth, but the data are insufficient to determine whether this property is related to microbial virulence and induction of disease.

AVOIDANCE OF INNATE HOST DEFENSES

As microbes have probably interacted with mucosal/epithelial surfaces since the emergence of multicellular organisms, it is not surprising that multicellular hosts have a variety of innate surface defense mechanisms that can sense when pathogens are present and contribute to their elimination. The skin is acidic and is bathed with fatty acids toxic to many microbes. Successful skin pathogens such as staphylococci must tolerate these adverse conditions. Mucosal surfaces are covered by a barrier composed of a thick mucus layer that entraps microbes and facilitates their transport out of the body by such processes as mucociliary clearance, coughing, and urination. Mucous secretions, saliva, and tears contain antibacterial factors such as lysozyme and antimicrobial peptides as well as antiviral factors such as interferons. Gastric acidity is inimical to the survival of many ingested pathogens, and many mucosal surfaces—particularly the nasopharynx, the vaginal tract, and the gastrointestinal tract—contain a resident flora of commensal microbes that interfere with the ability of pathogens to colonize and infect a host.

Pathogens that survive these factors must still contend with host endocytic, phagocytic, and inflammatory responses as well as with host genetic factors that determine the degree to which a pathogen can survive and grow. The growth of viral pathogens entering skin or mucosal epithelial cells can be limited by a variety of host genetic factors, including production of interferons, modulation of receptors for viral entry, and age- and hormone-related susceptibility factors; by nutritional status; and even by personal habits such as smoking and exercise.

ENCOUNTERS WITH EPITHELIAL CELLS Over the past decade, many bacterial pathogens have been shown to enter epithelial cells (Fig. 105-2); the bacteria often use specialized surface structures that bind to receptors, with consequent internalization. However, the exact role and the importance of this process in infection and disease are not well defined for most of these pathogens. Bacterial entry into host epithelial cells is seen as a means for dissemination to adjacent or deeper tissues or as a route to sanctuary to avoid ingestion and killing by professional phagocytes. Epithelial cell entry appears, for instance, to be a critical aspect of dysentery induction by *Shigella*.

Curiously, the less virulent strains of many bacterial pathogens are more adept at entering epithelial cells than are more virulent strains; examples include pathogens that lack the surface polysaccharide capsule needed to cause serious disease. Thus, for *Haemophilus influenzae*, *Streptococcus pneumoniae*, *Streptococcus agalactiae* (group B *Streptococcus*), and *Streptococcus pyogenes*, isogenic mutants or variants lacking capsules enter epithelial cells better than the wild-type, encapsulated parental forms that cause disseminated disease. These observations have led to the proposal that epithelial cell entry may be a manifestation of host defense, resulting in bacterial clearance by both shedding of epithelial cells containing internalized bacteria and initiation of a subclinical inflammatory response. However, a consequence of this process would be the opening of a hole in the epithelium, potentially allowing uningested organisms to enter the submucosa.

FIGURE 105-2   Entry of bacteria into epithelial cells. *A.* Internalization of *P. aeruginosa* by cultured airway epithelial cells expressing wild-type cystic fibrosis transmembrane conductance regulator (CFTR), the cell receptor for bacterial ingestion. *B.* Entry of *P. aeruginosa* into murine tracheal epithelial cells after murine infection by the intranasal route.

This scenario has been documented in murine *Salmonella typhimurium* infections and in experimental bladder infections with uropathogenic *E. coli.* In the latter system, bacterial pili mediate cell attachment to integral membrane glycoproteins called *uroplakins* that coat the host cells, resulting in exfoliation of the cells with attached bacteria. Subsequently, infection is produced by residual bacterial cells that invade the denuded epithelium. Perhaps at low bacterial inocula epithelial cell ingestion and subclinical inflammation are efficient means to eliminate pathogens, while at higher inocula a proportion of surviving bacterial cells enter the host tissue through the damaged mucosal surface and multiply, producing disease. Alternatively, failure of the appropriate epithelial cell response to a pathogen may allow the organism to survive on a mucosal surface where, if it avoids other host defenses, it can grow and cause a local infection. Along these lines, as noted above, *P. aeruginosa* is taken into epithelial cells by CFTR, a protein missing or nonfunctional in most severe cases of cystic fibrosis. The major clinical consequence of this disease is chronic airway-surface infection with *P. aeruginosa* in 80 to 90% of patients with cystic fibrosis. The failure of airway epithelial cells to ingest and promote the removal of *P. aeruginosa* has been proposed as a key component of the hypersusceptibility of these patients to chronic airway infection.

ENCOUNTERS WITH PHAGOCYTES ■ **Phagocytosis and Inflammation**   Phagocytosis of microbes is a major innate host defense that limits the growth and spread of pathogens. Phagocytes appear rapidly at sites of infection in conjunction with the initiation of inflammation. Ingestion

of microbes by both tissue-fixed macrophages and migrating phagocytes probably accounts for the limited ability of most microbial agents to cause disease. A family of related molecules called *collectins, soluble defense collagens,* or *pattern-recognition molecules* are found in blood (mannose-binding lectins), in lung (surfactant proteins A and D), and most likely in other tissues as well and bind to carbohydrates on microbial surfaces to promote phagocyte clearance. Bacterial pathogens seem to be ingested principally by polymorphonuclear neutrophils (PMNs), while eosinophils are frequently found at sites of infection by protozoan or multicellular parasites. Successful pathogens, by definition, must avoid being cleared by professional phagocytes. One of several antiphagocytic strategies employed by bacteria and by the fungal pathogen *Cryptococcus neoformans* is to elaborate large-molecular-weight surface polysaccharide antigens, often in the form of a capsule that coats the cell surface. Most pathogenic bacteria produce such antiphagocytic capsules.

As activation of local phagocytes in tissues is a key step in initiating inflammation and migration of additional phagocytes into infected sites, much attention has been paid to microbial factors that initiate inflammation. Encounters with phagocytes are governed largely by the structure of the microbial constituents that elicit inflammation, and detailed knowledge of these structures for bacterial pathogens has contributed greatly to our understanding of molecular mechanisms of microbial pathogenesis (Fig. 105-3). One of the best-studied systems involves the interaction of LPS from gram-negative bacteria and the glycosylphosphatidylinositol (GPI)-anchored membrane protein CD14 found on the surface of professional phagocytes, including migrating and tissue-fixed macrophages and PMNs. A soluble form of CD14 is also found in plasma and on mucosal surfaces. A plasma protein, LPS-binding protein (LBP), transfers LPS to membrane-bound CD14 on myeloid cells and promotes binding of LPS to soluble CD14. Soluble CD14/LPS/LBP complexes bind to many cell types and may be internalized to initiate cellular responses to microbial pathogens. It has been shown that peptidoglycan and lipoteichoic acid from gram-positive bacteria and cell-surface products of mycobacteria and spirochetes can interact with CD14 (Fig. 105-3).

GPI-anchored receptors do not have intracellular signaling domains, and mammalian Toll-like receptors (TLRs) transduce signals for cellular activation due to LPS binding. TLRs initiate cellular activation through a series of signal-transducing molecules (Fig. 105-3) that lead to nuclear translocation of the transcription factor NF-κB, a master-switch for production of important inflammatory cytokines such as tumor necrosis factor α (TNF-α) and interleukin (IL) 1.

The initiation of inflammation can occur not only with LPS and peptidoglycan but also with viral particles and other microbial products such as polysaccharides, enzymes, and toxins. Bacterial flagella activate inflammation by binding to TLR5. Bacteria also produce a high proportion of DNA molecules with unmethylated CpG residues that activate inflammation through TLR9. TLR3 recognizes double-stranded RNA, a pattern-recognition molecule produced by many viruses during their replicative cycle. TLR1 and TLR6 associate with TLR2 to promote recognition of acylated microbial proteins and peptides.

The myeloid differentiation factor 88 (MyD88) molecule is a generalized adaptor protein that binds to the cytoplasmic domains of all known TLRs and also to receptors that are part of the IL-1 receptor (IL-1Rc) family. Numerous studies have shown that MyD88-mediated transduction of signals from TLRs and IL-1Rc is critical for innate resistance to infection. Mice lacking MyD88 are more susceptible than normal mice to infection with group B *Streptococcus, Listeria monocytogenes,* and *Mycobacterium tuberculosis.*

Additional Interactions of Microbial Pathogens and Phagocytes   Other ways that microbial pathogens avoid destruction by phagocytes include production of factors that are toxic to the phagocytes or that interfere with the chemotactic and ingestion function of phagocytes. Hemolysins,

FIGURE 105-3 Cellular signaling pathways for production of inflammatory cytokines in response to microbial products. Various microbial cell-surface constituents interact with CD14, which in turn interacts in a currently unknown fashion with Toll-like receptors (TLRs). Some microbial factors do not need CD14 to interact with TLRs. Associating with TLR4 (and to some extent with TLR2) is MD-2, a cofactor that facilitates the response to lipopolysaccharide (LPS). Both CD14 and TLRs contain extracellular leucine-rich domains. The cytoplasmic domains of TLRs are oligomerized for binding to the general adaptor protein MyD88, which also binds to members of the interleukin-1 receptor (IL-1Rc) transmembrane proteins because of homology in the intracellular domain. TIRAP (TIR domain-containing adaptor protein) participates in the transduction of signals from TLR4. The receptor complex clusters or oligomerizes; oligomerization is followed by activation of signal-transducing molecules such as IRAK-1/2 (IL-1Rc-associated kinase 1 or 2), TRAF-6 (tumor necrosis factor receptor–associated factor 6), TAK-1 (transforming growth factor β–activating kinase 1), and TAB1 (TAK1-binding protein 1)/NIK (Nck-interacting kinase). In addition to activating other signaling pathways leading to cytokine production and stress responses, such as the c-Jun N-terminal kinase (JNK) pathway and MAP kinase kinase kinase (MEKK1) pathway [via evolutionarily conserved signaling intermediate in Toll pathways (ECSIT)], TLR-mediated signaling leads to activation of the inducible kinase complex, IKK-α, -β, and -γ. IKK-γ is also called NEMO [nuclear factor κB (NF-κB) essential modulator]. These are part of a larger complex that phosphorylates the inhibitory portion (I) of NF-κB, resulting in release of IκB from NF-κB. Phosphorylated (PP) IκB is then degraded, and NF-κB translocates to the nucleus, where it binds to transcriptional sites on target genes, many of which encode inflammatory proteins. *(Figure courtesy of Dr. Terry Means and Dr. Douglas Golenbock.)*

leukocidins, and the like are microbial proteins that can kill phagocytes that are attempting to ingest organisms elaborating these substances. For example, staphylococcal hemolysins inhibit macrophage chemotaxis and kill these phagocytes. Streptolysin O made by *S. pyogenes* binds to cholesterol in phagocyte membranes and initiates a process of internal degranulation, with the release of normally granule-sequestered toxic components into the phagocyte's cytoplasm. *Entamoeba histolytica*, an intestinal protozoan that causes amebic dysentery, can disrupt phagocyte membranes after direct contact via the release of protozoal phospholipase A and pore-forming peptides.

Microbial Survival Inside Phagocytes Many important microbial pathogens use a variety of strategies to survive inside phagocytes (particularly macrophages) after ingestion. Inhibition of fusion of the phagocytic vacuole (the phagosome) containing the ingested microbe with the lysosomal granules containing antimicrobial substances (the lysosome) allows *M. tuberculosis*, *S. typhi*, and *Toxoplasma gondii* to survive inside macrophages. Some organisms, such as *L. monocytogenes*, escape into the phagocyte's cytoplasm to grow and eventually spread to other cells. Resistance to killing within the macrophage and subsequent growth are critical to successful infection by herpes-type

viruses, measles virus, poxviruses, *Salmonella*, *Yersinia*, *Legionella*, *Mycobacterium*, *Trypanosoma*, *Nocardia*, *Histoplasma*, *Toxoplasma*, and *Rickettsia*. *Salmonella* spp. use a master regulatory system, in which the *PhoP/PhoQ* genes control other genes, to enter and survive within cells, with intracellular survival entailing structural changes in the cell envelope LPS.

TISSUE INVASION AND TISSUE TROPISM

TISSUE INVASION Most viral pathogens cause disease by growth at skin or mucosal entry sites, but some pathogens spread from the initial site to deeper tissues. Virus can spread via the nerves (rabies virus) or plasma (picornaviruses) or within migratory blood cells (poliovirus, Epstein-Barr virus, and many others). Specific viral genes determine where and how individual viral strains can spread.

Bacteria may invade deeper layers of mucosal tissue via intracellular uptake by epithelial cells, traversal of epithelial cell junctions, or penetration through denuded epithelial surfaces. Among virulent *Shigella* strains and invasive *E. coli*, outer-membrane proteins are critical to epithelial cell invasion and bacterial multiplication. *Neisseria* and *Haemophilus* spp. penetrate mucosal cells by poorly understood mechanisms before dissemination into the bloodstream. Staphylococci and streptococci elaborate a variety of extracellular enzymes, such as hyaluronidase, lipases, nucleases, and hemolysins, that are probably important in breaking down cellular and matrix structures and allowing the bacteria access to deeper tissues and blood. Organisms that colonize the gastrointestinal tract can often translocate through the mucosa into the blood and, under circumstances in which host defenses are inadequate, cause bacteremia. *Yersinia enterocolitica* can invade the mucosa through the activity of the invasin protein. Some bacteria (e.g., *Brucella*) can be carried from a mucosal site to a distant site by phagocytic cells (e.g., PMNs) that ingest but fail to kill the bacteria.

Fungal pathogens almost always take advantage of host immunocompromise to spread hematogenously to deeper tissues. The AIDS epidemic has resoundingly illustrated this principle: the immunodeficiency of many HIV-infected patients permits the development of life-threatening fungal infections of the lung, blood, and brain. Other than the capsule of *C. neoformans*, specific fungal antigens involved in tissue invasion are not well characterized. Both fungal pathogens and protozoal pathogens (e.g., *Plasmodium* spp. and *E. histolytica*) undergo morphologic changes to spread within a host. Malarial parasites grow in liver cells as merozoites and are released into the blood to invade erythrocytes and become trophozoites. *E. histolytica* is found as both a cyst and a trophozoite in the intestinal lumen, through which this pathogen enters the host, but only the trophozoite form can spread systemically to cause amebic liver abscesses. Other protozoal pathogens, such as *T. gondii*, *Giardia lamblia*, and *Cryptosporidium*, also undergo extensive morphologic changes after initial infection to spread to other tissues.

TISSUE TROPISM The propensity of certain microbes to cause disease by infecting specific tissues has been known since the early days of bacteriology, yet the molecular basis for this propensity is understood somewhat better for viral pathogens than for other agents of infectious disease. Specific receptor-ligand interactions clearly underlie the ability of certain viruses to enter cells within tissues and disrupt normal tissue function, but the mere presence of a receptor for a virus on a target tissue is not sufficient for tissue tropism. Factors in the cell, route of viral entry, viral capacity to penetrate into cells, viral genetic elements that regulate gene expression, and pathways of viral spread in a tissue all affect tissue tropism. Some viral genes are best transcribed in specific target cells, such as hepatitis B genes in liver cells and Epstein-Barr virus genes in B lymphocytes. The route of inoculation of poliovirus determines its neurotropism, although the molecular basis for this circumstance is not understood.

The lesser understanding of the tissue tropism of bacterial and parasitic infections is exemplified by *Neisseria* spp. There is no well-accepted explanation of why *N. gonorrhoeae* colonizes and infects the human genital tract while the closely related species *N. meningitidis* principally colonizes the human oropharynx. *N. meningitidis* expresses a capsular polysaccharide, while *N. gonorrhoeae* does not; however, there is no indication that this property plays a role in the different tissue tropisms displayed by these two bacterial species. *N. gonorrhoeae* can use cytidine monophosphate *N*-acetylneuraminic acid from host tissues to add *N*-acetylneuraminic acid (sialic acid) to its lipooligosaccharide (LOS) O side chain, and this alteration appears to make the organism resistant to host defenses. Lactate, present at high levels on genital mucosal surfaces, stimulates sialylation of gonococcal LOS. Bacteria with sialic acid sugars in their capsules, such as *N. meningitidis*, *E. coli* K1, and group D streptococci, have a propensity to cause meningitis, but this generalization has many exceptions. For example, all recognized serotypes of group B streptococci contain sialic acid in their capsules, but only one serotype (III) is responsible for most cases of group B streptococcal meningitis. Moreover, both *H. influenzae* and *S. pneumoniae* can readily cause meningitis, but these organisms do not have sialic acid in their capsules.

TISSUE DAMAGE AND DISEASE

Disease is a complex phenomenon resulting from tissue invasion and destruction, toxin elaboration, and host response. Viruses cause much of their damage by exerting a cytopathic effect on host cells and inhibiting host defenses. The growth of bacterial, fungal, and protozoal parasites in tissue, which may or may not be accompanied by toxin elaboration, can also compromise tissue function and lead to disease. For some bacterial and possibly some fungal pathogens, toxin production is one of the best-characterized molecular mechanisms of pathogenesis, while host factors such as IL-1, TNF-α, kinins, inflammatory proteins, products of complement activation, and mediators derived from arachidonic acid metabolites (leukotrienes) and cellular degranulation (histamines) readily contribute to the severity of disease.

VIRAL DISEASE Viral pathogens are well known to inhibit host immune responses by a variety of mechanisms. Immune responses can be affected by downregulating production of most major histocompatibility complex (MHC) molecules (adenovirus E3 protein), by diminishing cytotoxic T-cell recognition of virus-infected cells (Epstein-Barr virus EBNA1 antigen and cytomegalovirus IE protein), by producing virus-encoded complement receptor proteins that protect infected cells from complement-mediated lysis (herpesvirus and vaccinia virus), by making proteins that interfere with the action of interferon (influenza virus and poxvirus), and by elaborating superantigen-like proteins (mouse mammary tumor virus and related retroviruses, rabies nucleocapsid, and possibly the Nef protein of HIV). Superantigens activate large populations of T cells that express particular subsets of the T cell receptor β protein, causing massive cytokine release and subsequent host reactions. Another molecular mechanism of viral virulence involves the production of peptide growth factors for host cells, which disrupt normal cellular growth, proliferation, and differentiation. In addition, viral factors can bind to and interfere with the function of host receptors for signaling molecules. Modulation of cytokine production during viral infection can stimulate viral growth inside cells with receptors for the cytokine, and virus-encoded cytokine homologues (e.g., the Epstein-Barr virus BCRF1 protein, which is highly homologous to the immunoinhibitory IL-10 molecule) can potentially prevent immune-mediated clearance of viral particles. Viruses can cause disease in neural cells by interfering with levels of neurotransmitters without necessarily destroying the cells, or they may induce either programmed cell death (apoptosis) to destroy tissues or inhibitors of apoptosis to allow for prolonged viral infection of cells. Overall, any disruption of normal cellular and tissue function due to viral infection can underlie the resultant clinical disease.

BACTERIAL TOXINS Among the first infectious diseases to be understood were those due to toxin-elaborating bacteria. Diphtheria, botulism, and tetanus toxins are responsible for the diseases associated with local infections due to *Corynebacterium diphtheriae*, *Clostridium botulinum*, and *Clostridium tetani*, respectively. Enterotoxins produced by *E. coli*, *Salmonella*, *Shigella*, *Staphylococcus*, and *V. cholerae* contribute to diarrheal disease caused by these organisms. Staphylococci, streptococci, *P. aeruginosa*, and *Bordetella* elaborate various toxins that cause or contribute to disease, including toxic shock syndrome toxin 1 (TSST-1); erythrogenic toxin; exotoxins A, S, and U; and pertussis toxin. A number of these toxins (e.g., cholera toxin, diphtheria toxin, pertussis toxin, *E. coli* heat-labile toxin, and *P. aeruginosa* exotoxin) have adenosine diphosphate (ADP)-ribosyltransferase activity; i.e., the toxins enzymatically catalyze the transfer of the ADP-ribosyl portion of nicotinamide adenine dinucleotide to target proteins and inactivate them. The staphylococcal enterotoxins, TSST-1, and the streptococcal pyogenic exotoxins behave as superantigens, stimulating certain T cells to proliferate without processing of the protein toxin by antigen-presenting cells. Part of this process involves stimulation of the antigen-presenting cells to produce IL-1 and TNF-α, which have been implicated in many of the clinical features of diseases like toxic shock syndrome and scarlet fever. A number of gram-negative pathogens (*Salmonella*, *Yersinia*, and *P. aeruginosa*) can inject toxins directly into host target cells by means of a complex set of proteins referred to as the type III secretion system. Loss or inactivation of this virulence system usually greatly reduces the capacity of a bacterial pathogen to cause disease.

ENDOTOXIN The lipid A portion of gram-negative LPS has potent biologic activities that cause many of the clinical manifestations of gram-negative bacterial sepsis, including fever, muscle proteolysis, uncontrolled intravascular coagulation, and shock. The effects of lipid A appear to be mediated by the production of potent cytokines due to LPS binding to CD14 and signal transduction via TLRs, particularly TLR4. Cytokines exhibit potent hypothermic activity through effects on the hypothalamus; they also increase vascular permeability, alter the activity of endothelial cells, and induce endothelial-cell procoagulant activity. Numerous therapeutic strategies aimed at neutralizing the effects of endotoxin are under investigation, but so far the results have been disappointing.

INVASION Many diseases are caused primarily by pathogens growing in tissue sites that are normally sterile. Pneumococcal pneumonia is mostly attributable to the growth of *S. pneumoniae* in the lung and the attendant host inflammatory response, although specific factors that enhance this process (e.g., pneumolysin) may be responsible for some of the pathogenic potential of the pneumococcus. Disease that follows bacteremia and invasion of the meninges by meningitis-producing bacteria such as *N. meningitidis*, *H. influenzae*, *E. coli* K1, and group B streptococci appears to be due solely to the ability of these organisms to gain access to these tissues, multiply in them, and provoke cytokine production leading to tissue-damaging host inflammation.

Specific molecular mechanisms accounting for tissue invasion by fungal and protozoal pathogens are less well described. Except for studies pointing to factors like capsule and melanin production by *C. neoformans* and possibly levels of cell wall glucans in some pathogenic fungi, the molecular basis for fungal invasiveness is not well defined. Melanism has been shown to protect the fungal cell against death caused by phagocyte factors such as nitric oxide, superoxide, and hypochlorite. Morphogenic variation and production of proteases (e.g., the *Candida* aspartyl proteinase) have been implicated in fungal invasion of host tissues.

If pathogens are effectively to invade host tissues (particularly the blood), they must avoid the major host defenses represented by complement and phagocytic cells. Bacteria most often avoid these defenses through their cell surface polysaccharides—either capsular polysaccharides or long O-side-chain antigens characteristic of the smooth LPS of gram-negative bacteria. These molecules can prevent the activation and/or deposition of complement opsonins or limit the access of phagocytic cells with receptors for complement opsonins to these molecules when they are deposited on the bacterial surface below the capsular layer. Another potential mechanism of microbial virulence is the ability of some organisms to present the capsule as an apparent self antigen through molecular mimicry. For example, the polysialic acid capsule of group B *N. meningitidis* is chemically identical to an oligosaccharide found on human brain cells.

Immunochemical studies of capsular polysaccharides have led to an appreciation of the tremendous chemical diversity that can result from the linking of a few monosaccharides. For example, three hexoses can link up in more than 300 different, potentially serologically distinct ways, while three amino acids have only six possible peptide combinations. Capsular polysaccharides have been used as effective vaccines against meningococcal meningitis as well as against pneumococcal and *H. influenzae* infections and may prove to be of value as vaccines against any organisms that express a nontoxic, immunogenic capsular polysaccharide. In addition, most encapsulated pathogens become virtually avirulent when capsule production is interrupted by genetic manipulation; this observation emphasizes the importance of this structure in pathogenesis.

HOST RESPONSE   The inflammatory response of the host is critical for interruption and resolution of the infectious process but also is often responsible for the signs and symptoms of disease. Infection promotes a complex series of host responses involving the complement, kinin, and coagulation pathways. The production of cytokines such as IL-1, TNF-α, and other factors regulated in part by the NF-κB transcription factor leads to fever, muscle proteolysis, and other effects, as noted above. An inability to kill or contain the microbe usually results in further damage due to the progression of inflammation and infection. For example, in many chronic infections, degranulation of host inflammatory cells can lead to release of host proteases, elastases, histamines, and other toxic substances that can degrade host tissues. Chronic inflammation in any tissue can lead to the destruction of that tissue and to clinical disease associated with loss of organ function, such as sterility from pelvic inflammatory disease caused by chronic infection with *N. gonorrhoeae*.

The nature of the host response elicited by the pathogen often determines the pathology of a particular infection. Local inflammation produces local tissue damage, while systemic inflammation, such as that seen during sepsis, can result in the signs and symptoms of septic shock. The severity of septic shock is associated with the degree of production of host effectors. Disease due to intracellular parasitism results from the formation of granulomas, wherein the host attempts to wall off the parasite inside a fibrotic lesion surrounded by fused epithelial cells that make up so-called multinucleated giant cells. A number of pathogens, particularly anaerobic bacteria, staphylococci, and streptococci, provoke the formation of an abscess, probably because of the presence of zwitterionic surface polysaccharides such as the capsular polysaccharide of *Bacteroides fragilis*. The outcome of an infection depends on the balance between an effective host response that eliminates a pathogen and an excessive inflammatory response that is associated with an inability to eliminate a pathogen and with the resultant tissue damage that leads to disease.

TRANSMISSION TO NEW HOSTS

As part of the pathogenic process, most microbes are shed from the host, often in a form infectious for susceptible individuals. However, the rate of transmissibility may not necessarily be high, even if the disease is severe in the infected individual, as these traits are not linked. Most pathogens exit via the same route by which they entered: respiratory pathogens by aerosols from sneezing or coughing or through salivary spread, gastrointestinal pathogens by fecal-oral spread, sexually transmitted diseases by venereal spread, and vector-borne organisms by either direct contact with the vector through a blood meal or indirect contact with organisms shed into environmental sources such as water. Microbial factors that specifically promote transmission are not well characterized. Respiratory shedding is facilitated by overproduction of mucous secretions, with consequently enhanced sneezing and coughing. Diarrheal toxins such as cholera toxin, *E. coli* heat-labile toxins, and *Shigella* toxins probably facilitate fecal-oral spread of microbial cells in the high volumes of diarrheal fluid produced during infection. The ability to produce phenotypic variants that resist hostile environmental factors (e.g., the highly resistant cysts of *E. histolytica* shed in feces) represents another mechanism of pathogenesis relevant to transmission. Blood parasites such as *Plasmodium* spp. change phenotype after ingestion by a mosquito—a prerequisite for the continued transmission of this pathogen. Venereally transmitted pathogens may undergo phenotypic variation due to the production of specific factors to facilitate transmission, but shedding of these pathogens into the environment does not result in the formation of infectious foci.

In summary, the molecular mechanisms used by pathogens to colonize, invade, infect, and disrupt the host are numerous and diverse. Each phase of the infectious process involves a variety of microbial and host factors interacting in a manner that can result in disease. Recognition of the coordinated genetic regulation of virulence factor elaboration when organisms move from their natural environment into the mammalian host emphasizes the complex nature of the host-parasite interaction. Fortunately, the need for diverse factors in successful infection and disease implies that a variety of therapeutic strategies may be developed to interrupt this process and thereby prevent and treat microbial infections.

FURTHER READING

Bassler BL: Small talk. Cell-to-cell communication in bacteria. Cell 17:421, 2002

Caroff M et al: Structural and functional analyses of bacterial lipopolysaccharides. Microbes Infect 4:915, 2002

Clapham PR, McKnight A: Cell surface receptors, virus entry and tropism of primate lentiviruses. J Gen Virol 83:1809, 2002

Dobrovolskaia MA, Vogel SN: Toll receptors, CD14, and macrophage activation and deactivation by LPS. Microbes Infect 4:903, 2002

Modlin RL: Mammalian Toll-like receptors. Ann Allergy Asthma Immunol 88:543, 2002

Portnoy DA: The cell biology of *Listeria monocytogenes* infection: The intersection of bacterial pathogenesis and cell-mediated immunity. J Cell Biol 5:409, 2002

Soll DR: *Candida* commensalism and virulence: The evolution of phenotypic plasticity. Acta Trop 81:101, 2002

Weiss RA: Virulence and pathogenesis. Trends Microbiol 10:314, 2002

106   APPROACH TO THE ACUTELY ILL INFECTED FEBRILE PATIENT
Tamar F. Barlam, Dennis L. Kasper

The physician treating the acutely ill febrile patient must be able to recognize infections that require emergent attention. If such infections are not adequately evaluated and treated at initial presentation, the opportunity to alter an adverse outcome may be lost. In this chapter, the clinical presentations of and approach to patients with relatively common infectious disease emergencies are discussed. These infectious processes are discussed in detail in other chapters. →*Noninfectious causes of fever are not covered in this chapter; information on the approach to fever of unknown origin, including that eventually shown to be of noninfectious etiology, is presented in Chap. 18.*

GENERAL CONSIDERATIONS

APPEARANCE A physician must have a consistent approach to acutely ill patients. Even before the history is elicited and a physical examination performed, an immediate assessment of the patient's general appearance yields valuable information. The perceptive physician's subjective sense that a patient is septic or toxic often proves accurate. Visible agitation or anxiety in a febrile patient can be a harbinger of critical illness.

HISTORY Presenting symptoms are frequently nonspecific. In addition to a general description of symptoms, it is important to obtain a sense of disease progression. Detailed questions should be asked about the onset and duration of symptoms and about changes in severity or rate of progression over time. Host factors and comorbid conditions may enhance the risk of infection with certain organisms or of a more fulminant course than is usually seen. Lack of splenic function, alcoholism with significant liver disease, intravenous drug use, HIV infection, diabetes, malignancy, and chemotherapy all predispose to specific infections and frequently to increased severity. The patient should be questioned about factors that might help identify a nidus for invasive infection, such as recent upper respiratory tract infections, influenza, or varicella; prior trauma; disruption of cutaneous barriers due to lacerations, burns, surgery, or decubiti; and the presence of foreign bodies, such as nasal packing after rhinoplasty, barrier contraceptives, tampons, arteriovenous fistulas, or prosthetic joints. Travel, contact with pets or other animals, or activities that might result in tick exposure can lead to diagnoses that would not otherwise be considered. Recent dietary intake, medication use, social or occupational contact with ill individuals, vaccination history, recent sexual contacts, and menstrual history may be relevant. A review of systems should focus on any neurologic signs or sensorium alterations, rashes or skin lesions, and focal pain or tenderness and should also include a general review of respiratory, gastrointestinal, or genitourinary symptoms. It is especially important to determine the duration and progression of these symptoms in order to gain an appreciation of the pace and urgency of the process.

PHYSICAL EXAMINATION A complete physical examination should be performed, with special attention to some areas that are sometimes given short shrift in routine examinations. Assessment of the patient's general appearance and vital signs, skin and soft tissue examination, and the neurologic evaluation are of particular importance.

The patient may appear either anxious and agitated or lethargic and apathetic. Fever is usually present, although elderly patients and compromised hosts (e.g., patients who are uremic or cirrhotic and those who are taking glucocorticoids or nonsteroidal anti-inflammatory agents) may be afebrile despite serious underlying infection. Measurement of blood pressure, heart rate, and respiratory rate helps determine the degree of hemodynamic and metabolic compromise. The patient's airway must be evaluated to rule out the risk of obstruction from an invasive oropharyngeal infection.

The etiologic diagnosis may become evident in the context of a thorough skin examination (see also Chap. 17). Petechial rashes are typically seen with meningococcemia or Rocky Mountain spotted fever (RMSF); erythroderma is usual with toxic shock syndrome (TSS) and drug fever. The soft tissue and muscle examination is critical. Areas of erythema or duskiness, edema, and tenderness may indicate underlying necrotizing fasciitis, myositis, or myonecrosis. The neurologic examination must include a careful assessment of mental status for signs of early encephalopathy. Evidence of nuchal rigidity or focal neurologic findings should be sought. Focal findings, depressed mental status, or papilledema should be evaluated by brain imaging prior to lumbar puncture, which, in this setting, could initiate herniation.

DIAGNOSTIC WORKUP After a quick clinical assessment, diagnostic material should be obtained rapidly and antibiotic and supportive treatment begun. Blood (for cultures; baseline complete blood count with differential; measurement of serum electrolytes, blood urea nitrogen, serum creatinine, and serum glucose; and liver function tests) can be obtained at the time an intravenous line is placed and before antibiotics are administered. For patients with possible acute endocarditis, three sets of blood cultures should be performed. Asplenic patients should have a blood smear examined to confirm the presence of Howell-Jolly bodies (indicating the absence of splenic function) and a buffy coat examined for bacteria; these patients can have $>10^6$ organisms per milliliter of blood (compared with 10^4/mL in patients with an intact spleen). Blood smears from patients at risk for severe parasitic disease, such as malaria or babesiosis, must be examined for the diagnosis and quantitation of parasitemia. Blood smears may also be diagnostic in ehrlichiosis.

Patients with possible meningitis should have cerebrospinal fluid (CSF) obtained before the initiation of antibiotic therapy. *If focal neurologic signs, abnormal mental status, or papilledema mandates brain imaging before a lumbar puncture, antibiotics should be administered prior to imaging but after blood for cultures has been drawn.* If CSF cultures are negative, laboratory examination of CSF by latex agglutination or immunoprecipitation can be attempted to make an etiologic diagnosis. However, blood cultures will provide the diagnosis in 50 to 70% of cases.

Focal abscesses necessitate immediate computed tomography or magnetic resonance imaging (MRI) as part of an evaluation for surgical intervention. Other diagnostic procedures, such as cultures of wounds or scraping of skin lesions, should not delay the initiation of treatment for more than minutes. Once emergent evaluation, diagnostic procedures, and (if appropriate) surgical consultation (see below) have been completed, other laboratory tests can be conducted. Appropriate radiography, computed axial tomography, MRI, urinalysis, erythrocyte sedimentation rate (ESR) determination, and transthoracic or transesophageal echocardiography may all prove important.

℞ TREATMENT

In the acutely ill patient, empirical antibiotic therapy is critical and should be administered without undue delay. Table 106-1 lists first-line treatments for the infections considered in this chapter. (For a more detailed discussion of treatment, see specific chapters.) In addition to the initiation of parenteral antibiotic therapy, several of these infections require urgent surgical attention. General surgery for possible necrotizing fasciitis or myonecrosis, neurosurgical evaluation for subdural empyema or spinal epidural abscess, otolaryngologic surgery for possible mucormycosis, and cardiothoracic surgery for critically ill patients with acute endocarditis are as important as the rapid commencement of antibiotic therapy. For infections such as necrotizing fasciitis and clostridial myonecrosis, rapid surgical intervention supersedes other diagnostic or therapeutic maneuvers.

Adjunctive treatments, such as intravenous immunoglobulin administration for TSS, can be considered after initial stabilization. Some adjunctive treatments, such as dexamethasone for bacterial meningitis or protein C replacement for meningococcemia, must be considered in conjunction with the initiation of antibiotic treatment.

SPECIFIC PRESENTATIONS

For most infections, there is time for careful evaluation, diagnostic testing, and consultation with other physicians before therapy commences. However, the infections considered below according to common clinical presentation can have rapidly catastrophic outcomes, and their immediate recognition and treatment can be life-saving. Recommended empirical therapeutic regimens are presented in Table 106-1.

SEPSIS WITHOUT AN OBVIOUS FOCUS OF PRIMARY INFECTION These patients initially have a brief prodrome of nonspecific symptoms and signs that progresses quickly to hemodynamic instability with hypotension, tachycardia, tachypnea, or respiratory distress. A patient may display altered mental status. Disseminated intravascular coagulation (DIC)

TABLE 106-1 *Common Infectious Disease Emergencies*

Clinical Syndrome	Possible Etiologies	Treatment	Comments	Reference(s)
SEPSIS WITHOUT A CLEAR FOCUS				
Gram-negative sepsis	*Pseudomonas* spp., gram-negative enteric bacilli	Piperacillin/tazobactam (3.75 g q4h) *or* Ceftazidime (2 g q8h) *plus* Tobramycin (5 mg/kg per day)	See Chap. 254.	136, 254
Gram-positive sepsis	*Staphylococcus* spp., *Streptococcus* spp.	Vancomycin (1 g q12h) *plus* Gentamicin (5 mg/kg per day)	If a β-lactam-sensitive strain is identified, antibiotics should be altered.	120, 121, 254
Overwhelming post-splenectomy sepsis	*Streptococcus pneumoniae, Haemophilus influenzae, Neisseria meningitidis*	Ceftriaxone (2 g q12h)[a]	If the isolate is penicillin-sensitive, penicillin is the drug of choice.	254
Babesiosis	*Babesia microti* (U.S.), *B. divergens* (Europe)	*Either:* Clindamycin (600 mg tid) *plus* Quinine (650 mg tid) *or* Atovaquone (750 mg q12h) *plus* Azithromycin (500-mg loading dose, then 250 mg/d)	Atovaquone and azithromycin have been shown to be as effective as clindamycin and quinine and are associated with fewer side effects. Treatment with doxycycline (100 mg bid) for potential coinfection with *Borrelia burgdorferi* or *Ehrlichia* spp. may be prudent.	193, 195
SEPSIS WITH SKIN FINDINGS				
Petechiae: Meningococcemia	*N. meningitidis*	Penicillin (4 mU q4h) *or* Ceftriaxone (2 g q12h)	Consider protein C replacement in fulminant meningococcemia.	127, 158
Rocky Mountain spotted fever	*Rickettsia rickettsii*	Doxycycline (100 mg bid)	If both meningococcemia and Rocky Mountain spotted fever are being considered, use chloramphenicol (50–75 mg/kg per day in four divided doses). *Do not add doxycycline to a regimen including a β-lactam agent.* If Rocky Mountain spotted fever is diagnosed, doxycycline is the proven superior agent.	
Purpura fulminans	*S. pneumoniae, H. influenzae, N. meningitidis*	Ceftriaxone (2 g q12h)[a]	If the isolate is penicillin-sensitive, penicillin is the drug of choice.	127, 254
Erythroderma: toxic shock syndrome	Group A *Streptococcus, Staphylococcus aureus*	Penicillin (2 mU q4h) *or* Oxacillin (2 g q4h) *plus* Clindamycin (600 mg q8h)	Site of toxigenic bacteria should be debrided; if necessary, intravenous immunoglobulin can be used in severe cases. The optimal dose of IVIG has not been determined, but the median dose in observational studies is 2 g/kg (total dose administered over 1–5 days).	120, 121
SEPSIS WITH SOFT TISSUE FINDINGS				
Necrotizing fasciitis	Group A *Streptococcus*, mixed aerobic/anaerobic flora	Penicillin (2 mU q4h) *plus* Clindamycin (600 mg q8h) *plus* Gentamicin (5 mg/kg per day)	Urgent surgical evaluation is critical.	110, 121
Clostridial myonecrosis	*Clostridium perfringens*	Penicillin (2 mU q4h) *plus* Clindamycin (600 mg q8h)	Urgent surgical evaluation is critical.	126
NEUROLOGIC INFECTIONS				
Bacterial meningitis	*S. pneumoniae, N. meningitidis*	Ceftriaxone (2 g q12h)[a]	If the isolate is penicillin-sensitive, penicillin is the drug of choice. If the patient is >50 years old, add ampicillin for *Listeria* coverage. Dexamethasone (10 mg q6h × 4 days) improves outcome in adult patients with meningitis (especially that due to *S. pneumoniae*) and cloudy CSF, positive CSF Gram's stain, or CSF leukocyte count >1000/µL.	360
Suppurative intracranial infections	*Staphylococcus* spp., *Streptococcus* spp., anaerobes, gram-negative bacilli	Oxacillin (2 g q4h)[b] *plus* Metronidazole (500 mg tid) *plus* Ceftriaxone (2 g q12h)	Urgent surgical evaluation is critical.	360
Brain abscess	*Streptococcus* spp., anaerobes, *Staphylococcus* spp.	Penicillin (4 mU q4h) *or* Oxacillin (2 g q4h)[b] *plus* Metronidazole (500 mg tid)	Surgical evaluation is essential.	360

(continued)

TABLE 106-1—(Continued)

Clinical Syndrome	Possible Etiologies	Treatment	Comments	Reference(s)
Cerebral malaria	*Plasmodium falciparum*	Quinine (650 mg tid for 3 days) ***plus*** Tetracycline (250 mg tid for 7 days)	Do not use glucocorticoids.	193, 195
Spinal epidural abscess	*Staphylococcus* spp.	Oxacillin (2 g q4h)[c]	Surgical evaluation is essential.	356
FOCAL INFECTIONS				
Acute bacterial endocarditis	*S. aureus*, β-hemolytic streptococci, HACEK group,[d] *Neisseria* spp., *S. pneumoniae*	Ceftriaxone (2 g q12h) ***plus*** Vancomycin (1 g q12h)	Adjust treatment when culture data become available. Surgical evaluation is essential.	109

[a] If resistant pneumococci are prevalent, add vancomycin (1 g q12h).
[b] Vancomycin (1 g q12h) should replace oxacillin if methicillin-resistant strains are highly prevalent.
[c] In HIV-infected intravenous drug users with suspected spinal epidural abscess, empirical therapy must cover gram-negative rods and methicillin-resistant *S. aureus*.

[d] *Haemophilus aphrophilus, H. paraphrophilus, H. parainfluenzae, Actinobacillus acti-nomycetemcomitans, Cardiobacterium hominis, Eikenella corrodens*, and *Kingella kingae*.
Note: References refer to chapters.

with clinical evidence of a hemorrhagic diathesis is a poor prognostic sign.

Septic Shock (See also Chap. 254)   Patients with bacteremia leading to septic shock may have a primary site of infection (e.g., pneumonia, pyelonephritis, or cholangitis) that is not evident initially. Elderly patients with comorbid conditions, hosts compromised by malignancy and neutropenia, or patients who have recently undergone a surgical procedure or hospitalization are at increased risk for an adverse outcome. Gram-negative bacteremia with organisms such as *Pseudomonas aeruginosa, Aeromonas hydrophila*, or *Escherichia coli* and gram-positive infection with organisms such as *Staphylococcus aureus* or group A streptococci can present as intractable hypotension and multiorgan failure. Treatment can usually be initiated empirically on the basis of the presentation (Table 254-4).

Overwhelming Infection in Asplenic Patients (See also Chap. 254)   Patients without splenic function are at risk for overwhelming bacterial sepsis. Asplenic adult patients succumb to sepsis at 58 times the rate of the general population; 50 to 70% of cases occur within the first 2 years after splenectomy, with a mortality rate of up to 80%. However, in the asplenic individual, an increased risk of overwhelming sepsis continues throughout life. In asplenia, encapsulated bacteria cause the majority of infections, and adults are at lower risk than children because they are more likely to have antibody to these organisms. *Streptococcus pneumoniae* infection is most common, causing 50 to 70% of cases, but the risk of infection with *Haemophilus influenzae* or *Neisseria meningitidis* is also high. Severe clinical manifestations of infections due to *E. coli, S. aureus*, group B streptococci, *P. aeruginosa, Capnocytophaga, Babesia*, and *Plasmodium* have been described.

Babesiosis (See also Chap. 195)   A history of recent travel to endemic areas should raise the possibility of infection with *Babesia*. Between 1 and 4 weeks after a tick bite, the patient experiences chills, fatigue, anorexia, myalgia, arthralgia, shortness of breath, nausea, and headache; ecchymosis and/or petechiae are occasionally seen. The tick that most commonly transmits *Babesia, Ixodes scapularis*, also transmits *Borrelia burgdorferi* (the agent of Lyme disease) and *Ehrlichia*, and co-infection can occur, resulting in more severe disease. Infection with the European species *Babesia divergens* is more frequently fulminant than that due to the U.S. species *Babesia microti*, causing a febrile syndrome with hemolysis, jaundice, hemoglobinemia, and renal failure and a mortality rate of >50%. Severe babesiosis is especially common in asplenic hosts but does occur in hosts with normal splenic function, particularly those >60 years of age. Complications include renal failure, acute respiratory failure, and DIC.

Other Sepsis Syndromes   Tularemia (Chap. 142) is seen throughout the United States but occurs primarily in Arkansas, Oklahoma, and Missouri. This disease is associated with wild rabbit, tick, and tabanid fly contact. The uncommon typhoidal form can be associated with gram-negative septic shock and a mortality rate of >30%. In the United States, plague (Chap. 143) occurs primarily in New Mexico, Arizona,

and Colorado after contact with ground squirrels, prairie dogs, or chipmunks. The septic form is particularly rare and is associated with shock, multiorgan failure, and a 30% mortality rate. These rare infections should be considered in the appropriate epidemiologic setting. Tularemia and plague, along with anthrax, are listed by the Centers for Disease Control and Prevention as important biological agents that might be intentionally used for bioterrorism (Table 106-2 and Chap. 205).

SEPSIS WITH SKIN MANIFESTATIONS (See also Chap. 17)   Maculopapular rashes may reflect early meningococcal or rickettsial disease but are usually associated with nonemergent infections. Exanthems are usually viral. It is noteworthy that primary HIV infection commonly presents with rash. Untreated, symptomatic HIV-seroconversion illness is associated with rapid progression to late-stage disease. The rash is typically maculopapular and involves the upper part of the body but can spread to the palms and soles. In addition, the patient is febrile and can have lymphadenopathy, severe headache, dysphagia, diarrhea, myalgias, and arthralgias. Recognition of this syndrome not only can prevent the spread of HIV to other individuals but also provides an opportunity for early treatment and improved prognosis.

Petechiae   Petechial rashes caused by viruses are seldom associated with hypotension or a toxic appearance, although severe measles can be an exception. In other settings, petechial rashes require more urgent attention.

MENINGOCOCCEMIA (See also Chap. 127)   Almost three-quarters of patients with bacteremic *N. meningitidis* infection have a rash. Meningococcemia most often affects young children (i.e., those 6 months to 5 years old, often in day care). However, sporadic cases and outbreaks occur in schools (grade school through college) and army barracks. Between 10 and 20% of all cases have a fulminant course, with shock, DIC, and multiorgan failure. Of these patients, 50 to 60% die, and survivors often require extensive debridement or amputation of gangrenous extremities. Patients may exhibit fever, headache, nausea, vomiting, myalgias, change in mental status, and meningismus. However, the rapidly progressive form of disease is not usually associated with meningitis. The rash is initially pink, blanching, and maculopapular, appearing on the trunk and extremities, but then becomes hemorrhagic, forming petechiae. Petechiae are first seen at the ankles, wrists, axillae, mucosal surfaces, and palpebral and bulbar conjunctiva, with subsequent spread to the lower extremities and trunk. A cluster of petechiae may be seen at pressure points—e.g., where a blood pressure cuff has been inflated. In rapidly progressive meningococcemia, the petechial rash quickly becomes purpuric (see Fig. 46-5) and patients develop DIC. Hypotension with petechiae for <12 h is associated with significant mortality. The mortality rate can exceed 90% among patients without meningitis who have rash, hypotension, and a normal or low white blood cell count and ESR. Cyanosis, coma, oliguria, metabolic acidosis, and elevated partial thromboplastin time are also associated with a fatal outcome. A better prognosis has been re-

Clinical Presentation	Agent	Signs and Symptoms	First-Line Treatment[b]	Comments	Reference Chapters
Sepsis without an obvious focus	Plague[c] Tularemia[d]	Fever, fatigue, headache, dyspnea, chest pain progressing to fulminant course of sepsis, shock, multiorgan failure, DIC	Streptomycin (1 g IM q12h) *or* Gentamicin (5 mg/kg per day) *plus* Ciprofloxacin (400 mg IV q12h)	Alternatives: Doxycycline (100 mg IV q12h) *or* Chloramphenicol (15 mg/kg IV q6h) *or* A different fluoroquinolone	142, 143, 180, 181, 205
	Smallpox[e] and hemorrhagic fevers[f]	Patients can present before rash develops with severe nonspecific febrile illness.			
Sepsis with skin manifestations	Hemorrhagic fevers	Viral prodrome, high fevers, myalgias, encephalitis, bleeding diatheses with progression to petechial rash and mucous membrane hemorrhages	Provide supportive care and begin ribavirin. Continue if an arenavirus or bunyavirus is identified.	Person-to-person transmission with arenaviruses, Ebola virus, and Marburg virus	180, 181, 205
	Smallpox	Fever, myalgias, toxicity. Rash begins on face, extremities—vesicular lesions in one crop progressing to deep pustules	Supportive care	Person-to-person transmission Petechial or hemorrhagic forms described	
Neurologic infections with/without septic shock	Botulism[g]	No fever, sensation intact, mental status normal, symmetric cranial-nerve palsies, symmetric descending flaccid paralysis starting in bulbar region	Supportive care and antitoxin	Distinguish from Guillain-Barré and poliomyelitis—no antecedent infection, normal CSF, no sensory signs	125, 205
	Anthrax	Hemorrhagic meningitis can be associated with presentation.	Include rifampin, penicillin, or chloramphenicol along with primary treatment below.		
Focal infection with fulminant course	Anthrax[h] (inhalational)	Fever, cough, sweats, chest pain, abnormal chest x-rays—mediastinal widening, effusions	Ciprofloxacin (400 mg IV q12h) *or* Doxycycline (100 mg q12h) *plus* 1−2 additional agents	Consider clindamycin (600 mg q8h) for possible inhibition of toxin production.	142, 143, 205
	Plague	Fever, cough, cyanosis; bloody, watery sputum	See above.		
	Tularemia	Fulminant pneumonia	See above.		

[a] For details, see Chap. 205. The Centers for Disease Control and Prevention has defined three categories of biological agents that can be used as weapons of terror on the basis of their ease of dissemination or transmission, potential for public health impact, potential for public panic, and requirements for preparedness. Category A agents are those of greatest concern.

[b] Recommendations for mass casualty situations and special populations differ. Consult appropriate consensus statements.

[c] Inglesby TV et al: Plague as a biological weapon. JAMA 283:2281, 2000.
[d] Dennis DT et al: Tularemia as a biological weapon. JAMA 285:2763, 2001.
[e] Henderson DA et al: Smallpox as a biological weapon. JAMA 281:2127, 1999.
[f] Borio L et al: Hemorrhagic fever viruses as biological weapons. JAMA 287:2391, 2002.
[g] Arnon SS et al: Botulinum toxin as a biological weapon. JAMA 285:1059, 2001.
[h] Inglesby TV et al: Anthrax as a biological weapon. JAMA 287:2236, 2002.

ported in cases where antibiotics are given before admission by the primary care provider. This observation suggests that early initiation of treatment may be life-saving. In addition, several small experimental and clinical studies have suggested that correction of the protein C deficiency that is evident in meningococcal purpura fulminans can improve outcome.

ROCKY MOUNTAIN SPOTTED FEVER (See also Chap. 158) RMSF occurs throughout the United States. A history of known tick bite is common; however, if such a history is lacking, a history of travel or outdoor activity (e.g., camping in tick-infested areas) can be ascertained. RMSF is caused by *Rickettsia rickettsii*. For the first 3 days, headache, fever, malaise, myalgias, nausea, vomiting, and anorexia are present. By day 3, half of patients have skin findings. Blanching macules develop initially on the wrists and ankles and then spread over the legs and trunk. The lesions become hemorrhagic and are frequently petechial. The rash spreads to palms and soles later in the course. The centripetal spread is a classic feature of RMSF. However, 10 to 15% of patients with RMSF never develop a rash. The patient can be hypotensive and develop noncardiogenic pulmonary edema, confusion, lethargy, and encephalitis progressing to coma. The CSF contains 10 to 100 cells/μL, usually with a predominance of mononuclear cells. The CSF glucose level is often normal; the protein concentration may be slightly elevated. Renal and hepatic injury and bleeding secondary to vascular damage are noted. Untreated infection has a mortality rate of 30%.

Purpura Fulminans (See also Chaps. 127 and 254) Purpura fulminans is the cutaneous manifestation of DIC and presents as large ecchymotic areas and hemorrhagic bullae. Progression of petechiae to purpura and ecchymoses is associated with congestive heart failure, septic shock, acute renal failure, acidosis, hypoxia, hypotension, and death. Purpura fulminans has been associated primarily with *N. meningitidis* but, in splenectomized patients, may be associated with *S. pneumoniae* and *H. influenzae*.

Ecthyma Gangrenosum Septic shock caused by *P. aeruginosa* and *A. hydrophila* can be associated with ecthyma gangrenosum (see Fig. 136-1): hemorrhagic vesicles surrounded by a rim of erythema with central necrosis and ulceration. These gram-negative bacteremias are most common among patients with neutropenia, extensive burns, and hypogammaglobulinemia.

Other Emergent Infections Associated with Rash *Vibrio vulnificus* and other noncholera *Vibrio* bacteremic infections (Chap. 140) can cause focal skin lesions and overwhelming sepsis in the host with liver disease. After ingestion of contaminated shellfish, there is a sudden onset of malaise, chills, fever, and hypotension. The patient develops bullous or hemorrhagic skin lesions, usually on the lower extremities, and 75% of patients have leg pain. The mortality rate can be as high as 50%. *Capnocytophaga canimorsus* can cause septic shock in asplenic patients. Infection with this fastidious gram-negative rod typically presents after a dog bite as fever, chills, myalgia, vomiting, diarrhea, dyspnea, confusion, and headache. Findings can include an exanthem or erythema multiforme (see Fig. 46-9), cyanotic mottling or peripheral cyanosis, petechiae, and ecchymosis. About 30% of patients with this fulminant form die of overwhelming sepsis and DIC, and survivors may require amputation because of gangrene.

Erythroderma TSS (Chaps. 120 and 121) is usually associated with erythroderma. The patient presents with fever, malaise, myalgias, nausea, vomiting, diarrhea, and confusion. There is a sunburn-type rash that may be subtle and patchy but is usually diffuse and is found on the face, trunk, and extremities. Erythroderma, which desquamates after 1 to 2 weeks, is more common in *Staphylococcus*-associated than in *Streptococcus*-associated TSS. Hypotension develops rapidly—often within hours—after the onset of symptoms. Multiorgan failure is seen. Commonly there is no indication of a primary focal infection, although possible cutaneous or mucosal portals of entry for the organism can be ascertained when a careful history is taken. Colonization rather than overt infection of the vagina or a postoperative wound, for example, is typical with staphylococcal TSS, and the mucosal areas appear hyperemic but not infected. Early renal failure may precede hypotension and distinguishes this syndrome from other septic shock syndromes. Clinical evaluation constitutes the diagnosis because TSS is defined by the clinical criteria of fever, rash, hypotension, and multiorgan involvement. The mortality rate is 5% for menstruation-associated TSS, 10 to 15% for nonmenstrual TSS, and 30 to 70% for streptococcal TSS.

SEPSIS WITH A SOFT TISSUE/MUSCLE PRIMARY FOCUS (See also Chap. 110) ■ **Necrotizing Fasciitis** This infection may arise at a site of minimal trauma or postoperative incision and may also be associated with recent varicella, childbirth, or muscle strain. The most common causes of necrotizing fasciitis are group A streptococci alone (Chap. 121) and a mixed facultative and anaerobic flora (Chap. 110). Diabetes mellitus, peripheral vascular disease, and intravenous drug use are associated risk factors. Use of nonsteroidal anti-inflammatory agents adversely affects granulocyte chemotaxis, phagocytosis, and bacterial killing, allowing progression of skin or soft tissue infections. The patient may have bacteremia and hypotension without other organ-system failure. Physical findings are minimal compared with the severity of pain and the degree of fever. The examination is often unremarkable except for soft tissue edema and erythema. The infected area is red, hot, shiny, swollen, and exquisitely tender. In untreated infection, the overlying skin develops blue-gray patches after 36 h, and cutaneous bullae and necrosis develop after 3 to 5 days. Necrotizing fasciitis due to a mixed flora, but not that due to group A streptococci, can be associated with gas production. Without treatment, pain decreases because of thrombosis of the small blood vessels and destruction of the peripheral nerves—an ominous sign. The mortality rate is >30% overall, >70% in association with TSS, and nearly 100% without surgical intervention. Life-threatening necrotizing fasciitis may also be due to *Clostridium perfringens* (Chap. 126); in this condition, the patient is extremely toxic and the mortality rate is high. Within 48 h, rapid tissue invasion and systemic toxicity associated with hemolysis and death ensue. The distinction between this entity and clostridial myonecrosis is made by muscle biopsy.

Clostridial Myonecrosis (See also Chap. 126) Myonecrosis is often associated with trauma or surgery but can be spontaneous. The incubation period is usually 12 to 24 h long, and massive necrotizing gangrene develops within hours of onset. Systemic toxicity, shock, and death can occur within 12 h. The patient's pain and toxic appearance are out of proportion to physical findings. On examination, the patient is febrile, apathetic, tachycardic, and tachypneic and may express a feeling of impending doom. Hypotension and renal failure

develop later, and hyperalertness is evident preterminally. The skin over the affected area is bronze-brown, mottled, and edematous. Bullous lesions with serosanguineous drainage and a mousy or sweet odor can be present. Crepitus can occur secondary to gas production in muscle tissue. The mortality rate is >65% with spontaneous myonecrosis, which is often associated with *Clostridium septicum* and underlying malignancy. The mortality rates associated with trunk and limb infection are 63 and 12%, respectively, and any delay in surgical treatment increases the risk of death.

NEUROLOGIC INFECTIONS WITH OR WITHOUT SEPTIC SHOCK ■ **Bacterial Meningitis** (See also Chap. 360) Bacterial meningitis is one of the most common infectious emergencies involving the central nervous system. Although hosts with cell-mediated immune deficiency (including transplant recipients, diabetic patients, elderly patients, and cancer patients treated with certain chemotherapeutic agents) are at particular risk for *Listeria monocytogenes* meningitis, most cases in adults are due to *S. pneumoniae* (30 to 50%) and *N. meningitidis* (10 to 35%). An early presentation of headache, meningismus, and fever is classic but is seen in only one-half to two-thirds of patients. The elderly can present without fever or meningeal signs despite lethargy and confusion. Cerebral dysfunction is evidenced by confusion, delirium, and lethargy that can progress to coma. The presentation is fulminant, with sepsis and brain edema, in some cases; papilledema at presentation is unusual and suggests another diagnosis (e.g., an intracranial lesion). Focal signs, including cranial nerve palsies (IV, VI, VII), can be seen in 10 to 20% of cases; 50 to 60% of patients have bacteremia. A poor outcome is associated with coma at any time during the course, hypotension, meningitis due to *S. pneumoniae*, or a CSF glucose level of <0.6 mmol/L (<10 mg/dL). Mortality is associated with coma, respiratory distress, shock, a CSF protein level of >2.5 g/L, a peripheral white blood cell count of <5000/μL, and a serum sodium level of <135 mmol/L.

Suppurative Intracranial Infections (See also Chap. 360) Other rare intracranial lesions that present with sepsis and hemodynamic instability are subdural empyema, septic cavernous sinus thrombosis, and septic superior sagittal sinus thrombosis. Rapid recognition of the toxic patient with central neurologic signs is crucial to improvement of the dismal prognosis of these entities.

SUBDURAL EMPYEMA This infection arises from the paranasal sinus in 60 to 70% of cases. Microaerophilic streptococci and staphylococci are the predominant etiologic organisms. The patient is toxic, with fever, headache, and nuchal rigidity. Of all patients, 75% have focal signs and 6 to 20% die. Despite improved survival rates, 15 to 44% of patients are left with permanent neurologic deficits.

SEPTIC CAVERNOUS SINUS THROMBOSIS This condition follows a facial or sphenoid sinus infection; 70% of cases are due to staphylococci and the remainder are due primarily to aerobic or anaerobic streptococci. A unilateral or retroorbital headache progresses to a toxic appearance and fever within days. Three-quarters of patients have unilateral periorbital edema that becomes bilateral and then progresses to ptosis, proptosis, ophthalmoplegia, and papilledema. The mortality rate is as high as 30%.

SEPTIC THROMBOSIS OF THE SUPERIOR SAGITTAL SINUS This infection spreads from the ethmoid or maxillary sinuses. Its bacterial causes include *S. pneumoniae*, other streptococci, and staphylococci. The fulminant course is characterized by headache, nausea, vomiting, rapid progression to confusion and coma, nuchal rigidity, and brainstem signs. If the sinus is totally thrombosed, the mortality rate exceeds 80%.

Brain Abscess (See also Chap. 360) Brain abscess often occurs without systemic signs. Almost half of patients are afebrile, and presentations are more consistent with a space-occupying lesion in the brain; 70% of patients have headache, 50% have focal neurologic signs, and 25% have papilledema. Abscesses can present as single or multiple lesions resulting from contiguous foci or hematogenous infection, such as unrecognized endocarditis. The infection progresses over several days from cerebritis to an abscess with a mature capsule. More than half of infections are polymicrobial, with an etiology consisting of aerobic bacteria (primarily streptococcal species) and anaerobes. Abscesses arising hematogenously are especially apt to rupture into the ventricular space, causing a sudden and severe deterioration in clinical status and high mortality. Otherwise, mortality is low but morbidity is high (30 to 55%). Patients presenting with stroke and a parameningeal infectious focus, such as sinusitis or otitis, may have a brain abscess, and physicians must maintain a high level of suspicion. Prognosis worsens in patients with a fulminant course, delayed diagnosis, abscess rupture into the ventricles, multiple abscesses, or abnormal neurologic status at presentation.

Cerebral Malaria (See also Chap. 195)   This entity should be urgently considered if patients who have recently traveled to areas endemic for malaria present with a febrile illness and lethargy or other neurologic signs. Fulminant malaria is caused by *Plasmodium falciparum* and is associated with temperatures of >40°C (>104°F), hypotension, jaundice, adult respiratory distress syndrome, and bleeding. By definition, any patient with a change in mental status or repeated seizure in the setting of fulminant malaria has cerebral malaria. In adults, this nonspecific febrile illness progresses to coma over several days; occasionally, coma occurs within hours and death within 24 h. Nuchal rigidity and photophobia are rare. On physical examination, symmetric encephalopathy is typical, and upper motor neuron dysfunction with decorticate and decerebrate posturing can be seen in advanced disease. Unrecognized infection results in a 20 to 30% mortality rate.

SPINAL EPIDURAL ABSCESSES (See also Chap. 356)   Patients with spinal epidural abscesses often present with back pain and develop neurologic deficits late in their course. At-risk patients include those with diabetes mellitus; intravenous drug use; chronic alcohol abuse; recent spinal trauma, surgery, or epidural anesthesia; and other comorbid conditions, such as HIV infection. The thoracic or lumbar spine is the most common location, and staphylococci are the most common etiologic agents; in HIV-infected intravenous drug users, therapy must cover gram-negative rods and methicillin-resistant *S. aureus*. If a patient gives a history of antecedent back pain and has new neurologic symptoms, this diagnosis must immediately be considered. Almost 60% of patients have fever and almost 90% have back pain. Paresthesia, bowel and bladder dysfunction, radicular pain, and weakness are frequent neurologic complaints, and examination of the patient may reveal abnormal reflexes and motor and sensory deficits. The ESR and leukocyte counts are usually elevated. Rapid recognition and treatment, including immediate drainage, can prevent or minimize permanent neurologic sequelae.

FOCAL SYNDROMES WITH A FULMINANT COURSE   Infection at virtually any primary focus (e.g., osteomyelitis, pneumonia, pyelonephritis, or cholangitis) can result in bacteremia and sepsis. TSS has been associated with focal infections such as septic arthritis, peritonitis, sinusitis, and wound infection. Death occurs secondary to septic shock or toxin production with hemodynamic instability and multiorgan failure. Rapid clinical deterioration and death can be associated with destruction of the primary site of infection, as is seen in endocarditis and in necrotizing infections of the oropharynx (in which edema suddenly compromises the airway).

Rhinocerebral Mucormycosis (See also Chap. 189)   Patients with diabetes or malignancy are at risk for invasive rhinocerebral mucormycosis. Patients present with low-grade fever, dull sinus pain, diplopia, decreased mental status, decreased ocular motion, chemosis, proptosis, dusky or necrotic nasal turbinates, and necrotic hard-palate lesions that respect the midline. Without rapid recognition and intervention, the process continues an inexorable invasive course with high mortality.

Acute Bacterial Endocarditis (See also Chap. 109)   This entity presents with a much more aggressive course than subacute endocarditis. Bacteria such as *S. aureus*, *S. pneumoniae*, *L. monocytogenes*, *Haemophilus* spp., and streptococci of groups A, B, and G attack native valves. Mortality rates range from 10 to 40%. The host may have comorbid conditions such as underlying malignancy, diabetes mellitus, intravenous drug use, or alcoholism. The patient presents with fever, fatigue, and malaise <2 weeks after onset of infection. On physical examination, a changing murmur and congestive heart failure may be noted. Hemorrhagic macules on palms or soles (*Janeway lesions*) sometimes develop. Petechiae, Roth's spots, splinter hemorrhages, and splenomegaly are unusual. Rapid valvular destruction, particularly of the aortic valve, results in pulmonary edema and hypotension. Myocardial abscesses can form, eroding through the septum or into the conduction system and causing life-threatening arrhythmias or high-degree conduction block. Large friable vegetations can result in major arterial emboli, metastatic infection, or tissue infarction. Emboli can lead to stroke, change in mental status, visual disturbances, aphasia, ataxia, headache, meningismus, brain abscess, cerebritis, spinal cord infarct with paraplegia, arthralgia, osteomyelitis, splenic abscess, septic arthritis, and hematuria. Older patients with *S. aureus* endocarditis are especially likely to present with nonspecific symptoms—a circumstance that delays diagnosis and worsens prognosis. Rapid intervention is crucial for a successful outcome.

Inhalational Anthrax (See also Chap. 205)   Inhalational anthrax, the most severe form of disease caused by *Bacillus anthracis*, had not been reported in the United States for more than 25 years until the recent use of this organism as an agent of bioterrorism (Table 106-2 and Chap. 205). Patients presented with malaise, fever, cough, nausea, drenching sweats, shortness of breath, and headache. Rhinorrhea was unusual. All patients had abnormal chest roentgenograms at presentation. Mediastinal widening, pulmonary infiltrates, and pleural effusions were the most common findings. All patients who developed fulminant disease before receiving antibiotics died. Hemorrhagic meningitis has been seen in up to 50% of patients in other large outbreaks. Without urgent intervention with antimicrobial agents and supportive care, inhalational anthrax progresses rapidly to hypotension, cyanosis, and death.

CONCLUSION

Acutely ill febrile patients, with the syndromes discussed in this chapter, require close observation, aggressive supportive measures, and—in most cases—admission to intensive care units. The most important task of the physician is to distinguish these patients from other infected febrile patients who will not progress to fulminant disease. The alert physician must recognize the acute infectious emergency and then proceed with appropriate urgency.

FURTHER READING

ALBERIO L et al: Protein C replacement in severe meningococcemia: Rationale and clinical experience. Clin Infect Dis 32:1338, 2001

ASTIZ ME et al: Septic shock. Lancet 351:1501, 1998

DE GANS J et al: Dexamethasone in adults with bacterial meningitis. N Engl J Med 347:1549, 2002

HENRETIG FM et al: Medical management of the suspected victim of bioterrorism: An algorithmic approach to the undifferentiated patient. Emerg Med Clin North Am 20:351, 2002

KRAUSE PJ: Babesiosis. Med Clin North Am 86:361, 2002

NEWTON CRJC et al: Cerebral malaria. J Neurol Neurosurg Psychiatry 69:433, 2000

SEXTON DJ et al: Rocky Mountain spotted fever. Med Clin North Am 86:351, 2002

STEVENS DL: Streptococcal toxic shock syndrome associated with necrotizing fasciitis. Annu Rev Med 51:271, 2000

SUMARAJU V et al: Infectious complications in asplenic hosts. Infect Dis Clin North Am 15:551, 2001

Most humans live their lives ignoring the certainty of their own mortality. Perhaps this fact explains why the adage "an ounce of prevention is worth a pound of cure" has so little effect on their everyday behavior. Even when it comes to acting to protect their young, parents are capable of ignoring the potential for the death of their children in the developed world and of accepting the certainty of childhood deaths in the developing world. In both settings, parents all too often fail to seek out and demand the best preventive measures available. Unless mandated by the law in wealthy societies or provided by benevolent organizations or governments in poor nations, universal immunization has invariably remained an unattained goal.

Vaccination is ranked as one of the greatest public health achievements of the twentieth century and is the principal factor contributing to the reduction of morbidity and mortality among children around the world. The integration of immunization practices (a major component of primary disease prevention) into routine health care services has provided caregivers with control over a substantial proportion of the disease and mortality that plagued the United States during the first half of the twentieth century (Table 107-1). For society today, immunization is one of the few cost-saving interventions to prevent infectious disease. At present, >50 biologic products are licensed in the United States. A total of 21 antigens, many in the form of combined vaccines, are used for routine immunization during the first 18 months of life, including diphtheria/tetanus/acellular pertussis (DTaP) vaccine, trivalent inactivated poliovirus vaccine (IPV), measles/mumps/rubella (MMR) vaccine, Haemophilus influenzae type b (Hib) vaccine, hepatitis B (HepB) and hepatitis A (HepA) vaccines, and varicella vaccine. Recently, a heptavalent pneumococcal vaccine has been recommended for routine use in children, as has influenza vaccine (given annually). Five vaccines are designed for routine use in adults: tetanus/diphtheria (Td) toxoids formulated for adult use; HepB vaccine; influenza virus vaccine; polyvalent pneumococcal polysaccharide vaccine; and varicella vaccine. Some preparations are designated as special-use vaccines for outbreak response, prophylaxis in travelers, or regional use (e.g., vaccines against Neisseria meningitidis, Japanese B encephalitis virus, yellow fever virus, and Salmonella typhi and HepA vaccine). Unfortunately, vaccines for eukaryotic pathogens (protozoa and helminths), which affect a large proportion of the world's population, have been difficult to develop and remain only a hope for the future.

Healthy People 2010 Objectives for the Nation includes a set of immunization indicators. By 2010, 80% of children should have received DTaP, poliovirus, MMR, Hib, and HepB vaccines, while 90% of adults are expected to have received influenza and pneumococcal vaccines.

IMPACT OF IMMUNIZATION The epidemiologically appropriate use of vaccines has resulted in the global eradication of smallpox and, until recently, the cessation of smallpox vaccination. Immunization has eliminated naturally transmitted poliomyelitis from the Western Hemisphere, Europe, and the Western Pacific. Similarly, measles, which had a nearly 100% infectivity rate in the prevaccination era, has been effectively eliminated from most of the Western Hemisphere by widespread immunization. Current debate centers around whether it is possible to eradicate an organism from the world and cease immunization or whether the best that can be hoped for is the elimination of clinical disease worldwide, with continued routine immunization. Already achieved in the United States are the virtual elimination of congenital rubella syndrome, tetanus, and diphthe-

ria as well as a dramatic reduction in pertussis, rubella, measles, and mumps. The introduction of Hib conjugate vaccines for immunization of infants has all but eliminated invasive Haemophilus infections (including meningitis and pneumonia) because this vaccine both elicits durable immunity by the time maternal-derived antibodies have dissipated and reduces nasopharyngeal carriage of Hib, thereby reducing the risk of transmission. Polyvalent pneumococcal polysaccharide conjugate vaccine is having a significant impact on invasive pneumococcal disease, including otitis media.

DEFINITIONS Vaccination and immunization are often used as interchangeable terms. However, the former denotes only the administration of a vaccine, whereas the latter describes the process of inducing or providing immunity by any means, whether active or passive. Thus, vaccination does not guarantee immunization. Active immunization refers to the induction of immune defenses by the administration of antigens in appropriate forms, whereas passive immunization involves the provision of temporary protection by the administration of exogenously produced immune substances (Table 107-2).

PRINCIPLES OF IMMUNIZATION Artificial induction of immunity closely follows two well-tested principles of nature. The first, active immunization, can be traced at least as far back as Thucydides, who noted that people surviving epidemics of plague in Athens were spared during later outbreaks of the same disease. The second, passive immunization, is a natural process as well and is exemplified by the transplacental transmission of maternal antibodies to the fetus to provide protection against several diseases during the first months of life. Use of the two measures together may produce a complementary effect (as with HepB vaccine plus hepatitis B immune globulin) or may actually interfere with the development of immunity (as when measles vaccine is administered within 6 weeks of measles immunoglobulin). Depending on whether there are multiple species or serotypes of an organism and—if so—whether there are common, cross-reactive, protective antigens, a specific vaccine may induce protection against all representative forms of an infectious agent or against the immunizing strain only. One of the intrinsic virtues of whole-organism vaccines is that they potentially contain all protective antigens of the organism. However, this virtue is counterbalanced by an inherent problem with such vaccines: the possibility of adverse responses to reactive but nonprotective antigens present in the mix. Because the immune response to specific antigens is controlled genetically, all individuals cannot be expected to respond identically to the same vaccine.

APPROACHES TO ACTIVE IMMUNIZATION The two standard approaches to active immunization are (1) the use of live, generally attenuated, in-

TABLE 107-1 *Reduction in Morbidity due to Vaccine-Preventable Diseases in the United States, 1900–2002*

Disease	Reporting Period	Annual Morbidity Prior to Vaccine	2001 Morbidity	2002 Morbidity[a]	Decrease, %[b]
Smallpox	1900–1904	48,164	0	0	100
Diphtheria	1920–1922	175,885	2	1	100
Pertussis	1922–1925	147,271	7580	8296	94.6
Tetanus	1922–1926	1314	27	23	98.1
Neonatal tetanus	1972–1985	785	29	1	98.1
Poliomyelitis (paralytic)	1951–1954	16,316	0	0	100
Measles	1958–1962	503,282	116	37	99.9
Mumps	1968	152,209	266	238	99.8
Rubella	1966–1968	47,745	23	14	99.9
Congenital rubella syndrome	1969	823	3	3	99.6
Haemophilus influenzae type b	Before 1985	20,000	27	27	99.9

[a] Provisional data.
[b] Average of figures for 2001 and 2002 compared with peak incidence.

TABLE 107-2 *Definitions of Immunizing Agents*

Term	Definition
Vaccine	A preparation of attenuated live or killed microorganisms or antigenic portions of these agents presented to a potential host to induce immunity and prevent disease
Toxoid	A modified bacterial toxin that has been made nontoxic but retains the capacity to stimulate the formation of antitoxin
Immune globulin	An antibody-containing protein fraction derived from human plasma and used primarily for maintenance of the immunity of persons with immunodeficiency disorders or for passive immunization when there is no opportunity for active immunization[a]
Antitoxin	An antibody derived from the serum of animals after stimulation with specific antigens and used to provide passive immunity to the toxin protein to which it is directed

[a] Both intramuscular and intravenous preparations are available.

fectious agents (e.g., measles virus); and (2) the use of inactivated agents or their constituents or products obtained by genetic recombination (e.g., acellular pertussis vaccines). For many diseases (e.g., poliomyelitis), both approaches have been employed.

Live attenuated vaccines consisting of selected or genetically altered organisms that are avirulent or dramatically attenuated, yet remain immunogenic, generally produce long-lasting immunity. These agents are expected to cause a subclinical illness and immunologic response mimicking natural infection (except for the lack of clinically significant disease). They offer the advantage of replication in vivo, which increases the antigenic load presented to the host's immune system; they may confer lifelong protection with one dose; they present all expressed antigens, thus overcoming immunogenetic restrictions in some hosts; they may reach the local sites most relevant to the induction of protective immunity; and they may produce important protective antigens in vivo that are not efficiently expressed in vitro.

Inactivated vaccines typically require multiple doses and periodic boosters thereafter for the maintenance of immunity. The exception to this rule is pure polysaccharide vaccine, whose effects cannot be boosted by additional exposures. Nonviable vaccines administered parenterally fail to elicit mucosal IgA-mediated immunity, as they lack a delivery system that can effectively transport them to local antigen-processing cells. However, killed vaccines can be extremely successful. For example, the nonviable HepA vaccine formulation appears to be close to 100% effective in inducing protective immunity. Currently available nonviable vaccines consist of inactivated whole organisms (e.g., plague vaccine); detoxified protein exotoxins (e.g., tetanus toxoid); recombinant protein antigens (e.g., HepB vaccine); or carbohydrate antigens, either present as soluble purified capsular material (e.g., *Streptococcus pneumoniae* polysaccharides) or conjugated to a protein carrier (e.g., Hib polysaccharide conjugated to diphtheria or tetanus toxoids).

Despite their advantages, live vaccines are not always preferable. For example, live oral poliovirus vaccine (OPV) is contraindicated for use in children with immune deficiency diseases or their adult contacts. In addition, even though killed poliovirus vaccine does not completely immunize the gut or immunize contacts of vaccine recipients, the United States has now switched to a four-dose schedule of this vaccine because of the rare but real risk of vaccine-associated polio posed by live OPV.

APPROACHES TO PASSIVE IMMUNIZATION Passive immunization is generally used to provide temporary immunity in an unimmunized subject exposed to an infectious disease when active immunization either is unavailable (e.g., for respiratory syncytial virus) or has not been implemented before exposure (e.g., for rabies). Passive immunization is

used in the treatment of certain disorders associated with toxins (e.g., diphtheria), in certain bites (those of snakes and spiders), and as a specific or nonspecific immunosuppressant [Rho(D) immune globulin and antilymphocyte globulin, respectively]. Three types of preparations are used in passive immunization: (1) standard human immune serum globulin for general use (e.g., γ globulin), administered intramuscularly or intravenously; (2) special immune serum globulins with a known content of antibody to specific agents [e.g., hepatitis B virus (HBV) or varicella-zoster immune globulin]; and (3) animal sera and antitoxins.

ROUTE OF ADMINISTRATION The route of administration in part determines the rapidity and nature of the immune responses to vaccines. Vaccines can be administered orally, intranasally, intradermally, subcutaneously, or intramuscularly. Parenterally administered vaccine may not induce mucosal secretory IgA, and mucosal immunization may not induce good systemic responses. Vaccines must be administered by the licensed route to ensure immunogenicity and safety. For example, administration of HepB vaccine into the gluteal rather than the deltoid muscle often fails to induce an adequate immune response, while subcutaneous rather than intramuscular administration of diphtheria/tetanus/pertussis vaccine (DTP) increases the risk of reactions.

AGE Because age influences the response to vaccines, schedules for immunization are based on age-dependent responses determined empirically from clinical trials. The presence of high levels of maternal antibody and/or the immaturity of the immune system in the early months of life impairs the initial immune response to some vaccines (e.g., measles or Hib polysaccharide) but not to others (e.g., HepB). In the elderly, vaccine responses may be diminished because of natural waning of the immune system. Hence, larger amounts of an antigen may be required to produce the desired response (e.g., in vaccination against influenza).

ADJUVANT POTENTIATION The immune response to some antigens is potentiated by the addition of adjuvants such as aluminum salts or, in the case of polysaccharides (e.g., the polyribose phosphate oligosaccharide of Hib), by conjugation to a carrier protein. Adjuvants—nonspecific boosters of immune responses—are used with inactivated products such as diphtheria and tetanus toxoids, acellular pertussis vaccine, and HepB vaccine. The mechanism for adjuvant enhancement of immunogenicity is not well defined but relates in part to the rendering of soluble antigens into a particulate form; the mobilization of phagocytes to the site of antigen deposition; and the slowing down of the release of antigens, which prolongs stimulation of the immune response.

THE IMMUNE RESPONSE While many constituents of infectious microorganisms and their products, such as exotoxins, are or can be made to be immunogenic, only a limited number stimulate a protective immune response. The immune system is complex, and antigen composition and presentation are critical for stimulation of the desired immune responses.

The Primary Response In the primary response to a vaccine antigen, an apparent latent period of several days precedes the detection of humoral and cell-mediated immunity. Although the immune response begins with initial recognition of the antigen by the immune system, measurable circulating antibodies do not appear for 7 to 10 days. The immunoglobulin class of the response also changes over time. The primary response is characterized by early-appearing IgM antibodies. These generally exhibit only low affinity for the antigen, whereas later-appearing IgG antibodies display high affinity. For "thymus-dependent" antigens, CD4+ T-helper lymphocytes control the switch from IgM to IgG. Some individuals do not respond, even when presented repeatedly with a vaccine antigen, often because they lack the major histocompatibility complex determinants required to recognize the antigen. This situation is known as *primary vaccine failure*.

The Secondary Response Heightened humoral or cell-mediated responses are elicited by a second exposure to the same antigen and occur rapidly, usually within 4 or 5 days. The secondary response depends on immunologic memory after the first exposure and is characterized by a marked proliferation of IgG antibody–producing B lymphocytes and/or effector T cells. Whereas polysaccharide vaccines, such as that for *S. pneumoniae*, evoke immune responses that are independent of T cells and are not enhanced by repeated administration, conjugation to proteins converts the polysaccharides to T cell–dependent antigens that induce immunologic memory and secondary responses to revaccination. Although levels of vaccine-induced antibodies may decline over time (*secondary vaccine failure*), revaccination or exposure to the organism generally elicits a rapid protective secondary response consisting of IgG antibodies with little or no detectable IgM. This anamnestic response indicates that immunity has persisted. Thus, lack of measurable antibody does not necessarily mean that the individual is unprotected. Furthermore, the mere presence of detectable antibodies after the administration of some vaccines and toxoids does not ensure clinical protection. A minimal circulating level of antibody is known to be required for protection from some diseases (e.g., 0.01 IU/mL for tetanus antitoxin).

Hypersensitivity Reactions Independent of antibody production, the stimulation of the immune system by vaccination may elicit unanticipated responses, especially hypersensitivity reactions. In the past, killed measles vaccine induced incomplete humoral immunity and cell-mediated hypersensitivity, resulting in the development of a syndrome of atypical measles in some children after subsequent exposure; thus this type of vaccine is no longer in use.

Mucosal Immunity Some pathogens are confined to and replicate only at mucosal surfaces (e.g., *Vibrio cholerae*), while others are able to penetrate the mucosa and replicate (e.g., poliovirus, rubella virus, and influenza virus). At the mucosal site, these organisms induce secretory IgA. The induction of secretory IgA by vaccines may be an efficient way to block the essential first steps in pathogenesis, whether the organism is restricted to mucosal surfaces or invades the host across mucosal surfaces.

Measurement of the Immune Response Immune responses to vaccines are often gauged by the concentration of specific antibody in serum. While seroconversion serves as a dependable indicator of an immune response, it measures only one immunologic parameter and does not necessarily indicate protection. The development of circulating antibodies after immunization often correlates directly with clinical protection (e.g., against measles or rubella). Some responses may not in themselves confer immunity but may be sufficiently associated with protection that they remain useful proxy measures of protective immunity (e.g., vibriocidal serum antibodies in cholera).

HERD IMMUNITY Vaccination provides direct protection against infection of individuals, thereby decreasing the percentage of susceptible persons within a population. At a definable prevalence of immunity in the population (*herd immunity*), an organism can no longer circulate freely among the susceptibles. This indirect protection of unvaccinated (nonimmune) persons is called the *herd immunity effect*. The level of vaccination coverage needed to elicit a herd immunity effect is dependent on the mixing patterns of the population and the biology of the specific infectious agents. For example, measles and varicella viruses have high transmission rates and therefore require a higher level of vaccine coverage to elicit herd immunity than do organisms with lower transmission rates, such as *S. pneumoniae*. Wherever herd immunity for poliomyelitis and measles has been induced with vaccines, transmission of infection has ceased. It is not surprising that herd immunity may wane if immunization programs are interrupted (as was the case for diphtheria in the former Soviet Union) or if a sufficient percentage of individuals refuse to be immunized (as occurred for pertussis in the United Kingdom and Japan because concern about infrequent—albeit severe—vaccine reactions came to exceed the fear of the disease itself). In each setting, loss of herd immunity led to renewed circulation of the organism and subsequent large outbreaks.

TARGET POPULATIONS AND TIMING OF IMMUNIZATION Different age groups have different disease attack rates, and the effectiveness of vaccines depends on a variety of factors, including the individual's responsiveness to vaccines, the demographic features of the populations at risk, and the duration and character of the immunologic response. In vaccination programs, which are as much community as individual endeavors, schedules for immunization are based on careful consideration of the variables affecting age-dependent responses and population interactions (e.g., school entry, college enrollment, military induction) as well as the feasibility of implementation.

For common and highly communicable childhood diseases like measles, the target population is the universe of susceptible individuals, and the time to immunize is as early in life as is feasible. Yet epidemiologic differences in measles transmission in different settings dictate different strategies for immunization. In the industrialized world, immunization with live-virus vaccine at 12 to 15 months of age has been the norm because the vaccine protects >95% of those immunized at this age and there is little measles morbidity or mortality among very young infants. In contrast, in the developing world, measles is a significant cause of death in young infants. Thus, it is desirable to immunize children earlier to narrow the window of vulnerability between the rapid decline of maternal antibody after 4 to 6 months and the development of vaccine-induced active immunity.

Hib causes meningitis, epiglottitis, and pneumonia in early childhood, with rates rising sharply after the disappearance of maternally derived antibody. The first Hib polysaccharide vaccines often failed when administered during infancy, mainly because of an age-related inability to respond to polysaccharide antigens. To overcome this problem, the protective polysaccharide was converted to a T cell–dependent antigen by conjugation to proteins to which infants could respond.

In contrast, rubella is primarily a threat to the fetus; young infants and children are not at risk of serious illness. An ideal strategy would be to immunize all women of reproductive age before pregnancy. Because it is difficult to systematically vaccinate adolescent and young-adult females and to assure the protection of as many women as possible, rubella is included in a combination vaccine (MMR vaccine) that is administered during infancy. Screening for rubella antibodies during pregnancy should be followed up with postpartum vaccination of seronegative individuals.

Some vaccines were originally formulated primarily for adults. For example, influenza virus and polyvalent pneumococcal polysaccharide vaccines are used to prevent pneumonia, hospitalizations, and deaths among the elderly. Unfortunately, these vaccines are underutilized, in part because physicians and otherwise-healthy individuals in the target group ignore the indications and in part because there is still a tendency to think about disease prevention with vaccines as a strategy for children. With the advent of pneumococcal conjugate vaccines and the cold-adapted influenza strain as well as of administration by nasal spray, infants can also be targeted to receive these vaccines.

THE DEVELOPMENT OF VACCINES

BIOLOGIC IMPEDIMENTS There are often major technical problems to overcome in vaccine development. Although just one major antigenic type of influenza virus is typically in circulation at any one time, the virus is characterized biologically by its antigenic drift. Thus, a new antigenic version capable of causing a global pandemic emerges regularly, and a new vaccine must be rapidly devised, produced, distributed, and administered. In contrast, many prevalent pneumococcal polysaccharide serotypes circulate at all times. Because immunity to the pneumococcus is serotype specific, an individual is susceptible to all serotypes against which he or she lacks antibody. Serotype-specific protection has made it more difficult to develop an effective pneumococcal vaccine than it was to develop a vaccine against *H. influenzae*, of which one capsular serotype (type b) is associated with nearly all cases of severe disease. To overcome this problem, pneumococcal vaccine currently includes 23 polysaccharides that represent ~80% of the virulent serotypes commonly encountered in the United States. Unfortunately, some serotypes are poorly immunogenic, and immunized individuals remain susceptible to the serotypes not included in the vaccine.

STRATEGY FOR VACCINE DEVELOPMENT Vaccine development depends on the systematic application of a four-phase strategy: (1) studies in animals to identify protective antigens, (2) determination of how to present this antigen effectively to the immune system, (3) assessment of the safety and immunogenicity of the preparation in small and then in large human populations at various ages, and (4) evaluation of safety and efficacy in the target population. Each of these steps is simple in concept but difficult in execution; failure at any level stops the process. Progress in immunology has taught us much about the organization and function of the immune system (Chap. 295); it has also taught us that the immune system is complex and that details of antigen composition and presentation are critical for stimulating desired immune responses.

Ultimately, vaccines for humans must be tested in humans. After initial animal studies and small phase 1 and 2 human studies to assess immune responses, optimal dosage, and safety, clinical trials of vaccine efficacy are performed with informed volunteers who are challenged with a virulent strain. Larger clinical effectiveness trials in the community, typically involving 1000 to 10,000 vaccinees, may lead to application for licensure. Because of their limited size, however, these trials cannot be expected to detect rare adverse effects. Thus, licensing does not guarantee that a new vaccine is completely safe, and postlicensing monitoring is needed to ensure effectiveness and to document the occurrence of adverse events of low frequency. In 1999, the recently licensed rhesus rotavirus vaccine was withdrawn because postmarketing surveillance suggested an association with a rare event in infants: intussusception of the bowel.

The development of vaccines goes beyond technology and proof of principle to issues such as development costs, manufacturers' liability and indemnity, perceived public health needs, and the likelihood that a product will be used or sold. Given the complex science required, the costs of vaccine development are high and success is uncertain, adding risk to the development decision. It is unfortunate that the one sure implication of uncertainty in vaccine development is increased cost. In addition, a rational assignment of costs for development between the public and private sectors in the United States has never been achieved.

VACCINE FORMULATIONS Studies of clinical immunology have shown that living and dead antigens do not induce the same immune responses and that the requirements for the development of protective immunity may differ with the organism. These insights, together with the refinement of epidemiologic concepts surrounding immunization, have changed the strategy of vaccine development. The goal is not only to select the correct antigens but also to ensure that the vaccines will result in the type of immune response needed for protection, whether T cell–mediated activation of macrophages or the generation of cytotoxic T cells, B cell–mediated secretory IgA, or a particular IgG subtype response to a specific polysaccharide epitope. To create a deliverable vaccine, constituents other than antigens are also required (Table 107-3). These constituents can affect the immunogenicity, efficacy, and safety of a vaccine and can render one formulation superior to another.

PRODUCTION OF VACCINES As products to be given to healthy individuals to prevent disease, vaccines must not only be efficacious but also cause no harm. In the United States, quality assurance is the responsibility of vaccine manufacturers. Standards of manufacture of biologics (known as good manufacturing practices, or GMPs) are regulated and supervised by the U.S. Food and Drug Administration (FDA). Proof of the safety, efficacy, sterility, and purity of products is required before licensure, and sterility and purity are continually monitored for

TABLE 107-3 *Constituents of Vaccines*

Constituent(s)	Examples/Purpose
Preservatives, stabilizers, antibiotics	These components are used to prevent deterioration of the vaccine before use, to inhibit or prevent bacterial growth, or to stabilize the vaccine. Any of these additions can cause allergic responses.
Adjuvants	This type of additive (e.g., aluminum salts, or alum) is intended to enhance the immune response (e.g., to toxoids, hepatitis B vaccine).
Suspending fluid	The suspending fluid can be sterile water, saline, buffer, or more complex fluids derived from the growth medium or biologic system in which the agent is produced (e.g., egg antigens, cell culture ingredients, serum proteins).

all lots of vaccine after licensure. Postmarketing studies of safety (phase 4 studies) are part of routine regulatory control. On rare occasions, either GMP or quality assurance breaks down; for example, the release of incompletely killed Salk polio vaccine in 1955 caused an outbreak of poliomyelitis in nearly 200 vaccine recipients and their contacts. Unregulated and/or uncontrolled manufacture of vaccines in developing countries has sometimes led to immunization with inactive products that fail to provide the expected protective immunity (e.g., tetanus toxoid produced in Bangladesh).

There is a serious new problem affecting the production of vaccines. For various reasons, including the high costs of vaccine development and the prospect of much higher profitability from investments in other products, the number of vaccine manufacturers in the United States has declined and the cost of some basic childhood vaccines has increased. These changes raise concerns about the future availability of these essential biologics for national use. Furthermore, pricing decisions made within the private-sector pharmaceutical industry can have a major impact on vaccine use. This situation has stimulated an initiative toward increased public involvement in supplying vaccine to individuals for whom price is an issue as well as in oversight of the vaccine supply and of price negotiations with industry.

ADMINISTRATION OF VACCINES Health care workers administering vaccines must take the precautions necessary to minimize the risk of spreading disease—for example, hand washing between immunizations. Different vaccines should not be mixed in the same syringe unless such a practice is specifically endorsed by licensure. Disposable needles and syringes must be safely discarded to prevent inadvertent needlestick injury or, in resource-poor settings, the reuse of these items.

The addition of new, individually injectable vaccines to the childhood immunization schedule has heightened parental concerns about multiple injections being administered at a single clinic visit. The development and use of combinations of vaccines are intended to mitigate these concerns. Even when multiple injections are required, providers must make every effort to administer all indicated vaccines at each visit.

Wherever effective primary health care systems ensure access to medical services for the majority and the population is educated about the need for and efficacy of vaccines, coverage rates for basic immunization are usually high, regardless of the route of vaccine administration or the number of doses necessary. However, without systematic attention to the completion of multiple-dose vaccine schedules, coverage rates for second, third, and booster doses may drop off significantly.

USE OF VACCINES

Several professional groups develop recommendations for vaccine use in the United States: the Advisory Committee on Immunization Practices, the American Academy of Pediatrics (AAP), the American Academy of Family Practice, the American College of Obstetricians and Gynecologists, the American College of Physicians, and the Infectious Diseases Society of America. These recommendations are the

Vaccine	Year Licensed	Type of Immunizing Agent	Protective Antibody	Route of Administration	Efficacy, %	Adverse Events
DT, Td (adult)	1949	Toxoid	Diphtheria and tetanus neutralizing antitoxins, 0.1 IU/mL each	IM	D: 95 T: 95	Local reactions; hypersensitivity to tetanus toxoid
aP	1991	Inactivated bacterial antigen	Not established	IM	80–90	Reduced local reactions compared with whole-cell pertussis vaccines; no serious reactions reported
DTaP	1996	Acellular	Not established	IM	80–90	
Hib	1987	Bacterial polysaccharide–protein conjugate	Antibody to capsular polysaccharide, 0.15 μg/mL	IM	90	Few local, no serious reactions reported
HepB	1981 1987	Inactivated serum-derived antigen Recombinant antigen	Antibody to surface antigen, 10 mIU/mL	IM	80–95	Few (? Guillain-Barré syndrome)
Influenza	1945	Inactivated virus or viral components	Neutralizing antibody	IM	40–60	? Guillain-Barré syndrome with swine influenza vaccine
MMR	1971	Live viruses	Neutralizing measles antibody, 200 mIU/mL; not known for mumps or rubella	SC	M: 95 Mu: 90 R: 95	Acute encephalopathy (measles) Rare parotitis or orchitis (mumps) Arthralgia and rare arthropathy (rubella)
Pneumococcal polysaccharide	1983	Capsular polysaccharide (23 types)	Antibody to polysaccharides	IM or SC	60–80	Local reactions; rare anaphylaxis
Pneumococcal conjugate	2000	Polysaccharide-protein conjugates (7–11 types)	Antibody to polysaccharides	IM	73–94	None thus far
IPV	1967	Inactivated virus of 3 types, enhanced immunogenicity	Neutralizing antibody	SC	95	No significant reactions
Varicella	1995	Live virus	Neutralizing antibody	SC	86–100	Local reaction; varicella-like rash

Abbreviations: DT, diphtheria and tetanus toxoids, adsorbed; Td, tetanus and diphtheria toxoids, adsorbed, for adult use; aP, acellular pertussis; DTaP, diphtheria/tetanus/acellular pertussis vaccine; Hib, *Haemophilus influenzae* type b; HepB, hepatitis B virus vaccine; MMR, measles/mumps/rubella; IPV, inactivated poliovirus vaccine.
Source: Recommendations of the Advisory Committee on Immunization Practices, the American Academy of Pediatrics, and the American College of Physicans.

result of a collaborative process among the recommending groups, the pharmaceutical industry, and the FDA.

Vaccines recommended in 2003 for routine administration to infants, children, and adults are shown in Table 107-4; vaccines recommended for special use are shown in Table 107-5; and schedules for immunization of children and adolescents and of adults are shown in Fig. 107-1 and Fig. 107-2, respectively. The recommendations on route, site, and dosages for vaccination have been derived from theoretical considerations, experimental trials, and clinical experience; deviation from these recommendations can result in inadequate protection. The administration of doses at intervals longer than those recommended does not diminish the ultimate protective response but merely delays it. In contrast, giving vaccines at shorter-than-recommended intervals may result in poor responses. When a scheduled dose is missed, it is not necessary to restart from the beginning or to add an extra dose (www.cdc.gov/nip/recs/child-catchup.pdf).

RECORDING AND REPORTING REQUIREMENTS Certain aspects of vaccine use are regulated by the National Childhood Vaccine Injury Act (NCVIA) of 1986 (modified in 1995 and 2002). The act requires that all mandated childhood vaccinations be recorded by health care providers in the child's permanent medical record, including date of administration, manufacturer and lot number, and name of the provider administering the vaccine. State-based immunization information systems and electronic registries have been developed to help public and private providers manage their immunization activities and particularly to address the problem of assessing immunization coverage when an individual's records are divided among multiple medical facilities. By permitting active and targeted recall of children who are overdue for immunization and by providing data on immunization status at the time of an office visit, these systems improve vaccination rates and offer important public health benefits.

Parents must be informed about the benefits and risks of immunization and should maintain an up-to-date immunization record on their children. Educational materials providing the required information (Vaccine Information Statements) are available from the AAP or the Centers for Disease Control and Prevention (CDC; www.cdc.gov/nip/publications/vis/). The National Network for Immunization Information

tion website (www.immunizationinfo.org) is an excellent source of authoritative information for parents.

VACCINES FOR ROUTINE USE ■ Infants and Children (See Fig. 107-1 and www.cdc.gov/nip/recs/child-catchup.pdf) It is current practice for all children in the United States to receive DTaP, poliovirus, MMR, Hib, HepB, varicella, and pneumococcal conjugate vaccines unless there are specific contraindications. The administration of HepA vaccine is currently recommended when there is a special risk of exposure to infection due to residence in communities with elevated rates of hepatitis A or travel to highly endemic countries. Influenza vaccine is recommended for children 6 to 24 months of age, especially those who have certain risk factors or who reside with persons with certain chronic disorders. In several European countries, meningococcal C conjugate vaccine is routinely recommended.

Adults (See Fig. 107-2) Immunization recommendations for adults (>18 years old) fall into four categories: (1) routine vaccines for all adults; (2) vaccines for high-risk exposure groups (health care and other institutional workers, prisoners, students, military personnel, travelers to endemic areas, injection drug users, men who have sex with men); (3) vaccines for persons at high risk for severe outcomes of infection (pregnant women; the elderly; persons with chronic medical conditions, including diabetes, alcoholism, immunodeficiency, and renal, hepatic, respiratory, or cardiac disease); and (4) vaccines for household contacts of persons in group 3. A substantial proportion of adults in the United States no longer have protective levels of antibodies against tetanus or diphtheria. All adults who completed the pediatric series should be boosted with Td (adult formulation) every 10 years (once after age 50). If not previously immunized, however, adults require a primary immunizing course of Td. Young adults without laboratory evidence or a reliable history of past vaccination or disease should be immunized against measles, mumps, rubella, and varicella. A second dose of MMR vaccine is recommended for groups with a higher risk of exposure and for health care workers with certain other indications. Unless they have documented proof of immunity, rubella vaccine should be given to all nonpregnant women of childbearing age. Rubella-susceptible pregnant women should be vacci-

TABLE 107-5 *Special Vaccines for Infants, Children, and Adults*

Vaccine	Year Licensed	Type of Immunizing Agent	Route of Administration	Indications	Efficacy	Adverse Events
Anthrax	1970	Inactivated avirulent bacteria	SC (6 doses primary; annual booster)	For high risk of exposure (e.g., persons in contact with or involved in manufacture of animal hides, furs, bone meal, wool, goat hair) and military risk of biowarfare exposure	90% antibody response; efficacy uncertain	No serious adverse effects known
Tuberculosis (BCG)	1950	Living bacteria (attenuated *Mycobacterium bovis*)	ID	PPD-negative individuals in prolonged contact with active TB patients	Controversial, maximal for children <15 years	Regional adenitis, disseminated BCG in immunocompromised hosts
HepA	1995	Killed virus antigen	IM	Travelers or persons living in high-risk areas	94%	Local reactions, mild
Cholera	1914	Inactivated whole bacteria	SC or IM	Not recommended for public health use because of limited efficacy; two new vaccines licensed in Europe	?50% (short duration)	Frequent fever and local reactions, pain, swelling
Meningococcus A, C, Y, W-135	1981	Bacterial polysaccharides from 4 serotypes, not type B	SC	Military personnel; travelers to endemic areas; college students in dormitories	90% for 2- to 3-year olds	Rare
Plague	1994	Inactivated bacteria	IM	Laboratory workers; foresters in endemic areas; ? travelers	90% antibody response; efficacy uncertain	10% local reactions; rare sterile abscesses and hypersensitivity
Rabies (human diploid)	1980	Inactivated virus grown in cell culture	IM or ID	Travelers; laboratory workers; veterinarians	Virtually 100%	25% local reactions; 6% arthropathy, arthritis, angioedema
Yellow fever	1978	Live attenuated virus	SC	Laboratory workers	High	Encephalitis, encephalopathy, death
Japanese B encephalitis	1992	Inactivated virus	SC	Travelers to endemic areas	80–90%	Anaphylactic/severe delayed allergic reactions common; recipient should be observed for 10 days
Typhoid	1952	Heat- or phenol-killed bacteria	IM	Not routinely recommended in U.S.; used for travelers, contacts of carriers	50–70% (short duration)	Frequent fever, local swelling, pain
		Purified Vi polysaccharide	IM	Travelers	70–75%	Local reactions, mild
Lyme disease	1998	Recombinant outer-membrane protein	IM	For high risk of exposure to infected ticks	76% (3 doses)	Local reactions

Abbreviations: SC, subcutaneous; BCG, bacille Calmette-Guérin; PPD, purified protein derivative; TB, tuberculosis.

Source: Recommendations of the Advisory Committee on Immunization Practices, the American Academy of Pediatrics, and the American College of Physicians.

nated as early as possible in the postpartum period. Live-virus vaccines, such as MMR and varicella vaccines, are contraindicated in pregnant women and immunosuppressed individuals. Routine immunization against polio is not recommended for adults unless they are at particular risk of exposure because of travel to the remaining endemic areas. College students, particularly freshmen living at close quarters, are at increased risk of meningococcal meningitis and should be offered the meningococcal polysaccharide vaccine for serogroups A, C, Y, and W-135.

Current recommendations also include influenza vaccine for routine annual administration to individuals with chronic illness at any age, to persons living in the same household as chronically ill individuals, and to all adults >50 years of age. Polyvalent pneumococcal polysaccharide vaccine is similarly recommended for adults ≥65 years of age and for all chronically ill persons. HepB vaccine is recommended for individuals at high risk from clinical, occupational, behavioral, and travel exposures, including patients undergoing hemodialysis, routine recipients of clotting factors, health care workers exposed to potentially infected blood or blood products, individuals living and working in institutions for the mentally handicapped, travelers to highly endemic countries, persons at elevated risk for sexually transmitted diseases, injection drug users, and household contacts of known carriers of hepatitis B surface antigen. HepA vaccine is recommended for these same groups and for persons with clotting dis-

orders or chronic liver disease. There are a number of other special-use vaccines whose administration is related to travel and occupational exposures (e.g., Japanese B encephalitis, typhoid, yellow fever, rabies); specific recommendations for the use of these vaccines in the United States can be found at www.cdc.gov/nip.

Adverse Events   Given the success of vaccination programs and the virtual disappearance of many vaccine-preventable diseases in the United States, concerns about vaccine safety have sometimes become inflated in conjunction with complacency about the consequences of infection. An *adverse reaction* or *vaccine side effect* is an untoward effect caused by a vaccine that is extraneous to its primary purpose (to produce immunity). In contrast, an *adverse event* can be either a true vaccine reaction or a coincidental event. A small number of highly publicized claims unsubstantiated by valid data have heightened the suspicion that some or all vaccines routinely cause unacceptable adverse events. Antivaccine advocacy groups actively encourage avoidance of immunization because of the unproven belief that vaccines can cause certain disorders (e.g., autism). Websites maintained by such groups commonly appear in the first 10 listings identified by search engines. This situation presents a challenge to physicians and public health officials who must educate parents about vaccine benefits and risks.

In fact, modern vaccines, while safe and effective, are associated with adverse events that range from infrequent and mild to rare and life-threatening. The decision to recommend the use of a vaccine involves an assessment of the risks of disease and the benefits and risks of vaccination. Because these factors may change over time, continual assessment of the balance between societal benefits and individual risks is essential. Valid and invalid contraindications to childhood immunization and appropriate precautions in the use of specific vaccines can be found at www.cdc.gov/nip/recs/contraindications.pdf.

Ironically, ongoing efforts to enhance vaccine safety through quality improvement and changes in vaccine policy (e.g., the decision to eliminate the mercury-based preservative thimerosol from vaccines) have actually led to an even greater awareness of the possible adverse events associated with routine vaccine administration. It has been claimed that increased rates of diabetes mellitus in the general pediatric population are due to an increase in exposure to vaccine antigens in childhood, although rigorous studies have refuted this hypothesis. A putative link of measles immunization to autism has been the subject of intense international controversy. The Institute of Medicine issued four recent reports whose findings (1) fail to support hypotheses that vaccines are associated with multiple sclerosis, neurodevelopmental disorders, or immune dysfunction; (2) provide no evidence for a temporal association of these conditions with vaccination; and (3) elucidate no biologically plausible basis for the purported relationships.

Within 9 months of the introduction of routine administration of the rhesus reassortant rotavirus vaccine (Rotashield) in the United States, cases of intussusception were reported by the CDC to be temporally associated with administration of the initial dose. This report led first to the cessation of the vaccine's use and subsequently to the withdrawal of the vaccine from the market and the discontinuation of its production. Although other analyses have failed to support the association, rotavirus vaccine has not been introduced into developing countries, where the risk of any real increase in intussusception would be dramatically outweighed by the benefit of decreased rotavirus mortality.

The ramifications of these events for future vaccine development and introduction have yet to be assessed. Vaccine components, including protective antigens, animal proteins introduced during vaccine production, and antibiotics or other preservatives or stabilizers, can certainly cause allergic reactions in some recipients. These reactions may be local or systemic and include urticaria and serious anaphylaxis. The most common extraneous allergen is egg protein introduced when vaccines such as those for measles, mumps, influenza, and yellow fever are prepared in embryonated eggs. Gelatin, which is used as a heat stabilizer, has been implicated in rare but severe allergic reactions. Local or systemic reactions (probably due to antigen-antibody complexes) can result from too-frequent administration of vaccines such as Td, diphtheria/tetanus vaccine, or rabies vaccine. Because live-virus vaccines can interfere with tuberculin test responses, necessary tuberculin testing should be done either on the day of immunization or at

FIGURE 107-1 Recommended childhood and adolescent immunization schedule—United States, 2003. Any dose not given at the recommended age should be given at any subsequent time when indicated and feasible. Green bars indicate age groups that warrant special efforts to administer those vaccines not previously given. Infants born to mothers positive for hepatitis B surface antigen (HBsAg) should receive hepatitis B vaccine (HepB) and 0.5 mL of hepatitis B immune globulin (HBIG) at separate sites within 12 h of birth. The second dose of HepB is recommended at at age 1 to 2 months. The last dose in the series should not be administered before age 6 months. Infants born to mothers whose HBsAg status is unknown should receive the first dose of the HepB series within 12 h of birth. The mother's HBsAg status should be tested as soon as possible; if positive, the infant should receive HBIG as soon as possible. The number of *Haemophilus influenzae* type b (Hib) conjugate vaccine doses depends on the vaccine used. PRP-OMP (PedvaxHIB or ComVax) is administered just twice: at ages 2 and 4 months. Diphtheria/tetanus/acellular pertussis (DtaP)/Hib combination products should not be used for primary immunization but can be used as boosters following a primary series with any Hib vaccine. Influenza vaccine is now recommended annually for children age ≥6 months with certain risk factors (including but not limited to asthma, cardiac disease, sickle cell disease, HIV infection, and diabetes mellitus) and household members of persons in groups at high risk; it can be administered to all others wishing to obtain immunity. If feasible, influenza vaccination of healthy children age 6 to 23 months is encouraged because of a substantially increased risk for influenza-related hospitalizations in this group. Children ≥12 years old should receive influenza vaccine in a dosage appropriate for their age. Children ≤8 years old who are receiving influenza vaccine for the first time should receive two doses separated by at least 4 weeks. Hepatitis A vaccine is recommended for children and adolescents in selected states and regions and for certain high-risk groups; hepatitis A immunization can begin during any visit, and the two doses should be administered at least 6 months apart. The heptavalent pneumococcal conjugate vaccine (PCV) is recommended for all children age 2 to 23 months. It is also recommended for certain children age 24 to 59 months. Pneumococcal polysaccharide vaccine (PPV) is recommended in addition to the conjugate vaccine for certain high-risk groups. Further information can be obtained via the National Immunization Program website (www.cdc.gov/nip) or at the National Immunization Information Hotline (800-232-2522 for English and 800-232-0233 for Spanish). MMR, measles/mumps/rubella vaccine; IPV, inactivated poliovirus vaccine; Td, tetanus and diphtheria toxoids, adsorbed, for adult use. (*Adapted from recommendations approved by the Advisory Committee on Immunization Practices, the American Academy of Pediatrics, and the American College of Family Physicians.*)

least 6 weeks later. When influenza vaccine is given to children <13 years old, only "split-virus" preparations should be used since whole-virus vaccines are associated with higher rates of adverse reactions in this age group.

The U.S. government conducts vaccine safety surveillance through a network of active and passive reporting. All detected adverse events whose occurrence is temporally related to vaccination must be reported to both the local health department and the vaccine manufacturer. For the purpose of postlicensure passive surveillance of vaccines, health care providers are required to report certain suspected adverse events following the administration of a mandated vaccine to the FDA's Vaccine Adverse Events Reporting System. The NCVIA has established criteria for reimbursable vaccine-related adverse events (www.hrsa.gov/osp/vicp/table.htm). Although a temporal relationship does not establish cause and effect, this surveillance system remains the only mechanism for collecting the data needed for analysis, conclusions, and decision-making. The CDC has established an active-surveillance system for ongoing evaluation of vaccine safety in large populations of vaccinated individuals. The Vaccine Safety Datalink is a population-based network in which four large health maintenance organizations (HMOs) continuously monitor immunization records linked to the medical records of 600,000 children <7 years of age. A

Vaccine ▼ / Age ▶	19–49 Years	50–64 Years	65 Years and Older
Tetanus, diphtheria (Td)	1 dose booster every 10 years[1]		
Influenza	1 dose annually for persons with medical or occupational indications, or household contacts of persons with indications[2]	1 annual dose	
Pneumococcal (polysaccharide)	1 dose for persons with medical or other indications (1 dose revaccination for immunosuppressive conditions)[3,4]		1 dose for unvaccinated persons[3] / 1 dose revaccination[4]
Hepatitis B	3 doses (0, 1–2, 4–6 months) for persons with medical, behavioral, occupational, or other indications[5]		
Hepatitis A	2 doses (0, 6–12 months) for persons with medical, behavioral, occupational, or other indications[6]		
Measles, mumps, rubella (MMR)	1 dose if measles, mumps, or rubella vaccination history is unreliable; 2 doses for persons with occupational or other indications[7]		
Varicella	2 doses (0, 4–8 weeks) for persons who are susceptible[8]		
Meningococcal (polysaccharide)	1 dose for persons with medical or other indications[9]		

☐ For all persons in this group   ☐ Catch-up on childhood vaccinations   ☐ For persons with medical/ exposure indications

FIGURE 107-2   Recommended adult immunization schedule—United States, 2002–2003. (1) *Tetanus and diphtheria (Td)*: A primary series for adults is 3 doses, with the first 2 doses at least 4 weeks apart and the third dose 6 to 12 months after the second. One dose suffices if a primary series was completed >10 years before. In addition to a teenage/young adult booster, adults >50 years of age who have completed the full series plus booster should receive one more dose. (2) *Influenza vaccination*: Indications include chronic cardiovascular or pulmonary disease, asthma, diabetes, renal disease, hemoglobinopathy, immunosuppression (due to medications or HIV infection), pregnancy (second or third trimester during the influenza season), health care employment, residence in a nursing home or another long-term-care facility, and high likelihood of transmitting influenza to those at high risk. (3) *Pneumococcal polysaccharide vaccination*: Indications include chronic cardiovascular or pulmonary disease (except asthma), diabetes, chronic liver disease, chronic renal failure or nephrotic syndrome, asplenia, immunosuppression, certain cancer chemotherapy, and long-term systemic glucocorticoid therapy. Vaccination is also indicated in Alaskan natives, certain Native American populations, and residents of nursing homes and other long-term-care facilities. (4) *Revaccination with pneumococcal polysaccharide vaccine*: One-time revaccination after age 5 is indicated for persons with chronic renal failure or nephrotic syndrome, asplenia, immunosuppression, certain cancer chemotherapy, or long-term systemic glucocorticoid therapy. Persons >65 years old should undergo one-time revaccination if their prior vaccination was at least 5 years before and was given before age 65. (5) *Hepatitis B vaccination*: Vaccination is indicated for hemodialysis patients, patients receiving clotting factor concentrates, health care workers and public safety workers exposed to blood, students in the health professions, injection drug users, persons with multiple sex partners within 6 months, patients with recent sexually transmitted disease (STD), clients of STD clinics, men who have sex with men, household contacts and sex partners of persons with chronic hepatitis B virus infection, clients and staff of institutions for the mentally disabled, inmates of correctional institutions, and international travelers to countries with high prevalence. (6) *Hepatitis A vaccination*: For the combined HepA/HepB vaccine, use 3 doses at 0, 1, and 6 months. Hepatitis A vaccination is indicated in persons with clotting factor disorders or chronic liver disease, men who have sex with men, users of injection and noninjection illegal drugs, persons working with hepatitis A virus–infected primates or working with the virus in a laboratory, and persons traveling to or working in countries with high prevalence. (7) *Measles/mumps/rubella vaccination (MMR)*: *Measles component*: Adults born before 1957 are considered immune to measles. Adults born after 1957 should have at least 1 dose of MMR vaccine barring a medical contraindication or documentation of prior immunization. A second dose is recommended for adults who have recently been exposed to measles in an outbreak setting, who have previously received killed measles vaccine, who were vaccinated with an unknown measles vaccine between 1963 and 1967, who are students at a college or university, who work in health care facilities, or who plan to travel internationally. *Mumps component*: 1 dose of MMR vaccine is adequate. *Rubella component*: 1 dose of MMR vaccine should be given to women whose history is unreliable, with counseling to avoid becoming pregnant for 4 weeks. The rubella immune status of women of childbearing age should be ascertained and counseling provided regarding congenital rubella. (8) *Varicella vaccination*: Vaccination is recommended for all persons without a reliable clinical history of varicella or serologic evidence of immunity, health care workers, family contacts of immunosuppressed persons, those who live or work in high-risk settings (teachers of young children, daycare workers, residents and staff members working in institutional settings), adolescents and adults living in households with children, and women who are not pregnant but intend to become pregnant in the future. (9) *Meningococcal vaccine, quadrivalent*: Vaccination should be considered for adults with terminal complement component deficiencies, those with anatomical or functional asplenia, college freshmen (especially those living in dormitories), and travelers to the "meningitis belt" in sub-Saharan Africa or to Mecca for the Hajj. High-risk persons can be revaccinated in 5 years. (*Adapted from recommendations approved by the Advisory Committee on Immunization Practices and accepted by the American College of Obstetricians and Gynecologists and the American Academy of Family Physicians.*)

similar system is in place for immunized adult members of four HMOs.

USE OF VACCINES IN SPECIAL CIRCUMSTANCES
■ Influenza Pandemic Preparedness
Influenza pandemics occur at irregular intervals and are characterized by excess deaths, hospitalizations, public concern, and social and economic disruption. A National Preparedness Plan has been developed to assess the incidence of disease and the antigenic characteristics of the prevalent strain and to promote flexibility in vaccine manufacture and vaccination. This plan is based on enhancement of current capacities for virologic surveillance, disease surveillance, and emergency medical responses.

Pregnancy Because of the theoretical risk to the fetus and the real risk of litigation to the practitioner, routine immunization of pregnant women is best avoided. However, wherever hygienic conditions during delivery cannot be guaranteed, it is essential to ensure that pregnant women are immune to tetanus because the transfer of maternal antitoxin is an important means of preventing neonatal tetanus. Pregnant women can safely receive tetanus as well as diphtheria toxoids. Live-virus vaccines, such as rubella, measles, mumps, and varicella, should be withheld during pregnancy. However, if the risk of exposure is great, polio and yellow fever vaccines may be safely administered. If indicated, some inactivated vaccines (e.g., HepB, influenza, and pneumococcal vaccines) may be given during the second and third trimesters of pregnancy (Fig. 107-3).

Breast Feeding Neither killed nor live vaccine affects the safety of breast feeding for either mother or infant. Breast-fed infants can be immunized on a normal schedule.

Occupational Exposure Immunization recommendations for most occupational groups remain to be developed. Specific practices are now mandated by the Occupational Safety and Health Administration for the immunization of health care workers against hepatitis B in the United States. Rubella is transmitted to and from health care workers in medical facilities, particularly in pediatric practice. Health care workers who might transmit rubella to pregnant patients should be immune to rubella; it is prudent to screen these employees for antibodies to rubella virus and to immunize susceptible individuals. Persons providing health care are also at greater risk from measles and varicella than the general public, and those who are likely to come into contact with measles- and varicella-infected patients should be immune. Persons employed in caring for patients with chronic diseases can transmit influenza; such workers should be vaccinated annually.

HIV Infection and Other Immunocompromised

States Limited studies in HIV-infected individuals have found no increase in the risk of adverse events from live or inactivated vaccines. However, immune responses may not be as vigorous in immunocompromised individuals as in those with a normal immune system. Persons known to be infected with HIV should be immunized with recommended vaccines in the same manner as individuals with a normal immune system and as early in the course of their disease as possible, before immune function becomes significantly impaired (Fig. 107-3). Live attenuated MMR vaccine can be administered to this group. When vaccination against polio is indicated, IPV should be administered to immunocompromised HIV-infected individuals and to their household contacts. Albeit prudent, it is not necessary in practice to test for HIV before making decisions about the immunization of asymptomatic individuals from known HIV risk groups.

Live attenuated vaccines are also contraindicated in other immunocompromised patients, including those with congenital immunodeficiency syndromes and those receiving immunosuppressive therapy. Passive immunization with immunoglobulin preparations or antitoxins can be considered in individual cases, either as postexposure prophylaxis or as part of the treatment of established infection.

Postexposure Immunization For certain infections, active or passive immunization soon after exposure prevents or attenuates disease expression. Recommended postexposure immunization regimens are compiled in Table 107-6. Measles immune globulin given within 6 days of exposure may prevent or modify infection, and measles vaccine given within the first few days after exposure may prevent symptomatic infection. Although clinical manifestations of rubella in pregnant women are minimized by postexposure passive immunization, this approach may not prevent maternal viremia, fetal infection, and congenital rubella syndrome. Therefore, the administration of immune globulin is recommended only for women developing rubella during pregnancy who will not consider abortion under any circumstances. Proper immunization for tetanus plays an important role in wound management. The need for active immunization—with or without passive immunization—depends on the condition of the wound and the patient's immunization history (Table 107-7). Rarely have cases of tetanus occurred in persons with a documented primary series of tetanus toxoid. Tetanus immune globulin is useful in patients with tetanus. Survivors with no history of tetanus immunization should receive a primary series of toxoid since disease does not produce protective levels of antitoxin. Administration of rabies immune globulin plus rabies vaccine in the immediate postexposure period is highly effective in preventing disease. Similarly, for persons who have not been actively immunized, the use of hepatitis A immune globulin within 2 weeks of exposure to hepatitis A is likely to prevent clinical illness. Sound data indicate the efficacy of human hepatitis B

immune globulin in preventing disease after exposure. While no high-titer preparation is available for postexposure protection against non-A, non-B hepatitis, standard human immune serum globulin is efficacious.

Simultaneous Administration of Multiple Vaccines There are no contraindications to the simultaneous administration of several vaccines. The use of combination vaccines can potentially reduce the required number of injections from 9 to 3 during a child's first 6 months of life and from 21 to 13 during the first 2 years. Simultaneous administration of the most widely used live and inactivated vaccines has not resulted in impaired antibody responses or in increased rates of adverse reactions. Moreover, this approach increases the probability that a child will ultimately be fully immunized. Simultaneous administration is useful in any age group when the potential exists for exposure to multiple infectious diseases during travel to endemic countries. Combination DTaP/Hib vaccines should not be used for primary immunization of infants because the result is a blunted, suboptimal response to Hib; however, the combination may be used for booster immunizations.

Medical conditions ▼	Vaccine ► Tetanus-Diphtheria (Td)	Influenza	Pneumococcal (Polysaccharide)	Hepatitis B	Hepatitis A	Measles, Mumps, Rubella (MMR)	Varicella
Pregnancy		A					
Diabetes, heart disease, chronic pulmonary disease, chronic liver disease, including chronic alcoholism		B	C		D		
Congenital immunodeficiency, leukemia, lymphoma, generalized malignancy, therapy with alkylating agents, antimetabolites, radiation or large amounts of glucocorticoids			E				F
Renal failure/end stage renal disease, recipients of hemodialysis or clotting factor concentrates			E	G			
Asplenia (including elective splenectomy) and terminal complement component deficiencies			E, H, I				
HIV infection			E, J			K	

For all persons in this group · Catch-up on childhood vaccinations · For persons with medical/exposure indications · Contraindicated

FIGURE 107-3 Recommended immunizations for adults with medical conditions—United States, 2002–2003. **A.** Vaccine may be given if pregnancy is at second or third trimester during influenza season. **B.** Although chronic liver disease and alcoholism are not indicator conditions for influenza vaccination, give 1 dose annually if the patient is ≥50 years old, has other indications for influenza vaccine, or requests vaccination. **C.** Asthma is an indicator condition for influenza vaccination but not for pneumococcal vaccination. **D.** Vaccinate all persons with chronic liver disease. **E.** Revaccinate once after ≥5 years have elapsed since initial vaccination. **F.** Persons with impaired humoral (but not cellular) immunity may be vaccinated [*MMWR* 1999; 48 (RR-06), 1–5]. **G.** *Hemodialysis patients:* Use special formulation of vaccine (40 μg/mL) or two 1.0-mL, 20-μg doses given at one site. Vaccinate early in the course of renal disease. Assess antibody titers to hepatitis B surface antigen annually; administer additional doses if titers decline to <10 mIU/mL. **H.** Also administer meningococcal vaccine. **I.** In persons undergoing elective splenectomy, vaccinate at least 2 weeks before surgery. **J.** Vaccinate as close to diagnosis as possible, when CD4+ cell counts are highest. **K.** Withhold MMR or other measles-containing vaccines from HIV-infected persons with evidence of severe immunosuppression [*MMWR* 1996; 45, 603–606; *MMWR* 1992; 41 (RR-17), 1–19]. (Approved by the Advisory Committee on Immunization Practices and accepted by the American College of Obstetricians and Gynecologists and the American Academy of Family Physicians.)

TABLE 107-6 *Recommended Postexposure Immunization with Immunoglobulin Preparations in the United States*

Disease	Indicated	Comments
Measles	Yes	Standard human immune globulin is recommended for exposed infants and adults with normal immunocompetence (but with a contraindication to measles vaccine) and for immunocompromised patients exposed to measles (regardless of immunization status). Patients should be actively immunized 3 to 6 months after immunoglobulin administration. Recommended dose: 0.25–0.50 mL/kg (40–80 mg of IgG/kg) IM; 80 mg of IgG/kg for immunocompromised contact; maximum, 15 mL.
Rubella	No	Efficacy is unreliable; therefore, standard human immune globulin is recommended for administration only to antibody-negative pregnant women in the first trimester who have a documented rubella exposure and will not consider terminating the pregnancy. Recommended dose is 0.55 mL/kg (90 mg of IgG/kg) IM.
Tetanus	Yes	Human tetanus immune globulin (TIG) has replaced equine tetanus antitoxin because of the risk of serum sickness with equine serum. Recommended dose for postexposure prophylaxis is 250–500 units of TIG (10–20 mg of IgG/kg) IM. Recommended dose for treatment of tetanus is 3000–6000 units of TIG IM.
Rabies	Yes	Human rabies immune globulin (RIG) is preferred over equine rabies antiserum because of the risk of serum sickness with equine serum. RIG or antiserum is recommended for nonimmunized individuals with animal bites in whom rabies cannot be ruled out and with other exposures to known rabid animals. Recommended dose of RIG is 20 IU/kg (22 mg of IgG/kg). Recommended dose of antiserum is 40 IU/kg. Rabies vaccine is given as well at 0, 3, 7, 14, and 28 days.
Hepatitis A	Yes	Standard immune serum globulin is given in a single dose of 0.02–0.04 mL/kg or (for continuous exposure) in a dose up to 0.06 mL/kg every 5 months. Postexposure treatment with hepatitis A immune globulin has not been studied.

When live-virus vaccines are not given together on the same day, an interval of at least 30 days should be allowed.

Because high doses of immune globulin may inhibit the efficacy of measles and rubella vaccines, an interval of at least 3 months is recommended between the administration of immune globulin and that of MMR vaccine or its components. Postpartum vaccination of rubella-susceptible women should not be delayed because of the administration of anti-Rho(D) immune globulin or any other blood product during the last trimester or at delivery. Should administration of an immune globulin preparation become necessary after vaccination, it should be postponed, if possible, for at least 14 days to allow time for vaccine-virus replication and development of immunity. In general, there is little interaction of immune globulin with inactivated vaccines, and postexposure passive prophylaxis can be given together with HepB vaccine or tetanus toxoid, resulting in both immediate and long-lasting protection.

Travel (See also Chap. 108) The International Sanitary Regulations allow countries to impose requirements for yellow fever and killed cholera vaccines as a condition for admission, even though the latter is not an effective public health tool. Travelers should know whether these vaccines are required for entry into the countries on their itinerary to avoid being turned back or immunized on the spot, with the inherent danger of unsafe injections. Infants, children, and adults should have all routine immunizations updated before traveling, with particular attention to polio, measles, and DTP/DTaP or Td vaccines. The use of HepA vaccine may be advisable for travelers to some locales. Special-use vaccines (Table 107-5), including rabies, meningococcal polysaccharide, typhoid, Japanese B encephalitis, and plague vaccines, should be considered for those individuals who expect to go beyond the usual tourist routes or to spend extended periods in rural areas in disease-endemic regions. Most U.S. cities have travel clinics that maintain up-to-date epidemiologic information and can provide the appropriate vaccines. The CDC also maintains a website for travelers (www.cdc.gov/travel).

DELIVERY OF VACCINES Over the past 25 years, considerable progress has been made to ensure that every child in the United States is fully immunized by the time of school entry. All 50 states now require immunization for school entry, and most have laws addressing attendance at preschools and day-care centers. Despite the dramatic impact of immunization and of other improvements in the health care provided to the American population on the incidence of vaccine-preventable illness (Table 107-1), many children are not fully immunized—both in poor communities (as a result of inadequate health services) and in affluent communities (where parental concern about potential adverse events may exceed concern about now-uncommon diseases). The failure to vaccinate preschool children was largely responsible for the resurgence of measles in the United States between 1989 and 1991, with >55,000 cases and >130 measles-related deaths. Outbreaks of pertussis, mumps, and congenital rubella syndrome have occurred wherever immunization rates among preschool children are low. While measles (36 cases in 2002) and rubella (14 cases in 2002) have reached historic lows, the risk of imported infection and spread to susceptibles persists.

ACCESS TO IMMUNIZATION Four major barriers to infant and childhood immunization have been identified within the health care system: (1) low public awareness and lack of public demand for immunization, (2) inadequate access to immunization services, (3) missed opportunities to administer vaccines, and (4) inadequate resources for public health and preventive programs. These problems are sources of public concern, and their solution must be a priority for national health policy in the United States. At the national level, outreach and educational campaigns promote parental awareness of the value of vaccination and encourage health care providers to use every opportunity to vaccinate the children in their care. At the state and local levels, community and business groups, religious and service groups, schools, and the media have joined together in community-based networks. Those who remain unvaccinated do so largely because health care practices and providers do not always perform optimally in delivering vaccines. The AFIX Program (Assessment of coverage, Feedback of diagnostic information, Incentives or recognition, and eXchange of information among providers) is one effort by the CDC to change the attitude of health care personnel who lack an appreciation of low immunization rates in their practices to one of awareness, concern, and knowledge. The CDC has also developed two approaches to immunization assessment: CASA (Clinic Assessment Software Application) and LQA (Lot Quality Assessment). CASA requires review of up to 200 immunization records to assess whether record keeping and documentation are adequate, whether children start their vaccine series on time, whether and when patients drop out of the system, whether recall is used effectively, and whether vaccines are given simultaneously. LQA requires the review of only 30 records and does not yield a precise immunization rate or a diagnosis of the problem. A National Immunization Week each April has been established to focus attention on the vac-

TABLE 107-7 *Tetanus Wound Management*

	Clean, Minor Wounds		All Other Wounds	
Vaccination History	Td	TIG	Td	TIG
Unknown or <3 doses	Yes	No	Yes	Yes
3 doses	No[a]	No	No[b]	No

[a] Yes, if >10 years since last dose.
[b] Yes, if >5 years since last dose.

TABLE 107-8   Standards for Immunization Practice

Pediatric Practice

1. Immunization services are readily available.
2. There are no barriers to or unnecessary prerequisites for the receipt of vaccines.
3. Immunization services are available free or for a minimal fee.
4. Providers use all clinical encounters to screen and, when indicated, immunize children.
5. Providers educate parents and guardians about immunization in general terms.
6. Providers question parents or guardians about contraindications and, before immunizing a child, inform them in specific terms about the risks and benefits of the immunizations their child is to receive.
7. Providers follow only true contraindications.
8. Providers administer simultaneously all vaccine doses for which a child is eligible at the time of each visit.
9. Providers use accurate and complete recording procedures.
10. Providers coschedule immunization appointments in conjunction with appointments for other child health services.
11. Providers report adverse events following immunization promptly, accurately, and completely.
12. Providers operate a tracking system.
13. Providers adhere to appropriate procedures for vaccine management.
14. Providers conduct semiannual audits to assess immunization coverage levels and to review immunization records for the patient populations they serve.
15. Providers maintain up-to-date, easily retrievable medical protocols at all locations where vaccines are administered.
16. Providers operate with patient-oriented and community-based approaches.
17. Vaccines are administered by properly trained individuals.
18. Providers receive ongoing education and training on current immunization recommendations.

Adult Practice

1. Appropriate vaccine use is promoted through information campaigns for health care practitioners and trainees, employers, and the public about the benefits of immunizations.
2. Providers are completely immunized to protect themselves and prevent transmission to patients.
3. Providers routinely determine the immunization status of their adult patients, offer vaccines to those for whom they are indicated, and maintain complete immunization records.
4. Providers identify high-risk patients in need of influenza vaccine and develop a system to recall them for annual immunization.
5. Providers and institutions identify high-risk adult patients in hospitals and other treatment centers and ensure that appropriate vaccination is considered either before discharge or as part of discharge planning.
6. Licensing/accreditation agencies support the development by health care institutions of comprehensive immunization programs for staff, trainees, volunteer workers, inpatients, and outpatients.
7. States establish preenrollment immunization requirements for colleges and other institutions of higher learning.
8. Institutions that train health care professionals, deliver health care, or provide laboratory or other medical support services require appropriate immunizations for persons at risk of contracting or transmitting vaccine-preventable diseases.
9. Health care benefit programs, third-party payers, and government health care programs provide coverage for adult immunization services.
10. A standard personal and institutional immunization record is adopted as a means of verifying the immunization status of patients and staff.

cination needs of infants and children. To improve the quality and quantity of vaccination services, expanded immunization-clinic hours and computerization of immunization records have been implemented as well. State-mandated school-entry immunity requirements have also helped to raise population immunity.

Although special vaccination target groups (e.g., college students, military personnel, and health care workers) have been successfully immunized, there has been only modest progress toward immunization goals for older adults in the United States. As many as 60,000 adults die each year of vaccine-preventable diseases for which effective vaccines are not being optimally used. More than 30% of persons >65 years of age do not receive influenza vaccine each year, and even fewer have ever received pneumococcal vaccine. Health care providers more often miss vaccination opportunities with adults than with infants and children. From 60 to 90% of adults hospitalized for or dying of influenza-associated respiratory disease have received medical care during the previous year and could have been immunized at that time. Medicare reimbursement for excess hospitalization during influenza epidemics ranges from $750 million to $1 billion. Additional efforts are required to ensure that adults receive Td and HepB vaccines as well.

A special setting for adult immunization is the administration of certain vaccines (e.g., tetanus toxoid) to pregnant women to enhance passive immunity in their offspring. In most cases, the mother herself derives important benefits as well. Immunization of the mother should be undertaken at least 6 weeks before delivery to allow for efficient transplacental transfer of antibody to the fetus.

Recent childhood vaccine shortages in the United States have prompted federal authorities to recommend deferring some vaccinations and have caused states to reduce vaccination requirements. Efforts to resolve supply-and-demand issues have yielded plans to increase national stockpiles of vaccines.

HANDLING OF VACCINES   Vaccines must be handled and stored with care. Vaccines should be kept at 2° to 8°C and, with the exception of varicella vaccine, should not be frozen. Varicella should be kept frozen at −15°C. Measles vaccine must be protected from light, which inactivates the virus.

STANDARDS FOR IMMUNIZATION PRACTICE   National standards of immunization for adult and pediatric practice have been established to define common policies and practices for public health clinics and physicians' private offices (Table 107-8). These standards highlight the need to distinguish between valid contraindications and conditions that are often considered to be but are not in fact contraindications (www.cdc.gov/nip/recs/contraindications.pdf). Among the valid contraindications applicable to all vaccines are a history of anaphylaxis or other serious allergic reactions to a vaccine or vaccine component and the presence of a moderate or severe illness, with or without fever. Infants who develop encephalopathy within 72 h of a dose of DTP or DTaP should not receive further doses; those who develop a "precaution" should not normally receive further doses. Because of theoretical risks to the fetus, pregnant women should not receive MMR or varicella vaccine. Diarrhea, minor respiratory illness (with or without fever), mild to moderate local reactions to a previous dose of vaccine, the concurrent or recent use of antimicrobial agents, mild to moderate malnutrition, and the convalescent phase of an acute illness are not valid contraindications to routine immunization. Failure to vaccinate children because of these conditions is increasingly viewed as a missed opportunity for immunization.

THE NATIONAL VACCINE INJURY COMPENSATION PROGRAM   The use of mandated vaccines benefits society as a whole by reducing morbidity and the cost of care for preventable diseases and by reducing childhood mortality. Thus, in the United States, society has assumed the obligation to care for those injured by the administration of mandated vaccines. The NCVIA of 1986 (modified in 1995 and 2002) is the instrument in use to ensure both fairness to injured persons and protection for federal, state, and local immunization programs; private immunization providers; and vaccine manufacturers. The act was designed to implement two vital public policies: (1) to provide prompt and fair compensation to the families of children who have died or have been injured as a result of routine mandated immunization; and (2) to reduce the adverse impact of the tort system on vaccine supply, cost, and innovation/development. The success of immunization programs in the United States depends upon the continued viability of the National Vaccine Injury Compensation Program.

CONTROL OF VACCINE-PREVENTABLE DISEASE

A continuing task of public health practice is to maintain individual and herd immunity. The job is not over once a population is fully vaccinated; rather, it is imperative to immunize each subsequent generation as long as the threat of the reintroduction of the disease from anywhere in the world persists. Ongoing surveillance and prompt reporting of disease to local or state health departments are essential to this goal, ensuring a continuing awareness of the possibility of vaccine-preventable illness. Nearly all vaccine-preventable diseases are notifiable, and individual case data are routinely forwarded to the CDC. These data are used to detect outbreaks or other unusual events that require investigation and to evaluate prevention and control policies, practices, and strategies.

RESEARCH ON VACCINES AND IMMUNIZATION

The potential to eliminate selected diseases and to build sustainable immunization programs that reach every child is not being fulfilled with existing vaccines and delivery technology. New vaccines or new formulations that will not only improve protective responses but also simplify the immunization schedule are needed. The ideal would be vaccines that can be administered orally early in life, that provide lifelong protection against multiple infections, that can be given as one or only a few doses, and that are less reactive and more heat stable than current vaccines. Diseases for which safe and effective vaccines have not been achieved represent the more difficult immunologic challenges and mark the frontiers of vaccine development. To attain these ambitious goals may take decades. However, progress is already being made in combining current vaccines to facilitate complete immunization, and prototypes of new vaccines are being assessed in early clinical trials. The results will be applicable to immunization programs in both developed and developing countries.

REEMERGENCE OF CONTROLLED DISEASE AND EMERGENCE OF NEW DISEASE

The emergence of new pathogens is fostered by the genetic potential of microbes to evolve and exchange genetic material as well as by rapid changes in human demographics and behavior and in global ecology that create new or more favorable niches and hosts. Proof of the need for continuing vaccine research is provided by the emergence of new infectious diseases, including HIV infection, Lyme borreliosis, hantavirus pulmonary syndrome, hepatitis C, and—most recently— the severe acute respiratory syndrome (SARS) caused by a coronavirus; the sudden outbreak of epidemic cholera due to a previously unknown serotype (O139 Bengal); and the increase in global incidence and drug resistance of familiar diseases that were once considered under control (e.g., tuberculosis and malaria). In addition, some common illnesses without a previously known etiology, such as peptic ulcer disease and cervical and nasopharyngeal cancer, have now been epidemiologically linked to specific infectious agents and thus, by definition, are vaccine-preventable conditions.

NEW VACCINE APPROACHES

The first generation of vaccines included whole killed bacteria, partially purified microbial products that induced protective antibodies (e.g., tetanus and diphtheria toxoids), or live attenuated microorganisms. The second generation of vaccines has taken advantage of molecular genetics and protein chemistry: purified proteins or subunits of organisms have been isolated and manipulated, and genetically engineered and attenuated live native organisms have been generated, as have cloned antigens expressed by harmless vector organisms. One conceptual leap is the production of edible transgenic plants (e.g., potatoes, bananas) that express protective vaccine antigens (as a result of insertion of the relevant microbial genes) and that, when eaten, induce mucosal and systemic immune responses to homologous infectious challenges. While the practical use of this technique awaits further refinement, the concept that protective immunity can be induced in this manner has been proved in both animals and humans. Ease of production, stability, ease of administration without equipment, and low cost are the obvious advantages.

TABLE 107-9 *Advantages and Disadvantages of DNA Vaccines*

Advantages	Disadvantages
Safe; cannot cause infection; stable and heat resistant	Potential risk of integration of viral genes from the vector
No need to express or purify antigens in vitro; no need for adjuvants; can be genetically engineered	Tumor promotion from integration near proto-oncogenes or tumor suppressor genes
Normal processing of gene product closely resembling native conformation	Possible induction of tolerance or autoimmunity by vaccine persistence
Persistence for prolonged periods; induction of durable immune response	Possible influence of strong promoters on expression of host genes, with adverse consequences
Induction of both humoral and cell-mediated immunity, including cytotoxic T cells	
Likely to be safe in pregnant women, immunosuppressed patients, or (in the presence of maternal antibody) infants	

Another conceptual leap has led to a third generation of vaccines, in which nucleic acids (either DNA or RNA) are used to induce immunity. The principle is simple and offers many advantages (Table 107-9). First, a DNA plasmid containing the gene sequence for the immunogenic protein or fragment of interest is assembled and placed under the control of a strong promoter and an appropriate transcription termination sequence. A single immunization with the plasmid by a number of possible routes results in DNA uptake into cells, where the gene is expressed and processed normally. The resulting protein product of the vaccine DNA induces an immune response. It should be possible to manipulate the DNA construct, its mode of administration, or the coadministration of cytokine genes to drive a T_H1, T_H2, or cytotoxic T cell response that optimizes the protective immune response. Recently, a technique known as *prime-boost* has been used to convert antibody responses to an antigen into cell-mediated responses. In prime-boost, a priming dose—most often naked DNA encoding the antigen of interest—is followed at the optimal interval by the same DNA inserted into a viral vector (e.g., the modified vaccinia virus vector MVA). DNA vaccines may be particularly useful for the induction of tumor immunity, for the treatment of allergy by suppression of IgE production, or for gene therapy. Because RNA is less stable and does not persist or integrate into the chromosome or result in insertional mutagenesis, the value of RNA vaccines would be to diminish concerns about adverse events associated with the effects of DNA integration into the chromosome (Table 107-9). These virtues of RNA paradoxically represent the hurdles to overcome in producing stable, inexpensive, and effective RNA vaccines.

INTERNATIONAL CONSIDERATIONS

Since the establishment of the Expanded Programme on Immunization (EPI) by the World Health Organization (WHO) in 1981 and the involvement of UNICEF in the program's implementation, levels of coverage for the recommended basic children's vaccines (bacille Calmette-Guérin, poliomyelitis, DTP/DTaP, and measles) have risen from 5 to ~80% worldwide, although coverage does not necessarily translate into protective immunity. Each year, at least 2.7 million deaths from measles, neonatal tetanus, and pertussis and 200,000 cases of paralysis due to polio are prevented by immunization. Despite the successes of this program, many vaccine-preventable diseases remain prevalent in the developing world. Measles, for example, continues to kill an estimated 800,000 children each year, and diphtheria, whooping cough, polio, and neonatal tetanus still occur at unacceptably high rates. An estimated 20 to 35% of all deaths of children <5 years old are still associated with vaccine-preventable diseases.

In addition to the antigens included in the EPI for routine use in the developing world, others (hepatitis B, Hib, Japanese B encephalitis, yellow fever, meningococcus, mumps, and rubella) are used regionally, depending on disease epidemiology and resources. The rationale for inclusion of HepB vaccine in Africa and Asia is to prevent the subsequent development of hepatocellular carcinoma, which is strongly linked with the persistence of HBV from early childhood. The delivery of vaccines in mass campaigns on national immunization days, superseding even civil wars and insurgencies, has resulted in the cessation of transmission of poliomyelitis and the virtual elimination of clinical measles from the Western Hemisphere. Periodic vaccination campaigns complement routine infant and childhood vaccination services under the rubric "catch up, follow up, and keep up." Despite these successes, ongoing concerns remain about inadequate long-term strategies to ensure continuity, the impact of vaccine campaigns on the provision of routine services, and unsafe injection practices.

Because infectious diseases know no geographic or political boundaries, uncontrolled disease anywhere in the world poses a threat to the United States, even without the threat of bioterrorism (Chap. 205). Although the expectation of eradicating infectious agents and ceasing immunization altogether no longer seems realistic, vaccines offer the opportunity to effectively control and even eliminate some diseases through individual and herd protection. Vaccines also represent the best societal hope for stopping the pandemic of HIV infection throughout the world and efficiently controlling malaria and tuberculosis. Issues of cost, liability, risk, and profitability limit the interest of the pharmaceutical industry in the development of vaccines (e.g., for malaria) that will be used primarily in poor developing countries. Global recognition of the powerful effect that vaccines have on reduction of the disease burden has led to the creation of the Global Alliance for Vaccines and Immunization, which coordinates partnerships in public research and privately funded vaccine development. WHO, UNICEF, and other organizations (such as the International AIDS Vaccine Initiative, Rotary International, the Bill and Melinda Gates Foundation, and the Rockefeller Foundation) have helped to move the process forward with new strategies, investment in development, and implementation or with new funding for basic research. New international collaborations are being considered by wealthy industrial nations to attract increasing interest from the private sector—for example, advance-purchase schemes in which the purchase of effective vaccines is guaranteed, ensuring the profitability that the marketplace has provided for industry in wealthy countries. The effectiveness of such approaches remains to be seen, but they offer much-needed hope for at-risk populations around the world.

SOURCES OF INFORMATION ON IMMUNIZATION

- Official vaccine package circulars and Vaccine Administration Statements from the CDC
- Report of the Committee on Infectious Diseases of the American Academy of Pediatrics ("Red Book")
- Recommendations of the Advisory Committee on Immunization Practices, CDC
- Guide for Adult Immunization, American College of Physicians
- Health Information for International Travel (published yearly) and Advisory Memoranda on Travel (published periodically), CDC
- Control of Communicable Diseases in Man, American Public Health Association
- Technical Bulletin of the College of Obstetrics and Gynecology
- National Network for Immunization Information, Infectious Diseases Society of America/Pediatric Infectious Diseases Society/American Academy of Pediatrics/American Nurses Association

FURTHER READING

AVERY RK: Immunizations in adult immunocompromised patients: Which to use and which to avoid. Cleve Clin J Med 68:337, 2001

DENNEHY PH: Active immunization in the United States: Developments over the past decade. Clin Microbiol Rev 14:872, 2001

HINMAN A: Eradication of vaccine-preventable diseases. Annu Rev Public Health 20:211, 1999

KELLER MA, STIEHM ER: Passive immunity in prevention and treatment of infectious diseases. Microbiol Rev 13:602, 2000

MAHONEY RT, MAYNARD JE: The introduction of new vaccines into developing countries. Vaccine 17:646, 1999

MUNOZ FM, ENGLUND JA: Vaccines in pregnancy. Infect Dis Clin North Am 15:253, 2001

PETER G, GARDNER P: Standards for immunization practice for vaccines in children and adults. Infect Dis Clin North Am 15:9, 2001

WILSON ME: Travel-related vaccines. Infect Dis Clin North Am 15:231, 2001

WEBSITES OF INTEREST: www.cdc.gov/nip; www.idsociety.org/vaccine/resources; www.immunizationinfo.org; www.genweb.com/Dnavax/dnavax

ZIMMERMAN RK, BALL JA: Adult vaccinations. Prim Care 28:763, 2001

108 HEALTH ADVICE FOR INTERNATIONAL TRAVEL
J.S. Keystone, P.E. Kozarsky

According to the World Tourism Organization, the number of international tourist arrivals in 2001 amounted to 693 million—the highest figure ever documented. Not only are more people traveling; travelers are seeking more exotic and remote destinations. In 1999, more than 75 million people traveled from industrialized to developing countries; this figure represents a 50% increase from 1993. Studies show that between 50 and 75% of short-term travelers to the tropics or subtropics report some health impairment. Most of these health problems are minor, with only 5% requiring medical attention and fewer than 1% requiring hospitalization. Although infectious agents contribute substantially to morbidity among travelers, these pathogens account for only ~1% of deaths in this population. Cardiovascular disease and injuries are the most frequent causes of death among travelers from the United States, accounting for 49 and 22% of deaths, respectively. Age-specific rates of death due to cardiovascular disease are similar among travelers and nontravelers. In contrast, rates of death due to injury (the majority from motor vehicle, drowning, or aircraft accidents) are several times higher among travelers. Figure 108-1 summarizes the monthly incidence of health problems during travel in developing countries.

GENERAL ADVICE

Staying healthy during travel requires familiarity with the various health risks that may be encountered at a given destination. However, health maintenance recommendations are based not only on the traveler's destination but also on risk assessment, which is determined by health status, specific itinerary, and lifestyle during travel. Detailed information regarding country-specific risks and recommendations may be obtained from the Centers for Disease Control and Prevention (CDC) publication *Health Information for International Travel* (www.cdc.gov/travel).

Fitness for travel is an issue of growing concern in view of the increased numbers of elderly and chronically ill individuals journeying to exotic destinations (see "Travel and Special Hosts," below). Since most commercial aircraft are pressurized to 2500 m (8000 ft) above sea level (corresponding to a Pa_{O_2} of ~55 mmHg), individuals with serious cardiopulmonary problems should be evaluated before travel. In addition, those who have recently had surgery, a myocardial infarction, a cerebrovascular accident, or a deep-vein thrombosis (among other events) may be at high risk for adverse events in flight. A summary of current recommendations regarding fitness to fly has been

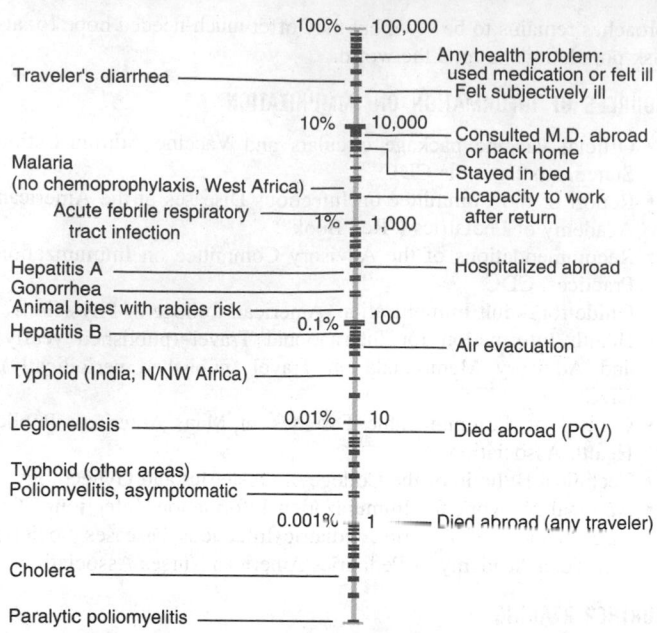

FIGURE 108-1 Incidence rate, per month, of health problems during a stay in developing countries. PCV, Peace Corps volunteer. (*From Steffen R, Lobel HO: Epidemiologic basis for the practice of travel medicine. J Wilderness Med 5:56, 1994. Reprinted with permission from Chapman and Hall, New York.*)

published by the Aerospace Medical Association Air Transport Medical Committee. A pretravel health assessment may also be advisable for individuals considering particularly adventurous recreational activities, such as mountain climbing and scuba diving.

TABLE 108-1 *Vaccines Commonly Used for Travel*

Vaccine	Primary Series	Booster Interval
Cholera, live oral (CVD 103 - HgR)	1 dose	6 months
Hepatitis A (Havrix), 1440 enzyme immunoassay U/mL	2 doses, 6–12 months apart, IM	None required
Hepatitis A (VAQTA, AVAXIM, EPAXAL)	2 doses, 6–12 months apart, IM	None required
Hepatitis A/B combined (Twinrix)	3 doses at 0, 1, and 6–12 months *or* 0, 7, and 21 days plus booster of B at 1 year, IM	None required *except* 12 months (once only, for accelerated schedule)
Hepatitis B (Engerix B): accelerated schedule	3 doses at 0, 1, and 2 months *or* 0, 7, and 21 days plus booster at 1 year, IM	12 months, once only
Hepatitis B (Engerix B or Recombivax): standard schedule	3 doses at 0, 1, and 6 months, IM	None required
Immune globulin (hepatitis A prevention)	1 dose IM	Intervals of 3–5 months, depending on initial dose
Japanese encephalitis (JEV, Biken)	3 doses, 1 week apart, SC	12–18 months (first booster), then 4 years
Meningococcus, quadrivalent	1 dose SC	>3 years (optimum booster schedule not yet determined)
Rabies (HDCV), rabies vaccine absorbed (RVA), or purified chick embryo cell vaccine (PCEC)	3 doses at 0, 7, and 21 or 28 days, IM	None required except with exposure
Typhoid Ty21a, oral live attenuated (Vivotif)	1 capsule every other day × 4 doses	5 years
Typhoid Vi capsular polysaccharide, injectable (Typhim Vi)	1 dose IM	2 years
Yellow fever	1 dose SC	10 years

IMMUNIZATIONS FOR TRAVEL Immunizations for travel fall into three broad categories: routine (childhood/adult boosters that are necessary regardless of travel), required (immunizations that are mandated by international regulations for entry into certain areas or for border crossings), and recommended (immunizations that are desirable because they confer protection against a variety of illnesses for which travel increases the risk). Vaccines commonly given to travelers are listed in Table 108-1.

Routine Immunizations ■ *Diphtheria, Tetanus, and Polio* Diphtheria continues to be a problem worldwide; large outbreaks have occurred over the past decade in the independent states formerly encompassed by the Soviet Union. Serosurveys show that tetanus antitoxin is lacking in many North Americans, especially in women over the age of 50. The risk of polio to the international traveler is extremely low, and wild poliovirus has been eradicated from the western hemisphere and Europe. However, studies in the United States have found varying levels of immunity in the general population, and data suggest that 12% of adult travelers from the United States are unprotected against at least one poliovirus serogroup. Foreign travel offers an ideal opportunity to have these immunizations updated.

Measles Measles (rubeola) continues to be a major cause of morbidity and mortality in the developing world (Chap. 176). Several outbreaks of measles in the United States have been linked to imported cases. The group at highest risk consists of persons born after 1956 and vaccinated before 1980, in many of whom primary vaccination failed. Travelers in this group should be reimmunized.

Influenza Influenza occurs year-round in the tropics and during the summer months in the southern hemisphere (coinciding with the winter months in the northern hemisphere). Vaccination should be considered for all travelers to these regions, particularly those who are elderly or chronically ill. The largest outbreak of travel-related influenza occurred in the summer of 1998 in Alaska and the Northwest Territories of Canada among cruise ship passengers and staff. Such outbreaks continue to occur; unfortunately, however, influenza vaccine is generally not available during the summer months in the United States (Chap. 171).

Pneumococcal Infection Pneumococcal vaccine should be administered routinely to persons at high risk of serious infection, such as individuals with chronic heart, lung, or renal disease and those who have been splenectomized or have sickle cell disease.

Required Immunizations ■ *Yellow Fever* Documentation of yellow fever vaccination may be required as a condition of entry into or passage through countries of sub-Saharan Africa and equatorial South America, where the disease is endemic or epidemic, or into countries that are at risk of having the infection introduced. This vaccine is given only by state-authorized yellow fever centers, and its administration must be documented on an official International Certificate of Vaccination. In Africa, the risk of yellow fever has been estimated to be as high as 1 case per 267 travelers per 2-week stay during epidemics and as low as 1 case per 2000 travelers per 2-week stay where the disease is endemic. The incidence of yellow fever among travelers is extremely low, probably because the vaccine is highly efficacious. However, recent data suggest that fewer than 50% of travelers entering areas endemic for yellow fever are immunized, and both American and European travelers have died of this very serious illness on their return home. It is also of concern that yellow fever–endemic areas may be expanding. Education about the importance of preventing this illness is crucial.

Cholera According to the World Health Organization, cholera vaccination should no longer be required for entry into any country. The inactivated injectable vaccine is no longer available in the United States.

Meningococcal Meningitis Protection against meningitis (using the quadrivalent polysaccharide vaccine) is required for entry into Saudi Arabia during the Hajj.

Recommended Immunizations ■ *Hepatitis A and B* Hepatitis A is the most frequent vaccine-preventable infection of travelers; Swiss data show that the incidence of symptomatic infection during a 1-month stay in a developing country ranges from 3 to 6 cases per 1000. The risk is six times greater for travelers who stray from the usual tourist routes. The results of a recent Canadian study showed that rates of hepatitis A among short-term vacationers to Mexico and the Caribbean were considerably lower (1 case per 10,000 to 20,000 travelers per month of stay). The mortality rate for hepatitis A increases with age, reaching almost 3% among symptomatic individuals over age 50. Of the four hepatitis A vaccines currently available in North America (two in the United States), all are interchangeable and have an efficacy rate of >95%. The monthly incidence of hepatitis B infection, both symptomatic and asymptomatic, is 80 to 240 cases per 100,000. For reasons that are not entirely clear, long-stay overseas workers are at considerable risk for hepatitis B infection. A combined hepatitis A and B vaccine is now available and has been approved for administration on a 3-week accelerated schedule in Canada and Europe.

Typhoid Fever The attack rate for typhoid fever is 1 case per 30,000 per month of travel to the developing world (Chap. 137). However, the attack rates in India, Senegal, and North Africa are tenfold higher; in these areas, rates are especially high among travelers to relatively remote destinations and among persons who are returning to their homelands to stay with relatives or friends. Between 1994 and 1999 in the United States, 77% of imported cases involved the latter group. The two available vaccines—one oral and the other injectable—have an efficacy rate of ~70%.

Meningococcal Meningitis Although the risk of meningococcal disease among travelers has not been quantified, it is likely to be higher among travelers who live with poor indigenous populations in overcrowded conditions. Meningococcal polysaccharide vaccine is recommended for persons traveling to sub-Saharan Africa during the dry season or to areas of the world where there are epidemics. The vaccine, which protects against serogroups A, C, Y, and W-135, has an efficacy rate of >90%.

Japanese Encephalitis The risk of Japanese encephalitis, an infection transmitted by mosquitoes in rural Asia and Southeast Asia, is ~1 case per 5000 travelers per month of stay in an endemic area. Most symptomatic infections among U.S. residents have involved military personnel or their families. The vaccine efficacy rate is >90%; serious allergic reactions sometimes occur. The vaccine is recommended for persons staying >1 month in rural endemic areas.

Cholera The risk of cholera is extremely low, with ~1 case per 500,000 journeys to endemic areas. Cholera vaccine, no longer available in the United States, was rarely recommended but was considered for aid and health care workers in refugee camps or in disaster/wartorn areas. A more effective oral cholera vaccine is available in other countries.

Rabies Many cases of rabies have been reported in travelers, but there are no data on the risk of infection. Domestic animals, primarily dogs, are the major transmitters of rabies in developing countries (Chap. 179). Several studies have shown that the risk of rabies posed by a dog bite in an endemic area ranges from 1 to 3.6 cases per 1000 travelers per month of stay. Countries where canine rabies is highly endemic include Mexico, the Philippines, Sri Lanka, India, Thailand, and Vietnam. The three vaccines available in the United States provide >90% protection. Rabies vaccine is recommended for long-stay travelers, particularly children, and persons who may be occupationally exposed to rabies in endemic areas.

PREVENTION OF MALARIA AND OTHER INSECT-BORNE DISEASES It is estimated that more than 30,000 American and European travelers develop malaria each year (Chap. 195). The risk of malaria is highest in Oceania and sub-Saharan Africa (estimated at 1:5 and 1:50 per month of stay, respectively, among persons not using chemoprophylaxis) and during the past decade has increased by more than fivefold for travelers to Kenya. The risk is intermediate (1:250 to 1:1000 per month) for travelers to malarious areas on the Indian subcontinent and in Southeast Asia and is low (1:2500 to 1:10,000 per month) for travelers to South and Central America. Of the more than 1000 cases of malaria reported annually in the United States, 90% of those due to *Plasmodium falciparum* occur in travelers returning or immigrating from Africa and Oceania. With the worldwide increase in chloroquine and multidrug-resistant falciparum malaria, decisions about chemoprophylaxis have become more difficult. In addition, the spread of malaria due to primaquine- and chloroquine-resistant strains of *Plasmodium vivax* has added to the complexity of treatment. The case-fatality rate of falciparum malaria in the United States is 4%; however, in only one-third of patients who die is the diagnosis of malaria considered before death.

Several recent studies indicate that fewer than 50% of travelers adhere to basic recommendations for malaria prevention. Keys to the prevention of malaria include both personal protection measures against mosquito bites, especially between dusk and dawn, and malaria chemoprophylaxis. The former measures include the use of DEET-containing insect repellents, permethrin-impregnated bed-nets and clothing, screened sleeping accommodations, and protective clothing. These practices also help prevent other insect-transmitted illnesses, such as dengue fever. Over the past decade, the incidence of dengue has increased, particularly in the Caribbean region, Latin America, and Southeast Asia. Dengue virus is transmitted by an urban-dwelling mosquito that bites at dawn and dusk.

The decision about whether to use malaria prophylaxis is based on the traveler's destination; the particular medication is determined by the destination as well as the traveler's preference and medical history. Table 108-2 lists the currently recommended drugs of choice for prophylaxis of malaria, by destination. Primaquine is an alternative medication used for prophylaxis by some physicians; although popular in parts of Europe, the chloroquine/proguanil combination is not recommended because of its low efficacy.

PREVENTION OF GASTROINTESTINAL ILLNESS Diarrhea, the leading cause of illness in travelers (Chap. 113), is usually a short-lived, self-limited condition; however, 40% of affected individuals need to alter their scheduled activities, and another 20% are confined to bed. The most important determinant of risk is the destination. Incidence rates per 2-week stay have been reported to be as low as 8% in industrialized countries and as high as 55% in parts of Africa, Central and South America, and Southeast Asia. Infants and young adults are at particularly high risk. The incidence of diarrhea is proportional to the num-

TABLE 108-2 *Malaria Chemosuppressive Regimens According to Geographic Area*[a]

Geographic Area	Drug of Choice	Alternatives
Central America (north of Panama), Haiti, Dominican Republic, Iraq, Egypt, Turkey, northern Argentina, and Paraguay	Chloroquine	Mefloquine Doxycycline Atovaquone/ proguanil
South America including Panama (except northern Argentina and Paraguay); Asia (including Southeast Asia); Africa; and Oceania	Mefloquine Doxycycline Atovaquone-proguanil (Malarone)	Primaquine
Thai, Myanmar, and Cambodian borders	Doxycycline Atovaquone-proguanil (Malarone)	

[a] See CDC's *Health Information for International Travel 2003–2004.*
Note: See also Chap. 195.

ber of dietary indiscretions. Studies of U.S. students in Mexico showed that eating meals in restaurants and cafeterias or consuming food from street vendors was associated with increased risk.

Etiology (See also Table 113-2)   The most frequently identified pathogen causing traveler's diarrhea is toxigenic *Escherichia coli*, although in some parts of the world (notably northern Africa and Southeast Asia) *Campylobacter* infections appear to predominate. Other common causative organisms include *Salmonella*, *Shigella*, rotavirus, and the Norwalk agent. Except for giardiasis, parasitic infections are uncommon causes of traveler's diarrhea. A growing problem for travelers is the development of antibiotic resistance by many bacterial pathogens, including strains of *Campylobacter* resistant to quinolones and strains of *E. coli*, *Shigella*, and *Salmonella* resistant to trimethoprim-sulfamethoxazole.

Precautions   Although the mainstay of prevention of traveler's diarrhea involves food and water precautions, the literature has repeatedly documented dietary indiscretions in 98% of travelers within the first 48 h after arrival at their destination. The maxim "Boil it, cook it, peel it, or forget it!" is easy to remember but apparently difficult to follow. General food and water precautions include eating foods piping hot; avoiding foods that are raw, poorly cooked, or sold by street vendors; and drinking only boiled or commercially bottled beverages, particularly those that are carbonated. Heating kills diarrhea-causing organisms, whereas freezing does not; therefore, ice cubes made from unpurified water should be avoided.

Self-Treatment (See also Table 113-4)   As traveler's diarrhea often occurs despite rigorous food and water precautions, travelers should carry medications for self-treatment. For mild to moderate diarrhea, loperamide and fluid replacement may be sufficient. An antibiotic is useful in reducing the frequency of bowel movements and duration of illness in moderate to severe diarrhea. The standard regimen is a 3-day course of a quinolone taken twice daily (or, in the case of some newer formulations, once daily). However, studies have shown that a single double dose of a quinolone may be equally effective, particularly if infection with a multidrug-resistant organism is not suspected. For diarrhea acquired in areas such as Thailand, where >90% of *Campylobacter* infections are quinolone resistant, azithromycin may be a better alternative.

Prophylaxis   Prophylaxis of traveler's diarrhea with bismuth subsalicylate is widely used but only ~60% effective. For certain individuals (e.g., athletes, persons with a repeated history of traveler's diarrhea, and persons with chronic diseases), a single daily dose of a quinolone during travel of <1 month's duration is highly effective.

Illness after Return   Although extremely common, acute traveler's diarrhea is usually self-limited or amenable to antibiotic therapy. Persistent bowel problems after the traveler returns home have a less well-defined etiology and may require medical attention from a specialist. Infectious agents appear to be responsible for only a small proportion of cases with persistent bowel symptoms. Of the pathogens detected in these instances, *Giardia lamblia* (Chap. 199) is by far the most common; *Cyclospora cayetanensis*, *Cryptosporidium* species, and *Entamoeba histolytica* are rarely isolated. Studies suggest that enteroadherent *E. coli* may be important. By far the most frequent causes of persistent diarrhea after travel are postinfectious sequelae, such as lactose intolerance or an irritable bowel syndrome. In the latter, intermittent diarrhea often alternates with constipation. When no infectious etiology can be identified, a trial of metronidazole therapy for presumed giardiasis, a strict lactose-free diet for 1 week, or a several-week trial of high-dose hydrophilic mucilloid (plus lactulose for persons with constipation) relieves the symptoms of many patients.

PREVENTION OF OTHER TRAVEL-RELATED PROBLEMS   Travelers are at high risk for *sexually transmitted diseases*. Surveys have shown that large numbers engage in casual sex, and there is a reluctance to use condoms

consistently. An increasing number of travelers are being diagnosed with *schistosomiasis*. Travelers should be cautioned to avoid bathing, swimming, or wading in freshwater lakes, streams, or rivers in parts of tropical South America, the Caribbean, Africa, and Southeast Asia where this infection can be acquired. Prevention of *travel-associated injury* depends mostly on common-sense precautions. Riding on motorcycles and in overcrowded public vehicles is not recommended; in particular, individuals should not travel by road after dark in rural areas. In addition to its association with motor vehicle accidents, excessive alcohol use has been a significant factor in drownings, assaults, and injuries. Travelers are cautioned to avoid walking barefoot because of the risk of hookworm and *Strongyloides* infections (Chap. 201) and snakebites (Chap. 378).

THE TRAVELER'S MEDICAL KIT   A traveler's medical kit is strongly advisable, particularly for long-stay travelers. The contents may vary widely, depending on the itinerary, duration of stay, style of travel, and local medical facilities. While many medications are available abroad, often over the counter, directions for their use may be nonexistent or in a foreign language, or a product may be outdated or counterfeit. Therefore, if possible, a complete supply of medications should accompany the traveler. In the kit, the short-term traveler should consider carrying an analgesic, an antidiarrheal agent, antihistamines, a laxative, oral rehydration salts, a sunscreen with a skin-protection factor of at least 30, a DEET-containing insect repellent for the skin, an insecticide for clothing (permethrin), and (if necessary) an antimalarial drug. To these medications the long-stay traveler might add a broad-spectrum general-purpose antibiotic (levofloxacin or azithromycin), an antibacterial eye and skin ointment, and a topical antifungal cream. Regardless of the duration of travel, a first-aid kit containing such items as scissors, tweezers, and bandages should be considered.

TRAVEL AND SPECIAL HOSTS

PREGNANCY AND TRAVEL   A woman's medical history and itinerary, the quality of medical care at her destinations, and her degree of flexibility determine whether travel is wise during pregnancy. According to the American College of Obstetrics and Gynecology, the safest part of pregnancy in which to travel is between 18 and 24 weeks, when there is the least danger of spontaneous abortion or premature labor. Some obstetricians prefer that women stay within a few hundred miles of home after the 28th week of pregnancy in case problems arise; in general, however, healthy women may be advised that it is acceptable to travel.

Despite this general recommendation, there are some relative contraindications to international travel during pregnancy, including certain obstetric risk factors: a history of miscarriage, premature labor, incompetent cervix, or toxemia. General medical problems such as diabetes, heart failure, severe anemia, or a history of thromboembolic disease should also prompt the pregnant woman to postpone her travels. Finally, regions in which the pregnant woman and her fetus may be at excessive risk (e.g., those at high altitudes and those where live-virus vaccines are required or where multidrug-resistant malaria is endemic) are not ideal destinations during any trimester.

Malaria   Malaria during pregnancy carries a significant risk of morbidity and death. Levels of parasitemia are highest and failure to clear the parasites after treatment is most frequent among primigravidae. Severe disease, with complications such as cerebral malaria, massive hemolysis, and renal failure, is especially likely in pregnancy. Fetal sequelae include spontaneous abortion, stillbirth, preterm delivery, and congenital infection.

Traveler's Diarrhea   Because dehydration due to traveler's diarrhea can lead to inadequate placental blood flow, pregnant travelers must be extremely cautious regarding their food and beverage intake. The exclusive consumption of bottled (carbonated) or boiled drinks without ice, the eating of well-cooked meats and pasteurized dairy products, and the avoidance of pre-prepared salad items should help protect against traveler's diarrhea due to the usual causes as well as against infections such as toxoplasmosis, hepatitis E, and listeriosis, which can have serious sequelae in pregnancy.

The mainstay of therapy for traveler's diarrhea is rehydration. Loperamide may be used if necessary, but many of the usual antibiotics are contraindicated during pregnancy. Ampicillin alone or with clavulanic acid may be used, but many strains of *E. coli* and other organisms implicated in traveler's diarrhea are resistant. Azithromycin may be the best option.

Because of the major problems encountered when infants are given local foods and beverages, women are strongly encouraged to breast-feed when traveling with a neonate. A nursing mother with traveler's diarrhea should not stop breast-feeding but should increase her fluid intake.

Air Travel and High-Altitude Destinations Commercial air travel is not a risk to the healthy pregnant woman or to the fetus. Fetal oxygenation is not adversely affected by decreased cabin pressures because of the fetal hemoglobin dissociation curve; the higher radiation levels reported at altitudes of >10,500 m (>35,000 ft) should pose no problem to the healthy pregnant traveler. Since each airline has a policy regarding pregnancy and flying, it is best to check with the specific carrier when booking reservations. Domestic air travel is usually permitted until the 36th week, whereas international air travel is generally curtailed after the 32nd week.

There are no known risks for pregnant women who travel to high-altitude destinations and stay for short periods. However, there are likewise no data on the safety of pregnant women at altitudes of >4500 m (15,000 ft). Because of the harsh conditions usually associated with such trips, they are generally contraindicated for other reasons.

THE HIV-INFECTED TRAVELER The traveler infected with HIV is at special risk of serious infections due to a number of pathogens that may be more prevalent at travel destinations than at home. However, the degree of risk depends primarily on the state of the immune system at the time of travel. For persons whose CD4+ cell counts are normal or >500/μL, no data suggest a greater risk during travel than for persons without HIV infection. Individuals with AIDS (CD4+ cell counts of <200/μL) and others who are symptomatic need special counseling and should visit a travel medicine practitioner before departure, especially when traveling to the developing world.

Several countries now routinely deny entry to HIV-positive individuals, even though no data show that these restrictions decrease rates of transmission of the virus. In general, HIV testing is required of those individuals who wish to stay abroad >3 months or who intend to work or study abroad. Some countries will accept an HIV serologic test done within 6 months of departure, whereas others will not accept a blood test done at any time in the traveler's home country. In addition, border officials often have the authority to make inquiries of individuals entering a country and to check the medications they are carrying. If a drug such as zidovudine is identified, the person may be barred from entering the country. Information on testing requirements for specific countries is available from consular offices but is subject to frequent change.

Health insurance policies should be checked to make sure they are valid for care in other countries. The HIV-positive traveler should strongly consider obtaining trip cancellation insurance and evacuation insurance in case of illness. It is ideal to have the name of a physician at the travel destination who is familiar with the treatment of patients with AIDS, as the clinical findings associated with infection may be atypical in a patient with AIDS, and several infections may exist simultaneously. The traveler should be encouraged to visit the physician promptly if problems arise.

Immunizations All of the HIV-infected traveler's routine immunizations should be up to date (Chap. 107). The response to immunization may be impaired at CD4+ cell counts of <200/μL (and in some cases at even higher counts). Thus HIV-infected persons should be vaccinated as early as possible to ensure adequate immune response to all vaccines. In patients receiving highly active antiretroviral therapy, at least 3 months must elapse before regenerated CD4+ cells can be considered fully functional; therefore, in these patients, vaccinations should be delayed, if possible, until the CD4+ cell count has been stable for this length of time. However, when the risk of illness is high or the sequelae of illness are serious, immunization is recommended. In certain circumstances, it may be prudent to check the adequacy of the serum antibody response before departure (e.g., yellow fever neutralization inhibition if exposure is unavoidable).

Because of the increased risk of infections due to *Streptococcus pneumoniae* and other bacterial pathogens that cause pneumonia following influenza, pneumococcal polysaccharide and influenza vaccines should be administered. The estimated rates of response to influenza vaccine are >80% among persons with asymptomatic HIV infection and <50% among those with AIDS.

In general, live attenuated vaccines are contraindicated for persons with immune dysfunction. Because measles (rubeola) can be a severe and lethal infection in HIV-positive patients, these patients should receive the measles vaccine (or the combination measles-mumps-rubella vaccine) unless they are severely immunocompromised (CD4+ cell count, <200/μL). Between 18 and 58% of symptomatic HIV-infected vaccinees develop adequate antibody titers, and between 50 and 100% of asymptomatic persons infected with HIV seroconvert. Immune globulin should be considered for measles-susceptible, severely immunosuppressed HIV-infected persons who are planning to travel to measles-endemic countries.

The decision of whether to administer any of the special vaccines to an HIV-infected traveler should be based on the individual's risk. Inactivated vaccines can be administered without concern for safety but with concern about adequate protection. For example, data suggest that HIV-infected persons do not have as strong an antibody response to the meningococcal meningitis vaccine as do uninfected persons. Moreover, few data are available on the efficacy of many of the other vaccines (e.g., those for hepatitis A and typhoid).

It is recommended that the live yellow fever vaccine not be given to HIV-infected travelers. Although the potential adverse affects of a live vaccine in an HIV-infected individual are always a consideration, there appear to have been no reported cases of illness in those who have inadvertently received this vaccine. Nonetheless, if the CD4+ count is <200/μL, an alternative itinerary that poses no risk of exposure to yellow fever is recommended. If the traveler is passing through or traveling to an area where the vaccine is required but the disease risk is low, a physician's waiver should be issued. Bacille Calmette-Guérin vaccine should not be given because of reports of disseminated infection in HIV-infected persons.

A transient increase in viremia (lasting days to weeks) has been demonstrated in HIV-infected individuals following immunization with vaccines for such diseases as influenza, pneumococcal infection, and tetanus (Chap. 173). However, at this point, there is no evidence that this transient increase in HIV levels in the bloodstream is detrimental over time. Furthermore, it is likely that immune activation associated with infection with the live organisms in question would result in increases in viremia of greater magnitude and duration than those associated with vaccination. Therefore, the vaccination recommendations discussed above need not be modified at this time.

Gastrointestinal Illness Decreased levels of gastric acid, abnormal gastrointestinal mucosal immunity, other complications of HIV infection, and medications taken by HIV-infected patients make traveler's diarrhea especially problematic in these individuals. Traveler's diarrhea is likely to occur more frequently, be more severe, and be more difficult to treat in association with HIV infection. *Salmonella*, *Shigella*, and *Campylobacter* infections are also more protracted and more often accompanied by bacteremia in HIV-infected persons.

Cryptosporidium (Chap. 199), a common cause of diarrhea in tropical countries, produces severe chronic diarrhea and cholecystitis with increased mortality among patients with AIDS. *Isospora belli* causes infections at high rates among AIDS patients in the developing world; this infection is associated with malabsorption, weight loss, and relapses after treatment. Persistent diarrhea due to microsporidiosis has been reported.

Because of these potential problems, the HIV-infected traveler must be careful to consume only appropriately prepared foods and beverages. In addition, this group of individuals may benefit from prophylaxis for traveler's diarrhea, using bismuth subsalicylate or a daily antibiotic (ideally a quinolone derivative) for short-term travel to the developing world. If the traveler is already taking a sulfonamide preparation for prophylaxis of *Pneumocystis* pneumonia, a regimen of self-treatment with a quinolone would be appropriate.

Other Travel-Related Infections   Data are lacking on the severity of many vector-borne diseases in HIV-infected individuals. Malaria is especially severe in asplenic and certain immunocompromised hosts, including those with AIDS. *Babesia* infection is known to cause serious illness and to recur in HIV-infected patients; this tick-transmitted illness occurs in parts of the United States but is not known to be a widespread problem.

Visceral leishmaniasis (Chap. 196) has been reported in numerous HIV-infected travelers. The diagnosis may be difficult to make, given that splenomegaly and hyperglobulinemia are often lacking and serologic results are frequently negative. This infection is difficult to treat, and its associated mortality is high. Even short-term travelers to southern Europe have developed the illness; thus the avoidance of sandfly bites is critical.

Certain respiratory illnesses, such as histoplasmosis and coccidioidomycosis, cause greater morbidity and mortality among patients with AIDS than in the general population. Although tuberculosis is common among HIV-infected persons (especially in developing countries), the acquisition of this infection by the short-term traveler is not a major concern. The possibility of acquiring *Legionella* infections from spas should be considered, although no data confirm an increase in the severity of such infections in AIDS.

Finally, the HIV-infected traveler should always be cautioned about safe sexual practices, which may help prevent both the transmission of HIV to others and the acquisition by the traveler of other sexually transmitted diseases that may be drug resistant or may result in serious sequelae (e.g., syphilis).

Medications   Adverse events due to medications and drug interactions are common and raise complex issues for HIV-infected persons. Rates of cutaneous reaction (e.g., increased cutaneous sensitivity to sulfonamides) are unusually high among patients with AIDS. Physicians advising HIV-infected travelers need to consider the problems that may arise from the use of agents such as antimalarial drugs, medications for altitude acclimation, or antidiarrheal compounds. Since zidovudine is metabolized by hepatic glucuronidation, inhibitors of this process may elevate serum levels of the drug. Concomitant administration of mefloquine and ritonavir may result in decreased plasma levels of ritonavir. In contrast, no significant influence of concomitant mefloquine administration on plasma levels of indinavir or nelfinavir was detected in two HIV-infected travelers.

CHRONIC ILLNESS, DISABILITY, AND TRAVEL   Chronic health problems should not prevent travel, but special measures can make the journey safer and more comfortable.

Heart Disease   Cardiovascular events are the main cause of deaths among travelers and of in-flight emergencies on commercial aircraft. Persons with underlying heart disease should review their itineraries with a physician prior to departure; travel in harsh environments or to remote destinations is not wise. Extra supplies of all medications should be kept in carry-on luggage, along with a copy of a recent electrocardiogram and the name and telephone number of the traveler's physician at home. Pacemakers are not affected by airport security

devices, but electronic telephone checks of pacemaker function cannot be transmitted by international satellites. The traveler may benefit from supplemental oxygen, which should be ordered by a physician (since oxygen delivery systems are not standard) 48 to 72 h before flight time. Personal oxygen tanks are not permitted aboard aircraft. Travelers should request aisle seating and should walk, perform stretching and flexing exercises, and remain hydrated during the flight to prevent venous thrombosis and pulmonary embolism.

Chronic Lung Disease   Chronic obstructive pulmonary disease is one of the most common diagnoses in patients who require emergency-room evaluation for symptoms occurring during airline flights. Patients with such disease experience dyspnea, edema, wheezing, cyanosis, and chest pain. The best predictor of the development of these symptoms is the sea level Pa_{O_2}. A Pa_{O_2} of at least 72 mmHg corresponds to an in-flight arterial Pa_{O_2} of ~55 mmHg when the cabin is pressurized to 2500 m (8000 ft). Therefore, if the traveler's baseline Pa_{O_2} is <72 mmHg, the provision of supplemental oxygen during the flight should be considered. Pulmonary function is also maximized by continuing bronchodilator treatment and the use of glucocorticoids as prescribed. Contraindications to flight include active bronchospasm, lower respiratory infection, lower-limb deep-vein phlebitis, pulmonary hypertension, and recent thoracic surgery (within the preceding 3 weeks) or pneumothorax. Consideration should be given to decreasing the amount of outdoor activity at the destination if there is excessive air pollution.

Diabetes Mellitus   Alterations in glucose control and changes in insulin requirements are common problems among patients with diabetes who travel. Changes in time zone, in the amount and timing of food intake, and in physical activity demand more vigilant assessment of metabolic control. The traveler with diabetes should pack medication (including a bottle of regular insulin for emergencies), insulin syringes and needles, equipment and supplies for glucose monitoring, and snacks in carry-on luggage. Insulin is stable for ~3 months at room temperature but should be kept as cool as possible. The name and telephone number of the home physician and a card and necklace listing the patient's medical problems and the type and dose of insulin used should accompany the traveler. When six or more time zones are crossed, insulin requirements may be temporarily altered, depending on food intake and physical activity. In traveling eastward (e.g., from the United States to Europe), the morning insulin dose on arrival may need to be decreased. The blood glucose can then be checked during the day to determine whether additional insulin is required. For flights westward, with lengthening of the day, an additional dose of regular insulin may be required. Comfortable footwear is essential for the traveler with diabetes.

Other Special Groups   Other groups for whom special travel measures are encouraged include patients undergoing dialysis, those with transplants, and those with other disabilities. Up to 13% of travelers have some disability, but few advocacy groups and tour companies dedicate themselves to this growing population. The key to safe travel in each case is adequate research ahead of time. Patients undergoing chronic ambulatory peritoneal dialysis may ship their dialysis solutions to their destinations before traveling. They should carry essential medical records as well as antibiotics for self-treatment of presumed peritonitis. Hemodialysis patients need to reserve appointments at dialysis centers prior to their departure from home. Travel by transplant recipients to distant destinations should ideally be scheduled at least 1 year after surgery, as most rejection episodes occur early. Medication interactions are a source of serious concern for these travelers, and appropriate medical information should be carried, along with the home physician's name and telephone number. Some travelers taking glucocorticoids carry stress doses in case they become ill. Immunization of these immunocompromised travelers may result in less than adequate protection against certain diseases. Thus the traveler and physician must carefully consider which destinations are appropriate.

The most common medical problems encountered by travelers after their return home are diarrhea, fever, respiratory illnesses, and skin diseases. Frequently ignored problems are fatigue and emotional stress, especially in long-stay travelers. The approach to diagnosis requires some knowledge of geographic medicine, in particular the epidemiology and clinical presentation of infectious disorders. A geographic history should focus on the traveler's exact itinerary, including dates of arrival and departure; exposure history (food indiscretions, drinking-water sources, freshwater contact, sexual activity, animal contact, insect bites); location and style of travel (urban vs. rural, first-class hotel accommodation vs. camping); immunization history; and use of antimalarial chemosuppression.

DIARRHEA See "Prevention of Gastrointestinal Illness," above.

FEVER Fever in a traveler who has returned from a malarious area should be considered a medical emergency because death from *P. falciparum* malaria can follow an illness of only several days' duration. Although "fever from the tropics" does not always have a tropical cause, malaria should be the first diagnosis considered. The risk of *P. falciparum* malaria is highest among travelers returning from Africa or Oceania and among those who become symptomatic within the first 2 months after return. Other important causes of fever after travel include viral hepatitis (hepatitis A and E), typhoid fever, bacterial enteritis, arbovirus infections (e.g., dengue fever), rickettsial infections (including tick and scrub typhus and Q fever), and—in rare instances—leptospirosis, acute HIV infection, and amebic liver abscess. In at least 25% of cases, no etiology can be found, and the illness resolves spontaneously. Clinicians should keep in mind that no present-day antimalarial agent guarantees protection from malaria and that some immunizations (notably, that against typhoid fever) are only partially protective.

As noted above, the approach to the febrile returned traveler begins with a detailed medical and geographic history. Knowing exact dates of arrival and departure from tropical areas enables the physician to ascertain the shortest and longest possible incubation periods for illnesses in the differential diagnosis. For example, a traveler who develops fever <1 week after arrival in a malarious area cannot have malaria because the incubation period is too short, whereas a fever whose onset comes >2 weeks after departure from an endemic area cannot be dengue fever because the incubation period is too long. In the physical examination, particular attention should be given to the skin so as not to miss a subtle rash or eschar.

When no specific diagnosis is forthcoming, the following investigations, where applicable, are suggested: complete blood count, liver function tests, thick/thin blood films for malaria (repeated twice if necessary), urinalysis, urine and blood cultures (repeated once), chest x-ray, and collection of an acute-phase serum sample to be held for subsequent examination along with a paired convalescent-phase serum sample.

SKIN DISEASES Pyodermas, sunburn, insect bites, skin ulcers, and cutaneous larva migrans are the most common skin conditions encountered in travelers after their return home. In those with persistent skin ulcers, a diagnosis of cutaneous leishmaniasis, mycobacterial infec-

tion, or fungal infection should be considered. Careful, complete inspection of the skin is important in detecting the rickettsial eschar in a febrile patient or the central breathing hole in a "boil" due to myiasis.

EMERGING INFECTIOUS DISEASES In recent years, travel and commerce have fostered the worldwide spread of HIV infection, led to the reemergence of cholera as a global health threat, and created considerable fear about the possible spread of Ebola virus infection and severe acute respiratory syndrome (SARS). For travelers, there are more realistic concerns. One of the largest outbreaks of dengue fever ever documented is now raging in Latin America; schistosomiasis is being described in previously unaffected lakes in Africa; and antibiotic-resistant strains of sexually transmitted and enteric pathogens are emerging at an alarming rate in the developing world. In addition, concerns have been raised regarding the potential for bioterrorism involving not only standard strains of unusual agents but mutant strains as well. Time will tell whether travelers (as well as persons at home) will routinely be vaccinated against diseases such as anthrax and smallpox. As Nobel Laureate Dr. Joshua Lederberg pointed out, "The microbe that felled one child in a distant continent yesterday can reach yours today and seed a global pandemic tomorrow." The vigilant clinician understands that the importance of a thorough travel history cannot be overemphasized.

FURTHER READING

AEROSPACE MEDICAL ASSOCIATION AIR TRANSPORT MEDICINE COMMITTEE: Medical guidelines for air travel. Aviat Space Environ Med 67(Suppl 10):b1, 1996

CAUMES E et al: Dermatoses associated with travel to tropical countries: A prospective study of the diagnosis and management of 269 patients presenting to a tropical disease unit. Clin Infect Dis 20:542, 1995

CENTERS FOR DISEASE CONTROL AND PREVENTION: *Health Information for International Travel 2003-2004.* HHS publication no (CDC) 92-8280. Washington, DC, Government Printing Office, 2003 (www.cdc.gov/travel/yb/index.htm)

ERICSSON CD: Travelers' diarrhea: Epidemiology, prevention and self-treatment. Infect Dis Clin North Am 12:285, 1998

FRADIN MS: Mosquitoes and mosquito repellents: A clinician's guide. Ann Intern Med 128:931, 1998

KAIN KC et al: Malaria chemoprophylaxis in the age of drug resistance. I. Currently recommended drug regimens. Clin Infect Dis 33:226, 2001

KEYSTONE JS et al: *Travel Medicine.* Mosby, Philadelphia, 2004

———— et al: Internet and computer-based resources for travel medicine practitioners. Clin Infect Dis 32:757, 2001

————: GIDEON computer program for diagnosing and teaching geographic medicine. J Travel Med 6:152, 1999

MILENO MD, BIA FJ: The compromised traveler. Infect Dis Clin North Am 12:369, 1998

RYAN ET et al: Illness after international travel. N Engl J Med 347:505, 2002

————, KAIN KC: Health advice and immunizations for travelers. N Engl J Med 342:1716, 2000

SAMUEL B, BARRY M: The pregnant traveler. Infect Dis Clin North Am 12:323, 1998

SPIRA A: Assessment of travellers who return. Lancet 361:1459, 2003

————: Preparing the traveller. Lancet 361:1368, 2003

WEBSITES OF INTEREST: Chronic renal failure: www.kidney.org. Diabetes: www.diabetesmonitor.com/other-14.htm. Dialysis: www.dialysisfinder.com. Disability: www.access-able.com. HIV: www.aegis.com

Section 2 Clinical Syndromes: Community-Acquired Infections

109 INFECTIVE ENDOCARDITIS
Adolf W. Karchmer

The proliferation of microorganisms on the endothelium of the heart results in infective endocarditis. The prototypic lesion at the site of infection, the *vegetation* (Fig. 109-1), is a mass of platelets, fibrin, microcolonies of microorganisms, and scant inflammatory cells. Infection most commonly involves heart valves (either native or prosthetic) but may also occur on the low-pressure side of the ventricular septum at the site of a defect, on the mural endocardium where it is damaged by aberrant jets of blood or foreign bodies, or on intracardiac devices themselves. The analogous process involving arteriovenous shunts, arterioarterial shunts (patent ductus arteriosus), or a coarctation of the aorta is called *infective endarteritis.*

Endocarditis may be classified according to the temporal evolution

FIGURE 109-1 Vegetations (*arrows*) due to viridans streptococcal endocarditis involving the mitral valve.

of disease, the site of infection, the cause of infection, or a predisposing risk factor such as injection drug use. While each classification criterion provides therapeutic and prognostic insight, none is sufficient alone. The classification of endocarditis as acute and subacute was initially used to describe the illness and the time elapsed until death; presently it is applied to the features and progression of infection until diagnosis. *Acute endocarditis* is a hectically febrile illness, rapidly damages cardiac structures, hematogenously seeds extracardiac sites, and, if untreated, progresses to death within weeks. *Subacute endocarditis* follows an indolent course; causes structural cardiac damage only slowly, if at all; rarely causes metastatic infection; and is gradually progressive unless complicated by a major embolic event or ruptured mycotic aneurysm.

In developed countries, the incidence of endocarditis ranges from 1.5 to 6.2 cases per 100,000 population per year. In the late 1980s in a metropolitan area of the United States (Philadelphia), endocarditis occurred in 9.3 persons per 100,000 population per year. However, half of these cases arose as a consequence of injection drug use. The incidence of endocarditis is notably increased among the elderly. The cumulative rate of prosthetic valve endocarditis is 1.5 to 3.0% at 1 year after valve replacement and 3 to 6% at 5 years; the risk is greatest during the first 6 months after valve replacement.

ETIOLOGY Many species of bacteria and fungi have been reported to cause sporadic episodes of endocarditis; nevertheless, a small number of bacterial species cause the majority of cases (Table 109-1). The causative microorganisms vary somewhat among the major clinical types of endocarditis, in part because of the different portals of entry. The oral cavity, skin, and upper respiratory tract are the respective primary portals for the viridans streptococci, staphylococci, and HACEK organisms (*Haemophilus, Actinobacillus, Cardiobacterium, Eikenella,* and *Kingella*) causing community-acquired native valve endocarditis. *Streptococcus bovis* originates from the gastrointestinal tract, where it is associated with polyps and colonic tumors, and enterococci enter the bloodstream from the genitourinary tract. Nosocomial native valve endocarditis is largely the consequence of bacteremia arising from intravascular catheters and less commonly from nosocomial wound and urinary tract infection. Endocarditis complicates 6 to 25% of episodes of catheter-associated *Staphylococcus aureus* bacteremia; the higher rates are detected by careful transesophageal echocardiography (TEE) screening (see "Echocardiography," below).

Prosthetic valve endocarditis arising within 2 months of valve surgery is generally the result of intraoperative contamination of the prosthesis or a bacteremic postoperative complication. The nosocomial nature of these infections is reflected in their primary microbial causes: coagulase-negative staphylococci, *S. aureus,* facultative gram-negative bacilli, diphtheroids, and fungi. The portals of entry and organisms causing cases beginning >12 months after surgery are similar to those in community-acquired native valve endocarditis. Epidemiologic evidence suggests that prosthetic valve endocarditis due to coagulase-negative staphylococci that presents between 2 and 12 months after surgery is often nosocomial in origin but with a delayed onset. At least 85% of coagulase-negative staphylococci that cause prosthetic valve endocarditis within 12 months of surgery are methicillin-resistant; the rate of methicillin resistance decreases to 25% among coagulase-negative staphylococci causing prosthetic endocarditis that presents >1 year after valve surgery.

Transvenous pacemaker lead– and/or implanted defibrillator–associated endocarditis is usually a nosocomial infection. The majority of episodes occur within weeks of implantation or generator change and are caused by *S. aureus* or coagulase-negative staphylococci.

Endocarditis occurring among injection drug users, especially when infection involves the tricuspid valve, is commonly caused by *S. aureus* strains, many of which are methicillin-resistant. Left-sided valve infections in addicts have a more varied etiology and involve abnormal valves, often ones damaged by prior episodes of endocarditis. A number of these cases are caused by *Pseudomonas aeruginosa*

TABLE 109-1 *Organisms Causing Major Clinical Forms of Endocarditis*

	Percent of Cases							
	Native Valve Endocarditis		**Prosthetic Valve Endocarditis at Indicated Time of Onset (Months) after Valve Surgery**			**Endocarditis in Injection Drug Users**		
Organism	Community-Acquired (n = 683)	Nosocomial (n = 82)	< 2 (n = 144)	2–12 (n = 31)	> 12 (n = 194)	Right-Sided (n = 346)	Left-Sided (n = 204)	Total (n = 675)
Streptococci[a]	32	7	1	9	31	5	15	12
Pneumococci	1	—	—	—	—	—	—	—
Enterococci	8	16	8	12	11	2	24	9
Staphylococcus aureus	35	55	22	12	18	77	23	57
Coagulase-negative staphylococci	4	10	33	32	11	—	—	—
Fastidious gram-negative coccobacilli (HACEK group)[b]	3	—	—	—	6	—	—	—
Gram-negative bacilli	3	5	13	3	6	5	13	7
Candida spp.	1	4	8	12	1	—	12	4
Polymicrobial/miscellaneous	6	1	3	6	5	8	10	7
Diphtheroids	—	—	6	—	3	—	—	0.1
Culture-negative	5	2	5	6	8	3	3	3

[a] Includes viridans streptococci; *Streptococcus bovis*; other non–group A, groupable streptococci; and *Abiotrophia* spp. (nutritionally variant, pyridoxal-requiring streptococci).

[b] Includes *Haemophilus* spp., *Actinobacillus actinomycetemcomitans, Cardiobacterium hominis, Eikenella* spp., and *Kingella kingae.*
Note: Data are compiled from multiple studies.

and *Candida* species, and sporadic cases are due to unusual organisms such as *Bacillus*, *Lactobacillus*, and *Corynebacterium* species. Polymicrobial endocarditis occurs more frequently in injection drug users than in patients who do not inject drugs. The presence of HIV in this population does not significantly impact the causes of endocarditis.

From 5 to 15% of patients with endocarditis have negative blood cultures; in one-third to one-half of these cases, cultures are negative because of prior antibiotic exposure. The remainder of these patients are infected by fastidious organisms, such as pyridoxal-requiring streptococci (now designated *Abiotrophia* species), the gram-negative coccobacillary HACEK organisms, *Bartonella henselae*, or *Bartonella quintana*. Some fastidious organisms that cause endocarditis have characteristic epidemiologic settings (e.g., *Coxiella burnetii* in Europe, *Brucella* species in the Middle East). *Tropheryma whipplei* causes an indolent, culture-negative, afebrile form of endocarditis.

PATHOGENESIS   Unless it is injured, the normal endothelium is resistant to infection by most bacteria and to thrombus formation. Endothelial injury (e.g., at the site of impact of high-velocity jets or on the low-pressure side of a cardiac structural lesion) causes aberrant flow and allows either direct infection by virulent organisms or the development of an uninfected platelet-fibrin thrombus—a condition called *nonbacterial thrombotic endocarditis* (NBTE). The thrombus subsequently serves as a site of bacterial attachment during transient bacteremia. The cardiac lesions most commonly resulting in NBTE are mitral regurgitation, aortic stenosis, aortic regurgitation, ventricular septal defects, and complex congenital heart disease. These lesions result from rheumatic heart disease (particularly in the developing world, where rheumatic fever remains prevalent), mitral valve prolapse, degenerative heart disease, and congenital malformations. NBTE also arises as a result of a hypercoagulable state; this phenomenon gives rise to the clinical entity of *marantic endocarditis* (uninfected vegetations seen in patients with malignancy and chronic diseases) and to bland vegetations complicating systemic lupus erythematosus and the antiphospholipid antibody syndrome.

Organisms that cause endocarditis generally enter the bloodstream from mucosal surfaces, the skin, or sites of focal infection. Except for more virulent bacteria (e.g., *S. aureus*) that can adhere directly to intact endothelium or exposed subendothelial tissue, microorganisms in the blood adhere to thrombi. If resistant to the bactericidal activity of serum and the microbicidal peptides released by platelets, the organisms proliferate and induce a procoagulant state at the site by eliciting tissue factor from adherent monocytes or, in the case of *S. aureus*, from monocytes and from intact endothelium. Fibrin deposition, resulting from tissue factor initiation of the coagulation cascade, combines with platelet aggregation, stimulated by tissue factor and independently by proliferating microorganisms, to generate an infected vegetation. The organisms that commonly cause endocarditis bear surface components that facilitate adherence to injured endothelium and host proteins or, in the case of *S. aureus*, to intact endothelial cells or to thrombi. Fibronectin-binding proteins present on many gram-positive bacteria, clumping factor (a fibrinogen- and fibrin-binding surface protein) on *S. aureus*, and glucans on streptococci facilitate adherence. Fibronectin-binding proteins are required for *S. aureus* invasion of intact endothelium; thus these surface proteins may facilitate infection of previously normal valves. In the absence of host defenses, organisms enmeshed in the growing platelet-fibrin vegetation proliferate to form dense microcolonies. Organisms deep in vegetations are metabolically inactive (nongrowing) and relatively resistant to killing by antimicrobial agents. Proliferating surface organisms are shed into the bloodstream continuously, whereupon some are cleared by the reticuloendothelial system and others are redeposited on the vegetation and stimulate further vegetation growth.

The pathophysiologic consequences and clinical manifestations of endocarditis—other than constitutional symptoms, which are probably a result of cytokine production—arise from damage to intracardiac structures; embolization of vegetation fragments, leading to infection or infarction of remote tissues; hematogenous infection of sites during bacteremia; and tissue injury due to the deposition of circulating immune complexes or immune responses to deposited bacterial antigens.

CLINICAL MANIFESTATIONS   The clinical syndrome of infective endocarditis is highly variable and spans a continuum between acute and subacute presentations. Native valve endocarditis (whether acquired in the community or nosocomially), prosthetic valve endocarditis, and endocarditis due to injection drug use share clinical and laboratory manifestations (Table 109-2). Although the relationship is not absolute, the causative microorganism is primarily responsible for the temporal course of endocarditis. β-Hemolytic streptococci, *S. aureus*, and pneumococci typically result in an acute course, although *S. aureus* occasionally causes subacute disease. Endocarditis caused by *Staphylococcus lugdunensis* (a coagulase-negative species) or by enterococci may present acutely. Subacute endocarditis is typically caused by viridans streptococci, enterococci, coagulase-negative staphylococci, and the HACEK group. Endocarditis caused by *Bartonella* species and the agent of Q fever, *C. burnetii*, is exceptionally indolent.

The clinical features of endocarditis are nonspecific. However, these symptoms in a febrile patient with valvular abnormalities or a behavior pattern (injection drug use) that predisposes to endocarditis suggest the diagnosis, as do bacteremia with organisms that frequently cause endocarditis, otherwise-unexplained arterial emboli, and progressive cardiac valvular incompetence. In patients with subacute presentations, fever is typically low-grade and rarely exceeds 39.4°C (103°F); in contrast, temperatures between 39.4 and 40°C (103 and 104°F) are often noted in acute endocarditis. Fever may be blunted or absent in patients who are elderly or severely debilitated or who have marked cardiac or renal failure.

Cardiac Manifestations   Although heart murmurs are usually indicative of the predisposing cardiac pathology rather than of endocarditis, valvular damage and ruptured chordae may result in new regurgitant murmurs. In acute endocarditis involving a normal valve, murmurs are heard on presentation in only 30 to 45% of patients but ultimately are detected in 85%. Congestive heart failure develops in 30 to 40% of patients; it is usually a consequence of valvular dysfunction but occasionally is due to endocarditis-associated myocarditis or an intracardiac fistula. The temporal progression of heart failure is variable; failure due to aortic valve dysfunction progresses more rapidly than that due to mitral valve dysfunction. Extension of infection beyond valve leaflets into adjacent annular or myocardial tissue results in perivalvular abscesses, which in turn may cause fistulae (from the root of

TABLE 109-2   *Clinical and Laboratory Features of Infective Endocarditis*

Feature	Frequency, %
Fever	80–90
Chills and sweats	40–75
Anorexia, weight loss, malaise	25–50
Myalgias, arthralgias	15–30
Back pain	7–15
Heart murmur	80–85
New/worsened regurgitant murmur	10–40
Arterial emboli	20–50
Splenomegaly	15–50
Clubbing	10–20
Neurologic manifestations	20–40
Peripheral manifestations (Osler's nodes, subungual hemorrhages, Janeway lesions, Roth's spots)	2–15
Petechiae	10–40
Laboratory manifestations	
Anemia	70–90
Leukocytosis	20–30
Microscopic hematuria	30–50
Elevated erythrocyte sedimentation rate	>90
Rheumatoid factor	50
Circulating immune complexes	65–100
Decreased serum complement	5–40

the aorta into cardiac chambers or between cardiac chambers) with new murmurs. Abscesses may burrow from the aortic valve annulus through the epicardium, causing pericarditis. Extension of infection into paravalvular tissue adjacent to either the right or the noncoronary cusp of the aortic valve may interrupt the conduction system in the upper interventricular septum, leading to varying degrees of heart block. Although perivalvular abscesses arising from the mitral valve may potentially interrupt conduction pathways near the atrioventricular node or in the proximal bundle of His, such interruption occurs infrequently. Emboli to a coronary artery may result in myocardial infarction; nevertheless, embolic transmural infarcts are rare.

Noncardiac Manifestations   The classic nonsuppurative peripheral manifestations of subacute endocarditis are related to the duration of infection and, with early diagnosis and treatment, have become infrequent. In contrast, septic embolization mimicking some of these lesions (subungual hemorrhage, Osler's nodes) is common in patients with acute *S. aureus* endocarditis (Fig. 109-2). Musculoskeletal symptoms, including nonspecific inflammatory arthritis and back pain, usually remit promptly with treatment but must be distinguished from focal metastatic infection. Hematogenously seeded focal infection may involve any organ but most often is clinically evident in the skin, spleen, kidneys, skeletal system, and meninges. Arterial emboli are clinically apparent in up to 50% of patients. Vegetations >10 mm in diameter (as measured by echocardiography) and those located on the mitral valve are more likely to embolize than are smaller or nonmitral vegetations. Embolic events—often with infarction—involving the extremities, spleen, kidneys (Fig. 109-3), bowel, or brain are often noted at presentation. With antibiotic treatment, the frequency of embolic events decreases from 13 per 1000 patient-days during the initial week to 1.2 per 1000 patient-days after the third week. Emboli occurring late during or after effective therapy do not in themselves constitute evidence of failed antimicrobial treatment. Neurologic symptoms, most often resulting from embolic strokes, occur in up to 40% of patients. Other neurologic complications include aseptic or purulent meningitis, intracranial hemorrhage due to hemorrhagic infarcts or ruptured mycotic aneurysms, seizures, and encephalopathy. (*Mycotic aneurysms* are focal dilations of arteries occurring at points in the artery wall that have been weakened by infection in the vasa vasorum or where septic emboli have lodged.) Microabscesses in brain and meninges occur commonly in *S. aureus* endocarditis; surgically drainable abscesses are infrequent.

Immune complex deposition on the glomerular basement membrane causes diffuse hypocomplementemic glomerulonephritis and renal dysfunction, which typically improve with effective antimicrobial

FIGURE 109-3   Computed tomography of the abdomen showing large embolic infarcts in the spleen and left kidney of a patient with *Bartonella* endocarditis.

therapy. Embolic renal infarcts cause flank pain and hematuria but rarely cause renal dysfunction.

Manifestations of Specific Predisposing Conditions   In almost 50% of patients who have endocarditis associated with injection drug use, infection is limited to the tricuspid valve. These patients present with fever, faint or no murmur, and (in 75% of cases) prominent pulmonary findings, including cough, pleuritic chest pain, nodular pulmonary infiltrates, and occasionally pyopneumothorax. Infection involving valves on the left side of the heart presents with the typical clinical features of endocarditis.

Nosocomial endocarditis (defined as that which results from hospital care within the prior month and most commonly presenting as intravascular catheter–associated bacteremia), if not associated with a retained intracardiac device, has typical manifestations. Endocarditis associated with flow-directed pulmonary artery catheters is often cryptic, with symptoms masked by comorbid critical illness, and is commonly diagnosed at autopsy. Transvenous pacemaker lead– and/or implanted defibrillator–associated endocarditis commonly follows initial implantation or a generator unit change; may be associated with obvious or cryptic generator pocket infection; and results in fever, minimal murmur, and pulmonary symptoms similar to those encountered in addicts with tricuspid endocarditis.

Prosthetic valve endocarditis presents with typical clinical features. Cases arising within 60 days of valve surgery (early onset) lack peripheral vascular manifestations and may be obscured by comorbidity associated with recent surgery. In both early-onset and more delayed presentations, paravalvular infection is common and often results in partial valve dehiscence, regurgitant murmurs, congestive heart failure, or disruption of the conduction system.

DIAGNOSIS ■ The Duke Criteria   The diagnosis of infective endocarditis is established with certainty only when vegetations obtained at cardiac surgery, at autopsy, or from an artery (an embolus) are examined histologically and microbiologically. Nevertheless, a highly sensitive and specific diagnostic schema—known as the *Duke criteria*—has been developed on the basis of clinical, laboratory, and echocardiographic findings (Table 109-3). Documentation of two major criteria, of one major and three minor criteria, or of five minor criteria allows a clinical diagnosis of definite endocarditis. The diagnosis of endocarditis is rejected if an alternative diagnosis is established, if symptoms resolve and do not recur with ≤4 days of antibiotic therapy, or if surgery or autopsy after ≤4 days of antimicrobial therapy yields no histologic evidence of endocarditis. Illnesses not classified as definite endocarditis or rejected are considered cases of possible infective endocarditis when either one major and one minor criteria or three minor criteria are identified. Requiring the identification of clinical features of en-

FIGURE 109-2   Septic emboli with hemorrhage and infarction due to acute *Staphylococcus aureus* endocarditis. (*Courtesy of L. Baden.*)

docarditis for classification as possible infective endocarditis increases the specificity of the schema without significantly reducing its sensitivity.

The roles of bacteremia and echocardiographic findings in the diagnosis of endocarditis are appropriately emphasized in the Duke criteria. That multiple blood cultures obtained over time are positive is consistent with the known continuous low-density nature of bacteremia characteristic of patients with endocarditis ($\leq$100 organisms per milliliter). Among untreated endocarditis patients who ultimately have a positive blood culture, 95% of all blood cultures are positive, and in 98% of cases one of the initial two sets of cultures yields the microorganism. The diagnostic criteria attach significance to the species of organism isolated from blood cultures. To fulfill a major criterion, the isolation of an organism that causes both endocarditis and bacteremia in the absence of endocarditis (e.g., *S. aureus*, enterococci) must take place repeatedly (i.e., persistent bacteremia) and in the absence of a primary focus of infection. Organisms that rarely cause endocarditis but commonly contaminate blood cultures (e.g., diphtheroids, coagulase-negative species) must be isolated repeatedly if their isolation is to serve as a major criterion.

Blood Cultures Isolation of the causative microorganism from blood cultures is critical not only for diagnosis but also for determination of antimicrobial susceptibility and planning of treatment. In the absence of prior antibiotic therapy, a total of three blood culture sets, ideally with the first separated from the last by at least 1 h, should be obtained from different venipuncture sites over 24 h. If the cultures remain negative after 48 to 72 h, two or three additional blood cultures, including a lysis-centrifugation culture, should be obtained, and the laboratory should be asked to pursue fastidious microorganisms by prolonging incubation time and performing special subcultures. Empirical antimicrobial therapy should not be administered initially to hemodynamically stable patients with subacute endocarditis, especially those who have received antibiotics within the preceding 2 weeks; thus, if necessary, additional blood cultures can be obtained without the confounding effect of empirical treatment. Patients with acute endocarditis or with deteriorating hemodynamics that may require urgent surgery should be treated empirically immediately after the initial three sets of blood cultures are obtained.

Non-Blood-Culture Tests for the Etiologic Agent Serologic tests can be used to identify some organisms causing endocarditis that are difficult to recover by blood culture: *Brucella*, *Bartonella*, *Legionella*, and *C. burnetii*. Pathogens can also be identified in vegetations by culture, by microscopic examination with special stains (i.e., the periodic acid–Schiff stain for *T. whipplei*), and by use of polymerase chain reaction to recover unique microbial DNA or 16S rRNA.

Echocardiography Cardiac imaging with echocardiography allows anatomic confirmation of infective endocarditis, sizing of vegetations, detection of intracardiac complications, and assessment of cardiac function. A two-dimensional study with color flow and continuous as well as pulsed Doppler is optimal. Transthoracic echocardiography (TTE) is noninvasive and exceptionally specific; however, it cannot image vegetations <2 mm in diameter, and in 20% of patients it is technically inadequate because of emphysema or body habitus. Thus, TTE detects vegetations in only 65% of patients with definite clinical endocarditis (i.e., it has a sensitivity of 65%). Moreover, TTE is not adequate for evaluating prosthetic valves or detecting intracardiac complications. TEE is safe and significantly more sensitive than TTE. It detects vegetations in >90% of patients with definite endocarditis; nevertheless, false-negative studies are noted in 6 to 18% of endocarditis patients. TEE is the optimal method for the diagnosis of prosthetic endocarditis or the detection of myocardial abscess, valve perforation, or intracardiac fistulae.

Experts favor echocardiographic evaluation of all patients with a clinical diagnosis of endocarditis; however, the test should not be used to screen patients with otherwise-explained positive blood cultures or patients with unexplained fever. In patients with a low pretest likelihood of endocarditis (<5%), a high-quality TTE that is negative is sufficient to exclude endocarditis. For patients whose habitus makes them difficult to study with TTE and for those who may have prosthetic valve endocarditis or who are at high risk of intracardiac complications, TEE is the preferred imaging modality. For patients with a pretest probability of endocarditis ranging from 5 to 50%, initial evaluation by TEE—in lieu of a sequential strategy of TTE, which, if negative, will be followed by TEE—is cost-effective. A negative TEE when endocarditis is likely does not exclude the diagnosis but rather warrants repetition of the study in 7 to 10 days with optimal multiplanar technique.

Other Studies Many laboratory studies that do not aid in diagnostic evaluation are nevertheless important in the management of patients with endocarditis; these studies include complete blood counts, creatinine measurement, chest radiography, and electrocardiography. The erythrocyte sedimentation rate, C-reactive protein level, circulating immune complex titer, and rheumatoid factor concentration are commonly increased in endocarditis (Table 109-2). Cardiac catheterization is useful primarily to assess coronary artery patency in older individuals who are to undergo surgery for endocarditis.

 TREATMENT

ANTIMICROBIAL THERAPY It is difficult to eradicate bacteria from the avascular vegetation in infective endocarditis because this site is rel-

---

TABLE 109-3 *The Duke Criteria for the Clinical Diagnosis of Infective Endocarditis*

MAJOR CRITERIA

1. Positive blood culture
   - Typical microorganism for infective endocarditis from two separate blood cultures
     - Viridans streptococci, *Streptococcus bovis*, HACEK group, *Staphylococcus aureus*, or Community-acquired enterococci in the absence of a primary focus, *or*
   - Persistently positive blood culture, defined as recovery of a microorganism consistent with infective endocarditis from:
     - Blood cultures drawn >12 h apart; *or*
     - All of three or a majority of four or more separate blood cultures, with first and last drawn at least 1 h apart
     - Single positive blood culture for *Coxiella burnetii* or phase I IgG antibody titer of >1:800
2. Evidence of endocardial involvement
   - Positive echocardiogram
     - Oscillating intracardiac mass on valve or supporting structures or in the path of regurgitant jets or in implanted material, in the absence of an alternative anatomic explanation, *or*
     - Abscess, *or*
     - New partial dehiscence of prosthetic valve, *or*
   - New valvular regurgitation (increase or change in preexisting murmur not sufficient)

MINOR CRITERIA

1. Predisposition: predisposing heart condition or injection drug use
2. Fever $\geq$38.0°C ($\geq$100.4°F)
3. Vascular phenomena: major arterial emboli, septic pulmonary infarcts, mycotic aneurysm, intracranial hemorrhage, conjunctival hemorrhages, Janeway lesions
4. Immunologic phenomena: glomerulonephritis, Osler's nodes, Roth's spots, rheumatoid factor
5. Microbiologic evidence: positive blood culture but not meeting major criterion as noted previously[a] or serologic evidence of active infection with organism consistent with infective endocarditis

[a] Excluding single positive cultures for coagulase-negative staphylococci and diphtheroids, which are common culture contaminants, and organisms that do not cause endocarditis frequently, such as gram-negative bacilli.
Note: HACEK, *Haemophilus* spp., *Actinobacillus actinomycetemcomitans*, *Cardiobacterium hominis*, *Eikenella corrodens*, *Kingella kingae*.
Source: Adapted from Li et al., with permission from the University of Chicago Press.

atively inaccessible to host defenses and because the bacteria are non-growing and metabolically inactive. Since all bacteria in the vegetation must be killed, therapy for endocarditis must be bactericidal and must be given for prolonged periods. Antibiotics are generally given parenterally and must reach high serum concentrations that will, through passive diffusion, lead to effective concentrations in the depths of the vegetation. The choice of effective therapy requires precise knowledge of the susceptibility of the causative microorganisms. The initiation of treatment before a cause is defined must balance the need to establish a microbiologic diagnosis against the potential progression of disease or the need for urgent surgery (see "Blood Cultures," above). The individual vulnerabilities of the patient should be weighed in the selection of therapy—e.g., simultaneous infection at other sites (such as meningitis), allergies, end-organ dysfunction, interactions with concomitant medications, and risks of adverse events.

Although given for several weeks longer, the regimens recommended for the treatment of endocarditis involving prosthetic valves (except for staphylococcal infections) are similar to those used to treat native valve infection (Table 109-4). Recommended doses and duration of therapy should be adhered to unless alterations are required by adverse events.

Organism-Specific Therapies ■ *STREPTOCOCCI* Although most strains of viridans streptococci and *S. bovis* that cause endocarditis are susceptible to penicillin [minimum inhibitory concentration (MIC) ≤0.1 µg/mL], recent reports indicate increasing penicillin resistance among viridans streptococci recovered from blood cultures. In the selection of optimal therapy, the penicillin MIC must be determined (Table 109-4). The 2-

TABLE 109-4   *Antibiotic Treatment for Infective Endocarditis Caused by Common Organisms[a]*

Organism	Drug, Dose, Duration	Comments
Streptococci		
Penicillin-susceptible[b] streptococci, *S. bovis*	Penicillin G 2–3 million units IV q4h for 4 weeks	—
	Penicillin G 2–3 million units IV q4h *plus* gentamicin[c] 1 mg/kg IM or IV q8h, both for 2 weeks	Avoid penicillin plus gentamicin if risks of aminoglycoside toxicity are increased or case is complicated
	Ceftriaxone 2 g/d IV as single dose for 4 weeks	Can use ceftriaxone in patients with nonimmediate penicillin allergy
	Vancomycin[d] 15 mg/kg IV q12h for 4 weeks	Use vancomycin in patients with severe or immediate β-lactam allergy
Relatively penicillin-resistant[e] streptococci	Penicillin G 3 million units IV q4h for 4–6 weeks *plus* gentamicin[c] 1 mg/kg IV q8h for 2 weeks	Preferred for treatment of prosthetic valve endocarditis caused by penicillin-susceptible streptococci; continue penicillin for 6 weeks in this setting
Moderately penicillin-resistant[f] streptococci, pyridoxal-requiring streptococci (*Abiotrophia* spp.)	Penicillin G 3–4 million units IV q4h *plus* gentamicin[c] 1 mg/kg IV q8h, both for 4–6 weeks	—
Enterococci[g]	Penicillin G 3–4 million units IV q4h *plus* gentamicin[c] 1 mg/kg IV q8h, both for 4–6 weeks	Can use streptomycin 7.5 mg/kg q12h in lieu of gentamicin if there is not high-level resistance to streptomycin
	Ampicillin 2 g IV q4h *plus* gentamicin[c] 1 mg/kg IV q8h, both for 4–6 weeks	Do not use cephalosporins or carbapenems for treatment of enterococcal endocarditis
	Vancomycin[d] 15 mg/kg IV q12h *plus* gentamicin[c] 1 mg/kg IV q8h, both for 4–6 weeks	Use vancomycin plus gentamicin for penicillin-allergic patients or desensitize to penicillin
Staphylococci		
Methicillin-susceptible, infecting native valves (no foreign devices)	Nafcillin or oxacillin 2 g IV q4h for 4–6 weeks *plus* (optional) gentamicin[c] 1 mg/kg IM or IV q8h for 3–5 days	May use penicillin 3–4 million units q6h if isolate is penicillin-susceptible (does not produce β-lactamase)
	Cefazolin 2 g IV q8h for 4–6 weeks *plus* (optional) gentamicin[c] 1 mg/kg IM or IV q8h for 3–5 days	Can use cefazolin regimen for patients with nonimmediate penicillin allergy
	Vancomycin[d] 15 mg/kg IV q12h for 4–6 weeks	Use vancomycin for patients with immediate (urticarial) or severe penicillin allergy
Methicillin-resistant, infecting native valves (no foreign devices)	Vancomycin[d] 15 mg/kg IV q12h for 4–6 weeks	No role for routine use of rifampin
Methicillin-susceptible, infecting prosthetic valves	Nafcillin or oxacillin 2 g IV q4h for 6–8 weeks *plus* gentamicin[c] 1 mg/kg IM or IV q8h for 2 weeks *plus* rifampin[h] 300 mg PO q8h for 6–8 weeks	Use gentamicin during initial 2 weeks; determine susceptibility to gentamicin before initiating rifampin (see text); if patient is highly allergic to penicillin, use regimen for methicillin-resistant staphylococci; if β-lactam allergy is of the minor, nonimmediate type, can substitute cefazolin for oxacillin/nafcillin
Methicillin-resistant, infecting prosthetic valves	Vancomycin[d] 15 mg/kg IV q12h for 6–8 weeks *plus* gentamicin[c] 1 mg/kg IM or IV q8h for 2 weeks *plus* rifampin[h] 300 mg PO q8h for 6–8 weeks	Use gentamicin during initial 2 weeks; determine gentamicin susceptibility before initiating rifampin (see text)
HACEK organisms	Ceftriaxone 2 g/d IV as single dose for 4 weeks	May use another third-generation cephalosporin at comparable dosage
	Ampicillin 2 g IV q4h *plus* gentamicin[c] 1 mg/kg IM or IV q8h, both for 4 weeks	Determine ampicillin susceptibility; do not use ampicillin if β-lactamase is produced

[a] Doses are for adults with normal renal function. Doses of gentamicin, streptomycin, and vancomycin must be adjusted for reduced renal function. Ideal body weight is used to calculate doses per kilogram (men = 50 kg + 2.3 kg per inch over 5 feet; women = 45.5 kg + 2.3 kg per inch over 5 feet).

[b] MIC ≤ 0.1 µg/mL.

[c] Aminoglycosides should not be administered as single daily doses and should be introduced as part of the initial treatment. Target peak and trough serum concentrations of gentamicin 1 h after a 20- to 30-min infusion or IM injection are 3–5 µg/mL and ≤1 µg/mL, respectively; the target peak serum concentration of streptomycin (timing as with gentamicin) is 20–25 µg/mL.

[d] Desirable peak vancomycin level 1 h after completion of a 1-h infusion is 30–45 µg/mL.

[e] MIC > 0.1 µg/mL and <0.5 µg/mL.

[f] MIC ≥ 0.5 µg/mL and <8.0 µg/mL.

[g] Antimicrobial susceptibility must be evaluated; see text.

[h] Rifampin increases warfarin and dicumarol requirements for anticoagulation.

week penicillin/gentamicin regimen should not be used to treat complicated native valve infection or prosthetic valve endocarditis. Although small studies have suggested that a 2-week regimen of single daily doses of ceftriaxone (2 g IV) plus gentamicin (3 mg/kg) or netilmicin (4 mg/kg) is effective for penicillin-susceptible streptococcal endocarditis, the data are not sufficient to support routine use of this regimen. Penicillin/gentamicin is recommended for the treatment of endocarditis caused by group B streptococci.

ENTEROCOCCI Enterococci are resistant to oxacillin, nafcillin, and the cephalosporins and are inhibited only by penicillin, ampicillin, teicoplanin (not available in the United States), and vancomycin. To kill enterococci requires the synergistic interaction of a cell wall–active antibiotic (penicillin, ampicillin, vancomycin, or teicoplanin) that is effective at achievable serum concentrations and an aminoglycoside (gentamicin or streptomycin) to which the isolate does not exhibit high-level resistance. An isolate's resistance to cell wall–active agents or ability to replicate in the presence of gentamicin at ≥500 μg/mL or streptomycin at 2000 μg/mL—a phenomenon called *high-level aminoglycoside resistance*—indicates that the ineffective antimicrobial cannot participate in the interaction to produce killing. High-level resistance to gentamicin predicts that tobramycin, netilmicin, amikacin, and kanamycin will also be ineffective. In fact, even when enterococci are not highly resistant to gentamicin, it is difficult to predict the ability of these other aminoglycosides to participate in synergistic killing; consequently, they should not in general be used to treat enterococcal endocarditis.

Clearly, enterococci causing endocarditis must be tested for high-level resistance to streptomycin and gentamicin, β-lactamase production, and susceptibility to penicillin and ampicillin (MIC ≤ 16 μg/mL) and to vancomycin (MIC ≤ 8 μg/mL). If the isolate produces β-lactamase, ampicillin/sulbactam or vancomycin can be used as the cell wall–active component; if the penicillin/ampicillin MIC is >16 μg/mL, vancomycin can be considered; and if the vancomycin MIC is >8 μg/mL, penicillin or ampicillin may be considered. Based on the absence of high-level resistance, gentamicin or streptomycin should be used as the aminoglycoside. If there is high-level resistance to both these drugs, no aminoglycoside should be given; instead, an 8- to 12-week course of a single cell wall–active agent is suggested. If single-drug therapy fails or the isolate is resistant to all of the commonly used agents, surgical treatment is advised. The role of newer agents potentially active against multidrug-resistant enterococci (quinupristin/dalfopristin, linezolid, and daptomycin) in the treatment of endocarditis has not been established. Although the dose of gentamicin used to achieve bactericidal synergy in treating enterococcal endocarditis is smaller than that used in standard therapy, nephrotoxicity is not uncommon during treatment with recommended regimens for 4 to 6 weeks. Regimens wherein gentamicin treatment has been truncated at 2 to 3 weeks because of nephrotoxicity have been curative. Thus, discontinuation of gentamicin is recommended when progressive nephrotoxicity develops in patients with enterococcal endocarditis who have responded satisfactorily to therapy.

STAPHYLOCOCCI The regimens used to treat staphylococcal endocarditis are not based upon coagulase production but rather upon the presence or absence of a prosthetic valve or foreign device, the native valve(s) involved, and the resistance of the isolate to penicillin and methicillin. Penicillinase is produced by 95% of staphylococci; thus, all isolates should be considered penicillin-resistant until shown not to produce this enzyme. The addition of gentamicin (if the isolate is susceptible) to a β-lactam antibiotic to enhance therapy for native mitral or aortic valve endocarditis is optional. Its addition hastens eradication of bacteremia but does not improve survival rates. If added, gentamicin should be limited to the initial 3 to 5 days of therapy to avoid nephrotoxicity. Gentamicin generally is not added to the vancomycin regimen in this setting.

Methicillin-susceptible *S. aureus* endocarditis that is uncomplicated and limited to the tricuspid or pulmonic valve—a condition occurring almost exclusively in injection drug users—can often be treated with a 2-week course that combines oxacillin or nafcillin (but not vancomycin) with gentamicin. Prolonged fevers (≥5 days) during therapy suggest that these patients should receive standard therapy.

Staphylococcal prosthetic valve endocarditis is treated for 6 to 8 weeks with a multidrug regimen. Rifampin is an essential component because it kills staphylococci that are adherent to foreign material. Two other agents (selected on the basis of susceptibility testing) are combined with rifampin to prevent in vivo emergence of resistance. Because many staphylococci, particularly methicillin-resistant *S. aureus* and *S. epidermidis*, are resistant to gentamicin, the utility of gentamicin should be established before rifampin treatment is begun. If the isolate is resistant to gentamicin, another aminoglycoside or a fluoroquinolone (chosen in light of susceptibility results) should be substituted.

OTHER ORGANISMS Endocarditis caused by *Streptococcus pneumoniae*, with a penicillin MIC ≤ 1.0 can be treated with intravenous penicillin (4 million units every 4 h), ceftriaxone (2 g/d as a single dose), or cefotaxime (at a comparable dosage). Infection caused by strains with a penicillin MIC ≥ 2.0 should be treated with vancomycin. Until the strain's susceptibility to penicillin is established, therapy should consist of vancomycin plus ceftriaxone, especially if concurrent meningitis is suspected. *P. aeruginosa* endocarditis is treated with an antipseudomonal penicillin (ticarcillin or piperacillin) and high doses of tobramycin (8 mg/kg per day in three divided doses). Endocarditis caused by Enterobacteriaceae is treated with a potent β-lactam antibiotic plus an aminoglycoside. Corynebacterial endocarditis is treated with penicillin plus an aminoglycoside (if the organism is susceptible to the aminoglycoside) or with vancomycin, which is highly bactericidal for most strains. Therapy for *Candida* endocarditis consists of amphotericin B plus flucytosine and early surgery; long-term (if not indefinite) suppression with fluconazole is used increasingly.

Empirical Therapy In designing and executing therapy without culture data (i.e., before culture results are known or when cultures are negative), clinical and epidemiologic clues to etiology must be weighed, and both the pathogens associated with the specific endocarditis syndrome and the hazards of suboptimal therapy must be considered. Thus, empirical therapy for acute endocarditis in an injection drug user should cover methicillin-resistant *S. aureus* and gram-negative bacilli. The initiation of treatment with vancomycin plus gentamicin immediately after blood is obtained for cultures covers these as well as many other potential causes. In treating culture-negative episodes, marantic endocarditis must be excluded and fastidious organisms sought serologically. In the absence of confounding prior antibiotic therapy, it is unlikely that *S. aureus*, coagulase-negative staphylococcal, or enterococcal infection will present with negative blood cultures. Thus, in this situation, these organisms are not the determinants of therapy for subacute endocarditis. Blood culture–negative subacute native valve endocarditis is treated with ceftriaxone plus gentamicin; these two antimicrobials plus vancomycin should be used if prosthetic valves are involved.

Outpatient Antimicrobial Therapy Fully compliant patients who have sterile blood cultures, are afebrile during therapy, and have no clinical or echocardiographic findings that suggest an impending complication may complete therapy as outpatients. Careful follow-up and a stable home setting are necessary, as are predictable intravenous access and selection of antimicrobials that are stable in solution.

Monitoring Antimicrobial Therapy The serum bactericidal titer—the highest dilution of the patient's serum during therapy that kills 99.9% of the standard inoculum of the infecting organism—is no longer recommended for assessment of patients receiving standard regimens. However, in the treatment of endocarditis caused by unusual organisms, this measurement, although not standardized and difficult to interpret, may provide a patient-specific assessment of in vivo antibiotic effect. Serum concentrations of aminoglycosides and vancomycin should be monitored.

TABLE 109-5 *Indications for Cardiac Surgical Intervention in Patients with Endocarditis*

Surgery required for optimal outcome
 Moderate to severe congestive heart failure due to valve dysfunction
 Partially dehisced unstable prosthetic valve
 Persistent bacteremia despite optimal antimicrobial therapy
 Lack of effective microbicidal therapy (e.g., fungal or *Brucella* endocarditis)
 S. aureus prosthetic valve endocarditis with an intracardiac complication
 Relapse of prosthetic valve endocarditis after optimal antimicrobial therapy
Surgery to be strongly considered for improved outcome[a]
 Perivalvular extension of infection
 Poorly responsive *S. aureus* endocarditis involving the aortic or mitral valve
 Large (>10-mm diameter) hypermobile vegetations with increased risk of embolism
 Persistent unexplained fever (≥10 days) in culture-negative native valve endocarditis
 Poorly responsive or relapsed endocarditis due to highly antibiotic-resistant enterococci or gram-negative bacilli

[a] Surgery must be carefully considered; findings are often combined with other indications to prompt surgery.

Antibiotic toxicities, including allergic reactions, occur in 25 to 40% of patients and commonly arise during the third week of therapy. Blood tests to detect antibiotic-specific potential end-organ toxicity should be performed periodically.

In most patients, effective antibiotic therapy results in subjective improvement and resolution of fever within 5 to 7 days. Blood cultures should be repeated daily until sterile, rechecked if there is recrudescent fever, and performed again 4 to 6 weeks after therapy to document cure. Blood cultures become sterile within 2 days after the start of appropriate therapy when infection is caused by viridans streptococci, enterococci, or HACEK organisms. In *S. aureus* endocarditis, β-lactam therapy results in sterile cultures in 3 to 5 days, whereas positive cultures may persist for 7 to 9 days with vancomycin treatment. When fever persists for 7 days in spite of appropriate antibiotic therapy, patients should be evaluated for paravalvular abscess and for extracardiac abscesses (spleen, kidney) or complications (embolic events). Recrudescent fever raises the question of these complications but also of drug reactions or complications of hospitalization. Serologic abnormalities (e.g., erythrocyte sedimentation rate, rheumatoid factor) resolve slowly and do not reflect response to treatment. Vegetations become smaller with effective therapy, but at 3 months after cure half are unchanged and 25% are slightly larger.

SURGICAL TREATMENT Intracardiac and central nervous system complications of endocarditis are important causes of the morbidity and mortality associated with this infection. In some cases, effective treatment for these complications requires surgery. Most of the clinical indications for surgical treatment of endocarditis are not absolute (Table 109-5). The risks and benefits as well as the timing of surgical treatment must therefore be individualized (Table 109-6).

Intracardiac Surgical Indications Most surgical interventions are warranted by intracardiac findings, often detected by echocardiography. Because of the highly invasive nature of prosthetic valve endocarditis, as many as 40% of affected patients merit surgical treatment. In many patients, coincident rather than single intracardiac events necessitate surgery.

CONGESTIVE HEART FAILURE Moderate to severe refractory congestive heart failure caused by new or worsening valve dysfunction is the major indication for cardiac surgical treatment of endocarditis. Of patients with moderate to severe heart failure due to valve dysfunction who are treated medically, 60 to 90% die within 6 months. In the setting of similar hemodynamic dysfunction, surgical treatment is associated with mortality rates of 20 to 40% with native valve endocarditis and 35 to 55% with prosthetic valve infection. Surgery may be required to relieve functional stenosis due to large vegetations or to restore competence to damaged regurgitant valves.

PERIVALVULAR INFECTION This complication, which occurs in 10 to 15% of native valve and 45 to 60% of prosthetic valve infections, is suggested by persistent unexplained fever during appropriate therapy, new electrocardiographic conduction disturbances, and pericarditis. Extension can occur from any valve but is most common with aortic valve infection. TEE with color Doppler is the test of choice to detect perivalvular abscesses (sensitivity ≥ 85%). Although occasional perivalvular infections are cured medically, surgery is warranted when fever persists, fistulae develop, prostheses are dehisced and unstable, and invasive infection relapses after appropriate treatment. Cardiac rhythm must be monitored since high-grade heart block may require insertion of a pacemaker.

UNCONTROLLED INFECTION Continued positive blood cultures or otherwise-unexplained persistent fevers (in patients with either blood culture–positive or –negative endocarditis) despite optimal antibiotic therapy may reflect uncontrolled infection and warrant surgery. Surgical treatment is also advised for endocarditis caused by those organisms against which clinical experience indicates that effective antimicrobial

TABLE 109-6 *Timing of Cardiac Surgical Intervention in Patients with Endocarditis*

	Indication for Surgical Intervention	
Timing	Strong Supporting Evidence	Conflicting Evidence, but Majority of Opinions Favor Surgery
Emergent (same day)	Acute aortic regurgitation plus preclosure of mitral valve	
	Sinus of Valsalva abscess ruptured into right heart	
	Rupture into pericardial sac	
Urgent (within 1–2 days)	Valve obstruction by vegetation	Major embolus plus persisting large vegetation (>10 mm in diameter)
	Unstable (dehisced) prosthesis	
	Acute aortic or mitral regurgitation with heart failure (New York Heart Association class III or IV)	
	Septal perforation	
	Perivalvular extension of infection with/without new electrocardiographic conduction system changes	
	Lack of effective antibiotic therapy	
Elective (earlier usually preferred)	Progressive paravalvular prosthetic regurgitation	Staphylococcal PVE
	Valve dysfunction plus persisting infection after ≥7–10 days of antimicrobial therapy	Early PVE (≤2 months after valve surgery)
	Fungal (mold) endocarditis	Fungal endocarditis (*Candida* spp.)
		Antibiotic-resistant organisms

Abbreviation: PVE, prosthetic valve endocarditis.
Source: Adapted from I Olaison, G Pettersson: Infect Dis Clin North Am 16:453, 2002.

TABLE 109-7 *Procedures for which Endocarditis Prophylaxis Is Advised in Patients at High or Moderate Risk for Endocarditis[a]*

Dental procedures
  Extractions
  Periodontal procedures, cleaning causing gingival bleeding
  Implant placement, reimplantation of avulsed teeth
  Endodontic instrumentation (root canal) or surgery beyond the apex
  Subgingival placement of antibiotic fibers or strips
  Placement of orthodontic bands but not brackets
  Intraligamentary injections (anesthetic)
Respiratory procedures
  Operations involving the mucosa
  Bronchoscopy with rigid bronchoscope
Gastrointestinal procedures[b]
  Esophageal: Sclerotherapy of varices, stricture dilation
  Biliary tract: Endoscopic retrograde cholangiography with biliary obstruction, biliary tract surgery
  Intestinal tract: Surgery involving the mucosa
Genitourinary procedures
  Urethral dilation, prostate or urethral surgery
  Cystoscopy

[a] Prophylaxis is optional for high-risk patients undergoing bronchoscopy or gastrointestinal endoscopy with/without biopsy, vaginal delivery, vaginal hysterectomy, or transesophageal echocardiography.

[b] Prophylaxis is recommended for high-risk patients and optional for moderate-risk group (see Table 109-8).

Source: Adapted from AS Dajani et al: JAMA 277:1794, 1997; with permission.

therapy is lacking. This category includes infections caused by yeasts, fungi, *P. aeruginosa*, other highly resistant gram-negative bacilli, *Brucella* species, and probably *C. burnetii*.

S. AUREUS ENDOCARDITIS Mortality rates for *S. aureus* prosthetic valve endocarditis exceed 70% with medical treatment but are reduced to 25% with surgical treatment. In patients with intracardiac complications associated with *S. aureus* prosthetic valve infection, surgical treatment reduces mortality by twentyfold. Surgical treatment should be considered for patients with *S. aureus* native aortic or mitral valve infection who have TTE-demonstrable vegetations and remain septic during the initial week of therapy. Isolated tricuspid valve endocarditis, even with persistent fever, rarely requires surgery.

PREVENTION OF SYSTEMIC EMBOLI Mortality and persisting morbidity due to emboli are largely limited to patients suffering occlusion of cerebral or coronary arteries. Echocardiographic determination of vegetation size and anatomy, although predictive of patients at high risk of systemic emboli, does not identify those patients in whom the benefits of surgery to prevent emboli clearly exceed the risks of the surgical procedure and an implanted prosthetic valve. Net benefits favoring surgery are most likely when the risk of embolism is high and other surgical benefits can be achieved simultaneously—e.g., repair of a moderately dysfunctional valve or debridement of a paravalvular abscess. Reduced overall risks of surgical intervention (e.g., use of vegetation resection and valve repair to avoid insertion of a prosthesis) make the benefit-to-risk ratio more favorable and this intervention more attractive.

TABLE 109-8 *Cardiac Lesions for which Endocarditis Prophylaxis Is Advised*

High Risk	Moderate Risk
Prosthetic heart valves	Congenital cardiac malformations (other than high-/low-risk lesions), ventricular septal defect, bicuspid aortic valve
Prior bacterial endocarditis	
Complex cyanotic congenital heart disease; other complex congenital lesions after correction (see text)	
	Acquired aortic and mitral valve dysfunction
Patent ductus arteriosus	
Coarctation of the aorta	Hypertrophic cardiomyopathy (asymmetric septal hypertrophy)
Surgically constructed systemic-pulmonary shunts	Mitral valve prolapse with valvular regurgitation and/or thickened leaflets

TABLE 109-9 *Cardiac Conditions That Are Considered to Pose a Low Risk of Endocarditis and for which Antibiotic Prophylaxis Is Not Recommended*

Isolated secundum ASD
Surgically repaired ASD, VSD, PDA (without residual defect, >6 months after repair)
Prior coronary artery bypass graft
Mitral valve prolapse without regurgitation or thickened leaflets
Physiologic or functional murmur
Prior Kawasaki disease or acute rheumatic fever without valve dysfunction
Cardiac pacemakers or implanted defibrillators

Abbreviations: ASD, atrial septal defect; VSD, ventricular septal defect; PDA, patent ductus arteriosus.
Source: Adapted from AS Dajani et al: JAMA 277:1794, 1997; with permission.

Timing of Cardiac Surgery In general, when indications for surgical treatment of infective endocarditis are identified, surgery should not be delayed simply to permit additional antibiotic therapy, since this course of action increases the risk of death (Table 109-6). Delay is justified only when infection is controlled and congestive heart failure is fully compensated with medical therapy. Recrudescent endocarditis involving a prosthetic valve follows surgery in 2% of patients with culture-positive native valve endocarditis and in 6 to 15% of patients with active prosthetic valve endocarditis. These risks are more acceptable than the high mortality rates that result when surgery is inappropriately delayed or not performed.

Among patients who have experienced a neurologic complication of endocarditis, further neurologic deterioration can occur as a consequence of cardiac surgery. The risk of significant neurologic exacerbation is related to the interval between the complication and surgery. Where feasible, cardiac surgery should be delayed for 2 to 3 weeks after a nonhemorrhagic embolic stroke and for 4 weeks after a

TABLE 109-10 *Antibiotic Regimens for Prophylaxis of Endocarditis in Adults at Moderate or High Risk[a]*

I. Oral cavity, respiratory tract, or esophageal procedures[b]
  A. Standard regimen
    1. Amoxicillin 2.0 g PO 1 h before procedure
  B. Inability to take oral medication
    1. Ampicillin 2.0 g IV or IM within 30 min of procedure
  C. Penicillin allergy
    1. Clarithromycin 500 mg PO 1 h before procedure
    2. Cephalexin[c] or cefadroxil[c] 2.0 g PO 1 h before procedure
    3. Clindamycin 600 mg PO 1 h before procedure or IV 30 min before procedure
  D. Penicillin allergy, inability to take oral medication
    1. Cefazolin[c] 1.0 g IV or IM 30 min before procedure
II. Genitourinary and gastrointestinal tract[d] procedures
  A. High-risk patients
    1. Ampicillin 2.0 g IV or IM *plus* gentamicin 1.5 mg/kg (not to exceed 120 mg) IV or IM within 30 min of procedure; repeat ampicillin 1.0 g IV or IM or amoxicillin 1.0 g PO 6 h later
  B. High-risk, penicillin-allergic patients
    1. Vancomycin 1.0 g IV over 1–2 h *plus* gentamicin 1.5 mg/kg (not to exceed 120 mg) IV or IM within 30 min before procedure; no second dose recommended
  C. Moderate-risk patients
    1. Amoxicillin 2.0 g PO 1 h before procedure or ampicillin 2.0 g IV or IM within 30 min before procedure
  D. Moderate-risk, penicillin-allergic patients
    1. Vancomycin 1.0 g IV infused over 1–2 h and completed within 30 min of procedure

[a] Dosing for children: for amoxicillin, ampicillin, cephalexin, or cefadroxil, use 50 mg/kg PO; cefazolin, 25 mg/kg IV; clindamycin, 20 mg/kg PO, 25 mg/kg IV; clarithromycin, 15 mg/kg PO; gentamicin, 1.5 mg/kg IV or IM; and vancomycin, 20 mg/kg IV.
[b] For patients at high risk (Table 109-8), administer a half-dose 6 h after the initial dose.
[c] Do not use cephalosporins in patients with immediate hypersensitivity (urticaria, angioedema, anaphylaxis) to penicillin.
[d] Excludes esophageal procedures.
Source: Adapted from AS Dajani et al: JAMA 277:1794, 1997; with permission.

hemorrhagic embolic stroke. A ruptured mycotic aneurysm should be clipped and cerebral edema allowed to resolve prior to cardiac surgery.

Extracardiac Complications   Splenic abscess develops in 3 to 5% of patients with endocarditis. Effective therapy requires either computed tomography–guided percutaneous drainage or splenectomy. Mycotic aneurysms occur in 2 to 15% of endocarditis patients; half of these cases involve the cerebral arteries and present as headaches, focal neurologic symptoms, or hemorrhage. Cerebral aneurysms should be monitored by angiography. Some will resolve with effective antimicrobial therapy, but those that persist, enlarge, or leak should be treated surgically if possible. Extracerebral aneurysms present as local pain, a mass, local ischemia, or bleeding; generally these aneurysms are treated by resection.

OUTCOME   The outcome of infective endocarditis is affected by a variety of factors, some of which are interrelated. Factors with an adverse impact include older age, severe comorbid conditions, delayed diagnosis, involvement of prosthetic valves or the aortic valve, an invasive (*S. aureus*) or antibiotic-resistant (*P. aeruginosa*, yeast) pathogen, intracardiac complications, and major neurologic complications. Death and poor outcome often are related not to failure of antibiotic therapy but rather to the interactions of comorbidities and endocarditis-related end-organ complications. The overall survival rate for patients with native valve endocarditis caused by viridans streptococci, HACEK organisms, or enterococci (susceptible to synergistic therapy) ranges from 85 to 90%. For *S. aureus* native valve endocarditis in patients who do not inject drugs, survival rates are 55 to 70%, whereas 85 to 90% of injection drug users survive this infection. Prosthetic valve endocarditis beginning within 2 months of valve replacement results in mortality rates of 40 to 50%, whereas rates are only 10 to 20% in later-onset cases.

PREVENTION   Antibiotics have been administered in conjunction with selected procedures considered to entail a risk for bacteremia and endocarditis. The benefits of antibiotic prophylaxis are not established and in fact may be modest: only 50% of patients with native valve endocarditis know that they have a valve lesion predisposing to infection, most endocarditis cases do not follow a procedure, and 35% of cases are caused by organisms not targeted by prophylaxis. Dental treatments, the procedures most widely accepted as predisposing to endocarditis, are no more frequent during the 3 months preceding this diagnosis than in uninfected matched controls. Nevertheless, an expert committee of the American Heart Association, along with similar advisory groups in other developed countries, has identified procedures that may precipitate bacteremia with organisms that cause endocarditis (Table 109-7), patients who should receive prophylaxis based on the relative risk for developing endocarditis and the severity of subsequent infection (Table 109-8), patients who are at low risk and do not require prophylaxis (Table 109-9), and regimens that may be used for prophylaxis (Table 109-10). Except for an isolated secundum atrial septal defect and a totally corrected patent ductus arteriosus, ventricular septal defect, or pulmonary stenosis, patients with congenital heart defects continue to experience high rates of endocarditis despite total surgical correction of the defect. In vulnerable patients, maintaining good dental hygiene and aggressively treating local infections may reduce the risk of endocarditis.

FURTHER READING

ANDREWS MM, VON REYN CF: Patient selection criteria and management guidelines for outpatient parenteral antibiotic therapy for native valve infective endocarditis. Clin Infect Dis 33:203, 2001

BAYER AS et al: Diagnosis and management of infective endocarditis and its complications. Circulation 98:2936, 1998

DURACK DT (ed): Infective endocarditis. Infect Dis Clin North Am 16:255, 2002

KARCHMER AW: Infections of prosthetic valves and intravascular devices, in *Mandell, Douglas, and Bennett's Principles and Practice of Infectious Diseases*, 5th ed, GL Mandell et al (eds). New York, Churchill Livingstone, 2000, pp 903–917

———: Infective endocarditis, in *Heart Disease*, 6th ed, E Braunwald et al (eds). Philadelphia, Saunders, 2000

LI JS et al: Proposed modifications to the Duke criteria for the diagnosis of infective endocarditis. Clin Infect Dis 30:633, 2000

MYLONAKIS E, CALDERWOOD SB: Infective endocarditis in adults. N Engl J Med 345:1318, 2001

110   INFECTIONS OF THE SKIN, MUSCLE, AND SOFT TISSUES
Dennis L. Stevens

ANATOMICAL RELATIONSHIPS: CLUES TO THE DIAGNOSIS OF SOFT TISSUE INFECTIONS   Protection against infection of the epidermis is dependent on the mechanical barrier afforded by the stratum corneum, since the epidermis itself is devoid of blood vessels (Fig. 110-1). Disruption of this layer by burns or bites, abrasions, foreign bodies, primary dermatologic disorders (e.g., herpes simplex, varicella, and ecthyma gangrenosum), surgery, or vascular or pressure ulcer allows penetration of bacteria to the deeper structures. Similarly, the hair follicle can serve as a portal either for components of the normal flora (e.g., *Staphylococcus*) or for extrinsic bacteria (e.g., *Pseudomonas* in hot-tub folliculitis). Intracellular infection of the squamous epithelium with vesicle formation may arise from cutaneous inoculation, as in infection with herpes simplex virus (HSV) type 1; from the dermal capillary plexus, as in varicella and infections due to other viruses associated with viremia; or from cutaneous nerve roots, as in herpes zoster. Bacteria infecting the epidermis, such as *Streptococcus pyogenes*, may be translocated laterally to deeper structures via lymphatics, an event that results in the rapid superficial spread of erysipelas. Later, engorgement or obstruction of lymphatics causes flaccid edema of the epidermis, another characteristic of erysipelas.

The rich plexus of capillaries beneath the dermal papillae provides nutrition to the stratum germinativum, and physiologic responses of this plexus produce important clinical signs and symptoms. For ex-

FIGURE 110-1   Structural components of the skin and soft tissue, superficial infections, and infections of the deeper structures. The rich capillary network beneath the dermal papillae plays a key role in the localization of infection and in the development of the acute inflammatory reaction.

ample, infective vasculitis of the plexus results in petechiae, Osler's nodes, Janeway lesions, and palpable purpura, which, if present, are important clues to the existence of endocarditis (Chap. 109). In addition, metastatic infection within this plexus can result in cutaneous manifestations of disseminated fungal infection (Chap. 187), gonococcal infection (Chap. 128), *Salmonella* infection (Chap. 137), *Pseudomonas* infection (i.e., ecthyma gangrenosum; Chap. 136), meningococcemia (Chap. 127), and staphylococcal infection (Chap. 120). The plexus also provides access for bacteria to the circulation, thereby facilitating local spread or bacteremia. The postcapillary venules of this plexus are a major site of polymorphonuclear leukocyte sequestration, diapedesis, and chemotaxis to the site of cutaneous infection.

Exaggeration of these physiologic mechanisms by excessive levels of cytokines or bacterial toxins causes leukostasis, venous occlusion, and pitting edema. Edema with purple bullae, ecchymosis, and cutaneous anesthesia suggests loss of vascular integrity and necessitates exploration of the deeper structures for evidence of necrotizing fasciitis or myonecrosis. An early diagnosis requires a high level of suspicion in instances of unexplained fever and of pain and tenderness in the soft tissue, even in the absence of acute cutaneous inflammation.

INFECTIONS ASSOCIATED WITH VESICLES (Table 110-1) Vesicle formation due to infection is caused by viral proliferation within the epidermis. In varicella and variola, viremia precedes the onset of a diffuse centripetal rash that progresses from macules to vesicles, then to pustules, and finally to scabs over the course of 1 to 2 weeks. Vesicles of varicella have a "dewdrop" appearance and develop in crops randomly about the trunk, extremities, and face over 3 to 4 days (see Fig. 164-1). Herpes zoster occurs in a single dermatome; the appearance of vesicles is preceded by pain for several days (see Figs. 164-2 and 164-3). Zoster may occur in persons of any age but is most common among immunosuppressed individuals and elderly patients, whereas most cases of varicella occur in young children. Vesicles due to HSV are found on or around the lips (HSV-1) or genitals (HSV-2) but may appear on the head and neck of young wrestlers (herpes gladiatorum) or on the digits of health care workers (herpetic whitlow). Recurrent herpes labialis (HSV-1) and herpes genitalis are common following primary infection. Coxsackievirus A16 characteristically causes vesicles on the hands, feet, and mouth of children. Orf is caused by a DNA virus related to smallpox virus and infects the fingers of individuals who work around goats and sheep. Molluscum contagiosum virus induces flaccid vesicles on the skin of healthy and immunocompromised individuals. Although variola (smallpox) in nature was eradicated as of 1977, recent terrorist events have renewed interest in this devastat-

TABLE 110-1 *Skin and Soft Tissue Infections*

Lesion, Clinical Syndrome	Infectious Agent	Chapter(s)
Vesicles		
Smallpox	Variola virus	205
Chickenpox	Varicella-zoster virus	164
Shingles (herpes zoster)	Varicella-zoster virus	164
Cold sores, herpetic whitlow, herpes gladiatorum	Herpes simplex virus	163
Hand-foot-and-mouth disease	Coxsackievirus A16	175
Orf	Parapoxvirus	167
Molluscum contagiosum	Pox-like virus	167
Rickettsialpox	*Rickettsia akari*	158
Blistering distal dactylitis	*Staphylococcus aureus* or *Streptococcus pyogenes*	120, 121
Bullae		
Staphylococcal scalded-skin syndrome	*S. aureus*	120
Necrotizing fasciitis	*S. pyogenes, Clostridium* spp., mixed aerobes and anaerobes	148
Gas gangrene	*Clostridium* spp.	126
Halophilic vibrio	*Vibrio vulnificus*	140
Crusted lesions		
Bullous impetigo/ecthyma	*S. aureus*	120
Impetigo contagiosa	*S. pyogenes*	121
Ringworm	Superficial dermatophyte fungi	190
Sporotrichosis	*Sporothrix schenckii*	190
Histoplasmosis	*Histoplasma capsulatum*	183
Coccidioidomycosis	*Coccidioides immitis*	184
Blastomycosis	*Blastomyces dermatitidis*	185
Cutaneous leishmaniasis	*Leishmania* spp.	196
Cutaneous tuberculosis	*Mycobacterium tuberculosis*	150
Nocardiosis	*Nocardia asteroides*	146
Folliculitis		
Furunculosis	*S. aureus*	120
Hot-tub folliculitis	*Pseudomonas aeruginosa*	136
Swimmer's itch	*Schistosoma* spp	203
Acne vulgaris	*Propionibacterium acnes*	47
Papular and nodular lesions		
Fish-tank or swimming-pool granuloma	*Mycobacterium marinum*	152
Creeping eruption (cutaneous larva migrans)	*Ancylostoma braziliense*	200
Dracunculiasis	*Dracunculus medinensis*	202
Cercarial dermatitis	*Schistosoma mansoni*	203
Verruca vulgaris	Human papillomaviruses 1, 2, 4	169
Condylomata acuminata (anogenital warts)	Human papillomaviruses 6, 11, 16, 18	169
Onchocerciasis nodule	*Onchocerca volvulus*	202
Cutaneous myiasis	*Dermatobia hominis*	379
Verruca peruana	*Bartonella bacilliformis*	144
Cat-scratch disease	*Bartonella henselae*	144
Lepromatous leprosy	*Mycobacterium leprae*	151
Secondary syphilis (papulosquamous, nodular, and condylomata lata lesions)	*Treponema pallidum*	153
Tertiary syphilis (nodular gummatous lesions)	*T. pallidum*	153
Ulcers with or without eschars		
Anthrax	*Bacillus anthracis*	205
Ulceroglandular tularemia	*Francisella tularensis*	142, 205
Bubonic plague	*Yersinia pestis*	143, 205
Buruli ulcer	*Mycobacterium ulcerans*	152
Leprosy	*M. leprae*	151
Cutaneous tuberculosis	*M. tuberculosis*	150
Chancroid	*Haemophilus ducreyi*	130
Primary syphilis	*T. pallidum*	153
Erysipelas	*S. pyogenes*	121
Cellulitis	*Staphylococcus* spp., *Streptococcus* spp., various other bacteria	Various
Necrotizing fasciitis		
Streptococcal gangrene	*S. pyogenes*	121
Fournier's gangrene	Mixed aerobic and anaerobic bacteria	148
Myositis and myonecrosis		
Pyomyositis	*S. aureus*	120
Streptococcal necrotizing myositis	*S. pyogenes*	121
Gas gangrene	*Clostridium* spp.	126
Nonclostridial (crepitant) myositis	Mixed aerobic and anaerobic bacteria	148
Synergistic nonclostridial anaerobic myonecrosis	Mixed aerobic and anaerobic bacteria	148

ing infection (see Chap. 205). Viremia beginning after an incubation period of 12 days is followed by a diffuse maculopapular rash, with rapid evolution to vesicles, pustules, and then scabs. Secondary cases can occur among close contacts.

Rickettsialpox begins after mite-bite inoculation of *Rickettsia akari* into the skin. A papule with a central vesicle evolves to form a 1- to 2.5-cm painless crusted black eschar with an erythematous halo and proximal adenopathy. While more common in the northeastern United States and the Ukraine in 1940–1950, rickettsialpox has recently been described in Ohio, Arizona, and Utah. Blistering dactylitis is a painful, vesicular, localized *Staphylococcus aureus* or group A streptococcal infection of the pulps of the distal digits of the hands.

INFECTIONS ASSOCIATED WITH BULLAE (Table 110-1) Staphylococcal scalded-skin syndrome (SSSS) in neonates is caused by a toxin (exfoliatin) from phage group II *S. aureus*. SSSS must be distinguished from toxic epidermal necrolysis (TEN), which occurs primarily in adults, is drug-induced, and has a higher mortality. Punch biopsy with frozen section is useful in making this distinction since the cleavage plane is the stratum corneum in SSSS (Fig. 110-1) and the stratum germinativum in TEN. Intravenous γ-globulin is a promising treatment for TEN. Necrotizing fasciitis and gas gangrene also induce bulla formation (see "Necrotizing Fasciitis," below). Halophilic vibrio infection can be as aggressive and fulminant as necrotizing fasciitis; a helpful clue in its diagnosis is a history of exposure to waters of the Gulf of Mexico or the Atlantic seaboard or (in a patient with cirrhosis) the ingestion of raw seafood. The etiologic organism (*Vibrio vulnificus*) is highly susceptible to tetracycline.

INFECTIONS ASSOCIATED WITH CRUSTED LESIONS (Table 110-1) Impetigo contagiosa is caused by *S. pyogenes*, and bullous impetigo is due to *S. aureus* (see Fig. 121-2). Both skin lesions may have an early bullous stage but then appear as thick crusts with a golden-brown color. Streptococcal lesions are most common among children 2 to 5 years of age, and epidemics may occur in settings of poor hygiene, particularly among children of lower socioeconomic status in tropical climates. It is important to recognize impetigo contagiosa because of its relationship to poststreptococcal glomerulonephritis. Rheumatic fever is not a complication of skin infection caused by *S. pyogenes*. Superficial dermatophyte infection (ringworm) can occur on any skin surface, and skin scrapings with KOH staining are diagnostic. Primary infections with dimorphic fungi such as *Blastomyces dermatitidis* and *Sporothrix schenckii* can initially present as crusted skin lesions resembling ringworm. Disseminated infection with *Coccidioides immitis* can also involve the skin, and biopsy and culture should be performed on crusted lesions in patients from endemic areas. Crusted nodular lesions caused by *Mycobacterium chelonei* have been described in HIV-seropositive patients. Treatment with clarithromycin looks promising.

FOLLICULITIS (Table 110-1) Hair follicles serve as portals for a number of bacteria, although *S. aureus* is the most common cause of localized folliculitis. Sebaceous glands empty into hair follicles and ducts and, if blocked, form sebaceous cysts, which may resemble staphylococcal abscesses or may become secondarily infected. Infection of sweat glands (hidradenitis suppurativa) can also mimic infection of hair follicles, particularly in the axillae. Chronic folliculitis is uncommon except in acne vulgaris, where constituents of the normal flora (e.g., *Propionibacterium acnes*) may play a role.

Diffuse folliculitis occurs in two settings. "Hot-tub folliculitis" is caused by *Pseudomonas aeruginosa* in waters that are insufficiently chlorinated and maintained at temperatures between 37 and 40°C. Infection is usually self-limited, though bacteremia and shock have been reported. Swimmer's itch occurs when a skin surface is exposed to water infested with freshwater avian schistosomes. Warm water temperatures and alkaline pH are suitable for mollusks that serve as intermediate hosts between birds and humans. Free-swimming schistosomal cercariae readily penetrate human hair follicles or pores but

quickly die and elicit a brisk allergic reaction, causing intense itching and erythema.

PAPULAR AND NODULAR LESIONS (Table 110-1) Raised lesions of the skin occur in many different forms. *Mycobacterium marinum* infections of the skin may present as cellulitis or as raised erythematous nodules. Erythematous papules are early manifestations of cat-scratch disease (primary site of inoculation) and bacillary angiomatosis (*Bartonella henselae*). Raised serpiginous or linear eruptions are characteristic of cutaneous larva migrans, which is caused by burrowing larvae of dog or cat hookworms (*Ancylostoma braziliense*) and which humans acquire through contact with soil that has been contaminated with dog or cat feces. Similar burrowing raised lesions are present in dracunculiasis caused by migration of the adult female nematode *Dracunculus medinensis*. Nodules caused by *Onchocerca volvulus* may range from 1 to 10 cm in diameter and occur largely in persons bitten by *Simulium* flies in Africa. The nodules contain the adult worm encased in fibrous tissue. Migration of microfilariae into the eyes may result in blindness. Verruca peruana is caused by *Bartonella bacilliformis*, which is transmitted to humans by the sandfly *Phlebotomus*. This condition can take the form of single gigantic lesions (several centimeters in diameter) or multiple small lesions (several millimeters in diameter). Numerous subcutaneous nodules may also be present in cysticercosis caused by larvae of *Taenia solium*. Multiple erythematous papules develop in schistosomiasis; each represents a cercarial invasion site. Skin nodules as well as thickened subcutaneous tissue are prominent features of lepromatous leprosy. Large nodules or gummas are features of tertiary syphilis, whereas flat papulosquamous lesions are characteristic of secondary syphilis. Human papillomavirus may cause singular warts (verruca vulgaris) or multiple warts in the anogenital area (condylomata acuminata). The latter are major problems in HIV-infected individuals.

ULCERS WITH OR WITHOUT ESCHARS (Table 110-1) Cutaneous anthrax begins as a pruritic papule, which develops within days into an ulcer with surrounding vesicles and edema and then into an enlarging ulcer with a black eschar. Cutaneous anthrax may cause chronic nonhealing ulcers with an overlying dirty-gray membrane, although lesions may also mimic psoriasis, eczema, or impetigo. Ulceroglandular tularemia may have associated ulcerated skin lesions with painful regional adenopathy. Although buboes are the major cutaneous manifestation of plague, ulcers with eschars, papules, or pustules are also present in 25% of cases.

Mycobacterium ulcerans typically causes chronic skin ulcers on the extremities of individuals living in the tropics. *Mycobacterium leprae* may be associated with cutaneous ulcerations in patients with lepromatous leprosy related to Lucio's phenomenon, in which immune-mediated destruction of tissue bearing high concentrations of *M. leprae* bacilli occurs, usually several months after initiation of effective therapy. *Mycobacterium tuberculosis* may also cause ulcerations, papules, or erythematous macular lesions of the skin in both normal and immunocompromised patients.

Decubitus ulcers are due to tissue hypoxia secondary to pressure-induced vascular insufficiency and may become secondarily infected with components of the skin and gastrointestinal flora, including anaerobes. Ulcerative lesions on the anterior shins may be due to pyoderma gangrenosum, which must be distinguished from similar lesions of infectious etiology by histologic evaluation of biopsy sites. Ulcerated lesions on the genitals may be either painful (chancroid) or painless (primary syphilis).

ERYSIPELAS (Table 110-1) Erysipelas is due to *S. pyogenes* and is characterized by an abrupt onset of fiery-red swelling of the face or extremities. The distinctive features of erysipelas are well-defined indurated margins, particularly along the nasolabial fold; rapid progression; and intense pain (see Fig. 121-3). Flaccid bullae may develop during the second or third day of illness, but extension to deeper soft tissues is rare. Treatment with penicillin is effective; swelling may progress despite appropriate treatment, although fever, pain, and the intense red color diminish. Desquamation of the involved skin occurs 5 to 10 days into the illness. Infants and elderly adults are most commonly afflicted, and the severity of systemic toxicity varies.

CELLULITIS (Table 110-1)   Cellulitis is an acute inflammatory condition of the skin that is characterized by localized pain, erythema, swelling, and heat. Cellulitis may be caused by indigenous flora colonizing the skin and appendages (e.g., *S. aureus* and *S. pyogenes*) or by a wide variety of exogenous bacteria. Because the exogenous bacteria involved in cellulitis occupy unique niches in nature, a thorough history (including epidemiologic data) provides important clues to etiology. When there is drainage, an open wound, or an obvious portal of entry, Gram's stain and culture provide a definitive diagnosis. In the absence of these findings, the bacterial etiology of cellulitis is difficult to establish, and in some cases staphylococcal and streptococcal cellulitis may have similar features. Even with needle aspiration of the leading edge or a punch biopsy of the cellulitis tissue itself, cultures are positive in only 20% of cases. This observation suggests that relatively low numbers of bacteria may cause cellulitis and that the expanding area of erythema within the skin may be a direct effect of extracellular toxins or of the soluble mediators of inflammation elicited by the host.

Bacteria may gain access to the epidermis through cracks in the skin, abrasions, cuts, burns, insect bites, surgical incisions, and intravenous catheters. Cellulitis caused by *S. aureus* spreads from a central localized infection, such as an abscess, folliculitis, or an infected foreign body (e.g., a splinter, a prosthetic device, or an intravenous catheter). In contrast, cellulitis due to *S. pyogenes* is a more rapidly spreading, diffuse process frequently associated with lymphangitis and fever. Recurrent streptococcal cellulitis of the lower extremities may be caused by organisms of group A, C, or G in association with chronic venous stasis or with saphenous venectomy for coronary artery bypass surgery. Streptococci also cause recurrent cellulitis among patients with chronic lymphedema resulting from elephantiasis, lymph node dissection, or Milroy's disease. Recurrent staphylococcal cutaneous infections are more common among individuals who have eosinophilia and elevated serum levels of IgE (Job's syndrome) and among nasal carriers of staphylococci. Cellulitis caused by *Streptococcus agalactiae* (group B *Streptococcus*) occurs primarily in elderly patients and those with diabetes mellitus or peripheral vascular disease. *Haemophilus influenzae* typically causes periorbital cellulitis in children in association with sinusitis, otitis media, or epiglottitis. It is unclear whether this form of cellulitis will (like meningitis) become less common as a result of the impressive efficacy of the *H. influenzae* type b vaccine.

Many other bacteria also cause cellulitis. Fortunately, these organisms occur in such characteristic settings that a good history provides useful clues to the diagnosis. Cellulitis associated with cat bites and, to a lesser degree, with dog bites is commonly caused by *Pasteurella multocida*, although in the latter case *Staphylococcus intermedius* and *Capnocytophaga canimorsus* (formerly DF-2) must also be considered. Sites of cellulitis and abscesses associated with dog bites and human bites also contain a variety of anaerobic organisms, including *Fusobacterium*, *Bacteroides*, aerobic and anaerobic streptococci, and *Eikenella corrodens*. *Pasteurella* is notoriously resistant to dicloxacillin and nafcillin but is sensitive to all other β-lactam antimicrobials as well as to quinolones, tetracycline, and erythromycin. Ampicillin/clavulanate, ampicillin/sulbactam, and cefoxitin are good choices for the treatment of animal or human bite infections. *Aeromonas hydrophila* causes aggressive cellulitis in tissues surrounding lacerations sustained in fresh water (lakes, rivers, and streams). This organism remains sensitive to aminoglycosides, fluoroquinolones, chloramphenicol, trimethoprim-sulfamethoxazole, and third-generation cephalosporins; it is resistant to ampicillin, however.

P. aeruginosa causes three types of soft tissue infection: ecthyma gangrenosum in neutropenic patients, hot-tub folliculitis, and cellulitis following penetrating injury. Most commonly, *P. aeruginosa* is introduced into the deep tissues when a person steps on a nail. Treatment includes surgical inspection and drainage, particularly if the injury also involves bone or joint capsule. Choices for empirical treatment while antimicrobial susceptibility data are awaited include an aminoglycoside, a third-generation cephalosporin (ceftazidime, cefoperazone, or cefotaxime), a semisynthetic penicillin (ticarcillin, mezlocillin, or piperacillin), or a fluoroquinolone (although drugs of the last class are not indicated for the treatment of children <13 years old).

Gram-negative bacillary cellulitis, including that due to *P. aeruginosa*, is most common among hospitalized, immunocompromised hosts. Cultures and sensitivity tests are critically important in this setting because of multidrug resistance (Chap. 136).

The gram-positive aerobic rod *Erysipelothrix rhusiopathiae* is most often associated with fish and domestic swine and causes cellulitis primarily in bone renderers and fishmongers. *E. rhusiopathiae* remains susceptible to most β-lactam antibiotics (including penicillin), erythromycin, clindamycin, tetracycline, and cephalosporins but is resistant to sulfonamides, chloramphenicol, and vancomycin. Its resistance to vancomycin, which is unusual among gram-positive bacteria, is of potential clinical significance since this agent is sometimes used in empirical therapy for skin infection. Fish food containing the water flea *Daphnia* is sometimes contaminated with *M. marinum*, which can cause cellulitis or granulomas on skin surfaces exposed to the water in aquariums or injured in swimming pools. Rifampin plus ethambutol has been an effective therapeutic combination in some cases, although no comprehensive studies have been undertaken. In addition, some strains of *M. marinum* are susceptible to tetracycline or to trimethoprim-sulfamethoxazole.

NECROTIZING FASCIITIS (Table 110-1)   Necrotizing fasciitis, formerly called streptococcal gangrene, may be associated with group A *Streptococcus* or mixed aerobic-anaerobic bacteria or may occur as part of gas gangrene caused by *Clostridium perfringens*. Early diagnosis may be difficult when pain or unexplained fever is the only presenting manifestation. Swelling then develops and is followed by brawny edema and tenderness. With progression, dark red induration of the epidermis appears, along with bullae filled with blue or purple fluid. Later the skin becomes friable and takes on a bluish, maroon, or black color. By this stage, thrombosis of blood vessels in the dermal papillae (Fig. 110-1) is extensive. Extension of infection to the level of the deep fascia causes this tissue to take on a brownish-gray appearance. Rapid spread occurs along fascial planes, through venous channels and lymphatics. Patients in the later stages are toxic and frequently manifest shock and multiorgan failure.

Necrotizing fasciitis caused by mixed aerobic-anaerobic bacteria begins with a breach in the integrity of a mucous membrane barrier, such as the mucosa of the gastrointestinal or genitourinary tract. The portal can be a malignancy, diverticulum, hemorrhoid, anal fissure, or urethral tear. Other predisposing factors include peripheral vascular disease, diabetes mellitus, surgery, and penetrating injury to the abdomen. Leakage into the perineal area results in a syndrome called *Fournier's gangrene*, characterized by massive swelling of the scrotum and penis with extension into the perineum or the abdominal wall and legs.

Necrotizing fasciitis caused by *S. pyogenes* has increased in frequency and severity since 1985. It frequently begins deep at the site of a nonpenetrating minor trauma, such as a bruise or a muscle strain. Seeding of the site via transient bacteremia is likely, although most patients deny antecedent streptococcal infection. Alternatively, *S. pyogenes* may reach the deep fascia from a site of cutaneous infection or penetrating trauma. Toxicity is severe, and renal impairment may precede the development of shock. In 20 to 40% of cases, myositis occurs concomitantly, and, as in gas gangrene (see below), serum creatine phosphokinase values may be markedly elevated. Necrotizing fasciitis due to mixed aerobic-anaerobic bacteria may be associated with gas in the deep tissue, but gas is not usually present when the cause is *S. pyogenes*. Prompt surgical exploration down to the deep fascia and muscle is essential. Necrotic tissue must be surgically removed, and Gram's staining and culture of excised tissue are useful in establishing whether group A streptococci, mixed aerobic-anaerobic bacteria, or *Clostridium* species are present (see "Treatment," below).

MYOSITIS/MYONECROSIS (Table 110-1)   Muscle involvement can occur with viral infection (e.g., influenza, dengue, or coxsackievirus B infection) or parasitic invasion (e.g., trichinellosis, cysticercosis, or toxoplasmosis). Although myalgia can occur in most of these infections, severe muscle pain is the hallmark of pleurodynia (coxsackievirus B), trichinellosis, and bacterial infection. Acute rhabdomyolysis predictably occurs with clostridial and streptococcal myositis but may also be associated with influenza virus, echovirus, coxsackievirus, Epstein-Barr virus, and *Legionella* infection.

Pyomyositis is usually due to *S. aureus*, is common in tropical areas, and generally has no known portal of entry. Infection remains localized, and shock does not develop unless organisms produce toxic shock syndrome toxin 1 or certain enterotoxins and the patient lacks antibodies to the toxin produced by the infecting organisms. In contrast, *S. pyogenes* may induce primary myositis (referred to as *streptococcal necrotizing myositis*) in association with severe systemic toxicity. Myonecrosis occurs concomitantly with necrotizing fasciitis in ~50% of cases. Both are part of the streptococcal toxic shock syndrome.

Gas gangrene usually follows severe penetrating injuries that result in interruption of the blood supply and introduction of soil into wounds. Such cases of traumatic gangrene are usually caused by the clostridial species *C. perfringens*, *C. septicum*, or *C. histolyticum*. Rarely, latent or recurrent gangrene can occur years after penetrating trauma; dormant spores that reside at the site of previous injury are most likely responsible. Spontaneous nontraumatic gangrene among patients with neutropenia, gastrointestinal malignancy, diverticulosis, or recent radiation therapy to the abdomen is caused by several clostridial species, of which *C. septicum* is the most commonly involved. The tolerance of this anaerobe to oxygen probably explains why it can initiate infection spontaneously in normal tissue anywhere in the body.

Synergistic nonclostridial anaerobic myonecrosis, also known as necrotizing cutaneous myositis and synergistic necrotizing cellulitis, is a variant of necrotizing fasciitis caused by mixed aerobic and anaerobic bacteria with the exclusion of clostridial organisms (see "Necrotizing Fasciitis," above).

DIAGNOSIS   This chapter has emphasized the physical appearance and location of lesions within the soft tissues as important diagnostic clues. The temporal progression of the lesions as well as the patient's travel history, animal exposure or bite history, age, underlying disease status, and lifestyle are also crucial considerations in the formulation of a narrowed differential diagnosis. However, even the astute clinician may find it challenging to diagnose all infections of the soft tissues by history and inspection alone. Soft tissue radiography, computed tomography, and magnetic resonance imaging may be useful in determining the depth of infection and should be performed in patients with rapidly progressing lesions or in those with evidence of systemic inflammatory response syndrome. These tests are particularly valuable

TABLE 110-2   *Treatment of Common Infections of the Skin*

Diagnosis/Condition	Primary Treatment	Alternative Treatment	See Also Chap(s).
Animal bite (prophylaxis or early infection)[a]	Amoxicillin/clavulanate, 875/125 mg PO bid	Doxycycline, 100 mg PO bid	. . .
Animal bite[a] (established infection)	Ampicillin/sulbactam, 1.5–3.0 g IV q6h	Clindamycin, 600–900 mg IV q8h *plus* Ciprofloxacin, 400 mg IV q12h *or* Cefoxitin, 2 g IV q6h	. . .
Bacillary angiomatosis	Erythromycin, 500 mg PO qid	Doxycycline, 100 mg PO bid	144
Herpes simplex (primary genital)	Acyclovir, 400 mg PO tid for 10 days	Famciclovir, 250 mg PO tid for 5–10 days *or* Valacyclovir, 1000 mg PO bid for 10 days	163
Herpes zoster (immunocompetent host >50 years of age)	Acyclovir, 800 mg PO 5 times daily for 7–10 days	Famciclovir, 500 mg PO tid for 7–10 days *or* Valacyclovir, 1000 mg PO tid for 7 days	164
Cellulitis (staphylococcal or streptococcal[b,c])	Nafcillin or oxacillin, 2 g IV q4–6h	Cefazolin, 1–2 g q8h *or* Ampicillin/sulbactam, 1.5–3.0 g IV q6h *or* Erythromycin, 0.5–1.0 g IV q6h *or* Clindamycin, 600–900 mg IV q8h	120, 121
Necrotizing fasciitis (group A streptococcal[b])	Clindamycin, 600–900 mg IV q6–8h *plus* Penicillin G, 4 million units IV q4h	Clindamycin, 600–900 mg IV q6–8h *plus* Cephalosporin (first- or second-generation)	121
Necrotizing fasciitis (mixed aerobes and anaerobes)	Ampicillin, 2 g IV q4h *plus* Clindamycin, 600–900 mg IV q6–8h *plus* Ciprofloxacin, 400 mg IV q6–8h	Vancomycin, 1 g IV q6h *plus* Metronidazole, 500 mg IV q6h *plus* Ciprofloxacin, 400 mg IV q6–8h	148
Gas gangrene	Clindamycin, 600–900 mg IV q6–8h *plus* Penicillin G, 4 million units IV q4–6h	Clindamycin, 600–900 mg IV q6–8h *plus* Cefoxitin, 2 g IV q6h	126

[a] *Pasteurella multocida*, a species commonly associated with both dog and cat bites, is resistant to cephalexin, dicloxacillin, clindamycin, and erythromycin. *Eikenella corrodens*, a bacterium commonly associated with human bites, is resistant to clindamycin, penicillinase-resistant penicillins, and metronidazole but is sensitive to trimethoprim-sulfamethoxazole and fluoroquinolones.
[b] The frequency of erythromycin resistance in group A *Streptococcus* is currently ~5% in the United States but has reached 70 to 100% in some other countries. Most, but not all, erythromycin-resistant group A streptococci are susceptible to clindamycin. Approximately 90 to 95% of *Staphylococcus aureus* strains are sensitive to clindamycin.
[c] Severe hospital-acquired *S. aureus* infections or community-acquired *S. aureus* infections that are not responding to the β-lactam antibiotics recommended in this table may be caused by methicillin-resistant strains, requiring a switch to vancomycin or linezolid.

for defining a localized abscess or detecting gas in tissue. Unfortunately, they may reveal only soft tissue swelling and thus are not specific for fulminant infections such as necrotizing fasciitis or myonecrosis caused by group A *Streptococcus*, where gas is not found in lesions.

Aspiration of the leading edge or punch biopsy with frozen section may be helpful if the results are positive, but false-negative results occur in ~80% of cases. There is some evidence that aspiration alone may be superior to injection and aspiration using normal saline. Frozen sections are especially useful in distinguishing SSSS from TEN and are quite valuable in cases of necrotizing fasciitis. Open surgical inspection with debridement as indicated is clearly the best way to determine the extent and severity of infection and to obtain material for Gram's staining and culture. Such an aggressive approach is important and may be lifesaving if undertaken early in the course of fulminant infections where there is evidence of systemic toxicity.

℞ TREATMENT

A full description of the treatment of all the clinical entities described herein is beyond the scope of this chapter. As a guide to the clinician in selecting appropriate treatment, the antimicrobial agents useful in the most common and the most fulminant cutaneous infections are listed in Table 110-2.

Early and aggressive surgical exploration is essential in patients with suspected necrotizing fasciitis, myositis, or gangrene in order to (1) visualize the deep structures, (2) remove necrotic tissue, (3) reduce compartment pressure, and (4) obtain suitable material for Gram's staining and for aerobic and anaerobic cultures. Appropriate empirical antibiotic treatment for mixed aerobic-anaerobic infections could consist of ampicillin/sulbactam, cefoxitin, or the following combination: (1) clindamycin (600 to 900 mg intravenously every 8 h) or metronidazole (750 mg every 6 h) plus (2) ampicillin or ampicillin/sulbactam (2 to 3 g intravenously every 6 h) plus (3) gentamicin (1.0 to 1.5 mg/kg every 8 h). Group A streptococcal and clostridial infection of the fascia and/or muscle carries a mortality rate of 20 to 50% with penicillin treatment. In experimental models of streptococcal and clostridial necrotizing fasciitis/myositis, clindamycin has exhibited markedly superior efficacy, but no comparative trials have been performed in humans. Hyperbaric oxygen treatment may also be useful in gas gangrene due to clostridial species. Antibiotic treatment should be continued until all signs of systemic toxicity have resolved, all devitalized tissue has been removed, and granulation tissue has developed (Chaps. 121, 126, and 148).

In summary, infections of the skin and soft tissues are diverse in presentation and severity and offer a great challenge to the clinician. This chapter provides an approach to diagnosis and understanding of the pathophysiologic mechanisms involved in these infections. More in-depth information is found in chapters on specific infections.

FURTHER READING

BISNO AI, STEVENS DL: Streptococcal infections in skin and soft tissues. N Engl J Med 334:240, 1996

BREMAN JG, HENDERSON DA: Diagnosis and management of smallpox. N Engl J Med 346:1300, 2002

NORRBY-TEGLUND A, STEVENS DL: Novel therapies in streptococcal toxic shock syndrome: Attenuation of virulence factor expression and modulation of host response. Curr Opin Infect Dis 11:285, 1998

STEVENS DL: Streptococcal toxic shock syndrome associated with necrotizing fasciitis. Annu Rev Med 51:271, 2000

———: Necrotizing soft tissue infections. Curr Treat Opt Infect Dis 2:359, 2000

TALAN DA et al: Bacteriologic analysis of infected dog and cat bites. Emergency Medicine Animal Bite Infection Study Group. N Engl J Med 340:85, 1999

TRAYLOR KK, TODD JK: Needle aspirate culture method in soft tissue infections: Injection of saline vs. direct aspiration. Pediatr Infect Dis J 17:840, 1998

111 OSTEOMYELITIS
Jeffrey Parsonnet, James H. Maguire

Osteomyelitis, an infection of bone, is caused most commonly by pyogenic bacteria and mycobacteria. As a useful framework for evaluating the patient and planning treatment, cases are classified on the basis of the causative agent; the route, duration, and anatomical location of infection; and local and systemic host factors.

PATHOGENESIS AND PATHOLOGY Microorganisms enter bone by the hematogenous route, by direct introduction from a contiguous focus of infection, or by a penetrating wound. Trauma, ischemia, and foreign bodies enhance the susceptibility of bone to microbial invasion by exposing sites to which bacteria can bind. Phagocytes attempt to contain the infection and, in the process, release enzymes that lyse bone. Bacteria escape host defenses by adhering tightly to damaged bone, by entering and persisting within osteoblasts, and by coating themselves and underlying surfaces with a protective polysaccharide-rich biofilm. Pus spreads into vascular channels, raising intraosseous pressure and impairing the flow of blood; as the untreated infection becomes chronic, ischemic necrosis of bone results in the separation of large devascularized fragments (*sequestra*). When pus breaks through the cortex, subperiosteal or soft tissue abscesses form, and the elevated periosteum deposits new bone (an *involucrum*) around the sequestrum.

Microorganisms, infiltrates of neutrophils, and congested or thrombosed blood vessels are the principal histologic findings of acute osteomyelitis. The distinguishing feature of chronic osteomyelitis is necrotic bone, which is characterized by the absence of living osteocytes. Mononuclear cells predominate in chronic infections, and granulation and fibrous tissues replace bone that has been resorbed by osteoclasts. In the chronic stage, organisms may be too few to be seen on staining.

HEMATOGENOUS OSTEOMYELITIS Hematogenous infection accounts for ~20% of cases of osteomyelitis and primarily affects children, in whom the long bones are infected, and older adults and intravenous drug users, in whom the spine is the most common site of infection.

Acute Hematogenous Osteomyelitis Infection usually involves a single bone, most commonly the tibia, femur, or humerus in children and vertebral bodies in older adults and injection drug users. Bacteria settle in the well-perfused metaphysis of growing bones where functioning phagocytes are scarce, a network of venous sinusoids slows the flow of blood, and fenestrations in capillaries allow organisms to escape into the extravascular space. Because vascular anatomy changes with age, hematogenous infection of long bones is uncommon during adulthood and, when it occurs, usually involves the diaphysis.

On presentation, the child with osteomyelitis usually appears acutely ill, with high fever, chills, and localized pain and tenderness and often with restriction of movement or difficulty bearing weight. Cutaneous erythema and swelling indicate extension of pus through the cortex. During infancy and after puberty, infection may spread through the epiphysis into the joint space. In children of other ages, extension of infection through the cortex results in involvement of joints if the metaphysis is intracapsular. Thus, septic arthritis of the elbow, shoulder, and hip may complicate osteomyelitis of the proximal radius, humerus, and femur, respectively. In children, the source of bacteremia is usually inapparent. A history is often obtained of recent blunt trauma to the area involved; presumably, this event results in a small intraosseous hematoma or vascular obstruction. Adults with osteomyelitis may present in the context of an apparent infection elsewhere, such as the lung, sinuses, or urinary tract, or without an obvious source of bacteremia.

Plain radiographs obtained early in the course of infection may show soft tissue swelling, but the first change in bone—a periosteal reaction—is not evident until at least 10 days after the onset of infection. Lytic changes can be detected after 2 to 6 weeks, when 50 to 75% of bone density has been lost. Rarely, a well-circumscribed lytic lesion, or *Brodie's abscess*, is seen in a child who has been in pain for several months but has had no fever.

Vertebral Osteomyelitis   The vertebral bodies are the most common sites of acute hematogenous osteomyelitis in adults. Organisms reach the well-perfused vertebral body via spinal arteries and quickly spread from the end plate into the disk space and then to the adjacent vertebral body. The infection may originate in the urinary tract, and it does so particularly often among men men over age 50. Other sources of bacteremia include endocarditis, dental abscess, soft tissue infection, and a contaminated intravenous line; these sources may or may not be obvious. Diabetes mellitus, hemodialysis, and injection drug use carry an increased risk of spinal infection. Many patients have a history of degenerative joint disease involving the spine, and some report an episode of trauma preceding the onset of infection. Penetrating injuries and surgical procedures to the spine may cause nonhematogenous vertebral osteomyelitis or infection localized to the disk.

Most patients with vertebral osteomyelitis report neck or back pain; patients may describe atypical pain in the chest, the abdomen, or an extremity that is due to irritation of nerve roots. Symptoms are localized to the lumbar spine more often than to the thoracic spine (>50% vs. 35% of cases) or the cervical spine in pyogenic infections, but the thoracic spine is involved most commonly in tuberculous spondylitis (Pott's disease). More than 50% of patients experience a subacute illness in which a vague, dull pain gradually intensifies over 2 to 3 months. Fever is usually low grade or absent, but some patients recall having had an episode of fever and chills prior to or at the onset of pain. An acute presentation with high fever and toxicity is less common and suggests ongoing bacteremia. Percussion over the involved vertebra elicits tenderness, and physical examination may reveal spasm of the paraspinal muscles and limitation of motion.

Laboratory findings at the time of presentation include a normal or modestly elevated white blood cell count and, almost invariably, an increased erythrocyte sedimentation rate (ESR) and C-reactive protein (CRP) level. Blood cultures are positive only 20 to 50% of the time.

Usually, by the time the patient seeks medical attention, plain radiographs show irregular erosions in the end plates of adjacent vertebral bodies and narrowing of the intervening disk space. This radiographic pattern is virtually diagnostic of bacterial infection because tumors and other diseases of the spine rarely cross the disk space. Computed tomography (CT) or magnetic resonance imaging (MRI) may demonstrate epidural, paraspinal, retropharyngeal, mediastinal, retroperitoneal, or psoas abscesses that originate in the spine.

A spinal epidural abscess may evolve suddenly or over several weeks; the classic clinical presentation is spinal pain progressing to radicular pain and/or weakness. Irreversible paralysis may result from failure to recognize epidural abscess before the development of neurologic deficits. MRI is the best procedure for detection of epidural abscess and should be performed in all cases of vertebral osteomyelitis accompanied by subjective weakness or objective neurologic abnormalities.

Microbiology   More than 95% of cases of hematogenous osteomyelitis are caused by a single organism. *Staphylococcus aureus* accounts for 50% of isolates. Other common pathogens include group B streptococci and *Escherichia coli* during the newborn period and group A streptococci in early childhood. Vertebral osteomyelitis is due to *E. coli* and other enteric bacilli in ~25% of cases. *S. aureus*, *Pseudomonas aeruginosa*, and *Serratia* infections are associated with intravenous drug use in some parts of the United States and may involve the sacroiliac, sternoclavicular, or pubic joints as well as the spine. *Salmonella* spp. and *S. aureus* are the major causes of long-bone osteomyelitis complicating sickle cell anemia and other hemoglobinopathies. Tuberculosis and brucellosis affect the spine more often than

other bones. Other common sites of tuberculous osteomyelitis include the small bones of the hands and feet, the metaphyses of long bones, the ribs, and the sternum.

Unusual causes of hematogenous osteomyelitis include disseminated histoplasmosis, coccidioidomycosis, and blastomycosis in endemic areas. Immunocompromised persons on rare occasions develop osteomyelitis due to atypical mycobacteria, *Bartonella henselae*, or *Pneumocystis* or to species of *Candida*, *Cryptococcus*, or *Aspergillus*. Hematogenous osteomyelitis with *Mycobacterium bovis* has been reported following intravesicular instillation of bacille Calmette-Guérin (BCG) for cancer of the bladder. The etiology of chronic relapsing multifocal osteomyelitis, an inflammatory condition of children that is characterized by recurrent episodes of painful lytic lesions in multiple bones, has not been identified.

OSTEOMYELITIS SECONDARY TO A CONTIGUOUS FOCUS OF INFECTION ■ Clinical Features   This broad category of osteomyelitis accounts for ~80% of all cases and occurs most commonly in adults. It includes infections introduced by penetrating injuries, such as bites, puncture wounds, and open fractures; by surgical procedures; and by direct extension of infection from adjacent soft tissues. Generalized vascular insufficiency and the presence of a foreign body are important predisposing factors and make infection more difficult to cure.

Frequently, the diagnosis of this type of osteomyelitis is not made until the infection has already become chronic. The pain, fever, and inflammatory signs due to acute infection may be attributed to the original injury or to overlying soft tissue infection. An indolent infection may become apparent only weeks or months later, when a sinus tract develops, a surgical wound breaks down, or a fracture fails to heal. It may be impossible to distinguish radiographic abnormalities due to osteomyelitis from those due to the precipitating condition.

A special type of contiguous-focus osteomyelitis occurs in the setting of peripheral vascular disease and nearly always involves the small bones of the feet of adult diabetic patients. This type of infection is a major cause of morbidity and hospitalization for patients with diabetes and results in many thousands of amputations per year. Diabetic neuropathy exposes the foot to frequent trauma and pressure sores, and the patient may be unaware of infection as it spreads into bone. Poor tissue perfusion impairs normal inflammatory responses and wound healing and creates a milieu that is conducive to anaerobic infections. It is often during the evaluation of a nonhealing ulcer, a swollen toe, or acute cellulitis that a radiograph provides the first evidence of osteomyelitis. If bone is palpable during examination of the base of an ulcer with a blunt surgical probe, osteomyelitis is likely.

Microbiology   *S. aureus* is a pathogen in more than half of cases of contiguous-focus osteomyelitis. However, in contrast to hematogenous osteomyelitis, these infections are often polymicrobial and are more likely to involve gram-negative and anaerobic bacteria. Hence a mixture of staphylococci, streptococci, enteric organisms, and anaerobic bacteria may be isolated from a diabetic foot infection or pelvic osteomyelitis underlying a decubitus ulcer. Aerobic and anaerobic bacteria cause osteomyelitis following surgery or soft tissue infection of the oropharynx, paranasal sinuses, gastrointestinal tract, or female genital tract. A human bite may result in mixed infection of the hand, with anaerobes included among the etiologic agents. *S. aureus* is the principal cause of postoperative infections; coagulase-negative staphylococci are common pathogens after implantation of orthopedic appliances; and these organisms as well as gram-negative enteric bacilli, atypical mycobacteria, and *Mycoplasma* may cause sternal osteomyelitis after cardiac surgery. Infection with *P. aeruginosa* is frequently associated with puncture wounds of the foot (especially by a nail through a sneaker) or with thermal burns, and *Pasteurella multocida* infection commonly follows cat bites.

CHRONIC OSTEOMYELITIS   With prompt treatment, fewer than 5% of cases of acute hematogenous osteomyelitis progress to chronic osteomyelitis. Chronic osteomyelitis is more likely to develop in contiguous-focus than in hematogenous osteomyelitis. The presence of a foreign body makes establishment of chronic infection especially likely.

A protracted clinical course, long periods of quiescence, and recurrent exacerbations are characteristic of chronic osteomyelitis. Sinus tracts between bone and skin may drain purulent material and occasionally pieces of necrotic bone. An increase in drainage, pain, or ESR signals an exacerbation. Fever is unusual except when obstruction of a sinus tract leads to soft tissue infection. Rare late complications include pathologic fractures, squamous cell carcinoma of the sinus tract, and amyloidosis.

DIAGNOSIS Early diagnosis of acute osteomyelitis is critical because prompt antibiotic therapy may prevent the necrosis of bone. The ESR and CRP levels are elevated in most cases of active osteomyelitis, including those in which constitutional symptoms and leukocytosis are lacking. These findings are not specific to osteomyelitis, however, and the ESR is occasionally normal in early infections. Baseline values are often useful in monitoring the efficacy of treatment. A variety of radiologic tests are available for evaluation of osteomyelitis (Table 111-1). Evaluation usually begins with plain radiographs because of their ready availability, although they frequently show no abnormalities during early infection. Three-phase bone scans (^{99}Tc-monodiphosphonate) offer high sensitivity but often have low specificity, especially in the presence of underlying bony abnormalities. There is a lack of consensus over the optimal use of other radionuclide studies, and there is considerable variation between institutions in their use. Although the use of MRI (Fig. 111-1) is expanding because of high sensitivity and specificity, this modality is not available at all institutions.

The role of diagnostic imaging in chronic osteomyelitis is to detect active infection and delineate the extent of debridement necessary to

FIGURE 111-1 Osteomyelitis of the thoracic spine demonstrated on a sagittal, fat-suppressed T1-weighted magnetic resonance image after the administration of intravenous gadolinium. At T8–T9, there is involvement of the adjacent vertebral bodies and intervening disk. Abnormally enhancing inflammatory tissue extends from the disk space anteriorly (*white arrow*) as well as posteriorly into the epidural space, compressing the thecal sac (*black arrow*).

remove necrotic bone and abnormal soft tissues. Although plain films accurately reflect chronic changes, CT is more sensitive for the detection of sequestra, sinus tracts, and soft tissue abscesses. Both CT and ultrasound are useful for guiding percutaneous aspiration of subperiosteal and soft tissue fluid collections. Sequential technetium and gallium or indium scans may help determine whether infection is active and may distinguish infection from noninflammatory bone changes. MRI provides superior information about the anatomical extent of infection but does not always distinguish osteomyelitis from healing fractures and tumors. MRI is particularly useful in distinguishing cellulitis from osteomyelitis in the diabetic foot; however, no imaging modality consistently distinguishes infection from neuropathic osteopathy.

Appropriate samples for microbiologic studies should be obtained in all cases of suspected osteomyelitis before the initiation of antimicrobial therapy. Blood cultures are indicated in acute cases and are positive in more than one-third of cases of hematogenous osteomyelitis in children and in 25% of cases of vertebral osteomyelitis in adults. The presence of sepsis occasionally requires initiation of empirical therapy after blood samples alone have been obtained for culture. If blood cultures are negative, samples from needle aspiration of pus in bone or soft tissues or from a bone biopsy should be obtained for culture; in the case of vertebral osteomyelitis, these samples can usually be obtained with the guidance of fluoroscopy or CT scan.

The results of culture of specimens obtained by swabbing of a sinus tract or the base of an ulcer correlate poorly with the organisms infecting the bone. For this reason, in cases of chronic osteomyelitis and contiguous-focus osteomyelitis, samples for aerobic and anaerobic culture should be obtained from several sites by percutaneous needle aspiration, percutaneous biopsy, or intraoperative biopsy at the time of debridement. Isolates of coagulase-negative staphylococci and other organisms of low virulence should not automatically be disregarded as contaminants, especially in the presence of prosthetic materials. Special culture media may be necessary for the isolation of mycobacteria, fungi, and less common pathogens. In some cases, histopathologic examination of biopsy specimens may be the only way to make a diagnosis.

TABLE 111-1	*Diagnostic Imaging Studies for Osteomyelitis*
Type of Study	**Comments**
Plain radiographs	Insensitive, especially in early osteomyelitis. May show periosteal elevation after 10 days, lytic changes after 2–6 weeks. Useful to look for anatomical abnormalities (e.g., fractures, bony variants, or deformities), foreign bodies, and soft tissue gas.
Three-phase bone scan (^{99m}Tc-MDP)	Characteristic finding in osteomyelitis: increased uptake in all three phases of scan. Highly sensitive (~95%) in acute infection; somewhat less sensitive if blood flow to bone is poor. Specificity moderate if plain films are normal, but poor in presence of neuropathic arthropathy, fractures, tumor, infarction.
Other radionuclide scans	Examples: ^{67}Ga-citrate, ^{111}In-labeled WBCs. ^{111}In-WBCs more specific than gallium but not always available. Often used in conjunction with bone scan because its greater specificity for inflammation than ^{99m}Tc-MDP helps to distinguish infectious from noninfectious processes. Lack of consensus over role in routine evaluation.
Ultrasound	May detect subperiosteal fluid collection or soft tissue abscess adjacent to bone, but largely supplanted by CT and MRI.
CT	Limited role in acute osteomyelitis. In chronic osteomyelitis, excellent for detection of sequestra, cortical destruction, soft tissue abscesses, and sinus tracts. Use may be limited by metallic foreign body.
MRI	As sensitive as ^{99m}Tc-MDP bone scan for acute osteomyelitis (~95%); detects changes in water content of marrow before disruption of cortical bone. High specificity (~87%), with better anatomical detail than nuclear studies. Procedure of choice for vertebral osteomyelitis because of high sensitivity for epidural abscess. Use may be limited by metallic foreign body.

Abbreviations: CT, computed tomography; MDP, monodiphosphonate; MRI, magnetic resonance imaging; WBCs, white blood cells.

℞ TREATMENT

Antibiotic Therapy (Table 111-2) Antibiotics are administered only after appropriate specimens have been obtained for culture. The antibiotics selected should be bactericidal, should be given at a high dose, and—at least initially—should be given intravenously. When necessary, empirical therapy is guided by findings on Gram's staining of a specimen from the bone or abscess or is chosen to cover the most

| Organism | Suggested Regimen[a] | |
	Primary	Alternative[b]
Staphylococcus aureus		
Penicillin-resistant, methicillin-sensitive (MSSA)	Nafcillin or oxacillin, 2 g IV q4h	Cefazolin, 1 g IV q8h; ceftriaxone, 1 g IV q24h; clindamycin, 900 mg IV q8h[c]
Penicillin-sensitive	Penicillin 3–4 million U IV q4h	Cefazolin, ceftriaxone, clindamycin (as above)
Methicillin-resistant (MRSA)	Vancomycin, 15 mg/kg (up to 1 g) IV q12h	Clindamycin[c] (as above); linezolid, 600 mg IV or PO q12h[d]; daptomycin, 4–6 mg/kg per day IV[d]
Streptococci (including *S. milleri*, β-hemolytic streptococci)	Penicillin (as above)	Cefazolin, ceftriaxone, clindamycin (as above)
Gram-negative aerobic bacilli		
Escherichia coli, other "sensitive" species	Ampicillin, 2 g IV q4h; cefazolin, 1 g IV q8h	Ceftriaxone, 1 g IV q24h; parenteral or oral fluoroquinolone (e.g., ciprofloxacin, 400 mg IV or 750 mg PO q12h)[e]
Pseudomonas aeruginosa	Extended-spectrum β-lactam agent (e.g., piperacillin, 3–4 g IV q4–6h or ceftazidime, 2 g IV q12h) *plus* tobramycin, 5–7 mg/kg q24h[f]	May substitute parenteral or oral fluoroquinolone for β-lactam agent
Enterobacter spp., other "resistant" species	Extended-spectrum β-lactam agent IV or fluoroquinolone IV or PO[e] (as above)	
Mixed infections possibly involving anaerobic bacteria	Ampicillin/sulbactam, 1.5–3 g IV q6h; piperacillin/tazobactam 3.375 g IV q6h	Cefotetan, 1–2 g IV q12h; combination of fluoroquinolone plus clindamycin (as above)

[a] Duration of treatment is discussed in the text.

[b] Cephalosporins may be used for the treatment of patients allergic to penicillin whose reaction did not consist of anaphylaxis or urticaria (immediate-type hypersensitivity).

[c] Because of the possibility of inducible resistance, clindamycin must be used with caution for the treatment of strains resistant to erythromycin. Consult clinical microbiology laboratory.

[d] Experience is limited; there are anecdotal reports of efficacy.

[e] Oral fluoroquinolones must not be coadministered with divalent cations (calcium, magnesium, iron, aluminum), which block the drugs' absorption.

[f] Tobramycin levels and renal function must be monitored closely to minimize the risks of nephro- and ototoxicity.

likely pathogens. Empirical therapy in most cases should include high doses of an agent active against *S. aureus* (such as oxacillin, nafcillin, cefazolin, or vancomycin) and—if gram-negative organisms are likely to be involved—a third-generation cephalosporin, an aminoglycoside, or a fluoroquinolone.

Specific intravenous therapy is based on the in vitro susceptibility of the organism(s) isolated from bone or blood. At-home intravenous administration of antibiotics or oral therapy is appropriate for motivated and medically stable patients and represents a significant advance in management. Antibiotics that require infrequent dosing, such as ceftriaxone, may facilitate home therapy. Many antibiotics can be given automatically by portable infusion pump, which decreases the disruption otherwise caused by the frequent administration of drug. Use of a peripherally inserted central catheter (PICC line) also facilitates outpatient administration of antibiotics. Outpatient therapy requires close coordination of nursing, pharmacy, and physician care, with clear delineations of responsibility for monitoring safety and efficacy.

Children with acute hematogenous osteomyelitis routinely receive oral antibiotics after 5 to 10 days of parenteral therapy if signs of active infection have resolved; such treatment has been as successful as standard parenteral therapy. The doses of oral penicillins or cephalosporins required for the treatment of osteomyelitis are several times higher than the doses of these drugs given for common infections. Adults may not tolerate these high doses as well as children, and, except in the case of the fluoroquinolones and rifampin, few data support the use of oral antibiotics by adults. For treatment of osteomyelitis due to Enterobacteriaceae, oral administration of a fluoroquinolone has been as successful as intravenous administration of β-lactam antibiotics.

Caution should be exercised in the use of fluoroquinolones as the sole agents for treatment of infection due to *S. aureus* or *P. aeruginosa* because resistance may develop during therapy. Addition of rifampin to a fluoroquinolone or a β-lactam agent has yielded encouraging results in infections due to *S. aureus*, but potential drug toxicity and drug interactions make this option desirable only for selected patients, such as those with necrotic bone that cannot be adequately debrided. Oral administration of clindamycin (300 to 450 mg every 6 h) or metronidazole (500 mg every 8 h) results in high drug levels in serum and can take the place of intravenous regimens for the treatment of *Bacteroides* infections. Oral clindamycin has produced good results for continuation treatment of osteomyelitis due to *S. aureus*, but consultation with the microbiology laboratory is advised because of inducible resistance exhibited by some strains. The bacteriostatic drug linezolid (600 mg by mouth every 12 h) and the bactericidal drug daptomycin (4 to 6 mg/kg per day intravenously) have been used successfully in a small number of patients with infection caused by methicillin-resistant *S. aureus* and vancomycin-resistant *Enterococcus*, but data are currently insufficient to recommend their routine use. Data do not support the routine use of the serum minimal bactericidal concentration in guiding therapy.

Acute Hematogenous Osteomyelitis Early treatment of acute hematogenous osteomyelitis of childhood with 4 to 6 weeks of an appropriate antibiotic is usually successful; treatment for <3 weeks has resulted in a 10-fold greater rate of failure. Surgical intervention in childhood cases is indicated for intraosseous or subperiosteal abscesses, concomitant septic arthritis, and failure of the acute signs of infection to improve in 24 to 48 h. Acute hematogenous osteomyelitis of bones other than the spine in adults often requires surgical debridement.

Vertebral Osteomyelitis A 4- to 6-week course of treatment with an appropriate antibiotic is usually sufficient to cure vertebral osteomyelitis. Failure of the ESR to drop by two-thirds or more of its pretreatment level or of CRP to normalize is an indication for reevaluation and (possibly) longer treatment. Surgery is seldom necessary, even in cases of many months' duration, except in instances of spinal instability, new or progressive neurologic deficits, or large soft-tissue abscesses that cannot be drained percutaneously. All but small and asymptomatic epidural abscesses should be surgically drained. Patients should maintain bed rest until back pain has declined to the point at which ambulation is possible. Body casts are no longer used except for comfort.

Contiguous-Focus Osteomyelitis Even when diagnosed early, contiguous-focus osteomyelitis usually requires surgery in addition to 4 to 6 weeks of appropriate antibiotic therapy because of underlying soft tissue infection or damage to bone from an injury or surgery. A 2-week course of antibiotics following thorough debridement and soft tissue coverage has yielded excellent results in the treatment of superficial osteomyelitis involving only the outer cortex of bone.

Chronic Osteomyelitis The risks and benefits of aggressive therapy for chronic osteomyelitis should be weighed before any attempt is made to eradicate the infection. Some patients with extensive disease prefer to live with their infections rather than undergo multiple surgical procedures, take prolonged courses of antimicrobial therapy, and face the risk of loss of an extremity. Such persons often benefit from intermittent courses of oral antibiotics to suppress acute exacerbations.

Once the decision has been made to treat chronic osteomyelitis aggressively, the patient's nutritional and metabolic status should be optimized to expedite healing of soft tissues and bone. Antibiotic administration should be started several days before surgery to reduce inflammation if the etiology of the infection is known; if not, antibiotic therapy should be withheld until debridement. A 4- to 6-week course of appropriate antibiotic therapy is given postoperatively on the basis of the susceptibility pattern of organisms isolated from bone. The benefit of prolonged oral antibiotic therapy after 4 to 6 weeks of parenteral therapy remains unproven. There is insufficient information to recommend either the routine use of hyperbaric oxygen or the use of antibiotic-impregnated methacrylate beads or other depots to deliver high levels of antibiotics to the bone. The success of therapy for chronic osteomyelitis still rests largely on the complete surgical removal of necrotic bone and abnormal soft tissues. In the past, the inability to repair large defects in bone and soft tissue limited the extent of debridement. Muscle flaps and skin grafts are now used routinely to cover large soft-tissue defects and to fill dead space, and bone grafts and vascularized bone transfer may restore a seriously compromised bone to a functional state.

In infections of recent fractures, internal fixators are often left in place, and the infection is controlled by limited debridement and suppressive antibiotic therapy. Definitive surgical/antimicrobial therapy is delayed until after bony union of the fracture is achieved. If there is nonunion of the fracture or loosening of the fixator, the appliance must be removed, the bone debrided, and an external fixator or a new internal fixator applied.

Osteomyelitis of the small bones of the feet in persons with vascular disease usually requires surgical treatment. The effectiveness of the surgery is limited by the blood supply to the site and the body's ability to heal the wound. Revascularization of the extremity is indicated if the vascular disease involves large arteries. In cases of decreased perfusion due to small-vessel disease, foot-sparing surgery may fail, and the best option is often suppressive therapy or amputation. The duration of antibiotic therapy depends on the surgical procedure performed. When the infected bone is removed entirely but residual infection of soft tissues remains, antibiotic therapy should be given for 2 weeks; if amputation eliminates infected bone and soft tissue, standard surgical prophylaxis is given; otherwise, postoperative antibiotics must be given for 4 to 6 weeks.

FURTHER READING

KAIM AH et al: Imaging of chronic posttraumatic osteomyelitis. Eur Radiol 12:1193, 2002

KHATRI G et al: Effect of bone biopsy in guiding antimicrobial therapy for osteomyelitis complicating open wounds. Am J Med Sci 321:367, 2001

LEW DP, WALDVOGEL FA: Osteomyelitis. N Engl J Med 336:999, 1997

LIPSKY BA: Osteomyelitis of the foot in diabetic patients. Clin Infect Dis 25:1318, 1997

MADER JT et al: Staging and staging application in osteomyelitis. Clin Infect Dis 25:1303, 1997

MCHENRY MC et al: Vertebral osteomyelitis: Long-term outcome for 253 patients from 7 Cleveland-area hospitals. Clin Infect Dis 34:1342, 2002

REZAI AR et al: Contemporary management of spinal osteomyelitis. Neurosurgery 44:1018, 1999

RISSING JP: Antimicrobial therapy for chronic osteomyelitis in adults: Role of the quinolones. Clin Infect Dis 25:1327, 1997

TICE AD et al: Outcomes of osteomyelitis among patients treated with outpatient parenteral antimicrobial therapy. Am J Med 114:723, 2003

TSUKAYAMA DT: Pathophysiology of posttraumatic osteomyelitis. Clin Orthop 360:22, 1999

112 INTRAABDOMINAL INFECTIONS AND ABSCESSES
Dennis L. Kasper, Dori F. Zaleznik

Intraperitoneal infections generally arise because a normal anatomical barrier is disrupted. This disruption may occur when the appendix, a diverticulum, or an ulcer ruptures; when the bowel wall is weakened by ischemia, tumor, or inflammation (e.g., in inflammatory bowel disease); or with adjacent inflammatory processes, such as pancreatitis or pelvic inflammatory disease, in which enzymes (in the former case) or organisms (in the latter) may leak into the peritoneal cavity. Whatever the inciting event, once inflammation develops and organisms usually contained within the bowel or another organ enter the normally sterile peritoneal space, a predictable series of events takes place. Intraabdominal infections occur in two stages: peritonitis and—if the patient survives this stage and goes untreated—abscess formation. The types of microorganisms predominating in each stage of infection are responsible for the pathogenesis of disease.

PERITONITIS

Peritonitis is a life-threatening event that is often accompanied by bacteremia and sepsis syndrome (Chap. 254). The peritoneal cavity is large but is divided into compartments. The upper and lower peritoneal cavities are divided by the transverse mesocolon; the greater omentum extends from the transverse mesocolon and from the lower pole of the stomach to line the lower peritoneal cavity. The pancreas, duodenum, and ascending and descending colon are located in the anterior retroperitoneal space; the kidneys, ureters, and adrenals are found in the posterior retroperitoneal space. The other organs, including liver, stomach, gallbladder, spleen, jejunum, ileum, transverse and sigmoid colon, cecum, and appendix, are found within the peritoneal cavity itself. Normally the cavity is lined with a serous membrane that can serve as a conduit for fluids—a property utilized in peritoneal dialysis.

A small amount of fluid, sufficient to allow movement of organs, is normally present in the peritoneal space. This fluid is serous, with a protein content (consisting mainly of albumin) of <30 g/L and <300 white blood cells (WBCs, generally mononuclear cells) per microliter. In the presence of infection, some compartments collect fluid or pus more often than others. These compartments include the pelvis (the lowest portion), the subphrenic spaces on the right and left sides, and Morrison's pouch, which is a posterosuperior extension of the subhepatic spaces and is the lowest part of the paravertebral groove when a patient is recumbent. The falciform ligament separating the right and left subphrenic spaces appears to act as a barrier to the spread of infection; consequently, it is unusual to find bilateral subphrenic collections. In bacterial infections, leukocyte recruitment into the infected peritoneal cavity consists of an early influx of polymorphonuclear leukocytes (PMNs) and a prolonged subsequent phase of mononuclear cell migration. The phenotype of the infiltrating leukocytes during the course of inflammation is regulated primarily by resident-cell chemokine synthesis.

PRIMARY (SPONTANEOUS) BACTERIAL PERITONITIS Peritonitis is either primary (without an apparent source of contamination) or secondary. The types of organisms found and the clinical presentations of these two processes are different. In adults, primary bacterial peritonitis (PBP) occurs most commonly in conjunction with cirrhosis of the liver (frequently the result of alcoholism). However, the disease has been reported in adults with metastatic malignant disease, postnecrotic cirrhosis, chronic active hepatitis, acute viral hepatitis, congestive heart failure, systemic lupus erythematosus, and lymphedema as well as in patients with no underlying disease. PBP virtually always develops in patients with ascites. Nevertheless, it is not a common event, occurring in ≤10% of cirrhotic patients. The cause of PBP has not been established definitively but is believed to involve hematogenous spread of organisms in a patient in whom a diseased liver and altered portal circulation result in a defect in the usual filtration function. Organisms are able to multiply in ascites, a good medium for growth. The proteins of the complement cascade have been found in peritoneal fluid, with lower levels in cirrhotic patients than in patients with ascites of other etiologies. The opsonic and phagocytic properties of neutrophils are diminished in patients with advanced liver disease.

The presentation of PBP differs from that of secondary peritonitis. The most common manifestation is fever, which is reported in as many as 80% of patients. Ascites is found but virtually always predates infection. Abdominal pain, an acute onset of symptoms, and peritoneal irritation detected during physical examination can be helpful diagnostically, but the absence of any of these findings does not exclude this often-subtle diagnosis. It is vital to sample the peritoneal fluid of any cirrhotic patient with ascites and fever. The finding of >300 PMNs per microliter is diagnostic for PBP, according to Conn. This criterion does not apply to secondary peritonitis (see below). The microbiology of PBP is also distinctive. While enteric gram-negative bacilli such as *Escherichia coli* are most commonly encountered, gram-positive organisms such as streptococci, enterococci, or even pneumococci are sometimes found. In PBP, a single organism is typically isolated; anaerobes are found less frequently in PBP than in secondary peritonitis, in which a mixed flora including anaerobes is the rule. In fact, if PBP is suspected and multiple organisms including anaerobes are recovered from the peritoneal fluid, the diagnosis must be reconsidered and a source of secondary peritonitis sought.

The diagnosis of PBP is not easy. It depends on the exclusion of a primary intraabdominal source of infection. Contrast-enhanced computed tomography (CT) is very useful in identifying an intraabdominal source for infection. It may be difficult to recover organisms from cultures of peritoneal fluid, presumably because the burden of organisms is low. However, the yield can be improved if 10 mL of peritoneal fluid is placed directly into a blood culture bottle. Since bacteremia frequently accompanies PBP, blood should be cultured simultaneously. No specific radiographic studies are helpful in the diagnosis of PBP. A plain film of the abdomen would be expected to show ascites. Chest and abdominal radiography should be performed in patients with abdominal pain to exclude free air, which signals a perforation.

℞ TREATMENT

Treatment for PBP is directed at the isolate from blood or peritoneal fluid. Gram's staining of peritoneal fluid often gives negative results in PBP. Therefore, until culture results become available, empirical therapy should cover gram-negative aerobic bacilli and gram-positive cocci. Third-generation cephalosporins such as cefotaxime [2 g q8h, administered intravenously (IV)] provide reasonable initial coverage in moderately ill patients. Broad-spectrum antibiotics, such as penicillin/β-lactamase inhibitor combinations (e.g., piperacillin/tazobactam, 3.375 g q6h IV) or ceftriaxone (2 g q24h IV), are also options. Empirical coverage for anaerobes is not necessary. After the infecting organism is identified, therapy should be narrowed to target the specific pathogen. Patients with PBP usually respond within 72 h to appropriate antibiotic therapy. Antimicrobial therapy can be administered for as little as 5 days if rapid improvement occurs and blood cultures are negative, but a course of up to 2 weeks may be required for patients with bacteremia and for those whose improvement is slow. Persistence of leukocytes in the ascitic fluid after therapy should initiate a search for additional diagnoses.

Prevention PBP has a high rate of recurrence. Up to 70% of patients reportedly experience a recurrence within 1 year. Antibiotic prophylaxis reduces the rate of recurrence to <20%. Recommended prophylactic regimens include fluoroquinolones (ciprofloxacin, 750 mg weekly; norfloxacin, 400 mg/d) or trimethoprim-sulfamethoxazole (one double-strength tablet per day). However, long-term administration of broad-spectrum antibiotics in this setting has been shown to increase the risk of severe hospital-acquired staphylococcal infections and of high-level resistance to antibiotics.

SECONDARY PERITONITIS Secondary peritonitis develops when bacteria contaminate the peritoneum as a result of spillage from an intraabdominal viscus. The organisms found almost always constitute a mixed flora in which facultative gram-negative bacilli and anaerobes predominate, especially when the contaminating source is colonic. Early in the course of infection, when the host response is directed toward containment of the infection, exudate containing fibrin and PMNs is found. Early death in this setting is attributable to gram-negative bacillary sepsis and to potent endotoxins circulating in the bloodstream (Chap. 254). Gram-negative bacilli, particularly *E. coli*, are common bloodstream isolates, but *Bacteroides fragilis* bacteremia occurs as well. The severity of abdominal pain and the clinical course depend on the inciting process. The species of organisms isolated from the peritoneum also vary with the source of the initial process and the normal flora present at that site. Secondary peritonitis can result primarily from chemical irritation or bacterial contamination. For example, as long as the patient is not achlorhydric, a ruptured gastric ulcer will release low-pH gastric contents that will serve as a chemical irritant. The normal flora of the stomach comprises the same organisms found in the oropharynx (Chap. 148) but in lower numbers. The surfaces of teeth contain ~10^7 aerobic and 10^7 anaerobic organisms per milliliter of saliva; the normally acidic stomach contains an equal ratio of aerobic and anaerobic species, but in concentrations more in the range of 10^5/mL. After meals, when gastric acidity is highest, this number may fall to 10^3/mL. Thus, the bacterial burden in a ruptured gastric ulcer—or even a duodenal ulcer—is negligible compared with that in a ruptured appendix. The normal flora of the colon below the ligament of Treitz contains ~10^{11} anaerobic organisms per gram of feces but only 10^8 aerobes per gram; therefore, anaerobic species account for 99% of the bacteria. Leakage of colonic contents (pH 7 to 8) does not cause significant chemical peritonitis, but infection is intense because of the heavy bacterial load.

Depending on the inciting event, local symptoms may initially be found in secondary peritonitis—for example, epigastric pain from a ruptured gastric ulcer. In appendicitis (Chap. 281), the initial presenting symptoms are often vague, with periumbilical discomfort and nausea followed in a number of hours by pain more localized to the right lower quadrant. Unusual locations of the appendix (including a retrocecal position) can complicate this presentation further. Once infection has spread to the peritoneal cavity, however, pain increases, particularly with infection involving the parietal peritoneum, which is innervated extensively. Patients usually lie motionless, often with knees drawn up to avoid stretching the nerve fibers of the peritoneal cavity. Coughing and sneezing, which increase pressure within the peritoneal cavity, are associated with sharp pain. There may or may not be pain localized to the infected or diseased organ from which secondary peritonitis has arisen. Patients with secondary peritonitis generally have abnormal findings on abdominal examination, with marked voluntary and involuntary guarding of the anterior abdominal musculature. Later findings include tenderness, especially rebound tenderness. In addition, there may be localized findings in the area of the inciting event. In general, patients are febrile, with marked leukocytosis and a left shift of the WBCs to earlier granulocyte forms.

While recovery of organisms from peritoneal fluid is easier in secondary than in primary peritonitis, a tap of the abdomen is rarely the procedure of choice in secondary peritonitis. An exception is in cases involving trauma, where the possibility of a hemoperitoneum may need to be excluded early. Etiologic studies to find the source of peritoneal contamination should be undertaken.

℞ TREATMENT

Treatment for secondary peritonitis includes early administration of antibiotics aimed particularly at aerobic gram-negative bacilli and anaerobes (see below). Mild to moderate disease can be treated with many drugs covering these organisms, including broad-spectrum penicillin/β-lactamase inhibitor combinations (e.g., ticarcillin/clavulanate, 3.1 g q6h IV) or cefoxitin (2 g q24h IV). Patients requiring hospitalization in intensive care should receive imipenem (500 mg q6h IV), meropenem (1 g q8h IV), or combinations of drugs, such as ampicillin plus metronidizole plus ciprofloxacin. Secondary peritonitis usually requires both surgical intervention to address the inciting process and antibiotic administration to treat early bacteremia, to decrease the incidence of abscess formation and wound infection, and to prevent more distant spread of infection. Whereas surgery is rarely indicated in PBP in adults, it may be life-saving in secondary peritonitis.

PERITONITIS IN PATIENTS UNDERGOING CAPD A third type of peritonitis arises in patients who are undergoing continuous ambulatory peritoneal dialysis (CAPD). Unlike primary and secondary peritonitis, which are caused by endogenous bacteria, peritonitis in CAPD patients usually involves skin organisms. The pathogenesis of infection is similar to that of intravascular-device infection, in which skin organisms migrate along the catheter, which both serves as an entry point and exerts the effects of a foreign body. Exit-site or tunnel infection may or may not accompany CAPD peritonitis. Like PBP, CAPD peritonitis is usually caused by a single organism. Peritonitis is, in fact, the most common reason for discontinuation of CAPD. Improvements in equipment design, especially that of the Y-set connector, have resulted in a decrease from one case of peritonitis per 9 months of CAPD to one case per 15 months.

The clinical presentation of CAPD peritonitis resembles that of secondary peritonitis in that diffuse pain and peritoneal signs are common. The dialysate is usually cloudy and contains >100 WBCs per microliter, >50% of which are neutrophils. The most common etiologic organism is coagulase-negative *Staphylococcus*, which accounts for ~30% of cases. *Staphylococcus aureus* causes ~10% of cases, is more commonly identified among patients who are nasal carriers of the organism, and is the most frequent pathogen in those with an overt exit-site infection. Gram-negative bacilli and fungi such as *Candida* species are also found. Vancomycin-resistant enterococci (VRE) and vancomycin-intermediate *S. aureus* (VISA) have been reported to produce peritonitis in CAPD patients. The finding of more than one organism in dialysate culture should prompt a search for a cause of secondary peritonitis. As with primary peritonitis, culture of dialysate fluid in blood culture bottles improves the yield. To facilitate diagnosis, several hundred milliliters of removed dialysis fluid should be concentrated by centrifugation before culture.

℞ TREATMENT

Empirical therapy for CAPD peritonitis should be directed at *S. aureus*, coagulase-negative *Staphylococcus*, and gram-negative bacilli until the results of cultures are available. Since the advent of VRE and VISA, a first-generation cephalosporin such as cefazolin and a third-generation cephalosporin such as ceftazidime constitute the treatment of choice. A loading dose of cefazolin is administered intraperitoneally along with ceftazidime; doses depend on the dialysis method and the patient's renal function. If methicillin-resistant *S. aureus* is a relatively common isolate in a community, vancomycin may be a reasonable first choice for empirical therapy, especially in a toxic-appearing patient or a patient with an overt exit-site infection. The dose (2 g) is allowed to remain in the peritoneal cavity for 6 h. If the patient is severely ill, intravenous antibiotics similar to those in the dialysis bag should be added to the regimen at doses appropriate for the patient's degree of renal failure. The clinical response to an empirical treatment regimen should be rapid; if the patient has not responded after 48 h of treatment, catheter removal should be considered.

TUBERCULOUS PERITONITIS See Chap. 150.

FAMILIAL MEDITERRANEAN FEVER (See Chap. 279) Familial Mediterranean fever is an autosomal recessive disorder usually presenting with episodic bouts of peritonitis without an infectious etiology.

INTRAPERITONEAL ABSCESSES

Abscess formation is common in untreated peritonitis if overt gram-negative sepsis either does not develop or develops but is not fatal. In experimental models of abscess formation, mixed aerobic and anaerobic organisms have been implanted intraperitoneally. Without therapy directed at anaerobes, animals develop intraabdominal abscesses. As in humans, these experimental abscesses may stud the peritoneal cavity, lie within the omentum or mesentery, or even develop on the surface of or within viscera such as the liver.

PATHOGENESIS AND IMMUNITY There is often disagreement about whether an abscess represents a disease state or a host response. In a sense, it represents both: While an abscess is an infection in which viable infecting organisms and PMNs are contained in a fibrous capsule, it is also a process by which the host confines microbes to a limited space, thereby preventing further spread of infection. In any event, abscesses do cause significant symptoms, and patients with abscesses can be quite ill. Experimental work has helped to define both the host cells and the bacterial virulence factors responsible—most notably, in the case of *B. fragilis*. This organism, although accounting for only 0.5% of the normal colonic flora, is the anaerobe most frequently isolated from intraabdominal infections, is especially prominent in abscesses, and is the most common anaerobic bloodstream isolate. On clinical grounds, therefore, *B. fragilis* appears to be uniquely virulent. Moreover, *B. fragilis* acts alone to cause abscesses in animal models of intraabdominal infection, whereas most other *Bacteroides* species must act synergistically with a facultative organism to induce abscess formation.

Of the several virulence factors identified in *B. fragilis*, one is critical: the capsular polysaccharide complex (CPC) found on the bacterial surface. The CPC comprises at least eight distinct surface polysaccharides. Structural analysis of some of the polysaccharides in the CPC has shown an unusual motif of oppositely charged sugars. Polysaccharides having these *zwitterionic* characteristics, such as polysaccharide A (PS A), evoke a host response in the peritoneal cavity that localizes bacteria into abscesses. *B. fragilis* and PS A have been found to adhere to primary mesothelial cells in vitro; this adherence, in turn, stimulates the production of tumor necrosis factor α (TNF-α) and intercellular adhesion molecule 1 (ICAM-1) by peritoneal macrophages. Although abscesses characteristically contain PMNs, the process of abscess induction depends on the stimulation of T lymphocytes by these unique zwitterionic polysaccharides. The stimulated CD4+ lymphocytes secrete leukoattractant cytokines and chemokines. The alternative pathways of complement and fibrinogen also participate in abscess formation.

While antibodies to the CPC enhance bloodstream clearance of *B. fragilis*, CD4+ T cells are critical in immunity to abscesses. When administered subcutaneously, *B. fragilis* PS A has immunomodulatory characteristics and stimulates CD4+ T regulatory (Treg) cells via an interleukin (IL) 2–dependent mechanism to produce IL-10. IL-10 downregulates the inflammatory response, thereby preventing abscess formation.

CLINICAL PRESENTATION Most intraperitoneal abscesses result from fecal spillage from a colonic source, such as an inflamed appendix. Of all intraabdominal abscesses, 74% are intraperitoneal or retroperitoneal and are not visceral. Abscesses can also arise from a number of other processes. They usually form within weeks of the development of peritonitis and may be found in a variety of locations—from omentum to mesentery, pelvis to psoas muscles, and subphrenic space to a visceral organ such as the liver, where they may develop either on the surface of the organ or within it. Periappendiceal and diverticular abscesses occur commonly. Diverticular abscesses are least likely to rupture. Infections of the female genital tract and pancreatitis are also among the more common causative events. When abscesses occur in the female genital tract—either as a primary infection (e.g., tuboovarian abscess) or as an infection extending into the pelvic cavity or peritoneum—*B. fragilis* figures prominently among the organisms isolated. *B. fragilis* is not found in large numbers in the normal vaginal flora. It is encountered less commonly in pelvic inflammatory disease and endometritis, for example, without an associated abscess. In pancreatitis with leakage of damaging pancreatic enzymes, inflammation is prominent. Therefore, clinical findings such as fever, leukocytosis, and even abdominal pain do not distinguish pancreatitis itself from complications such as pancreatic pseudocyst, pancreatic abscess (Chap. 294), or intraabdominal collections of pus. Especially in cases of necrotizing pancreatitis, in which the incidence of local pancreatic infection may be as high as 30%, needle aspiration under CT guidance is performed as often as once a week to sample fluid for culture. Many centers prescribe prophylactic antibiotics to prevent infection in patients with necrotizing pancreatitis. Imipenem is the drug most frequently used for this purpose since it reaches high tissue levels in the pancreas (although it is not unique in this regard). If needle aspiration yields infected fluid, most experts agree that surgery is superior to percutaneous drainage.

DIAGNOSIS   A variety of scanning procedures have considerably facilitated the diagnosis of intraabdominal abscesses. Abdominal CT probably has the highest yield, although ultrasonography is particularly useful for the right upper quadrant, kidneys, and pelvis. Both indium-labeled WBCs and gallium tend to localize in abscesses and may be useful in finding a collection. Since gallium is taken up in the bowel, indium-labeled WBCs may have a slightly greater yield for abscesses near the bowel. Neither indium-labeled WBC nor gallium scans serve as a basis for a definitive diagnosis, however; both need to be followed by other, more specific studies, such as CT, if an area of possible abnormality is identified. Abscesses contiguous with or contained within outpouchings of bowel are particularly difficult to diagnose with scanning procedures. Occasionally, a barium enema may detect a diverticular abscess not diagnosed by other procedures, although barium should not be injected if a free perforation is suspected. If one study is negative, a second study sometimes reveals a collection. Although exploratory laparotomy has been less commonly used since the advent of CT, this procedure still must be undertaken on occasion if an abscess is strongly suspected on clinical grounds.

℞ TREATMENT

An algorithm for the management of patients with intraabdominal abscesses is presented in Fig. 112-1. The treatment of intraabdominal infections involves the determination of the initial focus of infection, the administration of broad-spectrum antibiotics targeted at organisms involved in the associated infection, and the performance of a drainage procedure if one or more definitive abscesses have already formed. Antimicrobial therapy, in general, is adjunctive to drainage and/or surgical correction of an underlying lesion or process in intraabdominal abscesses. Unlike the intraabdominal abscesses precipitated by most infections, for which drainage of some kind is generally required, abscesses associated with diverticulitis usually wall off locally after rupture of a diverticulum, so that surgical intervention is not routinely required.

A number of antimicrobial agents exhibit excellent activity against aerobic gram-negative bacilli. Since mortality in intraabdominal sepsis is linked to gram-negative bacteremia, empirical therapy for intraabdominal infection always needs to include adequate coverage of gram-negative aerobic, facultative, and anaerobic organisms. Even if anaerobes are not cultured from clinical specimens, they still must be

FIGURE 112-1   Algorithm for the management of patients with intraabdominal abscesses using percutaneous drainage. Antimicrobial therapy should be administered concomitantly. CT, computed tomography. [*Reprinted with permission from B Lorber (ed): Atlas of Infectious Diseases, vol VII: Intra-abdominal Infections, Hepatitis, and Gastroenteritis. Philadelphia, Current Medicine, 1995, pp 1–101, as adapted from OD Rotstein, RL Simmons, in SL Gorbach et al (eds): Infectious Diseases, Philadelphia, Saunders, 1992, p. 668.*]

covered by the therapeutic regimen. Broad-spectrum empirical antibiotic therapy should be the same as that discussed above for secondary peritonitis.

VISCERAL ABSCESSES ■ **Liver Abscesses**   The liver is the organ most subject to the development of abscesses. In one study of 540 intraabdominal abscesses over a 12-year period, 26% of these abscesses were visceral. Liver abscesses made up 13% of the total number of abscesses, or 48% of all visceral abscesses. Liver abscesses may be solitary or multiple; they may arise from hematogenous spread of bacteria or from local spread from contiguous sites of infection within the peritoneal cavity. In the past, appendicitis with rupture and subsequent spread of infection was the most common route for the development of a liver abscess. Currently, associated disease of the biliary tract is most often the etiology. Suppurative pylephlebitis (suppurative thrombosis of the portal vein), usually arising from infection in the pelvis but sometimes from infection elsewhere in the peritoneal cavity, is another common source for bacterial seeding of the liver.

Fever is the most common presenting sign of liver abscess. Some patients, particularly those with active associated disease of the biliary tract, have symptoms and signs localized to the right upper quadrant, including pain, guarding, punch tenderness, and even rebound tenderness. Nonspecific symptoms, such as chills, anorexia, weight loss, nausea, and vomiting, may also develop. Only 50% of patients with liver abscesses, however, have hepatomegaly, right-upper-quadrant tenderness, or jaundice; thus, half of patients have no symptoms or signs that would direct attention to the liver. Fever of unknown origin (FUO) may be the only presenting manifestation of liver abscess, especially in the elderly. Diagnostic studies of the abdomen, especially the right upper quadrant, should be a part of any FUO workup. The single most reliable laboratory finding is an elevated serum concentration of alkaline phosphatase, which is documented in 70% of patients with liver abscesses. Other tests of liver function may yield normal results, but 50% of patients have elevated serum levels of bilirubin, and 48% have elevated concentrations of aspartate aminotransferase. Other associated laboratory findings include leukocytosis in 77% of patients, anemia (usually normochromic, normocytic) in 50%, and hypoalbuminemia in 33%. Concomitant bacteremia is found in one-third of patients. A liver abscess is sometimes suggested by chest radiography, especially if a new elevation of the right hemidiaphragm is seen; other suggestive findings include a right basilar infiltrate and a right pleural effusion.

Imaging studies are the most reliable methods for diagnosing liver abscesses. These studies include ultrasonography, CT (Fig. 112-2), indium-labeled WBC or gallium scans, and magnetic resonance im-

FIGURE 112-2 Multilocular liver abscess on computed tomography scan. Multiple or multilocular abscesses are more common than solitary abscesses. [*Reprinted with permission from B Lorber (ed): Atlas of Infectious Diseases, Vol VII: Intra-abdominal Infection, Hepatitis, and Gastroenteritis. Philadelphia, Current Medicine, 1996, Fig. 1-70.*]

aging. In an occasional case, more than one such study may be required. Organisms recovered from liver abscesses vary with the etiology. In liver infection arising from the biliary tree, enteric gram-negative aerobic bacilli and enterococci are common isolates. Unless previous surgery has been performed, anaerobes are not generally involved in liver abscesses arising from biliary infections. In contrast, in liver abscesses arising from pelvic and other intraperitoneal sources, a mixed flora including both aerobic and anaerobic species is common; *B. fragilis* is the species most frequently isolated. With hematogenous spread of infection, usually only a single organism is encountered; this species may be *S. aureus* or a streptococcal species such as *S. milleri*. Results of cultures obtained from drain sites are not reliable for defining the etiology of infections. Liver abscesses may also be caused by *Candida* species; such abscesses usually follow fungemia in patients receiving chemotherapy for cancer and often present when neutrophils return after a period of neutropenia. However, the recovery of *Candida* from a drain site does not necessarily implicate this organism as a cause of infection. Amebic liver abscesses are not an uncommon problem (Chap. 194). Amebic serologic testing gives positive results in >95% of cases; thus, a negative result helps to exclude this diagnosis.

℞ TREATMENT

While drainage—either percutaneous (with a pigtail catheter kept in place) or surgical—remains the mainstay of therapy for intraabdominal abscesses (including liver abscesses), there is growing interest in medical management alone for pyogenic liver abscesses. The drugs used for empirical broad-spectrum antibiotic therapy include the same ones used in intraabdominal sepsis and secondary bacterial peritonitis. Usually, a diagnostic aspirate of abscess contents should be obtained before the initiation of empirical therapy, with antibiotic choices adjusted when the results of Gram's staining and culture become available. Cases treated without definitive drainage generally require longer courses of antibiotic therapy. When percutaneous drainage was compared with open surgical drainage, the average length of hospital stay for the former was almost twice that for the latter, although both the time required for fever to resolve and the mortality rate were the same for the two procedures. Mortality was appreciable despite treatment, averaging 15%. Several factors may predict the failure of percutaneous drainage and therefore may favor primary surgical intervention. These factors include the presence of multiple, sizable abscesses; viscous abscess contents that tend to plug the catheter; associated disease (e.g., disease of the biliary tract) that requires surgery; or the lack of a clinical response to percutaneous drainage in 4 to 7 days.

Treatment of candidal liver abscesses usually entails lengthy ad-

ministration of amphotericin B, although reports have described successful maintenance therapy with fluconazole after an initial course of amphotericin (Chap. 187).

Splenic Abscesses Splenic abscesses are much less common than liver abscesses. The incidence of splenic abscesses has ranged from 0.14 to 0.7% in various autopsy series. The clinical setting and the organisms isolated usually differ from those for liver abscesses. The degree of clinical suspicion for splenic abscess needs to be high, as this condition is frequently fatal if left untreated. Even in the most recently published series, diagnosis was made only at autopsy in 37% of cases. While splenic abscesses may arise occasionally from contiguous spread of infection or from direct trauma to the spleen, hematogenous spread of infection is the usual mode of development. Bacterial endocarditis is the most common associated infection (Chap. 109). Splenic abscesses can develop in patients who have received extensive immunosuppressive therapy (particularly those with malignancy involving the spleen) and in patients with hemoglobinopathies or other hematologic disorders (especially sickle cell anemia).

While ~50% of patients with splenic abscesses have abdominal pain, the pain is localized to the left upper quadrant in only half of these cases. Splenomegaly is found in ~50% of cases. Fever and leukocytosis are generally present; the development of fever preceded diagnosis by an average of 20 days in one series. Left-sided chest findings may include abnormalities to auscultation, and chest radiographic findings may include an infiltrate or a left-sided pleural effusion. When splenic abscesses are being considered in a differential diagnosis, CT scan of the abdomen has been the most sensitive diagnostic tool. Ultrasonography can yield the diagnosis, but cases have been missed with this modality. Liver-spleen scan or gallium scan may also be useful. Streptococcal species are the most common bacterial isolates from splenic abscesses, and *S. aureus* is the next most common; presumably these prevalences reflect the bacterial cause of the associated endocarditis. An increase in the frequency of isolation of gram-negative aerobic organisms from splenic abscesses has been reported; these organisms often derive from a urinary tract focus, with associated bacteremia, or from another intraabdominal source. *Salmonella* species are seen fairly commonly, especially in patients with sickle cell hemoglobinopathy. Anaerobic species accounted for only 5% of isolates in the largest collected series, but the reporting of a number of "sterile abscesses" may indicate that optimal techniques for the isolation of anaerobes were not employed.

℞ TREATMENT

Because of the high mortality figures reported for splenic abscesses, the treatment of choice is splenectomy with adjunctive antibiotics. However, percutaneous drainage has been successful. The most important factor in successful treatment of splenic abscesses is early consideration of the diagnosis.

Perinephric and Renal Abscesses Perinephric and renal abscesses are not common: The former accounted for only ~0.02% of hospital admissions and the latter for ~0.2% in Altemeier's series of 540 intraabdominal abscesses. While liver abscesses generally arise from contiguous foci of infection or track from other intraabdominal sources and splenic abscesses usually arise from hematogenous spread (e.g., spread from bacterial endocarditis), perinephric and renal abscesses have a different pathogenesis. Before antibiotics became available, most renal and perinephric abscesses were hematogenous in origin, with *S. aureus* most commonly recovered. Now, in contrast, >75% of perinephric and renal abscesses arise from an initial urinary tract infection. Infection ascends from the bladder to the kidney, with pyelonephritis occurring first. Bacteria may directly invade the renal parenchyma from medulla to cortex. Local vascular channels within the kidney may also facilitate the transport of organisms. Areas of abscess developing within the parenchyma may rupture into the perinephric space. The kidneys and adrenal glands are surrounded by a layer of perirenal fat that, in turn, is surrounded by Gerota's fascia, which extends superiorly to the diaphragm and inferiorly to the pelvic fat. When abscesses extend into the perinephric space, tracking may occur through Gerota's fascia into the psoas or transversalis muscles, into the anterior peritoneal cavity, superiorly to the subdiaphragmatic space, or inferiorly to the pelvis. Of the several risk factors that have been associated with the development of perinephric abscesses, the most important is the presence of concomitant nephrolithiasis producing local obstruction to urinary flow. Of patients with perinephric abscess, 20 to 60% have renal stones. In addition, other structural abnormalities of the urinary tract, a history of urologic surgery, trauma, and diabetes mellitus have all been identified as risk factors.

The organisms most frequently encountered in perinephric and renal abscesses are *E. coli*, *Proteus* species, and *Klebsiella* species. *E. coli*, the aerobic species most commonly found in the colonic flora, seems to have unique virulence properties in the urinary tract, including factors promoting adherence to uroepithelial cells. The urease of *Proteus* species splits urea, thereby creating a more alkaline and more hospitable environment for bacterial proliferation. *Proteus* species are frequently found in association with large struvite stones caused by the precipitation of magnesium ammonium sulfate in an alkaline environment. These stones serve as a nidus for recurrent urinary tract infection. While a single bacterial species is usually recovered from a perinephric or renal abscess, multiple species may also be found. If a urine culture is not contaminated with periurethral flora and is found to contain more than one organism, a perinephric abscess or renal abscess should be considered in the differential diagnosis. Urine cultures may also be polymicrobial in cases of bladder diverticulum.

Candida species should be considered in the etiology of renal abscesses. This fungus may spread to the kidney via the hematogenous route or by ascension from the bladder. The hallmark of the latter route of infection is ureteral obstruction with large fungal balls.

The presentation of perinephric and renal abscesses is quite nonspecific. Flank pain and abdominal pain are common. At least 50% of patients are febrile. Pain may be referred to the groin or leg, particularly with extension of infection. The diagnosis of perinephric abscess, like that of splenic abscess, is frequently delayed, and the mortality rate in some series is appreciable, although lower than in the past. Perinephric or renal abscess should be most seriously considered when a patient presents with symptoms and signs of pyelonephritis and remains febrile after 4 or 5 days, by which time the fever should have resolved. Moreover, when a urine culture yields a polymicrobial flora, when a patient is known to have renal stone disease, or when fever and pyuria coexist with a sterile urine culture, the diagnosis of perinephric or renal abscess should be entertained.

Renal ultrasonography and abdominal CT are the most useful diagnostic modalities. If a renal abscess or perinephric abscess is diagnosed, nephrolithiasis should be excluded, especially when a high urinary pH suggests the presence of a urea-splitting organism.

℞ TREATMENT

Treatment for perinephric or renal abscesses, like that for other intraabdominal abscesses, includes drainage of pus and antibiotic therapy directed at the organism(s) recovered. For perinephric abscesses, percutaneous drainage is usually successful.

Psoas Abscesses   The psoas muscle is another location in which abscesses are encountered. Psoas abscesses may arise from a hematogenous source, by contiguous spread from an intraabdominal or pelvic process, or by contiguous spread from nearby bony structures (e.g., vertebral bodies). Associated osteomyelitis due to spread from bone to muscle or from muscle to bone is common in psoas abscesses. When Pott's disease was common, *Mycobacterium tuberculosis* was a frequent cause of psoas abscess. Currently, either *S. aureus* or a mixture of enteric organisms including aerobic and anaerobic gram-negative bacilli is usually isolated from psoas abscesses in the United States. *S. aureus* is most likely to be isolated when a psoas abscess arises from hematogenous spread or a contiguous focus of osteomyelitis; a mixed enteric flora is the most likely etiology when the abscess has an intraabdominal or pelvic source. Patients with psoas abscesses frequently present with fever, lower abdominal or back pain, or pain referred to the hip or knee. CT is the most useful diagnostic technique.

℞ TREATMENT

Treatment includes surgical drainage and the administration of an antibiotic regimen directed at the inciting organism(s).

Pancreatic Abscesses   See Chap. 294.

FURTHER READING

Bassi C et al: Controlled clinical trial of pefloxacin versus imipenem in severe acute pancreatitis. Gastroenterology 115:1513, 1998

Campillo B et al: Epidemiology of severe hospital-acquired infections in patients with liver cirrhosis: Effect of long-term administration of norfloxacin. Clin Infect Dis 26:1066,1998

Finegold SM: Anaerobic bacteria: General concepts, in *Principles and Practice of Infectious Diseases*, 5th ed, GL Mandell et al (eds). New York, Churchill Livingstone, 2000, pp 2519–2537

Gibson FC III et al: Cellular mechanism of intraabdominal abscess formation by *Bacteroides fragilis*. J Immunol 160:5000, 1998

Levison ME, Bush LM: Peritonitis and other intra-abdominal infections, in *Principles and Practice of Infectious Diseases*, 5th ed, GL Mandell et al (eds). New York, Churchill Livingstone, 2000, pp 821–856

Robson RI et al: Differential regulation of chemokine production in human peritoneal mesothelial cells: IFN-gamma controls neutrophil migration across the mesothelium in vitro and in vivo. J Immunol 167:1028, 2001

Solomkin JS et al: Guidelines for the selection of anti-infective agents for complicated intra-abdominal infections. Clin Infect Dis 37:997, 2003

———— et al: Results of a randomized trial comparing sequential intravenous/ oral treatment with ciprofloxacin plus metronidazole to imipenem/cilastatin for intra-abdominal infections. Ann Surg 223:303, 1996

Tzianabos AO et al: T cells activated by zwitterionic molecules prevent abscesses induced by pathogenic bacteria. J Biol Chem 275:6733, 2000

---

113 ACUTE INFECTIOUS DIARRHEAL DISEASES AND BACTERIAL FOOD POISONING
Joan R. Butterton, Stephen B. Calderwood

Ranging from mild annoyances during vacations to devastating dehydrating illnesses that can kill within hours, acute gastrointestinal illnesses rank second only to acute upper respiratory illnesses as the most common diseases worldwide. In children <5 years old, attack rates range from 2 to 3 illnesses per child per year in developed countries to as high as 10 to 18 illnesses per child per year in developing countries. In Asia, Africa, and Latin America, acute diarrheal illnesses are not only a leading cause of morbidity in children—with an estimated 1 billion cases per year—but also a major cause of mortality, being responsible for 4 to 6 million deaths per year, or a sobering total of 12,600 deaths per day. In some areas, >50% of childhood deaths are directly attributable to acute diarrheal illnesses. In addition, by contributing to malnutrition and thereby reducing resistance to other infectious agents, gastrointestinal illnesses may be indirect factors in a far greater burden of disease.

The wide range of clinical manifestations of acute gastrointestinal illnesses is matched by the wide variety of infectious agents involved, including viruses, bacteria, and parasitic pathogens (Table 113-1). This chapter will discuss factors that enable gastrointestinal pathogens to cause disease, will review host defense mechanisms, and will delineate an approach to the evaluation and treatment of patients presenting with acute diarrhea. Individual organisms causing acute gastrointestinal illnesses are discussed in detail in subsequent chapters.

PATHOGENIC MECHANISMS Enteric pathogens have developed a variety of tactics to overcome host defenses. Understanding the virulence factors employed by these organisms is important in the diagnosis and treatment of clinical disease.

Inoculum Size The number of microorganisms that must be ingested to cause disease varies considerably from species to species. For *Shigella*, enterohemorrhagic *Escherichia coli*, *Giardia lamblia*, or *Entamoeba*, as few as 10 to 100 bacteria or cysts can produce infection, while 10^5 to 10^8 *Vibrio cholerae* organisms must be ingested orally to cause disease. The infective dose of *Salmonella* varies widely, depending on the species, host, and food vehicle. The ability of organisms to overcome host defenses has important implications for transmission; *Shigella*, enterohemorrhagic *E. coli*, *Entamoeba*, and *Giardia* can spread by person-to-person contact, whereas under some circumstances *Salmonella* may have to grow in food for several hours before reaching an effective infectious dose.

Adherence Many organisms must adhere to the gastrointestinal mucosa as an initial step in the pathogenic process; thus, organisms that can compete with the normal bowel flora and colonize the mucosa have an important advantage in causing disease. Specific cell-surface proteins involved in attachment of bacteria to intestinal cells are important virulence determinants. *V. cholerae*, for example, adheres to the brush border of small-intestinal enterocytes via specific surface adhesins, including the toxin-coregulated pilus and other accessory colonization factors. Different pathogenic varieties of *E. coli* have different adherence mechanisms. Enterotoxigenic *E. coli*, which causes watery diarrhea, produces an adherence protein called *colonization factor antigen* that is necessary for colonization of the upper small intestine by the organism prior to the production of enterotoxin. Enteropathogenic *E. coli*, an agent of diarrhea in young children, and enterohemorrhagic *E. coli*, which causes hemorrhagic colitis and the hemolytic-uremic syndrome, produce virulence determinants that allow these organisms to attach to and efface the brush border of the intestinal epithelium.

Toxin Production The production of one or more exotoxins is important in the pathogenesis of numerous enteric organisms. Such toxins include *enterotoxins*, which cause watery diarrhea by acting directly on secretory mechanisms in the intestinal mucosa; *cytotoxins*, which cause destruction of mucosal cells and associated inflammatory diarrhea; and *neurotoxins*, which act directly on the central or peripheral nervous system. Some exotoxins act by more than one mechanism; *Shigella dysenteriae* type 1, for example, produces an exotoxin that has both enterotoxic and cytotoxic activities.

The prototypical enterotoxin is cholera toxin, a heterodimeric protein composed of one A and five B subunits. The A subunit contains the enzymatic activity of the toxin, while the B subunit pentamer binds holotoxin to the enterocyte surface receptor, the ganglioside G_{M1}. After the binding of holotoxin, a fragment of the A subunit is translocated

TABLE 113-1 *Gastrointestinal Pathogens Causing Acute Diarrhea*

Mechanism	Location	Illness	Stool Findings	Examples of Pathogens Involved
Noninflammatory (enterotoxin)	Proximal small bowel	Watery diarrhea	No fecal leukocytes; mild or no increase in fecal lactoferrin	*Vibrio cholerae*, enterotoxigenic *Escherichia coli* (LT and/or ST), *Clostridium perfringens*, *Bacillus cereus*, *Staphylococcus aureus*, *Aeromonas hydrophila*, *Plesiomonas shigelloides*, rotavirus, Norwalk-like viruses, enteric adenoviruses, *Giardia lamblia*, *Cryptosporidium* spp., *Cyclospora* spp., microsporidia
Inflammatory (invasion or cytotoxin)	Colon or distal small bowel	Dysentery or inflammatory diarrhea	Fecal polymorphonuclear leukocytes; substantial increase in fecal lactoferrin	*Shigella* spp., *Salmonella* spp., *Campylobacter jejuni*, enterohemorrhagic *E. coli*, enteroinvasive *E. coli*, *Yersinia enterocolitica*, *Vibrio parahaemolyticus*, *Clostridium difficile*, ?*A. hydrophila*, ?*P. shigelloides*, *Entamoeba histolytica*
Penetrating	Distal small bowel	Enteric fever	Fecal mononuclear leukocytes	*Salmonella typhi*, *Y. enterocolitica*, ?*Campylobacter fetus*

Abbreviations: LT, heat-labile enterotoxin; ST, heat-stable enterotoxin.
Source: After Guerrant and Steiner.

across the eukaryotic cell membrane into the cytoplasm, where it catalyzes the ADP-ribosylation of a GTP-binding protein and causes persistent activation of adenylate cyclase. The end result is an increase of cyclic AMP in the intestinal mucosa, which increases Cl⁻ secretion and decreases Na⁺ absorption, leading to loss of fluid and the production of diarrhea.

Enterotoxigenic strains of *E. coli* may produce a protein called *heat-labile enterotoxin* (LT) that is similar to cholera toxin and causes secretory diarrhea by the same mechanism. Alternatively, enterotoxigenic strains of *E. coli* may produce *heat-stable enterotoxin* (ST), one form of which causes diarrhea by activation of guanylate cyclase and elevation of intracellular cyclic GMP. Some enterotoxigenic strains of *E. coli* produce both LT and ST.

Bacterial cytotoxins, in contrast, destroy intestinal mucosal cells and produce the syndrome of dysentery, with bloody stools containing inflammatory cells. Enteric pathogens that produce such cytotoxins include *S. dysenteriae* type 1, *Vibrio parahaemolyticus*, and *Clostridium difficile*. Shiga toxin–producing strains of *E. coli* (a group that includes enterohemorrhagic strains and whose most common serotype in the United States is O157:H7) produce potent cytotoxins that are highly related to the Shiga toxin of *S. dysenteriae* type 1. Such strains of *E. coli* have been associated with outbreaks of hemorrhagic colitis and hemolytic-uremic syndrome.

Neurotoxins are usually produced by the responsible organism outside the host and therefore cause symptoms soon after ingestion. Included are the staphylococcal and *Bacillus cereus* toxins, which act on the central nervous system to produce vomiting.

Invasion Dysentery may result not only from the production of cytotoxins but also from bacterial invasion and destruction of intestinal mucosal cells. Infections due to *Shigella* and enteroinvasive *E. coli*, for example, are characterized by the organisms' invasion of mucosal epithelial cells, intraepithelial multiplication, and subsequent spread to adjacent cells. *Salmonella*, on the other hand, causes inflammatory diarrhea by invasion of the bowel mucosa but generally is not associated with the destruction of enterocytes or the full clinical syndrome of dysentery. *Salmonella typhi* and *Yersinia enterocolitica* can penetrate intact intestinal mucosa, multiply intracellularly in Peyer's patches and intestinal lymph nodes, and then disseminate through the

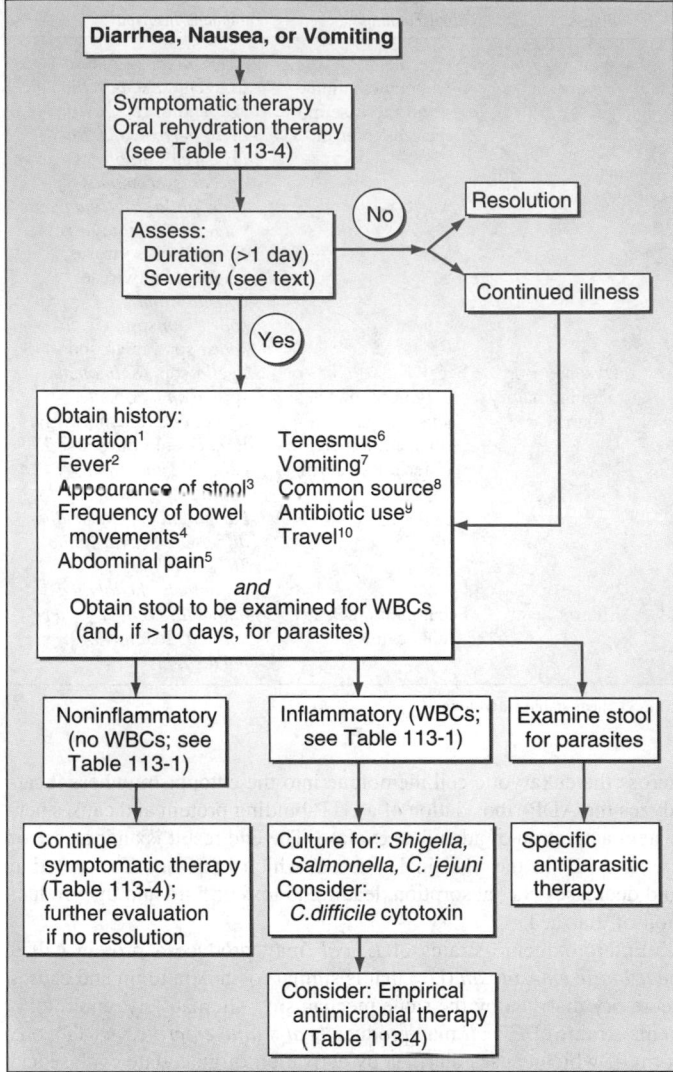

FIGURE 113-1 Clinical algorithm for the approach to patients with community-acquired infectious diarrhea or bacterial food poisoning. Key to superscripts: 1. Diarrhea lasting >2 weeks is generally defined as chronic; in such cases, many of the causes of acute diarrhea are much less likely, and a new spectrum of causes needs to be considered. 2. Fever often implies invasive disease, although fever and diarrhea may also result from infection outside the gastrointestinal tract, as in malaria. 3. Stools that contain blood or mucus indicate ulceration of the large bowel. Bloody stools without fecal leukocytes should alert the laboratory to the possibility of infection with Shiga toxin–producing enterohemorrhagic *Escherichia coli*. Bulky white stools suggest a small-intestinal process that is causing malabsorption. Profuse "rice-water" stools suggest cholera or a similar toxigenic process. 4. Frequent stools over a given period can provide the first warning of impending dehydration. 5. Abdominal pain may be most severe in inflammatory processes like those due to *Shigella*, *Campylobacter*, and necrotizing toxins. Painful abdominal muscle cramps, caused by electrolyte loss, can develop in severe cases of cholera. Bloating is common in giardiasis. An appendicitis-like syndrome should prompt a culture for *Yersinia enterocolitica* with cold enrichment. 6. Tenesmus (painful rectal spasms with a strong urge to defecate but little passage of stool) may be a feature of cases with proctitis, as in shigellosis or amebiasis. 7. Vomiting implies an acute infection (e.g., a toxin-mediated illness or food poisoning) but can also be prominent in a variety of systemic illnesses (e.g., malaria) and in intestinal obstruction. 8. Asking patients whether anyone else they know is sick is a more efficient means of identifying a common source than is constructing a list of recently eaten foods. If a common source seems likely, specific foods can be investigated. See text for a discussion of bacterial food poisoning. 9. Current antibiotic therapy or a recent history of treatment suggests *Clostridium difficile* diarrhea (Chap. 114). Stop antibiotic treatment if possible and consider tests for *C. difficile* toxins. Antibiotic use may increase the risk of other infections, such as salmonellosis. 10. See text (and Chap. 108) for a discussion of traveler's diarrhea. (*After Guerrant and Steiner; RL Guerrant, DA Bobak: N Engl J Med 325:327, 1991; with permission.*)

bloodstream to cause enteric fever, a syndrome characterized by fever, headache, relative bradycardia, abdominal pain, splenomegaly, and leukopenia.

HOST DEFENSES   Given the enormous number of microorganisms ingested with every meal, the normal host must possess effective defense mechanisms to combat a constant influx of potential enteric pathogens. Studies of infections in patients with alterations in these defenses have led to a greater understanding of the variety of ways in which the normal host can protect itself against disease.

Normal Flora   The large numbers of bacteria that normally inhabit the intestine act as an important host defense by preventing colonization by potential enteric pathogens. Persons with fewer intestinal bacteria, such as infants who have not yet developed normal enteric colonization or patients receiving antibiotics, are at significantly greater risk of developing infections with enteric pathogens. The composition of the intestinal flora is as important as the number of organisms present. More than 99% of the normal colonic flora is made up of anaerobic bacteria, and the acidic pH and volatile fatty acids produced by these organisms appear to be critical elements in resistance to colonization.

Gastric Acid   The acidic pH of the stomach is an important barrier to enteric pathogens, and an increased frequency of infections due to *Salmonella*, *G. lamblia*, and a variety of helminths has been reported among patients who have undergone gastric surgery or are achlorhydric for some other reason. Neutralization of gastric acid with antacids or H_2 blockers—common among hospitalized patients—similarly increases the risk of enteric colonization. Some microorganisms, however, can survive the extreme acidity of the gastric environment; rotavirus, for example, is highly stable to acidity.

Intestinal Motility   Normal peristalsis is the major mechanism for clearance of bacteria from the proximal small intestine, although gastric acidity and secreted immunoglobulins also play a role in limiting the number of organisms present. When intestinal motility is impaired—for example, by treatment with opiates or other antimotility drugs, anatomic abnormalities (diverticula, fistulas, or afferent-loop stasis following surgery), or hypomotility states (as in diabetes mellitus or scleroderma)—the frequency of bacterial overgrowth and infection of the small bowel with enteric pathogens is much increased. Some patients in whom *Shigella* infection is treated with diphenoxylate hydrochloride with atropine (Lomotil) experience prolonged fever and shedding of organisms, while patients treated with opiates for mild *Salmonella* gastroenteritis have a higher frequency of bacteremia than those not treated with opiates.

Immunity   Both cellular immune responses and antibody production play important roles in protecting susceptible hosts from enteric infections. The wide spectrum of viral, bacterial, parasitic, and fungal gastrointestinal infections in patients with AIDS highlights the significance of cell-mediated immunity in protecting the normal host from these pathogens. Humoral immunity is also important and consists of systemic IgG and IgM as well as secretory IgA. Growing evidence supports the concept of a mucosal immune system for secretory IgA in which binding of bacterial antigens to the luminal surface of M cells in the distal small bowel and subsequent presentation of antigens to subepithelial lymphoid tissue lead to the proliferation of sensitized lymphocytes. These lymphocytes circulate and populate all of the mucosal tissues of the body as IgA-secreting plasma cells.

APPROACH TO THE PATIENT

The approach to the patient with possible infectious diarrhea or bacterial food poisoning is shown in Fig. 113-1.

History   The answers to questions with high discriminating value can quickly narrow the range of potential causes of diarrhea and help determine whether treatment is needed. Important elements of the narrative history are detailed in Fig. 113-1.

Physical Examination The examination of patients for signs of dehydration provides essential information about the severity of the diarrheal illness and the need for rapid therapy. Mild dehydration is indicated by thirst, dry mouth, decreased axillary sweat, decreased urine output, and slight weight loss. Signs of moderate dehydration include an orthostatic fall in blood pressure, skin tenting, and sunken eyes (or, in infants, a sunken fontanelle). Signs of severe dehydration range from hypotension and tachycardia to confusion and frank shock.

Diagnostic Approach After the severity of illness is assessed, the most important distinction that the clinician must make is between *inflammatory* and *noninflammatory* disease. Using the history and epidemiologic features of the case as guides in making this distinction, the clinician can rapidly evaluate the need for further efforts to define a specific etiology and for therapeutic intervention. Examination of a stool sample is an important supplement to the narrative history. Grossly bloody or mucoid stool suggests an inflammatory process. A test for fecal leukocytes (preparation of a thin smear of stool on a glass slide, addition of a drop of methylene blue, and examination of the wet mount) can suggest inflammatory disease in patients presenting with diarrhea, although the predictive value of this test is still debated. A test for fecal lactoferrin, which is a marker of fecal leukocytes, is more sensitive and is available in latex agglutination and enzyme-linked immunosorbent assay formats. Causes of acute infectious diarrhea, categorized as inflammatory and noninflammatory, are listed in Table 113-1.

TABLE 113-2 *Epidemiology of Traveler's Diarrhea*

Etiologic Agent	Approximate Percentage of Cases	Comments
Enterotoxigenic *Escherichia coli*	15–50	Single most important agent, particularly in summertime in semitropical areas; percentage of cases ranges from 15% in Asia to 50% in Latin America
Enteroaggregative *E. coli*	10–20	May cause one-third of culture-negative cases
Shigella and enteroinvasive *E. coli*	10–25	Major causes of fever and dysentery
Salmonella	5–10	Causes fever and dysentery
Campylobacter jejuni	3–15	More common in winter in semitropical areas; more common in Asia
Aeromonas	5	Important in Thailand
Plesiomonas	5	Related to tropical travel and seafood consumption
Vibrio cholerae	0–10	Most common in India and Asia; also common in Central and South America
Rotavirus and Norwalk-like virus	10–40	Latin America, Asia, and Africa; Norwalk-like virus associated with seafood ingestion on cruise ships
Entamoeba histolytica	5	Particularly important in Mexico and Thailand
Giardia lamblia	<2	Zoonotic reservoirs in northern United States; affects hikers and campers who drink from freshwater streams; contaminates water supplies in Russia
Cryptosporidium	2	Affects travelers to Russia, Mexico, and Africa; causes large-scale urban outbreaks in United States
Cyclospora	<1	Affects travelers to Nepal, Haiti, and Peru; contaminates water or food
Unknown	20	Illness improves with antibacterial therapy, implicating bacterial diarrhea

Source: After Dupont

EPIDEMIOLOGY ■ Travel History Of the several million people who travel from temperate industrialized countries to tropical regions of Asia, Africa, and Central and South America each year, 20 to 50% experience a sudden onset of abdominal cramps, anorexia, and watery diarrhea; thus *traveler's diarrhea* is the most common travel-related illness (Chap. 108). The time of onset is usually 3 days to 2 weeks after the traveler's arrival in a tropical area; most cases begin within the first 3 to 5 days. The illness is generally self-limited, lasting 1 to 5 days. The high rate of diarrhea among travelers to underdeveloped areas is related to the ingestion of contaminated food or water.

The organisms that cause traveler's diarrhea vary considerably with location (Table 113-2). In all areas, enterotoxigenic *E. coli* is the most common isolate from persons with the classic secretory traveler's diarrhea syndrome.

Location Day-care centers have particularly high attack rates of enteric infections. Rotavirus is most common among children <2 years old, with attack rates of 75 to 100% among those exposed. *G. lamblia* is more common among older children, with somewhat lower attack rates. Other common organisms, often spread by fecal-oral contact, are *Shigella*, *Campylobacter jejuni*, and *Cryptosporidium*. A characteristic feature of infection among children attending day-care centers is the high rate of secondary cases among family members.

Similarly, hospitals are sites in which enteric infections are concentrated. In medical intensive-care units and pediatric wards, diarrhea is among the most common nosocomial infections. *C. difficile* is the predominant cause of nosocomial diarrhea among adults in the United States; viral pathogens, especially rotavirus, can spread rapidly in pediatric wards. Enteropathogenic *E. coli* has been associated with outbreaks of diarrhea in nurseries for newborns. One-third of elderly patients in chronic-care institutions develop a significant diarrheal illness each year. Surveillance stool cultures suggest that 25% of the residents of these institutions harbor cytotoxin-producing *C. difficile*, which causes more than half of all cases of diarrhea in this population. Antimicrobial therapy can predispose to pseudomembranous colitis by altering the normal colonic flora and allowing the multiplication of *C. difficile* (Chap. 114).

Age Most of the morbidity and mortality from enteric pathogens involves children <5 years of age. Breast-fed infants are protected from contaminated food and water and derive some protection from maternal antibodies, but their risk of infection rises dramatically when they begin to eat solid foods. Infants and younger children are more likely than adults to develop rotavirus disease, while older children and adults are more commonly infected with Norwalk-like viruses. Other organisms with higher attack rates among children than among adults include enterotoxigenic, enteropathogenic, and enterohemorrhagic *E. coli*; *C. jejuni*; and *G. lamblia*. In children, the incidence of *Salmonella* infections is highest among those <1 year of age, while the attack rate for *Shigella* infections is greatest among those 6 months to 4 years of age.

Bacterial Food Poisoning If the history and the stool examination indicate a noninflammatory etiology of diarrhea and there is evidence of a common-source outbreak, questions concerning the ingestion of specific foods and the time of onset of the diarrhea after a meal can provide clues to the bacterial cause of the illness. Potential causes of bacterial food poisoning are shown in Table 113-3.

Bacterial disease caused by an enterotoxin elaborated outside the host, such as that due to *Staphylococcus aureus* or *B. cereus*, has the shortest incubation period (1 to 6 h) and generally lasts <12 h. Most cases of staphylococcal food poisoning are caused by contamination from infected human carriers. Staphylococci can multiply at a wide range of temperatures; thus, if food is left to cool slowly and remains at room temperature after cooking, the organisms will have the opportunity to form enterotoxin. Outbreaks following picnics where potato salad, mayonnaise, and cream pastries have been served offer classic examples of staphylococcal food poisoning. Diarrhea,

TABLE 113-3 Bacterial Food Poisoning

Incubation Period, Organisms	Symptoms	Common Food Sources
1 TO 6 H		
Staphylococcus aureus	Nausea, vomiting, diarrhea	Ham, poultry, potato or egg salad, mayonnaise, cream pastries
Bacillus cereus	Nausea, vomiting, diarrhea	Fried rice
8 TO 16 H		
Clostridium perfringens	Abdominal cramps, diarrhea (vomiting rare)	Beef, poultry, legumes, gravies
B. cereus	Abdominal cramps, diarrhea (vomiting rare)	Meats, vegetables, dried beans, cereals
>16 H		
Vibrio cholerae	Watery diarrhea	Shellfish
Enterotoxigenic Escherichia coli	Watery diarrhea	Salads, cheese, meats, water
Enterohemorrhagic E. coli	Bloody diarrhea	Ground beef, roast beef, salami, raw milk, raw vegetables, apple juice
Salmonella spp.	Inflammatory diarrhea	Beef, poultry, eggs, dairy products
Campylobacter jejuni	Inflammatory diarrhea	Poultry, raw milk
Shigella spp.	Dysentery	Potato or egg salad, lettuce, raw vegetables
Vibrio parahaemolyticus	Dysentery	Mollusks, crustaceans

nausea, vomiting, and abdominal cramping are common, while fever is less so.

B. cereus can produce either a syndrome with a short incubation period—the *emetic* form, mediated by a staphylococcal type of enterotoxin—or one with a longer incubation period (8 to 16 h)—the *diarrheal* form, caused by an enterotoxin resembling *E. coli* LT, in which diarrhea and abdominal cramps are characteristic but vomiting is uncommon. The emetic form of *B. cereus* food poisoning is associated with contaminated fried rice; the organism is common in uncooked rice, and its heat-resistant spores survive boiling. If cooked rice is not refrigerated, the spores can germinate and produce toxin. Frying before serving may not destroy the preformed, heat-stable toxin.

Food poisoning due to *Clostridium perfringens* also has a slightly longer incubation period (8 to 14 h) and results from the survival of heat-resistant spores in inadequately cooked meat, poultry, or legumes. After ingestion, toxin is produced in the intestinal tract, causing moderately severe abdominal cramps and diarrhea; vomiting is rare, as is fever. The illness is self-limited, rarely lasting for more than 24 h.

Not all food poisoning has a bacterial cause. Diagnostic confusion can result from diarrhea caused by nonbacterial agents of short-incubation food poisoning, including capsaicin, which is found in hot peppers, and a variety of toxins found in fish and shellfish (Chap. 378).

LABORATORY EVALUATION Many cases of noninflammatory diarrhea are self-limited or can be treated empirically, and in these instances the clinician may not need to determine a specific etiology. Potentially pathogenic *E. coli* cannot be distinguished from normal fecal flora by routine culture. Special tests to detect LT and ST are not available in most clinical laboratories. In situations in which cholera is a concern, stool should be cultured on thiosulfate–citrate–bile salts–sucrose (TCBS) agar. A latex agglutination test has made the rapid detection of rotavirus in stool practical for many laboratories, while reverse-transcriptase polymerase chain reaction and specific antigen enzyme immunoassays have been developed for the identification of Norwalk-like viruses. At least three stool specimens should be examined for *Giardia* cysts or stained for *Cryptosporidium* if the level of clinical suspicion regarding the involvement of these organisms is high.

All patients with fever and evidence of inflammatory disease acquired outside the hospital should have stool cultured for *Salmonella*, *Shigella*, and *Campylobacter*. *Salmonella* and *Shigella* can be selected on MacConkey's agar as non-lactose-fermenting (colorless) colonies or can be grown on *Salmonella-Shigella* agar or in selenite enrichment broth, both of which inhibit most organisms except these pathogens. Evaluation of nosocomial diarrhea should initially focus on *C. difficile*; stool culture for other pathogens in this setting has an extremely low yield and is not cost-effective. Pathogenic strains of *C. difficile* generally produce two toxins, A and B. Toxin B can be detected with a cytotoxin assay; if the toxin is present, a monolayer culture of fibroblasts will show cytopathic effects within 6 to 24 h. Rapid enzyme immunoassays and latex agglutination tests for both toxin A and toxin B have been developed (Chap. 114). Isolation of *C. jejuni* requires inoculation of fresh stool onto selective growth medium and incubation at 42°C in a microaerophilic atmosphere. In many laboratories in the United States, *E. coli* O157:H7 is among the most common pathogens isolated from visibly bloody stools. Strains of this enterohemorrhagic serotype can be identified in specialized laboratories by serotyping but also can be identified presumptively in hospital laboratories as lactose-fermenting, indole-positive colonies of sorbitol nonfermenters (white colonies) on sorbitol MacConkey plates. Fresh stools should be examined for amebic cysts and trophozoites.

℞ TREATMENT

In many cases, a specific diagnosis is not necessary or not available to guide treatment. The clinician can proceed with the information obtained from the history, stool examination, and evaluation of the severity of dehydration. Empirical regimens for the treatment of traveler's diarrhea are listed in Table 113-4.

The mainstay of treatment is adequate rehydration. The treatment of cholera and other dehydrating diarrheal diseases was revolutionized by the promotion of oral rehydration solutions, the efficacy of which depends on the fact that glucose-facilitated absorption of sodium and water in the small intestine remains intact in the presence of cholera toxin. The use of oral rehydration solutions has reduced mortality due to cholera from >50% (in untreated cases) to <1%. The World Health Organization recommends a solution containing 3.5 g sodium chloride, 2.5 g sodium bicarbonate, 1.5 g potassium chloride, and 20 g glucose (or 40 g sucrose) per liter of water. Oral rehydration solutions containing rice or cereal as the carbohydrate source may be even more effective than glucose-based solutions. Patients who are severely dehydrated or in whom vomiting precludes the use of oral therapy should receive intravenous solutions such as Ringer's lactate.

Although most secretory forms of traveler's diarrhea—usually due to enterotoxigenic *E. coli*—can be treated effectively with rehydration, bismuth subsalicylate, or antiperistaltic agents, antimicrobial agents can shorten the duration of illness from between 3 and 4 days to between 24 and 36 h.

The antibiotic treatment of children who present with bloody diarrhea raises special concerns. Laboratory studies of enterohemorrhagic *E. coli* strains have demonstrated that a number of antibiotics induce replication of Shiga toxin–producing lambdoid bacteriophages, significantly increasing toxin production by these strains. Clinical studies have supported these laboratory results, and antibiotics are not recommended for the treatment of enterohemorrhagic *E. coli* infections in children.

PROPHYLAXIS Improvements in hygiene to limit fecal-oral spread of enteric pathogens will be necessary if the prevalence of diarrheal diseases is to be significantly reduced in developing countries. Travelers

Clinical Syndrome	Suggested Therapy
Watery diarrhea (no blood in stool, no fever), 1 or 2 unformed stools per day without distressing enteric symptoms	Oral fluids (Pedialyte, Lytren, or flavored mineral water) and saltine crackers
Watery diarrhea (no blood in stool, no fever), 1 or 2 unformed stools per day with distressing enteric symptoms	Bismuth subsalicylate (for adults): 30 mL or 2 tablets (262 mg/tablet) every 30 min for 8 doses; or loperamide[a]: 4 mg initially followed by 2 mg after passage of each unformed stool, not to exceed 8 tablets (16 mg) per day (prescription dose) or 4 caplets (8 mg) per day (over-the-counter dose); drugs can be taken for 2 days
Watery diarrhea (no blood in stool, no distressing abdominal pain, no fever), >2 unformed stools per day	Antibacterial drug[b] plus (for adults) loperamide[a] (see dose above)
Dysentery (passage of bloody stools) or fever (>37.8°C)	Antibacterial drug[b]
Vomiting, minimal diarrhea	Bismuth subsalicylate (for adults; see dose above)
Diarrhea in infants (<2 y old)	Fluids and electrolytes (Pedialyte, Lytren); continue feeding, especially with breast milk; seek medical attention for moderate dehydration, fever lasting >24 h, bloody stools, or diarrhea lasting more than several days
Diarrhea in pregnant women	Fluids and electrolytes; can consider attapulgite, 3 g initially, with dose repeated after passage of each unformed stool or every 2 h (whichever is earlier), for a total dosage of 9 g/d; seek medical attention for persistent or severe symptoms
Diarrhea despite trimethoprim-sulfamethoxazole prophylaxis	Fluoroquinolone—with loperamide[a] (see dose above) if no fever and no blood in stool, alone in cases of fever/dysentery
Diarrhea despite fluoroquinolone prophylaxis	Bismuth subsalicylate (see dose above) for mild to moderate disease; consult physician for moderate to severe disease or if disease persists

[a] Loperamide should not be used by patients with fever or dysentery; its use may prolong diarrhea in patients with infection due to *Shigella* or other invasive organisms.

[b] The recommended antibacterial drugs are as follows:
Travel to high-risk country other than Thailand:
Adults: A fluoroquinolone, such as ciprofloxacin, 500 mg bid; levofloxacin, 500 mg/d; norfloxacin, 400 mg bid; or ofloxacin, 400 mg bid on day 1; repeat on days 2 and 3 if diarrhea persists. Alternative agent: azithromycin, 500 mg on day 1, 250 mg on days 2 and 3 if diarrhea persists.
Children: Azithromycin, 10 mg/kg on day 1, 5 mg/kg on days 2 and 3 if diarrhea persists. Alternative agent: furazolidone, 7.5 mg/kg per day in four divided doses for 5 days.

Travel to Thailand (with risk of fluoroquinolone-resistant *Campylobacter*):
Adults: Azithromycin (at above dose for adults). Alternative agent: a fluoroquinolone (at above doses for adults).
Children: Same as for children traveling to other areas (see above).
All patients should take oral fluids (Pedialyte, Lytren, or flavored mineral water) plus saltine crackers. If diarrhea becomes moderate or severe, if fever persists, or if bloody stools or dehydration develops, the patient should seek medical attention.
Source: After Dupont.

can reduce their risk of diarrhea by eating only hot, freshly cooked food; by avoiding raw vegetables, salads, and unpeeled fruit; and by drinking only boiled or treated water and avoiding ice. In one cross-sectional epidemiologic survey, fewer than 3% of all European and North American travelers to Jamaica adhered to prescribed dietary restrictions, and travel health advice had no impact on the incidence of traveler's diarrhea; overall, the diarrhea attack rate among these travelers was 23.6%, with classic traveler's diarrhea in 11.7%.

Bismuth subsalicylate is an inexpensive agent for the prophylaxis of traveler's diarrhea; it is taken at a dosage of 2 tablets (525 mg) four times a day. Treatment appears to be effective and safe for up to 3 weeks. Prophylactic antimicrobial agents, although effective, are not generally recommended for the prevention of traveler's diarrhea, except when travelers are immunosuppressed or have other underlying illnesses that place them at high risk for morbidity from gastrointestinal infection. The risk of side effects and the possibility of developing an infection with a drug-resistant organism or with more harmful, invasive bacteria make it more reasonable to institute an empirical short course of treatment if symptoms develop.

The possibility of exerting a major impact on the worldwide morbidity and mortality associated with diarrheal diseases has led to intense efforts to develop effective vaccines against the common bacterial and viral enteric pathogens. Recent research has shown promising advances in the development of vaccines against rotavirus, *Shigella*, *V. cholerae*, *S. typhi*, and enterotoxigenic *E. coli*.

FURTHER READING

ANSDELL VE, ERICSSON CD: Prevention and empiric treatment of traveler's diarrhea. Med Clin North Am 83:945, 1999

BARTLETT JG: Clinical practice. Antibiotic-associated diarrhea. N Engl J Med 346:334, 2002

DUPONT HL: Travelers' diarrhea, in *Infections of the Gastrointestinal Tract*, 2d ed, MJ Blaser et al (eds). Philadelphia, Lippincott Williams & Wilkins, 2002, Chap 19

GUERRANT RL, STEINER TS: Principles and syndromes of enteric infection, in *Mandell, Douglas and Bennett's Principles and Practice of Infectious Diseases*, 5th ed, GL Mandell et al (eds). Philadelphia, Churchill Livingstone, 2000, Chap 81

RYAN ET et al: Illness after international travel. N Engl J Med 347:505, 2002

TALAN D et al: Etiology of bloody diarrhea among patients presenting to United States emergency departments: Prevalence of *Escherichia coli* O157:H7 and other enteropathogens. Clin Infect Dis 32:573, 2001

TAUXE RV et al: Foodborne disease, in *Mandell, Douglas and Bennett's Principles and Practice of Infectious Diseases*, 5th ed, GL Mandell et al (eds). Philadelphia, Churchill Livingstone, 2000, Chap 87

WONG CS et al: The risk of the hemolytic-uremic syndrome after antibiotic treatment of *Escherichia coli* O157:H7 infections. N Engl J Med 342:1930, 2000

DEFINITION *Clostridium difficile*–associated disease (CDAD) is a unique colon infection that is acquired almost exclusively in association with antimicrobial use and the consequent disruption of the normal colonic flora. The most commonly diagnosed diarrheal illness acquired in the hospital, CDAD results from the ingestion of spores of *C. difficile* that vegetate, multiply, and secrete toxins, causing diarrhea and pseudomembranous colitis (PMC).

ETIOLOGY AND EPIDEMIOLOGY *C. difficile* is an obligately anaerobic, gram-positive, spore-forming bacillus whose spores are found widely in nature, particularly in the environment of hospitals and chronic care facilities. CDAD occurs most frequently in hospitals and nursing homes where the level of antimicrobial use is high and the environment is contaminated by *C. difficile* spores.

Clindamycin, ampicillin, and cephalosporins were the first antibiotics associated with CDAD; the second- and third-generation cephalosporins, particularly cefotaxime, ceftriaxone, cefuroxime, and ceftazidime, are now the agents most frequently responsible for this condition. Penicillin/β-lactamase-inhibitor combinations such as ticarcillin/clavulanate and piperacillin/tazobactam pose significantly less risk. However, all antibiotics, including vancomycin and metronidazole (the agents most commonly used to treat CDAD), have been found to carry a risk of subsequent CDAD.

C. difficile is acquired exogenously, most frequently in the hospital, and is carried in the stool of symptomatic and asymptomatic patients. The rate of fecal colonization is often ≥20% among adult patients hospitalized for >1 week; in contrast, the rate is 1 to 3% among community residents. The risk of *C. difficile* acquisition increases in proportion to length of hospital stay. Asymptomatic fecal carriage of *C. difficile* in healthy neonates is very common, often exceeding 50% during the first 6 months of life. Spores of *C. difficile* are found on environmental surfaces (where the organism can persist for months) and on the hands of hospital personnel who fail to practice good hand hygiene. Hospital epidemics of CDAD have been attributed to a single *C. difficile* strain and to multiple strains present simultaneously. Other identified risk factors for CDAD include older age, greater severity of illness, use of electronic rectal thermometers, enteral tube feeding, antacid treatment, and gastrointestinal surgery.

PATHOLOGY AND PATHOGENESIS Spores of toxigenic *C. difficile* are ingested, survive gastric acidity, germinate in the small bowel, and colonize the lower intestinal tract, where they elaborate two large toxins: toxin A, an enterotoxin, and toxin B, a cytotoxin. These toxins initiate processes resulting in the disruption of epithelial-cell barrier function, diarrhea, and pseudomembrane formation. Toxin A is a potent neutrophil chemoattractant, and both toxins glucosylate the GTP-binding proteins of the Rho subfamily that regulate the actin cell cytoskeleton. Disruption of the cell cytoskeleton results in loss of cell shape, adherence, and tight junctions, with resultant fluid leakage. The pseudomembranes of PMC are confined to the colonic mucosa and initially appear as 1- to 2-mm whitish-yellow plaques. The intervening mucosa appears unremarkable, but, as the disease progresses, the pseudomembranes coalesce to form larger plaques and become confluent over the entire colon wall (Fig. 114-1). The whole colon is usually involved, but 10% of patients have rectal sparing. Viewed microscopically, the pseudomembranes have a mucosal attachment point and contain necrotic leukocytes, fibrin, mucus, and cellular debris. The epithelium is eroded and necrotic in focal areas, with neutrophil infiltration of the mucosa.

Patients colonized with *C. difficile* were initially thought to be at high risk for CDAD. However, four prospective studies have shown that colonized patients actually have a decreased risk of subsequent CDAD. At least three events are proposed as essential for the devel-

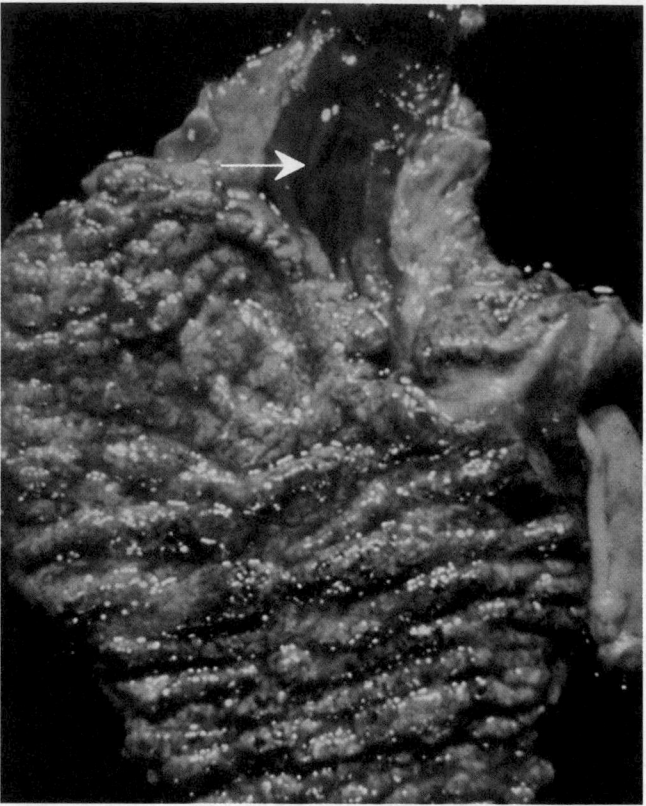

FIGURE 114-1 Autopsy specimen showing confluent pseudomembranes covering the cecum of a patient with pseudomembranous colitis. Note the sparing of the terminal ileum (*arrow*).

opment of CDAD (Fig. 114-2). Exposure to antimicrobial agents is the first event and establishes susceptibility to *C. difficile* infection. The second event is exposure to toxigenic *C. difficile*. Given that the majority of patients do not develop CDAD after the first two events, a third event is clearly essential for its occurrence. Candidate third

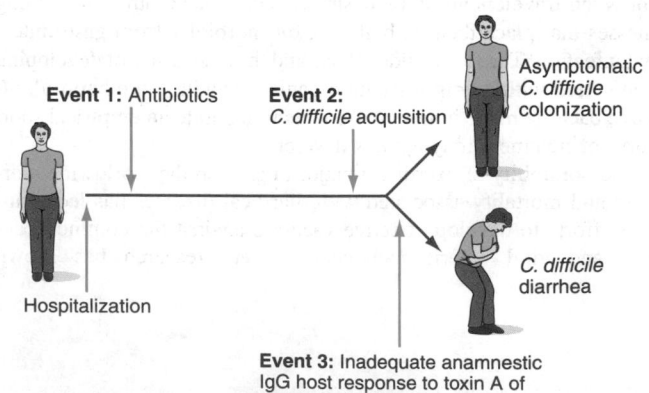

FIGURE 114-2 Pathogenesis model for hospital-acquired *Clostridium difficile*–associated diarrhea (CDAD). At least three events are integral to *C. difficile* pathogenesis. Exposure to antibiotics establishes susceptibility to infection. Once susceptible, the patient may acquire nontoxigenic (nonpathogenic) or toxigenic strains of *C. difficile* as a second event. Acquisition of toxigenic *C. difficile* may be followed by asymptomatic colonization or CDAD, depending on one or more additional events, including an inadequate host anamnestic IgG response to *C. difficile* toxin A.

events include exposure to a *C. difficile* strain of particular virulence, exposure to antimicrobial agents especially likely to cause CDAD, and an inadequate host immune response. The host anamnestic serum IgG antibody response to toxin A of *C. difficile* is the most likely third event that determines which patients will develop diarrhea and which patients will remain asymptomatic. The majority of humans first develop antibody to *C. difficile* toxins when colonized asymptomatically during the first year of life. Infants are thought not to develop symptomatic CDAD because they lack suitable mucosal toxin receptors that develop later in life. In adulthood, levels of antitoxin A IgG in serum increase more in response to infection in individuals who become asymptomatic carriers than in those who develop CDAD. For persons who develop CDAD, higher levels of antitoxin A correlate with a lower risk of recurrence of CDAD.

TABLE 114-1 *Relative Sensitivity and Specificity of Diagnostic Tests for Clostridium difficile–Associated Disease (CDAD)*

Type of Test	Relative Sensitivity[a]	Relative Specificity[a]	Comment
Stool culture for *C. difficile*	++++	+++	Most sensitive test; specificity is ++++ if the *C. difficile* isolate tests positive for toxin; with clinical data, is diagnostic of CDAD
Cell culture cytotoxin test on stool	+++	++++	With clinical data, is diagnostic of CDAD; highly specific but not as sensitive as stool culture
Enzyme immunoassay for toxin A or toxins A and B in stool	++ to +++	+++	With clinical data, is diagnostic of CDAD; rapid but not as sensitive as stool culture or cell culture cytotoxin test; rapid results
Latex test for *C. difficile* antigen in stool	++	+++	Detects glutamate dehydrogenase found in toxigenic and nontoxigenic strains of *C. difficile* and other stool organisms; less sensitive and specific than other tests; rapid results
Colonoscopy or sigmoidoscopy	+	++++	Highly specific if pseudomembranes are seen; insensitive compared with other tests

[a] According to both clinical and test-based criteria.
Note: ++++, >90%; +++, 71–90%; ++, 51–70%; +, ~50%.

CLINICAL MANIFESTATIONS Diarrhea is the most common symptom caused by *C. difficile*. Stools are almost never grossly bloody and range from soft and unformed to watery or mucoid in consistency, with a characteristic odor. Patients may have as many as 20 bowel movements per day. Clinical and laboratory findings include fever in 28% of cases, abdominal pain in 22%, and leukocytosis in 50%. When adynamic ileus (which is seen on x-ray in ~20% of cases) results in cessation of stool passage, the diagnosis of CDAD is frequently overlooked. A clue to the presence of unsuspected CDAD in these patients is unexplained leukocytosis with ≥15,000 cells/mm³. Such patients are at high risk for complications of *C. difficile* infection, particularly toxic megacolon and sepsis.

C. difficile diarrhea recurs after treatment in ~20% of cases. Recurrences may represent either relapses due to the same strain or reinfections with a new strain. Recurrence of clinical CDAD is likely to be a result of continued disruption of the normal fecal flora by the antibiotic used to treat CDAD.

DIAGNOSIS The diagnosis of CDAD is based on a combination of clinical criteria: (1) diarrhea (≥3 unformed stools per 24 h for ≥2 days), with no other recognized cause; plus (2) toxin A or B detected in the stool, toxin-producing *C. difficile* detected by stool culture, or pseudomembranes seen in the colon. PMC is a more advanced form of CDAD and is visualized at endoscopy in only ~50% of patients with diarrhea who have a positive stool culture and toxin assay for *C. difficile* (Table 114-1). Endoscopy is a rapid diagnostic tool in seriously ill patients with suspected PMC and an acute abdomen, but a negative result in this examination does not rule out CDAD.

Despite the array of tests available for *C. difficile* and its toxins (Table 114-1), no single test has high sensitivity, high specificity, and rapid turnaround. The turnaround time for reporting of a positive result in the cell cytotoxicity test can be shortened to <24 h if cell cultures are examined at intervals as short as 4 h. However, this approach is labor intensive, and observation for 48 h is required for a conclusive test result. Most laboratory tests for toxins lack sensitivity; thus, if the first specimen is negative and diarrhea persists, testing of additional stool specimens increases the likelihood of diagnosis. Empirical treatment is appropriate if CDAD is strongly suspected on clinical grounds. Testing of asymptomatic patients is not recommended except for epidemiologic study purposes. In particular, so-called "tests of cure" of asymptomatic treated patients are not recommended because many patients continue to harbor the organism and toxin after diarrhea has ceased and test results do not correlate with recurrence of CDAD. These test results should not be used to restrict placement of patients in long-term-care or nursing home facilities.

℞ TREATMENT

PRIMARY CDAD CDAD resolves in 15 to 23% of patients within 2 to 3 days after administration of the precipitating antimicrobial agent is discontinued, but most patients require specific treatment. General treatment guidelines include hydration and the avoidance of antiperistaltic agents and opiates, which may mask symptoms and possibly worsen disease. However, antiperistaltic agents have been used safely with vancomycin or metronidazole for mild to moderate CDAD. As mentioned above, test-of-cure cultures or toxin assays after treatment are not recommended; their results are not predictive of recurrence, and treatment of asymptomatic patients does not eradicate *C. difficile* from the stool.

Prospective randomized clinical trials show no statistical differences among the major therapeutic agents for the primary outcome end point of CDAD treatment: cessation of diarrhea (Table 114-2). The clinical response rate for bacitracin is 10 to 20% lower than that for vancomycin; therefore, bacitracin use for first-line therapy is discouraged. All drugs, particularly vancomycin, should be given orally if possible. When metronidazole is given intravenously, fecal bactericidal drug concentrations are achieved during acute diarrhea, and CDAD treatment has been successful; however, in the presence of adynamic ileus, intravenous metronidazole treatment of PMC has

TABLE 114-2 *Expected Treatment Outcomes Based on Randomized Comparative Trials of Oral Therapy for Initial Episodes of Clostridium difficile–Associated Diarrhea (CDAD)*

Treatment or Medication	Dose and Duration	Expected Resolution of Diarrhea, %	Expected Recurrence, %
Placebo or discontinuation of offending antibiotics	None	21	Unknown
Metronidazole	250 mg qid × 10 d	95	5
	500 mg tid × 10 d	94	17
Vancomycin[a]	500 mg tid × 10 d	94	17
	500 mg qid × 10 d	100	15
	125 mg qid × 7 d	86	33
	125 mg qid × 5 d	75	Unknown
Teicoplanin	400 mg bid × 10 d	96	7
	100 mg bid × 10 d	96	8
Fusidic acid	500 mg tid × 10 d	93	28
Bacitracin	25,000 U qid × 10 d	80	42

[a] Vancomycin treatment for first episodes of CDAD is discouraged because of possible development of vancomycin resistance in other nosocomial bacteria, such as enterococci.

failed. Diarrhea response rates to oral therapy with vancomycin or metronidazole are ≥94%. The mean interval to resolution of diarrhea is 2 to 4 days. Treatment should not be deemed a failure until a drug has been given for at least 6 days. On the basis of data for shorter courses of vancomycin (Table 114-2), it is recommended that treatment be given for 10 days, although no controlled comparisons are available. Metronidazole, although not approved by the U.S. Food and Drug Administration (FDA) for the treatment of CDAD, is the drug of first choice and the least expensive agent. Metronidazole-resistant isolates have been reported rarely, but treatment failure has not been attributed to resistance. Vancomycin as first-line treatment is discouraged because it may increase the incidence of vancomycin-resistant enterococci in hospitals.

Recurrent CDAD   In all, 15 to 25% of patients experience recurrences of CDAD, either as relapses caused by the original organism or as reinfections following treatment (Table 114-2). Re-treatment with metronidazole is recommended for first recurrences of CDAD. There is no standard treatment for multiple recurrences. Approaches include the administration of vancomycin, metronidazole, or bacitracin followed by the yeast *Saccharomyces boulardii* or *Lactobacillus* GG; the administration of vancomycin followed by synthetic fecal bacterial enema; and the intentional colonization of the patient with a nontoxigenic strain of *C. difficile*. None of these biotherapeutic agents is available in the United States as an FDA-approved pharmaceutical for treating CDAD. Other approaches include the use of vancomycin in tapering doses over 21 days, with subsequent pulse-dosing every several days for 21 days; the administration of vancomycin followed by that of the anion-exchange binding resin cholestyramine; and combined treatment with vancomycin and rifampin—the approach the authors favor (vancomycin, 125 mg four times daily, and rifampin, 300 mg twice daily, for 10 days). In antibody-deficient children, intravenous immunoglobulin has been used successfully to treat CDAD.

Fulminant CDAD   Fulminant CDAD is the most difficult treatment challenge in the rare patients who present with or develop toxic megacolon or ileus. These patients often do not have diarrhea, and their illness mimics an acute surgical abdomen. Sepsis (hypotension, fever, tachycardia, leukocytosis) may result from severe CDAD. An acute abdomen (with or without toxic megacolon) may include signs of obstruction, ileus, bowel-wall thickening, and ascites on abdominal computed tomography (CT), often with peripheral-blood leukocytosis (≥25,000 cells/mm³). Whether or not the patient has diarrhea, the differential diagnosis of an acute abdomen, sepsis, or toxic megacolon should include CDAD if the patient has received antibiotics in the past

2 months. Cautious sigmoidoscopy or colonoscopy to visualize PMC and an abdominal CT examination are the best diagnostic tests in patients without diarrhea.

Medical management of fulminant CDAD is suboptimal because of the difficulty of delivering metronidazole or vancomycin to the colon by the oral route in the presence of ileus. Six patients with severe ileus have been successfully treated by the authors with vancomycin—given via nasogastric tube and by retention enema—plus intravenous metronidazole. Surgical intervention is indicated for patients with suspected perforation of the colon or fulminant CDAD that does not respond to medical management. The incidence of fulminant CDAD requiring colectomy may be increasing, and surgical mortality may be >50% in this setting.

PROGNOSIS   The mortality rate attributed to CDAD is 0.6 to 3.5%, with the highest figures among the elderly. Most patients recover, but some have recurrences over months or years.

PREVENTION AND CONTROL   Strategies for the prevention of CDAD are of two types: those aimed at preventing transmission of the organism to the patient and those aimed at reducing the risk of CDAD if the organism is transmitted. Transmission of *C. difficile* in clinical practice has been prevented by gloving of personnel and elimination of the use of contaminated electronic thermometers. CDAD outbreaks have been most successfully controlled by restricting use of specific antibiotics, such as clindamycin and second- and third-generation cephalosporins. Outbreaks of CDAD due to clindamycin-resistant strains have resolved promptly when clindamycin use was restricted.

FURTHER READING

BIGNARDI GE: Risk factors for *Clostridium difficile* infection. J Hosp Infect 40:1, 1998

DALLAL RM et al: Fulminant *Clostridium difficile*: An underappreciated and increasing cause of death and complications. Ann Surg 235:363, 2002

FEKETY R: Guidelines for the diagnosis and management of *Clostridium difficile*–associated diarrhea and colitis. Am J Gastroenterol 92:739, 1997

GERDING DN et al: Society for Healthcare Epidemiology of America position paper on *Clostridium difficile*–associated diarrhea and colitis. Infect Control Hosp Epidemiol 16:459, 1995

JOHNSON S, GERDING DN: *Clostridium difficile* infection. Clin Infect Dis 26:1027, 1998

KYNE L et al: Association between antibody response to toxin A and protection against recurrent *Clostridium difficile* diarrhea. Lancet 357:189, 2001

WANAHITA A et al: Conditions associated with leukocytosis in a tertiary care hospital, with particular attention to the role of infection caused by *Clostridium difficile*. Clin Infect Dis 34:1585, 2002

WENISCH C et al: Comparison of vancomycin, teicoplanin, metronidazole, and fusidic acid for the treatment of *Clostridium difficile*–associated diarrhea. Clin Infect Dis 22:813, 1996

115 | SEXUALLY TRANSMITTED DISEASES: OVERVIEW AND CLINICAL APPROACH
King K. Holmes

CLASSIFICATION AND EPIDEMIOLOGY

Certain sexually transmitted diseases (STDs), such as syphilis, gonorrhea, HIV infection, hepatitis B, and chancroid, are most concentrated within "core populations" having high rates of partner change, concurrent partners, or "dense" sexual networks—for example, prostitutes and their clients, some homosexual men, and persons involved in the use of illicit drugs, particularly crack cocaine and methamphetamine. Other STDs are distributed more evenly throughout society. For example, chlamydial infections, genital infections with human papillomavirus (HPV), and genital herpes can spread efficiently in relatively low-risk populations.

In general, the product of three factors determines the initial rate of spread of any sexually transmitted infection (STI) within a population: rate of exposure of susceptible to infectious people, efficiency of transmission per exposure, and duration of infectivity of those in-

fected. Efforts to prevent and control STIs attempt to decrease the duration of infectivity (through early diagnosis and curative or suppressive treatment), to decrease the efficiency of transmission (e.g., through promotion of condom use and safer sexual practices), and to decrease the rate of exposure of susceptibles to infected persons (e.g., through individual counseling and efforts to change the norms of sexual behavior).

In all societies, STDs rank among the most common of all infectious diseases, with >30 infections now classified as predominantly sexually transmitted or as frequently sexually transmissible (Table 115-1). In developing countries, with three-quarters of the world's population and 90% of the world's STDs, such factors as population growth (especially in adolescent and young-adult age groups), rural-to-urban migration, wars, and poverty create exceptional vulnerability to disease resulting from risky sexual behaviors. During the 1990s, in

China, Russia, the other states of the former Soviet Union, and South Africa, internal social structures changed rapidly as borders opened to the West, unleashing enormous new epidemics of HIV infection and other STDs. HIV has become the leading cause of death in some developing countries, and HPV and hepatitis B virus (HBV) remain important causes of cervical and hepatocellular carcinoma, respectively—two of the most common malignancies in the developing world. Sexually transmitted herpes simplex virus (HSV) infections now cause most genital ulcer disease throughout the world and an increasing proportion of cases of genital herpes in developing countries with generalized HIV epidemics, where the positive feedback loop between HSV and HIV transmission is a growing, intractable problem. Globally, five curable STDs—gonorrhea, chlamydial infections, syphilis, chancroid, and trichomoniasis—caused ~350 million new infections annually in the mid-1990s. Up to 50% of women of reproductive age in developing countries have bacterial vaginosis (arguably acquired sexually). All six of these curable infections have been associated with increased risk of HIV transmission or acquisition.

In the industrialized countries, fear of HIV infection since the mid-1980s, coupled with widespread behavioral interventions and better-organized systems of care for the curable STDs, have helped curb the transmission of the latter diseases. Nonetheless, foci of hyperendemic transmission persist in the southeastern United States and in most large U.S. cities. Rates of gonorrhea and syphilis remain higher in the United States than in any other Western industrialized country. The remarkable resurgence of gonorrhea and syphilis among homosexual and bisexual men in many parts of the United States and Europe since the 1990s reflects increased risk-taking since the advent of potent antiretroviral therapy and has been accompanied by increasing HIV transmission in this group. The prevalence of antibody to HSV-2 has begun to fall only recently (since the mid-1990s), and genital HPV remains the most common sexually transmitted pathogen, infecting one-third of a cohort of U.S. college women within 2 years in a study conducted during the 1990s.

MANAGEMENT OF COMMON STD SYNDROMES

Although other chapters discuss management of specific STIs, delineating treatment based on diagnosis of a specific infection, most patients are actually managed (at least initially) on the basis of presenting symptoms and signs and associated risk factors, even in industrialized countries. Table 115-2 lists some of the most common clinical STD syndromes and their microbial etiologies. Strategies for their management are outlined below. →*Chapters 172 and 173 address the management of infections with human retroviruses.*

STD care and management begin with risk assessment and proceed to clinical assessment, diagnostic testing or screening, treatment, and prevention. Indeed, the routine care of any patient begins with risk assessment (e.g., for risk of heart disease, cancer). STD/HIV risk assessment is important in primary care, urgent care, and emergency care settings as well as in specialty clinics providing adolescent, prenatal, and family planning services. STD/HIV risk assessment guides interpretation of symptoms that could reflect an STD; decisions on screening or prophylactic/preventive treatment; risk reduction counseling and intervention (e.g., hepatitis B vaccination); and notification of partners of patients with known infections. Consideration of routine demographic data (e.g., gender, age, marital status, area of residence) is a simple first step in STD/HIV risk assessment. For example, national guidelines now recommend routine screening of sexually active fe-

males ≤25 years of age for *Chlamydia trachomatis* infection. Table 115-3 provides a set of 10 STD/HIV risk-assessment questions that clinicians can pose verbally or that health care systems can adapt (with yes/no responses) into a routine self-administered questionnaire for use in clinics. The initial framing statement gives permission to discuss taboo topics.

Risk assessment is followed by clinical assessment (elicitation of information on specific current symptoms and signs of STDs). Confirmatory diagnostic tests (for persons with symptoms or signs) or screening tests (for those without symptoms or signs) may involve microscopic examination, culture, antigen detection tests, genetic probe or amplification tests, or serology. Initial syndrome-based treatment should cover the most likely causes. For certain syndromes, results of rapid tests can narrow the spectrum of this initial therapy (e.g., wet mount of vaginal fluid for women with vaginal discharge, Gram's stain of urethral discharge for men with urethral discharge, rapid plasma reagin test for genital ulcer). After the institution of treatment, STD management proceeds to the "4 C's" of prevention and control: contact tracing (see "Prevention and Control of STDs," below), ensuring compliance with therapy, and counseling on risk reduction, including condom promotion and provision.

URETHRITIS IN MEN During the 1990s, the incidence of reported gonorrhea among men in the United States fell to 126 cases per 100,000 population; the incidence figures then leveled off through 2002. The incidence of reported *C. trachomatis* infections among men has been increasing steadily (with increased testing), reaching 130 cases per 100,000 in 2002. Until recently, *C. trachomatis* caused ~30 to 40% of cases of nongonococcal urethritis (NGU); however, the proportion of cases due to this organism may have declined in some populations served by effective chlamydial-control programs. HSV and *Trichomonas vaginalis* each cause a small proportion of NGU cases in the United States. Recently, multiple studies have consistently implicated *Mycoplasma genitalium* as a probable cause of many *Chlamydia*-negative cases, while fewer studies than in the past have implicated *Ureaplasma urealyticum*. Coliform bacteria can cause urethritis in men who practice insertive anal intercourse. The initial diagnosis of urethritis in men currently includes specific tests only for *Neisseria gonorrhoeae*

TABLE 115-1 Sexually Transmitted and Sexually Transmissible Microorganisms

Bacteria	Viruses	Other[a]
TRANSMITTED IN ADULTS PREDOMINANTLY BY SEXUAL INTERCOURSE		
Neisseria gonorrhoeae	HIV (types 1 and 2)	*Trichomonas vaginalis*
Chlamydia trachomatis	Human T-cell lymphotropic virus type I	*Phthirus pubis*
Treponema pallidum	Herpes simplex virus type 2	
Haemophilus ducreyi	Human papillomavirus (multiple genotypes)	
Calymmatobacterium granulomatis	Hepatitis B virus[b]	
Ureaplasma urealyticum	Molluscum contagiosum virus	
SEXUAL TRANSMISSION REPEATEDLY DESCRIBED BUT NOT WELL DEFINED OR NOT THE PREDOMINANT MODE		
Mycoplasma hominis	Cytomegalovirus	*Candida albicans*
Mycoplasma genitalium	Human T-cell lymphotropic virus type II	*Sarcoptes scabiei*
Gardnerella vaginalis and other vaginal bacteria	(?) Hepatitis C, D viruses	
Group B *Streptococcus*	Herpes simplex virus type 1	
Mobiluncus spp.	(?) Epstein-Barr virus	
Helicobacter cinaedi	Kaposi's sarcoma–associated herpesvirus[c]	
Sporothrix fennelliae	Transfusion-transmitted virus	
TRANSMITTED BY SEXUAL CONTACT INVOLVING ORAL-FECAL EXPOSURE; OF DECLINING IMPORTANCE IN HOMOSEXUAL MEN		
Shigella spp.	Hepatitis A virus	*Giardia lamblia*
Campylobacter spp.		*Entamoeba histolytica*

[a] Includes protozoa, ectoparasites, and fungi.
[b] Among U.S. patients for whom a risk factor can be ascertained, most hepatitis B virus infections are transmitted sexually or by injection drug use.
[c] Human herpesvirus type 8.

TABLE 115-2 *Major STD Syndromes and Sexually Transmitted Microbial Etiologies*

Syndrome	ST Microbial Etiologies
AIDS	HIV types 1 and 2
Urethritis: males	*Neisseria gonorrhoeae, Chlamydia trachomatis, Mycoplasma genitalium, Ureaplasma urealyticum, Trichomonas vaginalis,* HSV
Epididymitis	*C. trachomatis, N. gonorrhoeae*
Lower genital tract infections: females	
Cystitis/urethritis	*C. trachomatis, N. gonorrhoeae,* HSV
Mucopurulent cervicitis	*C. trachomatis, N. gonorrhoeae, M. genitalium*
Vulvitis	*Candida albicans,* HSV
Vulvovaginitis	*C. albicans, T. vaginalis*
Bacterial vaginosis (BV)	BV-associated bacteria (see text)
Acute pelvic inflammatory disease	*N. gonorrhoeae, C. trachomatis,* BV-associated bacteria, group B streptococci, *M. genitalium*
Infertility	*N. gonorrhoeae, C. trachomatis,* BV-associated bacteria
Ulcerative lesions of the genitalia	HSV-1, HSV-2, *Treponema pallidum, Haemophilus ducreyi, C. trachomatis* (LGV strains), *Calymmatobacterium granulomatis*
Complications of pregnancy/puerperium	Several agents implicated
Intestinal infections	
Proctitis	*C. trachomatis, N. gonorrhoeae,* HSV, *T. pallidum*
Proctocolitis or enterocolitis	*Campylobacter* spp., *Shigella* spp., *Entamoeba histolytica,* other enteric pathogens
Enteritis	*Giardia lamblia*
Acute arthritis with urogenital infection or viremia	*N. gonorrhoeae* (e.g., DGI), *C. trachomatis* (e.g., Reiter's syndrome), HBV
Genital and anal warts	HPV (30 genital types)
Mononucleosis syndrome	CMV, HIV, EBV
Hepatitis	Hepatitis viruses, *T. pallidum,* CMV, EBV
Neoplasias	
Squamous cell dysplasias and cancers of the cervix, anus, vulva, vagina, or penis	HPV (especially types 16, 18, 31, 45)
Kaposi's sarcoma, body-cavity lymphomas	HHV-8
T cell leukemia	HTLV-I
Hepatocellular carcinoma	HBV
Tropical spastic paraparesis	HTLV-I
Scabies	*Sarcoptes scabiei*
Pubic lice	*Phthirus pubis*

Note: HSV, herpes simplex virus; LGV, lymphogranuloma venereum; DGI, disseminated gonococcal infection; HPV, human papillomavirus; CMV, cytomegalovirus; EBV, Epstein-Barr virus; HBV, hepatitis B virus; HTLV, human T-cell lymphotropic virus; HHV-8, human herpesvirus type 8.

and *C. trachomatis.* The following summarizes the approach to the patient with suspected urethritis:

1. *Establish the presence of urethritis.* If proximal-to-distal "milking" of the urethra does not express a purulent or mucopurulent discharge, even after the patient has not voided for several hours or preferably overnight, a Gram's-stained smear of overt discharge or of an anterior urethral specimen obtained by passage of a small urethrogenital swab 2 to 3 cm into the urethra usually reveals ≥5 neutrophils per 1000× field in areas containing cells; in gonococcal infection, such a smear usually reveals gram-negative intracellular diplococci as well. Alternatively, the centrifuged sediment

of the first 20 to 30 mL of voided urine can be examined for inflammatory cells, either by microscopy showing ≥10 leukocytes per high-power field or by the leukocyte esterase test. Patients with symptoms who lack objective evidence of urethritis may have functional rather than organic problems and generally do not benefit from repeated courses of antibiotics.

2. *Evaluate for complications or alternative diagnoses.* A brief history and examination will exclude epididymitis and systemic complications, such as disseminated gonococcal infection (DGI) and Reiter's syndrome. Although digital examination of the prostate gland seldom contributes to the evaluation of sexually active young men with urethritis, men with dysuria who lack evidence of urethritis as well as sexually inactive men with urethritis should undergo prostate palpation, urinalysis, and urine culture to exclude bacterial prostatitis and cystitis.

3. *Evaluate for gonococcal and chlamydial infection.* An absence of typical gram-negative diplococci on Gram's-stained smear of urethral exudate containing inflammatory cells warrants a preliminary diagnosis of NGU and should lead to testing of the urethral specimen for *C. trachomatis.* Culture or DNA detection tests for *N. gonorrhoeae* may be positive when Gram's staining is negative; certain strains of *N. gonorrhoeae* can result in negative urethral Gram's stains in up to 30% of cases of urethritis. Results of tests for gonococcal and chlamydial infection predict the patient's prognosis (with greater risk for recurrent NGU if neither chlamydiae nor gonococci are found than if either is detected) and can

TABLE 115-3 *Ten-Question STD/HIV Risk Assessment*

Framing Statement:
In order to provide the best care for you today and to understand your risk for certain infections, it is necessary for us to talk about your sexual behavior.

Screening Questions:
(1) Do you have any reason to think you might have a sexually transmitted disease? If so, what reason?
(2) For all adolescents <18 years old: Have you begun having any kind of sex yet?

STD History:
(3) Have you ever had any sexually transmitted diseases or any genital infections? If so, which ones?

Sexual Preference:
(4) Have you had sex with men, women, or both?

Injection Drug Use:
(5) Have you ever injected yourself ("shot up") with drugs? (If yes, have you ever shared needles or injection equipment?)
(6) Have you ever had sex with a gay or bisexual man or with anyone who had ever injected drugs?

Characteristics of Partner(s):
(7) Has your sex partner(s) had any sexually transmitted infections? If so, which ones?

STD Symptoms Checklist:
(8) Have you recently developed any of these symptoms?

For Men	For Women
(a) Discharge of pus (drip) from the penis	(a) Abnormal vaginal discharge (increased amount, abnormal odor, abnormal yellow color)
(b) Genital sores (ulcers) or rash	(b) Genital sores (ulcers), rash, or itching

Sexual Practices, Past 2 Months (for patients answering yes to any of the above questions, to guide examination and testing):
(9) Now I'd like to ask what parts of your body may have been sexually exposed to an STD (e.g., your penis, mouth, vagina, anus)?
Query about Interest in STD Screening Tests (for patients answering no to all of the above questions):
(10) Would you like to be tested for HIV or any other STDs today? (If yes, clinician can explore which STD and why.)

Source: Adapted from JR Curtis, KK Holmes, in KK Holmes et al (eds): *Sexually Transmitted Diseases,* 3d ed. New York, McGraw-Hill, 1999.

TABLE 115-4 *Management of Urethral Discharge in Men*

Usual causes	Usual initial evaluation
Chlamydia trachomatis	Demonstration of urethral discharge or pyuria
Neisseria gonorrhoeae	
Ureaplasma urealyticum	Exclusion of local or systemic complications
Trichomonas vaginalis	
Herpes simplex virus	Urethral Gram's stain to confirm urethritis, detect gram-negative diplococci
Mycoplasma genitalium	
	Test for *N. gonorrhoeae, C. trachomatis*

INITIAL TREATMENT FOR PATIENT AND PARTNERS

Treat gonorrhea (unless excluded):	plus	Treat chlamydial infection:
Cefpodoxime, 400 mg PO; *or*		Azithromycin, 1 g PO; *or*
Ceftriaxone, 125 mg IM; *or*		
Fluoroquinolone (e.g., cipro-floxacin, 500 mg PO)		Doxycycline, 100 mg bid for 7 days

MANAGEMENT OF RECURRENCE

Confirm objective evidence of urethritis. If patient was reexposed to untreated or new partner, repeat treatment of patient and partner. If patient was not reexposed, consider infection with *T. vaginalis*[a] or doxycycline-resistant *Ureaplasma*, and consider treatment with metronidazole or azithromycin.

[a] In men, the diagnosis of *T. vaginalis* infection requires culture (or nucleic acid amplification test, where available) of early-morning first-voided urine sediment or of a urethral swab specimen obtained before voiding.

guide both the counseling given to the patient and the management of the patient's sexual partner(s).

4. *Treat urethritis.*

Table 115-4 summarizes the steps in management of sexually active men with symptoms of urethral discharge and/or dysuria.

℞ TREATMENT

In practice, if Gram's stain does not reveal gonococci, urethritis is treated with a regimen effective for NGU, such as azithromycin (1.0 g orally in a single dose) or doxycycline (100 mg orally bid for 7 days). If gonococci are demonstrated by Gram's stain or if no diagnostic tests are performed to definitively exclude gonorrhea, treatment should include a single-dose regimen for gonorrhea (Chap. 128) plus azithromycin or doxycycline treatment for *C. trachomatis*. Sexual partners should be tested for gonorrhea and chlamydial infection and should receive the same regimen given to the male index case. Patients with confirmed persistence or recurrence of urethritis after treatment should be re-treated with the initial regimen if they did not comply with the original treatment or were reexposed to an untreated partner. Otherwise, an intraurethral swab specimen and a first-voided urine sample should be cultured for *T. vaginalis*. If compliance with initial treatment is confirmed and reexposure excluded, treatment with metronidazole (2 g orally in a single dose) plus erythromycin base (500 mg orally qid for 7 days) is recommended.

EPIDIDYMITIS Acute epididymitis, almost always unilateral, must be differentiated from testicular torsion, tumor, and trauma. Torsion, a surgical emergency, usually occurs in the second or third decade of life and produces a sudden onset of pain, elevation of the testicle within the scrotal sac, rotation of the epididymis from a posterior to an anterior position, and absence of blood flow on Doppler examination or ^{99m}Tc scan. Persistence of symptoms after a course of therapy for epididymitis suggests the possibility of testicular tumor. In sexually active men under age 35, acute epididymitis is caused most frequently by *C. trachomatis* and less commonly by *N. gonorrhoeae* and is usually associated with overt or subclinical urethritis. Acute epididymitis occurring in older men or following urinary tract instrumentation is usually caused by urinary pathogens. Similarly, epididymitis in men who have practiced insertive rectal intercourse is often caused by En-

terobacteriaceae. These men usually have no urethritis but do have bacteriuria.

℞ TREATMENT

Ceftriaxone (250 mg as a single dose IM) followed by doxycycline (100 mg orally bid for 10 days) is effective for epididymitis caused by *N. gonorrhoeae* or *C. trachomatis*. Alternatively, ofloxacin (300 mg orally bid for 10 days) or levofloxacin (500 mg orally once daily for 10 days) is also effective for syndrome-based treatment of epididymitis because of effectiveness against Enterobacteriaceae as well as *N. gonorrhoeae* and *C. trachomatis*; however, emerging gonococcal resistance to fluoroquinolones now limits the use of these drugs in some areas.

URETHRITIS AND THE URETHRAL SYNDROME IN WOMEN *C. trachomatis, N. gonorrhoeae,* and occasionally HSV cause symptomatic urethritis—known as the urethral syndrome in women—characterized by "internal" dysuria (usually without urinary urgency or frequency) and pyuria, with *Escherichia coli* or other uropathogens not present in urine at counts of ≥10^2/mL. In contrast, the dysuria associated with vulvar herpes or vulvovaginal candidiasis (and perhaps with trichomoniasis) is often described as "external," being caused by painful contact of urine with the inflamed or ulcerated labia or introitus. Acute onset, association with urinary urgency or frequency, hematuria, or suprapubic bladder tenderness suggests bacterial cystitis. Among women with symptoms of acute bacterial cystitis, costovertebral pain and tenderness or fever suggests acute pyelonephritis. →*The management of bacterial urinary tract infection (UTI) is discussed in Chap. 269.*

Signs of vulvovaginitis, coupled with symptoms of external dysuria, suggest vulvar infection (e.g., with HSV or *Candida albicans*). Among dysuric women without signs of vulvovaginitis, bacterial UTI must be differentiated from the urethral syndrome by assessment of risk, evaluation of the pattern of symptoms and signs, and specific microbiologic testing. An STD etiology of the urethral syndrome is suggested by young age, more than one current sexual partner, a new partner within the past month, a partner with urethritis, or coexisting mucopurulent cervicitis (see below). The finding of a single urinary pathogen, such as *E. coli* or *Staphylococcus saprophyticus*, at a concentration of ≥10^2/mL in a properly collected specimen of midstream urine from a dysuric woman with pyuria indicates probable bacterial UTI, whereas pyuria with <10^2 conventional uropathogens per milliliter of urine ("sterile" pyuria) suggests acute urethral syndrome due to *C. trachomatis* or *N. gonorrhoeae*. Gonorrhea and chlamydial infection should be sought by specific tests (e.g., nucleic acid amplification tests on the first 10 mL of voided urine). Among dysuric women with sterile pyuria caused by infection with *N. gonorrhoeae* or *C. trachomatis*, appropriate treatment alleviates dysuria.

VULVOVAGINAL INFECTIONS ■ **Abnormal Vaginal Discharge** If directly questioned about vaginal discharge during routine health checkups, many women acknowledge having nonspecific symptoms of vaginal discharge that do not correlate with objective signs of inflammation or with actual infection. However, unsolicited reporting of abnormal vaginal discharge does suggest bacterial vaginosis or trichomoniasis. Specifically, an abnormally increased amount or an abnormal odor of the discharge is associated with one or both of these conditions. Cervical infection with *N. gonorrhoeae* or *C. trachomatis* does not appear to cause an increased amount or abnormal odor of discharge, but cervicitis, like trichomoniasis, can include the production of an increased number of neutrophils in vaginal fluid, resulting in a yellow color. Vulvar conditions such as genital herpes or vulvovaginal candidiasis can cause vulvar pruritus, burning, irritation, or lesions as well as external dysuria (as urine passes over the inflamed vulva) or vulvar dyspareunia.

Certain vulvovaginal infections may have serious sequelae. Trichomoniasis, bacterial vaginosis, and vulvovaginal candidiasis have all been associated with increased risk of acquisition of HIV infection. Vaginal trichomoniasis and bacterial vaginosis early in pregnancy independently predict premature onset of labor. Bacterial vaginosis can also lead to anaerobic bacterial infection of the endometrium and salpinges. Vaginitis may be an early and prominent feature of toxic shock syndrome, and recurrent or chronic vulvovaginal candidiasis develops with increased frequency among women with systemic illnesses, such as diabetes mellitus or HIV-related immunosuppression (although only a very small proportion of women with recurrent vulvovaginal candidiasis in the United States actually have a serious predisposing illness).

Thus vulvovaginal symptoms or signs warrant careful evaluation, including pelvic examination, simple rapid diagnostic tests, and appropriate therapy specific for the anatomical site and type of infection. Unfortunately, a recent survey in the United States indicated that clinicians seldom perform the tests required to establish the cause of such symptoms. Further, comparison of telephone and office management of vulvovaginal complaints has documented the inaccuracy of the former, and comparison of evaluations by nurse-midwives with those by physician-practitioners showed that the practitioners' clinical evaluations correlated poorly both with the nurses' evaluations and with diagnostic tests. The diagnosis and treatment of the three most common types of vaginal infection are summarized in Table 115-5.

Inspection of the vulva and perineum may reveal tender genital ulcerations (typically due to HSV infection, occasionally due to chancroid) or fissures (typically due to vulvovaginal candidiasis) or discharge visible at the introitus before insertion of a speculum (suggestive of bacterial vaginosis or trichomoniasis). Speculum examination permits the clinician to discern whether the discharge in fact looks abnormal and whether any abnormal discharge in the vagina emanates from the cervical os (mucoid and, if abnormal, yellow) or from the vagina (not mucoid, since the vaginal epithelium does not produce mucus). Symptoms or signs of abnormal vaginal discharge should prompt testing of vaginal fluid for pH, fishy odor when mixed with 10% KOH, and microscopic features when mixed with saline and with 10% KOH. Additional objective laboratory tests useful for establishing the cause of abnormal vaginal discharge include Gram's staining to

TABLE 115-5   *Diagnostic Features and Management of Vaginal Infection*

Feature	Normal Vaginal Examination	Vulvovaginal Candidiasis	Trichomonal Vaginitis	Bacterial Vaginosis
Etiology	Uninfected; lactobacilli predominant	*Candida albicans*	*Trichomonas vaginalis*	Associated with *Gardnerella vaginalis*, various anaerobic bacteria, and mycoplasmas
Typical symptoms	None	Vulvar itching and/or irritation	Profuse purulent discharge; vulvar itching	Malodorous, slightly increased discharge
Discharge				
Amount	Variable; usually scant	Scant	Often profuse	Moderate
Color[a]	Clear or white	White	White or yellow	White or gray
Consistency	Nonhomogeneous, floccular	Clumped; adherent plaques	Homogeneous	Homogeneous, low viscosity; uniformly coats vaginal walls
Inflammation of vulvar or vaginal epithelium	None	Erythema of vaginal epithelium, introitus; vulvar dermatitis common	Erythema of vaginal and vulvar epithelium; colpitis macularis	None
pH of vaginal fluid[b]	Usually ≤4.5	Usually ≤4.5	Usually ≥5.0	Usually >4.5
Amine ("fishy") odor with 10% KOH	None	None	May be present	Present
Microscopy[c]	Normal epithelial cells; lactobacilli predominant	Leukocytes, epithelial cells; mycelia or pseudomycelia in up to 80% of *C. albicans* culture-positive persons with typical symptoms	Leukocytes; motile trichomonads seen in 80 to 90% of symptomatic patients, less often in the absence of symptoms	Clue cells; few leukocytes; no lactobacilli or only a few outnumbered by profuse mixed flora, nearly always including *G. vaginalis* plus anaerobic species on Gram's stain
Usual treatment	None	Azole cream, tablet, or suppository—e.g., miconazole 100-mg vaginal suppository or clotrimazole 100-mg vaginal tablet, once daily for 7 days Fluconazole, 150 mg orally (single dose)	Metronidazole, 2 g orally (single dose) Metronidazole, 500 mg PO bid for 7 days	Metronidazole, 500 mg PO bid for 7 days Clindamycin, 2% cream, one full applicator vaginally each night for 7 days Metronidazole gel, 0.75%, one full applicator vaginally twice daily for 5 days Metronidazole, 2 g PO (single dose)[d]
Usual management of sexual partner	None	None; topical treatment if candidal dermatitis of penis is detected	Examination for STD; treatment with metronidazole, 2 g PO (single dose)	Examination for STD; no treatment if normal

[a] Color of discharge is best determined by examination against the white background of a swab.

[b] pH determination is not useful if blood is present.

[c] To detect fungal elements, vaginal fluid is digested with 10% KOH prior to microscopic examination; to examine for other features, fluid is mixed (1:1) with physiologic saline.

Gram's stain is also excellent for detecting yeasts and pseudomycelia and for distinguishing normal flora from the mixed flora seen in bacterial vaginosis, but it is less sensitive than the saline preparation for detection of *T. vaginalis*.

[d] Single-dose regimen is less effective than 7-day metronidazole regimen.

detect alterations in the vaginal flora; card tests for bacterial vaginosis, as described below; and a new DNA probe test (the Affirm test) to detect *T. vaginalis* and *C. albicans* as well as the increased concentrations of *Gardnerella vaginalis* associated with bacterial vaginosis.

℞ TREATMENT

Patterns of treatment for vaginal discharge vary widely. In developing countries, where clinics or pharmacies often dispense treatment based on symptoms alone without examination or testing, oral treatment with metronidazole—either as a 2-g single dose or as a 7-day regimen—provides reasonable coverage against both trichomoniasis and bacterial vaginosis, the usual causes of symptoms of vaginal discharge; metronidazole treatment of sex partners prevents reinfection of women with trichomoniasis, even though it does not help prevent the recurrence of bacterial vaginosis. Guidelines promulgated during the 1990s by the World Health Organization suggested treatment for cervical infection and for vulvovaginal candidiasis in women with symptoms of abnormal vaginal discharge; in retrospect, these recommendations were faulty, since these conditions seldom produce such symptoms.

In industrialized countries, clinicians treating symptoms and signs of abnormal vaginal discharge should at least differentiate between bacterial vaginosis and trichomoniasis, because optimal management of patients and partners differs for these two conditions (as discussed briefly below).

Vaginal Trichomoniasis (See also Chap. 199) Symptomatic trichomoniasis characteristically produces a profuse, yellow, purulent, homogeneous vaginal discharge and vulvar irritation, often with visible inflammation of the vaginal and vulvar epithelium and petechial lesions on the cervix (the so-called strawberry cervix, usually evident only by colposcopy). The pH of vaginal fluid usually rises to ≥5.0. In women with typical symptoms and signs of trichomoniasis, microscopic examination of vaginal discharge mixed with saline reveals motile trichomonads in most culture-positive cases. However, in the absence of symptoms or signs, culture is often required for detection of the organism. Polymerase chain reaction (PCR) tests for *T. vaginalis* compare favorably with culture, and PCR testing of urine is now disclosing surprisingly high prevalences of this pathogen among men at several STD clinics in the United States. Treatment of asymptomatic as well as symptomatic cases reduces rates of transmission and prevents later development of symptoms.

℞ TREATMENT

Only nitroimidazoles consistently cure trichomoniasis. Tinidazole and ornidazole have longer half-lives than metronidazole but do not give better results than a single 2-g oral dose of metronidazole, which is much less expensive. Treatment of male sexual partners—often facilitated by dispensing metronidazole to the female patient to give to her partner(s), with a warning about avoiding the concurrent use of alcohol—significantly reduces both the risk of reinfection and the reservoir of infection. Treatment with 0.75% metronidazole gel intravaginally, although moderately effective for bacterial vaginosis, is not reliable for vaginal trichomoniasis. Systemic use of metronidazole is not recommended during the first trimester of pregnancy but is considered safe thereafter. In a large randomized trial, metronidazole treatment of trichomoniasis during pregnancy did not reduce the frequency of perinatal morbidity.

Bacterial Vaginosis This syndrome (formerly termed *nonspecific vaginitis*, *Haemophilus vaginitis*, *anaerobic vaginitis*, or *Gardnerella-associated vaginal discharge*) is characterized by symptoms of vaginal malodor and a slightly to moderately increased white discharge, which appears homogeneous, is low in viscosity, and smoothly coats the vaginal mucosa. An interesting observation is that new genital HPV infection in young women is associated with increased subsequent risk of developing bacterial vaginosis. Other risk factors include multiple sexual partners and recent intercourse with a new partner, but metro-

nidazole treatment of male partners has not reduced the rate of recurrence among affected women.

The vaginal fluid of women with bacterial vaginosis is characterized by markedly increased prevalences and concentrations of *G. vaginalis*, *Mycoplasma hominis*, and several anaerobic bacteria [e.g., *Mobiluncus* spp., *Prevotella* spp. (formerly *Bacteroides* spp.), and some *Peptostreptococcus* spp.]. The vaginal fluid usually lacks hydrogen peroxide–producing *Lactobacillus* spp., which constitute most of the normal vaginal flora and perhaps help protect against certain cervical and vaginal infections. Vaginal douching, use of intravaginal nonoxynol-9 spermicide, and new sexual partners can all result in loss of vaginal colonization by hydrogen peroxide–producing lactobacilli.

Bacterial vaginosis is conventionally diagnosed clinically with the Amsel criteria, which include any three of the following four clinical abnormalities: (1) objective signs of increased white homogeneous vaginal discharge; (2) a vaginal discharge pH of >4.5; (3) liberation of a distinct fishy odor (attributable to volatile amines such as trimethylamine) immediately after vaginal secretions are mixed with a 10% solution of KOH; and (4) microscopic demonstration of "clue cells" (vaginal epithelial cells coated with coccobacillary organisms giving them a granular appearance and indistinct borders; Fig. 115-1) on a wet mount prepared by mixing vaginal secretions with normal saline in a ratio of ~1:1. A diagnostic card test facilitates screening of vaginal fluid for pH > 4.5 and amines, and a dipstick test detects proline aminopeptidase, an enzyme associated with this syndrome.

℞ TREATMENT

The standard dosage of metronidazole for the treatment of bacterial vaginosis is 500 mg orally bid for 7 days. The single 2-g oral dose of metronidazole recommended for trichomoniasis produces somewhat

FIGURE 115-1 *A.* Vaginal epithelial "clue cells." Note granular appearance due to adherent *Gardnerella vaginalis* and indistinct cell margins (400×). *B.* Normal vaginal epithelial cells. The cell margins are distinct and lack granularity.

lower short-term cure rates. Intravaginal treatment with 2% clindamycin cream [one full applicator (5 g containing 100 mg of clindamycin phosphate) each night for 7 nights] or with 0.75% metronidazole gel [one full applicator (5 g containing 37.5 mg of metronidazole) twice daily for 5 days] is also approved for use in the United States and does not elicit systemic adverse reactions. Oral clindamycin (300 mg bid for 7 days) and clindamycin ovules (100 g intravaginally once at bedtime for 3 days) have also been approved. Unfortunately, long-term recurrence (i.e., several months later) is distressingly common after either oral or intravaginal treatment. Treatment of male partners with metronidazole does not prevent recurrence of bacterial vaginosis.

No controlled data support the use of currently available vaginal or oral preparations of lactobacilli for the treatment or prevention of recurrence of bacterial vaginosis. In a randomized trial, repeated intravaginal inoculation of a vaginal peroxide-producing *Lactobacillus* species following treatment of bacterial vaginosis with metronidazole did not reduce the frequency of recurrence. A meta-analysis of 18 studies concluded that bacterial vaginosis during pregnancy substantially increased the risk of preterm delivery and of spontaneous abortion. Although intravaginal treatment of bacterial vaginosis during pregnancy has not reduced perinatal morbidity, oral clindamycin treatment of this syndrome early in pregnancy significantly reduced the risk of late miscarriage and of preterm delivery. Oral antimicrobial treatment of bacterial vaginosis for ≥7 days early in pregnancy may reduce the risk of preterm delivery for women with a history of this pregnancy outcome.

Vulvovaginal Pruritus, Burning, or Irritation   Vulvovaginal candidiasis produces vulvar pruritus, burning, or irritation, generally without symptoms of increased vaginal discharge or malodor. Genital herpes can produce similar symptoms, with lesions sometimes difficult to distinguish from the fissures caused by candidiasis. Signs of vulvovaginal candidiasis include vulvar erythema, edema, fissures, and tenderness. With candidiasis, a white scanty vaginal discharge sometimes takes the form of white thrush-like plaques or cottage cheese–like curds adhering loosely to the vaginal mucosa. *C. albicans* accounts for nearly all cases of symptomatic vulvovaginal candidiasis, which probably arise from endogenous strains of *C. albicans* that have colonized the vagina or the intestinal tract. Complicated vulvovaginal candidiasis includes cases that recur four or more times per year; are unusually severe; are caused by non-*albicans Candida* spp.; or occur in women with uncontrolled diabetes, debilitation, immunosuppression, or pregnancy.

The diagnosis of vulvovaginal candidiasis usually involves the demonstration of pseudohyphae or hyphae by microscopic examination of vaginal fluid mixed with saline or 10% KOH or subjected to Gram's staining. Microscopic examination is less sensitive than culture but correlates better with symptoms.

Rx TREATMENT

Symptoms and signs of vulvovaginal candidiasis warrant treatment, usually intravaginal administration of any of several imidazole antibiotics (e.g., miconazole or clotrimazole) for 3 to 7 days. Over-the-counter marketing of such preparations has reduced the cost of care and made treatment more convenient for many women with recurrent yeast vulvovaginitis. However, most women who purchase these preparations do not have vulvovaginal candidiasis, while many do have other vaginal infections that require different treatment. Therefore, only women with classic symptoms of vulvar pruritus and a history of previous episodes of yeast vulvovaginitis documented by an experienced clinician should self-treat. Single-dose oral treatment with fluconazole (150 mg) is also effective and is preferred by many patients. Management of complicated cases (see above) and those that do not respond to the usual intravaginal or single-dose oral therapy often involves prolonged or periodic oral therapy; this situation is discussed extensively in the *2002 STD Treatment Guidelines* published

by the Centers for Disease Control and Prevention (CDC). Treatment of sexual partners is not routinely indicated.

Other Causes of Vaginal Discharge or Vaginitis   In the ulcerative vaginitis associated with staphylococcal toxic shock syndrome, *Staphylococcus aureus* should be promptly identified in vaginal fluid by Gram's stain and by culture. In desquamative inflammatory vaginitis, smears of vaginal fluid reveal neutrophils, massive vaginal epithelial-cell exfoliation with increased numbers of parabasal cells, and gram-positive cocci; this syndrome may respond to treatment with 2% clindamycin cream. Additional causes of vaginitis and vulvovaginal symptoms include retained foreign bodies (e.g., tampons), cervical caps, vaginal spermicides, vaginal antiseptic preparations or douches, vaginal epithelial atrophy (in postmenopausal women or during prolonged breast-feeding in the postpartum period), allergic reactions to latex condoms, vaginal aphthae associated with HIV infection or Behçet's syndrome, and vestibulitis (a poorly understood syndrome).

MUCOPURULENT CERVICITIS   Mucopurulent cervicitis (MPC) refers to inflammation of the columnar epithelium and subepithelium of the endocervix and of any contiguous columnar epithelium that lies exposed in an ectopic position on the exocervix. MPC in women represents the "silent partner" of urethritis in men, being equally common and often caused by the same agents (*N. gonorrhoeae, C. trachomatis*, or—in a significant association shown by two recent case-control studies—*M. genitalium*); however, MPC is more difficult to recognize. As the most common manifestation of these serious bacterial infections in women, MPC can be a harbinger or sign of upper genital tract infection, also known as pelvic inflammatory disease (PID; see below). In pregnant women, MPC can lead to obstetric complications. More than half of all cases of MPC in the United States today remain idiopathic.

The diagnosis of MPC rests on the detection of yellow mucopurulent discharge from the cervical os or of increased numbers of polymorphonuclear leukocytes (PMNs) in Gram's-stained or Papanicolaou-stained smears of endocervical mucus. MPC due to *C. trachomatis* can also produce edematous cervical ectopy (see below) and endocervical bleeding upon gentle swabbing. Unlike the endocervicitis produced by gonococcal or chlamydial infection, cervicitis caused by HSV produces ulcerative lesions on the stratified squamous epithelium of the exocervix as well as on the columnar epithelium. Yellow cervical mucus on a white swab removed from the endocervix indicates the presence of PMNs. The mucus should be rolled thinly on a slide for Gram's staining. The presence of ≥20 polymorphonuclear cells per 1000× microscopic field within strands of cervical mucus not contaminated by vaginal squamous epithelial cells or vaginal bacteria indicates endocervicitis (Fig. 115-2). Detection of intracellular gram-negative diplococci in carefully collected endocervical mucus is quite specific but ≤50% sensitive for gonorrhea. Therefore, specific and sensitive tests for *N. gonorrhoeae* as well as *C. trachomatis* are also indicated in the evaluation of MPC.

Rx TREATMENT

Although the above criteria for MPC are neither highly specific nor highly predictive of gonococcal or chlamydial infection in many settings, current CDC guidelines call for consideration of empirical treatment for MPC, pending test results, "for a patient who has suspected gonorrhea or chlamydial infection, if (a) the prevalences of these infections are high in the patient population, and (b) the patient might be difficult to locate after treatment." In this situation, therapy should include a single-dose regimen effective for gonorrhea plus treatment for chlamydial infection, as outlined in Table 115-4 for the treatment of urethritis. In settings where gonorrhea is much less common than chlamydial infection, initial therapy for chlamydial infection alone suffices, pending test results for gonorrhea. The etiology and potential benefit of treatment of endocervicitis not associated with gonorrhea or chlamydial infection remain undefined. Although the antimicrobial susceptibility of *M. genitalium* is not yet well defined, it currently seems reasonable to use azithromycin to treat possible *M. genitalium*

FIGURE 115-2 Gram's stain of cervical mucus, showing a strand of cervical mucus containing many polymorphonuclear leukocytes. This picture is typical of mucopurulent cervicitis. Note that leukocytes are not seen in areas of the slide containing vaginal epithelial cells, adjacent to the mucus strands.

infection in such cases. Sexual partner(s) of a woman with MPC should be examined and given a regimen similar to that chosen for the woman unless results of tests for gonorrhea or chlamydial infection in either partner warrant different therapy or no therapy.

CERVICAL ECTOPY Cervical ectopy, often mislabeled "cervical erosion," is easily confused with infectious endocervicitis. Ectopy represents the presence of the one-cell-thick columnar epithelium extending from the endocervix out onto the visible ectocervix. In ectopy, the cervical os may contain clear or slightly cloudy mucus but usually not yellow mucopus. Colposcopy shows intact epithelium. Normally found during adolescence and early adulthood, ectopy gradually recedes through the second and third decades of life, as squamous metaplasia replaces the ectopic columnar epithelium. Oral contraceptive use favors the persistence or reappearance of ectopy, while smoking apparently accelerates squamous metaplasia. Cauterization of ectopy is not warranted. Ectopy may render the cervix more susceptible to infection with *N. gonorrhoeae*, *C. trachomatis*, or HIV.

PELVIC INFLAMMATORY DISEASE The term *pelvic inflammatory disease* usually refers to infection that ascends from the cervix or vagina to involve the endometrium and/or fallopian tubes. Infection can extend beyond the reproductive tract to cause pelvic peritonitis, generalized peritonitis, perihepatitis, or pelvic abscess. In rare instances, infection extends secondarily to the pelvic organs from adjacent foci of inflammation (e.g., appendicitis, regional ileitis, or diverticulitis), as a result of hematogenous dissemination (e.g., of tuberculosis), or as a rare complication of certain tropical diseases (e.g., schistosomiasis). Intrauterine infection can be primary (spontaneously occurring and usually sexually transmitted) or secondary to invasive intrauterine surgical procedures [e.g., dilatation and curettage, termination of pregnancy, insertion of an intrauterine device (IUD), or hysterosalpingography] or to parturition.

Etiology The agents most often implicated in acute PID include those that are primary causes of endocervicitis (*N. gonorrhoeae* and *C. trachomatis*) and those that can be regarded as components of an altered vaginal flora. In general, PID is most often associated with gonorrhea where there is a high incidence of gonorrhea—e.g., in developing countries and in indigent, inner-city populations in the United States.

In recent case-control studies, detection of *M. genitalium* by PCR in endometrial specimens has also been significantly associated with histopathologic diagnoses of endometritis.

Anaerobic and facultative organisms (especially *Prevotella* species, peptostreptococci, *E. coli*, *Haemophilus influenzae*, and group B streptococci) as well as genital mycoplasmas have been isolated from specimens obtained at laparoscopy from the peritoneal fluid or fallopian tubes in a varying proportion (typically one-fourth to one-third) of women with PID studied in the United States. The difficulty of determining the exact microbial etiology of an individual case of PID has implications for the approach to empirical antimicrobial treatment of this infection.

Epidemiology In the United States in 2002, women 15 to 44 years of age made ~200,000 initial visits to physician's offices for PID, and an estimated 66,000 women were hospitalized for acute PID. Important risk factors for acute PID include the presence of endocervical infection or bacterial vaginosis, a history of salpingitis or of recent vaginal douching, and the use of an IUD (especially among nulliparous women, during the first few months after IUD insertion, and among women with multiple sex partners). Certain other iatrogenic factors, such as dilatation and curettage or cesarean section, can increase the risk of PID, especially among women with endocervical gonococcal or chlamydial infection or bacterial vaginosis. The onset of symptoms of *N. gonorrhoeae*–associated and *C. trachomatis*–associated PID often occurs during or soon after the menstrual period; this timing suggests that menstruation is a risk factor in women with endocervical infection. Experimental inoculation of the fallopian tubes of lower primates has shown that repeated exposure to *C. trachomatis* leads to the greatest degree of tissue inflammation and damage; thus, immunopathology probably contributes to the pathogenesis of chlamydial salpingitis. Women using oral contraceptives appear to be at decreased risk of symptomatic PID, and tubal sterilization reduces the risk of salpingitis by preventing intraluminal spread of infection into the tubes.

Clinical Manifestations ■ *ENDOMETRITIS: A CLINICAL PATHOLOGIC SYNDROME* A study of women with clinically suspected PID who were undergoing both endometrial biopsy and laparoscopy showed that those with endometritis alone differed from those who also had salpingitis in that they significantly less often had lower quadrant, adnexal, or cervical motion or abdominal rebound tenderness; fever; or elevated C-reactive protein levels. In addition, women with endometritis alone differed from those with neither endometritis nor salpingitis in that they more often had gonorrhea, chlamydial infection, and risk factors such as douching or IUD use. Thus, women with endometritis alone were intermediate between those with neither endometritis nor salpingitis and those with salpingitis with respect to risk factors, clinical manifestations, cervical infection prevalence, and elevated C-reactive protein.

SALPINGITIS Symptoms of nontuberculous salpingitis classically evolve from a yellow or malodorous vaginal discharge caused by MPC and/or bacterial vaginosis to midline abdominal pain and abnormal vaginal bleeding caused by endometritis and then to bilateral lower abdominal and pelvic pain caused by salpingitis, with nausea, vomiting, and increased abdominal tenderness caused by peritonitis.

The abdominal pain in nontuberculous salpingitis is usually described as dull or aching. In some cases, pain is lacking or is atypical, but active inflammatory changes are found in the course of an unrelated evaluation or procedure, such as a laparoscopic evaluation for infertility. Abnormal uterine bleeding precedes or coincides with the onset of pain in ~40% of women with PID, symptoms of urethritis (dysuria) occur in 20%, and symptoms of proctitis (anorectal pain, tenesmus, and rectal discharge or bleeding) are occasionally seen in women with gonococcal or chlamydial infection.

Speculum examination shows evidence of MPC (yellow endocervical discharge, easily induced endocervical bleeding) in the majority of women with gonococcal or chlamydial PID. Cervical motion tenderness is produced by stretching of the adnexal attachments on the side toward which the cervix is pushed. Bimanual examination reveals uterine fundal tenderness due to endometritis and abnormal adnexal tenderness due to salpingitis that is usually, but not necessarily, bilateral. Adnexal swelling is palpable in about one-half of women with acute salpingitis, but evaluation of the adnexae in a patient with marked tenderness is not reliable. The initial temperature is >38°C in only about one-third of patients with acute salpingitis. Laboratory findings include elevation of the erythrocyte sedimentation rate (ESR) in 75% of patients with acute salpingitis and elevation of the peripheral white blood cell count in up to 60%.

Unlike nontuberculous salpingitis, genital tuberculosis often occurs in older women, many of whom are postmenopausal. Presenting symptoms include abnormal vaginal bleeding, pain (including dysmenorrhea), and infertility. About one-quarter of these women have had adnexal masses. Endometrial biopsy shows tuberculous granulomas and provides optimal specimens for culture.

PERIHEPATITIS AND PERIAPPENDICITIS Pleuritic upper abdominal pain and tenderness (usually localized to the right upper quadrant) develop in 3 to 10% of women with acute PID. Symptoms of perihepatitis arise during or after the onset of symptoms of PID and may overshadow lower abdominal symptoms, thereby leading to a mistaken diagnosis of cholecystitis. In perhaps 5% of cases of acute salpingitis, early laparoscopy reveals perihepatic inflammation ranging from edema and erythema of the liver capsule to exudate with fibrinous adhesions between the visceral and parietal peritoneum. When treatment is delayed and laparoscopy is performed late, dense "violin-string" adhesions can be seen over the liver; chronic exertional or positional right upper quadrant pain ensues when traction is placed on the adhesions. Although perihepatitis, also known as the *Fitz-Hugh–Curtis syndrome*, was for many years specifically attributed to gonococcal salpingitis, most cases are now attributed to chlamydial salpingitis. In patients with chlamydial salpingitis, serum titers of microimmunofluorescent antibody to *C. trachomatis* are typically much higher when perihepatitis is present than when it is absent.

Physical findings include right upper quadrant tenderness and usually include adnexal tenderness and cervicitis, even in patients whose symptoms do not suggest salpingitis. Results of liver function tests and right upper quadrant ultrasonography are nearly always normal. The presence of MPC and pelvic tenderness in a young woman with subacute pleuritic right upper quadrant pain and normal ultrasonography of the gallbladder points to a diagnosis of perihepatitis.

Periappendicitis (appendiceal serositis without involvement of the intestinal mucosa) has been found in ~5% of patients undergoing appendectomy for suspected appendicitis and can occur as a complication of gonococcal or chlamydial salpingitis.

Among women with salpingitis, HIV infection is associated with increased severity of salpingitis and with tuboovarian abscess requiring hospitalization and surgical drainage. Nonetheless, among women with HIV infection and salpingitis, the clinical reponse to conventional antimicrobial therapy (coupled with drainage of tuboovarian abscess, when found) has been satisfactory.

Diagnosis Treatment appropriate for PID must not be withheld from patients who have an equivocal diagnosis; it is better to err on the side of overdiagnosis and overtreatment. On the other hand, it is essential to differentiate between salpingitis and other pelvic pathology, particularly surgical emergencies such as appendicitis and ectopic pregnancy.

Nothing short of laparoscopy definitively identifies salpingitis, but routine laparoscopy to confirm suspected salpingitis is generally impractical. Most patients with acute PID have lower abdominal pain of <3 weeks' duration, pelvic tenderness on bimanual pelvic examination, and evidence of lower genital tract infection (e.g., MPC). Approximately 60% of such patients have salpingitis at laparoscopy, and perhaps 10 to 20% have endometritis alone. Among the patients with

these findings, a rectal temperature >38°C, a palpable adnexal mass, and elevation of the ESR to >15 mm/h also raise the probability of salpingitis, which has been found at laparoscopy in 68% of patients with one of these additional findings, 90% of patients with two, and 96% of patients with three. However, only 17% of all patients with laparoscopy-confirmed salpingitis have had all three additional findings.

In a woman with pelvic pain and tenderness, increased numbers of PMNs (30 per 1000× microscopic field in strands of cervical mucus) increase the predictive value of a clinical diagnosis of acute PID, as do onset with menses, history of recent abnormal menstrual bleeding, presence of an IUD, history of salpingitis, and sexual exposure to a male with urethritis. Appendicitis or another disorder of the gut is favored by the early onset of anorexia, nausea, or vomiting; the onset of pain later than day 14 of the menstrual cycle; or unilateral pain limited to the right or left lower quadrant. Whenever the diagnosis of PID is being considered, serum assays for human β-chorionic gonadotropin should be performed; these tests are usually positive with ectopic pregnancy. Ultrasonography and magnetic resonance imaging (MRI) can be useful for the identification of tuboovarian or pelvic abscess. MRI of the tubes can also show increased tubal diameter, intratubal fluid, or tubal wall thickening in cases of salpingitis.

The primary and uncontested value of laparoscopy in women with lower abdominal pain is for the exclusion of other surgical problems. Some of the most common or serious problems that may be confused with salpingitis (e.g., acute appendicitis, ectopic pregnancy, corpus luteum bleeding, ovarian tumor) are unilateral. Unilateral pain or pelvic mass, although not incompatible with PID, is a strong indication for laparoscopy unless the clinical picture warrants laparotomy instead. Atypical clinical findings, such as the absence of lower genital tract infection, a missed menstrual period, a positive pregnancy test, or failure to respond to appropriate therapy, are other common indications for laparoscopy. Endometrial biopsy is relatively sensitive and specific for the diagnosis of endometritis, which correlates well with the presence of salpingitis.

Endocervical swab specimens should be examined by Gram's staining for PMNs and gram-negative diplococci and by nucleic acid amplification tests for *N. gonorrhoeae* and *C. trachomatis*. The clinical diagnosis of PID made by expert gynecologists is confirmed by laparoscopy or endometrial biopsy in ~90% of women who also have cultures positive for *N. gonorrhoeae* or *C. trachomatis*. Even among women with no symptoms suggestive of acute PID who were attending an STD clinic or gynecology clinic in Pittsburgh, endometritis was significantly associated with endocervical gonorrhea or chlamydial infection or bacterial vaginosis, being detected in 26, 27, and 15% of women with these conditions, respectively.

Rx TREATMENT

Women with PID can be treated as either outpatients or inpatients. In the multicenter Pelvic Inflammatory Disease Evaluation and Clinical Health (PEACH) trial, 831 women with mild to moderately severe symptoms and signs of PID were randomized to receive either inpatient treatment with intravenous (IV) cefoxitin and doxycycline or outpatient treatment with a single intramuscular (IM) dose of cefoxitin plus oral doxycycline. Short-term clinical and microbiologic outcomes and long-term outcomes were equivalent in the two groups. Nonetheless, hospitalization should be considered when (1) the diagnosis is uncertain and surgical emergencies such as appendicitis and ectopic pregnancy cannot be excluded, (2) pelvic abscess is suspected, (3) severe illness or nausea and vomiting preclude outpatient management, (4) the patient has HIV infection, (5) the patient is assessed as unable to follow or tolerate an outpatient regimen, or (6) the patient has failed to respond to outpatient therapy. Some experts also prefer to hospitalize adolescents with PID for initial therapy.

Recommended combination regimens for ambulatory or parenteral management of PID are presented in Table 115-6. Women managed as outpatients should receive a combined regimen with broad activity,

TABLE 115-6 *Combination Antimicrobial Regimens Recommended for Outpatient Treatment or for Parenteral Treatment of PID*

Outpatient Regimens	Parenteral Regimens
Regimen A Ofloxacin 400 mg PO bid for 14 days *or* Levofloxacin 500 mg PO once daily for 14 days *plus*[a] Metronidazole 500 mg PO bid for 14 days	Initiate parenteral therapy with either of the following regimens; continue parenteral therapy until 48 h after clinical improvement; then change to outpatient therapy, as described in text.
Regimen B Ceftriaxone 250 mg IM once *plus* Doxycycline 100 mg PO bid for 14 days *plus*[a] Metronidazole 500 mg PO bid for 14 days	**Regimen A** Cefotetan 2 g IV q12h *or* Cefoxitin 2 g IV q6h *plus* Doxycycline 100 mg IV or PO q12h **Regimen B** Clindamycin 900 mg IV q8h *plus* Gentamicin, loading dose of 2 mg/kg IV or IM, then maintenance dose of 1.5 mg/kg q8h

[a] The addition of metronidazole is recommended by some experts.
Source: Adapted from Centers for Disease Control and Prevention: MMWR 51(RR-6):1, 2002.

such as ceftriaxone followed by doxycycline. Metronidazole can be added, if tolerated, to enhance activity against anaerobes. Alternatively, oral ofloxacin or levofloxacin, each continued for 14 days and given with or without metronidazole, provides good coverage of the major pathogens. Although few methodologically sound clinical trials (especially with prolonged follow-up) have been conducted, one meta-analysis suggested a benefit of providing good coverage against anaerobes.

The following two parenteral regimens have given nearly identical results in a multicenter randomized trial:

1. Doxycycline (100 mg bid, given IV or by mouth) plus cefotetan (2.0 g IV every 12 h) or cefoxitin (2.0 g IV every 6 h). Administration of these drugs should be continued by the IV route for at least 48 h after the patient's condition improves and then followed with doxycycline (100 mg bid by mouth) to complete 14 days of therapy.

2. Clindamycin (900 mg IV every 8 h) plus gentamicin (2.0 mg/kg IV or IM, followed by 1.5 mg/kg every 8 h) in patients with normal renal function. Once-daily dosing of gentamicin (with combination of the total daily dose into a single daily dose) has not been evaluated in PID but has been efficacious in other serious infections and could be substituted.

Treatment with these drugs should be continued for at least 48 h after the patient's condition improves and then followed with oral doxycycline (100 mg bid by mouth) or clindamycin (450 mg qid by mouth) to complete 14 days of therapy. In cases with tuboovarian abscess, clindamycin rather than doxycycline for continued therapy may provide better coverage for anaerobic infection.

FOLLOW-UP Hospitalized patients should show substantial clinical improvement within 3 to 5 days. Women treated as outpatients should be clinically reevaluated within 72 h. A follow-up telephone survey of women seen in an emergency room and given a prescription for 10 days of oral doxycycline for PID found that 28% never filled the prescription and 41% stopped taking medication early (after an average of 4.1 days), often because of persistent symptoms, lack of symptoms, or side effects. Women not responding favorably to ambulatory therapy should be hospitalized. After completion of treatment, tests for persistent or recurrent infection with *N. gonorrhoeae* or *C. trachomatis* should be performed if symptoms persist or recur or if the patient has not complied with therapy or has been reexposed to an untreated sex partner.

SURGERY Surgery is necessary for the treatment of salpingitis only in the face of life-threatening infection (such as rupture or threatened rupture of a tuboovarian abscess) or for drainage of an abscess. Conservative surgical procedures are usually sufficient. Pelvic abscesses can often be drained by posterior colpotomy, and peritoneal lavage can be used if there is generalized peritonitis.

Prognosis Among 900 women in Sweden who underwent long-term follow-up for a mean period of 8 years after successful treatment of an acute episode of PID with various regimens (that today would often not be considered to provide optimal broad antimicrobial activity), late sequelae included infertility due to bilateral tubal occlusion, ectopic pregnancy due to tubal scarring without occlusion, chronic pelvic pain, and recurrent salpingitis. The postsalpingitis risk of infertility due to tubal occlusion among sexually active women not using contraceptives was 14% at 15 to 24 years of age and 26% at 25 to 34 years of age; the risk for women of all ages combined was 11% after one episode of salpingitis, 23% after two episodes, and 54% after three or more episodes. A study at the University of Washington found a sevenfold increase in the risk of ectopic pregnancy and an eightfold increase in the rate of hysterectomy after PID.

Prevention A randomized controlled trial designed to determine whether selective screening for chlamydial infection reduced the risk of subsequent PID showed that women randomized to undergo screening had a 56% lower rate of PID over the following year than did women receiving the usual care without screening. This report helped to prompt the establishment of U.S. national guidelines for risk-based chlamydial screening of young women as a highly effective way to reduce the incidence of PID and the prevalence of post-PID sequelae, while also reducing sexual transmission of *C. trachomatis*.

ULCERATIVE GENITAL LESIONS Genital ulceration reflects a set of important STIs, most of which sharply increase the risk of sexual acquisition and shedding of HIV. In a 1996 study of genital ulcers in 10 of the U.S. cities with the highest rates of primary syphilis, PCR testing of ulcer specimens demonstrated HSV in 62% of patients, *Treponema pallidum* in 13%, and *Haemophilus ducreyi* in 12 to 20%.

In Asia and Africa, chancroid (Fig. 115-3) was once considered the most common type of genital ulcer, followed in frequency by primary

FIGURE 115-3 Chancroid: multiple, painful, punched-out ulcers with undermined borders on the labia occurring after autoinoculation.

FIGURE 115-4   Lymphogranuloma venereum: striking tender lymphadenopathy occurring at the femoral and inguinal lymph nodes, separated by a groove made by Poupart's ligament.

FIGURE 115-5   Donovanosis, ulcerovegetative type: extensive granulation-tissue formation, ulceration, and scarring of the perineum, scrotum, and penis.

syphilis and then genital herpes. With increased efforts to control chancroid and syphilis, together with more frequent recurrences or persistence of genital herpes attributable to HIV infection, PCR testing of genital ulcers now clearly implicates genital herpes as the most common cause of genital ulceration in many developing countries. Lymphogranuloma venereum (LGV; Fig. 115-4) and donovanosis (granuloma inguinale; Fig. 115-5) continue to cause genital ulceration in developing countries but rarely occur today in North America or Europe. Other causes of genital ulcer include (1) candidiasis and traumatized genital warts—both readily recognized; (2) lesions due to genital involvement of more widespread dermatoses; and (3) cutaneous manifestations of systemic diseases, such as genital mucosal ulceration in Stevens-Johnson syndrome or Behçet's disease.

Diagnosis   Although most genital ulcerations cannot be diagnosed confidently on clinical grounds alone, clinical findings plus epidemiologic considerations (Table 115-7) can usually guide initial management (Table 115-8) pending results of further tests. Clinicians should order a rapid serologic test for syphilis in all cases of genital ulcer and a dark-field or direct immunofluorescence test (or PCR test, where available) for *T. pallidum* in all lesions except those highly characteristic of infection with HSV (i.e., those with herpetic vesicles). All patients presenting with genital ulceration should be asked to undergo serologic testing for HIV infection.

Typical vesicles or pustules or a cluster of painful ulcers preceded by vesiculopustular lesions suggests genital herpes. These typical clinical presentations make detection of the virus optional; however, many patients want confirmation of the diagnosis, and differentiation of HSV-1 from HSV-2 has prognostic implications, since the latter causes more frequent genital recurrences.

Painless, nontender, indurated ulcers with firm, nontender inguinal adenopathy suggest primary syphilis. If dark-field examination and a rapid serologic test for syphilis are initially negative and the patient will comply with follow-up and sexual abstinence, the performance of two more dark-field examinations on successive days before treatment is begun will improve the sensitivity of the diagnosis of syphilis. Repeated serologic testing for syphilis 1 or 2 weeks after treatment of seronegative primary syphilis usually demonstrates seroconversion.

TABLE 115-7   *Clinical Features of Genital Ulcers*

Feature	Syphilis	Herpes	Chancroid	Lymphogranuloma Venereum	Donovanosis
Incubation period	9–90 days	2–7 days	1–14 days	3 days–6 weeks	1–4 weeks (up to 6 months)
Early primary lesions	Papule	Vesicle	Pustule	Papule, pustule, or vesicle	Papule
No. of lesions	Usually one	Multiple, may coalesce	Usually multiple, may coalesce	Usually one	Variable
Diameter	5–15 mm	1–2 mm	Variable	2–10 mm	Variable
Edges	Sharply demarcated, elevated, round, or oval	Erythematous	Undermined, ragged, irregular	Elevated, round, or oval	Elevated, irregular
Depth	Superficial or deep	Superficial	Excavated	Superficial or deep	Elevated
Base	Smooth, nonpurulent, relatively nonvascular	Serous, erythematous, nonvascular	Purulent, bleeds easily	Variable, nonvascular	Red and velvety, bleeds readily
Induration	Firm	None	Soft	Occasionally firm	Firm
Pain	Uncommon	Frequently tender	Usually very tender	Variable	Uncommon
Lymphadenopathy	Firm, nontender, bilateral	Firm, tender, often bilateral with initial episode	Tender, may suppurate, loculated, usually unilateral	Tender, may suppurate, loculated, usually unilateral	None; pseudobuboes

Source: From RM Ballard, in KK Holmes et al (eds): *Sexually Transmitted Diseases*, 3d ed. New York, McGraw-Hill, 1999.

TABLE 115-8 *Initial Management of Genital Ulcer*

Usual causes
　Herpes simplex virus (HSV)
　Treponema pallidum (primary syphilis)
　Haemophilus ducreyi (chancroid)
Usual initial laboratory evaluation
　Dark-field exam, direct FA, or PCR for *T. pallidum*; RPR test (if
　negative but primary syphilis suspected, repeat RPR in 1 week);
　culture, direct FA, ELISA, or PCR for HSV. In chancroid-endemic
　area: PCR or culture for *H. ducreyi*

INITIAL TREATMENT

Herpes confirmed or suspected (history or sign of vesicles):
　Treat for genital herpes with acyclovir, valacyclovir, or famciclovir
Syphilis confirmed (dark-field, FA, or PCR showing *T. pallidum*, or
　RPR reactive):
　Benzathine penicillin 2.4 million units IM once to patient, recent (e.g.
　within 3 months) seronegative partner(s), and every seropositive
　partner
Chancroid confirmed or suspected (diagnostic test positive, or HSV
　and syphilis excluded, and lesion persists):
　Ciprofloxacin 500 mg PO as single dose　*or*
　Ceftriaxone 250 mg IM as single dose　*or*
　Azithromycin 1 g PO as single dose

Note: FA, fluorescent antibody; PCR, polymerase chain reaction; RPR, rapid plasma reagin; ELISA, enzyme-linked immunosorbent assay; HSV, herpes simplex virus.

"Atypical" or clinically trivial ulcers may be more common manifestations of genital herpes than classic vesiculopustular lesions. Specific tests for HSV in such lesions are therefore indicated (Chap. 163). Type-specific serologic tests for serum antibody to HSV-2, now commercially available, may give negative results, especially when patients present early with the initial episode of genital herpes or when HSV-1 is the cause of genital herpes (as is often the case today). Furthermore, a positive test for HSV-2 antibody does not prove that the current lesions are herpetic, since nearly one-fourth of the general population of the United States becomes seropositive for HSV-2 during early adulthood. Nonetheless, a positive HSV-2 serology does enable the clinician to tell the patient that he or she has had genital herpes, should learn to recognize symptoms, should avoid sex during recurrences, and should consider use of condoms or suppressive antiviral therapy, both of which can reduce transmission to a sexual partner.

Demonstration of *H. ducreyi* by culture (or by PCR test, when available) is most useful when ulcers are painful and purulent, especially if inguinal lymphadenopathy with fluctuance or overlying erythema is noted; if chancroid is prevalent in the community; or if the patient has recently had a sexual exposure elsewhere in a chancroid-endemic area (e.g., a developing country). Enlarged, fluctuant lymph nodes should be aspirated for culture or PCR tests to detect *H. ducreyi* as well as for Gram's staining and culture to rule out the presence of other pyogenic bacteria.

When genital ulcers persist beyond the natural history of initial episodes of herpes (2 to 3 weeks) or of chancroid or syphilis (up to 6 weeks) and do not resolve with syndrome-based antimicrobial therapy, then—in addition to the usual tests for herpes, syphilis, and chancroid—biopsy is indicated to exclude donovanosis, carcinoma, and other nonvenereal dermatoses. HIV serology should also be undertaken, since chronic, persistent genital herpes is common in AIDS.

℞ TREATMENT

Immediate syndrome-based treatment for acute genital ulcerations (after collection of all necessary diagnostic specimens) is often appropriate before all test results become available, because patients with typical initial or recurrent episodes of genital or anorectal herpes can benefit from prompt oral antiviral therapy (Chap. 163); because early treatment of sexually transmitted causes of genital ulcers decreases further transmission; and because some patients do not return for test results and treatment. The patient with nonvesicular ulcerative lesions who may not return for follow-up or may continue sexual activity should receive initial treatment for syphilis, together with empirical therapy for chancroid if there has been an exposure in an area where chancroid occurs or if regional lymph node suppuration is evident. In resource-poor settings lacking ready access to diagnostic tests, this approach to syndromic treatment for syphilis and chancroid has helped bring these two diseases under control. Finally, empirical antimicrobial therapy may be indicated if ulcers persist and the diagnosis remains unclear after a week of observation despite attempts to diagnose herpes, syphilis, and chancroid.

PROCTITIS, PROCTOCOLITIS, ENTEROCOLITIS, AND ENTERITIS　Sexually acquired *proctitis*, with inflammation limited to the rectal mucosa (the distal 10 to 12 cm), results from direct rectal inoculation of typical STD pathogens. In contrast, inflammation extending from the rectum to the colon (*proctocolitis*), involving both the small and the large bowel (*enterocolitis*), or involving the small bowel alone (*enteritis*) can result from ingestion of typical intestinal pathogens through oral-anal exposure during sexual contact. Anorectal pain and mucopurulent, bloody rectal discharge suggest proctitis or proctocolitis. Proctitis commonly produces tenesmus (causing frequent attempts to defecate, but not true diarrhea) and constipation, whereas proctocolitis and enterocolitis more often cause true diarrhea. In all three conditions, anoscopy usually shows mucosal exudate and easily induced mucosal bleeding (i.e., a positive "wipe test"), sometimes with petechiae or mucosal ulcers. Exudate should be sampled for Gram's staining and other microbiologic studies. Sigmoidoscopy or colonoscopy shows inflammation limited to the rectum in proctitis or disease extending at least up into the sigmoid colon in proctocolitis.

The AIDS era brought an extraordinary shift in the clinical and etiologic spectrum of intestinal infections among homosexual men. The number of cases of the acute intestinal STIs described above fell as high-risk sexual behaviors became less common in this group. At the same time, the number of AIDS-related opportunistic intestinal infections increased rapidly, many associated with chronic or recurrent symptoms. The incidence of these infections has since fallen with increasingly effective antiretroviral therapy.

Acquisition of *N. gonorrhoeae*, HSV, or *C. trachomatis* during receptive anorectal intercourse causes most cases of infectious proctitis in women or homosexual men. Primary and secondary syphilis can also produce anal or anorectal lesions, with or without symptoms. Gonococcal or chlamydial proctitis typically involves the most distal rectal mucosa and the anal crypts and is clinically mild, without systemic manifestations. In contrast, primary proctitis due to HSV and proctocolitis due to the strains of *C. trachomatis* that cause LGV usually produce severe anorectal pain and often cause fever. Perianal ulcers and inguinal lymphadenopathy, most commonly due to HSV, can also occur in LGV or syphilis. Sacral nerve root radiculopathies, usually presenting as urinary retention, laxity of the anal sphincter, or constipation, may complicate primary herpetic proctitis. In LGV, rectal biopsy typically shows crypt abscesses, granulomas, and giant cells—findings resembling those in Crohn's disease; such findings should always prompt rectal culture and serology for LGV, which is a curable infection. Syphilis can also produce rectal granulomas, usually in association with infiltration by plasma cells or other mononuclear cells. Syphilis, LGV, and HSV infection involving the rectum can produce perirectal adenopathy that is sometimes mistaken for malignancy; syphilis, LGV, HSV infection, and chancroid involving the anus can produce inguinal adenopathy, because anal lymphatics drain to inguinal lymph nodes.

Diarrhea and abdominal bloating or cramping pain without anorectal symptoms and with normal findings on anoscopy and sigmoidoscopy occur with inflammation of the small intestine (enteritis) or with proximal colitis. In homosexual men without HIV infection, enteritis is often attributable to *Giardia lamblia*. Sexually acquired proctocolitis is most often due to *Campylobacter* or *Shigella* spp.

R̲x̲ TREATMENT

Acute proctitis in persons who have practiced receptive intercourse is usually sexually acquired. Such patients should undergo anoscopy to detect rectal ulcers or vesicles and petechiae after swabbing of the rectal mucosa; to examine rectal exudates for PMNs and gram-negative diplococci; and to obtain rectal swab specimens for testing for rectal gonorrhea, chlamydial infection, herpes, and syphilis. Pending test results, patients with proctitis should receive empirical syndromic treatment—e.g., with ceftriaxone (a single IM dose of 125 mg for gonorrhea) plus doxycycline (100 mg bid by mouth for 7 days for possible chlamydial infection) plus treatment for herpes or syphilis if indicated.

PREVENTION AND CONTROL OF STDS

Prevention and control of STDs require (1) reduction of the average rate of sexual exposure through alteration of behaviors and behavioral norms among both susceptible and infected persons in all population groups; (2) reduction of the efficiency of transmission through the promotion of safer sexual practices, the use of condoms during casual or commercial sex, hepatitis B immunization, and many other approaches (e.g., early detection and treatment of other STIs to reduce the efficiency of sexual transmission of HIV); and (3) shortening of the duration of infectivity of STDs through early detection and curative or suppressive treatment of patients and their sexual partners.

Financial and time constraints imposed by managed-care practice patterns often curtail screening and prevention services. As outlined in Fig. 115-6, the success of clinicians' efforts to detect and treat STDs depends in part on societal efforts to teach young people how to recognize symptoms of STDs; to motivate those with symptoms to seek care promptly; and to make such care accessible, affordable, and acceptable, especially to the young indigent patients most likely to acquire an STD.

Since many infected individuals develop no symptoms or fail to recognize and report symptoms, clinicians should routinely perform an STI risk assessment for teenagers and young adults as a guide to selective screening. U.S. Preventive Services Task Force Guidelines recommend screening sexually active female patients ≤25 years of age for *C. trachomatis* whenever they present for health care (at least once a year); older women should be tested if they have more than one sexual partner, have begun a new sexual relationship since the previous test, or have another STD diagnosed. In the United States, widespread selective screening of young women for cervical *C. trachomatis* infection in some regions has been associated with a 50 to 60% drop in prevalence, and such screening also protects the individual woman from PID. Sensitive urine-based genetic amplification tests permit expansion of screening to men, teenage boys, and girls in settings where examination is not planned or is impractical (e.g., during pre-participation sports examinations).

Although gonorrhea is now substantially less common than chlamydial infection in industrialized countries, screening tests for *N. gonorrhoeae* are still appropriate for women and teenage girls attending STD clinics and for sexually active teens and young women from areas of high gonorrhea prevalence. However, multiplex nucleic acid amplification tests that combine screening for *N. gonorrhoeae* and *C. trachomatis* in a single low-cost assay may facilitate the prevention and control of both infections in populations at high risk.

All patients with newly detected STIs or at high risk for STIs according to routine risk assessment as well as all pregnant women should be encouraged to undergo serologic testing for syphilis and HIV infection, with appropriate HIV counseling before and after testing. Randomized trials have shown that risk-reduction counseling of patients with STDs significantly lowers subsequent risk of acquiring an STD; such counseling should now be considered a standard component of STD management. Preimmunization serologic testing for antibody to HBV is indicated for unvaccinated persons who are known to be at high risk, such as homosexually active men and injection drug users. In most young persons, however, it is more cost-effective to vaccinate against HBV without serologic screening.

Partner notification is the process of identifying and informing partners of infected patients of possible exposure to an STI and of examining, testing, and treating partners as appropriate. In a series of 22 reports concerning partner notification during the 1990s, index patients with gonorrhea or chlamydial infection named a mean of 0.75 to 1.6 partners, of whom one-fourth to one-third were infected; those with syphilis named 1.8 to 6.3 partners, with one-third to one-half infected; and those with HIV infection named 0.76 to 5.31 partners, with up to one-fourth infected. Persons who transmit infection or who have recently been infected and are still in the incubation period usually have no symptoms or only mild symptoms and seek medical attention only when notified of their exposure. Therefore, the clinician must encourage patients to participate in partner notification, must ensure that exposed persons are notified, and must guarantee confidentiality to all involved. In the United States, local health departments often offer assistance in partner notification, treatment, and/or counseling. It seems both feasible and most useful to notify those partners exposed within the patient's likely period of infectiousness, which is often considered the preceding 1 month for gonorrhea, 1 to 2 months for chlamydial infection, and up to 3 months for early syphilis.

Persons with a new-onset STD always have a *source* contact who gave them the infection; in addition, they may have a *secondary* (*spread* or *exposed*) contact with whom they had sex after becoming infected. The identification and treatment of these two types of contacts have different objectives. Treatment of the source contact (often a casual contact) benefits the community by preventing further transmission; treatment of the recently exposed secondary contact (typically a spouse or another steady sexual partner) prevents both the development of serious complications (such as PID) in the partner and reinfection of the index patient. A recent survey of a random sample of U.S. physicians found that most instructed patients to abstain from sex during treatment, to use condoms, and to inform their sex partners after being diagnosed with gonorrhea, chlamydial infection, or syphilis; physicians sometimes gave the patients drugs for their partners. However, follow-up of the partners by physicians was infrequent. A recent randomized trial compared patients' delivery of therapy to partners exposed to gonorrhea or chlamydial infection with conventional notification and advice to partners to seek evaluation for STD; patients' delivery of therapy to their partners significantly reduced rates of re-

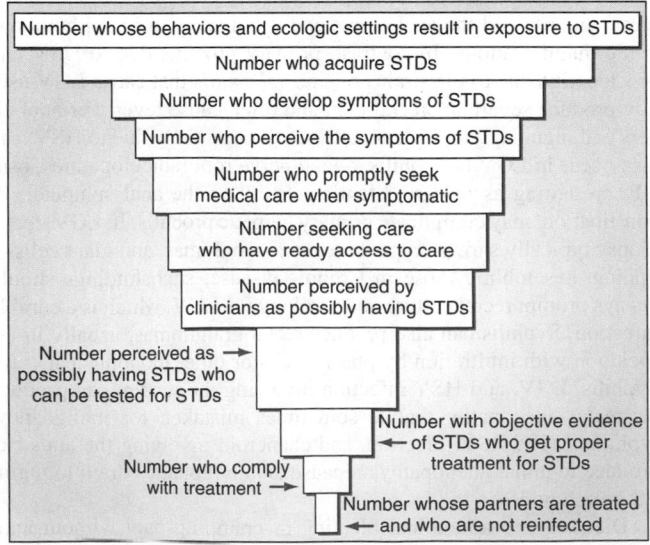

FIGURE 115-6 Critical control points for preventive and clinical interventions against sexually transmitted diseases (STDs). [*Adapted from HT Waller and MA Piot: Bull World Health Organ 41:75, 1969 and 43:1, 1970; and from "Resource allocation model for public health planning—a case study of tuberculosis control," Bull World Health Organ 84(Suppl) 1973.*]

infection of the index patient. State-by-state variations in regulations on this approach have not been well defined.

In summary, clinicians and public health agencies share responsibility for the prevention and control of STDs. In the managed-care era, the role of primary care clinicians has become increasingly important in prevention as well as in diagnosis and treatment.

FURTHER READING

ALLEN-DAVIS JT et al: Assessment of vulvovaginal complaints: Accuracy of telephone triage and in-office diagnosis. Obstet Gynecol 99:18, 2002

CENTERS FOR DISEASE CONTROL AND PREVENTION: Sexually transmitted diseases treatment guidelines 2002. MMWR 51(RR-6):1, 2002

———: Incorporating HIV prevention into the medical care of persons living with HIV. MMWR 52(RR-12):1, 2003

DALABETTA G et al (eds): Syndromic management of sexually transmitted diseases. Sex Transm Dis 74(Suppl 1):S1, 1998

ECKERT LO et al: Endometritis: The clinical-pathologic syndrome. Am J Obstet Gynecol 186:690, 2002

GROSSKURTH H et al: Impact of improved treatment of sexually transmitted diseases on HIV infection in rural Tanzania: Randomized controlled trial. Lancet 346:530, 1995

KAMB ML et al: Efficacy of risk-reduction counseling to prevent human immunodeficiency virus and sexually transmitted diseases: A randomized controlled trial. Project RESPECT Study Group. JAMA 280:1161, 1998

MCCREE DH et al: National survey of doctors' actions following the diagnosis of a bacterial STD. Sex Transm Infect 79:254, 2003

NESS RB et al: Effectiveness of inpatient and outpatient treatment strategies for women with pelvic inflammatory disease: Results from the Pelvic Inflammatory Disease Evaluation and Clinical Health (PEACH) Randomized Trial. Am J Obstet Gynecol 186:929, 2002

TAO G et al: Missed opportunities to assess sexually transmitted diseases in U.S. adults during routine medical checkups. Am J Prev Med 18:109, 2000

Section 3   Clinical Syndromes: Nosocomial Infections

116   HOSPITAL-ACQUIRED INFECTIONS
Robert A. Weinstein

The costs of nosocomial (hospital-acquired) infections are great. It is estimated that nosocomial infections affect more than 2 million patients, cost $4.5 billion, and contribute to 88,000 deaths in U.S. hospitals annually. Efforts to lower infection risks have been challenged by the growing numbers of immunocompromised patients, antibiotic-resistant bacteria, fungal and viral superinfections, and invasive devices and procedures. Nevertheless, evidence-based guidelines for prevention and control are now available (Table 116-1); according to some estimates, the consistent application of these guidelines may reduce the risk of nosocomial infection by more than one-third. This chapter reviews hospital-acquired and device-related infections and the basic surveillance, prevention, and control and treatment activities that have been developed to deal with these problems.

ORGANIZATION AND RESPONSIBILITIES OF INFECTION-CONTROL PROGRAMS The standards of the Joint Commission on Accreditation of Healthcare Organizations require all accredited hospitals to have an active program for surveillance, prevention, and control of nosocomial infections. A multidisciplinary infection-control committee usually oversees the program. The agents of the committee are the chairperson, who is preferably an infectious disease physician, and the infection-control practitioners, who are usually trained in nursing or medical technology and in epidemiology and public health. Education of physicians in infection control and hospital epidemiology is required in infectious disease fellowship programs and is available in courses provided by professional societies, primarily the Society for Healthcare Epidemiology of America.

Diagnosis-related reimbursement has led hospital administrators to place increased emphasis on cost containment and on documentation of the cost-effectiveness of infection control. The quality-improvement movements and the Joint Commission have redirected infection-control attention, in part, beyond the mere writing of policies and procedures to improvement of the actual processes and optimization of outcomes. In many hospitals, epidemiology programs have taken on additional pharmacoepidemiologic and antibiotic-use review responsibilities as well as broader quality-assurance activities under the rubric "patient safety." All programs must respond to governmental regulation of hospital waste and to standards mandated by the Occupational Safety & Health Administration for protecting health care workers from occupational exposure to bloodborne pathogens and tuberculosis.

SURVEILLANCE Traditionally, infection-control practitioners have surveyed inpatients for infections acquired in hospitals (defined as those neither present nor incubating at the time of admission). Surveillance involves a review of microbiology laboratory results, "shoe-leather" epidemiology on the nursing wards, application of standardized defi-

TABLE 116-1 *Sources of Infection-Control Guidance and Oversight*

Organization	Role	Major Constituents	Web Site
JCAHO	Regulatory	Hospitals, long-term-care facilities, laboratories	www.jcaho.org
CAP	Regulatory	Laboratories	www.cap.org
OSHA	Regulatory	Workers	www.osha.gov
CMS (formerly HCFA)	Regulatory	Medicare/Medicaid providers	www.cms.hhs.gov
CDC			
DHQP	Advisory	Health care facilities and personnel	www.cdc.gov/ncidod/hip/default.htm
HICPAC	Advisory	Health care facilities and personnel	www.cdc.gov/ncidod/hip/HICPAC/hicpac.htm
NIOSH	Advisory	Workers	www.cdc.gov/niosh/homepage.htm
AHRQ	Advisory	Broad (e.g., health care personnel)	www.ahrq.org
NQF	Advisory	Broad (e.g., health care personnel)	www.qualityforum.org
IOM	Advisory	Broad (e.g., health care personnel)	www.iom.edu
IDSA	Professional society	Infectious disease physicians/researchers	www.idsociety.org
SHEA	Professional society	Hospital epidemiologists	www.shea-online.org
APIC	Professional society	Infection-control practitioners	www.apic.org

Abbreviations: JCAHO, Joint Commission on Accreditation of Healthcare Organizations; CAP, College of American Pathologists; OSHA, Occupational Safety & Health Administration; CMS, Centers for Medicare & Medicaid Services; HCFA, Health Care Financing Administration; CDC, Centers for Disease Control and Prevention; DHQP, Division of Healthcare Quality Promotion; HICPAC, Healthcare Infection Control Practices Advisory Committee; NIOSH, National Institute for Occupational Safety and Health; AHRQ, Agency for Healthcare Research and Quality; NQF, National Quality Forum; IOM, Institute of Medicine; IDSA, Infectious Diseases Society of America; SHEA, Society for Healthcare Epidemiology of America, Inc.; APIC, Association for Professionals in Infection Control and Epidemiology, Inc.

nitions of infection, ongoing dialogue with hospital workers, and common sense. Some innovative infection-control programs have taken advantage of the increased use of computerized pharmacy, microbiology, and other databases in hospitals to create algorithm-driven surveillance.

Most hospitals aim surveillance at infections that (1) are associated with a high level of morbidity [e.g., intensive care unit (ICU)–related infections and nosocomial pneumonia]; (2) are costly (e.g., cardiac surgical wound infections); (3) are difficult to treat (e.g., infections due to antibiotic-resistant bacteria); (4) pose recurrent epidemic problems (e.g., *Clostridium difficile*–related diarrhea); and (5) are potentially preventable (e.g., vascular access–related infections). Quality-assurance activities in infection control have led to increased surveillance of the compliance of personnel with infection-control policies (e.g., monitoring of actual adherence to hand hygiene recommendations).

The results of surveillance are expressed as rates; in general, 5 to 10% of patients develop nosocomial infections. Such overall statistics have little value unless qualified by duration of risk, by site of infection, by patient population, and by exposure to risk factors. Meaningful denominators for infection rates include the number of patients exposed to a specific risk (e.g., rates of pneumonia among patients using mechanical ventilators) and the number of intervention days (e.g., rates of pneumonia per 1000 patient-days on a ventilator).

Temporal trends in rates should be reviewed, and rates should be compared with regional and national norms. However, even comparison rates generated by the ongoing National Nosocomial Infections Surveillance System [a program of the Centers for Disease Control and Prevention (CDC)], which collects data from more than 350 hospitals that use standardized definitions of nosocomial infections, have not been validated independently and represent a nonrandom sample of hospitals. Interhospital comparisons are easily confounded by the wide range in risk factors and in severity of underlying illnesses; unless rates are adjusted for these factors, comparisons may be misleading. Unfortunately, systems for making such adjustments either are rudimentary or have not been well validated.

The ongoing analysis of an individual hospital's infection rates helps to determine whether control efforts are succeeding and where increased education and control measures should be focused. Knowledge of infection rates is also useful in discussions with the hospital administration regarding areas to which additional resources should be directed.

EPIDEMIOLOGIC BASIS AND GENERAL MEASURES FOR PREVENTION AND CONTROL

Nosocomial infections follow basic epidemiologic patterns that can help to direct prevention and control measures. Nosocomial pathogens have reservoirs, are transmitted by predictable routes, and require susceptible hosts. Reservoirs and sources exist in the inanimate environment (e.g., tap water contaminated with *Legionella*) and in the animate environment (e.g., infected or colonized health care workers, patients, and hospital visitors). The mode of transmission most often is either cross-infection (e.g., indirect spread of pathogens from one patient to another on the inadequately cleaned hands of hospital personnel) or autoinoculation (e.g., aspiration of oropharyngeal flora into the lung along an endotracheal tube). Occasionally, pathogens (e.g., group A streptococci and many respiratory viruses) are spread indirectly from person to person via infectious droplets released by coughing or sneezing. Much less common—but often devastating in terms of epidemic risk—is true airborne spread of droplet nuclei (as in nosocomial chickenpox) or common-source spread by contaminated materials (e.g., iodophors contaminated with *Pseudomonas*). Factors that increase host susceptibility include underlying conditions and the many medical-surgical interventions and procedures that bypass or compromise normal host defenses.

Through its program, the hospital's infection-control committee must determine the general and specific measures used to control infections

and must review and recommend specific antiseptics and disinfectants for hospital use. Given the prominence of cross-infection, hand hygiene is the single most important preventive measure in hospitals (Table 116-2). Health care workers' rates of adherence to hand-hygiene recommendations are abysmally low (<50%). Reasons cited include inconvenience, time pressures, and skin damage from frequent washing. Sinkless alcohol rubs are quick and highly effective and actually improve hand condition since they contain emollients and allow the retention of natural protective oils that are removed with repeated rinsing. Use of alcohol hand rubs between patient contacts is now recommended for all health care workers except when the hands are visibly soiled, in which case washing with soap and water is still required.

NOSOCOMIAL AND DEVICE-RELATED INFECTIONS   The fact that 25 to 50% of nosocomial infections are due to the combined effect of the patient's own flora and invasive devices highlights the importance of improvements in the use and design of such devices. Intensive educational programs can be associated with at least a temporary reduction in infection rates through improved asepsis in handling and earlier removal of invasive devices, but the maintenance of such gains is often difficult. Of particular note, shortages of trained personnel jeopardize safe and effective patient care and have been associated with increased rates of infection and death among patients.

Urinary Tract Infections   Urinary tract infections (UTIs) account for as many as 40 to 45% of nosocomial infections; up to 3% of bacteriuric patients develop bacteremia. Although UTIs contribute only 10 to 15% to prolongation of hospital stay and to extra costs, these infections are important reservoirs and sources for spread of antibiotic-resistant bacteria in hospitals. Almost all nosocomial UTIs are associated with preceding instrumentation or indwelling bladder catheters, which create a 3 to 10% risk of infection each day. UTIs generally are caused by pathogens that spread up the periurethral space from the patient's perineum or gastrointestinal tract—the most common pathogenesis in women—or via intraluminal contamination of urinary catheters, usually due to cross-infection by caregivers who are irrigating catheters or emptying drainage bags. Pathogens occasionally come from inadequately disinfected urologic equipment and rarely come from contaminated supplies (e.g., dilute aqueous benzalkonium chloride, an ineffective disinfectant).

The most important measures for preventing nosocomial UTIs are (1) the placement of catheters only when absolutely necessary and not solely for the convenience of caregivers, (2) the use of aseptic technique for catheter insertion and for urinary tract instrumentation, (3) the manipulation and opening of drainage systems as infrequently as possible, and (4) the removal of catheters as soon as feasible. Hospitals

---

TABLE 116-2   *Examples of Ways in which Physicians Can Contribute to Infection-Control Efforts*

- Act as role models for other personnel by paying careful attention to hand-hygiene recommendations and barrier precautions during contact with patients and by observing posted isolation precautions.
- Give corrective feedback to caregivers who do not adhere to hand-hygiene recommendations or isolation precautions.
- Place invasive devices based on clinical need (not just on convenience).
- Remove invasive devices promptly when they are no longer needed clinically.
- Limit surgical antimicrobial prophylaxis to the perioperative period.
- Exercise care in initial empirical antibiotic selection (avoid "shotgun" approaches).
- Narrow the spectrum of antibiotic therapy once a pathogen is recovered.
- Discontinue antibiotic therapy in a timely fashion.
- Become familiar with the hospital's bloodborne pathogen and tuberculosis control plans.
- Order appropriate isolation precautions promptly for infected patients.
- During patient rounds, alert nursing staff to lapses in asepsis (e.g., soiled dressings at sites of intravascular catheters) and to infection-predisposing situations (e.g., aspiration-prone positioning of patients).
- Notify infection-control practitioners of potential infection-control problems (e.g., surgical wound infections that manifest after a patient's discharge).

should develop criteria for and closely monitor these four performance measures.

Sealed catheter–drainage tube junctions can help to prevent breaks in the system. Approaches to the prevention of UTIs also have included the use of topical meatal antimicrobials, drainage bag disinfectants, and anti-infective catheters. A meta-analysis and more recent studies suggest that silver alloy–coated catheters may reduce the incidence of bacteriuria, at least during short-term catheterization. However, because of conflicting study results, none of the latter three measures is considered routine.

Systemic antimicrobials given for other purposes decrease the risk of UTI during the first 4 days of catheterization, after which resistant bacteria or yeasts emerge as pathogens. Selective decontamination of the gut is also associated with a reduced risk. Again, however, neither approach is routine.

Irrigation of catheters, with or without antimicrobials, may actually increase the risk of infection. A condom catheter for men without bladder obstruction may be more acceptable than an indwelling catheter, but the infection risks with the two types are similar unless the condom catheter is carefully maintained. The role of suprapubic catheters in preventing infection is not well defined.

Treatment of UTIs is based on the results of quantitative cultures of urine (see Chap. 269); the most common pathogens are *Escherichia coli*, nosocomial gram-negative bacilli, enterococci, and *Candida*. Several caveats apply in the treatment of institutionally acquired infection. First, in patients with chronic indwelling bladder catheters, especially those in long-term-care facilities, the "catheter flora"—microorganisms living in the biofilm or on encrustations within the catheter lumen—may differ from the actual urinary tract pathogens. Therefore, for suspected infection in the setting of chronic catheterization (especially in women), it is useful to replace the bladder catheter and to obtain a freshly voided urine specimen. Second, as in all nosocomial infections, at the time treatment is initiated on the basis of a positive culture, it is useful to repeat the culture to verify the persistence of infection. Third, the frequency with which UTIs occur may lead to the erroneous assumption that this site alone is the source of infection in a febrile hospitalized patient. Thus, in the treatment of nosocomial UTIs, it is important to assess the patient for symptoms, especially of upper-pole infection (e.g., flank pain in conscious patients), and for signs of abnormal urinary sediment. Since nosocomial UTIs usually occur in the setting of catheterization or recent instrumentation, lower-tract symptoms (e.g., dysuria) may not be reliable. Fourth, recovery of *Staphylococcus aureus* from urine cultures may result from hematogenous seeding and may indicate an occult systemic infection. Finally, although *Candida* is now the most common pathogen in nosocomial UTIs in ICU patients, it is not clear that candiduria in the absence of upper-pole invasion, obstruction, neutropenia, or immunosuppression warrants treatment.

Pneumonia   Pneumonia accounts for 15 to 20% of nosocomial infections but has been responsible for 24% of extra hospital days and 39% of extra costs—i.e., 6 days and $6000 (based on 1992 dollars) per episode. Almost all cases of bacterial nosocomial pneumonia are caused by aspiration of endogenous or hospital-acquired oropharyngeal (and occasionally gastric) flora. Nosocomial pneumonias are associated with more deaths than are infections at any other body site. However, attributable mortality for ventilator-associated pneumonia—the most common and lethal form of nosocomial pneumonia—is in the 6 to 14% range; this figure suggests that the risk of dying from nosocomial pneumonia is affected greatly by other factors, including comorbidities, inadequate antibiotic treatment, and the involvement of specific pathogens (particularly *Pseudomonas aeruginosa* and *Acinetobacter*). Surveillance and accurate diagnosis of pneumonia are often problematic in hospitals because many patients, especially those in the ICU, have abnormal chest roentgenographs, fever, and leukocytosis potentially attributable to multiple causes. →*Viral pneumonias, which are particularly important in pediatric and immunocompromised patients, are discussed in the virology section and in Chap. 239.*

Risk factors for nosocomial pneumonia, particularly ventilator-associated pneumonia, include those events that increase the risk of colonization by potential pathogens (e.g., prior antimicrobial therapy, contaminated ventilator circuits or equipment, or decreased gastric acidity); those that heighten the possibility of aspiration of oropharyngeal contents into the lower respiratory tract (e.g., intubation, decreased levels of consciousness, or presence of a nasogastric tube); and those that reduce host defense mechanisms in the lung and permit overgrowth of aspirated pathogens (e.g., chronic obstructive pulmonary disease, old age, or upper abdominal surgery).

Control measures for pneumonia are aimed at the remediation of risk factors in general patient care (e.g., minimizing aspiration-prone supine positioning) and at meticulous aseptic care of respirator equipment (e.g., disinfecting or sterilizing all inline reusable components such as nebulizers, replacing tubing circuits at intervals of >48 h—rather than more frequently—to lessen the number of breaks in the system, and teaching aseptic technique for suctioning). In a large multicenter trial, sucralfate, which provides stress-ulcer prophylaxis without altering gastric pH, did not reduce the risk of ventilator-associated pneumonia, despite the theoretical advantage of lessened risk for gastric colonization by gram-negative bacilli. The benefits of selective decontamination of the oropharynx and gut with nonabsorbable antimicrobials and/or use of short-course postintubation systemic antibiotics have been controversial. Among the logical preventive measures that require further investigation are the use of endotracheal tubes that provide channels for subglottic drainage of secretions and the use of noninvasive mechanical ventilation whenever feasible. Of note, even interventions that have reduced the rate of ventilator-associated pneumonia most often have not reduced overall ICU mortality; this fact suggests that this infection is a marker for patients with an otherwise-heightened risk of death.

The most likely pathogens for nosocomial pneumonia and treatment options are discussed in Chap. 239. Several considerations regarding diagnosis and treatment are worth emphasizing. Clinical criteria for diagnosis (e.g., fever, leukocytosis, development of purulent secretions, new or changing radiographic infiltrates, change in oxygen requirement or ventilator settings) have high sensitivity but relatively low specificity. These criteria are most useful for selecting patients for bronchoscopic or nonbronchoscopic procedures that yield lower respiratory tract samples protected from upper-tract contamination; quantitative cultures of such specimens have diagnostic sensitivities in the range of 80%. Early-onset nosocomial pneumonia, which manifests within the first 4 days of hospitalization, is most often caused by community-acquired pathogens, such as *Streptococcus pneumoniae* and *Haemophilus* species. Late-onset pneumonias most commonly are due to *S. aureus*, *P. aeruginosa*, *Enterobacter* species, *Klebsiella pneumoniae*, or *Acinetobacter*—a pathogen of increasing concern in many ICUs. When invasive techniques are used to diagnose ventilator-associated pneumonia, the proportion of isolates accounted for by gram-negative bacilli decreases from 50–70% to 35–45%. Infection is polymicrobial in as many as 20 to 40% of cases. The role of anaerobic bacteria in ventilator-associated pneumonia is not well defined. The appropriate duration of therapy for nosocomial pneumonia, although generally stated to be in the 10- to 21-day range, is not well studied. Finally, in febrile patients (particularly those who have endotracheal and/or nasogastric tubes), more occult sources of respiratory tract infection, especially bacterial sinusitis and otitis media, should be considered.

Surgical Wound Infections   Wound infections account for up to 20 to 30% of nosocomial infections but contribute up to 57% of extra hospital days and 42% of extra costs. Because the average wound infection has an incubation period of 5 to 7 days, which is longer than many postoperative stays, and because many procedures now are performed on an outpatient basis, the incidence of wound infections has become difficult to assess. These infections usually are caused by the patient's endogenous or hospital-acquired skin and mucosal flora and occasionally are due to airborne spread of skin squames that may be shed into the wound from members of the operating-room team. True airborne spread of infection through droplet nuclei is rare in operating rooms unless there is a "disseminator" (e.g., of group A streptococci or staphylococci) among the staff. In general, the most common risks for postoperative wound infection are deficits in the surgeon's technical skill, the patient's underlying diseases (e.g., diabetes mellitus, obesity), and inappropriate timing of antibiotic prophylaxis. Additional risk factors include the presence of drains, prolonged preoperative hospital stays, shaving of the operative site the day before surgery, a long duration of surgery, and infection at remote sites (e.g., untreated UTI).

The substantial literature related to risk factors for surgical-site infections and the recognized morbidity and cost of these infections have led to careful evaluation of a number of interventions. The most important control measures include the use of antimicrobial prophylaxis at the start of high-risk procedures (see Chap. 118), attention to technical surgical issues and operating-room asepsis (e.g., not shaving the operative site until surgery and avoiding open or prophylactic drains), and preoperative therapy for active infection. Reporting of surveillance results to surgeons has been associated with reductions in infection rates. Measures that improve patients' resistance to infection are rare; thus the reductions in postoperative wound-infection rates associated with use of supplemental oxygen, maintenance of normothermia, or improved perioperative glucose control in recent studies are particularly exciting. The increasingly extensive review of infection rates by regulatory agencies and third-party payers emphasizes the importance of stratifying rates by patient-related risk factors and of developing meaningful systems for interhospital comparisons and for wound surveillance after the patient's discharge from the hospital or clinic (when more than 50% of infections first become apparent). The epidemic of mad cow disease, centered in the United Kingdom, and associated cases of variant Creutzfeldt-Jakob disease in humans (Chap. 362) caused by disinfection-resistant prion agents are leading to new recommendations for decontamination of surgical instruments, especially those used for operations on the central nervous system or in patients with a dementing illness of unknown etiology.

The process of diagnosing and treating wound infections begins with a careful assessment of the surgical site in the febrile postoperative patient. Clinical findings range from obvious cellulitis or abscess formation to subtle clues such as a sternal "click" following open heart surgery. Diagnosis of deeper organ-space infections or subphrenic abscesses requires a high index of suspicion and the use of computed tomography or magnetic resonance imaging. Diagnosis of infections of prosthetic devices, such as orthopedic implants, may be particularly difficult and often requires the use of interventional radiographic techniques to obtain periprosthetic specimens for culture. The most common pathogens in postoperative wound infections are S. aureus, coagulase-negative staphylococci, and enteric and anaerobic bacteria. In rapidly progressing postoperative infections, which manifest within 24 to 48 h of a surgical procedure, the level of suspicion regarding group A streptococcal or clostridial infection (Chaps. 121 and 126) should be high. Treatment of postoperative wound infections requires drainage or surgical excision of infected or necrotic material and antibiotic therapy aimed at the most likely or laboratory-confirmed pathogens.

Infections Related to Vascular Access and Monitoring   Intravascular devices are common causes of local site infection and cause up to 50% of nosocomial bacteremias; central vascular catheters account for 80 to 90% of these infections. National estimates indicate that as many as 250,000 bloodstream infections associated with central vascular catheters occur each year in the United States, with an attributable mortality of 12 to 25% and an estimated cost of $25,000 per episode; one-third to one-half of these episodes occur in ICUs. With increasing care of seriously ill patients in the community, vascular catheter–associated bloodstream infections acquired by outpatients are receiving more at-

tention than in the past. A recent study of bacteremia patients at three hospitals showed that the numbers of patients being treated for device-associated bacteremia acquired in the hospital or in the community setting (e.g., home or clinic intravascular therapy) were similar. This finding emphasizes the need to broaden surveillance activities.

Catheter-related bloodstream infections derive largely from the cutaneous microflora of the insertion site, with pathogens migrating extraluminally to the catheter tip, usually during the first week after insertion. In addition, contamination of hubs of central vascular catheters may lead to intraluminal infection over longer periods, particularly with surgically implanted or cuffed catheters. Intrinsic contamination of infusate, although rare, is the most common cause of epidemic device-related bloodstream infection; extrinsic contamination may cause up to half of endemic bacteremias related to arterial infusions used for hemodynamic monitoring. The most common pathogens isolated from vascular device–associated bacteremias include coagulase-negative staphylococci, S. aureus (with up to 50% of isolates potentially resistant to methicillin), enterococci, nosocomial gram-negative bacilli, and Candida.

Infections related to vascular catheters and monitoring devices may be the most preventable of nosocomial infections. Evidence-based control measures include implementing educational programs with didactic and interactive components for persons who insert and maintain catheters, using maximal sterile barrier precautions (e.g., gowns, gloves, masks, and large drapes) during catheter placement, using chlorhexidine for skin antisepsis prior to catheter placement, and ensuring that "idle catheters" are removed. Hospitals should periodically monitor adherence to these performance indicators. Use of antimicrobial- or antiseptic-impregnated central venous catheters is a reasonable control measure for adults whose catheters are expected to remain in place for >5 days if, after implementation of the performance measures just listed, the rates of catheter-related bloodstream infection remain above the goals set by individual institutions based on benchmark national rates and local factors. Additional control measures for infections associated with vascular access include avoiding the femoral site for catheterization because of an unusually high risk of infection (most likely related to the density of the skin flora); moving peripheral catheters to a new site at specified intervals (e.g., every 72 to 96 h), which may be facilitated by use of an intravenous therapy team; and applying disposable transducers for pressure monitoring and aseptic technique for accessing transducers or other vascular ports. Improvements in composition of semitransparent access-site dressings and potential nursing benefits (ease of bathing and site inspection, protection of site from secretions) favor the use of such coverings. Unresolved issues include the best frequency for rotation of central vascular catheter sites (given that guidewire-assisted catheter changes at the same site do not lessen infection risk); the appropriate role of mupirocin ointment, a topical antibiotic with excellent antistaphylococcal activity, in site care; the relative degrees of risk posed by peripherally inserted central catheters (PICC lines); and the risk-benefit of prophylactic use of heparin to avoid catheter thrombi, which may be associated with increased risk of infection.

Vascular device–related infection is suspected on the basis of the appearance of the catheter site or the presence of fever or bacteremia without another source in patients with vascular catheters. The diagnosis is confirmed by the recovery of the same species of microorganism from peripheral-blood cultures (preferably two cultures drawn from peripheral veins by separate venipunctures) and from semiquantitative or quantitative cultures of the vascular catheter tip. Less commonly used diagnostic measures include differential time to positivity (>2 h) for blood drawn through the vascular access device compared with a sample from a peripheral vein or differences in quantitative cultures (a 5- to 10-fold or greater "step-up") for blood samples drawn simultaneously from a peripheral vein and from a central vascular catheter. When infusion-related sepsis is considered (e.g., because of the abrupt onset of fever or shock temporally related to infusion therapy), a sample of the infusate or blood product should be retained for culture.

Therapy for vascular access–related infection is directed at the pathogen recovered from the blood and/or infected site. Important considerations in treatment are the need for an echocardiogram (to evaluate the patient for bacterial endocarditis), the duration of therapy, and the need to remove potentially infected catheters. In one report, approximately one-fourth of patients with intravascular catheter–associated *S. aureus* bacteremia studied by transesophageal echocardiography had evidence of endocarditis; the implication is that this test may be useful in determining the appropriate duration of treatment. Detailed consensus guidelines for the management of intravascular catheter–related infections have been published and recommend catheter removal in most cases of bacteremia or fungemia due to nontunneled central venous catheters. When attempting to salvage a potentially infected catheter, some clinicians use the "antibiotic lock" technique (instillation of concentrated antibiotic solution into the catheter lumen) in addition to systemic antimicrobial therapy. In one study of hemodialysis catheters, only about one third of salvage attempts were successful, although delayed removal did not appear to increase the risk of complications. When feasible, a potentially infected central vascular catheter may be exchanged over a guidewire. If cultures of the removed catheter tip are positive, the replacement catheter will be moved to a new site; if the tip cultures are negative, the replacement catheter can remain in the original site. For patients with track-site infection, successful therapy without catheter removal is unusual. For patients with suppurative venous thrombophlebitis, excision of the affected vein is required. The authors of the consensus guidelines advise that the decision to remove a tunneled catheter or implanted device suspected to be the source of bacteremia or fungemia should be based on the severity of the patient's illness, the strength of the evidence that the device is infected, an assessment of the specific pathogens, and the presence of local or systemic complications.

ISOLATION TECHNIQUES Written policies for the isolation of infectious patients are a standard component of infection-control programs. In 1996, the CDC revised its isolation guidelines to make them simpler; to recognize the importance of all body fluids, secretions, and excretions in the transmission of nosocomial pathogens; and to focus precautions on the major routes of infection transmission.

The revised guidelines contain two tiers of precautions. *Standard precautions* are designed for the care of all patients in hospitals to reduce the risk of transmission of microorganisms from both recognized and unrecognized sources of infection. These precautions include gloving as well as hand cleansing for potential contact with (1) blood; (2) all other body fluids, secretions, and excretions, whether or not they contain visible blood; (3) nonintact skin; and (4) mucous membranes. Depending on exposure risks, standard precautions also include use of masks, eye protection, and gowns.

In the second tier are precautions for the care of patients with suspected or diagnosed colonization or infection with transmissible pathogens. These transmission-based guidelines collapse the older category- and disease-specific isolation guidelines into three sets of precautions based on probable routes of transmission: *airborne precautions*, *droplet precautions*, and *contact precautions*. Sets of precautions may be combined for diseases that have more than one route of transmission (e.g., varicella). Potentially contagious clinical syndromes, such as acute diarrhea, are included in the revised guidelines.

Because some prevalent antibiotic-resistant pathogens, particularly vancomycin-resistant enterococci (VRE), may be present on *intact* skin of patients in hospitals, some experts recommend gloving for all contact with patients who are acutely ill and/or from high-risk units, such as ICUs. In recent trials, wearing gloves did not replace the need for hand hygiene because hands occasionally became contaminated during wearing or removal of gloves. Some studies have suggested that use of gowns and gloves compared with routine care of patients (i.e., using neither of these barriers) decreases the risk of nosocomial infection; however, more recent evaluation suggests that gowning by personnel does not add benefit beyond that conferred by gloving and hand hygiene. Nevertheless, requiring increased precaution levels can improve the compliance of health care workers with isolation recommendations by 30%.

EPIDEMIC AND EMERGING PROBLEMS Outbreaks and emerging pathogens are always big news but probably account for fewer than 5% of nosocomial infections. Concern about emerging pathogens often prompts authorities to require hospitals to develop contingency and response plans. The investigation and control of nosocomial epidemics require that infection-control personnel develop a case definition, confirm that an outbreak really exists (since many apparent epidemics are actually pseudo-outbreaks due to surveillance or laboratory artifacts), review aseptic practices and disinfectant use, determine the extent of the outbreak, perform an epidemiologic investigation to determine modes of transmission, work closely with microbiology personnel to culture for common sources or personnel carriers as appropriate and to type epidemiologically important isolates, and heighten surveillance to judge the effect of control measures. Control measures generally include the early reinforcement of routine aseptic practices and hand hygiene during a search for compliance problems that may have fostered the outbreak, the ensuring of the appropriate isolation of cases (and the institution of cohort isolation and nursing if needed), and the implementation of further controls on the basis of the investigation's findings. Examples of some emerging and potential epidemic problems follow.

Chickenpox When health care workers are exposed to chickenpox in the community or through patients with initially unrecognized infections, or when these employees work during the 24 h before developing chickenpox, infection-control practitioners institute a varicella exposure investigation and control plan. The names of exposed workers and patients are obtained; medical histories are reviewed, and (if necessary) serologic tests for immunity are conducted; physicians are notified of susceptible exposed patients; postexposure prophylaxis with varicella-zoster immune globulin (VZIG) is considered for immunocompromised or pregnant contacts (see Table 164-1); preemptive use of acyclovir is considered as an alternative strategy in some susceptible persons; and susceptible exposed employees are furloughed during the at-risk period for disease (8 to 21 days, or 28 days if VZIG has been administered). Routine varicella vaccination of children and susceptible employees can markedly decrease risk and frequency of exposures.

Tuberculosis The resurgence of pulmonary tuberculosis in the United States since 1987 and a series of nosocomial outbreaks of infection with multidrug-resistant strains—primarily involving patients with AIDS and their caregivers—led to a successful revamping of tuberculosis control. Important control measures include prompt recognition, isolation, and treatment of cases; recognition of atypical presentations (e.g., lower-lobe infiltrates without cavitation); use of negative-pressure, 100% exhaust, private isolation rooms with closed doors and 6 to 12 or more air changes per hour; use of face masks ("respirators") approved by the National Institute for Occupational Safety and Health) by caregivers entering isolation rooms; possible use of high-efficiency particulate air filter units and/or ultraviolet lights for disinfecting air when other engineering controls are not feasible or reliable; and follow-up skin-testing of susceptible personnel who have been exposed to infectious patients before isolation.

Group A Streptococci The potential for a group A streptococcal outbreak should be considered when even a single nosocomial case occurs. Most outbreaks involve surgical wounds and are due to the presence of an asymptomatic carrier in the operating room. Investigation can be confounded by carriage at extrapharyngeal sites such as the rectum and vagina. Health care workers in whom carriage has been linked to nosocomial transmission of group A streptococci are removed from the patient-care setting and are not permitted to return until carriage has been eliminated by antimicrobial therapy.

Aspergillus Fungal spores are common in the environment, particularly on dusty surfaces. When hospital ceiling tiles are removed to provide access for repairs or when dusty areas are disturbed during hospital renovation, the spores become airborne. Inhalation of spores by immunosuppressed (especially neutropenic) patients creates a risk of pulmonary and/or paranasal sinus infection and disseminated aspergillosis. Routine surveillance among neutropenic patients for infections with filamentous fungi, such as *Aspergillus* and *Fusarium*, helps hospitals to determine whether they have unduly large environmental risks. As a matter of routine, hospitals should inspect and clean air-handling equipment, review all planned renovations with infection-control personnel and subsequently construct appropriate barriers, remove immunosuppressed patients from renovation sites, and consider the use of high-efficiency particulate air intake filters for rooms housing immunosuppressed patients.

Legionella Sporadic and epidemic cases of nosocomial *Legionella* pneumonia are most often due to the contamination of potable water and predominantly affect immunosuppressed patients, particularly those receiving glucocorticoid medication. The risk varies greatly within and among geographic regions, depending on the extent of hospital hot-water contamination, on the presence or absence of high-risk patient populations, and on specific hospital practices (e.g., inappropriate use of nonsterile water in respiratory therapy equipment). Laboratory-based surveillance for nosocomial *Legionella* should be performed, and a diagnosis of legionellosis should probably be considered more often than it is. If cases are detected, environmental samples (e.g., tap water) should be cultured. If cultures yield *Legionella* and if typing of clinical and environmental isolates reveals a correlation, eradication measures should be pursued (Chap. 132). An alternative approach is to periodically culture tap water in wards housing high-risk patients. If *Legionella* is found, a concerted effort should be made to culture samples from all patients with nosocomial pneumonia for *Legionella*.

Antibiotic-Resistant Bacteria Outbreaks of antibiotic resistance can depend on any of the following events: Darwinian selection of bacterial chromosomal mutations, spread of plasmid- and/or transposon-borne resistance among bacterial species, and (re)admission to the hospital of patients chronically infected with resistant bacteria. After the introduction of resistant strains, dissemination occurs by cross-infection on contaminated hands of caregivers or, occasionally, via personnel carriage and/or environmental contamination. Outbreak control (Table 116-3) depends on close laboratory surveillance, with early detection of problems; on the reinforcement of routine asepsis (e.g., hand hygiene); on the implementation of barrier precautions for all colonized and/or infected patients; on the use of patient-surveillance cultures to more fully ascertain the extent of patient colonization; and on the timely initiation of an epidemiologic investigation when rates increase. Colonized personnel who are implicated in nosocomial transmission and patients who pose a threat may be decontaminated; for example, colonization with methicillin-resistant *S. aureus* may be controlled

with oral antibiotics, including trimethoprim-sulfamethoxazole and rifampin, and with topical agents, including hexachlorophene or chlorhexidine and mupirocin. In a few ICUs, selective decontamination has been used successfully as a temporary emergency control measure for outbreaks of infection due to gram-negative bacilli.

An emerging bacterial-resistance problem to plague hospitals is the presence of VRE. Initially an ICU problem, VRE have now spread onto general wards in many hospitals. VRE are particularly problematic because of a substantial "iceberg" effect (i.e., the fact that, for each individual with a clinical infection, many other patients are colonized); the occurrence of both gastrointestinal and skin colonization (reflecting fecal contamination on the skin of ill, hospitalized patients); and the propensity for these organisms to contaminate the patient's environment, which may increase the risk of cross-infection. Control of VRE requires strict attention to hand hygiene by personnel, concerted use of barrier precautions or cohort nursing for patients known to be colonized or infected, and emphasis on thorough cleaning of the rooms of these patients.

Spread of vancomycin resistance to *S. aureus* is a major concern. Clinical infections with methicillin-resistant *S. aureus* strains that exhibit high-level vancomycin resistance due to VRE-derived plasmids have now been reported in the setting of prolonged or repeated treatment with vancomycin and/or VRE colonization. The detection of these strains appears to be readily accomplished in clinical microbiology laboratories and should trigger an aggressive epidemiologic investigation and infection-control measures.

Because the excessive use of broad-spectrum antibiotics underlies many resistance problems, aggressive antibiotic-control policies must be considered a cornerstone of resistance-control efforts. Although the efficacy of antibiotic-control measures in reducing rates of antimicrobial resistance has not been proved in prospective controlled trials, it seems worthwhile to restrict the use of particular agents to narrowly defined indications or possibly to cycle the use of antibiotic classes to limit selective pressure on the nosocomial flora.

Bioterrorism Preparedness The terrorist attack on the World Trade Center in New York City; other horrific events of September 11, 2001; and the subsequent mailings of anthrax spores in the United States have made bioterrorism a prominent source of concern to hospital

---

TABLE 116-3 *Controlling Antibiotic Resistance: Approaches to Consider*

- Conduct surveillance for antibiotic resistance.
- Perform molecular typing (e.g., pulsed-field gel electrophoresis) when rates increase.
- For clonal expansion (e.g., single-strain outbreaks): Stress hand hygiene (alcohol hand rub and universal gloving); monitor adherence and give feedback.
- For polyclonal expansion (e.g., multistrain outbreaks): Stress antibiotic prudence (consider antibiotic rotation for ICUs); monitor adherence and give feedback.
- For continued problems: Obtain patient-surveillance cultures and isolate or provide cohort nursing for colonized/infected patients.
- Control device-related infections.
- Enlist administrative support proactively.

Source: Adapted from: RA Weinstein, *Emerg Infect Dis* 7:188, 2001.

TABLE 116-4 *Highlights of Hospital Preparedness for Bioterrorism*

Emergency Department: Educate staff regarding bioterrorism diagnoses, case definitions, and appropriate syndrome-based isolation precautions.
Laboratory: Identify protocols and laboratory safety procedures for agents of bioterrorism.
Pharmacy: Develop medication and vaccine par stock, allocation, and delivery plans.
Nursing: Assess bed and isolation surge capacity; help develop contingency plans to free bed space by early discharges and deferred admissions.
Hospital Police: Plan for responsibilities as first responders and providers of risk assessment.
Mailroom: Plan for risk assessment and need/indications-for-use of personal protective equipment as appropriate.
Engineering/Buildings and Grounds: Evaluate air-handling systems and ensure familiarity with shutoffs and controls; educate staff about environmental decontamination.
Outpatient Areas: Develop plans for family and community evaluation and staging for delivery of prophylactic medications and/or vaccines.
Public Health: Ascertain local public health resources and open lines of communication, education, and surveillance.
The Community: Plan for infection-control practitioners to serve as liaisons/links/facilitators for emergency departments, laboratories, and community providers.
Administration: Perform resource assessment for medical supplies, transportation capabilities, potable water, sanitation facilities, provider backup, bed-space backup, etc. Oversee development of an incident command system.
"Morale Officer": Establish this position to help survey and keep staff functioning.

infection-control programs. The essentials for hospital preparedness (Table 116-4) entail education, internal and external communication, and risk assessment. Among the category A agents of bioterrorism (Chap. 205), smallpox is of major concern to the U.S. intelligence community. Consequently, in December 2002, the President of the United States recommended smallpox vaccination of a core group of military and hospital personnel; up-to-date information on a variety of vaccination-related and other bioterrorism-associated issues is available from the CDC (see www.bt.cdc.gov).

EMPLOYEE HEALTH SERVICE ISSUES   An institution's employee health service is a critical component of its infection-control efforts. New employees should be processed through the service, where a contagious-disease history can be taken; evidence of immunity to a variety of diseases, such as hepatitis B, chickenpox, measles, and rubella, can be sought; immunizations for hepatitis B, measles, rubella, and varicella can be given as needed and a reminder about the need for yearly influenza immunization can be imparted; baseline and "booster" purified protein derivative of tuberculin skin-testing can be performed; and education about personal responsibility for infection control can be initiated. Evaluations of employees should be codified to meet the requirements of accrediting and regulatory agencies.

The employee health service must have protocols for dealing with workers who have been exposed to contagious diseases, such as those percutaneously or mucosally exposed to the blood of patients infected with HIV or hepatitis B or C virus. For example, postexposure HIV prophylaxis with a combination of two or three antiretroviral agents is recommended; free consultation is available from the CDC PEPLine (1-888-HIV-4911). Protocols are also needed for dealing with caregivers who have common contagious diseases, such as chickenpox, group A streptococcal infections, respiratory infections, and infectious diarrhea, and for those who have less common but high-visibility public health problems, such as chronic hepatitis B or C or HIV infection, for which exposure-control guidelines have been published by the CDC and by the Society for Healthcare Epidemiology of America.

FURTHER READING

CENTERS FOR DISEASE CONTROL AND PREVENTION: Guideline for hand hygiene in health-care settings: Recommendations of the Healthcare Infection Control Practices Advisory Committee and the HICPAC/SHEA/APIC/IDSA Hand Hygiene Task Force. MMWR 51(RR-16):1, 2002

———: Guidelines for preventing opportunistic infections among hematopoietic stem cell transplant recipients: Recommendations of CDC, the Infectious Diseases Society of America, and the American Society of Blood and Marrow Transplantation. MMWR 49(RR-10):1, 2000

HUBMAYR RD: Statement of the 4th International Consensus Conference in Critical Care on ICU-Acquired Pneumonia. Intensive Care Med 28:1521, 2002

MAKI DG, WEINSTEIN RA: Nosocomial infection in the intensive care unit, in *Critical Care Medicine—Principles of Diagnosis and Management in the Adult*, 2d ed, JE Parillo, RP Dellinger (eds). Saunders, Philadelphia, 2001, pp 981–1046

MERMEL LA et al: Guidelines for the management of intravascular catheter–related infections. Clin Infect Dis 32:1249, 2001

O'GRADY NP et al: Guidelines for the prevention of intravascular catheter–related infections. Clin Infect Dis 35:1281, 2002

SCHWARTZ DS, WEINSTEIN RA: Fever in hospitalized patients, in *Clinical Infectious Diseases: A Practical Approach*, R Root et al (eds). Oxford, New York, 1999, pp 449–458

WEINSTEIN RA, BONTEN M (eds): *Infection Control in the ICU Environment.* Boston, Kluwer, 2002

---

117   INFECTIONS IN TRANSPLANT RECIPIENTS
Robert Finberg, Joyce Fingeroth

The evaluation of infections in transplant recipients involves consideration of both the donor and the recipient of the transplanted organ. Infections following transplantation are complicated by the use of drugs that are necessary to enhance the likelihood of survival of the transplanted organ but that also cause the host to be immunocompromised. Thus what might have been a latent or asymptomatic infection in an immunocompetent donor or in the recipient prior to therapy becomes a life-threatening problem when the recipient becomes immunosuppressed.

A variety of organisms have been transmitted by organ transplantation (Table 117-1). Careful attention to the sterility of the medium used to process the organ combined with meticulous microbiologic evaluation reduces rates of transmission of bacteria that may be present or grow in the organ culture medium. From 2% to >20% of donor kidneys are estimated to be contaminated with bacteria—in most cases, with the organisms that colonize the skin or grow in the tissue culture medium used to bathe the donor kidney while it awaits implantation. The reported rate of bacterial contamination of transplanted bone marrow is as high as 17% but is most commonly ~1%. The use of enrichment columns and monoclonal-antibody depletion procedures results in a higher incidence of contamination. Approximately 2% of cryopreserved marrow and peripheral-blood stem cells transfused as part of treatment for cancer are contaminated. In one series of patients receiving contaminated products, 14% had fever or bacteremia, but none died. Results of cultures performed at the time of cryopreservation and at the time of thawing were helpful in guiding therapy for the recipient.

In many transplantation centers, transmission of infections that may be latent or clinically inapparent in the donor organ has resulted in the development of specific donor-screening protocols. In addition to ordering serologic studies focusing on viruses such as herpes-group viruses [herpes simplex virus (HSV) 1, HSV-2], varicella-zoster virus (VZV), cytomegalovirus (CMV), human herpesvirus (HHV) type 6, Epstein-Barr virus (EBV), HHV-8, hepatitis B and C viruses, HIV, and human T-cell lymphotropic virus (HTLV) type I and on parasites such as *Toxoplasma gondii*, clinicians caring for organ donors should consider assessing stool (for parasites) and should perform skin testing for *Mycobacterium tuberculosis*. An investigation of the patient's dietary habits (e.g., consumption of raw meat or fish or of unpasteurized dairy products), occupations or avocations (e.g., gardening or spelunking), and travel history (e.g., travel to areas with endemic fungi) is mandatory. It is expected that the recipient will have been likewise assessed. This chapter considers aspects of infection unique to various transplantation settings.

INFECTIONS IN BONE MARROW AND HEMATOPOIETIC STEM CELL TRANSPLANT RECIPIENTS

Bone marrow or hematopoietic stem cell transplantation for either immunodeficiency or cancer results in a transient state of complete immune incompetence. Immediately after transplantation, both phagocytes and immune cells (T and B cells) are absent, and the host is extremely susceptible to infection. The reconstitution that follows transplantation has been likened to maturation of the immune system in neonates. The analogy does not entirely predict infections seen in bone marrow transplant (BMT) and hematopoietic stem cell transplant (HSCT) recipients because the new marrow matures in an old host who has several latent infections already. Nevertheless, infections occur in a predictable time frame after transplantation (Table 117-2).

BACTERIAL INFECTIONS   In the first month after bone marrow or hematopoietic stem cell transplantation, infectious complications are similar to those in granulocytopenic patients receiving chemotherapy for acute leukemia (Chap. 72). Because of the anticipated 1- to 4-week duration

TABLE 117-1 *Organisms Transmitted by Organ Transplantation and Sites of Reactivation Disease[a]*

	Blood	Lungs	Heart	Brain	Liver	Skin
Viruses						
Cytomegalovirus[b]	+	+	+/−	+	+	+
Epstein-Barr virus[c]	+	+	+	+	+	+
Herpes simplex virus		+			+	+
Human herpesvirus type 6	+	+		+		+
Human herpesvirus type 8[b]	+	+/−			+/−	+
Hepatitis B and C viruses					+	
Bovine spongiform encephalopathy (prion)[d]				+		
Rabies virus[e]				+		
West Nile virus				+		
Fungi						
Candida albicans	+	+			+	+
Histoplasma capsulatum	+	+			+	
Cryptococcus neoformans	+	+		+		+
Parasites						
Toxoplasma gondii[f]		+	+	+		
Strongyloides stercoralis[g,h]		+				
Trypanosoma cruzi[h]			+			
Plasmodium falciparum[h]	+					

[a] +, well documented; ±, probably occurs.

[b] Cytomegalovirus reactivation is prone to occur in the transplanted organ. The same may be true for human herpesvirus type 8 (Kaposi's sarcoma–associated herpesvirus).

[c] Epstein-Barr virus reactivation usually presents as an extranodal proliferation of transformed B cells and can be present either as a diffuse disease or as a mass lesion in a single organ.

[d] Bovine spongiform encephalopathy, a prion-mediated disease, can be transmitted with organs.

[e] Rabies has been transmitted through corneal transplants.

[f] *T. gondii* usually causes disease in the brain. In bone marrow transplant recipients, acute pulmonary disease may also occur. Heart transplant recipients develop disease in the allograft.

[g] *Strongyloides* "hyperinfection" may present with pulmonary disease—often associated with gram-negative bacterial pneumonia.

[h] While transmission with organs has been described, it is unusual.

of neutropenia and the high rate of bacterial infection in this population, many centers give prophylactic antibiotics to patients upon initiation of chemotherapy. Levofloxacin decreases the incidence of gram-negative bacteremia among these patients. Bacterial infections are common in the first few days after bone marrow transplantation.

The organisms involved are predominantly aerobic bacteria found in the bowels (*Escherichia coli*, *Klebsiella*, *Pseudomonas*) and those found on the skin or in intravenous catheters (*Staphylococcus aureus*, coagulase-negative staphylococci). Beyond the first few days of neutropenia, infections with filamentous bacteria (*Nocardia* and the organisms that cause actinomycosis) become more common. Episodes of bacteremia due to encapsulated organisms mark the late posttransplantation period (>6 months after bone marrow reconstitution).

FUNGAL INFECTIONS Beyond the first week after transplantation, fungal infections become increasingly common. As in most granulocytopenic patients, *Candida* infections are most commonly seen in this setting. With increased use of prophylactic fluconazole, infections with resistant fungi, such as *Candida glabrata* and *Aspergillus*, have become more common. In patients with graft-versus-host disease (GVHD) who require prolonged or indefinite courses of glucocorticoids and other immunosuppressive agents [e.g., cyclosporine, tacrolimus, mycophenolate mofetil, rapamycin, alemtuzumab (an antilymphocyte and antimonocyte antibody)], there is a high risk of fungal infection (usually with *Candida* or *Aspergillus*), even after engraftment and resolution of neutropenia. These patients are also at high risk of reactivation of fungal infection (histoplasmosis, coccidioidomycosis, blastomycosis) in areas where endemic fungi reside and if they are involved in activities such as spelunking or gardening.

PARASITIC INFECTIONS Because of the high and prolonged risk of *Pneumocystis* pneumonia (especially among patients being treated for hematologic malignancies), most patients should receive maintenance prophylaxis with trimethoprim-sulfamethoxazole (TMP-SMX) starting 1 month after engraftment and continuing for at least 1 year. Such prophylaxis may also protect patients seropositive for *T. gondii*, which may cause pneumonia as well as central nervous system (CNS) lesions. The advantages of maintaining patients on daily TMP-SMX for 1 year after transplantation include protection against *Listeria monocytogenes* and nocardial disease as well as late infections with *Streptococcus pneumoniae* and *Haemophilus influenzae*, which are a consequence of the inability of the immature bone marrow to respond to polysaccharide antigens.

VIRAL INFECTIONS BMT/HSCT recipients are susceptible to infection with a variety of viruses, including reactivation syndromes caused by most HHVs (Table 117-3) and infections caused by viruses that circulate in the community.

Herpes Simplex Virus Within the first 2 weeks after transplantation, most patients who are seropositive for HSV-1 excrete the virus from the oropharynx. The ability to isolate HSV declines with time. Administration of prophylactic acyclovir (or valacyclovir) to seropositive BMT/HSCT recipients has been shown to reduce mucositis and prevent HSV pneumonia (a rare condition reported almost exclusively in BMT recipients). Both esophagitis (usually due to HSV-1) and anogenital disease (commonly induced by HSV-2) may be prevented with acyclovir prophylaxis. →*For further discussion, see Chap. 163.*

Varicella-Zoster Virus Reactivation of herpes zoster may occur within the first month but more commonly occurs several months after transplantation. Reactivation rates are ~40% for allogeneic recipients and 25% for autologous recipients. Localized zoster can spread locally in an immunosuppressed patient. Fortunately, disseminated disease can usually be controlled with high doses of acyclovir. Because of the high incidence of dissem-

TABLE 117-2 *Infections After Bone Marrow Transplantation*

	Period after Transplantation		
Infection Site	Early (<1 Month)	Middle (1–4 Months)	Late (>6 Months)
Disseminated	Bacteria (aerobic gram-negative, gram-positive)	Bacteria (*Nocardia*, agents of actinomycosis) Fungi (*Candida*, *Aspergillus*)	Encapsulated bacteria (*Streptococcus pneumoniae*, *Haemophilus influenzae*, *Neisseria meningitidis*)
Skin and mucous membranes	Herpes simplex virus	Human herpesvirus type 6	Varicella-zoster virus
Lungs	Herpes simplex virus	Viruses (cytomegalovirus, human herpesvirus type 6) Parasites (*Toxoplasma gondii*) Fungi (*Pneumocystis*)	
Kidneys			Viruses (BK)
Brain			Parasites (*T. gondii*) Viruses (JC)

Virus	Reactivation Disease
Herpes simplex virus type 1	Oral lesions, may be associated with pneumonia, described only in BMT recipients Hepatitis
Herpes simplex virus type 2	Severe and/or persistent anogenital lesions Hepatitis
Varicella-zoster virus	Zoster (potentially disseminated)
Cytomegalovirus	Associated with graft rejection, fever, bone marrow failure, pneumonitis, gastrointestinal disease, other
Epstein-Barr virus	B cell lymphoproliferative disease Oral hairy leukoplakia (rare)
Human herpesvirus type 6	Fever, rash,[a] pneumonitis, bone marrow suppression, encephalitis (manifestations controversial)
Human herpesvirus type 7	Undefined
Kaposi's sarcoma–associated herpesvirus/human herpesvirus type 8	Kaposi's sarcoma Primary effusion lymphoma (rare) Multicentric Castleman's disease (rare)

[a] A rash may be seen with primary infections, but it is difficult to distinguish from other rashes seen in these patients.
Note: BMT, bone marrow transplant.

ination of herpes zoster among patients with skin lesions, acyclovir is given prophylactically in some centers to prevent severe disease. Low doses of acyclovir (400 mg orally, three times daily) appear to be effective in preventing reactivation of VZV. However, acyclovir also inhibits the development of VZV-specific immunity. Thus, its administration for only 6 months after transplantation does not prevent zoster from occurring when treatment is stopped. Some data suggest that administration of low doses of acyclovir for an entire year after transplantation is effective and may eliminate most cases of posttransplantation zoster. →*For further discussion, see Chap. 164.*

Cytomegalovirus The onset of CMV disease (interstitial pneumonia, bone marrow suppression, or graft failure) usually comes between 30 and 90 days after transplantation, when the granulocyte count is adequate but immunologic reconstitution has not occurred. CMV disease rarely develops earlier than 14 days after transplantation and may become evident as late as 4 months after the procedure. It is of great concern in the second month after transplantation, particularly in allogeneic BMT/HSCT recipients. In cases in which the donor marrow is depleted of T cells (to prevent GVHD or eliminate a T cell tumor), the disease may be manifested earlier. The use of αCD52 antibody (alemtuzumab) to prevent GVHD in nonmyeloablative transplantation has been associated with an increase in CMV disease. Patients who receive ganciclovir (for prophylaxis, preemptive treatment, or treatment; see below) may develop CMV infection even later than 4 months after transplantation; treatment appears to delay the development of the normal immune response to CMV infection. Although CMV disease may present as isolated fever, granulocytopenia, or gastrointestinal disease, the foremost cause of death from CMV infection in this setting is pneumonia.

With the standard use of CMV-negative or filtered blood products, primary CMV infection should be a risk in allogeneic transplantation only when the donor is CMV-seropositive and the recipient is CMV-seronegative. Reactivation disease or superinfection with another strain from the donor is also common in CMV-positive recipients, and most seropositive patients who undergo bone marrow transplantation excrete CMV, with or without clinical findings. Serious CMV disease is much more common among allogeneic than autologous recipients and is often associated with GVHD. In addition to pneumonia and marrow suppression (and, less often, graft failure), manifestations of CMV disease in BMT/HSCT recipients include fever with or without arthralgias, myalgias, and esophagitis. CMV ulcerations occur in both the lower and the upper gastrointestinal tract, and it may be difficult to distinguish diarrhea due to GVHD from that due to CMV infection.

The finding of CMV in the liver of a patient with GVHD does not necessarily mean that CMV is responsible for hepatic enzyme abnormalities.

Management of CMV disease in BMT/HSCT recipients includes strategies directed at prophylaxis, suppression, preemptive therapy, or treatment. Prophylaxis results in a lower incidence of disease at the cost of treating many patients who otherwise would not require therapy. Because of the high fatality rate associated with CMV pneumonia in these patients and the difficulty of early diagnosis of CMV infection, prophylactic intravenous ganciclovir (or oral valganciclovir) has been used in some centers and has been shown to abort CMV disease during the period of maximal vulnerability (from engraftment to day 120 after transplantation). The foremost problem with the administration of ganciclovir relates to adverse effects, which include dose-related bone marrow suppression (thrombocytopenia, leukopenia, anemia, and pancytopenia). Because the frequency of CMV pneumonia is lower among autologous BMT recipients (2 to 7%) than among allogeneic BMT recipients (10 to 40%), prophylaxis in the former group will not become the rule until a less toxic antiviral agent becomes available.

Like prophylaxis, suppressive treatment, which targets patients with polymerase chain reaction evidence of CMV or urine cultures positive for CMV, entails the unnecessary treatment of many individuals (on the basis of a laboratory test that is not highly predictive of disease) with drugs that have adverse effects. Currently, because of the neutropenia associated with ganciclovir in BMT/HSCT recipients, a preemptive approach—treatment of those patients in whose blood CMV is detected by an antigen or DNA test—is used at most centers. This approach is almost as effective as prophylaxis or suppression and causes less toxicity. Quantitative viral load assays, which are not dependent on circulating polymorphonuclear leukocytes, have supplanted antigen-based assays and are used by most centers. A positive test (or increase in titer) prompts the initiation of preemptive therapy.

Treatment of CMV pneumonia in BMT/HSCT recipients requires both intravenous immune globulin (IVIg) and ganciclovir. In patients who cannot tolerate ganciclovir, foscarnet is a useful alternative, although it may produce nephrotoxicity and electrolyte imbalance. Transfusion of CMV-specific T cells from the donor decreased viral load in a small series of patients; this result suggests that immunotherapy may play a role in the treatment of this disease in the future. →*For further discussion, see Chap. 166.*

Human Herpesviruses 6 and 7 HHV-6, the cause of roseola in children, is a ubiquitous herpesvirus that reactivates (as determined by culture of the virus from the blood) in ~50% of transplant recipients between 2 and 4 weeks after surgery. In some cases, reactivation of HHV-6 appears to be associated with neutropenia; since, like CMV, this virus can be found in marrow cells, it is possible that HHV-6 reactivation is responsible for some of the neutropenia that follows bone marrow transplantation. Although encephalitis developing after transplantation has been associated with HHV-6 in cerebrospinal fluid (CSF), the causality of the association is not well defined. HHV-6 DNA is sometimes found in lung samples after transplantation. However, its role in pneumonitis is unclear. While HHV-6 has been shown to be susceptible to foscarnet (and possibly to ganciclovir) in vitro, the efficacy of antiviral treatment has not been well studied. Little is known about the related herpesvirus HHV-7 or its role in posttransplantation infection. →*For further discussion, see Chap. 166.*

Epstein-Barr Virus Primary EBV infection can be fatal to transplant recipients; EBV reactivation can cause EBV–B cell lymphoproliferative disease (LPD), which may also be fatal to patients taking immunosuppressive drugs. The localization of EBV to B cells leads to several interesting phenomena in BMT/HSCT recipients. The marrow ablation that occurs as part of the BMT/HSCT procedure may eliminate latent EBV from the host. Infection can then be reacquired immediately after transplantation by transfer of infected donor B cells.

Rarely, transplantation from a seronegative donor may result in cure. The recipient is then at risk for a second primary infection.

EBV-LPD can develop in the recipient's B cells (if any should survive marrow ablation) but is more likely to be a consequence of outgrowth of infected donor cells. Both lytic and latent EBV replication are more likely during immunosuppression (e.g., they are associated with GVHD and the use of antibodies to T cells). Although less likely in autologous transplantation, reactivation can occur in T cell–depleted autologous recipients (e.g., patients being given antibodies to T cells for the treatment of a T cell lymphoma with marrow depletion). EBV-LPD, which can become apparent as soon as 1 to 3 months after engraftment, causes high fevers and cervical adenopathy resembling the symptoms of infectious mononucleosis but more commonly presents as an extranodal mass. The incidence of 0.6% among allogeneic BMT/HSCT recipients contrasts with figures of ~5% for renal transplant recipients and up to 20% for cardiac transplant patients. In all cases, EBV-LPD is more likely to occur with continued immunosuppression (especially that caused by the use of antibodies to T cells and cyclosporine or other T cell–suppressive agents).

EBV-specific T cells generated from the donor have been used experimentally to prevent and to treat EBV-LPD in the allogeneic recipient. Administration of a monoclonal antibody to CD20 (rituximab) for the treatment of B cell lymphomas that express this surface protein has elicited dramatic responses and currently constitutes first-line therapy for EBV-LPD, although long-term suppression of new antibody responses accompanies therapy. The role of antivirals is uncertain because no available agents have been documented to have activity against latent EBV infection. Ganciclovir has been postulated to have activity on the basis of its ability to inhibit proliferation of B cells, but this activity is associated with toxicity. High-dose zidovudine shows promise for the treatment of EBV-positive CNS lymphomas—another EBV-associated complication of transplantation. Both interferon α and retinoic acid have been used in the treatment of EBV-LPD, as has IVIg, but no large studies have assessed the efficacy of these agents. Chemotherapeutic regimens have been used as a last resort, even though patients' tolerance and long-term results have been disappointing in this setting. →*For further discussion, see Chap. 165.*

Human Herpesvirus 8 The EBV-related gamma herpesvirus HHV-8, which is causally associated with Kaposi's sarcoma, with primary effusion lymphoma, and sometimes with multicentric Castleman's disease, has rarely resulted in disease in BMT/HSCT recipients. The reasons may be a relatively low seroprevalence in the population and the limited duration of profound T cell suppression after bone marrow/hematopoietic stem cell transplantation. →*For further discussion, see Chap. 166.*

Other (Nonherpes) Viruses The diagnosis of pneumonia in BMT/HSCT recipients poses some special problems. Because patients have undergone treatment with multiple chemotherapeutic agents and sometimes radiation, their differential diagnosis should include—in addition to bacterial pneumonia—CMV pneumonitis, pneumonia of other viral or fungal etiology, parasitic pneumonia, diffuse alveolar hemorrhage, and chemical- or radiation-associated pneumonitis. Since fungal disease and viruses such as respiratory syncytial virus (RSV), parainfluenza virus (types 1, 2, and 3), influenza A and B viruses, and adenovirus are also causes of pneumonia in this setting, it is important to diagnose CMV specifically (see above). *M. tuberculosis* has been an uncommon cause of pneumonia among BMT/HSCT recipients in Western countries (<0.1 to 0.2%) but is common in Hong Kong (5.5%) and in countries where the prevalence of tuberculosis is high. The exposure history of the recipient is clearly critical in an assessment of posttransplantation infections.

Both RSV and parainfluenza viruses, particularly type 3, can cause severe or even fatal pneumonia in BMT recipients. Infections with both of these agents sometimes occur as disastrous nosocomial epidemics. Therapy with aerosolized ribavirin as well as RSV immuno-

globulin or monoclonal antibody to RSV (palivizumab) has been reported to lessen the severity of RSV disease, but there are no large studies to prove efficacy. Influenza also occurs in BMT recipients and generally mirrors the presence of infection in the community. Several drugs are available for the treatment of influenza (amantadine/rimantadine, ribavirin?) but have limited effects, primarily reducing symptoms and shortening the duration of illness. The neuraminidase inhibitors (oseltamivir and zanamivir) are active against both influenza A virus and influenza B virus and are a reasonable treatment option. Adenovirus can be isolated from BMT recipients at rates varying from 5 to 18%. Although hemorrhagic cystitis, pneumonia, and fatal disseminated infection have been reported, adenovirus infection, which (like CMV infection) usually occurs in the first or second month after transplantation, is often asymptomatic. Cidofovir has proved effective in animal models and in case reports. Infections with parvovirus B19 (presenting as anemia or occasionally as pancytopenia) and enteroviruses (sometimes fatal) can occur. Parvovirus infection can be treated with IVIg (Chap. 168). Pleconaril, a capsid-binding agent, is being studied for the treatment of enterovirus infection. Rotaviruses are a common cause of gastroenteritis in BMT/HSCT recipients. Polyomavirus BK is found at high titers in the urine of patients who are highly immunosuppressed. BK viruria may be associated with hemorrhagic cystitis. Progressive multifocal leukoencephalopathy caused by JC virus is rare among BMT/HSCT recipients compared with the rate among patients with impaired T cell function due to HIV infection. There is no known treatment for this disease. When transmitted by mosquitoes or by blood transfusion, West Nile virus can cause encephalitis and death after bone marrow transplantation.

INFECTIONS IN SOLID ORGAN TRANSPLANT RECIPIENTS

Morbidity and mortality among solid organ transplant recipients have been reduced by the use of more effective antibiotics. The organisms that cause infections in recipients of solid organ transplants are different from those that infect BMT/HSCT recipients because solid organ recipients do not go through a period of neutropenia. As the transplantation procedure involves surgery, however, solid organ recipients are subject to infections at anastomotic sites and to wound infections. Compared with BMT/HSCT recipients, organ transplant patients are immunosuppressed for longer periods (often permanently). Thus they are susceptible to the same organisms as patients with chronically impaired T cell immunity (Chap. 72, especially Table 72-1).

During the early period (<1 month after transplantation), infections are most commonly caused by extracellular bacteria (staphylococci, streptococci, *E. coli*, other gram-negative organisms), which often originate in surgical wound or anastomotic sites. The spectrum of infection is largely determined by the type of transplant.

In subsequent weeks, the consequences of the administration of agents that suppress cell-mediated immunity and of the acquisition or reactivation (from the transplanted organ) of viruses and parasites become apparent. CMV infection is often a problem in the first 6 months after transplantation and may present as severe systemic disease or as infection of the transplanted organ. HHV-6 reactivation (assessed by blood culture) occurs within the first 2 to 4 weeks after transplantation and may be associated with fever and granulocytopenia. Data suggest that HHV-6 and HHV-7 may exacerbate CMV-induced disease. CMV is associated not only with generalized immunosuppression but also with organ-specific, rejection-related syndromes: glomerulopathy in kidney transplant recipients, bronchiolitis obliterans in lung transplant recipients, vasculopathy in heart transplant recipients, and the vanishing bile duct syndrome in liver transplant recipients. A complex interplay between increased CMV replication and enhanced graft rejection is well established: Increasing immunosuppression leads to increased CMV replication, which is associated with graft rejection. For this reason, considerable attention has been focused on the diagnosis, treatment, and prophylaxis of CMV infection in organ transplant recipients. Early transmission of West Nile virus to transplant recipients from an organ donor has been reported.

Beyond 6 months after transplantation, infections characteristic of patients with defects in cell-mediated immunity—e.g., infections with *Listeria*, *Nocardia*, various fungi, and other intracellular pathogens—may be a problem. Elimination of these late infections will not be possible until specific tolerance to the transplanted organ can be achieved without the administration of drugs that lead to generalized immunosuppression. Meanwhile, vigilance, prophylaxis/preemptive therapy (when indicated), and rapid diagnosis and treatment of infections can be lifesaving in solid organ transplant recipients, who, unlike most BMT recipients, continue to be immunosuppressed.

Solid organ transplant recipients are susceptible to EBV-LPD from as early as 2 months to many years after transplantation. The prevalence of this complication is increased by potent and prolonged use of T cell–suppressive drugs. The condition may be reversed (in some cases) by decreasing the degree of immunosuppression. Among organ transplant patients, those with heart and lung transplants—who receive the most intensive immunosuppressive regimens—are most likely to develop EBV-LPD, particularly in the lungs. Although the disease usually originates in recipient B cells, several cases of donor origin have been reported. There is a notable tendency for EBV-LPD to develop in the transplanted organ. High organ-specific content of B lymphoid tissues (i.e., bronchial-associated lymphoid tissue in the lung), anatomical factors (i.e., lack of access of host T cells to the transplanted organ because of disturbed lymphatics), and differences in major histocompatibility loci between the host T cells and the organ (i.e., lack of cell migration or lack of effective T cell/macrophage cooperation) may result in defective elimination of EBV-infected B cells. Solid organ transplant recipients are also highly susceptible to the development of Kaposi's sarcoma and to B cell proliferative disorders associated with Kaposi's sarcoma–associated herpesvirus (KSHV) (primary effusion lymphoma, multicentric Castleman's disease). Kaposi's sarcoma can develop very rapidly after transplantation and can occur in the allograft. However, because the seroprevalence of KSHV is very low in Western countries, Kaposi's sarcoma is infrequent in these areas.

KIDNEY TRANSPLANTATION (See Table 117-4) ■ **Early Infections** Infections developing soon after kidney transplantation are often caused by bacteria associated with skin or wound infections. There is a role for perioperative antibiotic prophylaxis, and many centers give cephalosporins to decrease the risk of postoperative complications. Urinary tract infections developing soon after transplantation are usually related to anatomical alterations resulting from surgery. Such early infections may require prolonged treatment (e.g., 6 weeks of antibiotic administration for pyelonephritis). Urinary tract infections that occur >6 months after transplantation do not seem to be associated with the high rate of pyelonephritis or relapse seen with infections that occur in the first 3 months and may be treated for shorter periods.

Prophylaxis with TMP-SMX [1 double-strength tablet (800 mg of sulfamethoxazole, 160 mg of trimethoprim) per day] for the first 4 months after transplantation decreases the incidence of early and middle-period infections (see below and Tables 117-4 and 117-5).

Middle-Period Infections Because of continuing immunosuppression, kidney transplant recipients are predisposed to lung infections char-

acteristic of those in patients with T cell deficiency (i.e., infections with intracellular bacteria, mycobacteria, nocardiae, fungi, viruses, and parasites). The high mortality associated with *Legionella pneumophila* infection (Chap. 132) led to the closing of renal transplant units in hospitals with endemic legionellosis.

About 50% of all renal transplant recipients presenting with fever 1 to 4 months after transplantation have evidence of CMV disease; CMV itself accounts for the fever in more than two-thirds of cases and thus is the predominant pathogen during this period. CMV infection (Chap. 166) may also present as arthralgias or myalgias. During this period, this infection may represent primary disease (in the case of a seronegative recipient of a kidney from a seropositive donor) or may present as reactivation disease or superinfection. Patients may have atypical lymphocytosis. Unlike immunocompetent patients, however, they often do not have lymphadenopathy or splenomegaly. Therefore, clinical suspicion and laboratory confirmation are necessary for diagnosis. The clinical syndrome may be accompanied by bone marrow suppression (particularly leukopenia). CMV also causes glomerulopathy and is associated with an increased incidence of other opportunistic infections. Because of the frequency and severity of CMV disease, a considerable effort has been made to prevent and treat it in renal transplant recipients. Administration of an immune globulin preparation enriched with antibodies to CMV decreases the incidence in the group at highest risk for severe infections (seronegative recipients of

TABLE 117-4 *Infections After Kidney Transplantation*

Infection Site	Early (<1 Month)	Middle (1–4 Months)	Late (>6 Months)
	Period after Transplantation		
Urinary tract	Bacteria (*Escherichia coli*, *Klebsiella*, Enterobacteriaceae, *Pseudomonas*, *Enterococcus*) associated with bacteremia and pyelonephritis, *Candida*	Cytomegalovirus (CMV; fever alone is common)	Bacteria; late infections usually not associated with bacteremia
Lungs	Bacteria (*Legionella* in endemic settings)	CMV diffuse interstitial pneumonitis, *Pneumocystis*, *Aspergillus*, *Legionella*	*Nocardia*, *Aspergillus*, *Mucor*
Central nervous system		*Listeria* meningitis, CMV encephalitis, *Toxoplasma gondii*	CMV retinitis, *Listeria* meningitis, cryptococcal meningitis, *Aspergillus*, *Nocardia*

TABLE 117-5 *Prophylaxis of Infections in Transplant Recipients*

Risk Factor	Organism	Prophylactic Antibiotics	Examinations
Travel to or residence in area with known risk of fungal infection	Coccidioidomycosis, histoplasmosis, blastomycosis	Imidazoles (fluconazole, itraconazole, voriconazole)	Chest radiography
Latent viruses	HSV, VZV, EBV, CMV	Acyclovir after bone marrow transplantation for HSV and VZV; ganciclovir in some settings	Serologic test for HSV, VZV, CMV, HHV-6, EBV, HHV-8
Latent parasites	*Pneumocystis*, *Toxoplasma gondii*	Trimethoprim-sulfamethoxazole or dapsone plus pyrimethamine	Serologic test for *Toxoplasma*
History of exposure to tuberculosis or latent tuberculosis	*Mycobacterium tuberculosis*	Isoniazid if recent conversion for positive chest x-ray and no previous treatment	PPD skin test and chest radiography

Note: CMV, cytomegalovirus; EBV, Epstein-Barr virus; HHV, human herpesvirus; HSV, herpes simplex virus; PPD, purified protein derivative; VZV, varicella-zoster virus.

seropositive kidneys). Ganciclovir is useful for prophylaxis and the treatment of serious CMV disease. One study showed a significant (50%) reduction in CMV disease and rejection at 6 months in patients who received prophylactic valacyclovir (an acyclovir congener) for the first 90 days after renal transplantation. The availability of valganciclovir and valacyclovir has allowed most centers to move to oral prophylaxis for transplant recipients.

Infection with the other herpes-group viruses may become evident within 6 months after transplantation or later. Early after transplantation, HSV may cause either oral or anogenital lesions that are usually responsive to acyclovir. Large ulcerating lesions in the anogenital area may lead to bladder and rectal dysfunction as well as predisposing to bacterial infection. VZV may cause fatal disseminated infection in nonimmune kidney transplant recipients, but in immune patients reactivation zoster usually does not disseminate outside the dermatome; thus disseminated VZV infection is a less fearsome complication in kidney transplantation than in bone marrow transplantation. HHV-6 may reactivate and (although usually asymptomatic) may be associated with fever, rash, marrow suppression, or encephalitis.

EBV reactivation disease is more serious; it may present as an extranodal proliferation of B cells that invade the CNS, nasopharynx, liver, small bowel, heart, and transplanted kidney. The disease is diagnosed by the finding of a proliferation of EBV-positive B cells. The incidence of EBV-LPD is higher among patients given high doses of cyclosporine, tacrolimus, or other immunosuppressive agents (including anti–T cell antibodies). Disease may regress once immunocompetence is restored. HHV-8 infection can be transmitted with the donor kidney and is associated with the development of Kaposi's sarcoma in the recipient. Kaposi's sarcoma (primary vs. reactivation of HHV-8) often appears within 1 year after transplantation, although the range of onset times is wide (1 month to ~20 years).

The papovaviruses BK and JC (polyomavirus hominis types 1 and 2) have been cultured from the urine of kidney transplant recipients (as they have from that of BMT recipients). The excretion of BK virus is associated with ureteral strictures, BK nephropathy, and—in rare instances—vasculopathy. JC virus is associated with progressive multifocal leukoencephalopathy (rare). Adenoviruses may persist with continued immunosuppression in these patients.

Kidney transplant recipients are also subject to infections with other intracellular organisms. These patients may develop pulmonary infections with *Nocardia*, *Aspergillus*, and *Mucor* as well as infections with other pathogens in which the T cell/macrophage axis plays an important role. In patients without intravenous catheters, *L. monocytogenes* is a common cause of bacteremia ≥1 month after renal transplantation and should be seriously considered in renal transplant recipients presenting with fever and headache. Kidney transplant recipients may develop *Salmonella* bacteremia, which can lead to endovascular infections and require prolonged therapy. Pulmonary infections with *Pneumocystis* are common unless the patient is maintained on TMP-SMX prophylaxis. *Nocardia* infection (Chap. 146) may present in the skin, bones, and lungs or in the CNS, where it usually takes the form of single or multiple brain abscesses. *Nocardia* infection generally occurs ≥1 month after transplantation and may follow immunosuppressive treatment for an episode of rejection. Pulmonary findings are nonspecific: localized disease with or without cavities is most common, but the disease may disseminate. The diagnosis is made by culture of the organism from sputum or from the involved nodule. As with *Pneumocystis*, prophylaxis with TMP-SMX is often efficacious in the prevention of disease. The occurrence of *Nocardia* infections >2 years after transplantation suggests that a long-term prophylactic regimen may be justified.

Toxoplasmosis can occur in seropositive patients but is less common than in other transplant settings, usually developing in the first few months after kidney transplantation. Again, TMP-SMX is helpful in prevention. In endemic areas, histoplasmosis, coccidioidomycosis, and blastomycosis may cause pulmonary infiltrates or disseminated disease.

Late Infections Late infections (>6 months after kidney transplantation) include CMV retinitis and a variety of CNS complications. Patients (particularly those whose immunosuppression has been increased) are at risk for subacute meningitis due to *Cryptococcus neoformans*. Cryptococcal disease may present in an insidious manner (sometimes as a skin infection before the development of clear CNS findings). *Listeria* meningitis may have an acute presentation and requires prompt therapy to avoid a fatal outcome.

Patients who continue to take glucocorticoids are predisposed to infection. "Transplant elbow" is a recurrent bacterial infection in and around the elbow that is thought to result from a combination of poor tensile strength of the skin of steroid-treated patients and steroid-induced proximal myopathy that requires patients to push themselves up with their elbows to get out of chairs. Bouts of cellulitis (usually caused by *S. aureus*) recur until patients are provided with elbow protection.

Kidney transplant recipients are susceptible to invasive fungal infections—such as those due to *Aspergillus* and *Rhizopus*, which may present as superficial lesions before dissemination. Mycobacterial infection (particularly that with *Mycobacterium marinum*) can be diagnosed by skin examination. Infection with *Prototheca wickerhamii* (an achlorophyllic alga) has been diagnosed by skin biopsy. Warts caused by human papillomaviruses (HPVs) are a late consequence of persistent immunosuppression; imiquimod or other forms of local therapy are usually satisfactory.

HEART TRANSPLANTATION ■ **Early Infections** Sternal wound infection and mediastinitis are early complications of heart transplantation. An indolent course is common, with fever or a mildly elevated white blood cell count preceding the development of site tenderness or drainage. Clinical suspicion based on evidence of sternal instability and failure to heal may lead to the diagnosis. Although common microbial residents of the skin (e.g., *S. aureus* and *Staphylococcus epidermidis*) as well as gram-negative organisms (e.g., *Pseudomonas aeruginosa*) and fungi (e.g., *Candida*) are often involved, mediastinitis in heart transplant recipients (in rare cases) can also be due to *Mycoplasma hominis* (Chap. 159). Since this organism requires an anaerobic environment for growth and may be difficult to see on conventional medium, the laboratory should be alerted that *M. hominis* infection is suspected. *M. hominis* mediastinitis has been cured with a combination of surgical debridement (sometimes requiring muscle-flap placement) plus clindamycin and tetracycline. Organisms associated with mediastinitis may be cultured from accompanying pericardial fluid.

Middle-Period Infections *T. gondii* (Chap. 198) resident in the heart of a seropositive donor may be transmitted to a seronegative recipient. Thus serologic screening for *T. gondii* infection is important before and in the months after cardiac transplantation. Rarely, active disease can be introduced at the time of transplantation. The overall incidence of toxoplasmosis is so high in this setting that some prophylaxis is always warranted. Although alternatives are available, the most frequently used agent is TMP-SMX, which prevents infection with *Pneumocystis* as well as with *Nocardia* and other bacterial pathogens. CMV has also been transmitted by heart transplantation. CNS infections can be caused by *Toxoplasma*, *Nocardia*, and *Aspergillus*. *L. monocytogenes* meningitis should be considered in heart transplant recipients with fever and headache.

CMV infection is associated with poor outcomes after heart transplantation. The virus is usually cultivable 1 to 2 months after transplantation, causes early signs and laboratory abnormalities (usually fever and atypical lymphocytosis or leukopenia and thrombocytopenia) at 2 to 3 months, and produces severe disease (e.g., pneumonia) at 3 to 4 months. Seropositive recipients usually develop cultivable virus faster than patients whose primary CMV infection is a consequence of transplantation. Between 40 and 70% of patients develop symptomatic CMV disease in the form of (1) CMV pneumonia, the most likely form of CMV disease to be fatal; (2) CMV esophagitis and gastritis, sometimes accompanied by abdominal pain with or without ulcerations and bleeding; and (3) the CMV syndrome, consisting of CMV in the blood along with fever, leukopenia, thrombocytopenia, and hepatic enzyme abnormalities. Ganciclovir is efficacious in the treatment of CMV infection; prophylaxis with ganciclovir or possibly with other antivirals, as described for renal transplantation, may reduce the incidence of CMV-related disease.

Late Infections EBV infection usually presents as a lymphoma-like proliferation of B cells late after heart transplantation, particularly in patients maintained on heavy immunosuppression. A subset of heart and heart-lung transplant recipients may develop early (within 2 months) fulminant EBV-LPD. Treatment includes the reduction of immunosuppression if possible and the consideration of B cell antibodies (rituximab), immunomodulatory agents, or chemotherapy, as discussed earlier under bone marrow/hematopoietic stem cell transplantation. HHV-8-associated disease, including primary effusion lymphoma, has been reported in heart transplant recipients. Prophylaxis for *Pneumocystis* infection is required for these patients (see below).

LUNG TRANSPLANTATION ■ Early Infections It is not surprising that lung transplant recipients are predisposed to the development of pneumonia. The combination of ischemia and the resulting mucosal damage together with accompanying denervation and lack of lymph drainage probably contributes to the high rate of pneumonia (66% in one series). The prophylactic use of high doses of broad-spectrum antibiotics for the first 3 or 4 days after surgery decreases the incidence of pneumonia. Gram-negative pathogens (Enterobacteriaceae and *Pseudomonas* species) are troublesome in the first 2 weeks after surgery (the period of maximal vulnerability). Pneumonia can also be caused by *Candida* (possibly as a result of colonization of the donor lung), *Aspergillus*, and *Cryptococcus*.

Mediastinitis may occur at an even higher rate among lung transplant recipients than among heart transplant recipients and most commonly develops within 2 weeks of surgery. Pneumonitis due to CMV (which may be transmitted as a consequence of transplantation) usually presents between 2 weeks and 3 months after surgery, with primary disease occurring later than reactivation disease.

Middle-Period Infections The incidence of CMV infection, either reactivated or primary, is between 75 and 100% if either the donor or the recipient is seropositive for CMV. CMV-induced disease appears to be most severe in recipients of lung and heart-lung transplants. Whether this severity relates to the mismatch in lung antigen-presenting and host immune cells or is attributable to other (nonimmune) factors is not known. More than half of lung transplant recipients with symptomatic CMV disease have pneumonia. Difficulty in distinguishing the radiographic picture of CMV infection from organ rejection further complicates therapy. CMV can also cause bronchiolitis obliterans in lung transplants. The development of pneumonitis related to HSV has led to the prophylactic use of acyclovir. Such prophylaxis may also decrease rates of CMV disease, but ganciclovir is more active against CMV and is also active against HSV. Prophylaxis of CMV infection with intravenous ganciclovir (or with valganciclovir, the oral alternative) is recommended for lung transplant recipients.

Late Infections The incidence of *Pneumocystis* infection (which may present with a paucity of findings) is high among lung and heart-lung transplant recipients. Some form of prophylaxis for *Pneumocystis* pneumonia is indicated in all organ transplant situations (Table 117-5). TMP-SMX prophylaxis for 12 months after transplantation may be sufficient to prevent *Pneumocystis* disease in patients whose degree of immunosuppression is not increased.

As in other transplant recipients, infection with EBV may cause either a mononucleosis-like syndrome or LPD. The tendency of the B cell blasts to present in the lung appears to be greater after lung transplantation than after the transplantation of other organs. Reduction of

immunosuppression causes remission in some cases, but airway compression can be fatal and more rapid intervention may therefore become necessary. The approach to EBV-LPD is similar to that described in other sections.

LIVER TRANSPLANTATION ■ Early Infections As in other types of transplantation, early bacterial infections are a major problem after liver transplantation. Many centers administer systemic broad-spectrum antibiotics for the first 5 days after surgery, even in the absence of documented infection. However, despite prophylaxis, infectious complications are common and are correlated with the duration of the surgical procedure and the type of biliary drainage. An operation lasting >12 h is associated with an increased likelihood of infection. Patients who have a choledochojejunostomy with drainage of the biliary duct to a Roux-en-Y jejunal bowel loop have more fungal infections than those whose bile is drained via a choledochocholedochostomy with anastomosis of the donor common bile duct to the recipient common bile duct.

Peritonitis and intraabdominal abscesses are common complications of liver transplantation. Bacterial peritonitis may result from biliary leaks and primary or secondary infection after leakage of bile. Peritonitis in liver transplant recipients is often polymicrobial, commonly involving enterococci, aerobic gram-negative bacteria, staphylococci, anaerobes, or *Candida*. Only one-third of patients with intraabdominal abscesses have bacteremia. Abscesses within the first month after surgery may occur not only over the liver but also in the spleen, pericolic area, and pelvis. Treatment includes antibiotic administration and drainage as necessary.

Liver transplant patients have a high incidence of fungal infections, and the occurrence of fungal infection (often candidiasis) correlates with preoperative use of glucocorticoids, a long duration of treatment with antibacterial agents, and posttransplantation use of immunosuppressive agents.

Middle-Period Infections The development of postsurgical biliary stricture predisposes patients to cholangitis. These patients may lack the characteristic signs and symptoms of cholangitis: fever, abdominal pain, and jaundice. Alternatively, these findings may be present but may suggest graft rejection. The diagnosis of cholangitis in liver transplant recipients therefore requires documentation of bacteremia or demonstration of aggregated neutrophils in bile duct biopsy specimens. Unfortunately, invasive studies of the biliary tract (either T-tube cholangiography or endoscopic retrograde cholangiopancreatography) may themselves lead to cholangitis. For this reason, many clinicians recommend prophylaxis with antibiotics covering gram-negative organisms and anaerobes when these procedures are performed in liver transplant recipients.

Viral hepatitis is a common complication of liver transplantation (Chap. 285). Reactivation of hepatitis B and C infections, for which transplantation may be performed, is problematic. To prevent hepatitis B infection, high-dose intravenous hepatitis B immune globulin is administered. The long-term efficacy of lamivudine (3TC) and adefovir in inhibiting hepatitis B viral replication after transplantation is being studied. A combination of interferon α and ribavirin is being tested for treatment/prophylaxis of hepatitis C infection.

As in other transplantation settings, reactivation disease with herpes-group viruses is common (Table 117-3). Herpesviruses can be transmitted in donor organs. Although CMV hepatitis occurs in ~4% of liver transplant recipients, it is usually not so severe as to require retransplantation. CMV disease develops in the majority of seronegative recipients of organs from CMV-positive donors, but fatality rates are lower among liver transplant recipients than among lung or heart-lung transplant recipients. Disease due to CMV is associated with the vanishing bile duct syndrome after liver transplantation. Patients respond to treatment with ganciclovir; prophylaxis with CMV immune globulin and acyclovir or oral ganciclovir may modify disease. A role for HHV-6 in posttransplantation fever and leukopenia has been proposed. HHV-6 and HHV-7 appear to exacerbate CMV disease in this setting. EBV-LPD after liver transplantation shows a propensity for involvement of the liver, and such disease may be of donor origin.

PANCREAS TRANSPLANTATION Transplantation of the pancreas can be complicated by early abdominal infection. To prevent contamination of the allograft with enteric bacteria and yeasts, some surgeons, instead of draining the pancreas through the bowel, drain secretions into the urinary tract or bladder. A cuff of duodenum is used in the anastomosis between the pancreatic graft and either the bladder or the gut. In addition to bicarbonate loss, bladder drainage causes a high rate of urinary tract infection and sterile cystitis. Prophylactic antimicrobials are commonly used at the time of surgery. An alternative method—the transplantation of islet cells only—may eliminate the problems characteristically posed by wound and urinary tract sepsis in pancreas transplant recipients.

Issues related to the development of CMV infection, EBV-LPD, and infections with opportunistic pathogens in patients receiving a pancreas are similar to those in other solid organ transplant recipients.

MISCELLANEOUS INFECTIONS IN SOLID ORGAN TRANSPLANTATION ■ Indwelling Intravenous Catheter Infections The prolonged use of indwelling intravenous catheters for administration of medications, blood products, and nutrition is common in diverse transplantation settings and poses a risk of local and bloodstream infection. Significant insertion-site infection is most commonly caused by *S. aureus*. Bloodstream infection most frequently develops within a week of catheter placement or in patients who become neutropenic. Coagulase-negative staphylococci are the most common isolates from the blood. →*For further discussion of differential diagnosis and therapeutic options, see Chap. 72.*

Tuberculosis The incidence of tuberculosis occurring within 12 months after solid organ transplantation ranges broadly worldwide (0.35 to 15%), reflecting prevalences in local populations. Nonrenal transplantation, GVHD within 6 months, and intensity of immunosuppression are predictive of tuberculosis reactivation and development of disseminated disease in a host with latent disease. The use of antibodies to tumor necrosis factor is associated with the development of active tuberculosis. Tuberculosis has rarely been transmitted from the donor organ. In contrast to the low mortality in BMT/HSCT recipients, mortality in solid organ transplant patients is reported to be 29%. Isoniazid toxicity has not been a significant problem except in the liver transplantation setting.

Virus-Associated Malignancies In addition to malignancy associated with gammaherpesvirus infection (EBV, HHV-8) and simple warts (HPV), other tumors that are virus-associated or suspected of being virus-associated are more likely to develop in transplant recipients, particularly those who require long-term immunosuppression, than in the general population. The interval to tumor development is usually >1 year. Transplant recipients develop nonmelanoma skin or lip cancers that, in contrast to de novo skin cancers, have a high ratio of squamous cells to basal cells. HPV appears to play a major role in these lesions. Cervical and vulvar carcinomas, quite clearly associated with HPV, develop with increased frequency in female transplant recipients. Among renal transplant recipients, rates of melanoma are modestly increased and rates of cancers of the kidney and bladder are increased.

VACCINATION OF TRANSPLANT RECIPIENTS

In addition to receiving antibiotic prophylaxis, transplant recipients should be vaccinated against likely pathogens (Table 117-6). In the case of BMT recipients, optimal responses cannot be achieved until after immune reconstitution, despite previous immunization of both donor and recipient. Recipients of allogeneic BMTs must be reimmunized if they are to be protected against pathogens. The situation is less clear-cut in the case of autologous transplantation. T and B cells in the peripheral blood may reconstitute the immune response if they

TABLE 117-6 *Vaccination for Bone Marrow or Solid Organ Transplant Recipients*

Vaccine	Type of Transplantation	
	Bone Marrow	Solid Organ
Streptococcus pneumoniae, Haemophilus influenzae, Neisseria meningitidis	Immunize after transplantation (optimal timing not established); preimmunize graft[a]	Immunize before transplantation and every 5 years for Pneumovax (others not established)
Seasonal influenza	Vaccinate in the fall; vaccinate close contacts	Vaccinate in the fall
Poliomyelitis	Administer inactivated vaccine	Administer inactivated vaccine
Measles/mumps/ rubella	Immunize 24 months after transplantation if patient does not have graft-versus-host disease	Immunize before transplantation
Tetanus, diphtheria	Reimmunize after transplantation	Immunize before transplantation; give boosters at 10 years or as required; a new primary series is not required

[a] Studies indicate that it is possible to "immunize the graft" before transplantation.

are transferred in adequate numbers. However, cancer patients (particularly those with Hodgkin's disease, in whom vaccination has been extensively studied) who are undergoing chemotherapy do not respond normally to immunization, and titers of antibodies to infectious agents fall more rapidly than in healthy individuals. Therefore, even immunosuppressed patients who have not had marrow transplants may need booster vaccine injections. If memory cells are specifically eliminated as part of a marrow "cleanup" procedure, it will be necessary to reimmunize the recipient with a new primary series. Optimal times for immunizations of different transplant populations are being evaluated. Immunization of household and other contacts (including health care personnel) against influenza every season is likely to benefit the patient by preventing local spread.

In the absence of compelling data as to optimal timing, it is reasonable to administer the pneumococcal and *H. influenzae* type b conjugate vaccines to both autologous and allogeneic BMT recipients 12 months after transplantation and again 12 months later (since the response to the initial vaccine dose is weak in the early posttransplantation period). Recent studies indicate that the use of the pneumococcal conjugate vaccines will be more effective than previous products. The pneumococcal and *H. influenzae* type b vaccines are particularly important for patients who have undergone splenectomy. In addition, *Neisseria meningitidis* polysaccharide vaccine, diphtheria vaccine, tetanus vaccine, and inactivated polio vaccine can all be given at these same intervals (12 and 24 months after transplantation). Some authorities recommend a new primary series for tetanus/diphtheria and inactivated polio vaccine (vaccination 12, 14, and 16 months after transplantation). Because of the risk of spread, household contacts of BMT recipients (or of patients immunosuppressed as a result of chemotherapy) should receive only inactivated polio vaccine. Live-virus measles/mumps/rubella (MMR) vaccine can be given to autologous BMT recipients 24 months after transplantation and to most allogeneic BMT recipients at the same point if they are not receiving maintenance therapy with immunosuppressive drugs and do not have ongoing GVHD. The risk of spread from a household contact is lower for MMR vaccine than for polio vaccine. Neither patients nor household contacts of patients should be vaccinated with vaccinia unless they have been exposed to the smallpox virus. In patients who have active GVHD and/or are taking high maintenance doses of glucocorticoids, it may be prudent to avoid all live-virus vaccines. In the absence of detectable antibody titers, vaccination to prevent hepatitis B and hepatitis A also seems advisable.

In the case of solid organ transplant recipients, administration of all the usual vaccines and of the indicated booster doses should be completed before immunosuppression, if possible, to maximize responses. For patients taking immunosuppressive agents, the administration of pneumococcal vaccine should be repeated every 5 years. No data are available for meningococcal polysaccharide vaccine, but it is probably reasonable to administer it along with the pneumococcal vaccine or more frequently (every 3 years for persons with significant exposure risk). *H. influenzae* conjugate vaccine is safe and should be efficacious in this population; therefore, its administration before transplantation is recommended. Booster doses of this vaccine are not recommended for adults. Solid organ transplant recipients who continue to receive immunosuppressive drugs (glucocorticoids, cyclosporine) should not receive live-virus vaccines. A person in this group exposed to measles should be given immune globulin. Similarly, an immunocompromised patient who is seronegative for varicella and who comes into contact with a person who has chickenpox should be given varicella-zoster immune globulin as soon as possible (and certainly within 96 h) or, if this is not possible, should be started immediately on a 10- to 14-day course of acyclovir therapy. Susceptible household contacts of transplant recipients should receive live attenuated VZV vaccine, but vaccinees should avoid direct contact with the patient if a rash develops.

Immunocompromised patients who travel may benefit from some but not all vaccines. In general, they should receive any killed or inactivated vaccine preparation appropriate to the area they are visiting; this recommendation includes the vaccines for Japanese encephalitis, hepatitis A and B, poliomyelitis, meningococcal infection, and typhoid. The live typhoid vaccines are not recommended for use in most immunocompromised patients, but inactivated typhoid or the purified polysaccharide vaccine can be used. Live yellow fever vaccine should not be administered. Phenol-inactivated cholera vaccine is probably of little use in this setting. On the other hand, immunization with the purified-protein hepatitis B vaccine is indicated if patients are likely to be exposed. Patients who will reside for >6 months in areas where hepatitis B is common (Africa, Southeast Asia, the Middle East, Eastern Europe, parts of South America, and the Caribbean) should receive hepatitis B vaccine. Inactivated hepatitis A vaccine should be used in the appropriate setting (Chap. 107). If hepatitis A vaccine is not administered, travelers should consider receiving passive protection with immune globulin (the dose depending on the duration of travel in the high-risk area).

FURTHER READING

Cone RW et al: Human herpesvirus 6 infections after bone marrow transplantation: Clinical and virologic manifestations. J Infect Dis 179:311, 1999
Euvrard S et al: Skin cancers after organ transplantation. N Engl J Med 348:1681, 2003
Fehr T et al: Disseminated varicella infection in adult renal allograft recipients: Four cases and a review of the literature. Transplantation 73:608, 2002
Hirsch HH et al: Prospective study of polyomavirus type BK replication and nephropathy in renal transplant recipients. N Engl J Med 347:488, 2002
Lo C-M et al: Prophylaxis and treatment of recurrent hepatitis B after liver transplantation. Transplantation 75:S41, 2003
Molrine DC et al: Donor immunization with pneumococcal conjugate vaccine and early protective antibody responses following allogeneic hematopoietic cell transplantation. Blood 101:831, 2003
Mylonakis E et al: Combination antiviral therapy for ganciclovir-resistant cytomegalovirus infection in solid-organ transplant recipients. Clin Infect Dis 34:1337, 2002
Singh N et al: Safety and efficacy of isoniazid chemoprophylaxis administered during liver transplant candidacy for the prevention of posttransplant tuberculosis. Transplantation 74:892, 2002

Section 4 Approach to Therapy for Bacterial Diseases

118 TREATMENT AND PROPHYLAXIS OF BACTERIAL INFECTIONS
Gordon L. Archer, Ronald E. Polk

The development of vaccines and drugs that prevent and cure bacterial infections was one of the twentieth century's major contributions to human longevity and quality of life. Antibacterial agents are among the most commonly prescribed drugs of any kind worldwide. Used appropriately, these drugs are lifesaving. However, their indiscriminate use drives up the cost of health care, leads to a plethora of side effects and drug interactions, and fosters the emergence of bacterial resistance, rendering previously valuable drugs useless. The rational use of antibacterial agents depends on an understanding of their mechanisms of action, pharmacokinetics, pharmacodynamics, toxicities, and interactions; bacterial strategies for resistance; and bacterial susceptibility in vitro. In addition, patient-associated parameters, such as the site of infection and the immune and excretory status of the host, are critically important to appropriate therapeutic decisions. This chapter provides specific data required for making an informed choice of antibacterial agent.

MECHANISMS OF ACTION

Antibacterial agents, like all antimicrobial drugs, are directed against unique targets not present in mammalian cells. The goal is to limit toxicity to the host and maximize chemotherapeutic activity affecting invading microbes only. *Bactericidal drugs* kill the bacteria that are within their spectrum of activity; *bacteriostatic drugs* only inhibit bacterial growth. While bacteriostatic activity is adequate for the treatment of most infections, bactericidal activity may be necessary for cure in patients with altered immune systems (e.g., neutropenia), protected infectious foci (e.g., endocarditis or meningitis), or specific infections (e.g., complicated *Staphylococcus aureus* bacteremia). The mechanisms of action of the antibacterial agents to be discussed in this section are summarized in Table 118-1 and are depicted in Fig. 118-1.

INHIBITION OF CELL-WALL SYNTHESIS One major difference between bacterial and mammalian cells is the presence in bacteria of a rigid wall external to the cell membrane. The wall protects bacterial cells from osmotic rupture, which would result from the cell's usual marked hyperosmolarity (by up to 20 atm) relative to the host environment. The structure conferring cell-wall rigidity and resistance to osmotic lysis in both gram-positive and gram-negative bacteria is peptidoglycan, a large, covalently linked sacculus that surrounds the bacterium. In gram-positive bacteria, peptidoglycan is the only layered structure external to the cell membrane and is thick (20 to 80 nm); in gram-negative bacteria, there is an outer membrane external to a very thin (1-nm) peptidoglycan layer.

Chemotherapeutic agents directed at any stage of the synthesis, export, assembly, or cross-linking of peptidoglycan lead to inhibition of bacterial cell growth and, in most cases, to cell death. Peptidoglycan is composed of (1) a backbone of two alternating sugars, *N*-acetylglucosamine and *N*-acetylmuramic acid; (2) a chain of four amino acids that extends down from the backbone (stem peptides); and (3) a peptide bridge that cross-links the peptide chains. Peptidoglycan is formed by the addition of subunits (a sugar with its five attached amino acids) that are assembled in the cytoplasm and transported through the cytoplasmic membrane to the cell surface. Subsequent cross-linking is

Letter for Fig. 118-1	Antibacterial Agent[a]	Major Cellular Target	Mechanism of Action	Major Mechanisms of Resistance
A	β-Lactams (penicillins and cephalosporins)	Cell wall	Inhibit cell-wall cross-linking	1. Drug inactivation (β-lactamase) 2. Insensitivity of target (altered penicillin-binding proteins) 3. Decreased permeability (altered gram-negative outer-membrane porins) 4. Active efflux
B	Vancomycin	Cell wall	Interferes with addition of new cell-wall subunits (muramyl pentapeptides)	Alteration of target (substitution of terminal amino acid of peptidoglycan subunit)
	Bacitracin	Cell wall	Prevents addition of cell-wall subunits by inhibiting recycling of membrane lipid carrier	Not defined
C	Macrolides (erythromycin)	Protein synthesis	Bind to 50S ribosomal subunit	1. Alteration of target (ribosomal methylation and mutation of 23S rRNA) 2. Active efflux
	Lincosamides (clindamycin)	Protein synthesis	Bind to 50S ribosomal subunit	Alteration of target (ribosomal methylation)
D	Chloramphenicol	Protein synthesis	Binds to 50S ribosomal subunit	1. Drug inactivation (chloramphenicol acetyltransferase) 2. Active efflux
E	Tetracycline	Protein synthesis	Binds to 30S ribosomal subunit	1. Decreased intracellular drug accumulation (active efflux) 2. Insensitivity of target
F	Aminoglycosides (gentamicin)	Protein synthesis	Bind to 30S ribosomal subunit	1. Drug inactivation (aminoglycoside-modifying enzyme) 2. Decreased permeability through gram-negative outer membrane 3. Active efflux
G	Mupirocin	Protein synthesis	Inhibits isoleucine tRNA synthetase	Mutation of gene for target protein or acquisition of new gene for drug-insensitive target
H	Quinupristin/ dalfopristin (Synercid)	Protein synthesis	Bind to 50S ribosomal subunit	1. Alteration of target (ribosomal methylation: dalfopristin) 2. Active efflux (quinupristin) 3. Drug inactivation (quinupristin and dalfopristin)
I	Linezolid	Protein synthesis	Bind to 50S ribosomal subunit	Alteration of target (mutation of 23S rRNA)
J	Sulfonamides and trimethoprim	Cell metabolism	Competitively inhibit enzymes involved in two steps of folic acid biosynthesis	Production of insensitive targets [dihydropteroate synthetase (sulfonamides) and dihydrofolate reductase (trimethoprim)] that bypass metabolic block
K	Rifampin	Nucleic acid synthesis	Inhibits DNA-dependent RNA polymerase	Insensitivity of target (mutation of polymerase gene)
L	Metronidazole	Nucleic acid synthesis	Intracellularly generates short-lived reactive intermediates that damage DNA by electron transfer system	Not defined
M	Quinolones (ciprofloxacin)	DNA synthesis	Inhibit DNA gyrase (A subunit) and topoisomerase IV	1. Insensitivity of target (mutation of gyrase genes) 2. Decreased intracellular drug accumulation (active efflux)
	Novobiocin	DNA synthesis	Inhibits DNA gyrase (B subunit)	Not defined
N	Polymyxins (polymyxin B)	Cell membrane	Disrupt membrane permeability by charge alteration	Not defined
	Gramicidin	Cell membrane	Forms pores	Not defined

[a] Compounds in parentheses are major representatives for the class.

driven by cleavage of the terminal stem-peptide amino acid. Antibacterial agents act to inhibit cell-wall synthesis in several ways, as described below.

Bacitracin   Bacitracin, a cyclic peptide antibiotic, inhibits the conversion to its active form of the lipid carrier that moves the water-soluble cytoplasmic peptidoglycan subunits through the cell membrane to the cell exterior. Cell-wall subunits accumulate in the cytoplasm and cannot be added to the growing peptidoglycan chain.

Glycopeptides   Glycopeptides (vancomycin and teicoplanin) are high-molecular-weight antibiotics that bind to the terminal D-alanine–D-alanine component of the stem peptide while the subunits are external to the cell membrane but still linked to the lipid carrier. This binding sterically inhibits the addition of subunits to the peptidoglycan backbone.

β-Lactam Antibiotics   β-Lactam antibiotics (penicillins, cephalosporins, carbapenems, and monobactams; Table 118-2) are characterized by a four-membered β-lactam ring and prevent the cross-linking reaction called *transpeptidation*. The energy for attaching a peptide cross-bridge from the stem peptide of one peptidoglycan subunit to another is derived from the cleavage of a terminal D-alanine residue from the subunit stem peptide. The cross-bridge amino acid is then attached to the penultimate D-alanine by transpeptidase enzymes. The β-lactam ring of the antibiotic forms an irreversible covalent acyl bond with the transpeptidase enzyme (probably because of the antibiotic's steric similarity to the enzyme's D-alanine–D-alanine target), preventing the cross-linking reaction. Transpeptidases and similar enzymes involved in cross-linking are called *penicillin-binding proteins* (PBPs) because they all have active sites that bind β-lactam antibiotics.

Virtually all the antibiotics that inhibit bacterial cell-wall synthesis are bactericidal. That is, they eventually result in the cell's death due to osmotic lysis. However, much of the loss of cell-wall integrity following treatment with cell wall–active agents is due to the bacteria's own cell-wall remodeling enzymes (autolysins) that cleave peptido-

Mechanisms of Action

Mechanisms of Resistance

2 Detergent action on lipid gram ⊖ outer membrane.

3 Penetration of hydrophilic drugs through porin channels in gram ⊖ outer membrane.

4 Free diffusion through gram ⊕ cell envelope with binding to cell wall PG **or**

5 Binding to cell membrane PBP. Drug confined to space external to IM.

6 Diffusion or transport of drugs with intracellular target through IM.

7 Binding to ribosomal target for protein synthesis inhibition.

8 Antibiotic interaction with target protein leading to metabolic (DHFR, DHPS), protein synthetic (tRNA synthetase), or nucleic acid (DNA gyrase, RNA polymerase) abnormalities.

9 Direct interaction of reactive intermediates with nucleic acid.

1 **Intrinsic resistance:** Inability of antibiotic to penetrate gram ⊖ envelope (e.g., vancomycin).

3 Mutant porin channels **decrease** antimicrobial **penetration**.

4 **Production of insensitive target** by acquired gene mediating production of altered peptidoglycan.

5a **Production of β-lactam-insensitive PBP target** by mutation of gene or acquisition of new gene.

5b **Inactivation** of β-lactam antibiotic by β-lactamases in periplasm (gram ⊖) or surrounding medium (gram ⊕).

6 **Active efflux** of drugs from cytoplasm or from gram ⊖ periplasm.

7a Decreased ribosomal binding due to **target site alteration**.

7b **Inactivation** of drug by chemical modification leading to decreased ribosomal interaction.

8 Mutation of target gene or acquisition of new gene producing a **drug-insensitive target** protein.

FIGURE 118-1 Mechanisms of action of and resistance to antibacterial agents. Black lines trace the routes of drug interaction with bacterial cells, from entry to target site. The letters in each figure indicate specific antibacterial agents or classes of agents, as shown in Table 118-1. The numbers correspond to mechanisms listed beneath each panel. Abbreviations: LPS, lipopolysaccharide; OM, outer membrane; PG, peptidoglycan; PBP, penicillin-binding protein; IM, inner (cytoplasmic) membrane; 50s and 30s, large and small ribosome subunits; DHFR, dihydrofolate reductase; DHPS, dihydropteroate synthetase; Ac, acetylation; Ad, adenylation; P, phosphorylation.

glycan bonds in the normal course of cell growth. In the presence of antibacterial agents that inhibit cell-wall growth, autolysis proceeds without normal cell-wall repair; weakness and eventual cellular lysis occur.

INHIBITION OF PROTEIN SYNTHESIS Most of the antibacterial agents that inhibit protein synthesis interact with the bacterial ribosome. The difference between the composition of bacterial and mammalian ribosomes gives these compounds their selectivity.

Aminoglycosides Aminoglycosides (gentamicin, kanamycin, tobramycin, streptomycin, netilmicin, neomycin, and amikacin) are a group of structurally related compounds containing three linked hexose sugars. They exert a bactericidal effect by binding irreversibly to the 30S subunit of the bacterial ribosome and blocking initiation of protein synthesis. The reason for the lethal effect of aminoglycosides, as opposed to the largely bacteriostatic effect of other protein synthesis–

inhibiting antibacterial drugs, is not completely understood. Uptake of aminoglycosides and their penetration through the cell membrane constitute an aerobic, energy-dependent process. Thus, aminoglycoside activity is markedly reduced in an anaerobic environment. *Spectinomycin*, an aminocyclitol antibiotic, also acts on the 30S ribosomal subunit but has a different mechanism of action from the aminoglycosides and is bacteriostatic rather than bactericidal.

Macrolide Antibiotics Macrolide antibiotics (erythromycin, clarithromycin, and azithromycin) consist of a large lactone ring to which sugars are attached. *Ketolide antibiotics*, including telithromycin, replace the cladinose sugar on the macrolactone ring with a ketone group. These drugs bind specifically to the 50S portion of the bacterial ribosome. After attachment of mRNA to the initiation site of the 30S ribosomal subunit (the process blocked by aminoglycosides), the 50S subunit becomes bound to the 30S component to form the 70S ribosomal com-

TABLE 118-2 *Classification of β-Lactam Antibiotics*

| | Route of Administration | |
Class	Parenteral	Oral
Penicillins		
β-Lactamase–susceptible		
Narrow-spectrum	Penicillin G	Penicillin V
Enteric-active	Ampicillin	Amoxicillin, ampicillin
Enteric-active and antipseudomonal	Ticarcillin	None
β-Lactamase–resistant		
Antistaphylococcal	Methicillin, oxacillin, nafcillin	Cloxacillin, dicloxacillin
Combined with β-lactamase inhibitors	Ticarcillin plus clavulanic acid, ampicillin plus sulbactam, piperacillin plus tazobactam	Amoxicillin plus clavulanic acid
Cephalosporins		
First-generation	Cefazolin, cephalothin, cephapirin	Cephalexin, cephradine, cefadroxil
Second-generation		
Haemophilus-active	Cefamandole, cefuroxime, cefonicid, ceforanide	Cefaclor, cefuroxime axetil, ceftibuten, cefdinir, cefprozil, cefpodoxime,[a] loracarbef
Bacteroides-active	Cefoxitin, cefotetan, cefmetazole	None
Third-generation		
Extended-spectrum	Ceftriaxone, cefotaxime, ceftizoxime	None
Extended-spectrum and antipseudomonal	Ceftazidime, cefepime	None
Carbapenems	Imipenem-cilastatin, meropenem, ertapenem	None
Monobactams	Aztreonam	None

[a] Some sources classify cefpodoxime as a third-generation oral agent because of a marginally broader spectrum.

Mupirocin Mupirocin (pseudomonic acid) is produced by the bacterium *Pseudomonas fluorescens*. Its mechanism of action is unique: the drug inhibits isoleucine tRNA synthetase by competing with bacterial isoleucine for its binding site on the enzyme. Inhibition of this enzyme depletes cellular stores of isoleucine-charged tRNA and therefore leads to a cessation of protein synthesis. Mupirocin is selective for bacteria because mammalian isoleucine tRNA synthetase lacks affinity for the compound.

INHIBITION OF BACTERIAL METABOLISM The *antimetabolites* are all synthetic compounds that interfere with bacterial synthesis of folic acid. Products of the folic acid synthesis pathway function as coenzymes for the one-carbon transfer reactions that are essential for the synthesis of thymidine, all purines, and several amino acids. Inhibition of folate synthesis leads to cessation of bacterial cell growth and, in some cases, to bacterial cell death. The principal antibacterial antimetabolites are sulfonamides (sulfisoxazole, sulfadiazine, and sulfamethoxazole) and trimethoprim.

plex, and protein chain elongation proceeds. When these drugs bind to the 50S ribosomal subunit, protein chain elongation is inhibited.

Although structurally unrelated to the macrolides, *lincosamides* (clindamycin and lincomycin) bind to a site on the 50S ribosome nearly identical to the binding site for macrolides. Although the mechanism and site of action of macrolides and lincosamides are similar, the number and types of bacteria against which these two groups of agents are active differ.

Streptogramins Streptogramins [quinupristin (streptogramin B) and dalfopristin (streptogramin A)], which are supplied as a combination in Synercid, are peptide macrolactones that also bind to the 50S ribosomal subunit and block protein synthesis. Streptogramin B binds to a ribosomal site similar to the binding site for macrolides and lincosamides, whereas streptogramin A binds to a different ribosomal site, blocking the late phase of protein synthesis. The two streptogramins act synergistically to kill bacteria if the strain is susceptible to both components.

Chloramphenicol Chloramphenicol consists of a single aromatic ring and a short side chain. This antibiotic binds reversibly to the 50S portion of the bacterial ribosome at a site close to but not identical with the binding sites for the macrolides and lincosamides. The ribosomal binding of chloramphenicol inhibits peptide bond formation.

Linezolid Linezolid is the first drug in a new, completely synthetic class of antimicrobial agents, the oxazolidinones. Linezolid binds to the 50S ribosomal subunit and blocks the initiation of protein synthesis.

Tetracyclines Tetracyclines (tetracycline, doxycycline, and minocycline) consist of four aromatic rings with various substituent groups. They interact reversibly with the bacterial 30S ribosomal subunit, blocking the binding of aminoacyl tRNA to the mRNA-ribosome complex. This mechanism is markedly different from that of the aminoglycosides, which also bind to the 30S subunit. The specificity of tetracyclines for bacteria depends both on their selectivity for bacterial ribosomes and on their requirement for active, energy-dependent transport into the bacterial cell by a system not found in mammalian cell membranes.

Sulfonamides Sulfonamides are structural analogues of *p*-aminobenzoic acid (PABA), one of the three structural components of folic acid (the other two being pteridine and glutamate). The first step in the synthesis of folic acid is the addition of PABA to pteridine by the enzyme dihydropteroic acid synthetase. Sulfonamides compete with PABA as substrates for the enzyme. The selective effect of sulfonamides is due to the fact that bacteria synthesize folic acid, while mammalian cells cannot synthesize the cofactor and must have exogenous supplies. However, the activity of sulfonamides can be greatly reduced by the presence of excess PABA or by the exogenous addition of end products of one-carbon transfer reactions (e.g., thymidine and purines). High concentrations of the latter substances may be present in some infections as a result of tissue and white cell breakdown, compromising sulfonamide activity.

Trimethoprim Trimethoprim is a diaminopyrimidine, a structural analogue of the pteridine moiety of folic acid. Trimethoprim is a competitive inhibitor of dihydrofolate reductase; this enzyme is responsible for reduction of dihydrofolic acid to tetrahydrofolic acid—the essential final component in the folic acid synthesis pathway that is necessary for all one-carbon transfer reactions. Like the sulfonamides, trimethoprim is bactericidal in the absence of thymine but is only bacteriostatic when this pyrimidine is present in high concentration. The selective antibacterial activity of trimethoprim is based on the much (~50,000-fold) greater sensitivity of bacterial dihydrofolate reductase than of the mammalian enzyme to inhibition by this drug.

INHIBITION OF NUCLEIC ACID SYNTHESIS OR ACTIVITY Numerous antibacterial compounds have disparate effects on nucleic acids. The *quinolones*, including nalidixic acid and its fluorinated derivatives (ciprofloxacin, levofloxacin, gatifloxacin, and moxifloxacin), are synthetic compounds that inhibit the activity of the A subunit of the bacterial enzyme DNA gyrase as well as topoisomerase IV. DNA gyrase and topoisomerases are responsible for negative supercoiling of DNA—an essential conformation for DNA replication in the intact cell. Inhibition of the activity of DNA gyrase and topoisomerase IV is lethal to bacterial cells. The antibiotic *novobiocin* also interferes with the activity of DNA gyrase, but it interferes with the B subunit.

Rifampin Rifampin, used primarily against *Mycobacterium tuberculosis*, is also active against a variety of other bacteria. Rifampin binds tightly to the B subunit of bacterial DNA-dependent RNA polymerase, thus inhibiting transcription of DNA into RNA. Mammalian-cell RNA polymerase is not sensitive to this compound.

Nitrofurantoin Nitrofurantoin, a synthetic compound, causes DNA damage. The nitrofurans, compounds containing a single five-membered ring, are reduced by a bacterial enzyme to highly reactive, short-lived intermediates that are thought to cause DNA strand breakage, either directly or indirectly.

Metronidazole Metronidazole, a synthetic imidazole, is active against a wide range of anaerobic bacteria and protozoa. Its activity is totally dependent on its anaerobic electron-transport system for energy production. In the presence of this system, the nitro group of metronidazole is reduced to a series of transiently produced, reactive intermediates that are thought to cause DNA damage. The unique redox system of anaerobes accounts for the selective antibacterial activity of metronidazole. This compound is also a mutagen and a radiosensitizer of hypoxic mammalian cells.

ALTERATION OF CELL-MEMBRANE PERMEABILITY
The *polymyxins* (polymyxin B and colistin, or polymyxin E) are cyclic, basic polypeptides. They behave as cationic, surface-active compounds that disrupt the permeability of both the outer and the cytoplasmic membranes of gram-negative bacteria.

Gramicidin A is a polypeptide of 15 amino acids that acts as an ionophore, forming pores or channels in lipid bilayers.

MECHANISMS OF RESISTANCE

Some bacteria exhibit *intrinsic resistance* to certain classes of antibacterial agents (e.g., obligate anaerobic bacteria to aminoglycosides and gram-negative bacteria to vancomycin). In addition, bacteria that are ordinarily susceptible to antibacterial agents can acquire resistance. *Acquired resistance* is one of the major limitations to effective antibacterial chemotherapy. Resistance can develop by mutation of resident genes or by acquisition of new genes. New genes mediating resistance are usually spread from cell to cell by way of mobile genetic elements such as plasmids, transposons, and bacteriophages. The resistant bacterial populations flourish in areas of high antimicrobial use, where they enjoy a selective advantage over susceptible populations.

The major mechanisms used by bacteria to resist the action of antimicrobial agents are inactivation of the compound, alteration or overproduction of the antibacterial target through mutation of the target protein's gene, acquisition of a new gene that encodes a drug-insensitive target, decreased permeability of the cell envelope to the agent, and active efflux of the compound from the periplasm or interior of the cell. Specific mechanisms of bacterial resistance to the major antibacterial agents are outlined below, summarized in Table 118-1, and depicted in Fig. 118-1.

β-LACTAMS
Bacteria develop resistance to β-lactam antibiotics by a variety of mechanisms. Most common is the destruction of the drug by β-lactamases. The β-lactamases of gram-negative bacteria are confined to the periplasm, between the inner and outer membranes, while gram-positive bacteria secrete their β-lactamases into the surrounding medium. These enzymes have a higher affinity for the antibiotic than the antibiotic has for its target. Binding results in hydrolysis of the β-lactam ring. Genes encoding β-lactamases have been found in both chromosomal and extrachromosomal locations and in both gram-positive and gram-negative bacteria; these genes are often on mobile genetic elements. Many "advanced-generation" β-lactam antibiotics, such as ceftriaxone and ceftazidime, are stable in the presence of plasmid-mediated β-lactamases and are active against bacteria resistant to earlier-generation β-lactam antibiotics. However, some β lactamases either acquired by gram-negative bacteria (e.g., *Klebsiella pneumoniae* and *Escherichia coli*) on mobile genetic elements or present as stable chromosomal genes in other gram-negative species (e.g., *Enterobacter*

spp.) have a broad substrate specificity, hydrolyzing virtually all penicillins and cephalosporins. One strategy that has been devised for circumventing resistance mediated by β-lactamases is to combine the β-lactam agent with an inhibitor that avidly binds the inactivating enzyme, preventing its attack on the antibiotic. Unfortunately, the inhibitors (e.g., clavulanic acid, sulbactam, and tazobactam) do not bind all chromosomal β-lactamases (e.g., *Enterobacter* chromosomal β-lactamase) and thus cannot be depended on to prevent the inactivation of β-lactam antibiotics by such enzymes. No β-lactam antibiotic or inhibitor has been produced that can resist all of the many β-lactamases that have been identified.

A second mechanism of bacterial resistance to β-lactam antibiotics is an alteration in PBP targets so that the PBPs have a markedly reduced affinity for the drug. While this alteration may occur by mutation of existing genes, the acquisition of new PBP genes (as in staphylococcal resistance to methicillin) or of new pieces of PBP genes (as in streptococcal, gonococcal, and meningococcal resistance to penicillin) is more important.

A final resistance mechanism is the coupling, in gram-negative bacteria, of a decrease in outer-membrane permeability with rapid efflux of the antibiotic from the periplasm to the cell exterior. Mutations of genes encoding outer-membrane protein channels called *porins* decrease the entry of β-lactam antibiotics into the cell, while additional proteins form channels that actively pump β-lactams out of the cell. Resistance of Enterobacteriaceae to some cephalosporins and resistance of *Pseudomonas* spp. to cephalosporins and ureidopenicillins are the best examples of this mechanism.

VANCOMYCIN
Clinically important resistance to vancomycin was first described among enterococci in France in 1988. Vancomycin-resistant enterococci have subsequently become disseminated worldwide. The genes encoding resistance are carried on plasmids that can transfer themselves from cell to cell and on transposons that can jump from plasmids to chromosomes. Resistance is mediated by enzymes that substitute D-lactate for D-alanine on the peptidoglycan stem peptide so that there is no longer an appropriate target for vancomycin binding. This alteration does not appear to affect cell-wall integrity, however. This type of acquired vancomycin resistance was confined for 14 years to enterococci—more specifically, to *Enterococcus faecium* rather than the more common pathogen *E. faecalis*. However, in 2002, *S. aureus* isolates that were highly resistant to vancomycin were recovered from two patients in the United States. Both isolates contained the gene that mediated vancomycin resistance in enterococci. In addition, since 1996, a few isolates of both *S. aureus* and *S. epidermidis* that display a four- to eightfold reduction in susceptibility to vancomycin have been found worldwide, and many more isolates may contain subpopulations with reduced vancomycin susceptibility. These isolates have not acquired the genes that mediate vancomycin resistance in enterococci but are mutant bacteria with markedly thickened cell walls. These mutants were apparently selected in patients who were undergoing prolonged vancomycin therapy. The failure of vancomycin therapy in some patients infected with *S. aureus* or *S. epidermidis* strains exhibiting only intermediate susceptibility to this drug is thought to have been a result of this resistance.

AMINOGLYCOSIDES
The most common aminoglycoside resistance mechanism is inactivation of the antibiotic. Aminoglycoside-modifying enzymes, usually encoded on plasmids, transfer phosphate, adenyl, or acetyl residues from intracellular molecules to hydroxyl or amino side groups on the antibiotic. The modified antibiotic is less active because of diminished binding to its ribosomal target. Modifying enzymes that can inactivate any of the available aminoglycosides have been found in both gram-positive and gram-negative bacteria.

A second aminoglycoside resistance mechanism, which has been identified predominantly in clinical isolates of *Pseudomonas aeruginosa*, is decreased antibiotic uptake, presumably due to alterations in the bacterial outer membrane.

MACROLIDES, KETOLIDES, LINCOSAMIDES, AND STREPTOGRAMINS Resistance in gram-positive bacteria, which are the usual target organisms for macrolides, lincosamides, and streptogramins, can be due to the production of an enzyme—most commonly plasmid-encoded—that methylates ribosomal RNA, interfering with binding of the antibiotics to their target. Methylation mediates resistance to erythromycin, clarithromycin, azithromycin, clindamycin, and streptogramin B. Resistance to streptogramin B converts quinupristin/dalfopristin from a bactericidal to a bacteriostatic antibiotic. Streptococci can also actively cause the efflux of macrolides, and staphylococci can cause the efflux of clindamycin and streptogramin A. In addition, staphylococci can inactivate streptogramin A by acetylation and streptogramin B by either acetylation or hydrolysis. Finally, mutations in 23S ribosomal RNA that alter macrolide binding to their targets have been found in both staphylococci and streptococci. Ketolides retain activity against most isolates of *Streptococcus pneumoniae* resistant to macrolides.

CHLORAMPHENICOL Most bacteria resistant to chloramphenicol produce a plasmid-encoded enzyme, chloramphenicol acetyltransferase, that inactivates the compound by acetylation.

TETRACYCLINES The most common mechanism of tetracycline resistance in gram-negative bacteria is a plasmid-encoded active-efflux pump that is inserted into the cytoplasmic membrane and extrudes antibiotic from the cell. Resistance in gram-positive bacteria is due either to active efflux or to ribosomal alterations that diminish binding of the antibiotic to its target. Genes involved in ribosomal protection are found on mobile genetic elements.

MUPIROCIN Although the topical compound mupirocin was introduced into clinical use relatively recently, resistance is already becoming widespread in some areas. The mechanism appears to be either mutation of the target isoleucine tRNA synthetase so that it is no longer inhibited by the antibiotic or plasmid-encoded production of a form of the target enzyme that binds mupirocin poorly.

TRIMETHOPRIM AND SULFONAMIDES The most prevalent mechanism of resistance to trimethoprim and the sulfonamides in both gram-positive and gram-negative bacteria is the acquisition of plasmid-encoded genes that produce a new, drug-insensitive target—specifically, an insensitive dihydrofolate reductase for trimethoprim and an altered dihydropteroate synthetase for sulfonamides.

QUINOLONES Resistance to the newer fluoroquinolones emerged rapidly among *Staphylococcus* and *Pseudomonas* spp. after the introduction of these agents. Widespread use of fluoroquinolones in the community has resulted in increasing rates of resistance in *S. pneumoniae*. The most common mechanism is the development of one or more mutations in target DNA gyrases and topoisomerase IV that prevent the antibacterial agent from interfering with the activity of the enzyme. Some gram-negative bacteria develop mutations that both decrease outer-membrane porin permeability and cause active drug efflux from the cytoplasm. Mutations that result in active quinolone efflux are also found in gram-positive bacteria.

RIFAMPIN Bacteria rapidly become resistant to rifampin by developing mutations in the B subunit of RNA polymerase that render the enzyme unable to bind the antibiotic. The rapid selection of resistant mutants is the major limitation to the use of this antibiotic against otherwise-susceptible staphylococci and requires that the drug be used in combination with another antistaphylococcal agent.

LINEZOLID Enterococci, streptococci, and staphylococci become resistant to linezolid in vitro by mutation of the 23S rRNA binding site. Clinical isolates of *E. faecium* and *E. faecalis* acquire resistance to linezolid readily by this mechanism, often during therapy, but linezolid-resistant staphylococcal and streptococcal isolates are rare.

MULTIPLE ANTIBIOTIC RESISTANCE The acquisition by one bacterium of resistance to multiple antibacterial agents is becoming increasingly common. The two major mechanisms are the acquisition of multiple unrelated resistance genes and the development of mutations in a single gene or gene complex that mediate resistance to a series of unrelated compounds. The construction of multiresistant strains by acquisition of multiple genes occurs by sequential steps of gene transfer and environmental selection in areas of high-level antimicrobial use. In contrast, mutations in a single gene can conceivably be selected in a single step. Bacteria that are multiresistant by virtue of the acquisition of new genes include hospital-associated gram-negative bacteria, enterococci, and staphylococci and community-acquired strains of salmonellae, gonococci, and pneumococci. Mutations that confer resistance to multiple unrelated antimicrobial agents occur in the genes encoding outer-membrane porins and efflux proteins of gram-negative bacteria. These mutations decrease bacterial intracellular and periplasmic accumulation of β-lactams, quinolones, tetracyclines, chloramphenicol, and aminoglycosides. Multiresistant bacterial isolates pose increasing problems in U.S. hospitals; strains resistant to all available antibacterial chemotherapy have already been identified.

PHARMACOKINETICS OF ANTIBIOTICS

The *pharmacokinetic profile* of an antibacterial agent refers to concentrations in serum and tissue versus time and reflects the processes of absorption, distribution, metabolism, and excretion. Important characteristics include peak and trough serum concentrations and mathematically derived parameters such as half-life, clearance, and distribution volume. Pharmacokinetic information is useful for estimating the appropriate antibacterial dose and frequency of administration, for adjusting dosages in patients with impaired excretory capacity, and for comparing one drug with another. In contrast, the *pharmacodynamic profile* of an antibiotic refers to the relationship between serum and tissue concentrations of the antibiotic and its minimal inhibitory concentrations (MICs) for bacteria. →*For further discussion of basic pharmacokinetic principles, see Chap. 3.*

ABSORPTION Antibiotic *absorption* refers to the rate and extent of a drug's systemic bioavailability after oral, intramuscular, or intravenous administration.

Oral Administration Most patients with infection are treated with oral antibacterial agents in the outpatient setting. Advantages of oral therapy over parenteral therapy include lower cost, generally fewer adverse effects (including complications of indwelling lines), and greater acceptance by patients. The percentage of an orally administered antibacterial agent that is absorbed (i.e., its *bioavailability*) ranges from as little as 10 to 20% (erythromycin and penicillin G) to nearly 100% [amoxicillin, clindamycin, metronidazole, doxycycline, trimethoprim-sulfamethoxazole (TMP-SMX), linezolid, and most fluoroquinolones]. These differences in bioavailability are not clinically important as long as drug concentrations at the site of infection are sufficient to inhibit or kill the pathogen. However, therapeutic efficacy may be compromised when absorption is reduced as a result of physiologic or pathologic conditions (such as the presence of food for some drugs or the shunting of blood away from the gastrointestinal tract in patients with hypotension), drug interactions (such as that of quinolones and metal cations), or noncompliance. The oral route is usually used for patients with relatively mild infections in whom absorption is not thought to be compromised by the preceding conditions. In addition, the oral route can often be used in more severely ill patients after they have responded to parenteral therapy ("switch" therapy).

Intramuscular Administration Although the intramuscular route of administration usually results in 100% bioavailability, it is not as widely used in the United States as the oral and intravenous routes, in part because of the pain often associated with intramuscular injections and the relative ease of intravenous access in the hospitalized patient. Intramuscular injection may be suitable for specific indications requiring an "immediate" and reliable effect (e.g., with long-acting forms of penicillin, including benzathine and procaine, and with single doses of ceftriaxone for acute otitis media or uncomplicated gonococcal infection).

Intravenous Administration The intravenous route is appropriate when oral antibacterial agents are not effective against a particular pathogen, when bioavailability is uncertain, or when larger doses are required than are feasible with the oral route. After intravenous administration, bioavailability is 100%; serum concentrations are maximal at the end of the infusion. For many patients in whom long-term antimicrobial therapy is required and oral therapy is not feasible, outpatient parenteral antibiotic therapy, including the use of convenient portable pumps, may be cost-effective and safe. Alternatively, some oral antibacterial drugs (e.g., fluoroquinolones) are sufficiently active against Enterobacteriaceae to provide potency equal to that of parenteral therapy; their use may allow the patient to return home from the hospital earlier or to avoid hospitalization entirely.

DISTRIBUTION To be effective, an antibacterial agent must exceed the pathogen's MIC. Serum concentrations usually exceed the MIC for susceptible bacteria, but since most infections are extravascular, the antibiotic must also distribute to the site of the infection. Concentrations of most antibacterial agents in interstitial fluid are similar to free-drug concentrations in serum. However, when the infection is located in a "protected" site where penetration is poor, such as cerebrospinal fluid (CSF), the eye, the prostate, or infected cardiac vegetations, high parenteral doses or local administration for prolonged periods may be required for cure. In addition, even though an antibacterial agent may penetrate to the site of infection, its activity may be antagonized by factors in the local environment, such as an unfavorable pH or inactivation by cellular degradation products. For example, since the activity of aminoglycosides is reduced at acidic pH, the acidic environment in many infected tissues may be partly responsible for the relatively poor efficacy of aminoglycoside monotherapy. In addition, the abscess milieu reduces the penetration and local activity of many antibacterial compounds, so that surgical drainage may be required for cure.

Most bacteria that cause human infections are located extracellularly. Intracellular pathogens such as *Legionella*, *Chlamydia*, *Brucella*, and *Salmonella* may persist or cause relapse if the antibacterial agent does not enter the cell. In general, β-lactams, vancomycin, and aminoglycosides penetrate cells poorly, whereas macrolides, ketolides, tetracyclines, metronidazole, chloramphenicol, rifampin, TMP-SMX, and quinolones penetrate cells well.

METABOLISM AND ELIMINATION Like other drugs, antibacterial agents are disposed of by hepatic elimination (metabolism or biliary elimination), by renal excretion of the unchanged or metabolized form, or by a combination of the two processes. For most antibacterial drugs, metabolism leads to loss of in vitro activity, although some agents, such as cefotaxime, rifampin, rifabutin, and clarithromycin, have bioactive metabolites that may contribute to their overall efficacy.

The most practical application of knowing the mode of excretion of an antibacterial agent is adjustment of the dosage when elimination capability is impaired (Table 118-3). Direct, nonidiosyncratic toxicity from antibacterial drugs may result from failure to reduce the dosage in a patient with impaired elimination. For agents that are primarily cleared intact by glomerular filtration, drug clearance is linearly correlated with creatinine clearance. Unfortunately, for drugs whose elimination is primarily hepatic, no simple marker (such as serum creatinine) is useful for dosage adjustment in patients with liver disease. Even in patients with severe hepatic disease, residual metabolic capability is usually sufficient to preclude accumulation and toxic effects.

PRINCIPLES OF ANTIBACTERIAL CHEMOTHERAPY

The choice of an antibacterial compound for a particular patient and a specific infection involves more than just a knowledge of the agent's pharmacokinetic profile and in vitro activity. The basic tenets of chemotherapy, to be elaborated below, include the following: When appropriate, material containing the infecting organism(s) should be obtained before the start of treatment so that presumptive identification can be made by microscopic examination of stained specimens and

TABLE 118-3 *Antibacterial Drug Dose Adjustments in Patients with Renal Impairment*

Antibiotic	Major Route of Excretion	Dosage Adjustment with Renal Impairment
Aminoglycosides	Renal	Yes
Azithromycin	Biliary	No
Cefazolin	Renal	Yes
Cefepime	Renal	Yes
Ceftazidime	Renal	Yes
Ceftriaxone	Renal/biliary	Modest reduction in severe renal impairment
Ciprofloxacin	Renal/biliary	Only in severe renal insufficiency
Clarithromycin	Renal/biliary	Only in severe renal insufficiency
Erythromycin	Biliary	Only when given in high IV doses
Levofloxacin	Renal	Yes
Linezolid	Metabolism	No
Metronidazole	Biliary	No
Nafcillin	Biliary	No
Penicillin G	Renal	Yes (when given in high IV doses)
Piperacillin	Renal	Only with Cl_{cr} of <40 mL/min
Quinupristin/ dalfopristin	Metabolism	No
Ticarcillin	Renal	Yes
TMP-SMX	Renal/biliary	Only in severe renal insufficiency
Vancomycin	Renal	Yes

Abbreviations: Cl_{cr}, creatinine clearance rate; TMP-SMX, trimethoprim-sulfamethoxazole.

the organism can be grown for definitive identification and susceptibility testing. Awareness of local susceptibility patterns is useful when the patient is treated empirically. Once the organism is identified and its susceptibility to antibacterial agents is determined, the regimen with the narrowest effective spectrum should be chosen. The choice of antibacterial agent is guided by the pharmacokinetic and adverse-reaction profile of active compounds, the site of infection, the immune status of the host, and evidence of efficacy from well-performed clinical trials. If all other factors are equal, the least expensive antibacterial regimen should be chosen.

SUSCEPTIBILITY OF BACTERIA TO ANTIBACTERIAL DRUGS IN VITRO Determination of the susceptibility of the patient's infecting organism to a panel of appropriate antibacterial agents is an essential first step in devising a chemotherapeutic regimen. Standard susceptibility testing is designed to estimate the susceptibility of a bacterial isolate to an antibacterial drug under standardized conditions. These conditions favor rapidly growing aerobic or facultative organisms and assess bacteriostasis only. Specialized testing is required for the assessment of bactericidal antimicrobial activity; for the detection of resistance among such fastidious organisms as obligate anaerobes, *Haemophilus* spp., and pneumococci; and for the determination of resistance phenotypes with variable expression, such as resistance to methicillin or oxacillin among staphylococci. Antimicrobial susceptibility testing is important when susceptibility is unpredictable, most often as a result of increasing acquired resistance among hospitalized patients.

PHARMACODYNAMICS: RELATIONSHIP OF PHARMACOKINETICS AND IN VITRO SUSCEPTIBILITY TO CLINICAL RESPONSE Bacteria are often considered to be *susceptible* to a drug if the achievable peak serum concentration exceeds the MIC by approximately fourfold. The *breakpoint* is the concentration of the antibiotic that separates susceptible from resistant bacteria (Fig. 118-2). When a majority of the isolates of a given bacterial species are inhibited at concentrations below the breakpoint, the species is considered to be within the spectrum of the antibiotic (see "Choice of Antibacterial Therapy," below).

The pharmacodynamic profile of an antibiotic refers to the quantitative relationships between the time course of antibiotic concentrations in serum and tissue, in vitro susceptibility, and microbial response (inhibition of growth or rate of killing). Three pharmacodynamic parameters quantify these relationships: the ratio of the area

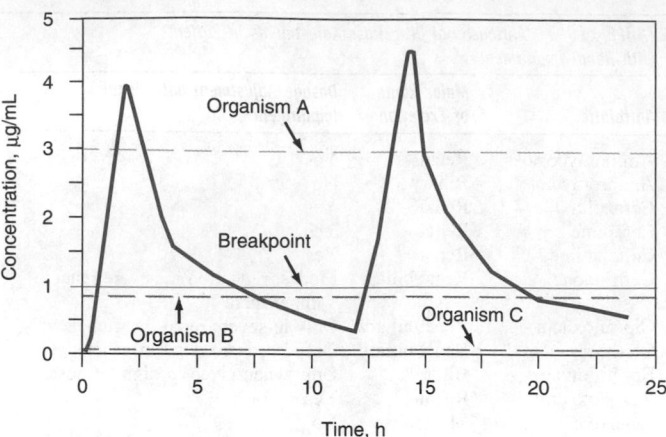

FIGURE 118-2 Relationship between pharmacokinetics of an antibiotic and susceptibility. Organism A is resistant, organism B is moderately susceptible, and organism C is very susceptible.

under the curve for the plasma concentration vs. time curve to MIC (AUC/MIC), the ratio of the maximal serum concentration to the MIC (C_{max}/MIC), and the time during a dosing interval that plasma concentrations exceed the MIC ($t >$ MIC). The pharmacodynamic profile of an antibiotic class is characterized as either *concentration dependent* (fluoroquinolones, aminoglycosides), such that the increase in antibiotic concentration leads to a more rapid rate of bacterial death, or *time dependent* (β-lactams), such that the reduction in bacterial density is proportional to the time that concentrations exceed the MIC. For concentration-dependent antibiotics, the C_{max}/MIC or AUC/MIC ratio correlates best with the reduction in microbial density in vitro and in animal investigations. Dosing strategies attempt to maximize these ratios by the administration of a large dose relative to the MIC for anticipated pathogens, often at long intervals (relative to the serum half-life). Once-daily dosing of aminoglycoside antibiotics is the most practical consequence of these relationships. In contrast, dosage strategies for time-dependent antibiotics emphasize the administration of doses sufficient to maintain serum concentrations above the MIC for a critical portion of the dose interval. Response to β-lactam antibiotics, measured as the decline in bacterial density at the site of infection, appears to be maximal when serum and tissue concentrations are maintained above the MIC for 30 to 50% of the dose interval. For example, the use of high-dose amoxicillin (90 to 100 mg/kg per day) in the treatment of acute otitis media increases not only the penetration of amoxicillin into the inner ear but also the duration of time that concentrations exceed the MIC for pneumococci. This approach provides effective therapy in most patients, including those whose pneumococcal isolates are penicillin resistant. The clinical implications of these pharmacodynamic relationships are in the early stages of investigation; their elucidation should eventually result in more rational antibacterial dosage regimens. Table 118-4 summarizes the pharmacodynamic properties of the major antibiotic classes.

STATUS OF THE HOST Various host factors must be considered in the devising of antibacterial chemotherapy. The host's antibacterial *immune function* is of importance, particularly as it relates to opsonophagocytic function. Since the major host defense against acute, overwhelming bacterial infection is the polymorphonuclear leukocyte, patients with neutropenia must be treated aggressively and empirically with bactericidal drugs for suspected infection (Chap. 72). Likewise, patients who have deficient humoral immunity (e.g., those with chronic lymphocytic leukemia and multiple myeloma) and individuals with surgical or functional asplenia (e.g., those with sickle cell disease) should be treated empirically for infections with encapsulated organisms, especially the pneumococcus.

Pregnancy increases the risk of toxicity of certain antibacterial drugs for the mother (e.g., hepatic toxicity of tetracycline), affects drug

disposition and pharmacokinetics, and—because of the risk of fetal toxicity—severely limits the choice of agents for treating infections. Certain antibacterial agents are contraindicated in pregnancy either because their safety has not been established or because they are known to be toxic. These agents include all fluoroquinolones, clarithromycin, erythromycin estolate (but not erythromycin base), and tetracyclines (Table 118-5). Data on the safety of many other antibacterial drugs are limited, but these drugs may be used cautiously when there is no suitable alternative and the perceived benefit outweighs the risk. These agents include the aminoglycosides, azithromycin, clindamycin, imipenem, metronidazole, trimethoprim, and vancomycin. Nitrofurantoin and the sulfonamides are contraindicated in the third trimester but can be used cautiously in the first two trimesters.

In patients with *concomitant viral infections*, the incidence of adverse reactions to antibacterial drugs may be unusually high. For example, persons with infectious mononucleosis and those infected with HIV react more often to ampicillin and folic acid synthesis inhibitors, respectively.

In addition, the patient's age, sex, racial heritage, genetic background, and excretory status all determine the incidence and type of side effects that can be expected with certain antibacterial agents.

SITE OF INFECTION The location of the infected site may play a major role in the choice and dose of antimicrobial drug. Patients with suspected *meningitis* should receive drugs that can cross the blood-CSF barrier; in addition, because of the relative paucity of phagocytes and opsonins at the site of infection, the agents should be bactericidal. Chloramphenicol, an older drug but occasionally useful in the treatment of meningitis, is bactericidal for common organisms causing meningitis (i.e., meningococci, pneumococci, and *Haemophilus influenzae*, but *not* enteric gram-negative bacilli), is highly lipid-soluble, and enters the CSF well. However, β-lactam drugs, the mainstay of therapy for most of these infections, do not normally reach high levels in CSF. Their efficacy is based on the increased permeability of the blood-brain and blood-CSF barriers to hydrophilic molecules during inflammation and the extreme susceptibility of most infectious organisms to even small amounts of β-lactam drug.

The vegetation, which is the major site of infection in *bacterial endocarditis*, is also a focus that is protected from normal host-defense mechanisms. Antibacterial therapy needs to be bactericidal, with the selected agent administered parenterally over a long period and at a dose that produces serum levels at least eight times higher than the minimal bactericidal concentration (MBC) for the infecting organism. Likewise, *osteomyelitis* involves a site that is somewhat resistant to opsonophagocytic removal of infecting bacteria; furthermore, avascular bone (sequestrum) represents a foreign body that thwarts normal host-defense mechanisms. *Chronic prostatitis* is exceedingly difficult to cure because most antibiotics do not penetrate through the capillaries serving the prostate, especially when acute inflammation is absent. *Intraocular infections*, especially endophthalmitis, are difficult to treat because retinal capillaries lacking fenestration hinder drug penetration into the vitreous from blood. Inflammation does little to disrupt this barrier. Thus, direct injection into the vitreous is necessary in many cases. Antibiotic penetration into *abscesses* is usually poor, and local conditions (e.g., low pH or the presence of enzymes that hydrolyze the drug) may further antagonize antibacterial activity.

TABLE 118-4	*Pharmacodynamic Parameters of Major Antimicrobial Classes*
Parameter Predicting Response	**Drug or Drug Class**
Time above the MIC	Penicillins, cephalosporins, carbapenems, aztreonam
24-h AUC/MIC	Aminoglycosides, fluoroquinolones, tetracyclines, vancomycin, macrolides, clindamycin, quinupristin/dalfopristin
Peak to MIC	Aminoglycosides, fluoroquinolones

Abbreviations: MIC, minimal inhibitory concentration; AUC, area under the concentration curve.

In contrast, *urinary tract infections*, when confined to the bladder, are relatively easy to cure, in part because of the higher concentration of most antibiotics in urine than in blood. Since blood is the usual reference fluid in defining susceptibility (Fig. 118-2), even organisms found to be resistant to achievable serum concentrations may be susceptible to achievable urine concentrations. For drugs that are used only for the treatment of urinary tract infections, such as nitrofurantoin and methenamine salts, achievable urine concentrations are used to determine susceptibility.

TABLE 118-5 *Antibacterial Drugs in Pregnancy*

Antibacterial Drug	Toxicity in Pregnancy	Recommendation
Aminoglycosides	Possible 8th nerve toxicity	Caution[a]
Chloramphenicol	Gray syndrome in newborn	Caution at term
Fluoroquinolones	Arthropathy in immature animals	Caution
Clarithromycin	Teratogenicity in animals	Contraindicated
Ertapenem	Decreased weight in animals	Caution
Erythromycin estolate	Cholestatic hepatitis	Contraindicated
Imipenem/cilastatin	Toxicity in some pregnant animals	Caution
Linezolid	Embryonic and fetal toxicity in rats	Caution
Meropenem	Unknown	Caution
Metronidazole	None known, but carcinogenic in rats	Caution
Nitrofurantoin	Hemolytic anemia in newborns	Caution; contraindicated at term
Quinupristin/dalfopristin	Unknown	Caution
Sulfonamides	Hemolysis in newborn with G6PD[b] deficiency; kernicterus in newborn	Caution; contraindicated at term
Tetracyclines	Tooth discoloration, inhibition of bone growth in fetus; hepatotoxicity	Contraindicated
Vancomycin	Unknown	Caution

[a] Use only for strong clinical indication in the absence of a suitable alternative.
[b] G6PD, glucose-6-phosphate dehydrogenase.
Source: *Medical Letter Handbook of Antimicrobial Therapy*, 16th ed, 2002.

COMBINATION CHEMOTHERAPY One of the tenets of antibacterial chemotherapy is that if the infecting bacterium has been identified, the most specific chemotherapy possible should be used. The use of a single agent with a narrow spectrum of activity against the pathogen diminishes the alteration of normal flora and thus limits the overgrowth of resistant nosocomial organisms (e.g., *Candida albicans*, enterococci, *Clostridium difficile*, or methicillin-resistant staphylococci), avoids the potential toxicity of multiple-drug regimens, and reduces cost. However, certain circumstances call for the use of more than one antibacterial agent. These are summarized below.

1. *Prevention of the emergence of resistant mutants.* Spontaneous mutations occur at a detectable frequency in certain genes encoding the target proteins for some antibacterial agents. The use of these agents can eliminate the susceptible population, select out resistant mutants at the site of infection, and result in the failure of chemotherapy. Resistant mutants are usually selected when the MIC of the antibacterial agent for the infecting bacterium is close to achievable levels in serum or tissues and/or when the site of infection limits the access or activity of the agent. Among the most common examples are rifampin for staphylococci, imipenem for *Pseudomonas*, and fluoroquinolones for staphylococci and *Pseudomonas*. Small-colony variants of staphylococci resistant to aminoglycosides also emerge during monotherapy with these antibiotics. A second antibacterial agent with a mechanism of action different from that of the first is added to prevent the emergence of these resistant mutants (e.g., imipenem plus an aminoglycoside for systemic *Pseudomonas* infections). However, since resistant mutants have emerged following combination chemotherapy, this approach clearly is not uniformly successful.

2. *Synergistic or additive activity.* Synergistic or additive activity involves a lowering of the MIC or MBC of each or all of the drugs tested in combination against a specific bacterium. In *synergy*, each agent is more active when combined with a second drug than it would be alone, and the drugs' combined activity is therefore greater than the sum of the individual activities of each drug. In an *additive relationship*, the combined activity of the drugs is equal to the sum of their individual activities. Among the best examples of a synergistic or additive effect, confirmed both in vitro and by animal studies, are the enhanced bactericidal activities of certain β-lactam/aminoglycoside combinations against enterococci, viridans streptococci, and *P. aeruginosa*. The synergistic or additive activity of these combinations has also been demonstrated against selected isolates of enteric gram-negative bacteria and staphylococci. The combination of trimethoprim and sulfamethoxazole has synergistic or additive activity against many enteric gram-negative bacteria. Most other antimicrobial combinations display indifferent activity (i.e., the combination is *no better* than the more active of the two agents alone), and some combinations (e.g.,

penicillin plus tetracycline against pneumococci) may be antagonistic (i.e., the combination is *worse* than either drug alone).

3. *Therapy directed against multiple potential pathogens.* For certain infections, either a mixture of pathogens is suspected or the patient is desperately ill with an as-yet-unidentified infection (see "Empirical Therapy," below). In these situations, the most important of the likely infecting bacteria must be covered by therapy until culture and susceptibility results become available. Examples of the former infections are intraabdominal or brain abscesses and infections of limbs in diabetic patients with microvascular disease. The latter situations include fevers in neutropenic patients, acute pneumonia from aspiration of oral flora by hospitalized patients, and septic shock or sepsis syndrome.

EMPIRICAL THERAPY In many situations, antibacterial therapy is begun before a specific bacterial pathogen has been identified. The choice of agent is guided by the results of studies identifying the usual pathogens at that site or in that clinical setting, by pharmacodynamic considerations, and by the resistance profile of the expected pathogens in a particular hospital or geographic area. Situations in which empirical therapy is appropriate include the following:

1. *Life-threatening infection.* Any suspected bacterial infection in a patient with a life-threatening illness should be treated presumptively. Therapy is usually begun with more than one agent and is later tailored to a specific pathogen if one is eventually identified.

2. *Treatment of community-acquired infections.* In many situations, it is appropriate to treat non-life-threatening infections without obtaining cultures. These situations include outpatient infections such as community-acquired upper and lower respiratory tract infections, cystitis, cellulitis or local wound infection, urethritis, and prostatitis. However, if any of these infections recurs or fails to respond to initial therapy, every effort should be made to obtain cultures to guide retreatment.

CHOICE OF ANTIBACTERIAL THERAPY

The antibacterial spectrum of specific agents and the infections for which they represent the treatment of choice are detailed below. No attempt has been made to include all the potential situations in which antibacterial agents may be used. A more detailed discussion of specific bacteria and infections that they cause can be found elsewhere in this volume.

β-LACTAMS (Table 118-2) All *penicillins* (except for the semisynthetic, penicillinase-resistant antistaphylococcal agents) are hydrolyzed by β-lactamases and are ineffective against isolates that produce these enzymes. Penicillin G has a spectrum that includes spirochetes

(*Treponema pallidum*, *Borrelia*, and *Leptospira*), streptococci (groups A and B, viridans, and many strains of *S. pneumoniae*), *E. faecalis*, most *Neisseria* spp., a few staphylococci, many fastidious oral bacteria (including many *Porphyromonas* and *Prevotella* spp., streptococci, *Actinomyces*, and *Fusobacterium*), *Clostridium* spp. (except *C. difficile*), *Pasteurella multocida*, *Erysipelothrix rhusiopathiae*, and *Streptobacillus moniliformis*. However, penicillin G resistance is widespread among staphylococci; is increasing rapidly among gonococci and pneumococci; and is emerging among meningococci, viridans streptococci, and oral anaerobes such as *Porphyromonas* and *Prevotella*. Penicillin G is the *drug of choice* for syphilis, yaws, leptospirosis, group A and B streptococcal infections, actinomycosis, oral and periodontal infections, meningococcal meningitis and meningococcemia, viridans streptococcal endocarditis, clostridial myonecrosis, tetanus, anthrax, rat-bite fever, *P. multocida* infections, and erysipeloid (*E. rhusiopathiae*).

Ampicillin extends the spectrum of penicillin G to some gram-negative rods. It is active against some isolates of *Escherichia coli*, *Proteus mirabilis*, *Salmonella*, *Shigella*, and *H. influenzae* and is one of the *drugs of choice* for susceptible organisms causing salmonellosis, acute otitis media, *H. influenzae* meningitis and epiglottitis, and *Listeria monocytogenes* meningitis. *E. faecalis* is usually susceptible, and amoxicillin is the *drug of choice* for urinary tract infections caused by this organism. High rates of resistance have lessened the value of ampicillin and amoxicillin as empirical therapy in some situations. For example, >80% of isolates of *E. coli* and *P. mirabilis* are resistant in many hospitals, as are ~30% of isolates of *H. influenzae*; moreover, in some outbreaks of infection due to salmonellae, all isolates are resistant to ampicillin.

The *penicillinase-resistant penicillins* are used solely for the treatment of staphylococcal infections and are the *drugs of choice* for systemic or deep staphylococcal infections caused by susceptible organisms. Unfortunately, on average, ~40% of *S. aureus* isolates and >70% of coagulase-negative staphylococcal isolates acquired in U.S. hospitals are resistant to these agents (i.e., methicillin-resistant). The spectrum of these agents also includes most of the same gram-positive bacteria that are susceptible to penicillin G.

The spectrum of the *antipseudomonal penicillins* includes the bacteria covered by ampicillin as well as some nonpseudomonal enteric gram-negative bacilli. For example, piperacillin is active against many indole-positive *Proteus*, *Enterobacter*, *Klebsiella*, *Providencia*, and *Serratia* spp. However, the susceptibility of these penicillins to β-lactamase markedly limits their utility as empirical therapy when infections caused by gram-negative enteric organisms are suspected. The "antipseudomonal penicillins" are no longer commercially available or have been formulated in combination with β-*lactamase inhibitors*. The addition of a β-lactamase inhibitor (clavulanic acid, sulbactam, or tazobactam) to ampicillin, amoxicillin, ticarcillin, or piperacillin extends the spectrum of the β-lactam agent to include many organisms that are resistant by virtue of β-lactamase production. These organisms include many strains of *E. coli*, *Klebsiella* spp., all *Proteus* spp., *H. influenzae*, *Moraxella catarrhalis*, *Providencia* spp., and anaerobes (including *Bacteroides* spp.). Such combinations are also active against staphylococci that produce β-lactamase but are not resistant to methicillin. However, the efficacy of these combinations in serious staphylococcal infections has not been adequately proven. Furthermore, *Serratia*, indole-positive *Proteus*, *Citrobacter*, *Enterobacter*, *Pseudomonas*, *Acinetobacter*, and various enteric gram-negative isolates either produce chromosomal β-lactamases that are not inhibited by these compounds or develop resistance attributable to non-β-lactamase-mediated mechanisms.

The *first-generation cephalosporins* have a spectrum that includes penicillinase-producing, methicillin-susceptible staphylococci and penicillin-susceptible streptococci. While these drugs may be used when infections with gram-positive bacteria are suspected, they are *not* the drugs of choice for such infections. They have excellent activity against many isolates of *E. coli*, *Klebsiella pneumoniae*, and *P. mirabilis* and are among the *drugs of choice* in presumptive therapy for community-acquired urinary tract infections. They have no activity against *Bacteroides fragilis*, enterococci, methicillin-resistant staphylococci, *Pseudomonas*, *Acinetobacter*, *Enterobacter*, indole-positive *Proteus*, and *Serratia* and only poor activity against *H. influenzae*.

The *parenteral second-generation cephalosporins* extend the gram-negative spectrum of first-generation compounds. The various second-generation agents have differing activities. Cefuroxime retains activity against gram-positive cocci and is also active against *H. influenzae*, *Neisseria*, and indole-positive *Proteus* but exhibits poor activity against *B. fragilis*. Cefoxitin and cefotetan have reasonably good activity against *B. fragilis*, but cefotetan is less effective against some other *Bacteroides* spp. (Chaps. 112 and 148). Both of the latter drugs display poor activity against gram-positive cocci and *Enterobacter*. No second-generation cephalosporin is active against *Pseudomonas* or *Acinetobacter*.

Oral second- and third-generation cephalosporins have fair activity against gram-positive cocci and *H. influenzae* and are widely used in outpatient therapy for otitis media, sinusitis, and lower respiratory tract infections, although cheaper agents that are equally effective are preferable. Cefditoren, cefdinir, and cefpodoxime have good activity against most respiratory pathogens and methicillin-susceptible *S. aureus*.

Third-generation parenteral cephalosporins all have a broad spectrum of activity against enteric gram-negative rods and are especially useful for treating hospital-acquired infections caused by multiresistant organisms. In addition, ceftazidime and cefepime have good antipseudomonal activity; the other drugs have poor activity. Since resistance to third-generation cephalosporins is increasing among all nosocomial gram-negative rods, the use of these agents should be guided by susceptibility testing. The gram-positive spectrum of the third-generation cephalosporins is variable. All are less active than first-generation cephalosporins against methicillin-susceptible staphylococci; ceftazidime has the least antistaphylococcal activity of this group. However, ceftriaxone and cefotaxime have excellent activity against streptococci, especially *S. pneumoniae*. Ceftazidime is not recommended for treatment of streptococcal infections.

Ceftriaxone has an excellent gram-negative spectrum; is active against *Haemophilus*, most *S. pneumoniae* strains, and penicillin-resistant *Neisseria*; has a long serum half-life; and reaches high serum and CSF levels (with inflammation). Thus it has become one of the *drugs of choice* for empirical therapy for bacterial meningitis (except that caused by *Listeria* and by highly penicillin-resistant pneumococcal strains), all gonococcal infections, salmonellosis, and typhoid fever. The third-generation cephalosporins are among the *drugs of choice* for nonpseudomonal hospital-acquired pneumonia. Cefepime is more resistant to chromosomal β-lactamase produced by *Enterobacter* spp. than are other third-generation cephalosporins and is more active against methicillin-susceptible *S. aureus*. Third-generation cephalosporins have poor activity against *Bacteroides* and no activity against methicillin-resistant staphylococci, *Enterococcus*, *Acinetobacter*, or *Stenotrophomonas*.

The *carbapenems* currently available in the United States are imipenem, meropenem, and ertapenem. Imipenem is marketed in combination with the renal dipeptidase inhibitor cilastatin, which enables imipenem to escape renal inactivation and thus to reach higher urinary levels. Imipenem and meropenem have excellent activity in vitro against virtually all bacterial pathogens except *Stenotrophomonas*, methicillin-resistant staphylococci, and *E. faecium*. Imipenem has dose-related central nervous system side effects that are less frequent with meropenem. Resistance to imipenem and meropenem is a problem among nosocomial isolates of *P. aeruginosa*, ~20% of which are resistant. Ertapenem has poor activity against enterococci, *P. aeruginosa*, and *Acinetobacter* but exhibits activity similar to that of meropenem against Enterobacteriaceae. Because of their broad spectrum, imipenem and meropenem can be used as empirical therapy for serious nosocomial infections thought to be caused by multiple bacterial species or multiresistant organisms. Imipenem and meropenem are often used to treat hospital-acquired infections caused by *Enterobacter* spp. because these organisms produce inducible β-lactamases that inactivate third-generation cephalosporins but not the carbapenems. The latter antibiotics are often held in reserve as therapy for nosocomial infections due to gram-negative pathogens that are resistant to third-generation cephalosporins.

The only *monobactam* currently available is aztreonam. This antibiotic has a spectrum limited to gram-negative enteric bacilli. It has no activity against any gram-positive or anaerobic bacterium. Its gram-negative spectrum is similar to that of ceftazidime, with equally good activity against *Pseudomonas*. Aztreonam's primary advantages are its theoretical ability to preserve the normal gram-positive and anaerobic flora and the lack of cross-reactive immediate hypersensitivity in patients who have had this type of reaction to other β-lactam antibiotics.

VANCOMYCIN The spectrum of vancomycin is limited to gram-positive cocci, especially enterococci, streptococci, and staphylococci. Vancomycin serves as second-line therapy for most gram-positive bacterial infections but is the *drug of choice* for infections caused by methicillin-resistant staphylococci or *Corynebacterium jeikeium* and for serious infections in penicillin-allergic patients. Given orally (a route by which it is not absorbed), vancomycin can be used to treat antibiotic-associated pseudomembranous colitis caused by *C. difficile* in patients who have failed to respond to metronidazole—the *drug of choice*. Vancomycin has also been recommended as initial empirical therapy for presumed pneumococcal meningitis because of increasing pneumococcal resistance to penicillins and cephalosporins. Resistance to vancomycin is increasing rapidly among isolates of *E. faecium* in large hospitals, particularly in areas of high vancomycin use. In addition, *S. aureus* isolates with both high-level resistance and reduced susceptibility to vancomycin have now been detected. Because of the growing threat of vancomycin-resistant enterococci and the potential for increasing resistance among staphylococci, a national advisory committee has established guidelines for appropriate and limited use of this antibiotic (Table 118-6).

AMINOGLYCOSIDES The aminoglycosides are rapidly bactericidal in vitro at low concentrations, with activity limited to gram-negative bacteria and staphylococci. They have no activity against anaerobic bacteria and are not effective in environments that are acidic or have a low oxygen tension. However, their spectrum includes virtually all gram-negative bacteria that are not strict anaerobes, and they are among the *drugs of choice* for any suspected gram-negative bacteremic infection, particularly in neutropenic patients. Aminoglycosides are synergistically bactericidal in combination with a penicillin for the treatment of staphylococcal, enterococcal, or viridans streptococcal endocarditis and are usually combined with a β-lactam antibiotic for the treatment of gram-negative bacteremia. Aminoglycosides are also among the *drugs of choice* for severe infections of the upper urinary tract. The major limitations to use of aminoglycosides are their renal and otic toxicity, their diminished activity at certain sites of infection (e.g., abscesses and the central nervous system), and the resistance of target bacteria. Among the available agents, gentamicin and tobramycin are generally preferred because of their low cost. Tobramycin has slightly greater activity against *P. aeruginosa*, and amikacin retains activity against many tobramycin- and gentamicin-resistant gram-negative bacteria because it is inactivated by fewer aminoglycoside-modifying enzymes. Streptomycin is still one of the *drugs of choice* in initial therapy for tularemia, plague, glanders, and brucellosis and is a second-line agent for the treatment of *tuberculosis*.

MACROLIDES AND KETOLIDES Erythromycin has broad-spectrum activity against gram-positive bacteria, with additional activity against *Legionella*, *Mycoplasma*, *Campylobacter*, *Bordetella pertussis*, and some *Chlamydia* isolates. It is the *drug of choice* for infections due to *Legionella*, *Campylobacter*, and *Mycoplasma* and is among the *drugs of choice* for community-acquired pneumococcal pneumonia and group A streptococcal pharyngitis in penicillin-allergic patients. However, resistance to erythromycin among group A streptococci and especially pneumococci is increasing dramatically in some areas. Erythromycin also appears to be one of the *drugs of choice* for infections caused by the agent of bacillary angiomatosis (*Bartonella henselae*) in immunocompromised patients. Clarithromycin and azithromycin have an antibacterial spectrum similar to that of erythromycin in vitro. However, azithromycin has greater activity against *Chlamydia*. Clarithromycin, in combination with a proton pump inhibitor, has been designated a *drug of choice* for the treatment of gastric infections due to *Helicobacter pylori* (gastritis, gastric and duodenal ulcers). Both azithromycin and clarithromycin are active against nontuberculous mycobacteria, and both appear to have fewer gastrointestinal side effects than does erythromycin. Bacteria that are resistant to erythromycin are also resistant to clarithromycin and azithromycin. Telithromycin is a ketolide antibiotic that is similar to erythromycin in structure, spectrum of activity, and mechanism of action. However, telithromycin is active against most macrolide-resistant strains of *S. pneumoniae*.

LINCOSAMIDES The only lincosamide used in the United States is clindamycin. It shares the gram-positive coccal spectrum of erythromycin but is more active (in some cases showing bactericidal activity) against susceptible staphylococci. However, resistance among staphylococci and some streptococci, mediated by the same genes responsible for macrolide resistance, limits clindamycin's usefulness against gram-positive cocci. In general, all staphylococci resistant to erythromycin should be considered resistant to clindamycin regardless of the results of in vitro susceptibility testing. However, at least half of the streptococci resistant to erythromycin are truly susceptible to clindamycin. In these bacteria, resistance is mediated by a drug-efflux pump that removes macrolides but not lincosamides. Despite increasing resistance, clindamycin remains useful for most anaerobic infections because of its broad spectrum of activity against most gram-positive and gram-negative strict anaerobes. It is also a *drug of choice* for the treatment of severe, invasive group A streptococcal infections. In contrast, clindamycin, like erythromycin, has no clinically significant activity against facultative gram-negative enteric bacilli. The appropriate use of clindamycin is limited only by resistance or the development of pseudomembranous colitis, the major serious side effect of this drug.

CHLORAMPHENICOL Chloramphenicol has a broad spectrum of activity against gram-positive and gram-negative bacteria, although plasmid-mediated resistance has diminished its effective spectrum. This antibiotic is rarely used in adult infections because of the rare idiosyncratic side effect of irreversible bone-marrow aplasia and the availability of other agents with similar activity. It remains one of the *drugs of choice* for the treatment of typhoid fever and plague and is still useful for the treatment of brucellosis and both pneumococcal and meningococcal meningitis in patients with severe penicillin allergy.

TABLE 118-6 *Guidelines for Appropriate and Limited Use of Vancomycin*

Acceptable Use	Discourage Use
Infection with methicillin-resistant *Staphylococcus aureus*	When culture reveals a β-lactam-susceptible organism
Infection with gram-positive bacteria in penicillin-allergic patient (where vancomycin is one of the drugs of choice)	Continued empirical use without indication (e.g., no evidence of infection)
Antibiotic-associated colitis unresponsive to metronidazole	Coagulase-negative staphylococcal bacteremia, single positive culture
Endocarditis prophylaxis during dental procedures for patients allergic to β-lactam antibiotics	Routine empirical therapy
Cardiovascular surgical prophylaxis (with unusually high rates of postoperative infection with β-lactam-resistant organisms)	Routine surgical prophylaxis or prophylaxis in the dialysis patient

TETRACYCLINES   Tetracyclines have a broad spectrum of bacteriostatic activity against gram-positive and gram-negative bacteria and are widely used in a variety of community-acquired infections. These agents are among the *drugs of choice* for acute bacterial exacerbations of chronic bronchitis, granuloma inguinale, brucellosis (with streptomycin), tularemia, glanders, melioidosis, spirochetal infections caused by *Borrelia* (Lyme disease and relapsing fever; doxycycline), infections caused by *Vibrio vulnificus*, some *Aeromonas* infections, infections due to *Stenotrophomonas* (minocycline), plague, ehrlichiosis, chlamydial infections (doxycycline), and granulomatous skin infections due to *Mycobacterium marinum* (minocycline). The tetracyclines are also used in penicillin-allergic patients for the treatment of leptospirosis, syphilis, actinomycosis, and skin and soft tissue infections caused by gram-positive cocci. Doxycycline is also among the drugs recommended for the treatment of community-acquired pneumonia, although clinical data are few and resistance in *S. pneumoniae* is increasing.

SULFONAMIDES AND TRIMETHOPRIM   The folic acid synthesis inhibitors have a broad spectrum of bacteriostatic activity individually; in combination, they can be bactericidal against facultative gram-negative bacteria and staphylococci. The fixed combination of sulfamethoxazole and trimethoprim, the major folic acid synthesis inhibitors used in therapy for bacterial infections, has modest activity against some streptococci and no activity against strict anaerobes. However, resistance to TMP-SMX is common among methicillin-resistant staphylococci and penicillin-resistant pneumococci and is increasing among *E. coli* strains that cause urinary tract infections. The individual sulfonamides are rarely used in the treatment of bacterial infections but are among the *drugs of choice* for the treatment of nocardial infections, leprosy (dapsone, a sulfone), and toxoplasmosis (sulfadiazine). Although increasing resistance has been reported among gram-negative organisms, TMP-SMX remains one of the *drugs of choice* for the treatment of uncomplicated urinary tract infections (except for those caused by enterococci) and had been used in the treatment of otitis media. It can be used in therapy for upper respiratory tract infections in which *S. pneumoniae*, *H. influenzae*, or *M. catarrhalis* is suspected (although resistance in *S. pneumoniae* is now common in some areas); for gonococcal and meningococcal infections; for chancroid; and for infections thought to be caused by *Aeromonas*, *Stenotrophomonas*, *Burkholderia cepacia*, *Acinetobacter*, and *Yersinia enterocolitica*. For nosocomial infections due to *Stenotrophomonas*, TMP-SMX is the *drug of choice*.

FLUOROQUINOLONES   The fluoroquinolones have excellent activity against most facultative gram-negative rods and variable activity against gram-positive cocci. The quinolones are the oral agents with greatest activity against *P. aeruginosa*; ciprofloxacin is the most active against this species, although a high rate of acquired resistance limits its utility in many hospitals. All the quinolones except norfloxacin are well absorbed orally; ciprofloxacin, levofloxacin, moxifloxacin, and gatifloxacin are also administered as intravenous formulations. The quinolones are among the *drugs of choice* for urinary tract infections, bacterial gastroenteritis, community-acquired pneumonia, and enteric fever and are useful for serious hospital-acquired infections caused by gram-negative organisms. While older quinolones (such as ciprofloxacin) have limited activity against gram-positive bacteria, the newer quinolones have an expanded spectrum of activity against gram-positive cocci, including staphylococci (methicillin-susceptible) and streptococci (especially *S. pneumoniae*). Quinolones can also be used as prophylaxis for persons at risk for meningococcal meningitis. However, use of quinolones should be coupled with the realization that, in conjunction with rapidly expanding usage, resistance is being reported increasingly among all bacteria targeted by these drugs, including *S. pneumoniae*, *Neisseria gonorrhoeae*, *E. coli*, and *P. aeruginosa*.

RIFAMPIN   Rifampin has been used in combinations for the treatment of serious infections due to methicillin-resistant staphylococci (e.g.,

coagulase-negative staphylococcal foreign-body infections). Because the spontaneous selection of rifampin-resistant mutants occurs rapidly, rifampin should never be used alone in the treatment of staphylococcal infections. Rifampin is also used for chemoprophylaxis in persons at risk of meningococcal meningitis and for the treatment of *Legionella* pneumonia.

METRONIDAZOLE   Metronidazole has a spectrum limited to anaerobic bacteria, especially gram-negative species (e.g., *Bacteroides* spp.). It is less active against anaerobic gram-positive cocci (e.g., *Peptostreptococcus* and *Peptococcus* spp.). Because of its spectrum and its ability to penetrate into the area of infection, metronidazole is one of the *drugs of choice* for the treatment of any abscess in which the involvement of obligate anaerobes is suspected (e.g., lung, brain, or intraabdominal abscesses). Other antibacterial agents should be used in combination with metronidazole if facultative and aerobic pathogens are also thought to be involved. Metronidazole is the *drug of choice* for the treatment of bacterial vaginosis and antibiotic-associated pseudomembranous colitis.

LINEZOLID   This antibacterial agent has a spectrum limited to gram-positive bacteria and is indicated for the treatment of infections caused by streptococci, staphylococci, and enterococci. Because there is very little preexisting resistance to linezolid, the drug is active against gram-positive bacteria that are resistant to other antibacterial agents. In particular, it is active against vancomycin-resistant enterococci (both *E. faecium* and *E. faecalis*) and is one of the *drugs of choice* for treating infections due to these organisms. However, since this drug has only bacteriostatic activity, it has limited utility in treating complicated *S. aureus* infections.

POLYMYXINS   Polymyxins B and E have a broad spectrum of activity that includes virtually all gram-negative bacteria. However, while polymyxin B is still used as a component of topical preparations (see "Topical Antibacterial Agents," below), polymyxin E (colistin) has been used little since the early 1980s because of the high incidence of severe renal toxicity associated with its systemic use. The occurrence in recent years of nosocomial infections caused by strains of bacteria such as *P. aeruginosa*, *Acinetobacter baumanii*, and *Stenotrophomonas maltophilia* that are resistant to all available therapy but susceptible to colistin has prompted a reexamination of its use in certain patients for whom there are no other options. Recent data suggest that colistin is reasonably safe and effective when used with caution.

STREPTOGRAMINS   The combination of streptogramin B (quinupristin) and streptogramin A (dalfopristin) has a spectrum that is limited to gram-positive bacteria and is indicated for the treatment of infections caused by staphylococci, streptococci, and *E. faecium*. It is not active against *E. faecalis*. Quinupristin/dalfopristin is used primarily as therapy for infections caused by vancomycin-resistant *E. faecium*. The agent has bactericidal activity against isolates of *S. aureus* and *S. epidermidis* that are susceptible to both components. However, since ~80% of oxacillin (methicillin)-resistant *S. aureus* and *S. epidermidis* and 20 to 40% of oxacillin-susceptible staphylococci are resistant to streptogramin A (dalfopristin) as a result of ribosomal methylation, quinupristin/dalfopristin has only bacteriostatic activity against most hospital-acquired staphylococci. It is *not*, therefore, a drug of choice for serious nosocomial staphylococcal infections and should be used for complicated *S. aureus* infections only when complete susceptibility to both components can be demonstrated.

URINARY TRACT ANTISEPTICS   Urinary tract antiseptics are active only in the lower urinary tract and cannot be used for the treatment of upper urinary tract or systemic infections. The available agents in this category include nitrofurantoin and methenamine salts, which are most active against susceptible gram-negative enteric bacteria. Nitrofurantoin is often active against vancomycin-resistant enterococci and is a less expensive alternative to linezolid for the treatment of lower urinary tract infections.

TOPICAL ANTIBACTERIAL AGENTS   Mupirocin is available only as a topical preparation for use against staphylococci and streptococci. Its major applications are for impetigo and eradication of the staphylococcal carrier state. It is the *drug of choice* for the elimination of nasal carriage of both methicillin-susceptible and methicillin-resistant staphylococci. Unfortunately, the emergence of resistance is limiting its usefulness in some hospitals.

Although their efficacy has never been well documented, topical preparations that include sulfonamides, polymyxin B, neomycin, bacitracin, gramicidin, and novobiocin in a variety of combinations are widely used as eyedrops, irrigation solutions, and ointments for superficial skin infections.

ADVERSE REACTIONS

Adverse drug reactions are frequently classified by mechanism as either dose-related ("toxic") effects or unpredictable reactions. Unpredictable reactions are either idiosyncratic or allergic. Dose-related reactions include aminoglycoside-induced nephrotoxicity, linezolid-induced thrombocytopenia, penicillin-induced seizures, and vancomycin-induced anaphylactoid reactions. Many of these reactions can be avoided by reducing dosage, limiting the duration of therapy, or reducing the frequency or rate of administration. Adverse reactions to antibacterial agents are a common cause of morbidity, requiring alteration in therapy and additional expense, and they occasionally result in death. The elderly, often those with the more severe infections, may be especially prone to certain adverse reactions. →*For further discussion of adverse drug reactions, see Chap. 3.*

β-LACTAMS The therapeutic index for β-lactam antibiotics is broad, and dose-related adverse reactions are uncommon and largely preventable. The greatest concern is allergic reactions. All types can occur, including anaphylaxis (type 1, immediate-hypersensitivity reactions), nephritis and Coombs-positive hemolytic anemia (type 2, cytotoxic reactions), drug fever and serum sickness (type 3, immune-complex formation), contact dermatitis (type 4, cell-mediated effects), and maculopapular eruption (type 5, idiopathic reactions). Approximately 1 to 4% of treatment courses result in an allergic reaction, and ~0.004 to 0.015% of treatment courses result in anaphylaxis. Only 10 to 20% of the patients who claim an allergy to penicillin react to skin testing with the major and minor determinants (penicilloyl-polylysine and benzylpenicillin degradation products, respectively); those with negative skin tests only rarely react adversely to subsequent therapeutic doses. Generally, a suitable alternative to β-lactams is available for patients who have a severe allergy, and penicillin desensitization can be carefully undertaken if there is no suitable alternative. A small proportion (<2%) of persons who are allergic to penicillin react similarly when a cephalosporin is administered; thus, cephalosporins are contraindicated in patients with a history of an immediate reaction to penicillin, although they are often used in patients with a history of mild reactions. The same precaution applies to carbapenems, but aztreonam is antigenically distinct and can be administered safely to the penicillin-allergic patient.

Other reactions thought to have an allergic basis include nephritis (associated with methicillin and occasionally nafcillin), hepatitis (related to oxacillin), leukopenia (following high doses of most β-lactams administered for prolonged periods), and severe skin rashes (toxic epidermal necrolysis and Stevens-Johnson syndrome). These reactions are not IgE-mediated, and skin testing is not predictive of their occurrence. For unclear reasons, most patients who have infectious mononucleosis or cytomegalovirus infection develop a rash when given ampicillin or amoxicillin.

Miscellaneous reactions to β-lactams include gastrointestinal side effects ranging in severity from mild diarrhea (5 to 10%) to pseudomembranous colitis (<1%). Although the probability of antibiotic-associated colitis is low, a large number of cases occur because β-lactams are so commonly prescribed. Drugs excreted to a large extent through the bile, such as ampicillin and ceftriaxone, may be especially prone to cause diarrhea. The addition of clavulanic acid to amoxicillin further increases the frequency of diarrhea. Ceftriaxone, because of extremely high concentrations in bile, can cause "sludging"

in the gallbladder and occasionally produces symptoms compatible with acute cholecystitis.

In high doses—and most often in patients with renal impairment who receive an excessive dose—penicillins (especially ticarcillin and penicillin G) can cause bleeding from impaired platelet aggregation. Seizures are occasionally observed with β-lactams, especially penicillin G and imipenem. This reaction is most common when excessive doses relative to renal function are administered or when the patient has a history of seizures.

VANCOMYCIN When vancomycin was first used clinically in 1956, local intolerance at the infusion site was common, as were systemic reactions, including ototoxicity and nephrotoxicity. Current formulations are of higher purity and, when proper dosage guidelines are followed, are very safe, although phlebitis can still be troublesome. The most common adverse reaction is called *red man syndrome* and is characterized by pruritus, flushing, and erythema of the head and upper torso. This anaphylactoid reaction usually follows the first dose, is dependent on dose size and infusion time, and results from vancomycin-induced release of histamine. The reaction is usually mild in adult patients who receive 1 g over 60 min and diminishes with repeated doses. If vancomycin is mistakenly given as a bolus, severe hypotension may result. In unusually sensitive patients, extending the infusion time or administering H_1 receptor antagonists is usually effective in preventing this reaction or reducing its severity. Patients with this reaction must not be mislabeled as having an allergy to vancomycin, since vancomycin may be the only effective treatment for certain infections (e.g., those due to methicillin-resistant staphylococci).

Nephrotoxicity from vancomycin is mild and uncommon. Although some data suggest that aminoglycosides and vancomycin are synergistically nephrotoxic, this point is difficult to prove, and the simultaneous use of these agents should not be avoided if clinically indicated, as in the treatment of enterococcal endocarditis in penicillin-allergic patients.

Ototoxicity from vancomycin is rare as long as doses are appropriately reduced in patients with renal insufficiency. Other uncommon adverse reactions include leukopenia, skin rashes, and true allergy. Serum concentrations of vancomycin are of little use in predicting toxicity but may be of value in selecting dosages for patients with unstable renal function.

AMINOGLYCOSIDES Aminoglycoside antibiotics have a narrow therapeutic index. The two most common adverse reactions are nephrotoxicity and ototoxicity. Rarely, respiratory depression is observed. Nephrotoxicity results from accumulation of the aminoglycoside in the peritubular space, with damage to the proximal tubule and a corresponding reduction in the glomerular filtration rate. The incidence of nephrotoxicity, defined as an increase of >0.5 mg/dL over baseline in the serum creatinine level, is ~5 to 10% among adult patients who receive therapy for 10 to 14 days. However, many cofactors also influence the frequency of toxicity, such as extremes of age (toxicity is uncommon among children, more common among the elderly), concomitant drug therapy, and hydration status. Nephrotoxicity is manifested clinically by a gradual rise in serum creatinine levels after a few days of therapy and is reversible if the dosage is reduced or treatment is discontinued. Serum creatinine levels should be monitored every 3 to 5 days or more often if changes are seen. There is not an important difference among the most useful agents (gentamicin, tobramycin, and amikacin) in terms of the frequency of nephrotoxicity; streptomycin is a rare cause of nephrotoxicity. Some data suggest that once-daily administration of aminoglycosides may cause less nephrotoxicity than more frequent administration.

Ototoxicity from aminoglycoside therapy presents as either auditory or vestibular damage. Since the aminoglycosides can destroy hair cells in the inner ear, ototoxicity may be permanent. The risk of ototoxicity increases with prolonged therapy, higher serum concentrations (especially in patients with renal impairment), hypovolemia, and concurrent treatment with other ototoxins, especially ethacrynic acid. There is evidence of a genetic predisposition to ototoxicity in some persons. Clinically apparent ototoxicity, manifested by diminished acuity or vestibular imbalance, is uncommon (probably occurring in <1% of cases) when the duration of therapy is kept to a minimum. With more sensitive monitoring (e.g., audiograms), asymptomatic high-tone hearing loss is more commonly noted. There are no clinically important differences among the aminoglycosides in the overall frequency of ototoxicity.

Neuromuscular depression from aminoglycosides is caused by reduced acetylcholine activity at postsynaptic membranes and can result in rare but severe respiratory depression. Risk factors include hypocalcemia, peritoneal administration, use of neuromuscular blockers, and preexisting respiratory depression. This complication can be largely avoided if the aminoglycoside is administered intravenously over 30 min or by intramuscular injection; if respiratory depression occurs, it is reversed by the administration of calcium.

Fear of toxicity should not prevent the use of aminoglycosides for a legitimate indication, since toxicity is usually mild and reversible. The value of measuring serum concentrations is controversial; these measurements are usually unnecessary when the patient is receiving once-daily therapy, especially when the duration is <7 to 10 days.

MACROLIDES　Serious adverse reactions to the macrolide antibiotics are very rare. Gastrointestinal effects, such as burning, nausea, and vomiting, are the most common adverse reactions to the macrolides; depending on dosage, these reactions may occur in up to 50% of patients, occasionally requiring early discontinuation of therapy. The mechanism is thought to be the binding of erythromycin to motilin receptors, with a consequent increase in gastrointestinal motility. Gastrointestinal side effects appear equally common for all the oral formulations and also occur with intravenous administration. Clarithromycin and azithromycin are better tolerated than erythromycin, although gastrointestinal distress is still their most common adverse effect.

Less common reactions include hepatotoxicity and ototoxicity. Hepatotoxicity is a rare, nonfatal complication that is usually associated with erythromycin estolate and presents as an allergic cholestatic jaundice. Ototoxicity is rare after oral administration but may occur in a dose-dependent pattern in up to 20% of adults who receive intravenous erythromycin (4 g/d) and have audiograms performed. Ototoxicity is usually reversible and mild. Allergic cutaneous reactions are observed in rare cases. Macrolides are among the many drugs that can prolong the QT$_c$ interval in some patients. The clinical significance of this effect continues to be investigated. The limited data suggest that the ketolide telithromycin has adverse effects similar to those of erythromycin.

LINCOSAMIDES　The most common adverse effect of clindamycin is gastrointestinal distress. Diarrhea has been reported in up to 20% of patients and pseudomembranous colitis in 0.01 to 10%. The mechanism of pseudomembranous colitis is production of a toxin by C. difficile (Chap. 114). C. difficile colonizes the gastrointestinal tract and may produce a toxin when the normal flora is suppressed by clindamycin and other antibiotics, especially β-lactams. This toxin causes mucosal damage that results in cramps, pain, and diarrhea that may be bloody. Pseudomembranous colitis may follow both intravenous and oral administration and may not become manifest until after completion of therapy. Oral metronidazole or oral vancomycin is effective in treating symptomatic patients with toxin-positive stools, but some spores may survive, and relapse is frequent. Metronidazole is the *drug of choice* since oral treatment with vancomycin can select for vancomycin-resistant enterococci. Although diarrhea and pseudomembranous colitis can be caused by most antibacterial agents, the incidence in relation to the amount used may be highest for clindamycin. Allergic reactions (such as rashes and fever), hepatotoxicity, and neutropenia are observed only rarely.

CHLORAMPHENICOL　Chloramphenicol causes two types of bone marrow suppression: a dose-related, reversible suppression of all elements, which occurs commonly during therapy at the maximal recommended doses (4 g/d in adults), and an idiosyncratic, irreversible aplastic anemia, which occurs in ~1 of every 25,000 to 40,000 exposures. The irreversible form has been reported to follow all types of chloramphenicol treatment, including ocular administration, and often develops months after therapy is discontinued.

In premature neonates and infants, chloramphenicol can cause a dose-related "gray syndrome" that is characterized by cyanosis, hypotension, and death and that results from an inability of the newborn to metabolize the drug. These potentially serious toxicities and the availability of newer drugs have substantially reduced the indications for chloramphenicol use.

TETRACYCLINES　Gastrointestinal effects are the most common adverse reactions to the tetracyclines. These problems may be related to a direct irritant effect, since tetracyclines can also cause esophageal ulceration when they dissolve before reaching the stomach. It is important that nighttime doses be taken with sufficient fluid. Concurrent food intake may improve tolerance, but absorption of tetracycline HCl is impaired when the drug is taken with food.

Hepatotoxicity has been reported after administration of >2 g of tetracycline intravenously and at lower doses during pregnancy. There are currently no indications for intravenous tetracycline treatment in pregnancy. All tetracyclines can cause phototoxic skin reactions; these reactions are most common with doxycycline. Other dermal reactions, including rash, are uncommon. Tetracyclines are contraindicated in children <8 years of age because of mottling of the permanent teeth; doxycycline may be less likely than the other tetracyclines to cause this problem. Worsening of renal function in patients with preexisting renal dysfunction has been reported with use of tetracycline. Doxycycline and perhaps minocycline appear to be free from these renal side effects. Alternative effective agents are nearly always available for use in patients with renal dysfunction. Minocycline can cause vertigo in up to 70% of women receiving therapeutic doses and in a lower percentage of men.

SULFONAMIDES AND TRIMETHOPRIM　The sulfonamides are generally safe, but the list of possible adverse reactions is very long. These compounds occasionally cause a number of allergic reactions, from relatively minor skin rashes (including maculopapular rashes and urticarial reactions typically appearing after a week of therapy) to severe or even life-threatening reactions such as erythema multiforme, Stevens-Johnson syndrome, and toxic epidermal necrolysis. The severe hypersensitivity reactions have occurred most commonly after treatment with the long-acting sulfonamides, such as sulfamethoxypyridazine, which are no longer used. Pyrimethamine plus sulfadoxine (Fansidar), used for malaria prophylaxis, may cause severe allergic reactions, including hepatic and hematologic toxicities, in addition to dermatologic toxicity. Photosensitivity reactions are also relatively common with sulfonamides.

Many patients infected with HIV who receive TMP-SMX have adverse dermatologic reactions. These reactions are usually not life-threatening and appear to regress in many cases despite continuation of therapy. In high doses, trimethoprim interferes with the renal secretion of potassium. Hyperkalemia is relatively common among HIV-positive patients and is most often found after 7 days of TMP-SMX therapy for pneumonia caused by *Pneumocystis*.

Sulfonamides and trimethoprim may also cause severe hematologic complications, including agranulocytosis, hemolytic and megaloblastic anemia, and thrombocytopenia. These dose-related side effects may be more frequent and more severe in patients with renal insufficiency. Hemolytic anemia is most common in patients with glucose-6-phosphate dehydrogenase deficiency who take long-acting compounds; TMP-SMX rarely causes hemolysis in such subjects. Granulocytopenia from TMP-SMX is especially common among HIV-infected patients, occurring in 10 to 50% of this group.

Renal insufficiency, caused by crystals of the relatively insoluble acetyl metabolite, is observed primarily with the long-acting sulfonamides. Many cases of crystalluria in HIV-infected patients taking sulfadiazine for toxoplasmosis have been reported. A high level of fluid intake may prevent this complication.

It is recommended that sulfonamides not be administered to newborns because of concerns that bilirubin may be displaced from protein-binding sites, with subsequent jaundice and kernicterus.

In addition to the preceding problems, sulfonamides may occasionally cause drug fever with serum sickness, hepatic toxicity (including necrosis), and systemic lupus erythematosus.

FLUOROQUINOLONES Fluoroquinolones are relatively safe; adverse reactions rarely require discontinuation of therapy. The most common reactions include gastrointestinal distress, such as nausea or diarrhea (<5%), and central nervous system effects, including insomnia and dizziness (<5%). Phototoxicity is occasionally severe. Rarely, hepatic and renal dysfunction and anaphylactoid and allergic reactions are observed. Quinolones can cause tendon rupture in rare instances. The use of these drugs is currently contraindicated in patients <18 years of age because of evidence in animals of cartilage damage in developing joints. In carefully selected situations in which the perceived benefits outweigh the risks (e.g., in adolescent patients with cystic fibrosis who have pulmonary exacerbations), fluoroquinolones may be useful for short-term therapy. They are contraindicated in pregnancy because of concern for the developing fetus. Quinolones can also increase the QT_c interval; it is unclear whether the currently available quinolones differ in a clinically important way in this respect. Hypo- and hyperglycemia have been reported and may be more common with gatifloxacin. As of 2003, a number of fluoroquinolones—including temafloxacin, sparfloxacin, grepafloxacin, and trovafloxacin—have been removed from the U.S. market because of rare but severe adverse effects. It may be prudent to limit the use of the newest drugs in this class until their safety has been fully established.

RIFAMPIN Rifampin is generally well tolerated but has several important side effects. Some patients have transient rises in hepatic aminotransferases, but these levels usually return to normal without discontinuation of the drug. Although hepatitis from rifampin itself develops only rarely, the drug is thought by some investigators to potentiate the hepatic toxicity of concomitantly administered isoniazid. Intermittent administration of rifampin (usually fewer than three times per week) has been associated with signs and symptoms that seem to have an immunologic basis. These include flulike symptoms and (rarely) hemolysis, thrombocytopenia, shock, and renal failure. Minor gastrointestinal side effects, skin rashes, and interstitial nephritis have also been reported. Patients should be warned that rifampin and its metabolites cause secretions such as urine, tears, sweat, and saliva to turn orange and that contact lenses may be stained.

METRONIDAZOLE Serious adverse reactions to metronidazole are uncommon. Gastrointestinal side effects such as nausea are most frequent but rarely necessitate discontinuation of therapy. Pseudomembranous colitis in association with metronidazole has been reported but is very rare. A metallic taste is relatively common, and stomatitis and glossitis are occasionally reported. Peripheral neuropathy develops in some patients, and seizures and encephalopathy have been reported after high doses and in patients with hepatic failure.

Concerns about mutagenicity and carcinogenicity from metronidazole have led to recommendations that it not be used in pregnancy (especially during the first trimester) when alternative agents are available. Although retrospective studies have found no association between metronidazole and carcinogenesis, long-term administration of high doses should be avoided when therapeutic alternatives exist.

LINEZOLID The most common adverse events accompanying linezolid therapy include gastrointestinal upset (nausea, vomiting, and diarrhea) and headache. Of most concern is a reversible myelosuppression that is directly related to the duration of therapy. Thrombocytopenia is the most likely hematologic abnormality, although anemia and leukopenia are also observed. If the duration of therapy is expected to exceed 1 week, then weekly complete blood counts are recommended.

QUINUPRISTIN/DALFOPRISTIN Quinupristin/dalfopristin is not well tolerated. In particular, venous irritation is a frequent and potentially serious adverse effect when the drug is given by peripheral intravenous infusion. Administration via a central line is often required to complete a course of therapy. In addition, arthralgia and myalgia are substan-

TABLE 118-7 *Interactions of Antibacterial Agents with Other Drugs*

Antibiotic	Interacts with	Potential Consequence (Clinical Significance[a])
Erythromycin/clarithromycin/ telithromycin	Theophylline	Theophylline toxicity (1)
	Carbamazepine	CNS depression (1)
	Digoxin	Digoxin toxicity (2)
	Triazolam/midazolam	CNS depression (2)
	Ergotamine	Ergotism (1)
	Warfarin	Bleeding (2)
	Cyclosporine/tacrolimus	Nephrotoxicity (1)
	Cisapride	Cardiac arrhythmias (1)
	Statins[b]	Rhabdomyolysis (2)
	Valproate	Valproate toxicity (2)
	Vincristine/vinblastine	Excess neurotoxicity (2)
Quinupristin/dalfopristin	Similar to erythromycin[c]	
Fluoroquinolones[d]	Theophylline	Theophylline toxicity (2)
	Antacids/sucralfate/iron	Subtherapeutic antibiotic levels (1)
Tetracycline	Antacids/sucralfate/iron	Subtherapeutic antibiotic levels (1)
Trimethoprim-sulfamethoxazole	Phenytoin	Phenytoin toxicity (2)
	Oral hypoglycemics	Hypoglycemia (2)
	Warfarin	Bleeding (1)
	Digoxin	Digoxin toxicity (2)
Metronidazole	Ethanol	Disulfiram-like reactions (2)
	Fluorouracil	Bone marrow suppression (1)
	Warfarin	Bleeding (2)
Rifampin	Warfarin	Clot formation (1)
	Oral contraceptives	Pregnancy (1)
	Cyclosporine/tacrolimus	Rejection (1)
	HIV-1 protease inhibitors	Increased viral load, resistance (1)
	Nonnucleoside reverse-transcriptase inhibitors	Increased viral load, resistance (1)
	Glucocorticoids	Loss of steroid effect (1)
	Methadone	Narcotic withdrawal symptoms (1)
	Digoxin	Subtherapeutic digoxin levels (1)
	Itraconazole	Subtherapeutic itraconazole levels (1)
	Phenytoin	Loss of seizure control (1)
	Statins	Hypercholesterolemia (1)
	Diltiazem	Subtherapeutic diltiazem levels (1)
	Verapamil	Subtherapeutic verapamil levels (1)

[a] 1 = a well-documented interaction with clinically important consequences; 2 = an interaction of uncertain frequency but of potential clinical importance.
[b] Lovastatin and simvastatin are most affected; pravastatin and atorvastatin are less prone to clinically important effects.
[c] The macrolide antibiotics and quinupristin/dalfopristin inhibit the same human metabolic enzyme, CYP3A4, and similar interactions are anticipated.
[d] Ciprofloxacin only. Levofloxacin, moxifloxacin, and gatifloxacin do not inhibit theophylline metabolism.
Note: New interactions are commonly reported after marketing. Consult the most recent prescribing information for updates.
Abbreviation: CNS, central nervous system.

TABLE 118-8 *Prophylaxis of Bacterial Infections in Adults*

Condition	Antibacterial Agent	Timing or Duration of Prophylaxis
Nonsurgical		
Cardiac lesions susceptible to bacterial endocarditis	Amoxicillin[a]	Before and after procedures causing bacteremia
Recurrent *S. aureus* infections	Mupirocin	5 days (intranasal)
Contact with patient with meningococcal meningitis	Rifampin Fluoroquinolone	2 days Single dose
Bite wounds[b]	Penicillin V or amoxicillin/clavulanic acid	3–5 days
Recurrent cystitis	Trimethoprim-sulfamethoxazole or a fluoroquinolone or nitrofurantoin	3 times per week for up to 1 year or after sexual intercourse
Surgical		
Clean (cardiac, vascular, neurologic, or orthopedic surgery)	Cefazolin (vancomycin)[c]	Before and during procedure
Ocular	Topical combinations and subconjunctival cefazolin	During and at end of procedure
Clean-contaminated (head and neck, high-risk gastroduodenal or biliary tract surgery; high-risk cesarean section; hysterectomy)	Cefazolin (or clindamycin for head and neck)	Before and during procedure
Clean-contaminated (vaginal or abdominal hysterectomy)	Cefazolin or cefoxitin or cefotetan	Before and during procedure
Clean-contaminated (high-risk genitourinary surgery)	Fluoroquinolone	Before and during procedure
Clean-contaminated (colorectal surgery or appendectomy)	Cefoxitin or cefotetan (add oral neomycin + erythromycin for colorectal)	Before and during procedure
Dirty[b] (ruptured viscus)	Cefoxitin or cefotetan ± gentamicin (clindamycin + gentamicin) or another appropriate regimen directed at anaerobes and gram-negative aerobes	Before and for 3–5 days after procedure
Dirty[b] (traumatic wound)	Cefazolin	Before and for 3–5 days after trauma

[a] Gentamicin should be added to the amoxicillin regimen for high-risk gastrointestinal and genitourinary procedures; vancomycin should be used in penicillin-allergic patients.

[b] In these cases, use of antibacterial agents actually constitutes treatment of infection rather than prophylaxis.

[c] Vancomycin is recommended only in institutions that have a high incidence of infection with methicillin-resistant staphylococci.

tially more common among patients treated with quinupristin/dalfopristin than among those receiving other antimicrobial agents. Other side effects include rash, elevated serum bilirubin levels, and gastrointestinal distress.

DRUG INTERACTIONS

Antimicrobial drugs are a common cause of drug-drug interactions. Table 118-7 lists the most common and best-documented interactions of antibacterial agents with other drugs and characterizes the clinical relevance of these interactions. Coadministration of drugs paired in the tables does not necessarily result in clinically important adverse consequences. Recognition of the potential for an interaction before the administration of an antibacterial agent is crucial to the rational use of these drugs, since adverse consequences can often be prevented if the interaction is anticipated. Table 118-7 is intended only to heighten awareness of the potential for an interaction. Additional sources should be consulted to identify appropriate options. →*For further discussion of drug interactions, see Chap. 3.*

MACROLIDES AND KETOLIDES Erythromycin, clarithromycin, and telithromycin inhibit the P450 enzyme CYP3A4 and thus the metabolism of many other drugs, including cyclosporine, certain statins (lovastatin, simvastatin), theophylline, carbamazepine, warfarin, certain antineoplastic agents (e.g., vincristine, irinotecan), and ergot alkaloids. When erythromycin and other inhibitors of CYP3A4 are given to patients receiving terfenadine, astemizole, cisapride, and pimozide, cardiac arrhythmias (including torsades de pointes) can occur; the availability of the latter drugs has been severely restricted or they have been removed from the U.S. market. Azithromycin has little effect on the metabolism of other drugs. In ~10% of patients receiving digoxin, concentrations increase when these drugs are given.

QUINUPRISTIN/DALFOPRISTIN Quinupristin/dalfopristin is an inhibitor of CYP3A4. Its interactions with other drugs should be similar to those of erythromycin.

LINEZOLID Linezolid is a monoamine oxidase inhibitor. Its concomitant administration with sympathomimetics such as phenylpropanolamine, with selective serotonin reuptake inhibitors, and with foods with high concentrations of tyramine should be avoided.

TETRACYCLINES The most important interaction involving tetracyclines is the reduction in absorption when these drugs are coadministered with divalent and trivalent cations, such as antacids, iron compounds, or dairy products. Food also adversely affects absorption of most tetracyclines. Inducers of hepatic isoenzymes, such as phenytoin and rifampin, increase the clearance of doxycycline; although the clinical significance of this effect is unknown, use of an alternative antibiotic may be appropriate.

SULFONAMIDES Sulfonamides, including sulfamethoxazole, increase the hypoprothrombinemic effect of warfarin by inhibition of its metabolism and possibly by protein-binding displacement. Sulfonamides may also potentiate the effects of oral hypoglycemic agents and phenytoin through reduction in metabolism or displacement from serum protein.

FLUOROQUINOLONES There are two clinically important drug interactions involving fluoroquinolones. First, like tetracyclines, all fluoroquinolones are chelated by divalent and trivalent cations, which prevent most of the dose from being absorbed. Second, certain fluoroquinolones, including ciprofloxacin, inhibit hepatic enzymes that metabolize theophylline, with consequent theophylline toxicity. The same mechanism accounts for increases in serum caffeine concentrations, but the clinical significance of this interaction is unknown. Scattered case reports suggest that quinolones can also potentiate the effects of warfarin, but this effect has not been observed in most controlled trials.

RIFAMPIN Rifampin is an excellent inducer of many cytochrome P450 enzymes and increases the hepatic clearance of a number of drugs, including the following (with the indicated predictable outcomes): HIV-1 protease inhibitors (loss of viral suppression), oral contraceptives (pregnancy), warfarin (decreased prothrombin times), cyclosporine and prednisone (organ rejection or exacerbations of any underlying inflammatory condition), and verapamil and diltiazem (increased dosage requirements). Before rifampin is prescribed for any patient, a review of concomitant drug therapy is essential.

METRONIDAZOLE Metronidazole can cause a disulfiram-like syndrome when alcohol is ingested; thus, patients taking metronidazole should be instructed to avoid alcohol. Inhibition of the metabolism of warfarin by metronidazole leads to significant rises in prothrombin times.

Antibacterial agents are occasionally indicated for use in patients who have no evidence of infection but who have been or are expected to be exposed to bacterial pathogens under circumstances that constitute a major risk of infection. The basic tenets of antimicrobial prophylaxis are as follows: (1) the risk or potential severity of infection should be greater than the risk of side effects from the antibacterial agent, (2) the antibacterial agent should be given for the shortest period necessary to prevent target infections, and (3) the antibacterial agent should be given before the expected period of risk (e.g., surgical prophylaxis) or as soon as possible after contact with an infected individual (e.g., prophylaxis for meningococcal meningitis).

Table 118-8 lists the major indications for antibacterial prophylaxis in adults. (The use of antibacterial agents in children to prevent rheumatic fever and otitis media under certain circumstances is also common practice.) The table includes only those indications that are widely accepted, supported by well-designed studies, or recommended by expert panels. Prophylaxis is also used but is less widely accepted for recurrent cellulitis in conjunction with lymphedema, recurrent pneumococcal meningitis in conjunction with deficiencies in humoral immunity or CSF leaks, traveler's diarrhea, gram-negative sepsis in conjunction with neutropenia, and spontaneous bacterial peritonitis in conjunction with ascites.

The major use of antibacterial prophylaxis in the United States is for infections following surgical procedures. Antibacterial agents are administered just before the surgical procedure—and, for long operations, during the procedure as well—to ensure high levels in serum and tissues during surgery. The objective is to eradicate bacteria originating from the air of the operating suite, the skin of the surgical team, or the patient's own flora that may contaminate the wound. In all but colorectal surgical procedures, prophylaxis is predominantly directed against staphylococci. Prophylaxis is intended to prevent wound infection or infection of implanted devices, not all infections that may occur during the postoperative period (e.g., urinary tract infections or pneumonia). Prolonged prophylaxis merely alters the normal flora and favors infections with organisms resistant to the antibacterial agents used.

DURATION OF THERAPY AND TREATMENT FAILURE

It is often difficult to determine the proper duration of therapy for bacterial infections. There are few infections for which trials have established the appropriate treatment duration. Table 118-9 lists those common bacterial infections for which guidelines have been established or for which there is sufficient clinical experience to establish treatment durations. The ultimate test of cure for a bacterial infection is the absence of relapse when therapy is discontinued. *Relapse* is defined as a recurrence of infection with the identical organism that caused the first infection. In general, therefore, the duration of therapy should be long enough to prevent relapse yet not excessive. Therapy extended beyond the limit of effectiveness will increase side effects of medication and encourage the selection of resistant bacteria. The art of treating bacterial infections lies in the ability to determine the appropriate duration of therapy for infections that are not covered by established guidelines. Re-treatment of infections for which therapy has failed usually requires a prolonged course (>4 weeks) with combinations of antibacterial agents.

ANTIBACTERIAL COSTS AND INAPPROPRIATE USE

Use of antibacterial agents in U.S. hospitals can represent the largest expenditure for any single pharmacologic class. It is not unusual for the purchase cost of a newer parenteral antibiotic (in 2003 dollars) to be $1000 to $2000 for a 10- to 14-day course of treatment. Therapy for 5 to 10 days with a new oral antibiotic can easily cost $60 to $100, compared with a few dollars for older drugs such as doxycycline and amoxicillin. Administration costs, monitoring costs, and pharmacy charges must be added to these figures. While some newer antibacterial agents undeniably represent important advances in therapy, many newer drugs offer no advantage over older, less expensive agents. With

TABLE 118-9 *Duration of Therapy for Bacterial Infections*

Duration of Therapy	Infections
Single dose	Gonococcal urethritis, streptococcal pharyngitis (penicillin G benzathine), primary and secondary syphilis (penicillin G benzathine)
3 days	Cystitis in young women, community- or travel-acquired diarrhea
7–10 days	Community-acquired pneumonia, community-acquired meningitis (pneumococcal or meningococcal), antibiotic-associated diarrhea (10 days), *Giardia* enteritis, cellulitis, epididymitis
2 weeks	*Helicobacter pylori*–associated peptic ulcer, neurosyphilis (penicillin IV), penicillin-susceptible viridans streptococcal endocarditis (penicillin plus aminoglycoside), disseminated gonococcal infection with arthritis, acute pyelonephritis, uncomplicated *S. aureus* catheter-associated bacteremia
3 weeks	Lyme disease, septic arthritis (nongonococcal)
4 weeks	Acute and chronic prostatitis, infective endocarditis (penicillin-resistant streptococcal)
>4 weeks	Acute and chronic osteomyelitis, *S. aureus* endocarditis, foreign-body infections (prosthetic-valve and joint infections), relapsing pseudomembranous colitis

rare exceptions, newer drugs are usually found to be no more effective than the comparison antibiotic in controlled trials, despite the "high prevalence of resistance" often touted to market the advantage of the new antibiotic over older therapies.

Clinicians are understandably confused by the bewildering array of available drugs and their competing claims of superiority. Numerous surveys have reported that ~50% of antibiotic use is in some way "inappropriate." Aside from the monetary cost of unnecessary antibiotics, there are the costs of excess morbidity from adverse effects and drug interactions and the eventual costs of treating more resistant organisms. The following suggestions are intended to provide guidance through the antibiotic maze.

First, objective evidence regarding the merits of newer drugs is available through publications such as *The Medical Letter* (including periodic updates of the *Drugs of Choice*) and through online references such as those on the Johns Hopkins website (http://hopkins-abxguide.org), which offers much current information. Second, clinicians should become comfortable using a few drugs recommended by independent experts and professional organizations and should resist the temptation to use a new drug unless the merits are clear. A new antibacterial agent with a "broader spectrum and greater potency," a "longer half-life and higher tissue levels," or a "higher serum concentration-to-MIC ratio" does not necessarily translate into greater clinical efficacy. Third, clinicians should become familiar with local bacterial susceptibility profiles. It may not be necessary to use a new drug with "improved activity against *P. aeruginosa*" if that pathogen is rarely encountered or if it retains full susceptibility to older drugs. Finally, with regard to inpatient use of antibacterial drugs, appropriate empirical treatment with one or more broad-spectrum agents may often be simplified, with use of a narrower-spectrum agent or even an oral drug, once the results of cultures and susceptibility tests become available. While there is an understandable temptation not to alter effective therapy, switching to a more specific agent once the patient has improved clinically does not compromise outcome. A promising and active area of research includes shorter durations of antimicrobial therapy. Many antibiotics that once were given for 7 to 14 days can probably be given for 3 to 7 days. As these clinical trials of shorter duration and equal efficacy are published, prompt adoption of the shorter courses by the clinical community may be an effective counter to the problems of increasing resistance. Adoption of these guidelines will not undermine the care of patients, many unnecessary complications and expenses will be avoided, and the useful life of valuable drugs will be extended.

FURTHER READING

ANTIMICROBIAL PROPHYLAXIS IN SURGERY. Med Lett Drugs Ther 43:92, 2001

AVORN J, SOLOMON DH: Cultural and economic factors that (mis)shape antibiotic use: The nonpharmacologic basis of therapeutics. Ann Intern Med 133:128, 2000

CRAIG WA: Does the dose matter? Clin Infect Dis 33(Suppl 3):S233, 2001

HOSPITAL INFECTION CONTROL PRACTICES ADVISORY COMMITTEE: Recommendations for preventing the spread of vancomycin resistance. Infect Control Hosp Epidemiol 16:105, 1995

LEVIN AS et al: Intravenous colistin as therapy for nosocomial infections caused by multidrug-resistant Pseudomonas aeruginosa and Acinetobacter baumanii. Clin Infect Dis 28:1008, 1999

THE CHOICE OF ANTIBACTERIAL DRUGS. Med Lett Drugs Ther 43:69, 2001

Section 5   Diseases Caused by Gram-Positive Bacteria

119   PNEUMOCOCCAL INFECTIONS
Daniel M. Musher

Streptococcus pneumoniae (the pneumococcus) was recognized as the major cause of pneumonia in the 1880s and has been a central focus of study leading to the modern understanding of humoral immunity. The name *Diplococcus pneumoniae* was assigned to the organism in 1926 because of its appearance in Gram-stained sputum. In 1974, the organism was renamed *Streptococcus pneumoniae* because it grows in chains in liquid medium. Around 1900, pneumococcal serotypes were recognized when the injection of killed organisms into a rabbit stimulated the production of serum antibody that agglutinated the immunizing strain and protected rabbits against challenge with that strain and with some but not all other pneumococcal isolates. Ninety serotypes have now been identified, each possessing a unique polysaccharide capsule.

MICROBIOLOGY   Pneumococci are identified in the clinical laboratory as gram-positive cocci that grow in chains and are catalase-negative. They produce pneumolysin, a toxin that breaks down hemoglobin into a greenish degradation product, thereby causing α-hemolysis on blood agar. More than 98% of pneumococcal isolates are susceptible to ethylhydrocupreinc (optochin), and virtually all pneumococcal colonies are dissolved by bile salts; these reactions are the basis for laboratory identification.

Peptidoglycan and teichoic acid are the principal constituents of the pneumococcal cell wall. The cell wall's integrity depends on the presence of numerous peptide side chains cross-linked by the activity of enzymes such as trans- and carboxypeptidases. β-Lactam antibiotics inactivate these enzymes by covalently binding their active site. Unique to *S. pneumoniae* and present in all strains is C (for "cell-wall") substance, a polysaccharide consisting of teichoic acid with a phosphorylcholine residue. Surface-exposed choline residues serve as a site of attachment for potential virulence factors, such as pneumococcal surface protein A (PspA), which may prevent phagocytosis. Except for strains that cause conjunctivitis, nearly every clinical isolate of *S. pneumoniae* has a polysaccharide capsule.

There are two systems for numbering the 90 known distinct capsules of *S. pneumoniae*. In the American system, serotypes are numbered in the order in which they were identified. The strains that most frequently cause human disease were generally the earliest to be identified and thus tend to have lower numbers. The more widely accepted Danish system places serotypes into groups based on antigenic similarities; for example, Danish group 19 includes types 19F ("first recognized"), 19A, 19B, and 19C, which in the American system would be types 19, 57, 58, and 59, respectively. Serotyping was clinically relevant in the 1930s, when type-specific antisera were administered as therapy, and again in the 1990s, when it was used to track the spread of antibiotic-resistant isolates (although this method has largely been replaced by molecular biologic techniques such as pulsed-field gel electrophoresis and multilocus sequence typing). Capsule switching has been documented and further limits the epidemiologic reliability of serotyping.

EPIDEMIOLOGY   *S. pneumoniae* colonizes the nasopharynx and, on any single occasion, can be isolated from 5 to 10% of healthy adults and from 20 to 40% of healthy children. Once the organisms have colonized an adult, they are likely to persist for 4 to 6 weeks but may persist for as long as 6 months. Pneumococci spread from one individual to another by direct or droplet transmission as a result of close contact; transmission may be enhanced by crowding or poor ventilation. Day-care centers have been a site of spread, especially of penicillin-resistant strains of serotypes 6B, 14, 19F, and 23F. Outbreaks occur among adults in crowded living conditions—e.g., in military barracks, prisons, and shelters for the homeless—as well as among susceptible populations in settings such as nursing homes. The risk of pneumococcal pneumonia is not increased by contact in schools or workplaces (including hospitals).

The incidence of bacteremic pneumococcal infection is relatively high among infants up to 2 years of age and low among teenagers and young adults; rates increase with increasing age beginning at around age 55. A surveillance study in South Carolina showed the incidences of pneumococcal bacteremia among infants, young adults, and persons ≥70 years of age to be 160, 5, and 70 cases per 100,000 population, respectively. (These results antecede implementation of vaccination for infants and young children.) Most cases of pneumococcal bacteremia in adults are due to pneumonia, and there are three to four cases of nonbacteremic pneumonia for every bacteremic case. Thus an estimated 20 cases of pneumococcal pneumonia per 100,000 young adults and 280 cases per 100,000 persons over the age of 70 occur annually. The incidence of pneumococcal bacteremia among adults exhibits a distinct midwinter peak and a striking dip in summer. In children, the incidence of bacteremia is relatively constant throughout the year except for a marked dip in midsummer. For reasons that are unclear but probably are multifactorial, Native Americans, Native Alaskans, and African Americans are unusually susceptible to invasive pneumococcal disease. This enhanced susceptibility is thought to have a genetic basis that thus far remains unelucidated.

PATHOGENETIC MECHANISMS   *S. pneumoniae* attaches to human nasopharyngeal cells through the specific interaction of bacterial surface adhesins, such as pneumococcal surface antigen A or choline-binding proteins (including PspA), with epithelial cell receptors. Epithelial cell glycoconjugates containing the disaccharide GlcNAcβ1-4Gal or asialo-GM1 glycolipid are possible binding sites. Pneumococcal phase variation, in which organisms may form transparent or opaque colonies, may also play a role in adherence. Organisms from opaque colonies have relatively little peptidoglycan and large capsules; those from transparent colonies have much more phosphorylcholine (which contributes to their capacity to adhere to mammalian cells) and less capsular polysaccharide. When pneumococci are inoculated intranasally into an experimental animal, organisms that form transparent colonies persist; in contrast, after intraperitoneal inoculation, organisms that yield transparent colonies are rapidly cleared from the blood, whereas those that make opaque colonies resist clearance.

Once the nasopharynx has been colonized, infection results if the organisms are carried into anatomically contiguous areas such as the eustachian tubes or the nasal sinuses and if their clearance is hindered, for example, by mucosal edema due to allergy or viral infection. Similarly, pneumonia ensues if organisms are inhaled or aspirated into the bronchioles or alveoli and then are not cleared—especially, for example, if viral infection or cigarette smoke or other toxic substances have increased mucus production and/or damaged ciliary action. A mechanism by which pneumococci may bind to pneumocytes after viral infection has been suggested. Pneumocytes activated by cytokines express the receptor for platelet-activating factor, which binds the phosphorylcholine residue of pneumococcal C substance, enhancing the adherence of pneumococci. Pneumococci may invade tissues by penetrating mucosal layers; the clinical significance of this finding remains to be determined.

Once pneumococci reach an area where they do not naturally belong, they activate complement by classic and alternative pathways and stimulate cytokine production, which leads to the attraction of polymorphonuclear leukocytes (PMNs). The polysaccharide capsule, however, renders the organisms resistant to phagocytosis. In the absence of anticapsular antibody, phagocytic cells such as alveolar macrophages have a limited capacity to ingest and kill pneumococci; a large bacterial inoculum and/or a compromise of phagocytic function allows the initiation of lung infection. Infection of the meninges, joints, bones, and peritoneal cavity may result from the spread of pneumococci through the bloodstream, usually but not always from a respiratory tract focus of infection.

The capacity to cause disease reflects the capacities of pneumococci to escape ingestion and killing by host phagocytic cells, on the one hand, and to stimulate an inflammatory response and damage tissues, on the other. Encapsulated pneumococci are poorly ingested and killed in vivo in the immunologically naïve host or in vitro by mammalian phagocytic cells in the absence of anticapsular antibody and complement. Unencapsulated pneumococci virtually never cause invasive disease (although they can cause conjunctivitis), and mutants lacking a capsule are essentially avirulent in mice. Symptoms of disease are largely attributable to the generation of an inflammatory response that may cause pain by increasing pressure (as in sinusitis or otitis media) or may interfere with vital bodily functions by preventing oxygenation of blood (as in pneumonia) or by inhibiting blood flow (as in vasculitis due to meningitis). Cell-wall constituents of *S. pneumoniae*, including teichoic acid, C substance, and (in particular) peptidoglycan, activate complement by the alternative pathway; the reaction between cell-wall structures and antibody that is present in all humans also activates the classic complement pathway. The result is the release of C5a, a potent attractant for PMNs, into the surrounding medium. Peptidoglycan can also directly stimulate the release of proinflammatory cytokines such as interleukin (IL) 1β, tumor necrosis factor (TNF) α, and IL-6 that activate a cascade of inflammation mediators. These cytokines increase expression of selectins on endothelial cells and integrins on leukocytes, thereby enhancing PMN migration. Pneumolysin, a thiol-activated toxin, exerts a variety of effects on ciliary cells and PMNs and also activates the classic complement pathway by direct binding of C1q. Injection of pneumolysin into the lungs of experimental animals produces the histologic features of pneumonia; in mice, immunization with this substance or challenge with genetically engineered mutants that do not produce it is associated with a significant reduction in virulence. Autolysin may contribute to the pathogenesis of pneumococcal disease by lysing bacteria, thereby releasing their constituents and heightening the reaction with human tissues. Inflammation in the central nervous system (CNS) during meningitis is a major contributor to neuronal cell injury. The release of matrix metalloproteinases, reactive oxygen species, and reactive nitrogen intermediates in neuronal tissue also contributes to damage caused by meningitis.

HOST DEFENSE MECHANISMS Mechanisms of host defense may be immunologically nonspecific or specific. Nonspecific mechanisms that protect against pneumonia include laminar airflow across mucous layers that filter inspired air, the glottal reflex, laryngeal closure, the cough reflex, clearance of organisms from the lower airways by ciliated cells, and ingestion by pulmonary macrophages and PMNs of small bacterial inocula that manage to reach alveolar spaces. Respiratory virus infection, chronic pulmonary disease, or heart failure compromises these mechanisms, predisposing to the development of pneumococcal pneumonia.

Anticapsular antibody provides the best specific protection against pneumococcal infection. Most healthy adults lack IgG antibody to the majority of pneumococcal capsular polysaccharides. Antibody appears after colonization, infection, or vaccination. In the first few weeks after colonization, nonspecific mechanisms probably protect the host from infection. Thereafter, newly developed anticapsular antibody provides a high degree of specific protection. Adults who are at risk of aspirating pharyngeal contents and/or who have diminished mechanisms of lower airway clearance are at risk of developing pneumonia before antibody is produced. Similarly, children whose nasal mucosal membranes become acutely congested around the time of colonization are at risk of developing otitis media. Persons with a diminished capacity to form antibody remain susceptible for as long as they are colonized. Antibody to PspA and other pneumococcal constituents, such as pneumolysin, is prevalent in the population and may contribute to immunity that is immunologically specific but not type specific.

The risk of serious pneumococcal infection is greatly increased in persons with conditions that compromise IgG synthesis and/or the phagocytic function of PMNs and macrophages; this risk is also elevated in the presence of conditions associated with debilitation or malnutrition. Nearly all adults who are hospitalized for pneumococcal pneumonia have at least one predisposing condition and/or fall into a group known to be at high risk epidemiologically (Table 119-1). Prior hospitalization either predisposes to or serves as a strong marker for subsequent pneumococcal infection. The susceptibility of elderly individuals to pneumococcal pneumonia is multifactorial, reflecting diminished clearance mechanisms as well as debilitation, malnutrition, and the presence of comorbid diseases. Although IgG responses to

TABLE 119-1 *Conditions That Commonly Predispose to Pneumococcal Infection*

Increased risk of exposure	Defective complement function
Day-care centers	Defective clearance of
Military training camps	pneumococcal bacteremia[a]
Prisons	Congenital asplenia,
Shelters for the homeless	hyposplenia
Respiratory infection,	Splenectomy
inflammation	Sickle cell disease
Influenza, other viral	Multifactorial conditions
respiratory infections	Infancy and aging
Air pollution	Chronic disease, hospitalization
Allergies	Alcoholism
Cigarette smoking	Malnutrition
Chronic obstructive pulmonary	HIV infection
disease	Chronic lung disease
Other causes of chronic	Glucocorticoid treatment
pulmonary inflammation or	Cirrhosis of the liver
obstruction	Renal insufficiency
Anatomical disruption of	Diabetes mellitus
meninges (dural tear)	Anemia
Defective antibody formation	Coronary artery disease
Common variable	Fatigue, stress, and/or exposure
hypogammaglobulinemia	to cold
Selective IgG subclass	
deficiency	
Multiple myeloma	
Chronic lymphocytic leukemia	
Lymphoma	

[a] The absence of a spleen predisposes to more fulminant infection (see text).

some capsular polysaccharides, as measured by enzyme-linked immunosorbent assay (ELISA), are more or less normal in elderly persons, postvaccination levels of antibody to others are reduced, and the functional capacity of the antibody appears to be decreased. A remarkably high incidence of pneumococcal infection—perhaps 100-fold above baseline—among persons with AIDS is largely related to poor formation of antibody to capsular polysaccharides.

Once a pneumococcal infection has been initiated, the absence of a spleen predisposes to fulminant disease. The liver is able to remove opsonized (antibody-coated) pneumococci from the circulation; in the absence of antibody, however, only the slow passage of blood through the splenic sinuses and prolonged contact with reticuloendothelial cells in the cords of Billroth allow time for bacterial clearance. Patients without spleens may die of pneumococcal pneumonia and sepsis at such an early stage of the illness that pulmonary consolidation is not evident on x-ray but rather is found only at autopsy.

SPECIFIC INFECTIONS CAUSED BY S. PNEUMONIAE

S. pneumoniae causes infections of the middle ear, sinuses, trachea, bronchi, and lungs (Table 119-2) by direct spread from the nasopharyngeal site of colonization. Infections of the CNS, heart valves, bones, joints, and peritoneal cavity usually arise by hematogenous spread; peritoneal infection also results from ascent via the fallopian tubes. The CNS may also be infected by contiguous spread of organisms, as in patients who have a tear in the dura. Primary pneumococcal bacteremia—i.e., the presence of pneumococci in the blood with no apparent source—occurs commonly in children <2 years of age and as a small percentage of all pneumococcal bacteremias in adults; if no therapy is given, a source and/or a secondary site of infection may become apparent. Pleural infection results either from direct extension of pneumonia to the visceral pleura or from hematogenous spread of bacteria from a pulmonary or extrapulmonary focus to the pleural space; the route cannot be determined in any individual case. Infections listed after meningitis in Table 119-2 are uncommon or rare.

Otitis Media and Sinusitis   When fluid from the middle ear is cultured during acute otitis media or fluid from a paranasal sinus is cultured during acute sinusitis, S. pneumoniae is the most common isolate or is second only to nontypable Haemophilus influenzae. Whether in adults or in children, pneumococci are identified in ~40 to 50% of cases of otitis in which an etiologic agent is isolated. Prior infection by a respiratory virus or allergy is thought to contribute significantly to these pneumococcal infections by causing congestion of the openings to the eustachian tubes or the paranasal sinuses. Prospective studies of young children have shown that colonization precedes infection in most cases. For reasons that are unclear, serotypes 6B, 14, 19F, and 23F predominate both as colonizing and as infecting organisms of children.

Pneumonia   The distinctive symptoms and signs of pneumonia, whether due to the pneumococcus or to other bacteria, are (1) cough and sputum production, which reflect the proliferation of bacteria and the resulting inflammatory response in the alveoli; (2) fever; and (3) radiographic detection of an infiltrate.

TABLE 119-2 *Most Common Infections Caused by Streptococcus pneumoniae in Adults*

Acute sinusitis	Septic arthritis
Pneumonia	Peritonitis
Acute purulent tracheobronchitis	Endocarditis
Otitis media	Pericarditis
Empyema	Endometritis
Meningitis	Cellulitis
Primary bacteremia	Brain abscess
Osteomyelitis	

Note: The order of the list very roughly approximates the order of frequency among adults, from most to least common.

PREDISPOSING CONDITIONS   Pneumococcal pneumonia is most common at the extremes of age. Despite the undisputed role of S. pneumoniae as a major pathogenic bacterium for humans, the great majority of adults with pneumococcal pneumonia have underlying diseases that predispose them to infection. Otherwise-healthy military recruits involved in outbreaks of infection may be an exception to this rule; however, many of those affected have an exposure to stress and/or an antecedent viral-type illness that may reduce normal host resistance. In addition to prior viral respiratory illness, the most common predisposing conditions are alcoholism, malnutrition, chronic pulmonary disease of any kind, cigarette smoking, infection with HIV, diabetes mellitus, cirrhosis of the liver, anemia, prior hospitalization for any reason, renal insufficiency, and coronary artery disease (with or without recognized congestive heart failure). HIV infection is such an important predisposing factor that some authorities recommend that any young adult with pneumococcal pneumonia be tested for antibody to HIV.

PRESENTING SYMPTOMS   Patients often present with a preexisting respiratory condition that has distinctly deteriorated. If a viral respiratory illness is the predisposing factor, the patient may have felt unwell for several days, with coryza or a nonproductive cough and low-grade fever. At the time of onset of pneumonia, the patient feels distinctly worse. The temperature may rise to 38.9 to 39.4°C (102 to 103°F); however, one series of cases documented temperatures from 33.3 to 40.5°C (92 to 104.9°F), with only one-third of bacteremic patients having a temperature of ≥37.5°C (≥99.5°F) at admission. Sputum production may become prominent; in a patient who has chronic bronchitis, the sputum may increase in volume and may become yellow or green and thicker than usual. In a small proportion of cases, the onset of disease follows a hyperacute pattern in which the patient suddenly has a single episode of shaking chills followed by sustained fever and a cough productive of blood-tinged sputum. This clinical picture is unfortunately called "classic," a vague term that is best avoided because many physicians believe that it means "most common," which is clearly not the case. In elderly subjects, the onset of disease may be especially insidious and may not suggest pneumonia at all. Elderly patients may have minimal cough, no sputum production, and no fever, instead appearing tired or confused. Nausea and vomiting or diarrhea, sometimes quite prominent, occur in up to 20% of cases of pneumococcal pneumonia. Symptoms of myocardial ischemia or an actual infarction may be present in 5% of cases. The most abrupt progression of pneumococcal disease is seen in patients who have undergone splenectomy; given their defective clearance of pneumococci from the bloodstream, these individuals may go from apparent good health to death in as little as 24 h. An inapparent pulmonary focus is often responsible. In pneumonia, pleuritic chest pain may result from extension of the inflammatory process to the visceral pleura; persistence of this pain, especially after the first day or two of treatment, raises concern about empyema (see "Complications," below). Clearly, the range of symptoms is sufficiently broad that no characteristic presentation distinguishes pneumococcal from other types of bacterial pneumonia (or from some types of nonbacterial pneumonia).

PHYSICAL FINDINGS   Patients with pneumococcal pneumonia usually appear ill and have a grayish, anxious appearance that differs from that of persons with viral or mycoplasmal pneumonia. Temperature, pulse, and respiratory rate are typically elevated. Elderly patients may have only a slight temperature elevation or may be afebrile. Hypothermia is associated with increased morbidity and mortality. Herpes labialis appears in a small percentage of cases. Pain may cause diminished respiratory excursion (splinting) on the affected side. Dullness to percussion is noted in about half of cases, and vocal fremitus is increased. Breath sounds may be bronchial or tubular, and crackles are heard in most cases if enough air is being moved to generate them. Flatness to percussion at the lung base, absent fremitus, and lack of the expected degree of diaphragmatic motion suggest the presence of pleural fluid, which raises the possibility that empyema is present. The finding of a heart murmur, certainly if new, raises concern about endocarditis, a rare but serious complication. Hypoxia or the generalized response to pneumonia may cause the patient to be confused, but the appearance of confusion should also raise concern about meningitis. Obtundation or neck stiffness should lead to an immediate consideration of this complication.

RADIOGRAPHIC FINDINGS Pneumococcal pneumonia involves only one lung segment or a portion thereof in one-fourth of cases; it involves more than one segment but only one lobe or a portion thereof in another one-fourth of instances. Thus multilobar disease is seen in half of cases. Air-space consolidation is the predominant finding and is detected in 80% of cases (Fig. 119-1). Air bronchogram (visualization of the air-filled bronchus against a background of consolidation in the alveoli) is evident in fewer than half of cases and is more common in bacteremic than in nonbacteremic disease. In rare instances, pneu-

FIGURE 119-1 A retrocardiac infiltrate in a patient with pneumococcal pneumonia. Consolidation is apparent on posterior-anterior view (left) but is better visualized on lateral view of the chest (right).

mococcal pneumonia leads to a lung abscess; an underlying malignancy may be present, and co-infection with a mixture of anaerobic and microaerophilic organisms may be documented as well. Although some pleural fluid may actually be present in half of cases, no more than 20% of patients have a sufficient volume of fluid to allow aspiration, and in only a minority of these patients is empyema documented.

GENERAL LABORATORY FINDINGS Anemia (a hemoglobin level of <10 g/dL) is present in 25% of cases. The peripheral-blood white blood cell (WBC) count exceeds 12,000/μL in the great majority of patients with pneumococcal pneumonia. However, the count is <6000/μL in 5 to 10% of persons hospitalized for pneumococcal pneumonia. Such a low count is strongly associated with lethal disease and is often but not always associated with bone marrow suppression due to alcohol ingestion. The serum bilirubin level is modestly elevated in one-third of cases; hypoxia, inflammatory changes in the liver, and breakdown of red blood cells in the lung are all thought to contribute to this increase. A serum albumin level of <2.5 g/dL in 30% of cases may indicate predisposing malnutrition or may be secondary to sepsis. About 20% of patients have serum sodium concentrations of ≤130 meq/L, and another 20% have serum creatinine concentrations of ≥2 mg/dL. →*Abnormalities of pleural fluid in empyema are reviewed in Chap. 239.*

DIFFERENTIAL DIAGNOSIS Patients who present with community-acquired pneumonia may actually have infection due to one of many organisms. The extensive list includes the following: *H. influenzae* or *Moraxella catarrhalis* in persons with little to predispose them other than chronic or acute inflammation of the airways; *Staphylococcus aureus* in persons who take glucocorticoids or who have major anatomical disruption of the airways; *Streptococcus pyogenes*; *Neisseria meningitidis*; anaerobic species in persons who have seizures or who may have aspirated oropharyngeal contents for some other reason; *Legionella*; *Pasteurella multocida* in dog or cat owners; gram-negative bacilli, especially in persons with severely damaged lungs who are taking glucocorticoids; viruses, especially influenza virus (in season), adenovirus, or respiratory syncytial virus; *Mycobacterium tuberculosis*; fungi, including *Pneumocystis* (depending on epidemiologic factors and the possible presence of HIV infection); *Mycoplasma*; *Chlamydia pneumoniae*, especially in older adults; and *Chlamydia psittaci* in bird owners. Many older men with lung cancer present with pneumonia, as

do persons who have acute-onset inflammatory pulmonary conditions of uncertain etiology or those with pulmonary embolus and infarction. The breadth of this list vividly illustrates the deficiency of empirical therapy for community-acquired pneumonia (Table 119-3). Many of these diseases require evaluation, and specific therapy is available for an increasing number. Moreover, pneumococci—perhaps the most common cause of community-acquired pneumonia—are increasingly resistant to available antibiotics. Taken together, these factors favor precise determination of the etiology of a pneumonia syndrome whenever possible.

DIAGNOSTIC MICROBIOLOGY An etiologic role for the pneumococcus in pneumonia is strongly suggested by the microscopic demonstration of large numbers of PMNs and slightly elongated gram-positive cocci in pairs and chains in the sputum (Fig. 119-2). Capsules may be seen surrounding the bacterial forms. Examined areas of the slide must be free of buccal epithelial cells, which indicate the admixture of saliva with sputum; saliva may contain viridans streptococci at counts of >10⁷/mL. When characteristic microscopic findings are noted, the identification of *S. pneumoniae* in sputum culture strongly indicates pneumococcal infection of the lower respiratory tract. In the absence of such microscopic findings, the identification of pneumococci by culture may be nonspecific, reflecting colonization of the upper airways. Culture is, however, more sensitive than microscopic exami-

TABLE 119-3 Causes of a Pneumonia Syndrome Leading to Hospitalization of Adults in Houston, Texas[a]

Common	Less Common
Streptococcus pneumoniae	*Moraxella catarrhalis*
Haemophilus influenzae	*Staphylococcus aureus*
Lung cancer	*Legionella* species
Mycobacterium tuberculosis	Pulmonary infarction
Pneumocystis	*Klebsiella pneumoniae*
Influenza (seasonal)	Respiratory syncytial virus
	Microaerophilic and anaerobic mouth flora
	Pseudomonas aeruginosa
	Chlamydia pneumoniae
	Cryptococcus, *Histoplasma*
	Hamman-Rich syndrome, others

[a] Pneumonia was defined as a syndrome consisting of fever, increased cough, sputum production, and an abnormal pulmonary shadow on chest x-ray.

FIGURE 119-2 Gram-stained sputum from a patient with pneumococcal pneumonia shows polymorphonuclear cells with no epithelial cells, indicating the origin of the sample in inflammatory exudate without contamination. Slightly pleomorphic grampositive coccobacilli appear, generally in pairs. Displacement of stained proteinaceous background material outlines a capsule surrounding some of the organisms. When obtained from a patient with pneumonia, a sample like this one is highly specific in identifying the pneumococcus as the etiologic agent.

nation for identifying pneumococci. Since most pneumococci do not produce distinctively mucoid colonies, their identification in the laboratory depends on the ability to select putative pneumococcal colonies for further study from among α-hemolytic streptococci of the mouth. In short, laboratory diagnosis by sputum culture depends on the quality of the specimen provided, the care with which the relevant purulent component is separated for study, and the assiduity with which α-hemolytic colonies are studied. Prior treatment with antibiotics can also rapidly clear pneumococci from sputum. These factors need to be considered when sputum cultures from patients who appear to have pneumococcal pneumonia are said to yield only "normal mouth flora" and when the medical literature describes what appear to be poor results of sputum culture. Because of the central role of microscopic examination in diagnosis, physicians may wish to view the slides with the microbiologist. Blood cultures yield *S. pneumoniae* in ~25% of cases of pneumococcal pneumonia, often within 12 h after the sample is obtained.

COMPLICATIONS Empyema is the most common complication of pneumococcal pneumonia, occurring in ~2% of cases. Some fluid appears in the pleural space in a substantial proportion of cases of pneumococcal pneumonia, but this parapneumonic effusion usually reflects an inflammatory response to infection that has been contained within the lung, and its presence is self-limited. When bacteria reach the pleural space—either hematogenously or as a result of contiguous spread, possibly across lymphatics of the visceral pleura—empyema results. The finding of frank pus, a positive result on Gram's staining, or the presence of fluid with a pH of ≤7.1 indicates the need for aggressive and complete drainage, preferably by prompt insertion of a chest tube, with verification by computed tomography (CT) that fluid has been removed. Failure to drain most or all of the fluid usually indicates the need for thoracotomy. Persistence of fever (even if low-grade) and leukocytosis after 4 or 5 days of appropriate antibiotic treatment for pneumococcal pneumonia suggests empyema. In this setting, the diagnosis is exceedingly likely if the x-ray shows pleural fluid; at this stage, thoracotomy is often needed for cure. Aggressive drainage is likely to reduce morbidity and mortality from empyema (Chap. 245).

Meningitis Except during outbreaks of meningococcal infection, *S. pneumoniae* is the most common cause of bacterial meningitis in adults. Because of the remarkable success of *H. influenzae* type b vac-

cine, *S. pneumoniae* now predominates among cases in infants and toddlers as well (but not among those in newborns). Meningitis develops either by the direct extension of infection from the sinuses or the middle ear or as a result of seeding of meningeal endothelial cells or the choroid plexus during bacteremia. Favoring the former pathogenesis are the association between acute otitis media or sinusitis and meningitis and the role of *S. pneumoniae* as the most common cause of recurrent meningitis associated with head trauma, cerebrospinal fluid (CSF) leak, and/or dural tear. Favoring the latter are the association between pneumococcal bacteremia from any source and meningitis as well as an autopsy study of temporal bone from children who died of bacterial meningitis, which yielded no evidence of extension from the middle ear. In adults, meningitis is usually a complication of bacteremia, which in turn is attributable, in the great majority of cases, to pneumonia.

In the meninges and subarachnoid space, pneumococcal peptidoglycan stimulates an intense inflammatory response mediated by the release of proinflammatory cytokines such as IL-8 and macrophage inflammatory protein (MIP)-1, which are detectable in the CSF of patients with meningitis. The ensuing inflammatory response results in raised intracranial pressure, brain edema, and decreased blood flow leading to meningismus, drowsiness, or coma. Activated leukocytes migrate across the blood-brain barrier and release matrix metalloproteases and reactive oxygen and nitrogen species that damage neurons. Focal neurologic signs may result from vasculitis with venous or arterial thrombosis, cranial neuropathy due to entrapment or infarction, local cerebritis, subdural effusion, or brain herniation (Chap. 360).

No distinctive clinical or laboratory feature differentiates meningitis due to *S. pneumoniae* from that due to other bacteria. Patients note the sudden onset of fever, headache, and stiffness or pain in the neck. Without treatment, there is a progression over 24 to 48 h to confusion and then obtundation. On physical examination, the patient looks acutely ill and has a rigid neck. In such cases lumbar puncture should not be delayed for CT of the head unless papilledema or focal neurologic signs are evident. Typical CSF findings consist of pleocytosis (500 to 10,000 cells/μL) with ≥85% PMNs, an elevated protein level (100 to 500 mg/dL), and a decrease in glucose content (<30 mg/dL). If antibiotics have not been given, large numbers of pneumococci can be seen in a Gram-stained specimen of CSF in all cases, and specific therapy can be administered, although, because of its similar appearance, *Listeria* may be misidentified as the pneumococcus. If an effective antibiotic has already been given, the number of bacteria may be greatly decreased and microscopic examination of a Gram-stained specimen may yield negative results. In this situation, immunologic methods for the detection of pneumococcal capsule in the CSF may be positive in up to two-thirds of cases, although these methods have fallen out of favor.

OTHER SYNDROMES The appearance of pneumococcal infection at other, ordinarily sterile body sites indicates hematogenous spread, usually during frank pneumonia or, in a small proportion of cases, from an inapparent focus of infection. A case of pneumococcal endocarditis is seen every few years at large tertiary-care hospitals. Purulent pericarditis, occurring as a separate entity or together with endocarditis, is even rarer. Septic arthritis can arise spontaneously in a natural or prosthetic joint or as a complication of rheumatoid arthritis. Osteomyelitis in adults tends to involve vertebral bones. Pneumococcal peritonitis occurs by one of three pathogenetic pathways: (1) hematogenous spread when ascites or other preexisting peritoneal disease is present; (2) local spread from a perforated viscus (usually appendicitis or perforated ulcer); or (3) transit via the fallopian tubes. Salpingitis may be recognized with or without accompanying peritonitis. Epidural and brain abscesses arise as a complication of sinusitis or mastoiditis. Cellulitis develops most often in persons who have connective tissue diseases or HIV infection. The appearance of any of these unusual pneumococcal infections may suggest that tests for HIV infection should be undertaken. Finally, for reasons that are unclear, unencapsulated (but not encapsulated) pneumococci cause sporadic or epidemic conjunctivitis.

Antibiotic Susceptibility β-Lactam antibiotics, the cornerstone of therapy for serious pneumococcal infection, bind covalently to the active site and thereby block the action of enzymes (endo-, trans-, and carboxypeptidases) needed for cell-wall synthesis. Because these enzymes were identified by their reaction with radiolabeled penicillin, they are called *penicillin-binding proteins*. In the 1960s, virtually all clinical isolates of *S. pneumoniae* were susceptible to penicillin (i.e., were inhibited in vitro by concentrations of <0.06 μg/mL). During the past two decades, an increasing number of isolates have shown some degree of resistance to penicillin. Resistance results when spontaneous mutation or acquisition of new genetic material alters penicillin-binding proteins in a manner that reduces their affinity for penicillin, thereby necessitating a higher concentration of penicillin for their saturation. The genetic information that renders pneumococci resistant to penicillin is generally acquired from oral streptococci and conveys resistance to other antibiotics as well. Selection of antibiotic-resistant strains in the United States— especially in areas of high antibiotic use, such as day-care centers—and importation of strains from other countries where antibiotics are available without prescription have contributed to the prevalence of multidrug resistance.

At present, ~20% of pneumococcal isolates in the United States are intermediately susceptible to penicillin [minimal inhibitory concentration (MIC) 0.1 to 1.0 μg/mL], and 15% are resistant (MIC ≥2.0 μg/mL; Fig. 119-3). These definitions were based on drug levels achievable in CSF during treatment of meningitis, whereas levels reached in the bloodstream, lungs, and sinuses are actually much higher. Thus the MIC needs to be interpreted in light of the infection being treated. Pneumonia caused by a penicillin-resistant strain is likely to respond to 24 million units of penicillin daily, whereas meningitis will not. The recently revised definition of amoxicillin resistance (susceptible, MIC ≤2 μg/mL; intermediately resistant, MIC = 4 μg/mL; resistant, MIC ≥8 μg/mL) is based on serum levels, assuming that no physician would knowingly treat meningitis with this oral medication. Pneumonia due to an intermediately amoxicillin-resistant strain may not respond to treatment with this drug, and that due to a resistant strain is likely not to respond. On the assumption that antibiotic concentrations in middle-ear fluid or sinus cavities approach those in serum, similar inferences can be made about the treatment of otitis or sinusitis.

Penicillin-susceptible pneumococci are susceptible to all commonly used cephalosporins. Penicillin-intermediate strains tend to be resistant to all first- and many second-generation cephalosporins (of which cefuroxime retains the best efficacy), but most are susceptible to certain third-generation cephalosporins, including cefotaxime, ceftriaxone, cefepime, and cefpodoxime. One-half of highly penicillin-resistant pneumococci are also resistant to cefotaxime, ceftriaxone, and cefepime, and nearly all are resistant to cefpodoxime. Just as in the case of penicillin, susceptibility to cefotaxime and ceftriaxone is defined on the basis of achievable CSF levels. Thus pneumonia caused by intermediately resistant strains (MIC = 2 μg/mL) will respond well to usual doses of these drugs, and pneumonia due to a resistant organism (MIC ≥ 4 μg/mL) is likely to respond. Meningitis due to inter-

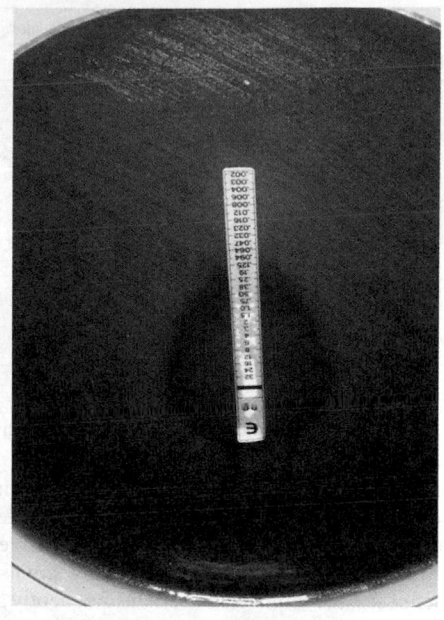

FIGURE 119-3 The e-strip method currently used by most laboratories to determine the susceptibility of *S. pneumoniae* to antibiotics. After the plate is streaked with a suspension of pneumococci, a strip that has been impregnated with graded concentrations of the antibiotic under study (penicillin in the example shown) is placed on the surface, and the plate is incubated overnight at 37°C. The organism on the left is inhibited by a penicillin concentration of 0.016 μg/mL and is fully susceptible to this drug. The organism on the right is inhibited only by a penicillin concentration of 0.25 μg/mL and is intermediately resistant to this agent.

mediately resistant strains may not respond, and meningitis due to a resistant strain is likely not to respond to treatment with cefotaxime or ceftriaxone.

About one-quarter of all pneumococcal isolates in the United States are resistant to erythromycin and the newer macrolides, including azithromycin and clarithromycin, with much higher rates of resistance in penicillin-resistant strains. This resistance will certainly affect empirical therapy for bronchitis, sinusitis, and pneumonia. In the United States, the majority of macrolide-resistant pneumococci bear the so-called M phenotype (erythromycin MIC = 1 to 8 μg/mL) and are susceptible to clindamycin. In this case, resistance is mediated by an efflux pump mechanism; to some extent, M-type resistance can be overcome by clinically achievable levels of macrolides. In Europe, most macrolide resistance is due to a mutation in *ermB*, which confers high-level resistance not only to macrolides but also to clindamycin; more than 90% of pneumococcal isolates in the United States are susceptible to clindamycin. Rates of doxycycline resistance among pneumococci of varying susceptibility to penicillin are similar to those observed for macrolides. One-third of pneumococcal isolates exhibit reduced susceptibility to trimethoprim-sulfamethoxazole. The newer fluoroquinolones remain highly effective against pneumococci, with equal efficacy against penicillin-susceptible and -resistant strains; the rate of resistance is generally <1% but approaches 2 to 3% in areas where quinolones are widely used and is increasing. Ketolides appear to be uniformly effective against pneumococci, as does vancomycin, although it is feared that the acquisition of vancomycin resistance by enterococci and other gram-positive bacteria may eventually lead to pneumococcal transformation to resistance. Oxazolidinones and glycopeptides also appear to be effective in vitro, with MICs no higher for drug-resistant *S. pneumoniae* strains than for penicillin-susceptible strains. Resistance to streptogramins parallels that to macrolides, limiting the usefulness of these drugs for the treatment of pneumonia.

Pneumococcal susceptibility patterns vary greatly between and even within individual communities, and the data are in a state of flux. It does appear, however, that the constant trend is toward more widespread antibiotic resistance.

Otitis Media and Acute Sinusitis (Table 119-4) Current treatment recommendations for otitis media and acute sinusitis—conditions whose pathogenesis and microbial etiology are similar—are based on the

TABLE 119-4 Regimens for the Treatment of Pneumococcal Otitis Media or Sinusitis in Adults[a]

Regimen	Drug, Dose	Duration	Comments
First-line	Amoxicillin, 1 g q8h	Otitis: 3–5 days after clinical response, not to exceed 7 days total; sinusitis: 7–10 days after clinical response, not to exceed 2 weeks total	If this regimen fails, try second-line regimen.
Second-line	Amoxicillin, 1 g q8h, plus clavulanic acid[b]	Same as above	If this regimen fails, try third-line regimen.
Third-line	Ceftriaxone, 1 g qd	3–5 days for otitis; longer for sinusitis	If this regimen fails, consider complications; consult otolaryngologist and/or infectious disease specialist.

[a] Treatment for otitis media or sinusitis is empirical, since aspiration of the involved area to establish an etiologic diagnosis is rarely undertaken, except under the conditions of a research protocol.
[b] Give half as amoxicillin alone and half as amoxicillin with clavulanic acid.

following points: (1) Acute otitis media is the most common infection for which antibiotics are prescribed in the United States. (2) As noted above, *S. pneumoniae* is the most likely treatable cause; taken together, *H. influenzae* and *M. catarrhalis*, many strains of which produce β-lactamases, are implicated nearly as frequently as pneumococci. (3) In the absence of diagnostic tympanocentesis, the etiologic diagnosis is nearly always presumptive. (4) Because penetration into a closed space is required, high serum levels of an effective antibiotic are required to treat otitis caused by intermediately or fully resistant pneumococci. (5) *S. pneumoniae* is more likely than *Haemophilus* to cause progression to serious complications without specific therapy. (6) Antibiotics that are effective against pneumococci and yet resist β-lactamases tend to be very expensive compared with amoxicillin.

As a result of these considerations, the Otitis Media Working Group of the Centers for Disease Control and Prevention (CDC) recommended that initial therapy be amoxicillin in a high dosage—e.g., 80 to 90 mg/kg per day in two or three divided doses for infants and toddlers or 1 g three times daily for adults. If this regimen fails, highly penicillin-resistant pneumococci or β-lactamase-producing bacteria may be responsible, and amoxicillin may be given at the same total dosage but with one-half of the dose in the form of amoxicillin/clavulanic acid. If this regimen fails, three doses of ceftriaxone at daily intervals are likely to be curative. A quinolone or ketolide may also be tried in adults. Patients must be monitored closely for a response. Despite the detection (by molecular analysis) of pneumococcal DNA in middle-ear fluid, chronic serous otitis ("glue ear") is probably not due to active infection and does not require antibiotic therapy. Treatment for otitis is recommended for a total of 5 to 7 days; treatment for acute sinusitis is given for 10 to 14 days.

Pneumonia (Table 119-5) This section will deal primarily with the treatment of pneumonia that is known to be due to *S. pneumoniae*. The broader issue of empirical therapy for community-acquired pneumonia is covered in detail elsewhere (Chap. 239). However, a few general comments on empirical therapy apply. Without a good sputum sample that can be Gram-stained and examined microscopically, the etiologic agent is not known at the time when treatment needs to be initiated and is not likely to become known later. Empirical therapy in such cases must be effective against *S. pneumoniae*, which remains the most likely causative agent of community-acquired pneumonia, unless epidemiologic, clinical, and radiologic findings strongly favor another etiologic entity. In the past, when pneumococci were uniformly susceptible to nearly all antibiotics, it did not matter which drug was selected. Now that pneumococci are resistant, it clearly makes a difference. If a good sputum sample reveals only organisms consistent with *S. pneumoniae*, therapy can be focused on this organism, although additional treatment may be added for organisms that are not visualized microscopically—e.g., influenza virus in a patient hospitalized during an influenza outbreak. Even if the pneumococcus is suspected, a certain degree of empiricism is required, because the antibiotic susceptibility of the strain involved will not be known for 1 or 2 days.

There has been increased emphasis on outpatient therapy in patients who are at low risk (as determined by PORT score according to criteria described by the Pneumonia Outcomes Research Team; Chap. 239). This approach appears to be safe. However, if the physician is in doubt about the severity of illness, the social circumstances, or the likelihood of compliance with the prescribed antibiotic regimen, it may be best to hospitalize the patient, at least briefly. Predictions based on PORT score have been validated for pneumococcal pneumonia.

OUTPATIENT THERAPY Amoxicillin (1 g three times daily) effectively treats all cases of pneumococcal pneumonia except those caused by the most highly penicillin-resistant isolates. Neither cefuroxime nor cefpodoxime offers any advantages over amoxicillin since these drugs are less likely, even at high dosages, to be active against highly resistant pneumococcal strains. One of the newer fluoroquinolones or a ketolide in an accepted dosage for pneumonia is highly likely to be effective. Clindamycin will be effective in 90% and doxycycline, azithromycin, or clarithromycin in 75% of cases—levels of resistance that make their use questionable unless the organism is known to be susceptible. Because one-third of all isolates are now resistant to trimethoprim-sulfamethoxazole, this agent can no longer be recommended. Since none of these therapies ensures the kind of antibiotic coverage that it would have in the past, patients should be instructed to remain in close contact with the prescribing physician, especially if there is any deterioration in their condition.

INPATIENT THERAPY Pneumonia caused by penicillin-susceptible or intermediately penicillin-resistant pneumococcal isolates is readily treatable with β-lactam antibiotics. The dosages that follow are acceptable against intermediately resistant strains and against many or most fully resistant isolates, although they are excessive for use against susceptible isolates. Lower doses, however, cannot be recommended initially because susceptibility is usually not known until 48 to 72 h after treatment is begun. Patients who are sick enough to be hospitalized should

TABLE 119-5 Regimens for the Treatment of Pneumococcal Pneumonia in Adults[a]

Route, Drug	Dose, Schedule[b]
ORAL THERAPY	
Amoxicillin	1 g q8h
Quinolone, e.g., gatifloxacin	400 mg q24h
PARENTERAL THERAPY	
Penicillin[c]	3–4 mU q4h
Ampicillin[d]	1–2 g q6h
Ceftriaxone	1 g q12–24h
Cefotaxime	1–2 g q6–8h
Quinolone, e.g., gatifloxacin	400 mg q24h
Imipenem	500 mg q6h
Vancomycin[e]	500 mg q6h

[a] These regimens are recommended for treatment after a presumptive diagnosis is made on the basis of examination of a Gram-stained sputum sample or as a replacement for more broad-spectrum empirical therapy after a diagnosis of pneumococcal pneumonia is proven by culture. When a valid sputum specimen cannot be obtained, concern for other likely pathogens should prompt the selection of more all-inclusive therapeutic regimens.
[b] Therapy should continue for 5 days after defervescence, not to exceed 7–10 days total. A switch from parenteral to oral drug administration may be made as soon as the patient can tolerate oral medications.
[c] This regimen is listed more for historic than for practical reasons. The spectrum is overly narrow, although perfectly acceptable if a Gram-stained sputum specimen shows only pneumococci. However, the need for frequent administration, mandated by the short half-life of penicillin, renders this regimen impractical.
[d] Usually given in the form of ampicillin/sulbactam.
[e] Not proven to be effective by the extensive clinical experience that applies to the other regimens.

be treated promptly. Most physicians favor parenteral antibiotics, although oral administration of well-absorbed drugs may be acceptable if the patient is not vomiting or hypotensive. Recommended regimens include ceftriaxone (1 g every 12 to 24 h) or cefotaxime (1 to 2 g every 6 to 8 h); the lower doses should suffice except against highly resistant strains. Ampicillin (1 to 2 g every 6 h) is also widely used, usually in the form of ampicillin/sulbactam. Quinolones are effective against all but a small percentage of pneumococcal strains and can be given parenterally or orally. Clindamycin is effective against ~90% of isolates. On the basis of in vitro considerations, vancomycin (500 mg every 6 h) is likely to be uniformly effective against pneumococci, and this drug or a quinolone should be used together with a third-generation cephalosporin for initial therapy in a patient who is likely to be infected with a highly antibiotic-resistant strain or in one who has had a severe allergic reaction to penicillins and cephalosporins. As noted above, there have always been treatment failures unrelated to the antimicrobial susceptibility of the organism; nevertheless, the failure of a patient to respond promptly should raise the question of resistance, and another drug should be given until the susceptibility of the infecting strain has been documented. Of course, evidence for loculated infections (such as empyema) and/or other causes of fever should be sought and addressed appropriately.

DURATION OF THERAPY The optimal duration of treatment for pneumococcal pneumonia is uncertain. Penicillin-susceptible strains begin to disappear from the sputum within several hours of the first dose of penicillin, and a single dose of procaine penicillin, which results in the maintenance of an effective antimicrobial level for 24 h, was said to cure pneumococcal pneumonia in otherwise-healthy young adults at the time when all isolates were susceptible. Most older physicians treated pneumococcal pneumonia for 5 to 7 days. In the absence of reports of therapy failure, younger physicians have tended to treat the infection for 10 to 14 days. Prolongation of therapy is a two-edged sword, especially in debilitated patients, because the risk of complications increases with each day of antibiotic treatment, particularly in the hospital setting. A few days of close observation and parenteral therapy followed by an oral antibiotic—with the entire course of treatment continuing for no more than 5 days after the patient becomes afebrile—may be the best approach.

Meningitis (Table 119-6) Pneumococcal meningitis should be treated initially with ceftriaxone (1 to 2 g every 12 h) plus vancomycin (500 mg every 6 h or 1 g every 12 h). At this time, studies in experimental animals suggest benefits of the addition of rifampin, but in vitro studies indicate antagonism between this drug and ceftriaxone or vancomycin. This author does not recommend that rifampin be added. Two drugs are given initially because the cephalosporin is likely to be effective against most isolates and readily penetrates the blood-brain barrier, whereas, although all isolates are susceptible to vancomycin, this drug has a somewhat unpredictable capacity to cross the blood-brain barrier. If the isolate is shown to be susceptible or intermediately resistant, treatment can be continued with ceftriaxone, and vancomycin may be discontinued. If the organism is resistant, continued treatment with two drugs is indicated. Cefotaxime (2 g every 6 h) may be used instead of ceftriaxone. Imipenem (500 mg every 6 h) may be used in patients who have had life-threatening reactions to β-lactam antibiotics. As noted above, the author of this chapter does not recommend the addition of rifampin. The total duration of therapy for pneumococcal meningitis is 10 days. Consistent with the central pathogenic role of inflammation in meningitis, a recent study demonstrates clear benefit from the addition of glucocorticoids; heretofore, relevant data were conflicting (Chap. 360). Meningitis should be treated in an intensive care unit and with the participation of appropriate consultants, generally including a neurologist and a specialist in infectious diseases.

Endocarditis Pneumococcal endocarditis is associated with rapid destruction of heart valves. Pending results of susceptibility studies, treatment should be initiated with ceftriaxone or cefotaxime; as the prevalence of highly resistant strains increases, it might be prudent to add vancomycin until results of susceptibility studies are available.

TABLE 119-6 *Treatment of Pneumococcal Meningitis*

Circumstance	Appropriate Course[a]
Diagnosis of pneumococcal meningitis; antibiotic susceptibility unknown	Treat with ceftriaxone, 1–2 g q12h, plus vancomycin, 500 mg q6h, until antibiotic susceptibility of organism is known.
Susceptibility results available	Continue treatment with ceftriaxone alone if organism is susceptible or intermediate; continue both ceftriaxone and vancomycin if organism is resistant.
Life-threatening penicillin allergy	Treat with imipenem, 500 mg q6h, rather than a β-lactam antibiotic.

[a] Treatment should be administered for 5–7 days after defervescence or for a total of 10 days.

There is no clear evidence that adding another antibiotic to the regimen is beneficial; aminoglycosides are somewhat synergistic and rifampin or quinolones are antagonistic with β-lactams. Patients with endocarditis should probably be treated in an intensive care unit in collaboration with an infectious disease consultant, a cardiologist, and a cardiovascular surgeon.

Other Therapeutic Modalities A variety of agents that block the action of TNF α, IL-1, or platelet-activating factor have conferred no benefit and may even have had a detrimental effect on pneumococcal sepsis. Similar results have been obtained with glucocorticoids except in cases of meningitis.

PREVENTION Pneumococcal polysaccharide vaccine contains 25 μg of capsular polysaccharide from the 23 most prevalent serotypes of *S. pneumoniae*; vaccination stimulates antibody to most serotypes in most recipients. In adults <55 years old, protection rates are at least 85% even 5 years or longer after vaccination (Table 119-7). The level and duration of protection decrease with advancing age, perhaps because of a diminished avidity of the antibody for the capsular polysaccharide. As a result, 50% of persons in their eighties are protected for up to 3 years, with very little or no protection thereafter. In subgroups of the population at high risk (e.g., debilitated elderly persons and individuals with severe chronic lung disease), vaccine has not been shown conclusively to be effective. Persons who most need the vaccine because of poor IgG responses are not likely to respond to immunization with significant increases in antibody level. Nevertheless, in light of the safety and low cost of the vaccine, some experts believe that the poor average rate of response should not deter physicians from administering vaccine to individual patients who are at increased risk of pneumococcal infection.

The CDC's Immunization Practices Advisory Committee has broadened its recommendations for pneumococcal vaccination to include all persons over the age of 2 years who are at substantially increased risk of developing pneumococcal infection and/or of having

TABLE 119-7 *Protective Efficacy of Polyvalent Pneumococcal Polysaccharide Vaccine[a]*

Age, Years	No. of Subject Pairs	Years since Last Vaccination		
		<3	3–5	>5
<55	125	93	89	85
55–64	149	88	82	75
65–74	213	80	71	58
75–84	188	67	53	32
≥85	133	46	22	−13

[a] Results of a case-control study involving all cases of invasive pneumococcal disease in Connecticut during 7 years (1984–1990). Vaccinated subjects were matched with controls, and the rate of invasive pneumococcal disease was related to age and time since vaccination. The data, showing protective efficacy, suggest that, within 5 years of vaccination, protection rates decline with age—i.e., from ~90% in persons <65 years of age to <50% in persons ≥85 years old. Protection also declines with increasing time from vaccination to infection, and this decline is more prominent in older patients.

Source: *Data adapted Ed Shapiro et al: N Engl J Med 325:1453, 1991; with permission.*

a serious complication of such an infection. Perhaps most important are those with anatomical or functional asplenia who are at risk for overwhelming, life-threatening infections. Others who might fall within these recommendations are persons (1) over the age of 65; (2) with CSF leak, diabetes mellitus, alcoholism, cirrhosis, chronic renal insufficiency, chronic pulmonary disease, or advanced cardiovascular disease; (3) who have an immunocompromising condition associated with increased risk of pneumococcal disease, such as multiple myeloma, lymphoma, Hodgkin's disease, HIV infection, organ transplantation, or chronic use of glucocorticoids; (4) who are genetically at increased risk, such as Native Americans and Alaskans; or (5) who live in environments where outbreaks are particularly likely to occur, such as nursing homes.

Recommendations regarding revaccination seem to be somewhat inconsistent. A single revaccination is advocated for persons over the age of 65 if more than 5 years have transpired since the first vaccination. Since antibody levels decline and there is no anamnestic response, it seems more reasonable simply to recommend revaccination at 5-year intervals, especially in persons over the age of 65, who tend to have almost no adverse reaction to vaccination, and in splenectomized patients, who are most in need.

Pneumococcal polysaccharide vaccine is not useful in children <2 years of age, whose immune system does not respond well to polysaccharide antigens. Conjugating the polysaccharide to a protein alters the form in which the antigen is presented to immune-processing cells, yielding an effective immunogen. A heptavalent protein-conjugate pneumococcal polysaccharide vaccine, approved for use in 2000, protects infants and young children against pneumococcal otitis media, pneumonia, bacteremia, and meningitis; efficacy for serotypes contained in the vaccine, which are responsible for about two-thirds of all cases of pneumococcal disease in young children, is 67% for otitis and 97% for bacteremia and meningitis. The rate of nasopharyngeal carriage of vaccine serotypes is also reduced. By its "herd effect" (i.e., the effect on nonvaccinated members of the population), widespread use of this vaccine appears to have decreased the overall incidence of invasive pneumococcal disease in the population. Protein conjugate vaccines that contain antigen from the 11 most common infecting serotypes are being studied. The usefulness of these products may ultimately be limited because they may lead to replacement of serotypes contained in the vaccine with nonvaccine serotypes. Vaccines that contain surface-expressed proteins present in all pneumococci, such as pneumococcal surface protein A (PspA) and surface adhesin A (PsaA), are in the early phases of investigation. Conjugate vaccines do not appear to offer any advantage over polysaccharide vaccine in healthy or diseased adults, although a subpopulation of persons who, on a genetic basis, fail to respond to pneumococcal polysaccharide vaccine may respond to a conjugate vaccine.

FURTHER READING

BARTLETT JG et al: Practice guidelines for the management of community-acquired pneumonia in adults. Clin Infect Dis 31:347, 2000

FEDSON DS, MUSHER DM: Pneumococcal vaccine, in *Vaccines,* 4th ed, SA Plotkin, EA Mortimer Jr (eds). Philadelphia, Saunders, 2003

HAUSDORFF WP et al: The contribution of specific pneumococcal serogroups to different disease manifestations: Implications for conjugate vaccine formulation and use, part II. Clin Infect Dis 30:122, 2000

MUSHER DM et al: A fresh look at the definition of susceptibility of *Streptococcus pneumoniae* to beta-lactam antibiotics. Arch Intern Med 161:2538, 2001

——— et al: Bacteremic and nonbacteremic pneumococcal pneumonia: A prospective study. Medicine 79:210, 2000

———: *Streptococcus pneumoniae,* in *Principles and Practice of Infectious Diseases,* 6th ed, GL Mandell et al (eds). New York, Churchill Livingstone, 2004 (in press)

THORNSBERRY C et al: Regional trends in antimicrobial resistance among clinical isolates of *Streptococcus pneumoniae, Haemophilus influenzae,* and *Moraxella catarrhalis* in the United States: Results from the TRUST Surveillance Program, 1999–2000. Clin Infect Dis 34(Suppl 1):S4, 2002

TUOMANEN EI et al: Pathogenesis of pneumococcal infection. N Engl J Med 332:1280, 1995

WATANAKUNAKORN C et al: Adult bacteremic pneumococcal pneumonia in a community teaching hospital, 1992–1996. A detailed analysis of 108 cases. Arch Intern Med 157:1965, 1997

120 | STAPHYLOCOCCAL INFECTIONS
Franklin D. Lowy

Staphylococcus aureus, the most virulent of the many staphylococcal species, has demonstrated its versatility by remaining a major cause of morbidity and mortality despite the availability of numerous effective antistaphylococcal antibiotics. *S. aureus* is a pluripotent pathogen, causing disease through both toxin-mediated and non-toxin-mediated mechanisms. This organism is responsible for both nosocomial and community-based infections that range from relatively minor skin and soft tissue infections to life-threatening systemic infections.

The "other" staphylococci, collectively designated *coagulase-negative staphylococci* (CoNS), are considerably less virulent than *S. aureus* but remain important pathogens in selected clinical settings. These include but are not limited to infections associated with prosthetic devices.

MICROBIOLOGY AND TAXONOMY

The 33 staphylococcal species (with additional staphylococcal species under review) are pathogenic members of the family Micrococcaceae. A simple strategy for identification of the more clinically important species is outlined in Fig. 120-1. Automated diagnostic systems as well as kits are available for biochemical characterization of all the staphylococcal species. 16S ribosomal RNA analysis has proved a reliable method for distinguishing among species. With few exceptions, *S. aureus* is distinguished from other staphylococcal species by its production of coagulase, a surface enzyme that converts fibrinogen to fibrin. Most other clinically relevant staphylococci are coagulase-negative. *S. aureus* also ferments mannitol, is positive for protein A, and produces DNase. On blood agar plates, *S. aureus* tends to form golden β-hemolytic colonies; in contrast, CoNS produce white nonhemolytic colonies.

Staphylococci are gram-positive cocci that form grapelike clusters on Gram's stain (Fig. 120-2). They are catalase-positive (unlike streptococcal species), nonmotile, aerobic, and facultatively anaerobic. These hardy organisms are capable of prolonged survival on environmental surfaces in varying conditions.

Determining whether multiple isolates (especially of CoNS) from a particular patient are the same or different is often an important factor in distinguishing contaminants from genuine pathogens. Determining whether multiple isolates from different patients are the same or different is relevant when there is concern that a nosocomial outbreak may have been due to a common point source (e.g., a contaminated medical instrument). Biochemical tests, often performed in conjunction with antimicrobial susceptibility testing, have been used as a relatively simple means of distinguishing among staphylococcal species or strains. More discriminating molecular typing techniques, such as pulsed-field gel electrophoresis, have also been used for this purpose.

S. AUREUS INFECTIONS

EPIDEMIOLOGY *S. aureus* is a part of the normal human flora. The anterior nares is the most frequent site of human colonization, although the skin (especially when damaged), vagina, axilla, perineum, and oropharynx may also be colonized. Approximately 25 to 50% of healthy persons may be persistently or transiently colonized with *S. aureus.* The rate of colonization is higher among insulin-dependent diabetics, HIV-infected patients, injection drug users, patients under-

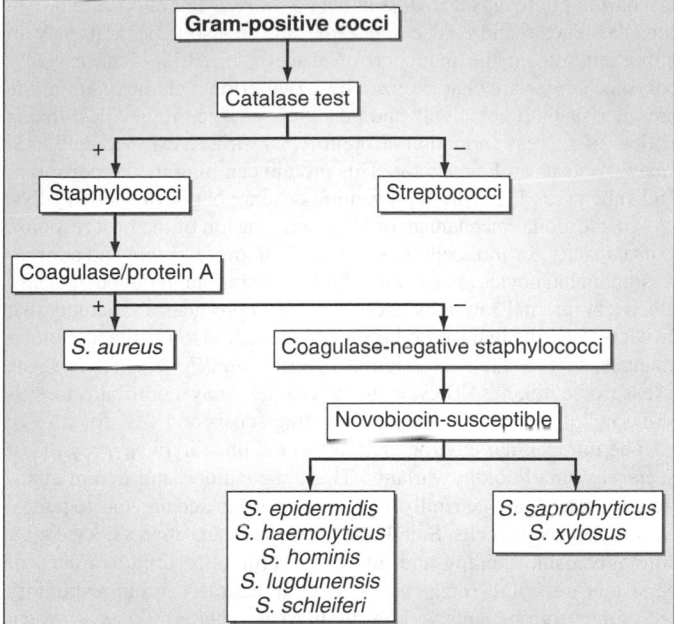

FIGURE 120-1 Biochemical characterization of staphylococci: algorithm of biochemical tests used to discriminate among the clinically important staphylococci. Additional tests are necessary to identify all of the different species.

going hemodialysis, and individuals with skin damage. Sites of colonization serve as a reservoir of strains for future *S. aureus* infections, and persons colonized with *S. aureus* are at greater risk of subsequent infection (with their colonizing strain) than are uncolonized individuals.

Overall, *S. aureus* is a leading cause of nosocomial infections. It is the most common cause of surgical wound infections and is second only to CoNS as a cause of primary bacteremia. Increasingly, nosocomial isolates are resistant to multiple drugs. In the community, *S. aureus* remains an important cause of skin and soft tissue infections, respiratory infections, and (among injection drug users) infective endocarditis. As the number of patients receiving home infusion therapy increases, so does the number of community-acquired staphylococcal infections.

Several reports have described community-acquired infections (in

FIGURE 120-2 Gram's stain of *S. aureus* in a sputum sample with polymorphonuclear leukocytes. (*From Lowy, 1998; with permission of the New England Journal of Medicine. Copyright 1998 Massachusetts Medical Society. All rights reserved.*)

both rural and urban settings) caused by methicillin-resistant *S. aureus* (MRSA) in individuals with no prior medical exposure. In contrast to hospital-acquired MRSA strains, these community isolates have remained susceptible to many non-β-lactam antibiotics. Of concern has been the apparent capacity of community-acquired MRSA strains to cause serious disease in immunocompetent individuals. This ability may be due to the presence of different toxin-producing genes in these strains as well as the use of β-lactam agents for empirical treatment of patients infected with these strains.

Most individuals who develop *S. aureus* infections do so with their own colonizing strains. However, *S. aureus* may also be acquired from other people or from environmental exposures. Transmission most frequently results from transient colonization of the hands of hospital personnel, who then transfer strains from one patient to another. Spread of staphylococci in aerosols of respiratory or nasal secretions from heavily colonized individuals has also been reported.

PATHOGENESIS ■ General Concepts *S. aureus* is a pyogenic pathogen known for its capacity to induce abscess formation at sites of both local and metastatic infections. This classic pathologic response to *S. aureus* defines the framework within which the infection will progress. The bacteria elicit an inflammatory response characterized by an initial intense polymorphonuclear leukocyte (PMN) response and the subsequent infiltration of macrophages and fibroblasts. Either the host cellular response (including the deposition of fibrin and collagen) contains the infection, or infection spreads to the adjoining tissue or the bloodstream.

In toxin-mediated staphylococcal disease, the clinical infection is not invariably present. For example, once toxin has been elaborated into food, staphylococcal food poisoning can develop in the absence of viable bacteria. In the staphylococcal toxic shock syndrome (TSS), conditions that allow elaboration of toxin at sites of colonization (e.g., the presence of a superabsorbent tampon) are sufficient for initiation of clinical illness.

The *S. aureus* Genome The entire genome has been sequenced for several strains of *S. aureus*. Among the interesting revelations are the following: (1) There is a high degree of nucleotide sequence similarity among the different strains. (2) A relatively large amount of genetic information is acquired by horizontal transfer from other bacterial species. (3) *S. aureus* contains a number of unique "pathogenicity" or "genomic" islands. These islands are mobile genetic elements that contain clusters of enterotoxin and exotoxin genes or antimicrobial resistance determinants. (4) Among the genes contained in these islands are those carrying *mecA*, the gene responsible for methicillin resistance. These methicillin resistance–containing islands have been designated *staphylococcal cassette chromosomes* (SCC*mec*) and range in size from ~20 to 60 kb. To date, four SCC*mec*s have been identified. The type 4 SCC*mec* has been associated with the community-acquired MRSA strains that have been responsible for numerous outbreaks.

Regulation of Virulence Gene Expression In both toxin-mediated and nontoxin-mediated diseases due to *S. aureus*, the expression of virulence determinants associated with infection is dependent on a series of regulatory genes [e.g., accessory gene regulator (*agr*) and staphylococcal accessory regulator (*sar*)] that coordinately control the expression of the virulence genes. The regulatory gene *agr* is part of a quorum-sensing signal transduction pathway that senses and responds to bacterial density. Staphylococcal surface proteins are synthesized during the bacterial exponential growth phase in vitro. In contrast, secreted proteins, such as α toxin, the enterotoxins, and assorted enzymes, are released during the postexponential growth phase.

It has been hypothesized that these regulatory genes serve a similar function in vivo. Successful invasion requires the sequential expression of these different bacterial elements. Bacterial adhesins are needed to initiate colonization of host tissue surfaces. The subsequent release of various enzymes enables the colony to obtain nutritional support and permits bacteria to spread to adjacent tissues. Studies using mutant strains with these regulatory genes inactivated show reduced virulence in several animal models of *S. aureus* infection.

Pathogenesis of Invasive *S. aureus* Infection Staphylococci are opportunists. For these organisms to invade the host and cause infection, some or all of the following steps are necessary: inoculation and local colonization of tissue surfaces, invasion, evasion of the host response, and metastatic spread. The initiation of staphylococcal infection requires a breach in cutaneous or mucosal barriers. Colonizing strains or strains transferred from other individuals are inoculated into damaged skin, a wound, or the bloodstream. Except under these circumstances, staphylococci generally persist as harmless commensals.

In *S. aureus* infections, recurrences develop relatively frequently, apparently because of the capacity of these pathogens to survive, to persist in a quiescent state in various tissues, and then to cause recrudescent infections when suitable conditions arise.

Nasal Colonization The anterior nares are the principal site of staphylococcal colonization in humans. Surprisingly little is known about the biology of this colonization process. It appears to involve the attachment of *S. aureus* to both nasal mucin and keratinized epithelial cells of the anterior nares. Other factors that may contribute to colonization include the influence of other resident nasal flora and their bacterial density, nasal mucosal damage (e.g., that resulting from inhalational drug use), the antimicrobial properties of nasal secretions, and host genetic factors [e.g., human leukocyte antigen (HLA) type].

Inoculation and Colonization of Tissue Surfaces Staphylococci may be introduced into tissue as a result of minor abrasions, administration of medications such as insulin, or establishment of intravenous access with catheters. After their introduction into a tissue site, bacteria replicate and colonize the host tissue surface. A family of structurally related *S. aureus* surface proteins referred to as MSCRAMMs (microbial surface components recognizing adhesive matrix molecules) plays an important role as a mediator of adherence to these sites. MSCRAMMs such as fibronectin-binding protein, clumping factor, and collagen-binding protein enable the bacteria to colonize different tissue surfaces; these proteins contribute to the pathogenesis of invasive infections such as endocarditis and arthritis by facilitating the adherence of *S. aureus* to surfaces with exposed fibronectin, fibrinogen, or collagen.

Although CoNS are classically known for their ability to elaborate a biofilm and colonize prosthetic devices, *S. aureus* also possesses the genes responsible for biofilm formation—the intercellular adhesion (*ica*) locus. Binding to these devices often involves staphylococcal adherence to serum constituents that have coated the device surface. As a result, *S. aureus* is frequently isolated from biomedical-device infections.

Invasion After colonization, staphylococci replicate at the initial site of infection, elaborating enzymes that include serine proteases, hyaluronidases, thermonucleases, and lipases. These enzymes facilitate bacterial survival and local spread across tissue surfaces, although their precise role in infections is still not well defined. The lipases may also facilitate survival in lipid-rich areas such as the hair follicles, where *S. aureus* infections are often initiated. The *S. aureus* toxin Panton-Valentine leukocidin is cytolytic to PMNs, macrophages, and monocytes. Strains elaborating this toxin have been epidemiologically linked with cutaneous infections such as furuncles and carbuncles as well as with serious pulmonary infections in adolescents.

Constitutional findings may result from either localized or systemic infections. The cell wall—consisting of alternating N-acetyl muramic acid and N-acetyl glucosamine units in combination with an additional cell wall component, lipoteichoic acid—can initiate an inflammatory response that includes the sepsis syndrome. Staphylococcal α toxin, which causes pore formation in various eukaryotic cells, can also initiate an inflammatory response with findings suggestive of sepsis.

Evasion of Host Defense Mechanisms Evasion of host defense mechanisms is critical to invasion. Staphylococci possess an antiphagocytic polysaccharide microcapsule. Most human *S. aureus* infections are due to capsular types 5 and 8. The *S. aureus* capsule also appears to play an important role in the induction of abscess formation. The capsular polysaccharides are characterized by a zwitterionic charge pattern (the presence of both negatively and positively charged molecules) that is critical to abscess formation. Protein A, an MSCRAMM unique to *S. aureus*, acts as an Fc receptor. This protein can bind the Fc portion of IgG subclasses 1, 2, and 4, preventing opsonophagocytosis by PMNs.

An additional mechanism of *S. aureus* evasion of the host response is its capacity for intracellular survival. Both professional and nonprofessional phagocytes are capable of internalizing staphylococci. Staphylococcal internalization by endothelial cells provides a sanctuary that protects bacteria against the host's defenses. It also results in cellular changes, such as the expression of integrins and Fc receptors and the release of cytokines. These cellular changes may contribute to systemic manifestations of disease, including sepsis and vasculitis.

The intracellular environment favors the phenotypic expression of *S. aureus* small-colony variants. These menadione and hemin auxotrophic mutants are generally deficient in α toxin and are able to persist within endothelial cells. Small-colony variants are often selected after aminoglycoside therapy and are more commonly found in sites of persistent infections (e.g., chronic bone infections) and in respiratory secretions from patients with cystic fibrosis. These variants represent another mechanism for prolonged staphylococcal survival that may enhance the likelihood of recurrences. Finally, *S. aureus* can survive within PMNs and may use these cells to spread and to seed other tissue sites.

Host Response to *S. aureus* Infection The primary host response to *S. aureus* infection is the PMN. PMNs are attracted to sites of infection by bacterial components such as formylated peptides or peptidoglycan. These cells are also attracted by the cytokines tumor necrosis factor (TNF) and interleukins (ILs) 1 and 6, which are released by activated macrophages and endothelial cells.

Although most individuals have antistaphylococcal antibodies, it is not clear that the antibody levels are qualitatively or quantitatively sufficient to protect against infection. Anticapsular and anti-MSCRAMM antibodies facilitate opsonization in vitro and have been protective against infection in several animal models.

Groups at Increased Risk of Infection Some diseases appear to entail multiple risk factors for *S. aureus* infection; diabetes, for example, entails an increased rate of colonization with *S. aureus*, the use of injectable insulin, and the possibility of impaired leukocyte function. Individuals with congenital or acquired qualitative or quantitative defects in PMNs are at increased risk of *S. aureus* infections; these include neutropenic patients (e.g., those receiving chemotherapeutic agents), individuals with defective intracellular killing of staphylococci (e.g., chronic granulomatous disease), and persons with Job's syndrome or Chédiak-Higashi syndrome. Other groups at risk include individuals with abnormalities of the skin (e.g., eczema) and those with prosthetic devices.

Pathogenesis of Toxin-Mediated Disease *S. aureus* produces three types of toxin: cytotoxins (discussed above), pyrogenic-toxin superantigens, and exfoliative toxins. Both epidemiologic and animal data suggest that the presence of antitoxin antibodies is protective against illness in TSS, staphylococcal food poisoning, and staphylococcal scalded-skin syndrome (SSSS). Illness develops after synthesis and absorption of the toxin followed by the toxin-initiated host response.

Enterotoxin and Toxic Shock Syndrome Toxin 1 (TSST-1) The pyrogenic toxin superantigens are a family of small-molecular-size, structurally similar proteins that are responsible for two diseases: TSS and food poisoning. TSS results from the ability of enterotoxins and TSST-1 to function as T cell mitogens. In the normal process of antigen presentation, the antigen is first processed within the cell, and peptides are then presented in the major histocompatibility complex (MHC) class II groove, initiating a measured T cell response. In contrast, enterotoxins bind directly to the invariant region of MHC—outside the MHC class II groove. The enterotoxins can then bind T cell receptors via the vβ chain, resulting in a dramatic overexpansion of T cell clones (up to 20% of the total T cell population).

As a result of this T cell expansion, there is the equivalent of a "cytokine storm," with the release of inflammatory mediators that include interferon (IFN) γ, IL-1, IL-6, TNF-α, and TNF-β. The result is a multisystem disease that produces a constellation of findings, including myalgias, fever, rash, and hypotension. These findings mimic those found in endotoxin shock; however, the pathogenic mechanisms differ. It has been hypothesized that a contributing factor to TSS is the release of endotoxin from the gastrointestinal tract, which may synergistically enhance the effects of the toxin.

A different region of the enterotoxin molecule is responsible for the symptoms of food poisoning. The enterotoxins are heat stable and can survive conditions that kill the bacteria. Illness results from the ingestion of preformed toxin. As a result, the incubation period is short (1 to 6 h). The toxin stimulates the vagus nerve and the vomiting center of the brain. It also appears to stimulate intestinal peristaltic activity.

Exfoliative Toxins and the Staphylococcal Scalded-Skin Syndrome   The exfoliative toxins are responsible for SSSS. The toxins that produce disease in humans have been divided into two serotypes: ETA and ETB. These toxins disrupt the desmosomes that link adjoining cells. Although the mechanism of this disruption remains uncertain, studies suggest that the toxins possess serine protease activity, which—through as-yet-undefined mechanisms—triggers exfoliation. The result is a split in the epidermis at the granular level, and this event is responsible for the superficial desquamation of the skin that typifies this illness.

DIAGNOSIS   *S. aureus* infections are readily diagnosed by Gram's stain (Fig. 120-2) and microscopic examination of abscess contents or of infected tissue. Staphylococci appear as large gram-positive cocci that are present singly, in pairs, or in clusters. Routine culture of infected material usually yields positive results, and blood cultures are sometimes positive even when infections are localized to extravascular sites. Polymerase chain reaction (PCR)–based assays have been applied to the rapid diagnosis of *S. aureus* infection and are increasingly being used in clinical microbiology laboratories. To date, serologic assays have not proved useful for the diagnosis of staphylococcal infections. Determining whether patients with documented *S. aureus* bacteremia also have infective endocarditis or a metastatic focus of infection remains a diagnostic challenge (see "Bacteremia, Sepsis, and Infective Endocarditis," below).

CLINICAL SYNDROMES (Table 120-1) ▪ **Skin and Soft Tissue Infections**   *S. aureus* causes a variety of cutaneous infections. Common predisposing factors include skin diseases, damage to the skin (e.g., insect bites, minor trauma), injections (e.g., in diabetes, injection drug use), and poor personal hygiene. These infections are characterized by the formation of pus-containing blisters, which often begin in hair follicles and spread to adjoining tissues. *Folliculitis* is a superficial infection that involves the hair follicle, with a central area of purulence (pus) surrounded by induration and erythema. *Furuncles* (boils) are more extensive, painful lesions that tend to occur in hairy, moist regions of the body and extend from the hair follicle to become a true abscess with an area of central purulence. *Carbuncles* are most often located in the lower neck and are even more severe and painful, resulting from the coalescence of other lesions that extend to a deeper layer of the subcutaneous tissue. In general, furuncles and carbuncles are readily apparent, with pus often expressible or discharging from the abscess.

Mastitis develops in 1 to 3% of nursing mothers. The infection, which generally presents within 2 to 3 weeks after delivery, is characterized by findings that range from cellulitis to abscess formation. Systemic signs, such as fever and chills, are often present in more severe cases.

Other cutaneous *S. aureus* infections include impetigo, cellulitis, and hidradenitis suppurativa (recurrent follicular infections in regions such as the axilla). *S. aureus* is also one of the most common causes of surgical wound infection.

TABLE 120-1   *Common Illnesses Caused by Staphylococcus aureus*

Skin and Soft Tissue Infections
  Folliculitis
  Furuncle, carbuncle
  Cellulitis
  Impetigo
  Mastitis
  Surgical wound infections
  Hidradenitis suppurativa
Musculoskeletal Infections
  Septic arthritis
  Osteomyelitis
  Pyomyositis
  Psoas abscess
Respiratory Tract Infections
  Ventilator-associated or nosocomial pneumonia
  Septic pulmonary emboli
  Postviral pneumonia (e.g., influenza)
  Empyema
Bacteremia and Its Complications
  Sepsis, septic shock
  Metastatic foci of infection (kidney, joints, bone, lung)
  Infective endocarditis
Infective Endocarditis
  Injection drug use–associated
  Native-valve
  Prosthetic-valve
  Nosocomial
Device-Related Infections (e.g., intravascular catheters, prosthetic joints)
Toxin-Mediated Illnesses
  Toxic shock syndrome
  Food poisoning
  Staphylococcal scalded-skin syndrome

Musculoskeletal Infections   *S. aureus* is among the most common causes of bone infections—both those resulting from hematogenous dissemination and those arising from contiguous spread from a soft tissue site.

Hematogenous osteomyelitis in children most often involves the long bones. Infections present with fever and bone pain or with a child's reluctance to bear weight. The white blood cell count and erythrocyte sedimentation rate are often elevated. Blood cultures are positive in ~50% of cases. When necessary, bone biopsies for culture and histopathologic examination are usually diagnostic. Routine x-rays may be normal for up to 14 days after the onset of symptoms. ^{99m}Tc-phosphonate scanning often detects early evidence of infection. Magnetic resonance imaging (MRI) is more sensitive than other techniques in establishing a radiologic diagnosis.

In adults, hematogenous osteomyelitis involving the long bones is less common. However, *vertebral osteomyelitis* is among the more common clinical presentations. These infections are most often seen in patients with endocarditis, those undergoing hemodialysis, diabetics, and injection drug users. Vertebral bone infections may present with intense back pain and fever but may also be clinically occult, presenting with chronic back pain and low-grade fever. *S. aureus* is the most common cause of epidural abscess, a complication that can result in neurologic compromise. Patients complain of difficulty voiding or walking and of radicular pain in addition to the symptoms associated with their osteomyelitis. Surgical intervention in this setting often constitutes a medical emergency. MRI most reliably establishes the diagnosis (Fig. 120-3).

Bone infections that result from contiguous spread tend to develop from soft tissue infections, such as those associated with diabetic or vascular ulcers, surgery, or trauma. Exposure of bone, a draining fistulous tract, failure to heal, or continued drainage suggests involvement of underlying bone. Bone involvement is established by bone culture and histopathologic examination. Contamination of culture material from adjacent tissue can make the diagnosis of osteomyelitis difficult in the absence of pathologic confirmation. In addition, it is

A   **B**

FIGURE 120-3 *S. aureus* vertebral osteomyelitis involving the thoracic disk between T8 and T9 in a 63-year-old man. *A.* The lower end plate is damaged (*arrow*), and there is an adjacent paraspinal mass (*arrowhead*). *B.* Sagittal T2-weighted magnetic resonance image of the spine, illustrating anterior wedging of the body of T8. (*From MA Artinian et al: Images in clinical medicine. Vertebral osteomyelitis. N Engl J Med 329:399, 1993. Copyright 1993 Massachusetts Medical Society. All rights reserved. Reprinted with permission.*)

sometimes difficult to distinguish radiologically between osteomyelitis and overlying soft tissue infection with underlying osteitis.

S. aureus is the most common cause of *septic arthritis* in children. This infection is rapidly progressive and may be associated with extensive joint destruction if left untreated. It presents with intense pain on motion of the affected joint, swelling, and fever. Aspiration of the joint reveals turbid fluid, with >50,000 PMNs/μL and gram-positive cocci in clusters on Gram's stain. In adults, arthritis may result from trauma, surgery, or hematogenous dissemination. The most commonly involved joints include the knees, shoulders, hips, and phalanges. Infection frequently develops in joints previously damaged by osteoarthritis or rheumatoid arthritis. Iatrogenic infections resulting from aspiration or injection of agents into the joint also occur. In these settings, the patient experiences increased pain and swelling in the involved joint in association with fever.

Pyomyositis is an unusual infection of skeletal muscles that is seen primarily in tropical climates. In addition to occurring in seriously immunocompromised patients, it has recently been reported in HIV-infected individuals. Pyomyositis presents with fever, swelling, and pain overlying the involved muscle. Aspiration of fluid from the involved tissue reveals pus containing numerous white blood cells and gram-positive bacteria in clusters. Although a history of trauma may be associated with the infection, its pathogenesis is poorly understood.

Respiratory Tract Infections Respiratory tract infections caused by *S. aureus* occur in selected clinical settings. *S. aureus* is a cause of serious infections in newborns and infants; these infections present with shortness of breath, fever, and respiratory failure. Chest x-ray may reveal pneumatoceles (shaggy, thin-walled cavities). Pneumothorax and empyema are recognized complications of this type of infection.

In adults, nosocomial *S. aureus* pulmonary infections are commonly seen in intubated patients on intensive care units. The clinical presentation is no different from that encountered in pulmonary infections of other bacterial etiologies. Patients produce increased volumes of purulent sputum and develop respiratory distress, fever, and new pulmonary infiltrates. Distinguishing bacterial pneumonia from other causes of respiratory failure or new pulmonary infiltrates in critically ill patients is often difficult and relies on a constellation of clinical, radiologic, and laboratory findings.

Community-acquired respiratory tract infections due to *S. aureus* are most commonly seen as postviral infections or as a result of septic pulmonary emboli (e.g., in injection drug users). Influenza is the most common cause of the former type of presentation. Patients may present with fever, bloody sputum production, and midlung field pneumatoceles or multiple, patchy pulmonary infiltrates. Diagnosis is made by sputum Gram's stain and culture. Blood cultures, although useful, are usually negative.

Bacteremia, Sepsis, and Infective Endocarditis *S. aureus* bacteremia may be complicated by sepsis, endocarditis, vasculitis, or metastatic seeding (establishment of suppurative collections at other tissue sites). The frequency of metastatic seeding during bacteremia has been estimated to be as high as 31%. Among the more commonly seeded tissue sites are bones, joints, kidneys, and lungs.

Recognition that these complications have developed is often difficult if clinical and laboratory diagnostic methods alone are used. Comorbid conditions that are frequently seen in association with *S. aureus* bacteremia and that increase the risk of complications include diabetes, HIV infection, and renal insufficiency. Other host factors associated with an increased risk of complications include presentation with community-acquired *S. aureus* bacteremia (except in injection drug users), lack of an identifiable primary focus, and presence of prosthetic devices.

Clinically, *S. aureus* sepsis presents in a manner similar to that documented for sepsis due to other bacteria. The well-described progression of hemodynamic changes—beginning with respiratory alkalosis and clinical findings of hypotension and fever—is commonly seen. The microbiologic diagnosis is established by positive blood cultures.

The overall incidence of *S. aureus* endocarditis has increased over the past 20 years. Depending on the series, *S. aureus* now accounts for 25 to 35% of all cases of bacterial endocarditis. This increase is due, at least in part, to the increased use of intravascular devices; the incidence of infective endocarditis among patients with *S. aureus* bacteremia and intravascular catheters was 25% when studied with transesophageal echocardiography. Other factors associated with an increased risk of endocarditis are injection drug use, hemodialysis, the presence of intravascular prosthetic devices, and immunosuppression. Despite the availability of effective antibiotics, mortality from these infections continues to range from 20 to 40%, depending on both the host and the nature of the infection. Complications of *S. aureus* endocarditis include cardiac valvular insufficiency, peripheral emboli, metastatic seeding, and central nervous system involvement. *S. aureus* brain abscess is a recognized complication of left-sided endocarditis.

S. aureus endocarditis is encountered in four clinical settings: (1) right-sided endocarditis in association with injection drug use, (2) left-sided native-valve endocarditis, (3) prosthetic-valve endocarditis, and (4) nosocomial endocarditis. In each of these settings, the diagnosis is established by recognition of clinical stigmata suggestive of endocarditis. These findings include cardiac manifestations such as new or changing cardiac valvular murmurs; cutaneous evidence of endocarditis such as vasculitic lesions, Osler's nodes, or Janeway lesions; evidence of embolic disease; and a history suggesting a risk for *S. aureus* bacteremia. In the absence of antecedent antibiotic therapy, blood cultures are almost uniformly positive. Transthoracic echocardiography, while less sensitive than transesophageal echocardiography, is less invasive and often establishes the presence of valvular vegetations.

Acute right-sided tricuspid valvular *S. aureus* endocarditis is most often seen in injection drug users. The classic presentation includes a high fever, a toxic clinical appearance, pleuritic chest pain, and the production of purulent (sometimes bloody) sputum. Chest x-rays reveal evidence of septic pulmonary emboli (small, peripheral, circular lesions that may cavitate with time). A high percentage of the affected patients have no history of antecedent valvular damage. At the outset of their illness, patients may present with fever alone, without cardiac or other localizing findings. As a result, a high index of clinical suspicion is essential to the diagnosis.

Individuals with antecedent cardiac valvular damage more commonly present with left-sided native-valve endocarditis involving the previously affected valve. These patients tend to be older than those with right-sided endocarditis, their prognosis is worse, and their incidence of complications (including peripheral emboli, cardiac decompensation, and metastatic seeding) is higher.

S. aureus is one of the more common causes of prosthetic-valve endocarditis. This infection is especially fulminant in the early postoperative period and is associated with a high mortality rate. In most instances, medical therapy alone is not sufficient and urgent valve replacement is necessary. Patients are prone to develop valvular insufficiency or myocardial abscesses originating from the region of valve implantation.

The increased frequency of nosocomial endocarditis (15 to 30% of cases, depending on the study) reflects in part the increased use of intravascular devices. This form of endocarditis is most commonly caused by *S. aureus*; because patients often are critically ill, are receiving antibiotics for various other indications, and have comorbid conditions, the diagnosis is not easily recognized.

Urinary Tract Infections Urinary tract infections are infrequently caused by *S. aureus*. In contrast with that of most other urinary pathogens, the presence of *S. aureus* in the urine is suggestive of hematogenous dissemination. Ascending *S. aureus* infections occasionally result from instrumentation of the genitourinary tract.

Prosthetic Device–Related Infections *S. aureus* accounts for a large proportion of prosthetic device–related infections. These infections often involve intravascular catheters, prosthetic valves, orthopedic devices, peritoneal or intraventricular catheters, and vascular grafts. Recently, *S. aureus* isolates have also been responsible for a sizable proportion of infections of left-ventricular-assist devices. In contrast with the more indolent presentation of CoNS infections, *S. aureus* device-related infections often present more acutely, with both localized and systemic manifestations. The latter infections also tend to be more rapidly progressive. It is relatively common for a pyogenic collection to be present at the device site. Aspiration of these collections and performance of blood cultures are important components in establishing a diagnosis. *S. aureus* infections tend to occur more commonly in the early postimplantation period unless the device is used for access (e.g., intravascular or hemodialysis catheters). In the latter instance, infections can occur as long as the device is used. As in most prosthetic-device infections, successful therapy usually involves removal of the device. Left in place, the device is a potential nidus for either persistent or recurrent infections.

Toxin-Mediated Diseases ■ *Toxic Shock Syndrome* TSS was first recognized as a disease in children in 1978. The disease gained national attention in the early 1980s, when a nationwide outbreak occurred among young, otherwise healthy, menstruating women. Epidemiologic investigation demonstrated that these cases were strongly associated with menstruation and the use of a highly absorbent tampon that had recently been introduced to the market. Subsequent studies established the role of TSST-1 in these illnesses. Withdrawal of the tampon from the market resulted in a rapid decline in the incidence of this disease. However, menstrual and nonmenstrual cases continue to be reported.

The clinical presentation is similar in menstrual and nonmenstrual TSS, although the nature of the risk clearly differs. Evidence of a clinical *S. aureus* infection is not a prerequisite for the development of the illness. TSS results from the elaboration of an enterotoxin or the structurally related enterotoxin-like TSST-1. More than 90% of menstrual cases are caused by TSST-1, whereas a high percentage of nonmenstrual cases are caused by enterotoxins.

TSS begins with relatively nonspecific flulike symptoms. In men-

strual cases, the onset usually comes 2 or 3 days after the start of menstruation. Patients present with fever, hypotension, and erythroderma of variable intensity. Mucosal involvement is common (e.g., conjunctival hyperemia). The illness can rapidly progress to symptoms that include vomiting, diarrhea, confusion, myalgias, and abdominal pain. These symptoms reflect the multisystemic nature of the disease, with involvement of the liver, kidneys, gastrointestinal tract, and/or central nervous system. Desquamation of the skin occurs during convalescence, usually 1 or 2 weeks after the onset of illness. Laboratory findings may include azotemia, leukocytosis, hypoalbuminemia, thrombocytopenia, and liver function abnormalities.

Diagnosis of TSS still depends on the presence of a constellation of findings rather than on one specific finding (Table 120-2). Part of the case definition is the absence of laboratory evidence of other illnesses that are often included in the differential (e.g., Rocky Mountain spotted fever, rubeola, leptospirosis). Other diagnoses to be considered are drug toxicities, viral exanthems, sepsis, and Kawasaki disease. Illness occurs only in persons who lack antibody to TSST-1. Recurrences are possible if antibody fails to develop after the illness.

Food Poisoning *S. aureus* is among the most common causes of foodborne outbreaks of infection in the United States. *S. aureus* food poisoning results from the inoculation of toxin-producing *S. aureus* into food by colonized food handlers. Toxin is then elaborated in such growth-promoting food as custards, potato salad, or processed meats. Even if the bacteria are killed by warming, the heat-stable toxin is not destroyed. The onset of illness is rapid and explosive, occurring within 1 to 6 h of ingestion. The illness is characterized by nausea and vomiting, although diarrhea, hypotension, and dehydration may also occur. The differential diagnosis includes diarrhea of other etiologies, especially that caused by similar toxins (e.g., the toxins elaborated by *Bacillus cereus*). The rapidity of onset, the absence of fever, and the epidemic nature of the presentation arouse suspicion regarding this diagnosis. Symptoms generally resolve within 8 to 10 h. The diagnosis can be established by the demonstration of bacteria or the documentation of enterotoxin in the implicated food. Treatment is entirely supportive.

Staphylococcal Scalded-Skin Syndrome SSSS most often affects newborns and children. The illness may vary from localized blister formation to exfoliation of much of the skin surface. The skin is usually fragile and often tender, with thin-walled, fluid-filled bullae. Gentle pressure results in rupture of the lesions, leaving denuded underlying skin (Ni-

---

TABLE 120-2 Case Definition of S. aureus Toxic Shock Syndrome

1. Fever: temperature of ≥38.9°C (≥102°F)
2. Hypotension: systolic blood pressure of ≤90 mmHg, or orthostatic hypotension (orthostatic drop in diastolic blood pressure by ≥15 mmHg, orthostatic syncope, or orthostatic dizziness)
3. Diffuse macular rash with subsequent desquamation in 1 to 2 weeks after onset (including the palms and soles)
4. Multisystem involvement
   a. Hepatic: bilirubin or aminotransferase levels ≥2 times normal
   b. Hematologic: platelet count ≤100,000/μL)
   c. Renal: blood urea nitrogen or serum creatinine level ≥2 times the normal upper limit
   d. Mucous membranes: vaginal, oropharyngeal, or conjunctival hyperemia
   e. Gastrointestinal: vomiting or diarrhea at onset of illness
   f. Muscular: severe myalgias or serum creatine phosphokinase level ≥2 times the upper limit
   g. Central nervous system: disorientation or alteration in consciousness without focal neurologic signs and in the absence of fever and hypotension
5. Negative serologic or other tests for measles, leptospirosis, and Rocky Mountain spotted fever as well as negative blood or cerebrospinal fluid cultures for organisms other than *S. aureus*

Source: M Wharton et al: Case definitions for public health surveillance. MMWR 39:1, 1990; with permission.

kolsky's sign; Fig. 120-4). The mucous membranes are usually spared. In more generalized infection, there are often constitutional symptoms, including fever, lethargy, and irritability with poor feeding. Significant amounts of fluid can be lost in more extensive cases. Illness usually follows localized infection at one of a number of possible sites. SSSS is much less common among adults but can follow infections caused by exfoliative toxin–producing strains.

PREVENTION   Prevention of the spread of *S. aureus* infections in the hospital setting involves hand washing and careful attention to appropriate isolation procedures. Through strict isolation practices, some Scandinavian countries have been remarkably successful at preventing the introduction and dissemination of MRSA in hospitals. Other countries, such as the United States and Great Britain, have been less successful.

The use of topical antimicrobial agents (e.g., mupirocin) to eliminate nasal colonization with *S. aureus* and to prevent subsequent infection has been investigated in a number of clinical settings. Elimination of nasal carriage of *S. aureus* has reduced the incidence of infections among patients undergoing hemodialysis and peritoneal dialysis. A randomized, placebo-controlled study attempted to reduce rates of wound infection among patients undergoing surgery with the prophylactic application of topical mupirocin to the nares. The results failed to demonstrate an overall benefit from the use of mupirocin but did suggest that the incidence of infections might be reduced if the use of mupirocin were limited to patients nasally colonized with *S. aureus*.

The ability of a capsular polysaccharide–protein conjugate vaccine to prevent staphylococcal infections in hemodialysis patients was studied. The results, while inconclusive, did show promise. Other potential vaccine candidates, including those incorporating the ligand-binding domains of several MSCRAMMs, are also under investigation.

COAGULASE-NEGATIVE STAPHYLOCOCCAL INFECTIONS

CoNS, although considerably less virulent than *S. aureus*, are among the most common causes of prosthetic-device infections. Approximately half of the 32 identified CoNS species have been associated with human infections. Of these species, *S. epidermidis* is the most common human pathogen overall; this component of the normal human flora is found on the skin (where it is the most abundant bacterial species) as well as in the oropharynx and vagina. *S. saprophyticus*, a novobiocin-resistant species, is a pathogen in urinary tract infections.

PATHOGENESIS   Among CoNS, *S. epidermidis* is the species most commonly associated with prosthetic-device infections. Infection is a two-

FIGURE 120-4   Evidence of staphylococcal scalded-skin syndrome in a 6-year-old boy. Nikolsky's sign, with separation of the superficial layer of the outer epidermal layer, is visible. (*From LA Schenfeld et al: Images in clinical medicine. Staphylococcal scalded skin syndrome. N Engl J Med 42:1178, 2000. Copyright 2000 Massachusetts Medical Society. All rights reserved. Reprinted with permission.*)

step process, with initial adhesion to the device followed by colonization. *S. epidermidis* is uniquely adapted to colonize these devices by its capacity to elaborate the extracellular polysaccharide (slime) that facilitates formation of a protective biofilm on the device surface.

Implanted prosthetic material is often coated with host serum or tissue constituents such as fibrinogen or fibronectin. These molecules serve as potential bridging ligands, facilitating bacterial attachment to the device surface. The surface-associated staphylococcal enzyme autolysin (AtlE) may play a role in attachment to either modified or unmodified prosthetic surfaces. In addition to AtlE, other surface molecules, such as fibrinogen-binding protein and cell wall teichoic acid, appear to mediate adherence to fibrinogen and fibronectin, respectively. The polysaccharide intercellular adhesin facilitates subsequent staphylococcal colonization and accumulation on the device surface. The genes responsible for synthesis of this polysaccharide (the *ica* genes) are also present in *S. aureus*, although their role in the two species may differ. In *S. epidermidis*, the *ica* genes are more commonly found in strains associated with device infections than in strains associated with colonization of mucosal surfaces. Biofilm appears to act as a barrier protecting bacteria from host defense mechanisms as well as from antibiotics, while providing a suitable environment for bacterial survival.

Two additional staphylococcal species, *S. lugdunensis* and *S. schleiferi*, produce more serious infections (native-valve endocarditis and osteomyelitis) than do other CoNS. The basis for this enhanced virulence is not known, although both species appear to share more virulence determinants with *S. aureus* (e.g., clumping factor and lipase) than do other CoNS.

The capacity of *S. saprophyticus* to cause urinary tract infections in young women appears to be related to its enhanced capacity to adhere to uroepithelial cells. A 160-kDa hemagglutinin/adhesin may contribute to this affinity.

DIAGNOSIS   While the detection of CoNS at sites of infection or in the bloodstream is not difficult by standard microbiologic culture methods, interpretation of these results is frequently problematic. Since these organisms are present in large numbers on the skin, they often contaminate cultures. It has been estimated that only 10 to 25% of blood cultures positive for CoNS reflect true bacteremia. Similar problems arise with cultures of other sites. Among the clinical findings suggestive of true bacteremia are fever, evidence of local infection (e.g., erythema or purulent drainage at the intravenous catheter site), leukocytosis, and systemic signs of sepsis. Laboratory findings suggestive of true bacteremia include multiple positive cultures of the same strain (i.e., the same species with the same antibiogram or a closely related DNA fingerprint) from separate cultures, growth of the strain within 48 h, and bacterial growth in both aerobic and anaerobic bottles.

CLINICAL SYNDROMES   CoNS cause diverse prosthetic device–related infections, including those that involve prosthetic cardiac valves and joints, vascular grafts, intravascular devices, and central nervous system shunts. In all of these settings, the clinical presentation is similar. The signs of localized infection are often subtle, the rate of disease progression is slow, and the systemic findings are often limited. Signs of infection such as purulent drainage, pain at the site, or loosening of prosthetic implants are sometimes evident. Fever is frequently but not always present, and there may be mild leukocytosis.

Infections that are not associated with prosthetic devices are infrequent, although native-valve endocarditis due to CoNS has accounted for ~5% of cases in some reviews. *S. lugdunensis* appears to be a more aggressive pathogen in this setting, causing greater mortality and rapid valvular destruction with abscess formation.

℞ TREATMENT

General Principles of Therapy   In addition to the selection of appropriate antimicrobial therapy for staphylococcal infections, surgical incision and drainage of all suppurative collections are necessary. Prosthetic-device infections are unlikely to be successfully managed unless the device is removed. In the limited number of situations in which removal is not possible or the infection is due to CoNS, an initial attempt at medical therapy without device removal may be warranted. Because of the well-recognized risk of complications associated with *S. aureus* bacteremia, therapy is generally prolonged (4 to 8 weeks) unless the patient is identified as being one of the small percentage of individuals who are at low risk for complications—e.g., immunocompetent patients and patients whose *S. aureus* infection is associated with a removable focus (such as an intravenous catheter) and whose device is promptly removed.

Duration of Antimicrobial Therapy Debate continues regarding the duration of therapy for bacteremic *S. aureus* infections. No carefully controlled, prospective study has addressed this question. A meta-analysis reviewing studies relevant to this issue concluded that insufficient information was currently available to determine which patients were candidates for short-course therapy (2 weeks rather than 4 to 8 weeks).

Among the findings associated with an increased risk of complicated bacteremia are persistently positive blood cultures 48 to 96 h after institution of therapy, acquisition of the infection in the community, a removable focus of infection (i.e., intravascular catheters) that is not removed, and cutaneous or embolic manifestations of infection. In those immunocompetent patients for whom short-course therapy is planned, a transesophageal echocardiogram to rule out endocarditis is warranted since neither clinical nor laboratory findings are adequate to detect cardiac involvement. In addition, an aggressive radiologic investigation to identify potential metastatic collections is indicated. All symptomatic sites need to be carefully evaluated.

Choice of Antimicrobial Agents The choice of antimicrobial agents to treat both coagulase-positive staphylococcal and CoNS infections has become increasingly problematic because of the prevalence of multidrug-resistant strains. Data collected by the Centers for Disease Control and Prevention from intensive care units in the United States (1988 to 1998) show a dramatic increase in the number of isolates that are now susceptible only to vancomycin. This trend is even more apparent with CoNS: more than 80% of nosocomial isolates are resistant to methicillin, and these MRSA strains are usually resistant to most other antibiotics as well. Because the selection of antimicrobial agents for the treatment of *S. aureus* infections is similar to that for CoNS infections, treatment options for these pathogens are discussed together and are summarized in Table 120-3.

As a result of the widespread dissemination of plasmids containing the enzyme penicillinase, few strains of staphylococci (<5%) remain susceptible to penicillin. However, against susceptible strains, penicillin remains the drug of choice. Penicillin-resistant isolates are treated with semisynthetic penicillinase-resistant penicillins (SPRPs) such as oxacillin or nafcillin. Methicillin, the first of the SPRPs, is now used infrequently. Cephalosporins are alternative therapeutic agents for these infections. Second- and third-generation cephalosporins do not have a therapeutic advantage over first-generation cephalosporins for the treatment of staphylococcal infections. The carbapenem imipenem has excellent activity against methicillin-sensitive *S. aureus* (MSSA) but not MRSA.

The isolation of MRSA was reported within 1 year of the introduction of methicillin. The prevalence of MRSA has since increased steadily. In many hospitals, 40 to 50% of *S. aureus* isolates are now resistant to methicillin. Resistance to methicillin indicates resistance to all SPRPs as well as all cephalosporins. Many MRSA isolates are also resistant to other antimicrobial families, including aminoglycosides, quinolones, and macrolides.

Production of a novel penicillin-binding protein (PBP 2a or 2′) is responsible for methicillin resistance. This protein is synthesized by the *mecA* gene, which (as stated above) is part of a large mobile genetic element—a pathogenicity or genomic island—called the staphylococcal cassette chromosome (SCC*mec*). It is hypothesized that acquisition of this genetic material resulted from horizontal transfer from a related staphylococcal species, such as *S. sciuri*. Phenotypic expression of methicillin resistance may be constitutive (i.e., expressed in all organisms in a population) or heterogeneous (i.e., displayed by only a proportion of the total organism population). Detection of methicillin resistance in the clinical microbiology laboratory can be difficult if the strain expresses heterogeneous resistance. Therefore, susceptibility studies are routinely performed at reduced temperatures (30° to 35°C for 24 h), with increased concentrations of salt in the medium to enhance the expression of resistance. In addition to PCR-based techniques, a number of rapid methods for the detection of methicillin resistance have recently been developed.

Vancomycin is the drug of choice for the treatment of methicillin-resistant staphylococcal infections. Because it is less bactericidal than the β-lactams, it should be used only after careful consideration in patients with a history of β-lactam allergies. In 1997, an *S. aureus* strain with reduced susceptibility to vancomycin (VISA) was reported from Japan. Subsequently, additional clinical isolates of VISA were reported from geographically disparate locations. These strains were all resistant to methicillin and many other antimicrobial agents. The VISA strains appear to evolve (under vancomycin selective pressure) from strains that are susceptible to vancomycin but are heterogeneous, with a small proportion of the bacterial population expressing the resistance phenotype. The mechanism of VISA resistance is uncertain but appears to be an abnormal cell wall, which was first noted by electron microscopy. Vancomycin is trapped by the abnormal peptidoglycan cross-linking and is unable to gain access to its target site.

In 2002, the first clinical isolate of fully vancomycin-resistant *S. aureus* was reported. Resistance in this and one subsequently reported clinical isolate was due to the presence of *vanA*, the gene responsible for expression of vancomycin resistance in enterococci. This observation suggested that resistance was acquired as a result of horizontal conjugal transfer from a vancomycin-resistant strain of *Enterococcus faecalis*. The patients had both MRSA and vancomycin-resistant enterococci cultured from sites of infection. The isolates remained susceptible to chloramphenicol, linezolid, minocycline, quinupristin/dalfopristin, and trimethoprim-sulfamethoxazole (TMP-SMX). The *vanA* gene is responsible for the synthesis of the dipeptide D-Ala-D-Lac in place of D-Ala-D-Ala. Vancomycin is not able to bind to the altered peptide.

Alternatives to the β-lactams and vancomycin have less antistaphylococcal activity. Although the quinolones have reasonable in vitro activity against staphylococci, the frequency of fluoroquinolone resistance has increased progressively, especially among methicillin-resistant isolates. Methicillin-susceptible staphylococci have remained more susceptible to the fluoroquinolones than have methicillin-resistant strains. Of particular concern in methicillin-resistant strains is the possible emergence of quinolone resistance during therapy. Resistance to the quinolones is most commonly chromosomal and results from mutations of the topoisomerase IV or DNA gyrase genes, although multidrug efflux pumps may also contribute. While the newer quinolones exhibit increased in vitro activity against staphylococci, it is uncertain whether this increase translates into enhanced in vivo activity. Other antibiotics such as minocycline and TMP-SMX have been successfully used to treat methicillin-resistant staphylococcal infections in the face of vancomycin toxicity or intolerance.

Among the newer antistaphylococcal agents, the parenteral streptogramin quinupristin/dalfopristin displays bactericidal activity against all staphylococci, including VISA strains. This drug has been used successfully to treat serious MRSA infections. In cases of erythromycin or clindamycin resistance, it is bacteriostatic against staphylococci.

Linezolid—the first member of a new drug family, the oxazolidinones—is bacteriostatic against staphylococci, has been well tolerated, and offers the advantage of comparable bioavailability after oral or parenteral administration. Cross-resistance with other inhibitors of protein synthesis has not been reported. Resistance to linezolid has been limited, although at least one resistant clinical isolate has been reported. The efficacy of linezolid in the treatment of deep-seated infections such as osteomyelitis has not yet been established. There are currently insufficient data on the efficacy of either quinupristin/dalfopristin or linezolid for the treatment of infective endocarditis. Dap-

TABLE 120-3 Antimicrobial Therapy for Serious S. aureus Infections[a]

Sensitivity/Resistance of Isolate	Drug of Choice	Alternative(s)	Comments
Sensitive to penicillin	Penicillin G (4 mU q4h)	Nafcillin (2 g q4h) or oxacillin (2 g q4h), cefazolin (2 g q8h), vancomycin (1 g q12h[b])	Fewer than 5% of isolates are sensitive to penicillin.
Sensitive to methicillin	Nafcillin or oxacillin (2 g q4h)	Cefazolin (2 g q8h[b]), vancomycin (1 g q12h[b])	Patients with penicillin allergy can be treated with a cephalosporin if the allergy does not involve an anaphylactic or accelerated reaction; vancomycin is the alternative. Desensitization to β-lactams may be indicated in selected cases of serious infection where maximal bactericidal activity is needed (e.g., prosthetic-valve endocarditis[c]). Type A β-lactamase may rapidly hydrolyze cefazolin and reduce its efficacy in endocarditis.
Resistant to methicillin	Vancomycin (1 g q12h[b])	TMP-SMX (TMP, 5 mg/kg q12h[b]), minocycline (100 mg PO q12h[b]), ciprofloxacin (400 mg q12h[b]), levofloxacin (500 mg q24h[b]), quinupristin/dalfopristin (7.5 mg/kg q8h), linezolid (600 mg q12h except: 400 mg q12h for uncomplicated skin infections); daptomycin (4 mg/kg q24h[b]) for complicated skin infections; investigational drugs: oritavancin, tigecycline	Sensitivity testing is necessary before an alternative drug is used. Adjunctive drugs (those that should be used only in combination with other antimicrobial agents) include gentamicin (1 mg/kg q8h[b]), rifampin (300 mg PO q8h), and fusidic acid (500 mg q8h; not readily available in the United States). Quinupristin/dalfopristin is bactericidal against methicillin-resistant isolates unless the strain is resistant to erythromycin or clindamycin. The newer quinolones may retain in vitro activity against ciprofloxacin-resistant isolates; resistance may develop during therapy. The efficacy of adjunctive therapy is not well established in many settings. Both linezolid and quinupristin/dalfopristin have had in vitro activity against most VISA and VRSA strains. See footnote for treatment of prosthetic-valve endocarditis.[c]
Resistant to methicillin with intermediate or complete resistance to vancomycin[d]	Uncertain	Same as for methicillin-resistant strains; check antibiotic susceptibilities	Same as for methicillin-resistant strains; check antibiotic susceptibilities
Not yet known (i.e., empirical therapy)	Vancomycin (1 g q12h)	—	Empirical therapy is given when the susceptibility of the isolate is not known. Vancomycin with or without an aminoglycoside is recommended for suspected community- or hospital-acquired S. aureus infections because of the increased frequency of methicillin-resistant strains in the community.

[a] Recommended dosages are for adults with normal renal and hepatic function. The route of administration is intravenous unless otherwise indicated.

[b] The dosage must be adjusted in patients with reduced creatinine clearance.

[c] For the treatment of prosthetic-valve endocarditis, the addition of gentamicin (1 mg/kg q8h) and rifampin (300 mg PO q8h) is recommended, with adjustment of the gentamicin dosage if the creatinine clearance rate is reduced.

[d] Vancomycin-resistant S. aureus isolates from clinical infections have recently been reported.

Source: Modified with permission of the *New England Journal of Medicine* (Lowy, 1998). Copyright 1998 Massachusetts Medical Society. All rights reserved.

Note: TMP-SMX, trimethoprim-sulfamethoxazole; VISA, vancomycin-intermediate *S. aureus*; VRSA, vancomycin-resistant *S. aureus*.

tomycin, a new parenteral bactericidal agent with antistaphylococcal activity, was recently approved for the treatment of complicated skin infections. This drug disrupts the cytoplasmic membrane. Oritavancin, a new glycopeptide, is undergoing clinical trials.

Combinations of antistaphylococcal agents are sometimes used to enhance bactericidal activity in the treatment of serious infections such as endocarditis or osteomyelitis. In selected instances (e.g., right-sided endocarditis), drug combinations are also used to shorten the duration of therapy. Among the antimicrobial agents used in combinations are rifampin, aminoglycosides (e.g., gentamicin), and fusidic acid (which is not readily available in the United States). While these agents are not effective singly because of the frequent emergence of resistance, they have proved useful in combination with other agents because of their bactericidal activity against staphylococci.

In vitro studies have demonstrated synergy against staphylococci with the following combinations: (1) β-lactams and aminoglycosides; (2) vancomycin and gentamicin; (3) vancomycin, gentamicin, and rifampin (against CoNS); and (4) vancomycin and rifampin. In several instances, these in vitro observations have been supported by studies using the experimental animal model of endocarditis.

Antimicrobial Therapy for Selected Settings For uncomplicated skin and soft tissue infections, the use of oral antistaphylococcal agents is usually successful. For other infections, parenteral therapy is indicated.

S. aureus endocarditis is usually an acute, life-threatening infection. Thus blood cultures need to be obtained promptly and followed by the immediate institution of empirical antimicrobial therapy. For *S. aureus* native-valve endocarditis, a combination of antimicrobial agents is often used. In a large prospective study, an SPRP combined with an aminoglycoside did not alter the clinical outcome but did reduce the duration of *S. aureus* bacteremia. As a result, many clinicians begin therapy for life-threatening infections with a 3- to 5-day course of a β-lactam and an aminoglycoside (gentamicin, 1 mg/kg intravenously every 8 h). If a MRSA strain is isolated, vancomycin (30 mg/kg every 24 h, given in two equal doses up to a total of 2 g) is recommended. Patients are treated for 4 to 6 weeks, depending on the clinical response.

In prosthetic-valve endocarditis, surgery in addition to antibiotic therapy is often necessary. The combination of a β-lactam agent—or, if the isolate is β-lactam resistant, vancomycin (30 mg/kg every 24 h, given in two equal doses up to a total of 2 g)—with an aminoglycoside (gentamicin, 1 mg/kg intravenously every 8 h) and rifampin (300 mg orally every 8 h) is recommended. This combination is used to avoid the possible emergence of rifampin resistance during therapy if only two drugs are used.

For hematogenous osteomyelitis or septic arthritis in children, a 4-week course of therapy is usually adequate. In adults, treatment is often more prolonged. For chronic forms of osteomyelitis, surgical debridement is necessary in combination with antimicrobial therapy. For joint infections, a critical component of therapy is the repeated aspiration or arthroscopy of the affected joint to prevent damage from leukocytes.

The combination of rifampin with ciprofloxacin has been used successfully to treat prosthetic-joint infections, especially when the device cannot be removed. The efficacy of this combination may reflect the enhanced activity against staphylococci in biofilms as well as the attainment of effective intracellular concentrations.

The choice of empirical therapy for staphylococcal infections depends in part on susceptibility data for the local geographic area. Increasingly, vancomycin (in combination with an aminoglycoside or rifampin for serious infections) is the drug of choice for both community- and hospital-acquired infections.

Therapy for Toxic Shock Syndrome Supportive therapy with reversal of hypotension is the mainstay of therapy for TSS. Both fluids and pressors may be necessary. Tampons or other packing material should be promptly removed. The role of antibiotics is less clear. Some investigators recommend a combination of clindamycin and a semisynthetic penicillin. Clindamycin is advocated because, as a protein synthesis inhibitor, it reduces toxin synthesis in vitro. A semisynthetic penicillin is suggested to eliminate any potential focus of infection as well as to eradicate persistent carriage that might increase the likelihood of recurrent illness. Anecdotal reports document the successful use of intravenous immunoglobulin to treat TSS. The role of glucocorticoids in the treatment of this disease is uncertain at present.

Therapy for Other Toxin-Mediated Diseases Therapy for staphylococcal food poisoning is entirely supportive. For SSSS, antistaphylococcal therapy targets the primary site of infection.

FURTHER READING

BABA T et al: Genome and virulence determinants of high virulence community-acquired MRSA. Lancet 359:1819, 2002

CHAMBERS HF: Methicillin resistance in staphylococci: Molecular and biochemical basis and clinical implications. Clin Microbiol Rev 10:781, 1997

FOWLER VG JR et al: Role of echocardiography in evaluation of patients with *Staphylococcus aureus* bacteremia: Experience in 103 patients. J Am Coll Cardiol 30:1072, 1997

HIRAMATSU K et al: The emergence and evolution of methicillin-resistant *Staphylococcus aureus*. Trends Microbiol 9:486, 2001

ING MB et al: Bacteremia and infective endocarditis: Pathogenesis, diagnosis, and complications, in *The Staphylococci in Human Disease*, KB Crossley, GL Archer (eds). New York, Churchill Livingstone, 1997, pp 331–354

LOWY FD: Antimicrobial resistance: The example of *Staphylococcus aureus*. J Clin Invest 111:1265, 2003

———: *Staphylococcus aureus* infections. N Engl J Med 339:520, 1998

MCCORMICK JK et al: Toxic shock syndrome and bacterial superantigens: An update. Annu Rev Microbiol 55:77, 2001

MYLOTTE JM, TAYARA A: *Staphylococcus aureus* bacteremia: Predictors of 30-day mortality in a large cohort. Clin Infect Dis 31:1170, 2000

VON EIFF C et al: Pathogenesis of infections due to coagulase-negative staphylococci. Lancet Infect Dis 2:677, 2002

121 STREPTOCOCCAL AND ENTEROCOCCAL INFECTIONS
Michael R. Wessels

Many varieties of streptococci are found as part of the normal human flora colonizing the respiratory, gastrointestinal, and genitourinary tracts. Several species are important causes of human disease. Group A *Streptococcus*, or *S. pyogenes*, is responsible for streptococcal pharyngitis, one of the most common bacterial infections of school-age children, and for the postinfectious syndromes of acute rheumatic fever and poststreptococcal glomerulonephritis. Group B *Streptococcus*, or *S. agalactiae*, is the leading cause of bacterial sepsis and meningitis in newborns and a major cause of endometritis and fever in parturient women. Enterococci are important causes of urinary tract infection, nosocomial bacteremia, and endocarditis. Viridans streptococci are the most common cause of bacterial endocarditis.

Streptococci are gram-positive bacteria of spherical to ovoid shape that characteristically form chains when grown in liquid media. Most streptococci that cause human infections are facultative anaerobes, although some are strict anaerobes. Streptococci are relatively fastidious organisms, requiring enriched media for growth in the laboratory. No single scheme for classification of streptococci is entirely satisfactory. Consequently, clinicians and clinical microbiologists often identify streptococci by any of several classification systems, including hemolytic pattern, Lancefield group, species name, and common or trivial name. Many of the streptococci associated with human infection produce a zone of complete hemolysis around the bacterial colony when cultured on blood agar, a pattern known as *β hemolysis*. The β-hemolytic streptococci can be classified by the Lancefield system, a serologic grouping based on the reaction of specific antisera with cell-wall carbohydrate antigens of the bacteria. With rare exceptions, organisms belonging to Lancefield groups A, B, C, and G are all β-hemolytic streptococci, and each is associated with characteristic patterns of human infection. Other streptococci produce a zone of partial (α) hemolysis, often imparting a greenish appearance to the agar. These α-hemolytic streptococci are further identified by biochemical testing and include *S. pneumoniae*, an important cause of pneumonia, meningitis, and other infections, and several species of streptococci referred to collectively as the *viridans streptococci*, which are part of

the normal oral flora and are important as agents of subacute bacterial endocarditis. Finally, some streptococci are nonhemolytic, a pattern sometimes called γ hemolysis. The classification of the major groups of streptococci responsible for human infections is outlined in Table 121-1. Among the organisms classified serologically as group D streptococci, the enterococci are now considered to constitute a separate genus on the basis of DNA homology studies. Thus species previously designated as *S. faecalis* and *S. faecium* have been renamed *Enterococcus faecalis* and *E. faecium*, respectively. →*For further discussion of pneumococcal infections, see Chap. 119.*

GROUP A STREPTOCOCCI

Lancefield's group A consists of a single species, *S. pyogenes*. As its species name implies, this organism is associated with a variety of suppurative infections. In addition, group A streptococci can trigger the postinfectious syndromes of acute rheumatic fever (which is uniquely associated with *S. pyogenes* infection; Chap. 302) and poststreptococcal glomerulonephritis (Chap. 264).

PATHOGENESIS Group A streptococci elaborate a number of cell-surface components and extracellular products important both in the pathogenesis of infection and in the immune response of the human host. The cell wall contains a carbohydrate antigen that may be released by treatment with acid. The reaction of such acid extracts with group A–specific antiserum is the basis for the definitive identification of a streptococcal strain as *S. pyogenes*. The major surface protein of group A streptococci is M protein, which occurs in more than 100 antigenically distinct types and is the basis for the serotyping of strains with specific antisera. The M protein molecules are fibrillar structures anchored in the cell wall of the organism that extend as hairlike projections away from the cell surface. The amino acid sequence of the distal or amino-terminal portion of the M protein molecule is quite variable, accounting for the antigenic variation of the different M types, while more proximal regions of the protein are relatively conserved. A newer technique for assignment of M type to group A streptococcal isolates uses the polymerase chain reaction to amplify the

TABLE 121-1 Classification of Streptococci

Lancefield Group	Representative Species	Hemolytic Pattern	Typical Infections
A	S. pyogenes	β	Pharyngitis, impetigo, cellulitis, scarlet fever
B	S. agalactiae	β	Neonatal sepsis and meningitis, puerperal infection, urinary tract infection, diabetic ulcer infection, endocarditis
C	S. equisimilis	β	Cellulitis, bacteremia, endocarditis
D	Enterococci: E. faecalis; E. faecium	Usually nonhemolytic	Urinary tract infection, nosocomial bacteremia, endocarditis
	Nonenterococci: S. bovis	Usually nonhemolytic	Bacteremia, endocarditis
G	S. canis	β	Cellulitis, bacteremia, endocarditis, septic arthritis
Variable or nongroupable	Viridans streptococci: S. sanguis; S. mitis	α	Endocarditis, dental abscess, brain abscess
	Intermedius, milleri, or anginosus group: S. intermedius, S. anginosus, S. constellatus	Variable	Brain abscess, visceral abscess
	Anaerobic streptococci: Peptostreptococcus magnus	Usually nonhemolytic	Sinusitis, pneumonia, empyema, brain abscess, liver abscess

variable region of the M protein gene. DNA sequence analysis of the amplified gene segment can be compared with an extensive database [developed at the Centers for Disease Control and Prevention (CDC)] for assignment of M type. This method eliminates the need for typing sera, which are available in only a few reference laboratories. The presence of M protein on a group A streptococcal isolate correlates with its capacity to resist phagocytic killing in fresh human blood; this phenomenon appears to be due, at least in part, to the binding of plasma fibrinogen to M protein molecules on the streptococcal surface, which interferes with complement activation and deposition of opsonic complement fragments on the bacterial cell. This resistance to phagocytosis may be overcome by M protein–specific antibodies; thus individuals with antibodies to a given M type acquired as a result of prior infection are protected against subsequent infection with organisms of the same M type but not against that with different M types.

Group A streptococci also elaborate, to varying degrees, a polysaccharide capsule composed of hyaluronic acid. The production of large amounts of hyaluronic acid capsule by certain strains lends a characteristic mucoid appearance to the bacterial colonies. The capsular polysaccharide also plays an important role in protecting the organisms from ingestion and killing by phagocytes. In contrast to M protein, the hyaluronic acid capsule is a weak immunogen, and antibodies to hyaluronate have not been shown to be important in protective immunity; the presumed explanation is the apparent structural identity between streptococcal hyaluronic acid and the hyaluronic acid of mammalian connective tissues. The capsular polysaccharide may also play a role in group A streptococcal colonization of the pharynx by binding to CD44, a hyaluronic acid–binding protein expressed on human pharyngeal epithelial cells.

Group A streptococci produce a large number of extracellular products that may be important in local and systemic toxicity and in the spread of infection through tissues. These products include streptolysins S and O, toxins that damage cell membranes and account for the hemolysis produced by the organisms; streptokinase; DNases; protease; and pyrogenic exotoxins A, B, and C. The pyrogenic exotoxins, previously known as erythrogenic toxins, cause the rash of scarlet fever. Since the mid-1980s, pyrogenic exotoxin–producing strains of group A *Streptococcus* have been linked to unusually severe invasive infections, including necrotizing fasciitis and a systemic syndrome termed the *streptococcal toxic shock syndrome*. Several extracellular products stimulate specific antibody responses useful in the serodiagnosis of recent streptococcal infection. Tests for these antibodies are used primarily for the detection of preceding streptococcal infection in cases of suspected acute rheumatic fever or poststreptococcal glomerulonephritis.

CLINICAL MANIFESTATIONS ■ Pharyngitis

Although seen in patients of all ages, group A streptococcal pharyngitis is one of the most common bacterial infections of childhood, accounting for 20 to 40% of all cases of exudative pharyngitis in children; it is rare among those under the age of 3. Younger children may manifest streptococcal infection with a syndrome of fever, malaise, and lymphadenopathy without exudative pharyngitis. Infection is acquired through contact with another individual carrying the organism. Respiratory droplets are the usual mechanism of spread, although other routes, including food-borne outbreaks, have been well described.

The incubation period is 1 to 4 days. Symptoms include sore throat, fever and chills, malaise, and sometimes abdominal complaints and vomiting, particularly in children. Both symptoms and signs are quite variable, ranging from mild throat discomfort with minimal physical findings to high fever and severe sore throat associated with intense erythema and swelling of the pharyngeal mucosa and the presence of purulent exudate over the posterior pharyngeal wall and tonsillar pillars. Enlarged, tender anterior cervical lymph nodes commonly accompany exudative pharyngitis.

The differential diagnosis of streptococcal pharyngitis includes the many other bacterial and viral causes of pharyngitis (Table 121-2). Streptococcal infection is unlikely to be the cause of pharyngitis when symptoms and signs suggestive of viral infection are prominent (conjunctivitis, coryza, cough, hoarseness, or discrete ulcerative lesions of

TABLE 121-2 Infectious Etiologies of Acute Pharyngitis

Organism	Associated Clinical Syndrome(s)
VIRUSES	
Rhinovirus	Common cold
Coronavirus	Common cold
Adenovirus	Pharyngoconjunctival fever
Influenza virus	Influenza
Parainfluenza virus	Cold, croup
Coxsackievirus	Herpangina, hand-foot-and-mouth disease
Herpes simplex virus	Gingivostomatitis (primary infection)
Epstein-Barr virus	Infectious mononucleosis
Cytomegalovirus	Mononucleosis-like syndrome
HIV	Acute (primary) infection syndrome
BACTERIA	
Group A streptococci	Pharyngitis, scarlet fever
Group C or G streptococci	Pharyngitis
Mixed anaerobes	Vincent's angina
Arcanobacterium haemolyticum	Pharyngitis, scarlatiniform rash
Neisseria gonorrhoeae	Pharyngitis
Treponema pallidum	Secondary syphilis
Francisella tularensis	Pharyngeal tularemia
Corynebacterium diphtheriae	Diphtheria
Yersinia enterocolitica	Pharyngitis, enterocolitis
Yersinia pestis	Plague
Chlamydiae	
Chlamydia pneumoniae	Bronchitis, pneumonia
Chlamydia psittaci	Psittacosis
Mycoplasmas	
Mycoplasma pneumoniae	Bronchitis, pneumonia

the buccal or pharyngeal mucosa). Other infections commonly producing exudative pharyngitis include infectious mononucleosis and adenovirus infection. Now rare in the United States, the pseudomembrane of diphtheria may give a similar appearance. The coryneform organism *Arcanobacterium haemolyticum* may cause pharyngitis, often in association with a scarlet fever–like rash (Chap. 122). Other causes of pharyngitis, usually without a purulent exudate, include coxsackievirus, influenza virus, mycoplasmas, and *Neisseria gonorrhoeae* and acute infection with HIV. Because of the range of clinical presentations of streptococcal pharyngitis and the large number of other agents that can produce the same clinical picture, diagnosis of streptococcal pharyngitis on clinical grounds alone is not reliable.

The throat culture remains the diagnostic "gold standard." Culture of a throat specimen that is properly collected (i.e., by vigorous rubbing of a sterile swab over both tonsillar pillars) and properly processed is the most sensitive and specific means available to make a definitive diagnosis. A rapid diagnostic kit for latex agglutination or enzyme immunoassay of swab specimens can serve as a useful adjunct to the throat culture. While precise figures on sensitivity and specificity vary among studies, the rapid diagnostic kits generally are >95% specific. Thus a positive result can be relied upon for definitive diagnosis and eliminates the need for a throat culture. However, because the rapid diagnostic tests are less sensitive than throat culture (with a relative sensitivity ranging from 55 to 90% in comparative studies), a negative result should be confirmed with a throat culture.

℞ TREATMENT

In the usual course of uncomplicated streptococcal pharyngitis, symptoms resolve after 3 to 5 days. The course is shortened little by treatment, which is given primarily to prevent suppurative complications and rheumatic fever. Prevention of rheumatic fever depends on eradication of the organism from the pharynx, not simply on resolution of symptoms, and requires 10 days of penicillin treatment—either a single intramuscular dose of benzathine penicillin G or a 10-day course of oral penicillin (Table 121-3). Erythromycin may be substituted for penicillin in the treatment of individuals allergic to penicillin. Once-daily azithromycin is a more convenient but expensive alternative. Although azithromycin is approved for a 5-day course of treatment, only limited data support equivalent efficacy to a standard 10-day treatment course. Resistance to erythromycin and other macrolides is common in isolates from several countries, including Spain, Italy, Finland, Japan, and Korea. Macrolide resistance may be becoming more prevalent elsewhere with the increasing use of this class of antibiotics. In areas in which resistance rates exceed 5 to 10%, macrolides should be avoided unless results of susceptibility testing are known. Follow-up culture after treatment is no longer routinely recommended but may be warranted in selected cases, such as those involving patients or families with frequent streptococcal infections or those occurring in situations in which the risk of rheumatic fever is thought to be high (e.g., when cases of rheumatic fever have recently been reported in the community).

COMPLICATIONS Suppurative complications of streptococcal pharyngitis have become uncommon with the widespread use of antibiotics for most cases of symptomatic streptococcal infection. The complications result from the spread of infection from the pharyngeal mucosa to deeper tissues by direct extension or by the hematogenous or lymphatic route and may include cervical lymphadenitis, peritonsillar or retropharyngeal abscess, sinusitis, otitis media, meningitis, bacteremia, endocarditis, and pneumonia. Local complications, such as abscess formation in the peritonsillar or parapharyngeal space, should be considered in a patient with unusually severe or prolonged symptoms or localized pain associated with high fever and a toxic appearance. Nonsuppurative complications include acute rheumatic fever (Chap. 302) and poststreptococcal glomerulonephritis (Chap. 264), both of which are thought to result from immune responses to streptococcal infection. Penicillin treatment of streptococcal pharyngitis has been shown to reduce the likelihood of acute rheumatic fever but not that of poststreptococcal glomerulonephritis.

Bacteriologic Treatment Failure and the Asymptomatic Carrier State Surveillance cultures have shown that up to 20% of individuals in certain populations may have asymptomatic pharyngeal colonization with group A streptococci. There are no definitive guidelines for management of these asymptomatic carriers or of asymptomatic individuals who still have a positive throat culture after a full course of treatment for symptomatic pharyngitis. A reasonable course of action is to give a single 10-day course of penicillin for symptomatic pharyngitis and, if positive cultures persist, not to re-treat unless symptoms recur. Studies of the natural history of streptococcal carriage and infection have shown that the risk both of developing rheumatic fever and of transmitting infection to others is substantially lower among asymptomatic carriers than among individuals with symptomatic pharyngitis. Therefore, overly aggressive attempts to eradicate carriage are probably not justified under most circumstances. An exception is the situation in which an asymptomatic carrier is a potential source of infection to others. Outbreaks of food-borne infection and nosocomial puerperal infection have been traced to asymptomatic carriers who may harbor the organisms in the throat, on the skin, or in the vagina or anus.

℞ TREATMENT

In cases in which a carrier is transmitting infection to others, attempts to eradicate carriage are warranted, although data are limited on the best regimen to use to clear the organism after penicillin alone has failed. The combination of penicillin V (500 mg four times daily for 10 days) and rifampin (600 mg twice daily for the last 4 days) has been used to eliminate pharyngeal carriage. A 10-day course of oral vancomycin (250 mg four times daily) and rifampin (600 mg twice daily) has eradicated rectal colonization. However, experience is not extensive with any regimen.

Scarlet Fever Scarlet fever consists of streptococcal infection, usually pharyngitis, accompanied by a characteristic rash (Fig. 121-1). The rash arises from the effects of one of three toxins, currently designated streptococcal pyrogenic exotoxins A, B, and C, and previously known as erythrogenic or scarlet fever toxins. In the past, scarlet fever was thought to reflect infection of an individual lacking toxin-specific immunity with a toxin-producing strain of group A *Streptococcus*. Susceptibility to scarlet fever was correlated with results of the Dick test, in which a small amount of erythrogenic toxin injected intradermally produced local erythema in susceptible individuals but elicited no re-

TABLE 121-3 *Treatment of Group A Streptococcal Infections*

Infection	Treatment[a]
Pharyngitis	Benzathine penicillin G, 1.2 mU IM; *or* penicillin V, 250 mg PO tid or 500 mg PO bid × 10 days (Children <27 kg: Benzathine penicillin G, 600,000 units IM; *or* penicillin V, 250 mg PO bid or tid × 10 days)
Impetigo	Same as pharyngitis
Erysipelas/cellulitis	Severe: Penicillin G, 1–2 mU IV q4h Mild to moderate: Procaine penicillin, 1.2 mU IM bid
Necrotizing fasciitis/myositis	Surgical debridement; *plus* penicillin G, 2–4 mU IV q4h; *plus* clindamycin,[b] 600–900 mg q8h
Pneumonia/empyema	Penicillin G, 2–4 mU IV q4h; *plus* drainage of empyema
Streptococcal toxic shock syndrome	Penicillin G, 2–4 mU IV q4h; *plus* clindamycin,[b] 600–900 mg q8h; *plus* intravenous immunoglobulin,[b] 2 g/kg as a single dose

[a] Penicillin allergy: Erythromycin (10 mg/kg PO qid up to a maximum of 250 mg per dose) may be substituted for oral penicillin. Alternative agents for parenteral therapy include first-generation cephalosporins—if the nature of the allergy is not an immediate hypersensitivity reaction (anaphylaxis or urticaria) or another potentially life-threatening manifestation (e.g., severe rash and fever)—or vancomycin.

[b] Efficacy unproven, but recommended by several experts. See text for discussion.

FIGURE 121-1 Scarlet fever exanthem. Finely punctated erythema has become confluent (scarlatiniform); petechiae can occur and have a linear configuration within the exanthem in body folds (Pastia's lines). *(From Fitzpatrick, Johnson, Wolff: Color Atlas and Synopsis of Clinical Dermatology, 4th ed., New York, McGraw-Hill, 2001, with permission.)*

action in those with specific immunity. Subsequent studies have suggested that development of the scarlet fever rash may reflect a hypersensitivity reaction requiring prior exposure to the toxin. For reasons that are not clear, scarlet fever has become less common in recent years, although strains of group A streptococci that produce pyrogenic exotoxins continue to be prevalent in the population.

The symptoms of scarlet fever are the same as those of pharyngitis alone. The rash typically begins on the first or second day of illness over the upper trunk, spreading to involve the extremities but sparing the palms and soles. The rash is made up of minute papules, giving a characteristic "sandpaper" feel to the skin. Associated findings include circumoral pallor, "strawberry tongue" (enlarged papillae on a coated tongue, which later may become denuded), and accentuation of the rash in the skin folds (Pastia's lines). Subsidence of the rash in 6 to 9 days is followed after several days by desquamation of the palms and soles. The differential diagnosis of scarlet fever includes other causes of fever and generalized rash, such as measles and other viral exanthems, Kawasaki disease, toxic shock syndrome, and systemic allergic reactions (e.g., drug eruptions).

Skin and Soft Tissue Infections Group A streptococci—and occasionally other streptococcal species—cause a variety of infections involving the skin, subcutaneous tissues, muscles, and fascia. While several clinical syndromes, recognized according to the tissues involved, offer a useful means for classification of skin and soft tissue infections, not all cases fit exactly into a single category. The classic syndromes should be considered as general guides to predicting the level of tissue involvement in a particular patient, the probable clinical course, and the likelihood that surgical intervention or aggressive life-support will be required.

IMPETIGO (PYODERMA) Impetigo is a superficial infection of the skin caused primarily by group A streptococci and occasionally by other streptococci or by *Staphylococcus aureus*. Impetigo is seen most often in young children, tends to occur during the warmer months, and is more common in semitropical or tropical climates than in cooler regions. Infection is more common among children living under conditions of poor hygiene. Prospective studies have shown that colonization of unbroken skin with group A streptococci precedes the de-

velopment of clinical infection. Minor trauma, such as a scratch or an insect bite, may then serve to inoculate organisms into the skin. Impetigo is best prevented, therefore, by attention to adequate hygiene. The usual sites of involvement are the face (particularly around the nose and mouth) and the legs, although lesions may occur at other locations. Individual lesions begin as red papules, which evolve quickly into vesicular and then pustular lesions that break down and coalesce to form characteristic honeycomb-like crusts (Fig. 121-2). Lesions are generally not painful, and patients do not appear ill. Fever is not a feature of impetigo and, if present, suggests either infection extending to deeper tissues or another diagnosis.

The classic presentation of impetigo usually poses little diagnostic difficulty. Cultures of impetiginous lesions often yield *S. aureus* as well as group A streptococci, but longitudinal studies have shown that, in almost all cases, streptococci can be isolated initially, with staphylococci appearing later, presumably as secondary colonizing flora. In the past, penicillin was nearly always effective against these infections; in recent years, however, penicillin treatment failures have become more common, an observation suggesting that *S. aureus* infection may have become more prominent as a cause of impetigo. *Bullous impetigo due to S. aureus* is distinguished from typical streptococcal infection by the presence of more extensive, bullous lesions that break down and leave thin paper-like crusts instead of the thick amber crusts of streptococcal impetigo. Other skin lesions that may be confused with impetigo include herpetic lesions—either those of orolabial herpes simplex or those of chickenpox or zoster. Herpetic lesions can generally be distinguished by their appearance as more discrete, grouped vesicles and by a positive Tzanck test. In difficult cases, cultures of vesicular fluid should yield group A streptococci in impetigo and the responsible virus in *Herpesvirus* infections.

R_x TREATMENT

Treatment of streptococcal impetigo is the same as that for streptococcal pharyngitis. In view of evidence that *S. aureus* has become a relatively frequent cause of impetigo, empirical regimens should cover both streptococci and *S. aureus*. For example, either dicloxacillin or cephalexin can be given at a dose of 250 mg four times daily for 10 days. Topical mupirocin ointment is also effective. Rheumatic fever is not a sequela to streptococcal skin infections, although poststreptococcal glomerulonephritis may follow either skin or throat infection. The reason for this difference is not known. One hypothesis is that the immune response necessary for development of rheumatic fever occurs only after infection of the pharyngeal mucosa. In addition, the strains of group A streptococci that cause pharyngitis are generally of different M protein types than those associated with skin infections; thus the strains that cause pharyngitis may have rheumatogenic potential, while the skin-infecting strains may not.

FIGURE 121-2 Impetigo contagiosa is a superficial streptococcal or *Staphylococcus aureus* infection consisting of honey-colored crusts and erythematous weeping erosions. Occasionally, bullous lesions may be seen. *(Courtesy of Mary Spraker, MD.)*

CELLULITIS Inoculation of organisms into the skin may lead to infection involving the skin and subcutaneous tissues, or *cellulitis*. The portal of entry may be a traumatic or surgical wound, an insect bite, or any other break in skin integrity. Often, no entry site is apparent.

One form of streptococcal cellulitis, *erysipelas*, is characterized by a bright red appearance of the involved skin, which forms a plateau sharply demarcated from surrounding normal skin (Fig. 121-3). The lesion is warm to the touch, may be tender, and appears shiny and swollen. The skin often has a *peau d' orange* texture, which is thought to reflect involvement of superficial lymphatics; superficial blebs or bullae may form, usually 2 or 3 days after onset. The lesion typically develops over a few hours and is associated with fever and chills. Erysipelas tends to occur in certain characteristic locations: the malar area of the face (often with extension over the bridge of the nose to the contralateral malar region) and the lower extremities. After one episode, recurrence at the same site—sometimes years later—is not uncommon.

Classic cases of erysipelas, with the typical features described above, are almost always due to β-hemolytic streptococci, usually those of group A and occasionally those of group C or G. Often, however, the appearance of streptococcal cellulitis is not sufficiently distinctive to permit a specific diagnosis on clinical grounds. The area of involvement may not be one of the typical sites for erysipelas, the lesion may be less intensely red than usual and may fade into surrounding skin, and/or the patient may appear only mildly ill. In such cases, it is prudent to broaden the spectrum of empiric antimicrobial therapy to include other pathogens, particularly *S. aureus*, that can produce cellulitis with the same appearance. Staphylococcal infection should be suspected if cellulitis develops around a wound or an ulcer.

Streptococcal cellulitis tends to develop at anatomic sites in which normal lymphatic drainage has been disrupted, such as sites of prior episodes of cellulitis, the arm ipsilateral to a mastectomy and axillary lymph node dissection, a lower extremity previously involved in deep venous thrombosis or chronic lymphedema, or the leg from which a saphenous vein has been harvested for coronary artery bypass grafting. The organism may enter via a breach in the dermal barrier at a location some distance from the eventual site of clinical cellulitis. For example, some patients with recurrent episodes of leg cellulitis following saphenous vein removal stop having recurrent episodes only after treatment of tinea pedis on the affected extremity. Fissures in the skin presumably serve as a portal of entry for streptococci, which then produce infection more proximally in the leg at the site of previous injury. Streptococcal cellulitis may also involve recent surgical wounds. Group A streptococci are among the few bacterial pathogens that typically produce signs of wound infection and surrounding cellulitis within the first 24 h after surgery. These wound infections are usually associated with a thin exudate and may spread rapidly, either as cellulitis in the skin and subcutaneous tissue or as a deeper tissue infection (see below). Streptococcal wound infection or localized cellulitis may also be associated with *lymphangitis*, manifested by red streaks extending proximally along superficial lymphatics from the site of infection.

FIGURE 121-3 Erysipelas is a streptococcal infection of the superficial dermis and consists of well-demarcated, erythematous, edematous, warm plaques.

Rx TREATMENT

See Table 121-3 and Chap. 110.

Deep Soft-Tissue Infections *Necrotizing fasciitis*, also referred to as *hemolytic streptococcal gangrene*, is an infection involving the superficial and/or deep fascia investing the muscles of an extremity or the trunk. The source of the infection is either the skin, with organisms introduced into the tissue as a result of trauma (sometimes trivial), or the bowel flora, with organisms released during abdominal surgery or from an occult enteric source, such as a diverticular or appendiceal abscess. The site of inoculation in both forms of necrotizing fasciitis may be inapparent and is often some distance from the site of clinical involvement; e.g., the introduction of organisms via minor trauma to the hand may be associated with clinical infection of the tissues overlying the shoulder or chest. In cases associated with the bowel flora, the infection is usually polymicrobial, involving a mixture of anaerobic bacteria (such as *Bacteroides fragilis* or anaerobic streptococci) and facultative organisms (usually gram-negative bacilli). Cases unrelated to contamination from bowel organisms are most commonly caused by group A streptococci, either alone or in combination with other organisms (most often *S. aureus*). Overall, group A streptococci are implicated in about 60% of cases of necrotizing fasciitis. The onset of symptoms is usually quite acute and is marked by severe pain at the site of involvement, malaise, fever, chills, and a toxic appearance. The physical findings, particularly early in the illness, may not be striking, with only minimal erythema of the overlying skin. Pain and tenderness are usually severe; in contrast, in more superficial cellulitis, the skin appearance is more abnormal, but pain and tenderness are only mild or moderate. As the infection progresses (often in a matter of several hours), the severity and extent of symptoms worsen, and skin changes become more evident, with the appearance of dusky or mottled erythema and edema. The marked tenderness of the involved area may evolve into anesthesia as the spreading inflammatory process produces infarction of cutaneous nerves.

Although myositis is more commonly due to *S. aureus* infection, group A streptococci occasionally produce abscesses in skeletal muscles (*streptococcal myositis*), with little or no involvement of the surrounding fascia or overlying skin. The presentation is usually subacute, but a fulminant form has been described in association with severe systemic toxicity, bacteremia, and a high mortality rate. The fulminant form may reflect the same basic disease process as that seen in necrotizing fasciitis, but with the necrotizing inflammatory process extending into the muscles themselves rather than remaining limited to the fascial layers.

Rx TREATMENT

Once necrotizing fasciitis is suspected, early surgical exploration is both diagnostically and therapeutically indicated. Surgery reveals necrosis and inflammatory fluid tracking along the fascial planes above and between muscle groups, without involvement of the muscles themselves. The process usually extends beyond the area of clinical involvement, and extensive debridement is required. Drainage and debridement are central to the management of necrotizing fasciitis; antibiotic treatment is a useful adjunct (Table 121-3), but surgery is life-saving.

Treatment for streptococcal myositis consists of surgical drainage—usually by an open procedure that permits evaluation of the extent of the infection and ensures adequate debridement of involved tissues—and high-dose penicillin (Table 121-3).

Pneumonia and Empyema Group A streptococci are an occasional cause of pneumonia, generally in previously healthy individuals. The onset of symptoms may be abrupt or gradual. Pleuritic chest pain, fever, chills, and dyspnea are the characteristic symptoms. Cough is usually present but may not be prominent. Approximately one-half of patients with group A streptococcal pneumonia have an accompanying pleural effusion. In contrast to the sterile parapneumonic effusions typical of pneumococcal pneumonia, those complicating streptococcal pneumonia are almost always infected. The empyema fluid is usually visible by chest radiography on initial presentation and may enlarge rapidly. These pleural collections should be drained early, as they tend to become loculated rapidly, resulting in a chronic fibrotic reaction that may require thoracotomy for removal.

Bacteremia, Puerperal Sepsis, and Streptococcal Toxic Shock Syndrome Group A streptococcal bacteremia is usually associated with an identifiable local infection. Bacteremia occurs rarely with otherwise uncomplicated pharyngitis, occasionally with cellulitis or pneumonia, and relatively frequently with necrotizing fasciitis. Bacteremia without an identified source raises the possibility of endocarditis, an occult abscess, or osteomyelitis. A variety of focal infections may arise secondarily from streptococcal bacteremia, including endocarditis, meningitis, septic arthritis, osteomyelitis, peritonitis, and visceral abscesses.

Group A streptococci are occasionally implicated in infectious complications of childbirth, usually endometritis and associated bacteremia. In the preantibiotic era, puerperal sepsis was commonly caused by group A streptococci, but currently it is more often caused by group B streptococci. Several nosocomial outbreaks of puerperal infection due to group A streptococci have been traced to an asymptomatic carrier, usually an individual present at the delivery of the infant. The site of carriage may be the skin, throat, anus, or vagina.

Beginning in the late 1980s, several reports described patients who had group A streptococcal infections associated with shock and multisystem organ failure. This syndrome has been called the streptococcal toxic shock syndrome (TSS) because it shares certain features with staphylococcal TSS. In 1993, a case definition for group A streptococcal TSS was formulated by a group of clinicians, microbiologists, and epidemiologists in conjunction with the CDC (Table 121-4). The general features of the illness include fever, hypotension, renal impairment, and respiratory distress syndrome. Various types of rash have been described, but rash usually does not develop. Laboratory abnormalities include a marked shift to the left in the white blood cell differential, with many immature granulocytes; hypocalcemia; hypoalbuminemia; and thrombocytopenia, which usually becomes more pronounced on the second or third day of illness. In contrast to those with staphylococcal TSS, the majority of patients with streptococcal TSS are bacteremic. The most common associated infection is a soft tissue infection—necrotizing fasciitis, myositis, or cellulitis—although a variety of other associated local infections have been described, including pneumonia, peritonitis, osteomyelitis, and myometritis. Streptococcal TSS is associated with a mortality rate of 30%, with most deaths secondary to shock and respiratory failure. Because of its rapidly progressive and lethal course, early recognition of the syndrome is essential. Patients should be given aggressive supportive care in the form of fluid resuscitation, pressors, and mechanical ventilation in addition to antimicrobial therapy and, in cases associated with necrotizing fasciitis, surgical debridement. Exactly why certain patients develop this fulminant syndrome is not known. Early studies of the streptococcal strains isolated from these patients demonstrated a strong association with the production of pyrogenic exotoxin A. This association has been inconsistent in subsequent cases series. Pyrogenic exotoxin A and several other streptococcal exotoxins act as superantigens to trigger release of inflammatory cytokines from T lymphocytes. Fever, shock, and organ dysfunction in streptococcal TSS may reflect, in part, the systemic effects of superantigen-mediated cytokine release.

TABLE 121-4   *Proposed Case Definition for the Streptococcal Toxic Shock Syndrome*[a]

I. Isolation of group A streptococci (*Streptococcus pyogenes*)
   A. From a normally sterile site (e.g., blood, cerebrospinal fluid, pleural or peritoneal fluid, tissue biopsy, surgical wound)
   B. From a nonsterile site (e.g., throat, sputum, vagina, superficial skin lesion)
II. Clinical signs of severity
   A. Hypotension: Systolic blood pressure of ≤90 mmHg in adults or in the 5th percentile for age in children *and*
   B. Two or more of the following signs:
     1. Renal impairment: Serum creatinine level of ≥177 μmol/L (≥2 mg/dL) for adults or at least twice the upper limit of normal for age; in patients with preexisting renal disease, elevation over baseline by a factor of at least 2
     2. Coagulopathy: Platelet count of ≤100 × 10^9/L (100,000/μL) *or* disseminated intravascular coagulation, defined by prolonged clotting times, low fibrinogen level, and the presence of fibrin degradation products
     3. Liver involvement: Alanine aminotransferase (SGOT), aspartate aminotransferase (SGPT), or total bilirubin level at least twice the upper limit of normal for age; in patients with preexisting liver disease, elevation over baseline by a factor of at least 2
     4. Adult respiratory distress syndrome, defined by acute onset of diffuse pulmonary infiltrates and hypoxemia in the absence of cardiac failure; *or* evidence of diffuse capillary leak manifested by acute onset of generalized edema; *or* pleural or peritoneal effusions with hypoalbuminemia
     5. Generalized erythematous macular rash that may desquamate
     6. Soft tissue necrosis, including necrotizing fasciitis or myositis; *or* gangrene

[a] An illness fulfilling criteria IA, IIA, and IIB is defined as a *definite* case. An illness fulfilling criteria IB, IIA, and IIB is defined as a *probable* case if no other etiology for the illness is identified.

Source: Working Group on Severe Streptococcal Infections, 1993.

Rx TREATMENT

In light of the possible role of pyrogenic exotoxins or other streptococcal toxins in streptococcal TSS, treatment of the affected patients with clindamycin has been advocated by some authorities, who argue that, through its direct action on protein synthesis, clindamycin is more effective in rapidly terminating toxin production than penicillin—a cell-wall agent (Table 121-3). Support for this view comes from studies of an experimental model of streptococcal myositis, in which mice treated with clindamycin had a higher rate of survival than those given penicillin. Comparable data on the treatment of human infections are not available. Although clindamycin resistance in group A streptococci is uncommon (<2% among U.S. isolates), it has been documented. Thus, if clindamycin is used for initial treatment of a critically ill patient, penicillin should be given as well until the antibiotic susceptibility of the streptococcal isolate is known.

Intravenous immunoglobulin has been used as adjunctive therapy for streptococcal TSS; pooled immunoglobulin preparations contain antibodies capable of neutralizing the effects of streptococcal toxins (Table 121-3). Anecdotal reports and case series have suggested favorable clinical responses to intravenous immunoglobulin, but no prospective controlled trials of this modality of therapy have yet been reported.

STREPTOCOCCI OF GROUPS C AND G

Group C and group G streptococci are β-hemolytic bacteria that occasionally cause human infections similar to those caused by group A streptococci, including pharyngitis, cellulitis and soft-tissue infections, pneumonia, bacteremia, endocarditis, and septic arthritis. Puerperal sepsis, meningitis, epidural abscess, intraabdominal abscess, urinary tract infection, and neonatal sepsis have also been reported. Group C streptococci are a common cause of infection in domesticated animals, especially horses and cattle, and some human infections have been acquired through contact with animals or through consumption of unpasteurized milk. Bacteremia and septic arthritis more frequently involve group G than group C streptococci. Group C or G streptococcal bacteremia occurs most often in patients who are elderly or chronically ill and, in the absence of an obvious local infection, is likely to reflect endocarditis. Septic arthritis, sometimes involving multiple joints, may complicate endocarditis or develop in its absence.

Rx TREATMENT

Penicillin is the drug of choice for treatment of infections due to group C or G streptococci. Antibiotic treatment is the same as for patients with similar syndromes due to group A *Streptococcus* (Table 121-3). Patients with bacteremia or septic arthritis should receive intravenous penicillin (2 to 4 mU every 4 h). All group C and G streptococci are sensitive to penicillin; nearly all are inhibited in vitro by concentrations of ≤ 0.03 μg/mL. Occasional isolates exhibit tolerance: although inhibited by low concentrations of penicillin, they are killed only by significantly higher concentrations. The clinical significance of tolerance is unknown. Because of the poor clinical response of some patients to penicillin alone, the addition of gentamicin (1 mg/kg every 8 h for patients with normal renal function) is recommended by some authorities for treatment of endocarditis or septic arthritis due to group C or G streptococci; however, combination therapy has not been shown to be superior to treatment with penicillin alone. Patients with joint infections often require repeated aspiration or open drainage and debridement for cure; the response to treatment may be slow, particularly in debilitated patients and those with involvement of more than one joint. Infection of prosthetic joints almost always requires removal of the prosthesis in addition to antibiotic therapy.

GROUP B STREPTOCOCCI

Identified first as a cause of mastitis in cows, streptococci belonging to Lancefield's group B have since been recognized as a major cause of sepsis and meningitis in human neonates. Group B streptococci are also a frequent cause of peripartum fever in women and an occasional cause of serious infection in nonpregnant adults. Lancefield group B consists of a single species, *S. agalactiae*, which is definitively identified with specific antiserum to the group B cell wall–associated carbohydrate antigen. A streptococcal isolate can be classified presumptively as belonging to group B on the basis of biochemical tests, including hydrolysis of sodium hippurate (in which 99% of isolates are positive), hydrolysis of bile esculin agar (in which 99 to 100% are negative), bacitracin susceptibility (in which 92% are resistant), and production of CAMP factor (in which 98 to 100% are positive). CAMP factor is a phospholipase produced by group B streptococci that results in synergistic hemolysis with β lysin produced by certain strains of *S. aureus*. Its presence can be demonstrated by cross-streaking of the test isolate and an appropriate staphylococcal strain on a blood agar plate. Group B streptococci causing human infections are encapsulated by one of nine antigenically distinct polysaccharides. The capsular polysaccharide has been shown experimentally to be important in the virulence of the organism. Antibodies to the capsular polysaccharide afford protection against group B streptococci of the same (but not of a different) capsular type.

INFECTION IN NEONATES   Two general types of group B streptococcal infection in infants are defined by the age of the patient at presentation. *Early-onset infections* occur within the first week of life, with a median age of 20 h at the onset of illness. Approximately half of these infants have signs of group B streptococcal disease at birth. The infection is acquired during or shortly before birth from organisms colonizing the maternal genital tract. Surveillance studies have shown that 5 to 40% of women are vaginal or rectal carriers of group B streptococci. Approximately 50% of infants delivered vaginally by carrier mothers become colonized, although only 1 to 2% of those colonized develop clinically evident infection. Prematurity and maternal risk factors (prolonged labor, obstetric complications, and maternal fever) are often involved. The presentation of early-onset infection is the same as that of other forms of neonatal sepsis. Typical findings include respiratory distress, lethargy, and hypotension. Essentially all infants with early-onset disease are bacteremic, one-third to one-half have pneumonia and/or respiratory distress syndrome, and one-third have meningitis.

Late-onset infections occur in infants between 1 week and 3 months of age, with a mean age at onset of 3 to 4 weeks. The infecting organism may be acquired during delivery (as in early-onset cases) or during later contact with a colonized mother, nursery personnel, or another source. Meningitis is the most common manifestation of late-onset infection and in most cases is associated with a strain of capsular type III of the organism. Infants present with fever, lethargy or irritability, poor feeding, and seizures. The various other types of late-onset infection include bacteremia without an identified source, osteomyelitis, septic arthritis, and facial cellulitis associated with submandibular or preauricular adenitis.

Rx TREATMENT

Penicillin is the treatment of choice for all group B streptococcal infections. Empiric broad-spectrum therapy for suspected bacterial sepsis, consisting of ampicillin and gentamicin, is generally administered until culture results become available. If cultures yield group B streptococci, many pediatricians continue to administer gentamicin, along with ampicillin or penicillin, for a few days until clinical improvement becomes evident. Infants with bacteremia or soft-tissue infection should receive penicillin at a dosage of 200,000 units/kg per day in divided doses; those with meningitis should receive 400,000 units/kg per day. Meningitis should be treated for at least 14 days because of the risk of relapse with shorter courses.

Prevention   The incidence of group B streptococcal infection is unusually high among infants of women with risk factors: preterm delivery, early rupture of membranes (>24 h before delivery), prolonged labor, fever, or chorioamnionitis. Because the usual source of the organisms infecting a neonate is the mother's birth canal, efforts have been made to prevent group B streptococcal infections by the identification of high-risk carrier mothers and their treatment with various forms of antibiotic or immunoprophylaxis. Prophylactic administration of ampicillin or penicillin to such patients during delivery has been shown to reduce the risk of infection in the newborn. This approach has been hampered by the logistical difficulties of identifying colonized women before delivery, since the results of vaginal cultures early in pregnancy are poor predictors of carrier status at delivery. The CDC has recommended that women be screened for anogenital colonization at 35 to 37 weeks of pregnancy by means of a swab culture of the lower vagina and anorectum; intrapartum chemoprophylaxis is recommended for women who are culture-positive and to all women, regardless of culture status, who have previously given birth to an infant with group B streptococcal infection or who have a history of group B streptococcal bacteriuria during pregnancy. Women whose culture status is unknown and who develop premature labor (<37 weeks), prolonged rupture of membranes (>18 h), or intrapartum fever should also receive intrapartum chemoprophylaxis. The recommended regimen for chemoprophylaxis is 5 million units of penicillin G followed by 2.5 million units every 4 h until delivery. Cefazolin is an alternative for women with a history of penicillin allergy who are thought not to be at high risk for anaphylaxis. For women with a history of an immediate hypersensitivity reaction, clindamycin or erythromycin may be substituted, but only if the colonizing isolate has been demonstrated to be susceptible. If susceptibility testing results are not available or indicate resistance, vancomycin should be used in this situation.

Treatment of all pregnant women who are colonized or who have risk factors for neonatal infection will result in exposure of 15 to 25% of pregnant women and newborns to antibiotics, with the attendant risks of allergic reactions and selection for resistant organisms. Although still in the developmental stages, a group B streptococcal vaccine may ultimately offer a better solution to prevention. Because transplacental passage of maternal antibodies produces protective antibody levels in the newborn, efforts are under way to develop a vaccine against group B streptococci that can be given to childbearing women before or during pregnancy. Results of phase 1 clinical trials of group B streptococcal capsular polysaccharide–protein conjugate vaccines suggest that a multivalent conjugate vaccine would be safe and highly immunogenic.

INFECTION IN ADULTS   The majority of group B streptococcal infections in adults are related to pregnancy and parturition. Peripartum fever, the most common manifestation, is sometimes accompanied by symptoms and signs of endometritis or chorioamnionitis (abdominal distention and uterine or adnexal tenderness). Blood cultures are often positive, as are cultures of vaginal swabs. Bacteremia is usually transitory but occasionally results in meningitis or endocarditis. Infections in adults that are not associated with the peripartum period generally involve individuals who are elderly or have some underlying chronic illness, such as diabetes mellitus or a malignancy. Among the infections that develop with some frequency in adults are cellulitis and soft tissue infection (including infected diabetic skin ulcers), urinary tract infection, pneumonia, endocarditis, and septic arthritis. Other reported infections include meningitis, osteomyelitis, and intraabdominal or pelvic abscesses.

℞ TREATMENT

Group B streptococci are less sensitive to penicillin than group A organisms, requiring somewhat higher doses. Adults with serious localized infections (pneumonia, pyelonephritis, abscess) should receive doses in the range of 12 million units of penicillin G daily, while patients with endocarditis or meningitis should receive 18 to 24 million units per day in divided doses. Vancomycin is an acceptable alternative for patients allergic to penicillin.

ENTEROCOCCI AND NONENTEROCOCCAL GROUP D STREPTOCOCCI

ENTEROCOCCI   Lancefield group D includes the enterococci, organisms now classified in a separate genus from other streptococci, and nonenterococcal group D streptococci. Enterococci are distinguished from nonenterococcal group D streptococci by their ability to grow in the presence of 6.5% sodium chloride and by the results of other biochemical tests. The enterococcal species that are significant pathogens for humans are *E. faecalis* and *E. faecium*. These organisms tend to produce infection in patients who are elderly or debilitated or in whom mucosal or epithelial barriers have been disrupted or the balance of the normal flora altered by antibiotic treatment. Urinary tract infections due to enterococci are quite common, particularly among patients who have received antibiotic treatment or undergone instrumentation of the urinary tract. Enterococci are a frequent cause of nosocomial bacteremia in patients with intravascular catheters. These organisms account for 10 to 20% of cases of bacterial endocarditis on both native and prosthetic valves. The presentation of enterococcal endocarditis is usually subacute but may be acute, with rapidly progressive valve destruction. Enterococci are frequently cultured from bile and are involved in infectious complications of biliary surgery and in liver abscesses. Moreover, enterococci are often isolated from polymicrobial infections arising from the bowel flora (e.g., intraabdominal abscesses), from abdominal surgical wounds, and from diabetic foot ulcers. While such mixed infections are frequently cured by antimicrobials not active against enterococci, specific therapy directed against enterococci is warranted when these organisms are the predominant species or are isolated from blood cultures.

℞ TREATMENT

Unlike streptococci, enterococci are not reliably killed by penicillin or ampicillin alone at concentrations achieved clinically in the blood or tissues. Ampicillin reaches sufficiently high urinary concentrations to constitute adequate monotherapy for uncomplicated urinary tract infections. Because in vitro testing has shown evidence of synergistic killing of most enterococcal strains by the combination of penicillin or ampicillin with an aminoglycoside, combined therapy is recommended for enterococcal endocarditis and meningitis; the regimen is penicillin (3 to 4 million units every 4 h) or ampicillin (2 g every 4 h) plus moderate-dose gentamicin (1 mg/kg every 8 h for patients with normal renal function). Enterococcal endocarditis should be treated for

a minimum of 4 weeks and for 6 weeks if symptoms have been present for ≥3 months or if the infection involves a prosthetic heart valve. For nonendocarditis bacteremia and other serious enterococcal infections, it is not known whether the efficacy of single-agent β-lactam therapy is improved by the addition of gentamicin, but many infectious disease specialists use combination therapy for such infections, especially in critically ill patients. Vancomycin, in combination with gentamicin, may be substituted for penicillin in allergic patients. Enterococci are resistant to all cephalosporins; therefore, this class of antibiotics should not be used for treatment of enterococcal infections.

Antimicrobial susceptibility testing should be performed routinely on enterococcal isolates from patients with serious infections, and therapy should be adjusted according to the results (Table 121-5). Most enterococci are resistant to streptomycin, and this drug should not be used for treatment of enterococcal infection unless in vitro testing of the strain indicates susceptibility. Though less widespread than streptomycin resistance, high-level resistance to gentamicin—with a minimum inhibitory concentration (MIC) of >2000 μg/mL—has become common. Gentamicin-resistant enterococci should be tested for susceptibility to streptomycin; occasional gentamicin-resistant enterococci are sensitive to streptomycin. If the isolate is resistant to all aminoglycosides, treatment with penicillin or ampicillin alone may be successful. The prolonged administration (i.e., for at least 6 weeks) of high-dose ampicillin (e.g., 12 g/d) is recommended for endocarditis due to these highly resistant enterococci.

Enterococci may be resistant to penicillins via two distinct mechanisms. The first is the production of β-lactamase (mediating resistance to penicillin and ampicillin), which has been reported for *E. faecalis* isolates from several locations in the United States and other countries. Because the amount of β-lactamase produced by enterococci may be insufficient for detection by routine antibiotic susceptibility testing, isolates from serious infections should be screened specifically for β-lactamase production with use of a chromogenic cephalosporin or by another method. For the treatment of β-lactamase-producing strains, vancomycin, ampicillin/sulbactam, amoxicillin/clavulanate, or imipenem may be used in combination with gentamicin.

The second mechanism of penicillin resistance is not mediated by β-lactamase and may be due to altered penicillin-binding proteins. This intrinsic penicillin resistance is common among *E. faecium* isolates, which routinely are more resistant to β-lactam antibiotics than are isolates of *E. faecalis*. Moderately resistant enterococci (MICs of penicillin and ampicillin, 16 to 64 μg/mL) may be susceptible to high-dose penicillin or ampicillin plus gentamicin, but strains with MICs of ≥200 μg/mL must be considered resistant to clinically achievable levels of β-lactam antibiotics, including imipenem. Vancomycin plus gentamicin is the recommended regimen for infections due to enterococci with high-level intrinsic resistance to β-lactams.

Vancomycin-resistant enterococci, first reported from clinical sources in the late 1980s, have become common in many hospitals.

TABLE 121-5   *Treatment Options for Antibiotic-Resistant Enterococcal Infections*

Resistance Pattern	Recommended Therapy
β-Lactamase production	Gentamicin plus ampicillin/sulbactam, amoxicillin/clavulanate, imipenem, or vancomycin
β-Lactam resistance, but no β-lactamase production	Gentamicin plus vancomycin
High-level gentamicin resistance	Streptomycin-sensitive isolate: Streptomycin plus ampicillin or vancomycin Streptomycin-resistant isolate: No proven therapy (continuous-infusion ampicillin, prolonged treatment)
Vancomycin resistance	Ampicillin plus gentamicin
Vancomycin and β-lactam resistance	No uniformly bactericidal drugs; linezolid (all enterococci) or quinupristin/dalfopristin (*E. faecium* only)

Three major vancomycin resistance phenotypes have been described: VanA, VanB, and VanC. The VanA phenotype is associated with high-level resistance to vancomycin and to teicoplanin, a related glycopeptide antibiotic not currently available in the United States. VanB and VanC strains are resistant to vancomycin but susceptible to teicoplanin, although teicoplanin resistance may develop during treatment in VanB strains. For enterococci resistant to both vancomycin and β-lactams, there are no established therapies that provide uniformly bactericidal activity. Regimens that have been tried with some success in individual cases or experimentally include ciprofloxacin plus rifampin plus gentamicin; ampicillin plus vancomycin (particularly if in vitro testing shows synergistic bacteriostatic activity); and chloramphenicol or tetracycline (if the strain is susceptible in vitro). Two newer agents with activity against vancomycin-resistant enterococci are quinupristin/dalfopristin and linezolid, which were approved for use in the United States in 1999 and 2000, respectively. Quinupristin/dalfopristin is a streptogramin combination with in vitro bacteriostatic activity against *E. faecium*, including vancomycin-resistant isolates, but not against *E. faecalis* or other enterococcal species. Favorable clinical responses have been obtained in approximately three-quarters of patients treated with this agent. Linezolid is an oxazolidinone antibiotic with good bacteriostatic activity against nearly all enterococci, including vancomycin-resistant enterococci. Limited clinical experience suggests that linezolid is at least as efficacious as quinupristin/dalfopristin.

OTHER GROUP D STREPTOCOCCI   The main nonenterococcal group D streptococcal species that causes human infections is *S. bovis*. *S. bovis* endocarditis is often associated with neoplasms of the gastrointestinal tract—most frequently a colon carcinoma or polyp—but is also reported in association with other bowel lesions. When occult gastrointestinal lesions are carefully sought, abnormalities are found in $\geq$60% of patients with *S. bovis* endocarditis. In contrast to the enterococci, nonenterococcal group D streptococci like *S. bovis* are reliably killed by penicillin as a single agent, and penicillin is the treatment of choice for *S. bovis* infections.

VIRIDANS AND OTHER STREPTOCOCCI

VIRIDANS STREPTOCOCCI   Consisting of multiple species of α-hemolytic streptococci, the viridans streptococci are a heterogeneous group of organisms that are important as agents of bacterial endocarditis (Chap. 109). Several species of viridans streptococci, including *S. salivarius*, *S. mitis*, *S. sanguis*, and *S. mutans*, are part of the normal flora of the mouth, where they live in close association with the teeth and gingiva. Some species contribute to the development of dental caries. The transient viridans streptococcal bacteremia induced by eating, tooth-brushing, flossing, and other sources of minor trauma, together with adherence to biologic surfaces, is thought to account for the predilection of these organisms to cause endocarditis (see Fig. 109-1). Viridans streptococci are also isolated, often as part of a mixed flora, from sites of sinusitis, brain abscess, and liver abscess.

Viridans streptococcal bacteremia occurs relatively frequently in neutropenic patients, particularly after bone marrow transplantation or high-dose chemotherapy for cancer. Some of these patients develop a sepsis syndrome with high fever and shock. Risk factors for viridans streptococcal bacteremia include chemotherapy with high-dose cytosine arabinoside, prior treatment with trimethoprim-sulfamethoxazole or a fluoroquinolone, treatment with antacids or histamine antagonists, mucositis, and profound neutropenia.

The *S. milleri* group (also referred to as the *S. intermedius* or *S. anginosus* group) includes three species that cause human disease: *S. intermedius*, *S. anginosus*, and *S. constellatus*. These organisms are often considered viridans streptococci, although they differ somewhat from other viridans streptococci in both their hemolytic pattern (they may be α-, β-, or nonhemolytic) and the disease syndromes they cause. This group commonly produces suppurative infections, particularly

abscesses of brain and abdominal viscera, and infections related to the oral cavity or respiratory tract, such as peritonsillar abscess, lung abscess, and empyema.

TREATMENT

Isolates from neutropenic patients with bacteremia are often resistant to penicillin; thus these patients should be treated presumptively with vancomycin until the results of susceptibility testing become available. Viridans streptococci isolated in other clinical settings usually are sensitive to penicillin.

ABIOTROPHIA SPECIES (NUTRITIONALLY VARIANT STREPTOCOCCI)

Occasional isolates cultured from the blood of patients with endocarditis fail to grow when subcultured on solid media. These *nutritionally variant streptococci* require supplemental thiol compounds or active forms of vitamin B$_6$ (pyridoxal or pyridoxamine) for growth in the laboratory. The nutritionally variant streptococci are generally grouped with the viridans streptococci because they cause similar types of infections. However, they have been reclassified on the basis of 16S ribosomal RNA sequence comparisons into a separate genus, *Abiotrophia*, with two species: *A. defectivus* and *A. adjacens*.

TREATMENT

Treatment failure and relapse appear to be more common in cases of endocarditis due to nutritionally variant streptococci than in those due to the usual viridans streptococci. Thus the addition of gentamicin (1 mg/kg every 8 h for patients with normal renal function) to the penicillin regimen is recommended in therapy for endocarditis due to the nutritionally variant organisms.

OTHER STREPTOCOCCI

S. suis is an important pathogen in swine and has been reported to cause meningitis in humans, usually in individuals with occupational exposure to pigs. Strains of *S. suis* associated with human infections have generally reacted with Lancefield group R typing serum and sometimes with group D typing serum as well. Isolates may be α- or β-hemolytic and are sensitive to penicillin. *S. iniae*, a pathogen of fish, has been associated with infections in humans who have handled live or freshly killed fish. Cellulitis of the hand is the most common form of human infection, although bacteremia and endocarditis have been reported. *Anaerobic streptococci*, or *peptostreptococci*, are part of the normal flora of the oral cavity, bowel, and vagina. Infections caused by the anaerobic streptococci are discussed in Chap. 148.

FURTHER READING

BISNO AL, STEVENS DL: Streptococcal infections of skin and soft tissues. N Engl J Med 334:240, 1996

——— et al: Practice guidelines for the diagnosis and management of group A streptococcal pharyngitis. Clin Infect Dis 35:113, 2002

BRUCKNER LB et al: High incidence of penicillin resistance among α-hemolytic streptococci isolated from the blood of children with cancer. J Pediatr 140:20, 2002

CENTERS FOR DISEASE CONTROL AND PREVENTION: Prevention of perinatal group B streptococcal disease. MMWR 51(RR-11):1, 2002

EDWARDS MS, BAKER CJ: *Streptococcus agalactiae* (group B *Streptococcus*), in *Principles and Practice of Infectious Diseases*, 5th ed, GL Mandell et al (eds). New York, Churchill Livingstone, 2000

GOLD HS: Vancomycin-resistant enterococci: Mechanism and clinical observations. Clin Infect Dis 33:210, 2001

JACKSON LA et al: Risk factors for group B streptococcal disease in adults. Ann Intern Med 123:415, 1995

KAUL R et al: Intravenous immunoglobulin therapy for streptococcal toxic shock syndrome—a comparative observational study. The Canadian Streptococcal Study Group. Clin Infect Dis 28:800, 1999

ZURAWSKI CA et al: Invasive group A streptococcal disease in metropolitan Atlanta: A population-based assessment. Clin Infect Dis 27:150, 1998

DIPHTHERIA

DEFINITION Diphtheria is a localized infection of mucous membranes or skin that is caused by *Corynebacterium diphtheriae* and may be associated with a characteristic pseudomembrane at the site of infection (Fig. 122-1). Some strains of *C. diphtheriae* produce diphtheria toxin, a protein that can cause myocarditis, polyneuropathy, and other systemic toxic effects. Respiratory diphtheria is usually caused by toxinogenic (tox+) *C. diphtheriae*, but infections of the skin (cutaneous diphtheria) and other anatomical sites are often caused by nontoxinogenic (tox−) *C. diphtheriae*. Respiratory diphtheria caused by either tox+ or tox− isolates of *C. diphtheriae*—but not cutaneous diphtheria—is a nationally notifiable infectious disease in the United States.

ETIOLOGY *C. diphtheriae* is an aerobic, nonmotile, nonsporulating, irregularly staining, gram-positive rod. The bacteria are club-shaped and are often arranged in clusters (*Chinese letters*) or parallel arrays (*palisades*). Selective media containing either tellurite or colistin plus nalidixic acid are recommended for cultivation of *C. diphtheriae*. The gravis, mitis, and intermedius biotypes are distinguished by colonial morphology and laboratory tests. Both tox+ and tox− strains are infectious, but tox+ strains can produce toxemic diphtheria and are more likely to cause pseudomembranes. Diphtheria toxin is encoded by specific corynephages, and tox− *C. diphtheriae* (or other *Corynebacterium* species, such as *C. ulcerans* and *C. pseudotuberculosis*) can acquire the ability to produce diphtheria toxin by infection with tox+ phages (*phage conversion*). Growth of *C. diphtheriae* under low-iron conditions that mimic the environment of host tissues induces production of diphtheria toxin and expression of systems for siderophore-dependent iron uptake, utilization of iron from heme, and several other iron-regulated functions.

IMMUNOLOGY Treatment of diphtheria toxin with formaldehyde converts it to a nontoxic but immunogenic product (*diphtheria toxoid*). Immunization with toxoid elicits antibody (*antitoxin*) that neutralizes the toxin and prevents diphtheria. The attack rate and mortality rate

FIGURE 122-1 Pseudomembrane of diphtheria. Diphtheria is now a rare cause of exudative pharyngitis in the United States, but outbreaks continue to occur in underimmunized countries and regions. The pharyngitis has an acute onset, is characterized by severe dysphagia, and is accompanied by a thick, tenacious, gray-white exudate on the tonsils, uvula, and pharynx. As the exudate coagulates, it forms a so-called pseudomembrane, which may result in respiratory obstruction. [*From Upper Respiratory and Head and Neck Infections, Vol. IV, I. Brook (ed), in Atlas of Infectious Diseases, GL Mandell (ed). Philadelphia, Current Medicine, Inc., with permission.*]

for diphtheria are low in immune individuals with antitoxin titers of >0.01 unit per milliliter. Antitoxin neither prevents colonization by *C. diphtheriae* nor eradicates the *carrier state*. When most individuals in a population have protective levels of antitoxin (*herd immunity*), the carrier rate for tox+ strains of *C. diphtheriae* falls to a low level, and the risk that susceptible individuals will be exposed to tox+ *C. diphtheriae* decreases dramatically. Susceptible individuals may contract diphtheria if they travel to regions where the disease is present or if tox+ strains of *C. diphtheriae* are introduced into their community.

EPIDEMIOLOGY AND IMMUNITY Humans are the principal reservoir for *C. diphtheriae*. Transmission occurs primarily by close personal contact. The risk that *C. diphtheriae* will be transmitted to susceptible individuals from patients with diphtheria is greater than the risk that it will be transmitted to them from carriers. The incubation period for respiratory diphtheria is typically 2 to 5 days (range, 1 to 10 days). Cutaneous diphtheria is usually a secondary infection whose signs develop an average of 7 days (range, 1 to >21 days) after the appearance of other primary dermatologic lesions.

In temperate climates, diphtheria primarily involves the respiratory tract. It occurs throughout the year, with a peak incidence in colder months, and it is usually caused by tox+ *C. diphtheriae*. Before immunization was introduced, diphtheria was primarily a disease of children; it affected up to 10% of individuals in this group and sometimes caused devastating epidemics. Most young infants were immune because of transplacental transfer of maternal IgG antitoxin, but children became susceptible by 6 to 12 months of age. Approximately 75% of individuals became immune by 10 years of age as a result of contact with *C. diphtheriae*. Mortality rates of 30 to 40% were common in untreated disease and were sometimes >50% in epidemics. Treatment with antitoxin reduced the case-fatality rate to 5 to 10%.

Routine immunization of children in the United States resulted in a progressive decrease of diphtheria from the peak of 206,939 cases (incidence rate, 191 cases per 100,000 population) in 1921 to ≤5 cases per year since 1980. Circulation of tox+ strains of *C. diphtheriae* among the population decreased dramatically throughout this period, but endemic foci of clonally related tox+ and tox− strains, belonging predominantly to the ET215 complex, have persisted for the past 25 years in South Dakota and Ontario. As the incidence of diphtheria decreased, a higher proportion of cases occurred in older persons (who were never immunized or whose immunity waned because they did not receive booster doses of vaccine or did not have contact with *C. diphtheriae*), but the case-fatality ratio remained unchanged at 5 to 10%. High rates of immunization are achieved by school entry (>96%), but immunization rates for younger children are substantially lower. Immunity to diphtheria among adults declines gradually with increasing age, and only 30% of men in the 60- to 69-year-old age group have protective levels of diphtheria antitoxin. Among adults immunity to diphtheria is typically lower among women than among men; likewise, it is lower among Mexican-Americans than among other racial or ethnic groups. The most recent large diphtheria outbreak in the United States (about 1100 cases) occurred in Seattle, Washington, between 1972 and 1982. Alcoholism, low socioeconomic status, crowded living conditions, and Native-American ethnic background were significant risk factors in this outbreak.

A massive diphtheria epidemic (>157,000 cases and >5000 deaths) occurred during the 1990s in Russia and the newly independent states of the former Soviet Union and accounted for >80% of diphtheria cases reported worldwide during that decade. The epidemic began in 1990 with 1436 cases (0.49 per 100,000 population) and peaked in 1995 with 50,425 cases (17.29 per 100,000 population). Clonally related tox+ *C. diphtheriae* stains of the ET8 complex, which constituted only a small percentage of archival *C. diphtheriae* isolates from Russia before that epidemic, increased dramatically in prevalence, accounting for >80% of isolates by 1994. Molecular analysis of *tox* gene alleles from isolates of the ET8 complex demonstrated that the existing diphtheria toxoid vaccine remained appropriate for ongoing use as a protective immunogen, and a mass vaccination program succeeded in reducing the number of cases to 2720 in 1998 (0.93 per 100,000 population). A majority of cases throughout this epidemic occurred in persons ≥15 years old, and adults from 40 to 49 years old had very high incidence and death rates. In 1994, case-fatality rates varied from 2.8% in the Russian Federation to 23% in Lithuania and Turkmenistan. Factors that facilitated the spread of this epidemic included large-scale population movements, socioeconomic instability, deteriorating health infrastructure, delayed implementation of aggressive control measures in response to the epidemic, inadequate information for physicians and the public, and frequent shortages of supplies for prevention and treatment of the disease. The most important risk factor for diphtheria in the Republic of Georgia was lack of vaccination (matched odds ratio, 19.?), but household diphtheria exposure, exposure to skin lesions, the presence of tonsils, a history of eczema, preceding fever with myalgia, sharing a bed, sharing glasses and cups, and taking a bath less often than weekly were also significant risk factors. Although small numbers of imported cases from this epidemic occurred in western European countries, none resulted in secondary transmission of diphtheria, notwithstanding a high proportion of susceptible adults in countries with imported cases. Inadequate primary immunization of children in the states of the former Soviet Union in the years preceding the epidemic, along with failure to maintain adequate immunity in adults by booster immunization, appear to have been primary factors in the development of the massive diphtheria epidemic in this region.

In the tropics, cutaneous diphtheria is more common than respiratory diphtheria, occurs throughout the year, and often develops as a secondary infection complicating other dermatoses. Isolates of *C. diphtheriae* from skin lesions are more often tox⁻ than tox⁺. Cutaneous diphtheria is increasingly recognized in temperate climates and accounted for 86% of the 1100 cases in the Seattle epidemic of 1972 to 1982. Since 1980, cutaneous diphtheria has not been a reportable disease in the United States, and recent health statistics include only respiratory diphtheria.

During the 1990s, tox⁻ strains of *C. diphtheriae* were associated with new types of infections. In the United Kingdom, these strains caused symptomatic pharyngitis, predominantly among homosexual men, that was sometimes accompanied by tonsillar exudate. In Switzerland, strains with a high potential for invasiveness were isolated from 38 intravenous drug users and shown by ribotyping to be clonally related. The latter strains caused infections of the skin (15 cases), respiratory tract (10 cases), and blood (13 cases). Among the patients with bloodstream infections, 9 had endocarditis, and 4 of these 9 patients died.

PATHOLOGY AND PATHOGENESIS *C. diphtheriae* infects mucous membranes, most commonly in the respiratory tract, and also invades open skin lesions resulting from insect bites or trauma. In infections caused by tox⁺ *C. diphtheriae*, initial edema and hyperemia are often followed by epithelial necrosis and acute inflammation. Coagulation of the dense fibrinopurulent exudate produces a pseudomembrane (Fig. 122-1), and the inflammatory reaction accompanied by vascular congestion extends into the underlying tissues. The pseudomembrane contains large numbers of *C. diphtheriae* organisms, but the bacteria are rarely isolated from the blood or internal organs.

Diphtheria toxin acts both locally and systemically, and the lethal dose for humans is ~0.1 µg/kg. Toxin contributes locally to pseudomembrane formation; systemically, it can cause myocarditis, polyneuropathy, and focal necrosis in various organs, including the kidneys, liver, and adrenal glands. Changes in the myocardium include cloudy swelling of muscle fibers and interstitial edema. These changes are followed within weeks by hyaline and granular degeneration (sometimes with fatty degeneration), progressing to myolysis and finally to the replacement of lost muscle by fibrosis. Thus, diphtheria can cause permanent cardiac damage. In diphtheritic polyneuropathy, pathologic changes include patchy breakdown of myelin sheaths in peripheral and autonomic nerves, but recovery of nerve damage is the rule if the patient survives.

Diphtheria toxin is produced by *C. diphtheriae* as an extracellular polypeptide. Proteolytic cleavage of the intact toxin forms nicked toxin consisting of fragments A and B. Fragment B binds to a plasma-membrane receptor (a precursor of a heparin-binding growth factor resembling epidermal growth factor), and the bound toxin is internalized by receptor-mediated endocytosis. Fragment A is translocated across the membrane of acidified endosomes and released into the cytoplasm, where it catalyzes the transfer of the adenosine diphosphate ribose moiety from nicotinamide adenine dinucleotide (NAD) to a modified histidine residue (diphthamide) on elongation factor 2 (EF-2), thereby inactivating EF-2 and inhibiting protein synthesis. One molecule of fragment A in the cytoplasm can kill a cell. Other metabolic alterations are secondary to inhibition of protein synthesis.

CLINICAL MANIFESTATIONS ■ Respiratory Diphtheria The current epidemiologic case definition of diphtheria used by the Centers for Disease Control and Prevention (CDC) is based on both a clinical syndrome [upper respiratory tract illness with sore throat, low-grade fever, and an adherent membrane of the tonsil(s), pharynx, and/or nose] and laboratory criteria (isolation of *C. diphtheriae* from a clinical specimen or a histopathologic diagnosis of diphtheria). Clinically compatible cases are classified as *confirmed* if they are either confirmed by the laboratory or epidemiologically linked to a laboratory-confirmed case and as *probable* if they are neither confirmed by the laboratory nor linked to a laboratory-confirmed case. By these criteria, both asymptomatic individuals and patients with respiratory findings but no pseudomembrane are classified as *carriers* if *C. diphtheriae* is isolated from the respiratory tract. On clinical grounds, diphtheria is graded as *tonsillar* if pseudomembranes are localized to the tonsils, as *combined types* or *delayed diagnosis* if more extensive pseudomembranes are present, and as *severe* if cervical adenopathy or cervical edema is also present. Onset is often gradual, but most patients seek medical care within a few days of becoming ill. Fever [a temperature of 37.8° to 38.9°C (100° to 102°F)], sore throat, and weakness are the most common symptoms, while dysphagia, headache, and change of voice occur in fewer than half of patients. Neck edema and difficulty breathing are noted in ≤10% of patients and are associated with an increased risk of death. Systemic manifestations are due primarily to toxic effects of diphtheria toxin. Patients without toxicity exhibit discomfort and malaise associated with local infection, whereas severely toxic patients may develop listlessness, pallor, and tachycardia that can progress rapidly to vascular collapse.

Primary infection in the respiratory tract is most often tonsillopharyngeal but may also be (in decreasing order of frequency) laryngeal, nasal, and tracheobronchial. Multiple sites are frequently involved, and secondary spread of pharyngeal infection upward to the nasal mucosa or downward to the larynx and tracheobronchial tree is much more common than primary infection at those sites. Systemic toxicity is usually most severe when extensive pseudomembrane extends from the tonsils and pharynx into contiguous regions. A small percentage of patients present with malignant or "bull-neck" diphtheria, with extensive pseudomembrane formation, foul breath, massive swelling of the tonsils and uvula, thick speech, cervical lymphadenopathy, striking edematous swelling of the submandibular region and anterior neck, and severe toxicity.

In tonsillopharyngeal diphtheria, isolated spots of gray or white exudate may appear first. These spots often extend and coalesce within a day to form a confluent, sharply demarcated pseudomembrane (Fig. 122-1) that becomes progressively thicker, more tightly adherent to the underlying tissue, and darker gray in color. Unlike the exudate in streptococcal pharyngitis, the diphtheritic pseudomembrane often extends beyond the margin of the tonsils onto the tonsillar pillars, palate, or uvula. Dislodging the membrane is likely to cause bleeding. Laryngeal diphtheria often presents as hoarseness and cough. Demonstration of laryngeal pseudomembrane by laryngoscopy helps distinguish diphtheria from other infectious forms of laryngitis. Patients with nasal diphtheria may present with unilateral or bilateral serosanguineous nasal discharge associated with irritation of the nares or lip. Primary or secondary diphtheritic infection occasionally involves other mucous membranes, including the conjunctiva and the membranes of the genitourinary and gastrointestinal tracts.

Cutaneous Diphtheria Cutaneous diphtheria usually presents as an infection by *C. diphtheriae* of preexisting dermatoses involving the lower extremities, upper extremities, head, or trunk. The clinical features are similar to those of other secondary cutaneous bacterial infections. In the tropics, cutaneous diphtheria may present as a primary cutaneous lesion, typically with morphologically distinct "punched-out" ulcers that are covered by necrotic slough or membrane and have well-demarcated edges.

Other Clinical Presentations *C. diphtheriae* is an occasional cause of invasive infections, including endocarditis and septic arthritis. Risk factors for such infections include preexisting cardiac abnormalities, abuse of intravenous drugs, and alcoholic cirrhosis.

COMPLICATIONS Obstruction of the respiratory tract can be caused by extensive pseudomembrane formation and swelling early in the disease or by sloughed pseudomembrane that becomes lodged in the airways later in the disease. The risk is greater when infection involves the larynx or the tracheobronchial tree and in children because of the small size of the airways.

Myocarditis and polyneuropathy are the prominent toxic manifestations of diphtheria. The risk of each is proportional to the severity of local disease. Myocarditis occurred in 22% and neuropathy in 5% of 656 hospitalized patients (54% female, 70% ≥15 years old) with diphtheria in the Kyrgyz Republic in 1995; 7% of patients with myocarditis and 2% of patients without myocarditis died. The median interval from hospitalization to death was 4.5 days (range, 0 to 13 days). Manifestations of diphtheritic myocarditis include various dysrhythmias, conduction disturbances, and dilated cardiomyopathy. Although complete heart block from diphtheritic myocarditis was almost always fatal before temporary cardiac pacemakers were developed, approximately one-fourth of patients with this complication have recently been treated successfully.

Polyneuropathy typically begins 3 to 5 weeks after onset of diphtheria and has a slow course. It appears earliest in patients who experience the most severe and prolonged neurologic abnormalities. The initial presentation commonly involves gingival, lingual, or facial numbness as well as dysphonia, dysphagia, and paresthesias of the extremities. These findings may be followed by cranial motor nerve pareses, respiratory and abdominal muscle weakness that may require artificial ventilation, quadriparesis or quadriplegia, peripheral sensory disturbances, sensory ataxia, pain in the extremities, and a variety of autonomic disturbances. Cranial nerve dysfunction typically appears earlier than motor disturbances of the trunk and extremities. In severely affected patients, paresis or paralysis of the trunk and extremities may become worse during the second month, as cranial nerve dysfunction is improving, and peak at 7 to 9 weeks after the onset of polyneuropathy. Severe arterial hypotension attributable to autonomic dysfunction may occur from 4 to 7 weeks after the onset of polyneuropathy and last from 3 to 10 days. Polyneuropathy usually resolves completely in patients who survive.

Pneumonia occurs in more than one-half of fatal cases of diphtheria. Less common complications include renal failure, encephalitis, cerebral infarction, pulmonary embolism, and bacteremia or endocarditis due to invasive infection by *C. diphtheriae*. Serum sickness may result from antitoxin therapy.

COURSE AND PROGNOSIS Most cases of diphtheria develop in nonimmunized patients. The attack rate, severity of disease, and risk of complications are much lower in immunized patients. The pseudomembrane may continue to increase in size during the first day after administration of antitoxin. During the next several days to a week, it becomes softer, less adherent, and nonconfluent and eventually disappears. In the preantibiotic era, *C. diphtheriae* persisted in the throat for ~2 weeks in one-half of patients and for ≥1 month in about one-fifth. Mortality increases with the severity of local disease, the extent of pseudomembrane formation, and the delay between onset of local disease and administration of antitoxin. The death rate is highest during the first week of illness; among patients with bull-neck diphtheria; among patients with myocarditis who develop ventricular tachycardia, atrial fibrillation, or complete heart block; among patients with laryngeal or tracheobronchial involvement; among infants and patients >60 years of age; and among alcoholics. Both the mortality rate and the risk of myocarditis or peripheral neuropathy are significantly lower in cutaneous diphtheria than in respiratory diphtheria.

DIAGNOSIS A characteristic pseudomembrane (Fig. 122-1) on the mucosa of the tonsils, palate, oropharynx, nasopharynx, nose, or larynx suggests diphtheria but is not uniformly present. Diphtheritic pseudomembrane must be distinguished from other pharyngeal exudates, including those of group A β-hemolytic streptococcal infections, infectious mononucleosis, viral pharyngitis, fusospirochetal infection, and candidiasis. Diphtheria should be considered in patients with sore throat, cervical adenopathy or swelling, and low-grade fever, especially when these manifestations are accompanied by systemic toxicity, hoarseness, stridor, palatal paralysis, or serosanguineous nasal discharge with or without demonstrable pseudomembrane. Treatment with diphtheria antitoxin should begin as soon as the clinical diagnosis of diphtheria is made.

Definitive diagnosis of respiratory diphtheria is based on compatible clinical findings supported by the isolation of *C. diphtheriae* from local lesions or by histopathology. Rarely, respiratory diphtheria may be caused by infection with tox⁺ *C. ulcerans*, and such cases should be managed like cases caused by *C. diphtheriae*. *C. pseudodiphtheriticum*, a tox⁻ organism that is often part of the normal throat flora, can be associated with pseudomembranous pharyngitis or lower respiratory tract infection; however, unlike. *C. diphtheriae*, it does not pose a significant risk to contacts of infected patients. Specimens from the nose, throat, and membrane (and, when possible, from beneath the membrane) should be submitted for culture. The laboratory should be notified that diphtheria is suspected to ensure that one appropriate selective medium, such as cysteine-tellurite blood agar or Tinsdale medium, is used in addition to a nonselective medium (e.g., sheep blood agar) for primary plating of the specimens. Biochemical tests needed to differentiate *C. diphtheriae* from corynebacteria of the normal flora (diphtheroids) require several days. Group A β-hemolytic streptococci and *Staphylococcus aureus* are also isolated frequently from patients with diphtheria. All laboratory isolates of *C. diphtheriae*, whether or not they are associated with disease, should be submitted to the Diphtheria Laboratory, National Center for Infectious Diseases, CDC, for confirmation of biotype and toxinogenicity and for other specialized tests.

Cutaneous diphtheria may present as a characteristic "punched-out" ulcer with a membrane, but it is more often indistinguishable from other inflammatory dermatoses. Diagnosis depends on a high degree of suspicion and on culture of cutaneous lesions on laboratory media appropriate for isolation of *C. diphtheriae*. Throat samples from all patients with cutaneous diphtheria should be cultured for *C. diphtheriae*.

℞ TREATMENT

Administration of diphtheria antitoxin is the most import element in the treatment of respiratory diphtheria. The decision to administer diphtheria antitoxin must be based on the clinical diagnosis of respiratory diphtheria, without waiting for definitive laboratory confirmation. Since antitoxin cannot neutralize toxin that is already bound to tissues, each day of delay in initiating treatment with antitoxin is associated with a significant increase in mortality risk. Because diphtheria antitoxin is produced in horses, it is necessary to question patients about possible allergy to horse serum and to perform a conjunctival or intracutaneous test with diluted antitoxin for immediate hypersensitivity. Epinephrine must be available for immediate administration to patients with severe allergic reactions. Patients with immediate hypersensitivity should be desensitized before a full therapeutic dose of antitoxin is given. The risk of serum sickness associated with administration of equine antitoxin is acceptable because of the established therapeutic value of antitoxin in decreasing mortality from respiratory diphtheria. Since 1997, diphtheria antitoxin has been available in the United States only from the CDC and is distributed under an Investigational New Drug (IND) protocol. Physicians should promptly notify their state health departments of suspected diphtheria cases. To obtain diphtheria antitoxin and consultation on its use, physicians should promptly contact staff at the National Immunization Program at (404) 639-8255 during office hours from 8:00 A.M. to 4:30 P.M. eastern standard time or through the CDC operator at (404) 639-2889 or (404) 639-2888 at any time.

Antibiotics have little demonstrated effect on the healing of local infection in diphtheria patients treated with antitoxin. The primary goal of antibiotic therapy for patients or carriers is therefore to eradicate *C. diphtheriae* and prevent its transmission from the patient to susceptible contacts. Regimens currently recommended by the CDC for the treatment of patients with respiratory diphtheria are erythromycin given orally or by injection for 14 days (40 mg/kg per day; maximum, 2 g/d) or procaine penicillin G given intramuscularly for 14 days (300,000 U/d for patients weighing ≤10 kg and 600,000 U/d for those weighing >10 kg). Rifampin or clindamycin has also been used successfully and is an acceptable alternative for treating patients who cannot take penicillin G or erythromycin. Eradication of *C. diphtheriae* should be documented by negative cultures of samples taken on two or three successive days at least 24 h after the completion of antibiotic therapy. Some authorities also recommend a repeat throat culture 2 weeks later. The small percentage of patients who continue to be infected with *C. diphtheriae* after treatment with penicillin or erythromcyin should receive an additional 10-day course of oral erythromycin followed by a repeat culture for *C. diphtheriae*. Plasmid-mediated resistance to erythromycin emerged transiently in *C. diphtheriae* during the Seattle epidemic, but its frequency declined dramatically after the routine use of erythromycin was discontinued.

Patients with respiratory or cutaneous diphtheria caused by tox+ *C. diphtheriae* or by *C. diphtheriae* strains of unknown toxinogenicity should be hospitalized, kept in bed initially, handled with isolation procedures appropriate for the site of infection, and given supportive care as needed. Respiratory and cardiac function must be monitored closely. Early intubation or tracheostomy is recommended when the larynx is involved or signs of impending airway obstruction are detected. Tracheobronchial membrane can sometimes be removed mechanically via the endotracheal tube or tracheostomy. Primary or secondary pneumonia should be diagnosed and treated promptly. Sedative or hypnotic drugs that may mask respiratory symptoms are contraindicated. Close electrocardiographic monitoring, treatment of arrhythmias, and electrical pacing for heart block are essential. Congestive heart failure should be treated as described in Chap. 216. Glucocorticoids do not reduce the risk of diphtheritic myocarditis or polyneuropathy. Ulcerative or ecthymatous cutaneous lesions should be treated with Burow's solution applied on wet compresses after debridement of necrotic areas, and treatment for associated conditions such as pediculosis, scabies, or underlying dermatoses should be instituted. Recovery from diphtheria does not always confer active immunity, and initiation of an immunization regimen for diphtheria that is appropriate for the patient's age should be an integral part of the treatment plan.

PREVENTION DTaP (diphtheria and tetanus toxoids and acellular pertussis vaccine adsorbed) is currently recommended for all doses in the primary immunization schedule for children up to age 7 years who do not have contraindications. Td (tetanus and diphtheria toxoids adsorbed; for adult use) is currently recommended for routine booster immunizations at 10-year intervals in adults who do not have contraindications. Td is also recommended for adults who require prophylactic booster immunizations for tetanus-prone wounds. Currently recommended schedules for primary immunization of children and adults against diphtheria and for maintenance of immunity by periodic booster doses of appropriate vaccines throughout life are summarized in Chap. 107.

Close contacts of patients with respiratory diphtheria, especially household contacts, should have throat and nasal specimens collected and cultured for *C. diphtheriae*, should receive a 7- to 10-day course of either benzathine penicillin G (600,000 U for persons <6 years old or 1,200,000 U for persons ≥6 years old) or oral erythromycin (40 mg/kg per day for children and 1 g/d for adults), and should promptly receive diphtheria antitoxin if they become ill. Contacts whose immunization status is inadequate should receive a booster dose of diphtheria toxoid appropriate for their age. In situations where surveillance of contacts cannot be maintained, the benzathine penicillin G regimen should be used for treatment to ensure compliance. Contacts of patients with cutaneous diphtheria should be treated similarly, except that ongoing investigation of contacts can be discontinued if the strain of *C. diphtheriae* from the patient is found to be nontoxinogenic. Identified carriers of *C. diphtheriae* in the community should also be treated with the recommended regimen for contacts.

OTHER CORYNEBACTERIAL INFECTIONS

DEFINITION Medically important coryneform bacteria include 36 of 59 currently recognized species in the genus *Corynebacterium* plus numerous other taxonomically related organisms that share specific 16S rDNA signature nucleotides and belong to the high-guanosine-plus-cytosine lineage of gram-positive bacteria. They include environmental organisms and members of the normal flora that cause opportunistic infections, human pathogens of relatively low virulence, and animal pathogens that cause zoonotic infections. Reported infections caused by coryneform bacteria have increased substantially in number over the past several decades. Isolates of *C. jeikeium* and *C. urealyticum* are often resistant to multiple antibiotics.

ETIOLOGY AND LABORATORY DIAGNOSIS Because coryneform bacteria are potential pathogens, it is important not to dismiss them arbitrarily as components of the normal flora or as contaminants when they are found in clinical specimens. Coryneform bacteria should be identified to the species level when they are isolated from normally sterile body sites (unless only one of several specimens is positive for growth), when they represent the predominant organisms in appropriately collected clinical specimens, and when they are present as the only organism in urine at a count of >10⁴/mL or as the predominant organisms in urine with a total bacterial count of >10⁵/mL.

The coryneform bacteria are a large, heterogeneous group of gram-positive, pleomorphic, irregularly staining bacilli or coccobacilli that superficially resemble *C. diphtheriae*, have widely varying guanosine-plus-cytosine contents (from 46 to 74% guanosine plus cytosine) for members of the genus *Corynebacterium*, and are often difficult to identify and classify. Club-shaped rod forms are observed only for true *Corynebacterium* species. The genus *Corynebacterium* is currently divided into three groups: the nonlipophilic, fermentative corynebacteria (including *C. diphtheriae*, *C. ulcerans*, *C. pseudotuberculosis*, *C. xerosis*, *C. striatum*, *C. minutissimum*, and others); the nonlipophilic, nonfermentative corynebacteria (including *C. pseudodiphtheriticum* and others); and the lipophilic corynebacteria (including *C. jeikeium*, *C. urealyticum*, and others). The coryneform group includes additional genera, such as *Arcanobacterium* and *Rhodococcus*. Classification of coryneform bacteria is based on routine and molecular genetics–based diagnostic methods; these are often supplemented by chemotaxonomic methods that include identification of the short-chain mycolic acids present in most *Corynebacterium* species but absent in other coryneform bacteria, determination of the specific diamino acid present in peptidoglycan, and characterization of the major cellular fatty acids. The classification system for coryneform bacteria is evolving rapidly, with 14 new species defined in the past 5 years. All coryneform bacteria that are clinically significant but cannot be readily identified in routine diagnostic laboratories should be submitted to an appropriate reference laboratory experienced in this area.

ECOLOGY AND EPIDEMIOLOGY

Humans are the probable natural reservoir for *C. xerosis*, *C. pseudodiphtheriticum*, *C. striatum*, *C. minutissimum*, *C. jeikeium*, *C. urealyticum*, and *Arcanobacterium haemolyticum*. Animals are the probable natural reservoir for *Arcanobacterium pyogenes* (cows, sheep, pigs), *C. ulcerans* (cows, horses), and *C. pseudotuberculosis* (sheep, horses, goats, cattle). The natural reservoir for *Rhodococcus equi* is soil. The ecologic niches for many other coryneform bacteria of medical importance are not well defined.

Corynebacterial species that are found frequently as components of the normal human flora include *C. pseudodiphtheriticum* (pharynx, skin), *C. xerosis* (conjunctival sac, nasopharynx, skin), *C. auris* (external auditory canal), and *C. striatum* (anterior nares, skin). Corynebacterial species that commonly colonize the skin of hospitalized patients include *C. jeikeium* (axilla, groin, perineum) and *C. urealyticum*. *C. jeikeium* most often colonizes patients with malignancies or severe immunodeficiency; it is also isolated from environmental sources (surfaces, air) in hospitals and from the hands of ward staff. *C. ulcerans* infections are acquired by consumption of raw milk. *C. pseudotuberculosis* infections are acquired by contact with animals or animal products or by consumption of raw milk.

PATHOGENESIS AND CLINICAL MANIFESTATIONS

C. ulcerans infections of humans usually present as pharyngitis and can mimic respiratory diphtheria, whereas infections caused by *C. pseudotuberculosis* typically present as suppurative granulomatous lymphadenitis. Some strains of *C. ulcerans* and *C. pseudotuberculosis* can produce diphtheria toxin, but infections of humans with tox$^-$ strains have been reported only for *C. ulcerans*. *C. ulcerans* infections that are presumed on clinical grounds to be caused by tox$^+$ strains should be managed like diphtheria, and diphtheria antitoxin should be administered. *C. pseudodiphtheriticum*, a tox$^-$ commensal of low virulence, is an uncommon cause of pneumonia in men with AIDS and of pharyngitis. It has also been associated with necrotizing tracheitis, tracheobronchitis, endocarditis, and urinary tract infection in patients without known immune deficiencies. Pharyngeal infections associated with *C. pseudodiphtheriticum* can be confused with diphtheria until the bacteriologic diagnosis is established; however, unlike diphtheria, these infections do not pose a danger to contacts. *C. xerosis* and *C. striatum* are constituents of the normal human flora that are of low virulence and rarely cause human infections.

C. jeikeium causes severe infections primarily in patients with hematologic malignancies and neutropenia. Skin colonization precedes clinical infection. Risk factors for nosocomial *C. jeikeium* sepsis include prolonged hospitalization, breaks in the integument, chronic intravascular catheterization, and prior treatment with broad-spectrum antibiotics. Other presentations of *C. jeikeium* infection include endocarditis, device-related infections, pulmonary infiltrates, cutaneous septic emboli, soft tissue infections, and rashes. Endocarditis due to *C. jeikeium* occurs primarily in patients with prosthetic heart valves. *C. jeikeium* is a rare cause of central nervous system infections in patients with ventricular shunts.

C. urealyticum is a significant cause of nosocomial urinary tract infections, including acute and chronic cystitis and pyelonephritis. The organism closely resembles *C. jeikeium* but differs from the latter by producing urease and failing to convert glucose to acidic metabolites. Hydrolysis of urea by urease causes alkalinization of the urine and formation of ammonium magnesium phosphate (struvite) stones. *C. urealyticum* is a cause of alkaline-encrusted cystitis in patients with preexisting bladder lesions that serve as foci for precipitation of struvite crystals. Risk factors associated with symptomatic urinary tract infections include preexisting immunosuppression, recent urologic procedures (including renal transplantation), underlying disorders of the genitourinary tract, and a history of urinary tract infections.

C. minutissimum is frequently isolated from the lesions of erythrasma, a common superficial skin infection characterized by the presence in intertriginous areas of reddish-brown, scaly, pruritic, macular patches that exhibit coral-red fluorescence under a Wood's light. The etiology of erythrasma appears to be polymicrobial; infection of the skin by *C. minutissimum* follows the onset of maceration and scaling. Deep infections caused by *C. minutissimum*, which are rare, include abscesses, bacteremia, endocarditis, peritonitis, pyelonephritis, and infection of central venous catheters.

A. haemolyticum causes pharyngitis and chronic skin ulcers. Less frequently, it causes a variety of deep tissue infections, septicemia, and endocarditis. Some 90% of *A. haemolyticum* infections occur in patients between 10 and 30 years old. *A. haemolyticum* pharyngitis in this age group is 5 to 13% as frequent as *Streptococcus pyogenes* pharyngitis. An erythematous rash is present in 30 to 67% of cases. The rash is usually scarlatiniform and most pronounced on the trunk and proximal extremities, but it sometimes resembles urticaria or erythema multiforme. Because rash is more frequent in *A. haemolyticum* infections than in *S. pyogenes* infections, *A. haemolyticum* should be considered as a possible etiology in older children and adults who present with the scarlet fever syndrome. Infection due to *A. haemolyticum* can also present as extensive pharyngeal exudate and can mimic diphtheria. *A. haemolyticum* occasionally causes peritonsillar abscess, sepsis, endocarditis, or meningitis.

A. pyogenes causes bovine mastitis, a disease transmitted by flies. Yearly epidemics of leg ulcers infected with *A. pyogenes* among schoolchildren in Thailand occurred between 1979 and 1984 and were postulated to have resulted from introduction of the organism into traumatic skin lesions by flies. Reported *A. pyogenes* infections in adults in Denmark have included abscesses, cystitis, intraabdominal infections, and mastoiditis with bacteremia.

R. equi, which causes bronchopneumonia in horses and occasional infections in other animals, has emerged as an important intracellular opportunistic pathogen in immunocompromised patients. Most reported cases are necrotizing pulmonary infections that resemble tuberculosis or nocardiosis in patients with severely defective cell-mediated immunity, including those with AIDS.

DIAGNOSIS

Pharyngitis caused by tox$^+$ strains of *C. ulcerans* may be clinically indistinguishable from diphtheria. The presentations of infections caused by other coryneform bacteria are not pathognomonic, and diagnosis of these infections is based on a high index of suspicion, identification of the organism by culture in appropriate clinical specimens, and exclusion of other likely causes of infection. Sheep blood agar containing fosfomycin (100 μg/mL) or colistin–nalidixic acid blood agar is useful as a selective medium for most coryneform bacteria, and medium containing 0.1 to 1% Tween 80 is useful for isolation of lipophilic coryneform bacteria.

Since *C. urealyticum* is often undetected by routine urine cultures; it is necessary to incubate cultures for 24 to 48 h on blood agar or on special media for selected patients (especially elderly men with preexisting genitourinary abnormalities) with alkaline urine, ammonium magnesium phosphate stones, gram-positive bacilli in the urine, or negative standard urine cultures despite clinical evidence of bacteriuria. Other microbes that can cause urinary tract infections with alkaline urine include *Proteus*, *Ureaplasma*, and some staphylococci and streptococci. Alkaline-encrusted cystitis is an anatomic diagnosis made by cystoscopy.

The differential diagnosis of *A. haemolyticum* pharyngitis with rash includes scarlet fever; rubella; staphylococcal and streptococcal toxic shock syndromes; infections caused by Epstein-Barr virus, cytomegalovirus, and enteroviruses (especially coxsackieviruses); disseminated gonococcal infection; secondary syphilis; and drug allergy. Routine diagnostic methods for throat cultures are not ideal for the detection of *A. haemolyticum*, nor is this organism detected by the rapid tests for *S. pyogenes* that are sometimes substituted for throat cultures. Pharyngitis caused by *A. haemolyticum* in adolescents and

adults is likely to remain underdiagnosed until improved tests for the organism are developed and used by diagnostic laboratories.

Erythrasma is diagnosed clinically. Because of uncertainty about the etiologic role of *C. minutissimum*, culture of erythrasma lesions is not currently recommended.

℞ TREATMENT

Since prediction of susceptibility patterns on the basis of isolate identification to the species level is not necessarily reliable, antimicrobial susceptibility testing should be performed on all isolates of clinically significant coryneform bacteria. In light of the emergence and spread of vancomycin resistance in several gram-positive bacterial species as well as the observation of intrinsic vancomycin resistance in some species of coryneform bacteria (e.g., *Microbacterium resistens*), some authorities have recently recommended that glycopeptide antibiotics not be used as first-line agents to treat infections caused by coryneform bacteria. Physicians treating infections caused by coryneform bacteria that are likely to exhibit resistance to multiple antibiotics should obtain expert consultation concerning current treatment recommendations.

Strains of *C. jeikeium* are typically resistant to most antibiotics. Vancomycin has been recommended most often as the drug of choice for empirical treatment of infections caused by this organism, although antimicrobial susceptibility testing may reveal other antibiotic options for some isolates. For device-related *C. jeikeium* infections, removal of the infected device is usually required in addition to appropriate antibiotic therapy.

C. urealyticum is often resistant to the antibiotics used commonly for the treatment of urinary tract infections. Empirical treatment with vancomycin has often been recommended pending the results of antimicrobial susceptibility testing. Several courses of antibiotic therapy may be necessary for bacteriologic cure. Patients with alkaline-encrusted cystitis require resection of the encrusted lesions in addition to antibiotic therapy.

No controlled trials of treatment for *A. haemolyticum* infections have been performed. In vitro tests usually demonstrate susceptibility to penicillins, erythromycin, azithromycin, clindamycin, doxycycline, ciprofloxacin, and vancomycin, but treatment failures have been reported with appropriate doses of penicillins. Limited data suggest that

the clinical course of *A. haemolyticum* pharyngitis may be shortened by treatment with erythromycin.

Infections with *C. ulcerans* that present like diphtheria or are known to be caused by tox$^+$ strains should be treated like diphtheria. Oral erythromycin is usually effective for treatment of erythrasma. For infections caused by *R. equi*, vancomycin has often been recommended as the drug of choice. Possible alternatives include erythromycin, rifampin, aminoglycosides, and chloramphenicol; the combination of erythromycin and rifampin is attractive because of possible synergy. Penicillins should not be used, because *R. equi* rapidly develops resistance. Many weeks of antibiotic treatment, sometimes supplemented by surgical intervention, are often needed for infections caused by *R. equi*. Suppressive therapy with antibiotics should be continued indefinitely in patients with AIDS after initial treatment of infections caused by *R. equi*. Initial treatment of infections caused by other coryneform bacteria should be based on the identity of the organism and published data regarding antibiotic susceptibility. Therapy should be modified, when necessary, in light of the results of antibiotic susceptibility tests.

FURTHER READING

BROWN AE: Other corynebacteria and *Rhodococcus*, in *Mandell, Douglas, and Bennett's Principles and Practice of Infectious Diseases*, vol 2, 5th ed, GL Mandell et al (eds). Philadelphia, Churchill Livingstone, 2000, pp 2198–2208

FUNKE G, BERNARD KA: Coryneform gram-positive rods, in *Manual of Clinical Microbiology*, 8th ed, PR Murray et al (eds). Washington, DC, ASM Press, 2003, pp 472–501

HADFIELD TL: The pathology of diphtheria. J Infect Dis 181(Suppl 1):S116, 2000

HOLMES RK: Biology and molecular epidemiology of diphtheria toxin and the *tox* gene. J Infect Dis 181(Suppl 1):S156, 2000

KADIROVA R et al: Clinical characteristics and management of 676 hospitalized diphtheria cases, Kyrgyz Republic, 1995. J Infect Dis 181(Suppl 1):S110, 2000

MCQUILLAN GM et al: Serologic immunity to diphtheria and tetanus in the United States. Ann Intern Med 136:660, 2002

OHUABUNOWO CJ et al: Diphtheria, in *Centers for Disease Control and Prevention. Manual for the Surveillance of Vaccine-Preventable Diseases*, 3d ed, M Wharton et al (eds). 2002, pp 1-1–1-8 [http://www.cdc.gov/nip/publications/surv-manual/default.htm]

123 INFECTIONS CAUSED BY *LISTERIA MONOCYTOGENES*
Anne Schuchat, Claire V. Broome

Listeria monocytogenes is a gram-positive rod that can be isolated from soil, vegetation, and many animal reservoirs. Human disease due to *L. monocytogenes* generally occurs in the setting of pregnancy or of immunosuppression caused by illness or medication. Increasing evidence suggests that a substantial portion of cases of human listeriosis are attributable to the food-borne transmission of *L. monocytogenes*. Unlike most food-borne pathogens, which cause primarily gastrointestinal illness, *L. monocytogenes* causes invasive syndromes, such as meningitis, sepsis, chorioamnionitis, and stillbirth.

ETIOLOGY Listeriae are aerobic or facultatively anaerobic, nonsporulating gram-positive bacilli that grow at 1 to 45°C and typically have tumbling motility when cultured at 20 to 25°C. Characteristics that help distinguish *L. monocytogenes* from other *Listeria* spp. include the formation of a narrow zone of β hemolysis on sheep blood agar and the production of acid from glucose, maltose, L-rhamnose, and α-methyl-D-mannoside but not from D-xylose. Determination of the serotype of *L. monocytogenes* is based on somatic (O) and flagellar (H) antigens. Most cases of human disease are caused by serotypes 1/2a, 1/2b, and 4b. Subtyping, especially by pulsed-field gel electrophoresis, has made it easier to discriminate among strains of *Listeria* and thus to link environmental or food isolates with clinical infections.

PATHOGENESIS *L. monocytogenes* is an intracellular pathogen—a characteristic consistent with its predilection for causing illness in persons with deficient cell-mediated immunity. The organism can be found as part of the gastrointestinal flora in healthy individuals. Lack of gastric acidity and abnormal gastrointestinal functioning may increase the risk of invasive disease following exposure to the organism in the gastrointestinal tract. The increased risk of *L. monocytogenes* infection in pregnant women may be due to both systemic and local immunologic changes associated with pregnancy. For example, local immunosuppression at the maternal-fetal interface of the placenta may facilitate intrauterine infection following transient maternal bacteremia.

The molecular pathogenesis of *L. monocytogenes* has been elucidated. The cell-surface protein internalin interacts with specific receptors to induce phagocytosis. Both listeriolysin O and phospholipase permit the organism to escape from the phagosome into the cytosol while avoiding intracellular killing. Through the surface protein ActA, *L. monocytogenes* uses actin-based motility to move to the cell membrane. Efficient cell-to-cell spread is accomplished by both actin filament formation and phospholipase production. Genetic determinants of these proteins have been characterized. Because the organism is adapted for both intracellular survival and direct cell-to-cell spread, it is not eliminated by antibodies.

EPIDEMIOLOGY Long recognized as a veterinary pathogen, *L. monocytogenes* causes basilar meningitis ("circling disease") and stillbirth in sheep and cattle. The occurrence of listeriosis among humans has received increasing attention as the role of contaminated foods in the pathogenesis of epidemic listeriosis has been recognized and reports of disease associated with the expanding immunosuppressed population have accumulated.

Invasive listeriosis—confirmed by culture of blood or cerebrospinal fluid (CSF)—occurs in approximately 3 to 5 individuals per million population annually in the United States. Perinatal listeriosis complicates 9 births per 100,000. A 40% decline in incidence since the period from 1986 through 1990 may be attributable to aggressive food regulation and industrial clean-up efforts. Incidence further declined by 35% from 1996 through 2001. Multistate surveillance for sporadic listeriosis suggests that 20% of infections are fatal or result in stillbirth, although higher case-fatality rates have been reported during listeriosis epidemics and were described in early series. Most cases of disease due to *L. monocytogenes* are sporadic; however, investigation of several outbreaks of listeriosis since 1980 has demonstrated common-source food-borne transmission as a cause of human illness and has shown that the incubation period for disease following consumption of contaminated food can be 2 to 6 weeks. The largest North American outbreak, which took place in Los Angeles in 1985, involved more than 100 cases and 48 deaths or stillbirths. A nationwide outbreak in France in 1992 involved 279 cases and 63 deaths. Foods implicated in outbreaks of listeriosis include contaminated coleslaw, pasteurized milk, soft cheeses, pâté, ready-to-eat turkey and pork products, hot dogs, butter, and prepared salads; epidemiologic studies have implicated undercooked chicken, uncooked hot dogs, soft cheeses, and food from store delicatessen counters in sporadic disease. Listerial contamination of foods is relatively common. Among foods contaminated with the organism, those that are purchased ready to eat, are contaminated with serotype 4b, and are contaminated at a relatively high level may be the most likely to cause illness. The long incubation period associated with listeriosis contributes to the difficulty of implicating specific foods as the cause of either common-source outbreaks or sporadic cases.

Although food-borne transmission appears to be the foremost cause of epidemic and sporadic disease, several clusters of late-onset neonatal infection suggest nosocomial transmission of *L. monocytogenes*. Contaminated multiuse materials and equipment have been suggested as causes of some nosocomial clusters. Listeriosis has been reported in veterinarians and other persons in close contact with infected animals.

CLINICAL PRESENTATION *Pregnancy-associated listeriosis* may occur during any stage of pregnancy, although most infections are detected during the third trimester, possibly because of failure to obtain specimens for bacterial culture earlier during gestation in instances of abortion and stillbirth. One-half to two-thirds of pregnant women with perinatal listeriosis experience a mild illness characterized by fever, myalgias, malaise, and backache, which sometimes are accompanied by diarrhea, abdominal pain, nausea, and/or vomiting during the bacteremic phase. Blood cultures should be used for diagnosis. Transplacental spread of the organism results in intrauterine infection, which can lead to chorioamnionitis, premature labor, intrauterine fetal demise, or early-onset disease of the newborn. Women with listeriosis diagnosed during pregnancy have a favorable clinical outcome after antibiotic therapy or delivery. Although often included in the differential diagnosis of recurrent spontaneous abortion, infection with *L. monocytogenes* appears to cause fewer than 2% of stillbirths.

Neonatal listeriosis can be classified under the same categories used for group B streptococcal infection (Chap. 121), with early-onset disease evident during the first week of life and late-onset disease developing thereafter. Infants may be symptomatic at birth; most infants with early-onset disease are symptomatic by the second day of life. Aspiration of infected amniotic fluid contributes to pathogenesis. Early-onset disease may include sepsis, respiratory distress, skin lesions, and the syndrome called *granulomatosis infantisepticum*, which is characterized by disseminated abscesses involving the liver, spleen, adrenal glands, lungs, and other sites. Infants with late-onset neonatal disease are more likely than those with early-onset disease to develop meningitis. While early-onset disease is often associated with obstetric complications such as premature delivery and chorioamnionitis, late-onset disease typically affects infants born at term by uncomplicated deliveries. Infants may acquire *L. monocytogenes* during passage through the birth canal; except in several clusters of late-onset neonatal infections linked to nosocomial transmission, the pathogenesis of late-onset disease is not well understood.

Listeriosis not associated with pregnancy usually affects persons with immunosuppressive conditions, although invasive disease can also affect immunocompetent adults, particularly elderly persons. The most common underlying conditions in nonpregnant adults with listeriosis are chronic glucocorticoid therapy, solid or hematologic malignancies (particularly in fludarabine-treated patients), diabetes mellitus, renal disease, liver disease, and AIDS. Although the prevalence of listeriosis among persons infected with HIV is much higher than that in the general population, listeriosis is a relatively uncommon opportunistic infection in AIDS.

Sepsis Clinical studies have shown that bacteremic infection without an evident focus is the most common clinical manifestation of listeriosis among immunocompromised hosts, while infection of the central nervous system (CNS) ranks second in frequency. Listerial sepsis cannot be distinguished clinically from bacteremia involving other organisms. Patients are usually febrile, often appear extremely ill, and may have prodromal symptoms including myalgia, nausea, vomiting, and diarrhea. Immunocompromised patients with listeriosis are less likely than other *Listeria*-infected adults to present with CNS infection, possibly because they are more likely to have blood cultured during febrile episodes and thus to have transient listerial bacteremia recognized.

CNS Infection The most common presentation of CNS infection due to *L. monocytogenes* is meningitis, which can present as either an acute or (less often) a subacute illness. Presenting symptoms include fever, headache, and an altered level of consciousness. Examination of CSF usually reveals pleocytosis, increased protein concentrations, and normal glucose levels, although other patterns are sometimes found. Gram's stain is positive in only 25% of cases. The diagnosis is made when *L. monocytogenes* is identified on culture. Despite its name, *L. monocytogenes* is rarely associated with monocytosis of either CSF or blood. Other syndromes seen in CNS infection include meningoencephalitis; cerebritis; and brainstem, spinal cord, or intracranial abscesses. The unusual syndrome of rhombencephalitis includes asymmetric cranial-nerve palsies, altered consciousness, cerebellar signs, and motor or sensory loss. Symptoms of other nonmeningitic CNS infections include fever, ataxia, seizures, personality changes, and coma. Nuchal rigidity is rare in nonmeningitic infections. CSF cultures may be sterile; blood cultures are usually diagnostic.

Endocarditis Like most forms of bacterial endocarditis, listerial endocarditis typically occurs in patients with prosthetic or previously damaged valves. The organism has a predilection for the left side of the heart. Endocarditis due to *L. monocytogenes* is often associated with systemic embolization.

Focal Infections Other focal infections that can follow unrecognized bacteremia include endophthalmitis, peritonitis, osteomyelitis, visceral abscess, pleuropulmonary infection, and cholecystitis. Cutaneous lesions may develop without systemic involvement and have been reported in veterinarians and poultry workers.

Gastrointestinal Illness Several common-source outbreaks of acute febrile gastroenteritis suggest that *L. monocytogenes* can cause an acute diarrheal syndrome in persons without immunocompromising conditions. The importance of *L. monocytogenes* in sporadic diarrheal illness is unclear. Although the organism is not identified by the culture methods routinely used for stool specimens, studies using selective enrichment media for evaluation of consecutive specimens from patients hospitalized with acute diarrhea have suggested that *L. monocytogenes* is not a major cause of sporadic diarrhea.

Recurrences Recurrent infection with *L. monocytogenes* has been reported but is rare. Many recurrences are due to the subtype responsible for the initial infection. The implication is that such recurrences result either from insufficient treatment of a focus of primary infection or from repeated exposure to a persistently contaminated source.

DIAGNOSIS Invasive listeriosis is diagnosed when the organism is cultured from a site that is usually sterile, such as blood, CSF, or amniotic fluid. The organism grows readily within 36 h on routine culture media, but morphologic similarities between *Listeria* and diphtheroids make it necessary to use biochemical tests to identify the species. Serologic assays with whole-cell antigens have not been useful for the diagnosis of listeriosis, both because exposure to the organism (and thus the presence of antibody) may be common and because infected individuals may not produce antibody. Assays for antibody to listeriolysin O have been applied in epidemiologic investigations and, retrospectively, in the diagnosis of culture-negative CNS infection. Culture of the organism from nonsterile sites such as the vagina and rectum is not useful for clinical diagnosis, as the organism may be carried at these sites by ~5% of healthy individuals.

Differential diagnosis of prematurity, spontaneous abortion, or stillbirth includes infectious diseases such as group B streptococcal infection, congenital syphilis, and toxoplasmosis; pathogens such as group B streptococci and *Escherichia coli* are more common than *L. monocytogenes* as causes of meningitis and sepsis in the newborn period. Listerial infection should always be considered in the differential diagnosis of meningitis in immunosuppressed persons, particularly transplant recipients and others undergoing glucocorticoid treatment, patients with hematologic malignancy, and HIV-infected patients. Among healthy adults, meningitis is much more likely to be caused by *Neisseria meningitidis*, *Streptococcus pneumoniae*, or viral pathogens than by *L. monocytogenes*.

℞ TREATMENT

The treatment of choice for listeriosis is intravenous administration of either ampicillin or penicillin, often in combination with an aminoglycoside for synergy. Trimethoprim-sulfamethoxazole is bactericidal against *L. monocytogenes* and has been used successfully in the treatment of patients with penicillin allergy. *L. monocytogenes* is susceptible in vitro to penicillin G, ampicillin, erythromycin, trimethoprim-sulfamethoxazole, chloramphenicol, rifampin, tetracyclines, aminoglycosides, and imipenem. However, chloramphenicol and rifampin may antagonize the bactericidal effect of penicillins. Because *L. monocytogenes* is not sensitive to cephalosporins, these agents should not be used for single-agent empirical treatment of neonatal sepsis or of meningitis in newborns or immunocompromised hosts.

Dosages and durations of therapy have not been subjected to controlled trials. For nonpregnant adults with listeriosis, the regimen of choice is either ampicillin (12 g intravenously per day in six divided doses) or penicillin G (15 to 20 million units intravenously per day in six divided doses); for immunosuppressed patients with meningitis, some experts add gentamicin (1.3 mg/kg intravenously every 8 h) for synergy. Penicillin-allergic patients may be treated with trimethoprim-sulfamethoxazole (15/75 mg/kg intravenously per day in three equal portions every 8 h). Meningitis in an immunocompetent patient may require 2 to 3 weeks of antibiotic therapy after defervescence. Meningitis, bacteremia, endocarditis, and nonmeningitic listeriosis in immunosuppressed patients should be treated longer, probably for 4 to 6 weeks. Neonatal listeriosis can be treated with a 2-week course of ampicillin. Infants weighing <2000 g should receive 100 mg/kg per day in two equal doses during the first week of life and 150 mg/kg per day during the second week. Infants weighing ≥2000 g should receive 150 mg/kg per day in three equal doses during the first week of life and 200 mg/kg per day during the second week. The addition of an aminoglycoside should be considered for neonatal infection (genta-

TABLE 123-1 *Dietary Recommendations for the Prevention of Food-Borne Listeriosis*

Recommendations to all individuals
1. Thoroughly cook raw food from animal sources, such as beef, pork, and poultry.
2. Wash raw vegetables thoroughly before eating them.
3. Keep uncooked meats separate from vegetables and from cooked and ready-to-eat foods.
4. Avoid raw (unpasteurized) milk or foods made from raw milk.
5. Wash hands, knives, and cutting boards after handling uncooked foods.

Additional recommendations to high-risk individuals[a]
6. Avoid soft cheeses such as Mexican-style, feta, Brie, Camembert, and blue-veined cheese. There is no need to avoid hard cheeses, cream cheese, cottage cheese, or yogurt.
7. Leftover foods or ready-to-eat foods, such as hot dogs, should be reheated until steaming hot before being eaten.
8. Although the risk of listeriosis associated with foods from delicatessen counters is relatively low and poorly characterized, pregnant women and immunosuppressed persons may choose to avoid these foods or to thoroughly reheat cold cuts before eating them.

[a] Persons immunocompromised by illness or medications; pregnant women.

micin, 5 mg/kg per day in two divided doses during the first week of life; 7.5 mg/kg per day in three equal doses during the second week). For listeriosis in pregnant women, a 2-week course of ampicillin (4 to 6 g per day in four equal doses) is recommended. During the last month of pregnancy, infected women with serious penicillin allergies may be treated with erythromycin.

PROGNOSIS Treatment of maternal bacteremia during pregnancy can prevent neonatal infection. Antibiotic therapy for the newborn can limit sequelae, although the widely disseminated disease characteristic of granulomatosis infantisepticum is frequently fatal regardless of treatment. Early-onset disease carries a higher mortality risk than late-onset infection, and immunocompromised hosts have a worse prognosis than do otherwise-healthy adults with listeriosis.

PREVENTION *L. monocytogenes* is frequently isolated from food; the Food and Drug Administration, the U.S. Department of Agriculture, and manufacturers are pursuing further measures to reduce *L. monocytogenes* contamination of foods that have been subjected to listericidal processing. Prevention of listeriosis requires dietary counseling of persons at increased risk of disease (Table 123-1). There is no role for the administration of prophylaxis to contacts of patients with listeriosis. Clinicians are encouraged to report cases of listeriosis to local or state health departments. Case reporting and subtyping of clinical isolates can facilitate early recognition of outbreaks and prevention of subsequent cases.

FURTHER READING

Aureli P et al: An outbreak of febrile gastroenteritis associated with corn contaminated by *Listeria monocytogenes*. N Engl J Med 342:1236, 2000

Pinner RW et al: Role of foods in sporadic listeriosis: II. Microbiologic and epidemiologic investigation. JAMA 267:2046, 1992

Ryser ET, Marth EH (eds): *Listeria, Listeriosis, and Food Safety*, 2d ed. New York, Marcel Dekker, 1999

Schlech WF III: Foodborne listeriosis. Clin Infect Dis 31:770, 2000

Schuchat A et al: Role of foods in sporadic listeriosis: I. Case-control study of dietary risk factors. JAMA 267:2041, 1992

Slutsker L et al: Listeriosis, in *Emerging Infections 4*, W Scheld et al (eds). Washington, DC, ASM Press, 2000, pp 83–106

Southwick FS, Purich DL: Intracellular pathogenesis of listeriosis. N Engl J Med 334:770, 1996

Tappero JW et al: Reduction in the incidence of human listeriosis in the United States—effectiveness of prevention efforts? JAMA 273:1118, 1995

124 | TETANUS
Elias Abrutyn

DEFINITION Tetanus is a neurologic disorder, characterized by increased muscle tone and spasms, that is caused by tetanospasmin, a powerful protein toxin elaborated by *Clostridium tetani*. Tetanus occurs in several clinical forms, including generalized, neonatal, and localized disease.

ETIOLOGIC AGENT *C. tetani* is an anaerobic, motile gram-positive rod that forms an oval, colorless, terminal spore and thus assumes a shape resembling a tennis racket or drumstick. The organism is found worldwide in soil, in the inanimate environment, in animal feces, and occasionally in human feces. Spores may survive for years in some environments and are resistant to various disinfectants and to boiling for 20 min. Vegetative cells, however, are easily inactivated and are susceptible to several antibiotics (metronidazole, penicillin, and others).

Tetanospasmin is formed in vegetative cells under plasmid control. It is a single polypeptide chain. With autolysis, the single-chain toxin is released and cleaved to form a heterodimer consisting of a heavy chain (100 kDa), which mediates binding to nerve-cell receptors and entry into these cells, and a light chain (50 kDa), which acts to block neurotransmitter release. The genome sequence of *C. tetani* has been reported. The amino acid structures of the two most powerful toxins known, botulinum toxin and tetanus toxin, are partially homologous.

EPIDEMIOLOGY Tetanus occurs sporadically and almost always affects nonimmunized persons, partially immunized persons, or fully immunized individuals who fail to maintain adequate immunity with booster doses of vaccine. Although tetanus is entirely preventable by immunization, the burden of disease is large worldwide. The disease is common in areas where soil is cultivated, in rural areas, in warm climates, during summer months, and among males. In countries without a comprehensive immunization program, tetanus occurs predominantly in neonates and other young children. It is noteworthy that international programs to eliminate neonatal tetanus have been in place for some time. In the United States and other nations with successful immunization programs, neonatal tetanus is rare (only one case was reported in the United States during the period 1998–2000), and the disease affects other age groups and groups inadequately covered by immunization (such as nonwhites). The success of immunization in the United States is depicted in Fig. 124-1. Since 1976, fewer than 100 cases have been reported yearly; this figure contrasts remarkably with that of 500 to 600 cases reported annually in the late 1940s, when vaccine administration became routine and tetanus became notifiable. In 1947, the incidence of tetanus was 3.9 cases per 1 million population. In contrast, the average annual incidence rate for 1998–2000 was

FIGURE 124-1 Tetanus: Reported cases by year—United States, 1970–2000. [From *Centers for Disease Control and Prevention: Summary of notifiable diseases, United States, 2000. MMWR 49(53):74, 2000.*]

0.16 per 1 million population. The risk for the development of tetanus is highest among the elderly. A large-scale national serologic survey for tetanus and diphtheria antibody performed in 1988–1994 showed that, overall, 72% of Americans over the age of 6 years were protected against tetanus. Whereas 91% of children 6 to 11 years old were protected, the percentage protected fell with age: only 30% of persons >70 years old (men, 45%; women, 21%) had adequate antibody levels. Notably, individuals 20 to 49 years old now account for a large proportion of cases, because fewer cases occurred in the elderly without a similar reduction among young and middle-aged adults.

In the United States, most cases of tetanus follow an acute injury, such as a puncture wound, laceration, or abrasion. Tetanus is acquired indoors or during farming, gardening, and other outdoor activities. The injury may be major but often is trivial, so that medical attention is not sought; in some instances no injury can be identified. The disease may complicate chronic conditions such as skin ulcers, abscesses, and gangrene. Tetanus is also associated with burns, frostbite, middle-ear infection, surgery, abortion, childbirth, body piercing, and drug abuse, notably "skin popping." In some patients no portal of entry for the organism can be identified.

PATHOGENESIS Contamination of wounds with spores of *C. tetani* is probably a frequent occurrence. Germination and toxin production, however, take place only in wounds with low oxidation-reduction potential, such as those with devitalized tissue, foreign bodies, or active infection. *C. tetani* does not itself evoke inflammation, and the portal of entry retains a benign appearance unless infection with other organisms is present.

Toxin released in the wound binds to peripheral motor neuron terminals, enters the axon, and is transported to the nerve-cell body in the brainstem and spinal cord by retrograde intraneuronal transport. The toxin then migrates across the synapse to presynaptic terminals, where it blocks release of the inhibitory neurotransmitters glycine and γ-aminobutyric acid (GABA). The blocking of neurotransmitter release by tetanospasmin, a zinc metalloprotease, involves the cleavage of protein(s) critical to proper function of the synaptic vesicle release apparatus. With diminished inhibition, the resting firing rate of the α motor neuron increases, producing rigidity. With lessened activity of reflexes that limit polysynaptic spread of impulses (a glycinergic activity), agonists and antagonists may be recruited rather than inhibited, with the consequent production of spasms. Loss of inhibition may also affect preganglionic sympathetic neurons in the lateral gray matter of the spinal cord and produce sympathetic hyperactivity and high circulating catecholamine levels. Tetanospasmin, like botulinum toxin, may block neurotransmitter release at the neuromuscular junction and produce weakness or paralysis; recovery requires sprouting of new nerve terminals.

In local tetanus, only the nerves supplying the affected muscles are involved. Generalized tetanus occurs when toxin released in the wound enters the lymphatics and bloodstream and is spread widely to distant nerve terminals; the blood-brain barrier blocks direct entry into the central nervous system. If it is assumed that intraneuronal transport times are equal for all nerves, short nerves are affected before long nerves: this fact explains the sequential involvement of nerves of the head, trunk, and extremities in generalized tetanus.

CLINICAL MANIFESTATIONS *Generalized tetanus*, the most common form of the disease, is characterized by increased muscle tone and generalized spasms. The median time of onset after injury is 7 days; 15% of cases occur within 3 days and 10% after 14 days.

Typically, the patient first notices increased tone in the masseter muscles (trismus, or lockjaw). Dysphagia or stiffness or pain in the neck, shoulder, and back muscles appears concurrently or soon thereafter. The subsequent involvement of other muscles produces a rigid abdomen and stiff proximal limb muscles; the hands and feet are relatively spared. Sustained contraction of the facial muscles results in a grimace or sneer (risus sardonicus), and contraction of the back muscles produces an arched back (opisthotonos). Some patients develop paroxysmal, violent, painful, generalized muscle spasms that may cause cyanosis and threaten ventilation. These spasms occur repetitively and may be spontaneous or provoked by even the slightest stimulation. A constant threat during generalized spasms is reduced ventilation or apnea or laryngospasm. The severity of illness may be mild (muscle rigidity and few or no spasms), moderate (trismus, dysphagia, rigidity, and spasms), or severe (frequent explosive paroxysms). The patient may be febrile, although many have no fever; mentation is unimpaired. Deep tendon reflexes may be increased. Dysphagia or ileus may preclude oral feeding.

Autonomic dysfunction commonly complicates severe cases and is characterized by labile or sustained hypertension, tachycardia, dysrhythmia, hyperpyrexia, profuse sweating, peripheral vasoconstriction, and increased plasma and urinary catecholamine levels. Periods of bradycardia and hypotension may also be documented. Sudden cardiac arrest sometimes occurs, but its basis is unknown. Other complications include aspiration pneumonia, fractures, muscle rupture, deep-vein thrombophlebitis, pulmonary emboli, decubitus ulcer, and rhabdomyolysis.

Neonatal tetanus usually occurs as the generalized form and is usually fatal if left untreated. It develops in children born to inadequately immunized mothers, frequently after unsterile treatment of the umbilical cord stump. Its onset generally comes during the first 2 weeks of life. Poor feeding, rigidity, and spasms are typical features of neonatal tetanus. *Local tetanus* is an uncommon form in which manifestations are restricted to muscles near the wound. The prognosis is excellent. *Cephalic tetanus*, a rare form of local tetanus, follows head injury or ear infection. Trismus and dysfunction of one or more cranial nerves, often the seventh nerve, are found. The incubation period is a few days and the mortality is high.

DIAGNOSIS   The diagnosis of tetanus is based entirely on clinical findings. Tetanus is unlikely if a reliable history indicates the completion of a primary vaccination series and the receipt of appropriate booster doses. Wounds should be cultured in suspected cases. However, *C. tetani* can be isolated from wounds of patients without tetanus and frequently cannot be recovered from wounds of those with tetanus. The leukocyte count may be elevated. Cerebrospinal fluid examination yields normal results. Electromyograms may show continuous discharge of motor units and shortening or absence of the silent interval normally seen after an action potential. Nonspecific changes may be evident on the electrocardiogram. Muscle enzyme levels may be raised. Serum antitoxin levels of ≥ 0.15 U/mL are considered protective and make tetanus unlikely, although cases developing despite protective antitoxin levels have been reported.

The differential diagnosis includes local conditions also producing trismus, such as alveolar abscess, strychnine poisoning, dystonic drug reactions (e.g., to phenothiazines and metoclopramide), and hypocalcemic tetany. Other conditions sometimes confused with tetanus include meningitis/encephalitis, rabies, and an acute intraabdominal process (because of the rigid abdomen). Markedly increased tone in central muscles (face, neck, chest, back, and abdomen) with superimposed generalized spasms and relative sparing of the hands and feet strongly suggests tetanus.

℞ TREATMENT

General Measures   The goals of therapy are to eliminate the source of toxin, neutralize unbound toxin, and prevent muscle spasms, monitoring the patient's condition and providing support—especially respiratory support—until recovery. Patients should be admitted to a quiet room in an intensive care unit, where observation and cardiopulmonary monitoring can be maintained continuously but stimulation can be minimized. Protection of the airway is vital. Wounds should be explored, carefully cleansed, and thoroughly debrided.

Antibiotic Therapy   Although of unproven value, antibiotic therapy is administered to eradicate vegetative cells—the source of toxin. The use of penicillin (10 to 12 million units intravenously, given daily for 10 days) has been recommended, but metronidazole (500 mg every 6 h or 1 g every 12 h) is preferred by some experts on the basis of this drug's excellent antimicrobial activity, a survival rate higher than that obtained with penicillin in one nonrandomized trial, and the absence of activity antagonistic to GABA, as seen with penicillin. Clindamycin and erythromycin are also alternatives for the treatment of penicillin-allergic patients. Additional specific antimicrobial therapy should be given for active infection with other organisms.

Antitoxin   Given to neutralize circulating toxin and unbound toxin in the wound, antitoxin effectively lowers mortality; toxin already bound to neural tissue is unaffected. Human tetanus immune globulin (TIG) is the preparation of choice and should be given promptly. The dose is 3000 to 6000 units intramuscularly, usually in divided doses because the volume is large. The optimal dose is not known, however, and results from one study indicated that a 500-unit dose was as effective as higher doses. Pooled intravenous immunoglobulin may be an alternative to TIG, but the specific antitoxin concentration in this formulation is not standardized. It may be best to administer antitoxin before manipulating the wound; the value of injecting a dose proximal to the wound or infiltrating the wound is unclear. Additional doses are unnecessary because the half-life of antitoxin is long. Antibody does not penetrate the blood-brain barrier. Intrathecal administration should be considered experimental. Equine tetanus antitoxin (TAT) is not available in the United States but is used elsewhere. It is cheaper than human antitoxin, but its half-life is shorter and its administration commonly elicits hypersensitivity and serum sickness.

Control of Muscle Spasms   Many agents, alone and in combination, have been used to treat the muscle spasms of tetanus, which are painful and can threaten ventilation by causing laryngospasm or sustained contraction of ventilatory muscles. The ideal therapeutic regimen would abolish spasmodic activity without causing oversedation and hypoventilation. Diazepam, a benzodiazepine and GABA agonist, is in wide use. The dose is titrated, and large doses (≥ 250 mg/d) may be required. Lorazepam, with a longer duration of action, and midazolam, with a short half-life, are other options. Barbiturates and chlorpromazine are considered second-line agents. Therapeutic paralysis with a nondepolarizing neuromuscular blocking agent and mechanical ventilation may be required for the treatment of spasms unresponsive to medication or spasms that threaten ventilation. However, prolonged paralysis after the discontinuation of therapy with such agents has been described, and both the need for continued paralysis and the occurrence of complications should be assessed daily. Alternative agents include propofol, which is expensive; dantrolene and intrathecal baclofen, which are being investigated in the hope of shortening the period of therapeutic paralysis; succinylcholine, which has been associated with hyperkalemia; and magnesium sulfate, which requires monitoring of neurologic (patellar reflex) and respiratory function as well as daily measurement of serum magnesium levels.

Respiratory Care   Intubation or tracheostomy, with or without mechanical ventilation, may be required for hypoventilation due to oversedation or laryngospasm or for the avoidance of aspiration by patients with trismus, disordered swallowing, or dysphagia. The need for these procedures should be anticipated, and they should be undertaken electively and early.

Autonomic Dysfunction   The optimal therapy for sympathetic overactivity has not been defined. Agents that have been considered include labetalol (an α- and β-adrenergic blocking agent that is recommended by some experts but that reportedly has caused sudden death), esmolol administered by continuous infusion (a beta blocker whose short half-life may be advantageous in the event of severe hypertension from unopposed α-adrenergic activity), clonidine (a central-acting antiadrenergic drug), and morphine sulfate. Parenteral magnesium sulfate and continuous spinal or epidural anesthesia have been used but may be more difficult to administer and monitor. The relative efficacy of these modalities has yet to be determined. Hypotension or bradycardia may require volume expansion, use of vasopressors or chronotropic agents, or pacemaker insertion.

Vaccine Patients recovering from tetanus should be actively immunized (see below) because immunity is not induced by the small amount of toxin that produces disease.

Additional Measures Additional therapeutic measures include hydration to control insensible and other fluid losses, which may be significant; the meeting of the patient's increased nutritional requirements by enteral or parenteral means; physiotherapy to prevent contractures; and administration of heparin or another anticoagulant to prevent pulmonary emboli. Bowel, bladder, and renal function must be monitored. Gastrointestinal bleeding and decubitus ulcers must be prevented, and intercurrent infection should be treated.

PREVENTION ■ **Active Immunization** All partially immunized and unimmunized adults should receive vaccine, as should those recovering from tetanus. The primary series for adults consists of three doses: the first and second doses are given 4 to 8 weeks apart, and the third dose is given 6 to 12 months after the second. A booster dose is required every 10 years and may be given at mid-decade ages—35, 45, and so on. Combined tetanus and diphtheria toxoid, adsorbed (Td, for adult use)—rather than single-antigen tetanus toxoid—is preferred for persons >7 years of age. Adsorbed vaccine is preferred because it produces more persistent antibody titers than fluid vaccine. In response to a vaccine shortage in 2001, the Centers for Disease Control and Prevention recommended that routine booster doses of Td for adolescents and adults be deferred until 2002, pending a better supply, but that all other existing recommendations for vaccine use be followed.

Wound Management Proper wound management requires consideration of the need for (1) passive immunization with TIG and (2) active immunization with vaccine, preferably Td in persons over age 7 (Table 124-1). The dose of TIG for passive immunization of persons with wounds of average severity is 250 units intramuscularly, which produces a protective antibody level in the serum for at least 4 to 6 weeks; the appropriate dose of TAT, an equine-derived product, is 3000 to 6000 units. Vaccine and TAT should be administered at separate sites with separate syringes.

Neonatal Tetanus Measures aimed at preventing neonatal tetanus include maternal vaccination, even during pregnancy; efforts to increase the proportion of births that take place in the hospital; and the provision of training for nonmedical birth attendants.

PROGNOSIS The application of methods to monitor and support oxygenation has markedly improved the prognosis in tetanus; mortality rates as low as 10% have been reported from units accustomed to handling such cases. In the United States during the periods 1995–

TABLE 124-1 Wound Care: Administration of Tetanus Toxoid and Tetanus Immune Globulin

History of Adsorbed Tetanus Toxoid	Clean Minor Wound		All Other Wounds[a]	
	Td[b]	TIG	Td[b]	TIG
Unknown or <3 doses	Yes	No	Yes	Yes
3 doses[c]	No, unless >10 years since last dose	No	No, unless >5 years since last dose	No

[a] Such as, but not limited to, wounds contaminated with dirt, feces, soil, and saliva; puncture wounds; avulsions; and wounds resulting from missile or crushing injuries, burns, and frostbite.
[b] For children <7 years old, DTP (or DT, if pertussis vaccine is contraindicated) is preferred to tetanus toxoid alone. Td is preferred to tetanus toxoid alone in adults.
[c] If only three doses of fluid toxoid have been received, then a fourth dose of toxoid—preferably an adsorbed toxoid—should be given.
Note: DT, diphtheria and tetanus vaccine; DTP, diphtheria, tetanus, and pertussis vaccine; Td, tetanus-diphtheria toxoid, adsorbed; TIG, tetanus immune globulin.
Source: Modified from Centers for Disease Control and Prevention: Diphtheria, tetanus, and pertussis: Recommendations for vaccine use and other preventive measures: Recommendations of the Immunization Practices Advisory Committee (ACIP). MMWR 40(RR-10):1, 1991.

1997 and 1998–2000, the case-fatality rates were 11% and 16%, respectively. In the latter period, there were 20 deaths among the 113 cases with known outcome (total, 130 cases). The outcome is poor in neonates and the elderly and in patients with a short incubation period, a short interval from the onset of symptoms to admission, or a short period from the onset of symptoms to the first spasm (period of onset). Outcome is also related to the extent of prior vaccination.

The course of tetanus extends over 4 to 6 weeks, and patients may require prolonged ventilator support. Increased tone and minor spasms can last for months, but recovery is usually complete.

FURTHER READING

ABRUTYN E, BERLIN JA: Intrathecal therapy of tetanus: A meta-analysis. JAMA 266:2262, 1991

AHMADSYAH I, SALIM A: Treatment of tetanus: An open study to compare the efficacy of procaine penicillin and metronidazole. BMJ 291:648, 1985

BLECK TP: *Clostridium tetani* (tetanus), in *Principles and Practice of Infectious Diseases*, 5th ed, GL Mandell et al (eds). New York, Churchill Livingstone, 2000, pp 2537–2543

BRUGGEMANN H et al: The genome sequence of *Clostridium tetani*, the causative agent of tetanus disease. Proc Natl Acad Sci USA 100:1316, 2003

CENTERS FOR DISEASE CONTROL AND PREVENTION: Tetanus—Puerto Rico, 2002. MMWR 51:613, 2002

———: Tetanus surveillance—United States, 1998–2000. Surveillance summaries, June 20, 2003. MMWR 52(SS-3):1, 2003

COOK TM et al: Tetanus: A review of the literature. Br J Anaesth 87:477, 2001

HSU SS et al: Tetanus in the emergency department: A current review. J Emerg Med 20:357, 2001

MCQUILLAN CM et al: Serologic immunity to diphtheria and tetanus in the United States. Ann Intern Med 136:660, 2002

TURTON K et al: Botulinum and tetanus neurotoxins: Structure, function and therapeutic utility. Trends Biochem Sci 27:552, 2002

125 BOTULISM
Elias Abrutyn

DEFINITION Botulism is a paralytic disease caused by potent protein neurotoxins elaborated by *Clostridium botulinum*. Illness begins with cranial nerve involvement, and progression proceeds caudally to involve the extremities. Cases may be classified as (1) *food-borne botulism*, from ingestion of preformed toxin in food contaminated with *C. botulinum*; (2) *wound botulism*, from toxin produced in wounds contaminated with the organism; and (3) *intestinal botulism*, from in-

gestion of spores and production of toxin in the intestine of infants (infant botulism) or adults. Botulinum toxin, because of its extraordinary potency, has long been considered a threat as an agent of bioterrorism or biological warfare (see Chap. 205).

ETIOLOGIC AGENT *C. botulinum*, a species encompassing a heterogeneous group of anaerobic gram-positive organisms that form subterminal spores, is found in soil and marine environments throughout the world and elaborates the most potent bacterial toxin known. Organisms of types A through G have been distinguished by the antigenic specificities of their toxins; a classification system based on physiologic characteristics has also been described. Rare strains of other clostridial species—*C. butyricum* and *C. baratii*—have also been found to produce toxin. *C. botulinum* strains with proteolytic activity can digest food and produce a spoiled appearance; nonproteolytic types leave the appearance of food unchanged.

Of the eight distinct toxin types described (A, B, C_1, C_2, D, E, F, and G), all except C_2 are neurotoxins; C_2 is a cytotoxin of unknown clinical significance. Botulinum neurotoxin, whether ingested, inhaled, or produced in the intestine or a wound, enters the vascular system and is transported to peripheral cholinergic nerve terminals, including neuromuscular junctions, postganglionic parasympathetic nerve endings, and peripheral ganglia. The central nervous system is not involved. Active neurotoxin (150 kDa) is composed of a heavy chain (a 100-kDa fragment responsible for neurospecific binding and translocation in the nerve cell) and a light chain (a 50-kDa fragment responsible for intracellular catalytic activity). The steps involved in neurotoxin activity include (1) specific binding to presynaptic nerve cells at the myoneural junction, (2) internalization of the toxin inside the nerve cell in endocytic vesicles, (3) translocation of the toxin into the cytosol, and (4) proteolysis by toxin (a zinc endopeptidase) of components of the neuroexocytosis apparatus curtailing release of the neurotransmitter acetylcholine. Cure follows sprouting of new nerve terminals.

Toxin is heat-labile, but spores are highly heat-resistant; both can be inactivated under appropriate conditions (see "Prevention," below). In the gastrointestinal tract, toxin is complexed with nontoxin proteins and resists degradation. Toxin types A, B, E, and (rarely) F cause human disease; type G (from *C. argentinense*) has been associated with sudden death, but not with neuroparalytic illness, in a few patients in Switzerland; and types C and D cause animal disease.

EPIDEMIOLOGY Human botulism occurs worldwide. In the United States, the geographic distribution of cases by toxin type parallels the distribution of organism types found in the environment. Type A predominates west of the Rocky Mountains; type B is generally distributed but is more common in the East; and type E is found in the Pacific Northwest, Alaska, and the Great Lakes area. In the United States, food-borne botulism has been associated primarily with home-canned food, particularly vegetables, fruit, and condiments, and less commonly with meat and fish. Type E outbreaks are frequently associated with fish products. Commercial products occasionally cause outbreaks, but some of these outbreaks have resulted from improper handling after purchase. Outbreaks in restaurants, schools, and private homes have been traced to uncommon sources (commercial potpies, beef stew, turkey loaf, sautéed onions, baked potatoes, and chopped garlic in oil). Food-borne botulism can occur when (1) a food to be preserved is contaminated with spores, (2) preservation does not inactivate the spores but kills other putrefactive bacteria that might inhibit growth of *C. botulinum* and provides anaerobic conditions at a pH and temperature that allow germination and toxin production, and (3) food is not heated to a temperature that destroys toxin before being eaten.

CLINICAL MANIFESTATIONS ■ **Food-Borne Botulism** After ingestion of food containing toxin, illness varies from a mild condition for which no medical advice is sought to very severe disease that can result in death within 24 h. The incubation period is usually 18 to 36 h but, depending on toxin dose, can extend from a few hours to several days. Symmetric descending paralysis is characteristic and can lead to respiratory failure and death. Cranial nerve involvement, which almost always marks the onset of symptoms, usually produces diplopia, dysarthria, dysphonia, and/or dysphagia. Weakness progresses, often rapidly, from the head to involve the neck, arms, thorax, and legs; occasionally, weakness is asymmetric. Nausea, vomiting, and abdominal pain may precede or follow the onset of paralysis. Dizziness, blurred vision, dry mouth, and very dry, occasionally sore throat are common. Patients are generally alert and oriented, but they may be drowsy, agitated, and anxious. Typically, they have no fever. Ptosis is frequent; the pupillary reflexes may be depressed, and fixed or dilated pupils are noted in half of patients. The gag reflex may be suppressed, and deep tendon reflexes may be normal or decreased. Sensory findings are usually absent. Paralytic ileus, severe constipation, and urinary retention are common.

Wound Botulism Wound botulism occurs when the spores contaminating a wound germinate and form vegetative organisms that produce toxin. This rare condition resembles food-borne illness except that the incubation period is longer, averaging about 10 days, and gastrointestinal symptoms are lacking. Wound botulism has been documented after traumatic injury involving contamination with soil; in injection drug users, for whom black-tar heroin use has been identified as a risk factor; and after cesarean delivery. The illness has occurred even after antibiotics have been given to prevent wound infection. When present, fever is probably attributable to concurrent infection with other bacteria. The wound may appear benign.

Intestinal Botulism In intestinal botulism, toxin is produced in and absorbed from the intestine after the germination of ingested spores. Infant botulism is the most common form of botulism. The severity ranges from mild illness with failure to thrive to fulminant severe paralysis with respiratory failure. Infant botulism may be one cause of sudden infant death. The identification of contaminated honey as one source of spores has led to the recommendation that honey not be fed to children <12 months of age. Most cases cannot be attributed to a particular food source. The factors permitting intestinal colonization with *C. botulinum* are not fully defined, but cases usually involve infants <6 months of age; susceptibility may decrease as the normal intestinal flora develops. Intestinal botulism involving adults is uncommon. The patient may have a history of gastrointestinal disease, gastrointestinal surgery, or recent antibiotic therapy. Toxin and organisms may be identified in the stool.

Bioterrorism and Biological Warfare (See also Chap. 205) Botulinum toxin could be dispersed as an aerosol (producing inhalational botulism) or as a contaminant in material to be ingested (producing food-borne botulism). Inhalational botulism resembles food-borne illness, but gastrointestinal symptoms are absent. Botulism follows adsorption of toxin from mucosal surfaces (gut, lung) and wounds, but the toxin does not penetrate intact skin. As a toxin-mediated illness, botulism is noncommunicable, and standard isolation precautions are sufficient unless bacterial meningitis is being considered. Features suggestive of an outbreak due to deliberate release of botulinum toxin are shown in Table 125-1.

DIAGNOSIS A diagnosis of botulism must be considered in patients with symmetric descending paralysis who are afebrile and mentally intact. The bulbar musculature is involved initially, but sensory findings are absent and, early on, deep tendon reflexes remain intact. The differential diagnosis of botulism and differentiating features are listed in Table 125-2.

The demonstration of toxin in serum by bioassay in mice is definitive, but this test may be negative, particularly in wound and infant botulism. It is performed only by specific laboratories, which can be identified through regional public health authorities. Other assays are

---

TABLE 125-1 *Features of Outbreaks Suggesting Deliberate Release of Botulinum Toxin*[a]

- Outbreak of large number of cases of acute flaccid paralysis with prominent bulbar palsies
- Outbreak with an unusual botulinum toxin type (i.e., type C, D, F, or G or type E toxin not associated with food of aquatic origin)
- Outbreak with a common geographic factor among cases (e.g., airport, work location) but without a common dietary exposure (i.e., features suggesting an aerosol attack)
- Multiple simultaneous outbreaks with no common source

[a] A careful travel and activity history, as well as a dietary history, should be taken in any suspected botulism outbreak. Patients should also be asked whether they know of other persons with similar symptoms.

Source: Reproduced with permission of the publisher from Arnon et al, 2002

TABLE 125-2 *Selected Mimics That May Lead to Misdiagnosis of Botulism*

Condition	Features Distinguishing Condition from Botulism
COMMON MISDIAGNOSES	
Guillain-Barré syndrome[a] and its variants, especially Miller-Fisher variant	History of antecedent infection; paresthesias; often ascending paralysis; early areflexia; eventual CSF protein increase; EMG findings
Myasthenia gravis[a]	Recurrent paralysis; EMG findings; sustained response to anticholinesterase
Stroke[a]	Paralysis often asymmetric; abnormal CNS image
Intoxication with depressants (e.g., acute alcohol intoxication), organophosphates, carbon monoxide, or nerve gas	History of exposure; excessive drug levels detected in body fluids
Lambert-Eaton syndrome	Increased strength with sustained contraction; evidence of lung carcinoma; EMG findings similar to botulism
Tick paralysis	Paresthesias; ascending paralysis; tick attached to skin
OTHER MISDIAGNOSES	
Poliomyelitis	Antecedent febrile illness; asymmetric paralysis; CSF pleocytosis
CNS infections, especially of the brainstem	Mental status changes; CSF and EEG abnormalities
CNS tumor	Paralysis often asymmetric; abnormal CNS image
Streptococcal pharyngitis[b]	Absence of bulbar palsies; positive rapid antigen test result or throat culture
Psychiatric illness[a]	Normal EMG in conversion paralysis
Viral syndrome[a]	Absence of bulbar palsies and flaccid paralysis
Inflammatory myopathy[a]	Elevated creatine kinase level
Diabetic complications[a]	Sensory neuropathy; few cranial nerve palsies
Hyperemesis gravidarum[a]	Absence of bulbar palsies and acute flaccid paralysis
Hypothyroidism[a]	Abnormal thyroid function tests
Laryngeal trauma[a]	Absence of flaccid paralysis; dysphonia without flaccid paralysis
Overexertion[a]	Absence of bulbar palsies and acute flaccid paralysis

[a] Misdiagnoses made in a large outbreak of botulism (St. Louis ME et al: Botulism from chopped garlic: Delayed recognition of a major outbreak. Ann Intern Med 108:363, 1988).

[b] Pharyngeal erythema can occur in botulism.

Note: CNS, central nervous system; CSF, cerebrospinal fluid; EEG, electroencephalogram; EMG, electromyogram.

Source: Reproduced with the permission of the publisher from Arnon et al, 2002.

being developed and remain experimental. The demonstration of the organism or its toxin in vomitus, gastric fluid, or stool is strongly suggestive of the diagnosis, because intestinal carriage is rare. Isolation of the organism from food without toxin is insufficient grounds for the diagnosis. Wound cultures yielding the organism are suggestive of botulism. The edrophonium chloride (Tensilon) test for myasthenia gravis may be falsely positive in botulism but is usually less dramatically positive than in the former condition. Nerve conduction velocity is normal, but compound muscle action potentials on routine nerve stimulation studies are decreased with a supramaximal stimulus, and facilitation is evident after repetitive stimulation at high frequency. Single-fiber electromyography may be helpful. The white blood cell count and erythrocyte sedimentation rate are normal.

℞ TREATMENT

Patients should be hospitalized and monitored closely, both clinically and by spirometry, pulse oximetry, and measurement of arterial blood gases for incipient respiratory failure. Intubation and mechanical ventilation should be strongly considered when the vital capacity is <30% of predicted, especially when paralysis is progressing rapidly and hypoxemia with absolute or relative hypercarbia is documented (Chap. 252). Serial measurements of the maximal static inspiratory pressure may be useful in predicting respiratory failure.

In food-borne illness, equine antitoxin should be administered as soon as possible after specimens are obtained for laboratory analysis. Treatment should not await laboratory analyses, which may take days. The previous trivalent antitoxin (types A, B, and E) preparation is no longer available. Instead, a bivalent preparation containing toxin types A and B and an investigational monovalent type E preparation can be obtained. The bivalent preparation is given routinely; monovalent type E antitoxin is given in addition when exposure to type E toxin is suspected (after seafood ingestion, for example). In the United States, antitoxin as well as help in clinical management and laboratory confirmation are available at *any* time from state health departments or from the Centers for Disease Control and Prevention (CDC: 404-639-2206; emergency number, 404-639-2888). A limited supply of an investigational heptavalent antitoxin (types A through G) is maintained by the U.S. military for emergency use.

After testing for hypersensitivity to horse serum, antitoxin is given as recommended by the CDC; repeated doses are not considered necessary. Anaphylaxis and serum sickness are risks inherent in use of the equine product, and desensitization of allergic patients may be required. If there is no ileus, cathartics and enemas may be given to purge the gut of toxin; emetics or gastric lavage can also be used if the time since ingestion is brief (only a few hours). Neither the use of antibiotics to eliminate an intestinal source for possible continued toxin production nor the administration of guanidine hydrochloride and other drugs to reverse paralysis is of proven value.

Treatment of infant botulism requires supportive care and administration of human botulism immune globulin (obtainable at all times from the California Department of Health Services at 510-540-2646). Neither equine antitoxin nor antibiotics have been shown to be beneficial. In wound botulism, equine antitoxin is administered. The wound should be thoroughly explored and debrided, and an antibiotic such as penicillin should be given to eradicate *C. botulinum* from the site, even though the benefit of this therapy is unproven. Results of wound cultures should guide the use of other antibiotics.

Botulinum toxins have been approved for therapeutic use. Botulinum toxin type A has been approved for the treatment of strabismus, blepharospasm, cervical dystonia, and glabellar lines; therapy appears safe and effective. Botulinum toxin type B has been approved for the treatment of cervical dystonia. The value of these preparations in many other conditions is being evaluated. Generalized botulism-like weakness complicating therapy has been reported but is rare.

PROGNOSIS Type A disease is generally more severe than type B, and mortality from botulism is higher among patients above age 60 than among younger patients. With improved respiratory and intensive care, the case-fatality rate in food-borne illness has been reduced to ~7.5% and is low in infant botulism as well. Artificial respiratory support may be required for months in severe cases. Some patients experience residual weakness and autonomic dysfunction for as long as a year after disease onset.

PREVENTION A pentavalent vaccine (A–E) is available for use in highly exposed individuals. Spores can be inactivated by exposure to high temperature (116° to 121°C) and pressure, as in steam sterilizers or pressure cookers used in accordance with the manufacturer's instructions. Toxin can be inactivated by exposure to a temperature of 100°C for 10 min. Newly identified cases should be reported immediately to public health authorities.

ANGULO FJ et al: Large outbreak of botulism: The hazardous baked potato. Clin Infect Dis 178:172, 1998

ARNON SS et al: Botulinum toxin as a biological weapon, in *Bioterrorism: Guidelines for Medical and Public Health Management*, DA Henderson et al (eds). Chicago, AMA Press, 2002, pp 141–165

CHERINGTON M: Clinical spectrum of botulism. Muscle Nerve 21:701, 1998

HATHEWAY CL: Botulism: The present status of disease. Curr Top Microbiol Immunol 195:55, 1995

LONG SS: Infant botulism. Pediatr Infect Dis J 20:707, 2001

MEUNIER FA et al: Botulinum neurotoxins: From paralysis to recovery of functional neuromuscular transmission. J Physiol Paris, 96:105, 2002

SHAPIRO RL et al: Botulism in the United States: A clinical and epidemiologic review. Ann Intern Med 129:221, 1998

WERNER SB et al: Wound botulism in California, 1951–1998: Recent epidemic in heroin injectors. Clin Infect Dis 31:1018, 2000

126 GAS GANGRENE AND OTHER CLOSTRIDIAL INFECTIONS
Dennis L. Kasper, Lawrence C. Madoff

DEFINITION Bacteria of the genus *Clostridium* are gram-positive, spore-forming, obligate anaerobes that are ubiquitous in nature. There are >60 recognized species of clostridia, many of which are generally considered saprophytic. Some of these species are pathogenic for humans and animals, particularly under conditions of lowered oxidation-reduction potential. Infections associated with these organisms range from localized wound contamination to overwhelming systemic disease. The four major disease categories for which clostridia are responsible are intestinal disorders, suppurative deep-tissue infections, skin and soft tissue infections, and bacteremia. Toxins play a major role in some of these syndromes. →*Colitis caused by C. difficile is discussed in Chap. 114.*

ETIOLOGY In humans, clostridia normally reside in the gastrointestinal tract and in the female genital tract, although they occasionally are isolated from the skin or the mouth. Of the known species of the genus *Clostridium*, at least 30 have been isolated from human infections. Like several other pathogenic anaerobic bacterial species, clostridia are quite aerotolerant, but they do not grow on artificial media in the presence of oxygen. Clostridia characteristically produce abundant gas in artificial media and form subterminal endospores. *C. perfringens*, one of the most important species, is encapsulated and nonmotile and rarely sporulates in artificial media; the spores can usually be destroyed by boiling. →*C. tetani and C. botulinum are discussed in detail in Chaps. 124 and 125, respectively.*

Clostridia are present in the normal colonic flora at concentrations of 10^9 to 10^{10}/g. Of the >30 species that normally colonize humans, *C. ramosum* is the most abundant and is followed in frequency by *C. perfringens*. These organisms are universally present in soil at concentrations of up to 10^4/g. *C. perfringens* strains are classified (on the basis of their production of several lethal toxins) into five types, designated A through E. Type A predominates in fecal flora of humans as well as in soil, whereas the habitats of types B through E are thought to be the intestinal tracts of other animals. Although clostridia are gram-positive organisms, many species may appear to be gram-negative in clinical specimens or stationary-phase cultures. Therefore, the results of Gram's staining of cultures or clinical material should be interpreted with great care.

C. perfringens is the most common of the clostridial species isolated from tissue infections and bacteremias; next in frequency are *C. novyi* and *C. septicum*. In the category of enteric infections, *C. difficile* is an important cause of antibiotic-associated colitis, and *C. perfringens* is associated with food poisoning (type A) and enteritis necroticans (type C).

PATHOGENESIS Despite the isolation of clostridial species from many serious traumatic wounds, the prevalence of severe infections due to these organisms is low. Two factors that appear to be essential to the development of severe disease are tissue necrosis and a low oxidation-reduction potential. *C. perfringens* requires about 14 amino acids and at least 6 additional growth factors for optimal growth. These nutrients are not found in appreciable concentrations in normal body fluids but are present in necrotic tissue. When *C. perfringens* grows in necrotic tissue, a zone of tissue damage due to the toxins elaborated by the

organism allows progressive growth. In contrast, when only a few bacteria leak into the bloodstream from a small defect in the intestinal wall, the organisms do not have the opportunity to multiply rapidly because blood as a medium for growth is relatively deficient in certain amino acids and growth factors. Therefore, in a patient without tissue necrosis, bacteremia is usually benign.

C. perfringens possesses at least 17 possible virulence factors, including 12 active tissue toxins and enterotoxins. The enterotoxins include four major lethal toxins: α, β, ϵ, and ι. The α *toxin* is a phospholipase C (lecithinase) that splits lecithin into phosphorylcholine and diglyceride. It has been associated with gas gangrene and is known to be hemolytic, to destroy platelets and polymorphonuclear leukocytes (PMNs), and to cause widespread capillary damage. When injected intravenously, it causes massive intravascular hemolysis and damages liver mitochondria. The α toxin may be important in the initiation of muscle infections that may progress to gas gangrene. Experimentally, the higher the concentration of α toxin in the culture fluid, the smaller the dose of *C. perfringens* required to produce infection. The protective effect of antiserum is directly proportional to its content of α antitoxin. Studies suggest that θ *toxin*, a thiol-activated cytolysin that is also called *perfringolysin O*, may also play an important role in pathogenesis by promoting vascular leukostasis, endothelial cell injury, and regional tissue hypoxia. The resulting perfusion defects extend the anaerobic environment and contribute to rapidly advancing tissue destruction. A characteristic pathologic finding in gas gangrene is the near absence of PMNs despite extensive tissue destruction. Experimental data indicate that both α and θ toxins are essential in the leukocyte aggregation that occurs at the margins of tissue injury instead of the expected infiltration of these cells into the area of damage. Genetically altered strains induce less leukocyte aggregation when α toxin is absent and none when θ toxin is missing. The other major toxins, β, ϵ, and ι, are known to increase capillary permeability.

CLINICAL MANIFESTATIONS ■ **Intestinal Disorders** ■ *FOOD POISONING* *C. perfringens*, primarily type A, is the second or third most common cause of food poisoning in the United States (Chap. 113). The responsible toxin is thought to be a cytotoxin produced by >75% of strains isolated from cases of foodborne disease. The cytotoxin binds to a receptor on the small-bowel brush border and induces a calcium ion–dependent alteration in permeability. The associated loss of ions alters intracellular metabolism, resulting in cell death. Outbreaks generally have resulted from problems in the cooling and storage of food cooked in bulk. The food sources primarily involved are meat, meat products, and poultry. Generally, the implicated meats have been cooked, allowed to cool, and then recooked the following day, often in a stew or hash. Strains of *C. perfringens* that contaminate meat manage to survive initial cooking. During reheating, the organisms sporulate and germinate. The disease is associated with an attack rate that is often as high as 70%. Symptoms of food poisoning from type A strains develop 8 to 24 h after ingestion of foods heavily contaminated with the organism. The primary symptoms include epigastric pain, nausea, and watery diarrhea usually lasting 12 to 24 h. Fever and vomiting are uncommon. Molecular methods including ribotyping and pulsed-field gel electrophoresis have been used to detect fecal cytotoxin in outbreaks of food poisoning caused by *C. perfringens*.

C. perfringens has also been implicated in a more severe form of diarrhea than that of classic food poisoning. This more severe disease tends to occur in the elderly and has been associated with antibiotic use in hospitalized populations. In this form of disease, diarrhea is generally more profuse, of longer duration, and accompanied by abdominal pain. Blood and mucus have been detected in the feces of the affected patients. In one hospital-based study of a cluster of cases, widespread environmental contamination with *C. perfringens* spores was documented.

ENTERITIS NECROTICANS   Necrotizing enteritis (enteritis necroticans, or *pigbel*) is caused by β toxin produced by type C strains of *C. perfringens* following ingestion of a high-protein meal in conjunction with trypsin inhibitors (e.g., in sweet potatoes) by a susceptible host who has limited intestinal proteolytic activity. This disease has been reported among children and adults in New Guinea. A similar disease, *darmbrand*, was epidemic in Germany after World War II. Clinical features of pigbel include acute abdominal pain, bloody diarrhea, vomiting, shock, and peritonitis; 40% of patients die. Pathologic studies reveal an acute ulcerative process of the bowel restricted to the small intestine. The mucosa is lifted off the submucosa, with the formation of large denuded areas. Pseudomembranes composed of sloughed epithelium are common, and gas may dissect into the submucosa. The source of the organisms may be the patient's own intestinal flora; cultures of ingested pork have failed to yield the organism. Antibodies to the β toxin of *C. perfringens* have been of considerable benefit in changing the course of established disease. In a large-scale trial, children immunized with *C. perfringens* β toxoid were protected.

NEUTROPENIC ENTEROCOLITIS (TYPHLITIS)   See Chaps. 72 and 148.

Suppurative Deep Tissue Infections   Clostridia are frequently recovered from various suppurative conditions in conjunction with other anaerobic and aerobic bacteria but can also be the only organisms isolated. These suppurative conditions, which exist with severe local inflammation but usually without the characteristic systemic signs induced by clostridial toxins, include intraabdominal sepsis, empyema, pelvic abscess, subcutaneous abscess, frostbite with gas gangrene, infection of a stump in an amputee, brain abscess, prostatic abscess, perianal abscess, conjunctivitis, infection of a renal cell carcinoma, and infection of an aortic graft.

Clostridia are isolated from approximately two-thirds of patients with intraabdominal infections resulting from intestinal perforation. *C. ramosum*, *C. perfringens*, and *C. bifermentans* are the most commonly isolated species. The presence of clostridial species does not affect the clinical presentation or outcome of these infections (Chap. 148).

An association has been made between malignancy and the isolation of *C. septicum* in the absence of grossly contaminated deep traumatic wounds. A major site for such a malignancy is the gastrointestinal tract, particularly the colon. An association with leukemia or with other solid tumors has also been noted, and one case of fatal myonecrosis has been reported in a patient with ovarian cancer. Some of these patients present with *C. septicum* bacteremia; these cases have a fulminant clinical course (discussed below). Others develop localized suppurative infection in the abdomen or the abdominal wall without bacteremia. Presumably, this infection arises from a silent perforation that leads to intraabdominal abscess formation.

Clostridia have been isolated from suppurative infections of the female genital tract, particularly tuboovarian and pelvic abscesses. The major species involved has been *C. perfringens*. Most of these are mild suppurative infections without evidence of uterine gangrene. *C. perfringens* has been isolated from as many as 20% of diseased gallbladders at surgery. One clinical syndrome, *emphysematous cholecystitis*, is caused by clostridial species at least 50% of the time. In this syndrome, gas forms in the biliary radicles and the wall of the gallbladder.

Emphysematous cholecystitis is seen most often in diabetic patients. Although the mortality rate in this entity is higher than in more common forms of cholecystitis, there is no evidence of myonecrosis.

Clostridia are among the many organisms found in empyema fluid or isolated by transtracheal aspiration from patients with lung abscesses. There is no unique clinical clue to the presence of clostridia (as opposed to other organisms) in these infections. *C. perfringens* has been reported as a cause of empyema arising from aspiration pneumonia, pulmonary emboli, and infarction. However, the majority of cases of clostridial empyema are secondary to trauma.

Skin and Soft Tissue Infections   Various categories of traumatic wound infections due to clostridia have been described: simple contamination, anaerobic cellulitis, fasciitis with or without systemic manifestations, and anaerobic myonecrosis.

SIMPLE CONTAMINATION   Clostridia are cultured most often from wounds in the absence of clinical signs of sepsis. As many as 30% of battle wounds are contaminated by clostridia without signs of suppuration, and 16% of penetrating abdominal wounds yield clostridia on culture despite treatment with cephalothin and kanamycin. In cases of trauma, clostridia are isolated with equal frequency from suppurative and well-healing wounds. Thus the diagnosis of clostridial infection should be based on clinical rather than bacteriologic criteria.

LOCALIZED INFECTION OF THE SKIN AND SOFT TISSUE WITHOUT SYSTEMIC SIGNS   This condition, originally referred to as *anaerobic cellulitis*, is a localized infection involving the skin and soft tissue and is due to clostridia alone or with other bacteria. There are no systemic signs of toxicity, although the infection may invade locally, producing necrosis. These infections tend to be relatively indolent, spreading slowly to contiguous areas. Localized infections are relatively free of pain and edema. Perhaps because of the lack of edema, gas that is limited to the wound and the immediately surrounding tissue may be more evident than in gas gangrene. In these localized infections, gas is never found intramuscularly. Cellulitis, perirectal abscesses, and diabetic foot ulcers are typical infections from which clostridial species can be isolated. If inadequately treated, these localized infections advance by extension through subcutaneous tissue and fascial planes into muscle and may produce severe systemic disease with signs of toxemia.

A localized form of suppurative myositis has been described in heroin addicts. These patients develop local pain and tenderness in discrete areas (particularly the thigh and forearm), with the subsequent appearance of fluctuance and crepitance that require surgical drainage. The unusual aspect of these infections is that they remain localized without systemic signs of toxicity. Moreover, the affected local areas are not necessarily sites of trauma or heroin injection. Pathologic examination reveals subcutaneous abscesses, purulent myositis, and fasciitis from which clostridia are recovered in pure culture; on occasion, mixed infections involving aerobes and anaerobes are found. Wound botulism has been reported in association with the injection of black tar heroin.

SPREADING CELLULITIS AND FASCIITIS WITH SYSTEMIC TOXICITY   This condition involves diffuse spreading cellulitis and fasciitis, without myonecrosis and with only mild inflammation in muscle. Patients present with the abrupt onset of a syndrome that progresses rapidly (within hours) through the fascial planes. In cases with suppuration and gas in soft tissues as well as overwhelming toxemia, the infection is rapidly fatal. On physical examination there is subcutaneous crepitation but little localized pain. Surgery is of no proven value because there are no discretely involved tissues amenable to resection, as may be the case in myonecrosis. However, in rapidly advancing fasciitis, incision of the affected area is still the cornerstone of therapy. The initial local lesion may be quite innocuous and arises from an area involved by tumor or other infection and not by injury. The systemic toxic effects include hemolysis and injury of capillary membranes. Usually, this infection is fatal within 48 h, despite intensive therapy involving antitoxin and exchange transfusion. This syndrome is seen most commonly in patients with carcinoma, especially of the sigmoid or the cecum. Presumably, the tumor invades the fascia, and colonic contents leak into the abdominal wall. Patients present with extreme toxicity and occasionally with total-body crepitation. The syndrome differs from necrotizing fasciitis caused by other organisms in three respects: (1) rapid mortality, (2) rapid tissue invasion, and (3) the systemic effects of the toxin, typified by massive hemolysis.

GAS GANGRENE (CLOSTRIDIAL MYONECROSIS) Gas gangrene is characterized by rapid and extensive necrosis of muscle accompanied by gas formation and systemic toxicity and occurs when bacteria invade healthy muscle from adjacent traumatized muscle or soft tissue. The infection originates in a wound contaminated with clostridia. Although >30% of deep wounds are infected with clostridia, the incidence of clostridial myonecrosis is quite low. These infections occur in both military and civilian settings. An essential factor in the genesis of gas gangrene appears to be trauma, particularly involving deep muscle laceration. The entity of clostridial myonecrosis is relatively uncommon after simple, through-and-through bullet wounds without shattering of bone and is relatively common following shrapnel fragmentation wounds, particularly when deep muscle is involved. In civilian cases, gas gangrene can follow trauma, surgery, or intramuscular injection. The trauma need not be severe; however, the wound must be deep, necrotic, and without communication to the surface.

The incubation period of gas gangrene is usually short: almost always <3 days and frequently <24 h. Some 80% of cases are caused by *C. perfringens*, while *C. novyi*, *C. septicum*, and *C. histolyticum* cause most of the remaining cases. Typically, gas gangrene begins with the sudden onset of pain in the region of the wound, which helps to differentiate it from spreading cellulitis. Once established, the pain increases steadily in severity but remains localized to the infected area and spreads only if the infection spreads. Soon after pain develops, local swelling and edema—accompanied by a thin, often hemorrhagic exudate—appear. Patients frequently develop marked tachycardia, but elevation in temperature may be only minimal. Gas is usually not obvious at this early stage and may be completely absent. Frothiness of the wound exudate may be noted. The skin is tense, white, often marbled with blue, and cooler than normal. The symptoms progress rapidly; swelling, edema, and toxemia increase, and a profuse serous discharge, which may have a peculiar sweetish smell, appears. Gram's staining of the wound exudate shows many gram-positive rods with relatively few inflammatory cells.

At surgery, muscle may appear pale because of the intensity of edema, but it does not contract when probed with a scalpel. When dissected, the muscle is beefy red and nonviable and can progress to become black, friable, and gangrenous. It is important to establish a diagnosis early, preferably by frozen-section biopsy of muscle.

Despite hypotension, renal failure, and (often) body crepitation, patients with myonecrosis frequently have a heightened awareness of their surroundings until just before death, when they lapse into toxic delirium and coma. In untreated cases, as the local wounds progress, the skin becomes bronzed; bullae appear, become filled with dark red fluid, and are accompanied by dark patches of cutaneous gangrene. Gas appears in later phases (Fig. 126-1) but may not be as obvious as in anaerobic cellulitis. Jaundice is rare in wound gas gangrene (in contrast to uterine infections) and, when it does appear, is almost invariably associated with hemoglobinuria, hemoglobinemia, and septicemia. Cases of clostridial myonecrosis without a history of trauma have been reported. These patients have bullous lesions and crepitation of the skin; they present with a rapidly worsening course that includes myonecrosis, especially of the extremities.

FIGURE 126-1 Spontaneous gas gangrene. Radiographs of the elbow (*A*) and shoulder (*B*) show gas in tissue. The patient developed spontaneous gas gangrene of the hand, which spread rapidly up the arm and onto the thorax. *C. septicum* was grown from blood and necrotic tissue of the arm. *[Reprinted with permission from DL Stevens (ed): Atlas of Infectious Diseases, vol II: Skin, Soft Tissue, Bone and Joint Infections. Philadelphia, Current Medicine, 1995.]*

Bacteremia and Clostridial Sepsis The relatively common entity of transient clostridial bacteremia can arise in any hospitalized patient but is most common with a predisposing focus in the gastrointestinal tract, biliary tract, or uterus. Fever frequently resolves within 24 to 48 h without therapy. Despite the finding of clostridial bacteremia following septic abortions and the frequent isolation of clostridia from the lochia, most of the patients involved do not have evidence of sepsis. In one series of 60 patients with clostridial bacteremia, half had an infected site that could be associated with the bacteremia, while the other half had a totally unrelated illness, such as tuberculous pneumonia, meningitis, or benign gastroenteritis. By the time blood culture reports are returned, patients frequently are completely well and sometimes have been discharged. Therefore, when a blood culture is positive for clostridia, the patient must be assessed clinically rather than simply treated on the basis of the culture result.

Clostridial sepsis is an uncommon but almost invariably fatal illness following clostridial infection—primarily that of the uterus, colon, or biliary tract. This entity must be differentiated from transient clostridial bacteremia, which is much more common. *C. perfringens* causes the majority of cases of both sepsis and transient bacteremia. *C. septicum*, *C. sordellii*, and *C. novyi* account for most of the remainder of cases. Clostridia account for 1 to 2.5% of all positive blood cultures in major hospital centers.

The majority of cases of clostridial sepsis originate from the female genital tract and follow septic abortion. Introduction of a foreign body is a common antecedent event. In the uterus, residual necrotic fetal and placental tissues and traumatized endometrium may allow the growth of clostridia. Only a small fraction of cases of septic abortion (1%) are followed by serious sepsis. In these patients, sepsis, fever, and chills begin from 1 to 3 days after the attempted abortion. The initial signs are malaise, headache, severe myalgias, abdominal pain, nausea, vomiting, and occasionally diarrhea. Frequently, a bloody or brown vaginal discharge is noted. Patients may rapidly develop oliguria, hypotension, jaundice, and hemoglobinuria. The hemolysis, which is secondary to *C. perfringens* α toxin, causes a characteristic bronzing of the skin. As in myonecrosis, the mental status of severely ill patients is characterized by increased alertness and apprehension. Local examination of the pelvis reveals foul cervical discharge, occasionally with gas. Frequently, laceration marks around the cervix or perforation of the cervical segment is evident. If the infection involves the myometrium or has spread to the adnexa, extreme tenderness, guarding, and an adnexal mass may be found.

Laboratory studies in patients with sepsis reveal an elevated white blood cell count and may show pink, hemoglobin-tinged plasma. Anemia is proportional to the degree of hemolysis, and the hematocrit may be extremely low. Platelet counts may be reduced, and there is often evidence of disseminated intravascular coagulation (DIC). Oliguria or anuria, increasingly refractory hypotension, and hemorrhage and bruising may develop.

Clostridia may enter the bloodstream from the gastrointestinal or biliary tract. This occurrence is associated with ulcerative lesions or obstruction of the small or large intestine, necrotic or infiltrating malignancy, bowel surgery, or various abdominal catastrophes. The patient may present with an acute febrile illness, with chills and fever but no other signs of localized infection. Intravascular hemolysis occurs in as many as half of such cases. Biliary or gastrointestinal symptoms, if present, may be the only clue to the etiology. Positive blood cultures provide the definitive clue to the diagnosis.

Patients with malignant disease can also develop rapidly fatal clostridial sepsis, particularly from a gastrointestinal focus. The most common species in this setting is *C. septicum*. Characteristic signs and symptoms include fever, tachycardia, hypotension, abdominal pain or tenderness, nausea, vomiting, and (preterminally) coma. The tachycardia may be out of proportion to the fever. Only ~20 to 30% of patients develop hemolysis. A striking feature of this syndrome is the rapidity of death, which frequently occurs in <12 h.

DIAGNOSIS The diagnosis of clostridial disease, in association with positive cultures, must be based primarily on clinical findings. Because of the presence of clostridia in many wounds, their mere isolation from any site, including the blood, does not necessarily indicate severe disease. Smears of wound exudates, uterine scrapings, or cervical discharge may show abundant large gram-positive rods as well as other organisms. Cultures should be placed in selective media and incubated anaerobically for identification of clostridia. The diagnosis of clostridial myonecrosis can be established by frozen-section biopsy of muscle.

The urine of patients with severe clostridial sepsis may contain protein and casts, and some patients may develop severe uremia. Profound alterations of circulating erythrocytes are seen in severely toxemic patients. Patients have hemolytic anemia, which develops extremely rapidly, along with hemoglobinemia, hemoglobinuria, and elevated levels of serum bilirubin. Spherocytosis, increased osmotic and mechanical red blood cell fragility, erythrophagocytosis, and methemoglobinemia have been described. DIC may develop in patients with severe infection. In patients with severe sepsis, Wright's or Gram's staining of a smear of peripheral blood or buffy coat may demonstrate clostridia.

X-ray examination sometimes provides an important clue to the diagnosis by revealing gas in muscles, subcutaneous tissue, or the uterus. However, the finding of gas is not pathognomonic for clostridial infection. Other anaerobic bacteria, frequently mixed with aerobic organisms, may produce gas.

℞ TREATMENT (Table 126-1)

Traumatic wounds should be thoroughly cleansed and debrided. Traditionally, the antibiotic treatment of choice for severe clostridial infection has been penicillin G (20 million units per day in adults). Penicillin G treatment of gas gangrene has become more controversial because of increasing resistance to this drug and data obtained from animal models of infection. In a mouse model of gas gangrene, antibiotics inhibiting toxin synthesis appeared to be preferable to cell wall–active drugs; clindamycin treatment enhanced survival more than therapy with penicillin; and the combination of clindamycin and penicillin was superior to penicillin alone. For severe clostridial sepsis, clindamycin may be used at a dose of 600 mg every 6 h in combination with high-dose penicillin (3 to 4 million units every 4 h). Although no clinical trials validate this choice, it is gaining acceptance in the infectious disease community.

In cases of penicillin sensitivity or allergy, other antibiotics should be considered, but all should be tested for in vitro activity because of the occasional isolation of resistant strains. Clostridia are frequently, but not universally, susceptible in vitro to cefoxitin, carbenicillin, chloramphenicol, clindamycin, metronidazole, doxycycline, imipenem, minocycline, tetracycline, third-generation cephalosporins, and vancomycin. For severe clostridial infections, sensitivity testing should be done before an antimicrobial agent with unpredictable activity is used. Simple contamination of a wound with clostridia should not be treated with antibiotics. Localized skin and soft tissue infection can be managed by debridement rather than with systemic antibiotics. Drugs are required when the process extends into adjacent tissue or when fever and systemic signs of sepsis are present. Surgery is a mainstay of therapy for gas gangrene. Amputation is often required for rapidly spreading infection involving a limb, as the process frequently fails to respond to antibiotics. Hysterectomy is required for uterine myonecrosis. Abdominal wall myonecrosis usually continues despite initial aggressive surgery and antibiotic therapy and requires repeated surgical debridement of all involved muscle.

Suppurative infections should be treated with antibiotics. Frequently, broad-spectrum antibiotics must be used because of the mixed flora involved in these infections. Aminoglycosides can be used for the aerobic gram-negative bacteria involved in mixed infections.

The use of a polyvalent gas gangrene antitoxin is still recommended by some authorities. At present, no such antitoxin is produced in the United States, and most centers have discontinued its use in the management of patients with suspected gas gangrene or clostridial postabortion sepsis because of questionable efficacy and the substantial risk of hypersensitivity to horse serum, from which the antitoxin is derived.

The use of hyperbaric oxygen in the treatment of gas gangrene is also controversial. Studies in humans are not well designed to an-

TABLE 126-1 *Treatment of Clostridial Infections*[a]

Condition	Antibiotic Treatment	Penicillin Allergy	Adjunctive Treatment/Note
Contamination	None	—	—
Gas gangrene	Penicillin, 3 to 4 million units IV q4h, *plus* Clindamycin, 600 mg IV q6h	Chloramphenicol, metronidazole, imipenem, doxycycline (see text)[b]	Surgical debridement with wide excision is essential; consider hyperbaric oxygen
Clostridial sepsis	Penicillin, 3 to 4 million units IV q4h, *plus* Clindamycin, 600 mg IV q6h	Chloramphenicol, metronidazole, imipenem, doxycycline (see text)[b]	Transient bacteremia may be clinically insignificant
Suppurative deep-tissue infections (e.g., abdominal wall, gynecologic)	Penicillin, 3 to 4 million units IV q4h, *plus* Gentamicin, 5 mg/kg IV q24h, *or* A third-generation cephalosporin (e.g., ceftriaxone, 2 g IV q12h)	As above, plus gentamicin or a quinolone	Empirical therapy should be given; therapy should be based on Gram's stain and culture results when available

[a] Treatment recommendations for *C. difficile* colitis, tetanus, and botulism are found in Chaps. 114, 124, and 125, respectively.
[b] Perform sensitivity testing; consider desensitization.

swer questions on efficacy, but several knowledgeable authors believe that hyperbaric oxygen therapy has contributed to dramatic clinical improvement. Such therapy may, however, be associated with untoward effects due to oxygen toxicity and high atmospheric pressure. Some centers without hyperbaric chambers have reported acceptable mortality rates; thus expert surgical and medical management and control of complications are probably the most important factors in the treatment of gas gangrene. Fasciotomy should not be delayed for hyperbaric oxygen therapy.

ACKNOWLEDGMENT

The authors acknowledge the contributions of Dori F. Zaleznik, MD, to this chapter in earlier editions.

FURTHER READING

BORRIELLO SP: Clostridial disease of the gut. Clin Infect Dis 20:S242, 1995

LORBER B: Gas gangrene and other *Clostridium*-associated diseases, in *Principles and Practice of Infectious Diseases*, 5th ed, GL Mandell et al (eds). New York, Churchill Livingstone, 2000, pp 2549–2560

PRINSSEN HM et al: *Clostridium septicum* myonecrosis and ovarian cancer: A case report and review of literature. Gynecol Oncol 72:116, 1999

ROOD JI: Virulence genes of *Clostridium perfringens*. Annu Rev Microbiol 52:333, 1998

STEVENS DL, BRYANT AE: The role of clostridial toxins in the pathogenesis of gas gangrene. Clin Infect Dis 35:S93, 2002

WANG C et al: Hyperbaric oxygen for treating wounds: A systematic review of the literature. Arch Surg 138:272, 2003

Section 6   Diseases Caused by Gram-Negative Bacteria

127   MENINGOCOCCAL INFECTIONS
David S. Stephens, Robert S. Munford, Lee M. Wetzler

DEFINITION *Neisseria meningitidis* is the etiologic agent of two life-threatening diseases: meningococcal meningitis and fulminant meningococcemia. Meningococci also cause pneumonia, septic arthritis, pericarditis, urethritis, and conjunctivitis. Most cases are potentially preventable by vaccination.

ETIOLOGIC AGENT Meningococci are gram-negative aerobic diplococci. Unlike the other neisseriae, they have a polysaccharide capsule. They are transmitted among humans—their only known habitat—via respiratory secretions. Colonization of the nasopharynx or pharynx is much more common than invasive disease.

MICROBIOLOGY AND CLASSIFICATION On the basis of genome sequencing, *N. meningitidis* is categorized as a β-proteobacterium related to *Bordetella*, *Burkholderia*, *Kingella*, and *Methylomonas* and—more distantly—to *Vibrio*, *Haemophilus*, and *Escherichia coli*. Meningococci are traditionally classified by serologic typing systems based on structural differences in capsule (serogroup), major outer-membrane protein (OMP) porins (serotype), other OMPs (serosubtype), and lipooligosaccharide (LOS; immunotype). Thus, the meningococcal strain designation B:2b:P1.5:L3,7,9 reflects the serogroup (B), serotype (2b), serosubtype (P1.5), and immunotype (L3,7,9).

Meningococci are classified into serogroups according to the antigenicity of their capsular polysaccharides, which reflects structural differences in these carbohydrates. Five serogroups (A, B, C, Y, and W-135) are responsible for >90% of cases of meningococcal disease worldwide. Serogroup A strains, which caused most of the large epidemics of meningococcal disease during the first half of the twentieth century, are now associated with recurring epidemics in sub-Saharan Africa and other locales in the developing world. Serogroups B and C cause most cases of sporadic and epidemic meningococcal disease in industrialized countries. In the United States and Canada during the 1990s, serogroup B was the most common cause of sporadic disease, while serogroup C was a more frequent cause of outbreaks. Serogroup Y has recently been isolated from almost one-third of cases of meningococcal disease in the United States. In general, patients with serogroup Y disease are older and more likely to be African American or to have a chronic underlying illness than are patients with disease caused by other serogroups. Serogroups Y and W-135 are isolated more often than the other serogroups from patients with pneumonia.

One limitation of the serogroup classification is that the genes for capsule biosynthesis can be transferred from one strain to another, with consequent changes in the capsule structure of the recipient strain and therefore in its serogroup. Other methods for tracking meningococcal strains have thus become increasingly useful. Meningococcal serotypes and subtypes are defined by antigenic differences in specific OMPs, whereas multilocus enzyme electrophoresis classifies bacteria into electrophoretic types (ETs). Other techniques for establishing strain identity or nonidentity are pulsed-field gel electrophoresis and amplification of bacterial genomic sequences by polymerase chain reaction (PCR). These techniques are used for the identification of the strains associated with outbreaks of disease. For example, the virulent III-1 clonal complex of serogroup A was first recognized in Nepal in 1983 to 1984; it spread to Mecca, then to sub-Saharan Africa, and subsequently to temperate Africa. The serogroup B ET-5 complex was first identified in Norway in the 1970s and later caused outbreaks in Europe, Cuba, and South and North America (most recently, in the Pacific Northwest). Serogroup C ET-24 (the ET-37 complex) has caused sporadic cases and outbreaks in Canada and the United States; in some analyses, it has been associated with high rates of mortality and morbidity.

EPIDEMIOLOGY Meningococcal disease occurs worldwide as isolated (sporadic) cases, institution- or community-based outbreaks, and large epidemics. Despite effective antibiotics and partially effective vaccines, *N. meningitidis* is still a leading global cause of meningitis and rapidly fatal sepsis, often in otherwise-healthy individuals.

N. meningitidis is unique among the major bacterial agents of meningitis in that it causes epidemic as well as endemic (sporadic) disease. In all, 300,000 to 500,000 cases of meningococcal disease occur worldwide each year—numbers that frequently are increased by large epidemics. The annual incidence of meningococcal disease is 1 to 2 cases per 100,000 population for sporadic disease, 5 to 10 per 100,000 for hypersporadic disease (localized outbreaks and case clusters), and 10 to >1000 per 100,000 for pandemic and epidemic disease (e.g., serogroup A epidemics). The African meningitis belt (i.e., sub-Saharan Africa) continues to have high levels of sporadic disease and major outbreaks. In the largest meningococcal epidemic outbreak recorded, >300,000 cases and 30,000 deaths occurred in sub-Saharan Africa in 1996 to 1997 due to serogroup A *N. meningitidis*. Large serogroup B epidemics and/or outbreaks of serogroup A or C meningococcal disease have also occurred in Europe, the United States, Canada, China, Nepal, Mongolia, New Zealand, Cuba, Brazil, Chile, Saudi Arabia, and South Africa since 1980. In 2000, 2001, and 2002, worldwide epidemics of serogroup W-135 meningococcal disease occurred in association with the Muslim pilgrimage to Mecca (the Hajj) and in the meningitis belt of sub-Saharan Africa.

In the United States, the attack rate for sporadic meningococcal disease is ~1 case per 100,000 persons per year. Disease attack rates are highest among infants 3 to 9 months of age (10 to 15 cases per

100,000 infants per year). Attack rates are higher among children than among adults, and there is a second peak of incidence among teenagers, in whom outbreaks have often been tied to residence in barracks, dormitories, or other crowded conditions. Although the age-specific incidence is much lower among adults (<1 case per 100,000 persons per year), one-third to one-half of all cases of sporadic meningococcal disease occur in individuals ≥18 years of age. Peak disease incidence coincides with the winter peak of respiratory viral illnesses. During epidemics, disease incidence increases disproportionately among teenagers and young adults. In sub-Saharan Africa, epidemic outbreaks occur with the dry season and the coming of the dry dusty winds of the harmattan.

Meningococcal disease occurs more commonly among the household contacts of primary cases than in the general population. The secondary attack rate is 400 to 1000 per 100,000 household members. School-based clusters of cases have also been described; the attack rate among school contacts of cases has been estimated at 2 to 4 cases per 100,000 exposed individuals. In outbreaks on college campuses, attack rates have been highest among students living in dormitories. Most secondary cases occur within 2 weeks of the primary case, although some cases may develop as long as several months later. Secondary cases account for <2% of all cases reported each year in the United States.

Meningococcal colonization of the nasopharynx (asymptomatic carriage) can persist for months. In nonepidemic periods, ~10% of healthy individuals are colonized. Factors that predispose individuals to colonization with *N. meningitidis* include residence in the same household with a person who has meningococcal disease or is a carrier, household or institutional crowding, active or passive exposure to tobacco smoke, and a recent history of a viral upper respiratory infection. These factors have also been associated with an increased risk of meningococcal disease.

PATHOGENESIS (Fig. 127-1)   Meningococci that colonize the upper respiratory tract are internalized by nonciliated mucosal cells and may traverse them to enter the submucosa, from which they can make their way into the bloodstream. While meningococcal colonization occurs often in healthy humans, bloodstream infection is an infrequent event that is not essential for the organisms' survival and spread. The pro-

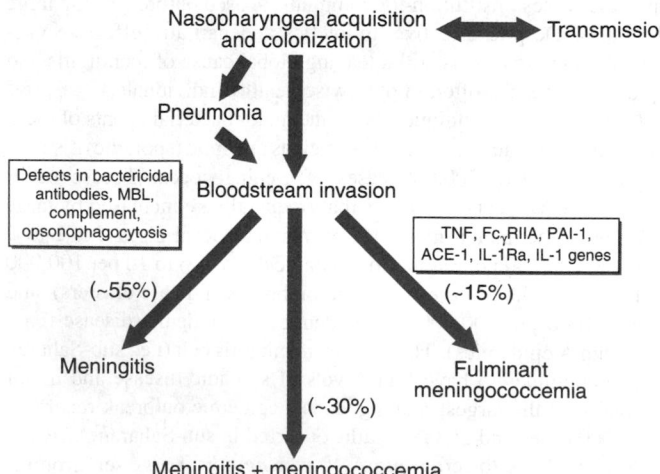

FIGURE 127-1   Meningococcal disease pathogenesis, susceptibility, and severity. After human-to-human transmission, environmental factors (smoking, coinfections), polymorphisms in innate immunity or other genes, and absence of mucosal antibodies may confer susceptibility to meningococcal invasion from the nasopharynx into the bloodstream. In individuals who lack bactericidal antibodies, terminal or alternative pathway complement-deficiency states and other genetic polymorphisms may influence the severity of the ensuing host response and the clinical presentation. Although each of these gene associations has been reported, most of them require confirmation in different ethnic groups. MBL, mannose-binding lectin; TNF, tumor necrosis factor; FcγRIIA, FcγRIIA R131 allele; PAI-1, plasminogen activator inhibitor 1; ACE-1, angiotensin-converting enzyme 1; IL, interleukin.

duction of human disease has no obvious evolutionary advantage for either pathogen or host. Although some strains of *N. meningitidis* are thought to cause more severe disease in humans than do other strains, the basis for this difference is not understood. Meningococci may undergo important phenotypic changes when they adapt to growth in vivo; presumed virulence traits include the antiphagocytic capsular polysaccharide, an ability to sialylate LOS so that it mimics host-cell carbohydrate moieties, the secretion of IgA protease, and mechanisms for iron acquisition. The ET-5 strain of serogroup B *N. meningitidis* has been associated with high case-fatality rates in some populations but not in others; this discrepancy suggests that host factors also contribute importantly to disease pathogenesis.

A meningococcus that enters the bloodstream from the nasopharynx and survives host defenses generally has one of two fates. If multiplication occurs slowly, the bacteria eventually may seed local sites, such as the meninges and/or (less commonly) the joints or the pericardium. More rapid multiplication in the bloodstream is associated with the clinical features of meningococcemia, with petechiae, purpura, disseminated intravascular coagulation (DIC), and shock, which usually causes symptoms before local sites become infected. Thus compartmentalization of bacterial growth and host inflammation either in the blood or at a local site (usually the meninges) can occur.

Outer-Membrane Components Associated with Virulence   Invasive meningococcal strains are characterized by the expression of capsular polysaccharide and other outer-membrane structures, including LOS (endotoxin). Outer-membrane blebbing, meningococcal autolysis, molecular mimicry, genome plasticity, horizontal DNA exchange, and phase and/or antigenic variation are all important in meningococcal virulence.

CAPSULE   The polysaccharide capsule is a major—if not the major—virulence factor of *N. meningitidis*. As stated above, meningococci isolated from the blood or cerebrospinal fluid (CSF) of patients with invasive meningococcal disease most often express capsules of serogroups A, B, C, Y, and W-135. Isolates from asymptomatic nasopharyngeal carriers are nongroupable or express B, Y, X, Z, or 29E capsular serogroups. Capsules impart antiphagocytic and antibactericidal properties to the meningococcus and thus enhance meningococcal survival during invasion of the bloodstream or CSF. Capsules also provide protective properties (e.g., preventing desiccation and phagocytic killing) and antiadherent properties; these properties promote meningococcal transmission, spread, and survival externally and within intracellular compartments such as phagocytic vacuoles.

Except in serogroup A, the major meningococcal capsular polysaccharides associated with invasive disease are composed of sialic acid (*N*-acetyl neuraminic acid, NANA) derivatives. The serogroup B capsule is composed of $(\alpha2\rightarrow8)$-linked NANA, the serogroup C capsule of $(\alpha2\rightarrow9)$-linked NANA, the serogroup Y capsule of alternating D-glucose and NANA, and the serogroup W-135 capsule of D-galactose and NANA. The differences in sialic acid capsule composition are derived from the distinct polysialyltransferases encoded by the fourth gene of the capsule biosynthesis operon, which is also used as a basis for capsule-specific PCR diagnosis. A four-gene operon encoding the capsule transport apparatus (ctr) is conserved among different serogroups and is also used in PCR diagnosis. The serogroup A capsule is composed of repeating units of (α)-linked *N*-acetyl-mannosamine-1-phosphate and is encoded by a four-gene biosynthesis cassette unique for this serogroup.

OUTER-MEMBRANE PROTEINS   Meningococci isolated from sites of colonization or invasive disease are piliated. Pili are complex outer-membrane, protein-based organelles that facilitate adhesion—the first step in meningococcal host-cell interactions. Meningococci express two major OMP porins, PorA and PorB. Human opsonins and bactericidal antibodies induced during meningococcal disease have been shown to recognize PorA and PorB. Vaccines based on PorA-containing outer-membrane vesicles are under development. Another OMP, Opc, is involved in cell attachment and is also a target of bactericidal antibodies. Meningococci encounter iron-restricted environments during infection. The majority of host iron is presented intracellularly as hemoglobin and extracellularly as human transferrin and lactoferrin. Meningococci have evolved systems for acquisition of these iron-carrying molecules.

LIPOOLIGOSACCHARIDE Meningococcal LOS is structurally related to the lipopolysaccharide (LPS) expressed by many gram-negative bacilli. However, LOS does not have repeating O-antigen subunits of sugars. The lipid A moiety of LOS, which has been classically termed *endotoxin* (as opposed to the bacterial exotoxins), is the portion that mediates the induction of inflammatory cytokines often seen in disease. The effect of lipid A is due to an interaction with the innate immune receptor Toll-like receptor 4 (TLR4) in association with the membrane protein MD2. TLR4 and MD2 are found mainly on macrophages/monocytes, dendritic cells, and other phagocytes. The morbidity and mortality of meningococcal bacteremia and meningitis have been directly correlated with the amount of circulating meningococcal endotoxin.

Other Virulence Mechanisms The outer-membrane components of *N. meningitidis* (e.g., pili, LOS, Opa proteins, Opc, capsule) vary in expression or structure at high frequencies (10^{-2} to 10^{-4} per cell per generation). Variation is the result of genetic switches that turn expression of a component on or off, regulate the amount of a component, or alter the structure of a component. Genetic events leading to phase and structural variation allow immune escape and create variability in the structures that are important in pathogenesis (on and off expression of attachment ligands, protection against serum killing, invasion determinants). The serogroup B capsule provides an example of how meningococci downregulate the human immune response through the expression of host-like antigens. The ($\alpha2 \rightarrow 8$)-linked polysialic acid capsule of serogroup B meningococci is identical to structures on the human neural cell adhesion molecule N-CAM. Meningococci are also characterized by frequent vesiculation (blebbing) of the outer membrane, and the amount of blebbing may vary between strains. Blebs may contribute to the rapid initiation of the inflammatory and clotting cascades. They may also be related to the natural autolysis of meningococci that results in DNA release and facilitates genetic transformation.

Specific disease manifestations of meningococcal infections have specific virulence and pathogenic mechanisms as described below for fulminant meningococcemia and meningitis.

Fulminant Meningococcemia (Purpura Fulminans) Fulminant meningococcemia is perhaps the most rapidly lethal form of septic shock experienced by humans. It differs from most other forms of septic shock by the prominence of hemorrhagic skin lesions (petechiae, purpura; see Fig. 46-5) and the consistent development of DIC.

The dominant proinflammatory molecule in the meningococcal cell wall is the endotoxin or LOS, and the outer membrane that contains it is poorly tethered to the underlying peptidoglycan. This structural peculiarity seems to account for the fact that meningococci shed LOS-containing membrane blebs as they grow. The bacteria can multiply to very high concentrations in the blood. The concentrations of endotoxin detected in the blood of patients with fulminant meningococcemia are 10- to 1000-fold higher than those found in the blood of patients with bacteremia due to other gram-negative bacteria. The bacteria and endotoxin-containing blebs stimulate monocytes, neutrophils, and endothelial cells, which then release cytokines and other mediators that can activate many distant targets, including other leukocytes, platelets, and endothelial cells. In addition, meningococci can invade the vascular endothelium. When activated, the endothelium produces molecules that can be procoagulant as well as adhesive for leukocytes.

Patients with fulminant meningococcemia usually have extremely high blood levels of both proinflammatory mediators—i.e., tumor necrosis factor (TNF), interleukin (IL) 1, interferon γ, and IL-8—and anti-inflammatory mediators—i.e., IL-1 receptor antagonist (IL-1Ra), soluble IL-1 receptors, soluble TNF receptors, and IL-10. The plasma of patients with meningococcal shock can decrease the responses of normal leukocytes to stimuli such as LOS; the implication is that anti-inflammatory mediators predominate in the blood late in infection.

Procoagulant, antifibrinolytic forces are also active in the blood of patients with fulminant meningococcemia (Fig. 127-2). Monocytes express large amounts of tissue factor. Fibrinopeptide A and thrombin-antithrombin levels are high, reflecting active clotting, while antithrombin and fibrinogen levels are low. Although the tissue factor–regulated ("extrinsic") arm of coagulation predominates, the contact system (factors XII and XI, prekallikrein, high-molecular-weight kininogen) is also activated. Striking deficiencies of antithrombin and proteins C and S can occur; studies have found a strong negative correlation between protein C activity and both the size of purpuric skin lesions and the mortality rate. Plasminogen levels are decreased, while plasmin-antiplasmin complexes and plasminogen activator inhibitor 1 (PAI-1) levels in the blood are very high. PAI-1 levels have been correlated with mortality risk.

Fibrin deposition is therefore favored both by the procoagulant tendency (promoted through activation of tissue factor and deficiencies of proteins C and S and antithrombin) and by an antifibrinolytic tendency (favored by excessive PAI-1). Both platelets and leukocytes doubtless contribute to the formation of microthrombi and to the vascular injury that ensues. Thrombosis of small to mid-sized arteries can produce peripheral necrosis and gangrene necessitating limb or digit amputation.

Meningitis Meningococcal bacteremia can result in the seeding of the meninges, pericardium, and large joints. Up to one-third of patients with meningococcal disease present with meningitis or other closed-space infections without signs of sepsis. How meningococci traverse the blood-brain barrier and enter the CSF or reach other closed sites is unclear. Meningococci have been shown to invade endothelial cells both experimentally and in vivo. The choroid plexus is also a potential site of meningococcal entry into the CSF. Meningococcal pili may bind CD46, a complement-regulatory protein that is expressed by the choroid plexus and meningeal epithelia. Upon meningococcal entry into the CSF, a vigorous local inflammatory response ensues, probably triggered by endotoxin-containing meningococcal membranes. Both bacterial growth and the inflammatory response occur within the CSF, where levels of endotoxin, IL-6, TNF, IL-1β, IL-1Ra, and IL-10 exceed the concentrations found in plasma by 100- to 1000-fold. The inflammatory response is largely confined to the subarachnoid space and contiguous structures. The inflammatory cytokines TNF and IL-1 released in meningococcal bacteremia may also enhance the permeability of the blood-brain barrier. Meningitis and other closed-space infections (e.g., arthritis, pericarditis) are the result of bacterial survival and multiplication at these sites. For example, meningitis and its sequelae are due to the induction of local inflammatory cytokines and other mediators (e.g., nitric oxide), leukocyte infiltration across the blood-brain barrier, breakdown of the blood-brain barrier with edema,

FIGURE 127-2 The pathogenesis of fibrin deposition in patients with fulminant meningococcemia. PAI-1, plasminogen activator inhibitor 1. (*Adapted from M Levi et al: Eur J Clin Invest 27:3, 1997.*)

release of metalloproteases, induction of cellular apoptosis, coagulation of vessels, and ischemia.

Patients who develop meningitis without meningococcemia may be individuals in whom meningococci do not grow rapidly in or have been cleared from the blood; may have antibodies or phagocytes that slow meningococcal growth; or may lack the (unknown) factors that allow *N. meningitidis* to multiply rapidly in vivo. If disease is recognized early, the prognosis of patients with meningococcal meningitis is substantially better than that of patients with fulminant meningococcemia.

HOST DEFENSE MECHANISMS   Preventing meningococcal growth in blood requires bactericidal and opsonic antibodies, complement, and phagocytes (Fig. 127-3). The major bactericidal antibodies are IgM and IgG, which (except for serogroup B) bind to the capsular polysaccharide. Immunity to meningococci is therefore serogroup specific. Antibodies to other surface (subcapsular) antigens may confer cross-serogroup protection. PorA, PorB, Opc, and LOS appear to be major targets of cross-reactivity and of serogroup B bactericidal antibodies. Infants are protected from meningococcal disease during the first months of life by passively transferred maternal IgG antibodies. As maternal antibody levels wane, the attack rate increases, peaking from 3 to 9 months of age. Disease incidence declines as protective antibodies are induced by colonization with nonpathogenic bacteria that have cross-reactive antigens. In addition to *Neisseria lactamica*, which frequently colonizes young children, some enteric bacteria have antigens that cross-react with those of meningococci. One theory relates the occurrence of some cases of meningococcal disease to the presence of high levels of IgA antibodies to meningococci, since these antibodies can block the bactericidal activity of IgM.

Complement is required for bactericidal activity and for efficient opsonophagocytosis. Individuals deficient in any of the late complement components (C5 to C9) cannot assemble the membrane-attack complex (MAC) needed to kill *Neisseria*. These persons typically develop less severe meningococcal disease than complement-sufficient individuals, do so at an older age, and tend to have disease due to uncommon serogroups (W-135, X, Y, Z, and 29E). Although only one-half of individuals with known late-complement-component deficiency ever experience meningococcal disease, some affected persons have several episodes. Deficiency of each of the terminal complement components is inherited in an autosomal recessive fashion. Properdin deficiency, in contrast, is X-linked; some affected males develop overwhelming meningococcal disease, an observation indicating that the alternative complement pathway is also needed for antimeningococcal host defense. Disease onset in properdin-deficient individuals typically occurs in the teens or twenties. There is also recent evidence that inherited differences in the mannose-binding lectin (MBL) pathway of complement activation may influence the risk of acquiring meningococcal disease in childhood. Alleles that decrease MBL synthesis have been associated with increased risk in the few studies reported to date.

Activation of the classic pathway of complement by antigen-antibody complexes or of the alternative pathway by LOS or capsular polysaccharide is important for producing and maintaining C3b (Fig. 127-3). Without C3b, neither bactericidal lysis nor phagocytosis can proceed effectively. When C3b is generated, meningococcal growth is probably checked by the MAC, which produces bacterial lysis, and by robust phagocytosis. Most IgG antibodies to the meningococcal polysaccharide are of the IgG$_2$ isotype; a phagocytic cell defect (the FcγRIIA R131 allele) that impairs the phagocytosis of IgG$_2$-coated particles has been associated with more severe meningococcal disease. This allele has also been associated with a more severe clinical course in patients with late-complement-component deficiency; thus effective phagocytosis may contribute to the relatively mild meningococcal disease usually observed in these individuals.

The available studies of gene polymorphism–disease associations are summarized in Figs. 127-1 and 127-3. In individuals who lack bactericidal antibodies, protection from acquiring meningococcal bacteremia may be provided, at least in part, by innate immune mechanisms such as the MBL pathway for activating complement, complement factor C4b, and the TLR4 pathway for LOS recognition. Other genes may influence meningococcal survival in vivo [FcγIIA (CD32)], while still others seem to regulate the host inflammatory (IL-1β, IL-1Ra, TNF, angiotensin-converting enzyme) and clotting (PAI-1) responses to invading meningococci. Although many of these associations await confirmation in other populations of patients, in sum they point to important genetic influences on the acquisition and severity of meningococcal disease. This conclusion is supported by the overrepresentation of ABO blood group nonsecretors among patients with meningococcal disease and by the striking variability in meningococcal disease incidence among different racial groups.

CLINICAL MANIFESTATIONS ■ Upper Respiratory Tract Infections   Although many patients who develop meningococcal meningitis or meningococcemia report having had throat soreness or other upper respiratory symptoms during the preceding week, it is uncertain whether these symptoms are due to infection with meningococci. Meningococcal pharyngitis is rarely diagnosed. Adult patients with *N. meningitidis* bacteremia more often have clinically apparent disease of the respiratory tract (pneumonia, sinusitis, tracheobronchitis, conjunctivitis) than do younger patients.

Meningococcemia   Patients with meningococcal disease may have both meningococcemia and meningitis. These conditions have a wide clinical spectrum, with many overlapping features.

Approximately 10 to 30% of patients with meningococcal disease have meningococcemia without clinically apparent meningitis. Although meningococcal bacteremia may occasionally be transient and asymptomatic, in most individuals it is associated with fever, chills, nausea, vomiting, and myalgias. Prostration is common. The most distinctive feature is rash. Erythematous macules rapidly become petechial and, in severe cases, purpuric (see Fig. 46-5). Although the lesions are typically found on the trunk and lower extremities, they may also occur on the face, arms, and mucous membranes. The petechiae may coalesce into hemorrhagic bullae or may undergo necrosis and ulcerate. Patients with severe coagulopathy may develop ischemic extremities or digits, often with a sharp line of demarcation between normal and ischemic tissue.

In many patients with fulminant meningococcemia, the CSF may be normal and the CSF culture negative. Indeed, the absence of meningitis in a patient with meningococcemia is a poor prognostic sign; it suggests that the bacteria have multiplied so rapidly in the blood that meningeal seeding has not yet occurred or had time to elicit in-

FIGURE 127-3   Protection from meningococcal disease involves both antimeningococcal immunoglobulins and complement. Activation of complement by antimeningococcal IgM or IgG promotes bacterial lysis via the membrane attack complex (C5–C9), while C3b [produced by alternative, mannose-binding lectin (MBL), or classic pathway activation] and antimeningococcal IgG$_2$ cooperate to produce effective opsonophagocytosis. A neutrophil defect in binding IgG$_2$ (the FcγRIIA R131 allele) has been associated with more severe meningococcal disease. CR1, complement receptor 1; LOS, lipooligosaccharide.

flammation in the CSF. Most of these patients also lack evidence of an acute-phase response; i.e., the erythrocyte sedimentation rate is normal, and the C-reactive protein concentration in blood is low.

The *Waterhouse-Friderichsen syndrome* is a dramatic example of DIC-induced microthrombosis, hemorrhage, and tissue injury. Although overt adrenal failure is infrequently documented in patients with fulminant meningococcemia, patients may have partial adrenal insufficiency and be unable to mount the normal hypercortisolemic response to severe stress or cosyntropin stimulation. Almost all patients who die from fulminant meningococcemia have adrenal hemorrhages at autopsy.

Chronic meningococcemia (Fig. 127-4) is a rare syndrome of episodic fever, rash, and arthralgias that can last for weeks to months. The rash may be maculopapular; it is occasionally petechial. Splenomegaly may develop. If untreated or if treated with glucocorticoids, chronic meningococcemia may evolve into meningitis, fulminant meningococcemia, or (rarely) endocarditis.

Meningitis (See also Chap. 360) Patients with meningococcal meningitis have usually been sick for ≥24 h before they seek medical attention. Common presenting symptoms include nausea and vomiting, headache, neck stiffness, lethargy, and confusion. The symptoms and signs of meningococcal meningitis cannot be distinguished from those elicited by other meningeal pathogens. Many patients with meningococcal meningitis have concurrent meningococcemia, however, and petechial or purpuric skin lesions (Fig. 46-5) may suggest the correct diagnosis. CSF findings are consistent with those of purulent meningitis: hypoglycorrhachia, an elevated protein concentration, and a neutrophilic leukocytosis. A Gram's stain of CSF is usually positive (see "Diagnosis," below); when this finding is unaccompanied by CSF leukocytosis, the prognosis for normal recovery is often poor.

Other Manifestations Arthritis occurs in ~10% of patients with meningococcal disease. When arthritis develops during the first few days of the patient's illness, it usually reflects direct meningococcal invasion of the joint. Arthritis that begins later in the course is thought to be due to immune complex deposition. Primary meningococcal pneumonia occurs principally in adults, often in military populations, and is often due to serogroup Y. While meningococcal pericarditis is occasionally seen, endocarditis due to *N. meningitidis* is now exceedingly rare. Primary meningococcal conjunctivitis can be complicated by meningococcemia; systemic therapy is therefore warranted when this condition is diagnosed. Meningococcal urethritis has been reported in individuals who practice oral sex.

Complications Patients with meningococcal meningitis may develop cranial nerve palsies, cortical venous thrombophlebitis, and cerebral edema. Children may develop subdural effusions. Permanent sequelae

FIGURE 127-4 Erythematous papular lesions are seen on the leg of this patient with chronic meningococcemia. (*Courtesy of Kenneth M. Kaye, M.D., and Elaine T. Kaye, M.D.*)

can include mental retardation, deafness, and hemiparesis. The major long-term morbidity of fulminant meningococcemia is the loss of skin, limbs, or digits that results from ischemic necrosis and infarction.

DIAGNOSIS Few clinical clues help the physician distinguish the patient with early meningococcal disease from patients with other acute systemic infections. The most useful clinical finding is the petechial or purpuric rash (see Fig. 46-5), but it must be differentiated from the petechial lesions seen with gonococcemia (see Fig. 128-1), Rocky Mountain spotted fever (see Fig. 158-1), hypersensitivity vasculitis (see Fig. 46-4), endemic typhus, and some viral infections. In one case series, one-half of the adults with meningococcal bacteremia had neither meningitis nor a rash.

The definitive diagnosis is established by recovering *N. meningitidis*, its antigens, or its DNA from normally sterile body fluids, such as blood, CSF, or synovial fluid, or from skin lesions. Meningococci grow best on Mueller-Hinton or chocolate blood agar at 35°C in an atmosphere that contains 5 to 10% CO_2. Specimens should be plated without delay. *N. meningitidis* bacteria are oxidase-positive, gram-negative diplococci that typically utilize maltose and glucose.

A Gram's stain of CSF reveals intra- or extracellular organisms in ~85% of patients with meningococcal meningitis. The latex agglutination test for meningococcal polysaccharides is less sensitive. PCR amplification of DNA in buffy coat or CSF samples is more sensitive than either of these tests; like the latex agglutination test, this method is unaffected by prior antibiotic therapy.

Throat or nasopharyngeal specimens should be cultured on Thayer-Martin medium, which suppresses the competing oral flora. Throat or nasopharyngeal cultures are recommended only for research or epidemiologic purposes, since a positive result merely confirms the carrier state and does not establish the existence of systemic disease.

℞ TREATMENT (Table 127-1)

A third-generation cephalosporin, such as cefotaxime (2 g intravenously every 4 h) or ceftriaxone (2 g intravenously every 12 h), is preferred for initial therapy. One of these cephalosporins in combination with other agents may cover other bacteria (such as *Streptococcus pneumoniae* and *Haemophilus influenzae*) that can cause the same syndromes (Chap. 360). Penicillin G (18 to 24 million units intravenously per day) remains an acceptable alternative for confirmed invasive meningococcal disease in most countries. However, the prevalence of meningococci with reduced susceptibility to penicillin has been increasing, and high-level penicillin resistance has been reported. Other options include meropenem (1 g intravenously every 8 h). In the patient who is allergic to β-lactam drugs, chloramphenicol (75 to 100 mg/kg per day) is a suitable alternative; chloramphenicol-resistant meningococci have been reported from Vietnam and France. The newer fluoroquinolones gatifloxacin, moxifloxacin, and gemifloxacin have excellent in vitro activity against *N. meningitidis*, with measurable CNS penetration, and appear promising in animal models. Patients with meningococcal meningitis should be given antimicrobial therapy for at least 5 days. While glucocorticoid therapy for meningitis in adults is controversial, many experts administer dexamethasone, beginning if possible before antibiotic therapy is initiated; the schedule is 10 mg intravenously 15 to 20 min before the first antibiotic dose and then every 6 h for 4 days.

Patients with fulminant meningococcemia often experience diffuse leakage of fluid into extravascular spaces, shock, and multiple-organ dysfunction (Chaps. 253 and 254). Myocardial depression may be prominent. Supportive therapy, although never studied in randomized, placebo-controlled trials, is recommended. Standard measures include vigorous fluid resuscitation (often requiring several liters over the first 24 h), elective ventilation, and pressors. Some authorities recommend early hemodialysis or hemofiltration. Fresh-frozen plasma is often given to patients who are bleeding extensively or who have severely deranged clotting parameters. Many European experts have adminis-

ANTIBIOTIC TREATMENT[a]

1. Ceftriaxone 2 g IV q12h (100 mg/kg per day) or cefotaxime 2 g IV q4h
2. For penicillin-sensitive *N. meningitidis*: Penicillin G 18–24 million units per day in divided doses q4h (250,000 units/kg per day)
3. Chloramphenicol 75–100 mg/kg per day in divided doses q6h
4. Meropenem 1.0 g (children, 40 mg) IV q8h
5. In an outbreak setting in developing countries: Long-acting chloramphenicol in oil suspension (Tifomycin), single dose
    Adults: 3.0 g (6 mL)
    Children 1–15 years old: 100 mg/kg
    Children <1 year old: 50 mg/kg

CHEMOPROPHYLAXIS[b]

Rifampin (oral)
　Adults: 600 mg bid for 2 days
　Children ≥1 month old: 10 mg/kg bid for 2 days
　Children <1 month old: 5 mg/kg bid for 2 days
Ciprofloxacin (oral)
　Adults: 500 mg, 1 dose
Ofloxacin (oral)
　Adults: 400 mg, 1 dose
Ceftriaxone (IM)
　Adults: 250 mg, 1 dose
　Children <15 years old: 125 mg, 1 dose
Azithromycin (oral)
　500 mg, 1 dose

VACCINATION[c]

A, C, Y, W-135 vaccine (Memomune, Aventis Pasteur) or A, C vaccine
　Single 0.5-mL subcutaneous injection
New C; A, C; and A, C, Y, W-135 meningococcal conjugate vaccines[d]

[a] Patients with meningococcal meningitis should receive antimicrobial therapy for at least 5 days.
[b] Use is recommended for close contacts of cases.
[c] At present, use is generally limited to the control of epidemics and to individuals with increased risk of meningococcal disease. Vaccine efficacy wanes after 3–5 years, and vaccine is not effective in recipients <2 years of age.
[d] These vaccines appear to provide immunity in young children, a prolonged immune response, and herd immunity (decreased transmission and colonization).

tered antithrombin III to such patients. Patients with fulminant meningococcemia in whom shock persists despite vigorous fluid resuscitation should receive supplemental glucocorticoid treatment (hydrocortisone, 1 mg/kg every 6 h) pending tests of adrenal reserve.

Although it has not been formally tested in patients with fulminant meningococcemia, activated protein C (drotrecogin alfa, Xigris) is approved for use in patients with severe sepsis and dysfunction of more than one organ (APACHE II score, >25). Because of the pathophysiology, patients with meningococcemia may represent a group most likely to benefit from administration of activated protein C. The recommended dose is 24 μg/kg per hour, given as a continuous intravenous infusion for 96 h. Drotrecogin alfa is contraindicated when the peripheral-blood platelet count is <50,000/μL, however, and when there is active bleeding or a high risk of bleeding. Clotting parameters should be monitored closely while the drug is being infused; its administration should be discontinued 4 to 6 h before the performance of an invasive procedure. Drotrecogin alfa should not be used in patients with meningitis pending further evidence that it does not induce intracranial bleeding when the meninges are inflamed.

PROGNOSIS When patients are first evaluated, the clinical features most strongly associated with a fatal outcome are shock, a purpuric or ecchymotic rash, a low or normal blood leukocyte count, an age of ≥60 years, and coma. The absence of meningitis, the presence of thrombocytopenia, low blood concentrations of antithrombin or proteins S and C, high blood levels of PAI-1, and a low erythrocyte sedimentation rate (or C-reactive protein level) have also been associated with increased mortality from meningococcal disease. In contrast, the receipt of antibiotics before hospital admission has been associated with lower mortality rates in some studies.

PREVENTION ■ Meningococcal Polysaccharide Vaccines A single injection of quadrivalent meningococcal polysaccharide vaccine (serogroups A, C, W-135, and Y) immunizes ~80 to 95% of immunocompetent adults (Table 127-1). Children ≥3 months of age can be vaccinated to prevent serogroup A disease, but multiple doses are required; the vaccine is otherwise ineffective in children <2 years old. The duration of vaccine-induced immunity in adults is probably <5 years. There is currently no vaccine for serogroup B; its polysaccharide is a sialic acid homopolymer that is poorly immunogenic in humans. In addition to individuals with late-complement-component or properdin deficiency, persons with sickle cell anemia, asplenia, or splenectomy should receive the quadrivalent vaccine. Vaccination is also recommended for military recruits, pilgrims on the Hajj, and individuals traveling to sub-Saharan Africa during the dry months (June to December) or to other areas with epidemic meningococcal disease. The Advisory Committee on Immunization Practices (ACIP) of the Centers for Disease Control and Prevention (CDC) recommends vaccination of incoming college freshmen who will live in dormitories. In general, the vaccine should be given only to persons >2 years of age.

New meningococcal capsular oligosaccharide and polysaccharide conjugate vaccines (C; A and C; A, C, Y, and W-135) are being developed; some are currently undergoing clinical trials, and some are now in use in Europe and Canada. These vaccines are based on the approach used for the highly successful *H. influenzae* type b conjugate vaccines. Covalent linkage of the polysaccharide to a carrier protein converts the polysaccharide to a thymus-dependent antigen enhancing IgG anticapsular antibodies and memory B cells. Because levels of antibody in mucosal secretions are much higher after the administration of a conjugate vaccine than after vaccination with an unconjugated preparation, a major benefit of these vaccines may be the introduction of herd immunity. Memory response to meningococcal polysaccharide also appears to be an important effect of the conjugate vaccines. Meningococcal conjugate vaccines are not yet licensed in the United States. However, in the United Kingdom, serogroup C conjugate vaccines introduced in 2000 have had a marked impact on the incidence of serogroup C disease in the population vaccinated. If conjugate meningococcal vaccines prove to be capable of providing durable antibody or memory responses (particularly in infants and young children), their integration into the routine childhood immunization schedule would appear warranted. Vaccines for serogroup B meningococcal disease remain elusive; none of the group B vaccines studied in clinical trials has proven to be broadly effective, but these products have a role in the control of serogroup B epidemics. The identification of new meningococcal protective antigens and the development of better meningococcal vaccines are areas of continued research and hold promise for the prevention of diseases due to *N. meningitidis*.

Screening tests for complement-component deficiency should be conducted in patients who have a family history of meningococcal or disseminated gonococcal disease; in patients who have a recurrence; in patients whose first case occurs at ≥15 years of age; in patients with cases caused by serogroups other than A, B, or C; and in family members of patients found to have a complement deficiency.

Antimicrobial Chemoprophylaxis The attack rate for meningococcal disease among household or other close contacts of cases is >400-fold greater than that in the population as a whole. Close contacts of cases should receive chemoprophylaxis with rifampin, ciprofloxacin, ofloxacin, or azithromycin (Table 127-1). A single intramuscular injection of ceftriaxone is also effective. Close contacts include persons who live in the same household, day-care center contacts, and anyone directly exposed to a patient's oral secretions. Casual contacts are not at increased risk. Chemoprophylaxis should be administered as soon as possible after the case is identified.

Isolation Precautions The CDC recommends that patients with meningococcal disease who are hospitalized be placed in respiratory isolation for the first 24 h.

Outbreak Control An organization- or community-based outbreak of meningococcal disease is defined as the occurrence of three or more cases within ≤3 months in persons who have a common affiliation or reside in the same area but who are not close contacts of one another; in addition, the primary disease attack rate must exceed 10 cases per 100,000 persons, and the case strains of *N. meningitidis* must be of the same molecular type. Mass vaccination should be considered when such outbreaks occur, and mass chemoprophylaxis may be used to control school- or other institution-based outbreaks. Consultation with public health authorities is recommended when such campaigns are contemplated.

FURTHER READING

BRANDTZAEG P et al: Net inflammatory capacity of human septic shock plasma evaluated by a monocyte-based target cell assay: Identification of interleukin-10 as a major functional deactivator of human monocytes. J Exp Med 184:51, 1996

CENTERS FOR DISEASE CONTROL AND PREVENTION: Prevention and control of meningococcal disease: Recommendations of the Advisory Committee on Immunization Practices (ACIP). MMWR 49(RR-7):1, 2000

FIJEN CA et al: Assessment of complement deficiency in patients with meningococcal disease in the Netherlands. Clin Infect Dis 28:98, 1999

HIBBERD ML et al: Association of variants of the gene for mannose-binding lectin with susceptibility to meningococcal disease. Lancet 353:1049, 1999

JOHANSSON L et al: CD46 in meningococcal disease. Science 301:373, 2003

MACDONALD NE et al: Induction of immunologic memory by conjugated vs plain meningococcal C polysaccharide vaccine in toddlers—a randomized controlled trial. JAMA 280:1685, 1998

PLATONOV AE et al: Meningococcal disease and polymorphism of FcγRIIA (CD32) in late complement component–deficient individuals. Clin Exp Immunol 111:97, 1998

ROSENSTEIN NE et al: Meningococcal disease. N Engl J Med 344:1378, 2001

SMIRNOVA I et al: Assay of locus-specific genetic load implicates rare Toll-like receptor 4 mutations in meningococcal susceptibility. Proc Natl Acad Sci USA 100:6075, 2003

128 GONOCOCCAL INFECTIONS
Sanjay Ram, Peter A. Rice

DEFINITION Gonorrhea is a sexually transmitted infection of epithelium and commonly manifests as cervicitis, urethritis, proctitis, and conjunctivitis. If untreated, infections at these sites can lead to local complications such as endometritis, salpingitis, tuboovarian abscess, bartholinitis, peritonitis, and perihepatitis in the female; periurethritis and epididymitis in the male; and ophthalmia neonatorum in the newborn. Disseminated gonococcemia is an uncommon event whose manifestations include skin lesions, tenosynovitis, arthritis, and (in rare cases) endocarditis or meningitis.

Neisseria gonorrhoeae is a gram-negative, nonmotile, non-spore-forming organism that grows in pairs (diplococci). Each individual organism is shaped like a coffee bean, with adjacent concave sides seen on Gram's stain. Gonococci, like all other *Neisseria* spp., are oxidase positive. They are distinguished from other neisseriae by their ability to grow on selective media and to utilize glucose but not maltose, sucrose, or lactose.

EPIDEMIOLOGY The incidence of gonorrhea has declined significantly in the United States, but there were still ~362,000 newly reported cases in 2002. Gonorrhea remains a major public health problem worldwide, is a significant cause of morbidity in developing countries, and may play a role in enhancing transmission of HIV.

Gonorrhea predominantly affects young, nonwhite, unmarried, less educated members of urban populations. The number of reported cases probably represents half of the true number of cases—a discrepancy resulting from underreporting, self-treatment, and nonspecific treatment without a culture-proven diagnosis. The number of reported cases of gonorrhea in the United States rose from ~250,000 in the early 1960s to a high of 1.01 million in 1978. The peak recorded incidence of gonorrhea in modern times was reported in 1975, with 468 cases per 100,000 population in the United States. This peak was attributable to the interaction of several variables, including improved accuracy of diagnosis, changes in patterns of contraceptive use, and changes in sexual behavior. The incidence of the disease has since gradually declined and is currently estimated at 120 cases per 100,000, a figure that is still the highest among industrialized countries. A further decline in the overall incidence of gonorrhea in the United States over the past decade may reflect increased condom use resulting from public health efforts to curtail HIV transmission. Presently, the attack rate in the United States is highest in the 20- to 24-year age group, in which 75% of all cases occur. With adjustment for sexual experience, the risk is highest among sexually active 15- to 19-year-old women. In terms of ethnicity, rates are highest among African Americans and lowest among persons of Asian or Pacific Island descent.

The incidence of gonorrhea is highest in developing countries. The exact incidence of any of the sexually transmitted diseases (STDs) is difficult to ascertain in developing countries because of limited surveillance and variable diagnostic criteria. For example, in Kenya, it was estimated in 1987 that 10% of all live births were adversely affected by STDs, and gonococcal ophthalmia neonatorum reportedly affected 4% of all live-born infants. The median prevalence of gonorrhea in unselected populations of pregnant women has been estimated at 10% in Africa, 5% in Latin America, and 4% in Asia. Studies in Africa have clearly demonstrated that nonulcerative STDs such as gonorrhea are an independent risk factor for the transmission of HIV (Chap. 173).

Gonorrhea is transmitted from males to females more efficiently than in the opposite direction. The rate of transmission to a woman following a single unprotected sexual encounter with an infected man is on the order of 40 to 60%. Oropharyngeal gonorrhea occurs in ~20% of women who practice fellatio with infected partners. Transmission in either direction by cunnilingus is rare.

There exists in any population a small minority of individuals who have high rates of new-partner acquisition. These "core-group members" or "high-frequency transmitters" are vital in sustaining STD transmission at the population level. Another instrumental factor in sustaining gonorrhea in the population is the large number of infected individuals who are asymptomatic or have minor symptoms that are ignored. These persons, unlike symptomatic individuals, do not cease sexual activity and therefore continue to transmit the disease. This situation underscores the importance of contact tracing and empirical treatment of sex partners of index cases.

PATHOGENESIS, IMMUNOLOGY, AND ANTIMICROBIAL RESISTANCE ■ **Outer-Membrane Proteins** ■ *PILI* Fresh clinical isolates of *N. gonorrhoeae* initially form piliated (fimbriated) colonies distinguishable on translucent agar. Pilus expression is rapidly switched off with unselected subculture because of rearrangements in pilus genes. This change is a basis for phase variation of gonococci. Piliated strains adhere better to cells derived from human mucosal surfaces and are more virulent in organ culture models and human inoculation experiments than nonpiliated variants. In a fallopian tube explant model, pili mediate gonococcal attachment to nonciliated columnar epithelial cells. This event initiates gonococcal phagocytosis and transport through these cells to intercellular spaces near the basement membrane or directly into the subepithelial tissue. Damage to nearby ciliated columnar epithelial cells, which is caused by the release of cytokines, results in loss of cilia and sloughing of ciliated cells and diminishes the integrity of the fallopian tube. Nonpiliated gonococci cause epithelial damage at a much slower rate. CD46 (membrane cofactor protein) is present on urogenital epithelial cells in both men and women and has been determined to be a receptor for PilC; this subunit is located at the tip of the pilus molecule and is critical in mediating adherence. Pili are also essential for genetic competence and transformation of *N. gonorrhoeae*, which permit horizontal transfer of genetic material between different gonococcal lineages in vivo.

OPACITY-ASSOCIATED PROTEIN   Another gonococcal surface protein that is important in adherence to epithelial cells is opacity-associated protein (Opa, formerly called protein II). Opa contributes to intergonococcal adhesion, which is responsible for the opaque nature of gonococcal colonies on translucent agar and the organism's adherence to a variety of eukaryotic cells, including polymorphonuclear leukocytes (PMNs). Certain Opa variants promote invasion of epithelial cells, and this effect has been linked with the ability of Opa to bind vitronectin, glycosaminoglycans, and several members of the carcinoembryonic antigen–related cell adhesion molecule (CEACAM, previously known as CD66) receptor family. Each strain of *N. gonorrhoeae* possesses as many as 11 different *opa* genes, but usually no more than three types are expressed at any given time. Isolates from normally sterile sites such as the fallopian tube and synovial fluid usually fail to express Opa, while isolates from mucosal sites usually form opaque colonies. Female commercial sex workers with antibodies to Opa may be less likely to develop pelvic inflammatory disease (PID) than women without such antibodies. *N. gonorrhoeae* Opa proteins that bind CEACAM 1, which is expressed by primary CD4+ T lymphocytes, suppress the activation and proliferation of these lymphocytes. This phenomenon may serve to explain the transient decrease in CD4+ T-lymphocyte counts associated with gonococcal infection.

PORIN   Porin (previously designated protein I) is the most abundant gonococcal surface protein, accounting for >50% of the organism's total outer-membrane protein. Porin molecules exist as trimers that provide anion aqueous channels through the otherwise-hydrophobic outer membrane. Porin shows stable interstrain antigenic variation and forms the basis for gonococcal serotyping. Two main serotypes have been identified: Por1A strains are often associated with disseminated gonococcal infection (DGI), while Por1B strains usually cause local genital infections only. DGI strains are generally resistant to the killing action of normal human serum, do not incite a significant local inflammatory response, and therefore may not cause symptoms at genital sites. These characteristics may be related to the ability of Por1A strains to bind to complement-downregulatory molecules, resulting in a diminished inflammatory response. Porin can translocate to the cytoplasmic membrane of host cells—a process that could initiate gonococcal endocytosis and invasion. In addition, porin is an immunologic target of bactericidal and opsonophagocytic antibodies that may arise in response to immune stimulation resulting from infection or immunization with porin-containing vaccine candidates.

OTHER OUTER-MEMBRANE PROTEINS   Other notable outer-membrane proteins include H.8, a lipoprotein that is present in high concentration on the surface of all gonococcal strains and is an excellent target for antibody-based diagnostic testing. Transferrin-binding proteins (Tbp1 and Tbp2) and lactoferrin-binding protein are required for scavenging iron from transferrin and lactoferrin in vivo. Transferrin and iron have been shown to increase attachment of iron-deprived *N. gonorrhoeae* to human endometrial cells. Studies with volunteers have demonstrated that gonococci deficient in transferrin- and lactoferrin-binding proteins cannot establish infection in men. IgA1 protease is produced by *N. gonorrhoeae* and may protect the organism from the action of mucosal IgA.

Lipooligosaccharide   Gonococcal lipooligosaccharide (LOS) consists of a lipid A and a core oligosaccharide that lacks the repeating O-carbohydrate antigenic side chain seen in other gram-negative bacteria (Chap. 105). Gonococcal LOS possesses marked endotoxic activity and contributes to the local cytotoxic effect in the fallopian tube model. LOS core sugars undergo a high degree of antigenic variation under different conditions of growth; this variation reflects genetic regulation

and expression of glycotransferase genes that dictate the carbohydrate structure of LOS. These phenotypic changes may affect interactions of *N. gonorrhoeae* with elements of the humoral immune system (antibodies and complement) and may also influence direct binding of organisms to both professional phagocytes and nonprofessional phagocytes (epithelial cells). For example, gonococci that are sialylated at their LOS sites bind complement factor H and downregulate the alternative pathway of complement. LOS sialylation may also mask bactericidal antibody–binding epitopes on LOS and porin and may decrease opsonophagocytosis and inhibit the oxidative burst in PMNs. While sialylation of LOS confers on the bacteria the ability to attenuate the inflammatory response and evade the innate immune system, experiments in male volunteers suggest that sialylated gonococci may be less capable of establishing infection than their unsialylated counterparts. This difference could be explained by the observation that the unsialylated terminal lactosamine residue of LOS binds to an asialoglycoprotein receptor on male epithelial cells that would otherwise facilitate binding and subsequent gonococcal invasion of these cells.

Host Factors   In addition to gonococcal structures that interact with epithelial cells, host factors seem to be important in mediating entry of gonococci into nonphagocytic cells. Activation of phosphatidylcholine-specific phospholipase C and acidic sphingomyelinase by *N. gonorrhoeae*, which results in the release of diacylglycerol and ceramide, is a requirement for the entry of *N. gonorrhoeae* into epithelial cells. Ceramide accumulation within cells leads to apoptosis, which may disrupt epithelial integrity and facilitate entry of gonococci into subepithelial tissue. Release of chemotactic factors as a result of complement activation contributes to inflammation, as does the toxic effect of LOS in provoking the release of inflammatory cytokines.

The importance of humoral immunity in host defenses against neisserial infections is best illustrated by the predisposition of persons deficient in terminal complement components (C5 through C9) to recurrent bacteremic gonococcal infections and to recurrent meningococcal meningitis or meningococcemia. Gonococcal porin induces T cell–proliferative responses in persons with urogenital gonococcal disease. A significant increase in porin-specific interleukin (IL) 4–producing CD4+ as well as CD8+ lymphocytes is seen in individuals with mucosal gonococcal disease. A portion of these lymphocytes that show a porin-specific T_H2-type response could traffic to mucosal surfaces and play a role in immune protection against the disease. Few data clearly indicate that protective immunity is acquired from a previous gonococcal infection, although bactericidal and opsonophagocytic antibodies to porin and LOS may offer partial protection. On the other hand, women who are infected and acquire high levels of antibody to another outer-membrane protein, Rmp (reduction modifiable protein, formerly called protein III), may be especially likely to become reinfected with *N. gonorrhoeae* because Rmp antibodies block the effect of bactericidal antibodies to porin and LOS. Rmp shows little, if any, interstrain antigenic variation; therefore, Rmp antibodies potentially may block antibody-mediated killing of all gonococci. The mechanism of blocking has not been fully characterized, but Rmp antibodies noncompetitively inhibit binding of porin and LOS antibodies because of the proximity of these structures in the gonococcal outer membrane. Less well understood is how blocking antibody may divert complement binding to the gonococcal surface or otherwise hasten inactivation of complement. In male volunteers who have no history of gonorrhea, the net effect of these events may influence the outcome of experimental challenge with *N. gonorrhoeae*. Because Rmp bears extensive homology to enterobacterial OmpA and meningococcal class 4 proteins, it is possible that these blocking antibodies result from prior exposure to cross-reacting proteins from these species and also play a role in first-time infection with *N. gonorrhoeae*.

Gonococcal Resistance to Antimicrobial Agents   It is no surprise that *N. gonorrhoeae*, with its remarkable capacity to alter its antigenic structure and adapt to changes in the microenvironment, has become resistant to numerous antibiotics. The first effective agents against gonorrhea were the sulfonamides, which were introduced in the 1930s. Within a decade, antibiotic resistance emerged, resulting in treatment failures in one-third of patients. Penicillin was then employed as the drug of choice for the treatment of gonorrhea. By 1965, 42% of gonococcal isolates had developed low-level resistance to penicillin G. To prevent treatment failures, the Centers for Disease Control and Prevention (CDC) at that time recommended doubling the dose of penicillin for the treatment of gonorrhea. Resistance due to the production of penicillinase arose later.

Gonococci become fully resistant to antibiotics either by chromosomal mutations or by acquisition of R factors (plasmids). Two types of chromosomal mutations have been described. The first type, which is drug specific, is a single-step mutation leading to high-level resistance. The second type involves mutations at several chromosomal loci that combine to determine the level as well as the pattern of resistance. Strains with mutations in chromosomal genes were first observed in the late 1950s. As recently as 1997, strains with chromosomal resistance (CMRNG) accounted for resistance to penicillin, tetracycline, or both in ~20% of strains surveyed in the United States.

β-Lactamase (penicillinase)–producing strains of *N. gonorrhoeae* (PPNG) carrying plasmids with the Pc^r determinant were seen almost simultaneously in the United States, England, western Africa, and the Philippines in the late 1970s. PPNG strains have since spread worldwide and by the early 1980s accounted for >50% of all gonococcal isolates in some parts of the developing world. The average prevalence of PPNG in the United States dropped by two-thirds after most penicillin use was discontinued and is now on the order of 4%, with higher rates reported from certain areas. *N. gonorrhoeae* strains with plasmidborne tetracycline resistance (TRNG) can mobilize some β-lactamase plasmids, and PPNG and TRNG occur together, sometimes along with CMRNG. Penicillin, ampicillin, and tetracycline are no longer reliable agents for the treatment of gonorrhea and should not be used. Thirdgeneration cephalosporins have remained highly effective as singledose therapy for gonorrhea. Even though the minimal inhibitory concentrations (MICs) of ceftriaxone for certain strains may reach 0.015 to 0.125 mg/L (higher than MICs of 0.0001 to 0.008 mg/L for fully susceptible strains), these levels are greatly exceeded in blood, the urethra, and the cervix when the routinely recommended ceftriaxone and cefixime regimens are administered (see below). These regimens almost always result in an effective cure.

Quinolone-containing regimens are also recommended for treatment of gonococcal infections; the fluoroquinolones offer the advantage of antichlamydial activity when administered for 7 days. Serum concentrations following therapeutic dosages of the quinolones exceed the MIC for *N. gonorrhoeae* by ~100-fold. However, quinolone-resistant *N. gonorrhoeae* (QRNG) appeared soon after these agents were first used to treat gonorrhea, particularly in Southeast Asia. QRNG strains have been reported recently in the United States, mostly in the far western states. Alterations in DNA gyrase and topoisomerase IV have been implicated as mechanisms of fluoroquinolone resistance.

Resistance to spectinomycin, which is used as an alternative agent, has been reported, but resistance to this agent is usually not associated with resistance to other antibiotics. Therefore, spectinomycin can be reserved for use against multiresistant strains of *N. gonorrhoeae*. Nevertheless, outbreaks caused by strains resistant to spectinomycin have been documented in Korea and England when the drug was used as a primary agent to treat gonorrhea.

CLINICAL MANIFESTATIONS ■ Gonococcal Infection in Males Acute urethritis is the most common clinical manifestation of gonorrhea in males. The usual incubation period following exposure is 2 to 7 days, although the interval can be longer and some men remain asymptomatic. Strains of the Por1A serotype, with nutritional requirements for arginine, hypoxanthine, and uracil (i.e., the AHU auxotype), tend to cause a greater proportion of cases of mild and asymptomatic urethritis than Por1B strains. Urethral discharge and dysuria, usually without urinary frequency or urgency, are the major symptoms. The discharge initially is scant and mucoid but becomes profuse and purulent within a day

or two. The clinical manifestations of gonococcal urethritis are usually more severe and overt than those of nongonococcal urethritis, including urethritis caused by *Chlamydia trachomatis* (Chap. 160); however, exceptions are common, and it is often impossible to differentiate the causes of urethritis on clinical grounds alone. The majority of cases of urethritis seen in the United States today are not caused by *N. gonorrhoeae* and/or *C. trachomatis*. Although a number of other organisms may be responsible, most cases do not have a specific etiologic agent identified. Most symptomatic males with gonorrhea seek treatment and cease to be infectious. The remaining men, who are largely asymptomatic, accumulate in number over time and constitute about two-thirds of all infected men at any point in time. Together with men incubating the organism (who shed the organism but are asymptomatic), they serve as the source of spread of infection. Prior to the antibiotic era, symptoms of urethritis persisted for about 8 weeks. Epididymitis is now an uncommon complication, and gonococcal prostatitis occurs rarely, if at all. Other unusual local complications of gonococcal urethritis include edema of the penis due to dorsal lymphangitis or thrombophlebitis, submucous inflammatory "soft" infiltration of the urethral wall, periurethral abscess or fistulae, inflammation or abscess of Cowper's gland, and seminal vesiculitis. Balanitis may develop in uncircumcised men. After a decline in gonococcal infections among homosexual men early in the era of AIDS, a disturbing increase in gonorrhea was observed among young homosexual men in the 1990s, probably related to decreased condom use. The clinical features of anorectal and pharyngeal gonorrhea are discussed below.

Gonococcal Infections in Females ■ *GONOCOCCAL CERVICITIS* Mucopurulent cervicitis is the most common STD diagnosis in American women and may be caused by *N. gonorrhoeae*, *C. trachomatis*, and other organisms. Cervicitis may coexist with candidal or trichomonal vaginitis. *N. gonorrhoeae* primarily infects the cervical os but can also infect more peripheral areas of the cervix where columnar epithelium meets stratified squamous epithelium. Except in rare instances, the vaginal mucosa, which is lined by stratified squamous epithelium, does not become infected. Bartholin's glands occasionally become infected.

Women infected with *N. gonorrhoeae* usually develop symptoms. However, the women who either remain asymptomatic or have only minor symptoms may delay in seeking medical attention. These symptoms may include scant discharge from the vagina that may issue forth from the inflamed cervix (not vaginitis or vaginosis per se) and dysuria (often without urgency or frequency) that may be associated with gonococcal urethritis. Although the incubation period of gonorrhea is less well defined in women than in men, symptoms usually develop within 10 days of infection and are more acute and intense than those of chlamydial cervicitis.

The physical examination may reveal a mucopurulent discharge (mucopus) issuing from the cervical os. The examiner may check for mucopurulent discharge by swabbing a sample of mucus from the endocervix and observing its color against the white background of the swab; yellow or green mucus suggests mucopus. However, only 35% of women with gonococcal cervicitis actually have a mucopurulent discharge defined by these criteria. Because Gram's stain is not sensitive for the diagnosis of gonorrhea in women, specimens should be submitted for culture or a nonculture assay (see below). Edematous and friable cervical ectopy as well as endocervical bleeding induced by gentle swabbing are more often seen in chlamydial infection.

N. gonorrhoeae may be recovered from the urethra and rectum of women with cervicitis, but these are rarely the sole infected sites. Urethritis in women may produce symptoms of internal dysuria, which is often attributed to "cystitis." Pyuria in the absence of bacteriuria seen on Gram's stain of unspun urine, accompanied by urine cultures that fail to yield >10^5 colonies of bacteria usually associated with urinary tract infection, signifies the possibility of urethritis due to *C. trachomatis*. Urethral infection with *N. gonorrhoeae* may also occur in this context, but in this instance urethral cultures will usually be positive. Compression of the urethra through the anterior vaginal wall against the symphysis pubis may express urethral exudate.

COMPLICATIONS OF GONOCOCCAL CERVICITIS   Gonococcal infection may extend deep enough to produce dyspareunia and lower abdominal or back pain. In such cases, it is imperative to consider a diagnosis of PID and to administer treatment for that disease (Chap. 115). Ascending infection of the genital tract follows ~20% of cases of gonococcal cervicitis and may result in acute endometritis accompanied by abnormal menstrual bleeding, midline lower abdominal pain and tenderness, and dyspareunia. Spread to the fallopian tubes results in acute salpingitis, whose symptoms may be accompanied by signs of cervical motion tenderness and abnormal adnexal mass on pelvic examination. Patients may be febrile, and leukocytosis and an elevated erythrocyte sedimentation rate or C-reactive protein level may be detected. Co-infection with C. trachomatis may increase the risk of PID, which is the clinical counterpart of endometritis and salpingitis. Tubal scarring leading to infertility is the most devastating sequela of salpingitis; the increased risk of ectopic pregnancy is also significant. Prompt and appropriate antibiotic therapy for gonococcal salpingitis (prior to the development of an adnexal mass) can prevent tubal infertility in nearly all cases. Bilateral tubal damage occurs in ~20% of women with an adnexal mass. More than half of women with tubal infertility give no history of PID. These women with "silent salpingitis" may report abdominal or pelvic discomfort (such as dysmenorrhea or dyspareunia) that may be attributed to other diagnoses (such as endometriosis). Spread of infection to the pelvis may result in pelvic peritonitis characterized by nausea and vomiting. Spread of gonococci—or, more commonly, of chlamydiae—via the peritoneal cavity to the upper abdomen may cause perihepatitis (Fitz-Hugh–Curtis syndrome; Chap. 115).

GONOCOCCAL VAGINITIS   The vaginal mucosa of healthy women is lined by stratified squamous epithelium and is usually not infected by N. gonorrhoeae. However, gonococcal vaginitis can occur in anestrogenic women (e.g., prepubertal girls and postmenopausal women), in whom the vaginal stratified squamous epithelial layers are often thinned down to the basilar layer, which can be infected by N. gonorrhoeae. The intense inflammation of the vagina makes the physical (speculum and bimanual) examination extremely painful. The vaginal mucosa is red and edematous, and an abundant purulent discharge is present. Infection in the urethra and in Skene's and Bartholin's glands often accompanies gonococcal vaginitis. Inflamed cervical erosion or abscesses in nabothian cysts may also occur. Coexisting cervicitis may result in pus in the cervical os.

Differential Diagnosis of Genital Gonococcal Infections   The clinical features of uncomplicated gonococcal infections closely resemble those of genital infections caused by C. trachomatis. Although the symptoms produced by chlamydial infections tend to be milder, the two infections are often indistinguishable on clinical grounds alone. Co-infection with N. gonorrhoeae and C. trachomatis is seen in up to 40% of cases. →*The differential diagnosis of urethritis, epididymitis, and proctitis in men; of cervicitis and PID in women; and of vaginitis in prepubertal girls is discussed in Chap. 115.*

Anorectal Gonorrhea   Because the female anatomy permits the spread of cervical exudate to the rectum, N. gonorrhoeae is sometimes recovered from the rectum of women with uncomplicated gonococcal cervicitis. The rectum is the sole site of infection in only 5% of women with gonorrhea. Such women are usually asymptomatic but occasionally have acute proctitis manifested by anorectal pain or pruritus, tenesmus, purulent rectal discharge, and rectal bleeding. Among homosexual men, the frequency of gonococcal infection, including rectal infection, fell by ≥90% throughout the United States in the early 1980s, but a resurgence of gonorrhea among homosexual men was documented in several cities during the 1990s. Gonococcal isolates from the rectum of homosexual men tend to be more resistant than other gonococcal

isolates to antimicrobials. Gonococcal isolates with a mutation in mtrR (multiple transferable resistance repressor) or in the promoter region of the gene that encodes for this transcriptional repressor develop increased resistance to antimicrobial hydrophobic agents such as bile acids and fatty acids in feces and thus are found with increased frequency in homosexual men. The mutation, which curtails the production of a DNA-binding protein called MtrR, results in derepression of the expression of other *mtr* genes that encode the production of an energy-dependent efflux pump, thereby resulting in increased resistance to hydrophobic agents. This situation may have been responsible for higher rates of failure of treatment for rectal gonorrhea with older regimens consisting of penicillin or tetracyclines.

Pharyngeal Gonorrhea   Pharyngeal gonorrhea is usually mild or asymptomatic, although symptomatic pharyngitis does occasionally occur with cervical lymphadenitis. The mode of acquisition is oral-genital sexual exposure, with fellatio being a more efficient means of transmission than cunnilingus. It is important to solicit a sexual history as part of the evaluation of pharyngitis so that appropriate cultures for N. gonorrhoeae can be performed. Acute HIV infection should also be considered in the differential diagnosis of pharyngitis in persons with appropriate risk factors. Most cases resolve spontaneously, and transmission from the pharynx to sexual contacts is rare. Pharyngeal infection almost always coexists with genital infection. Swabs from the pharynx should be plated directly onto gonococcal selective media. Because pharyngeal colonization with N. meningitidis needs to be differentiated from that with other Neisseria species, the diagnosis of pharyngeal gonorrhea is more expensive and difficult than that of anogenital gonorrhea.

Ocular Gonorrhea in Adults   Ocular gonorrhea in an adult usually results from autoinoculation from an infected genital site. As in genital infection, the manifestations range from severe to occasionally mild or asymptomatic disease. The variability in clinical manifestations may result from differences in the ability of the infecting strain to elicit an inflammatory response.

Infection may result in a markedly swollen eyelid, severe hyperemia and chemosis, and a profuse purulent discharge. The massively inflamed conjunctiva may be draped over the cornea and limbus. Lytic enzymes from the infiltrating PMNs occasionally cause corneal ulceration and rarely cause perforation.

Prompt recognition and treatment of this condition are of paramount importance. Gram's stain and culture of the purulent discharge establish the diagnosis. Genital cultures should also be performed.

Gonorrhea in Pregnant Women, Neonates, and Children   Gonorrhea in pregnancy can have serious consequences for both the mother and the infant. Therefore, early detection and eradication of the disease in the mother are extremely important. Recognition of gonorrhea early in pregnancy also identifies a population at risk for other STDs, particularly chlamydial infection and syphilis. These women should be monitored closely for these infections throughout pregnancy. The incidence of gonorrhea in pregnancy ranges from rare to ~10%, depending upon the population surveyed. Salpingitis and PID can occur during the first trimester and are associated with a high rate of fetal loss. In the second and third trimesters, the relative impermeability of the cervical mucus (under the influence of progesterone) and the obliteration of the intrauterine cavity (resulting from the attachment of the chorion to the endometrial decidua by around the twelfth week of gestation) pose physical barriers that usually prevent ascending infection. Pharyngeal infection, most often asymptomatic, may be more common during pregnancy because of altered sexual practices. Acquisition of gonococcal infection late in pregnancy can adversely affect labor and delivery as well as the well-being of the fetus. Prolonged rupture of the membranes, premature delivery, chorioamnionitis, funisitis (infection of the umbilical cord stump), and sepsis in the infant (with N. gonorrhoeae detected in the gastric aspirate of the newborn during delivery) are common complications of maternal gonococcal infection at term. Hazards to the fetus include spontaneous abortion, perinatal death, premature delivery, perinatal distress, and premature rupture of membranes. Other microorganisms and conditions, including *Mycoplasma hominis, Ureaplasma urealyticum, C. trachomatis,* and bacterial vaginosis, have been associated with similar complications.

The most common form of gonorrhea in neonates is ophthalmia neonatorum, which results from exposure to infected cervical secretions during parturition. Ocular neonatal instillation of a prophylactic agent (e.g., 1% silver nitrate eyedrops or ophthalmic preparations containing erythromycin or tetracycline) is a cost-effective measure for the prevention of ophthalmia neonatorum but is not effective for its treatment, which requires systemic antibiotics. The clinical manifestations are acute and begin 2 to 5 days after birth. A small inoculum of organisms, low virulence of the infecting strain, or partial suppression by ophthalmic prophylaxis can result in a more indolent course. Therefore, gonococcal infection must be ruled out by culture in every case of conjunctivitis in infants. An initial nonspecific conjunctivitis with a serosanguineous discharge is followed by tense edema of both eyelids, chemosis, and a profuse, thick, purulent discharge. Corneal ulcerations that result in nebulae or perforation may lead to anterior synechiae, anterior staphyloma, panophthalmitis, and blindness. Infections described at other mucosal sites in infants, including vaginitis, rhinitis, and anorectal infection, are likely to be asymptomatic. Pharyngeal colonization has been demonstrated in 35% of infants with gonococcal ophthalmia, and coughing is the most prominent symptom in these cases. Septic arthritis (see below) is the most common manifestation of systemic infection or DGI in the newborn. The primary focus of DGI in most of these cases is uncertain. The onset usually comes at 3 to 21 days of age, and polyarticular involvement is common. Sepsis, meningitis, and pneumonia are seen in rare instances.

Any STD in children beyond the neonatal period raises the possibility of sexual abuse. In most cases of abuse, the perpetrator is a male assailant known to the child. Gonococcal vulvovaginitis is the most common manifestation of gonococcal infection in children beyond infancy. Anorectal and pharyngeal infections are common in these children and are frequently asymptomatic. The urethra, Bartholin's and Skene's glands, and the upper genital tract are rarely involved. All children with gonococcal infection should also be evaluated for chlamydial infection, syphilis, and possibly HIV infection. All cases of suspected and confirmed child abuse should be reported to the appropriate social service agency in the county where the child resides.

Gonococcal Arthritis (DGI) DGI or gonococcal arthritis results from gonococcal bacteremia. In the 1970s, DGI occurred in ~0.5 to 3% of persons with untreated gonococcal mucosal infection. The lower incidence at present is probably attributable to a decline in the prevalence of particular strains that are likely to disseminate and has resulted in fewer cases that present in the bacteremic stage of the disease (see below). DGI strains resist the bactericidal action of human serum and generally do not incite inflammation at genital sites, probably because of limited generation of chemotactic factors. These strains are often of the Por1A serotype, are highly susceptible to penicillin, and have special growth requirements (i.e., the AHU auxotype) that makes the organism more fastidious and more difficult to isolate. Menstruation is a risk factor for dissemination, and approximately two-thirds of cases of DGI are in women. In about half of affected women, symptoms of DGI begin within 7 days of onset of menses. Complement deficiencies, especially of the components involved in the assembly of the membrane attack complex (C5 through C9), predispose to neisserial bacteremia. Up to 13% of patients with DGI have complement deficiencies, and persons with more than one episode of DGI should be screened with an assay for total hemolytic complement activity.

The clinical manifestations of DGI have sometimes been classified into two stages: a bacteremic stage, which is less common today, and a joint-localized stage with suppurative arthritis. A clear-cut progression usually is not evident. Patients in the bacteremic stage have higher temperatures, and their fever is more frequently accompanied by chills. Painful joints are common and often occur in conjunction with tenosynovitis and skin lesions. Polyarthralgias usually include the knees,

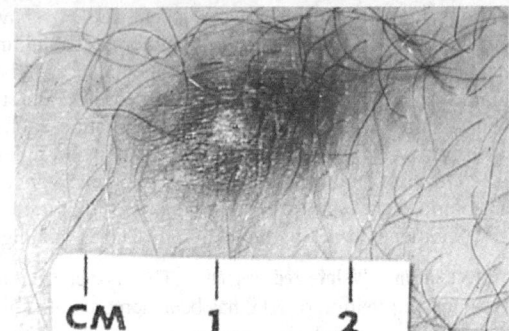

FIGURE 128-1 Disseminated gonococcemia in the skin is seen as hemorrhagic papules and pustules with purpuric centers in a centrifugal distribution.

elbows, and more distal joints; the axial skeleton is generally spared. Skin lesions are seen in ~75% of patients and include papules and pustules, often with a hemorrhagic component (Fig. 128-1). These lesions are usually on the extremities and number between 5 and 40. The differential diagnosis of the bacteremic stage of DGI includes Reiter's syndrome, acute rheumatoid arthritis, sarcoidosis, erythema nodosum, drug-induced arthritis, and viral infections (e.g., hepatitis B and acute HIV infection). The distribution of joint symptoms in Reiter's syndrome differs from DGI (Fig. 128-2), as do the skin and genital manifestations (Chap. 305).

Suppurative arthritis involves one or two joints, most often (in decreasing order of frequency) the knees, wrists, ankles, and elbows. The occurrence of arthritis in the absence of signs and symptoms of the bacteremic stage has led to the suggestion that these are separate syndromes. Other joints, such as the small joints of the hands and feet and the sternoclavicular and temporomandibular joints, are occasionally involved. Most patients who develop gonococcal septic arthritis do so without prior polyarthralgias or skin lesions; in the absence of symptomatic genital infection, this disease cannot be distinguished from septic arthritis caused by other pathogens. The differential diagnosis of acute arthritis in young adults is discussed in Chap. 314. Rarely, osteomyelitis complicates septic arthritis involving small joints of the hand.

Although it has been postulated that the initial arthritis and skin lesions are due to direct tissue invasion by *N. gonorrhoeae*, the organism has been recovered from <5% of skin lesions cultured. This low isolation rate has been attributed to either a small inoculum of infecting organisms or the fastidious growth requirements of *N. gon-*

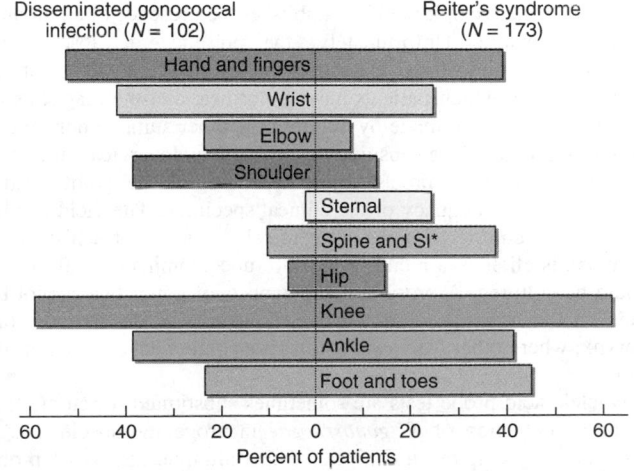

FIGURE 128-2 Distributions of joints with arthritis in 102 patients with disseminated gonococcal infection and 173 patients with Reiter's syndrome. "Sternal" includes the sternoclavicular joints. *SI denotes the sacroiliac joint. (*Reprinted with permission from M Kousa et al: Sex Transm Dis 5:57, 1978; with permission.*)

orrhoeae strains that disseminate. Gonococcal antigens have been identified in "sterile" skin lesions by immunofluorescent staining techniques. There is also evidence that immune-mediated or hypersensitivity phenomena caused by gonococcal antigens account for skin lesions. Other manifestations of noninfectious dermatitis, such as nodular lesions, urticaria, and erythema multiforme, have been described. Gonococcal endocarditis, although rare today, was relatively common in the preantibiotic era, causing about one-quarter of reported cases of endocarditis. Another unusual complication of DGI is meningitis.

Gonococcal Infection in HIV-Infected Persons The association between gonorrhea and the acquisition of HIV has been demonstrated in several well-controlled studies, mainly in Kenya and Zaire. The nonulcerative STDs enhance the transmission of HIV by three- to fivefold, possibly because of increased viral shedding in persons with urethritis or cervicitis (Chap. 173). HIV has been detected by polymerase chain reaction (PCR) more commonly in ejaculates from HIV-positive men with gonococcal urethritis than in those from HIV-positive men with nongonococcal urethritis. PCR positivity diminishes by twofold following appropriate therapy for urethritis. Not only does gonorrhea enhance the transmission of HIV, it may also increase the individual's risk for acquisition of HIV. A proposed mechanism is the significantly greater number of CD4+ lymphocytes and dendritic cells that can be infected by HIV in endocervical secretions of women with nonulcerative STDs than in those of women with ulcerative STDs.

LABORATORY DIAGNOSIS A rapid diagnosis of gonococcal infection in men may be obtained by Gram's staining of urethral exudates. The detection of gram-negative intracellular diplococci is usually highly specific and sensitive in diagnosing gonococcal urethritis in symptomatic males but is only ~50% sensitive in diagnosing gonococcal cervicitis. Samples should be collected with Dacron or rayon swabs. Part of the sample should be inoculated onto a plate of modified Thayer-Martin or other gonococcal selective medium for culture. It is important to process all samples immediately because gonococci do not tolerate drying. If plates cannot be incubated immediately, they can be held safely for several hours at room temperature in candle extinction jars prior to incubation. If processing is to occur within 6 h, transport of specimens may be facilitated by the use of nonnutritive swab transport systems such as Stuart or Amies medium. For longer holding periods (e.g., when specimens for culture are to be mailed), culture media with self-contained CO_2-generating systems (such as the JEMBEC or Gono-Pak systems) may be used. Specimens should also be obtained for the diagnosis of chlamydial infection.

PMNs are often seen in the endocervix on a Gram's stain, and an abnormally increased number [≥30 PMNs per field in five 1000X oil-immersion (microscopic) fields] establishes the presence of an inflammatory discharge. Unfortunately, the presence or absence of gram-negative intracellular diplococci in cervical smears does not accurately predict which patients have gonorrhea, and the diagnosis in this setting should be made by culture or another suitable nonculture diagnostic method. The sensitivity of a single endocervical culture is ~80 to 90%, with the precise figure depending on the quality of the medium and the adequacy of the clinical specimen. The yield can be enhanced by culture of a second cervical specimen. If a history of rectal sex is elicited, a rectal wall swab (uncontaminated with feces) should be cultured. A presumptive diagnosis of gonorrhea cannot be made on the basis of gram-negative diplococci in smears from the pharynx, where other *Neisseria* species are components of the normal flora.

Nucleic acid probe tests are sometimes substituted for culture for the direct detection of *N. gonorrhoeae* in urogenital specimens. A common assay employs a nonisotopic chemiluminescent DNA probe that hybridizes specifically with gonococcal 16S ribosomal RNA. Studies assessing the utility of the nucleic acid probe system in high-risk outpatients undergoing screening for STDs have revealed that it is at least as sensitive as conventional culture techniques and may be

a cost-effective alternative to culture, especially in high-risk males. A disadvantage of non-culture-based assays in general is that specimens submitted in probe-transport systems cannot be cultured subsequently. Therefore, a culture-confirmatory test is not possible, and formal antimicrobial susceptibility testing, if needed, cannot be performed. Low-cost point-of-care tests are under development for use in resource-poor settings, where specific diagnosis often gives way to syndromic management. Nucleic acid amplification tests (NAATs, including Roche Amplicor, Gen-Probe APTIMA, and BDProbeTec) have been cleared by the U.S. Food and Drug Administration (FDA) and offer the advantage of testing urine samples with a sensitivity similar to that of culture and other non-NAATs on urethral or cervical swab samples.

Because of the legal implications, the preferred method for the diagnosis of gonococcal infection in children is a standardized culture. Two positive NAATs, each targeting a different nucleic acid sequence, may be substituted for culture of the cervix or the urethra as legal evidence of infection; however, cervical specimens are not recommended for prepubertal girls. Nonculture tests for gonococcal infection have not been approved by the FDA for use with specimens obtained from the pharynx and rectum of infected children. Cultures should be obtained from the pharynx and anus of both girls and boys, the vagina of girls, and the urethra of boys. For boys with a urethral discharge, a meatal specimen of the discharge is adequate for culture. Presumptive colonies of *N. gonorrhoeae* should be identified definitively by at least two independent methods (e.g., biochemical, enzyme substrate, or serologic).

Blood should be cultured in suspected cases of DGI. The use of Isolator blood culture tubes may enhance the yield. The probability of positive blood cultures decreases after 48 h of illness. Synovial fluid should be inoculated into blood culture broth medium and plated onto chocolate agar rather than selective medium because this fluid is not likely to be contaminated with commensal bacteria. Gonococci are infrequently recovered from early joint effusions containing <20,000 leukocytes/μL but may be recovered from effusions containing >80,000 leukocytes/μL. The organisms are seldom recovered from blood and synovial fluid of the same patient.

℞ TREATMENT

Although clinical isolates of *N. gonorrhoeae* vary in their antimicrobial susceptibility patterns in different parts of the world, they remain susceptible to a wide variety of agents. Because failure of treatment can lead to continued transmission and the emergence of antibiotic resistance, the importance of adequate treatment with a regimen that the patient will adhere to cannot be overemphasized. Thus highly effective single-dose regimens have been developed for the treatment of uncomplicated gonococcal infections. The 2002 CDC treatment guidelines for gonococcal infections are summarized in Table 128-1; the recommendations for uncomplicated gonorrhea apply to HIV-infected as well as HIV-uninfected patients.

The third-generation cephalosporins cefixime (given orally) and ceftriaxone (given intramuscularly), both as a single dose, have been the mainstay of therapy with this class of antibiotics for uncomplicated gonococcal infection of the urethra, cervix, rectum, or pharynx. The recent discontinuation of cefixime production in the United States has prompted further examination of alternative oral options for urogenital and pharyngeal gonococcal infections. To be considered as a recommended treatment for uncomplicated gonorrhea, an antimicrobial regimen should cure >95% of urogenital infections. (The therapeutic efficacy for anorectal infection is typically comparable to that for urogenital infection.) Studies documenting efficacy should have sufficient sample size so that the lower limit of the confidence interval (CI) of the cure rate is also >95%. The available data do not demonstrate that any single-dose oral antimicrobial regimen other than cefixime or a fluoroquinolone (see below) meets these efficacy criteria for urogenital gonococcal infection; published data on the efficacy of alternative oral regimens in treating pharyngeal gonococcal infection are even more limited. Single doses of ciprofloxacin, ofloxacin, or levofloxacin are effective first-line regimens. Other quinolones, such as gatifloxacin, norfloxacin, and lomefloxacin, are probably efficacious for treating uncomplicated gonorrhea, but data regarding their use are also limited, and they offer no advantage over the other recommended quinolones. Because of resistance to fluoroquinolones in several parts of Asia and the Pacific (including Hawaii), these agents should not be used to treat gonorrhea acquired in these regions. Several states, including California, are now recommending the curtailment of quinolone treatment for gonorrhea infection altogether, and in these regions ceftriaxone should be used.

Because co-infection with *C. trachomatis* occurs frequently, initial treatment regimens must incorporate an agent (e.g., azithromycin or doxycycline) effective against chlamydial infection. Routine dual therapy without testing for *Chlamydia* can be cost-effective for populations where chlamydial infection accompanies 10 to 30% of gonococcal infections. Pregnant women with gonorrhea should receive concurrent treatment with a macrolide antibiotic for possible chlamydial infection; doxycycline should not be used during pregnancy. A single 1-g dose of azithromycin, which is effective therapy for uncomplicated chlamydial infections, results in an unacceptably low cure rate (93%) for gonococcal infections and should not be used alone.

Uncomplicated gonococcal infections in penicillin-allergic persons who cannot tolerate quinolones may be treated with a single dose of spectinomycin.

Persons with uncomplicated infections who receive a recommended regimen need not return for a test of cure. Cultures for *N. gonorrhoeae* should be performed if symptoms persist after therapy with an established regimen, and any gonococci isolated should be tested for antimicrobial susceptibility.

Symptomatic gonococcal pharyngitis is more difficult to eradicate than genital infection. Few regimens result in cure rates of >90%. Persons who cannot tolerate cephalosporins or quinolones can be treated with spectinomycin, but this agent results in a cure rate of ≤52%. Therefore, persons given spectinomycin should have a pharyngeal culture performed 3 to 5 days after treatment as a test of cure.

Treatments for gonococcal epididymitis and PID are discussed in Chap. 115. Ocular gonococcal infections in older children and adults should be managed with a single dose of ceftriaxone combined with saline irrigation of the conjunctivae (both undertaken expeditiously), and patients should undergo a careful ophthalmologic evaluation that includes a slit-lamp examination.

DGI may require higher dosages and longer durations of therapy (Table 128-1). Hospitalization is indicated if the diagnosis is uncertain, if the patient has localized joint disease that requires aspiration, or if the patient cannot be relied on to comply with treatment. Open drainage is necessary only occasionally—e.g., for management of hip infections that may be difficult to drain percutaneously. Nonsteroidal anti-inflammatory agents may be indicated to alleviate pain and hasten improvement of affected joints. Gonococcal meningitis and endocarditis should be treated in the hospital with high-dose intravenous ceftriaxone (1 to 2 g every 12 h); therapy should continue for 10 to 14 days for meningitis and for at least 4 weeks for endocarditis. All persons who experience more than one episode of DGI should be evaluated for complement deficiency.

PREVENTION AND CONTROL Condoms, if properly used, provide effective protection against the transmission and acquisition of gonorrhea as well as other infections that are transmitted to and from genital mucosal surfaces. Spermicidal preparations used with a diaphragm or cervical sponges impregnated with nonoxynol 9 offer some protection against gonorrhea and chlamydial infection. However, the frequent use of preparations that contain nonoxynol 9 is associated with mucosal disruption that paradoxically may enhance the risk of HIV infection

TABLE 128-1 Recommended Treatment for Gonococcal Infections: 2002 Guidelines of the Centers for Disease Control and Prevention

Diagnosis	Treatment of Choice
Uncomplicated gonococcal infection of the cervix, urethra, pharynx, or rectum[a]	
First-line regimens	Ceftriaxone (125 mg IM, single dose) *or* Ciprofloxacin (500 mg PO, single dose)[b] *or* Ofloxacin (400 mg PO, single dose)[b] *or* Levofloxacin (250 mg PO, single dose)[b] *or* Cefixime (400 mg PO, single dose)[c] *plus* If chlamydial infection is not ruled out: Azithromycin (1 g PO, single dose) *or* Doxycycline (100 mg PO bid for 7 days)
Alternative regimens	Spectinomycin (2 g IM, single dose) *or* Ceftizoxime (500 mg IM, single dose) *or* Cefotaxime (500 mg IM, single dose) *or* Cefotetan (1 g IM, single dose) plus probenecid (1 g PO, single dose) *or* Cefoxitin (2 g IM, single dose) plus probenecid (1 g PO, single dose)
Epididymitis	See Chap. 115
Pelvic inflammatory disease	See Chap. 115
Gonococcal conjunctivitis in an adult	Ceftriaxone (1 g IM, single dose)[d]
Ophthalmia neonatorum[e]	Ceftriaxone (25–50 mg/kg IV, single dose, not to exceed 125 mg)
Disseminated gonococcal infection[f] Initial therapy[g]	
Patient tolerant of β-lactam drugs	Ceftriaxone (1 g IM or IV q24h; recommended) *or* Cefotaxime (1 g IV q8h) *or* Ceftizoxime (1 g IV q8h)
Patients allergic to β-lactam drugs	Ciprofloxacin (500 mg IV q12h)[b] *or* Ofloxacin (400 mg IV q12h)[b] *or* Levofloxacin (500 mg IV q24h)[b] *or* Spectinomycin (2 g IM q12h)
Continuation therapy	Ciprofloxacin (500 mg PO bid)[b] *or* Ofloxacin (400 mg PO bid)[b] *or* Levofloxacin (500 mg PO qd)[b] *or* Cefixime (400 mg PO bid)[c]
Meningitis or endocarditis	See text[h]

[a] True failure of treatment with a recommended regimen is rare and should prompt an evaluation for reinfection or consideration of an alternative diagnosis. In cases of quinolone failure, the isolate should be tested for drug resistance if possible.

[b] Quinolones should not be used for infections acquired in Asia or the Pacific, including Hawaii and California. The use of quinolones is also inadvisable for treating infections acquired in other areas where the prevalence of quinolone-resistant *N. gonorrhoeae* (QRNG) is >1%, or in areas that are reporting increasing numbers of QRNG strains.

[c] Cefixime, a first-line recommendation for treatment of uncomplicated gonococcal infection (or continuation therapy for DGI), is currently unavailable in the United States.

[d] Plus lavage of the infected eye with saline solution (once).

[e] Prophylactic regimens are discussed in the text.

[f] Hospitalization is indicated if the diagnosis is uncertain, if the patient has frank arthritis with an effusion, or if the patient cannot be relied on to adhere to treatment.

[g] All initial regimens should be continued for 24 to 48 h after clinical improvement begins, at which time therapy may be switched to one of the continuation regimens to complete a full week of antimicrobial treatment.

[h] Hospitalization is indicated to exclude suspected meningitis or endocarditis.

in the event of exposure. All patients should be instructed to refer sex partners for evaluation and treatment. All sex partners of persons with gonorrhea should be evaluated and treated for *N. gonorrhoeae* and *C. trachomatis* infections if their last contact with the patient took place within 60 days before the onset of symptoms or the diagnosis of infection in the patient. If the patient's last sexual encounter was >60 days before onset of symptoms or diagnosis, the patient's most recent sex partner should be treated. Patients should be instructed to abstain from sexual intercourse until therapy is completed and until they and their sex partners no longer have symptoms. Greater emphasis must be placed on prevention by public health education, individual patient counseling, and behavior modification. Sexually active persons, especially adolescents, should be offered screening for STDs. For males, a NAAT on urine or a urethral swab may be used for screening. Preventing the spread of gonorrhea may help reduce the transmission of HIV. No effective vaccine for gonorrhea is yet available, but efforts to test a porin vaccine candidate are under way.

ACKNOWLEDGMENT

The authors acknowledge the contributions of Dr. King K. Holmes and Dr. Stephen A. Morse to the chapter on this subject in earlier editions of Harrison's.

FURTHER READING

CENTERS FOR DISEASE CONTROL AND PREVENTION: Annual Report; Gonococcal Isolate Surveillance Project (GISP); *www.cdc.gov/ncidod/dastlr/gcdir/Resist/gisp.html*

———: 2002 Sexually transmitted diseases treatment guidelines. MMWR 51(RR-6):1, 2002

———: Screening tests to detect *Chlamydia trachomatis* and *Neisseria gonorrhoeae* infections—2002. MMWR 51 (RR-15):1, 2002

HOOK EW III, HOLMES KK: Gonococcal infections. Ann Intern Med 102:229, 1985

LAGA M et al: Non-ulcerative sexually transmitted diseases as risk factors for HIV-1 transmission in women: Results from a cohort study. AIDS 7:95, 1993

O'BRIEN JP et al: Disseminated gonococcal infection: A prospective analysis of 49 patients and a review of pathophysiology and immune mechanisms. Medicine (Baltimore) 62:395, 1983

129　*MORAXELLA CATARRHALIS* AND OTHER *MORAXELLA* SPECIES
Daniel M. Musher

MORAXELLA CATARRHALIS

The gram-negative coccus *Moraxella catarrhalis* is a component of the normal bacterial flora of the upper airways and has been increasingly recognized as a cause of otitis media, sinusitis, and bronchopulmonary infection. Over the past several decades, this organism has been variously designated as *Micrococcus catarrhalis*, *Neisseria catarrhalis*, and *Branhamella catarrhalis*.

BACTERIOLOGY AND IMMUNITY　On Gram's staining, *M. catarrhalis* organisms appear as gram-negative cocci, sometimes occurring in pairs and retaining the side-by-side kidney-bean configuration of *Neisseria* (Fig. 129-1). These cocci tend to retain crystal violet during the decolorizing step and may be confused with *Staphylococcus aureus*. *Moraxella* colonies grow well on blood or chocolate agar but may be overlooked because of their resemblance to *Neisseria* spp. (a major component of the normal pharyngeal flora). *Moraxella* is readily distinguishable from *Neisseria* spp. by biochemical tests.

Strains of *M. catarrhalis* show a surprising degree of homogeneity in terms of their outer-membrane proteins. Antibody to some of these proteins is generally present in serum of children >4 years old; however, colonizing or disease-causing isolates may survive in serum despite this naturally present antibody and complement. Bactericidal antibody emerges after natural infection and may be directed against one or more conserved outer-membrane proteins—a property of potential value in vaccine development. The presence of certain outer-membrane proteins is associated with virulence in mice, and antibody may be protective. Antibody to lipooligosaccharide may also provide some degree of protection. These and other bacterial constituents are under investigation for use as vaccines.

EPIDEMIOLOGY　With repeated cultures and the use of selective media, *M. catarrhalis* can be isolated from the upper respiratory tract or saliva of 50% of healthy schoolchildren and of up to 7% of healthy adults. When conventional microbiologic techniques are used, *Moraxella* can be isolated from sputum of about 10% of persons who have chronic bronchitis and 25% of those who have bronchiectasis in the absence of acute infection. Investigators in both the northern and southern hemispheres have reported a striking seasonal variation in the isolation of this organism from clinical specimens, with a peak in late winter/early spring and a nadir in late summer/early fall. Direct contact has not been shown to contribute to community-acquired infection, but nosocomial spread of infection has been documented occasionally.

CLINICAL MANIFESTATIONS ■ Otitis Media and Sinusitis　*M. catarrhalis* has repeatedly been shown to be the third most common bacterial isolate from middle-ear fluid of children who have otitis media, being surpassed only by *Streptococcus pneumoniae* and nontypable *Haemophilus influenzae*. Recent studies have shown that this organism is also a prominent isolate from sinus cavities in acute and chronic sinusitis.

Purulent Tracheobronchitis and Pneumonia　*M. catarrhalis* causes acute exacerbations of chronic bronchitis (increased production and/or purulence of sputum), purulent tracheobronchitis (the latter also involving fever and leukocytosis), and pneumonia; acquisition of a new bacterial strain is often responsible. The great majority of infected persons are >50 years old and have a long history of cigarette smoking and underlying chronic obstructive pulmonary disease (COPD); many have lung cancer as well. In one study, 76% of affected persons had COPD (severe in many cases), and one-third of those with COPD had lung cancer; most patients also had clinical evidence of malnutrition. In one extensive series of cases, *M. catarrhalis* pneumonia did not occur in otherwise-healthy hosts.

Symptoms of *M. catarrhalis* infection have been regarded as modest in severity. Both cough and the amount and purulence of sputum are usually increased above baseline. Chills are reported in one-quarter

FIGURE 129-1　Gram-stained sputum from a patient with acute purulent tracheobronchitis. Many polymorphonuclear neutrophils and a few macrophages are seen along with many gram-negative cocci (*Moraxella catarrhalis*), a few of which appear as pairs. Nearly all organisms are cell associated and probably have been taken up by phagocytes, consistent with the notion that *Moraxella* is a lower-grade pathogen than organisms such as *Streptococcus pneumoniae*.

of patients, pleuritic pain in one-third, and malaise in 40%. Most patients have peak temperatures of <38.3°C (<101°F), and peripheral white blood cell counts are <10,000/μL in nearly one-quarter of cases. Microscopic examination of a good sputum specimen following Gram's staining regularly reveals profuse organisms, and quantitative culture yields ~ 2×10^8 colony-forming units per milliliter. The radiologic appearance is variable; in one study, 43% of subjects had segmental or lobar infiltrates, and the remainder had a mixed pattern of subsegmental, segmental, interstitial, and diffuse involvement. These clinical, laboratory, and radiographic findings do not differ from those of pneumococcal or *Haemophilus* pneumonia in an older patient population. However, a far lesser degree of bloodstream invasion occurs in *M. catarrhalis* infection; in one series, none of 25 patients with *M. catarrhalis* pneumonia had bacteremia. Nevertheless, pneumonia due to *M. catarrhalis* is a marker for severe underlying disease: nearly half of patients die within 3 months of onset.

Other Syndromes Local extension causing empyema is very uncommon, and, as might be inferred from the low rate of bacteremia, metastatic complications of *M. catarrhalis* pneumonia, such as septic arthritis, are exceedingly rare. As of 1995, 58 cases of bacteremic infection due to *M. catarrhalis* had been reported, mainly in children <10 years old or adults >60 years old; most of these patients had severe underlying lung disease and/or were immunocompromised. The syndromes reported have included bacteremia with no apparent focus, pneumonia, endocarditis, and meningitis. A petechial or purpuric rash, reminiscent of that observed in meningococcal sepsis and associated with disseminated intravascular coagulation, has been described in a few cases.

DIAGNOSIS Microscopic examination of Gram-stained sputum yields characteristic findings (Fig. 129-1). The presence of many polymorphonuclear leukocytes without epithelial cells indicates that the sputum sample is of good quality; since most patients with *Moraxella* infection have chronic lung disease, it is usually not difficult to obtain a good specimen. Large numbers of *Moraxella* organisms are seen as gram-negative cocci, often lining up side by side and thus resembling pairs of kidneys.

℞ TREATMENT

Treatment of *M. catarrhalis* infection with a penicillin/clavulanic acid combination seems highly appropriate. Penicillin resistance first appeared in isolates in the mid-1970s and is now found in 94% of clinical isolates. Resistance is mediated by two closely related β-lactamases, BRO-1 and BRO-2, which are present in 90% and 10% of resistant isolates, respectively. These enzymes are active against penicillin, ampicillin, and amoxicillin but less so against cephalosporins, especially third-generation cephalosporins, and they bind avidly to clavulanic acid and sulbactam. Thus a β-lactam/β-lactamase inhibitor combination offers an effective mode of treatment. Cephalosporins, especially those of the second and third generations, are effective alternatives. Isolates in the United States are also nearly uniformly susceptible to tetracycline, newer macrolides, ketolides, trimethoprim-sulfamethoxazole (TMP-SMX), quinolones, and chloramphenicol. A 5-day course of therapy has been shown to cure respiratory infection, although a longer course is required in sinusitis.

Treatment of sinusitis or otitis media is empirical, as appropriate specimens are usually obtained only in research studies. In the treatment of pneumonia during the period between the identification of gram-negative cocci in a Gram-stained specimen and the final identification of the organisms by culture, the severity of the condition and the potential presence of other infecting organisms should guide antibiotic selection. For example, an exacerbation of bronchitis caused by *M. catarrhalis* might be treated with tetracycline or TMP-SMX; however, in a patient with pneumonia, the possibility that pneumo-

---

TABLE 129-1 *Moraxella* Species

Moraxella Species	Number of Isolates	Common Sites/ Clinical Association	Number (Percent) for Each Site
M. osloensis[a]	199	Blood	44 (22)
		CSF	18 (9)
		Urine	17 (9)
		Respiratory tract	24 (12)
M. nonliquefaciens	356	Blood	27 (8)
		CSF	6 (2)
		Respiratory tract	196 (55)
M. canis	74	Dog-bite wound	53 (72)
M-6	47	Blood, bone	15 (32)
M. lacunata	33	Conjunctivitis, keratitis	23 (70)
M. urethralis	28	Urine	16 (57)
		Genital tract	3 (11)
M. phenylpyruvica	73	Blood	19 (26)
		CSF	8 (11)
		Urine	12 (16)
M. atlantae	44	Blood	20 (45)
		CSF	5 (11)

[a] Some of these isolates would now be distinguished as a new species, *Moraxella lincolnii*.
Note: CSF, cerebrospinal fluid.
Source: Adapted from a summary of CDC experience (Graham et al).

cocci resistant to these agents also might be present dictates the choice of ampicillin/sulbactam, a third-generation cephalosporin, or a quinolone, at least until culture results become available.

OTHER *MORAXELLA* SPECIES

Other *Moraxella* species cause a wide range of infections, including bronchitis, pneumonia, empyema, endocarditis, meningitis, conjunctivitis, endophthalmitis, urinary tract infection, septic arthritis, and wound infection. In a report on all *Moraxella* isolates submitted to the Centers for Disease Control and Prevention (CDC) between 1953 and 1980, certain clinical associations were apparent (Table 129-1). *M. osloensis* and *M. nonliquefaciens*, the most commonly isolated species, were cultured from a wide range of normally sterile body sites, including blood, cerebrospinal fluid, and joints. *M. osloensis* was the *Moraxella* species most frequently isolated from blood; *M. nonliquefaciens* tended to be isolated from the ears, nose, or throat (47%) or the sputum (8%) and has since been implicated as a cause of conjunctivitis and keratitis. *M. urethralis* was isolated most often from urine and the genital tract and probably represents the *Moraxella* species implicated previously in urethritis. More than half of isolates of *M. phenylpyruvica* and *M. atlantae* were obtained from normally sterile sites. A recent study found *Moraxella* spp., including *M. catarrhalis*, in 35% of infected wounds following cat bites and in 10% of those following dog bites. The clinical features of infections due to *Moraxella* spp. other than *M. catarrhalis* and the nature of the hosts in which they occur have not been fully characterized.

FURTHER READING

GRAHAM D et al: Infections caused by *Moraxella*, *Moraxella urethralis*, *Moraxella*-like groups M-5 and M-6, and *Kingella kingae* in the United States, 1953–1980. Rev Infect Dis 12:423, 1990

IOANNIDIS JPA et al: Spectrum and significance of bacteremia due to *Moraxella catarrhalis*. Clin Infect Dis 21:390, 1995

SETHI S et al: New strains of bacteria and exacerbations of chronic obstructive pulmonary disease. N Engl J Med 347:465, 2002

TALAN DA et al: Bacteriologic analysis of infected dog and cat bites. N Engl J Med 340:85, 1999

VERDUIN CM et al: *Moraxella catarrhalis*: From emerging to established pathogen. Clin Microbiol Rev 15:125, 2002

WRIGHT PW et al: A descriptive study of 42 cases of *Branhamella catarrhalis* pneumonia. Am J Med 88(Suppl 5A):2S, 1990

130 HAEMOPHILUS INFECTIONS
Timothy F. Murphy

HAEMOPHILUS INFLUENZAE

MICROBIOLOGY *Haemophilus influenzae* was first recognized in 1892 by Pfeiffer, who erroneously concluded that the bacterium was the cause of influenza. The bacterium is a small (1- by 0.3-μm) gram-negative organism of variable shape; hence, it is often described as a pleomorphic coccobacillus. In clinical specimens such as cerebrospinal fluid (CSF) and sputum, it frequently stains only faintly with phenosafranin and therefore can easily be overlooked.

H. influenzae grows both aerobically and anaerobically. Its aerobic growth requires two factors: hemin (X factor) and nicotinamide adenine dinucleotide (V factor). These requirements are used in the clinical laboratory to identify the bacterium. Six major serotypes of *H. influenzae* have been identified; designated *a* through *f*, they are based on antigenically distinct polysaccharide capsules. In addition, some strains lack a polysaccharide capsule and are referred to as *nontypable* strains. Type b and nontypable strains are the most relevant strains clinically (Table 130-1), although encapsulated strains other than type b can cause disease. *H. influenzae* was the first free-living organism to have its entire genome sequenced.

The antigenically distinct type b capsule is a linear polymer composed of ribosyl-ribitol phosphate. Strains of *H. influenzae* type b (Hib) cause disease primarily in infants and children under the age of 6 years. Nontypable strains are primarily mucosal pathogens, although these strains occasionally cause invasive disease.

EPIDEMIOLOGY AND TRANSMISSION *H. influenzae* is an exclusively human pathogen. The organism is spread by airborne droplets or by direct contact with secretions or fomites. Nontypable strains colonize the upper respiratory tract of up to three-fourths of healthy adults. Colonization with nontypable *H. influenzae* is a dynamic process; new strains are acquired and other strains are replaced periodically.

The widespread use of Hib conjugate vaccines has resulted in striking decreases in the rate of nasopharyngeal colonization by Hib and the incidence of Hib infection (Fig. 130-1). Invasive Hib disease now occurs predominantly in underimmunized children and in infants who have not completed the primary immunization series.

Certain population groups have a higher incidence of invasive Hib disease than the general population. The incidence of meningitis due to Hib has been three to four times higher among black children than among white children in several studies. In some Native American groups, the incidence of invasive Hib disease is 10 times higher than that in the general population. Although this increased incidence has not yet been accounted for, several factors may be relevant, including age at exposure to the bacterium, socioeconomic conditions, and genetic differences in the ability to mount an immune response.

PATHOGENESIS Hib strains cause systemic disease by invasion and hematogenous spread to distant sites such as the meninges, bones, and

FIGURE 130-1 Estimated incidence (rate per 100,000) of invasive disease due to *Haemophilus influenzae* type b among children <5 years of age: 1987–2000. (*Data from the Centers for Disease Control and Prevention.*)

joints. The type b polysaccharide capsule is an important virulence factor affecting the bacterium's ability to avoid opsonization and cause systemic disease.

Nontypable strains cause disease by local invasion of mucosal surfaces. Otitis media results when bacteria reach the middle ear by way of the eustachian tube. Adults with chronic bronchitis experience recurrent lower respiratory tract infection due to nontypable strains. The incidence of invasive disease caused by nontypable strains is low.

IMMUNE RESPONSE Antibody to capsule is important in protection from infection by Hib strains. The level of (maternally acquired) serum antibody to the capsular polysaccharide, which is a polymer of polyribitol ribose phosphate (PRP), declines from birth to 6 months of age and, in the absence of vaccination, remains low until around 2 or 3 years of age. The age at the antibody nadir correlates with that of the peak incidence of type b disease. Antibody to PRP then appears partly as a result of exposure to Hib or cross-reacting antigens. Systemic Hib disease is unusual after the age of 6 years because of the presence of protective antibody. Vaccines in which PRP is conjugated to protein carrier molecules have been developed and are now used widely. These vaccines generate an antibody response to PRP in infants and are effective in preventing invasive infections in infants and children.

Since nontypable strains lack a capsule, the immune response to infection is directed at noncapsular antigens. These noncapsular antigens of *H. influenzae* have generated considerable interest as targets of the human immune response and as potential vaccine components. The human immune response to nontypable strains appears to be strain-specific, accounting in part for the propensity of these strains to cause recurrent otitis media and recurrent exacerbations of chronic bronchitis in immunocompetent hosts.

CLINICAL MANIFESTATIONS ■ **Hib** The most serious manifestation of infection with Hib is meningitis. The age of peak incidence varies somewhat among populations, depending in part on the use of vaccine, but this infection primarily affects infants <2 years of age. The clinical manifestations of meningitis caused by Hib are similar to those of meningitis caused by other bacterial pathogens. Fever and altered central nervous system function are the most common features at presentation. Nuchal rigidity may or may not be evident. Subdural effusion, the most common complication, is suspected when, despite 2 or 3 days of appropriate antibiotic therapy, the infant has seizures, hemiparesis, or continued obtundation. The overall mortality from meningitis caused by Hib is ~5%, and the rate of morbidity is high. Of survivors, 6% have permanent sensorineural hearing loss, and about one-fourth have a significant handicap of some type. If more subtle handicaps are sought, up to half of survivors are found to have some neurologic sequelae, such as partial hearing loss and delay in language development.

Epiglottitis is a life-threatening infection involving cellulitis of the epiglottis and supraglottic tissues. It can lead to acute upper airway obstruction. Its unique epidemiologic features are its occurrence in an older age group (2 to 7 years old) than other Hib infections and its absence among Navajo Indians and Alaskan Eskimos. Sore throat and

TABLE 130-1 *Characteristics of Type b and Nontypable Strains of Haemophilus influenzae*

Feature	Type b Strains	Nontypable Strains
Capsule	Ribosyl-ribitol phosphate	Unencapsulated
Pathogenesis	Invasive infections due to hematogenous spread	Mucosal infections due to contiguous spread
Clinical manifestations	Meningitis and invasive infections in incompletely immunized infants and children	Otitis media in infants and children; lower respiratory tract infections in adults with chronic bronchitis
Evolutionary history	Basically clonal	Genetically diverse
Vaccine	Highly effective conjugate vaccines	None available; under development

fever rapidly progress to dysphagia, drooling, and airway obstruction. Epiglottitis also occurs in adults.

Cellulitis due to Hib occurs in young children. The most common location is on the head or neck, and the involved area sometimes takes on a characteristic bluish-red color. Most patients have bacteremia, and 10% have an additional focus of infection.

Hib causes *pneumonia* in infants. The infection is clinically indistinguishable from other types of bacterial pneumonia (e.g., pneumococcal pneumonia) except that Hib is more likely to involve the pleura.

Several less common invasive conditions can be important clinical manifestations of Hib infection in children. These include osteomyelitis, septic arthritis, pericarditis, orbital cellulitis, endophthalmitis, urinary tract infection, abscesses, and bacteremia without an identifiable focus. As has already been mentioned, infections due to Hib are unusual among patients older than 6 years.

Nontypable *H. influenzae* Nontypable *H. influenzae* is a common cause of community-acquired bacterial pneumonia in adults. Nontypable *H. influenzae* pneumonia is especially common among patients with chronic obstructive pulmonary disease (COPD) or AIDS. The clinical features of pneumonia due to *H. influenzae* are similar to those of other types of bacterial pneumonia (including pneumococcal pneumonia). Patients present with fever, cough, and purulent sputum, usually of several days' duration. Chest radiography reveals alveolar infiltrates in a patchy or lobar distribution. Gram-stained sputum contains a predominance of small, pleomorphic, coccobacillary gram-negative bacteria.

Exacerbations of COPD caused by nontypable *H. influenzae* are characterized by increased cough, sputum production, and shortness of breath. Fever is low-grade, and no infiltrates are evident on chest x-ray.

Nontypable *H. influenzae* is one of the three most common causes of childhood otitis media (the other two being *Streptococcus pneumoniae* and *Moraxella catarrhalis*). Infants are febrile and irritable, while older children report ear pain. Symptoms of viral upper respiratory infection often precede otitis media. The diagnosis is made by pneumatic otoscopy. An etiologic diagnosis, although not routinely sought, can be established by tympanocentesis and culture of middle-ear fluid.

Nontypable *H. influenzae* also causes puerperal sepsis and is an important cause of neonatal bacteremia. These nontypable strains tend to be of biotype IV and cause invasive disease after colonizing the female genital tract.

Nontypable *H. influenzae* causes sinusitis in adults and children. In addition, the bacterium is a less common cause of various invasive infections that are reported primarily as small-series descriptions and case reports. These infections include empyema, adult epiglottitis, pericarditis, cellulitis, septic arthritis, osteomyelitis, endocarditis, cholecystitis, intraabdominal infections, urinary tract infections, mastoiditis, aortic graft infection, and bacteremia without a detectable focus.

DIAGNOSIS The most reliable method for establishing a diagnosis of Hib infection is recovery of the organism in culture. The CSF of a patient in whom meningitis is suspected should be subjected to Gram's staining and culture. The presence of gram-negative coccobacilli in Gram-stained CSF is strong evidence for Hib meningitis. Recovery of the organism from CSF confirms the diagnosis. Cultures of other normally sterile body fluids, such as blood, joint fluid, pleural fluid, pericardial fluid, and subdural effusion, are confirmatory in other infections.

Detection of PRP is an important adjunct to culture in rapid diagnosis. Immunoelectrophoresis, latex agglutination, coagglutination, and enzyme-linked immunosorbent assay are effective in detecting PRP. These assays are particularly helpful when patients have received prior antimicrobial therapy and thus are especially likely to have negative cultures.

Before the early 1980s, nontypable strains of *H. influenzae* were frequently misidentified as Hib because of their autoagglutination when serotypes were determined in agglutination assays. Since nontypable *H. influenzae* is primarily a mucosal pathogen, it is a component of a mixed flora; this situation makes etiologic diagnosis challenging. Nontypable *H. influenzae* infection is strongly suggested by the predominance of gram-negative coccobacilli among abundant polymorphonuclear leukocytes in a Gram-stained sputum specimen from a patient in whom pneumonia or tracheobronchitis is suspected. A sputum culture is helpful when interpreted along with the results of Gram's staining. Although bacteremia is detectable in a small proportion of patients with pneumonia due to nontypable *H. influenzae*, most such patients have negative blood cultures.

A diagnosis of otitis media is based on the detection by pneumatic otoscopy of fluid in the middle ear. An etiologic diagnosis requires tympanocentesis but is not routinely sought. An invasive procedure is also required to determine the etiology of sinusitis; thus, treatment is often empirical once the diagnosis is suspected in light of clinical symptoms and sinus radiographs.

℞ TREATMENT

Initial therapy for meningitis due to Hib should consist of a cephalosporin such as ceftriaxone or cefotaxime. For children, the dosage of ceftriaxone is 75 to 100 mg/kg daily given in two doses 12 h apart. The pediatric dosage of cefotaxime is 200 mg/kg daily given in four doses 6 h apart. Adult dosages are 2 g every 12 h for ceftriaxone and 2 g every 4 to 6 h for cefotaxime. An alternative regimen for initial therapy is ampicillin (200 to 300 mg/kg daily in four divided doses) plus chloramphenicol (75 to 100 mg/kg daily in four divided doses). Therapy should continue for a total of 1 to 2 weeks.

Administration of glucocorticoids to patients with Hib meningitis reduces the incidence of neurologic sequelae. The presumed mechanism is reduction of the inflammation induced by bacterial cell-wall mediators of inflammation when cells are killed by antimicrobial agents. Dexamethasone (0.6 mg/kg per day intravenously in four divided doses for 2 days) is recommended for the treatment of Hib meningitis in children >2 months of age.

Invasive infections other than meningitis are treated with the same antimicrobial agents. For epiglottitis, the dosage of ceftriaxone is 50 mg/kg daily, and the dosage of cefotaxime is 150 mg/kg daily, given in three divided doses 8 h apart. Epiglottitis constitutes a medical emergency, and maintenance of an airway is critical. The duration of therapy is determined by the clinical response. A course of 1 to 2 weeks is usually appropriate.

Many infections caused by nontypable strains of *H. influenzae*, such as otitis media, sinusitis, and exacerbations of COPD, can be treated with oral antimicrobial agents. Approximately 25% of nontypable strains produce β-lactamase and are resistant to ampicillin. Infections caused by ampicillin-resistant strains can be treated with a variety of agents, including trimethoprim-sulfamethoxazole, amoxicillin/clavulanic acid, various extended-spectrum cephalosporins, and newer macrolides (azithromycin and clarithromycin). Fluoroquinolones are highly active against *H. influenzae* but are not currently recommended for the treatment of children or pregnant women because of possible effects on articular cartilage.

PREVENTION ■ **Vaccination** (See also Chap. 107) The development of conjugate vaccines that prevent invasive infections with Hib in infants and children has been a dramatic success. Three such vaccines are licensed in the United States. In addition to eliciting protective antibody, these vaccines prevent disease by reducing pharyngeal colonization with Hib.

All children should be immunized with an Hib conjugate vaccine, receiving the first dose at ~2 months of age, the rest of the primary series between 2 and 6 months of age, and a booster dose at 12 to 15 months of age. Specific recommendations vary for the different conjugate vaccines. The reader is referred to the recommendations of the American Academy of Pediatrics. Currently, no vaccines are available for the prevention of disease caused by nontypable *H. influenzae*.

Chemoprophylaxis The risk of secondary disease is greater than normal among household contacts of patients with Hib disease. The attack rate is as high as 4% among susceptible infants. Therefore, all children and adults (except pregnant women) in households with at least one contact <4 years of age who is incompletely immunized should receive prophylaxis with oral rifampin. (This rule does not apply when all household contacts under the age of 4 years have been completely immunized with conjugate vaccine.) Children <12 years old should receive rifampin at a dose of 20 mg/kg once daily for 4 days, and adults should receive 600 mg daily for 4 days. The index case should receive rifampin before or at the time of discharge from the hospital because antimicrobial agents used for the treatment of meningitis do not reliably eradicate Hib from the nasopharynx.

When two or more cases of invasive Hib disease have occurred within 60 days at a child-care facility attended by incompletely vaccinated children, administration of rifampin to all attendees and personnel is indicated, as is recommended for household contacts. Chemoprophylaxis is not indicated in nursery and child-care contacts of a single index case. The reader is referred to the recommendations of the American Academy of Pediatrics.

HAEMOPHILUS INFLUENZAE BIOGROUP AEGYPTIUS

H. influenzae biogroup aegyptius was formerly called *Haemophilus aegyptius* because of phenotypic characteristics distinct from those of *H. influenzae*. However, later studies involving DNA hybridization and DNA transformation demonstrated that *H. aegyptius* and *H. influenzae* are members of the same species.

H. influenzae biogroup aegyptius has long been associated with conjunctivitis. Moreover, this strain is now known to be the cause of Brazilian purpuric fever (BPF), which was first recognized in 1984 in the rural Brazilian town of Promissao. The sharing of many phenotypic and genotypic characteristics by the various strains of *H. influenzae* biogroup aegyptius that cause BPF indicates that these strains represent a clone of *H. influenzae*. The age of peak incidence of BPF is 1 to 4 years, with a range of 3 months to 8 years. The illness can occur sporadically or in outbreaks. Typically, after an episode of purulent conjunctivitis, high fever occurs in association with vomiting and abdominal pain. Within 12 to 48 h after onset, the patient develops petechiae, purpura, and peripheral necrosis and experiences vascular collapse. The characteristic laboratory features are thrombocytopenia, prolonged prothrombin time, uniformly unrevealing CSF findings, and blood cultures positive for *H. influenzae* biogroup aegyptius. Initial reports cited high mortality (70%), but subsequent studies have indicated that milder forms of the illness exist. Most patients have resolved or resolving purulent conjunctivitis, and culture of the conjunctiva is positive in approximately one-third of cases. BPF has been seen in several towns in Brazil and on two occasions in Australia.

HAEMOPHILUS DUCREYI

Haemophilus ducreyi is the etiologic agent of chancroid (Chap. 115), a sexually transmitted disease characterized by genital ulceration and inguinal adenitis. *H. ducreyi* poses a significant health problem in developing countries. Although this infection is less common in the United States, its incidence has increased dramatically in the past several years. In addition to being a cause of morbidity in itself, chancroid is associated with infection with HIV because of the role of genital ulceration in the transmission of HIV.

MICROBIOLOGY *H. ducreyi* is a highly fastidious coccobacillary gram-negative bacterium whose growth requires X factor (hemin). Although, in light of this requirement, the bacterium has been classified in the genus *Haemophilus*, DNA homology and chemotaxonomic studies have established substantial differences between *H. ducreyi* and other *Haemophilus* species. Taxonomic reclassification of the organism is likely in the future but awaits further study.

The histology of the genital ulcer of chancroid is characterized by perivascular and interstitial infiltrates of macrophages and of CD4+ and CD8+ lymphocytes. The appearance is consistent with a delayed-type hypersensitivity, cell-mediated immune response. The presence of CD4+ cells and macrophages in the ulcer may explain, in part, the facilitation of transmission of HIV in patients with chancroid.

EPIDEMIOLOGY AND PREVALENCE Chancroid is a common cause of genital ulcers in developing countries. In the United States, chancroid is now endemic in some regions, and several large outbreaks have occurred since 1981. Recurring epidemiologic themes have been apparent in these outbreaks: (1) transmission has been predominantly heterosexual; (2) males have outnumbered females by ratios of 3:1 to 25:1; (3) prostitutes have been important in transmission of the infection; and (4) chancroid has been strongly associated with illicit drug use. The incidence of chancroid in the United States will likely increase in the coming years, and the genital ulcers associated with this infection will continue to play a role in the transmission of HIV.

CLINICAL MANIFESTATIONS Infection is acquired as the result of a break in the epithelium during sexual contact with an infected individual. After an incubation period of 4 to 7 days, the initial lesion—a papule with surrounding erythema—appears. In 2 to 3 days, the papule evolves into a pustule, which spontaneously ruptures and forms a sharply circumscribed ulcer that is generally not indurated (Fig. 130-2). The ulcers are painful and bleed easily; little or no inflammation of the surrounding skin is evident. Approximately half of patients develop enlarged, tender inguinal lymph nodes, which frequently become fluctuant and spontaneously rupture. Patients usually seek medical care after 1 to 3 weeks of painful symptoms.

The presentation of chancroid does not usually include all of the typical clinical features and is sometimes atypical. Multiple ulcers can coalesce to form giant ulcers. Ulcers can appear and then resolve, with inguinal adenitis (Fig. 130-2) and suppuration following 1 to 3 weeks later; this clinical picture can be confused with that of lymphogranuloma venereum. Multiple small ulcers can resemble folliculitis. Other differential diagnostic considerations include the various infections causing genital ulceration, such as primary syphilis, condyloma latum of secondary syphilis, genital herpes, and donovanosis. In rare cases chancroid lesions become secondarily infected with bacteria; the result is extensive inflammation.

DIAGNOSIS Clinical diagnosis of chancroid is often inaccurate, and laboratory confirmation should be attempted in suspected cases. Gram's staining of a swab of the lesion may reveal a predominance of characteristic gram-negative coccobacilli, but the presence of other bacteria often makes it difficult to interpret this result. An accurate diagnosis of chancroid relies on cultures of *H. ducreyi* from the lesion. In addition, aspiration and culture of suppurative lymph nodes should be considered. Since the organism can be difficult to grow, the use of selective and supplemented media is necessary. A new multiplex

FIGURE 130-2 Chancroid with characteristic penile ulcers and associated left inguinal adenitis (bubo).

polymerase chain reaction (PCR) assay has been developed to amplify simultaneously DNA targets from *H. ducreyi*, *Treponema pallidum*, and herpes simplex virus types 1 and 2. When this assay becomes commercially available, it will be a useful diagnostic method with which to identify the etiology of genital ulcers.

℞ TREATMENT

The treatment regimen recommended by the Centers for Disease Control and Prevention is a single 1-g oral dose of azithromycin. Alternative regimens include ceftriaxone (250 mg intramuscularly in a single dose), ciprofloxacin (500 mg orally twice a day for 3 days), or erythromycin base (500 mg orally three times a day for 7 days). Isolates from patients who do not respond promptly to treatment should be tested for antimicrobial susceptibility. In patients with HIV infection, healing may be slow and longer courses of treatment may be necessary. Clinical treatment failure in HIV-seropositive patients may reflect co-infection, especially with herpes simplex virus. Contacts of patients with chancroid should be identified and treated whether or not symptoms are present if they had sexual contact with the patient during the 10 days preceding the patient's onset of symptoms.

OTHER *HAEMOPHILUS* SPECIES

Haemophilus species are often recovered as components of the flora of the normal human upper respiratory tract. However, these bacteria are infrequent causes of infection because of their low pathogenic potential. *Haemophilus* species have fastidious growth requirements and are generally rather slow-growing. The species implicated in human infections include *H. parainfluenzae*, *H. aphrophilus*, and *H. paraphrophilus* (Chap. 131); *H. parahaemolyticus*; *H. haemolyticus*; and *H. segnis*. *Haemophilus* species are differentiated from one another by several characteristics, primarily their requirements for X and V factors. Species designated *para-* require V factor but not X factor for growth, whereas the others require either X and V or X only.

Haemophilus species, particularly *H. parainfluenzae*, are an increasingly recognized cause of endocarditis and should be considered as such, especially when initial blood cultures are negative but clinical suspicion of endocarditis is high. Blood cultures should be incubated for 2 weeks to increase the likelihood of isolating slow-growing *Hae-*

mophilus species. Endocarditis due to *Haemophilus* species usually presents with a subacute course, but the presentation varies.

A variety of other infections involving almost all organ systems can be caused by *Haemophilus* species. Most of these unusual manifestations have been reported as single cases and small series.

℞ TREATMENT

The antimicrobial susceptibility characteristics of other *Haemophilus* species are similar to those of *H. influenzae*. Some strains produce β-lactamase and are thereby resistant to ampicillin. Other strains are sensitive to ampicillin, and this agent has been used successfully to treat many infections. Alternative agents with good activity against most *Haemophilus* species include trimethoprim-sulfamethoxazole, third-generation cephalosporins, tetracycline, chloramphenicol, and aminoglycosides. Endocarditis caused by ampicillin-sensitive strains should be treated with ampicillin plus an aminoglycoside.

FURTHER READING

BONG CT et al: *Haemophilus ducreyi*: Clinical features, epidemiology, and prospects for disease control. Microbes Infect 4:1141, 2002

COMMITTEE ON INFECTIOUS DISEASES: *Haemophilus influenzae* infections, in *2000 Red Book, Report of the Committee on Infectious Diseases,* LK Pickering et al (eds). Elk Grove Village, IL, American Academy of Pediatrics, 2000

FOXWELL AR et al: Nontypeable *Haemophilus influenzae*: Pathogenesis and prevention. Microbiol Mol Biol Rev 62:294, 1998

HOBAN DJ et al: Worldwide prevalence of antimicrobial resistance in *Streptococcus pneumoniae*, *Haemophilus influenzae*, and *Moraxella catarrhalis* in the SENTRY antimicrobial surveillance program, 1997–1999. Clin Infect Dis 32(Suppl):S81, 2001

PELTOLA H: Worldwide *Haemophilus influenzae* type b disease at the beginning of the 21st century: Global analysis of the disease burden 25 years after the use of the polysaccharide vaccine and a decade after the advent of conjugates. Clin Microbiol Rev 13:302, 2000

SARANGI J et al: Invasive *Haemophilus influenzae* disease in adults. Epidemiol Infect 124:441, 2000

SETHI S et al: New strains of bacteria and exacerbations of chronic obstructive pulmonary disease. N Engl J Med 347:465, 2002

131 INFECTIONS DUE TO HACEK GROUP AND MISCELLANEOUS GRAM-NEGATIVE BACTERIA
Dennis L. Kasper, Tamar F. Barlam

HACEK GROUP ORGANISMS

HACEK organisms are a group of fastidious, slow-growing, gram-negative bacteria whose growth requires an atmosphere of carbon dioxide. Species belonging to this group include several *Haemophilus* species, *Actinobacillus actinomycetemcomitans*, *Cardiobacterium hominis*, *Eikenella corrodens*, and *Kingella kingae*. HACEK bacteria normally reside in the oral cavity and have been associated with local infections in the mouth. They are also known to cause severe systemic infections, most often bacterial endocarditis (Chap. 109).

Of the HACEK group, the *Haemophilus* species, *A. actinomycetemcomitans*, and *C. hominis* are most frequently associated with endocarditis, which can develop on either native or prosthetic valves. In large series, up to 3% of cases of infective endocarditis are attributable to HACEK organisms. The clinical course of HACEK endocarditis tends to be subacute; however, embolization is common. The overall prevalence of major emboli associated with HACEK endocarditis ranges from 28 to 71% in different series. On echocardiography, valvular vegetations are seen in up to 85% of patients. The vegetations are frequently large, although vegetation size has not been directly correlated with risk of embolization. Cultures of blood from patients with suspected HACEK endocarditis may require up to 30 days to

become positive, and the microbiology laboratory should be alerted if a HACEK organism is being considered. However, most cultures that ultimately yield a HACEK organism become positive within the first week, especially with improved culture systems such as BACTEC. In addition, polymerase chain reaction techniques are facilitating the diagnosis of HACEK infections. Because of the organisms' slow growth, antimicrobial testing may be difficult, and strains producing β-lactamase may not be identified accurately. This factor should be considered in the selection of a therapeutic regimen. E-test methodology may improve the accuracy of susceptibility testing.

Native-valve endocarditis should be treated for 4 weeks with antibiotics, whereas prosthetic-valve endocarditis requires 6 weeks of therapy. The cure rates for HACEK prosthetic-valve endocarditis appear to be high. Unlike prosthetic-valve endocarditis caused by other gram-negative organisms, HACEK endocarditis is often cured with antibiotic treatment alone—i.e., without surgical intervention. Recommendations for the treatment of HACEK endocarditis are presented in Table 131-1.

***HAEMOPHILUS* SPECIES** *Haemophilus* species cause more than half of all cases of HACEK endocarditis. *H. aphrophilus* and *H. parainfluenzae* are most common; *H. paraphrophilus* is less common. Up to 50%

TABLE 131-1 *Treatment of Endocarditis Caused by HACEK Group Organisms*[a]

Organism	Initial Therapy	Alternative Agents	Comments
Haemophilus species	Ceftriaxone (2 g/d)	Fluoroquinolones,[b] ampicillin/ sulbactam	Ampicillin ± aminoglycoside can be used if organism does not produce β-lactamase.
Actinobacillus actinomycetemcomitans	Ceftriaxone (2 g/d)	Semisynthetic penicillins (e.g., mezlocillin), TMP-SMX, fluoroquinolones,[b] azithromycin	Limited data exist on efficacy of regimens other than semisynthetic penicillins or third-generation cephalosporins.
Cardiobacterium hominis	Penicillin (16–18 mU/d in 6 divided doses) ± gentamicin (5–6 mg/kg/ d in 3 divided doses)	Ceftriaxone, ampicillin/sulbactam	Value of aminoglycoside has not been proven. Organism is usually pan-sensitive, but high-level resistance to penicillin has been reported.
Eikenella corrodens	Ampicillin (2 g q4h)	Ceftriaxone, fluoroquinolones[b]	Organism is resistant to clindamycin and metronidazole.
Kingella kingae	Ceftriaxone (2 g/d) or ampicillin/ sulbactam (3 g of ampicillin q6h)	Fluoroquinolones,[b] vancomycin, clindamycin, macrolides, TMP-SMX	Prevalence of β-lactamase-producing strains is increasing. Efficacy for invasive infections is best demonstrated for first-line treatments.

[a] Susceptibility testing should be performed to guide therapy.
[b] Fluoroquinolones are not recommended for treatment of children <17 years of age.

Note: TMP-SMX, trimethoprim-sulfamethoxazole.

of patients with native-valve endocarditis due to *Haemophilus* species report a history of cardiac valvular disease, 60% have been ill for <2 months before presentation, and 50% are anemic at presentation. Some 19% to 50% of these patients develop congestive heart failure. Mortality rates as high as 30% to 50% have been reported in older series, with most deaths attributed to cerebral embolism; however, recent studies have documented mortality rates of <5%. In rare cases, *H. parainfluenzae* has been isolated from other infections, such as meningitis; brain, dental, and liver abscess; pneumonia; and septicemia.

 TREATMENT

See Table 131-1.

ACTINOBACILLUS ACTINOMYCETEMCOMITANS *A. actinomycetemcomitans*, another slow-growing inhabitant of the oral cavity, can be isolated from soft tissue infections and abscesses in association with *Actinomyces israelii*. About 30% of actinomycotic lesions also yield *A. actinomycetemcomitans* on culture. *A. actinomycetemcomitans* has been associated with severe destructive periodontal disease, characterized by loss of alveolar bone of the molars and incisors, in both children and adults. Patients who develop endocarditis with this organism typically have severe periodontal disease and underlying cardiac valvular damage as well as high rates of embolic phenomena. *A. actinomycetemcomitans* has been isolated from patients with brain abscess, meningitis, parotitis, osteomyelitis, urinary tract infection, pneumonia, and empyema, among other infections.

 TREATMENT

See Table 131-1.

CARDIOBACTERIUM HOMINIS *C. hominis* primarily causes endocarditis in patients with underlying valvular heart disease or with prosthetic valves. Unlike other HACEK bacteria, *C. hominis* most frequently affects the aortic valve. Many patients have signs and symptoms of long-standing infection before diagnosis and have evidence of arterial embolization, vasculitis, cerebrovascular accidents, immune complex glomerulonephritis, or arthritis at presentation. As in endocarditis due to other HACEK organisms, embolization, mycotic aneurysms, and congestive heart failure are frequent.

 TREATMENT

See Table 131-1.

EIKENELLA CORRODENS *E. corrodens*, a fastidious, facultative gram-negative organism, is part of the endogenous flora of the mouth and nasopharynx. It is most frequently recovered from sites of infection in conjunction with other bacterial species. Clinical sources of *E. corrodens* include sites of human bite wounds (clenched-fist injuries), endocarditis, soft tissue infections of the head and neck, soft tissue infections in injection drug users, osteomyelitis, respiratory infections, chorioamnionitis, gynecologic infections associated with intrauterine devices, meningitis and brain abscesses, and visceral abscesses.

 TREATMENT

See Table 131-1.

KINGELLA KINGAE *K. kingae* is a β-hemolytic, fastidious, nonmotile gram-negative rod. Because of improved microbiologic methodology, isolation of this organism is increasingly common. In recent series, *K. kingae* was the cause of up to half of all cases of previously undiagnosed osteomyelitis and septic arthritis in children <2 years old. *K. kingae* has been the third most common cause of septic arthritis in children <24 months of age; staphylococcal and streptococcal species remain most prevalent. In children <4 years of age, there is evidence for prolonged nasopharyngeal colonization, with carriage rates of 10%. Invasive *K. kingae* infections with bacteremia are associated with stomatitis. Both *K. kingae* colonization and primary herpes—a major cause of stomatitis—peak in children 6 to 48 months of age. *K. kingae* bacteremia can present with a petechial rash similar to that seen with *Neisseria meningitidis* sepsis.

Infective endocarditis, unlike other infections with *K. kingae*, occurs in older children and adults. The majority of patients have pre-existing valvular disease. As in endocarditis caused by the other HACEK organisms, there is a high incidence of complications, including arterial emboli, cerebrovascular accidents, tricuspid insufficiency, and congestive heart failure with cardiovascular collapse.

 TREATMENT

See Table 131-1.

OTHER GRAM-NEGATIVE BACTERIA
ACINETOBACTER SPECIES See Chap. 134.

ACHROMOBACTER XYLOSOXIDANS Previously known as *Alcaligenes xylosoxidans*, this gram-negative bacillus is probably part of the endogenous intestinal flora and has been isolated from water sources. Immunocompromised hosts appear to be at increased risk for infection with this organism. Nosocomial sources to which outbreaks of infection with *A. xylosoxidans* have been attributed include contaminated intravenous fluids, pressure transducers, and disinfectants. Clinical illness has been associated with isolates from many sites, including blood (often in the setting of infected intravascular devices), urine, respiratory secretions, cerebrospinal fluid, peritoneal and pleural fluids, and endocarditic prosthetic valves. Community-acquired bacteremia with *A. xylosoxidans* usually occurs in the setting of pneumonia. Metastatic skin lesions are present in one-fifth of cases. The reported mortality rate is 67%, similar to rates for other bacteremic gram-negative pneumonias.

℞ TREATMENT

In vitro susceptibility testing of all clinically relevant isolates is essential to the selection of appropriate therapy.

AGROBACTERIUM RADIOBACTER (TUMEFACIENS) This organism has been associated with intravascular catheter–related infections in immunocompromised hosts, especially individuals infected with HIV. Clinically important infections associated with *A. radiobacter* include prosthetic-joint and prosthetic-valve infections, bacteremia, peritonitis, and urinary tract infections.

℞ TREATMENT

Antibiotic sensitivity testing is essential in the choice of therapy.

CAPNOCYTOPHAGA SPECIES This genus of fusiform, long, thin, gram-negative coccobacilli is facultatively anaerobic and requires an atmosphere enriched in carbon dioxide for optimal growth. *C. ochracea*, *C. gingivalis*, and *C. sputigena* are inhabitants of the healthy human oral cavity and have been isolated from the female genital tract. Their isolation has also been reported from blood, cerebrospinal fluid, and respiratory fluids (including pleural collections). These organisms have been associated with sepsis in immunocompromised hosts; particularly at risk are neutropenic patients with acute myelogenous leukemia or acute lymphocytic leukemia. In the immunocompetent host, these three species probably play a role in localized juvenile periodontitis; however, they have been isolated from many other sites as well, usually as part of a polymicrobial infection. In vitro sensitivity testing of these organisms is difficult because they are slow-growing and fastidious.

C. canimorsus and *C. cynodegmi* are endogenous to the canine mouth. Patients infected with these species frequently have a history of dog bites or of exposure to dogs without scratches or bites. Asplenia, glucocorticoid therapy, and alcohol abuse are predisposing conditions and are associated with relatively fulminant infections. The interval from dog bite to presentation averages 5 days but ranges from 1 day to 1 month. *C. canimorsus* causes a wide range of infections, including severe sepsis with shock and disseminated intravascular coagulation, meningitis, endocarditis, cellulitis, and septic arthritis. In the asplenic individual who has recently sustained a dog bite, infection with this organism must be considered early because of a potentially rapid progression to death.

℞ TREATMENT

Although penicillin has been considered first-line therapy for infections due to *C. ochracea*, *C. gingivalis*, and *C. sputigena*, an increasing number of isolates reportedly produce β-lactamase. Fluoroquinolone resistance is also increasing. Clindamycin (600 to 900 mg every 6 to 8 h) or drug combinations including a penicillin derivative plus a β-lactamase inhibitor—such as ampicillin/sulbactam (1.5 to 3.0 g of ampicillin every 6 h)—are currently recommended for empirical therapy. Penicillin (12 to 18 million units daily in 6 divided doses) is the drug of choice for documented infections with *C. canimorsus*. This regimen or ampicillin/sulbactam should also be given prophylactically to asplenic patients sustaining dog-bite injuries. Patients with suspected infection due to *C. canimorsus* should be treated empirically, because identification of this organism and determination of its antibiotic sensitivity can take many days. Other drugs to which *C. canimorsus* is reportedly susceptible include clindamycin, imipenem, quinolones, and third-generation cephalosporins.

CHROMOBACTERIUM VIOLACEUM This organism is rarely a human pathogen but reportedly has been responsible for life-threatening infections

with severe sepsis and metastatic abscesses, particularly in children. A slender, slightly curved, gram-negative rod that is facultatively anaerobic, *C. violaceum* inhabits tropical water and soil and causes infection after contamination of skin wounds. Patients with defective neutrophil function (e.g., those with chronic granulomatous disease) are infected by this organism with unusual frequency. The mortality rate in the United States from infection with *C. violaceum* has been reported at >60%.

℞ TREATMENT

C. violaceum is generally susceptible to ciprofloxacin (500 mg every 12 h orally or 400 mg every 12 h intravenously), trimethoprim-sulfamethoxazole (TMP-SMX), gentamicin, and chloramphenicol.

CHRYSEOBACTERIUM SPECIES *C. meningosepticum* and *C. indologenes* were previously classified as *Flavobacterium* species. *C. meningosepticum* is a ubiquitous organism and an important cause of nosocomial infections. It has been associated with outbreaks due to contaminated fluids, such as disinfectants, arterial catheter flush solutions, and aerosolized antibiotics, and with sporadic infections due to indwelling devices, vials, sink traps, feeding tubes, and other fluid-associated apparatus. Patients with nosocomial *C. meningosepticum* infection usually have underlying immunosuppression (e.g., related to malignancy). *C. meningosepticum* has been reported to cause meningitis (primarily in neonates), sepsis, endocarditis, bacteremia, soft tissue infections, and pneumonia. *C. indologenes* has caused bacteremia, sepsis, and pneumonia, typically in immunocompromised patients with indwelling devices.

℞ TREATMENT

Antibiotic treatment should be based on susceptibility results because of the high likelihood that a *C. meningosepticum* isolate will produce β-lactamase. Early reports suggested that vancomycin might be efficacious, but more recent data refute this conclusion.

PLESIOMONAS SHIGELLOIDES This freshwater organism is a cause of acute diarrhea (Chap. 113) and occasionally of serious extraintestinal disease. *P. shigelloides* is transmitted to humans via contaminated water or food. This motile, facultatively anaerobic gram-negative rod most often produces mild, watery diarrhea. Severe extraintestinal infections have been reported, most commonly in immunocompromised hosts, and include bacteremia, cellulitis, neonatal sepsis and meningitis, and septic arthritis.

℞ TREATMENT

There is great variability among strains in terms of antibiotic sensitivity patterns, and isolates must be tested before appropriate therapy can be selected.

AEROMONAS SPECIES Five species of *Aeromonas* are known to be associated with disease in humans, but more than 85% of these *Aeromonas* infections are caused by *A. hydrophila*, *A. caviae*, and *A. veronii* biovar *sobria*. *Aeromonas* proliferates in potable and fresh water and in soil. It remains controversial whether *Aeromonas* is a cause of bacterial gastroenteritis. Although many case reports have associated *Aeromonas* with gastroenteritis, no clear outbreaks with a single isolate have been documented, no conclusive animal model exists, and asymptomatic colonization of the intestinal tract with *Aeromonas* occurs frequently. However, rare cases of hemolytic-uremic syndrome following bloody diarrhea have been shown to be secondary to the presence of *Aeromonas*. In addition, identification of an enterotoxin (different from the Shiga-like toxin produced by *Escherichia coli* O157:H7) in these cases supports the hypothesis that *Aeromonas* causes gastroenteritis.

Aeromonas causes sepsis and bacteremia in infants with multiple medical problems and in immunocompromised hosts, particularly those with cancer or hepatobiliary disease. *Aeromonas* infection and sepsis can occur in trauma patients with myonecrosis or in burn patients exposed to *Aeromonas* by environmental contamination of their wounds from fresh water or soil sources. Mortality ranges from 25% among immunocompromised adults with sepsis to >90% among patients with myonecrosis. *Aeromonas* can produce skin lesions resembling the ecthyma gangrenosum lesions seen in *Pseudomonas aeruginosa* infection. These lesions are hemorrhagic vesicles surrounded by a rim of erythema with central necrosis and ulceration.

Aeromonas wound infections can occur in healthy adults who sustain minor trauma with environmental contamination, usually water-related; after severe trauma and crush injuries with sepsis and environmental exposure, usually to soil; and in nosocomial infections related to catheters, surgical incisions, or use of leeches. Other clinical manifestations include meningitis, peritonitis, pneumonia, and ocular infections.

℞ **TREATMENT**

Treatment should be guided by antimicrobial susceptibility testing. *Aeromonas* species are generally susceptible to fluoroquinolones (e.g., ciprofloxacin at a dosage of 500 mg every 12 h orally or 400 mg every 12 h intravenously), TMP-SMX (at a trimethoprim dosage of 10 mg/kg per day in 3 or 4 divided doses), third-generation cephalosporins, and aminoglycosides. However, resistance is increasing.

MISCELLANEOUS ORGANISMS   Many other gram-negative rods have been reported to cause occasional infections in hosts who are immunologically unprepared to deal with relatively avirulent organisms or who are unfortunate enough to encounter an exceptionally large inoculum. Such organisms include *Weeksella* species; various CDC groups, such as EF-4, Ve-2 (*Flavimonas* species), IVc-2, NO-1, WO-1, and Gilardi Group WO-1; *Sphingobacterium* species; *Protomonas* species; *Ochrobactrum anthropi*; *Oligella urethralis*; and *Shewanella putrefaciens*. The reader is advised to consult subspecialty texts and references for further guidance on these organisms.

FURTHER READING

BROUQUI P, RAOULT D: Endocarditis due to rare and fastidious bacteria. Clin Microbiol Rev 14:177, 2001

DARRAS-JOLY C et al: *Haemophilus* endocarditis: Report of 42 cases in adults and review. Clin Infect Dis 24:1087, 1997

DAS M et al: Infective endocarditis caused by HACEK microorganisms. Annu Rev Med 48:25, 1997

JANDA JM et al: Evolving concepts regarding the genus *Aeromonas*: An expanding panorama of species, disease presentations, and unanswered questions. Clin Infect Dis 27:332, 1998

MARTINO R et al: Bacteremia caused by *Capnocytophaga* species in patients with neutropenia and cancer: Results of a multicenter study. Clin Infect Dis 33:E20, 2001

PAUL K, PATEL SS: *Eikenella corrodens* infections in children and adolescents: Case report and review of the literature. Clin Infect Dis 33:54, 2001

SHIGEMATSU M et al: An epidemiological study of *Plesiomonas shigelloides* diarrhoea among Japanese travelers. Epidemiol Infect 125:523, 2000

YAGUPSKY P, DAGAN R: Population-based study of invasive *Kingella kingae* infections. Emerg Infect Dis 6:85, 2000

132 *LEGIONELLA* INFECTION
Feng-Yee Chang, Victor L. Yu

DEFINITION   *Legionellosis* refers to the two clinical syndromes caused by bacteria of the genus *Legionella*. *Pontiac fever* is an acute, febrile, self-limited illness that has been serologically linked to *Legionella* species, whereas *Legionnaires' disease* is the designation for pneumonia caused by these species.

HISTORY   Legionnaires' disease was first recognized in 1976, when an outbreak of pneumonia took place at a hotel in Philadelphia during the American Legion Convention. The causative agent proved to be a newly discovered bacterium, *Legionella pneumophila*, that was isolated from lung specimens obtained from the victims at autopsy.

MICROBIOLOGY   The family Legionellaceae comprises 41 species with 64 serogroups. The species *L. pneumophila* causes 80 to 90% of human infections and includes at least 14 serogroups; serogroups 1, 4, and 6 are most commonly implicated in human infections. To date, 17 species other than *L. pneumophila* have been associated with human infections, among which *L. micdadei* (Pittsburgh pneumonia agent), *L. bozemanii*, *L. dumoffii*, and *L. longbeachae* are the most common.

Members of the Legionellaceae are aerobic gram-negative bacilli that do not grow on routine microbiologic media. Buffered charcoal yeast extract (BCYE) agar is the medium used to grow *Legionella*. Antibiotics added to the medium suppress the growth of competing flora from nonsterile sites, and dyes color the colonies and assist in identification.

The direct fluorescent antibody (DFA) test can definitively identify a number of individual species. In *L. pneumophila*, lipopolysaccharide is a prominent constituent of the outer membrane, and the serogroup-specific antigen and antibodies detected by immunofluorescence are directed primarily at the lipopolysaccharide. Both polyclonal and monoclonal DFA reagents are commercially available. The monoclonal antibody reagent is less cross-reactive but is specific for *L. pneumophila*.

ECOLOGY AND TRANSMISSION   The natural habitats for *L. pneumophila* are aquatic bodies, including lakes and streams. *L. longbeachae* has been isolated from soil. *Legionella* can survive under a wide range of environmental conditions; for example, the organisms can live for years in refrigerated water samples. Natural bodies of water contain only small numbers of *Legionella*. However, once the organisms enter human-constructed aquatic reservoirs (such as water-distribution systems), they can grow and proliferate. Factors known to enhance colonization by and amplification of legionellae include warm temperatures (25° to 42°C), stagnation, and scale and sediment. *L. pneumophila* can form microcolonies within biofilms; its eradication from water-distribution systems requires disinfectants that can penetrate the biofilm. The presence of symbiotic microorganisms, including algae, amebas, ciliated protozoa, and other water-dwelling bacteria, promotes the growth of *L. pneumophila*. *Legionella* can invade and multiply within free-living protozoa.

Hot-water tanks colonized with *L. pneumophila* are significantly more likely than uncolonized tanks to be cooler, to have a vertical configuration, to be older, and to have higher concentrations of calcium and magnesium. Vertical tanks, especially those that are electric coil–heated rather than gas-heated, have a pronounced temperature stratification and thick sediment accumulation at the bottom.

The source of *Legionella* is water. Early investigations that implicated cooling towers antedated the discovery that the organism could also exist in potable-water distribution systems. It is now known that, in most previously reported outbreaks, cases of Legionnaires' disease continued to occur despite disinfection of cooling towers and the potable water supply was the actual source. Koch's postulates have been fulfilled in epidemiologic studies using molecular fingerprinting methods to link potable water sources (rather than cooling towers) to *Legionella* infection in humans. Community-acquired Legionnaires' disease has also been linked to colonization of residential and industrial water supplies.

Multiple modes of transmission of *Legionella* to humans exist, including aerosolization, aspiration, and direct instillation into the lung during respiratory tract manipulations. Aspiration is the predominant mode of transmission, but it is unclear whether *Legionella* enters the lung via oropharyngeal colonization or directly via the drinking of contaminated water. Nasogastric tubes have been linked to nosocomial Legionnaires' disease in several reports; microaspiration of contaminated water was the hypothesized mode of transmission. Surgery with general anesthesia is a known risk factor that is consistent with aspiration. Especially compelling is the reported 30% incidence of postoperative *Legionella* pneumonia among patients undergoing head and neck surgery at a hospital with a contaminated water supply; aspiration is a recognized sequela in such cases. Studies of patients with hospital-acquired Legionnaires' disease have shown that these individuals underwent endotracheal intubation significantly more often and for a significantly longer duration than patients with nosocomial pneumonia of other etiologies.

Aerosolization of *Legionella* by devices filled with tap water, including nebulizers and humidifiers, has been implicated in disease causation. An ultrasonic mist machine in the produce section of a grocery store was implicated in a community outbreak. Pontiac fever has been linked to *Legionella*-containing aerosols from water-using machinery, a cooling tower, air-conditioners, and whirlpools.

EPIDEMIOLOGY The incidence of Legionnaires' disease depends on the degree of contamination of the aquatic reservoir, the immune status of the persons exposed to water from that reservoir, the intensity of exposure, and the availability of specialized laboratory tests on which the correct diagnosis can be based.

Numerous prospective studies have ranked *Legionella* among the top four microbial causes of community-acquired pneumonia (with *Streptococcus pneumoniae*, *Haemophilus influenzae*, and *Chlamydia pneumoniae* usually ranked first, second, and third, respectively), accounting for 3 to 15% of cases. On the basis of a multihospital study of community-acquired pneumonia in Ohio, it is estimated that only 3% of sporadic cases of Legionnaires' disease are correctly diagnosed. *Legionella* is responsible for 10 to 50% of nosocomial pneumonias when a hospital's water system is colonized with the organisms. One situation in which the diagnosis of Legionnaires' disease should be considered is that in which the presenting patient has been hospitalized within 10 days before the onset of symptoms.

The most common risk factors for Legionnaires' disease are cigarette smoking, chronic lung disease, advanced age, and immunosuppression (including receipt of glucocorticoids). However, in a large prospective study of community-acquired pneumonia, 28% of patients with Legionnaires' disease did not have these classic risk factors. Surgery is a prominent predisposing factor in hospital-acquired infection, with transplant recipients at highest risk. Hospital-acquired cases are now being recognized among neonates and children with immunosuppression or underlying pulmonary disease.

Pontiac fever occurs in epidemics. The high attack rate (>90%) reflects airborne transmission.

PATHOGENESIS AND IMMUNITY *Legionella* enters the lungs through aspiration or direct inhalation. Attachment of the bacteria to host cells is mediated by type IV pili, heat-shock protein Hsp60, and the major outer-membrane protein. *Legionella* binds to complement CR1 and CR3 integrin receptors on the surface of the host cell. Because the organisms possess pili that may mediate adherence to respiratory tract epithelial cells, conditions that impair mucociliary clearance, including cigarette smoking, lung disease, or alcoholism, predispose to Legionnaires' disease.

Cell-mediated immunity is the primary mechanism of host defense against *Legionella*, as it is against other intracellular pathogens, including *Mycobacterium tuberculosis*, *Listeria*, and *Toxoplasma*. Alveolar macrophages readily phagocytose *Legionella*. The attachment of the bacteria to phagocytes is mediated via Fc receptors and complement receptors, which attach to the bacterial major outer-membrane protein. Binding to these receptors promotes phagocytosis but fails to trigger an oxidative burst. The *L. pneumophila* phagosome resists acidification and evades fusion with late endocytic compartments and ly-

sosomes. Although many *Legionella* organisms are killed, some proliferate intracellularly until the cells rupture; the bacteria are then phagocytosed again by newly recruited phagocytes, and the cycle begins anew.

Two general types of bacterial virulence genes required for intracellular growth have been identified: those that affect trafficking of the bacterial phagosome (establishment factors) and those that affect replication after trafficking (maintenance factors). Establishment factor mutants exhibit severe intracellular-growth defects because they cannot alter phagosome trafficking to inhibit fusion with lysosomes. Genes of the *L. pneumophila* chromosome that harbor this phenotype, referred to as *dot* (defective organelle trafficking) or *icm* (intracellular multiplication) genes, play an essential role in redirecting phagosome trafficking and establishing an intracellular site for bacterial growth. The Dot/Icm apparatus is hypothesized to be a translocase that exports effector molecules into host cells. *Legionella* does not require this transporter for growth once a replicative niche has been established. Among the *L. pneumophila* maintenance factors is the macrophage infectivity potentiator protein (Mip), which is exported to the bacterial surface and is involved in establishing intracellular infection. *L. pneumophila* Mip mutants have macrophage uptake and replicative phagosome formation kinetics that are similar to those of wild-type bacteria. However, these activities are delayed once the replicative phagosome is established.

Legionnaires' disease is more common and its manifestations are more severe among patients with depressed cell-mediated immunity, including transplant recipients, patients infected with HIV, and patients receiving glucocorticoids. The disease also occurs with unusual frequency among patients with hairy cell leukemia (which is characterized by monocyte deficiency and dysfunction) but not among patients with other types of leukemia.

The role of neutrophils in immunity appears to be minimal: neutropenic patients are not predisposed to Legionnaires' disease. Although *L. pneumophila* is susceptible to oxygen-dependent microbiologic systems in vitro, it resists killing by neutrophils.

The humoral immune system is active against *Legionella*. Type-specific IgM and IgG antibodies are measurable within weeks of infection. In vitro, antibodies promote killing of *Legionella* by phagocytes (neutrophils, monocytes, and alveolar macrophages). Immunized animals develop a specific antibody response, with subsequent resistance to *Legionella* challenge. However, antibodies neither enhance lysis by complement nor inhibit intracellular multiplication within phagocytes.

Some *L. pneumophila* strains are clearly more virulent than others, although the precise factors mediating virulence remain uncertain. For example, although multiple strains may colonize water-distribution systems, only a few cause disease in patients exposed to water from these systems. At least one surface epitope of *L. pneumophila* serogroup 1 is associated with virulence. *L. pneumophila* serogroup 6 is more commonly involved in hospital-acquired Legionnaires' disease and is more likely to be associated with a poor outcome.

PATHOLOGY The consistent pathologic features of Legionnaires' disease are confined to the lungs. Multifocal pneumonia with patchy lobular inflammation and extensive multilobar consolidation has been observed. Visible abscesses with central necrosis were seen in 20% of autopsied cases in one study. On histologic examination, fibrinopurulent pneumonia with intensive alveolitis and bronchiolitis is evident. Lesions of longer standing can have a nodular appearance with a central area of necrosis surrounded by macrophages and other cells. The alveoli are filled with fibrin, neutrophils, and alveolar macrophages. The direct fluorescent stain is not only specific but also the most sensitive option for visualization of the organism in tissues. Polyvalent DFA stains but not monoclonal DFA stain can be used for formalinized specimens. Culture is the preferred method for diagnosis based on clinical specimens.

CLINICAL AND LABORATORY FEATURES ■ Pontiac Fever Pontiac fever is an acute, self-limiting, flulike illness with a 24- to 48-h incubation period. Pneumonia does not develop. Malaise, fatigue, and myalgias are the most frequent symptoms, occurring in 97% of cases. Fever (usually with chills) develops in 80 to 90% of cases and headache in 80%. Other symptoms (seen in fewer than 50% of cases) include arthralgias, nausea, cough, abdominal pain, and diarrhea. Modest leukocytosis with a neutrophilic predominance is sometimes detected. Complete recovery takes place within only a few days without antibiotic therapy; a few patients may experience lassitude for many weeks thereafter. The diagnosis is established by antibody seroconversion.

Legionnaires' Disease (Pneumonia) Legionnaires' disease is often included in the differential diagnosis of "atypical pneumonia," along with infection due to *C. pneumoniae*, *Chlamydia psittaci*, *Mycoplasma pneumoniae*, *Coxiella burnetii*, and some viruses. The clinical similarities among these types of pneumonia include a relatively nonproductive cough and a low incidence of grossly purulent sputum. However, the clinical manifestations of Legionnaires' disease are usually more severe than those of most "atypical" pneumonias, and the course and prognosis of *Legionella* pneumonia more closely resemble those of bacteremic pneumococcal pneumonia than those of pneumonia due to other "atypical" pathogens. Patients with community-acquired Legionnaires' disease are significantly more likely than patients with pneumonia of other etiologies to be admitted to an intensive care unit on presentation.

The incubation period for Legionnaires' disease is 2 to 10 days. The symptoms and signs may range from a mild cough and a slight fever to stupor with widespread pulmonary infiltrates and multisystem failure. Nonspecific symptoms—malaise, fatigue, anorexia, and headache—are seen early in the illness. Myalgias and arthralgias are uncommon but are prominent in a few patients. Upper respiratory symptoms, including coryza, are rare.

The mild cough of Legionnaires' disease is only slightly productive. Sometimes the sputum is streaked with blood. Chest pain—either pleuritic or nonpleuritic—can be a prominent feature and, when coupled with hemoptysis, can lead to an incorrect diagnosis of pulmonary embolism. Shortness of breath is reported by one-third to one-half of patients.

Gastrointestinal difficulties are often pronounced; abdominal pain, nausea, and vomiting affect 10 to 20% of patients. Diarrhea (watery rather than bloody) is reported in 25 to 50% of cases. The most common neurologic abnormalities are confusion or changes in mental status; however, the multitudinous neurologic symptoms reported range from headache and lethargy to encephalopathy.

Patients with Legionnaires' disease virtually always have fever. Temperatures in excess of 40.5°C (104.9°F) were recorded in 20% of the cases in one series. Relative bradycardia has been overemphasized as a useful diagnostic finding; it occurs primarily in older patients with severe pneumonia. Chest examination reveals rales early in the course and evidence of consolidations as the disease progresses. Abdominal examination may reveal generalized or local tenderness.

Although the clinical manifestations often considered classic for Legionnaires' disease (Table 132-1) may suggest the diagnosis, pro-

---

TABLE 132-1 *Clinical Clues Suggestive of Legionnaires' Disease*

Diarrhea
High fever (>40°C or >104°F))
Numerous neutrophils but no organisms revealed by Gram's staining of
   respiratory secretions
Hyponatremia (serum sodium level of <131 meq/L)
Failure to respond to β-lactam drugs (penicillins or cephalosporins) and
   aminoglycoside antibiotics
Occurrence of illness in an environment in which the potable water
   supply is known to be contaminated with *Legionella*
Onset of symptoms within 10 days after discharge from the hospital

---

spective comparative studies have shown that clinical manifestations are generally nonspecific and that Legionnaires' disease is not readily distinguishable from pneumonia of other etiologies. In a review of 13 studies of community-acquired pneumonia, clinical manifestations that occurred significantly more often in Legionnaires' disease included diarrhea, neurologic findings (including confusion), and a temperature of >39°C. Hyponatremia, elevated values in liver function tests, and hematuria also occurred more frequently in Legionnaires' disease. Other laboratory abnormalities include creatine phosphokinase elevation, hypophosphatemia, serum creatinine elevation, and proteinuria.

Extrapulmonary Legionellosis Since the portal of entry for *Legionella* is the lung in virtually all cases, extrapulmonary manifestations usually result from bloodborne dissemination from the lung. In a prospective survey of patients with Legionnaires' disease diagnosed by isolation of the organism from sputum, *Legionella* was isolated from the blood by a special culture method in 38% of cases.

Legionella has been identified in lymph nodes, spleen, liver, or kidneys in autopsied cases of Legionnaires' disease. The most common extrapulmonary site of legionellosis is the heart; numerous reports have described myocarditis, pericarditis, postcardiotomy syndrome, and prosthetic-valve endocarditis. Most cases have been hospital-acquired. In some patients who have not had overt evidence of pneumonia, the organisms may have gained entry through a postoperative sternal wound exposed to contaminated tap water or through a mediastinal-tube insertion site. Sinusitis, peritonitis, pyelonephritis, skin and soft tissue infection, septic arthritis, and pancreatitis have been seen predominantly in immunosuppressed patients.

Chest Radiographic Abnormalities Virtually all patients with Legionnaires' disease have abnormal chest radiographs showing pulmonary infiltrates at the time of clinical presentation. In a few cases of hospital-acquired disease, fever and respiratory tract symptoms have preceded the appearance of the infiltrate on chest radiography. Findings on chest radiography are useful for assessing the severity of illness in that they identify multilobar involvement and permit monitoring of disease progression. However, these findings are nonspecific and do not serve to distinguish Legionnaires' disease from pneumonias of other etiologies. Pleural effusion is evident in 28 to 63% of cases on hospital admission. In immunosuppressed patients, especially those receiving glucocorticoids, distinctive rounded nodular opacities may be seen; these lesions may expand and cavitate (Fig. 132-1). Likewise, pulmonary abscesses can occur in immunosuppressed hosts. The progression of infiltrates and pleural effusion on chest radiography despite appropriate antibiotic therapy within the first week is common, and radiographic improvement lags behind clinical improvement by several days. Complete clearing of infiltrates requires 1 to 4 months.

DIAGNOSIS The diagnosis of Legionnaires' disease requires special microbiologic tests (Table 132-2). The sensitivity of bronchoscopy specimens is approximately the same as that of sputum samples for culture on selective media; if sputum is not available, bronchoscopy specimens may yield the organism. Bronchoalveolar lavage fluid gives higher yields than bronchial wash specimens. Thoracentesis should be performed if pleural effusion is found, and the fluid should be evaluated by DFA staining, culture, and the antigen assay designed for use with urine.

Staining Gram's staining of material from normally sterile sites, such as pleural fluid or lung tissue, occasionally suggests the diagnosis; efforts to detect *Legionella* in sputum by Gram's staining typically reveal numerous leukocytes but no organisms. When they are visualized, the organisms appear as small, pleomorphic, faint, gram-negative bacilli. *L. micdadei* organisms can be detected as weakly or partially acid-fast bacilli in clinical specimens. Modified acid-fast staining substitutes 1% sulfuric acid for the traditional 3% hydrochloric acid; the less aggressive decolorizer increases the yield of *L. micdadei*. *Legionella*-infected patients have occasionally been treated empirically with

FIGURE 132-1 Chest radiographic findings in a 52-year-old man who presented with pneumonia subsequently diagnosed as Legionnaires' disease. The patient was a cigarette smoker with chronic obstructive pulmonary disease and alcoholic cardiomyopathy; he had received glucocorticoids. *L. pneumophila* was identified by DFA staining and culture of sputum. *Left:* Baseline chest radiograph showing long-standing cardiomegaly. *Center:* Admission chest radiograph showing now rounded opacities. *Right:* Chest radiograph taken 3 days after admission, during treatment with erythromycin.

antituberculosis medications because of false positive acid-fast smears.

The DFA test is rapid and highly specific but is less sensitive than culture because large numbers of organisms are required for microscopic visualization. This test is more likely to be positive in advanced than in early disease.

Culture The definitive method for diagnosis of *Legionella* infection is isolation of the organism from respiratory secretions or other specimens. Multiple selective BCYE media are required for maximal sensitivity. Colonies grow slowly, requiring 3 to 5 days to become grossly visible. When culture plates are overgrown with other microflora, pretreatment of the specimen with acid or heat can markedly improve the yield. *L. pneumophila* is often isolated from sputum that is not grossly or microscopically purulent; sputum containing more than 25 epithelial cells per high-power field (a finding that classically suggests contamination) may still yield *L. pneumophila.*

Antibody Detection Antibody testing of both acute- and convalescent-phase sera is necessary. A fourfold rise in titer is diagnostic; 12 weeks are often required for the detection of an antibody response. A single titer of 1:128 in a patient with pneumonia constitutes presumptive (but not definitive) evidence for Legionnaires' disease. Serology is of use primarily in epidemiologic studies. The specificity of serology for *Legionella* species other than *L. pneumophila* is uncertain; there is cross-reactivity with *Legionella* spp. and some gram-negative bacilli.

Urinary Antigen The assay for *Legionella* soluble antigen in urine (Binax, Portland, ME) is rapid, relatively inexpensive, easy to perform, second only to culture in terms of sensitivity, and highly specific. Its use in every clinical laboratory is recommended. The test is available only for *L. pneumophila* serogroup 1, which, as has been mentioned, causes about 80% of *Legionella* infections. Cross-reactivity with other *L. pneumophila* serogroups and other *Legionella* species has been detected in up to 22% of urine samples from patients with culture-proven cases. Antigen in urine is detectable 3 days after the onset of clinical disease, and urinary antigen positivity persists for several weeks. The test is not affected by antibiotic administration.

Molecular Methods Polymerase chain reaction (PCR) with DNA probes is theoretically more sensitive and specific than other methods, but the results have been disappointing to date. PCR has proved useful in the identification of *Legionella* from environmental water specimens.

TREATMENT

Since *Legionella* is an intracellular pathogen, antibiotics that can reach intracellular concentrations exceeding the minimal inhibitory concentration are most likely to be efficacious in the clinical setting. The dosages for various drugs used in the treatment of *Legionella* infection are listed in Table 132-3.

The newer macrolides (especially azithromycin) and respiratory tract quinolones (levofloxacin, gemifloxacin, moxifloxacin) are now the antibiotics of choice and are effective as monotherapy. Compared with erythromycin, the newer macrolides have superior in vitro activity, display greater intracellular activity, and reach higher concentrations in respiratory secretions and in lung tissue. The pharmacokinetics of the newer macrolides and quinolones also allow once- or twice-daily dosing. Finally, the large fluid volume required for intravenous administration, symptomatic ototoxicity, and gastrointestinal side effects have rendered erythromycin obsolete for the treatment of *Legionella* infection. Quinolones are the preferred antibiotics for transplant recipients because both macrolides and rifampin interact

TABLE 132-2 Utility of Special Laboratory Tests for the Diagnosis of Legionnaires' Disease

Test	Sensitivity, %	Specificity, %
Culture		
Sputum[a]	80	100
Transtracheal aspirate	90	100
DFA staining of sputum	50–70	96–99
Urinary antigen testing[b]	70	100
Antibody serology[c]	40–60	96–99

[a] Use of multiple selective media with dyes.
[b] Serogroup 1 only.
[c] IgG and IgM testing of both acute- and convalescent-phase sera. A single titer of ≥1:256 is considered presumptive, while fourfold seroconversion is considered definitive.

TABLE 132-3 Antibiotic Therapy for Legionella Infection

Antimicrobial Agent	Dosage[a]
Macrolides	
Azithromycin	500 mg[b] PO or IV[c] q24h
Clarithromycin	500 mg PO or IV[c] q12h
Quinolones	
Levofloxacin	750 mg IV q24h
	500 mg[b] PO q24h
Ciprofloxacin	400 mg IV q8h
	750 mg PO q12h
Ofloxacin	400 mg PO or IV q12h
Moxifloxacin	400 mg[b] PO q24h
Tetracyclines	
Doxycycline	100 mg[b] PO or IV q12h
Minocycline	100 mg[b] PO or IV q12h
Tetracycline	500 mg PO or IV q6h
Others	
Trimethoprim-sulfamethoxazole	160/800 mg IV q8h
	160/800 mg PO q12h
Rifampin[d]	300–600 mg PO or IV q12h

[a] Dosages are derived from clinical experience.
[b] We recommend doubling the first dose.
[c] Intravenous formulation is not available in some countries.
[d] Rifampin should be used only in combination with a macrolide or a quinolone.

pharmacologically with cyclosporine and tacrolimus. One uncontrolled retrospective study has suggested that complications are fewer and clinical response is more rapid in patients receiving quinolones than in those receiving macrolides. Alternative agents include tetracycline and its analogues doxycycline and minocycline. Anecdotal reports have described both successes and failures with trimethoprim-sulfamethoxazole, imipenem, and clindamycin. For severely ill patients with extensive pulmonary infiltrates, a combination of rifampin with a newer macrolide or quinolone can be used for initial treatment.

Initial therapy should be given by the intravenous route. A clinical response usually occurs within 3 to 5 days, after which oral therapy can be substituted. The total duration of therapy in the immunocompetent host is 10 to 14 days; a longer course (3 weeks) may be appropriate for immunosuppressed patients and those with advanced disease. For azithromycin, with its long half-life, a 5- to 10-day course is sufficient.

Pontiac fever requires only symptom-based treatment, not antimicrobial therapy.

PROGNOSIS Mortality rates for Legionnaires' disease vary, depending on the patient's underlying disease and its severity, the patient's immune status, the severity of pneumonia, and the timing of administration of appropriate antimicrobial therapy. Mortality rates are highest (80%) among immunosuppressed patients who do not receive appropriate antimicrobial therapy early in the course of illness. With appropriate and timely antibiotic treatment, mortality from community-acquired Legionnaires' disease among immunocompetent patients ranges from 0 to 11%; without treatment, the figure may be as high as 31%. In an observational study of survivors of an outbreak of community-acquired Legionnaires' disease, sequelae of fatigue, neurologic symptoms, and weakness were found in 63% to 75% of patients 17 months after receipt of antibiotics.

PREVENTION Routine environmental culture of the hospital water supply is recommended as an approach to the prevention of hospital-acquired Legionnaires' disease. Positive cultures from the water supply mandate the use of specialized laboratory tests (especially culture on selective media and urinary antigen assay) for patients with hospital-acquired pneumonia. Studies have shown that neither a high degree of outward cleanliness nor routine application of maintenance measures decreases the frequency or intensity of *Legionella* colonization. Thus, engineering guidelines and building codes, although routinely advocated as preventive measures, have little impact on *Legionella* colonization.

Disinfection of the water supply is now feasible. Two methods have proven reliable and cost-effective. The superheat-and-flush method requires heating of the water so that the distal-outlet temperature is 70 to 80°C and flushing of the distal outlets with hot water for at least 30 min. This method is ideal for emergency situations. A commercial copper and silver ionization method has proved effective in numerous hospitals. Hyperchlorination is no longer recommended because of its expense, carcinogenicity, corrosive effects on piping, and unreliable efficacy.

FURTHER READING

FIORE AE et al: A survey of methods used to detect nosocomial legionellosis among participants in the NNIS system. Infect Control Hosp Epidemiol 20: 412, 1999

FORMICA N et al: The impact of diagnosis by *Legionella* urinary antigen test on the epidemiology and outcomes of Legionnaires' disease. Epidemiol Infect 127:275, 2001

MARRE R et al: *Legionella*. Washington, DC, ASM Press, 2002

MUDER R, YU VL: Infection due to *Legionella* species other than *L. pneumophila*. Clin Infect Dis 35:990, 2002

MULAZIMOGLU L, YU VL: Can Legionnaires' disease be diagnosed by clinical criteria? A critical review. Chest 120:1049, 2001

PEDRO-BOTET ML et al: Legionnaires' disease contracted from patient homes: The coming of the third plague? Eur J Clin Microbiol Infect Dis 21:699, 2002

SABRIA M, YU VL: Hospital-acquired legionellosis: Solutions for preventable infection. Lancet Infect Dis 2:368, 2002

STOUT JE, YU VL: Experience of the first 16 hospitals using copper-silver ionization for *Legionella* control: Implications for the evaluation of other disinfection modalities. Infect Control Hosp Epidemiol 24:563, 2003

——: Current concepts: Legionellosis. N Engl J Med 337:682, 1997

SWANSON MS, HAMMER BK: *Legionella pneumophila* pathogenesis: A fateful journey from amoebae to macrophages. Annu Rev Microbiol 54:567, 2000

TAN MJ et al: The radiologic manifestations of Legionnaire's disease. Chest 116:398, 2000

YU VL: Resolving the controversy on environmental cultures for *Legionella*. Infect Control Hosp Epidemiol 19:893, 1998

133 PERTUSSIS AND OTHER *BORDETELLA* INFECTIONS
Scott A. Halperin

Pertussis is an acute infection of the respiratory tract caused by *Bordetella pertussis*. The name *pertussis* means "violent cough," which aptly describes the most consistent and prominent feature of the illness. The inspiratory sound made at the end of an episode of paroxysmal coughing gives rise to the common name for the illness, "whooping cough"; however, this feature is variable, being uncommon in infants ≤6 months of age and frequently absent in older children and adults. The Chinese name for pertussis is "the 100-day cough," which accurately describes the clinical course of the illness. The identification of *B. pertussis* was first reported by Bordet and Gengou in 1906, and vaccines were produced over the following two decades.

MICROBIOLOGY Six species have been identified in the genus *Bordetella*: *B. pertussis*, *B. parapertussis*, *B. bronchiseptica*, *B. avium*, *B. holmesii*, and *B. hinzii*. *B. pertussis* infects only humans and is the most important *Bordetella* species causing human disease. *B. parapertussis* causes an illness in humans that is similar to pertussis but is typically milder; coinfections with *B. parapertussis* and *B. pertussis* have been documented. *B. bronchiseptica* is an important pathogen of domestic animals that causes kennel cough in dogs, atrophic rhinitis and pneumonia in pigs, and pneumonia in cats. Both respiratory infection and opportunistic infection are occasionally reported in humans. *B. avium* is an important cause of respiratory illness in turkeys. The remaining two species, *B. hinzii* and *B. holmesii*, have been recognized as unusual causes of bacteremia. Both of these species have been isolated from patients with sepsis, most often from those who are immunocompromised.

Bordetella species are gram-negative pleomorphic aerobic bacilli that share common genotypic characteristics. *B. pertussis* and *B. parapertussis* are the most similar of the species but differ in that *B. parapertussis* does not express the gene coding for pertussis toxin. *B. pertussis* is a slow-growing fastidious organism that requires selective medium and forms small glistening bifurcated colonies. Suspicious colonies are presumptively identified as *B. pertussis* by direct fluorescent antibody testing or by agglutination with species-specific antiserum. *B. pertussis* is further differentiated from other *Bordetella* species by biochemical and motility characteristics.

B. pertussis produces a wide array of toxins and biologically active products that are important in its pathogenesis and in immunity. Most of these virulence factors are under the control of a single genetic locus that regulates their production, resulting in antigenic modulation and phase variation. Although these processes occur both in vitro and in vivo, their importance in the pathobiology of the organism is unknown; they may play a role in intracellular persistence and person-to-person spread. The organism's most important virulence factor is *pertussis toxin*, which is composed of a B oligomer–binding subunit and an enzymatically active A protomer that ADP-ribosylates a guanine nucleotide-binding regulatory protein (G protein) in target cells, producing a variety of biologic effects. Pertussis toxin has important mitogenic activity, affects the circulation of lymphocytes, and serves as an adhesin for bacterial binding to respiratory ciliated cells. In animal models, the toxin's effects include histamine sensitization, lymphocytosis promotion, and insulin secretion. Another virulence factor is *filamentous hemagglutinin*, a component of the cell wall and a bacterial adhesin. *Pertactin* is an outer-membrane protein and another important adhesin. *Fimbriae* are bacterial appendages that also play a role in bacterial attachment; they are the major antigens against which agglutinating antibodies are directed. These agglutinating antibodies have historically been the primary means of serotyping *B. pertussis* strains. Other virulence factors include tracheal cytotoxin, which causes respiratory epithelial damage; adenylate cyclase toxin, which impairs host immune-cell function; dermonecrotic toxin, which may contribute to respiratory mucosal damage; and lipooligosaccharide, which has properties similar to those of other gram-negative bacterial endotoxins.

PATHOGENESIS Infection with *B. pertussis* is initiated by attachment of the organism to the ciliated epithelial cells of the nasopharynx. Attachment is mediated by surface adhesins (e.g., pertactin and filamentous hemagglutinin), which bind to the integrin family of cell-surface proteins, probably in conjunction with pertussis toxin. The role of fimbriae in adhesion or maintenance of infection has not been fully delineated. At the site of attachment, the organism multiplies, producing a variety of other toxins that cause local mucosal damage (tracheal cytotoxin, dermatonecrotic toxin). Impairment of host defense by *B. pertussis* is mediated by pertussis toxin and adenylate cyclase toxin. There is local cellular invasion, with intracellular bacterial persistence; however, systemic dissemination does not occur. Systemic manifestations (lymphocytosis) result from the effects of the toxins.

The pathogenesis of the clinical manifestations of pertussis is poorly understood. It is not known what causes the paroxysmal cough that is the hallmark of pertussis. A pivotal role for pertussis toxin has been proposed. Proponents of this position point to the efficacy of preventing clinical symptoms with a vaccine containing only pertussis toxoid. Detractors counter that pertussis toxin is not the critical factor because paroxysmal cough also occurs in patients infected with *B. parapertussis*, which does not produce pertussis toxin. It is thought that the neurologic events observed in pertussis, such as seizures and encephalopathy, are due to hypoxia from coughing paroxysms or apnea rather than to the effects of specific bacterial products. *B. pertussis* pneumonia, which occurs in up to 10% of infants with pertussis, is usually a diffuse bilateral primary infection. In older children and adults with pertussis, pneumonia is often due to secondary bacterial infection with streptococci or staphylococci.

IMMUNITY Both humoral and cell-mediated immunity are thought to be important in pertussis. Antibodies to pertussis toxin, filamentous hemagglutinin, pertactin, and fimbriae are all protective in animal models. Pertussis agglutinins were correlated with protection in early studies of whole-cell pertussis vaccines. Serologic correlates of protection conferred by acellular pertussis vaccines have not been established, although antibody to pertactin, fimbriae, and (to a lesser degree) pertussis toxin correlated best with protection in two acellular pertussis vaccine efficacy trials. The duration of immunity after whole-cell pertussis vaccination is short-lived, with little protection remaining after 10 to 12 years. Data on the duration of protection after acellular pertussis vaccination are still being collected. Although immunity after natural infection has been said to be lifelong, seroepidemiologic evidence suggests that it may not be and that subsequent episodes of clinical pertussis are prevented by intermittent subclinical infection.

EPIDEMIOLOGY Pertussis is a highly communicable disease, with attack rates of 80 to 100% among unimmunized household contacts and 20% within households in well-immunized populations. The infection has a worldwide distribution, with cyclical outbreaks every 3 to 5 years (a pattern that has persisted despite widespread immunization). Pertussis occurs in all months; however, in North America, pertussis activity peaks in the summer and autumn.

Before the institution of widespread immunization programs, pertussis was one of the most common infectious causes of morbidity and death. In the United States prior to the 1940s, between 115,000 and 270,000 cases of pertussis were reported annually, with an average yearly rate of 150 cases per 100,000 population. With universal childhood immunization, the number of reported cases fell by >95%, with even more dramatic decreases in mortality. Only 1010 cases of pertussis were reported in 1976. Since that time, however, rates have slowly increased. In 2000, more than 7800 cases of pertussis were reported in the United States.

Although thought of as a disease of childhood, pertussis can affect people of all ages and is increasingly being identified as a cause of prolonged coughing illness in adolescents and adults. In unimmunized populations, pertussis incidence peaks in the preschool years, and well over half of children have the disease before reaching adulthood. In highly immunized populations such as those in North America, the peak incidence is among infants <1 year of age who have not completed the three-dose primary immunization series. Recent trends, however, show an increasing incidence of pertussis among adolescents and adults. In the United States in 2000, 24% of patients were <7 months of age, 36% were adolescents, and 20% were adults. The figures for adolescents and adults are probably underestimates because of a greater degree of underrecognition and underreporting in these age groups. A number of studies of prolonged coughing illness suggest that pertussis may be the etiologic agent in 12 to 30% of adults with cough that does not improve within 2 weeks. In a recent study of the efficacy of an acellular pertussis vaccine in adolescents and adults, the incidence of pertussis in the placebo group was 3.7 to 4.5 cases per 1000 person-years. Although this prospective cohort study yielded a lower estimate than the studies of cough illness, its results still translate to between 600,000 and 800,000 cases of pertussis in adults annually in the United States. Severe morbidity and mortality, however, are virtually restricted to infants. In Canada, there were 10 deaths from pertussis between 1991 and 1998; all those who died were infants ≤6 months of age. Although school-age children are the source of infection for most households, adults are the likely source for high-risk infants and may serve as the reservoir of infection between epidemic years. In developing countries, pertussis remains an important cause of infant morbidity and mortality. The World Health Organization estimated that in 1995 over 40 million people worldwide were infected by *B. pertussis* and that 355,000 children died of pertussis.

CLINICAL MANIFESTATIONS Pertussis is a prolonged coughing illness with clinical manifestations that vary by age (Table 133-1). Classic pertussis is most often seen in preschool and school-age children, although it is not uncommon among adolescents and adults. After an incubation

TABLE 133-1 *Clinical Features of Pertussis, by Age Group and Diagnostic Status*

	Percentage of Patients		
	Adolescents and Adults		
Feature	Laboratory Confirmation	No Laboratory Confirmation	Children
Cough	95–100	95–100	95–100
Prolonged	60–80	60–80	60–95
Paroxysmal	60–90	50–90	80–95
Sleep-disturbing	50–80	50–80	90–100
Whoop	10–40	5–30	40–80
Posttussive vomiting	20–50	5–30	80–90

period averaging 7 to 10 days, an illness develops that is indistinguishable from the common cold and is characterized by coryza, lacrimation, mild cough, low-grade fever, and malaise. After 1 to 2 weeks, this *catarrhal phase* evolves into the *paroxysmal phase*: the cough becomes more frequent and spasmodic with repetitive bursts of 5 to 10 coughs, often within a single expiration. Posttussive vomiting is frequent, with a mucous plug occasionally expelled at the end of an episode. The episode may be terminated by an audible whoop, which occurs upon rapid inspiration against a closed glottis at the end of a paroxysm. During a spasm, there may be impressive neck-vein distension, bulging eyes, tongue protrusion, and cyanosis. Paroxysms may be precipitated by noise, eating, or physical contact. Between attacks, the patient's appearance is normal but increasing fatigue is evident. The frequency of paroxysmal episodes varies widely, from several per hour to 5 to 10 per day. Episodes are often worse at night and interfere with sleep. Weight loss is not uncommon as a result of the illness's interference with eating. Most complications occur during the paroxysmal stage. Fever is uncommon and suggests bacterial superinfection.

After 2 to 4 weeks, the coughing episodes become less frequent and less severe—changes heralding the onset of the *convalescent phase*. This phase can last from 1 to 3 months and is characterized by a gradual resolution of the coughing episodes. For 6 months to a year, intercurrent viral infections may be associated with a recrudescence of paroxysmal cough.

Not all individuals who develop pertussis have classic disease. The clinical manifestations in adolescents and adults are more often atypical. In a German study of pertussis in adults, more than two-thirds had paroxysmal cough and more than one-third had whoop. Adult illness in North America differs from this experience: the cough may be severe and prolonged but is less frequently paroxysmal, and a whoop is uncommon. Vomiting with cough is the best predictor of a diagnosis of pertussis as the cause of a prolonged cough in adults. Other features predictive of this diagnosis are a cough at night and exposure to other individuals with a prolonged coughing illness.

COMPLICATIONS Complications are frequently associated with pertussis and are more common among infants than among older children or adults. Subconjunctival hemorrhages, abdominal and inguinal hernias, pneumothoraces, and facial and truncal petechiae can result from increased intrathoracic pressure generated by severe fits of coughing. Weight loss can follow decreased caloric intake. In a series of more than 1100 children <2 years of age who were hospitalized with pertussis, 27.1% had apnea, 9.4% had pneumonia, 2.6% had seizures, and 0.4% had encephalopathy; 10 children (0.9%) died. Pneumonia is reported in <5% of adolescents and adults and increases in frequency after 50 years of age. In contrast to the primary *B. pertussis* pneumonia that develops in infants, pneumonia in adolescents and adults with pertussis is usually caused by a secondary infection with encapsulated organisms such as *Streptococcus pneumoniae* or *Haemophilus influenzae*. Pneumothorax, severe weight loss, inguinal hernia, rib fracture, carotid artery aneurysm, and cough syncope have all been reported in adolescents and adults with pertussis.

DIAGNOSIS If the classic symptoms of pertussis are present, clinical diagnosis is not difficult. However, particularly in older children and adults, it is difficult to differentiate infections caused by *B. pertussis* and *B. parapertussis* from other respiratory tract infections on clinical grounds. Therefore, laboratory confirmation should be attempted in all cases. Lymphocytosis (absolute lymphocyte count, $>10 \times 10^9$/L) is common among young children (in whom it is unusual with other infections) but not among adolescents and adults. Culture of nasopharyngeal secretions remains the "gold standard" of diagnosis; the best specimen is collected by nasopharyngeal aspiration, in which a fine flexible plastic catheter attached to a 10-mL syringe is passed into the nasopharynx and withdrawn while gentle suction is applied. Since *B. pertussis* is highly sensitive to drying, secretions should be inoculated without delay onto appropriate media (Bordet-Gengou or Regan-

Lowe) or the catheter should be flushed with a phosphate-buffered saline solution. An alternative is a nasopharyngeal culture with a calcium alginate swab; again, inoculation of culture plates should be immediate or an appropriate transport medium (such as Regan-Lowe charcoal medium) should be used. Cultures become positive by day 5 of incubation, and *B. pertussis* and *B. parapertussis* can be differentiated by agglutination with specific antisera or by direct immunofluorescence.

Nasopharyngeal cultures in untreated pertussis remain positive for a mean of 3 weeks after the onset of illness; these cultures become negative within 5 days of the institution of appropriate antimicrobial therapy. Since much of the period during which the organism can be recovered from the nasopharynx falls into the catarrhal phase, when the etiology of the infection is not suspected, there is only a small window of opportunity for culture-proven diagnosis. Cultures from infants and young children are more frequently positive than those from older children and adults; this difference may reflect earlier presentation of the former age group for medical care. The increasing availability of the polymerase chain reaction for pertussis in diagnostic laboratories is enhancing the sensitivity of the organism's detection. This method may further laboratory confirmation but does not solve problems related to the long delays in specimen procurement that often are encountered in pertussis cases. Direct fluorescent antibody tests of nasopharyngeal secretions for direct diagnosis may still be available in some laboratories but should not be used because of poor sensitivity and specificity.

As a result of the difficulties with laboratory diagnosis of pertussis in adolescents, adults, and any patient who has been symptomatic for >4 weeks, increasing attention is being given to serologic diagnosis. Enzyme immunoassays detecting IgA and IgG antibodies to pertussis toxin, filamentous hemagglutinin, pertactin, and fimbriae have been developed and assessed for reproducibility. Two- or fourfold increases in antibody titer are suggestive of pertussis, although cross-reactivity of some antigens (such as filamentous hemagglutinin and pertactin) among *Bordetella* species makes it difficult to depend diagnostically on seroconversion involving a single type of antibody. Late presentation for medical care and prior immunization also complicate serologic diagnosis because the first sample obtained may in fact be a convalescent-phase specimen. Proposed criteria for serologic diagnosis based on a single serum specimen call for comparison of the patient's antibody levels with established population values; for example, a patient with serologically confirmed pertussis might be required to have a titer greater than two or three standard deviations above the mean titer for a normal population. However, at present, no antibody test is widely or commercially available, and no specific serologic criteria are universally accepted.

DIFFERENTIAL DIAGNOSIS A child presenting with paroxysmal cough, posttussive vomiting, and whoop is likely to have an infection caused by *B. pertussis* or *B. parapertussis*; lymphocytosis increases the likelihood of a *B. pertussis* etiology. Viruses such as respiratory syncytial virus and adenovirus have been isolated from patients with clinical pertussis but probably represent coinfection. In adolescents and adults, among whom paroxysmal cough and whoop are frequently absent, the differential diagnosis of a prolonged coughing illness is more extensive. Pertussis should be suspected in anyone with a cough that does not improve within 14 days, a paroxysmal cough of any duration, or any respiratory symptoms after contact with a laboratory-confirmed case of pertussis. Other etiologies to consider include infections caused by *Mycoplasma pneumoniae*, *Chlamydia pneumoniae*, adenovirus, influenza virus, and other respiratory viruses. Use of angiotensin-converting enzyme (ACE) inhibitors, reactive airway disease, and gastroesophageal reflux disease are well-described noninfectious causes of prolonged cough in adults.

℞ **TREATMENT**

Antibiotics   The purpose of antibiotic therapy for pertussis is to eradicate the infecting bacteria from the nasopharynx; therapy does not substantially alter the clinical course unless given early in the catarrhal phase. Macrolide antibiotics are the drugs of choice for treatment of pertussis (Table 133-2); a macrolide-resistant *B. pertussis* strain has been reported from a single case in an outbreak in Arizona. Trimethoprim-sulfamethoxazole is recommended as an alternative for individuals allergic to macrolides.

Supportive Care Young infants have the highest rates of complication and death from pertussis; therefore, most infants and older children with severe disease should be hospitalized. A quiet environment may decrease the stimulation that can trigger paroxysmal episodes. Use of β-adrenergic agonists and/or glucocorticoids has been advocated by some authorities but has not been proved to be effective. Cough suppressants are not effective and play no role in the management of pertussis.

Infection Control Measures Hospitalized patients with pertussis should be placed in respiratory isolation, with the use of precautions appropriate for pathogens spread by large respiratory droplets. Isolation should continue for 5 days after initiation of erythromycin therapy or for 3 weeks (i.e., until nasopharyngeal cultures are consistently negative) in those individuals unable to tolerate antimicrobial therapy.

PREVENTION ■ Chemoprophylaxis Because the risk of transmission of *B. pertussis* within households is high, chemoprophylaxis is widely recommended for household contacts of pertussis cases. The effectiveness of chemoprophylaxis, although unproven, is supported by several epidemiologic studies of institutional and community outbreaks of pertussis. In the only randomized placebo-controlled study, erythromycin estolate (50 mg/kg per day in three divided doses; maximum dose, 1 g/d) was effective in reducing the incidence of bacteriologically confirmed pertussis by 67%; however, there was no decrease in the incidence of clinical disease. Despite these disappointing results, many authorities continue to recommend chemoprophylaxis, particularly in households with members at high risk of severe disease (children <1 year of age). Data are not yet available on use of the newer macrolides for chemoprophylaxis.

Immunization (See also Chap. 107) The mainstay of pertussis prevention is active immunization. Pertussis vaccine has been available for over 70 years and became widely used in North America after 1940; reported cases of pertussis have since fallen by >90%. Whole-cell pertussis vaccines are prepared through the heating, chemical inactivation, and purification of whole *B. pertussis* organisms. Although effective (average efficacy estimate, 85%, with results in various studies of different products ranging from 30 to 100%), whole-cell pertussis vaccines are associated with adverse events—both common (fever; injection-site pain, erythema, and swelling; irritability) and uncommon (febrile seizures, hypotonic hyporesponsive episodes). Alleged associations of whole-cell pertussis vaccine with encephalopathy, sudden infant death syndrome, and autism, although not substantiated, have spawned an active anti-immunization lobby. The development of acellular pertussis vaccines, which are effective but less reactogenic, has greatly alleviated concerns about the inclusion of pertussis vaccine in the combined infant immunization series. Although whole-cell vaccines are still extensively used worldwide, acellular pertussis vaccines are used exclusively for childhood immunization in the United States and elsewhere (Canada, Sweden, Germany, Japan). In North America, acellular pertussis vaccines are given as a three-dose primary series at 2, 4, and 6 months of age, with a reinforcing dose between 15 and 18 months of age and a booster dose at 4 to 6 years of age.

TABLE 133-2 Antimicrobial Therapy for Pertussis

Drug	Adult Daily Dose	Frequency	Duration (Days)	Comments
Erythromycin estolate	1–2 g	3 divided doses	7–14	Frequent gastrointestinal side effects
Clarithromycin	500 mg	2 divided doses	7	
Azithromycin	500 mg on day 1, 250 mg subsequently	1 daily dose	5	
Trimethoprim-sulfamethoxazole	160 mg of trimethoprim, 800 mg of sulfamethoxazole	2 divided doses	14	For patients allergic to macrolides; data on effectiveness limited

A wide variety of acellular pertussis vaccines have been developed, although not all are available in every country. All acellular pertussis vaccines currently available contain pertussis toxoid. Only one monovalent pertussis toxoid vaccine has been licensed in the United States; the remainder of the fully developed vaccines contain filamentous hemagglutinin as well as toxoid. At least four acellular pertussis vaccines also contain pertactin, and two products also contain one or more types of fimbriae. All of the licensed acellular pertussis vaccines have undergone phase 3 efficacy testing. Although differences in study design make direct comparisons difficult, an effort to standardize case definitions and the similarity of some of the studies, which used common vaccine arms to allow "bridging" of the data between studies, have permitted some general conclusions. Even though some would still disagree, most experts have concluded that two-component acellular pertussis vaccines are more effective than monocomponent vaccines and that the addition of pertactin further increases efficacy. The further addition of fimbriae appears to provide some additional protective efficacy against milder disease. In two studies, protection against pertussis by vaccines correlated best with the production of antibody to pertactin, fimbriae, and pertussis toxin.

The development of acellular pertussis vaccines has sparked interest in the potential for control of pertussis in adolescents and adults and in the possibility that pertussis control in those groups will enhance the protection of infants too young to be immunized. Whole-cell pertussis vaccine is contraindicated in individuals ≥7 years of age because of their poor toleration of possible adverse events. However, adult formulations of acellular pertussis vaccines, both alone and in combination with adult-formulation diphtheria-tetanus toxoid, have been demonstrated to be safe, immunogenic, and efficacious in clinical trials in adolescents and adults and are now recommended for routine immunization of adolescents in several countries. Further epidemiologic studies will help public health authorities and advisory committees determine the role of pertussis immunization in the control of pertussis in adults.

FURTHER READING

DE SERRES G et al: Morbidity of pertussis in adolescents and adults. J Infect Dis 182:174, 2000

HALPERIN SA et al: A randomized, placebo-controlled trial of erythromycin estolate chemoprophylaxis for household contacts of children with culture-positive *Bordetella pertussis* infection. Pediatrics 104:e42, 1999

———— et al: Epidemiological features of pertussis in hospitalized patients in Canada, 1991–1997: Report of the Immunization Monitoring Program—Active (IMPACT). Clin Infect Dis 28:1238, 1999

SENZILET LD et al: Pertussis is a frequent cause of prolonged cough illness in adults and adolescents. Clin Infect Dis 32:1691, 2001

SKOWRONSKI DM et al: The changing age and seasonal profile of pertussis in Canada. J Infect Dis 185:1448, 2002

WIRSING VON KÖNIG CH et al: Pertussis in adults: Frequency of transmission after household exposure. Lancet 346:1326, 1995

YIH WK et al: The increasing incidence of pertussis in Massachusetts adolescents and adults, 1989–1998. J Infect Dis 182:1409, 2000

Extraintestinal infections are the predominant presentation of disease caused by gram-negative bacilli (GNB) belonging to medically important genera of the family Enterobacteriaceae (*Escherichia, Klebsiella, Proteus, Enterobacter, Serratia, Citrobacter, Morganella, Providencia,* and *Edwardsiella*) and by the genus *Acinetobacter* from the family Neisseriaceae. However, certain strains of *Escherichia coli* have evolved to be strictly intestinal pathogens, causing gastroenteritis by a variety of unique pathogenic mechanisms. The virulence traits of intestinal pathogenic *E. coli* are for the most part distinct from those of extraintestinal pathogenic *E. coli* and other GNB that cause disease outside the bowel. This difference reflects site-dependent differences in host environments and defense mechanisms.

E. COLI AS AN INTESTINAL PATHOGEN

Certain strains of *E. coli* are capable of causing intestinal infection. Other important intestinal pathogens are discussed in Chaps. 113, 126, and 137–140.

ETIOLOGY, EPIDEMIOLOGY, AND MANIFESTATIONS Intestinal pathogenic strains of *E. coli* are rarely encountered in the fecal flora of healthy hosts and instead appear to be essentially obligate pathogens. These strains have evolved a special ability to cause enteritis, enterocolitis, and colitis whenever ingested in sufficient quantities by a naive host. At least six distinct "pathotypes" of intestinal pathogenic *E. coli* exist: (1) Shiga toxin–producing *E. coli* (STEC)/enterohemorrhagic *E. coli* (EHEC), (2) enterotoxigenic *E. coli* (ETEC), (3) enteropathogenic *E. coli* (EPEC), (4) enteroinvasive *E. coli* (EIEC), (5) enteroaggregative *E. coli* (EAEC), and (6) diffusely adherent *E. coli* (DAEC). Organisms of these pathotypes are acquired via the fecal-oral route. Transmission occurs predominantly via contaminated food and water for ETEC, STEC, EIEC, EAEC, and DAEC and by person-to-person spread for EPEC (and occasionally STEC). Humans appear to be the major reservoir (except for STEC), since the host range appears to be dictated by species-specific attachment factors. Although there is some overlap, each pathotype possesses a unique combination of virulence traits that results in a distinctive intestinal pathogenic mechanism (Table 134-1); however, these strains are largely incapable of causing disease outside the intestinal tract. Except in the case of STEC, disease due to this group of pathogens occurs primarily in developing countries.

Shiga Toxin–Producing E. coli STEC strains constitute an emerging group of pathogens that can cause hemorrhagic colitis and the hemolytic-uremic syndrome (HUS). Several large outbreaks resulting from the consumption of undercooked ground beef and other foods have received significant attention from the media. O157:H7 is the most prominent serotype, but O6, O26, O55, O91, O103, O111, O113, and OX3 have also been associated with these syndromes. The ability to produce Shiga toxins (Stx2 and/or Stx1) or related toxins is the critical factor dictating whether a bacterium can cause the STEC syndrome. *Shigella dysenteriae* strains that produce the closely related Shiga toxin Stx can cause the same syndrome. Stx2 appears to be more important than Stx1 in the development of HUS and other severe disease. All Shiga toxins studied to date consist of an enzymatically active A subunit and five identical B subunits that mediate binding to globoceramides. The A subunit cleaves an adenine from the 28S rRNA, which irreversibly inhibits ribosomal function. Therefore, Shiga toxins belong to the class of toxins known as *ribosome-inactivating proteins* (RIPs).

Additional factors, such as acid tolerance and adherence, are necessary for maximal pathogenicity of STEC. The genomes of the majority of isolates responsible for disease possess the locus for enterocyte effacement (LEE). This pathogenicity island was first described in EPEC strains and contains genes that mediate adherence to intestinal epithelial cells. It has been proposed that the subgroup of STEC strains that possess stx_1 and/or stx_2 as well as LEE be termed *enterohemorrhagic E. coli* (EHEC).

Domesticated ruminant animals, particularly cattle and young calves, serve as the major reservoir for STEC. Ground beef—the most common food source of STEC strains—is often contaminated during processing. Furthermore, manure from cattle or other animals that is used as fertilizer can contaminate produce (potatoes, lettuce, sprouts, fallen apples) and water (fecal runoff). It is estimated that <10^3 CFU (colony-forming units) of STEC can cause disease. Therefore, not only can low levels of food or environmental contamination (e.g., in water swallowed while swimming) result in disease, but person-to-person transmission (e.g., at day-care centers and in institutions) becomes an important vehicle for secondary spread. Laboratory-associated infections also take place. Both outbreaks and sporadic cases are attributable to this group of pathogens, with a seasonal peak in the summer months.

In contrast to the other pathotypes, STEC causes infections more frequently in developed countries, where the consumption of processed foods is more common than in developing regions. O157 strains are the fourth most commonly reported cause of bacterial diarrhea in the United States (after *Campylobacter, Salmonella,* and *Shigella*). Colonization of the colon and perhaps the ileum results in symptoms after an incubation period of 3 or 4 days. Colonic edema and an initial secretory diarrhea may develop into the STEC syndrome's hallmark trait of grossly bloody diarrhea (detected by history or examination) in >90% of cases. Significant abdominal pain and fecal leukocytes are commonly present (70% of cases), but fever is usually absent. Occasionally, *Clostridium difficile, Campylobacter,* and *Salmonella* infection present in a similar fashion, as do noninfectious diseases (e.g., inflammatory bowel disease). STEC disease is usually self-limited, lasting 5 to 10 days. This infection can be complicated by HUS, which occurs 2 to 14 days after diarrhea in 2 to 8% of cases, most often affecting the very young and the elderly. It is estimated that >50% of all cases of HUS in the United States are caused by STEC. This complication is probably mediated by the systemic translocation of Shiga toxins. Erythrocytes may serve as carriers of Stx to small-vessel renal and cerebral endothelial cells. The subsequent development of thrombotic microangiopathy (perhaps with direct toxin-mediated effects on various cells) most commonly results in some combination of fever, thrombocytopenia, renal failure, and encephalopathy. Although the mortality rate with dialysis support is <10%, residual renal dysfunction and neurologic sequelae may persist.

Enterotoxigenic E. coli In tropical or developing countries, ETEC is a major cause of endemic diarrhea. After weaning, children experience several episodes of ETEC infection during the first 3 years of life. The incidence of disease diminishes with age, a pattern that correlates with the development of mucosal immunity to colonization factors. In industrialized countries, infection usually follows travel to endemic areas. ETEC is the most common agent of traveler's diarrhea, causing 25 to 75% of cases. The incidence of infection is decreased by the prudent avoidance of potentially contaminated fluids and foods (Chap. 108). ETEC infection is uncommon in the United States, but outbreaks secondary to consumption of food products imported from endemic areas have occurred. A large inoculum (10^6 to 10^{10} CFU) is needed to produce disease. After ingestion of contaminated water or food (particularly items poorly cooked, unpeeled, or unrefrigerated), colonization factor–mediated intestinal adherence occurs over 12 to 72 h.

Disease is mediated primarily by heat-labile toxin (LT-1) and/or a heat-stable toxin (STa) that causes net fluid secretion via activation of adenylate cyclase (LT-1) and/or guanylate cyclase (STa) in the jejunum and ileum; the result is watery diarrhea accompanied by cramps. LT-1 consists of an A and a B subunit and is structurally and functionally similar to cholera toxin. Strong binding of the B subunit to the GM_1 ganglioside leads to the intracellular translocation of the A subunit, which functions as an ADP-ribosyltransferase. The mature STa toxin is an 18- or 19-amino-acid secreted peptide whose biologic activity is mediated by binding to the guanylate cyclase C found in the brush-border membrane of intestinal epithelial cells; this binding results in increased intracellular concentrations of cyclic GMP. Characteristically absent are histopathologic changes of the small bowel; mucus, blood, and inflammatory cells in stool; and fever. The disease spectrum ranges from a mild illness to a life-threatening cholera-like illness. Although symptoms are usually self-limited (typically lasting for 3 days), infection may result in significant morbidity and mortality when health care is poor and when small and/or undernourished children are affected.

Enteropathogenic *E. coli* EPEC causes disease primarily in young children, including neonates. The first *E. coli* pathotype recognized as an agent of diarrheal disease, EPEC was responsible for outbreaks of infantile diarrhea (including some outbreaks in hospital nurseries) in industrialized countries in the 1940s and 1950s. At present, however, infection due to EPEC is uncommon in developed countries. In contrast, EPEC is an important cause of infant diarrhea (both sporadic and epidemic) in developing countries. Breast-feeding diminishes the incidence of EPEC infection. Rapid person-to-person spread may occur. Upon colonization of the small bowel, symptoms develop after a brief incubation period (1 or 2 days). Initial localized adherence leads to a characteristic effacement of microvilli, with the formation of cuplike, actin-rich pedestals. Diarrheal stool often contains mucus but no blood. Although usually self-limited (lasting for 5 to 15 days), EPEC diarrhea may persist for weeks.

Enteroinvasive *E. coli* EIEC, a relatively uncommon cause of diarrhea, is rarely identified in the United States, although a few food-related outbreaks have been described. In developing countries, sporadic disease is infrequently recognized in children and travelers. EIEC shares many genetic and clinical features with *Shigella*; however, unlike *Shigella*, EIEC produces disease only at a large inoculum (10^8 to 10^{10} CFU), with onset generally occurring after an incubation period of 1 to 3 days. Initially, enterotoxins are believed to induce secretory small-bowel diarrhea. Subsequently, colonization and invasion of the colonic mucosa, followed by replication therein and cell-to-cell spread, result in the development of inflammatory colitis characterized by fever, abdominal pain, tenesmus, and scant stool containing mucus, blood, and inflammatory cells. Symptoms are usually self-limited (7 to 10 days).

Enteroaggregative and Diffusely Adherent *E. coli* EAEC and DAEC have been described primarily in developing countries and in young children. These strains can cause traveler's diarrhea. A large inoculum is required for infection. In vitro, the organisms exhibit a diffuse or "stacked-brick" adherence pattern. Clinical disease has been associated with prolonged watery diarrhea.

DIAGNOSIS A practical approach to the evaluation of diarrhea is to distinguish noninflammatory from inflammatory cases (Chap. 113). ETEC, EPEC, EAEC, and DAEC are uncommon causes of noninflammatory diarrhea in the United States. Their diagnosis requires specialized assays that are not routinely available and whose use is rarely indicated since these diseases are self-limited. ETEC causes the majority of cases of noninflammatory traveler's diarrhea; EAEC and DAEC cause a minority of these cases. Definitive diagnosis generally is not necessary, and empirical antimicrobial treatment is a reasonable approach. If diarrhea persists despite treatment, *Giardia* or *Cryptosporidium* should be sought. The diagnosis of infection with EIEC, a rare

cause of inflammatory diarrhea in the United States, also requires specialized assays. However, evaluation for STEC infection, particularly when bloody diarrhea is reported or observed, is appropriate. Although screening for *E. coli* strains that do not ferment sorbitol and subsequent serotyping for O157 constitute the most common method presently used to detect STEC, testing for Shiga toxins or toxin genes is more sensitive, specific, and rapid. The latter approach offers another advantage as well: it detects both non-O157 strains and sorbitol-fermenting strains of O157, which otherwise are difficult to identify. DNA-based, enzyme-linked immunosorbent, and cytotoxicity assays are in various stages of development and are likely to emerge as the diagnostic standards in time.

R̳x̳ TREATMENT

The mainstay of treatment for all diarrheal syndromes is the appropriate replacement of water and electrolytes (Chap. 113). The use of prophylactic antibiotics to prevent traveler's diarrhea should be discouraged, especially in light of high rates of antibiotic resistance. When stools are free of mucus and blood, early patient-initiated treatment of traveler's diarrhea with a quinolone decreases the duration of illness, and the use of loperamide may halt symptoms within a few hours (Chap. 113). Although dysentery caused by EIEC is self-limited, treatment hastens the resolution of symptoms, particularly in severe cases. Treatment of STEC infection should be avoided since antibiotics may increase the incidence of HUS (possible via increased release of Stx).

EXTRAINTESTINAL PATHOGENS

GENERAL FEATURES AND PRINCIPLES ■ **Epidemiology** Extraintestinal pathogenic *E. coli*, *Klebsiella*, *Proteus*, *Enterobacter*, *Serratia*, *Citrobacter*, *Morganella*, *Providencia*, *Edwardsiella*, and *Acinetobacter* are components of the normal animal and human colonic flora and/or of the flora of a variety of environmental habitats (including long-term-care facilities and hospitals). In healthy humans, *E. coli* is the predominant gram-negative bacillus in the colonic flora. GNB (primarily *E. coli*, *Klebsiella*, and *Proteus*) only transiently colonize the oropharynx and skin of healthy individuals. In contrast, in long-term-care and hospital settings, a variety of GNB emerge as the dominant colonizing flora of both mucosal and skin surfaces, particularly with antimicrobial use, severe illness, and extended length of stay. Acquisition of the GNB (from various reservoirs) leads to infection.

Pathogenesis Multiple bacterial traits are required for various aspects of the pathogenesis of GNB. The possession of specialized virulence genes is what defines pathogens and enables them to infect the host efficiently. As more is learned about these genes, it is becoming clear

---

TABLE 134-1 *Intestinal Pathogenic E. coli*

Pathotype[a]	Clinical Syndrome(s)[b]	Defining Molecular Trait	Responsible Genetic Element[c]
STEC	Hemorrhagic colitis, hemolytic-uremic syndrome	Shiga toxin	Lambda-like Stx1 or Stx2 encoding bacteriophage
ETEC	Traveler's diarrhea	Heat-stable and -labile enterotoxins, colonization factors	Virulence plasmid(s)
EPEC	Watery diarrhea in young children	Localized adherence, attaching and effacing lesion on intestinal epithelium	EPEC adherence factor plasmid pathogenicity island (locus for enterocyte effacement)
EIEC	Dysentery	Invasion of colonic epithelial cells, intracellular multiplication, cell-to-cell spread	Multiple genes contained primarily in large virulence plasmid
EAEC/DAEC	Traveler's diarrhea, persistent diarrhea	Aggregative/diffuse adherence	Chromosomal or plasmid-associated adherence genes

[a] STEC, Shiga toxin–producing *E. coli*; ETEC, enterotoxigenic *E. coli*; EPEC, enteropathogenic *E. coli*; EIEC, enteroinvasive *E. coli*; EAEC, enteroaggregative *E. coli*; DAEC, diffusely adherent *E. coli*.
[b] Classic syndromes; see text for details on spectrum of disease.
[c] Pathogenesis is multigenic and requires genes in addition to those listed.

TABLE 134-2 *Interactions of Extraintestinal Pathogenic* E. coli *with the Human Host: A Paradigm for Extracellular, Extraintestinal Gram-Negative Bacterial Pathogens*

Bacterial Goal	Host Obstacle	Bacterial Solution
Extraintestinal attachment	Flow of urine, mucociliary blanket	Multiple adhesins (e.g., type 1 fimbriae, Sfa/Foc, P pili)
Nutrient acquisition for growth	Nutrient sequestration (e.g., iron via intracellular storage and extracellular scavenging via lactoferrin and transferrin)	Cellular lysis (e.g., hemolysin); multiple mechanisms for competing for extracellular iron (e.g., siderophores) and other nutrients
Initial avoidance of host bactericidal activity	Complement, phagocytic cells, antimicrobial peptides	Capsular polysaccharide, lipopolysaccharide
Transmission	?	Irritant tissue damage resulting in increased excretion (e.g., toxins such as hemolysin)
Late avoidance of host bactericidal activity	Acquired immunity (e.g., specific antibodies), treatment with antibiotics	? Cell entry, acquisition of antimicrobial resistance

that hosts and their cognate pathogens have been coadapting throughout evolutionary history. In fact, it has been speculated that infection is just a point on the spectrum of evolutionary development between microbes and hosts. At one end of this spectrum is a commensal/symbiotic interaction (e.g., mitochondria—formerly bacteria—within eukaryotic cells); at the other end is a lethal outcome that results in a "dead-end relationship" (e.g., Ebola virus). During this host-pathogen "chess match" over time, various and redundant solutions have emerged both in pathogens and in their hosts that enable these partners to maintain their coexistence (Table 134-2).

Extraintestinal pathogenic strains of *E. coli* (ExPEC) and the other genera discussed in this chapter cause infection outside the bowel. All are extracellular pathogens and therefore share certain pathogenic features. Innate defense systems (complement, antimicrobial peptides, professional phagocytes) and humoral immunity are the most critical host-defense components. As a result, both susceptibility to and severity of infection are increased with dysfunction or deficiencies of these components (e.g., neutrophils) (Chap. 104).

A given pathogen usually possesses multiple adhesins for binding to a variety of host cells (e.g., in *E. coli*: type 1 fimbriae, Sfa/Foc, P pili). Nutrient acquisition (e.g., iron via siderophores) requires many genes that are necessary but not sufficient for pathogenesis. The ability to resist the bactericidal activity of complement and professional phagocytes in the absence of antibody [e.g., conferred by capsule or O antigen of lipopolysaccharide (LPS)] is one of the defining traits of an extracellular pathogen. Tissue damage (e.g., hemolysis in the case of *E. coli*) may facilitate spread. Many important virulence genes await identification, and our understanding of many aspects of the pathogenesis of GNB is in its infancy (Chap. 105).

The ability to induce septic shock is another defining feature of these genera. GNB are the most common cause of this dangerous complication. The lipid A moiety of LPS (via interaction with host Toll-like receptors) and probably other bacterial factors as well (including capsule) stimulate a proinflammatory host response, which, if overexuberant, results in shock (Chap. 254).

Lastly, many serotypes exist in most genera of GNB; for example, there are >100 O-specific antigens and >80 capsular antigens in *E. coli*. This antigenic variability, which permits immune evasion and successful recurrent infection by strains of the same species, has also impeded vaccine development (Chap. 107).

Infectious Syndromes Depending on both the host and the pathogen, nearly every organ or body cavity can be infected with GNB. *E. coli* and, to a lesser degree, *Klebsiella* and *Proteus* account for the majority of infections and are the most virulent pathogens of this group. However, the other genera are becoming increasingly important, particularly among persons in long-term care and hospitalized patients. This expanding role is in large part due to the innate or acquired resistance of these organisms to antimicrobial agents and to the increasing number of immunocompromised hosts. The mortality rate is significant in many GNB infections and correlates with the severity of illness. Especially problematic are pneumonia and bacteremia from any source complicated by severe sepsis (with or without shock); these conditions have associated mortality rates of 20 to 50%.

Diagnosis Isolation of GNB from ordinarily sterile sites almost always implies infection. Their isolation from nonsterile sites, particularly from soft-tissue and respiratory cultures, requires clinical correlation to differentiate colonization from infection. Results of an assessment of lactose fermentation (described for each genus below) are usually available before final identification of the organism and its antimicrobial susceptibilities and may assist in guiding empirical therapy.

℞ TREATMENT

The antimicrobial resistance of GNB is variable and is influenced by both geographic location and regional antibiotic use. Empirical antimicrobial choices should be based on local susceptibility patterns. Extended-spectrum β-lactamases (ESBLs, class A) and AmpC β-lactamases (class C) are responsible for the majority of multidrug resistance in GNB. The acquisition of ESBLs via transferable plasmids is increasing. To date, ESBLs are most prevalent in *Klebsiella* and *E. coli*, but they have also been described (and are probably underrecognized) in *Enterobacter* and other enteric GNB. Plasmids encoding for ESBLs confer resistance to third-generation cephalosporins and aztreonam and frequently contain linked resistance determinants for aminoglycosides, tetracyclines, and trimethoprim-sulfamethoxazole (TMP-SMX). Up to 50% of strains expressing ESBLs have associated fluoroquinolone resistance. Outbreaks due to strains possessing ESBLs have been associated with extensive institutional use of third-generation cephalosporins, particularly ceftazidime. The carbapenems (e.g., imipenem) are the only β-lactam agents that are reliably efficacious against strains expressing an ESBL.

Derepression of inducible chromosomal AmpC β-lactamases, another important resistance mechanism, may be preexisting or may develop during therapy. This determinant confers resistance to second- and third-generation cephalosporins, to aztreonam, and often to β-lactam/β-lactamase inhibitor combinations. Chromosomal AmpC β-lactamases occur in *Enterobacter*, *Serratia*, *Citrobacter*, *Proteus vulgaris*, *Proteus penneri*, *Providencia*, *Morganella*, and *Acinetobacter*. In addition, some strains of *E. coli*, *Klebsiella pneumoniae*, and other Enterobacteriaceae that carry chromosomal AmpC β-lactamases have acquired plasmids that contain AmpC β-lactamases.

Although relevant data are suboptimal or conflicting, combination therapy may increase antibiotic efficacy (particularly for serious infections, such as pneumonia) and diminish the emergence of resistance. Furthermore, drainage of abscesses and removal of infected foreign bodies are often needed for cure.

GNB are commonly involved in polymicrobial infections, in which it is difficult to determine the role of each specific pathogen (Chap. 148). Although some GNB are more pathogenic than others, it is usually prudent, if possible, to design an antimicrobial regimen that includes activity against all of the GNB identified, since each is capable of pathogenicity in its own right.

Prevention Diligent hand hygiene by health care personnel and avoidance of inappropriate antimicrobial use are key in preventing infection and the further development of antimicrobial resistance.

ESCHERICHIA COLI INFECTIONS ■ Commensal Strains
Commensal *E. coli* variants, which constitute the major portion of the normal facultative intestinal flora in most humans, for the most part confer benefits (such as resistance to colonization) to their hosts. These strains generally

lack the specialized virulence traits that enable intestinal and extraintestinal pathogenic *E. coli* strains to cause disease within and outside the gastrointestinal tract, respectively. However, commensal *E. coli* are sometimes involved in extraintestinal infections when an aggravating factor is present, such as a foreign body (e.g., a urinary catheter), host compromise (e.g., local anatomical or functional abnormalities such as urinary or biliary tract obstruction or immunocompromise), or an inoculum that is large or contains a mixture of bacterial species (e.g., fecal contamination of the peritoneal cavity).

Extraintestinal Pathogenic Strains (ExPEC)   The majority of *E. coli* isolates from symptomatic infections of the urinary tract, bloodstream, cerebrospinal fluid, respiratory tract, and peritoneum (spontaneous bacterial peritonitis) are distinct from commensal and intestinal pathogenic strains of *E. coli* by virtue of their functionally similar virulence factor profiles (Table 134-2) and clonal background. It has recently been proposed that these extraintestinal strains of *E. coli* be termed *ExPEC*. Evaluation of a limited number of strains has established that ExPEC can also cause surgical wound infection, osteomyelitis, and myositis, but the number of cases evaluated to date is too small for a reliable assessment of proportions. Studies on the nature of *E. coli* strains responsible for other extraintestinal infections are in progress.

Like commensal *E. coli* (but in contrast to intestinal pathogenic *E. coli*), ExPEC strains are often found in the normal intestinal flora and do not cause gastroenteritis in humans. Although acquisition of an ExPEC strain by the host is a prerequisite for ExPEC infection, it is not the rate-limiting step, which instead is entry of a colonizing ExPEC strain from its site of colonization (e.g., the colon, vagina, or oropharynx) into a normally sterile extraintestinal site (e.g., the urinary tract, peritoneal cavity, or lungs). ExPEC strains have acquired genes encoding diverse extraintestinal virulence factors that enable the bacteria to cause infections outside the gastrointestinal tract in both normal and compromised hosts (Table 134-2). These virulence genes are, for the most part, distinct from those that enable intestinal pathogenic strains to cause intestinal disease. All age groups, all types of hosts, and nearly all organs and sites are susceptible to infection by ExPEC. Previously healthy hosts infected with ExPEC can become severely ill and even die; however, adverse outcomes are more prevalent in the presence of coincidental disease and abnormalities in host defenses. *E. coli* is the most common enteric gram-negative species to cause extraintestinal infection in ambulatory, long-term-care, and hospital settings. The diversity and the medical and economic impact of ExPEC infections are evident from a review of the following specific syndromes.

Infectious Syndromes ■ *URINARY TRACT INFECTION (UTI)*   The urinary tract is the site most frequently infected by ExPEC. A common infection among ambulatory patients, UTI accounts for 1% of ambulatory care visits in the United States and is second only to lower respiratory tract infection among infections responsible for hospitalization. UTIs are best considered by clinical syndrome (e.g., uncomplicated cystitis, catheter-associated) within the context of specific hosts (e.g., premenopausal women, compromised host; Chap. 269). *E. coli* is the single most prevalent pathogen for all UTI syndrome/host group combinations. Each year in the United States, for example, *E. coli* causes 85 to 95% of an estimated 6 to 8 million episodes of uncomplicated cystitis in premenopausal women, with an estimated $1 billion in direct health care costs. Furthermore, 20% of women with an initial infection develop frequent recurrences (0.3 to >20 per year). Except in the first year of life, acceptance of the diagnosis of UTI in males requires clear documentation since such infection is unusual in the absence of a history of instrumentation or anal intercourse.

Uncomplicated urethritis or cystitis occurs most commonly and is characterized by symptoms of dysuria, frequency, and suprapubic pain. Fever and/or back pain suggests progression to pyelonephritis. Pregnant women are at unusually high risk for this complication, which can adversely affect the outcome of pregnancy. As a result, prenatal screening for bacteriuria, with treatment when the results are

positive, is the standard of care. Fever may take 5 to 7 days to resolve completely in appropriately treated patients with pyelonephritis but should fall over time. Persistently elevated or increasing fever and neutrophil counts should prompt evaluation for intrarenal or perinephric abscess and/or obstruction. Renal parenchymal damage and loss of renal function occur primarily in the setting of obstruction. Prostatic infection is generally a complication of UTI in men with a history of instrumentation and/or prostatic hypertrophy. The diagnosis and treatment of UTI are detailed in Chap. 269 and are tailored according to the individual host, the nature and site of infection, and the local pattern of antimicrobial susceptibility.

ABDOMINAL AND PELVIC INFECTION   The abdomen/pelvis is the second most frequent site of extraintestinal infection due to *E. coli*. A wide variety of clinical syndromes occur in this location, including acute peritonitis secondary to fecal contamination, spontaneous bacterial peritonitis, peritoneal dialysis–associated peritonitis, diverticulitis, appendicitis, intraperitoneal or visceral abscesses (hepatic, pancreatic, splenic), infected pancreatic pseudocysts, and septic cholangitis and/or cholecystitis. In intraabdominal infections, *E. coli* can be isolated either alone or (as is often the case) along with other facultative and/or anaerobic members of the intestinal flora (Chap. 112).

PNEUMONIA   *E. coli* is not usually considered a cause of pneumonia (Chap. 239). Indeed, enteric GNB account for only 2 to 5% of cases of community-acquired pneumonia (CAP), in part because these organisms only transiently colonize the oropharynx of a minority of healthy individuals. In contrast, rates of oral colonization with *E. coli* and other GNB increase with the severity of illness and with antibiotic use. Thus, GNB are a common cause of pneumonia among residents of long-term-care institutions and are the most frequent cause (60 to 70% of cases) of hospital-acquired pneumonia (Chap. 116), particularly among postoperative and intensive care patients. Infection is usually acquired by small-volume aspiration but occasionally occurs via hematogenous spread, in which case multifocal nodular infiltrates can be seen. Tissue necrosis, probably due to cytotoxins produced by GNB, is common. Despite significant institutional variation, *E. coli* is generally the third or fourth most commonly isolated gram-negative bacillus in these settings, accounting for 5 to 8% of episodes in both U.S.- and European-based studies. Regardless of the host, pneumonia due to enteric GNB is a serious disease, with high crude and attributable mortality rates (20 to 60% and 10 to 20%, respectively).

MENINGITIS (See also Chap. 360)   *E. coli* is one of the two leading causes of neonatal meningitis (the other being group B *Streptococcus*). The majority of responsible strains possess the K1 capsular serotype. Outside this setting, meningitis due to *E. coli* is uncommon, occurring predominantly in the setting of disruption of the meninges due to craniotomy or trauma or in the presence of cirrhosis. In these instances, the meninges are presumably seeded from poorly cleared portal-source episodes of bacteremia or via direct extension from an otogenic or sinus source.

CELLULITIS/MUSCULOSKELETAL INFECTION   Infections of decubitus ulcers and the lower extremities in diabetic patients (or other hosts with neurovascular compromise) are usually polymicrobial. *E. coli* contributes frequently to decubitus infections and occasionally to lower-extremity infections in these patients. In addition, *E. coli* may occasionally cause cellulitis or burn-site or surgical-wound infection, particularly when the infection originates close to the perineum. Osteomyelitis secondary to contiguous spread can occur in these settings. Hematogenously acquired osteomyelitis, particularly of vertebral bodies, is more commonly caused by *E. coli* than is generally appreciated; this organism accounts for 10% of cases in some series (Chap. 111). *E. coli* occasionally causes orthopedic device–associated infection or septic arthritis and is a rare cause of hematogenously acquired myositis. Myositis or fasciitis of the upper leg should prompt an evaluation for an abdominal source with contiguous spread.

ENDOVASCULAR INFECTION Despite being one of the most common causes of bacteremia, *E. coli* rarely seeds native heart valves and is an uncommon cause of prosthetic-valve endocarditis. Likewise, *E. coli* infections of aneurysms and vascular grafts are uncommon.

MISCELLANEOUS INFECTIONS *E. coli* can cause infection in nearly every organ and site. It is responsible for 8% of surgical site infections (superficial, deep tissue, or organ/space—e.g., mediastinitis), occasional cases of complicated sinusitis, and uncommon cases of endophthalmitis or brain abscess.

BACTEREMIA *E. coli* bacteremia can arise from primary infection at any extraintestinal site. In addition, primary *E. coli* bacteremia can arise from percutaneous intravascular devices or can result from the increased intestinal mucosal permeability seen in neonates and in the settings of neutropenia and chemotherapy-induced mucositis, trauma, and burns. Roughly equal proportions of bacteremia cases originate in the community and in the hospital. *E. coli* and *Staphylococcus aureus* are the most common clinically significant blood isolates; *E. coli*, which is isolated in 17 to 37% of cases, is the gram-negative bacillus most often isolated from the blood in the ambulatory setting as well as in most long-term-care and hospital settings. Isolation of *E. coli* from the blood is almost always clinically significant and typically is accompanied by the sepsis syndrome, severe sepsis (sepsis-induced dysfunction of at least one organ or system), or septic shock (Chap. 254). Calculations based on a conservative estimate for severe *E. coli* sepsis (i.e., 17% of all cases of severe sepsis) translate into an estimated 40,000 deaths among the affected patients in the United States in 2001.

The urinary tract is the most common source of *E. coli* bacteremia, accounting for two-thirds of episodes. Bacteremia from a urinary tract source is particularly common with pyelonephritis, urinary tract obstruction, or instrumentation in the presence of infected urine. The abdomen is the second most common source, accounting for 25% of episodes. Although obstructive biliary tract disease (stones, tumor) and overt disruption of bowel are responsible for many of these cases, some abdominal sources (e.g., abscesses) are remarkably silent clinically and require identification via imaging studies (e.g., computed tomography). Therefore, the physician should be cautious in designating the urinary tract as the source of *E. coli* bacteremia in the absence of appropriate signs and symptoms. Soft tissue, bone, and pulmonary infections are the next most common sources for bacteremia.

Diagnosis Strains of *E. coli* that cause extraintestinal infections usually grow both aerobically and anaerobically within 24 h on standard diagnostic media and are easily identified by the clinical microbiology laboratory according to standard biochemical criteria. More than 90% of ExPEC strains are rapid lactose fermenters.

℞ TREATMENT

In the past, *E. coli* has typically been highly susceptible to antibiotics and readily eradicated with antibiotic therapy. Unfortunately, this situation has changed. In general, the frequency of ampicillin resistance precludes its empirical use, even in community-acquired infections. Rates of resistance to first-generation cephalosporins and TMP-SMX are increasing among community-acquired strains in the United States (with current rates of 10 to 40%) and are even higher in Europe and developing countries. Until recently, TMP-SMX was the drug of choice for the treatment of uncomplicated cystitis in many locales. Although continued empirical use of TMP-SMX will predictably result in ever-diminishing cure rates, a wholesale switch to alternative agents (e.g., fluoroquinolones) will just as predictably accelerate the widespread emergence of resistance to these antimicrobial classes, as has already occurred in some areas. It is not surprising that rates of resistance among isolates from long-term-care facilities and hospitals are particularly high. Significant resistance (30 to 40%) to amoxicillin/clavulanic acid and piperacillin has been increasingly reported. For-

tunately, rates of resistance to cephalosporins (second-, third-, and fourth-generation), quinolones, monobactams (e.g., aztreonam), carbapenems (e.g., imipenem), and aminoglycosides are generally <10%. [The mean rate of resistance to third-generation cephalosporins was 3.2% among isolates reported to the National Nosocomial Infections Surveillance (NNIS) system in 1998.] An exception involves settings where extensive use of quinolone prophylaxis has led to the emergence of significant quinolone resistance (e.g., in patients with leukemia, transplant recipients, and patients with cirrhosis). Whatever the current rates, the frequency of acquisition of plasmids containing ESBLs and other resistance determinants is likely to increase.

KLEBSIELLA **INFECTIONS** *K. pneumoniae* is the most important *Klebsiella* species from a medical standpoint, causing community-acquired, long-term-care, and nosocomial infections. *K. oxytoca* is primarily a pathogen in long-term-care and hospital settings. *K. rhinoscleromatis* and *K. ozaenae* are usually isolated from patients in tropical climates. *Klebsiella* species are broadly prevalent in the environment and colonize mucosal surfaces of mammals. In healthy humans, *K. pneumoniae* colonization rates range from 5 to 35% in the colon and from 1 to 5% in the oropharynx; the skin is usually colonized only transiently. In long-term-care facilities and hospitals, colonization occurs with *K. oxytoca* as well, and carriage rates are significant among both workers and patients. Person-to-person spread is thought to be the predominant mode of acquisition. Classically, *Klebsiella* is associated with CAP, primarily in alcoholics. However, the majority of *Klebsiella* infections now occur in long-term-care facilities and hospitals. *Klebsiella* causes a spectrum of extraintestinal infections similar to that caused by *E. coli*. However, extraintestinal infections due to *Klebsiella* occur at a lower incidence in all sites except the respiratory tract. These variances in infection rates are probably due to differences in colonization and site-specific virulence traits. Antibiotic-resistant strains have been responsible for a number of nosocomial outbreaks of infection in intensive care units (ICUs) and neonatal nurseries. The most common clinical syndromes are pneumonia, UTI, abdominal infection, surgical site infection, soft tissue infection, and subsequent bacteremia. *K. rhinoscleromatis* is the causative agent of rhinoscleroma, a slowly progressive (months to years) mucosal upper respiratory infection that causes necrosis and occasional obstruction of the nasal passages. *K. ozaenae* has been implicated as a cause of chronic atrophic rhinitis.

Infectious Syndromes ■ *PNEUMONIA* *K. pneumoniae* causes only a small proportion of cases of CAP (Chap. 239). This infection occurs primarily in hosts with underlying disease, such as alcoholics, diabetics, and individuals with chronic lung disease. As in all pneumonias due to enteric GNB, purulent sputum production and "airspace" disease on x-ray are typical. Presentation with earlier, less extensive infection is more common than that with the classic lobar infiltrate with a bulging fissure. Pulmonary necrosis, pleural effusion, and empyema occur with progression. Pulmonary infection in residents of long-term-care facilities and in hospitalized patients is especially frequent because of increased oropharyngeal colonization rates. Mechanical ventilation is an important risk factor.

UTI The incidence of *K. pneumoniae* UTI among healthy adults is only 1 to 2%. However, in complicated UTIs (including those associated with indwelling bladder catheters), the incidence of *Klebsiella* infection increases to 5 to 17%.

ABDOMINAL INFECTION *Klebsiella* causes a spectrum of abdominal infections similar to that caused by *E. coli* but is less frequently isolated from these infections.

OTHER INFECTIONS *Klebsiella* cellulitis or soft tissue infection occurs most frequently in devitalized tissue (e.g., decubitus ulcers, diabetes, burn sites) or in immunocompromised hosts. *Klebsiella* causes a significant minority of surgical site infections, hematogenously derived endophthalmitis cases, and nosocomial sinusitis cases as well as occasional cases of osteomyelitis contiguous to soft tissue infection, temperate myositis, and neonatal meningitis or meningitis associated with neurosurgery.

Klebsiella infection at any site can result in bacteremia. Infections of the urinary tract, respiratory tract, and abdomen each account for 15 to 30% of *Klebsiella* bacteremias. Intravascular device–related infection is another important source (5 to 15%). Surgical site infection and other miscellaneous infections account for the rest. *Klebsiella* is one of the agents that causes sepsis neonatorum and bacteremia with fever and neutropenia. Like enteric GNB in general, *Klebsiella* rarely causes endocarditis or endovascular infection.

Diagnosis Except for *K. rhinoscleromatis* and *K. ozaenae*, klebsiellae are readily isolated and identified by the laboratory and usually ferment lactose.

℞ TREATMENT

K. pneumoniae and *K. oxytoca* have similar antibiotic resistance profiles. They are intrinsically resistant to ampicillin and ticarcillin. NNIS data from 1998 indicated that 10.7% of ICU patients were infected with strains resistant to third-generation cephalosporins. This increasing degree of resistance is primarily mediated by plasmids containing genes that encode ESBLs. In addition, these plasmids usually possess linked resistance determinants for aminoglycosides, tetracyclines, and TMP-SMX. In specific hospitals or geographic locales (e.g., Brooklyn, NY), the prevalence of ESBL-containing isolates is significantly higher. Resistance to β-lactam/β-lactamase inhibitor combinations and second-generation cephalosporins independent of ESBL-containing plasmids has also been increasingly described. Up to 50% of ESBL-containing strains have displayed associated fluoroquinolone resistance. At this time, rates of resistance to quinolones, cephamycins (e.g., cefoxitin), fourth-generation cephalosporins (e.g., cefepime), and amikacin are generally <10%, but these rates will probably increase. Carbapenems (e.g., imipenem) remain the most active antibiotic class against *Klebsiella*.

PROTEUS INFECTIONS *P. mirabilis* causes 90% of *Proteus* infections. These infections occur in the community, in long-term-care facilities, and in hospitals. *P. vulgaris* and *P. penneri* are isolated primarily from infections contracted in long-term-care facilities or hospitals. *Proteus* species are part of the colonic flora of a wide variety of mammals, birds, fish, and reptiles. Their ability to generate histamine from contaminated fish has implicated these GNB in the pathogenesis of scombroid (fish) poisoning (Chap. 378). *P. mirabilis* colonizes healthy humans (prevalence, 50%), but *P. vulgaris* and *P. penneri* are isolated primarily from individuals with underlying disease. The urinary tract is overwhelmingly the favored site of *Proteus* infection, with adhesins, flagella, IgA protease, and urease as the important virulence factors. However, *Proteus* less commonly causes infection in a variety of extraintestinal sites.

Infectious Syndromes ■ *UTI* *P. mirabilis* causes only 1 to 2% of cases of UTI in healthy women, and *Proteus* species cause only 5% of cases of hospital-acquired UTI. However, *Proteus* is responsible for 10 to 15% of cases of complicated UTI, primarily those associated with catheterization; in the setting of long-term catheterization, their prevalence rate ranges from 20 to 45%. This high prevalence is due in part to the ability of *Proteus* to produce high levels of urease, which hydrolyzes urea to ammonia and results in alkalization of the urine. This situation, in turn, leads to precipitation of organic and inorganic compounds, with the formation of struvite and carbonate-apatite crystals, biofilm formation on catheters, and/or the development of calculi. *Proteus* becomes associated with the stones and can usually be eradicated only by complete stone removal. Over time, staghorn calculi may form and lead to obstruction and renal failure. Therefore, an unexplained alkaline urine should be cultured for *Proteus*, and identification of a *Proteus* species should prompt an evaluation for calculi.

OTHER INFECTIONS Although the majority of *Proteus* infections arise from the urinary tract, these bacteria occasionally cause pneumonia (primarily in long-term-care or hospitalized patients), nosocomial si-

nusitis, intraabdominal abscesses, biliary tract infection, surgical site infection, soft tissue infection (especially decubitus and diabetic ulcers), and osteomyelitis (primarily contiguous); they rarely cause temperate myositis. In addition, *Proteus* occasionally causes neonatal meningitis (with the umbilicus often implicated as the source), which is often complicated by the development of a cerebral abscess. Otogenic brain abscess is also seen.

BACTEREMIA The majority of *Proteus* bacteremias originate from the urinary tract; however, any of the less common sites of infection are also potential sources. Infection of intravascular devices should also be considered. Endovascular infection is rare. *Proteus* species are occasional agents of sepsis neonatorum and bacteremia with fever and neutropenia.

Diagnosis *Proteus* is readily isolated and identified by the laboratory. The majority of strains are lactose negative, and most demonstrate characteristic "swarming" motility on agar plates.

℞ TREATMENT

P. mirabilis remains susceptible to most antimicrobial agents except tetracycline. Resistance to ampicillin and first-generation cephalosporins has been acquired by 10 to 50% of strains. Overall, 5% of *P. mirabilis* isolates in the United States now possess an ESBL. *P. vulgaris* and *P. penneri* are more resistant than *P. mirabilis*. Resistance to ampicillin and first-generation cephalosporins is the rule for these species. Derepression of an inducible chromosomal AmpC β-lactamase (not present in *P. mirabilis*) occurs in up to 30% of strains. Imipenem, fourth-generation cephalosporins (e.g., cefepime), aminoglycosides, TMP-SMX, and quinolones have excellent activity (90 to 100%).

ENTEROBACTER INFECTIONS *E. cloacae* and *E. aerogenes* are responsible for most *Enterobacter* infections (65 to 75% and 15 to 25%, respectively); *E. agglomerans*, *E. sakazakii*, and *E. gergoviae* are less commonly isolated (5%, 1%, and <1%, respectively). These organisms cause primarily health care–related or hospital-related infections. They are widely prevalent in foods, environmental sources (including health care facility equipment), and a wide variety of animals. Only a minority of healthy humans are colonized, but the percentage increases significantly in the setting of long-term care or hospitalization. Although colonization is an important prelude to infection, direct introduction via intravenous lines (e.g., contaminated intravenous fluids, pressure monitors) also occurs. Significant antibiotic resistance has developed in *Enterobacter* species and has contributed to their emergence as prominent nosocomial pathogens. Individuals who have received prior antibiotic treatment, who have comorbid disease, and who are patients in ICUs are at greatest risk for infection. *Enterobacter* causes a spectrum of extraintestinal infections similar to that described for other GNB in this chapter.

Infectious Syndromes Pneumonia, UTI (particularly catheter-related), intravascular device–related infection, surgical site infection, and abdominal infection (primarily postoperative or device-related—e.g., biliary stents) are the most common syndromes encountered. Nosocomial sinusitis, meningitis related to neurosurgical procedures (including use of pressure monitors), osteomyelitis, and endophthalmitis after eye surgery are less frequent. *E. sakazakii* is commonly responsible for neonatal meningitis/sepsis (particularly in premature infants); contaminated formula has been implicated as a source of this infection, which is often complicated by brain abscess or ventriculitis. Bacteremia can result from infection at any of these sites. In the setting of *Enterobacter* bacteremia, contamination of intravenous fluids or medications, blood components or plasma derivatives, catheter-flushing fluids, pressure monitors, and dialysis equipment should always be considered, particularly with epidemic infection. *Enterobacter* can also cause bacteremia in patients with fever and neutropenia. *Enterobacter* endocarditis is rare, occurring primarily in association with intravenous drug abuse or prosthetic valves.

Diagnosis   *Enterobacter* is readily isolated and identified by the laboratory. Most strains are lactose positive.

℞ TREATMENT

Significant antimicrobial resistance exists among *Enterobacter* strains. Ampicillin and the first- and second-generation cephalosporins have little or no activity. The extensive use of third-generation cephalosporins has resulted in the selection of strains that produce high levels of AmpC β-lactamase, which confers resistance to second- and third-generation cephalosporins, monobactams (e.g., aztreonam), and (frequently) β-lactam/β-lactamase inhibitor combinations. Resistant isolates may emerge during therapy; their presence should be considered a possibility when clinical deterioration follows several days of improvement. A 34% resistance rate to third-generation cephalosporins was reported in ICU isolates in 1998 (NNIS data). Imipenem, fourth-generation cephalosporins (e.g., cefepime), aminoglycosides (amikacin > gentamicin), TMP-SMX, and quinolones have retained excellent activity (90 to 99%). However, increasing resistance to quinolones, in conjunction with the increased use of these agents, is a concern.

ACINETOBACTER INFECTIONS   *A. baumannii* is responsible for the majority of *Acinetobacter* infections; a minority are due to *A. calcoaceticus*, *A. junii*, and *Acinetobacter* genospecies 3 and 13TU. *Acinetobacter* is highly prevalent in the environment. It is found in most water and soil samples and has a wide habitat. *Acinetobacter* has been cultured from the moist skin of healthy humans; increased colonization of the skin and the respiratory and gastrointestinal tracts occurs in individuals in long-term-care facilities and hospitals. Reservoirs for acquisition in these settings include health care personnel, medical equipment, food, and the surrounding environment. The overwhelming majority of infections are acquired in the hospital or in long-term-care facilities. The spectrum of extraintestinal infections caused by *Acinetobacter* is similar to that caused by other GNB. *Acinetobacter* species account for 1 to 3% of hospital-acquired infections and primarily affect immunocompromised hosts and patients with comorbid disease. ICUs are a prominent site of *Acinetobacter* infection. In some centers, the incidence of *Acinetobacter* infections, particularly those due to antibiotic-resistant strains, is increasing. Both sporadic and epidemic infections occur, usually after the first week of hospitalization.

Infectious Syndromes   The respiratory tract (particularly in ventilated patients) and intravascular devices (particularly for non–*A. baumannii* species) are the favored sites of infection. *A. baumannii* uncommonly causes severe CAP, usually in compromised hosts (e.g., alcoholics), with the preponderance of cases reported from warm, humid geographic locales. Infections of a catheterized urinary tract, postoperative sites, burn sites, biliary stents, and sinuses (with tube-related ostial obstruction) are less common, as are neurosurgical infections (site- or device-associated—e.g., pressure monitors). Uncommon infections include contiguous osteomyelitis, peritonitis associated with continuous ambulatory peritoneal dialysis, and ophthalmic infection. The respiratory tract and intravascular devices are the most common sources for bacteremia.

Diagnosis   On Gram's stain, *Acinetobacter* organisms usually appear as short GNB or coccobacilli. They are strictly aerobic, nonfermenting, and readily isolated and identified.

℞ TREATMENT

Many strains of *Acinetobacter* are highly resistant to antimicrobial agents. Empirical combination therapy is prudent pending susceptibility studies. Ampicillin, aztreonam, and the first- and second-generation cephalosporins possess little or no activity against these species. Resistance rates are 20 to 50% for mezlocillin, piperacillin,

quinolones, third-generation cephalosporins, and gentamicin. Imipenem is presently the most active antimicrobial (>95% sensitivity); β-lactam/β-lactamase inhibitor combinations, cefepime, and amikacin are often active.

SERRATIA INFECTIONS   *S. marcescens* causes the majority of *Serratia* infections (>90%), and *S. liquefaciens* is occasionally isolated. Serratiae are found primarily in the environment (including health care institutions) and particularly in moist foci. Although strains have been isolated from a variety of animals, healthy humans are rarely colonized. In long-term-care facilities or hospitals, diverse reservoirs for the organisms include health care personnel, food, milk in neonatal units, sinks, respiratory and other hospital equipment, pressure monitors, intravenous solutions, multiply accessed medication vials, blood products (e.g., platelets), lotions, irrigation solutions, and even disinfectants. Infection results from either direct inoculation (e.g., via intravenous fluid) or colonization (primarily of the respiratory tract) and subsequent infection. Sporadic infection is most common, but occasional epidemics and common-source outbreaks occur. The spectrum of extraintestinal infections caused by *Serratia* is similar to that for other GNB. *Serratia* species account for 1 to 3% of hospital-acquired infections.

Infectious Syndromes   The respiratory tract, the genitourinary tract, intravascular devices, and surgical wounds are the most common sites of *Serratia* infection and sources of *Serratia* bacteremia. Soft tissue infections, including myositis, osteomyelitis, abdominal and biliary tract infection (postprocedural), contact lens–associated keratitis, endophthalmitis, septic arthritis (primarily with intraarticular injections), and infusion-related bacteremias occur less commonly. Serratiae are uncommon causes of neonatal or postsurgical meningitis and bacteremia associated with fever and neutropenia. Endocarditis is rare.

Diagnosis   Serratiae are readily cultured and identified by the laboratory and are usually lactose negative. A minority of *S. marcescens* strains are red-pigmented.

℞ TREATMENT

A high proportion of *Serratia* strains (>80%) are resistant to ampicillin and the first-generation cephalosporins. Although derepression of inducible chromosomal AmpC β-lactamases may be preexistent or may develop during therapy, >90% of isolates are susceptible to other GNB-appropriate antibiotics.

CITROBACTER INFECTIONS   *C. freundii* and *C. koseri* (formerly *C. diversus*) cause the majority of human *Citrobacter* infections, which are similar epidemiologically and clinically to *Enterobacter* and *Acinetobacter* infections. *Citrobacter* organisms are commonly present in water, food, soil, and the intestinal tracts of animals. *Citrobacter* is part of the normal fecal flora in a minority of healthy humans, but colonization rates increase in long-term-care facilities and hospitals—the settings in which nearly all infections occur. *Citrobacter* species account for 1 to 2% of nosocomial infections. The affected hosts are usually immunocompromised or have comorbid disease. *Citrobacter* causes extraintestinal infections whose spectrum is similar to that described for other GNB.

Infectious Syndromes   The urinary tract is the site of 40 to 50% of infections due to *Citrobacter*. Less commonly infected sites include the biliary tree (particularly with stones or obstruction), the respiratory tract, surgical sites, soft tissue (e.g., decubitus ulcers), the peritoneum, and intravascular devices. Osteomyelitis (usually contiguous), neurosurgery-related infection, and myositis occur rarely. *Citrobacter* is also an uncommon cause of neonatal meningitis; *C. koseri* accounts for 90% of cases due to this genus. A frequent and devastating complication of this infection (occurring in 50 to 80% of cases) is the development of brain abscesses. Bacteremia is most commonly due to UTI, biliary or abdominal infection, or intravascular devices. *Citrobacter* is an uncommon cause of bacteremia in the setting of fever and neutropenia. Endocarditis or endovascular infection is rare.

Diagnosis *Citrobacter* species are readily isolated and identified, often as part of a polymicrobial culture; 35 to 50% of isolates are lactose positive.

℞ TREATMENT

C. freundii is generally more resistant to antibiotics than *C. koseri*. Ampicillin and the first- and second-generation cephalosporins display poor activity against *Citrobacter*. Resistance is variable but increasing to ticarcillin, mezlocillin, piperacillin, aztreonam, quinolones, gentamicin, and third-generation cephalosporins; such resistance may evolve during therapy. The β-lactamase inhibitors usually do not improve susceptibility to β-lactam agents. Imipenem, amikacin, and the fourth-generation cephalosporins are most active, with >90% of strains sensitive.

MORGANELLA AND PROVIDENCIA INFECTIONS *M. morganii* (formerly *Proteus morganii*), *P. stuartii*, and (less frequently) *P. rettgeri* (formerly *Proteus rettgeri*) are the members of these genera that are responsible for human infections. The epidemiologic, pathogenic, and clinical manifestations of these organisms are similar to those of *Proteus* species; however, *Morganella* and *Providencia* are almost exclusively pathogens of persons in long-term-care facilities and, to a lesser degree, hospitalized patients.

Infectious Syndromes These species are primarily urinary tract pathogens, most often associated with long-term (>30-day) catheterization. UTI in uncatheterized or short-term-catheterized individuals is uncommon. Biofilm formation or encrustation of the catheter usually develops and may lead to catheter obstruction. Likewise, infection may result in the development of struvite bladder or renal stones, which, in turn, may lead to renal obstruction and serve as foci for relapse. Other infectious syndromes occur less commonly but include surgical site infection, soft tissue infection (primarily decubitus and diabetic ulcers), burn site infection, pneumonia (particularly ventilator-associated), intravascular device infection, and intraabdominal infection. Rarely, the other extraintestinal infections described for GNB also occur. Bacteremia is uncommon; although any infected site can serve as the source, the urinary tract accounts for the majority of cases, with surgical site and soft tissue infections less frequently responsible.

Diagnosis *M. morganii* and *Providencia* are readily isolated and identified. Nearly all isolates are unable to ferment lactose.

℞ TREATMENT

Morganella and *Providencia* may be highly resistant to antimicrobial agents. Ampicillin and the first-generation cephalosporins exhibit poor activity against these organisms. Of *Providencia* isolates, 40% are resistant to fluoroquinolones. Variable resistance is emerging (and may evolve during therapy) against ticarcillin, mezlocillin, piperacillin, aztreonam, gentamicin, TMP-SMX, and the second- and third-generation cephalosporins. The β-lactamase inhibitor tazobactam (but not sulbactam or clavulanic acid) somewhat improves susceptibility to β-lactam agents. Imipenem, amikacin, and the fourth-generation cephalosporins are most active, with >90% of strains susceptible. Removal of an infected catheter or stones is critical for eradication of the organisms from the urinary tract.

EDWARDSIELLA INFECTION *E. tarda* is the only member of this genus associated with human disease. This organism is found predominantly in both freshwater and marine environments and in the animals that live in these environments. Human acquisition occurs primarily during interaction with these reservoirs. *E. tarda* infection is rare in the United States; most recently reported cases are from Southeast Asia. This pathogen shares some of the clinical features of both *Salmonella* species and *Vibrio vulnificus*.

Infectious Syndromes Gastroenteritis is the predominant infectious syndrome reported (50 to 80% of infections). Self-limiting watery diarrhea is most frequent; however, cases of severe colitis responding to therapy have also been described. The most common extraintestinal infection is wound infection due to direct inoculation, which is often associated with freshwater, marine, or snake-related injuries. Other infectious syndromes appear to be due to invasion of the gastrointestinal tract and subsequent bacteremia. The majority of afflicted hosts have either liver disease or an iron-overload state (e.g., sickle cell disease). A primary bacteremic syndrome, sometimes complicated by meningitis, has been described and has a 40% case-fatality rate. Visceral (primarily hepatic) or intraperitoneal abscesses have also been reported.

Diagnosis Although *E. tarda* can readily be isolated and identified, most laboratories do not routinely identify it from stool.

℞ TREATMENT

E. tarda is sensitive to most GNB-appropriate antimicrobial agents. Gastroenteritis is generally self-limiting, but treatment with TMP-SMX or a quinolone may expedite its resolution. In the setting of overwhelming sepsis, quinolones, third- or fourth-generation cephalosporins, imipenem, and aminoglycosides—alone or in combination—are the safest choices pending susceptibility information.

INFECTIONS CAUSED BY MISCELLANEOUS GENERA Species from genera of GNB such as *Hafnia*, *Kluyvera*, *Cedecea*, *Pantoea*, and *Ewingella* are occasionally isolated from a variety of clinical specimens, including blood, sputum, cerebrospinal fluid, joint fluid, biliary drainage, and wounds. Although their role in disease has not always been defined, these strains appear to be rare and usually opportunistic human pathogens. The primary medical literature should be consulted for details on their potential role as infectious agents.

FURTHER READING

DONNENBERG M (ed): *Escherichia coli: Virulence Mechanisms of a Versatile Pathogen*. San Diego, Academic Press, 2002

GRANSDEN WR et al: Bacteremia due to *Escherichia coli*: A study of 861 episodes. Rev Infect Dis 12:1008, 1990

HEJAZI A, FALKINER FR: *Serratia marcescens*. J Med Microbiol 46:903, 1997

LEVISON ME: Plasmid-mediated extended-spectrum β-lactamases in organisms other than *Klebsiella pneumoniae* and *Escherichia coli*: A hidden reservoir of transferable resistance genes. Curr Infect Dis Rep 4:181, 2002

PODSCHUN R, ULLMANN U: *Klebsiella* spp. as nosocomial pathogens: Epidemiology, taxonomy, typing methods, and pathogenicity factors. Clin Microbiol Rev 11:589, 1998

SANDERS WE JR, SANDERS CC: *Enterobacter* spp.: Pathogens poised to flourish at the turn of the century. Clin Microbiol Rev 10:220, 1997

SHIH CC et al: Bacteremia due to *Citrobacter* species: Significance of primary intraabdominal infection. Clin Infect Dis 23:543, 1996

SLAVEN EM et al: Myonecrosis caused by *Edwardsiella tarda*: A case report and case series of extraintestinal *E. tarda* infections. Clin Infect Dis 32:1430, 2001

WATANAKUNAKORN C, PERNI SC: *Proteus mirabilis* bacteremia: A review of 176 cases during 1980–1992. Scand J Infect Dis 26:361, 1994

DEFINITION *Helicobacter pylori* persistently colonizes the human stomach and is of etiologic importance in peptic ulcer disease (Chap. 274) and gastric malignancy (Chap. 77). Other gastric *Helicobacter* species colonize animals, some with a narrow range and others with a broad range of host species specificity. Those with broad specificity are occasionally found in humans, probably as zoonoses. The two most common of these species among isolates from humans are *Helicobacter bizzozeronii* (formerly known as *Helicobacter heilmannii* or *Gastrospirillum hominis*) and *Helicobacter felis*. It is unclear whether these helicobacters cause human disease. Numerous species of nongastric helicobacters are found in humans and animals and have been increasingly recognized as causes of human disease, especially in immunocompromised hosts.

ETIOLOGIC AGENT *H. pylori* is a gram-negative, spiral, flagellated bacillus that has naturally colonized humans for at least tens of thousands of years. It is noninvasive, living in gastric mucus; a small proportion of the bacterial cells are adherent to the mucosa. Its spiral shape and flagella render *H. pylori* motile in the mucus environment. This organism has several acid-resistance mechanisms, most notably a highly expressed urease that catalyzes urea hydrolysis to produce buffering ammonia. In vitro, *H. pylori* is microaerophilic and slow-growing and requires complex growth media. Publication of the complete genomic sequence of *H. pylori* in 1997 led to significant advances in the understanding of the organism's biology.

EPIDEMIOLOGY The prevalence of *H. pylori* is ~30% in the United States and other developed countries as opposed to >80% in most developing countries. In the United States, prevalence varies with age: ~50% of 60-year-old persons and 20% of 30-year-old persons are colonized. *H. pylori* is usually acquired in childhood. The age association is due mostly to a birth-cohort effect whereby current 60-year-olds were more commonly colonized as children than current 30-year-olds. Spontaneous acquisition or loss of the bacterium in adulthood is uncommon. Other than age, the main risk factor for *H. pylori* positivity is low socioeconomic status; crowding and markers of poor hygiene in childhood are particularly strong risk factors. Thus, the falling incidence among children is likely due, at least in part, to improvements in living standards and increased use of antibiotics.

Humans are the only important reservoir of *H. pylori*. Members of a family may carry the same strain, and colonization is particularly common in childhood institutions. These findings imply direct person-to-person spread, but whether transmission takes place by the fecal-oral or the oral-oral route is unknown. *H. pylori* is easily cultured from vomitus and gastroesophageal refluxate and is less easily cultured from stool.

PATHOLOGY AND PATHOGENESIS *H. pylori* colonization induces chronic superficial gastritis, which includes both mononuclear and polymorphonuclear cell infiltration of the mucosa. (The term *gastritis* should be used specifically to describe histologic features; it also has been used to describe endoscopic appearances and even symptoms, which do not correlate closely with microscopic findings or with the presence of *H. pylori*.) The immune response to *H. pylori* includes both the production of antibody (local and systemic) and a cell-mediated response but is ineffective in clearing the bacterium. The pattern of gastric inflammation is associated with disease risk: antral-predominant gastritis is most closely linked with duodenal ulceration, whereas pangastritis is linked with gastric ulceration and adenocarcinoma. This probably explains why patients with duodenal ulceration rarely develop gastric adenocarcinoma later, despite being colonized by *H. pylori*. Longitudinal analyses of gastric biopsy specimens taken years apart from the same patient show that inflammation may progress stepwise through atrophy, intestinal metaplasia, and dysplasia to carcinoma. Continuous proton pump inhibitor (PPI) therapy—for example,

for gastroesophageal reflux disease (GERD)—may speed progression to atrophy when *H. pylori* is present, but it remains unclear whether this situation increases cancer risk.

Most *H. pylori*–colonized persons do not develop clinical sequelae. That some persons develop overt disease whereas others do not is probably due to a combination of bacterial strain differences, host susceptibility to disease, and environmental factors. Several *H. pylori* virulence factors are more common in disease-associated strains. The *cag* PaI is a group of genes including those that encode a secretion system through which a specific protein, CagA, is translocated into epithelial cells. CagA interferes with host cell signaling, causing proliferation and cytoskeletal changes. The secretion system also induces a proinflammatory cytokine response, which results in enhanced inflammation. The CagA protein is highly immunogenic, and patients with peptic ulcer disease or gastric adenocarcinoma are more likely than persons without these conditions to have antibodies to CagA. However, patients with severe reflux esophagitis, the premalignant condition Barrett's esophagus, or esophageal adenocarcinoma are less likely to harbor *cag*+ strains than are persons with a normal esophagus. The *H. pylori* vacuolating cytotoxin VacA occurs in several forms that exhibit different levels of toxicity. Strains with the more toxic forms are more commonly isolated from patients with peptic ulcer disease or gastric carcinoma than from persons without these conditions. BabA, an adhesin expressed by only some strains, is associated with increased gastric inflammation and with increased risk of peptic ulceration and gastric adenocarcinoma.

The best-characterized host determinant of disease is the possession of genetic polymorphisms leading to enhanced *H. pylori*–stimulated secretion of the proinflammatory cytokine interleukin 1β. If they are *H. pylori*–positive, individuals with these polymorphisms are at increased risk of hypochlorhydria and gastric adenocarcinoma. Environmental cofactors are also important in pathogenesis. Smoking increases ulcer and cancer risk in *H. pylori*–positive individuals. Diets high in salt and preserved foods increase cancer risk, whereas diets high in antioxidants and vitamin C are protective.

The pathogenesis of duodenal ulceration is becoming clearer. Antral *H. pylori* colonization diminishes the number of somatostatin-producing cells. Since somatostatin inhibits gastrin release, gastrin levels are higher than normal in *H. pylori*–positive persons. Individuals with antral-predominant gastritis (and thus a normally functioning acid-producing gastric corpus) develop increased acid secretion, which induces protective gastric metaplasia in the duodenum; the duodenum becomes colonized by *H. pylori*, inflamed, and then ulcerated. The pathogenesis of gastric ulceration is less well understood. These ulcers usually occur at the junction of antral and corpus-type mucosa, and this region is particularly inflamed. Gastric cancer probably stems from progressive DNA damage and the survival of abnormal epithelial cell clones. The DNA damage is thought to be due principally to reactive oxygen and nitrogen species arising from inflammatory cells and perhaps from other bacteria that survive in the achlorhydric stomachs in which gastric malignancies occur.

CLINICAL MANIFESTATIONS Essentially all *H. pylori*–colonized persons have gastric inflammation, but fewer than 10% of these individuals develop associated illnesses such as peptic ulceration, gastric adenocarcinoma, or gastric lymphoma (Fig. 135-1).

More than 80% of duodenal ulcers and 60% of gastric ulcers are related to *H. pylori* colonization (Chap. 274), most of the remainder being due to aspirin or nonsteroidal anti-inflammatory drugs (NSAIDs). The main lines of evidence for an ulcer-promoting role of *H. pylori* are (1) that the presence of the organism is a risk factor for the development of ulcers, (2) that (non-NSAID-induced) ulcers rarely develop in the absence of *H. pylori*, (3) that eradication of *H. pylori* markedly reduces rates of ulcer relapse, and (4) that experimental *H. pylori* infection of gerbils causes gastric ulceration.

Prospective nested case-control studies have shown that *H. pylori* colonization is a risk factor for adenocarcinomas of the distal stomach (Chap. 77). Long-term experimental infection of gerbils also may result in gastric adenocarcinoma. The presence of *H. pylori* is strongly associated with gastric lymphoma, although this is a rarer condition. Many low-grade gastric B cell lymphomas arising from mucosa-associated lymphoid tissue (MALT) are driven by T cell stimulation, which in turn is driven by *H. pylori* antigen stimulation; *H. pylori* antigen–driven tumors may regress either fully or partially after *H. pylori* eradication.

Many patients have upper gastrointestinal symptoms but normal results in upper gastrointestinal endoscopy (so-called functional or nonulcer dyspepsia; Chap. 274). Because *H. pylori* is common, some of these patients will be positive for the organism. *H. pylori* eradication leads to symptom resolution more commonly than does placebo treatment, but only by a little (<10%). Whether such patients have peptic ulcers in remission at the time of endoscopy or whether a subgroup of patients with true functional dyspepsia respond to *H. pylori* treatment is unclear.

Much interest has focused on a possible protective role for *H. pylori* against GERD (Chap. 273) and adenocarcinoma of the esophagus and gastric cardia (Chap. 77). The main lines of evidence for this role are (1) that there is a temporal relationship between a falling prevalence of *H. pylori* colonization and a rising incidence of these conditions; (2) that in most studies, the prevalence of *H. pylori* colonization (especially with proinflammatory *cagA*⁺ strains) is significantly lower among patients with these esophageal diseases than among control subjects; and (3) that in some studies, eradication of *H. pylori* leads to the development or worsening of GERD. The mechanism underlying this protective effect appears to be *H. pylori*–induced hypochlorhydria. Since—at the individual level—GERD symptoms may decrease, worsen, or remain unchanged after *H. pylori* treatment, concerns about GERD should not affect treatment decisions where a definite indication exists.

H. pylori has a less-well-established role in other gastric pathologies. *H. pylori* may be one initial precipitant of autoimmune gastritis and pernicious anemia and also may predispose to iron deficiency in some patients through hypochlorhydria and reduced iron absorption. In addition, several extragastrointestinal pathologies have been linked epidemiologically with *H. pylori* colonization, the most notable being ischemic heart disease and cerebrovascular disease. However, the strength of these associations is reduced if confounding factors are considered, and most authorities consider them to be noncausal.

DIAGNOSIS Tests for *H. pylori* can be divided into two groups: invasive tests, which require upper gastrointestinal endoscopy and are based on the analysis of gastric biopsy specimens, and noninvasive tests (Table 135-1). Endoscopy often is not performed in the initial management of young dyspeptic patients without worrying symptoms but is commonly used in older people to exclude malignancy. If endoscopy is performed, the most convenient biopsy-based test is the biopsy urease test, in which one large or two small antral biopsy specimens are placed into a gel containing urea and an indicator. The presence of *H. pylori* urease elicits a color change, which often occurs within minutes but can require up to 24 h. Histologic examination of biopsy specimens is accurate, provided that a special stain (e.g., a modified Giemsa or silver stain) permitting optimal visualization of *H. pylori* is used. If biopsies from both antrum and corpus are obtained, histologic study yields additional information, including the degree and pattern of inflammation, atrophy, metaplasia, and dysplasia. Microbiologic culture is most specific but may be insensitive because of difficulty with *H. pylori* isolation. Once cultured, the identity of *H. pylori* can be confirmed by its typical appearance on Gram's stain and its positive reactions in oxidase, catalase, and urease tests. Moreover, the organism's antibiotic sensitivities can be determined. The occasional biopsy specimens containing the less common non-*pylori* helicobacters give only weakly positive results in the biopsy urease test.

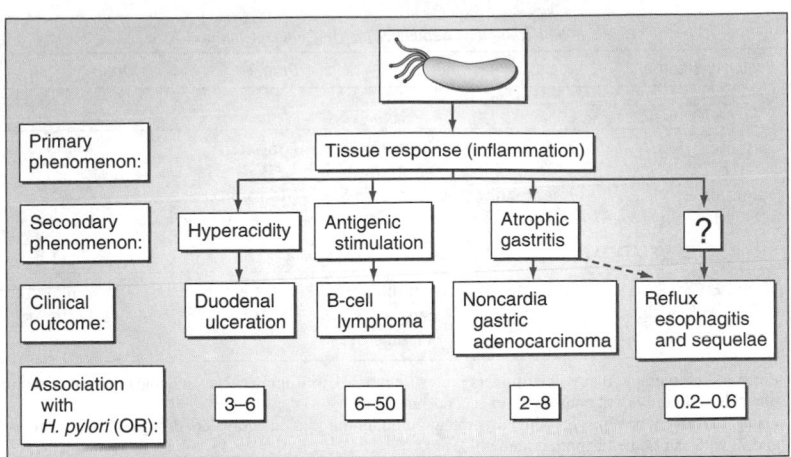

FIGURE 135-1 Schematic of the relationships between colonization with *Helicobacter pylori* and diseases of the upper gastrointestinal tract among persons in developed countries. Essentially all persons colonized with *H. pylori* develop a host response, which is generally termed *chronic gastritis*. The nature of the interaction of the host with the particular bacterial population determines the clinical outcome. *H. pylori* colonization increases the lifetime risk of peptic ulcer disease, noncardia gastric cancer, and B cell non-Hodgkin's gastric lymphoma [odds ratios (ORs) for all, >3]. In contrast, a growing body of evidence indicates that *H. pylori* colonization (especially with *cag*⁺ strains) protects against adenocarcinoma of the esophagus (and the related gastric cardia) and premalignant lesions such as Barrett's esophagus (OR, <1). While the incidences of peptic ulcer disease (cases not due to nonsteroidal anti-inflammatory drugs) and noncardia gastric cancer are declining in developed countries, the incidence of adenocarcinoma of the esophagus is rapidly increasing. (*Adapted from Blaser 1999, with permission.*)

Positive identification of these bacteria requires visualization of the characteristic long, tight spiral bacteria in histologic sections.

Noninvasive *H. pylori* testing is now the norm if gastric cancer does not need to be excluded. The most consistently accurate test is the urea breath test. In this simple test, the patient drinks a labeled urea solution and then blows into a tube. The urea is labeled with either the nonradioactive isotope ¹³C or a minute dose of the radioactive isotope ¹⁴C. If *H. pylori* urease is present, the urea is hydrolyzed and labeled carbon dioxide is detected in breath samples. The stool antigen test is another simple assay that is dependent on the detection of *H. pylori* antigens in stool. It is more convenient and less expensive than the urea breath test but has been slightly less accurate in some

TABLE 135-1 Tests Commonly Used to Detect *Helicobacter pylori*

Test	Advantages	Disadvantages
INVASIVE (BASED ON ENDOSCOPIC BIOPSY)		
Biopsy urease test	Quick, simple	Some commercial tests not fully sensitive before 24 h
Histology	May give additional histologic information	Sensitivity dependent on experience and use of special stains
Culture	Permits determination of antibiotic susceptibility	Sensitivity dependent on experience
NONINVASIVE		
Serology	Inexpensive and convenient	Cannot be used for early follow-up; some commercial kits inaccurate
¹³C or ¹⁴C urea breath test	Inexpensive and simpler than endoscopy; useful for follow-up after treatment	Low-dose irradiation in ¹⁴C test
Stool antigen test	Inexpensive and convenient; useful for follow-up after treatment; may be useful in children	New test; role not fully established; appears less accurate than urea breath test

TABLE 135-2 *Recommended Treatment Regimens for Helicobacter pylori*

Regimen, Duration	Drug 1	Drug 2	Drug 3	Drug 4
FIRST-LINE TREATMENT				
Regimen 1: OCA (7 days)[a]	Omeprazole[b] (20 mg bid)	Clarithromycin (500 mg bid)	Amoxicillin (1 g bid)	—
Regimen 2: OCM (7 days)	Omeprazole[b] (20 mg bid)	Clarithromycin (500 mg bid)	Metronidazole (500 mg bid)	—
SECOND-LINE TREATMENT[c]				
Regimen 3: OBTM (14 days)[d]	Omeprazole[b] (20 mg bid)	Bismuth subsalicylate (2 tabs qid)	Tetracycline HCl (500 mg qid)	Metronidazole (500 mg tid)

[a] For first-line therapy, many practitioners prefer Regimen 1 to Regimen 2, as it avoids the use of metronidazole—an important constituent of second-line therapy.

[b] Omeprazole may be replaced with any protein pump inhibitor at an equivalent dosage or, in Regimens 1 and 2, with ranitidine bismuth citrate (400 mg).

[c] An alternative to this second-line therapy is to culture *H. pylori* and to be guided by antibiotic susceptibility data. Patients in whom second-line therapy fails should undergo endoscopy for *H. pylori* culture and antibiotic susceptibility testing.

[d] Data supporting this regimen come mainly from Europe and are based on the use of bismuth subcitrate and metronidazole (400 mg tid).

comparative studies. The urea breath test, the stool antigen test, and biopsy-based tests can all be used to assess the success of treatment. However, because these tests are dependent on *H. pylori* load, their use <4 weeks after treatment may lead to false-negative results. These tests are also unreliable if performed within 4 weeks of intercurrent treatment with antibiotics or bismuth compounds or within 2 weeks of the discontinuation of PPI treatment. In the assessment of treatment success, noninvasive tests are normally preferred; however, after gastric ulceration, endoscopy should be repeated to ensure healing and to exclude gastric carcinoma by further histologic sampling.

The simplest tests for ascertaining *H. pylori* status are serologic assays measuring specific IgG levels in serum by enzyme-linked immunosorbent assay (ELISA) or immunoblot. The best of these tests are as accurate as other diagnostic methods, but many commercial tests, especially rapid office tests, perform poorly. In quantitative tests, a defined drop in antibody titer between matched serum samples taken before and 6 months after treatment (no sooner because of the slow decline in titer) accurately indicates that *H. pylori* has been eradicated. However, serologic tests are not commonly used in this context because of the inconvenient wait and the logistics. Although serology can distinguish between *cag*+ and *cag*− strains, this technique is not yet commercially available in the United States.

℞ TREATMENT

The most clear-cut indications for treatment are *H. pylori*–related duodenal or gastric ulceration and low-grade gastric B cell lymphoma. *H. pylori* should be eradicated in patients with documented ulcer disease, whether or not the ulcers are currently active, to reduce the likelihood of relapse. Many guidelines now recommend *H. pylori* treatment in uninvestigated simple dyspepsia following noninvasive diagnosis; others also recommend treatment in functional dyspepsia, in case the patient is one of the perhaps 5 to 10% to benefit (beyond placebo effects) from such treatment. People with a strong family history of gastric cancer should be treated for *H. pylori* in the hope that this therapy will reduce their risk. For many reasons, widespread community screening for and treatment of *H. pylori* as primary prophylaxis for gastric cancer and peptic ulcers are not currently recommended. It is unclear whether treatment of *H. pylori* (as opposed to never having acquired the organism) reduces cancer risk, except in certain high-risk populations. Treatment has side effects, which are severe in rare cases. Antibiotic resistance may arise in *H. pylori* or other incidentally carried bacteria. Otherwise healthy people may become anxious, especially if treatment is unsuccessful. Finally, there is a possible risk of provoking or worsening GERD.

Although *H. pylori* is susceptible to a wide range of antibiotics in vitro, monotherapy has been disappointing in vivo, probably because of inadequate antibiotic delivery to the full locus of colonization. Failure of monotherapy has led to the development of multidrug regimens, the most successful of which are triple and quadruple combinations that produce *H. pylori* eradication rates of >90% in many trials and >75% in clinical practice. Current regimens consist of a PPI or ranitidine bismuth citrate and two or three antimicrobial agents given for 7 to 14 days (Table 135-2).

The two most important goals in *H. pylori* eradication are to obtain the patient's close compliance with the dosing regimen and to use drugs to which *H. pylori* has not acquired resistance. Treatment failure following minor lapses in compliance is common and often leads to acquired resistance to metronidazole or clarithromycin. To stress the importance of compliance, written instructions should be given to the patient, and minor side effects of the regimen should be explained. Resistance to metronidazole and clarithromycin is of growing concern. Clarithromycin resistance is less prevalent but, if present, usually results in treatment failure. Metronidazole-resistant strains of *H. pylori* are more common, but infections with these strains may still respond to metronidazole-containing regimens. Assessment of antibiotic susceptibilities before treatment would be optimal but is not usually undertaken. In the absence of susceptibility information, a history of antibiotic use should be obtained, and, even if only distant exposure is identified (e.g., previous metronidazole consumption for giardiasis or trichomoniasis), use of the agent should be avoided if possible. If initial *H. pylori* treatment fails, two strategies are commonly used. One is re-treatment with a quadruple drug regimen (Table 135-2). The second is endoscopy and biopsy culture plus treatment based on documented antibiotic sensitivities. If re-treatment fails, susceptibility testing should always be performed.

Clearance of non-*pylori* gastric helicobacters following the use of bismuth compounds alone or triple-therapy regimens has been described. However, in the absence of trials, it is unclear whether this result represents successful treatment or natural clearance of the bacterium.

PREVENTION Carriage of *H. pylori* has considerable public health significance in developed countries, where it is associated with peptic ulcer disease and gastric adenocarcinoma, and in developing countries, where gastric adenocarcinoma is an even more common cause of cancer death late in life. However, given that *H. pylori* has co-evolved with its human host over millennia, preventing or eliminating colonization on a population basis may have distinct disadvantages. For example, absence of *H. pylori* has been reported to increase the risk of diarrheal diseases and, as has been mentioned, appears to increase the risk of GERD and esophageal adenocarcinoma. If mass prevention were contemplated, vaccination would be the most obvious method, and experimental immunization of animals has given promising results. However, in the United States and other developed countries, rates of *H. pylori* carriage, peptic ulceration, and gastric adenocarcinoma are falling. Thus, prevention of colonization in these countries may be unnecessary or even unwise.

FURTHER READING

BLASER MJ: Hypothesis: The changing relationships of *Helicobacter pylori* and humans: Implications for health and disease. J Infect Dis 179:1523, 1999

GHOSE C et al: East Asian genotypes of *Helicobacter pylori* strains in Amerindians provide evidence for its ancient human carriage. Proc Natl Acad Sci USA 99:15107, 2002

HANSSON LE et al: The risk of stomach cancer in patients with gastric or duodenal ulcer disease. N Engl J Med 335:242, 1996

KUIPERS E et al: Atrophic gastritis and *Helicobacter pylori* infection in patients with reflux esophagitis treated with omeprazole or fundoplication. N Engl J Med 334:1018, 1996

PARSONNET J et al: *Helicobacter pylori* infection and gastric lymphoma. N Engl J Med 330:1267, 1994

PEEK RM JR, BLASER MJ: *Helicobacter pylori* and gastrointestinal tract adenocarcinomas. Nat Rev Cancer 2:28, 2002

UEMURA N et al: *Helicobacter pylori* infection and the development of gastric cancer. N Engl J Med 345:784, 2001

ZUCCA E et al: Molecular analysis of the progression from *Helicobacter pylori*—associated chronic gastritis to mucosa-associated lymphoid-tissue lymphoma of the stomach. N Engl J Med 338:804, 1998

136 INFECTIONS DUE TO *PSEUDOMONAS* SPECIES AND RELATED ORGANISMS
Christopher A. Ohl, Matthew Pollack

Pseudomonas species and phylogenetically related bacteria are ubiquitous, free-living, opportunistic gram-negative pathogens. *Pseudomonas aeruginosa*, the most common human pathogen in this group, is the primary subject of this chapter. Also discussed are *Burkholderia cepacia* (formerly *Pseudomonas cepacia*), *Stenotrophomonas maltophilia* (formerly *Xanthomonas maltophilia*), and *Burkholderia pseudomallei* and *Burkholderia mallei* (the causative agents of melioidosis and glanders, respectively).

INFECTIONS DUE TO *P. AERUGINOSA*

MICROBIOLOGY *P. aeruginosa* is a small, nonsporulating, aerobic gram-negative rod belonging to the family Pseudomonadaceae. It is motile by virtue of its single polar flagellum. More than half of all clinical isolates produce the blue-green pigment pyocyanin; this pigment is helpful in the identification of the organism and accounts for the species name *aeruginosa*, which refers to the distinctive color of copper oxide. The organism, which can easily be identified in culture by the clinical laboratory, is differentiated from enteric gram-negative bacilli by its ability to oxidize indophenol and its inability to ferment lactose.

EPIDEMIOLOGY *P. aeruginosa* is widespread in nature, inhabiting soil, water, plants, and animals (including humans). It has a predilection for moist environments. This organism occasionally colonizes the skin, external ear, upper respiratory tract, or large bowel of healthy humans. Rates of carriage are relatively low, however, except among patients who have serious underlying disease, whose host defenses have been naturally or iatrogenically compromised, who have previously received antibiotic therapy, and/or who have been exposed to the hospital environment. Under these circumstances, colonization with *P. aeruginosa* frequently precedes infection, and factors that predispose to the former also increase the likelihood of the latter.

Most *P. aeruginosa* infections are acquired in the hospital, where intensive care units (ICUs) account for higher rates of infection than other hospital units. According to the National Nosocomial Infections Surveillance (NNIS) System, between 1992 and 1999, *P. aeruginosa* was the second most common cause of pneumonia, the fourth most common cause of urinary tract infection, and the sixth most common bloodstream isolate in ICUs. Many potential reservoirs of infection have been identified in the hospital environment, including respiratory equipment, cleaning solutions, disinfectants, sinks, vegetables, flowers, endoscopes, and physiotherapy pools. Most reservoirs are associated with moisture. While some infecting strains of *P. aeruginosa* appear to be endemic within the hospital, others are traced to a common source associated with a specific outbreak or epidemic. Nosocomial outbreaks of *Pseudomonas* infection have been specifically traced to the hands and fingernails of health care workers, and the majority of instances of patient-to-patient transmission in the hospital are thought to occur via this route. Epidemiologic investigation of health care—associated outbreaks is facilitated by the use of molecular techniques such as pulsed-field gel electrophoresis.

PATHOGENESIS The pathogenesis of *Pseudomonas* disease is complex, as is suggested by the clinical diversity of the infections related to this organism and by the multiplicity of putative virulence factors it produces. *P. aeruginosa* rarely causes disease in the healthy host but is highly virulent for persons in whom the normal cutaneous or mucosal barriers have been breached or bypassed, the immunologic defense mechanisms have been compromised, or the protective function of the normal bacterial flora has been disrupted (Table 136-1). The organism's ubiquity, flexible nutritional and metabolic requirements, invasive capacity, toxinogenicity, and innate antibiotic resistance help account for the frequency and success with which it acts as an opportunistic pathogen.

Infections caused by *P. aeruginosa* usually begin with bacterial attachment and superficial colonization of cutaneous or mucosal surfaces and progress to localized bacterial invasion and damage to underlying tissues. The infection may remain anatomically localized or may spread by direct extension to contiguous structures. This process may continue with bloodstream invasion, dissemination, the systemic inflammatory response syndrome (SIRS), multiple-organ dysfunction, and ultimately death. Not only is local infection more likely to occur in immunocompromised hosts (e.g., those with profound neutropenia), it is also more likely to culminate in bloodstream invasion and dissemination in these patients. Both intrinsic and extrinsic virulence factors appear to play roles in the pathogenicity of *P. aeruginosa* (Table 136-2). The organism's 6.3-million base-pair genome has been sequenced in its entirety, and a number of genes with specific regulatory, catabolic, and transport functions have been identified. These findings will undoubtedly increase our understanding of the pathogenicity and virulence of *P. aeruginosa*.

The production and secretion of many of the extracellular virulence factors of *P. aeruginosa* as well as the assembly and maturation of its biofilm are under the regulatory control of a complex cell-to-cell signaling system termed *quorum sensing*. Through lactones and other signal molecules secreted by each individual bacterium, the entire population of *P. aeruginosa* in a biofilm, colonized mucosa, or infected tissue senses its environment, communicates, and discerns its own cell density. This regulatory system may conceivably allow the bacteria to produce extracellular virulence factors in a coordinated manner that depends on cell density and thus may give the pathogen an appreciable advantage over host defense mechanisms.

Some of the exotoxins produced by *P. aeruginosa* (ExoS, ExoT, ExoU, and ExoY) are introduced directly from the bacterial cytosol into the host cell cytoplasm via a complex array of transmembrane proteins that together make up the *type III secretion apparatus*. This

---

TABLE 136-1   *Factors Predisposing to Pseudomonas aeruginosa Infections*

DISRUPTION OF CUTANEOUS OR MUCOSAL BARRIERS	
Burn injury	Endotracheal intubation
Cystic fibrosis	Indwelling central venous catheterization
Dermatitis	
Penetrating trauma	Urinary bladder catheterization
Surgery	Injection drug use

IMMUNOSUPPRESSION	
Neutropenia	Extremes of age
Qualitative white blood cell defects	Diabetes mellitus
	Steroid therapy
Hypogammaglobulinemia	Cancer
Defective cell-mediated immunity	AIDS

DISRUPTION OF NORMAL BACTERIAL FLORA
Broad-spectrum antibiotic therapy
Exposure to the hospital environment

TABLE 136-2 *Putative Virulence Factors of Pseudomonas aeruginosa*

Virulence Factor	Function(s)
Pili or fimbriae	Attachment to epithelial cells
Mucoid exopolysaccharide (alginate)	Attachment to epithelial cells, inhibition of mucociliary and opsonophagocytic clearance, biofilm formation
Alkaline protease	Tissue breakdown, proteolysis of immunoglobulin and complement
Elastase	Destruction of elastic tissues, including lamina of blood vessels
Phospholipase C (a hemolysin)	Breakdown of lipids and lecithin, tissue necrosis
Lipopolysaccharide (LPS or endotoxin)	Fever, leukocytosis or leukopenia, hypotension, shock; disseminated intravascular coagulation; adult respiratory distress syndrome; systemic inflammatory response syndrome
Exotoxins	
ExoA	Inhibition of protein synthesis through interference with adenosine diphosphate ribosylation of elongation factor-2
ExoS	Ribosylation of guanosine triphosphate binding proteins; disruption of cellular actin cytoskeleton
ExoT	Disruption of cellular actin cytoskeleton
ExoU	Acute cytotoxicity
ExoY	Increase in intracellular cyclic adenosine monophosphate

system requires direct cell contact and allows the injection of virulence factors from the bacterium into host cells without interference from humoral immune defenses.

CLINICAL MANIFESTATIONS AND DIAGNOSIS ■ **Respiratory Tract Infections** *Primary pneumonia* or *nonbacteremic pneumonia* results from the aspiration of upper respiratory tract secretions and often develops in patients with previous antibiotic use who are exposed to the hospital environment, particularly the ICU. It is a common cause of ventilator-associated pneumonia and is noted especially often in patients with chronic lung disease, congestive heart failure, or AIDS. Community-aquired pneumonia due to *P. aeruginosa* is uncommon among normal hosts. Fever, chills, severe dyspnea, cyanosis, productive cough, apprehension, confusion, and other signs of severe systemic toxicity characterize this acute, often life-threatening infection. Chest roentgenograms typically show bilateral bronchopneumonia with nodular infiltrates and small areas of radiolucency; pleural effusions are common; empyema is relatively uncommon; and lobar consolidation is occasionally seen. Cavitary lesions are unusually common among AIDS patients with *P. aeruginosa* pneumonia. Pathologic lesions include alveolar necrosis, focal hemorrhages, and microabscesses.

Bacteremic pneumonia due to *P. aeruginosa* begins as a respiratory infection. However, unlike primary pneumonia, it is typically associated with neutropenia, subsequent bloodstream invasion, and metastatic spread that produces characteristic lesions in the lungs and other viscera. Alveolar hemorrhage and necrosis are common. The signs and symptoms of this fulminant disease include those described for nonbacteremic pneumonia caused by this organism as well as those associated with gram-negative sepsis. Chest roentgenograms characteristically demonstrate a rapid progression from pulmonary vascular congestion to interstitial edema, then to alveolar edema, and finally to diffuse necrotizing bronchopneumonia with cavity formation. The patient typically dies 3 or 4 days after initial presentation.

Chronic infection of the lower respiratory tract with *P. aeruginosa* is caused almost exclusively by mucoid strains that produce alginate and is prevalent among older children and young adults with cystic fibrosis as well as in some patients with bronchiectasis or AIDS. In patients with cystic fibrosis, mucoid strains invariably colonize and infect patients with increasing prevalence over time and contribute to

the acute exacerbations and chronic progression that characterize pulmonary disease in these individuals. Airway obstruction appears to begin with bronchiolitis, which causes mucus plugging and predisposes to *P. aeruginosa* infection. The latter produces more mucus plugging, chronic suppuration, bronchiectasis, atelectasis, and ultimately fibrosis. This process progresses to pulmonary insufficiency, hypoxemia, and alterations in cardiopulmonary dynamics resulting in pulmonary hypertension and cor pulmonale.

Clinical manifestations of lower respiratory tract infections due to *P. aeruginosa* in patients with cystic fibrosis vary with the severity and duration of underlying lung disease, the frequency and intensity of acute episodes, and the presence of co-infecting pathogens such as *B. cepacia* (Chap. 241). Early in the disease, patients may experience recurrent upper respiratory symptoms followed by a lingering cough. Episodes of pneumonia develop later, with persistent cough between acute episodes. Eventually, patients exhibit a chronic productive cough, wheezing, diminished appetite, weight loss, growth retardation, and decreased activity. Acute exacerbations are typically accompanied by low-grade fever and heightened respiratory symptoms. Physical signs include evidence of malnutrition, an increase in anteroposterior diameter, intercostal retractions, cyanosis, inspiratory and expiratory wheezing, rhonchi, moist rales, abdominal distention, and clubbing of the fingers and toes. Laboratory abnormalities include leukocytosis with a left shift and hypoxemia with or without hypercarbia. Tests of pulmonary function demonstrate obstructive and restrictive defects. Chest roentgenograms reveal overaeration, patchy atelectasis, peribronchial fibrosis, and patchy infiltrates associated with pneumonia. In more advanced disease, there may be evidence of severe overaeration, depressed diaphragm, further increased anteroposterior diameter, extensive peribronchial infiltration, generalized bronchiectasis, and cyst formation.

Bacteremia *P. aeruginosa* remains an important cause of life-threatening bloodstream infection in immunocompromised patients, particularly those with hematologic malignancies complicated by neutropenia. Bacteremia is frequently iatrogenic and is usually seen in hospitalized patients with various comorbid conditions (Table 136-1). Bloodstream infection may be primary (with no identifiable source) or secondary to a discrete focus of infection. Common primary sites of infection include the urinary and gastrointestinal tracts, lungs, skin and soft tissues, and intravascular foci, including indwelling central venous catheters.

The clinical features of *P. aeruginosa* bacteremia are similar to those of other forms of bacteremia. Fever, tachypnea, tachycardia, and prostration are common. Disorientation, confusion, or obtundation may be evident. Hypotension can progress to refractory shock. Renal failure, adult respiratory distress syndrome, disseminated intravascular coagulation, and other manifestations of SIRS occur as complications.

Pathognomonic skin lesions termed *ecthyma gangrenosum* (Fig. 136-1) develop in a relatively small minority of patients with *P. aeruginosa* bacteremia. The lesions begin as small hemorrhagic vesicles

FIGURE 136-1 Ecthyma gangrenosum in a neutropenic patient with *Pseudomonas aeruginosa* bacteremia.

surrounded by a rim of erythema and undergo central necrosis with subsequent ulceration. They occur singly or in small numbers on the perineum, buttocks, and extremities; in the axillae; and elsewhere. Bacterial invasion of blood vessels, documented histologically, is the sine qua non of ecthyma lesions. Bacteria are visible on Gram's staining or are recoverable by culture of aspirated material from lesions.

Endocarditis (See also Chap. 109) *P. aeruginosa* infects the native heart valves of intravenous drug users as well as prosthetic heart valves. The source of *P. aeruginosa* strains infecting drug users appears to be standing water contaminating drug paraphernalia. Foreign materials mixed with heroin may cause injury to valve leaflets or mural endocardium, with resulting fibrosis and an increased risk for valve infection. Exposure of the tricuspid valve to both trauma and bacteria apparently accounts for the high incidence of tricuspid involvement in association with intravenous drug use.

The tricuspid, pulmonic, mitral, or aortic valve and the mural endocardium of either atrium may be affected in *P. aeruginosa* endocarditis. Multiple-valve infections are common. Tricuspid or right-sided involvement is often associated with septic pulmonary emboli. Right-sided *P. aeruginosa* endocarditis usually presents subacutely, while the appearance of left-sided disease is likely to be more acute or even fulminant. Fever is virtually invariable, and murmurs are usually detectable at initial presentation or shortly thereafter. Septic pulmonary emboli associated with right-sided disease result in cough, pleuritic chest pain, sputum production, pulmonary infiltration (with or without abscess formation), and pleural effusion. Left-sided infections may present as intractable heart failure or large systemic emboli. Mycotic aneurysms, cerebritis, or brain abscess may occur; septic infarcts are occasionally found in the spleen. Skin and soft tissue manifestations, including Janeway lesions, Osler's nodes, and ecthyma gangrenosum, are relatively uncommon.

The diagnosis of *P. aeruginosa* endocarditis is based on positive blood culture in the absence of an extracardiac source; an indication of valvular dysfunction or vegetation on an echocardiogram; evidence of septic pulmonary lesions on a chest roentgenogram (in right-sided disease); and the actual demonstration of infected heart valves at the time of surgery.

Central Nervous System Infections *P. aeruginosa* infections of the central nervous system include meningitis and brain abscess. These infections follow extension from a contiguous parameningeal structure such as the ear, mastoid, or paranasal sinus; direct inoculation into the subarachnoid space or brain through head trauma, surgery, or diagnostic procedures; or bacteremic spread from infection at a distant site. Like *P. aeruginosa* infections at other anatomical sites, central nervous system infections are documented almost exclusively in patients with compromised local or systemic immune-defense mechanisms. Mortality rates from these infections are high.

The clinical signs of *P. aeruginosa* meningitis, like those of other forms of acute bacterial meningitis, include fever, headache, stiff neck, confusion, and obtundation. The onset of illness may be acute or even fulminant, particularly in bacteremic patients, with a precipitous downhill course, shock, coma, and early death. In nonbacteremic patients, *P. aeruginosa* meningitis or brain abscess may present more insidiously, with a paucity of systemic symptoms. This presentation is especially common in infections resulting from recent neurosurgery, cancer of the head and neck, or direct extension from a parameningeal focus of chronic infection. Occasionally, *P. aeruginosa* meningitis runs a subacute or relapsing course that is thought to be related to the intermittent release of bacteria from a loculated site of infection.

Ear Infections *P. aeruginosa* is often found in the external auditory canal, particularly under moist conditions and in the presence of inflammation or maceration (as in "swimmer's ear"). Moreover, this organism is the predominant pathogen associated with external otitis, a usually benign inflammatory process affecting the external auditory canal. The ear is painful or merely itchy, there is a purulent discharge, and pain is elicited by pulling on the pinna. The external canal appears edematous and is filled with detritus that often prevents visualization of the tympanic membrane.

P. aeruginosa occasionally penetrates the epithelium overlying the floor of the external auditory canal at the junction between bone and cartilage and invades underlying soft tissue. The ensuing invasive process, which involves soft tissue, cartilage, and cortical bone, is typically slow but destructive. Termed *malignant external otitis*, this condition occurs predominantly in elderly diabetic patients but is reported occasionally in infants with other underlying diseases and rarely in elderly nondiabetic patients. Virtually all cases of malignant external otitis are caused by *P. aeruginosa*. From the external ear, the infection advances to the retromandibular area or parotid space and enters the mastoid air cells and temporal bone. Advancing osteomyelitis at the base of the skull often involves the seventh, ninth, tenth, and eleventh cranial nerves. The cavernous sinus can become involved, as can the contralateral petrous apex. The middle ear is commonly spared; meningitis and brain abscess are relatively rare complications.

Otorrhea and severe otalgia are common presenting symptoms of malignant external otitis. Facial-nerve paralysis tends to occur early, while other cranial-nerve palsies appear later. There may be a loss of hearing. Constitutional symptoms such as fever and weight loss are relatively uncommon. Physical examination almost always reveals remarkable tenderness of the pinna and abnormalities of the external auditory canal, including swelling, erythema, purulent discharge, debris, and granulation tissue in the canal wall. The tympanic membrane is often hidden from view and is sometimes perforated. Inflammation may involve the pinna as well as the periauricular, retromandibular, and mastoid areas.

Peripheral leukocytosis is relatively infrequent in malignant external otitis, while the erythrocyte sedimentation rate (ESR) is usually markedly elevated. Cerebrospinal fluid occasionally exhibits pleocytosis and an elevation in the protein level. Computed tomography (CT) or magnetic resonance imaging (MRI) of the mastoid or temporal bone typically reveals bony erosions and new bone formation, while the floor of the skull may have soft tissue densities associated with areas of cellulitis. In addition, technetium 99m bone scans and gallium 67 scans frequently give positive results. Cultures of samples from the external auditory canal and of surgical specimens are almost always positive for *P. aeruginosa*.

Eye Infections (See also Chap. 25) *P. aeruginosa* causes bacterial keratitis or corneal ulcer and endophthalmitis in the human eye. Keratitis due to *P. aeruginosa* may result from even minor corneal injury, which interrupts the integrity of the superficial epithelial surface and permits bacterial access to the underlying stroma. Corneal ulcer may complicate contact lens use, particularly when extended-wear soft contact lenses are involved. Contact lens solutions or the lenses themselves may be the source of the organism, which is probably inoculated into the eye at sites of minor lens-induced corneal damage. Patients who have sustained serious burns, have undergone ocular irradiation or tracheostomy, have been exposed to the intensive care environment, and/or are in a coma are also susceptible to *P. aeruginosa*–associated corneal ulcers. Contaminated eye medications are occasionally implicated in these infections. *P. aeruginosa* keratitis usually starts as a small central ulcer; spreads concentrically to involve a large portion of the cornea, sclera, and underlying stroma; and in some cases progresses to posterior corneal perforation.

The clinical manifestations of *P. aeruginosa* keratitis include a rapidly expanding, necrotic stromal infiltrate in the bed of an epithelial injury; surrounding epithelial edema; an anterior chamber reaction; and mucopurulent discharge adherent to the ulcer's surface. Corneal ulcer due to *P. aeruginosa* may advance rapidly to involve the entire cornea in ≤2 days or may evolve subacutely over several days. Systemic symptoms are uncommon. Complications include corneal perforation, anterior chamber involvement, and endophthalmitis.

P. aeruginosa endophthalmitis is typically a rapidly progressive, sight-threatening condition that demands immediate therapeutic intervention. It may complicate penetrating injuries of the eye, intraocular surgery, hematogenous spread from other sites of *Pseudomonas* infection, or posterior perforation of corneal ulcers. Clinical manifestations may include eye pain, conjunctival hyperemia, chemosis, lid edema, decreased visual acuity, hypopyon, severe anterior uveitis, and signs of possible vitreous involvement. Panophthalmitis may result from this intraocular infection.

Bone and Joint Infections   Sternoclavicular pyarthrosis caused by *P. aeruginosa* is often a complication of injection drug use and is rarely associated with *P. aeruginosa* endocarditis. Joint involvement is usually monarticular, with the sternoclavicular joint more often affected than sternochondral joints. Patients present with acute or chronic pain in the anterior chest wall, often associated with fever and restricted movement of the homolateral shoulder. Physical examination reveals tenderness, erythema, and swelling over the affected joint. Leukocytosis is common, and the ESR is almost invariably elevated. Roentgenograms show soft tissue edema, bone demineralization, lytic lesions, and periosteal elevation of the clavicular head, rib, or sternum. Material obtained by arthrocentesis or synovial biopsy yields *P. aeruginosa* in culture.

P. aeruginosa infections of the symphysis pubis are associated with pelvic surgery and injection drug use. The symphysis pubis, like other fibrocartilaginous joints, exhibits a peculiar susceptibility to bloodborne infection with *P. aeruginosa*. Affected patients report pain in the groin, hip, thigh, and/or lower abdomen that is made worse by walking. Fever is variable, and the duration of symptoms before diagnosis ranges from days to months. The ESR is markedly elevated. Roentgenograms or CT scans show irregularities of the pubic margins, separation of the symphysis pubis, and osteomyelitic abnormalities of the pubic rami that may be extensive. Bone scans are usually positive. Needle aspiration or biopsy is necessary to obtain material for culture. A positive culture is particularly important for the discrimination of *P. aeruginosa* infections and other pyogenic infections from osteitis pubis, which is thought to be a noninfectious condition complicating pelvic surgery, childbirth, or trauma.

P. aeruginosa is the most common cause of osteochondritis of the foot following plantar puncture wounds. This infection is seen primarily in children and is usually acquired via the direct inoculation of *P. aeruginosa* that inhabits the moist environment found in the soles of shoes. The organism infects the small joints and bones, including the proximal phalanges, metatarsals, metatarsophalangeal joints, tarsal bones, and calcaneus. On average, local pain and swelling last for several weeks, and systemic symptoms are usually lacking. There may be plantar cellulitis over the involved area or tenderness upon deep palpation. Results of roentgenograms and bone scans are generally positive. Aspiration of the affected joint frequently yields purulent material in which *P. aeruginosa* can be demonstrated by Gram's staining and by culture.

Vertebral osteomyelitis due to *P. aeruginosa* is associated with complicated urinary tract infection, genitourinary instrumentation or surgery, and injection drug use. Vertebral infections that are associated with a urinary tract source most often develop in the elderly and usually affect the lumbosacral spine. Presumably the route of infection in these patients is a shared venous plexus between the pelvis and spine. Drug use–related infections typically occur in younger patients and may affect the cervical or lumbosacral spine. *P. aeruginosa* vertebral osteomyelitis is usually an indolent disease. Accordingly, symptoms may develop weeks or even months before diagnosis. Back or neck pain is generally reported, while fever and systemic symptoms are relatively uncommon. Local tenderness and decreased range of motion of the affected spine are typical. Leukocytosis may be noted, the ESR is almost always markedly elevated, and blood cultures are sometimes positive. Roentgenograms reveal loss of bone density, narrowed intervertebral space, destruction of vertebral end plates, lytic lesions of

vertebral bodies, sclerosis, and possible osteophyte formation. MRI or CT is the most sensitive and specific means of defining lesions. Technetium bone scans and gallium scans usually yield positive results but have lower specificity. An etiologic diagnosis requires the culture of material obtained by needle aspiration or biopsy of the affected spine under fluoroscopic guidance; open biopsy is occasionally needed.

P. aeruginosa is one of the most common causative agents in a variety of other, less specific syndromes involving nonhematogenous infections of bones and joints and collectively referred to as *chronic contiguous osteomyelitis*. These infections may result, for example, from compound fractures, contamination associated with open reduction and fixation of closed fractures, sternotomy performed in conjunction with cardiac surgery, contiguous spread from infected ischemic ulcers related to peripheral vascular disease or diabetes mellitus, and cellulitis in general. The chronicity, indolence, and heterogeneity of these infections explain their varied clinical manifestations and the frequent need for complicated long-term management.

Urinary Tract Infections   *P. aeruginosa* is one of the most common causes of complicated and nosocomial infections of the urinary tract. These infections may result from urinary tract catheterization, instrumentation, surgery (including renal transplantation), or obstruction; they may arise from persistent foci (e.g., the prostate or stones) and may be chronic or recurrent. The urinary tract may be a target for bloodborne infection in patients with *P. aeruginosa* bacteremia but more often is the source of bacteremia. Chronic *P. aeruginosa* infections of the urinary tract are relatively common among patients with indwelling bladder catheters, altered urinary tract anatomy secondary to diversionary procedures, and paraplegia. Chronic or recurrent urinary tract infection caused by *Pseudomonas* often involves multidrug-resistant (MDR) strains.

The clinical features of urinary tract infections due to *P. aeruginosa* are usually indistinguishable from those of other bacterial infections. However, *P. aeruginosa* infections exhibit a propensity for persistence, chronicity, and recurrence. More unusual forms of urinary tract involvement peculiar to *P. aeruginosa* include (1) ulcerative lesions of the renal pelvis, ureters, and bladder that cause sloughing of vesical membranes in the urine; and (2) ecthyma-like lesions of the renal cortex that are seen in association with *Pseudomonas* sepsis.

Skin and Soft Tissue Infections (See also Chap. 110)   As indicated above, *P. aeruginosa* bacteremia may be associated with the disseminated skin lesions of ecthyma gangrenosum (Fig. 136-1). Less common skin manifestations of *P. aeruginosa* sepsis include vesicular or pustular lesions, bullae, subcutaneous nodules, deep abscesses, and cellulitis. Metastatic lesions of the skin or mucous membranes complicate *Pseudomonas* sepsis and occasionally produce massive necrosis or gangrene of the extremities, perineum, face, or oropharynx.

Primary *P. aeruginosa* pyoderma occurs when the skin breaks down secondary to surgery, trauma, burn injury, dermatitis, or ulcers related to peripheral vascular disease or pressure sores. Moist conditions and neutropenia may predispose to this condition. The clinical appearance of primary *P. aeruginosa* pyoderma, which frequently includes hemorrhage and necrosis, resembles that of metastatic *P. aeruginosa* skin lesions. Histologic studies document vascular invasion by bacteria in both diseases. A rare distinguishing feature of *P. aeruginosa* pyoderma is its association with a characteristic fruity odor and an exudate of blue-green hue (due to pyocyanin) that is occasionally noted on dressings or bandages rather than on the wound itself.

P. aeruginosa wound infection complicating extensive third-degree burn injuries typically occurs at least 1 to 2 weeks after the injury and results from colonization of the burn site or burn eschar. Invasion of the subeschar space and underlying dermis, vascular invasion, and systemic spread may occur and are associated with an elevated mortality rate. The development and progression of *P. aeruginosa* burn wound sepsis are facilitated by the injury-associated breakdown of normal skin, selection of antibiotics with inadequate coverage for this pathogen, and burn-related immune defects. Local manifestations include black, dark brown, or violaceous discoloration of the burn eschar; degeneration of underlying granulation tissue, hemorrhage, and premature eschar separation; edema, hemorrhage, and necrosis of skin adjacent to the burn site; and erythematous nodular lesions in unburned skin. Systemic manifestations include fever or hypothermia and other signs of sepsis, SIRS, or multiple-organ system failure. The diagnosis of *P. aeruginosa* burn sepsis is based on these local and systemic clinical manifestations and on a burn wound biopsy that reveals both >10^5 colony-forming units of *P. aeruginosa* per gram of tissue and histologic evidence of bacterial invasion of unburned tissue, vasculitis, or intense inflammation at the burn margin.

P. aeruginosa causes diffuse, pruritic, maculopapular, and vesiculopustular rashes associated with exposure to contaminated hot tubs, spas, whirlpools, and swimming pools. Most cases of *P. aeruginosa* dermatitis have occurred as part of a common-source outbreak. At least two nosocomial common-source outbreaks—one related to a physiotherapy pool—have been reported. Skin rashes may be limited to areas covered by swimsuits or may be more diffuse, sparing only the head and neck. Low-grade fever or other associated symptoms are uncommon. The illness is usually self-limited, and the rash resolves without specific therapy after cessation of exposure. A related benign condition has been reported in children exposed to *P. aeruginosa*–contaminated wading pools. Termed *pseudomonas hot-foot syndrome*, this infection presents with painful nodules on the plantar aspect of the foot.

P. aeruginosa Infections in Patients with AIDS During the 1980s and 1990s, *P. aeruginosa* infections were increasingly associated with AIDS. The vast majority of these infections are currently seen in patients with advanced AIDS, previous opportunistic infections, and CD4+ lymphocyte counts <100/μL (often <50/μL). The specific immunologic factors that lead to *P. aeruginosa* infections in patients with AIDS are not well understood but are thought to result from a loss of mucosal integrity, defects in cellular and humoral immunity, and qualitative leukocyte abnormalities. Notably, the majority of *P. aeruginosa* infections in this population are community-acquired, in contrast to the nosocomial transmission observed for most infections in non-AIDS patients.

Pneumonia accounts for a substantial proportion of *P. aeruginosa* infections in patients with AIDS. In most instances, pneumonia presents as a necrotizing infection of the pulmonary parenchyma, frequently with cavitary lesions, or as a chronic relapsing bronchopulmonary infection reminiscent of the bronchopulmonary disease seen in patients with cystic fibrosis. Also observed are bloodstream infections, including those associated with indwelling central venous catheters, and infections of the paranasal sinuses, skin and soft tissue, and urinary tract. Bacteremia, either primary or secondary to infection at a remote site, is often recurrent, associated with high mortality, and occasionally accompanied by skin manifestations similar to those seen in non-AIDS patients.

Because *P. aeruginosa* infections occur in patients with advanced AIDS, survival after recovery from the initial infection may be limited to a few months. However, with the widespread use of highly active antiretroviral therapy and the resultant increase in CD4+ cell count, the incidence of *P. aeruginosa* infection among patients with AIDS appears to have declined and the natural history of infection to have been modified. For example, a small number of patients with recalcitrant, relapsing *P. aeruginosa* bronchopulmonary infections have reportedly experienced the resolution of infection soon after initiation of intensive antiretroviral therapy. For those patients infected with HIV that has developed antiretroviral resistance, the risk of *Pseudomonas* infection remains elevated.

R~x~ TREATMENT

Approach to Therapy Table 136-3 lists antimicrobial agents available in the United States that are generally active against *P. aeruginosa*. Table 136-4 outlines suggested antibiotic choices and an approach to therapy for infections at selected sites. The initial antibiotic selection should take into account the local patterns of antimicrobial susceptibility, and

the susceptibilities of the isolate from a particular case should guide definitive antibiotic therapy (see below).

In most severe or life-threatening infections due to *P. aeruginosa*, two antipseudomonal antibiotics to which the infecting strain is (or is likely to be) sensitive should be administered together. The putative benefits of this combined therapy, as determined by in vitro studies, are to increase efficacy, to achieve additive or synergistic killing, and to prevent the emergence of antibiotic resistance. Despite widespread acceptance of combination therapy for *P. aeruginosa* infections, there are few clinical data collected since the advent of newer β-lactam antibiotics to document that combination therapy is in fact more efficacious than monotherapy or that it actually forestalls the acquisition of antimicrobial resistance. Nevertheless, combination therapy continues to be recommended—at least as initial treatment—for most fulminant infections, as outlined in Table 136-4.

The appropriate duration of antibiotic therapy for disease caused by *P. aeruginosa* depends on the type, location, and severity of infection. In general, chronic infections associated with extensive tissue injury, disruption of normal anatomy, foreign or prosthetic material, or suboptimal antibiotic accessibility require therapy for weeks or even months rather than days. More acute infections may be treated aggressively but for shorter periods.

P. aeruginosa infections of the lower respiratory tract in cystic fibrosis pose a special challenge because of their long-standing nature (Chap. 241). In general, antibiotic therapy for acute exacerbations results in short-term clinical improvement, while periodic expectant courses of antimicrobial therapy may limit disease progression. The clinical response to antimicrobial therapy may have little relation to the identity and antimicrobial susceptibility of cultured sputum isolates. A more novel approach to antimicrobial treatment—the use of intermittent, cyclical inhaled tobramycin—has been shown to improve pulmonary function, decrease the risk of hospitalization, and reduce the density of *P. aeruginosa* in sputum of older patients with cystic fibrosis. In addition, lung transplantation has been employed with good results in selected cystic fibrosis patients with severe, progressive lower respiratory tract infections due to *P. aeruginosa*.

Antimicrobial Resistance Antibiotic resistance in *P. aeruginosa* is both intrinsic (as reflected by the relative paucity of antibiotics with inherent activity against wild-type strains) and acquired (as defined by high-level resistance to agents that normally would be expected to exhibit antimicrobial activity). Acquired resistance is rapidly increasing among isolates of *P. aeruginosa*, particularly those associated with cystic fibrosis and with ICUs. Escalating resistance among ICU isolates is especially alarming. Data from NNIS and the Intensive Care Antimicrobial Resistance Epidemiology (ICARE) project on the resistance of *P. aeruginosa* between 1998 and 2002 show that the pooled mean figures for resistance to piperacillin, ceftazidime, imipenem, and ciprofloxacin increased from previous years and represented 14.3, 10.5, 13.7, and 28.9% of ICU-associated isolates, respectively. Factors responsible for this increase may include the expanding use of immunosuppressive therapies, the increased severity of illness in hospitalized patients, inadequate infection-control procedures, and growing antibiotic use. Resistant organisms can be transmitted directly to patients from the hospital staff, other patients, or the environment, or they may arise de novo during therapy with any given agent. The emergence of MDR strains has been associated with increases in secondary bacteremia and mortality and has led in some cases to longer hospital stays and increased hospitalization costs. Therapy for resistant *P. aeruginosa* infections should consist of antimicrobial agents selected on the basis of extended susceptibility testing and may involve increased treatment duration as well as surgical drainage or removal of infected tissues. Infections due to strains resistant to all commonly available antimicrobial agents may respond to parenteral or inhaled therapy with the relatively toxic antibiotics polymyxin B and colistin.

Agent	Dose,[a] Route	Comments
ANTIPSEUDOMONAL PENICILLINS		
Piperacillin	3–4 g q4–6h IV	Drugs in class are listed in order of decreasing in
Piperacillin/tazobactam	3.375 g q4h IV	vitro activity. Piperacillin/tazobactam or ticarcil-
Mezlocillin	3 g q4h IV	lin/clavulanate has little more activity against *P.*
Ticarcillin	3 g q3–6h IV	*aeruginosa* than piperacillin or ticarcillin alone.
Ticarcillin/clavulanate	3.1 g q4–6h IV	Monotherapy should not be used for serious in- fections.
ANTIPSEUDOMONAL CEPHALOSPORINS		
Ceftazidime[b]	2 g q8–12h IV	Use more frequent indicated doses for CNS infec-
Cefoperazone[b]	2 g q6h IV	tions or infections in neutropenic or severely im-
Cefepime	2 g q8–12h IV	munocompromised patients. The antipseudomonal activity of cefepime is equivalent to that of cefta- zidime, with less potential for β-lactamase induc- tion in gram-negative enteric bacteria.
CARBAPENEMS[b,c]		
Imipenem/cilastatin	0.5 g q6h IV	Class is active against strains producing β-lacta-
Meropenem	1 g q8h IV	mases. Imipenem may cause seizures in patients with renal failure (avoid by reducing dose) or CNS infections or lesions. Meropenem is slightly more active in vitro against *P. aeruginosa* than imipenem.
MONOBACTAMS		
Aztreonam	2 g q6–8h IV	Drug can usually be administered to patients with β-lactam hypersensitivity.
AMINOGLYCOSIDES[b]		
Tobramycin	MD: 2 mg/kg load, then 1.7 mg/kg q8h IV ODD: 5–7 mg/kg q24h IV	Tobramycin has greater in vitro activity against *P.* *aeruginosa* than gentamicin, but the drugs' clini- cal efficacies are probably equivalent. Some *P.*
Gentamicin	MD: Same as tobramycin ODD: Same as tobramycin	*aeruginosa* isolates that are resistant to tobramy- cin or gentamicin may be susceptible to amikacin.
Amikacin	MD: 7.5 mg/kg load, then 7.5 mg/kg q12h IV ODD: 15 mg/kg q24h IV	Except in urinary tract infection, this class should not be used for monotherapy. ODD may reduce adverse effects. Serum levels must be monitored.
FLUOROQUINOLONES[b,d]		
Ciprofloxacin	0.4 g q12h IV or 0.5–0.75 g bid PO	Ciprofloxacin is the most active of the available quinolones against *P. aeruginosa*. Serum levels
Levofloxacin	0.75 g q24h IV or PO	attained with oral therapy approximate those after IV therapy; thus oral formulations are useful for long-duration therapy in selected patients.
OTHER AGENTS		
Polymyxin B	0.75–1.25 mg/kg q12h IV	These drugs are reserved for use in multidrug-resis-
Colistin	1.5 mg/kg q8h IV	tant infections. Nephrotoxicity and neurotoxicity occur. Colistin inhalational therapy consists of 75 mg in 3 mL of normal saline via nebulizer, given twice daily.

[a] Indicated dosages are for the treatment of infections due to *P. aeruginosa* in adults. Doses should be adjusted in renal insufficiency. Higher doses may be required in patients with cystic fibrosis, and lower doses may be adequate for the treatment of
uncomplicated urinary tract infections.
[b] Some strains of *P. aeruginosa* may rapidly develop resistance to these agents during therapy.
[c] Ertapenem, an additional drug in this class, has less in vitro activity and should not be used for the treatment of *Pseudomonas*
infections.
[d] Trovafloxacin, an additional fluoroquinolone with antipseudomonal activity, has limited usefulness because of its hepatotoxicity.
Gatifloxacin and moxifloxacin have in vitro activity against *P. aeruginosa* (albeit less than ciprofloxacin and levofloxacin), but
there are no clinical studies to support their use in *Pseudomonas* or nosocomial infections.
Abbreviations: MD, multidose; ODD, once-daily dosing; CNS, central nervous system.

INFECTIONS CAUSED BY OTHER *PSEUDOMONAS* SPECIES AND RELATED BACTERIA

Burkholderia cepacia Like *P. aeruginosa*, *B. cepacia* is primarily an opportunistic pathogen that is implicated in both sporadic endemic infections and occasional nosocomial outbreaks. *B. cepacia* is actually a complex of closely related bacteria, and the species is now divided into nine distinct genomovars based on molecular sequencing and bio-chemical analysis. Hospital epidemics are most frequently associated with a liquid reservoir or a moist environmental surface. Colonization by this organism precedes infection, and distinction between the two is often difficult. *B. cepacia* has been reported to cause pneumonia,

urinary tract infections, meningitis, peritonitis, surgical and burn wound infections, bacteremia, and endocarditis related to injection drug use. In addition, *B. cepacia* has been implicated as a cause of chronic lower respiratory tract infections in patients with chronic granulomatous disease, in patients with sickle cell hemoglobinopathies, and—together with *P. aeruginosa*—in patients with cystic fibrosis. For cystic fibrosis patients, chronic *B. cepacia* respiratory infection (especially that involving genomovar III) is of special concern, as it portends an unusually rapid decline in pulmonary function and a poor clinical prognosis. Moreover, in some patients with cystic fibrosis, *B. cepacia* has been associated with fulminant necrotizing pneumonia, bacteremia, and a rapid downhill course.

℞ TREATMENT

The treatment of *B. cepacia* infections typically is complicated by intrinsic resistance of the organism to several antimicrobial drugs, including many β-lactam agents, the aminoglycosides, colistin, and polymyxin B. Trimethoprim-sulfamethoxazole (TMP-SMX; 15 to 20 mg/kg per day for patients with normal renal function) is preferred for the treatment of *B. cepacia* infections, although acquired resistance to this agent has been reported. Carbapenems, third-generation cephalosporins, fluoroquinolones, minocycline, and chloramphenicol may offer activity against sensitive strains. For infections with MDR strains or those not responding to a single antibiotic, combinations of agents may display in vitro synergy and clinical efficacy. Some cystic fibrosis centers segregate patients infected with *B. cepacia* in an attempt to reduce horizontal transmission to uninfected patients. In addition, many centers consider lung transplantation contraindicated in patients with chronic infection due to genomovar III because of an unacceptably high mortality rate following surgery.

Stenotrophomonas maltophilia A ubiquitous free-living opportunistic bacterium, *S. maltophilia* has emerged as an important pathogen among hospitalized patients, particularly at cancer centers and in ICUs. Most infections are sporadic; however, nosocomial outbreaks of *S. maltophilia* infection have been linked to contaminated respiratory and inhalational equipment and water faucets. As with *P. aeruginosa* and *B. cepacia*, infection can be difficult to discriminate from colonization. Risk factors for either include prolonged hospitalization, malignancy, chemotherapy-induced mucositis and neutropenia, instrumentation (e.g., urinary, peritoneal, and central venous catheterization), and prior administration of broad-spectrum antibiotics. Intrinsic antibiotic resistance of *S. maltophilia*, based on both low outer-membrane permeability and inducible β-lactamases, is at least partly responsible for the emergence of this organism as a nosocomial pathogen under the selective pressure of antibiotic treatment.

Anatomical Site or Diagnosis	Preferred Therapy[a,b]	Alternative Therapy[a,b]	Comments
Bacteremia, endocarditis, wound infections, or pneumonia	Antipseudomonal penicillin *plus* aminoglycoside	Antipseudomonal penicillin *plus* ciprofloxacin (IV) *or* Antipseudomonal cephalosporin, aztreonam, or carbapenem *plus* aminoglycoside *or* ciprofloxacin (IV)	Bacteremia due to infection of an indwelling central venous catheter usually necessitates catheter removal. Monotherapy with an antipseudomonal penicillin, cephalosporin, carbapenem, or fluoroquinolone may be acceptable for patients without neutropenia, concomitant *Pseudomonas* pneumonia, septic shock, or life-threatening co-morbidity. Endocarditis: Use highest indicated doses from Table 136-3. MD is preferable to ODD for aminoglycosides. Serum aminoglycoside levels should be 10 times the MBC for the isolate. Valve replacement is often required. Wounds: Debridement is required. Pneumonia: Combination therapy should initially be employed for severe pneumonia if *P. aeruginosa* is highly suspected or confirmed by culture. Repeated or prolonged therapy may be required in patients with AIDS. Inhalational therapy for cystic fibrosis: Give 300 mg of tobramycin inhalation solution (TOBI) q12h via jet nebulizer.
Central nervous system	Ceftazidime *plus or minus* aminoglycoside	Cefepime[c] or ciprofloxacin (IV)[c] or aztreonam[c] or meropenem[c]	Aminoglycosides should be administered intrathecally for central nervous system infections not responding to initial IV therapy. Brain abscesses >2 cm in diameter require drainage.
Bone and joint	Antipseudomonal penicillin *plus* either aminoglycoside or ciprofloxacin	Antipseudomonal cephalosporin *or* aztreonam *or* fluoroquinolone *or* carbapenem	A 4- to 6-week course of therapy is often suggested. Limited data suggest that prolonged therapy with an oral fluoroquinolone may be equivalent to IV administration. Surgical debridement is often required for osteomyelitis that is chronic or associated with trauma, direct inoculation of bone, or extension from adjacent tissues.
Malignant external otitis	Antipseudomonal cephalosporin *or* carbapenem *or* ciprofloxacin (IV or PO)	Antipseudomonal penicillin or cephalosporin *plus* aminoglycoside	Surgical debridement is usually required. At least 4–6 weeks of therapy is suggested. Oral ciprofloxacin can be used with close follow-up for limited disease or after initial IV therapy.
Eye Keratitis and corneal ulcer	Tobramycin (14 mg/mL, topical solution[d]) *plus or minus* piperacillin or ticarcillin (6–12 mg/mL topical solution[d])	Ciprofloxacin *or* ofloxacin (0.3% topical solution[d])	Fortified aminoglycoside eyedrops require pharmacy preparation. Systemic antibiotics are reserved for severe infections with impending perforation or extension beyond the cornea (see endophthalmitis). If combination therapy is used, the second agent should be administered at least 5 min after the first.
Endophthalmitis	Same as for corneal ulcer above *plus* intravitreal amikacin (0.4 mg in 0.1 mL) *or* ceftazidime (2.25 mg in 0.1 mL)	Same as for corneal ulcer above *plus* intravitreal amikacin (0.4 mg in 0.1 mL) *or* ceftazidime (2.25 mg in 0.1 mL)	Surgical vitrectomy is usually indicated. Addition of systemic therapy with ceftazidime or an antipseudomonal penicillin plus ciprofloxacin or an aminoglycoside and subconjunctival injection of an intravitreal agent may be beneficial.
Urinary tract	Ciprofloxacin (PO or IV)	Aminoglycoside, *or* antipseudomonal penicillin or cephalosporin, *or* carbapenem	Relieve obstructions and remove foreign bodies (e.g., chronic urinary catheters and stones). Monotherapy is usually sufficient.
Dermatitis or folliculitis	None	None	Diffuse folliculitis related to spas, whirlpools, or hot tubs does not require therapy in normal hosts.

[a] Susceptibility testing should be performed on all significant *Pseudomonas* isolates in order to direct definitive therapy. Empirical antibiotic therapy for suspected *Pseudomonas* infections should take into account the institution's antimicrobial susceptibility patterns.

[b] Dosages for individual agents from each antimicrobial class are listed in Table 136-3.

[c] Clinical experience is limited for treatment of this infection with this agent. Addition of a second antipseudomonal agent is advised.

[d] 1 drop q5min X 1 h, then q15–30min for 24–48 h; frequency can then be gradually decreased.

Abbreviations: MD, multidose; ODD, once-daily dosing; MBC, minimal bactericidal concentration.

S. maltophilia has most commonly been associated with pneumonia but also causes bacteremia, urinary tract infection, wound infection, peritonitis, cholangitis, meningitis, and (rarely) endocarditis. Acute *S. maltophilia* pneumonia, an uncommon but devastating disease associated with bacteremia, is usually seen in debilitated patients in ICUs. Bacteremia is most often related to central venous catheter infection, although it may arise secondary to any focal *S. maltophilia* infection.

℞ TREATMENT

TMP-SMX is the drug of choice for the treatment of most *S. maltophilia* infections. Other agents include ticarcillin/clavulanate, minocycline, or doxycycline, either alone or in combination with TMP-SMX. The third-generation cephalosporins cefoperazone and ceftazidime and the fluoroquinolones are occasionally active against *S. maltophilia*, but in vitro susceptibility data may not reflect the clinical efficacy of these agents. The aminoglycosides and carbapenems are almost always inactive. Indwelling catheters or appliances that are associated with infection should be removed.

Melioidosis ■ *ETIOLOGY AND EPIDEMIOLOGY* Infections caused by *B. pseudomallei* (formerly *P. pseudomallei*) constitute a broad spectrum of acute and chronic, local and systemic, clinical and subclinical disease processes collectively called *melioidosis. B. pseudomallei* and the infections it causes are found mainly in the tropics and are endemic in Southeast Asia, northern Australia, and—to a lesser extent—southern Asia and southern China. Melioidosis is sometimes seen outside of these regions, however, in immigrants or travelers arriving from endemic areas.

B. pseudomallei is a free-living, small, motile, aerobic gram-negative bacillary saprophyte normally found in soil, ponds, and rice paddies and on produce from endemic areas. It is occasionally a pathogen for animals, but zoonotic transmission to humans is rare. Humans contract the disease during contact with *B. pseudomallei*–contaminated soil or water through exposure of abraded skin, percutaneous inoculation, nasal instillation, inhalation, or possibly ingestion. Unlike *B. cepacia*, *B. pseudomallei* does not cause colonization without infection and is only rarely transmitted from person to person. *B. pseudomallei* is listed as a category B biological agent by the Centers for Disease Control and Prevention (CDC) because of its potential to cause considerable morbidity and mortality if deliberately disseminated as a weapon of mass destruction.

MANIFESTATIONS Melioidosis presents in different forms. The infection may be acute, subacute, or chronic. High rates of seropositivity in endemic areas such as Vietnam, Thailand, and Malaysia suggest that many infections are clinically inapparent. The occasional diagnosis based solely on abnormal routine chest roentgenography represents asymptomatic pneumonitis. Acute pulmonary infections are the most common manifestation of melioidosis and may result from hematogenous spread or originate in the respiratory tract; these infections vary from mild bronchitis to extensive necrotizing pneumonia. Their onset may be sudden or gradual. Fever, rigors, productive cough, and marked tachypnea are common. More chronic pulmonary infections may present as productive cough, hemoptysis, and indolent fever with night sweats mimicking tuberculosis. Chest roentgenograms typically reveal upper-lobe infiltrates, occasionally with thin-walled cavities. Another common manifestation of melioidosis is an acute, localized skin infection with ulceration or abscess that is associated with nodular lymphangitis and regional lymphadenitis. Melioidosis may also present as suppurative parotitis, particularly in children. More rarely, *B. pseudomallei* may cause liver or splenic abscesses, septic arthritis, osteomyelitis, or genitourinary or central nervous system infection. Recrudescent disease arising from inactive sites of infection and perhaps triggered by intercurrent illness or other events may present in an acute or chronic form.

Either acute suppurative infections or pulmonary disease may give rise to hematogenous dissemination and the acute septicemic form of melioidosis. This progression is more likely in chronically debilitated patients, such as those with diabetes mellitus, chronic renal disease, or alcoholism. Septicemic patients may present with severe tachypnea, confusion, headache, pharyngitis, diarrhea, and pustular lesions of the head, trunk, and extremities. The skin may be flushed or cyanotic, signs of meningitis or arthritis may be apparent, the liver and spleen may be enlarged, and muscle tenderness may be striking. Chest roentgenograms show diffuse nodular densities that may expand, coalesce, and finally cavitate. The acute septicemic form of melioidosis usually follows a rapid downhill course, ending in early death. Mortality rates remain high despite optimal therapy.

DIAGNOSIS The diagnosis of melioidosis should be entertained when a febrile patient who has been in an endemic area presents with an acute lower respiratory tract illness, parotitis, lymphadenitis, or unusual skin or subcutaneous lesions or has a chest roentgenogram suggesting tuberculosis in the absence of sputum-associated tubercle bacilli. An etiologic diagnosis is suggested by the microscopic demonstration in exudate material of small, bipolar, irregularly staining, gram-negative rods with a characteristic "safety-pin" appearance and is confirmed by a culture positive for *B. pseudomallei* and/or a fourfold or greater rise in the titer of serum antibody to the organism.

℞ TREATMENT

The mainstay of treatment for melioidosis is antibiotic administration combined with appropriate surgical drainage of abscesses and aggressive support for patients with septicemic forms of the disease. The guidelines for antibiotic therapy are somewhat imprecise. Ceftazidime or carbapenems such as imipenem or meropenem appear to be the agents of choice for clinical disease, including severe infections. TMP-SMX, cefotaxime, and amoxicillin/clavulanate are possible alternatives. Fluoroquinolones are not active against *B. pseudomallei* and

have no role in the treatment of melioidosis. Combination therapy with ceftazidime or imipenem plus TMP-SMX may be indicated in severe forms of melioidosis, including septicemia. Unfortunately, the increasing resistance of many strains of *B. pseudomallei* to TMP-SMX, particularly in Southeast Asia, is of concern. Patients with acute pulmonary infections who are treated with either ceftazidime or carbapenems should receive antibiotics until they show definite evidence of clinical improvement (often in 10 to 30 days), at which time they can be switched to oral maintenance or eradication therapy with a combination of chloramphenicol, TMP-SMX, and doxycycline or with the single agent amoxicillin/clavulanate for 12 to 20 weeks. Chronic disease associated with persistently positive sputum cultures and extrapulmonary suppurative disease may require treatment for up to 1 year.

Glanders ■ *ETIOLOGY AND EPIDEMIOLOGY* Glanders is primarily a systemic equine disease that is caused by *B. mallei*. Once widespread, glanders was eradicated from North America in 1938 through the extensive culling of infected or exposed horses. The disease still occurs sporadically, however, in Africa, Asia, and South America. Historically, glanders was occasionally transmitted to humans during close contact with infected horses, mules, or donkeys. *B. mallei* is believed to have been used deliberately as an agent of biological warfare during World War I, an effort resulting in the infection of large numbers of Russian horses and mules. Research on *B. mallei* as an agent of biological warfare may have continued into more recent times, including work to develop an antibiotic-resistant aerosolized form of the bacterium. The first human case of glanders since 1949 was reported in the United States in 2001 and was acquired through laboratory exposure to *B. mallei* during the course of research on defense against agents of biological warfare and terrorism. Like *B. pseudomallei*, *B. mallei* has been classified by the CDC as a category B biological agent.

MANIFESTATIONS Glanders can assume the following forms in humans: acute localized suppurative infection, acute pulmonary infection, acute septicemic infection, and chronic suppurative infection. Disease develops several days or weeks after the inoculation of *B. mallei* into the skin, usually of the hand or arm. A localized skin nodule or suppurative focus is associated with regional lymphadenitis, fever, malaise, and prostration. Mucous membrane infection results in the production of a mucopurulent discharge from the eye, nose, or lips, with the subsequent development of granulomatous ulcers. Inhalation of the organism is accompanied by the typical symptoms and signs of pneumonia. The acute septicemic form of the infection may follow local infection and is characterized by signs of sepsis frequently associated with shock and multiorgan system failure. Evidence of acute *B. mallei* dissemination may include lymphadenopathy, splenomegaly, lung abscesses, lobar consolidation, liver and splenic abscesses, and a diffuse papular or pustular eruption resembling smallpox. Mortality rates from septicemic and acute disseminated disease are high. Chronic suppurative glanders presents as multiple subcutaneous, intramuscular, and visceral abscesses. Any form of glanders could follow aerosolized dissemination of the organism—e.g., in a bioterrorist event.

DIAGNOSIS The diagnosis of glanders may be suggested by the epidemiology and clinical setting of the infection together with evidence of irregularly staining, small, bipolar, gram-negative rods in suppurative exudates. *B. mallei* can be cultured and identified with standard bacteriologic media but may be misidentified as *Pseudomonas fluorescens* or *P. putida* by automated identification systems. Molecular methods, such as 16S rRNA gene sequencing, can be used for rapid identification of *B. mallei* from culture and can discriminate this organism from closely related organisms, including *B. pseudomallei*. A single high titer of serum antibody or a fourfold increase in titer suggests recent infection. A diagnosis of glanders in the absence of close contact with an infected equine should raise suspicion regarding the deliberate, bioterrorism-related dissemination of *B. mallei*.

℞ TREATMENT

Treatment of glanders includes appropriate supportive measures for sepsis and the surgical drainage of abscesses. Optimal antimicrobial therapy for glanders has not been adequately defined because of a lack of human infections in the antibiotic era. Ceftazidime, gentamicin, imipenem, doxycycline, and ciprofloxacin all have in vitro activity against *B. mallei*. A recent laboratory-acquired case of human glanders responded to a combination of imipenem and doxycycline, and experimental glanders in primates responds to a combination of sulfamonomethoxine (not available in the United States) and trimethoprim. It has been suggested that rational therapy for glanders should consist of the same antibiotics recommended for the treatment of melioidosis, with the specific agent chosen on the basis of in vitro susceptibility testing. As in melioidosis, long-term antimicrobial therapy is probably necessary. The antimicrobial susceptibilities of *B. mallei* organisms disseminated in the context of bioterrorism or biowarfare may not be predictable, given the possibility of bioengineered antimicrobial resistance.

Other Species *P. fluorescens* occasionally causes human disease; it is implicated particularly often in infections related to the administration of contaminated (stored) blood products and in pseudoinfections. Additional bacterial species that are associated only rarely with human infections include *P. putida*, *Pseudomonas luteola*, *Pseudomonas stutzeri*, *Pseudomonas alcaligenes*, *Pseudomonas pseudoalcaligenes*, and (all formerly *Pseudomonas* species) *Burkholderia gladioli*, *Burkholderia pickettii*, *Comamonas acidovorans*, *Comamonas testosteroni*, *Brevundimonas diminuta*, and *Brevundimonas vesicularis*.

FURTHER READING

ACHARYA A, PATERSON DL: *Pseudomonas aeruginosa*, in *Antimicrobial Therapy and Vaccines*, 2d ed, VL Yu et al (eds). New York, Apple Trees Productions, 2002, pp 549–562

BALTCH AL, SMITH RP (eds): *Pseudomonas aeruginosa Infections and Treatment*. New York, Marcel Dekker, 1994

MORRISON AF, WENZEL RP: Epidemiology of infections due to *Pseudomonas aeruginosa*. Rev Infect Dis 6(Suppl):S267, 1984

NEUHAUSER MM et al: Antibiotic resistance among gram-negative bacilli in US intensive care units: Implications for fluoroquinolone use. JAMA 289: 885, 2003

OHL CA, POLLACK M: *Pseudomonas aeruginosa* and related bacteria, in *Infectious Diseases*, 3d ed, SL Gorbach et al (eds). New York, Lippincott Williams & Wilkins, 2004, pp 1703–1717

SHEPP DH et al: Serious *Pseudomonas aeruginosa* infection in AIDS. J Acquir Immun Defic Syndr 7:823, 1994

SIMPSON AJ et al: Comparison of imipenem and ceftazidime as therapy for severe melioidosis. Clin Infect Dis 29:381, 1999

SMITH RS, IGLEWSKI BH: *P. aeruginosa* quorum-sensing systems and virulence. Curr Opin Microbiol 6:56, 2003

VARTIVARIAN S, ANAISSIE E: *Stenotrophomonas maltophilia* and *Burkholderia cepacia*, in *Principles and Practice of Infectious Diseases*, 5th ed, GL Mandell et al (eds). New York, Churchill Livingstone, 2000, pp 2335–2339

WHITE NJ: Melioidosis. Lancet 361:1715, 2003

137 SALMONELLOSIS
Cammie F. Lesser, Samuel I. Miller

Salmonellae constitute a genus of more than 2300 serotypes that are highly adapted for growth in both humans and animals and that cause a wide spectrum of disease. The growth of *S. typhi* and *S. paratyphi* is restricted to human hosts, in whom these organisms cause enteric (typhoid) fever. The remainder of *Salmonella* serotypes, referred to as nontyphoidal *Salmonella*, can colonize the gastrointestinal tracts of a broad range of animals, including mammals, reptiles, birds, and insects. More than 200 of these serotypes are pathogenic to humans, in whom they often cause gastroenteritis and can also be associated with localized infections and/or bacteremia.

ETIOLOGY Salmonellae make up a large genus of gram-negative bacilli within the family Enterobacteriaceae. In 1983, more than 2000 bacterial strains exhibiting a high degree of DNA similarity among their genomes were grouped into one species, *S. choleraesuis*. This species was further divided into seven subgroups based on host range specificity and additional DNA similarity. Almost all the strains pathogenic for humans are in subgroup 1 (*enterica* or *choleraesuis*) except for those causing rare infections [subgroups 3a (*S. arizonae*) and 3b]. The nomenclature of this large species is quite complex. For example, the correct taxonomic name for the organism that causes enteric fever is *Salmonella choleraesuis* ssp. *choleraesuis* (or subgroup 1), serovar *typhi*. A simplified system is commonly used in which the species name that predated the reclassification is accepted. For example, *S. choleraesuis* ssp. *choleraesuis*, serovar *typhi*, is referred to by its common name, *S. typhi*.

The initial identification of *Salmonella* in the clinical microbiology laboratory is based on growth characteristics. Salmonellae, like other Enterobacteriaceae, produce acid on glucose fermentation, reduce nitrates, and do not produce cytochrome oxidase. They are facultatively anaerobic and do not form spores. In addition, all salmonellae except *S. gallinarum-pullorum* are motile by means of peritrichous flagella, and all but *S. typhi* produce gas (H_2S) on sugar fermentation. Notably, only 1% of clinical isolates ferment lactose; a high level of suspicion must be maintained to detect these rare clinical lactose-fermenting isolates.

The genus *Salmonella* can be further divided into serovars based on the detection of three major antigenic determinants: the somatic O antigen [lipopolysaccharide (LPS) cell-wall components], the surface Vi antigen (restricted to *S. typhi* and *S. paratyphi* C), and the flagellar H antigen. In general, clinical laboratories initially divide *Salmonella* into serogroups (A, B, C_1, C_2, D, and E) based on reactivity to somatic O-antigen antisera. These initial groupings provide only limited clinical information since there is a high degree of cross-reactivity. Additional biochemical and serologic tests are needed to identify specific serotypes. Bacteriophage typing, plasmid profile determination, and pulsed-field gel electrophoresis analyses are used to determine whether a specific *Salmonella* strain within a serovar is responsible for an outbreak.

PATHOGENESIS All *Salmonella* infections begin with ingestion of organisms in contaminated food or water. The infectious dose of *Salmonella* varies from 10^3 to 10^6 colony-forming units. This variability probably reflects the ability of salmonellae to resist the low pH of the stomach—a powerful component of host defense. Conditions that decrease stomach acidity (an age of <1 year, antacid ingestion, or achlorhydric disease) or conditions that decrease intestinal integrity (inflammatory bowel disease, history of gastrointestinal surgery, or alteration of the intestinal flora by antibiotic administration) increase susceptibility to *Salmonella* infection.

Once salmonellae reach the small intestines, the bacteria again encounter numerous host defenses, including bile salts, lysozyme, complement, and cationic antimicrobial peptides—all components of the host's innate immune response. The salmonellae next penetrate the mucous layer of the gut and subsequently traverse the intestinal layer through phagocytic microfold (M) cells that reside within Peyer's patches. Salmonellae can also trigger the formation of membrane ruffles in normally nonphagocytic epithelial cells. These ruffles reach out and enclose adherent bacteria within large vesicles by a process referred to as *bacteria-mediated endocytosis* (BME). BME is dependent on the direct delivery of *Salmonella* proteins into the cytoplasm of epithelial cells by a specialized bacterial secretion system (*type III secretion*). These bacterial proteins mediate alterations in the actin cytoskeleton that are required for *Salmonella* uptake.

After crossing the epithelial layer of the small intestine, *S. typhi* and *S. paratyphi*, which cause enteric (typhoid) fever, are phagocytosed by macrophages. Once internalized, the salmonellae are protected from polymorphonuclear leukocytes (PMNs), the complement system, and the acquired immune response (antibodies). However, these bacteria must survive the antimicrobial environment of the macrophage, which includes the production of reactive oxygen and nitrogen species, antimicrobial peptides, and hydrolytic enzymes. Environmental signals within the macrophage trigger alterations in regulatory systems of the phagocytosed bacteria. The best-characterized regulatory system is PhoP/PhoQ, a two-component regulon that senses changes in bacterial location and alters bacterial protein expression. For example, PhoP/PhoQ triggers the expression of outer-membrane proteins and mediates modifications in LPS so that the bacteria's outer surface can resist microbicidal activities and potentially alter host cell signaling. In addition, salmonellae encode a second type III secretion system that directly delivers bacterial proteins from the phagosome into the macrophage cytoplasm. This secretion system is essential for survival within macrophages.

Once phagocytosed, salmonellae disseminate throughout the body in macrophages via the lymphatics and colonize reticuloendothelial tissues (liver, spleen, lymph nodes, and bone marrow). Patients have relatively few or no signs and symptoms during this initial incubation stage. Signs and symptoms, including fever and abdominal pain, probably result from secretion of cytokines by macrophages when a critical number of organisms have replicated. For example, the development of hepatosplenomegaly is likely to be related to the recruitment of mononuclear cells and the development of a cell-mediated immune response to *S. typhi* colonization. The recruitment of additional mononuclear cells and lymphocytes to Peyer's patches during the several weeks after initial colonization/infection can result in marked enlargement and necrosis of the Peyer's patches.

In contrast to enteric fever, which is characterized by an infiltration of mononuclear cells into the small-bowel mucosa, nontyphoidal *Salmonella* gastroenteritis is characterized by massive PMN infiltration into both the large- and the small-bowel mucosa. This response appears to depend on the induction of interleukin (IL) 8, a strong neutrophil chemotactic factor, which is secreted by intestinal cells. The degranulation and release of toxic substances by neutrophils may result in damage to the intestinal mucosa, causing the inflammatory diarrhea observed with nontyphoidal gastroenteritis.

It is not yet known why *S. typhi* and *S. paratyphi* cause systemic disease and are host restricted, whereas the vast majority of pathogenic *Salmonella* strains cause gastroenteritis in a broad range of hosts. Recently generated genome sequences show that *S. typhi* contains more than 200 pseudogenes, which appear to be functional genes in *S. typhimurium*. These pseudogenes may have been dispensable for *S. typhi* growth in humans.

ENTERIC (TYPHOID) FEVER

Typhoid fever is a systemic disease characterized by fever and abdominal pain caused by dissemination of *S. typhi* or *S. paratyphi*. The disease was initially called *typhoid fever* because of its clinical similarity to typhus. However, in the early 1800s, typhoid fever was clearly defined pathologically as a unique illness on the basis of its association with enlarged Peyer's patches and mesenteric lymph nodes. In 1869, given the anatomical site of infection, the term *enteric fever* was proposed as an alternative designation to distinguish typhoid fever from typhus. However, to this day, the two designations are used interchangeably.

EPIDEMIOLOGY In contrast to other *Salmonella* serotypes, the etiologic agents of enteric fever—*S. typhi* and *S. paratyphi*—have no known hosts other than humans. Thus, enteric fever is transmitted only through close contact with acutely infected individuals or chronic carriers. While direct person-to-person transmission through the fecal-oral route has been documented, it is quite rare. Rather, most cases of disease result from ingestion of contaminated food or water. Health care workers occasionally acquire enteric fever after exposure to infected patients, while laboratory workers can acquire the disease after laboratory accidents.

Over the past four decades, with the advent of improvements in food handling and water/sewage treatment, enteric fever has become a rare occurrence in developed nations. Over the past 10 years, ~400 cases of typhoid fever and even fewer cases of paratyphoid fever have been reported annually in the United States. In contrast, enteric fever continues to be a global health problem, with an estimated 13 to 17 million cases worldwide resulting in ~600,000 deaths per year. Children <1 year of age appear to be most susceptible to initial infection and to the development of severe disease.

Enteric fever is endemic in most developing regions, especially the Indian subcontinent, South and Central America, and Asia, and is related to rapid population growth, increased urbanization, inadequate human waste treatment, limited water supply, and overburdened health care systems. These conditions most likely account for the recent epidemics of typhoid fever in Eastern Europe. Antibiotic resistance among salmonellae is also a rising concern and has been linked to antibiotic use in livestock. Many *S. typhi* strains contain plasmids encoding resistance to chloramphenicol, ampicillin, and trimethoprim—antibiotics that have long been used to treat enteric fever. In addition, resistance to ciprofloxacin, either chromosomally or plasmid encoded, has been observed in Asia (India and Vietnam). Morbidity and mortality are increased in outbreaks associated with antibiotic-resistant strains, presumably because of inadequate or delayed treatment.

The high worldwide prevalence of enteric fever serves as a reservoir for cases in the United States. More than 70% of U.S. cases are related to international travel within 30 days before onset. Only 3% of travelers diagnosed with enteric fever give a history of vaccination against *S. typhi* within the previous 2 years. Of U.S. cases of internationally acquired enteric fever, 80% can be linked to travel in six countries: Mexico (28%), India (25%), the Philippines (10%), Pakistan (8%), El Salvador (5%), and Haiti (4%). While the percentage of cases associated with travel to Mexico is declining, travel to the Indian subcontinent is becoming much riskier, with an incidence 18 times higher than for any other area. The trend toward an increased incidence of multidrug-resistant (MDR) *Salmonella* (see "Treatment," below) in developing countries is reflected by the increase in the proportion of U.S. cases caused by MDR strains from 0.6% in 1985–1989 to 12% in 1990–1994.

Almost 30% of the reported cases of enteric fever in the United States are domestically acquired. Although the majority of these cases (80%) are sporadic, large outbreaks do occur. In 1993, 47 culture-proven and 24 potential cases were linked to contaminated orange juice at a resort in New York. Evaluation of this outbreak led to the identification of a previously unknown chronic carrier. Similarly, evaluation of 25% of the 571 cases of domestically acquired enteric fever reported between 1985 and 1994 led to the identification of previously unknown chronic carriers.

CLINICAL COURSE Enteric fever is a misnomer, in that the hallmark features of this disease—fever and abdominal pain—are variable. While fever is documented at presentation in more than 75% of cases, abdominal pain is reported in only 20 to 40%. Thus, a high index of suspicion for this potentially lethal systemic illness is necessary when a person presents with fever and a history of recent travel to a developing country.

The incubation period for *S. typhi* ranges from 3 to 21 days. This variability is most likely related to the size of the initial inoculum and the health and immune status of the host. The most prominent symptom of this systemic infection is prolonged fever (38.8° to 40.5°C, or 101.8° to 104.9°F). A prodrome of nonspecific symptoms often precedes fever and includes chills, headache, anorexia, cough, weakness, sore throat, dizziness, and muscle pains. Gastrointestinal symptoms are quite variable. Patients can present with either diarrhea or constipation; diarrhea is more common among patients with AIDS and among children <1 year of age. As stated above, only 20 to 40% of patients present with abdominal pain, although the majority have abdominal tenderness over the course of the disease. In general, the symptoms associated with *S. typhi* are more severe than those associated with *S. paratyphi*.

Early physical findings of enteric fever include rash ("rose spots"), hepatosplenomegaly, epistaxis, and relative bradycardia. Rose spots (Fig. 137-1) make up a faint, salmon-colored, blanching, maculopapular rash located primarily on the trunk and chest. The rash is evident in ~30% of patients at the end of the first week and resolves after 2 to 5 days without leaving a trace. Patients can have two or three crops of lesions, and *Salmonella* can be cultured from punch biopsies of these lesions. The faintness of the rash makes it difficult to detect in dark-skinned patients. On occasion, patients who remain toxic manifest neuropsychiatric symptoms described as a "muttering delirium" or "coma vigil," with picking at bedclothes or imaginary objects.

Late complications, occurring in the third and fourth weeks of infection, are most common in untreated adults and include intestinal perforation and/or gastrointestinal hemorrhage. These complications can develop despite clinical improvement and presumably result from necrosis at the initial site of *Salmonella* infiltration at the Peyer's patches of the small intestine. Both complications are life-threatening and require immediate medical and surgical interventions, with broadened antibiotic coverage for polymicrobial peritonitis (Chap. 112) and treatment of gastrointestinal hemorrhages, including bowel resection.

Rare complications whose incidences are reduced by prompt antibiotic treatment include pancreatitis, hepatic and splenic abscesses, endocarditis, pericarditis, orchitis, hepatitis, meningitis, nephritis, myocarditis, pneumonia, arthritis, osteomyelitis, and parotitis. Despite prompt antibiotic treatment, relapse rates remain at ~10% in immunocompetent hosts.

Approximately 1 to 5% of patients with enteric fever become long-term, asymptomatic, chronic carriers who shed *S. typhi* in either urine or stool for >1 year. The incidence of chronic carriage is higher among women and among persons with biliary abnormalities (e.g., gallstones, carcinoma of the gallbladder) and gastrointestinal malignancies. The anatomical abnormalities associated with these conditions presumably allow prolonged colonization.

DIAGNOSIS Since the clinical presentation of typhoid fever is relatively nondescript, the diagnosis needs to be considered in any febrile traveler returning from a developing country, especially the Indian subcontinent, the Philippines, or Latin America. Other diagnoses that should be considered in this patient population include malaria, hepatitis, bacterial enteritis, dengue fever, rickettsial infections, leptospi-

rosis, amebic liver abscesses, and acute HIV infection (Chap. 108). Other than a positive culture, no specific laboratory test is diagnostic for enteric fever. In 15 to 25% of cases, leukopenia and neutropenia are detectable. In the majority of cases, the white blood cell count is normal despite high fever. However, leukocytosis can develop in typhoid fever (especially in children) during the first 10 days of the illness, or later if the disease course is complicated by intestinal perforation or secondary infection. Other nonspecific laboratory results include moderately elevated values in liver function tests (aminotransferases, alkaline phosphatase, and lactate dehydrogenase). In addition, nonspecific ST and T wave abnormalities can be seen on electrocardiograms.

The diagnostic "gold standard" is a culture positive for *S. typhi* or *S. paratyphi*. The yield of blood cultures is quite variable: it can be as high as 90% during the first week of infection and decrease to 50% by the third week. A low yield is related to low numbers of *Salmonella* (<15 organisms per milliliter) in infected patients and/or to recent antibiotic treatment. Centrifugation to isolate and culture the buffy coat, which contains abundant blood mononuclear cells associated with the bacteria, decreases time to isolation but does not affect culture sensitivity.

A diagnosis can also be based on positive cultures of stool, urine, rose spots, bone marrow, and gastric or intestinal secretions. Unlike blood cultures, bone marrow cultures remain highly (90%) sensitive despite ≤5 days of antibiotic therapy. Culture of intestinal secretions (best obtained by a noninvasive duodenal string test) can be positive despite a negative bone marrow culture. If blood, bone marrow, and intestinal secretions are all cultured, the yield of a positive culture is >90%. Stool cultures, while negative in 60 to 70% of cases during the first week, can become positive during the third week of infection in untreated patients. Although the majority of patients (90%) clear bacteria from the stool by the eighth week, a small percentage become chronic carriers and continue to have positive stool cultures for at least 1 year.

Several serologic tests, including the classic Widal test for "febrile agglutinins," are available; however, given high rates of false-positivity and false-negativity, these tests are not clinically useful. Polymerase chain reaction and DNA probe assays are being developed.

℞ TREATMENT

In the preantibiotic era, the mortality rate from typhoid fever was as high as 15%. The introduction of treatment with chloramphenicol in 1948 greatly altered the disease course, decreasing mortality to <1% and the duration of fever from 14–28 days to 3–5 days. Chloramphenicol remained the standard treatment for enteric fever until the emergence of plasmid-mediated resistance to this drug in the 1970s. Given the increased mortality associated with resistance to chloramphenicol and the rare chloramphenicol-induced bone marrow toxicity, ampicillin (1 g orally every 6 h) and trimethoprim-sulfamethoxazole (TMP-SMX; one double-strength tablet twice daily) became the mainstays of treatment.

In 1989, MDR *S. typhi* emerged. These bacteria are resistant to chloramphenicol, ampicillin, trimethoprim, streptomycin, sulfonamides, and tetracycline. Like chloramphenicol resistance, resistance to ampicillin and trimethoprim is plasmid-encoded. In 1994, 12% of *S. typhi* isolates in the United States were MDR. Thus either quinolones or third-generation cephalosporins are currently recommended for empirical antibiotic treatment (Table 137-1). Despite efficient in vitro killing of *Salmonella*, first- and second-generation cephalosporins as well as aminoglycosides are ineffective in treating clinical infections.

Quinolones are the only available oral antibiotics for the treatment of MDR *S. typhi* infections. The greatest experience has been gained for ciprofloxacin (500 mg orally twice a day for 10 days). Shorter courses of ofloxacin (10 to 15 mg/kg in divided doses twice daily for 2 to 3 days) have also been successful. Limited data suggest that treatment with fluoroquinolones is associated with fewer treatment failures

FIGURE 137-1 "Rose spots," the rash of enteric fever due to *S. typhi* or *S. paratyphi*.

TABLE 137-1 *Antibiotic Therapy Options for Typhoid Fever*

Antibiotic	Dosage
First-line	
Ciprofloxacin	500 mg PO bid for 10 days
Ceftriaxone	1–2 g IV or IM for 10–14 days
Alternative (NARST[a])	
Azithromycin	1 g PO daily for 5 days
Ciprofloxacin	10 mg/kg PO bid for 10 days

[a] Nalidixic acid—resistant *S. typhi*.

and more rapid resolution of symptoms than treatment with β-lactam agents. However, quinolone resistance is emerging. In 1993, an outbreak of nalidixic acid–resistant *S. typhi* (NARST) infections in Vietnam was linked to chromosomal mutations in the gene encoding DNA gyrase (the target of the quinolones). NARST strains have also been isolated in India. Thus, all strains of *S. typhi* must be screened for resistance to nalidixic acid and tested for sensitivity to a clinically appropriate quinolone. Patients infected with NARST strains need to be treated with higher doses of ciprofloxacin (10 mg/kg twice a day for 10 days) or longer courses of ofloxacin (10 to 15 mg/kg in divided doses twice daily for 7 to 10 days) or with other antibiotics to which the strains are sensitive.

Ceftriaxone (1 to 2 g intravenously or intramuscularly) for 10 to 14 days is equivalent to oral or intravenous chloramphenicol in the treatment of susceptible strains. An alternative agent shown to be effective in an open-label study for the treatment of NARST strains is azithromycin (1 g orally once a day for 5 days or 1 g orally on day 1 followed by 500 mg orally for 6 days).

In cases of severe typhoid fever (fever; an abnormal state of consciousness—i.e., delirium, obtundation, stupor, or coma—or septic shock; and a positive culture for *S. typhi* or *S. paratyphi* A), dexamethasone treatment should be considered. In a single trial in Jakarta in the early 1980s in chloramphenicol-treated patients, treatment with dexamethasone (a single dose of 3 mg/kg followed by eight doses of 1 mg/kg, given every 6 h) decreased the mortality rate from 56% to 10%.

The 1 to 4% of patients who develop chronic carriage of *Salmonella* can be treated for 6 weeks with an appropriate antibiotic. Treatment with oral amoxicillin, TMP-SMX, ciprofloxacin, or norfloxacin has been shown to be ~80% effective in eradicating chronic carriage of susceptible organisms. However, in cases of anatomical abnormality (e.g., biliary or kidney stones), eradication of the infection often cannot be achieved by antibiotic therapy alone and requires surgical correction of the abnormalities.

PREVENTION AND CONTROL   Theoretically, it is possible to eliminate salmonellae that cause enteric fever since the bacteria survive only in human hosts and are spread by contaminated food and water. However, given the high prevalence of the disease in developing countries that lack good facilities for sewage disposal and water treatment, this goal is currently unrealistic. Thus, travelers to developing countries should be advised to monitor their food and water intake carefully and to consider vaccination.

Three vaccine alternatives are currently available: (1) a heat-killed, phenol-extracted, whole-cell vaccine (two parenteral doses); (2) Ty21a, an attenuated *S. typhi* vaccine (four oral doses); and (3) ViCPS, consisting of purified Vi polysaccharide from the bacterial capsule (one parenteral dose). In addition, an acetone-killed whole-cell vaccine is available only for use by the U.S. military. The minimal ages for vaccination with the Ty21a, ViCPS, and Vi-rEPA (see below) vaccines are 6 years, 2 years, and 6 months, respectively. A large-scale meta-analysis of vaccine trials comparing the whole-cell vaccine, Ty21a, and ViCPS in populations of endemic areas indicates that, while all three vaccines have similar efficacy for the first year, the 3-year cumulative efficacy of the whole-cell vaccine (73%) exceeds that of both

Ty21a (51%) and purified Vi (55%). In addition, the heat-killed whole-cell vaccine maintains its efficacy for 5 years, while Ty21a and ViCPS most likely maintain their efficacy for 4 and 2 years, respectively. However, the whole-cell vaccine is associated with a much higher incidence of side effects than the other two vaccines: 16% of whole-cell vaccine recipients develop fever and 10% miss a day of work or school, while only 1 to 2% of persons receiving the alternative vaccines have any fever. A fourth vaccine, Vi-rEPA, has been developed. This vaccine consists of Vi polysaccharide bound to a nontoxic recombinant protein that is identical to *Pseudomonas aeruginosa* exotoxin A; two parenteral doses are given. Coupling of the Vi polysaccharide to exotoxin A results in impressive T cell responses. In a trial in 2- to 5-year-old children, the vaccine provided 90% efficacy and was very well tolerated, with no serious adverse reactions. Trials of this vaccine in adults and infants are under way.

Although data on typhoid vaccines in travelers are limited, some evidence suggests that efficacy may be substantially lower than that for populations in endemic areas. The Centers for Disease Control and Prevention (CDC) currently recommends vaccination for persons traveling to developing countries who will have prolonged exposure to contaminated food and water or close contact with indigenous populations in rural areas. The only recommendations for domestic vaccination include people who have intimate or household contact with a chronic carrier or laboratory workers who frequently work with *S. typhi*. Given their decreased incidence of side effects and their similar short-term efficacy, the current bias is toward the use of Ty21a or ViCPS for vaccination of travelers.

Enteric fever is a reportable disease in the United States. Individual health departments have their own guidelines for allowing food handlers or health care workers to return to work. The reporting system enables public health departments to track down potential source patients and thus to identify and treat chronic carriers in order to prevent further outbreaks. In addition, since 1 to 4% of patients with *S. typhi* infection become chronic carriers, it is important to monitor patients (especially those employed in child care or food handling) for chronic carriage and to treat this condition if indicated.

NONTYPHOIDAL SALMONELLOSIS

EPIDEMIOLOGY   The incidence of nontyphoidal salmonellosis has doubled in the United States over the past two decades. Currently, the CDC estimates that there are 2 million cases annually, with 500 to 2000 deaths. Although more than 200 serovars of *Salmonella* are considered to be human pathogens, the majority of the reported cases in the United States are caused by *S. typhimurium* or *S. enteritidis*. The incidence of salmonellosis is highest during the rainy season in tropical climates and during the warmer months in temperate climates, coinciding with the peak in food-borne outbreaks. Morbidity and mortality associated with salmonellosis are highest among the elderly, infants, and immunocompromised individuals, including those with hemoglobinopathies and those infected with HIV or with pathogens that cause blockade of the reticuloendothelial system (e.g., patients with bartonellosis, malaria, schistosomiasis, or histoplasmosis).

Unlike *S. typhi* and *S. paratyphi*, whose only reservoir is humans, nontyphoidal salmonellosis is acquired from multiple animal reservoirs. The main mode of transmission is from food products contaminated with animal products or waste—most commonly eggs and poultry but also undercooked meat, unpasteurized dairy products, seafood, and fresh produce.

S. enteritidis associated with chicken eggs is emerging as a major cause of food-borne disease. *S. enteritidis* causes infection of the ovaries and upper oviduct tissue of hens, resulting in contamination of the contents of eggs prior to shell deposition. Approximately 1 in 20,000 eggs is thought to be infected with *S. enteritidis*. Between 1974 and 1994, there was a fivefold increase (from 5% to 25%) in the isolation of *S. enteritidis* from eggs in the United States; in 1998, the U.S. Department of Agriculture estimated that 80% of all salmonellosis cases were caused by infected eggs. Eradication of *S. enteritidis* from hens has proved difficult, given that infection is spread to egg-laying hens both vertically from breeding flocks and horizontally through contact with rodents and manure. Transmission via contaminated eggs can be prevented by cooking of eggs such that the liquid yolk is solidified or through pasteurization of egg products.

Another factor in the increasing incidence of nontyphoidal salmonellosis in developed countries, including the United States, is related to the centralization of food processing and widespread distribution. For example, a 1994 outbreak of ~250,000 cases was linked to a pasteurized ice-cream premix most likely contaminated in tanker trucks that had previously carried unpasteurized eggs. Similar outbreaks have been traced to manufactured foods including pasteurized milk, infant formula, powdered-milk products, paprika-powdered potato chips, and a ready-to-eat savory snack. In addition, large outbreaks have been linked to fresh produce, including alfalfa sprouts, cantaloupe, fresh-squeezed orange juice, and sliced tomatoes, contaminated by manure or water at a single site and then broadly distributed.

A less common source of nontyphoidal *Salmonella* infections is exposure to pets, especially reptiles. Fecal carriage rates in reptiles can be >90%. In the 1970s, 14% of cases of salmonellosis were attributed to small turtles; the U.S. Food and Drug Administration subsequently prohibited the distribution of these pets, with a resultant decline in rates of reptile-associated salmonellosis. However, since 1986, an increase in the popularity of nonbanned reptiles, including iguanas, has been followed by increases in rates of *Salmonella* infections. Other pets, including African hedgehogs, snakes, birds, rodents, baby chicks, ducklings, dogs, and cats, can also serve as potential vectors.

Antibiotic resistance is an increasing phenomenon among nontyphoidal *Salmonella* serovars. In particular, *S. typhimurium* of definitive phage type 104 (DT104)—a serotype resistant to ampicillin, chloramphenicol, streptomycin, sulfonamides, and tetracyclines—has become prominent in the United Kingdom. This serotype is associated with greater mortality and morbidity than other nontyphoidal *Salmonella* serotypes. Its acquisition is associated with exposure to ill farm animals and to a variety of meat products. The prevalence of *S. typhimurium* DT104 in the United States increased from 0.6% in 1979–1980 to 34% in 1996. Of concern is the isolation in the United Kingdom in 1996 of *S. typhimurium* DT104 strains resistant to ciprofloxacin (14%) or trimethoprim (24%).

Also of concern is the recent increase in ceftriaxone- and fluoroquinolone-resistant nontyphoidal *Salmonella* strains in the United States. The CDC reported that the prevalence of ceftriaxone-resistant strains increased from 0 to 0.5% from 1995 to 1998. Each resistant strain appears to be an independent isolate. The majority of resistant strains have been isolated from children, where the clinical use of fluoroquinolones is limited. The likely source of resistant strains appears to be cattle and chickens treated with ceftiofur, since 2% of *S. typhimurium* strains isolated from these livestock in the United States are also resistant to ceftriaxone. In addition, at least two outbreaks of fluoroquinolone-resistant *S. typhimurium* have been reported in this country. In each instance, the index case presumably originated in the Philippines. Fluoroquinolone-resistant *S. choleraesuis* has also been documented in Taiwan. One outbreak was associated with fluoroquinolone-treated swine; thus the source of these resistant strains also appears to be livestock treated with antibiotics.

CLINICAL MANIFESTATIONS ■ Gastroenteritis Infection with nontyphoidal *Salmonella* most often results in gastroenteritis indistinguishable from that caused by other bacterial and viral pathogens. Nausea, vomiting, and diarrhea occur 6 to 48 h after the ingestion of contaminated food or water. Patients often experience abdominal cramping and fever (38° to 39°C, or 100.5° to 102.2°F). The diarrhea is usually characterized as loose, nonbloody stools of moderate volume. However, large-volume watery stools, bloody stools, or symptoms of dysentery do not rule out the diagnosis. Rarely, *Salmonella* causes a syndrome of pseudoappendicitis or an illness that mimics inflammatory bowel disease.

Gastroenteritis caused by nontyphoidal *Salmonella* is usually self-limited. Diarrhea resolves within 3 to 7 days and fever within 72 h. Stool cultures remain positive for 4 to 5 weeks after infection and—

in rare cases of chronic carriage (<1%)—remain positive for >1 year. Antibiotic treatment usually is not recommended and in some studies has prolonged carriage of *Salmonella*. Neonates, the elderly, and the immunosuppressed (e.g., HIV-infected patients) with nontyphoidal *Salmonella* gastroenteritis are especially susceptible to dehydration and dissemination and may require hospitalization and antibiotic therapy.

Bacteremia and Endovascular Infections Up to 5% of patients with nontyphoidal *Salmonella* gastroenteritis have positive blood cultures, and 5 to 10% of these bacteremic persons develop localized infections. Bacteremia is particularly common and persistent among infants, the elderly, and patients with severe underlying infection or immunosuppression (e.g., transplant recipients, HIV-infected patients). Salmonellae have a propensity for infection of vascular sites; if >50% of three or more blood cultures are positive, an endovascular infection should be suspected. Preexisting valvular heart disease is a strong risk factor for the development of endocarditis, while atherosclerotic plaque, prosthetic grafts, and aortic aneurysms are associated with arteritis. Arteritis should be suspected in elderly patients who have a history of prolonged fever with associated back, chest, or abdominal pain preceded by gastroenteritis. Endocarditis and arteritis are rare (<1% of cases) but are associated with potentially morbid complications. Endocarditis can be complicated by cardiac valve perforation or by ring or septal abscesses, while arteritis can be associated with mycotic aneurysms, ruptured aneurysms, or vertebral osteomyelitis.

Unlike most nontyphoidal *Salmonella* serotypes, *S. choleraesuis* and *S. dublin* are frequently associated with sustained bacteremia and fever, often in the absence of a history of gastroenteritis. Similarly, these serotypes appear to be especially invasive and are often associated with metastatic infection.

Localized Infections ■ INTRAABDOMINAL INFECTIONS Intraabdominal infections due to nontyphoidal *Salmonella* are rare and usually manifest as hepatic or splenic abscesses or as cholecystitis. Involvement of the pancreas and adrenals and even an infected pheochromocytoma have been reported. Risk factors include anatomical abnormalities of the hepatobiliary system, including gallstones; abdominal malignancy; and sickle cell disease (especially with splenic abscesses). Eradication of the infection often requires surgical correction of anatomical abnormalities and drainage of abscesses.

CENTRAL NERVOUS SYSTEM INFECTIONS *Salmonella* infections of the central nervous system usually manifest as meningitis, although cerebral abscesses have been found. Meningitis is usually seen in neonates (<4 months old) and is associated with severe sequelae, including residual seizures, hydrocephalus, ventriculitis, abscess formation, subdural empyema, and permanent disability (e.g., mental retardation and paralysis).

PULMONARY INFECTIONS Nontyphoidal *Salmonella* pulmonary infections usually present as lobar pneumonia, sometimes complicated by lung abscesses, empyemas, pleural effusions, and bronchopleural fistulas. The majority of cases occur in patients with a preexisting abnormality of lung or pleura, including malignancy. Additional risk factors include sickle cell disease and glucocorticoid use. It is important to determine whether the pulmonary infection is in fact due to *Salmonella* or whether it is a secondary infection.

URINARY AND GENITAL TRACT INFECTIONS Urinary tract infections caused by nontyphoidal salmonellae present as either cystitis or pyelonephritis, usually in association with malignancy, urolithiasis, structural abnormalities, or immunosuppression (HIV infection, renal transplantation). Genital infections due to these bacteria are rare and present as ovarian and testicular abscesses, prostatitis, or epididymitis. Like other focal infections, both genital and urinary tract infections can be complicated by abscess formation.

BONE, JOINT, AND SOFT TISSUE INFECTIONS *Salmonella* osteomyelitis most commonly affects the femur, tibia, humerus, or lumbar vertebrae and is most often seen in association with sickle cell disease, hemoglobin-opathies, or preexisting bone disease (e.g., fractures). Prolonged antibiotic treatment is recommended to decrease the incidence of relapse and chronic osteomyelitis. Septic arthritis occurs in the same patient population as osteomyelitis and usually presents in the knee, hip, or shoulder joints. Reactive arthritis (Reiter's syndrome) can follow *Salmonella* gastroenteritis and is seen most frequently in persons with the HLA-B27 histocompatibility antigen. *Salmonella* can cause rare soft tissue infections, usually at sites of local trauma in immunosuppressed patients.

DIAGNOSIS Nontyphoidal *Salmonella* gastroenteritis is diagnosed when *Salmonella* is cultured from stool. All salmonellae isolated in clinical laboratories should be sent to local public health departments. In cases where there is concern about bacteremia (i.e., those including prolonged or recurrent fever), blood cultures are indicated. Once bacteremia is documented, it is important to determine whether it is high-grade (>50% of three or more blood cultures positive); if so, endovascular infection is possible and further evaluation to identify the source is indicated. In addition, depending on clinical symptoms and on whether metastatic disease is suspected, other body fluids, such as joint fluid or cerebrospinal fluid, should be cultured.

℞ TREATMENT

Antibiotic treatment is not generally recommended for *Salmonella* gastroenteritis. The symptoms are usually self-limited and have not been demonstrated to be altered by short courses of antibiotics. In addition, in case-control and double-blind placebo-controlled trials, antibiotic treatment has been associated with increased rates of relapse and prolonged gastrointestinal carriage. Dehydration secondary to diarrhea should be treated with fluid and electrolyte replacement.

However, preemptive antibiotic treatment should be considered in patients at increased risk for metastatic infection. These patients include neonates (probably up to 3 months of age); persons >50 years old (because of the high risk of atherosclerotic plaque or aneurysm); transplant recipients; and patients with lymphoproliferative disease, HIV infection, prosthetic joints, vascular grafts, significant joint disease, or underlying sickle cell disease. This group should receive a course of oral or intravenous antibiotics lasting for 2 or 3 days or until defervescence in immunologically normal patients. Limited data exist regarding the treatment of highly immunocompromised individuals; however, these individuals may require a longer course of therapy—perhaps 7 to 14 days, depending on the clinical scenario. Rare cases of chronic nontyphoidal *Salmonella* carriage should be treated with a prolonged antibiotic course, as described above for chronic carriage of *S. typhi*.

Focal infections or life-threatening bacteremia with nontyphoidal *Salmonella* should be treated with antibiotics (at the same doses used for enteric fever). Given the increasing prevalence of antibiotic resistance, empirical therapy should include a third-generation cephalosporin or a quinolone. If the bacteremia is low-grade (<50% of blood cultures positive), the patient should be treated for 7 to 14 days. Patients with AIDS and *Salmonella* bacteremia should receive 1 to 2 weeks of intravenous antibiotic therapy followed by 4 weeks of oral therapy with quinolones. Patients who relapse after this regimen should receive long-term suppressive therapy with a quinolone or TMP-SMX, as indicated by bacterial sensitivities.

If the patient has an endovascular infection or endocarditis, treatment for 6 weeks with intravenous β-lactam antibiotics is indicated. Chloramphenicol treatment has been associated with high failure rates and is not recommended. Limited case reports have described the successful treatment of *Salmonella* endovascular infections with quinolones, which may prove an alternative approach in cases caused by sensitive strains. However, concern remains about the development of quinolone resistance during prolonged therapy. Surgical resection of infected aneurysms or other infected endovascular sites is often required. If surgical resection is not possible, lifelong suppressive antibiotic therapy may be indicated. For extraintestinal nonvascular infections, 2 to 4 weeks of antibiotic therapy (depending on the site) are usually recommended. In cases of chronic osteomyelitis, abscesses, and urinary or biliary tract abnormality, surgical interventions may be required in addition to prolonged antibiotic therapy to eradicate infection.

PREVENTION AND CONTROL The incidence of nontyphoidal salmonellosis continues to rise along with rates of emergence of antibiotic-resistant strains. The increased centralization of food production plays a prominent role in the growing incidence, as one oversight can result in rapid, widespread distribution of contaminated food. Thus, it is important to monitor every step of food production, from handling of raw products to preparation of finished foods. In particular, with the increasing prevalence of *S. enteritidis* in egg-laying hens, it is recommended that pasteurized eggs be substituted for bulk-pooled eggs at all nursing homes, hospitals, and commercial food-service establishments. All cases of nontyphoidal salmonellosis should be reported to public health departments, since tracking and monitoring of these cases result in the identification of the sources of local outbreaks and help authorities anticipate large-scale international outbreaks. Lastly, the prudent use of antimicrobial agents in both humans and animals is necessary to minimize the further emergence of antibiotic-resistant strains.

FURTHER READING
COHEN JI et al: Extra-manifestations of *Salmonella* infections. Medicine 66: 349, 1987

GLYNN MK et al: Emergence of multidrug-resistant *Salmonella enterica* serotype *typhimurium* DT104 infections in the United States. N Engl J Med 338:1333, 1998

LIN FY et al: The efficacy of a *Salmonella typhi* Vi conjugate vaccine in two-to-five-year-old children. N Engl J Med 344:1263, 2001

MERMIN JH et al: Typhoid fever in the United States, 1985–1994: Changing risks of international travel and increasing antimicrobial resistance. Arch Intern Med 158:633, 1998

OHL ME, MILLER, SI: *Salmonella*: A model for bacterial pathogenesis. Annu Rev Med 52:259, 2001

TAUXE RV: Emerging foodborne diseases: An evolving public health challenge. Emerg Infect Dis 3:425, 1997

138 | SHIGELLOSIS
Gerald T. Keusch, Dennis J. Kopecko

DEFINITION *Shigellosis* is an acute infectious inflammatory colitis due to one of the members of the genus *Shigella*. Although the disease is often referred to as "bacillary dysentery," many patients have only mild watery diarrhea and never develop dysenteric symptoms. Less severe illness predominates in industrialized countries such as the United States, whereas more severe, often fatal dysentery occurs commonly in patients in developing countries.

ETIOLOGIC AGENT Shigellae are small, gram-negative, nonmotile bacilli and are members of the family Enterobacteriaceae and the tribe Escherichieae. They are so closely related to *Escherichia coli* that the two genera cannot be distinguished by DNA hybridization methods. In fact, shigellae are now thought to be differentiated pathogenic *E. coli*. The four *Shigella* species (*S. dysenteriae*, *S. flexneri*, *S. boydii*, and *S. sonnei*) are defined on the basis of somatic O antigens and carbohydrate fermentation patterns. Overall, there are 43 O serotypes of *Shigella*; *S. sonnei* is the only species that exists as a single serotype. Because acquired immunity is serotype-specific, an individual can be infected multiple times by different serotypes. Shigellae are classically lactose-negative; the exception is *S. sonnei*, which is a late, weak lactose fermenter. All shigellae produce acid but not gas from glucose; the result is a typical acid butt and alkaline slant in triple sugar iron agar without H_2S production. The genus is characterized by its ability to invade intestinal epithelial cells and to cause infection and illness in humans with a very small number of ingested bacteria, from a few hundred to a few thousand organisms.

EPIDEMIOLOGY Worldwide, it is estimated that at least 200 million clinical cases and more than 650,000 deaths due to shigellosis occur annually, primarily in developing countries and especially among children <5 years old. Shigellae are ubiquitous but have no known animal hosts other than higher primates. Poor environmental sanitation and crowding facilitate transmission from person to person. For example, a major outbreak took place in the makeshift camps for refugees fleeing the Rwandan civil war in 1994, with thousands of cases and high mortality.

The Centers for Disease Control and Prevention (CDC) maintain a national *Shigella* surveillance system based on data collected by state public health laboratories. In 2001, 10,598 isolates (primarily *S. sonnei*) were reported to the CDC, representing an apparent 45% decrease from 1991; this figure translates to an isolation rate in 2001 of 3.8/100,000 population—down from 6/100,000 a decade earlier. As in the past, the young were most susceptible, with one-fourth of isolates obtained from children <5 years old and another one-fourth from persons 5 to 19 years old. However, the reporting system seriously underestimates the number of infections occurring in the United States, both because some individuals are not sick enough to seek care and because no culture is performed in some instances when care is sought. Thus, the CDC-estimated number of *Shigella* infections in the United States approaches half a million per year. Rates are similar among males and females except among women aged 20 to 39; in this group, the rate is almost twice that among males, presumably because of greater contact with young children, especially those in day care. Cases are detected most commonly in counties with a relatively high proportion of low-income minority-group residents, including African Americans, Hispanics, and Native Americans; rates are especially high in poor urban communities, in day-care centers, and among retarded children in custodial care. Incidence rates in communities bordering Mexico are 228% higher than those in nonborder states; even so, they are several hundred times lower than those recorded among young children in many developing countries.

Since the discovery of the genus *Shigella* in 1896, major unexplained global shifts in the prevalence of its four species have been noted. Until World War I, *S. dysenteriae* type 1 was the predominant isolate, frequently causing devastating epidemics with high mortality until it was replaced by *S. flexneri*. Since World War II, *S. flexneri* has been steadily replaced by *S. sonnei* in industrialized countries. Since 1969, epidemic *S. dysenteriae* type 1 has reappeared in Latin America, in the Indian subcontinent and elsewhere in Asia, and in sub-Saharan Africa and has been associated with relatively high mortality rates due to multidrug resistance and inadequate diagnosis and case management. In contrast, *S. boydii*, the fourth species, has remained largely confined to the Indian subcontinent. The reasons for these epidemiologic trends are not clear. *Shigella* is highly host-adapted and is a natural pathogen only of humans and higher primates. It is transmitted from feces to the mouth, generally via direct person-to-person contact, although intermediate vectors such as food, water, flies, and fomites can be involved. In the United States, imported herbs and salads have recently caused multistate outbreaks. *Shigella* infection can also be transmitted during participation in recreational water sports in poorly chlorinated pools or lakes fecally contaminated by infected infants and young children and can spread rapidly among confined populations in close contact—for example, in day-care centers, in institutions for the mentally retarded, on cruise ships, or on military bases. Moreover, *Shigella* is transmitted by anal-oral sexual practices among gay men; although these infections were previously caused primarily by *S. flexneri*, *S. sonnei* now accounts for two-thirds of isolates. Similar trends are reported from Canada, Australia, and New Zealand. Rates of *Shi-*

gella infection and recurrent disease among HIV-infected individuals greatly exceed those in the HIV-uninfected population (Chap. 173).

Shigellosis is associated with a high rate of secondary household transmission. As many as 40% of children and 20% of adults who are household contacts of a case (generally a preschool child) develop *Shigella* infection. The infection is often symptomatic in children but asymptomatic in adults, presumably because of acquired immunity in adults. In contrast, epidemic disease due to newly introduced strains affects all ages, with severe and fatal cases occurring primarily in the very young and the very old. Prolonged asymptomatic carriage of *Shigella* in humans is uncommon; unless there is underlying malnutrition, the organisms are generally cleared rapidly. However, veterinary reports suggest that long-term asymptomatic carriage of *Shigella* by non-human primates is not uncommon.

PATHOGENESIS AND PATHOLOGY Shigellae enter the host via the mouth. Because they are genetically equipped to survive low pH, they readily pass the gastric acid barrier. An essential step in pathogenesis is invasion of the colonic mucosa and cell-to-cell spread of infection. It was originally thought that shigellae invade the host across the absorptive epithelial cells. However, the luminal surface of colonic cells appears to be resistant to invasion. More recent experimental studies show that *Shigella* uptake occurs primarily through the antigen-sampling M cells, resulting in initial limited penetration of the lamina propria, where the organisms encounter and are ingested by resident macrophages. Shigellae multiply within and trigger apoptosis of the infected macrophage, but not before initiating the production of the proinflammatory cytokine interleukin (IL) 1β. Viable shigellae released from dead macrophages then invade the basolateral surface of the colonic epithelium, spread from cell to cell via a novel host actin-based propulsion mechanism, and provoke the synthesis of IL-8 from the epithelium. IL-8 is a chemokine that induces the migration of polymorphonuclear neutrophils (PMNs) through the epithelial cell layer into the intestinal lumen; the tight junctions are damaged as the PMNs traverse the mucosa, and this damage allows further *Shigella* invasion and exacerbates inflammation. The consequences are mucosal ulcerations and characteristic dysenteric small-volume stools consisting of mucus, cellular debris, neutrophil exudates, and blood. The host inflammatory response is essential to disease pathogenesis, and its blockade by any number of interventions interrupts the cascade from invasion to illness.

After attaching to the colonic epithelium, shigellae induce their own uptake via a host endocytic mechanism (i.e., a phagocytosis-like process) in which the bacteria are initially engulfed within plasma membrane–enclosed endosomes. Subsequently, the bacteria dissolve the endosomal vacuole and are released into the nutrient-rich cytoplasm—a step that is essential for their intracellular replication. This intracellular existence also provides the organism with a means to evade extracellular host defenses, to move within the cell to the plasma membrane, and to spread directly from cell to cell via protrusions it creates at the interface between adjacent cells.

Many of the microbial virulence features as well as the host cell biologic responses occurring during pathogenesis have been defined during the past decade, and this information has led to the following understanding of this complex process: Virulence requires the function of multiple genes and regulatory elements encoded both on the chromosome and on a large (180- to 210-kilobase pair) plasmid present in all virulent shigellae as well as in enteroinvasive *E. coli* (EIEC, which causes a *Shigella*-like disease). Some of these gene products convey acid resistance, some mediate the endocytic cell invasion process, others underlie the subsequent escape from the endosomal vacuole, and still others underlie the movement of the organism to the plasma membrane, leading to cell-to-cell transfer. The plasmid-borne invasion genes encode a type III bacterial secretion system that, upon contact with the host cell, injects invasion effectors into that cell via needle-like microbial structures. These effectors cause an actin-dependent rearrangement of the local plasma membrane, which engulfs the attached bacterium into a plasma membrane–bound endosome.

Shigellae lack flagella and are nonmotile. To move within the cell, they have evolved a novel mechanism involving the formation of a growing tail of polymerized host actin created by the microbial protein IcsA (an ATPase) localized to one pole of the bacterium. Actin polymerization and cross-linking at one end of the bacterium propel it randomly through the cytosol. Some organisms reach the plasma membrane, where they form protrusions into the adjacent cell. When these protrusions are pinched off and the resulting double host-cell membrane surrounding the organism is lysed, the bacterium lies within the cytoplasm of the newly invaded cell, and the process is repeated. Inactivation of IcsA by host phosphorylases may serve as a molecular host-defense mechanism to modulate virulence by limiting microbial spread. Another important host protein essential for cell-to-cell spread is the cadherin L-CAM. Mutations in L-CAM alter the long finger-like protrusions induced by shigellae at the plasma membrane and impair their subsequent fusion with the adjacent cell. Once a single *Shigella* organism has invaded a host epithelial cell, the entire process of bacterial escape from the endosome into the host cell's cytoplasm, multiplication, and cell-to-cell spread can take place without exposure of the bacterium to the extracellular milieu and host immune defenses. Invaded host epithelial cells ultimately die.

Another property of apparent importance in the virulence of *S. dysenteriae* type 1 (which causes the most clinically severe form of shigellosis) is the ability to produce Shiga toxin, a protein encoded by the iron-regulated chromosomal gene *stx*. Related members of this toxin family are produced by some strains of *E. coli*, including serotype O157:H7. Such strains, designated Shiga toxin–producing *E. coli* (STEC), cause hemorrhagic colitis and hemolytic-uremic syndrome (HUS). Shiga toxins are composed of two distinct peptide subunits, each with highly conserved active regions. The first, located on the larger A subunit, is an *N*-glycosidase that hydrolyzes adenine from specific sites of ribosomal RNA of the mammalian 60S ribosomal subunit, irreversibly inhibiting protein synthesis. The second conserved region is a binding site on the B subunit that recognizes the receptor glycolipid Gb3 on host cells. Receptor specificity is determined by a terminal galactose $\alpha1\rightarrow4$-galactose disaccharide. Wild-type toxigenic *S. dysenteriae* causes more severe illness than does an isogenic toxin-negative mutant in an experimental monkey model. The related Shiga toxins all target endothelial cells and appear to play a role in the pathogenesis of the microangiopathic complications associated with toxin-producing shigellae and *E. coli*: HUS and thrombotic thrombocytopenic purpura (TTP). Two other *Shigella* enterotoxins, ShET-1 and -2, have been described; the former is restricted almost exclusively to *S. flexneri* 2a, whereas the latter is distributed more widely (e.g., in the physiologically similar EIEC). These two enterotoxins, encoded by chromosomal and plasmid-encoded genes, respectively, alter electrolyte transport by gut segments in vitro and cause net fluid secretion in ligated rabbit ileal loops in vivo. Although both toxins induce antibody in infected humans, their role (if any) in the pathogenesis of the watery-diarrhea phase of shigellosis remains uncertain.

The characteristic pathology of human bacillary dysentery is extensive ulceration of the epithelial surface of the colonic mucosa, with an exudate consisting of desquamated colonic cells, PMNs, and erythrocytes that may resemble a pseudomembrane in severely affected areas. Marked mucus depletion and increased mitotic activity are evident in the crypt regions and presumably reflect a response to the loss of surface colonic cells. The lamina propria is edematous and hemorrhagic and is infiltrated by neutrophils and plasma cells. There is also swelling of capillary and venular endothelial cells, with margination of neutrophils. At the ultrastructural level, intraepithelial-cell bacteria can be seen within endosomes as well as free in the cytoplasm. Histologic examination of colon from dysenteric humans shows an alteration of mucosal endothelial cells similar to that induced by endotoxin (lipopolysaccharide, LPS). Shiga toxin also targets endothelial cells, especially when toxin receptor expression is upregulated by exposure to LPS or proinflammatory cytokines. Circulating LPS is detectable in human shigellosis and is present in blood at especially high levels in *S. dysenteriae* type 1 infection, even without detectable bacteremia. Variation in the lipid A component of LPS is related to virulence—an observation that further suggests the importance of LPS in pathogenesis. One likely mechanism involves the ability of LPS to induce cytokine gene transcription and the strong association of cytokine secretion and inflammation. However, bacterial invasion of the colonic mucosa itself activates the transcription factor NF-κB, which is involved in regulation of cytokine synthesis. Cytokine-producing cells are present in the colonic mucosa of patients infected with *S. dysenteriae* or *S. flexneri* and in their stools as well. In fact, the number of cells producing IL-1, IL-6, interferon γ, and transforming growth factor β is directly related to the severity of inflammation. These inflammatory processes persist longer in children than in adults; this difference may reflect the lesser efficacy of the immune responses of the young in clearing the offending pathogen. Resolution of disease symptoms probably involves clearance of the organisms by both nonspecific immune defenses (i.e., PMNs and accelerated intestinal cell turnover) and specific immune defenses, with down-modulation of inflammation and repair of damaged mucosa.

Epidemiologic evidence indicates that protective immunity develops and is serotype-specific (i.e., LPS-related). Despite much effort, the precise nature of this immunity has not been elucidated. Common surface outer-membrane proteins involved in invasion elicit serum antibodies that, although cross-reactive among *Shigella* species and serotypes, do not seem to be protective. The serotype-specific determinants are likely to be the somatic antigens, as serum antibody to LPS predicts resistance to infection and evidence exists for IgA-mediated mucosal responses to LPS during convalescence from shigellosis.

CLINICAL MANIFESTATIONS Shigellosis in the United States, due primarily to *S. sonnei*, is typically a pediatric ambulatory disease, presenting as a self-limited nonbloody but inflammatory watery diarrhea containing many neutrophils. The clinical spectrum of shigellosis was clearly shown in an experiment in which adult volunteers ingested 10,000 virulent *S. flexneri* type 2a organisms. Approximately one-fourth of the volunteers never became ill. However, over the first 24 to 48 h, one-fourth developed transient fever, another one-fourth had fever and self-limited watery diarrhea, and the remaining one-fourth had fever and watery diarrhea that progressed to bloody diarrhea and dysentery. In young children in particular, body temperature can rise rapidly to 40° to 41°C, sometimes resulting in generalized seizures; however, they rarely recur or result in serious sequelae. Fever is part of a cytokine-mediated response to infection that includes anorexia and muscle catabolism initiating negative nitrogen balance; additional energy is consumed in raising body temperature. This response is of significance in patients who are already poorly nourished, sometimes precipitating severe protein-energy malnutrition that can lead to later death. Dysentery is a syndrome characterized by frequent passage (usually 10 to 30 times per day) of small-volume stools consisting of blood, mucus, and pus; this diarrhea is accompanied by severe abdominal cramps and tenesmus—the painful straining with stooling that may lead to rectal prolapse (especially in young children, in whom the ligamentous support of the rectum is still poorly developed). Severe dysentery most likely involves infection due to *S. dysenteriae* type 1, occurs less commonly with *S. flexneri*, and is least likely with *S. sonnei* or *S. boydii*. Patients with mild disease generally recover without specific therapy in a few days to a week. Severe shigellosis can progress to toxic dilatation and colonic perforation, either of which may be fatal. In developing countries, shigellosis almost doubles the risk of persistent diarrhea; the mortality rate increases by tenfold when persistent *Shigella* diarrhea develops.

Endoscopy shows the mucosa to be hemorrhagic, with mucous discharge and focal ulcerations and sometimes an overlying exudate resembling a pseudomembrane. The majority of lesions are in the distal colon, with progressively fewer in the more proximal segments of large bowel. Mild dehydration is common among patients with watery diarrhea; severe dehydration is very rare. With extensive colonic involvement, protein-losing enteropathy can occur and can have important adverse nutritional consequences, especially for already poorly nourished children. The majority of extraintestinal complications of shigellosis arise in patients in developing countries and are related both to the prevalence of infections caused by *S. dysenteriae* type 1 and *S. flexneri* and to the poor nutritional state of the hosts. For example, bacteremia, thought to occur relatively infrequently among patients with shigellosis in the United States, develops in up to 8% of patients hospitalized for shigellosis in Dacca, Bangladesh. The causative *Shigella* species is isolated from half of these patients, while other Enterobacteriaceae are found in the remainder. Bacteremia is associated with higher-than-usual mortality and is more common among infants (<1 year old) and among persons with protein-energy malnutrition. Persistent and clinically severe *Shigella* bacteremia has been encountered in the United States only in patients with AIDS (Chap. 173).

HUS may occur with *S. dysenteriae* type 1 infection. In the United States, STEC strains (such as *E. coli* O157:H7) producing high levels of Shiga-family toxins are the most likely causes of HUS. Manifestations of HUS usually develop toward the end of the first week of shigellosis, when dysentery is already resolving. Oliguria and a marked drop in hematocrit (by as much as 10% within 24 h) are the first signs and may progress to anuria with renal failure and to severe anemia with congestive heart failure, respectively. Even with advanced therapy, 5 to 10% of patients with HUS die of the acute illness. In addition, renal damage progresses slowly over several decades in survivors, some of whom will develop significant renal failure and require long-term dialysis or renal transplantation for survival. Leukemoid reactions, with leukocyte counts of <50,000/μL, usually accompany HUS; thrombocytopenia, with 30,000 to 100,000 platelets/μL, is common and in adults can lead to TTP, which is part of the spectrum of the toxin-mediated microangiopathy. Profound hyponatremia and severe hypoglycemia are also encountered, especially in developing countries, and may underlie central nervous system abnormalities such as seizures and altered consciousness. *S. flexneri* is associated with a rare toxic encephalopathy that is manifested by bizarre posturing and lethal cerebral edema.

Reactive arthritis is a less common extraintestinal manifestation that is usually associated with *S. flexneri* strains. In patients expressing histocompatibility antigen HLA-B27, the full triad of Reiter's syndrome sometimes develops weeks to months after diarrheal illness (Chap. 305). Pneumonia, meningitis, vaginitis (in prepubertal girls), keratoconjunctivitis, and "rose spot" rashes are rare events.

DIAGNOSIS AND LABORATORY FINDINGS Shigellosis is the principal bacterial cause of dysentery and should be considered whenever a patient presents with bloody diarrhea. However, in the United States, because *S. sonnei* is the most common infecting *Shigella* species, most patients present with fever and nonbloody watery diarrhea that are indistinguishable from the signs caused by other bacterial or viral agents of mild to moderate diarrhea. In this country, many patients with bloody diarrhea have STEC or *Campylobacter jejuni* identified as the cause. The specific diagnosis is based on culture of *Shigella* from the stool; sensitive and specific diagnostic methods based on the polymerase chain reaction have been developed but are not yet widely available. A commercial enzyme immunoassay to detect Shiga-family toxins in stool can identify most patients infected with *S. dysenteriae* type 1 (rare in the United States) or STEC within 3 h. The yield of *Shigella* in culture is increased if the patient has fecal leukocytes or bloody diarrhea. The organism is very labile and must be transferred quickly to plates or holding media (such as buffered glycerol saline) if it is to be isolated. Stool samples are preferable to swabs; when the latter are used, a rectal sample should be obtained. More than one differential selective medium should be used for culture—i.e., MacConkey and one other medium, such as Hektoen enteric or xylose-lysine-deoxycholate. Stool cultures to diagnose nonbloody watery diarrhea have a very low yield of positives and are not considered to be cost-effective in the United States.

Serologic tests can be performed, since antibodies to somatic antigens develop early in the acute phase of disease. However, the reagents for such tests generally are not available, even in the United

States, and serologic assessments are usually used only for epidemiologic studies.

The differential diagnosis includes inflammatory colitis due to other microbial agents: STEC, EIEC, *C. jejuni*, *Salmonella enteritidis*, *Yersinia enterocolitica*, *Clostridium difficile*, and the protozoan *Entamoeba histolytica*. Ulcerative colitis and Crohn's colitis are among the "noninfectious" conditions that should be considered (Chap. 276). All these infections except that due to *E. histolytica* are associated with the presence of large numbers of fecal leukocytes. Amebiasis can be diagnosed by the detection of erythrophagocytic trophozoites in the stool or by immunoassay (Chap. 194).

Other laboratory studies are nonspecific and may disclose neutrophilic leukocytosis, anemia due to blood loss with hemorrhagic diarrhea, prerenal azotemia, or (if watery diarrhea has been pronounced) hyperchloremic acidosis. Laboratory findings in shigellosis complicated by HUS are discussed above.

R_x TREATMENT

The mild to moderate dehydration in shigellosis is readily corrected with oral rehydration solutions (Chap. 140). The role of antibiotic therapy depends on the bacterial species involved and the severity of disease. Since *S. sonnei* infection is usually self-limited, culture results generally do not become available until the patient is better and there is little clinical need for further therapy. The use of antibiotics in severe cases with bloody diarrhea or dysentery reduces the duration of illness and can shorten the carriage state. Resistance to sulfonamides, streptomycin, chloramphenicol, and tetracyclines is almost universal, and many shigellae are now resistant to ampicillin and trimethoprim-sulfamethoxazole (TMP-SMX) as well. Knowledge of the pattern of resistance in a given population, which can change with time, is essential. In the United States, multiresistant strains are most likely to be acquired during travel abroad; therefore, for domestically acquired infection, either ampicillin or TMP-SMX remains the drug of choice unless resistance is known to be prevalent in particular communities (Table 138-1). Amoxicillin should not be substituted for ampicillin; it is ineffective because it is too well absorbed proximally and does not reach bacteria in the colonic lumen. Similarly, nonabsorbable antibiotics are ineffective because they do not reach the mucosal bacterial population. Short courses of treatment (1 or 3 days) or even single doses of a fluoroquinolone such as ciprofloxacin or the macrolide azithromycin have been employed with success. In developing countries, where resistance to ampicillin and TMP-SMX is commonplace, the drug of choice for the treatment of multiresistant *S. dysenteriae* type 1 infections is nalidixic acid; however, resistance to the latter agent is increasing in prevalence with its increasing use. The fluoroquinolones (e.g., ciprofloxacin, ofloxacin) are highly effective against all strains (Chap. 118) but are currently too costly for use in the developing world and are not yet approved for use in children <17 years old in the United States; these drugs have caused cartilage damage in young rodents during toxicity tests, although there is no evidence for a similar effect at therapeutic doses in humans. Alternative drugs shown to be effective include oral pivamdinocillin (amdinocillin, pivoxil, pivmecillinam; still not available in the United States), azithromycin, and intravenous ceftriaxone (50 mg/kg per day for 5 days). In small-scale clinical trials, 2 to 5 days of cefixime treatment resulted in the resolution of clinical symptoms due to *S. sonnei*, but the relapse rate was 20 to 24%. (Cefixime is not currently available in the United States.) Single doses of ceftriaxone may be effective, but more clinical data are needed. No antibiotic treatment is recommended for the convalescent carrier state, which usually lasts no more than a few weeks—i.e., for a much shorter period than is seen with nontyphoidal *Salmonella* or *Salmonella typhi*. Patients with AIDS can develop chronic carriage of *Shigella* and may be subject to relapsing infection with bacteremia (Chap. 173). This cycle can be interrupted by several weeks of treatment with a quinolone.

The role of antimotility agents such as atropine sulfate and di-

TABLE 138-1 Options for Oral Antibiotic Treatment of Shigellosis

Drug	Dose/Duration		Daily Cost ($US)[a]	Comments
	Children	Adults		
UNITED STATES				
Ampicillin	100 mg/kg q6h × 5 d	500 mg q6h × 5 d	$0.12/kg, liquid form $0.88, capsule form	Resistance varies with locale and is very common when infection is acquired abroad. Diarrhea is a frequent side effect.
Trimethoprim-sulfamethoxazole	10/50 mg/kg bid × 3–5 d	160/800 mg (1 DS tablet) bid × 3–5 d	$0.26/kg, liquid form $0.64, tablet form	Resistance varies with locale and is very common when infection is acquired abroad.
Ciprofloxacin	15 mg/kg q12h × 3–5 d; 500 mg max/dose	500 mg bid × 3 d	$0.17/kg, liquid form $10.80, tablet form	Resistance rates are low. Regimen is not licensed for use in children <17 years old, but there is no evidence of toxicity.
Azithromycin	12 mg/kg on day 1 (max, 500 mg), 6 mg/kg on days 2–5 (max, 250 mg/d)	1 g (single dose)	$0.37/kg day 1 (liquid) $27.00, adult tablet form	Single-dose regimen for adults is attractive but has not been tested in children.
Cefixime[b]	8 mg/kg (max, 400 mg) once daily × 5 d	400 mg/d × 5 d	$0.30/kg, liquid form $8.80, adult tablet form	Efficacy differs in different studies. Some studies show bacteriologic relapse rates of 20–24%.
DEVELOPING COUNTRIES				
Naladixic acid	55 mg/kg, divided into daily dose × 5 d	1 g qid × 5 d	$0.20/kg, children $16.00/d, adults	This is not an FDA-approved indication for either children or adults. Prices are likely to be lower in developing countries.

[a] Redbook 2003 average wholesale prices; for comparison only, as actual cost to pharmacies and charges to patients vary greatly.

[b] Cefixime is not currently available in the United States.
Note: DS, double strength; FDA; U.S. Food and Drug Adminstration.

phenoxylate (Lomotil) and loperamide (Imodium) in the early phases of shigellosis is controversial. Loperamide, in particular, may reduce diarrhea volume and in one study was highly effective in combination with antimicrobial therapy. However, antimotility drugs are suspected of enhancing the severity of disease by delaying excretion of organisms and facilitating further invasion of the mucosa, potentially increasing the likelihood of complicating toxic megacolon. Therefore, they are contraindicated in infants and young children. In adults, these agents are contraindicated for use in the dysenteric phase of disease.

Unique therapies are also being tested. Hyperimmune bovine colostrum containing high titers of antibody to *S. dysenteriae* type 1 LPS did not alter the clinical course of disease when coadministered with an effective antibiotic. An energy-dense diet did not improve the outcome of acute shigellosis in malnourished children but appeared to hasten the resolution of rectal prolapse. An interesting experimental approach is the use of engineered avirulent bacteria hyperexpressing Shiga toxin receptors to bind and prevent the biologic effects of the toxin.

Treatment of complications of shigellosis often differs in developed and developing countries. For example, antibiotic-unresponsive toxic megacolon, with or without perforation, is often managed by colectomy and ileostomy in the United States. Surgery is less often employed in developing countries because of a lack of surgical services or difficulties in ileostomy management; instead, management concentrates on antibiotic administration and conservative fluid and electrolyte support. HUS often requires dialysis; however, in developing countries, the threshold for dialysis may be higher than in the United States because azotemia is slow to develop and the risk of significant hyperkalemia is often diminished by a preexisting deficiency in total-body potassium due to malnutrition and wasting of lean body mass. The management of hyponatremia, usually caused by inappropriate secretion of antidiuretic hormone (vasopressin), is governed by the severity of the condition and the symptomatic state of the patient, as outlined in Chap. 41. Infusion of glucose can reverse clinical manifestations caused by hypoglycemia, and responses can be monitored by finger-stick blood glucose tests if no biochemistry laboratory is available. In developing countries, optimal nutritional management is needed to correct deficiencies due to underlying malnutrition as well as the superimposed catabolic stress and protein-losing enteropathy of shigellosis. Nutritional support should begin during the acute illness and is required for months thereafter (Chap. 63).

PREVENTION There are no licensed vaccines against *Shigella*, although considerable effort is being directed toward the development of a safe

and effective vaccine. Direct-contact transmission of shigellosis can be prevented by appropriate environmental and personal hygiene. Hand washing with soap and water when caring for infected infants, handling diapers, or preparing food is effective, and efficacy can be enhanced by the use of a triclosan antibacterial soap. Safe water supplies and sanitary latrines or toilets significantly reduce the primary and secondary transmission of *Shigella* infection. In highly endemic developing countries, infants are protected during the period of exclusive breast-feeding, which should be encouraged wherever HIV transmission via breast-feeding is not a consideration. Any measures that reduce the burden of malnutrition also reduce the burden of shigellosis in the population. Stool precautions should be instituted for hospitalized infected patients to ensure safe disposal of infected excreta and linens, and hospital personnel must wash and disinfect their hands and medical instruments (such as stethoscopes) after each contact with an infected patient. In the United States, cohorting of asymptomatic infected children, use of antibiotics to reduce infectiousness, and scrupulous attention to hygiene are usually successful in nosocomial outbreaks. Children in day care must be kept at home while clinically ill and ideally should have one negative stool culture before returning to the day-care facility. Likewise, food handlers who develop shigellosis should be culture-negative before returning to work. Antibiotic treatment is not indicated for the asymptomatic carrier state.

FURTHER READING

AHMED F et al: Epidemiology of postshigellosis persistent diarrhea in young children. Pediatr Infect Dis J 20:525, 2001

D'HAUTEVILLE H et al: Two msbB genes encoding maximal acylation of lipid A are required for invasive *Shigella flexneri* to mediate inflammatory rupture and destruction of the intestinal epithelium. J Immunol 168:5240, 2002

KOTLOFF KL et al: Global burden of *Shigella* infection: Implications for vaccine development and implementation of control strategies. Bull World Health Organ 77:651, 1999

LOPEZ EL et al: *Shigella* and Shiga toxin–producing *Escherichia coli* causing bloody diarrhea in Latin America. Infect Dis Clin North Am 14:41, 2000

MEAD PS et al: Food-related illness and death in the United States. Emerg Infect Dis 5:607, 1999

SHANE AL et al: Sharing *Shigella*: Risk factors for a multicommunity outbreak of shigellosis. Arch Pediatr Adolesc Med 157:601, 2003

ZIMBABWE, BANGLADESH, SOUTH AFRICA DYSENTERY STUDY GROUP: Multicenter, randomized, double blind clinical trial of short course versus standard course oral ciprofloxacin for *Shigella dysenteriae* type 1 dysentery in children. Pediatr Infect Dis J 21:1136, 2002

DEFINITION Bacteria of the genus *Campylobacter* and of the related genera *Arcobacter* and *Helicobacter* (Chap. 135) cause a variety of inflammatory conditions. Although acute diarrheal illnesses are most common, these organisms may cause infections in virtually all parts of the body, especially in compromised hosts, and these infections may have late nonsuppurative sequelae. The designation *Campylobacter* comes from the Greek for "curved rod" and refers to the organism's vibrio-like morphology.

ETIOLOGY Campylobacters are motile, non-spore-forming, curved gram-negative rods. Originally known as *Vibrio fetus*, these bacilli were reclassified as a new genus in 1973, after it was recognized that they were quite dissimilar to other vibrios. Since then, >15 species have been identified. These species are currently divided into three genera: *Campylobacter*, *Arcobacter*, and *Helicobacter*. Not all of the species are pathogens of humans. The human pathogens can be divided into two major groups: those that primarily cause diarrheal disease and those that cause extraintestinal infection. The principal diarrheal pathogen is *C. jejuni*, which accounts for 80 to 90% of all cases of recognized illness due to campylobacters. Other organisms that cause diarrheal disease include *C. coli*, *C. upsaliensis*, *C. lari*, and *C. fetus*. The major species causing extraintestinal illnesses is *C. fetus*; however, any of the diarrheal agents may cause systemic or localized infection as well. Neither aerobes nor strict anaerobes, these microaerophilic organisms are adapted for survival in the gastrointestinal mucous layer. This chapter will focus on *C. jejuni* and *C. fetus* as the major pathogens and prototypes for their groups; the key features of infection are listed by species (excluding *C. jejuni*, described in detail in the text below) in Table 139-1.

EPIDEMIOLOGY Campylobacters are found in the gastrointestinal tract of many animals used for food (including poultry, cattle, sheep, and swine) and of many household pets (including birds, dogs, and cats). These microorganisms usually do not cause illness in their animal hosts. In most cases, campylobacters are transmitted to humans in raw or undercooked food products or through direct contact with infected animals. In the United States and other developed countries, ingestion of contaminated poultry that has not been sufficiently cooked is the most common means of acquiring infection (50 to 70% of cases). Other modes of transmission include ingestion of raw (unpasteurized) milk or untreated water, contact with infected household pets, travel to developing countries (campylobacters being among the causes of traveler's diarrhea; Chap. 113), oral-anal sexual contact, and (occasionally) contact with an index case who is incontinent of stool.

Campylobacter infections are common. Several studies indicate that, in the United States, diarrheal disease due to campylobacters is more common than that due to *Salmonella* and *Shigella* combined. Infections occur throughout the year, but their incidence peaks during summer and early autumn. Persons of all ages are affected; however, attack rates for *C. jejuni* are highest among young children and young adults, while those for *C. fetus* are highest at the extremes of age. Systemic infections due to *C. fetus* (and to other *Campylobacter* and related species) are most common in compromised hosts. Persons at increased risk include those with AIDS, hypogammaglobulinemia, neoplasia, liver disease, diabetes mellitus, and generalized atherosclerosis as well as neonates and pregnant women. However, apparently healthy nonpregnant persons occasionally develop transient *Campylobacter* bacteremia as part of a gastrointestinal illness.

In developing countries, *C. jejuni* infections are hyperendemic, with the highest rates among children <2 years old. Infection rates fall with age, as does the illness-to-infection ratio; these observations suggest that frequent exposure to *C. jejuni* leads to the acquisition of immunity.

PATHOLOGY AND PATHOGENESIS Many *C. jejuni* infections are subclinical, especially in hosts in developing countries who have had multiple prior infections and thus are partially immune. Most illnesses occur within 2 to 4 days (range, 1 to 7 days) of exposure to the organism in food or water. The sites of tissue injury include the jejunum, ileum, and colon. Biopsies show an acute nonspecific inflammatory reaction, with neutrophils, monocytes, and eosinophils in the lamina propria, as

TABLE 139-1 *Clinical Features Associated with Infection Due to "Atypical" Campylobacter and Related Species Implicated as Causes of Human Illness*

Species	Common Clinical Features	Less Common Clinical Features	Additional Information
Campylobacter coli	Fever, diarrhea, abdominal pain	Bacteremia[a]	Clinically indistinguishable from *C. jejuni*
Campylobacter fetus	Bacteremia,[a] sepsis, meningitis, vascular infections	Diarrhea, relapsing fevers	Not usually isolated from media containing cephalothin or incubated at 42°C
Campylobacter upsaliensis	Watery diarrhea, low-grade fever, abdominal pain	Bacteremia, abscesses	Difficult to isolate because of cephalothin susceptibility
Campylobacter lari	Abdominal pain, diarrhea	Colitis, appendicitis	Seagulls frequently colonized; organism often transmitted to humans via contaminated water
Campylobacter hyointestinalis	Watery or bloody diarrhea, vomiting, abdominal pain	Bacteremia	Causes proliferative enteritis in swine
Helicobacter fennelliae	Chronic mild diarrhea, abdominal cramps, proctitis	Bacteremia[a]	Best treated with fluoroquinolones
Helicobacter cinaedi	Chronic mild diarrhea, abdominal cramps, proctitis	Bacteremia[a]	Best treated with fluoroquinolones; identified in healthy hamsters
Campylobacter jejuni subspecies *doylei*	Diarrhea	Chronic gastritis, bacteremia[b]	Uncertain role as human pathogen
Arcobacter cryaerophila	Diarrhea	Bacteremia	Cultured under aerobic conditions
Arcobacter butzleri	Fever, diarrhea, abdominal pain, nausea	Bacteremia, appendicitis	Cultured under aerobic conditions; enzootic in nonhuman primates
Campylobacter sputorum	Pulmonary, perianal, groin, and axillary abscesses	Bacteremia	Three clinically relevant biovars: *C. sputorum* subspecies *sputorum*, *C. sputorum* subspecies *bubulus*, and *Campylobacter mucosalis*

[a] In immunocompromised hosts, especially HIV-infected persons.
[b] In children.

Source: Adapted from Allos and Blaser.

well as damage to the epithelium, including loss of mucus, glandular degeneration, and crypt abscesses. Biopsy findings may be consistent with Crohn's disease or ulcerative colitis, but these "idiopathic" chronic inflammatory diseases should not be diagnosed unless infectious colitis, *specifically including* that due to infection with *Campylobacter* species and related organisms, has been ruled out.

The high frequency of *C. jejuni* infections and their severity and recurrence among hypogammaglobulinemic patients suggest that antibodies are important in protective immunity. The pathogenesis of infection is uncertain. Both the motility of the strain and its capacity to adhere to host tissues appear to favor disease, but classic enterotoxins and cytotoxins (although described and including cytolethal distending toxin, or CLDT) appear not to play any substantial role in tissue injury or disease production. The organisms have been visualized in the epithelium, albeit in low numbers. The documentation of a significant tissue response and occasionally of *C. jejuni* bacteremia further suggests that tissue invasion is clinically significant.

The pathogenesis of *C. fetus* infections is better defined. Virtually all clinical isolates of *C. fetus* possess a proteinaceous capsule-like structure (an S-layer) that renders the organism resistant to complement-mediated killing and opsonization. As a result, *C. fetus* can cause bacteremia and can seed sites beyond the intestinal tract. The ability of the organism to switch the S-layer proteins expressed, a phenomenon that results in antigenic variability, may contribute to the chronicity and high rate of recurrence of these infections in compromised hosts.

CLINICAL MANIFESTATIONS OF *C. JEJUNI* AND *C. FETUS* INFECTIONS The clinical features of infections due to all of the *Campylobacter* and related species causing enteric disease appear to be highly similar. There is often a prodrome, with fever, headache, myalgia, and/or malaise, 12 to 48 h before the onset of diarrheal symptoms. The most common signs and symptoms of the intestinal phase are diarrhea, abdominal pain, and fever. The degree of diarrhea varies from several loose stools to grossly bloody stools; most patients presenting for medical attention have 10 or more bowel movements on the worst day of illness. Abdominal pain usually consists of cramping and may be the most prominent symptom. Pain is usually generalized but may become localized; *C. jejuni* infection may cause pseudoappendicitis. Fever may be the only initial manifestation of *C. jejuni* infection, a situation mimicking the early stages of typhoid fever. Febrile young children may develop convulsions. *Campylobacter* enteritis is generally self-limited; however, symptoms persist for >1 week in 10 to 20% of patients seeking medical attention, and relapses occur in 5 to 10% of untreated patients.

C. fetus may cause a diarrheal illness similar to that due to *C. jejuni*, especially in normal hosts, or may cause either intermittent diarrhea or nonspecific abdominal pain without localizing signs. Sequelae are uncommon, and outcome is benign. *C. fetus* may also cause a prolonged relapsing systemic illness (with fever, chills, and myalgias) that has no obvious primary source; this manifestation is especially common in compromised hosts. Secondary seeding of an organ (e.g., meninges, brain, bone, urinary tract, or soft tissue) complicates the course, which may be fulminant. *C. fetus* infections have a tropism for vascular sites: endocarditis, mycotic aneurysm, and septic thrombophlebitis may all occur. Infection during pregnancy often leads to fetal death. *H. cinaedi* causes recurrent cellulitis with fever and bacteremia in immunocompromised hosts.

COMPLICATIONS Except in the case of infection with *C. fetus*, bacteremia is uncommon, developing most often in immunocompromised hosts and at the extremes of age. Three patterns of extraintestinal infection have been noted: (1) transient bacteremia in a normal host with enteritis (benign course, no specific treatment needed); (2) sustained bacteremia or focal infection in a normal host (bacteremia originating from enteritis, with patients responding well to antimicrobial therapy); and (3) sustained bacteremia or focal infection in a compromised host. Enteritis may not be clinically apparent. Antimicrobial therapy, possibly prolonged, is necessary for suppression or cure of the infection.

Campylobacter infections in patients with AIDS or hypogammaglobulinemia may be severe, persistent, and extraintestinal; relapse after cessation of therapy is common. Hypogammaglobulinemic patients may also develop osteomyelitis and an erysipelas-like rash.

Local suppurative complications of infection include cholecystitis, pancreatitis, and cystitis; distant complications include meningitis, endocarditis, arthritis, peritonitis, cellulitis, and septic abortion. All are rare. Hepatitis, interstitial nephritis, and the hemolytic-uremic syndrome occasionally complicate acute infection. Reactive arthritis and other rheumatologic complaints may develop several weeks after infection, especially in persons with the HLA-B27 phenotype. Guillain-Barré syndrome follows *Campylobacter* infections uncommonly (i.e., in 1 of every 1000 to 2000 cases). For certain *C. jejuni* serotypes, such as O19, Guillain-Barré syndrome may occur once following 100 or 200 cases. Because of their high incidence, it is now estimated that *Campylobacter* infections may trigger 20 to 40% of all cases of Guillain-Barré syndrome.

DIAGNOSIS In patients with *Campylobacter* enteritis, peripheral leukocyte counts reflect the severity of the inflammatory process. However, stools from nearly all *Campylobacter*-infected patients presenting for medical attention in the United States contain leukocytes or erythrocytes. Fecal smears should be treated with Gram's or Wright's stain and examined in all suspected cases. When the diagnosis of *Campylobacter* enteritis is suspected on the basis of findings indicating inflammatory diarrhea (fever, fecal leukocytes), clinicians can ask the laboratory to attempt the visualization of organisms with characteristic vibrioid morphology by direct microscopic examination of stools with Gram's staining or to use phase-contrast or dark-field microscopy to identify the organisms' characteristic "darting" motility. Confirmation of the diagnosis of *Campylobacter* infection is based on identification of an isolate from cultures of stool, blood, or another site. *Campylobacter*-specific media should be used to culture stools from all patients with inflammatory or bloody diarrhea. Since all *Campylobacter* species are fastidious, they will not be isolated unless selective media or other selective techniques are used. Not all media are equally useful for isolation of the broad array of campylobacters; therefore, failure to isolate campylobacters from stool does not entirely rule out their presence. The detection of the organisms in stool almost always implies infection; there is a brief period of postconvalescent fecal carriage and no commensalism in humans. In contrast, *C. sputorum* and related organisms found in the oral cavity are commensals with rare pathogenic significance.

DIFFERENTIAL DIAGNOSIS The symptoms of *Campylobacter* enteritis are not sufficiently unusual to distinguish this illness from that due to *Salmonella*, *Shigella*, or *Yersinia*, among other pathogens. The combination of fever and fecal leukocytes or erythrocytes is indicative of inflammatory diarrhea, and definitive diagnosis is based on culture or demonstration of the characteristic organisms on stained fecal smears. Similarly, extraintestinal *Campylobacter* illness is diagnosed by culture. Infection due to *Campylobacter* should be suspected in the setting of septic abortion and that due to *C. fetus* specifically in the setting of septic thrombophlebitis. It is important to reiterate that the presentation of *Campylobacter* enteritis may mimic that of ulcerative colitis or Crohn's disease, that *Campylobacter* enteritis is much more common than either of the latter (especially among young adults), and that biopsy may not be able to distinguish among these entities. Thus a diagnosis of inflammatory bowel disease should not be made until *Campylobacter* infection has been ruled out, especially in persons with a history of foreign travel, significant animal contact, immunodeficiency, or exposure incurring a high risk of transmission.

℞ TREATMENT

Fluid and electrolyte replacement is central to the treatment of diarrheal illnesses (Chap. 113). Even among patients presenting for medical attention with *Campylobacter* enteritis, fewer than half will clearly benefit from specific antimicrobial therapy. Indications for such therapy include high fever, bloody diarrhea, severe diarrhea, persistence for >1 week, and worsening of symptoms. A 5- to 7-day course of erythromycin (250 mg orally four times daily or—for children—30 to 50 mg/kg per day, in divided doses) is the regimen of choice. Although no relevant clinical trials have been conducted, the in vitro susceptibility of *Campylobacter* species to macrolides such as clarithromycin and azithromycin suggests that these antibiotics would also be useful therapeutic agents. An alternative regimen for adults is ciprofloxacin (500 mg orally twice daily) or another fluoroquinolone for 5 to 7 days, but resistance to this class of agents is increasing. Other alternatives include tetracycline and furazolidone. Use of antimotility agents, which may prolong the duration of symptoms and has been associated with toxic megacolon and with death, is not recommended.

For systemic infections, treatment with gentamicin (1.7 mg/kg intravenously every 8 h after a loading dose of 2 mg/kg), imipenem (500 mg intravenously every 6 h), or chloramphenicol (50 mg/kg intravenously each day in three or four divided doses) should be started empirically, but susceptibility testing should then be performed. Ciprofloxacin and amoxicillin/clavulanate are alternative agents for susceptible strains. In the absence of immunocompromise or endovascular infections, therapy should be administered for 14 days. For immunocompromised patients with systemic infections due to *C. fetus* and for patients with endovascular infections, prolonged therapy (for up to 4 weeks) is usually necessary.

PROGNOSIS Nearly all patients recover fully from *Campylobacter* enteritis, either spontaneously or after antimicrobial therapy. Volume depletion likely contributes to the few deaths that are reported. As stated above, occasional patients develop reactive arthritis or Guillain-Barré syndrome. Systemic infection with *C. fetus* is much more often fatal than that due to related species; this higher mortality reflects in part the population affected. Prognosis is dependent on the rapidity with which appropriate therapy is begun. Otherwise healthy hosts usually survive *C. fetus* infections without sequelae. Compromised hosts often have recurrent infections.

FURTHER READING

ALLOS BM, BLASER MJ: *Campylobacter jejuni* and the expanding spectrum of related infections. Clin Infect Dis 20:1092, 1995

LANG DR et al (eds): Development of Guillain-Barré syndrome following *Campylobacter* infection. J Infect Dis 176(Suppl 2):S91, 1997

MEAD PS et al: Food-related illness and death in the United States. Emerg Infect Dis 5:607, 1999

NACHAMKIN I, BLASER MJ (eds): *Campylobacter jejuni*, 2d ed. Washington, American Society for Microbiology, 2000

SMITH KE et al: Quinolone-resistant *Campylobacter jejuni* infections in Minnesota, 1992–1998. Investigation Team. N Engl J Med 340:1525, 1999

140 CHOLERA AND OTHER VIBRIOSES
Matthew K. Waldor, Gerald T. Keusch

Members of the genus *Vibrio* cause a number of important infectious syndromes. Classic among them is cholera, a devastating diarrheal disease caused by *V. cholerae* that has been responsible for seven global pandemics and much suffering over the past two centuries. Epidemic cholera remains a significant public health concern in the developing world today. Other vibrioses have also been described, including syndromes of diarrhea, soft tissue infection, or primary sepsis caused by additional named species in the genus *Vibrio*.

All members of the genus are highly motile, facultatively anaerobic, curved gram-negative rods with one or more flagella. Except for *V. cholerae* and *V. mimicus*, all vibrios are halophilic (i.e., require salt for growth). In nature, vibrios most commonly reside in tidal rivers and bays under conditions of moderate salinity. They proliferate in the summer months when water temperatures exceed 20°C. As might be expected, the illnesses they cause also increase in frequency during the warm months.

CHOLERA

DEFINITION Cholera is an acute diarrheal disease that can, in a matter of hours, result in profound, rapidly progressive dehydration and death. Accordingly, cholera gravis (the severe form of cholera) is a much-feared disease, particularly in its epidemic presentation. Fortunately, prompt aggressive fluid repletion and supportive care can obviate the high mortality that cholera has historically wrought. While the term *cholera* has occasionally been applied to any severely dehydrating secretory diarrheal illness, whether infectious in etiology or not, it has generally referred to disease caused by *V. cholerae* serogroup O1. In 1992, however, a new serogroup (O139) that causes epidemic cholera emerged on the Indian subcontinent and has since killed thousands of people.

MICROBIOLOGY AND EPIDEMIOLOGY The species *V. cholerae* comprises a host of organisms classified on the basis of the carbohydrate determinants of their lipopolysaccharide (LPS) O antigens. Some 200 serogroups have now been recognized. They are divided into those that agglutinate in antisera to the O1 group antigen (*V. cholerae* O1) and those that do not (non-O1 *V. cholerae*). Although some non-O1 *V. cholerae* serogroups have occasionally caused sporadic outbreaks of diarrhea, serogroup O1 was, until the emergence of serogroup O139, the exclusive cause of epidemic cholera.

Two biotypes of *V. cholerae* O1, *classical* and *El Tor*, are distinguished. Each biotype is further subdivided into two serotypes, termed *Inaba* and *Ogawa*.

The natural habitat of *V. cholerae* is coastal salt water and brackish estuaries, where the organism lives in close relation to plankton and where it may survive in a viable but nonculturable form. Humans become infected incidentally but, once infected, can act as vehicles for spread. Ingestion of water contaminated by human feces is the most common means of acquisition of *V. cholerae*. Consumption of contaminated food can also contribute to spread. There is no known animal reservoir. While the infectious dose is relatively high, it is markedly reduced in hypochlorhydric persons, in those using antacids, and when gastric acidity is buffered by a meal. Cholera is predominantly a pediatric disease in endemic areas, but it affects adults and children equally when newly introduced into a population. In endemic areas, the disease is more common in the summer and fall months. While this seasonality has not been explained fully, it may be due to environmental conditions that affect the multiplication of vibrios or to seasonal alterations in human behavior that affect contact with water. In endemic areas, children <2 years of age are less likely to develop severe cholera than are older children, perhaps because of passive immunity acquired from breast milk. For unexplained reasons, susceptibility to cholera is significantly influenced by ABO blood group status; those with type O blood are at greatest risk, while those with type AB are at least risk.

Cholera is native to the Ganges delta in the Indian subcontinent. Since 1817, seven global pandemics have occurred. The current (seventh) pandemic—the first due to the El Tor biotype—began in Indonesia in 1961 and spread throughout Asia as *V. cholerae* El Tor displaced the endemic classical strain in many areas. In the early 1970s, El Tor cholera exploded in Africa, causing major epidemics before becoming a persistent endemic problem. Its recent history in Africa has been punctuated by severe outbreaks, often fed by the chaos of war and genocide. Such was the case in the camps for Rwandan refugees set up in 1994 around Goma, Zaire. Tens of thousands of cases occurred and mortality was high. In 1995, the occurrence of hundreds of cases in Romania and the Black Sea states of the former Soviet Union demonstrated the potential of this organism to cause epidemics whenever public health measures break down.

Since 1973, sporadic endemic infections due to vibrios related to the seventh-pandemic strain have been recognized along the U.S. Gulf Coast of Louisiana and Texas. These infections are typically associated with the consumption of contaminated, locally harvested shellfish. Occasionally, cases in U.S. locations remote from the Gulf Coast have been linked to shipped-in Gulf Coast seafood.

It was not until 1991 that the current cholera pandemic reached Latin America. Beginning along the Peruvian coast in January 1991, the disease spread in an explosive epidemic to virtually all of South and Central America and to Mexico (Fig. 140-1). About 400,000 cases were reported in the first year of the outbreak, and >1 million had been reported by the end of 1994. While the cumulative mortality rate has been <1%, the mortality rate approached 30% in the communities first affected, where a lack of familiarity with the disease led initially to the deployment of ineffective treatment. Intensive education of health care providers and of the community at large has enhanced awareness of the disease and its appropriate management and has greatly diminished mortality. As it did in Africa two decades earlier, the epidemic El Tor strain proved capable of establishing itself in inland waters rather than in its classic niche of coastal salt waters; the organism has already become endemic in many of the Latin American countries into which it was recently introduced. Cases linked to the Latin American epidemic have occurred (via importation of contaminated seafood) in the United States. Although secondary spread of this strain has not taken place in the United States, these events underscore the need for vigilance among health care professionals, even in locations remote from an epidemic.

In October 1992, a large-scale outbreak of clinical cholera occurred in southeastern India. The etiologic agent proved to be a novel strain of *V. cholerae* belonging neither to the O1 serogroup that typically causes epidemic cholera nor to any of the 137 other serogroups known at the time. This strain spread rapidly up and down the coast of the Bay of Bengal, reaching Bangladesh in December 1992. There alone, it caused more than 100,000 cases of cholera in the first 3 months of 1993. It subsequently spread across the Indian subcontinent and to neighboring countries, affecting Pakistan, Nepal, western China, Thailand, and Malaysia by the end of 1994 (Fig. 140-2). The organism has since been designated *V. cholerae* O139 Bengal in recognition of its novel O antigen and its geographic origin. The clinical manifestations and epidemiologic features of the disease caused by *V. cholerae* O139

Initial Epidemic, October 1992

——— March 1993

——— October 1994

FIGURE 140-2   Spread of *Vibrio cholerae* O139 in the Indian subcontinent and elsewhere in Asia, 1992–1994. *(Courtesy of Dr. Robert V. Tauxe, Centers for Disease Control and Prevention, Atlanta.)*

Bengal are indistinguishable from those of O1 cholera. Immunity to the latter, however, is not protective against the former. Because naturally acquired immunity to *V. cholerae* O1 does not cross-protect against *V. cholerae* O139 Bengal, vaccines being developed against the former are unlikely to be effective against the latter.

Some authorities believed that the emergence of *V. cholerae* O139 signaled the beginning of the eighth global cholera pandemic. Indeed, just as O1 El Tor replaced the classical biotype that preceded it, O139 Bengal in 1993 rapidly replaced O1 El Tor as the most common environmental isolate and the predominant cause of clinical cholera in the areas in which it had appeared. However, by the beginning of 1994, O1 El Tor resumed its dominance in Bangladesh. Currently, in most regions of Southest Asia, O1 *V. cholerae* remains dominant; in others, O139 periodically reemerges.

PATHOGENESIS   In the final analysis, cholera is a toxin-mediated disease. Its characteristic watery diarrhea is due to the action of cholera toxin (CT), a potent protein enterotoxin elaborated by the organism following its colonization of the small intestine. For *V. cholerae* to colonize the small intestine and produce CT, it must first recognize, contend with, and traverse several hostile environments. The first of these is the acidic milieu of the stomach. To elude the bactericidal effects of gastric acidity, *V. cholerae* relies, at least in part, on a relatively large inoculum size (compared to that needed for colonization by *Shigella*, for instance). The organism must next traverse the mucous layer lining the small bowel. *V. cholerae* chemotaxis and motility and a variety of proteases may allow the organism to traverse this gel covering the intestinal epithelium. Adherence to the intestinal epithelium is believed to be mediated by the toxin-coregulated pilus (TCP), so named because its synthesis is regulated in parallel with that of CT. CT, TCP, and several other virulence factors are coordinately regulated by the *toxR* gene product. The ToxR protein modulates the expression of virulence genes in response to environmental signals via a cascade of regulatory proteins. Additional regulatory processes, including the density of the bacterial population (in a phenomenon known as *quorum sensing*), control the virulence of *V. cholerae*.

Once established in the human small bowel, the organism produces CT, which consists of a monomeric enzymatic moiety (the A subunit) and a pentameric binding moiety (the B subunit). The B pentamer binds to G_{M1} ganglioside, a glycolipid on the surface of epithelial cells that serves as the toxin receptor and makes possible the delivery of

Initial Epidemics January 1991

- - - - August 1991

——— February 1992

——— November 1994

FIGURE 140-1   Spread of *Vibrio cholerae* O1 in the Americas, 1991–1994. *(Courtesy of Dr. Robert V. Tauxe, Centers for Disease Control and Prevention, Atlanta.)*

the A subunit to its cytosolic target. The activated A subunit (A_1) irreversibly transfers ADP-ribose from nicotinamide adenine dinucleotide to its specific target protein, the GTP-binding regulatory component of adenylate cyclase in intestinal epithelial cells. The ADP-ribosylated G protein upregulates the activity of adenylate cyclase; the result is the intracellular accumulation of high levels of cyclic AMP. In intestinal epithelial cells, cyclic AMP inhibits the absorptive sodium transport system in villus cells and activates the secretory chloride transport system in crypt cells, and these events lead to the accumulation of sodium chloride in the intestinal lumen. Since water moves passively to maintain osmolality, isotonic fluid accumulates in the lumen. When the volume of that fluid exceeds the capacity of the rest of the gut to resorb it, watery diarrhea results. Unless the wasted fluid and electrolytes are adequately replaced, shock (due to profound dehydration) and acidosis (due to loss of bicarbonate) follow. Although perturbation of the adenylate cyclase pathway is the primary mechanism by which CT causes excess fluid secretion, it is not the only one. Increasing evidence indicates that CT also enhances intestinal secretion via prostaglandins and/or neural histamine receptors.

The genes encoding CT (*ctxAB*) are part of the genome of a bacteriophage designated CTXΦ. The receptor for this phage on the *V. cholerae* surface is the essential *V. cholerae* intestinal colonization factor TCP. After the infection of TCP+ *ctxAB*− *V. cholerae* cells, the CTXΦ genome stably integrates at a specific site on the *V. cholerae* chromosome. Since *ctxAB* is part of a mobile genetic element (CTXΦ), horizontal transfer of this bacteriophage may account for the emergence of new toxigenic *V. cholerae* serogroups. Many of the other genes important for *V. cholerae* pathogenicity, including the genes encoding the biosynthesis of TCP, those encoding accessory colonization factors, and those regulating virulence gene expression, are clustered together in the *V. cholerae* pathogenicity island. Similar clustering of virulence genes is found in other bacterial pathogens. It is believed that pathogenicity islands are acquired by horizontal gene transfer.

V. cholerae O139 Bengal is closely related to the O1 El Tor strains of the seventh pandemic and seems to have arisen from them by horizontal gene transfer. It shares the virulence attributes and general pathogenic mechanisms of O1 vibrios. *V. cholerae* O139 Bengal is in fact virtually identical to the seventh-pandemic strains of *V. cholerae* O1 El Tor except for two important differences: production of the novel O139 LPS and of an immunologically related O-antigen polysaccharide capsule. The ability to produce the O139 LPS is due to a replacement of a 22-kb DNA segment encoding O1 antigen biosynthesis with a 35-kb segment containing the genes encoding O139 LPS and capsule biosynthesis. Encapsulation is not a feature of O1 strains and may explain the resistance of O139 strains to human serum in vitro as well as the occasional development of O139 bacteremia.

CLINICAL MANIFESTATIONS After a 24- to 48-h incubation period, cholera begins with the sudden onset of painless watery diarrhea that may quickly become voluminous and is often followed shortly by vomiting. In severe cases, stool volume can exceed 250 mL/kg in the first 24 h. If fluids and electrolytes are not replaced, hypovolemic shock and death ensue. Fever is usually absent. Muscle cramps due to electrolyte disturbances are common. The stool has a characteristic appearance: a nonbilious, gray, slightly cloudy fluid with flecks of mucus, no blood, and a somewhat sweet, inoffensive odor. It has been called "rice-water" stool because of its resemblance to the water in which rice has been washed. Clinical symptoms parallel volume contraction: At losses of 3 to 5% of normal body weight, thirst develops; at 5 to 8%, postural hypotension, weakness, tachycardia, and decreased skin turgor are documented; and at >10%, oliguria, weak or absent pulses, sunken eyes (and, in infants, sunken fontanelles), wrinkled ("washerwoman") skin, somnolence, and coma are characteristic. Complications derive exclusively from the effects of volume and electrolyte depletion and include renal failure due to acute tubular necrosis. Thus, if the patient is adequately treated with fluid and electrolytes, complications are averted and the process is self-limited, resolving in a few days.

Laboratory data usually reveal an elevated hematocrit (due to hemoconcentration) in nonanemic patients; mild neutrophilic leukocytosis; elevated levels of blood urea nitrogen and creatinine consistent with prerenal azotemia; normal sodium, potassium, and chloride levels; a markedly reduced bicarbonate level (<15 mmol/L); and an elevated anion gap (due to increases in serum lactate, protein, and phosphate). Arterial pH is usually low (about 7.2).

DIAGNOSIS The clinical suspicion of cholera can be confirmed by the identification of *V. cholerae* in stool; however, the organism must be specifically sought. With experience, it can be detected directly by dark-field microscopy on a wet mount of fresh stool, and its serotype can be discerned by immobilization with Inaba- or Ogawa-specific antiserum. Laboratory isolation of the organism requires the use of a selective medium. The best of these is thiosulfate–citrate–bile salts–sucrose (TCBS) agar, on which the organism grows as a flat yellow colony. If a delay in sample processing is expected, Carey-Blair transport medium and/or alkaline-peptone water-enrichment medium should be inoculated as well. In endemic areas there is little need for biochemical confirmation and characterization, although these tasks may be worthwhile in places where *V. cholerae* is an uncommon isolate. Standard microbiologic biochemical testing for Enterobacteriaceae will suffice for identification of *V. cholerae*. All vibrios are oxidase-positive.

The yield of stool cultures for the diagnosis of *V. cholerae* infection declines late in the course of the illness or when effective antibacterial therapy is initiated. Although not generally performed in clinical laboratories, measurement of serum vibriocidal antibody titers can be used to confirm the diagnosis in non-cholera-endemic regions of the world. Monoclonal antibody–based diagnostic kits and methods based on the polymerase chain reaction and on DNA probes have also been developed for detection of *V. cholerae* O1 and O139.

℞ TREATMENT

Cholera is simple to treat; only the rapid and adequate replacement of fluids, electrolytes, and base is required. The mortality rate for appropriately treated disease is usually <1%. However, analysis of a large outbreak of cholera among airline travelers from an endemic country to the United States revealed frequent misdiagnoses by U.S. health professionals and poor appreciation on their part of the principles of management. It has been proved conclusively that fluid may be given orally. This approach takes advantage of the hexose-Na^+ cotransport mechanism to move Na^+ across the gut mucosa together with an actively transported molecule such as glucose. Since Na^+ losses in the stool are high, a fluid containing Na^+ at 90 mmol/L has been recommended by the World Health Organization (WHO) (Table 140-1). This amount of Na^+ is higher than that needed to treat diarrhea due to most other causes. The solution is safe, even for infants, if its intake is alternated with the consumption of sodium-free fluids such as breast milk or water. For the sake of simplicity, WHO advises routine use of

TABLE 140-1 *Composition of World Health Organization Oral Rehydration Solution (ORS)*[a,b]

Constituent	Concentration, mmol/L
Na^+	90
K^+	20
Cl^-	80
Citrate[c]	10
Glucose	110

[a] Contains (per package, to be added to 1 L of drinking water): NaCl, 3.5 g; $Na_3C_6H_5O_7 \cdot 2H_2O$, 2.9 g; KCl, 1.5 g; and glucose, 20 g

[b] If prepackaged ORS is unavailable, a simple homemade alternative can be prepared by combining 5 g NaCl (about 1 level teaspoon) with either 50 g precooked rice cereal or 40 g sucrose in 1 L of drinking water. In that case, potassium must be supplied separately (e.g., in orange juice or coconut water).

[c] 10 mmol citrate per liter, which supplies 30 mmol HCO_3/L.

this single solution for diarrheal disease rather than attempts to choose among multiple formulations according to etiology.

Cereal-based formulations are receiving increased attention as alternative oral rehydration solutions. Because of their lower osmolarity, they may reduce stool output. A mixture with a lower sugar and salt content has also been evaluated in cholera patients, with favorable results. However, concerns have been raised over the safety of its use—in particular, whether it could cause significant hyponatremia in patients with moderate or severe diarrhea. Because commercial oral rehydration solutions also contain concentrations of glucose and sodium lower than those of the WHO formulation, they should not yet be used routinely to treat cholera.

For initial management of severely dehydrated patients, intravenous fluid replacement is preferable, if available. Because profound acidosis (pH < 7.2) is common in this group, Ringer's lactate is the best choice among commercial products (Table 140-2). It must be used with additional potassium supplements, preferably given by mouth. The total fluid deficit in severely dehydrated patients (≥10% of body weight) can be replaced safely within the first 4 h of therapy, half within the first hour. Thereafter, oral therapy can usually be initiated, with the goal of maintaining fluid intake equal to fluid output. However, patients with continued large-volume diarrhea may require prolonged intravenous treatment to keep up with gastrointestinal fluid losses. Severe hypokalemia can develop but will respond to potassium given either intravenously or orally. In the absence of adequate staff to monitor the patient's progress, the oral route of rehydration and potassium replacement is safer than the intravenous route.

Although not necessary for cure, the use of an antibiotic to which the organism is susceptible will diminish the duration and volume of fluid loss and will hasten clearance of the organism from the stool. Single-dose tetracycline (2 g) or doxycycline (300 mg) is effective in adults but is not recommended for children <8 years of age because of possible deposition in bone and developing teeth. Emerging drug resistance is an ever-present concern. For adults with cholera in areas where tetracycline resistance is prevalent, ciprofloxacin—either in a single dose (30 mg/kg, not to exceed a total dose of 1 g) or in a short course (15 mg/kg twice daily for 3 days, not to exceed a total daily dose of 1 g)—or erythromycin (a total of 40 mg/kg daily in three divided doses for 3 days) is a clinically effective substitute. Both drugs are highly effective in reducing total stool output, and each is significantly better than trimethoprim-sulfamethoxazole. Because of the high cost of quinolones, WHO recommends erythromycin as the first alternative to tetracycline. For children, furazolidone has been the recommended agent and trimethoprim-sulfamethoxazole the second choice. Because of cost and/or toxicity issues related to the other drugs, erythromycin is a good choice for pediatric cholera.

CONTROL   In outbreaks, efforts should first be made to identify case contacts and to treat incubating carriers. Next, epidemiologic studies should be undertaken to establish the modes of transmission in order to define the best strategy to interrupt them. Both the establishment of rehydration centers and instruction in rehydration techniques are essential to the reduction of mortality.

TABLE 140-2 *Electrolyte Composition of Cholera Stool and of Intravenous Rehydration Solution*

Substance	Concentration, mmol/L			
	Na+	K+	Cl−	Base
Stool				
Adult	135	15	90	30
Child	100	25	90	30
Ringer's lactate	130	4a	109	28

a Potassium supplements, preferably administered by mouth, are required to replace the usual potassium losses from stool.

PREVENTION   Provision of safe water and facilities for sanitary disposal of feces, improved nutrition, and attention to food preparation and storage in the household could significantly reduce the incidence of cholera. Much effort has been devoted to the development of an effective cholera vaccine over the past two decades, with a particular focus on oral vaccine strains. Traditional killed cholera vaccine given intramuscularly provides little protection to nonimmune subjects and predictably causes adverse effects, including pain at the injection site, malaise, and fever. The vaccine's limited efficacy is at least partially due to its failure to induce a local immune response at the intestinal mucosal surface.

Two types of oral cholera vaccines are under development. The first is a killed whole-cell (WC) vaccine. Two formulations of the killed WC vaccine have been prepared: one that also contains the nontoxic B subunit of CT (WC/BS) and one composed solely of killed bacteria. In field trials in Bangladesh, both of the killed vaccines were compared with placebo and conferred ~50% protection over a 3-year evaluation period. The protective efficacy of WC/BS was superior to that of WC during the initial 8 months of follow-up (69 versus 41%) but equivalent or inferior thereafter. Immunity was relatively sustained in persons vaccinated at an age of >5 years but was not well sustained in younger vaccinees. The WC/BS vaccine is now available in Europe but not in the United States.

The second approach is that of a live attenuated vaccine strain developed, for example, by the isolation or creation of mutants lacking the genes encoding CT. Strain CVD 103-HgR, an oral live cholera vaccine licensed for immunization of travelers in Europe, is derived from a classical biotype strain of *V. cholerae* and contains a deletion of the CT A subunit gene. This strain has been extensively tested in volunteers; although it is poorly excreted in the stool of human vaccinees, a single dose produces a significant increase in the titer of vibriocidal antibody in ~75% of recipients, including children between the ages of 2 and 4 years, with almost no side effects. Unfortunately, in a large field trial in Indonesian children, this vaccine failed to induce protection against clinical cholera. Other live attenuated vaccine candidate strains have been prepared from El Tor and O139 *V. cholerae* and are now undergoing clinical trials. Because of the minimal efficacy of existing parenteral vaccines, cholera immunization is recommended for U.S. travelers only if it is mandated by the countries they plan to visit.

OTHER *VIBRIO* SPECIES

The genus *Vibrio* includes several human pathogens that do not cause clinical cholera. Abundant in coastal waters throughout the world, noncholera vibrios can reach high concentrations in the tissues of filter-feeding mollusks. As a result, human infection commonly follows the ingestion of seawater or of raw or undercooked shellfish (Table 140-3). Most noncholera vibrios can be cultured on blood or MacConkey agar, which contains enough salt to support the growth of these halophilic species. In the microbiology laboratory, the species of noncholera vibrios are distinguished by standard biochemical tests. The most important of these organisms are *V. parahaemolyticus* and *V. vulnificus*.

The two major types of syndromes for which these species are responsible are gastrointestinal illness (due to *V. parahaemolyticus*, non-O1 *V. cholerae*, *V. mimicus*, *V. fluvialis*, *V. hollisae*, and *V. furnissii*) and soft tissue infections (due to *V. vulnificus*, *V. alginolyticus*, and *V. damsela*). *V. vulnificus* is also a cause of primary sepsis in some compromised individuals. *V. parahaemolyticus* causes rare cases of wound infection and otitis and very rare cases of sepsis.

SPECIES ASSOCIATED PRIMARILY WITH GASTROINTESTINAL ILLNESS ■ *V. parahaemolyticus*   Widespread in marine environments, *V. parahaemolyticus* grows in saline concentrations up to 8 to 10%. This species was originally implicated in enteritis in Japan in 1953, accounting for 24% of reported cases in one study—a rate that presumably was due to the common practice of eating raw seafood in that country. *V. parahaemolyticus* has since been identified as a significant intestinal pathogen in many regions of the world. In the United States, common-source outbreaks of diarrhea caused by this organism have been linked to the consumption of undercooked or improperly handled seafood or of other foods contaminated by seawater. Since the mid-1990s, the incidence of *V. parahaemolyticus* infections has increased in several countries, including the United States. Serotypes O3:K6, O4:K68, and O1:K-untypable, which are genetically related to one another, account for this increase. The enteropathogenicity of *V. parahaemolyticus* is closely linked to its ability to cause hemolysis on Wagatsuma agar (i.e., the *Kanagawa phenomenon*). The genome sequence of *V. parahaemolyticus* contains a pathogenicity island—a cluster of likely virulence-associated genes. Although the mechanism by which the organism causes diarrhea remains unclear, it should be considered a possible etiologic agent in all cases of diarrhea that can be linked epidemiologically to seafood consumption or to the sea itself.

TABLE 140-3   *Features of Selected Noncholera Vibrioses*

Organism	Vehicle or Activity	Host at Risk	Syndrome
V. parahaemolyticus	Shellfish, seawater	Normal	Gastroenteritis
	Seawater	Normal	Wound infection
Non-O1 *V. cholerae*	Shellfish, travel	Normal	Gastroenteritis
	Seawater	Normal	Wound infection, otitis media
V. vulnificus	Shellfish	Immunosuppressed[a]	Sepsis, secondary cellulitis
	Seawater	Normal	Wound infection, cellulitis
V. alginolyticus	Seawater	Normal	Wound infection, cellulitis, otitis
	Seawater	Burned, other immunosuppressed	Sepsis

[a] Especially with liver disease or hemochromatosis.
Source: Table 161-3 in *Harrison's Principles of Internal Medicine*, 14th edition.

Infections with *V. parahaemolyticus* can result in two distinct gastrointestinal presentations. The more common of the two presentations (including nearly all cases in North America) is characterized by watery diarrhea, usually occurring in conjunction with abdominal cramps, nausea, and vomiting and accompanied in ~25% of cases by fever and chills. After an incubation period of 4 h to 4 days, symptoms develop and persist for a median of 3 days. Dysentery, the less common presentation, is characterized by severe abdominal cramps, nausea, vomiting, and bloody or mucoid stools. This syndrome is reported from India and Bangladesh.

Most cases of *V. parahaemolyticus*–associated gastrointestinal illness, regardless of the presentation, are self-limited and require neither antimicrobial treatment nor hospitalization. Deaths are extremely rare. Severe infections are associated with underlying diseases, including diabetes, preexisting liver disease, iron-overload states, or immunosuppression. The occasional severe case should be treated with fluid replacement and antibiotics, as described above for cholera.

Non-O1 *V. cholerae*   The heterogeneous non-O1 *V. cholerae* organisms cannot be distinguished from *V. cholerae* O1 by routine biochemical tests but do not agglutinate in O1 antiserum. Non-O1 strains have caused several well-studied food-borne outbreaks of gastroenteritis and have also been responsible for sporadic cases of otitis media, wound infection, and bacteremia. Like other vibrios, non-O1 *V. cholerae* organisms are widely distributed in marine environments. In most instances, recognized cases in the United States have been associated with the consumption of raw oysters or with recent travel, typically to Mexico. The broad clinical spectrum of diarrheal illness caused by these organisms is probably due to the group's heterogeneous virulence attributes. *V. cholerae* O139 Bengal, although technically a non-O1 *vibrio*, is not grouped with these pathogens because it can cause epidemic cholera.

In the United States, about half of all non-O1 *V. cholerae* isolates are from stool samples. The typical incubation period for gastroenteritis due to these organisms is <2 days, and the illness lasts for ~2 to 7 days. Patients' stools may be copious and watery or may be partly formed, less voluminous, and bloody or mucoid. Diarrhea can result in severe dehydration. Many cases include abdominal cramps, nausea, vomiting, and fever. Like those with cholera, patients who are seriously dehydrated should receive oral or intravenous fluids; the value of antibiotics is not clear.

Extraintestinal infections due to non-O1 *V. cholerae* commonly follow occupational or recreational exposure to seawater. Around 10% of non-O1 *V. cholerae* isolates come from cases of wound infection, 10% from cases of otitis media, and 20% from cases of bacteremia (which is particularly likely to develop in patients with liver disease). Extraintestinal infections should be treated with antibiotics. Information to guide agent selection and dosing is limited, but most strains are sensitive in vitro to tetracycline, ciprofloxacin, and third-generation cephalosporins.

SPECIES ASSOCIATED PRIMARILY WITH SOFT TISSUE INFECTION OR BACTEREMIA
(See also Chap. 110)   ■ ***V. vulnificus***   *V. vulnificus* is the most common cause of severe *Vibrio* infections in the United States. Like most vibrios, this organism proliferates in the warm summer months and requires a saline environment for growth. In this country, infections in humans typically occur in coastal states between May and October and most commonly affect men >40 years of age. *V. vulnificus* has been linked unequivocally to two distinct syndromes: primary sepsis, which usually occurs in patients with underlying liver disease, and primary wound infection, which generally affects people without underlying disease. Some authors have suggested that *V. vulnificus* also causes gastroenteritis independent of other clinical manifestations. *V. vulnificus* is endowed with a number of virulence attributes, including a capsule that confers resistance to phagocytosis and to the bactericidal activity of human serum as well as a cytolysin. Measured as the 50% lethal dose in mice, the organism's virulence is considerably increased under conditions of iron overload; this observation is consistent with the propensity of *V. vulnificus* to infect patients who have hemochromatosis.

Primary sepsis most often develops in patients who have cirrhosis or hemochromatosis. However, *V. vulnificus* bacteremia can also affect individuals who have hematopoietic disorders or chronic renal insufficiency, those who are using immunosuppressive medications or alcohol, or (in rare instances) those who have no known underlying disease. After a median incubation period of 16 h, the patient develops malaise, chills, fever (mean temperature, 39.8°C), and prostration. One-third of patients develop hypotension, which is often apparent at admission. Cutaneous manifestations develop in most cases (usually within 36 h of onset) and characteristically involve the extremities (the lower more often than the upper). In a common sequence, erythematous patches are followed by ecchymoses, vesicles, and bullae. In fact, sepsis and bullous skin lesions suggest the diagnosis in appropriate settings. Necrosis and sloughing may also be evident. Laboratory studies reveal leukopenia more often than leukocytosis, thrombocytopenia, or elevated levels of fibrin split products. *V. vulnificus* can be cultured from blood or cutaneous lesions. The mortality rate approaches 50%, with most deaths due to uncontrolled sepsis. Accordingly, prompt treatment is critical and should include empirical antibiotic administration, aggressive debridement, and general supportive care. *V. vulnificus* is sensitive in vitro to a number of antibiotics, including tetracycline, fluoroquinolones, and third-generation cephalosporins. Data from animal models suggest that either a fluoroquinolone or the combination of minocycline and cefotaxime should be used in the treatment of *V. vulnificus* septicemia.

V. vulnificus can infect either a fresh or an old wound that comes into contact with seawater; the patient may or may not have underlying disease. After a short incubation period (4 h to 4 days; mean, 12 h), the disease begins with swelling, erythema, and (in many cases) intense pain around the wound. These signs and symptoms are followed by cellulitis, which spreads rapidly and is sometimes accompanied by vesicular, bullous, or necrotic lesions. Metastatic events are uncommon. Most patients have a fever (median temperature, 38.9°C) and leukocytosis. *V. vulnificus* can be cultured from skin lesions and occasionally from the blood. Prompt antibiotic therapy and debridement are usually curative.

V. alginolyticus First identified as a pathogen of humans in 1973, *V. alginolyticus* occasionally causes eye, ear, and wound infections. This species is the most salt-tolerant of the vibrios and can grow in salt concentrations of >10%. Most clinical isolates come from superinfected wounds that presumably become contaminated at the beach. Although severity varies, *V. alginolyticus* infection tends not to be serious and generally responds well to antibiotic therapy and drainage. A few cases of otitis externa, otitis media, and conjunctivitis due to this pathogen have been described. Tetracycline treatment usually results in cure. *V. alginolyticus* is a rare cause of bacteremia in immunocompromised hosts.

ACKNOWLEDGMENT
The authors gratefully acknowledge the valuable contributions of Dr. Robert Deresiewicz, a coauthor of this chapter for the 14th edition of Harrison's.

FURTHER READING

COLWELL RR: Global climate and infectious disease: The cholera paradigm. Science 274:2025, 1996

DANIELS NA et al: *Vibrio parahaemolyticus* infections in the United States, 1973–1998. J Infect Dis 181:1661, 2000

MAKINO K et al: Genome sequence of *Vibrio parahaemolyticus*: A pathogenic mechanism distinct from that of *V. cholerae*. Lancet 361:743, 2003

MILLER MB et al: Parallel quorum sensing systems converge to regulate virulence in *Vibrio cholerae*. Cell 110:303, 2002

RAMAKRISHNA BS et al: Amylase-resistant starch plus oral rehydration solution for cholera. N Engl J Med 342:308, 2000

RAUFMAN JP: Cholera. Am J Med 104:386, 1998

RYAN ET, CALDERWOOD SB: Cholera vaccines. Clin Infect Dis 31:561, 2000

TANG HJ et al: In vitro and in vivo activities of newer fluoroquinolones against *Vibrio vulnificus*. Antimicrob Agents Chemother 46:3580, 2002

141 BRUCELLOSIS
Michael J. Corbel, Nicholas J. Beeching

DEFINITION Brucellosis is a bacterial zoonosis transmitted directly or indirectly to humans from infected animals, predominantly domesticated ruminants and swine. The disease is known colloquially as *undulant fever* because of its remittent character. Its distribution is worldwide apart from the few countries where it has been eradicated from the animal reservoir (see "Epidemiology," below). Although brucellosis commonly presents as an acute febrile illness, its clinical manifestations can be quite varied, and definitive signs to indicate the diagnosis can be lacking. Thus the clinical diagnosis must usually be supported by the results of bacteriologic and/or serologic tests.

ETIOLOGIC AGENT Human brucellosis is caused by strains of *Brucella*, a bacterial genus considered on genetic grounds to comprise a single species, *Brucella melitensis*, with a number of biologic variants that exhibit particular host preferences. For the sake of convenience, the traditional classification into nomen species is still in general use; this scheme, which closely follows the epidemiologic patterns of the infection, recognizes *B. melitensis*, which is the commonest cause of symptomatic disease in humans and for which the main sources are sheep, goats, and camels; *B. abortus*, which is usually acquired from cattle or buffalo: *B. suis*, which is generally acquired from swine except for one variant enzootic in reindeer and caribou and another enzootic in rodents; and *B. canis*, which is most often acquired from dogs. *B. ovis*, which causes reproductive disease in sheep, and *B. neotomae*, which is specific for desert rodents, have not been clearly implicated in human disease. Other brucellae have been isolated from marine mammals and probably correspond to at least three distinctive nomen species. At least one case of laboratory-acquired human disease due to these marine types has been described, and apparent cases of natural infection have been reported.

All brucellae are small, gram-negative, unencapsulated, nonsporulating rods or coccobacilli. They grow aerobically on peptone-based media incubated at 37°C; the growth of some types is enhanced by supplementary CO_2. In vivo, brucellae behave as facultative intracellular parasites. The organisms are sensitive to sunlight, ionizing radiation, and moderate heat; they are killed by boiling and pasteurization but are resistant to freezing and drying. Their resistance to drying renders brucellae stable in aerosol form and facilitates airborne transmission. Brucellae can survive for up to 2 months in soft cheeses made from goat or sheep milk; for at least 6 weeks in dry soil contaminated with infected urine, vaginal discharge, or placental or fetal tissues; and for at least 6 months in damp soil or liquid manure kept under cool, dark conditions. The bacteria are easily killed by a wide range of common disinfectants used under optimal conditions but are likely to be much more resistant at low temperatures or in the presence of heavy organic contamination.

EPIDEMIOLOGY Brucellosis is a zoonosis whose occurrence is closely related to its prevalence in domesticated animals. The true global prevalence of human brucellosis is unknown because of the imprecision of diagnosis and the inadequacy of reporting and surveillance systems in many countries. Even in developed countries, the true incidence may be 10 to 20 times higher than the reported figures. Bovine brucellosis has been the subject of control programs in many parts of the world and has been eradicated from the cattle populations of Australia, New Zealand, Bulgaria, Canada, Cyprus, Great Britain (including the Channel Islands), Japan, Luxembourg, Romania, the Scandinavian countries, Switzerland, and the Czech and Slovak Republics. Its incidence in cattle has been reduced to a low level in the United States and most Western European countries, with a varied picture in other parts of the world. There is evidence of some resurgence of brucellosis in cattle in Eastern Europe following economic changes in recent years. Efforts to eradicate *B. melitensis* infection from sheep and goat populations have been much less successful. These efforts have relied heavily on vaccination programs, which have tended to fluctuate with changing economic and political conditions. In some countries, such as Israel, *B. melitensis* has caused serious outbreaks in cattle. Brucellosis still represents a major public health problem in Mediterranean countries; in western, central, and southern Asia; and in parts of Africa and South and Central America.

Human brucellosis is usually associated with occupational or domestic exposure to infected animals or their products. Farmers, shepherds, goatherds, veterinarians, and workers in slaughterhouses and meat-processing plants in endemic areas are occupationally exposed to infection. Family members (including children) of individuals involved in animal husbandry may also be at risk, although it is often difficult to differentiate food-borne infection from environmental contamination under these circumstances. Laboratory workers involved in handling cultures or infected samples are also at risk. Travelers and urban dwellers usually acquire the infection through consumption of contaminated foods. In countries that have eradicated the disease, new cases are most often acquired abroad. Dairy products, especially soft cheeses, unpasteurized milk, and ice cream, are the most frequently implicated sources; raw meat and bone marrow may be sources of infection under exceptional circumstances. Infection resulting from contact with cosmetic products containing infected fetal materials has been recorded. Person-to-person transmission is extremely rare, as is transfer of infection by blood or tissue donation. Although brucellosis is a chronic intracellular infection, there is no evidence for increased prevalence or severity among individuals with HIV infection or other forms of immune deficiency or immune suppression.

Brucellosis may be acquired by ingestion or inhalation or through mucosal or percutaneous exposure. *B. melitensis* and *B. suis* are known to have been developed as biological weapons by several countries and could be exploited as weapons of bioterrorism (Chap. 205). This possibility should be borne in mind in the event of sudden unexplained outbreaks.

IMMUNITY AND PATHOGENESIS The mechanisms of protective immunity against human brucellosis are presumed to be similar to those documented in laboratory animals. Exposure to infection generates both humoral and cell-mediated immune responses. Although antibodies promote clearance of extracellular brucellae by bactericidal action and through the facilitation of phagocytosis by polymorphonuclear phagocytes, the antibody response cannot eradicate the infection. Organisms taken up by macrophages and other cell types can establish persistent intracellular infections. Early in the course of infection, cytokines such as interleukin (IL) 12 promote production of interferon γ, which drives T_H1-type responses and stimulates macrophage activation. Activated macrophages can kill intracellular brucellae (probably mainly through the production of reactive oxygen intermediates) and can clear the infection. Tumor necrosis factor α (TNF-α) is produced early in the immune response and stimulates cytotoxic lymphocytes, which can achieve partial clearance; however, the ability of virulent *Brucella* cells to suppress the TNF-α response may explain its limited role in protection. Inflammatory cytokines, including IL-6 and IL-10, downregulate the protective response. As in other types of intracellular infection, it is assumed that initial replication of brucellae takes place within cells of the lymph nodes draining the point of entry. Subsequent hematogenous spread may result in chronic localizing infection at almost any site, although the reticuloendothelial system, musculoskeletal tissues, and the genitourinary system are most frequently involved. Both acute and chronic inflammatory responses develop in brucellosis, and the local tissue response may include granuloma formation, with or without necrosis and caseation. Abscesses may also develop, especially in chronic localized infection.

The determinants of pathogenicity of *Brucella* have not been fully characterized, and the mechanisms underlying the manifestations of brucellosis are incompletely understood. The survival strategy of the organism is centered on processes that enable it to persist within monocytic cells. The smooth *Brucella* lipopolysaccharide, which has an unusual O-chain composition, possesses endotoxin activity and plays a key role in pyrogenicity and in resistance to phagocytosis and serum killing in the nonimmune host. Specific exotoxins have not been isolated, but a type IV secretion system responsible for secreting proteins that regulate intracellular survival and trafficking has been identified. This system is activated by low pH, and brucellae produce acid-stable proteins that facilitate survival in phagosomes and depress activation of the oxidative burst. Macrophage apoptosis and phagosome-lysosome fusion are also suppressed. Virulent brucellae are resistant to defensins and produce a Cu-Zn superoxide dismutase that enhances resistance to reactive oxygen intermediates.

CLINICAL FEATURES Brucellosis almost invariably causes fever, which may be associated with profuse sweats, especially at night. In endemic areas, brucellosis may be difficult to distinguish from the many other causes of fever. However, two features were recognized in the nineteenth century to distinguish brucellosis from other tropical fevers, such as typhoid and malaria: (1) Left untreated, the fever of brucellosis shows an undulating pattern that persists for weeks before the commencement of an afebrile period that may be followed by relapse, and (2) the fever of brucellosis is associated with musculoskeletal symptoms and signs in about one-half of all patients.

The clinical syndromes caused by the different nomen species are similar, although *B. melitensis* tends to be associated with a more acute and aggressive presentation and *B. suis* with focal abscess induction. *B. abortus* infections may be more insidious in onset and more likely to become chronic.

The incubation period varies from 1 week to several months, and the onset of fever and other symptoms may be abrupt or insidious. In addition to fever and sweats, patients become increasingly apathetic and fatigued; lose appetite and weight; and have nonspecific myalgia, headache, and chills. Overall, the presentations of brucellosis often fit into one of three patterns: febrile illness that resembles typhoid but is less severe; fever and acute monarthritis, typically of hip or knee, in a young child; or long-lasting fever, misery, and low-back pain or hip pain in an older man. In an endemic area (e.g., much of the Middle East), a patient with fever and difficulty walking into the clinic would be regarded as having brucellosis until it was proved otherwise.

Diagnostic clues in the patient's history include travel to an endemic area, employment in a diagnostic microbiology laboratory, consumption of unpasteurized milk products (including soft cheeses), contact with animals, and—in an endemic setting—a history of similar illness in the family (documented in almost 50% of cases).

Focal features are present in the majority of patients. The most common is musculoskeletal pain and physical findings in the peripheral and axial skeleton (~40% of cases). Osteomyelitis more commonly involves the lumbar and lower thoracic vertebrae than the cervical and high thoracic spine. Individual joints that are most commonly affected by septic arthritis are the knee, hip, sacroiliac, shoulder, and sternoclavicular joints, and the pattern may be one of either monarthritis or polyarthritis. Osteomyelitis may also accompany septic arthritis.

In addition to the usual causes of vertebral osteomyelitis or septic arthritis, the most important differential diagnosis is tuberculosis. This point has an impact on the therapeutic approach as well as on the prognosis, given that several antimicrobial agents used to treat brucellosis are also used to treat tuberculosis. Septic arthritis in brucellosis progresses slowly, starting with small pericapsular erosions. In the vertebrae, anterior erosions of the superior end plate are typically the first features to become evident, with eventual involvement and sclerosis of the whole vertebra. Anterior osteophytes eventually develop, but vertebral destruction or impingement on the spinal cord is rare and usually suggests tuberculosis (Table 141-1).

Other systems may be involved in a manner that resembles typhoid. About one-quarter of patients have a dry cough, usually with few changes visible on the chest x-ray, although pneumonia, empyema, intrathoracic adenopathy, or lung abscess can occur. One-quarter of patients have hepatosplenomegaly, and 10 to 20% have significant lymphadenopathy; the differential diagnosis includes glandular fever-like illness such as that caused by Epstein-Barr virus, *Toxoplasma*, and cytomegalovirus; HIV infection; or tuberculosis. Up to 10% of men have acute epididymoorchitis, which must be distinguished from that due to mumps or surgical problems such as torsion. Prostatitis, inflammation of the seminal vesicles, salpingitis, and pyelonephritis all occur. There is an increased incidence of fetal loss among infected pregnant women, although teratogenicity has not been described and

TABLE 141-1 *Radiology of the Spine: Differentiation of Brucellosis from Tuberculosis*

	Brucellosis	Tuberculosis
Site	Lumbar and others	Dorsolumbar
Vertebrae	Multiple or contiguous	Contiguous
Diskitis	Late	Early
Body	Intact until late	Morphology lost early
Canal compression	Rare	Common
Epiphysitis	Anterosuperior	General: upper, lower disk region, central, subperiosteal
Osteophyte	Anterolateral	Unusual
Deformity	Wedging uncommon	Anterior wedge, gibbus
Recovery	Sclerosis, whole body	Variable
Paravertebral abscess	Small, well-localized	Common and discrete loss, transverse process
Psoas abscess	Rare	More likely

the tendency to cause abortions is much less pronounced in humans than in farm animals.

Neurologic involvement is common, with depression and lethargy whose severity may not be fully appreciated by either the patient or the physician until after treatment. A small proportion of patients develop lymphocytic meningoencephalitis that mimics neurotuberculosis or noninfectious conditions and that may be complicated by intracerebral abscess, a variety of cranial nerve deficits, and ruptured mycotic aneurysms.

Endocarditis occurs in ~1% of cases, most often affecting the aortic valve (natural or prosthetic). Any site in the body may be involved in metastatic abscess formation or inflammation; the female breast and the thyroid gland are affected particularly often. Nonspecific maculopapular rashes and other skin manifestations are uncommon and are rarely noticed by the patient even if they are present.

DIAGNOSIS   Because the clinical picture of brucellosis is not distinctive, the diagnosis must be based on a history of potential exposure, a presentation consistent with the disease, and supporting laboratory findings. Routine biochemical assays are usually within normal limits, although serum levels of hepatic enzymes and bilirubin may be elevated. Peripheral leukocyte counts are usually normal or low, with relative lymphocytosis. Mild anemia may be documented. Thrombocytopenia and disseminated intravascular coagulation with raised levels of fibrinogen degradation products can develop. The erythrocyte sedimentation rate and C-reactive protein levels are often normal but may be raised.

In body fluids such as cerebrospinal fluid (CSF) or joint fluid, lymphocytosis and low glucose levels are the norm. Elevated CSF levels of adenosine deaminase cannot be used to distinguish tubercular meningitis, as they may also be found in brucellosis. Biopsied samples of tissues such as lymph node or liver may show noncaseating granulomas (Fig. 141-1) without acid/alcohol-fast bacilli. The radiologic features of bony disease develop late in brucellosis and are much more subtle than those of tuberculosis or septic arthritis of other etiologies, with less bone and joint destruction. Isotope scanning is more sensitive than plain x-ray and continues to give positive results long after successful treatment.

Isolation of brucellae from blood, CSF, bone marrow, or joint fluid or from a tissue aspirate or biopsy sample is definitive, and attempts at isolation are usually successful in 50 to 70% of cases. Duplicate cultures (in air and 10% CO_2, respectively) should be incubated for up to 6 weeks. Concentration and lysis of buffy coat cells before culture may increase the isolation rate. Cultures in modern nonradiometric or similar signaling systems (e.g., BACTEC) usually become positive within 7 to 10 days but should be maintained for at least 3 weeks before the results are declared negative.

FIGURE 141-1   Liver biopsy specimen from a patient with brucellosis shows a noncaseating granuloma. [From Mandell's Atlas of Infectious Diseases, Vol II, in DL Stevens (ed): Skin, Soft Tissue, Bone and Joint Infections, Fig. 5-9; with permission.]

Nucleic acid amplification techniques are not yet widely available for the diagnosis of human brucellosis, and no single standardized procedure has been adopted. The peripheral blood–based polymerase chain reaction (PCR) has enormous potential to detect bacteremia, to predict relapse, and to exclude "chronic brucellosis" (see "Prognosis and Follow-Up," below); PCR is probably more sensitive and is certainly quicker than blood culture, and it does not carry the attendant biohazard risk posed by culture. Primers for the spacer region between the genes encoding the 16S and 23S ribosomal RNAs (*rrs–rrl*), outer-membrane protein Omp2, insertion sequence IS711, or protein BCSP31 are sensitive and specific. Blood or other tissues are the most suitable samples for PCR testing.

Serologic examination often provides the only positive laboratory findings in brucellosis. In acute infection, IgM antibodies appear early and are followed by IgG and IgA antibodies. All these antibodies are active in agglutination tests, whether performed by tube, plate, or microagglutination methods. The majority of patients have detectable agglutinins at this stage. As the disease progresses, IgM levels decline, and the avidity and subclass distribution of IgG and IgA change. The result is reduced or undetectable agglutinin titers. However, the antibodies are detectable by alternative tests, including the complement fixation test, Coombs' antiglobulin test, and enzyme-linked immunosorbent assay. There is no clear cutoff value for a diagnostic titer. Rather, serologic results must be interpreted in the context of exposure history and clinical presentation. In endemic areas or in settings of potential occupational exposure, agglutinin titers of ≥1:320 to 1:640 are considered diagnostic; in nonendemic areas, a titer of ≥1:160 is considered significant. Repetition of tests after 2 to 4 weeks may demonstrate a rising titer.

In most centers, the standard agglutination test (SAT) is still the mainstay of serologic diagnosis, although some investigators rely on the rose bengal test, which has not been fully validated for human diagnostic use. Dipstick assays for anti-*Brucella* IgM are useful for the diagnosis of acute infection but are less sensitive for infection with symptoms of several months' duration. In an endemic setting, >90% of patients with acute bacteremia have SAT titers of at least 1:320.

Antibody to the *Brucella* lipopolysaccharide O chain—the dominant antigen—is detected by all the conventional tests that employ smooth *B. abortus* cells as antigen. Since *B. abortus* cross-reacts with *B. melitensis* and *B. suis*, there is no advantage in replicating the tests with these antigens. Cross-reactions also occur with the O chains of some other gram-negative bacteria, including *Escherichia coli* O157, *Francisella tularensis*, *Salmonella enterica* group N, *Stenotrophomonas maltophilia*, and *Vibrio cholerae*. Cross-reactions do not occur with the cell-surface antigens of rough *Brucella* strains such as *B. canis* or *B. ovis*; serologic tests for these nomen species must employ an antigen prepared from either one. Most protein antigens are shared by all *Brucella* strains, and some are also common to *Ochrobactrum* species.

℞ TREATMENT

The broad aims of antimicrobial therapy for brucellosis are to treat current infection and relieve its symptoms and to prevent relapse. Focal disease presentations may require surgical intervention (e.g., cardiac valve replacement, abscess drainage, joint replacement) in addition to more prolonged and tailored antibiotic therapy. In addition, tuberculosis must always be excluded, or—to prevent the emergence of resistance—the regimen must be tailored to specifically exclude monotherapy with agents active against tuberculosis (e.g., rifampin) or to include a full antituberculous regimen.

Early experience with streptomycin monotherapy for brucellosis showed that relapse was common; thus dual therapy with streptomycin and tetracyclines became the norm. This is still the most effective combination, but alternatives may be used, with the options depending on local or national policy about the use of rifampin for the treatment of nonmycobacterial infection. Antimicrobial efficacy can usually be predicted by in vitro testing. The efficacy of fluoroquinolone monotherapy has been disappointing, with a high relapse rate, despite the good in vitro activity and white-cell penetration of most agents of this class.

For adults with acute nonfocal brucellosis (duration, <1 month), a 6-week course of therapy incorporating at least two antimicrobial agents is required. Complex or focal disease necessitates ≥3 months of therapy. Adherence to the therapeutic regimen is very important, and poor compliance underlies almost all cases of apparent treatment failure; such failure is rarely due to the emergence of drug resistance, although increasing resistance to trimethoprim-sulfamethoxazole (TMP-SMX) has been reported at one center. There is good retrospective evidence that a 3-week course of two agents is as good as a 6-week course for treatment and prevention of relapse in children, but this point has not yet been proved in prospective studies.

The "gold standard" for the treatment of brucellosis in adults is intramuscular streptomycin (750 mg to 1 g daily for 14 to 21 days) together with doxycycline (100 mg twice daily for 6 weeks). In both clinical trials and observational studies, relapse follows such treatment in 5 to 10% of patients. The usual alternative regimen (and the current World Health Organization recommendation) is rifampin (600 to 900 mg/d) plus doxycycline (100 mg twice daily) for 6 weeks. In trial conditions, the relapse/failure rate is ~10%, but this rate rises to >20% in many nontrial situations, possibly because doxycycline levels are reduced and clearance rates increased by concomitant rifampin administration. Patients who cannot tolerate or receive tetracyclines (children, pregnant women) can be given high-dose TMP-SMX instead (2 or 3 standard-strength tablets twice daily for adults, depending on weight).

Evidence is beginning to accumulate that other aminoglycosides can be substituted for streptomycin—e.g., netilmicin or gentamicin given at a dosage of 5 to 6 mg/kg per day for at least 2 weeks. (Shorter courses have been associated with high failure rates in adults.) A 5- to 7-day course of therapy with gentamicin (and a 3-week course of TMP-SMX) is probably adequate for children with uncomplicated disease. Early experience with fluoroquinolone monotherapy was disappointing, but high-dose ofloxacin (400 mg twice daily) or ciprofloxacin (500 mg twice daily), given for 6 weeks with rifampin, may become accepted as an alternative to the other 6-week regimens for adults.

Significant neurologic disease due to Brucella requires prolonged treatment (i.e., for 6 to 12 months), usually with ceftriaxone supplementation of a standard regimen. Brucella endocarditis is treated with at least three drugs (an aminoglycoside, a tetracycline, and rifampin), and many experts add ceftriaxone and/or a fluoroquinolone to reduce the need for valve replacement. Treatment is usually given for at least 6 months, and clinical end points for its discontinuation are often difficult to define. Surgery is still required for the majority of cases of infection of prosthetic heart valves and prosthetic joints.

There is no evidence base to guide prophylaxis after exposure to brucellae in the laboratory, inadvertent immunization with live vaccine intended for use in animals, or exposure to deliberately released brucellae. Most authorities recommend the administration of rifampin plus doxycycline for 3 weeks after a low-risk exposure (e.g., a nonspecific laboratory accident) and for 6 weeks after a major exposure to aerosol or injected material.

PROGNOSIS AND FOLLOW-UP Relapse occurs in up to 30% of poorly compliant patients. Thus patients ideally should be followed clinically for up to 2 years to detect relapse, which responds to a prolonged course of the same therapy that was originally used. The general well-being and body weight of the patient are more useful guides than serology to lack of relapse. IgG antibody levels detected by SAT and variants of this test can remain in the diagnostic range for >2 years after successful treatment. Complement fixation titers usually fall to normal within 1 year of cure. Immunity is not solid; patients can be reinfected after repeated exposures. Fewer than 1% of patients die of brucellosis. When the outcome of this infection is fatal, death is usually a consequence of cardiac involvement; more rarely, it results from severe neurologic disease. Despite the low mortality rate, recovery from brucellosis is slow, and the illness in humans can cause prolonged inactivity, with consequent domestic difficulties and economic losses.

The existence of a prolonged chronic brucellosis state after successful treatment remains controversial. Evaluation of patients in whom this state is considered (often those with work-related exposure to brucellae) includes careful exclusion of malingering, nonspecific chronic fatigue syndromes and other causes of excessive sweating, such as alcohol abuse and obesity. In the future, the availability of more sensitive assays to detect Brucella antigen or DNA may help to identify patients with ongoing infection.

PREVENTION Vaccines based on live attenuated Brucella strains, such as B. abortus strain 19BA or 104M, have been used in some countries to protect high-risk populations but have displayed only short-term efficacy and a high incidence of local and systemic side effects (local inflammation, pain, lymphadenopathy, fever, malaise, nausea). Subunit vaccines have been developed but are of uncertain value and cannot be recommended at present. Interest in biodefense has stimulated research in this area (Chap. 205). The mainstay of veterinary prevention is a national commitment to testing and slaughter of infected herds and flocks (with compensation for owners), control of animal movement, and active immunization of animals. These measures are usually sufficient to control human disease as well. In their absence, pasteurization of all milk products before consumption is sufficient to prevent animal-to-human transmission. All cases of Brucella infection in animals and humans should be reported to the appropriate public health authorities.

FURTHER READING

ALMUNEEF M, MEMISH ZA: Prevalence of brucella antibodies after acute brucellosis. J Chemother 15:148, 2003

CORBEL MJ, MACMILLAN AP: Brucellosis, in Topley and Wilson's Microbiology and Microbial Infections, vol 3, Bacterial Infections, WJ Hausler Jr, M Sussman (eds). London, Arnold, 1999, pp 819–847

———, BANAI M: Genus Brucella Meyer and Shaw 1920,173AL, in Bergey's Manual of Systematic Bacteriology, 2d ed, vol 2. Berlin, Springer-Verlag, 2004 (in press)

HALLING SM, BOYLE SM (eds): Brucellosis [special issue]. Vet Microbiol 90: Issues 1–4, 2003

KHAN MY et al: Brucellosis in pregnant women. Clin Infect Dis 32:1172, 2000

MEMISH Z et al: Brucella bacteraemia: Clinical and laboratory observations in 160 patients. J Infect 40:59, 2000

MONTEJO JM et al: Open, randomized therapeutic trial of six antimicrobial regimens in the treatment of human brucellosis. Clin Infect Dis 16:671, 1993

142 TULAREMIA
Richard F. Jacobs

DEFINITION Tularemia is a zoonosis caused by Francisella tularensis. Humans of any age, sex, or race are universally susceptible to this systemic infection. Tularemia is primarily a disease of wild animals and persists in contaminated environments, ectoparasites, and animal carriers. Human infection is incidental and usually results from interaction with biting or blood-sucking insects, wild or domestic animals, or the environment. Tularemia is common in Arkansas, Oklahoma, and Missouri, where more than 50% of the cases in the United States occur. An increasing number of cases of tularemia have been reported from the Scandinavian countries, eastern Europe, and Siberia. The illness is characterized by various clinical syndromes, the most common of which consists of an ulcerative lesion at the site of inoculation, with regional lymphadenopathy and lymphadenitis. Systemic manifestations, including pneumonia, typhoidal tularemia, and fever without localizing findings, pose a greater diagnostic challenge.

ETIOLOGY AND EPIDEMIOLOGY With rare exceptions, tularemia is the only disease produced by F. tularensis—a small (0.2 μm by 0.2 to 0.7 μm), gram-negative, pleomorphic, nonmotile, non-spore-forming bacillus. Bipolar staining results in a coccoid appearance. The organism is a thinly encapsulated, nonpiliated strict aerobe that invades host cells. In nature, *F. tularensis* is a hardy organism that persists for weeks or months in mud, water, and decaying animal carcasses. Dozens of biting and blood-sucking insects, especially ticks and tabanid flies, serve as vectors. Ticks and wild rabbits are the source for most of the human cases in the endemic areas of the southeastern and Rocky Mountain states. In Utah, Nevada, and California, tabanid flies are the most common vectors. Animal reservoirs include wild rabbits, squirrels, birds, sheep, beavers, muskrats, and domestic dogs and cats. Humans become infected by various modes, including bites by infected arthropods; handling of infected animal tissues or fluids; direct contact with or ingestion of contaminated water, food, or soil; and inhalation of infected aerosols.

The two main biovars of *F. tularensis*—*tularensis* (type A) and *palearctica* (type B)—are both found in the United States. Type A produces more serious disease in humans; without treatment, the associated fatality rate is ~5%. Type B produces a milder, often subclinical infection that is usually contracted from water or marine mammals. Although all strains appear serologically identical, individual strains may possess varying degrees of virulence. *F. tularensis* does not produce an exotoxin, but an endotoxin similar to that of other gram-negative bacilli has been identified. The progression of illness depends on the organism's virulence, the inoculum size, the portal of entry, and the host's immune status.

Ticks pass the organism to their offspring via a transovarian route. The organism is found in tick feces but not in large quantities in tick salivary glands. In the United States, the disease can be carried by *Dermacentor andersoni* (Rocky Mountain wood tick), *D. variabilis* (American dog tick), *D. occidentalis* (Pacific coast dog tick), and *Amblyomma americanum* (Lone Star tick). *F. tularensis* is transmitted frequently during blood meals taken by embedded ticks following hours of attachment. It is the taking of a blood meal through a fecally contaminated field that transmits the organism. Tularemia is more common among men than among women. Person-to-person transmission is rare or nonexistent. Transmission of the organism by ticks and tabanid flies takes place mainly in the spring and summer. However, continued transmission in the winter months by trapped or hunted animals has been documented. The organism is extremely infectious. Biosafety level 2 is recommended for clinical laboratory work with material whose contamination is suspected, and biosafety level 3 is required for culture of the organism in large quantities. Issues related to the intentional spread of tularemia through ingestion or inhalation are discussed in Chap. 205.

PATHOGENESIS AND PATHOLOGY   The most common portal of entry for human infection is through skin or mucous membranes, either directly—through the bite of ticks, other arthropods, or other animals—or via inapparent abrasions. Inhalation or ingestion of *F. tularensis* can also result in infection. Although more than 10^8 organisms are usually required to produce infection via the oral route (oropharyngeal or gastrointestinal tularemia), fewer than 50 organisms will result in infection when injected into the skin (ulceroglandular/glandular tularemia) or inhaled (pneumonia). After inoculation into the skin, the organism multiplies locally; within 2 to 5 days (range, 1 to 10 days), it produces an erythematous, tender, or pruritic papule. The papule rapidly enlarges and forms an ulcer with a black base (chancriform lesion). The bacteria spread to regional lymph nodes, producing lymphadenopathy (buboes), and, with bacteremia, may spread to distant organs.

Tularemia is characterized by mononuclear cell infiltration with pyogranulomatous pathology. The histopathologic findings can be quite similar to those in tuberculosis, although tularemia develops more rapidly. As a facultatively intracellular bacterium, *F. tularensis* can parasitize both phagocytic and nonphagocytic host cells and survive intracellularly for prolonged periods. In the acute phase of infection, the primary organs affected (skin, lymph nodes, liver, and spleen) include areas of focal necrosis, initially surrounded by polymorphonuclear leukocytes (PMNs). Subsequently, granulomas form, with epithelioid cells, lymphocytes, and multinucleated giant cells surrounded by areas of necrosis. These areas may resemble caseation necrosis but later coalesce to form abscesses.

Conjunctival inoculation can result in infection of the eye, with regional lymph node enlargement (preauricular lymphadenopathy, Parinaud's complex). Aerosolization and inhalation or hematogenous spread of organisms can result in pneumonia. In the lung, an inflammatory reaction develops, including foci of alveolar necrosis and cell infiltration (initially polymorphonuclear and later mononuclear) with granulomas. Chest roentgenograms usually reveal bilateral patchy infiltrates rather than large areas of consolidation. Pleural effusions are common and may contain blood. Lymphadenopathy occurs in regions draining infected organs. Therefore, in pulmonary infection, mediastinal adenopathy may be evident, whereas patients with oropharyngeal tularemia develop cervical lymphadenopathy. In gastrointestinal or typhoidal tularemia, mesenteric lymphadenopathy may follow the ingestion of large numbers of organisms. The term *typhoidal tularemia* may be used to describe severe bacteremic disease, irrespective of the mode of transmission or portal of entry. Meningitis has been reported as a primary or secondary manifestation of bacteremia. Patients may also present with fever and no localizing signs.

IMMUNOLOGY   Infection with *F. tularensis* stimulates the host to produce antibodies. However, this antibody response probably plays only a minor role in the containment of infection. In contrast, cell-mediated immunity, which develops over 2 to 4 weeks, plays a major role in containment and eradication. Macrophages, once activated, can kill *F. tularensis*. Recovery from infection generally renders the patient resistant to reinfection; this point is not completely understood.

Immunospecific protection against tularemia can be afforded either by natural infection or by vaccination with live attenuated strains of *F. tularensis*. Killed vaccines, on the other hand, induce no protection against virulent *F. tularensis*. After natural infection or vaccination, serum antibodies to surface-exposed carbohydrate antigens predominate, whereas T cell determinants are located on membrane proteins beneath the bacterial capsule. T cell responses are thought to be due to priming by the organism. The anamnestic T cell response to *F. tularensis* seems to involve a multitude of microbial proteins, each with a distinct set of T cell determinants. A predominant role for CD4+ T cells is supported by the results of experiments in mice, which indicated that resistance to infection was restricted at the level of the major histocompatibility complex (MHC) class II determinants. Humans primed to *F. tularensis* (like those primed to *Mycobacterium tuberculosis*) show a T_H1-like response. T cell proliferation is associated with the production of interleukin (IL) 2 and interferon γ but with little or no production of IL-4. Recent evidence indicates that the percentage of $\gamma\delta$ T cells expressing tumor necrosis factor α is decreased during the first 7 to 40 days after infection. This decrease may reflect the modulation of an inflammatory response. Investigations of neutrophils in tularemia suggest that PMNs are needed for defense against primary infection. PMNs may restrict the growth of *F. tularensis* before the organism becomes intracellular.

CLINICAL MANIFESTATIONS   Tularemia often starts with a sudden onset of fever, chills, headache, and generalized myalgias and arthralgias (Table 142-1). This onset takes place when the organism penetrates the skin, is ingested, or is inhaled. An incubation period of 2 to 10 days is followed by the formation of an ulcer at the site of penetration, with local inflammation. The ulcer may persist for several months as organisms are transported via the lymphatics to the regional lymph nodes. These nodes enlarge and may become necrotic and suppurative. If the organism enters the bloodstream, widespread dissemination as well as signs and symptoms of endotoxemia may result.

In the United States, most patients with tularemia (75 to 85%) acquire the infection by inoculation of the skin. In adults, the most

TABLE 142-1 *Clinical Presentation of Tularemia*

Sign or Symptom	Rate of Occurrence, %	
	Children	Adults
Lymphadenopathy	96	65
Fever (≥38.3°C or ≥101°F)	87	21
Ulcer/eschar/papule	45	51
Myalgias/arthralgias	39	2
Headache	9	5
Cough	9	5
Pharyngitis	43	—
Diarrhea	43	—

Source: Adapted from Jacobs and Narain (1985).

common localized form is inguinal/femoral lymphadenopathy; in children, it is cervical lymphadenopathy. About 20% of patients develop a generalized maculopapular rash, which occasionally becomes pustular. Erythema nodosum occurs infrequently. The clinical manifestations of tularemia have been divided into various syndromes, which are listed in Table 142-2.

Ulceroglandular/Glandular Tularemia These two forms of tularemia account for ~75 to 85% of cases. The predominant form in children involves cervical or posterior auricular lymphadenopathy and is usually related to tick bites on the head and neck. In adults, the most common form is inguinal/femoral lymphadenopathy resulting from insect and tick exposures on the lower limbs. In cases related to wild game, the usual portal of entry for *F. tularensis* is either an injury sustained while skinning or cleaning an animal carcass or a bite (usually on the hand). Epitrochlear lymphadenopathy/lymphadenitis is common in patients with bite-related injuries.

In ulceroglandular tularemia, the ulcer is erythematous, indurated, and nonhealing, with a punched-out appearance that lasts from 1 to 3 weeks. The papule may begin as an erythematous lesion that is tender or pruritic; it evolves over several days into an ulcer with sharply demarcated edges and a yellow exudate. The ulcer gradually develops a black base, and simultaneously the regional lymph nodes become tender and severely enlarged (Fig. 142-1). The affected lymph nodes may become fluctuant and drain spontaneously, but usually the condition resolves with effective treatment. Late suppuration of lymph nodes has been described in up to 25% of patients with ulceroglandular/glandular tularemia. Examination of material taken from these late fluctuant nodes after successful antimicrobial treatment has revealed sterile necrotic tissue. In 5 to 10% of patients, the skin lesion may be inapparent, with lymphadenopathy plus systemic signs and symptoms the only physical findings (*glandular tularemia*). Conversely, a tick or deerfly bite on the trunk may result in an ulcer without evident lymphadenopathy.

Oculoglandular Tularemia In ~1% of patients, the portal of entry for *F. tularensis* is the conjunctiva. Usually, the organism reaches the conjunctiva through contact with contaminated fingers. The inflamed conjunctiva is painful, with numerous yellowish nodules and pinpoint ulcers. Purulent conjunctivitis with regional lymphadenopathy (preauricular, submandibular, or cervical) is evident. Because of debilitating pain, the patient may seek medical attention before regional

TABLE 142-2 *Clinical Syndromes of Tularemia*

Syndrome	Rate of Occurrence, %	
	Children	Adults
Ulceroglandular	45	51
Glandular	25	12
Pulmonary (pneumonia)	14	18
Oropharyngeal	4	—
Oculoglandular	2	—
Typhoidal	2	12
Unclassified	6	11

Source: Adapted from Jacobs and Narain (1985).

FIGURE 142-1 An ulcerative lesion (*lower arrow*) with adjacent lymphadenitis (*upper arrow*) on the lateral chest wall of a patient with ulceroglandular tularemia.

lymphadenopathy develops. Painful preauricular lymphadenopathy is unique to tularemia and distinguishes it from cat-scratch disease, tuberculosis, sporotrichosis, and syphilis. Corneal perforation may occur.

Oropharyngeal and Gastrointestinal Tularemia Rarely, tularemia follows the ingestion of contaminated undercooked meat, the oral inoculation of *F. tularensis* from the hands in association with the skinning and cleaning of animal carcasses, or the consumption of contaminated food or water. Oral inoculation may result in acute, exudative, or membranous pharyngitis associated with cervical lymphadenopathy or in ulcerative intestinal lesions associated with mesenteric lymphadenopathy, diarrhea, abdominal pain, nausea, vomiting, and gastrointestinal bleeding. Infected tonsils become enlarged and develop a yellowish-white pseudomembrane, which can be confused with that of diphtheria. The clinical severity of gastrointestinal tularemia varies from mild, unexplained, persistent diarrhea with no other symptoms to a fulminant, fatal disease. In fatal cases, the extensive intestinal ulceration found at autopsy suggests an enormous inoculum.

Pulmonary Tularemia Tularemia pneumonia presents as variable parenchymal infiltrates that are unresponsive to treatment with β-lactam antibiotics. Tularemia must be considered in the differential diagnosis of atypical pneumonia in a patient with a history of travel to an endemic area. The disease can result from either inhalation of an infectious aerosol or can spread to the lungs and pleura after bloodstream dissemination. Inhalation-related pneumonia has been described in laboratory workers after exposure to contaminated materials and is associated with a relatively high mortality rate. Exposure to *F. tularensis* in aerosols from live domestic animals or dead wildlife (including birds) has been reported to cause pneumonia. Hematogenous dissemination to the lungs occurs in 10 to 15% of cases of ulceroglandular tularemia and in about half of cases of typhoidal tularemia. Previously, tularemia pneumonia was thought to be a disease of older patients, but as many as 10 to 15% of children with clinical manifestations of tularemia have parenchymal infiltrates detected by chest roentgenography. Patients with pneumonia usually have a nonproductive cough and may have dyspnea or pleuritic chest pain. Roentgenograms of the chest usually reveal bilateral patchy infiltrates (described as ovoid or lobar densities), lobar parenchymal infiltrates, and cavitary lesions. Pleural effusions may have a predominance of mononuclear

Glandular	Oropharyngeal	Typhoidal	Pneumonia
Pyogenic bacterial infection[a]	Group A streptococcal pharyngitis	Typhoid fever	*Mycoplasma pneumoniae* pneumonia
Nontuberculous mycobacterial infection	*Arcanobacterium haemolyticum* pharyngitis	Other *Salmonella* bacteremias	*Chlamydia pneumoniae* pneumonia
Sporotrichosis	Diphtheria	Rocky Mountain spotted fever	Psittacosis
Tuberculosis	Infectious mononucleosis	Human monocytotropic ehrlichiosis	*Legionella pneumophila* pneumonia
Syphilis	Various viruses[b]	Human granulocytotropic ehrlichiosis	Q fever
Anthrax			Histoplasmosis
Rat-bite fever		Infectious mononucleosis	Blastomycosis
Scrub typhus		Brucellosis	Coccidioidomycosis
Plague		Toxoplasmosis	Various viruses[c]
Lymphogranuloma venereum		Tuberculosis	
Cat-scratch disease		Sarcoidosis	
		Malignancy[d]	

[a] *Staphylococcus aureus, Streptococcus pyogenes.*
[b] Adenovirus, enteroviruses, parainfluenza virus, influenza virus A and B, respiratory syncytial virus.
[c] Influenza virus A and B, parainfluenza virus, respiratory syncytial virus, adenovirus, enteroviruses, hantavirus.
[d] Hematologic and reticuloendothelial malignancies.

leukocytes or PMNs and sometimes red blood cells. Empyema may develop. Blood cultures may be positive for *F. tularensis.*

Typhoidal Tularemia   The typhoidal presentation is now considered rare in the United States. The source of infection in typhoidal tularemia is usually associated with pharyngeal and/or gastrointestinal inoculation or bacteremic disease. Fever usually develops without apparent skin lesions or lymphadenopathy. Some patients have cervical and mesenteric lymphadenopathy. In the absence of a history of possible contact with a vector, diagnosis can be extremely difficult. Blood cultures may be positive and patients may present with classic sepsis or septic shock in this acute systemic form of the infection. Typhoidal tularemia is usually associated with a huge inoculum or with a preexisting compromising condition. High continuous fevers, signs of endotoxemia, and severe headache are common. The patient may be delirious and may develop prostration and shock. If presumptive antibiotic therapy in culture-negative cases does not include an aminoglycoside, the mortality rate can approach 30%.

Other Manifestations   *F. tularensis* infection has been associated with meningitis, pericarditis, hepatitis, peritonitis, endocarditis, osteomyelitis, and sepsis and septic shock with rhabdomyolysis and acute renal failure. In the rare cases of tularemia meningitis, a predominantly lymphocytic response is demonstrated in cerebrospinal fluid.

DIFFERENTIAL DIAGNOSIS   When patients in endemic areas present with fever, chronic ulcerative skin lesions, and large tender lymph nodes (Fig. 142-1), a diagnosis of tularemia should be made presumptively, and confirmatory diagnostic testing and appropriate therapy should be undertaken. When the possibility of tularemia is considered in a nonendemic area, an attempt should be made to identify contact with a potential animal vector. The level of suspicion should be especially high in hunters, trappers, game wardens, veterinarians, laboratory workers, and individuals exposed to an insect or another animal vector. However, up to 40% of patients with tularemia have no known history of epidemiologic contact with an animal vector.

The characteristic presentation of ulceroglandular tularemia does not pose a diagnostic problem, but a less classic progression of regional lymphadenopathy or glandular tularemia must be differentiated from other diseases (Table 142-3). The skin lesion of tularemia may resemble those seen in various other diseases but is generally accompanied by more impressive regional lymphadenopathy. In children, the differentiation of tularemia from cat-scratch disease is made more difficult by the chronic papulovesicular lesion associated with *Bartonella henselae* infection (Chap. 144). Oropharyngeal tularemia can resemble and must be differentiated from pharyngitis due to other bacteria or viruses. Tularemia pneumonia may resemble any atypical pneumonia. Typhoidal tularemia may resemble a variety of other infections.

LABORATORY DIAGNOSIS   Direct microscopic examination of polychromatically stained tissue smears or clinical specimens reveals *F. tularensis* organisms, singly and in groups, both intra- and extracellularly. Gram's staining of clinical or biopsy material is of little value, as the small, weakly staining organisms cannot be readily distinguished from the background. An indirect fluorescent antibody test with commercially available antisera can be useful, although false-positive results due to *Legionella* spp. have been reported.

The diagnosis of tularemia is most frequently confirmed by serologic testing. In the standard tube agglutination test, a single titer of ≥1:160 is interpreted as a presumptive positive result. A fourfold increase in titer between paired serum samples collected 2 to 3 weeks apart is considered diagnostic. False-negative serologic responses are obtained early in infection; up to 30% of patients infected for 3 weeks have sera that test negative. Late in infection, titers into the thousands are common, and titers of 1:20 to 1:80 may persist for years. A microagglutination test that may be as much as 100-fold more sensitive than the standard tube agglutination test has been described and is currently being used in many clinical microbiology laboratories. Enzyme-linked immunosorbent assays have proved useful for the detection of both antibodies and antigens. Analysis of urine for *F. tularensis* antigen has yielded promising results in clinical trials, but facilities for this type of analysis are not widely available. A skin test for delayed hypersensitivity to *F. tularensis* turns positive during the first week of illness and remains positive for years. The skin-test antigen, which is not commercially available, can boost titers of agglutinating antibody.

Culture and isolation of *F. tularensis* are difficult. In one study the organism was isolated in only 10% of more than 1000 human cases, 84% of which were confirmed by serology. The medium of choice is cysteine-glucose-blood agar. *F. tularensis* can be isolated directly from infected ulcer scrapings, lymph-node biopsy specimens, gastric washings, sputum, and blood cultures. Colonies are blue-gray, round, smooth, and slightly mucoid. On media containing blood, a small zone of α hemolysis usually surrounds the colony. Slide agglutination tests or direct fluorescent antibody tests with commercially available antisera can be applied directly to culture suspensions for identification.

The polymerase chain reaction (PCR) has been used to detect *F. tularensis* DNA in multiple clinical specimens. During one outbreak, a multiplex PCR was used to target 16S rRNA and to diagnose ulceroglandular tularemia with DNA extracted from wound swabs; the PCR result was positive in 29 (73%) of 40 serologically confirmed cases. However, this test has not been shown to be more sensitive than direct culture and at present remains a research tool.

℞ TREATMENT

F. tularensis cannot be subjected to standardized antimicrobial susceptibility testing because the organism will not grow on the media used. A wide variety of antibiotics, including all β-lactam antibiotics and the newer cephalosporins, are ineffective for the treatment of this infection. Several studies indicated that third-generation cephalosporins were active against *F. tularensis* in vitro, but clinical case reports suggested a nearly universal failure rate of ceftriaxone in pediatric patients with tularemia. Although in vitro data indicate that imipenem may be active, therapy with imipenem, sulfanilamides, and macrolides is not presently recommended because of the lack of relevant clinical data. Fluoroquinolones have shown promise in terms of their relatively low toxicity and their potential for oral administration. With intracellular activity, fluoroquinolones have been used for successful treatment of tularemia and are candidates for primary or alternative therapy, pending clinical trials. The use of these agents should also be considered when patients are allergic or intolerant to other treatments. When used, ciprofloxacin should be given for a total of 10 days. Chloramphenicol and tetracycline have been used successfully for treatment of the acute stages of tularemia but have been associated with higher relapse rates (up to 20%) than conventionally used agents. Oral chloramphenicol is no longer available in the United States.

Streptomycin, given intramuscularly at a dose of 7.5 to 10 mg/kg every 12 h, is considered the drug of choice for adults. In severe cases, 15 mg/kg every 12 h may be used for the first 48 to 72 h. Streptomycin is also considered the drug of choice for children; the appropriate dose is 30 to 40 mg/kg daily in two divided doses administered intramuscularly. In children, after a clinical response is demonstrated at 3 to 5 days, the dose can be reduced to 10 to 15 mg/kg daily in two divided doses. Therapy is typically continued for 7 to 10 days; however, in mild to moderate cases of tularemia in which the patient becomes afebrile within the first 48 to 72 h of streptomycin treatment, a 5 to 7-day course has been successful.

Gentamicin, at a dose of 1.7 mg/kg given intravenously or intramuscularly every 8 h, is also effective and may be more readily available. The published experience in adults consists of two reports describing, respectively, nine and eight patients who were treated effectively with gentamicin. The eight patients in one of the reports all had fever before treatment, and all eight became afebrile within 24 to 72 h. In a pediatric study, other symptoms, such as tender lymphadenitis and pharyngitis, also responded within 24 to 72 h of the start of gentamicin therapy.

Virtually all strains of *F. tularensis* are susceptible to streptomycin and gentamicin. In successfully treated patients, defervescence usually occurs within 2 days, but skin lesions and lymph nodes may take 1 to 2 weeks to heal. When therapy is not initiated within the first several days of illness, defervescence may be delayed. Relapses are uncommon with streptomycin or gentamicin therapy. Late lymph-node suppuration, however, occurs in ~40% of children, regardless of the treatment received. These nodes have typically been found to contain sterile necrotic tissue without evidence of active infection. Patients with fluctuant nodes should receive several days of antibiotic therapy before drainage to minimize the risk to hospital personnel. Unlike streptomycin and gentamicin, tobramycin is ineffective in the treatment of tularemia and should not be used.

PROGNOSIS   If tularemia goes untreated, symptoms usually last 1 to 4 weeks but may continue for months. The mortality rate from severe untreated infection (including all cases of untreated tularemia pneu-monia and typhoidal tularemia) can be as high as 30%. However, the overall mortality rate for untreated tularemia is <8%. Mortality is <1% with appropriate treatment. Poor outcomes are often associated with long delays in diagnosis and treatment. Lifelong immunity usually follows tularemia.

PREVENTION   The prevention of tularemia is based on avoidance of exposure to biting and blood-sucking insects, especially ticks and deer-flies. An intradermal vaccine made from live attenuated *F. tularensis* is available from the Centers for Disease Control and Prevention. This vaccine is effective in reducing the frequency and severity of infection. Vaccination of high-risk individuals working with large quantities of cultured organisms is recommended. Others who come into contact with the organisms, such as veterinarians, hunters, or game wardens, should consider vaccination, particularly if they live in endemic areas. The avoidance of skinning wild animals, especially rabbits, and the wearing of gloves while handling animal carcasses decrease the risk of transmission. Use of insect repellents and preparations that prevent tick attachment as well as prompt removal of ticks can be helpful. Prophylaxis of tularemia has not proved effective in patients with embedded ticks or insect bites. However, in patients who are known to have been exposed to large quantities of organisms (e.g., in the laboratory) and who have incubating infection with *F. tularensis*, early treatment can prevent the development of significant clinical disease.

FURTHER READING

CENTERS FOR DISEASE CONTROL AND PREVENTION: Tularemia—United States, 1990–2000. MMWR 51:181, 2002

DENNIS DT et al: Tularemia as a biological weapon: Medical and public health management. JAMA 285:2763, 2001

ENDERLIN G et al: Streptomycin and alternative agents for the treatment of tularemia: Review of the literature. Clin Infect Dis 19:42, 1994

FELDMAN KA et al: Outbreak of primary pneumonic tularemia on Martha's Vineyard. N Engl J Med 345:1601, 2001

JACOBS RF, NARAIN JP: Tularemia in adults and children: A changing presentation. Pediatrics 76:818, 1985

PENN RL, KINASEWITZ GT: Factors associated with a poor outcome in tularemia. Arch Intern Med 147:265, 1987

SCHEEL O et al: Treatment of tularemia with ciprofloxacin. Eur J Microbiol Infect Dis 11:447, 1992

TAYLOR JP et al: Epidemiologic characteristics of human tularemia in the southwest-central states, 1981–1987. Am J Epidemiol 133:1032, 1991

143   PLAGUE AND OTHER *YERSINIA* INFECTIONS
David T. Dennis, Grant L. Campbell

PLAGUE

DEFINITION   Plague is an acute, febrile, zoonotic disease caused by infection with *Yersinia pestis*. Although human cases are infrequent and are curable with antibiotics, plague is one of the most virulent and potentially lethal bacterial diseases known. The plague bacterium occurs in widely scattered foci in Asia, Africa, and the Americas, where its usual hosts are various wild rodents and human-associated rats. Infection is transmitted to humans typically by flea bite and less commonly by direct contact with infected animal tissues or by airborne droplet. The principal clinical forms of plague are bubonic, septicemic, and pneumonic. Although most cases are now sporadic, occurring singly or in small clusters, the potential for outbreaks and epidemic spread remains. Because of its virulence and transmissibility, *Y. pestis* is considered an important potential agent of biological terrorism that requires special countermeasures to protect the public's health (Chap. 205).

ETIOLOGIC AGENT   *Y. pestis* is a gram-negative coccobacillus in the family Enterobacteriaceae. Genomic analysis suggests that it has recently evolved from *Y. pseudotuberculosis*. *Y. pestis* is microaerophilic, non-motile, nonsporulating, oxidase and urease negative, and biochemically unreactive. The organism is nonfastidious and infective for laboratory rodents. It grows well, if slowly, on routinely used microbiologic media (e.g., sheep blood agar, brain-heart infusion broth, and MacConkey agar). *Y. pestis* can multiply within a wide range of temperatures ($-2°C$ to $45°C$) and pH values (5.0 to 9.6), but optimal growth occurs at $28°C$ and at pH ~7.4. When stained with a polychromatic stain (e.g., Wayson or Giemsa), *Y. pestis* isolated from clinical specimens exhibits a characteristic bipolar appearance, resembling closed safety pins. The bacterium is nonencapsulated but when grown at $\geq 30°C$ produces a plasmid-expressed envelope glycoprotein, fraction 1 (F1) antigen—a virulence factor that serves as the principal immunodiagnostic marker of infection.

HISTORIC BACKGROUND   Plague's deadly epidemic potential is notorious and well documented. The Justinian pandemic (542 to 767 A.D.) spread from central Africa to the Mediterranean littoral and thence to Asia Minor, causing an estimated 40 million deaths. The second pandemic began in central Asia, was carried to Sicily by ship from Constantinople in 1347, and within a few years swept through Europe and the British Isles; successive epidemics of lesser magnitude occurred over the next four centuries. At its height, the second plague pandemic killed as many as a quarter of the affected population and became known as the Black Death. In the third (modern) pandemic, plague appeared in Yunnan, China, in the latter half of the nineteenth century; established itself in Hong Kong in 1894; and spread by ship to Bombay in 1896 and subsequently to major port cities throughout the world, including San Francisco and several other West Coast and Gulf Coast ports in the United States. The plague bacillus was first cultured by Alexandre Yersin in Hong Kong in 1894. In 1898, Paul-Louis Simond, a French scientist sent to investigate epidemic bubonic plague in Bombay, identified the bacillus in the tissues of dead rats and proposed transmission by rat fleas. Waldemar Haffkine, also in Bombay at that time, developed a crude vaccine.

By 1910, plague had circled the globe and was established in rodent populations on all inhabited continents other than Australia. After 1920, however, the spread of plague was largely halted by international regulations that mandated control of rats in harbors and inspection and rat-proofing of ships. Before subsiding, the third pandemic had resulted in an estimated 26 million plague cases and >12 million deaths, the vast majority in India. By 1950, plague outbreaks around the world had become isolated, sporadic, and manageable with modern techniques of surveillance, flea and rat control, and antimicrobial treatment of patients. Plague has nearly disappeared from cities and now occurs mostly in rural and semirural areas, where it is maintained in various rodents and their fleas. In the United States, the last outbreak of urban plague occurred in Los Angeles in 1924 and 1925, and human cases since then have, with very few exceptions, resulted from exposures in rural areas of western states.

Plague remains one of three quarantinable diseases subject to international health regulations (the other two being cholera and yellow fever). The alarm that plague is still able to evoke was highlighted by the public panic and exaggerated official responses to reported outbreaks of bubonic and pneumonic plague in India in 1994. The plague bacillus is considered to have a high potential for use in biological terrorism; the agent is available around the world, has been "weaponized" for airborne delivery, and would be expected to cause a high primary fatality rate as well as secondary spread among an affected population (Chap. 205).

EPIDEMIOLOGY *Y. pestis* is maintained in well-established "silent" enzootic cycles involving relatively resistant wild rodents and their fleas in remote, lightly populated areas of Asia, Africa, and the Americas and in limited rural foci in extreme southeastern Europe near the Caspian Sea. Humans and mammals other than rodents are incidental hosts. Outbreaks (epizootics) of plague in susceptible rodent populations may result in widespread die-offs of these animals, an avid search by their fleas for new hosts, and an increased risk of spread of infection to humans. In the United States, the principal epizootic hosts are various ground squirrels, prairie dogs, and chipmunks; a variety of burrowing rodents act as epizootic hosts in rural areas elsewhere in the world. *Y. pestis* occasionally spills over from wild rodents to rat species that inhabit cultivated fields and adjacent homes, villages, and towns. The organism can then be transported from towns to cities by these highly adaptable rats and their fleas.

Plague in populated areas is most likely to develop when sanitation is poor and rats are numerous—especially the common black or roof rat (*Rattus rattus*), its close relatives, and the larger brown sewer or Norway rat (*R. norvegicus*). The cosmopolitan oriental rat flea *Xenopsylla cheopis* and (in southern Africa and Brazil) the related species *X. brasiliensis* are efficient vectors of the plague bacillus from rat to rat and from rats to humans. *Y. pestis* multiplies to enormous numbers in the foregut (proventriculus) of these fleas, resulting in a bolus of organisms and clotted blood that blocks the passage of subsequent

blood meals. This situation occurs only at temperatures of ≤28°C and depends on a single protease expressed by the plasminogen activator (*pla*) gene of a 9.5-kb plasmid of *Y. pestis*. Regurgitation by a "blocked" flea while it feeds facilitates transmission of the plague bacillus to the new host. Except for large outbreaks of pneumonic plague in Manchuria in the early part of the twentieth century, person-to-person respiratory transmission of plague has since occurred only sporadically and has been limited to clusters of close, direct contacts of pneumonic plague patients, such as household members and caregivers.

International health regulations require that national authorities immediately report plague cases to the World Health Organization. From 1987 through 2001, 36,876 human plague cases (mean, 2458 cases per year) and 2847 deaths (mortality, 8%) were reported by 24 countries. In the same 15-year period, the United States reported 125 cases and 12 deaths (mortality, 10%). Cases reported by the United States are confirmed by the plague laboratory of the Centers for Disease Control and Prevention (CDC). Animal plague occurs in 17 contiguous western states, extending from the Great Plains states and eastern Texas to the Pacific Coast; around 80% of human cases in this country now occur in New Mexico, Arizona, and Colorado and around 10% in California. The arid Native American reservations of New Mexico and Arizona are active plague foci, and Native Americans account for a disproportionately high percentage of plague cases in the United States. Although plague is a rural disease in this country, >50% of cases are thought to be caused by peridomestic exposures, especially in the southwestern states, where homes are often situated in natural surroundings that provide a favorable habitat for plague-susceptible animals (such as rock squirrels and wood rats) and their fleas. In the Sierra Nevadas of California and Nevada, epizootic plague in chipmunks and ground squirrels poses a risk to visitors in public parks. Hikers, campers, and hunters in natural areas throughout the western states are at a small but finite risk of exposure to plague, especially in the summer months.

Plague can be transmitted during the skinning and handling of carcasses of wild animals such as rabbits and hares, prairie dogs, wildcats, and coyotes. Such direct inoculation of mammal-adapted organisms expressing the F1 antigen is associated with primary septicemia and high mortality. Pharyngeal plague can result from the ingestion of undercooked contaminated meat, from inhaling respiratory droplets, and perhaps from the manual transfer of infected fluids to the mouth during the handling of infected animal tissues.

Carnivores, including dogs and cats, can become infected with *Y. pestis* by eating infected rodents and possibly by being bitten by infective fleas. Although clinical plague commonly develops in infected cats, it rarely does so in infected dogs. Both dogs and cats may transport infected fleas from rodent-infested areas to the home environment.

From 1947 through 2001, 421 plague cases were reported in the United States. Of the 409 evaluable cases, 349 cases (85%) presented as primary lymphadenitic (bubonic) plague, almost all of them thought to be associated with flea bites; 55 cases (13%) presented as primary septicemic plague, many of them following direct animal exposures; and 8 cases (2%) presented as primary pneumonic plague, 6 resulting from the inhalation of respiratory droplets released by infected cats and 2 from unknown sources. The last case of human-to-human plague transmission in the United States occurred in Los Angeles in 1924.

PATHOGENESIS AND PATHOLOGY *Y. pestis* is highly invasive and pathogenic. The mechanisms by which the organism causes disease are incompletely understood, but both chromosome- and plasmid-encoded gene products as well as altered cell-mediated immune responses are involved. Three plasmids encode for a variety of known or presumed virulence factors; these include the F1 envelope antigen and various *Yersinia* outer-membrane proteins (Yops), which confer bacterial resistance to phagocytosis; the V antigen, which is essential for virulence and immunocompromises the host by suppressing the synthesis of various proinflammatory cytokines (e.g, interferon γ and tumor necrosis factor α); pesticin, which interferes with iron uptake; a protease that

FIGURE 143-1   Plague patient in the southwestern United States with a left axillary bubo and an unusual plague ulcer and eschar at the site of the infective flea bite.

activates plasminogen and degrades serum complement and is thought to enhance dissemination of *Y. pestis* following inoculation of the skin; a coagulase; and a fibrinolysin. A chromosomally encoded lipopolysaccharide endotoxin is important in sepsis, triggering the systemic inflammatory response syndrome and its complications.

Y. pestis organisms inoculated through the skin or mucous membranes are typically carried to regional lymph nodes via lymphatic channels, although direct bloodstream inoculation and dissemination may take place. Mononuclear phagocytes, which can phagocytize *Y. pestis* organisms without destroying them, may play a role in dissemination of the infection to distant sites. Plague can involve almost any organ, and untreated plague generally results in widespread and massive tissue destruction. In the early stages, infected lymph nodes (*buboes*, Fig. 143-1) are characterized by edema and congestion without inflammatory infiltrates or apparent vascular injury. Fully developed buboes contain huge numbers of infectious plague organisms and show distorted or obliterated lymph node architecture with loss of vascular integrity, hemorrhage, necrosis, infiltration of polymorphonuclear neutrophils (PMNs), and extensive serosanguineous effusion. The effusion typically involves perinodal tissues. If several adjacent lymph nodes are involved, a boggy edematous mass can result.

Primary septicemic plague consists of sepsis in the absence of a bubo; secondary septicemic plague is a complication of bubonic or pneumonic plague that occurs when local host defenses are breached. In fatal septicemic plague, multifocal hepatic and splenic necrosis is

common. Diffuse interstitial myocarditis with cardiac dilatation is sometimes found. If disseminated intravascular coagulation (DIC) ensues, vascular necrosis may lead to widespread cutaneous, mucosal, and serosal ecchymoses and petechiae. Acral ischemia and resulting gangrene sometimes develop.

Primary plague pneumonia generally begins as a lobular process and then extends by confluence, becoming lobar and then multilobar (Fig. 143-2). Plague organisms are typically most numerous in the alveoli. Secondary plague pneumonia begins more diffusely, with organisms at first most numerous in the interstitium. In advanced cases of both primary and secondary plague pneumonia, affected lung tissue is characterized by edema, hemorrhagic necrosis, and infiltration by neutrophilic leukocytes.

MANIFESTATIONS   Plague is characterized by a rapid onset of fever and other systemic manifestations of gram-negative bacterial infection. If it is not quickly and correctly treated, plague can follow a toxic course, resulting in shock, multiple-organ failure, and death. In humans, the three principal forms of plague are bubonic, septicemic, and pneumonic. Bubonic plague, the most common form, is almost always caused by the bite of an infected flea but occasionally results from direct contact with infectious materials. Septicemic and pneumonic plague can be either primary or secondary to metastatic spread. Unusual forms include plague meningitis, endophthalmitis, and lymphadenitis at multiple sites. Primary plague pharyngitis has been documented by culture of organisms from throat swabs and can result from respiratory exposure or ingestion of undercooked flesh of infected animals.

Bubonic Plague   Bubonic plague has a usual incubation period of 2 to 6 days. Patients experience chills; fever, with temperatures that rise within hours to ≥38°C; myalgias; arthralgias; headache; and a feeling of weakness. Soon—usually within 24 h—the patient notices tenderness and pain in one or more regional lymph nodes proximal to the site of inoculation of the plague bacillus (Fig. 143-1). Because fleas most often bite the legs, femoral and inguinal nodes are most commonly involved; axillary and cervical nodes are next most commonly affected. Within hours, the enlarging bubo becomes progressively painful and tender, sometimes exquisitely so. The patient usually guards against palpation and limits movement, pressure, and stretch around the bubo. The surrounding tissue often becomes edematous, sometimes markedly so, and the overlying skin may be erythematous, warm, and tense. Inspection of the skin surrounding or distal to the bubo sometimes reveals the site of a flea bite marked by a papule, pustule, or ulcer. The ulcer may be covered by an eschar (Fig. 143-1). A list of lymphadenitic conditions that could be confused with bubonic plague includes *Staphylococcus aureus* and group A β-hemolytic streptococcal infections, cat-scratch disease, tularemia, and—in filariasis endemic areas—acute filarial lymphadenitis. The bubo of plague

FIGURE 143-2   Sequential chest radiographs of a patient with fatal primary plague pneumonia. *Left*: Upright posteroanterior film taken at admission to hospital emergency department on third day of illness, showing segmental consolidation of right upper lobe. *Center*: Portable anteroposterior film taken 8 h after admission, showing extension of pneumonia to right middle and right lower lobes. *Right*: Portable anteroposterior film taken 13 h after admission (when patient had clinical adult respiratory distress syndrome), showing diffuse infiltration throughout right lung and patchy infiltration of left lower lung. A cavity later developed at the site of initial right-upper-lobe consolidation.

is distinguishable from lymphadenitis of most other causes, however, by its rapid onset, its extreme tenderness, the accompanying signs of toxemia, and the absence of cellulitis or obvious ascending lymphangitis. The pain and swelling of bubonic plague can be confused with a strangulated hernia or trauma.

Treated in the uncomplicated state with an appropriate antibiotic, bubonic plague usually responds quickly, with resolution of fever and alleviation of other systemic manifestations over 2 to 5 days. Buboes often remain enlarged and tender for a week or more after the initiation of treatment and can become fluctuant. Without effective antimicrobial treatment, patients with typical bubonic plague manifest an increasingly toxic state of fever, tachycardia, lethargy leading to prostration, agitation and confusion, and (occasionally) convulsions and delirium. Secondary plague sepsis may result in an alarmingly rapid and refractory cascade of DIC, bleeding, shock, and organ failure. Mild forms of bubonic plague, called *pestis minor*, have been described in South America and other plague endemic areas; in these cases, the patients are ambulatory, are only mildly febrile, and have subacute buboes.

Septicemic Plague Septicemic plague is a progressive, overwhelming gram-negative infection. Primary septicemia develops in the absence of a bubo, and the diagnosis is often not suspected until preliminary blood culture results are reported to be positive by the laboratory. *Y. pestis*, however, can also be cultured from the blood of most bubonic plague patients, and bacteremia should be distinguished from septicemia, in which the patient is desperately ill and requires aggressive care. Septic patients often present with gastrointestinal symptoms of nausea, vomiting, diarrhea, and abdominal pain, which may further confound the correct diagnosis. If not treated early with appropriate antibiotics, septicemic plague can be fulminant and fatal. In the United States in 1947 through 2001, 55 cases of primary septicemic plague with 13 deaths were reported, for a case-fatality rate of 24%. Petechiae, ecchymoses, bleeding from puncture wounds and orifices, and gangrene of acral parts are manifestations of DIC; refractory hypotension, renal shutdown, obtundation, and other signs of shock are preterminal events. Adult respiratory distress syndrome (ARDS), which can occur at any stage of septicemic plague, is sometimes confused with other conditions, such as hantavirus pulmonary syndrome. The differential diagnosis of septicemic plague includes sepsis of other gram-negative bacterial etiology, meningococcemia, and acute severe viral infections such as hantavirus illness.

Pneumonic Plague Of all forms of the disease, pneumonic plague develops most rapidly and is most frequently fatal. The incubation period for primary pneumonic plague is usually 3 to 5 days (range, 1 to 7 days). The onset is most often sudden, with chills, fever, headache, myalgias, weakness, and dizziness. Pulmonary signs, including tachypnea and dyspnea, cough, sputum production, and chest pain, typically arise on the second day of illness and may be accompanied by hemoptysis, increasing respiratory distress, cardiopulmonary insufficiency, and circulatory collapse. In primary plague pneumonia, the sputum is most often watery or mucoid, frothy, and blood-tinged, but it may become frankly bloody. Pulmonary signs in primary pneumonic plague may indicate involvement of a single lobe in the early stage, with rapidly developing segmental consolidation before bronchopneumonic spread to other lobes of the same and opposite lungs (Fig. 143-2). Liquefaction necrosis and cavitation may occur early in areas of consolidation and may or may not leave significant residual scarring.

Secondary plague pneumonia, which occurs in 10 to 15% of bubonic plague cases in the United States, typically manifests first as a diffuse interstitial pneumonitis in which sputum production is scant; since the sputum is more likely to be inspissated and tenacious in character than the sputum found in primary pneumonia, it may be less infectious. In the United States in 1947 through 2001, 46 cases of secondary pneumonic plague and 8 cases of primary pneumonic plague were described, with no known transmission to contacts and an overall case-fatality rate of 41%. Observers in the early twentieth century remarked on the relative lack of auscultatory findings, the usual presence of toxemia, and the frequency of sudden death among patients with pneumonic plague as compared to patients with other bacterial pneumonias.

The differential diagnosis of pneumonic plague includes acute community-acquired pneumonia of another bacterial or a viral etiology, tularemia, coccidioidomycosis, *Pneumocystis* pneumonia, and Q fever.

Plague Meningitis Meningitis is an unusual manifestation of plague. In the United States, there were 17 meningitis cases among the 409 evaluable plague cases reported in 1947 through 2001. All cases of meningitis were complications of bubonic plague, and all but three patients survived. Although meningitis may be a part of the initial presentation of plague, its onset is often delayed and is a manifestation of insufficient treatment. Recent cases in the United States have occurred in association with treatment of bubonic plague with tetracyclines, which are bacteriostatic against *Y. pestis*. Chronic relapsing meningeal plague over periods of weeks or even months was described in the preantibiotic era. The affected patients typically present with fever, headache, meningismus, and neutrophilic pleocytosis.

Plague Pharyngitis Plague pharyngitis presents as fever, sore throat, cervical lymphadenitis, and headache and is often indistinguishable clinically from pharyngitis and tonsillitis of other infectious etiologies, especially streptococcal pharyngitis. Plague pharyngitis can be difficult to distinguish from cervical bubonic plague arising from an infective flea bite on the head and neck region. Caregivers working in endemic areas must be alert to plague in the differential diagnosis of pharyngitis to avoid delayed and/or inappropriate treatment.

LABORATORY FINDINGS AND DIAGNOSIS Since plague is a rare disease in the United States, a high index of clinical suspicion as well as the elicitation of a thorough clinical and epidemiologic history and a careful physical examination are required for timely diagnosis and prompt institution of specific therapy. When the diagnosis of plague is delayed or missed altogether, a high case-fatality rate results; infected travelers who seek medical care after they have left endemic areas (peripatetic plague cases) are at especially high risk. Plague must be considered in the differential diagnosis of acute regional lymphadenitis, sepsis, or acute severe pneumonia in an otherwise-healthy person who has a history of recent travel to or residence in the rural western United States. When the diagnosis of plague is being considered, close communication between clinicians and the diagnostic laboratory and between the diagnostic laboratory and a qualified reference laboratory is essential. Tests for plague are highly reliable when conducted by laboratory personnel experienced with *Y. pestis*, but such expertise is usually limited to selected reference laboratories, including state health department laboratories in some plague-endemic states and the CDC plague laboratory (Fort Collins, Colorado; tel. 970-221-6400).

When plague is suspected, specimens should be collected promptly for laboratory studies, chest roentgenograms should be obtained, and specific antimicrobial therapy should be initiated pending confirmation. Appropriate diagnostic specimens for smear and culture include citrated or heparinized whole blood from all patients with suspected plague; lymph node aspirates from those with suspected buboes; sputum samples, pharyngeal swabs, and tracheal or pulmonary alveolar aspirates from those with suspected pneumonic plague; and cerebrospinal fluid (CSF) from those with suspected plague meningitis. Since early buboes are often exquisitely tender and are seldom fluctuant or necrotic, these lesions usually require aspiration under local anesthesia following the injection of 1 to 2 mL of normal saline (sterile but nonbacteriostatic) into the bubo with a 20- to 22-gauge needle. Typically, aspiration produces a scant amount of serosanguineous fluid. A variety of appropriate culture media (including brain-heart infusion broth, sheep blood agar, and MacConkey agar) should be inoculated with a portion of each specimen. Moreover, for each specimen, at least one smear should be examined immediately with Wayson or Giemsa stain and at least one with Gram's stain; a smear should also be submitted to a reference laboratory for direct fluorescent antibody testing, antigen-capture enzyme-linked immunosorbent assay (ELISA), polymerase chain reaction (PCR) analysis, or testing by another rapid detection method (e.g., immunochromatographic hand-held assay). An acute-phase serum specimen should be tested for antibody to *Y. pestis*; whenever possible, a convalescent-phase serum specimen collected 3 to 4 weeks later should also be tested. When a patient dies and plague is suspected, appropriate autopsy tissues for culture, direct fluorescent antibody testing, and immunohistochemical staining include buboes, all solid organs (especially liver, spleen, and lung), and bone marrow. If culture of such specimens is to be attempted, they should be sent to the laboratory either fresh or frozen on dry ice, not in preservatives or fixatives. If necessary, Cary-Blair or a similar medium can be used to transport *Y. pestis*–infected tissues.

Laboratory confirmation of plague depends on the isolation of *Y. pestis* from cultures of body fluids or tissues. Cultures of three blood samples taken over a 45-min period before treatment will usually result in isolation of the bacterium. *Y. pestis* strains are readily distinguished from those of the closely related species *Y. pseudotuberculosis* by differences in biochemical profile, temperature-dependent susceptibility to lysis by a *Y. pestis*–specific bacteriophage, and motility. Automated bacteriologic test systems can be used to assist in the identification of isolates as *Y. pestis*, but *Y. pestis* can be misidentified (e.g., as *Y. pseudotuberculosis*) or overlooked if these systems are improperly programmed.

In the absence of *Y. pestis* isolation, plague cases can be confirmed either by the demonstration of seroconversion (a fourfold or greater titer rise) to *Y. pestis* F1 antigen in passive hemagglutination tests of acute- and convalescent-phase serum specimens or by detection of an antibody titer of >128 in a single serum sample from a patient with a plague-compatible illness who has not received plague vaccine. The specificity of a positive passive-hemagglutination test requires confirmation with the F1 antigen hemagglutination-inhibition test. A few plague patients seroconvert to F1 antigen as early as 5 days after the onset of illness; most seroconvert between 1 and 2 weeks after onset; a few seroconvert >3 weeks after onset; and a few (<5%) fail to seroconvert at all. Early, specific antibiotic treatment may delay seroconversion by several weeks. After seroconversion, positive serologic titers diminish gradually over months to years. ELISAs for IgM and IgG antibodies to *Y. pestis* are replacing hemagglutination tests in some laboratories. Other new test methods include those mentioned above: antigen-capture ELISAs, PCR, and immunochromatographic hand-held assays for rapid identification of *Y. pestis* in aspirates, sputum, and other infected body fluids or tissues. The hand-held assays can be used at the bedside in the remote rural settings where most plague cases occur and could prove important in responding to bioterrorism (Chap. 205).

Patients with plague typically have white blood cell (WBC) counts of 10,000 to 25,000/μL, with a predominance of PMNs and a left shift. Leukemoid reactions with WBC counts as high as 100,000/μL can occur. Modest thrombocytopenia is usually documented, and fibrin-fibrinogen split products are often detected even in patients without frank DIC. Serum levels of aminotransferases and bilirubin may be elevated. In plague pneumonia, stained respiratory secretions usually contain PMNs and characteristic bipolar-staining bacilli. In *Y. pestis* septicemia, visualization of the characteristic bacilli in a routine blood smear or a buffy-coat smear is an uncommon but grave prognostic sign (Fig. 143-3). In patients with plague meningitis, PMN pleocytosis is typical, and the bacilli are usually visible in stained CSF smears.

℞ TREATMENT

Left untreated, plague is fatal in >50% of cases of bubonic disease and in nearly all cases of septicemic and pneumonic disease. The overall mortality rate for plague cases in the United States since 1950 has been ~14%; deaths are almost always due to delays in seeking treatment, misdiagnosis, delays in the institution of treatment, or incorrect treatment. Rapid diagnosis and appropriate antimicrobial therapy are essential.

FIGURE 143-3   Peripheral blood smear from a patient with fatal plague septicemia and shock, showing characteristic bipolar-staining *Y. pestis* bacilli (Wright's stain, oil immersion).

Guidelines for the treatment of plague are given in Table 143-1. Although streptomycin is the drug of choice, gentamicin is increasingly used for the treatment of plague in the United States because of its ready availability; it is probably as effective as streptomycin and less toxic, although results of controlled studies in humans have not been published. Alternative antibiotics include the tetracyclines and chloramphenicol; these agents are usually given orally with initial loading doses but may be given intravenously to critically ill patients and to patients unable to tolerate oral medication. Doxycycline is considered the tetracycline of choice. Penicillins, cephalosporins, and macrolides are suboptimal and should not be used. Trimethoprim-sulfamethoxazole (TMP-SMX) has been used successfully to treat bubonic plague but is not considered a first-line agent. Chloramphenicol may be indicated for the treatment of plague meningitis, pleuritis, endophthalmitis, and myocarditis because of its superior tissue penetration; it is used alone or in combination with streptomycin or another first-line agent. In general, antimicrobial treatment should be continued for 7 to 10 days or for at least 3 days after the patient has become afebrile and has made a clinical recovery. Patients initially given intravenous antibiotics may be switched to oral regimens upon clinical improvement. Such improvement is usually evident 2 or 3 days after the start of treatment, even though fever may continue for several days. National bioterrorism-response protocols propose gentamicin, ciprofloxacin, and doxycycline as antimicrobial agents of first choice for treatment and postexposure prophylaxis in the event of an attack using *Y. pestis* (Chap. 205).

Consequences of delayed treatment of plague include DIC, ARDS, and other complications of gram-negative sepsis. Patients with these

TABLE 143-1   *Guidelines for the Treatment of Plague*

Drug	Daily Dosage	Interval, h	Route(s) of Administration
Streptomycin			
Adults	2 g	12	IM
Children	30 mg/kg	12	IM
Gentamicin			
Adults	3–5 mg/kg[a]	8	IM or IV
Children	6.0–7.5 mg/kg	8	IM or IV
Infants/neonates	7.5 mg/kg	8	IM or IV
Tetracycline			
Adults	2 g	6	PO or IV
Children ≥8 y	25–50 mg/kg	6	PO or IV
Doxycycline			
Adults	200 mg	12 or 24	PO or IV
Children ≥8 y	4.4 mg/kg	12 or 24	PO or IV
Chloramphenicol			
Adults	50 mg/kg[b]	6	PO or IV
Children ≥1 y	50 mg/kg[b]	6	PO or IV

[a] Dosage should be reduced to 3 mg/kg daily as soon as clinically indicated.
[b] For meningitis, up to 100 (mg/kg)/d initially.

disorders require intensive monitoring and close physiologic support, as outlined elsewhere (Chaps. 102 and 251). Buboes may require surgical drainage. Abscessed nodes can cause recurrent fever in patients who have apparently recovered; the cause may be occult if intrathoracic or intraabdominal nodes are involved. Although *Y. pestis* is considered to be genetically stable, a multidrug-resistant strain was recently isolated from a plague patient in Madagascar. This strain exhibited resistance (mediated by a transferable plasmid) to principal first-line antibiotics used for treatment and prophylaxis of plague.

PREVENTION AND CONTROL Persons at greatest risk for plague in the United States are individuals who live, work, and participate in outdoor recreational activities in areas of those western states in which plague is enzootic. Surveillance, education, and environmental management are the cornerstones of prevention and control. A network of biologists and public health specialists coordinates these activities through local and state health departments and the CDC. Personal protective measures include the avoidance of areas with known epizootic plague (in which warning signs may be posted) and of sick or dead animals; the use of repellents, insecticides, and protective clothing when at risk of exposure to rodents' fleas; and the wearing of gloves when handling animal carcasses. Short-term antibiotic prophylaxis (Table 143-2) is recommended for persons known to have had close contact with a patient with suspected or confirmed pneumonic plague and occasionally for persons who are unable to avoid an area where a plague outbreak is in progress or who may be caring for patients with plague. Patients in whom respiratory plague is suspected should be managed under isolation, with use of respiratory-droplet precautions until pneumonia has been ruled out or until 48 h of effective antimicrobial therapy has been administered, after which standard infection-control precautions are adequate. Masks are considered to be protective against respiratory transmission of plague and would be expected to be an important tool to prevent secondary plague spread in the event of bioterrorism (Chap. 205).

Rodent food (garbage, pet food) and habitats (brush piles, junk heaps, woodpiles) should be eliminated in domestic, peridomestic, and working environments; buildings and food stores should be rodent-proofed. The control of fleas with insecticides is a key public health measure in situations where epizootic plague activity places humans at high risk; this effort includes dusting and spraying of rodent burrows, rodent runs, and other sites where rodents and their fleas are found. In plague-endemic areas of the western United States, persons should keep their dogs and cats free of fleas and restrained. The decision to control plague by killing rodents should be left to public health authorities, and such a program should be carried out only in conjunction with effective flea control. Killing of rodents has no lasting benefit without environmental sanitation.

TABLE 143-2 *Guidelines for Plague Prophylaxis*

Drug	Daily Dosage	Interval, h	Route of Administration
Tetracycline			
Adults	1–2 g	6 or 12	PO
Children ≥8 y	25–50 mg/kg	6 or 12	PO
Doxycycline			
Adults	100–200 mg	12 or 24	PO
Children ≥8 y	2–4 mg/kg	12 or 24	PO
Trimethoprim-sulfamethoxazole			
Adults	320 mg[a]	12	PO
Children ≥2 mo	8 mg/kg[a]	12	PO
Ciprofloxacin[b]			
Adults	1 g	12	PO
Children	40 mg/kg	12	PO

[a] Trimethoprim component.
[b] Recommended as an alternative to doxycycline in bioterrorism-response plans.

The previously used killed, whole-cell plague vaccine is no longer available in the United States. New and improved vaccines are being evaluated that use recombinant F1 and V antigens to induce protective antibodies. In the United States, the indications for use of these newer vaccines would probably be similar to those for the previously available killed vaccine, which was mostly limited to protecting laboratory personnel who routinely worked with *Y. pestis* and some persons whose vocations brought them into regular contact with wild rodents and their fleas in areas with enzootic or epizootic plague. In addition, a vaccine might be useful in protecting selected persons at risk from biowarfare or bioterrorism.

OTHER *YERSINIA* INFECTIONS

DEFINITION Yersiniosis is an uncommon bacterial zoonosis caused primarily by infection with either of two enteropathogenic *Yersinia* species: *Y. enterocolitica* or *Y. pseudotuberculosis*. Reservoir hosts of these bacteria include swine and other wild and domestic animals, and transmission to humans is predominantly via the oral route. Both sporadic cases and common-source outbreaks occur. The most frequent acute clinical manifestations are (1) enteritis or enterocolitis with self-limited diarrhea (especially with *Y. enterocolitica*) and (2) mesenteric adenitis and terminal ileitis (especially with *Y. pseudotuberculosis*), which can be confused with acute appendicitis. Septicemia and metastatic focal infections are less common. Yersiniosis can be complicated by nonsuppurative, extraintestinal, inflammatory sequelae—e.g., reactive arthritis (Chap. 305) and erythema nodosum (Chap. 17). Other nonplague *Yersinia* species, including *Y. intermedia*, *Y. frederiksenii*, and *Y. kristensenii*, have been associated with enteritis or enterocolitis in humans (particularly immunocompromised adults), but little is known about their pathogenicity, public health importance, or clinical management.

ETIOLOGIC AGENTS *Y. enterocolitica* and *Y. pseudotuberculosis* are pleomorphic gram-negative bacilli in the family Enterobacteriaceae. They can multiply within a wide temperature range ($-1°C$ to 45°C). Pathogenic *Y. enterocolitica* isolates are most commonly identified by biotyping based on biochemical profiles and serotyping according to somatic O and H antigens. Six biotypes and >60 serotypes of *Y. enterocolitica* are recognized. A separate serotyping system for *Y. pseudotuberculosis* (also based on somatic antigens) has distinguished six major serotypes (I through VI) and their subtypes.

EPIDEMIOLOGY ■ **Yersinia enterocolitica** *Y. enterocolitica* is distributed worldwide and has been isolated from soil, fresh water, contaminated foodstuffs (e.g., meat, milk, and vegetables), and a wide variety of wild and domestic animals. Many serotypes isolated from environmental sources, however, evidently are not human pathogens. Most human infections have been caused by *Y. enterocolitica* serotypes O:3, O:5,27, O:8, and O:9, which are primarily associated with wild and domestic mammals. The recognized incidence of these infections and their sequelae is highest in Scandinavia and some other northern European countries, but reliable population-based estimates of incidence are unavailable.

All age groups are susceptible to *Y. enterocolitica* infections, but the majority of cases of enterocolitis are in children aged 1 to 4. Moreover, these infections show a modest predilection for males. Mesenteric adenitis and terminal ileitis are most common among older children and young adults. Risk factors for *Y. enterocolitica* septicemia and metastatic focal infections include chronic liver disease, malignancy, diabetes mellitus, immunosuppressive therapy, alcoholism, malnutrition, advanced age, iron overload (see below), and hemolytic anemias (including the thalassemias). The nonsuppurative sequelae of yersiniosis are most common among adults. HLA-B27 is expressed in 70 to 80% of patients who develop reactive arthritis associated with yersiniosis. HLA-B27 is not a risk factor for *Yersinia*-induced erythema nodosum; females with this condition outnumber males by 2 to 1.

Among *Y. enterocolitica* strains isolated from patients in recent decades, serotypes O:3 and O:9 have predominated in Europe, while serotype O:3 has predominated in Canada, Japan, and the United States. The apparent incidence of *Yersinia*-induced nonsuppurative sequelae reportedly is 10 to 30% in Scandinavia and much lower in most other countries, including the United States.

Common-source outbreaks of *Y. enterocolitica* enteritis have been traced to such vehicles as raw milk, contaminated pasteurized milk, and foods prepared with contaminated fresh water. Because *Y. enterocolitica* commonly colonizes the gastrointestinal tracts of swine, sporadic human cases and outbreaks of yersiniosis have also been associated with the preparation or ingestion of raw pork products (e.g., chitterlings). In some cases of yersiniosis, circumstantial evidence suggests transmission via contact with dogs and cats or their feces. Several nosocomial outbreaks of *Y. enterocolitica* infection have been described; fecal-oral transmission from person to person was suspected. Fecal-oral transmission among family members may also explain occasional secondary cases in households. In a prospective study of 50 children with *Y. enterocolitica* enteritis, fecal excretion of the organism persisted for an average of 27 days (range, 4 to 79 days) after the cessation of symptoms. A chronic carrier state, however, has not been demonstrated. *Y. enterocolitica* is a rare but often lethal cause of transfusion-associated septicemia. The explanation is that blood donors occasionally have transient, occult *Y. enterocolitica* bacteremia and that this organism can slowly multiply to high concentrations in blood refrigerated for at least 10 days.

Yersinia pseudotuberculosis The ecology of *Y. pseudotuberculosis* seems to parallel that of *Y. enterocolitica* closely. *Y. pseudotuberculosis* is also widespread in wild and domestic animals and is isolated from many environmental sources. Human infections with *Y. pseudotuberculosis*, however, appear to be rare. Swine appear to be an important reservoir for pathogenic strains of *Y. pseudotuberculosis*.

PATHOGENESIS AND PATHOLOGY With rare exceptions (e.g., transmission via contaminated blood products or direct cutaneous inoculation), the enteropathogenic yersiniae are thought to enter the host via the oral route. The incubation period averages 5 days (range, 1 to 11 days). Studies of animals have shown that the organisms initially invade the ileal epithelium, then are translocated via M cells into the lamina propria, and finally enter Peyer's patches, where they are able to replicate. They subsequently drain into the mesenteric lymph nodes, which undergo hyperplasia and from which the bacteria can be disseminated. The mesenteric lymph nodes can become intensely swollen and matted and are occasionally detected on physical examination as a tender right-lower-quadrant mass. Intestinal inflammation (most commonly of the distal ileum and less commonly of the ascending colon) develops and may be accompanied by mucosal ulcerations and by the shedding of PMNs and red blood cells into the intestinal lumen. In relatively severe cases, thrombosis of mesenteric blood vessels, intestinal hemorrhage, and necrosis can occur. In patients with enteropathogenic yersinial infections who undergo exploratory laparotomy, the appendix usually is histologically normal or shows only lymphoid hyperplasia, but frank suppuration is sometimes evident.

A plasmid of ~70 kb is essential for virulence of the enteropathogenic yersiniae because it encodes at least six Yops, which confer a variety of pathogenic properties—e.g., cytotoxicity; resistance to phagocytosis by PMNs; and the ability to cause monocyte apoptosis (programmed cell death), to suppress the host's expression of tumor necrosis factor α, and to interfere with platelet aggregation and host complement activation. A chromosomal gene (*inv*) encodes for the surface protein invasin, which is necessary for yersinial invasion of nonphagocytic host cells (e.g., epithelial cells) in vitro and which facilitates the translocation of bacteria across the intestinal epithelium. Both *Y. enterocolitica* and *Y. pseudotuberculosis* can express at least one protein superantigen that selectively stimulates the proliferation of T cells. Many strains of *Y. enterocolitica* produce a heat-stable enterotoxin that is similar to *Escherichia coli* enterotoxin. The cell walls of *Y. enterocolitica* and *Y. pseudotuberculosis* contain a lipopolysaccharide (endotoxin). Some *Yersinia* strains are unable to synthesize bacterial iron chelators called *siderophores*. However, they can

exploit host-chelated iron stores and the drug deferoxamine (a siderophore produced by *Streptomyces pilosus*). Therefore, iron overload (e.g., caused by hemodialysis or multiple transfusions) and deferoxamine therapy appear to be independent risk factors for *Y. enterocolitica* bacteremia, especially that involving serotypes O:3 and O:9, and to a lesser degree for *Y. pseudotuberculosis* bacteremia.

Immunogenetic factors and cell-mediated immune responses are clearly involved in the pathogenesis of reactive arthritis following infection with the enteropathogenic yersiniae. As noted above, most patients with *Yersinia*-induced reactive arthritis express HLA-B27. In addition, *Y. pseudotuberculosis* shares at least one cross-reactive epitope with HLA-B27, and *Y. enterocolitica* infection alters the expression of serologic HLA-B27 epitopes on lymphocytes and monocytes. In patients with reactive arthritis following *Y. enterocolitica* infection, yersinial antigens are commonly detectable in synovial fluid cells in the apparent absence of whole organisms. Thus, it is unknown whether the arthritis results from occult bacterial persistence through self-tolerance of HLA-B27 with a failure of cross-reactive immune responses to yersiniae, from an immune response to common antigenic determinants shared by the bacteria and host HLA-B27 (i.e., molecular mimicry), or from other mechanisms. The pathogenesis of *Yersinia*-induced erythema nodosum is obscure.

In some assays, patients with Graves' disease have an increased prevalence of serum antibodies to *Y. enterocolitica*, and the immunoglobulins of patients recovering from *Y. enterocolitica* infections react with the human thyroid-stimulating hormone receptor. However, a link between *Y. enterocolitica* infection and the subsequent development of autoimmune thyroiditis has not been convincingly demonstrated.

MANIFESTATIONS ■ *Yersinia enterocolitica* The principal clinical manifestations of *Y. enterocolitica* infection are enteritis, enterocolitis, mesenteric adenitis, and terminal ileitis. Less common manifestations include exudative pharyngitis, septicemia, metastatic focal infections, reactive polyarthritis, and erythema nodosum. When age groups are combined, the most common presentation of *Y. enterocolitica* infection is acute diarrhea from enteritis or enterocolitis. Low-grade fever and cramping abdominal pain occur in most cases, nausea and vomiting in 15 to 40%, hematochezia in up to 30%, and a generalized maculopapular skin rash in a few cases. Diarrhea persists for an average of 2 weeks (range, 1 day to many months), during which the frequency of bowel movements diminishes. Uncommonly, enteritis or enterocolitis can be complicated by severe abdominal pain and high fever. Rare (and sometimes fatal) complications include diffuse inflammation, ulceration, hemorrhage, and necrosis of the small bowel and colon; intestinal perforation; peritonitis; ascending cholangitis; mesenteric vein thrombosis; diverticulitis; toxic megacolon; and ileocecal intussusception.

The syndrome of mesenteric adenitis and terminal ileitis without diarrhea is easily confused with appendicitis. Low-grade fever and right-lower-quadrant pain, tenderness, guarding, and rebound tenderness are common. During six recognized common-source outbreaks in the United States, 10% of 444 patients with symptomatic undiagnosed *Y. enterocolitica* infections underwent laparotomy for suspected appendicitis; surgical incisions became infected with *Y. enterocolitica* in a few of these cases.

Acute pharyngitis and pharyngotonsillitis, with or without cervical adenitis or intestinal illness, are less common but potentially lethal manifestations of *Y. enterocolitica* infection, particularly in adults. *Y. enterocolitica* septicemia generally presents as a severe illness with fever and leukocytosis, often with abdominal pain and jaundice and without localized signs of infection. Metastatic focal *Y. enterocolitica* infections can occur with or without clinically apparent bacteremia and can affect almost any organ system. Examples include abscess formation (e.g., in liver, spleen, kidney, lung, skeletal muscle, lymph node, or cutaneous tissue), osteomyelitis, meningitis, peritonitis, urinary tract infection, pneumonia, empyema, endocarditis, pericarditis, mycotic aneurysm, septic arthritis, suppurative conjunctivitis, panophthalmitis, Parinaud's oculoglandular syndrome, and cutaneous pustules or bullae.

In Scandinavia, the incidence of reactive arthritis following *Y. enterocolitica* infection among adults is estimated to be at least 10%. About 80% of these patients have preceding symptoms such as fever, diarrhea, or abdominal pain. Typically, these symptoms precede the arthritis by 1 week and are of short duration. The most commonly affected joints are the knees and ankles, but other joints can be involved. Typically, multiple (two to eight) joints become involved sequentially and asymmetrically over a period of a few days to 2 weeks, after which no additional joints are affected. Monarticular arthritis occurs less commonly. In two-thirds of cases, the acute arthritis remits spontaneously within 1 to 3 months. Chronic joint disease is documented in a minority of cases. A few HLA-B27-positive patients with *Y. enterocolitica*–induced arthritis have subsequent ankylosing spondylitis, but this development is best explained by the fact that HLA-B27 is a major risk factor for each of these diseases. Mild, self-limited myocarditis accompanies ~10% of cases of *Yersinia*-induced arthritis and can occur independently. Typical manifestations include cardiac murmurs and transient electrocardiographic abnormalities, such as prolongation of the PR interval and nonspecific ST-segment and T-wave changes. The syndrome of *Yersinia*-induced arthritis and carditis can be confused with acute rheumatic fever. In Scandinavia, erythema nodosum occurs in 15 to 20% of patients with yersiniosis, usually within a few days to 3 weeks after the onset of intestinal illness. Lesions typically are located on the lower extremities and resolve within 1 month. Less commonly reported nonsuppurative sequelae of *Y. enterocolitica* infections include reactive uveitis, iritis, conjunctivitis, urethritis, and glomerulonephritis. The complete triad of Reiter's syndrome (arthritis, conjunctivitis, and urethritis) is seen in 5 to 10% of patients with *Yersinia*-induced arthritis.

Yersinia pseudotuberculosis The most common clinical presentation of *Y. pseudotuberculosis* infection is fever and abdominal pain caused by mesenteric adenitis; diarrheal illness is less common than in *Y. enterocolitica* infection. Systemic manifestations, including septicemia, focal infections, reactive arthritis, and erythema nodosum, are generally similar to those associated with *Y. enterocolitica* infection. In addition, *Y. pseudotuberculosis* has been associated with a scarlet fever–like syndrome, acute interstitial nephritis, and hemolytic-uremic syndrome.

LABORATORY FINDINGS AND DIAGNOSIS Results of routine laboratory tests in most patients with yersiniosis are nonspecific. Leukocyte counts are usually normal or slightly elevated, often with a modest left shift. Standard microbiologic methods are sufficient to isolate *Y. enterocolitica* and *Y. pseudotuberculosis* from otherwise-sterile sites, such as blood, CSF, lymph node tissue, and peritoneal fluid, and from abscesses. Isolation of these organisms from feces is impeded by their slow growth and the overgrowth of normal fecal flora on culture media routinely used to select for enteric bacteria. The yield from feces and other grossly contaminated specimens can be increased by the use of *Yersinia*-selective [e.g., cefsulodin-Irgasan-novobiocin (CIN)] agar and by cold enrichment. Because bacteriologic procedures designed to isolate yersiniae from feces are not considered cost-effective, many laboratories undertake them by special request only.

The results of serologic tests can be used to support a diagnosis of yersiniosis. Agglutination tests or ELISAs are used most commonly; immunoblotting has also been used. The existence of multiple serotypes makes routine serologic tests laborious; thus these tests are generally conducted only in research laboratories or large commercial laboratories. Since these tests are experimental and are neither standardized nor well validated, and since some strains of *Yersinia* cross-react with other bacteria (e.g., *Brucella, Salmonella,* and *Vibrio*) and with serum from some patients with thyroiditis, results should be interpreted with caution. In typical uncomplicated cases of yersiniosis,

agglutinin titers begin to rise within the first week of illness, peak in the second week, and then gradually diminish and return to normal within 3 to 6 months, although agglutinating antibody may remain detectable for several years in some cases. Because an initial serum specimen is often collected a week or more after the onset of illness, when agglutinin titers are already high, it is usually impossible to document a fourfold or greater rise in titer between paired specimens (although a fourfold or greater fall in titer may be found). Immunohistochemical techniques and PCR tests to detect yersinial antigens and DNA, respectively, in clinical specimens are experimental at this time.

In patients with *Yersinia*-induced reactive arthritis, synovial fluid is sterile and the leukocyte count ranges from a few hundred to 60,000/μL, with a majority of PMNs. The erythrocyte sedimentation rate is often >100 mm/h. Rheumatoid factor and antinuclear antibodies are usually absent. The diagnosis of *Yersinia*-induced reactive arthritis or other nonsuppurative inflammatory sequelae can be difficult, especially when triggering infections are asymptomatic or clinically mild or occur several weeks before the diagnosis is attempted. Because the isolation of a pathogenic *Yersinia* strain from feces is the most specific diagnostic test in such cases, it should be attempted. Since culture is of limited sensitivity in this clinical setting, a high index of suspicion and positive results of serologic tests for *Y. enterocolitica* or *Y. pseudotuberculosis* are usually required for diagnosis.

℞ TREATMENT

The effectiveness of antimicrobial agents in the treatment of yersinial enteritis, enterocolitis, mesenteric adenitis, or terminal ileitis has not been established. These conditions are usually self-limited, and their treatment is symptom-based and supportive. In uncomplicated cases, diarrhea should be treated with fluid and electrolyte replacement, with the route of delivery dependent on clinical severity. Enteric precautions are advisable for patients hospitalized with yersinial diarrhea. In general, antimicrobial treatment should be reserved for patients with septicemia, metastatic focal infections, or immunosuppression and enterocolitis. Controlled clinical comparisons of antimicrobial agents in the treatment of severe cases of yersiniosis have not yet been conducted. In such cases, drug selection should ultimately be guided by clinical response and bacterial sensitivity patterns. Clinical isolates of *Y. enterocolitica* and *Y. pseudotuberculosis* are usually susceptible in vitro to aminoglycosides, third-generation cephalosporins, chloramphenicol, quinolones, tetracyclines, and TMP-SMX. In laboratory animals infected with enteropathogenic yersiniae, the fluoroquinolones have exerted the strongest bactericidal effects in vivo; clinical experience with these drugs against these pathogens in humans is promising but limited. Because they produce β-lactamases, isolates typically are resistant to penicillin, ampicillin, carbenicillin, and first-generation and most second-generation cephalosporins. Optimal dosages and durations of therapy have not been established. Mortality from *Y. enterocolitica* septicemia is ~10% despite treatment. Focal extraintestinal infections may require at least 3 weeks of therapy. No role for antimicrobial agents in the management of the nonsuppurative inflammatory manifestations of yersiniosis has been established. Patients with reactive arthritis may benefit from treatment with nonsteroidal anti-inflammatory drugs, intraarticular steroid injections, and physical therapy.

PREVENTION AND CONTROL The importance of safe food-handling and food-preparation practices in the prevention of yersiniosis cannot be overemphasized. Caution is particularly warranted in the case of pork and other animal products. The consumption of raw or undercooked meats, especially pork, should be avoided. Increased efforts to prevent the spread of enteric pathogens in household, pet-care, day-care, and hospital settings and in the food industry would be likely to decrease the incidence of yersiniosis. Current regulations of the U.S. Food and Drug Administration require visual inspection of packed red cell units before transfusion, with the discarding of units in which bacterial contamination is suspected on the basis of darkening (reflecting decreased oxygen saturation and hemolysis). Since the risk is minimal, more specific measures to further decrease the likelihood of transfusion of *Y. enterocolitica*–contaminated blood products (e.g., limiting the period for which red cells can be stored before transfusion) have not been widely implemented.

Yersiniosis is not routinely reportable to public health authorities in most jurisdictions. However, clinicians who suspect a common-source outbreak (e.g., because they have documented a familial case cluster) or some other public health threat (e.g., because they have found *Y. enterocolitica* bacteremia in a recent blood donor) should consult promptly with local public health officials.

FURTHER READING

BOTTONE EJ: *Yersinia enterocolitica*: Overview and epidemiologic correlates. Microbes Infect 1:323, 1999

CENTERS FOR DISEASE CONTROL AND PREVENTION: Imported plague—New York City, 2002. MMWR 52:725, 2003

———: *Yersinia enterocolitica* gastroenteritis among infants exposed to chitterlings—Chicago, Illinois, 2002. MMWR 52:956, 2003

CHANTEAU S et al: Development and testing of a rapid diagnostic test for bubonic and pneumonic plague. Lancet 361:211, 2003

INGLESBY TV et al: Plague as a biological weapon: Medical and public health management. JAMA 283:2281, 2000

LOFTUS CG et al: Clinical features of patients with novel *Yersinia* species. Dig Dis Sci 47:2805, 2002

RATSITORAHINA M et al: Epidemiological and diagnostic aspects of the outbreak of pneumonic plague in Madagascar. Lancet 355:111, 2000

SMEGO RA et al: Yersiniosis I: Microbiological and clinicoepidemiological aspects of plague and non-plague *Yersinia* infections. Eur J Clin Microbiol Infect Dis 18:1, 1999

144 BARTONELLA INFECTIONS, INCLUDING CAT-SCRATCH DISEASE
Lucy Stuart Tompkins

Bartonella species, including *B. bacilliformis*, *B. henselae*, and *B. quintana*, are tiny gram-negative bacilli that can adhere to and invade mammalian cells, including endothelial cells and erythrocytes. Previously classified as *Rochalimaea* species within the rickettsia group, *Bartonella* species have now been removed from the order Rickettsiales on the grounds that they are not obligate intracellular parasites. These agents cause a wide spectrum of clinical illnesses, including trench fever, cat-scratch disease (CSD), bacillary angiomatosis, peliosis hepatis, endocarditis, Oroya fever, and verruga peruana. The pathologic manifestations of *Bartonella* disease vary with the immune status of the host. Key features of major *Bartonella* infections are summarized in Table 144-1.

OROYA FEVER AND VERRUGA PERUANA

DEFINITION AND ETIOLOGY Oroya fever and verruga peruana are caused by *B. bacilliformis*. Oroya fever is characterized by fever, profound anemia, and—unless antibiotic treatment is given—high mortality. The lesions referred to as verruga peruana may develop during the convalescent phase of Oroya fever or during chronic infection with *B. bacilliformis*. In 1885 Daniel Carrion, a Peruvian medical student, inoculated himself with material from a patient with verruga peruana and subsequently died of Oroya fever, thus proving that a single agent causes both diseases.

EPIDEMIOLOGY Infection with *B. bacilliformis* follows the bite of the sandfly vector *Phlebotomus*, an insect found in the river valleys of the Andes Mountains at altitudes of 600 to 2500 m. Oroya fever develops in nonimmune individuals who are not residents of the endemic region, whereas verruga peruana occurs in persons who apparently have been exposed in the past, including those who have recently had Oroya fever. The infection has not been acquired in the United States.

PATHOLOGY During initial infection in the nonimmune host, *B. bacilliformis* cells adhere to erythrocytes and produce indentations in the cell membrane; the bacteria subsequently enter the erythrocytes and cause persistent deformation of the cytoskeleton. The parasitized erythrocytes are ultimately phagocytosed and destroyed. Although the life span of infected erythrocytes is markedly shortened, not all of this

TABLE 144-1 Bartonella Infections: Clinical Syndromes, Risk Factors, and Therapy

Bartonella Species	Clinical Syndrome	Risk Factors	Therapy[a]
Bartonella henselae	Cat-scratch disease	Cat scratch or bite	Azithromycin for 5 days (500 mg on day 1, 250 mg on days 2–5); or variable duration of rifampin (300 mg daily or bid), doxycycline (100 mg/d), or ciprofloxacin (500 mg/d)
	Bacillary angiomatosis/peliosis	Cat scratch or bite	Erythromycin (500 mg qid) or doxycycline (100 mg/d) for 3–6 weeks
	Endocarditis	Cat exposure	If patient is *Bartonella* culture-positive or seropositive: Give azithromycin (250 mg/d) or doxycycline (100 mg/d) for 4–6 months (surgery may be required)
			If *Bartonella* is suspected but unconfirmed: Treat for culture-negative endocarditis with ceftriaxone (2 g/d IV) plus gentamicin for 6–8 weeks[b]
Bartonella quintana	Trench fever	Homelessness; alcoholism; body lice	Doxycycline (100 mg bid) or azithromycin (500 mg/d) for 4–6 weeks
	Bacillary angiomatosis	Homelessness ± body lice; HIV infection	Same as for bacillary angiomatosis due to *B. henselae*
	Endocarditis	Same as for other *B. quintana* infections	Same as for endocarditis due to *B. henselae*
Bartonella bacilliformis	Oroya fever	Lack of immunity; sandfly bite	Chloramphenicol for 10 days (in South America); ampicillin (1 g q6h IV or PO) or cephalexin (500 mg qid PO) for 10–14 days
	Verruga peruana	Previous exposure to *B. bacilliformis*	Rifampin (300 mg bid) or ciprofloxacin (500 mg/d) for 7–10 days

[a] Azithromycin therapy for cat-scratch disease is based on clinical-trial data; all other recommendations are based on case reports or case series.

[b] If culture results confirm *Bartonella* infection, ceftriaxone may be discontinued and therapy with azithromycin or doxycycline given for a prolonged period.

change can be attributed to the mechanical fragility induced by the internalization of bacteria. Decreased bone marrow erythropoiesis also contributes to anemia.

CLINICAL MANIFESTATIONS   The onset of symptoms in Oroya fever may be either insidious or abrupt, after an incubation period of ~3 weeks. The subacute presentation may include low-grade fever, malaise, headache, and anorexia. Sudden-onset disease commences with high fever, chills, diaphoresis, headaches, and changes in mental status. These manifestations are followed by the sudden development of profound anemia, which is due to a marked decrease in erythrocyte numbers and is associated with macrocytic changes, poikilocytosis, Howell-Jolly bodies, nucleated erythrocytes, and immature myeloid cells. The leukocyte differential usually shifts to the left, although the total leukocyte count may be normal. The erythrocyte count may fall to extremely low levels. In eosin/thiazine-stained peripheral-blood smears, numerous microorganisms can be seen adhering to most erythrocytes.

During the acute phase, muscle and joint pain and headache may be severe; central nervous system changes include insomnia, delirium, and a decreased level of consciousness. Thrombocytopenic purpura may develop. If the patient survives, a convalescent phase ensues, characterized by the sudden disappearance of bacteria from blood smears, declining fever, and an increase in the erythrocyte count. Although much of the mortality associated with Oroya fever is due to profound anemia and toxicity, secondary bacterial infections (including salmonellosis and other enteric infections, malaria, and tuberculosis) are often an important contributing factor.

After convalescence from acute Oroya fever, nodular dermal eruptions known as *verrugas*, *verruga peruana*, or *Peruvian warts* may develop. These red or purple cutaneous lesions may be either tiny and sessile or large, pedunculated, and nodular. They bear a marked resemblance to the lesions of bacillary angiomatosis and to Kaposi's sarcoma.

DIAGNOSIS   During acute infection, bacteria can be cultured from the blood on agar containing rabbit blood, with incubation at 28°C. The hallmark of verruga peruana is the formation of new blood vessels (angiogenesis) at the sites of bacterial replication.

℞ **TREATMENT**

Oroya fever responds to a variety of antimicrobial agents, including chloramphenicol, tetracyclines, penicillin, and streptomycin. In South America, chloramphenicol is used most often because of its simultaneous efficacy against most *Salmonella* infections (which may develop intercurrently). Ampicillin (1 g every 6 h) has also been used, as has cephalexin (500 mg every 6 h). Verruga peruana may respond similarly; rifampin (300 mg twice a day) and ciprofloxacin (500 mg/d) have also been used. Failure to respond to therapy and relapse are common and require the reinstitution of prolonged therapy.

CAT-SCRATCH DISEASE

DEFINITION AND ETIOLOGY   Typical CSD is manifest by painful regional lymphadenopathy persisting for several weeks or months after a cat scratch. Occasionally, infection may disseminate and produce more generalized lymphadenopathy and systemic manifestations, which may be confused with the manifestations of lymphoma. *B. henselae* is the causative agent of CSD. There is no evidence that other *Bartonella* species cause CSD. The role of *Afipia felis* (originally proposed as the agent of CSD) is unclear inasmuch as only a few cases are associated with its isolation. Several reports suggest that *B. clarridgeiae* may cause feline lymphadenopathy.

EPIDEMIOLOGY   Acquisition of *B. henselae* has been significantly associated with exposure to young cats infested with fleas (*Ctenocephalides felis*). The finding that a high proportion of cats with fleas

have persistent asymptomatic *B. henselae* bacteremia suggests that the domestic cat is the animal reservoir of this microorganism. The flea can serve as a transmitting vector in the cross-infection of cats, but its role in human infection is not clear. Regions of the United States where fleas are endemic have higher rates of CSD. Approximately 60% of cases occur in children.

MICROBIOLOGY   *B. henselae* may be isolated from blood and rarely from lymph nodes or other tissues. Co-cultivation with endothelial cell monolayers has been employed to detect growth. Colonies develop after prolonged incubation (1 to 4 weeks) with 5 to 10% CO_2 at 37°C on blood-containing media (rabbit blood is preferred); the colonies pit the agar. Bacterial cells are gram-negative.

CLINICAL MANIFESTATIONS   A localized papule, progressing to a pustule that often crusts over, develops 3 to 5 days after a cat scratch. Tender regional lymphadenopathy develops within 1 to 2 weeks after inoculation; by this time, the papule may have healed spontaneously. Scratches are most often sustained on the hands or face, producing epitrochlear, axillary, pectoral, or cervical lymph node involvement. The involved nodes occasionally become suppurative; bacterial superinfection with staphylococci or other cutaneous pathogens may develop. Although most patients do not have fever, systemic symptoms are frequent and include malaise, anorexia, and weight loss. Without treatment, lymphadenopathy persists for weeks or even months and may be confused with lymphatic malignancy. Other manifestations in apparently immunocompetent patients include encephalitis, seizures and coma (especially in children), meningitis, transverse myelitis, granulomatous hepatitis and splenitis, osteomyelitis, and disseminated infection. Conjunctival inoculation may cause Parinaud's oculoglandular syndrome, with conjunctivitis and periauricular lymphadenopathy. *B. henselae* is considered the most common cause of acute neuroretinitis. This condition may present as an acute change in vision associated with a stellate macular lesion; other pathologic changes of the retina may also occur.

PATHOLOGY   The histopathologic hallmark of CSD is granulomatous inflammation with stellate necrosis but no evidence of angiogenesis. Infection by *B. henselae* can produce two entirely different pathologic reactions, depending on the immune status of the host: granulomatous inflammation or angiogenesis.

DIAGNOSIS   CSD should be suspected if the patient has a history of exposure to cats and develops lymphadenopathy and a skin lesion. The diagnosis can be confirmed by pathologic examination of the involved nodes. Tiny bacilli in clusters can sometimes be seen in biopsy samples stained with Warthin-Starry silver. The CSD skin test, in which lymph node material obtained from patients with CSD serves as an antigen, is no longer used. Specific serologic tests have been developed and produce positive results in 70 to 90% of patients with intact immunity. These tests are commercially available. The identification of *B. henselae* 16S ribosomal RNA genes in biopsy material by polymerase chain reaction (PCR) amplification with specific oligonucleotide primers can also be diagnostically useful; however, these methods are not commercially available. Cultures of lymph nodes, cerebrospinal fluid, or other tissues are rarely positive.

℞ **TREATMENT**

Although CSD is generally self-limited, tender regional lymphadenopathy and systemic symptoms may be debilitating. Patients with encephalitis or other serious manifestations should be treated with antibiotics. A randomized, double-blind, placebo-controlled trial demonstrated significant clinical benefit of treatment with oral azithromycin for 5 days in cases of typical CSD (regimen for adults weighing >100 lb: one dose of 500 mg on day 1, 250 mg on days 2 through 5). Several reports suggest that aminoglycoside treatment (e.g., intravenous gentamicin at standard doses calculated to result in therapeutic levels) is effective in patients with encephalitis and other systemic infections. On the basis of case reports and case series, the oral agents that appear to be useful are those that also are most effective for the treatment of bacillary angiomatosis; they include doxycycline (100 mg/d), rifampin (300 mg daily or twice daily), and azithromycin (250 mg/d). Unlike bacillary angiomatosis, CSD may also respond to treatment with ciprofloxacin (500 mg/d). The necessary duration of therapy is variable. Antibiotic treatment of neuroretinitis is followed by partial or complete resolution.

TRENCH FEVER

DEFINITION AND ETIOLOGY   Trench fever was first described as a debilitating febrile illness associated with prolonged *B. quintana* bacteremia in soldiers fighting in Europe during World War I. Cases have since occurred throughout the world. In recent years, trench fever has re-emerged in the United States and France among urban homeless patients.

EPIDEMIOLOGY   Although trench fever was once thought to have disappeared from the United States, recent cases have been diagnosed in homeless persons with alcohol abuse. Similar epidemiologic features have been noted in Marseilles, France. An outbreak of infection occurred in Seattle, Washington, in 1993, and few cases have been documented subsequently. In World War I, *B. quintana* was transmitted from person to person by the human body louse, and recent cases in Seattle and Marseilles have also been associated with lice.

CLINICAL MANIFESTATIONS   Trench fever is characterized by the sudden onset of headache, aseptic meningitis, persistent or relapsing fever (which can be high-grade and is commonly paroxysmal), malaise, weight loss, and other nonspecific symptoms. Some patients may have an indolent course with minimal clinical manifestations. The incubation period is 3 to 38 days. Severe musculoskeletal pain is more common among immunocompetent than among immunocompromised patients. Bacteremia can persist for days or weeks, and relapses have followed short courses of antibiotic therapy. Localized findings are uncommon.

DIAGNOSIS   The infection is diagnosed by the finding of sustained bacteremia. *B. quintana* grows slowly, and colonies may develop on rabbit blood agar after 1 to 4 weeks of incubation under conditions of increased CO_2. The infection may also be detected serologically, although these tests are not standardized.

℞ TREATMENT

A prolonged course (4 to 6 weeks) of antimicrobial therapy may be required. Agents that can cross the mammalian cell membrane are most effective, including doxycycline (100 mg by mouth twice daily), erythromycin (2 g/d), or azithromycin (500 mg/d). Data on the efficacy of these agents come from a limited number of case reports.

BACILLARY ANGIOMATOSIS

DEFINITION AND ETIOLOGY   Bacillary angiomatosis was initially described as a condition occurring primarily in patients with AIDS and characterized by vascular cutaneous lesions resembling verruga peruana and Kaposi's sarcoma. The disease can disseminate to involve virtually any organ system, including the liver (peliosis hepatis). Immunocompromised individuals, especially those infected with HIV, are at particularly high risk for bacillary angiomatosis, although in rare instances the patient is not obviously immunosuppressed. Both *B. henselae* and *B. quintana* produce bacillary angiomatosis in persons with immunodeficiency.

EPIDEMIOLOGY   A case-control study revealed that *B. henselae* and *B. quintana* differ significantly in terms of epidemiologic risk factors. All cases of *B. henselae* infection were associated with exposure to cats and their fleas and occurred sporadically, whereas the cases of *B. quintana* bacillary angiomatosis occurred in clusters and were associated with low socioeconomic status, homelessness, and exposure to body lice. Direct transmission of *B. henselae* from cats to their owners,

presumably through cutaneous trauma, was supported by the matching DNA fingerprint patterns of isolates from the two sources.

PATHOGENESIS AND PATHOLOGY   Bacillary angiomatosis is characterized by a lobular proliferation of new blood vessels (angiogenesis) and a neutrophilic inflammatory response to myriad bacilli located within collagen-rich microscopic and macroscopic nodules. The organisms can be visualized with Warthin-Starry silver stain. The endothelial cells lining the vascular spaces have a typical epithelioid appearance, and the lesions may resemble Kaposi's sarcoma histopathologically, although the characteristic spindle cell of the latter disease is usually absent. The bacterial and eukaryotic host factors that elicit the pathologic response are unknown.

CLINICAL MANIFESTATIONS   The skin lesions of bacillary angiomatosis (also called *epithelioid angiomatosis*) are vascular nodules, papules, or tumors that range from tiny lesions resembling cherry angiomas or pyogenic granulomas to large, pedunculated, exophytic masses (Fig. 144-1). Characteristically, the lesions are red or purple, resembling Kaposi's sarcoma; they may be surrounded by an epithelial collarette, may be located anywhere on the skin, and may involve mucous membranes. The overlying epidermis may be focally ulcerated, and the underlying bone may be invaded and destroyed.

Dissemination of *B. henselae* infection occurs primarily in patients with cellular immune defects. Clinical manifestations accompanying dissemination are often nonspecific and include persistent fever, abdominal pain, weight loss, and malaise. Although the liver, spleen, bone marrow, and lymph nodes are primarily affected, HIV-infected patients may also develop central nervous system abnormalities (including psychiatric disorders and brain lesions), which are responsive to antibiotic therapy. Skin lesions usually are not evident in disseminated infection. Involvement of the liver or spleen may produce bacillary peliosis hepatis. Patients with the latter condition may report localized pain on palpation of the abdomen. Nodular lesions of variable size can be demonstrated by computed tomography or magnetic resonance imaging, with or without contrast agents. As these lesions are associated with neovascularization, percutaneous biopsy may lead to hemorrhage.

In a case-control study of bacillary angiomatosis (see "Epidemiology" above), only *B. henselae* was associated with hepatosplenic disease (peliosis hepatis) and displayed a predilection for lymph nodes. *B. quintana*, in contrast, was associated with osseous and subcutaneous infection.

DIAGNOSIS   The diagnosis of bacillary angiomatosis is based primarily on the typical histopathologic findings of angiomas in association with clumps of tiny bacilli revealed by Warthin-Starry silver stain. Infection can also be established by blood cultures performed with a lysis-centrifugation system or by identification of specific DNA sequences. Bacilli picked from new colonies growing on blood agar but not subcultured may not stain, even with acridine orange; they stain weakly with

FIGURE 144-1   Characteristic skin lesion of bacillary angiomatosis in an HIV-positive young woman. This large, pedunculated tumor exhibits the typical angiomatous appearance. The patient was treated with oral erythromycin, with nearly complete resolution of the lesion; however, on discontinuation of antibiotic therapy after a 4-week course, the lesion recurred.

safranin. Identification of *B. henselae* and *B. quintana* is based primarily on cellular fatty-acid analysis and PCR-based restriction fragment length polymorphism analysis. Definitive identification of *Bartonella* species depends on DNA sequence analysis of 16S ribosomal RNA genes. The sensitivity and specificity of serologic tests have not been determined.

DIFFERENTIAL DIAGNOSIS The differential diagnosis of cutaneous bacillary angiomatosis includes Kaposi's sarcoma, angiomas, and pyogenic granulomas. These conditions can be distinguished by histopathologic examination of biopsied material. AIDS patients may have both Kaposi's sarcoma lesions and bacillary angiomatosis lesions simultaneously; thus biopsy is essential to differentiate the two.

Rx TREATMENT

Cutaneous lesions have been treated with a wide variety of antimicrobial drugs, including macrolides, tetracyclines, and antituberculous agents; *B. henselae* is susceptible to most antibiotics in vitro. Erythromycin (2 g/d), given orally for 3 weeks, is usually effective, as are newer macrolides; however, relapse may require prolonged therapy (3 weeks to 2 months) with an antibiotic that reaches an intracellular compartment, such as a macrolide or doxycycline (100 mg/d). Patients with peliosis hepatis should be treated with intravenous antibiotics, and those with disseminated disease or bacteremia should be treated with a prolonged course of a systemic antibiotic. In a case-control study of bacillary angiomatosis, treatment with a macrolide was associated with a therapeutic response and sterile tissue samples and may have been protective, whereas treatment with trimethoprim-sulfamethoxazole, ciprofloxacin, penicillins, or cephalosporins had no protective effect. Cutaneous lesions may or may not regress spontaneously, perhaps depending on the status of the host's immunity. The safety of ciprofloxacin in pregnant or lactating women has not been established. No antimicrobial agent has been studied prospectively, and information on efficacy comes only from case reports.

OTHER *BARTONELLA* INFECTIONS, INCLUDING CULTURE-NEGATIVE ENDOCARDITIS

The application of molecular methods to the detection of microorganisms that are difficult to cultivate in the laboratory has revealed new *Bartonella* species and has established *Bartonella* species as a cause of endocarditis cases previously classified as being of unknown etiology. *B. quintana* is the *Bartonella* species most frequently isolated from patients with endocarditis. Two other species, *B. elizabethae* and *B. clarridgeiae*, as well as *B. henselae* have also been identified as agents of subacute and chronic endocarditis.

The diagnosis of *Bartonella* endocarditis is confirmed by blood cultures. A presumptive diagnosis can be made on the basis of epidemiologic history and by serology. Infection may elicit antibodies that cross-react with *Chlamydia pneumoniae*, and *Coxiella burnetii* infection (Q fever) elicits antibodies that cross-react with *B. quintana*.

In culture-positive or seropositive endocarditis, initial treatment with azithromycin (250 mg/d) or doxycycline (100 mg/d) for 4 to 6 months is recommended. A third-generation cephalosporin or an aminoglycoside may be added for the initial 2 to 3 weeks of therapy. If *Bartonella* infection is suspected but not yet confirmed, therapy for culture-negative endocarditis with ceftriaxone (2 g/d by the intravenous route) plus an aminoglycoside for 6 to 8 weeks is recommended. If culture results prove positive, ceftriaxone administration may be discontinued and treatment with a macrolide (azithromycin) or doxycycline given for a prolonged period.

FURTHER READING

BASS JW et al: Prospective randomized double blind placebo-controlled evaluation of azithromycin for treatment of cat-scratch disease. Pediatr Infect Dis J 17:447, 1998

BROUQUI P et al: Chronic *Bartonella quintana* bacteremia in homeless patients. N Engl J Med 340:184, 1999

CARITHERS HA: Cat scratch disease: An overview based on a study of 1,200 patients. Am J Dis Child 139:1124, 1985

COCKERELL DJ, LEBOIT PE: Bacillary angiomatosis: A newly characterized, pseudoneoplastic, infectious, cutaneous vascular disorder. J Am Acad Dermatol 22:501, 1990

FOURNIER P-E et al: Epidemiologic and clinical characteristics of *B. quintana* and *B. henselae* endocarditis. Medicine 80:245, 2001

MAGUINA C et al: Bartonellosis (Carrion's disease) in the modern era. Clin Infect Dis 33:772, 2001

OHL ME, SPACH DH: *Bartonella quintana* and urban trench fever. Clin Infect Dis 31:131, 2000

SPACH DH et al: *Bartonella (Rochalimaea) quintana* bacteremia in inner-city patients with chronic alcoholism. N Engl J Med 332:425, 1995

---

145 DONOVANOSIS
Gavin Hart

Donovanosis is a chronic, progressively destructive bacterial infection of the genital region that is generally regarded as sexually transmitted. The disease has been known by many other names, the most common of which are granuloma inguinale and granuloma venereum.

ETIOLOGY Donovanosis is caused by *Calymmatobacterium granulomatis*, an intracellular, gram-negative, pleomorphic, encapsulated (when mature) bacterium measuring 1.5 by 0.7 μm. *C. granulomatis* shares many morphologic and serologic characteristics and >99% homology at the nucleotide level with *Klebsiella* species that are pathogenic to humans. Polymerase chain reaction (PCR) amplification of the *phoE* gene shows it to be closely related to that in *Klebsiella pneumoniae*, *K. rhinoscleromatis*, and *K. ozaenae*. Electron microscopy shows typical gram-negative morphology and a large capsule but no flagella. Filiform or vesicular protrusions occur on a corrugated cell wall.

EPIDEMIOLOGY Donovanosis is endemic among Aborigines in central Australia as well as in Papua New Guinea, southeastern India, southern Africa, and the Caribbean and adjacent areas of South America. In the first half of the twentieth century, the disease was endemic in parts of the United States (with an estimated 5000 to 10,000 cases in 1947); small epidemics still occur in this country and in other developed countries. The decline in the United States to fewer than 20 reported cases annually in the past decade has probably resulted from lower transmission rates due to earlier presentation for increasingly effective antibiotic therapy. Over 70% of cases involve persons 20 to 40 years of age. The infection is predominantly sexually transmitted, but extragenital skin lesions can follow transmission from concurrent genital lesions via the fingers or through other nonsexual contact, and autoinoculation may produce new lesions from contact with adjacent skin ("kissing" lesions). Infants born to infected mothers have acquired infection at birth.

The classification of donovanosis as a sexually transmitted disease (STD) has been disputed because of cases in young children and occasionally in sexually inactive individuals, transmission by direct body contact and via inanimate intermediaries, and the low and variable prevalence of donovanosis among sexual partners (0.4 to 52%). The dominance of sexual transmission is suggested by the combined factors of lesions predominantly affecting the genitalia, the highest prevalence among persons in age and socioeconomic groups that are most

FIGURE 145-1 Multiple granulomatous lesions of the penis in a patient with donovanosis.

TABLE 145-1 Differential Diagnosis of Donovanosis

Disease (Chapter)	Distinguishing Features
Secondary syphilis: condylomata lata (153)	White or pale moist plaques in anogenital region (as opposed to bright red donovanosis lesions); lesions subside within 1 week of treatment with benzathine penicillin, 2.4 mU (whereas donovanosis lesions remain unchanged)
Squamous cell carcinoma (73)	Histologic appearance
Penile amebiasis (194)	Microscopic identification of *Entamoeba histolytica*
Chancroid: pseudogranuloma inguinale (130)	Culture of *Haemophilus ducreyi*
Tuberculosis (150)	Histologic features of bony lesions
Actinomycosis (147)	Microscopic identification of sulfur granules
Rhinoscleroma (134)	Histologic features
Leishmaniasis (196)	Histologic features
Histoplasmosis (183)	Histologic features

often affected by STDs, and the predictable occurrence of disease in visitors to areas of endemicity following sexual exposure.

CLINICAL MANIFESTATIONS The incubation period is usually 1 to 4 weeks but may extend to 1 year. Skin lesions have been detected in infants 6 weeks to 6 months after birth. The disease begins as one or more subcutaneous nodules that erode through the skin to produce clean, granulomatous, sharply defined, usually painless lesions (Fig. 145-1). These lesions, which bleed readily on contact, slowly enlarge. The genitalia are involved in 90% of cases, the inguinal region in 10%, and the anal region in 5 to 10%. Genital swelling, particularly of the labia, is a common feature and occasionally progresses to pseudoelephantiasis. Phimosis and paraphimosis are common local complications, and progressive erosion of affected tissues may completely destroy the penis or other organs. Less common clinical variants include a hypertrophic form (cauliflower- or wartlike lesions), a necrotic form (destructive lesions with foul-smelling exudate, often resembling amebiasis), and a sclerotic or cicatricial form, which has a dry base with extensive scar tissue.

Extragenital lesions occur in at least 6% of cases. Oral donovanosis, the most common extragenital manifestation, presents as pain or bleeding in the mouth, lesions on the lips, or extensive swelling of the gums and palate. Donovanosis may affect most bones, and sometimes many bones are affected at the same time; the tibia is involved in over 50% of such cases. Bony lesions are associated with constitutional symptoms (weight loss, fever, night sweats, and malaise) and are usually found in women. More than 50% of women with donovanosis have primary lesions on the cervix. Prompt pelvic examinations and early diagnosis are likely to substantially decrease the morbidity and mortality (likely outcomes in misdiagnosed spinal lesions) associated with extragenital donovanosis in women.

DIAGNOSIS ■ Laboratory Diagnosis The preferred diagnostic method involves demonstration of typical intracellular Donovan bodies within large mononuclear cells visualized in smears prepared from lesions or biopsy specimens. With typical beefy lesions, a small piece of tissue is removed with forceps and scalpel, and a crush impression of the deep surface is made on a glass slide. The smear is air-dried, heatfixed, and stained with Giemsa, Leishman's, or Wright's stain. For dry, flat, or necrotic lesions, a punch-biopsy specimen should be obtained from the advancing edge. This specimen can be used to prepare a smear or embedded for histologic examination (with a silver stain). Histologic examination shows epithelial proliferation, often simulating

neoplasia, with a heavy inflammatory infiltrate of plasma cells, some neutrophils, and few if any lymphocytes. The large mononuclear cells are 25 to 90 μm in diameter, with a vesicular or pyknotic nucleus. Up to 20 intracytoplasmic vacuoles contain pleomorphic Donovan bodies in either young unencapsulated forms (which often resemble closed safety pins) or mature encapsulated forms. *C. granulomatis* has never been grown on artificial solid media but has been cultured in chicken embryonic yolk sacs, on human monocytes, and on human epithelial (HEp-2) cells. A diagnostic PCR test has been developed and incorporated into a colorimetric detection system for *C. granulomatis*. A serologic test, based on indirect immunofluorescence, is more useful in confirming the diagnosis in cases with long-standing lesions than in early disease.

Differential Diagnosis The differential diagnosis of donovanosis is summarized in Table 145-1. Syphilis and donovanosis frequently coexist because syphilis is usually highly prevalent in areas where donovanosis is endemic; thus positive syphilis serology does not exclude a diagnosis of donovanosis. Genital ulcers are a risk factor for HIV acquisition in developing countries, and patients with donovanosis should be tested for HIV infection.

℞ TREATMENT

Table 145-2 shows the most effective regimens for treating donovanosis. Doxycycline offers the advantage of convenient administration and has been widely used in developed countries, but azithromycin is increasingly being used as first-choice therapy. Extensive lesions have been cured with oral azithromycin at a dosage of 500 mg/d, but the more convenient dose of 1 g weekly is also effective. Although chlor-

TABLE 145-2 The Most Effective Antibiotic Regimens for Treatment of Donovanosis[a]

Antibiotic	Oral Dosage
Azithromycin	1 g weekly or 500 mg/d
Erythromycin	500 mg qid
Tetracycline	500 mg qid
Doxycycline	100 mg bid
Trimethoprim-sulfamethoxazole	1 double-strength tablet[b] bid
Chloramphenicol	500 mg tid

[a] Patients should be examined weekly, and therapy should be continued until lesions have healed (3 to 5 weeks, except in severe cases).
[b] 160 mg/800 mg.

amphenicol is the drug of choice in some developing countries, it is unlikely to be acceptable in developed countries because of bone marrow toxicity. Penicillin is not effective for treating donovanosis. Patients should be examined weekly, and therapy should be continued until lesions have healed (3 to 5 weeks, except in severe cases). If antibiotic therapy is stopped earlier, lesions often continue to heal, but the relapse rate is higher. If the lesions are unchanged after 2 weeks of treatment, an alternative antibiotic regimen should be used.

The treatment regimens listed in Table 145-2 are usually adequate in HIV-infected patients without immunosuppression, but an increas-ing failure rate has been reported in immunosuppressed patients, for whom daily administration of azithromycin is recommended if other regimens fail to elicit a response.

FURTHER READING

See www.stdservices.on.net/std/donovanosis/Default.htm for an illustrated lec-ture and a comprehensive bibliography on donovanosis.
CARTER JS, KEMP DJ: A colorimetric detection system for Calymmatobac-terium granulomatis. Sex Trans Infect 76:134, 2000
HART G: Donovanosis (granuloma inguinale), in *Atlas of Infectious Diseases*, vol V: *Sexually Transmitted Diseases*, MF Rein (ed). Philadelphia, Church-ill Livingstone, 1996, pp 17.1–17.10
———: Donovanosis. Clin Infect Dis 25:24, 1997
O'FARRELL N: Donovanosis: An update. Int J STD AIDS 12:423, 2001

Section 7   Miscellaneous Bacterial Infections

146 | NOCARDIOSIS
Gregory A. Filice

Nocardiosis refers to disease associated with members of the genus *Nocardia*. Of several distinctive syndromes associated with these bac-teria, pneumonia and disseminated disease are most common. Others include cellulitis, lymphocutaneous syndrome, actinomycetoma, and keratitis.

MICROBIOLOGY Nocardiae are saprophytic aerobic actinomycetes that are common worldwide in soil, where they contribute to decay of organic matter. Nocardial taxonomy is complex and incompletely un-derstood. Seven species have been clearly associated with human dis-ease: *N. asteroides*, *N. brasiliensis*, *N. otitidis-caviarum* (formerly *N. caviae*), *N. farcinica*, *N. nova*, *N. transvalensis*, and *N. pseudobrasi-liensis*. In addition, two newly described species have been associated with disease in humans: *N. abscessus* from soft-tissue abscesses and *N. africana* from respiratory secretions of patients in the Sudan with pneumonia.

N. asteroides is the species most commonly associated with inva-sive disease. *N. farcinica* disease is less common, but this species is more virulent and prone to dissemination. *N. pseudobrasiliensis* is most often associated with invasive disease, and *N. brasiliensis* is usu-ally associated with disease limited to the skin. *N. transvalensis* is generally associated with pulmonary or systemic disease in immuno-suppressed persons or with *actinomycetoma*, an indolent, slowly pro-gressive disease of skin and underlying tissues with nodular swellings and draining sinuses.

EPIDEMIOLOGY Approximately 1000 cases of nocardial infection are diagnosed annually in the United States, 85% of them pulmonary and/or systemic. The disease is more common among adults than among children and among males than among females. Nearly all cases are sporadic, but outbreaks have been associated with contamination of the hospital environment, solutions, or drug injection equipment. Per-son-to-person spread is not well documented. There is no known sea-sonality.

The risk of pulmonary or disseminated disease is greater than usual among persons with deficient cell-mediated immunity, especially that associated with lymphoma, transplantation, glucocorticoid therapy, or AIDS. In AIDS, nocardiosis usually affects persons with <250 CD4+ lymphocytes/μL. Nocardiosis has also been associated with pulmo-nary alveolar proteinosis, tuberculosis and other mycobacterial dis-eases, chronic granulomatous disease, and interleukin 12 deficiency.

N. brasiliensis, *N. asteroides*, *N. otitidis-caviarum*, and *N. trans-valensis* are associated with actinomycetoma. Cases occur mainly in tropical and subtropical regions, especially those of Mexico, Central and South America, Africa, and India. The most important risk factor is frequent contact with soil or vegetable matter.

PATHOLOGY AND PATHOGENESIS Pneumonia and disseminated disease are both thought to follow inhalation of fragmented bacterial mycelia. The characteristic histologic feature of nocardiosis is an abscess with ex-tensive neutrophil infiltration and prominent necrosis. Granulation tis-sue usually surrounds the lesions, but extensive fibrosis or encapsu-lation is uncommon. Actinomycetoma is characterized by suppurative inflammation with sinus tract formation. Granules—microcolonies composed of dense masses of bacterial filaments extending radially from a central core—are occasionally observed in histologic prepa-rations. They are frequently found in discharges from lesions of acti-nomycetoma but almost never from lesions in other forms of nocar-diosis. Infrequently, nocardiae and other indolent pathogens, including fungi or mycobacteria, are isolated from the same patient.

Nocardiae have evolved a number of properties that enable them to survive within phagocytes, including neutralization of oxidants, pre-vention of phagosome-lysosome fusion, and prevention of phagosome acidification. Neutrophils phagocytose the organisms and limit their growth but do not kill them efficiently. Cell-mediated immunity is important for definitive control and elimination of nocardiae.

CLINICAL MANIFESTATIONS ■ **Respiratory Tract Disease** Pneumonia is by far the most common respiratory tract nocardial disease. Nocardial pneumonia is typically subacute; symptoms have usually been present for days or weeks at presentation. The onset is more acute in some immunosuppressed patients. Cough is prominent and produces small amounts of thick, purulent sputum that is not malodorous. Fever, an-orexia, weight loss, and malaise are common; dyspnea, pleuritic pain, and hemoptysis are less common. Remissions and exacerbations over several weeks are frequent.

Roentgenographic patterns vary, but some are highly suggestive of nocardial pneumonia. Infiltrates vary in size and are typically of at least moderate density. Single or multiple nodules are common, some-times suggesting tumor metastases (Fig. 146-1). Infiltrates and nodules tend to cavitate. Empyema is present in one-third of cases.

Nocardiosis may spread directly from the lungs to adjacent tissues. Pericarditis, mediastinitis, and the superior vena cava syndrome have all been reported. Nocardial laryngitis, tracheitis, and bronchitis are much less common than pneumonia. In the major airways, disease often presents as a nodular or granulomatous mass. A few cases of sinusitis have been reported.

Nocardiae are sometimes isolated from respiratory secretions of patients without apparent nocardial disease. Most of these patients have chronic pulmonary disease with abnormal airways or parenchyma and do not necessarily require treatment for nocardiosis (see "Diag-nosis," below).

Extrapulmonary Disease In half of all cases of pulmonary nocardiosis, disease appears outside the lungs. In one-fifth of cases of disseminated disease, lung disease is not apparent. The most common site of dis-semination is the brain. Other common sites include the skin and sup-

FIGURE 146-1 Nocardial pneumonia. *Top:* Three large nodules with apparent cavitation are apparent on the anterior-posterior chest roentgenograph. *Bottom:* A computed tomographic scan of the same patient confirms the presence of bilateral nodules and cavitation in the nodule in the left midlung field.

porting structures, kidneys, bone, and muscle, but almost any organ can be involved. Peritonitis has been reported. Nocardiae have been recovered from blood in a few cases of pneumonia or disseminated disease. Nocardial endocarditis occurs rarely and can affect either native or prosthetic valves. A few cases of nocardial bacteremia associated with infected central venous catheters have been reported.

The typical manifestation of extrapulmonary dissemination is a subacute abscess. A minority of abscesses outside the lungs or central nervous system (CNS) form fistulae and discharge small amounts of pus.

In CNS infections, brain abscesses are usually supratentorial, are often multiloculated, and may be single or multiple (Fig. 146-2). Brain abscesses tend to burrow into the ventricles or extend out into the subarachnoid space. The symptoms and signs are somewhat more indolent than those of other types of bacterial brain abscess. Meningitis is uncommon and is usually due to spread from a nearby brain abscess. Nocardiae are not easily recovered from cerebrospinal fluid (CSF).

Disease Following Transcutaneous Inoculation   Disease following transcutaneous nocardial inoculation usually takes one of three forms: cellulitis, lymphocutaneous syndrome, or actinomycetoma.

Cellulitis generally begins 1 to 3 weeks after a recognized breach of the skin, often with soil contamination. Subacute cellulitis with pain, swelling, erythema, and warmth develops over days to weeks. The

lesions are usually firm and nonfluctuant. Disease may progress to involve underlying muscle, tendon, bones, or joints. Dissemination is rare. *N. asteroides* is common in colder climates, while *N. brasiliensis* predominates in warmer climates.

Lymphocutaneous disease usually begins with a pyodermatous lesion at the site of inoculation, with central ulceration and purulent or honey-colored drainage. Subcutaneous nodules often appear along lymphatics that drain the primary lesion. The lymphangitic form closely resembles lymphocutaneous sporotrichosis (Chap. 190). Most cases of the lymphocutaneous syndrome are associated with *N. brasiliensis*.

Actinomycetoma usually begins with a nodular swelling, sometimes at a site of local trauma. Lesions typically develop on the feet or hands but may involve the posterior part of the neck, the upper back, the head, and other sites. The nodule eventually breaks down and a fistula appears, which is then accompanied by others. The fistulas tend to come and go, with new ones forming as old ones disappear. The discharge is serous or purulent, may be bloody, and often contains 0.1- to 2-mm white granules consisting of masses of mycelia. The lesions spread slowly along fascial planes to involve adjacent areas of skin, subcutaneous tissue, and bone. Over months or years, there may be extensive deformation of the affected part. Lesions involving soft tissues are only mildly painful; those affecting bones or joints are more so. Systemic symptoms are absent or minimal. Infection rarely disseminates from actinomycetoma, and lesions on the hands and feet usually cause only local disability. Lesions on the head, neck, and trunk can invade locally to involve deep organs and result in severe disability or death.

Keratitis   *Nocardia* species, usually *N. asteroides*, are uncommon causes of subacute keratitis. The infection usually follows eye trauma. Nocardial infection of lacrimal glands has been reported. Endophthalmitis and other diseases involving deeper eye structures are usually manifestations of dissemination.

DIAGNOSIS   The first step in diagnosis is examination of sputum or pus for crooked, branching, beaded, gram-positive filaments 1 μm wide and up to 50 μm long. Most nocardiae are acid-fast in direct smears if a weak acid is used for decolorization (e.g., in the modified Kinyoun, Ziehl-Neelsen, and Fite-Faraco methods). The organisms often take up silver stains. Nocardiae grow relatively slowly; colonies may take

FIGURE 146-2   Nocardial abscesses in the right cerebellum. The appearance suggests one large abscess and multiple daughter abscesses.

TABLE 146-1 *Treatment for Nocardiosis*

Disease	Duration	Drugs (Daily Dose)[a]
Pulmonary or systemic		Systemic therapy
Intact host defenses	6–12 mo	Oral
Deficient host defenses	12 mo[b]	1. Sulfonamides (6–8 g) or combination of
CNS disease	12 mo[c]	trimethoprim (10–20 mg/kg) and
Cellulitis, lympho-		sulfamethoxazole (50–100 mg/kg)
cutaneous syndrome	2 mo	2. Minocycline (200–400 mg)
Osteomyelitis, arthritis,		Parenteral
laryngitis, sinusitis	4 mo	1. Amikacin (10–15 mg/kg)
Actinomycetoma	6–12 mo after	2. Cefotaxime (6 g), ceftizoxime (6 g),
	clinical cure	ceftriaxone (2 g), imipenem (2 g)
Keratitis	Topical: Until apparent cure	1. Sulfonamide drops
		2. Amikacin drops
	Systemic: Until 2–4 mo after apparent cure	Drugs for systemic therapy as listed above

[a] For each category, choices are numbered in order of preference.

[b] In some patients with AIDS or chronic granulomatous disease, therapy for pulmonary or systemic disease must be continued indefinitely.

[c] If all apparent CNS disease has been excised, the duration of therapy may be reduced to 6 months.

℞ TREATMENT

Sulfonamides are the drugs of choice for nocardiosis (Table 146-1). Initially, 6 to 8 g/d of sulfadiazine or sulfisoxazole in four divided doses should be used. After disease is controlled, 4 g/d can be used to complete therapy. In difficult cases, sulfonamide levels should be measured and dosages adjusted to keep serum levels between 100 and 150 μg/mL. The combination of sulfamethoxazole (SMX) and trimethoprim (TMP) is probably equivalent to sulfonamides; some authorities believe that the combination may in fact be more effective, but it also poses a modestly greater risk of hematologic toxicity. At the outset, 10 to 20 mg of TMP per kg and 50 to 100 mg of SMX per kg should be given each day in two divided doses. Later, the daily doses can be decreased to as little as 5 mg/kg and 25 mg/kg, respectively. In persons with sulfonamide allergies, desensitization usually allows continuation of therapy with these effective and inexpensive drugs.

Minocycline is the best-established alternative oral drug and should be given in doses of 100 to 200 mg twice a day. Other tetracyclines are usually ineffective. *N. nova* infections can be treated with erythromycin (500 to 750 mg four times a day) and/or ampicillin (1 g four times a day), but other *Nocardia* species are often resistant to both drugs. Amoxicillin (500 mg) combined with clavulanic acid (125 mg), given three times a day, has been effective in a few cases but should be avoided in cases due to *N. nova*, in which clavulanate induces β-lactamase production. Ofloxacin (400 mg twice a day) and clarithromycin (500 mg twice a day) have each been successful in a few cases. Linezolid is active in vitro against most *Nocardia* isolates, but there is little clinical experience with this drug as nocardiosis therapy.

Amikacin, the best-established parenteral drug, is given in doses of 5 to 7.5 mg/kg every 12 h. Serum levels should be monitored during prolonged therapy in patients with diminished renal function and in the elderly. Newer β-lactam antibiotics, including cefotaxime, ceftizoxime, ceftriaxone, and imipenem, are usually effective. These agents may be less effective in some cases caused by *N. farcinica*.

In vitro, strains of *N. farcinica* differ from most in that they are usually resistant to cephalosporins and in one-fifth of cases are resistant to imipenem. *N. pseudobrasiliensis* strains often exhibit resistance to minocycline or amoxicillin/clavulanic acid and susceptibility to ciprofloxacin or clarithromycin. *N. transvalensis* displays increased resistance to many antimicrobial agents, including amikacin, tobramycin, cefotaxime, ceftriaxone, and amoxicillin/clavulanic acid. *N. nova* isolates appear to be susceptible to ampicillin and erythromycin in vitro but also produce β-lactamase constitutively or in the presence of a β-lactam.

Use of SMX and TMP in high-risk populations to prevent *Pneumocystis carinii* disease or urinary tract infections appears to reduce the risk of nocardiosis as well. However, the incidence of nocardiosis is infrequent enough that prophylaxis of this disease is not recommended.

In patients with nocardiosis who need immunosuppressive therapy for an underlying disease or prevention of transplant rejection, such therapy should be continued. In many cases, two or more antimicrobial agents have been used to treat nocardiosis, often in combinations including drugs that are usually effective by themselves, like a sulfonamide or minocycline. Whether such combination therapy is better than monotherapy is not known, and it certainly increases the risk of toxicity.

Surgical management of nocardial disease is similar to that of other bacterial diseases. Brain abscesses should be aspirated, drained, or excised if the diagnosis is unclear, if an abscess is large and accessible,

up to 2 weeks to appear and may not develop their characteristic appearance for up to 4 weeks. Several blood culture systems support nocardial growth. Yield is enhanced when blood cultures are incubated aerobically for up to 4 weeks and when blind subcultures are performed. Nocardial growth is so different from that of more common pathogens that the laboratory should be alerted when nocardiosis is suspected to maximize the likelihood of isolation. Since nocardiae are among the few aerobic microorganisms that use paraffin as a carbon source, paraffin baiting can be used to isolate the organisms from mixed cultures.

In cases of pneumonia, sputum smears are often negative. Unless the diagnosis can be made in these cases by sampling lesions in other, more accessible sites, bronchoscopy or lung aspiration is usually necessary. Transtracheal aspiration should be avoided, as it frequently leads to nocardial cellulitis in tissues around the puncture wound.

In patients with nocardial pneumonia, a careful history should be obtained and a thorough physical examination performed to evaluate the possibility of dissemination. Suggestive symptoms or signs should be pursued with further diagnostic tests. Computed tomography or magnetic resonance imaging of the head, with and without contrast material, should be undertaken if signs or symptoms suggest brain involvement. Some authorities recommend brain imaging in all cases of pulmonary or disseminated disease.

When clinically indicated, CSF or urine should be concentrated and then cultured. In actinomycetoma cases, granules should be sought in the discharge. Suspect particles should be washed in saline, examined microscopically, and cultured.

Isolation of nocardiae from sputum or blood occasionally represents colonization, transient infection, or contamination. In typical cases of respiratory tract colonization, Gram-stained specimens are negative and cultures are only intermittently positive. A positive sputum culture in an immunosuppressed patient usually reflects disease. When nocardiae are isolated from an immunocompetent patient without apparent nocardial disease, the patient should be observed carefully without treatment. A patient with a host-defense defect that increases the risk of nocardiosis should usually receive antimicrobial treatment.

Nocardia spp. are difficult to differentiate from one another with standard biochemical tests, and isolates from patients with systemic or severe disease should be sent to a reference laboratory for definitive identification and antimicrobial susceptibility testing. Susceptibility results, which help differentiate species, are of less certain clinical value but sometimes guide therapy in difficult cases.

Several presumptive diagnostic tests for nocardial infection have been studied, including tests for antibodies, nocardial metabolites, and nocardial DNA. None is ready for clinical use at this time.

or if an abscess fails to respond to chemotherapy. Brain abscesses that are small or inaccessible should be treated medically; in these cases, clinical improvement should be noticeable within 1 to 2 weeks. Brain imaging should be repeated to document the resolution of lesions, although abatement on images often lags behind clinical improvement.

Antimicrobial therapy usually suffices for nocardial actinomycetoma. In deep or extensive cases, drainage or excision of heavily involved tissue may facilitate healing, but structure and function should be preserved whenever possible.

Nocardial infections tend to relapse (particularly in patients with chronic granulomatous disease), and long courses of antimicrobial therapy are necessary. If disease is unusually extensive, if the patient is immunosuppressed, or if the response to therapy is slow, the recommendations in Table 146-1 should be exceeded.

The mortality rate for pulmonary or disseminated nocardiosis outside the CNS should be <5%. CNS disease carries a higher mortality rate. Patients should be followed carefully for at least 6 months after therapy has ended. Any child with nocardiosis and no known cause of immunosuppression should undergo tests to determine the adequacy of the phagocytic respiratory burst.

FURTHER READING

CHOUCIÑO C et al: Nocardial infections in bone marrow transplant recipients. Clin Infect Dis 23:1012, 1996

HAMID ME et al: *Nocardia africana* sp. nov., a new pathogen isolated from patients with pulmonary infections. J Clin Microbiol 39:625, 2001

KONTOYIANNIS DP et al: *Nocardia* bacteremia. Report of 4 cases and review of the literature. Medicine 77:255, 1998

MINAMOTO GY, SORDILLO EM: Disseminated nocardiosis in a patient with AIDS: Diagnosis by blood and cerebrospinal fluid cultures. Clin Infect Dis 26:242, 1998

SMEGO RA JR et al: Lymphocutaneous syndrome. A review of non-sporothrix causes. Medicine 78:38, 1999

UTTAMCHANDANI RB et al: Nocardiosis in 30 patients with advanced human immunodeficiency virus infection: Clinical features and outcome. Clin Infect Dis 18:348, 1994

WATSON A et al: *Nocardia asteroides* native valve endocarditis. Clin Infect Dis 32:660, 2001

YASSIN AF et al: *Nocardia abscessus* sp. nov. Int J Syst Evol Microbiol 50:1487, 2000

147 ACTINOMYCOSIS
Thomas A. Russo

Actinomycosis is an indolent, slowly progressive infection caused by anaerobic or microaerophilic bacteria, primarily of the genus *Actinomyces*, that colonize the mouth, colon, and vagina. Mucosal disruption may lead to infection at virtually any site in the body. In vivo growth of actinomycetes usually results in the formation of characteristic clumps called *grains* or *sulfur granules*. The clinical presentations of actinomycosis are myriad. Common in the preantibiotic era, actinomycosis has diminished in incidence, as has its timely recognition. Actinomycosis has been called "the most misdiagnosed disease," and it has been said that "no disease is so often missed by experienced clinicians." Thus this entity remains a diagnostic challenge. Three clinical presentations that should prompt consideration of this unique infection are (1) the combination of chronicity, progression across tissue boundaries, and mass-like features (mimicking malignancy, with which it is often confused); (2) the development of a sinus tract, which may spontaneously resolve and recur; and (3) a refractory or relapsing infection after a short course of therapy, since cure of established actinomycosis requires prolonged treatment. An awareness of the full spectrum of the disease will expedite its diagnosis and treatment and will minimize the unnecessary surgical interventions, morbidity, and mortality that are reported all too often.

ETIOLOGIC AGENTS Actinomycosis is most commonly caused by *A. israelii*. *A. naeslundii*, *A. odontolyticus*, *A. viscosus*, *A. meyeri*, *A. gerencseriae*, and *Propionibacterium propionicum* are established but less common causes of the disease. Most if not all actinomycotic infections are polymicrobial. *Actinobacillus actinomycetemcomitans*, *Eikenella corrodens*, Enterobacteriaceae, and species of *Fusobacterium*, *Bacteroides*, *Capnocytophaga*, *Staphylococcus*, and *Streptococcus* are commonly isolated with actinomycetes in various combinations, depending on the site of infection. The contribution of these other species to the pathogenesis of actinomycosis is uncertain.

Comparative 16S rRNA gene sequencing has led to the identification of *A. europaeus*, *A. neuii*, *A. radingae*, *A. graevenitzii*, *A. turicensis*, and *A. funkei* in clinical specimens. Increasing data suggest that these species may also cause actinomycosis.

EPIDEMIOLOGY Actinomycosis occurs throughout life, with a peak incidence in the middle decades. Males have a threefold higher incidence of infection than females, possibly because of poorer dental hygiene and/or more frequent trauma. Likely contributing factors to the decrease in the incidence of actinomycosis since the preantibiotic era include improved dental hygiene and the initiation of antimicrobial treatment early on—before the full development of the disease. Individuals who do not seek or have access to health care are undoubtedly at higher risk.

PATHOGENESIS AND PATHOLOGY The etiologic agents of actinomycosis are members of the normal oral flora and are often cultured from the bronchi, the gastrointestinal tract, and the female genital tract. The critical step in the development of actinomycosis is disruption of the mucosal barrier. Local infection may consequently ensue. Once established, actinomycosis spreads contiguously in a slow progressive manner, ignoring tissue planes. Although acute inflammation may initially develop at the site of infection, the hallmark of actinomycosis is the characteristic chronic, indolent phase. This stage is manifested by lesions that usually appear as single or multiple indurations. Central necrosis consisting of neutrophils and sulfur granules develops and is virtually diagnostic of this disease. The fibrotic walls of the mass are typically described as "wooden." The responsible bacterial and/or host factors have not yet been identified. Over time, sinus tracts to the skin, adjacent organs, or bone may develop. In rare instances, distant hematogenous seeding may occur. As mentioned above, these unique features of actinomycosis mimic malignancy, with which it is often confused.

Foreign bodies appear to facilitate infection. This association most frequently involves intrauterine contraceptive devices (IUCDs). In addition, an increasing number of reports have described an association of actinomycosis with HIV infection, transplantation, and radio- or chemotherapy. Ulcerative mucosal infections (e.g., by herpes simplex virus or cytomegalovirus) and abnormalities in host defenses may facilitate the development of actinomycosis in the latter settings.

CLINICAL MANIFESTATIONS ■ **Oral-Cervicofacial Disease** Actinomycosis occurs most frequently at an oral, cervical, or facial site, usually as a soft tissue swelling, abscess, or mass lesion that is often mistaken for a neoplasm. The angle of the jaw is generally involved, but a diagnosis of actinomycosis should be considered with any mass lesion or relapsing infection in the head and neck (Chap. 27). Otitis, sinusitis, and canaliculitis can also develop. Pain, fever, and leukocytosis are variably reported. Contiguous extension to the cranium, cervical spine, or thorax is a potential sequela.

Thoracic Disease Thoracic actinomycosis usually follows an indolent progressive course, with involvement of the pulmonary parenchyma and/or the pleural space. Chest pain, fever, and weight loss are common. A cough, when present, is variably productive. The usual radiographic appearance is either a mass lesion or pneumonia. On computed tomography (CT), central areas of low attenuation and ringlike rim

FIGURE 147-1 Thoracic actinomycosis. *Top*: A chest wall mass from extension of pulmonary infection. *Bottom*: Pulmonary infection is complicated by empyema (*open arrow*) and extension to the chest wall (*closed arrow*). (*Courtesy of Dr. C. B. Hsiao, Division of Infectious Diseases, Department of Medicine, State University of New York at Buffalo.*)

enhancement may be seen. Cavitary disease or hilar adenopathy may develop. More than 50% of cases include pleural thickening, effusion, or empyema (Fig. 147-1). Rarely, pulmonary nodules or endobronchial lesions occur. Pulmonary lesions suggestive of actinomycosis may cross fissures or pleura; may involve the mediastinum, contiguous bone, or chest wall; or may be associated with a sinus tract. In the absence of these findings, thoracic actinomycosis is usually mistaken for a neoplasm or for pneumonia due to more usual causes.

Mediastinal infection is uncommon, usually arising from thoracic extension but rarely resulting from perforation of the esophagus, from trauma, or from head and neck or abdominal disease. The structures within the mediastinum and the heart can be involved in various combinations; consequently, the possible presentations are diverse. Primary endocarditis and isolated disease of the breast have been described.

Abdominal Disease Abdominal actinomycosis poses a great diagnostic challenge. Months or years usually pass from the inciting event (e.g., appendicitis, diverticulitis, peptic ulcer disease, foreign-body perforation, bowel surgery, or ascension from IUCD-associated pelvic disease) to clinical recognition. Because of the flow of peritoneal fluid and/or the direct extension of primary disease, virtually any abdominal organ, region, or space can be involved. The disease usually presents as an abscess, a mass, or a mixed lesion that is often fixed to underlying tissue and mistaken for a tumor. On CT, enhancement is most often heterogeneous and adjacent bowel is thickened. Sinus tracts to the abdominal wall, to the perianal region, or between the bowel and other organs may develop and mimic inflammatory bowel disease. Recurrent disease or a wound or fistula that fails to heal suggests actinomycosis.

Hepatic infection usually presents as single or multiple abscesses or masses. Isolated disease presumably develops via hematogenous seeding from cryptic foci. Presently available imaging and percutaneous techniques have resulted in improved diagnosis and treatment.

All levels of the urogenital tract can be infected. Renal disease usually presents as pyelonephritis and/or renal and perinephric abscess. Bladder involvement, usually due to extension of pelvic disease, may result in ureteral obstruction or fistulas to bowel, skin, or uterus. *Actinomyces* can be detected in urine with use of appropriate stains and cultures.

Pelvic Disease Actinomycotic involvement of the pelvis occurs most commonly in association with an IUCD. Pelvic symptoms when an IUCD is in place or has recently been removed should prompt consideration of actinomycosis. Although the risk has not yet been quantified, it appears to be small. The disease rarely develops when the IUCD has been in place for <1 year, but the risk increases with time. Actinomycosis can also present months after the removal of the device. Symptoms are typically indolent; fever, weight loss, abdominal pain, and abnormal vaginal bleeding or discharge are the most common. The earliest stage of disease—often endometritis—commonly progresses to pelvic masses or a tuboovarian abscess (Fig. 147-2). Unfortunately, because the diagnosis is often delayed, a "frozen pelvis" mimicking malignancy or endometriosis can develop by the time of recognition.

An unresolved issue is whether screening of cervical or endometrial specimens for *Actinomyces*-like organisms (ALOs) can predict or prevent IUCD-associated disease. Although the risk appears to be small, the consequences of infection are significant. Therefore, until more quantitative data become available, it would appear prudent to remove the IUCD in the presence of symptoms that cannot be accounted for, regardless of whether ALOs or immunofluorescence-positive organisms are detected, and—if advanced disease is excluded—to initiate a 14-day course of empirical treatment for possible early pelvic actinomycosis. The detection of ALOs or immunofluorescence-positive organisms in the absence of symptoms warrants education of the patient and close follow-up but not removal of the IUCD unless an equally suitable means of contraception can be agreed upon.

Central Nervous System Disease Actinomycosis of the central nervous system is rare. Single or multiple brain abscesses are most common. An abscess usually appears on CT as a ring-enhancing lesion with a thick wall that may be irregular or nodular. Meningitis, epidural or subdural space infection, and cavernous sinus syndrome have also been described.

FIGURE 147-2 Computed tomogram showing pelvic actinomycosis associated with an intrauterine contraceptive device. The device is encased by endometrial fibrosis (*solid arrow*); also visible are paraendometrial fibrosis (*open triangular arrowhead*) and an area of suppuration (*open arrow*).

Musculoskeletal and Soft Tissue Infection Actinomycotic infection of the bone is usually due to adjacent soft-tissue infection but may be associated with trauma (e.g., fracture of the mandible) or hematogenous spread. Because of slow disease progression, new bone formation and bone destruction are seen concomitantly. Infection of an extremity is uncommon and is usually a result of trauma. Skin, subcutaneous tissue, muscle, and bone (with periostitis or acute or chronic osteomyelitis) are involved alone or in various combinations. Cutaneous sinus tracts frequently develop.

Disseminated Disease Hematogenous dissemination of disease from any location rarely results in multiple-organ involvement. The lungs and liver are most commonly affected, with the presentation of multiple nodules mimicking disseminated malignancy. The clinical presentation may be surprisingly indolent given the extent of disease.

DIAGNOSIS The diagnosis of actinomycosis is rarely considered. All too often, the first mention of actinomycosis is by the pathologist after extensive surgery has been performed. Since medical therapy alone is often sufficient for cure, the challenge for the clinician is to consider the possibility of actinomycosis in time to diagnose it in the least invasive fashion and to avoid unnecessary surgery. The clinical and radiographic presentations that suggest actinomycosis have been discussed above. Aspirations and biopsies (with or without CT or ultrasound guidance) are being used successfully to obtain clinical material for diagnosis, although surgery may be required. The diagnosis is most commonly made by microscopic identification of sulfur granules (an in vivo matrix of bacteria, calcium phosphate, and host material) in pus or tissues. Occasionally these granules can be grossly identified from draining sinus tracts or pus. Although sulfur granules are a defining characteristic of actinomycosis, granules are also found in mycetoma (Chaps. 146 and 190) and botryomycosis (a chronic suppurative bacterial infection of soft tissue or, in rare cases, visceral tissue that produces clumps of bacteria resembling granules); however, these entities can easily be differentiated from actinomycosis with appropriate histopathologic and microbiologic studies. Microbiologic identification of actinomycetes is often precluded by the administration of prior antimicrobial therapy or the failure to perform appropriate microbiologic cultures. For optimal yield, the avoidance of even a single dose of antibiotics is mandatory. Primary isolation usually requires 5 to 7 days but may take as long as 2 to 4 weeks. Immunofluorescence testing for *A. israelii*, *A. naeslundii*, and *P. propionicum* (available through the Centers for Disease Control and Prevention in Atlanta) is a useful diagnostic alternative. Although 16S rRNA gene amplification and sequencing would be predicted to have increased diagnostic sensitivity, this method apparently has not been used so far. Because these organisms are components of the normal oral and genital-tract flora, their identification in the absence of sulfur granules in sputum, bronchial washings, and cervicovaginal secretions is of little significance.

℞ TREATMENT

Decisions about treatment are based on the collective clinical experience of the past 50 years. Actinomycosis must be treated with high doses of antimicrobials for a prolonged period. The need for this intensive treatment is presumably due to difficulty encountered by antimicrobial agents in penetrating the thick-walled masses that commonly occur in this infection and/or the sulfur granules themselves. Although therapy needs to be individualized, the intravenous administration of 18 to 24 million units of penicillin daily for 2 to 6 weeks, followed by oral therapy with penicillin or amoxicillin for 6 to 12 months, is a reasonable guideline for serious infections. Less extensive disease, particularly that involving the oral-cervicofacial region, may require less intensive therapy. If therapy is extended beyond the point

TABLE 147-1 *Appropriate and Inappropriate Antibiotic Therapy for Actinomycosis*[a]

Category	Agent
Agents for which there is extensive successful clinical experience[b]	Penicillin: 18–24 mU/d IV q4h, 1–2 g/d PO q6h Amoxicillin: 1.5 g/d PO q8h Erythromycin: 2–4 g/d IV q6h, 1–2 g/d PO q6h Tetracycline: 1–2 g/d PO q6h Doxycycline: 200 mg/d IV or PO q12–24 h Minocycline: 200 mg/d IV or PO q12h Clindamycin: 2.7 g/d IV q8h, 1.2–1.8 g/d PO q6–8h
Agents for which there is anecdotal successful clinical experience	Ceftriaxone Ceftizoxime Imipenem Ciprofloxacin
Agents that should be avoided	Metronidazole Aminoglycosides Oxacillin Dicloxacillin Cephalexin

[a] Additional coverage for concomitant "companion" bacteria may be required.
[b] Controlled evaluations have not been performed. Dosing regimens require individualization according to the site and extent of infection. As a general rule, parenteral administration of the maximal antimicrobial dose for 2 to 6 weeks followed by oral therapy, for a total duration of 6 to 12 months, is required for most infections.

of resolution of measurable disease, the risk of relapse—a clinical hallmark of this infection—will be minimized; CT and magnetic resonance imaging (MRI) are generally the most sensitive and objective techniques by which to accomplish this goal. A similar approach is reasonable for immunocompromised patients, although refractory disease has been described in HIV-infected individuals. Suitable alternative antimicrobial agents and those deemed unreliable are listed in Table 147-1. Although the role played by "companion" microbes in actinomycosis is unclear, many isolates are pathogens in their own right, and a regimen covering these organisms during the initial treatment course is reasonable.

Combined medical-surgical therapy is still advocated by some authorities. However, an increasing body of literature now supports an initial attempt at cure with medical therapy alone, even in extensive disease. CT and MRI should be used to monitor the response to therapy. In most cases, either surgery can be avoided or a less extensive procedure can be used. This approach is particularly valuable in sparing critical organs, such as the bladder or the reproductive organs in women of child-bearing age. For a well-defined abscess, percutaneous drainage in combination with medical therapy is a reasonable approach. When a critical location is involved (e.g., the epidural space, the central nervous system) or when suitable medical therapy fails, surgical intervention may be appropriate.

FURTHER READING

DE FEITER PW, SOETERS PB: Gastrointestinal actinomycosis: An unusual presentation with obstructive uropathy: Report of a case and review of the literature. Dis Colon Rectum 44:1521, 2001

LEE YC et al: Computed tomography guided core needle biopsy diagnosis of pelvic actinomycosis. Gynecol Oncol 79:318, 2000

MILLER M, HADDAD AJ: Cervicofacial actinomycosis. Oral Surg Oral Med Oral Pathol Oral Radiol Endod 85:496, 1998

RUSSO TA: Actinomycosis, in *Principles and Practice of Infectious Diseases*, 5th ed, GL Mandell et al (eds). New York, Churchill Livingstone, 2000, pp 2645–2654

SMEGO RA, FOGLIA G: Actinomycosis. Clin Infect Dis 26:1255, 1998

DEFINITIONS *Anaerobic bacteria* are organisms that require reduced oxygen tension for growth, failing to grow on the surface of solid media in 10% CO_2 in air. (In contrast, *microaerophilic bacteria* can grow in an atmosphere of 10% CO_2 in air or under anaerobic or aerobic conditions, although they grow best in the presence of only a small amount of atmospheric oxygen, and *facultative bacteria* can grow in the presence or absence of air.) This chapter describes infections caused by nonsporulating anaerobic bacteria. In general, anaerobes associated with human infections are relatively aerotolerant. They can survive for as long as 72 h in the presence of oxygen, although generally they will not multiply in this environment. A far smaller number of pathogenic anaerobic bacteria (which are also part of the normal flora) die after brief contact with oxygen, even in low concentrations.

The nonsporulating anaerobic bacteria exist as components of the normal flora on the mucosal surfaces of humans and animals. The major reservoirs of these bacteria are the mouth, lower gastrointestinal tract, skin, and female genital tract. Among the constituents of the oral flora, anaerobes are the predominant commensal organisms, ranging in concentration from 10^9/mL in saliva to 10^{12}/mL in gingival scrapings. In the oral cavity, the ratio of anaerobic to aerobic bacteria ranges from 1:1 on the surface of a tooth to 1000:1 in the gingival crevice. Anaerobic bacteria are not found in appreciable numbers in the normal upper intestine until the distal ileum. In the colon, the proportion of anaerobes increases significantly, as does the overall bacterial count. For example, in the colon there are 10^{11} to 10^{12} organisms per gram of stool, with an anaerobe-to-aerobe ratio of ~1000:1. In the female genital tract, there are ~10^9 organisms per milliliter of secretions, with an anaerobe-to-aerobe ratio of ~10:1.

It is becoming clear that anaerobes play a key role in maintaining the balance between the host and its colonizing organisms. Hundreds of species of anaerobic bacteria have been identified as part of the normal flora of humans. Identification of as many as 500 different anaerobic species in fecal specimens reflects the diversity of the anaerobic flora. Despite the complex array of bacteria in the normal flora, relatively few species are isolated commonly from human infection. Anaerobic infections occur when the harmonious relationship between the host and the bacteria is disrupted. Any site in the body is susceptible to infection with these indigenous organisms when a mucosal barrier or the skin is compromised by surgery, trauma, tumor, or ischemia or necrosis, all of which can reduce local tissue redox potentials. Because the sites that are colonized by anaerobes contain many species of bacteria, disruption of anatomical barriers allows the penetration of many organisms, resulting in mixed infections involving multiple species of anaerobes combined with facultative or microaerophilic organisms. Such mixed infections are seen in the head and neck (chronic sinusitis, chronic otitis media, Ludwig's angina, and periodontal abscesses). Brain abscesses and subdural empyema are the most common anaerobic infections of the central nervous system. Anaerobes are responsible for pleuropulmonary diseases such as aspiration pneumonia, necrotizing pneumonia, lung abscess, and empyema. These organisms also play an important role in various intraabdominal infections, such as peritonitis and intraabdominal and liver abscesses (Chap. 112). They are isolated frequently in female genital tract infections, such as salpingitis, pelvic peritonitis, tuboovarian abscess, vulvovaginal abscess, septic abortion, and endometritis (Chap. 115). Anaerobic bacteria are also found often in infections of the skin, soft tissues, and bones and in bacteremia.

ETIOLOGY The taxonomic classification of anaerobes is a rapidly evolving field, with frequent changes in nomenclature based on newly discovered relationships among bacterial species. The major anaerobic gram-positive cocci that produce disease are *Peptostreptococcus* spp. The major species of this genus that are involved in infections are *Peptostreptococcus micros*, *P. magnus*, *P. asaccharolyticus*,

P. anaerobius, and *P. prevotii*. Clostridia (Chap. 126) are gram-positive rods that are isolated from wounds, abscesses, sites of abdominal infection, and blood. The principal anaerobic gram-negative bacilli found in human infections are the *Bacteroides fragilis* group as well as *Fusobacterium*, *Prevotella*, and *Porphyromonas* spp. Other members of the Bacteroidaceae family include *Bilophila wadsworthia*, an organism that has been isolated from infected sites and has been reported to cause serious infections, including bacteremia, necrotizing fasciitis, and abscesses; this organism is frequently resistant to several antimicrobial agents, including imipenem, cefoxitin, and other β-lactam drugs. Gram-positive anaerobic non-spore-forming bacilli are uncommon as etiologic agents of human infection. *Propionibacterium acnes*, a rare cause of foreign-body infections, is one of the few nonclostridial gram-positive rods associated with infections.

The *B. fragilis* group contains the anaerobic pathogens most frequently isolated from clinical infections. Members of this group are part of the normal bowel flora; they include several distinct species, such as *B. fragilis*, *B. thetaiotaomicron*, *B. distasonis*, *B. vulgatus*, *B. uniformis*, and *B. ovatus*. Of this group, *B. fragilis* is the most important clinical isolate. However, *B. fragilis* is isolated from the normal fecal flora in lower numbers than some of the other *Bacteroides* spp.

A second major group of phenotypically similar organisms is part of the indigenous oral flora. Thus these organisms are found at infected sites that can be seeded with oral microflora. Many of these species are pigment-producing bacteria previously classified as *Bacteroides melaninogenicus*. The nomenclature of this group has changed so that two distinct genera, *Prevotella* and *Porphyromonas*, are now recognized; these genera comprise several pathogenic species, including *Porphyromonas gingivalis*, *Porphyromonas asaccharolytica*, and *Prevotella oralis*. *Porphyromonas* and *Prevotella* spp. cause localized infections that can spread contiguously.

In female genital tract infections, organisms normally colonizing the vagina, such as *Prevotella bivia* and *Prevotella disiens*, are the most frequent isolates, although *B. fragilis* is not uncommon. The *Fusobacterium* species *Fusobacterium necrophorum*, *F. nucleatum*, and *F. varium*, which reside primarily in the oral cavity and the gastrointestinal tract, are also isolated from clinical infections, including necrotizing pneumonia and abscesses.

Infections caused by anaerobic bacteria most frequently are due to more than one organism. These polymicrobial infections may be caused by one or several anaerobic species or by a combination of anaerobic organisms and microaerophilic or facultative bacteria acting synergistically.

APPROACH TO THE PATIENT

The physician must consider several points when approaching the patient with presumptive infection due to anaerobic bacteria.

1. Most of the organisms colonizing mucosal sites are harmless commensals; very few cause disease.

2. For anaerobes to cause tissue infection, they must spread beyond the normal mucosal barriers.

3. Conditions favoring the propagation of these bacteria, particularly a lowered oxidation-reduction potential, are necessary. These conditions exist at sites of trauma, tissue destruction, compromised vascular supply, and complications of preexisting infection, which produce necrosis.

4. There is a complex array of infecting flora. For example, as many as 12 different types of organisms can be isolated from a suppurative site.

5. Anaerobic organisms tend to be found in abscess cavities or in necrotic tissue. The failure of an abscess to yield organisms on routine culture is a clue that the abscess is likely to contain

anaerobic bacteria. Often smears of this "sterile pus" are found to be teeming with bacteria when Gram's stain is applied. Malodorous pus suggests anaerobic infection. Although some facultative organisms, such as *Staphylococcus aureus*, are also capable of causing abscesses, abscesses in organs or deeper body tissues should call to mind anaerobic infection.

6. Gas is found in many anaerobic infections of deep tissues.

7. Some species (the best example being the *B. fragilis* group) require specific therapy. However, many synergistic infections can be cured with antibiotics directed at some but not all of the organisms involved. Antibiotic therapy, combined with debridement and drainage, disrupts the interdependent relationship among the bacteria, and some species that are resistant to the antibiotic do not survive without the coinfecting organisms.

8. Manifestations of disseminated intravascular coagulation are unusual in patients with purely anaerobic infection.

EPIDEMIOLOGY Difficulties in the performance of appropriate cultures, contamination of cultures by aerobic bacteria or components of the normal flora, and the lack of readily available, reliable culture techniques have made it impossible to obtain accurate incidence or prevalence data. However, anaerobic infections are encountered frequently in hospitals with active surgical, trauma, and obstetric and gynecologic services. In some centers, anaerobic bacteria, particularly *B. fragilis*, account for ~4% of positive blood cultures.

PATHOGENESIS Anaerobic bacterial infections usually occur when an anatomical barrier becomes disrupted and constituents of the local flora enter a site that was previously sterile. Because of the specific growth requirements of anaerobic organisms and their presence as commensals on mucosal surfaces, conditions must arise that allow these organisms to penetrate mucosal barriers and enter tissue with a lowered oxidation-reduction potential. Therefore, tissue ischemia, trauma, surgery, perforated viscus, shock, and aspiration provide environments conducive to the proliferation of anaerobes. In the case of a perforated viscus, hundreds of species of anaerobic bacteria are spilled into the peritoneal cavity, but many of these organisms are unable to survive because the highly vascularized tissue provides a sufficiently high redox potential. The entry of oxygen into the environment results in the selection of the more aerotolerant anaerobic organisms.

The ability of an organism to adhere to host tissues is important to the establishment of infection. Some oral species adhere to crevicular epithelium in the oral cavity. *Prevotella melaninogenica* actually attaches to other microorganisms; *P. gingivalis* is a common isolate in periodontal disease. These organisms have fimbriae that facilitate attachment. Some unencapsulated *Bacteroides* strains appear to be piliated, a characteristic that may account for their ability to adhere.

The most extensively studied virulence factor of the nonsporulating anaerobes is the polysaccharide capsule of *B. fragilis*. This polysaccharide possesses distinct biologic properties, such as the ability (owing to a unique zwitterionic motif of charged sugars) to promote abscess formation. Intraabdominal abscess induction is related to the capacity of the polysaccharide to stimulate the release of cytokines and chemokines—in particular interleukin (IL) 8, IL-17, and tumor necrosis factor (TNF) α—from resident peritoneal cells. The release of cytokines and chemokines results in the chemotaxis of polymorphonuclear neutrophils (PMNs) into the peritoneum, where they adhere to mesothelial cells induced by TNF-α to upregulate their expression of intercellular adhesion molecule 1 (ICAM-1). PMNs adherent to ICAM-1-expressing cells probably represent the nidus for an abscess. Prophylactic or therapeutic administration of the polysaccharide or a zwitterionic mimetic to experimental animals confers protection against abscess induction following challenge with intestinal microorganisms capable of inducing abscesses. This protection is mediated by T cells controlling cytokine release; IL-10 appears to be the cytokine primarily responsible for downregulating the tissue response of abscess formation. Although abscesses constitute a host response

that localizes and contains infecting bacteria, abscess formation in patients with sepsis often results in severe and chronic illness that requires surgical drainage in combination with antimicrobial therapy.

Anaerobic bacteria produce a number of exoproteins that are capable of enhancing the organisms' virulence. The collagenase produced by *P. gingivalis* may enhance tissue destruction. An enterotoxin has been identified in *B. fragilis* strains associated with diarrheal disease in animals and young children. This 20-kDa zinc-dependent metalloprotease reversibly alters the morphology of the tight junctional complexes of intestinal epithelial cells. Both *B. fragilis* and *P. melaninogenica* possess lipopolysaccharides (endotoxins) that are less biologically potent than endotoxins associated with aerobic gram-negative bacteria. This relative biologic inactivity may account for the lower frequency of disseminated intravascular coagulation and purpura in *Bacteroides* bacteremia than in facultative and aerobic gram-negative bacillary bacteremia.

CLINICAL MANIFESTATIONS ■ **Anaerobic Infections of the Mouth, Head, and Neck** (See also Chap. 27) Infections of the mouth can arise from either the supragingival or the subgingival dental plaque. Supragingival plaque formation begins with the adherence of gram-positive bacteria to the tooth surface. This form of plaque is influenced by salivary and dietary components, oral hygiene, and local host factors. Once the supragingival plaque is established, the acquisition of pathogenic bacteria and an increase in the amount of plaque are responsible for the ultimate development of gingivitis. Early bacteriologic changes in the supragingival plaque initiate an inflammatory response in the gingiva, including edema, swelling, and increased gingival fluid, and cause the development of caries and endodontic (pulp) infections. In addition, these changes contribute to the subsequent pathogenic alteration in the subgingival plaque that arises from poor or inadequate oral hygiene.

Subgingival plaque is associated with periodontal disease and disseminated infection arising from the oral cavity. Bacteria that colonize the subgingival area are primarily anaerobic. The black-pigmented gram-negative anaerobic bacilli (principally *P. gingivalis*, *P. asaccharolytica*, and *P. melaninogenica*) are the most important. Infections in this area are frequently mixed and involve both anaerobic and aerobic bacteria. After establishment of local infection either in root canals or in the periodontal area, infection may extend into the mandible, causing osteomyelitis of the maxillary sinuses, or to local tissues in the submandibular or submental spaces, depending on which teeth are involved. Periodontitis may also result in spreading infection that can involve adjacent bone or soft tissues.

NECROTIZING ULCERATIVE GINGIVITIS Gingivitis may become a necrotizing infection (trench mouth, Vincent's stomatitis). The onset of disease is usually sudden and is associated with tender bleeding gums, foul breath, and a bad taste. The gingival mucosa, especially the papillae between the teeth, becomes ulcerated and may be covered by a gray exudate, which is removable with gentle pressure. Patients may become systemically ill, developing fever, cervical lymphadenopathy, and leukocytosis. Occasionally, ulcerative gingivitis can spread to the buccal mucosa, the teeth, and the mandible or maxilla, resulting in widespread destruction of bone and soft tissue. This infection is termed *acute necrotizing ulcerative mucosis* (cancrum oris, noma). It destroys tissue rapidly, causing the teeth to fall out and large areas of bone—or even the whole mandible—to be sloughed. A strong putrid odor is frequently detected, although the lesions are not painful. The gangrenous lesions eventually heal, leaving large disfiguring defects. This infection most commonly follows a debilitating illness or affects severely malnourished children. It has been known to complicate leukemia or to develop in individuals with a genetic deficiency of catalase.

ACUTE NECROTIZING INFECTIONS OF THE PHARYNX These infections usually occur in association with ulcerative gingivitis. Symptoms include an extremely sore throat, foul breath, and a bad taste accompanied by fever and a sensation of choking. Examination of the pharynx demonstrates that the tonsillar pillars are swollen, red, ulcerated, and covered with a grayish membrane that peels easily. Lymphadenopathy and leukocytosis are common. The disease may last for only a few days or, if not treated, may persist for weeks. Lesions begin unilaterally but may spread to the other side of the pharynx or the larynx. Aspiration of the infected material by the patient can result in lung abscesses. Soft tissue infection of the oral-facial area may or may not be odontogenic. Ludwig's angina, a periodontal infection usually arising from the tissues surrounding the third molar, may produce submandibular soft tissue infection that results in marked local swelling of tissues, with pain, trismus, and superior and posterior displacement of the tongue. Submandibular swelling of the neck can impair swallowing and cause respiratory obstruction. In some cases, tracheotomy may be life-saving.

FASCIAL INFECTIONS   These infections arise from the spread of organisms originating in the upper airways to potential spaces formed by the fascial planes of the head and neck. Perimandibular space infection most commonly involves the submandibular, peritonsillar, and parapharyngeal spaces. Peritonsillar abscesses occur in association with pharyngitis. Complicated dental infections spread to the submandibular and buccal spaces. Entry of organisms by either portal can result in parapharyngeal space infections. Although there are few well-documented reports on the microbiology of these syndromes, anaerobes from the oral flora have been implicated in many cases. Fascial infections associated with *S. aureus* or *Streptococcus pyogenes* may arise from boils or impetigo, whereas anaerobes are associated with space infections either occurring spontaneously or arising from diseases of the mucous membranes or from dental manipulations.

SINUSITIS AND OTITIS   The role of anaerobic bacteria in acute sinusitis may be underestimated because of improper collection of specimens. In a study of chronic sinusitis, anaerobic bacteria were found in 52% of specimens collected during external frontoethmoidotomy or radical antrotomy. However, antibiotic therapy against anaerobes alone is not usually curative. Anaerobic bacteria are much more easily implicated in chronic suppurative otitis media than in acute otitis media. Purulent exudate from chronically draining ears has been found to contain anaerobes, particularly *Bacteroides* spp., in up to 50% of cases. *B. fragilis* has been isolated from up to 28% of patients with chronic otitis media.

COMPLICATIONS OF ANAEROBIC HEAD AND NECK INFECTIONS   Contiguous craniad spread of these infections may result in osteomyelitis of the skull or mandible or in intracranial infections such as brain abscess and subdural empyema. Caudad spread can produce mediastinitis or pleuropulmonary infection. Hematogenous complications may also result from anaerobic infections of the head and neck. Bacteremia, which occasionally is polymicrobial, can lead to endocarditis or other distant infections. Lemierre syndrome, which has been uncommon in the antimicrobial era, is an acute oropharyngeal infection with secondary septic thrombophlebitis of the internal jugular vein and frequent metastatic infections (see also "Bone and Joint Infections," below). *F. necrophorum* is the usual cause. This infection typically begins with pharyngitis, which is followed by local invasion in the lateral pharyngeal space with resultant internal jugular vein thrombophlebitis. The most common site for metastatic infection is the lungs. A typical clinical triad seen in recent series is pharyngitis, a tender/swollen neck, and noncavitating pulmonary infiltrates.

Central Nervous System Infections   Brain abscesses are frequently associated with anaerobic bacteria (Chap. 360). If optimal bacteriologic techniques are employed, as many as 85% of brain abscesses yield anaerobic bacteria—most often anaerobic gram-positive cocci (especially peptostreptococci), which are followed in frequency by *Fusobacterium* and *Bacteroides* spp. Facultative or microaerophilic streptococci and coliforms are often are part of a mixed infecting flora in brain abscesses.

Pleuropulmonary Infections   Anaerobic pleuropulmonary infections result from the aspiration of oropharyngeal contents, often in the context of an altered state of consciousness or an absent gag reflex. Four clinical syndromes are associated with anaerobic pleuropulmonary infection produced by aspiration: simple aspiration pneumonia, necrotizing pneumonia, lung abscess, and empyema.

ASPIRATION PNEUMONITIS   Aspiration pneumonitis must be distinguished from two other clinical syndromes associated with aspiration that are not of bacterial etiology. One syndrome results from aspiration of solids, usually food. Obstruction of major airways typically results in atelectasis and moderate nonspecific inflammation. Therapy consists of removal of the foreign body.

The second aspiration syndrome is more easily confused with bacterial aspiration. *Mendelson's syndrome* results from regurgitation of stomach contents and aspiration of chemical material, usually gastric juices. Pulmonary inflammation—including the destruction of the alveolar lining, with transudation of fluid into the alveolar space—occurs with remarkable rapidity. Typically this syndrome develops within hours, often following anesthesia when the gag reflex is depressed. The patient becomes tachypneic, hypoxic, and febrile. The leukocyte count may rise, and the chest x-ray may evolve suddenly from normal to a complete bilateral "whiteout" within 8 to 24 h. Sputum production is minimal. The pulmonary signs and symptoms can resolve quickly with symptom-based therapy or can culminate in respiratory failure, with the subsequent development of bacterial superinfection over a period of days. Antibiotic therapy is not indicated unless bacterial infection supervenes. The signs of bacterial infection include sputum production, persistent fever, leukocytosis, and clinical evidence of sepsis.

In contrast to these syndromes, bacterial aspiration pneumonia develops more slowly. It is seen in patients who are hospitalized and have a depressed gag reflex, impaired swallowing, or a tracheal or nasogastric tube; elderly patients; or those with transiently impaired consciousness in the wake of seizures, cerebrovascular accidents, or alcoholic blackouts. Patients who enter the hospital with this syndrome typically have been ill for several days and generally report low-grade fever, malaise, and sputum production. Usually the history reveals factors predisposing to aspiration, such as alcohol overdose or residence in a nursing home. Sputum characteristically is not malodorous unless the process has been underway for at least a week. A mixed bacterial flora with many PMNs is evident on Gram's staining of sputum. The most commonly encountered anaerobes in sputum in these infections are pigmented and nonpigmented *Prevotella* spp., *F. nucleatum*, *Peptostreptococcus* spp., and *Bacteroides* spp. Cultures are reliable only if contamination with the normal oral flora is avoided—that is, if specimens are obtained by open lung biopsy. In general, this procedure is not indicated in the evaluation of these patients. Chest x-rays show consolidation in dependent pulmonary segments: in the basilar segments of the lower lobes if the patient has aspirated while upright and in either the posterior segment of the upper lobe (usually on the right side) or the superior segment of the lower lobe if the patient has aspirated while supine. The organisms isolated from the lungs reflect the pharyngeal flora; *P. melaninogenica*, *Fusobacterium* spp., and anaerobic cocci are the most common isolates. The patient who aspirates in the hospital may also have a mixed infection involving enteric gram-negative rods.

NECROTIZING PNEUMONITIS   This form of anaerobic pneumonitis is characterized by numerous small abscesses that spread to involve several pulmonary segments. The process can be indolent or fulminating. This syndrome is less common than either aspiration pneumonia or lung abscess and includes features of both types of infection.

ANAEROBIC LUNG ABSCESSES   These abscesses result from subacute anaerobic pulmonary infection. The clinical syndrome typically involves a history of constitutional symptoms, including malaise, weight loss, fever, chills, and foul-smelling sputum, perhaps over a period of weeks (Chap. 239). Patients who develop lung abscesses characteristically have dental infection and periodontitis, but lung abscesses in edentulous patients have been reported. Abscess cavities may be single or multiple and generally occur in dependent pulmonary segments (Fig. 148-1). Anaerobic abscesses must be distinguished from those associated with tuberculosis, neoplasia, and other conditions. Oral anaerobes predominate, although *B. fragilis* is isolated in up to 10% of cases. *S. aureus* may be found as well.

EMPYEMA Empyema is a manifestation of long-standing anaerobic pulmonary infection. The clinical presentation, which includes the presence of foul-smelling sputum, resembles that of other anaerobic pulmonary infections. Patients may report pleuritic chest pain and marked chest-wall tenderness.

Empyema may be masked by overlying pneumonitis and should be considered especially in cases of persistent fever despite antibiotic therapy. Diligent physical examination and the use of ultrasound to localize a loculated empyema are important diagnostic tools. The collection of a foul-smelling exudate by thoracentesis is typical. Cultures of infected pleural fluid yield an average of 3.5 anaerobes and 0.6 facultative or aerobic bacterial species. Drainage is required. Defervescence, a return to a feeling of well-being, and resolution of the process may require several months.

Extension from a subdiaphragmatic infection may also result in anaerobic empyema. Septic pulmonary emboli may originate from intraabdominal or female genital tract infections and can produce anaerobic pneumonia.

Intraabdominal Infections Enterotoxigenic *B. fragilis* has been associated with watery diarrhea in a small number of young children and adults. In case-control studies of children with undiagnosed diarrheal disease, enterotoxigenic *B. fragilis* was isolated from significantly more children with diarrhea than children in the control group. This organism may play a role in a small proportion of childhood diarrhea cases. Neutropenic enterocolitis (typhlitis) has been associated with anaerobic infection of the cecum but—in the setting of neutropenia (Chap. 72)—may involve the entire bowel. Patients usually present with fever; abdominal pain, tenderness, and distention; and watery diarrhea. The bowel wall is edematous with hemorrhage and necrosis. The primary pathogen is thought by some authorities to be *Clostridium septicum*, but other clostridia and mixed anaerobic infections have also been implicated. More than 50% of patients developing early clinical signs can benefit from antibiotic therapy and bowel rest. Surgery is sometimes required to remove gangrenous bowel. →*See Chap. 112 for a complete discussion of intraabdominal infections.*

Pelvic Infections The vagina of a healthy woman is one of the major reservoirs of anaerobic and aerobic bacteria. In the normal flora of the female genital tract, anaerobes outnumber aerobes by a ratio of ~10:1 and include anaerobic gram-positive cocci and *Bacteroides* spp. Anaerobes are isolated from most women with genital tract infections that are not caused by a sexually transmitted pathogen. The major anaerobic pathogens are *B. fragilis*, *P. bivia*, *P. disiens*, *P. melaninogenica*, anaerobic cocci, and *Clostridium* spp. Anaerobes are frequently encountered in tuboovarian abscess, septic abortion, pelvic abscess, endometritis, and postoperative wound infection, particularly following hysterectomy. Although these infections are often of mixed etiology, involving both anaerobes and coliforms, pure anaerobic infections without coliform or other facultative bacterial species occur more often in pelvic than in intraabdominal sites and are characterized by drainage of foul-smelling pus or blood from the uterus, generalized uterine or local pelvic tenderness, and continued fever and chills. Suppurative thrombophlebitis of the pelvic veins may complicate the infections and lead to repeated episodes of septic pulmonary emboli.

Anaerobic bacteria have been thought to be contributing factors in the etiology of bacterial vaginosis. This syndrome of unknown etiology is characterized by a profuse malodorous discharge and an increase in the number of bacteria in the vagina, including *Gardnerella vaginalis*, *Prevotella* spp., *Mobiluncus* spp., peptostreptococci, and genital mycoplasmas. Anaerobic bacteria are thought to play a role in the etiology of pelvic inflammatory disease (Chap. 115), and several investigations have shown an association between bacterial vaginosis and the development of pelvic inflammatory disease.

Pelvic infections due to *Actinomyces* spp. have been associated with use of intrauterine devices (Chap. 147).

Skin and Soft Tissue Infections Injury to skin, bone, or soft tissue by trauma, ischemia, or surgery creates a suitable environment for anaerobic infections. These infections are most frequently found in sites prone to contamination with feces or with upper airway secretions—for example, wounds associated with intestinal surgery, decubitus ulcers, or human bites. Anaerobic bacteria can be isolated in cases of crepitant cellulitis, synergistic cellulitis, or gangrene and necrotizing fasciitis (Chaps. 110 and 126). Moreover, these organisms have been isolated from cutaneous abscesses, rectal abscesses, and axillary sweat gland infections (hidradenitis suppurativa). Anaerobes are frequently cultured from foot ulcers in diabetic patients.

These soft tissue or skin infections are usually polymicrobial. A mean of 4.8 bacterial species are isolated, with an anaerobe-to-aerobe ratio of ~3:2. The most frequently isolated organisms include *Bacteroides* spp., peptostreptococci, enterococci, clostridia, and *Proteus* spp. The involvement of anaerobes in these types of infections is associated with a higher frequency of fever, foul-smelling lesions, gas in the tissues, and visible foot ulcer.

Anaerobic bacterial *synergistic gangrene* (*Meleney's gangrene*) is characterized by exquisite pain, redness, and swelling followed by induration. Erythema surrounds a central zone of necrosis. A granulating ulcer forms at the original center as necrosis and erythema extend outward. Symptoms are limited to pain; fever is not typical. These infections usually involve a combination of *Peptostreptococcus* spp. and *S. aureus*; the usual site of infection is an abdominal surgical wound or the area surrounding an ulcer on an extremity. Treatment includes surgical removal of necrotic tissue and antimicrobial administration.

Necrotizing fasciitis, a rapidly spreading destructive disease of the fascia, is usually attributed to group A streptococci (Chap. 121) but can also be a mixed infection involving anaerobes and aerobes. The most frequently isolated anaerobes in these infections are *Peptostreptococcus* and *Bacteroides* spp. Gas may be found in the tissues. Similarly, myonecrosis can be associated with mixed anaerobic infection. *Fournier's gangrene* consists of cellulitis involving the scrotum, perineum, and anterior abdominal wall, with mixed anaerobic organisms spreading along deep external fascial planes and causing extensive loss of skin.

Bone and Joint Infections Although actinomycosis (Chap. 147) accounts on a worldwide basis for most anaerobic infections in bone, organisms including peptostreptococci or microaerophilic cocci, *Bacteroides* spp., *Fusobacterium* spp., and *Clostridium* spp. can also be found. These infections frequently arise adjacent to soft tissue infections. Hematogenous seeding of bone is uncommon. *Prevotella* and *Porphyromonas* spp. are detected in infections involving the maxilla and

FIGURE 148-1 Chest radiograph of right-lower-lobe lung abscess in a 60-year-old alcoholic. [*From GL Mandell (ed): Atlas of Infectious Diseases, Vol VI. Philadelphia, Current Medicine Inc, Churchill Livingstone, 1996; with permission.*]

mandible, whereas *Clostridium* spp. have been reported as anaerobic pathogens in cases of osteomyelitis of the long bones following fracture or trauma. Fusobacteria have been isolated in pure culture from sites of osteomyelitis adjacent to the perinasal sinuses. Peptostreptococci and microaerophilic cocci have been reported as significant pathogens in infections involving the skull, mastoid, and prosthetic implants placed in bone. In patients with osteomyelitis (Chap. 111), the most reliable culture specimen is a bone biopsy sample free of normal uninfected skin and subcutaneous tissue. In patients with anaerobic osteomyelitis, a mixed flora is frequently isolated from a bone biopsy specimen.

In cases of anaerobic septic arthritis, the most common isolates are *Fusobacterium* spp. Most of the patients involved have uncontrolled peritonsillar infections progressing to septic cervical venous thrombophlebitis (Lemierre syndrome) and resulting in hematogenous dissemination with a predilection for the joints. Unlike anaerobic osteomyelitis, anaerobic pyoarthritis in most cases is not polymicrobial and may be acquired hematogenously. Anaerobes are important pathogens in infections involving prosthetic joints; in these infections, the causative organisms (such as *Peptostreptococcus* spp. and *P. acnes*) are part of the normal skin flora.

Bacteremia Transient bacteremia is a well-known event in healthy people whose anatomical mucosal barriers have been injured (e.g., during dental extractions or dental scaling). These bacteremic episodes, which are often due to anaerobes, have no pathologic consequences. However, anaerobic bacteria are found in cultures of blood from clinically ill patients when proper culture techniques are used. *B. fragilis* is the single most common anaerobic isolate from the bloodstream.

In recent years, the rate of isolation of anaerobic bacteria from blood cultures has been decreasing. Studies from the 1970s and early 1980s found that 10 to 15% of positive blood cultures yielded anaerobes, while more recent surveys have found rates as low as 4%. The cause of this change is unknown but may be related to the administration of antibiotic prophylaxis before intestinal surgery, the earlier recognition of localized infections, and the empirical use of broad-spectrum antibiotics for presumed infection.

Once the organism has been identified, both the portal of bloodstream entry and the underlying problem that probably led to seeding of the bloodstream can often be deduced from an understanding of the organism's normal site of residence. For example, mixed anaerobic bacteremia including *B. fragilis* usually implies colonic pathology with mucosal disruption from neoplasia, diverticulitis, or some other inflammatory lesion. The initial manifestations are determined by the portal of entry and reflect the localized condition. When bloodstream invasion occurs, patients can become extremely ill, with rigors and hectic fevers ranging up to 40.6°C (105°F). The clinical picture may be quite similar to that seen in sepsis involving aerobic gram-negative bacilli. Although other complications of anaerobic bacteremia, such as septic thrombophlebitis and septic shock, have been reported, the incidence of these complications in association with anaerobic bacteremia is low. Anaerobic bacteremia is potentially fatal and requires rapid diagnosis and appropriate therapy. Mortality appears to increase with the age of the patient (with reported rates of >66% among patients >60 years old), with the isolation of multiple species from the bloodstream, and with the failure to surgically remove a focus of infection.

Endocarditis and Pericarditis (See also Chap. 109) Endocarditis due to anaerobes is uncommon. However, anaerobic streptococci, which are often classified incorrectly, are responsible for this disease more frequently than is generally appreciated. Gram-negative anaerobes are unusual causes of endocarditis. Signs and symptoms of anaerobic endocarditis are similar to those of endocarditis due to facultative organisms. The mortality rate for anaerobic endocarditis has been reported at 21 to 43%.

Anaerobes, particularly *B. fragilis* and *Peptostreptococcus* spp., are uncommonly found in infected pericardial fluids. Anaerobic pericarditis is associated with a mortality rate of >50%.

DIAGNOSIS There are three critical steps in the diagnosis of anaerobic infection: (1) proper specimen collection; (2) rapid transport of the specimens to the microbiology laboratory, preferably in anaerobic transport media; and (3) proper handling of the specimens by the laboratory. Specimens must be collected by meticulous sampling of infected sites, with avoidance of contamination by the normal flora. When such contamination is likely, the specimen is unacceptable. Examples of specimens unacceptable for anaerobic culture include sputum collected by expectoration or nasal tracheal suction, bronchoscopy specimens, samples collected directly through the vaginal vault, urine collected by voiding, and feces. Specimens that can be cultured for anaerobes include blood, pleural fluid, transtracheal aspirates, pus obtained by direct aspiration from an abscess cavity, fluid obtained by culdocentesis, suprapubic bladder aspirates, cerebrospinal fluid, and lung puncture specimens.

Because even brief exposure to oxygen may kill some anaerobic organisms and result in failure to isolate them in the laboratory, air must be expelled from the syringe used to aspirate the abscess cavity, and the needle must be capped with a sterile rubber stopper. Proper precautions should be used in the handling of contaminated needles. Specimens can be injected into transport bottles containing a reduced medium or taken immediately in syringes to the laboratory for direct culture on anaerobic media. In general, swabs should not be used. If a swab must be used, it should be placed in a reduced semisolid carrying medium before transport to the laboratory. Delays in transport may lead to a failure to isolate anaerobes due to exposure to oxygen or overgrowth of facultative organisms, which may eliminate or obscure any anaerobes that are present. All clinical specimens from suspected anaerobic infections should be Gram-stained and examined for organisms with characteristic morphology. It is not unusual for organisms to be observed on Gram's staining but not isolated in culture. If purulent materials are found to be sterile or organisms are seen on Gram's staining but do not grow in the culture, the involvement of anaerobes should be suspected.

Because of the time and difficulty involved in the isolation of anaerobic bacteria, diagnosis of anaerobic infections must frequently be based on presumptive evidence. Certain sites (such as avascular necrotic tissues) with lowered oxidation-reduction potential favor the diagnosis of an anaerobic infection. When infections occur in proximity to mucosal surfaces normally harboring an anaerobic flora, such as the gastrointestinal tract, female genital tract, or oropharynx, anaerobes should be considered as potential etiologic agents. A foul odor is often indicative of anaerobes, which produce certain organic acids as they proliferate in necrotic tissue. Although these odors are nearly pathognomonic for anaerobic infection, the absence of odor does not exclude an anaerobic etiology. Because anaerobes often coexist with other bacteria to cause mixed or synergistic infection, Gram's staining of exudate frequently reveals numerous pleomorphic cocci and bacilli suggestive of anaerobes. Sometimes these organisms have morphologic characteristics associated with specific species.

The presence of gas in tissues is highly suggestive, but not diagnostic, of anaerobic infection. When cultures of obviously infected sites yield no growth, streptococci only, or a single aerobic species (such as *Escherichia coli*) and Gram's staining reveals a mixed flora, the implication is that the anaerobic microorganisms failed to grow because of inadequate transport and/or culture techniques. Failure of a patient to respond to antibiotics that are not active against anaerobes (e.g., aminoglycosides and—in some circumstances—penicillin, cephalosporins, or tetracyclines) suggests anaerobic infection.

℞ **TREATMENT**

Successful therapy for anaerobic infections requires the administration of a combination of appropriate antibiotics, surgical resection, debridement of devitalized tissues, and drainage. Perforations must be closed promptly, closed spaces drained, tissue compartments decompressed, and an adequate blood supply established. Abscess cavities should be drained as soon as fluctuation or localization occurs. Surgery was formerly required to establish drainage; however, computed tomography (CT), magnetic resonance imaging (MRI), and ultrasound now allow diagnostic radiologists to drain many abscess sites percutaneously.

Antibiotic Therapy and Resistance Decisions about the treatment of anaerobic infections with antibiotics are usually based on known resistance patterns in certain species, on the likelihood of encountering a given species in the case at hand, and on Gram's stain findings. Antibiotics active against *Bacteroides* spp., penicillin-resistant *Prevotella* and *Porphyromonas* spp., and *Fusobacterium* spp. can be grouped into four categories on the basis of their predicted activity against anaerobes (Table 148-1). (Nearly all the drugs listed have toxic side effects, which are described in detail in Chap. 118.) In many infections, anaerobes are mixed with coliforms and other facultative organisms. The best therapeutic regimens, therefore, are usually those active against both aerobic and anaerobic bacteria. The choice of empirical antibiotics for the anaerobes in mixed infections can nearly always be made reliably, since patterns of antimicrobial susceptibility are usually predictable (Chap. 118 and Table 148-1).

Antibiotic susceptibility testing of anaerobic bacteria has been difficult and controversial. Owing to the slow growth rate of many anaerobes, the lack of standardized testing methods and of clinically relevant standards for resistance, and the generally good results obtained with empirical therapy, there has been limited interest in testing these organisms for antibiotic susceptibility. However, a recent study found mortality rates of 45 and 16% among antibiotic-treated patients with *Bacteroides* blood isolates deemed resistant and sensitive, respectively, to the agent used. These figures suggest that in vitro susceptibility testing should be performed for *Bacteroides* isolates from hospitalized patients with bacteremia and that the results of this testing should guide treatment.

Clinically important *Bacteroides* spp. are essentially all resistant to penicillin, and penicillin resistance rates among *Porphyromonas*, *Prevotella*, and *Fusobacterium* spp. are increasing rapidly. Failures of therapy are common when documented *Bacteroides* (especially *B. fragilis*) infection is treated with penicillin or first-generation cephalosporins. The number of antimicrobial agents effective against *Bacteroides* spp. has expanded, and there are currently several useful choices (Table 148-1). In general, cure rates of >80% can be attained in patients with *Bacteroides* infection by means of appropriate antimicrobial therapy and drainage.

Resistance to metronidazole has been reported only rarely in *Bacteroides* spp. This well-tolerated drug, which reaches significant levels in serum and can also be found at high concentrations in abscess cavities, should be considered first-line therapy against *Bacteroides* infection. However, if metronidazole is used to treat mixed anaerobic and aerobic infections, it is imperative that other appropriate antibiotics be used in conjunction. Metronidazole is inactive against aerobic and facultative bacteria, *Actinomyces* spp., and *Propionibacterium* spp. The sensitivity of peptostreptococci to metronidazole is unpredictable, and penicillin remains the drug of choice.

If a patient fails to respond to one of the category 1 or category 2 drugs (Table 148-1), consideration should be given to alternative therapy and to determination of the resistance patterns among *Bacteroides* isolates. Although in vitro resistance of *Bacteroides* spp. to chloramphenicol has not been reported, this drug may not be as effective as other category 1 drugs. Ampicillin/sulbactam, ticarcillin/clavulanic acid, piperacillin/tazobactam, imipenem, and meropenem have been effective in the treatment of *B. fragilis* infection. Some newer quinolones, such as moxifloxacin, appear to be highly active in vitro against certain anaerobes, including *B. fragilis*, but not against all members of the *B. fragilis* group; consideration of their use must await appropriate clinical trials.

TABLE 148-1 Antimicrobial Therapy for Infections Involving Commonly Encountered Anaerobic Gram-Negative Rods

Category 1 (<2% Resistance)	Category 2 (<15% Resistance)	Category 3 (Variable Resistance)	Category 4 (Resistance)
Imipenem	Cefoxitin	Penicillin	Aminoglycosides
Meropenem	Clindamycin	Cephalosporins	Quinolones[b]
Metronidazole[a]	High-dose antipseudomonal penicillins	Tetracycline	Monobactams
Ampicillin/ sulbactam		Vancomycin	
Ticarcillin/ clavulanic acid		Erythromycin	
Piperacillin/ tazobactam			
Chloramphenicol[c]			

[a] Usually needs to be given in combination with aerobic bacterial coverage. For infections originating below the diaphragm, aerobic gram-negative coverage is essential. For infections from an oral source, aerobic gram-positive coverage is added. Metronidazole also is not active against *Actinomyces*, *Propionibacterium*, or other gram-positive non-spore-forming bacilli (e.g., *Eubacterium*, *Bifidobacterium*) and is unreliable against peptostreptococci.
[b] Moxifloxacin appears to have in vitro activity against many anaerobes.
[c] Chloramphenicol is probably not as effective as other category 1 antimicrobials in treating anaerobic infections.

Treatment of Infections at Specific Sites In clinical situations, specific regimens must be tailored to the initial site of infection. The duration of therapy also depends on the infection site; the reader is referred to specific chapters on sites of infection for recommendations.

β-Lactamase production has been reported in anaerobic strains that are usually isolated from infections originating above the diaphragm. Up to 60% of clinical isolates classified as *Prevotella* or *Porphyromonas* spp., non-*B. fragilis* species of *Bacteroides*, or *Fusobacterium* spp. reportedly produce β-lactamase. The clinical significance of resistance in these organisms has been suggested by studies showing clindamycin to be superior to penicillin (which for many years was considered the therapeutic "gold standard") for the treatment of lung abscesses. Presumably, the success of clindamycin is attributable to a broader spectrum of activity against oral anaerobes; thus, a combination of penicillin and metronidazole or another antibiotic combination that is active against both oral anaerobes and aerobes is likely to be as effective as clindamycin. Bronchoscopy in lung abscess is indicated only to rule out airway obstruction and does not enhance drainage; in any event, it should be delayed until the antimicrobial regimen has begun to affect the disease process so that the procedure does not spread the infection. Surgery is almost never indicated because of the danger of spilling the abscess contents into the lungs.

Although many oral anaerobic infections and most cases of anaerobic pneumonia still respond to penicillin therapy, some infections due to oral organisms fail to respond to this drug, and in these cases the use of a drug that is effective against penicillin-resistant anaerobes is recommended (Table 148-1). Life-threatening infections involving the anaerobic flora of the mouth, such as space infections of the head and neck, should be treated empirically as if penicillin-resistant anaerobes are involved. Less serious infections involving the oral microflora can be treated with penicillin alone; metronidazole can be added (or clindamycin can be substituted) if the patient responds poorly to penicillin therapy. Combinations of antibiotics used to treat mixed infections of oral origin must include drugs active against the gram-positive aerobic flora of the mouth.

Chloramphenicol has been used successfully against anaerobic central nervous system infections at doses of 30 to 60 mg/kg per day, with the exact dose depending on the severity of illness. However, penicillin G and metronidazole also cross the blood-brain barrier and are bactericidal for many anaerobic organisms (Chap. 360).

Anaerobic infections arising below the diaphragm (e.g., colonic and intraabdominal infections) must be treated specifically with agents active against *Bacteroides* spp. (Table 148-1). In intraabdominal sepsis (Chap. 112), the use of antibiotics effective against penicillin-resistant anaerobes has clearly reduced the incidence of postoperative infections and serious infectious complications. Specifically, a drug from cate-

TABLE 148-2 *Doses and Schedules for Treatment of Serious Infections Due to Commonly Encountered Anaerobic Gram-Negative Rods*

First-Line Therapy	Dose	Schedule[a]
Metronidazole[b]	500 mg	q6h
Ticarcillin/clavulanic acid	3.1 g	q4h
Piperacillin/tazobactam	3.375 g	q6h
Imipenem	0.5 g	q6h
Meropenem	1.0 g	q8h

[a] See disease-specific chapters for recommendations on duration of therapy.

[b] Should generally be used in conjunction with drugs active against aerobic or facultative organisms.

Note: All drugs are given by the intravenous route.

gory 1 (Table 148-1) must be included for broad-spectrum coverage. Recommended doses for commonly used category 1 drugs are given in Table 148-2. Therapy for intraabdominal sepsis must also include drugs active against the gram-negative aerobic flora of the bowel. If the involvement of gram-positive bacteria such as enterococci is suspected, either ampicillin or vancomycin should be added.

Cases of anaerobic osteomyelitis in which a mixed flora is isolated from a bone biopsy specimen should be treated with a regimen that covers all the isolates. When an anaerobic organism is recognized as a major or sole pathogen infecting a joint, the duration of treatment should be similar to that used for arthritis caused by aerobic bacteria (Chap. 314). Therapy includes the management of underlying disease states, the administration of appropriate antimicrobial agents, temporary joint immobilization, percutaneous drainage of effusions, and (usually) the removal of infected prostheses or internal fixation devices. Surgical drainage and debridement procedures such as sequestrectomy are essential for the removal of necrotic tissue that can sustain anaerobic infections.

The outcome of anaerobic bacteremia is significantly better in patients either initially given or switched to appropriate therapy based on known antibiotic susceptibilities.

Failure of Therapy   Anaerobic infections that fail to respond to treatment or that relapse should be reassessed. Consideration should be given to additional surgical drainage or debridement. Superinfections with resistant gram-negative facultative or aerobic bacteria should be ruled out. The possibility of drug resistance must be entertained; if resistance is involved, repeated cultures may yield the pathogenic organism.

Supportive Measures   Other supportive measures in the management of anaerobic infections include careful attention to fluid and electrolyte balance (since extensive local edema may lead to hypoalbuminemia), hemodynamic support for septic shock, immobilization of infected extremities, maintenance of adequate nutrition during chronic infections by parenteral hyperalimentation, relief of pain, and anticoagulation with heparin for thrombophlebitis. For patients with severe anaerobic infections of soft tissues, hyperbaric oxygen therapy is advocated by some experts, but its value has not been proven in controlled trials.

FURTHER READING

ALDRIDGE KE et al: Bacteremia due to *Bacteroides fragilis* group: Distribution of species, beta-lactamase production and antimicrobial susceptibility patterns. Antimicrob Agents Chemother 47:148, 2003

CITRON DM et al: 2001: An anaerobe odyssey. Clin Infect Dis 35;S1, 2002

FINEGOLD SM: Anaerobic bacteria: General concepts, in *Principles and Practice of Infectious Diseases*, 5th ed, GL Mandell et al (eds). New York, Churchill Livingstone, 2000, pp 2519–2537

————: Overview of clinically important anaerobes. Clin Infect Dis 20:S205, 1995

NGUYEN MH et al: Antimicrobial resistance and clinical outcome of *Bacteroides* bacteremia: Findings of a multicenter prospective observational trial. Clin Infect Dis 30:870, 2000

SALONEN JH et al: Clinical significance and outcome of anaerobic bacteremia. Clin Infect Dis 26:1413, 1998

SOLOMKIN JS et al: Guidelines for the selection of anti-infective agents for complicated intra-abdominal infections. Clin Infect Dis 37:997, 2003

TZIANABOS AO et al: Role of T cells in abscess formation, in *Current Opinion in Microbiology*, J Davies, P Cossart (eds). London, Elsevier Science, 2002, pp 92–96

Section 8   Mycobacterial Diseases

149   ANTIMYCOBACTERIAL AGENTS
Richard J. Wallace, Jr., David E. Griffith

The physician is greatly challenged to provide optimal therapy for mycobacterial illnesses because of the increase in both drug-susceptible and multidrug-resistant tuberculosis; the increasing number of pathogenic nontuberculous mycobacteria (NTM); drug-related toxicities and drug-drug interactions (especially in patients who have AIDS, with their complex antiretroviral drug regimens); and the plethora of new antibiotics with antimycobacterial potential. This chapter reviews the therapeutic agents used for treatment of tuberculosis, leprosy (Hansen's disease), and diseases caused by NTM, including *Mycobacterium avium-intracellulare* (MAI), *M. kansasii*, the rapidly growing mycobacteria, and *M. marinum*. The use of antimycobacterial agents in patients with renal or hepatic disease and in pregnant women is summarized in Table 149-1. The effects of antimycobacterial agents on the levels, activity, and toxicity of other commonly used drugs are summarized in Table 149-2.

TUBERCULOSIS

Drugs used to treat tuberculosis have been classified into first-line and second-line agents. *First-line essential* antituberculous agents are the most effective and are a necessary component of any short-course therapeutic regimen. The three drugs in this category are rifampin, isoniazid, and pyrazinamide. The *first-line supplemental* agents, which are highly effective and infrequently toxic, include ethambutol and streptomycin. Favorable experience in patients with tuberculosis resistant to first-line essential drugs suggests that rifabutin and the fluoroquinolones ciprofloxacin and levofloxacin are important additions to multidrug antituberculous regimens; thus these agents have now been added to the list of first-line supplemental drugs. *Second-line* antituberculous drugs are clinically much less effective than first-line agents and elicit severe reactions much more frequently. These drugs are rarely used in therapy and then only by caregivers experienced with their use. The older agents include para-aminosalicylic acid (PAS), ethionamide, cycloserine, amikacin, and capreomycin. *Newer* antituberculous drugs, which have not yet been placed in the above categories, include rifapentine and the 8-methoxyfluoroquinolones gatifloxacin and moxifloxacin.

FIRST-LINE ESSENTIAL ANTITUBERCULOUS DRUGS ■ **Rifampin**   Rifampin, a semisynthetic derivative of *Streptomyces mediterranei*, is considered the most important and potent antituberculous agent. It is also active against a wide spectrum of other organisms, including some gram-positive and gram-negative bacteria, *Legionella* spp., *M. kansasii*, and *M. marinum*.

MECHANISM OF ACTION   Rifampin has both intracellular and extracellular bactericidal activity. It blocks RNA synthesis by specifically binding and inhibiting DNA-dependent RNA polymerase. Susceptible strains

| | | Use in Indicated Circumstances | | |
| | | Renal Disease: Creatinine Clearance Rate | | |
Agent	Severe Hepatic Disease	>30 mL/min	≤30 mL/min	Pregnancy[a]
Azithromycin	No change	No change	?Decrease dose	No evidence of risk (B)
Clarithromycin	No change	No change	Decrease dose	Risk cannot be ruled out (C)
Ethambutol	No change	No change	No change	Risk cannot be ruled out (C)
Isoniazid	Avoid use or decrease dose	No change	Decrease dose	Risk cannot be ruled out (C)
Pyrazinamide	Avoid use or decrease dose	No change	Decrease dose[b]	Risk cannot be ruled out (C)[c]
Rifabutin	No change	No change	No change	No evidence of risk (B)
Rifampin	Avoid use or decrease dose	No change	No change	Risk cannot be ruled out (C)
Rifapentine	Avoid use or decrease dose	No change	No change	Risk cannot be ruled out (C)
Streptomycin	No change	Decrease dose	Decrease dose and frequency	Definite evidence of risk (D)

[a] Based on Food and Drug Administration pregnancy categories of A–D, X.
[b] Prudent but not absolutely necessary.
[c] Use in pregnancy is recommended by international organizations outside the United States.

of *M. tuberculosis* as well as *M. kansasii* and *M. marinum* are inhibited by ≤1 μg/mL.

PHARMACOLOGY Rifampin is a fat-soluble complex macrocyclic antibiotic that is absorbed readily after either oral or intravenous administration. Serum levels of 10 to 20 μg/mL follow a standard adult oral dose of 600 mg. Rifampin distributes well throughout most body tissues, including inflamed meninges. The fact that rifampin turns body fluids (urine, saliva, sputum, tears) a red-orange color makes it simple and inexpensive to check on patients' compliance with therapy. Rifampin is excreted primarily through the bile and the enterohepatic circulation, while 30 to 40% of a dose is excreted via the kidneys. The drug is administered either twice weekly or daily at a dose of 600 mg for adults (10 mg/kg) and 10 to 20 mg/kg for children. As mentioned above, rifampin is also available for intravenous administration.

TABLE 149-2 Effects of Major Antimycobacterial Agents on Levels/Activity/Toxicity of Other Commonly Used Drugs[a]

Rifampin/rifabutin[b]	Isoniazid
Acetaminophen ($\downarrow$)	Alcohol ($\uparrow$ in risk of hepatitis)
Antiarrhythmics ($\downarrow$)	Carbamazepine ($\uparrow$)
Anticonvulsants ($\downarrow$)	Diphenylhydantoin ($\uparrow$)
Azole antifungals ($\downarrow$)	Enflurane ($\uparrow$ in risk of renal failure)
Barbiturates ($\downarrow$)	Warfarin ($\uparrow$)
β Blockers ($\downarrow$)	**Clarithromycin**
Calcium channel blockers ($\downarrow$)	Astemizole ($\uparrow$)
Chloramphenicol ($\downarrow$)	Carbamazepine ($\uparrow$)
Clarithromycin ($\downarrow$)	Digoxin ($\uparrow$)
Cyclosporine ($\downarrow$)	Rifabutin ($\uparrow$)
Dapsone ($\downarrow$)	Ritonavir ($\uparrow$)
Delavirdine ($\downarrow$)	Terfenadine ($\uparrow$)
Diazepam ($\downarrow$)	Zidovudine ($\downarrow$)
Digoxin ($\downarrow$)	
Doxycycline ($\downarrow$)	
Fluoroquinolones ($\downarrow$)	
Glucocorticoids ($\downarrow$)	
Halothane ($\downarrow$)	
Hormonal contraceptives ($\downarrow$)	
Narcotics ($\downarrow$)	
NNRTIs[c] ($\downarrow$)	
Oral hypoglycemics ($\downarrow$)	
Probenecid ($\downarrow$)	
Protease inhibitors ($\downarrow$)	
Quinidine ($\downarrow$)	
Theophylline ($\downarrow$)	
Tricyclic antidepressants ($\downarrow$)	
Warfarin ($\downarrow$)	
Zidovudine ($\downarrow$)	

[a] The following antimycobacterial agents have no or minimal effects on other drugs: amikacin, azithromycin, capreomycin, ethambutol, streptomycin, pyrazinamide.
[b] Rifabutin, which induces the cytochrome P450 system, has the same effects ($\downarrow$) as rifampin but to a lesser degree. All drugs whose half-life is decreased by rifampin induction of hepatic microsomal enzymes may be subject to the same effect when coadministered with rifabutin; however, this point has not yet been studied.
[c] NNRTIs, nonnucleoside reverse transcriptase inhibitors.

ADVERSE EFFECTS (Table 149-3) Rifampin is generally well tolerated; the most common adverse event is gastrointestinal upset. Patients with chronic liver disease, especially those with alcoholism and the elderly, appear to be at unusually high risk for the most serious adverse drug reaction: hepatitis. Other adverse effects of rifampin include rash (0.8%), hemolytic anemia (<1%), thrombocytopenia, and immunosuppression of unknown clinical importance. Rifampin is a potent inducer of the hepatic microsomal enzymes and thereby decreases the half-life of a number of drugs, including digoxin, warfarin, prednisone, cyclosporine, methadone, oral contraceptives, clarithromycin, the HIV protease inhibitors, the HIV nonnucleoside reverse transcriptase inhibitors, and quinidine (Table 149-2). The dose of rifampin generally does not require reduction in patients with renal failure, especially those receiving intermittent rifampin administration (Table 149-1).

RESISTANCE Resistance to rifampin results from spontaneous point mutations that alter the β subunit of the RNA polymerase (*rpoB*) gene. Studies have shown that 96% of rifampin-resistant strains have a missense mutation within a 91-bp central core region of the gene. Rifampin-resistant strains of *M. leprae* have similar mutations that alter a single serine residue (Ser-425) in the same core region of the *rpoB* gene.

Isoniazid After rifampin, isoniazid is considered the best antituberculous drug currently available. Isoniazid should be included in all tuberculosis treatment regimens unless the organism is resistant. Isoniazid is inexpensive, readily synthesized, available worldwide, highly selective for mycobacteria, and well tolerated, with only 5% of patients exhibiting adverse effects.

MECHANISM OF ACTION Isoniazid is the hydrazide of isonicotinic acid, a small, water-soluble molecule that easily penetrates the cell. Its mechanism of action involves inhibition of mycolic acid cell-wall synthesis via oxygen-dependent pathways such as the catalase-peroxidase reaction. Isoniazid is bacteriostatic against resting bacilli and bactericidal against rapidly multiplying organisms, both extracellularly and intracellularly. The minimal inhibitory concentrations (MICs) of isoniazid for wild-type (untreated) strains of *M. tuberculosis* are <0.1 μg/mL, while those for *M. kansasii* are usually 0.5 to 2.0 μg/mL. The MICs of this drug for other NTM are often higher.

PHARMACOLOGY Both oral and intramuscular preparations of isoniazid are readily absorbed. The standard adult daily oral dose of 300 mg produces peak serum levels of 3 to 5 μg/mL. Isoniazid diffuses well throughout the body and reaches therapeutic concentrations in serum, cerebrospinal fluid (CSF), and infected tissue, including caseous granulomas. Isoniazid is metabolized in the liver via acetylation and hydrolysis; its metabolites are excreted into the urine. The rate of acetylation is genetically controlled. The recommended daily dose for the treatment of tuberculosis in the United States is 5 mg/kg for adults and 10 to 20 mg/kg for children, with a maximal daily dose of 300 mg for both groups. (Tuberculosis organizations outside the United States have recommended 5 mg/kg daily for both groups.) For inter-

TABLE 149-3 *Monitoring Side Effects of Common Antituberculous Drugs*

Drug	Side Effect	Management
Rifampin	Rash	Observe patient/stop drug if significant
	Liver dysfunction	Monitor AST/limit alcohol consumption/monitor for hepatitis symptoms
	Flulike syndrome	Administer at least twice weekly/limit dose to 10 mg/kg (adults)
	Red-orange urine	Reassure patient
	Drug interactions	Consider monitoring levels of other drugs affected by rifampin, especially with contraceptives, anticoagulants, and digoxin/avoid use with protease inhibitors
	Fever, chills	Stop drug
Isoniazid	Hepatitis	Monitor AST/limit alcohol consumption/monitor for hepatitis symptoms/educate patient/stop drug at first symptoms of hepatitis (nausea, vomiting, anorexia, flulike syndrome)
	Peripheral neuritis	Administer vitamin B_6
	Optic neuritis	Administer vitamin B_6/stop drug
	Seizures	Administer vitamin B_6
Pyrazinamide	Hepatitis	Monitor AST/limit daily dosage to 15–30 mg/kg/discontinue with signs or symptoms of hepatitis
	Hyperuricemia	Monitor uric acid level only in cases of gout or renal failure
Ethambutol	Optic neuritis	Use 25 mg/kg daily only for first 2 months (except in drug-resistant tuberculosis), then use lower daily dose (15 mg/kg) when possible/monitor visual acuity (eye chart) and red-green color vision (Ishihara Color Book) at baseline and with any visual complaint/educate patient/stop drug at first change in vision, get ophthalmologic evaluation
Streptomycin, amikacin, capreomycin	Ototoxicity, renal toxicity	Limit dose and duration of therapy as much as possible/avoid daily therapy in patients >50 years old/monitor BUN and serum creatinine levels and possibly conduct audiometry before and as needed during therapy/question patient regularly about tinnitus, dizziness, vertigo, and decreased hearing/measure serum drug levels if possible/educate patient/stop drug at first development of adverse effect (usually tinnitus)

Note: AST, aspartate aminotransferase; BUN, blood urea nitrogen.

mittent therapy (usually directly observed), a maximal dose of 900 mg twice or thrice weekly is used. Even in moderate to severe renal failure, the adult dose rarely needs to be reduced below 200 mg/d. Although not approved by the Food and Drug Administration (FDA), intravenous isoniazid can be given in an urgent situation.

ADVERSE EFFECTS (Table 149-3) The two most important adverse effects of isoniazid therapy are hepatotoxicity and peripheral neuropathy. Other adverse reactions are either rare or less significant and include rash (2%), fever (1.2%), anemia, acne, arthritic symptoms, a systemic lupus erythematosus–like syndrome, optic atrophy, seizures, and psychiatric symptoms. Isoniazid-associated hepatitis is idiosyncratic and increases in incidence with age, daily alcohol consumption, concomitant rifampin administration, and HIV infection as well as in women who are pregnant or in the immediate (3 months) postpartum period. Appropriate clinical monitoring of patients receiving isoniazid includes at least monthly questioning about hepatitis-related symptoms and filling of prescriptions for no more than 1 month's worth of medication. Clinical monitoring is essential for all patients since discontinuation of the drug at the onset of hepatitis symptoms reduces the risk of progression to fatal hepatitis. The Centers for Disease Control and Prevention (CDC) and the American Thoracic Society (ATS) recommend that serum concentrations of aspartate aminotransferase (AST) or alanine aminotransferase (ALT) be determined at baseline in patients with liver disorders or HIV infection, in women who are pregnant or in the immediate postpartum period (3 months), in persons with a history of liver disease (e.g., hepatitis B or C, alcoholic hepatitis, or cirrhosis), in persons who use alcohol regularly, and in other individuals at risk for chronic liver disease who are receiving isoniazid for treatment of latent tuberculosis. Baseline testing is no longer routinely indicated in persons >35 years of age. Routine laboratory monitoring during isoniazid treatment is indicated for patients whose baseline liver function tests yield abnormal results and for persons at risk for hepatic disease, including the groups just mentioned. Measurement of the ALT or AST level is certainly mandatory whenever a patient notices the onset of symptoms suggestive of isoniazid-associated hepatitis (e.g., fever, anorexia, nausea, vomiting, and/or a flulike syndrome including fever and myalgias), and treatment should be discontinued until the relationship between therapy and symptoms is ascertained. Several studies have demonstrated that many patients with isoniazid intolerance can be desensitized. The CDC/ATS recommends that discontin-

uation of isoniazid be strongly considered whenever an asymptomatic elevation of the AST or ALT level exceeds 150 to 200 IU (three to five times the upper limit of normal) in high-risk patients whose baseline values were normal. In one study, only 11 (0.1%) of 11,141 patients had hepatotoxic reactions to isoniazid during preventive treatment.

Peripheral neuritis associated with isoniazid is uncommon and probably relates to interference with pyridoxine (vitamin B_6) metabolism. The risk of isoniazid-related neurotoxicity is greatest for patients with preexisting disorders that also pose a risk of neuropathy, such as diabetes, alcohol abuse, or malnutrition. In these patients, the prophylactic administration of 25 to 50 mg of pyridoxine daily should be considered.

RESISTANCE Isoniazid-resistant mutants of *M. tuberculosis* occur spontaneously at a rate of 1 in 10^5 to 10^6 organisms. The molecular sites of isoniazid resistance have been detailed. Most isoniazid-resistant strains have amino acid changes in either the catalase-peroxidase gene (*katG*) or the promoter of a two-gene locus known as *inhA*. Missense mutations or deletion of *katG* is also associated with reduced catalase and peroxidase activity. Rates of primary isoniazid resistance in untreated patients are much higher in many foreign-born populations than in populations born in the United States.

Pyrazinamide A derivative of nicotinic acid, pyrazinamide is an important bactericidal drug used in short-course therapy for tuberculosis.

MECHANISM OF ACTION Pyrazinamide is similar to isoniazid in its narrow spectrum of antibacterial activity, which essentially includes only *M. tuberculosis*. The drug is bactericidal to slowly metabolizing organisms located within the acidic environment of the phagocyte or caseous granuloma; it is active only at a pH of <6.0. Pyrazinamide is considered a prodrug and is converted by the tubercle bacillus to the active form pyrazinoic acid. The target for this compound is thought to be a fatty acid synthase gene (*fasI*). Susceptible strains of *M. tuberculosis* are inhibited by 20 µg/mL.

PHARMACOLOGY Pyrazinamide is well absorbed after oral administration, with a plasma concentration range of 20 to 60 µg/mL 1 to 2 h after oral ingestion of the currently recommended adult daily dose of 15 to 30 mg/kg (maximum, 2 g/d). The drug is well distributed throughout the body. Levels in CSF are excellent, reaching 50 to 100% of levels in serum. The serum half-life of the drug is 9 to 11 h. Pyrazinamide is metabolized by at least two major pathways and one minor pathway in the liver; its several metabolites include pyrazinoic acid, 5-hydroxy-pyrazinamide, and 5-hydroxypyrazinoic acid. Pyrazinamide is not available in a parenteral formulation.

ADVERSE EFFECTS (Table 149-3) At the high dosages used in the past, hepatotoxicity was a prominent complication of pyrazinamide therapy. However, at the currently recommended dosages, the frequency of hepatotoxicity is no higher than that for concomitant isoniazid and rifampin therapy. Although pyrazinamide is recommended by international tuberculosis organizations for routine use in pregnancy, it is not recommended in the United States because of inadequate teratogenicity data (Table 149-1). The combination of rifampin/pyrazinamide once recommended for treatment of latent tuberculosis has recently been shown to have an unacceptably high rate of hepatitis. Hyperuricemia is a common adverse effect of pyrazinamide therapy, the incidence is probably reduced by concurrent rifampin therapy. Clinical gout is seen only rarely. Polyarthralgias are encountered fairly commonly but are not related to the hyperuricemia.

RESISTANCE Resistance to pyrazinamide is associated with loss of pyrazinamidase activity such that pyrazinamide is no longer converted to pyrazinoic acid. More than 90% of isolates with MICs of >100 μg/mL have mutations in the *pncA* gene, which encodes for pyrazinamidase. All strains of *M. bovis* are naturally resistant to pyrazinamide and have a point substitution within the *pncA* gene.

FIRST-LINE SUPPLEMENTAL DRUGS ■ Ethambutol

A derivative of ethylenediamine, ethambutol is a water-soluble compound that is active only against mycobacteria. Susceptible species include *M. tuberculosis*, *M. marinum*, *M. kansasii*, and MAI. Among first-line drugs, ethambutol is the least potent against *M. tuberculosis*. It is used most often with rifampin for treatment of tuberculosis in patients who cannot tolerate isoniazid or who are thought or known to be infected with isoniazid-resistant organisms.

MECHANISM OF ACTION Ethambutol at standard doses is bacteriostatic against *M. tuberculosis*. Its primary mechanism of action appears to be inhibition of an arabinosyltransferase that mediates the polymerization of arabinose into arabinogalactan within the cell wall.

PHARMACOLOGY After oral administration, 75 to 80% of a dose of ethambutol is absorbed from the gastrointestinal tract. Peak serum levels of 2 to 4 μg/mL are achieved 2 to 4 h after the standard adult daily dose of 15 mg/kg. The drug's distribution throughout the body is adequate except in the CSF, where it reaches only low levels. However, ethambutol can reach CSF levels up to 50% as high as peak plasma levels when administered at a daily dosage of 25 mg/kg (which may be given in one daily dose) for the first 2 months, with subsequent reduction to 15 mg/kg. In cases of drug-resistant tuberculosis or where re-treatment is necessary, the higher dose may be given for the duration. For intermittent therapy, the dosage is 50 mg/kg twice weekly or 30 mg/kg thrice weekly. The dosage must be lowered for patients with renal insufficiency (a creatinine clearance rate of <50 mL/min) to prevent drug accumulation and toxicity.

ADVERSE EFFECTS (Table 149-3) Ethambutol is usually well tolerated. Retrobulbar optic neuritis is the most serious adverse effect; axial or central neuritis—the only form reported in patients taking doses of <30 mg/kg—involves the papillomacular bundle of fibers and results in reduced visual acuity, central scotoma, and loss of ability to see green. Symptoms of ocular toxicity typically develop several months after initiation of therapy, but rapid-onset optic neuritis has been reported. The risk of optic neuritis depends on the dose and duration of therapy: this reaction develops in 5% of patients receiving a daily dose of 25 mg/kg but in fewer than 1% of patients given a daily dose of 15 mg/kg. Patients taking the lower dose should be tested at baseline and whenever there is a subjective visual change for visual acuity and red-green color discrimination. Patients taking the higher dose should be tested at baseline, monthly thereafter, and whenever there is subjective

visual change. Intermittent (three times weekly) administration of ethambutol at 25 mg/kg per dose appears to be better tolerated than daily administration of 15 mg/kg, especially in elderly populations being treated for *M. avium* complex infection. Optic neuritis with associated visual loss is usually reversible, but recovery may take >6 months.

Other adverse effects of ethambutol are infrequent. Hyperuricemia occurs but is usually asymptomatic. Peripheral sensory neuropathy occurs in rare instances. Optic neuritis is rare at the low dose in children; however, the use of ethambutol in very young children is problematic because visual complications are difficult to monitor.

RESISTANCE Ethambutol resistance in *M. tuberculosis* most commonly relates to missense mutations in the *embB* gene that encodes for arabinosyltransferase. Such mutations have been found in 70% of resistant strains and involve amino acid replacements at position 306 or 406 in ~90% of cases. Species of NTM that are intrinsically resistant to ethambutol have variant amino acids in this region of the gene, while susceptible species have the same amino acid sequences as *M. tuberculosis*.

Streptomycin An aminoglycoside isolated from *Streptomyces griseus*, streptomycin is available for intramuscular and intravenous administration only. In the United States, it is the least-used first-line supplemental drug for tuberculosis because of its toxicity, the difficulty in obtaining adequate CSF levels, and the inconvenience of parenteral administration. In developing countries, however, streptomycin is frequently used because of its low cost. The drug is active against untreated strains of *M. tuberculosis*, *M. kansasii*, and *M. marinum* and against some strains of the *M. avium* complex at achievable serum levels.

MECHANISM OF ACTION Streptomycin inhibits protein synthesis by disruption of ribosomal function.

PHARMACOLOGY Serum levels of streptomycin peak at 25 to 40 μg/mL after a 1.0-g dose. Streptomycin is bactericidal for rapidly dividing extracellular mycobacteria but is ineffective in the acidic environment within the macrophage. It diffuses poorly into the meninges and, in patients with meningitis, reaches CSF levels that are only 20% of serum levels.

The usual adult dose of streptomycin for a 70-kg patient is 0.5 to 1.0 g (10 to 15 mg/kg) given intramuscularly daily or five times per week; the pediatric dose is 20 to 40 mg/kg daily, with a maximum of 1 g/d. Because streptomycin is eliminated almost exclusively by the kidneys, the dosage must be lowered and the frequency of administration reduced (to only two or three times per week) in most patients >50 years of age and in any patient with renal impairment (Table 149-1) or reduced body weight. Although this approach is not approved by the FDA, streptomycin can be given intravenously.

ADVERSE EFFECTS (Table 149-3) Adverse reactions to streptomycin therapy occur in 10 to 20% of recipients. Ototoxicity and renal toxicity are the most common and the most serious. Renal toxicity, usually manifested as nonoliguric renal failure, is less common with streptomycin than with other frequently used aminoglycosides, such as gentamicin. Ototoxicity involves both hearing loss and vestibular dysfunction. The latter is more common and includes loss of balance, vertigo, and tinnitus. Patients receiving streptomycin must be monitored carefully for these adverse effects. Less serious reactions include perioral paresthesia, eosinophilia, rash, and drug fever.

RESISTANCE Spontaneous resistance to streptomycin occurs in 1 in 10^5 to 10^7 organisms. In two-thirds of streptomycin-resistant strains of *M. tuberculosis*, mutations have been identified in one of two targets: a 16S rRNA gene (*rrs*) or the gene encoding ribosomal protein S12 (*rpsL*). Both targets are believed to be involved in streptomycin ribosomal binding. No mutational change has been identified in the other one-third of resistant isolates. Strains of *M. tuberculosis* resistant to streptomycin are not cross-resistant to capreomycin or amikacin.

SECOND-LINE ANTITUBERCULOUS DRUGS   Second-line and/or newer anti-tuberculosis agents are used either when tuberculosis is drug resistant or when first-line supplemental drugs are not available. The more important second-line drugs are discussed below in their general (descending) order of usefulness.

Quinolones   A surprisingly large number of fluorinated quinolones are being developed and studied as inhibitors of mycobacteria. Their mode of action presumably is the prevention of DNA synthesis through the inhibition of DNA gyrase. Ofloxacin, levofloxacin, ciprofloxacin, gatifloxacin, and moxifloxacin are active against many mycobacteria, including *M. tuberculosis*, *M. leprae*, *M. marinum*, *M. kansasii*, and *M. fortuitum*. These drugs are well absorbed orally, reach high serum levels, and distribute well to body tissues and fluids. While not approved for antituberculous therapy in the United States, ofloxacin—used in combination with isoniazid and rifampin for the treatment of pulmonary tuberculosis—has been as active and safe as ethambutol in initial trials. Adverse effects are relatively uncommon, occurring in 0.5 to 10% of cases and consisting mostly of benign reactions such as gastrointestinal intolerance, rashes, dizziness, and headache. However, more serious adverse effects are being reported and include confusion, seizures, interstitial nephritis, skin vasculitis, and acute renal failure. The quinolones are rapidly becoming some of the most important and effective drugs for the treatment of tuberculosis resistant to first-line essential drugs. Some experts would classify the quinolones as first-line supplemental agents. The quinolones can also be administered intravenously.

Mycobacterial resistance to the fluoroquinolones develops rapidly. Its molecular basis is complex; only some strains exhibit missense mutations in the A subunit (*gyrA* gene) of DNA gyrase. Fluoroquinolone-resistant tuberculosis is a source of growing concern. Antituberculous therapy with quinolones should be reserved for patients with multidrug resistance and for those who cannot tolerate first-line drugs.

Capreomycin   Capreomycin, a complex cyclic polypeptide antibiotic derived from *Streptomyces capreolus*, is similar to streptomycin in terms of dosing, mechanism of action, pharmacology, and toxicity. It is administered only by the intramuscular route in doses of 10 to 15 mg/kg daily or five times per week (maximal daily dose, 1 g), with peak blood levels of 20 to 40 μg/mL. After 2 to 4 months, the dosage should be reduced to 1 g two or three times a week. Cross-resistance to kanamycin and amikacin—but not to streptomycin—is common. After streptomycin, capreomycin is the injectable drug of choice for tuberculosis.

Rifabutin   Rifabutin, a semisynthetic rifamycin spiropiperidyl derivative, shares many characteristics with rifampin, including its activity against *M. tuberculosis*. Rifabutin is also active against some strains of rifampin-resistant *M. tuberculosis* and is more active than rifampin against the *M. avium* complex and other NTM. To date, rifabutin has been most useful in the prophylaxis of disseminated MAI infection and in the treatment of drug-resistant tuberculosis. Because it seems to exhibit more antituberculous activity than rifampin in vitro and in animals, its possible clinical advantages over rifampin are being evaluated. In a multinational trial in which either rifampin (600 mg/d) or rifabutin (150 mg/d) was administered in combination with isoniazid plus a 2-month regimen of pyrazinamide and ethambutol, the two rifamycins were equally effective and well tolerated in the treatment of newly diagnosed pulmonary tuberculosis. Rifabutin is recommended in place of rifampin for the treatment of HIV-positive individuals who are also taking a protease inhibitor because its effect on these agents is less pronounced (Table 149-2).

MECHANISM OF ACTION   In *Escherichia coli* and *Bacillus subtilis*, rifabutin inhibits DNA-dependent RNA polymerase in the same manner as rifampin. Its mode of action against mycobacteria is believed to be the same.

PHARMACOLOGY   The pharmacology of rifabutin is dramatically different from that of rifampin. Rifabutin is readily absorbed after a single oral dose of 300 mg and reaches peak serum levels (0.35 μg/mL) in 2 to 4 h. This lipophilic drug distributes best to tissues: tissue levels are 5 to 10 times higher than plasma levels. CSF concentrations are 30 to 70% of plasma levels in HIV-infected patients who have meningitis. The drug's slow clearance via hepatic metabolism and renal excretion results in a mean serum half-life of 45 h, which is much longer than the 3- to 5-h half-life of rifampin. Clarithromycin (but not azithromycin) and fluconazole appear to block the hepatic metabolism of rifabutin, with consequent increases in serum levels. When rifabutin is administered orally with food, its rate of absorption is slowed but the extent of absorption is unchanged. Adjustment of dosage is usually unnecessary in elderly patients and in patients with reduced hepatic or renal function (Table 149-1).

ADVERSE EFFECTS   The majority of rifabutin's adverse effects are dose related and occur most frequently in patients receiving >300 mg/d. Discontinuation of therapy because of adverse drug reactions is reported in 16% of patients receiving rifabutin as opposed to 8% of those receiving a placebo. The most common symptoms are gastrointestinal; other reactions include rash, headache, asthenia, chest pain, myalgia, and insomnia. Like those taking rifampin, most patients taking rifabutin have discolored (orange to tan) urine and other body fluids. Less common adverse reactions include fever, chills, a flulike syndrome, hepatitis, *Clostridium difficile*–associated diarrhea, a diffuse polymyalgia syndrome, and a yellow skin discoloration ("pseudojaundice"). After a rifabutin dose of 450 or 600 mg in combination with clarithromycin, anterior uveitis is reported in up to 40% of patients; also common at these high doses are hyperpigmentation and the polymyalgia/arthralgia syndrome. All of these conditions are reversible when treatment is discontinued. Laboratory abnormalities include neutropenia, leukopenia, thrombocytopenia, and increased levels of liver enzymes.

Rifabutin induces the hepatic cytochrome P450 enzymes but does so much less strongly than rifampin. Drugs whose metabolism is enhanced by rifabutin include anticoagulants, quinidine, oral contraceptives, sulfonylureas, analgesics, dapsone, narcotics, glucocorticoids, clarithromycin, zidovudine, protease inhibitors, nonnucleoside reverse transcriptase inhibitors, and cardiac glycosides.

RESISTANCE   Resistance to rifabutin is attributable to the same mechanism as that to rifampin—i.e., mutations involving the *rpoB* gene. However, of the 14 mutant *rpoB* alleles that confer resistance to rifampin, only 9 confer high-level resistance to rifabutin, while the remaining 5 result in only small changes in rifabutin MICs, which remain at ≤0.5 μg/mL. The MIC of rifabutin for susceptible strains of *M. tuberculosis* is low (<0.06 μg/mL), and the drug is considered clinically active against partially resistant strains that are inhibited by plasma levels of ≤0.5 μg/mL. Thus rifabutin inhibits about one-quarter of rifampin-resistant strains of *M. tuberculosis*.

Amikacin   This well-known aminoglycoside is bactericidal to extracellular organisms. Amikacin is active against *M. tuberculosis* and several of the nontuberculous species, including the rapidly growing mycobacteria, *M. kansasii*, *M. leprae*, and the *M. avium* complex. The usual adult dosage is 7 to 10 mg/kg intramuscularly or intravenously three to five times per week (generally no more than 500 to 750 mg/d). Resistance relates to a single A → G base-pair change at position 1408 in the 16S ribosomal RNA gene.

Ethionamide   Like isoniazid and pyrazinamide, ethionamide is a derivative of isonicotinic acid. This agent is bacteriostatic against metabolizing *M. tuberculosis* and some NTM. It is most useful in the treatment of multidrug-resistant tuberculosis. However, its use is severely limited by its toxicity and frequent side effects, which include intense gastrointestinal intolerance (anorexia, vomiting, and dysgeusia), serious neurologic reactions, reversible hepatitis (5% of cases), hypersensitivity reactions, and hypothyroidism. Ethionamide is well absorbed orally and is widely distributed throughout the body at sites including the CSF.

Para-Aminosalicylic Acid   PAS as a calcium or sodium salt inhibits the growth of *M. tuberculosis* by impairing folate synthesis. It is rarely indicated for the treatment of tuberculosis because of its low level of antituberculous activity and its high level of gastrointestinal toxicity (manifesting as nausea, vomiting, and diarrhea). Enteric-coated PAS granules (4 g every 8 h) may be better tolerated than other formulations and produce higher therapeutic blood levels. PAS is well absorbed after oral administration but reaches only low concentrations in the CSF. The drug has a short half-life (1 h), and 80% of the dose is excreted in the urine.

Cycloserine   Cycloserine (D-4-amino-3-isoxazolidinone) is produced by *Streptomyces orchidaceus* and is active against a broad spectrum of bacteria, including *M. tuberculosis*. Cycloserine is well absorbed after oral administration and is widely distributed throughout body fluids, including the CSF. Serious side effects limit the use of this drug and include psychosis (with suicide in some cases), seizures, peripheral neuropathy, headaches, somnolence, and allergic reactions. Cycloserine should not be given to patients with epilepsy, active alcohol abuse, severe renal insufficiency, or a history of depression or psychosis.

NEWER ANTITUBERCULOUS DRUGS   A number of drugs are being evaluated for their antituberculous activity. This group includes rifapentine, the newer 8-methoxyfluoroquinolones gatifloxacin and moxifloxacin, clarithromycin, linezolid and other oxazolidinones, and rifamycins not yet approved by the FDA, such as KRM-1648 (benzoxazinorifamycin).

Rifapentine   A semisynthetic cyclopentyl rifamycin antibiotic, rifapentine has received accelerated approval from the FDA for the treatment of tuberculosis. It is the first new drug approved for tuberculosis in the United States in 25 years. While similar to rifampin, rifapentine is lipophilic and longer acting—characteristics that enhance patient compliance; the drug can be administered at a dose of 600 mg once or twice weekly. It is active against *M. tuberculosis* but has undergone only minimal testing against NTM. Rifapentine has not yet been approved for the treatment of patients with HIV disease because rifapentine/rifampin monoresistance frequently develops in HIV-positive patients receiving isoniazid plus once-weekly rifapentine. Like rifampin, rifapentine is active against many nonmycobacterial organisms, including *Haemophilus influenzae*, *Bordetella pertussis*, *Bordetella parapertussis*, *Brucella* spp., *Legionella* spp., *Neisseria* spp., streptococci, and staphylococci.

In a randomized comparative study, 672 Chinese patients received isoniazid plus either rifapentine or rifampin. The isoniazid/rifapentine group had a higher relapse rate than the isoniazid/rifampin group (10% vs 5%). Nevertheless, this disadvantage was considered acceptable in light of the lower rate of adverse effects and the less frequent administration for isoniazid/rifapentine.

MECHANISM OF ACTION   Rifapentine exerts its bactericidal effect by inhibiting DNA-dependent RNA polymerase in susceptible bacteria. The MICs of rifapentine for rifampin-susceptible strains of *M. tuberculosis* range from 0.03 to 0.12 μg/mL.

PHARMACOLOGY   Food enhances the oral absorption of rifapentine, whereas antacids impair its absorption. After oral administration with food, this drug reaches peak serum concentrations in 5 to 6 h and achieves a steady state in 10 days. The half-life of rifapentine and its active metabolite 25-desacetyl rifapentine is ~13 h. The administered dose is excreted via the liver (70%). Oral clearance is more rapid in males than in females (2.51 vs 1.69 L/h), but the clinical significance of this difference is unknown.

ADVERSE EFFECTS   Rifapentine demonstrates an adverse-event pattern similar to that of rifampin. Both drugs are frequently associated with hyperuricemia when administered with pyrazinamide and with elevated hepatocellular enzyme levels in 3 to 4% of patients when ad-

ministered with other antituberculous agents. Liver enzyme levels should be monitored in patients receiving rifapentine who already have elevated liver enzyme concentrations or known liver disease. Like rifampin, rifapentine causes an orange-red discoloration of body fluids, including urine, saliva, and tears, and stains contact lenses.

Rifapentine induces the hepatic cytochrome P450 enzymes CYP3A4 and 2C8/9. Current induction studies suggest that its potential for drug-drug interaction may be less than that of rifampin but greater than that of rifabutin. Other drugs potentially affected by concomitant administration of rifapentine are listed in Table 149-2.

Rifapentine is in category C for use in pregnancy (Table 149-1) because of its teratogenesis in rats and rabbits. There are insufficient data concerning use of this drug in pregnant and breast-feeding patients.

RESISTANCE   Strains of *M. tuberculosis* resistant to rifapentine, rifampin, and rifabutin all involve spontaneous point mutations in the *rpoB* gene. All strains resistant to rifampin are also resistant to rifapentine.

LEPROSY (HANSEN'S DISEASE)

Therapy for leprosy remains difficult, especially in developing countries. Obstacles include the long courses of drug therapy required, the high cost and low availability of most drugs, the frequency of adverse drug reactions, the difficulty of determining a treatment endpoint, and (given that *M. leprae* still cannot be grown in vitro) the difficulty of conducting susceptibility testing. While many drugs are active against *M. leprae*, efficacy in the treatment of leprosy has been established only for dapsone, rifampin, clofazimine, and ethionamide. Initiation of multidrug treatment has reduced the problem of acquired drug resistance seen previously with dapsone monotherapy.

Rifampin   Rifampin is considered the most active agent for the treatment of leprosy. Its worldwide use is limited only by its cost. This drug is highly bactericidal against *M. leprae* and reduces the number of viable bacilli in patients' tissues faster than any other available agent. Rifampin must be combined with other antileprosy drugs to forestall resistance. For cost reasons, the drug dose of 600 mg is given once a month (supervised) outside the United States, but it is given daily in the United States. For details on pharmacology, adverse events, and resistance, see relevant sections under "Tuberculosis." Allergic interstitial nephritis is a rare but significant complication of rifampin use in Hansen's disease.

Dapsone   Dapsone (4,4'-diaminodiphenylsulfone) inhibits bacterial folic acid synthesis. It is now considered the second most active drug (after rifampin) in the treatment of Hansen's disease because of its ready availability, low cost, and low toxicity and the susceptibility of untreated strains of *M. leprae* to low concentrations.

PHARMACOLOGY   Dapsone is well absorbed orally and distributes well throughout the body. The usual daily dosage is 100 mg for adults and 0.9 to 1.4 mg/kg for children. Plasma concentrations peak within 1 to 3 h. The median elimination half-life is 22 h. Dapsone is cleared by acetylation in the liver, with genetic variation similar to that documented for the acetylation of isoniazid. The drug is 70% bound to plasma protein. Usual daily doses produce serum concentrations of 10 to 15 μg/mL, which far exceed the MIC for *M. leprae* (0.01 to 0.001 μg/mL).

ADVERSE EFFECTS   Hemolysis and methemoglobinemia are common untoward reactions to dapsone. Patients should be screened for glucose-6-phosphate dehydrogenase deficiency to prevent serious drug-induced hemolysis. However, most patients tolerate dapsone therapy well with adequate clinical and laboratory supervision. Other side effects include gastrointestinal intolerance, headache, pruritus, peripheral neuropathies, nephrotic syndrome, fever, and rash. In lepromatous and borderline lepromatous leprosy, erythema nodosum leprosum (ENL) may occur. ENL and other reactions of leprosy may be difficult to distinguish from drug reactions and the infectious mononucleosis–like syndrome due to dapsone.

Clofazimine   A phenazine iminoquinone dye, clofazimine is weakly bactericidal against *M. leprae*. It is useful in treating dapsone-resistant leprosy and may lessen the severity of ENL. Clofazimine's mode of action is not well understood, but the drug may inhibit DNA binding. It is absorbed orally and distributed to the fatty tissues and the reticuloendothelial system. Its serum half-life is ~60 to 70 days; only a small proportion of the dose is excreted daily into the urine or bile. Bactericidal activity is very slow and is evident for ~50 days after administration. The usual adult dosage is 50 to 100 mg/d, 100 mg three times a week, or (for treatment of ENL) 300 mg/d. Untoward effects include skin discoloration and, less commonly, gastrointestinal intolerance. Clofazimine was reported to be responsible for a case of cardiotoxicity induced via ventricular arrhythmia. Even though clofazimine-resistant disease has been reported only rarely when this agent is used alone, it should be used with other effective antibiotics. Clofazimine is active in vitro against some NTM species, including MAI, *M. kansasii*, *M. simiae*, and *M. abscessus*.

Ethionamide   While ethionamide (250 mg/d) has not been approved by the FDA for the treatment of leprosy, it is sometimes used in the United States in combination with rifampin (600 mg/d) to treat dapsone-resistant leprosy in patients who cannot accept the skin-pigmentation effect of clofazimine. Because resistance to ethionamide develops quickly when the drug is used alone, it must be used with other effective agents. Patients should be monitored closely for hepatotoxicity when taking ethionamide (especially in combination with rifampin), and treatment should be discontinued if the patient's ALT levels exceed 2.5 times the normal value. Prothionamide, a congener of ethionamide that is not available in the United States, has pharmacologic properties similar to those of ethionamide and is widely used throughout the world.

Other Agents   A number of other drugs exhibit significant activity against *M. leprae*, but clinical experience with these agents is lacking. Thalidomide is now approved by the FDA for treatment of ENL. This drug is sedating and extremely teratogenic and should *never* be taken by anyone who is or may become pregnant. Physicians wishing to prescribe thalidomide must register with the System for Thalidomide Education and Prescription Safety (S.T.E.P.S) at 1-888-423-5436 (Celgene Corporation); the sole exceptions to this registration requirement are physicians at Hansen's disease clinics that are receiving medication support from the national Hansen's disease program. It is noteworthy that ENL may be a presenting feature of Hansen's disease *before* treatment. It is not considered an adverse drug reaction but may be confused with drug reactional states.

The newer macrolide antibiotics (particularly clarithromycin), minocycline (a long-acting tetracycline), and a number of fluoroquinolones (including ofloxacin, sparfloxacin, and pefloxacin) have shown promising bactericidal activity against *M. leprae*. Ofloxacin and minocycline are being investigated with rifampin in short-course regimens for lepromatous disease. All of these newer leprosy drugs have low toxicity profiles, modes of action different from those of the established agents, and bactericidal activity against *M. leprae*. However, their levels of bactericidal activity are lower than that of rifampin.

NONTUBERCULOUS MYCOBACTERIA

Although less pathogenic than *M. tuberculosis*, NTM can cause pulmonary, skin, bone, joint, lymph node, and soft tissue infection as well as disseminated disease in immunocompromised hosts, including patients with AIDS. MAI and *M. kansasii* are the two most common causes of NTM pulmonary infection. Up to 40% of AIDS patients with CD4+ cell counts of <50/μL develop disseminated infected disease due to *M. avium* unless they are receiving specific *M. avium* prophylaxis.

Clarithromycin   Clarithromycin (6-0-methylerythromycin) is a newer macrolide that is similar to erythromycin in its mechanism of action. It is well absorbed with or without meals and elicits little gastrointestinal intolerance at low doses. Clarithromycin distributes well into body tissues and fluids and is highly concentrated in macrophages. The drug is metabolized in the liver, with ~30% of a given dose excreted in the urine. The dosage should be reduced if the creatinine clearance rate is ≤30 mL/min. Like erythromycin, clarithromycin binds with plasma proteins (65 to 70%) and can raise the levels of drugs such as theophylline and carbamazepine. Serum levels of clarithromycin are reduced by rifampin and, to a lesser degree, by rifabutin; clarithromycin increases serum levels of rifabutin and some antihistamines (e.g., terfenadine), thus potentially increasing their toxicity. Clarithromycin and (probably) azithromycin are the most active agents for the treatment of MAI infections; one of these drugs is considered an essential component of any regimen for this purpose. However, because of the risk of mutational drug resistance, clarithromycin should be given in combination with other agents, such as ethambutol and rifampin or rifabutin. The drug is also highly active against almost all other NTM, including *M. marinum*, *M. kansasii*, *M. haemophilum*, *M. genavense*, *M. xenopi*, *M. abscessus*, *M. chelonae*, and most isolates of *M. fortuitum* Standard antimycobacterial doses have been 500 mg twice daily or, in the case of MAI pulmonary disease, three times weekly. The more common side effects of high doses include nausea, vomiting, and (occasionally) abnormal liver function tests. A bitter taste is common even with routine doses. Most gastrointestinal side effects can be minimized by reducing the dose. Clarithromycin is teratogenic in laboratory animals and is in category C for use in pregnancy (Table 149-1). Resistance results from point mutations involving adenine at positions 2058 or 2059 in the 23S ribosomal RNA gene macrolide binding site. Mutational resistance occurs in 1 in 10^8 to 10^9 organisms and develops with monotherapy, especially for all slowly growing species and the rapid growers *M. chelonae* and *M. abscessus*, which have only a single copy of the ribosomal genes.

Azithromycin   Azithromycin is a macrolide that belongs to the family of azalides. This drug reaches much lower serum levels than clarithromycin (usually ≤0.5 μg/mL), but its high tissue and macrophage concentrations and longer half-life suggest the feasibility of intermittent therapy. Azithromycin is involved in few drug interactions since it does not affect the cytochrome P450 system. The usual doses are 250 to 500 mg three times weekly (MAI therapy) or 1200 mg once a week (prophylaxis for disseminated *M. avium*). No alteration in dose is required in renal failure. The most common side effects are gastrointestinal symptoms and reversible hearing loss. Azithromycin appears to be less active than clarithromycin for both pulmonary and disseminated MAI disease. Resistance to azithromycin develops by the same mechanism as that to clarithromycin, with cross-resistance between the two macrolides.

Therapy for Specific NTM Infections ■ *MAI*   Therapy for MAI lung disease in the adult usually involves the administration of clarithromycin (500 mg morning and night), ethambutol (25 mg/kg), and rifampin (600 mg) on a Monday-Wednesday-Friday schedule. Therapy is generally continued until cultures have been negative for 12 months.

For disseminated disease in AIDS, daily administration of one of the newer macrolides (clarithromycin or azithromycin) and ethambutol (15 mg/kg) is considered an essential component of any treatment regimen, with rifabutin (300 mg) a commonly used third drug. Other alternative drugs include streptomycin and amikacin. Clofazimine appears to increase mortality and should be avoided. For prophylaxis of disseminated MAI disease, rifabutin (300 mg/d), clarithromycin (500 mg twice daily), and azithromycin (1200 mg once weekly) have all been demonstrated to be effective in controlled or comparative clinical trials. Once-weekly azithromycin is the drug most often used.

MYCOBACTERIUM KANSASII   *M. kansasii* is usually susceptible to most antituberculous drugs except for pyrazinamide. Current ATS recommendations for the treatment of *M. kansasii* pulmonary disease are 18 to 24 months of daily isoniazid (300 mg), rifampin (600 mg), and ethambutol (15 mg/kg). In patients taking protease inhibitors, rifabutin (150 mg/d) or clarithromycin (500 mg twice daily) should be substituted for rifampin. The potential advantages of the highly active rifabutin and the newer macrolides in immunocompetent patients have not been studied.

RAPIDLY GROWING MYCOBACTERIA The *M. fortuitum* group, *M. abscessus*, and *M. chelonae* account for more than 80% of cases of clinical disease due to rapidly growing mycobacteria. These organisms are resistant to antituberculous agents other than amikacin but are variably susceptible to several traditional antibiotics Clarithromycin has dramatically changed the approach to therapy for infection with these organisms, as it inhibits all rapidly growing mycobacteria (except for 20% of *M. fortuitum* strains and most *M. smegmatis* strains) at concentrations of ≤4 µg/mL. Other drugs with good activity include amikacin (which inhibits 80 to 100% of strains), cefoxitin (80% of *M. abscessus* and *M. fortuitum* strains), doxycycline (50% of *M. fortuitum* strains), imipenem (100% of *M. fortuitum* strains, 70% of *M. chelonae* strains, and 70% of *M. abscessus* strains), the fluorinated quinolones (100% of *M. fortuitum* strains), sulfonamides (90% of *M. fortuitum* strains), and linezolid (>90% of isolates of *M. chelonae* and *M. fortuitum*).

MYCOBACTERIUM MARINUM *M. marinum*, a cause of posttraumatic localized skin infection, is typically susceptible to minocycline, rifampin, ethambutol, clarithromycin, and trimethoprim-sulfamethoxazole and is resistant to isoniazid.

MYCOBACTERIUM HAEMOPHILUM Infection due to *M. haemophilum* occurs most commonly as disseminated cutaneous disease in immunocompromised patients with or without AIDS. Isolates typically show in vitro resistance to most drugs but may be susceptible to rifampin, rifabutin, quinolones, and clarithromycin.

MYCOBACTERIUM XENOPI In the United States, *M. xenopi* is best known as a cause of nosocomial pseudoinfections associated with contamination of the hospital's hot-water system. Drug therapy for *M. xenopi* infection is difficult. *M. xenopi* is often resistant to first-line antituberculous agents but susceptible to the newer macrolides, quinolones, streptomycin, and ethionamide. Patients usually respond to multidrug regimens that include clarithromycin, but relapses are common.

MYCOBACTERIUM GENAVENSE *M. genavense* is a fastidious organism that grows only in liquid media, such as BACTEC 12B or 13A, after prolonged incubation. This organism almost exclusively infects AIDS patients, causing disseminated disease and being isolated from blood, bone marrow, liver, lymph node, spleen, and intestinal cultures. The in vitro susceptibility profile of *M. genavense* has not been well established. Some isolates are susceptible to amikacin, clarithromycin, ofloxacin, rifampin, and rifabutin. Isolates generally respond to macrolide-containing regimens similar to those used for disseminated *M. avium* infection.

MYCOBACTERIUM SIMIAE *M. simiae* is a cause of chronic lung disease, especially in Texas and other southwestern states. It is highly drug resistant, and no satisfactory treatment regimen has yet been established.

FURTHER READING

ALANGADEN GJ, LERNER SA: The clinical use of fluoroquinolones for the treatment of mycobacterial disease. Clin Infect Dis 25:1213, 1997

AMERICAN THORACIC SOCIETY: Targeted tuberculin testing and treatment of latent tuberculosis infection. Am J Respir Crit Care Med 161:S221, 2000

AMERICAN THORACIC SOCIETY/CENTERS FOR DISEASE CONTROL AND PREVENTION/INFECTIOUS DISEASES SOCIETY OF AMERICA: Treatment of tuberculosis. Am J Respir Crit Care Med 167:603–622, 2003 [special issue]

BOCK NN et al: A prospective, randomized, double-blind study of the tolerability of rifapentine 600, 900, and 1,200 mg plus isoniazid in the continuation phase of tuberculosis treatment. Am J Respir Crit Care Med 165:1526, 2002

MUSSER JM: Antimicrobial agent resistance in mycobacteria: Molecular genetic insights. Clin Microbiol Rev 8:496, 1995

JASMER RM et al: Short-course rifampin and pyrazinamide compared with isoniazid for latent tuberculosis infection: A multicenter clinical trial. Ann Intern Med 137:640, 2002

WALLACE RJ JR et al: American Thoracic Society Statement: Diagnosis and treatment of disease caused by nontuberculous mycobacteria. Am J Respir Crit Care Med 156:S1, 1997

WHO EXPERT COMMITTEE ON LEPROSY: Seventh Report. Geneva, World Health Organization, 1998, Technical Report Series, No. 874

150 TUBERCULOSIS
Mario C. Raviglione, Richard J. O'Brien

DEFINITION Tuberculosis, one of the oldest diseases known to affect humans, is caused by bacteria belonging to the *Mycobacterium tuberculosis* complex. The disease usually affects the lungs, although in up to one-third of cases other organs are involved. If properly treated, tuberculosis caused by drug-susceptible strains is curable in virtually all cases. If untreated, the disease may be fatal within 5 years in more than half of cases. Transmission usually takes place through the airborne spread of droplet nuclei produced by patients with infectious pulmonary tuberculosis.

ETIOLOGIC AGENT Mycobacteria belong to the family Mycobacteriaceae and the order Actinomycetales. Of the pathogenic species belonging to the *M. tuberculosis* complex, the most frequent and important agent of human disease is *M. tuberculosis*. The complex includes *M. bovis* (the bovine tubercle bacillus, once an important cause of tuberculosis transmitted by unpasteurized milk and currently the cause of a small percentage of cases in developing countries), *M. africanum* (isolated from cases in West, Central, and East Africa), *M. microti* (the "vole" bacillus, a less virulent and rarely encountered organism), and *M. canettii* (a very rare isolate in African cases).

M. tuberculosis is a rod-shaped, non-spore-forming, thin aerobic bacterium measuring 0.5 µm by 3 µm. Mycobacteria, including *M. tuberculosis*, are often neutral on Gram's staining. However, once stained, the bacilli cannot be decolorized by acid alcohol, a characteristic justifying their classification as acid-fast bacilli (AFB; Fig. 150-1). Acid fastness is due mainly to the organisms' high content of mycolic acids, long-chain cross-linked fatty acids, and other cell-wall lipids. Microorganisms other than mycobacteria that display some acid fastness include species of *Nocardia* and *Rhodococcus*, *Legionella micdadei*, and the protozoa *Isospora* and *Cryptosporidium*. In the mycobacterial cell wall, lipids (e.g., mycolic acids) are linked to underlying arabinogalactan and peptidoglycan. This structure confers very low permeability of the cell wall, thus reducing effectiveness of most antibiotics. Another molecule in the mycobacterial cell wall, lipoarabinomannan, is involved in the pathogen-host interaction and facilitates the survival of *M. tuberculosis* within macrophages. The several proteins characteristic of *M. tuberculosis* include those in purified protein derivative (PPD) tuberculin, a precipitate of non-species-specific molecules obtained from filtrates of heat-sterilized, concentrated broth cultures. The complete genome sequence of *M. tuberculosis* comprises ~4000 genes and has a high guanine-plus-cytosine content. A large proportion of genes are devoted to the production of enzymes involved in cell wall metabolism.

EPIDEMIOLOGY More than 3.8 million new cases of tuberculosis—all forms (pulmonary and extrapulmonary), 90% of them from developing countries—were reported to the World Health Organization (WHO) in 2001. However, because of a low level of case detection and incomplete notifications, reported cases represent only a fraction of the total. It is estimated that 8.5 million new cases of tuberculosis occurred worldwide in 2001, 95% of them in developing countries of Asia (5 million), Africa (2 million), the Middle East (0.6 million), and Latin

FIGURE 150-1   Acid-fast bacillus (AFB) smear showing *M. tuberculosis* bacilli. (*Courtesy of the CDC, Atlanta.*)

America (0.4 million). It is also estimated that 1.8 million deaths from tuberculosis occurred in 2000, 98% of them in developing countries. Estimates of tuberculosis incidence rates (per 100,000 population) and numbers of tuberculosis-related deaths in 2001 are depicted in Fig. 150-2 and Fig. 150-3, respectively.

After an increase in the late 1980s, numbers of cases have declined during the past few years in several industrialized countries, including the United States. The increases in the 1980s were largely related to immigration from countries with a high prevalence of tuberculosis; infection with HIV; social problems, such as poverty, homelessness, and drug abuse; and dismantling of tuberculosis services. In the United States, with the implementation of stronger control programs, the decrease resumed in 1993. In 2002, 15,075 cases of tuberculosis (5.2 cases per 100,000 population) were reported to the U.S. Centers for Disease Control and Prevention (CDC)—a 43% decrease from the 1992 peak.

In the United States, tuberculosis is uncommon among young adults of European descent, who have only rarely been exposed to *M. tuberculosis* infection during recent decades. In contrast, because of a

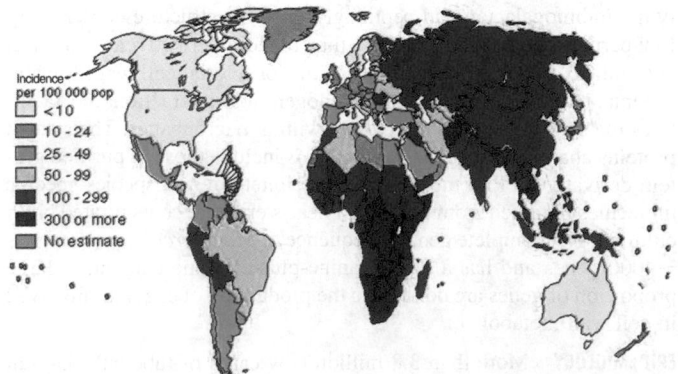

FIGURE 150-2   Map of the world showing the estimated tuberculosis incidence rates (per 100,000 population) in 2001. The designations employed and the presentation of material on this map do not imply the expression of any opinion whatsoever on the part of the WHO concerning the legal status of any country, territory, city or area or of its authorities, or concerning the delimitation of its frontiers or boundaries. White lines on maps represent approximate border lines for which there may not yet be full agreement. (*Courtesy of the Stop TB Department, WHO.*)

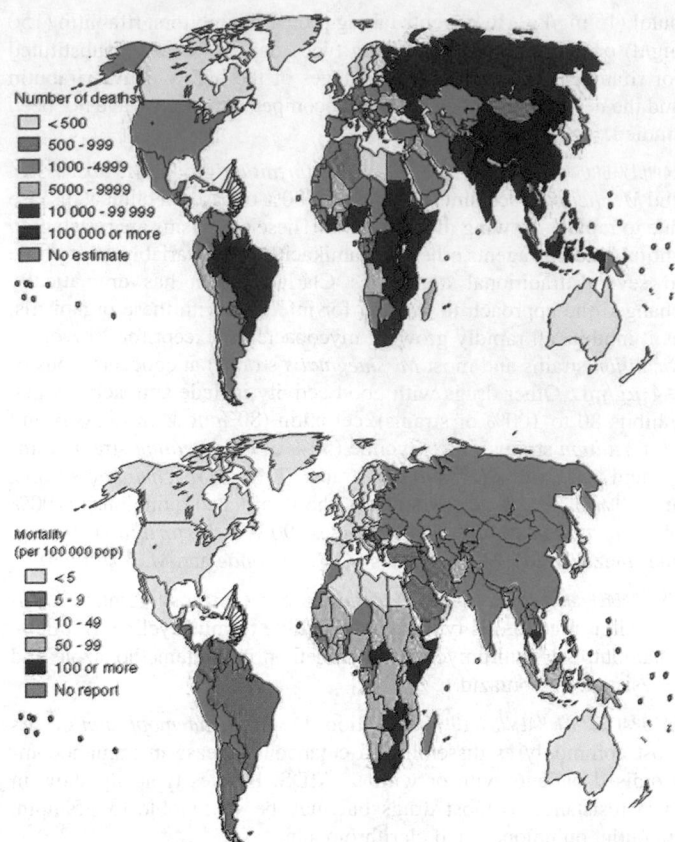

FIGURE 150-3   Maps of the world showing the estimated number of tuberculosis-related deaths and estimated tuberculosis mortality figures in 2001. (*See also disclaimer in Fig. 150-2. Courtesy of the Stop TB Department, WHO.*)

high risk in the past, the prevalence of *M. tuberculosis* infection is relatively high among elderly Caucasians, who remain at increased risk of developing active tuberculosis. Tuberculosis in the United States is also a disease of young adult members of the HIV-infected, immigrant, and disadvantaged/marginalized populations. Similarly, in Europe, tuberculosis has reemerged as an important public health problem, mainly as a result of cases among immigrants from high-prevalence countries.

Recent tuberculosis trends in developing countries indicate a stable situation, with almost no decline. There are two exceptions. First, in sub-Saharan Africa, the spread of the HIV epidemic has resulted in doubling or tripling of the number of reported cases of tuberculosis during the past 15 years. Second, in countries of the former Soviet Union and in Romania, numbers of cases have increased by two- or threefold in the past 10 years, largely as the result of deterioration in socioeconomic conditions and the health care infrastructure.

From Exposure to Infection   *M. tuberculosis* is most commonly transmitted from a patient with infectious pulmonary tuberculosis to other persons by droplet nuclei, which are aerosolized by coughing, sneezing, or speaking. The tiny droplets dry rapidly; the smallest ($<10~\mu m$ in diameter) may remain suspended in the air for several hours and may gain direct access to the terminal air passages when inhaled. There may be as many as 3000 infectious nuclei per cough. Other routes of transmission of tubercle bacilli, such as through the skin or the placenta, are uncommon and of no epidemiologic significance.

The probability of contact with a case of tuberculosis, the intimacy and duration of that contact, the degree of infectiousness of the case, and the shared environment of the contact are all important determinants of transmission. Several studies of close contacts have clearly demonstrated that tuberculosis patients whose sputum contains AFB visible by microscopy play the greatest role in the spread of infection. These patients often have cavitary pulmonary disease or tuberculosis of the respiratory tract (endobronchial or laryngeal tuberculosis) and produce sputa containing as many as 10^5 AFB/mL. Patients with sputum smear−negative/culture-positive tuberculosis are less infectious, and those with culture-negative pulmonary disease and extrapulmonary tuberculosis are essentially noninfectious. The frequent absence of cavities among HIV-infected patients may reduce their infectiousness. Crowding in poorly ventilated rooms is one of the most important factors in the transmission of tubercle bacilli, since it increases the intensity of contact with a case.

In short, the risk of acquiring *M. tuberculosis* infection is determined mainly by exogenous factors. Because of delays in seeking care and in diagnosis, it is estimated that up to 20 contacts may be infected by each AFB-positive case before detection in high-prevalence settings.

From Infection to Disease Unlike the risk of acquiring infection with *M. tuberculosis*, the risk of developing disease after being infected depends largely on endogenous factors, such as the individual's innate susceptibility to disease and level of function of cell-mediated immunity. Clinical illness directly following infection is classified as *primary tuberculosis* and is common among children up to 4 years of age. Although this form may be severe and disseminated, it is usually not transmissible. When infection is acquired later in life, the chance is greater that the immune system will contain it, at least temporarily. The majority of infected individuals who ultimately develop tuberculosis do so within the first year or two after infection. Dormant bacilli, however, may persist for years before reactivating to produce *secondary* (or *postprimary*) *tuberculosis*, which is often infectious. Overall, it is estimated that ~10% of persons infected in their youth will eventually develop active tuberculosis. This risk, however, is greatly increased among HIV-infected persons. Reinfection of a previously infected individual, which is common in areas with high rates of tuberculosis transmission, may also favor the development of disease. Molecular typing and comparison of strains of *M. tuberculosis* have suggested that up to one-third of cases of active tuberculosis in U.S. inner-city communities are due to recent transmission rather than to reactivation of latent infection.

Age is an important determinant of the risk of disease after infection. Among infected persons, the incidence of tuberculosis is highest during late adolescence and early adulthood; the reasons are unclear. The incidence among women peaks at 25 to 34 years of age. In this age group rates among women are usually higher than those among men, while at older ages the opposite is true. The risk may increase in the elderly, possibly because of waning immunity and comorbidity.

A variety of diseases and conditions favor the development of active tuberculosis (Table 150-1). The most potent risk factor for tuberculosis among infected individuals is clearly HIV co-infection, which suppresses cellular immunity. The risk that latent *M. tuberculosis* infection will proceed to active disease is directly related to the patient's degree of immunosuppression. In a study of HIV-infected, PPD-positive persons, this risk varied from 2.6 to 13.3 cases per 100 person-years and depended upon the CD4+ cell count.

TABLE 150-1 *Risk Factors for Active Tuberculosis among Persons Who Have Been Infected with Tubercle Bacilli*

Factor	Relative Risk/Odds[a]
Recent infection (<1 year)	12.9
Fibrotic lesions (spontaneously healed)	2–20
Comorbidity	
HIV infection	100
Silicosis	30
Chronic renal failure/hemodialysis	10–25
Diabetes	2–4
Intravenous drug use	10–30
Immunosuppressive treatment	10
Gastrectomy	2–5
Jejunoileal bypass	30–60
Posttransplantation period (renal, cardiac)	20–70
Malnutrition and severe underweight	2

[a] Old infection = 1.

NATURAL HISTORY OF DISEASE Studies conducted in various countries before the advent of chemotherapy showed that untreated tuberculosis is often fatal. About one-third of patients died within 1 year after diagnosis, and one-half died within 5 years. Five-year mortality among sputum smear−positive cases was 65%. Of the survivors at 5 years, ~60% had undergone spontaneous remission, while the remainder were still excreting tubercle bacilli.

With effective, timely, and proper chemotherapy, patients have a very high chance of being cured. However, improper use of antituberculosis drugs, while reducing mortality, may also result in large numbers of chronic infectious cases, often with drug-resistant bacilli.

PATHOGENESIS AND IMMUNITY The interaction of *M. tuberculosis* with the human host begins when droplet nuclei containing microorganisms from infectious patients are inhaled. While the majority of inhaled bacilli are trapped in the upper airways and expelled by ciliated mucosal cells, a fraction (usually <10%) reach the alveoli. There, nonspecifically activated alveolar macrophages ingest the bacilli. Invasion of macrophages by mycobacteria may result in part from association of C2a with the bacterial cell wall followed by C3b opsonization of the bacteria and recognition by the macrophages. The balance between the bactericidal activity of the macrophage and the number and virulence of the bacilli (with virulence partially linked to the bacterium's lipid-rich cell wall and to its glycolipid capsule, both of which confer resistance to complement and free radicals of the phagocyte) determines the events following phagocytosis.

Several genes thought to confer virulence to *M. tuberculosis* have been identified; *katG* encodes for catalase, an enzyme protective against oxidative stress; *rpoV* is the main sigma factor initiating transcription of several genes. Defects in these two genes result in loss of virulence. The *erp* gene, encoding a protein required for multiplication, also contributes to virulence. Outbreaks of tuberculosis in Tennessee and Kentucky in 1994 through 1996 exemplify how infection with virulent strains can result in enhanced transmission with high rates of disease. Strains of the Beijing/W genotype family have been identified in outbreak conditions in a variety of settings worldwide and have been associated with high mortality and drug resistance.

Several observations suggest that genetic factors play a key role in innate nonimmune resistance to infection with *M. tuberculosis*. The existence of this resistance is suggested by the differing degrees of susceptibility to tuberculosis in different populations. In mice, a gene called *Nramp1* (natural resistance−associated macrophage protein 1) has a regulatory role in resistance/susceptibility to mycobacteria. The human homologue NRAMP1, cloned to chromosome 2q, may have a role in determining susceptibility to tuberculosis, as is suggested by a study among West Africans.

In the initial stage of host-bacterium interaction, either the host's macrophages contain bacillary multiplication by producing proteolytic enzymes and cytokines or the bacilli begin to multiply. If the bacilli multiply, their growth quickly kills the macrophages, which lyse. Nonactivated monocytes attracted from the bloodstream to the site by various chemotactic factors ingest the bacilli released from the lysed macrophages. These initial stages of infection are usually asymptomatic.

About 2 to 4 weeks after infection, two additional host responses to *M. tuberculosis* develop: a tissue-damaging response and a macrophage-activating response. The *tissue-damaging response* is the result of a delayed-type hypersensitivity (DTH) reaction to various bacillary antigens; it destroys nonactivated macrophages that contain multiplying bacilli. The *macrophage-activating response* is a cell-mediated phenomenon resulting in the activation of macrophages that are capable of killing and digesting tubercle bacilli. Although both of these responses can inhibit mycobacterial growth, it is the balance between the two that determines the form of tuberculosis that will develop subsequently.

With the development of specific immunity and the accumulation of large numbers of activated macrophages at the site of the primary lesion, granulomatous lesions (tubercles) are formed. These lesions consist of lymphocytes and activated macrophages, such as epithelioid cells and giant cells. Initially, the newly developed tissue-damaging response is the only event capable of limiting mycobacterial growth within macrophages. This response, mediated by various bacterial products, not only destroys macrophages but also produces early solid necrosis in the center of the tubercle. Although *M. tuberculosis* can survive, its growth is inhibited within this necrotic environment by low oxygen tension and low pH. At this point, some lesions may heal by fibrosis and calcification, while others undergo further evolution.

Cell-mediated immunity is critical at this early stage. In the majority of infected individuals, local macrophages are activated when bacillary antigens processed by macrophages stimulate T lymphocytes to release a variety of lymphokines. These activated cells aggregate around the lesion's center and effectively neutralize tubercle bacilli without causing further tissue destruction. In the central part of the lesion, the necrotic material resembles soft cheese (*caseous necrosis*)—a phenomenon that may also be observed in other conditions, such as neoplasms. Even when healing takes place, viable bacilli may remain dormant within macrophages or in the necrotic material for years or even throughout the patient's lifetime. These "healed" lesions in the lung parenchyma and hilar lymph nodes may later undergo calcification.

In a minority of cases, the macrophage-activating response is weak, and mycobacterial growth can be inhibited only by intensified DTH reactions, which lead to tissue destruction. The lesion tends to enlarge further, and the surrounding tissue is progressively damaged. At the center of the lesion, the caseous material liquefies. Bronchial walls as well as blood vessels are invaded and destroyed, and cavities are formed. The liquefied caseous material, containing large numbers of bacilli, is drained through bronchi. Within the cavity, tubercle bacilli multiply well and spread into the airways and the environment through expectorated sputum.

In the early stages of infection, bacilli are usually transported by macrophages to regional lymph nodes, from which they disseminate widely to many organs and tissues. The resulting lesions may undergo the same evolution as those in the lungs, although most tend to heal. In young children with poor natural immunity, hematogenous dissemination may result in fatal miliary tuberculosis or tuberculous meningitis.

Cell-mediated immunity confers partial protection against *M. tuberculosis*, while humoral immunity has no defined role in protection. Two types of cells are essential: macrophages, which directly phagocytize tubercle bacilli, and T cells (mainly CD4+ lymphocytes), which induce protection through the production of lymphokines, especially interferon γ (IFN-γ).

After infection with *M. tuberculosis*, alveolar macrophages secrete a number of cytokines: interleukin (IL) 1 contributes to fever; IL-6 contributes to hyperglobulinemia; and tumor necrosis factor α (TNF-α) contributes to the killing of mycobacteria, the formation of granulomas, and a number of systemic effects, such as fever and weight loss. Macrophages are also critical in processing and presenting antigens to T lymphocytes; the result is a proliferation of CD4+ lymphocytes, which are crucial to the host's defense against *M. tuberculosis*. Qualitative and quantitative defects of CD4+ T cells explain the inability of HIV-infected individuals to contain mycobacterial proliferation. Reactive CD4+ lymphocytes produce cytokines of the T_H1 pattern and participate in MHC class II–restricted killing of cells infected with *M. tuberculosis*. T_H1 CD4+ cells produce IFN-γ and IL-2 and promote cell-mediated immunity. T_H2 cells produce IL-4, IL-5, and IL-10 and promote humoral immunity. The interplay of these various cytokines and their cross-regulation determine the host's response. The role of cytokines in promoting intracellular killing of mycobacteria has not been entirely elucidated. IFN-γ may induce release of nitric oxide, and TNF-α also seems to be important. Obser-

vations in transgenic knockout mice suggest that other T cell subsets (especially CD8+ cells) restricted by alternative antigen-presenting molecules containing a β_2-microglobulin subunit may play an important role. Lipids have been involved in mycobacterial recognition by the innate immune system, and lipoproteins have been proven to trigger potent signals through Toll-like receptors. Finally, a recently described subset of T cells capable of recognizing lipid elements of the bacillus presented by CD1 molecules may be implicated in protection.

M. tuberculosis possesses various protein antigens. Some are present in the cytoplasm and cell wall; others are secreted. That the latter are more important in eliciting a T lymphocyte response is suggested by experiments documenting the appearance of protective immunity in animals after immunization with live, protein-secreting mycobacteria. Among the antigens with a potential protective role are the 30-kDa (or 85B) and the ESAT-6 antigens. Protective immunity is probably the result of reactivity to a large number of different mycobacterial antigens.

Coincident with the appearance of immunity, DTH to *M. tuberculosis* develops. This reactivity is the basis of the PPD skin test, which is used primarily for the detection of *M. tuberculosis* infection in persons without symptoms. The cellular mechanisms responsible for PPD reactivity are related mainly to previously sensitized CD4+ lymphocytes, which are attracted to the skin-test site. There, they proliferate and produce cytokines.

While DTH is associated with protective immunity (PPD-positive persons being less susceptible to a new *M. tuberculosis* infection than PPD-negative persons), it by no means guarantees protection against reactivation. In fact, severe cases of active tuberculosis are often accompanied by strongly positive skin-test reactions.

CLINICAL MANIFESTATIONS Tuberculosis is classified as pulmonary or extrapulmonary. Before the recognition of HIV infection, >80% of all cases of tuberculosis were limited to the lungs. However, up to two-thirds of HIV-infected patients with tuberculosis may have both pulmonary and extrapulmonary disease or extrapulmonary disease alone.

Pulmonary Tuberculosis Pulmonary tuberculosis can be categorized as primary or postprimary (secondary).

PRIMARY DISEASE Primary pulmonary tuberculosis results from an initial infection with tubercle bacilli. In areas of high tuberculosis prevalence, this form of disease is often seen in children and is frequently localized to the middle and lower lung zones. The lesion forming after infection is usually peripheral and accompanied by hilar or paratracheal lymphadenopathy, which may not be detectable on chest radiography. In the majority of cases, the lesion heals spontaneously and may later be evident as a small calcified nodule (*Ghon lesion*).

In children and in persons with impaired immunity (e.g., those with malnutrition or HIV infection), primary pulmonary tuberculosis may progress rapidly to clinical illness. The initial lesion increases in size and can evolve in different ways. Pleural effusion, a frequent finding, results from the penetration of bacilli into the pleural space from an adjacent subpleural focus. In severe cases, the primary site rapidly enlarges, its central portion undergoes necrosis, and acute cavitation develops (progressive primary tuberculosis). Tuberculosis in young children is almost invariably accompanied by hilar or mediastinal lymphadenopathy due to the spread of bacilli from the lung parenchyma through lymphatic vessels. Enlarged lymph nodes may compress bronchi, causing obstruction and subsequent segmental or lobar collapse. Partial obstruction may cause obstructive emphysema, and bronchiectasis may also develop. Hematogenous dissemination, which is common and is often asymptomatic, may result in the most severe manifestations of primary *M. tuberculosis* infection. Bacilli reach the bloodstream from the pulmonary lesion or the lymph nodes and disseminate into various organs, where they may produce granulomatous lesions. Although healing frequently takes place, immunocompromised persons (e.g., patients with HIV infection) may develop miliary tuberculosis and/or tuberculous meningitis.

POSTPRIMARY DISEASE Also called adult-type, reactivation, or secondary tuberculosis, postprimary disease results from endogenous reactivation of latent infection and is usually localized to the apical and posterior segments of the upper lobes, where the high oxygen concentration favors mycobacterial growth. In addition, the superior segments of the lower lobes are frequently involved. The extent of lung parenchymal involvement varies greatly, from small infiltrates to extensive cavitary disease. With cavity formation, liquefied necrotic contents are ultimately discharged into the airways, resulting in satellite lesions within the lungs that may in turn undergo cavitation (Fig. 150-4). Massive involvement of pulmonary segments or lobes, with coalescence of lesions, produces tuberculous pneumonia. While up to one-third of untreated patients reportedly succumb to severe pulmonary tuberculosis within a few weeks or months after onset, others undergo a process of spontaneous remission or proceed along a chronic, progressively debilitating course ("consumption"). Under these circumstances, some pulmonary lesions become fibrotic and may later calcify, but cavities persist in other parts of the lungs. Individuals with such chronic disease continue to discharge tubercle bacilli into the environment. Most patients respond to treatment, with defervescence, decreasing cough, weight gain, and a general improvement in well-being within several weeks.

Early in the course of disease, symptoms and signs are often nonspecific and insidious, consisting mainly of fever and night sweats, weight loss, anorexia, general malaise, and weakness. However, in the majority of cases, cough eventually develops—often initially nonproductive and subsequently accompanied by the production of purulent sputum. Blood streaking of the sputum is frequently documented. Massive hemoptysis may ensue as a consequence of the erosion of a fully patent vessel located in the wall of a cavity. Hemoptysis, however, may also result from rupture of a dilated vessel in a cavity (*Rasmussen's aneurysm*) or from aspergilloma formation in an old cavity. Pleuritic chest pain sometimes develops in patients with subpleural parenchymal lesions but can also result from muscle strain due to persistent coughing. Extensive disease may produce dyspnea and (occasionally) adult respiratory distress syndrome (ARDS).

Physical findings are of limited use in pulmonary tuberculosis. Many patients have no abnormalities detectable by chest examination, while others have detectable rales in the involved areas during inspiration, especially after coughing. Occasionally, rhonchi due to partial bronchial obstruction and classic amphoric breath sounds in areas with

FIGURE 150-4 Chest radiograph showing bilateral upper-lobe infiltrates and cavities in a patient with active tuberculosis. (*Courtesy of L. Richeldi, G. Ferrera, and L. M. Fabbri, University of Modena and Reggio Emilia, Italy.*)

large cavities may be heard. Systemic features include fever (often low-grade and intermittent) and wasting. In some cases, pallor and finger clubbing develop. The most common hematologic findings are mild anemia and leukocytosis. Hyponatremia due to the syndrome of inappropriate secretion of antidiuretic hormone (SIADH) has also been reported.

Extrapulmonary Tuberculosis In order of frequency, the extrapulmonary sites most commonly involved in tuberculosis are the lymph nodes, pleura, genitourinary tract, bones and joints, meninges, peritoneum, and pericardium. However, virtually all organ systems may be affected. As a result of hematogenous dissemination in HIV-infected individuals, extrapulmonary tuberculosis is seen more commonly today than in the past.

LYMPH-NODE TUBERCULOSIS (TUBERCULOUS LYMPHADENITIS) The most common presentation of extrapulmonary tuberculosis (documented in >25% of cases), lymph-node disease is particularly frequent among HIV-infected patients. In the United States, children and women (particularly non-Caucasians) also seem to be especially susceptible. Once caused mainly by *M. bovis*, tuberculous lymphadenitis is today due largely to *M. tuberculosis*. Lymph-node tuberculosis presents as painless swelling of the lymph nodes, most commonly at cervical and supraclavicular sites (a condition often referred to as *scrofula*). Lymph nodes are usually discrete in early disease but may be inflamed and have a fistulous tract draining caseous material. Systemic symptoms are usually limited to HIV-infected patients, and concomitant lung disease may or may not be present. The diagnosis is established by fine-needle aspiration or surgical biopsy. AFB are seen in up to 50% of cases, cultures are positive in 70 to 80%, and histologic examination shows granulomatous lesions. Among HIV-infected patients, granulomas are usually not seen. Differential diagnosis includes a variety of infectious conditions as well as neoplastic diseases such as lymphomas or metastatic carcinomas.

PLEURAL TUBERCULOSIS Involvement of the pleura is common in primary tuberculosis and results from penetration by tubercle bacilli into the pleural space. Depending on the extent of reactivity, the effusion may be small, remain unnoticed, and resolve spontaneously or may be sufficiently large to cause symptoms such as fever, pleuritic chest pain, and dyspnea. Physical findings are those of pleural effusion: dullness to percussion and absence of breath sounds. A chest radiograph reveals the effusion and, in no more than one-third of cases, also shows a parenchymal lesion. Thoracentesis is required to ascertain the nature of the effusion. The fluid is straw colored and at times hemorrhagic; it is an exudate with a protein concentration >50% of that in serum, a normal to low glucose concentration, a pH that is generally <7.2, and detectable white blood cells (usually 500 to 2500/μL). Neutrophils may predominate in the early stage, while mononuclear cells are the typical finding later. Mesothelial cells are generally rare or absent. AFB are very rarely seen on direct smear, but cultures may be positive for *M. tuberculosis* in up to one-third of cases. Needle biopsy of the pleura is often required for diagnosis and reveals granulomas and/or yields a positive culture in up to 70% of cases. This form of pleural tuberculosis responds well to chemotherapy and may resolve spontaneously. The usefulness of glucocorticoids is debatable.

Tuberculous empyema is a less common complication of pulmonary tuberculosis. It is usually the result of the rupture of a cavity, with delivery of a large number of organisms into the pleural space, or of a bronchopleural fistula from a pulmonary lesion. A chest radiograph may show pyopneumothorax with an air-fluid level. The effusion is purulent and thick and contains large numbers of lymphocytes. An acid-fast smear of pleural fluid is often found to be positive when examined by microscopy, as is culture of the pleural fluid. Surgical drainage is usually required as an adjunct to chemotherapy. Tuberculous empyema may result in severe pleural fibrosis and restrictive lung disease.

TUBERCULOSIS OF THE UPPER AIRWAYS   Nearly always a complication of advanced cavitary pulmonary tuberculosis, tuberculosis of the upper airways may involve the larynx, pharynx, and epiglottis. Symptoms include hoarseness and dysphagia in addition to chronic productive cough. Findings depend on the site of involvement, and ulcerations may be seen on laryngoscopy. Acid-fast smear of the sputum is often positive, but biopsy may be necessary in some cases to establish the diagnosis. Cancer may have similar features but is usually painless.

GENITOURINARY TUBERCULOSIS   Genitourinary tuberculosis accounts for ~15% of all extrapulmonary cases, may involve any portion of the genitourinary tract, and is usually due to hematogenous seeding following primary infection. Local symptoms predominate. Urinary frequency, dysuria, hematuria, and flank pain are common presentations. However, patients may be asymptomatic and the disease discovered only after severe destructive lesions of the kidneys have developed. Urinalysis gives abnormal results in 90% of cases, revealing pyuria and hematuria. The documentation of culture-negative pyuria in acidic urine raises the suspicion of tuberculosis. An intravenous pyelogram helps in diagnosis. Calcifications and ureteral strictures are suggestive findings. Culture of three morning urine specimens yields a definitive diagnosis in nearly 90% of cases. Severe ureteral strictures may lead to hydronephrosis and renal damage.

Genital tuberculosis is diagnosed more commonly in female than in male patients. In female patients, it affects the fallopian tubes and the endometrium and may cause infertility, pelvic pain, and menstrual abnormalities. Diagnosis requires biopsy or culture of specimens obtained by dilatation and curettage. In male patients, tuberculosis preferentially affects the epididymis, producing a slightly tender mass that may drain externally through a fistulous tract; orchitis and prostatitis may also develop. In almost half of cases of genitourinary tuberculosis, urinary tract disease is also present. Genitourinary tuberculosis responds well to chemotherapy.

SKELETAL TUBERCULOSIS   In the United States, tuberculosis of the bones and joints is responsible for ~10% of extrapulmonary cases. In bone and joint disease, pathogenesis is related to reactivation of hematogenous foci or to spread from adjacent paravertebral lymph nodes. Weight-bearing joints (spine, hips, and knees—in that order) are affected most commonly. Spinal tuberculosis (Pott's disease or tuberculous spondylitis; Fig. 150-5) often involves two or more adjacent vertebral bodies. While the upper thoracic spine is the most common site of spinal tuberculosis in children, the lower thoracic and upper lumbar vertebrae are usually affected in adults. From the anterior superior or inferior angle of the vertebral body, the lesion reaches the adjacent body, also destroying the intervertebral disk. With advanced disease, collapse of vertebral bodies results in kyphosis (*gibbus*). A paravertebral "cold" abscess may also form. In the upper spine, this abscess may track to the chest wall as a mass; in the lower spine, it

FIGURE 150-5   Computed tomography scan demonstrating destruction of the right pedicle of T10 due to Pott's disease. The patient, a 70-year-old Asian woman, presented with back pain and weight loss and had biopsy-proven tuberculosis. (*Courtesy of Charles L. Daley, M.D., University of California, San Francisco.*)

may reach the inguinal ligaments or present as a psoas abscess. Computed tomography (CT) or magnetic resonance imaging (MRI) reveals the characteristic lesion and suggests its etiology, although the differential diagnosis includes other infections and tumors. Aspiration of the abscess or bone biopsy confirms the tuberculous etiology, as cultures are usually positive and histologic findings highly typical. A catastrophic complication of Pott's disease is paraplegia, which is usually due to an abscess or a lesion compressing the spinal cord. Paraparesis due to a large abscess is a medical emergency and requires abscess drainage. Tuberculosis of the hip joints causes pain and limping; tuberculosis of the knee produces pain and swelling and sometimes follows trauma. If the disease goes unrecognized, the joints may be destroyed. Skeletal tuberculosis responds to chemotherapy, but severe cases may require surgery.

TUBERCULOUS MENINGITIS AND TUBERCULOMA   Tuberculosis of the central nervous system accounts for ~5% of extrapulmonary cases. It is seen most often in young children but also develops in adults, especially those who are infected with HIV. Tuberculous meningitis results from the hematogenous spread of primary or postprimary pulmonary disease or from the rupture of a subependymal tubercle into the subarachnoid space. In more than half of cases, evidence of old pulmonary lesions or a miliary pattern is found on chest radiography. The disease may present subtly as headache and mental changes or acutely as confusion, lethargy, altered sensorium, and neck rigidity. Typically, the disease evolves over 1 or 2 weeks, a course longer than that of bacterial meningitis. Paresis of cranial nerves (ocular nerves in particular) is a frequent finding, and the involvement of cerebral arteries may produce focal ischemia. Hydrocephalus is common. Lumbar puncture is the cornerstone of diagnosis. In general, examination of the cerebrospinal fluid (CSF) reveals a high leukocyte count (usually with a predominance of lymphocytes but often with a predominance of neutrophils in the early stage), a protein content of 1 to 8 g/L (100 to 800 mg/dL), and a low glucose concentration; however, any of these three parameters can be within the normal range. AFB are seen on direct smear of CSF sediment in only 20% of cases, but repeated lumbar punctures increase the yield. Culture of CSF is diagnostic in up to 80% of cases. Imaging studies (CT and MRI) may show hydrocephalus and abnormal enhancement of basal cisterns or ependyma. If unrecognized, tuberculous meningitis is uniformly fatal. This disease responds to chemotherapy; however, neurologic sequelae are documented in 25% of treated cases, in most of which the diagnosis has been delayed. Clinical trials have demonstrated that patients treated with adjunctive glucocorticoids experience a significantly faster resolution of CSF abnormalities and elevated CSF pressure. Adjunctive glucocorticoids (e.g., dexamethasone, up to 12 mg/d for 4 to 6 weeks) enhance the chances of survival and reduce the frequency of neurologic sequelae.

Tuberculoma, an uncommon manifestation of tuberculosis, presents as one or more space-occupying lesions and usually causes seizures and focal signs. CT or MRI reveals contrast-enhanced ring lesions, but biopsy is necessary to establish the diagnosis.

GASTROINTESTINAL TUBERCULOSIS   Any portion of the gastrointestinal tract may be affected by tuberculosis. Various pathogenetic mechanisms are involved: swallowing of sputum with direct seeding, hematogenous spread, or (although rare today) ingestion of milk from cows affected by bovine tuberculosis. The terminal ileum and the cecum are the sites most commonly involved. Abdominal pain (at times similar to that associated with appendicitis), diarrhea, obstruction, hematochezia, and a palpable mass in the abdomen are common findings at presentation. Fever, weight loss, and night sweats are also frequent. With intestinal-wall involvement, ulcerations and fistulae may simulate Crohn's disease. Anal fistulae should prompt an evaluation for rectal tuberculosis. As surgery is required in most cases, the diagnosis can be established by histologic examination and culture of specimens obtained intraoperatively.

Tuberculous peritonitis follows either the direct spread of tubercle bacilli from ruptured lymph nodes and intraabdominal organs or hematogenous seeding. Nonspecific abdominal pain, fever, and ascites should raise the suspicion of tuberculous peritonitis. The coexistence of cirrhosis (Chap. 288) in patients with tuberculous peritonitis complicates the diagnosis. In tuberculous peritonitis, paracentesis reveals an exudative fluid with a high protein content and leukocytosis that is usually lymphocytic (although neutrophils occasionally predominate). The yield of direct smear and culture is relatively low; culture of a large volume of ascitic fluid can increase the yield, but peritoneal biopsy is often needed to establish the diagnosis.

PERICARDIAL TUBERCULOSIS (TUBERCULOUS PERICARDITIS) Due to direct progression of a primary focus within the pericardium, to reactivation of a latent focus, or to rupture of an adjacent lymph node, pericardial tuberculosis has often been a disease of the elderly in countries with low tuberculosis prevalence but also develops frequently in HIV-infected patients. Case-fatality rates are as high as 40% in some series. The onset may be subacute, although an acute presentation, with fever, dull retrosternal pain, and a friction rub, is possible. An effusion eventually develops in many cases; cardiovascular symptoms and signs of cardiac tamponade may ultimately appear (Chap. 222). In the presence of effusion detected on chest radiography, tuberculosis must be suspected if the patient belongs to a high-risk population (HIV-infected, originating in a high-prevalence country), if there is evidence of previous tuberculosis or disease in other organs, or if echocardiography shows thick strands crossing the pericardial space. Diagnosis can be facilitated by pericardiocentesis under echocardiographic guidance. The pericardial fluid must be submitted for biochemical, cytologic, and microbiologic study. The effusion is exudative in nature, with a high count of leukocytes (predominantly mononuclear cells). Hemorrhagic effusion is frequent. Culture of the fluid reveals *M. tuberculosis* in ~30% of cases, while biopsy has a higher yield. High levels of adenosine deaminase and IFN-γ may also suggest a tubercular etiology. Without treatment, pericardial tuberculosis is usually fatal. Even with treatment, complications may develop, including chronic constrictive pericarditis with thickening of the pericardium, fibrosis, and sometimes calcification, which may be visible on a chest radiograph. A course of glucocorticoid treatment (e.g., prednisone, 20 to 60 mg/d for up to 6 weeks) is useful in the management of acute disease, reducing effusion, facilitating hemodynamic recovery, and thus decreasing mortality. Progression to chronic constrictive pericarditis, however, seems unaffected by such therapy.

MILIARY OR DISSEMINATED TUBERCULOSIS Miliary tuberculosis is due to hematogenous spread of tubercle bacilli. Although in children it is often the consequence of a recent primary infection, in adults it may be due to either recent infection or reactivation of old disseminated foci. Lesions are usually yellowish granulomas 1 to 2 mm in diameter that resemble millet seeds (thus the term *miliary*, coined by nineteenth-century pathologists).

Clinical manifestations are nonspecific and protean, depending on the predominant site of involvement. Fever, night sweats, anorexia, weakness, and weight loss are presenting symptoms in the majority of cases. At times, patients have a cough and other respiratory symptoms due to pulmonary involvement as well as abdominal symptoms. Physical findings include hepatomegaly, splenomegaly, and lymphadenopathy. Eye examination may reveal choroidal tubercles, which are pathognomonic of miliary tuberculosis, in up to 30% of cases. Meningismus occurs in <10% of cases.

A high index of suspicion is required for the diagnosis of miliary tuberculosis. Frequently, chest radiography reveals a miliary reticulonodular pattern (more easily seen on underpenetrated film), although no radiographic abnormality may be evident early in the course and among HIV-infected patients. Other radiologic findings include large infiltrates, interstitial infiltrates (especially in HIV-infected patients), and pleural effusion. A sputum smear is negative in 80% of cases. Various hematologic abnormalities may be seen, including anemia with leukopenia, neutrophilic leukocytosis and leukemoid reactions, and polycythemia. Disseminated intravascular coagulation has been reported. Elevation of alkaline phosphatase levels and other abnormal values in liver function tests are detected in patients with severe hepatic involvement. The PPD test may be negative in up to half of cases, but reactivity may be restored during chemotherapy. Bronchoalveolar lavage and transbronchial biopsy are more likely to permit bacteriologic confirmation, and granulomas are evident in liver or bone-marrow biopsy specimens from many patients. If it goes unrecognized, miliary tuberculosis is lethal; with proper treatment, however, it is amenable to cure.

A rare presentation seen in the elderly is *cryptic miliary tuberculosis*, which has a chronic course characterized by mild intermittent fever, anemia, and—ultimately—meningeal involvement preceding death. An acute septicemic form, *nonreactive miliary tuberculosis*, occurs very rarely and is due to massive hematogenous dissemination of tubercle bacilli. Pancytopenia is common in this form of disease, which is rapidly fatal. At postmortem examination, multiple necrotic but nongranulomatous ("nonreactive") lesions are detected.

LESS COMMON EXTRAPULMONARY FORMS Tuberculosis may cause choriorctinitis, uveitis, panophthalmitis, and painful hypersensitivity-related phlyctenular conjunctivitis. Tuberculous otitis is rare and presents as hearing loss, otorrhea, and tympanic membrane perforation. In the nasopharynx, tuberculosis may simulate Wegener's granulomatosis. Cutaneous manifestations of tuberculosis include primary infection due to direct inoculation, abscesses and chronic ulcers, scrofuloderma, lupus vulgaris, miliary lesions, and erythema nodosum. Adrenal tuberculosis is a manifestation of advanced disease presenting as signs of adrenal insufficiency. Finally, congenital tuberculosis results from transplacental spread of tubercle bacilli to the fetus or from ingestion of contaminated amniotic fluid. This rare disease affects the liver, spleen, lymph nodes, and various other organs.

HIV-Associated Tuberculosis (See also Chap. 173) Tuberculosis is an important opportunistic disease among HIV-infected persons worldwide. In some African countries, the rate of HIV infection among tuberculosis patients may reach 70 to 80% in certain urban settings. A person with skin test–documented *M. tuberculosis* infection who acquires HIV infection has a 3 to 15% annual risk of developing active tuberculosis.

Tuberculosis can appear at any stage of HIV infection, and its presentation varies with the stage. When cell-mediated immunity is only partially compromised, pulmonary tuberculosis presents as a typical pattern (Fig. 150-4) of upper lobe infiltrates and cavitation, without significant lymphadenopathy or pleural effusion. In late stages of HIV infection, a primary tuberculosis–like pattern, with diffuse interstitial or miliary infiltrates, little or no cavitation, and intrathoracic lymphadenopathy, is more common. Overall, sputum smears may be positive less frequently among tuberculosis patients with HIV infection than among those without; thus the diagnosis of tuberculosis may be unusually difficult, especially in view of the variety of HIV-related pulmonary conditions mimicking tuberculosis.

Extrapulmonary tuberculosis is common among HIV-infected patients. In various series, extrapulmonary tuberculosis—alone or in association with pulmonary disease—has been documented in 40 to 60% of all cases in HIV co-infected individuals. The most common forms are lymphatic, disseminated, pleural, and pericardial. Mycobacteremia and meningitis are also frequent, particularly in advanced HIV disease.

The diagnosis of tuberculosis in HIV-infected patients may be difficult not only because of the increased frequency of sputum-smear negativity (up to 40% in culture-proven pulmonary cases) but also because of atypical radiographic findings, a lack of classic granuloma formation in the late stages, and negative results in PPD skin tests. Delays in treatment may prove fatal.

Recommendations for the prevention and treatment of tuberculosis in HIV-infected individuals are provided below.

DIAGNOSIS The key to the diagnosis of tuberculosis is a high index of suspicion. Diagnosis is not difficult with a high-risk patient—e.g., a homeless alcoholic who presents with typical symptoms and a classic chest radiograph showing upper lobe infiltrates with cavities (Fig.

150-4). On the other hand, the diagnosis can easily be missed in an elderly nursing-home resident or a teenager with a focal infiltrate.

Often, the diagnosis is first entertained when the chest radiograph of a patient being evaluated for respiratory symptoms is abnormal. If the patient has no complicating medical conditions that favor immunosuppression, the chest radiograph may show the typical picture of upper lobe infiltrates with cavitation (Fig. 150-4). The longer the delay between the onset of symptoms and the diagnosis, the more likely is the finding of cavitary disease. In contrast, immunosuppressed patients, including those with HIV infection, may have "atypical" findings on chest radiography—e.g., lower-zone infiltrates without cavity formation.

AFB Microscopy A presumptive diagnosis is commonly based on the finding of AFB on microscopic examination of a diagnostic specimen such as a smear of expectorated sputum or of tissue (for example, a lymph node biopsy). Most modern laboratories processing large numbers of diagnostic specimens use auramine-rhodamine staining and fluorescence microscopy. The more traditional method—light microscopy of specimens stained with Kinyoun or Ziehl-Neelsen basic fuchsin dyes—is satisfactory, although more time-consuming. For patients with suspected pulmonary tuberculosis, three sputum specimens, preferably collected early in the morning, should be submitted to the laboratory for AFB smear and mycobacteriology culture. If tissue is obtained, it is critical that the portion of the specimen intended for culture not be put in formaldehyde. The use of AFB microscopy on urine or gastric lavage fluid is limited by the presence of mycobacterial commensals, which can cause false-positive results.

Mycobacterial Culture Definitive diagnosis depends on the isolation and identification of *M. tuberculosis* from a diagnostic specimen—in most cases, a sputum specimen obtained from a patient with a productive cough. Specimens may be inoculated onto egg- or agar-based medium (e.g., Löwenstein-Jensen or Middlebrook 7H10) and incubated at 37°C under 5% CO_2. Because most species of mycobacteria, including *M. tuberculosis*, grow slowly, 4 to 8 weeks may be required before growth is detected. Although *M. tuberculosis* may be presumptively identified on the basis of growth time and colony pigmentation and morphology, a variety of biochemical tests have traditionally been used to speciate mycobacterial isolates. In today's laboratories, the use of liquid media for isolation and speciation by nucleic acid probes or high-pressure liquid chromatography of mycolic acids has replaced the traditional methods of isolation on solid media and identification by biochemical tests. These new methods have decreased the time required for bacteriologic confirmation to 2 to 3 weeks.

Nucleic Acid Amplification Several test systems based on amplification of mycobacterial nucleic acid are available. These systems permit the diagnosis of tuberculosis in as little as several hours. However, their applicability is limited by low sensitivity (lower than culture, but higher than AFB smear microscopy) and high cost. At present, these tests are most useful for the rapid confirmation of tuberculosis in persons with AFB-positive sputa. However, they may also have utility for the diagnosis of AFB-negative pulmonary and extrapulmonary tuberculosis in selected patients.

Drug Susceptibility Testing In general, the initial isolate of *M. tuberculosis* should be tested for susceptibility to isoniazid, rifampin, and ethambutol. In addition, expanded susceptibility testing is mandatory when resistance to one or more of these drugs is found or the patient either fails to respond to initial therapy or has a relapse after the completion of treatment (see below). Susceptibility testing may be conducted directly (with the clinical specimen) or indirectly (with mycobacterial cultures) on solid or liquid medium. Results are obtained most rapidly by direct susceptibility testing on liquid medium, with an average reporting time of 3 weeks. With indirect testing on solid medium, results may not be available for ≥8 weeks. Molecular methods for the rapid identification of drug resistance are becoming available. One of the most promising uses polymerase chain reaction (PCR) to detect mutations in the *rpoB* gene associated with resistance to rifampin.

Radiographic Procedures As noted above, the initial suspicion of pulmonary tuberculosis is often based on abnormal chest radiographic findings in a patient with respiratory symptoms. Although the "classic" picture is that of upper lobe disease with infiltrates and cavities (Fig. 150-4), virtually any radiographic pattern—from a normal film or a solitary pulmonary nodule to diffuse alveolar infiltrates in a patient with ARDS—may be seen. In the era of AIDS, no radiographic pattern can be considered pathognomonic.

PPD Skin Testing and Diagnosis of Latent Tuberculosis Infection In 1891, Robert Koch discovered components of *M. tuberculosis* in a concentrated liquid culture medium. Subsequently named "old tuberculin" (OT), this material was initially believed to be useful in the treatment of tuberculosis (although this idea was later disproved). It soon became clear that OT was capable of eliciting a skin reaction when injected subcutaneously into patients with tuberculosis. In 1932, Seibert and Munday purified this product by ammonium sulfate precipitation. The result was an active protein fraction known as *tuberculin PPD*. However, the complexity and diversity of the constituents of PPD rendered its standardization difficult. PPD-S, developed by Seibert and Glenn in 1941, was chosen as the international standard. Later, the WHO and UNICEF sponsored large-scale production of a master batch of PPD, termed *RT23*, and made it available for general use. The greatest limitation of PPD is its lack of mycobacterial species specificity, a property that is due to the large number of proteins in this product that are highly conserved in the various species of mycobacteria.

Skin testing with PPD is most widely used in screening for *M. tuberculosis* infection (see below). The test is of limited value in the diagnosis of active tuberculosis because of its low sensitivity and specificity. False-negative reactions are common in immunosuppressed patients and in those with overwhelming tuberculosis. Positive reactions are obtained when patients have been infected with *M. tuberculosis* but do not have active disease and when persons have been sensitized by nontuberculous mycobacteria (Chap. 152) or bacille Calmette-Guérin (BCG) vaccination. Although BCG vaccine is not used in the United States for tuberculosis prevention, many immigrants will have received it. In the absence of a history of BCG vaccination, a positive skin test may provide additional support for the diagnosis of tuberculosis in culture-negative cases.

Because results of anergy testing in HIV-infected populations do not seem useful to clinicians making decisions about preventive therapy, anergy testing based on other DTH antigens is no longer recommended as a routine component of tuberculosis screening among HIV-infected persons. However, some experts support the use of anergy testing to help guide individual decisions regarding preventive therapy, and some recommend that PPD skin testing be performed for patients previously classified as anergic if evidence indicates that these patients' immune systems have responded to therapy with antiretroviral drugs.

Cytokine Release Assays A commercially available whole-blood cytokine assay, the QuantiFERON-TB test (Cellestis Ltd), has been approved by the U.S. Food and Drug Administration (FDA) as an aid in the diagnosis of latent tuberculosis infection. The test requires overnight incubation of a peripheral-blood sample with PPD and control antigens followed by measurement of IFN-γ released by sensitized lymphocytes in an enzyme-linked immunosorbent assay (ELISA). A multicenter study conducted by the CDC indicated good agreement between this assay and the PPD skin test, although the assay's ability to predict the development of active tuberculosis is not known. At present, the QuantiFERON-TB test is recommended for screening for latent tuberculosis infection in populations at low to moderate risk of tuberculosis. Studies are under way to assess the performance of this test in contact investigations, persons with suspected tuberculosis disease, HIV-infected persons, and children. The test's performance will probably be enhanced by the use of antigens such as ESAT-6 and CPF-

10 that are present in *M. tuberculosis* but absent from BCG strains and most nontuberculous mycobacteria.

Additional Diagnostic Procedures Other diagnostic tests may be used when pulmonary tuberculosis is suspected. Sputum induction by ultrasonic nebulization of hypertonic saline may be useful for patients unable to produce a sputum specimen spontaneously. Frequently, patients with radiographic abnormalities that are consistent with other diagnoses (e.g., bronchogenic carcinoma) undergo fiberoptic bronchoscopy with bronchial brushings or transbronchial biopsy of the lesion. Bronchoalveolar lavage of a lung segment containing an abnormality may also be performed. In all cases, it is essential that specimens be submitted for AFB smear and mycobacterial culture. For the diagnosis of primary pulmonary tuberculosis in children, who often do not expectorate sputum, specimens from early-morning gastric lavage may yield positive cultures.

Invasive diagnostic procedures are indicated for patients with suspected extrapulmonary tuberculosis. In addition to specimens of involved sites (e.g., CSF for tuberculous meningitis, pleural fluid and biopsy samples for pleural disease), bone marrow and liver biopsy and culture have a good diagnostic yield in disseminated (miliary) tuberculosis, particularly in HIV-infected patients, who also have a high frequency of positive blood cultures.

In some cases, cultures will be negative, but a clinical diagnosis of tuberculosis will be supported by consistent epidemiologic evidence (e.g., a history of close contact with an infectious patient), a positive PPD skin test, and a compatible clinical and radiographic response to treatment. In the United States and other industrialized countries with low rates of tuberculosis, some patients with limited abnormalities on chest radiographs and sputum positive for AFB are infected with organisms of the *M. avium* complex or *M. kansasii* (Chap. 152). Factors favoring the diagnosis of nontuberculous mycobacterial disease over tuberculosis include an absence of risk factors for tuberculosis, a negative PPD skin test, and underlying chronic obstructive pulmonary disease.

Patients with HIV-associated tuberculosis pose several diagnostic problems, as noted above in the description of clinical manifestations. Moreover, HIV-infected patients with sputum culture–positive and AFB-positive tuberculosis may present with a normal chest radiograph. With the advent of highly active antiretroviral therapy (HAART), the occurrence of disseminated *M. avium* complex disease that can be confused with tuberculosis has become much less common.

Adjunctive Diagnostic Tests A number of methods have been evaluated as adjuncts to standard laboratory diagnosis. The most thoroughly investigated is serologic diagnosis based on detection of antibody to a variety of mycobacterial antigens. However, tests with most of the target antigens have a low predictive value when used in a population with a low probability of disease. Tests aimed at detection of mycobacterial antigen by serologic methods have generally been insufficiently sensitive to be useful.

℞ TREATMENT

The two aims of tuberculosis treatment are to interrupt tuberculosis transmission by rendering patients noninfectious and to prevent morbidity and mortality by curing patients with tuberculosis disease. Chemotherapy for tuberculosis became possible with the discovery of streptomycin in the mid-1940s. Randomized clinical trials clearly indicated that the administration of streptomycin to patients with chronic tuberculosis reduced mortality and led to cure in the majority of cases. However, monotherapy with streptomycin was frequently associated with the development of resistance to this drug and the attendant failure of treatment. With the discovery of para-aminosalicylic acid (PAS) and isoniazid, it became axiomatic that cure of tuberculosis required the concomitant administration of at least two agents to which the organism was susceptible. Furthermore, early clinical trials demonstrated that a long period of treatment—i.e., 12 to 24 months—was required to prevent the recurrence of tuberculosis.

The introduction of rifampin in the early 1970s heralded the era of effective short-course chemotherapy, with a treatment duration of <12 months. The discovery that pyrazinamide, which was first used in the 1950s, augmented the potency of isoniazid/rifampin regimens led to the use of a 6-month course of this triple-drug regimen as standard therapy.

DRUGS Four major drugs are considered the first-line agents for the treatment of tuberculosis: isoniazid, rifampin, pyrazinamide, and ethambutol (Table 150-2). These drugs are well absorbed after oral administration, with peak serum levels at 2 to 4 h and nearly complete elimination within 24 h. These agents are recommended on the basis of their bactericidal activity (ability to rapidly reduce the number of viable organisms and render patients noninfectious), their sterilizing activity (ability to kill all bacilli and thus sterilize the affected organ, measured in terms of the ability to prevent relapses), and their low rate of induction of drug resistance. Rifapentine and rifabutin, two drugs related to rifampin, are also available in the United States and are useful for selected patients. →*For a detailed discussion of the drugs used for the treatment of tuberculosis, see Chap. 149.*

Because of a lower degree of efficacy and a higher degree of intolerability and toxicity, a number of second-line drugs are generally used only for the treatment of patients with tuberculosis resistant to first-line drugs. Included in this group are the injectable drugs streptomycin (formerly a first-line agent), kanamycin, amikacin, and capreomycin and the oral agents ethionamide, cycloserine, and PAS. Recently, fluoroquinolone antibiotics have become the most commonly used second-line drugs. Of available agents, ofloxacin is the most widely used, but levofloxacin, gatifloxacin, and moxifloxacin are the most active. Other drugs of doubtful efficacy that have been used in the treatment of patients with resistance to most of the first- and second-line agents include clofazimine, amithiozone (thiacetazone, still used in less wealthy countries but not marketed in North America or Europe), amoxicillin/clavulanic acid, and linezolid.

REGIMENS Short-course regimens are divided into an initial, or bactericidal, phase and a continuation, or sterilizing, phase. During the initial phase, the majority of the tubercle bacilli are killed, symptoms resolve, and the patient becomes noninfectious. The continuation phase is required to eliminate persisting mycobacteria and prevent relapse.

The treatment regimen of choice for virtually all forms of tuberculosis in both adults and children consists of a 2-month initial phase of isoniazid, rifampin, pyrazinamide, and ethambutol followed by a 4-month continuation phase of isoniazid and rifampin (Table 150-3). Treatment may be given daily throughout the course or intermittently (either three times weekly throughout the course or twice weekly following an initial phase of daily therapy). A continuation phase of once-weekly rifapentine and isoniazid is equally effective for HIV-

TABLE 150-2 *Recommended Dosage for Initial Treatment of Tuberculosis in Adults*[a]

Drug	Dosage	
	Daily Dose	Thrice-Weekly Dose[b]
Isoniazid	5 mg/kg, max 300 mg	15 mg/kg, max 900 mg
Rifampin	10 mg/kg, max 600 mg	10 mg/kg, max 600 mg
Pyrazinamide	20–25 mg/kg, max 2 g	30–40 mg/kg, max 3 g
Ethambutol[c]	15–20 mg/kg	25–30 mg/kg

[a] Dosages for children are similar, except that some authorities recommend higher doses of isoniazid (10–15 mg/kg daily; 20–30 mg/kg intermittent) and rifampin (10–20 mg/kg).
[b] Dosages for twice-weekly administration are the same for isoniazid and rifampin but are higher for pyrazinamide (50 mg/kg, with a maximum of 4 g/d) and ethambutol (40–50 mg/d).
[c] In certain settings, streptomycin (15 mg/kg daily, with a maximum dose of 1 g; or 25–30 mg/kg thrice weekly, with a maximum dose of 1.5 g) can replace ethambutol in the initial phase of treatment. However, streptomycin is no longer considered a first-line drug by the ATS, the IDSA, or the CDC.
Source: Based on American Thoracic Society, Infectious Diseases Society of America, and Centers for Disease Control and Prevention.

TABLE 150-3 *Recommended Antituberculosis Treatment Regimens*

	Initial Phase		Continuation Phase	
Indication	Duration, Months	Drugs	Duration, Months	Drugs
New smear- or culture-positive cases	2	HRZE[a,b]	4	HR[a,c,d]
New culture-negative cases	2	HRZE[a]	2	HR[a]
Pregnancy	2	HRE[e]	7	HR
Failure and relapse[f]	—	—	—	—
Resistance (or intolerance) to H	Throughout (6)	RZE[g]		
Resistance to H + R	Throughout (18–24)	ZEQ + S (or another injectable agent[h])		
Resistance to all first-line drugs	Throughout (24)	1 injectable agent[h] + 3 of these 4: ethionamide, cycloserine, Q, PAS		
Standardized re-treatment (susceptibility testing unavailable)	3	HRZES[i]	5	HRE
Drug intolerance to R	Throughout (12)[j]	HZE		
Drug intolerance to Z	2	HRE	7	HR

[a] All drugs can be given daily or intermittently (three times weekly throughout or twice weekly after 2 to 8 weeks of daily therapy during the initial phase).

[b] Streptomycin can be used in place of ethambutol but is no longer considered to be a first-line drug by ATS/IDSA/CDC.

[c] The continuation phase should be extended to 7 months for patients with cavitary pulmonary tuberculosis who remain sputum culture–positive after the initial phase of treatment.

[d] HIV-negative patients with noncavitary pulmonary tuberculosis who have negative sputum AFB smears after the initial phase of treatment can be given once-weekly rifapentine/isoniazid in the continuation phase.

[e] The 6-month regimen with pyrazinamide can probably be used safely during pregnancy and is recommended by the WHO and the International Union Against Tuberculosis and Lung Disease. If pyrazinamide is not included in the initial treatment regimen, the minimum duration of therapy is 9 months.

[f] Regimen is tailored according to the results of drug susceptibility tests.

[g] A fluoroquinolone (Q) may strengthen the regimen for patients with extensive disease.

[h] Amikacin, kanamycin, or capreomycin. All these agents should be discontinued after 2 to 6 months, depending upon tolerance and response.

[i] Streptomycin should be discontinued after 2 months. This regimen is less effective for patients in whom treatment has failed, who have an increased probability of rifampin-resistant disease. In such cases, the re-treatment regimen might include second-line drugs chosen in light of the likely pattern of drug resistance.

[j] Streptomycin for the initial 2 months or a fluoroquinolone might strengthen the regimen for patients with extensive disease.

Note: H, isoniazid; R, rifampin; Z, pyrazinamide; E, ethambutol; S, streptomycin; Q, a quinolone antibiotic; PAS, para-aminosalicylic acid.

seronegative patients with noncavitary pulmonary tuberculosis who have negative sputum cultures at 2 months. Intermittent treatment is especially useful for patients whose therapy is being directly observed (see below). Patients with cavitary pulmonary tuberculosis and delayed sputum-culture conversion (i.e., those who remain culture-positive at 2 months) should have their treatment extended by 3 months, for a total course of 9 months. For patients with sputum culture–negative pulmonary tuberculosis, the duration of treatment may be reduced to a total of 4 months. To prevent isoniazid-related neuropathy, pyridoxine (10 to 25 mg/d) should be added to the regimen given to persons at high risk of vitamin B6 deficiency (e.g., alcoholics; malnourished persons; pregnant and lactating women; and patients with conditions such as chronic renal failure, diabetes, and HIV infection or AIDS, which are also associated with neuropathy). A full course of therapy (completion of treatment) is defined more accurately by the total number of doses taken than by the length of treatment. Specific recommendations on the required numbers of doses for each of the various treatment regimens have been published jointly by the American Thoracic Society (ATS), the Infectious Diseases Society of America (IDSA), and the CDC.

Lack of adherence to treatment is recognized worldwide as the most important impediment to cure. Moreover, the tubercle bacilli infecting patients who do not adhere to the prescribed regimen are likely to become drug resistant. Both patient- and provider-related factors may affect compliance. Patient-related factors include a lack of belief that the illness is significant and/or that treatment will have a beneficial effect; the existence of concomitant medical conditions (notably substance abuse); lack of social support; and poverty, with attendant joblessness and homelessness. Provider-related factors that may promote compliance include the education and encouragement of patients, the offering of convenient clinic hours, and the provision of incentives and enablers such as meals and bus tokens.

In addition to specific measures addressing noncompliance, two other strategic approaches are used: direct observation of treatment and provision of fixed-drug-combination (FDC) products. Because it is difficult to predict which patients will adhere to the recommended treatment, all patients should have their therapy directly supervised, especially during the initial phase. In the United States, personnel to supervise therapy are usually available through tuberculosis control programs of local public health departments. Supervision increases the proportion of patients completing treatment and greatly lessens the chances of relapse and acquired drug resistance. FDC products (e.g., isoniazid/rifampin, isoniazid/rifampin/pyrazinamide, and isoniazid/rifampin/pyrazinamide/ethambutol) are available (except, in the United States, for the four-drug FDC) and strongly recommended as a means of minimizing the likelihood of prescription error and of the development of drug resistance as the result of monotherapy. In some formulations of these combination products, the bioavailability of rifampin has been found to be substandard. In North America and Europe, regulatory authorities ensure that combination products are of good quality; however, this type of quality assurance cannot be assumed to take place in less affluent countries. Alternative regimens for patients who exhibit drug intolerance or adverse reactions are listed in Table 150-3. However, severe side effects prompting discontinuation of any of the first-line drugs and use of these alternative regimens are uncommon.

MONITORING TREATMENT RESPONSE AND DRUG TOXICITY Bacteriologic evaluation is the preferred method of monitoring the response to treatment for tuberculosis. Patients with pulmonary disease should have their sputum examined monthly until cultures become negative. With the recommended regimen, >80% of patients will have negative sputum cultures at the end of the second month of treatment. By the end of the third month, virtually all patients should be culture-negative. In some patients, especially those with extensive cavitary disease and large numbers of organisms, AFB smear conversion may follow culture conversion. This phenomenon is presumably due to the expectoration and microscopic visualization of dead bacilli. As noted above, patients with cavitary disease who do not achieve sputum culture conversion by 2 months require extended treatment. When a patient's sputum cultures remain positive at ≥3 months, treatment failure and drug resistance should be suspected (see below). A sputum specimen should be collected by the end of treatment to document cure. If mycobacterial cultures are not practical, then monitoring by AFB smear examination should be undertaken at 2, 5, and 6 months. Smears positive after 5 months are indicative of treatment failure.

Bacteriologic monitoring of patients with extrapulmonary tuberculosis is more difficult and often is not feasible. In these cases, the response to treatment must be assessed clinically.

Monitoring of the response to treatment during chemotherapy by serial chest radiographs is not recommended, as radiographic changes may lag behind bacteriologic response and are not highly sensitive. After the completion of treatment, neither sputum examination nor chest radiography is recommended for follow-up purposes. However, a chest radiograph may be obtained at the end of treatment and used for comparative purposes should the patient develop symptoms of recurrent tuberculosis months or years later. Patients should be instructed to report promptly for medical assessment should they develop any such symptoms.

During treatment, patients should be monitored for drug toxicity (Table 149-3). The most common adverse reaction of significance is hepatitis. Patients should be carefully educated about the signs and symptoms of drug-induced hepatitis (e.g., dark urine, loss of appetite) and should be instructed to discontinue treatment promptly and see their health care provider should these symptoms occur. Although biochemical monitoring is not routinely recommended, all adult patients should undergo baseline assessment of liver function (e.g., measurement of serum levels of hepatic aminotransferases and serum bilirubin). Older patients, those with concomitant diseases, those with a history of hepatic disease, and those using alcohol daily should be monitored especially closely (i.e., monthly), with repeated measurements of aminotransferases, during the initial phase of treatment. Up to 20% of patients have small increases in aspartate aminotransferase (up to three times the upper limit of normal) that are accompanied by no symptoms and are of no consequence. For patients with symptomatic hepatitis and those with marked (five- to sixfold) elevations in serum levels of aspartate aminotransferase, treatment should be stopped and drugs reintroduced one at a time after liver function has returned to normal.

Hypersensitivity reactions usually require the discontinuation of all drugs and rechallenge to determine which agent is the culprit. Because of the variety of regimens available, it is usually not necessary—although it is possible—to desensitize patients. Hyperuricemia and arthralgia caused by pyrazinamide can usually be managed by the administration of acetylsalicylic acid; however, pyrazinamide treatment should be stopped if the patient develops gouty arthritis. Individuals who develop autoimmune thrombocytopenia secondary to rifampin therapy should not receive the drug thereafter. Similarly, the occurrence of optic neuritis with ethambutol is an indication for permanent discontinuation of this drug. Other common manifestations of drug intolerance, such as pruritus and gastrointestinal upset, can generally be managed without the interruption of therapy.

TREATMENT FAILURE AND RELAPSE As stated above, treatment failure should be suspected when a patient's sputum cultures remain positive after 3 months or when AFB smears remain positive after 5 months. In the management of such patients, it is imperative that the current isolate be tested for susceptibility to first- and second-line agents. When the results of susceptibility testing are expected to become available within a few weeks, changes in the regimen can be postponed until that time. However, if the patient's clinical condition is deteriorating, an earlier change in regimen may be indicated. A cardinal rule in the latter situation is always to add more than one drug at a time to a failing regimen: at least two and preferably three drugs that have never been used and to which the bacilli are likely to be susceptible should be added. The patient may continue to take isoniazid and rifampin along with these new agents pending the results of susceptibility tests.

The mycobacterial strains infecting patients who experience a relapse after apparently successful treatment are less likely to have acquired drug resistance (see below) than are strains from patients in whom treatment has failed. However, if the regimen administered initially does not contain rifampin (and thus is not a short-course regimen), the probability of isoniazid resistance is high. Acquired resistance is uncommon among strains from patients who relapse after completing a short-course regimen. However, it is prudent to begin the treatment of all relapses with all five first-line drugs pending the results of susceptibility testing. In less affluent countries and other settings where facilities for culture and drug susceptibility testing are not available, a standard regimen should be used in all instances of relapse and treatment failure (Table 150-3).

HIV-ASSOCIATED TUBERCULOSIS In general, the standard treatment regimens are equally efficacious in HIV-negative and HIV-positive patients. However, adverse drug effects may be more pronounced in HIV-infected patients. Since these effects may include serious or even fatal skin reactions to amithiozone (thiacetazone), this drug, which has been used in place of ethambutol in developing countries, is no longer recommended by WHO.

There are three important considerations relevant to tuberculosis treatment in HIV-infected patients: an increased frequency of paradoxical reactions, drug interactions between HAART and rifamycins, and development of rifampin monoresistance with widely spaced intermittent treatment. Exacerbations in symptoms, signs, and laboratory or radiographic manifestations of tuberculosis—termed *paradoxical reactions*—have been associated with the administration of HAART regimens. The presumed pathogenesis of paradoxical reactions is an immune response to antigens released as bacilli are killed by effective chemotherapy. In patients in whom HAART has recently been started, paradoxical reactions may be due to improving immune function. The first priority in the management of a possible paradoxical reaction is to ensure that the clinical syndrome does not represent a failure of tuberculosis treatment or the development of another infection. Mild paradoxical reactions can be managed with symptom-based treatment. Glucocorticoids have been used for more severe reactions, although this practice has not been formally evaluated in clinical trials.

Most HIV-infected tuberculosis patients are candidates for HAART, although the optimal timing for antiretroviral treatment is not known. Rifampin, a potent inducer of enzymes of the cytochrome P450 system, lowers serum levels of many HIV protease inhibitors and some nonnucleoside reverse transcriptase inhibitors, essential drugs used in HAART regimens. In such cases, rifabutin, which has much less enzyme-inducing activity, has been recommended in place of rifampin. However, dose adjustments for rifabutin and/or the antiretroviral drugs may be necessary. Because recommendations are frequently updated, consultation of the CDC website is advised (www.cdc.gov/nchstp/tb).

Several clinical trials of HIV-associated tuberculosis have found that patients with advanced immunosuppression (CD4+ cell counts of <100) are prone to treatment failure and relapse with rifampin-resistant organisms when treated with "highly intermittent" (i.e., once- or twice-weekly) rifamycin-containing regimens. Consequently, it is recommended that these patients receive daily or thrice-weekly therapy for the entire course.

DRUG-RESISTANT TUBERCULOSIS Strains of *M. tuberculosis* resistant to individual drugs arise by spontaneous point mutations in the mycobacterial genome, which occur at low but predictable rates. Because there is no cross-resistance among the commonly used drugs, the probability that a strain will be resistant to two drugs is the product of the probabilities of resistance to each drug and thus is low. The development of drug-resistant tuberculosis is invariably the result of monotherapy—i.e., the failure of the health care provider to prescribe at least two drugs to which tubercle bacilli are susceptible or of the patient to take properly prescribed therapy.

Drug-resistant tuberculosis may be either primary or acquired. Primary drug resistance is that in a strain infecting a patient who has not previously been treated. Acquired resistance develops during treatment with an inappropriate regimen. In North America and Europe, rates of primary resistance are generally low, and isoniazid resistance is most common. In the United States, while primary isoniazid resistance was stable at about 7 to 8% between 1993 and 2002, the rate of primary multidrug-resistant (MDR) tuberculosis declined from 2.5% to 1%. Resistance rates are higher among foreign-born and HIV-infected patients. Worldwide, MDR tuberculosis is a serious problem in some regions, especially in the former Soviet Union and parts of Asia. As noted above, drug-resistant tuberculosis can be prevented by adherence to the principles of sound therapy: the inclusion of at least two bactericidal drugs to which the organism is susceptible and the verification that patients complete the prescribed course.

Although the 6-month regimen described in Table 150-3 is generally effective for patients with initial isoniazid-resistant disease, it is prudent to include ethambutol and pyrazinamide for the full 6 months. In such cases, isoniazid probably does not contribute to a successful outcome and should be omitted. MDR tuberculosis is more difficult to manage than is disease caused by a drug-susceptible organism, especially because resistance to other first-line drugs as well as to isoniazid and rifampin is common. For strains resistant to isoniazid and rifampin, combinations of a fluoroquinolone, ethambutol, pyrazinamide, and streptomycin (or, for those resistant to streptomycin as well, another injectable agent such as amikacin), given for 18 to 24 months and for at least 9 months after sputum culture conversion, may be effective. For patients with bacilli resistant to all of the first-line agents, cure may be attained with a combination of four second-line drugs, including one injectable agent (Table 150-3). The optimal duration of treatment in this situation is not known; however, a duration of 24 months is recommended. For patients with localized disease and sufficient pulmonary reserve, lobectomy or pneumonectomy may be helpful. Because the management of patients with MDR tuberculosis is complicated by both social and medical factors, care of these patients should be restricted to specialists and tuberculosis control programs.

SPECIAL CLINICAL SITUATIONS   Although comparative clinical trials of treatment for extrapulmonary tuberculosis are limited, the available evidence indicates that most forms of disease can be treated with the 6-month regimen recommended for patients with pulmonary disease. The American Academy of Pediatrics recommends that children with bone and joint tuberculosis, tuberculous meningitis, or miliary tuberculosis receive 9 to 12 months of treatment.

Treatment for tuberculosis may be complicated by underlying medical problems that require special consideration (Table 149-1). As a rule, patients with chronic renal failure should not receive aminoglycosides and should receive ethambutol only if serum levels can be monitored. Isoniazid, rifampin, and pyrazinamide may be given in the usual doses in cases of mild to moderate renal failure, but the dosages of isoniazid and pyrazinamide should be reduced for all patients with severe renal failure except those undergoing hemodialysis. Patients with hepatic disease pose a special problem because of the hepatotoxicity of isoniazid, rifampin, and pyrazinamide. Patients with severe hepatic disease may be treated with ethambutol and streptomycin and, if required, with isoniazid and rifampin under close supervision. The use of pyrazinamide by patients with liver failure should be avoided. Silicotuberculosis necessitates the extension of therapy by at least 2 months. The regimen of choice for pregnant women (Tables 149-1 and 150-3) is 9 months of treatment with isoniazid and rifampin supplemented by ethambutol for the first 2 months. When required, pyrazinamide may be given, although there are no data concerning its safety in pregnancy. Streptomycin is contraindicated because it is known to cause eighth-cranial-nerve damage in the fetus. Treatment for tuberculosis is not a contraindication to breast feeding; most of the drugs administered will be present in small quantities in breast milk, albeit at concentrations far too low to provide any therapeutic or prophylactic benefit to the child.

PREVENTION   By far the best way to prevent tuberculosis is to diagnose infectious cases rapidly and administer appropriate treatment until cure. Additional strategies include BCG vaccination and treatment of persons with latent tuberculosis infection who are at high risk of developing active disease.

BCG Vaccination   BCG was derived from an attenuated strain of *M. bovis* and was first administered to humans in 1921. Many BCG vaccines are available worldwide; all are derived from the original strain, but the vaccines vary in efficacy. In fact, estimates of efficacy from randomized, placebo-controlled trials have ranged from 80% to nil. A similar range of efficacy was found in recent observational studies (case-control, historic cohort, and cross-sectional) in areas where infants are vaccinated at birth. These studies also found higher rates of efficacy in the protection of infants and young children from relatively serious forms of tuberculosis, such as tuberculous meningitis and miliary tuberculosis.

BCG vaccine is safe and rarely causes serious complications. The local tissue response begins 2 to 3 weeks after vaccination, with scar formation and healing within 3 months. Side effects—most commonly, ulceration at the vaccination site and regional lymphadenitis—occur in 1 to 10% of vaccinated persons. Some vaccine strains have caused osteomyelitis in ~1 case per million doses administered. Disseminated BCG infection and death have occurred in 1 to 10 cases per 10 million doses administered, although this problem is restricted almost exclusively to persons with impaired immunity, such as children with severe combined immunodeficiency syndrome or adults with HIV infection. BCG vaccination induces PPD reactivity, which tends to wane with time. The presence or size of PPD skin-test reactions after vaccination does not predict the degree of protection afforded.

BCG vaccine is recommended for routine use at birth in countries with high tuberculosis prevalence. However, because of the low risk of transmission of tuberculosis in the United States and the unreliable protection afforded by BCG, the vaccine has never been recommended for general use in the United States. The CDC has recommended that HIV-infected adults and children not receive BCG vaccine, although the WHO has recommended that asymptomatic HIV-infected children residing in tuberculosis-endemic areas receive BCG.

Treatment of Latent Tuberculosis Infection   A major component of tuberculosis control in the United States is the treatment of selected persons with latent tuberculosis infection to prevent active disease. This intervention (formerly called preventive chemotherapy or chemoprophylaxis) is based on the results of a large number of randomized, placebo-controlled clinical trials demonstrating that a 6- to 12-month course of isoniazid reduces the risk of active tuberculosis in infected people by ≥90%. Analysis of available data indicates that the optimal duration of treatment is 9 to 10 months. In the absence of reinfection, the protective effect is believed to be lifelong. Clinical trials have also shown that isoniazid reduces rates of tuberculosis among PPD-positive persons with HIV infection. Studies in HIV-infected patients have demonstrated the effectiveness of shorter courses of rifampin-based treatment.

In most cases, candidates for treatment of latent tuberculosis (Table 150-4) are identified by PPD skin testing of persons in defined high-risk groups. For skin testing, 5 tuberculin units of polysorbate-stabilized PPD should be injected intradermally into the volar surface of the forearm (Mantoux method). Multipuncture tests, which may be useful for screening large populations, are not recommended for this purpose; any positive reaction to a multipuncture test must be confirmed by Mantoux testing. Reactions are read at 48 to 72 h as the transverse diameter in millimeters of induration; the diameter of erythema is not considered. In some persons, PPD reactivity wanes with time but can be recalled by a second skin test administered ≥1 week after the first (i.e., two-step testing). For persons undergoing periodic

TABLE 150-4   *Tuberculin Reaction Size, Treatment of Latent Tuberculosis Infection*

Risk Group	Tuberculin Reaction Size, mm
HIV-infected persons or persons receiving immunosuppressive therapy	≥5
Close contacts of tuberculosis patients	≥5[a]
Persons with fibrotic lesions on chest radiography	≥5
Recently infected persons (≤2 years)	≥10
Persons with high-risk medical conditions[b]	≥10
Low-risk persons[c]	≥15

[a] Tuberculin-negative contacts, especially children, should receive prophylaxis for 2 to 3 months after contact ends and should then be retested with PPD. Those whose results remain negative should discontinue prophylaxis. HIV-infected contacts should receive a full course of treatment regardless of PPD results.

[b] Includes diabetes mellitus, some hematologic and reticuloendothelial diseases, injection drug use (with HIV seronegativity), end-stage renal disease, and clinical situations associated with rapid weight loss.

[c] Decision to treat should be based on individual risk/benefit considerations.

PPD skin testing, such as health care workers and individuals admitted to long-term-care institutions, initial two-step testing may preclude subsequent misclassification of persons with boosted reactions as PPD converters.

The cutoff for a positive skin test (and thus for treatment) is related both to the probability that the reaction represents true infection and to the likelihood that the individual, if truly infected, will develop tuberculosis (Table 150-4). Thus positive reactions for close contacts of infectious cases, persons with HIV infection, persons receiving drugs that suppress the immune system, and previously untreated persons whose chest radiograph is consistent with healed tuberculosis are defined as an area of induration ≥5 mm in diameter. A 10-mm cutoff is used to define positive reactions in most other at-risk persons. For persons with a very low risk of developing tuberculosis if infected, a cutoff of 15 mm is used. Treatment should be considered for persons from tuberculosis-endemic countries who have a history of BCG vaccination.

Some PPD-negative individuals are also candidates for treatment. Infants and children who have come into contact with infectious cases should be treated and should have a repeat skin test 2 or 3 months after contact ends. Those whose test results remain negative should discontinue treatment. HIV-infected persons who have been exposed to an infectious tuberculosis patient should receive treatment regardless of the PPD test result.

Isoniazid is administered at a daily dose of 5 mg/kg (up to 300 mg/d) for 9 months (Table 150-5). On the basis of cost-benefit analyses, a 6-month period of treatment has been recommended in the past and may be considered for HIV-negative adults with normal chest radiographs when financial considerations are important. When supervised treatment is desirable and feasible, isoniazid may be given at a dose of 15 mg/kg (up to 900 mg) twice weekly. An alternative regimen for adults is 4 months of daily rifampin. A previously recommended regimen of 2 months of rifampin and pyrazinamide has been associated with serious and fatal hepatotoxicity and is now generally not recommended for use. The rifampin regimen should be considered for persons who are likely to have been infected with an isoniazid-resistant strain.

Isoniazid should not be given to persons with active liver disease. All persons at increased risk of hepatotoxicity (e.g., those abusing alcohol daily and those with a history of liver disease) should undergo baseline and then monthly assessment of liver function. All patients should be carefully educated about hepatitis and instructed to discontinue use of the drug immediately should any symptoms develop. Moreover, patients should be seen and questioned monthly during therapy about adverse reactions and should be given no more than 1 month's supply of drug at each visit.

It may be more difficult to ensure compliance when treating persons with latent infection than when treating those with active tuberculosis. If family members of active cases are being treated, compliance and monitoring may be easier. When feasible, twice-weekly supervised therapy may increase the likelihood of completion. As in active cases, the provision of incentives may also be helpful.

BASICS OF CONTROL The highest priority in any tuberculosis control program is the prompt detection of cases and the provision of short-course chemotherapy to all tuberculosis patients under proper case-management conditions, including directly observed therapy, with emphasis on the cure of sputum smear–positive cases. In addition, in low-prevalence countries with adequate resources, screening of high-risk groups (such as immigrants from high-prevalence countries and HIV-seropositive persons) is recommended. Identification of active cases of tuberculosis should be followed by treatment. PPD-positive high-risk persons should be treated for latent infection. Contact investigation is an important component of efficient tuberculosis control. In the United States, a great deal of attention has been given to the transmission of tuberculosis (particularly in association with HIV infection) in institutional settings such as hospitals, homeless shelters, and prisons. Measures to limit such transmission include respiratory isolation of persons with suspected tuberculosis until they are proven to be noninfectious (i.e., by sputum AFB smear negativity), proper ventilation in rooms of patients with infectious tuberculosis, use of ultraviolet lights in areas of increased risk of tuberculosis transmission, and

TABLE 150-5 *Revised Drug Regimens for Treatment of Latent Tuberculosis Infection (LTBI) in Adults*

Drug	Interval and Duration	Comments[a]	Rating[b] (Evidence[c]) HIV-Negative	Rating[b] (Evidence[c]) HIV-Infected
Isoniazid	Daily for 9 months[d,e]	In HIV-infected persons, isoniazid may be administered concurrently with nucleoside reverse transcriptase inhibitors, protease inhibitors, or nonnucleoside reverse transcriptase inhibitors (NNRTIs).	A (II)	A (II)
	Twice weekly for 9 months[d,e]	Directly observed therapy (DOT) must be used with twice-weekly dosing.	B (II)	B (II)
	Daily for 6 months[e]	Regimen is not indicated for HIV-infected persons, those with fibrotic lesions on chest radiographs, or children.	B (I)	C (I)
	Twice weekly for 6 months[e]	DOT must be used with twice-weekly dosing.	B (II)	C (I)
Rifampin[f]	Daily for 4 months	Regimen is used for contacts of patients with isoniazid-resistant, rifampin-susceptible tuberculosis. In HIV-infected persons, most protease inhibitors and delavirdine should not be administered concurrently with rifampin. Rifabutin, with appropriate dose adjustments, can be used with protease inhibitors (saquinavir should be augmented with ritonavir) and NNRTIs (except delavirdine). Clinicians should consult web-based updates for the latest specific recommendations.	B (II)	B (III)
Rifampin plus pyrazinamide (RZ)	Daily for 2 months	Regimen generally should not be offered for treatment of LTBI in either HIV-infected or HIV-negative persons.	D (II)	D (II)
	Twice weekly for 2–3 months		D (III)	D (III)

[a] Interactions with HIV-related drugs are updated frequently and are available at http://www.aidsinfo.nih.gov/guidelines.
[b] Strength of the recommendation: A. Both strong evidence of efficacy and substantial clinical benefit support recommendation for use. Should always be offered. B. Moderate evidence for efficacy or strong evidence for efficacy, but only limited clinical benefit, supports recommendation for use. Should generally be offered. C. Evidence for efficacy is insufficient to support a recommendation for or against use, or evidence for efficacy might not outweigh adverse consequences (e.g., drug toxicity, drug interactions) or cost of the treatment or alternative approaches. Optional. D. Moderate evidence for lack of efficacy or for adverse outcome supports a recommendation against use. Should generally not be offered. E. Good evidence for lack of efficacy or for adverse outcome supports a recommendation against use. Should never be offered.
[c] Quality of evidence supporting the recommendation: I. Evidence from at least one properly randomized controlled trial. II. Evidence from at least one well-designed clinical trial without randomization, from cohort or case-controlled analytic studies (preferably from more than one center), from multiple time-series studies, or from dramatic results in uncontrolled experiments. III. Evidence from opinions of respected authorities based on clinical experience, descriptive studies, or reports of expert committees.
[d] Recommended regimen for persons aged <18 years.
[e] Recommended regimen for pregnant women.
[f] The substitution of rifapentine for rifampin is not recommended because rifapentine's safety and effectiveness have not been established for patients with LTBI.
Source: Adapted from CDC: Targeted tuberculin testing and treatment of latent tuberculosis infection. MMWR 49(RR-6), 2000

periodic screening of personnel who may come into contact with known or unsuspected cases of tuberculosis. In the past, radiographic surveys, especially those conducted with portable equipment and miniature films, were advocated for case finding. Today, however, the prevalence of tuberculosis in industrialized countries is sufficiently low that "mass miniature radiography" is not cost-effective.

In high-prevalence countries, tuberculosis control programs should be based on the following key elements defining the DOTS strategy promoted by the WHO: (1) political commitment by the government to sustained tuberculosis control; (2) case detection through microscopic examination of sputum from patients who present to health care facilities with cough of >2 to 3 weeks' duration; (3) administration of standard short-course chemotherapy to all sputum smear–positive patients under proper case-management conditions, including direct observation of drug ingestion; (4) establishment and maintenance of a system of regular drug supply; and (5) establishment and maintenance of an effective surveillance and monitoring system that allows assessment of treatment outcomes (e.g., cure, completion of treatment without bacteriologic proof of cure, death, treatment failure, and default) in all cases registered and notified.

FURTHER READING

AMERICAN THORACIC SOCIETY, CENTERS FOR DISEASE CONTROL AND PREVENTION: Targeted tuberculin testing and treatment of latent tuberculosis infection. Am J Respir Crit Care Med 161:S221, 2000

———, INFECTIOUS DISEASES SOCIETY OF AMERICA, CENTERS FOR DISEASE CONTROL AND PREVENTION: Treatment of tuberculosis. Am J Respir Crit Care Med 167:603, 2003

BURMAN WG, JONES BE: Treatment of HIV associated tuberculosis in the era of effective antiretroviral therapy. Am J Respir Crit Care Med 164:7, 2002

CEGIELSKI JP et al: The global tuberculosis situation: Progress and problems in the 20th century, prospects for the 21st century. Infect Dis Clin North Am 16:1, 2002

CORBETT EL et al: The growing burden of tuberculosis: Global trends and interaction with the HIV epidemic. Arch Intern Med 163:1009, 2003

TUBERCULOSIS TRIALS CONSORTIUM: Rifapentine and isoniazid once a week versus rifampicin and isoniazid twice a week for treatment of drug-susceptible pulmonary tuberculosis in HIV-negative patients: A randomized clinical trial. Lancet 360:528, 2002

WORLD HEALTH ORGANIZATION: *Treatment of Tuberculosis*. Guidelines for National Programmes. Geneva, World Health Organization, 2003

YOUNG DB: Ten years of research progress and what's to come. Tuberculosis 83:77, 2003

151 LEPROSY (HANSEN'S DISEASE)
Robert H. Gelber

Leprosy, first described in ancient Indian texts from the sixth century B.C., is a nonfatal, chronic infectious disease caused by *Mycobacterium leprae*, whose clinical manifestations are largely confined to the skin, peripheral nervous system, upper respiratory tract, eyes, and testes. The unique tropism of *M. leprae* for peripheral nerves (from large nerve trunks to microscopic dermal nerves) and certain immunologically mediated reactional states are the major causes of morbidity in leprosy. The propensity of the disease, when untreated, to result in characteristic deformities and the recognition in most cultures that the disease is communicable from person to person have resulted historically in a profound social stigma. Today, with early diagnosis and the institution of appropriate and effective antimicrobial therapy, patients can lead productive lives in the community, and deformities and other visible manifestations can largely be prevented.

ETIOLOGY *M. leprae* is an obligate intracellular bacillus (0.3 to 1 μm wide and 1 to 8 μm long) that is acid-fast, indistinguishable microscopically from other mycobacteria, and ideally detected in tissue sections by a modified Fite stain. Strain variability was recently discovered in this organism. *M. leprae* produces no known toxins and is well adapted to penetrate and reside within macrophages, yet it may survive outside the body for months. In untreated patients, only ~1% of *M. leprae* organisms are viable. The morphologic index (MI), a measure of the number of acid-fast bacilli (AFB) in skin scrapings that stain uniformly bright, correlates with viability. The bacteriologic index (BI), a logarithmic-scaled measure of the density of *M. leprae* in the dermis, may be as high as 4+ to 6+ in untreated patients, falling by one unit per year during effective therapy; the rate of fall is independent of the relative potency of effective antimicrobial therapy. A rising MI or BI suggests relapse and perhaps—if the patient is being treated—drug resistance; the latter possibility can be confirmed or excluded in the mouse model.

As a result of reductive evolution, almost half of the *M. leprae* genome contains nonfunctional genes; only 1605 genes encode for proteins. In contrast, *M. tuberculosis* uses 91% of its genome to encode for 4000 proteins. Among the lost genes in *M. leprae* are those for catabolic and respiratory pathways; transport systems; purine, methionine, and glutamine synthesis; and nitrogen regulation. The genome of *M. leprae* provides a metabolic rationale for its obligate intracellular existence and reliance on host biochemical support, a template for targets of drug development, and ultimately a pathway to cultivation. The recent finding of strain variability among *M. leprae* isolates provides a powerful tool with which to address anew the organism's epidemiology and pathobiology. The bacterium's complex cell wall has a peptidoglycan backbone, which is linked to arabinogalactan and mycolic acids. Lipoarabinomannan is a key component of the cell membrane, and the outer capsule contains large amounts of an *M. leprae*–specific phenolic glycolipid (PGL-1), which is detected in serologic tests.

Among the mycobacteria, *M. leprae* is unique in exhibiting dopa oxidase activity and an acid-fastness that is pyridine-extractable. Although it was the first bacterium to be etiologically associated with human disease, *M. leprae* remains one of the few bacterial species that still has not been cultivated on artificial medium or tissue culture. The multiplication of *M. leprae* in mouse footpads (albeit limited, with a doubling time of ~2 weeks) has provided a means to evaluate antimicrobial agents, monitor clinical trials, and screen vaccines. *M. leprae* grows best in cooler tissues (the skin, peripheral nerves, anterior chamber of the eye, upper respiratory tract, and testes), sparing warmer areas of the skin (the axilla, groin, scalp, and midline of the back).

EPIDEMIOLOGY ■ Demographics Leprosy is almost exclusively a disease of the developing world, affecting areas of Asia, Africa, Latin America, and the Pacific. While Africa has the highest disease prevalence, Asia has the most cases. More than 80% of the world's cases occur in a few countries: India, China, Myanmar, Indonesia, Brazil, Nigeria, Madagascar, and Nepal. Within endemic locales, the distribution of leprosy is quite uneven, with areas of high prevalence bordering on areas with little or no disease. In Brazil the majority of cases occur in the Amazon basin and two western states, while in Mexico leprosy is mostly confined to the Pacific coast. Except as imported cases, leprosy is largely absent from the United States, Canada, and northwestern Europe. In the United States, ~4000 persons have leprosy and 100 to 200 new cases are reported annually, most of them in California, Texas, New York, and Hawaii among immigrants from Mexico, Southeast Asia, the Philippines, and the Caribbean.

The global prevalence of leprosy is difficult to assess, given that many of the locales with high prevalence lack a significant medical or public health infrastructure. Estimates range from 0.6 to 8 million affected individuals. The lower estimate includes only persons who have not completed chemotherapy, excluding those who may be physically or psychologically damaged from leprosy and who may yet relapse or develop immune-mediated reactions; the higher figure includes patients whose infections probably are already cured and many who have no leprosy-related deformity or disability. Although the figures on the worldwide prevalence of leprosy are debatable, it is generally agreed that the annual incidence of new cases is rising (529,000 estimated new cases in 1995 and 719,000 in 2001, with 60% of the latter number from India alone).

Leprosy is associated with poverty and rural residence. It appears not to be associated with AIDS, perhaps because of leprosy's long incubation period. Most people appear to be naturally immune to leprosy and do not develop disease manifestations following exposure. The time of peak onset is in the second and third decades of life. The most severe polar form of leprosy is twice as common among men as among women and is rarely encountered in children. The frequency of the polar forms of leprosy in different countries varies widely and may in part be genetically determined; certain HLA associations are known for both polar forms of leprosy (see below). In India and Africa, 90% of cases are tuberculoid; in Southeast Asia, 50% are tuberculoid and 50% lepromatous; and in Mexico, 90% are lepromatous. (For definitions of disease types, see Table 151-1 and "Clinical, Histologic, and Immunologic Spectrum," below).

Transmission The route of transmission of leprosy remains uncertain and may be multiple; nasal droplet infection, contact with infected soil, and even insect vectors have been considered the prime candidates. Aerosolized *M. leprae* can cause infection in immunosuppressed mice, and a sneeze from an untreated lepromatous patient may contain $>10^{10}$ AFB. Furthermore, both IgA antibody to *M. leprae* and genes of *M. leprae*—demonstrable by polymerase chain reaction (PCR)—have been found in the nose of individuals without signs of leprosy from endemic areas and in 19% of occupational contacts of lepromatous patients.

Several lines of evidence implicate soil transmission of leprosy: (1) in endemic countries such as India, leprosy is primarily a rural and not an urban disease; (2) *M. leprae* products have been demonstrated to be resident in soil in endemic locales; and (3) direct dermal inoculation (e.g., during tattooing) may transmit *M. leprae*, and common sites of leprosy in children are the buttocks and thighs, suggesting that microinoculation of infected soil may transmit the disease.

Evidence for insect vectors of leprosy includes the demonstration that bedbugs and mosquitoes in the vicinity of leprosaria regularly harbor *M. leprae* and that experimentally infected mosquitoes can transmit infection to mice. Skin-to-skin contact is generally not considered an important route of transmission.

In endemic countries, ~50% of leprosy patients have a history of intimate contact with an infected person (often a household member), while, for unknown reasons, leprosy patients in nonendemic locales can identify such contact only 10% of the time. Moreover, household contact with an infected lepromatous case carries an eventual risk of disease acquisition of ~10% in endemic areas as opposed to only 1% in nonendemic locales. Contact with a tuberculoid case carries a very low risk. Physicians and nurses caring for leprosy patients and the co-workers of these patients are not at risk for leprosy.

M. leprae causes disease primarily in humans. However, in Texas and Louisiana, 15% of nine-banded armadillos are infected, and armadillo contact occasionally results in human disease; armadillos develop a disseminated infection following intravenous inoculation of live *M. leprae*.

CLINICAL, HISTOLOGIC, AND IMMUNOLOGIC SPECTRUM The incubation period prior to manifestation of clinical disease can vary between 2 and 40 years, although it is generally 5 to 7 years in duration. Leprosy presents as a spectrum of clinical manifestations that have bacteriologic, pathologic, and immunologic counterparts. The spectrum from polar tuberculoid (TT) to borderline tuberculoid (BT) to mid-borderline (BB, which is rarely encountered) to borderline lepromatous (BL) to polar lepromatous (LL) disease is associated with an evolution from asymmetric localized macules and plaques to nodular and indurated symmetric generalized skin manifestations, an increasing bacterial

TABLE 151-1 *Clinical, Bacteriologic, Pathologic, and Immunologic Spectrum of Leprosy*

Clinical and Histologic Features	Tuberculoid (TT) Leprosy	Borderline Tuberculoid (BT) Leprosy	Mid-Borderline (BB) Leprosy	Borderline Lepromatous (BL) Leprosy	Lepromatous (LL) Leprosy
Skin Lesions	Up to 3 in number; sharply defined asymmetric macules or plaques with tendency toward central clearing, elevated borders	Smaller or larger than in TT; potentially more numerous than in TT; usually annular lesions with sharp margination on exterior and interior borders; borders not as elevated as in TT	Dimorphic lesions intermediate between BT and BL	LL-type lesions; ill-defined plaques with an occasional sharp margin; few or many in number, shiny appearance	Symmetric, poorly marginated, multiple infiltrated nodules and plaques or diffuse infiltration; xanthoma-like or dermatofibroma papules; leonine facies and eyebrow alopecia
Nerve lesions	Skin lesions anesthetic early; nerve near lesions sometimes enlarged	Skin lesions anesthetic early; nerve trunk palsies asymmetric; nerve abscesses most common in BT	Anesthetic skin lesions; nerve trunk palsies	Skin lesions usually hypoesthetic, may be anesthetic; nerve trunk palsies common and frequently symmetric	Hypesthesia a late sign; nerve palsies variable; acral, distal, symmetric anesthesia common
Acid-fast bacilli (BI)	3	0–1+	3–4+	4–5+	4–6+
Lymphocytes	3+	2+	1+	1+	0–1+
Macrophage differentiation	Epithelioid	Epithelioid	Epithelioid	Usually undifferentiated; epithelioid foci sometimes present; may show foamy change	Foamy change the rule; may be undifferentiated in early lesions
Langhans' giant cells	1–3+	2+	—	—	—
Lepromin skin test	+++	+++	—	—	—
Lymphocyte transformation test	95%	40%	10%	1–2%	1–2%
CD4+/CD8+ T-cell ratio in lesions	1.35	1.11	NT	0.48	0.50
M. leprae PGL-1 antibodies	1+ (60%+)	2+	2+	3+	3+ (95%+)

Abbreviations: BI, bacteriologic index; PGL-1, phenolic glycolipid 1.

load, and loss of *M. leprae*–specific cellular immunity (Table 151-1). Distinguishing dermatopathologic characteristics include the number of lymphocytes, giant cells, and AFB as well as the nature of epithelioid cell differentiation. Where a patient presents on the clinical spectrum largely determines prognosis, complications, reactional states, and the intensity of antimicrobial therapy required.

Tuberculoid Leprosy   At the less severe end of the spectrum is tuberculoid leprosy, which encompasses TT and BT disease. In general, these forms of leprosy result in symptoms confined to the skin and peripheral nerves. The skin lesions of tuberculoid leprosy consist of one or a few hypopigmented macules or plaques that are sharply demarcated and hypesthetic, often have erythematous or raised borders, and are devoid of the normal skin organs (sweat glands and hair follicles) and thus are dry, scaly, and anhidrotic. AFB are generally absent or few in number. Tuberculoid leprosy patients may have asymmetric enlargement of one or a few peripheral nerves. Indeed, leprosy and certain rare hereditary neuropathies are the only human diseases associated with peripheral-nerve enlargement. Although any peripheral nerve may be enlarged (including small digital and supraclavicular nerves), those most commonly affected are the ulnar, posterior auricular, peroneal, and posterior tibial nerves, with associated hypesthesia and myopathy. TT leprosy is the most common form of the disease encountered in India and Africa but is virtually absent in Southeast Asia, where BT leprosy is frequent.

In tuberculoid leprosy, T cells breach the perineurium, and destruction of Schwann cells and axons may be evident, resulting in fibrosis of the epineurium, replacement of the endoneurium with epithelial granulomas, and occasionally caseous necrosis. Such invasion and destruction of nerves in the dermis by T cells are pathognomonic for leprosy.

Circulating lymphocytes from patients with tuberculoid leprosy readily recognize *M. leprae* and its constituent proteins, and patients have positive lepromin skin tests (see "Diagnosis," below). In tuberculoid leprosy tissue, there is a 2:1 predominance of helper CD4+ over CD8+ T lymphocytes. Tuberculoid tissues are rich in the mRNAs of the proinflammatory T_H1 family of cytokines: interleukin (IL) 2, interferon γ (IFN-γ), and IL-12; in contrast, IL-4, IL-5, and IL-10 mRNAs are scarce.

Lepromatous Leprosy   Lepromatous leprosy patients present with symmetrically distributed skin nodules, raised plaques, or diffuse dermal infiltration, which, when on the face, results in leonine facies. Late manifestations include loss of eyebrows (initially the lateral margins only; Fig. 151-1) and eyelashes, pendulous earlobes, and dry scaling skin, particularly on the feet. In LL leprosy, bacilli are numerous in the skin (as many as 10^9/g), where they are often found in large clumps (*globi*), and in peripheral nerves, where they initially invade Schwann cells, resulting in foamy degenerative myelination and axonal degeneration and later in Wallerian degeneration. In addition, bacilli are plentiful in circulating blood and in all organ systems except the lungs and the central nervous system. Nevertheless, patients are afebrile, and there is no evidence of major organ system dysfunction. Almost exclusively found in western Mexico and the Caribbean is a form of lepromatous leprosy without visible skin lesions but with diffuse dermal infiltration and a demonstrably thickened dermis, termed *diffuse lepromatosis*. In lepromatous leprosy, nerve enlargement and damage tend to be symmetric, result from actual bacillary invasion, and are more insidious but ultimately more extensive than in tuberculoid leprosy. Patients with LL leprosy have acral, distal, symmetric peripheral neuropathy and a tendency toward symmetric nerve-trunk enlargement. They may also have signs and symptoms related to involvement of the upper respiratory tract, the anterior chamber of the eye, and the testes.

In untreated LL patients, lymphocytes regularly fail to recognize either *M. leprae* or its protein constituents, and lepromin skin tests are negative (see "Diagnosis," below). This loss of protective cellular im-

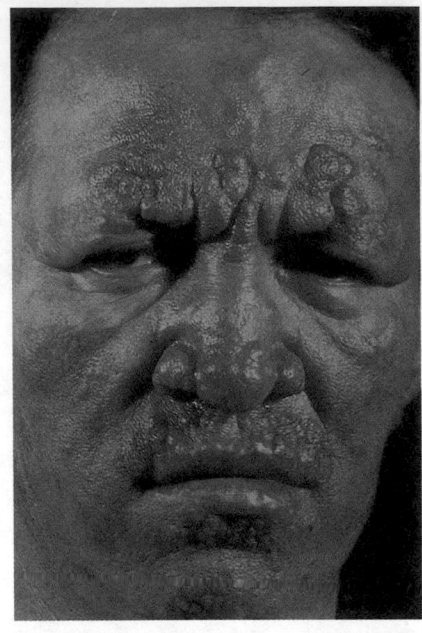

FIGURE 151-1 A patient with features of polar lepromatous leprosy: multiple nodular skin lesions, particularly of the forehead, and loss of eyebrows.

munity appears to be antigen-specific, as patients are not unusually susceptible to opportunistic infections, cancer, or AIDS and maintain delayed-type hypersensitivity to *Candida*, *Trichophyton*, mumps, tetanus toxoid, and even purified protein derivative of tuberculin. At times, *M. leprae*–specific anergy is reversible with effective chemotherapy. In LL tissues, there is a 2:1 ratio of CD8+ to CD4+ T lymphocytes. LL tissues demonstrate a T_H2 cytokine profile, being rich in mRNAs for IL-4, IL-5, and IL-10 and poor in those for IL-2, IFN-γ, and IL-12. It appears that cytokines mediate a protective tissue response in leprosy, as injection of IFN-γ or IL-2 into lepromatous lesions causes a loss of AFB and histopathologic conversion toward a tuberculoid pattern. Macrophages of lepromatous leprosy patients appear to be functionally intact; circulating monocytes exhibit normal microbicidal function and responsiveness to IFN-γ.

Reactional States   Lepra reactions comprise several common immunologically mediated inflammatory states that cause considerable morbidity. Some of these reactions precede diagnosis and the institution of effective antimicrobial therapy. Indeed, these reactions may precipitate presentation for medical attention and diagnosis; others occur after the initiation of appropriate chemotherapy. In the latter circumstances, patients often lose confidence in conventional therapy, perceiving that their leprosy is worsening. Only by warning patients of the potential for these reactions and describing their manifestations can physicians treating leprosy patients ensure continued credibility.

TYPE 1 LEPRA REACTIONS (DOWNGRADING AND REVERSAL REACTIONS)   These reactions occur in almost half of patients with borderline forms of leprosy but not in patients with polar disease. Manifestations include classic signs of inflammation within previously involved macules, papules, and plaques and, on occasion, the appearance of new skin lesions, neuritis, and (less commonly) fever—generally low-grade. The nerve trunk most commonly involved in this process is the ulnar nerve at the elbow, which may be painful and exquisitely tender. If patients with affected nerves are not treated promptly with glucocorticoids (see below), irreversible nerve damage may result in as little as 24 h. The most dramatic manifestation is footdrop, which occurs when the peroneal nerve is involved.

When type 1 lepra reactions precede the initiation of appropriate antimicrobial therapy, they are termed *downgrading reactions*, and the case becomes histologically more lepromatous; when they occur after the initiation of therapy, they are termed *reversal reactions*, and the case becomes more tuberculoid. Reversal reactions often occur in the first months or years after the initiation of therapy but may also develop several years thereafter.

Edema is the most characteristic microscopic feature of type 1 lepra lesions, whose diagnosis is primarily clinical. Reversal reactions are typified by a T_H1 cytokine profile, with an influx of CD4+ helper cells and increased levels of IFN-γ and IL-2. In addition, type 1 reactions are associated with large numbers of T cells bearing γ/∂ receptors—a unique feature of leprosy.

TYPE 2 LEPRA REACTIONS (ERYTHEMA NODOSUM LEPROTICUM, ENL) ENL occurs exclusively in patients near the lepromatous end of the leprosy spectrum (BL-LL), affecting nearly 50% of this group. Although ENL may precede leprosy diagnosis and initiation of therapy—sometimes, in fact, prompting the diagnosis—in 90% of cases it follows the institution of chemotherapy, generally within 2 years. The most common features of ENL are crops of painful erythematous papules that resolve spontaneously in a few days to a week but may recur; malaise; and fever that can be profound. However, patients may also experience symptoms of neuritis, lymphadenitis, uveitis, orchitis, and glomerulonephritis and may develop anemia, leukocytosis, and abnormal liver function tests, particularly increased aminotransferase levels. Individual patients may have either a single bout of ENL or chronic recurrent manifestations. Bouts may be either mild or severe and generalized; in rare instances, ENL results in death.

Skin biopsy of ENL papules reveals vasculitis or panniculitis, sometimes with many lymphocytes but characteristically with polymorphonuclear leukocytes as well.

Elevated levels of circulating tumor necrosis factor (TNF) have been demonstrated in ENL; thus, TNF may play a central role in the pathobiology of this syndrome. ENL is thought to be a consequence of immune complex deposition, given its T_H2 cytokine profile and its high levels of IL-6 and IL-8. However, in ENL tissue, the presence of HLA Dr framework antigen of epidermal cells—considered a marker for a delayed-type hypersensitivity response—and evidence for higher levels of IL-2 and IFN-γ than are usually seen in polar lepromatous disease suggest an alternative mechanism.

LUCIO'S PHENOMENON This unusual reaction is seen exclusively in patients from the Caribbean and Mexico who have the diffuse lepromatosis form of lepromatous leprosy, most often those who are untreated. Patients with this reaction develop recurrent crops of large, sharply marginated, ulcerative lesions—particularly on the lower extremities—that may be generalized and, when so, are frequently fatal as a result of secondary infection and consequent septic bacteremia. Histologically, the lesions are characterized by ischemic necrosis of the epidermis and superficial dermis, heavy parasitism of endothelial cells with AFB, and endothelial proliferation and thrombus formation in the larger vessels of the deeper dermis. Like ENL, the Lucio phenomenon is probably mediated by the immune complex.

Complications ■ *THE EXTREMITIES* Complications of the extremities in leprosy patients are primarily a consequence of neuropathy leading to insensitivity and myopathy. Insensitivity affects fine touch, pain, and heat receptors but generally spares position and vibration appreciation. The most commonly affected nerve trunk is the ulnar nerve at the elbow, whose involvement results in clawing of the fourth and fifth fingers, loss of dorsal interosseous musculature in the affected hand, and loss of sensation in these distributions. Median nerve involvement in leprosy impairs thumb opposition and grasp, while radial nerve dysfunction, though rare in leprosy, leads to wristdrop. Tendon transfers can restore hand function but should not be performed until 6 months after the initiation of antimicrobial therapy and the conclusion of episodes of acute neuritis.

Plantar ulceration, particularly at the metatarsal heads, is probably the most frequent complication of leprous neuropathy. Therapy requires careful debridement; administration of appropriate antibiotics; avoidance of weight-bearing until ulcerations are healed, with slowly progressive ambulation thereafter; and wearing of specialized shoes to prevent recurrence.

Footdrop as a result of peroneal nerve palsy should be treated with a simple nonmetallic brace within the shoe or surgical correction attained by tendon transfers. Although uncommon, Charcot's joints, particularly of the foot and ankle, may result from leprosy.

The loss of distal digits in leprosy is a consequence of insensitivity, trauma, secondary infection, and—in lepromatous patients—a poorly understood and sometimes profound osteolytic process. Conscientious protection of the extremities during cooking and work and the early institution of therapy have substantially reduced the frequency and severity of distal digit loss in recent times.

THE NOSE In lepromatous leprosy, bacillary invasion of the nasal mucosa can result in chronic nasal congestion and epistaxis. Saline nose drops may relieve these symptoms. Long-untreated LL leprosy may further result in destruction of the nasal cartilage, with consequent saddle-nose deformity or anosmia (more common in the preantibiotic era than at present). Nasal reconstructive procedures can ameliorate significant cosmetic defects.

THE EYE Owing to cranial nerve palsies, lagophthalmus and corneal insensitivity may complicate leprosy, resulting in trauma, secondary infection, and (without treatment) corneal ulcerations and opacities. For patients with these conditions, eyedrops during the day and ointments at night provide some protection from such consequences. Furthermore, in LL leprosy, the anterior chamber of the eye is invaded by bacilli, and ENL may result in uveitis, with consequent cataracts and glaucoma. Thus leprosy is a major cause of blindness in the developing world. Slit-lamp evaluation of LL patients often reveals "corneal beading," representing globi of *M. leprae*.

THE TESTES *M. leprae* invades the testes, while ENL may cause orchitis. Thus males with lepromatous leprosy often manifest mild to severe testicular dysfunction, with an elevation of luteinizing and follicle-stimulating hormones, decreased testosterone, and aspermia or hypospermia in 85% of LL patients but in only 25% of BL patients. LL patients may become impotent and infertile. Impotence is sometimes responsive to testosterone replacement.

AMYLOIDOSIS Secondary amyloidosis is a complication of LL leprosy and ENL that is encountered infrequently in the antibiotic era. This complication may result in abnormalities of hepatic and particularly renal function.

NERVE ABSCESSES Patients with various forms of leprosy, but particularly those with the BT form, may develop abscesses of nerves (most commonly the ulnar) with an adjacent cellulitic appearance of the skin. In such conditions, the affected nerve is swollen and exquisitely tender. Although glucocorticoids may reduce signs of inflammation, rapid surgical decompression is necessary to prevent irreversible sequelae.

DIAGNOSIS Leprosy most commonly presents with both characteristic skin lesions and skin histopathology. Thus the disease should be suspected when a patient from an endemic area has suggestive skin lesions or peripheral neuropathy; the diagnosis should be confirmed by histopathology. In tuberculoid leprosy, lesional areas—preferably the advancing edge—must be biopsied because normal-appearing skin does not have pathologic features. In lepromatous leprosy, nodules, plaques, and indurated areas are optimal biopsy sites, but biopsies of normal-appearing skin are also generally diagnostic. Lepromatous leprosy is associated with diffuse hyperglobulinemia, which may result in false-positive serologic tests (e.g., VDRL, RA, ANA) and therefore may cause diagnostic confusion. On occasion, tuberculoid lesions may not (1) appear typical, (2) be hypesthetic, and (3) contain granulomas but only nonspecific lymphocytic infiltrates. In such instances, two of these three characteristics are considered sufficient for a diagnosis. It is preferable to overdiagnose leprosy rather than to allow a patient to remain untreated.

IgM antibodies to PGL-1 are found in 95% of untreated lepromatous leprosy patients; the titer decreases with effective therapy. However, in tuberculoid leprosy—the form of disease most often associated with diagnostic uncertainty owing to the absence or paucity of AFB—patients have significant antibodies to PGL-1 only 60% of the time; moreover, in endemic locales, exposed individuals without clinical leprosy may harbor antibodies to PGL-1. Thus PGL-1 serology is of little diagnostic utility in tuberculoid leprosy. Heat-killed *M. leprae* (lepromin) has been used as a skin test reagent. It generally elicits a reaction in tuberculoid leprosy patients, may do so in individuals without leprosy, and gives negative results in lepromatous leprosy patients; consequently, it is likewise of little diagnostic value. Unfortunately, PCR of the skin for *M. leprae*, although positive in LL and BL leprosy, yields negative results in 50% of tuberculoid leprosy cases, again offering little diagnostic assistance.

Included in the differential diagnosis of lesions that resemble leprosy are sarcoidosis, leishmaniasis, lupus vulgaris, lymphoma, syphilis, yaws, granuloma annulare, and various other disorders causing hypopigmentation. Sarcoidosis may result in perineural inflammation, but actual granuloma formation within dermal nerves is pathognomonic for leprosy. In lepromatous leprosy, sputum specimens may be loaded with AFB—a finding that can be inappropriately interpreted as representing pulmonary tuberculosis.

℞ TREATMENT

Antimicrobial Therapy ▪ *ACTIVE AGENTS*   Established agents used to treat leprosy include dapsone (50 to 100 mg/d), clofazimine (50 to 100 mg/d, 100 mg three times weekly, or 300 mg monthly), and rifampin (600 mg daily or monthly). Of these drugs, only rifampin is bactericidal. The sulfones (folate antagonists), the foremost of which is dapsone, were the first antimicrobials found to be effective for the treatment of leprosy and are still the mainstay of therapy. With sulfone treatment, skin lesions resolve and numbers of viable bacilli in the skin are reduced. Although primarily bacteriostatic, dapsone monotherapy results in only a 2.5% resistance-related relapse rate; after ≥18 years of therapy and subsequent discontinuation, only another 10% of patients relapse, developing new, usually asymptomatic, shiny, "histoid" nodules. Dapsone is generally safe and inexpensive. Individuals with glucose-6-phosphate dehydrogenase deficiency who are treated with dapsone may develop severe hemolysis; those without this deficiency also have reduced red cell survival and a hemoglobin decrease averaging 1 g/dL. Dapsone's usefulness is limited occasionally by allergic dermatitis and rarely by the sulfone syndrome (including high fever, anemia, exfoliative dermatitis, and a mononucleosis-type blood picture). It must be remembered that rifampin induces microsomal enzymes, necessitating increased doses of medications such as glucocorticoids and oral birth control regimens. Clofazimine is often cosmetically unacceptable to light-skinned leprosy patients because it causes a red-black skin discoloration that accumulates, particularly in lesional areas, and makes the patient's diagnosis obvious to members of the community.

Other antimicrobial agents active against *M. leprae* in animal models and at the usual daily doses used in clinical trials include ethionamide/prothionamide; the aminoglycosides streptomycin, kanamycin, and amikacin (but not gentamicin or tobramycin); minocycline; clarithromycin; and several fluoroquinolones, particularly ofloxacin. Next to rifampin, minocycline, clarithromycin, and ofloxacin appear to be most bactericidal for *M. leprae*, but these drugs have not been used extensively in leprosy control programs. Most recently, rifapentine and moxifloxacin have been found to be especially potent against *M. leprae*.

CHOICE OF REGIMENS   Antimicrobial therapy for leprosy must be individualized, depending on the clinical/pathologic form of the disease encountered. Tuberculoid leprosy, which is associated with a low bacterial burden and a protective cellular immune response, is the easier form to treat and can be reliably cured with a finite course of chemotherapy. In contrast, lepromatous leprosy may have a higher bacillary load than any other human bacterial disease, and the absence of a salutary T cell repertoire requires prolonged or even lifelong chemotherapy. Hence, careful classification of disease prior to therapy is important. In developed countries, clinical experience with leprosy

classification is limited; fortunately, however, the resources needed for skin biopsy are highly accessible and pathologic interpretation is readily available. In developing countries, clinical expertise is greater but is now waning substantially as the care of leprosy patients is integrated into general health services. In addition, access to dermatopathology services is often limited. In such instances, skin smears may prove useful, but in many locales access to the resources needed for their preparation and interpretation may also be unavailable. Use of skin smears is no longer encouraged by the World Health Organization (WHO) and is often replaced by mere counting of lesions, which, together with the lack of histopathology, may negatively affect decisions about chemotherapy, increase the potential for reactions, and worsen the ultimate prognosis.

A reasoned approach to the treatment of leprosy is confounded by these and several other issues:

1. Even without therapy, TT leprosy may heal spontaneously, and prolonged dapsone monotherapy (even for LL leprosy) is generally curative in 80% of cases.

2. In tuberculoid disease, there are often no bacilli found in the skin prior to therapy, and thus there is no objective measure of therapeutic success. Furthermore, despite adequate treatment, TT and particularly BT lesions often resolve little or incompletely, while relapse and late type 1 lepra reactions can be difficult to distinguish.

3. LL leprosy patients commonly harbor viable persistent *M. leprae* organisms after prolonged intensive therapy; the propensity of these organisms to initiate clinical relapse is unclear. Because relapse in LL patients after discontinuation of rifampin-containing regimens usually begins only after 7 to 10 years, follow-up over the very long term is necessary to assess ultimate clinical outcomes.

4. Even though primary dapsone resistance is exceedingly rare and multidrug therapy is generally recommended (at least for lepromatous leprosy), there is a paucity of information from experimental animals and clinical trials on the optimal combination of antimicrobials, dosing schedule, or duration of therapy.

In 1982, the WHO made recommendations for "the chemotherapy of leprosy for control programs." These recommendations came on the heels of the demonstration of the relative success of long-term dapsone monotherapy and in the context of concerns about dapsone resistance. Other complicating considerations included the limited resources available for leprosy care in the very areas where it is most prevalent and the frustration and discouragement of patients and program managers with the previous requirement for lifelong therapy for many leprosy patients. The WHO delineated for the first time a finite duration of therapy for all forms of leprosy and—given the prohibitive cost of daily rifampin treatment in developing countries—encouraged the monthly administration of this agent as part of a multidrug regimen.

Over the ensuing years, these WHO recommendations have been broadly implemented, and the duration of therapy required, particularly for lepromatous leprosy, has been progressively shortened. For treatment purposes, the WHO classifies patients as paucibacillary and multibacillary. Previously, patients without demonstrable AFB in the dermis were classified as paucibacillary and those with AFB as multibacillary. Currently, owing to the perceived unreliability of skin smears in the field, patients are classified as multibacillary if they have six or more skin lesions and as paucibacillary if they have fewer. The WHO recommends that paucibacillary adults be treated with 100 mg of dapsone daily and 600 mg of rifampin monthly (supervised) for 6 months (Table 151-2). For patients with single-lesion paucibacillary leprosy, the WHO recommends as an alternative a single dose of rifampin (600 mg), ofloxacin (400 mg), and minocycline (100 mg). Multibacillary adults should be treated with 100 mg of dapsone plus 50 mg of clofazimine daily (unsupervised) and with 600 mg of rifampin plus 300 mg of clofazimine monthly (supervised). Originally, the WHO recommended that lepromatous patients be treated for 2 years or until smears became negative (generally in ~5 years); subsequently,

TABLE 151-2 Antimicrobial Regimens Recommended for the Treatment of Leprosy in Adults

Form of Leprosy	More Intensive Regimen	WHO Recommended Regimen (1982)
Tuberculoid (paucibacillary)	Dapsone (100 mg/d) for 5 years	Dapsone (100 mg/d, unsupervised) *plus* rifampin (600 mg/month, supervised) for 6 months
Lepromatous (multibacillary)	Rifampin (600 mg/d) for 3 years *plus* dapsone (100 mg/d) indefinitely	Dapsone (100 mg/d) *plus* clofazimine (50 mg/d), unsupervised; *and* rifampin (600 mg) *plus* clofazimine (300 mg) monthly (supervised) for 1–2 years

Note: See text for discussion and comparison of WHO recommendations and more intensive approach as well as alternative WHO regimen for single-lesion paucibacillary leprosy.

the acceptable course was reduced to 1 year—a change that remains especially controversial in the absence of supporting clinical trials.

Several factors have caused many authorities to question the WHO recommendations and to favor a more intensive approach. Among these factors are—for multibacillary patients—a high (double-digit) relapse rate in three locales (reaching 20 to 40% in one locale, with the rate directly related to the initial bacterial burden) and—for paucibacillary patients—demonstrable lesional activity for years in fully half of patients after the completion of therapy. The more intensive approach (Table 151-2) calls for tuberculoid leprosy to be treated with dapsone (100 mg/d) for 5 years and for lepromatous leprosy to be treated with rifampin (600 mg/d) for 3 years and with dapsone (100 mg/d) throughout life.

On effective antimicrobial therapy, new skin lesions and signs and symptoms of peripheral neuropathy cease appearing. Nodules and plaques of lepromatous leprosy noticeably flatten in 1 to 2 months and resolve in 1 year or a few years, while tuberculoid skin lesions may disappear, improve, or remain relatively unchanged. Although the peripheral neuropathy of leprosy may improve somewhat in the first few months of therapy, rarely is it significantly ameliorated by treatment.

Therapy for Reactions ■ *TYPE 1* Type 1 lepra reactions are best treated with glucocorticoids (e.g., prednisone, initially at doses of 40 to 60 mg/d). As the inflammation subsides, the glucocorticoid dose can be tapered, but steroid therapy must be continued for at least 3 months lest recurrence supervene. Because of the myriad toxicities of prolonged glucocorticoid therapy, the indications for its initiation are strictly limited to lesions whose intense inflammation poses a threat of ulceration; lesions at cosmetically important sites, such as the face; and cases in which neuritis is present. Mild to moderate lepra reactions that do not meet these criteria should be tolerated and glucocorticoid treatment withheld. Thalidomide is ineffective against type 1 lepra reactions; clofazimine (200 to 300 mg/d) is of questionable benefit but in any event is far less efficacious than glucocorticoids.

TYPE 2 Treatment of ENL must be individualized. If ENL is mild (i.e., without fever or other organ involvement, with occasional crops of only a few skin papules), it may be treated with antipyretics alone. However, in cases with many skin lesions, fever, malaise, and other tissue involvement, brief courses (1 to 2 weeks) of glucocorticoids (initially 40 to 60 mg/d) are often effective. With or without therapy, individual inflamed papules last for >1 week. Successful therapy is defined by the cessation of skin lesion development and the disappearance of other systemic signs and symptoms. If, despite two courses of glucocorticoid therapy, ENL appears to be recurring and persisting, treatment with thalidomide (100 to 300 mg nightly) should be initiated, with the dose depending on the initial severity of the reaction. Because even a single dose of thalidomide administered early in pregnancy may result in severe birth defects, including phocomelia, the use of this drug in the United States for the treatment of fertile female patients is tightly regulated and requires informed consent, prior pregnancy testing, and maintenance of birth control measures. Although the mech-

anism of thalidomide's dramatic action against ENL is not entirely clear, the drug's efficacy is probably attributable to its reduction of TNF levels and IgM synthesis and its slowing of polymorphonuclear leukocyte migration. After the reaction is controlled, lower doses of thalidomide (50 to 200 mg nightly) are effective in preventing relapses of ENL. Clofazimine in high doses (300 mg nightly) has some efficacy against ENL, but its use permits only a modest reduction of the glucocorticoid dose necessary for ENL control.

LUCIO'S PHENOMENON Neither glucocorticoids nor thalidomide is effective against this syndrome. Optimal wound care and therapy for bacteremia are indicated. Ulcers tend to be chronic and heal poorly. In severe cases, exchange transfusion may prove useful.

PREVENTION AND CONTROL Vaccination at birth with bacille Calmette-Guérin (BCG) has proved variably effective in preventing leprosy: the results have ranged from total inefficacy to 80% efficacy. The addition of heat-killed *M. leprae* to BCG does not increase vaccine efficacy. Because whole mycobacteria contain large amounts of lipids and carbohydrates that have proven in vitro to be immunosuppressive for lymphocytes and macrophages, *M. leprae* proteins may prove to be superior vaccines. Data from a mouse model support this possibility.

Chemoprophylaxis with dapsone may reduce the number of cases of tuberculoid leprosy but not of lepromatous leprosy and hence is not recommended, even for household contacts. Because leprosy transmission appears to require close prolonged household contact, hospitalized patients need not be isolated.

In 1992, the WHO—on the basis of that organization's treatment recommendations—launched a landmark campaign to eliminate leprosy as a public health problem by the year 2000 (goal, <1 case per 10,000 population). The campaign mobilized and energized nongovernmental organizations and national health services to treat leprosy with multiple drugs and to clean up outdated registries; in these respects, the effort has proven hugely successful, with >6 million patients completing therapy. However, the target of leprosy elimination has not yet been reached. In fact, the success of the WHO campaign in reducing the number of cases worldwide has been largely attributable to the redefinition of what constitutes a case of leprosy: Formerly calculated by disease prevalence, the case count is now limited to those not yet treated with multiple drugs. In each of the 23 countries with the largest number of leprosy cases, the annual incidence of leprosy is stable or actually rising. Furthermore, after the completion of therapy, when a patient is no longer considered to represent a "case," half of all patients continue to manifest disease activity for years; relapse rates (at least for multibacillary patients) are unacceptably high; disabilities and deformities go unchecked; and the social stigma of the disease persists.

During most of the twentieth century, nongovernmental organizations, particularly Christian missionaries, provided a medical infrastructure devoted to the care and treatment of leprosy patients—the envy of those with other medical priorities in the developing world. With the public perception that leprosy is near eradication, resources for patient care are rapidly being diverted, and the burden of patient care is being transferred to nonexistent or overloaded national health services and to health workers who lack the tools and skills needed for disease diagnosis, classification, and nuanced therapy (particularly in cases of reactional neuritis). Thus the prerequisites for a salutary outcome are increasingly unmet.

FURTHER READING

BAOHONG JI: Does there exist a subgroup of MB patients at greater risk of relapse after MDT? Lepr Rev 72:3, 2001

COLE ST et al: Massive gene decay in the leprosy bacillus. Nature 409:1007, 2001

GELBER RH: Chemotherapy of lepromatous leprosy: Recent developments and prospects for the future. Eur J Clin Microbiol Infect Dis 13:942, 1994

———— et al: Vaccination of mice with a soluble protein fraction of *Mycobac-*

terium leprae provides consistent and long-term protection against *M. leprae* infection. Infect Immun 60:1840, 1992

JAMET P et al: Marchoux Chemotherapy Study Group. Relapse after long-term follow up of multibacillary patients treated by WHO multidrug regimen. Int J Lepr 63:195, 1995

LOCKWOOD D: Leprosy elimination—a virtual phenomenon or a reality? BMJ 324:1516, 2002

MODLIN RL, REA TH: Immunology of leprosy granulomas. Springer Semin Immunopathol 10:359, 1998

RIDLEY DS: Histological classification and the immunological spectrum of leprosy. Bull World Health Organ 51:451, 1974

SHEPARD CC: The experimental disease that follows injection of human leprosy bacilli into foot pads of mice. J Exp Med 112:445, 1960

WHO EXPERT COMMITTEE ON LEPROSY: Seventh Report. WHO Tech Rep Ser No. 874. Geneva, World Health Organization, 1998

152 NONTUBERCULOUS MYCOBACTERIA
C. Fordham von Reyn

The designation *nontuberculous mycobacteria* (NTM) encompasses the mycobacterial species other than organisms of the *Mycobacterium tuberculosis* complex and *M. leprae*. The NTM are distributed widely in the environment, are typically acquired from environmental sources, and therefore are also referred to as *environmental mycobacteria*. Most species are less virulent for humans than is *M. tuberculosis*. Thus symptomatic infections are often associated with local or generalized defects in host defenses. Because isolation of an NTM species from a clinical specimen may represent true infection, colonization, or environmental contamination, strict criteria are required to assess the clinical significance of a positive culture. Although the >90 species of NTM have been associated with a wide variety of infections, most NTM infections are due to a relatively limited number of species that cause characteristic patterns of disease (Table 152-1).

MICROBIOLOGY Similar to *M. tuberculosis*, NTM organisms resist decolorization after staining and are referred to as *acid-fast bacilli* (AFB). NTM have conventionally been characterized by the time required for clinical specimens to yield visible growth on solid media. Rapidly growing NTM species, such as *M. abscessus*, *M. fortuitum*, and *M. chelonae*, appear within 7 days. These organisms grow on standard microbiologic media and thus may be reported even when the clinician has not explicitly requested cultures for mycobacteria. Slow-growing species, in contrast, often take 2 to 3 weeks to grow on solid media and require special mycobacterial media such as Lowenstein-Jensen or Middlebrook. Accordingly, slow-growing NTM species are usually isolated only when the clinician specifically requests cultures for mycobacteria. Representative species include *M. avium*, *M. kansasii*, *M. ulcerans*, and *M. marinum*. Automated broth culture systems are now used in many laboratories and may permit isolation of slow-growing NTM organisms within 10 to 14 days, thus tending to blur species distinctions based on growth rate.

Further classification based on colony pigmentation (Runyon classification) has been replaced by the use of DNA probes for identification of common species such as *M. avium*, *M. intracellulare*, *M. gordonae* (which is rarely pathogenic), and *M. kansasii*. Less common species may be identified rapidly on the basis of fatty acid composition or DNA sequencing. Molecular strain typing ("fingerprinting") based on analysis of polymorphisms among large restriction fragments can be used to determine whether two or more isolates are genotypically—and, by implication, epidemiologically—related. This technique has been useful for identifying common-source outbreaks of infection or contamination.

Antibiotic susceptibility testing should be performed for rapidly growing NTM species. However, susceptibility testing of slow-growing species is of limited value: testing methods are not well standardized, and the relevance of the results to outcome is uncertain since patients are usually treated with multiple-drug regimens. Testing of *M. avium* or *M. kansasii* for susceptibility to specific drugs may be useful in certain situations (see below).

DISTRIBUTION NTM have a waxy, hydrophobic, triple-layered cell wall that renders them unusually resistant to physical conditions and chemical agents (including disinfectants such as chlorine at concentrations used in drinking water). These organisms can make use of a wide variety of carbon and nitrogen sources and can survive in nutrient-poor environments. Thus they are widely distributed in water, biofilms, and soil as well as in numerous animal species. Optimal growth temperatures vary and may influence distribution. For example, *M. avium* and *M. intracellulare* are often isolated from potable hot-water sources, whereas *M. marinum* is found in the cooler water of fish tanks. Most species of NTM are obligate aerobes and grow best at acid pH. Soil and natural water samples from most regions of the world contain numerous species of NTM, which are as common in northern regions (e.g., Finland) as they are in more temperate areas (e.g., the southern United States).

EPIDEMIOLOGY Asymptomatic infections with NTM are common in humans and are probably acquired most often from childhood contact with soil, water, and possibly animals. Studies with skin tests derived from NTM indicate that 30 to 40% of adults in the northern and southern United States have had prior unrecognized or asymptomatic infection with NTM—most often with organisms of the *M. avium* complex (MAC). Since latent infection is not a recognized characteristic of NTM, most symptomatic infections are thought to represent recent exposure. Molecular methods have identified clusters of infections and pseudoinfections associated with potable water as well as with clinical procedures such as endoscopy and surgery. Environmental exposures are assumed to cause most symptomatic infections; however, this point has been difficult to document by molecular methods, presumably because there are many potential exposures (some of which are sporadic) and because a specific NTM species may be present only transiently or in low numbers in any given source.

TABLE 152-1   *Main Species of NTM and Patterns of Disease*

Species	Growth on Solid Media	Environmental Reservoir	Patterns of Disease[a]			
			Cutaneous	Pulmonary	Disseminated	Other
M. avium	Slow	Hot water systems, natural water, soil	−	++	+++	Lymphadenitis
M. intracellulare	Slow	Hot water systems, natural water, soil	−	+++	+	Lymphadenitis
M. kansasii	Slow	Potable and natural water	−	+++	++	−
M. abscessus, M. chelonae, M. fortuitum	Rapid	Potable and natural water, soil	++	+	−	Sporotrichoid spread
M. marinum	Slow	Fish tanks, salt water	++	−	−	Sporotrichoid spread
M. ulcerans	Slow	Natural water	++	−	−	"Buruli ulcer," osteomyelitis

[a] Symbols indicate relative prevalence among NTM infections of the indicated species and pattern of disease: +++, most common; ++, common; +, reported but uncommon; −, rare or not reported.

PATHOGENESIS NTM may be acquired through cutaneous, respiratory, gastrointestinal, or (rarely) parenteral exposure. Organisms are ingested by host macrophages and may survive within these cells to replicate and cause symptomatic infection. Disease manifestations in immunocompetent hosts are due to host cellular immune responses and the formation of granulomas. Intracellular killing of mycobacteria, with ultimate control of infection, requires the action of cellular immune mechanisms including proliferation of CD4+ T lymphocytes and elaboration of interferon γ (IFN-γ) and interleukin 12. Deficiencies in CD4+ T cell function due to HIV infection and inherited deficiencies in the production of or response to IFN-γ are associated with disseminated NTM infection (Chap. 173).

There is no convincing evidence that NTM can establish latent infection with subsequent clinical reactivation—a pattern characteristic of *M. tuberculosis.* Asymptomatic infection with NTM in a healthy host may induce beneficial immunity; persons with skin-test reactivity to NTM antigens (e.g., *M. intracellulare*) are at decreased risk for the subsequent development of tuberculosis. Likewise, immunization with bacille Calmette-Guérin (BCG) from *M. bovis* provides protection against childhood cervical adenitis due to NTM.

CLINICAL SYNDROMES ■ **Cutaneous Disease** NTM can cause a variety of cutaneous disease syndromes when directly inoculated from an environmental source into an area of open or diseased skin or into a surgical wound. *M. abscessus, M. fortuitum, M. chelonae, M. marinum,* and *M. ulcerans* are the most commonly involved species. Cutaneous disease may be nodular or ulcerating, sometimes with reddish-blue discoloration and typically with minimal drainage. Lesions may be single, or the infection may spread proximally up the lymphatics, producing additional nodules (sporotrichoid spread). In compromised hosts, disseminated lesions may appear as a result of bacteremic spread. Clinical suspicion of NTM infection is based on chronicity, the absence of bacterial growth on routine culture, and the failure to respond to standard antibacterial therapy. Biopsies often reveal granuloma formation, and acid-fast stains may be positive.

Pulmonary Disease NTM species cause chronic progressive pulmonary infection both in normal hosts and in those with underlying pulmonary disease. The clinical features may resemble slowly progressive pulmonary tuberculosis, which is often the initial diagnosis in patients with positive AFB smears. Among patients born in the United States, pulmonary disease due to acid-fast organisms is more likely to be due to NTM than to *M. tuberculosis.*

The diagnosis of pulmonary NTM infection is complicated by the variability in clinical and radiologic manifestations, the frequent presence of significant prior pulmonary disease, and the fact that isolation of NTM from the sputum may represent harmless colonization of the lower respiratory tract. The diagnosis should be based on specific, validated criteria that emphasize a compatible clinical syndrome, characteristic findings on computed tomography (CT), and repeated isolation of NTM from the sputum or growth of NTM from a lung biopsy (Table 152-2).

In normal hosts, infection may result in the onset of chronic cough, dyspnea, and fatigue; fever is unusual. Pathologic and radiologic manifestations of NTM pulmonary infection include the formation of solitary or multiple nodules, chronic pneumonitis, bronchiectasis, cavity formation, or a combination of these features. In some patients with NTM pulmonary disease, CT shows the characteristic formation of small cylindrical bronchiectasis and multiple small (<5-mm) nodules and fibrosis. Patients with these findings and negative results of routine sputum cultures for mycobacteria should have bronchoscopy and transbronchial biopsy performed in an attempt to identify granulomas and acid-fast organisms. In patients with chronic pulmonary disease, the superimposition of infection with NTM may not be associated with easily recognizable changes in symptoms or radiologic features.

MAC organisms (especially *M. intracellulare*) are the most common cause of pulmonary disease due to NTM in developed countries; next in frequency are *M. kansasii* (United States, Europe, South Africa), *M. abscessus* (United States), *M. xenopi* (Europe, Canada), and

TABLE 152-2 *Criteria for the Diagnosis of Pulmonary Disease Due to NTM[a]*

Category	Requirement
Clinical	Compatible symptoms (e.g., fever, cough), *and* deterioration in clinical status (if underlying lung disease present), *and* reasonable exclusion of other disease
Radiologic	Chest radiograph: Infiltrates with or without nodules, either persistent (≥2 months) or progressive; *or* cavitation; *or* multiple nodules alone
	High-resolution CT: Multiple small nodules; *or* multifocal bronchiectasis, with or without small nodules
Bacteriologic	Sputum/bronchial wash: At least 3 positive cultures in 1 year
	Bronchial wash only: At least 1 positive culture with moderate growth or positive AFB smear
	Lung biopsy: Positive culture

[a] Diagnosis requires clinical criteria plus one radiologic criterion and one bacteriologic criterion.
Abbreviations: AFB, acid-fast bacilli; CT, computed tomography.
Source: Adapted from RJ Wallace et al: Am Rev Respir Crit Care Med 156:S1, 1997.

M. malmoense (United Kingdom, northern Europe). However, isolation of NTM from the sputum must be considered in the context of clinical manifestations. For example, NTM (most prominently MAC organisms, less commonly *M. abscessus*) can be cultured from 13% of cystic fibrosis patients in the United States (Chap. 241); however, not all of these patients appear to have invasive NTM disease. Although invasive disease is particularly strongly suspected when the same NTM species is isolated on multiple occasions from a patient with lung disease, even persistent organisms may represent colonization or slowly progressive disease apparent only on long-term followup. Additional laboratory tests (e.g., immunologic assessments) are of no value in the diagnosis.

Although treatment should be considered in patients who meet clinical, radiologic, and microbiologic criteria for disease (Table 152-2), several other factors require consideration. For example, species such as *M. kansasii* are usually pathogenic, and a single isolate may be significant, while species such as *M. gordonae* are rarely pathogenic, even when isolated repeatedly. In addition, in some patients with true invasive disease, infection may progress so slowly that it is unlikely to have much impact on longevity determined by such factors as age or comorbid illness. Since therapy for NTM requires prolonged administration of multiple drugs and is associated with significant side effects, the decision to institute treatment in patients with noncavitary disease who do not have clearly progressive pulmonary disease should be made with careful deliberation after a period of clinical and radiologic follow-up.

Disseminated Disease Patients with impaired cellular immunity—most notably, patients with advanced HIV disease (Chap. 173)—are susceptible to disseminated disease due to NTM. Other conditions that predispose patients to this syndrome include treatment with glucocorticoids or other immunosuppressive agents (e.g., for organ transplantation), lymphoma and leukemia (especially hairy cell leukemia), and heritable disorders of IFN-γ production and function. *M. avium* and *M. kansasii* are the species most commonly isolated in disseminated disease, but numerous other organisms (e.g., *M. genavense, M. haemophilum*) have also been recovered.

Patients with disseminated infection present with fever, weight loss, and fatigue and sometimes with hepatosplenomegaly or lymphadenopathy. Chest radiographs are typically normal in infection with *M. avium* (although they may show a miliary pattern) but are usually abnormal in that with *M. kansasii.* Laboratory studies may demonstrate anemia and an elevated level of alkaline phosphatase in serum. Disseminated disease is characterized by the widespread presence of foamy macrophages with AFB, which may be demonstrated in biopsy samples of bone marrow, intestine, or liver. Granulomas are typically absent in patients with impaired cellular immunity. In most cases, the diagnosis can be established by one or two sets of mycobacterial blood cultures, which will be positive for the etiologic mycobacteria in 2 to 3 weeks. Treatment requires long-term administration of a multiple-drug antimycobacterial regimen and attempts to ameliorate the defect in cellular immunity (e.g., institution of antiretroviral therapy, discontinuation of glucocorticoid administration).

Other Disease NTM species have been associated with disease at numerous other anatomical locations, including ocular infections, mastoiditis, sinusitis, mastitis, catheter site infections, endocarditis, meningitis, peritonitis, appendicitis, pericarditis, pyelonephritis, prostatitis, tenosynovitis, bursitis, septic arthritis, osteomyelitis, and lymphadenitis (especially in children). Accumulating data support an association between infection with *M. avium* subspecies *paratuberculosis* and Crohn's disease.

ORGANISMS

M. AVIUM COMPLEX ■ **Pulmonary Disease** MAC organisms (*M. avium, M. intracellulare*, and genetically related unnamed species) are more common than *M. tuberculosis* as a cause of mycobacterial pulmonary disease among persons born in the United States. Epidemiologic data support a marked increase in the incidence of MAC infection over the past two to three decades. Two patterns of MAC disease are recognized: a primary form in apparently healthy nonsmokers and a secondary form in patients with preexisting pulmonary disease (Table 152-3). The description of subtle defects in cellular immune responses and body morphotype in patients with primary disease raises the possibility of an as-yet-undefined immune defect predisposing to MAC infection. Patients with secondary disease include those with chronic obstructive pulmonary disease, prior tuberculosis, cystic fibrosis, or pulmonary alveolar proteinosis. The sources of infection have not been identified.

CLINICAL FEATURES AND DIAGNOSIS Symptoms and diagnostic studies are described above (see "Clinical Syndromes"). CT identifies characteristic cylindrical bronchiectasis with nodule formation, documents the extent of disease, and establishes a baseline for possible treatment. Standard diagnostic criteria should be applied (Table 152-2), and antibiotic susceptibility testing should be reserved for patients with prolonged prior macrolide exposure and for those in whom treatment fails.

℞ **TREATMENT**

Treatment should be initiated in most patients with cavitary disease and those with documented progression of a pulmonary process who meet diagnostic criteria for NTM infection. A period of observation prior to consideration of treatment may be useful when there is no evidence of an otherwise-explainable progressive pulmonary process

TABLE 152-3 *Typical Features of Primary and Secondary Pulmonary Disease Due to the M. avium Complex*

Feature	Primary	Secondary
Age	>50 years	30–70 (mean, 60) years
Sex	F > M	M > F
Underlying disease	None definitively identified; subtle defect in cellular immunity postulated	Chronic obstructive pulmonary disease, cystic fibrosis, prior tuberculosis, alveolar proteinosis
Clinical features	Early disease may be limited to cylindrical bronchicctasis, <5-mm nodules, and midzone involvement on chest radiography	Infiltrates, <5-mm nodules, cavities

and when the patient's age or underlying disease is likely to be the critical determinant of survival over the next few years.

Recommended treatment for pulmonary disease includes daily ethambutol and rifabutin plus a macrolide (either daily clarithromycin or thrice-weekly azithromycin; Table 152-4). Concomitant streptomycin therapy for the first 2 months should be considered in patients with extensive or cavitary disease. As many as 30% of patients treated with standard drugs and doses are unable to tolerate therapy, generally because of gastrointestinal side effects. Rifabutin appears to have the highest rate of side effects. Thus, doses often need to be reduced or drugs eliminated or replaced with alternatives. A fluoroquinolone may be considered as a substitute drug, although clinical data on this option are limited.

For patients with positive sputum cultures who receive a macrolide-containing regimen, treatment should be continued for at least 12 months after cultures revert to negative—typically for ≥18 months. The duration of therapy with other regimens may need to be extended to 24 months. In some cases, cough and radiographic findings may improve after several months; in others, treatment may serve only to prevent the progression of disease. Approximately 20% of patients experience treatment failure or relapse; some apparent treatment failures may actually represent reinfection. Surgical resection is an option for patients with localized disease who are intolerant or unresponsive to multiple-drug therapy; however, this approach is associated with postoperative complications in as many as 20% of patients and should be undertaken only by surgeons who have considerable experience with this intervention.

Disseminated Disease Disseminated MAC disease occurs principally among patients with advanced HIV disease who live in developed countries but are not receiving antiretroviral therapy. Almost all cases occur at CD4+ T cell counts of <100/μL, and the risk is ~20% per year for untreated patients with CD4+ T cell counts of <50/μL. The risk of disease is essentially eliminated for patients given highly active antiretroviral therapy (HAART) who have an increase in CD4+ T cell count to >100/μL for 3 months. Most cases are due to *M. avium*, and molecular studies indicate that as many as 25% of disseminated infections involve more than one strain. Strains causing bacteremia differ genetically from those typically isolated from respiratory sources or the environment. Molecular techniques have documented nosocomial acquisition from potable hot water and have demonstrated common genotypes among isolates from humans and those from peat used in potting soil. Epidemiologic studies have demonstrated an increased risk associated with consumption of untreated spring water and of raw or partially cooked fish or shellfish and a decreased risk associated with showering. Overall, sources of acquisition appear to be diverse and exposure is probably unavoidable; at this time, no specific behavioral changes are recommended for at-risk patients.

CLINICAL FEATURES AND DIAGNOSIS Disseminated *M. avium* infection in AIDS is associated with fever, weakness, and weight loss and usually presents as a wasting syndrome in patients who are not receiving HAART or chemoprophylaxis for *M. avium* (Chap. 173). Untreated disease shortens the survival period of patients with advanced AIDS by 4 to 5 months. Laboratory findings may include anemia, hypoalbuminemia, and elevated serum levels of alkaline phosphatase and lactate dehydrogenase. HIV-infected patients with prior disseminated MAC infection or unrecognized or subclinical MAC infection may experience an immune reconstitution syndrome when they start to receive HAART (Chap. 173). This syndrome presents 1 to 12 weeks after the institution of HAART and manifests as localized (or generalized) culture-positive lymphadenitis with negative blood cultures for *M. avium*.

℞ **TREATMENT**

Disseminated *M. avium* disease requires treatment with the combination of clarithromycin and ethambutol, with or without rifabutin (Table

152-4), along with HAART for HIV. Antimycobacterial treatment should be continued for at least 12 months and until the CD4+ T cell count has been >100/μL for at least 6 months. The immune reconstitution syndrome should be treated with initiation or continuation of the same antimycobacterial regimen.

PREVENTION Chemoprophylaxis is highly effective for the prevention of disseminated *M. avium* infection in AIDS. Weekly azithromycin administration should be instituted when the CD4+ T cell count is <50/μL or when a patient with HIV infection has had an AIDS-defining opportunistic infection (e.g., *Pneumocystis* infection). Chemoprophylaxis may be discontinued when the CD4+ T cell count has been >100/μL for >6 months.

M. KANSASII ▪ Pulmonary Disease

Pulmonary disease due to *M. kansasii* has been reported from many areas of the world, including North America, Europe, and South Africa. In the United States, *M. kansasii* is the second most common cause of lung disease due to NTM and is distributed largely in central and southern states and California. The average age of onset is 60 years, and most patients have predisposing factors, such as chronic obstructive pulmonary disease, carcinoma of the lung, silicosis, or prior tuberculosis. However, pulmonary infection sometimes occurs in persons without predisposing disease and has also been associated with poverty. Disease may sometimes wax and wane over many years; this pattern is assumed to represent chronic infection rather than reactivation. Localized pulmonary infection has been described in South African miners with early HIV infection and preserved CD4+ T cell counts. The source of infection has not been identified, although *M. kansasii* has been isolated from both potable and natural water sources.

CLINICAL FEATURES AND DIAGNOSIS *M. kansasii* is the most pathogenic nontuberculous mycobacterial species affecting the lung, and the clinical features of *M. kansasii* disease resemble those of tuberculosis. Most cases include cough and sputum production; 30% include frank hemoptysis. Systemic signs and symptoms, including fever, night sweats, and weight loss, are reported by as many as 50% of patients. However, symptoms may be subtle or absent in patients with underlying malignancy. Chest radiographs show cavitation in 50% of patients, pleural scarring in 40%, and infiltrates in 30%; abnormalities are most prominent in the apices. Clinical and radiographic effects progress in the absence of treatment.

Sputum samples should be obtained for AFB staining and mycobacterial culture. The isolation of *M. kansasii* sometimes represents colonization; the diagnostic criteria in Table 152-2 are useful when multiple sputum samples can be obtained. However, the growth of *M. kansasii* from even a single sputum culture should be considered to have potential clinical significance, especially in HIV-positive patients. Testing of *M. kansasii* isolates for susceptibility to rifampin is recommended.

℞ TREATMENT

For susceptible strains of *M. kansasii*, rifampin is the foundation of a multiple-drug regimen. The recommended regimen consists of daily rifampin (600 mg), isoniazid (300 mg), and ethambutol (25 mg/kg for the initial 2 months, 15 mg/kg subsequently) for at least 18 months. Sputum cultures almost always become negative by 4 months; patients with delayed conversion should be treated for at least 12 months after the last positive culture. Resistance to rifampin may develop, in which case clarithromycin or azithromycin may be substituted

Disseminated Disease Disseminated *M. kansasii* disease occurs principally among patients with advanced AIDS and CD4+ T cell counts

TABLE 152-4 *Regimens for Prevention and Treatment of Disease Due to the M. avium Complex*

Category	Regimen	Indication and Duration
Pulmonary disease treatment	Clarithromycin 500 mg bid (or azithromycin 600 mg 3 times/week), ethambutol 15 mg/kg/d, and rifabutin 150–300 mg/d; consider adding streptomycin 500–1000 mg 2 or 3 times/week for first 2 months	Treat for 18 months or until 12 months after conversion of sputum culture.
Disseminated disease Treatment	Clarithromycin 500 mg PO bid (or azithromycin 500 mg/d[a]) plus ethambutol 15 mg/kg per day[b]	Treat when MAC blood culture is positive or MAC organism is isolated from ordinarily sterile site. Continue with secondary prevention.
Primary prevention	Azithromycin 1200 mg PO weekly[a] or clarithromycin 500 mg PO bid	Treat when CD4+ T cell count is <50/μL. Discontinue if CD4+ T cell count exceeds 100/μL for >3 months during HAART.
Secondary prevention	Clarithromycin 500 mg PO bid (or azithromycin 500 mg/d[a]) plus ethambutol 15 mg/kg per day[b]	Discontinue if disease resolves with >12 months of MAC therapy and CD4+ T cell count exceeds 100/μL for >6 months during HAART.

[a] Azithromycin is preferred to clarithromycin in pregnancy.
[b] Concomitant rifabutin (150–300 mg/d) may protect against the development of clarithromycin resistance and improve survival but can cause interactions with antiretroviral therapy.
Abbreviations: HAART, highly active antiretroviral therapy.

of <100/μL. It has also been reported in patients with leukemia, lymphoma, or solid-organ transplantation.

CLINICAL FEATURES AND DIAGNOSIS Symptoms are similar to those reported for disseminated MAC infection, although cough is more common with disseminated *M. kansasii* infection and chest radiographs often demonstrate alveolar or interstitial infiltrates or cavities. An immune reconstitution syndrome may occur after the institution of HAART in HIV-infected patients and manifests as cervical or mediastinal lymphadenitis (Chap. 173).

The diagnosis is established by the isolation of *M. kansasii* from a normally sterile parenchymal site or from blood. In one series of cases, concurrent disseminated infection with a second NTM species (most often *M. avium*), was found in one-third of patients. The isolation of *M. kansasii* from sputum from a patient with advanced HIV disease suggests possible disseminated infection and is an indication for mycobacterial blood culture.

℞ TREATMENT

Antimycobacterial treatment of disseminated *M. kansasii* disease is the same as that for pulmonary disease due to this organism. Patients with AIDS who are receiving HAART should have rifabutin (150 mg/d) or clarithromycin (500 mg twice daily) substituted for rifampin because of drug interactions. Untreated disease is associated with shortened survival, and the response to treatment is good in patients who do not have rapidly progressive HIV infection. HIV-positive patients who experience clearing of systemic symptoms and have positive cultures with sustained recovery of the CD4+ T cell count can probably have treatment discontinued (as described above for *M. avium* infection), although there are no clinical data on this point. Azithromycin prophylaxis for disseminated *M. avium* infection may also be effective in preventing disseminated *M. kansasii* infection.

M. ABSCESSUS, M. CHELONAE, AND M. FORTUITUM

Three rapidly growing NTM species are prominent in reports of human infection and colonization: *M. abscessus*, *M. chelonae*, and *M. fortuitum*. These organisms are acquired from water, soil, or nosocomial sources. The most common clinical manifestation of infection is disseminated cutaneous disease in patients who have defects in cellular immunity or are receiving glucocorticoid therapy. Normal hosts develop localized cutaneous infection in surgical or traumatic wounds, from contaminated injections, or after body piercing. Cutaneous lesions are cellulitic or nodular; are typically erythematous, indurated, and tender; and may progress to ulceration and purulent drainage. Proximal sporotrichoid spread has also been reported. Pulmonary infections (usually due to *M. abscessus*) are the next most common manifestation and occur principally in patients with underlying lung disease, such as cystic fibrosis.

The rapidly growing NTM species may be isolated from clinical specimens submitted for routine microbiologic testing. However, reliable evaluation requires inoculation onto special mycobacterial media and an extended incubation period. Because rapidly growing NTM species are also common laboratory contaminants, numerous false alarms in the form of pseudoepidemics have been reported.

Rx TREATMENT

Treatment varies with the patient group and with the species of rapidly growing NTM. Susceptibility tests should be performed and used to guide antibiotic selection. All three species are usually susceptible to clarithromycin and amikacin; *M. abscessus* and *M. fortuitum* are also susceptible to cefoxitin. Other agents that may be active include imipenem, doxycycline, and fluoroquinolones. Patients with localized cutaneous disease may respond to a single active agent (e.g., clarithromycin, 500 mg twice daily by mouth for ≥2 weeks). Up to 6 months of therapy may be optimal for bacteremic or disseminated cutaneous disease, and a second agent should be added on the basis of susceptibility tests. Pulmonary disease is especially difficult to treat since prolonged therapy is required and the most active drugs require parenteral administration. Current recommendations are to administer intravenous amikacin (5 to 7.5 mg/kg every 12 h) and cefoxitin (3 g every 6 h) with oral clarithromycin (500 mg twice daily) and to continue treatment for 6 to 12 months. Surgery can be considered for localized disease.

M. MARINUM *M. marinum* is widely distributed in water and causes chronic cutaneous infection when an open cutaneous lesion is exposed to a colonized water source. Most infections are due to hand or upper-extremity exposure to fish tanks, and some are due to shellfish or marine exposures. Swimming pools are no longer a common source of infection because of current chlorination standards. *M. marinum* grows optimally at 30°C—a lower temperature than is optimal for most pathogenic mycobacteria. After a median incubation period of 21 days (≥30 days in 35% of cases), a granulomatous or ulcerating skin lesion develops at the site of entry with subsequent sporotrichoid spread in many cases. In some patients, especially those with serious underlying disease and those receiving immunosuppressive therapy, infection may extend to deeper structures, producing tenosynovitis or osteomyelitis. The diagnosis is established by mycobacterial culture of a biopsied lesion or by demonstration of granulomas or AFB in a biopsy sample from a patient with a compatible exposure history.

Rx TREATMENT

Treatment consists of the combination of clarithromycin and ethambutol, with administration continuing for 1 to 2 months after resolution of lesions—typically 3 to 4 months in total. Surgical debridement may be necessary in extensive or deep disease; however, in contrast to pyogenic infections, routine incision and drainage are not helpful. Persons with occupational or avocational exposure to fish tanks or salt water should wear waterproof gloves to prevent infection of open cutaneous lesions.

M. ULCERANS *M. ulcerans* causes cutaneous infection ("Buruli ulcer") in endemic regions of Central and West Africa, Central and South America, Malaysia, Indonesia, Papua New Guinea, and Australia. The organism is closely related to *M. marinum*, has a similar temperature for optimal growth, and has been isolated from natural bodies of water. Most cases of human infection occur on the bare arms or legs of children or young adults living near rivers, lakes, or swamps. Transmission is thought to result from minor trauma or the bite of an aquatic insect. The initial lesion is a small painless nodule that progresses to a deep ulcer. The ulcer expands, resulting in sloughing of skin and subcutaneous tissue; osteomyelitis may also occur. Stellate scarring and deforming contractures may result from extensive necrosis.

Biopsy analyses demonstrate extracellular AFB in early lesions, with a limited inflammatory reaction. Tissue destruction extends beyond the area of demonstrable bacterial infection and has been attributed to a unique mycobacterial toxin, mycolactone.

Rx TREATMENT

Antimicrobial therapy has not yet been shown to be beneficial, although rifampin, dapsone, clarithromycin, streptomycin, and amikacin display in vitro activity against *M. ulcerans*. Surgical treatment is primary and may require skin grafting. Immunization with BCG reduces the risk of disease by ~50%.

OTHER NTM SPECIES Numerous other NTM species have been associated with human disease, although they may represent contaminants in clinical specimens. Species and sites of possible infection include *M. celatum* (lung, lymph nodes), *M. genavense* (disseminated), *M. gordonae* (skin, contaminant), *M. haemophilum* (skin, disseminated), *M. malmoense* (lung), *M. simiae* (lung, disseminated), *M. scrofulaceum* (lymphadenitis), *M. szulgai* (skin, lung), and *M. xenopi* (lung, disseminated).

FURTHER READING

CENTERS FOR DISEASE CONTROL AND PREVENTION: Guidelines for preventing opportunistic infections among HIV-infected persons—2002 recommendations of the U.S. Public Health Service and the Infectious Diseases Society of America. MMWR 51(RR-8):10, 2002

FALKINHAM JO: Nontuberculous mycobacteria in the environment. Clin Chest Med 23:529, 2002

HAVLIR DV et al: Prophylaxis against disseminated *Mycobacterium avium* complex with weekly azithromycin, daily rifabutin, or both. N Engl J Med 335:392, 1996

HORSBURGH CR et al: Disseminated *Mycobacterium avium* complex disease among patients infected with human immunodeficiency virus, 1985–2000. Clin Infect Dis 33:1938, 2001

JERNIGAN JA, FARR BM: Incubation period and sources of exposure for cutaneous *Mycobacterium marinum* infection: A case report and review of the literature. Clin Infect Dis 31:439, 2000

VON REYN CF et al: Skin test reactions to *Mycobacterium tuberculosis* purified protein derivative and *Mycobacterium avium* sensitin among health care workers and medical students in the United States. Int J Tuberc Lung Dis 5:1122, 2001

WITZIG RS et al: Clinical manifestations and implications of coinfection with *Mycobacterium kansasii* and human immunodeficiency virus type 1. Clin Infect Dis 21:77, 1995

153 | SYPHILIS
Sheila A. Lukehart

DEFINITION Syphilis, a chronic systemic infection caused by *Treponema pallidum* subspecies *pallidum*, is usually sexually transmitted and is characterized by episodes of active disease interrupted by periods of latency. After an incubation period averaging 2 to 6 weeks, a primary lesion appears, often associated with regional lymphadenopathy. A secondary bacteremic stage, associated with generalized mucocutaneous lesions and generalized lymphadenopathy, is followed by a latent period of subclinical infection lasting many years. In about one-third of untreated cases, the tertiary stage is characterized by progressive destructive mucocutaneous, musculoskeletal, or parenchymal lesions; aortitis; or symptomatic central nervous system (CNS) disease.

ETIOLOGY The Spirochaetales include three genera that are pathogenic for humans and for a variety of other animals: *Leptospira*, which causes human leptospirosis (Chap. 155); *Borrelia*, which causes relapsing fever and Lyme disease (Chaps. 156 and 157); and *Treponema*, which causes the diseases known as treponematoses (see also Chap. 154). The genus *Treponema* includes *T. pallidum* subspecies *pallidum*, which causes venereal syphilis; *T. pallidum* subspecies *pertenue*, which causes yaws; *T. pallidum* subspecies *endemicum*, which causes endemic syphilis or bejel; and *T. carateum*, which causes pinta. Until recently, the subspecies were distinguished primarily by the clinical syndromes they produce. Researchers have now identified molecular signatures that can differentiate *T. pallidum* subspecies *pallidum* from the other pathogenic *T. pallidum* subspecies by culture independent, polymerase chain reaction (PCR)–based methods. Other *Treponema* species found in the human mouth, genital mucosa, and gastrointestinal tract have no proven pathogenic role in human disease. These spirochetes can be confused with *T. pallidum* on dark-field examination.

T. pallidum subspecies *pallidum* (hereafter referred to in this chapter simply as *T. pallidum*), a thin delicate organism with 6 to 14 spirals and tapered ends, measures 6 to 15 μm in total length and 0.2 μm in width. The cytoplasm is surrounded by a trilaminar cytoplasmic membrane, which in turn is surrounded by a delicate peptidoglycan layer providing some structural rigidity. This layer is surrounded by a lipid-rich outer membrane that contains relatively few integral membrane proteins. Endoflagella wind around the cell body in the periplasmic space and appear to be responsible for motility.

The sequencing of the genome of *T. pallidum* has yielded information about the organism's metabolic capabilities. *T. pallidum* lacks the genes required to synthesize enzyme cofactors, fatty acids, and nucleotides de novo. In addition, it lacks genes encoding the enzymes of the Krebs cycle and oxidative phosphorylation. To compensate, the organism contains numerous genes predicted to code for transporters of amino acids, carbohydrates, and cations. In addition, the genome analyses and other studies have revealed the existence of a 12-member gene family (called *tpr*) that bears similarities to variable outer-membrane antigens of other spirochetes. One member, TprK, has discrete variable (V) regions that are targets of the humoral immune response. Data suggest that sequence variation occurs in TprK during infection and that this variation is a mechanism for immune invasion.

The only known natural host for *T. pallidum* is the human. *T. pallidum* can infect many mammals, but only humans, higher apes, and a few laboratory animals regularly develop syphilitic lesions. Virulent strains of *T. pallidum* are grown and maintained in rabbits, as none of the pathogenic treponemes has been successfully cultured.

EPIDEMIOLOGY Nearly all cases of syphilis are acquired by sexual contact with infectious lesions (i.e., the chancre, mucous patch, skin rash, or condyloma latum). Less common modes of transmission include nonsexual personal contact, infection in utero, and blood transfusion.

The total number of cases of syphilis reported annually in the United States declined from 575,593 in 1943 to a low of 31,575 in 2000—a 95% decrease. This downward trend was interrupted by an epidemic peaking in 1990. Surveillance of the number of new cases of infectious syphilis—a better indicator of disease activity—has revealed four cycles of 7 to 10 years, each with a rapid rise and fall in incidence (with peaks in 1965, 1975, 1982, and 1990). From 1990 to 2000, the number of reported cases of infectious syphilis declined by >88%. In 1997, however, the number of cases of early syphilis began to rise in Seattle, Washington, marking the beginning of a trend that, by 2000, included Los Angeles and San Francisco. Infectious syphilis rates have also begun to rise in the southern region of the United States.

The populations at highest risk for acquiring syphilis have changed. Between 1977 and 1982, approximately half of all patients with early syphilis in the United States were homosexual or bisexual men. The epidemic of syphilis that peaked in 1990 predominantly involved African-American heterosexual men and women and occurred largely in urban areas, where infectious syphilis has been correlated significantly with the exchange of sex for crack cocaine. Since 1996, syphilis rates have declined steadily among African Americans but remain higher than those for other racial/ethnic groups. Foci of syphilis still exist in a small number of counties in the southern United States, and rates are still increasing there. The current outbreak of syphilis in large cities on the West Coast of the United States is focused in men who have sex with men; a high proportion of the individuals in this group who have syphilis are also infected with HIV.

The incidence of congenital syphilis roughly parallels that of infectious syphilis in females. The number of reported cases of congenital syphilis in infants ≤1 year of age was lowest (107 cases) in 1978, when infectious syphilis was most prevalent among homosexual and bisexual men. The dramatic increase in the incidence of primary and secondary syphilis among women from 1986 to 1990 resulted in a proportionate increase in the number of infants born with congenital syphilis—to 4424 infants in 1991. The incidence of early syphilis among women has declined since 1991, as has the number of reported cases of congenital syphilis in infants (with 529 cases in 2000). It is important to note that the case definition for congenital syphilis was broadened in 1989 and now includes all live or stillborn infants delivered to women with untreated or inadequately treated syphilis at delivery.

Approximately one of every two individuals named as sexual contacts of persons with infectious syphilis becomes infected. Many sexual contacts will already have developed manifestations of syphilis when they are first seen, and ~30% of apparently uninfected contacts who are examined within 30 days of exposure actually have incubating infection and will later develop infectious syphilis if not treated. Thus, the identification and "epidemiologic" treatment of all recently exposed sexual contacts constitute an important aspect of syphilis control. Also important is the identification of infected persons by serologic testing of pregnant women, persons admitted to hospitals, military inductees, and persons undergoing examination in physicians' offices. Still controversial are laws and regulations requiring routine premarital serologic testing for syphilis, where—though national data are not available—the yield is undoubtedly lower.

NATURAL COURSE AND PATHOGENESIS OF UNTREATED SYPHILIS *T. pallidum* rapidly penetrates intact mucous membranes or microscopic abrasions in skin and within a few hours enters the lymphatics and blood to produce systemic infection and metastatic foci long before the appearance of a primary lesion. Blood from a patient with incubating or early syphilis is infectious. The generation time of *T. pallidum* during early active disease in vivo is estimated to be 30 to 33 h, and the incubation period of syphilis is inversely proportional to the number of organisms inoculated. The concentration of treponemes generally reaches at least $10^7/g$ of tissue before the appearance of a clinical lesion. On the basis of intradermal injection of graded doses of *T. pallidum* into eight volunteers, the 50% infectious dose was calculated to be 57 organisms. The median incubation period in humans ($\sim$21 days) suggests an average inoculum of 500 to 1000 infectious organisms for naturally acquired disease. The incubation period (from inoculation until the primary lesion becomes discernible) rarely exceeds 6 weeks. Subcurative therapy during the incubation period may delay the onset of the primary lesion, but it is not certain that such treatment reduces the probability that symptomatic disease will ultimately develop.

The primary lesion appears at the site of inoculation, usually persists for 4 to 6 weeks, and then heals spontaneously. Histopathologic examination of primary lesions shows perivascular infiltration, chiefly by lymphocytes (including CD8+ and CD4+ cells), plasma cells, and macrophages, with capillary endothelial proliferation and subsequent obliteration of small blood vessels. The cellular infiltration displays a T_H1-type cytokine profile consistent with the activation of macrophages. At this time *T. pallidum* is demonstrable in the chancre in spaces between epithelial cells; within invaginations or phagosomes of epithelial cells, fibroblasts, plasma cells, and the endothelial cells of small capillaries; within lymphatic channels; and in the regional lymph nodes. Phagocytosis of organisms by activated macrophages ultimately causes their destruction, which results in spontaneous resolution of the chancre.

The generalized parenchymal, constitutional, and mucocutaneous manifestations of secondary syphilis usually appear about 6 to 8 weeks after healing of the chancre, although 15% of patients with secondary syphilis still have persisting or healing chancres. In other patients, secondary lesions may appear several months after the chancre has healed, and some patients may enter the latent stage without ever recognizing secondary lesions. The histopathologic features of secondary maculopapular skin lesions are hyperkeratosis of the epidermis; capillary proliferation with endothelial swelling in the superficial corium; and dermal papillae with transmigration of polymorphonuclear leukocytes and, in the deeper corium, perivascular infiltration by CD8+ lymphocytes, CD4+ lymphocytes and macrophages, and plasma cells. Treponemes are found in many tissues, including the aqueous humor of the eye and the cerebrospinal fluid (CSF). Invasion of the CNS by *T. pallidum* occurs during the first weeks or months of infection, and CSF abnormalities are detected in as many as 40% of patients during the secondary stage. Clinical hepatitis and immune complex–induced membranous glomerulonephritis are relatively rare but recognized manifestations of secondary syphilis; liver function tests may yield abnormal results in up to a quarter of patients with early syphilis. Generalized nontender lymphadenopathy is noted in 85% of patients with secondary syphilis. The paradoxical appearance of secondary manifestations despite high titers of antibody (including immobilizing antibody) to *T. pallidum* is unexplained but may result from changes in expression of surface antigens. Secondary lesions subside within 2 to 6 weeks, and the infection enters the latent stage, which is detectable only by serologic testing. In the preantibiotic era, up to 25% of untreated patients experienced at least one generalized or localized mucocutaneous relapse, usually during the first year; therefore, identification and examination of sexual contacts are most important for patients with syphilis of <1 year's duration. Recurrent generalized rash is now rare.

In the preantibiotic era, about one-third of patients with untreated latent syphilis developed clinically apparent tertiary disease; today, in industrialized countries, specific treatment and coincidental therapy for early and latent syphilis have all but eliminated tertiary disease except for sporadic cases of neurosyphilis in persons infected with HIV. In the past, the most common type of tertiary disease was the gumma, a usually benign granulomatous lesion. Today, gummas are very uncommon. Cardiovascular syphilis, now also rare, is caused by obliterative small-vessel endarteritis, usually involving the vasa vasorum of the ascending aorta and resulting in aneurysm. Asymptomatic CNS involvement is demonstrable in up to 25% of patients with late latent syphilis. The factors that contribute to the development and progression of tertiary disease are unknown.

The course of untreated syphilis was studied retrospectively in a group of nearly 2000 patients with primary or secondary disease diagnosed clinically (the Oslo Study, 1891–1951) and was assessed prospectively in 431 African-American men with seropositive latent syphilis of $\geq$3 years' duration (the notorious Tuskegee Study, 1932–1972). In the Oslo Study, 24% of patients developed relapsing secondary lesions within 4 years, and 28% eventually developed one or more manifestations of tertiary syphilis. Cardiovascular syphilis, including aortitis, was detected in 10% of patients, none of whom had been infected before age 15; 7% of patients developed symptomatic neurosyphilis, and 16% developed benign tertiary syphilis (gummas of the skin, mucous membranes, and skeleton). Syphilis was the primary cause of death in 15% of men and 8% of women. Cardiovascular syphilis was documented in 35% of men and 22% of women who eventually came to autopsy. In general, serious late complications were nearly twice as common among men as among women.

The Tuskegee Study showed that the death rate among untreated African-American men with syphilis (25 to 50 years old) was 17% higher than that among uninfected subjects and that 30% of all deaths were attributable to cardiovascular or CNS syphilis. By far the most important factor in increased mortality was cardiovascular syphilis. Anatomic evidence of aortitis was found in 40 to 60% of autopsied subjects with syphilis (vs. 15% of control subjects), whereas CNS syphilis was found in only 4%. Rates of hypertension were also higher among the infected subjects. The ethical issues eventually raised by this study, begun in the preantibiotic era but continuing into the early 1970s, had a major influence on the development of current guidelines for human medical experimentation, and the history of the study may still contribute to a reluctance of some African Americans to participate as subjects in clinical research.

These two studies both showed that about one-third of patients with untreated syphilis develop clinical or pathologic evidence of tertiary syphilis, that about one-fourth die as a direct result of tertiary syphilis, and that there is additional excess mortality not directly attributable to tertiary syphilis.

MANIFESTATIONS ■ Primary Syphilis The typical primary chancre usually begins as a single painless papule that rapidly becomes eroded and usually becomes indurated, with a characteristic cartilaginous consistency on palpation of the edge and base of the ulcer. In heterosexual men the chancre is usually located on the penis (Fig. 153-1), whereas in homosexual men it is often found in the anal canal or rectum, in the mouth, or on the external genitalia. In women, common primary

FIGURE 153-1 Primary syphilis with a firm, nontender chancre.

FIGURE 153-2 Secondary syphilis demonstrating the papulosquamous truncal eruption.

FIGURE 153-4 Condylomata lata are moist, somewhat verrucous intertriginous plaques seen in secondary syphilis.

sites are the cervix and labia. Consequently, primary syphilis goes unrecognized in women and homosexual men more often than in heterosexual men. Multiple primary lesions may be more common among men with concurrent HIV infection.

Atypical primary lesions are common. The clinical appearance depends on the number of treponemes inoculated and on the immunologic status of the patient. A large inoculum produces a dark-field-positive ulcerative lesion in nonimmune volunteers but may produce a small dark-field-negative papule, an asymptomatic but seropositive latent infection, or no response at all in individuals with a history of syphilis. A small inoculum may produce only a papular lesion, even in nonimmune individuals. Therefore, syphilis should be considered even in the evaluation of trivial or atypical dark-field-negative genital lesions. The genital lesions that most commonly must be differentiated from those of primary syphilis include those caused by herpes simplex virus infection (Chap. 163), chancroid (Chap. 130), traumatic injury, and donovanosis (Chap. 145). *Primary genital herpes* may produce inguinal adenopathy, but the nodes are tender and the lesions consist of multiple painful vesicles, which later ulcerate and are often accompanied by systemic symptoms, including fever. *Recurrent genital herpes* typically begins with a unilateral cluster of painful vesicles, usually without associated adenopathy. *Chancroid* produces painful, superficial, exudative, nonindurated ulcers, more often multiple than in syphilis (see Fig. 130-2); adenopathy is common, can be either unilateral or bilateral, is tender, and may be suppurative. Donovanosis, which is rare in the United States and Europe, is usually seen as a granulomatous ulcer that, although painless, is friable.

Regional lymphadenopathy usually accompanies the primary syphilitic lesion, appearing within 1 week of the onset of the lesion. The

FIGURE 153-3 Secondary syphilis commonly affects the palms and soles with scaling, firm, red-brown papules.

nodes are firm, nonsuppurative, and painless. Inguinal lymphadenopathy is bilateral and may occur with anal as well as with external genital chancres. The chancre generally heals within 4 to 6 weeks (range, 2 to 12 weeks), but lymphadenopathy may persist for months.

Secondary Syphilis   The protean manifestations of the secondary stage usually include localized or diffuse symmetric mucocutaneous lesions and generalized nontender lymphadenopathy. The healing primary chancre is still present in 15% of cases, and the stages may overlap more frequently in persons with concurrent HIV infection than in those without this co-infection. The skin rash consists of macular, papular, papulosquamous, and occasionally pustular syphilides; often more than one form is present simultaneously. The eruption may be very subtle. Approximately 25% of patients with a discernible rash of secondary syphilis may be unaware that they have dermatologic manifestations. Initial lesions are bilaterally symmetric, pale red or pink, nonpruritic, discrete, round macules that measure 5 to 10 mm in diameter and are distributed on the trunk and proximal extremities. After several days or weeks, red papular lesions 3 to 10 mm in diameter also appear (Fig. 153-2). These lesions, which may progress to necrotic lesions (resembling pustules) in association with increasing endarteritis and perivascular mononuclear infiltration, are distributed widely, frequently involve the palms and soles (Fig. 153-3), and may occur on the face and scalp. Tiny papular *follicular syphilides* involving hair follicles may result in patchy alopecia, with loss of scalp hair, eyebrows, or beard in up to 5% of cases.

In warm, moist, intertriginous body areas, including the perianal area, vulva, scrotum, inner thighs, axillae, and skin under pendulous breasts, papules can enlarge and become eroded to produce broad, moist, pink or gray-white, highly infectious lesions called *condylomata lata* (Fig. 153-4); these lesions develop in 10% of patients with secondary syphilis. Superficial mucosal erosions, called *mucous patches*, occur in 10 to 15% of patients and may involve the lips, oral mucosa, tongue (Fig. 153-5), palate, pharynx, vulva and vagina, glans penis, or inner prepuce. The typical mucous patch is a painless silver-gray erosion surrounded by a red periphery. During relapses of secondary syphilis, condylomata lata are particularly common, and skin lesions tend to be asymmetrically distributed and more infiltrated, resembling skin lesions of late syphilis. These characteristics may reflect increasing cellular immunity.

Constitutional symptoms that may accompany or precede secondary syphilis include sore throat (15 to 30%), fever (5 to 8%), weight loss (2 to 20%), malaise (25%), anorexia (2 to 10%), headache (10%), and meningismus (5%). *Acute meningitis* occurs in only 1 to 2% of cases, but numbers of cells and levels of protein in CSF are increased

FIGURE 153-5 Mucous patches on the tongue of a patient with secondary syphilis. (*Courtesy of Ron Roddy.*)

in ≥30% of cases. *T. pallidum* has been recovered from CSF during primary and secondary syphilis in 30% of cases; this finding is often but not always associated with other CSF abnormalities.

Less common complications of secondary syphilis include hepatitis, nephropathy, gastrointestinal involvement (hypertrophic gastritis, patchy proctitis, ulcerative colitis, or a rectosigmoid mass), arthritis, and periostitis. Ocular findings that suggest secondary syphilis include otherwise-unexplained pupillary abnormalities, optic neuritis, and a retinitis pigmentosa syndrome as well as the classic iritis (especially granulomatous iritis) or uveitis. The diagnosis of secondary syphilis is often considered in such patients only after they fail to respond to steroid therapy. Anterior uveitis has been reported in 5 to 10% of patients with secondary syphilis, and *T. pallidum* has been demonstrated in the aqueous humor from such patients. Hepatic involvement is common in syphilis; although it is usually asymptomatic, at least 25% of patients may have abnormal liver function tests. Frank *syphilitic hepatitis* is distinguished by an unusually high serum level of alkaline phosphatase and by a nonspecific histologic appearance that is unlike that of viral hepatitis and includes moderate inflammation with polymorphonuclear leukocytes and lymphocytes, some hepatocellular damage, and no cholestasis. *Renal involvement* produces proteinuria associated with an acute nephrotic syndrome (or rarely with hemorrhagic glomerulonephritis) and is characterized by subepithelial electron-dense deposits and glomerular immune complexes—findings suggesting immune-complex glomerulonephritis. Like those of primary syphilis, the manifestations of the secondary stage resolve spontaneously, usually within 1 to 6 months.

Latent Syphilis Positive serologic tests for syphilis, together with a normal CSF examination and the absence of clinical manifestations of syphilis, indicate a diagnosis of latent syphilis. The diagnosis is often suspected on the basis of a history of primary or secondary lesions, a history of exposure to syphilis, or the delivery of an infant with congenital syphilis. A previous negative serologic test or a history of lesions or exposure may help establish the duration of latent infection, which is an important factor in the selection of appropriate therapy. *Early latent* syphilis encompasses the first year after infection, whereas *late latent* syphilis (beginning ≥1 year after infection in the untreated patient) is associated with relative immunity to infectious relapse. *T. pallidum* may still seed the bloodstream intermittently during the latent stage, and pregnant women with latent syphilis may infect the fetus in utero. Moreover, syphilis has been transmitted through the transfusion of blood from patients with latent syphilis of many years' duration. It was previously thought that untreated late latent syphilis had three

possible outcomes: (1) it could persist throughout the lifetime of the infected individual; (2) it could end in the development of late syphilis; or (3) it could end with the spontaneous cure of infection, with reversion of serologic tests to negative. It is now apparent, however, that the more sensitive treponemal antibody tests rarely, if ever, become negative without treatment. About 70% of untreated patients with latent syphilis never develop clinically evident late syphilis, but the occurrence of spontaneous cure is in doubt.

Involvement of the Central Nervous System Traditionally, neurosyphilis has been considered to be a late manifestation of syphilis, but this view is inaccurate. CNS syphilis represents a continuum encompassing early invasion (usually within the first weeks or months of infection), months to years of asymptomatic involvement, and, in some cases, development of early or late neurologic manifestations.

ASYMPTOMATIC NEUROSYPHILIS The diagnosis of asymptomatic neurosyphilis is made in patients who lack neurologic symptoms and signs but who have CSF abnormalities including mononuclear pleocytosis, increased protein concentrations, or a reactive Venereal Disease Research Laboratory (VDRL) slide test. Such abnormalities are found in up to one-quarter of patients with untreated latent syphilis, and these are the patients who are known to be at risk for neurologic complications. In primary and secondary syphilis, such abnormalities may be found in up to 40% of untreated patients, and *T. pallidum* can be isolated from CSF of 30% of patients even in the absence of other CSF abnormalities. Although the therapeutic implications of these findings in early syphilis are uncertain, it seems appropriate to conclude that even patients with early syphilis who have such findings do indeed have asymptomatic neurosyphilis and should be treated for neurosyphilis. In patients with untreated asymptomatic neurosyphilis, the overall cumulative probability of progression to clinical neurosyphilis is about 20% in the first 10 years but increases with time; the likelihood is highest among patients with the greatest degree of pleocytosis or protein elevation. Patients with untreated latent syphilis and normal CSF probably run no risk of subsequent neurosyphilis. In one study, neurosyphilis was associated with a rapid plasma reagin (RPR) titer of ≥1:32, regardless of clinical stage or HIV infection status.

SYMPTOMATIC NEUROSYPHILIS Although mixed features are common, the major clinical categories of symptomatic neurosyphilis include meningeal, meningovascular, and parenchymatous syphilis. The last category includes general paresis and tabes dorsalis. The onset of symptoms usually comes <1 year after infection for meningeal syphilis, at 5 to 10 years for meningovascular syphilis, at 20 years for general paresis, and at 25 to 30 years for tabes dorsalis. However, symptomatic neurosyphilis, particularly in the antibiotic era, often presents not as a classic picture but rather as mixed and subtle or incomplete syndromes.

Meningeal syphilis may involve either the brain or the spinal cord, and patients may present with headache, nausea, vomiting, neck stiffness, cranial nerve involvement, seizures, and changes in mental status. This condition may be concurrent with or may follow the secondary stage. Patients presenting with uveitis or iritis frequently have meningeal syphilis. *Meningovascular syphilis* reflects diffuse inflammation of the pia and arachnoid together with evidence of focal or widespread arterial involvement of small, medium, or large vessels. The most common presentation is a stroke syndrome involving the middle cerebral artery of a relatively young adult; however, unlike the usual thrombotic or embolic stroke syndrome of sudden onset, meningovascular syphilis often becomes manifest after a subacute encephalitic prodrome (with headaches, vertigo, insomnia, and psychological abnormalities), which is followed by a gradually progressive vascular syndrome.

The manifestations of *general paresis* reflect widespread late parenchymal damage and include abnormalities corresponding to the mnemonic *paresis:* *p*ersonality, *a*ffect, *r*eflexes (hyperactive), *e*ye (e.g., Argyll Robertson pupils), *s*ensorium (illusions, delusions, hallucinations), *i*ntellect (a decrease in recent memory and in the capacity for orientation, calculations, judgment, and insight), and *s*peech. *Tabes* *dorsalis* is also a late manifestation of syphilis that presents as symptoms and signs of demyelination of the posterior columns, dorsal roots, and dorsal root ganglia. Symptoms include ataxic wide-based gait and footslap; paresthesia; bladder disturbances; impotence; areflexia; and loss of position, deep pain, and temperature sensations. Trophic joint degeneration (Charcot's joints) and perforating ulceration of the feet can result from loss of pain sensation. The small, irregular Argyll Robertson pupil, a feature of both tabes dorsalis and paresis, reacts to accommodation but not to light. *Optic atrophy* also occurs frequently in association with tabes.

Other Manifestations of Late Syphilis The slowly progressive inflammatory disease leading to tertiary manifestations begins early during the pathogenesis of syphilis, although these manifestations may not become clinically apparent for years. Early syphilitic aortitis becomes evident soon after secondary lesions subside, and treponemes that trigger the development of gummas may have seeded the tissue years earlier.

CARDIOVASCULAR SYPHILIS Cardiovascular manifestations are attributable to endarteritis obliterans of the vasa vasorum, which provide the blood supply to large vessels. This condition results in uncomplicated aortitis, aortic regurgitation, saccular aneurysm, or coronary ostial stenosis, with symptoms usually appearing 10 to 40 years after infection. In the preantibiotic era, symptomatic cardiovascular complications developed in ~10% of persons with late untreated syphilis, although syphilitic aortitis was demonstrated at autopsy in about one-half of African-American men with untreated syphilis.

Linear calcification of the ascending aorta on chest x-ray films suggests asymptomatic syphilitic aortitis, as arteriosclerosis seldom produces this sign. Syphilitic aneurysms—usually saccular, occasionally fusiform—do not lead to dissection. Only 1 in 10 aortic aneurysms of syphilitic origin involves the abdominal aorta.

LATE BENIGN SYPHILIS (GUMMA) Gummas may be multiple or diffuse but are usually solitary lesions that range from microscopic in size to several centimeters in diameter. Histologic examination shows a granulomatous inflammation with a central area of necrosis. Although rarely demonstrated microscopically, *T. pallidum* has reportedly been recovered from these lesions. The most commonly involved sites include the skin and skeletal system, the mouth and upper respiratory tract, the larynx, the liver, and the stomach; however, any organ may be involved. Gummas of the skin produce painless and indurated nodular, papulosquamous, or ulcerative lesions that are usually indolent. These lesions may resemble those of many other chronic granulomatous conditions, including tuberculosis and sarcoidosis, leprosy, and deep fungal infections. Skeletal gummas most frequently involve the long bones of the legs, although any bone may be affected. Radiographic abnormalities with advanced gummas of bone include periostitis or destructive or sclerosing osteitis. Upper respiratory gummas can lead to perforation of the nasal septum or palate.

Because the histologic changes may be suggestive but are nonspecific, the diagnosis of late benign syphilis is confirmed by serologic testing and by therapeutic trial. Treatment with penicillin results in rapid healing of active gummatous lesions.

Congenital Syphilis Transmission of *T. pallidum* from a syphilitic woman to her fetus across the placenta may occur at any stage of pregnancy, but the lesions of congenital syphilis generally have their onset after the fourth month of gestation, when fetal immunologic competence begins to develop. This timing suggests that the pathogenesis of congenital syphilis depends on the immune response of the host rather than on a direct toxic effect of *T. pallidum*. The risk of infection of the fetus during untreated early maternal syphilis is estimated to be 75 to 95%, decreasing to about 35% for maternal syphilis of >2 years' duration. Adequate treatment of the mother before the 16th week of pregnancy should prevent fetal damage. Untreated maternal infection may result in a rate of fetal loss of up to 40% (with stillbirth more common than abortion because of the late onset of fetal pathology), prematurity, neonatal death, or nonfatal congenital syph-

ilis. Among infants born alive, only fulminant congenital syphilis is clinically apparent at birth, and these babies have a very poor prognosis. The most common clinical problem is the healthy-appearing baby born to a mother with a positive serologic test. Routine serologic testing in early pregnancy is considered cost-effective in virtually all populations, even in areas with a low prenatal prevalence of syphilis. Where the prevalence of syphilis is high or when the patient is at high risk, serologic testing should be repeated in the third trimester and at delivery.

The manifestations of congenital syphilis can be divided into three types according to their timing: (1) early manifestations, which appear within the first 2 years of life (often between 2 and 10 weeks of age), are infectious and resemble the manifestations of severe secondary syphilis in the adult; (2) late manifestations, which appear after 2 years and are noninfectious; and (3) residual stigmata. The earliest sign of congenital syphilis is usually rhinitis, or "snuffles" (23%), which is soon followed by other mucocutaneous lesions (35 to 41%). These may include bullae (syphilitic pemphigus), vesicles, superficial desquamation, petechiae, and (later) papulosquamous lesions, mucous patches, and condylomata lata. The most common early manifestations are bone changes (61%), including osteochondritis, osteitis, and periostitis. Hepatosplenomegaly (50%), lymphadenopathy (32%), anemia (34%), jaundice (30%), thrombocytopenia, and leukocytosis are common. *T. pallidum* can be isolated, by rabbit inoculation, from the CSF of 22% of infected neonates without prior antibiotic exposure.

Neonatal congenital syphilis must be differentiated from other generalized congenital infections, including rubella, cytomegalovirus or herpes simplex virus infection, and toxoplasmosis, as well as from erythroblastosis fetalis. Neonatal death is usually due to pulmonary hemorrhage, secondary bacterial infection, or severe hepatitis.

Late congenital syphilis is that which remains untreated after 2 years of age. In 60% of cases, the infection remains subclinical; the clinical spectrum in the remainder of cases differs in certain respects from that of acquired late syphilis in the adult. For example, cardiovascular syphilis rarely develops in late congenital syphilis, whereas interstitial keratitis is much more common and occurs between the ages of 5 and 25. Other manifestations include eighth-nerve deafness and recurrent arthropathy. Bilateral knee effusions are known as *Clutton's joints*. Asymptomatic neurosyphilis is present in about one-third of untreated patients, and clinical neurosyphilis occurs in one-quarter of untreated individuals >6 years old. Gummatous periostitis occurs between the ages of 5 and 20 and, as in nonvenereal endemic syphilis, tends to cause destructive lesions of the palate and nasal septum.

Characteristic stigmata include *Hutchinson's teeth*—centrally notched, widely spaced, peg-shaped upper central incisors—and "mulberry" molars—sixth-year molars with multiple, poorly developed cusps. The abnormal facies of patients with congenital syphilis include frontal bossing, saddle nose, and poorly developed maxillae. Saber shins, characterized by anterior tibial bowing, are rare. *Rhagades* are linear scars at the angles of the mouth and nose that are caused by secondary bacterial infection of the early facial eruption.

LABORATORY EXAMINATIONS ■ Demonstration of the Organism *T. pallidum* cannot be detected by culture; therefore, other tests are necessary. Dark-field microscopic examination of lesion exudate is useful in evaluating moist cutaneous lesions, such as the chancre of primary syphilis or the condylomata lata of secondary syphilis. The identification of a single characteristic motile organism by a trained observer is sufficient for diagnosis. Examination of oral lesions and anal ulcers by this method is not recommended, as it is difficult to differentiate *T. pallidum* from other spirochetes that may be present.

Most syphilis is diagnosed in settings where dark-field microscopy is not available. The direct fluorescent antibody *T. pallidum* (DFA-TP) test, an alternative available at central laboratories, uses fluorescein-conjugated polyclonal antitreponemal antibody for the detection of *T. pallidum* in fixed smears prepared from suspect lesions. More sensitive PCR tests have been developed but are available only in research laboratories.

T. pallidum can be found in tissue with appropriate silver stains, although these results should be interpreted with caution because artifacts resembling *T. pallidum* are often seen. Treponemes can be demonstrated more reliably in tissue by immunofluorescence or immunohistochemical methods using specific monoclonal or polyclonal antibodies to *T. pallidum*.

Serologic Tests for Syphilis There are two types of serologic test for syphilis: nontreponemal and treponemal. Both types of test are reactive in persons with any treponemal infection, including yaws, pinta, and endemic syphilis.

The nontreponemal tests measure IgG and IgM directed against a cardiolipin-lecithin-cholesterol antigen complex. The most widely used nontreponemal antibody tests for syphilis are the RPR test, which can be automated (ART), and the VDRL slide test. The RPR test is easier to perform and uses unheated serum; it is the test of choice for rapid serologic diagnosis in a clinic or office setting. The VDRL test, however, remains the standard for use with CSF.

The RPR and VDRL tests are equally sensitive and may be used for initial screening or for quantitation of serum antibody. The titer reflects the activity of the disease. Titers rise during the evolution of early syphilis; VDRL titers usually reach 1:32 or higher in secondary syphilis. A persistent fall by two dilutions (fourfold) or more after treatment of early syphilis provides essential evidence of an adequate response to therapy. VDRL titers do not correspond directly to RPR titers, and sequential quantitative testing (as for response to therapy) must employ a single test.

Two standard treponemal tests are used for confirmation of reactive nontreponemal results: the fluorescent treponemal antibody–absorbed (FTA-ABS) test and the agglutination assays for antibodies to *T. pallidum*. The microhemagglutination assay for *T. pallidum* (MHA-TP) has been replaced by the Serodia TP-PA test (Fujirebio, Tokyo), which is more sensitive for primary syphilis. The *T. pallidum* hemagglutination test (TPHA) is widely used in Europe but is not available in the United States. Both the agglutination assays and the FTA-ABS test are very specific and, when used for confirmation of positive nontreponemal tests, have a very high positive predictive value for the diagnosis of syphilis. However, even these tests give false-positive results at rates as high as 1 to 2% when used for the screening of normal populations. New enzyme-linked immunosorbent assays have also been approved as confirmatory tests.

The relative sensitivities of the VDRL and RPR tests, the FTA-ABS test, and the TP-PA test in the various stages of untreated syphilis are shown in Table 153-1. The nontreponemal tests may be nonreactive in very early primary syphilis, and the detection of antibody can be maximized by the performance of a treponemal test. All treponemal and nontreponemal tests are reactive during secondary syphilis, and a nonreactive result virtually excludes syphilis in a patient with otherwise-compatible mucocutaneous lesions. (Fewer than 1% of patients with secondary syphilis have a VDRL test that is nonreactive or weakly reactive with undiluted serum but is positive at higher serum dilutions—the *prozone phenomenon*.) Although the nontreponemal tests will become nonreactive or will be reactive at lower titers after therapy for early syphilis, the treponemal tests often remain reactive after therapy and therefore are not helpful in determining the infection status of persons with past syphilis. Treatment of early primary syphilis may result in seroreversion in treponemal tests.

For practical purposes, most clinicians need to be familiar with the three uses of serologic tests for syphilis: (1) testing of large numbers of sera for screening or diagnostic purposes (e.g., the RPR or VDRL test), (2) quantitative measurement of antibody titer to assess the clinical activity of syphilis or to monitor the response to therapy (e.g., the RPR or VDRL test), and (3) confirmation of the diagnosis of syphilis in a patient with a positive nontreponemal antibody test or with a

TABLE 153-1 *Sensitivity of Serodiagnostic Tests in Untreated Syphilis*

| Test[a] | Mean Percentage Positive (Range) at Indicated Stage of Disease[b] | | | |
	Primary	Secondary	Latent	Tertiary
VDRL, RPR	78 (74–87)	100	95 (88–100)	71 (37–94)
FTA-ABS	84 (70–100)	100	100	96
TP-PA[c]	89	100	100	NA

[a] The specificity for each of these tests is 94 to 99%.
[b] In CDC studies.
[c] Limited numbers of sera have been evaluated by TP-PA.
Source: Modified from SA Larsen et al: Clin Microbiol Rev 8:1, 1995; and V Pope et al: J Clin Microbiol 38:2543, 2000.

suspected clinical diagnosis of syphilis (e.g., the FTA-ABS test or the Serodia TP-PA test).

For measurement of IgM in neonates in whom congenital syphilis is suspected, the syphilis Captia-M test (Trinity Biotech, Jamestown, NY) and the 19S IgM FTA-ABS test are available.

False-Positive Serologic Tests for Syphilis Because the antigen used in nontreponemal tests is found in other tissues, the tests may be reactive in persons without treponemal infection, although rarely do titers exceed 1:8 in such patients. In a population selected for screening because of clinical suspicion, history of exposure, or increased risk for sexually transmitted infections, fewer than 1% of reactive tests are falsely positive. The modern VDRL and RPR tests are 97 to 99% specific, and false-positive reactions are now limited largely to those conditions listed in Table 153-2. False positivity is common among persons with autoimmune disorders. The prevalence of false-positive nontreponemal tests increases with advancing age; 10% of people >70 years of age have false-positive reactions. In the patient with a false-positive nontreponemal test, syphilis is excluded by a nonreactive treponemal test.

Evaluation for Neurosyphilis Involvement of the CNS is detected by examination of CSF for pleocytosis (>5 white blood cells/mm^3), increased protein concentration (>45 mg/dL), or VDRL reactivity. CSF abnormalities can be demonstrated in up to 40% of cases of primary or secondary syphilis and in 25% of cases of latent syphilis. In older asymptomatic seropositive individuals, the yield of lumbar puncture is relatively low. *T. pallidum* has been recovered by CSF inoculation into rabbits from up to 30% of patients with primary or secondary syphilis but rarely from those with latent syphilis. The demonstration of *T. pallidum* in CSF is often associated with other CSF abnormalities; however, organisms can be recovered from patients with otherwise-normal CSF. Before the advent of penicillin, the risk of developing clinical neurosyphilis was roughly proportional to the intensity of CSF changes. CSF examination is recommended by the Centers for Disease Control and Prevention (CDC) in the evaluation of any sero-

TABLE 153-2 *Causes of False-Positive Reactions in Nontreponemal Serologic Tests for Syphilis*

Cause	Rate of False-Positive Reactions, %[a]
ACUTE FALSE-POSITIVE REACTION (<6 MONTHS)	
Recent viral illness or immunization	1–2
Genital herpes	4
Human immunodeficiency virus infection	1–4
Malaria	11
Parenteral drug use	20–25
CHRONIC FALSE-POSITIVE REACTION (≥6 MONTHS)	
Aging	9–11
Autoimmune disorders	1–20
Systemic lupus erythematosus	11–20
Rheumatoid arthritis	5
Parenteral drug use	20–25

[a] Data were collected from a variety of published reports.

positive patient with neurologic signs and symptoms, patients with other late syphilis, cases of suspected treatment failure, and HIV-infected patients with untreated syphilis of unknown duration or of >1 year's duration. The possibility of asymptomatic neurosyphilis in some patients with early disease is not addressed by these recommendations. Because standard therapy with penicillin G benzathine (benzathine benzylpenicillin) for early syphilis fails to result in treponemicidal drug levels in the CSF, some experts also advise lumbar puncture in early syphilis, particularly in patients with HIV infection or with non-treponemal test titers of ≥1:32.

The CSF VDRL test is highly specific but is insensitive and may be non-reactive even in cases of progressive symptomatic neurosyphilis. The degree of sensitivity is highest in meningovascular syphilis and paresis and is lower in asymptomatic neurosyphilis and tabes dorsalis. The unabsorbed FTA test on CSF is reactive far more often than the CSF VDRL test in all stages of syphilis, but FTA reactivity may reflect passive transfer of serum antibody into the CSF. A nonreactive CSF FTA test, however, may be used to rule out neurosyphilis.

TABLE 153-3 *Recommendations for the Treatment of Syphilis[a]*

Stage of Syphilis	Patients without Penicillin Allergy	Patients with Confirmed Penicillin Allergy
Primary, secondary, or early latent	Penicillin G benzathine (single dose of 2.4 mU IM)	Tetracycline hydrochloride (500 mg PO qid) or doxycycline (100 mg PO bid) for 2 weeks
Late latent (or latent of uncertain duration), cardiovascular, or benign tertiary	Lumbar puncture CSF normal: Penicillin G benzathine (2.4 mU IM weekly for 3 weeks) CSF abnormal: Treat as neurosyphilis	Lumbar puncture CSF normal and patient not infected with HIV: Tetracycline hydrochloride (500 mg PO qid) or doxycycline (100 mg PO bid) for 4 weeks CSF normal and patient infected with HIV: Desensitization and treatment with penicillin if compliance cannot be ensured CSF abnormal: Treat as neurosyphilis
Neurosyphilis (asymptomatic or symptomatic)	Aqueous penicillin G (18–24 mU/d IV, given as 3–4 mU q4h or continuous infusion) for 10–14 days *or* Aqueous penicillin G procaine (2.4 mU/d IM) plus oral probenecid (500 mg qid), both for 10–14 days	Desensitization and treatment with penicillin
Syphilis in pregnancy	According to stage	Desensitization and treatment with penicillin

[a] See text for full discussion of syphilis therapy in HIV-infected individuals.
Abbreviation: mU, million units.
Source: These recommendations are based on those issued by the Centers for Disease Control and Prevention in 2002.

Evaluation for Syphilis in Patients Infected with HIV
Because persons at highest risk for syphilis (inner-city populations, homosexually active men, and people in many developing countries) are also at increased risk for HIV infection, these two infections frequently coexist. There is evidence that syphilis and other genital-ulcer diseases may be important risk factors for the acquisition and transmission of HIV infection.

The manifestations of syphilis may be altered in patients with concurrent HIV infection, and multiple cases of neurologic relapse after standard therapy have been reported in HIV-infected patients. *T. pallidum* has been isolated from the CSF of several patients after therapy for early syphilis with penicillin G benzathine. A multicenter U.S. study of early syphilis found similar clinical responses to therapy in persons with and without concurrent HIV infection, although the study lacked sufficient statistical power to exclude an effect of HIV and 41% of subjects were lost to follow-up. Serologically defined treatment failure was more common among HIV-infected patients than among those without this co-infection. This investigation confirmed the high rate of CNS invasion in early syphilis and the persistence of *T. pallidum* after standard therapy: 11 of 43 HIV-infected patients and 21 of 88 HIV-uninfected patients had *T. pallidum* detectable in CSF before therapy; 7 of the 35 patients who underwent lumbar puncture after therapy (some HIV-infected and others uninfected) still had *T. pallidum* detectable in CSF.

There is no clear evidence that the sensitivity of serologic tests for syphilis differs in HIV-infected versus HIV-uninfected patients. Rates of decline of serologic titers appear to be slower in HIV-infected individuals. The clinical significance of this observation is unclear.

Persons with newly diagnosed HIV infection should be tested for syphilis; conversely, all patients with newly diagnosed syphilis should be tested for HIV infection. Some authorities, persuaded by reports of the persistence of *T. pallidum* in the CSF of HIV-infected persons after standard penicillin benzathine therapy for early syphilis, recommend examination of CSF for evidence of neurosyphilis for all co-infected patients, regardless of the clinical stage of syphilis, with treatment for neurosyphilis if CSF abnormalities are found or if CSF examination is not performed. Others do not recommend routine CSF examination for HIV-co-infected patients with early syphilis and believe that standard therapy is sufficient. Serologic testing after treatment is important for all patients with syphilis, particularly those also infected with HIV.

Rx TREATMENT

Treatment of Acquired Syphilis The CDC's 2002 guidelines for the treatment of syphilis are summarized in Table 153-3 and are discussed below. Penicillin G is the drug of choice for all stages of syphilis. *T. pallidum* is killed by very low concentrations of penicillin G, although a long period of exposure to penicillin is required because of the unusually slow rate of multiplication of the organism. The efficacy of penicillin against syphilis remains undiminished after 50 years of use. Other antibiotics effective in syphilis include the tetracyclines, erythromycin, and the cephalosporins. Aminoglycosides and spectinomycin inhibit *T. pallidum* only in very large doses, and the sulfonamides and the quinolones are inactive. Azithromycin shows significant promise as an effective oral agent against *T. pallidum*.

Serum levels of penicillin G of ≥0.03 μg/mL for at least 7 days are considered necessary for the cure of early syphilis. Recurrence rates for a given regimen increase as infection progresses from incubating to seronegative primary to seropositive primary to secondary to late syphilis. Therefore, it is probable, but unproven, that a longer duration of therapy is required to effect cure as the infection progresses.

PATIENTS WITH EARLY SYPHILIS AND THEIR CONTACTS Preventive (abortive, "epidemiologic") treatment is recommended for seronegative individuals without signs of syphilis who have been exposed to infectious syphilis within the previous 3 months. Before treatment is given, every effort should be made to establish a diagnosis by examination and serologic testing. *The regimens recommended for prevention are the same as those recommended for early syphilis.*

Penicillin G benzathine is the most widely used agent for the treatment of early syphilis, although it is more painful on injection than penicillin G procaine. A single dose of 2.4 million units cures more than 95% of cases of primary syphilis. Because the drug's efficacy in secondary syphilis may be slightly lower, some physicians administer a second dose of 2.4 million units 1 week after the initial dose at this stage of disease. Clinical relapse can follow treatment with penicillin G benzathine in patients with both HIV infection and early syphilis. Because the risk of neurorelapse may be higher in HIV-infected patients, examination of CSF from HIV-seropositive individuals with syphilis of any stage is recommended by some experts; therapy appropriate for neurosyphilis should be given if there is any evidence of CNS syphilis.

For penicillin-allergic patients with early syphilis, a 2-week course of therapy with doxycycline or tetracycline is recommended. These regimens appear to be effective, although no well-controlled studies have been performed and poor compliance may be problematic. Limited studies suggest that ceftriaxone (1 g/d, given intramuscularly or intravenously, for 8 to 10 days) and azithromycin (a single oral dose of 2 g) may be effective against early syphilis. These nonpenicillin regimens have not been evaluated in HIV-infected individuals and should be used with caution.

LATE LATENT AND LATE SYPHILIS   If CSF abnormalities are found, the patient should be treated for neurosyphilis. The recommended treatment for late latent syphilis with normal CSF, for cardiovascular syphilis, and for late benign syphilis (gumma) is penicillin G benzathine, 2.4 million units intramuscularly once a week for 3 successive weeks (7.2 million units total). Doxycycline or tetracycline (given for 4 weeks) offers an untested alternative for penicillin-allergic patients with latent or late syphilis and normal CSF. Penicillin-allergic HIV-infected persons with late latent or late syphilis should be desensitized and treated with penicillin if compliance and follow-up cannot be ensured. The clinical response to treatment for benign tertiary syphilis is usually impressive; however, responses to therapy for cardiovascular syphilis are not dramatic because aortic aneurysm and aortic regurgitation cannot be reversed by antibiotic treatment.

NEUROSYPHILIS   Penicillin G benzathine, given in total doses of up to 7.2 million units to adults, or 50,000 units/kg to infants, does not produce detectable concentrations of penicillin G in CSF, and asymptomatic neurosyphilis may relapse in patients treated with 2.4 million units; the risk may be higher in HIV-infected patients. Therefore, the use of penicillin G benzathine alone for the treatment of neurosyphilis is not recommended. On the other hand, administration of intravenous penicillin G in recommended doses is thought to ensure treponemicidal concentrations of penicillin G in CSF. The clinical response to penicillin therapy for meningeal syphilis is dramatic, but the response to treatment for parenchymal neurosyphilis is variable. In general, treatment of neurosyphilis with existing damage may produce no clinical change but may arrest disease progression.

Several recent publications have reported neurologic relapse after high-dose intravenous penicillin therapy for neurosyphilis in HIV-infected patients. No alternative therapies have been explored, but careful follow-up is essential, and re-treatment is warranted in such patients.

No data support the use of antibiotics other than penicillin G for the treatment of neurosyphilis; however, some of the third-generation cephalosporins and azithromycin may deserve further evaluation. In patients with penicillin allergy demonstrated by skin testing, desensitization and treatment with penicillin is the recommended course.

MANAGEMENT OF SYPHILIS IN PREGNANCY   Every pregnant woman should undergo a nontreponemal test at her first prenatal visit, and women at high risk of exposure should have a repeat test in the third trimester and at delivery. In the untreated pregnant patient with presumed syphilis, expeditious evaluation and initiation of treatment appropriate to the stage of the disease are essential. Patients should be warned of the risk of a Jarisch-Herxheimer reaction, which may be associated with mild premature contractions but rarely results in premature delivery.

Penicillin is the only recommended therapy for syphilis in pregnancy. If the patient has a well-documented penicillin allergy, desensitization and penicillin therapy should be undertaken according to the CDC's 2002 treatment guidelines. After treatment, a quantitative nontreponemal test should be repeated monthly throughout pregnancy. Treated women whose titers rise by fourfold or who do not show a fourfold decrease in titer over a 3-month period should be re-treated.

Evaluation and Management of Congenital Syphilis   Newborn infants of mothers with reactive serologic tests may themselves have reactive tests, whether or not they have become infected, because of transplacental transfer of maternal IgG antibody. Rising or persistent titers indicate infection, and the infant should be treated. Neonatal IgM antibody can be detected in cord or neonatal serum with the syphilis Captia-M or 19S IgM FTA-ABS test; its detection indicates active infection. For asymptomatic infants born to women treated adequately with penicillin during pregnancy, monthly quantitative nontreponemal tests may be performed to monitor for appropriate declines in titer.

An infant should be treated at birth if the seropositive mother has received penicillin therapy in the third trimester, inadequate penicillin treatment, or therapy with a drug other than penicillin; if her treatment status is unknown; or if the infant may be difficult to follow. It is unwise to require proof of diagnosis before treatment in such cases. The CSF should be examined to obtain baseline values before treatment. Penicillin is the only recommended drug for syphilis in infants. The penicillin dosage used for the treatment of the patient with late congenital syphilis is calculated in the same way as for the infant, until dosage based on weight reaches that used for adult neurosyphilis. Specific recommendations for the treatment of infants are included in the CDC's 2002 guidelines.

Jarisch-Herxheimer Reaction   A dramatic though usually mild reaction consisting of fever (average temperature elevation, 1.5°C), chills, myalgias, headache, tachycardia, increased respiratory rate, increased circulating neutrophil count, and vasodilation with mild hypotension may follow the initiation of treatment for syphilis. This reaction occurs in ~50% of patients with primary syphilis, 90% of those with secondary syphilis, and 25% of those with early latent syphilis, and defervescence takes place within 12 to 24 h. The reaction is more delayed in neurosyphilis, with fever peaking after 12 to 14 h. In patients with secondary syphilis, erythema and edema of the mucocutaneous lesions may increase. Patients should be warned to expect such symptoms, which can be managed with symptom-based treatment. Steroid and other anti-inflammatory therapy is not required for this mild transient reaction.

Follow-Up Evaluation of Responses to Therapy   The response of syphilis to treatment should be determined by monitoring of the quantitative VDRL or RPR titer (Table 153-4). More frequent serologic examination is recommended for patients concurrently infected with HIV. Because the FTA-ABS and agglutination tests remain positive in most patients treated for seropositive syphilis, these tests are not useful in following the response to therapy. After successful treatment of seropositive first-episode primary or secondary syphilis, the VDRL titer progressively declines, becoming negative by 12 months in 40 to 75% of seropositive primary cases and in 20 to 40% of secondary cases. Patients with a history of syphilis have less rapid declines in titer and are less likely to become VDRL- or RPR-negative. Re-treatment should be considered if serologic responses are not adequate or if clinical signs persist or recur. Every effort should be made to differentiate treatment failure from reinfection, and the CSF should be examined. Patients in whom treatment failure is suspected, especially those with abnormal CSF, should be treated for neurosyphilis. If the patient remains seropositive but asymptomatic after such re-treatment, no further therapy is necessary. Patients treated for late latent syphilis frequently have low initial VDRL or RPR titers and may not have a fourfold drop after therapy with penicillin; about half of these patients remain seropositive (with low titers) for years after therapy. Re-treat-

TABLE 153-4 *Recommended Follow-Up Evaluation after Therapy for Syphilis*

Stage of Syphilis	Tests to Perform	When to Perform	Re-Treatment[a] Considered If:
Primary or secondary	Quantitative RPR or VDRL[b]	HIV-uninfected: 6 and 12 months HIV-infected: 3, 6, 9, and 12 months	1. Titer increases by fourfold *or* 2. Titer fails to decline by fourfold or test fails to become nonreactive by 6 months *or* 3. Clinical signs persist or recur
Latent or late	Quantitative RPR or VDRL[b]	6, 12, and 24 months	1. Titer increases by fourfold *or* 2. Initial titer of $\geq$1:32 fails to decline by fourfold by 6 months *or* 3. New clinical signs develop
Neurosyphilis (asymptomatic or symptomatic)	1. If CSF pleocytosis was documented initially, repeat CSF exam. 2. Monitor decline in CSF protein and CSF-VDRL. (Note: Rate of decline may be slow.) 3. Quantitative RPR or VDRL[b]	1. Every 6 months until CSF cell count is normal 2. Until normal 3. At 6, 12, 18, and 24 months	1. CSF cell count has not decreased at 6 months *or* 2. CSF is not normal after 2 years

[a] Try to distinguish between reinfection and treatment failure. If evidence of treatment failure exists, perform CSF examination. If CSF is normal, treat as for late latent syphilis (Table 153-3). If CSF is abnormal, treat as for neurosyphilis (Table 153-3).

[b] VDRL and RPR titers cannot be compared; use the same test for each follow-up sample.

ment is not warranted unless the titer rises or signs and symptoms of syphilis appear.

The activity of neurosyphilis correlates best with CSF pleocytosis, and this measure provides the most sensitive index of response to treatment. An elevated CSF cell count falls to normal in 3 to 12 months in adequately treated HIV-uninfected patients. The persistence of mild pleocytosis in HIV-infected patients may be due to the presence of HIV in CSF; this scenario may be difficult to distinguish from treatment failure. Elevated levels of CSF protein fall more slowly, and the CSF VDRL titer declines gradually over a period of several years.

IMMUNITY TO AND PREVENTION OF SYPHILIS The rate of development of acquired resistance to *T. pallidum* after natural or experimental infection is related to the size of the antigenic stimulus, which depends on both the size of the infecting inoculum and the duration of infection before treatment. The role of serum antibody in conferring immunity to syphilis remains undefined, although antibodies have been implicated in strain-specific immunity. Cellular immunity is considered to be of major importance in immunity and in the healing of early lesions. The cellular infiltration, predominantly T lymphocytes and macrophages, produces a T_H1 cytokine milieu consistent with the clearance of organisms by activated macrophages. Specific antibody enhances phagocytosis and is required for macrophage-mediated killing of *T. pallidum*. Recent unpublished studies indicate that sequence variation

of TprK occurs during *T. pallidum* infection. This observation suggests a role for antigenic variation in the persistence of infection and in susceptibility to reinfection with another strain.

FURTHER READING

CENTERS FOR DISEASE CONTROL AND PREVENTION: 2002 sexually transmitted diseases treatment guidelines. MMWR 51(RR-6):18, 2002

HOOK EW III et al: A randomized, comparative pilot study of azithromycin versus benzathine penicillin G for treatment of early syphilis. Sex Transm Dis 29:486, 2002

LUKEHART SA et al: Invasion of the central nervous system by *Treponema pallidum*: Implications for diagnosis and treatment. Ann Intern Med 109: 855, 1988

MARRA CM et al: Risk factors for neurosyphilis (late-breaker abstract). 2002 National STD Prevention Conference (http://www.cdc.gov/nchstp/dstd/2002ConfAbstracts/2002ConfAbLatebreaker.htm)

MCBROOM RL et al: Secondary syphilis in persons infected with and not infected with HIV-1: A comparative immunohistologic study. Am J Dermatopathol 21:432, 1999

MICHELOW IC et al: Central nervous system infection in congenital syphilis. N Engl J Med 346:1792, 2002

ROLFS RT et al: A randomized trial of enhanced therapy for early syphilis in patients with and without human immunodeficiency virus infection. N Engl J Med 337:307, 1997

ROMPALO AM et al: Modification of syphilitic genital ulcer manifestations by coexistent HIV infection. Sex Transm Dis 28:448, 2001

154 ENDEMIC TREPONEMATOSES
Sheila A. Lukehart

The endemic, or nonvenereal, treponematoses are bacterial infections that are caused by close relatives of *Treponema pallidum* subspecies *pallidum*, the etiologic agent of venereal syphilis (Chap. 153). Yaws, pinta, and endemic syphilis are distinguished from venereal syphilis by mode of transmission, age of acquisition, geographic distribution, and clinical features. These infections are limited primarily to rural areas of developing nations and are seen in the United States and Europe only in recent immigrants from endemic regions. Much of our "knowledge" about the endemic treponematoses is based upon impressions and observations of health care workers who have visited endemic areas; virtually no well-designed studies of the natural history, diagnosis, or treatment of these infections have been conducted. The treponemal infections are compared and contrasted in Table 154-1.

EPIDEMIOLOGY The endemic treponematoses are chronic diseases acquired during childhood and, like syphilis, can cause severe late manifestations years after initial infection. These infections were very com-

mon in Africa, Asia, and South America when the World Health Organization (WHO) and UNICEF embarked on a highly successful mass eradication campaign. From 1952 to 1969, it is estimated that over 160 million people were examined for treponemal infections and over 50 million cases, contacts, and latent infections were treated. This categorical program is one of WHO's outstanding successes in that the prevalence of active yaws was reduced from >20% to <1% in many rural areas and endemic syphilis was eradicated in Bosnia. In the decades since the eradication programs, lack of focused surveillance and diversion of resources to other pressing needs have resulted in a resurgence of these infections in some regions, particularly in Africa. The estimated geographic distribution of the endemic treponematoses in the 1990s is shown in Fig. 154-1. In the early 1980s, WHO sponsored a series of regional meetings on the endemic treponematoses, and areas of resurgent yaws morbidity were identified in West Africa (Ivory Coast, Ghana, Togo, Benin) and extending into the Central African Republic and rural Democratic Republic of Congo (formerly Zaire). The prevalence of endemic syphilis is estimated to be >10% in some regions of Mali, Niger, Burkina Faso, and Senegal. In Asia and the western Pacific, yaws is still prevalent in Indonesia,

TABLE 154-1 *Comparison of the Treponemes and Associated Diseases*

Feature	Venereal Syphilis	Yaws	Endemic Syphilis	Pinta
Organism	*T. pallidum* subspecies *pallidum*	*T. pallidum* subspecies *pertenue*	*T. pallidum* subspecies *endemicum*	*T. carateum*
Mode of transmission	Sexual, transplacental	Skin-to-skin	Household contacts: mouth-to-mouth or via shared drinking/eating utensils	Skin-to-skin
Usual age of acquisition	Adulthood	Early childhood	Early childhood	Late childhood
Primary lesion	Cutaneous ulcer (chancre)	Papilloma, often ulcerative	Rarely seen	Nonulcerating papule with satellites, pruritic
Location	Genital, oral, anal	Extremities	Oral	Extremities, face
Secondary lesions	Mucocutaneous lesions; condylomata lata	Cutaneous papulo-squamous lesions; osteoperiostitis	Florid mucocutaneous lesions (mucous patch, split papule, condyloma latum); osteoperiostitis	Pintides, pigmented, pruritic
Infectious relapses	~25%	Common	Unknown	None
Late complications	Gummas, cardiovascular and CNS involvement[a]	Destructive gummas of skin, bone, cartilage	Destructive gummas of skin, bone, cartilage	Nondestructive, dyschromic, achromic macules

[a] CNS involvement in the endemic treponematoses has been postulated by some investigators (see text).

Papua New Guinea, and the Solomon Islands; cases have also been identified in Laos and Kampuchea. In the Americas, foci of yaws persist in Haiti and other Caribbean islands, Peru, Colombia, Ecuador, Brazil, Guyana, and Surinam. Pinta is limited to Central America and northern South America, where it is found rarely and only in remote villages. No accurate prevalence data are available for any of the endemic treponematoses because of a lack of active surveillance for these diseases. WHO estimates that there are 2.6 million cases overall, of which 460,000 are infectious.

MICROBIOLOGY The etiologic agents of the endemic treponematoses are *T. pallidum* subspecies *pertenue* (yaws), *T. pallidum* subspecies *endemicum* (endemic syphilis), and *T. carateum* (pinta). These little-studied organisms are morphologically identical to *T. pallidum* subspecies *pallidum*, and no antigenic differences among the pathogenic treponemes have been identified to date. A controversy has existed about whether the treponematoses are caused by different organisms or by the same organism, with clinical manifestations and routes of transmission defined by the climate of the region and the culture of

the population. Three of the four organisms have been placed in the same species because of their genetic similarity; the fourth (*T. carateum*) remains a separate species simply because no organisms have been available for genetic studies. However, a molecular signature has been defined that can be used to differentiate *T. pallidum* subspecies *pallidum* from the nonvenereal subspecies of *T. pallidum*, and unpublished studies have identified a number of distinct differences in the *tpr* gene family between venereal and nonvenereal treponemes. Whether these differences are related to the different clinical courses has not yet been determined.

CLINICAL FEATURES All of the treponemal infections are characterized by defined disease stages, with a localized primary lesion, disseminated secondary lesions, periods of latency, and possible late lesions. Primary and secondary stages are more frequently overlapping in yaws and endemic syphilis, and the late manifestations of pinta are very mild relative to the destructive lesions of the other treponematoses. The current preference is to divide the clinical course of the endemic treponematoses into "early" and "late" stages.

The major clinical features differing between venereal syphilis and the nonvenereal infections are the apparent lack of congenital transmission and the lack of central nervous system (CNS) involvement in the nonvenereal infections. It is not known whether these distinctions are accurate. Because of the high degree of genetic relatedness among the organisms, there is little biologic reason to think that *T. pallidum* subspecies *endemicum* and *T. pallidum* subspecies *pertenue* would be unable to cross the blood-brain barrier or to invade the placenta. These organisms obviously can disseminate from the site of primary infection to other tissues, and they can persist for decades. In this respect, they are like *T. pallidum* subspecies *pallidum*. The lack of recognized congenital infection may be due to the fact that the nonvenereal treponematoses are usually acquired during childhood. By the time an infected girl becomes sexually mature, she would be at low risk for

Pinta
Yaws–Pian
Endemic syphilis–Syphilis endémique

WHO 92522

FIGURE 154-1 Geographic distribution of endemic treponematoses in the 1990s. *(Courtesy of the World Health Organization.)*

transplacental transmission. Neurologic involvement may not have been recognized in nonvenereal treponemal infection because of the lack of trained medical personnel in endemic regions, the lag of years to decades between acquisition of infection and possible CNS manifestations, or a low rate of symptomatic CNS disease.

Some published evidence supports congenital transmission as well as cardiovascular, ophthalmologic, and CNS involvement in yaws. Although the case is strong, particularly for CNS involvement, most studies that have shown a relatively high incidence (average, 24.9%) of cerebrospinal fluid (CSF) abnormalities in patients with yaws were not controlled for other possible causes of CSF abnormalities, did not include treponeme-specific tests, or did not follow patients for resolution of abnormalities after antitreponemal therapy. Thus, while no firm conclusions can be drawn about the invasion of the CNS and placenta by the non-*pallidum* treponemes, it may be erroneous to accept unquestioningly the frequently repeated belief that these organisms fail to cause such manifestations.

Yaws Also known as *pian*, *framboesia*, or *bouba*, yaws is a chronic infection that is usually acquired in childhood and is caused by *T. pallidum* subspecies *pertenue*. The disease is characterized by the development of one or several primary lesions (called the "mother yaw"), followed by the appearance of multiple disseminated skin lesions. The early lesions may persist for many months, are infectious, and usually recur several times within the early years of infection. Late manifestations are destructive and can involve skin, bone, and joints.

The infection is transmitted by direct contact with infectious lesions, and transmission may be enhanced by disruption of the skin by insect bites or abrasions. Children with open lesions and without covering clothing are most likely to transmit infection during play or group sleeping. After an average incubation period estimated at 3 to 4 weeks, the first lesion begins as a papule, usually on an extremity, and then enlarges (particularly during moist warm weather) to become papillomatous or "raspberry-like" (thus the name "framboesia") (Fig. 154-2). Regional lymphadenopathy develops, and the lesion usually heals within 6 months; dissemination is thought to occur during the early weeks and months of infection. A generalized secondary eruption, accompanied by generalized lymphadenopathy, appears either concurrent with or following the primary lesion, may take several forms (macular, papular, or papillomatous), and may become secondarily infected with other bacteria. Painful papillomatous lesions on the soles of the feet result in a painful crablike gait ("crab yaws"), and periostitis may result in nocturnal bone pain and polydactylitis. All early skin lesions are infectious, and cutaneous relapses are common during the first 5 years. Late yaws is recognized in ~10% of untreated patients and is manifested by gummas of the skin and long bone, hyperkeratoses of the palms and soles, osteitis and periostitis, and hydrarthrosis. The late gummatous lesions are characteristically very destructive and extensive. Destruction of the nose, maxilla, palate, and pharynx is termed *gangosa* and is similar to the destructive lesions seen in leprosy and leishmaniasis.

Endemic Syphilis Endemic syphilis, also called *bejel*, *siti*, *dichuchwa*, *njovera*, or *skerljevo*, is a chronic infection caused by *T. pallidum* subspecies *endemicum*. Like other endemic treponematoses, endemic syphilis is chronic and is acquired in childhood. The early lesions are primarily localized to the mucocutaneous and mucosal surfaces, and the infection may be transmitted by direct contact, by kissing, or by sharing drinking and eating utensils. A role for insects in transmission has been suggested but is unproved. The initial lesion, usually an intraoral papule (Fig. 154-2), often goes unrecognized and is followed by mucous patches on the oral mucosa and mucocutaneous lesions resembling the condylomata lata of secondary syphilis. This eruption may last for months or even years, and treponemes can readily be demonstrated in early lesions. Periostitis and regional lymphadenopathy are common. After a variable period of latency, late manifestations may appear, including osseous and cutaneous gummas. Destructive gummas, osteitis, and gangosa are more common in endemic syphilis than in late yaws. Gummas of the nipples develop in women who have previously had endemic syphilis and who breast-feed infants with oral lesions. Thus, it appears that the late lesion may result from repeated exposure of a sensitized host.

Pinta Pinta (also called *mal del pinto*, *carate*, *azul*, or *purupuru*) is the most benign of the treponemal infections and is caused by *T. carateum*. This disease has three stages that are characterized by marked changes in skin color (Fig. 154-2), but it does not appear to cause destructive lesions or to involve other tissues. Transmission occurs by direct contact, usually during late childhood. The initial papule is most often located on the extremities or face and is pruritic. After one to many months of infection, numerous disseminated secondary lesions (*pintides*) appear. These lesions are initially red but become deeply pigmented, ultimately turning a dark slate blue. The secondary lesions are infectious and highly pruritic and may persist for years. Late pigmented lesions are called *dyschromic macules* and contain treponemes. Over time, most pigmented lesions show varying degrees of depigmentation, becoming brown and eventually white and giving the skin a mottled appearance. White achromic lesions are characteristic of the late stage.

DIAGNOSIS Diagnosis of the endemic treponematoses is based upon clinical manifestations and, when available, dark-field microscopy and serologic testing. The same tests that are used for venereal syphilis (Chap. 153) become reactive during all treponemal infections, and there is no serologic test that can discriminate among the different infections. The nonvenereal treponemal infections should be considered in the evaluation of a reactive syphilis serology in any person who has emigrated from an endemic area.

FIGURE 154-2 Clinical manifestations of endemic treponematoses. *Left*: Papillomatous primary lesion of yaws. *Center*: Split papules of early endemic syphilis. *Right*: Pigmented macules of pinta. *(From PL Perine et al.)*

Rx TREATMENT

The recommended therapy for patients and their contacts is benzathine penicillin at a dose of 1.2 million units intramuscularly; the dose for children <10 years of age is 600,000 units. There have been no controlled studies to show that the recommended lower dose (which is half the dose recommended for patients and contacts in early venereal syphilis) is effective in stopping relapse or progression to late disease. Definitive evidence of resistance to penicillin is lacking. However, because failure to heal existing lesions and frequent relapse following treatment for yaws have been described in Papua New Guinea, some health workers have suggested doubling the recommended dose of benzathine penicillin. Limited data suggest the efficacy of tetracycline for the treatment of yaws, but no such data exist for other endemic treponematoses. Solely on the basis of experience with venereal syphilis, it is thought that doxycycline, tetracycline, and erythromycin (at doses appropriate for syphilis; Chap. 153) are therapeutic alternatives for patients allergic to penicillin. A Jarisch-Herxheimer reaction (Chap. 153) may follow treatment of endemic treponematoses. Nontreponemal serologic titers [in the Venereal Disease Research Laboratory (VDRL) slide test or the rapid plasma reagin (RPR) test] usually decline after effective therapy, but patients may not become seronegative.

CONTROL   The endemic treponematoses can be controlled with inexpensive therapy. However, remote locations of affected populations can limit the availability of medical care. Although the mass treatment programs of three decades ago were widely successful, time has shown that sustained control requires vigilance in regular screening and in the investigation of outbreaks—luxuries that are often impossible in countries with more pressing medical needs. There is concern that, as HIV spreads throughout developing countries, it may markedly affect the manifestations and transmission of the endemic treponematoses.

FURTHER READING

ANTAL GM et al: The endemic treponematoses. Microbes Infect 4:83, 2002

BACKHOUSE JL et al: Failure of penicillin treatment of yaws on Karkar Island, Papua New Guinea. Am J Trop Med 59:388, 1998

CENTURION-LARA A et al: The flanking region sequences of the 15 kD lipoprotein gene differentiate pathogenic treponemes. J Infect Dis 177:1036, 1998

——— et al: Multiple alleles of *Treponema pallidum* repeat gene D in *Treponema pallidum* isolates. J Bacteriol 182:2332, 2000

ENGELKENS HJH et al: Nonvenereal treponematoses in tropical countries. Clin Dermatol 17:143, 1999

PARISH JL: Treponemal infections in the pediatric population. Clin Dermatol 18:687, 2000

WALKER SL et al: Yaws—a review of the last 50 years. Int J Dermatol 39:258, 2000

155 | LEPTOSPIROSIS
Peter Speelman

Leptospirosis is an emerging infectious disease, as illustrated by recent large outbreaks in Asia, Central and South America, and the United States. The disease is caused by pathogenic leptospires and characterized by a broad spectrum of clinical manifestations, varying from inapparent infection to fulminant, fatal disease. In its mild form, leptospirosis may present as an influenza-like illness with headache and myalgias. Severe leptospirosis, characterized by jaundice, renal dysfunction, and hemorrhagic diathesis, is referred to as *Weil's syndrome*.

ETIOLOGIC AGENTS   Leptospires are spirochetes belonging to the order Spirochaetales and the family Leptospiraceae. Traditionally, the genus *Leptospira* comprised two species: the pathogenic *L. interrogans* and the free-living *L. biflexa*. Although 16 genomospecies of pathogenic leptospires are now recognized on the basis of their DNA relatedness, it is more practical clinically and epidemiologically to use a classification based on serologic differences. The pathogenic leptospires are divided into serovars according to their antigenic composition. More than 200 serovars make up the 25 serogroups.

Leptospires are coiled, thin, highly motile organisms with hooked ends and two periplasmic flagella that permit burrowing into tissue (Fig. 155-1). These organisms are 6 to 20 μm long and ~0.1 μm wide; they stain poorly but can be seen microscopically by dark-field examination and after silver impregnation staining. Leptospires require special media and conditions for growth; it may take weeks for cultures to become positive.

EPIDEMIOLOGY   Leptospirosis is an important zoonosis with a worldwide distribution that affects at least 160 mammalian species. Rodents, especially rats, are the most important reservoir, although other wild mammals as well as domestic and farm animals may also harbor these microorganisms. Leptospires establish a symbiotic relationship with their host and can persist in the renal tubules for years. Some serovars are generally associated with particular animals—e.g., icterohaemorrhagiae/copenhageni with rats, grippotyphosa with voles, hardjo with cattle, canicola with dogs, and pomona with pigs—but may occur in other animals as well.

Transmission of leptospires may follow direct contact with urine, blood, or tissue from an infected animal or exposure to a contaminated environment; human-to-human transmission is rare. Since leptospires are excreted in the urine and can survive in water for many months, water is an important vehicle in their transmission. Epidemics of leptospirosis may result from exposure to flood waters contaminated by urine from infected animals, as has been reported from Nicaragua. Leptospirosis occurs most commonly in the tropics because the climate as well as the sometimes poor hygienic conditions favor the pathogen's survival. In many developing countries, leptospirosis is an underestimated problem. Reliable data on morbidity and mortality from leptospirosis have gradually started to appear. In 1999, more than 500,000 cases were reported from China, with case-fatality rates ranging from 0.9 to 7.9%. In Brazil, more than 28,000 cases were reported in the same year.

Humans are not commonly infected with leptospires. However, in the United States, the 40 to 120 cases reported annually to the Centers for Disease Control and Prevention (CDC) surely represent a significant underestimation of the total number. Certain occupational groups

FIGURE 155-1   Scanning electron micrograph of leptospires.

are at especially high risk; included are veterinarians, agricultural workers, sewage workers, slaughterhouse employees, and workers in the fishing industry. Such individuals may acquire leptospirosis through direct exposure to or contact with contaminated water and soil. Leptospirosis has also been recognized in deteriorating inner cities where rat populations are expanding. One report described leptospirosis in urban residents of Baltimore who were sporadically exposed to rat urine.

Recreational exposure and domestic-animal contact are also prominent sources of leptospirosis. Recreational water activities, such as canoeing, windsurfing, swimming, and waterskiing, place persons at risk for leptospirosis. In 1998, a large outbreak occurred among athletes and community residents after a triathlon in Illinois. Among athletes, the ingestion of one or more swallows of lake water was a prominent risk factor for illness. Heavy rains that preceded the triathlon, with consequent agricultural runoff, are likely to have increased the level of leptospiral contamination in the lake water.

Sometimes leptospirosis is acquired during travel abroad. In a study in the Netherlands, 14% of patients with confirmed leptospirosis had acquired the infection while traveling in tropical countries, mostly in Southeast Asia. Transmission via laboratory accidents has been reported but is rare. Leptospirosis develops occasionally after unanticipated immersion in contaminated water (e.g., in an automobile accident) and rarely after an animal bite. Most cases occur in men, with a peak incidence during the summer and fall in Western countries and during the rainy season in the tropics.

PATHOGENESIS The pathogenesis of leptospirosis is incompletely understood. Leptospires may enter the host through abrasions in the skin or through intact mucous membranes, especially the conjunctiva and the lining of the oro- and nasopharynx. Drinking of contaminated water may introduce leptospires through the mouth, throat, or esophagus. After entry of the organisms, leptospiremia develops, with subsequent spread to all organs. Multiplication takes place in blood and in tissues, and leptospires can be isolated from blood and cerebrospinal fluid (CSF) during the first 4 to 10 days of illness. CSF examination during this period documents pleocytosis in the majority of instances, but only a minority of patients develop symptoms and signs of meningitis at this point. All forms of leptospires can damage the wall of small blood vessels; this damage leads to vasculitis with leakage and extravasation of cells, including hemorrhages. The most important known pathogenic properties of leptospires are adhesion to cell surfaces and cellular toxicity.

Vasculitis is responsible for the most important manifestations of the disease. Although leptospires mainly infect the kidneys and liver, any organ may be affected. In the kidney, leptospires migrate to the interstitium, renal tubules, and tubular lumen, causing interstitial nephritis and tubular necrosis. Hypovolemia due to dehydration or altered capillary permeability may contribute to the development of renal failure. In the liver, centrilobular necrosis with proliferation of Kupffer cells may be found. However, severe hepatocellular necrosis is not a feature of leptospirosis. Pulmonary involvement is the result of hemorrhage and not of inflammation. Invasion of skeletal muscle by leptospires results in swelling, vacuolation of the myofibrils, and focal necrosis. In severe leptospirosis, vasculitis may ultimately impair the microcirculation and increase capillary permeability, resulting in fluid leakage and hypovolemia.

When antibodies are formed, leptospires are eliminated from all sites in the host except the eye, the proximal renal tubules, and perhaps the brain, where they may persist for weeks or months. The persistence

FIGURE 155-2 Biphasic nature of leptospirosis and relevant investigations at different stages of disease. Specimens 1 and 2 for serology are acute-phase serum samples; specimen 3 is a convalescent-phase serum sample that may facilitate detection of a delayed immune response; and specimens 4 and 5 are follow-up serum samples that can provide epidemiologic information, such as the presumptive infecting serogroup. [*Reprinted as adapted by Levett (from Turner LH: Leptospirosis. BMJ 1:231, 1969) with permission from the American Society for Microbiology and the BMJ Publishing Group.*]

of leptospires in the aqueous humor occasionally causes chronic or recurrent uveitis. The systemic immune response is effective in eliminating the organism but may also produce symptomatic inflammatory reactions. A rise in antibody titer coincides with the development of meningitis; this association suggests that an immunologic mechanism is responsible.

After the start of antimicrobial treatment for leptospirosis, a Jarisch-Herxheimer reaction similar to that seen in other spirochetal diseases may develop. Although frequently described in older publications, this reaction seems to be a rare event in leptospirosis and is certainly less frequent in this infection than in other spirochetal diseases.

CLINICAL MANIFESTATIONS (Fig. 155-2) It is important to try to obtain a history of exposure to contaminated materials. Serologic evidence of past inapparent infection is found in 15 to 40% of persons who have been exposed but have not become ill. In symptomatic cases of leptospirosis, clinical manifestations vary from mild to serious or even fatal. More than 90% of symptomatic persons have the relatively mild and usually anicteric form of leptospirosis, with or without meningitis. Severe leptospirosis with profound jaundice (Weil's syndrome) develops in 5 to 10% of infected individuals. The idea that distinct clinical syndromes are associated with specific serogroups has been refuted.

The incubation period is usually 1 to 2 weeks but ranges from 2 to 20 days (Fig. 155-2). Typically, an acute leptospiremic phase is followed by an immune leptospiruric phase. The distinction between the first and second phases is not always clear, and milder cases do not always include the second phase.

Anicteric Leptospirosis Leptospirosis may present as an acute influenza-like illness, with fever, chills, severe headache, nausea, vomiting, and myalgias. Muscle pain, which especially affects the calves, back, and abdomen, is an important feature of leptospiral infection. Less common features include sore throat and rash. The patient usually has an intense headache (frontal or retroorbital) and sometimes develops photophobia. Mental confusion may be evident. Pulmonary involvement, manifested in most cases by cough and chest pain and in a few cases by hemoptysis, is not uncommon.

The most common finding on physical examination is fever with conjunctival suffusion. Less common findings include muscle tenderness, lymphadenopathy, pharyngeal injection, rash, hepatomegaly, and splenomegaly. The rash may be macular, maculopapular, erythematous, urticarial, or hemorrhagic. Mild jaundice may be present.

Most patients become asymptomatic within 1 week. After an interval of 1 to 3 days, the illness recurs in a number of cases. The start of this second (immune) phase coincides with the development of antibodies. Symptoms are more variable than during the first (leptospiremic) phase. Usually the symptoms last for only a few days, but occasionally they persist for weeks. Often the fever is less pronounced and the myalgias are less severe than in the leptospiremic phase. An important event during the immune phase is the development of aseptic meningitis. Although no more than 15% of all patients have symptoms and signs of meningitis, many patients have CSF pleocytosis. Meningeal symptoms usually disappear within a few days but may persist for weeks. Similarly, pleocytosis generally disappears within 2 weeks but occasionally persists for months. Aseptic meningitis is more common among children than among adults. Iritis, iridocyclitis, and chorioretinitis—late complications that may persist for years—can become apparent as early as the third week but often present several months after the initial illness. One epidemic of uveitis among patients with leptospirosis has been reported. Mortality in anicteric leptospirosis is almost nil, although death as a result of pulmonary hemorrhage occurred in 2.4% of cases in a Chinese outbreak.

Severe Leptospirosis (Weil's Syndrome)   Weil's syndrome, the most severe form of leptospirosis, is characterized by jaundice, renal dysfunction, hemorrhagic diathesis, and a mortality rate ranging from 5 to 15%. In Europe, this syndrome is frequently but not exclusively associated with infection due to serovar icterohaemorrhagiae/copenhageni. The onset of illness is no different from that of less severe leptospirosis; however, after 4 to 9 days, jaundice as well as renal and vascular dysfunction generally develop. Although some degree of defervescence may be noted after the first week of illness, a biphasic disease pattern like that seen in anicteric leptospirosis is lacking. The jaundice of Weil's syndrome, which can be profound and give an orange cast to the skin, is usually not associated with severe hepatic necrosis. Death is rarely due to liver failure. Hepatomegaly and tenderness in the right upper quadrant are usually detected. Splenomegaly is found in 20% of cases.

Renal failure may develop, often during the second week of illness. Hypovolemia and decreased renal perfusion contribute to the development of acute tubular necrosis with oliguria or anuria. Dialysis is sometimes required, although a fair number of cases can be managed without dialysis. Renal function may be completely regained.

Pulmonary involvement occurs frequently; in some clusters of cases, it is a major manifestation, resulting in cough, dyspnea, chest pain, and blood-stained sputum and sometimes in hemoptysis or even respiratory failure. Hemorrhagic manifestations are seen in Weil's syndrome: epistaxis, petechiae, purpura, and ecchymoses are found commonly, while severe gastrointestinal bleeding and adrenal or subarachnoid hemorrhage are detected rarely.

Rhabdomyolysis, hemolysis, myocarditis, pericarditis, congestive heart failure, cardiogenic shock, adult respiratory distress syndrome, necrotizing pancreatitis, and multiorgan failure have all been described during severe leptospirosis.

LABORATORY AND RADIOLOGIC FINDINGS   (Fig. 155-2) The kidneys are invariably involved in leptospirosis. Related findings range from urinary sediment changes (leukocytes, erythrocytes, and hyaline or granular casts) and mild proteinuria in anicteric leptospirosis to renal failure and azotemia in severe disease.

The erythrocyte sedimentation rate is usually elevated. In anicteric leptospirosis, peripheral leukocyte counts range from 3000 to 26,000/μL, with a left shift; in Weil's syndrome, leukocytosis is often marked. Mild thrombocytopenia occurs in up to 50% of patients and is associated with renal failure.

In contrast to patients with acute viral hepatitis, those with leptospirosis typically have elevated serum levels of bilirubin and alkaline phosphatase as well as mild increases (up to 200 U/L) in serum levels of aminotransferases. In Weil's syndrome, the prothrombin time may be prolonged but can be corrected with vitamin K. Levels of creatine phosphokinase, which are elevated in up to 50% of patients with leptospirosis during the first week of illness, may help to differentiate this infection from viral hepatitis.

When a meningeal reaction develops, polymorphonuclear leukocytes predominate initially and the number of mononuclear cells increases later. The protein concentration in the CSF may be elevated; CSF glucose levels are normal.

In severe leptospirosis, pulmonary radiographic abnormalities are more common than would be expected on the basis of physical examination. These abnormalities most frequently develop 3 to 9 days after the onset of illness. The most common radiographic finding is a patchy alveolar pattern that corresponds to scattered alveolar hemorrhage. Radiographic abnormalities most often affect the lower lobes in the periphery of the lung fields.

DIAGNOSIS   (Fig. 155-2) A definite diagnosis of leptospirosis is based either on isolation of the organism from the patient or on seroconversion or a rise in antibody titer in the microscopic agglutination test (MAT). In the United States, the MAT is performed only at the CDC. In cases with strong clinical evidence of infection, a single antibody titer of 1:400 to 1:800 (depending on whether the case occurs in a low- or high-endemic area) in the MAT is required. Preferably, a fourfold or greater rise in titer is detected between acute- and convalescent-phase serum specimens. Antibodies generally do not reach detectable levels until the second week of illness. The antibody response can be affected by early treatment.

The MAT, which uses a battery of live leptospiral strains, and the enzyme-linked immunosorbent assay (ELISA), which uses a broadly reacting antigen, are the standard serologic procedures. These tests usually are available only in specialized laboratories and are used for determination of the antibody titer and for tentative identification of the serogroup—and in some cases the serovar—involved (thus the importance of using antigens representative of the serovars prevalent in the particular geographic area). Since cross-reactions occur frequently, however, it is often impossible to identify the infecting serogroup or serovar. Serologic testing cannot be used as the basis for a decision about whether to start treatment.

In addition to the MAT and the ELISA, various other tests with diagnostic value have been developed. Some tests, such as an indirect hemagglutination test and a microcapsule agglutination test, are commercially available. A recent advance is the development of rapid serologic assays that apply lateral flow, latex agglutination, or ELISA methodology with reasonable sensitivity and specificity. These methods do not require culture or MAT facilities. However, in endemic areas, pooled serum samples from the local population are required as positive and negative controls. Polymerase chain reaction (PCR) techniques have been developed but so far have not found widespread use outside research and reference laboratories.

Leptospires can be isolated from blood and/or CSF during the first 10 days of illness and from urine for several weeks beginning at around 1 week. Cultures most often become positive after 2 to 4 weeks, with a range of 1 week to 4 months. Sometimes urine cultures remain positive for months or years after the start of illness. For isolation of leptospires from body fluids or tissues, Ellinghausen-McCullough-Johnson-Harris (EMJH) medium is useful; other possibilities are Fletcher medium and Korthof medium. Specimens can be mailed to a reference laboratory for culture, since leptospires remain viable in anticoagulated blood (heparin, EDTA, or citrate) for up to 11 days. Isolation of leptospires is important since it is the only way the infecting serovar can be correctly identified. Dark-field examination of blood or urine frequently results in misdiagnosis and should not be used.

DIFFERENTIAL DIAGNOSIS   Leptospirosis should be differentiated from other febrile illnesses associated with headache and muscle pain, such as dengue, malaria, enteric fever, viral hepatitis, *Hantavirus* infections, and rickettsial diseases. In light of the strong similarity in epidemiology and clinical presentation between leptospirosis and *Hantavirus* infections and given the reported occurrence of dual infections, it is advisable to conduct serologic testing for *Hantavirus* in cases of suspected leptospirosis. When patients have a flulike disease with disproportionately severe myalgia or aseptic meningitis, a diagnosis of leptospirosis should be considered.

℞ TREATMENT

The effectiveness of antimicrobial therapy for the mild febrile form of leptospirosis is controversial, but such treatment is indicated for more severe forms. Treatment should be initiated as early as possible; nevertheless, contrary to previous reports, treatment started after the first 4 days of illness is effective.

For severe cases of leptospirosis, intravenous administration of penicillin G, amoxicillin, ampicillin, or erythromycin is recommended (Table 155-1). In milder cases, oral treatment with tetracycline, doxycycline, ampicillin, or amoxicillin should be considered. Although several other antibiotics, including newer cephalosporins, are highly active against leptospires in vitro, no clinical experience has yet been gained with these drugs.

In rare cases, a Jarisch-Herxheimer reaction develops within hours after the start of antimicrobial therapy (see "Pathogenesis" above). Although so far the only effective mode of management is supportive, the role of antibodies to tumor necrosis factor in the treatment of this reaction deserves further study. A beneficial effect of the use of such antibodies for the modulation of the reaction has been demonstrated in patients with louse-borne relapsing fever. Patients with severe leptospirosis and renal failure may require dialysis. Those with Weil's syndrome may need transfusions of whole blood and/or platelets. Intensive care may be necessary.

PROGNOSIS Most patients with leptospirosis recover. Mortality is highest among patients who are elderly and those who have Weil's syndrome. Leptospirosis during pregnancy is associated with high fetal mortality. Long-term follow-up of patients with renal failure and hepatic dysfunction has documented good recovery of renal and hepatic function.

PREVENTION Individuals who may be exposed to leptospires through their occupations or their involvement in recreational water activities should be informed about the risks. Measures for controlling leptospirosis include avoidance of exposure to urine and tissues from infected animals, vaccination of animals, and rodent control. The animal

TABLE 155-1 *Treatment and Chemoprophylaxis of Leptospirosis*

Purpose of Drug Administration	Regimen
Treatment	
Mild leptospirosis	Doxycycline, 100 mg orally bid *or* Ampicillin, 500–750 mg orally qid *or* Amoxicillin, 500 mg orally qid
Moderate/severe leptospirosis	Penicillin G, 1.5 million units IV qid *or* Ampicillin, 1 g IV qid *or* Amoxicillin, 1 g IV qid *or* Erythromycin, 500 mg IV qid
Chemoprophylaxis	Doxycycline, 200 mg orally once a week

Note: All regimens used for treatment are administered for 7 days.

vaccine used in a given area should contain the serovars known to be present in that area. Unfortunately, some vaccinated animals still excrete leptospires in their urine. Vaccination of humans against a specific serovar prevalent in an area has been undertaken in some European and Asian countries and has proved effective. Although a large-scale trial of vaccine in humans has been reported from Cuba, no conclusions can be drawn about efficacy and adverse reactions because of insufficient details on study design. Chemoprophylaxis with doxycycline (200 mg once a week) has appeared to be efficacious to some extent but is indicated only in rare instances of sustained short-term exposure (Table 155-1).

FURTHER READING

CHU KM et al: Identification of *Leptospira* species in the pathogenesis of uveitis and determination of clinical ocular characteristics in south India. J Infect Dis 177:1314, 1998

LEVETT PN: Leptospirosis. Clin Microbiol Rev 14: 296, 2001

MORGAN J et al: Outbreak of leptospirosis among triathlon participants and community residents in Springfield, Illinois, 1998. Clin Infect Dis 34:1593, 2002

SEHGAL SC et al: Randomized controlled trial of doxycycline prophylaxis against leptospirosis in an endemic area. Int J Antimicrob Agents 13:249, 2000

TREVEJO RT et al: Epidemic leptospirosis associated with pulmonary hemorrhage Nicaragua. J Infect Dis 178:1457, 1998

VINETZ JM: Leptospirosis. Curr Opin Infect Dis 14:527, 2001

WORLD HEALTH ORGANIZATION/INTERNATIONAL LEPTOSPIROSIS SOCIETY: *Human Leptospirosis: Guidance for Diagnosis, Surveillance and Control.* Geneva, World Health Organization, 2003, 109 pp

156 RELAPSING FEVER
David T. Dennis, Edward B. Hayes

DEFINITION The term *relapsing fever* describes two distinct diseases. *Tick-borne (endemic) relapsing fever* (TBRF) is a zoonosis that is transmitted principally from rodents to humans by the bite of various soft ticks. *Louse-borne (epidemic) relapsing fever* (LBRF) is a disease of humans that is transmitted from one person to another by the body louse. Both are characterized by recurrent acute episodes of spirochetemia and fever alternating with spontaneous spirochetal clearance and apyrexia.

ETIOLOGY Relapsing fever is caused by infection with spirochetal gram-negative bacteria of the genus *Borrelia* (family Spirochaetaceae). The borreliae are helical in shape and average 0.2 to 0.5 μm in width and 5 to 20 μm in length. They comprise an outer membrane, an intermediate peptidoglycan layer, and an inner cytoplasmic membrane, which encloses the protoplasmic cylinder. A variable number of periplasmic flagella are situated beneath the outer membrane. Relapsing-

fever borreliae are slow-growing and microaerophilic; they grow best at 30° to 35°C in Barbour-Stoenner-Kelly (BSK II) medium.

B. recurrentis is the only species that causes LBRF. Most of the several species of *Borrelia* that cause TBRF are named after the species of *Ornithodoros* tick responsible for their transmission. In North America, *B. hermsii* and *B. turicatae* cause almost all cases of TBRF; *B. duttoni* is the most common cause of TBRF in sub-Saharan Africa, an area of high endemicity. Borreliae are unique among bacteria in having a genome composed of a linear chromosome and a series of linear and circular plasmids. The sequences of both the flagellin and the 16S ribosomal RNA genes are homogeneous among LBRF strains; in contrast, there is considerable heterogeneity of these genes between Old World and New World TBRF strains. A unique process of DNA rearrangement within *vmp* genes located on linear plasmids results in extensive variation in the expression of the surface antigens in relapsing-fever borreliae. These *vmp* genes encode variable major proteins (VMPs) found on the spirochete's outer-membrane surface. The antigenic variation generated by sequential expression of previously silent *vmp* genes allows the borreliae to intermittently escape the immune response of the host and results in the febrile relapses that are characteristic of infection with these organisms.

EPIDEMIOLOGY ■ Louse-Borne Relapsing Fever

Body lice (*Pediculus humanus* var. *corporis*) become infected with *B. recurrentis* by feeding on spirochetemic humans, the only reservoirs of infection. In lice, *B. recurrentis* spirochetes are found almost exclusively in the hemolymph; humans acquire infection when infected body lice are crushed and their fluids contaminate mucous membranes or breaks in the skin (such as abrasions caused by scratching of pruritic louse bites). Spirochetes are *not* transmitted directly by the bite of a louse (anterior station transmission) or by inoculation of louse feces (posterior station transmission). Lice have a life span of only a few weeks, feed at frequent intervals, and survive only a few days off the human host. Head lice do not appear to be vectors of LBRF.

LBRF has severely affected military and civilian populations disrupted by war and other disasters. In the nineteenth century, the disease was common among slum dwellers, prisoners, and others living in impoverished, overcrowded, and unhygienic conditions. In the first half of the twentieth century, during periods of war and famine, both LBRF and louse-borne typhus were epidemic in eastern Europe, the Balkans, and the former Soviet Union. The global distribution and incidence of LBRF were substantially reduced following improvements in standards of living, sanitation, and hygiene; LBRF is now an important disease only in northeastern Africa, especially the highlands of Ethiopia, where an estimated 10,000 cases occur annually. In Ethiopia, the disease affects mostly homeless men crowded together in unhygienic circumstances, especially during the cool rainy season, when washing and changing clothing is more difficult. LBRF has repeatedly spilled out of Ethiopia into populations of displaced persons in neighboring Somalia and Sudan. During the Second World War, the spread of LBRF from Ethiopia and the Sudan to western Africa was pandemic.

Short-term visitors to endemic areas (e.g., tourists) are at almost no risk of LBRF, but persons who have close contact with LBRF populations (such as relief workers) can acquire the disease from lice, accidental needle sticks, or other direct contact with contaminated blood.

Tick-Borne Relapsing Fever Argasid ticks of the genus *Ornithodoros* transmit TBRF through their saliva and excreta when they feed on humans. As a rule, the ticks become infected with TBRF borreliae as part of a zoonotic cycle when they feed on spirochetemic rodents and lagomorphs; the exception to this rule is *O. moubata*, a tick species that acquires *B. duttoni* by feeding on infected humans. Ticks transmit TBRF borreliae vertically from one stage to the next; in some species, infection is transmitted transovarially over several generations. Soft ticks are hardy and can survive for 10 years with only an occasional blood meal. These ticks feed painlessly, relatively quickly (for 20 to 45 min), and usually at night while hosts are sleeping. Thus patients with TBRF are often unaware of tick exposures.

TBRF borreliae are widely distributed throughout the world. Human infection with these organisms is generally underrecognized and underreported. TBRF is most highly endemic in sub-Saharan Africa but is also found in countries of the Mediterranean littoral, Middle Eastern states, southern Russia, the Indian subcontinent, Central Asia, and China and at low frequency in North, Central, and South America. The disease typically occurs sporadically or in small—often familial—clusters. Infected soft ticks may cause repeated infections among persons living or sleeping in the same dwelling. In sub-Saharan Africa, *O. moubata*, the vector of *B. duttoni*, infests native huts and rest houses, hiding in crevices of floors and walls during the day and emerging at night to feed on sleeping inhabitants.

In the United States, TBRF disease occurs west of the Mississippi River, especially in forested mountainous areas of far western states, where *B. hermsii* is the causative agent. Less commonly, persons are infected with *B. turicatae* following exposures in tick-infested caves in semidesert areas of the Southwest. On average, ~35 cases of TBRF are reported annually in the United States. *B. hermsii* infections most often occur during spring and summer months among persons sleeping in rustic mountain cabins and vacation homes and occasionally in permanent residences and in outdoor settings. Infections of humans are sometimes precipitated by the disappearance of rodents (e.g., as a result of epizootic plague) that nest in foundations, wall spaces, and attics and that serve as the usual maintenance hosts for *O. hermsii* ticks. Outbreaks caused by *B. hermsii* have taken place among persons staying in cabins along the north rim of the Grand Canyon and in the mountains of California, Idaho, and Colorado. In North America, most recent cases have been reported from Washington, California, Colorado, Idaho, Oregon, and British Columbia.

PATHOGENESIS AND PATHOLOGY

In humans, relapsing-fever borreliae pass through the skin or mucous membranes, multiply in the blood, and circulate in great numbers during febrile periods. The organisms have also been found in the liver, spleen, bone marrow, and central nervous system and may be sequestered at these sites during periods of remission. The disease tends to be more severe when spirochete density in the blood is high. Even though the pathophysiologic manifestations of the disease resemble responses to endotoxin, and although plasma from some patients with relapsing fever coagulates *Limulus* amebocyte lysates, borreliae and other spirochetes have not been shown to express a true lipopolysaccharide (endotoxin) molecule. Infection with *B. recurrentis* has been shown, however, to activate protein mediators of inflammation, such as Hageman factor (factor XII), prekallikrein, and proteins of the complement system; furthermore, a spirochetal heat-stable pyrogenic factor stimulates mononuclear phagocytes to express increased amounts of leukocyte pyrogen and thromboplastin.

The treatment of relapsing fever with antibiotics may provoke a Jarisch-Herxheimer reaction (see "Treatment," below). In patients with LBRF, this reaction has been associated with a release of various cytokines into the plasma, including interleukin 6, interleukin 8, C-reactive protein, and large amounts of tumor necrosis factor a (TNF-α). Pretreatment of LBRF patients with antibody to TNF-α suppressed Jarisch-Herxheimer reactions following penicillin treatment and reduced the plasma concentrations of certain other cytokines.

Death due to TBRF is rare. In contrast, fatality rates of 20% have been recorded during outbreaks of LBRF in malnourished and stressed populations. Relapsing fever in pregnancy can result in abortion, stillbirth, and fatal neonatal infections. Autopsies of patients with relapsing fever most often reveal hepatosplenomegaly and variable edema and swelling of other organs, including brain, lungs, and kidneys. On microscopic examination, the spleen is congested and contains multiple microabscesses composed of mononuclear cells that replace the white pulp, the myocardium displays diffuse histiocytic inflammation and interstitial edema, and the liver has areas of midzonal necrosis. Petechial hemorrhages are commonly evident over the surfaces of the meninges, pleura, heart, spleen, liver, kidneys, and mesentery. Subcapsular and parenchymal hemorrhagic infarcts of the spleen, heart, liver, and brain are sometimes grossly visible.

CLINICAL MANIFESTATIONS

The clinical manifestations of LBRF and TBRF are similar. The common signs and symptoms of TBRF, as documented in North America, are listed in Table 156-1. The mean incubation period is 7 days (range, 2 to 18 days), and the onset of illness is sudden, with fever, headache, shaking chills, sweats, myalgias, and arthralgias. The arthralgia of relapsing fever can be severe, involving small and large joints, but there is no evidence of arthritis. Dizziness, nausea, and vomiting are common. Sleep may be difficult and is sometimes accompanied by disturbing dreams. The patient is coherent but withdrawn, thirsty, and uninterested in food and other outside stimuli. The fever is high from the first, with temperature usually reaching ≥40°C (≥104°F) and then becoming irregular in pattern. High fever is sometimes accompanied by delirium. Patients are usually

TABLE 156-1 *Manifestations of Tick-Borne Relapsing Fever Acquired in the Northwestern United States and Southwestern British Columbia*

Sign or Symptom	%	Sign or Symptom	%
Headache	94	Photophobia	25
Myalgia	92	Neck pain	24
Chills	88	Rash	18
Nausea	76	Dysuria	13
Arthralgia	73	Jaundice	10
Vomiting	71	Hepatomegaly	10
Abdominal pain	44	Splenomegaly	6
Confusion	38	Conjunctival injection	5
Dry cough	27	Eschar	2
Eye pain	26	Meningitis	2
Diarrhea	25	Nuchal rigidity	2
Dizziness	25		

Source: From a review of 182 cases reported in the period 1980–1995 (Dworkin et al.).

tachycardic and mildly tachypneic and become prostrate as the disease progresses. Some patients have meningismus. The conjunctivae are often injected, and photophobia is common. The sclerae may become icteric, particularly in the later stages of illness. The mucous membranes may be dry, and patients are often dehydrated. Scattered petechiae develop on the trunk, extremities, and mucous membranes in one-third or more of patients with LBRF but in a smaller proportion of patients with TBRF. A nonproductive cough is common, but chest sounds are usually normal; pleuritic pain and an accompanying pleuritic rub are sometimes noted. Cardiac findings are compatible with a high-output state; tachycardia and summation gallop are common. Tender enlargement of the spleen and liver frequently occurs in the acute phase of illness.

Epistaxis and blood-tinged sputum are common complications, and gastrointestinal and central nervous system hemorrhage can occur. Because of this coagulopathy, one LBRF outbreak in southern Sudan was thought to be viral hemorrhagic fever. Other complications of variable incidence include iridocyclitis, optic neuritis, lymphocytic meningitis, coma, isolated cranial-nerve palsy, pneumonitis, myocarditis, and rupture of the spleen. Life-threatening complications are unusual in otherwise healthy persons given supportive care, especially if the illness is diagnosed and treated early. Children generally have a milder course of illness than adults.

Without treatment, symptoms intensify over a 2- to 7-day period (average, 5 days in LBRF and 3 days in TBRF), ending in a spontaneous crisis that coincides with the disappearance of spirochetes from the circulation. The crisis comprises two phases over several hours: a *chill phase*, characterized by rigors, rising temperature, and hypermetabolism, and a *flush phase* of falling temperature, diaphoresis, and a decreased effective circulating blood volume. The pathophysiologic events associated with this crisis are magnified when precipitated by antibiotic treatment and are indistinguishable from the Jarisch-Herxheimer reaction of treated syphilis (see "Treatment," below). The crisis is followed by a period of exhaustion, sleep, and an uneventful recovery. Orthostatic hypotension is typical in the early recovery phase. Not uncommonly, in the first week of convalescence, the patient experiences 1 or 2 days of mild fever unassociated with detectable spirochetemia. In untreated patients, spirochetemia and symptoms may recur after a period of several days or weeks (average interval to first relapse, 9 days in LBRF and 7 days in TBRF). Only one or two relapses characteristically occur in untreated patients with LBRF, whereas as many as 10 (average, three) can occur in untreated patients with TBRF. In most cases, the illness becomes shorter and milder and the afebrile intervals longer with each relapse. Because of the great antigenic variation among *Borrelia* strains, infection confers only partial immunity, and repeated infections of the same individual have been recorded.

Diseases that should be considered in the differential diagnosis of relapsing fever or that may complicate relapsing fever include typhus fever, typhoid fever, nontyphoid salmonellosis, malaria, dengue and other arboviral illnesses, tuberculosis, leptospirosis, and viral hemorrhagic fevers. In the United States, the geographic distribution of Colorado tick fever (Chap. 180) overlaps that of TBRF, and the two diseases have similar manifestations early in their courses.

LABORATORY FINDINGS AND DIAGNOSIS The diagnosis of relapsing fever is confirmed most easily by the detection of spirochetes in blood, bone marrow aspirates, or cerebrospinal fluid. Motile spirochetes can be seen when specimens are examined by dark-field microscopy. Fixed organisms are clearly visible in Wright-, Giemsa-, or acridine orange–stained preparations of thin or dehemoglobinized thick smears of peripheral blood or buffy-coat preparations (Fig. 156-1). Organisms are most numerous in specimens taken during periods of high temperature preceding the crisis; smears of peripheral blood are positive in ≥70% of patients with LBRF and in a lower percentage of patients with TBRF. In reference laboratories, relapsing-fever spirochetes are cultured from blood by the inoculation of BSK II medium or by the intraperitoneal inoculation of immature laboratory mice. Serum antibodies to *Borrelia* can be detected by enzyme immunoassays, indirect fluorescent antibody (IFA) assay, and western immunoblotting using whole-cell sonicates as antigen; however, these tests are unstandardized and subject to insensitivity and cross-reactivity with other spirochetal agents, including *B. burgdorferi* (the agent of Lyme disease) and *Treponema pallidum*. A recently developed western immunoblot test employing species-specific recombinant glycerophosphodiester phosphodiesterase (GlpQ) as antigen has been shown to be more sensitive and specific than the whole-cell sonicate IFA or enzyme-linked immunosorbent assay (ELISA) tests.

Other laboratory findings in relapsing fever are nonspecific. The leukocyte count is normal or moderately elevated, with an unremarkable cell differential. Serum bilirubin levels are generally only slightly elevated. Thrombocytopenia commonly occurs in relapsing-fever patients during the acute phase of the illness; platelet counts rebound during early convalescence. Prothrombin and partial thromboplastin times are often moderately prolonged during acute illness, as are standardized bleeding times. Fibrinogen concentrations in the blood are normal, and fibrinolysis is mild or absent. Results of the Rumpel-

FIGURE 156-1 Photomicrograph of tick-borne relapsing fever spirochete (*B. hermsii*) in a Wright-Giemsa-stained peripheral blood film.

Leede tourniquet test for capillary fragility are negative, despite the presence of petechiae.

Rx TREATMENT

Relapsing-fever borreliae are exquisitely sensitive to antibiotics. Treatment with doxycycline (or another tetracycline), erythromycin, or chloramphenicol produces rapid clearance of spirochetes and a remission of symptoms (Table 156-2). The response to a single dose of penicillin may be delayed and incomplete. Although a single dose of doxycycline (or another tetracycline), erythromycin, or chloramphenicol is highly effective in the treatment of LBRF, less is known about the efficacy of single-dose treatment of TBRF. Empirical treatment of TBRF for 7 days is therefore recommended to reduce the risk of persisting or relapsing borreliosis. For children <8 years of age and for pregnant women, erythromycin or penicillin may be preferred, given the potential adverse effects of tetracyclines.

Treatment of LBRF with a rapidly acting antibiotic regularly precipitates a Jarisch-Herxheimer-like reaction within 1 to 4 h of the first dose. This reaction, which occurs in more than 50% of treated TBRF patients in North America, tends to be more severe when the patient has LBRF rather than TBRF and when high numbers of spirochetes are circulating in the bloodstream. In the chill phase of the reaction, rigors and rising fever are accompanied by an increasing metabolic rate, alveolar hyperventilation, high cardiac output, increasing peripheral vascular resistance, and decreased pulmonary arterial pressure. The body temperature commonly rises to $\geq41°C$ ($\geq105.8°F$). This high fever is accompanied often by agitation and confusion and sometimes by delirium. Fever can be partially controlled by the use of a cooling blanket and ice packs and by sponging of the patient with tepid water and alcohol. The chill phase terminates after 10 to 30 min, giving way to a flush phase characterized by a fall in body temperature, drenching sweats, and sometimes (more commonly in LBRF) a potentially dangerous fall in systemic arterial pressure and rise in pulmonary arterial pressure. Although cardiac output is maintained at high levels, the effective circulating blood volume decreases as peripheral vascular resistance falls. Vital signs must be monitored carefully during this period of the reaction, which usually lasts ≤8 h. Clinical and electrocardiographic evidence of myocarditis and myocardial dysfunction includes a prolonged QT_c interval, a third heart sound (S_3), elevated central venous pressure, arterial hypotension, and rare pulmonary congestion. The use of delayed-release intramuscular penicillin may prolong or delay the clearance of spirochetes and thereby attenuate the accompanying Jarisch-Herxheimer reaction, but this response is not predictable; furthermore, single-dose penicillin treatment sometimes results in relapse of spirochetemia and symptoms. Glucocorticoids and nonsteroidal anti-inflammatory agents do not prevent or significantly modify the cardiopulmonary disturbances of the Jarisch-Herxheimer reaction, although hydrocortisone and acetaminophen given at the same time as antibiotics reduce peak body temperature. Although pretreatment with antibody to TNF-α may moderate the Jarisch-Herxheimer reaction in treated patients with LBRF, its use in LBRF is impractical and its use in TBRF (whose treatment is associated with a relatively mild Jarisch-Herxheimer reaction) is not warranted. Close monitoring of fluid balance, arterial and venous pressures, and myocardial function is advised in supportive management of the Jarisch-Herxheimer reaction in patients with LBRF.

The management of patients with relapsing fever–induced myocardial dysfunction requires caution in the administration of intravenous fluids and, in some cases, use of short-term inotropic therapy. The inability of heparin to control bleeding in LBRF suggests that disseminated intravascular coagulation is not important in its causation. Vitamin K and other soluble vitamins are sometimes given to counter dietary deficiencies in patients with LBRF. Because postural hypotension is often pronounced during the acute phase of relapsing fever and in the early stage of recovery, patients should be assisted when arising from bed.

Untreated LBRF has a high case-fatality rate, especially among persons in otherwise poor health, such as those in famine-affected populations. The fatality rate among treated persons is usually <5%. In general, TBRF is a milder disease than LBRF: the spontaneous crisis and the Jarisch-Herxheimer reactions are less pronounced and the case-fatality rates are lower for TBRF than for LBRF.

PREVENTION AND CONTROL LBRF can be prevented by addressing socioeconomic circumstances that promote louse infestation (crowding, poverty, homelessness), by applying hygienic practices that reduce numbers of body lice (washing clothes, drying clothes in direct sunlight, changing clothes at frequent intervals), and by using acaricides. Spread of infection can be controlled by early case detection and treatment of infected persons and close contacts. Historically, outbreaks of LBRF have been controlled by mass delousing. In situations like those in refugee camps, individuals, their clothes, and their bedding should be deloused with appropriate acaricides, such as 0.5% permethrin dust. Impregnation of clothing with liquid permethrin, a residual acaricide, can provide long-term protection against infestation. In outbreaks of fever that involve louse-infested populations, empirical single-dose treatment with doxycycline will be effective against typhus as well as LBRF. *B. recurrentis* has a fragile life cycle and is eradicable.

TBRF can be prevented by the avoidance of rodent- and tick-infested dwellings and infested natural sites. Limiting rodent access to the foundations and attics of homes and vacation cabins and eliminating harborage for rodents in and around these dwellings reduce the potential for tick exposure. Rodents and rodent nests should be removed from infested buildings and their surroundings. Tick harborages of infested buildings or other circumscribed sites, such as rodent burrows and nests in hollow logs surrounding dwellings and in rodent-infested caves, can be chemically treated by pest-control specialists using various acaricides, such as carbaryl, diazinon, chlorpyrifos, pyrethrins, and malathion. Persons who enter tick-infested sites can protect themselves by wearing clothing that denies ticks access to the skin, by applying repellents to exposed skin and to clothing, and by applying an acaricide containing permethrin to clothing. Reporting of suspected cases of relapsing fever to public health authorities is important so that an epidemiologic investigation and control measures can be initiated promptly. Prompt diagnosis and treatment of relapsing fever in pregnant women is important in avoiding the potentially severe consequences of fetal or neonatal infection acquired in utero.

TABLE 156-2 *Antibiotic Treatment of Louse-Borne and Tick-Borne Relapsing Fever in Adults*

Medication	Louse-Borne Relapsing Fever (Single Dose)	Tick-Borne Relapsing Fever (7-Day Schedule)
Oral		
Erythromycin	500 mg	500 mg q6h
Tetracycline	500 mg	500 mg q6h
Doxycycline	100 mg	100 mg q12h
Chloramphenicol	500 mg	500 mg q6h
Parenteral[a]		
Erythromycin	500 mg	500 mg q6h
Tetracycline	250 mg	250 mg q6h
Doxycycline	100 mg	100 mg q12h
Chloramphenicol	500 mg	500 mg q6h
Penicillin G (procaine)	600,000 IU	600,000 IU daily

[a]For tick-borne relapsing fever, parenteral therapy is used only until oral treatment is tolerated.

FURTHER READING

BARBOUR AG, RESTREPO BI: Antigenic variation in vector-borne pathogens. Emerg Infect Dis 6:449, 2000

CADAVID D, BARBOUR AG: Neuroborreliosis during relapsing fever: Review of clinical manifestations, pathology, and treatment of infections in humans and experimental animals. Clin Infect Dis 26:151, 1998

CUTLER SJ et al: *Borrelia recurrentis* characterization and comparison with relapsing fever, Lyme-associated, and other *Borrelia* spp. Int J Syst Bacteriol 47:958, 1997

DWORKIN MS et al: Tick-borne relapsing fever in North America. Med Clin North Am 86:417, 2002

HORTON JM, BLASER MJ: The spectrum of relapsing fever in the Rocky Mountains. Arch Intern Med 145:871, 1985

PAUL WS et al: Outbreak of tick-borne relapsing fever at the north rim of the Grand Canyon: Evidence for effectiveness of preventive measures. Am J Trop Med Hyg 66:71, 2002

157 LYME BORRELIOSIS
Allen C. Steere

DEFINITION Lyme borreliosis is caused by a spirochete, *Borrelia burgdorferi, sensu lato*, that is transmitted by ticks of the *Ixodes ricinus* complex. The infection usually begins with a characteristic expanding skin lesion, erythema migrans (EM; stage 1, localized infection). After several days or weeks, the spirochete may spread hematogenously to many different sites (stage 2, disseminated infection). Possible manifestations of disseminated infection include secondary annular skin lesions, meningitis, cranial or peripheral neuritis, carditis, atrioventricular nodal block, or migratory musculoskeletal pain. Months to years later (usually after periods of latent infection), intermittent or chronic arthritis, chronic encephalopathy or polyneuropathy, or acrodermatitis may develop (stage 3, persistent infection). Most patients experience early symptoms of the illness during the summer, but the infection may not become symptomatic until it progresses to stage 2 or 3. Despite regional variations, the basic stages of the illness are similar worldwide.

Lyme disease was recognized as a separate entity in 1976 because of geographic clustering of children in Lyme, Connecticut, who were thought to have juvenile rheumatoid arthritis. The rural setting of the case clusters and the identification of EM as a feature of the illness suggested that the disorder was transmitted by an arthropod. It became apparent that Lyme disease was a multisystem illness that affected primarily the skin, nervous system, heart, and joints. Epidemiologic studies of patients with EM implicated certain *Ixodes* ticks as vectors of the disease. Early in the twentieth century, EM had been described in Europe and attributed to *I. ricinus* tick bites. In 1982, a previously unrecognized spirochete, now called *Borrelia burgdorferi*, was recovered from *Ixodes scapularis* ticks and then from patients with Lyme disease. The entity is now called Lyme disease or Lyme borreliosis.

ETIOLOGIC AGENT *B. burgdorferi*, the causative agent of Lyme disease, is a fastidious, microaerophilic bacterium. The spirochete's genome is quite small ($\sim$1.5 Mb) and consists of a highly unusual linear chromosome of 950 kb as well as 9 linear and 12 circular plasmids. *B. burgdorferi* contains many immunogenic proteins, including a number of differentially expressed lipoproteins, most of which are encoded by plasmid DNA. To date, three groups of pathogenic *B. burgdorferi* organisms, together referred to as *B. burgdorferi sensu lato*, have been identified. All North American strains have belonged to the first group, *B. burgdorferi sensu stricto*. Although all three of the identified groups have been found in Europe, most isolates there have been strains of group 2 (*B. garinii*) or group 3 (*B. afzelii*), and only the latter two groups have been found in Asia. These differences may well account for the clinical variations in the disease in different geographic regions.

EPIDEMIOLOGY Lyme borreliosis in all locations is transmitted by ticks of the *I. ricinus* complex: *I. scapularis* (also called *I. dammini*), *I. pacificus*, *I. ricinus*, and *I. persulcatus*. *I. scapularis* is the principal vector in the northeastern United States from Maine to Maryland and in the midwestern states of Wisconsin and Minnesota. *I. pacificus* is the vector in the western states of California and Oregon. The disease is acquired throughout Europe (from Great Britain to Scandinavia to European Russia), where *I. ricinus* is the vector, and in Asian Russia, China, and Japan, where *I. persulcatus* is the vector. These ticks may transmit other diseases as well. In the United States, *I. scapularis* also

transmits babesiosis and human anaplasmosis; in Europe and Asia, *I. ricinus* and *I. persulcatus* also transmit tick-borne encephalitis.

Ticks of the *I. ricinus* complex have larval, nymphal, and adult stages; they require a blood meal at each stage. The risk of infection in a given area depends largely on the density of these ticks as well as their feeding habits and animal hosts, which have evolved differently in different locations. For *I. scapularis* in the northeast, the white-footed mouse is the preferred host of the immature larval and nymphal ticks. It is critical that both of the tick's immature stages feed on the same host, because the life cycle of the spirochete depends on horizontal transmission: in early summer from infected nymphs to mice and in late summer from infected mice to larvae, which then molt to become the infected nymphs that will begin the cycle again the following year. It is the tiny nymphal tick that is primarily responsible for transmission of the disease to humans during the early summer months. White-tailed deer, which are not involved in the life cycle of the spirochete, are the preferred host for the adult stage of *I. scapularis* and seem to be critical to the tick's survival.

Lyme disease is now the most common vector-borne infection in the United States. Since surveillance was begun by the Centers for Disease Control and Prevention (CDC) in 1982, the number of cases has increased dramatically. More than 15,000 new cases are now reported each summer. In Europe, Lyme borreliosis is widely established in forested areas; there, the highest reported frequencies of the disease are in the middle of the continent and in Scandinavia. Cases have occurred in persons who reside in endemic suburban, wooded, or rural areas and in persons who visit, hike, camp, or hunt in these areas.

PATHOGENESIS To maintain its complex enzootic cycle, *B. burgdorferi* must adapt to two markedly different environments: the tick and the mammalian host. The spirochete expresses outer-surface proteins A and B (OspA and OspB) in the midgut of the tick, whereas OspC is upregulated as the organism travels to the tick's salivary gland and thence to the mammalian host. The tick must usually be attached for at least 24 h for transmission of *B. burgdorferi*.

After injection into the human skin, *B. burgdorferi* may migrate outward, producing EM, and may spread hematogenously to other organs. A number of mechanisms may aid in spirochetal dissemination. For example, the sequences of OspC vary considerably among strains, and only a few groups of sequences are associated with disseminated disease. Spread through the skin and other tissue matrices may be facilitated by the binding of human plasminogen and its activators to the surface of the spirochete. During its dissemination and homing to specific sites, the organism attaches to certain host integrins, matrix glycosaminoglycans, and extracellular matrix proteins. For example, *Borrelia* decorin-binding proteins A and B bind decorin, a glycosaminoglycan on collagen fibrils; this binding may explain why the organism is commonly aligned with collagen fibrils in the extracellular matrix in the heart, nervous system, or joints. The only known virulence factors of *B. burgdorferi* are surface proteins that allow the spirochete to attach to mammalian cells.

Inflammatory innate immune responses are critical in the control of early disseminated infection. Spirochetal lipoproteins, which bind to the CD14 molecule and toll-like receptor 2 on macrophages, are potent activators of the innate immune response, leading to the production of macrophage-derived inflammatory cytokines. After the first several weeks of infection, T cells, which are part of the adaptive immune response, generally exhibit heightened responsiveness to *B.*

burgdorferi antigens, and evidence of B-cell hyperactivity is found, including elevated total serum IgM levels, cryoprecipitates, and circulating immune complexes. Titers of specific IgM antibody to *B. burgdorferi* peak between the third and sixth week after disease onset. The specific IgG response develops gradually over months, with response to an increasing array of at least 12 spirochetal polypeptides and maximal expansion during the period of arthritis. Histologic examination of all affected tissues reveals an infiltration of lymphocytes, macrophages, and plasma cells with some degree of vascular damage (including mild vasculitis or hypervascular occlusion), suggesting that the spirochete may have been present in or around blood vessels.

Despite the innate and adaptive immune responses, *B. burgdorferi* may sometimes survive in certain sites. The ability of the spirochete to downregulate the expression of surface-exposed protein antigens is one important mechanism of immune evasion. In addition, during disseminated infection, a surface-exposed lipoprotein called VlsE undergoes extensive antigenic variation. However, the organism does not have mechanisms that help to protect it from antibiotic therapy. For example, *B. burgdorferi* has only been seen extracellularly in affected tissues; it has not been shown to "hide out" in intracellular locations, thereby evading antibiotic exposure.

CLINICAL MANIFESTATIONS   ■   **Early Infection: Stage 1 (Localized Infection)**
After an incubation period of 3 to 32 days, EM, which occurs at the site of the tick bite, usually begins as a red macule or papule that expands slowly to form a large annular lesion. As the lesion increases in size, it often develops a bright red outer border and partial central clearing. Because of the small size of ixodid ticks, most patients do not remember the preceding tick bite. The center of the lesion sometimes becomes intensely erythematous and indurated, vesicular, or necrotic. In other instances, the expanding lesion remains an even, intense red; several red rings are found within an outside ring; or the central area turns blue before the lesion clears. Although EM can be located anywhere, the thigh, groin, and axilla are particularly common sites. The lesion is warm but not often painful. Approximately 20% of patients do not exhibit this characteristic skin manifestation. In Europe, EM is often an indolent localized infection of the skin; in contrast, in the United States, this lesion is associated with more intense inflammation and signs that often suggest dissemination of the spirochete.

Early Infection: Stage 2 (Disseminated Infection)   In cases in the United States, *B. burgdorferi* often spreads hematogenously to many sites within days or weeks after the onset of EM. In these cases, patients may develop secondary annular skin lesions similar in appearance to the initial lesion. Skin involvement is commonly accompanied by severe headache, mild stiffness of the neck, fever, chills, migratory musculoskeletal pain, arthralgias, and profound malaise and fatigue. Less common manifestations include generalized lymphadenopathy or splenomegaly, hepatitis, sore throat, nonproductive cough, conjunctivitis, iritis, or testicular swelling. Except for fatigue and lethargy, which are often constant, the early signs and symptoms of Lyme disease are typically intermittent and changing. Even in untreated patients, the early symptoms usually become less severe or disappear within several weeks. In ~15% of patients, the infection presents with these nonspecific systemic symptoms.

Symptoms suggestive of meningeal irritation may develop early in Lyme disease when EM is present but usually are not associated with cerebrospinal fluid (CSF) pleocytosis or an objective neurologic deficit. After several weeks or months, ~15% of untreated patients develop frank neurologic abnormalities, including meningitis, subtle encephalitic signs, cranial neuritis (including bilateral facial palsy), motor or sensory radiculoneuropathy, mononeuritis multiplex, cerebellar ataxia, or myelitis—alone or in various combinations. In the United States, the usual pattern consists of fluctuating symptoms of meningitis accompanied by facial palsy and peripheral radiculoneuropathy. Lymphocytic pleocytosis (~100 cells per μL) is found in CSF, often along with elevated protein levels and normal or slightly low glucose concentrations. In Europe and Asia, the first neurologic sign is characteristically radicular pain, which is followed by the development of CSF pleocytosis (called meningopolyneuritis or *Bannwarth's syndrome*), but meningeal or encephalitic signs are frequently absent. In children, the optic nerve may be affected because of inflammation or increased intracranial pressure, which may lead to blindness. These early neurologic abnormalities usually resolve completely within months, but in rare cases, chronic neurologic disease may occur later.

Within several weeks after the onset of illness, ~8% of patients develop cardiac involvement. The most common abnormality is a fluctuating degree of atrioventricular block (first-degree, Wenckebach, or complete heart block). Some patients have more diffuse cardiac involvement, including electrocardiographic changes indicative of acute myopericarditis, left ventricular dysfunction evident on radionuclide scans, or (in rare cases) cardiomegaly or pancarditis. Cardiac involvement usually lasts for only a few weeks but may recur. Chronic cardiomyopathy caused by *B. burgdorferi* has been reported in Europe.

During this stage, musculoskeletal pain is common. The typical pattern consists of migratory pain in joints, tendons, bursae, muscles, or bones (usually without joint swelling) lasting for hours or days and affecting one or two locations at a time.

Late Infection: Stage 3 (Persistent Infection)   Months after the onset of infection, ~60% of patients in the United States who have received no antibiotic treatment develop frank arthritis. The typical pattern comprises intermittent attacks of oligoarticular arthritis in large joints (especially the knees), lasting for weeks to months in a given joint. Small joints and periarticular sites also may be affected, primarily during early attacks. The number of patients who continue to have recurrent attacks decreases each year. However, in a small percentage of cases, involvement of large joints—usually one or both knees—becomes chronic and may lead to erosion of cartilage and bone. These patients have a higher frequency of the class II major histocompatibility complex alleles associated with rheumatoid arthritis, particularly HLA-DRBI*0401 or *0101 alleles, than patients with brief Lyme arthritis. Moreover, they may have persistent arthritis for months or even several years after the apparent eradication of spirochetes from the joints with antibiotic therapy. In these genetically susceptible individuals, it has been postulated that autoimmunity may develop within the proinflammatory milieu of the joints because of molecular mimicry between a dominant T-cell epitope of OspA and a similar sequence in a human protein.

White cell counts in joint fluid range from 500 to 110,000/μL (average, 25,000/μL); most of these cells are polymorphonuclear leukocytes. Tests for rheumatoid factor or antinuclear antibodies usually give negative results. Examination of synovial biopsy samples reveals fibrin deposits, villous hypertrophy, vascular proliferation, microangiopathic lesions, and a heavy infiltration of lymphocytes and plasma cells.

Although less common, chronic neurologic involvement may also become apparent months or years after the onset of infection, sometimes following long periods of latent infection. The most common form of chronic central nervous system involvement is subtle encephalopathy affecting memory, mood, or sleep and often accompanied by axonal polyneuropathy manifested as either distal paresthesia or spinal radicular pain. Patients with encephalopathy frequently have evidence of memory impairment in neuropsychological tests and abnormal results in CSF analyses. In cases with polyneuropathy, electromyography generally shows extensive abnormalities of proximal and distal nerve segments. Encephalomyelitis or leukoencephalitis, a rare manifestation of Lyme borreliosis associated primarily with *B. garinii* infection in Europe, is a severe neurologic disorder that may include spastic paraparesis, upper motor-neuron bladder dysfunction, and lesions in the periventricular white matter. The prolonged course of chronic neuroborreliosis following periods of latent infection is reminiscent of tertiary neurosyphilis.

Acrodermatitis chronica atrophicans, the late skin manifestation of the disorder, has been associated primarily with *B. afzelii* infection in Europe and Asia. It has been observed mostly in elderly women. The skin lesions, which are usually found on the acral surface of an arm or leg, begin insidiously with reddish-violaceous discoloration; they become sclerotic or atrophic over a period of years.

DIAGNOSIS The culture of *B. burgdorferi* in Barbour-Stoenner-Kelly (BSK) medium permits definitive diagnosis, but this complex method has been used only in research studies. Moreover, with a few exceptions, positive cultures have been obtained only early in the illness—primarily from biopsy samples of EM skin lesions, less often from plasma samples, and occasionally from CSF samples. Later in the infection, polymerase chain reaction (PCR) is greatly superior to culture for the detection of *B. burgdorferi* DNA in joint fluid, and this has been the major use for PCR testing in Lyme disease. In one study, *B. burgdorferi* DNA was detected by PCR in synovial fluid samples from 75 (85%) of 88 patients and in none of 64 control samples. However, the sensitivity of PCR determinations in CSF from patients with neuroborreliosis has been much lower. There seems to be little if any role for PCR in the detection of *B. burgdorferi* DNA in blood or urine samples. Moreover, this procedure, which must be carefully controlled to prevent contamination, is not routinely available.

Because of the problems associated with direct detection of *B. burgdorferi*, Lyme disease is usually diagnosed by the recognition of a characteristic clinical picture with serologic confirmation. Although serologic testing may yield negative results during the first several weeks of infection, most patients have a positive antibody response to *B. burgdorferi* after that time. The limitation of serologic tests is that they do not clearly distinguish between active and inactive infection. Patients with previous Lyme disease—particularly in cases progressing to late stages—often remain seropositive for years, even after adequate antibiotic treatment. In addition, about 10% of patients are seropositive because of asymptomatic infection. If these individuals subsequently develop another illness, the positive serologic test for Lyme disease may cause diagnostic confusion. Conversely, in rare instances, patients who receive inadequate antibiotic therapy during the first several weeks of infection may subsequently develop subtle joint or neurologic symptoms but are seronegative. The important point is that seronegative Lyme disease is usually a mild, attenuated illness that responds well to standard courses of antibiotic therapy. According to an algorithm published by the American College of Physicians (Table 157-1), serologic testing for Lyme disease is recommended only for patients with at least an intermediate pretest probability of Lyme disease, such as those with oligoarticular arthritis. It should not be used as a screening procedure in patients with pain or fatigue syndromes. In such patients, the probability of a false-positive serologic result is higher than that of a true-positive result.

For serologic analysis of Lyme disease in the United States, the CDC recommends a two-step approach in which samples are first tested by enzyme-linked immunosorbent assay (ELISA) and equivocal or positive results are then tested by western blotting. During the first month of infection, both IgM and IgG responses to the spirochete should be determined, preferably in both acute- and convalescent-phase serum samples. Approximately 20 to 30% of patients have a positive response detectable in acute-phase samples, whereas about 70 to 80% have a positive response during convalescence (2 to 4 weeks later). After 1 month of infection, by which time most patients with active Lyme disease have disseminated infection, the sensitivity and specificity of the IgG response to the spirochete are both very high—in the range of 95% to 99%—as determined by the two-test approach of ELISA and western blot. At this point and thereafter, a single test (that for IgG) is usually sufficient. In persons with illness of >1 month's duration, a positive IgM test result alone is likely to be false-positive and therefore should not be used to support the diagnosis. According to current criteria adopted by the CDC, an IgM western blot is considered positive if two of the following three bands are present: 23, 39, and 41 kDa. However, the combination of the 23- and

41-kDa bands may still represent a false-positive result. An IgG blot is considered positive if 5 of the following 10 bands are present: 18, 23, 28, 30, 39, 41, 45, 58, 66, and 93 kDa. In European cases, there is less expansion of the antibody response, and no single set of criteria for the interpretation of immunoblots results in high levels of sensitivity and specificity in all countries.

Several second-generation tests that use recombinant spirochetal proteins or synthetic peptides have shown promising results. For example, an IgG ELISA employing a 26-mer peptide from invariant region 6 (IR$_6$) of the VlsE lipoprotein has a sensitivity and a specificity similar to those achieved with the IgM and IgG two-test approach using sonicated whole spirochetes. However, the IR$_6$ ELISA has a limitation similar to that affecting standard serology, in that a positive test result does not distinguish clearly between active and past infection. The IR$_6$ ELISA may be of value with regard to European as well as American strains of the spirochete.

DIFFERENTIAL DIAGNOSIS Classic EM is a slowly expanding erythema, often with partial central clearing. If the lesion expands little, it may represent the red papule of an uninfected tick bite. If the lesion expands rapidly, it may represent cellulitis (e.g., streptococcal cellulitis) or an allergic reaction, perhaps to tick saliva. Patients with secondary annular lesions may be thought to have erythema multiforme, but neither the development of blistering mucosal lesions nor the involvement of the palms or soles is a feature of *B. burgdorferi* infection. In the southeastern United States, an EM-like skin lesion, sometimes with mild systemic symptoms, may be associated with *Amblyomma americanum* tick bites, but the cause of this illness has not yet been identified.

In the United States, *I. scapularis* ticks may transmit not only *B. burgdorferi* but also *Babesia microti*, a red blood cell parasite (Chap. 195), or *Anaplasma phagocytophila*, the agent of human anaplasmosis (formerly called the agent of human granulocytotropic ehrlichiosis; Chap. 158). Although babesiosis and anaplasmosis are most often asymptomatic, infection with any of these three agents may cause nonspecific systemic symptoms, and coinfected patients may have more severe or persistent symptoms than patients infected with a single agent. Standard blood counts may yield clues regarding the presence of coinfection. Anaplasmosis may cause leukopenia or thrombocytopenia, and babesiosis may cause thrombocytopenia or (in severe cases) hemolytic anemia. However, IgM serologic responses may confuse the diagnosis. For example, *A. phagocytophila* may elicit a positive IgM response to *B. burgdorferi*. The frequency of coinfection in different studies has been variable. In one prospective study, 4% of patients with EM had evidence of coinfection.

Facial palsy caused by *B. burgdorferi*, which occurs in the early disseminated phase of the infection (often in July, August, or September), is usually recognized by its association with EM. However, facial palsy without EM may be the presenting manifestation of Lyme disease. In such cases, both the IgM and IgG responses to the spirochete are usually positive. The most common infectious agents that cause

TABLE 157-1 *Algorithm for Testing for and Treating Lyme Disease*

Pretest Probability	Example	Recommendation
High	Patients with erythema migrans	Empirical antibiotic treatment without serologic testing
Intermediate	Patients with oligoarticular arthritis	Serologic testing and antibiotic treatment if test results are positive
Low	Patients with nonspecific symptoms (myalgias, arthralgias, fatigue)	Neither serologic testing nor antibiotic treatment

Source: Adapted from the recommendations of the American College of Physicians (G Nichol et al: Ann Intern Med 128:37, 1998, with permission).

facial palsy are herpes simplex virus type 1 (Bell's palsy; Chap. 163) and varicella-zoster virus (Ramsay-Hunt syndrome; Chap. 164).

Later in the infection, oligoarticular Lyme arthritis most resembles reactive arthritis in an adult or the pauciarticular form of juvenile rheumatoid arthritis in a child. Patients with Lyme arthritis usually have the highest IgG antibody responses seen in the infection, with reactivity to many spirochetal proteins.

The most common problem in diagnosis is to mistake Lyme disease for chronic fatigue syndrome (Chap. 370) or fibromyalgia (Chap. 315). This difficulty is compounded by the fact that a small percentage of patients do in fact develop these chronic pain or fatigue syndromes in association with or soon after Lyme disease. Compared with Lyme disease, chronic fatigue syndrome or fibromyalgia tends to produce more generalized and disabling symptoms, including marked fatigue, severe headache, diffuse musculoskeletal pain, multiple symmetric tender points in characteristic locations, pain and stiffness in many joints, diffuse dysesthesia, difficulty with concentration, and sleep disturbances. Patients with chronic fatigue syndrome or fibromyalgia lack evidence of joint inflammation; they have normal results in neurologic tests; and they usually have a greater degree of anxiety and depression than patients with chronic neuroborreliosis.

℞ TREATMENT

As outlined in the algorithm in Fig. 157-1, the various manifestations of Lyme disease can usually be treated successfully with orally administered antibiotics; the exceptions are objective neurologic abnormalities and third-degree atrioventricular heart block, which seem to require intravenous therapy. For early Lyme disease, doxycycline is effective in men and in nonpregnant women. An advantage of this regimen is that it is also effective against *A. phagocytophila*, which is

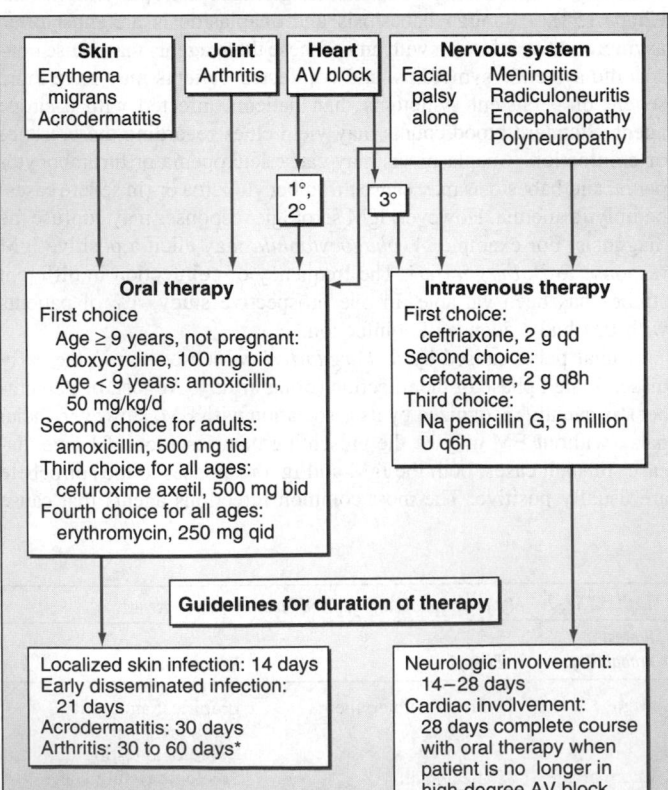

FIGURE 157-1 *Algorithm for the treatment of the various acute or chronic manifestations of Lyme borreliosis. AV, atrioventricular. *For Lyme arthritis, intravenous ceftriaxone, 2 g given once a day for 14 to 28 days, is also effective and may elicit a response more quickly than oral therapy; however, compared with oral treatment, this regimen is less convenient to administer, has more side effects, and is more expensive.*

transmitted by the same tick that transmits the Lyme disease agent. Amoxicillin, cefuroxime axetil, and erythromycin or its congeners are second-, third-, and fourth-choice alternatives, respectively. In children, amoxicillin is effective (not more than 2 g/d); in cases of penicillin allergy, cefuroxime axetil or erythromycin may be used. In contrast to second- or third-generation cephalosporin antibiotics, first-generation cephalosporins, such as cephalexin, are not effective. For patients with infection localized to the skin, a 14-day course of therapy is generally sufficient; in contrast, for patients with disseminated infection, a 21-day course is recommended. Approximately 15% of patients experience a Jarisch-Herxheimer-like reaction during the first 24 h of therapy. In multicenter studies, more than 90% of patients whose early Lyme disease was treated with these regimens had satisfactory outcomes. Although some patients reported symptoms after treatment, objective evidence of persistent infection or relapse was rare, and retreatment was usually unnecessary.

One of these oral antibiotic regimens, when given for 30 to 60 days, or intravenous ceftriaxone, given for 14 to 28 days, is effective for the treatment of Lyme arthritis. Oral therapy is easier to administer, is associated with fewer side effects, and is considerably less expensive. However, the response to oral therapy may be slower than that to intravenous therapy, and some patients given oral therapy have subsequently developed overt neuroborreliosis, which may require intravenous therapy for a successful outcome. In the small percentage of patients with arthritis in whom arthritic symptoms persist for months or even years after the apparent eradication of spirochetes from the joints with antimicrobial therapy, treatment with anti-inflammatory agents or synovectomy may be successful.

For objective neurologic abnormalities (with the possible exception of facial palsy alone), parenteral antibiotic therapy seems to be necessary. Intravenous ceftriaxone, given for 14 to 28 days, is most commonly used for this purpose, but intravenous cefotaxime or intravenous penicillin G for the same duration may also be effective. In patients with high-degree atrioventricular block or a PR interval of >0.3 s, intravenous therapy for at least part of the course and cardiac monitoring are recommended, but the insertion of a permanent pacemaker is not necessary.

It is unclear how and whether asymptomatic infection should be treated, but patients with such infection are often given a course of oral antibiotics. Because maternal-fetal transmission of *B. burgdorferi* seems to occur rarely, if at all, standard therapy for the manifestations of the illness is recommended for pregnant women. Long-term persistence of *B. burgdorferi* has not been documented in any large series of patients after treatment with currently recommended regimens. Therefore, there is no indication for multiple, repeated antibiotic courses in the treatment of Lyme disease.

After appropriately treated Lyme disease, a small percentage of patients continue to have subjective symptoms, primarily musculoskeletal pain, neurocognitive difficulties, or fatigue. This so-called chronic Lyme disease or post–Lyme disease syndrome is a disabling condition that is similar to chronic fatigue syndrome or fibromyalgia. In a large study, one group of patients with post–Lyme disease syndrome received intravenous ceftriaxone for 30 days followed by oral doxycycline for 60 days, while another group received intravenous and oral placebo preparations for the same durations. No significant differences were found between groups in the numbers of patients reporting that their symptoms had improved, become worse, or stayed the same. Such patients are best treated for the relief of symptoms rather than with prolonged courses of antibiotics.

The risk of infection with *B. burgdorferi* after a recognized tick bite is so low that antibiotic prophylaxis is not routinely indicated. However, if an attached, engorged *I. scapularis* nymph is found or if follow-up is anticipated to be difficult, a single 200-mg dose of doxycycline, which effectively prevents Lyme disease when given within 72 h after the tick bite, may be administered.

PROGNOSIS   The response to treatment is best early in the disease. Later treatment of Lyme borreliosis is still effective, but the period of convalescence may be longer. Eventually, most patients recover with minimal or no residual deficits.

REINFECTION Reinfection may occur after EM when patients are treated with antimicrobial agents. In such cases, the immune response is not adequate to provide protection from subsequent infection. However, patients who develop an expanded immune response to the spirochete over a period of months (such as those with Lyme arthritis) have protective immunity for a period of years and do not acquire the infection again.

PREVENTION Protective measures for the prevention of Lyme disease may include the avoidance of tick-infested areas, the use of repellents and acaricides, tick checks, and modification of landscapes in or near residential areas. Although a vaccine for Lyme disease used to be available, the manufacturer has discontinued its production. Therefore, no vaccine is now commercially available for the prevention of this infection.

FURTHER READING

BARBOUR AG, HAYES SF: Biology of *Borrelia* species. Microbiol Rev 50: 381, 1986

KLEMPNER MS et al: Two controlled trials of antibiotic treatment in patients with persistent symptoms and a history of Lyme disease. N Engl J Med 345:85, 2001

LIANG FT et al: Sensitive and specific serodiagnosis of Lyme disease by enzyme-linked immunosorbent assay with a peptide based on an immunodominant conserved region of *Borrelia burgdorferi* VlsE. J Clin Microbiol 37:3990, 1999

NADELMAN RB et al: Prophylaxis with single-dose doxycycline for the prevention of Lyme disease after *Ixodes scapularis* tick bite. N Engl J Med 345:79, 2001

STEERE AC: Lyme disease. N Engl J Med 345:115, 2001

WORMSER GP et al: Guidelines from the Infectious Diseases Society of America: Practice guidelines for the treatment of Lyme disease. Clin Infect Dis 31(Suppl 1):S1, 2000

Section 10   Diseases Caused by Rickettsia, Mycoplasma, and Chlamydia

158   RICKETTSIAL DISEASES
David H. Walker, Didier Raoult, J. Stephen Dumler, Thomas Marrie

The rickettsiae make up a family of gram-negative coccobacilli and short bacilli that grow strictly in eukaryotic cells. Characteristics of these organisms include their obligately intracellular location and persistence. The pathogenic rickettsiae move through mammalian reservoirs; they are transmitted by insect or tick vectors. Except for louse-borne typhus, humans are incidental hosts. Among rickettsiae, *Coxiella burnetii* (the agent of Q fever) is notorious for its ability to survive for an extended period outside of the reservoir or vector and for its extreme infectiousness: inhalation of a single microorganism can cause pneumonia. Clinical infections with rickettsiae can be classified into five general groups: (1) tick-, louse-, flea-, and gamasid mite–borne, spotted fever group (SFG) and typhus group rickettsial diseases; (2) chigger-borne scrub typhus; (3) tick-borne ehrlichioses and anaplasmosis; (4) neorickettsiosis (sennetsu fever); and (5) Q fever. The rickettsiae that cause spotted fevers, typhus, and scrub typhus are listed along with their vectors, geographic ranges, and associated diseases in Table 158-1.

TICK-, MITE-, AND FLEA-BORNE SPOTTED FEVERS

ROCKY MOUNTAIN SPOTTED FEVER Rocky Mountain spotted fever (RMSF), the most severe of the rickettsial diseases, is caused by *Rickettsia rickettsii*. This organism possesses two major immunodominant surface-exposed proteins, OmpA and OmpB, which have species-specific conformational epitopes. OmpA functions as an adhesin for the host cell; OmpB, the most abundant outer-membrane protein, shares genetic sequences and limited antigens with typhus group rickettsiae. This small (0.3 μm by 1.0 μm) bacillus has a gram-negative cell wall

---

TABLE 158-1 *Features of Selected Rickettsial Infections*

Disease	Organism	Vector(s)	Geographic Range	Incubation Period	Duration
Rocky Mountain spotted fever	*Rickettsia rickettsii*	*Dermacentor andersoni* *D. variabilis* *Amblyomma cajennense* *Rhipicephalus sanguineus*	United States United States Central/South America Mexico	2–14 days	10–20 days
Mediterranean spotted fever[a]	*R. conorii*	*R. sanguineus*	Southern Europe, Africa, Middle East, Central Asia	5–7 days	7–14 days
African tick-bite fever	*R. africae*	*A. hebraeum, A. variegatum*	Sub-Saharan Africa, West Indies	4–10 days	?
Rickettsialpox[a]	*R. akari*	*Liponyssoides sanguineus*	United States, Ukraine, Croatia	10–17 days	3–11 days
Cat-flea typhus	*R. felis*	*Ctenocephalides felis*	North and South America, Europe	8–16 days	8–16 days
Epidemic typhus	*R. prowazekii*	*Pediculus humanus corporis*	Worldwide	7–14 days	10–18 days
Brill-Zinsser disease	*R. prowazekii*	—[b]	Worldwide	Years	7–11 days
Murine typhus	*R. typhi*	*Xenopsylla cheopis*	Worldwide	8–16 days	8–16 days
Scrub typhus[a]	*Orientia tsutsugamushi*	*Leptotrombidium deliense*	Asia, Australia, New Guinea, Pacific Islands	6–21 days	6–21 days

[a] Eschar is usually present at the bite site.   [b] Brill-Zinsser disease represents a recrudescence of latent epidemic typhus.

structure; its lipopolysaccharide shares antigens mainly within the SFG and is not endotoxic in the quantities found in human infections.

Discovered in the American West in the late nineteenth century, RMSF is at present documented in 48 states (with the highest prevalences in the south-central and southeastern states) as well as in Canada, Mexico, Costa Rica, Panama, Colombia, Argentina, and Brazil. It is transmitted by *Dermacentor variabilis*, the American dog tick, in the eastern two-thirds of the United States and in California; by *D. andersoni*, the Rocky Mountain wood tick, in the western United States; by *Rhipicephalus sanguineus* in Mexico; and by *Amblyomma cajennense* in Central and South America. Maintained principally by transovarian transmission from one generation of ticks to the next, *R. rickettsii* can be acquired by uninfected ticks through the ingestion of a blood meal from rickettsemic small mammals.

Humans become infected during the active season of the vector tick species. In northern areas, cases occur mainly in the spring; in warmer southern states, most cases occur from May to September, although some cases are reported in the winter. Although 4% of *D. variabilis* ticks contain rickettsiae, the vast majority of these are nonpathogenic species such as *R. montanensis* and *R. bellii*. The likelihood of an individual tick's containing *R. rickettsii* is remote. From 1971 to 2001, the reported incidence of RMSF was in the range of 0.16 to 0.50 cases per 100,000 population in the United States. In 2001, 0.20 persons per 100,000 in the United States developed RMSF. This rate is probably an underestimate, since the diagnosis is difficult and reporting incomplete. The 5- to 9-year-old age group has the highest incidence. The mortality rate was 20 to 25% in the preantibiotic era and now remains at ~3 to 5% because of delayed diagnosis and treatment. The case-fatality ratio increases with each decade of life above age 20.

Pathogenesis *R. rickettsii* organisms are inoculated into the dermis along with secretions of the tick's salivary glands after ≥6 h of feeding. Rickettsiae spread lymphohematogenously throughout the body, attach via OmpA to the endothelial cell membrane, and induce their own engulfment. Once intracellularly located, they escape rapidly from the phagosome, replicate in the cytosol by binary fission, and spread from cell to cell, propelled by polar polymerization of the host cell's actin. The result is numerous foci of contiguous infected endothelial cells that are extensive enough to manifest clinically after a dose-dependent incubation period of ~1 week (range, 2 to 14 days). *R. rickettsii* is more invasive than other rickettsiae, routinely spreading to infect vascular smooth-muscle cells. Despite frequent statements to the contrary, occlusive thrombosis and ischemic necrosis are not the fundamental pathologic basis for tissue and organ injury in RMSF. Instead, increased vascular permeability, with resulting edema, hypovolemia, and ischemia, is responsible. Indeed, immunohistologic studies of severely infected humans and animals have demonstrated numerous zones of infected endothelium, only a small proportion of which contain thrombi. The thrombi are usually located to one side of the lumen, which is not occluded. These hemostatic plugs appear to be an appropriate host response rather than a pathogenic process. Consumption of platelets results in thrombocytopenia in 32 to 52% of patients, but disseminated intravascular coagulation with hypofibrinogenemia is rare. Activation of platelets, generation of thrombin, and activation of the fibrinolytic system all appear to be homeostatic physiologic responses to endothelial injury.

Clinical Manifestations The incubation period averages 7 days. Early in the illness, when medical attention usually is first sought, RMSF is difficult to distinguish from many self-limiting viral illnesses. Fever, headache, malaise, myalgia, nausea, vomiting, and anorexia are the most frequent symptoms during the first 3 days. The patient becomes progressively more ill as vascular infection and injury advance. In one large series, only one-third of patients were diagnosed with presumptive RMSF early in the clinical course and treated appropriately as outpatients. In the tertiary care setting, RMSF is all too often recog-

nized only when its late severe manifestations, developing at the end of the first week or during the second week of illness in patients without appropriate treatment, prompt admission to the intensive care unit.

The progressive nature of the infection is clearly manifested in the skin. Rash is evident in only 14% of patients on the first day of illness and in only 49% during the first 3 days. Macules (1 to 5 mm) appear first on the wrists and ankles and then on the remainder of the extremities and the trunk. Later, more severe vascular damage results in frank hemorrhage at the center of the maculopapule, a petechia that does not disappear upon compression (Fig. 158-1). This sequence of events is sometimes delayed or aborted by effective treatment. In fact, rash appears on day 6 or later in 20% of cases and does not appear at all in 9 to 16% of cases, including some with severe visceral lesions that result in death. Petechiae occur in 41 to 59% of cases, appearing on or after day 6 in 74% of cases that include a rash. Involvement of the palms and soles, often considered diagnostically important, usually occurs relatively late in the course (after day 5 in 43% of cases) and does not occur at all in 18 to 64% of cases.

The microcirculation, both systemic and pulmonary, is the target of intracellular rickettsial infection, and the clinical manifestations reflect the ensuing vascular changes. Widespread increased vascular permeability results in edema, decreased plasma volume, hypoalbuminemia, reduced serum oncotic pressure, and prerenal azotemia. Hypotension occurs in 17% of cases. Extensive infection of the pulmonary microcirculation is associated with noncardiogenic pulmonary edema. Cardiac involvement is most frequently manifested as dysrhythmia, which is detected in 7 to 16% of cases. Pulmonary involvement, often a major factor in fatal cases, is observed in 17% of cases, of which 12% are considered to represent severe respiratory disease and 8% require mechanical ventilation.

FIGURE 158-1 *Top:* Petechial lesions of Rocky Mountain spotted fever on the lower legs and soles of a young, otherwise-healthy patient. *Bottom:* Close-up of lesions from the same patient. (*Photos courtesy of Dr. Lindsey Baden.*)

Central nervous system (CNS) involvement is the other important determinant of the outcome of RMSF. Encephalitis, presenting as confusion or lethargy, is apparent in 26 to 28% of cases. Progressively severe encephalitis manifests as stupor or delirium in 21 to 26% of cases, as ataxia in 18%, as coma in 9 to 10%, and as seizures in 8%. Cranial nerve palsy, hearing loss, severe vertigo, nystagmus, dysarthria, aphasia, unilateral corticospinal signs, ankle clonus, extensor toe signs, hyperreflexia, spasticity, fasciculations, athetosis, neurogenic bladder, hemiplegia, paraplegia, and complete paralysis have been reported. Meningoencephalitis results in cerebrospinal fluid (CSF) pleocytosis in 34 to 38% of cases; usually there are 10 to 100 cells per microliter with a mononuclear predominance, but occasionally there are more than 100 cells per microliter and a polymorphonuclear predominance. The CSF protein concentration is increased in 30 to 35% of cases, but the CSF glucose concentration is usually normal.

Renal failure, which occurs in more severely ill patients, is often reversible with rehydration. However, in the most severe cases, shock results in acute tubular necrosis–induced renal failure, which often requires hemodialysis.

Hepatic injury is manifested in 38% of cases as mildly or moderately increased serum aminotransferase concentrations and is due to focal death of individual hepatocytes, but hepatic failure does not occur. Jaundice is recognized in 8 to 9% of cases and an elevated serum bilirubin concentration in 18 to 30%. Marked hyperbilirubinemia occasionally occurs, probably as a consequence of both hemolysis and hepatocytic injury.

Bleeding is a potentially life-threatening effect of severe vascular damage. Anemia develops in 30% of cases and is severe enough to require red blood cell transfusions in 11%. Blood is detected in the stools or vomitus of 10% of patients, and death has followed massive upper gastrointestinal hemorrhage.

Other characteristic clinical laboratory findings include a normal white blood cell count with increased numbers of immature myeloid cells, increased plasma levels of proteins of the acute-phase response (C-reactive protein, fibrinogen, ferritin, and others), and hyponatremia (in 56% of cases) due to the appropriate secretion of antidiuretic hormone in response to the hypovolemic state. Skeletal muscle injury, clinically manifested as myositis, has been documented in several individual cases by the detection of marked elevations in serum creatine kinase or of histopathologic evidence of vascular injury in skeletal muscle and multifocal rhabdomyonecrosis. Ocular involvement includes conjunctivitis in 30% of cases and retinal vein engorgement, flame hemorrhages, arterial occlusion, and papilledema with normal CSF pressure in some instances.

In untreated cases, death usually occurs 8 to 15 days after the onset of illness. A rare presentation, fulminant RMSF, is fatal within 5 days after onset. This fulminant presentation has been associated with RMSF in black males who have a glucose-6-phosphate dehydrogenase (G6PD) deficiency and is thought to be related to an undefined effect of hemolysis on the rickettsial infection. Although survivors of RMSF usually appear to return to their previous state of health, permanent sequelae, including neurologic deficits and amputation of gangrenous extremities, may follow severe illness.

Diagnosis The diagnosis of RMSF during the acute stage is more difficult than is generally appreciated. Clinical and epidemiologic considerations are more important than laboratory features early in the illness. The most important epidemiologic factor is a history of exposure within the 12 days preceding disease onset to a potentially tick-infested environment during a season of possible tick activity. However, only 60% of patients actually recall being bitten by a tick during the incubation period.

The differential diagnosis for early clinical manifestations of RMSF (fever, headache, and myalgia without a rash) includes influenza, enteroviral infection, infectious mononucleosis, viral hepatitis, leptospirosis, typhoid fever, gram-negative or gram-positive bacterial sepsis, human monocytotropic or granulocytotropic ehrlichiosis or anaplasmosis, murine typhus, sylvatic flying-squirrel typhus, and rickettsialpox. Enterocolitis may be suggested by nausea, vomiting, and abdominal pain; prominence of abdominal tenderness has resulted in exploratory laparotomy. CNS involvement may masquerade as bacterial and viral meningoencephalitis, with seizures, coma, neurologic signs, and CSF abnormalities. Cough, pulmonary signs, and chest roentgenographic opacities may lead to a diagnostic consideration of bronchitis or pneumonia.

At presentation during the first 3 days of illness, only 3% of patients exhibit the classic triad of fever, rash, and history of tick exposure. When a rash appears, a diagnosis of RMSF should certainly be considered. However, many illnesses considered in the differential diagnosis may also be associated with a rash, including rubeola, rubella, meningococcemia, disseminated gonococcal infection, secondary syphilis, toxic shock syndrome, drug hypersensitivity, idiopathic thrombocytopenic purpura, thrombotic thrombocytopenic purpura, Kawasaki syndrome, and immune complex vasculitis. Conversely, any person in an endemic area with a provisional diagnosis of one of the above illnesses may have RMSF.

The most common serologic test for confirmation of the diagnosis is the indirect immunofluorescence assay. Between 7 and 10 days after onset, a diagnostic titer of ≥1:64 is usually detectable. Latex agglutination and a solid-state enzyme immunoassay are also available commercially. Latex agglutination usually yields a diagnostic titer of ≥1:128 at 7 to 9 days after onset. The sensitivity and specificity of the indirect immunofluorescence assay are 94 to 100% and 100%, respectively, and the latex agglutination test has a sensitivity of 71 to 94% and a specificity of 96 to 99%. The performance of the solid-state immunoassay has not been reported. It is important to understand that serologic tests for RMSF are usually negative at the time of presentation for medical care and that treatment should not be delayed while a positive serologic result is awaited.

The only diagnostic test that is useful during the acute illness is immunohistologic examination (immunofluorescence or immunoenzyme staining) of a cutaneous biopsy of a rash lesion for *R. rickettsii*. Examination of a 3-mm punch biopsy of such a lesion is 70% sensitive and 100% specific. Polymerase chain reaction (PCR) amplification and detection of *R. rickettsii* DNA in peripheral blood is a relatively insensitive approach except in the preterminal state; rickettsiae are present in large quantities in heavily infected foci of endothelial cells but in relatively low quantities in the circulation. Cultivation of rickettsiae in cell culture is technically feasible but is seldom undertaken because of biohazard and technologic concerns.

℞ TREATMENT

The drug of choice for the treatment of both children and adults with RMSF is doxycycline, except when the patient is pregnant or allergic to the drug. Because of the severity of RMSF, immediate empirical administration of doxycycline should be strongly considered in any patient with a consistent clinical presentation in the appropriate epidemiologic setting. Doxycycline is administered orally (or, in the presence of coma or vomiting, intravenously) at 200 mg/d in two divided doses. For children with suspected RMSF infection, up to five courses of doxycycline may be administered with minimal risk of dental staining. Other regimens include oral tetracycline (25 to 50 mg/kg per day) in four divided doses. The antirickettsial drug should be administered until the patient has been afebrile and improving clinically for 2 or 3 days. β-Lactam antibiotics, erythromycin, and aminoglycosides have no role in the treatment of RMSF, and sulfa-containing drugs are likely to exacerbate this infection. There is not enough clinical experience to comment on the use of fluoroquinolones in this setting. The most seriously ill patients are managed in intensive care units, with careful administration of fluids to achieve optimal tissue perfusion without precipitating noncardiogenic pulmonary edema. In some severely ill patients, hypoxemia requires intubation and mechanical ventilation; oliguric or anuric acute renal failure requires hemodialysis; seizures

TABLE 158-2 *Laboratory Diagnosis and Treatment of Selected Rickettsial Diseases*

Disease	Laboratory Diagnosis	Treatment
Mediterranean spotted fever, Japanese spotted fever, Queensland tick typhus, Flinders Island spotted fever, African tick-bite fever	Isolation of rickettsiae by shell-vial culture; serology, IFA (IgM, ≥1:64; or IgG, ≥1:128); skin biopsy immunohistochemical detection of rickettsiae; PCR amplification of DNA from tissue specimens	Doxycycline (100 mg bid PO for 1–5 days) *or* Ciprofloxacin (750 mg bid PO for 5 days) *or* Chloramphenicol (500 mg qid PO for 7–10 days) *or* (in pregnancy) Josamycin*ᵃ* (3 g/d PO for 5 days)
Rickettsialpox	IFA: seroconversion to a titer of ≥1:64 or a single titer of ≥1:128; cross-adsorption to eliminate antibodies to shared antigens necessary for a specific diagnosis of the spotted fever rickettsial species; skin biopsy immunohistochemistry	Doxycycline (100 mg bid PO for 1–5 days) *or* Ciprofloxacin (750 mg bid PO for 5 days) *or* Chloramphenicol (500 mg qid PO for 7–10 days) *or* (in pregnancy) Josamycin*ᵃ* (3 g/d PO for 5 days)
Endemic (murine) typhus	IFA: fourfold rise to a titer of ≥1:64 or a single titer of ≥1:128; immunohistology: skin biopsy; PCR amplification of *R. typhi* or *R. felis* DNA from blood; dot ELISA and immunoperoxidase methods also available	Doxycycline (100 mg bid PO for 7–15 days) *or* Chloramphenicol (500 mg qid PO for 7–15 days)
Epidemic typhus	IFA: titer of ≥1:128; necessary to use clinical and epidemiologic data to distinguish among louse-borne epidemic typhus, flying-squirrel typhus, and Brill-Zinsser disease	Doxycycline (200 mg PO as a single dose or until patient is afebrile for 24 h)
Scrub typhus	IFA: titer of ≥1:200; PCR amplification of *O. tsutsugamushi* DNA from blood of febrile patients	Doxycycline*ᵇ* (100 mg bid PO for 7–15 days) *or* Chloramphenicol (500 mg qid PO for 7–15 days *or* (for children) Chloramphenicol (150 mg/kg per day for 5 days)

ᵃ Not approved by the U.S. Food and Drug Administration.
ᵇ Azithromycin is more effective than doxycycline in vitro against both doxycycline-susceptible and doxycycline-resistant strains of *O. tsutsugamushi*.
Abbreviations: IFA, indirect immunofluorescence assay; PCR, polymerase chain reaction; ELISA, enzyme-linked immunosorbent assay.

necessitate the use of antiseizure medication; anemia or severe hemorrhage necessitates transfusions of packed red blood cells; and bleeding with severe thrombocytopenia requires platelet transfusions. Heparin is not a useful component of treatment, and there is no evidence that glucocorticoids, although frequently administered, affect outcome.

Prevention Avoidance of tick bites is the only available preventive approach. Protective clothing and tick repellents, which could reduce the risk, are seldom actually used. After possible tick exposure, it is wise to inspect the body once or twice a day and remove ticks before they can inoculate rickettsiae.

MEDITERRANEAN SPOTTED FEVER (BOUTONNEUSE FEVER) AND OTHER TICK-BORNE SPOTTED FEVERS

The etiologic agent of Mediterranean spotted fever, *R. conorii*, is prevalent in southern Europe (below the 45th parallel), all of Africa, and southwestern and south-central Asia. The tick vector and reservoir is *R. sanguineus*, the brown dog tick. The name of this disease varies with the region in which it occurs; examples include Kenya tick typhus, Indian tick typhus, Israeli spotted fever, and Astrakhan spotted fever. Whatever the designation, the disease is characterized by a high fever, rash, and—in most geographic locales—an inoculation eschar (*tâche noire*) at the site of the tick bite. A severe form of the disease, associated with a 50% mortality rate, has been observed in patients with diabetes, alcoholism, or heart failure.

African tick-bite fever, which is caused by *R. africae* and has been recognized since the beginning of the twentieth century, was first documented in the modern era in Zimbabwe in 1992. The disease occurs in rural areas and follows bites by ticks of cattle and wild animals. *R. africae* is prevalent in *Amblyomma hebraeum* and *A. variegatum* ticks, which readily feed on humans. Cases occur throughout sub-Saharan Africa and in the Caribbean islands. The average incubation period is 7 days (range, 4 to 10 days). The illness is mild and consists of headache, fever, eschar at the tick bite site, and regional lymphadenopathy. *Amblyomma* ticks often feed in groups, and several ticks may be found on one patient, with the subsequent development of multiple eschars. Rash is frequently lacking or transient and may be vesicular. African tick-bite fever is the most prevalent rickettsiosis worldwide, and—because of tourism in sub-Saharan Africa—is the most frequently occurring imported rickettsiosis in Europe and North America.

Rickettsia japonica causes *Japanese spotted fever*. Patients present with fever, cutaneous eruption, and an inoculation eschar. A similar disease in northern Asia is caused by *R. sibirica*. In Australia, two spotted fevers have been described. *Queensland tick typhus* is due to *R. australis* and is transmitted by *Ixodes holocyclus*. The skin rash in this disease is usually maculopapular but is sometimes vesicular, and there is an inoculation eschar. *Flinders Island spotted fever*, observed also on nearby Tasmania, is due to *R. honei*. In Europe, patients infected with *R. slovaca* after a *Dermacentor* tick bite manifest an eschar and regional lymphadenopathy.

Diagnosis The diagnosis of these tick-borne spotted fevers is based on clinical and epidemiologic findings and is confirmed by cell-culture isolation of rickettsiae, by PCR of skin biopsies (a method not available in most laboratories), or by serology. The serologic identification of infection with a specific species requires cross-adsorption (Table 158-2). In an endemic area, patients presenting with fever, rash, and/or a skin lesion consisting of a black necrotic area or a crust surrounded by erythema should be considered to have one of these rickettsial spotted fevers.

 TREATMENT

See Table 158-2.

RICKETTSIALPOX Rickettsialpox was first described in 1946 by a general practitioner in New York City and soon afterwards was shown to be caused by a distinct species, *R. akari*. This organism was isolated from mice and their mites (*Liponyssoides sanguineus*), which maintain the organisms by transovarian transmission. *R. akari* shares lipopolysaccharide antigens with other members of the SFG.

Epidemiology More than 100 cases of rickettsialpox were diagnosed annually in the northeastern United States in the late 1940s and the 1950s, and outbreaks occurred in the Ukraine in the 1950s. However, few cases are diagnosed currently. Recently, a culture-confirmed case of rickettsialpox was documented in southern Europe; this case was initially misdiagnosed as Mediterranean spotted fever on the basis of the development of serum antibodies cross-reactive with *R. conorii*. Investigation of eschars suspected to represent bioterrorism-associated cutaneous anthrax has resulted in the diagnosis of cases of rickettsialpox in the United States and has revealed that its occurrence is more widespread than was previously realized. Rickettsialpox is recognized principally in New York City, but cases have also been reported in North Carolina, Virginia, Maryland, Arizona, Utah, and Ohio.

Clinical Manifestations A papule forms at the site of the mite bite. This lesion develops a central vesicle that becomes a 1- to 2.5-cm painless black crusted eschar surrounded by an erythematous halo (Fig. 158-2). Enlargement of the lymph nodes draining the region of the eschar suggests initial lymphogenous spread. After an incubation period of 10 to 17 days, during which the eschar and regional lymphadenopathy frequently go unnoticed, the onset of illness is marked by malaise, chills, fever, headache, and myalgia. A macular rash appears 2 to 6 days after onset and evolves sequentially into papules, vesicles, and crusts that heal without scarring (Fig. 158-3). In some cases the rash remains macular or maculopapular. Some patients suffer nausea, vomiting, abdominal pain, cough, conjunctivitis, or photophobia. Untreated rickettsialpox is not fatal, with fever lasting 6 to 10 days.

Diagnosis and Treatment See Table 158-2.

CAT FLEA–ASSOCIATED RICKETTSIOSIS An emerging rickettsiosis caused by *R. felis* has been documented in North and South America and Europe. Transmitted and maintained transovarially in the geographically widespread cat flea *Ctenocephalides felis*, the infection has been described as moderately severe, with fever, rash, headache, and CNS and gastrointestinal signs. However, the clinical spectrum and frequency of the various clinical manifestations have yet to be determined.

FLEA- AND LOUSE-BORNE TYPHUS GROUP RICKETTSIOSES

ENDEMIC MURINE TYPHUS (FLEA-BORNE) Murine typhus was postulated to be a distinct disease, with rats as the reservoir and fleas as the vector, by Maxcy in 1926. Dyer isolated the etiologic agent, *R. typhi*, from rats and fleas in 1931. By the end of World War II, murine typhus was known to be a global disease.

Epidemiology *R. typhi* is maintained in mammalian host/flea cycles, with rats (*Rattus rattus* and *R. norvegicus*) and the Oriental rat flea (*Xenopsylla cheopis*) as the classic zoonotic niche. Fleas acquire *R. typhi* from rickettsemic rats and carry the organism throughout the rest of their life span. Nonimmune rats and humans are infected when rickettsia-laden flea feces are "scratched" into pruritic bite lesions; less frequently, the flea bite itself transmits the organisms. Yet another possible route of transmission is the inhalation of aerosolized flea feces. Infected rats appear healthy, although they are rickettsemic for ~2 weeks.

Currently, <100 cases of endemic typhus are reported annually in the United States. These cases occur mainly in southern Texas and southern California, where the classic rat/flea cycle is absent and an opossum/cat flea (*C. felis*) cycle is prominent. Cases of endemic typhus occur year-round, mainly in warm (often coastal) areas. This infection has also been reported from Greece, Spain, and Indonesia. The prevalence peaks from April through June in southern Texas and during

FIGURE 158-2 Eschar at the site of the mite bite in a patient with rickettsialpox. (*Reprinted from A Krusell et al: Emerg Infect Dis 8:727, 2002. Photo obtained by Dr. Kenneth Kaye.*)

FIGURE 158-3 *Top:* Papulovesicular lesions on the trunk of the patient with rickettsialpox shown in Fig. 158-2. *Bottom:* Close-up of lesions from the same patient. (*Reprinted from A Krusell et al: Emerg Infect Dis 8:727, 2002. Photos obtained by Dr. Kenneth Kaye.*)

the warm months of summer and early fall in other geographic locations. Patients seldom recall a flea bite or exposure to fleas, although exposure to animals such as cats, opossums, raccoons, skunks, and rats is reported by nearly 40% of those who are questioned.

Clinical Manifestations The incubation period of experimental murine typhus in volunteers averages 11 days, with a range of 8 to 16 days. Close observation during this period reveals prodromal symptoms of headache, myalgia, arthralgia, nausea, and malaise developing 1 to 3 days before the abrupt onset of chills and fever. Nearly all patients experience nausea and vomiting early in the illness.

The duration of untreated illness averages 12 days, with a range of 9 to 18 days. Rash is present in only 13% of patients at the time of presentation for medical care (usually ~4 days after onset of symptoms), appearing an average of 2 days later in half of the remaining patients and never appearing in the other half. The initial macular rash is often detected by careful inspection of the axilla or the inner surface of the arm. Subsequently, the rash becomes maculopapular, involving the trunk more often than the extremities; it is seldom petechial and rarely involves the face, palms, or soles. A rash is detected in only 20% of patients with dark brown or black skin.

Pulmonary involvement is frequently prominent in murine typhus; 35% of patients have a hacking, nonproductive cough, and 23% of patients who undergo chest radiography have pulmonary densities due to interstitial pneumonia, pulmonary edema, and pleural effusions. Bibasilar rales are the most common pulmonary sign. Less common clinical symptoms and signs include abdominal pain, confusion, stupor, seizures, ataxia, coma, and jaundice. Clinical laboratory studies frequently reveal anemia and leukopenia early in the course, leukocytosis late in the course, thrombocytopenia, hyponatremia, hypoalbuminemia, mildly increased serum levels of hepatic aminotransferases, and prerenal azotemia. Complications may include respiratory failure requiring intubation and mechanical ventilation, hematemesis, cerebral hemorrhage, and hemolysis (in patients with G6PD deficiency and some hemoglobinopathies). The illness is severe enough to necessitate the admission of 10% of hospitalized patients to an intensive care unit. Greater severity is generally associated with old age, underlying disease, and treatment with a sulfonamide drug; the case-fatality rate is 1%. In a study of children with murine typhus, 50% suffered only nocturnal fevers, feeling well enough for active daytime play.

Diagnosis and Treatment   See Table 158-2.

EPIDEMIC TYPHUS (LOUSE-BORNE)   Epidemic typhus due to infection with *R. prowazekii* is transmitted by the human body louse (*Pediculus humanus corporis*), which lives on clothes and is found in poor hygienic conditions (especially in jails, where the disease it causes is called *jail fever*) and usually in cold areas. Lice acquire *R. prowazekii* when they ingest a blood meal from a rickettsemic patient. The rickettsiae multiply in the midgut epithelial cells of the louse and spill over into the louse feces. The infected louse defecates during its blood meal, and the patient autoinoculates the organisms by scratching. The fact that the louse abandons dead hosts and patients with high fever (>40°C) improves its efficiency as a vector. Since the louse does not pass *R. prowazekii* to its offspring, the disease is usually spread from person to person by the louse-borne route. Lice die within 1 to 2 weeks after infection, turning red because of intestinal perforation just prior to death—hence the name *red louse disease*. This epidemic form of typhus is related to poverty, cold weather, war, and disasters and is currently prevalent in mountainous areas of Africa, South America, and Asia. A large outbreak involving 100,000 people in refugee camps in Burundi occurred in 1997, a small focus was reported in Russia in 1998, sporadic cases have been reported from Algeria, and annual outbreaks have occurred in Peru. The global reemergence of the disease is due to proliferation of body lice. In the United States, sporadic cases of epidemic typhus are transmitted by flying-squirrel fleas. Eastern flying-squirrel (*Glaucomys volans*) lice and fleas have been found to be infected with *R. prowazekii*. The flying-squirrel fleas occasionally bite humans.

Brill-Zinsser disease is a recrudescent, mild form of epidemic typhus occurring years after the acute disease, probably as a result of immunosuppression or old age. Nathan Brill first identified recrudescent typhus in New York in 1898. In 1933 Hans Zinsser noted that >90% of patients with recrudescent typhus had emigrated from typhus-endemic areas of Europe. Strains of *R. prowazekii* indistinguishable from classic strains were isolated from patients with recrudescent typhus. Furthermore, *R. prowazekii* was isolated from the lymph nodes of patients undergoing elective surgery who had had typhus years earlier. Thus the typhus rickettsiae can remain dormant for years and can reactivate with waning immunity.

Rickettsiae, particularly *R. prowazekii*, are potential agents of bioterrorism (Chap. 205). *R. prowazekii* and *R. rickettsii* have a high case-fatality ratio, cause diseases that are difficult to diagnose, and can be engineered to display complete antimicrobial resistance. A strain of tetracycline-resistant *R. prowazekii* was developed in the former Soviet Union. *R. prowazekii* and *R. typhi* have dormant forms that survive extracellularly for long periods, and all rickettsiae are highly infectious when inhaled as aerosols.

Clinical Manifestations   After an incubation period of ~1 week (range, 7 to 14 days), the onset of illness is abrupt, with prostration, severe headache, and fever rising rapidly to 38.8° to 40.0°C (102° to 104°F). Cough is frequently prominent, occurring in 70% of patients. Myalgias are usually severe. In the outbreak in Burundi, the disease was referred to as *sutama* ("crouching"), the myalgias being so severe that patients crouched in an attempt to alleviate the pain. A rash begins on the upper trunk, usually on the fifth day, and then becomes generalized, involving all of the body except the face, palms, and soles. Initially, this rash is macular; without treatment, it becomes maculopapular, petechial, and confluent. The rash is frequently absent or not detected on black skin in Africa, where 60% of patients have *spotless epidemic typhus*. Photophobia, with considerable conjunctival injection and eye pain, is frequent. The tongue may be dry, brown, and furred. Confusion and coma are common. Skin necrosis and gangrene of the digits as well as interstitial pneumonia have been noted in severe cases. Untreated disease is fatal in 7 to 40% of cases, with outcome depending primarily on the condition of the host. Patients with untreated infections develop renal insufficiency and multiorgan involvement in which neurologic manifestations are frequently prominent. Overall, 12% of patients with epidemic typhus have neurologic involvement. North American *R. prowazekii* infection transmitted by flying-squirrel ectoparasites is a milder illness; whether this milder disease is due to host factors (e.g., better health status) or organism factors (e.g., attenuated virulence) is unknown.

Diagnosis and Treatment   See Table 158-2. Epidemic typhus is sometimes misdiagnosed as typhoid fever in tropical countries (Chap. 137).

Prevention   Prevention of epidemic typhus involves control of body lice. Clothes should be changed regularly, and insecticides should be used every 6 weeks to control the louse population.

SCRUB TYPHUS

The etiologic agent of scrub typhus is a small, obligately intracellular bacterium of the family Rickettsiaceae that differs substantially from other family members in its genetic makeup and in the composition of its cell wall (which, for example, lacks lipopolysaccharide and peptidoglycan). Consequently, this organism has been classified as a species in a separate genus, *Orientia tsutsugamushi*.

O. tsutsugamushi is maintained in nature by transovarian transmission in trombiculid mites, mainly of the genus *Leptotrombidium*. After hatching, infected larval mites (chiggers, the only stage that feeds on an animal host) inoculate organisms into the skin while feeding. Scrub typhus is found in environments that harbor the infected chiggers, particularly areas of heavy scrub vegetation—e.g., where the forest is regrowing after being cleared and along riverbanks. Infections occur during the wet season, when the mites lay their eggs. The disease is endemic in eastern and southern Asia, northern Australia, and islands of the western Pacific Ocean. Scrub typhus is also found in tropical areas of India, Sri Lanka, Bangladesh, Myanmar, Thailand, Malaysia, Laos, Vietnam, Kampuchea, China, Taiwan, the Philippines, Indonesia, Papua New Guinea, northern Australia, and islands of the South Pacific Ocean; in temperate areas of Japan, Korea, far-eastern Russia, Tadzhikistan, the mountains of northern India, Pakistan, and Nepal; and in nontropical areas of China, such as Tibet and Shangdong Province. Those infected include indigenous rural workers, residents of suburban areas, and westerners visiting endemic areas for professional or recreational purposes. Infections are more prevalent than the number of clinical diagnoses would suggest; in some areas >3% of the population is infected or reinfected each month. Immunity wanes over 1 to 3 years, and there is remarkable antigenic diversity.

Clinical Manifestations   The illness varies in severity from mild and self-limiting to fatal. After an incubation period of 6 to 21 days (usually 8 to 10 days), the onset of disease is characterized by fever, headache, myalgia, cough, and gastrointestinal symptoms. Some patients develop no further signs or symptoms and recover spontaneously after a few days. The classic case description includes an eschar at the site of chigger feeding, regional lymphadenopathy, and a maculopapular rash—signs that are seldom observed in indigenous patients. Fewer than 50% of Westerners develop an eschar, and <40% develop a rash (on day 4 to 6 of illness). Severe cases typically include prominent encephalitis and interstitial pneumonia as key features of vascular injury. Severe illness in persons with G6PD deficiency has been accompanied by hemolysis. The case-fatality rate for untreated classic cases

FIGURE 158-4 *Ehrlichia chaffeensis* microcolonies (morulae) within cytoplasmic vacuoles manifest as two morphologic forms: reticulate cells (r) and dense-core cells (d). Bar = 1 μm. *(Photo courtesy of Dr. Vsevolod L. Popov.)*

is 7% but would probably be lower if all relatively mild cases (which are underdiagnosed) were included.

Diagnosis and Treatment   See Table 158-2. Some cases of scrub typhus in Thailand are caused by *O. tsutsugamushi* strains that are resistant to doxycycline or chloramphenicol. These strains are susceptible to rifampin, and azithromycin and clarithromycin have been used successfully in small numbers of patients.

EHRLICHIOSES AND ANAPLASMOSIS

Ehrlichiae are small, obligately intracellular bacteria with a gram-negative-type cell wall that grow in cytoplasmic vacuoles to form clusters called *morulae* (Fig. 158-4). Two distinct *Ehrlichia* species and one *Anaplasma* species cause human infections that can be severe and frequent (Table 158-3). *E. chaffeensis*, the agent of human monocytotropic ehrlichiosis (HME), infects predominantly mononuclear phagocytic cells in tissues and blood monocytes. *E. ewingii* and *A. phagocytophila* infect cells of myeloid lineage, particularly neutrophils. Confusion may arise from the facts that *Anaplasma phagocytophila* is the agent of the disease originally designated human granulocytotropic ehrlichiosis (HGE) and *Ehrlichia ewingii* is a human granulocytotropic pathogen. Such confusion can be avoided through use of the terms *human anaplasmosis* and *ehrlichiosis ewingii*, with avoidance of the ambiguous *HGE*. Both *E. chaffeensis* and *E. ewingii* are transmitted mainly by the Lone Star tick *Amblyomma americanum* and cause persistent infections in the same reservoir, the white-tailed deer. *A. phagocytophila* is transmitted, with little geographic overlap, by *Ixodes scapularis* in the northeastern and upper midwestern states and by *I. ricinus* in Europe. In California, both HME and *A. phagocytophila* infection have been documented, with apparent partial overlap of their vectors. In Eurasia, reports of human infection caused by an *I. persulcatus*–transmitted *E. muris*–like agent and of *A. phagocytophila* associated with *I. persulcatus* are beginning to appear. The worldwide prevalence of ehrlichioses and anaplasmoses is an important issue in the field of emerging infectious diseases.

Ehrlichiae were discovered by veterinarians

during the investigation of hemolytic anemia of cattle before 1910. Researchers thereafter discerned that "marginal points" visible within erythrocytes were infectious and named the agent *Anaplasma marginale*. Subsequently, several other species generally considered to be ehrlichiae were detected as veterinary infectious agents, including *E. ruminantium*, *E. canis*, *E. ewingii*, *A. phagocytophila*, and *Neorickettsia risticii*.

The current taxonomic positions are determined by nucleic acid sequences of conserved and unique genes among these species. By analysis of 16S ribosomal RNA and other sequences, the family Anaplasmataceae can be divided into four genera: *Ehrlichia*, *Anaplasma*, *Wolbachia*, and *Neorickettsia*. Given the lack of transovarian transmission in ticks, the natural maintenance of the tick-borne ehrlichiae and anaplasmae clearly depends in part on prolonged or persistent infections in wild and feral mammalian reservoirs. Thus, *Ehrlichia* and *Anaplasma* are propagated by horizontal transmission that relies on a tick-mammal-tick cycle; humans are inadvertently infected when they impinge on the natural habitats occupied by the ticks and the reservoir hosts. Wolbachiae are associated with human diseases caused by filariae, with symbiosis in some instances. The wolbachiae are important for filarial viability and pathogenicity. Treatment of wolbachiae is now a strategy in the control of filariasis. Neorickettsiae parasitize flukes that in turn are parasites of aquatic snails, fish, and insects. Although only a single human neorickettsiosis, *sennetsu fever*, has been described, others may be discovered. Probably in association with the ingestion of raw fish containing *N. sennetsu*–infected flukes, patients develop an infectious mononucleosis–like illness that was first identified in 1953.

HUMAN MONOCYTOTROPIC EHRLICHIOSIS ■ **Epidemiology**   More than 1363 cases of infections caused by *E. chaffeensis* had been reported to the Centers for Disease Control and Prevention (CDC) as of September 2002. However, since HME is not a reportable disease in most states, this figure is a gross underestimate. Most *E. chaffeensis* infections have been identified in the south-central, southeastern, and mid-Atlantic states, but cases have also been recognized in California. The vector is the Lone Star tick (*A. americanum*), which in all its life stages feeds on white-tailed deer—a major reservoir host. Dogs and coyotes have been discovered to be subclinically infected and may also be an important reservoir. Tick bites and exposures are reported by patients, frequently in rural areas and especially in the months May through July. The median age of HME patients is 44 years, and 75% of the affected individuals are male; however, severe and fatal infections in children are also well recognized. Active prospective surveillance has revealed that in rural areas inhabited by abundant deer and Lone Star ticks, HME is a common disease, with an incidence as high as 1000 cases per 1 million population.

TABLE 158-3   *Comparison of Three Human Ehrlichioses: Human Monocytotropic Ehrlichiosis (HME), Anaplasmosis, and Human Ehrlichiosis Ewingii*

Variable	HME	Human Anaplasmosis	Ehrlichiosis Ewingii
Etiologic agent	*E. chaffeensis*	*A. phagocytophila*	*E. ewingii*
Tick vector(s)	*Amblyomma americanum*, *Dermacentor variabilis* (dog tick)	*Ixodes scapularis* (deer tick), *I. ricinus*, *I. pacificus*	*A. americanum*
Seasonality	April through September	Year-round (peak: May, June, and July)	April through September
Major target cell	Monocyte	Granulocyte	Neutrophil
Morulae seen	Rarely	Frequently	Rarely
Antigen used in IFA test	*E. chaffeensis*	*A. phagocytophila*	*E. chaffeensis* as surrogate
Diagnostic titer	Fourfold rise or a single titer of ≥1:128; cutoff for negative titer, 1:64	Fourfold rise; cutoff for negative titer, 1:80	No established criteria
Treatment of choice	Doxycycline	Doxycycline	Doxycycline
Mortality	2–3%	<1%	None reported

Note: IFA, indirect immunofluorescence assay.

Clinical Manifestations *E. chaffeensis* is inoculated into the dermal blood pool created by the feeding tick and subsequently disseminates via the blood to tissues. After a median incubation period of 8 days, illness develops. The classic clinical manifestations are not specific and include fever (97% of cases), headache (81%), myalgia (68%), and malaise (84%); less frequently observed are gastrointestinal involvement (nausea, vomiting, diarrhea; 25 to 68%), cough (25%), rash (36% overall, 6% at presentation), and confusion (20%). HME may be severe: 62% of patients with documented cases are hospitalized, and ~3% die. Severe complications include a toxic shock–like or septic shock–like syndrome, respiratory insufficiency and adult respiratory distress, meningoencephalitis, fulminant infection (in immunocompromised patients), severe opportunistic and nosocomial infections, and hemorrhage. Laboratory findings may be of value in the differential diagnosis; 60 to 74% of patients with HME have leukopenia (initially lymphopenia, later neutropenia), 72% have thrombocytopenia, and nearly 90% have elevations in serum levels of hepatic aminotransferases. With effective therapy, rebound lymphocytosis (mainly γ/δ T cells) is common. In spite of abnormal blood counts, examinations reveal hypercellular bone marrow, and noncaseating granulomas may be present. Vasculitis is not a component of HME.

Diagnosis Because HME can be fatal, empirical antibiotic therapy should be instituted on the basis of a clinical diagnosis. This diagnosis may be suggested by fever in the setting of known tick exposure during the preceding 3 weeks, leukopenia and/or thrombocytopenia, and increased aminotransferase concentrations in serum. Morulae are rarely demonstrated in peripheral blood smears unless an intensive examination is performed; even then, an experienced microscopist is required. The active phase of HME may be diagnosed by PCR amplification of *E. chaffeensis* nucleic acids from EDTA-anticoagulated blood obtained before the start of doxycycline therapy. Retrospective serologic diagnosis requires a consistent clinical picture and detection of a fourfold increase in *E. chaffeensis* antibody titer (to ≥1:64) by indirect immunofluorescence in paired serum samples obtained ~3 weeks apart. It must be underscored that separate specific diagnostic tests for HME and HGE are necessary.

EHRLICHIOSIS EWINGII *Ehrlichia ewingii*, originally identified as a neutrophil pathogen that causes febrile lameness in dogs, resembles HME in many respects, including its tick vector (*A. americanum*) and its vertebrate hosts (white-tailed deer and dogs). The illness caused by *E. ewingii* is similar to HME but is somewhat less severe. The majority of cases have been diagnosed in immunocompromised patients.

℞ TREATMENT

Tetracycline is effective therapy for HME or ehrlichiosis ewingii. Either tetracycline (250 to 500 mg given orally every 6 h) or doxycycline (100 mg given orally or intravenously twice daily) is associated with a lowered rate of hospitalization and a shortened duration of fever. The use of chloramphenicol is controversial, and *E. chaffeensis* is not susceptible to this drug in vitro. While a few reports document the persistence of *E. chaffeensis* in patients after the acute phase of illness, such persistence is very infrequent; most infections are cured by relatively short courses of tetracycline therapy (continuing for 3 to 5 days after defervescence).

Prevention HME and ehrlichiosis ewingii are prevented by the avoidance of ticks in endemic areas. The use of protective clothing and tick repellents, careful tick searches after exposures, and prompt removal of attached ticks are practices that markedly diminish risk.

HUMAN ANAPLASMOSIS ■ Epidemiology As of 2002, 1278 cases of HGE had been reported to the CDC, most of them from upper midwestern and northeastern states; the distribution of cases was similar to that for Lyme disease. Most cases were identified within the range of various

I. persulcatus–complex ticks, particularly *I. scapularis*. White-footed deer mice and white-tailed deer in the United States as well as red deer in Europe appear to play a role in maintaining HGE in nature. The incidence of HGE peaks in May, June, and July, but the disease may occur throughout the year in conjunction with human exposure to *Ixodes* ticks. HGE affects predominantly males (79%) and older persons (median age, 58 years).

Clinical Manifestations Because of high seroprevalence rates in endemic regions, it seems likely that only a minority of infected individuals develop clinical manifestations. The incubation period for HGE varies between 4 and 8 days, and the disease manifests as fever (94 to 100% of cases), myalgia (78 to 98%), headache (61 to 85%), and malaise (98%)—findings suggestive of an influenza-like illness. A minority of patients develop gastrointestinal involvement, including nausea, vomiting, or diarrhea (22 to 39%); rash (2 to 11%); cough (27%); and confusion (17%). Severe complications occur most often in the elderly, but even children may be severely affected. Respiratory insufficiency, with adult respiratory distress syndrome, a toxic shock–like syndrome, and life-threatening opportunistic infections, are the most worrisome complications. Meningoencephalitis has not yet been conclusively recognized with HGE. The case-fatality rate is probably <1%, but nearly 7% of ill patients may require intensive care. As in HME, laboratory findings are of great assistance; most patients develop leukopenia and/or thrombocytopenia with increased serum levels of hepatic aminotransferases. The pancytopenia observed in HGE presumably relates to sequestration or destruction of platelets and leukocytes, since the bone marrow is ordinarily normo- or hypercellular. Vasculitis is not a component of HGE. Unlike HME, HGE is not associated with granulomas. While clear evidence exists for co-infections with *Borrelia burgdorferi* and *Babesia microti*, which are transmitted by the same tick vector(s), there is little evidence of comorbidity or of a persistent or chronic phase for HGE.

Diagnosis HGE should be included in the differential diagnosis for patients who have been exposed to ticks and who develop an influenza-like illness during the season of *Ixodes* tick activity (May through December). The concurrent detection of thrombocytopenia, leukopenia, and/or elevations in serum aminotransferase activities further increases the likelihood of HGE. A substantial proportion of patients with HGE develop serologic reactions considered diagnostic of Lyme disease in the absence of clear clinical findings consistent with that diagnosis. Thus, HGE should be considered in the differential diagnosis of atypical severe presentations of Lyme disease. Although not highly sensitive, a thorough peripheral blood film examination for morulae in neutrophils may identify 20 to 75% of infections. PCR testing of EDTA-anticoagulated blood collected before the initiation of tetracycline therapy from patients with active disease is a sensitive and specific method for early confirmation. Serodiagnosis is based mostly upon the retrospective demonstration of a fourfold increase in *A. phagocytophila* group antibody titer to a minimum of 1:80 in paired serum samples obtained ~1 month apart. IgM antibodies may be detected in many patients within the first 1.5 months after illness. Approximately 15 to 40% of infected persons have a detectable antibody titer at presentation, but, in regions where seroprevalence is high, a single acute-phase polyvalent titer may be misleading.

℞ TREATMENT

Doxycycline (100 mg by mouth twice daily) is an effective therapeutic agent, while rifampin has been associated with clinical improvement in pregnant patients with HGE. No prospective studies of any therapy for HGE have been conducted. Most treated patients defervesce within 24 to 48 h.

Prevention Prevention of HGE requires tick avoidance. The Lyme disease vaccine offers no protection against HGE, and no other vaccine is available.

Q fever results from infection with *C. burnetii*. This small gram-negative microorganism (0.2 μm by 0.7 μm) exists in two antigenic forms: phase I and phase II. When *C. burnetii* is passaged in cell cultures or embryonated eggs, its lipopolysaccharide undergoes truncation that results in an antigenic change called *phase variation*. The phase I form is extremely infectious and exists in humans and other animals. Passage in cell culture or embryonated eggs results in a shift to the phase II form, which is avirulent. The ability of *C. burnetii* to form spores allows the organism to survive in harsh environments. Indeed, it can survive for >40 months in skim milk at room temperature and is readily recovered from soil up to 1 month after contamination. Three different plasmids have been described in various isolates of *C. burnetii*. Q fever encompasses two broad clinical syndromes: acute and chronic infection. It is likely that the host's immune response (rather than characteristics of the infecting strain) determines whether or not chronic Q fever develops. Attachment of the virulent form (phase I) of *C. burnetii* to monocytes requires $\alpha_v \beta_3$ integrin only, whereas attachment of the avirulent form (phase II) requires both $\alpha_v \beta_3$ and CR_3 integrins. The transendothelial migration of monocytes infected by virulent *C. burnetii* is impaired, while that of monocytes infected by the avirulent form is not. Production of tumor necrosis factor (TNF) by monocytes is initiated by virulent *C. burnetii* through a mechanism involving both $\alpha_v \beta_3$ integrin and interaction with bacterial lipopolysaccharide. *C. burnetii* survives in monocytes from patients with chronic Q fever but not in monocytes from patients with acute Q fever or from seronegative control subjects. Impairment of the bactericidal activity of the *C. burnetii*–infected monocyte seems to be due to dysregulation of the cytokine network, as TNF in monocyte supernatants from these patients depresses the microbicidal activity of monocytes. The soluble TNF receptor TNF-R75 is upregulated in monocytes from patients with chronic Q fever. This upregulation is due to overproduction of interleukin 10, antibodies to which restore the microbicidal activity of these monocytes in vitro. The CD4+/CD8+ ratio is decreased in patients with Q fever endocarditis. All of the above findings translate into the observations that very few organisms and a strong cellular response are seen in patients with acute Q fever, while many organisms and a moderate cellular response are seen in patients with chronic Q fever.

Epidemiology   Q fever is a zoonosis. The primary sources of human infection are infected cattle, sheep, and goats. However, infected cats, rabbits, pigeons, and dogs have also been shown to transmit *C. burnetii* to humans. The extensive wildlife reservoir for *C. burnetii* includes mammals, birds, and ticks. In the infected female mammal, *C. burnetii* localizes to the uterus and the mammary glands. Infection is reactivated during pregnancy, and high concentrations of *C. burnetii* are found in the placenta. At parturition, *C. burnetii* is dispersed as an aerosol, and infection follows inhalation of aerosolized organisms by a susceptible host. Soil is contaminated during parturition, and *C. burnetii* aerosols can be generated weeks to months later during wind storms. Individuals up to 18 km from the source may be infected. Infected female animals shed the organism in milk for weeks to months after parturition. In rare instances, human-to-human transmission has followed delivery of an infant to an infected woman or autopsy on an infected individual. *C. burnetii* has been transmitted via blood transfusion. Persons who are at risk for Q fever include abattoir workers, veterinarians, and other individuals who have vocational or avocational contact with infected animals. Exposure to infected newborn animals or to infected products of conception poses the highest risk. Sexual transmission has been demonstrated experimentally in mice, as has transmission during artificial insemination in cattle. Some evidence suggests that *C. burnetii* can be sexually transmitted among humans. The ingestion of contaminated milk in some areas probably represent a major route of transmission to humans, although the experimental evidence on this point is contradictory. In any event, the vast majority of Q fever cases result from inhalation of contaminated

aerosols. Q fever in children is uncommon, accounting for only 1 to 2% of cases.

Infections due to *C. burnetii* occur in most countries. Indeed, the only areas known to be free of *C. burnetii* are New Zealand and Antarctica. The primary manifestation of acute Q fever differs from place to place. For example, the primary manifestation is pneumonia in Nova Scotia (Canada), granulomatous hepatitis in Marseille (France), and both of these conditions in the Basque region of Spain. These differences may reflect the route of infection; i.e., the ingestion of contaminated milk may result in hepatitis and the inhalation of contaminated aerosols in pneumonia.

In New South Wales, Australia, 2351 cases of Q fever were reported in 1991 to 2000, and the number of cases per 100,000 persons varied from 6.7 in 1996 to 1.8 in 2000. Males accounted for 84% of the cases and children for 1.5%. In Australia each year, Q fever costs the meat industry almost $1 million and >1700 weeks of time lost from work.

Clinical Manifestations ■ *ACUTE Q FEVER*   The incubation period for acute Q fever ranges from 3 to 30 days. The clinical presentations include flulike syndromes, prolonged fever, pneumonia, hepatitis, pericarditis, myocarditis, meningoencephalitis, and infection during pregnancy. A study of 1383 cases of Q fever from southern France gives an indication of the spectrum of the clinical manifestations of Q fever. Among the 1070 patients with acute Q fever, 40% had hepatitis, 20% had both pneumonia and hepatitis, 17% had pneumonia, 14% had isolated fever, 2% had central nervous system involvement, 1% had pericarditis, and 1% had myocarditis; in 3% of patients, the clinical presentation was not defined.

The symptoms of acute Q fever are nonspecific; common among them are fever, extreme fatigue, and severe headache. Other symptoms include chills, sweats, nausea, vomiting, and diarrhea, which occur in 5 to 20% of patients. Cough develops in about half of patients with Q fever pneumonia. Neurologic manifestations of acute Q fever are uncommon; however, in one outbreak in the West Midlands, United Kingdom, 23% of 102 patients had neurologic signs and symptoms as the major manifestation. A nonspecific rash may be evident in 4 to 18% of patients. The white blood cell count is usually normal. Thrombocytopenia is detected in ~25% of patients, and reactive thrombocytosis [with platelet counts of up to 1 million/μL (1×10^{12}/L)] frequently develops during recovery. This thrombocytosis may account for cases of deep vein thrombophlebitis complicating acute Q fever in some series. Uncommon manifestations of acute Q fever include optic neuritis, extrapyramidal neurologic disease, Guillain-Barré syndrome, inappropriate secretion of antidiuretic hormone, epididymitis, orchitis, priapism, hemolytic anemia, hemolytic-uremic syndrome, mediastinal lymphadenopathy mimicking lymphoma, spontaneous rupture of the spleen, pancreatitis, erythema nodosum, and mesenteric panniculitis. Chest radiography may show an opacity that is indistinguishable from that seen in pneumonia of other etiologies. Multiple rounded opacities are common; in the appropriate epidemiologic setting (e.g., exposure to a parturient cat), they are highly suggestive of Q fever pneumonia. However, right-sided endocarditis resulting in septic pulmonary emboli can produce the same radiographic appearance.

Up to 70% of the uncommon cases of Q fever in children are asymptomatic. Symptomatic cases in children result in a spectrum of disease similar to that in adults, although only a few cases of Q fever endocarditis in children have been reported.

In Australia and the United Kingdom, a prolonged fatigue state (lasting 5 to 10 years) has followed Q fever in some cases. Low levels of *C. burnetii* DNA have been noted in the affected patients 0.75 to 5 years after infection.

CHRONIC Q FEVER   Chronic Q fever, which is uncommon, almost always implies endocarditis. This infection usually occurs in patients with previous valvular heart disease, immunosuppression, or chronic renal insufficiency. Fever is usually absent or low grade. Patients may have nonspecific symptoms for up to 1 year before diagnosis. Valvular vegetations have been seen in only 12% of patients with transthoracic echocardiograms, but the rate of detection may be higher with the use of transesophageal echocardiography. The vegetations in chronic Q fever endocarditis are different from those in bacterial endocarditis, manifesting as nodules on the valve. A high index of suspicion is necessary for a correct diagnosis. The disease should be suspected in all patients with culture-negative endocarditis. In addition, all patients with valvular heart disease and an unexplained purpuric eruption, renal insufficiency, stroke, and/or progressive heart failure should be tested for *C. burnetii* infection. Patients with chronic Q fever have hepatomegaly and/or splenomegaly. These two findings, especially in combination with positive rheumatoid factor, high erythrocyte sedimentation rate, high C-reactive protein level, and/or increased γ-globulin concentrations (up to 60 to 70 g/L), suggest this diagnosis. Other manifestations of chronic Q fever include infection of vascular prostheses, aneurysms, and bone and as well as chronic sternal wound infection.

Diagnosis *C. burnetii* can be isolated from buffy-coat blood samples or tissue specimens by a shell-vial technique; however, most laboratories are not permitted to attempt the isolation of *C. burnetii* since it is considered highly infectious. PCR can be used to amplify *C. burnetii* DNA from tissue or biopsy specimens. This technique can also be used on paraffin-embedded tissues. Serology, however, is the most commonly used diagnostic tool. Three techniques are available: complement fixation, indirect immunofluorescence, and enzyme-linked immunosorbent assay. Indirect immunofluorescence is sensitive and specific and is the method of choice. Rheumatoid factor should be adsorbed from the specimen before testing. An IgG titer of ≥1:800 to phase I antigen is suggestive of chronic Q fever. In almost all instances of chronic Q fever, the antibody titer to phase I antigen is much higher than that to phase II antigen. The reverse is true in acute Q fever. In addition, in acute Q fever, it is usually possible to demonstrate a fourfold rise in titer between acute- and convalescent-phase serum samples.

R_X TREATMENT

Treatment of acute Q fever with doxycycline (100 mg twice daily for 14 days) is usually successful. Quinolones are also effective. If Q fever

is diagnosed during pregnancy, treatment with trimethoprim-sulfamethoxazole is recommended for the duration of the pregnancy. Treatment of chronic Q fever should include at least two antibiotics active against *C. burnetii*. Rifampin (300 mg once daily) combined with doxycycline (100 mg twice daily) or ciprofloxacin (750 mg twice daily) has been used with success. The optimal duration of antibiotic therapy for chronic Q fever remains undetermined. We recommend at least 3 years of treatment, with discontinuation only if the phase I IgA antibody titer is ≤1:50 and the IgG phase I titer is ≤1:200. Another therapeutic option under investigation is the combination of doxycycline (100 mg twice daily) with hydroxychloroquine (600 mg once daily). With this combination, therapy can be completed in 18 months. It is necessary to monitor hydroxychloroquine levels and to adjust the dosage to maintain a plasma concentration of 0.8 to 1.2 μg/mL. In vitro, the addition of 1 mg of hydroxychloroquine/mL renders doxycycline bactericidal against *C. burnetii*. Resistance to ciprofloxacin has been associated with substitution of glutamine for lysine at the position corresponding to amino acid 87 in resistant strains of *Escherichia coli*.

Prevention A vaccine has been shown to be effective in preventing Q fever in abattoir workers in Australia.

FURTHER READING

ARCHIBALD LK, SEXTON DJ: Long-term sequelae of Rocky Mountain spotted fever. Clin Infect Dis 20:1122, 1995

BAKKEN JS et al: Human granulocytic ehrlichiosis in the upper midwest United States. A new species emerging? JAMA 272:212, 1994

BULLER RS et al: *Ehrlichia ewingii*, a newly recognized agent of human ehrlichiosis. N Engl J Med 341:148, 1999

DALTON MJ et al: National surveillance for Rocky Mountain spotted fever, 1981–1982: Epidemiologic summary and evaluation of risk factors for fatal outcome. Am J Trop Med Hyg 52:405, 1995

DUMLER JS, BAKKEN JS: Human ehrlichioses. Newly recognized infections transmitted by ticks. Annu Rev Med 49:201, 1998

RAOULT D et al: Outbreak of epidemic typhus associated with trench fever in Burundi. Lancet 352:353, 1998

——— et al: Treatment of Q fever endocarditis. Comparisons of 2 regimens containing doxycycline and ofloxacin or hydroxychloroquine. Arch Intern Med 159:167, 1999

——— et al: Q fever 1985–1998. Clinical and epidemiologic features of 1,383 infections. Medicine (Baltimore) 79:109, 2000

——— et al: Q fever during pregnancy. Arch Intern Med 162:701, 2002

159 INFECTIONS DUE TO MYCOPLASMAS
William M. McCormack

Mycoplasmas, the smallest free-living organisms known, are prokaryotes that are bounded only by a plasma membrane. Their lack of a cell wall is associated with cellular pleomorphism and resistance to cell wall–active antimicrobial agents, such as penicillins and cephalosporins. The organisms' small genome limits biosynthesis and explains the difficulties encountered with in vitro cultivation. Mycoplasmas typically colonize mucosal surfaces of the respiratory and urogenital tracts of many animal species. Sixteen species of mycoplasmas have been recovered from humans. Most are commensals. *Mycoplasma pneumoniae* causes upper and lower respiratory tract infections. *M. genitalium* and *Ureaplasma urealyticum* are established causes of urethritis and have been implicated in other genital conditions. *M. hominis* and *U. urealyticum* are part of the complex microbial flora of bacterial vaginosis (Chap. 115).

MECHANISMS OF PATHOGENICITY

Adherence of mycoplasmas to the surface of the host cell is necessary for colonization and infection. Some pathogenic mycoplasmas are flask-shaped, with specialized tips that enhance adherence. *M. pneu-*

moniae adheres via a network of interactive adhesins and accessory proteins and produces hydrogen peroxide, which may cause injury to host cells. *M. hominis* metabolizes arginine, with the production of potentially cytotoxic amounts of ammonia. Ureaplasmas have been placed in a separate genus because of their unique urease activity; the metabolism of urea also produces ammonia. *M. pneumoniae* may evoke IgM autoantibodies that agglutinate human erythrocytes at 4°C. These cold agglutinins can cause anemia and other complications.

MYCOPLASMA PNEUMONIAE

EPIDEMIOLOGY *M. pneumoniae* causes upper and lower respiratory tract symptoms in all age groups, with the highest attack rates in 5- to 20-year-olds. The infection is acquired by inhalation of aerosols. The incubation period is 2 to 3 weeks, considerably longer than that of most other respiratory infections. Although epidemics have taken place in closed populations, such as schools and military installations, most cases occur sporadically or in families. In families, cases typically occur serially, with 2- to 3-week intervals between cases. Infections in adults are often the result of contact with children.

Infection with *M. pneumoniae* is worldwide. Cases occur throughout the year, with epidemics every few years. Some studies have noted an increase in the number of cases during the autumn months in temperate climates. Although pneumonia is the classic presentation, non-pneumonic infection is considerably more common. In very young children, most infections result only in upper respiratory symptoms, whereas children >5 years of age and adults may have bronchitis and pneumonia.

CLINICAL PRESENTATION After a prolonged incubation period, fever and constitutional symptoms develop along with headache and cough, both of which can be prominent and distressing. Symptoms typically progress less rapidly than those of viral respiratory tract infections. In the minority (perhaps 5 to 10%) of infected individuals who develop tracheobronchitis or pneumonia, cough becomes more prominent. Sputum, if produced at all, is usually white and may be tinged with blood. The temperature seldom rises above 38.9° to 39.4°C (102° to 103°F). Shaking chills, myalgias, and gastrointestinal symptoms (e.g., nausea, vomiting, and diarrhea) are unusual. Chest muscle soreness may result from frequent and prolonged coughing, but true pleuritic pain is uncommon.

Pharyngeal injection is often noted. Cervical lymph node enlargement is unusual. Ear pain due to bullous myringitis (blisters on the tympanic membrane) is a unique but uncommon manifestation. As in other "atypical" pneumonias, findings on auscultation of the lung may be normal or nearly normal despite striking radiographic abnormalities. Pleural effusions develop in fewer than 20% of patients.

M. pneumoniae infection may be particularly severe in patients who have sickle cell disease and other hemoglobin S–related hemoglobinopathies. The functional asplenia seen in sickle cell disease may contribute to severe mycoplasmal disease as it does in pneumococcal infection. Severe respiratory distress and large pleural effusions may occur.

EXTRAPULMONARY MANIFESTATIONS A broad array of extrapulmonary abnormalities have been associated with *M. pneumoniae* infection. Although these events are unusual, they complicate other respiratory diseases even more rarely and often provide the only clue that an otherwise-unremarkable respiratory infection may be mycoplasmal.

Erythema multiforme (Stevens-Johnson syndrome; see Fig. 46-9) typically occurs in young male patients with *M. pneumoniae* infection. Other dermatologic manifestations, such as maculopapular and vesicular exanthems, erythema nodosum, and urticaria, have been reported, but none is as clearly linked to *M. pneumoniae* as is erythema multiforme. Digital necrosis has been seen in patients with sickle cell disease who develop very high titers of cold agglutinins.

Cardiac abnormalities reported in conjunction with *M. pneumoniae* infection include myocarditis and pericarditis, which may result in abnormalities of conduction. Of the wide variety of neurologic conditions associated with *M. pneumoniae*, most have been documented in case reports, where establishment of a cause-and-effect relationship is problematic. Central nervous system abnormalities that have been associated with *M. pneumoniae* include encephalitis, cerebellar ataxia, Guillain-Barré syndrome, transverse myelitis, and peripheral neuropathies. Arthralgias are not unusual in patients who have mycoplasmal pneumonia; mycoplasmal arthritis is rare except in patients who have hypogammaglobulinemia. Hematologic abnormalities associated with *M. pneumoniae* include hemolytic anemia and coagulopathies.

The pathogenesis of the extrapulmonary manifestations of *M. pneumoniae* infection is controversial. Occasional reports have described the identification of *M. pneumoniae* or its nucleic acids in involved tissues. The fact that most attempts at detection have yielded negative results, however, suggests that these extrapulmonary complications have an immunologic basis. Mycoplasmas, including *M. pneumoniae*, can nonspecifically stimulate B lymphocytes. *M. pneumoniae*–infected individuals can develop autoantibodies, including those reactive with brain, heart, and muscle.

DIAGNOSIS Most infections with *M. pneumoniae* are not diagnosed, as they are indistinguishable from upper and lower respiratory tract infections caused by myriad other viral and bacterial pathogens. When the diagnosis is suspected, it is usually because illness is prolonged or extrapulmonary manifestations develop. The white blood cell count is generally somewhat elevated, with few immature cells. Gram's stain

of sputum shows leukocytes without a predominance of any bacterial morphologic type. Since *M. pneumoniae* lacks a cell wall, it cannot be detected on Gram's stain. In patients who have pneumonia, the chest radiograph may show reticulonodular or interstitial infiltration, primarily in the lower lobes. As in other "atypical" pneumonias, radiographic abnormalities may be more prominent than would be predicted by auscultation of the chest.

M. pneumoniae can be grown on artificial media, but the process is exacting, requires special media, and takes upwards of 2 weeks. Thus, mycoplasmal cultures do not provide timely information to aid in patient management. The same, unfortunately, is true of serologic diagnosis. Specific antibodies can be detected by enzyme-linked immunoassays, indirect immunofluorescence, or complement fixation but do not develop early enough to guide decisions regarding treatment. As with most serologic tests, examination of paired acute- and convalescent-phase serum specimens is required for good sensitivity and specificity.

Cold agglutinins are nonspecific but develop within the first 7 to 10 days in more than half of patients with *M. pneumoniae* pneumonia and may be detectable when the patient presents to a health care provider. In a patient with a compatible clinical picture, a cold agglutinin titer of ≥1:32 supports the diagnosis of mycoplasmal pneumonia. Cold agglutinin determinations are readily available from diagnostic laboratories. The test can also be performed at the bedside by the addition of 1 mL of the patient's blood to a tube containing anticoagulant (e.g., a tube used to collect blood for determination of prothrombin activity). Before cooling, the nonaggregated red blood cells coat the sides of the inverted tube. The blood is cooled to 4°C when the tube is placed in an ice bath for 3 to 5 min or in a standard refrigerator. In a positive test, clumps of red blood cells can be observed when the tube is inverted. Rewarming of the sample to 37°C in an incubator or by exposure to body heat should reverse the agglutination. A positive "bedside" cold agglutinin test is equivalent to a laboratory titer of ≥1:64.

The lack of sensitive, specific, and timely diagnostic tests has prompted the development of a variety of antigen detection tests that do not involve serology or the cultivation of live organisms. Such tests include antigen capture, indirect enzyme immunoassays, DNA probing, and nucleic acid amplification. Since many viral and bacterial infections result in clinical presentations similar to that caused by *M. pneumoniae*, examination of specimens for single antigens is unlikely to be useful. Rather, tests that examine an individual specimen for multiple antigens are needed. Multiplex nucleic acid amplification tests that examine a single throat swab or sputum sample for all of the most likely causative microorganisms are feasible with current technology. Prototype multiplex polymerase chain reaction (PCR) assays have already been developed. If such tests become available clinically, more precise etiologic diagnosis of upper and lower respiratory tract infections will be possible.

℞ TREATMENT

Pneumonia due to *M. pneumoniae* is usually self-limited and is seldom life-threatening. Effective antimicrobial agents do shorten the duration of illness and, by reducing coughing, may conceivably render the patient less infectious. Although symptoms are alleviated by antimicrobial treatment, the organism usually is not eradicated. Cultures positive for *M. pneumoniae* may persist for months despite clinically effective antimicrobial therapy. The beneficial effects, if any, of such treatment on extrapulmonary manifestations of *M. pneumoniae* infection are unknown.

Because most mycoplasmal infections are not specifically diagnosed, management is directed at one of two syndromes: upper respiratory tract infection or community-acquired pneumonia. Upper respiratory infections, whether caused by viruses or by *M. pneumoniae*, do not require antimicrobial treatment. Community-acquired pneumonia (Chap. 239) may be caused by bacteria such as *Strepto-coccus pneumoniae* and *Haemophilus influenzae* or by "atypical" agents such as *Chlamydia pneumoniae*, *Legionella pneumophila*, and *M. pneumoniae*. Recommended treatment regimens are detailed in Tables 159-1 and 159-2. Treatment of documented *M. pneumoniae* pneumonia is usually continued for 14 to 21 days.

GENITAL MYCOPLASMAS (See also Chap. 115)

EPIDEMIOLOGY *M. hominis* and *U. urealyticum* are the most prevalent genital mycoplasmas. Infants may become colonized with one or both of these organisms during passage through a colonized birth canal. Neonatal colonization tends not to persist. Only ~10% of prepubertal girls and even fewer prepubertal boys are colonized with ureaplasmas. After puberty, colonization occurs mainly as a result of sexual activity. Among adults, disadvantaged populations have higher colonization rates. Ureaplasmas can be cultured from the vaginas of ~80% of women cared for in public clinics and about half of women cared for by private obstetricians and gynecologists. Similarly, vaginal *M. hominis* is found in ~50% of women attending public clinics and in ~20% of private patients. Men have somewhat lower rates of genital colonization than women. In short, both *U. urealyticum* and *M. hominis* are frequently detected in genital specimens from healthy, sexually experienced adults. Evaluation of the role of these organisms in human disease must take into account their high prevalence among healthy people.

M. fermentans colonizes both the respiratory and genital tracts in more than 20% of adults. There is no convincing evidence that *M. fermentans* causes human disease; although it had been implicated as a possible determinant of HIV-1 disease progression, more recent data do not support such a role. *M. genitalium* is a fastidious organism that is difficult to cultivate. PCR studies have identified the organism more successfully. Little is known about the epidemiology of *M. genitalium*.

ASSOCIATION WITH HUMAN DISEASE ■ Nongonococcal Urethritis (NGU)
Chlamydia trachomatis is the organism most firmly implicated in the etiology of NGU. There is no doubt that sexually transmitted *U. urealyticum* and *M. genitalium* also cause some cases of NGU. The ubiquity of ureaplasmas among men who do not have urethritis and the difficulty of identifying *M. genitalium* do not allow precise estimation of the proportion of cases of NGU caused by each of these mycoplasmas. *U. urealyticum* and *M. genitalium* do, however, appear to cause most of the nonchlamydial cases.

Epididymitis and Prostatitis Ureaplasmas may be an occasional cause of epididymitis. *M. hominis* has not been implicated in this disease. Neither organism has been convincingly associated with prostatitis.

Pelvic Inflammatory Disease (PID) *M. hominis* and *U. urealyticum* are both prominent components of the complex microbial flora of bacterial vaginosis. Since bacterial vaginosis is associated with PID, it is difficult to determine whether either organism plays an independent role in this condition. Although *M. genitalium* is not associated with bacterial vaginosis, preliminary studies have linked it to PID in women

TABLE 159-1 *Oral Antimicrobial Agents for the Treatment of Ambulatory Patients with Community-Acquired Pneumonia*

Agent	Dose and Schedule
Doxycycline	100 mg bid
Erythromycin	500 mg qid
Clarithromycin	500 mg bid
Azithromycin	500 mg qd
Levofloxacin	500 mg qd
Gatifloxacin	400 mg qd
Moxifloxacin	400 mg qd

Note: Treatment of documented *M. pneumoniae* pneumonia is usually continued for 14 to 21 days.

TABLE 159-2 *Antimicrobial Agents for the Treatment of Hospitalized Patients with Community-Acquired Pneumonia*

1. Intravenous ceftriaxone (1.0 g/d) *or*
   Intravenous cefotaxime (1.0 g q8h) *or*
   Intravenous ampicillin/sulbactam (1.5–3.0 g q6h)
   plus
   Intravenous or oral erythromycin (500 mg qid) *or*
   Intravenous or oral azithromycin (500 mg qd) *or*
   Oral clarithromycin (500 mg bid)
2. Intravenous or oral levofloxacin (500 mg qd)
3. Intravenous or oral gatifloxacin (400 mg qd)
4. Intravenous or oral moxifloxacin (400 mg qd)

Note: Treatment of documented *M. pneumoniae* pneumonia is usually continued for 14 to 21 days.

who are not infected with either *Neisseria gonorrhoeae* or *C. trachomatis*.

Disorders of Reproduction Ureaplasmas have been considered as causes of involuntary infertility in both men and women, but there is no convincing evidence for such an association. These organisms have been associated with chorioamnionitis and late abortion. Given the close association of ureaplasmas with bacterial vaginosis, a condition that is strongly associated with chorioamnionitis and late abortion, it is difficult to define an independent role for ureaplasmas in this condition. In infants of very low birth weight, ureaplasmas have been shown to cause pneumonia and chronic lung disease.

Extragenital Infections Sexually acquired reactive arthritis and Reiter's syndrome may be triggered by ureaplasmas, although *C. trachomatis* is the usual triggering agent. Patients who have hypogammaglobulinemia may develop chronic arthritis due to ureaplasmas and some other mycoplasmal species. *M. hominis* has been identified in patients with postthoracotomy sternal wound infection and in rare instances of prosthetic heart valve and prosthetic joint infection.

DIAGNOSIS There is seldom any reason to examine specimens from the lower genital tract (vagina, male urethra) for mycoplasmas. The ubiquity of the organisms among healthy individuals makes a positive result uninterpretable. The organisms should be sought only in specimens from normally sterile areas, such as joint fluid with evidence of inflammation and cultures negative for conventional microorganisms.

M. hominis can replicate in many routine blood culture media without changing the appearance of the media; although it forms nonhemolytic pinpoint colonies on blood agar, organisms cannot be visualized in gram-stained smears of these colonies. Neither *U. urealyticum* nor *M. genitalium* will grow in ordinary microbiologic media.

Microbiologic diagnosis of genital mycoplasmal infection requires specially prepared media and is beyond the capability of all but reference and research laboratories. Nucleic acid amplification tests such as PCR have been developed and may become commercially available.

℞ TREATMENT

Ureaplasmas, *M. genitalium*, and *M. hominis* are usually susceptible to tetracyclines (e.g., doxycycline). Infections caused by tetracycline-resistant ureaplasmas can be treated with erythromycin, while those due to tetracycline-resistant strains of *M. hominis* respond to treatment with clindamycin. As noted above, a specific microbiologic diagnosis of mycoplasmal infection is seldom made. Appropriate treatment provides antimicrobial coverage for the organisms that cause the particular syndrome. Accordingly, NGU is treated with doxycycline (100 mg orally twice a day for 7 days) or azithromycin (1.0 g as a single oral dose) to provide activity against *C. trachomatis*, *U. urealyticum*, and *M. genitalium*. Recommended regimens for the treatment of PID provide antimicrobial activity against gonococci, chlamydiae, and anaerobes as well as genital mycoplasmas.

FURTHER READING

BARTLETT JG et al: Practice guidelines for the management of community-acquired pneumonia in adults. Clin Infect Dis 31:347, 2000

BASEMAN JB, TULLY JG: Mycoplasmas: Sophisticated, reemerging, and burdened by their notoriety. Emerg Infect Dis 3:21, 1997

HAMMERSCHLAG MR: *Mycoplasma pneumoniae* infections. Curr Opin Infect Dis 14:181, 2001

HICKMAN-DAVIS JM: Role of innate immunity in respiratory *Mycoplasma* infection. Front Biosci 7:d1347, 2002

MURRAY HW et al: The protean manifestations of *Mycoplasma pneumoniae* in adults. Am J Med 58:229, 1975

TAYLOR-ROBINSON D: *Mycoplasma genitalium*—an update. Int J STD AIDS 13:145, 2002

————, FURR PM: Update on sexually transmitted mycoplasmas. Lancet 351(Suppl 3):12, 1998

160 CHLAMYDIAL INFECTIONS
Walter E. Stamm

The genus *Chlamydia* contains three species that infect humans: *Chlamydia psittaci*, *C. trachomatis*, and *C. pneumoniae* (formerly the TWAR agent). *C. psittaci* is widely distributed in nature, producing genital, conjunctival, intestinal, or respiratory infections in many mammalian and avian species. Genital infections with *C. psittaci* have been well characterized in several species and cause abortion and infertility. Although mammalian strains of *C. psittaci* are not known to infect humans, avian strains occasionally do so, causing pneumonia and the systemic illness known as *psittacosis*.

C. pneumoniae is a fastidious chlamydial species that appears to be a common cause of upper respiratory tract infection and pneumonia, primarily in children and young adults, and is a cause of recurrent respiratory infections in older adults. Studies have also linked *C. pneumoniae* infection to atherosclerotic cardiovascular disease and perhaps to asthma and sarcoidosis. No animal reservoir has been identified for *C. pneumoniae*; it appears to be an exclusively human pathogen spread via the respiratory route through close personal contact. To date, all strains of *C. pneumoniae* studied have been serologically homologous.

C. trachomatis is also an exclusively human pathogen and was identified as the cause of trachoma in the 1940s. Since then, *C. trachomatis* has been recognized as a major cause of sexually transmitted and perinatal infection.

Chlamydiae are obligate intracellular bacteria that are classified in their own order (Chlamydiales). They possess both DNA and RNA, have a cell wall and ribosomes similar to those of gram-negative bacteria, and are inhibited by antibiotics such as tetracycline.

A unique feature of all chlamydiae is their complex reproductive cycle. Two forms of the microorganism—the extracellular elementary body and the intracellular reticulate body—participate in this cycle. The elementary body is adapted for extracellular survival and is the infective form transmitted from one person to another. Elementary bodies attach to susceptible target cells (usually columnar or transitional epithelial cells) and enter the cells inside a phagosome. Within 8 h of cell entry, the elementary bodies reorganize into reticulate bodies, which are adapted to intracellular survival and multiplication. They undergo binary fission, eventually producing numerous replicates contained within the intracellular membrane-bound "inclusion body," which occupies much of the infected host cell. Chlamydial inclusions resist lysosomal fusion until late in the developmental cycle. After 24 h, the reticulate bodies condense and form elementary bodies still contained within the inclusion. The inclusion then ruptures, releasing elementary bodies from the cell to initiate infection of adjacent cells or transmission to another person.

Studies with monoclonal antibodies to and nucleotide sequencing of the major outer membrane protein have delineated at least 20 serotypes of *C. trachomatis*. According to the classification of Wang and Grayston, strains associated with trachoma have generally been those of the A, B, Ba, and C serovars, while serovars D through K have largely been associated with sexually transmitted and perinatally acquired infections. Serovars L_1, L_2, and L_3 produce lymphogranuloma venereum (LGV) and hemorrhagic proctocolitis. The LGV strains demonstrate unique biologic behavior in that they are more invasive than the other serovars, produce disease in lymphatic tissue, grow readily in cell culture systems and macrophages, and are lethal when inoculated intracerebrally into mice and monkeys. Non-LGV strains of *C. trachomatis* characteristically produce infections involving the superficial columnar epithelium of the eye, genitalia, and respiratory tract.

C. trachomatis has been reported as an infrequent cause of endocarditis, peritonitis, pleuritis, and possibly periappendicitis and may occasionally cause respiratory infections in older children and adults. Some immunosuppressed patients with pneumonia have had either serologic or cultural evidence of *C. trachomatis* infection, but more data are necessary to define a pathogenic role for *Chlamydia* in these patients.

C. TRACHOMATIS INFECTIONS

C. TRACHOMATIS GENITAL INFECTIONS Genital infections caused by *C. trachomatis* represent the most common bacterial sexually transmitted diseases (STDs) in the United States (Chap. 115). An estimated 4 million cases occur each year. In adults, the clinical spectrum of sexually transmitted *C. trachomatis* infections parallels that of gonococcal infections. Both infections have been associated with urethritis, proctitis, and conjunctivitis in both sexes; with epididymitis in men; and with mucopurulent cervicitis (MPC), acute salpingitis, bartholinitis, and the Fitz-Hugh–Curtis syndrome (perihepatitis) in women. Moreover, both types of infection can be associated with septic arthritis. In general, however, chlamydial infections produce fewer symptoms and signs than corresponding gonococcal infections at the same anatomic site; in fact, chlamydial infections are often totally asymptomatic. Increasing evidence suggests that many chlamydial infections of the genital tract, especially in women, persist for months without producing symptoms. Simultaneous infection with *C. trachomatis* often occurs in women with cervical gonococcal infection and in heterosexual men with gonococcal urethritis.

Epidemiology Infections due to *C. trachomatis* have been reportable in the United States since 1985, and national incidence data show steadily rising numbers of reported infections, undoubtedly reflecting both increased testing and increased reporting. Most testing to date has focused upon women, and thus the reported incidence is severalfold greater among women than among men; this difference likely represents a surveillance artifact.

The age of peak incidence of genital *C. trachomatis* infections, as of other sexually transmitted infections, is the late teens and early twenties. The prevalence of chlamydial urethral infection among young men is at least 3 to 5% for those seen in general medical settings or in urban high schools, >10% for asymptomatic soldiers undergoing routine physical examination, and 15 to 20% for heterosexual men seen in STD clinics. In areas where chlamydial control programs have been implemented, prevalence may be markedly reduced. In short, prevalence varies widely with the population group studied and with the geographic locale. With the newer, more sensitive nucleic acid amplification tests such as polymerase chain reaction (PCR) and ligase chain reaction (LCR), prevalences in most populations have been 10 to 30% higher than those measured with older, less sensitive tests.

The prevalence of cervical infection among women is ~5% for asymptomatic college students and prenatal patients in the United States, >10% for women seen in family planning clinics, and >20% for women seen in STD clinics. As in men, prevalence varies substantially by geographic locale, with the highest rates in the southeast. However, substantial prevalences (~8%) of asymptomatic chlamydial infection have been demonstrated among young female military recruits from all parts of the United States. In this country, the prevalence of *C. trachomatis* in the cervix of pregnant women is 5 to 10 times higher than that of *Neisseria gonorrhoeae*. The prevalence of genital infection with either agent is highest among individuals who are between the ages of 18 and 24, single, and non-Caucasian (e.g., African American or Latino). Recurrent chlamydial infections occur frequently in these same risk groups, often acquired from untreated sexual partners. Oral contraceptive pill use and the presence of cervical ectopy also confer an increased risk of chlamydial infection. The proportion of infections that are asymptomatic appears to be higher for *C. trachomatis* than for *N. gonorrhoeae*, and symptomatic *C. trachomatis* infections are clinically less severe. Mild or asymptomatic chlamydial infections of the fallopian tubes nonetheless cause ongoing tubal damage and infertility. Furthermore, because the total number of *C. trachomatis* infections exceeds the total number of *N. gonorrhoeae* infections in industrialized countries, the total morbidity caused by *C. trachomatis* genital infections in these countries equals or exceeds that caused by *N. gonorrhoeae*. The prevalence of *C. trachomatis* is higher than that of *N. gonorrhoeae* in industrialized countries, in part because measures such as treatment of sex partners and routine cultures for case detection in asymptomatic individuals have been applied much longer and more effectively to the control of gonorrhea than to the control of *C. trachomatis* infection.

Pathogenesis   *C. trachomatis* preferentially infects the columnar epithelium of the eye and the respiratory and genital tracts. The infection induces an immune response but often persists for months or years in the absence of antimicrobial therapy. Serious sequelae often occur in association with repeated or persistent infections. The precise mechanism through which repeated infection elicits an inflammatory response that leads to tubal scarring and damage in the female upper genital tract is not yet clear. One antigen, the chlamydial 60-kDa heat-shock protein, may be involved in inducing the pathologic immune response or may elicit antibodies that cross-react with human heat-shock proteins. The recent sequencing of the chlamydial genome may soon offer further insights into the pathogenic mechanisms of *C. trachomatis*.

Clinical Manifestations ■ *NONGONOCOCCAL AND POSTGONOCOCCAL URETHRITIS* Nongonococcal urethritis (NGU) is a diagnosis of exclusion that is applied to men with symptoms and/or signs of urethritis who do not have gonorrhea. Postgonococcal urethritis (PGU) refers to nongonococcal urethritis developing in men 2 to 3 weeks after treatment of gonococcal urethritis with single doses of agents such as amoxicillin or cephalosporins that lack antimicrobial activity against chlamydiae. Since current treatment regimens for gonorrhea also include tetracycline, doxycycline, or azithromycin for possible concomitant chlamydial infection, both the incidence of PGU and the causative role of chlamydiae in this syndrome have declined. *C. trachomatis* causes 20 to 40% of cases of NGU in heterosexual men but is less commonly isolated from homosexual men with this syndrome. The cause of most of the remaining cases is uncertain; considerable evidence suggests that *Ureaplasma urealyticum* and *Mycoplasma genitalium* cause many cases of NGU, while *Trichomonas vaginalis* and herpes simplex virus (HSV) cause some cases.

NGU is diagnosed by documentation of a leukocytic urethral exudate and by exclusion of gonorrhea by Gram's staining or culture. *C. trachomatis* urethritis is generally less severe than gonococcal urethritis, although in an individual patient these two forms of urethritis cannot be reliably differentiated solely on clinical grounds. Symptoms include urethral discharge (often whitish and mucoid rather than frankly purulent), dysuria, and urethral itching. Physical examination may reveal meatal erythema and tenderness and a urethral exudate that is often demonstrable only by stripping of the urethra.

At least one-third of males with *C. trachomatis* urethral infection have no demonstrable signs or symptoms of urethritis. Use of nucleic acid amplification assays on first-void urine specimens to diagnose chlamydial infections in men has facilitated more broadly based testing for asymptomatic infection in males. As a result, asymptomatic chlamydial urethritis has been demonstrated in 5 to 10% of sexually active adolescent males screened in school-based clinics or community centers. Such patients generally have first-glass pyuria (≥15 leukocytes per 400× microscopic field in the sediment of first-void urine), a positive leukocyte esterase test, or an increased number of leukocytes on Gram-stained smear prepared from a urogenital swab inserted 1 to 2 cm into the anterior urethra. For the enumeration of leukocytes, the smear is first scanned at low power to identify areas of the slide containing the highest concentration of leukocytes. These areas are then examined under oil immersion (1000×). An average of four or more leukocytes in at least three of five 1000× (oil-immersion) fields is indicative of urethritis and correlates with the recovery of *C. trachomatis*. To differentiate between true urethritis and functional symptoms among symptomatic patients or to make a presumptive diagnosis of *C. trachomatis* infection in "high-risk" but asymptomatic men (e.g., male patients in STD clinics, sex partners of women with nongonococcal salpingitis or MPC, fathers of children with inclusion conjunctivitis), the examination of an endourethral specimen for increased leukocytes is useful if specific diagnostic tests for chlamydiae are not available. Alternatively, noninvasive screening for urethritis can be accomplished by testing of a first-void urine sample for pyuria, either by microscopy or by the leukocyte esterase test. Urine can also be directly tested for chlamydiae or gonococci by DNA amplification methods, as described below.

EPIDIDYMITIS   *C. trachomatis* is the foremost cause of epididymitis in sexually active heterosexual men <35 years of age, accounting for ~70% of cases. *N. gonorrhoeae* causes most of the remaining cases, and some men have simultaneous infections with both pathogens, usually accompanied by asymptomatic urethritis as defined above. In homosexual men, sexually transmitted coliform infection acquired via insertive rectal intercourse may cause epididymitis. Coliform bacteria and *Pseudomonas aeruginosa*, usually in association with preceding urologic instrumentation or surgery, are the most common causes of epididymitis in men over 35. Men with chlamydial epididymitis typically present with unilateral scrotal pain, fever, and epididymal tenderness or swelling on examination. The illness may be mild enough to treat on an outpatient basis with oral antibiotics or severe enough to require hospitalization and parenteral therapy. Testicular torsion should be excluded promptly by radionuclide scan, Doppler flow study, or surgical exploration in a teenager or young adult who presents with acute unilateral testicular pain without urethritis. The possibility of testicular tumor or chronic infection (e.g., tuberculosis) should be excluded when a patient with unilateral intrascrotal pain and swelling does not respond to appropriate antimicrobial therapy.

REITER'S SYNDROME   Reiter's syndrome consists of conjunctivitis, urethritis (or cervicitis in females), arthritis, and characteristic mucocutaneous lesions (Chap. 305). *C. trachomatis* has been recovered from the urethra of up to 70% of men with untreated nondiarrheal Reiter's syndrome and associated urethritis. In the absence of overt urethritis, it is important to exclude subclinical urethritis in the men in whom this diagnosis is suspected.

The pathogenesis of Reiter's syndrome remains obscure. However, since more than 80% of affected patients have the HLA-B27 phenotype and since other mucosal infections (with *Salmonella*, *Shigella*, or *Campylobacter*, for example) produce an identical syndrome, chlamydial infection is thought to initiate an aberrant and hyperactive immune response that produces inflammation at the involved target organs in these genetically predisposed individuals. Evidence of exaggerated cell-mediated and humoral immune responses to chlamydial antigens in Reiter's syndrome supports this hypothesis. The presumptive demonstration of chlamydial elementary bodies and chlamydial DNA in the joint fluid and synovial tissue of patients with Reiter's syndrome suggests that chlamydiae may actually spread from genital to joint tissues in these patients, perhaps in macrophages.

PROCTITIS *C. trachomatis* strains of either the genital immunotypes D through K or the LGV immunotypes cause proctitis in homosexual men who practice receptive anorectal intercourse. In the United States, the vast majority of cases are due to immunotypes D through K and present either as asymptomatic infection or as mild proctitis not unlike gonococcal proctitis. These infections may develop in heterosexual women as well. Patients present with mild rectal pain, mucous discharge, tenesmus, and (occasionally) bleeding. Nearly all have neutrophils in their rectal Gram's stain. Anoscopy in these non-LGV cases of chlamydial proctitis reveals mild, patchy mucosal friability and mucopurulent discharge, and the disease process is limited to the distal rectum. LGV strains produce more severe ulcerative proctitis or proctocolitis that can be confused clinically with HSV proctitis (severe rectal pain, bleeding, discharge, and tenesmus) and that histologically resembles Crohn's disease in that giant cell formation and granulomas can be seen (Chap. 276). In the United States, these cases occur almost exclusively in homosexual men.

MUCOPURULENT CERVICITIS Although many women with *C. trachomatis* infection of the cervix have no symptoms or signs, a careful speculum examination reveals evidence of MPC in 30 to 50% of cases. As is discussed more fully in Chap. 115, MPC is associated with yellow mucopurulent endocervical discharge and with ≥ 20 neutrophils per $1000\times$ microscopic field within strands of cervical mucus on a thinly smeared, Gram-stained preparation of endocervical exudate. Other characteristic findings include edema of the zone of cervical ectopy and a propensity of the mucosa to bleed on minor trauma—e.g., when specimens are collected with a swab. A Pap smear shows increased numbers of neutrophils as well as a characteristic pattern of mononuclear inflammatory cells, including plasma cells, transformed lymphocytes, and histiocytes. Cervical biopsy shows a predominantly mononuclear cell infiltrate of the subepithelial stroma, often with follicular cervicitis.

PELVIC INFLAMMATORY DISEASE (PID) (See also Chap. 115) In the United States, *C. trachomatis* has been identified in the fallopian tubes or endometrium of up to 50% of women with PID, and its role as an important etiologic agent in this syndrome is well accepted. PID occurs via ascending intraluminal spread of *C. trachomatis* from the lower genital tract. MPC is thus followed by endometritis, endosalpingitis, and finally pelvic peritonitis. Evidence of MPC is usually found in women with laparoscopically verified salpingitis. Similarly, endometritis, demonstrated by endometrial biopsy showing plasma cell infiltration of the endometrial epithelium, is documented in most women with laparoscopically verified chlamydial (or gonococcal) salpingitis. Chlamydial endometritis can also occur in the absence of clinical evidence of salpingitis: ~40 to 50% of women with MPC have plasma cell endometritis. Histologic evidence of endometritis has been correlated with an "endometritis syndrome" consisting of vaginal bleeding, lower abdominal pain, and uterine tenderness in the absence of adnexal tenderness. Chlamydial salpingitis produces milder symptoms than does gonococcal salpingitis and may be associated with less marked adnexal tenderness. Thus mild adnexal or uterine tenderness in sexually active women with cervicitis suggests PID.

Infertility associated with fallopian-tube scarring has been strongly linked to antecedent *C. trachomatis* infection in serologic studies. Since many infertile women with tubal scarring and antichlamydial antibody have no history of PID, it appears that subclinical tubal infection ("silent salpingitis") may produce scarring. Studies in animals and humans with salpingitis and tubal scarring suggest the continuing presence of persistent, slowly replicating chlamydial infection in tubal tissue. While the pathogenesis of *Chlamydia*-induced tubal scarring remains poorly understood, antibodies to the chlamydial 60-kDa heat-shock protein have been correlated with tubal infertility, ectopic pregnancy, and Fitz-Hugh–Curtis syndrome (see below). Thus this antigen may initiate an immune-mediated process that ultimately damages the fallopian tube. Host genetic susceptibility, as defined by HLA type, may also play an important role.

Perihepatitis, or the Fitz-Hugh–Curtis syndrome, was originally described as a complication of gonococcal PID. The syndrome should be suspected whenever a young, sexually active woman presents with an illness resembling cholecystitis (fever and right-upper-quadrant pain of subacute or acute onset). Symptoms and signs of salpingitis may be minimal. Cultural and/or serologic evidence of *C. trachomatis* infection is found in three-quarters of women with this syndrome.

URETHRAL SYNDROME IN WOMEN In the absence of infection with uropathogens such as coliforms or *Staphylococcus saprophyticus*, *C. trachomatis* is the pathogen most commonly isolated from college women with dysuria, frequency, and pyuria (Chap. 269). *Chlamydia* can also be isolated from the urethra of women without symptoms of urethritis, and up to 25% of female STD clinic patients with chlamydial urogenital infection have cultures positive for *C. trachomatis* from the urethra only.

C. TRACHOMATIS INFECTION IN PREGNANCY AND THE NEONATAL PERIOD Studies in the United States have demonstrated that 5 to 25% of pregnant women have *C. trachomatis* infections of the cervix. In these studies, approximately one-half to two-thirds of children exposed during birth have acquired *C. trachomatis* infection. Roughly half of the infected infants (or 25% of the group exposed) have developed clinical evidence of inclusion conjunctivitis. In addition to infecting the eye, *C. trachomatis* has been isolated frequently and persistently from the nasopharynx, rectum, and vagina of such infants, occasionally for periods exceeding 1 year in the absence of treatment. Pneumonia develops in ~10% of children infected perinatally, and otitis media may in some cases result from perinatally acquired chlamydial infection.

Neonatal chlamydial conjunctivitis has an acute onset 5 to 14 days after birth and often produces a profuse mucopurulent discharge. However, it is impossible to differentiate chlamydial conjunctivitis from other forms of neonatal conjunctivitis (such as that due to *N. gonorrhoeae*, *Haemophilus influenzae*, *Streptococcus pneumoniae*, or HSV) on clinical grounds; thus laboratory diagnosis is required. Inclusions within epithelial cells are often detected in Giemsa-stained conjunctival smears, but these smears are considerably less sensitive than cultures, antigen detection tests, or nucleic acid hybridization tests for chlamydiae. Gram-stained smears may show gonococci or occasional small gram-negative coccobacilli in *Haemophilus* conjunctivitis, but smears should be accompanied by cultures for these agents.

C. trachomatis causes a distinctive pneumonia syndrome in infants. Recent epidemiologic studies have linked chlamydial pulmonary infection in infants with increased occurrence of subacute lung disease (bronchitis, asthma, wheezing) in later childhood.

Lymphogranuloma Venereum ■ *DEFINITION* LGV is a sexually transmitted infection caused by *C. trachomatis* strains of the L$_1$, L$_2$, and L$_3$ serovars. In the United States, most cases are caused by L$_2$ organisms. Acute LGV is characterized by a transient primary genital lesion followed by multilocular suppurative regional lymphadenopathy. Patients exposed via insertive rectal intercourse may develop hemorrhagic proctitis with regional lymphadenitis. Acute LGV is almost always associated with systemic symptoms such as fever and leukocytosis but is rarely associated with systemic complications such as meningoencephalitis. After a period of years, late complications include genital elephantiasis due to lymphatic involvement; strictures; and fistulas of the penis, urethra, and rectum.

EPIDEMIOLOGY LGV is usually sexually transmitted, but occasional transmission by nonsexual personal contact, fomites, or laboratory accidents has been documented. Laboratory work involving the creation of aerosols of LGV organisms (e.g., sonication, homogenization) must be conducted only with appropriate measures for biologic containment.

The peak incidence of LGV corresponds to the age of greatest sexual activity: the second and third decades of life. The worldwide incidence of LGV is falling, but the disease is still endemic and a major cause of morbidity in Asia, Africa, South America, and parts of the Caribbean. In the Bahamas, an apparent outbreak of LGV has been described in association with a concurrent increase in heterosexual infection with HIV. However, the reported incidence of LGV in the United States has been only 0.1 case per 100,000 persons for more than a decade.

The frequency of infection following exposure is believed to be much lower than that for gonorrhea and syphilis. Early manifestations are recognized far more often in men than in women, who usually present with late complications. In the United States, where the reported male-to-female ratio of cases is 3.4:1, most cases have involved homosexually active men and persons returning from abroad (travelers, sailors, and military personnel). The main reservoir of infection, although it has not been directly demonstrated, is presumed to be asymptomatically infected individuals.

CLINICAL MANIFESTATIONS   A *primary genital lesion* develops from 3 days to 3 weeks after exposure. It is a small, painless vesicle or nonindurated ulcer or papule located on the penis in men and on the labia, posterior vagina, or fourchette in women. The primary lesion is noticed by fewer than one-third of men with LGV and only rarely by women. It heals in a few days without scarring and, even when noticed, is usually recognized as LGV only in retrospect. LGV strains of *C. trachomatis* have occasionally been recovered from genital ulcers and from the urethra of men and the endocervix of women who present with inguinal adenopathy; these areas may be the primary site of infection in some cases.

Primary anal or *rectal infection* develops after receptive anorectal intercourse. In women, rectal infection with LGV (or non-LGV) strains of *C. trachomatis* presumably can also arise by the contiguous spread of infected secretions along the perineum (as in rectal gonococcal infections in women) or perhaps by spread to the rectum via the pelvic lymphatics.

From the site of the primary urethral, genital, anal, or rectal infection, the organism spreads via the regional lymphatics. Penile, vulvar, or anal infection can lead to inguinal and femoral lymphadenitis. Rectal infection produces hypogastric and deep iliac lymphadenitis. Upper vaginal or cervical infection results in enlargement of the obturator and iliac nodes.

The most common presenting picture in heterosexual men is the *inguinal syndrome*, which is characterized by painful inguinal lymphadenopathy beginning 2 to 6 weeks after presumed exposure; in rare instances, the onset comes after a few months. The inguinal adenopathy is unilateral in two-thirds of cases, and palpable enlargement of the iliac and femoral nodes is often evident on the same side as the enlarged inguinal nodes. The nodes are initially discrete, but progressive periadenitis results in a matted mass of nodes that becomes fluctuant and suppurative. The overlying skin becomes fixed, inflamed, and thin and finally develops multiple draining fistulas. Extensive enlargement of chains of inguinal nodes above and below the inguinal ligament ("the sign of the groove") is not specific and, although not uncommon, is documented in only a minority of cases. On histologic examination, infected nodes are initially found to have characteristic small stellate abscesses surrounded by histiocytes. These abscesses coalesce to form large, necrotic, suppurative foci. Spontaneous healing usually takes place after several months; inguinal scars or granulomatous masses of various sizes persist for life. Massive pelvic lymphadenopathy may lead to exploratory laparotomy.

As cultures and serologic tests for *C. trachomatis* are being used more often, increasing numbers of cases of LGV proctitis are being recognized in homosexual men. Such patients present with anorectal pain and mucopurulent, bloody rectal discharge. Although these patients may complain of diarrhea, they are often referring not to diarrhea but rather to frequent, painful, unsuccessful attempts at defecation (tenesmus). Sigmoidoscopy reveals ulcerative proctitis or proctocolitis, with purulent exudate and mucosal bleeding. The histopathologic findings in the rectal mucosa include granulomas with giant cells, crypt

abscesses, and extensive inflammation. These clinical, sigmoidoscopic, and histopathologic findings may closely resemble those of Crohn's disease of the rectum.

Constitutional symptoms are common during the stage of regional lymphadenopathy and, in cases of proctitis, may include fever, chills, headache, meningismus, anorexia, myalgias, and arthralgias. These findings in the presence of lymphadenopathy are sometimes mistakenly interpreted as representing malignant lymphoma. Other systemic complications are infrequent but include arthritis with sterile effusion, aseptic meningitis, meningoencephalitis, conjunctivitis, hepatitis, and erythema nodosum. Chlamydiae have been recovered from the cerebrospinal fluid and in one case were isolated from the blood of a patient with severe constitutional symptoms—a result indicating the dissemination of infection. Laboratory-acquired infections suspected of being due to the inhalation of aerosols have been associated with mediastinal lymphadenitis, pneumonitis, and pleural effusion.

Complications of untreated anorectal infection include perirectal abscess; fistula in ano; and rectovaginal, rectovesical, and ischiorectal fistulas. Secondary bacterial infection probably contributes to these complications. Rectal stricture is a late complication of anorectal infection and usually develops 2 to 6 cm from the anal orifice—i.e., at a site within reach on digital rectal examination. Proximal extension of the stricture for several centimeters may lead to a mistaken clinical and radiographic diagnosis of carcinoma.

A small percentage of cases of LGV in men present as chronic progressive infiltrative, ulcerative, or fistular lesions of the penis, urethra, or scrotum. Associated lymphatic obstruction may produce elephantiasis. When urethral stricture occurs, it usually involves the posterior urethra and causes incontinence or difficulty with urination.

Approach to the Diagnosis and Treatment of *C. trachomatis* Genital Infections

Four types of laboratory procedure are available to confirm *C. trachomatis* infection: direct microscopic examination of tissue scrapings for typical intracytoplasmic inclusions or elementary bodies; isolation of the organism in cell culture; detection of chlamydial antigens or nucleic acid by immunologic or hybridization methods; and detection of antibody in serum or in local secretions.

Except in conjunctivitis, direct microscopic examination of Giemsa-stained cell scrapings for typical inclusions has an unacceptably low degree of sensitivity, and false-positive interpretations by inexperienced observers are common. Even for conjunctivitis, this approach has been replaced by direct fluorescent antibody staining of conjunctival smears to identify chlamydial elementary bodies with specific monoclonal antibodies (see below).

Cell culture techniques for isolation of *C. trachomatis* are available in most large medical centers but not in other clinical settings. In addition to limited availability, other disadvantages of cell culture include its low and variable level of sensitivity (60 to 80%), its requirement for rigorous transport conditions, and its high cost and technically demanding nature. Therefore, nonculture alternatives involving antigen detection or nucleic acid hybridization have been developed. In the direct immunofluorescent antibody (DFA) slide test, potentially infected genital or ocular secretions are smeared onto a slide, fixed, and stained with fluorescein-conjugated monoclonal antibody specific for chlamydial antigens. The observation of fluorescing elementary bodies confirms the diagnosis. Enzyme-linked immunosorbent assay (ELISA) techniques for the detection of chlamydial antigens provide another alternative to culture. The reported sensitivity and specificity of these tests for genital infections (as compared with culture) have been 60 to 80% and 97 to 99%, respectively, in high-risk populations. Assays with nucleic acid probes have also been developed for chlamydial diagnosis. One such test uses DNA-RNA hybridization and appears to be approximately equal to the best ELISAs in terms of sensitivity and specificity. Nucleic acid probes have also been developed for use in amplification assays such as LCR and PCR. These tests are now the most sensitive chlamydial diagnostic methods available, being the first nonculture assays to surpass culture itself in sensitivity. In addition, the ability of these tests to detect chlamydial genes in urine with a high degree of sensitivity and specificity allows—for the first time—the use of urine specimens rather than conventional urethral and cervical swabs. The use of urine specimens is particularly appealing for public-health chlamydial screening programs because of the ease of sample collection, even in community-based settings.

Serologic tests are of limited usefulness in the diagnosis of chlamydial oculogenital infections. The complement fixation test with heat-stable, genus-specific antigen has been used with some success to diagnose LGV but is insensitive in infections due to non-LGV strains of *C. trachomatis*. The microimmunofluorescence (micro-IF) test with *C. trachomatis* antigens is more sensitive but is generally available only in research laboratories. The test measures antibodies by serovar specificity and by immunoglobulin class (IgM, IgG, IgA, secretory IgA) in both serum and local secretions. Serologic diagnosis by the micro-IF test may be useful in infant pneumonia (in which high-titer IgM antibody and/or fourfold rises in titer are often demonstrated), in chlamydial salpingitis (especially Fitz-Hugh–Curtis syndrome), and in LGV. In all of these more invasive syndromes, high antibody levels are present.

Table 160-1 summarizes the diagnostic tests of choice for patients with suspected *C. trachomatis* infection. It is clear that, in most settings and for most purposes, sensitivity and specificity will be greatest with nucleic acid amplification techniques. For patients to whom medicolegal considerations may apply (victims of sexual or child abuse), cultures or nucleic acid amplification methods should always be used. In men with suspected urethritis, PCR or LCR testing of a first-void urine specimen offers a more sensitive and noninvasive diagnostic method than the use of urethral swabs. For the diagnosis of urogenital (cervical or urethral) infections in women, testing of a first-void urine specimen by nucleic acid amplification methods is at least as sensitive as testing of a cervical swab. Patient-collected vaginal swabs tested by PCR or LCR have also been used successfully. Since chlamydial diagnostic testing has become more widely available and is now more sensitive and specific than in the past, its use for specific diagnosis in patients with suspected chlamydial syndromes (such as MPC, NGU, and PID) and their partners should be promoted. High priority should also be given to the screening of asymptomatic high-risk women who would not otherwise receive treatment for presumptive chlamydial infection, especially those seen in high-risk settings (e.g., STD clinics or abortion clinics) and those with a high-risk profile (e.g., sexually active and ≤21 years of age, new sex partner within the preceding 2 months, or more than one current sex partner). Similar screening programs should be used to detect and treat asymptomatic urethritis in high-risk adolescent males. Where implemented, screening programs of this type have been associated with reductions in the prevalence of chlamydial infection and of its complications, such as PID.

℞ TREATMENT

Until the introduction of azithromycin, chlamydial infections could not be eradicated by single-dose or short-term antimicrobial regimens. In most uncomplicated infections in adults, a 7-day course of treatment

---

TABLE 160-1 *Diagnostic Tests for Sexually Transmitted and Perinatal Chlamydia trachomatis Infection*

Infection	Suggestive Signs/Symptoms	Presumptive Diagnosis[a]	Confirmatory Test of Choice
MEN			
NGU, PGU	Discharge, dysuria	Gram's stain with >4 neutrophils per oil-immersion field; no gonococci	Urethral culture or nonculture test for *C. trachomatis*; urine or urethral NAAT for *C. trachomatis*
Epididymitis	Unilateral intrascrotal swelling, pain, tenderness; fever; NGU	Gram's stain with >4 neutrophils per oil-immersion field; no gonococci; urinalysis with pyuria	Urethral culture or nonculture test for *C. trachomatis*; urine or urethral NAAT for *C. trachomatis*
WOMEN			
Cervicitis	Mucopurulent cervical discharge, bleeding and edema of the zone of cervical ectopy	Cervical Gram's stain with ≥20 neutrophils per oil-immersion field in cervical mucus	Cervical culture or nonculture test for *C. trachomatis*; urine or cervical NAAT for *C. trachomatis*
Salpingitis	Lower abdominal pain, cervical motion tenderness, adnexal tenderness or masses	*C. trachomatis* always potentially present in salpingitis	Cervical culture or nonculture test for *C. trachomatis*; urine or cervical NAAT for *C. trachomatis*
Urethritis	Dysuria and frequency without urgency or hematuria	MPC; sterile pyuria; negative routine urine culture	Urethral and cervical cultures or nonculture test for *C. trachomatis*; urine NAAT for *C. trachomatis*
ADULTS OF EITHER SEX			
Proctitis	Rectal pain, discharge, tenesmus, bleeding; history of receptive anorectal intercourse	Negative gonococcal culture and Gram's stain; at least 1 neutrophil per oil-immersion field in rectal Gram's stain	Rectal culture or direct immunofluorescence test for *C. trachomatis*
Reiter's syndrome	NGU, arthritis, conjunctivitis, typical skin lesions	Gram's stain with >4 neutrophils per oil-immersion field; lack of gonococci indicative of NGU	Urethral culture or nonculture test for *C. trachomatis*
LGV	Regional adenopathy, primary lesion, proctitis, systemic symptoms	None	Isolation of LGV strain from node or rectum, occasionally from urethra or cervix; LGV CF titer, ≥1:64; micro-IF titer, ≥1:512
NEONATES			
Conjunctivitis	Purulent conjunctival discharge 6 to 18 days postdelivery	Negative culture and Gram's stain for gonococci, *Haemophilus* spp., pneumococci, staphylococci	Conjunctival culture or nonculture test for *C. trachomatis*; FA-stained scraping of conjunctival material
Infant pneumonia	Afebrile, staccato cough, diffuse rales, bilateral hyperinflation, interstitial infiltrates	None	Chlamydial culture of sputum, pharynx, eye, rectum; micro-IF antibody to *C. trachomatis*—fourfold change in IgG or IgM antibody titer

[a] A presumptive diagnosis of chlamydial infection is often made in the syndromes listed when gonococci are not found. A positive test for *Neisseria gonorrhoeae* does not exclude the involvement of *C. trachomatis*, which often is present in patients with gonorrhea.

Note: CF, complement-fixing; FA, fluorescent antibody; LGV, lymphogranuloma venereum; micro-IF, microimmunofluorescence; MPC, mucopurulent cervicitis; NAAT, nucleic acid amplification test; NGU, nongonococcal urethritis; PGU, postgonococcal urethritis.

with doxycycline or tetracycline must be given for genital infections. A 2-week course is recommended for complicated chlamydial infections (e.g., PID, epididymitis) and at least a 3-week course of doxycycline (100 mg orally bid) or erythromycin base (500 mg orally qid) for LGV. Failure of treatment of genital infections with a tetracycline usually indicates poor compliance or reinfection rather than the involvement of a drug-resistant strain. To date, clinically significant drug resistance has not been observed in *C. trachomatis* infection.

Therapy for *C. trachomatis* urethritis is more efficacious than therapy for nonchlamydial NGU. *C. trachomatis* is eradicated from the urethra in nearly all cases by treatment with tetracycline hydrochloride (500 mg qid for 7 days) or doxycycline (100 mg by mouth bid for 7 days).

Eradication of *C. trachomatis* from the cervix by tetracycline and doxycycline, with doses and durations similar to those specified above for urethritis, has been demonstrated. Erythromycin base (500 mg qid for 10 to 14 days) is the regimen of choice for pregnant women with *C. trachomatis* infection. Amoxicillin (500 mg tid for 10 days) has also been used successfully in pregnant women. Tetracycline hydrochloride (500 mg qid) or doxycycline (100 mg bid) for 14 days produces clinical and microbiologic cure of epididymitis and PID associated with *C. trachomatis* infection, but in this situation a tetracycline should always be used together with a drug that is highly effective against gonorrhea.

Azithromycin is highly active against *C. trachomatis*, exhibits prolonged bioavailability, is concentrated intracellularly, and has made possible single-dose therapy for chlamydial infection for the first time. In comparative trials, a 1-g single dose of azithromycin has been as effective as 7 days of doxycycline therapy for uncomplicated chlamydial infection. Azithromycin causes fewer adverse gastrointestinal reactions than do older macrolides such as erythromycin. The single-dose regimen of azithromycin has great appeal for the treatment of patients with uncomplicated chlamydial infection (especially those without symptoms and those with a likelihood of poor compliance) and of sexual partners of infected patients. These advantages must be weighed against the considerably greater cost of azithromycin. Whenever possible, the single 1-g dose should be given as directly observed therapy. Although not approved by the U.S. Food and Drug Administration for the treatment of pregnant women, the 1-g single-dose regimen of azithromycin appears to be safe and effective for this purpose.

Of the newer fluoroquinolones, ofloxacin (300 mg by mouth bid for 7 days) has been shown to be as effective as doxycycline for the treatment of chlamydial infection and appears to be safe and well tolerated. It cannot be used in pregnancy.

Treatment of Sex Partners   The continued high prevalence of chlamydial infections in most parts of the United States is due primarily to the failure to diagnose—and therefore treat—patients with symptomatic or asymptomatic infection and their sex partners. *C. trachomatis* urethral or cervical infection has been well documented in a high proportion of the sex partners of patients with NGU, epididymitis, Reiter's syndrome, salpingitis, or endocervicitis. If possible, confirmatory laboratory tests for *Chlamydia* should be undertaken in these individuals, but even those without positive tests or evidence of clinical disease who have recently been exposed to proven or possible chlamydial infection (e.g., NGU) should be offered therapy.

Treatment of Neonates and Infants   In neonates with conjunctivitis or infants with pneumonia, erythromycin ethylsuccinate or estolate can be given orally in a dose of 50 mg/kg per day, preferably in four divided doses, for 2 weeks. Careful attention must be given to compliance with therapy—a frequent problem. Relapses of eye infection are common following treatment with topical erythromycin or tetracycline ophthalmic ointment and may also occur after oral erythromycin therapy. Thus follow-up cultures should be performed after treatment. Both parents should be examined for *C. trachomatis* infec-

tion and, if diagnostic testing is not readily available, should be treated with doxycycline or azithromycin.

Prevention   Efforts to develop a vaccine for chlamydial infection have not yet been successful. Early diagnosis and treatment shorten the duration of infectiousness and therefore constitute primary prevention of chlamydial infection. By the early 1990s, one of the 10 regions of the United States (Region X, the Pacific Northwest) had formally undertaken a chlamydial control program involving widespread screening of women attending family planning clinics. Approximately 500,000 tests per year were conducted at 150 such clinics throughout the region in women meeting the criteria for high risk. Within 5 years, the prevalence of chlamydial infection had been reduced by >30% in this population. While most regions of the United States have now initiated similar programs, some family planning and STD clinics still do not offer chlamydial testing. The availability of highly sensitive and specific diagnostic tests that can be done with urine specimens and of single-dose therapy makes it feasible to mount an effective chlamydial control program nationwide, with screening of high-risk persons both in traditional health care settings and in novel community- and school-based settings.

TRACHOMA AND ADULT INCLUSION CONJUNCTIVITIS ■ Definition   Trachoma is a chronic conjunctivitis associated with infection by *C. trachomatis* serovar A, B, Ba, or C. It has been responsible for an estimated 20 million cases of blindness throughout the world and remains an important cause of preventable blindness. Inclusion conjunctivitis is an acute ocular infection caused by sexually transmitted *C. trachomatis* strains (usually serovars D through K) in adults exposed to infected genital secretions and in their newborn offspring.

Epidemiology   In trachoma-endemic areas where the classic eye disease is seen, transmission is from eye to eye via hands, flies, towels, and other fomites and usually involves serovar A, B, Ba, or C. The worldwide incidence and severity of trachoma have decreased dramatically during the past 35 years, mainly as a result of improving hygienic and economic conditions. Endemic trachoma is still the major cause of preventable blindness in northern Africa, sub-Saharan Africa, the Middle East, and parts of Asia. Transmission occurs primarily through close personal contact, particularly among young children in rural communities with limited water supplies. In endemic areas, trachoma is associated with repeated exposure and reinfection, but the infection can also become chronic and persistent. Acute relapse of old trachoma occasionally follows treatment with cortisone eye ointment or develops in very old persons who were exposed in their youth.

Clinical Manifestations   Both endemic trachoma and adult inclusion conjunctivitis present initially as a conjunctivitis characterized by small lymphoid follicles in the conjunctiva. In regions with hyperendemic classic blinding trachoma, the disease usually starts insidiously before the age of 2 years. Reinfection is common and probably contributes to the pathogenesis of trachoma. Studies using PCR techniques indicate that chlamydial DNA is often present in the ocular secretions of patients with trachoma, even in the absence of positive cultures. Thus persistent infection may be more common than was previously thought.

The cornea becomes involved, with inflammatory leukocytic infiltrations and superficial vascularization (pannus formation). As the inflammation continues, conjunctival scarring eventually distorts the eyelids, causing them to turn inward so that the inturned lashes constantly abrade the eyeball (trichiasis and entropion); eventually the corneal epithelium is abraded and may ulcerate, with subsequent corneal scarring and blindness. Destruction of the conjunctival goblet cells, lacrimal ducts, and lacrimal gland may produce a "dry-eye" syndrome, with resultant corneal opacity due to drying (xerosis) or secondary bacterial corneal ulcers.

Communities with blinding trachoma often experience seasonal epidemics of conjunctivitis due to *H. influenzae* that contribute to the intensity of the inflammatory process. In such areas the active infectious process usually resolves spontaneously in affected persons between 10 and 15 years of age, but the conjunctival scars continue to shrink, producing trichiasis and entropion and subsequent corneal scarring in adults. In areas with milder and less prevalent disease, the process may be much slower, with active disease continuing into adulthood; blindness is rare in these cases.

Eye infection with genital *C. trachomatis* strains in sexually active young adults presents as the acute onset of unilateral follicular conjunctivitis and preauricular lymphadenopathy similar to that seen in acute adenovirus or herpesvirus conjunctivitis. If untreated, the disease may persist for 6 weeks to 2 years. It is frequently associated with corneal inflammation in the form of discrete opacities ("infiltrates"), punctate epithelial erosions, and minor degrees of superficial corneal vascularization. Very rarely, conjunctival scarring and eyelid distortion occur, particularly in patients treated for many months with topical glucocorticoids. Recurrent eye infections develop most often in patients whose sexual consorts are not treated with antimicrobials.

Diagnosis The clinical diagnosis of classic trachoma can be made if two of the following signs are present: (1) lymphoid follicles on the upper tarsal conjunctiva; (2) typical conjunctival scarring; (3) vascular pannus; or (4) limbal follicles or their sequelae, Herbert's pits.

The clinical diagnosis of endemic trachoma should be confirmed by laboratory tests in children with more marked degrees of inflammation. Intracytoplasmic chlamydial inclusions are found in 10 to 60% of Giemsa-stained conjunctival smears in such populations, but chlamydial PCR or LCR is more sensitive and is often positive when smears or cultures are negative. Follicular conjunctivitis in adult Europeans or Americans living in trachomatous regions is rarely due to trachoma.

℞ TREATMENT

Public health control programs for endemic trachoma have consisted of the mass application of tetracycline or erythromycin ointment to the eyes of all children in affected communities for 21 to 60 days or on an intermittent schedule. These programs also include surgical correction of inturned eyelids by a mobile surgical team that visits each locale. Mass treatment of entire villages with single dose azithromycin may be an alternative approach.

Adult inclusion conjunctivitis responds well to treatment with full doses of oral tetracycline or erythromycin administered for 3 weeks. Simultaneous treatment of all sexual consorts of the patient is also necessary to prevent ocular reinfection and to avoid genital disease due to chlamydial infection. Topical antibiotic treatment is not required for patients who receive systemic antibiotics.

Prevention Efforts to develop a trachoma vaccine have not yet been successful. General hygienic measures associated with improved living standards are effective in the elimination of endemic trachoma. An adequate water supply for personal cleanliness may be a key factor. In some areas the reduction of numbers of flies in the household is important.

C. PSITTACI INFECTIONS

Definition Psittacosis is primarily an infectious disease of birds and mammals that is caused by *C. psittaci*. Transmission of infection from birds to humans results in a febrile illness characterized by pneumonitis and systemic manifestations. Inapparent infections or mild influenzalike illnesses may also occur. The term *ornithosis* is sometimes applied to infections contracted from birds other than parrots or parakeets, but *psittacosis* is the preferred generic term for all forms of the disease.

Epidemiology Almost any avian species can harbor *C. psittaci*. Psittacine birds (parrots, parakeets, budgerigars) are most commonly infected, but human cases have been traced to contact with pigeons, ducks, turkeys, chickens, and many other birds. Psittacosis may be considered an occupational disease of pet-shop owners, poultry workers, pigeon fanciers, taxidermists, veterinarians, and zoo attendants. During the past 20 years, there has been an increase in incidence, with cases and outbreaks occurring primarily among employees of poultry-

processing plants. It is suspected that many cases go undiagnosed and unreported.

The agent is present in nasal secretions, excreta, tissues, and feathers of infected birds. Although the disease can be fatal, infected birds frequently show only minor evidence of illness, such as ruffled feathers, lethargy, and anorexia. Asymptomatic avian carriers are common, and complete recovery may be followed by continued shedding of the organism for many months.

Psittacosis is almost always transmitted to humans by the respiratory route. On rare occasions the disease may be acquired from the bite of a pet bird. Prolonged contact is not essential for transmission of the disease; a few minutes spent in an environment previously occupied by an infected bird has resulted in human infection. In one outbreak, gardening rather than direct exposure to birds was associated with infection. A psittacosis-like agent has been transmitted among hospital personnel, with severe and sometimes fatal infections. There is evidence that these "human" strains are more virulent than avian organisms. There is no record of infection acquired by the ingestion of poultry products.

Pathogenesis The psittacosis agent gains entrance to the body through the upper part of the respiratory tract, spreads via the bloodstream, and eventually localizes in the pulmonary alveoli and in the reticuloendothelial cells of the spleen and liver. Invasion of the lung probably takes place by way of the bloodstream rather than by direct extension from the upper air passages. A lymphocytic inflammatory response occurs on both the interstitial and the respiratory surfaces of the alveoli as well as in the perivascular spaces. The alveolar walls and interstitial tissues of the lung are thickened, edematous, necrotic, and occasionally hemorrhagic. Histologic examination of the affected areas reveals alveolar spaces filled with fluid, erythrocytes, and lymphocytes. The picture is not pathognomonic of psittacosis unless macrophages containing characteristic cytoplasmic inclusion bodies (Levinthal-Coles-Lillie bodies) can be identified. The respiratory epithelium of the bronchi and bronchioles usually remains intact.

Clinical Manifestations The clinical manifestations and course of psittacosis are extremely variable. After an incubation period of 7 to 14 days or longer, the disease may start abruptly with shaking chills and fever, with temperatures ranging as high as 40.5°C (105°F); however, the onset is often gradual, with fever increasing over a 3- to 4-day period. Headache is almost always a prominent symptom; it is usually diffuse and excruciating and is often the patient's chief complaint.

Many patients present with a dry hacking cough that is usually nonproductive, but small amounts of mucoid or bloody sputum may be raised as the disease progresses. Cough may begin early in the course of the disease or as late as 5 days after the onset of fever. Chest pain, pleurisy with effusion, or a friction rub may all occur but are rare. Pericarditis and myocarditis have been reported. Most patients have a normal or slightly increased respiratory rate; marked dyspnea with cyanosis occurs only in severe psittacosis with extensive pulmonary involvement. In psittacosis, as in mycoplasmal pneumonias, the physical signs of pneumonitis tend to be less prominent than symptoms and x-ray findings would suggest. The initial examination may reveal fine sibilant rales, or clinical evidence of pneumonia may be completely lacking. Rales usually become audible and more numerous as the illness progresses. Signs of frank pulmonary consolidation are usually absent. Symptoms of upper respiratory tract infection are not prominent, although mild sore throat, pharyngitis, and cervical adenopathy are often documented; on occasion, the last may be the only manifestation of illness. Epistaxis is encountered early in the course of nearly one-fourth of cases. Photophobia is also a common complaint.

Patients often report generalized myalgia, and spasm and stiffness of the muscles of the back and neck may lead to an erroneous diagnosis of meningitis. Lethargy, mental depression, agitation, insomnia, and disorientation have been prominent features of the illness in some epidemics but not in others; delirium and stupor develop near the end of the first week in severe cases. Occasional patients are comatose when first seen, and the diagnosis of psittacosis may be elusive in these cases. Gastrointestinal manifestations such as abdominal pain, nausea, vomiting, or diarrhea are noted in some cases; constipation and abdominal distention sometimes occur as late complications. Icterus, the result of severe hepatic involvement, is a rare and ominous finding. A faint macular rash (Horder's spots) resembling the rose spots of typhoid fever has been described.

Patients without cough or other clinical evidence of respiratory involvement present with fever of unknown origin (Chap. 18). The pulse rate is slow in relation to the fever. When splenomegaly is noted in a patient with acute pneumonitis, psittacosis should be considered; the reported incidence of splenomegaly in this disease ranges from 10 to 70%. Nontender hepatic enlargement also occurs, but jaundice is rare. Thrombophlebitis is not unusual during convalescence; indeed, pulmonary infarction is sometimes a late complication and may be fatal.

In untreated cases of psittacosis, sustained or mildly remittent fever persists for 10 days to 3 weeks or occasionally for as long as 3 months. Over this period, the respiratory manifestations gradually abate. Psittacosis contracted from parrots or parakeets is more likely to be a severe, prolonged illness than infection acquired from pigeons or barnyard fowl. Relapses occur but are rare. Occasional patients develop endocarditis, and C. psittaci infection should be considered in cases of culture-negative endocarditis. Secondary bacterial infections are uncommon. Immunity to reinfection is probably permanent.

Laboratory Findings The chest x-ray in psittacosis is nonspecific and may show pneumonic lesions that are usually patchy in appearance but can be hazy, diffuse, homogeneous, lobar, atelectatic, wedge-shaped, nodular, or miliary. The white blood cell count is normal or moderately decreased in the acute phase of the disease but may rise in convalescence. The erythrocyte sedimentation rate frequently is not elevated. Transient proteinuria is common. The cerebrospinal fluid sometimes contains a few mononuclear cells but is otherwise normal. Despite hepatomegaly, the results of liver function tests are generally normal or only mildly elevated.

The diagnosis can be confirmed only by isolation of the causative microorganism or by serologic studies. The agent is present in the blood during the acute phase of the disease and in the bronchial secretions for weeks or sometimes years after infection, but it is difficult to isolate. Further, the organism is hazardous to work with in the laboratory, and most clinical laboratories do not offer culture for C. psittaci. Thus psittacosis is most readily diagnosed by the demonstration of a rising titer of complement fixation antibody in the serum of a patient with a compatible clinical syndrome. Both an acute-phase and a convalescent-phase specimen should always be tested. C. trachomatis, C. psittaci, and C. pneumoniae all share a genus-specific "group" antigen, which is the basis of the complement fixation test. Thus acute infections with C. trachomatis or C. pneumoniae can also produce titer rises in this test. However, these three species have different major outer-membrane proteins that are the principal antigens in the micro-IF test. If there is doubt as to the interpretation of the complement fixation test, the micro-IF test can be used to differentiate among these antigens. The prompt initiation of treatment with tetracycline has been shown to delay an antibody rise in convalescence for several weeks or months.

Differential Diagnosis A history of exposure to birds may be the only clinical basis for differentiating psittacosis from a variety of infectious and noninfectious febrile disorders. The list of pulmonary diseases that may be confused with psittacosis includes Mycoplasma pneumonia, C. pneumoniae pneumonia, legionellosis, viral pneumonia, Q fever, coccidioidomycosis, tuberculosis, enterovirus infection, carcinoma of the lung with bronchial obstruction, and common bacterial pneumonias. In the early stages, before pneumonitis appears, psittacosis may be mistaken for influenza, typhoid fever, miliary tuberculosis, or infectious mononucleosis.

℞ TREATMENT

The tetracyclines are consistently effective in the treatment of psittacosis. Defervescence and alleviation of symptoms usually take place within 24 to 48 h after the institution of therapy with 2 g daily in four divided doses. To avoid relapse, treatment should probably be continued for at least 7 to 14 days after defervescence. In severe cases, hospitalization and pulmonary intensive care may be indicated. Sulfonamides are not active against C. psittaci. Erythromycin can be used in patients allergic to or intolerant of tetracyclines.

C. PNEUMONIAE INFECTIONS

Definition A third chlamydial species that causes disease in humans, C. pneumoniae, has been described in the past quarter century. C. pneumoniae can be distinguished from the other two species on the basis of DNA hybridization and elementary body morphology. Although C. pneumoniae can be grown in a variety of cell cultures, it is considerably more difficult to culture than other chlamydiae, especially from clinical specimens. HL cells appear to be the most effective cell line for isolation of C. pneumoniae.

Epidemiology Knowledge of the epidemiology of C. pneumoniae infections has been derived primarily from serologic studies. Infections begin to occur in late childhood, achieve peak incidence in young adults, but continue throughout adult life. Seroprevalence in the many adult populations that have been tested throughout the world exceeds 40%—a figure suggesting that C. pneumoniae infections are ubiquitous. Secondary episodes (reinfections) appear to occur commonly in older adults throughout life. C. pneumoniae also produces epidemics of pneumonia and respiratory illness, especially in close residential quarters such as military barracks. The incidence of infections outside of epidemics remains poorly defined. Transmission appears to be from person to person, probably primarily in schools and family units.

Pathogenesis Little is known about the pathogenesis of C. pneumoniae infection. The infection begins in the upper respiratory tract and in many persons is a long-lived asymptomatic condition of the upper respiratory mucosal surfaces. However, in at least some individuals, the organism is transported to distant sites—perhaps within macrophages—since evidence exists for replication within arteries and synovial membranes of joints. A C. pneumoniae outer-membrane protein may induce host immune responses whose cross-reaction with human proteins results in an autoimmune reaction.

Clinical Manifestations The clinical spectrum of C. pneumoniae infection includes acute pharyngitis, sinusitis, bronchitis, and pneumonitis, primarily in young adults. The clinical manifestations of primary infection appear to be more severe and prolonged than those of reinfection. The pneumonitis resembles that of M. pneumoniae pneumonia in that leukocytosis is frequently lacking and patients often have prominent antecedent upper respiratory tract symptoms, fever, nonproductive cough, a mild to moderate degree of illness, minimal findings on chest auscultation, and small segmental infiltrates on chest x-ray. In elderly patients, pneumonia due to C. pneumoniae can be especially severe and may necessitate hospitalization and respiratory support.

Epidemiologic studies have demonstrated an association between serologic evidence of C. pneumoniae infection and atherosclerotic disease of the coronary and other arteries. In addition, C. pneumoniae has been identified in atherosclerotic plaques by electron microscopy, DNA hybridization, and immunocytochemistry. The organism has been recovered in culture from atheromatous plaque—a result indicating the presence of viable replicating bacteria in vessels. Evidence from animal models supports the hypothesis that C. pneumoniae infection of the upper respiratory tract is followed by recovery of the organism from atheromatous lesions in the aorta and that the infection accelerates the process of atherosclerosis, especially in hypercholesterolemic animals. Antimicrobial treatment of the infected animals reverses the increased risk of atherosclerosis. In humans, two small trials in patients with unstable angina or recent myocardial infarction also suggested that antibiotics reduce subsequent untoward cardiac events. Larger trials have been initiated to determine more definitively whether antibiotics affect the risk of atherosclerosis.

Diagnosis Diagnosis of *C. pneumoniae* infection is currently difficult because cell culture techniques are not available for routine clinical use and nonculture tests using antigen detection methods or DNA probes have not been developed for commercial use. Acute- and convalescent-phase sera can be tested for chlamydial complement fixation antibody to make a retrospective diagnosis. However, this test does not distinguish *C. pneumoniae* infection from infection due to *C. trachomatis* or *C. psittaci*.

℞ TREATMENT

Although controlled treatment trials have not been conducted, *C. pneumoniae* is inhibited in vitro by erythromycin and tetracycline. Recommended therapy consists of 2 g per day of either agent for 10 to 14 days. Other macrolides, such as azithromycin, and some fluoroquinolones, such as levofloxacin, also appear to be effective.

FURTHER READING

ADIMORA AA: Treatment of uncomplicated genital *Chlamydia trachomatis* infections in adults. Clin Infect Dis 35(Suppl 2):S183, 2002

GILBERT DN, GRAYSTON JT (eds): The potential etiologic role of *Chlamydia pneumoniae* in atherosclerosis: A multidisciplinary meeting to promote collaborative research. J Infect Dis 181(Suppl 3):S383, 2000

GRAYSTON JT: Infections caused by *Chlamydia pneumoniae*, strain TWAR. Clin Infect Dis 15:757, 1992

HOLMES KK, STAMM WE: Lower genital tract infections in women: Cystitis, urethritis, vulvovaginitis, and cervicitis, in *Sexually Transmitted Diseases*, 3d ed, KK Holmes et al (eds). New York, McGraw-Hill, 1999

MARRAZZO JM, STAMM WE: New approaches to the diagnosis, treatment, and prevention of chlamydial infection. Curr Clin Top Infect Dis 18:37, 1998

STAMM WE: Expanding efforts to prevent chlamydial infection. N Engl J Med 339:768, 1998

————: *Chlamydia trachomatis* infections in adults, in *Sexually Transmitted Diseases*, 3d ed, KK Holmes et al (eds). New York, McGraw-Hill, 1999

————: *Chlamydia trachomatis*: The persistent pathogen. Sex Transm Dis 13: 684, 2001

US PREVENTIVE SERVICE TASK FORCE: Chlamydial infection. Screening 2001. Guide to clinical preventive services. Alexandria, VA, International Medical Publishing, 2001, pp 325–332

Section 11   Viral Diseases: General Considerations

161 MEDICAL VIROLOGY
Fred Wang, Elliott Kieff

DEFINING A VIRUS

Viruses consist of a nucleic acid surrounded by one or more proteins. Some viruses also have an outer-membrane envelope. Viruses are obligate intracellular parasites: they can replicate only within cells since their nucleic acids do not encode the many enzymes necessary for protein, carbohydrate, or lipid metabolism and for the generation of high-energy phosphates. Typically, viral nucleic acids encode proteins necessary for replicating and packaging the nucleic acids within the biochemical milieu of host cells.

Viruses differ from viroids, prions, and virusoids. *Virusoids* are nucleic acids that depend on helper viruses to package their nucleic acids into virus-like particles. *Viroids* are naked, cyclical, mostly double-stranded, small RNAs. Viroids, which appear to be restricted to plants, spread from cell to cell and are replicated by cellular RNA polymerase II. *Prions* (Chap. 362) are abnormal protein molecules that can spread and change the structure of their normal counterparts (cellular proteins). Prions have been implicated in neurodegenerative conditions such as Creutzfeldt-Jakob disease, Gerstmann-Sträussler disease, kuru, and human bovine spongiform encephalopathy ("mad cow disease").

VIRAL STRUCTURE

Viruses have from a few to several hundred genes. These genes may be in a single-strand or double-strand DNA genome or in a single-strand sense, a single-strand or segmented antisense, or a double-strand segmented RNA genome. Sense-strand RNA genomes can be translated directly into protein. Sense and antisense genomes are also referred to as positive-strand and negative-strand genomes, respectively. The viral nucleic acid is usually associated with one or more virus-encoded nucleoproteins in the core of the viral particle. The viral nucleic acid and nucleoproteins are almost always enclosed in a protein shell called a *capsid*. Because of the limited genetic complexity of viruses, their capsids are usually composed of multimers of identical capsomers. Capsomers are in turn composed of one or a few proteins. Capsids have icosahedral or helical symmetry. Icosahedral structures approximate spheres but have two-, three-, and fivefold axes of sym-

metry, while helical structures have only a twofold axis of symmetry. The entire structural unit of nucleic acid, nucleoprotein(s), and capsid is called a *nucleocapsid*. Many human viruses are simply composed of a core and a capsid. For these viruses, the outer surface of the capsid mediates contact with uninfected cells. Other viruses are more complex and have an outer lipid-containing envelope derived from virus-modified membranes of the infected cell. The piece of infected-cell membrane that becomes the viral envelope has usually been modified during infection by the insertion of virus-encoded glycoproteins. Virus-encoded glycoproteins usually mediate contact of enveloped viruses with uninfected cells. Matrix or tegument proteins fill the space between the nucleocapsid and the envelope in many enveloped viruses. In general, enveloped viruses are sensitive to lipid solvents and nonionic detergents that can dissolve the envelope, while viruses that consist only of nucleocapsids are somewhat resistant. A schematic diagram for large and complex herpesviruses is shown in Fig. 161-1. Prototypical pathogenic human viruses are listed in Table 161-1. The relative sizes and structures of typical pathogenic human viruses are shown in Fig. 161-2.

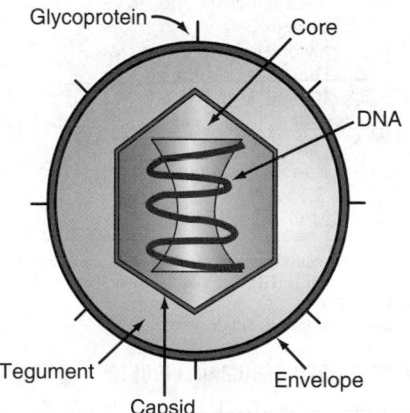

FIGURE 161-1 Schematic diagram of an enveloped herpesvirus with an icosahedral nucleocapsid. The approximate respective dimensions of the nucleocapsid and the enveloped particles are 110 and 180 nm. The capsid is composed of 162 capsomeres: 150 with sixfold and 12 with fivefold axes of symmetry.

TABLE 161-1 *Virus Families Pathogenic for Humans*

Family	Representative Viruses	Type of RNA/DNA	Lipid Envelope
RNA VIRUSES			
Picornaviridae	Poliovirus Coxsackievirus Echovirus Enterovirus Rhinovirus Hepatitis A virus	(+) RNA	No
Caliciviridae	Norwalk agent Hepatitis E virus	(+) RNA	No
Togaviridae	Rubella virus Eastern equine encephalitis virus Western equine encephalitis virus	(+) RNA	Yes
Flaviviridae	Yellow fever virus Dengue virus St. Louis encephalitis virus West Nile virus Hepatitis C virus Hepatitis G virus	(+) RNA	Yes
Coronaviridae	Coronaviruses[a]	(+) RNA	Yes
Rhabdoviridae	Rabies virus Vesicular stomatitis virus	(−) RNA	Yes
Filoviridae	Marburg virus Ebola virus	(−) RNA	Yes
Paramyxoviridae	Parainfluenza virus Respiratory syncytial virus Newcastle disease virus Mumps virus Rubeola (measles) virus	(−) RNA	Yes
Orthomyxoviridae	Influenza A, B, and C viruses	(−) RNA, 8 segments	Yes
Bunyaviridae	Hantavirus California encephalitis virus Sandfly fever virus	(−) RNA, 3 circular segments	Yes
Arenaviridae	Lymphocytic choriomeningitis virus Lassa fever virus South American hemorrhagic fever virus	(−) RNA, 2 circular segments	Yes
Reoviridae	Rotavirus Reovirus Colorado tick fever virus	ds RNA, 10–12 segments	No
Retroviridae	Human T-lymphotropic virus types I and II Human immunodeficiency virus types 1 and 2	(+) RNA, 2 identical segments	Yes
DNA VIRUSES			
Hepadnaviridae	Hepatitis B virus	ds DNA with ss portions	Yes
Parvoviridae	Parvovirus B19	ss DNA	No
Papovaviridae	Human papillomaviruses JC virus BK virus	ds DNA	No
Adenoviridae	Human adenoviruses	ds DNA	No
Herpesviridae	Herpes simplex virus types 1 and 2[b] Varicella-zoster virus[c] Epstein-Barr virus[d] Cytomegalovirus[e] Human herpesvirus 6 Human herpesvirus 7 Kaposi's sarcoma–associated herpesvirus[f]	ds DNA	Yes
Poxviridae	Variola (smallpox) virus Orf virus Molluscum contagiosum virus	ds DNA	Yes

[a] Including the coronavirus causing severe acute respiratory syndrome (SARS).
[b] Also called human herpesvirus (HHV) 1 and 2, respectively; [c] also called HHV-3; [d] also called HHV-4; [e] also called HHV-5; [f] also called HHV-8
Abbreviations: ds, double-strand; ss, single-strand.

TAXONOMY OF PATHOGENIC HUMAN VIRUSES

As is apparent from Table 161-1 and Fig. 161-2, the classification of viruses into orders and families is based on nucleic acid composition, nucleocapsid size and symmetry, and presence or absence of an envelope. Viruses of a single family have similar types of genomes and are often morphologically indistinguishable in electron micrographs.

Further subclassification into genus is dependent on similarities in epidemiology and biologic effects and on the degree of colinear nucleic acid sequence homology. Most human viruses have a common name related to their pathologic effects or the circumstances of their discovery. Formal species names have been assigned by the International Committee on Taxonomy of Viruses. The latter designation consists of the name of the host followed by the family or genus of the virus and a number. This dual terminology has created a confusing situation in which viruses are referred to and referenced by either name—e.g., varicella-zoster virus (VZV) or human herpesvirus (HHV) 3.

VIRAL INFECTION IN VITRO

STAGES OF VIRAL INFECTION AT THE CELLULAR LEVEL

■ **Viral Interactions with the Cell Surface and Cell Entry**   Viral infection is initiated by adsorption of the virus to the cell surface. Adsorption results from the molecular interaction of viral surface proteins with receptors on the cell's plasma membrane. For example, a poliovirus capsid protein binds to a cell plasma-membrane protein of the immunoglobulin superfamily type. A rhinovirus capsid protein binds to intracellular adhesion molecule 1. An echovirus capsid protein binds to an integrin. The influenza A virus envelope hemagglutinin protein binds to sialic acid. The HIV envelope glycoprotein binds to CD4 and then engages one of several chemokine receptors that function as coreceptors for the virus. Herpes simplex virus (HSV) envelope glycoproteins bind to heparan sulfate on cell surfaces and then engage one of several immunoglobulin superfamily or tumor necrosis factor (TNF) receptors. Epstein-Barr virus (EBV) glycoprotein gp350 binds to the B lymphocyte complement receptor CD21. Adsorption characteristically proceeds almost as well at 4°C as at 37°C. Adsorbed virus can still be neutralized by antibody. Adsorption frequently initiates changes in virion surface proteins that destabilize the viral surface proteins and prepare the way for the next stage of entry into the cell.

After adsorption, viruses penetrate the cell membrane by fusing with the membrane. The fusion reaction results in the virus's partial decomposition. The virus becomes insensitive to neutralizing antibody as it penetrates, becomes uncoated, and enters the cytoplasm. Penetration and uncoating result in viral nucleocapsid or nucleoprotein entry into the cytoplasm. Penetration and uncoating as well as subsequent steps in viral replication depend on the cell's energy metabolism and on biochemical changes in the cell's plasma membrane and cytoskeleton. Therefore, penetration proceeds slowly at temperatures <37°C. Interaction of viral surface proteins with cell receptors can induce receptor aggregation at the site of adsorption. Receptor aggregation can trigger signaling events within the cytoplasm and changes in the plasma membrane. The cell frequently misperceives that the receptor has encountered its "normal ligand." Aggregated receptor may be internalized with the attached virus in an endocytic process. Viral endocytosis may proceed through clathrin-coated pits. Endocytosis is important in the entry of viruses as diverse as picornaviruses, influenza viruses, HIV, adenoviruses, and herpesviruses. In many cases, entry of the virus into the cytoplasm depends on acidification of the viral endosome.

One of the best-studied examples of the effect of low pH on viral penetration is influenza virus. Influenza hemagglutinin mediates adsorption, receptor aggregation, and endocytosis. In low-pH endosomes, changes in the conformation of the hemagglutinin expose amphipathic domains that interact chemically with the cell membrane and initiate fusion of the viral and cellular membranes. The HIV envelope glycoprotein undergoes similar conformational changes after interaction with CD4 and chemokine receptors. For influenza virus, the M2 membrane protein also plays a key role in the uncoating of the viral envelope by providing an ion channel in the envelope. Fusion of viral and cell membranes results in the mixture of viral envelope lipids and proteins with cell membrane lipids and proteins and the penetration of the influenza nucleocapsid into the cytoplasm. With more complex viruses, such as herpesviruses, different glycoproteins interact with specific receptors on different cell types or on different surfaces of polarized epithelial cells. Viral glycoproteins other than the protein that mediates initial adsorption may be critical in mediating envelope fusion with cell membranes. The fusion of viral proteins with cell membranes is a crucial step in viral infection, which involves hydrophobic interactions. Hydrophobic interactions can be susceptible to chemical inhibition or blockade.

Viral Gene Expression and Replication   After uncoating and release of viral nucleoprotein into the cytoplasm, the viral genome is transported to a site for expression and replication. In order to produce infectious progeny, viruses must (1) produce proteins necessary to replicate their nucleic acid, (2) produce structural proteins, and (3) assemble the nucleic acid and proteins into progeny virions. Different viruses use different strategies and gene repertoires to accomplish these goals. DNA viruses, except for poxviruses, replicate their nucleic acid and assemble into nucleocapsid complexes in the cell nucleus. RNA viruses, except for influenza viruses, transcribe and replicate their nucleic acid and assemble entirely in the cytoplasm. Thus, the replication strategies of DNA and RNA viruses are presented separately below. Positive-strand and negative-strand RNA viruses are discussed separately. Medically important viruses of each group are used for illustrative purposes.

POSITIVE-STRAND RNA VIRUSES   Medically important positive-strand RNA viruses include picornaviruses, flaviviruses, togaviruses, caliciviruses, and coronaviruses. Genomic RNA from positive-strand RNA viruses is released into the cytoplasm without associated enzymes. Cell ribosomes recognize and associate with an internal ribosome entry sequence in the viral genomic RNA and translate a polyprotein that is a fusion of many or all of the viral proteins. The viral RNA polymerase and other viral proteins are cleaved from the polyprotein by protease components of the polyprotein. Antigenomic RNA is then transcribed from the genomic RNA template. Positive-strand genomes and mRNAs are next transcribed from the antigenomic RNA by the viral RNA polymerase. Positive-strand genomic RNA is encapsidated in the cytoplasm.

NEGATIVE-STRAND RNA VIRUSES   Medically important negative-strand RNA viruses include rhabdoviruses, filoviruses, paramyxoviruses, myxoviruses, and bunyaviruses. Negative-strand RNA virus genomes are released into the cytoplasm with an associated RNA polymerase and one or more accessory proteins. Some of these genomes are segmented. Except for influenza viruses, negative-strand RNA viruses replicate entirely in the cytoplasm. The viral RNA polymerase transcribes mes-

Positive-strand RNA viruses

	Picornaviridae	Caliciviridae	Togaviridae	Flaviviridae	Coronaviridae
Genome size (kb)	7.2-8.4	8	12	10	16-21
Envelope	No	No	Yes	Yes	Yes
Capsid symmetry	Icosahedral	Icosahedral	Icosahedral	Icosahedral	Helical

Negative-strand RNA viruses

	Rhabdoviridae	Filoviridae	Paramyxoviridae
Genome size (kb)	13-16	13	16-20
Envelope	Yes	Yes	Yes
Capsid symmetry	Helical	Helical	Helical

Segmented negative-strand RNA viruses   **Segmented double-strand RNA viruses**

	Orthomyxoviridae	Bunyaviridae	Arenaviridae	Reoviridae
Genome size (kb)	14	13-21	10-14	16-27
Envelope	Yes	Yes	Yes	No
Capsid symmetry	Helical	Helical	Helical	Icosahedral

Retroviruses

	Retroviridae
Genome size (kb)	3-9
Envelope	Yes
Capsid symmetry	Icosahedral

DNA viruses

	Parvoviridae	Papovaviridae	Adenoviridae	Herpesviridae	Poxviridae
Genome size (kb)	5	5-9	36-38	100-250	240
Envelope	No	No	No	Yes	Yes
Capsid symmetry	Icosahedral	Icosahedral	Icosahedral	Icosahedral	Complex

100 nm

FIGURE 161-2   Schematic diagrams of the major virus families including species that infect humans. The viruses are grouped by genome type and are drawn approximately to scale. Prototype viruses of each family that cause human disease are listed in Table 161-1.

senger RNAs (mRNAs) as well as full-length antigenomic RNA, which is the template for replication of genomic RNA. These mRNAs encode for the viral RNA polymerase and accessory factors as well as for viral structural proteins. Influenza virus is an unusual negative-strand RNA virus that transcribes its mRNAs and antigenomic RNAs in the cell's nucleus. The influenza genome RNA snatches cellular mRNA cap sequences to enhance translation of viral mRNAs and uses cell splicing machinery to encode additional viral mRNAs. All negative-strand RNA viruses, including influenza viruses, assemble in the cytoplasm.

DOUBLE-STRAND SEGMENTED RNA VIRUSES   These viruses, which are taxonomically grouped in the reovirus family, have 10 to 12 RNA segments that make up their genome. The medically important viruses in this group are rotaviruses and Colorado tick fever virus. Reovirus virions include an RNA polymerase complex. Reoviruses replicate and assemble in the cytoplasm.

DNA VIRUSES   Medically important DNA viruses include parvoviruses, papovaviruses (e.g., human papillomaviruses, or HPVs, and polyomaviruses), adenoviruses, herpesviruses, and poxviruses. Other than poxviruses, most DNA viruses must get to the cell's nucleus for DNA transcription by cellular RNA polymerase II. For example, after receptor binding and fusion, herpesvirus nucleocapsids are released into the cytoplasm along with tegument proteins. The complex is then transported along microtubules to nuclear pores, and the DNA is released into the nucleus.

Transcriptional regulation and mRNA processing for nuclear DNA viruses depend on both viral and cellular proteins. For herpesviruses, the viral tegument protein activates transcription of viral immediate-early genes, a class of genes expressed immediately after infection. Transcription of immediate-early genes requires the viral tegument protein and preexisting cellular transcription factors. One of the key preexisting cellular factors for HSV-1 immediate-early gene transcription is docked in the cytoplasm in neurons. Nuclear absence of this critical cell factor important for viral gene transcription may explain why HSV-1 goes into a latent state in neurons and how lytic infection is activated by signaling in a latently infected cell.

DNA virus gene transcription is usually regulated and proceeds in an organized cascade. Transcription and expression of adenovirus and herpesvirus immediate-early genes turn on the promoters for early genes in a sequential fashion, whereas poxvirus virions carry all the factors necessary for early-gene transcription. Smaller DNA viruses are not as dependent on transactivators encoded from the viral genome for early-gene transcription. Most early genes encode proteins that are necessary for viral DNA synthesis and for the turn on of late-gene transcription. Late genes encode mostly viral structural proteins or viral proteins necessary for the assembly and egress of the virus from the infected cell. Late-gene transcription is continuously dependent on DNA replication. Therefore, inhibitors of DNA replication also stop late-gene transcription.

Each DNA virus family uses unique mechanisms for replicating its DNA. Herpesvirus DNAs are linear in the virion but circularize in the infected cell. In lytic virus infection, circular herpesvirus genomes are replicated into linear concatemers through a "rolling-circle" mechanism. Herpesviruses encode a DNA polymerase and at least six other viral proteins necessary for viral DNA replication; these viruses also encode several enzymes that increase the pool of precursor deoxynucleotide triphosphates. Adenovirus genomes are linear in the virion and are replicated into complementary linear copies by a virus-encoded DNA polymerase and an initiator protein complex. The double-strand circular papovavirus genomes are replicated into progeny circular DNA molecules by cellular DNA replication enzymes. Two viral early proteins contribute to viral DNA replication and to the persistence of papovavirus DNA in latently infected cells. Early papovavirus proteins stimulate cells to remain in cycle, thus facilitating viral DNA replication. Occasionally, HPVs integrate into the host chromosome; overexpression of viral early proteins and excessive stimulation of cellular growth can result. Sometimes the consequence is the development of malignancies such as cervical cancer (see "Persistent Viral Infections and Cancer," below).

Parvoviruses are the smallest DNA viruses: their genomes are half the size of the papovavirus genomes and include only two genes. Parvoviruses have negative single-strand DNA genomes. The replication of autonomous parvoviruses, such as B19, depends on cellular DNA replication and requires the virus-encoded Rep protein. Other parvoviruses, such as adeno-associated virus (AAV), are not autonomous and require helper viruses of the adenovirus or herpesvirus family for their replication. AAV has been touted as a potentially safe human gene therapy vector because its Rep protein causes its integration at a single chromosomal site.

Poxviruses are the largest DNA viruses and are unique among DNA viruses in replicating and assembling in the cytoplasm. Poxviruses encode transcription factors and an RNA polymerase as well as enzymes for RNA capping and polyadenylation and for DNA synthesis. Poxvirus DNA also has a unique structure. The two strands of the double-strand linear DNA are covalently linked at the ends so that the genome is also a covalently closed single-strand circle. In addition, there are inverted repeats at the ends of the DNA. During DNA replication, the genome is cleaved within the terminal inverted repeat, and the inverted repeats self-prime complementary-strand synthesis by the virus-encoded DNA polymerase. Like herpesviruses, poxviruses encode several enzymes that increase deoxynucleotide triphosphate precursor levels and thus facilitate viral DNA synthesis.

VIRUSES WITH BOTH RNA AND DNA GENOMES Retroviruses and hepatitis B virus (HBV) are not purely RNA or DNA viruses. Retroviruses are enveloped RNA viruses with two identical sense-strand genomes and associated reverse transcriptase and integrase enzymes. Retroviruses differ from all other viruses in that they reverse-transcribe themselves into partially duplicated double-strand DNA copies and then routinely integrate into the host genome as part of their replication strategy. Cellular RNA polymerase II and transcription factors regulate transcription from the integrated provirus genome. Some retroviruses also encode for regulators of transcription and RNA processing, such as Tax and Rex in human T-lymphotropic virus (HTLV) types I and II and Tat and Rev in HIV-1 and HIV-2. HIV genomes also encode for the additional accessory proteins Vpr, Vpu, and Vif, which are important for efficient infection and immune escape. Full-length proviral transcripts are made from a promoter in the viral terminal repeat and serve as both genomic RNAs that will be packaged in the nucleocapsids and mRNAs that encode for the viral Gag protein, polymerase/integrase protein, and envelope glycoprotein. The Gag protein includes a protease that cleaves it into several components, including a viral matrix protein that coats the viral RNA. Viral RNA polymerase/integrase, matrix protein, and cellular tRNA are key components of the viral nucleocapsid. The HIV Gag protease has been an important target for inhibition of HIV replication. Remnants and even complete copies of simple retroviral DNA in the human genome indicate that there may be replication-competent simple human retroviruses. However, replication has not been documented or associated with any disease. Integrated retroviral DNAs are also present in other animal species, such as pigs. These porcine retroviruses are a potential cause for concern in xenotransplantation because retroviral replication could cause disease in humans. Since the retroviral DNA is integrated into the porcine genome, special pathogen-free breeding practices cannot cleanse the donor herd of retroviral infection.

HBV is unique because virion DNA expression in infected cells results in the packaging of reverse transcriptase and genomic RNA in the virion. The genomic RNA is then copied into an incomplete double-strand circular DNA genome before the virion matures and is released from the infected cell. On entry of HBV into the cytoplasm of an infected cell, the virion reverse transcriptase/DNA polymerase completes DNA synthesis, and the covalently closed circular genome resides in the nucleus. Viral mRNAs are transcribed from the closed circular viral episome by cellular RNA polymerase II. A capped and polyadenylated, full-genome-length, terminally redundant transcript is packaged into virus core particles in the cytoplasm of infected cells. This RNA associates with the viral reverse transcriptase. The reverse transcriptase converts the full-length, terminally redundant, core-particle, encapsidated RNA genome into partially double-strand DNA. HBV is believed to mature by budding through the cell's plasma membrane, which has been modified by the insertion of viral surface antigen protein.

Viral Assembly and Egress   For most viruses, nucleic acid and structural protein synthesis are accompanied by the assembly of protein and nucleic acid complexes. The assembly and egress of mature infectious virus mark the end of the eclipse phase of infection, during which infectious virus cannot be recovered from the infected cell. Nucleic acids from RNA viruses and poxviruses assemble into nucleocapsids in the cytoplasm. For all DNA viruses except poxviruses, viral DNA assembles into nucleocapsids in the nucleus. In general, the capsid proteins of viruses with icosahedral nucleocapsids can self-assemble into densely packed and highly ordered capsid structures. Herpesviruses require an assemblin protein as a scaffold for capsid assembly. Viral nucleic acid then spools into the assembled capsid. For herpesviruses, a full unit of the viral DNA genome is packaged into the capsid, and a capsid-associated nuclease cleaves the viral DNA at both ends. In the case of viruses with helical nucleocapsids, the protein component appears to assemble around the nucleic acid, which contributes to capsid organization.

Viruses must egress from the infected cell and not bind back to the outer surface of the plasma membrane. In many cases, enveloped viruses simply egress and acquire their envelope by budding through the cell's plasma membrane. Excess viral membrane glycoproteins are synthesized to saturate cell receptors and facilitate virus separation from the infected cell. Some viruses encode membrane proteins with enzymatic activity for receptor destruction. Influenza virus, for example, encodes a glycoprotein with neuraminidase activity, which destroys sialic acid on the infected cell's plasma membrane. Herpesvirus nucleocapsids acquire their initial envelope by assembling in the nucleus and then budding through the nuclear membrane into the endoplasmic reticular space. The enveloped herpesvirus is then released from the cell either by maturation in cytoplasmic vesicles, which fuse with the plasma membrane and release the virus by exocytosis, or by "de-envelopment" into the cytoplasm and "re-envelopment" at the plasma membrane. In most instances, nonenveloped viruses appear to depend on the death and dissolution of the infected cell for their release.

FIDELITY OF VIRAL REPLICATION Cells grow by doubling their genome and dividing, whereas viruses typically make large quantities of viral nucleic acid and structural proteins, and thousands of progeny may be produced from a single virus-infected cell. Many particles partially assemble and never mature into virions. Many mature-appearing virions are imperfect and have only incomplete or nonfunctional genomes. Despite the inefficiency of assembly, a typical virus-infected cell releases 10 to 1000 infectious progeny. Some of these progeny may contain genomes that differ from those of the virus that infected the cell. Smaller, "defective" virus genomes have been noted with the replication of many RNA and DNA viruses. Virions with defective genomes can be produced in large numbers through packaging of incompletely synthesized nucleic acid. Adenovirus packaging is notoriously inefficient, and a high particle-to-infectious virus ratio may limit the amount of recombinant adenovirus that can be administered for gene therapy. Mutant viral genomes are also produced and can be of medical significance. In general, viral nucleic acid replication is more error-prone than cellular nucleic acid replication. RNA polymerases and reverse transcriptases are significantly more error-prone than DNA polymerases. Mutant viruses can be virulent and may preferentially cause disease through evasion of the host immune response or through resistance to antiviral drugs. Persistent hepatitis C virus (HCV) infection appears to be due to genome mutation and persistent immune escape. Viral nucleic acids can also mutate by recombination or reassortment between two related viruses in a single cell. While this occurrence is unusual under most circumstances of natural infection, the changes can be substantial and can significantly alter virulence or epidemiology. Reassortment of an avian or mammalian influenza A hemagglutinin gene into a human influenza background is believed to play a role in the emergence of new epidemic influenza A strains.

VIRAL GENES NOT REQUIRED FOR VIRAL REPLICATION Viruses frequently have genes encoding proteins that are not directly involved in replication or packaging of the viral nucleic acid, in virion assembly, or in regulation of the transcription of viral genes involved in those processes. Most of these proteins fall into five classes: (1) proteins that directly or indirectly alter cell growth; (2) proteins that inhibit cellular RNA or protein synthesis so that viral mRNA can be efficiently transcribed or translated; (3) proteins that promote cell survival or inhibit apoptosis so that progeny virus can mature and escape from the infected cell; (4) proteins that inhibit the host interferon response; and (5) proteins that downregulate host inflammatory or immune responses so that virus infection can proceed in an infected person to the maximum extent consistent with the survival of the virus and its efficient transmission to a new host. More complex viruses of the poxvirus or herpesvirus family encode many proteins that serve these functions. Some of these viral proteins have motifs similar to those of cell proteins, while others are quite novel. Virology has increasingly focused on these more sophisticated strategies evolved by viruses to permit the establishment of long-term infection in humans and other animals. These strategies often provide unique insights into the control of cell growth, cell survival, macromolecular synthesis, proteolytic processing, immune or inflammatory suppression, immune resistance, cytokine mimicry, or cytokine blockade.

HOST RANGE The concept of host range was originally based on the cell types in which a virus replicated in tissue culture. For the most part, the host range is limited by specific cell-surface proteins required for viral adsorption or penetration. Another common basis for host-range limitation is transcription from viral promoters. Most DNA viruses depend not only on cellular RNA polymerase II and the basal components of the cellular transcription complex but also on activated components and transcriptional accessory factors, both of which differ among differentiated tissues, among cells at various phases of the cell cycle, and between resting and cycling cells.

The concept of host range for virus infection in humans includes these factors and others since (1) most viruses infect more than one cell type in vivo, and (2) the viral life cycle and extent of viral replication can be affected by the differentiation and activation state of a given cell type. This point is particularly relevant for human papovavirus, herpesvirus, and lentivirus infections, in which vigorous replication during initial infection may be followed by quiescent or latent infection—a situation that allows the virus to persist.

VIRAL CYTOPATHIC EFFECTS AND INHIBITORS OF APOPTOSIS The replication of almost all viruses has adverse effects on the infected cell, inhibiting cellular synthesis of DNA, RNA, or proteins. This inhibitory effect probably stems from the viruses' need to prevent or limit nonspecific, innate host resistance factors, including interferon (IFN). Most commonly, viruses specifically inhibit host protein synthesis by attacking a component of the translational initiation complex—frequently, a component that is not required for efficient translation of viral RNAs. Poliovirus protease 2A, for example, cleaves a cellular component of the complex that ordinarily facilitates translation of cell mRNAs by interacting with their cap structure. Poliovirus RNA is efficiently translated without a cap since it has an internal ribosome entry sequence. Influenza virus inhibits the processing of mRNA by snatching cap structures from nascent cell RNAs and using them as primers in the synthesis of viral mRNA. HSV has a virion tegument protein that inhibits cellular mRNA translation.

Apoptosis is the expected consequence of virus-induced inhibition of cellular macromolecular synthesis and viral nucleic acid replication. While the induction of apoptosis may be important for the release of some viruses (particularly nonenveloped viruses), many viruses have acquired genes or parts of genes that enable them to forestall infected-cell apoptosis. This delay may be advantageous in allowing the completion of viral replication. Adenoviruses and herpesviruses encode analogues of the cellular Bcl2 protein, which blocks mitochondrial enhancement of proapoptotic stimuli. Poxviruses and some herpesviruses encode caspase inhibitors. Many viruses, including HPVs and adenoviruses, encode proteins that inhibit p53 or its downstream proapoptotic effects.

VIRAL INFECTION IN VIVO

The capsid and envelope of a virus protect its genome and permit its efficient transmission from cell to cell and to prospective hosts. Most common viral infections are spread by aerosolized particles, by ingestion of contaminated water or food, or by direct contact. In all these situations, infection begins on an epithelial or mucosal surface and spreads along it or from it to deeper tissues. Infection may then spread through the body via the bloodstream, lymphatics, or neural circuits. Parenteral inoculation also serves to transmit some viral infections among humans or from animals, including insects, to humans.

PRIMARY INFECTION The first (primary) episode of viral infection usually lasts from several days to several weeks. During this period, the concentration of virus at sites of infection rises and then falls, usually to unmeasurable levels. The rate at which the intensity of viral infection rises and falls at a given site depends on the accessibility of that organ or tissue to both the virus and systemic immune effectors, the intrinsic ability of the virus to replicate at that site, and endogenous nonspecific and specific resistance. Typically, infections with enterovirus, mumps virus, measles virus, rubella virus, rotavirus, influenza virus, AAV, adenovirus, HSV, and VZV are cleared from almost all sites within 3 to 4 weeks. Some of these viruses are especially proficient in altering or evading the innate and acquired immune responses; thus primary infection with AAV, EBV, or cytomegalovirus (CMV) can last for several months. Characteristically extending beyond several weeks are primary infections due to HBV, HCV, hepatitis D virus (HDV), HIV, HPV, and molluscum contagiosum virus. For some of these viruses (e.g., HPV, HBV, HCV, HDV, and molluscum contagiosum virus), the primary phase of infection is almost indistinguishable from the persistent phase.

Disease manifestations usually arise as a consequence of viral replication and the resultant inflammatory response at a specific site but do not necessarily correlate with levels of replication at that site. For example, the clinical manifestations of limited infection with poliovirus, enterovirus, rabies virus, measles virus, mumps virus, or HSV in neural cells are severe relative to the level of viral replication at mucosal surfaces. Similarly, significant morbidity may accompany in utero fetal infection with rubella virus or CMV.

Primary infections are cleared by nonspecific innate and specific adaptive immune responses. Thereafter, an immunocompetent host is usually immune to the disease manifestations of reinfection by the same virus. Immunity frequently does not prevent transient surface colonization on reexposure, persistent colonization, or even limited deeper infection.

PERSISTENT AND LATENT INFECTIONS Relatively few viruses cause persistent or latent infections. HBV, HCV, rabies virus, measles virus, HIV, HTLV, HPV, HHV, and some poxviruses are notable exceptions. The mechanisms for persistent infection vary widely. In persistent HCV infection and to a lesser extent in HIV infection, the high mutation rates in viral genome replication or reverse transcription significantly facilitate persistent infection, continuously yielding mutant viruses that have lost antigenic determinants to which the host has developed effective immune responses. HIV is also directly immunosuppressive, depleting CD4+ T lymphocytes and compromising CD8+ cytotoxic T-cell immune responsiveness. Moreover, HIV encodes a Nef protein that downmodulates major histocompatibility complex (MHC) class I expression, rendering HIV-infected cells partially resistant to immune CD8+ cytolysis. The high mutation rate and the magnitude of the viral load conspire to promote persistent infection with drug-resistant HIV mutants.

In contrast, DNA viruses have much lower mutation rates. Their persistence is due to their ability to establish latent infection and to reactivate from latency. In this instance, latency is defined as a state of infection in which the virus is not replicating. The complete viral genome is present and may be replicated by cellular DNA polymerase in conjunction with the cell genome replication. Viral genes associated with lytic infection are not expressed and infectious virus is not made. HPVs establish latent infection in basal epithelial cells, which replicate. Some of the progeny cells provide a stable supply of latently infected basal cells, while others go on to squamous differentiation and, in the process, become permissive for lytic viral infection. For herpesviruses, latent infection is established in nonreplicating neural cells (HSV and VZV) or in replicating cells of hematopoietic lineages [EBV and probably CMV, HHV-6, HHV-7, and Kaposi's sarcoma–associated herpesvirus (KSHV, also known as HHV-8)]. Reactivation from neural latency appears to be an intermittent process provoked by external stimuli, whereas reactivation from hematopoietic precursors appears to be a more continuous process. In their latent stage, HPV and herpesvirus genomes are largely hidden from the normal immune response. It is still not fully understood how partially latent and reactivated HPV and herpesvirus infections escape immediate and effective immune responses in highly immune hosts. HPV, HSV, and VZV may be somewhat protected because of their replication in middle and upper layers of the squamous epithelium—sites not routinely visited by immune and inflammatory cells. HSV and CMV are also known to encode proteins that downregulate MHC class I expression and antigenic peptide presentation on infected cells, thereby enabling these cells to escape CD8+ T lymphocyte cytotoxicity. Latent infection and intermittent reactivation perpetuate herpesvirus infections in human populations by allowing the viruses to persist in immune hosts and to be transmitted to the next generation of naive hosts.

Like other poxviruses, molluscum contagiosum virus cannot establish latent infection but rather causes persistent infection in hypertrophic lesions that last for months or years. This virus encodes a chemokine homologue that probably blocks inflammatory responses and an MHC class I analogue that may block cytotoxic T lymphocyte attack.

PERSISTENT VIRAL INFECTIONS AND CANCER Persistent viral infection is estimated to be the root cause of as many as 20% of human malignancies. For the most part, cancer is an accidental and highly unusual or long-term effect of infection with oncogenic human viruses. In these malignancies, viral infection is a critical and ultimately determinative early step, putting infected cells into cycle and enhancing their survival. An unusual virus-infected cell undergoes the subsequent genetic changes that permit the enhanced autonomous growth and survival characteristic of a highly malignant cell.

Most hepatocellular carcinoma is now believed to be caused by chronic inflammatory, immune, and regenerative responses to HBV or HCV infection. Epidemiologic data firmly link HBV and HCV infection to hepatocellular carcinoma. Studies in murine experimental models indicate that chronic liver injury and repair induced by virus-encoded proteins can result in hepatocellular cancer. In rare instances, HBV DNA integrates into cellular DNA—an event that probably contributes to the development of some tumors.

Almost all cervical carcinoma is caused by long-term persistent replication of "high-risk" genital HPV strains. Persistent, high-level HPV replication can result in the integration of a small fragment of the HPV genome encoding the HPV E6 and E7 proteins into chromosomal DNA. Integrations that result in overexpression of HPV type 16 or 18 E6 and E7 cause the loss of at least two major tumor-suppressive functions mediated by pRb and p53. This loss in turn causes profound changes in cell growth and survival. Nevertheless, subsequent chromosomal changes must occur over ensuing cycles of cell growth if a sufficiently malignant cell is to invade the surrounding tissues.

Similarly, long-term EBV infection and expression of the EBV oncogene LMP1 in latently infected epithelial cells appear to be critical early steps in the evolution of anaplastic nasopharyngeal carcinoma, a common malignancy in Chinese and North African populations. High-level LMP1 expression is also a hallmark of many cases of Hodgkin's disease. Among younger age groups, >50% of Hodgkin's disease tumors are clonally derived from an EBV-infected cell. The HTLV-I Tax and Rex proteins appear to be critical to the initiation of cutaneous adult T cell lymphoma/leukemias that may occur long after primary HTLV-I infection.

The EBV-related herpesvirus KSHV was identified in a search for the postulated sexually transmitted etiologic agent of Kaposi's sarcoma in HIV-infected individuals. Molecular data confirm the presence of KSHV DNA in all Kaposi's tumors, including those associated with HIV infection, transplantation, and familial transmission. KSHV infection is also etiologically implicated in pleural-effusion lymphomas and multicentric Castleman's disease, which are more common among HIV-infected than among HIV-uninfected people.

Evidence supporting a causal role of viral infection in these malignancies includes epidemiologic data, the presence of viral DNA in all tumor cells, the ability of the viruses to transform human cells in culture, the results of in vitro assays for transforming effects of specific viral genes on cell growth, and pathologic data indicating the expression of transforming viral genes in premalignant or malignant cells in vivo.

EBV is a unique example of a human virus that relies on the normal immune response to contain the potentially unrestrained growth of infected cells. In the initial stages of normal primary EBV infection, EBV "latently" infects B lymphocytes and expresses at least eight viral proteins that play no role in viral replication but cause the expansion of latently infected cells. These infected cells can grow indefinitely. Most of the viral proteins that cause this proliferative state are highly antigenic. These virus-infected cells, which can transiently constitute 10% of the circulating B lymphocyte population, are met with an overwhelming helper and cytotoxic T cell response during primary infection. The number of virus-infected cells then falls rapidly, and the one EBV-infected cell in a million that persists does not express most of the viral proteins that cause B cell proliferation. These persisting cells are the site of normal latent infection. Breakthrough growth of the EBV-infected B lymphocytes almost never occurs in immunocompetent hosts. However, in immunosuppressed AIDS patients or organ transplant recipients, EBV-infected B lymphocytes expressing the full set of growth-transforming genes may grow and cause self-sustained and potentially fatal lymphoproliferative disease. Clinical investigation has resulted in novel strategies for treating these virus-induced malignancies with EBV-specific T cells or with antibody to B cells.

RESISTANCE TO VIRAL INFECTIONS Resistance to viral infection is initially provided by factors that are not virus-specific. Physical protection is afforded by the cornified layers of the skin and by mucous secretions that continuously sweep over mucosal surfaces. Once the first cell is infected, viral infection induces IFNs, which are important local resistance factors. Viral infection may also trigger the release of other cytokines from infected cells; these cytokines may be chemotactic to inflammatory and immune cells. Viral protein epitopes expressed on the cell surface in the context of MHC class I and II HLA proteins attract T cells with appropriate receptors. Cytokines, inflammatory agents, and antigens released by virus-induced cell death further attract inflammatory cells, dendritic cells, granulocytes, natural killer (NK) cells, and B lymphocytes to the sites of initial infection and to draining lymph nodes. IFNs and NK cells are particularly important in containing viral infection for the first several days. Granulocytes and macrophages are also important in the phagocytosis and degradation of viruses, especially after an initial antibody response.

Some 7 to 10 days after infection, virus-specific antibody responses, virus-specific HLA class II–restricted CD4+ helper T lymphocyte responses, and virus-specific HLA class I–restricted CD8+ cytotoxic T lymphocyte responses emerge. These responses, whose magnitude typically increases over the second and third weeks of infection, are important in rapid recovery. Between the second and third weeks of infection, the antibody type usually changes from IgM to IgG; IgA antibody can then be detected at initially infected mucosal surfaces. Antibody may directly neutralize virus by binding to its surface and preventing its adsorption or penetration. Complement usually enhances antibody-mediated virus neutralization. Antibody and complement can also lyse virus-infected cells that express viral proteins on their surface. A cell infected with an enveloped virus usually expresses viral envelope glycoprotein components on its surface and is subject to destruction by antibodies and complement.

Antibody and CD4+/CD8+ T lymphocyte responses tend to persist for several months after primary infection. Antibody-producing lymphocytes persist in small numbers as memory cells and begin to proliferate rapidly in response to a second infection, providing an early barrier to reinfection with the same virus. Immunologic memory for T cell responses appears to be shorter-lived. Redevelopment of T cell immunity may take longer than secondary antibody responses, particularly when many years have elapsed between primary infection and reexposure. Persistent or latent and reactivating viral infections can result in sustained high-level T cell responses.

Some viruses have genes that alter innate and acquired host defenses. Adenoviruses encode small RNAs that inhibit IFN shutoff of infected-cell protein synthesis. Adenovirus E1A inhibits IFN-mediated changes in cell gene transcription. Adenovirus E3 proteins prevent TNF-induced cytolysis and block HLA class I antigen synthesis by the infected cell. HSV ICP47 and CMV US11 block class I antigen presentation. EBV encodes an interleukin (IL) 10 homologue that inhibits NK and T cell responses. Vaccinia virus B15R is an IL-1 receptor decoy. Vaccinia virus B8R is a soluble TNF receptor that blocks the effects of TNF. Vaccinia virus CrmA inhibits the ability of CD8+ cytotoxic cells to kill virus-infected cells. Some poxviruses and herpesviruses encode blockers of chemokines and thereby inhibit cellular inflammatory responses. The adoption of these strategies by viruses highlights the importance of these host resistance factors in containing viral infection as well as the importance of redundancy in host resistance. The ultimate success of a virus requires a live host to help it disseminate infection.

Much has been written about the role of specific aspects of the host immune response in containment of specific virus infections. Certainly, T lymphocyte disorders and T cell immunosuppression for the purpose of transplantation or as a consequence of HIV infection are associated with severe primary and reactivated herpesvirus infections. Antibody responses are important in most viral infections and may be fully protective in many RNA virus infections. Specific immunoglobulin therapy can ameliorate even herpesvirus infections. T lymphocyte responses may play a significant role in resistance to RNA virus infections. Cytotoxic T cells specific for influenza virus nucleoprotein may provide a measure of protection that is independent of viral changes in hemagglutinin.

Host resistance does not come without a price. Clearly, aspects of the host response contribute to the pathophysiologic manifestations and symptoms of viral infection. Inflammation at sites of viral infection can increase rates of local cell death. Moreover, immune responses to viral infection could, in principle, result in immune attack of related epitopes on normal cells, with consequent autoimmunity. While such effects have been demonstrated in experimental models, their role in the autoimmune manifestations of primary or recurrent human viral infections is uncertain.

INTERFERONS All human cells can synthesize IFN-α or -β in response to viral infection. These IFN responses are usually induced by the presence of double-strand viral RNA, which can be made by both RNA and DNA viruses. IFN-γ is not highly related to IFN-α or -β and is produced mainly by NK cells and by immune T lymphocytes responding to IL-12. IFN-α and -β bind to the IFN-α receptor, while IFN-γ binds to a different but related receptor. Both receptors signal through receptor-associated JAK kinases and other cytoplasmic proteins, including "STAT" proteins. STAT proteins are tyrosine-phosphorylated by JAK kinases, translocate to the nucleus, and transactivate promoters for specific cell genes. Three types of antiviral effects are induced by IFN at the transcriptional level. The first effect is attributable to the induction of 2'-5' oligo(A) synthetases, which require double-strand RNA for their activation. Activated synthetase polymerizes oligo(A) and thereby activates RNAse L, which in turn degrades single-strand RNA. The second effect takes place through the induction of PKR, a serine and threonine kinase that is also activated by double-strand RNA. PKR phosphorylates and negatively regulates the translational initiation factor eIF2-α, shutting down protein synthesis in the infected cell. A third effect is initiated through the induction of Mx proteins, a family of GTPases that is particularly important in inhibiting the replication of influenza virus and vesicular stomatitis virus (VSV). None of these IFN effects is directed specifically against the virus; infected-cell RNA and protein synthesis are globally inhibited by inhibiting cell protein synthesis. IFN probably contributes to the death of the infected cell.

DIAGNOSTIC VIROLOGY A wide variety of methods are now used to diagnose viral infection. Serology and viral isolation in tissue culture remain important standards. Acute- and convalescent-phase sera with rising titers of antibody to virus-specific antigens and a shift from IgM to IgG antibodies are generally accepted as diagnostic of acute viral infection. Traditionally, virus-specific antibodies have been detected by hemadsorption, hemagglutination, or indirect immunofluorescence. Immunofluorescence assays use fixed virus-infected cells as a target for serum antibodies. Hemadsorption and hemagglutination assays measure the ability of serum antibodies to inhibit RNA virus–induced erythrocyte adsorption or agglutination. Serologic diagnosis is based on a greater-than-fourfold rise in IgG antibody concentration when acute- and convalescent-phase serum samples are analyzed at the same time. A simultaneous fall in IgM antibody confirms recent primary viral infection. Immunofluorescence, hemadsorption, and hemagglutination assays for antiviral antibodies are labor intensive and are being replaced by enzyme-linked immunosorbent assays (ELISAs). ELISAs generally use specific viral proteins purified from virus-infected cells or produced by recombinant DNA technology. These viral antigens are attached to a solid phase, where they can be incubated with serum, washed to eliminate nonspecific antibodies, and reacted with an enzyme-linked reagent to detect human IgG or IgM antibody specifically adhering to the viral antigen on the solid phase. The amount of antibody can then be quantitated by the intensity of a color reaction mediated by the linked enzyme. ELISAs can be sensitive and automated. Western blots can confirm the presence of antibody to multiple specific viral proteins simultaneously. The proteins are separated by size and transferred to an inert membrane, where they are incubated with serum antibodies. Western blots have an internal specificity control, since the level of reactivity for viral proteins can be compared with that for cellular proteins in the same sample. Western blots require individual evaluation and are inherently difficult to quantitate or automate.

Virus isolation in tissue culture is dependent on the infection of susceptible cells and amplification by viral replication in infected cells. Virus growing in tissue culture cells can frequently be identified by its effect under light microscopy. For example, HSV produces a typical cytopathic effect in rabbit kidney cells within 3 days. Other viral cytopathic effects may not be as diagnostically useful. Identification may require confirmation by staining with virus-specific monoclonal antibodies. Viruses growing in tissue culture can also be identified by hemadsorption or by interference; e.g., rubella virus–infected cells resist lysis by echovirus. Electron microscopy can identify the type of virus in tissue or tissue culture (assuming that the specimen has altered cell morphology, as observed by ordinary light microscopy).

The efficiency and speed of virus identification can be enhanced by combining short-term culture with immune detection. In assays with "shell vials" of tissue culture cells growing on a coverslip, viral infection can be detected by staining of the culture with a monoclonal antibody to a specific viral protein expressed early in viral replication. Thus, virus-infected cells can be detected within hours or days of inoculation; several rounds of infection would be required to produce a visible cytopathic effect.

Virus isolation in tissue culture depends on the collection of specimens from the appropriate site and the rapid transport of these specimens in the appropriate medium to the virology laboratory. Rapid transport maintains viral viability and limits bacterial and fungal overgrowth. Lipid-enveloped viruses are generally much more sensitive to freezing and thawing than nonenveloped viruses. The most appropriate site for culture depends on the pathogenesis of the virus in question. Nasopharyngeal, tracheal, or endobronchial aspirates are most appropriate for the identification of respiratory viruses. Sputum cultures generally are less appropriate because bacterial contamination and vis-

cosity threaten tissue-culture cell viability. Aspirates of vesicular fluid are useful for isolation of HSV and VZV. Nasopharyngeal aspirates and stool specimens may be useful when the patient has fever and a rash and an enteroviral infection is suspected. Adenoviruses can be cultured from the urine of patients with hemorrhagic cystitis. CMV can frequently be isolated from cultures of urine or buffy coat. Biopsy material can be effectively cultured when viruses infect major organs, as in HSV encephalitis or adenovirus pneumonia. Virus isolation does not necessarily establish disease causality. Viruses can persistently or intermittently colonize normal human mucosal surfaces. Saliva can be positive for herpesviruses, and normal urine samples can be positive for CMV. Isolations from blood, cerebrospinal fluid (CSF), or tissue are more often diagnostic of significant viral infection.

Another method aimed at increasing the speed of viral diagnosis is direct testing for antigen or cytopathic effects. Virus-infected cells from the patient may be detected by staining with virus-specific monoclonal antibodies; e.g., epithelial cells obtained by nasopharyngeal aspiration can be stained with a variety of monoclonal antibodies to respiratory viruses. The Tzanck preparation can be used to detect multinucleated giant cells in HSV- or VZV-induced lesions. Tzanck preparations can be enhanced by the use of HSV- or VZV-specific monoclonal antibodies. Monoclonal antibodies can also be used in histopathology to identify virus-infected cells.

Advances in nucleic acid technology are revolutionizing diagnostic virology. The speed and sensitivity of tests that directly amplify minute amounts of viral nucleic acids present in specimens mean that detection no longer depends on viable virus and its replication. For example, amplification and detection of HSV nucleic acids in the CSF of patients with HSV encephalitis is a more sensitive detection method than culture of virus from CSF. The extreme sensitivity of these tests can be a problem, since subclinical infection or contamination can lead to false-positive results. Detection of viral nucleic acids does not necessarily indicate virus-induced disease. Herpesviruses can cause persistent asymptomatic infection.

Measurement of the amount of viral RNA or DNA in peripheral blood is becoming an important means for determining which patients are at increased risk for virus-induced disease and for evaluating clinical responses to antiviral chemotherapy. Nucleic acid technologies for RNA quantification are routinely used in AIDS patients to evaluate responses to antiviral agents and to detect resistance to or noncompliance with therapy. Viral-load measurements may also be useful for evaluating the treatment of patients with HBV and HCV infections. Direct staining with CMV-specific monoclonal antibodies to quantitate virus-infected cells in the peripheral blood or CMV antigenemia can be useful in identifying which immunosuppressed patients may be at risk for CMV-induced disease. CMV assays employing nucleic acid technologies for the same purpose have been approved for clinical use.

DRUG TREATMENT FOR VIRAL INFECTIONS Specific antiviral drugs have revolutionized treatment of herpes and HIV infections. Effective drugs have also been developed for influenza A and moderately effective drugs for respiratory syncytial virus and HCV infections. However, the emergence of drug-resistant strains in treated patients can limit therapeutic efficacy. The increased number of antiviral agents with different viral targets has made the identification of drug-resistant viruses clinically relevant, especially for HIV infection. Drug resistance in herpesviruses is a more unusual problem. HIV genotyping is a new method for the rapid identification of drug-resistant viruses. Resistance to reverse transcriptase or protease inhibitors has been associated with specific mutations in the reverse transcriptase or protease genes. Identification of these mutations by polymerase chain reaction amplification and nucleic acid sequencing can be clinically useful for determining which antiviral agents may still be effective. HCV genotyping may also identify patients who can benefit from combination chemotherapy.

IMMUNIZATION FOR THE PREVENTION OF VIRAL INFECTIONS Viral vaccines are among the outstanding accomplishments of medical science. Smallpox has been eradicated except as a potential weapon of biological warfare or bioterrorism (Chap. 205). Poliovirus eradication may soon follow. Measles can be contained or eliminated. Excess mortality due to influenza virus epidemics can be prevented, and the threat of influenza pandemics has decreased. Widespread HBV vaccination has dramatically lessened the frequency of acute and chronic hepatitis and is expected to lead to a dramatic decrease in the incidence of hepatocellular carcinoma. Rubella, mumps, and chickenpox viruses have been attenuated in culture, formulated into vaccines, and widely administered in the developed world. Purified proteins, genetically engineered live virus vaccines, and recombinant DNA-based strategies will make it possible to prevent severe infections with many other viruses. The evolutionary divergence of HIV and HCV and repeated high-level exposure in some populations complicate the development of effective vaccines for these agents. Immunogens that incorporate multiple B and T cell epitopes are likely to be useful for low-level exposures. Concerns about the use of smallpox and other viruses as weapons may create a need to maintain immunity to agents that are not naturally encountered.

VIRUSES AS NOVEL THERAPEUTIC AGENTS   Viruses are being experimentally developed for the delivery of biotherapeutics or novel vaccines. Foreign genes can be inserted into viral nucleic acids, and the recombinant virus vectors can be used to infect the patient or the patient's cells ex vivo. Retroviruses integrate into the cell genome and have been used to functionally replace the abnormal gene in T cells of patients with severe combined immunodeficiency (SCID), thereby restoring immune function. Recombinant adenovirus, AAV, and retroviruses are being explored for use in diseases due to single-gene defects, such as cystic fibrosis and hemophilia. Recombinant poxviruses and adeno-

viruses are also being used experimentally as vaccine vectors. Viral vectors are being experimentally tested for expressing cytokines to improve immunity against tumor cells or for expressing proteins that can increase the sensitivity of tumor cells to chemotherapy.

For improved safety, nonreplicating viruses are frequently employed in clinical trial settings. Potential adverse events associated with virus-mediated gene transfer include the induction of inflammatory and antiviral immune responses. Adenoviruses contain many immunogenic proteins, and, since wild-type adenovirus infection is prevalent, immunity to adenovirus infection may reduce the efficacy of or enhance inflammatory responses to adenovirus gene therapy. Integration, another complication of virus-mediated gene therapy, is useful for permanent gene therapy, but integrations can induce disease by enhancing or interrupting the expression of important cellular genes.

FURTHER READING

FIELDS BN et al (eds): *Virology*, 4th ed. New York, Lippincott Williams & Wilkins, 2000

HACEIN-BEY-ABINA S et al: Sustained correction of X-linked severe combined immunodeficiency by ex vivo gene therapy. N Engl J Med 346:1185, 2002

HOLMES KV: SARS-associated coronavirus. N Engl J Med 348:1948, 2003

JOHNSON WE, DESROSIERS RC: Viral persistence: HIV's strategies of immune system evasion. Annu Rev Med 53:499, 2002

KATZE MG et al: Viruses and interferon: A fight for supremacy. Nat Rev Immunol 2:675, 2002

LENNETTE EH, SMITH TF (eds): *Laboratory Diagnosis of Viral Infections*. New York, Marcel Dekker, 1999

ROULSTON A et al: Viruses and apoptosis. Annu Rev Microbiol 53:577, 1999

162 ANTIVIRAL CHEMOTHERAPY, EXCLUDING ANTIRETROVIRAL DRUGS
Lindsey R. Baden, Raphael Dolin

The development of drugs for antiviral chemotherapy and chemoprophylaxis is a relatively recent but extremely active area of biomedical research. Significant progress has been made in recent years on new drugs for several viral infections. Despite these advances, the field of antiviral therapy—both the number of antiviral drugs and our understanding of their optimal use—continues to lag behind the field of antibacterial drug treatment, in which more than 60 years of experience have now been accumulated.

The development of antiviral drugs poses several challenges. Viruses replicate intracellularly and often employ host cell enzymes, macromolecules, and organelles for synthesis of viral particles. Therefore, useful antiviral compounds must discriminate between host and viral functions with a high degree of specificity; agents without such selectivity are likely to be too toxic for clinical use.

The development of laboratory assays to assist clinicians in the appropriate use of antiviral drugs is also in its infancy. Phenotypic and genotypic assays for resistance to antiviral drugs are becoming more widely available, and correlations of laboratory results with clinical outcomes in various settings are beginning to be defined. Of particular note has been the development of highly sensitive and specific methods to measure the concentration of virus in blood (*virus load*), which permit direct assessment of the antiviral effect of a given drug regimen in the host. Virus load measurements have been useful in recognizing the risk of disease progression in patients with certain viral infections and in identifying patients in whom antiviral chemotherapy might be of greatest benefit. Like any in vitro laboratory test, these tests yield results that are highly dependent on (and likely to vary with) the laboratory techniques employed.

Information regarding the pharmacokinetics of some antiviral drugs, particularly in diverse clinical settings, is limited. Assays to measure the concentrations of these drugs, especially of their active moieties within cells, are primarily research procedures and are not

widely available to clinicians. Thus, there are relatively few guidelines for adjusting dosages of antiviral agents to maximize antiviral activity and minimize toxicity. Clinical use of antiviral drugs must therefore be accompanied by particular vigilance with regard to unanticipated adverse effects.

Like that of other infections, the course of viral infections is profoundly affected by an interplay of the pathogen with a complex set of host defenses. The presence or absence of preexisting immunity and the ability to mount humoral and/or cell-mediated immune responses are important determinants of the outcome of viral infections. The state of the host's defenses needs to be considered when antiviral agents are utilized or evaluated.

As with any therapy, the optimal use of antiviral compounds requires a specific and timely diagnosis. For some viral infections, such as herpes zoster, the clinical manifestations are so characteristic that a diagnosis can be made on clinical grounds alone. For other viral infections, such as influenza A, epidemiologic information (e.g., the documentation of a community-wide outbreak) can be used to make a presumptive diagnosis with a high degree of accuracy. However, for most other viral infections, including herpes simplex encephalitis, cytomegaloviral infections other than retinitis, and enteroviral infections, diagnosis on clinical grounds alone cannot be accomplished with certainty. For such infections, rapid viral diagnostic techniques are of great importance. Considerable progress has been made in recent years in the development of such tests, which are now widely available for a number of viral infections.

Despite these complexities, the efficacy of a number of antiviral compounds has been clearly established in rigorously conducted and controlled studies. As summarized in Table 162-1, this chapter reviews the antiviral drugs that are currently approved or are likely to be considered for approval in the near future for use against viral infections other than those caused by HIV. Antiretroviral drugs are reviewed in Chap. 173.

TABLE 162-1 *Antiviral Chemotherapy and Chemoprophylaxis*

Infection	Drug	Route	Dosage	Comment
Influenza A and B Prophylaxis	Amantadine[a] or rimantadine[a]	Oral	Adults: 200 mg/d for period at risk Children ≤9 yrs: 5 mg/kg per day (maximum, 150 mg/d) Children ≥13 yrs: 75 mg/d	Therapy must continue for duration of outbreak. Dosage should be reduced for amantadine and rimantadine in patients with renal failure and the elderly. Drugs can be administered along with inactivated vaccine.
Treatment	Oseltamivir Zanamivir	Oral Inhaled orally	10 mg q12h for 5 days in adults and children ≥7 yrs old	Zanamivir and oseltamivir reduce symptoms by 1.0–1.5 and 1.3 days, respectively, in uncomplicated disease when started within 2 days of onset and are under study in complicated disease. Zanamivir may exacerbate bronchospasm in patients with asthma. Oseltamivir's side effects of nausea and vomiting can be reduced in frequency by administration with food. Both amantadine and rimantadine are effective in uncomplicated influenza. None of the above drugs has been thoroughly studied in complicated cases (e.g., pneumonia).
	Oseltamivir	Oral	75 mg bid for 5 days in adults and 2 mg/kg for 5 days up to a total of 45 mg bid in children 1–12 yrs old	
	Amantadine[a]	Oral	100–200 mg/d in adults and dosage for children as above for 5–7 days	
	Rimantadine[a]	Oral	100–200 mg/d for 5–7 days in adults	
RSV infection	Ribavirin	Small-particle aerosol	Administered continuously from reservoir containing 20 mg/mL for 3–6 days	Ribavirin is used for treatment of infants and young children hospitalized with RSV pneumonia and bronchiolitis.
CMV retinitis in immunocompromised host (AIDS)	Ganciclovir	IV	5 mg/kg bid for 14–21 days; then 5 mg/kg per day as maintenance dose	Ganciclovir, valganciclovir, foscarnet, and cidofovir are approved for treatment of CMV retinitis in patients with AIDS. They are also used for colitis, pneumonia, or ''wasting'' syndromes associated with CMV and for prevention of CMV disease in transplant recipients. Valganciclovir has largely supplanted oral ganciclovir and is frequently used in place of IV ganciclovir. Foscarnet is not myelosuppressive and is active against acyclovir- and ganciclovir-resistant herpesviruses.
		Oral	1 g tid as maintenance dose	
	Valganciclovir	Oral	900 mg bid for 21 days; then 900 mg/d as maintenance dose	
	Foscarnet	IV	60 mg/kg q8h for 14–21 days; then 90–120 mg/kg per day as maintenance dose	
	Cidofovir	IV	5 mg/kg once weekly for 2 weeks, then once every other week; given with probenecid	
Varicella Immunocompetent host	Acyclovir	Oral	20 mg/kg (maximum, 800 mg) 4 or 5 times daily for 5 days	Treatment confers modest clinical benefit when administered within 24 h of rash onset.
Immunocompromised host	Acyclovir	IV	500 mg/m^2 q8h for 7 days	A change to oral valacyclovir can be considered once fever has subsided and there is no evidence of visceral involvement.
Herpes simplex encephalitis	Acyclovir	IV	10 mg/kg q8h for 14–21 days	Results are optimal when therapy is initiated early. Some authorities recommend treatment for 21 days to prevent relapses.
Neonatal herpes simplex	Acyclovir	IV	10 mg/kg q8h for 14–21 days	Serious morbidity is frequent despite therapy. Prolonged oral administration of acyclovir after initial IV therapy has been suggested because of long-term sequelae associated with cutaneous recurrences of HSV infection.
Genital herpes simplex Primary (treatment)	Acyclovir	IV	5 mg/kg q8h for 5–10 days	The IV route is preferred for infections severe enough to warrant hospitalization or with neurologic complications.
		Oral	200 mg 5 times daily for 10 days	The oral route is preferred for patients whose condition does not warrant hospitalization. Adequate hydration must be maintained.
		Topical	5% ointment; 4–6 applications daily for 7–10 days	Topical use—largely supplemented by oral therapy—may obviate systemic administration to pregnant women. Systemic symptoms and untreated areas are not affected.
	Valacyclovir	Oral	1 g bid for 10 days	Valacyclovir appears to be as effective as acyclovir but can be administered less frequently.
	Famciclovir	Oral	250 mg bid for 5–10 days[b]	Famciclovir appears to be similar in effectiveness to acyclovir.
Recurrent (treatment)	Acyclovir Famciclovir Valacyclovir	Oral Oral Oral	200 mg 5 times daily for 5 days 125 mg bid for 5 days 500 mg bid for 3 days	Clinical effect is modest and is enhanced if therapy is initiated early. Treatment does not affect recurrence rates.

(continued)

TABLE 162-1—(Continued)

Infection	Drug	Route	Dosage	Comment
Recurrent (suppression)	Acyclovir Valacyclovir Famciclovir	Oral Oral Oral	400 mg bid for ≥12 months 500–1000 mg daily 125–250 mg bid	Suppressive therapy is recommended only for patients with at least 6–10 recurrences per year. "Breakthrough" occasionally takes place, and asymptomatic shedding of virus occurs. The need for suppressive therapy should be reevaluated after 1 year. Suppression with valacyclovir reduces transmission of genital HSV among discordant couples.
Mucocutaneous herpes simplex in immuno-compromised host Treatment	Acyclovir Valacyclovir Famciclovir	IV Oral Topical Oral Oral	250 mg/m² q8h for 7 days 400 mg 5 times daily for 10 days 5% ointment; 4–6 applications daily for 7 days or until healed 1 g tid for 7 days[b] 500 mg bid for 4 days[c]	Choice of IV or oral route depends on severity of infection and patient's ability to take oral medication. Oral or IV treatment has supplanted topical therapy except for small, easily accessible lesions. Foscarnet is used for acyclovir-resistant viruses.
Prevention of recurrences during intense immunosuppression	Acyclovir Valacyclovir Famciclovir	Oral IV Oral Oral	200 mg qid 5 mg/kg q12h 1 g tid[b] 500 mg bid[b]	Treatment is administered during periods when intense immunosuppression is expected—e.g., during antitumor chemotherapy or after transplantation—and is usually continued for 2–3 months.
Herpes simplex orolabialis (recurrent)	Penciclovir Valacyclovir Famciclovir[b] Docosanol[d]	Topical Oral Oral Topical	1.0% cream applied q2h during waking hours for 4 days 2 g q12h for 1 day 500 mg tid for 5 days 10% cream 5 times daily until healed	Treatment shortens healing time and symptoms by 0.5–1.0 day (compared with placebo). Therapy begun at earliest symptom reduces disease duration by 1 day. Therapy begun 48 h after UV light exposure decreases time to healing by 2 days. Application at initial symptoms reduces healing time by 1 day.
Herpes simplex keratitis	Trifluridine Vidarabine	Topical Topical	1 drop of 1% ophthalmic solution q2h while awake (maximum, 9 drops daily) 0.5-in. ribbon of 3% ophthalmic ointment 5 times daily	Therapy should be undertaken in consultation with an ophthalmologist.
Herpes zoster Immunocompromised host	Acyclovir Famciclovir	IV Oral Oral	500 mg/m² q8h for 7 days 800 mg 5 times daily for 7 days 500 mg tid for 10 days[b]	Effectiveness in localized zoster is most marked when treatment is given early. Foscarnet may be used for VZV infections that are resistant to acyclovir.
Immunocompetent host	Valacyclovir Famciclovir Acyclovir	Oral Oral Oral	1 g tid for 7 days 500 mg q8h for 7 days 800 mg 5 times daily for 7–10 days	Valacyclovir may be more effective than acyclovir for pain relief; otherwise, it has a similar effect on cutaneous lesions and should be given within 72 h of rash onset. The duration of postherpetic neuralgia is shorter than with placebo. Famciclovir showed overall efficacy similar to that of acyclovir in a comparative trial. It should be given ≤72 h of rash onset. Acyclovir causes faster resolution of skin lesions than placebo and provides some relief of acute symptoms if given within 72 h of rash onset. Combined with tapering doses of prednisone, acyclovir improves quality-of-life outcomes.
Herpes zoster ophthalmicus	Acyclovir	Oral	600 mg 5 times daily for 10 days	Treatment reduces ocular complications, including ocular keratitis and uveitis.
Condyloma acuminatum	IFN-α2b IFN-αn3	Intralesional Intralesional	1 million units per wart (maximum of 5) thrice weekly for 3 weeks 250,000 units per wart (maximum of 10) twice weekly for up to 8 weeks	Intralesional treatment frequently results in regression of warts, but lesions often recur. Parenteral administration may be useful if lesions are numerous.
Chronic hepatitis B	IFN-α2b Lamivudine	SC or IM Oral	5 million units daily or 10 million units thrice weekly for 16 weeks 100 mg/d for 12–18 months; 150 mg bid as part of therapy	Hepatitis B e antigen and DNA are eliminated in 33–37% of cases. Histopathologic improvement is also seen. Efficacy similar to that of IFN but better tolerated. Resistance develops in 24% of recipients.

(continued)

TABLE 162-1 *Antiviral Chemotherapy and Chemoprophylaxis—(Continued)*

Infection	Drug	Route	Dosage	Comment
	Adefovir dipivoxil	Oral	10 mg/d for 12 months	A return of ALT levels to normal is documented in 48–72% of recipients, improved liver histopathology in 53–64%. Adefovir is effective in lamivudine-resistant hepatitis B. Renal functions should be monitored.
Chronic hepatitis C	IFN-α2a or -α2b	SC or IM	3 million units thrice weekly for 12–18 months	A return of ALT levels to normal is documented in 54% of recipients but is sustained in only 28%. Improvement in liver histopathology is seen.
	IFN-α2b/ribavirin	SC or IM (IFN)/ oral (ribavirin)	3 million units thrice weekly (IFN)/1000–1200 mg daily (ribavirin) for 6–12 months	Combination therapy results in sustained responses in up to 40–50% of all recipients.
	Pegylated-IFN-α2b	SC	1 μg/kg weekly for 12–24 months	The slower clearance of pegylated IFNs than of standard IFNs permits once-weekly administration. The pegylated formulations appear to be superior to standard IFNs in tolerability and efficacy, both as monotherapy and in combination with ribavirin. Sustained virologic responses were seen in 42–46% of genotype 1 patients and in 76–82% of those with genotype 2 or 3.
	Pegylated-IFN-α2a	SC	180 μg/kg weekly for 12–24 months	
	Pegylated-IFN-α2b/ribavirin	SC (IFN)/oral (ribavirin)	1 μg/kg weekly (IFN)/800–1200 mg daily (ribavirin) for 12–24 months	
	Pegylated-IFN-α2a/ribavirin	SC (IFN)/oral (ribavirin)	180 μg/kg weekly (IFN)/1000–1200 mg daily (ribavirin) for 12–24 months	
	IFN alfacon	SC	9–15 μg thrice weekly for 6–12 months	Doses of 9 and 15 μg are equivalent to IFN-α2a or -α2b doses of 3 million units and 5 million units, respectively.
Chronic hepatitis D	IFN-α2a or -α2b	SC or IM	9 million units thrice weekly for 12 months	The overall efficacy and the optimal regimen and duration of therapy have not been established. Responses are usually not sustained when therapy is stopped.

[a] Influenza A only.
[b] Not approved for this indication by the U.S. Food and Drug Administration (FDA).
[c] Approved by the FDA for treatment of HIV-infected individuals.
[d] Active ingredient: behenyl alcohol. Available without prescription.
Abbreviations: ALT, alanine aminotransferase; CMV, cytomegalovirus; HSV, herpes simplex virus; IFN, interferon; RSV, respiratory syncytial virus; UV, ultraviolet.

ANTIVIRAL DRUGS ACTIVE AGAINST RESPIRATORY INFECTIONS

AMANTADINE AND RIMANTADINE Amantadine and the closely related compound rimantadine are primary symmetric amines. Their antiviral activity is limited to influenza A viruses, whose replication they inhibit by interfering with the uncoating of virus after infection of the cell. This interference is attributable to the agents' interaction with the influenza A M2 matrix protein, during which the ion channel function of M2 is inhibited. A substitution of a single amino acid at critical sites in the M2 protein can result in a virus that is resistant to amantadine and rimantadine.

Amantadine and rimantadine have been demonstrated to be effective in the prophylaxis of influenza A in large-scale studies of young adults and in less extensive studies of children and elderly subjects. In such studies, efficacy rates of 55 to 80% in the prevention of influenza-like illness were noted, and even higher rates were reported when virus-specific attack rates were calculated. Amantadine and rimantadine have also been demonstrated to be effective in the treatment of influenza A infection in studies involving predominantly young adults and, to a lesser extent, children. Administration of these compounds within 24 to 72 h after the onset of illness has resulted in a reduction of the duration of signs and symptoms by ~50% from that in a placebo-treated group. The effect on signs and symptoms of illness is superior to that of commonly used antipyretic-analgesics. Only anecdotal reports are available concerning the efficacy of amantadine or rimantadine in the prevention or treatment of complications of influenza (e.g., pneumonia).

Amantadine and rimantadine are available only in oral formulations and are ordinarily administered to adults once or twice daily, with a dosage of 100 to 200 mg/d. Despite their structural similarities, the pharmacokinetics of the two compounds are different. Amantadine is not metabolized and is excreted almost entirely by the kidney, with a half-life of 12 to 17 h and peak plasma concentrations of 0.4 μg/mL. Rimantadine is extensively metabolized to hydroxylated derivatives

and has a half-life of 30 h. Only 30 to 40% of an orally administered dose is recovered in the urine. The peak plasma levels of rimantadine are approximately half those of amantadine, but rimantadine is concentrated in respiratory secretions to a greater extent than amantadine. For prophylaxis, the compounds must be administered daily for the period at risk (i.e., the peak duration of the outbreak). For therapy, amantadine or rimantadine is generally administered for 5 to 7 days.

Although these compounds are generally well tolerated, 5 to 10% of amantadine recipients experience mild central nervous system side effects consisting primarily of dizziness, anxiety, insomnia, and difficulty in concentrating. These effects are rapidly reversible upon cessation of the drug's administration. At a dose of 200 mg/d, rimantadine is better tolerated than amantadine; in a large-scale study of young adults, adverse effects were no more frequent among rimantadine recipients than among placebo recipients. Seizures and worsening of congestive heart failure have also been reported in patients treated with amantadine, although a causal relationship has not been established. The dosage of amantadine should be reduced to ≤100 mg/d in patients with renal insufficiency [i.e., a creatinine clearance (Cr_{Cl}) rate of <50 mL/min] and in the elderly. A rimantadine dose of 100 mg/d should be used for patients with a Cr_{Cl} of <10 mL/min and in the elderly. Resistance to amantadine and rimantadine can be induced readily in vitro. The emergence and probable transmission of virus resistant to these drugs have also been noted in vivo after their use for the treatment of children or adults. In the United States, both amantadine and rimantadine are approved for the prophylaxis and treatment of influenza A in adults and for prophylaxis in children. Amantadine is also approved for the treatment of influenza A in children.

ZANAMIVIR AND OSELTAMIVIR Influenza viral neuraminidase is essential for release of the virus from infected cells and for its subsequent spread throughout the respiratory tract of the infected host. The enzyme cleaves terminal sialic acid residues, thus destroying the cellular receptors recognized by the viral hemagglutinin. Zanamivir, a sialic acid analogue, is a highly active and specific inhibitor of the neuraminidases of influenza A and B viruses. Oseltamivir is another neuraminidase inhibitor that is a transition-state analogue of sialic acid cleavage. Its antineuraminidase activity is similar to that of zanamivir. Oseltamivir phosphate is an ethyl ester prodrug that is converted to oseltamivir carboxylate by esterases in the liver. Both zanamivir and oseltamivir act through competitive and reversible inhibition of the active site of influenza A and B viral neuraminidases and have relatively little effect on mammalian cell enzymes. As would be expected from their different mechanisms of action, zanamivir and oseltamivir are active against strains of influenza A virus that are resistant to amantadine and rimantadine.

Zanamivir has low oral bioavailability. It is inhaled orally via a hand-held inhaler. By this route, ~15% of the dose is deposited in the lower respiratory tract, and low plasma levels of the drug are detected. Orally administered oseltamivir has a bioavailability of >60% and a plasma half-life of 7 to 9 h. The drug is excreted unmetabolized, primarily by the kidneys.

Intranasal inhaled zanamivir is generally well tolerated, although exacerbations of asthma may occur. The toxicities most frequently encountered with orally administered oseltamivir are nausea, gastrointestinal discomfort, and (less commonly) vomiting. Gastrointestinal discomfort is usually transient and is less likely if the drug is administered with food. No serious clinical or laboratory toxicities have yet been reported with zanamivir or oseltamivir in clinical trials.

Inhaled zanamivir and orally administered oseltamivir have been effective in the treatment of naturally occurring influenza A or B in otherwise-healthy adults. In placebo-controlled studies, illness has been shortened by 1 to 1.5 days of therapy with either of these drugs when administered within 2 days of onset. Once-daily inhaled zanamivir or orally administered oseltamivir provides effective prophylaxis against laboratory-documented influenza A–associated illness. The emergence of viruses resistant to zanamivir or oseltamivir appears to be infrequent in clinical studies carried out thus far.

Zanamivir and oseltamivir have been approved by the U.S. Food and Drug Administration (FDA) for treatment of influenza in adults and in children (those ≥7 years old for zanamivir and those ≥1 year old for oseltamivir) who have been symptomatic for ≤2 days. Oseltamivir is approved for prophylaxis of influenza in individuals ≥13 years of age.

RIBAVIRIN   Ribavirin is a synthetic nucleoside analogue that inhibits a wide range of RNA and DNA viruses. The mechanism of action of ribavirin is not completely defined and may be different for different groups of viruses. Ribavirin-5'-monophosphate blocks the conversion of inosine-5'-monophosphate to xanthosine-5'-monophosphate and interferes with the synthesis of guanine nucleotides as well as that of both RNA and DNA. Ribavirin-5'-monophosphate also inhibits capping of virus-specific messenger RNA in certain viral systems. In studies demonstrating the effectiveness of ribavirin in the treatment of respiratory syncytial virus (RSV) infection in infants, the compound has been administered as a small-particle aerosol. It has been used less extensively to treat parainfluenza virus infections in children and influenza A and B virus infections in young adults. In infants with RSV infection who were given ribavirin by continuous aerosol for 3 to 6 days, illness and lower respiratory tract signs resolved more rapidly and arterial oxygen desaturation was less pronounced than in placebo-treated groups. Ribavirin has also had a beneficial clinical effect in infants with RSV infection who require mechanical ventilation. Aerosolized ribavirin has been administered to older children and adults with severe RSV and parainfluenza virus infections (including immunosuppressed patients), but the benefit of this treatment, if any, is unclear. In RSV infections in immunosuppressed patients, ribavirin is often given in combination with immunoglobulins.

Orally administered ribavirin has not been effective in the treatment of influenza A virus infections. Intravenous or oral ribavirin has reduced mortality among patients with Lassa fever; it has been partic-

ularly effective in this regard when given within the first 6 days of illness. Intravenous ribavirin has been reported to be of clinical benefit in the treatment of hemorrhagic fever with renal syndrome caused by Hantaan virus and as therapy for Argentinian hemorrhagic fever. Moreover, oral ribavirin has been recommended for the treatment and prophylaxis of Congo-Crimean hemorrhagic fever. Intravenous ribavirin is being evaluated as therapy for the hemorrhagic fever with pulmonary syndrome caused by newly described hantaviruses in the United States. Oral administration of ribavirin reduces serum aminotransferase levels in patients with chronic hepatitis C virus (HCV) infection; since it appears not to reduce serum HCV RNA levels, the mechanism of this effect is unclear. The drug provides an added beneficial effect when given by mouth in doses of 800 to 1200 mg/d in combination with interferon (IFN) α2b or α2a (see below), and the ribavirin/IFN combination has been approved for the treatment of patients with chronic HCV infection.

Large doses of ribavirin administered orally (800 to 1000 mg/d) have been associated with reversible hematopoietic toxicity. This effect has not been observed with aerosolized ribavirin, apparently because little drug is absorbed systemically. Aerosolized administration of ribavirin is generally well tolerated but occasionally is associated with bronchospasm, rash, or conjunctival irritation. Aerosolized ribavirin has been licensed for treatment of RSV infection in infants and should be administered under close supervision—particularly in the setting of mechanical ventilation, where precipitation of the drug is possible. Health care workers exposed to the drug have experienced minor toxicity, including eye and respiratory tract irritation. Because ribavirin is mutagenic, teratogenic, and embryotoxic, its use is generally contraindicated in pregnancy. Its administration as an aerosol poses a risk to pregnant health care workers.

PLECONARIL   Pleconaril is an investigational drug active in vitro against picornavirus replication, including >90% of the most commonly isolated enterovirus types and 80% of rhinovirus serotypes. Its mechanism of action is through binding to a specific hydrophobic pocket in the viral capsid, which prevents attachment and/or uncoating of the virus. Pleconaril is poorly water soluble and is formulated as an oral suspension. It is generally well tolerated; the most frequently reported adverse effects are headache, nausea, diarrhea, and gastrointestinal discomfort, which have occurred at rates similar to those among placebo recipients. Pleconaril treatment of adults with enterovirus meningitis decreased the overall duration of illness and headache and reduced the use of analgesics from that by placebo recipients. A large-scale clinical study demonstrated a mild therapeutic effect on rhinovirus-associated colds, but pleconaril was deemed to be of insufficient benefit to gain approval by an FDA advisory panel.

ANTIVIRAL DRUGS ACTIVE AGAINST HERPESVIRUS INFECTIONS

ACYCLOVIR AND VALACYCLOVIR   Acyclovir is a highly potent and selective inhibitor of the replication of certain herpesviruses, including herpes simplex virus (HSV) types 1 and 2, varicella-zoster virus (VZV), and Epstein-Barr virus (EBV). It is relatively ineffective in the treatment of human cytomegalovirus (CMV) infections; however, some studies have indicated its effectiveness in the prevention of CMV-associated disease in immunosuppressed patients. Valacyclovir, the L-valyl ester of acyclovir, is converted almost entirely to acyclovir by intestinal and hepatic hydrolysis after oral administration. Valacyclovir has pharmacokinetic advantages over orally administered acyclovir: it exhibits significantly greater oral bioavailability, results in higher blood levels, and can be given less frequently than acyclovir (two or three rather than five times daily).

The high degree of selectivity of acyclovir is related to its mechanism of action, which requires that the compound first be phosphorylated to acyclovir monophosphate. This phosphorylation occurs efficiently in herpesvirus-infected cells by means of a virus-coded thymidine kinase. In uninfected mammalian cells, little phosphorylation of acyclovir occurs, and the drug is therefore concentrated in herpesvirus-infected cells. Acyclovir monophosphate is subsequently converted by host cell kinases to a triphosphate that is a potent inhibitor of virus-induced DNA polymerase but has relatively little effect on host cell DNA polymerase. Acyclovir triphosphate can also be incorporated into viral DNA, with early chain termination.

Acyclovir is available in intravenous, oral, and topical forms, while valacyclovir is available in an oral formulation. Intravenous acyclovir is markedly effective in the treatment of mucocutaneous HSV infections in immunocompromised hosts, reducing time to healing, duration of pain, and virus shedding. When administered prophylactically during periods of intense immunosuppression (e.g., related to chemotherapy for leukemia or transplantation) and before the development of lesions, intravenous acyclovir reduces the frequency of HSV-associated disease. After prophylaxis is discontinued, HSV lesions recur. Intravenous acyclovir is also effective in the treatment of HSV encephalitis; two comparative trials have indicated that acyclovir is more effective than vidarabine for this indication (see below). Because VZV is generally less sensitive to acyclovir than is HSV, higher doses of acyclovir must be used to treat VZV infections. In immunocompromised patients with herpes zoster, intravenous acyclovir reduces the frequency of cutaneous dissemination and visceral complications and—in one comparative trial—was more effective than vidarabine. Acyclovir, administered orally at doses of 800 mg five times a day, had a modest beneficial effect on localized herpes zoster lesions in both immunocompromised and immunocompetent patients. Combination of acyclovir with a tapering regimen of prednisone appeared to be more effective than acyclovir alone in terms of quality-of-life outcomes in immunocompetent herpes zoster patients over age 50. A comparative study of acyclovir (800 mg orally five times daily) and valacyclovir (1 g orally tid) in immunocompetent patients with herpes zoster indicated that the latter drug may be more effective in eliciting the resolution of zoster-associated pain. Orally administered acyclovir (600 mg five times a day) reduced complications of herpes zoster ophthalmicus in a placebo-controlled trial.

In normal children with chickenpox, acyclovir—administered at 20 mg/kg (up to a maximum of 800) four times daily, within 24 h of the onset of rash—resulted in a modest overall clinical benefit. Intravenous acyclovir has also been reported to be effective in the treatment of immunocompromised children with chickenpox.

The most widespread use of acyclovir is in the treatment of genital HSV infections. Intravenous or oral acyclovir or oral valacyclovir has shortened the duration of symptoms, reduced virus shedding, and accelerated healing when employed for the treatment of primary genital HSV infections. Oral acyclovir and valacyclovir have also had a modest effect in treatment of recurrent genital HSV infections. However, the failure of treatment of either primary or recurrent disease to reduce the frequency of subsequent recurrences has indicated that acyclovir is ineffective in eliminating latent infection. Chronic oral administration of acyclovir 1 to 6 years or longer or of valacyclovir for 1 year or longer has reduced the frequency of recurrences markedly during therapy; once the drug is discontinued, lesions recur. In one study, suppressive therapy with valacyclovir (500 mg once daily for 8 months) reduced transmission of HSV-2 genital infections among discordant couples by 50%. A modest effect on herpes labialis (i.e., a reduction of disease duration by 1 day) was seen when valacyclovir was administered upon detection of the first symptom of a lesion at a dose of 2 g every 12 h for 1 day. In AIDS patients, chronic or intermittent administration of acyclovir has been associated with the development of HSV and VZV strains resistant to the action of the drug and with clinical failures. The most common mechanism of resistance is a deficiency of the virus-induced thymidine kinase. Patients with HSV or VZV infections resistant to acyclovir have frequently responded to foscarnet.

With the availability of the oral and intravenous forms, there are few indications for topical acyclovir, although treatment with this formulation has been modestly beneficial in primary genital HSV infections and in mucocutaneous HSV infections in immunocompromised hosts.

Overall, acyclovir is remarkably well tolerated and is generally free of toxicity. The most frequently encountered form of toxicity is renal dysfunction, particularly after rapid intravenous administration or with inadequate hydration. Central nervous system changes, including lethargy and tremors, are occasionally reported, primarily in immunosuppressed patients. However, whether these changes are related to acyclovir, to concurrent administration of other therapy, or to underlying infection remains unclear. Acyclovir is excreted primarily unmetabolized by the kidney, via both glomerular filtration and tubular secretion. Approximately 15% of a dose of acyclovir is metabolized to 9-[(carboxymethoxy)methyl]guanine or other minor metabolites. Reduction in dosage is indicated in patients with a Cr_{Cl} of <50 mL/min per 1.73 m². The half-life of acyclovir is ~3 h in normal adults, and the peak plasma concentration after a 1-h infusion of a dose of 5 mg/kg is 9.8 μg/mL. Approximately 22% of an orally administered acyclovir dose is absorbed, and peak plasma concentrations of 0.3 to 0.9 μg/mL are attained after administration of a 200-mg dose. Acyclovir penetrates relatively well into the cerebrospinal fluid (CSF), with concentrations approaching half of those found in plasma.

Acyclovir causes chromosomal breakage at high doses, but its administration to pregnant women has not been associated with fetal abnormalities. Nonetheless, the potential risks and benefits of acyclovir should be carefully assessed before the drug is used in pregnancy.

Valacyclovir exhibits three to five times greater bioavailability than acyclovir. The concentration-time curve for valacyclovir, given as 1 g by mouth three times daily, is similar to that for acyclovir, given as 5 mg/kg intravenously every 8 h. The safety profiles of valacyclovir and acyclovir are similar, although thrombotic thrombocytopenic purpura/hemolytic-uremic syndrome has been reported in immunocompromised patients who have received high doses (8 g/day) of valacyclovir. Valacyclovir is approved for the treatment of herpes zoster and for initial and recurrent episodes of genital HSV infections in immunocompetent adults as well as for suppressive treatment of genital herpes. Although it has not been extensively studied in other herpesvirus infections, many consultants use valacyclovir rather than oral acyclovir in clinical settings where the latter has been approved because of valacyclovir's superior pharmacokinetics and more convenient dosing schedule.

CIDOFOVIR Cidofovir is a phosphonate nucleotide analogue of cytosine. Its major use is in CMV infections, particularly retinitis, but it is active against a broad range of herpesviruses, including HSV, human herpesvirus (HHV) type 6, HHV-8, and certain other DNA viruses such as polyomaviruses, papillomaviruses, adenoviruses, and poxviruses, including variola (smallpox) and vaccinia. Cidofovir does not require initial phosphorylation by virus-induced kinases; the drug is phosphorylated by host cell enzymes to cidofovir diphosphate, which is a competitive inhibitor of viral DNA polymerases and, to a lesser extent, of host cell DNA polymerases. Incorporation of cidofovir diphosphate slows or terminates nascent DNA chain elongation. Cidofovir is active against HSV isolates that are resistant to acyclovir because of absent or altered thymidine kinase and against CMV isolates that are resistant to ganciclovir because of UL97 mutations. Cidofovir is usually active against foscarnet-resistant CMV, although cross-resistance to foscarnet as well as to ganciclovir has been described.

Cidofovir has poor oral availability and is administered intravenously. It is excreted primarily by the kidney and has a plasma half-life of 2.6 h. Cidofovir diphosphate's intracellular half-life of >48 h is the basis for the recommended dosing regimen of 5 mg/kg once a week for the initial 2 weeks and then 5 mg/kg every other week. The major toxic effect of cidofovir is proximal renal tubular injury, as manifested by elevated serum creatinine levels and proteinuria. The risk of nephrotoxicity can be reduced by vigorous saline hydration and by concomitant oral administration of probenecid. Neutropenia, rashes, and gastrointestinal tolerance may also occur.

Intravenous cidofovir has been approved for the treatment of CMV retinitis in AIDS patients who are intolerant of ganciclovir or foscarnet or in whom those drugs have failed. In a controlled study, a maintenance dosage of 5 mg/kg a week administered to AIDS patients reduced the progression of CMV retinitis from that seen at 3 mg/kg. Intravenous cidofovir has been reported anecdotally to be effective therapy for acyclovir-resistant mucocutaneous HSV infections. Likewise, topically administered cidofovir is reportedly beneficial against these infections in HIV patients; it is also being studied for the treatment of anogenital warts. Intravenous cidofovir is being evaluated as therapy for progressive multifocal leukoencephalopathy and for Kaposi's sarcoma. An ophthalmic formulation is being studied as treatment for adenoviral keratoconjunctivitis. Intravitreal cidofovir has been used to treat CMV retinitis but has been associated with significant toxicity.

FOMIVIRSEN Fomivirsen is the first antisense oligonucleotide approved by the FDA for therapy in humans. This phosphorothioate oligonucleotide, 21 nucleotides in length, inhibits CMV replication through interaction with CMV messenger RNA. Fomivirsen is complementary to messenger transcripts of the major immediate early region 2 (IE2) of CMV, which codes for proteins regulating viral gene expression. In addition to its antisense mechanism of action, fomivirsen may exert activity against CMV through inhibition of viral adsorption to cells as well as direct inhibition of viral replication. Because of its different mechanism of action, fomivirsen is active against CMV isolates that are resistant to nucleoside or nucleotide analogues, such as ganciclovir, foscarnet, or cidofovir.

Fomivirsen has been approved for intravitreal administration in the treatment of CMV retinitis in AIDS patients who have failed to respond to other treatments or cannot tolerate them. Injections of 330 mg every 2 weeks have resulted in significant reductions in the rate of progression of CMV retinitis. The major toxicity is ocular inflammation, including vitritis and iritis, which usually responds to topically administered glucocorticoids.

GANCICLOVIR AND VALGANCICLOVIR An analogue of acyclovir, ganciclovir is active against HSV and VZV and is markedly more active than acyclovir against CMV. Ganciclovir triphosphate inhibits CMV DNA polymerase and can be incorporated into CMV DNA, whose elongation it eventually terminates. In HSV- and VZV-infected cells, ganciclovir is phosphorylated by virus-encoded thymidine kinases; in CMV-infected cells, it is phosphorylated by a viral kinase encoded by the UL97 gene. Ganciclovir triphosphate is present in tenfold higher concentrations in CMV-infected cells than in uninfected cells. Ganciclovir is approved for the treatment of CMV retinitis in immunosuppressed patients and for the prevention of CMV disease in transplant recipients. It is widely used for the treatment of other CMV-associated syndromes, including pneumonia, esophagogastrointestinal infections, hepatitis, and "wasting" illness.

Ganciclovir is available for intravenous or oral administration. Because its oral bioavailability is low (5 to 9%), relatively large doses (1 g three times daily) must be administered by this route. Oral ganciclovir has largely been supplanted by valganciclovir, which is the L-valyl ester of ganciclovir. Valganciclovir is well absorbed orally, with a bioavailability of 60%, and is rapidly hydrolyzed to ganciclovir in the intestine and liver. The area under the curve for a 900-mg dose of valganciclovir is equivalent to that for 5 mg/kg of ganciclovir given intravenously, although peak serum concentrations are ~40% lower for valganciclovir. The serum half-life is 3.5 h after intravenous administration of ganciclovir and 4.0 h after oral administration of valganciclovir. Ganciclovir is excreted primarily by the kidneys in unmetabolized form, and its dosage should be reduced in cases of renal failure. The most commonly employed dosage for initial intravenous therapy is 5 mg/kg every 12 h for 14 to 21 days; this regimen is followed by an intravenous maintenance dose of 5 mg/kg per day or five times per week, possibly for as long as immunosuppression persists. For oral therapy with valganciclovir, the dose is 900 mg twice daily for 21 days followed by 900 mg once a day for maintenance,

with dose adjustment in patients with renal dysfunction. Intraocular ganciclovir, given by either intravitreal injection or intraocular implantation, has also been used to treat CMV retinitis.

Ganciclovir is effective as prophylaxis against CMV-associated disease in organ and bone marrow transplant recipients. Oral ganciclovir administered prophylactically to AIDS patients with CD4+ cell counts of <100/μL has provided protection against the development of CMV retinitis. However, the long-term benefits of this approach to prophylaxis in AIDS patients have not been established, and most experts do not recommend the use of oral ganciclovir for this purpose. As already mentioned, valganciclovir has supplanted oral ganciclovir in settings where oral prophylaxis or therapy is considered.

The administration of ganciclovir has been associated with profound bone marrow suppression, particularly neutropenia, which significantly limits the drug's use in many patients. Bone marrow toxicity is potentiated when other bone marrow suppressants, such as zidovudine, are used concomitantly.

Resistance has been noted in CMV isolates obtained after therapy with ganciclovir, especially in patients with AIDS. Such resistance may develop through a mutation in either the viral UL97 gene or the viral DNA polymerase. Ganciclovir-resistant isolates are usually sensitive to foscarnet (see below) or cidofovir (see above).

FAMCICLOVIR AND PENCICLOVIR Famciclovir is the diacetyl 6-deoxyester of the guanosine analogue penciclovir. Famciclovir is well absorbed orally, has a bioavailability of 77%, and is rapidly converted to penciclovir by deacetylation and oxidation in the intestine and liver. Penciclovir's spectrum of activity and mechanism of action are similar to those of acyclovir; thus penciclovir is usually not active against acyclovir-resistant viruses. Penciclovir is phosphorylated initially by a virus-encoded thymidine kinase and subsequently by cellular kinases to penciclovir triphosphate, which inhibits HSV-1, HSV-2, and VZV DNA polymerases as well as hepatitis B virus (HBV). The serum half-life of penciclovir is 2 h, but the intracellular half-life of penciclovir triphosphate is 7 to 20 h— markedly longer than that of acyclovir triphosphate. The latter is the basis for the less frequent (twice-daily) dosing schedule for famciclovir than for acyclovir. Penciclovir is eliminated primarily in the urine by both glomerular filtration and tubular secretion. The usually recommended dosage interval should be adjusted for renal insufficiency.

Clinical trials involving immunocompetent adults with herpes zoster showed that famciclovir was superior to placebo in eliciting the resolution of skin lesions and virus shedding and in shortening the duration of postherpetic neuralgia; moreover, it was at least as effective as acyclovir administered orally at a dose of 800 mg five times daily. Famciclovir was also effective in the treatment of herpes zoster in immunosuppressed patients. Clinical trials have demonstrated its effectiveness in the suppression of genital HSV infections for up to 1 year and in the treatment of initial and recurrent episodes of genital herpes. Famciclovir is effective as therapy for mucocutaneous HSV infections in HIV-infected patients. Application of a 1% penciclovir cream reduces the duration of signs and symptoms of herpes labialis in immunocompetent patients (by 0.5 to 1.0 day) and has been approved for that purpose by the FDA. Famciclovir is generally well tolerated, with occasional headache, nausea, and diarrhea reported in frequencies similar to those among placebo recipients. The administration of high doses of famciclovir for 2 years was associated with an increased incidence of mammary adenocarcinomas in female rats, but the clinical significance of this effect is unknown. Intravenous penciclovir is being investigated for the treatment of mucocutaneous HSV infections in immunosuppressed patients.

FOSCARNET Foscarnet (phosphonoformic acid) is a pyrophosphate-containing compound that potently inhibits herpesviruses, including CMV. This drug inhibits DNA polymerases at the pyrophosphate binding site at concentrations that have relatively little effect on cellular polymerases. Foscarnet does not require phosphorylation to exert its antiviral activity and is therefore active against HSV and VZV isolates that are resistant to acyclovir because of deficiencies in thymidine kinase as well as against most ganciclovir-resistant strains of CMV. Foscarnet also inhibits the reverse transcriptase of HIV and is active against HIV in vivo.

Foscarnet is poorly soluble and must be administered intravenously via an infusion pump in a dilute solution over 1 to 2 h. The plasma half-life of foscarnet is 3 to 5 h and increases with decreasing renal function, since the drug is eliminated primarily by the kidneys. It has been estimated that 10 to 28% of a dose may be deposited in bone, where it can persist for months. The most common initial dosage of foscarnet—60 mg/kg every 8 h for 14 to 21 days—is followed by a maintenance dose of 90 to 120 mg/kg once a day.

Foscarnet is approved for the treatment of CMV retinitis in patients with AIDS and of acyclovir-resistant mucocutaneous HSV infections. In a comparative clinical trial, the drug appeared to be about as efficacious as ganciclovir against CMV retinitis but was associated with a longer survival period, possibly because of its anti-HIV activity. Intraocular foscarnet has been used to treat CMV retinitis. Foscarnet has also been employed to treat acyclovir-resistant HSV and VZV infections as well as ganciclovir-resistant CMV infections, although resistance to foscarnet has been reported in CMV isolates obtained during therapy.

The major form of toxicity associated with foscarnet is renal impairment. Thus renal function should be monitored closely, particularly during the initial phase of therapy. Since foscarnet binds divalent metal ions, hypocalcemia, hypomagnesemia, hypokalemia, and hypo- or hyperphosphatemia can develop. Saline hydration and slow infusion appear to protect the patient against nephrotoxicity and electrolyte disturbances. Although hematologic abnormalities have been documented (most commonly anemia), foscarnet is not generally myelosuppressive and may be administered concomitantly with myelosuppressive medications such as zidovudine.

TRIFLURIDINE Trifluridine is a pyrimidine nucleoside active against HSV-1, HSV-2, and CMV. Trifluridine monophosphate irreversibly inhibits thymidylate synthetase, and trifluridine triphosphate inhibits viral and, to a lesser extent, cellular DNA polymerases. Because of systemic toxicity, its use is limited to topical therapy. Trifluridine is approved for treatment of HSV keratitis, for which trials have shown that it is more effective than topical idoxuridine but similarly effective to topical vidarabine. The drug has benefited some patients with HSV keratitis who have failed to respond to idoxuridine or vidarabine. Topical application of trifluridine to sites of acyclovir-resistant HSV mucocutaneous infections has also been beneficial in some cases.

VIDARABINE Vidarabine is a purine nucleoside analogue with activity against HSV-1, HSV-2, VZV, and EBV. Vidarabine inhibits viral DNA synthesis through its 5′-triphosphorylated metabolite, although its precise molecular mechanisms of action are not completely understood. Intravenously administered vidarabine has been shown to be effective in the treatment of herpes simplex encephalitis, mucocutaneous HSV infections, herpes zoster in immunocompromised patients, and neonatal HSV infections. Its use has been supplanted by that of intravenous acyclovir, which is more effective and easier to administer. Production of the intravenous preparation has been discontinued by the manufacturer, but vidarabine is available as an ophthalmic ointment, which is effective in the treatment of HSV keratitis.

ANTIVIRAL DRUGS ACTIVE AGAINST HEPATITIS VIRUSES

LAMIVUDINE Lamivudine is a pyrimidine nucleoside analogue that is used primarily in combination therapy against HIV infection (Chap. 173). It is also active against HBV through inhibition of the viral DNA polymerase and has been approved for the treatment of chronic HBV infection. At doses of 100 mg/d for 1 year, lamivudine was well tolerated and results in suppression of HBV DNA levels, normalization of serum aminotransferase levels in 50 to 70% of patients, and reduc-

tion of hepatic inflammation and fibrosis in 50 to 60% of patients. Loss of hepatitis B e antigen (HBeAg) occurred in 30% of patients. Resistance to lamivudine develops in 24% of patients treated for 1 year and is associated with changes in the YMDD motif of HBV DNA polymerase. This is an important limitation of monotherapy with the drug. Studies of lamivudine as a component of combination therapy for hepatitis B are under way. Lamivudine also appears to be useful in the prevention or suppression of HBV infection associated with liver transplantation.

ADEFOVIR Adefovir dipivoxil is an acyclic nucleotide analogue of adenosine monophosphate that has activity against HBV, HIV, HSV, and CMV. It is phosphorylated by cellular kinases to the active triphosphate moiety, which is a competitive inhibitor of HBV DNA polymerase and results in chain termination after incorporation into nascent viral DNA. Adefovir is administered orally and is eliminated primarily by the kidneys, with a plasma half-life of 7.5 h. In clinical studies, therapy with adefovir at a dose 10 μg/d for 48 weeks resulted in normalization of alanine aminotransferase (ALT) levels in 48 to 72% of patients and improved liver histology in 53 to 64%; it also resulted in a $3.6-\log_{10}$ reduction in the number of HBV DNA copies per milliliter of plasma. Adefovir was effective in treatment naive patients as well as in those infected with lamivudine-resistant HBV. This agent was generally well tolerated. Significant nephrotoxicity attributable to adefovir was uncommon at the dose employed in the treatment of HBV infections (10 μg/d) but was a treatment-limiting adverse effect at the higher doses used in the treatment of HIV infections (30 to 120 μg/d). In any case, renal function should be monitored in patients taking adefovir, even at the lower dose. Adefovir is approved only for treatment of chronic hepatitis B infection.

TENOFOVIR Tenofovir disoproxil fumarate is a nucleotide analogue with activity against both retroviruses and hepadnaviruses. In one small study of patients coinfected with HIV and HBV, tenofovir reduced HBV loads by $>10^4$ copies/mL at 24 weeks. The drug is approved only for treatment of HIV infection, but its use should be considered in HIV/HBV-coinfected patients. →*For a more detailed discussion of tenofovir, see Chap. 173.*

INTERFERONS

Interferons are cytokines that exhibit a broad spectrum of antiviral activities as well as immunomodulating and antiproliferative properties. The IFNs are not available for oral administration but must be given intramuscularly, subcutaneously, or intravenously. Early studies with human leukocyte IFN demonstrated an effect in the prophylaxis of experimentally induced rhinovirus infections in humans and in the treatment of VZV infections in immunosuppressed patients. DNA recombinant technology has made available highly purified α, β, and γ IFNs that have been evaluated in a variety of viral infections. Results of such trials have confirmed the effectiveness of intranasally administered IFN in the prophylaxis of rhinovirus infections, although its use has been associated with nasal mucosal irritation. Studies have also demonstrated a beneficial effect of intralesionally or systemically administered IFNs on genital warts. The effect of systemic administration consists primarily of a reduction in the size of lesions, and this mode of therapy may be useful in persons who have numerous warts that cannot easily be treated by individual intralesional injections. However, lesions frequently recur after either intralesional or systemic IFN therapy is discontinued.

Interferons have undergone extensive study in the treatment of chronic HBV infection. The administration of IFN-α2b (5 million units daily or 10 million units three times a week for 16 weeks) to patients with stable chronic HBV infection resulted in loss of markers of HBV replication, such as HBeAg and HBV DNA, in 33 to 37% of cases; 8% of patients also became negative for hepatitis B surface antigen. In >80% of patients who lose HBeAg and HBV DNA markers, serum aminotransferases return to normal levels, and both short- and long-term improvements in liver histopathology have been described. Predictors of a favorable response to therapy include low pretherapy levels of HBV DNA, high pretherapy serum levels of ALT, a short duration of chronic HBV infection, and active inflammation in liver histopathology. Poor responses are seen in immunosuppressed patients, including those with HIV infection. Adverse effects of the above dose of IFN are common and include fever, chills, myalgia, fatigue, neurotoxicity (primarily manifested as somnolence and confusion), and leukopenia. Approximately 25% of patients receiving a daily dose of 5 million units require dose reduction, but <5% require discontinuation of therapy.

Several IFN preparations, including IFN-α2a, IFN-α2b, IFN-alfacon-1, and IFN-αm1 (lymphoblastoid), have been studied as therapy for chronic HCV infections. A variety of regimens have been employed, of which the most common is IFN-α2b or -α2a at 3 million units three times per week for 12 to 18 months. The addition of oral ribavirin to IFN-α2b—either as initial therapy or after failure of interferon therapy alone—results in significantly higher rates of sustained virologic and/or serum ALT responses (40 to 50%) than were obtained with monotherapy. *Pegylated* IFN-α2b or -α2a, in which the IFNs are covalently linked with monomethoxy polyethylene glycol, have been approved by the FDA for the treatment of chronic HCV infection. These interferons have a markedly reduced clearance rate and can therefore be administered less frequently than standard IFNs (i.e., once a week). Comparative studies indicate that pegylated IFN therapy may be more effective than standard IFN treatment against chronic HCV infection. The combination of intramuscular pegylated IFN and oral ribavirin appears to be a particularly convenient and effective regimen for treatment of chronic hepatitis C. Prognostic factors for a favorable response include an age of <45 years, a short duration of disease, low levels of HCV RNA, and infection with HCV genotypes other than 1. IFN alfacon, a synthetic "consensus" α interferon, appears to produce response rates similar to those elicited by IFN-α2a or -α2b alone and is also approved in the United States for the treatment of chronic hepatitis C. In early clinical trials, pegylated IFN alfas also appear promising as therapy for hepatitis B.

Treatment of acute hepatitis C with IFN has been investigated relatively little. In one study, the administration of IFN-α2b to patients recently infected with HCV (with a dose of 5 million units per day for 4 weeks followed by 3 million units per week for 20 weeks) resulted in clearance of HCV from blood and normalization of ALT levels in 43 of 44 patients at 48 weeks. Additional studies are required to establish the role of IFN therapy in this setting.

The efficacy of IFN-α treatment for chronic hepatitis D remains unestablished. Anecdotal reports suggested that doses of 5 million units daily to 9 million units three times per week for 12 months elicited biochemical and virologic responses. Results from small controlled trials have been inconsistent, and observed responses have not generally been sustained.

FURTHER READING

BALFOUR HH: Antiviral drugs. N Engl J Med 340:1255, 1999

BEUTNER KR et al: Valaciclovir compared with acyclovir for improved therapy for herpes zoster in immunocompetent adults. Antimicrob Agents Chemother 39:1546, 1995

COUCH RB: Drug therapy: Prevention and treatment of influenza. N Engl J Med 343:1778, 2000

CRUMPACKER CS: Ganciclovir. N Engl J Med 335:721, 1996

DOLIN R et al: A controlled trial of amantadine and rimantadine in the prophylaxis of influenza A infection. N Engl J Med 307:580, 1982

HALL CB et al: Aerosolized ribavirin treatment of infants with respiratory syncytial viral infection: A randomized double-blind study. N Engl J Med 308:1443, 1983

LALEZARI JP et al: Randomized controlled study of the safety and efficacy of intravenous cidofovir for the treatment of relapsing cytomegalovirus retinitis in patients with AIDS. J AIDS 17:339, 1998

LOK AS et al: Management of hepatitis B: 2000—summary of a workshop. Gastroenterology 120:1828, 2001

MARTIN DF et al: A controlled trial of valganciclovir as induction therapy for cytomegalovirus retinitis. N Engl J Med 346:1119, 2002

National Institutes of Health Consensus Development Conference Statement: Management of hepatitis C. September 12, 2002 (available at www.niaid.nih.gov)

WHITLEY RJ et al: Herpes simplex encephalitis: Adenine arabinoside versus acyclovir therapies. N Engl J Med 314:144, 1986

Section 12   Infections Due to DNA Viruses

163   HERPES SIMPLEX VIRUSES
Lawrence Corey

DEFINITION Herpes simplex viruses (HSV-1, HSV-2; *Herpesvirus hominis*) produce a variety of infections involving mucocutaneous surfaces, the central nervous system (CNS), and—on occasion—visceral organs. Prompt recognition and treatment reduce the morbidity and mortality of HSV infections.

ETIOLOGIC AGENT The genome of HSV is a linear, double-stranded DNA molecule (molecular weight, $\sim100 \times 10^6$ units) that encodes >90 transcription units with 84 identified proteins. The genomic structures of the two HSV subtypes are similar, and the overall sequence homology between HSV-1 and HSV-2 is $\sim50\%$. The homologous sequences are distributed over the entire genome map, and most of the polypeptides specified by one viral type are antigenically related to polypeptides of the other viral type. Many type-specific regions unique to HSV-1 and HSV-2 proteins do exist, however, and a number of them appear to be important in host immunity. These type-specific regions have been used to develop serologic assays that distinguish between the two viral subtypes. Either restriction endonuclease analysis of viral DNA or DNA sequencing can be used to distinguish between the two subtypes and among strains of each subtype. The variability of nucleotide sequences from clinical strains of HSV-1 and HSV-2 is such that HSV isolates obtained from two individuals can be differentiated by restriction enzyme patterns or genomic sequences unless the isolates are from epidemiologically related sources, such as sexual partners, mother-infant pairs, or persons involved in a common-source outbreak.

The viral genome is packaged in a regular icosahedral protein shell (capsid) composed of 162 capsomers. The outer covering of the virus is a lipid-containing membrane (envelope) derived from modified cell membrane and acquired as the DNA-containing capsid buds through the inner nuclear membrane of the host cell. Between the capsid and lipid bilayer of the envelope is the tegument. Viral replication has both nuclear and cytoplasmic phases. Attachment and fusion between the viral envelope and the cell membrane involve several ubiquitous heparin-like surface receptors. Replication is highly regulated. After fusion and entry, the nucleocapsid enters the cytoplasm and several viral proteins are released from the virion. Some of these viral proteins shut off host protein synthesis (by increasing cellular RNA degradation), while others "turn on" the transcription of early genes of HSV replication. These early gene products, designated α *genes*, are required for synthesis of the subsequent polypeptide group, the β polypeptides, many of which are regulatory proteins and enzymes required for DNA replication. Most current antiviral drugs interfere with β proteins, such as the viral DNA polymerase enzyme. The third (γ) class of HSV genes requires viral DNA replication for expression and constitutes most of the structural proteins specified by the virus.

After replication of the viral genome and synthesis of structural proteins, nucleocapsids are assembled in the nucleus of the cell. Envelopment occurs as the nucleocapsids bud through the inner nuclear membrane into the perinuclear space. In some cells, viral replication in the nucleus forms two types of inclusion bodies: type A basophilic Feulgen-positive bodies that contain viral DNA and an eosinophilic inclusion body that is devoid of viral nucleic acid or protein and represents a "scar" of viral infection. Virions are then transported via the endoplasmic reticulum and the Golgi apparatus to the cell surface.

HSV infection of some neuronal cells does not result in cell death. Instead, viral genomes are maintained by the cell in a repressed state compatible with survival and normal activities of the cell, a condition called *latency*. Latency is associated with transcription of only a limited number of virus-encoded proteins. Subsequently, the viral genome may become activated; its activation results in the normal pattern of regulated viral gene expression, replication, and release of HSV. The release of virus from the neuron and its subsequent entry into epithelial cells result in viral replication and reappearance of virus on mucosal surfaces. This process is termed *reactivation*. Whereas infectious virus is rarely recovered from sensory or autonomic nervous system ganglia dissected from cadavers, maintenance and growth of the neural cells in tissue culture result in production of infectious virions (*explantation*) and in subsequent permissive infection of susceptible cells (*co-cultivation*). The mechanisms by which latency is established, maintained, or recovered are incompletely understood. Two RNA "latency-associated" transcripts that overlap the immediate early (α) gene products, called *ICP-O*, are found in abundance in the nuclei of latently infected neurons. Deletion mutants of this region that can become latent have been made. However, the efficiency of their later reactivation is reduced; thus, the antisense transcripts may play a role in maintaining rather than in establishing latency. Data from animal models suggest that HSV-specific T cell immunity may influence the process of reactivation in neuronal cells. At present, strategies to interrupt latency or to maintain molecular latency in neurons are not available. In experimental animals, ultraviolet light, systemic and local immunosuppression, and trauma to the skin or ganglia are associated with reactivation.

PATHOGENESIS Exposure to HSV at mucosal surfaces or abraded skin sites permits entry of the virus and initiation of its replication in cells of the epidermis and dermis. HSV infections are usually acquired subclinically. Both clinical acquisition and subclinical acquisition are associated with sufficient viral replication to permit infection of either sensory or autonomic nerve endings. On entry into the neuronal cell, the virus—or, more likely, the nucleocapsid—is transported intraaxonally to the nerve cell bodies in ganglia. In humans, the interval from inoculation of virus in peripheral tissue to spread to the ganglia is unknown. During the initial phase of infection, viral replication occurs in ganglia and contiguous neural tissue. Virus then spreads to other mucosal skin surfaces through centrifugal migration of infectious virions via peripheral sensory nerves. This mode of spread helps explain the large surface area involved, the high frequency of new lesions distant from the initial crop of vesicles that is characteristic in patients with primary genital or oral-labial HSV infection, and the recovery of virus from neural tissue distant from neurons innervating the inoculation site. Contiguous spread of locally inoculated virus also may take place and allow further mucosal extension of disease.

Analysis of the DNA from sequentially isolated strains of HSV or from isolates from multiple infected ganglia in any one individual has revealed similar, if not identical, restriction endonuclease or DNA sequence patterns in most persons. Occasionally (most frequently in immunocompromised persons), multiple strains of the same viral subtype are detected in one individual. As exposure to mucosal shedding is relatively common during a person's lifetime, these data suggest that exogenous infection with different strains of the same subtype is possible, albeit very uncommon.

IMMUNITY Host responses to infection with HSV influence the acquisition of disease, the severity of infection, resistance to the development of latency, the maintenance of latency, and the frequency of recurrences. Both antibody-mediated and cell-mediated reactions are clinically important. Immunocompromised patients with defects in cell-mediated immunity experience more severe and more extensive HSV infections than those with deficits in humoral immunity, such as agammaglobulinemia. Experimental ablation of lymphocytes indicates that T cells play a major role in preventing lethal disseminated disease, although antibodies help reduce virus titers in neural tissue. Some of the clinical manifestations of HSV disease appear to be related to the host immune response (e.g., stromal opacities associated with recurrent herpetic keratitis). The surface viral glycoproteins have been shown to be antigens recognized by antibodies mediating neutralization and immune-mediated cytolysis (antibody-dependent cell-mediated cytotoxicity). Monoclonal antibodies specific for each of the known viral glycoproteins have, in experimental infections, conferred protection against subsequent neurologic disease or ganglionic latency. However, the use of subunit glycoprotein vaccines in humans has been, up to the present, only partially successful in reducing acquisition of infection. Multiple cell populations, including natural killer cells, macrophages, and a variety of T lymphocytes, play a role in host defenses against HSV infections, as do lymphokines generated by T lymphocytes. In animals, passive transfer of primed lymphocytes confers protection from subsequent challenge. Maximum protection usually requires the activation of multiple T cell subpopulations, including cytotoxic T cells and T cells responsible for delayed hypersensitivity. The latter cells may confer protection by the antigen-stimulated release of lymphokines (e.g., interferons), which may have a direct antiviral effect and may activate and enhance a variety of specific and nonspecific effector cells. Increasing evidence suggests that HSV-specific CD8+ T cell responses are critical for clearance of virus from lesions. In addition, immunosuppressed patients with frequent and prolonged HSV lesions have fewer functional CD8+ T cells directed at HSV. The HSV virion contains a variety of genes that are directed at the inhibition of host responses. These include gene no. 12 (*US-12*), which can bind to the cellular transporter-activating protein TAP-1 and reduce the ability of this protein to bind HSV peptides to HLA class I, thereby reducing recognition of viral proteins by cytotoxic T cells of the host. This effect can be overcome by the addition of interferon γ, but this reversal requires 24 to 48 h; thus, the virus has time to replicate and invade other host cells. Prior HSV-1 infection appears not to reduce the frequency of acquisition of HSV-2, as measured by seroconversion. However, persons with prior HSV-1 infection who acquire HSV-2 appear to have a higher frequency of subclinical acquisition. These data suggest that type-specific immune responses are central to the control of HSV infection.

EPIDEMIOLOGY Seroepidemiologic studies have documented HSV infections worldwide. Serologic assays with whole-virus antigen preparations, such as complement fixation, neutralization, indirect immunofluorescence, passive hemagglutination, radioimmunoassay, and enzyme-linked immunosorbent assay, are useful for differentiating uninfected (seronegative) persons from those with past HSV-1 or HSV-2 infection, but they do not reliably distinguish between the two viral subtypes. Serologic assays that identify antibodies to type-specific surface proteins (epitopes) of the two viral subtypes have been developed and can distinguish reliably between the human antibody responses to HSV-1 and HSV-2. The most commonly used assays are those that measure antibodies to glycoprotein G of HSV-1 (gG1) and HSV-2 (gG2). A western blot assay that can detect several HSV type-specific proteins can also be used.

Infection with HSV-1 is acquired more frequently and earlier than infection with HSV-2. More than 90% of adults have antibodies to HSV-1 by the fifth decade of life. In populations of low socioeconomic status, most persons acquire HSV-1 infection before the third decade of life.

Antibodies to HSV-2 are not detected routinely until puberty. Antibody prevalence rates correlate with past sexual activity and vary greatly among different population groups. Serosurveys indicate that

~20% of the U.S. population has antibodies to HSV-2. In most routine obstetric and family planning clinics, 25% of women have HSV-2 antibodies, although only 10% report a history of genital lesions. As many as 50% of heterosexual adults attending sexually transmitted disease clinics have antibodies to HSV-2. A wide variety of serologic surveys have indicated a similar or even higher seroprevalence of HSV-2 in most parts of Europe, Central and South America, and Africa. Antibody prevalence rates average ~5% higher among women than among men. Several studies suggest that much of this "asymptomatic" infection is largely unrecognized: when "asymptomatic" seropositive persons are shown pictures of genital lesions, more than 60% subsequently identify episodes of symptomatic reactivation. Most important, these asymptomatic seropositive persons with reactivation shed virus on mucosal surfaces as frequently as those with symptomatic disease. The large reservoir of unidentified carriers of HSV-2 and the frequent asymptomatic reactivation of virus from the genital tract have fostered the continued spread of genital herpes throughout the world. HSV-2 infection is an independent risk factor for the acquisition and transmission of infection with HIV type 1. Among coinfected persons, HIV-1 virions can be shed from herpetic lesions of the genital region. This shedding may facilitate the spread of HIV through sexual contact.

HSV infections occur throughout the year. Transmission can result from contact with persons with active ulcerative lesions or with persons without clinical manifestations of infection who are shedding HSV or on whose mucosal surfaces the virus is replicating. Studies using the polymerase chain reaction (PCR) have shown that HSV reactivation on mucosal surfaces is much more frequent than previously recognized. Among immunocompetent adults, HSV-2 can be isolated by culture from the genital tract on 2 to 10% of days, and HSV DNA can be detected on 20 to 30% of days by PCR. Corresponding figures for HSV-1 in oral secretions are similar. Shedding rates are highest during the initial years after acquisition, and viral shedding may occur on as many as 30 to 50% of days during this period. Immunosuppressed patients shed HSV on mucosal sites at even higher frequency (20 to 70% of days). Daily antiviral chemotherapy can markedly reduce shedding rates, as measured by PCR. These data indicate that potential exposure to HSV from sexual or other close contact (kissing, sharing of glasses or silverware) is common, and these high rates of mucosal reactivation are consistent with the continuing spread and high seroprevalence of HSV infections worldwide.

CLINICAL SPECTRUM HSV has been isolated from nearly all visceral and mucocutaneous sites. The clinical manifestations and course of HSV infection depend on the anatomical site involved, the age and immune status of the host, and the antigenic type of the virus. Primary HSV infections (i.e., first infections with either HSV-1 or HSV-2 in which the host lacks HSV antibodies in acute-phase serum) are frequently accompanied by systemic signs and symptoms. Primary infections involve both mucosal and extramucosal sites; compared with recurrent episodes of disease, they are characterized by a longer duration of symptoms and virus isolation from lesions as well as a higher rate of complications. The incubation period ranges from 1 to 26 days (median, 6 to 8 days). Both viral subtypes can cause genital and oral-facial infections, and the infections caused by the two subtypes are clinically indistinguishable. However, the frequency of reactivation of infection is influenced by anatomical site and virus type. Genital HSV-2 infection is twice as likely to reactivate and recurs 8 to 10 times more frequently than genital HSV-1 infection. Conversely, oral-labial HSV-1 infection recurs more frequently than oral-labial HSV-2 infection. Asymptomatic shedding rates follow the same pattern.

Oral-Facial Infections Gingivostomatitis and pharyngitis are the most frequent clinical manifestations of first-episode HSV-1 infection, while recurrent herpes labialis is the most frequent clinical manifestation of reactivation HSV infection. HSV pharyngitis and gingivostomatitis usually result from primary infection and are most commonly seen in children and young adults. Clinical symptoms and signs, which include fever, malaise, myalgias, inability to eat, irritability, and

cervical adenopathy, may last from 3 to 14 days. Lesions may involve the hard and soft palate, gingiva, tongue, lip, and facial area. HSV-1 or HSV-2 infection of the pharynx usually results in exudative or ulcerative lesions of the posterior pharynx and/or tonsillar pillars. Lesions of the tongue, buccal mucosa, or gingiva may occur later in the course in one-third of cases. Fever lasting from 2 to 7 days and cervical adenopathy are common. It can be difficult to differentiate HSV pharyngitis clinically from bacterial pharyngitis, *Mycoplasma pneumoniae* infections, and pharyngeal ulcerations of noninfectious etiologies (e.g., Stevens-Johnson syndrome). No substantial evidence suggests that reactivation oral-labial HSV infection is associated with symptomatic recurrent pharyngitis.

Reactivation of HSV from the trigeminal ganglia may be associated with asymptomatic virus excretion in the saliva, development of intraoral mucosal ulcerations, or herpetic ulcerations on the vermilion border of the lip or external facial skin. About 50 to 70% of seropositive patients undergoing trigeminal nerve root decompression and 10 to 15% of those undergoing dental extraction develop oral-labial HSV infection a median of 3 days after these procedures.

In immunosuppressed patients, infection may extend into mucosal and deep cutaneous layers. Friability, necrosis, bleeding, severe pain, and inability to eat or drink may result. The lesions of HSV mucositis are clinically similar to mucosal lesions caused by cytotoxic drug therapy, trauma, or fungal or bacterial infections. Persistent ulcerative HSV infections are among the most common infections in patients with AIDS. HSV and *Candida* infections often occur concurrently. Systemic antiviral therapy speeds the rate of healing and relieves the pain of mucosal HSV infections in immunosuppressed patients. The frequency of HSV reactivation during the early phases of transplantation or induction chemotherapy is high (50 to 90%), and prophylactic systemic antiviral agents such as intravenous acyclovir or penciclovir are used to reduce reactivation rates. Patients with atopic eczema may also develop severe oral-facial HSV infections (eczema herpeticum), which may rapidly involve extensive areas of skin and occasionally disseminate to visceral organs. Extensive eczema herpeticum has resolved promptly with the administration of intravenous acyclovir. Erythema multiforme may also be associated with HSV infections (see Fig. 46-9); some evidence suggests that HSV infection is the precipitating event in ~75% of cases of cutaneous erythema multiforme. HSV antigen has been demonstrated both in circulatory immune complexes and in skin lesion biopsy samples from these cases. Patients with severe HSV-associated erythema multiforme are candidates for chronic suppressive oral antiviral therapy.

HSV-1 and varicella-zoster virus (VZV) have been implicated in the etiology of Bell's palsy (flaccid paralysis of the mandibular portion of the facial nerve). Although uniform recommendations for treatment of this entity are not available, recent evidence suggests that antiviral chemotherapy, usually with a short course of glucocorticoids, may improve outcome.

Genital Infections First-episode primary genital herpes is characterized by fever, headache, malaise, and myalgias. Pain, itching, dysuria, vaginal and urethral discharge, and tender inguinal lymphadenopathy are the predominant local symptoms. Widely spaced bilateral lesions of the external genitalia are characteristic (Fig. 163-1). Lesions may be present in varying stages, including vesicles, pustules, or painful erythematous ulcers. The cervix and urethra are involved in >80% of women with first-episode infections. First episodes of genital herpes in patients who have had prior HSV-1 infection are associated with less frequent systemic symptoms and faster healing than primary genital herpes. The clinical courses of acute first-episode genital herpes among patients with HSV-1 and HSV-2 infections are similar. However, the recurrence rates of genital disease differ with the viral subtype: the 12-month recurrence rates among patients with first-episode HSV-2 and HSV-1 infections are ~90% and ~55%, respectively (median number of recurrences, 4 and <1, respectively). Recurrence rates

FIGURE 163-1   Bilateral serpiginous ulcerative lesions of the labia minora and majora in a woman with extensive primary genital HSV-2 infection.

for genital HSV-2 infections vary greatly among individuals and over time within the same individual. HSV has been isolated from the urethra and urine of men and women without external genital lesions. A clear mucoid discharge and dysuria are characteristics of symptomatic HSV urethritis. HSV has been isolated from the urethra of 5% of women with the dysuria-frequency syndrome. Occasionally, HSV genital tract disease is manifested by endometritis and salpingitis in women and by prostatitis in men. About 15% of cases of HSV-2 acquisition are associated with these nonlesional clinical syndromes, such as aseptic meningitis, cervicitis, or urethritis. →*A more complete discussion of the differential diagnosis of genital herpes is presented in Chap. 115.*

Both HSV-1 and HSV-2 can cause symptomatic or asymptomatic rectal and perianal infections. HSV proctitis is usually associated with rectal intercourse. However, subclinical perianal shedding of HSV is detected both in heterosexual men and in women who report no rectal intercourse. This phenomenon is due to the establishment of latency in the sacral dermatome from prior genital tract infection, with subsequent reactivation in epithelial cells in the perianal region. Such reactivations are often subclinical. Symptoms of HSV proctitis include anorectal pain, anorectal discharge, tenesmus, and constipation. Sigmoidoscopy reveals ulcerative lesions of the distal 10 cm of the rectal mucosa. Rectal biopsies show mucosal ulceration, necrosis, polymorphonuclear and lymphocytic infiltration of the lamina propria, and (in occasional cases) multinucleated intranuclear inclusion–bearing cells. Perianal herpetic lesions are also found in immunosuppressed patients receiving cytotoxic therapy. Extensive perianal herpetic lesions and/or HSV proctitis is common among patients with HIV infection.

Herpetic Whitlow   Herpetic whitlow—HSV infection of the finger—may occur as a complication of primary oral or genital herpes by inoculation of virus through a break in the epidermal surface or by direct introduction of virus into the hand through occupational or some other type of exposure. Clinical signs and symptoms include the abrupt onset of edema, erythema, and localized tenderness of the infected finger. Vesicular or pustular lesions of the fingertip that are indistinguishable from lesions of pyogenic bacterial infection are seen. Fever, lymphadenitis, and epitrochlear and axillary lymphadenopathy are common. The infection may recur. Prompt diagnosis (to avoid unnecessary and potentially exacerbating surgical therapy and/or transmission) is essential. Antiviral chemotherapy (to speed the healing of the process) is usually recommended (see below).

Herpes Gladiatorum   HSV may infect almost any area of skin. Mucocutaneous HSV infections of the thorax, ears, face, and hands have been described among wrestlers. Transmission of these infections is facilitated by trauma to the skin sustained during wrestling. Several recent outbreaks of this infection have illustrated the importance of prompt diagnosis and therapy, which are required to contain the spread of this infection.

Eye Infections   HSV infection of the eye is the most frequent cause of corneal blindness in the United States. HSV keratitis presents with an acute onset of pain, blurring of vision, chemosis, conjunctivitis, and characteristic dendritic lesions of the cornea. Use of topical glucocorticoids may exacerbate symptoms and lead to involvement of deep structures of the eye. Debridement, topical antiviral treatment, and/or interferon therapy hastens healing. However, recurrences are common, and the deeper structures of the eye may sustain immunopathologic injury. Stromal keratitis due to HSV appears to be related to T cell–dependent destruction of deep corneal tissue. An HSV-1 epitope that is autoreactive with T cell–targeting corneal antigens has been postulated to be a factor in this infection. Chorioretinitis, usually a manifestation of disseminated HSV infection, may occur in neonates or in patients with HIV infection. HSV and VZV can cause acute necrotizing retinitis as an uncommon but severe manifestation.

Central and Peripheral Nervous System Infections   HSV accounts for 10 to 20% of all cases of sporadic viral encephalitis in the United States. The estimated incidence is ~2.3 cases per 1 million persons per year. Cases are distributed throughout the year, and the age distribution appears to be biphasic, with peaks at 5 to 30 and >50 years of age. Subtype 1 virus causes >95% of cases of HSV encephalitis.

The pathogenesis of HSV encephalitis varies. In children and young adults, primary HSV infection may result in encephalitis; presumably, exogenously acquired virus enters the CNS by neurotropic spread from the periphery via the olfactory bulb. However, most adults with HSV encephalitis have clinical or serologic evidence of mucocutaneous HSV-1 infection before the onset of the CNS symptoms. In ~25% of the cases examined, the HSV-1 strains from the oropharynx and brain tissue of the same patient differ; thus some cases may result from reinfection with another strain of HSV-1 that reaches the CNS. Two theories have been proposed to explain the development of actively replicating HSV in localized areas of the CNS in persons whose ganglionic and CNS isolates are similar. Reactivation of latent HSV-1 infection in trigeminal or autonomic nerve roots may be associated with extension of virus into the CNS via nerves innervating the middle cranial fossa. HSV DNA has been demonstrated by DNA hybridization in brain tissue obtained at autopsy—even from healthy adults. Thus, reactivation of long-standing latent CNS infection may be another mechanism for the development of HSV encephalitis.

The clinical hallmark of HSV encephalitis has been the acute onset of fever and focal neurologic symptoms and signs, especially in the temporal lobe (Fig. 163-2). Clinical differentiation of HSV encephalitis from other viral encephalitides, focal infections, or noninfectious processes is difficult. The most sensitive noninvasive method for early diagnosis of HSV encephalitis is the demonstration of HSV DNA in cerebrospinal fluid (CSF) by PCR. Although titers of CSF and serum antibodies to HSV increase in most cases of HSV encephalitis, they rarely do so earlier than 10 days into the illness and therefore, while useful retrospectively, are generally not helpful in establishing an early clinical diagnosis. Demonstration of HSV antigen, HSV DNA, or HSV replication in brain tissue obtained by biopsy is highly sensitive and has a low complication rate; examination of such tissue also provides the best opportunity to identify alternative, potentially treatable causes of encephalitis. Antiviral chemotherapy reduces the rate of death from HSV encephalitis. Intravenous acyclovir is more effective than vidarabine. Even with therapy, however, neurologic sequelae are frequent, especially in persons >50 years of age. Most authorities recommend the administration of intravenous acyclovir to patients with presumed HSV encephalitis until the diagnosis is confirmed or an alternative diagnosis is made. Among proven cases of HSV encephalitis, intravenous therapy is usually recommended until HSV DNA levels in CSF are substantially reduced or at nearly undetectable levels.

HSV DNA has been detected in CSF from 3 to 15% of persons presenting to the hospital with aseptic meningitis. HSV meningitis, which is usually seen in association with primary genital HSV infection, is an acute, self-limited disease manifested by headache, fever, and mild photophobia and lasting from 2 to 7 days. Lymphocytic pleocytosis in the CSF is characteristic. Neurologic sequelae of HSV meningitis are rare. HSV is the most commonly identified cause of recurrent lymphocytic meningitis (Mollaret's meningitis). Demonstration of HSV antibodies in CSF or persistence of HSV DNA in CSF can establish the diagnosis. For persons with frequent recurrences of HSV meningitis, antiviral therapy has been successful in reducing the frequency of such episodes.

FIGURE 163-2 Computed tomographic and diffusion-weighted magnetic resonance scans of the brain of a patient with left-temporal-lobe HSV encephalitis.

Autonomic nervous system dysfunction, especially of the sacral region, has been reported in association with both HSV and VZV infections. Numbness, tingling of the buttocks or perineal areas, urinary retention, constipation, CSF pleocytosis, and (in males) impotence may occur. Symptoms appear to resolve slowly over days to weeks. Occasionally, hypesthesia and/or weakness of the lower extremities may persist for many months. Rarely, transverse myelitis manifested by a rapidly progressive symmetric paralysis of the lower extremities or a Guillain-Barré syndrome may follow HSV infection. Similarly, peripheral nervous system involvement (Bell's palsy) or cranial polyneuritis may also be related to reactivation of HSV-1 infection. Transitory hypesthesia of the area of skin innervated by the trigeminal nerve and vestibular system dysfunction as measured by electronystagmography are the predominant signs of disease. Studies to determine whether antiviral chemotherapy may abort these signs or reduce their frequency and severity are unavailable.

Visceral Infections   HSV infection of visceral organs usually results from viremia, and multiple-organ involvement is common. Occasionally, however, the clinical manifestations of HSV infection involve only the esophagus, lung, or liver. HSV esophagitis may result from direct extension of oral-pharyngeal HSV infection into the esophagus or may occur de novo by reactivation and spread of HSV to the esophageal mucosa via the vagus nerve. The predominant symptoms of HSV esophagitis are odynophagia, dysphagia, substernal pain, and weight loss. There are multiple oval ulcerations on an erythematous base with or without a patchy white pseudomembrane. The distal esophagus is most commonly involved. With extensive disease, diffuse friability may spread to the entire esophagus. Neither endoscopic nor barium examination can reliably differentiate HSV esophagitis from *Candida* esophagitis or from esophageal ulcerations due to thermal injury, radiation, or corrosives. Endoscopically obtained secretions for cytologic examination and culture provide the most useful material for diagnosis. Systemic antiviral chemotherapy usually reduces symptoms and heals esophageal ulcerations.

HSV pneumonitis is uncommon except in severely immunosuppressed patients and may result from extension of herpetic tracheobronchitis into lung parenchyma. Focal necrotizing pneumonitis usually ensues. Hematogenous dissemination of virus from sites of oral or genital mucocutaneous disease may also occur and produce bilateral interstitial pneumonitis. Bacterial, fungal, and parasitic pathogens are commonly present in HSV pneumonitis. The mortality rate from untreated HSV pneumonia in immunosuppressed patients is high (>80%). HSV has also been isolated from the lower respiratory tract of persons with adult respiratory distress syndrome. However, the re-

lationship between the isolation of HSV and the pathogenesis of this syndrome is unclear.

HSV is an uncommon cause of hepatitis in immunocompetent patients. HSV infection of the liver is associated with fever, abrupt elevations of bilirubin and serum aminotransferase levels, and leukopenia (<4000 white blood cells per microliter). Disseminated intravascular coagulation may also develop.

Other reported complications of HSV infection include monarticular arthritis, adrenal necrosis, idiopathic thrombocytopenia, and glomerulonephritis. Disseminated HSV infection in immunocompetent patients is rare. In immunocompromised, burned, or malnourished patients, HSV occasionally disseminates to other visceral organs, such as the adrenal glands, pancreas, small and large intestines, and bone marrow. Rarely, primary HSV infection in pregnancy disseminates and may be associated with the death of both mother and fetus. This uncommon event is usually related to the acquisition of primary infection in the third trimester.

Neonatal HSV Infection   Of all HSV-infected populations, neonates (infants younger than 6 weeks) have the highest frequency of visceral and/or CNS infection. Without therapy, the overall rate of death from neonatal herpes is 65%; <10% of neonates with CNS infection develop normally. Although skin lesions are the most commonly recognized features of disease, many infants do not develop lesions until well into the course of disease. Neonatal infection is usually acquired perinatally from contact with infected genital secretions at the time of delivery. Congenitally infected infants have been reported. In most series, 30% of neonatal HSV infections are due to HSV-1 and 70% to HSV-2. The risk of developing neonatal HSV infection is 10 times higher for an infant born to a mother who has recently acquired HSV than for other infants. Neonatal HSV-1 infections may also be acquired through postnatal contact with immediate family members who have symptomatic or asymptomatic oral-labial HSV-1 infection or through nosocomial transmission within the hospital. All neonates with presumed neonatal herpes should be treated with intravenous acyclovir (see below). Antiviral chemotherapy has reduced the rate of death from neonatal herpes to 25%. However, the rate of morbidity, especially among infants with HSV-2 infection involving the CNS, is still very high.

DIAGNOSIS   Both clinical and laboratory criteria are useful for establishing the diagnosis of HSV infections. A clinical diagnosis can be made accurately when characteristic multiple vesicular lesions on an erythematous base are present. However, it is increasingly being recognized that herpetic ulcerations may clinically resemble skin ulcerations of other etiologies. Mucosal HSV infections may also present as urethritis or pharyngitis without cutaneous lesions. Thus, laboratory studies to confirm the diagnosis and to guide therapy are recommended. While staining of scrapings from the base of the lesions with Wright's, Giemsa's (Tzanck preparation), or Papanicolaou's stain to detect giant cells or intranuclear inclusions of *Herpesvirus* infection is a well-described procedure, few clinicians are skilled in these techniques. Moreover, these cytologic methods do not differentiate between HSV and VZV infections.

HSV infection is best confirmed in the laboratory by isolation of the virus in tissue culture or by demonstration of HSV antigens or DNA in scrapings from lesions. HSV causes a discernible cytopathic effect in a variety of cell culture systems, and this effect can be identified within 48 to 96 h after inoculation. Spin-amplified culture with subsequent staining for HSV antigen has shortened the time needed to identify HSV to <24 h. Increasingly, PCR is being used for the detection of HSV DNA, and several studies have shown this assay to be more sensitive than culture for detection of HSV in CSF and at mucosal sites. The sensitivity of viral isolation and of antigen or DNA detection depends on the stage of the lesions (with higher sensitivity in vesicular than in ulcerative lesions), on whether the patient has a first or a recurrent episode of the disease (with higher sensitivity in first than in recurrent episodes), and on whether the sample is from an immunosuppressed or an immunocompetent patient (with more antigen in immunosuppressed patients). Laboratory confirmation permits subtyping of the virus; information on subtype may be useful epidemiologically and may help to predict the frequency of reactivation after first-episode oral-labial or genital HSV infection.

Acute- and convalescent-phase serum can be useful in demonstrating seroconversion during primary HSV-1 or HSV-2 infection. However, only 5% of patients with recurrent mucocutaneous HSV infections have a fourfold or greater rise in titer of antibody to HSV in the interval between the collection of the first and second samples. Serologic assays, especially type-specific assays, should be used to identify asymptomatic carriers of HSV-1 or HSV-2 infection.

Several studies have shown that persons seropositive for HSV-2 to whom the clinical manifestations of HSV have been explained are able to identify symptomatic reactivations. Individuals seropositive for HSV-2 should be told about the high frequency of subclinical reactivation in mucosal surfaces not visible to the eye (e.g., cervix, urethra, perianal skin) or in microscopic ulcerations that may not be clinically symptomatic. Transmission of infection during such episodes is well established. HSV-2-seropositive persons should be educated about the high likelihood of subclinical shedding and the role condoms (male or female) may play in reducing transmission. Antiviral therapy with the drug valacyclovir (500 mg once daily) has been shown to reduce the transmission of HSV-2 between sexual partners.

℞ TREATMENT

Many aspects of mucocutaneous and visceral HSV infections are amenable to antiviral chemotherapy. For mucocutaneous infections, acyclovir and its congeners famciclovir and valacyclovir have been the mainstay of therapy. Several antiviral agents are available for topical use in HSV eye infections: idoxuridine, trifluorothymidine, topical vidarabine, and cidofovir. For HSV encephalitis and neonatal herpes, intravenous acyclovir is the treatment of choice.

All licensed antiviral agents for use against HSV inhibit the viral DNA polymerase. One class of drugs, typified by the drug acyclovir, is made up of substrates for the HSV enzyme thymidine kinase. Acyclovir, ganciclovir, famciclovir, and valacyclovir are all selectively phosphorylated to the monophosphate form in virus-infected cells. Cellular enzymes convert the monophosphate form of the drug to the triphosphate, which is then incorporated into the viral DNA chain.

Acyclovir is the most frequently used agent for the treatment of HSV infections and is available in intravenous, oral, and topical formulations. Valacyclovir is the valyl ester of acyclovir and offers greater bioavailability than acyclovir. Famciclovir, the oral formulation of penciclovir, is clinically effective in the treatment of a variety of HSV-1 and HSV-2 infections. Ganciclovir is active against both HSV-1 and HSV-2; however, it is more toxic than acyclovir, valacyclovir, and famciclovir and generally is not recommended for the treatment of HSV infections.

All three recommended compounds—acyclovir, valacyclovir, and famciclovir—have proven effective in shortening the duration of symptoms and lesions of mucocutaneous HSV infections in both immunocompromised and immunocompetent patients (Table 163-1). Intravenous and oral formulations prevent reactivation of HSV in seropositive immunocompromised patients during induction chemotherapy or in the period immediately after bone marrow or solid organ transplantation. Chronic daily suppressive therapy reduces the frequency of reactivation disease among patients with frequent genital or oral-labial herpes. Only valacyclovir has been shown to reduce transmission of HSV-2 infection between sexual partners.

Intravenous acyclovir (30 mg/kg per day, given as a 10-mg/kg infusion over 1 h at 8-h intervals) is effective in reducing rates of death and morbidity from HSV encephalitis. Early initiation of therapy is a critical factor in outcome. The major side effect associated with intravenous acyclovir is transient renal insufficiency, usually due to crystallization of the compound in the renal parenchyma. This adverse reaction can be avoided if the medication is given slowly over 1 h and the patient is well hydrated. Because CSF levels of acyclovir average only 30 to 50% of plasma levels, the dosage of acyclovir used for treatment of CNS infection (30 mg/kg per day) is double that used for treatment of mucocutaneous or visceral disease (15 mg/kg per day). Even higher doses of intravenous acyclovir are used for neonatal HSV infection (60 mg/kg per day in 3 divided doses).

Among immunocompetent patients, recent studies have shown the effectiveness of short-course oral therapy to reduce the signs and symptoms of oral and genital HSV infection. These regimens include valacyclovir (1 or 3 days) for oral-labial HSV and acyclovir (2 days) or valacyclovir (3 days) for recurrent-episode genital herpes (Table 163-1).

Suppression of Mucocutaneous Herpes   Recognition of the high frequency of subclinical reactivation has provided an ever-greater rationale for the use of daily antiviral therapy to suppress reactivations of HSV, especially in persons with frequent clinical reactivations (e.g., those with recently acquired genital HSV infection). Immunosuppressed persons, including those with HIV infection, may also benefit from daily antiviral therapy. Of the various regimens used, famciclovir (500 mg twice daily) and valacyclovir (1 g twice daily) are two of the most common; valacyclovir at a dose of 4 g daily was associated with thrombotic thrombocytopenic purpura in one study of HIV-infected persons.

Reduction in Transmission of HSV to Sexual Partners   Once-daily valacyclovir (500 mg) has been shown to reduce transmission of HSV-2 between sexual partners. Transmission rates are higher from males to females and among persons with frequent HSV-2 reactivation. Serologic screening can be used to identify at-risk couples.

Acyclovir Resistance   Acyclovir-resistant strains of HSV have been identified. Most of these strains have an altered substrate specificity for phosphorylating acyclovir. Thus, cross-resistance to famciclovir and valacyclovir is usually found. Occasionally, an isolate with altered thymidine kinase (TK) specificity arises and is sensitive to famciclovir but not to acyclovir. In some patients infected with TK-deficient virus, higher doses of acyclovir are associated with clearing of lesions. In others, clinical disease progresses despite high-dose therapy. Almost all clinically significant acyclovir resistance has been seen in immunocompromised patients, and HSV-2 isolates are more often resistant than HSV-1 strains. A study by the Centers for Disease Control and Prevention indicated that ~5% of HSV-2 isolates from HIV-positive persons exhibit some degree of in vitro resistance to acyclovir. Among immunocompetent patients attending sexually transmitted disease clin-

TABLE 163-1 *Antiviral Chemotherapy for HSV Infection*

I. Mucocutaneous HSV infections
  A. Infections in immunosuppressed patients:
    1. Acute symptomatic first or recurrent episodes: IV acyclovir (5 mg/kg q8h) or oral acyclovir (400 mg qid), famciclovir (500 mg tid), or valacyclovir (500 mg bid). Treatment duration may vary from 7 to 14 days.
    2. Suppression of reactivation disease: IV acyclovir (5 mg/kg q8h) or oral valacyclovir (500 mg bid) or acyclovir (400–800 mg 3–5 times per day) prevents recurrences during the 30-day period immediately after transplantation. Longer-term HSV suppression is often used for persons with continued immunosuppression. In bone marrow and renal transplant recipients, oral valacyclovir (2 g/d) is also effective in preventing cytomegalovirus infection. Oral valacyclovir at a dose of 4 g/d has been associated with thrombotic thrombocytopenic purpura after extended use in HIV-positive persons. In HIV-infected persons, oral famciclovir (500 mg bid) is effective in reducing clinical and subclinical reactivations of HSV-1 and HSV-2.
  B. Genital herpes:
    1. First episodes: Oral acyclovir (200 mg 5 times per day or 400 mg tid), valacyclovir (1 g bid), or famciclovir (250 mg bid) for 10–14 days is effective. IV acyclovir (5 mg/kg q8h for 5 days) is given for severe disease or neurologic complications such as aseptic meningitis.
    2. Symptomatic recurrent genital herpes: Oral acyclovir (200 mg 5 times per day for 5 days, 800 mg tid for 2 days), valacyclovir (500 mg bid for 3 or 5 days), or famciclovir (125 mg bid for 5 days) is effective in shortening lesion duration.
    3. Suppression of recurrent genital herpes: Oral acyclovir (200-mg capsules tid or qid, 400 mg bid, or 800 mg qd), famciclovir (250 mg bid), or valacyclovir (500 mg or 1 g qd or 500 mg bid) prevents symptomatic reactivation. Persons with frequent reactivation but <9 episodes per year can take valacyclovir (500 mg PO daily); those with >9 episodes per year should take 1 g PO daily or 500 mg PO bid.
  C. Oral-labial HSV infections:
    1. First episode: Oral acyclovir (200 mg) is given 4 or 5 times per day. Oral famciclovir (250 mg bid) or valacyclovir (1 g bid) has been used clinically.
    2. Recurrent episodes: Oral valacyclovir (1 g bid for 1 day or 500 mg bid for 3 days) is effective in reducing pain and speeding healing. Self-initiated therapy with 6-times-daily topical penciclovir cream is effective in speeding the healing of oral-labial HSV. Topical acyclovir cream has also been shown to speed healing.
    3. Suppression of reactivation of oral-labial HSV: Oral acyclovir (400 mg bid), if started before exposure and continued for the duration of exposure (usually 5–10 days), will prevent reactivation of recurrent oral-labial HSV infection associated with severe sun exposure.
  D. Herpetic whitlow: Oral acyclovir (200 mg) is given 5 times daily for 7–10 days.
  E. HSV proctitis: Oral acyclovir (400 mg 5 times per day) is useful in shortening the course of infection. In immunosuppressed patients or in patients with severe infection, IV acyclovir (5 mg/kg q8h) may be useful.
  F. Herpetic eye infections: In acute keratitis, topical trifluorothymidine, vidarabine, idoxuridine, acyclovir, penciclovir, and interferon are all beneficial. Debridement may be required; topical steroids may worsen disease.
II. CNS HSV infections
  A. HSV encephalitis: IV acyclovir (10 mg/kg q8h; 30 mg/kg per day) for at least 10 days.
  B. HSV aseptic meningitis: No studies of systemic antiviral chemotherapy exist. If therapy is to be given, IV acyclovir (15–30 mg/kg per day) should be used.
  C. Autonomic radiculopathy: No studies are available. Most authorities recommend a trial of IV acyclovir.
III. Neonatal HSV infections
  Oral acyclovir (60 mg/kg per day, divided into 3 doses) is given. The recommended duration of treatment is 21 days. Monitoring for relapse should be undertaken, and some authorities recommend continued suppression with oral acyclovir suspension for 3 to 4 months.
IV. Visceral HSV infections
  A. HSV esophagitis: IV acyclovir (15 mg/kg per day). In some patients with milder forms of immunosuppression, oral therapy with valacyclovir or famciclovir is effective.
  B. HSV pneumonitis: No controlled studies exist. IV acyclovir (15 mg/kg per day) should be considered.
V. Disseminated HSV infections
  No controlled studies exist. Intravenous acyclovir nevertheless should be tried. No definite evidence indicates that therapy will decrease the risk of death.
VI. Erythema multiforme–associated HSV
  Anecdotal observations suggest that oral acyclovir (400 mg bid or tid) or valacyclovir (500 mg bid) will suppress erythema multiforme.
VII. Surgical prophylaxis
  Several surgical procedures (e.g., laser skin resurfacing, trigeminal nerve root decompression, and lumbar disk surgery) have been associated with HSV reactivation. Intravenous or oral acyclovir (800 mg bid) or oral valacyclovir (500 mg bid) or famciclovir (250 mg bid) is effective in reducing reactivation. Therapy should be initiated 48 h before surgery and continued for 3–7 days.
VIII. Infections due to acyclovir-resistant HSV
  IV foscarnet (40 mg/kg q8h) should be given until lesions heal. The optimal duration of therapy and the usefulness of its continuation to suppress lesions are unclear. Some patients may benefit from cutaneous application of trifluorothymidine or 5% cidofovir gel.

ics, <0.5% of HSV-2 isolates show reduced in vitro sensitivity to acyclovir. The lack of appreciable change in the frequency of detection of such isolates in the past 20 years probably reflects the reduced transmission of TK-deficient mutants. Isolation of HSV from lesions persisting despite adequate dosages and blood levels of acyclovir should raise the suspicion of acyclovir resistance. Therapy with the antiviral drug foscarnet is useful (Chap. 162). Because of its toxicity and cost, this drug is usually reserved for patients with extensive mucocutaneous infections. Cidofovir is a nucleotide analogue and exists as a phosphonate or monophosphate form. Most TK-deficient strains of HSV are sensitive to cidofovir. Cidofovir ointment speeds healing of acyclovir-resistant lesions. No well-controlled trials of systemic cidofovir have been reported. True TK-negative variants of HSV appear to have a reduced capacity to spread because of altered neurovirulence—a feature important in the relatively infrequent presence of such strains in immunocompetent populations, even with increasing use of antiviral drugs.

PREVENTION The success of efforts to control HSV disease on a population basis through suppressive antiviral chemotherapy and/or educational programs will be limited.

Barrier forms of contraception (especially condoms) decrease the likelihood of transmission of HSV infection, particularly during periods of asymptomatic viral excretion. When lesions are present, HSV infection may be transmitted by skin-to-skin contact despite the use of a condom. Nevertheless, the available data suggest that consistent condom use is an effective means of reducing the risk of genital HSV-2 transmission. Recent studies have shown that chronic daily antiviral therapy with valacyclovir can also be partially effective in reducing acquisition of HSV-2, especially among susceptible women. There are no comparative efficacy studies of valacyclovir versus condom use. Most authorities suggest both approaches. Several candidate HSV vaccines are under investigation.

Prevention of neonatal HSV requires the prevention of acquisition of HSV by women in the third trimester of pregnancy. Identification of women or couples susceptible to acquisition of HSV in pregnancy through serologic screening is receiving increasing attention, and such screening is being used with increasing frequency.

FURTHER READING

BROWN ZA et al: The acquisition of herpes simplex virus during pregnancy. N Engl J Med 337:509, 1997

CHILUKURI S, ROSEN T: Management of acyclovir-resistant herpes simplex virus. Dermatol Clin 21:311, 2003

LANGENBERG AGM et al: A prospective study of new infections with herpes simplex virus type 1 and herpes simplex virus type 2. N Engl J Med 341:1532, 1999

LEONE PA et al: Valacyclovir for episodic treatment of genital herpes: A shorter 3-day treatment course compared with 5-day treatment. Clin Infect Dis 34:958, 2002

RABORN GW et al: Effective treatment of herpes simplex labialis with pen-ciclovir cream: Combined results of two trials. J Am Dent Assoc 133:303, 2002

REYES M et al: Acyclovir-resistant genital herpes among persons attending sexually transmitted disease and human immunodeficiency virus clinics. Arch Intern Med 163:76, 2003

SCHACKER T et al: Frequent recovery of HIV-1 from genital herpes simplex virus lesions in HIV-1-infected men. JAMA 280:61, 1998

SPRUANCE SL et al: High-dose, short-duration, early valacyclovir therapy for episodic treatment of cold sores: Results of two randomized, placebo-controlled, multicenter studies. Antimicrob Agents Chemother 47:1072, 2003

WALD A et al: Effect of condoms on reducing the transmission of herpes simplex virus type 2 from men to women. JAMA 285:3100, 2002

——— et al: Frequent genital herpes simplex virus 2 shedding in immuno-competent women: Effect of acyclovir treatment. J Clin Invest 99:1092, 1997

184   VARICELLA-ZOSTER VIRUS INFECTIONS
Richard J. Whitley

DEFINITION   Varicella-zoster virus (VZV) causes two distinct clinical entities: varicella (chickenpox) and herpes zoster (shingles). Chickenpox, a ubiquitous and extremely contagious infection, is usually a benign illness of childhood characterized by an exanthematous vesicular rash. With reactivation of latent VZV (which is most common after the sixth decade of life), herpes zoster presents as a dermatomal vesicular rash, usually associated with severe pain.

ETIOLOGY   A clinical association between varicella and herpes zoster has been recognized for nearly 100 years. Early in the twentieth century, similarities in the histopathologic features of skin lesions resulting from varicella and herpes zoster were demonstrated. Viral isolates from patients with chickenpox and herpes zoster produced similar alterations in tissue culture—specifically, the appearance of eosinophilic intranuclear inclusions and multinucleated giant cells. These results suggested that the viruses were biologically similar. Restriction endonuclease analyses of viral DNA from a patient with chickenpox who subsequently developed herpes zoster verified the molecular identity of the two viruses responsible for these different clinical presentations.

VZV is a member of the family Herpesviridae, sharing with other members such structural characteristics as a lipid envelope surrounding a nucleocapsid with icosahedral symmetry, a total diameter of ~180 to 200 nm, and centrally located double-stranded DNA that is ~125,000 bp in length.

PATHOGENESIS AND PATHOLOGY   ■   **Primary Infection**   Transmission is most likely to take place by the respiratory route; the subsequent localized replication of the virus at an undefined site (presumably the nasopharynx) leads to seeding of the reticuloendothelial system and ultimately to the development of viremia. Viremia in patients with chickenpox is reflected in the diffuse and scattered nature of the skin lesions and can be verified in selected cases by the recovery of VZV from the blood or routinely by polymerase chain reaction (PCR). Vesicles involve the corium and dermis, with degenerative changes characterized by ballooning, the presence of multinucleated giant cells, and eosinophilic intranuclear inclusions. Infection may involve localized blood vessels of the skin, resulting in necrosis and epidermal hemorrhage. With the evolution of disease, the vesicular fluid becomes cloudy because of the recruitment of polymorphonuclear leukocytes and the presence of degenerated cells and fibrin. Ultimately, the vesicles either rupture and release their fluid (which includes infectious virus) or are gradually reabsorbed.

Recurrent Infection   The mechanism of reactivation of VZV that results in herpes zoster is unknown. Presumably, the virus infects the dorsal root ganglia during chickenpox, where it remains latent until reactivated. Histopathologic examination of representative dorsal root ganglia during active herpes zoster demonstrates hemorrhage, edema, and lymphocytic infiltration.

Active replication of VZV in other organs, such as the lung or the brain, can occur during either chickenpox or herpes zoster but is uncommon in the immunocompetent host. Pulmonary involvement is characterized by interstitial pneumonitis, multinucleated giant cell formation, intranuclear inclusions, and pulmonary hemorrhage. Central nervous system (CNS) infection leads to histopathologic evidence of perivascular cuffing similar to that encountered in measles and other viral encephalitides. Focal hemorrhagic necrosis of the brain, characteristic of herpes simplex virus encephalitis, is uncommon in VZV infection.

EPIDEMIOLOGY AND CLINICAL MANIFESTATIONS   ■   **Chickenpox**   Humans are the only known reservoir for VZV. Chickenpox is highly contagious, with an attack rate of at least 90% among susceptible (seronegative) individuals. Persons of both sexes and all races are infected equally often. The virus is endemic in the population at large; however, it becomes epidemic among susceptible individuals during seasonal peaks—namely, late winter and early spring in the temperate zone. Historically, children between the ages of 5 and 9 are most commonly affected and account for 50% of all cases. Most other cases involve children aged 1 to 4 and those aged 10 to 14. Approximately 10% of the population of the United States over the age of 15 is susceptible to infection. VZV vaccination during the second year of life is dramatically changing the epidemiology of infection.

The incubation period of chickenpox ranges from 10 to 21 days but is usually between 14 and 17 days. Secondary attack rates in susceptible siblings within a household are between 70 and 90%. Patients are infectious ~48 h prior to the onset of the vesicular rash, during the period of vesicle formation (which generally lasts 4 to 5 days), and until all vesicles are crusted.

Clinically, chickenpox presents as a rash, low-grade fever, and malaise, although a few patients develop a prodrome 1 to 2 days before onset of the exanthem. In the immunocompetent patient, this is usually a benign illness that is associated with lassitude and with body temperatures of 37.8° to 39.4°C (100° to 103°F) of 3 to 5 days' duration. The skin lesions—the hallmark of the infection—include maculopapules, vesicles, and scabs in various stages of evolution (Fig. 164-1). These lesions, which evolve from maculopapules to vesicles over hours to days, appear on the trunk and face and rapidly spread to involve other areas of the body. Most are small and have an erythematous base with a diameter of 5 to 10 mm. Successive crops appear over a 2- to 4-day period. Lesions can also be found on the mucosa of the pharynx and/or the vagina. Their severity varies from one person to another. Some individuals have very few lesions, while others have

FIGURE 164-1   Numerous varicella lesions at various stages of evolution: vesicles on an erythematous base, umbilical vesicles, and crusts.

as many as 2000. Younger children tend to have fewer vesicles than older individuals. Secondary and tertiary cases within families are associated with a relatively large number of vesicles. Immunocompromised patients—both children and adults, particularly those with leukemia—have lesions (often with a hemorrhagic base) that are more numerous and take longer to heal than those of immunocompetent patients. Immunocompromised individuals are also at greater risk for visceral complications, which occur in 30 to 50% of cases and are fatal 15% of the time in the absence of antiviral therapy.

The most common infectious complication of varicella is secondary bacterial superinfection of the skin, which is usually caused by *Streptococcus pyogenes* or *Staphylococcus aureus*. This complication may result from excoriation of skin lesions after scratching. Gram's staining of skin lesions should help clarify the etiology of unusually erythematous and pustulated lesions.

The most common extracutaneous site of involvement in children is the CNS. The syndrome of acute cerebellar ataxia and meningeal irritation generally appears ~21 days after the onset of the rash and rarely develops in the preeruptive phase. The cerebrospinal fluid (CSF) contains lymphocytes and elevated levels of protein. CNS involvement is a benign complication of VZV infection in children and generally does not require hospitalization. Aseptic meningitis, encephalitis, transverse myelitis, Guillain-Barré syndrome, and Reye's syndrome can also occur. Encephalitis is reported in 0.1 to 0.2% of children with chickenpox. Other than supportive care, no specific therapy is available for patients with CNS involvement.

Varicella pneumonia is the most serious complication following chickenpox, developing more commonly in adults (up to 20% of cases) than in children. It usually has its onset 3 to 5 days into the illness and is associated with tachypnea, cough, dyspnea, and fever. Cyanosis, pleuritic chest pain, and hemoptysis are frequent. Roentgenographic evidence of disease consists of nodular infiltrates and interstitial pneumonitis. Resolution of pneumonitis parallels improvement of the skin rash; however, patients may have persistent fever and compromised pulmonary function for weeks.

Other complications of chickenpox include myocarditis, corneal lesions, nephritis, arthritis, bleeding diatheses, acute glomerulonephritis, and hepatitis. Hepatic involvement, distinct from Reye's syndrome and usually asymptomatic, is common in chickenpox and is generally characterized by elevated levels of liver enzymes, particularly aspartate and alanine aminotransferases.

Perinatal varicella is associated with a high mortality rate when maternal disease develops within 5 days before delivery or within 48 h thereafter. Because the newborn does not receive protective transplacental antibodies and has an immature immune system, the illness may be unusually severe. The reported mortality rate has been as high as 30% in this group. *Congenital varicella*, with clinical manifestations of limb hypoplasia, cicatricial skin lesions, and microcephaly at birth, is extremely uncommon.

Herpes Zoster   Herpes zoster, a sporadic disease, is the consequence of reactivation of latent VZV from the dorsal root ganglia. Most patients have no history of recent exposure to other individuals with VZV infection. Herpes zoster occurs at all ages, but its incidence is highest (5 to 10 cases per 1000 persons) among individuals in the sixth decade of life and beyond. Recurrent herpes zoster is exceedingly rare except in immunocompromised hosts, especially those with AIDS.

Herpes zoster, also called shingles, is characterized by a unilateral vesicular eruption within a dermatome, often associated with severe pain. The dermatomes from T3 to L3 are most frequently involved. If the ophthalmic branch of the trigeminal nerve is involved, zoster ophthalmicus results. The factors responsible for the reactivation of VZV are not known. In children reactivation is usually benign, whereas in adults it can be debilitating. The continuum of pain from onset to resolution is known as *zoster-associated pain*. The onset of disease is heralded by pain within the dermatome that may precede lesions by 48 to 72 h; an erythematous maculopapular rash evolves rapidly into vesicular lesions (Fig. 164-2). In the normal host, these lesions may remain few in number and continue to form only for a period of 3 to 5 days. The total duration of disease is generally between 7 and 10 days; however, it may take as long as 2 to 4 weeks for the skin to return to normal. Patients with herpes zoster can transmit infection to seronegative individuals, with consequent chickenpox. In a few patients, characteristic localization of pain to a dermatome with serologic evidence of herpes zoster has been reported in the absence of skin lesions. When branches of the trigeminal nerve are involved, lesions may appear on the face, in the mouth, in the eye, or on the tongue. Zoster ophthalmicus is usually a debilitating condition that can result in blindness in the absence of antiviral therapy. In the Ramsay Hunt syndrome, pain and vesicles appear in the external auditory canal, and patients lose their sense of taste in the anterior two-thirds

FIGURE 164-2   Close-up of lesions of disseminated zoster. Note lesions at different stages of evolution, including pustules and crusting. (*Photo courtesy of Lindsey Baden.*)

of the tongue while developing ipsilateral facial palsy. The geniculate ganglion of the sensory branch of the facial nerve is involved.

The most debilitating complication of herpes zoster, in both the normal and the immunocompromised host, is pain associated with acute neuritis and postherpetic neuralgia. Postherpetic neuralgia is uncommon in young individuals; however, at least 50% of patients over age 50 with zoster report some degree of pain in the involved dermatome months after the resolution of cutaneous disease. Changes in sensation in the dermatome, resulting in either hypo- or hyperesthesia, are common.

CNS involvement may follow localized herpes zoster. Many patients without signs of meningeal irritation have CSF pleocytosis and moderately elevated levels of CSF protein. Symptomatic meningoencephalitis is characterized by headache, fever, photophobia, meningitis, and vomiting. A rare manifestation of CNS involvement is granulomatous angiitis with contralateral hemiplegia, which can be diagnosed by cerebral arteriography. Other neurologic manifestations include transverse myelitis with or without motor paralysis.

Like chickenpox, herpes zoster is more severe in the immunocompromised host than in the normal individual. Lesions continue to form for over a week, and scabbing is not complete in most cases until 3 weeks into the illness. Patients with Hodgkin's disease and non-Hodgkin's lymphoma are at greatest risk for progressive herpes zoster. Cutaneous dissemination (Fig. 164-3) develops in ~40% of these patients. Among patients with cutaneous dissemination, the risk of pneumonitis, meningoencephalitis, hepatitis, and other serious complications is increased by 5 to 10%. However, even in immunocompromised patients, disseminated zoster is rarely fatal.

Patients who have received a bone marrow transplant are at particularly high risk of VZV infection. Thirty percent of cases of posttransplantation VZV infection occur within 1 year (50% of these within 9 months); 45% of the patients involved have cutaneous or visceral dissemination. The mortality rate in this situation is 10%. Postherpetic neuralgia, scarring, and bacterial superinfection are especially frequent in VZV infections occurring within 9 months of transplantation. Among infected patients, concomitant graft-versus-host disease increases the chance of dissemination and/or death.

DIFFERENTIAL DIAGNOSIS   The diagnosis of chickenpox is not difficult. The characteristic rash and a history of recent exposure should lead to a prompt diagnosis. Other viral infections that can mimic chickenpox include disseminated herpes simplex virus infection in patients with atopic dermatitis and the disseminated vesiculopapular lesions sometimes associated with coxsackievirus infection, echovirus infection, or atypical measles. However, these rashes are more commonly morbil-

FIGURE 164-3   Herpes zoster is seen in this HIV-infected patient as hemorrhagic vesicles and pustules on an erythematous base grouped in a dermatomal distribution.

liform with a hemorrhagic component rather than vesicular or vesiculopustular. Rickettsialpox (Chap. 158) can be confused with chickenpox; however, it can be distinguished easily by detection of the "herald spot" at the site of the mite bite and the development of a more pronounced headache. Serologic testing is also useful in differentiating rickettsialpox from varicella. Concern about smallpox has recently increased because of the threat of bioterrorism (Chap. 205). The lesions of smallpox are larger than those of chickenpox and are all at the same stage of evolution.

Unilateral vesicular lesions in a dermatomal pattern should lead rapidly to the diagnosis of herpes zoster, although the occurrence of shingles without a rash has been reported. Both herpes simplex virus infections and coxsackievirus infections can cause dermatomal vesicular lesions. Supportive diagnostic virology and fluorescent staining of skin scrapings with monoclonal antibodies are helpful in ensuring the proper diagnosis. In the prodromal stage of herpes zoster, the diagnosis can be exceedingly difficult and may be made only after lesions have appeared or by retrospective serologic assessment.

LABORATORY FINDINGS   Unequivocal confirmation of the diagnosis is possible only through the isolation of VZV in susceptible tissue-culture cell lines, the demonstration of either seroconversion or a fourfold or greater rise in antibody titer between convalescent- and acute-phase serum specimens, or the detection of VZV DNA by PCR. A rapid impression can be obtained by a Tzanck smear, with scraping of the base of the lesions in an attempt to demonstrate multinucleated giant cells, although the sensitivity of this method is low (~60%). PCR technology for the detection of viral DNA in vesicular fluid is available in a limited number of diagnostic laboratories. Direct immunofluorescent staining of cells from the lesion base or detection of viral antigens by other assays (such as the immunoperoxidase assay) is also useful, although these tests are not commercially available. The most frequently employed serologic tools for assessing host response are the immunofluorescent detection of antibodies to VZV membrane antigens, the fluorescent antibody to membrane antigen (FAMA) test, immune adherence hemagglutination, and enzyme-linked immunosorbent assay (ELISA). The FAMA test and the ELISA appear to be the most sensitive.

R̲x̲ **TREATMENT**

Medical management of chickenpox in the immunologically normal host is directed toward the prevention of avoidable complications. Obviously, good hygiene includes daily bathing and soaks. Secondary bacterial infection of the skin can be avoided by meticulous skin care, particularly with close cropping of fingernails. Pruritus can be decreased with topical dressings or the administration of antipruritic drugs. Tepid water baths and wet compresses are better than drying lotions for the relief of itching. Aluminum acetate soaks for the management of herpes zoster can be both soothing and cleansing. Administration of aspirin to children with chickenpox should be avoided because of the association of aspirin derivatives with the development of Reye's syndrome. Acyclovir therapy (800 mg by mouth five times daily for 5 to 7 days) is recommended for adolescents and adults with chickenpox of ≤24 h duration. Likewise, acyclovir therapy may be of benefit to children <12 years of age if initiated early in the disease (<24 h) at a dose of 20 mg/kg every 6 h.

Patients with herpes zoster benefit from oral antiviral therapy, as evidenced by accelerated healing of lesions and resolution of zoster-associated pain with acyclovir, valacyclovir, or famciclovir. Acyclovir, now off patent, is administered at a dosage of 800 mg five times daily for 7 to 10 days. Famciclovir, the prodrug of penciclovir, is at least as effective as acyclovir and perhaps more so. One study showed twofold faster resolution of postherpetic neuralgia in famciclovir-treated patients with zoster than in recipients of placebo. The dose is 500 mg by mouth three times daily for 7 days. Valacyclovir, the prodrug of acyclovir, accelerates healing and resolution of zoster-associated pain more promptly than acyclovir. The dose is 1 g by mouth three times daily for 5 to 7 days. Both famciclovir and valacyclovir offer the advantage of a lower dosing frequency than acyclovir.

In the immunocompromised host, both chickenpox and herpes zoster (including disseminated disease) should be treated with intravenous acyclovir, which reduces the occurrence of visceral complications but has no effect on healing of skin lesions or pain. The dose is 10 to 12.5 mg/kg every 8 h for 7 days. Oral acyclovir therapy is not recommended for the treatment of VZV infections in immunocompromised patients. Concomitant with the administration of intravenous acyclovir, it is desirable to attempt to wean these patients from immunosuppressive treatment.

Patients with varicella pneumonia may require removal of bronchial secretions and ventilatory support. Persons with zoster ophthalmicus should be referred immediately to an ophthalmologist. Therapy for this condition consists of the administration of analgesics for severe pain and the use of atropine. Acyclovir accelerates healing.

The management of acute neuritis and/or postherpetic neuralgia can be particularly difficult. In addition to the judicious use of analgesics, ranging from nonnarcotics to narcotic derivatives, drugs such as gabapentin, amitriptyline hydrochloride, lidocaine patches, and fluphenazine hydrochloride have been reported to be beneficial for pain relief. In one study, glucocorticoid therapy administered early in the course of localized herpes zoster significantly accelerated such quality-of-life improvements as a return to usual activity and termination of analgesia. The dose of prednisone administered orally was 60 mg/d on days 1 through 7, 30 mg/d on days 8 through 14, and 15 mg/d on days 15 through 21. This regimen is appropriate only for relatively healthy elderly persons who have moderate or severe pain at presentation. Patients with osteoporosis, diabetes mellitus, glycosuria, or hypertension may not be appropriate candidates. Glucocorticoids should not be used without concomitant antiviral therapy.

PREVENTION Three methods are used for the prevention of VZV infections. First, a live attenuated varicella vaccine (OKA) is recommended for all children >1 year of age (up to 12 years of age) who have not had chickenpox and for adults known to be seronegative for VZV. A single dose of vaccine is administered to children, whereas adults require two doses. The vaccine is both safe and efficacious. Breakthrough cases are mild and may result in spread of the vaccine virus to susceptible contacts. The universal vaccination of children is resulting in a decreased incidence of chickenpox in sentinel communities. Furthermore, inactivation of the vaccine virus significantly decreases the occurrence of herpes zoster after human stem-cell transplantation. A vaccine study is being performed in individuals >60 years of age to determine its impact on the incidence and severity of shingles.

A second approach is to administer varicella-zoster immune globulin (VZIg) to individuals who are susceptible, are at high risk for developing complications of varicella, and have had a significant exposure. This product should be given within 96 h (preferably within 72 h) of the exposure. Indications for administration of VZIg appear in Table 164-1.

Lastly, antiviral therapy can be given as prophylaxis to individuals at high risk who are ineligible for vaccine or beyond the 96-h window after direct contact. While the initial studies have used acyclovir, similar benefit can be anticipated with either valacyclovir or famciclovir. Therapy is instituted 7 days after intense exposure. At this time, the host is midway into the incubation period. This approach significantly decreases disease severity, if not totally preventing disease.

TABLE 164-1 *Recommendations for VZIg Administration*

Exposure criteria
1. Exposure to person with chickenpox or zoster
   a. Household: residence in the same household
   b. Playmate: face-to-face indoor play
   c. Hospital
      Varicella: same 2- to 4-bed room or adjacent beds in large ward, face-to-face contact with infectious staff member or patient, visit by a person deemed contagious
      Zoster: intimate contact (e.g., touching or hugging) with a person deemed contagious
   d. Newborn infant: onset of varicella in the mother ≤5 days before delivery or ≤48 h after delivery; VZIg is not indicated if the mother has zoster
2. Patient should receive VZIg as soon as possible but not >96 h after exposure

Candidates (provided they have significant exposure) include:
1. Immunocompromised susceptible children without history of varicella or varicella immunization
2. Susceptible pregnant women
3. Newborn infants whose mother had onset of chickenpox within 5 days before or within 48 h after delivery
4. Hospitalized premature infant (≥28 weeks of gestation) whose mother lacks a reliable history of chickenpox or serologic evidence of protection against varicella
5. Hospitalized premature infant (<28 weeks of gestation or ≤1000-g birth weight), regardless of maternal history of varicella or varicella-zoster virus serologic status

Source: Adapted from American Academy of Pediatrics, *Red Book, Report of the Committee on Infectious Diseases,* G Peter (ed), Elk Grove Village, IL, American Academy of Pediatrics, 2003, pp 678–679; with permission.

FURTHER READING

BEUTNER KR et al: Valacyclovir compared with acyclovir for improved therapy for herpes zoster in immunocompetent adults. Antimicrob Agents Chemother 39:1547, 1995

DUNKLE LM et al: A controlled trial of acyclovir for chickenpox in normal children. N Engl J Med 325:1539, 1991

GNANN JW, WHITLEY RJ: Herpes zoster. N Engl J Med 347:340, 2002

IZURIETA HS et al: Postlicensure effectiveness of varicella vaccine during an outbreak in a child care center. JAMA 278:1495, 1997

ROWBOTHAM M et al: Gabapentin for the treatment of postherpetic neuralgia. A randomized controlled trial. JAMA 280:1837, 1998

SHEPP D et al: Treatment of varicella-zoster virus in severely immunocompromised patients: A randomized comparison of acyclovir and vidarabine. N Engl J Med 314:208, 1987

TYRING S et al: Famciclovir for the treatment of acute herpes zoster. Effects on acute disease and postherpetic neuralgia: A randomized, double-blind, placebo-controlled trial. Ann Intern Med 123:89, 1995

WHITLEY RJ et al: Disseminated herpes zoster in the immunocompromised host: A comparative trial of acyclovir and vidarabine. J Infect Dis 165:450, 1992

——— et al: Acyclovir with and without prednisone for the treatment of herpes zoster: A randomized, placebo-controlled trial. Ann Intern Med 125:376, 1996

WOOD MJ et al: A randomized trial of acyclovir for 7 days or 21 days with and without prednisolone for treatment of acute herpes zoster. N Engl J Med 330:896, 1994

DEFINITION Epstein-Barr virus (EBV) is the cause of heterophile-positive infectious mononucleosis (IM), which is characterized by fever, sore throat, lymphadenopathy, and atypical lymphocytosis. EBV is also associated with several human tumors, including nasopharyngeal carcinoma, Burkitt's lymphoma, Hodgkin's disease, and (in patients with immunodeficiencies) B cell lymphoma. The virus, a member of the family Herpesviridae, consists of a linear DNA core surrounded by a nucleocapsid and an envelope that contains glycoproteins. The two types of EBV that are widely prevalent in nature are not distinguishable by conventional serologic tests.

EPIDEMIOLOGY EBV infections occur worldwide. These infections are most common in early childhood, with a second peak during late adolescence. By adulthood, more than 90% of individuals have been infected and have antibodies to the virus. IM is usually a disease of young adults. In lower socioeconomic groups and in areas of the world with lower standards of hygiene (e.g., developing countries), EBV tends to infect children at an early age, and symptomatic IM is uncommon. In areas with higher standards of hygiene, infection with EBV is often delayed until adulthood, and IM is more prevalent.

EBV is spread by contact with oral secretions. The virus is frequently transmitted from asymptomatic adults to infants and among young adults by transfer of saliva during kissing. Transmission by less intimate contact is rare. EBV has been transmitted by blood transfusion and by bone marrow transplantation. More than 90% of asymptomatic seropositive individuals shed the virus in oropharyngeal secretions.

PATHOGENESIS EBV is transmitted by salivary secretions. The virus infects the epithelium of the oropharynx and the salivary glands and is shed from these cells. While B cells may become infected after contact with epithelial cells, studies suggest that lymphocytes in the tonsillar crypts can be infected directly. The virus then spreads through the bloodstream. The proliferation and expansion of EBV-infected B cells along with reactive T cells during IM result in enlargement of lymphoid tissue. Polyclonal activation of B cells leads to the production of antibodies to host-cell and viral proteins. During the acute phase of IM, up to 1 in every 100 B cells in the peripheral blood is infected by EBV, while after recovery, about 1 in every million B cells is infected. During IM there is an inverted CD4+/CD8+ T cell ratio. The percentage of CD4+ T cells decreases, while there are large clonal expansions of CD8+ T cells; up to 40% of CD8+ T cells are directed against EBV antigens during acute infection. Data suggest that memory B cells, not epithelial cells, are the reservoir for EBV in the body. When patients are treated with acyclovir, shedding of EBV from the oropharynx stops but the virus persists in B cells.

The EBV receptor (CD21), present on the surface of B cells, is also the receptor for the C3d component of complement. EBV infection of epithelial cells results in viral replication and production of virions. When B cells are infected by EBV in vitro, they become transformed and can proliferate indefinitely. During latent infection of B cells, only the EBV nuclear antigens (EBNAs), latent membrane proteins (LMPs), and small EBV RNAs are expressed in vitro. EBV-transformed B cells secrete immunoglobulin; only a small fraction of cells produce virus.

Cellular immunity is more important than humoral immunity in controlling EBV infection. In the initial phase of infection, suppressor T cells, natural killer cells, and nonspecific cytotoxic T cells are important in controlling the proliferation of EBV-infected B cells. Levels of markers of T cell activation and serum interferon γ are elevated. Later in infection, HLA-restricted cytotoxic T cells that recognize EBNAs and LMPs and destroy EBV-infected cells are generated. Studies have shown that one of the late genes expressed during EBV replication, *BCRF1*, is a homologue of interleukin 10 and can inhibit the production of interferon γ by mononuclear cells in vitro.

If T cell immunity is compromised, EBV-infected B cells may begin to proliferate. When EBV is associated with lymphoma, virus-induced proliferation is but one step in a multistep process of neoplastic transformation. In many EBV-containing tumors, LMP-1 mimics members of the tumor necrosis factor receptor family (e.g., CD40), transmitting growth-proliferating signals.

CLINICAL MANIFESTATIONS Most EBV infections in infants and young children either are asymptomatic or present as mild pharyngitis with or without tonsillitis. In contrast, up to 75% of infections in adolescents present as IM.

Signs and Symptoms The incubation period for IM in young adults is ~4 to 6 weeks. A prodrome of fatigue, malaise, and myalgia may last for 1 to 2 weeks before the onset of fever, sore throat, and lymphadenopathy. Fever is usually low-grade and is most common in the first 2 weeks of the illness; however, it may persist for >1 month. Common signs and symptoms are listed along with their frequencies in Table 165-1. Lymphadenopathy and pharyngitis are most prominent during the first 2 weeks of the illness, while splenomegaly is more prominent during the second and third weeks. Lymphadenopathy most often affects the posterior cervical nodes but may be generalized. Enlarged lymph nodes are frequently tender and symmetric but are not fixed in place. Pharyngitis, often the most prominent sign, can be accompanied by enlargement of the tonsils with an exudate resembling that of streptococcal pharyngitis. A morbilliform or papular rash, usually on the arms or trunk, develops in ~5% of cases. Most patients treated with ampicillin develop a macular rash; this rash is not predictive of future adverse reactions to penicillins. Erythema nodosum and erythema multiforme have also been described (Chap. 48). Most patients have symptoms for 2 to 4 weeks, but malaise and difficulty concentrating can persist for months.

Symptomatic IM is uncommon in infants and young children. IM in the elderly presents relatively often as nonspecific symptoms, including prolonged fever, fatigue, myalgia, and malaise; in contrast, pharyngitis, lymphadenopathy, splenomegaly, and atypical lymphocytes are relatively rare in elderly patients.

Laboratory Findings The white blood cell count is usually elevated and peaks at 10,000 to 20,000/μL during the second or third week of illness. Lymphocytosis is usually demonstrable, with >10% atypical lymphocytes. The latter cells are enlarged lymphocytes that have abundant cytoplasm, vacuoles, and indentations of the cell membrane. CD8+ cells predominate among the atypical lymphocytes. Low-grade neutropenia and thrombocytopenia are common during the first month

TABLE 165-1 *Signs and Symptoms of Infectious Mononucleosis*

Manifestation	Median Percentage of Patients (Range)
Symptoms	
Sore throat	75 (50–87)
Malaise	47 (42–76)
Headache	38 (22–67)
Abdominal pain, nausea, or vomiting	17 (5–25)
Chills	10 (9–11)
Signs	
Lymphadenopathy	95 (83–100)
Fever	93 (60–100)
Pharyngitis or tonsillitis	82 (68–90)
Splenomegaly	51 (43–64)
Hepatomegaly	11 (6–15)
Rash	10 (0–25)
Periorbital edema	13 (2–34)
Palatal enanthem	7 (3–13)
Jaundice	5 (2–10)

of illness. Liver function is abnormal in more than 90% of cases. Serum levels of aminotransferases and alkaline phosphatase are usually mildly elevated; the serum concentration of bilirubin is elevated in ~40% of cases.

Complications Most cases of IM are self-limited. Deaths are very rare and most often are due to central nervous system (CNS) complications, splenic rupture, upper airway obstruction, or bacterial superinfection.

When CNS complications develop, they usually do so during the first 2 weeks of EBV infection; in some patients, especially children, they are the only clinical manifestations of IM. Heterophile antibodies and atypical lymphocytes may be absent. Meningitis and encephalitis are the most common neurologic abnormalities, and patients may present with headache, meningismus, or cerebellar ataxia; acute hemiplegia and psychosis have also been described. The cerebrospinal fluid (CSF) contains mainly lymphocytes, with occasional atypical lymphocytes. Most cases resolve without neurologic sequelae. Acute EBV infection has also been associated with cranial nerve palsies (especially ones involving cranial nerve VII), Guillain-Barré syndrome, acute transverse myelitis, and peripheral neuritis.

Autoimmune hemolytic anemia occurs in ~2% of cases during the first 2 weeks. In most cases the anemia is Coombs'-test positive, with cold agglutinins directed against the i red blood cell antigen. Most patients with hemolysis have mild anemia that lasts for 1 or 2 months, but some patients have severe disease with hemoglobinuria and jaundice. Nonspecific antibody responses may also include rheumatoid factor, antinuclear antibodies, anti–smooth muscle antibodies, antiplatelet antibodies, and cryoglobulins. IM has been associated with red-cell aplasia, severe granulocytopenia, thrombocytopenia, pancytopenia, and hemophagocytic syndrome. The spleen ruptures in fewer than 0.5% of cases. Splenic rupture is more common among males than among females and may be manifest as abdominal pain, referred shoulder pain, or hemodynamic compromise.

Hypertrophy of lymphoid tissue in the tonsils or adenoids can result in upper airway obstruction, as can inflammation and edema of the epiglottis, pharynx, or uvula. About 10% of patients with IM develop streptococcal pharyngitis after their initial sore throat resolves.

Other rare complications associated with acute EBV infection include hepatitis (which can be fulminant), myocarditis or pericarditis with electrocardiographic changes, pneumonia with pleural effusion, interstitial nephritis, genital ulcerations, and vasculitis.

OTHER DISEASES ASSOCIATED WITH EBV INFECTION EBV-associated lymphoproliferative disease has been described in patients with congenital or acquired immunodeficiency, including those with severe combined immunodeficiency, AIDS, and recipients of bone marrow or organ transplants who are receiving immunosuppressive drugs (especially cyclosporine). Proliferating EBV-infected B cells infiltrate lymph nodes and multiple organs, and patients present with fever and lymphadenopathy or gastrointestinal symptoms. Pathologic studies show B cell hyperplasia or poly- or monoclonal lymphoma. The X-linked lymphoproliferative syndrome (Duncan's disease) is a recessive disorder of young boys who have a normal response to childhood infections but develop fatal lymphoproliferative disorders after infection with EBV. The gene mutated in this syndrome, *SAP* or *SH2D1A*, has been identified; its product binds to a protein that mediates interactions of B and T cells. Most patients with this syndrome die of acute IM; others develop hypogammaglobulinemia, malignant B cell lymphomas, aplastic anemia, or agranulocytosis. IM has also proved fatal to some patients with no obvious preexisting immune abnormality.

Oral hairy leukoplakia (Fig. 165-1) is an early manifestation of infection with HIV in adults (Chap. 173). Most patients present with raised, white corrugated lesions on the tongue (and occasionally on the buccal mucosa) that contain EBV DNA. Children infected with HIV can develop lymphoid interstitial pneumonitis; EBV DNA is often found in lung tissue from these patients.

Patients with the chronic fatigue syndrome may have titers of antibody to EBV that are elevated but are not significantly different from those in healthy EBV-seropositive adults. While some patients have

FIGURE 165-1 Oral hairy leukoplakia often presents as white plaques on the lateral surface of the tongue and is associated with Epstein-Barr virus infection.

malaise and fatigue that persist for weeks or months after IM, persistent EBV infection is not a cause of the chronic fatigue syndrome. Chronic active EBV infection is very rare and is distinct from the chronic fatigue syndrome. The affected patients have an illness lasting >6 months with markedly elevated titers of antibody to EBV and evidence of organ involvement, including hepatosplenomegaly, lymphadenopathy, and pneumonitis, uveitis, or neurologic disease.

EBV is associated with several malignancies. About 15% of cases of Burkitt's lymphoma in the United States and ~90% of those in Africa are associated with EBV (Chap. 97). African patients with Burkitt's lymphoma have high levels of antibody to EBV, and their tumor tissue usually contains viral DNA. EBV-containing Burkitt's lymphoma also occurs in patients with AIDS. Anaplastic nasopharyngeal carcinoma is uniformly associated with EBV; the affected tissues contain viral DNA and antigens. Patients with nasopharyngeal carcinoma often have elevated titers of antibody to EBV (Chap. 74).

EBV has been associated with Hodgkin's disease, especially the mixed-cellularity type (Chap. 97). Patients with Hodgkin's disease often have elevated titers of antibody to EBV, and in about half of cases viral DNA and antigens are found in Reed-Sternberg cells. In some cases, EBV DNA has been detected in tonsillar carcinoma, angioimmunoblastic lymphadenopathy, angiocentric nasal NK/T cell immunoproliferative lesions, T cell lymphoma, thymoma, gastric carcinoma, and CNS lymphoma from patients with no underlying immunodeficiency. Studies have demonstrated viral DNA in leiomyosarcomas from AIDS patients and in smooth-muscle tumors from organ transplant recipients. Virtually all CNS lymphomas in AIDS patients are associated with EBV. While serologic studies have shown higher levels of antibodies to EBV before the onset of multiple sclerosis, other studies (including measurement of EBV antibody titers in the CSF) are needed to ascertain a possible causal relationship.

DIAGNOSIS ■ Serologic Testing The heterophile test is used for the diagnosis of IM in children and adults (Table 165-2). In the test for this antibody, human serum is absorbed with guinea pig kidney, and the heterophile titer is defined as the greatest serum dilution that agglutinates sheep, horse, or cow erythrocytes. Although heterophile antibody binds to certain animal erythrocytes, it does not interact with EBV proteins. A titer of 40-fold or greater is diagnostic of acute EBV infection in a patient who has symptoms compatible with IM and atypical lymphocytes. Tests for heterophile antibodies are positive in 40% of patients with IM during the first week of illness and in 80 to 90% during the third week. Therefore, repeated testing may be necessary, especially if the initial test is performed early. Tests usually remain positive for 3 months after the onset of illness, but heterophile antibodies can persist for up to 1 year. These antibodies usually are not detectable in children <5 years of age, in the elderly, or in patients presenting with symptoms not typical of IM. The commercially available monospot test for heterophile antibodies is somewhat more sensitive than the classic heterophile test. The monospot test is ~75%

TABLE 165-2 *Serologic Features of EBV-Associated Diseases*

Condition	Heterophile	Anti-VCA		Anti-EA		Anti-EBNA
		IgM	IgG	EA-D	EA-R	
Acute infectious mononucleosis	+	+	++	+	−	−
Convalescence	±	−	+	−	±	+
Past infection	−	−	+	−	−	+
Reactivation with immunodeficiency	−	−	++	+	+	±
Burkitt's lymphoma	−	−	+++	±	++	+
Nasopharyngeal carcinoma	−	−	+++	++	±	+

[a] VCA, viral capsid antigen; EA, early antigen; EA-D antibody, antibody to early antigen in diffuse pattern in nucleus and cytoplasm of infected cells; EA-R antibody, antibody to early antigen restricted to the cytoplasm; and EBNA, Epstein-Barr nuclear antigen.

Source: Adapted from Okano, 1988.

sensitive and ~90% specific compared with EBV-specific serologies. False-positive monospot results are more common in persons with connective tissue disease, lymphoma, viral hepatitis, and malaria.

EBV-specific antibody testing is used for patients with suspected acute EBV infection who lack heterophile antibodies and for patients with atypical infections (Table 165-2). Serologic tests are particularly useful in young children, who often do not develop heterophile antibodies. Titers of IgM and IgG antibodies to viral capsid antigen (VCA) are elevated in the serum of more than 90% of patients at the onset of disease. IgM antibody to VCA is most useful for the diagnosis of acute IM because it is present at elevated titers only during the first 2 to 3 months of the disease; in contrast, IgG antibody to VCA is usually not useful for diagnosis of IM but is often used to assess exposure to EBV in the past because it persists for life. Seroconversion to EBNA positivity is also useful for the diagnosis of acute infection with EBV. Antibodies to EBNA are detectable relatively late (3 to 6 weeks after the onset of symptoms) in nearly all cases of acute EBV infection and persist for the lifetime of the patient. These antibodies may be lacking in immunodeficient patients and in those with chronic active EBV infection.

Titers of other antibodies may also be elevated in IM; however, these elevations are less useful for diagnosis. Antibodies to early antigens (EAs) are found either in a diffuse pattern in the nucleus and cytoplasm of infected cells (EA-D antibody) or restricted to the cytoplasm (EA-R antibody). These antibodies are detectable 3 to 4 weeks after the onset of symptoms in patients with IM. About 70% of individuals with IM have EA-D antibodies during the course of illness; the presence of EA-D antibodies is especially likely in those with relatively severe disease. These antibodies usually persist for only 3 to 6 months. Levels of EA-D antibodies are also elevated in patients with nasopharyngeal carcinoma or chronic active EBV infection. EA-R antibodies are only occasionally detected in patients with IM but are often found at elevated titers in patients with African Burkitt's lymphoma or chronic active EBV infection. IgA antibodies to EBV antigens have proved useful for the identification of patients with nasopharyngeal carcinoma and of persons at high risk for the disease.

TABLE 165-3 *Treatment Options for Posttransplantation EBV Lymphoproliferative Disease*

1. Reduction of immunosuppression, when possible
2. Excision of localized lesions
3. Interferon α
4. Monoclonal antibody to CD20 (rituximab)
5. Radiation therapy (especially for CNS lesions)
6. For stem cell transplant recipients: donor lymphocyte infusions or donor EBV-specific cytotoxic T cell infusions[a]
7. For solid organ transplant recipients: autologous or HLA-matched, EBV-specific, cytotoxic T cell infusions[a]
8. Cytotoxic chemotherapy

[a] Infused T cells must be HLA matched; lymphoproliferative lesions are usually of donor origin for stem cell transplant recipients and of recipient origin for solid organ transplant recipients.

Other Studies Detection of EBV DNA, RNA, or proteins has been valuable in demonstrating the association of the virus with various malignancies. The polymerase chain reaction has been used to detect EBV DNA in the CSF of some AIDS patients with lymphomas and to monitor the amount of EBV DNA in the blood of patients with lymphoproliferative disease. Culture of EBV from throat washings or blood is not helpful in the diagnosis of acute infection, since EBV commonly persists in the oropharynx and in B cells for the lifetime of the infected individual.

Differential Diagnosis The differential diagnosis of IM and atypical lymphocytosis includes acute infection with cytomegalovirus, *Toxoplasma*, HIV, human herpesvirus 6, and hepatitis viruses as well as drug hypersensitivity reactions. Cytomegalovirus is the most common cause of heterophile-negative mononucleosis, usually involves older patients, and is associated with a lower frequency of sore throat, splenomegaly, and lymphadenopathy than IM due to EBV. Other diseases that share some of the features of IM include rubella, acute infectious lymphocytosis in children, and lymphoma or leukemia.

℞ TREATMENT

Therapy for IM consists of supportive measures, with rest and analgesia. Excessive physical activity during the first month should be avoided to reduce the possibility of splenic rupture. If splenic rupture occurs, splenectomy is required. Glucocorticoid therapy is not indicated for uncomplicated IM and in fact may predispose to bacterial superinfection. Prednisone (40 to 60 mg/d for 2 to 3 days, with subsequent tapering of the dose over 1 to 2 weeks) has been used for the prevention of airway obstruction in patients with severe tonsillar hypertrophy, for autoimmune hemolytic anemia, and for severe thrombocytopenia. Glucocorticoids have also been used in a few selected patients with severe malaise and fever and in patients with severe CNS or cardiac disease.

Acyclovir has had no significant clinical impact on IM in controlled trials. In one study, the combination of acyclovir and prednisolone had no significant effect on the duration of symptoms of IM. Acyclovir, at a dosage of 400 to 800 mg five times daily, has been effective for the treatment of oral hairy leukoplakia (despite common relapses) and some cases of chronic active EBV disease. The posttransplantation EBV lymphoproliferative syndrome (Chap. 117) generally does not respond to antiviral therapy. When possible, therapy should be directed toward reduction of immunosuppression (Table 165-3). Interferon α or antibody to CD20 has been effective in some cases. Infusions of donor lymphocytes are often effective for stem cell transplant recipients, although graft-versus-host disease can occur. Infusions of EBV-specific cytotoxic T cells have been used to prevent EBV lymphoproliferative disease in high-risk settings as well as to treat the disease.

The isolation of patients with IM is unnecessary. Vaccines directed against the major EBV glycoprotein have been effective in animal studies and are undergoing small-scale clinical trials.

FURTHER READING

AUWAERTER PG: Infectious mononucleosis in middle age. JAMA 281:454, 1999

CHIEN Y-C et al: Serologic markers of Epstein-Barr virus infection and nasopharyngeal carcinoma in Taiwanese men. N Engl J Med 345:1877, 2001

COHEN JI: Epstein-Barr virus infection. N Engl J Med 343:481, 2000

GOTTSCHALK S et al: Treatment of Epstein-Barr virus–associated malignancies with specific T cells. Adv Cancer Res 84:175, 2002

LEVIN LI et al: Multiple sclerosis and Epstein-Barr virus. JAMA 289:1533, 2003

OKANO M et al: Epstein-Barr virus and human diseases: Recent advances in diagnosis. Clin Microbiol Rev 1:300, 1988

PAPADOPOULOS EB et al: Infusions of donor leukocytes to treat Epstein-Barr virus–associated lymphoproliferative disorders after allogeneic bone marrow transplantation. N Engl J Med 330:1185, 1994

PAYA CV et al: Epstein-Barr virus–induced posttransplant lymphoproliferative disorders. Transplantation 68:1517, 1999

RICKINSON AB, KIEFF E: Epstein-Barr virus, in *Fields Virology*, 4th ed, DM Knipe, PM Howley (eds). Philadelphia, Lippincott Williams & Wilkins, 2001

SAYOS J et al: The X-linked lymphoproliferative-disease gene product SAP

regulates signals induced through the co-receptor SLAM. Nature 395:462, 1998

TYNELL E et al: Acyclovir and prednisolone treatment of acute infectious mononucleosis: A multicenter, double-blind, placebo-controlled study. J Infect Dis 174:324, 1996

166 CYTOMEGALOVIRUS AND HUMAN HERPESVIRUS TYPES 6, 7, AND 8
Martin S. Hirsch

CYTOMEGALOVIRUS

DEFINITION Cytomegalovirus (CMV), which was initially isolated from patients with congenital cytomegalic inclusion disease, is now recognized as an important pathogen in all age groups. In addition to inducing severe birth defects, CMV causes a wide spectrum of disorders in older children and adults, ranging from an asymptomatic, subclinical infection to a mononucleosis syndrome in healthy individuals to disseminated disease in immunocompromised patients. Human CMV is one of several related species-specific viruses that cause similar diseases in various animals. All are associated with the production of characteristic enlarged cells—hence the name *cytomegalovirus*.

CMV is a member of the β-herpesvirus group and has double-strand DNA, four species of mRNA, a protein capsid, and a lipoprotein envelope. Like other herpesviruses, CMV demonstrates icosahedral symmetry, replicates in the cell nucleus, and can cause either a lytic and productive or a latent infection. CMV can be distinguished from other herpesviruses by certain biologic properties, such as host range and type of cytopathology induced. Viral replication is associated with the production of large intranuclear inclusions and smaller cytoplasmic inclusions. The virus appears to replicate in a variety of cell types in vivo; in tissue culture it grows preferentially in fibroblasts. Although there is little evidence that CMV is oncogenic in vivo, the virus does transform fibroblasts in rare instances, and genomic transforming fragments have been identified.

EPIDEMIOLOGY CMV has a worldwide distribution. Approximately 1% of newborns in the United States are infected with CMV, and the percentage is higher in many less-developed countries. Communal living and poor personal hygiene facilitate early spread. Perinatal and early childhood infections are common. Virus may be present in breast milk, saliva, feces, and urine. Transmission of CMV has been identified among young children in day-care centers and has been traced from infected toddler to pregnant mother to developing fetus. When an infected child introduces CMV into a household, 50% of susceptible family members seroconvert within 6 months.

The virus is not readily spread by casual contact but requires repeated or prolonged intimate exposure for transmission. In late adolescence and young adulthood, CMV is often transmitted sexually, and asymptomatic viral carriage in semen or cervical secretions is common. CMV antibody is present at detectable levels in nearly 100% of female prostitutes and sexually active homosexual men. Sexually active adults may harbor several strains of CMV simultaneously. Transfusion of whole blood or certain blood products containing viable leukocytes may also transmit CMV, with a frequency of 0.14 to 10% per unit transfused.

Once infected, an individual probably carries CMV for life. The infection usually remains latent. However, CMV reactivation syndromes develop frequently when T lymphocyte–mediated immunity is compromised—for example, after organ transplantation or in association with lymphoid neoplasms and certain acquired immunodeficiencies (in particular, infection with HIV; Chap. 173). Most primary CMV infections in organ transplant recipients (Chap. 117) result from transmission of the virus in the graft itself. In CMV-seropositive transplant recipients, infection results from reactivation of latent virus or, less commonly, from reinfection by a new strain of CMV. CMV infection may be associated with coronary artery stenosis following heart transplantation or coronary angioplasty, but this association requires further validation.

PATHOGENESIS Congenital CMV infection can result from either primary or reactivation infection of the mother. However, clinical disease in the fetus or newborn is almost exclusively related to primary maternal infection (Table 166-1). The factors determining the severity of congenital infection are unknown; a deficient capacity to produce precipitating antibodies and to mount T cell responses to CMV is associated with relatively severe disease.

Primary infection in late childhood or adulthood is often associated with a vigorous T lymphocyte response that may contribute to the development of a mononucleosis syndrome similar to that observed following Epstein-Barr virus (EBV) infection (Chap. 165). The hallmark of such infection is the appearance of atypical lymphocytes in the peripheral blood; these cells are predominantly activated CD8+ T lymphocytes. Polyclonal activation of B cells by the virus contributes to the development of rheumatoid factors and other autoantibodies during CMV mononucleosis.

Once acquired by symptomatic or asymptomatic primary infection,

TABLE 166-1 *CMV in the Immunocompromised Host*

Population	Risk Factors	Principal Syndromes	Treatment	Prevention
Fetus	Primary maternal infection/early pregnancy	Cytomegalic inclusion disease	None (?ganciclovir)	Avoidance of exposure
Organ transplant recipient	Seropositive donor, seronegative recipient; intensive immunosuppression, particularly with antilymphocyte globulins, cyclosporine	Febrile leukopenia; pneumonia; gastrointestinal disease	Ganciclovir or valganciclovir	Donor matching; CMV immunoglobulin; ganciclovir or high-dose acyclovir
Bone marrow transplant recipient	Graft-vs.-host disease; older age; seropositive recipient; viremia	Pneumonia; gastrointestinal disease	Ganciclovir plus CMV immunoglobulin	Ganciclovir or high-dose acyclovir
Person with AIDS	<100 CD4+ cells per microliter; CMV seropositivity	Retinitis; gastrointestinal disease; neurologic disease	Foscarnet, ganciclovir, valganciclovir, or cidofovir	Oral ganciclovir

CMV persists indefinitely in tissues of the host. The sites of persistent or latent infection probably include multiple cell types and various organs. Transmission following blood transfusion or organ transplantation is due to silent infections in these tissues. Autopsy studies suggest that salivary glands and bowel may be areas of latent infection.

If the host's T cell responses become compromised by disease or by iatrogenic immunosuppression, latent virus can be reactivated to cause a variety of syndromes. Chronic antigenic stimulation in the presence of immunosuppression (for example, following tissue transplantation) appears to be an ideal setting for CMV activation and CMV-induced disease. Certain particularly potent suppressants of T cell immunity, such as antithymocyte globulin, are associated with a high rate of clinical CMV syndromes, which may follow either primary or reactivation infection. CMV may itself contribute to further T lymphocyte hyporesponsiveness, which often precedes superinfection with other opportunistic pathogens, such as *Pneumocystis*. CMV and *Pneumocystis* are frequently found together in immunosuppressed patients with severe interstitial pneumonia.

PATHOLOGY   Cytomegalic cells in vivo (presumed to be infected epithelial cells) are two to four times larger than surrounding cells and often contain an 8- to 10-μm intranuclear inclusion that is eccentrically placed and is surrounded by a clear halo, producing an "owl's eye" appearance. Smaller granular cytoplasmic inclusions are demonstrated occasionally. Cytomegalic cells are found in a wide variety of organs, including salivary gland, lung, liver, kidney, intestine, pancreas, adrenal gland, and the central nervous system.

The cellular inflammatory response to infection consists of plasma cells, lymphocytes, and monocyte-macrophages. Granulomatous reactions occasionally develop, particularly in the liver. Immunopathologic reactions may contribute to CMV disease. Immune complexes have been detected in infected infants, sometimes in association with CMV-related glomerulopathies. Immune-complex glomerulopathy has been observed in some CMV-infected patients after renal transplantation.

CLINICAL MANIFESTATIONS ■ Congenital CMV Infection   Fetal infections range from inapparent to severe and disseminated. Cytomegalic inclusion disease develops in ~5% of infected fetuses and is seen almost exclusively in infants born to mothers who develop primary infections during pregnancy. Petechiae, hepatosplenomegaly, and jaundice are the most common presenting features (60 to 80% of cases). Microcephaly with or without cerebral calcifications, intrauterine growth retardation, and prematurity are reported in 30 to 50% of cases. Inguinal hernias and chorioretinitis are less common. Laboratory abnormalities include elevated alanine aminotransferase levels, thrombocytopenia, conjugated hyperbilirubinemia, hemolysis, and elevated cerebrospinal fluid protein levels. The prognosis for severely infected infants is poor; the mortality rate is 20 to 30%, and few of the patients who survive escape intellectual or hearing difficulties later in childhood. The differential diagnosis of cytomegalic inclusion disease in infants includes syphilis, rubella, toxoplasmosis, infection with herpes simplex virus or enterovirus, and bacterial sepsis.

Most congenital CMV infections are clinically inapparent at birth. Between 5 and 25% of asymptomatically infected infants develop significant psychomotor, hearing, ocular, or dental abnormalities over the next several years.

Perinatal CMV Infection   The newborn may acquire CMV at the time of delivery by passage through an infected birth canal or by postnatal contact with breast milk or other maternal secretions. Approximately 40 to 60% of infants who are breast-fed for >1 month by seropositive mothers become infected. Iatrogenic transmission can also result from neonatal blood transfusion. Screening of blood products before they are transfused into low-birth-weight seronegative infants or into seronegative pregnant women decreases the risk of infection.

The great majority of infants infected at or after delivery remain asymptomatic. However, protracted interstitial pneumonitis has been associated with perinatally acquired CMV infection, particularly in premature infants, and occasionally has been accompanied by infection with *Chlamydia trachomatis*, *Pneumocystis*, or *Ureaplasma urealyticum*. Poor weight gain, adenopathy, rash, hepatitis, anemia, and atypical lymphocytosis may also be found, and CMV excretion often persists for months or years.

CMV Mononucleosis   The most common clinical manifestation of CMV infection in normal hosts beyond the neonatal period is a heterophil antibody–negative mononucleosis syndrome. This manifestation may develop spontaneously or may follow the transfusion of leukocyte-containing blood products. Although the syndrome occurs at all ages, it most often involves sexually active young adults. Incubation periods range from 20 to 60 days, and the illness generally lasts for 2 to 6 weeks. Prolonged high fevers, sometimes accompanied by chills, profound fatigue, and malaise, characterize this disorder. Myalgias, headache, and splenomegaly are frequent, but in CMV mononucleosis (as opposed to infectious mononucleosis caused by EBV), exudative pharyngitis and cervical lymphadenopathy are rare. Occasional patients develop rubelliform rashes, often after exposure to ampicillin. Less commonly observed are interstitial or segmental pneumonia, myocarditis, pleuritis, arthritis, and encephalitis. In rare cases, Guillain-Barré syndrome complicates CMV mononucleosis. The characteristic laboratory abnormality is relative lymphocytosis in peripheral blood, with more than 10% atypical lymphocytes. Total leukocyte counts may be low, normal, or markedly elevated. Although significant jaundice is uncommon, serum aminotransferase and alkaline phosphatase levels are often moderately elevated. Heterophil antibodies are absent; however, transient immunologic abnormalities are common and may include the presence of cryoglobulins, rheumatoid factors, cold agglutinins, and antinuclear antibodies. Hemolytic anemia, thrombocytopenia, and granulocytopenia complicate recovery in rare instances.

Most patients recover without sequelae, although postviral asthenia may persist for months. The excretion of CMV in urine, genital secretions, and/or saliva often continues for months or years. Rarely, CMV infection is fatal in immunocompetent hosts; even when such patients survive, they can have recurrent episodes of fever and malaise that are sometimes associated with autonomic nervous system dysfunction (e.g., attacks of sweating or flushing).

CMV Infection in the Immunocompromised Host (See also Table 166-1)   CMV appears to be the most common and important viral pathogen complicating organ transplantation (Chap. 117). In recipients of kidney, heart, lung, and liver transplants, CMV induces a variety of syndromes, including fever and leukopenia, hepatitis, pneumonitis, esophagitis, gastritis, colitis, and retinitis. CMV disease may be an independent risk factor for both graft loss and death. The period of maximal risk is between 1 and 4 months after transplantation, although retinitis may be a later complication. Disease likelihood and levels of viral replication generally are greater after primary infection than after reactivation. In addition, molecular studies indicate that seropositive transplant recipients are susceptible to reinfection with donor-derived, genotypically variant CMV, and such infection often results in disease. Reactivation infection, although frequent, is less likely than primary infection to be important clinically. The risk of clinical disease is related to various factors, such as the degree of immunosuppression; the use of antibodies to T cell receptors; and co-infection with other pathogens, such as human herpesvirus type 6. The transplanted organ is particularly vulnerable as a target for CMV infection; thus, there is a tendency for CMV hepatitis to follow liver transplantation and for CMV pneumonitis to follow lung transplantation.

CMV pneumonia occurs in 15 to 20% of bone marrow transplant recipients, with a case-fatality rate of 84 to 88%. The risk is greatest between 5 and 13 weeks after transplantation, and the several risk factors identified include certain types of immunosuppressive therapy, acute graft-versus-host disease, older age, viremia, and seropositivity before transplantation.

CMV is recognized as an important pathogen in patients with advanced HIV infection (Chap. 173), in whom it often causes retinitis or disseminated disease, particularly when peripheral-blood CD4+ cell counts fall below 50 to 100/μL. As treatment for underlying HIV infection has improved, the incidence of serious CMV infections (e.g., retinitis) has decreased. However, institution of highly active antiretroviral regimens sometimes leads to acute flare-ups of CMV retinitis during the first few weeks of therapy.

Syndromes produced by CMV in the immunocompromised host often begin with prolonged fever, malaise, anorexia, fatigue, night sweats, and arthralgias or myalgias. Liver function abnormalities, leukopenia, thrombocytopenia, and atypical lymphocytosis may be observed during these episodes. The development of tachypnea, hypoxia, and unproductive cough signals respiratory involvement. Radiologic examination of the lung often reveals bilateral interstitial or reticulonodular infiltrates, which begin in the periphery of the lower lobes and spread centrally and superiorly; localized segmental, nodular, or alveolar patterns are less common. The differential diagnosis includes infection with *Pneumocystis*; infections due to other viral, bacterial, or fungal pathogens; pulmonary hemorrhage; and injury secondary to irradiation or to treatment with cytotoxic drugs.

Gastrointestinal CMV involvement may be localized or extensive and almost exclusively affects compromised hosts. Ulcers of the esophagus, stomach, small intestine, or colon may result in bleeding or perforation. CMV infection may lead to exacerbations of underlying ulcerative colitis. Hepatitis occurs frequently, particularly following liver transplantation, and CMV-associated acalculous cholecystitis and adrenalitis have been described.

CMV rarely causes meningoencephalitis in otherwise-healthy individuals. Two forms of CMV encephalitis are seen in patients with AIDS. One resembles HIV encephalitis and presents as progressive dementia; the other is a ventriculoencephalitis characterized by cranial-nerve deficits, nystagmus, disorientation, lethargy, and ventriculomegaly. In immunocompromised patients, CMV can also cause subacute progressive polyradiculopathy, which is often reversible if recognized and treated promptly.

CMV retinitis is an important cause of blindness in immunocompromised patients, particularly patients with advanced AIDS (Chap. 173). Early lesions consist of small, opaque, white areas of granular retinal necrosis that spread in a centrifugal manner and are later accompanied by hemorrhages, vessel sheathing, and retinal edema (Fig. 166-1). CMV retinopathy must be distinguished from that due to other conditions, including toxoplasmosis, candidiasis, and herpes simplex virus infection.

Fatal CMV infections are often associated with persistent viremia and the involvement of multiple organ systems. Progressive pulmonary infiltrates, pancytopenia, hyperamylasemia, and hypotension are characteristic features that are frequently found in conjunction with a terminal bacterial, fungal, or protozoan superinfection. Extensive ad-

renal necrosis with CMV inclusions is often documented at autopsy, as is CMV involvement of many other organs.

DIAGNOSIS The diagnosis of CMV infection usually cannot be made reliably on clinical grounds alone. Isolation of the virus or detection of CMV antigens or DNA from appropriate clinical specimens is the preferred diagnostic approach. Virus excretion or viremia is readily detected by culture of appropriate specimens on human fibroblast monolayers. If viral titers are high, as is frequently the case in congenital disseminated infection or in patients with AIDS, characteristic cytopathic effects may be detected within a few days. However, in some situations—such as CMV mononucleosis—viral titers are low, and cytopathic effects may take several weeks to appear. Many laboratories expedite diagnosis with an overnight tissue-culture method (shell vial assay) involving centrifugation and an immunocytochemical detection technique employing monoclonal antibodies to an immediate-early CMV antigen. Isolation of virus from urine or saliva does not, by itself, constitute proof of acute infection, since excretion from these sites may continue for months or years after illness. Detection of CMV viremia is a better predictor of acute infection.

Detection of CMV antigens (pp65) in peripheral-blood leukocytes or of CMV DNA in blood or tissues may hasten the diagnosis of CMV disease in certain populations, including organ transplant recipients and persons with AIDS. Such assays may yield a positive result several days earlier than culture methods. The most sensitive way to detect CMV in blood or other fluids may be by amplifying CMV DNA by polymerase chain reaction (PCR) assays. PCR detection of CMV DNA in blood may predict the risk for disease progression, and PCR detection of CMV DNA in cerebrospinal fluid is useful in the diagnosis of CMV encephalitis or polyradiculopathy.

A variety of serologic assays are available to detect increases in titers of antibody to CMV antigens. An increased antibody level may not be detectable for up to 4 weeks after primary infection, and titers often remain high for years after infection. For this reason, single-sample antibody determinations are of no value in assessing the acuteness of infection. Detection of CMV-specific IgM is sometimes useful in the diagnosis of recent or active infection; circulating rheumatoid factors may result in occasional false-positive IgM tests.

Rx TREATMENT

Several prophylactic measures are useful for the prevention of CMV infection in patients at high risk. The use of blood from seronegative donors or of blood that has been frozen, thawed, and deglycerolized greatly decreases the rate of transfusion-associated transmission of CMV. Similarly, matching of organ or bone marrow transplants by CMV serology, with exclusive use of organs from seronegative donors in seronegative recipients, reduces rates of primary infection following transplantation. Both live attenuated and CMV subunit vaccines have been evaluated, but neither is close to approval for general use.

CMV immune globulin has been reported to reduce rates of CMV-associated syndromes and of fungal or parasitic superinfections among seronegative renal transplant recipients. Studies in bone marrow transplant recipients have produced conflicting results. Prophylactic acyclovir or valacyclovir may reduce rates of CMV infection and disease in certain seronegative renal transplant recipients, although neither drug is effective in the treatment of active CMV disease.

Ganciclovir is a guanosine derivative that has considerably more activity against CMV than its congener acyclovir. After intracellular conversion by a viral phosphotransferase encoded by CMV gene region UL97, ganciclovir triphosphate is a selective inhibitor of CMV DNA polymerase. Several clinical studies have indicated response rates of 70 to 90% among patients with AIDS given ganciclovir for the treatment of CMV retinitis or colitis. In bone marrow transplant recipients with CMV pneumonia, ganciclovir is less effective when given alone, but it elicits a favorable clinical response 50 to 70% of the time when it is combined with CMV immune globulin. Prophy-

FIGURE 166-1 Cytomegalovirus in a patient with AIDS appears as an arcuate zone of retinitis with hemorrhages and optic disk swelling. Often CMV is confined to the retinal periphery, beyond view of the direct ophthalmoscope.

lactic or suppressive ganciclovir may be useful in high-risk bone marrow or organ transplant recipients (e.g., those who are CMV-seropositive before transplantation or who are CMV culture–positive afterward). In many patients with AIDS, persistently low CD4+ cell counts, and CMV disease, clinical and virologic relapses occur promptly if treatment with ganciclovir is discontinued. Therefore, prolonged maintenance regimens are recommended for such patients. Resistance to ganciclovir is common among patients treated for >3 months and is usually related to mutations in the CMV UL97 gene.

Valganciclovir is an orally bioavailable prodrug that is rapidly metabolized to ganciclovir in intestinal tissues and the liver. Approximately 60% of an oral dose of valganciclovir is absorbed. An oral valganciclovir dose of 900 mg results in ganciclovir blood levels similar to those obtained with an intravenous ganciclovir dose of 5 mg/kg. Oral valganciclovir appears to be as effective as intravenous ganciclovir for both CMV retinitis induction and maintenance regimens. Furthermore, the adverse-event profiles and rates of resistance development for the two drugs are similar.

Ganciclovir or valganciclovir therapy for CMV retinitis consists of a 14- to 21-day induction course (5 mg/kg intravenously twice daily for ganciclovir or 900 mg twice daily for valganciclovir) followed by a prolonged maintenance regimen. For parenteral maintenance, the ganciclovir dose is 5 mg/kg daily or 6 mg/kg 5 days per week; for oral maintenance, 900 mg of valganciclovir once daily is recommended. Peripheral-blood neutropenia develops in 16 to 29% of treated patients but may be ameliorated by granulocyte colony-stimulating factor or granulocyte-macrophage colony-stimulating factor. Discontinuation of maintenance therapy should be considered in patients with AIDS who, while receiving antiretroviral therapy, have a sustained (>6-month) increase in CD4 cell counts to >100–150/μL.

Foscarnet (sodium phosphonoformate) also acts against CMV infection by inhibiting viral DNA polymerase. Because this agent does not require phosphorylation to be active, it is also effective against most ganciclovir-resistant CMV isolates. Foscarnet is less well tolerated than ganciclovir and causes considerable toxicity, including renal dysfunction, hypomagnesemia, hypokalemia, hypocalcemia, genital ulcers, dysuria, nausea, and paresthesia. Moreover, foscarnet administration requires the use of an infusion pump and close clinical monitoring. With aggressive hydration and dose adjustments for renal dysfunction, the toxicity of foscarnet can be reduced. The use of foscarnet should be avoided when a saline load cannot be tolerated (e.g., in cardiomyopathy). The approved induction regimen is 60 mg/kg every 8 h for 2 weeks, although 90 mg/kg every 12 h is equally effective and no more toxic. Maintenance infusions should deliver 90 to 120 mg/kg once daily; no oral preparation is available. Foscarnet-resistant viruses may emerge during extended therapy.

Ganciclovir may also be administered via a slow-release pellet sutured into the eye. Although this intraocular device provides good local protection, contralateral eye disease and disseminated disease are not affected, and early retinal detachment is possible. A combination of intraocular and systemic therapy may be better than the intraocular implant alone.

Cidofovir is a nucleotide analogue with a long intracellular half-life that allows intermittent intravenous administration. Induction regimens of 5 mg/kg weekly for 2 weeks are followed by maintenance regimens of 3 to 5 mg/kg every 2 weeks. Cidofovir can cause severe nephrotoxicity through dose-dependent proximal tubular cell injury; however, this adverse effect can be ameliorated somewhat by saline hydration and probenecid.

It is still not clear whether universal prophylaxis or preemptive therapy in immunocompromised hosts with CMV seropositivity is the preferable approach. For patients with advanced HIV infection (CD4 cell counts of <50/μL), some authorities have advocated prophylaxis with oral ganciclovir or valganciclovir. However, side effects, lack of proven benefit, possible induction of viral resistance, and cost have precluded the wide acceptance of this practice. Similar questions have arisen concerning prophylaxis in organ transplant recipients. As techniques for identifying individuals at risk improve (e.g., quantification of CMV DNA by PCR), it may become possible to preemptively treat those at highest risk to prevent end-organ disease.

HUMAN HERPESVIRUS TYPES 6, 7, AND 8

Human herpesvirus (HHV) type 6 was first isolated in 1986 from peripheral-blood leukocytes of six persons with various lymphoproliferative disorders. The virus has a worldwide distribution, and two genetically distinct variants (HHV-6A and HHV-6B) are now recognized.

Infection with HHV-6 frequently develops during infancy as maternal antibody wanes. Congenital infections have also been described. HHV-6 (mostly variant B) can cause exanthem subitum (roseola infantum), a common illness characterized by fever with subsequent rash. This virus is also a major cause of febrile seizures without rash during infancy. In older age groups, HHV-6 has been associated with mononucleosis syndromes, focal encephalitis, and (in immunocompromised hosts) pneumonitis and disseminated disease. In transplant recipients, HHV-6 infection may be associated with graft dysfunction. As many as 80% of adults are seropositive for HHV-6. The virus may be transmitted by saliva and possibly by genital secretions. Like many other viruses, HHV-6 has been implicated in the pathogenesis of multiple sclerosis, although further study is needed to distinguish between association and etiology.

HHV-7 was isolated in 1990 from T lymphocytes from the peripheral blood of a healthy 26-year-old man. Other isolates have since been obtained. It appears that the virus is frequently acquired during childhood and is commonly present in the saliva of healthy adults. No human disease has yet been definitively linked to HHV-7, although some cases of exanthem subitum, other childhood febrile illnesses, and neurologic syndromes (encephalitis, flaccid paralysis) have been associated with HHV-7 infection. An association has been made between HHV-7 and pityriasis rosea, but further studies must confirm this relationship.

HHV-6, HHV-7, and CMV infections may cluster in transplant recipients, making it difficult to sort out the roles of the various agents in individual clinical syndromes. HHV-6 and HHV-7 appear to be susceptible to ganciclovir and foscarnet, although definitive evidence of clinical responses is lacking.

Unique herpesvirus-like DNA sequences were reported during 1994 and 1995 in tissues derived from Kaposi's sarcoma (KS) and body cavity–based lymphoma occurring in patients with AIDS. The virus from which these sequences were derived has now been cultured and is designated HHV-8 or Kaposi's sarcoma–associated herpesvirus (KSHV). HHV-8, which infects certain B lymphocytes and endothelium-derived spindle cells, appears to be causally related not only to KS but also to a subgroup of AIDS-related B-cell body-cavity-based lymphomas and to multicentric Castleman's disease, a lymphoproliferative disorder of B cells.

Unlike other herpesvirus infections, HHV-8 infection is more common in some geographic areas (e.g., central and southern Africa) than in others (North America, Asia, northern Europe). Concurrent epidemics of HIV-1 and HHV-8 infections among certain populations (e.g., homosexual and bisexual men) in the late 1970s and early 1980s appear to have resulted in the frequent association of AIDS and KS. Both viruses appear to be sexually transmitted, and HHV-8 may be transmitted in saliva as well. Transmission of HHV-8 may also be associated with organ transplantation and injection drug use. Among individuals with intact immunity, asymptomatic infection is the rule, and neoplastic disorders develop only after immunocompromise. Effective antiretroviral therapy for HIV-infected individuals has led to a marked reduction in rates of KS among individuals dually infected with HHV-8 and HIV in resource-rich areas. HHV-8 itself is susceptible in vitro to ganciclovir, foscarnet, and cidofovir, although clinical evidence for benefit of these agents is lacking.

FURTHER READING

CANNON MJ et al: Blood-borne and sexual transmission of human herpesvirus 8 in women with or at risk for human immunodeficiency virus infection. N Engl J Med 344:637, 2001

CENTERS FOR DISEASE CONTROL AND PREVENTION: Guidelines for preventing opportunistic infections among HIV-infected persons—2002. MMWR 51(RR-8):1, 2002

GOODMAN AD et al: Human herpesvirus 6 genome and antigen in acute multiple sclerosis lesions. J Infect Dis 187:1365, 2003

LUPPI M et al: Bone marrow failure associated with human herpesvirus 8 infection after transplantation. N Engl J Med 343:1378, 2000

LURAIN NS et al: Analysis and characterization of antiviral drug-resistant cytomegalovirus isolates from solid organ transplant recipients. J Infect Dis 186:760, 2002

MARTIN DF et al: A controlled trial of valganciclovir as induction therapy for cytomegalovirus retinitis. N Engl J Med 346:1119, 2002

NOKTA MA et al: Cytomegalovirus (CMV) polymerase chain reaction profiles in individuals with advanced human immunodeficiency virus infection: Relationship to CMV disease. J Infect Dis 185:1717, 2002

PAUK J et al: Mucosal shedding of human herpesvirus 8 in men. N Engl J Med 343:1369, 2000

PAYA CV: Prevention of cytomegalovirus disease in recipients of solid-organ transplants. Clin Infect Dis 32:596, 2001

RENWICK N et al: Seroconversion for human herpesvirus 8 during HIV infection is highly predictive of Kaposi's sarcoma. AIDS 12:2481, 1998

WALSH JC et al: Increasing survival in AIDS patients with cytomegalovirus retinitis treated with combination antiretroviral therapy including protease inhibitors. AIDS 12:613, 1998

167 MOLLUSCUM CONTAGIOSUM AND OTHER POXVIRUSES, EXCLUDING SMALLPOX VIRUS
Fred Wang

The poxviruses include a large number of related DNA viruses that infect various vertebrate hosts. The poxviruses responsible for infections in humans, along with the main manifestations of these infections, are listed in Table 167-1. Systemic human disease can result from infection with smallpox (variola major) virus, a poxvirus that infects only humans (Chap. 205), or from zoonotic infection with monkeypox virus. Other poxvirus infections cause primarily localized skin disease in humans. Molluscum contagiosum virus (MCV) is an obligate human pathogen that causes distinctive proliferative skin lesions; molluscum contagiosum is the most frequent human disease resulting from poxvirus infection. Exposure to animals infected with other poxviruses can also cause localized skin disease in humans.

MOLLUSCUM CONTAGIOSUM

Molluscum contagiosum is generally a benign disease consisting of pearly, flesh-colored, umbilicated skin lesions 2 to 5 mm in diameter with a characteristic dimple at the center (Fig. 167-1). A relative lack of inflammation and necrosis distinguishes these proliferative lesions from other poxvirus lesions. The lesions occur singly or in clusters. MCV is a human poxvirus that is transmitted by close contact, including sexual intercourse. Swimming pools are a common vector for transmission. Atopy and compromise of skin integrity increase the risk of infection. Lesions may be found anywhere on the body except the palms and soles and may be associated with an eczematous rash. The incubation period ranges from 2 weeks to 6 months, with an average of 2 to 7 weeks. In most cases, the disease is self-limited and regresses spontaneously after 3 to 4 months in immunocompetent hosts. There are no systemic complications, but skin lesions may persist for 3 to 5 years. Molluscum contagiosum develops especially often in association with the advanced stages of HIV infection, with a prevalence of

FIGURE 167-1 Molluscum contagiosum is a cutaneous poxvirus infection characterized by multiple umbilicated flesh-colored or hypopigmented papules.

5 to 18% among HIV-infected patients (Chap. 173). The disease is often more generalized, severe, and persistent in AIDS patients than in other groups, frequently involving the face and upper body. Extensive molluscum contagiosum has also been reported in conjunction with other types of immunodeficiency.

The diagnosis of molluscum contagiosum is typically made by its clinical presentation and can be confirmed by histologic demonstration of the cytoplasmic eosinophilic inclusions, or *molluscum bodies*, that are characteristic of poxvirus replication. MCV cannot be propagated in vitro, but electron microscopy and molecular studies can be used for its identification.

There is no specific systemic treatment for molluscum contagiosum, but a variety of techniques for physical ablation have been used. Molluscum contagiosum may respond to effective control of HIV infection with highly active antiretroviral therapy. Cidofovir displays in vitro activity against many poxviruses, including smallpox virus and MCV, and case reports suggest that parenteral or topical cidofovir may have some efficacy in the treatment of recalcitrant molluscum contagiosum in immunosuppressed hosts.

ZOONOTIC POXVIRUS INFECTIONS

Monkeypox virus naturally infects nonhuman primates in the tropical rain forests of western and central Africa and can infect humans who come into direct contact with infected animals. Human disease is rare and is characterized by a systemic illness and vesicular rash similar to those of variola. A large outbreak of monkeypox occurred between February 1996 and October 1997 in central Africa, with a case-fatality ratio of 3%. The prolonged period of active cases suggested a potential

TABLE 167-1 *Poxviruses and Human Infections*

Genus	Species	Human Disease
Orthopoxvirus	Variola[a]	Smallpox, systemic
	Monkeypox	Smallpox-like, systemic
	Vaccinia	Local pox lesion, occasionally systemic
	Cowpox	Local pox lesions
Molluscipoxvirus	Molluscum contagiosum	Molluscum contagiosum, multiple cutaneous lesions
Parapoxvirus	Orf	Contagious pustular dermatitis, local pox lesions
	Pseudocowpox	Milker's nodule, local pox lesions
Yatapoxvirus	Tanapox	Local pox lesions

[a] See Chap. 205.

for sustained person-to-person transmission, and the higher proportion of younger case-patients suggested the possible consequences of discontinued smallpox vaccination. Clinical presentations were occasionally confused with the more common varicella-zoster virus infection. Compared with the lesions of this herpesvirus infection, monkeypox lesions tend to be more uniform (i.e., in the same stage of development at the same time), diffuse, and peripheral in distribution.

The first outbreak of monkeypox infection in the Western Hemisphere occurred in the midwestern United States during May and June 2003. Monkeypox virus infections were diagnosed in several people who had close contact with ill prairie dogs, a Gambian rat, and a rabbit purchased as pets from a common animal distributor. Patients presented most frequently with fever, respiratory symptoms, and lymphadenopathy ~12 days after exposure. The typical vesicular rash developed with or shortly (1 to 3 days) after the fever. The Centers for Disease Control and Prevention recommended smallpox vaccination for persons having close or intimate contact with a documented case of human or animal monkeypox infection in order to reduce the risk of spread. Vaccination can be given up to 14 days after exposure.

Orf virus and pseudocowpox virus are parapoxviruses that naturally infect sheep and cattle. Direct contact with infected animals can result in infections in humans, typically on the hands, with the development of a nodular, highly vascular proliferative lesion that may ulcerate. Human orf virus infection is also called *ecthyma contagiosum*, and human pseudocowpox virus infection causes "milker's nodules." Zoonotic infection with cowpox virus, an orthopoxvirus, causes painful hemorrhagic lesions, mostly on the hands or face, with fever or flulike symptoms and lymphadenitis. Lesions generally resolve in 6 to 8 weeks. Human infection with tanapox virus occurs after contact with infected monkeys. In most cases, a febrile prodrome is followed by eruption of a single nodular lesion on the exposed area, but multiple lesions have also been reported. The lesions are relatively large, often break down to form an ulcer, and resolve in 5 to 6 weeks.

FURTHER READING

BERTHISTLE K, CARRINGTON D: Molluscum contagiosum virus. J Infect 34: 21, 1997

CENTERS FOR DISEASE CONTROL AND PREVENTION: Human monkeypox—Kasai Oriental, Zaire, 1996–1997. MMWR 46:304, 2002

———: Update: Multistate outbreak of monkeypox—Illinois, Indiana, Kansas, Missouri, Ohio, and Wisconsin, 2003. MMWR 52:642, 2003

DECLERCQ E: Cidofovir in the treatment of poxvirus infections. Antiviral Res 55:1, 2002

168 | PARVOVIRUS
Neil R. Blacklow

DEFINITION   The parvovirus group includes several species-specific viruses of animals. One parvovirus, designated B19, is known to be a human pathogen. B19 is a small (diameter, 20 to 25 nm), icosahedral, nonenveloped, single-stranded DNA virus with an outer capsid formed by two structural proteins. Individual virus particles contain DNA strands of positive or negative polarity. The virus is stable and retains infectivity after incubation at 60°C for 16 h. It has failed to grow in conventional cell culture lines and animal model systems but does replicate in vitro in erythroid progenitor cells derived from human bone marrow, umbilical cord, peripheral blood, or fetal liver sources.

During the 1980s, it was discovered that B19 causes a variety of disorders ranging from erythema infectiosum and acute arthropathy in otherwise healthy hosts to transient aplastic crisis and chronic anemia in compromised patients to fetal infection manifested by death or hydrops fetalis. Many of the severe manifestations of B19 viremia relate to the propensity of the virus to infect and lyse erythroid precursor cells in the bone marrow. The name B19 is derived from the code number of the human serum in which the virus was discovered.

PATHOGENESIS   Two studies of adult volunteers have provided a basis for understanding the pathogenesis of B19 infection, which has two phases. The first phase is characterized by viremia that develops approximately 6 days after intranasal inoculation of B19 into susceptible individuals who lack serum antibodies to the virus (Fig. 168-1). The viremia lasts about 1 week; its clearance is correlated with the development of IgM antibodies to B19, which remain detectable for up to a few months. IgG antibodies develop several days later and persist indefinitely. Nonspecific systemic symptoms lasting 2 or 3 days occur early during the viremic phase; these symptoms include headache, malaise, myalgia, fever, chills, and pruritus and are accompanied by reticulocytopenia and excretion of the virus from the respiratory tract. Several days after the onset of symptoms, a clinically insignificant decline in hemoglobin concentration is noted; the decreased level is maintained for 7 to 10 days, during which time examination of bone marrow samples reveals a marked depletion of erythroid precursor cells. Transient mild lymphopenia, neutropenia, and a drop in platelet count also may be found. A second phase of illness begins around 17 or 18 days after virus inoculation (after the clearance of viremia, the cessation of viral shedding in throat secretions, and the resolution of reticulocytopenia). This illness mimics erythema infectiosum in adults, with 2 or 3 days of fine maculopapular rash accompanied by arthralgias and arthritis that last another 1 or 2 days. This phase occurs in the presence of rising serum titers of antibody to B19.

The studies just described indicate that B19 disease in the otherwise *healthy host*, manifested by self-limited erythema infectiosum and/or arthropathy, is almost certainly an immune-complex disorder. This concept is supported by the induction of erythema infectiosum through the infusion of immunoglobulins into chronically viremic patients. In contrast, B19 disease in the *compromised host* (chronic hemolytic disease or immunodeficiency syndromes) is often serious, resulting from the destruction by B19 of erythroid precursor cells. Normal hosts can tolerate 7 to 10 days of shutoff of erythropoiesis; however, patients with hemolytic disease who require increased production of erythrocytes do not tolerate erythroid cell destruction and thus usually develop severe transient aplastic crisis. Patients who are immunodeficient may fail to clear B19 viremia, the results being persistent infection of red blood cells and chronic severe anemia. The fetus requires a higher level of red cell production than do adults and has an immature immune system; both these factors could explain B19-induced hydrops fetalis.

B19 binds specifically to a cellular receptor, erythrocyte P antigen; this specific binding explains the tropism of B19 for erythroid progenitor cells, particularly pronormoblasts and normoblasts. The few persons who lack P antigen cannot be infected with B19.

EPIDEMIOLOGY   Although B19 infections occur year-round, they appear most commonly as outbreaks of erythema infectiosum in schools during winter and spring months. Between 20 and 60% of children in outbreaks are symptomatic, and many are asymptomatically infected. Seroepidemiologic studies indicate that approximately half of adults possess serum antibodies to B19. Antibody prevalence (reflecting prior exposure and probable immunity to the virus) rises rapidly between the ages of 5 and 18 years and continues to increase with age—a pattern probably indicating ongoing exposure during adulthood. B19 can be detected in throat swabbings, respiratory tract secretions, and serum, and its detection at these sites probably correlates with infectiousness. Patients with transient aplastic crisis have viremia and shed virus and therefore are highly infectious. Their infectivity has been firmly documented as the source of one well-defined nosocomial outbreak of erythema infectiosum among nurses. In contrast, individuals with erythema infectiosum are much less infectious. The usual route of viral transmission under natural conditions is unknown but may be respiratory or through direct contact. B19 can be transmitted during therapy with clotting factor concentrate and other plasma derivatives, even after exposure to detergent, steam, or dry heat. It has been recommended that polymerase chain reaction (PCR) testing for B19 be used for screening and that potentially infectious material be discarded.

CLINICAL MANIFESTATIONS ■ Erythema Infectiosum

Erythema infectiosum is the most common manifestation of B19 infection and occurs predominantly in children. This entity is also called *fifth disease* because it was classified in the late nineteenth century as the fifth in a series of six exanthems of childhood. Normally a mild illness, erythema infectiosum typically presents as a facial rash with a "slapped-cheek" appearance that is sometimes preceded by low-grade fever. The rash may develop quickly on the arms and legs and usually has a lacy, reticular, erythematous appearance (Fig. 168-2). The trunk, palms, and soles are less commonly involved. Occasionally, the rash appears with maculopapular, morbilliform, vesicular, purpuric, or pruritic characteristics. The typical rash resolves in about a week but can recur intermittently for several weeks, particularly after stress, exercise, exposure to sunlight, bathing, or change in environmental temperature. Arthralgia and arthritis are uncommon among children but are frequent among adults, in whom the rash is often absent or nonspecific, with a lack of the characteristic facial erythema.

Arthropathy B19 infection in adults most commonly presents as acute arthralgias and arthritis, sometimes accompanied by rash. The arthritis is characteristically symmetric and peripheral, involving the wrists, hands, and knees most frequently. It normally resolves in about 3 weeks and is nondestructive. However, a small percentage of patients have arthritis persisting for months or even (in rare cases) for years. It is not known whether these individuals have persistent infection or an abnormal immune response to the virus.

FIGURE 168-1 Features of primary parvovirus infection in a seronegative volunteer inoculated with B19 virus intranasally on day 0. Asterisks indicate days on which immune complexes and virus excretion are detected. Lines refer to the time frame in which the symptoms are detected. *(From Anderson et al, with permission.)*

Transient Aplastic Crisis B19 infection is the cause in most instances of transient aplastic crisis developing suddenly in patients with chronic hemolytic disease. Nearly all hemolytic conditions can be affected by B19 infection, including sickle cell disease, erythrocyte enzyme deficiencies, hereditary spherocytosis, thalassemias, paroxysmal nocturnal hemoglobinuria, and autoimmune hemolysis. B19-induced aplastic crisis can also occur in the setting of acute blood loss. Patients present with weakness, lethargy, pallor, and severe anemia, a syndrome often preceded by a few days of nonspecific symptoms. These patients have intense reticulocytopenia lasting 7 to 10 days, and their bone marrow contains no erythroid precursor cells despite a normal myeloid series. Transient aplastic crisis can produce life-threatening anemia and may require urgent transfusion therapy. Unlike patients with erythema infectiosum or arthropathy, those with transient aplastic crisis are viremic and can readily transmit B19 infection to other people.

Chronic Anemia in Immunodeficient Patients Immunodeficient patients may be unable to eliminate B19 infection, probably because they cannot produce adequate levels of virus-specific IgG antibodies. The result is persistent infection with destruction of erythroid precursor cells in the bone marrow and chronic transfusion-dependent anemia. This condition has been described occasionally in patients with immunodeficiency related to infection with HIV, congenital immunodeficiencies, and acute lymphoblastic leukemia during maintenance chemotherapy

as well as in recipients of bone marrow, heart, liver, lung, and kidney transplants. In addition, some cases of idiopathic pure red-cell aplasia probably are caused by persistent B19 infection. B19-induced chronic anemia may be the presenting finding of an otherwise unrecognized immunodeficiency. Chronic anemia may fluctuate in intensity over time and may be cured or controlled by immunoglobulin therapy. Both the spectrum of immunodeficiencies associated with B19-induced chronic anemia and the frequency of the association remain to be determined.

Fetal and Congenital Infection Maternal B19 infections usually do not adversely affect the fetus. More often than not, in fact, the fetus remains uninfected. Therefore, couples in which the pregnant woman is infected should be counseled as to the relatively low risk of fetal infection. It is estimated that fewer than 10% of maternal B19 infections in the first 20 weeks of pregnancy lead to fetal death; when fetal death does occur, it is usually attributable to the development of nonimmune hydrops fetalis, wherein the fetus succumbs to severe anemia and congestive heart failure. In these instances, B19 can be detected in fetal tissues, with predominant infection of erythroblasts. One unconfirmed report suggests that B19 causes late second-trimester and third-trimester nonhydropic fetal deaths. Pregnant women with known exposure to B19 should have their serum monitored for IgM antibodies to the virus and for elevated levels of α-fetoprotein and human chorionic gonadotropin; ultrasonic examinations of the fetus for hydrops should

FIGURE 168-2 Lacy reticular rash of erythema infectiosum (fifth disease).

also be conducted. Some hydropic fetuses survive B19 infection and appear normal at delivery. Rarely, fetal infection with hydrops results in congenital anemia and hypogammaglobulinemia that is unresponsive to immunoglobulin therapy.

Possible Clinical Associations   Case studies suggest a link—as yet inconclusive—between B19 and several rheumatic diseases, most notably rheumatoid arthritis but also vasculitis (including polyarteritis, Wegener's granulomatosis, Raynaud's phenomenon, and giant cell arteritis), lupus erythematosus, dermatomyositis, and juvenile rheumatoid arthritis. Other associations include those involving multiple systems: cardiac (myocarditis), hematologic (hemophagocytic syndrome, idiopathic thrombocytopenic purpura), hepatic (fulminant hepatitis), neurologic (meningoencephalitis), renal (glomerulonephritis), and respiratory (pneumonia).

DIAGNOSIS   Diagnosis most commonly relies on measurements of B19-specific IgM and IgG antibodies, which can be detected with commercially available immunoassay kits. The virus, its DNA, or its antigens are also detected in the serum or infected tissues of some patients. Acute infection can be proven by B19-compatible symptoms and the presence of IgM antibodies or virus itself, whereas past infection is documented by IgG antibodies. Individuals with erythema infectiosum and acute arthropathy usually have IgM antibodies without detectable virus in serum. Those with transient aplastic crisis may have IgM antibodies but typically possess high titers of virus and its DNA in serum; the bone marrow of these patients shows characteristic giant

pronormoblasts and hypoplasia. Immunodeficient patients with anemia often lack readily detectable antibodies but have viral particles and DNA detectable by PCR in serum. Fetal infection may be recognized by hydrops fetalis and the presence of B19 DNA in amniotic fluid or fetal blood in association with maternal IgM antibodies to B19.

℞ TREATMENT

Erythema infectiosum usually requires no treatment; the same is true for many cases of arthropathy. More severe cases of arthritis, particularly those involving chronic symptoms, can be treated with nonsteroidal anti-inflammatory agents. Transient aplastic crisis is usually treated with erythrocyte transfusions. In immunodeficient anemic patients, B19 infection should be treated with commercial intravenous immunoglobulin, which is known to contain IgG antibodies to B19. This therapy controls and may cure B19 infection.

PROPHYLAXIS   Prophylaxis of B19 infection with immunoglobulin should be considered for patients with chronic hemolysis or immunodeficiency and for pregnant women. The risk of infection for these persons may be reduced by hand washing before eating or after contact with respiratory or other secretions when B19 is known to be present in a community. Patients with transient aplastic crisis or chronic B19 infection (but not those with erythema infectiosum or arthropathy) pose a serious risk for nosocomial transmission of infection. They should be hospitalized in a private room with contact and respiratory isolation precautions. It is not known whether pre- or postexposure administration of immunoglobulin prevents infection. No vaccine for B19 is currently available; however, noninfectious B19 capsid proteins have been given safely to healthy volunteers, who developed high levels of B19-specific neutralizing antibodies.

FURTHER READING

ABKOWITZ JL et al: Clinical relevance of parvovirus B19 as a cause of anemia in patients with human immunodeficiency virus infection. J Infect Dis 176: 269, 1997

ANDERSON MJ et al: Experimental parvoviral infection in humans. J Infect Dis 152:257, 1985

BARAH F et al: Association of human parvovirus B19 infection with acute meningoencephalitis. Lancet 358:729, 2001

HAREL L et al: Raynaud's phenomenon as a manifestation of parvovirus B19 infection: Case reports and review of parvovirus B19 rheumatic and vasculitic syndromes. Clin Infect Dis 30:500, 2000

MILLER E et al: Immediate and long term outcome of human parvovirus B19 infection in pregnancy. Br J Obstet Gynaecol 105:174, 1998

MORI Y et al: Association of parvovirus B19 infection with acute glomerulonephritis in healthy adults: Case report and review of the literature. Clin Nephrol 57:69, 2002

WEIGEL-KELLEY KA et al: Recombinant human parvovirus B19 vectors: Erythrocyte P antigen is necessary but not sufficient for successful transduction of human hematopoietic cells. J Virol 75:4110, 2001

169 HUMAN PAPILLOMAVIRUS INFECTIONS
Richard C. Reichman

DEFINITION   Human papillomaviruses (HPVs) selectively infect the epithelium of skin and mucous membranes. These infections may be asymptomatic, produce warts, or be associated with a variety of both benign and malignant neoplasias.

ETIOLOGIC AGENT   Papillomaviruses are members of the family Papillomaviridae. They are nonenveloped, measure 50 to 55 nm in diameter, have icosahedral capsids composed of 72 capsomeres, and contain a double-stranded circular DNA genome of ~7900 base pairs. The genomic organization of all papillomaviruses is similar and consists of an early (E) region, a late (L) region, and a noncoding upstream regulatory region (URR). Oncogenic HPV types can immortalize human

keratinocytes, and this activity has been mapped to products of early genes E6 and E7. E6 protein facilitates the degradation of the p53 tumor-suppressor protein, and E7 protein binds the retinoblastoma gene product and related proteins. The E1 and E2 proteins modulate viral DNA replication and regulate gene expression. The L1 gene codes for the major capsid protein, which makes up 80% of the virion mass. L2 codes for a minor capsid protein. Type-specific conformational antigenic determinants are located on the virion surface. Papillomavirus types are distinguished from one another by the degree of nucleic acid sequence homology. Distinct types share <90% of their DNA sequences in L1. More than 100 HPV types are recognized, and individual types are associated with specific clinical manifestations. For example, HPV-1 causes plantar warts, HPV-6 causes anogenital warts, and HPV-16 infection can produce cervical dysplasia and invasive cervical cancer. HPVs are species-specific and have not been propagated in tissue culture or in common experimental animals. However, some HPV types have been produced in human tissues implanted in immunodeficient mice.

EPIDEMIOLOGY There are few good studies of the incidence or prevalence of human warts in well-defined populations. Common warts (verruca vulgaris) are found in as many as 25% of some groups and are most prevalent among young children. Plantar warts (verruca plantaris) are also widely prevalent; they occur most often among adolescents and young adults. Condyloma acuminatum (anogenital warts) is one of the most common sexually transmitted diseases in the United States. HPV infection of the uterine cervix produces the squamous cell abnormalities most frequently detected on Papanicolaou smears.

Most anogenital HPV infections are transmitted through direct contact with infectious lesions. However, characteristics of infectious lesions, including appearance, have not been defined, and individuals without obvious disease may transmit infection. Close personal contact is also assumed to play a role in the transmission of most cutaneous warts; the importance of fomites in this setting is not clear. Minor trauma at the site of inoculation may facilitate transmission. Recurrent respiratory papillomatosis in young children is an uncommon disease that is acquired from maternal genital tract infection; in adults, orogenital sexual contact may transmit the disease.

According to a consensus panel gathered by the World Organization, a large body of epidemiologic and biologic data has established that some HPV infections cause cervical cancer. For example, >95% of cervical cancers contain HPV DNA of oncogenic (high-risk) types, such as 16, 18, 31, 33, and 45. HPV DNA is also present in the precursor lesions of cervical cancer (cervical intraepithelial neoplasias). Such lesions containing DNA of oncogenic types are more likely to progress than those associated with low-risk HPV types, such as 6 and 11. HPV DNA is transcribed in tumor tissues, and many epidemiologic studies have confirmed a strong relationship between HPV infection (with or without cofactors) and the development of cervical cancer. However, it is important to realize that most cervical HPV infections, including those caused by high-risk types, are self-limited. Infection with specific HPV types has also been associated with squamous cell carcinomas and dysplasias of the penis, anus, vagina, and vulva. In patients with epidermodysplasia verruciformis, squamous cell cancers develop frequently at sites infected with specific HPV types, including 5 and 8.

Serologic studies employing virus-like particles as antigens have demonstrated type-specific antibodies in most patients with HPV genital tract infections.

CLINICAL MANIFESTATIONS The clinical manifestations of HPV infection depend on the location of lesions and the type of virus. Common warts usually occur on the hands as flesh-colored to brown, exophytic, and hyperkeratotic papules. Plantar warts may be quite painful; they can be differentiated from calluses by paring of the surface to reveal thrombosed capillaries. Flat warts (verruca plana) are most common among children and occur on the face, neck, chest, and flexor surfaces of the forearms and legs.

Anogenital warts develop on the skin and mucosal surfaces of external genitalia and perianal areas (Fig. 169-1). Among circumcised men, warts are most commonly found on the penile shaft. Lesions frequently occur at the urethral meatus and may extend proximally. Receptive anal intercourse predisposes both men and women to the development of perianal warts, but such lesions occasionally develop without such a history. In women, warts appear first at the posterior introitus and adjacent labia. They then spread to other parts of the vulva and commonly involve the vagina and cervix. External warts in both sexes are suggestive of the presence of internal lesions, although internal lesions may be present without external warts, particularly among women. The differential diagnosis of anogenital warts includes condylomata lata of secondary syphilis, molluscum contagiosum, hirsutoid papillomatosis (pearly penile papules), fibroepitheliomas, and a variety of benign and malignant mucocutaneous neoplasms. Respiratory papillomatosis in young children, which may be life-threaten-

FIGURE 169-1 Condylomata acuminata are lesions produced by human papillomavirus and in this patient are seen as multiple verrucous papules coalescing into plaques.

ing, presents as hoarseness, stridor, or respiratory distress. The disease in adults is usually milder.

Immunosuppressed patients, particularly those undergoing organ transplantation, often develop pityriasis versicolor–like lesions, from which DNA of several HPV types has been extracted. Occasionally, such lesions appear to undergo malignant transformation. Patients infected with HIV frequently have severe clinical manifestations of HPV infection and appear to be at unusually high risk for cervical and anal dysplasia as well as for potentially invasive cancer. HPV disease in patients with HIV infection is difficult to treat and often recurs.

Epidermodysplasia verruciformis is a rare autosomal recessive disease characterized by an inability to control HPV infection. Patients are often infected with unusual HPV types and frequently develop cutaneous squamous cell malignancies, particularly in sun-exposed areas. The lesions resemble flat warts or macules similar to those of pityriasis versicolor.

The complications of warts include itching and occasionally bleeding. In rare cases warts become secondarily infected with bacteria or fungi. Large masses of warts may cause mechanical problems, such as obstruction of the birth canal. Dysplasias of the uterine cervix are generally asymptomatic until frank carcinoma develops. Patients with anogenital HPV disease may develop serious psychological symptoms due to anxiety and depression over this condition.

PATHOGENESIS The incubation period of HPV disease is usually 3 to 4 months (range, 1 month to 2 years). All types of squamous epithelium can be infected by HPV, and the gross and histologic appearances of individual lesions vary with the site of infection and the type of virus. The replication of HPV begins with the infection of basal cells. As cellular differentiation proceeds, HPV DNA replicates and is transcribed. Ultimately, virions are assembled in the nucleus and released when keratinocytes are shed. This process is associated with proliferation of all epidermal layers except the basal layer and produces acanthosis, parakeratosis, and hyperkeratosis. Koilocytes—large round cells with pyknotic nuclei—appear in the granular layer. Histologically normal epithelium may contain HPV DNA, and residual DNA after treatment can be associated with recurrent disease.

Episomal HPV DNA is present in the nuclei of infected cells in benign lesions caused by HPV. However, in severe dysplasias and cancers, HPV DNA is generally integrated, with disruption of the E1/E2 open reading frames. This disruption leads to upregulation of E6 and E7 and subsequent interference with cellular tumor-suppressor proteins.

Host defense responses to HPV infection are incompletely understood, and immune correlates of protection from infection and resolution of disease have not been established. Because patients with defects in cell-mediated immune responses, including transplant recipients and patients with HIV infection, frequently develop severe HPV disease, such responses are probably important for the control of virus replication. Histologic studies demonstrating an epidermal lymphomonocytic infiltrate in resolving warts suggest that local immunity may be of particular importance in the resolution of disease. HPV infection can also elicit a serologic response; antibodies to the viral capsid have been found in sera of patients with anogenital warts, cutaneous warts, and respiratory papillomatosis. Antibodies to E-region proteins, most notably E7, have been detected among patients with cervical carcinoma. In one prophylactic vaccine study, induction of a serologic response was associated with protection from cervical HPV infection in a group of immunocompetent young women.

DIAGNOSIS   Most warts that are visible to the naked eye can be diagnosed correctly by history and physical examination alone. The use of a colposcope is invaluable in assessing vaginal and cervical lesions and is helpful in the diagnosis of oral and cutaneous HPV disease as well. Application of 3 to 5% solutions of acetic acid may aid in the visualization of lesions, although the sensitivity and specificity of this procedure are unknown. Papanicolaou smears prepared from cervical or anal scrapings often show cytologic evidence of HPV infection. Persistent or atypical lesions should be biopsied and examined by routine histologic methods. The most sensitive and specific methods of virologic diagnosis entail the use of techniques such as the polymerase chain reaction or the hybrid capture assay to detect HPV nucleic acids and to identify specific virus types. Such tests may be useful in the diagnosis and management of cervical HPV disease, although their utility may vary according to the prevalence of disease and the availability of traditional cytologic and histologic testing. Serologic techniques to diagnose HPV infection are not helpful in individual cases and are not widely available.

℞ **TREATMENT** (Table 169-1)

Decisions regarding the initiation of therapy should be made with the knowledge that currently available modes of treatment are not completely effective and some have significant side effects. In addition, treatment may be expensive, and many HPV lesions resolve spontaneously. Frequently used therapies include cryosurgery, application of caustic agents, electrodesiccation, surgical excision, and ablation with a laser. Topical antimetabolites such as 5-fluorouracil have also been used. Both failure and recurrence have been well documented with all of these methods of treatment. Cryosurgery is the initial treatment of choice for condyloma acuminatum. Topically applied podophyllum preparations as well as podofilox may also be used. Various interferon preparations have been employed with modest success in the treatment of respiratory papillomatosis and condyloma acuminatum. A topically applied interferon inducer, imiquimod, is also of benefit in the treatment of condyloma acuminatum. The diagnosis and management of

TABLE 169-1   *Treatment of External, Exophytic Anogenital Warts*

I. Administered by provider
    A. Cryotherapy with liquid nitrogen or cryoprobe weekly
    B. Podophyllin resin, 10–25% weekly for up to 4 weeks
    C. Trichloroacetic acid or bichloroacetic acid, 80–90% weekly
    D. Surgical excision
    E. Other regimens
       1. Intralesionally administered interferon
       2. Laser surgery
II. Administered by patient
    A. Podofilox, 0.5% solution or gel twice daily for 3 days, followed by 4 days without therapy. This cycle may be repeated four times.
    B. Imiquimod, 5% cream 3 times per week for up to 16 weeks

Source: Modified from Centers for Disease Control and Prevention: MMWR 51(RR-6):1, 2002 (*http://www.cdc.gov/mmwr/PDF/RR/RR5106.pdf*).

anogenital dysplasias and of internal anogenital warts require special skills and resources, and patients with such lesions should be referred to a qualified specialist.

PREVENTION   Apart from the avoidance of contact with infectious lesions, no effective methods for the prevention of HPV infections are available at present. Barrier methods of contraception may be helpful in preventing transmission of condyloma acuminatum and other anogenital HPV-associated diseases. Vaccines consisting of virus-like particles (VLPs) can prevent papillomavirus disease in animal models. One study of an HPV-16 VLP vaccine in uninfected women has shown protection from cervical infection with the homologous virus. More extensive clinical trials of these preparations are likely to demonstrate reductions in rates of cervical HPV disease.

FURTHER READING

BALDWIN SB et al: Human papillomavirus infection in men attending a sexually transmitted disease clinic. J Infect Dis 187:1064, 2003

BONNEZ W, REICHMAN RC: Papillomaviruses, in *Principles and Practice of Infectious Diseases*, 6th ed, GL Mandell et al (eds). Churchill Livingstone, New York, 2004

BOSCH FX et al: The causal relationship between human papillomavirus and cervical cancer. J Clin Pathol 55:244, 2002

CENTERS FOR DISEASE CONTROL AND PREVENTION: Sexually transmitted diseases treatment guidelines—2002. MMWR 51(RR-6):1, 2002

EVANS TG et al: A phase I study of a recombinant virus-like particle vaccine against human papillomavirus type 11 in healthy adult volunteers. J Infect Dis 183:1485, 2001

FRISCH M et al: Human papillomavirus–associated cancers in patients with human immunodeficiency virus infection and acquired immunodeficiency syndrome. J Natl Cancer Inst 92:1500, 2000

KOUTSKY LA et al: A controlled trial of a human papillomavirus type 16 vaccine. N Engl J Med 347:1645, 2002

LUQUE AE et al: Association of human papillomavirus infection and disease with magnitude of human immunodeficiency virus type 1 (HIV-1) RNA plasma level among women with HIV-1 infection. J Infect Dis 179:1405, 1999

MUNOZ N et al: Epidemiologic classification of human papillomavirus types associated with cervical cancer. N Engl J Med 348:518, 2003

WRIGHT TC JR et al: ASCCP-Sponsored Consensus Conference: 2001 consensus guidelines for the management of women with cervical cytological abnormalities. JAMA 287:2120, 2002

170 COMMON VIRAL RESPIRATORY INFECTIONS AND SEVERE ACUTE RESPIRATORY SYNDROME (SARS)
Raphael Dolin

GENERAL CONSIDERATIONS   Acute viral respiratory illnesses are among the most common of human diseases, accounting for one-half or more of all acute illnesses. The incidence of acute respiratory disease in the United States is from 3 to 5.6 cases per person per year. The rates are highest among children <1 year old (6.1 to 8.3 cases per year) and remain high until age 6, when a progressive decrease begins. Adults have 3 to 4 cases per person per year. Morbidity from acute respiratory illnesses accounts for 30 to 50% of time lost from work by adults and for 60 to 80% of time lost from school by children. The use of antibacterial agents to treat viral respiratory infections represents a major source of abuse of that category of drugs.

It has been estimated that two-thirds to three-fourths of cases of acute respiratory illnesses are caused by viruses. More than 200 antigenically distinct viruses from 9 different genera have been reported to cause acute respiratory illness, and it is likely that additional agents will be described in the future. The vast majority of these viral infections involve the upper respiratory tract, but lower respiratory tract disease can also develop, particularly in younger age groups and in certain epidemiologic settings.

The illnesses caused by respiratory viruses traditionally have been divided into multiple distinct syndromes, such as the "common cold," pharyngitis, croup (laryngotracheobronchitis), tracheitis, bronchiolitis, bronchitis, and pneumonia. Each of these general categories of illness has a certain epidemiologic and clinical profile; for example, croup occurs exclusively in very young children and has a characteristic clinical course. Some types of respiratory illness are more likely to be associated with certain viruses (e.g., the common cold with rhinoviruses), while others occupy characteristic epidemiologic niches (e.g., adenovirus infections in military recruits). The syndromes most commonly associated with infections with the major respiratory virus groups are summarized in Table 170-1. Most respiratory viruses clearly have the potential to cause more than one type of respiratory illness, and frequently features of several types of illness are found in the same patient. Moreover, the clinical illnesses induced by these viruses are rarely sufficiently distinctive to permit an etiologic diagnosis on clinical grounds alone, although the epidemiologic setting increases the likelihood that one group of viruses rather than another is involved. In general, laboratory methods must be relied on to establish a specific viral diagnosis.

This chapter reviews viral infections caused by six of the major groups of respiratory viruses:

rhinoviruses, coronaviruses, respiratory syncytial viruses, metapneumoviruses, parainfluenza viruses, and adenoviruses. The recent extraordinary outbreaks of lower respiratory tract disease associated with coronaviruses (severe acute respiratory syndrome, or SARS) are also discussed. Influenza viruses, which are a major cause of mortality as well as morbidity, are reviewed in Chap. 171. Herpesviruses, which occasionally cause pharyngitis and which also cause lower respiratory tract disease in immunosuppressed patients, are reviewed in Chap. 163. Enteroviruses, which account for occasional respiratory illnesses during the summer months, are reviewed in Chap. 175.

RHINOVIRUS INFECTIONS

ETIOLOGIC AGENT   Rhinoviruses are members of the Picornaviridae family, small (15 to 30 nm) nonenveloped viruses that contain a single-stranded RNA genome. In contrast to other members of the picornavirus family, such as enteroviruses, rhinoviruses are acid-labile and are almost completely inactivated at pH ≤ 3. Rhinoviruses grow preferentially at 33° to 34°C—the temperature of the human nasal passages—rather than at the higher temperature (37°C) of the lower respiratory tract. A total of 102 distinct serotypes of rhinovirus are recognized. Of these serotypes, 91 use intercellular adhesion molecule 1 (ICAM-1) as a cellular receptor and comprise the "major" receptor

TABLE 170-1   *Illnesses Associated with Respiratory Viruses*

Virus	Frequency of Respiratory Syndromes		
	Most Frequent	**Occasional**	**Infrequent**
Rhinoviruses	Common cold	Exacerbation of chronic bronchitis and asthma	Pneumonia in children
Coronaviruses[a]	Common cold	Exacerbation of chronic bronchitis and asthma	Pneumonia and bronchiolitis
Respiratory syncytial virus	Pneumonia and bronchiolitis in young children	Common cold in adults	Pneumonia in elderly and immunosuppressed patients
Parainfluenza viruses	Croup and lower respiratory tract disease in young children	Pharyngitis and common cold	Tracheobronchitis in adults; lower respiratory tract disease in immunosuppressed patients
Adenoviruses	Common cold and pharyngitis in children	Outbreaks of acute respiratory disease in military recruits[b]	Pneumonia in children; lower respiratory tract and disseminated disease in immunosuppressed patients
Influenza A viruses	Influenza[c]	Pneumonia and excess mortality in high-risk patients	Pneumonia in healthy individuals
Influenza B viruses	Influenza[c]	Rhinitis and pharyngitis alone	Pneumonia
Enteroviruses	Acute undifferentiated febrile illnesses[d]	Rhinitis and pharyngitis	Pneumonia
Herpes simplex viruses	Gingivostomatitis in children; pharyngotonsillitis in adults	Tracheitis and pneumonia in immunocompromised patients	Disseminated infection in immunocompromised patients
Human metapneumoviruses[e]	—	—	—

[a] SARS-associated coronavirus (SARS-CoV) caused epidemics of pneumonia from November 2002 to July 2003 (see text).
[b] Serotypes 4 and 7.
[c] Fever, cough, myalgia, malaise.
[d] May or may not have a respiratory component.
[e] Newly recognized human metapneumoviruses that cause upper and lower respiratory tract illnesses; their relative frequency has not yet been established.

group, 10 use the low-density lipoprotein receptor and comprise the "minor" receptor group, and 1 uses a sialoprotein cellular receptor.

EPIDEMIOLOGY Rhinoviruses are a major cause of the common cold and have been isolated from 15 to 40% of adults with common cold–like illnesses. Overall rates of infection with rhinoviruses are higher among infants and young children and decrease with increasing age. Rhinovirus infections occur throughout the year, with seasonal peaks in early fall and spring in temperate climates. These infections are most often introduced into families by preschool or grade-school children <6 years old. Between 25 and 70% of initial illnesses in family settings are followed by secondary cases, with the highest attack rates among the youngest siblings at home. Attack rates also increase with family size.

Rhinoviruses appear to spread through direct contact with infected secretions, usually respiratory droplets. In some studies of volunteers, transmission was most efficient by hand-to-hand contact, with subsequent self-inoculation of the conjunctival or nasal mucosa. In other studies, transmission by large- or small-particle aerosol was demonstrated. Virus can also be recovered from plastic surfaces inoculated 1 to 3 h previously; this observation suggests that environmental surfaces contribute to transmission. In studies of married couples in which neither partner had detectable serum antibody, transmission was associated with prolonged contact ($\geq$122 h) during a 7-day period. Transmission was infrequent unless virus was recoverable from the donor's hands and nasal mucosa, at least 1000 TCID$_{50}$ of virus was present in nasal washes from the donor, and the donor was at least moderately symptomatic with the "cold." Despite anecdotal observations, exposure to cold temperatures, fatigue, or sleep deprivation has not been associated with increased rates of rhinovirus-induced illness in volunteers, although some studies have suggested that psychologically defined "stress" may contribute to development of symptoms.

Infection with rhinoviruses is worldwide in distribution. By the time they reach adulthood, nearly all individuals have neutralizing antibodies to multiple serotypes, although the prevalence of antibody to any one serotype varies widely. Multiple serotypes circulate simultaneously, and generally no single serotype or group of serotypes has been more prevalent than the others.

PATHOGENESIS Rhinoviruses infect cells through attachment to specific cellular receptors; as mentioned above, most serotypes attach to ICAM-1, while a few use the low-density lipoprotein receptor. Relatively limited information is available on the histopathology and pathogenesis of acute rhinovirus infections in humans. Examination of biopsy specimens obtained during experimentally induced and naturally occurring illness indicates that the nasal mucosa is edematous, is often hyperemic, and—during acute illness—is covered by a mucoid discharge. There is a mild infiltrate with inflammatory cells, including neutrophils, lymphocytes, plasma cells, and eosinophils. Mucus-secreting glands in the submucosa appear hyperactive; the nasal turbinates are engorged, a condition that may lead to obstruction of nearby openings of sinus cavities. Several mediators, such as bradykinin, lysylbradykinin, prostaglandins, histamine, and interleukins 1, 6, and 8, have been linked to the development of signs and symptoms in rhinovirus-induced colds.

The incubation period for rhinovirus illness is short, generally 1 or 2 days. Virus shedding coincides with the onset of illness or may begin shortly before symptoms develop. The mechanisms of immunity to rhinovirus are not well worked out. In some studies, the presence of homotypic antibody has been associated with significantly reduced rates of subsequent infection and illness, but data conflict regarding the relative importance of serum and local antibody in protection from rhinovirus infection.

CLINICAL MANIFESTATIONS The most common clinical manifestations of rhinovirus infections are those of the common cold. Illness usually begins with rhinorrhea and sneezing accompanied by nasal congestion. The throat is frequently sore, and in some cases sore throat is the initial complaint. Systemic signs and symptoms, such as malaise and headache, are mild or absent, and fever is unusual. Illness generally lasts for 4 to 9 days and resolves spontaneously without sequelae. In children, bronchitis, bronchiolitis, and bronchopneumonia have been reported; nevertheless, it appears that rhinoviruses are not major causes of lower respiratory tract disease in children. Rhinoviruses may cause exacerbations of asthma and chronic pulmonary disease in adults. The vast majority of rhinovirus infections resolve without sequelae, but complications related to obstruction of the eustachian tubes or sinus ostia, including otitis media or acute sinusitis, can develop. In immunosuppressed patients, particularly bone marrow transplant recipients, severe and even fatal pneumonias have been associated with rhinovirus infections.

DIAGNOSIS Although rhinoviruses are the most frequently recognized cause of the common cold, similar illnesses are caused by a variety of other viruses, and the etiologic diagnosis cannot be made on clinical grounds alone. Rather, rhinovirus infection is diagnosed by isolation of the virus from nasal washes or nasal secretions in tissue culture. In practice, this procedure is rarely undertaken because of the benign, self-limited nature of the illness. In most settings, detection of rhinovirus RNA by polymerase chain reaction (PCR) is more sensitive than that by tissue culture; however, this PCR is largely a research procedure. Given the many serotypes of rhinovirus, diagnosis by serum antibody tests is currently impractical. Likewise, common laboratory tests, such as white cell count and sedimentation rate, are not helpful.

Rx TREATMENT

Rhinovirus infections are generally mild and self-limited, so treatment is not usually necessary. Therapy in the form of first-generation antihistamines and nonsteroidal anti-inflammatory drugs may be beneficial in patients with particularly pronounced symptoms, and an oral decongestant may be added if nasal obstruction is particularly troublesome. Reduction of activity is prudent in instances of significant discomfort or fatigability. Antibacterial agents should be used only if bacterial complications such as otitis media or sinusitis develop. Specific antiviral therapy is not available.

PREVENTION Application of interferon sprays intranasally has been effective in the prophylaxis of rhinovirus infections but is also associated with local irritation of the nasal mucosa. Studies of the prevention of rhinovirus infection by administration of antibodies to ICAM-1 or by the soluble purified receptors themselves have yielded disappointing results. Experimental vaccines to certain rhinovirus serotypes have been generated, but their usefulness is questionable because of the myriad serotypes and the uncertainty about mechanisms of immunity. Thorough hand washing, environmental decontamination, and protection against autoinoculation may help to reduce rates of transmission of infection.

CORONAVIRUS INFECTIONS, INCLUDING SARS

ETIOLOGIC AGENT Coronaviruses are pleomorphic, single-strand RNA viruses that measure 100 to 150 nm in diameter. The name derives from the crownlike appearance produced by the club-shaped projections that stud the viral envelope. Coronaviruses infect a wide variety of animal species and have been divided into three antigenic groups. Previously recognized coronaviruses that infect humans fell into two of these groups (I and II), which are represented by prototype isolates HCoV-229E and HCoV-OC43, respectively. The coronavirus associated with SARS (SARS-CoV) appears to be of a novel and distinct group (Fig. 170-1). To date, the SARS-CoV strains that have been fully sequenced have shown only minimal variation.

In general, human coronaviruses have been difficult to cultivate in vitro, and some strains grow only in human tracheal organ cultures rather than in tissue culture. SARS-CoV is an exception whose ready growth in African green monkey kidney (Vero E6) cells greatly facilitates its study.

EPIDEMIOLOGY Generally, human coronavirus infections are present throughout the world. Seroprevalence studies of strains HCoV-229E and HCoV-OC43 have demonstrated that serum antibodies are acquired early in life and increase in prevalence with advancing age, so that >80% of adult populations have antibodies as measured by enzyme-linked immunosorbent assay (ELISA). Overall, coronaviruses account for 10 to 35% of common colds, depending on the season. Coronavirus infections appear to be particularly prevalent in late fall, winter, and early spring—times when rhinovirus infections are less common.

The epidemic of the coronavirus-associated illness known as SARS apparently began in Guangdong Province of China in November 2002 and possibly originated from contact with semidomesticated animals such as the palm civet or the dog raccoon. These animals are prized as edible delicacies in the area and harbor infections with coronaviruses related to SARS CoV. Between November 16, 2002, and February 28, 2003, 792 cases of apparent SARS were noted in Guangdong, and it was recognized that health care workers and their contacts accounted for many of the cases. A physician from Guangdong who traveled to Hong Kong to visit his family 5 days after the onset of his illness may represent the index case that introduced SARS into Hong Kong. In March 2003, a large number of cases of severe respiratory disease were reported to the World Health Organization (WHO) from Hong Kong. Many of the patients had had contact with the putative index case, had stayed at the hotel where he resided, or had had contact with secondary cases. At nearly the same time, similar cases were noted in Singapore, Thailand, Vietnam, Taiwan, and Toronto (Canada), initially in travelers from Hong Kong or Guangdong. Ultimately, 8422 cases were identified by WHO in 28 countries of Asia, Europe, and North America, although ~90% of cases occurred in China and Hong Kong. Case-fatality rates varied among the outbreaks, with an overall figure of ~11%. The disease appeared to be somewhat milder in cases in the United States and was clearly less severe among children (see below).

The mechanisms of transmission of SARS are incompletely understood. Clusters of cases suggest that spread may occur by both large and small aerosols and perhaps by the fecal-oral route as well. The outbreak of illness in a large apartment complex in Hong Kong suggested that environmental sources, such as sewage or water, may also play a role in transmission. Some ill individuals appeared to be hyperinfectious ("super-spreaders") and were capable of transmitting infection to 10 to 40 contacts, although most infections resulted in spread either to no one or to up to three individuals.

PATHOGENESIS Coronaviruses that cause the common cold (e.g., strains HCoV-229E and HCoV-OC43) infect ciliated epithelial cells in the nasopharynx. Viral replication leads to damage of ciliated cells and induction of chemokines and interleukins, which result in common-cold symptoms similar to those induced by rhinoviruses.

The pathogenesis of SARS is that of a systemic illness in which virus likely enters and infects cells of the respiratory tract but is also found in the bloodstream, in the urine, and (for up to 2 months) in the stool. Virus persists in the respiratory tract for 2 to 3 weeks, and titers peak ~10 days after the onset of systemic illness. Pulmonary pathology consists of hyaline membrane formation, desquamation of pneumocytes in alveolar spaces, and an interstitial infiltrate consisting of lymphocytes and mononuclear cells. Giant cells are frequently seen, and coronavirus particles have been detected in type II pneumocytes.

CLINICAL MANIFESTATIONS After an incubation period that generally lasts 2 to 7 days (range, 1 to 10 days), SARS usually begins as a systemic illness marked by the onset of fever, which is often accompanied by malaise, headache, and myalgias and is followed in 1 to 2 days by a nonproductive cough and dyspnea. Approximately 25% of patients have diarrhea. Chest x-rays can show a variety of infiltrates, including patchy areas of consolidation—most frequently in peripheral and lower lung fields—or interstitial infiltrates, which can progress to diffuse involvement (Fig. 170-2).

FIGURE 170-1 Electron micrograph of SARS-associated coronavirus (SARS-CoV) isolated in fetal rhesus kidney tissue culture from a lung biopsy sample from a patient with SARS. Viral particles are 55 to 90 mm in diameter. [*Reprinted with permission from Elsevier (JSM Peiris et al., Lancet 361:1319, 2003).*]

In severe cases, respiratory function may worsen during the second week of illness and progress to frank adult respiratory distress syndrome (ARDS) accompanied by multiorgan dysfunction. Risk factors for severity of disease include an age of >50 and comorbidities such as cardiovascular disease, diabetes, or hepatitis. Illness in pregnant women may be particularly severe, but SARS-CoV infection appears to be milder in children than in adults.

The clinical features of common colds caused by human coronaviruses are similar to those of illness caused by rhinoviruses. In studies of volunteers, the mean incubation period of colds induced by coronaviruses (3 days) is somewhat longer than that of illness caused by rhinoviruses, and the duration of illness is somewhat shorter (mean, 6 to 7 days). In some studies, the amount of nasal discharge was somewhat greater in colds induced by coronaviruses than in those induced by rhinoviruses. Coronaviruses other than SARS-CoV have been recovered occasionally from infants with pneumonia and from military recruits with lower respiratory tract disease and have been associated with worsening of chronic bronchitis.

LABORATORY FINDINGS AND DIAGNOSIS Laboratory abnormalities in SARS include lymphopenia, which is present in ~50% of cases and which mostly affects CD4+ T cells but also involves CD8+ T cells and NK cells. Total white blood cell counts are normal or slightly low, and thrombocytopenia may develop as the illness progresses. Elevated serum levels of aminotransferases, creatine kinase, and lactate dehydrogenase have been reported.

The WHO and the Centers for Disease Control and Prevention have developed case definitions for diagnosis of SARS. These definitions include clinical, epidemiologic, and laboratory features, which are being refined as additional information on SARS is gathered. SARS-CoV can be grown from respiratory tract samples by inoculation into Vero E6 tissue culture cells, in which a cytopathic effect can be seen within days. A rapid diagnosis can be made by reverse-transcriptase PCR (RT-PCR) of respiratory tract samples and plasma early in illness and of urine and stool later on. RT-PCR appears to be more sensitive than tissue culture, but only around one-third of cases are positive by PCR at initial presentation. Serum antibodies can be detected by ELISA or immunofluorescence, and nearly all patients develop detectable serum antibodies within 28 days after the onset of illness.

Laboratory diagnosis of coronavirus-induced colds is rarely required. Coronaviruses that cause those illnesses are frequently difficult to cultivate in vitro but can be detected in clinical samples by ELISA or immunofluorescence assays or by RT-PCR for viral RNA. These research procedures can be used to detect coronaviruses in unusual clinical settings.

FIGURE 170-2 Chest x-rays of a 46-year-old man with SARS. The left lower lung infiltrate seen initially (*A*) progressed to multiple bilateral opacities (*B*). (*Reprinted with permission from L Lee et al. © 2003 Massachusetts Medical Society.*)

℞ TREATMENT

There is no specific therapy of established efficacy for SARS. Although ribavirin has frequently been used, it has little if any activity against SARS-CoV in vitro, and no beneficial effect on the course of illness has been demonstrated. Because of suggestions that immunopathology may contribute to the disease, glucocorticoids have also been widely used, but their benefit, if any, is likewise unestablished. Supportive care to maintain pulmonary and other organ system functions remains the mainstay of therapy.

The approach to the treatment of common colds caused by coronaviruses is similar to that discussed above for rhinovirus-induced illnesses.

PREVENTION The recognition of SARS led to a worldwide mobilization of public health resources to apply infection control practices and thus to contain the disease. Case definitions were established, travel advisories were proposed, and quarantines were imposed in certain locales. In line with criteria based on the absence of new cases for 30 days (three times the estimated incubation period of 10 days for the disease), all travel advisories have been lifted as of this writing (February 2004). It remains unknown whether the disappearance of cases is a result of the above control measures, whether it is part of a seasonal or otherwise unexplained epidemiologic pattern of SARS, and when or whether SARS might reemerge. The frequent transmission of the disease to health care workers makes it mandatory that strict infection control practices be employed by health care facilities to prevent airborne, droplet, and contact transmission from any suspected cases of SARS in the fruture.

Vaccines have been developed against several animal coronaviruses but not against known human coronaviruses. The emergence of SARS-CoV has emphasized the importance of the development of vaccines against such agents.

RESPIRATORY SYNCYTIAL VIRUS INFECTIONS

ETIOLOGIC AGENT Respiratory syncytial virus (RSV) is a member of the Paramyxoviridae family (genus *Pneumovirus*). RSV, an enveloped virus ~150 to 300 nm in diameter, is so named because its replication in vitro leads to the fusion of neighboring cells into large multinucleated syncytla. The single-stranded RNA genome codes for 11 virus-specific proteins. Viral RNA is contained in a helical nucleocapsid surrounded by a lipid envelope bearing two glycoproteins: the G protein, by which the virus attaches to cells, and the F (fusion) protein, which facilitates entry of the virus into the cell by fusing host and viral

membranes. RSV was once considered to be of a single antigenic type, but two distinct groups (A and B) and multiple subtypes within each group have now been described. Antigenic diversity is reflected by differences in the G protein, while the F protein is highly conserved. Both antigenic groups can circulate simultaneously in outbreaks, although the relative proportions of each vary. Infections with group B viruses may be somewhat milder than those with group A viruses.

EPIDEMIOLOGY RSV is the major respiratory pathogen of young children and the foremost cause of lower respiratory disease in infants. Infection with RSV is seen throughout the world in annual epidemics that occur in late fall, winter, or spring and last up to 5 months. The virus is rarely encountered during the summer. Rates of illness are highest among infants 1 to 6 months of age, peaking between 2 and 3 months of age. The attack rates among susceptible infants and children are extraordinarily high, approaching 100% in settings such as day-care centers where large numbers of susceptible infants are present. By age 2, virtually all children will have been infected with RSV. RSV accounts for 20 to 25% of hospital admissions of young infants and children for pneumonia and for up to 75% of cases of bronchiolitis in this age group. It has been estimated that more than half of infants who are at risk will become infected during an RSV epidemic.

In older children and adults, reinfection with RSV is frequent but disease is milder than in infancy. A common cold–like syndrome is the illness most commonly associated with RSV infection in adults. Severe lower respiratory tract disease with pneumonitis can occur in elderly (often institutionalized) adults and in patients with immuno-compromising disorders or treatment, including recipients of bone-marrow and solid-organ transplants. RSV is also an important nosocomial pathogen; during an outbreak, it can infect pediatric patients and up to 25 to 50% of the staff on pediatric wards. The spread of virus among families is efficient: up to 40% of siblings may become infected when RSV is introduced into the family setting.

RSV is transmitted primarily by close contact with contaminated fingers or fomites and by self-inoculation of the conjunctiva or anterior nares. Virus may also be spread by coarse aerosols produced by coughing or sneezing, but it is inefficiently spread by fine-particle aerosols. The incubation period is ~4 to 6 days, and virus shedding may last for ≥2 weeks in children and for shorter periods in adults. In immunosuppressed patients, shedding can be prolonged for multiple weeks.

PATHOGENESIS Little is known about the histopathology of minor RSV infection. Severe bronchiolitis or pneumonia is characterized by necrosis of the bronchiolar epithelium and a peribronchiolar infiltrate of lymphocytes and mononuclear cells. Interalveolar thickening and filling of alveolar spaces with fluid can also be found. The correlates of protective immunity to RSV are incompletely understood. Because reinfection occurs frequently and is often associated with illness, the immunity that develops after single episodes of infection clearly is not complete or long-lasting. However, the cumulative effect of multiple reinfections is to temper subsequent disease and to provide some temporary measure of protection against infection. Studies of experimentally induced disease in healthy volunteers indicate that the presence of nasal IgA neutralizing antibody correlates more closely with protection than does the presence of serum antibody. Studies in infants, however, suggest that maternally acquired antibody provides some protection from lower respiratory tract disease, although illness can be severe even in infants who have moderate levels of maternally derived serum antibody. The relatively severe disease observed in immuno-suppressed patients and experimental animal models indicates that cell-mediated immunity is an important mechanism of host defense against RSV. Evidence suggests that class I MHC-restricted cytotoxic T cells may be particularly important in this regard.

CLINICAL MANIFESTATIONS RSV infection leads to a wide spectrum of respiratory illnesses. In infants, 25 to 40% of infections result in lower respiratory tract involvement, including pneumonia, bronchiolitis, and tracheobronchitis. In this age group, illness begins most frequently with rhinorrhea, low-grade fever, and mild systemic symptoms, often accompanied by cough and wheezing. Most patients recover gradually over 1 to 2 weeks. In more severe illness, tachypnea and dyspnea develop, and eventually frank hypoxia, cyanosis, and apnea can ensue. Physical examination may reveal diffuse wheezing, rhonchi, and rales. Chest radiography shows hyperexpansion, peribronchial thickening, and variable infiltrates ranging from diffuse interstitial infiltrates to segmental or lobar consolidation. Illness may be particularly severe in children born prematurely and in those with congenital cardiac disease, bronchopulmonary dysplasia, nephrotic syndrome, or immunosuppression. One study documented a 37% mortality rate for infants with RSV pneumonia and congenital cardiac disease.

In adults, the most common symptoms of RSV infection are those of the common cold, with rhinorrhea, sore throat, and cough. Illness is occasionally associated with moderate systemic symptoms such as malaise, headache, and fever. RSV has also been reported to cause lower respiratory tract disease with fever in adults, including severe pneumonia in the elderly—particularly in nursing-home residents, among whom its impact can rival that of influenza. RSV pneumonia can be a significant cause of morbidity and mortality in patients undergoing bone-marrow and solid-organ transplantation, where case-fatality rates of 20 to 80% have been reported. Sinusitis, otitis media, and worsening of chronic obstructive and reactive airway disease have also been associated with RSV infection.

LABORATORY FINDINGS AND DIAGNOSIS The diagnosis of RSV infection can be suspected on the basis of a suggestive epidemiologic setting—that is, severe illness among infants during an outbreak of RSV in the community. Infections in older children and adults cannot be differentiated with certainty from those caused by other respiratory viruses. The specific diagnosis is established by isolation of RSV from respiratory secretions, such as sputum, throat swabs, or nasopharyngeal washes. Virus is isolated in tissue culture and is identified specifically by immunofluorescence, ELISA, or other immunologic techniques. Rapid viral diagnosis is available by immunofluorescence techniques or ELISA of nasopharyngeal washes, aspirates, and (less satisfactorily) nasopharyngeal swabs. In children, these techniques have sensitivities and specificities of 80 to 95%; they are somewhat less sensitive in specimens from adults. Serologic diagnosis may be made by comparison of acute- and convalescent-phase serum specimens by ELISA, neutralization, or complement-fixation tests. These tests may be useful in older children and adults but are less sensitive in children <4 months of age.

℞ TREATMENT

Treatment of upper respiratory tract RSV infection is aimed primarily at the alleviation of symptoms and is similar to that for other viral infections of the upper respiratory tract. For lower respiratory tract infections, respiratory therapy, including hydration, suctioning of secretions, and administration of humidified oxygen and antibronchospastic agents, is given as needed. In severe hypoxia, intubation and ventilatory assistance may be required. Studies of infants with RSV infection who were given aerosolized ribavirin, a nucleoside analogue active in vitro against RSV, have demonstrated a beneficial effect on the resolution of lower respiratory tract illness, including alleviation of blood-gas abnormalities. Treatment with aerosolized ribavirin is recommended for infants who are severely ill or who are at high risk

for complications of RSV infection; included are premature infants and those with bronchopulmonary dysplasia, congenital heart disease, or immunosuppression. The efficacy of ribavirin in older children and adults with RSV pneumonia, including those with immunosuppression, has not been established. Administration of standard immunoglobulin, immunoglobulin with high antibody titers to RSV (RSVIg), or chimeric mouse-human monoclonal IgG against RSV (palivizumab) has not been found to be beneficial in the treatment of RSV pneumonia. Combined therapy with aerosolized ribavirin and palivizumab is being evaluated in the treatment of immunosuppressed patients with RSV pneumonia.

PREVENTION Monthly administration of RSVIg or palivizumab has been approved as prophylaxis against RSV for children <2 years of age who have bronchopulmonary dysplasia or were born prematurely. Considerable interest exists in the development of vaccines against RSV. Inactivated whole-virus vaccines have been ineffective; in one study, they actually potentiated the disease in infants. Other approaches include immunization with purified F and G surface glycoproteins of RSV or generation of stable, live attenuated virus vaccines. In settings such as pediatric wards where rates of transmission are high, barrier methods for the protection of hands and conjunctivae may be useful in reducing the spread of virus.

METAPNEUMOVIRUS INFECTIONS

Human metapneumovirus (HMPV) is a newly described viral respiratory pathogen that has been assigned to the Paramyxoviridae family (genus *Metapneumovirus*). Its morphology and genomic organization are similar to those of avian metapneumoviruses, which are recognized respiratory pathogens of turkeys. HMPV particles may be spherical, filamentous, or pleomorphic in shape and measure 60 to 280 nm in diameter. Particles contain 15-nm projections from the surface that are similar in appearance to those of other Paramyxoviridae. Studies of the RNA genome indicate that there are at least two genetic subgroups or genotypes of HMPV.

HMPV was initially detected in nasal aspirates from 28 children hospitalized with lower respiratory tract illnesses over a 20-year period (1981–2001) in the Netherlands. HMPV infections have since been reported in a wide variety of age groups, including elderly adults, and in both immunocompetent and immunosuppressed hosts. Initial sero-epidemiologic studies suggest that HMPV infections are worldwide in distribution, are most frequent during the winter, and occur early in life, so that serum antibodies to the virus are present in nearly all children by the age of 5. The spectrum of clinical illnesses associated with HMPV is similar to that associated with RSV and includes both upper and lower respiratory tract illnesses, such as bronchiolitis, croup, and pneumonia.

HMPV can be detected in nasal aspirates and respiratory secretions by PCR or by growth in rhesus monkey kidney (LLC-MK2) tissue cultures. Serologic diagnosis can be made by ELISA, which utilizes HMPV-infected tissue culture lysates as sources of antigens.

Preliminary studies indicate that HMPV infections account for 4% of respiratory tract illnesses requiring hospitalization of children and for 2 to 4% of acute respiratory illnesses in ambulatory adults and elderly patients. HMPV has been detected in a few cases of SARS, but its role (if any) in these illnesses has not been established. Assessment of the overall significance of HMPV infections awaits the conduct of large-scale epidemiologic studies.

PARAINFLUENZA VIRUS INFECTIONS

ETIOLOGIC AGENT Parainfluenza viruses belong to the Paramyxoviridae family (genera *Respirovirus* and *Rubulavirus*). They are 150 to 200 nm in diameter, are enveloped, and contain a single-stranded RNA genome. The envelope is studded with two glycoproteins: one possesses both hemagglutinin and neuraminidase activity and the other contains fusion activity. The viral RNA genome is enclosed in a helical nucleocapsid and codes for six structural and several accessory proteins. All four distinct serotypes of parainfluenza viruses share certain antigens with other members of the Paramyxoviridae family, including mumps and Newcastle disease viruses.

EPIDEMIOLOGY Parainfluenza viruses are distributed throughout the world; infection with type 4 (subtypes 4A and 4B) has been reported less widely, probably because type 4 is more difficult to grow in tissue culture. Infection is acquired in early childhood, so that by 5 years of age most children have antibodies to serotypes 1, 2, and 3. Types 1 and 2 cause epidemics during the fall, often occurring in an alternate-year pattern. Type 3 infection has been detected during all seasons of the year, but epidemics have occurred annually in the spring.

The contribution of parainfluenza infections to respiratory disease varies with both the location and the year. In studies conducted in the United States, parainfluenza virus infections have accounted for 4.3 to 22% of respiratory illnesses in children. In adults, parainfluenza infections are generally mild and account for <10% of respiratory illnesses. The major importance of parainfluenza viruses is as a cause of respiratory illness in young children, in whom they rank second only to RSV as causes of lower respiratory tract illness. Parainfluenza virus type 1 is the most frequent cause of croup (laryngotracheobronchitis) in children, while serotype 2 causes similar, although generally less severe, disease. Type 3 is an important cause of bronchiolitis and pneumonia in infants, while illnesses associated with type 4 have generally been mild. Unlike types 1 and 2, type 3 frequently causes illness during the first month of life, when passively acquired maternal antibody is still present. Parainfluenza viruses are spread through infected respiratory secretions, primarily by person-to-person contact and/or by large droplets. The incubation period has varied from 3 to 6 days in experimental infections but may be somewhat shorter for naturally occurring disease in children.

PATHOGENESIS Immunity to parainfluenza viruses is incompletely understood, but evidence suggests that immunity to infections with serotypes 1 and 2 is mediated by local IgA antibodies in the respiratory tract. Passively acquired serum neutralizing antibodies also confer some protection against infection with types 1, 2, and—to a lesser degree—3. Studies in experimental animal models and in immunosuppressed patients suggest that T cell–mediated immunity may also be important in parainfluenza virus infections.

CLINICAL MANIFESTATIONS Parainfluenza virus infections occur most frequently among children, in whom initial infection with serotype 1, 2, or 3 is associated with an acute febrile illness 50 to 80% of the time. Children may present with coryza, sore throat, hoarseness, and cough that may or may not be croupy. In severe croup, fever persists, with worsening coryza and sore throat. A brassy or barking cough may progress to frank stridor. Most children recover over the next 1 or 2 days, although progressive airway obstruction and hypoxia ensue occasionally. If bronchiolitis or pneumonia develops, progressive cough accompanied by wheezing, tachypnea, and intercostal retractions may occur. In this setting, sputum production increases modestly. Physical examination shows nasopharyngeal discharge and oropharyngeal injection, along with rhonchi, wheezes, or coarse breath sounds. Chest x-rays can show air trapping and occasionally interstitial infiltrates.

In older children and adults, parainfluenza infections tend to be milder, presenting most frequently as a common cold or as hoarseness, with or without cough. Lower respiratory tract involvement in older children and adults is uncommon, but tracheobronchitis in adults has been reported. Severe, prolonged, and even fatal parainfluenza infection has been reported in children and adults with severe immunosuppression, including bone-marrow and solid-organ transplant recipients.

LABORATORY FINDINGS AND DIAGNOSIS The clinical syndromes caused by parainfluenza viruses (with the possible exception of croup in young children) are not sufficiently distinctive to be diagnosed on clinical grounds alone. A specific diagnosis is established by detection of virus in respiratory tract secretions, throat swabs, or nasopharyngeal washings. Viral growth in tissue culture is detected either by hemagglutination or by a cytopathic effect. Rapid viral diagnosis may be made by identification of parainfluenza antigens in exfoliated cells from the respiratory tract with immunofluorescence or ELISA, although these techniques appear to be less sensitive than tissue culture. Highly specific and sensitive PCR assays have also been described. Serologic diagnosis can be established by hemagglutination inhibition, complement-fixation, or neutralization tests of acute- and convalescent-phase specimens. However, as frequent heterotypic responses occur among the parainfluenza serotypes, the serotype causing illness often cannot be identified by serologic techniques alone.

Acute epiglottitis caused by *Haemophilus influenzae* type b must be differentiated from viral croup. Influenza A virus is also a common cause of croup during epidemic periods.

℞ TREATMENT

For upper respiratory tract illness, symptoms can be treated as discussed for other viral respiratory tract illnesses. If complications such as sinusitis, otitis, or superimposed bacterial bronchitis develop, appropriate antibiotics should be administered. Mild cases of croup should be treated with bed rest and moist air generated by vaporizers. More severe cases require hospitalization and close observation for the development of respiratory distress. If acute respiratory distress develops, humidified oxygen and intermittent racemic epinephrine are usually administered. Aerosolized or systemically administered glucocorticoids are beneficial; the latter have a more profound effect. No specific antiviral therapy is available, although ribavirin is active against parainfluenza viruses in vitro and anecdotal reports describe its use clinically, particularly in immunosuppressed patients. Effective vaccines against parainfluenza viruses have not been developed.

ADENOVIRUS INFECTIONS

ETIOLOGIC AGENT Adenoviruses are complex DNA viruses that measure 70 to 80 nm in diameter. Human adenoviruses belong to the genus *Mastadenovirus*, which includes 51 serotypes. Adenoviruses have a characteristic morphology consisting of an icosahedral shell composed of 20 equilateral triangular faces and 12 vertices. The protein coat (capsid) consists of hexon subunits with group-specific and type-specific antigenic determinants and penton subunits at each vertex primarily containing group-specific antigens. A fiber with a knob at the end projects from each penton; this fiber contains type-specific and some group-specific antigens. Human adenoviruses have been divided into six subgenera (A through F) on the basis of the homology of DNA genomes and other properties. The adenovirus genome is a linear double-stranded DNA that codes for structural and nonstructural polypeptides. The replicative cycle of adenovirus may result either in lytic infection of cells or in the establishment of a latent infection (primarily involving lymphoid cells). Some adenovirus types can induce oncogenic transformation, and tumor formation has been observed in rodents; however, despite intensive investigation, adenoviruses have not been associated with tumors in humans.

EPIDEMIOLOGY Adenovirus infections most frequently affect infants and children. Infections occur throughout the year but are most common from fall to spring. Adenoviruses account for ~10% of acute respiratory infections in children but for <2% of respiratory illnesses in civilian adults. Nearly 100% of adults have serum antibody to multiple serotypes—a finding indicating that infection is common in childhood. Types 1, 2, 3, and 5 are the most frequent isolates from children. Certain adenovirus serotypes—particularly 4 and 7 but also 3, 14, and 21—are associated with outbreaks of acute respiratory disease in military recruits in winter and spring. Adenovirus infection can be transmitted by inhalation of aerosolized virus, by inoculation of virus into conjunctival sacs, and probably by the fecal-oral route as well. Type-specific antibody generally develops after infection and is associated with protection, albeit incomplete, against infection with the same serotype.

CLINICAL MANIFESTATIONS In children, adenoviruses cause a variety of clinical syndromes. The most common is an acute upper respiratory tract infection, with prominent rhinitis. On occasion, lower respiratory tract disease, including bronchiolitis and pneumonia, also develops. Adenoviruses, particularly types 3 and 7, cause pharyngoconjunctival fever, a characteristic acute febrile illness of children that occurs in outbreaks, most often in summer camps. The syndrome is marked by bilateral conjunctivitis in which the bulbar and palpebral conjunctivae have a granular appearance. Low-grade fever is frequently present for the first 3 to 5 days, and rhinitis, sore throat, and cervical adenopathy develop. The illness generally lasts for 1 to 2 weeks and resolves spontaneously. Febrile pharyngitis without conjunctivitis has also been associated with adenovirus infection. Adenoviruses have been isolated from cases of whooping cough with or without *Bordetella pertussis*; the significance of adenovirus in that disease is unknown.

In adults, the most frequently reported illness has been acute respiratory disease caused by adenovirus types 4 and 7 in military recruits. This illness is marked by a prominent sore throat and the gradual onset of fever, which often reaches 39°C (102.2°F) on the second or third day of illness. Cough is almost always present, and coryza and regional lymphadenopathy are frequently seen. Physical examination may show pharyngeal edema, injection, and tonsillar enlargement with little or no exudate. If pneumonia has developed, auscultation and x-ray of the chest may indicate areas of patchy infiltration.

Adenoviruses have been associated with a number of non–respiratory tract diseases, including acute diarrheal illness caused by types 40 and 41 in young children and hemorrhagic cystitis caused by types 11 and 21. Epidemic keratoconjunctivitis, caused most frequently by types 8, 19, and 37, has been associated with contaminated common sources such as ophthalmic solutions and roller towels. Adenoviruses have also been implicated in disseminated disease and pneumonia in immunosuppressed patients, including recipients of solid-organ or bone-marrow transplants. In bone-marrow transplant recipients, adenovirus infections have manifested as pneumonia, hepatitis, nephritis, colitis, encephalitis, and hemorrhagic cystitis. In solid-organ transplant recipients, adenovirus infection may involve the organ transplanted (e.g., hepatitis in liver transplants, nephritis in renal transplants) but can disseminate to other organs as well. In patients with AIDS, high-numbered and intermediate adenovirus serotypes have been isolated, usually in the setting of low CD4+ cell counts, but their isolation frequently has not been clearly linked to disease manifestations. Adenovirus nucleic acids have been detected in myocardial cells from patients with "idiopathic" myocardiopathies, and adenoviruses have been suggested as causative agents in some cases.

LABORATORY FINDINGS AND DIAGNOSIS Adenovirus infection should be suspected in the epidemiologic setting of acute respiratory disease in military recruits and in certain of the clinical syndromes (such as pharyngoconjunctival fever or epidemic keratoconjunctivitis) in which outbreaks of characteristic illnesses occur. In most cases, however, illnesses caused by adenovirus infection cannot be differentiated from those caused by a number of other viral respiratory agents and *Mycoplasma pneumoniae*. A definitive diagnosis of adenovirus infection is established by detection of the virus in tissue culture (as evidenced by cytopathic changes) and by specific identification with immunoflu-

orescence or other immunologic techniques. Rapid viral diagnosis can be established by immunofluorescence or ELISA of nasopharyngeal aspirates, conjunctival or respiratory secretions, urine, or stool. Highly sensitive and specific PCR assays or nucleic acid hybridization is also available. Adenovirus types 40 and 41, which have been associated with diarrheal disease in children, require special tissue-culture cells for isolation, and these serotypes are most commonly detected by direct ELISA of stool. Serum antibody rises can be demonstrated by complement-fixation or neutralization tests, ELISA, radioimmunoassay, or (for those adenoviruses that hemagglutinate red cells) hemagglutination inhibition tests.

℞ TREATMENT

Only symptom-based treatment and supportive therapy are available for adenovirus infections, and no clinically useful antiviral compounds have been identified. Ribavirin and cidofovir have activity in vitro against adenoviruses, and anecdotes of their use in disseminated infection have been reported.

PREVENTION Live vaccines have been developed against adenovirus types 4 and 7 and have been used to control illness in military recruits. These vaccines consist of live, unattenuated virus administered in enteric-coated capsules. Infection of the gastrointestinal tract with types 4 and 7 does not cause disease but stimulates local and systemic antibodies that are protective against subsequent acute respiratory disease due to those serotypes. This vaccine has not been produced since 1999, and outbreaks of acute respiratory illness caused by adenovirus types 4 and 7 have emerged again among military recruits. Vaccines prepared from purified subunits of adenovirus are being investigated. Adenoviruses are also being studied as live-virus vectors for the delivery of vaccine antigens and for gene therapy.

FURTHER READING

BAUM SG: Adenoviruses, in *Principles and Practice of Infectious Diseases*, 5th ed, GF Mandell et al (eds). New York, Saunders, 2000, pp 1624–1629

COMMITTEE ON INFECTIOUS DISEASES: Use of ribavirin in the treatment of respiratory syncytial virus infection. Pediatrics 92:501, 1993

CRAWFORD-MIKSZU XX et al: Seroepidemiology of new AIDS-associated adenoviruses among the San Francisco Men's Health Study. J Med Virol 50:230, 1996

ENGLUND JA et al: Respiratory syncytial virus infection in immunocompromised adults. Ann Intern Med 109:203, 1988

GLEZEN WP et al: Impact of respiratory virus infections on persons with chronic underlying conditions. JAMA 283:499, 2000

GRAHAM BS et al: Respiratory syncytial virus immunobiology and pathogenesis. Virology 297:1, 2002

GWALTNEY JM: Rhinoviruses, in *Principles and Practice of Infectious Diseases*, 5th ed, GF Mandell et al (eds). New York, Saunders, 2000, pp 1940–1948

HOLMES KH: Coronaviruses, in *Virology*, 4th ed, DN Knipe, PM Howley (eds). Philadelphia, Lippincott Williams & Wilkins, 2001, pp 1187–1204

LEE N et al: A major outbreak of severe acute respiratory syndrome in Hong Kong. N Engl J Med 348:1986, 2003

PEIRIS JSM et al: Coronavirus as a possible cause of severe acute respiratory syndrome. Lancet 361:1319, 2003

PERET T et al: Characterization of human metapneumoviruses isolated from patients in North America. J Infect Dis 185:1660, 2002

STOCKTON J et al: Human metapneumovirus as a cause of community-acquired respiratory illness. Emerg Infect Dis 8:897, 2002

WRIGHT PF: Parainfluenza viruses, in *Viral Infections of the Respiratory Tract*, R Dolin, PF Wright (eds). New York, Marcel Dekker, 1999

DEFINITION Influenza is an acute respiratory illness caused by infection with influenza viruses. The illness affects the upper and/or lower respiratory tract and is often accompanied by systemic signs and symptoms such as fever, headache, myalgia, and weakness. Outbreaks of illness of variable extent and severity occur nearly every winter. Such outbreaks result in significant morbidity in the general population and in increased mortality rates among certain high-risk patients, mainly as a result of pulmonary complications.

ETIOLOGIC AGENT Influenza viruses are members of the Orthomyxoviridae family, of which influenza A, B, and C viruses constitute three separate genera. The designation of influenza viruses as type A, B, or C is based on antigenic characteristics of the nucleoprotein (NP) and matrix (M) protein antigens. Influenza A viruses are further subdivided (subtyped) on the basis of the surface hemagglutinin (H) and neuraminidase (N) antigens (see below); individual strains are designated according to the site of origin, isolate number, year of isolation, and subtype—for example, influenza A/Moscow/10/99 (H3N2). Influenza A has 15 distinct H and 9 distinct N subtypes, of which only H1, H2, H3, N1, and N2 have been associated with extensive outbreaks of disease in humans. Influenza B and C viruses are similarly designated, but H and N antigens from these viruses do not receive subtype designations, since intratypic variations in influenza B antigens are less extensive than those in influenza A viruses and may not occur with influenza C virus.

Influenza A and B viruses are major human pathogens and the most extensively studied of the Orthomyxoviridae. The type A and type B viruses are morphologically similar. The virions are irregularly shaped spherical particles, 80 to 120 nm in diameter, and have a lipid envelope from the surface of which the H and N glycoproteins project (Fig. 171-1). The hemagglutinin is the site by which virus binds to cell receptors, whereas the neuraminidase degrades the receptor and plays a role in the release of virus from infected cells after replication has taken place. Influenza viruses enter cells by receptor-mediated endocytosis, forming a virus-containing endosome. The viral hemagglutinin mediates fusion of the endosomal membrane with the virus envelope, and viral nucleocapsids are subsequently released into the cytoplasm. Antibodies to the H antigen are the major determinants of immunity to influenza virus, while those to the N antigen limit viral spread and contribute to reduction of the infection. The inner surface of the lipid envelope contains the M proteins M1 and M2, which are involved in stabilization of the lipid envelope and in virus assembly. The virion also contains the NP antigen, which is associated with the viral genome, as well as three polymerase (P) proteins that are essential for transcription and synthesis of viral RNA. Two nonstructural proteins function as an interferon antagonist and posttranscriptional regulator (NS1) and a nuclear export factor (NS2 or NEP).

The genomes of influenza A and B viruses consist of eight single-stranded RNA segments, which code for the structural and nonstructural proteins. Because the genome is segmented, the opportunity for gene reassortment during infection is high; reassortment often occurs during infection of cells with more than one influenza A virus.

EPIDEMIOLOGY Influenza outbreaks are recorded virtually every year, although their extent and severity vary widely. Localized outbreaks take place at variable intervals, usually every 1 to 3 years. Except in the past 25 years, global epidemics or pandemics have occurred approximately every 10 to 15 years since the 1918–1919 pandemic (Table 171-1).

The most extensive and severe outbreaks are caused by influenza A viruses, in part because of the remarkable propensity of the H and N antigens of these viruses to undergo periodic antigenic variation. Major antigenic variations, called *antigenic shifts*, may be associated with pandemics and are restricted to influenza A viruses. Minor variations are called *antigenic drifts*. These types of antigenic variation may involve the hemagglutinin alone or both the hemagglutinin and the neuraminidase. An example of an antigenic shift involving both the hemagglutinin and the neuraminidase is that of 1957, when the predominant influenza A virus subtype shifted from H1N1 to H2N2; this shift resulted in a severe pandemic, with an estimated 70,000 excess deaths (i.e., deaths in excess of the number expected without an influenza epidemic) in the United States alone. In 1968, an antigenic shift involving only the hemagglutinin occurred (H2N2 to H3N2); the subsequent pandemic was less severe than that of 1957. In 1977, an H1N1 virus emerged and caused a pandemic that primarily affected younger individuals (i.e., those born after 1957). As can be seen in Table 171-1, H1N1 viruses circulated from 1918 to 1956; thus, individuals born prior to 1957 would be expected to have some degree of immunity to H1N1 viruses. During most outbreaks of influenza A, a single subtype has circulated at a time. However, since 1977, H1N1 and H3N2 viruses have circulated simultaneously, resulting in outbreaks of varying severity. In some outbreaks, influenza B viruses have also circulated simultaneously with influenza A viruses.

The origin of pandemic strains is unknown. Given the marked differences between the primary structures of the hemagglutinins of different subtypes of influenza A viruses (H1, H2, and H3), it seems unlikely that antigenic shifts result from spontaneous mutations in the hemagglutinin gene. Because the segmented genome of influenza viruses may result in high rates of reassortment, it has been suggested that pandemic strains may emerge by reassortment of genes between human and animal influenza A viruses that are known to have a broad host range of infection. There was concern that such reassortment might have occurred in 1997 in Hong Kong, where cases of infection caused by influenza virus A/H5N1 were detected in humans during an extensive outbreak of avian influenza A/H5N1 in poultry. However, only a few cases of A/H5N1 influenza in humans were documented, and the infection did not spread into the community. Recently, H9N2 viruses, which circulate in poultry and swine, have also been associated with limited infections in humans. Influenza B viruses have a much more restricted host range and do not undergo antigenic shifts, although they do undergo antigenic drift.

TABLE 171-1 *Emergence of Antigenic Subtypes of Influenza A Virus Associated with Pandemic or Epidemic Disease*

Years	Subtype	Extent of Outbreak
1889–90	H2N8[a]	Severe pandemic
1900–03	H3N8[a]	?Moderate epidemic
1918–19	H1N1[b] (formerly HswN1)	Severe pandemic
1933–35	H1N1[b] (formerly H0N1)	Mild epidemic
1946–47	H1N1	Mild epidemic
1957–58	H2N2	Severe pandemic
1968–69	H3N2	Moderate pandemic
1977–78[c]	H1N1	Mild pandemic

[a] As determined by retrospective serologic survey of individuals alive during those years ("seroarcheology").

[b] Hemagglutinins formerly designated as Hsw and H0 are now classified as variants of H1.

[c] From this time until the present (2002–2003), viruses of the H1N1 and H3N2 subtypes have circulated either in alternating years or concurrently.

FIGURE 171-1 An electron micrograph of influenza A virus (×140,000).

Pandemics provide the most dramatic evidence of the impact of influenza. However, illnesses that occur between pandemics account for greater total mortality and morbidity, albeit over a longer period. From 1972 through the present, influenza has been associated with at least 20,000 excess deaths during more than half of the interpandemic epidemics in the United States; >40,000 influenza-associated deaths occurred in each of six of these epidemics. Influenza A viruses that circulate between pandemics demonstrate antigenic drifts in the H antigen. These antigenic drifts apparently result from point mutations involving the RNA segment that codes for the hemagglutinin, which occurs most frequently in five hypervariable regions. Epidemiologically significant strains—that is, those with the potential to cause widespread outbreaks—exhibit changes in amino acids in at least two of the major antigenic sites in the hemagglutinin molecule. Since two point mutations are unlikely to occur simultaneously, it is believed that antigenic drifts result from point mutations occurring sequentially during the spread of virus from person to person. Antigenic drifts have been reported nearly annually since 1977 for H1N1 viruses and since 1968 for H3N2 viruses.

Influenza A epidemics begin abruptly, peak over a 2- to 3-week period, generally last for 2 to 3 months, and often subside almost as rapidly as they began. The first indication of influenza activity in a community is an increase in the number of children with febrile respiratory illnesses who present for medical attention. This increase is followed by increases in rates of influenza-like illnesses among adults and eventually by an increase in hospital admissions for patients with pneumonia, worsening of congestive heart failure, and exacerbations of chronic pulmonary disease. Rates of absence from work and school also rise at this time. An increase in the number of deaths caused by pneumonia and influenza is generally a late observation in an outbreak. Attack rates have been highly variable from outbreak to outbreak but most commonly are in the range of 10 to 20% of the general population. During the pandemic of 1957, it was estimated that the attack rate of clinical influenza exceeded 50% in urban populations and that an additional 25% or more of individuals in these populations may have been subclinically infected with influenza A virus. Among institutionalized populations and in semiclosed settings with many susceptible individuals, even higher attack rates have been reported.

Epidemics of influenza occur almost exclusively during the winter months in the temperate zones of the northern and southern hemispheres. In those locations, it is highly unusual to detect influenza A virus at other times, although serologic rises or even outbreaks have been noted rarely during warm-weather months. In contrast, influenza virus infections occur throughout the year in the tropics. Where or how influenza A virus persists between outbreaks in temperate zones is unknown. It is possible that influenza A viruses are maintained in the human population on a worldwide basis by person-to-person transmission and that large population clusters support a low level of interepidemic transmission. Alternatively, human strains may persist in animal reservoirs. Convincing evidence to support either explanation is not available. In the modern era, rapid transportation may contribute to the transmission of viruses among widespread geographic locales.

The factors that result in the inception and termination of outbreaks of influenza are incompletely understood. A major determinant of the extent and severity of an outbreak is the level of immunity in the population at risk. With the emergence of an antigenically novel influenza virus to which little or no antibody is present in a community, extensive outbreaks may occur. When the absence of antibody is worldwide, epidemic disease may spread around the globe, resulting in a pandemic. Such pandemic waves can continue for several years, until immunity in the population reaches a high level. In the years following pandemic influenza, antigenic drifts among influenza viruses result in outbreaks of variable severity in populations with high levels of immunity to the pandemic strain that circulated earlier. This situation persists until another antigenically novel pandemic strain emerges. On the other hand, outbreaks sometimes end despite the persistence of a large pool of susceptible individuals in the population.

Occasionally, the emergence of a significantly different antigenic variant will result only in a localized outbreak. The swine influenza outbreak of 1976 in the United States, caused by an A/H1N1 virus antigenically similar to the virus that circulated in 1918–1919, may be an example, although this outbreak may have represented simply the introduction of a swine influenza virus into a crowded human population without spread beyond that setting. The cluster of human infections with influenza A/H5N1 in Hong Kong in 1997 may also be an example of this phenomenon. It has been suggested that certain viruses, such as recently circulating A/H1N1 strains, may be intrinsically less virulent and cause less severe disease than other variants, even in immunologically virgin subjects. If so, then other (undefined) factors besides the level of preexisting immunity must play a role in the epidemiology of influenza.

Influenza B virus causes outbreaks that are generally less extensive and are associated with less severe disease than those caused by influenza A virus. The hemagglutinin and neuraminidase of influenza B virus undergo less frequent and less extensive variation than those of influenza A viruses; this characteristic may account, in part, for the lesser extent of disease. Influenza B outbreaks are seen most frequently in schools and military camps, although outbreaks in institutions in which elderly individuals reside have also been noted on occasion. The most serious complication of influenza B virus infection is Reye's syndrome (Chap. 290). In contrast to influenza A and B viruses, influenza C virus appears to be a relatively minor cause of disease in humans. It has been associated with common cold–like symptoms and occasionally with lower respiratory tract illness. The wide prevalence of serum antibody to this virus indicates that asymptomatic infection may be common.

The morbidity and mortality caused by influenza outbreaks continue to be substantial. Most individuals who die in this setting have underlying diseases that place them at high risk for complications of influenza. Excess hospitalizations for adults and children with high-risk medical conditions have ranged from 56 to 1900 per 100,000 during recent outbreaks of influenza. The most prominent high-risk conditions are chronic cardiac and pulmonary diseases and old age. Mortality among individuals with chronic metabolic, renal, and certain immunosuppressive diseases has also been elevated, although lower than that among patients with chronic cardiopulmonary diseases. The morbidity attributable to influenza in the general population is considerable. It is estimated that interpandemic outbreaks of influenza currently incur annual costs of $12 billion in the United States. If a pandemic were to occur, it is estimated that annual costs would range from $71 to $167 billion for attack rates of 15 to 35%.

PATHOGENESIS AND IMMUNITY   The initial event in influenza is infection of the respiratory epithelium with influenza virus acquired from respiratory secretions of acutely infected individuals. In all likelihood, transmission occurs via aerosols generated by coughs and sneezes, although hand-to-hand contact, other personal contact, and even fomite transmission may take place. Experimental evidence suggests that infection by a small-particle aerosol (particle diameter $<10~\mu m$) is more efficient than that by larger droplets. Initially, viral infection involves the ciliated columnar epithelial cells, but it may also involve other respiratory tract cells, including alveolar cells, mucous gland cells, and macrophages. In infected cells, virus replicates within 4 to 6 h, after which infectious virus is released to infect adjacent or nearby cells. In this way, infection spreads from a few foci to a large number of respiratory cells over several hours. In experimentally induced infection, the incubation period of illness has ranged from 18 to 72 h, depending on the size of the viral inoculum. Histopathologic study reveals degenerative changes, including granulation, vacuolization, swelling, and pyknotic nuclei, in infected ciliated cells. The cells eventually become necrotic and desquamate; in some areas, previously columnar epithelium is replaced by flattened and metaplastic epithelial cells. The severity of illness is correlated with the quantity of virus shed in secretions; thus, the degree of viral replication itself may be an important factor in pathogenesis. Despite the frequent development of systemic signs and symptoms such as fever, headache, and myalgias, influenza virus has only rarely been detected in extrapulmonary sites (including the bloodstream). Evidence suggests that the pathogenesis of systemic symptoms in influenza may be related to the induction of certain cytokines, particularly tumor necrosis factor α, interferon α, and interleukin 6, in respiratory secretions and in the bloodstream.

The host response to influenza infections involves a complex interplay of humoral antibody, local antibody, cell-mediated immunity, interferon, and other host defenses. Serum antibody responses, which can be detected by the second week after primary infection, are measured by a variety of techniques: hemagglutination inhibition (HI), complement fixation (CF), neutralization, enzyme-linked immunosorbent assay (ELISA), and antineuraminidase antibody assay. Antibodies directed against the hemagglutinin appear to be the most important mediators of immunity; in several studies, HI titers of ≥ 40 have been associated with protection from infection. Secretory antibodies produced in the respiratory tract are predominantly of the IgA class and also play a major role in protection against infection. Secretory antibody neutralization titers of ≥ 4 have also been associated with protection. A variety of cell-mediated immune responses, both antigen-specific and antigen-nonspecific, can be detected early after infection and depend on the prior immune status of the host. These responses include T-cell proliferative, T-cell cytotoxic, and natural killer cell activity. In humans, CD8+, HLA class I–restricted cytotoxic T cells (CTLs) are directed at conserved regions of internal proteins (NP, M, and polymerases) as well as against the surface proteins (H and N). Interferons can be detected in respiratory secretions shortly after the shedding of virus has begun, and rises in interferon titers coincide with decreases in virus shedding.

The host defense factors responsible for cessation of virus shedding and resolution of illness have not been defined specifically. Virus shedding generally stops within 2 to 5 days after symptoms first appear, at a time when serum and local antibody responses often are not detectable by conventional techniques (although antibody rises may be detected earlier by use of highly sensitive techniques, particularly in individuals with previous immunity to the virus). It has been suggested that interferon, cell-mediated immune responses, and/or nonspecific inflammatory responses all contribute to the resolution of illness. CTL responses may be particularly important in that regard.

MANIFESTATIONS Influenza has most frequently been described as an illness characterized by the abrupt onset of systemic symptoms, such as headache, feverishness, chills, myalgia, or malaise, and accompanying respiratory tract signs, particularly cough and sore throat. In many cases, the onset is so abrupt that patients can recall the precise time they became ill. However, the spectrum of clinical presentations is wide, ranging from a mild, afebrile respiratory illness similar to the common cold (with either a gradual or an abrupt onset) to severe prostration with relatively few respiratory signs and symptoms. In most of the cases that come to a physician's attention, the patient has a fever, with temperatures of 38° to 41°C (100.4° to 105.8°F). A rapid temperature rise within the first 24 h of illness is generally followed by a gradual defervescence over a 2- to 3-day period, although, on occasion, fever may last for as long as a week. Patients report a feverish feeling and chilliness, but true rigors are rare. Headache, either generalized or frontal, is often particularly troublesome. Myalgias may involve any part of the body but are most common in the legs and lumbosacral area. Arthralgias may also develop.

Respiratory complaints often become more prominent as systemic symptoms subside. Many patients have a sore throat or persistent cough, which may last for a week or more and which is often accompanied by substernal discomfort. Ocular signs and symptoms include pain on motion of the eyes, photophobia, and burning of the eyes.

Physical findings are usually minimal in cases of uncomplicated influenza. Early in the illness, the patient appears flushed and the skin is hot and dry, although diaphoresis and mottled extremities are sometimes evident, particularly in older patients. Examination of the pharynx may yield surprisingly unremarkable results despite a severe sore throat, but injection of the mucous membranes and postnasal discharge are apparent in some cases. Mild cervical lymphadenopathy may be noted, especially in younger individuals. The results of chest examination are largely negative in uncomplicated influenza, although rhonchi, wheezes, and scattered rales have been reported with variable frequency in different outbreaks. Frank dyspnea, hyperpnea, cyanosis, diffuse rales, and signs of consolidation are indicative of pulmonary complications. Patients with apparently uncomplicated influenza have been reported to have a variety of mild ventilatory defects and increased alveolar-capillary diffusion gradients; thus, subclinical pulmonary involvement may be more frequent than is appreciated.

In uncomplicated influenza, the acute illness generally resolves over a 2- to 5-day period, and most patients have largely recovered in 1 week, although cough may persist for 1 to 2 weeks longer. In a significant minority (particularly the elderly), however, symptoms of weakness or lassitude (postinfluenzal asthenia) may persist for several weeks and may prove troublesome for persons who wish to resume their full level of activity promptly. The pathogenetic basis for this asthenia is unknown, although pulmonary function abnormalities may persist for several weeks after uncomplicated influenza.

COMPLICATIONS Complications of influenza occur most frequently in patients >64 years old and in those with certain chronic disorders, including cardiac or pulmonary diseases, diabetes mellitus, hemoglobinopathies, renal dysfunction, and immunosuppression. Pregnancy in the second or third trimester also predisposes to complications with influenza. The most significant complication of influenza is pneumonia: "primary" influenza viral pneumonia, secondary bacterial pneumonia, or mixed viral and bacterial pneumonia. Primary influenza viral pneumonia is the least common but most severe of the pneumonic complications. It presents as acute influenza that does not resolve but instead progresses relentlessly, with persistent fever, dyspnea, and eventual cyanosis. Sputum production is generally scanty, but the sputum can contain blood. Few physical signs may be evident early in the illness. In more advanced cases, diffuse rales may be noted, and chest x-ray findings consistent with diffuse interstitial infiltrates and/or acute respiratory distress syndrome may be present. In such cases, arterial blood-gas determinations show marked hypoxia. Viral cultures of respiratory secretions and lung parenchyma, especially if samples are taken early in illness, yield high titers of virus. In fatal cases of primary viral pneumonia, histopathologic examination reveals a marked inflammatory reaction in the alveolar septa, with edema and infiltration by lymphocytes, macrophages, occasional plasma cells, and variable numbers of neutrophils. Fibrin thrombi in alveolar capillaries, along with necrosis and hemorrhage, have also been noted. Eosinophilic hyaline membranes can be found lining alveoli and alveolar ducts.

Primary influenza viral pneumonia has a predilection for individuals with cardiac disease, particularly those with mitral stenosis, but has also been reported in otherwise-healthy young adults as well as in older individuals with chronic pulmonary disorders. In some epidemics of influenza (notably those of 1918 and 1957), pregnancy increased the risk of primary influenza pneumonia. Subsequent epidemics of influenza have been associated with increased rates of hospitalization among pregnant women.

Secondary bacterial pneumonia follows acute influenza. Improvement of the patient's condition over 2 to 3 days is followed by a reappearance of fever along with clinical signs and symptoms of bacterial pneumonia, including cough, production of purulent sputum, and physical and x-ray signs of consolidation. The most common bacterial pathogens in this setting are *Streptococcus pneumoniae*, *Staphylococcus aureus*, and *Haemophilus influenzae*—organisms that can colonize the nasopharynx and that cause infection in the wake of changes in bronchopulmonary defenses. The etiology can often be determined by Gram's staining and culture of an appropriately obtained sputum specimen. Secondary bacterial pneumonia occurs most frequently in high-risk individuals with chronic pulmonary and cardiac disease and in elderly individuals. Patients with secondary bacterial pneumonia often respond to antibiotic therapy when it is instituted promptly.

Perhaps the most common pneumonic complications during outbreaks of influenza have mixed features of viral and bacterial pneumonia. Patients may experience a gradual progression of their acute illness or may show transient improvement followed by clinical exacerbation, with eventual manifestation of the clinical features of bacterial pneumonia. Sputum cultures may contain both influenza A virus and one of the bacterial pathogens described above. Patchy infiltrates or areas of consolidation may be detected by physical examination and chest x-ray. Patients with mixed viral and bacterial pneumonia generally have less widespread involvement of the lung than those with primary viral pneumonia, and their bacterial infections may respond to appropriate antibiotics. Mixed viral and bacterial pneumonia occurs primarily in patients with chronic cardiovascular and pulmonary diseases.

Other pulmonary complications associated with influenza include worsening of chronic obstructive pulmonary disease and exacerbation of chronic bronchitis and asthma. In children, influenza infection may present as croup. Sinusitis as well as otitis media (the latter occurring particularly often in children) may also be associated with influenza.

In addition to the pulmonary complications of influenza, a number of extrapulmonary complications may occur. These include *Reye's syndrome* (Chap. 290), a serious complication in children that is associated with influenza B and to a lesser extent with influenza A virus infection as well as with varicella-zoster virus infection. An epidemiologic association between Reye's syndrome and aspirin therapy for the antecedent viral infection has been noted, and the syndrome's incidence has decreased markedly with widespread warnings regarding aspirin use by children with acute viral respiratory infections.

Myositis, rhabdomyolysis, and myoglobinuria are occasional complications of influenza infection. Although myalgias are exceedingly common in influenza, true myositis is rare. Patients with acute myositis have exquisite tenderness of the affected muscles, most commonly in the legs, and may not be able to tolerate even the slightest pressure, such as the touch of bedsheets. In the most severe cases, there is frank swelling and bogginess of muscles. Serum levels of creatine phospho kinase and aldolase are markedly elevated, and an occasional patient has developed renal failure from myoglobinuria. The pathogenesis of influenza-associated myositis is also unclear, although the presence of influenza virus in affected muscles has been reported.

Myocarditis and pericarditis were reported in association with influenza virus infection during the 1918–1919 pandemic; these reports were based largely on histopathologic findings, and these complications have been reported only infrequently since that time. Electrocardiographic changes during acute influenza are common among patients who have cardiac disease but have been ascribed most often to exacerbations of the underlying cardiac disease rather than to direct involvement of the myocardium with influenza virus.

Central nervous system (CNS) diseases, including encephalitis, transverse myelitis, and Guillain-Barré syndrome, have been reported during influenza. The etiologic relationship of influenza virus to such CNS illnesses remains uncertain. Toxic shock syndrome associated with *S. aureus* or group A streptococcal infection following acute influenza infection has also been reported (Chaps. 120 and 121).

In addition to complications involving the specific organ systems described above, influenza outbreaks include a number of cases in which elderly and other high risk individuals develop influenza and subsequently experience a gradual deterioration of underlying cardiovascular, pulmonary, or renal function—changes that occasionally are irreversible and lead to death. These fatalities contribute to the overall excess mortality associated with influenza A outbreaks.

LABORATORY FINDINGS AND DIAGNOSIS Influenza virus may be isolated during acute influenza from throat swabs, nasopharyngeal washes, or sputum. Virus is usually detected by use of tissue culture or, less commonly, chick embryos within 48 to 72 h after inoculation. Most commonly, the diagnosis is established by the use of rapid viral tests that detect viral nucleoprotein or neuraminidase with high sensitivity and a specificity of 60 to 90% compared with that of tissue culture. Viral nucleic acids can be detected in clinical samples by reverse transcriptase polymerase chain reaction. The type of influenza virus (A or B) may be determined by either immunofluorescence or HI techniques, and the hemagglutinin subtype of influenza A virus (H1, H2, or H3) may be identified by HI with use of subtype-specific antisera. Serologic methods for diagnosis require comparison of antibody titers in sera obtained during the acute illness with those in sera obtained 10 to 14 days after the onset of illness and are useful primarily in retrospect. Fourfold or greater titer rises as detected by HI or CF or significant rises as measured by ELISA are diagnostic of acute infection. CF tests are generally less sensitive than other serologic techniques, but, as they detect type-specific antigens, they may be particularly useful when subtype-specific reagents are not available.

Other laboratory tests are generally not helpful in making a specific diagnosis of influenza virus infection. Leukocyte counts are variable, frequently being low early in illness and normal or slightly elevated later. Severe leukopenia has been described in overwhelming viral or bacterial infection, while leukocytosis with >15,000 cells/μL raises the suspicion of secondary bacterial infection.

DIFFERENTIAL DIAGNOSIS During a community-wide outbreak of influenza, a clinical diagnosis of influenza can be made with a high degree of certainty in patients who present to a physician's office with the typical febrile respiratory illness described above. In the absence of an outbreak (i.e., in sporadic or isolated cases), influenza may be difficult to differentiate on clinical grounds alone from an acute respiratory illness caused by any of a variety of respiratory viruses or by *Mycoplasma pneumoniae*. Severe streptococcal pharyngitis or early bacterial pneumonia may mimic acute influenza, although bacterial pneumonias generally do not run a self-limited course. Purulent sputum in which a bacterial pathogen can be detected by Gram's staining is an important diagnostic feature in bacterial pneumonia.

℞ TREATMENT

In uncomplicated cases of influenza, symptom-based therapy with acetaminophen for the relief of headache, myalgia, and fever may be considered, but the use of salicylates should be avoided in children <18 years of age because of the possible association of salicylates with Reye's syndrome. Since cough is ordinarily self-limited, treatment with cough suppressants generally is not indicated, although codeine-containing compounds may be employed if the cough is particularly troublesome. Patients should be advised to rest and maintain hydration during acute illness and to return to full activity only gradually after illness has resolved, especially if it has been severe.

Specific antiviral therapy is available for influenza: amantadine and rimantadine for influenza A and the neuraminidase inhibitors zanamivir and oseltamivir for both influenza A and influenza B. If begun within 48 h of the onset of illness, treatment with amantadine or rimantadine has reduced the duration of systemic and respiratory symptoms of influenza by ~50%. From 5 to 10% of individuals who receive amantadine experience mild CNS side effects, primarily jitteriness, anxiety, insomnia, or difficulty in concentrating. These side effects disappear promptly upon cessation of the drug. Rimantadine appears to be equally efficacious and is associated with less frequent CNS side effects than is amantadine. In adults, the usual dose of amantadine or rimantadine is 200 mg/d for 3 to 7 days. Since both drugs are excreted via the kidney, the dose should be reduced to ≤100 mg/d in elderly patients and in patients with renal insufficiency. Zanamivir, inhaled orally at a dose of 10 mg twice a day for 5 days, or oseltamivir, ingested orally at a dose of 75 mg twice a day for 5 days, has reduced the duration of signs and symptoms of influenza by 1 to 1.5 days if treatment is started within 2 days of the onset of illness. Zanamivir may exacerbate bronchospasm in asthmatic patients, and oseltamivir has been associated with nausea and vomiting, whose frequency can be reduced by drug administration with food. Resistant viruses emerge frequently during treatment with amantadine or rimantadine and can be transmitted among family members. The development of resistance appears to be infrequent with zanamivir or oseltamivir. Treatment of children is approved for amantadine and oseltamivir (≥ 1 year of age) and for zanamivir (≥ 7 years of age). Ribavirin is a nucleoside analogue with activity against influenza A and B viruses in vitro. It has been reported to be variably effective against influenza when administered as an aerosol but ineffective when administered orally. Its efficacy in the treatment of influenza A or B is unestablished.

Studies demonstrating the therapeutic efficacy of antiviral compounds in influenza have primarily involved young adults with uncomplicated disease; it is not known whether such compounds are effective in the treatment of influenza pneumonia or of other complications of influenza. Therapy for primary influenza pneumonia is directed at maintaining oxygenation and is most appropriately undertaken in an intensive care unit, with aggressive respiratory and hemodynamic support as needed. Bypass membrane oxygenators have been employed in this setting with variable results. When an acute respiratory distress syndrome develops, fluids must be administered cautiously, with close monitoring of blood gases and hemodynamic function.

Antibacterial drugs should be reserved for the treatment of bacterial complications of acute influenza, such as secondary bacterial pneumonia. The choice of antibiotics should be guided by Gram's staining and culture of appropriate specimens of respiratory secretions, such as sputum or transtracheal aspirates. If the etiology of a case of bacterial pneumonia is unclear from an examination of respiratory secretions, empirical antibiotics effective against the most common bacterial pathogens in this setting (*S. pneumoniae*, *S. aureus*, and *H. influenzae*) should be selected (Chaps. 119, 120, and 130).

PROPHYLAXIS   The major public health measure for prevention of influenza has been the use of inactivated influenza vaccines derived from influenza A and B viruses that circulated during the previous influenza season. If the vaccine virus and the currently circulating viruses are closely related, 50 to 80% protection against influenza would be expected. Presently available inactivated vaccines have been highly purified and are associated with few reactions. Up to 5% of individuals experience low-grade fever and mild systemic symptoms 8 to 24 h after vaccination, and up to one-third develop mild redness or tenderness at the vaccination site. Since the vaccine is produced in eggs, individuals with true hypersensitivity to egg products either should be desensitized or should not be vaccinated. Although the 1976 swine influenza vaccine appears to have been associated with an increased frequency of Guillain-Barré syndrome, influenza vaccines administered since 1976 generally have not been. Possible exceptions were noted during the 1992–1993 and 1993–1994 influenza seasons, when there may have been an excess risk of Guillain-Barré syndrome of slightly more than one case per million among vaccine recipients. However, the overall health risk following influenza outweighs the potential risk associated with vaccination.

The U.S. Public Health Service recommends influenza vaccination for any individual >6 months of age who is at an increased risk for complications of influenza, as noted earlier (Table 171-2). Since commercially available vaccines are inactivated ("killed"), they may be administered safely to immunocompromised patients. Influenza vaccination is not associated with exacerbations of chronic nervous-system diseases such as multiple sclerosis. Vaccine should be administered early in the autumn before influenza outbreaks occur and should then be given annually to maintain immunity against the most current influenza virus strains.

Recently, an advisory committee of the U.S. Food and Drug Administration recommended approval of a live attenuated influenza vaccine that is administered by intranasal spray. The vaccine is generated by reassortment of currently circulating strains of influenza A and B virus with a cold-adapted, attenuated master strain. The cold-adapted vaccine is well tolerated and highly efficacious (92% protective) in young children; in one study, it provided protection against a circulating influenza virus that had drifted antigenically away from the vaccine strain. The committee recommended approval of the cold-adapted vaccine for use in healthy children and adults from 5 to 49 years of age.

Chemoprophylaxis with amantadine or rimantadine, at dosages of 100 to 200 mg/d, has efficacy rates of 70 to 100% against illness associated with influenza A infection. Chemoprophylaxis with oseltamivir (75 mg/d by mouth) or zanamivir (10 mg/d inhaled) has resulted in efficacy rates of 84 to 89% against influenza A and B. Chemoprophylaxis is most likely to be used for high-risk individuals who have not received influenza vaccine or in a situation where the vaccines previously administered are relatively ineffective because of antigenic changes in the circulating virus. During an outbreak, antiviral chemoprophylaxis can be administered simultaneously with inactivated vaccine, since the drugs do not interfere with an immune response to the vaccine. In fact, there is evidence that the protective effects of chemoprophylaxis and vaccine may be additive. However, concurrent administration of chemoprophylaxis and the live attenuated vaccine may interfere with the immune response to the latter. Chemoprophylaxis may also be employed to control nosocomial outbreaks of influenza. For prophylaxis, administration should be instituted promptly when influenza activity is detected and must be continued daily for the duration of the outbreak. Amantadine and rimantadine are approved for prophylaxis in adults and in children ≥ 1 year old; oseltamivir is approved for prophylaxis in adults and in children ≥ 13 years old.

TABLE 171-2   *Recommendations for Influenza Vaccination*[a]

Persons at increased risk for complications
Persons ≥ 65 years of age
Residents of nursing homes and other chronic-care facilities that house persons of any age who have chronic medical conditions
Adults and children (≥ 6 months) who have chronic disorders of the pulmonary or cardiovascular systems, including asthma
Adults and children (≥ 6 months) who have required regular medical follow-up or hospitalization during the preceding year because of chronic metabolic diseases (including diabetes mellitus), renal dysfunction, hemoglobinopathies, or immunosuppression (including immunosuppression caused by medications or by HIV)
Children and adolescents (6 months to 18 years old) who are receiving long-term aspirin therapy and therefore may be at risk for developing Reye's syndrome after influenza infection
Women who will be in the second or third trimester of pregnancy during the influenza season
Persons 50 to 64 years of age
Included because of increased prevalence of high-risk conditions
Persons who can transmit influenza to those at high risk
Physicians, nurses, and other personnel in both hospital and outpatient-care settings, including medical emergency response workers (e.g., paramedics and emergency medical technicians)
Employees of nursing homes and chronic-care facilities who have contact with patients or residents
Employees of assisted-living and other residences for persons in groups at high risk
Persons who provide home care to individuals in groups at high risk
Household members (including children) of persons in groups at high risk

[a] Vaccination of healthy children 6 to 23 months of age is encouraged.
Source: Centers for Disease Control and Prevention.

FURTHER READING

CENTERS FOR DISEASE CONTROL AND PREVENTION: Prevention and control of influenza. MMWR 51(RR–3):1, 2002
DOLIN R et al: A controlled trial of amantadine and rimantadine in the prophylaxis of influenza A infection. N Engl J Med 307:580, 1982

GROSS PA et al: Association of influenza immunization with reduction in mortality in an elderly population: A prospective study. Arch Intern Med 148: 562, 1988

HAYDEN FG et al: Use of the selective oral neuraminidase inhibitor oseltamivir to prevent influenza. N Engl J Med 341:1336, 1999

MIST [MANAGEMENT OF INFLUENZA IN THE SOUTHERN HEMISPHERE TRIALISTS] STUDY GROUP: Randomized trial of efficacy and safety of inhaled zanamivir in treatment of influenza A and B infections. Lancet 352: 1871, 1998

NEUZIL KM et al: Influenza-associated morbidity and mortality in young and middle-aged women. JAMA 281:901, 1999

NICHOL KL et al: Effectiveness of live, attenuated intranasal influenza virus vaccine in healthy, working adults. JAMA 282:137, 1999

SIMONSEN L et al: Pandemic vs epidemic mortality: A pattern of changing age distribution. J Infect Dis 178:53, 1998

WRIGHT DF, WEBSTER RG: Orthomyxoviruses, in Virology, 4th ed, DM Knipe, PM Howley (eds). Philadelphia, Lippincott Williams & Wilkins, 2001, pp 1533–1580

Section 14 Infections Due to Human Immunodeficiency Virus and Other Human Retroviruses

172 THE HUMAN RETROVIRUSES
Dan L. Longo, Anthony S. Fauci

The retroviruses, which make up a large family (Retroviridae), infect mainly vertebrates. They have a unique replication cycle whereby their genetic information is encoded by RNA rather than DNA. Retroviruses contain an RNA-dependent DNA polymerase (a reverse transcriptase) that directs the synthesis of a DNA form of the viral genome after infection of a host cell. The designation *retrovirus* denotes that information in the form of RNA is transcribed into DNA in the host cell—a sequence that overturned a central dogma of molecular biology: that information passes unidirectionally from DNA to RNA to protein. The observation that RNA was the source of genetic information in the causative agents of certain animal tumors led to a number of paradigm-shifting biologic insights regarding not only the direction of genetic-information passage but also the viral etiology of certain cancers and the concept of oncogenes as normal host genes scavenged and altered by a viral vector.

The family Retroviridae includes three subfamilies (Table 172-1): Oncovirinae, of which human T-cell lymphotropic virus (HTLV) type I is the most important in humans; Lentivirinae, of which HIV is the most important in humans; and Spumavirinae, the "foamy" viruses, named for the pathologic appearance of infected cells. A number of spumaviruses have been isolated from humans; however, they are not associated with any known disease and therefore are not discussed further in this chapter.

The wide variety of interactions of a retrovirus with its host range from completely benign events (e.g., silent carriage of endogenous retroviral sequences in the germ-line genome of many animal species) to rapidly fatal infections (e.g., exogenous infection with an oncogenic virus such as Rous sarcoma virus in chickens). The ability of retroviruses to acquire and alter the structure and function of host cell sequences has revolutionized our understanding of molecular carcinogenesis. The viruses can insert into the germ-line genome of the host cell and behave as a transposable or movable genetic element. They can activate or inactivate genes near the site of integration into the genome. They can rapidly alter their own genome by recombination and mutation under selective environmental stimuli.

Most human viral diseases occur as a consequence of either tissue destruction by the virus itself or the host's response to the virus. Although these mechanisms are operative in retroviral infections, retroviruses have addi-tional mechanisms of inducing disease, including the malignant transformation of an infected cell and the induction of an immunodeficiency state that leads to opportunistic diseases (infections and neoplasms; Chap. 173).

STRUCTURE AND LIFE CYCLE Despite the wide range of biologic consequences of retroviral infection, all retroviruses are similar in structure, genome organization, and mode of replication. Retroviruses are 70 to 130 nm in diameter and have a lipid-containing envelope surrounding an icosahedral capsid with a dense inner core. The core contains two identical copies of the single-strand RNA genome. The RNA molecules are 8 to 10 kb long and are complexed with reverse transcriptase and tRNA. Other viral proteins, such as integrase, are also components of the virion particle. The RNA has features usually found in mRNA: a cap site at the 5′ end of the molecule, which is important in the initiation of mRNA translation, and a polyadenylation site at the 3′ end, which influences mRNA turnover (i.e., messages with shorter polyA tails turn over faster than messages with longer polyA tails). However, the retroviral RNA is not translated; instead it is transcribed into DNA. The DNA form of the retroviral genome is called a *provirus*.

The replication cycle of retroviruses proceeds in two phases (Fig. 172-1). In the first phase, the virus enters the cytoplasm after binding to a specific cell-surface receptor (with HIV, a cell-surface co-receptor is also utilized for binding and entry); the viral RNA and reverse transcriptase synthesize a double-strand DNA version of the RNA template; and the provirus moves into the nucleus and integrates into the host cell genome. This proviral integration is permanent. Although some animal retroviruses integrate into a single specific site of the host

TABLE 172-1 *Classification of Retroviruses: the Family Retroviridae*

Subfamily, Group[a]	Example	Feature
Oncovirinae (oncogenic viruses)		
Avian leukosis	Rous sarcoma virus	Contains *src* oncogene
Mammalian C-type	Abelson leukemia virus	Contains *abl* oncogene
B-type	Murine mammary tumor virus	Can be endogenous or exogenous
D-type	Mason-Pfizer monkey virus	—
HTLV-BLV	HTLV-I	Causes T-cell lymphoma and neurologic disease
Lentivirinae (slow viruses)	HIV-1, HIV-2	Causes AIDS
	Visna virus	Causes lung and brain diseases in sheep
	Feline immunodeficiency virus	Causes immunodeficiency in cats
Spumavirinae (foamy viruses)	Simian foamy virus, human foamy virus	Causes no known disease

[a] The Oncovirinae were originally grouped into types A–D on the basis of morphologic features (size, core location, budding) under electron microscopy; however, this system has been replaced by groupings based on relationships of genome structure and sequence.

Note: HTLV, human T-lymphotropic virus; BLV, bovine leukemia virus.

FIGURE 172-1 The life cycle of retroviruses. *A.* Overview of virus replication. The retrovirus enters a target cell by binding to a specific cell-surface receptor; once the virus is internalized, its RNA is released from the nucleocapsid and is reverse-transcribed into proviral DNA. The provirus is inserted into the genome and then transcribed into RNA; the RNA is translated; and virions assemble and are extruded from the cell membrane by budding. *B.* Overview of retroviral gene expression. The provirus is transcribed, capped, and polyadenylated. Viral RNA molecules then have one of three fates: They are exported to the cytoplasm, where they are packaged as the viral RNA in infectious viral particles; they are spliced to form the message for the envelope polyprotein; or they are translated into Gag and Pol proteins. Most of the messages for the Pol protein fail to initiate Pol translation because of a stop codon before its initiation; however, in a fraction of the messages, the stop codon is missed and the Pol proteins are translated. [*Modified from JM Coffin, in BN Fields, DM Knipe (eds): Fields Virology. New York, Raven, 1990, with permission.*]

genome in every infected cell, the four known human retroviruses (HTLV-I, HTLV-II, HIV-1, and HIV-2) integrate randomly. This first phase of replication depends entirely on gene products in the virus. The second phase includes the synthesis and processing of viral genomes, mRNAs, and proteins using host cell machinery, often under the influence of viral gene products. Virions are assembled and released from the cell by budding from the membrane; host cell membrane proteins are frequently incorporated into the envelope of the virus. Proviral integration occurs during the S-phase of the cell cycle; thus, in general, nondividing cells are resistant to retroviral infection. Only the lentiviruses are able to infect nondividing cells. Once a host cell is infected, it is infected for the life of the cell.

Retroviral genomes include both coding and noncoding sequences (Fig. 172-2). In general, noncoding sequences are important recognition signals for DNA or RNA synthesis or processing events and are located in the 5′ and 3′ terminal regions of the genome. All retroviral genomes are terminally redundant, containing identical sequences called *long terminal repeats* (LTRs). The ends of the retroviral RNA genome differ slightly in sequence from the integrated retroviral DNA.

In the latter, the LTR sequences are repeated in both the 5′ and the 3′ terminus of the virus. The LTRs contain sequences involved in initiating the expression of the viral proteins, the integration of the provirus, and the polyadenylation of viral RNAs. The primer binding site, which is critical for the initiation of reverse transcription, and the viral packaging sequences are located outside the LTR sequences. The coding regions include the *gag* (group-specific antigen, core protein), *pol* (RNA-dependent DNA polymerase), and *env* (envelope) genes. The *gag* gene encodes a precursor polyprotein that is cleaved to form three to five capsid proteins; a fraction of the Gag precursor proteins also contain a protease responsible for cleaving the Gag and Pol polyproteins. A Gag-Pol polyprotein gives rise to the protease that is responsible for cleaving the Gag-Pol polyprotein. The *pol* gene encodes three proteins: the reverse transcriptase, the integrase, and the protease. The reverse transcriptase functions to copy the viral RNA into the double-strand DNA provirus, which can attach to the host cell DNA via the action of integrase. The protease functions to cleave the Gag-Pol polyprotein into smaller protein products. The *env* gene encodes the envelope glycoproteins: one protein that binds to specific surface receptors and determines what cell types can be infected and a smaller transmembrane protein that anchors the complex to the envelope. The cartoon in Fig. 172-3 shows how the retroviral gene products make up the virus structure.

HTLVs have a region between *env* and the 3′ LTR that encodes at least two proteins in overlapping reading frames: Tax, a 40-kDa protein that does not bind to DNA but induces the expression of host cell transcription factors that alter host cell gene expression; and Rex, a 27-kDa protein that regulates the expression of viral mRNAs. These two proteins are produced from messages that are similar but that are spliced differently from overlapping but distinct exons.

The lentiviruses in general, and HIV-1 and -2 in particular, contain a larger genome than other pathogenic retroviruses. They contain an untranslated region between *pol* and *env* that encodes portions of several proteins, varying with the reading frame into which the mRNA is spliced. Tat is a 14-kDa protein that augments the expression of virus from the LTR. The Rev protein of HIV-1, similar to the Rex protein of HTLV, regulates RNA splicing and/or RNA transport. The Nef protein downregulates CD4, the cellular receptor for HIV; alters host T cell activation pathways; and enhances viral infectivity. The Vif protein is necessary for the proper assembly of the HIV nucleoprotein core in many types of cells; without Vif, proviral DNA is not efficiently produced in these infected cells. Vpr, Vpu (HIV-1 only), and Vpx (HIV-2 only) are viral proteins encoded by translation of the same message in different reading frames. As noted above, oncogenic retroviruses depend on cell proliferation for their replication; lentiviruses can infect nondividing cells, largely owing to effects mediated by Vpr. Vpr facilitates transport of the provirus into the nucleus and can induce other cellular changes, such as G_2 growth arrest and differentiation of some target cells. Vpx is structurally related to Vpr, but its functions are not fully defined. Vpu promotes the degradation of CD4 in the endoplasmic reticulum and stimulates the release of virions from infected cells.

Retroviruses can be either exogenously acquired by infection with a virion capable of replication or transmitted in the germ line as endogenous virus. Endogenous retroviruses are often replication-defective. The human genome contains endogenous retroviral sequences, but there are no known replication-competent endogenous retroviruses in humans.

In general, viruses that contain only the *gag*, *pol*, and *env* genes either are not pathogenic or take a long time to induce disease; these observations indicate the importance of the other regulatory genes in viral disease pathogenesis. The pathogenesis of neoplastic transformation by retroviruses relies on the chance integration of the provirus at a spot in the genome that will result in the expression of a cellular gene (proto-oncogene) that becomes transforming by virtue of its unregulated expression. For example, avian leukosis virus causes B cell leukemia by inducing the expression of *myc*. Some retroviruses possess captured and altered cellular genes near their integration site, and these viral oncogenes are capable of transforming the infected host cell. Viruses that have oncogenes often have lost a portion of their genome that is required for replication. Such viruses need helper viruses to reproduce, a feature that may explain why these acute transforming retroviruses are rare in nature. All human retroviruses identified to date are exogenous and are not acutely transforming (i.e., they lack a transforming oncogene).

These remarkable properties of retroviruses have led to experimental efforts to use them as vectors to insert specific genes into particular cell types, a process known as *gene therapy* or *gene transfer*. The process could be used to repair a genetic defect or to introduce a new property that could be used therapeutically; for example, a gene (e.g., thymidine kinase) that would make a tumor cell susceptible to killing by a drug (e.g., ganciclovir) could be inserted. One source of concern about the use of retroviral vectors in humans is that replication-competent viruses might rescue endogenous retroviral replication, with unpredictable results. This concern is not merely hypothetical: The detection of proteins encoded by endogenous retroviral sequences on the surface of cancer cells implies that the genetic events leading to the cancer were able to activate the synthesis of these usually silent genes.

FIGURE 172-2 Genomic structure of retroviruses. The murine leukemia virus MuLV has the typical three structural genes: *gag*, *pol*, and *env*. The *gag* region gives rise to three proteins: matrix (MA), capsid (CA), and nucleic acid–binding (NC) proteins. The *pol* region encodes both a protease (PR) responsible for cleaving the viral polyproteins and a reverse transcriptase (RT). In addition, HIV *pol* encodes an integrase (IN). The *env* region encodes a surface protein (SU) and a small transmembrane protein (TM). The human retroviruses have additional gene products translated in each of the three possible reading frames. HTLV-I and HTLV-II have *tax* and *rex* genes with exons on either side of the *env* gene. HIV-1 and HIV-2 have six accessory gene products: *tat, rev, vif, nef, vpr,* and either *vpu* (in HIV-1) or *vpx* (in HIV-2). The genes for these proteins are located mainly between the *pol* and *env* genes.

HUMAN T-CELL LYMPHOTROPIC VIRUS

HTLV-I was isolated in 1980 from a T-cell lymphoma cell line from a patient originally thought to have cutaneous T cell lymphoma. Later it became clear that the patient had a distinct form of lymphoma (originally reported in Japan) called *adult T-cell leukemia/lymphoma* (ATL). Serologic data have determined that HTLV-I is the cause of at least two important diseases: ATL and tropical spastic paraparesis, also called *HTLV-I-associated myelopathy* (HAM). HTLV-I may also play a role in infective dermatitis and uveitis syndromes.

Two years after the isolation of HTLV-I, HTLV-II was isolated from a patient with an unusual form of hairy cell leukemia that affected T cells. Although early epidemiologic studies of HTLV-II failed to reveal a consistent disease association, more recent studies suggest an association of HTLV-II with human disease (see "Associated Diseases" under "Features of HTLV-II Infection," below), particularly among injection drug users.

BIOLOGY AND MOLECULAR BIOLOGY Because the biology of HTLV-I and that of HTLV-II are similar, the following discussion will focus on HTLV-I.

The cellular receptor for HTLV-I has not yet been identified, but it maps to chromosome 17. Generally, only T cells are productively infected, but infection of B cells and other cell types is occasionally detected. The most common outcome of HTLV-I infection is latent carriage of randomly integrated provirus in CD4+ T cells. HTLV-I does not contain an oncogene and does not insert into a unique site in the genome. Indeed, most infected cells express no viral gene products. The only viral gene product that is routinely expressed in tumor cells transformed by HTLV-I in vivo is *tax*, and even *tax* is not expressed in the tumor cells of many ATL patients. Cells transformed in vitro, by contrast, actively transcribe HTLV-I RNA and produce infectious virions. Most HTLV-I-transformed cell lines are the result of the infection of a normal host T cell in vitro. It is difficult to establish cell lines derived from authentic ATL cells.

Although *tax* does not itself bind to DNA, it does induce the expression of a wide range of host cell gene products, including transcription factors (especially c-*rel*, *ets*-1 and -2, and members of the *fos/jun* family), cytokines [e.g., interleukin (IL) 2, granulocyte-macrophage colony-stimulating factor, and tumor necrosis factor (TNF)], and membrane proteins and receptors [major histocompatibility (MHC) molecules and IL-2 receptor α]. The genes activated by *tax* are generally controlled by transcription factors of the c-*rel* and cyclic AMP response element binding (CREB) protein families. It is unclear how this induction of host gene expression leads to neoplastic transformation; *tax* can interfere with G_1 and mitotic cell-cycle checkpoints, block apoptosis, and promote antigen-independent T cell proliferation. Induction of a cytokine-autocrine loop has been proposed; however, IL-2 is not the crucial cytokine. The involvement of IL-4, IL-7, and IL-15 has been proposed.

In light of the irregular expression of *tax* in ATL cells, it has been suggested that *tax* is important in the early phases of transformation

FIGURE 172-3 Schematic structure of human retroviruses. The surface glycoprotein (SU) is responsible for binding to receptors of host cells. The transmembrane protein (TM) anchors SU to the virus. NC is a nucleic acid–binding protein found in association with the viral RNA. A protease (PR) cleaves the polyproteins encoded by the *gag*, *pol*, and *env* genes into their functional components. RT is reverse transcriptase, and IN is an integrase present in some retroviruses (e.g., HIV-1) that facilitates insertion of the provirus into the host genome. MA is a Gag protein closely associated with the lipid of the envelope. The capsid protein (CA) forms the major internal structure of the virus, the core shell.

but is not essential for the maintenance of the transformed state. As is clear from the epidemiology of HTLV-I infection, transformation of an infected cell is a rare event and may depend on heterogeneous second, third, or fourth genetic hits. No consistent chromosomal abnormalities have been described in ATL; however, individual cases with p53 mutations and translocations involving the T cell receptor genes on chromosome 14 have been reported. *Tax* may repress certain DNA repair enzymes, permitting the accumulation of genetic damage that would normally be repaired. However, the molecular pathogenesis of HTLV-I-induced neoplasia is not fully understood.

FEATURES OF HTLV-I INFECTION ■ **Epidemiology** HTLV-I infection is transmitted in at least three ways: from mother to child, especially in breast milk; through sexual activity, more commonly from men to women; and through the blood—via contaminated transfusions or contaminated needles. The virus is most commonly transmitted perinatally. Compared with HIV, which can be transmitted in cell-free form, HTLV-I is less infectious, and its transmission usually requires cell-to-cell contact.

HTLV-I is endemic in southwestern Japan and Okinawa, where >1 million persons are infected. Antibodies to HTLV-I are present in the serum of up to 35% of Okinawans, 10% of residents of the Japanese island of Kyushu, and <1% of persons in nonendemic regions of Japan. Despite this high prevalence of infection, only ~500 cases of ATL are diagnosed in this area each year. Clusters of infection have been noted in other areas of the Orient, such as Taiwan; in the Caribbean basin, including northeastern South America; in central Africa; in Italy; in Israel; in the Arctic; and in the southeastern part of the United States.

A progressive spastic or ataxic myelopathy that develops in an individual who is HTLV-I positive (i.e., who has serum antibodies to HTLV-I) is likely to be due to direct nervous system infection with the virus; a similar disorder may result from infection with HIV or HTLV-II. In rare instances, patients with HAM are seronegative but have detectable antibody to HTLV-I in the cerebrospinal fluid (CSF).

The cumulative lifetime risk of developing ATL is 3% among HTLV-I-infected patients (the risk is three times greater in men than in women); a similar cumulative risk is projected for HAM. The distribution of the two diseases overlaps the distribution of HTLV-I, with >95% of affected patients showing serologic evidence of HTLV-I infection. The latent period between infection and the emergence of disease is 20 to 30 years for ATL. For HAM, the median latency period is ~3.3 years (range, 4 months to 30 years). The development of ATL is rare among persons infected by blood products; however, ~20% of patients with HAM acquire HTLV-I from contaminated blood.

Associated Diseases ■ *ATL* Four clinical types of HTLV-I-induced neoplasia have been described: acute, lymphomatous, chronic, and smoldering. All of these tumors are monoclonal proliferations of CD4+ post-thymic T cells with clonal proviral integrations and clonal T cell receptor gene rearrangements.

About 60% of patients who develop malignancy have classic acute ATL, which is characterized by a short clinical prodrome (~2 weeks between the first symptoms and the diagnosis) and an aggressive natural history (median survival period, 6 months). The clinical picture is dominated by rapidly progressive skin lesions, pulmonary involvement, hypercalcemia, and lymphocytosis with cells containing lobulated or "flower-shaped" nuclei (see Fig. 97-10). The malignant cells have monoclonal proviral integrations and express CD4, CD3, and CD25 (low-affinity IL-2 receptors) on their surface. Serum levels of CD25 can be used as a tumor marker. Anemia and thrombocytopenia are rare. The skin lesions may be difficult to distinguish from those in mycosis fungoides. Lytic bone lesions, which are common, do not contain tumor cells but rather are composed of osteolytic cells, usually

without osteoblastic activity. Despite the leukemic picture, bone marrow involvement is patchy in most cases.

The hypercalcemia of ATL is multifactorial; the tumor cells produce osteoclast-activating factors (TNF-α, IL-1, lymphotoxin) and can also produce a parathyroid hormone–like molecule. Affected patients have an underlying immunodeficiency that makes them susceptible to opportunistic infections similar to those seen in patients with AIDS (Chap. 173). The pathogenesis of the immunodeficiency is unclear. Pulmonary infiltrates in ATL patients reflect leukemic infiltration half the time and opportunistic infections with organisms such as *Pneumocystis* and other fungi the other half. Gastrointestinal symptoms are nearly always related to opportunistic infection. *Strongyloides stercoralis* is a gastrointestinal parasitic infection that has a pattern of endemic distribution similar to that of HTLV-I. HTLV-I-infected persons also infected with the parasite may develop ATL more often or more rapidly than those without *Strongyloides* infections. Serum concentrations of lactate dehydrogenase (LDH) and alkaline phosphatase are often elevated. About 10% of patients have leptomeningeal involvement leading to weakness, altered mental status, paresthesia, and/or headache. Unlike other forms of central nervous system (CNS) lymphoma, ATL may be accompanied by normal CSF protein levels. The diagnosis depends on finding ATL cells in the CSF (Chap. 97).

The lymphomatous type of ATL occurs in ~20% of patients and is similar to the acute form in its natural history and clinical course, except that circulating abnormal cells are rare and lymphadenopathy is evident. The histology of the lymphoma is variable but does not influence the natural history. In general, the diagnosis is suspected on the basis of the patient's birthplace and the presence of skin lesions and hypercalcemia. The diagnosis is confirmed by the detection of antibodies to HTLV-I in serum.

Patients with the chronic form of ATL generally have normal serum levels of calcium and LDH and no involvement of the CNS, bone, or gastrointestinal tract. The median duration of survival for these patients is 2 years. In some cases, chronic ATL progresses to the acute form of the disease.

Fewer than 5% of patients have the smoldering form of ATL. In this form, the malignant cells have monoclonal proviral integration; <5% of peripheral blood cells exhibit typical morphologic abnormalities; hypercalcemia, adenopathy, and hepatosplenomegaly do not develop; the CNS, the bones, and the gastrointestinal tract are not involved; and skin and pulmonary lesions may be present. The median survival period of this small subset of patients appears to be ≥5 years.

HAM (TROPICAL SPASTIC PARAPARESIS) In contrast to ATL, in which there is a slight predominance of male patients, HAM affects females disproportionately. HAM resembles multiple sclerosis in certain ways (Chap. 359). The onset is insidious. Symptoms include weakness or stiffness in one or both legs, back pain, and urinary incontinence. Sensory changes are usually mild, but peripheral neuropathy may develop. The disease generally takes the form of slowly progressive and unremitting thoracic myelopathy; one-third of patients are bedridden within 10 years of diagnosis, and one-half are unable to walk unassisted by this point. Patients display spastic paraparesis or paraplegia with hyperreflexia, ankle clonus, and extensor plantar responses. Cognitive function is usually spared; cranial nerve abnormalities are unusual.

Magnetic resonance imaging (MRI) reveals lesions in both the white matter and the paraventricular regions of the brain as well as in the spinal cord. Pathologic examination of the spinal cord shows symmetric degeneration of the lateral columns, including the corticospinal tracts; some cases involve the posterior columns as well. The spinal meninges and cord parenchyma contain an inflammatory infiltrate with myelin destruction.

HTLV-I is not usually found in cells of the CNS but may be detected in a small population of lymphocytes present in the CSF. In general, HTLV-I replication is greater in HAM than in ATL, and patients with HAM have a stronger immune response to the virus. Antibodies to HTLV-I are present in the serum and appear to be produced in the CSF of HAM patients, where titers are often higher than in the serum. The pathophysiology of HAM may involve the induction of autoimmune destruction of neural cells by T cells with specificity for viral components such as Tax or Env proteins. One theory is that susceptibility to HAM may be related to the presence of human leukocyte antigen (HLA) alleles capable of presenting viral antigens in a fashion that leads to autoimmunity. Insufficient data are available to confirm an HLA association.

It is unclear what factors influence whether HTLV-I infection will cause disease and, if it does, whether it will induce a neoplasm (ATL) or an autoimmune disorder (HAM). Differences in viral strains, in the susceptibility of particular MHC haplotypes, in the route of HTLV-I infection, in the viral load, and in the nature of the HTLV-I-related immune response are putative factors, but few definitive data are available.

OTHER PUTATIVE HTLV-I-RELATED DISEASES In areas where HTLV-I is endemic, diverse inflammatory and autoimmune diseases have been attributed to the virus, including uveitis, dermatitis, pneumonitis, rheumatoid arthritis, and polymyositis. However, a causal relationship between HTLV-I and these illnesses has not been rigorously established.

Prevention Women in endemic areas should not breast-feed their children, and blood donors should be screened for serum antibodies to HTLV-I. As in the prevention of HIV infection, the practice of safe sex and the avoidance of needle sharing are important.

℞ TREATMENT

For the small number of patients who develop HTLV-I-related disease, therapies are not curative. In patients with the acute and lymphomatous types of ATL, the disease progresses rapidly. Hypercalcemia is generally controlled by glucocorticoid administration and cytotoxic therapy directed against the neoplasm. The tumor is highly responsive to combination chemotherapy that is employed against other forms of lymphoma; however, patients are susceptible to overwhelming bacterial and opportunistic infections, and ATL relapses within 4 to 10 months after remission in most patients. The combination of interferon α and zidovudine may extend survival. Because viral replication is not clearly associated with ATL progression, zidovudine is probably effective through its cytotoxic effects (as a chain-terminating thymidine analogue) rather than its antiviral effects. An experimental approach using an yttrium 90–labeled or toxin-conjugated antibody to the IL-2 receptor appears promising but is not widely available. Patients with the chronic or smoldering form of ATL may be managed with an expectant approach: Treat any infections, and watch and wait for signs of progression to acute disease.

Patients with HAM may obtain some benefit from the use of glucocorticoids to reduce inflammation. Antiretroviral regimens have not been effective. In one study, danazol (200 mg three times daily) produced significant neurologic improvement in five of six treated patients, with resolution of urinary incontinence in two cases, decreased spasticity in three, and restoration of the ability to walk after confinement to a wheelchair in two. Physical therapy and rehabilitation are important components of management.

FEATURES OF HTLV-II INFECTION ■ Epidemiology HTLV-II is endemic in certain Native American tribes and in Africa. It is generally considered to be a New World virus that was brought from Asia to the Americas

10,000 to 40,000 years ago during the migration of infected populations across the Bering land bridge.

The mode of transmission of HTLV-II is probably the same as that of HTLV-I (see above). HTLV-II may be less readily transmitted sexually than HTLV-I.

Studies of large cohorts of injection drug users with serologic assays that reliably distinguish HTLV-I from HTLV-II indicate that the vast majority of HTLV-positive subjects are infected with HTLV-II. The seroprevalence of HTLV in a cohort of 7841 injection drug users from drug treatment centers in Baltimore, Chicago, Los Angeles, New Jersey (Asbury Park and Trenton), New York City (Brooklyn and Harlem), Philadelphia, and San Antonio was 20.9%, with >97% of cases due to HTLV-II. The seroprevalence of HTLV-II was higher in the Southwest and the Midwest than in the Northeast. In contrast, the seroprevalence of HIV-1 was higher in the Northeast than in the Southwest or the Midwest. Approximately 3% of the cohort members were infected with both HTLV-II and HIV-1. The seroprevalence of HTLV-II increased linearly with age. Women were significantly more likely to be infected with HTLV-II than were men; the virus is thought to be more efficiently transmitted from male to female than from female to male.

Associated Diseases Although HTLV-II was isolated from a patient with a T cell variant of hairy cell leukemia, this virus has not been consistently associated with a particular disease and in fact has been thought of as "a virus searching for a disease." However, evidence is accumulating that HTLV-II may play a role in certain neurologic, hematologic, and dermatologic diseases. These data require confirmation, particularly in light of the previous confusion regarding the relative prevalences of HTLV-I and HTLV-II among injection drug users.

Prevention Avoidance of needle sharing, safe-sex practices, screening of blood (by assays for HTLV-I, which also detect HTLV-II), and avoidance of breast-feeding by infected women are important principles in the prevention of spread of HTLV-II.

HUMAN IMMUNODEFICIENCY VIRUS

HIV-1 and HIV-2 are members of the lentivirus subfamily of Retroviridae and are the only lentiviruses known to infect humans. The lentiviruses are slow-acting by comparison with viruses that cause acute infection (e.g., influenza virus) but not by comparison with other retroviruses. The features of acute primary infection with HIV resemble those of more classic acute infections. The characteristic chronicity of HIV disease is consistent with the designation lentivirus. →*For a detailed discussion of HIV, see Chap. 173.*

FURTHER READING

BARNAK K et al: Human T cell leukemia virus type I–induced disease: Pathways to cancer and neurodegeneration. Virology 308:1, 2003

GALLO RC: Human retroviruses after 20 years: A perspective from the past and prospects for their future control. Immunol Rev 185:236, 2002

GATZA ML et al: Cellular transformation by the HTLV-I Tax protein, a jack-of-all-trades. Oncogene 22:5141, 2003

JACOBSON S: Immunopathogenesis of human T cell lymphotropic virus type-1–associated neurologic disease. J Infect Dis 186(Suppl 2):S187, 2002

LOWIS GW et al: Epidemiologic features of HTLV-II: Serologic and molecular evidence. Ann Epidemiol 12:46, 2001

POIESZ BJ et al: The human T-cell lymphoma/leukemia viruses. Cancer Invest 21:253, 2003

AIDS was first recognized in the United States in the summer of 1981, when the U.S. Centers for Disease Control and Prevention (CDC) reported the unexplained occurrence of *Pneumocystis carinii* pneumonia in five previously healthy homosexual men in Los Angeles and of Kaposi's sarcoma (KS) in 26 previously healthy homosexual men in New York and Los Angeles. Within months, the disease became recognized in male and female injection drug users (IDUs) and soon thereafter in recipients of blood transfusions and in hemophiliacs. As the epidemiologic pattern of the disease unfolded, it became clear that a microbe transmissible by sexual (homosexual and heterosexual) contact and blood or blood products was the most likely etiologic agent of the epidemic.

In 1983, human immunodeficiency virus (HIV) was isolated from a patient with lymphadenopathy, and by 1984 it was demonstrated clearly to be the causative agent of AIDS. In 1985, a sensitive enzyme-linked immunosorbent assay (ELISA) was developed, which led to an appreciation of the scope and evolution of the HIV epidemic at first in the United States and other developed nations and ultimately among developing nations throughout the world (see below). The staggering worldwide growth of the HIV pandemic has been matched by an explosion of information in the areas of HIV virology, pathogenesis (both immunologic and virologic) and treatment of HIV disease, treatment and prophylaxis of the opportunistic diseases associated with HIV infection, and vaccine development. The information flow related to HIV disease is enormous and continues to expand, and it has become almost impossible for the health care generalist to stay abreast of the literature. The purpose of this chapter is to present the most current information available on the scope of the epidemic; on its pathogenesis, treatment, and prevention; and on prospects for vaccine development. Above all, the aim is to provide a solid scientific basis and practical clinical guidelines for a state-of-the-art approach to the HIV-infected patient.

DEFINITION With the identification of HIV in 1983 and its proof as the etiologic agent of AIDS in 1984, and with the availability of sensitive and specific diagnostic tests for HIV infection, the case definition of AIDS has undergone several revisions over the years. The current CDC classification system for HIV-infected adolescents and adults categorizes persons on the basis of clinical conditions associated with HIV infection and CD4+ T lymphocyte counts. The system is based on three ranges of CD4+ T lymphocyte counts and three clinical categories and is represented by a matrix of nine mutually exclusive categories (Tables 173-1 and 173-2). Using this system, any HIV-infected individual with a CD4+ T cell count of <200/µL has AIDS by definition, regardless of the presence of symptoms or opportunistic diseases (Table 173-1). Once individuals have had a clinical condition in category B, their disease cannot again be classified as category A, even if the condition resolves; the same holds true for category C in relation to category B.

The definition of AIDS is indeed complex and comprehensive; however, the clinician should not focus on whether AIDS is present but should view HIV disease as a spectrum ranging from primary infection, with or without the acute syndrome, to the asymptomatic stage, to advanced disease (see below). The definition of AIDS was established not for the practical care of patients but for surveillance purposes.

TABLE 173-2 *Clinical Categories of HIV Infection*

Category A: Consists of one or more of the conditions listed below in an adolescent or adult (>13 years) with documented HIV infection. Conditions listed in categories B and C must not have occurred.
  Asymptomatic HIV infection
  Persistent generalized lymphadenopathy
  Acute (primary) HIV infection with accompanying illness or history of acute HIV infection

Category B: Consists of symptomatic conditions in an HIV-infected adolescent or adult that are not included among conditions listed in clinical category C and that meet at least one of the following criteria: (1) The conditions are attributed to HIV infection or are indicative of a defect in cell-mediated immunity; or (2) the conditions are considered by physicians to have a clinical course or to require management that is complicated by HIV infection. Examples include, but are not limited to, the following:
  Bacillary angiomatosis
  Candidiasis, oropharyngeal (thrush)
  Candidiasis, vulvovaginal; persistent, frequent, or poorly responsive to therapy
  Cervical dysplasia (moderate or severe)/cervical carcinoma in situ
  Constitutional symptoms, such as fever (38.5°C) or diarrhea lasting >1 month
  Hairy leukoplakia, oral
  Herpes zoster (shingles), involving at least two distinct episodes or more than one dermatome
  Idiopathic thrombocytopenic purpura
  Listeriosis
  Pelvic inflammatory disease, particularly if complicated by tuboovarian abscess
  Peripheral neuropathy
Category C: Conditions listed in the AIDS surveillance case definition.
  Candidiasis of bronchi, trachea, or lungs
  Candidiasis, esophageal
  Cervical cancer, invasive[a]
  Coccidioidomycosis, disseminated or extrapulmonary
  Cryptococcosis, extrapulmonary
  Cryptosporidiosis, chronic intestinal (>1 month's duration)
  Cytomegalovirus disease (other than liver, spleen, or nodes)
  Cytomegalovirus retinitis (with loss of vision)
  Encephalopathy, HIV-related
  Herpes simplex: chronic ulcer(s) (>1 month's duration); or bronchitis, pneumonia, or esophagitis
  Histoplasmosis, disseminated or extrapulmonary
  Isosporiasis, chronic intestinal (>1 month's duration)
  Kaposi's sarcoma
  Lymphoma, Burkitt's (or equivalent term)
  Lymphoma, primary, of brain
  Mycobacterium avium complex or *M. kansasii*, disseminated or extrapulmonary
  Mycobacterium tuberculosis, any site (pulmonary[a] or extrapulmonary)
  Mycobacterium, other species or unidentified species, disseminated or extrapulmonary
  Pneumocystis carinii pneumonia
  Pneumonia, recurrent[a]
  Progressive multifocal leukoencephalopathy
  Salmonella septicemia, recurrent
  Toxoplasmosis of brain
  Wasting syndrome due to HIV

[a] Added in the 1993 expansion of the AIDS surveillance case definition.
Source: MMWR 42(No. RR-17), December 18, 1992.

TABLE 173-1 *1993 Revised Classification System for HIV Infection and Expanded AIDS Surveillance Case Definition for Adolescents and Adults*[a]

CD4+ T Cell Categories	Clinical Categories		
	A Asymptomatic, Acute (Primary) HIV or PGL[b]	B Symptomatic, Not A or C Conditions	C AIDS-Indicator Conditions
>500/µL	A1	B1	C1
200–499/µL	A2	B2	C2
<200/µL	A3	B3	C3

[a] The shaded areas indicate the expanded AIDS surveillance case definition.
[b] PGL, progressive generalized lymphadenopathy.
Source: MMWR 42(No. RR-17), December 18, 1992.

The etiologic agent of AIDS is HIV, which belongs to the family of human retroviruses (Retroviridae) and the subfamily of lentiviruses (Chap. 172). Nononcogenic lentiviruses cause disease in other animal species, including sheep, horses, goats, cattle, cats, and monkeys. The four recognized human retroviruses belong to two distinct groups: the human T lymphotropic viruses (HTLV) I and HTLV-II, which are transforming retroviruses; and the human immunodeficiency viruses, HIV-1 and HIV-2, which are cytopathic viruses (Chap. 172). The most common cause of HIV disease throughout the world, and certainly in the United States, is HIV-1, which comprises several subtypes with different geographic distributions (see below). HIV-2 was first identified in 1986 in West African patients and was originally confined to West Africa. However, a number of cases that can be traced to West Africa or to sexual contacts with West Africans have been identified throughout the world. Both HIV-1 and HIV-2 are zoonotic infections. HIV-2 is more closely related phylogenetically to the simian immunodeficiency virus (SIV) found in sooty mangabeys than it is to HIV-1. HIV-1 likely originated from the *Pan troglodytes troglodytes* species of chimpanzees in whom the virus had co-evolved over centuries. The taxonomic relationship among primate lentiviruses is shown in Fig. 173-1.

MORPHOLOGY OF HIV   Electron microscopy shows that the HIV virion is an icosahedral structure (Fig. 173-2*A*) containing numerous external spikes formed by the two major envelope proteins, the external gp120 and the transmembrane gp41. The virion buds from the surface of the infected cell and incorporates a variety of host proteins, including major histocompatibility complex (MHC) class I and II antigens (Chap. 296), into its lipid bilayer. The structure of HIV-1 is schematically diagrammed in Fig. 173-2*B* (Chap. 172).

REPLICATION CYCLE OF HIV   HIV is an RNA virus whose hallmark is the reverse transcription of its genomic RNA to DNA by the enzyme *reverse transcriptase*. The replication cycle of HIV begins with the high-affinity binding of the gp120 protein via a portion of its V1 region near the N terminus to its receptor on the host cell surface, the CD4 molecule (Fig. 173-3). The CD4 molecule is a 55-kDa protein found predominantly on a subset of T lymphocytes that are responsible for helper or inducer function in the immune system (Chap. 295). It is also expressed on the surface of monocytes/macrophages and dendritic/Langerhans cells. Once gp120 binds to CD4, the gp120 undergoes a conformational change that facilitates binding to one of a group of co-receptors. The two major co-receptors for HIV-1 are CCR5 and CXCR4. Both receptors belong to the family of seven-transmembrane-domain G protein–coupled cellular receptors, and the use of one or the other or both receptors by the virus for entry into the cell is an important determinant of the cellular tropism of the virus (see below for details). Certain dendritic cells express a diversity of C-type lectin receptors on their surface, one of which is called *DC-SIGN*, that bind with high affinity to the HIV gp120 envelope protein, allowing the dendritic cell to facilitate the binding of virus to the CD4+ T cell upon engagement of dendritic cells with CD4+ T cells. Following binding of the envelope protein to the CD4 molecule, the conformation of the viral envelope changes dramatically, and fusion with the host cell membrane occurs via the newly exposed gp41 molecule penetrating the plasma membrane of the target cell and then coiling upon itself to bring the virion and target cell together. Following fusion (Fig. 173-4), the HIV ge-

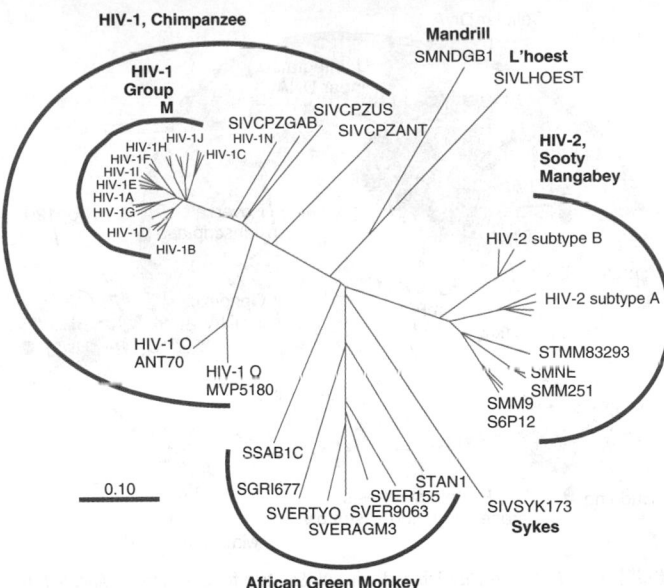

FIGURE 173-1   A phylogenetic tree, based on the complete genomes of primate immunodeficiency viruses. The scale at the bottom (0.10) indicates a 10% difference at the nucleotide level. (*Prepared by Brian Foley, PhD, of the HIV Sequence Database, Theoretical Biology and Biophysics Group, Los Alamos National Laboratory.*)

nomic RNA is uncoated and internalized into the target cell (Fig. 173-3). The reverse transcriptase enzyme, which is contained in the infecting virion, then catalyzes the reverse transcription of the genomic RNA into double-strand DNA. The DNA translocates to the nucleus, where it is integrated in a somewhat, but not completely, random fashion into the host cell chromosomes through the action of another virally encoded enzyme, *integrase*. Sites of HIV integration into the nuclear DNA are preferential for active genes and regional hotspots. This provirus may remain transcriptionally inactive (latent) or it may manifest varying levels of gene expression, up to active production of virus.

Cellular activation plays an important role in the life cycle of HIV and is critical to the pathogenesis of HIV disease (see below). Following initial binding and internalization of virions into the target cell, incompletely reverse-transcribed DNA intermediates are labile in quiescent cells and will not integrate efficiently into the host cell genome

FIGURE 173-2   *A.* Electron micrograph of HIV. Figure illustrates a typical virion following budding from the surface of a CD4+ T lymphocyte, together with two additional incomplete virions in the process of budding from the cell membrane. *B.* Structure of HIV-1, including the gp120 outer membrane, gp41 transmembrane components of the envelope, genomic RNA, enzyme reverse transcriptase, p18(17) inner membrane (matrix), and p24 core protein (capsid) (copyright by George V. Kelvin). (*Adapted from RC Gallo: Sci Am 256:46, 1987.*)

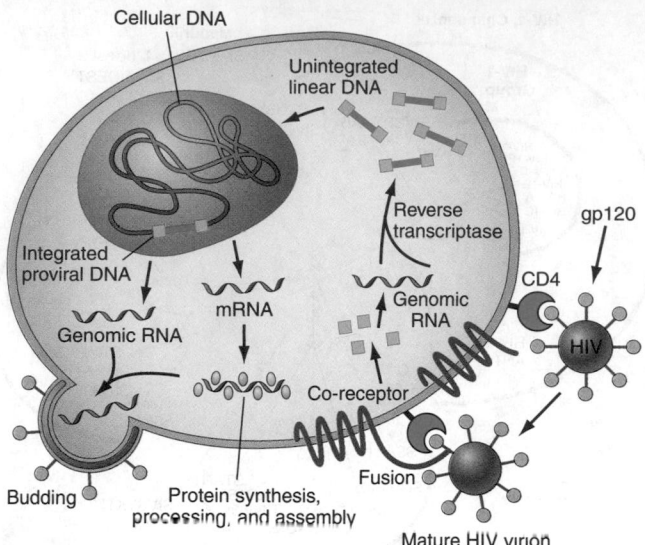

FIGURE 173-3   The replication cycle of HIV. See text for description. (*Adapted from Fauci, 1996.*)

unless cellular activation occurs shortly after infection. Furthermore, some degree of activation of the host cell is required for the initiation of transcription of the integrated proviral DNA into either genomic RNA or mRNA. This latter process may not necessarily be associated with the obvious expression of the classic cell surface markers of activation. In this regard, activation of HIV expression from the latent state depends on the interaction of a number of cellular and viral factors. Following transcription, HIV mRNA is translated into proteins that undergo modification through glycosylation, myristylation, phosphorylation, and cleavage. The viral particle is formed by the assembly of HIV proteins, enzymes, and genomic RNA at the plasma membrane of the cells. Budding of the progeny virion occurs through specialized regions in the lipid bilayer of the host cell membrane known as *lipid rafts*, where the core acquires its external envelope (Chap. 172). The virally encoded protease then catalyzes the cleavage of the gag-pol precursor (see below) to yield the mature virion. Progression through the virus replication cycle is profoundly influenced by a variety of viral regulatory gene products. Likewise, each point in the replication cycle of HIV is a real or potential target for therapeutic intervention (see below). Thus far, the reverse transcriptase and protease enzymes have proven clinically to be susceptible to pharmacologic disruption (see below). Recently, inhibitors of virus–target cell fusion have shown therapeutic promise, and inhibitors of the viral enzyme integrase are in clinical trials.

HIV GENOME   Figure 173-5 illustrates the arrangement of the HIV genome schematically. Like other retroviruses, HIV-1 has genes that encode the structural proteins of the virus: *gag* encodes the proteins that form the core of the virion (including p24 antigen); *pol* encodes the enzymes responsible for reverse transcription and integration; and *env* encodes the envelope glycoproteins. However, HIV-1 is more complex than other retroviruses, particularly those of the nonprimate group, in that it also contains at least six other genes (*tat, rev, nef, vif, vpr,* and *vpu*), which code for proteins involved in the regulation of gene expression (Chap. 172). Several of these proteins are felt to play a role in the pathogenesis of HIV disease; their various functions are listed in Fig. 173-5. Flanking these genes are the long terminal repeats (LTRs), which contain regulatory elements involved in gene expression (Fig. 173-5). The major difference between the genomes of HIV-1 and HIV-2 is the fact that HIV-2 lacks the *vpu* gene and has a *vpx* gene not contained in HIV-1.

MOLECULAR HETEROGENEITY OF HIV-1   Molecular analyses of various HIV isolates reveal sequence variations over many parts of the viral ge-

nome. For example, in different isolates, the degree of difference in the coding sequences of the viral envelope protein ranges from a few percent (very close) to 50%. These changes tend to cluster in hypervariable regions. HIV can evolve by several means, including simple base substitution, insertions and deletions, recombination, and gain and loss of glycosylation sites. The balance of immune pressure and functional constraints on proteins influences the regional level of variation within proteins. For example, Envelope, which is exposed on the surface of the virion and is under immune selective pressure from both antibodies and cytolytic T lymphocytes, is extremely variable, with clusters of mutations in hypervariable domains. In contrast, Reverse Transcriptase, with important enzymatic functions, is relatively conserved, particularly around the active site. The extraordinary variability of HIV-1 is in marked contrast to the relative stability of HTLV-I and -II.

There are three groups of HIV-1: group M (major), which is responsible for most of the infections in the world; group O (outlier), a relatively rare viral form found originally in Cameroon, Gabon, and France; and group N first identified in a Cameroonian woman with AIDS; only a few cases of the latter have been identified. Among primate lentiviruses, HIV-1 is most closely related to viruses isolated from chimpanzees. The M group comprises nine subtypes, or *clades*, designated A, B, C, D, F, G, H, J, and K, as well as a growing number of major circulating recombinant forms (CRFs). These CRFs range from highly prevalent forms such as the AE virus, CRF 01, which is predominant in southeast Asia and often referred to simply as E, despite the fact that the parental E virus has never been found, and AG from west and central Africa, to a large number of CRFs that are more or less rare. The subtypes and CRFs create the major lineages of the M group of HIV-1. The picture has been complicated somewhat when it was found that some subtypes are not equidistant from one another, while others contained sequences so diverse that they could not properly be considered to be the same subtype. Thus, the sub-subtype was introduced, and subtypes A and F are now subdivided into A1 and A2, F1 and F2. It has also been argued that subtypes B and D are really too close to be separate subtypes and should be considered sub-subtypes; it was decided, however, not to increase the confusion by renaming the clades (Fig. 173-6).

The global patterns of HIV-1 variation likely result from accidents of viral trafficking. Subtype B viruses, which now differ by up to 17% in their *env* coding sequences, are the overwhelmingly predominant viruses seen in the United States, Canada, certain countries in South America, western Europe, and Australia. Other subtypes are also present in these countries to varying degrees. It is thought that, purely by chance, subtype B was seeded into the United States in the late 1970s, thereby establishing an overwhelming founder effect. Subtype C viruses (of the M group) are the most common form worldwide; many countries have cocirculating viral subtypes that are giving rise

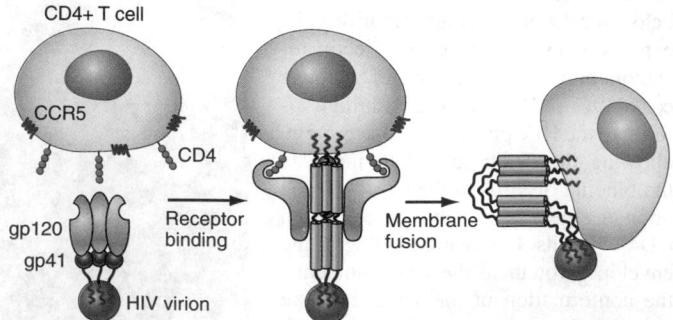

FIGURE 173-4   Binding and fusion of HIV-1 with its target cell. HIV-1 binds to its target cell via the CD4 molecule, leading to a conformational change in the gp120 molecule that allows it to bind to the co-receptor CCR5 (for R5-using viruses). The virus then firmly attaches to the host cell membrane in a coiled-spring fashion via the newly exposed gp41 molecule. Virus-cell fusion occurs as the transitional intermediate of gp41 undergoes further changes to form a hairpin structure that draws the two membranes into close proximity (see text for details). (*Adapted from D Montefiori, JP Moore: Science 283:336, 1999; with permission.*)

LTR: Long terminal repeat
Contains control regions that bind host transcription factors (NF-κB, NFAT, Sp.1, TBP)
Required for the initiation of transcription
Contains RNA trans-acting response element (TAR) that binds Tat

vif: Viral infectivity factor (p23)
Overcomes inhibitory effects of unidentified host factor, yielding more stable RT complexes

vpu: Viral protein U
Promotes CD4 degradation and influences virion release

env: gp 160 envelope protein
Cleaved in endoplasmic reticulum to gp 120 (SU) and gp41 (TM)
gp 120 mediates CD4 and chemokine receptor binding, while gp41 mediates fusion
Contains RNA response element (RRE) that binds Rev

nef: Negative effector (p24)
Promotes down-regulation of surface CD4 and MHC 1 expression
Blocks apoptosis
Enhance virion infectivity
Alters state of cellular activation
Progression to disease slowed significantly in absence of Nef

gag: Pr55^{gag}
Polyprotein processed by PR
MA, matrix (p17)
Undergoes myristylation that helps target gag polyprotein to lipids rafts; implicated in nuclear import of HIV preintegration complex (PIC)
CA, capsid (p24) Binds cyclophillin A
NC, nucleocapsid (p7) Zn finger, RNA-binding protein
p6
Interacts with Vpr; contain slate domain (PTAP) that binds TSG101 and participates in terminal stops of virion budding

pol: Polymerase
Encodes a variety of viral enzymes, including PR (p10), RT, and RNAase H (p66/51), and IN (p32) all processed by PR

vpr: Viral protein R (p15)
Promotes G2 cell-cycle arrest
Facilitates HIV infection of macrophages

rev: Regulator of viral gene expression (p19)
Binds RRE
Inhibits viral RNA splicing and promotes nuclear export of incompletely spliced viral RNAs

tat: Transcriptional activator (p14)
Binds TAR
In presence of host cyclin T1 and CDK9 enhances RNA Pol II elongation on the viral DNA template

FIGURE 173-5 Organization of the genome of the HIV provirus together with a summary description of its nine genes encoding 15 proteins. (*From Greene and Peterlin.*)

to CRFs. Figure 173-7 schematically diagrams the worldwide distribution of HIV-1 subtypes by region. The predominant subtype in Europe and the Americas is subtype B. In Africa, >75% of strains recovered to date have been of subtypes A, C, and D, with C being the most common. In Asia, HIV-1 isolates of the CRF01 (AE) lineage and subtypes C and B predominate. CRF01 (AE) accounts for most infections in southeast Asia, while subtype C is prevalent in India (see "HIV Infection and AIDS Worldwide," below). Sequence analyses of HIV-1 isolates from infected individuals indicate that recombination among viruses of different clades likely occurs as a result of infection of an individual with viruses of more than one subtype, particularly in geographic areas where subtypes overlap.

TRANSMISSION

HIV is transmitted by both homosexual and heterosexual contact; by blood and blood products; and by infected mothers to infants either intrapartum, perinatally, or via breast milk. After >20 years of scrutiny, there is no evidence that HIV is transmitted by casual contact or that the virus can be spread by insects, such as by a mosquito bite.

SEXUAL TRANSMISSION HIV infection is predominantly a sexually transmitted disease (STD) worldwide. Although in the United States ~42% of new HIV infections are among men who have sex with men and ~33% of new HIV infections are by heterosexual transmission, the most common mode of infection worldwide, particularly in developing countries, is clearly heterosexual transmission. Furthermore, the yearly incidence of new cases of AIDS attributed to heterosexual transmission of HIV is steadily increasing in the United States, mainly among minorities, particularly women in minority groups (Fig. 173-8).

HIV has been demonstrated in seminal fluid both within infected mononuclear cells and in the cell-free state. The virus appears to concentrate in the seminal fluid, particularly in situations where there are increased numbers of lymphocytes and monocytes in the fluid, as in genital inflammatory states such as urethritis and epididymitis, con-

ditions closely associated with other STDs (see below). The virus has also been demonstrated in cervical smears and vaginal fluid. There is a strong association of transmission of HIV with receptive anal intercourse, probably because only a thin, fragile rectal mucosal membrane separates the deposited semen from potentially susceptible cells in and beneath the mucosa and trauma may be associated with anal intercourse. Anal douching and sexual practices that traumatize the rectal mucosa also increase the likelihood of infection. It is likely that anal intercourse provides at least two modalities of infection: (1) direct inoculation into blood in cases of traumatic tears in the mucosa; and (2) infection of susceptible target cells, such as Langerhans cells, in the mucosal layer in the absence of trauma (see below). Although the vaginal mucosa is several layers thicker than the rectal mucosa and less likely to be traumatized during intercourse, it is clear that the virus can be transmitted to either partner through vaginal intercourse. In a 10-year prospective study in the United States of heterosexual transmission of HIV, male-to-female transmission was approximately eight times more efficient than female-to-male transmission. This difference may be due in part to the prolonged exposure to infected seminal fluid of the vaginal and cervical mucosa, as well as the endometrium (when

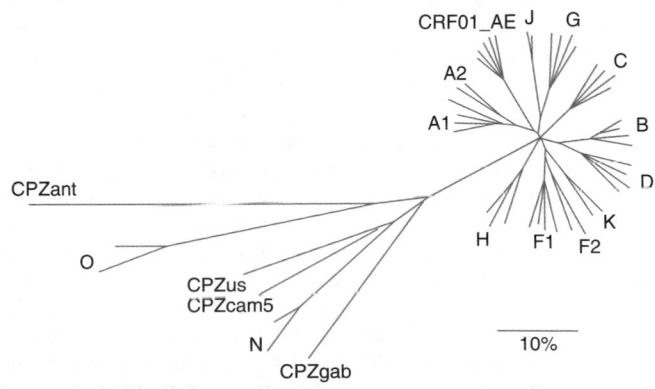

FIGURE 173-6 Phylogenetic tree constructed from representative viral envelope sequences of the subtypes and circulating recombinant forms (CRFs) in group M and some isolates from groups N and O (human) and CPZ (chimpanzee). The scale bar at the bottom indicates the genetic distances between the sequences. A1 and A2, F1 and F2 are subtypes; CRF01_AE is unique in the envelope gene, but similar to subtype A in the rest of the genome. (*Courtesy of Bette Korber, PhD, and Carla Kuiken, PhD, HIV Database, Los Alamos National Laboratory*).

FIGURE 173-7 Geographic distribution of HIV-1 subtypes, 2001. The prevalence of HIV-1 genetic subtypes varies by geographic region. The proportions of subtypes in different regions are indicated by pie charts. (*From S Osmanov et al: J Acquir Imm Def Syndr 29:184, 2002.*)

semen enters through the cervical os). By comparison, the penis and urethral orifice are exposed relatively briefly to infected vaginal fluid. Among various cofactors examined in this study, a history of STDs (see below) was most strongly associated with HIV transmission. In this regard, there is a close association between genital ulcerations and transmission, from the standpoints of both susceptibility to infection and infectivity. Infections with microorganisms such as *Treponema pallidum* (Chap. 153), *Haemophilus ducreyi* (Chap. 130), and herpes simplex virus (HSV; Chap. 163) are important causes of genital ulcerations linked to transmission of HIV. In addition, pathogens responsible for nonulcerative inflammatory STDs such as those caused by *Chlamydia trachomatis* (Chap. 160), *Neisseria gonorrhoeae* (Chap. 128), and *Trichomonas vaginalis* (Chap. 199) are also associated with an increased risk of transmission of HIV infection. Bacterial vaginosis, an infection related to sexual behavior, but not strictly an STD, may also be linked to an increased risk of transmission of HIV infection. Several studies suggest that treating other STDs and genital tract syndromes may help prevent transmission of HIV. This effect is most prominent in populations in which the prevalence of HIV infection is relatively low. In studies conducted in Uganda, the chief predictor of heterosexual transmission of HIV was the level of plasma viremia. In a cohort of couples in which one partner was HIV-infected and one was initially uninfected, the mean serum HIV RNA level was significantly higher among HIV-infected subjects whose partners seroconverted than among those whose partners did not seroconvert. In fact transmission was rare when the infected partner had a plasma level of <1500 copies of HIV RNA per milliliter. Of note, in that study, there were no seroconversions among 50 circumcised male partners. Furthermore, in a number of other studies, lack of circumcision has been strongly associated with a higher risk of HIV infection. This difference may be due to increased susceptibility of uncircumcised men to ulcerative STDs, as well as other factors such as microtrauma. In addition, the highly vascularized inner foreskin tissue contains a high density of Langerhans cells as well as increased numbers of CD4+ T cells, macrophages, and other cellular targets for HIV. Finally, the moist environment under the foreskin may promote the presence or persistence of microbial flora which, via inflammatory changes, may lead to even higher concentrations of target cells for HIV in the foreskin. In some studies the use of oral contraceptives was associated with an increase in incidence of HIV infection over and above that which might be expected by not using a condom for birth control.

Oral sex is a much less efficient mode of transmission of HIV than is receptive anal intercourse. A number of studies have reported that the incidence of transmission of infection by oral sex among couples discordant for HIV was extremely low; indeed, one study reported no cases among 239 men whose only risk was receptive oral intercourse where 28% knew that their partner was HIV-infected. However, there have been several reports of documented HIV transmission resulting solely from receptive fellatio and insertive cunnilingus. There are probably many more cases that go unreported because of the frequent practice of both oral sex and receptive anal intercourse by the same person. Therefore, the assumption that receptive oral sex is com-

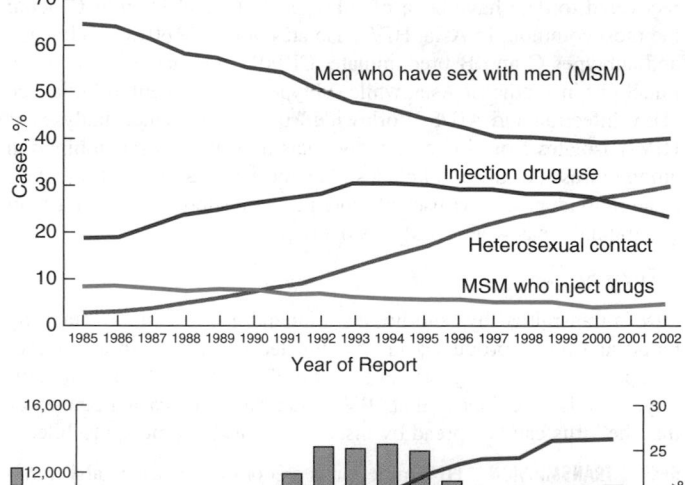

FIGURE 173-8 The changing face of the HIV/AIDS epidemic in the United States. *Upper.* Proportion of AIDS cases among U.S. adults and adolescents, by exposure category and year of diagnosis. *Lower.* The proportion of AIDS cases among women and adolescent girls (aged >13 years) increased from 8% in 1986 to 26% in 2002. (*From the Centers for Disease Control and Prevention, 2003.*)

pletely safe is not warranted. The association of alcohol consumption and illicit drug use with unsafe sexual behavior, both homosexual and heterosexual, leads to an increased risk of sexual transmission of HIV.

TRANSMISSION BY BLOOD AND BLOOD PRODUCTS HIV can be transmitted to individuals who receive HIV-tainted blood transfusions, blood products, or transplanted tissue as well as to IDUs who are exposed to HIV while sharing injection paraphernalia such as needles, syringes, the water in which drugs are mixed, or the cotton through which drugs are filtered. Parenteral transmission of HIV during injection drug use does not require intravenous puncture; subcutaneous ("skin popping") or intramuscular ("muscling") injections can transmit HIV as well, even though these behaviors are sometimes erroneously perceived as low-risk. Among IDUs, the risk of HIV infection increases with the duration of injection drug use; the frequency of needle sharing; the number of partners with whom paraphernalia are shared, particularly in the setting of "shooting galleries" where drugs are sold and large numbers of IDUs may share a limited number of "works"; comorbid psychiatric conditions such as antisocial personality disorder; the use of cocaine in injectable form or smoked as "crack"; and the use of injection drugs in a geographic location with a high prevalence of HIV infection, such as certain inner-city areas in the United States.

From the late 1970s until the spring of 1985, when mandatory testing of donated blood for HIV-1 was initiated, it has been estimated that >10,000 individuals in the United States were infected through transfusions of blood or blood products (Chap. 99). Approximately 9300 individuals in the United States who survived the illness for which they received HIV-contaminated blood transfusions, blood components, or transplanted tissue have developed AIDS. It is estimated that 90 to 100% of individuals who were exposed to such HIV-contaminated products became infected. Transfusions of whole blood, packed red blood cells, platelets, leukocytes, and plasma are all capable of transmitting HIV infection. In contrast, hyperimmune γ globulin, hepatitis B immune globulin, plasma-derived hepatitis B vaccine, and Rh$_o$ immune globulin have not been associated with transmission of HIV infection. The procedures involved in processing these products either inactivate or remove the virus.

In addition to the above, several thousand individuals in the United States with hemophilia or other clotting disorders were infected with HIV by receipt of HIV-contaminated fresh-frozen plasma or concentrates of clotting factors; ~5470 of these individuals have developed AIDS. Currently, in the United States and in most developed countries, the following measures have made the risk of transmission of HIV infection by transfused blood or blood products extremely small: (1) the screening of all blood for HIV nucleic acid, p24 antigen, and/or anti-HIV antibodies; (2) the self-deferral of donors on the basis of risk behavior; (3) the screening out of HIV-negative individuals with positive surrogate laboratory parameters of HIV infection, such as hepatitis B and C; and (4) serologic testing for syphilis. It is currently estimated that the risk of infection with HIV in the United States via transfused screened blood is approximately 1 in 725,000 to 1 in 835,000 donations. Therefore, among the 12 million donations collected in the United States each year, an estimated 16 infectious donations are available for transfusion. Thus, despite the best efforts of science, one cannot completely eliminate the risk of tranfusion-related transmission of HIV since current technology cannot detect HIV RNA for the first 1 to 2 weeks following infection due to the low levels of viremia. In this regard, two individuals in Florida recently contracted HIV from a single donor who had recently become infected; the blood collection system in question had used nucleic acid amplification testing to screen the blood. There have been several reports of sporadic breakdowns in routinely available screening procedures in certain countries, where contaminated blood was allowed to be transfused, resulting in small clusters of patients becoming infected. In China, a disturbingly large number of people have become infected by selling blood in situations where the collectors reused needles that were con-

taminated and in some instances mixed blood products from a number of people, separated the plasma, and re-infused red blood cells back into individual donors. It is estimated that >6% of China's HIV-infected population were infected while selling blood. There have been no reported cases of transmission of HIV-2 in the United States via donated blood, and, currently, donated blood is screened for both HIV-1 and HIV-2 antibodies. The chance of infection of a hemophiliac via clotting factor concentrates has essentially been eliminated because of the added layer of safety resulting from heat treatment of the concentrates.

Prior to the screening of donors, a small number of cases of transmission of HIV via semen used in artificial insemination and tissues used in organ transplantation were well documented. At present, donors of such tissues are prescreened for HIV infection.

OCCUPATIONAL TRANSMISSION OF HIV: HEALTH CARE WORKERS AND LABORATORY WORKERS There is a small, but definite, occupational risk of HIV transmission to health care workers and laboratory personnel and potentially others who work with HIV-containing materials, particularly when sharp objects are used. An estimated 600,000 to 800,000 health care workers are stuck with needles or other sharp medical instruments in the United States each year. Large, multi-institutional studies have indicated that the risk of HIV transmission following skin puncture from a needle or a sharp object that was contaminated with blood from a person with documented HIV infection is ~0.3% and after a mucous membrane exposure it is 0.09% (see "HIV and the Health Care Worker," p. 1136). HIV transmission after non-intact skin exposure has been documented, but the average risk for transmission by this route has not been precisely determined; however, it is estimated to be less than the risk for mucous membrane exposure. Transmission of HIV through intact skin has not been documented. An increased risk for HIV infection following percutaneous exposures to HIV-infected blood is associated with exposures involving a relatively large quantity of blood, as in the case of a device visibly contaminated with the patient's blood, a procedure that involves a needle placed directly in a vein or artery, or a deep injury. Factors that might be associated with mucocutaneous transmission of HIV include exposure to an unusually large volume of blood, prolonged contact, and a potential portal of entry. In addition, the risk increases for exposures to blood from patients with advanced-stage disease, probably owing to the higher titer of HIV in the blood as well as to other factors, such as the presence of more virulent strains of virus. The use of antiretroviral drugs as postexposure prophylaxis decreases the risk of infection compared to historic controls in occupationally exposed health care workers (see "HIV and the Health Care Worker"). The risk of hepatitis B virus (HBV) infection following a similar type of exposure is 6 to 30% in nonimmune individuals; if a susceptible worker is exposed to HBV, postexposure prophylaxis with hepatitis B immune globulin and initiation of HBV vaccine is >90% effective in preventing HBV infection. The risk of hepatitis C virus (HCV) infection following percutaneous injury is ~1.8% (Chap. 285).

Since the beginning of the HIV epidemic, there have been at least three reported instances in which transmission of infection from a health care worker to patients seemed highly probable. The first involved a dentist in Florida who apparently infected six of his patients, most likely through contaminated instruments. Another case involved an orthopedic surgeon in France who apparently infected a patient during placement of a total hip prosthesis. A third case involved the apparent transmission of HIV from a nurse to a surgical patient in France. An additional situation involved the apparent infection of four patients by an HIV-negative general surgeon in Australia during routine outpatient surgery. The cause of the transmission was felt to be a failure on the part of the surgeon to sterilize instruments properly between procedures following prior surgery on an infected patient. Despite these few cases, the risk of transmission from an infected health care worker to patients is extremely low; in fact, too low to be measured accurately. Indeed several epidemiologic studies have been performed tracing thousands of patients of HIV-infected dentists, physicians, surgeons, obstetricians, and gynecologists, and no other cases of HIV infection that could be linked to the health care providers were identified. The very occurrence of transmission of HIV as well as HBV and HCV to and from health care workers in the workplace underscores the importance of the use of universal precautions when caring for all patients (see below and Chap. 116).

MATERNAL-FETAL/INFANT TRANSMISSION HIV infection can be transmitted from an infected mother to her fetus during pregnancy, during delivery, or by breast-feeding. This is an extremely important form of transmission of HIV infection in developing countries, where the proportion of infected women to infected men is ~1:1. Virologic analysis of aborted fetuses indicate that HIV can be transmitted to the fetus as early as the first and second trimester of pregnancy. However, maternal transmission to the fetus occurs most commonly in the perinatal period. This conclusion is based on a number of considerations, including the time frame of identification of infection by the sequential appearance of classes of antibodies to HIV (i.e., the appearance of HIV-specific IgA antibody within 3 to 6 months after birth); a positive viral culture; the appearance of p24 antigenemia weeks to months after delivery, but not at the time of delivery; a polymerase chain reaction (PCR) assay of infant blood following delivery that is negative at birth and positive several months later; the demonstration that the firstborn twin of an infected mother is more commonly infected than is the second twin; and the evidence that cesarean section results in decreased transmission to the infant. Two studies performed in Rwanda and the former Zaire indicated that the relative proportions of mother-to-child transmissions were 23 to 30% before birth, 50 to 65% during birth, and 12 to 20% via breast-feeding.

In the absence of prophylactic antiretroviral therapy to the mother during pregnancy, labor, and delivery, and to the fetus following birth (see below), the probability of transmission of HIV from mother to infant/fetus ranges from 15 to 25% in industrialized countries and from 25 to 35% in developing countries. These differences may relate to the adequacy of prenatal care as well as to the stage of HIV disease and the general health of the mother during pregnancy. Higher rates of transmission have been reported to be associated with many factors; some of these are well proven by a number of studies, while others are considered to be potential factors since various studies may have given divergent results. The best-documented factor that is associated with higher rates of transmission is the presence of high maternal levels of plasma viremia. Low maternal CD4+ T cell counts have also been associated with higher rates of transmission; however, since low CD4+ T cell counts are often associated with high levels of plasma viremia, in one study using multivariate analysis including plasma viral load and CD4+ T cell count, only the level of plasma HIV RNA was significant. A prolonged interval between membrane rupture and delivery is another well-documented risk factor for transmission. Other conditions that are potential risk factors, but which have not been consistently demonstrated, are the presence of chorioamnionitis at delivery; STDs during pregnancy; hard drug use during pregnancy; cigarette smoking; preterm delivery; and obstetric procedures such as amniocentesis, amnioscopy, fetal scalp electrodes, and episeotomy. Vitamin A deficiency had been reported to be associated with higher transmission rates; however, vitamin A supplementation during pregnancy resulted in improved birth weight and neonatal growth and reduced anemia but did not affect perinatal transmission of HIV. With regard to levels of viremia, several studies indicate that the risk of transmission increases with the maternal plasma HIV RNA level. In one series of 552 singleton pregnancies in the United States, the rate of mother-to-baby transmission was 0% among women with <1000 copies of HIV RNA per milliliter of blood, 16.6% among women with 1000 to 10,000/mL, 21.3% among women with 10,001 to 50,000/mL, 30.9% among women with 50,001 to 100,000/mL, and 40.6% among

women with >100,000/mL. However, there may be no lower "threshold" below which transmission never occurs, since other studies have reported transmission by women with viral RNA levels <50 copies per milliliter. Finally, it has been speculated that if the mother experiences acute primary infection during pregnancy, there is a higher rate of transmission to the fetus, owing to the high levels of viremia that occur during primary infection. However, a study from Thailand reported no increased risk of transmission of HIV from mother-to-child in women who seroconverted during pregnancy. In that study, maternal viral loads at delivery were no different among women who seroconverted during pregnancy and those who were seropositive when first tested. In a study conducted in the United States, zidovudine treatment of HIV-infected pregnant women from the beginning of the second trimester through delivery and of the infant for 6 weeks following birth dramatically decreased the rate of intrapartum and perinatal transmission of HIV infection from 22.6% in the untreated group to <5%. The rate of mother-to-child transmission is approaching 1% or less in pregnant women who are receiving combination antiretroviral therapy for their HIV infection. Such treatment, combined with cesarean section delivery, has rendered mother-to-child transmission of HIV an unusual event in the United States and other developed nations. In developed countries, current recommendations to reduce perinatal transmission of HIV include universal voluntary HIV testing and counseling of pregnant women, antiretroviral prophylaxis with one or more drugs in cases in which the mother does not require therapy for her HIV infection, combination therapy for women who do require therapy, obstetric management that attempts to minimize exposure of the infant to maternal blood and genital secretions, and avoidance of breast-feeding. It is recommended that the choice of antiretroviral therapy for pregnant women should be based on the same considerations used for women who are not pregnant, with discussion of the recognized and unknown risks and benefits of such therapy during pregnancy. The cost and logistics of the above protocol are not currently feasible for developing countries, particularly those in sub-Saharan Africa where the per capita health care delivery allocation is often only a few dollars per year. Studies have demonstrated that truncated regimens of zidovudine alone or in combination with lamivudine given to the mother during the last few weeks of pregnancy or even only during labor and delivery, and to the infant for a week or less, reduced transmission to the infant by 50% compared to placebo. One important study in Uganda demonstrated that a single dose of nevirapine given to the mother at the onset of labor followed by a single dose to the newborn within 72 h of birth decreased transmission by 50% compared with a regimen of zidovudine to the mother that began at the onset of labor and continued throughout labor and to the infant for 1 week following birth. The cost of the nevirapine for the mother and infant was $4.00, thus making this regimen more affordable. Indeed, short-course nevirapine regimens increasingly are being utilized in developing nations for the prevention of mother-to-child transmission. It is estimated that the successful implementation of such regimens could potentially save 1000 babies per day from becoming infected with HIV, the vast majority of whom are in sub-Saharan Africa.

Breast-feeding is an important modality of transmission of HIV infection in developing countries, particularly where mothers continue to breast feed for prolonged periods. The risk factors for mother-to-child transmission of HIV via breast-feeding are not fully understood; factors that increase the likelihood of transmission include detectable levels of HIV in breast milk, the presence of mastitis, low maternal CD4+ T cell counts, and maternal vitamin A deficiency. The risk of HIV infection via breast-feeding is highest in the early months of breast-feeding. In addition, exclusive breast-feeding has been reported to carry a lower risk of HIV transmission than mixed feeding. Certainly, in developed countries breast-feeding by an infected mother should be avoided. However, there is disagreement regarding recommendations for breast-feeding in certain developing countries, where breast milk is the only source of adequate nutrition as well as immunity against potentially serious infections for the infant. Studies are being conducted to determine whether intermittent administration of nevirapine, which has a relatively long half-life, to uninfected babies born of infected mothers decreases the incidence of infection via breast-feeding. The optimal approach to prevent transmission by infected mothers who choose to breast-feed would be to provide continual treatment to the infected mother where feasible.

TRANSMISSION BY OTHER BODY FLUIDS Although HIV can be isolated typically in low titers from saliva of a small proportion of infected individuals, there is no convincing evidence that saliva can transmit HIV infection, either through kissing or through other exposures, such as occupationally to health care workers. Saliva contains endogenous antiviral factors; among these factors, HIV-specific immunoglobulins of IgA, IgG, and IgM isotypes are detected readily in salivary secretions of infected individuals. It has been suggested that large glycoproteins such as mucins and thrombospondin-1 sequester HIV into aggregates for clearance by the host. In addition, a number of soluble salivary factors inhibit HIV to various degrees in vitro, probably by targeting host cell receptors rather than the virus itself. Perhaps the best-studied of these, secretory leukocyte protease inhibitor (SLPI), blocks HIV infection in several cell culture systems, and it is found in saliva at levels that approximate those required for inhibition of HIV in vitro. In this regard, higher salivary levels of SLPI in breast-fed infants were associated with a decreased risk of HIV transmission through breast milk. It has also been suggested that submandibular saliva reduces HIV infectivity by stripping gp120 from the surface of virions, and that saliva-mediated disruption and lysis of HIV-infected cells occurs because of the hypotonicity of oral secretions. There have been outlier cases of suspected transmission by saliva, but these have probably been blood-to-blood transmissions. Transmission of HIV by a human bite can occur but is a rare event; at least four cases of such transmission have been reported. In addition, a most unusual form of HIV transmission from infected children to mothers in the former Soviet Union has been identified. In those cases, the children (infected through transfusion) were said to have bleeding sores in the mouth, and the mothers were said to have lacerations and abrasions on and around the nipples of the breast resulting from trauma from the children's teeth. Breast-feeding had been continued until the children were older than is usual in other developed countries.

Although virus can be identified, if not isolated, from virtually any body fluid, there is no evidence that HIV transmission can occur as a result of exposure to tears, sweat, and urine. However, there have been isolated cases of transmission of HIV infection by body fluids that may or may not have been contaminated with blood. Most of these situations occurred in the setting of a close relative providing intensive nursing care for an HIV-infected person without observing universal precautions. These cases underscore the importance of observing universal precautions in the handling of body fluids and wastes from HIV-infected individuals (see below).

EPIDEMIOLOGY

HIV INFECTION AND AIDS WORLDWIDE HIV infection/AIDS is a global pandemic, with cases reported from virtually every country. The current estimate of the number of cases of HIV infection among adults worldwide is ~37 million, two-thirds of whom are in sub-Saharan Africa; 50% of cases are women. In addition, an estimated 2.5 million children younger than age 15 are living with HIV/AIDS. The global distribution of these cases is illustrated in Fig. 173-9. According to the Joint United Nations Programme on HIV/AIDS (UNAIDS), in 2003 alone there were an estimated 5 million new cases of infection worldwide (>14,000 new infections each day) and 3 million deaths from AIDS, making it the fourth leading cause of mortality worldwide. The cumulative number of AIDS-related deaths worldwide through the year 2003 exceeds 20 million. The HIV epidemic has occurred in "waves" in different regions of the world, each wave having somewhat different characteristics depending on the demographics of the country and region in question and the timing of the introduction of HIV into the population. As noted above, different subtypes, or clades, of HIV-1 are prevalent in different regions of the world (see above and Fig. 173-7), increasing the difficulty in the development of vaccines and perhaps accounting for different degrees of virulence. It is unlikely that a single vaccine will be applicable to all regions of the world. In this regard, in addition to HIV-1 subtype B, the predominant subtype in the United States, HIV-1 subtypes A, AE, AG, C, D, and O have been detected in individuals in the United States, as might be expected given the degree of international travel that occurs.

Table 173-3 provides the statistics and demographic features of HIV/AIDS in different regions of the world. Although the epidemic was first recognized in the United States and shortly thereafter in western Europe, it very likely began in sub-Saharan Africa (see above), which has been particularly devastated by the epidemic, with the prevalance of infection in many cities in the double digits. In certain sub-Saharan African countries, such as Zimbabwe and Botswana, available seroprevalence data indicate >30% of the adult population aged 15 to 49 is HIV-infected. In addition, among high-risk individuals (e.g., commercial sex workers, patients attending STD clinics) who live in urban areas of sub-Saharan Africa, seroprevalence is now >50% in many countries. According to projections of the United Nations Pop-

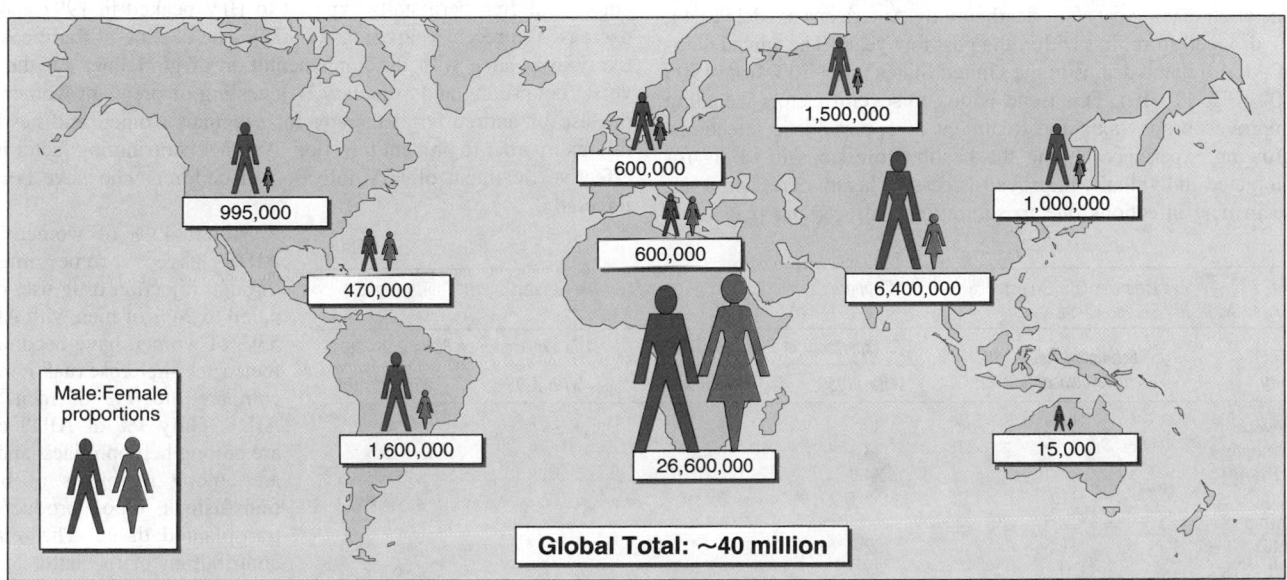

FIGURE 173-9   Estimated number of adults and children living with HIV infection as of December, 2003. (*From Joint United Nations Programme on HIV/AIDS.*)

TABLE 173-3 *Regional HIV/AIDS Statistics and Features, December, 2003*

Region	Epidemic Started	Adults and Children Living with HIV/AIDS	Adults and Children Newly Infected with HIV in 2003	Adult Prevalence Rate[a]	Adults and Child Deaths due to AIDS in 2003
Sub-Saharan Africa	Late '70s–Early '80s	26.6 million	3.2 million	8.0%	2.3 million
North Africa & Middle East	Late '80s	600,000	55,000	0.3%	42,500
South & Southeast Asia	Late '80s	6.4 million	855,000	0.6%	460,000
East Asia & Pacific	Late '80s	1.0 million	210,000	0.1%	45,000
Latin America	Late '70s–Early '80s	1.6 million	150,000	0.6%	59,500
Caribbean	Late '70s–Early '80s	470,000	62,500	2.5%	40,000
Eastern Europe & Central Asia	Early '90s	1.5 million	230,000	0.7%	30,000
Western Europe	Late '70s–Early '80s	600,000	35,000	0.3%	3,000
North America	Late '70s–Early '80s	995,000	45,000	0.6%	15,000
Australia & New Zealand	Late '70s–Early '80s	15,000	850	0.1%	<100
Total		**40 million**	**5 million**	**1.1%**	**3 million**

[a] The estimated proportion of adults (15–49 years) living with HIV/AIDS in December 2003.

Source: Joint United Nations Programme on HIV/AIDS (UNAIDS).

ulation Division, by the year 2015 life expectancy at birth in the seven countries in Africa with adult HIV prevalence rates >20% will be 32 years lower on average than the projected life expectancy in the absence of AIDS (Table 173-4). The epidemic in Asian countries, particularly India and China, has lagged temporally behind that in Africa; however, the number of new cases in this region is accelerating rapidly, and the magnitude of the epidemic is projected to exceed that of sub-Saharan Africa in the early part of the twenty-first century. The epidemic is also expanding rapidly in the Baltic States, the Russian Federation, and several Central Asian Republics. The major mode of transmission of HIV worldwide is unquestionably heterosexual sex; this is particularly true and has been so since the beginning of the epidemic in developing countries, where the numbers of infected men and women are approximately equal. The epidemic in most developed countries was first introduced among homosexual men and, to a greater or lesser degree (depending on the individual country), among IDUs. In this regard, the total numbers of AIDS cases in those countries still reflect a high proportion of cases among these high-risk groups. However, in most developed countries, including the United States (see below), there has been a gradual shift such that among new cases of AIDS, there is a greater total prevalence among heterosexuals and IDUs than among homosexual men.

AIDS IN THE UNITED STATES AIDS has had and will continue to have an extraordinary public health impact in the United States. As of January 1, 2003, an estimated 886,575 cumulative cases of AIDS had been diagnosed in adults and adolescents in the United States (Table 173-5) and ~502,000 AIDS-related deaths had occurred. In 2002, AIDS was the sixth leading cause of death among Americans aged 25 to 44, having dropped from first within the past few years. The annual number of AIDS-related deaths in the United States fell ~70% from 1995 to 2002 (Fig. 173-10). This trend is due to several factors including the improved prophylaxis and treatment of opportunistic infections, the growing experience among the health professions in caring for HIV-infected individuals, improved access to health care, and a decrease in new infections due to saturational effects and prevention

efforts. However, the most influential factor clearly has been the increased use of potent antiretroviral drugs, generally administered in a combination of three or four agents (see below). When one looks at the totality of data collected from the beginning of the epidemic, ~47% of all cases are among men who have had sex with men. However, since the mid-1980s the proportion of newly reported cases of AIDS in this population has declined from 65% of cases diagnosed in 1985 to 40% of cases diagnosed in 2002. Meanwhile, the proportion of new AIDS cases attributed to heterosexual contact has increased dramatically, from 3% in 1985 to 29% in 2002 (Fig. 173-8). Women are increasingly affected; the proportion of AIDS cases in the United States reported among adult and adolescent females has increased from <5% to 26% from 1985 to 2002 (Fig. 173-8). Most cases of transmission by injection drug use and heterosexual contact are reported from the northeast and southeast regions of the country, particularly among minorities. HIV infection and AIDS have disproportionately affected minority populations in the United States. The estimated rates of AIDS diagnoses per 100,000 population among adults and adolescents in 2002 were 76.4 for African Americans, 26.0 for Hispanics, 7.0 for whites, 11.2 for American Indians/Alaska Natives, and 4.9 for Asian/Pacific Islanders (Fig. 173-11).

As of January 1, 2003, an estimated 9,300 cases of AIDS in children ≤13 years old had been diagnosed, and ~55% of these children have died. Approximately 90% of these children were born to mothers who were HIV-infected or who were at risk for HIV infection and, in ~60% of those cases, the mother was either an IDU or the heterosexual partner of an IDU. The estimated number of AIDS cases diagnosed among children perinatally exposed to HIV peaked in 1992 and has decreased in recent years (Fig. 173-12). The decline of these cases is likely associated with the implementation of guidelines for the universal counseling and voluntary HIV testing of pregnant women and the use of antiretroviral therapy for pregnant women and newborn infants in order to prevent infection. Another contributing factor is the effective treatment of HIV infection in children who have become infected.

About 43% of women with AIDS have become infected through injection drug use, compared to 24% of men with AIDS; 53% of women have become infected by heterosexual contact, compared to 7% of men with AIDS. Only 1% of AIDS cases are among hemophiliacs, and 1% are among recipients of blood transfusions, blood products, or transplanted tissue. The relative contribution of the latter groups will gradually decrease, even though individuals infected pre-

Country	Estimated Adult HIV Seroprevalence, % 2002[a]	Life Expectancy at Birth, 2000–2005		Life Expectancy at Birth, 2010–2015	
		With AIDS	Without AIDS	With AIDS	Without AIDS
Botswana	38.8	39.7	68.1	31.6	70.7
Zimbabwe	33.7	33.1	67.6	31.8	70.5
Swaziland	33.4	34.4	62.2	30.3	66.3
Lesotho	31.0	35.1	59.0	32.2	63.0
Namibia	22.5	44.3	65.4	39.6	78.9
Zambia	21.5	32.4	53.4	35.3	57.4
South Africa	20.1	47.7	66.6	41.5	69.9

[a] Individuals ages 15–49.

Source: United Nations: *World Population Prospects: The 2002 Revision*; UNAIDS.

TABLE 173-5 *Estimated Numbers of AIDS Diagnoses, 2002 and Cumulative Through 2002, by Age at Diagnosis, Race/Ethnicity, and Exposure Category, United States*

	2002	Cumulative 1981–2002
Age at diagnosis (yrs)		
<13	92	9300
13–14	76	839
15–24	1833	35,460
25–34	9688	301,278
35–44	17,398	347,860
45–54	9488	138,386
55–64	2773	40,584
≥65	789	12,868
Race/ethnicity		
White, not Hispanic	11,929	364,458
Black, not Hispanic	21,169	347,491
Hispanic	8242	163,940
Asian/Pacific Islander	478	6924
American Indian/Alaska Native	206	2875
Exposure category		
Male adult or adolescent (≥13 years)		
Male-to-male sexual contact	16,944	420,790
Injection drug use	6945	172,351
Male-to-male sexual contact and injection drug use	1898	59,719
Heterosexual contact	4937	50,793
Other[a]	365	14,350
Subtotal	31,089	718,002
Female adult or adolescent (≥13 years)		
Injection drug use	3180	67,917
Heterosexual contact	7476	84,835
Other[a]	299	6519
Subtotal	10,955	159,271
Child (<13 years)		
Perinatal	90	8629
Other[b]	2	671
Subtotal	92	9300
Total[c]	42,136	886,575

[a] Includes hemophilia, blood transfusion, perinatal transmission, and risk not reported or identified.
[b] Includes hemophilia, blood transfusion, and risk not reported or identified.
[c] Cumulative total includes 887 persons of unknown or multiple race and 2 persons of unknown sex.
Source: Centers for Disease Control and Prevention, 2003.

viously through this mode of transmission will continue to develop AIDS. The risk of additional infections via this mode of transmission in the United States is extremely small (see above). In recent years, the incidence of AIDS has decreased considerably, with ~42,000 new cases in 2002 compared to ~60,000 in 1996 (Fig. 173-10). This trend likely reflects both reduced infection rates since the mid-1980s; more widespread use of prophylactic therapies, which delay the onset of AIDS; and the use of highly effective antiretroviral therapy early in

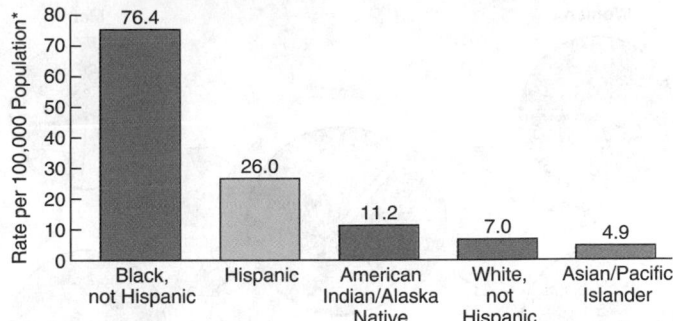

FIGURE 173-11 Rates of adult/adolescent AIDS cases per 100,000 population diagnosed in 2001 in various racial/ethnic groups in the United States. (*From Centers for Disease Control and Prevention, 2003.*)

the course of HIV infection (see below). Also, the demography of newly infected individuals has changed considerably since the mid-1980s (see below).

HIV PREVALENCE AND INCIDENCE IN THE UNITED STATES It is estimated that between 850,000 and 950,000 adults and adolescents in the United States are living with HIV infection, one-quarter of whom are unaware of their infection. This estimate results in an overall nationwide prevalence of HIV infection of ~0.3%. Prevalence is highest among young adults in their late twenties and thirties and among minorities. An estimated 3% of black men and 1% of black women in their thirties are living with HIV infection. The number of new infections per year is estimated to be ~40,000, and this number has remained stable for more than a decade. The estimated proportion of HIV infections has declined among white males, especially those >30, while the proportion of new HIV infections appears to have increased among young homosexual men and heterosexual women, especially in minority groups. Among newly infected persons in the United States, ~70% are men and ~30% are women (Fig. 173-13). Of these newly infected individuals, half are <25 years. Of new infections among men, the CDC estimates that ~60% were infected through homosexual sex, 25% through injection drug use, and 15% through heterosexual sex. Of new infections among women, ~75% were infected through heterosexual sex and 25% through injection drug use.

HIV infection and AIDS are widespread in the United States; although the epidemic on the whole is plateauing, it is spreading rapidly among certain populations, stabilizing in others, and decreasing in others. Similar to other STDs, HIV infection will not spread homogeneously throughout the population of the United States. However, it is clear that anyone who practices high-risk behavior is at risk for HIV infection. In addition, the increase in infections and AIDS cases among young homosexual men, heterosexuals (particularly sexual partners of IDUs, women, and adolescents) as well as the spread in

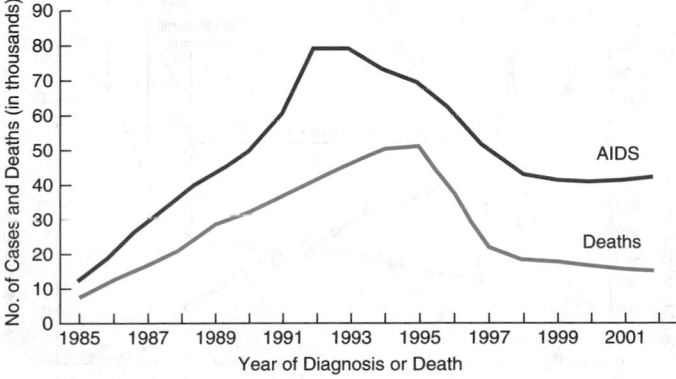

FIGURE 173-10 Estimated incidence of AIDS and deaths of adults and adolescents with AIDS, 1985–2002, United States. (*From the Centers for Diseases Control and Prevention, 2003.*)

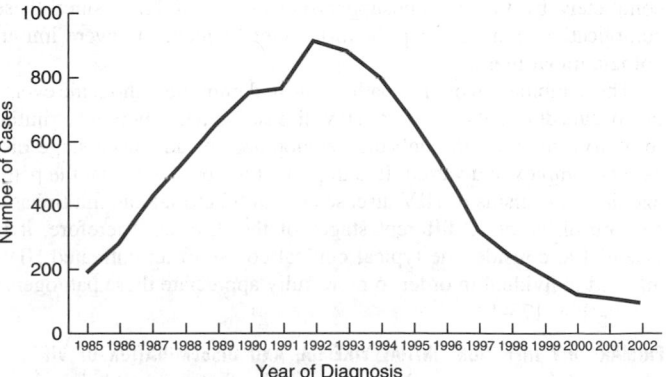

FIGURE 173-12 Perinatally acquired AIDS cases by year of diagnosis, 1985–2002, United States. (*From the Centers for Disease Control and Prevention, 2003.*)

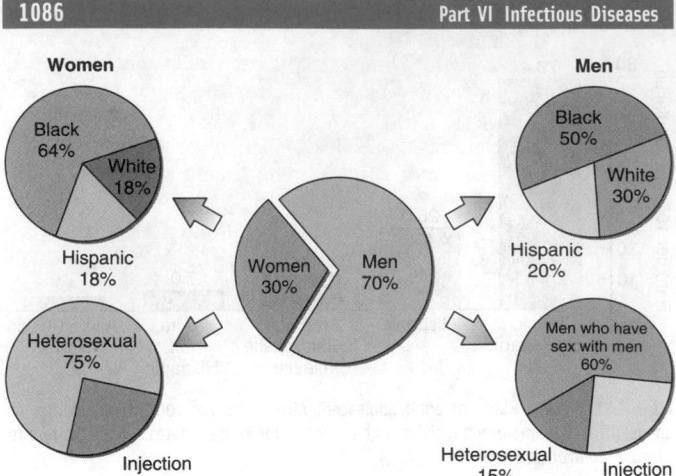

Women

Black 64%
White 18%
Hispanic 18%

Heterosexual 75%
Injection drug user 25%

Women 30%   Men 70%

Men

Black 50%
White 30%
Hispanic 20%

Men who have sex with men 60%
Heterosexual 15%
Injection drug user 25%

FIGURE 173-13   Estimated new HIV infections annually by race and risk in the United States. (*From the Centers for Disease Control and Prevention.*)

pockets of poverty in both urban and rural regions (particularly among underserved minority populations with inadequate access to health care) testifies to the fact that the epidemic of HIV infection in the United States is a public health problem of major proportions.

PATHOPHYSIOLOGY AND PATHOGENESIS

The hallmark of HIV disease is a profound immunodeficiency resulting primarily from a progressive quantitative and qualitative deficiency of the subset of T lymphocytes referred to as *helper T cells*, or *inducer T cells*. This subset of T cells is defined phenotypically by the presence on its surface of the CD4 molecule (Chap. 295), which serves as the primary cellular receptor for HIV. A co-receptor must also be present together with CD4 for efficient fusion and entry of HIV-1 into its target cells (Figs. 173-3 and 173-4). HIV uses two major co-receptors for fusion and entry; these co-receptors are also the primary receptors for certain chemoattractive cytokines termed *chemokines* and belong to the seven-transmembrane-domain G protein–coupled family of receptors. CCR5 and CXCR4 are the major co-receptors used by HIV (see above and below). Although a number of mechanisms responsible for cytopathicity and immune dysfunction of CD4+ T cells have been demonstrated in vitro, particularly direct infection and destruction of these cells by HIV and activation-induced cell death (see below), it remains unclear which mechanisms or combination of mechanisms are primarily responsible for their progressive depletion and functional impairment in vivo. When the number of CD4+ T cells declines below a certain level (see below), the patient is at high risk of developing a variety of opportunistic diseases, particularly the infections and neoplasms that are AIDS-defining illnesses. Some features of AIDS, such as KS and neurologic abnormalities (see below), cannot be explained completely by the immunosuppressive effects of HIV, since these complications may occur prior to the development of severe immunologic impairment.

The combination of viral pathogenic and immunopathogenic events that occurs during the course of HIV disease from the moment of initial (primary) infection through the development of advanced-stage disease is complex and varied. It is important to appreciate that the pathogenic mechanisms of HIV disease are multifactorial and multiphasic and are different at different stages of the disease. Therefore, it is essential to consider the typical clinical course of an untreated HIV-infected individual in order to more fully appreciate these pathogenic events (Fig. 173-14).

PRIMARY HIV INFECTION, INITIAL VIREMIA, AND DISSEMINATION OF VIRUS

The events associated with primary HIV infection are likely critical determinants of the subsequent course of HIV disease. In particular, the dissemination of virus to lymphoid organs is a major factor in the

establishment of a chronic and persistent infection (see below). The initial infection of susceptible cells may vary somewhat with the route of infection. Virus that enters directly into the bloodstream via infected blood or blood products (i.e., transfusions, use of contaminated needles for injecting drugs, sharp-object injuries, maternal-to-fetal transmission either intrapartum or perinatally, or sexual intercourse where there is enough trauma to cause bleeding) is likely cleared from the circulation to the spleen and other lymphoid organs, where it replicates to a critical level and then leads to a burst of viremia that disseminates virus throughout the body. Dendritic cells play an important role in the initiation of HIV infection. These cells express a diversity of C-type lectin receptors on their surface, one of which is called *DC-SIGN* (see above). DC-SIGN binds with high affinity to the HIV envelope gp120 and can retain infectious particles for days in vitro. Certain studies have demonstrated that following binding to DC-SIGN, HIV is internalized into a low pH nonlysosomal compartment that allows for the retention of infectivity. Upon encountering a susceptible CD4+ T cell target, the dendritic cell markedly enhances the infectivity of the virus for the target cell. This mechanism likely operates in humans when HIV enters "locally" (as opposed to directly into the blood) and encounters mucosal dendritic cells via the vagina, rectum, or urethra during intercourse or via the upper gastrointestinal tract from swallowed infected semen, vaginal fluid, or breast milk. In primary HIV infection, virus replication in CD4+ T cells intensifies prior to the initiation of an HIV-specific immune response (see below), leading to a burst of viremia (Fig. 173-14) and then to a rapid dissemination of virus to other lymphoid organs, the brain, and other tissues. Individuals who experience the "acute HIV syndrome," which occurs to varying degrees in ~50% of individuals with primary infection, have high levels of viremia measured in millions of copies of HIV RNA per milliliter that last for several weeks (see below). The acute mononucleosis-like symptoms are well correlated with the presence of viremia. Virtually all patients appear to develop some degree of viremia during primary infection, which contributes to virus dissemination throughout the lymphoid tissue, even though they may remain asymptomatic or not recall experiencing symptoms. A more detailed description of the role of lymphoid tissue in the immunopathogenesis of HIV disease is given below. It appears that the initial level of plasma viremia in primary HIV infection does not necessarily determine the rate of disease progression; however, the set point of the level of steady-state plasma viremia after ~1 year does seem to correlate with the rapidity of disease progression (see below).

ESTABLISHMENT OF CHRONIC AND PERSISTENT INFECTION ■ **Persistent Virus Replication**   HIV infection is unique among human viral infections. Despite the robust cellular and humoral immune responses that are mounted following primary infection (see below), once infection has been established the virus succeeds in escaping immune-mediated

FIGURE 173-14   Typical course of an HIV-infected individual. See text for detailed description. (*From A Fauci et al: Ann Intern Med 124:654, 1996.*)

clearance (see below) and is virtually never eliminated completely from the body. Rather, a chronic infection develops that persists with varying degrees of virus replication in the untreated patient for a median of ~10 years before the patient becomes clinically ill (see below). It is this establishment of a chronic, persistent infection that is the hallmark of HIV disease. Throughout the often protracted course of chronic infection, virus replication can almost invariably be detected in untreated patients, both by highly sensitive assays for plasma viremia as well as by demonstration of cell-associated HIV RNA in immunocompetent cells (predominantly CD4+ T cells and macrophages) in the circulation and in lymphoid tissue. In other human viral infections, with very few exceptions, if the host survives, the virus is completely cleared from the body and a state of immunity against subsequent infection develops. HIV infection very rarely kills the host during primary infection. Certain viruses, such as HSV (Chap. 163), are not completely cleared from the body after infection but instead enter a latent state; in these cases, clinical latency is accompanied by microbiologic latency. This is not the case with HIV infection, in which some degree of virus replication invariably occurs during the period of clinical latency (see below). Chronicity associated with persistent virus replication can also be seen in certain cases of HBV and HCV infections (Chap. 287); however, in these infections the immune system is not a target of the virus.

Evasion of Immune System Control   Inherent to the establishment of chronicity of HIV infection is the ability of the virus to evade elimination and control by the immune system. There are a number of mechanisms whereby the virus accomplishes this evasion. Paramount among these is the ability of the virus to mutate, which becomes particularly relevant after the establishment of chronic infection and which contributes to the maintenance of chronicity. The evolution of mutants that escape control by CD8+ cytolytic T lymphocytes (CTLs) is critical to the propagation and progression of HIV infection. The high rate of virus replication and the continual mutation of virus also contribute to the inability of neutralizing antibody to contain the virus quasispecies present in an individual at any given time. Molecular analysis of clonotypes has demonstrated that clones of CD8+ CTLs that expand greatly during primary HIV infection, and likely represent the high-affinity clones that would be expected to be most efficient in eliminating virus-infected cells, are no longer detectable after their initial burst of expansion. It is thought that the initially expanded clones may have been deleted owing to the overwhelming exposure to viral antigens during the initial burst of viremia, similar to the exhaustion of CD8+ CTLs that has been reported in the murine model of lymphocytic choriomeningitis virus (LCMV) infection. To compound this phenomenon, virus replication and thus saturation of antigen-presenting cells with viral antigen take place in the lymphoid tissue (see below), which is also the site of generation of HIV-specific CTLs. Another mechanism of evasion by HIV of immune system control is the downregulation of HLA class I molecules on the surface of HIV-infected cells by the Nef protein of HIV, resulting in the lack of ability of the CD8+ CTL to recognize and kill the infected target cell. Although this downregulation of HLA class I molecules would favor elimination of HIV-infected cells by natural killer (NK) cells, this latter mechanism does not seem to effectively remove HIV-infected cells (see below). An important mechanism of evasion of the humoral immune response is the avoidance by the virus of antibody-mediated neutralization through its conformational masking of receptor-binding sites.

CD4+ T cell help is critical for the integrity of antigen-specific immune responses, both humoral and cell-mediated. HIV preferentially infects HIV-specific CD4+ T cells, and so this loss of viral-specific helper T cell responses has potentially profound negative consequences for the immunologic control of HIV replication. Other means of escape of HIV-infected cells from elimination by CD8+ CTLs are the sequestration of infected cells in immunologically privileged sites such as the central nervous system (CNS) as well as the segregation of HIV-specific CTLs and CTL precursors in the periph-

eral blood where relatively little active virus replication takes place, rather than in the lymphoid tissue, which is the major site of virus replication and spread.

Finally, the escape of HIV from elimination during primary infection allows the formation of a large pool of latently infected cells that cannot be eliminated by virus-specific CTLs (see below). Thus, despite a potent immune response and the marked downregulation of virus replication following primary HIV infection, HIV succeeds in establishing a state of chronic infection with a variable degree of persistent virus replication. In most cases, during this period the patient makes the clinical transition from acute primary infection to a relatively prolonged state of clinical latency (see below).

Latent Reservoir of HIV-Infected Cells: Obstacle to the Eradication of Virus
There exists in virtually all HIV-infected individuals a pool of latently infected, resting CD4+ T cells that serves as at least one component of the persistent reservoir of virus. Such cells manifest postintegration latency in that the HIV provirus integrates into the genome of the cell and can remain in this state until an activation signal drives the expression of HIV transcripts and ultimately replication-competent virus. This form of latency is to be distinguished from preintegration latency, in which HIV enters a resting CD4+ T cell and, in the absence of an activation signal, only a limited degree of reverse transcription of the HIV genome occurs. This period of preintegration latency may last hours to days, and if no activation signal is delivered to the cell, the proviral DNA loses its capacity to initiate a productive infection. If these cells do become activated, reverse transcription proceeds to completion and the virus continues along its replication cycle (see above and Fig. 173-15). The pool of cells that are in the postintegration state of latency is established early during the course of primary HIV infection. Despite the suppression of plasma viremia to <50 copies of

FIGURE 173-15   Generation of latently infected, resting CD4+ T cells in HIV-infected individuals. See text for details. Ag, antigen; CTLs, cytolytic T lymphocytes. (*Courtesy of TW Chun.*)

HIV RNA per milliliter by potent combinations of several antiretroviral drugs for as long as 5 years, this pool of latently infected cells persists and can give rise to replication-competent virus. Modeling studies built on projections of decay curves (see below) have estimated that in a setting of prolonged suppression of plasma viremia to <50 copies of HIV RNA per milliliter by antiretroviral therapy (a goal that is difficult to maintain consistently over years), it would require from 7 to 70 years for the pool of latently infected cells to be completely eliminated. Furthermore, the reservoir of latently infected cells is replenished during minor rebounds of virus replication that may occur intermittently, even in patients who for the most part are treated successfully, and certainly during major rebounds of viremia in patients whose therapy is interrupted for a period of weeks or longer. Thus, this persistent pool of latently infected cells is a major obstacle to any goal of eradication of virus from infected individuals, despite the favorable clinical outcomes that have resulted from antiretroviral therapy (see below).

Viral Dynamics The dynamics of viral production and turnover have been quantified using mathematical modeling in the setting of the administration of reverse transcriptase and protease inhibitors to HIV-infected individuals in clinical studies. Treatment with these drugs resulted in a precipitous decline in the level of plasma viremia, which typically fell by well over 90% within 2 weeks. The number of CD4+ T cells in the blood increased concurrently, which suggested that the killing of CD4+ T cells was linked directly to the levels of replicating virus. However, it is generally agreed that a significant component of the early rise in CD4+ T cell numbers following the initiation of therapy is due to the redistribution of cells into the peripheral blood from other body compartments as a consequence of alterations in immune system activation. It was determined on the basis of modeling the kinetics of viral decline and the emergence of resistant mutants during therapy that 93 to 99% of the circulating virus originated from recently infected, rapidly turning over CD4+ T cells and that ~1 to 7% of circulating virus originated from longer-lived cells, likely monocyte/macrophages. A negligible amount of circulating virus originated from the pool of latently infected cells (see above) (Fig. 173-16). It was also determined that the half-life of a circulating virion was approximately 30 to 60 min and that of productively infected cells was 1 day. Given the relatively steady level of plasma viremia and of infected cells, it appears that extremely large amounts of virus (~10^{10} to 10^{11} virions) are produced and cleared from the circulation each day. In addition, data suggest that the minimum duration of the HIV-1 replication cycle in vivo is ~2 days. Other studies have demonstrated that the decrease in plasma viremia that results from antiretroviral therapy correlates closely with a decrease in virus replication in lymph nodes, further confirming that lymphoid tissue is the main site of HIV replication and the main source of plasma viremia.

The level of steady-state viremia, called the viral *set point*, at ~1

year has important prognostic implications for the progression of HIV disease. It has been demonstrated that HIV-infected individuals who have a low set point at 6 months to 1 year progress to AIDS much more slowly than individuals whose set point is very high at that time (Fig. 173-17). Levels of viremia generally increase as disease progresses. Measurement of the level of viremia is critical in guiding therapeutic decisions in HIV-infected individuals (see below).

Clinical Latency versus Microbiologic Latency With the exception of long-term nonprogressors (see below), the level of CD4+ T cells in the blood decreases progressively in HIV-infected individuals. The slope of this decline is usually a good predictor of the pattern of the clinical course and the development of advanced disease. The decline in CD4+ T cells may be gradual or abrupt, the latter usually reflecting a significant spike in the level of plasma viremia. Most patients are entirely asymptomatic while this progressive decline is taking place (see below) and are often described as being in a state of *clinical latency*. However, this term is misleading; it does not mean disease latency, since progression is generally relentless during this period. Furthermore, clinical latency should not be confused with microbiologic latency, since virus replication manifested by low-level viremia is present in the vast majority of patients during the period of clinical latency. Even in those rare patients who have <50 copies of HIV RNA per milliliter in the absence of therapy, there is virtually always some degree of ongoing virus replication, as determined by sensitive molecular methods such as PCR techniques that detect cell-associated viral RNA or that concentrate virus from large volumes of blood.

ADVANCED HIV DISEASE In untreated patients or in patients in whom therapy has not adequately controlled virus replication (see below), after a variable period, usually measured in years, the CD4+ T cell count falls below a critical level (<200/μL) and the patient becomes highly susceptible to opportunistic disease (Fig. 173-14). For this reason, the CDC case definition of AIDS includes all HIV-infected individuals with CD4+ T cell counts below this level (Table 173-1). Patients may experience constitutional signs and symptoms or may develop an opportunistic disease abruptly without any prior symptoms, although the latter scenario is unusual. The depletion of CD4+ T cells continues to be progressive and unrelenting in this phase. It is not uncommon for CD4+ T cell counts to drop as low as 10/μL or even to zero, yet such patients may survive for months or even years. This situation has become increasingly common as patients are treated more aggressively and are given prophylaxis against the common life-threatening opportunistic infections (see below). In this regard, control of plasma viremia by antiretroviral therapy, even in individuals with extremely low CD4+ T cell counts, has increased survival in these patients despite the fact that their CD4+ T cell counts may not significantly increase as a result of therapy. Ultimately, patients who

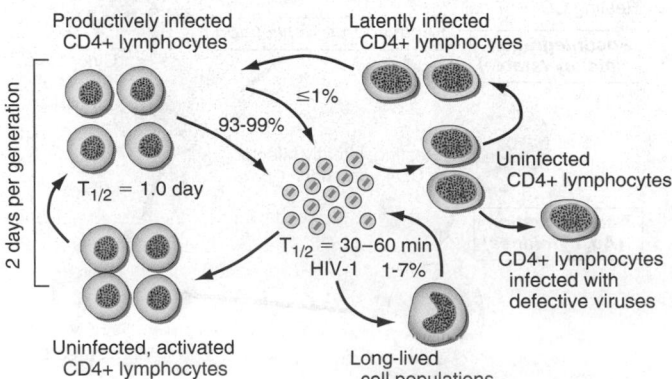

FIGURE 173-16 Dynamics of HIV infection in vivo. See text for detailed description. (*From AS Perelson et al: Science 271:1582, 1996.*)

FIGURE 173-17 Relationship between levels of virus and rates of disease progression. Kaplan-Meier curves for AIDS-free survival stratified by baseline HIV-1 RNA categories (copies per milliliter). (*From Mellors et al.*)

progress to this severest form of immunodeficiency usually succumb to opportunistic infections or neoplasms (see below).

LONG-TERM SURVIVORS AND LONG-TERM NONPROGRESSORS The prognosis for HIV-infected individuals who have access to health care and antiretroviral therapy has improved greatly since the beginning of the epidemic. The median time from primary HIV infection to the development of AIDS in untreated individuals in the developed world is ~10 years. This period has been markedly extended by the wide availability of combinations of antiretroviral drugs in the developed world; the full extent of this benefit has yet to be realized. It is important to distinguish between the terms *long-term survivor* and *long-term nonprogressor*. Long-term nonprogressors are by definition long-term survivors; however, the reverse is not always true. The definitions of these categories are empirical and continue to change as more data are collected from prospective cohort studies. Predictions from one study that antedated the availability of effective antiretroviral therapy estimated that ~13% of homosexual/bisexual men who were infected at an early age may remain free of clinical AIDS for >20 years. Originally, individuals were considered to be long-term survivors if they remained alive for 10 to 15 years after initial infection. Currently, individuals are considered to be long-term survivors if they remain alive for ≥20 years after initial infection. In most such individuals the disease has progressed, in that they have significant immunodeficiency, and many have experienced opportunistic diseases. Some of these individuals have CD4+ T cell counts that have decreased to ≤200/μL but have remained stable at that level for years. The mechanisms of this stabilization are not entirely clear but may relate to the beneficial effects of antiretroviral therapy and prophylaxis against opportunistic infections. In addition, a number of viral and/or host determinants likely contribute to the long-term survival of these individuals. Quantitative and qualitative aspects of the HIV-specific immune response, as well as recognized and unrecognized genetic factors (see below), may also contribute to the long-term survival of these individuals.

Definitions of long-term nonprogressors have varied considerably over the years, and so such individuals constitute a heterogeneous group. Originally, individuals considered to be long-term nonprogressors were those who had been infected with HIV for a long period (≥10 years), whose CD4+ T cell counts were in the normal range and remained stable over years, and who had not received antiretroviral therapy. Such patients had low, but usually detectable, levels of plasma viremia, generally normal immune function according to commonly measured parameters (skin tests, in vitro lymphocyte responses to various mitogens and antigens), and normal-appearing lymphoid tissue architecture as determined on lymph node biopsy. The definition rested more on the status of the immune system than on the absolute control of plasma viremia. In general, long-term nonprogressors manifested robust HIV-specific immune responses, both humoral (neutralizing antibodies) and cell-mediated (HIV-specific CTLs). However, this may also be true of some individuals early in the course of disease who ultimately progress to advanced disease. No qualitative abnormalities in the virus were detected in most of these patients. However, a small subset of patients did have defective virus; in particular, in one cohort of five long-term nonprogressors, the virus had a defect in the *nef* gene. In another report, a blood donor in Australia who was HIV-infected and a group of seven individuals who were infected by blood or blood products from that donor remained free of HIV-related disease and maintained normal and stable CD4+ T cell counts for several years after infection. Sequence analysis of viruses isolated from the donor and recipients revealed similar deletions in the *nef* gene and the region of overlap of *nef* and the U3 region of the HIV LTR (Fig. 173-5). The vast majority of these originally reported long-term nonprogressors have now gone on to progressive disease. More recently, cohorts of rare long-term nonprogressors have been described who have been infected for 20 years with normal CD4+ T cell counts and who typically maintain plasma viral RNA <50 copies per milliliter without antiretroviral therapy. When these more stringent definitions based

predominantly on levels of plasma viremia are applied, very strong associations with HLA B*5701 or HLA B*2705 alleles have been found. In addition, the HIV-specific CD8+ T cell response in these patients is highly focused on B5701-restricted peptides, suggesting that the B5701 molecule plays a direct role in restriction of virus replication in these individuals, although the precise mechanisms of this effect remain unclear.

A number of other host genetic factors exert more modest effects on restriction of HIV replication, yet they also may be associated with slower progression of disease (see "Genetic Factors in HIV Pathogenesis," below). The precise role of host factors in long-term nonprogression remains unclear. There is no obvious and consistent genetic determinant for nonprogression. However, several genetic mutations have been demonstrated to result in a delay in the progression of HIV disease. These include heterozygosity for the *CCR5-Δ32* deletion, heterozygosity for the *CCR2-64I* mutation, homozygosity for the *SDF1-3′A* mutation, and heterozygosity for the *RANTES*-28G mutation (see "Genetic Factors in HIV Pathogenesis," below). Since CCR5 is the major co-receptor for R5 or macrophage-tropic strains of HIV and since individuals who are homozygous for the *CCR5-Δ32* deletion are, with rare exceptions, protected against HIV infection, the potential mechanism for slow progression in heterozygotes is clear. In addition, certain single nucleotide polymorphisms in the *CCR5* promoter have been shown to be associated with slower progression of disease. The reason for the slowing of progression of HIV disease in individuals who are heterozygous for the *CCR2-64I* mutation is less clear; however, it has been demonstrated that CXCR4 can dimerize with the CCR2-64I mutant but not with wild-type CCR2. This dimerization may reduce the amount of CXCR4 on the cell surface and as a result inhibit infection with X4 viruses. Homozygosity for the *SDF1-3′A* mutation may upregulate the *SDF1* gene enabling SDF-1, which is the natural ligand for CXCR4, to compete more effectively with X4 or T cell tropic virus for the CXCR4 coreceptor. The *RANTES*-28G mutation increases RANTES expression, which is the natural ligand for CCR5 and may thus inhibit infection with R5 viruses. Finally, maximal HLA heterozygosity of class I loci (A, B, and C) has been shown to be associated with delayed progression of HIV disease. Although long-term nonprogressors have robust HIV-specific immune responses as well as competent CD8+ T cell suppressors of HIV replication, it is unclear whether these factors are directly responsible for the state of nonprogression. A substantial proportion of HIV-infected individuals manifest comparable immune responses early in the course of their disease and still experience disease progression. As noted above, long-term nonprogressors likely represent a heterogeneous group. The lack of disease progression may be explained in some by a defect in the virus; in others by any of a variety of host factors, including recognized and as yet unrecognized genetic factors; and in others by a combination of both.

LYMPHOID ORGANS AND HIV PATHOGENESIS Regardless of the portal of entry of HIV, lymphoid tissues are the major anatomic sites for the establishment and propagation of HIV infection (see above) Despite the use of measurements of plasma viremia to determine the level of disease activity, virus replication occurs mainly in lymphoid tissue and not in blood; indeed, the level of plasma viremia directly reflects virus production in lymphoid tissue.

Some patients experience progressive generalized lymphadenopathy (see below) early in the course of the infection; others experience varying degrees of transient lymphadenopathy. Lymphadenopathy reflects the cellular activation and immune response to the virus in the lymphoid tissue, which is generally characterized by follicular or germinal center hyperplasia. Lymphoid tissue involvement is a common denominator of virtually all patients with HIV infection, even those without easily detectable lymphadenopathy.

Simultaneous examinations of lymph tissue and peripheral blood in patients and monkeys during various stages of HIV and SIV infection, respectively, have led to substantial insight into the pathogenesis of HIV disease. Using a combination of PCR techniques for HIV DNA and HIV RNA in tissue and HIV RNA in plasma, in situ hybridization for HIV RNA, and light and electron microscopy, the following picture has emerged. During acute HIV infection, a high level of viral replication in individual cells is demonstrated in lymphoid tissue and is associated with a burst of plasma viremia. A profound degree of cellular activation occurs (see below) and is reflected in follicular or germinal center hyperplasia. At this time copious amounts of extracellular virions are trapped on the processes of the follicular dendritic cells (FDCs) in the germinal centers of the lymph nodes (Fig. 173-18A). Virions that have bound complement components on their surfaces attach to the surface of FDCs via interactions with complement receptors and likely via Fc receptors that bind to antibodies that are attached to the virions. In situ hybridization reveals expression of virus in individual cells of the paracortical area and, to a lesser extent, the germinal center (Fig. 173-18B). The persistence of trapped virus after the transition from acute to chronic infection likely reflects a steady state whereby trapped virus turns over and is replaced by fresh virions, which are continually produced to a greater or lesser degree in individual patients.

During early-stage HIV disease, the architecture of the germinal centers is generally preserved and may even be hyperplastic owing to in situ proliferation of cells (mostly B lymphocytes) and recruitment to the lymph nodes of a number of cell types (B cells, CD4+ and CD8+ T cells). Electron microscopy demonstrates a fine network of FDCs with many long, finger-like processes that envelop virtually every lymphocyte in the germinal center (Fig. 173-18C). Extracellular virions can be seen attached to the processes, yet the FDCs appear to be relatively healthy. The trapping of antigen is a physiologically normal function for the FDCs, which present antigen to B cells and contribute to the generation of B cell memory. However, in the case of HIV, the trapped virions serve as a persistent source of cellular activation, resulting in the secretion of proinflammatory cytokines such as interleukin (IL) 1β, tumor necrosis factor (TNF) α, and IL-6, which can upregulate virus replication in infected cells (see below). Furthermore, although trapped virus is coated by neutralizing antibodies, it has been demonstrated that these virions remain infectious for CD4+ T cells while attached to the processes of the FDCs. CD4+ T cells that migrate into the germinal center to provide help to B cells in the generation of an HIV-specific immune response are susceptible to infection by these trapped virions. Thus, in HIV infection, a normal physiologic function of the immune system, which contributes to the clearance of virus as well as to the generation of a specific immune response, can also have deleterious consequences. It is difficult to demonstrate infection of the FDCs at this point, or even in advanced disease; however, rare examples of virus budding off FDCs have been reported.

As the disease progresses, the architecture of the germinal centers begins to show disruption, and the trapping efficiency of the lymph node diminishes. Electron microscopy reveals swollen organelles, and the FDCs begin to undergo cell death. The mechanisms of FDC death remain unclear; there is no indication by electron microscopy of copious virus replication or budding of virions off the cell in great quantities. As the disease progresses to an advanced stage, there is complete disruption of the architecture of the germinal centers, accompanied by

FIGURE 173-18 HIV in the lymph nodes of HIV-infected individuals. *A.* Cervical lymph node from an asymptomatic individual with very low levels of plasma viremia. In situ hybridization using a molecular probe for HIV RNA reveals copious virus demarcating the numerous germinal centers (bright areas) of the node. The virus was extracellular and bound to the processes of the follicular dendritic cells (FDCs), which form a matrix within the confines of the germinal centers. Original ×25. *B.* Individual cells infected with HIV. Two cells in the paracortical area of the lymph node are shown expressing HIV RNA by in situ hybridization using a radiolabeled molecular probe. Original ×250. *C.* FDCs in cervical node of an asymptomatic HIV-infected individual. Electron microscopy reveals an FDC with a prominent nucleolus surrounded by several lymphocytes within the germinal center of the node. Higher magnification of several fields indicates that multiple processes of the FDCs are in contact with several lymphocytes. Original ×1920. *D.* Dissolution of FDCs in the germinal center of a cervical lymph node from a patient with advanced HIV disease. Widespread death of FDCs is associated with a loss of ability of the lymph node to trap virus late in the course of HIV disease. Original ×3744. (*A and B courtesy of Dr. Cecil Fox; C and D courtesy of Dr. Jan Orenstein. Adapted from G Pantaleo et al: N Engl J Med 328:327, 1993.*)

dissolution of the FDC network and massive dropout of FDCs (Fig. 173-18*D*). At this point, the lymph nodes are "burnt out." This destruction of lymphoid tissue compounds the immunodeficiency of HIV disease and contributes both to the inability to control HIV replication (leading usually to high levels of plasma viremia in the untreated or inadequately treated patient) and to the inability to mount adequate immune responses against opportunistic pathogens. The events from primary infection to the ultimate destruction of the immune system are illustrated in Fig. 173-19.

CELLULAR ACTIVATION AND HIV PATHOGENESIS

Activation of the immune system is an essential component of an appropriate immune response to a foreign antigen. The immune system is normally in a state of homeostasis, awaiting perturbation by foreign antigenic stimuli. Once the immune response deals with and clears the antigen, the system returns to relative quiescence (Chap. 295). In HIV infection, however, the immune system is chronically activated owing to the persistence of virus replication throughout the course of HIV disease, particularly in the untreated patient (see above) and to variable degrees even in certain patients receiving antiretroviral therapy whose level of plasma viremia is suppressed to below the level of detection by standard assays (see below). Aberrant immune activation is the hallmark of HIV infection and is a critical component of the pathogenesis of HIV disease. This activated state is reflected by hyperactivation of B cells leading to hypergammaglobulinemia; spontaneous lymphocyte proliferation; activation of monocytes; expression of activation markers on CD4+ and CD8+ T cells; lymph node hyperplasia, particularly early in the course of disease (see above); increased secretion of proinflammatory cytokines (see below); elevated levels of neopterin, β_2-microglobulin, acid-labile interferon, and soluble IL-2 receptors; and autoimmune phenomena (see below). Even in the absence of direct infection of a target cell, HIV envelope proteins can interact with cellular receptors (CD4 molecules and chemokine receptors) to deliver potent activation signals resulting in calcium flux, the phosphorylation of certain proteins involved in signal transduction, co-localization of cytoplasmic proteins including those involved in cell trafficking, immune dysfunction, and under certain circumstances, apoptosis (see below). The secretion of certain proinflammatory and immunoregulatory cytokines is both a consequence of the aberrant immune activation associated with HIV infection and a mechanism of propagation of the process of aberrant cellular activation (see below).

In addition to endogenous factors such as cytokines, a number of exogenous factors such as other microbes that are associated with heightened cellular activation can enhance HIV replication and thus may have important effects on HIV pathogenesis. Co-infection or simultaneous cotransfection of cells with HIV and other viruses or viral genes has demonstrated that certain viruses, such as HSV type 1, cytomegalovirus (CMV), human herpesvirus (HHV) 6, Epstein-Barr virus (EBV), HBV, adenovirus, pseudorabies virus, and HTLV-I can upregulate HIV expression. Other microbes, such as *Mycoplasma*, have been reported to contribute to the induction of HIV expression. In addition, infestation with nematodes has been shown to be associated with a heightened state of immune activaton that facilitates HIV replication; de-worming of the infected host results in a decrease in plasma viremia. *Mycobacterium tuberculosis* is a common opportunistic infection in HIV-infected individuals (see below and Chap. 150). In addition to the fact that HIV-infected individuals are more likely to develop active tuberculosis (TB) after exposure, it has been demonstrated that active TB can accelerate the course of HIV infection. It has also been shown that levels of plasma viremia are greatly elevated in HIV-infected individuals with active TB, compared to pre-TB levels

FIGURE 173-19 Events that transpire from primary HIV infection through the establishment of chronic persistent infection to the ultimate destruction of the immune system. See text for details; CTLs, cytolytic T lymphocytes.

and levels of viremia after successful treatment of the active TB. In vitro studies demonstrated that virus replication was markedly enhanced in lymphocytes of HIV-infected individuals who were skin test–positive for purified protein derivative (PPD) when PPD antigen was added to culture, resulting in cellular activation. Confirmatory evidence that antigen-induced activation was a major contributor to the accelerated viremia in HIV-infected individuals with active TB was provided by studies in which HIV-infected individuals were immunized with common recall antigens such as tetanus toxoid, influenza, or pneumococcal polysaccharide. Under these circumstances, a transient elevation of plasma viremia accompanied the cellular activation induced by the immunization. A greater degree of induction of virus was seen in those individuals with early-stage as opposed to advanced stage HIV disease, and the degree of virus induction correlated with the level of immune system activation.

Persistent immune activation may have several deleterious consequences. From a virologic standpoint, although quiescent CD4+ T cells can be infected with HIV, reverse transcription, integration, and virus spread are much more efficient in activated cells. Furthermore, cellular activation induces expression of virus in cells latently infected with HIV (see above). From an immunologic standpoint, chronic exposure of the immune system to a particular antigen over an extended period may ultimately lead to an inability to sustain an adequate immune response to the antigen in question. Furthermore, the ability of the immune system to respond to a broad spectrum of antigens may be compromised if immunocompetent cells are maintained in a state of chronic activation. In addition, activation of the immune system may favor the elimination of cells via programmed cell death (apoptosis) (see below) as well as the secretion of certain cytokines that can induce HIV expression (see below).

Apoptosis *Apoptosis* is a form of programmed cell death that is a normal mechanism for the elimination of effete cells in organogenesis as well as in the cellular proliferation that occurs during a normal immune response (Chap. 295). Apoptosis is strictly dependent on cellular activation, and the aberrant cellular activation associated with HIV disease (see above) is correlated with a heightened state of apoptosis. It has been hypothesized that, in HIV infection, sequential activation signals delivered to CD4+ T cells induce apoptosis. Cross-linking of the CD4 molecule by gp120 or gp120/anti-gp120 complexes delivers the first of two signals required for apoptosis. The second signal supposedly leading to cell death is delivered via the T cell receptor by antigen. According to this hypothesis, direct infection of CD4+ T cells is not required for apoptosis to occur, although it has been demonstrated that alterations in tyrosine kinase activity of HIV-infected cells may induce the cell to undergo apoptosis. HIV can trigger both Fas-dependent and Fas-independent pathways of apoptosis. Mechanisms involved in this process include upregulation of Fas and Fas ligand, upregulation of caspase-1 and caspase-6, downregulation of the anti-apoptotic Bcl-2 protein, and activation of cyclin-dependent kinases. Certain viral gene products have been associated with enhanced susceptibility to apoptosis including Envelope, Tat, and Vpr. In contrast, Nef has been shown to possess antiapoptotic properties. A number of studies, including those examining lymphoid tissue, have demonstrated that the rate of apoptosis is elevated in HIV infection and that apoptosis is seen in "bystander" cells such as CD8+ T cells and B cells as well as in CD4+ T cells. The intensity of apoptosis correlates with the general state of activation of the immune system and not with the stage of disease or with viral burden. The potential role of apoptosis in the pathogenesis of HIV disease is underscored by results from animal studies that show an increased frequency of apoptosis in CD4+ T cells in primates infected with pathogenic strains of SIV but not in primates infected with nonpathogenic strains of SIV. It is likely that apoptosis of immunocompetent cells contributes to the immune abnormalities in HIV disease; however, this is probably a nonspecific mechanism that merely reflects the aberrant state of immune activation.

Autoimmune Phenomena   The autoimmune phenomena that are common in HIV-infected individuals reflect, at least in part, chronic immune system activation as well as molecular mimickry by viral components. Although these phenomena usually occur in the absence of autoimmune disease, a wide spectrum of clinical manifestations that may be associated with autoimmunity have been described (see below). Autoimmune phenomena include antibodies to lymphocytes and, less commonly, to platelets and neutrophils. Antiplatelet antibodies have some clinical relevance, in that they may contribute to the thrombocytopenia of HIV disease (see below). Antibodies to nuclear and cytoplasmic components of cells have been reported, as have antibodies to cardiolipin; CD4 molecules; CD43 molecules, C1q-A; variable regions of the T cell receptor α, β, and γ chains; Fas; denatured collagen; and IL-2. In addition, autoantibodies to a range of serum proteins, including albumin, immunoglobulin, and thyroglobulin, have been reported. There is antigenic cross-reactivity between HIV viral proteins (gp120 and gp41) and MHC class II determinants, and anti-MHC class II antibodies have been reported in HIV infection. These antibodies could potentially lead to the elimination of MHC class II–bearing cells via antibody-dependent cellular cytotoxicity (ADCC) (Chap. 295). In addition, regions of homology exist between HIV envelope glycoproteins and IL-2 as well as MHC class I molecules.

THE CYTOKINE NETWORK IN HIV PATHOGENESIS   The immune system is homeostatically regulated by a complex network of immunoregulatory cytokines, which are pleiotropic and redundant and operate in an autocrine and paracrine manner. They are expressed continuously, even during periods of apparent quiescence of the immune system. On perturbation of the immune system by antigenic challenge, the expression of cytokines increases to varying degrees (Chap. 295). Cytokines that are important components of this immunoregulatory network have been demonstrated to play a major role in the regulation of HIV expression in vitro. Potent modulation of HIV expression has been demonstrated either by manipulating endogenous cytokines or by adding exogenous cytokines to culture. Cytokines that induce HIV expression in one or more of these systems include IL-1, IL-2, IL-3, IL-6, IL-12, TNF-α, TNF-β, macrophage colony-stimulating factor (M-CSF), and granulocyte-macrophage colony-stimulating factor (GM-CSF). Among these cytokines, the most consistent and potent inducers of HIV expression are the *proinflammatory cytokines* TNF-α, IL-1β, and IL-6. Interferon (IFN)-α and -β suppress HIV replication, whereas transforming growth factor (TGF) β, IL-4, IL-10, and IFN-γ can either induce or suppress HIV expression, depending on the system involved. The *CC-chemokines* RANTES, macrophage inflammatory protein (MIP) 1α, and MIP-1β (Chap. 295) inhibit infection by and spread of R5 (macrophage-tropic) HIV-1 strains, while *stromal cell–derived factor* (SDF) 1 inhibits infection by and spread of X4 (T cell–tropic) strains (see below). The alpha defensin family of cytokines has been

shown to inhibit both R5 and X4 viruses, and other soluble factors that have not yet been fully characeized have also been shown to suppress HIV replication. Blocking of endogenous HIV-inducing cytokines or addition of inhibitors of HIV suppressor cytokines in cultures of peripheral blood and lymph node mononuclear cells from HIV-infected individuals has demonstrated that HIV replication is controlled tightly by endogenous cytokines that act synergistically and in an autocrine and paracrine manner, similar to their physiologic function in the regulation of the immune system. Indeed, the net level of virus replication in an HIV-infected individual reflects at least in part a balance between inductive and suppressive host factors, mediated mainly by cytokines.

The molecular mechanisms of HIV regulation are best understood for TNF-α, which activates NF-κB proteins that function as transcriptional activators of HIV expression. The HIV-inducing effect of IL-1β is thought to occur at the level of viral transcription in an NF-κB-independent manner. IL-6, GM-CSF, and IFN-γ regulate HIV expression mainly by posttranscriptional mechanisms. Elevated levels of TNF-α and IL-6 have been demonstrated in plasma and cerebrospinal fluid (CSF), and increased expression of TNF-α, IL-1β, IFN-γ, and IL-6 has been demonstrated in the lymph nodes of HIV-infected individuals. The mechanisms whereby the CC-chemokines RANTES, MIP-1α, and MIP-1β inhibit infection of R5 strains of HIV involve blocking of the binding of the virus to its co-receptor, the CC-chemokine receptor CCR5 (see above and below). Of note is the fact that CC-chemokines that inhibit infection by R5 strains of virus actually enhance infection by X4 strains of virus by inducing intracellular signal transduction through the CCR5 and CD4 molecules. The mechanisms whereby other less well characterized factors (see above) inhibit HIV replication are not completely understood.

LYMPHOCYTE TURNOVER IN HIV INFECTION   The immune systems of patients with HIV infection are characterized by a profound increase in lymphocyte turnover that is immediately reduced with effective antiretroviral therapy. Studies utilizing in vivo or in vitro labelling of lymphocytes in the S-phase of the cell cycle have demonstrated a tight correlation between the degree of lymphocyte turnover and plasma levels of HIV RNA. This increase in turnover is seen in CD4+ and CD8+ T lymphocytes as well as B lymphocytes and can be observed in peripheral blood and lymphoid tissue. Mathematical models derived from these data suggest that one can view the lymphoid pool as consisting of dynamically distinct subpopulations of cells that are differentially affected by HIV infection. A major consequence of HIV infection appears to be a shift in cells from a more quiescent pool to a pool with a higher turnover rate. It is likely that a consequence of a higher rate of turnover is a higher rate of death. The role of the thymus in adult human T cell homeostasis and HIV pathogenesis is an area of controversy. While some data point to an important role for the thymus in maintaining T cell numbers and suggest that impairment of thymic function may be responsible for the declines in CD4+ T cells seen in the setting of HIV infection, other studies have concluded that the thymus plays a minor role in HIV pathogenesis. Among the data supporting an important role for the thymus are those that demonstrate an increase in the levels of T cell receptor excision circles (TRECs) following initiation of antiretroviral therapy. TRECs are a byproduct of T cell development and represent episomal fragments of DNA that are excised during T cell receptor gene rearrangement (Chap. 295). Levels of TRECs will be the net result of changes in thymic output and changes in T cell turnover. An increase in thymic output and/or a decrease in T cell turnover will lead to an increase in levels of TRECs. While it is clear that levels of TRECs increase following initiation of antiretroviral therapy, it is not clear whether this is a consequence of increased thymic output or decreased T cell turnover.

CELLULAR TROPISM FOR HIV: ROLE OF CO-RECEPTORS   HIV-1 utilizes two major co-receptors along with CD4 to bind to, fuse with, and enter target cells; these co-receptors are CCR5 and CXCR4, which are receptors for certain endogenous chemokines and belong to the seven-transmembrane-domain G protein–coupled family of receptors (see above). Strains of HIV that utilize CCR5 as a co-receptor are referred to as *R5 viruses*. Strains of HIV that utilize CXCR4 are referred to as *X4 viruses*. Many virus strains are *dual tropic* in that they utilize both CCR5 and CXCR4; these are referred to as *R5X4 viruses*. Other terminology that has been associated with R5 versus X4 viruses is *non-syncytium-inducing viruses* versus *syncytium-inducing viruses*, respectively, based on the observation that R5 viruses generally do not form syncytia in culture with certain T cell lines, whereas X4 viruses readily form syncytia. In reality, under certain conditions both R5 and X4 viruses are capable of forming syncytia in culture.

The natural chemokine ligands for the major HIV co-receptors can readily block entry of HIV. For example, the CC-chemokines RANTES, MIP-1α, and MIP-1β, which are the natural ligands for CCR5, block entry of R5 viruses, whereas SDF-1, the natural ligand for CXCR4, blocks entry of X4 viruses. The mechanism of inhibition of viral entry is a steric inhibition of binding that is not dependent on signal transduction (Fig. 173-20).

The transmitting virus is almost invariably an R5 virus that predominates during the early stages of HIV disease. In ~40% of HIV-infected individuals, there is a transition to a predominantly X4 virus that is associated with a relatively rapid progression of disease. However, at least 60% of infected individuals progress in their disease while maintaining predominance of an R5 virus. Other chemokine receptor family members may function as coreceptors for HIV and SIV entry, but to a much lesser extent than do CCR5 and CXCR4; these include CCR3, BOB/GPR15, Bonzo/STRL33/TYMSTR, CCR2, CCR8, CX$_3$CR1(V28), and GPR1.

The basis for the tropism of different envelope glycoproteins for either CCR5 or CXCR4 relates to the ability of the HIV envelope, particularly the third variable region (V3 loop) of gp120, to interact with these co-receptors. In this regard, binding of gp120 to CD4 induces a conformational change in gp120 that increases its affinity for CCR5. It appears that the interaction of gp120 with CXCR4 is less

FIGURE 173-20 Model for the role of co-receptors CXCR4 and CCR5 in the efficient binding and entry of X4 (*A*) and R5 (*B*) strains of HIV-1, respectively, into CD4+ target cells. Blocking of this initial event in the virus life cycle can be accomplished by inhibition of binding to the co-receptor by the normal ligand for the receptor in question. The ligand for CXCR4 is stromal cell–derived factor (SDF-1); the ligands for CCR5 are RANTES, MIP-1α, and MIP-1β.

dependent on the conformational change induced in gp120 by CD4. In fact, there are X4 strains of HIV that bind to CXCR4 in the absence of surface-bound or soluble CD4. Finally, R5 viruses are more efficient in infecting monocyte/macrophages and microglial cells of the brain (see "Neuropathogenesis," below).

CELLULAR TARGETS OF HIV Although the CD4+ T lymphocytes and CD4+ cells of monocyte lineage are the principal targets of HIV, virtually any cell that expresses the CD4 molecule together with co-receptor molecules (see above and below) can potentially be infected with HIV. Circulating dendritic cells have been reported to express low levels of CD4, and depending on their stage of maturation, these cells can be infected with HIV (see below). Epidermal Langerhans cells express CD4 and have been infected by HIV in vivo. In vitro, HIV has been reported also to infect a wide range of cells and cell lines that express low levels of CD4, no detectable CD4, or only CD4 mRNA; among these are FDCs; megakaryocytes; eosinophils; astrocytes; oligodendrocytes; microglial cells; CD8+ T cells; B cells; NK cells; renal epithelial cells; cervical cells; rectal and bowel mucosal cells such as enterochromaffin, goblet, and columnar epithelial cells; trophoblastic cells; and cells from a variety of organs, such as liver, lung, heart, salivary gland, eye, prostate, testis, and adrenal gland. Since the only cells that have been shown unequivocally to be infected with HIV and to support replication of the virus are CD4+ T lymphocytes and cells of monocyte/macrophage lineage, the relevance of the in vitro infection of these other cell types is questionable.

Of potentially important clinical relevance is the demonstration that thymic precursor cells, which were assumed to be negative for CD3, CD4, and CD8 molecules, actually do express low levels of CD4 and can be infected with HIV in vitro. In addition, human thymic epithelial cells transplanted into an immunodeficient mouse can be infected with HIV by direct inoculation of virus into the thymus. Since these cells may play a role in the normal regeneration of CD4+ T cells, it is possible that their infection and depletion contribute, at least in part, to the impaired ability of the CD4+ T cell pool to completely reconstitute itself in certain infected individuals in whom antiretroviral therapy has suppressed viral replication to <50 copies of HIV RNA per milliliter (see below). In addition, CD34+ monocyte precursor cells have been shown to be infected in vivo in patients with advanced HIV disease. It is likely that these cells express low levels of CD4, and therefore it is not essential to invoke CD4-independent mechanisms to explain the infection.

ABNORMALITIES OF MONONUCLEAR CELLS ■ CD4+ T Cells The range of T cell abnormalities in advanced HIV infection is broad. The defects are both quantitative and qualitative and affect virtually every limb of the immune system (see below), indicating the critical dependence of the integrity of the immune system on the inducer/helper function of CD4+ T cells. In advanced HIV disease, virtually all of the observed immune defects can ultimately be explained by the quantitative depletion of CD4+ T cells. However, T cell dysfunction (see below) can be demonstrated in patients early in the course of infection, even when the CD4+ T cell count is in the low-normal range. The degree and spectrum of dysfunctions increase as the disease progresses. One of the first abnormalities to be detected is a defect in response to remote recall antigens, such as tetanus toxoid and influenza, at a time when mononuclear cells can still respond normally to mitogenic stimulation. Defects in responses to soluble antigens are followed in time by the loss of T cell proliferative responses to alloantigens, and subsequently to mitogens. Essentially every T cell function has been reported to be abnormal at some stage of HIV infection. These abnormalities include defective T cell cloning and colony-forming efficiencies, impaired expression of IL-2 receptors, defective IL-2 production, and decreased IFN-γ production in response to antigens. The proportion of CD4+ T cells that express CD28, which is a major co-stimulatory molecule necessary for the normal activation of T cells, is reduced during HIV infection. Cells lacking expression of CD28 do not respond normally to activation signals and may express markers of terminal activation including HLA-DR, CD38, and CD45RO. CD4+ T cells from HIV-infected individuals express abnormally low levels of CD40 ligand, which may contribute to the dysregulation of B cell function observed in HIV disease.

It is difficult to explain completely the profound immunodeficiency noted in HIV-infected individuals solely on the basis of direct infection and quantitative depletion of CD4+ T cells. This is particularly apparent during the early stages of HIV disease, when CD4+ T cell numbers may be only marginally decreased. In this regard, it is likely that CD4+ T cell dysfunction results from a combination of depletion of cells due to direct infection of the cell and a number of virus-related but indirect effects on the cell (Table 173-6). Indeed, it has been demonstrated that patients with high levels of plasma viremia have a variety of subtle abnormalities of CD4+ T cell function, particularly involving aberrancies in signal transduction pathways. These abnormalities could be due either to aberrant activation induced by the cascade of cytokines that are expressed in viremic patients or by the direct effect of virus on the cell. In this regard, certain of these abnormalities can be reproduced by exposing CD4+ T cells of normal individuals to oligomeric HIV envelope proteins in vitro (see below).

Single-cell killing and the formation of syncytia between infected and uninfected cells have been demonstrated clearly in vitro, although the precise mechanisms of cell death in vivo have not been determined. Cytopathicity in an infected cell in vitro may result from a number of mechanisms, including copious budding of virions from the cell surface with resulting disruption of the integrity of the cell membrane; interference with cellular RNA processing or the accumulation of high levels of heterodisperse RNA molecules; disruption of cellular protein synthesis owing to high levels of viral RNA; accumulation of high levels of unintegrated viral DNA in the cell cytoplasm; induction of aberrant patterns of protein tyrosine phosphorylation; and the interaction between HIV gp120 and CD4 intracellularly. Strain differences in single-cell killing are determined largely by gp120 sequences, which supports the importance of the viral envelope in this process. *Syncytia formation* involves fusion of the cell membrane of an infected cell with the cell membranes of variable numbers of uninfected CD4+ cells. Although cell fusion has not been shown to be an important pathogenic process in vivo, a direct relationship between the presence of syncytia and the degree of cytopathic effect has been demonstrated in vitro, and a correlation has been reported between the presence of virus isolates that readily induce syncytia in vitro and a more aggressive clinical course in the patient. Humoral and cellular immune responses to HIV may contribute to protective immunity by eliminating virus and virus-infected cells (see below). However, since the main targets of HIV infection are immunocompetent cells, these responses may contribute to immune cell depletion and immunologic dysfunction by eliminating both infected cells and "innocent bystander" cells. Soluble viral proteins, particularly gp120, can bind with high affinity to the CD4 molecules on uninfected T cells and monocytes; in addition, virus and/or viral proteins can bind to dendritic cells or FDCs. HIV-specific antibody can recognize these bound molecules and potentially collaborate in the elimination of the cells by ADCC.

Nonpolymorphic determinants of MHC class I products share a degree of homology with gp120 and gp41 proteins of HIV. Such similarities may lead to the generation of autoantibodies to self-MHC determinants. In fact, anti-HLA-DR antibodies have been demonstrated in the sera of HIV-infected individuals (see "Autoimmune Phenomena," above). These antibodies could contribute to the elimination of HLA-DR–expressing cells by ADCC; in addition, it has been suggested that these antibodies may inhibit certain T cell functions that involve HLA-DR molecules.

HIV envelope glycoproteins gp120 and gp160 manifest high-affinity binding to CD4 as well as to various chemokine receptors (see above). Intracellular signals transduced by gp120 have been associated with a number of immunopathogenic processes including anergy, apoptosis, and abnormalities of cell trafficking. The molecular mechanisms responsible for these abnormalities include dysregulation of the T cell receptor–phosphoinositide pathway, p56lck activation, phosphorylation of focal adhesion kinase, activation of the MAP kinase and ras signaling pathways, and downregulation of the co-stimulatory molecules CD40 ligand and CD80.

Finally, the inexorable decline in CD4+ T cell counts that occurs in most HIV-infected individuals may result in part from the inability of the immune system to regenerate the rapidly turning over CD4+ T cell pool efficiently enough to compensate for both HIV-mediated and naturally occurring attrition of cells. At least two major mechanisms may contribute to the failure of the CD4+ T cell pool to reconstitute itself adequately over the course of HIV infection. The first is the destruction of lymphoid precursor cells, including thymic and bone marrow progenitor cells (see above); the other is the gradual disruption of the lymphoid tissue microenvironment, which is essential for efficient regeneration of immunocompetent cells (see above).

CD8+ T Cells A relative C8+ T lymphocytosis is generally associated with high levels of HIV plasma viremia and may in part reflect the expansion of clones of HIV-specific CD8+ CTLs. During the late stages of HIV infection, there may be a significant reduction in the numbers of CD8+ T cells despite the presence of high levels of viremia. HIV-specific CD8+ CTLs have been demonstrated in HIV-infected individuals early in the course of disease (see below). The emergence of HIV escape mutants may ultimately evade these HIV-specific CD8+ T cells. However, as the disease progresses, the functional capability of these cells may decrease and may be lost entirely. The cause of this loss of cytolytic activity is unclear. However, it has been demonstrated that, as disease progresses, CD8+ T cells assume an abnormal phenotype characterized by expression of activation markers such as HLA-DR with an absence of expression of the IL-2 receptor (CD25) and a loss of clonogenic potential. In this regard, it has been reported that nonprogressors can be distinguished from progressors by the maintenance in the former of a high proliferative capacity of their HIV-specific CD8+ T cells coupled to increases in perforin expression. It has been reported that the phenotype of CD8+ T cells in HIV-infected individuals may be of prognostic significance. Those individuals whose CD8+ T cells developed a phenotype of HLA-DR+/CD38− following seroconversion had stabilization of their CD4+ T cell counts, whereas those whose CD8+ T cells developed a phenotype of HLA-DR+/CD38+ had a more aggressive course and a poorer prognosis. In addition to the defects in HIV-specific CTLs, functional defects in other MHC-restricted CTLs, such as those directed against influenza and CMV, have been demonstrated. CD8+ T cells secrete a variety of soluble factors that inhibit HIV replication including the CC-chemokines RANTES, MIP-1α, MIP-1β, and the alpha defensins -1, -2, and -3, as well as one or more as yet poorly identified factors (see above). The presence of high levels of HIV viremia in vivo as well as exposure of CD8+ T cells in vitro to HIV envelope has been shown to be associated with a variety of cellular functional abnormalities. Finally, since the integrity of CD8+ T cell function depends in part on adequate inductive signals from CD4+ T cells, the defect in CD8+ CTLs is likely compounded by the quantitative loss and qualitative dysfunction of CD4+ T cells.

TABLE 173-6   *Mechanisms of CD4+ T Cell Dysfunction and Depletion*

Direct Mechanisms	Indirect Mechanisms
Loss of plasma membrane integrity due to viral budding	Aberrant intracellular signaling events
Accumulation of unintegrated viral DNA	Autoimmunity
Interference with cellular RNA processing	Innocent bystander killing of viral antigen–coated cells
Intracellular gp120-CD4 autofusion events	Apoptosis
	Inhibition of lymphopoiesis
Syncytia formation	Activation-induced cell death
	Elimination of HIV-infected cells by virus-specific immune responses

B Cells The predominant defect in B cells from HIV-infected individuals is one of aberrant cellular activation, which is reflected by spontaneous proliferation and immunoglobulin secretion and by increased spontaneous secretion of TNF-α and IL-6. In addition, B cells from HIV viremic patients manifest a decreased capacity to mount a proliferative response to ligation of the B cell antigen receptor (surface IgM) at the same time as they are capable of robust differentiation in response to a variety of stimuli. B cells from HIV-infected individuals manifest enhanced spontaneous in vitro transformation with EBV, a process that is likely due to defective T cell immune surveillance. The in vivo counterpart of this phenomenon is an increase in the incidence of EBV-related B cell lymphomas. Untransformed B cells cannot be infected with HIV. However, HIV or its products can activate B cells directly; portions of the HIV gp41 envelope protein have been reported to induce polyclonal B cell activation. In addition, it has been reported that products of the VH₃ genes on the surface of B cells can serve as a receptor for HIV. B cells from patients with high levels of viremia bind virions to their surface via the CD21 complement receptor. It is likely that in vivo activation of B cells by virus products during the viremic state accounts at least in part for the spontaneous activation of these cells noted ex vivo. B cells from HIV-infected individuals express abnormally low levels of HLA-DR and CD21 on their surface. Cognate B cell–CD4+ T cell interactions are abnormal in viremic HIV-infected individuals. B cells respond poorly to CD4+ T cell help; this is due at least in part to an intrinsic defect in responder B cells with regard to their inability to normally upregulate CD25 (IL-2 receptor) and thus to proliferate normally in response to IL-2; in addition, B cells fail to adequately upregulate CD80 and CD86 following stimulation with activated T cells. In vivo, the aberrant activated state of B cells manifests itself by hypergammaglobulinemia and by the presence of circulating immune complexes and autoantibodies (see above). HIV-infected individuals respond poorly to primary and secondary immunizations with protein and polysaccharide antigens. These B cell defects are likely responsible in part for the increase in certain bacterial infections seen in advanced HIV disease in adults, as well as for the important role of bacterial infections in the morbidity and mortality of HIV-infected children, who cannot mount an adequate humoral response to common bacterial pathogens. The absolute number of circulating B cells may be depressed in primary HIV infection; however, this phenomenon is usually transient and likely reflects in part a redistribution of cells out of the circulation and into the lymphoid tissue. In certain patients, the number of circulating B cells decreases in advanced-stage disease.

Monocyte/Macrophages Circulating monocytes are generally normal in number in HIV-infected individuals. Monocytes express the CD4 molecule and several co-receptors for HIV on their surface, including CCR5, CXCR4, and CCR3, and thus are targets of HIV infection. Of note is the fact that the degree of cytopathicity of HIV for cells of the monocyte lineage is low, and HIV can replicate extensively in cells of the monocyte lineage with little cytopathic effect. Hence, monocyte-lineage cells may play a role in the dissemination of HIV in the body and can serve as reservoirs of HIV infection, thus representing an obstacle to the eradication of HIV by antiretroviral drugs. In vivo infection of circulating monocytes is difficult to demonstrate; however, infection of tissue macrophages and macrophage-lineage cells in the brain (infiltrating macrophages or resident microglial cells) and lung (pulmonary alveolar macrophages) can be demonstrated easily. Tissue macrophages are an important source of HIV during opportunistic infections. Infection of monocyte precursors in the bone marrow may directly or indirectly be responsible for certain of the hematologic abnormalities in HIV-infected individuals. A number of abnormalities of circulating monocytes have been reported in HIV-infected individuals, including decreased secretion of IL-1 and IL-12; increased secretion of IL-10; defects in antigen presentation and induction of T cell responses due to decreased MHC class II expression; and abnormalities of Fc receptor function, C3 receptor–mediated clearance, oxidative burst responses, and certain cytotoxic functions such as ADCC,

possibly related to low levels of expression of Fc and complement receptors. Exposure of monocytes to viral proteins such as gp120 and Tat, as well as to certain cytokines, can cause abnormal activation, and this may play a role in cellular dysfunction (see above).

Dendritic and Langerhans Cells Dendritic cells play an important role in the initiation of HIV infection by virtue of the ability of HIV to bind to cell surface C-type lectin receptors, particularly DC-SIGN (see above). This allows efficient presentation of virus to CD4+ T cell targets that become infected; complexes of infected CD4+ T cells and dendritic cells provide an optimal microenvironment for virus replication. There has been considerable disagreement regarding the HIV infectibility and hence the depletion as well as the dysfunction of dendritic cells themselves. Depending on their state of maturation, dendritic cells express varying levels of CD4 as well as several chemokine receptors. In this regard, it appears that the ability of a dendritic cell to become infected depends in part on its state of maturation. Mature dendritic cells have been demonstrated to be infectable by both R5 and X4 isolates of HIV-1. Immature tissue dendritic cells have been less well studied in their native state. Even in those dendritic cells in which infection occurs, the efficiency of infection and level of productivity of infection is quite low compared to CD4+ T cells.

Natural Killer Cells The role of NK cells is to provide immunosurveillance against virus-infected cells, certain tumor cells, and allogeneic cells (Chap. 295). Functional abnormalities in NK cells have been observed throughout the course of HIV disease, and the severity of these abnormalities increases as disease progresses. Most studies report that NK cells are normal in number and phenotype in HIV-infected individuals; however, a numerical decrease in the CD16+/CD56+ subpopulation of NK cells has been reported together with an increase in activation markers. The abnormality in NK cell function is thought to result from a defect in postbinding lysis. However, the lytic machinery does not appear to be impaired, since NK cells from HIV-infected individuals mediate ADCC normally. The addition of either IL-2, IL-12, IL-15, or IFN-α to cultures improves the defective in vitro NK cell function of HIV-infected individuals. HIV-mediated down-regulation of HLA-A and -B, but not HLA-C and -D molecules may inhibit NK-mediated killing of HIV-infected target cells. NK cells serve as important sources of HIV-inhibitory CC-chemokines. NK cells isolated from HIV-infected individuals constitutively produce high levels of MIP-1α, MIP-1β, and RANTES. In addition, high levels of these chemokines are seen when NK cells are stimulated with IL-2 or IL-15 or when CD16 is cross-linked or during the process of lytic killing of target cells. HIV-infected patients with high levels of plasma viremia manifest a decreased ability, compared to HIV-infected individuals who are aviremic, of their NK cells to block HIV replication in vitro in assays of both cell contact and supernatant-mediated suppression of virus. In addition, viremic patients have a decrease in expression of activating receptors (responsible for killer activity) and an increase in certain inhibitory receptors (responsible for inhibition of killer activity) on NK cells, suggesting one potential mechanism whereby viremia might inhibit the ability of NK cells to kill HIV-infected target cells.

GENETIC FACTORS IN HIV PATHOGENESIS Several reports have described MHC alleles and other host factors that may influence the pathogenesis and course of HIV disease. These include associations with certain HIV-related manifestations, such as KS and diffuse lymphadenopathy, or with the type of clinical course, such as long-term survival or rapid progression (Table 173-7). A number of mechanisms have been proposed whereby MHC-encoded molecules might predispose an individual either to rapid progression or to nonprogression to AIDS. These proposed mechanisms include the ability to present certain immunodominant HIV T helper or CTL epitopes, leading to a relatively protective immune response against HIV and hence to slow progression of disease. In contrast, certain MHC class I or class II alleles might predispose an individual to an immunopathogenic response against

TABLE 173-7 *Genetic Factors Implicated in the Pathogenesis of HIV Disease*

Factor	Association
MAJOR HISTOCOMPATIBILITY LOCI-ENCODED GENES	
B35, C4, DR1, DQ1	Kaposi's sarcoma
DR1	Kaposi's sarcoma
DR2, DR5	Kaposi's sarcoma
DR5	Kaposi's sarcoma
Aw23, Bw49	Kaposi's sarcoma
B62	Fever, skin rash in primary HIV infection
Aw19	HIV seropositivity in individuals multiply exposed to HIV
A1, A24, C7, B8, DR3	Rapid progression to AIDS
DR4, DQB1*0302	Rapid progression to AIDS
DR3, DQ1	Rapid progression to AIDS
B*35	Rapid progression to AIDS
Cw*04	Rapid progression to AIDS
TAP2.1	Promotes HIV progression to AIDS
DR5	Thrombocytopenia and lymphadenopathy in HIV infection
DR5, DR6	Diffuse infiltrative CD8+ lymphocytosis with Sjögren-like syndrome in HIV infection
Bw4	Slow decline in CD4+ T cell count
B13, B27, B51, B57, DQB1*0302,0303	Protects from progression to AIDS
B*5701	Strong protection from progression to AIDS
A26, B38, TAP1 4, TAP2,3	Ability to clear HIV infection in transiently infected seronegative individuals
A28, Bw70, Aw69, B18	Protection from HIV infection
A32, B4, C2	Long-term survival in HIV infection
A11, A32, B13, C2, DQA1*0301, DQB1*0302, DRB1*0400, DRB4*0101	Long-term survival in HIV infection
Heterozygosity for class I loci (A, B, and C)	Delayed onset to AIDS
Homozygosity for class I loci (A, B, and C)	Rapid onset to AIDS and death
OTHER GENES	
p53 tumor-suppressor gene	Controls HIV replicative patterns and determinant of viral latency
CCR5 gene	Homozygous defect involving a 32-bp deletion corresponding to the second extracellular loop of the receptor results in resistance to infection; heterozygous defect appears to result in partial protection against disease progression. Also, several single nucleotide polymorphisms (SNPs) in the CCR5 promoter have been shown to be associated with variable rates of progression in AIDS.
CCR2 gene	Heterozygosity for CCR2-641 mutation is associated with delay in progression of HIV disease
CX3CR1 gene	Mutations in I249 and M280 associated with rapid progression to AIDS
RANTES gene	A mutation of the RANTES gene (RANTES-28G) results in increased transcription and expression of RANTES on mononuclear cells with resulting inhibition of infection with R5 strains of HIV and delay of disease progression. Three SNPs; 403A in the RANTES promoter, In1.1C in the first intron, and 3′222C in the 3′ untranslated region of the gene are associated with increased frequency of HIV-1 infection. The SNP In1.1C allele results in decreased RANTES production and correlates with rapid progression to AIDS.
IL-10 gene	Individuals carrying the IL10-5′-592A promoter allele were at increased risk for HIV infection and, once infected, progressed more rapidly than homozygotes for the alternative IL10-5′-592 C/C genotype
VDR gene	Homozygosity for vitamin D receptor gene polymorphism B (VDR-BB) correlates with rapid progression to AIDS
IL-4 gene	SNP IL-4-589T causes higher levels of IL-4 production in vivo, resulting in downregulation of CCR5. The presence of SNP IL-4-589T is modestly associated with protection from acquisition of HIV-1 by heterosexual contact. This SNP also correlates with slower disease progression and decreased viral load early in infection.
IL-1ra gene	Homozygosity IL-1ra gene*2 correlates with significantly lower viral loads.
TNF-α gene	SNP TNF-α-238A, but not the -308A allele correlates with a higher frequency of lipodystrophy.
IL-6 gene	Among HIV-positive men, homozygosity for SNP IL-6-174G carries an increased risk of development of Kaposi sarcoma; men with homozygosity for SNP IL-6-174C were less likely to develop Kaposi sarcoma.
GENE INTERACTIONS	
KIR gene with *HLA-B*	In the absence of HLA-B Bw4-80I, KIR3DS1 is strongly associated with rapid progression to AIDS. This effect is reversed by the presence of HLA-B Bw4-80I. Individuals carrying both genes have a delayed progression to AIDS; in the absence of KIR3DS1, HLA-B Bw4-80I has no effect on disease progression.

Sources: Adapted from BF Haynes et al: Science 271:324, 1996; O'Brien and Moore.

viral epitopes in certain tissues, such as the CNS or lungs, or against certain HIV-infected cell types, such as macrophages or dendritic cells/Langerhans cells. In addition, certain rare MHC class I and class II alleles might facilitate rapid recognition of HIV-infected cells from the infecting partner in primary HIV infection and promote rejection of these cells by alloreactive responses. Similarly, common MHC alleles could lead to less effective removal of HIV-infected allogeneic cells. It has been clearly demonstrated that maximal *HLA* heterozygosity for class I loci (A, B, and C) is associated with a delayed onset of AIDS among HIV-infected individuals, whereas homozygosity for these loci was associated with a more rapid progression to AIDS and death. This observation is likely due to the fact that individuals who are heterozygous at *HLA* loci are able to present a greater variety of antigenic peptides to cytotoxic T lymphocytes than are homozygotes, resulting in a more effective immune response against a number of pathogens including HIV. Of particular note is the fact that the HLA class I alleles B*35 and Cw*04 were consistently associated with rapid development of AIDS. Other data have indicated that transporter associated with antigen-presenting (TAP) genes play a role in determining the outcome of HIV infection. HLA profiles that reflect certain combinations of MHC-encoded TAP and class I and class II genes are strongly associated with different rates of progression to AIDS. A recent finding of genetic association with HIV disease progression has highlighted the role for NK cells in HIV disease. A single nucleotide polymorphism (SNP) in the killer immunoglobulin-like receptor (KIR) gene was shown to be strongly associated with rapid progression to AIDS. However, when the KIR3 DS1 SNP was present with HLA-B Bw4-80I, the resultant phenotype was delayed progression to AIDS, even though this HLA-B allele alone has no effect on HIV disease progression. Furthermore, the KIR3 DS1/HLA-B Bw4-80I-carrying individuals had a significantly reduced viral load, beginning early in the course of infection. This points to the potential role of NK cells in the maintenance of the viral set point, strongly suggesting that HLA-B Bw4-80I serves as the ligand activating this KIR receptor, resulting in the death of the target cell.

The most dramatic example of a genetic factor influencing HIV infection and/or pathogenesis relates to the gene that codes for the HIV cellular co-receptor CCR5. Rare individuals have been reported who had had repetitive sexual exposure to HIV in high-risk situations but remained uninfected. The peripheral blood mononuclear cells of two such individuals were found to be highly resistant to infection in vitro with R5 strains of HIV-1, but they were readily infected with X4 strains. Genetic analysis revealed that these two individuals inherited a homozygous defect in the gene that codes for CCR5, the cellular co-receptor for R5 strains of HIV-1. The defective *CCR5* allele contained a 32-bp deletion corresponding to the second extracellular loop of the receptor. The encoded protein was severely truncated, and the receptor was nonfunctional, explaining the refractoriness to infection with R5 strains of HIV-1. Population studies revealed that ~1% of the Caucasian population of western European ancestry possessed the homozygous defect. Up to 20% of this group had the heterozygous defect. Of note, cohort studies of hundreds of DNA samples originating from western and central Africa and Japan did not reveal a single mutant allele, suggesting that the allele is either absent or extremely rare in Africa and Japan. In a cohort of 1400 HIV-1–infected Caucasian individuals, no subject homozygous for the mutation was found, strongly supporting the concept that the homozygous defect confers protection against infection. This finding is particularly compelling in light of the fact that transmitting viruses are strongly biased towards R5 strains of HIV-1 (see above). Furthermore, there was a higher frequency of individuals heterozygous for the genetic defect among HIV-infected patients who were long-term nonprogressors compared to HIV-infected individuals who progressed more rapidly (see above). Of note, several individuals have been identified who were homozygous for the *CCR5*-Δ32 defect who in fact did become infected with HIV. These individuals were found to have an X4 strain of HIV that was associated in some cases with an accelerated course of disease. Slow progression of HIV disease is also seen in individuals who are heterozygous for the *CCR2-64I* mutation or SNP; this is felt to be due to dimerization of CXCR4 with the mutated CCR2-64I resulting in a decreased expression of CXCR4 on the cell surface. Delayed progression of disease is also seen in those individuals who have any of a number of SNPs in the *CCR5* promoter. In addition, individuals who carry a certain allele (IL-10-5-592A) of the IL-10 promoter are at increased risk of infection and, once infected, progress more rapidly than homozygotes for the alternative genotype. The mechanism of this effect is felt to be a downregulation of the inhibitory cytokine IL-10 resulting in facilitation of HIV replication. The SNP, IL-4-589T, increases IL-4 production. This allele associates with a slower progression to AIDS, presumably through the downregulation of CCR5 by higher and more sustained levels of IL-4. Separate SNPs have been found in the RANTES gene that correlate with either an increased or decreased expression of this chemokine (Table 173-7). As expected, based upon the effect of RANTES as an inhibitor of R5 HIV, RANTES-28G SNP upregulates RANTES and is associated with delayed progression to AIDS. The opposite effects are seen with SNP RANTES In1.1C. This SNP decreases RANTES expression and correlates strongly with rapid progression to AIDS. Other SNPs that decrease RANTES expression are associated with a higher rate of HIV infection, reinforcing the central role for R5 viruses in the establishment of HIV infection.

Additional genes have been found that are associated with rapid progression to AIDS or susceptibility to significant AIDS complication. Homozygosity for the vitamin D receptor form B correlates with rapid progression to AIDS. The mechanism is thought to relate to the known effects of vitamin D on immune modulation. The TNF-α SNP-238A is associated with a higher frequency of lipodystrophy. The underlying causes of this complication of AIDS remain to be defined, including the role of combination antiretroviral therapy. Finally, SNP IL-6-174G has been shown to lead to higher levels of IL-6. Homozygosity at this locus correlates with an increased risk of development of KS. Not surprisingly, homozygosity for SNP IL-6-174C, which results in lower levels of IL-6, was protective, correlating with significantly lower levels of KS.

NEUROPATHOGENESIS HIV-infected individuals can experience a variety of neurologic abnormalities due either to opportunistic infections and neoplasms (see below) or to direct effects of HIV or its products. With regard to the latter, HIV has been demonstrated in the brain and CSF of infected individuals with and without neuropsychiatric abnormalities. The main cell types that are infected in the brain in vivo are the perivascular macrophages and the microglial cells; monocytes that have already been infected in the blood can migrate into the brain, where they then reside as macrophages, or macrophages can be directly infected within the brain. The precise mechanisms whereby HIV enters the brain are unclear; however, they are felt to relate, at least in part, to the ability of virus-infected and immune-activated macrophages to induce adhesion molecules such as E-selectin and vascular cell adhesion molecule-1 (VCAM-1) on brain endothelium. Other studies have demonstrated that HIV gp120 enhances the expression of intercellular adhesion molecule-1 (ICAM-1) in glial cells; this effect may facilitate entry of HIV-infected cells into the CNS and may promote syncytia formation. Virus isolates from the brain are preferentially R5 strains as opposed to X4 strains (see above); in this regard, HIV-infected individuals who are heterozygous for *CCR5-δ32* appear to be relatively protected against the development of HIV encephalopathy compared to wild-type individuals. Distinct HIV envelope sequences are associated with the clinical expression of the AIDS dementia complex (see below). Although there have been reports of infrequent HIV infection of neuronal cells and astrocytes, there is no convincing evidence that brain cells other than those of monocyte/macrophage lineage can be productively infected in vivo.

HIV-infected individuals may manifest white matter lesions as well as neuronal loss. Given the relative absence of evidence of HIV infection of neurons either in vivo or in vitro, it is unlikely that direct infection of these cells accounts for their loss. Rather, the HIV-mediated effects on neurons and oligodendrocytes are felt to involve indirect pathways whereby viral proteins, particularly gp120 and Tat, trigger the release of endogenous neurotoxins from macrophages and to a lesser extent from astrocytes. In addition, it has been demonstrated that both HIV-1 Nef and Tat can induce chemotaxis of leukocytes, including monocytes, into the CNS. Neurotoxins can be released from monocytes as a consequence of infection and/or immune activation. Monocyte-derived neurotoxic factors have been reported to kill neurons via the *N*-methyl-D-aspartate (NMDA) receptor. In addition, HIV gp120 shed by virus-infected monocytes could cause neurotoxicity by antagonizing the function of vasoactive intestinal peptide (VIP), by elevating intracellular calcium levels, and by decreasing nerve growth factor levels in the cerebral cortex. A variety of monocyte-derived cytokines can contribute directly or indirectly to the neurotoxic effects in HIV infection; these include TNF-α, IL-1, IL-6, TGF-β, IFN-γ, platelet-activating factor, and endothelin. Furthermore, among the CC-chemokines, elevated levels of monocyte chemotactic protein (MCP)1 in the brain and CSF have been shown to correlate best with the presence and degree of HIV encephalopathy. In addition, infection and/or activation of monocyte-lineage cells can result in increased production of eicosanoids, nitric oxide, and quinolinic acid, which may contribute to neurotoxicity. Astrocytes may play diverse roles in HIV neuropathogenesis. Reactive gliosis or astrocytosis has been demonstrated in the brains of HIV-infected individuals, and TNF-α and IL-6 have been shown to induce astrocyte proliferation. In addition, astrocyte-derived IL-6 can induce HIV expression in infected cells in vitro. Furthermore, it has been suggested that astrocytes may downregulate macrophage-produced neurotoxins. It has been reported that HIV-infected individuals with the E4 allele for apolipoprotein E (apo E) are at increased risk for AIDS encephalopathy and peripheral neuropathy. The likelihood that HIV or its products are involved in neuropathogenesis is supported by the observation that neuropsychiatric abnormalities may undergo remarkable and rapid improvement upon the initiation of antiretroviral therapy; this is true of HIV-infected children as well as adults. In fact, there has been a remarkable decrease in the incidence of HIV encephalopathy in the era of successful combination antiretroviral therapy.

PATHOGENESIS OF KAPOSI'S SARCOMA There are at least four distinct epidemiologic forms of KS: (1) the classic form that occurs in older men of predominantly Mediterranean or eastern European Jewish backgrounds with no recognized contributing factors; (2) the equatorial African form that occurs in all ages, also without any recognized precipitating factors; (3) the form associated with organ transplantation and its attendent iatrogenic immunosuppressed state; and (4) the form associated with HIV-1 infection. In the latter two forms, KS is an opportunistic disease; in HIV-infected individuals, unlike typical opportunistic infections, its occurrence is not strictly related to the level of depression of CD4+ T cell counts (see below). The pathogenesis of KS is complex; fundamentally, it is an angioproliferative disease that is not a true neoplastic sarcoma, at least not in its early stages. It is a manifestation of excessive proliferation of spindle cells that are believed to be of vascular origin and have features in common with endothelial and smooth-muscle cells. In HIV disease the development of KS is dependent on the interplay of a variety of factors including HIV-1 itself, human herpes virus 8 (HHV-8), immune activation, and cytokine secretion. A number of epidemiologic and virologic studies have clearly linked HHV-8, which is also referred to as *Kaposi's sarcoma–associated herpesvirus* (KSHV), to KS not only in HIV-infected individuals but also in individuals with the other forms of KS. HHV-8 is a γ-herpesvirus related to EBV and herpesvirus saimiri. It encodes a homologue to human IL-6 and in addition to KS has been implicated in the pathogenesis of body cavity lymphoma, multiple myeloma, and monoclonal gammopathy of undetermined significance. Sequences of HHV-8 are found universally in the lesions of KS, and patients with KS are virtually all seropositive for HHV-8. HHV-8 DNA sequences can be found in the B cells of 30 to 50% of patients with KS and 7% of patients with AIDS without clinically apparent KS.

Between 1 and 2% of eligible blood donors are positive for antibodies to HHV-8, while the prevalence of HHV-8 seropositivity in HIV-infected men is 30 to 35%. The prevalence in HIV-infected women is ~4%. This finding is reflective of the lower incidence of KS in women. It has been debated whether HHV-8 is actually the transforming agent in KS; the bulk of the cells in the tumor lesions of KS are not neoplastic cells. However, it has been demonstrated that endothelial cells can be transformed in vitro by HHV-8. In this regard, HHV-8 possesses a number of genes including homologues of the IL-8 receptor, Bcl-2, and cyclin D, which can potentially transform the host cell. Despite the complexity of the pathogenic events associated with the development of KS in HIV-infected individuals, it is generally agreed that HHV-8 is indeed the etiologic agent of this disease. The initiation and/or propagation of KS requires an activated state and is mediated, at least in part, by cytokines. A number of factors, including TNF α, IL-1β, IL-6, GM-CSF, basic fibroblast growth factor, and oncostatin M, function in an autocrine and paracrine manner to sustain the growth and chemotaxis of the KS spindle cells. In this regard, KSHV-derived IL-6 has been demonstrated to induce proliferation of lymphoma cells and to inhibit the cytostatic effects of INF-α on

KSHV-infected lymphoma cells. It has been suggested that the HIV Tat protein plays a major role in the pathogenesis of KS. In this regard, it has been demonstrated that IFN-γ can induce endothelial cells to proliferate and to invade the extracellular matrix in response to HIV Tat. This occurs as a result of the upregulation by IFN-γ of the expression and activity of the receptors for Tat, which are the integrins $\alpha_5\beta_1$ and $\alpha_v\beta_3$. In addition, the HIV-1 Tat protein has been shown to act synergistically with basic fibroblast growth factor in the induction of lesions resembling KS lesions in mice by increasing matrix-metalloproteinase-2 secretion and activation in endothelial cells. Glucocorticoids have been shown to have a stimulatory effect, and human chorionic gonadotropin an inhibitory effect, on KS spindle cells, suggesting that modulation of the balance of autocrine factors may have therapeutic potential in KS. It has been demonstrated that HIV protease inhibitors have potent anti-angiogenic properties and, as such, promote regression of KS.

IMMUNE RESPONSE TO HIV

As detailed above and below, following the initial burst of viremia during primary infection, HIV-infected individuals mount a robust immune response that usually substantially curtails the levels of plasma viremia and likely contributes to delaying the ultimate development of clinically apparent disease for a median of 10 years. This immune response contains elements of both humoral and cell-mediated immunity (Table 173-8; Fig. 173-21). It is directed against multiple antigenic determinants of the HIV virion as well as against viral proteins expressed on the surface of infected cells. Ironically, those CD4+ T cells with T cell receptors specific for HIV are theoretically those CD4+ T cells most likely to bind to infected cells and themselves be infected and destroyed. Thus, an early consequence of HIV infection may be interference with the generation of an effective immune response through the elimination or compromise of HIV-specific CD4+ T lymphocytes.

Although a great deal of investigation has been directed toward delineating and better understanding the components of this immune response, it remains unclear which of these phenomena are most important in delaying progression of infection and which, if any, play a role in the pathogenesis of HIV disease. This lack of knowledge has also hampered the ability to develop an effective vaccine for HIV disease.

HUMORAL IMMUNE RESPONSE Antibodies to HIV usually appear within 6 weeks and almost invariably within 12 weeks of primary infection (Fig. 173-22); rare exceptions are individuals who have defects in the ability to produce HIV-specific antibodies. Detection of these antibodies forms the basis of most diagnostic screening tests for HIV infection. The appearance of HIV-binding antibodies detected by ELISA and western blot assays occurs prior to the appearance of neutralizing antibodies; the latter generally appear following the initial decreases in plasma viremia, which is more closely related to the appearance of HIV-specific CD8+ T lymphocytes. The first antibodies detected are

---

TABLE 173-8 *Elements of the Immune Response to HIV*

Humoral immunity
  Binding antibodies
  Neutralizing antibodies
    Type specific
    Group specific
  Antibodies participating in antibody-dependent cellular cytotoxicity
    (ADCC)
    Protective
    Pathogenic (bystander killing)
  Enhancing antibodies
Cell-mediated immunity
  Helper CD4+ T lymphocytes
  Class I MHC–restricted cytotoxic CD8+ T lymphocytes
  CD8+ T cell–mediated inhibition (noncytolytic)
  ADCC
  Natural killer cells

FIGURE 173-21 Schematic representation of the different immunologic effector mechanisms felt to be active in the setting of HIV infection. Detailed descriptions are given in the text. TCR, T cell receptor; ADCC, antibody dependent cellular cytotoxicity; MHC, major histocompatibility complex.

those directed against the structural or gag proteins of HIV, p24 and p17, and the gag precursor p55. The development of antibodies to p24 is associated with a decrease in the serum levels of free p24 antigen. Antibodies to the gag proteins are followed by the appearance of antibodies to the envelope proteins (gp160, gp120, p88, and gp41) and to the products of the *pol* gene (p31, p51, and p66). In addition, one may see antibodies to the low-molecular-weight regulatory proteins encoded by the HIV genes *vpr, vpu, vif, rev, tat,* and *nef.*

While antibodies to multiple antigens of HIV are produced, the precise functional significance of these different antibodies is unclear. The best studied have been the antibodies directed toward the envelope proteins of the virus. As noted above, the envelope of HIV consists of an outer envelope glycoprotein with a molecular mass of 120 kDa and a transmembrane glycoprotein with a molecular mass of 41 kDa. These are initially synthesized as a 160-kDa precursor that is cleaved by cellular proteases. Most of the antienvelope antibodies are directed either toward an epitope in the gp41 region comprising amino acids 579 to 613 or toward a hypervariable region in the gp120 molecule, known as the *V3 loop region,* comprising amino acids 303 through 338. This V3 region is a major site for the development of mutations that lead to variants of HIV that are not well recognized by the immune system.

Antibodies directed toward the envelope proteins of HIV have been characterized both as being protective and as possibly contributing to

the pathogenesis of HIV disease. Among the protective antibodies are those that function to neutralize HIV directly and prevent the spread of infection to additional cells, as well as those that participate in ADCC. *Neutralizing antibodies* may be a component of primary HIV infection, and some long-term nonprogressors have been reported to have increased titers of neutralizing antibodies. Neutralizing antibodies appear to be of two forms, type-specific and group-specific. *Type-specific neutralizing antibodies* are generally directed to the V3 loop region. These antibodies neutralize only viruses of a given strain and are present in low titer in most infected individuals. *Group-specific neutralizing antibodies* are capable of neutralizing a wide variety of HIV isolates. At least two forms of group-specific antibodies have been identified: those binding to amino acids 423 to 437 of gp120 and those binding to amino acids 728 to 745 of gp41. The other major class of protective antibodies are those that participate in ADCC, which is actually a form of cell-mediated immunity (Chap. 295) in which NK cells that bear Fc receptors are armed with specific anti-HIV antibodies that bind to the NK cells via their Fc portion. These armed NK cells then bind to and destroy cells expressing HIV antigens. Antibodies to both gp120 and gp41 have been shown to participate in ADCC-mediated killing of HIV-infected cells. The levels of antienvelope antibodies capable of mediating ADCC are highest in the earlier stages of HIV infection. In vitro, IL-2 can augment ADCC-mediated killing.

In addition to playing a role in host defense, HIV-specific antibodies have also been implicated in disease pathogenesis. Antibodies directed to gp41, when present in low titer, have been shown in vitro to be capable of facilitating infection of cells through an Fc receptor–mediated mechanism known as *antibody enhancement*. Thus, the same regions of the envelope protein of HIV that give rise to antibodies capable of mediating ADCC also elicit the production of antibodies that can facilitate infection of cells in vitro. In addition, it has been postulated that anti-gp120 antibodies that participate in the ADCC killing of HIV-infected cells might also kill uninfected CD4+ T cells if the uninfected cells had bound free gp120, a phenomenon referred to as *bystander killing*.

CELLULAR IMMUNE RESPONSE Given the fact that T cell–mediated immunity is known to play a major role in host defense against most viral infections (Chap. 295), it is generally thought to be an important component of the host immune response to HIV. T cell immunity can be divided into two major categories, mediated respectively by the *helper/inducer CD4+ T cells* and the *cytotoxic/immunoregulatory CD8+ T cells.*

HIV-specific CD4+ T cells can be detected in the majority of HIV-infected patients through the use of flow cytometry to measure single-

FIGURE 173-22 Relationship between antigenemia and the development of antibodies to HIV. Antibodies to HIV proteins are generally seen 6 to 12 weeks following infection and 3 to 6 weeks after the development of plasma viremia. Late in the course of illness, antibody levels to p24 decline, generally in association with a rising titer of p24 antigen.

cell IFN-γ production in response to HIV antigens, binding to MHC class II tetramers, or HIV p24 lymphocyte proliferation assays. Although these cells, with their high affinity for binding to HIV-infected cells, may be among the first to be infected and destroyed during HIV infection, they also are likely to undergo clonal expansions in response to HIV antigens and thus survive as a population of cells. No clear correlations exist between levels of HIV-specific CD4+ T lymphocytes and plasma HIV RNA levels; however, in the setting of high viral loads, CD4+ T cell responses to HIV antigens appear to shift from one of proliferaton to one of IFN-γ production. Thus, while a reverse correlation exists between the level of p24-specific proliferation and levels of plasma HIV viremia, the nature of the causal relationship between these parameters is unclear. Through the use of computer modeling, several regions of the HIV-1 envelope molecule have been identified that are structurally analogous to other known T cell epitopes by virtue of having structures known as *amphipathic helices*. Peptides from these envelope regions have been used to identify the presence of CD4+ T cells specific for these regions in the peripheral blood of HIV infected individuals. Other studies have demonstrated that peripheral blood T cells of some healthy, HIV-negative individuals also react to the envelope proteins of HIV. It is unclear whether or not this represents the presence of a degree of protective immunity in these individuals.

MHC class I–restricted, HIV-specific CD8+ T cells have been identified in the peripheral blood of patients with HIV-1 infection. These cells include CTLs and T cells that can be induced by HIV antigens to express cytokines such as IFN-γ. CTLs have been identified in the peripheral blood of patients within weeks of HIV infection. These CD8+ T lymphocytes, through their HIV-specific antigen receptors, bind to and cause the lytic destruction of target cells bearing autologous MHC class I molecules associated with HIV antigens. Two types of CTL activity can be demonstrated in the peripheral blood or lymph node mononuclear cells of HIV-infected individuals. The first type directly lyses appropriate target cells in culture without prior in vitro stimulation (*spontaneous CTL activity*). The other type of CTL activity reflects the *precursor frequency of CTLs* (CTLp); this type of CTL activity can be demonstrated by stimulation of CD8+ T cells in vitro with a mitogen such as phytohemagglutinin or anti-CD3 antibody. Following primary HIV infection, the qualitative nature of the HIV-specific CTL response is an important predictor of eventual clinical outcome. Patients who mount a broad CD8+ CTL response generally have a more favorable clinical course than do patients who mount a more restricted CTL response. These data are consistent with studies in the SIV model where deletion of CD8+ T cells leads to a more accelerated clinical course.

In addition to CTLs, CD8+ T cells capable of being induced by HIV antigens to express cytokines such as IFN-γ also appear in the setting of HIV-1 infection. It is not clear whether these are the same or different effector pools compared to those cells mediating cytotoxicity; in addition, the relative roles of each in host defense against HIV are not fully understood. It does appear that these CD8+ T cells are driven to in vivo expansion by HIV antigen. There is a direct correlation between levels of CD8+ T cells capable of producing IFN-γ in response to HIV antigens and plasma levels of HIV-1 RNA. Thus, while these cells are clearly induced by HIV-1 infection, their overall ability to control infection remains unclear. Multiple HIV antigens, including Gag, Env, Pol, Tat, Rev, and Nef, can elicit CD8+ T cell responses. Among patients who control viral replication in the absence of antiretroviural drugs are a subset of patients whose peripheral blood contains a population of CD8+ T cells that undergo substantial proliferation and perforin expression in response to HIV antigens. It is possible that these cells play an important role in HIV-specific host defense.

At least three other forms of cell-mediated immunity to HIV have been described: CD8+ T cell–mediated suppression of HIV replication, ADCC, and NK cell activity. *CD8+ T cell–mediated suppression*

of HIV replication refers to the ability of CD8+ T cells from an HIV-infected patient to inhibit the replication of HIV in tissue culture in a noncytolytic manner. There is no requirement for HLA compatibility between the CD8+ T cells and the HIV-infected cells. This effector mechanism is thus nonspecific and appears to be mediated by soluble factor(s) including the CC-chemokines RANTES, MIP-1α, and MIP-1β (see above) and the alpha defensin family of cytokines. The CC-chemokines are potent suppressors of HIV replication and operate at least in part via blockade of the co-receptor (CCR5) on peripheral blood mononuclear cells for R5 or macrophage-tropic strains of HIV (see above). The alpha defensins appear able to inhibit replication of either R5 or X4 viruses. The mechanism of this inhibition remains unclear. *ADCC*, as described above in relation to humoral immunity, involves the killing of HIV-expressing cells by NK cells armed with specific antibodies directed against HIV antigens. Finally, *NK cells* alone have been shown to be capable of killing HIV-infected target cells in tissue culture. This primitive cytotoxic mechanism of host defense is directed toward nonspecific surveillance for neoplastic transformation and viral infection through recognition of altered class I MHC molecules.

DIAGNOSIS AND LABORATORY MONITORING OF HIV INFECTION

The establishment of HIV as the causative agent of AIDS and related syndromes early in 1984 was followed by the rapid development of sensitive screening tests for HIV infection. By March, 1985, blood donors in the United States were routinely screened for antibodies to HIV. In June 1996, blood banks in the United States added the p24 antigen capture assay to the screening process to help identify the rare infected individuals who were donating blood in the time (up to 3 months) between infection and the development of antibodies. In 2002 the ability to detect early infection with HIV was further enhanced by the licensure of nucleic acid amplification testing as a routine part of blood donor screening. These refinements decreased the interval between infection and detection (window period) from 22 days for antibody testing to 16 days with p24 antigen testing and subsequently to 12 days with nucleic acid testing. The development of sensitive assays for monitoring levels of plasma viremia ushered in a new era of being able to monitor the progression of HIV disease more closely. Utilization of these tests, coupled with the measurement of levels of CD4+ T lymphocytes in peripheral blood, is essential in the management of patients with HIV infection.

DIAGNOSIS OF HIV INFECTION   The diagnosis of HIV infection depends upon the demonstration of antibodies to HIV and/or the direct detection of HIV or one of its components. As noted above, antibodies to HIV generally appear in the circulation 2 to 12 weeks following infection.

The standard screening test for HIV infection is the ELISA, also referred to as an enzyme immunoassay (EIA). This solid-phase assay is an extremely good screening test with a sensitivity of >99.5%. Most diagnostic laboratories use a commercial EIA kit that contains antigens from both HIV-1 and HIV-2 and thus are able to detect either. These kits use both natural and recombinant antigens and are continuously updated to increase their sensitivity to newly discovered species, such as group O viruses (Fig. 173-6). EIA tests are generally scored as positive (highly reactive), negative (nonreactive), or indeterminate (partially reactive). While the EIA is an extremely sensitive test, it is not optimal with regard to specificity. This is particularly true in studies of low-risk individuals, such as volunteer blood donors. In this latter population, only 10% of EIA-positive individuals are subsequently confirmed to have HIV infection. Among the factors associated with false-positive EIA tests are antibodies to class II antigens, autoantibodies, hepatic disease, recent influenza vaccination, and acute viral infections. For these reasons, anyone suspected of having HIV infection based upon a positive or inconclusive EIA result must have the result confirmed with a more specific assay. One can estimate whether or not an indvdual has a recent infection with HIV-1 by comparing the results on a standard assay that will score positive for all infected individuals to the results on an assay modified to be less sensitive ("detuned assay") that will only score positive for individuals with established HIV infection.

The most commonly used confirmatory test is the western blot (Fig. 173-23). This assay takes advantage of the fact that multiple HIV antigens of different, well-characterized molecular weights elicit the production of specific antibodies. These antigens can be separated on the basis of molecular weight, and antibodies to each component can be detected as discrete bands on the western blot. A negative western blot is one in which no bands are present at molecular weights corresponding to HIV gene products. In a patient with a positive or indeterminate EIA and a negative western blot, one can conclude with certainty that the EIA reactivity was a false positive. On the other hand, a western blot demonstrating antibodies to products of all three of the major genes of HIV (*gag*, *pol*, and *env*) is conclusive evidence of infection with HIV. Criteria established by the U.S. Food & Drug Administration (FDA) in 1993 for a positive western blot state that a result is considered positive if antibodies exist to two of the three HIV proteins: p24, gp41, and gp120/160. Using these criteria, ~10% of all blood donors deemed positive for HIV-1

A
1. Virus digested: digest separated into components by molecular weight
2. Proteins transferred to filter paper: reaction with test serum
3. Enzyme-conjugated antihuman antibody added
4. Substrate added and color noted

B
1. Positive HIV-1 infection
2. gp 160 immunization
3. Indeterminate (HIV-2 infection)
4. Indeterminate (cross-reacting antibody to p24)
5. Negative

FIGURE 173-23 *A.* Schematic representation of how a western blot is performed. *B.* Examples of patterns of western blot reactivity. In each instance the western blot strip contains antigens to HIV-1. The sera from the patient immunized to the HIV-1 envelope only contains antibodies to the HIV-1 envelope proteins. The sera from the patient with HIV-2 infection cross-reacts with both *reverse transcriptase* and *gag* gene products of HIV-1.

infection lacked an antibody band to the *pol* gene product p31. Some 50% of these blood donors were subsequently found to be false positives. Thus, the absence of the p31 band should increase the suspicion that one may be dealing with a false-positive test result. In this setting it is prudent to obtain additional confirmation with an RNA-based test and/or a follow-up western blot. By definition, western blot patterns of reactivity that do not fall into the positive or negative categories are considered "indeterminate." There are two possible explanations for an indeterminate western blot result. The most likely explanation in a low-risk individual is that the patient being tested has antibodies that cross-react with one of the proteins of HIV. The most common patterns of cross-reactivity are antibodies that react with p24 and/or p55. The least likely explanation in this setting is that the individual is infected with HIV and is in the process of mounting a classic antibody response. In either instance, the western blot should be repeated in 1 month to determine whether or not the indeterminate pattern is a pattern in evolution. In addition, one may attempt to confirm a diagnosis of HIV infection with the p24 antigen capture assay or one of the tests for HIV RNA (discussed below). While the western blot is an excellent confirmatory test for HIV infection in patients with a positive or indeterminate EIA, it is a poor screening test. Among individuals with a negative EIA and PCR for HIV, 20 to 30% may show one or more bands on western blot. While these bands are usually faint and represent cross-reactivity, their presence creates a situation in which other diagnostic modalities [such as DNA PCR, RNA PCR, the (b)DNA assay, or p24 antigen capture] must be employed to ensure that the bands do not indicate early HIV infection.

A guideline for the use of these serologic tests in attempting to make a diagnosis of HIV infection is depicted in Fig. 173-24. In patients in whom HIV infection is suspected, the appropriate initial test is the EIA. If the result is negative, unless there is strong reason to suspect early HIV infection (as in a patient exposed within the previous 3 months), the diagnosis is ruled out and retesting should be performed only as clinically indicated. If the EIA is indeterminate or positive, the test should be repeated. If the repeat is negative on two occasions, one can assume that the initial positive reading was due to a technical error in the performance of the assay and that the patient is negative. If the repeat is indeterminate or positive, one should proceed to the HIV-1 western blot. If the western blot is positive, the diagnosis is HIV-1

infection. If the western blot is negative, the EIA can be assumed to have been a false positive for HIV-1 and the diagnosis of HIV-1 infection is ruled out. It would be prudent at this point to perform specific serologic testing for HIV-2 following the same type of algorithm. If the western blot for HIV-1 is indeterminate, it should be repeated in 4 to 6 weeks; in addition, one may proceed to a p24 antigen capture assay, HIV-1 RNA assay, or HIV-1 DNA PCR and specific serologic testing for HIV-2. If the p24 and HIV RNA assays are negative and there is no progression in the western blot, a diagnosis of HIV-1 is ruled out. If either the p24 or HIV-1 RNA assay is positive and/or the HIV-1 western blot shows progression, a tentative diagnosis of HIV-1 infection can be made and later confirmed with a follow-up western blot demonstrating a positive pattern.

As mentioned above, a variety of laboratory tests are available for the direct detection of HIV or its components (Table 173-9; Fig. 173-25). These tests may be of considerable help in making a diagnosis of HIV infection when the western blot results are indeterminate. In addition, the tests detecting levels of HIV RNA can be used to determine prognosis and to assess the response to antiretroviral therapies. The

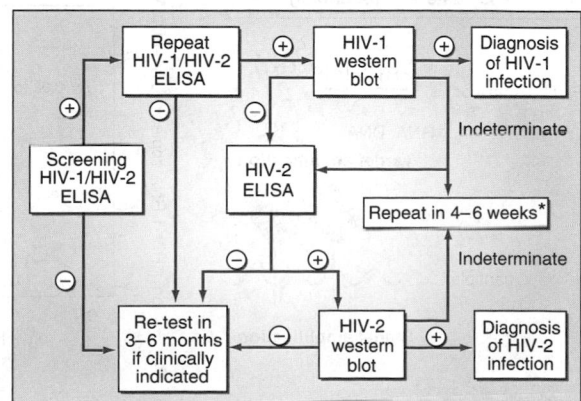

FIGURE 173-24 Algorithm for the use of serologic tests in the diagnosis of HIV-1 or HIV-2 infection. * Stable indeterminate western blot 4 to 6 weeks later makes HIV infection unlikely. However, it should be repeated twice at 3-month intervals to rule out HIV infection. Alternatively, one may test for HIV-1 p24 antigen or HIV RNA.

TABLE 173-9 *Characteristics of Tests for Direct Detection of HIV*

Test	Technique	Sensitivity[a]	Cost/Test
Immune complex–dissociated p24 antigen capture assay	Measurement of levels of HIV-1 core protein in an ELISA-based format following dissociation of antigen-antibody complexes by weak acid treatment	Positive in 50% of patients; detects down to 15 pg/mL of p24 protein	$1–2
HIV RNA by PCR	PCR amplification of cDNA generated from viral RNA (target amplification)	Reliable to 40 copies/mL of HIV RNA	$75–150
HIV RNA by bDNA	Measurement of levels of particle-associated HIV RNA in a nucleic acid capture assay employing signal amplification	Reliable to 75 copies/mL of HIV RNA	$75–150
HIV RNA by NASBA	Isothermic nucleic acid amplification with internal controls	Reliable to 176 copies/mL of HIV RNA	$75–150

[a] Sensitivity figures refer to those approved by the US FDA. Prices may be lower in large volume settings.
Note: ELISA, enzyme-linked immunosorbent assay; PCR, polymerase chain reaction; NASBA, nucleic acid sequence based assay.

While routinely used in the past, along with testing for HIV antibodies, to screen blood donors for HIV infection, this use of the p24 assay has been replaced by the use of nucleic acid testing. These tests are of value in making a diagnosis of HIV infection, in establishing intial prognosis and determining the need for therapy, and for monitoring the effects of therapy. In addition to these three commercially available tests, the *DNA PCR* is also employed by research laboratories for making a diagnosis of HIV infection by amplifying HIV proviral DNA from peripheral blood mononuclear cells. The commercially available RNA detection tests have a sensitivity of 50 to 75 copies of HIV RNA per milliliter of plasma, while the DNA PCR tests can detect proviral DNA at a frequency of one copy per 10,000 to 100,000 cells. Thus, these tests are extremely sensitive. One frequent consequence of a high degree of sensitivity is some loss of specificity, and false-positive results have been reported with each of these techniques. For this reason, a positive EIA with a confirmatory western blot remains the "gold standard" for a diagnosis of HIV infection, and the interpretation of other test results must be done with this in mind.

simplest of the direct detection tests is the *p24 antigen capture assay*. This is an EIA-type assay in which the solid phase consists of antibodies to the p24 antigen of HIV. It detects the viral protein p24 in the blood of HIV-infected individuals where it exists either as free antigen or complexed to anti-p24 antibodies. Overall, ~30% of individuals with untreated HIV infection have detectable levels of free p24 antigen. This increases to about 50% when samples are treated with a weak acid to dissociate antigen-antibody complexes. Throughout the course of HIV infection, an equilibrium exists between p24 antigen and anti-p24 antibodies. During the first few weeks of infection, before an immune response develops, there is a brisk rise in p24 antigen levels (Fig. 173-22). After the development of anti-p24 antibodies, these levels decline. Late in the course of infection, when circulating levels of virus are high, p24 antigen levels also increase, particularly when detected by techniques involving dissociation of antigen-antibody complexes. This assay has its greatest use as a screening test for HIV infection in patients suspected of having the acute HIV syndrome, as high levels of p24 antigen are present prior to the development of antibodies. In addition, it is currently used routinely along with the HIV EIA and nucleic acid test to screen blood donors in the United States for evidence of HIV infection. The ability to measure and monitor levels of HIV RNA in the plasma of patients with HIV infection has been of extraordinary value in furthering our understanding of the pathogenesis of HIV infection and in providing a diagnostic tool in settings where measurements of anti-HIV antibodies may be misleading, such as in acute infection and neonatal infection. Three assays are predominantly used for this purpose. They are the reverse transcriptase PCR (*RT-PCR*; Amplicor); the branched DNA (*bDNA*; VERSANT); and the nucleic acid sequenced based assay (*NASBA*; NucliSens).

available RNA detection tests have a sensitivity of 50 to 75 copies of HIV RNA per milliliter of plasma, while the DNA PCR tests can detect proviral DNA at a frequency of one copy per 10,000 to 100,000 cells. Thus, these tests are extremely sensitive. One frequent consequence of a high degree of sensitivity is some loss of specificity, and false-positive results have been reported with each of these techniques. For this reason, a positive EIA with a confirmatory western blot remains the "gold standard" for a diagnosis of HIV infection, and the interpretation of other test results must be done with this in mind.

In the RT-PCR technique, following DNase treatment, a cDNA copy is made of all RNA species present in plasma. Insofar as HIV is an RNA virus, this will result in the production of DNA copies of the HIV genome in amounts proportional to the amount of HIV RNA present in plasma. This cDNA is then amplified and characterized using standard PCR techniques, employing primer pairs that can distinguish genomic cDNA from messenger cDNA. The bDNA assay involves the use of a solid-phase nucleic acid capture system and signal amplification through successive nucleic acid hybridizations to detect small quantities of HIV RNA. Both tests can achieve a tenfold increase in sensitivity to 40 to 50 copies of HIV RNA per milliliter with a preconcentration step in which plasma undergoes ultracentrifugation to pellet the viral particles. The NASBA technique involves the isothermal amplification of a sequence within the gag region of HIV in the presence of internal standards and employs the production of multiple RNA copies through the action of T7-RNA polymerase. The lower limit of detection for the NASBA is 176 copies/mL.

In addition to being a diagnostic and prognostic tool, RT-PCR is also useful for amplifying defined areas of the HIV genome for sequence analysis and has become an important technique for studies of sequence diversity and microbial resistance to antiretroviral agents. In patients with a positive or indeterminate EIA test and an indeterminate western blot, and in patients in whom serologic testing may be unreliable (such as patients with hypogammaglobulinemia or advanced HIV disease), these tests for quantitating HIV RNA in plasma provide valuable tools for making a diagnosis of HIV infection; however, they should be used for diagnosis only when standard serologic testing has failed to provide a definitive result.

FIGURE 173-25 Comparison of RT-PCR and bDNA assays. *A.* Schematic representation of reverse transcriptase–polymerase chain reaction (RT-PCR) and bDNA assays. See text for detailed description. *B.* Scatter plot of $\log_{10}$ v3 bDNA versus $\log_{10}$ RT-PCR with the line of equity (solid) and the fitted regression line (hatched). The equation for the fitted regression line is given in the lower-right-hand corner. There is good agreement between the two assays. v3, version 3 of the bDNA assay. (*From HC Highbarger et al: J Clin Microbiol 37:3612, 1999.*)

$r = 0.98$ ($p < .0001$)

Line of equality

Predicted $\log_{10}$ v3-bDNA = $-0.0915 + 1.0052 * \log_{10}$ RT-PCR

LABORATORY MONITORING OF PATIENTS WITH HIV INFECTION The epidemic of HIV infection and AIDS has provided the clinician with new challenges for integrating clinical and laboratory data to effect optimal patient management.

The close relationship between clinical manifestations of HIV infection and CD4+ T cell count has made measurement of the latter a routine part of the evaluation of HIV-infected individuals. Determinations of CD4+ T cell counts and measurements of the levels of HIV RNA in serum or plasma provide a powerful set of tools for determining prognosis and monitoring response to therapy. While the CD4+ T cell count provides information on the current immunologic status of the patient, the HIV RNA level predicts what will happen to the CD4+ T cell count in the near future, and hence provides an important piece of prognostic information.

CD4+ T Cell Counts The CD4+ T cell count is the laboratory test generally accepted as the best indicator of the immediate state of immunologic competence of the patient with HIV infection. This measurement, which is the product of the percent of CD4+ T cells (determined by flow cytometry) and the total lymphocyte count [determined by the white blood cell count (WBC) and the differential percent] has been shown to correlate very well with the level of immunologic competence. Patients with CD4+ T cell counts <200/μL are at high risk of infection with *P. carinii*, while patients with CD4+ T cell counts <50/μL are at high risk of infection with CMV and mycobacteria of the *M. avium complex* (MAC) (Fig. 173-26). Patients with HIV infection should have CD4+ T cell measurements performed at the time of diagnosis and every 3 to 6 months thereafter. More frequent measurements should be made if a declining trend is noted. According to most guidelines, a CD4 T cell count <350/μL is an indication for consideration of initiating antiretroviral therapy, and a decline in CD4+ T cell count of >25% is an indication for considering a change in therapy. Once the CD4+ T cell count is <200/μL, patients should be placed on a regimen for *P. carinii* prophylaxis, and once the count is <50/μL, primary prophylaxis for MAC infection is indicated. As with any laboratory measurement, one may wish to obtain two determinations prior to any significant changes in patient management based upon CD4+ T cell count alone.

HIV RNA Determinations Facilitated by highly sensitive techniques for the precise quantitation of small amounts of nucleic acids, the measurement of serum or plasma levels of HIV RNA has become an essential component in the monitoring of patients with HIV infection. As discussed under diagnosis of HIV infection, the two most commonly used techniques are the RT-PCR assay and the bDNA assay. Both assays generate data in the form of number of copies of HIV RNA per milliliter of serum or plasma and, by employing a 1:10 concentration step with ultracentrifugation, can detect as few as 50 to 75 copies of HIV RNA per milliliter of plasma. Although earlier versions of the bDNA assay generated values that were ~50% of those of the RT-PCR assay, the more recent versions (version 3 or higher) provide numbers essentially identical to those of the RT-PCR test (Fig. 173-25). While it is common practice to describe levels of HIV RNA below these cut-offs as "undetectable," this is a term that should be avoided as it is imprecise and leaves the false impression that the level of virus is 0. By utilizing more sensitive, nested PCR techniques and by studying tissue levels of virus as well as plasma levels, HIV RNA can be detected in virtually every patient with HIV infection. Measurements of changes in HIV RNA levels over time have been of great value in delineating the relationship between levels of virus and rates of disease progression (Fig. 173-17), the rates of viral turnover, the relationship between immune system activation and viral replication, and the time to development of drug resistance. HIV RNA measurements are

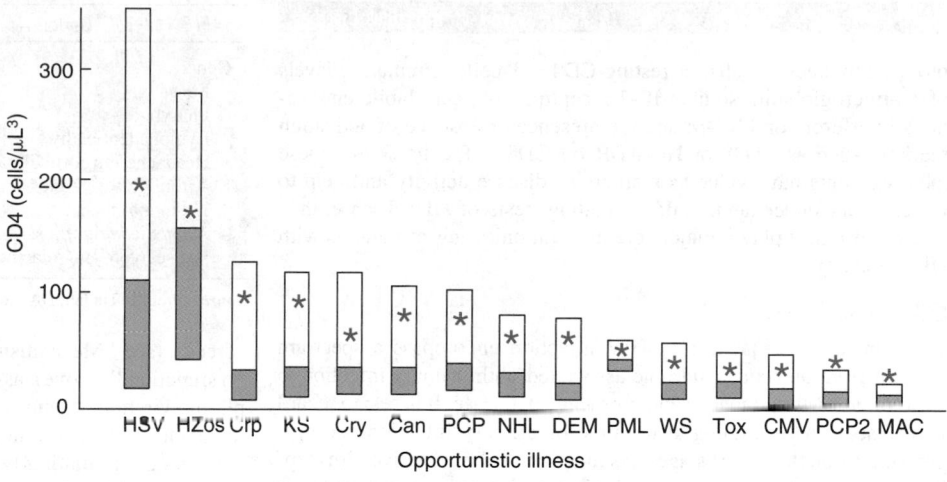

FIGURE 173-26 Relationship between CD4+ T cell counts and the development of opportunistic diseases. Boxplot of the median (line inside the box), first quartile (bottom of the box), third quartile (top of the box), and mean (asterisk) CD4+ lymphocyte count at the time of the development of opportunistic disease. Can, candidal esophagitis; CMV, cytomegalovirus infection; Crp, cryptosporidiosis; Cry, cryptococcal meningitis; DEM, AIDS dementia complex; HSV, herpes simplex virus infection; HZos, herpes zoster; KS, Kaposi's sarcoma; MAC, *Mycobacterium avium* complex bacteremia; NHL, non-Hodgkin's lymphoma; PCP, primary *Pneumocystis carinii* pneumonia; PCP2, secondary *Pneumocystis carinii* pneumonia; PML, progressive multifocal leukoencephalopathy; Tox, *Toxoplasma gondii* encephalitis; WS, wasting syndrome. (*From RD Moore, RE Chaisson: Ann Intern Med 124:633, 1996.*)

greatly influenced by the state of activation of the immune system and may fluctuate greatly in the setting of secondary infections or immunization. For these reasons, decisions based upon HIV RNA levels should never be made on a single determination. Measurements of plasma HIV RNA levels should be made at the time of HIV diagnosis and every 3 to 4 months thereafter in the untreated patient. In general, most guidelines suggest that therapy be considered in patients with >50,000 copies of HIV RNA per milliliter (see below). Following the initiation of therapy or any change in therapy, plasma HIV RNA levels should be monitored approximately every 4 weeks until the effectiveness of the therapeutic regimen is determined by the development of a new steady-state level of HIV RNA. In most instances of effective therapy this will be <50 copies per milliliter. This level of virus is generally achieved within 6 months of the initiation of effective treatment. During therapy, levels of HIV RNA should be monitored every 3 to 4 months to evaluate the continuing effectiveness of therapy.

HIV Resistance Testing The availability of multiple antiretroviral drugs as treatment options has generated a great deal of interest in the potential for measuring the sensitivity of an individual's HIV virus(es) to different antiretroviral agents. HIV resistance testing can be done through either genotypic or phenotypic measurements. In the genotypic assays, sequence analyses of the HIV genomes obtained from patients are compared to sequences of viruses with known antiretroviral resistance profiles. In the phenotypic assays, the in vivo growth of viral isolates obtained from the patient are compared to the growth of reference strains of the virus in the presence or absence of different antiretroviral drugs. A modification of this phenotypic approach utilizes a comparison of the enzymatic activities of the reverse transcriptase or protease genes obtained by molecular cloning of patients' isolates to the enzymatic activities of genes obtained from reference strains of HIV in the presence or absence of different drugs targeted to these genes. These tests are quite good in identifying those antiretroviral agents that have been utilized in the past in a given patient. In the hands of experts, resistance testing enhances the short-term ability to decrease viral load by ~0.5 log compared to changing drugs merely on the basis of drug history. While some have advocated the use of resistance testing in the selection of an initial treatment regimen, the value of resistance testing in this setting is unknown.

Other Tests A variety of other laboratory tests have been studied as potential markers of HIV disease activity. Among these are quantitative culture of replication-competent HIV from plasma, peripheral blood mononuclear cells, or resting CD4+ T cells; circulating levels of β_2-microglobulin, soluble IL-2 receptor, IgA, acid-labile endogenous interferon, or TNF-α; and the presence or absence of activation markers such as CD38 or HLA-DR on CD8+ T cells. While these measurements have value as markers of disease activity and help to increase our understanding of the pathogenesis of HIV disease, they do not currently play a major role in the monitoring of patients with HIV infection.

CLINICAL MANIFESTATIONS

The clinical consequences of HIV infection encompass a spectrum ranging from an acute syndrome associated with primary infection to a prolonged asymptomatic state to advanced disease. It is best to regard HIV disease as beginning at the time of primary infection and progressing through various stages. As mentioned above, active virus replication and progressive immunologic impairment occur throughout the course of HIV infection in most patients. With the exception of the rare true long-term nonprogressors (see above), HIV disease in untreated patients inexorably progresses even during the clinically latent stage. However, antiretroviral therapy has had a major impact on blocking or slowing the progression of disease over extended periods of time in a substantial proportion of adequately treated patients (see below).

THE ACUTE HIV SYNDROME   It is estimated that 50 to 70% of individuals with HIV infection experience an acute clinical syndrome approximately 3 to 6 weeks after primary infection (Fig. 173-27). Varying degrees of clinical severity have been reported, and although it has been suggested that symptomatic seroconversion leading to the seeking of medical attention indicates an increased risk for an accelerated course of disease, this has not been shown definitively. In fact, there does not appear to be a correlation between the level of the initial burst of viremia in acute HIV infection and the subsequent course of disease. The typical clinical findings in the acute HIV syndrome are listed in Table 173-10; they occur along with a burst of plasma viremia. It has been reported that several symptoms of the acute HIV syndrome (fever, skin rash, pharyngitis, and myalgia) occur less frequently in those infected by injection drug use versus those infected by sexual contact. The syndrome is typical of an acute viral syndrome and has been likened to acute infectious mononucleosis. Symptoms usually persist for 1 to several weeks and gradually subside as an immune response to HIV develops and the levels of plasma viremia decrease. Opportunistic infections have been reported during this stage of infection, reflecting the immunodeficiency that results from reduced numbers of CD4+ T cells and likely also from the dysfunction of CD4+ T cells owing to viral protein and endogenous cytokine-induced perturbations

TABLE 173-10   Clinical Findings in the Acute HIV Syndrome

General	Neurologic
Fever	Meningitis
Pharyngitis	Encephalitis
Lymphadenopathy	Peripheral neuropathy
Headache/retroorbital pain	Myelopathy
Arthralgias/myalgias	Dermatologic
Lethargy/malaise	Erythematous maculopapular rash
Anorexia/weight loss	Mucocutaneous ulceration
Nausea/vomiting/diarrhea	

Source: From B Tindall, DA Cooper: AIDS 5:1, 1991.

of cells (see "Mechanisms of CD4+ T Lymphocyte Depletion and Dysfunction," above) associated with the extremely high levels of plasma viremia. A number of immunologic abnormalities accompany the acute HIV syndrome, including multiphasic perturbations of the numbers of circulating lymphocyte subsets. The number of total lymphocytes and T cell subsets (CD4+ and CD8+) are initially reduced. An inversion of the CD4+/CD8+ T cell ratio occurs later because of a rise in the number of CD8+ T cells. In fact, there may be a selective and transient expansion of CD8+ T cell subsets, as determined by T cell receptor analysis (see above). The total circulating CD8+ T cell count may remain elevated or return to normal; however, CD4+ T cell levels usually remain somewhat depressed, although there may be a slight rebound towards normal. Lymphadenopathy occurs in ~70% of individuals with primary HIV infection. Most patients recover spontaneously from this syndrome and many are left with only a mildly depressed CD4+ T cell count that remains stable for a variable period before beginning its progressive decline (see below); in some individuals, the CD4+ T cell count returns to the normal range. Approximately 10% of patients manifest a fulminant course of immunologic and clinical deterioration after primary infection, even after the disappearance of initial symptoms. In most patients, primary infection with or without the acute syndrome is followed by a prolonged period of clinical latency.

THE ASYMPTOMATIC STAGE—CLINICAL LATENCY   Although the length of time from initial infection to the development of clinical disease varies greatly, the median time for untreated patients is ~10 years. As emphasized above, HIV disease with active virus replication is ongoing and progressive during this asymptomatic period. The rate of disease progression is directly correlated with HIV RNA levels. Patients with high levels of HIV RNA in plasma progress to symptomatic disease faster than do patients with low levels of HIV RNA (Fig. 173-17). Some patients referred to as long-term nonprogressors show little if any decline in CD4+ T cell counts over extended periods of time. These patients generally have extremely low levels of HIV RNA. Certain other patients remain entirely asymptomatic despite the fact that their CD4+ T cell counts show a steady progressive decline to extremely low levels. In these patients, the appearance of an opportunistic disease may be the first manifestation of HIV infection. During the asymptomatic period of HIV infection, the average rate of CD4+ T cell decline is ~50/μL per year. When the CD4+ T cell count falls to <200/μL, the resulting state of immunodeficiency is severe enough to place the patient at high risk for opportunistic infection and neoplasms, and hence for clinically apparent disease.

SYMPTOMATIC DISEASE   Symptoms of HIV disease can appear at any time during the course of HIV infection. Generally speaking, the spectrum of illness that one observes changes as the CD4+ T cell count declines. The more severe and life-threatening complications of HIV infection occur in patients with CD4+ T cells counts <200/μL. A diagnosis of AIDS is made in anyone with HIV infection and a CD4+ T cell count <200/μL and in anyone with HIV infection who develops one of the HIV-associated diseases considered to be indicative of a severe defect in cell-mediated immunity (category C, Table 173-2). While the causative agents of the secondary infections are characteristically opportunistic organisms such as *P. carinii*, atypical mycobacteria, CMV, and other organisms that do not ordinarily cause disease

FIGURE 173-27   The acute HIV syndrome. See text for detailed description. (*Adapted from G Pantaleo et al: N Engl J Med 328:327, 1993.*)

in the absence of a compromised immune system, they also include common bacterial and mycobacterial pathogens. Approximately 60% of deaths among AIDS patients are as a direct result of an infection other than HIV, with *P. carinii*, viral hepatitis, and non-AIDS-defining bacterial infections heading the list. Following the widespread use of combination antiretroviral therapy and implementation of guidelines for the prevention of opportunistic infections (Table 173-11), the incidence of secondary infections has decreased dramatically (Fig. 173-28). Overall, the clinical spectrum of HIV disease is constantly changing as patients live longer and new and better approaches to treatment and prophylaxis are developed. In general, it should be stressed that a key element of treatment of symptomatic complications of HIV disease, whether they are primary or secondary, is achieving good control of HIV replication through the use of combination antiretroviral therapy and instituting primary and secondary prophylaxis as indicated.

Disease of the Respiratory System Acute bronchitis and sinusitis are prevalent during all stages of HIV infection. The most severe cases tend to occur in patients with lower CD4+ T cell counts. Sinusitis presents as fever, nasal congestion, and headache. The diagnosis is made by computed tomography (CT) or magnetic resonance imaging (MRI). The maxillary sinuses are most commonly involved; however, disease is also frequently seen in the ethmoid, sphenoid, and frontal sinuses. While some patients may improve without antibiotic therapy, radiographic improvement is quicker and more pronounced in patients who have received antimicrobial therapy. It is postulated that this high incidence of sinusitis results from an increased frequency of infection with encapsulated organisms such as *H. influenzae* and *Streptococcus pneumoniae*. In patients with low CD4+ T cell counts one may see mucormycosis infections of the sinuses. In contrast to the course of this infection in other patient populations, mucormycosis of the sinuses in patients with HIV infection may progress more slowly. In this setting aggressive, frequent local debridement in addition to local and systemic amphotericin B may be needed for effective treatment.

Pulmonary disease is one of the most frequent complications of HIV infection. The most common manifestation of pulmonary disease is pneumonia. The two most common causes of pneumonia are bacterial infections and *P. carinii* infection. Other major causes of pulmonary infiltrates include mycobacterial infections, fungal infections, nonspecific interstitial pneumonitis, KS, and lymphoma.

Pneumonia is seen with an increased frequency in patients with HIV infection; they appear to be particularly prone to infections with encapsulated organisms. *S. pneumoniae* (Chap. 119) and *H. influenzae* (Chap. 130) are responsible for most cases of bacterial pneumonia in patients with AIDS. This may be a consequence of altered B cell function and/or defects in neutrophil function that may be secondary to HIV disease (see above). Pneumococcal infection may be the earliest serious infection to occur in patients with HIV disease. This can present as pneumonia, sinusitis, and/or bacteremia. Patients with HIV infection have a sixfold increase in the incidence of pneumococcal pneumonia and a 100-fold increase in the incidence of pneumococcal bacteremia. Pneumococcal disease may be seen in patients with relatively intact immune systems. In one study, the baseline CD4+ T cell count at the time of a first episode of pneumococcal pneumonia was ~300/μL. Of interest is the fact that the inflammatory response to pneumococcal infection appears proportional to the CD4+ T cell count. Due to this high risk of pneumococcal disease, immunization with pneumococcal polysaccharide is one of the generally recommended prophylactic measures for patients with HIV infection and CD4+ T cell counts >200/μL. It is less clear if this intervention is of benefit in patients with more advanced disease and high viral loads.

P. carinii pneumonia (PCP), once the hallmark of AIDS, has dramatically declined in incidence following the development of effective prophylactic regimens and the widespread use of combination antiretroviral therapy. It is, however, the single most common cause of pneumonia in patients with HIV infection in the United States and can be identified as a likely etiologic agent in 25% of cases of pneumonia in patients with HIV infection. Approximately 25% of cases of HIV-associated PCP occur in patients who are unaware of their HIV status. The risk of PCP is greatest among those who have experienced a previous bout of PCP and those who have CD4+ T cell counts of <200/μL. Overall, 79% of patients with PCP have CD4+ T cell counts <100/μL and 95% of patients have CD4+ T cell counts <200/μL. Recurrent fever, night sweats, thrush, and unexplained weight loss are also associated with an increased incidence of PCP. For these reasons, it is strongly recommended that all patients with CD4+ T cell counts <200/μL (or a CD4 percentage <15) receive some form of PCP prophylaxis. At present the incidence of PCP is approaching zero in patients with known HIV infection receiving appropriate antiretroviral therapy and prophylaxis. In the United States, primary PCP is now occurring at a median CD4+ T cell count of 36/μL, while secondary PCP is occurring at a median CD4+ T cell count of 10/μL. Patients with PCP generally present with fever and a cough that is usually nonproductive or productive of only scant amounts of white sputum. They may complain of a characteristic retrosternal chest pain that is worse on inspiration and is described as sharp or burning. HIV-associated PCP may have an indolent course characterized by weeks of vague symptoms and should be included in the differential diagnosis of fever, pulmonary complaints, or unexplained weight loss in any patient with HIV infection and <200 CD4+ T cells/μL. The most common finding on chest x-ray is either a normal film, if the disease is suspected early, or a faint bilateral interstitial infiltrate. The classic finding of a dense perihilar infiltrate is unusual in patients with AIDS. In patients with PCP who have been receiving aerosolized pentamidine for prophylaxis, one may see an x-ray picture of upper lobe cavitary disease, reminiscent of TB. Other less common findings on chest x-ray include lobar infiltrates and pleural effusions. Routine laboratory evaluation is usually of little help in the differential diagnosis of PCP. A mild leukocytosis is common, although this may not be obvious in patients with prior neutropenia. Arterial blood gases may indicate hypoxemia with a decline in Pa_{O_2} and an increase in the arterial-alveolar (a − A) gradient. Arterial blood gas measurements not only aid in making the diagnosis of PCP but also provide important information for staging the severity of the disease and directing treatment (see below). A definitive diagnosis of PCP requires demonstration of the trophozoite or cyst form of the organism in samples obtained from induced sputum, bronchoalveolar lavage, transbronchial biopsy, or open lung biopsy. PCR has been used to detect specific DNA sequences for *P. carinii* in clinical specimens where histologic examinations have failed to make a diagnosis.

In addition to pneumonia, a number of other clinical problems have been reported in HIV-infected patients as a result of infection with *P. carinii*. Otic involvement may be seen as a primary infection, presenting as a polypoid mass involving the external auditory canal. In patients receiving aerosolized pentamidine for prophylaxis against PCP one may see a variety of extrapulmonary manifestations of *P. carinii*. These include ophthalmic lesions of the choroid, a necrotizing vasculitis that resembles Burger's disease, bone marrow hypoplasia, and intestinal obstruction. Other organs that have been involved include lymph nodes, spleen, liver, kidney, pancreas, pericardium, heart, thyroid, and adrenals. Organ infection may be associated with cystic lesions that may appear calcified on CT or ultrasound.

The standard treatment for PCP or disseminated pneumocystosis is trimethoprim/sulfamethoxazole (TMP/SMX). A high incidence of side effects, particularly skin rash and bone marrow suppression, is seen with TMP/SMX in patients with HIV infection. Alternative treatments for mild to moderate PCP include dapsone/trimethoprim and clindamycin/primaquine. Intravenous pentamidine is the treatment of choice for severe disease in the patient unable to tolerate TMP/SMX. For patients with a Pa_{O_2} < 70 mmHg or with an a − A gradient >35 mmHg, adjunct glucocorticoid therapy should be used in addition to specific antimicrobials. Overall, treatment should be for 21 days and followed by secondary prophylaxis. Prophylaxis for PCP is indicated for any HIV-infected individual who has experienced a prior bout of

Pathogen	Indications	First Choice(s)	Alternatives
STRONGLY RECOMMENDED AS STANDARD OF CARE FOR PRIMARY AND SECONDARY PROPHYLAXIS			
Pneumocystis carinii	CD4 count <200/μL or Oropharyngeal candidiasis or Unexplained fever >2 weeks or Prior bout of PCP	Trimethoprim/sulfamethoxazole (TMP/SMZ), 1 DS tablet qd	Dapsone 50 mg bid PO or 100 mg/d PO
	May stop prophylaxis if CD4+ T cell count > 200/μL for 6 mo	TMP/SMZ, 1 SS tablet qd	Dapsone 50 mg/d PO+ Pyrimethamine 50 mg/wk PO+ Leucovorin 25 mg/wk PO Dapsone 200 mg PO+ Pyrimethamine 75 mg + Leucovorin 25 mg PO weekly Aerosolized pentamidine, 300 mg qm via Respirgard II nebulizer Atovoquone 1500 mg/d PO TMP/SMZ 1 DS tablet PO 3$\times$/wk
Mycobacterium tuberculosis Isoniazid sensitive	Skin test >5 mm or Prior positive test without treatment or Contact with case of active TB	Isoniazid 300 mg PO+ Pyridoxine 50 mg/d PO $\times$9 mo	Rifampin 600 mg/d PO or Rifabutin 300 mg/d PO+ Pyrazinamide 20 (mg/kg)/d PO $\times$2 mo
		Isoniazid 900 mg PO+ Pyridoxine 100 mg PO 2 $\times$/wk $\times$9 mo	Rifampin 600 mg/d PO or Rifabutin 300 mg/d PO $\times$4 mo
Isoniazid resistant	Same with high probability of exposure to isoniazid-resistant TB	Rifabutin 300 mg or Rifampin 600 mg; PO qd $\times$4 mo	Pyrazinamide 20 (mg/kg)/d PO $\times$2 mo + either Rifampin 600 mg/d or Rifabutin 300 mg/d PO $\times$4 mo
Multidrug resistant	Same with high probability of exposure to multidrug resistant TB	Consult local public health authorities	
Mycobacterium-avium complex	CD4 count <50/μL Prior documented disseminated disease	Azithromycin 1200 mg weekly PO Clarithromycin 500 mg bid PO	Rifabutin 300 mg/d PO Azithromycin 1200 mg weekly PO + Rifabutin 300 mg/d PO
	May stop prophylaxis if CD4+ T cell count > 100/μL for 6 mo	Clarithromycin 500 mg bid PO + Ethambutol 15 (mg/kg)/d PO +/− Rifabutin 300 mg/d PO	Azithromycin 500 mg/d PO + Ethambutol 15 (mg/kg)/d PO +/− Rifabutin 300 mg/d PO
Toxoplasma gondii	IgG antibody and CD4 count <100/μL	TMP/SMZ 1 DS tablet qd	TMP/SMZ 1 SS tablet qd Dapsone 50 mg/d PO + Pyrimethamine 50 mg weekly PO + Leucovorin 25 mg weekly PO Dapsone 200 mg PO + Pyrimethamine 75 mg PO + Leucovorin 25 mg PO weekly Atovaquone 1500 mg PO + Pyrimethamine 25 mg PO + Leucovorin 10 mg PO daily
	Prior toxoplasmic encephalitis	Sulfadiazine 500–1000 mg qid PO+ Pyrimethamine 25–50 mg/d PO+ Leucovorin 10–25 mg/d PO Atovaquone 750 mg PO q6–12 h +/− Pyrimethamine 25 mg/d + Leucovorin 10 mg/d PO	Clindamycin 300–450 mg q6–8h PO+ Pyrimethamine 25–75 mg/d PO+ Leucovorin 10–25 mg/d PO
Varicella zoster virus	Significant exposure to chickenpox or shingles in a patient with no history of immunization or prior exposure to either	Varicella zoster immune globulin 6.25 mL, IM, within 96 h	
Cryptococcus neoformans	Prior documented disease	Fluconazole 200 mg/d PO	Amphotericin B 0.6–1.0 mg/kg 3 $\times$/wk IV Itraconazole 200 mg/d PO
Histoplasma capsulatum	Prior documented disease	Itraconazole 200 mg bid PO	Amphotericin B 1.0 (mg/kg)/wk IV
Coccidioides immitis	Prior documented disease	Fluconazole 400 mg/d PO	Amphotericin B 1.0 (mg/kg)/wk IV Itraconazole 200 mg/d PO
Salmonella species	Prior bacteremia	Ciprofloxacin 500 mg bid PO for several months	
Cytomegalovirus	Prior end-organ disease May stop prophylaxis if CD4+ T cell count > 100/μL for 6 mo	Ganciclovir, 5–6 mg/kg 5–7 d/wk IV Ganciclovir 1000 mg tid PO Foscarnet 90–120 (mg/kg)/d IV	Cidofovir 5 mg/kg every other week IV + Probenecid Formivirsen 330 μg intravitreal q2–4 wk
	Prior retinitis	Ganciclovir implant q6–9 mo + Ganciclovir 1–1.5 g PO tid Ganciclovir sustained-release implant q6–9mo + Ganciclovir 1–1.5 g tid PO	Valganciclovir 900 mg PO daily Fomivirsen, 1 vial injected into the vitreous q2–4wk

(continued)

TABLE 173-11— *(Continued)*

Pathogen	Indications	First Choice(s)	Alternatives
IMMUNIZATIONS GENERALLY RECOMMENDED			
Hepatitis B virus	All susceptible (anti-HBc and anti-HBs negative) patients	Hepatitis B vaccine: 3 doses	
Hepatitis A virus	All susceptible (anti-HAV negative) patients with chronic hepatitis C or at increased risk for hepatitis A	Hepatitis A vaccine: 2 doses	
Influenza virus	All patients annually	Inactivated trivalent influenza virus vaccine 1 dose yearly Oseltamivir 75 mg PO qd Rimantadine or amantadine 100 mg PO qd	
Streptococcus pneumoniae	All patients	Pneumoccal vaccine 0.5 mL IM ×1 if CD4 count >200/μL Reimmunize patients initially immunized at a CD4 count <200/μL whose CD4 count then increases to >200/μL	
RECOMMENDED FOR PREVENTION OF SEVERE OR FREQUENT RECURRENCES			
Herpes simplex	Frequent/severe recurrences	Acyclovir 200 mg tid PO Acyclovir 400 mg bid PO Famciclovir 250 mg bid PO	Valacyclovir 500 mg PO bid
Candida	Frequent/severe recurrences	Fluconazole 100–200 mg/d PO	Itraconazole solution 200 mg/d PO

Note: DS, double strength; SS, single strength; PCP, *Pneumocystis carinii* pneumonia; TB, tuberculosis

PCP, any patient with a CD4+ T cell count of <200/μL or a CD4 percentage <15, any patient with unexplained fever for >2 weeks, and any patient with a history of oropharyngeal candidiasis. The preferred regimen for prophylaxis is TMP/SMX, one double-strength tablet daily. This regimen also provides protection against toxoplasmosis and some bacterial respiratory pathogens. For patients who cannot

tolerate TMP/SMX, alternatives include dapsone plus pyrimethamine plus leucovorin, aerosolized pentamidine administered by the Respirgard II nebulizer, and atovaquone. Primary or secondary prophylaxis for PCP can be discontinued in those patients treated with combination antiretroviral therapy who maintain good suppression of HIV (<500 copies per milliliter) and CD4+ T cell counts >200/μL for at least 3 to 6 months.

M. tuberculosis, once thought to be on its way to extinction in the United States, experienced a resurgence associated with the HIV epidemic (Chap. 150). Worldwide, approximately one-third of all AIDS-related deaths are associated with TB. In the United States ~5% of AIDS patients have active TB. HIV infection increases the risk of developing active TB by a factor of 100. For the patient with untreated HIV infection and a positive PPD skin test, the rate of reactivation TB is 7 to 10% per year. Untreated TB can accelerate the course of HIV infection. Levels of plasma HIV RNA increase in the setting of active TB and decline in the setting of successful TB treatment. Active TB is most common in patients 25 to 44 years of age, in African Americans and Hispanics, in patients in New York City and Miami, and in patients in developing countries. In these demographic groups, 20 to 70% of the new cases of active TB are in patients with HIV infection. The epidemic of TB embedded in the epidemic of HIV infection probably represents the greatest health risk to the general public and the health care profession associated with the HIV epidemic. In contrast to infection with atypical mycobacteria such as MAC, active TB often develops relatively early in the course of HIV infection and may be an early clinical sign of HIV disease. In one study, the median CD4+ T cell count at presentation of TB was 326/μL. The clinical manifestations of TB in HIV-infected patients are quite varied and generally show different patterns as a function of the CD4+ T cell count. In patients with relatively high CD4+ T cell counts, the typical pattern of pulmonary reactivation occurs in which patients present with fever, cough, dyspnea on exertion, weight loss, night sweats, and a chest x ray revealing cavitary apical disease of the upper lobes. In patients with lower CD4+ T cell counts, disseminated disease is more common. In these patients the chest x-ray may reveal diffuse or lower lobe bilateral reticulonodular infiltrates consistent with miliary spread, pleural effusions, and hilar and/or mediastinal adenopathy. Infection may be present in bone, brain, meninges, gastrointestinal tract, lymph nodes (particularly cervical lymph nodes), and viscera. Approximately 60 to 80% of patients have pulmonary disease, and 30 to 40% have extrapulmonary disease. Respiratory isolation and a negative-pressure room should be used for patients in whom a diagnosis of pulmonary

FIGURE 173-28   *A.* Decrease in the incidence of opportunistic infections and Kaposi's sarcoma in HIV-infected individuals with CD4+ T cell counts <100/μL from 1992 through 1998. [*Adapted and updated from Palella et al, and JE Kaplan et al: Clin Infect Dis 30(S1):S5, 2000, with permission.*] *B.* Quarterly incidence rates of cytomegalovirus (CMV), *Pneumocystis carinii* pneumonia (PCP), and *Mycobacterium avium* complex (MAC) from 1995–2001. (*From FJ Palella et al: AIDS 16:1617, 2002.*)

TB is being considered. This approach is critical to limit nosocomial and community spread of infection. Culture of the organism from an involved site provides a definitive diagnosis. Blood cultures are positive in 15% of patients. In the setting of fulminant disease one cannot rely upon the accuracy of a negative PPD skin test to rule out a diagnosis of TB. TB is one of the conditions associated with HIV infection for which cure is possible. Therapy for TB is generally the same in the HIV-infected patient as in the HIV-negative patient (Chap. 150). Due to pharmacokinetic interactions, rifabutin should be substituted for rifampin in patients receiving the HIV protease inhibitors or nonnucleoside reverse transcriptase inhibitors; both drugs should be avoided in patients receiving ritonavir. Treatment is most effective in programs that involve directly observed therapy. Effective prevention of active TB can be a reality if the health care professional is aggressive in looking for evidence of latent TB by making sure that all patients with HIV infection receive a PPD skin test. Anergy testing is not of value in this setting. HIV-infected individuals with a skin test reaction of >5 mm or those who are close household contacts of persons with active TB should receive treatment with 9 months of isoniazid.

Atypical mycobacterial infections are also seen with an increased frequency in patients with HIV infection. Infections with at least 12 different mycobacteria have been reported, including *M. bovis* and representatives of all four Runyon groups. The most common atypical mycobacterial infection is with *M. avium* or *M. intracellulare* species—MAC. Infections with MAC are seen mainly in patients in the United States and are rare in Africa. It has been suggested that prior infection with *M. tuberculosis* decreases the risk of MAC infection. MAC infections probably arise from organisms that are ubiquitous in the environment, including both soil and water. The presumed portals of entry are the respiratory and gastrointestinal tract. MAC infection is a late complication of HIV infection, predominantly occurring in patients with CD4+ T cell counts of <50/μL. The average CD4+ T cell count at the time of diagnosis is 10/μL. The most common presentation is disseminated disease with fever, weight loss, and night sweats. At least 85% of patients with MAC infection are mycobacteremic, and large numbers of organisms can often be demonstrated on bone marrow biopsy. The chest x-ray is abnormal in ~25% of patients, with the most common pattern being that of a bilateral, lower lobe infiltrate suggestive of miliary spread. Alveolar or nodular infiltrates and hilar and/or mediastinal adenopathy can also occur. Other clinical findings include endobronchial lesions, abdominal pain, diarrhea, and lymphadenopathy. The diagnosis is made by the culture of blood or involved tissue. The finding of two consecutive sputum samples positive for MAC is highly suggestive of pulmonary infection. Cultures may take 2 weeks to turn positive. Therapy consists of a macrolide, usually clarithromycin, with ethambutol. Some physicians elect to add a third drug from among rifabutin, ciprofloxacin, or amikacin in patients with extensive disease. Therapy is generally for life; however, with the advent of highly active antiretroviral therapy (HAART), it may be possible to discontinue therapy in patients with sustained suppression of HIV replication and CD4+ T cell counts >100/μL for >6 months. Primary prophylaxis for MAC is indicated in patients with HIV infection and CD4+ T cell counts <50/μL. This may be discontinued in patients in whom HAART induces a sustained suppression of viral replication and increases in CD4+ T cell counts to >100/μL for 3 to 6 months.

Rhodococcus equi is a gram-positive pleomorphic acid-fast non-spore-forming bacillus that can cause pulmonary and/or disseminated infection in patients with HIV infection. Fever and cough are the most common presenting signs. Radiographically one may see cavitary lesions and consolidation. Blood cultures are often positive. Treatment is based upon antimicrobial sensitivity testing.

Fungal infections of the lung, in addition to PCP, can be seen in patients with AIDS. Patients with pulmonary cryptococcal disease present with fever, cough, dyspnea, and in some cases, hemoptysis. A focal or diffuse interstitial infiltrate is seen on chest x-ray in >90% of patients. In addition, one may see lobar disease, cavitary disease, pleural effusions, and hilar or mediastinal adenopathy. Over half of patients are fungemic, and 90% of patients have concomitant CNS infection. *Coccidioides immitis* is a mold that is endemic in the southwest United States. It can cause a reactivation pulmonary syndrome in patients with HIV infection. Most patients with this condition will have CD4+ T cell counts <250/μL. Patients present with fever, weight loss, cough, and extensive, diffuse reticulonodular infiltrates on chest x-ray. One may also see nodules, cavities, pleural effusions, and hilar adenopathy. While serologic testing is of value in the immunocompetent host, serologies are negative in 25% of HIV-infected patients with coccidioidal infection. Invasive aspergillosis is not an AIDS-defining illness and is generally not seen in patients with AIDS in the absence of neutropenia or administration of glucocorticoids. *Aspergillus* infection may have an unusual presentation in the respiratory tract of patients with AIDS where it gives the appearance of a pseudomembranous tracheobronchitis. Primary pulmonary infection of the lung may be seen with *histoplasmosis*. The most common pulmonary manifestation of histoplasmosis, however, is in the setting of disseminated disease, presumably due to reactivation. In this setting respiratory symptoms are usually minimal, with cough and dyspnea occurring in 10 to 30% of patients. The chest x-ray is abnormal in ~50% of patients, showing either a diffuse interstitial infiltrate or diffuse small nodules.

Two forms of *idiopathic interstitial pneumonia* have been identified in patients with HIV infection: lymphoid interstitial pneumonitis (LIP) and nonspecific interstitial pneumonitis (NIP). LIP, a common finding in children, is seen in about 1% of adult patients with HIV infection. This disorder is characterized by a benign infiltrate of the lung and is felt to be part of the polyclonal activation of lymphocytes seen in the context of HIV and EBV infections. Transbronchial biopsy is diagnostic in 50% of the cases, with an open-lung biopsy required for diagnosis in the remainder of cases. This condition is generally self-limited and no specific treatment is necessary. Severe cases have been managed with brief courses of glucocorticoids. Although rarely a clinical problem since the use of HAART, evidence of NIP may be seen in up to half of all patients with untreated HIV infection. Histologically, interstitial infiltrates of lymphocytes and plasma cells in a perivascular and peribronchial distribution are present. When symptomatic, patients present with fever and nonproductive cough occasionally accompanied by mild chest discomfort. Chest x-ray is usually normal or may reveal a faint interstitial pattern. Similar to LIP, this is a self-limited process for which no therapy is indicated other than appropriate management of the underlying HIV infection.

Neoplastic diseases of the lung including KS and lymphoma are discussed below in the section on malignancies.

Diseases of the Cardiovascular System   Heart disease is a relatively common postmortem finding in HIV-infected patients (25 to 75% in autopsy series). Cardiovascular disease may be seen as a direct consequence of HIV infection or as a consequence of antiretroviral therapy as part of the lipodystrophy syndrome. As a primary conseqeunce of HIV infection, the most common clinically significant finding is a dilated cardiomyopathy associated with congestive heart failure referred to as *HIV-associated cardiomyopathy*. This generally occurs as a late complication of HIV infection and, histologically, displays elements of myocarditis. For this reason some have advocated treatment with intravenous Ig. HIV can be directly demonstrated in cardiac tissue in this setting, and there is debate over whether or not it plays a direct role in this condition. Patients present with typical findings of congestive heart failure, namely edema and shortness of breath. Patients with HIV infection may also develop cardiomyopathy as a side effect of IFN-α nucleoside analogue therapy, which is reversible once therapy is stopped. KS, cryptococcosis, Chagas disease, and toxoplasmosis can involve the myocardium, leading to cardiomyopathy. In one series, most patients with HIV infection and a treatable myocarditis were found to have myocarditis associated with toxoplasmosis. Most of these patients also had evidence of CNS toxoplasmosis. Thus, MRI or double-dose contrast CT scan of the brain should be included in the workup of any patient with advanced HIV infection and cardiomyopathy.

A variety of other cardiovascular problems are found in patients with HIV infection. Pericardial effusions may be seen in the setting of advanced HIV infection. Predisposing factors include TB, congestive heart failure, mycobacterial infection, cryptococcal infection, pulmonary infection, lymphoma, and KS. While pericarditis is quite rare, in one series 5% of patients with HIV disease had pericardial effusions that were considered to be moderate or severe. Tamponade and death have occurred in association with pericardial KS, presumably owing to acute hemorrhage. Nonbacterial thrombotic endocarditis has been reported and should be considered in patients with unexplained embolic phenomena. Intravenous pentamidine, when given rapidly, can result in hypotension as a consequence of cardiovascular collapse. A high percentage of patients have hypertriglyceridemia and elevations in serum cholesterol, and coronary artery disease has been a relatively frequent finding at autopsy. This problem appears to becoming even more prevalent as a side effect of HAART. While the clinical significance of these findings has not been precisely defined, recent data suggest a linear relationship between time on HAART and development of ischemic heart disease. In one large series the overall rate of myocardial infarction was 3.5/1000 years, 28% of these events were fatal, and myocardial infarction was responsible for 7% of all deaths in the cohort. The risk of myocardial infarction increased by 26% per year of HAART. This small increase in the risk of death from myocardial infarction in the setting of HAART has to be balanced against the marked increase in overall survival brought about by HAART.

Diseases of the Oropharynx and Gastrointestinal System   Oropharyngeal and gastrointestinal diseases are common features of HIV infection. They are most frequently due to secondary infections. In addition, oral and gastrointestinal lesions may occur with KS and lymphoma.

Oral lesions, including *thrush, hairy leukoplakia,* and *aphthous ulcers*, are particularly common in patients with untreated HIV infection. Thrush, due to *Candida* infection, and oral hairy leukoplakia, presumed due to EBV, are usually indicative of fairly advanced immunologic decline; they generally occur in patients with CD4+ T cell counts of <300/μL. In one study, 59% of patients with oral candidiasis went on to develop AIDS in the next year. Thrush appears as a white, cheesy exudate, often on an erythematous mucosa in the posterior oropharynx (see Fig. 187-1). While most commonly seen on the soft palate, early lesions are often found along the gingival border. The diagnosis is made by direct examination of a scraping for pseudohyphal elements. Culturing is of no diagnostic value, as most patients with HIV infection will have a positive throat culture for *Candida* even in the absence of thrush. Oral hairy leukoplakia presents as white, frondlike lesions, generally along the lateral borders of the tongue and sometimes on the adjacent buccal mucosa (see Fig. 165-1). Despite its name, oral hairy leukoplakia is not considered a premalignant condition. Lesions are associated with florid replication of EBV. While usually more disconcerting as a sign of HIV-associated immunodeficiency than a clinical problem in need of treatment, severe cases have been reported to respond to topical podophyllin or systemic therapy with anti-herpesvirus agents. Aphthous ulcers of the posterior oropharynx are also seen with regularity in patients with HIV infection. These lesions are of unknown etiology and can be quite painful and interfere with swallowing. Topical anesthetics provide immediate symptomatic relief of short duration. The fact that thalidomide is an effective treatment for this condition suggests that the pathogenesis may involve the action of tissue-destructive cytokines. Palatal, glossal, or gingival ulcers may also result from cryptococcal disease or histoplasmosis.

Esophagitis (Fig. 173-29) may present with odynophagia and retrosternal pain. Upper endoscopy is generally required to make an accurate diagnosis. Esophagitis may be due to *Candida*, CMV, or HSV. While CMV tends to be associated with a single large ulcer, HSV infection is more often associated with multiple small ulcers. The esophagus may also be the site of KS and lymphoma. Like the oral

FIGURE 173-29 Barium swallow of a patient with *Candida* esophagitis. The flow of barium along the mucosal surface is grossly irregular.

mucosa, the esophageal mucosa may have large, painful ulcers of unclear etiology that may respond to thalidomide. While achlorhydria is a common problem in patients with HIV infection, other gastric problems are generally rare. Among the conditions involving the stomach are KS and lymphoma. Infections of the small and large intestine leading to diarrhea, abdominal pain, and occasionally fever are among the most significant gastrointestinal problems in the HIV-infected patients. They include infections with bacteria, protozoa, and viruses.

Bacteria may be responsible for secondary infections of the gastrointestinal tract. Infections with enteric pathogens such as *Salmonella*, *Shigella*, and *Campylobacter* are more common in homosexual men and are often more severe and more apt to relapse in patients with HIV infection. Patients with untreated HIV have approximately a 20-fold increased risk of infection with *S. typhimurium*. They may present with a variety of nonspecific symptoms including fever, anorexia, fatigue, and malaise of several weeks' duration. Diarrhea is common but may be absent. Diagnosis is made by culture of blood and stool. Long-term therapy with ciprofloxacin is the recommended treatment. HIV-infected patients also have an increased incidence of *S. typhi* infection in areas of the world where typhoid is a problem. *Shigella* spp., particularly *S. flexneri*, can cause severe intestinal disease in HIV-infected individuals. Up to 50% of patients will develop bacteremia. *Campylobacter* infections occur with an increased frequency in patients with HIV infection. While *C. jejuni* is the strain most frequently isolated, infections with many other strains have been reported. Patients usually present with crampy abdominal pain, fever, and bloody diarrhea. Infection may present as proctitis. Stool examination reveals the presence of fecal leukocytes. Systemic infection can occur, with up to 10% of infected patients exhibiting bacteremia. Most strains are sensitive to erythromycin. Abdominal pain and diarrhea may be seen with MAC infection.

Fungal infections may also be a cause of diarrhea in patients with HIV infection. Histoplasmosis, coccidioidomycosis, and penicilliosis have all been identified as a cause of fever and diarrhea in patients with HIV infection. Peritonitis has been seen with *C. immitis*.

Cryptosporidia, microsporidia, and *Isospora belli* (Chap. 199) are the most common opportunistic protozoa that infect the gastrointestinal tract and cause diarrhea in HIV-infected patients. Cryptosporidial infection may present in a variety of ways, ranging from a self-limited or intermittent diarrheal illness in patients in the early stages of HIV infection to a severe, life-threatening diarrhea in severely immuno-deficient individuals. In patients with untreated HIV infection and CD4+ T cell counts of <300/μL, the incidence of cryptosporidiosis is ~1% per year. In 75% of cases the diarrhea is accompanied by crampy abdominal pain, and 25% of patients have nausea and/or vomiting. Cryptosporidia may also cause biliary tract disease in the HIV-infected patient, leading to cholecystitis with or without accompanying cholangitis. The diagnosis of cryptosporidial diarrhea is made by stool examination. The diarrhea is noninflammatory, and the characteristic finding is the presence of oocysts that stain with acid-fast dyes. Therapy is predominantly supportive, and marked improvements have been reported in the setting of effective antiretroviral therapy. Treatment with up to 2000 mg/d of nitazoxanide (NTZ) is associated with improvement in symptoms or a decrease in shedding of organisms in about half of patients. Its overall role in the management of this condition remains unclear. Patients can minimize their risk of developing cryptosporidiosis by avoiding contact with human and animal feces and by not drinking untreated water from lakes or rivers.

Microsporidia are small, unicellular, obligate intracellular parasites that reside in the cytoplasm of enteric cells (Chap. 199). The main species causing disease in humans is *Enterocytozoon bieneusi*. The clinical manifestations are similar to those described for cryptosporidia and include abdominal pain and diarrhea. The small size of the organism may make it difficult to detect; however, with the use of chromotrope-based stains, organisms can be identified in stool samples by light microscopy. Definitive diagnosis generally depends on electron microscopic examination of a stool specimen, intestinal aspirate, or intestinal biopsy specimen. In contrast to cryptosporidia, microsporidia have been noted in a variety of extraintestinal locations, including the eye, muscle, and liver, and have been associated with conjunctivitis and hepatitis. Albendazole, 400 mg bid, has been reported to be of benefit in some patients.

I. belli is a coccidian parasite (Chap. 199) most commonly found as a cause of diarrhea in patients from the Caribbean and Africa. Its cysts appear in the stool as large, acid-fast structures that can be differentiated from those of cryptosporidia on the basis of size, shape, and number of sporocysts. The clinical syndromes of *Isospora* infection are identical to those caused by cryptosporidia. The important distinction is that infection with *Isospora* is generally relatively easy to treat with TMP/SMX. While relapses are common, a thrice-weekly regimen, similar to that used to provide prophylaxis against PCP, appears adequate to prevent recurrence.

CMV colitis was once seen in 5 to 10% of patients with AIDS. It is much less common with the advent of HAART. CMV colitis presents as diarrhea, abdominal pain, weight loss, and anorexia. The diarrhea is usually nonbloody, and the diagnosis is achieved through endoscopy and biopsy. Multiple mucosal ulcerations are seen at endoscopy, and biopsies reveal characteristic intranuclear inclusion bodies. Secondary bacteremias may result as a consequence of thinning of the bowel wall. Treatment is with either ganciclovir or foscarnet for 3 to 6 weeks. Relapses are common, and maintenance therapy is typically necessary in patients whose HIV infection is poorly controlled. Patients with CMV disease of the gastrointestinal tract should be carefully monitored for evidence of retinitis.

In addition to disease caused by specific secondary infections, patients with HIV infection may also experience a chronic diarrheal syndrome for which no etiologic agent other than HIV can be identified. This entity is referred to as *AIDS enteropathy* or *HIV enteropathy*. It is most likely a direct result of HIV infection in the gastrointestinal tract. Histologic examination of the small bowel in these patients reveals low-grade mucosal atrophy with a decrease in mitotic figures, suggesting a hyporegenerative state. Patients often have decreased or absent small-bowel lactase and malabsorption with accompanying weight loss.

The initial evaluation of a patient with HIV infection and diarrhea

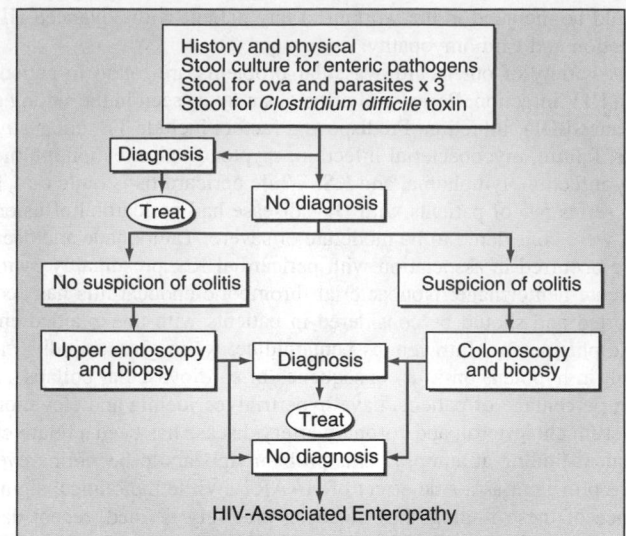

FIGURE 173-30   Algorithm for the evaluation of diarrhea in a patient with HIV infection. HIV-associated enteropathy is a diagnosis of exclusion and can be made only after other, generally treatable, forms of diarrheal illness have been ruled out.

should include a set of stool examinations, including culture, examination for ova and parasites, and examination for *Clostridium difficile* toxin. Approximately 50% of the time this workup will demonstrate infection with pathogenic bacteria, mycobacteria, or protozoa. If the initial stool examinations are negative, additional evaluation, including upper and/or lower endoscopy with biopsy, will yield a diagnosis of microsporidial or mycobacterial infection of the small intestine ~30% of the time. In patients for whom this diagnostic evaluation is nonrevealing, a presumptive diagnosis of HIV enteropathy can be made if the diarrhea has persisted for >1 month. An algorithm for the evaluation of diarrhea in patients with HIV infection is given in Fig. 173-30.

Rectal lesions are common in HIV-infected patients, particularly the perirectal ulcers and erosions due to the reactivation of HSV (Fig. 173-31). These may appear quite atypical, as denuded skin without vesicles, and they respond well to treatment with acyclovir, famciclovir, or foscarnet. Other rectal lesions encountered in patients with HIV infection include condylomata acuminata, KS, and intraepithelial neoplasia (see below).

FIGURE 173-31   Severe, erosive perirectal herpes simplex in a patient with AIDS.

Hepatobiliary Disease Diseases of the hepatobiliary system are a major problem in patients with HIV infection. It has been estimated that approximately one-third of the deaths of patients with HIV infection are in some way related to liver disease. While this is predominantly a reflection of the problems encountered in the setting of co-infection with hepatitis B or C, it is also a reflection of the hepatic injury, ranging from hepatic steatosis to hypersensitivity reactions to immune reconstitution, that can be seen in the context of antiretroviral therapy.

Approximately 95% of HIV-infected individuals have evidence of infection with HBV; 5 to 40% of patients are co-infected with HCV; and co-infection with hepatitis D, E, and/or G viruses is common. HIV infection has a significant impact on the course of hepatitis virus infection. It is associated with approximately a threefold increase in the development of persistent hepatitis B surface antigenemia. Patients infected with both HBV and HIV have decreased evidence of inflammatory liver disease. The presumption that this is due to the immunosuppressive effects of HIV infection is supported by the observations that this situation can be reversed, and one may see the development of more severe hepatitis following the initiation of effective antiretroviral therapy. In a study of the impact of HIV on hepatitis B infection a tenfold increase in liver-related mortality was noted in patients with HIV and active HBV infection compared to rates in patients with either infection alone. IFN-α is less successful as a treatment of HBV in patients with HIV co-infection, and lamivudine or adefovir/tenofovir is the treatment of choice. It is important to remember that these drugs are also potent antiretroviral agents in the setting of combination antiretroviral therapy. They should not be used as single agents in patients with HIV infection, even if it is only being used to treat HBV, in order to avoid the rapid development of resistant quasispecies of HIV. In contrast to the situation with HBV, HCV infection is more severe in the patient with HIV infection; however, it does not appear to affect overall mortality when other variables such as age, baseline CD4+ T cell count, and use of HAART are taken into account. In the setting of HIV and HCV co-infection, levels of HCV are approximately tenfold higher than in the HIV-negative patient with HCV infection and there is an increased rate of progression to cirrhosis. Treatment for HCV infection consists of pegylated IFN-α and ribavirin. If a 2-log drop in levels of HCV RNA is not seen within 12 weeks, it is unlikely that therapy will be of value. Hepatitis A virus infection is not seen with an increased frequency in patients with HIV infection. It is recommended that all patients with HIV infection who have not experienced natural infection be immunized with hepatitis A and/or hepatitis B vaccines. Infection with hepatits G virus, also known as GB virus C, is seen in ~50% of patients with HIV infection. For reasons that are currently unclear there are data to suggestion that patients with HIV infection co-infected with this virus have a decreased rate of progression to AIDS.

A variety of other infections may also involve the liver. Granulomatous hepatitis may be seen as a consequence of mycobacterial or fungal infections, particularly MAC infection. Hepatic masses may be seen in the context of TB, peliosis hepatis, or fungal infection. Among the fungal opportunistic infections *C. immitis* and *Histoplasma capsulatum* are those most likely to involve the liver. Biliary tract disease in the form of papillary stenosis or sclerosing cholangitis has been reported in the context of cryptosporidiosis, CMV infection, and KS.

Many of the drugs used to treat HIV infection are metabolized by the liver and can cause liver injury. Fatal hepatic reactions have been reported with a wide array of antiretrovirals including nucleoside analogues, nonnucleoside analogues, and protease inhibitors. Nucleoside analogues work by inhibiting DNA synthesis. This can result in toxicity to mitochondria, which can lead to disturbances in oxidative metabolism. This may be manifest as hepatic steatosis and, in severe cases, lactic acidosis and fulminant liver failure. It is important to be aware of this condition and to watch for it in patients with HIV infection receiving nucleoside analogues. It is reversible if diagnosed early and the offending agent(s) discontinued. Nevirapine has been associated with at times fatal fulminant and cholestatic hepatitis, hepatic necrosis, and hepatic failure. Indinavir may cause mild to moderate

elevations in serum bilirubin in 10 to 15% of patients in a syndrome similar to Gilbert's syndrome. A similar pattern of hepatic injury may be seen with atazanavir. In the patient receiving HAART with an unexplained increase in hepatic transaminases, strong consideration should be given to drug toxicity. *Pancreatic injury* is most commonly a consequence of drug toxicity, notably that secondary to pentamidine or dideoxynucleosides. While up to half of patients in some series have biochemical evidence of pancreatic injury, <5% of patients show any clinical evidence of pancreatitis that is not linked to a drug toxicity.

Diseases of the Kidney and Genitourinary Tract Diseases of the kidney or genitourinary tract may be a direct consequence of HIV infection, due to an opportunistic infection or neoplasm, or related to drug toxicity. *HIV-associated nephropathy* was first described in IDUs and was initially thought to be IDU nephropathy in patients with HIV infection; it is now recognized as a true direct complication of HIV infection. HIV-associated nephropathy can be an early manifestation of HIV infection and is also seen in children. Over 90% of reported cases have been in African-American or Hispanic individuals; the disease is not only more prevalent in these populations but also more severe. Proteinuria is the hallmark of this disorder. Overall, microalbuminuria is seen in ~20% of untreated HIV-infected patients; significant proteinuria is seen in closer to 2%. Edema and hypertension are rare. Ultrasound examination reveals enlarged, hyperechogenic kidneys. A definitive diagnosis is obtained through renal biopsy. Histologically, focal segmental glomerulosclerosis is present in 80%, and mesangial proliferation in 10 to 15% of cases. Prior to effective antiretroviral therapy, this disease was characterized by relatively rapid progression to end-stage renal disease. Treatment with prednisone, 60 mg/d, has been reported to be of benefit in some cases. The incidence of this disease in patients receiving adequate antiretroviral therapy has not been well defined; however, the impression is that it has decreased in frequency. It is the leading cause of end-stage renal disease in patients with HIV infection.

Among the drugs commonly associated with renal damage in patients with HIV disease are pentamidine, amphotericin, adefovir, cidofovir, and foscarnet. TMP/SMX may compete for tubular secretion with creatinine and cause an increase in the serum creatinine level. Sulfadiazine may crystallize in the kidney and result in an easily reversible form of renal shutdown. One of the most common drug-induced renal complications is indinavir-associated renal calculi. This condition is seen in ~10% of patients receiving this HIV protease inhibitor. It may present with a variety of manifestations, ranging from asymptomatic hematuria to renal colic. Adequate hydration is the mainstay of treatment and prevention for this condition.

Genitourinary tract infections are seen with a high frequency in patients with HIV infection; they present with dysuria, hematuria, and/or pyuria and are managed in the same fashion as in patients without HIV infection. Infections with *T. pallidum*, the etiologic agent of *syphilis*, play an important role in the HIV epidemic (Chap. 172). In HIV-negative individuals, genital syphilitic ulcers as well as the ulcers of chancroid are major predisposing factors for heterosexual transmission of HIV infection. While most HIV-infected individuals with syphilis have a typical presentation, a variety of formerly rare clinical problems may be encountered in the setting of dual infection. Among them are *lues maligna*, an ulcerating lesion of the skin due to a necrotizing vasculitis; unexplained fever; nephrotic syndrome; and neurosyphilis. The most common presentation of syphilis in the HIV-infected patient is that of *condylomata lata*, a form of secondary syphilis. Neurosyphilis may be asymptomatic or may present as acute meningitis, neuroretinitis, deafness, or stroke. The rate of neurosyphilis may be as high as 1% in patients with HIV infection. As a consequence of the immunologic abnormalities seen in the setting of HIV infection, diagnosis of syphilis through standard serologic testing may be challenging. On the one hand, a significant number of patients have false-positive Venereal Disease Research Laboratory (VDRL) tests mesenteric fat, a dorsocervical fat pad ("buffalo hump") reminiscent of patients with Cushing's syndrome, and enlargement of the breasts. The peripheral wasting or lipoatrophy is particularly noticeable in the face and buttocks and by the prominence of the veins in the legs. These changes may develop at any time ranging from ~6 weeks to several years following the initiation of HAART. The syndrome has been reported in association with regimens containing a variety of different drugs, and while initially reported in the setting of protease inhibitor therapy, it appears similar changes can also be induced by potent protease-sparing regimens. It has been suggested that the lipoatrophy changes are particularly severe in patients receiving thymidine analogues. National Cholesterol Education Program (NCEP) guidelines should be followed in the management of these lipid abnormalities (Chap. 225). Due to concerns regarding drug interactions, the most commonly utilized agents in this setting are gemfibrozil and atorvostatin. In addition to these abnormalities, patients with HIV infection treated with HAART have been found to have an increased incidence of osteonecrosis or avascular necrosis of the hip and shoulders. In a study of asymptomatic patients, 4.4% were found to have evidence of osteonecrosis on MRI. This complication was associated with the use of lipid-lowering agents, systemic glucocorticoids or testosterone; body-building exercise; and the presence of anticardiolipin antibodies. Lactic acidosis is also associated with antiretroviral therapy. This is most commonly seen with nucleoside reverse transcriptase inhibitors and can be fatal (see below).

FIGURE 173-32 Characteristics of lipodystrophy. *A*. Truncal obesity and buffalo hump. *B*. Facial wasting. *C*. Accumulation of intraabdominal fat on CT scan.

due to polyclonal B cell activation. On the other hand, the development of a new positive VDRL may be delayed in patients with new infections, and the anti-fluorescent treponema antibody (anti-FTA) test may be negative due to immunodeficiency. Thus, dark-field examination of appropriate specimens should be performed in any patient in whom syphilis is suspected, even if the patient has a negative VDRL. Similarly, any patient with a positive serum VDRL test, neurologic findings, and an abnormal spinal fluid examination should be considered to have neurosyphilis, regardless of the CSF VDRL result. In any setting, patients treated for syphilis need to be carefully monitored to ensure adequate therapy.

Vulvovaginal candidiasis is a common problem in women with HIV infection. Symptoms include pruritus, discomfort, dyspareunia, and dysuria. Vulvar infection may present as a morbilliform rash that may extend to the thighs. Vaginal infection is usually associated with a white discharge, and plaques may be seen along an erythematous vaginal wall. Diagnosis is made by microscopic examination of the discharge for pseudohyphal elements in a 10% potassium hydroxide solution. Mild disease can be treated with topical therapy. More serious disease can be treated with fluconazole. Other causes of vaginitis include *Trichomonas* and mixed bacteria.

Diseases of the Endocrine System and Metabolic Disorders A variety of endocrine and metabolic disorders are seen in the context of HIV infection. Between 33 and 75% of patients with HIV infection receiving HAART develop a syndrome often referred to as *lipodystrophy*, consisting of elevations in plasma triglycerides, total cholesterol, and apolipoprotein B, as well as hyperinsulinemia and hyperglycemia. Many of these patients have been noted to have a characteristic set of body habitus changes associated with fat redistribution, consisting of truncal obesity coupled with peripheral wasting (Fig. 173-32). Truncal obesity is apparent as an increase in abdominal girth related to increases in

Patients with advanced HIV disease may develop hyponatremia due to the syndrome of inappropriate antidiuretic hormone (vasopressin) secretion (SIADH) as a consequence of increased free water intake and decreased free water excretion. SIADH is usually seen in conjunction with pulmonary or CNS disease. Low serum sodium may also be due to adrenal insufficiency; concomitant high serum potassium should alert one to this possibility. Adrenal gland disease may be due to mycobacterial infections, CMV disease, cryptococcal disease, histoplasmosis, or ketoconazole toxicity.

Thyroid function is generally normal in patients with HIV infection although ~2 to 3% of patients may have elevations in thyroid-stimulating hormone (TSH). In the setting of HAART up to 10% of patients have been noted to have elevated TSH levels, suggesting that this may be a manifestation of immune reconstitution. In advanced HIV disease, infection of the thyroid gland may occur with opportunistic pathogens, including *P. carinii*, CMV, mycobacteria, *Toxoplasma gondii*, and *Cryptococcus neoformans*. These infections are generally associated with a nontender, diffuse enlargement of the thyroid gland. Thyroid function is usually normal. Diagnosis is made by fine-needle aspirate or open biopsy.

Advanced HIV disease is associated with *hypogonadism* in ~50% of men. While this is generally a complication of underlying illness, testicular dysfunction may also be a side effect of ganciclovir therapy. In some surveys, up to two-thirds of patients report decreased libido and one-third complain of impotence. Androgen replacement therapy should be considered in patients with symptomatic hypogonadism. HIV infection does not seem to have a significant effect on the menstrual cycle outside the setting of advanced disease.

Rheumatologic Diseases Immunologic and rheumatologic disorders are common in patients with HIV infection and range from excessive immediate-type hypersensitivity reactions (Chap. 298) to an increase in the incidence of reactive arthritis (Chap. 305) to conditions characterized by a diffuse infiltrative lymphocytosis. The occurrence of these phenomena is an apparent paradox in the setting of the profound immunodeficiency and immunosuppression that characterizes HIV infection. In addition, following the initiation of antiretroviral therapy, one may see a variety of exaggerated immune responses to existing opportunistic infections referred to as *immune reactivation syndromes*.

Drug allergies are the most significant allergic reactions occurring in HIV-infected patients and appear to become more common as the disease progresses. They occur in 65% of patients who receive therapy with TMP/SMX for PCP. In general, these drug reactions are characterized by erythematous, morbilliform eruptions that are pruritic, tend to coalesce, and are often associated with fever. Nonetheless, ~33% of patients can be maintained on the offending therapy, and thus these reactions are not an immediate indication to stop the drug. Anaphylaxis is extremely rare in patients with HIV infection, and patients who have a cutaneous reaction during a single course of therapy can still be considered candidates for future treatment or prophylaxis with the same agent. The one exception to this is the nucleoside analogue abacavir, where fatal hypersensitivity reactions have been reported with rechallenge. A hypersensitivity reaction to abacavir is an absolute contraindication to future therapy. For other agents, including TMP/SMX, desensitization regimens are moderately successful. While the mechanisms underlying these allergic-type reactions remain unknown, patients with HIV infection have been noted to have elevated IgE levels that increase as the CD4+ T cell count declines. The numerous examples of patients with multiple drug reactions suggest that a common pathway is involved.

HIV infection shares many similarities with a variety of autoimmune diseases, including a substantial polyclonal B cell activation that is associated with a high incidence of antiphospholipid antibodies, such as anticardiolipin antibodies, VDRL antibodies, and lupus-like anticoagulants. In addition, HIV-infected individuals have an increased incidence of antinuclear antibodies. Despite these serologic findings, there is no evidence that HIV-infected individuals have an increase in two of the more common autoimmune diseases, i.e., systemic lupus erythematosus and rheumatoid arthritis. In fact, it has been observed that these diseases may be somewhat ameliorated by the concomitant presence of HIV infection, suggesting that an intact CD4+ T cell limb of the immune response plays an integral role in the pathogenesis of these conditions. Similarly, there are anecdotal reports of patients with common variable immunodeficiency (Chap. 297), characterized by hypogammaglobulinemia, who have had a normalization of Ig levels following the development of HIV infection, suggesting a possible role for overactive CD4+ T cell immunity in certain forms of that syndrome. The one autoimmune disease that may occur with an increased frequency in patients with HIV infection is a variant of primary Sjögren's syndrome (Chap. 304). Patients with HIV infection may develop a syndrome consisting of parotid gland enlargement, dry eyes, and dry mouth that is associated with lymphocytic infiltrates of the salivary gland and lung. In contrast to Sjögren's syndrome, in which these infiltrates are composed predominantly of CD4+ T cells, in patients with HIV infection the infiltrates are composed predominantly of CD8+ T cells. In addition, while patients with Sjögren's syndrome are mainly women who have autoantibodies to Ro and La and who frequently have HLA-DR3 or -B8 MHC haplotypes, HIV-infected individuals with this syndrome are usually African-American men who do not have anti-Ro or anti-La and who most often are HLA-DR5. This syndrome appears to be less common with the increased use of effective antiretroviral therapy. The term *diffuse infiltrative lymphocytosis syndrome* (DILS) has been proposed to describe this entity and to distinguish it from Sjögren's syndrome.

Approximately one-third of HIV-infected individuals experience arthralgias; furthermore, 5 to 10% are diagnosed as having some form of reactive arthritis, such as Reiter's syndrome or psoriatic arthritis (Chap. 305). These syndromes occur with increasing frequency as the competency of the immune system declines. This association may be related to an increase in the number of infections with organisms that

may trigger a reactive arthritis with progressive immunodeficiency or to a loss of important regulatory T cells. Reactive arthritides in HIV-infected individuals generally respond well to standard treatment; however, therapy with methotrexate has been associated with an increase in the incidence of opportunistic infections and should be used with caution and only in severe cases.

HIV-infected individuals also experience a variety of joint problems without obvious cause that are referred to generically as *HIV- or AIDS-associated arthropathy*. This syndrome is characterized by subacute oligoarticular arthritis developing over a period of 1 to 6 weeks and lasting 6 weeks to 6 months. It generally involves the large joints, predominantly the knees and ankles, and is nonerosive with only a mild inflammatory response. X-rays of the joint are nonrevealing. Nonsteroidal anti-inflammatory drugs are only marginally helpful; however, relief has been noted with the use of intraarticular glucocorticoids. A second form of arthritis also thought to be secondary to HIV infection is called *painful articular syndrome*. This condition, found in as many as 10% of AIDS patients, presents as an acute, severe, sharp pain in the affected joint. It affects primarily the knees, elbows, and shoulders; lasts 2 to 24 h; and may be severe enough to require narcotic analgesics. The cause of this arthropathy is unclear; however, it is thought to result from a direct effect of HIV on the joint. This condition is reminiscent of the fact that other lentiviruses, in particular the caprine arthritis-encephalitis virus, are capable of directly causing arthritis.

A variety of other immunologic or rheumatologic diseases have been reported in HIV-infected individuals, either de novo or in association with opportunistic infections or drugs. Using the criteria of widespread musculoskeletal pain of at least 3 months' duration and the presence of at least 11 of 18 possible tender points by digital palpation, 11% of an HIV-infected cohort containing 55% IDUs were diagnosed as having *fibromyalgia* (Chap. 315). While the incidence of frank arthritis was less in this population than in other studied populations that consisted predominantly of homosexual men, these data support the concept that there are musculoskeletal problems that occur as a direct result of HIV infection. In addition there have been reports of leukocytoclastic vasculitis in the setting of zidovudine therapy. CNS angiitis and polymyositis have also been reported in HIV-infected individuals. Septic arthritis is surprisingly rare, especially given the increased incidence of staphylococcal bacteremias seen in this population. When septic arthritis has been reported, it has usually been due to systemic fungal infections with *C. neoformans*, *Sporothrix schenckii*, or *H. capsulatum*, or to systemic mycobacterial infection with *M. haemophilum*.

Following the initiation of effective antiretroviral therapy, a paradoxical worsening of preexisting, untreated, or partially treated opportunistic infections may be noted. These *immune reactivation syndromes* are particularly common in patients with underlying untreated mycobacterial infections. They appear to be related to a phenomenon similar to type IV hypersensitivity reactions and reflect the immediate improvements in immune function that occur as levels of HIV RNA drop and the immunosuppressive effects of HIV infection are controlled. In severe cases the use of immunosuppressive drugs such as glucocorticoids may be required to blunt the inflammatory component of these reactions while specific antimicrobial therapy takes effect.

Diseases of the Hematopoietic System Disorders of the hematopoietic system including lymphadenopathy, anemia, leukopenia, and/or thrombocytopenia are common throughout the course of HIV infection and may be the direct result of HIV, manifestations of secondary infections and neoplasms, or side effects of therapy (Table 173-12). Direct histologic examination and culture of lymph node or bone marrow tissue are often diagnostic. A significant percentage of bone marrow aspirates from patients with HIV infection have been reported to contain lymphoid aggregates, the precise significance of which is un-

TABLE 173-12 *Causes of Bone Marrow Suppression in Patients with HIV Infection*

HIV infection	Medications
Mycobacterial infections	Zidovudine
Fungal infections	Dapsone
B19 parvovirus infection	Trimethoprim/sulfamethoxazole
Lymphoma	Pyrimethamine
	5-Flucytosine
	Ganciclovir
	Interferon-α
	Trimetrexate
	Foscarnet

known. Initiation of HAART will lead to reversal of most hematologic complications that are the direct result of HIV infection.

Some patients, otherwise asymptomatic, may develop *persistent generalized lymphadenopathy* as an early clinical manifestation of HIV infection. This condition is defined as the presence of enlarged lymph nodes (>1 cm) in two or more extrainguinal sites for >3 months without an obvious cause. The lymphadenopathy is due to marked follicular hyperplasia in the node in response to HIV infection. The nodes are generally discrete and freely movable. This feature of HIV disease may be seen at any point in the spectrum of immune dysfunction and is not associated with an increased likelihood of developing AIDS. Paradoxically, a loss in lymphadenopathy or a decrease in lymph node size outside the setting of antiretroviral therapy may be a prognostic marker of disease progression. In patients with CD4+ T cell counts >200/μL, the differential diagnosis of lymphadenopathy includes KS, TB, and lymphoma. In patients with more advanced disease, lymphadenopathy may also be due to atypical mycobacterial infection, toxoplasmosis, systemic fungal infection, or bacillary angiomatosis. While indicated in patients with CD4+ T cell counts <200/μL, lymph node biopsy is not indicated in patients with early-stage disease unless there are signs and symptoms of systemic illness, such as fever and weight loss, or unless the nodes begin to enlarge, become fixed, or coalesce.

Anemia is the most common hematologic abnormality in HIV-infected patients. While generally mild, anemia can be quite severe and require chronic blood transfusions. Among the specific reversible causes of anemia in the setting of HIV infection are drug toxicity, systemic fungal and mycobacterial infections, nutritional deficiencies, and parvovirus B19 infections. Zidovudine may block erythroid maturation, prior to its effects on other marrow elements. A characteristic feature of zidovudine therapy is an elevated mean corpuscular volume (MCV). Another drug used in patients with HIV infection that has a selective effect on the erythroid series is dapsone. This drug can cause a serious hemolytic anemia in patients who are deficient in glucose-6-phosphate dehydrogenase and can create a functional anemia in others through induction of methemoglobinemia. Folate levels are usually normal in HIV-infected individuals; however, vitamin B_{12} levels may be depressed as a consequence of achlorhydria or malabsorption. True autoimmune hemolytic anemia is rare, although ~20% of patients with HIV infection may have a positive direct antiglobulin test as a consequence of polyclonal B cell activation. Infection with parvovirus B19 may also cause anemia. It is important to recognize this possibility given the fact that it responds well to treatment with intravenous immunoglobulin. Erythropoietin levels in patients with HIV infection and anemia are generally less than expected given the degree of anemia. Treatment with erythropoietin at doses of 100 μg/kg three times a week may result in an increase in hemoglobulin levels. An exception to this is a subset of patients with zidovudine-associated anemia in whom erythropoietin levels may be quite high.

During the course of HIV infection, neutropenia may be seen in approximately half of patients. In most instances it is mild; however, it can be severe and can put patients at risk of spontaneous bacterial infections. This is most frequently seen in patients with severely advanced HIV disease and in patients receiving any of a number of po-

tentially myelosuppressive therapies. In the setting of neutropenia, diseases that are not commonly seen in HIV-infected patients, such as aspergillosis or mucormycosis, may occur. The potential role of colony-stimulating factors in the management of patients with HIV infection has undergone extensive evaluation. Both granulocyte colony-stimulating factor (G-CSF) and GM-CSF increase neutrophil counts in patients with HIV infection regardless of the cause of the neutropenia. Earlier concerns about the potential of these agents to also increase levels of HIV were not confirmed in controlled clinical trials.

Thrombocytopenia may be an early consequence of HIV infection. Approximately 3% of patients with untreated HIV infection and CD4+ T cell counts ≥400/μL have platelet counts <150,000/μL. For untreated patients with CD4+ T cell counts <400/μL, this incidence increases to 10%. Thrombocytopenia is rarely a serious clinical problem in patients with HIV infection and generally responds well to antiretroviral therapy. Clinically, it resembles the thrombocytopenia seen in patients with idiopathic thrombocytopenic purpura (Chap. 101). Immune complexes containing anti-gp120 antibodies and anti-anti-gp120 antibodies have been noted in the circulation and on the surface of platelets in patients with HIV infection. Patients with HIV infection have also been noted to have a platelet-specific antibody directed towards a 25-kDa component of the surface of the platelet. Other data suggest that the thrombocytopenia in patients with HIV infection may be due to a direct effect of HIV on megakaryocytes. Whatever the cause, it is very clear that the most effective medical approach to this problem has been the use of HAART. For patients with platelet counts <20,000/μL a more aggressive approach combining intravenous Ig or anti-Rh Ig for an immediate response with antiretroviral therapy for a more lasting response is appropriate. Splenectomy is a rarely needed option and is reserved for patients refractory to medical management. Because of the risk of serious infection with encapsulated organisms, all patients with HIV infection about to undergo splenectomy should be immunized with pneumococcal polysaccharide. It should be noted that, in addition to causing an increase in the platelet count, removal of the spleen will result in an increase in the peripheral blood lymphocyte count, making CD4+ T cell counts unreliable. In this setting, the clinician should rely on the CD4+ T cell percent for making diagnostic decisions with respect to the likelihood of opportunistic infections. A CD4+ T cell percent of 15 is approximately equivalent to a CD4+ T cell count of 200/μL. In patients with early HIV infection, thrombocytopenia has also been reported as a consequence of classic thrombotic thrombocytopenic purpura (Chap. 101). This clinical syndrome, consisting of fever, thrombocytopenia, hemolytic anemia, and neurologic and renal dysfunction, is a rare complication of early HIV infection. As in other settings, the appropriate management is the use of salicylates and plasma exchange. Other causes of thrombocytopenia include lymphoma, mycobacterial infections, and fungal infections.

Dermatologic Diseases Dermatologic problems occur in >90% of patients with HIV infection. From the macular, roseola-like rash seen with the acute seroconversion syndrome to extensive end-stage KS, cutaneous manifestations of HIV disease can be seen throughout the course of HIV infection. Among the more common nonneoplastic problems are seborrheic dermatitis, eosinophilic pustular folliculitus, and opportunistic infections. Extrapulmonary pneumocystosis may cause a necrotizing vasculitis. Neoplastic conditions are covered below in the section on malignant diseases.

Seborrheic dermatitis occurs in 3% of the general population and in up to 50% of patients with HIV infection. Seborrheic dermatitis increases in prevalence and severity as the CD4+ T cell count declines. In HIV-infected patients, seborrheic dermatitis may be aggravated by concomitant infection with *Pityrosporum*, a yeastlike fungus; use of topical antifungal agents has been recommended in cases refractory to standard topical treatment.

Eosinophilic pustular folliculitis is a rare dermatologic condition that is seen with increased frequency in patients with HIV infection.

It presents as multiple, urticarial perifollicular papules that may co-alesce into plaquelike lesions. Skin biopsy reveals an eosinophilic in-filtrate of the hair follicle, which in certain cases has been associated with the presence of a mite. Patients typically have an elevated serum IgE level and may respond to treatment with topical anthelminthics. Patients with HIV infection have also been reported to develop a se-vere form of *Norwegian scabies* with hyperkeratotic psoriasiform le-sions.

Both *psoriasis* and *ichthyosis*, although they are not reported to be increased in frequency, may be particularly severe when they occur in patients with HIV infection. Preexisting psoriasis may become guttate in appearance and more refractory to treatment in the setting of HIV infection.

Reactivation herpes zoster (shingles) is seen in 10 to 20% of pa-tients with HIV infection. This reactivation syndrome of varicella-zoster virus indicates a modest decline in immune function and may be the first indication of clinical immunodeficiency. In one series, pa-tients who developed shingles did so an average of 5 years after HIV infection. In a cohort of patients with HIV infection and localized zoster, the subsequent rate of the development of AIDS was 1% per month. In that study, AIDS was more likely to develop if the outbreak of zoster was associated with severe pain, extensive skin involvement, or involvement of cranial or cervical dermatomes. The clinical mani-festations of reactivation zoster in HIV-infected patients, although in-dicative of immunologic compromise, are not as severe as those seen in other immunodeficient conditions. Thus, while lesions may extend over several dermatomes (see Fig. 164-5) and frank cutaneous dissem-ination may be seen, visceral involvement has not been reported. In contrast to patients without a known underlying immunodeficiency state, patients with HIV infection tend to have recurrences of zoster with a relapse rate of ~20%. Acyclovir or famciclovir is the treatment of choice. Foscarnet is of value in patients with acyclovir-resistant virus.

Infection with *herpes simplex virus* in HIV-infected individuals is associated with recurrent orolabial, genital, and perianal lesions as part of recurrent reactivation syndromes (Chap. 163). As HIV disease pro-gresses and the CD4+ T cell count declines, these infections become more frequent and severe. Lesions often appear as beefy red, are ex-quisitely painful, and have a tendency to occur high in the gluteal cleft (Fig. 173-31). Perirectal HSV may be associated with proctitis and anal fissures. HSV should be high in the differential diagnosis of any HIV-infected patient with a poorly healing, painful perirectal lesion. In addition to recurrent mucosal ulcers, recurrent HSV infection in the form of *herpetic whitlow* can be a problem in patients with HIV in-fection, presenting with painful vesicles or extensive cutaneous ero-sion. Acyclovir or famciclovir is the treatment of choice in these settings. Of note is the fact that even subclinical reactivation of herpes simplex may be associated with increases in plasma HIV RNA levels. Consideration should be given to chronic suppressive therapy in pa-tients with recurrent outbreaks of herpesvirus.

Diffuse skin eruptions due to *Molluscum contagiosum* may be seen in patients with advanced HIV infection. These flesh-colored, umbil-icated lesions may be treated with local therapy. They tend to regress with effective antiretroviral therapy. Similarly, *condyloma acumina-tum* lesions may be more severe and more widely distributed in pa-tients with low CD4+ T cell counts. Atypical mycobacterial infections may present as erythematous cutaneous nodules as may fungal infec-tions, *Bartonella*, *Acanthamoeba*, and KS.

The skin of patients with HIV infection is often a target organ for drug reactions (Chap. 50). Although most skin reactions are mild and not necessarily an indication to discontinue therapy, patients may have particularly severe cutaneous reactions, including erythroderma and *Stevens-Johnson syndrome*, as a reaction to drugs, particularly sulfa drugs, the nonnucleoside reverse transcriptase inhibitors, abacavir, and amprenavir. Similarly, patients with HIV infection are often quite pho-tosensitive and burn easily following exposure to sunlight or as a side effect of radiation therapy (Chap. 51).

HIV infection and its treatment may be accompanied by cosmetic changes of the skin that are not of great clinical importance but may be troubling to patients. Yellowing of the nails and straightening of the hair, particularly in African-American patients, have been reported as a consequence of HIV infection. Zidovudine therapy has been as-sociated with elongation of the eyelashes and the development of a bluish discoloration to the nails, again more common in African-Amer-ican patients. Therapy with clofazimine may cause a yellow-orange discoloration of the skin.

Neurologic Diseases   Clinical disease of the nervous system accounts for a significant degree of morbidity in a high percentage of patients with HIV infection (Table 173-13). The neurologic problems that oc-cur in HIV-infected individuals may be either primary to the patho-genic processes of HIV infection or secondary to opportunistic infections or neoplasms (see above). Among the more frequent op-portunistic diseases that involve the CNS are toxoplasmosis, crypto-coccosis, progressive multifocal leukoencephalopathy, and primary CNS lymphoma. Other less common problems include mycobacterial infections; syphilis; and infection with CMV, HTLV-I, *T. cruzi*, or *Acanthamoeba*. Overall, secondary diseases of the CNS occur in ap-proximately one-third of patients with AIDS. These data antedate the widespread use of combination antiretroviral therapy, and this fre-quency is considerably less in patients receiving effective antiretroviral drugs. Primary processes related to HIV infection of the nervous sys-tem are reminiscent of those seen with other lentiviruses, such as the Visna-Maedi virus of sheep. Neurologic problems occur throughout the course of disease and may be inflammatory, demyelinating, or degenerative in nature. While only one of these, the *AIDS dementia complex*, or *HIV encephalopathy*, is considered an AIDS-defining ill-ness, most HIV-infected patients have some neurologic problem dur-ing the course of their disease. As noted in the section on pathogenesis, damage to the CNS may be a direct result of viral infection of the CNS macrophages or glial cells or may be secondary to the release of neurotoxins and potentially toxic cytokines such as IL-1β, TNF-α, IL-6, and TGF-β. It has been reported that HIV-infected individuals with the E4 allele for apolipoprotein E (apo E) are at increased risk for AIDS encephalopathy and peripheral neuropathy. Virtually all patients with HIV infection have some degree of nervous system involvement with the virus. This is evidenced by the fact that CSF findings are abnormal in ~90% of patients, even during the asymptomatic phase of HIV infection. CSF abnormalities include pleocytosis (50 to 65% of patients), detection of viral RNA (~75%), elevated CSF protein (35%), and evidence of intrathecal synthesis of anti-HIV antibodies (90%). It is important to point out that evidence of infection of the CNS with HIV does not imply impairment of cognitive function. The neurologic function of an HIV-infected individual should be consid-ered normal unless clinical signs and symptoms suggest otherwise.

Aseptic meningitis may be seen in any but the very late stages of HIV infection. In the setting of acute primary infection patients may

---

TABLE 173-13 *Neurologic Diseases in Patients with HIV Infection*

Opportunistic infections	Myelopathy
Toxoplasmosis	Vacuolar myelopathy
Cryptococcosis	Pure sensory ataxia
Progressive multifocal	Paresthesia/dysesthesia
leukoencephalopathy	Peripheral neuropathy
Cytomegalovirus	Acute inflammatory demyelinating
Syphilis	polyneuropathy (Guillain-Barré
Mycobacterium tuberculosis	syndrome)
HTLV-I infection	Chronic inflammatory demyelinating
Neoplasms	polyneuropathy (CIDP)
Primary CNS lymphoma	Mononeuritis multiplex
Kaposi's sarcoma	Distal symmetric polyneuropathy
Result of HIV-1 infection	Myopathy
Aseptic meningitis	
HIV encephalopathy (AIDS	
dementia complex)	

experience a syndrome of headache, photophobia, and meningismus. Rarely, an acute encephalopathy due to encephalitis may occur. Cranial nerve involvement may be seen, predominantly cranial nerve VII but occasionally V and/or VIII. CSF findings include a lymphocytic pleocytosis, elevated protein level, and normal glucose level. This syndrome, which cannot be clinically differentiated from other viral meningitides (Chap. 361), usually resolves spontaneously within 2 to 4 weeks; however, in some patients, signs and symptoms may become chronic. Aseptic meningitis may occur any time in the course of HIV infection; however, it is rare following the development of AIDS. This fact suggests that clinical aseptic meningitis in the context of HIV infection is an immune-mediated disease.

C. neoformans is the leading infectious cause of meningitis in patients with AIDS (Chap. 186). It is the initial AIDS-defining illness in ~2% of patients and generally occurs in patients with CD4+ T cell counts <100/μL. Cryptococcal meningitis is particularly common in patients with AIDS in Africa, occurring in ~20% of patients. Most patients present with a picture of subacute meningoencephalitis with fever, nausea, vomiting, altered mental status, headache, and meningeal signs. The incidence of seizures and focal neurologic deficits is low. The CSF profile may be normal or may show only modest elevations in WBC or protein levels. In addition to meningitis, patients may develop cryptococcomas. Approximately one-third of patients also have pulmonary disease. Uncommon manifestations of cryptococcal infection include skin lesions that resemble *molluscum contagiosum*, lymphadenopathy, palatal and glossal ulcers, arthritis, gastroenteritis, myocarditis, and prostatitis. The prostate gland may serve as a reservoir for smoldering cryptococcal infection. The diagnosis of cryptococcal meningitis is made by identification of organisms in spinal fluid with India ink examination or by the detection of cryptococcal antigen. A biopsy may be needed to make a diagnosis of CNS cryptococcoma. Treatment is with intravenous amphotericin B, at a dose of 0.7 mg/kg daily, with flucytosine, 25 mg/kg qid for 2 weeks, followed by fluconazole, 400 mg/d orally for 10 weeks, and then fluconazole, 200 mg/d until the CD4+ T cell count has increased to >200 cells/μl for 6 months in response to HAART. Symptoms may recur with initiation of HAART as an immune reconstitution syndrome (see above). Other fungi that may cause meningitis in patients with HIV infection are *C. immitis* and *H. capsulatum*. Meningoencephalitis has also been reported due to *Acanthamoeba* or *Naegleria*.

HIV encephalopathy, also called HIV-associated dementia or AIDS dementia complex, consists of a constellation of signs and symptoms of CNS disease. While this is generally a late complication of HIV infection that progresses slowly over months it can be seen in patients with CD4 counts >350 cells/μl. A major feature of this entity is the development of dementia, defined as a decline in cognitive ability from a previous level. It may present as impaired ability to concentrate, increased forgetfulness, difficulty reading, or increased difficulty performing complex tasks. Initially these symptoms may be indistinguishable from findings of situational depression or fatigue. In contrast to "cortical" dementia (such as Alzheimer's disease), aphasia, apraxia, and agnosia are uncommon, leading some investigators to classify HIV encephalopathy as a "subcortical dementia" (see below). In addition to dementia, patients with HIV encephalopathy may also have motor and behavioral abnormalities. Among the motor problems are unsteady gait, poor balance, tremor, and difficulty with rapid alternating movements. Increased tone and deep tendon reflexes may be found in patients with spinal cord involvement. Late stages may be complicated by bowel and/or bladder incontinence. Behavioral problems include apathy and lack of initiative, with progression to a vegetative state in some instances. Some patients develop a state of agitation or mild mania. These changes usually occur without significant changes in level of alertness. This is in contrast to the finding of somnolence in patients with dementia due to toxic/metabolic encephalopathies.

HIV encephalopathy is the initial AIDS-defining illness in ~3% of patients with HIV infection and thus only rarely precedes clinical ev-

idence of immunodeficiency. Clinically significant encephalopathy eventually develops in approximately one-fourth of patients with AIDS. As immunologic function declines, the risk and severity of HIV encephalopathy increases. Autopsy series suggest that 80 to 90% of patients with HIV infection have histologic evidence of CNS involvement. Several classification schemes have been developed for grading HIV encephalopathy; a commonly used clinical staging system is outlined in Table 173-14.

The precise cause of HIV encephalopathy remains unclear, although the condition is thought to be a result of direct effects of HIV on the CNS. HIV has been found in the brains of patients with HIV encephalopathy by Southern blot, in situ hybridization, PCR, and electron microscopy. Multinucleated giant cells, macrophages, and microglial cells appear to be the main cell types harboring virus in the CNS. Histologically, the major changes are seen in the subcortical areas of the brain and include pallor and gliosis, multinucleated giant cell encephalitis, and vacuolar myelopathy. Less commonly, diffuse or focal spongiform changes occur in the white matter.

There are no specific criteria for a diagnosis of HIV encephalopathy, and this syndrome must be differentiated from a number of other diseases that affect the CNS of HIV-infected patients (Table 173-13) The diagnosis of dementia depends upon demonstrating a decline in cognitive function. This can be accomplished objectively with the use of a Mini-Mental Status Examination (MMSE) in patients for whom prior scores are available. For this reason, it is advisable for all patients with a diagnosis of HIV infection to have a baseline MMSE. However, changes in MMSE scores may be absent in patients with mild HIV encephalopathy. Imaging studies of the CNS, by either MRI or CT, often demonstrate evidence of cerebral atrophy (Fig. 173-33). MRI may also reveal small areas of increased density on T2-weighted images. Lumbar puncture is an important element of the evaluation of patients with HIV infection and neurologic abnormalities. It is generally most helpful in ruling out or making a diagnosis of opportunistic infections. In HIV encephalopathy, patients may have the nonspecific findings of an increase in CSF cells and protein level. While HIV RNA can often be detected in the spinal fluid and HIV can be cultured from the CSF, this finding is not specific for HIV encephalopathy. There

TABLE 173-14	*Clinical Staging of HIV Encephalopathy (AIDS Dementia Complex)*
Stage	**Definition**
Stage 0 (normal)	Normal mental and motor function
Stage 0.5 (equivocal/ subclinical)	Absent, minimal, or equivocal symptoms without impairment of work or capacity to perform activities of daily living. Mild signs (snout response, slowed ocular or extremity movements) may be present. Gait and strength are normal.
Stage 1 (mild)	Able to perform all but the more demanding aspects of work or activities of daily living but with unequivocal evidence (signs or symptoms that may include performance on neuropsychological testing) of functional, intellectual, or motor impairment. Can walk without assistance.
Stage 2 (moderate)	Able to perform basic activities of self-care but cannot work or maintain the more demanding aspects of daily life. Ambulatory, but may require a single prop.
Stage 3 (severe)	Major intellectual incapacity (cannot follow news or personal events, cannot sustain complex conversation, considerable slowing of all output) or motor disability (cannot walk unassisted, usually with slowing and clumsiness of arms as well).
Stage 4 (end-stage)	Nearly vegetative. Intellectual and social comprehension and output are at a rudimentary level. Nearly or absolutely mute. Paraparetic or paraplegic with urinary and fecal incontinence.

Source: Adapted from JJ Sidtis, RW Price, Neurology 40:197, 1990.

FIGURE 173-33 AIDS dementia complex. Postcontrast CT scan through the lateral ventricles of a 47-year-old man with AIDS, altered mental status, and dementia. The lateral and third ventricles and the cerebral sulci are abnormally prominent. Mild white matter hypodensity is also seen adjacent to the frontal horns of the lateral ventricles.

appears to be no correlation between the presence of HIV in the CSF and the presence of HIV encephalopathy. Elevated levels of β_2-microglobulin, neopterin, and quinolinic acid (a metabolite of tryptophan reported to cause CNS injury) have been noted in the CSF of patients with HIV encephalopathy. These findings suggest that these factors as well as inflammatory cytokines may be involved in the pathogenesis of this syndrome.

Combination antiretroviral therapy is of benefit in patients with HIV encephalopathy. Improvement in neuropsychiatric test scores has been noted for both adult and pediatric patients treated with antiretrovirals. The rapid improvement in cognitive function noted with the initiation of antiretroviral therapy suggests that at least some component of this problem is quickly reversible, again supporting at least a partial role of soluble mediators in the pathogenesis. It should also be noted that these patients have an increased sensitivity to the side effects of neuroleptic drugs. The use of these drugs for symptomatic treatment is associated with an increased risk of extrapyramidal side effects; therefore, patients with HIV encephalopathy who receive these agents must be monitored carefully.

Seizures may be a consequence of opportunistic infections, neoplasms, or HIV encephalopathy (Table 173-15). The seizure threshold is often lower than normal in these patients owing to the frequent presence of electrolyte abnormalities. Seizures are seen in 15 to 40% of patients with cerebral toxoplasmosis, 15 to 35% of patients with primary CNS lymphoma, 8% of patients with cryptococcal meningitis, and 7 to 50% of patients with HIV encephalopathy. Seizures may also be seen in patients with CNS tuberculosis, aseptic meningitis, and progressive multifocal leukoencephalopathy. Seizures may be the presenting clinical symptom of HIV disease. In one study of 100 patients with HIV infection presenting with a first seizure, cerebral mass lesions were the most common cause, responsible for 32 of the 100 new-onset seizures. Of these 32 cases, 28 were due to toxoplasmosis and 4 to lymphoma. HIV encephalopathy accounted for an additional 24 new-onset seizures. Cryptococcal meningitis was the third most common

diagnosis, responsible for 13 of the 100 seizures. In 23 cases, no cause could be found, and it is possible that these cases represent a subcategory of HIV encephalopathy. Of these 23 cases, 16 (70%) had two or more seizures, suggesting that anticonvulsant therapy is indicated in all patients with HIV infection and seizures unless a rapidly correctable cause is found. While phenytoin remains the initial treatment of choice, hypersensitivity reactions to this drug have been reported in >10% of patients with AIDS, and therefore the use of phenobarbital or valproic acid must be considered as alternatives.

Patients with HIV infection may present with *focal neurologic deficits* from a variety of causes. The most common causes are toxoplasmosis, progressive multifocal leukoencephalopathy, and CNS lymphoma. Other causes include cryptococcal infections (discussed above, also Chap. 186), stroke, and reactivation Chagas' disease.

Toxoplasmosis has been one of the most common causes of secondary CNS infections in patients with AIDS, but its incidence is decreasing in the era of HAART. It is most common in patients from the Caribbean and from France. Toxoplasmosis is generally a late complication of HIV infection and usually occurs in patients with CD4+ T cell counts <200/μL. Cerebral toxoplasmosis is thought to represent a reactivation syndrome. It is 10 times more common in patients with antibodies to the organism than in patients who are seronegative. Patients diagnosed with HIV infection should be screened for IgG antibodies to *T. gondii* during the time of their initial workup. Those who are seronegative should be counseled about ways to minimize the risk of primary infection including avoiding the consumption of undercooked meat and careful hand washing after contact with soil or changing the cat litter box. The most common clinical presentation of cerebral toxoplasmosis in patients with HIV infection is fever, headache, and focal neurologic deficits. Patients may present with seizure, hemiparesis, or aphasia as a manifestation of these focal deficits or with a picture more influenced by the accompanying cerebral edema and characterized by confusion, dementia, and lethargy, which can progress to coma. The diagnosis is usually suspected on the basis of MRI findings of multiple lesions in multiple locations, although in some cases only a single lesion is seen. Pathologically, these lesions generally exhibit inflammation and central necrosis and, as a result, demonstrate ring enhancement on contrast MRI (Fig. 173-34) or, if MRI is unavailable or contraindicated, on double-dose contrast CT. There is usually evidence of surrounding edema. In addition to toxoplasmosis, the differential diagnosis of single or multiple enhancing mass lesions in the HIV-infected patient includes primary CNS lymphoma (see below) and, less commonly, TB or fungal or bacterial abscesses.

TABLE 173-15	Causes of Seizures in Patients with HIV Infection	
Disease	Overall Contribution to First Seizure, %	Fraction of Patients Who Have Seizures, %
HIV encephalopathy	24–47	7–50
Cerebral toxoplasmosis	28	15–40
Cryptococcal meningitis	13	8
Primary central nervous system lymphoma	4	15–30
Progressive multifocal leukoencephalopathy	1	

Source: From DM Holtzman et al: Am J Med 87:173, 1989.

FIGURE 173-34 Central nervous system toxoplasmosis. A coronal postcontrast T1-weighted MR scan demonstrates a peripheral enhancing lesion in the left frontal lobe, associated with an eccentric nodular area of enhancement (*arrow*); this so-called "eccentric target sign" is typical of toxoplasmosis.

The definitive diagnostic procedure is brain biopsy. However, given the morbidity than can accompany this procedure, it is usually reserved for the patient who has failed 2 to 4 weeks of empirical therapy. If the patient is seronegative for *T. gondii*, the likelihood that a mass lesion is due to toxoplasmosis is <10%. In that setting, one may choose to be more aggressive and perform a brain biopsy sooner. Standard treatment is sulfadiazine and pyrimethamine with leucovorin as needed for a minimum of 4 to 6 weeks. Alternative therapeutic regimens include clindamycin in combination with pyrimethamine; atovaquone plus pyrimethamine; and azithromycin plus pyrimethamine plus rifabutin. Relapses are common, and it is recommended that patients with a history of prior toxoplasmic encephalitis receive maintenance therapy with sulfadiazine, pyrimethamine, and leucovorin. Patients with CD4+ T cell counts <100/μL and IgG antibody to *Toxoplasma* should receive primary prophylaxis for toxoplasmosis. Fortunately, the same daily regimen of a single double-strength tablet of TMP/SMX used for *P. carinii* prophylaxis provides adequate primary protection against toxoplasmosis. Secondary prophylaxis for toxoplasmosis may be discontinued in the setting of effective antiretroviral therapy and increases in CD4+ T cell counts to >200/μL for 6 months.

JC virus, a human polyomavirus that is the etiologic agent of *progressive multifocal leukoencephalopathy* (PML), is an important opportunistic pathogen in patients with AIDS (Chap. 361). While ~70% of the general adult population have antibodies to JC virus, indicative of prior infection, <10% of healthy adults show any evidence of ongoing viral replication. PML is the only known clinical manifestation of JC virus infection. It is a late manifestation of AIDS and is seen in ~4% of patients with AIDS. The lesions of PML begin as small foci of demyelination in subcortical white matter that eventually coalesce. The cerebral hemispheres, cerebellum, and brainstem may all be involved. Patients typically have a protracted course with multifocal neurologic deficits, with or without changes in mental status. Ataxia, hemiparesis, visual field defects, aphasia, and sensory defects may occur. MRI typically reveals multiple, nonenhancing white matter lesions that may coalesce and have a predeliction for the occipital and parietal lobes. The lesions show signal hyperintensity on T2-weighted images and diminished signal on T1-weighted images. Prior to the availability of potent antiretroviral combination therapy, the majority of patients with PML died within 3 to 6 months of the onset of symptoms. Paradoxical worsening of PML has been seen with initiation of HAART as an immune reactivation syndrome. There is no specific treatment for PML; however, regressions of >2.5 years in duration have been reported in patients with PML treated with HAART for their HIV disease. Studies with antiviral agents such as cidofovir have failed to show clear benefit. Factors influencing a favorable prognosis for PML in the setting of HIV infection include a CD4+ T cell count >100/μL at baseline and the ability to maintain an HIV viral load of <500 copies per milliliter. Baseline viral load does not have independent predictive value of survival. PML is one of the few opportunistic infections that continues to occur with some frequency despite the widespread use of HAART.

Reactivation American trypanosomiasis may present as acute meningoencephalitis with focal neurologic signs, fever, headache, vomiting, and seizures. In South America, reactivation of *Chagas' disease* is considered to be an AIDS-defining condition and may be the initial AIDS-defining condition. Lesions appear radiographically as single or multiple hypodense areas, typically with ring enhancement and edema. They are found predominantly in the subcortical areas, a feature that differentiates them from the deeper lesions of toxoplasmosis. *Trypanosoma cruzi* amastigotes, or trypanosomes, can be identified from biopsy specimens or CSF. Other CSF findings include elevated protein and a mild (<100 cells/μL) lymphocytic pleocytosis. Organisms can also be identified by direct examination of the blood. Treatment consists of benzimidazole (2.5 mg/kg bid) or nifurtimox (2 mg/kg qid) for at least 60 days, followed by maintenance therapy for life with either drug at a dose of 5 mg/kg three times a week. As is the case

with cerebral toxoplasmosis, successful therapy with antiretrovirals may allow discontinuation of therapy for Chagas' disease.

Stroke may occur in patients with HIV infection. In contrast to the other causes of focal neurologic deficits in patients with HIV infection, the symptoms of a stroke are sudden in onset. Among the secondary infectious diseases in patients with HIV infection that may be associated with stroke are vasculitis due to cerebral varicella zoster or neurosyphilis and septic embolism in association with fungal infection. Other elements of the differential diagnosis of stroke in the patient with HIV infection include atherosclerotic cerebral vascular disease, thrombotic thrombocytopenic purpura, and cocaine or amphetamine use.

Primary CNS lymphoma is discussed below in the section on neoplastic diseases.

Spinal cord disease, or myelopathy, is present in ~20% of patients with AIDS, often as part of HIV encephalopathy. In fact, 90% of the patients with HIV-associated myelopathy have some evidence of dementia, suggesting that similar pathologic processes may be responsible for both conditions. Three main types of spinal cord disease are seen in patients with AIDS. The first of these is a vacuolar myelopathy, as discussed above under HIV encephalopathy. This condition is pathologically similar to subacute combined degeneration of the cord such as occurs with pernicious anemia. Although vitamin B_{12} deficiency can be seen in patients with AIDS, it does not appear to be responsible for the myelopathy seen in the majority of patients. Vacuolar myelopathy is characterized by a subacute onset and often presents with gait disturbances, predominantly ataxia and spasticity; it may progress to include bladder and bowel dysfunction. Physical findings include evidence of increased deep tendon reflexes and extensor plantar responses. The second form of spinal cord disease involves the dorsal columns and presents as a pure sensory ataxia. The third form is also sensory in nature and presents with paresthesias and dysesthesias of the lower extremities. In contrast to the cognitive problems seen in patients with HIV encephalopathy, these spinal cord syndromes do not respond well to antiretroviral drugs, and therapy is mainly supportive.

One important disease of the spinal cord that also involves the peripheral nerves is a *myelopathy* and *polyradiculopathy* seen in association with CMV infection. This entity is generally seen late in the course of HIV infection and is fulminant in onset, with lower extremity and sacral paresthesias, difficulty in walking, areflexia, ascending sensory loss, and urinary retention. The clinical course is rapidly progressive over a period of weeks. CSF examination reveals a predominantly neutrophilic pleocytosis, and CMV DNA can be detected by CSF PCR. Therapy with ganciclovir or foscarnet can lead to rapid improvement, and prompt initiation of foscarnet or ganciclovir therapy is important in minimizing the degree of permanent neurologic damage. Combination therapy with both drugs should be considered in patients who have been previously treated for CMV disease. Other diseases involving the spinal cord in patients with HIV infection include HTLV-I-associated myelopathy (HAM) (Chap. 172), neurosyphilis (Chap. 153), infection with herpes simplex (Chap. 163) or varicella-zoster (Chap. 164), TB (Chap. 150), and lymphoma (Chap. 97).

Peripheral neuropathies are common in patients with HIV infection. They occur at all stages of illness and take a variety of forms. Early in the course of HIV infection, an acute inflammatory demyelinating polyneuropathy resembling Guillain-Barré syndrome may occur (Chap. 366). In other patients, a progressive or relapsing-remitting inflammatory neuropathy resembling chronic inflammatory demyelinating polyneuropathy (CIDP) has been noted. Patients commonly present with progressive weakness, areflexia, and minimal sensory changes. CSF examination often reveals a mononuclear pleocytosis, and peripheral nerve biopsy demonstrates a perivascular infiltrate suggesting an autoimmune etiology. Plasma exchange or intravenous immunoglobulin has been tried with variable success. Because of the immunosuppressive effects of glucocorticoids, they should be reserved for severe cases of CIDP refractory to other measures. Another autoimmune peripheral neuropathy seen in patients with AIDS is mononeuritis multiplex (Chaps. 366 and 306) due to a necrotizing arteritis of peripheral nerves. The most common peripheral neuropathy in patients with HIV infection is a *distal sensory polyneuropathy* that may be a direct consequence of HIV infection or a side effect of dideoxynucleoside therapy. Two-thirds of patients with AIDS may be shown by electrophysiologic studies to have some evidence of peripheral nerve disease. Presenting symptoms are usually painful burning sensations in the feet and lower extremities. Findings on examination include a stocking-type sensory loss to pinprick, temperature, and touch sensation and a loss of ankle reflexes. Motor changes are mild and are usually limited to weakness of the intrinsic foot muscles. Response of this condition to antiretrovirals has been variable, perhaps because antiretrovirals are responsible for the problem in some instances. When due to dideoxynucleoside therapy, patients with lower extremity peripheral neuropathy may complain of a sensation that they are walking on ice. Other entities in the differential diagnosis of peripheral neuropathy include diabetes mellitus, vitamin B₁₂ deficiency, and side effects from metronidazole or dapsone. For distal symmetric polyneuropathy that fails to resolve following the discontinuation of dideoxynucleosides, therapy is symptomatic; gabapentin, carbamazepine, tricyclics, or analgesics may be effective for dysesthesias. Treatment-naive patients may respond to combination antiretroviral therapy, and preliminary data suggest that nerve growth factor may benefit some cases.

Myopathy may complicate the course of HIV infection; causes include HIV infection itself, zidovudine, and the generalized wasting syndrome. HIV-associated myopathy may range in severity from an asymptomatic elevation in creatine kinase levels to a subacute syndrome characterized by proximal muscle weakness and myalgias. Quite pronounced elevations in creatine kinase may occur in asymptomatic patients, particularly after exercise. The clinical significance of this as an isolated laboratory finding is unclear. A variety of both inflammatory and noninflammatory pathologic processes have been noted in patients with more severe myopathy, including myofiber necrosis with inflammatory cells, nemaline rod bodies, cytoplasmic bodies, and mitochondrial abnormalities. Profound muscle wasting, often with muscle pain, may be seen after prolonged zidovudine therapy. This toxic side effect of the drug is dose-dependent and is related to its ability to interfere with the function of mitochondrial polymerases. It is reversible following discontinuation of the drug. Red ragged fibers are a histologic hallmark of zidovudine-induced myopathy.

Ophthalmologic Disease   Ophthalmologic problems occur in approximately half of patients with advanced HIV infection. The most common abnormal findings on funduscopic examination are cotton-wool spots. These are hard white spots that appear on the surface of the retina and often have an irregular edge. They represent areas of retinal ischemia secondary to microvascular disease. At times they are associated with small areas of hemorrhage and thus can be difficult to distinguish from CMV retinitis. In contrast to CMV retinitis, however, these lesions are not associated with visual loss and tend to remain stable or improve over time.

One of the most devastating consequences of HIV infection is CMV retinitis. Patients at high risk of CMV retinitis (CD4+ T cell count <100/μL) should undergo an ophthalmologic examination every 3 to 6 months. The majority of cases of CMV retinitis occur in patients with a CD4+ T cell count <50/μL. Prior to the availability of HAART, this CMV reactivation syndrome was seen in 25 to 30% of patients with AIDS. CMV retinitis usualy presents as a painless, progressive loss of vision. Patients may also complain of blurred vision, "floaters," and scintillations. The disease is usually bilateral, affecting one eye more than the other. The diagnosis is made on clinical grounds by an experienced ophthalmologist. The characteristic retinal appearance is that of perivascular hemorrhage and exudate (see Fig. 25-5). In situations where the diagnosis is in doubt due to an atypical presentation or an unexpected lack of response to therapy, vitreous or aqueous humor sampling with molecular diagnostic techniques may be of value. CMV infection of the retina results in a necrotic inflammatory process, and the visual loss that develops is irreversible. CMV retinitis may be complicated by rhegmatogenous retinal detachment as a consequence of retinal atrophy in areas of prior inflammation. Therapy for CMV retinitis consists of oral valganciclovir, intravenous ganciclovir, or intravenous foscarnet, with cidofovir as an alternative. Combination therapy with ganciclovir and foscarnet has been shown to be slightly more effective than either ganciclovir or foscarnet alone in the patient with relapsed CMV retinitis. A 3-week induction course is followed by maintenance therapy with oral valganciclovir. If CMV disease is limited to the eye, a ganciclovir-releasing intraocular implant, periodic injections of the antisense nucleic acid preparation formivirsen, or intravitreal injections of ganciclovir or foscarnet may be considered; some choose to combine intraocular implants with oral valganciclovir. Intravitreal injections of cidofovir are generally avoided due to the increased risk of uveitis and hypotony. Maintenance therapy is continued until the CD4+ T cell count remains >100 to 150/μL for >6 months. The majority of patients with HIV infection and CMV disease develop some degree of uveitis with the initiation of antiretroviral therapy. The etiology of this is unknown; however, it has been suggested that this may be due to the generation of an enhanced immune response to CMV as an immune reactivation syndrome. In some instances this has required the use of topical glucocorticoids.

Both HSV and varicella zoster virus can cause a rapidly progressing, bilateral necrotizing retinitis referred to as the *acute retinal necrosis syndrome* or progressive outer retinal necrosis (PORN). This syndrome, in contrast to CMV retinitis, is associated with pain, keratitis, and iritis. It is often associated with orolabial HSV or trigeminal zoster. Ophthalmologic examination reveals widespread pale gray peripheral lesions. This condition is often complicated by retinal detachment. It is important to recognize and treat this condition with intravenous acyclovir as quickly as possible to minimize the loss of vision.

Several other secondary infections may cause ocular problems in HIV-infected patients. *P. carinii* can cause a lesion of the choroid that may be detected as an incidental finding on ophthalmologic examination. These lesions are typically bilateral, are from half to twice the disc diameter in size, and appear as slightly elevated yellow-white plaques. They are usually asymptomatic and may be confused with cotton-wool spots. Chorioretinitis due to toxoplasmosis can be seen alone or, more commonly, in association with CNS toxoplasmosis. Kaposi's sarcoma may involve the eyelid or conjunctiva while lymphoma may involve the retina.

Additional Disseminated Infections and Wasting Syndrome   Infections with species of the small, gram-negative rickettsia-like organism *Bartonella* (Chap. 144) are seen with increased frequency in patients with HIV infection. While not considered an AIDS-defining illness by the CDC, many experts view infection with *Bartonella* as indicative of a severe defect in cell-mediated immunity. It is usually seen in patients with CD4+ T cell counts <100/μL. Among the clinical manifestations of *Bartonella* infection are bacillary angiomatosis, cat-scratch disease, and trench fever. *Bacillary angiomatosis* is usually due to infection with *B. henselae*. It is characterized by a vascular proliferation that leads to a variety of skin lesions that have been confused with the skin lesions of KS. In contrast to the lesions of KS, the lesions of bacillary angiomatosis generally blanch, are painful, and typically occur in the setting of systemic symptoms. Infection can extend to the lymph nodes, liver (peliosis hepatis), spleen, bone, heart, CNS, respiratory tract, and gastrointestinal tract. *Cat-scratch disease* generally begins with a papule at the site of inoculation. This is followed several weeks later by the development of regional adenopathy and malaise. Infection with *B. quintana* is transmitted by lice and has been associated with case reports of trench fever, endocarditis, adenopathy, and bacillary angiomatosis. The organism is quite difficult to culture, and diagnosis often relies upon identifying the organism in biopsy specimens using the Warthin-Starry or similar stains. Treatment is with either erythromycin or doxycycline for at least 3 months.

Histoplasmosis is an opportunistic infection that is seen most frequently in patients in the Mississippi and Ohio River valleys, Puerto Rico, the Dominican Republic, and South America. These are all areas in which infection with *H. capsulatum* is endemic (Chap. 183). Because of this limited geographic distribution, the percentage of AIDS cases in the United States with histoplasmosis is only ~0.5. Histoplasmosis is generally a late manifestation of HIV infection; however, it may be the initial AIDS-defining condition. In one study, the median CD4+ T cell count for patients with histoplasmosis and AIDS was 33/μL. While disease due to *H. capsulatum* may present as a primary infection of the lung, disseminated disease, presumably due to reactivation, is the most common presentation in HIV-infected patients. Patients usually present with a 4- to 8-week history of fever and weight loss. Hepatosplenomegaly and lymphadenopathy are each seen in about 25% of patients. CNS disease, either meningitis or a mass lesion, is seen in 15% of patients. Bone marrow involvement is common, with thrombocytopenia, neutropenia, and anemia occurring in 33% of patients. Approximately 7% of patients have mucocutaneous lesions consisting of a maculopapular rash and skin or oral ulcers. Respiratory symptoms are usually mild, with chest x-ray showing a diffuse infiltrate or diffuse small nodules in approximately half of cases. Diagnosis is made by culturing the organisms from blood, bone marrow, or tissue. Treatment is typically with amphotericin B, 0.7 to 1.0 mg/kg daily to a total dose of 1 g followed by maintenance therapy with itraconazole. In the setting of mild infection, it may be appropriate to treat with itraconazole alone.

Following the spread of HIV infection to southeast Asia, disseminated infection with the fungus *Penicillium marneffei* was recognized as a complication of HIV infection and is considered an AIDS-defining condition in those parts of the world where it occurs. *P. marneffei* is the third most common AIDS-defining illness in Thailand, following TB and cryptococcosis. It is more frequently diagnosed in the rainy than the dry season. Clinical features include fever, generalized lymphadenopathy, hepatosplenomegaly, anemia, thrombocytopenia, and papular skin lesions with central umbilication. Treatment is with amphotericin B followed by itraconazole.

Visceral leishmaniasis (Chap. 196) is recognized with increasing frequency in patients with HIV infection who live in or travel to areas endemic for this protozoal infection transmitted by sandflies. The clinical presentation is one of hepatosplenomegaly, fever, and hematologic abnormalities. Lymphadenopathy and other constitutional symptoms may be present. Organisms can be isolated from cultures of bone marrow aspirates. Histologic stains may be negative, and antibody titers are of little help. Patients with HIV infection usually respond well initially to standard therapy with pentavalent antimony compounds. Eradication of the organism is difficult, however, and relapses are common.

Generalized wasting is an AIDS-defining condition; it is defined as involuntary weight loss of >10% associated with intermittent or constant fever and chronic diarrhea or fatigue lasting >30 days in the absence of a defined cause other than HIV infection. It is the initial AIDS-defining condition in ~10% of patients with AIDS in the United States and is an indication for intiation of HAART. A constant feature of this syndrome is severe muscle wasting with scattered myofiber degeneration and occasional evidence of myositis. Glucocorticoids may be of some benefit; however, this approach must be carefully weighed against the risk of compounding the immunodeficiency of HIV infection. Androgenic steroids, growth hormone, and total parenteral nutrition have been used as therapeutic interventions with variable success.

Neoplastic Diseases The neoplastic diseases clearly seen with an increased frequency in patients with HIV infection are KS and non-Hodgkin's lymphoma. In addition, there also appears to be an increased incidence of Hodgkin's disease; multiple myeloma; leukemia; melanoma; and cervical, brain, testicular, oral, lung, and anal cancers. Recent years have witnessed a marked reduction in the incidence of KS (Fig. 173-28), felt to be primarily due to the use of potent antiretroviral therapy. Rates of non-Hodgkin's lymphoma have declined as well; however, this decline has not been as dramatic as the decline in rates of KS.

Kaposi's sarcoma is a multicentric neoplasm consisting of multiple vascular nodules appearing in the skin, mucous membranes, and viscera. The course ranges from indolent, with only minor skin or lymph node involvement, to fulminant, with extensive cutaneous and visceral involvement. In the initial period of the AIDS epidemic, KS was a prominent clinical feature of the first cases of AIDS, occurring in 79% of the patients diagnosed in 1981. By 1989 it was seen in only 25% of cases, by 1992 the number had decreased to 9%, and by 1997 the number was <1%. HHV-8 or KSHV has been strongly implicated as a viral cofactor in the pathogenesis of KS (see above).

Clinically, KS has varied presentations and may be seen at any stage of HIV infection, even in the presence of a normal CD4+ T cell count. The initial lesion may be a small, raised reddish-purple nodule on the skin, a discoloration on the oral mucosa, or a swollen lymph node (Fig. 173-35). Lesions often appear in sun-exposed areas, particularly the tip of the nose, and have a propensity to occur in areas of trauma (Koebner phenomenon). Because of the vascular nature of the tumors and the presence of extravasated red blood cells in the lesions, their color ranges from reddish to purple to brown and often take the appearance of a bruise, with yellowish discoloration and tattooing. Lesions range in size from a few millimeters to several centimeters in diameter and may be either discrete or confluent. KS lesions most commonly appear as raised macules; however, they also can be papular, particularly in patients with higher CD4+ T cell counts. Confluent lesions may give rise to surrounding lymphedema and may be disfiguring when they involve the face and disabling when they involve the lower extremities or the surfaces of joints. Apart from skin, lymph nodes, gastrointestinal tract, and lung are the organ systems most commonly affected by KS. Lesions have been reported in virtually every organ, including the heart and the CNS. In contrast to most malignancies, in which lymph node involvement implies metastatic spread and a poor prognosis, lymph node involvement may be seen very early in KS and is of no special clinical significance. In fact, some patients may present with disease limited to the lymph nodes. These are generally patients with relatively intact immune function and thus the patients with the best prognosis. Pulmonary involvement with KS generally presents with shortness of breath. Some 80% of patients with pulmonary KS also have cutaneous lesions. The chest x-ray characteristically shows bilateral lower lobe infiltrates that obscure the margins of the mediastinum and diaphragm (Fig. 173-36). Pleural effusions are seen in 70% of cases of pulmonary KS, a fact that is often helpful in the differential diagnosis. Gastrointestinal involvement is seen in 50% of patients and usually takes one of two forms. The first is mucosal involvement, which may lead to bleeding that can be

FIGURE 173-35 Kaposi's sarcoma in a patient with AIDS demonstrating patch, plaque, and tumor stages.

FIGURE 173-36 Chest x-ray of a patient with AIDS and pulmonary Kaposi's sarcoma. The characteristic findings include dense bilateral lower lobe infiltrates obscuring the heart borders and a pleural effusion.

severe. These patients sometimes also develop symptoms of gastrointestinal obstruction if lesions become large. The second gastrointestinal manifestation is due to biliary tract involvement. KS lesions may infiltrate the gallbladder and biliary tree, leading to a clinical picture of obstructive jaundice similar to that seen with sclerosing cholangitis. Several staging systems have been proposed for KS. One in common use was developed by the National Institute of Allergy and Infectious Diseases AIDS Clinical Trials Group; it distinguishes patients on the basis of tumor extent, immunologic function, and presence or absence of systemic disease (Table 173-16).

A diagnosis of KS is based upon biopsy of a suspicious lesion. Histologically one sees a proliferation of spindle cells and endothelial cells, extravasation of red blood cells, hemosiderin-laden macrophages, and, in early cases, an inflammatory cell infiltrate. Included in the differential diagnosis are lymphoma (particularly for oral lesions), bacillary angiomatosis, and cutaneous mycobacterial infections.

Management of KS (Table 173-17) should be carried out in consultation with an expert since definitive treatment guidelines do not exist. In the majority of cases effective antiretroviral therapy will go a long way in achieving control. Indeed, spontaneous regressions have been reported in the setting of HAART. For patients in whom tumor persists or in whom control of HIV replication is not possible, a variety of options exist. In some cases, lesions remain quite indolent, and many of these patients can be managed with no specific treatment. Fewer than 10% of AIDS patients with KS die as a consequence of their malignancy, and death from secondary infections is considerably more common. Thus, whenever possible one should avoid treatment regimens that may further suppress the immune system and increase susceptibility to opportunistic infections. Treatment is indicated under two main circumstances. The first is when a single lesion or a limited number of lesions are causing significant discomfort or cosmetic problems, such as with prominent facial lesions, lesions overlying a joint, or lesions in the oropharynx that interfere with swallowing or breathing. Under these circumstances, treatment with localized radiation, intralesional vinblastine, or cryotherapy may be indicated. It should be noted that patients with HIV infection are particularly sensitive to the side effects of radiation therapy. This is especially true with respect to the development of radiation-induced mucositis; doses of radiation directed at mucosal surfaces, particularly in the head and neck region, should be adjusted ac-

cordingly. The use of systemic therapy, either IFN-α or chemotherapy, should be considered in patients with a large number of lesions or in patients with visceral involvement. The single most important determinant of response appears to be the CD4+ T cell count. This relationship between response rate and baseline CD4+ T cell count is particularly true for IFN-α. The response rate for patients with CD4+ T cell counts >600/μL is ~80%, while the response rate for patients with counts <150/μL is <10%. In contrast to the other systemic therapies, IFN-α provides an added advantage of having antiretroviral activity; thus, it may be the appropriate first choice for single-agent systemic therapy for early patients with disseminated disease. A variety of chemotherapeutic agents have also been shown to have activity against KS. Three of them, liposomal daunorubicin, liposomal doxorubicin, and paclitaxel have been approved by the FDA for this indication. Liposomal daunorubicin is approved as first-line therapy for patients with advanced KS. It has fewer side effects than conventional chemotherapy. In contrast, liposomal doxorubicin and paclitaxel are approved only for KS patients who have failed standard chemotherapy. Response rates vary from 23 to 88%, appear to be comparable to what had been achieved earlier with combination chemotherapy regimens, and are greatly influenced by CD4+ T cell count.

Lymphomas occur with an increased frequency in patients with congenital or acquired T cell immunodeficiencies (Chap. 297). AIDS is no exception; at least 6% of all patients with AIDS develop lymphoma at some time during the course of their illness. This is a 120-fold increase in incidence compared to the general population. In contrast to the situation with KS, primary CNS lymphoma, and most opportunistic infections, the incidence of AIDS-associated systemic lymphomas has not experienced as dramatic a decrease as a consequence of the widespread use of effective antiretroviral therapy. Lymphoma occurs in all risk groups, with the highest incidence in patients with hemophilia and the lowest incidence in patients from the Caribbean or Africa with heterosexually acquired infection. Lymphoma is a late manifestation of HIV infection, generally occurring in patients with CD4+ T cell counts <200/μL. As HIV disease progresses, the risk of lymphoma increases. In contrast to KS, which occurs at a relatively constant rate throughout the course of HIV disease, the attack rate for lymphoma increases exponentially with increasing duration of HIV infection and decreasing level of immunologic function. At 3 years following a diagnosis of HIV infection, the risk of lymphoma is 0.8% per year; by 8 years after infection, it is 2.6% per year. As people with HIV infection live longer as a consequence of improved antiretroviral therapy and better treatment and prophylaxis of opportunistic infections, it is anticipated that the incidence of lymphomas may increase.

Three main categories of lymphoma are seen in patients with HIV infection: grade III or IV immunoblastic lymphoma, Burkitt's lym-

TABLE 173-16 *National Institute of Allergy and Infectious Diseases AIDS Clinical Trials Group TIS Staging System for Kaposi's Sarcoma*

Parameter	Good Risk (stage 0): All of the Following	Poor Risk (stage 1): Any of the Following
Tumor (T)	Confined to skin and/or lymph nodes and/or minimal oral disease	Tumor-associated edema or ulceration Extensive oral lesions Gastrointestinal lesions Nonnodal visceral lesions
Immune system (I) Systemic illness (S)	CD4+ T cell count ≥200/μL No B symptoms[a] Karnofsky performance status >70 No history of opportunistic infection, neurologic disease, lymphoma, or thrush	CD4+ T cell count <200/μL B symptoms[a] present Karnofsky performance status <70 History of opportunistic infection, neurologic disease, lymphoma, or thrush

[a] Defined as unexplained fever, night sweats, >10% involuntary weight loss, or diarrhea persisting for more than 2 weeks.

TABLE 173-17   *Management of AIDS-Associated Kaposi's Sarcoma*

Observation and optimization of antiretroviral therapy
Single or limited number of lesions
  Radiation
  Intralesional vinblastine
  Cryotherapy
Extensive disease
  Initial therapy
    Interferon-α (if CD4+ T cells >150/μL)
    Liposomal daunorubicin
  Subsequent therapy
    Liposomal doxorubicin
    Paclitaxel
  Combination chemotherapy with low-dose doxorubicin, bleomycin,
    and vinblastine (ABV)
  Radiation treatment

FIGURE 173-37   Diffuse histiocytic lymphoma involving the hard palate of a patient with AIDS.

phoma, and primary CNS lymphoma. Approximately 90% of these lymphomas are B cell in phenotype, and half contain EBV DNA. These tumors may be either monoclonal or oligoclonal in nature and are probably in some way related to the pronounced polyclonal B cell activation seen in patients with AIDS.

Immunoblastic lymphomas account for ~60% of the cases of lymphoma in patients with AIDS. These are generally high grade and would have been classified as diffuse histiocytic lymphomas in earlier classification schemes. This tumor is more common in older patients, increasing in incidence from 0% in HIV-infected individuals <1 year old to >3% in those >50. One variant of immunoblastic lymphoma is body cavity lymphoma. This malignancy presents with lymphomatous pleural, pericardial, and/or peritoneal effusions in the absence of discrete nodal or extranodal masses. The tumor cells do not express surface markers for B cells or T cells. HHV-8 DNA sequences have been found in the genome of the malignant cells (see above).

Small non-cleaved cell lymphoma (Burkitt's lymphoma) accounts for ~20% of the cases of lymphoma in patients with AIDS. It is most frequent in patients 10 to 19 years old and usually demonstrates characteristic c-*myc* translocations from chromosome 8 to chromosomes 14 or 22. Burkitt's lymphoma is not commonly seen in the setting of immunodeficiency other than HIV-associated immunodeficiency, and the incidence of this particular tumor is over 1000-fold higher in the setting of HIV infection than in the general population. In contrast to African Burkitt's lymphoma, where 97% of the cases contain EBV genome, only 50% of HIV-associated Burkitt's lymphomas are EBV-positive.

Primary CNS lymphoma accounts for ~20% of the cases of lymphoma in patients with HIV infection. In contrast to HIV-associated Burkitt's lymphoma, primary CNS lymphomas are usually positive for EBV. In one study, the incidence of Epstein-Barr positivity was 100%. This malignancy does not have a predilection for any particular age group. The median CD4+ T cell count at the time of diagnosis is ~50/μL. Thus, CNS lymphoma generally presents at a later stage of HIV infection than systemic lymphoma. This fact may at least in part explain the poorer prognosis for this subset of patients.

The clinical presentation of lymphoma in patients with HIV infection is quite varied, ranging from focal seizures to rapidly growing mass lesions in the oral mucosa (Fig. 173-37) to persistent unexplained fever. At least 80% of patients present with extranodal disease, and a similar percentage have B-type symptoms of fever, night sweats, or weight loss. Virtually any site in the body may be involved. The most common extranodal site is the CNS, which is involved in approximately one-third of all patients with lymphoma. Approximately 60% of these cases are primary CNS lymphoma. Primary CNS lymphoma generally presents with focal neurologic deficits, including cranial nerve findings, headaches, and/or seizures. MRI or CT generally reveals a limited number (one to three) of 3- to 5-cm lesions (Fig. 173-38). The lesions often show ring enhancement on contrast administra-

tion and may occur in any location. Locations that are most commonly involved with CNS lymphoma are deep in the white matter. Contrast enhancement is usually less pronounced than that seen with toxoplasmosis. The main diseases in the differential diagnosis are cerebral toxoplasmosis and cerebral Chagas' disease. In addition to the 20% of lymphomas in HIV-infected individuals that are primary CNS lymphomas, CNS disease is also seen in HIV-infected patients with systemic lymphoma. Approximately 20% of patients with systemic lymphoma have CNS disease in the form of leptomeningeal involvement. This fact underscores the importance of lumbar puncture in the staging evaluation of patients with systemic lymphoma.

Systemic lymphoma is seen at earlier stages of HIV infection than primary CNS lymphoma. In one series the mean CD4+ T cell count was 189/μL. In addition to lymph node involvement, systemic lymphoma may commonly involve the gastrointestinal tract, bone marrow, liver, and lung. Gastrointestinal tract involvement is seen in ~25% of patients. Any site in the gastrointestinal tract may be involved, and patients may complain of difficulty swallowing or abdominal pain. The diagnosis is usually suspected on the basis of CT or MRI of the abdomen. Bone marrow involvement is seen in ~20% of patients and may lead to pancytopenia. Liver and lung involvement are each seen in ~10% of patients. Pulmonary disease may present as either a mass lesion, multiple nodules, or an interstitial infiltrate.

Both conventional and unconventional approaches have been employed in an attempt to treat HIV-related lymphomas. Systemic lymphoma is generally treated by the oncologist with combination

FIGURE 173-38   Central nervous system lymphoma. Postcontrast T1-weighted MR scan in a patient with AIDS, an altered mental status, and hemiparesis. Multiple enhancing lesions, some ring-enhancing, are present. The left Sylvian lesion shows gyral and subcortical enhancement, and the lesions in the caudate and splenium (*arrowheads*) show enhancement of adjacent ependymal surfaces.

chemotherapy. Earlier disappointing figures are being replaced with more optimistic results for the treatment of systemic lymphoma following the availability of more effective combination antiretroviral therapy. As in most situations in patients with HIV disease, those with the higher CD4+ T cell counts tend to do better. Response rates as high as 72% and disease-free intervals >15 months have been reported. Treatment of primary CNS lymphoma remains a significant challenge. Treatment is complicated by the fact that this illness usually occurs in patients with advanced HIV disease. Palliative measures such as radiation therapy provide some relief. The prognosis remains poor in this group, with median survival <1 year.

Evidence of infection with *human papilloma virus* (HPV), associated with *intraepithelial dysplasia of the cervix or anus*, is approximately twice as common in HIV-infected individuals as in the general population and can lead to intraepithelial neoplasia and eventually invasive cancer. In two separate studies, HIV-infected men without anorectal symptoms were studied for evidence of dysplasia, and Papanicolaou (Pap) smears were found to be abnormal in 40%. These changes were persistent at 1 year follow-up, raising the possibility of a subsequent transition to a more malignant condition. While the incidence of an abnormal Pap smear of the cervix is ~5% in otherwise healthy women, the incidence of abnormal cervical smears in women with HIV infection is 60%. Based on this finding, *invasive cervical cancer* was added to the list of AIDS-defining conditions. Thus far, however, only small increases in the incidence of cervical or anal cancer have been seen as a consequence of HIV infection. However, given this high rate of dysplasia, a comprehensive gynecologic and rectal examination, including Pap smear, is indicated at the initial evaluation and 6 months later for all patients with HIV infection. If these examinations are negative at both time points, the patient should be followed with yearly evaluations. If an initial or repeat Pap smear shows evidence of severe inflammation with reactive squamous changes, the next Pap smear should be performed at 3 months. If, at any time, a Pap smear shows evidence of squamous intraepithelial lesions, colposcopic examination with biopsies as indicated should be performed. HAART has been found to reduce the rate of progression and in some instances to induce regression of HPV-induced dysplasia.

IDIOPATHIC CD4+ T LYMPHOCYTOPENIA

A syndrome was recognized in 1992 that was characterized by an absolute CD4+ T cell count of <300/μL or <20% of total T cells on more than one occasion; no evidence of HIV-1, HIV-2, HTLV-I, or HTLV-II on testing; and the absence of any defined immunodeficiency or therapy associated with decreased levels of CD4+ T cells. By mid-1993, ~100 patients had been described. After extensive multicenter investigations, a series of reports were published in early 1993, which together allowed a number of conclusions. Idiopathic CD4+ lymphocytopenia (ICL) is a very rare syndrome, as determined by studies of blood donors and cohorts of HIV-seronegative homosexual men. Cases were clearly identified as early as 1983, and cases remarkably similar to ICL had been identified decades ago. The definition of ICL based on CD4+ T cell counts coincided with the ready availability of testing for CD4+ T cells in patients suspected of being immunosuppressed. Although, as a result of immune deficiency, certain patients with ICL develop some of the opportunistic diseases (particularly cryptococcosis) seen in HIV-infected patients, the syndrome is demographically, clinically, and immunologically unlike HIV infection and AIDS. Fewer than half of the reported ICL patients had risk factors for HIV infection, and there were wide geographic and age distributions. The fact that a significant proportion of patients did have risk factors probably reflects a selection bias, in that physicians who take care of HIV-infected patients are more likely to monitor CD4+ T cells. Approximately one-third of the patients are women, compared to 16% of women among HIV-infected individuals in the United States. Many patients with ICL remained clinically stable, and their condition did not deteriorate progressively as is common with seriously immunodeficient HIV-infected patients. Certain patients with ICL even experienced spontaneous reversal of the CD4+ T lymphocytopenia.

Immunologic abnormalities in ICL are somewhat different from those of HIV infection. ICL patients often also have decreases in CD8+ T cells and in B cells. Furthermore, immunoglobulin levels were either normal or, more commonly, decreased in patients with ICL, compared to the usual hypergammaglobulinemia of HIV-infected individuals. Finally, virologic studies revealed no evidence of HIV-1, HIV-2, HTLV-I, or HTLV-II or of any other mononuclear cell–tropic virus. Furthermore, there was no epidemiologic evidence to suggest that a transmissible microbe was involved. The cases of ICL were widely dispersed, with no clustering. Close contacts and sexual partners who were studied were clinically well and were serologically, immunologically, and virologically negative for HIV. ICL is a heterogeneous syndrome, and it is highly likely that there is no common cause; however, there may be common causes among subgroups of patients that are currently unrecognized.

Patients who present with laboratory data consistent with ICL should be worked up for underlying diseases that could be responsible for the immune deficiency. If no underlying cause is detected, no specific therapy should be initiated. However, if opportunistic diseases occur, they should be treated appropriately (see above). Depending on the level of the CD4+ T cell count, patients should receive prophylaxis for the commonly encountered opportunistic infections.

℞ TREATMENT

General Principles of Patient Management The treatment of patients with HIV infection requires not only a comprehensive knowledge of the possible disease processes that may occur but also the ability to deal with the problems of a chronic, potentially life-threatening illness. Great advances have been made in the treatment of patients with HIV infection. The appropriate use of potent combination antiretroviral therapy and other treatment and prophylactic interventions is of critical importance in providing each patient with the best opportunity to live a long and healthy life despite the presence of HIV infection. In contrast to the earlier days of this epidemic, a diagnosis of HIV infection need no longer be equated with an inevitably fatal disease. In addition to medical interventions, the health care provider has a responsibility to provide each patient with appropriate counseling and education concerning their disease as part of a comprehensive care plan. Patients must be educated about the potential transmissibility of their infection and about the fact that while health care providers may refer to levels of the virus as "undetectable," this is more a reflection of the sensitivity of the assay being used to measure the virus than a comment on the presence or absence of the virus. It is important for patients to be aware that the virus is still present and capable of being transmitted at all stages of HIV disease. Thus, there need to be frank discussions concerning sexual practices and the sharing of needles. The treating physician must not only be aware of the latest medications available for patients with HIV infection but must also educate patients concerning the natural history of their illness and listen and be sensitive to their fears and concerns. As with other diseases, therapeutic decisions should be made in consultation with the patient, when possible, and with the patient's proxy if the patient is incapable of making decisions. In this regard, it is recommended that all patients with HIV infection, and in particular those with CD4+ T cell counts <200/μL, designate a trusted individual with durable power of attorney to make medical decisions on their behalf, if necessary.

No matter how well prepared a patient is for adversity, the discovery of a diagnosis of HIV infection is a devastating event. For this reason, it is recommended that anyone about to undergo testing have "pretest counseling" to prepare him or her at least partially should the results demonstrate the presence of HIV infection. Following a diagnosis of HIV infection, the health care provider should be prepared to activate support systems immediately for the newly diagnosed patient. These should include an experienced social worker or nurse who can spend time talking to the person and ensuring that he or she is emotionally stable. Most communities have HIV crisis centers that can be of great help in these difficult situations.

Following a diagnosis of HIV infection, there are several examinations and laboratory studies that should be performed to help determine the extent of disease and provide baseline standards for future reference (Table 173-18). In addition to routine chemistry and hematology screening panels and chest x-ray, one should also obtain a CD4+ T cell count, two separate plasma HIV RNA levels, a VDRL test, and an anti-*Toxoplasma* antibody titer. A PPD test should be done, and a MMSE performed and recorded. Patients should be immunized with pneumococcal polysaccharide and, if seronegative for these viruses, with hepatitis A and hepatitis B vaccines. The status of hepatitis C infection should be determined. In addition, patients should be counseled with regard to sexual practices and needle sharing, and counseling should be offered to those whom the patient knows or suspects may also be infected. Once these baseline activities are performed, short- and long-term medical management strategies should be developed based upon the most recent information available and modified as new information becomes available. The field of HIV medicine is changing rapidly, and it is difficult to remain fully up to date. Fortunately there are a series of excellent sites on the internet that are frequently updated, and they provide the most recent information on a variety of topics, including consensus panel reports on treatment (Table 173-19).

Antiretroviral Therapy   Combination antiretroviral therapy, or HAART, is the cornerstone of management of patients with HIV infection. Following the initiation of widespread use of HAART in the United States in 1995 to 1996, marked declines have been noted in the incidence of most AIDS-defining conditions (Fig. 173-28). Suppression of HIV replication is an important component in prolonging life as well as improving the quality of life in patients with HIV infection. Unfortunately, many of the most important questions related to the treatment of HIV disease currently lack definitive answers. Among them are the questions of when should therapy be started, what is the best initial regimen, when should a given regimen be changed, and what should it be changed to when a change is made. Notwithstanding these uncertainties, the physician and patient must come to a mutually agreeable plan based upon the best available data. In an effort to facilitate this process, the United States Department of Health and Human Services has published a series of frequently updated guidelines including the "*Principles of Therapy of HIV Infection,*" "*Guidelines for the Use of Antiretroviral Agents in HIV-Infected Adults and Adolescents,*" and "*Guidelines for the Prevention of Opportunistic Infections in Persons Infected with Human Immunodeficiency Virus.*" At present, an extensive clinical trials network, involving both clinical investigators and patient advocates, is in place attempting to develop improved approaches to therapy. Consortia comprising representatives of academia, industry, and the federal government are involved in the process of drug development, including a wide-ranging series of clinical trials. As a result, new therapies and new therapeutic strategies are contin-

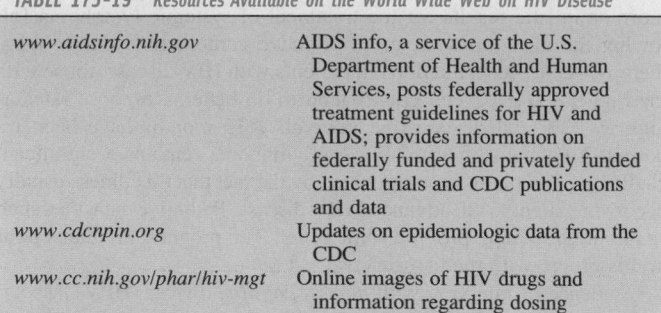

TABLE 173-19   *Resources Available on the World Wide Web on HIV Disease*

www.aidsinfo.nih.gov	AIDS info, a service of the U.S. Department of Health and Human Services, posts federally approved treatment guidelines for HIV and AIDS; provides information on federally funded and privately funded clinical trials and CDC publications and data
www.cdcnpin.org	Updates on epidemiologic data from the CDC
www.cc.nih.gov/phar/hiv-mgt	Online images of HIV drugs and information regarding dosing

Note: CDC, Centers for Disease Control and Prevention.

ually emerging. New drugs are often available through expanded access programs prior to official licensure. Given the complexity of this field, decisions regarding antiretroviral therapy are best made in consultation with experts. Currently licensed drugs for the treatment of HIV infection fall into three categories: those that inhibit the viral reverse transcriptase enzyme (Table 173-20, Fig. 173-39), those that inhibit the viral protease enzyme, and those that interfere with viral entry. There are numerous drug-drug interactions that one must take into consideration when using these agents (Table 173-21).

The FDA-approved reverse transcriptase inhibitors include the *nucleoside analogues* zidovudine, didanosine, zalcitabine, stavudine, lamivudine, abacavir, and emtricitabine; the *nucleotide analogue* tenofovir; and the *nonnucleoside reverse transcriptase inhibitors* nevirapine, delavirdine, and efavirenz (Fig. 173-39; Table 173-20). These were the first class of drugs that were licensed for the treatment of HIV infection. They are indicated for this use as part of combination regimens. It should be stressed that none of these drugs should be used as monotherapy for HIV infection. Thus, when lamivudine or tenofovir are used to treat hepatitis B infection in the setting of HIV infection, one should ensure that the patient is also on additional antiretroviral medication. The reverse transcriptase inhibitors block the HIV replication cycle at the point of RNA-dependent DNA synthesis, the reverse transcription step. While the nonnucleoside reverse transcriptase inhibitors are quite selective for the HIV-1 reverse transcriptase, the nucleoside and nucleotide analogues inhibit a variety of DNA polymerization reactions in addition to those of the HIV-1 reverse transcriptase. For this reason, serious side effects are more common with the nucleoside analogues and include mitochondrial damage that can lead to hepatic steatosis and lactic acidosis as well as peripheral neuropathy and pancreatitis. One of the more recently recognized problems that has been encountered with the widespread use of HAART therapy has been a syndrome of hyperlipidemia, glucose intolerance, and fat distribution often referred to as *lipodystrophy syndrome* (discussed above under metabolic abnormalities).

Zidovudine (AZT; 3'-azido-2',3'-dideoxythymidine) was the first drug approved for the treatment of HIV infection and is the prototype nucleoside analogue. These compounds, in which the hydroxyl group in the 3' position of the ribose moiety is substituted with a hydrogen or other chemical group, act as DNA chain terminators owing to their inability to form a 3'-5' phosphodiester linkage with another nucleoside. They bind much more avidly to the active site of the RNA-dependent DNA polymerase of HIV (reverse transcriptase) than to the active site of mammalian cell DNA polymerases; this explains their selective effect on HIV replication. Zidovudine also has a relatively high avidity for the DNA polymerase-γ of human mitochondria. This may contribute to the development of the fatty liver and the myopathy sometimes observed in patients taking zidovudine. As with all the nucleoside analogues, the active form of zidovudine is the triphosphate, and the rate of phosphorylation, a thymidine kinase–dependent pathway, may be different in different cells. This may explain why zidovudine is more effective at inhibiting HIV replication in some cells than others. The clinical efficacy of zidovudine was clearly established in 1986 in a phase II, randomized, placebo-controlled trial in patients

TABLE 173-18   *Initial Evaluation of the Patient with HIV Infection*

History and physical examination
Routine chemistry and hematology
CD4+ T lymphocyte count
Two plasma HIV RNA levels
RPR test
Anti-*Toxoplasma* antibody titer
PPD skin test
Mini-mental status examination
Serologies for hepatitis A, hepatitis B, and hepatitis C
Immunization with pneumococcal polysaccharide; influenza as indicated
Immunization with hepatitis A and hepatitis B if seronegative
Counseling regarding natural history and transmission
Help contacting others who might be infected

Note: VDRL, Venereal Disease Research Laboratory; PPD, purified protein derivative.

Drug	Status	Indication	Dose as Monotherapy	Dose in Combination	Supporting Data	Toxicity
REVERSE TRANSCRIPTASE INHIBITORS						
Zidovudine (AZT, azidothymidine, Retrovir, 3'azido-3'-deoxythymidine)	Licensed	Treatment of HIV infection in combination with other antiretroviral agents	Not indicated	200 mg q8h or 300 mg bid	19 vs 1 death in original placebo-controlled trial in 281 patients with AIDS or ARC. Decreased progression to AIDS in patients with CD4+ T cell counts <500/μL, $n = 2051$	Anemia, granulocytopenia, myopathy, lactic acidosis, hepatomegaly with steatosis, headache, nausea
		Prevention of maternal-fetal HIV transmission	*Mother:* 200 mg tid or 300 mg bid until the start of labor, then 2 mg/kg over 1 h IV, followed by 1 mg/kg per h IV until clamping of umbilical cord; *Infant:* 2 mg/kg q6h PO beginning within 12 h birth, or 1.5 mg/kg q6h IV over 30 min for 6 weeks		In pregnant women with CD4+ T cell count ≥200/μL, AZT PO beginning at weeks 14–34 of gestation plus IV drug during labor and delivery plus PO AZT to infant for 6 wk decreased transmission of HIV by 67.5% (from 25.5% to 8.3%), $n = 363$	
Didanosine (Videx, Videx EC, ddI, dideoxyinosine, 2',3'-dideoxyinosine)	Licensed	For treatment of HIV infection in combination with other antiretroviral agents	Not indicated	Buffered: Requires 2 tablets to achieve adequate buffering of stomach acid; should be administered on an empty stomach ≥60 kg: 200 mg bid <60 kg: 125 mg bid Enteric coated: ≥60 kg: 400 mg qd < 60 kg: 250 mg qd	Clinically superior to AZT as monotherapy in 913 patients with prior AZT therapy. Clinically superior to AZT and comparable to AZT + ddI and AZT + ddC in 1067 AZT-naive patients with CD4+ T cell counts of 200–500/μL	Pancreatitis, peripheral neuropathy, abnormalities on liver function tests, lactic acidosis, hepatomegaly with steatosis
Zalcitabine (ddC, HIVID, 2'3'-dideoxycytidine)	Licensed	In combination with other antiretroviral agents for the treatment of HIV infection	Not indicated	0.75 mg tid	Clinically inferior to AZT monotherapy as initial treatment. Clinically as good as ddI in advanced patients intolerant to AZT. In combination with AZT, was clinically superior to AZT alone in patients with AIDS or CD4+ T cell count <350/μL	Peripheral neuropathy, pancreatitis, lactic acidosis, hepatomegaly with steatosis, oral ulcers
Stavudine (d4T, Zerit, 2'3'-didehydro-3'-dideoxythymidine)	Licensed	Treatment of HIV-infected patients in combination with other antiretroviral agents	Not indicated	≥60 kg: 40 mg bid <60 kg: 30 mg bid	Superior to AZT with respect to changes in CD4+ T cell counts in 359 patients who had received ≥24 wk of AZT. Following 12 wk of randomization, the CD4+ T cell count had decreased in AZT-treated controls by a mean of 22/μL, while in stavudine-treated patients, it had increased by a mean of 22/μL	Peripheral neuropathy, pancreatitis, lactic acidosis, hepatomegaly with steatosis, ascending neuromuscular weakness, lipodystrophy
Lamivudine (Epivir, 2'3'-dideoxy-3'-thiacytidine, 3TC)	Licensed	In combination with other antiretroviral agents for the treatment of HIV infection	Not indicated	150 mg bid 300 mg qd	Superior to AZT alone with respect to changes in CD4 counts in 495 patients who were zidovudine-naive and 477 patients who were zidovudine-experienced. Overall CD4+ T cell counts for the zidovudine group were at baseline by 24 wk, while in the group treated with zidovudine plus lamivudine, they were 10–50 cells/μL above baseline. 54% decrease in progression to AIDS/death compared to AZT alone	

(continued)

Drug	Status	Indication	Dose as Monotherapy	Dose in Combination	Supporting Data	Toxicity
Emtricitabine (FTC, Emtriva)	Licensed	In combination with other antiretroviral agents for the treatment of HIV infection	Not indicated	200 mg qd	Comparable to d4T in combination with ddI and efavirenz in 571 treatment-naive patients. Similar to 3TC in combination with 2DV or d4T + NNRT1 or PI in 440 patients doing well for at least 12 weeks on a 3TC regimen.	
Abacavir (Ziagen)	Licensed	For treatment of HIV infection in combination with other antiretroviral agents	Not indicated	300 mg bid	Abacavir + AZT + 3TC equivalent to indinavir + AZT + 3TC with regard to viral load suppression (~60% in each group with <400 HIV RNA copies/mL plasma) and CD4 cell increase (~100/μL in each group) at 24 weeks	Hypersensitivity reaction (can be fatal); fever, rash, nausea, vomiting, malaise or fatigue, and loss of appetite
Tenofovir (Viread)	Licensed	For use in combination with other antiretroviral agents when treatment is indicated	Not indicated	300 mg qd	Reduction of ~0.6 log in HIV-1 RNA levels when added to background regimen in treatment-experienced patients	Potential for renal toxicity
Delavirdine (Rescriptor)	Licensed	For use in combination with appropriate antiretrovirals when treatment is warranted	Not indicated	400 mg tid	Delavirdine + AZT superior to AZT alone with regard to viral load suppression at 52 weeks	Skin rash, abnormalities in liver function tests
Nevirapine (Viramune)	Licensed	In combination with other antiretroviral agents for treatment of progressive HIV infection	Not indicated	200 mg/d × 14 days then 200 mg bid	Increases in CD4+ T cell count, decrease in HIV RNA when used in combination with nucleosides	Skin rash, hepatotoxicity
Efavirenz (Sustiva)	Licensed	For treatment of HIV infection in combination with other antiretroviral agents	Not indicated	600 mg qhs	Efavirenz + AZT + 3TC comparable to indinavir + AZT + 3TC with regard to viral load suppression (a higher percentage of the efavirenz group achieved viral load <50 copies/mL; however, the discontinuation rate in the indinavir group was unexpectedly high, accounting for most treatment "failures") and CD4 cell increase (~140/μL in each group) at 24 weeks	Rash, dysphoria, elevated liver function tests, drowsiness, abnormal dreams, depression
PROTEASE INHIBITORS						
Saquinavir mesylate (Invirase—hard gel capsule)	Licensed	In combination with other antiretroviral agents when therapy is warranted	Not indicated	600 mg q8h	Increases in CD4+ T cell counts, reduction in HIV RNA most pronounced in combination therapy with ddC. 50% reduction in first AIDS-defining event or death in combination with ddC compared to either agent alone	Diarrhea, nausea, headaches, hyperglycemia, fat redistribution, lipid abnormalities
(Fortovase—soft gel capsule)	Licensed	For use in combination with other antiretroviral agents when treatment is warranted	Not indicated	1200 mg tid	Reduction in the mortality rate and AIDS-defining events for patients who received hard-gel formulation in combination with ddC	Diarrhea, nausea, abdominal pain, headaches, hyperglycemia, fat redistribution, lipid abnormalities
Ritonavir (Norvir)	Licensed	In combination with other antiretroviral agents for treatment of HIV infection when treatment is warranted	Not indicated	600 mg bid	Reduction in the cumulative incidence of clinical progression or death from 34 to 17% in patients with CD4+ T cell count <100/μL treated for a median of 6 months	Nausea, abdominal pain, hyperglycemia, fat redistribution, lipid abnormalities, may alter levels of many other drugs, including saquinavir

(continued)

TABLE 173-20—(Continued)

Drug	Status	Indication	Dose as Monotherapy	Dose in Combination	Supporting Data	Toxicity
Indinavir sulfate (Crixivan)	Licensed	For treatment of HIV infection in combination with other antiretroviral agents when antiretroviral treatment is warranted	Not indicated	800 mg q8h	Increase in CD4+ T cell count by 100/μL and 2-log decrease in HIV RNA levels when given in combination with zidovudine and lamivudine. Decrease of 50% in risk of progression to AIDS or death when given with zidovudine and lamivudine compared with zidovudine and lamivudine alone	Nephrolithiasis, indirect hyperbilirubinemia, hyperglycemia, fat redistribution, lipid abnormalities
Nelfinavir mesylate (Viracept)	Licensed	For treatment of HIV infection in combination with other antiretroviral agents when antiretroviral therapy is warranted	Not indicated	750 mg tid or 1250 mg bid	2.0-log decline in HIV RNA when given in combination with stavudine	Diarrhea, loose stools, hyperglycemia, fat redistribution, lipid abnormalities
Amprenavir (Agenerase)	Licensed	In combination with other antiretroviral agents for treatment of HIV infection	Not indicated	1200 mg bid or 600 mg bid + Ritonavir 100 mg bid or 1200 mg qd + Ritonavir 200 mg qd	In treatment-naïve patients, amprenavir + AZT + 3TC superior to AZT + 3TC with regard to viral load suppression (53% vs 11% with <400 HIV RNA copies/mL plasma at 24 weeks), CD4+ T cell responses similar between treatment groups. In treatment-experienced patients, amprenavir + NRTIs similar to indinavir + NRTIs with regard to viral load suppression (43% vs 53% with <400 HIV RNA copies/mL plasma at 24 weeks). CD4+ T cell responses superior in the indinavir + NRTIs group	Nausea, vomiting, diarrhea, rash, oral paresthesias, elevated liver function tests, hyperglycemia, fat redistribution, lipid abnormalities
Fosamprenavir (Lexiva)	Licensed			1400 mg bid or 700 mg bid + Ritonavir 100 mg bid		
Lopinavir/ritonavir (Kaletra)	Licensed	For treatment of HIV infection in combination with other antiretroviral agents	Not indicated	400 mg/100 mg bid	In treatment of naïve patients, lopinavir/ritonavir + d4T + 3TC superior to nelfinavir + d4T + 3TC with regard to viral load suppression (79% vs 64% with <400 HIV RNA copies/mL at 40 weeks). CD4+ T cell increases similar in both groups.	Diarrhea, hyperglycemia, fat redistribution, lipid abnormalities
Atazanavir (Reyataz)	Licensed	For treatment of HIV infection in combination with other antiretroviral agents	Not indicated	400 mg qd or 300 mg qd + Ritonavir 100 mg qd when given with efavirenz	Comparable to efavirenz when given in combination with AZT + 3TC in a study of 810 treatment-naive patients. Comparable to nelfinavir when given in combination with d4T + 3TC in a study of 467 treatment-naive patients.	Hyperbilirubinemia, PR prolongation, nausea, vomiting, hyperglycemia, fat maldistribution
FUSION INHIBITOR						
Enfuvirtide (Fuzeon)	Licensed	In combination with other agents in treatment-experienced patients with evidence of HIV-1 replication despite ongoing antiretroviral therapy	Not indicated	90 mg SC bid	In treatment of experienced patients, superior to placebo when added to new optimized background (37% vs 16% with <400 HIV RNA copies/mL at 24 weeks; + 71 vs + 35 CD4+ T cells at 24 weeks)	Local injection reactions, hypersensitivity reactions, increased rate of bacterial pneumonia

Note: ARC, AIDS-related complex; NRTIs, nonnucleoside reverse transcriptase inhibitors.

with advanced HIV disease. However, while treatment of patients with early stages of HIV infection was associated with increases in CD4+ T cell count, it was not associated with a better overall outcome than waiting until later to treat. Subsequent trials established the ability of this drug to dramatically decrease the incidence of perinatal transmission of HIV from infected mother to infant. Eventually a series of studies demonstrated the superiority of combination antiretroviral regimens over zidovudine alone, and combination therapy (discussed below) remains the standard of treatment today. Among the side effects of zidovudine at the initiation of therapy are fatigue, malaise, nausea, and headache. These side effects often subside over time. Patients on zidovudine may develop a macrocytic anemia, myopathy, cardiomyopathy, and lactic acidosis associated with fatty infiltration of the liver. As with every antiretroviral drug, HIV has the ability to develop re-

Nucleoside Analogues

Zidovudine Didanosine Zalcitabine Abacavir

Stavudine Lamivudine Emtricitabine Tenofovir

Nonnucleoside Reverse Transcriptase Inhibitors

Delavirdine Nevirapine Efavirenz

FIGURE 173-39 Molecular structures of antiretroviral agents.

sistance to zidovudine. Zidovudine resistance has been reported to occur ~6 months following the initiation of zidovudine monotherapy. More recently, zidovudine-resistant viruses have been noted in patients with acute infection prior to the initiation of therapy, implying that zidovudine-resistant viruses can be transmitted from person to person. Resistance emerges more rapidly in late-stage patients, presumably as a consequence of a greater degree of viral replication and thus a greater opportunity for mutation. A variety of amino acid changes including substitutions, insertions, and deletions have been reported to confer zidovudine resistance (Fig. 173-40). One combination preparation, Combivir, consists of zidovudine and lamivudine, while another, Trizivir, consists of zidovudine, lamivudine, and abacavir.

Didanosine (ddI; 2′,3′-dideoxyinosine) was the second drug licensed for the treatment of HIV infection, followed shortly thereafter by zalcitabine. Didanosine is metabolized to dideoxyadenosine in vivo. It is best absorbed on an empty stomach at a high pH. For this reason, the formulations of didanosine either contain a buffer, and each dose must be administered in no fewer than two tablets to ensure adequate buffering of stomach acid, or are provided as an extended-release enteric-coated capsule. The toxicity profile of didanosine is quite different from that of zidovudine. The most common toxicity is a painful sensory peripheral neuropathy that occurs in ~30% of patients receiving >400 mg/d. It generally resolves with discontinuation of the drug and may not recur if the drug is resumed at a reduced dose. At higher doses than are currently used one may see pancreatitis in ~10% of patients. Pancreatitis associated with didanosine therapy can be fatal. Didanosine should be discontinued if a patient experiences abdominal pain consistent with pancreatitis or if an elevated serum amylase or lipase level is found in association with an edematous pancreas on ultrasound. Didanosine is contraindicated in patients with a prior history of pancreatitis, regardless of etiology.

Zalcitabine (ddC; 2′,3′-dideoxycytidine) is rarely used today in the management of patients with HIV infection. Among the nucleoside analogues licensed for the treatment of HIV infection, it is probably the weakest. The main toxicity of ddC is pancreatitis.

Stavudine (d4T; 2′,3′-didehydro-3′-deoxythymidine) was the

fourth drug licensed for the treatment of HIV infection. Like zidovudine, stavudine is a thymidine analogue. These two drugs are antagonistic in vitro and in vivo and should not be given together. Peripheral neuropathy and hepatic steatosis are the main toxicities of stavudine. It is commonly used with lamivudine as part of an initial treatment regimen.

Lamivudine (3TC; 2′,3′-dideoxy-3′-thiacytidine) is the fifth of the nucleoside analogues to be licensed in the United States. It is licensed for use in combination with zidovudine in situations where zidovudine is indicated. In actual practice, lamivudine is a frequent element of many different combination regimens currently in use. It is available either alone or in combination with zidovudine (Combivir). One reason behind the excellent synergy seen between lamivudine and the other nucleoside analogues may be that strains of HIV resistant to lamivudine (M184V substitution) appear to have enhanced sensitivity to other nucleosides, and thus development of dual resistance is quite difficult. In addition, there is a suggestion that 3TC-resistant strains of HIV may be less virulent and are less able to generate new mutants than are strains of HIV that are 3TC-sensitive. Lamivudine is among the best tolerated and least toxic nucleoside analogues.

Emtricitabine (FTC; 5-fluoro-1-(2R,5S)-[2-(hydroxymethyl)-1,3-oxathiolan-5-yl]cytosine) is the negative enantiomer of a thio analogue of cytidine with a fluorine in the 5 position. It is licensed for use in combination with other antiretroviral agents for treatment of HIV-1 infection in adults. Similar in activity to lamivudine, resistance to emtricitabine is associated with the M184V mutation in reverse transcriptase. Viruses showing the K65R mutation in reverse transcriptase may have reduced susceptibility to emtricitabine.

Abacavir {(1S,cis)-4-[2-amino-6-(cyclopropylamino)-9H-purin-9-yl]-2-cyclopentene-1-methanol sulfate (salt)(2:1)} is a synthetic carbocyclic analogue of the nucleoside guanosine. It is licensed to be used in combination with other antiretroviral agents for the treatment of HIV-1 infection. Hypersensitivity reactions have been reported in ~4% of patients treated with this drug, and patients developing signs or symptoms of hypersensitivity such as fever, skin rash, fatigue, and gastrointestinal symptoms should discontinue the drug and not restart it. Fatal hyper-

Ritonavir

Nelfinavir mesylate

Lopinavir

Saquinavir mesylate

Indinavir sulfate

Amprenavir

Atazanavir

Enfuvirtide

FIGURE 173-39— *(Continued)*

sensitivity reactions have been reported with rechallenge. Abacavir hypersensitiviy appears to occur with a higher frequency in patients who are HLA-B57. Abacavir-resistant strains of HIV are typically also resistant to lamivudine, didanosine, and zalcitabine.

Tenofovir disoproxil fumarate (9-[(R)-2-[[bis[[(isopropoxycarbonyl)oxy]methoxy]phosphinyl]methoxy]propyl]adenine fumarate (1:1)) is an acyclic nucleoside phosphonate diester analogue of adenosine monophosphate. It undergoes diester hydrolysis to form tenofovir and is the first nucleotide analogue to be licensed for treatment of HIV infection. It is indicated in combination with other antiretroviral agents for the treatment of HIV-1 infection. HIV isolates with increased resistance typically express a K65R mutation in reverse transcriptase and a three- to four-fold reduction in sensitivity to tenofovir. Tenofovir is primarily eliminated by the kidneys, and renal impairment with hypophosphatemia may occur. Tenofovir is contraindicated in patients with renal impairment. Coadministration with didanosine leads to a 60% increase in didanosine levels, and thus doses of didanosine need

to be adjusted and patients monitored carefully if these two drugs are used in combination.

Nevirapine, delavirdine, and *efavirenz* are nonnucleoside inhibitors of the HIV-1 reverse transcriptase. They are licensed for use in combination with nucleoside analogues for the treatment of HIV-infected adults. These agents inhibit reverse transcriptase by binding to regions of the enzyme outside the active site and causing conformational changes in the enzyme that render it inactive. Although these agents are active in the nanomolar range, they are also very selective for the reverse transcriptase of HIV-1, have no activity against HIV-2, and, when used as monotherapy, are associated with the rapid emergence of drug-resistant mutants (Table 173-20; Fig. 173-40). Efavirenz is administered once a day, nevirapine twice a day, and delavirdine three times a day. All three drugs are associated with the development of a maculopapular rash, generally seen within the first few weeks of therapy. While it is possible to treat through this rash, it is important to be sure that one is not dealing with a more severe eruption such as

TABLE 173-21 Drug-Drug Interactions Involving Antiretroviral Agents

Index Drug	Interacting Drug(s)	Mechanism/Effect	Recommendation
Amprenavir	Efavirenz	Induction of metabolism, decreased amprenavir AUC	Consider dosage increase to 1200 mg tid or add ritonavir 200 mg bid
	Indinavir	Inhibition of metabolism—drug levels increased 33%	No change
	Ritonavir	Inhibition of metabolism—amprenavir AUC increased 2.5-fold	Decrease to 600 mg bid
Amprenavir, indinavir, saquinavir, ritonavir, nelfinavir	Rifampin	Induction of metabolism—marked decrease in protease inhibitor drug levels	Avoid concomitant use
Antiarrhythmics (flecainaide, quinidine, propafenone, amiodarone)	Ritonavir	Inhibition of metabolism—potential for increased levels and toxicity	Use with caution or avoid concomitant use
Atorvastatin	Protease inhibitors	Inhibition of metabolism—increased drug levels	Use with caution
Atovaquone	Rifampin	Induction of metabolism—decreased drug levels	Concentrations may not be therapeutic—avoid or increase dose
Benzodiazepines (flurazepam, diazepam, midazolam, triazolam)	Protease inhibitors, delavirdine, efavirenz	Inhibition of metabolism—increased drug levels	Monitor for toxicity such as increased sedation, decrease dose, or use temazepam, lorazepam. Not recommended for use with triazolam
Bepridil	Ritomavir, amprenavir	Inhibition of metabolism—increased drug levels	Avoid concomitant use
Carbamazepine	Indinavir, ritonavir	Inhibition of metabolism—increased toxicity	Avoid concomitant use or monitor levels
Cidofovir	Nephrotoxic drugs (aminoglycosides, amphotericin, foscarnet)	Potential for increased side effects	Monitor renal function
Cisapride	Protease inhibitors, azole antifungals, macrolides, delavirdine, efavirenz	Inhibition of metabolism	Cardiotoxic life-threatening effects possible—avoid concomitant use
Clarithromycin	Efavirenz	Induction of metabolism—40% decrease in clarithromycin AUC	Clinical significance unknown, but clarithromycin effectiveness may be altered
	Nevirapine	Induction of metabolism—decrease in clarithromycin AUC by 30%, increase in 14-OH clarithromycin by 58%	No dosage adjustments necessary
	Delavirdine	Inhibition of metabolism—100% increase in clarithromycin	Adjust dose in renal failure
	Ritonavir Atazanavir	Inhibition of metabolism—drug levels increased 77%	No adjustment needed in normal renal function
	Agents that increase gastric pH—antacids, H₂ blockers, proton pump inhibitors, didanosine	Delavirdine absorption decreased with increased pH	Avoid concomitant use with H$_2$ blockers and proton pump inhibitors; separate from antacids by at least 2 h
	Rifabutin	Induction of metabolism—50–60% decrease in delavirdine levels	Clinical significance unknown; may require increased delavirdine dose
	Rifampin	Induction of metabolism—marked decrease in drug levels	Avoid concomitant use
Didanosine (ddI)	Allopurinol	Increased ddI AUC by 2-fold	Clinical significance unknown
	Methadone	Decrease in ddI AUC by 52%	No clinical data, but potential for decreased ddI efficacy
	Tenofovir	Increase in ddI AUC by 44%	Consider ddI dose reduction
	Ganciclovir	Increased ddI AUC by 111%	Monitor for ddI toxicity
Efavirenz	Fluconazole	Inhibition of metabolism—efavirenz AUC increased 15%	No dosage adjustment necessary
	Indinavir	Induction of hepatic metabolism—indinavir AUC decreased 35%	Consider increasing indinavir dose to 1000 mg q8h
	Nelfinavir	Nelfinavir AUC increased 21%	No dosage adjustment necessary
	Rifampin	Induction of metabolism—significant reduction in efavirenz AUC	Clinical significance unknown; increase in efavirenz dose may be required
	Rifampin	Induction of metabolism—efavirenz AUC decreased 26%	Clinical significance unknown
	Ritonavir	Inhibition of metabolism—efavirenz AUC increased 21%	No dosage adjustment necessary
Ergot alkaloids (ergotamine, dihydroergotamine, ergoloid mesylates)	Protease inhibitors, azole antifungals, macrolides, delavirdine, efavirenz	Inhibition of metabolism—potential for acute toxicity	Use with caution or avoid concomitant use; monitor for toxicity such as peripheral vasoconstriction, nausea and vomiting, and impaired mental status

(continued)

TABLE 173-21—(Continued)

Index Drug	Interacting Drug(s)	Mechanism/Effect	Recommendation
Ethinyl estradiol	Efavirenz	Inhibition of metabolism—37% increase in estradiol AUC	No dosage adjustment necessary
	Protease inhibitors, nevirapine	Induction of metabolism—decreased levels of oral contraceptive	Use alternative or additional method of contraception
Fluvastatin, lovastatin, simvastatin	Protease inhibitors, azole antifungals, macrolides, delavirdine	Inhibition of metabolism—potential for increased levels and toxicity	Potential for hypolipidemic toxicity (dizziness, headache, GI side effects); monitor patient closely and consider dose reduction or use pravastatin or atorvastatin
Foscarnet	Nephrotoxic drugs (aminoglycosides, amphotericin, cidofovir)	Potential for increased toxicity	Monitor renal function
Ganciclovir	Drugs causing bone marrow suppression (i.e., TMP/SMZ, zidovudine)	Potential for increased hematologic toxicity	Monitor for anemia and neutropenia—adjust/change doses and drugs if required; consider supportive therapy with G-CSF
	Tenofovir	Competition for tubular secretion	Monitor for renal toxicity
Indinavir, saquinavir, ritonavir, nelfinavir, amprenavir	Anticonvulsants (carbamazepine, phenytoin, phenobarbital)	Induction of metabolism— potential decrease in drug levels	Clinical effects unknown; monitor blood levels, consider dosage increase, or avoid concomitant use
Indinavir	Delavirdine	Increased indinavir levels	Consider reducing indinavir dose to 600 mg q8h
	St. John's wort	Decreased indinavir levels	Avoid use of St. John's wort
	Didanosine, antacids	ddI buffer decreases absorption of indinavir	Separate doses by at least 1 h
	Methadone	Indinavir C_{max} decreased 16–36%; indinavir C_{min} increased by 50–100%	No dosage adjustments necessary
	Nelfinavir	Inhibition of metabolism—indinavir drug levels increased by 51%, nelfinavir drug levels by 83%	Avoid concommitant use
	Nevirapine	Induction of metabolism—decreased drug levels of indinavir by 30%	Consider increasing indinavir dose to 1000 mg q8h
	Ritonavir	Inhibition of metabolism—indinavir AUC increased 3–7-fold	Consider 800 mg indinavir/200 mg ritonavir bid
	Efavirenz	Induction of metabolism—31% decrease in indinavir levels	Dose indinavir at 1000 mg q8h or add ritonavir
Lopinavir/ritonavir	Nevirapine, efavirenz	Induction of metabolism—40–55% decrease in lopinavir levels	Dose lopinavir/ritonavir at 533/133 mg bid
Meperidine	Ritonavir	Likely induction of metabolism—decrease in meperidine AUC 67%, increase in normeperidine 47%	Potential for decreased meperidine effectiveness—may require increased dose; caution with chronic dosing
Methadone	Abacavir	Methadone clearance decreased 22%	Low potential for opiate withdrawal; monitor closely and increase methadone dose as required to control symptoms
	Fluconazole	Inhibition of metabolism—drug levels increased 30%	Monitor for methadone toxicity such as respiratory depression, drop in blood pressure, and mental status changes; consider dosage adjustment
	Nevirapine, efavirenz, ritonavir	Induction of metabolism—substantial decrease in methadone levels	Potential for opiate withdrawal; monitor closely and increase methadone dose as required to control symptoms
Nelfinavir	Ritonavir	Inhibition of metabolism—increased drug levels of nelfinavir by 152%	Consider nelfinavir 500–750 mg bid + ritonavir 200–400 mg bid
Pentamidine	Drugs that cause pancreatitis (didanosine, zalcitabine)	Increased risk of pancreatitis	Monitor amylase, lipase
Quinolone antibiotics (ciprofloxacin, levofloxacin, ofloxaxin, etc)	Didanosine buffered tablet, antacids, iron products, calcium products, sucralfate	Chelation resulting in marked decrease in quinolone drug levels	Administer cation preparations at least 2 h after quinolone
Rifabutin	Amprenavir, atazanavir, ritonavir, indinavir, nelfinavir, lopinavir/ritonavir	Inhibition of metabolism—marked increase in rifabutin drug levels	Use 150 mg qd with indinavir, nelfinavir, amprenavir; increase nelfinavir to 1000 mg tid Use 150 mg every other day with ritonavir, lopinavir/ritonavir, atazanavir
	Delavirdine	Induction of delavirdine metabolism; inhibition of rifabutin metabolism	Avoid concomitant use
	Efavirenz	Induction of rifabutin metabolism—levels decrease 35%	Increase rifabutin to 450–600 mg qd
	Fluconazole	Inhibition of metabolism—marked increase in rifabutin drug levels	Monitor for rifabutin toxicity such as uveitis, nausea, neutropenia

(continued)

Index Drug	Interacting Drug(s)	Mechanism/Effect	Recommendation
Rifampin	Protease inhibitors, delavirdine, nevirapine	Induction of metabolism—decreased drug levels	Avoid concomitant use
	Efavirenz	Induction of metabolism	Increase efavirenz to 800 mg qd
Ritonavir	Delavirdine	Inhibition of metabolism—70% increase in ritonavir levels	No data to base recommendations
Saquinavir	Nevirapine	Induction of metabolism—drug levels decreased 27%	Clinical significance unknown—consider dosage increase of saquinavir or add ritonavir
	Ritonavir	Inhibition of metabolism—3-fold or higher increase in saquinavir drug levels	Various combinations used to optimize saquinavir therapy including 400 mg saquinavir/400 mg ritonavir
	Delavirdine	Inhibition of metabolism—5-fold increase in saquinavir drug levels	Dose saquinavir at 800 mg tid
	Nelfinavir	Inhibition of metabolism—3–5-fold increase in saquinavir drug levels	Dose saquinavir at 800 mg tid or 1200 mg bid
	Efavirenz	Induction of metabolism—saquinavir AUC decreased 62%	Avoid concomitant use unless saquinavir is administered with ritonavir
Sildenafil	Protease inhibitors, delavirdine	Inhibition of metabolism—sildenafil AUC increased 2–11-fold	Use 25-mg sildenafil dose and do not repeat for 48 h
St. John's Wort	Protease inhibitors, NRTIs	Induction of metabolism—decreased drug levels	Avoid concomitant use
Terfenadine, astemizole	Protease inhibitors, azole antifungals, macrolides, delavirdine, efavirenz	Inhibition of metabolism	Cardiotoxic life-threatening effects possible—avoid concomitant use
Theophylline	Ritonavir	Induction of metabolism—decreased blood levels	Monitor theophylline levels
Tipranavir	Ritonavir	Inhibition of metabolism—tipranavir AUC increased 7–45-fold	Combination under investigation to optimize tipranavir levels
TMP/SMZ	Rifampin	TMP AUC decreased 63%, SMX AUC decreased 23%	Clinical significance unknown
Zalcitabine, stavudine, didanosine	Drugs that cause peripheral neuropathy—INH, d4T, ddI, ddC	Potential for increased risk of peripheral neuropathy	Monitor for signs and symptoms such as numbness and tingling in extremities
Zidovudine	Drugs causing bone marrow suppression (i.e., TMP/SMX, ganciclovir, sulfadiazine)	Increased bone marrow suppression	Monitor for anemia, neutropenia—may require supportive therapy (EPO, G-CSF)

Note: AUC, area under the curve; *C*, concentration; EPO, erythropoietin; G-CSF, granulocyte colony stimulating factor; TMP/SMX, trimethoprim/sulfamethoxazole.

Stevens-Johnson syndrome by looking carefully for signs of mucosal involvement, significant fever, or painful lesions with desquamation. Severe, life-threatening, and in some cases fatal hepatotoxicity, including fulminant and cholestatic hepatitis, hepatic necrosis and hepatic failure, have been reported in patients treated with nevirapine. Many patients treated with efavirenz note a feeling of light-headedness, dizziness, or out of sorts following the initiation of therapy. Some complain of vivid dreams. These symptoms tend to disappear after several weeks of therapy. Aside from difficulties with dreams, taking efavirenz at bedtime may minimize the side effects. Nevirapine and efavirenz are both commonly used as part of initial treatment regimens in combination with two nucleoside analogues. Another common use of these drugs is as part of salvage regimens in patients whose current regimen is inadequate.

The introduction of the HIV-1 protease inhibitors (saquinavir, indinavir, ritonavir, nelfinavir, amprenavir, lopinavir/ritonavir, and atazanavir) to the therapeutic armamentarium of antiretrovirals has had a profound impact on the efficacy of antiretroviral therapy. When used as part of initial regimens in combination with reverse transcriptase inhibitors, these agents have been shown to be capable of suppressing levels of HIV replication to under 50 copies per milliliter in the majority of patients for a minimum of 5 years. HIV protease inhibitors appear to be good substrates for the drug transporters MDR-1 and MRP-2. Whether or not genetic variations in these genes will lead to variability in protease inhibitor activity remains to be determined. As in the case of reverse transcriptase inhibitors, resistance to protease inhibitors can develop rapidly in the setting of monotherapy, and thus these agents should only be used as part of combination therapeutic regimens. A summary of known resistance mutations for protease inhibitors is shown in Fig. 173-40.

Saquinavir was the first of the HIV-1 protease inhibitors to be licensed. Initially provided as a hard gel (Invirase) with poor bioavailability, the soft-gel formulation (Fortavase) provides good plasma levels of drug, particularly when administered in conjunction with ritonavir. Saquinavir is metabolized by the cytochrome P450 system, and ritonavir therapy results in inhibition of cytochrome P450 action. Thus, when both drugs are administered together there is the potential for increases in saquinavir levels. The use of low doses of ritonavir to provide pharmacodynamic boosting of other agents has become a fairly common strategy in HIV therapy. Saquinavir is among the best-tolerated protease inhibitors.

Ritonavir was the first protease inhibitor for which clinical efficacy was demonstrated. In a study of 1090 patients with CD4+ T cell counts $<100/\mu L$ who were randomized to receive either placebo or ritonavir in addition to any other licensed medications, patients receiving ritonavir had a reduction in the cumulative incidence of clinical progression or death from 34% to 17%. Mortality decreased from 10.1% to 5.8%. At full doses, ritonavir is poorly tolerated. Among the main side effects are nausea, diarrhea, abdominal pain, and circumoral paresthesia. Ritonavir has a high affinity for several isoforms of cytochrome P450, and its use can result in large increases in the plasma concentrations of drugs metabolized by this pathway. Among the agents affected in this manner are saquinavir, indinavir, macrolide antibiotics, R-warfarin, ondansetron, rifampin, most calcium channel blockers, glucocorticoids, and some of the chemotherapeutic agents used to treat KS. In addition, ritonavir may increase the activity of glucuronyltransferases, thus decreasing the levels of drugs metabolized by this pathway. Overall, great care must be taken when prescribing additional drugs to patients taking ritonavir. As mentioned above, the pharmacodynamic boosting property of ritonavir, seen with

MUTATIONS IN THE REVERSE TRANSCRIPTASE GENE ASSOCIATED WITH RESISTANCE TO REVERSE TRANSCRIPTASE INHIBITORS

Nucleoside and Nucleotide Reverse Transcriptase Inhibitors

Multi-nRTI Resistance: 151 Complex
```
        A              V  F              F    Q
        62             75 77             116  151
        V              I  L              Y    M
```

Multi-nRTI Resistance: 69 Insertion Complex
```
M       A      D ▼ K                          L  T  K
41      62     67 69 70                        210 215 219
L       V      N insert R                      W  Y  Q
                                                  F  E
                                                  T  K
```

Multi-nRTI Resistance: NAMs
```
M  E        D    K          V          L  T  K
41 44       67   70         118         210 215 219
L  D        N    R          I          W  Y  Q
                                           F  E
                                           T  K
```

Zidovudine
```
M  E        D    K          V          L  T  K
41 44       67   70         118         210 215 219
L  D        N    R          I          W  Y  Q
                                           F  E
                                           T  K
```

Stavudine
```
M  E        D    K          V          L  T  K
41 44       67   70         118         210 215 219
L  D        N    R          I          W  Y  Q
                                           F  E
```

Didanosine
```
        K         L
        65        74
        R         V
```

Zalcitabine
```
        K    T    L                M
        65   69   74               184
        R    D    V                V
```

Abacavir
```
        K         L       Y        M
        65        74      115      184
        R         V       F        V
```

Lamivudine
```
E                      V        M
44                     118      184
D                      I        V
                                I
```

Tenofovir
```
        K
        65
        R
```

Nonnucleoside Reverse Transcriptase Inhibitors

Multi-NNRTI Resistance
```
        K  V                   Y
        103 106                188
```

Multi-NNRTI Resistance: Accumulation of Mutations
```
        N  M                   L
        L  V              Y    G          M
        100    106        188  190        230
        I      A          C    S          L
                          I    A
```

Nevirapine
```
        L  K  V  V         Y    Y  G
        100 103 106 108    181  188 190
        I  N  A  I         C    C  A
              M            I    L
                                H
```

Delavirdine
```
        K  V              Y    Y               P
        103 106           181  188             236
        N  M              C    L               L
```

Efavirenz
```
        L  K  V  V         Y    Y  G       P
        100 103 106 108    181  188 190    225
        I  N  M  I         C    L  S       H
                           I       A
```

MUTATIONS IN THE GP41 ENVELOPE GENE ASSOCIATED WITH RESISTANCE TO ENTRY INHIBITORS

Enfuvirtide
```
        G  I  V  Q        N  N
        36 37 38 39       42 43      HRI Region
        D  V  A  R        T  D
        S     M
```

MUTATIONS

```
Amino Acid, Wild-Type ──────── L        Insertion
Amino Acid Position
Major (boldface type; ──────── 90       54
  protease only)
Amino Acid, Substitution ───── M

        Verticle pink lines    Minor (lightface type;
        indicate NAMs          protease only)
```

FIGURE 173-40 Amino acid substitutions conferring resistance to antiretroviral drugs. For each amino acid residue, the letter above the bar indicates the amino acid associated with wildtype virus and the letter(s) below indicate the substitution(s) that confer viral resistance. The number shows the position of the mutation in the protein. Mutations selected by protease inhibitors in Gag cleavage sites are not listed because their contribution to resistance is not yet fully defined. HR1 indicates first heptad repeat; NAMs indicates nRTI-associated mutations; nRTI indicates nucleoside reverse transcriptase inhibitor; NNRTI indicates nonnucleoside reverse transcriptase inhibitor; PI indicates protease inhibitor. Amino acid abbreviations: A, alanine; C, cysteine; D, aspartate; E, glutamine; F, phenylalenine; G, glycine; H, histidine; I, isoleucine; K, lysine; L, leucine; M, methionine; N, asparagine; P, proline; Q, glutamine; R, arginine; S, serine; T, threonine; V, valine; W, tryptophan; Y, tyrosine. (*Reprinted with permission from the International AIDS Society-USA. Johnson VA et al: Topics HIV Med 11:215, 2003. Accompanying usernotes, updates of the figure, and additional information available at http://www.iasusa.org.*)

Protease Inhibitors

Multi-PI Resistance: Accumulation of Mutations

Position	10	46	54	82	84	90
Wild-type	L	M	I	V	I	L
Mutations	F, I, R, V	I, L	V, M, L	A, F, T, S	V	M

Indinavir

Position	10	20	24	32	36	46	54	71	73	77	82	84	90
Wild-type	L	K	L	V	M	M	I	A	G	V	V	I	L
Mutations	I, R, V	M, R	I	I	I	I, L	V	V, T	S, A	I	A, F, T	V	M

Ritonavir

Position	10	20	32	33	36	46	54	71	77	82	84	90
Wild-type	L	K	V	L	M	M	I	A	V	V	V	L
Mutations	F, I, R, V	M, R	I	F	I	I, L	V, L	V, T	I	A, F, T, S	V	M

Saquinavir

Position	10	48	54	71	73	77	82	84	90
Wild-type	L	G	I	A	G	V	V	I	L
Mutations	I, R, V	V	V, L	V, T	S	I	A	V	M

Nelfinavir

Position	10	30	36	46	71	77	82	84	88	90
Wild-type	L	D	M	M	A	V	V	I	N	L
Mutations	F, I	N	I	I, L	V, T	I	A, F, T, S	V	D, S	M

Amprenavir

Position	10	32	46	47	50	54	73	84	90
Wild-type	L	V	M	I	I	I	G	I	L
Mutations	F, I, R, V	I	I, L	V	V	L, V, M	S	V	M

Lopinavir/Ritonavir

Position	10	20	24	32	33	46	47	50	53	54	63	71	73	82	84	90
Wild-type	L	K	L	V	L	M	I	I	F	I	L	A	G	V	I	L
Mutations	F, I, R, V	M, R	I	I	F	I, L	V	V	L	V, L	P	V, T	S	A, F, T, S	V	M

Atazanavir

Position	10	20	24	32	33	36	46	48	50	54	71	73	82	84	88	90
Wild-type	L	K	L	V	L	M	M	G	I	I	A	G	V	I	N	L
Mutations	F, I, R, V	M, R	I	I	I, F, V	I, L, V	I	V	L	L	V	C, S, S, T, A	A	V	S	M

Tipranavir/Ritonavir (expanded access)

Position	10	20	33	46	54	82	84	90
Wild-type	L	K	L	M	I	V	I	L
Mutations	I, V	M, L, T	I, F, V	I	V	A, F, T, S	V	M

FIGURE 173-40—(Continued)

doses as low as 100 to 200 mg twice a day, is often used in the setting of HIV infection to derive more convenient regimens. For example, when given with low-dose ritonavir, saquinavir and indinavir can both be given on twice-a-day schedules and taken with food.

Indinavir is among the best studied of the HIV-1 protease inhibitors. It was the first protease inhibitor used in combination with dual nucleoside therapy. The combination of zidovudine, lamivudine, and indinavir was the first "triple combination" shown to have a profound effect on HIV replication. The main side effects of indinavir are nephrolithiasis (seen in 4% of patients) and asymptomatic indirect hyperbilirubinemia (seen in 10%). Indinavir is predominantly metabolized by the liver. The dose should be lowered in patients with cirrhosis. Indinavir shares metabolic pathways with terfenadine, astemizole, cisapride, triazolam, and midazolam. To avoid the potential for cardiac arrhythmias or prolonged sedation, these drugs should not be administered to patients taking indinavir. Levels of indinavir are decreased during concurrent therapy with rifabutin or nevirapine and increased during concurrent therapy with ketoconazole, delavirdine, efavirenz, or ritonavir. Dosages should be modified appropriately in these circumstances (Table 173-21).

Nelfinavir was approved in 1997 and *amprenavir* was approved in 1999 for the treatment of adult or pediatric HIV infection when antiretroviral therapy is warranted. As with most of the newer antiretroviral agents, these approvals were based on randomized, controlled trials that demonstrated decreases in plasma HIV RNA levels and increases in CD4+ T cell counts. Both agents have unique resistance profiles. Nelfinavir resistance is associated with a D30N substitution in the protease gene. Viruses harboring this single mutation retain sensitivity to other protease inhibitors, and it has been suggested that for this reason nelfinavir is a good initial protease inhibitor. It is not clear, however, whether this theoretical consideration will be borne out in the results of clinical trials. Protease inhibitor resistance typically involves multiple amino acid substitutions and reduced susceptibility across the class. Amprenavir resistance is associated with a unique substitution at amino acid 50 (I50V), and it has been suggested that amprenavir may be of particular value in salvage regimens. This assumption also awaits verification in controlled clinical trials. Nelfinavir and amprenavir are both associated with gastrointestinal side effects. About 1% of patients receiving amprenavir have experienced severe and life-threatening skin reactions. An additional disadvantage

TABLE 173-22 *Principles of Therapy of HIV Infection*

1. Ongoing HIV replication leads to immune system damage and progression to AIDS.
2. Plasma HIV RNA levels indicate the magnitude of HIV replication and the rate of CD4+ T cell destruction. CD4+ T cell counts indicate the current level of competence of the immune system.
3. Rates of disease progression differ among individuals, and treatment decisions should be individualized based upon plasma HIV RNA levels and CD4+ T cell counts.
4. Maximal suppression of viral replication is a goal of therapy; the greater the suppression the less likely the appearance of drug-resistance quasispecies.
5. The most effective therapeutic strategies involve the simultaneous initiation of combinations of effective anti-HIV drugs with which the patient has not been previously treated and that are not cross-resistant with antiretroviral agents that the patient has already received.
6. The antiretroviral drugs used in combination regimens should be used according to optimum schedules and dosages.
7. The number of available drugs is limited. Any decisions on antiretroviral therapy have a long-term impact on future options for the patient.
8. Women should receive optimal antiretroviral therapy regardless of pregnancy status.
9. The same principals apply to children and adults. The treatment of HIV-infected children involves unique pharmacologic, virologic, and immunologic considerations.
10. Compliance is an important part of ensuring maximal effect from a given regimen. The simpler the regimen, the easier it is for the patient to be compliant.

Source: Modified from, *Principles of Therapy of HIV Infection*, USPHS and the Henry J. Kaiser Family Foundation.

of amprenavir is that the original formulation requires the patient to take 8 large capsules twice a day.

Fosamprenavir (Lexiva) is a recently licensed prodrug of amprenavir that is rapidly converted to amprenavir by cellular phosphatases. It is supplied as a 700-mg tablet. The recommended dosage is 1400 mg bid or 700 mg bid with ritonavir 100 mg bid or 1400 mg once a day with ritonavir 200 mg once a day.

Lopinavir/ritonavir (Kaletra) is a fixed dose combination of the protease inhibitors lopinavir (133.3 mg) and ritonavir (33.3 mg). It is indicated for treatment of HIV-1 infection in combination with other agents. A main advantage of this pill is that it combines the pharmacologic enhancement of low-dose ritonavir with a second protease inhibitor in a single capsule. In a randomized, controlled trial, this combination capsule was found to be superior to nelfinavir.

Atazanavir (Reytaz) is an azapeptide inhibitor of the HIV-1 protease. Initial studies suggest that total cholesterol and triglyceride levels may not increase as much with atazanavir as is seen with other protease inhibitors. Atazanavir is associated with increases in serum bilirubin and prolongations of the PR interval. Atazanavir-resistant isolates emerging in previously treatment-naïve individuals frequently harbor an I50L substitution. This mutation in some instances is associated with increased sensitivity to other protease inhibitors. Atazanavir is an inhibitor of cytochrome P3A and its use may be associated with increased levels of calcium channel blockers, HMB-CoA reductase inhibitors, and sildenafil.

The newest class of antiretroviral compounds are the entry inhibitors. These agents act by interfering with the binding of HIV to its receptor or co-receptor or by interfering with the process of fusion (see above). A variety of small molecules that bind to HIV-1 co-receptors are currently in clinical trials. The first drug in this class to be licensed is the fusion inhibitor enfuvirtide (Fuzeon), or T-20.

Enfuvirtide is a linear 36-amino acid synthetic peptide with the N-terminus acetylated and the C-terminus a carboxamide. It is composed of naturally occurring L-amino acid residues and interferes with the fusion of the viral and cellular membranes by binding to the HR1 region in the gp41 subunit of the HIV-1 envelope. This binding interferes with the coil-coil interaction required to approximate the two membranes. Resistant isolates of HIV exhibit amino acid changes in

positions 36 to 45 of gp41. In two independent studies, patients who had persistent viremia despite prior treatment with agents from all three available classes of drugs were randomized to receive an individualized regimen (based upon prior treatment history and resistance profile) with or without enfuvirtide. The change in plasma HIV-1 RNA from baseline was approximately 1 log greater (-1.53 vs. -0.68) in patients randomized to receive enfuvirtide. Among the drawbacks of this agent are the requirement for twice-a-day injection, the occurrence of injection site reactions in 98% of patients, and an increase in bacterial pneumonia in the enfuvirtide-treated patients compared to the patients in the control arm (4.68 vs. 0.61 events per 100 patient years) in the phase III studies.

The principles of therapy for HIV infection have been articulated by a panel sponsored by the U.S. Department of Health and Human Services and the Henry J. Kaiser Family Foundation. These principles are summarized in Table 173-22. As noted in these guidelines, eradication of HIV infection has not yet been possible. Treatment decisions must take into account the fact that one is dealing with a chronic infection. While early therapy is generally the rule in infectious diseases, immediate treatment of every HIV-infected individual upon diagnosis may not be prudent, and therapeutic decisions must take into account the balance between risks and benefits. At present, a reasonable course of action is to initiate antiretroviral therapy in anyone with the acute HIV syndrome; patients with symptomatic disease; patients with asymptomatic disease with CD4+ T cell counts $<250/\mu L$ or with $>50,000$ copies of HIV RNA per milliliter (Table 173-23). In addition, one may wish to administer a 6-week course of therapy to uninfected individuals immediately following a high-risk exposure to HIV (see below).

Once the decision has been made to initiate therapy, the health care provider must decide which drugs to use as the first regimen. The decision regarding choice of drugs not only will affect the immediate response to therapy but also will have implications regarding options for future therapeutic regimens. The initial regimen is usually the most effective insofar as the virus has yet to develop significant resistance. The two options for initial therapy most commonly in use today are two different three-drug regimens. The first regimen utilizes two nucleoside analogues (one of which is usually lamivudine) and a nonnucleoside reverse transcriptase inhibitor. The second regimen utilizes two nucleoside analogues and a protease inhibitor. Unfortunately there are no clear data at present on which to base distinctions between these two approaches. Following the initiation of therapy one should expect a 1 log (tenfold) reduction in plasma HIV RNA levels within 1 to 2 months and eventually a decline in plasma HIV RNA levels to <50 copies per milliliter. During this same time there should be a rise in the CD4+ T cell count of 100 to $150/\mu L$ that is particularly brisk during the first month of therapy. Many clinicians feel that failure to achieve this endpoint is an indication for a change in therapy. Other reasons for a change in therapy include a persistently declining CD4+

TABLE 173-23 *Indications for the Initiation of Antiretroviral Therapy in Patients with HIV Infection*

I. Acute infection syndrome
II. Chronic infection
   A. Symptomatic disease
   B. Asymptomatic diseases[a]
      1. CD4+ T cell count $<350/\mu L$ or decreasing
      2. HIV RNA $>50,000$ copies mL or increasing
III. Postexposure prophylaxis

[a] This is the area of greatest controversy. Some experts would wait until the CD4 cell count declines to $200/\mu L$, whereas others would treat everyone regardless of CD4+ T cell count.
Source: *Guidelines for the Use of Antiretroviral Agents in HIV-Infected Adults and Adolescents*. USPHS.

T cell count, clinical deterioration, or drug toxicity (Table 173-24). As in the case of initiating therapy, changing therapy may have a lasting impact on future therapeutic options. When changing therapy because of treatment failure (clinical progression or worsening laboratory parameters), it is important to attempt to provide a regimen with at least two new drugs. In the patient in whom a change is made for reasons of drug toxicity, a simple replacement of one drug is reasonable. It should be stressed that in attempting to sort out a drug toxicity it may be advisable to hold all therapy for a period of time to distinguish between drug toxicity and disease progression. Drug toxicity will usually begin to show signs of reversal within 1 to 2 weeks. Prior to changing a treatment regimen because of drug failure, it is important to ensure that the patient has been adherent to the prescribed regimen. As in the case of initial therapy, the simpler the therapeutic regimen, the easier it is for the patient to be compliant. Plasma HIV RNA levels and CD4+ T lymphocyte counts should be monitored every 3 to 4 months during therapy and more frequently if one is contemplating a change in regimen or immediately following a change in regimen.

In an attempt to determine an optimal therapeutic regimen, one may attempt to measure antiretroviral drug susceptibility through genotyping or phenotyping of HIV quasispecies and determine adequacy of dosing through measurement of drug levels. Genotyping may be done through dideoxynucleotide sequencing, DNA chip hybridization, or line probe assays. Phenotypic assays measure the performance of reverse transcriptase or protease in the presence or absence of different concentrations of different drugs. These assays will generally detect quasispecies present at a frequency of at least 10%. The precise role of resistance testing in the management of patients with HIV infection is not yet clear. While randomized studies have suggested that information regarding HIV resistance profiles may improve virologic outcomes in patients failing their current antiretroviral regimen, the degree of improvement thus far has been small and the duration of the benefit limited. Resistance testing may be of particular value in distinguishing drug-resistant virus from poor patient compliance; it may also be of value to help guide initial therapy in a setting where transmission of a drug-resistant isolate is felt to be likely. Measurement of plasma drug levels can also be used to tailor an individual treatment. The inhibitory quotient, defined as the trough blood level/IC50 of the patient's virus is used by some to determine the adequacy of dosing of a given treatment regimen.

In addition to the licensed medications discussed above, a large number of experimental agents are being evaluated as possible therapies for HIV infection. Therapeutic strategies are being developed that interfere with virtually every step of the replication cycle of the virus (Fig. 173-3). In addition, as more is discovered about the role of the immune system in controlling viral replication, additional strategies, generically referred to as "immune-based therapies," are being developed as a complement to antiviral therapy. Among the antiviral agents in early clinical trials are additional nucleoside and nucleotide analogues, additional protease inhibitors including nonpeptidomimetic compounds, additional fusion inhibitors, receptor and co-receptor antagonists, integrase inhibitors, and antisense nucleic acids. Among the immune-based therapies being evaluated are IFN-α, bone marrow transplantation, adoptive transfer of lymphocytes genetically modified to resist infection or enhance HIV-specific immunity, active immunotherapy with inactivated HIV or its components, and IL-2.

HIV AND THE HEALTH CARE WORKER

Health care workers, especially those who deal with large numbers of HIV-infected patients, have a small but definite risk of becoming infected with HIV as a result of professional activities. As of January 1, 2002, 57 health care workers in the United States had been documented as having seroconverted to HIV following occupational exposure; 26 have developed AIDS. The individuals who seroconverted include 19 laboratory workers (16 of whom were clinical laboratory workers), 24 nurses, 6 physicians, 2 surgical technicians, 1 dialysis technician, 1 respiratory therapist, 1 health aide, 1 embalmer/morgue technician, and 2 housekeeper/maintenance workers. The exposures included 48 percutaneous (puncture/cut injury), 5 mucocutaneous (mucous membrane and/or skin), 2 both percutaneous and mucocutaneous, and 2 unknown route of exposure. Forty-nine exposures were to HIV-infected blood, three to concentrated virus in a laboratory, one to visibly bloody fluid, and four to an unspecified fluid. As of January 1, 2002, there had been 138 other cases of HIV infection or AIDS among health care workers who have not reported other risk factors for HIV infection and who report a history of exposure to blood, body fluids, or HIV-infected laboratory material, but for whom seroconversion after exposure was not documented. The number of these workers who actually acquired their infection through occupational exposures is not known. Taken together, the data from several large studies suggest that the risk of HIV infection following a percutaneous exposure to HIV-contaminated blood is ~0.3%, and after a mucous membrane exposure, approximately 0.09%. Although episodes of HIV transmission after non-intact skin exposure have been documented, the average risk for transmission by this route has not been precisely quantified but is estimated to be less than the risk for mucous membrane exposures. The risk for transmission after exposure to fluids or tissues other than HIV-infected blood also has not been quantified but is probably considerably lower than for blood exposures. A seroprevalence survey of 3420 orthopedic surgeons, 75% of whom practiced in an area with a relatively high prevalence of HIV infection and 39% of whom reported percutaneous exposure to patient blood, usually through an accident involving a suture needle, failed to reveal any cases of possible occupational infection, suggesting that the risk of infection with a suture needle may be considerably less than that with a blood-drawing needle.

Most cases of health care worker seroconversion occur as a result of needle-stick injuries. When one considers the circumstances that result in needle-stick injuries, it is immediately obvious that adhering to the standard guidelines for dealing with sharp objects would result in a significant decrease in this type of accident. In one study, 27% of needle-stick injuries resulted from improper disposal of the needle (over half of these were due to recapping the needle), 23% occurred during attempts to start an intravenous line, 22% occurred during blood drawing, 16% were associated with an intramuscular or subcutaneous injection, and 12% were associated with giving an intravenous infusion.

Recommendations regarding postexposure prophylaxis must take into account that several circumstances determine the risk of transmission of HIV following occupational exposure. In this regard, several factors have been associated with an increased risk for occupational transmission of HIV infection including: deep injury, the presence of visible blood on the instrument causing the exposure, injury with a device that had been placed in the vein or artery of the

---

TABLE 173-24 *Indications for Changing Antiretroviral Therapy in Patients with HIV Infection*[a]

Less than a 1-log drop in plasma HIV RNA by 4 weeks following the initiation of therapy

A reproducible significant increase (defined as 3-fold or greater) from the nadir of plasma HIV RNA level not attributable to intercurrent infection, vaccination, or test methodology

Persistently declining CD4+ T cell numbers

Clinical deterioration

Side effects

[a] Generally speaking, a change should involve the initiation of at least 2 drugs felt to be effective in the given patient. The exception to this is when change is being made to manage toxicity, in which case a single substitution is reasonable.

Source: Guidelines for the Use of Antiretroviral Agents in HIV-Infected Adults and Adolescents. USPHS.

source patient, terminal illness in the source patient, and lack of post-exposure antiretroviral therapy in the exposed health care worker. Other important considerations include pregnancy in the health care worker and the possibility of exposure to drug-resistant virus. Regardless of the decision to use postexposure prophylaxis, the wound should be cleansed immediately and antiseptic applied. If a decision is made to offer postexposure prophylaxis, U.S. Public Health Service guidelines recommend (1) a combination of two nucleoside analogue reverse transcriptase inhibitors given for 4 weeks for routine exposures, or (2) a combination of two nucleoside analogue reverse transcriptase inhibitors plus a third drug given for 4 weeks for high-risk or otherwise complicated exposures, although most clinicians administer the latter regimen in all cases in which a decision is made to treat. Further details are available from the *Updated U.S. Public Health Service Guidelines for the Management of Occupational Exposures to HBV, HCV and HIV and Recommendations for Postexposure Prophylaxis* (CDC, 2001).

Health care workers can minimize their risk of occupational HIV infection by following the CDC guidelines of July 1991, which include adherence to universal precautions, refraining from direct patient care if one has exudative lesions or weeping dermatitis, and disinfecting and sterilizing reusable devices employed in invasive procedures. The premise of universal precautions is that every specimen should be handled as if it came from someone infected with a bloodborne pathogen. All samples should be double-bagged, gloves should be worn when drawing blood, and spills should be immediately disinfected with bleach.

In attempting to put this small but definite risk to the health care worker in perspective, it is important to point out that ~200 health care workers die each year as a result of occupationally acquired hepatitis B infection. The tragedy in this instance is that these infections and deaths due to HBV could be greatly decreased by more extended use of the HBV vaccine. The risk of HBV infection following a needlestick injury from a hepatitis antigen–positive patient is much higher than the risk of HIV infection (see "Transmission," above). There are multiple examples of needle-stick injuries where the patient was positive for both HBV and HIV and the health care worker became infected only with HBV. For these reasons, it is advisable, given the high prevalence of HBV infection in HIV-infected individuals, that all health care workers dealing with HIV-infected patients be immunized with the HBV vaccine.

TB is another infection common to HIV-infected patients that can be transmitted to the health care worker. For this reason, all health care workers should know their PPD status, have it checked yearly, and receive 1 year of isoniazid treatment if their skin test converts to positive. In addition, all patients in whom a diagnosis of TB is being entertained should be placed immediately in respiratory isolation, pending results of the diagnostic evaluation. The emergence of drug-resistant organisms has made TB an increasing problem for health care workers. This is particularly true for the health care worker with pre-existing HIV infection.

One of the most charged issues ever to come between health care workers and patients is that of transmission of infection from HIV-infected health care workers to their patients. This is discussed under "Occupational Transmission of HIV: Health Care Workers and Laboratory Workers." Theoretically, the same universal precautions that are used to protect the health care worker from the HIV-infected patient will also protect the patient from the HIV-infected health care worker.

VACCINES

Historically, vaccines have provided a safe, cost-effective, and efficient means of preventing illness, disability, and death from infectious diseases. Given the fact that human behavior, especially human sexual behavior, is extremely difficult to change, the best hope for preventing the spread of HIV infection rests with the development of a safe and effective vaccine. This task is problematic for a number of reasons, including the high mutability of the virus, the fact that the infection can be transmitted by cell-free or cell-associated virus, the likely need for the development of effective mucosal immunity, and the fact that it has been difficult to establish the precise correlates of protective immunity to HIV infection. Some HIV-infected individuals are long-term nonprogressors (see above), and a number of individuals have been exposed to HIV multiple times but remain uninfected; these facts suggest that there are protective elements of an HIV-specific immune response. In addition, studies using animal models, specifically SIV in the monkey and HIV-1 in the chimpanzee, have been encouraging and suggest that an HIV vaccine is possible. It should be pointed out that while the ideal goal of an HIV vaccine is to prevent infection, a vaccine given to an uninfected individual that significantly alters the course of disease or the infectivity of the individual, should that person become infected, could have an impact not only on the individual in question but also on the spread of infection in the community.

A number of clinical trials ranging from several small phase I trials to determine safety to fewer intermediate-sized phase II trials to determine safety and immunogenicity have taken place and are under way. The single completed phase III trial of a recombinant gp120 protein failed to show protection despite evidence of HIV-specific antibodies and CD4+ T cells in phase II. These results suggest the potential importance of CD8+ T cell immunity in host defense against HIV-1. The furthest advanced among the current phase II trials involves a combination approach using a live canarypox vector expressing one or multiple HIV epitopes given together with gp120 or using the gp120 as a boost. This approach has resulted in neutralizing antibodies in virtually all recipients and HIV-specific cytolytic T cells in ~30% of individuals at any given time during the course of the trial. Other work is exploring the effects of recombinant adenovirus or naked DNA in combination with protein immunization.

Other approaches currently being tested in phase I and/or phase II trials in humans include vaccines employing vectors such as modified vaccinia Ankara (MVA), salmonella, and Venezuela equine encephalitis (VEE) virus, among others; peptide and subunit vaccines; and pseudovirions (Fig. 173-41). Live attenuated HIV vaccines have not proceeded into human trials at this time because of safety concerns. It is clear that it will take several years of clinical trials to establish the efficacy or lack thereof of a candidate vaccine for HIV.

PREVENTION

Education, counseling, and behavior modification are the cornerstones of an HIV prevention strategy. Widespread voluntary testing of individuals who have practiced or are practicing high-risk behavior, together with counseling of infected individuals, is recommended. Information gathered from such an approach should serve as the basis for behavior-modification programs, both for infected individuals who may be unaware of their HIV status and who could infect others and for uninfected individuals practicing high-risk behavior. The practice of "safer sex" is the most effective way for sexually active uninfected individuals to avoid contracting HIV infection and for infected individuals to avoid spreading infection. Abstinence from sexual relations is the only absolute way to prevent sexual transmission of HIV infection. However, for many people this may not be feasible, and there are a number of relatively safe practices that can markedly decrease the chances of transmission of HIV infection. Partners engaged in monogamous sexual relationships who wish to be assured of safety should both be tested for HIV antibody. If both are negative, it must be understood that any divergence from monogamy puts both partners at risk; open discussion of the importance of honesty in such relationships should be encouraged. When the HIV status of either partner is not known, or when one partner is positive, there are a number of options. Use of condoms can markedly decrease the chance of HIV

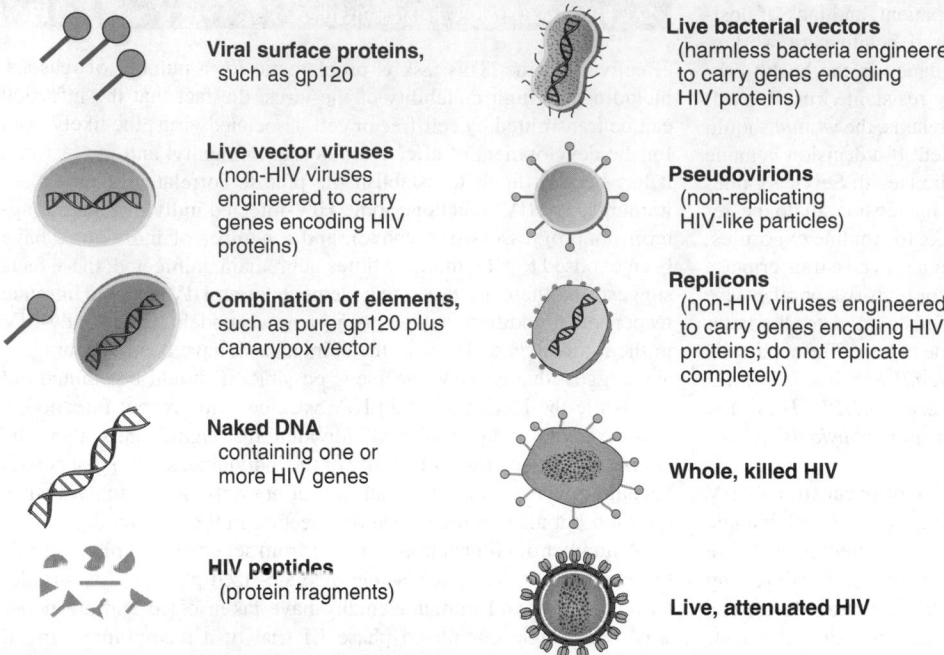

Viral surface proteins, such as gp120

Live vector viruses (non-HIV viruses engineered to carry genes encoding HIV proteins)

Combination of elements, such as pure gp120 plus canarypox vector

Naked DNA containing one or more HIV genes

HIV peptides (protein fragments)

Live bacterial vectors (harmless bacteria engineered to carry genes encoding HIV proteins)

Pseudovirions (non-replicating HIV-like particles)

Replicons (non-HIV viruses engineered to carry genes encoding HIV proteins; do not replicate completely)

Whole, killed HIV

Live, attenuated HIV

FIGURE 173-41 Candidate HIV vaccines. See text for detailed discussion. (*Adapted from D Baltimore, C Heilman: Sci Am 279:98, 1998. Copyright Slim Films.*)

transmission. It should be remembered that condoms are not 100% effective in preventing transmission of HIV infection, and there is an ~10% failure rate of condoms used for contraceptive purposes. Most condom failures result from breakage or improper usage, such as not wearing the condom for the entire period of intercourse. Latex condoms are preferable, since virus has been shown to leak through natural skin condoms. Petroleum-based gels should never be used for lubrication of the condom, since they increase the likelihood of condom rupture. There has been a tendency among homosexual men to practice fellatio as a "minimal risk" activity compared to receptive anal intercourse. It should be emphasized that receptive fellatio is definitely not safe sex, and although the incidence of transmission via fellatio is considerably less than that of rectal or vaginal intercourse, there has been documentation of transmission of HIV where receptive fellatio was the only sexual act performed (see "Transmission," above). Topical microbicides for vaginal and anal use are being pursued actively as a means by which individuals could avoid infection when the insertive partner cannot be relied on to use a condom. Kissing is considered safe, although there is a theoretical possibility of transmission via virus in saliva. The low concentration of virus in saliva of infected individuals, as well as the presence in saliva of HIV-inhibitory proteins (see above), lessens any risk of transmission by kissing.

The most effective way to prevent transmission of HIV infection among IDUs is to stop the use of injectable drugs. Unfortunately, that is extremely difficult to accomplish unless the individual enters a treatment program. For those who will not or cannot participate in a drug treatment program and who will continue to inject drugs, the avoidance of sharing of needles and other paraphernalia ("works") is the next best way to avoid transmission of infection. The cultural and social factors that contribute to the sharing of paraphernalia are complex and difficult to overcome. In addition, needles and syringes may be in short supply. Under these circumstances, paraphernalia should be cleaned after each usage with a virucidal solution, such as undiluted sodium hypochlorite (household bleach). Data from a number of studies have indicated that programs that provide sterile needles to addicts in exchange for used needles have resulted in a decrease in HIV transmission without increasing the use of injection drugs. It is important for IDUs to be tested for HIV infection and counseled, to avoid transmission to their sexual partners. Secondary and tertiary spread of HIV infection by the heterosexual route within settings of a high level of

injection drug use has increased greatly in the United States (see above).

Transmission of HIV via transfused blood or blood products has been decreased dramatically by a combination of screening of all blood donors for HIV infection by assays for both HIV antibody and p24 antigen and self-deferral of individuals at risk for HIV infection. In addition, clotting factor concentrates are heat-treated, essentially eliminating the risk to hemophiliacs who require these products. Autologous transfusions are preferable to transfusions from another individual. However, logistic constraints as well as the unpredictability of the need for most transfusions limit the feasibility of this approach. At present the risk of becoming HIV-infected from a contaminated blood transfusion is approximately 1 in 725,000 to 1 in 835,000 donations.

Treatment of an HIV-infected mother with antiretroviral therapy during pregnancy and the infant during the first weeks following birth has proven very effective in dramatically decreasing mother to child transmission of HIV. In situations such as that seen in certain developing countries where pregnant women frequently present to a health care system during labor, administration of a short course (as little as a single dose of one drug) of antiretroviral therapy to the mother during labor and to the infant within 48 h of birth has also been successful in decreasing the incidence of mother to child transmission of HIV.

HIV can be transmitted via breast milk and colostrum. The avoidance of breast-feeding may not be practical in developing countries, where nutritional concerns override the risk of HIV transmission. However, it is becoming appreciated that 5 to 15% of infants who were born of HIV-infected mothers and who were fortunate enough not to have been infected intrapartum or peripartum become infected via breast-feeding. Therefore, in developing countries, breast-feeding from an infected mother should be avoided if at all possible. Unfortunately, this is rarely the case, and given the disadvantages of withholding breast-feeding in developing countries (see above), health authorities in most developing countries continue to recommend breast-feeding despite the potential for HIV transmission. Treatment of the infected mother with antiretroviral therapy, in addition to decreasing perinatal mother-to-child transmission can also decrease transmission by breast-feeding. In developed countries such as the United States, where bottled formula and milk are readily accessible, breast-feeding is absolutely contraindicated when a mother is HIV positive.

FURTHER READING

ANTMAN K, CHANG Y: Kaposi's sarcoma. N Engl J Med 342:1027, 2000

AUERBACH JD, COATES TJ: HIV prevention research: Accomplishments and challenges for the third decade of AIDS. Am J Public Health 90:1029, 2000

CARDO DM et al: A case-control study of HIV seroconversion in health care workers after percutaneous exposure. N Engl J Med 337:1485, 1997

CENTERS FOR DISEASE CONTROL AND PREVENTION: HIV/AIDS Surveillance Report, 2002;14, 2003. Available at *http://www.cdc.gov/hiv/stats/hasrlink.HTM*

————: Updated U.S. Public Health Service guidelines for the management of occupational exposures to HBV, HCV, and HIV and recommendations for postexposure prophylaxis. MMWR 50 (RR11):1, 2001

————: Revised guidelines for HIV counseling, testing, and referral. MMWR Recomm Rep 50(RR-19):1, 2001

————; HEALTH RESOURCES AND SERVICES ADMINISTRATION; NATIONAL INSTITUTES OF HEALTH; HIV MEDICINE ASSOCIATION OF THE INFEC-

TIOUS DISEASES SOCIETY OF AMERICA: Incorporating HIV prevention into the medical care of persons living with HIV. MMWR Recomm Rep 52(RR-12):1–24, 2003

CHUN TW, FAUCI AS: Latent reservoirs of HIV: Obstacles to the eradication of virus. Proc Natl Acad Sci USA 96:10958, 1999

D'AQUILA RT et al: Drug resistance mutations in HIV-1. Top HIV Med 11: 92, 2003

DAVEY RT JR et al: HIV-1 and T cell dynamics after interruption of highly active antiretroviral therapy (HAART) in patients with a history of sustained viral suppression. Proc Natl Acad Sci USA 21:96,15109, 1999

DONG KL et al: Changes in body habitus and serum lipid abnormalities in HIV-positive women on highly active antiretroviral therapy. J Acquir Immune Defic Syndr 21:107, 1999

DYBUL M et al: Guidelines for using antiretroviral agents among HIV-infected adults and adolescents. Recommendations of the Panel on Clinical Practices for Treatment of HIV. MMWR Recomm Rep 51(RR-7):1, 2002. Updates available at http://www.aidsinfo.nih.gov

EGGLER M et al: Prognosis of HIV-1 infected patients starting highly active antiretroviral therapy: A collaborative analysis of prospective studies. Lancet 360:119, 2002

FAUCI AS: Host factors and the pathogenesis of HIV-induced disease. Nature 384:529, 1996

————: The AIDS epidemic—considerations for the 21st century. N Engl J Med 341:1046, 1999

GALLO RC: Human retroviruses after 20 years: A perspective from the past and prospects for their future control. Immunol Rev 185:236, 2002

GANDHI RT, WALKER BD: Immunologic control of HIV-1. Annu Rev Med 53:149, 2002

GAO F et al: Origin of HIV-1 in the chimpanzee *Pan troglodytes troglodytes*. Nature 397:436, 1999

GOEDERT JJ et al: Spectrum of AIDS-associated malignant disorders. Lancet 351:1833, 1998

GREENE WC, PETERLIN BM: Charting HIV's remarkable voyage through the cell: Basic science as a passport to future therapy. Nat Med 8:673, 2002

GULICK RM: New antiretroviral drugs. Clin Microbiol Infect 9:186, 2003

HO DD et al: Rapid turnover of plasma virions and CD4 lymphocytes in HIV infection. Nature 373:123, 1995

JOINT UNITED NATIONS PROGRAMME ON HIV/AIDS (UNAIDS): AIDS Epidemic Update, December, 2003.

JONES D, HAVLIR DV: Nontuberculous mycobacteria in the HIV infected patient. Clin Chest Med 3:665, 2002

KAPLAN JE et al: Guidelines for preventing opportunistic infections among HIV-infected persons—2002. Recommendations of the U.S. Public Health Service and the Infectious Diseases Society of America. MMWR Recomm Rep 51(RR-8):1, 2003. Updates available at http://www.aidsinfo.nih.gov

KINTER A et al: Chemokines, cytokines and HIV: A complex network of interactions that influence HIV pathogenesis. Immunol Rev 177:88, 2000

LOPEZ BERNALDO DE QUIROS JC et al: A randomized trial of the discontinuation of primary and secondary prophylaxis against *Pneumocystis carinii* pneumonia after highly active antiretroviral therapy in patients with HIV infection. N Engl J Med 344:159, 2001

MELLORS JW et al: Prognosis in HIV-1 infection predicted by the quantity of virus in plasma. Science 272:1167, 1996

MIGUELES SA: et al: HIV-specific CD*+ T cell proliferation is coupled to perforin expression and is maintained in nonprogressors. Nat Immunol 3: 1061, 2002

MILLER KD et al: High prevalence of osteonecrosis of the femoral head in HIV-infected adults. Ann Intern Med 137:17, 2002

MOFENSON LM et al: Risk factors for perinatal transmission of human immunodeficiency virus type 1 in women treated with zidovudine. N Engl J Med 334:385, 1999

———— et al: U.S. Public Health Service Task Force recommendations for use of antiretroviral drugs in pregnant HIV-1-infected women for maternal health and interventions to reduce perinatal HIV-1 transmission in the United States. MMWR Recomm Rep 51(RR-18):1, 2002. Updates available at http://www.aidsinfo.nih.gov

NABEL GJ: Challenges and opportunities for development of an AIDS vaccine. Nature 410(6831):1002, 2001

NAKASHIMA AK, FLEMING PL: HIV/AIDS surveillance in the United States, 1981–2001. J Acquir Immune Defic Syndr 32(Suppl 1):S68, 2003

O'BRIEN SJ, MOORE JP: The effect of genetic variation in chemokines and their receptors on HIV transmission and progression to AIDS. Immunol Rev 177:99, 2000

PANTALEO G, FAUCI AS: HIV infection is active and progressive in lymphoid tissue during the clinically latent stage of disease. Nature 362:355, 1993

QUINN TC et al: Viral load and heterosexual transmission of human immunodeficiency virus type 1. Rakai Project Group Study. N Engl J Med 342: 921, 2000

RAMRATNAM B et al: The decay of the latent reservoir of replication-competent HIV-1 is inversely correlated with the extent of residual viral replication during prolonged anti-retroviral therapy. Nat Med 6:82, 2000

ROWLAND-JONES SL: Timeline: AIDS pathogenesis: What have two decades of HIV research taught us? Nat Rev Immunol 3:343, 2002

SMITH KJ et al: Cutaneous findings in HIV-1 positive patients: A 42-month prospective study. J Am Acad Dermatol 31:746, 1994

STEVENSON M: HIV-1 pathogenesis. Nat Med 9:853, 2003

STOVER J et al: Can we reverse the HIV/AIDS pandemic with an expanded response? Lancet 360:73, 2002

TEDALDI EM et al: Influence of coinfection with hepatitis C virus on morbidity and mortality due to human immunodeficiency virus infection in the era of highly active antiretroviral therapy. Clin Infect Dis 36:363, 2003

THIO CL et al: HIV-1, hepatitis B virus, and risk of liver-related mortality in the Multicenter Cohort Study (MACS). Lancet 360:1921, 2002

U.S. PUBLIC HEALTH SERVICE: Updated U.S. Public Health Service Guidelines for the Management of Occupational Exposures to HBV, HCV, and HIV and Recommendations for Postexposure Prophylaxis. MMWR Recomm Rep 50(RR-11):1, 2001. Updates available at http://www.aidsinfo.nih.gov

VALDISERRI RO et al: Accomplishments in HIV prevention science: Implications for stemming the epidemic. Nat Med 9:881, 2003

VIALE P et al: HIV-associated community-acquired pneumonia in the highly active antiretroviral therapy era. AIDS 16:2361, 2002

WEI X et al: Viral dynamics in human immunodeficiency virus type 1 infection. Nature 373:117, 1995

174 | VIRAL GASTROENTERITIS
Umesh D. Parashar, Roger I. Glass

Acute infectious gastroenteritis is a common illness that affects persons of all ages worldwide. It is a leading cause of mortality among children in developing countries, accounting for an estimated 2.4 to 2.9 million deaths each year, and is responsible for up to 10 to 12% of all hospitalizations among children in industrialized countries, such as the United States. Elderly persons, especially those with debilitating health conditions, are also at risk of severe complications and death from acute gastroenteritis. Acute gastroenteritis rarely causes mortality among healthy young adults, but it incurs substantial medical and social costs, including those of time lost from work.

Several enteric viruses have been recognized as important etiologic agents of acute infectious gastroenteritis (Table 174-1). Illness caused by these viruses is characterized by the acute onset of vomiting and/or diarrhea, which may be accompanied by fever, nausea, abdominal cramps, anorexia, and malaise. As shown in Table 174-2, several features can help distinguish gastroenteritis caused by viruses from that caused by bacterial agents. However, the distinction based on clinical and epidemiologic parameters alone is often difficult, and laboratory tests may be required to confirm the diagnosis.

The Norwalk and related human caliciviruses affect both adults and children and are a leading cause of epidemics of gastroenteritis. Rotaviruses are the leading cause of severe childhood gastroenteritis worldwide. Enteric adenoviruses and astroviruses are recognized as less common causes of gastroenteritis, and the role of some viruses, such as toroviruses and picobirnaviruses, remains to be elucidated. A brief discussion of these agents of acute infectious gastroenteritis among humans follows.

NORWALK AND RELATED HUMAN CALICIVIRUSES ■ Etiologic Agent The
Norwalk virus is the prototype strain of a group of nonenveloped, small (27 to 40 nm), round, icosahedral viruses with relatively amorphous surface features on visualization by electron microscopy. These viruses are usually named after the geographic location of the gastroenteritis outbreak from which they were first identified (e.g., Norwalk virus, Hawaii virus, Toronto virus) and have been difficult to classify because they have not been adapted to cell culture, no animal models are available, and often they are shed in low titers for only a few days. Molecular cloning and characterization have demonstrated that these viruses have a single, positive-strand RNA genome that is ~7.5 kb in

length and that they possess a single virion-associated protein with a molecular mass of 60 kDa, similar to that of typical caliciviruses. On the basis of these molecular characteristics, these viruses are presently classified in two genera belonging to the family Caliciviridae: the *noroviruses* and the *sapoviruses* (previously called Norwalk-like viruses and Sapporo-like viruses, respectively).

Epidemiology Infections with the Norwalk and related human caliciviruses are common, and most adults have antibodies to these viruses. Antibody is acquired at an earlier age in developing countries—a pattern consistent with the presumed fecal-oral mode of transmission of these viruses. Infections occur year-round, although, in temperate climates, a distinct increase has been noted in cold-weather months.

Noroviruses may be the most common infectious agents of mild gastroenteritis in the community and affect all age groups, whereas sapoviruses primarily cause gastroenteritis in children. Noroviruses are also a cause of traveler's diarrhea, and outbreaks have occurred among military personnel deployed to various parts of the world. The etiologic role of noroviruses in moderate to severe gastroenteritis requiring a visit to a physician or hospitalization is still being studied, but data from industrialized countries indicate that norovirus may be the second most common viral agent (after rotavirus) among young children and the most common agent among older children and adults.

Noroviruses are also recognized as the major cause of epidemics of gastroenteritis worldwide. In the United States, more than 90% of outbreaks of nonbacterial gastroenteritis are caused by noroviruses. Epidemics occur throughout the year, in all age groups, and in a variety of settings, such as schools, camps and recreational facilities, nursing homes, cruise ships, swimming facilities, and restaurants. Food items contaminated either by infectious food handlers or at the source are often implicated in outbreaks of infection. Because of their capacity to concentrate virus through filtration, shellfish harvested from fecally contaminated waters pose a special risk.

Transmission occurs predominantly by the fecal-oral route, but virus is also present in vomitus. Because an inoculum with very few viruses can be infectious, transmission can occur by aerosolization, by contact with contaminated formites, and by person-to-person contact. Viral shedding and infectivity are greatest during the acute illness, but challenge studies of volunteers with Norwalk virus indicate that viral antigen may be shed by asymptomatically infected persons and also by symptomatic persons prior to the onset of symptoms and for up to 2 weeks after the resolution of illness.

Pathogenesis The exact sites and cellular receptors for attachment of viral particles have not been determined. Data suggest that carbohydrates that are similar to human histo-blood group antigens and are present on the gastroduodenal epithelium of individuals with the secretor phenotype may serve as ligands for the attachment of Norwalk virus. Additional studies must more fully elucidate norovirus-carbohydrate interactions, including potential strain-specific variations. After the infection of volunteers, reversible lesions are noted in the upper jejunum, with broadening and blunting of the villi, shortening of the microvilli, vacuolization of the lining epithelium, crypt hyperplasia, and infiltration of the lamina propria by polymorphonuclear cells and lymphocytes. The lesions persist for at least 4 days after the resolution of symptoms and are associated with malabsorption of carbohydrates and fats and a decreased level of brush-border enzymes. Adenylate cyclase activity is not altered. No histopathologic changes are seen in the stom-

TABLE 174-1   *Viral Causes of Gastroenteritis among Humans*

Virus	Family	Genome	Primary Age Group at Risk	Clinical Severity	Detection Assays[a]
Group A rotavirus	Reoviridae	Double-strand segmented RNA	Children <5 years	+++	EM, EIA (commercial), PAGE, RT-PCR
Norovirus	Caliciviridae	Positive-sense single-strand RNA	All ages	++	EM, EIA, RT-PCR
Sapovirus	Caliciviridae	Positive-sense single-strand RNA	Children <5 years	+	EM, EIA, RT-PCR
Astrovirus	Astroviridae	Positive-sense single-strand RNA	Children <5 years	+	EM, EIA, RT-PCR
Adenovirus (types 40 and 41)	Adenoviridae	Double-strand DNA	Children <5 years	+/++	EM, EIA (commercial), RT-PCR

[a] EIA, enzyme immunoassay; EM, electron microscopy; PAGE, polyacrylamide gel electrophoresis; RT-PCR, reverse-transcriptase polymerase chain reaction.

ach or colon, but gastric motor function is delayed, and this alteration is believed to contribute to the nausea and vomiting that are typical of this illness.

Clinical Manifestations Gastroenteritis caused by Norwalk and related human caliciviruses has a sudden onset, following an average incubation period of 24 h (range, 12 to 72 h). The illness generally lasts 12 to 60 h and is characterized by one or more of the following symptoms: nausea, vomiting, abdominal cramps, and diarrhea. Vomiting is more prevalent among children, whereas a greater proportion of adults develop diarrhea. Constitutional symptoms are common, including headache, fever, chills, and myalgias. Noroviruses appear to cause more severe illness than sapoviruses, although both illnesses are less severe than that due to rotavirus. The stools are characteristically loose and watery, without blood, mucus, or leukocytes. White cell counts are generally normal; rarely, leukocytosis with relative lymphopenia may be observed. Death is a rare outcome and usually results from severe dehydration in vulnerable persons (e.g., elderly patients with debilitating health conditions).

Immunity Approximately 50% of persons challenged with Norwalk virus become ill and acquire short-term immunity against the infecting strain. Immunity to Norwalk virus appears to correlate inversely with level of antibody; i.e., persons with higher levels of preexisting antibody to Norwalk virus are more susceptible to illness. This observation suggests that some individuals have a genetic predisposition to illness. Recent data indicate that specific ABO, Lewis, and secretor blood group phenotypes may influence susceptibility to Norwalk virus infection.

Diagnosis Cloning and sequencing of the genome of Norwalk and several other human caliciviruses have allowed the development of assays based on polymerase chain reaction (PCR) for detection of virus in stool and vomitus. Virus-like particles produced by expression of capsid proteins in a recombinant baculovirus vector have been used to develop enzyme immunoassays (EIAs) for detection of virus in stool or a serologic response to a specific viral antigen. These newer diagnostic techniques are considerably more sensitive than previous detection methods such as electron microscopy, immune electron microscopy, and EIAs based on reagents derived from humans. However, no currently available single assay can detect all human caliciviruses because of their great genetic and antigenic diversity. In addition, the assays are still cumbersome and are available primarily in research laboratories, although they are increasingly being adopted by public health laboratories for routine screening of fecal specimens from patients affected by outbreaks of gastroenteritis.

℞ TREATMENT

Treatment generally is not required because the disease is self-limited. If severe dehydration develops, oral or intravenous fluid therapy is indicated. No specific antiviral therapy is available.

Prevention Epidemic prevention relies on situation-specific measures, such as control of contamination of food and water, exclusion of ill food handlers, and reduction of person-to-person spread through good personal hygiene and disinfection of contaminated fomites. The role

TABLE 174-2 Characteristics of Gastroenteritis Caused by Viral and Bacterial Agents

Feature	Viral Gastroenteritis	Bacterial Gastroenteritis
Setting	Incidence similar in developing and developed countries	More common in settings with poor hygiene and sanitation
Infectious dose	Low (10–100 viral particles) for most agents	High (>10^5 bacteria) for *Escherichia coli, Salmonella, Vibrio*; medium (10^2–10^5 bacteria) for *Campylobacter jejuni*; low (10–100 bacteria) for *Shigella*
Seasonality	In temperate climates, winter seasonality for most agents; year-round occurrence in tropical areas	More common in summer or rainy months, particularly in developing countries with a high disease burden
Incubation period	1–3 days for most agents; can be shorter for norovirus	1–7 days for common agents (e.g., *Campylobacter, E. coli, Shigella, Salmonella*); few hours for bacteria producing preformed toxins (e.g., *Staphylococcus aureus, Bacillus cereus*)
Reservoir	Primarily humans	Depending on species, both human (e.g., *Shigella, Salmonella*) and animal (e.g., *Campylobacter, Salmonella, E. coli*) reservoirs exist.
Fever	Common with rotavirus and norovirus; uncommon with other agents	Common with agents causing inflammatory diarrhea (e.g., *Salmonella, Shigella*)
Vomiting	Prominent and can be the only presenting feature, especially in children	Common with bacteria producing preformed toxins; less prominent in diarrhea due to other agents
Diarrhea	Common; nonbloody in almost all cases	Prominent and frequently bloody with agents causing inflammatory diarrhea
Duration	1–3 days for norovirus and sapovirus; 2–8 days for other viruses	1–2 days for bacteria producing preformed toxins; 2–8 days for most other bacteria
Diagnosis	This is often a diagnosis of exclusion in clinical practice. Commercial enzyme immunoassays are available for detection of rotavirus and adenovirus, but identification of other agents is limited to research and public health laboratories.	Fecal examination for leukocytes and blood is helpful in differential diagnosis. Culture of stool specimens, sometimes on special media, can identify several pathogens. Molecular techniques are useful epidemiologic tools but are not routinely used in most laboratories.
Treatment	Supportive therapy to maintain adequate hydration and nutrition should be given. Antibiotics and antimotility agents are contraindicated.	Supportive hydration therapy is adequate for most patients. Antibiotics are recommended for patients with dysentery caused by *Shigella* or *Vibrio cholerae* and for some patients with *Clostridium difficile* colitis.

of immunoprophylaxis is not clear, given the lack of long-term immunity from natural disease and the paradoxic inverse association between the level of immune response and protection from disease.

ROTAVIRUS ■ Etiologic Agent Rotaviruses are members of the family Reoviridae. The viral genome consists of 11 segments of double-strand RNA that are enclosed in a triple-layered, nonenveloped, icosahedral capsid 75 nm in diameter. Viral protein 6 (VP6), the major structural protein, is the target of commercial immunoassays and determines the group specificity of rotaviruses. There are seven major groups of rotavirus (A through G); human illness is caused primarily by group A and, to a much lesser extent, by groups B and C. Two outer-capsid proteins, VP7 (G-protein) and VP4 (P-protein), determine serotype specificity, induce neutralizing antibodies, and form the basis of the binary classification of rotaviruses (G and P types). The segmented genome of rotavirus allows genetic reassortment (i.e., exchange of genome segments between viruses) during co-infection—a property that may play a role in viral evolution and has been utilized in the development of reassortant animal-human rotavirus–based vaccines.

Epidemiology Nearly all children are infected with rotavirus by 3 to 5 years of age. Neonatal infections are common but are often asymptomatic or mild, presumably because of protection from maternal antibody or breast-feeding. Nevertheless, rotavirus is known to cause disease in neonates, particularly in those admitted to intensive care units, and some data suggest that the clinical manifestations in full-term infants may differ from those in preterm infants. First infections after 3 months of age are likely to be symptomatic, and the incidence of disease peaks among children 4 to 23 months of age. Reinfections are common, but the severity of disease decreases with each repeat infection. Therefore, severe rotavirus infections are relatively uncommon in older children and adults. However, rotavirus can cause illness in parents and caretakers of children with rotavirus diarrhea, immunocompromised persons, travelers, and elderly individuals and should be considered in the differential diagnosis of gastroenteritis among adults.

In temperate climates, rotavirus disease occurs predominantly during the cooler fall and winter months. In the United States, the annual rotavirus epidemic begins in the Southwest in autumn (October through December) and migrates across the continent, peaking in the Northeast during spring (March through May). In tropical settings, rotavirus disease occurs year-round, with less pronounced seasonal peaks.

Rotavirus gastroenteritis is more frequently associated with dehydration than is gastroenteritis caused by other pathogens. Therefore, the proportion of gastroenteritis cases that are attributable to rotavirus increases with increasing severity of illness, ranging from a median of 8% of cases in the community to 18% of cases in outpatients and 30% of cases in hospitalized patients. Each year, rotavirus is estimated to cause ~500,000 childhood deaths worldwide.

During episodes of rotavirus-associated diarrhea, virus is shed in large quantities (10^7 to 10^{12}/g) in stool. Viral shedding detectable by EIA usually subsides within a week but may persist for >30 days in immunocompromised individuals. Viral shedding may be detected for longer periods by sensitive molecular assays, such as PCR. The virus is transmitted predominantly through the fecal-oral route. Spread through respiratory secretions, person-to-person contact, or contaminated environmental surfaces has also been postulated to explain the rapid acquisition of antibody in the first 3 years of life, regardless of sanitary conditions.

At least 10 different G serotypes of group A rotavirus have been identified in humans, but only 5 types (G1 through G4 and G9) are common. While human rotavirus strains that possess a high degree of genetic homology with animal strains have been identified, animal-to-human transmission appears to be uncommon. Group B rotaviruses have been associated with several large epidemics of severe gastroenteritis among adults in China since 1982 and have recently been identified in India but not in other parts of the world. Group C rotaviruses have been associated with a small proportion of pediatric gastroenteritis cases in several countries worldwide.

Pathogenesis Rotaviruses infect and ultimately destroy the mature enterocytes in the villous epithelium of the proximal small intestine. The loss of absorptive villous epithelium coupled with the proliferation of secretory crypt cells results in secretory diarrhea. Brush-border enzymes characteristic of differentiated cells are reduced, and this change leads to the accumulation of unmetabolized disaccharides and consequent osmotic diarrhea. Studies in mice indicate that a nonstructural rotavirus protein, NSP4, functions as an enterotoxin and contributes to secretory diarrhea by altering epithelial cell function and permeability. In addition, rotavirus may evoke fluid secretion through activation of the enteric nervous system in the intestinal wall. Recent data indicate that rotavirus antigen and RNA are present in serum of children with acute rotavirus infection; further investigations are needed to establish the significance of these findings in the pathogenesis of rotavirus disease.

Clinical Manifestations The clinical spectrum of rotavirus infection ranges from subclinical illness to severe gastroenteritis leading to the development of life-threatening dehydration. After an incubation period of 1 to 3 days, the illness has an abrupt onset, with vomiting frequently preceding the onset of diarrhea. Up to one-third of patients may have a temperature of >39°C. The stools are characteristically loose and watery and only infrequently contain red or white cells. The gastrointestinal symptoms generally resolve in 3 to 7 days.

Respiratory and neurologic features in children with rotavirus infection have been reported, but causal associations have not been proven. Rotavirus infection has been associated with a variety of other clinical syndromes (e.g., sudden infant death syndrome, necrotizing enterocolitis, intussusception, and diabetes mellitus type 1), but no causal relationship has been confirmed with any of these syndromes.

Rotavirus does not appear to be a major opportunistic pathogen in children with HIV infection. In severely immunodeficient children, rotavirus can cause protracted diarrhea with prolonged viral excretion and, in rare instances, can disseminate systemically. Persons who are immunosuppressed for bone marrow transplantation are also at risk for severe, or even fatal, rotavirus disease.

Immunity Protection against rotavirus disease is correlated with the presence of virus-specific secretory IgA antibodies in the intestine and, to some extent, the serum. Because virus-specific IgA production at the intestinal surface is short-lived, complete protection against disease is only temporary. However, each infection and subsequent reinfection confers progressively greater immunity, so severe disease is most common among young children with first or second infections. Immunologic memory is believed to be important in the attenuation of the severity of disease upon reinfection.

Diagnosis Illness caused by rotavirus is difficult to distinguish clinically from that caused by other enteric viruses. Because large quantities of virus are shed in feces, the diagnosis can usually be confirmed by a wide variety of commercially available EIAs or by techniques for detecting viral RNA, such as gel electrophoresis, probe hybridization, or PCR.

℞ TREATMENT

Rotavirus gastroenteritis can lead to severe dehydration. Thus appropriate treatment should be instituted early. Standard oral rehydration therapy is successful in most children who can take oral fluids, but intravenous fluid replacement may be required for patients who are severely dehydrated or are unable to tolerate oral therapy because of frequent vomiting. The therapeutic role of probiotics, bismuth salicylate, and enkephalinase inhibitors has been evaluated in clinical studies but is not clearly defined. Antibiotics and antimotility agents should be avoided. In immunocompromised children with chronic symptomatic rotavirus disease, orally administered immunoglobulins or colostrum may resolve symptoms, but the choice of agents and their doses have not been well studied and are often empirical.

Prevention Efforts to develop rotavirus vaccines were pursued because it was apparent—given the similar rates in less developed and industrialized nations—that improvements in hygiene and sanitation were unlikely to reduce disease incidence. In 1998, a rotavirus vaccine was licensed in the United States and was recommended for routine immunization of infants. However, this vaccine was withdrawn in 1999 because it was causally linked with intussusception, with an estimated 1 case per 11,000 vaccinated infants. Other rotavirus vaccines are being developed, including two leading multinational candidate vaccines whose safety and efficacy are currently being studied in large-scale clinical trials.

OTHER VIRAL AGENTS OF GASTROENTERITIS Enteric adenoviruses of serotypes 40 and 41 belonging to subgroup F are 70- to 80-nm viruses with double-strand DNA that cause ~2 to 12% of all diarrhea episodes in young children. Unlike adenoviruses that cause respiratory illness, enteric adenoviruses are difficult to cultivate in cell lines, but they can be detected with commercially available EIAs.

Astroviruses, 28- to 30-nm viruses with a characteristic icosahedral structure, contain a positive-sense, single-strand RNA. At least seven serotypes have been identified, of which serotype 1 is most common. Astroviruses are primarily pediatric pathogens, causing ~2 to 10% of cases of mild to moderate gastroenteritis in children. The availability of simple immunoassays to detect virus in fecal specimens and of molecular methods to confirm and characterize strains will permit more comprehensive assessment of the etiologic role of these agents.

Toroviruses are 100- to 140-nm, enveloped, positive-strand RNA viruses that are recognized as causes of gastroenteritis in horses (Berne virus) and cattle (Breda virus). Their role as a cause of diarrhea in humans is still unclear, but a study from Canada demonstrated an association between torovirus excretion and nosocomial gastroenteritis in pediatric patients. In this study, more than half of the patients with torovirus in stool also had a demonstrable immune response. Patients with torovirus infection were older and experienced less vomiting and more bloody diarrhea than did those with rotavirus or astrovirus infection. Further studies are required to confirm these findings.

Picobirnaviruses are small, bi-segmented, double-strand RNA viruses that cause gastroenteritis in a variety of animals. Their role as primary causes of gastroenteritis in humans remains unclear, but several studies have found an association between picobirnaviruses and gastroenteritis in HIV-infected adults.

The recently recognized severe acute respiratory syndrome–associated coronavirus (SARS-CoV) has been associated with gastroenteritis in 20 to 66% of affected patients. In one study of 138 SARS patients in Hong Kong, 20.3% presented with watery diarrhea, and up to 38.4% had diarrhea during their illness. Diarrhea was most common during the first week of illness, lasted for an average of 3.7 days, and was self-limiting in most instances. Studies of intestinal biopsy specimens showed minimal architectural disruption but also revealed active viral replication within both the small and the large intestine. SARS-CoV RNA could be detected in the stool of patients for >10 weeks after the onset of symptoms.

Several other viruses (e.g., enteroviruses, reoviruses, pestiviruses, and parvoviruses B) have been identified in the feces of patients with diarrhea, but their etiologic role in gastroenteritis has not been proved.

FURTHER READING

BLUTT SE et al: Rotavirus antigenaemia and viraemia: A common event? Lancet 362:1445, 2003

CUNLIFFE NA et al: Effect of concomitant HIV infection on presentation and outcome of rotavirus gastroenteritis in Malawian children. Lancet 358:550, 2001

FANKHAUSER RL et al: Epidemiologic and molecular trends of "Norwalk like viruses" associated with outbreaks of gastroenteritis in the United States. J Infect Dis 186:1, 2002

JAMIESON FB et al: Human torovirus: A new nosocomial gastrointestinal pathogen. J Infect Dis 178:1263, 1998

LEUNG WK et al: Enteric involvement of severe acute respiratory syndrome–associated coronavirus infection. Gastroenterology 125:1011, 2003

MURPHY TV et al: Intussusception among infants given an oral rotavirus vaccine. N Engl J Med 344:564, 2001

NAKAJIMA H et al: Winter seasonality and rotavirus diarrhoea in adults. Lancet 357:1950, 2001

PANG XL et al: Human caliciviruses in acute gastroenteritis of young children in the community. J Infect Dis 181:S288, 2000

175 ENTEROVIRUSES AND REOVIRUSES
Jeffrey I. Cohen

ENTEROVIRUSES

CLASSIFICATION AND CHARACTERIZATION Enteroviruses are so named because of their ability to multiply in the gastrointestinal tract. Despite their name, these viruses are not a prominent cause of gastroenteritis. Enteroviruses encompass 64 human serotypes: 3 serotypes of poliovirus, 23 serotypes of coxsackievirus A, 6 serotypes of coxsackievirus B, 28 serotypes of echovirus, and enteroviruses 68 through 71. Enterovirus surveillance conducted in the United States by the Centers for Disease Control and Prevention (CDC) in 2000 and 2001 revealed that echoviruses accounted for >60% of all enterovirus isolates (Table 175-1).

Human enteroviruses contain a single-stranded RNA genome surrounded by an icosahedral capsid comprising four viral proteins. These viruses have no lipid envelope and are stable in acidic environments, including the stomach. They are resistant to inactivation by standard disinfectants (e.g., alcohol, detergents) and can persist for days at room temperature.

PATHOGENESIS AND IMMUNITY Much of what is known about the pathogenesis of enteroviruses has been derived from studies of poliovirus infection. After ingestion, poliovirus is thought to infect epithelial cells in the mucosa of the gastrointestinal tract and then to spread to and replicate in the submucosal lymphoid tissue of the tonsils and Peyer's patches. The virus next spreads to the regional lymph nodes, a viremic phase ensues, and the virus replicates in organs of the reticuloendothelial system. In some cases, a second viremia occurs and the virus replicates further in various tissues, sometimes causing symptomatic disease.

It is uncertain whether poliovirus reaches the central nervous system (CNS) during viremia or whether it also spreads via peripheral nerves. Since viremia precedes the onset of neurologic disease in humans and in experimentally infected chimpanzees, it has been assumed that the virus enters the CNS via the bloodstream. The poliovirus receptor is a member of the immunoglobulin superfamily. Poliovirus infection is limited to primates, largely because of the ability of their cells to express the viral receptor. Studies demonstrating the poliovirus receptor in the end-plate region of muscle at the neuromuscular junction suggest that, if the virus enters the muscle during viremia, it could travel across the neuromuscular junction up the axon to the anterior horn cells. Studies of monkeys or transgenic mice expressing the poliovirus receptor show that, after intramuscular injection, poliovirus does not reach the spinal cord if the sciatic nerve is cut. Taken together, these findings suggest that poliovirus can spread directly from muscle to the CNS by neural pathways. Intercellular adhesion molecule 1 (ICAM-1) is a receptor for coxsackieviruses A13, A18, and A21; CAR for coxsackievirus B; VLA-2 integrin for echovirus types 1 and 8; and CD55 for enterovirus 70 and some serotypes of coxsackievirus B and echovirus.

Poliovirus can usually be cultured from the blood 3 to 5 days after infection, before the development of neutralizing antibodies. While viral replication at secondary sites begins to slow 1 week after infection, it continues in the gastrointestinal tract. Poliovirus is shed from the oropharynx for up to 3 weeks after infection and from the gastrointestinal tract for as long as 12 weeks; immunodeficient patients can shed poliovirus for more than 1 year. During replication in the gastrointestinal tract, attenuated oral poliovirus can mutate, reverting to a more neurovirulent phenotype within a few days. The clinical significance of this increased neurovirulence is unknown.

TABLE 175-1 *Frequency of the Most Common Non-Poliovirus Isolates of Enterovirus in the United States, 2000–2001*

Serotype	Percentage
Echovirus 18	22.0
Echovirus 13	20.8
Coxsackievirus B5	11.9
Coxsackievirus B2	6.3
Echovirus 6	6.1
Echovirus 11	4.5
Coxsackievirus A9	4.0
Echovirus 9	3.3
Coxsackievirus B4	3.2
Echovirus 4	3.1
All others	15.0

Source: Centers for Disease Control and Prevention, 2002.

Humoral and secretory immunity in the gastrointestinal tract is important for the control of enterovirus infections. Enteroviruses induce specific IgM, which usually persists for <6 months, and specific IgG, which persists for life. Capsid protein VP1 is the predominant target of neutralizing antibody, which generally confers lifelong protection against subsequent disease caused by the same serotype but does not prevent infection or virus shedding. Enteroviruses also induce cellular immunity, but the significance of this mechanism in limiting infection is uncertain. Patients with impaired cellular immunity are not known to develop unusually severe disease when infected with enteroviruses. In contrast, the severe infections in patients with agammaglobulinemia emphasize the importance of humoral immunity in controlling enterovirus infections. IgA antibodies are instrumental in reducing poliovirus replication in and shedding from the gastrointestinal tract. Breast milk contains IgA specific for enteroviruses and can protect humans from infection.

EPIDEMIOLOGY Enteroviruses have a worldwide distribution. More than 50% of nonpoliovirus enterovirus infections and more than 90% of poliovirus infections are subclinical. When symptoms do develop, they are usually nonspecific and occur in conjunction with fever; only a minority of infections are associated with specific clinical syndromes. The incubation period for most enterovirus infections ranges from 2 to 14 days but usually is <1 week.

Enterovirus infection is more common in socioeconomically disadvantaged areas, especially in those where conditions are crowded and in tropical areas where hygiene is poor. Infection is most common among infants and young children; serious illness develops most often during the first few days of life and in older children and adults. In developing countries, where children are infected at an early age, poliovirus infection has less often been associated with paralysis; in countries with better hygiene, older children and adults are more likely to be seronegative, become infected, and develop paralysis. Passively acquired maternal antibody reduces the risk of symptomatic infection in neonates. Young children are the most frequent shedders of enteroviruses and are usually the index cases in family outbreaks. In temperate climates, enterovirus infections occur most often in the summer and fall; no seasonal pattern is apparent in the tropics.

Most enteroviruses are transmitted primarily by the fecal-oral route from fecally contaminated fingers or inanimate objects. Patients are most infectious shortly before and after the onset of symptomatic disease, when virus is present in the stool and throat. The ingestion of virus-contaminated food or water can also cause disease. Certain enteroviruses (such as enterovirus 70, which causes acute hemorrhagic conjunctivitis) can be transmitted by direct inoculation from the fingers to the eye. Airborne transmission is important for some viruses that cause respiratory tract disease, such as coxsackievirus A21. Enteroviruses can be transmitted across the placenta from mother to fetus, causing severe disease in the newborn. The transmission of enteroviruses through blood transfusions or insect bites has not been documented. Nosocomial spread of coxsackievirus and echovirus has taken place in hospital nurseries.

CLINICAL FEATURES OF INFECTION WITH POLIOVIRUS Most infections with poliovirus are asymptomatic. After an incubation period of 3 to 6 days, ~5% of patients present with a minor illness (abortive poliomyelitis) manifested by fever, malaise, sore throat, anorexia, myalgias, and headache. This condition usually resolves in 3 days. About 1% of patients present with aseptic meningitis (nonparalytic poliomyelitis). Examination of cerebrospinal fluid (CSF) reveals lymphocytic pleocytosis, a normal glucose level, and a normal or slightly elevated protein level; CSF polymorphonuclear leukocytes may be present early. In some patients, especially children, malaise and fever precede the onset of aseptic meningitis.

The least common presentation is that of paralytic disease. After one or several days, signs of aseptic meningitis are followed by severe back, neck, and muscle pain and by the rapid or gradual development of motor weakness. In some cases the disease appears to be biphasic, with aseptic meningitis followed first by apparent recovery but then (1 or 2 days later) by the return of fever and the development of paralysis; this form is more common among children than among adults. Weakness is generally asymmetric, is proximal more than distal, and may involve the legs (most commonly); the arms; or the abdominal, thoracic, or bulbar muscles. Paralysis develops during the febrile phase of the illness and usually does not progress after defervescence. Urinary retention may also occur. Examination reveals weakness, fasciculations, decreased muscle tone, and reduced or absent reflexes in affected areas. Transient hyperreflexia sometimes precedes the loss of reflexes. Patients frequently report sensory symptoms, but objective sensory testing usually yields normal results. Bulbar paralysis may lead to dysphagia, difficulty in handling secretions, or dysphonia. Respiratory insufficiency due to aspiration, involvement of the respiratory center in the medulla, or paralysis of the phrenic or intercostal nerves may develop, and severe medullary involvement may lead to circulatory collapse. Most patients with paralysis recover some function weeks to months after infection. About two-thirds of patients have residual neurologic sequelae.

Paralytic disease is more common among older individuals, pregnant women, and persons exercising strenuously or undergoing trauma at the time of CNS symptoms. Tonsillectomy predisposes to bulbar poliomyelitis, and intramuscular injections increase the risk of paralysis in the involved limb(s).

Until recently, poliomyelitis due to live poliovirus vaccine occurred in the United States. The risk of developing poliomyelitis after oral vaccination is estimated at 1 case per 2.5 million doses. The risk is ~2000 times higher among immunodeficient persons, especially in persons with hypo- or agammaglobulinemia. Before 1997, an average of eight cases of vaccine-associated poliomyelitis occurred—in both vaccinees and their contacts—in the United States each year. With the change in recommendations first to a sequential regimen of inactivated poliovirus vaccine (IPV) and oral poliovirus vaccine (OPV) in 1997 and then to an all-IPV regimen in 2000, the number of cases of vaccine-associated poliovirus declined. From 1997 to 1999, six such cases were reported in the United States; no cases have been reported since 1999.

The *postpolio syndrome* presents as a new onset of weakness, fatigue, fasciculations, and pain with additional atrophy of the muscle group involved during the initial paralytic disease 20 to 40 years earlier. The syndrome is more common among women and with increasing time after acute disease. The onset is usually insidious, and weakness occasionally extends to muscles that were not involved during the initial illness. The prognosis is generally good; progression to further weakness is usually slow, with plateau periods that range from 1 to 10 years. The postpolio syndrome is thought to be due to progressive dysfunction and loss of motor neurons that compensated for the neurons lost during the original infection and not to persistent or reactivated poliovirus infection.

CLINICAL FEATURES OF INFECTION WITH COXSACKIEVIRUS, ECHOVIRUS, AND OTHER ENTEROVIRUSES An estimated 5 to 10 million cases of symptomatic disease due to enterovirus other than poliovirus occur in the United States each year. Enteroviruses are the most common cause of aseptic meningitis and nonspecific febrile illnesses of neonates. Certain clinical syndromes are more likely to be caused by certain serotypes (Table 175-2), but there is much overlap. In 2000–2001, 85% of enterovirus infections were caused by only 10 of the 64 human serotypes. Echoviruses 13 and 18 accounted for 43% of recognized enterovirus infections (Table 175-1).

Nonspecific Febrile Illness (Summer Grippe) The most common clinical manifestation of enterovirus infection is a nonspecific febrile illness. After an incubation period of 3 to 6 days, patients present with an acute onset of fever, malaise, and headache. Occasional cases are associated with upper respiratory symptoms, and some cases include nausea and vomiting. Symptoms often last for 3 to 4 days, and most cases resolve in a week. While infections with other respiratory viruses occur more often from late fall to early spring, enterovirus febrile illness frequently occurs in the summer and early fall.

Generalized Disease of the Newborn Most serious enterovirus infections in infants develop during the first week of life, although severe disease can occur up to 3 months of age. Neonates often present with an illness resembling bacterial sepsis, with fever, irritability, and lethargy. Laboratory abnormalities include leukocytosis with a left shift, thrombocytopenia, elevated values in liver function tests, and CSF pleocytosis. The illness can be complicated by myocarditis and hypotension, fulminant hepatitis and disseminated intravascular coagulation, meningitis or meningoencephalitis, or pneumonia. It may be difficult to distinguish enterovirus infection from bacterial sepsis, although a history of a recent virus-like illness in the mother provides a clue.

Aseptic Meningitis and Encephalitis Enteroviruses are the cause of up to 90% of cases of aseptic meningitis in children and young adults in which an etiologic agent can be identified. Patients with aseptic meningitis typically present with an acute onset of fever, chills, headache, photophobia, and pain on eye movement. Nausea and vomiting are also common. Examination reveals meningismus without localizing neurologic signs; drowsiness or irritability may also be apparent. In some cases, a febrile illness may be reported that remits but returns several days later in conjunction with signs of meningitis. Other systemic manifestations may provide clues to an enteroviral cause, including diarrhea, myalgias, rash, pleurodynia, myocarditis, and herpangina. Examination of the CSF invariably reveals pleocytosis; early in the course, polymorphonuclear leukocytes may be present or even predominant, raising the possibility of bacterial or other nonviral causes of meningitis. Partially treated bacterial meningitis may be particularly difficult to exclude in some instances. A useful rule is that the CSF cell count in enteroviral meningitis shows a shift to lymphocytic predominance within 24 h of presentation, and the total count generally does not exceed 1000 cells/μL. Additional CSF findings consist of a normal glucose content and a normal or only slightly elevated (by $\leq$100 mg/mL) level of protein. Enteroviruses and mumps virus may produce a similar picture of meningitis; a low CSF glucose level suggests mumps, whereas a normal CSF glucose level and transient CSF polymorphonuclear pleocytosis suggest enterovirus infection. Enteroviral meningitis is more frequent in summer and fall in temperate climates, while viral meningitis of other etiologies (e.g., mumps) is more common in winter and spring. Symptoms ordinarily resolve within a week, although CSF abnormalities can persist for several weeks. Enteroviral meningitis is often more severe in adults than in children. Neurologic sequelae are rare, and most patients have an excellent prognosis.

Enteroviral encephalitis is much less common than enteroviral aseptic meningitis. Occasional highly inflammatory cases of enteroviral meningitis may be complicated by a mild form of encephalitis that is recognized on the basis of progressive lethargy, disorientation, and sometimes seizures. Less commonly, severe primary encephalitis may develop. It is estimated that 10 to 20% of cases of viral encephalitis are due to enteroviruses. Immunocompetent patients generally have a good prognosis.

Patients with hypo- or agammaglobulinemia or severe combined immunodeficiency may develop chronic meningitis or encephalitis; about half of these patients have a dermatomyositis-like syndrome, with peripheral edema, rash, and myositis. They may also have chronic hepatitis. Patients may develop neurologic disease while receiving gamma globulin replacement therapy. Echoviruses (especially echovirus 11) are the most common pathogens in this situation.

TABLE 175-2 *Manifestations Commonly Associated with Enterovirus Serotypes*

Manifestation	Serotype(s) of Indicated Virus	
	Coxsackievirus	Echovirus (E) and Enterovirus (Ent)
Acute hemorrhagic conjunctivitis	A24	E70
Aseptic meningitis	A2, 4, 7, 9, 10; B1-5	E4, 6, 7, 9, 11, 13, 16, 18, 19, 30, 33; Ent70, 71
Encephalitis	A9; B1-5	E3, 4, 6, 9, 11, 25, 30; Ent71
Exanthem	A4, 5, 9, 10, 16; B1, 3-5	E4-7, 9, 11, 16-19, 25, 30; Ent71
Generalized disease of the newborn	B2-5	E4-6, 9, 11, 14, 16, 19
Hand-foot-and-mouth disease	A5, 7, 9, 10, 16; B2, 5	Ent71
Herpangina	A1-10, 16, 22; B1-5	E6, 9, 11, 16, 17, 25; Ent71
Myocarditis, pericarditis	A4, 9, 16; B1-5	E6, 9, 11, 22
Paralysis	A4, 7, 9; B1-5	E2, 4, 6, 9, 11, 30; Ent70, 71
Pleurodynia	A1, 2, 4, 6, 9, 10, 16; B1-6	E1-3, 6, 7, 9, 11, 12, 14, 16, 19, 24, 25, 30
Pneumonia	A9, 16; B1-5	E6, 7, 9, 11, 12, 19, 20, 30; Ent68, 71

Paralytic disease due to enteroviruses other than poliovirus occurs sporadically and is usually less severe than poliomyelitis. Most cases are due to enterovirus 70 or 71 or to coxsackievirus A7 or A9. Guillain-Barré syndrome is also associated with enterovirus infection. While some studies have suggested a link between enteroviruses and the chronic fatigue syndrome, most recent studies have not demonstrated such an association.

Pleurodynia (Bornholm Disease) Patients with pleurodynia present with an acute onset of fever and spasms of pleuritic chest or upper abdominal pain. Chest pain is more common in adults, and abdominal pain is more common in children. Paroxysms of severe, knifelike pain usually last 15 to 30 min and are associated with diaphoresis and tachypnea. Fever peaks within an hour after the onset of paroxysms and subsides when pain resolves. The involved muscles are tender to palpation, and a pleural rub may be detected. The white blood cell count and chest x-ray are usually normal. Most cases are due to coxsackievirus B and occur during epidemics. Symptoms resolve in a few days, and recurrences are rare. Treatment includes the administration of nonsteroidal anti-inflammatory agents or the application of heat to the affected muscles.

Myocarditis and Pericarditis Enteroviruses are estimated to cause up to one-third of cases of acute myocarditis. Coxsackievirus B and its RNA have been detected in pericardial fluid and myocardial tissue in some cases of acute myocarditis and pericarditis. Most cases of enteroviral myocarditis or pericarditis occur in newborns, adolescents, or young adults. More than two-thirds of patients are male. Patients often present with an upper respiratory tract infection that is followed by fever, chest pain, dyspnea, arrhythmias, and occasionally heart failure. A pericardial friction rub is documented in half of cases, and the electrocardiogram shows ST segment elevations or ST- and T-wave abnormalities. Serum levels of myocardial enzymes are often elevated. Neonates commonly have severe disease, while most older children and adults recover completely. Up to 10% of cases progress to chronic dilated cardiomyopathy. Chronic constrictive pericarditis may also be a sequela.

Exanthems Enterovirus infection is the leading cause of exanthems in children in the summer and fall. While exanthems are associated with many enteroviruses, certain types have been linked to specific syndromes. Echoviruses 9 and 16 have frequently been associated with exanthem and fever. Rashes may be discrete (rubelliform) or confluent (morbilliform), beginning on the face and spreading to the trunk and extremities. Echovirus 9 is the most common cause of rubelliform rash. Unlike the rash of rubella, the enteroviral rash occurs in the summer and is not associated with lymphadenopathy. Roseola-like rashes develop after defervescence, with macules and papules on the face and trunk. The Boston exanthem, caused by echovirus 16, is a roseola-like rash that often affects multiple members of a family. A variety of other rashes have been associated with enteroviruses, including erythema multiforme and vesicular, urticarial, petechial, or purpuric lesions. Enanthems also occur, including lesions that resemble the Koplik's spots seen with measles.

Hand-Foot-and-Mouth Disease   After an incubation period of 4 to 6 days, patients with hand-foot-and-mouth disease present with fever, anorexia, and malaise; these manifestations are followed by the development of sore throat and vesicles (Fig. 175-1) on the buccal mucosa and often on the tongue and then by the appearance of tender vesicular lesions on the dorsum of the hands, sometimes with involvement of the palms. The vesicles may form bullae and quickly ulcerate. About one-third of patients also have lesions on the palate, uvula, or tonsillar pillars, and one-third have a rash on the feet (including the soles) or on the buttocks. The disease is highly infectious, with attack rates of close to 100% among young children. The lesions usually resolve in 1 week. Most cases are due to coxsackievirus A16 or enterovirus 71.

An epidemic of enterovirus 71 infection in Taiwan in 1998 resulted in thousands of cases of hand-foot-and-mouth disease or herpangina. Severe complications included CNS disease, myocarditis, and pulmonary hemorrhage. About 90% of those who died were children ≤5 years old, and these deaths were associated with pulmonary edema or pulmonary hemorrhage. CNS disease included aseptic meningitis, flaccid paralysis (similar to poliomyelitis), or rhombencephalitis with myoclonus and tremor or ataxia. The mean age of patients with CNS complications was 2.5 years, and magnetic resonance imaging in cases with encephalitis usually showed brain-stem lesions.

Herpangina   Herpangina is usually caused by coxsackievirus A and presents as acute-onset fever, sore throat, dysphagia, and grayish-white papulovesicular lesions on an erythematous base that ulcerate. The lesions can persist for weeks; are present on the soft palate, anterior pillars of the tonsils, and uvula; and are concentrated in the posterior portion of the mouth. In contrast to herpes stomatitis, enteroviral herpangina is not associated with gingivitis. Acute lymphonodular pharyngitis associated with coxsackievirus A10 presents as white or yellow nodules surrounded by erythema in the posterior oropharynx. The lesions do not ulcerate.

Acute Hemorrhagic Conjunctivitis   Patients with acute hemorrhagic conjunctivitis present with an acute onset of severe eye pain, blurred vision, photophobia, and watery discharge from the eye. Examination reveals edema, chemosis, and subconjunctival hemorrhage and often shows punctate keratitis and conjunctival follicles as well. Preauricular adenopathy is often found. Epidemics and nosocomial spread have been associated with enterovirus 70 and coxsackievirus A24. Systemic symptoms, including headache and fever, develop in 20% of cases, and recovery is usually complete in 10 days. The sudden onset and short duration of the illness help to distinguish acute hemorrhagic conjunctivitis from other ocular infections such as those due to adenovirus and *Chlamydia*. Paralysis has been associated with some cases of acute hemorrhagic conjunctivitis due to enterovirus 70 during epidemics.

Other Manifestations   Enteroviruses are an infrequent cause of childhood pneumonia and the common cold. Coxsackievirus B has been isolated at autopsy from the pancreas of a few children presenting with insulin-dependent diabetes mellitus; however, most attempts to isolate the virus have been unsuccessful. Other diseases that have been associated with enterovirus infection include parotitis, bronchitis, bronchiolitis, croup, infectious lymphocytosis, polymyositis, acute arthritis, and acute nephritis.

DIAGNOSIS   Isolation of enterovirus in cell culture is the most common procedure for the diagnosis of infection. While cultures of stool, nasopharyngeal, or throat samples from patients with enterovirus diseases are often positive, isolation of the virus from these sites does not prove that it is directly associated with disease because these sites are frequently colonized for weeks in patients with subclinical infections. Isolation of virus from the throat is more likely to be associated with disease than isolation from the stool since virus is shed for shorter periods from the throat. Cultures of CSF, serum, fluid from body cavities, or tissues are positive less frequently, but a positive result is indicative of disease caused by enterovirus. In some cases the virus can be isolated only from the blood or only from the CSF; therefore, it is important to culture multiple sites. Cultures are more likely to be positive earlier than later in the course of infection. Most human enteroviruses can be detected within a week after inoculation of cell cultures. Cultures may be negative because of the presence of neutralizing antibody, lack of susceptibility of the cells used, or inappropriate handling of the specimen. Coxsackievirus A may require inoculation into special cell-culture lines or into suckling mice.

Identification of the serotype of an enterovirus is useful primarily for epidemiologic studies and, with a few exceptions, has little clinical utility. It is important to identify serious infections with enterovirus during epidemics and to distinguish the vaccine strain of poliovirus from the other enteroviruses in the throat or in the feces. Stool and throat samples for culture as well as acute- and convalescent-phase serum specimens should be obtained from all patients with suspected poliomyelitis. In the absence of a positive CSF culture, a positive culture of stool obtained within the first 2 weeks after the onset of symptoms is most often used to confirm the diagnosis of poliomyelitis. If poliovirus is isolated, it should be sent to the CDC in Atlanta for identification as either a wild-type or a vaccine virus.

The polymerase chain reaction (PCR) has been used to amplify viral nucleic acid from CSF, serum, urine, throat swabs, and tissues. A single pair of PCR primers can detect more than 92% of the serotypes that infect humans. With the proper controls, PCR of the CSF is highly sensitive (≥95%) and specific (>80%) and is more rapid than culture. PCR of serum is also highly sensitive and specific in the diagnosis of disseminated disease. PCR may be particularly helpful for the diagnosis and follow-up of enterovirus disease in immunodeficient patients receiving immunoglobulin therapy, whose viral cultures may be negative. Antigen detection and hybridization of enterovirus sequences in human tissues with a specific probe are additional options, but these techniques are generally less sensitive than PCR.

Serologic diagnosis of enterovirus infection is limited by the large

FIGURE 175-1   Tender vesicles and erosions in the mouth of a patient with hand-foot-and-mouth disease.

number of serotypes and the lack of a common antigen. Demonstration of seroconversion may be useful in rare cases for confirmation of culture results, but serologic testing is usually limited to epidemiologic studies. Serum should be collected and frozen soon after the onset of disease and again about 4 weeks later. Measurement of neutralizing titers is the most accurate method for antibody determination; measurement of complement-fixation titers is usually less sensitive. Titers of virus-specific IgM are elevated in both acute and chronic infection.

℞ TREATMENT

Most enterovirus infections are mild and resolve spontaneously; however, intensive supportive care may be needed for cardiac, hepatic, or CNS disease. Intravenous, intrathecal, or intraventricular immunoglobulin has been used with apparent success for the treatment of chronic enterovirus meningoencephalitis and dermatomyositis in patients with hypo- or agammaglobulinemia. The disease may stabilize or resolve during therapy; however, some patients decline inexorably despite therapy. Intravenous administration of immunoglobulin with high titers of antibody to the infecting virus has been used in the treatment of some cases of life-threatening infection in neonates, who may not have maternally acquired antibody. In one trial involving neonates with enterovirus infections, immunoglobulin containing very high titers of antibody to the infecting virus reduced rates of viremia; however, the study was too small to show a substantial clinical benefit. The level of enteroviral antibodies varies with the immunoglobulin preparation. Oral pleconaril, which binds to the enterovirus capsid, reduced symptoms in a placebo-controlled trial of enteroviral aseptic meningitis. In a review of compassionate-release pleconaril therapy in patients with potentially life-threatening enteroviral infections, ~75% of persons were judged to have a clinical response associated with therapy. These individuals included patients with chronic enteroviral meningoencephalitis, neonatal sepsis, myocarditis, and vaccine-associated paralytic poliomyelitis. Further study is needed to confirm these findings; pleconaril is available on a compassionate-use basis for patients with severe enteroviral infections. Glucocorticoids are contraindicated.

Good hand-washing practices and the use of gowns and gloves are important in limiting nosocomial transmission of enteroviruses during epidemics. Enteric precautions are indicated for 7 days after the onset of enterovirus infections.

PREVENTION AND ERADICATION OF POLIOVIRUS (See also Chap. 107)   After a peak of 57,879 cases of poliomyelitis in the United States in 1952, the introduction of inactivated vaccine in 1955 and of oral vaccine in 1961 ultimately eradicated disease due to wild-type poliovirus in the Western Hemisphere. Such disease has not been documented in the United States since 1979, when cases occurred among religious groups who had declined immunization. In the Western Hemisphere, paralysis due to wild-type poliovirus was last documented in 1991.

In 1988, the World Health Organization adopted a resolution to eradicate poliomyelitis by the year 2000. From 1988 to 2001, the number of cases worldwide decreased by >99%, with fewer than 1000 confirmed cases reported in 2001. In 2002, however, there were ~1900 cases of polio, with ~1500 reported in India. Wild-type poliovirus type 2 has not been detected in the world since 1999. The Americas were certified free of indigenous wild-type poliovirus transmission in 1994, the Western Pacific Region in 2000, and the European Region in 2002. In 2001, there were only 11 countries in which indigenous wild-type poliovirus was still being transmitted (Table 175-3). Polio is a source of concern for unimmunized or partially immunized travelers to these regions. Outbreaks of polio in Europe and North America have been traced to cases imported from the Indian subcontinent. Clearly, global eradication of polio is necessary to eliminate the risk of importation of wild-type virus. Outbreaks are thought to have been facilitated by suboptimal rates of vaccination, isolated pockets of unvaccinated children, poor sanitation and crowding, improper vaccine-storage conditions, and a reduced level of response to one of the serotypes in the vaccine.

TABLE 175-3   *Laboratory-Confirmed Cases of Poliomyelitis in Countries Where Wild-Type Poliovirus Was Endemic in 2001*

Country	Virus-Confirmed Cases in 2001
India	268
Pakistan	119
Nigeria	56
Afghanistan	11
Somalia	7
Niger	6
Egypt	5
Angola, Ethiopia, Sudan, Mauritania	1 case each
Total	476

Source: World Health Organization.

Outbreaks of poliomyelitis due to circulating vaccine-derived poliovirus have recently occurred. In the Dominican Republic and Haiti, 21 cases of vaccine-derived polio occurred in 2000 and 2001; 32 cases occurred in Egypt from 1988 to 1993, and 3 cases occurred in the Philippines in 2001. These OPV-derived viruses reverted to a more neurovirulent phenotype after undetected circulation (probably for >2 years). The epidemic in Hispaniola was rapidly terminated after intensive vaccination with OPV. These outbreaks emphasize the need for maintaining high levels of vaccine coverage and continued surveillance for circulating virus.

IPV is used in most industrialized countries and OPV in most developing countries, including those in which polio still is or recently was endemic. After several doses of OPV alone, the seropositivity rate for individual poliovirus serotypes may still be suboptimal for children in developing countries; one or more supplemental doses of IPV can increase the rate of seropositivity for these serotypes. While intramuscular injections of other vaccines (live or attenuated) can be given concurrently with OPV, unnecessary intramuscular injections should be avoided during the first month after vaccination because they increase the risk of vaccine-associated paralysis. Since 1988, an enhanced-potency inactivated poliovirus vaccine has been available in the United States.

OPV and IPV induce antibodies that persist for at least 5 years. Both vaccines induce IgG and IgA antibodies. Compared with recipients of IPV, recipients of OPV shed less virus and less frequently develop reinfection with wild-type virus after exposure to poliovirus. Although IPV is safe and efficacious, OPV offers the advantages of ease of administration, lower cost, and induction of intestinal immunity resulting in a reduction in the risk of community transmission of wild-type virus. Because of progress toward global eradication of polio (with a reduced risk of imported cases) and the continued occurrence of cases of vaccine-associated polio, an all-IPV regimen was recommended in 2000 for childhood poliovirus vaccination in the United States, with vaccine administration at 2, 4, and 6 to 18 months and 4 to 6 years of age. OPV will be used only in special circumstances: (1) for mass immunization campaigns to control outbreaks of polio; (2) for vaccination of unimmunized children who will be traveling to a polio-endemic area within 4 weeks; and (3) for children whose parents do not accept an all-IPV regimen. The latter children should receive at least two doses of IPV before receiving OPV. The risk of vaccine-associated polio should be discussed before administering OPV. Recommendations for vaccination of adults are listed in Table 175-4.

While it is hoped that endemic spread of poliovirus may be eliminated during the first decade of the 21st century, there are concerns about stopping vaccination. These include the observations that poliovirus is shed from some immunocompromised persons for several years, that vaccine-derived poliovirus can circulate and cause disease, and that wild-type poliovirus is present in a large number of laboratories. A national survey began in October 2002 to encourage laboratories to dispose of all unneeded wild-type poliovirus materials and to identify laboratories that have wild-type poliovirus or specimens (e.g., feces) that may contain the virus.

TABLE 175-4 *Recommendations for Poliovirus Vaccination of Adults*

1. Routine primary poliovirus vaccination is not indicated for unvaccinated adults residing in the United States, except for:
   a. travelers to areas where poliovirus is or may be epidemic or endemic;
   b. members of communities or population groups with disease caused by wild-type polioviruses;
   c. laboratory workers handling specimens that may contain wild-type polioviruses;
   d. health care workers in close contact with patients who may be excreting wild-type polioviruses.
2. Three doses of IPV are recommended for adults who need to be immunized. The second dose should be given 1 to 2 months after the first dose; the third dose should be given 6 to 12 months after the second dose.
3. Adults who are at increased risk of exposure to wild-type poliovirus and who have previously completed primary immunization should receive a single dose of IPV.

Abbreviation: IPV, inactivated poliovirus vaccine.
Source. Modified from 2000 Redbook, Report of the Committee on Infectious Diseases.

REOVIRUSES

Reoviruses are double-stranded RNA viruses encompassing three serotypes. Serologic studies indicate that most humans are infected with reoviruses during childhood; however, it has been difficult to establish a definite link of reovirus infection with a particular disease. It is likely that most infections either are asymptomatic or cause very mild disease. One outbreak of reovirus infection in children resulted in minor upper respiratory tract symptoms. Reovirus is considered a rare cause of mild gastroenteritis in infants and children. Speculation regarding an association of reovirus type 3 with idiopathic neonatal hepatitis and extrahepatic biliary atresia is based on an elevated prevalence of antibody to reovirus among some of these patients, detection of viral RNA by PCR in hepatobiliary tissues in some studies, and detection of virus in the porta hepatis in one case.

FURTHER READING

CENTERS FOR DISEASE CONTROL AND PREVENTION: Enterovirus surveillance—United States, 2000–2001. MMWR 51:1047, 2002
———: Progress toward global eradication of poliomyelitis, 2001. MMWR 51:253, 2002
HENDERSON DA: Countering the posteradication threat of smallpox and polio. Clin Infect Dis 34:79, 2002
HO M et al: An epidemic of enterovirus 71 infection in Taiwan. N Engl J Med 341:929, 1999
JUBELT B, AGRE JC: Characteristics and management of postpolio syndrome. JAMA 284:412, 2000
KEW O et al: Outbreak of poliomyelitis in Hispaniola associated with circulating type 1 vaccine-derived poliovirus. Science 296:356, 2002
ROTBART HA et al: Treatment of potentially life-threatening enterovirus infections with pleconaril. Clin Infect Dis 32:28, 2001

---

176 MEASLES (RUBEOLA)
Anne Gershon

DEFINITION   Measles (rubeola) is a highly contagious, acute, exanthematous respiratory disease with a characteristic clinical picture and a pathognomonic enanthem: Koplik's spots, an eruption on the buccal mucous membranes (Fig. 176-1). A successful live attenuated measles vaccine became available in 1963 in the United States and elsewhere, and measles is now an unusual disease in most developed countries where this vaccine is widely used. However, measles continues to occur sporadically in miniepidemics in the United States, and major epidemics in developing nations make this disease a persistent cause of childhood morbidity and mortality.

ETIOLOGIC AGENT   Measles virus is the only member of the genus *Morbillivirus* that infects humans. Part of the family Paramyxoviridae, it is closely related to the viruses causing canine and porcine distemper, rinderpest of cattle, morbilli of certain aquatic mammals, and *peste des petits ruminants* of goats and sheep. There is only one antigenic type. Measles virions are pleomorphic spherical structures having a diameter of 100 to 250 nm and consisting of six proteins. The inner capsid is composed of a coiled helix of RNA and three proteins, and the outer envelope consists of a matrix protein bearing two types of short surface-glycoprotein projections or peplomers. One peplomer is a conical hemagglutinin (H) and the other a dumbbell-shaped fusion (F) protein. Sequencing of the single-stranded genome has made it possible to distinguish vaccine-type measles virus from the wild type. The genetic variability of wild-type measles virus permits the identification of strains that are endemic within a given locale where measles cases have occurred. In all, 20 genotypes have been identified. The cellular receptors for measles virus are the CD46 and CD150 molecules expressed on human lymphocytes and many other human cell types.

EPIDEMIOLOGY   Measles has a worldwide distribution; humans are the only natural hosts, although other primates can be experimentally infected. During the prevaccination era in the United States, measles epidemics occurred every 2 to 5 years in the winter and spring. In an epidemic year, roughly half a million measles cases were reported; 99% of adults had serologic evidence of previous measles infection.

FIGURE 176-1   Koplik's spots, which manifest as white or bluish lesions with an erythematous halo on the buccal mucosa, usually occur in the first 2 days of measles symptoms and may briefly overlap the measles exanthem. The presence of the erythematous halo differentiates Koplik's spots from Fordyce's spots (ectopic sebaceous glands), which occur in the mouths of healthy individuals. *(Source: CDC. Photo selected by Dr. Kenneth Kaye.)*

After the live attenuated vaccine became available, the number of cases reported to the Centers for Disease Control and Prevention (CDC) fell, with a nadir of 1497 cases in 1983. After an upsurge to more than 27,000 cases (with 89 deaths) in 1990, the disease was once more brought under control, in part through the routine administration of two doses of vaccine. The foremost reason for the resurgence of measles was failure to immunize infants and young children, especially in inner-city areas. Primary vaccine failure (documented in about 5% of individuals) and secondary vaccine failure or waning immunity accounted for some cases.

In recent years, the majority of cases of measles have involved preschool children. Between 1993 and 1996, fewer than 1000 cases were reported annually in the United States; 309 cases were reported in 1995 and 116 cases in 2001. Molecular studies indicated interruption of transmission of indigenous measles in 1993. Most cases have since resulted from international importations of the virus. Mortality is highest among children under 2 years of age and among adults. Patients with impaired cell-mediated immunity are at especially high risk for severe or even fatal measles. The measles-associated mortality rate in the United States is about 0.3%; in developing countries, mortality frequently exceeds 1% and sometimes approaches 10%.

Measles virus is transmitted by respiratory secretions, predominantly through exposure to aerosols but also through direct contact with larger droplets. Patients are contagious from 1 or 2 days before the onset of symptoms until 4 days after the appearance of the rash. Infectivity peaks during the prodromal phase. The mean intervals from infection to onset of symptoms and to appearance of rash are 10 and 14 days, respectively.

PATHOGENESIS, IMMUNITY, AND PATHOLOGY Measles virus invades the respiratory epithelium and spreads via the bloodstream to the reticuloendothelial system, from which it infects all types of white blood cells, thereby establishing infection of the skin, respiratory tract, and other organs. Both viremia and viruria develop. Multinucleated giant cells with inclusion bodies in the nucleus and cytoplasm (Warthin-Finkeldey cells) are found in respiratory and lymphoid tissues and are pathognomonic for measles. Direct invasion of T lymphocytes and increased levels of suppressive cytokines, such as interleukin 4, may play a role in the temporary depression of cellular immunity that accompanies and transiently follows measles. The major infected cell in the blood is the monocyte. Infection of the entire respiratory tract accounts for the characteristic cough and coryza of measles and for the less frequent manifestations of croup, bronchiolitis, and pneumonia. Generalized damage to the respiratory tract, with resultant loss of cilia, predisposes to secondary bacterial infections such as pneumonia and otitis media.

Specific antibodies are not detectable before the onset of rash. Cellular immunity (consisting of cytotoxic T cells and possibly natural killer cells) plays a prominent role in host defense, and patients who are deficient in cellular immunity are at high risk for severe measles. Children with isolated agammaglobulinemia are not at increased risk. Immune reactions to the virus in the endothelial cells of dermal capillaries play a substantial role in the development of Koplik's spots (the pathognomonic enanthem) as well as in that of rash; in immunodeficient hosts, measles may be severe despite the absence of these manifestations. Measles antigens have been demonstrated in involved skin during early stages of the illness.

Pathologic changes in measles encephalitis include focal hemorrhage, congestion, and perivascular demyelination. Measles virus is rarely isolated from cerebrospinal fluid (CSF) in cases of encephalitis, which are thought to be due to the interaction of virus-infected cells with local cellular immune factors.

CLINICAL MANIFESTATIONS Measles begins with a 2- to 4-day respiratory prodrome of malaise, cough, coryza, conjunctivitis with lacrimation, nasal discharge, and increasing fever [with temperatures as high as 40.6°C (105°F), probably reflecting secondary viremia]. At this stage of the illness, in which the rash has not yet developed, influenza may be suspected. Just before the onset of the rash, Koplik's spots appear as 1- to 2-mm blue-white spots on a bright red background (Fig. 176-1). Without adequate illumination for examination, they may be overlooked. Koplik's spots are typically located on the buccal mucosa alongside the second molars and may be extensive; they are not associated with any other infectious disease. The spots wane after the onset of rash and soon disappear. The entire buccal and inner labial mucosa may be inflamed, and the lips may be reddened.

The characteristic erythematous, nonpruritic, maculopapular rash of measles begins at the hairline and behind the ears, spreads down the trunk and limbs to include the palms and soles, and often becomes confluent (Fig. 176-2). At this time, the patient is at the most severe point of the illness. By the fourth day, the rash begins to fade in the order in which it appeared. Brownish discoloration of the skin and

FIGURE 176-2 In measles, discrete erythematous lesions become confluent as the rash spreads downward. (Reprinted with permission from Fitzpatrick TB et al: Color Atlas & Synopsis of Clinical Dermatology, 4th ed. New York, McGraw-Hill, 2001, p 775.)

desquamation may occur later. Fever usually resolves by the fourth or fifth day after the onset of rash; prolonged fever suggests a complication of measles. Lymphadenopathy, diarrhea, vomiting, and splenomegaly are common features. The chest x-ray may be abnormal, even in uncomplicated measles, because of the propensity of this virus to invade the respiratory tract. The entire illness usually lasts about 10 days. The disease tends to be more severe in adults than in children, with higher fever, more prominent rash, and a higher incidence of complications.

Milder forms of the illness with less intense symptoms and a milder rash, termed *modified measles*, may occur in individuals with preexisting partial immunity induced by active or passive vaccination. These patients include infants under 1 year of age who retain some proportion of passively acquired maternal antibodies. On occasion, individuals with a history of immunization may develop modified measles.

COMPLICATIONS The complications of measles (Table 176-1) can conveniently be divided into three groups, according to the site involved: the respiratory tract, the central nervous system (CNS), and the gastrointestinal tract. Respiratory tract involvement, manifested as laryngitis, croup, or bronchitis, occurs in the majority of cases of uncomplicated measles. In young children, otitis media is the most common complication. Pneumonia is a frequent reason for hospitalization, especially of adults. The pneumonia is of viral origin in the majority of cases, but secondary bacterial infection (most commonly caused by streptococci, pneumococci, or staphylococci) also develops with some frequency. Primary giant cell (Hecht's) pneumonia is most often documented in immunocompromised and/or malnourished patients.

Encephalographic abnormalities in the absence of symptoms of CNS disease are extremely frequent in measles. Symptomatic CNS disease may present with fever, headache, drowsiness, coma, and/or seizures. Symptoms usually begin within days after the onset of rash but occasionally appear for the first time several weeks later. About 10% of patients do not survive acute measles encephalitis; a significant percentage of surviving patients develop permanent sequelae, such as mental retardation or epilepsy. Most cases appear to result from an immune-mediated response to myelin proteins (postinfectious encephalomyelitis) and not directly from viral infection of the CNS (Chap. 359). Rarely, transverse myelitis follows measles. Immunocompromised patients are at risk for progressive fatal encephalitis 1 to 6 months after measles; in some cases, even though prior measles has

TABLE 176-1 *Complications of Measles*

Complication	Comments
Otitis media	Very common in infants with measles
Pneumonia	May be primary viral pneumonia or bacterial superinfection; frequent reason for hospitalization of adults; measles rash sometimes lacking in immunocompromised patients with measles pneumonia
Croup	Occasionally severe, requiring intubation in infants
Gastroenteritis	Diarrhea can be life threatening in infants
Cervical adenitis	Due to lymphoid hyperplasia as host response to virus; common
Acute encephalitis	May be mild to severe/fatal; occurs in 1 in 1000 cases of measles; cerebral and cerebellar forms; immune-mediated pathogenesis
Subacute sclerosing panencephalitis (SSPE)	In 1 in 100,000 cases of measles, usually when measles occurred in infancy; seen 5–10 years later. In United States, most children with SSPE were born in another country where measles vaccine is not routinely used.

not been recognized, the virus is identified at autopsy. Subacute sclerosing panencephalitis (SSPE)—a protracted, chronic, extremely rare form of measles encephalitis—sometimes follows measles and is particularly common among children who have measles before the age of 2 years (Chap. 360). SSPE has virtually disappeared in the United States as a result of widespread vaccination. Typically, progressive dementia evolves over several months. SSPE is thought to be due to a complex interaction of the host with defective measles virus. It is associated with extremely high levels of antibodies to measles virus in the blood and CSF.

Gastrointestinal complications of measles include gastroenteritis, hepatitis, appendicitis, ileocolitis, and mesenteric adenitis. It is not uncommon to detect high levels of alanine and aspartate aminotransferases in the absence of gastrointestinal signs such as jaundice.

Other, rare complications include myocarditis, glomerulonephritis, and postinfectious thrombocytopenic purpura. Measles can exacerbate preexisting tuberculosis, presumably through depression of cellular immunity induced by the virus. Natural measles and immunization against measles can result in tuberculin skin-test anergy lasting for about 1 month.

ATYPICAL MEASLES An atypical form of measles has been reported in individuals who received formalin-inactivated measles vaccine (used in the United States from 1963 through 1967 and in Canada until 1970) and subsequently were exposed to measles virus. After a several-day prodrome of fever, myalgia, and headache, the rash appears (Fig. 176-3). Unlike the rash of typical measles, that of atypical measles begins peripherally and moves centrally; it can be urticarial, maculopapular, hemorrhagic, and/or vesicular. Fever is usually high and is accompanied by edema of the extremities, interstitial pulmonary infiltrates, hepatitis, and (on occasion) pleural effusion. The differential diagnosis often includes Rocky Mountain spotted fever, Henoch-Schönlein purpura, meningococcemia, drug allergy, toxic shock syndrome, and varicella. Despite the severity of atypical measles, patients invariably recover after a convalescence that may be prolonged. Measles virus is not isolated from these patients, and they do not spread the virus to others. This disease is believed to be due to hypersensitivity to measles virus induced by the inactivated vaccine. Formalin inactivation destroys the antigenicity of the F protein, antibodies to which are important in preventing spread of the virus from one cell to another. The role of cellular immunity in this process is unknown. Extremely high convalescent titers of antibody to measles virus (e.g., 1:1,000,000) are diagnostic of atypical measles. To prevent this syndrome, adults who

received formalin-inactivated measles vaccine should be reimmunized with at least one dose of live attenuated measles vaccine. Because inactivated measles vaccine has not been available for more than 25 years, atypical measles has now virtually disappeared.

MEASLES IN THE IMMUNOCOMPROMISED HOST Patients with defects in cell-mediated immunity are at risk for severe protracted and fatal measles. Included in this category are patients with congenital cellular immune defects or malignancy, recipients of immunosuppressive therapy, or persons infected with HIV. In these patients, measles may not be accompanied by a rash. Complications are primary measles (giant cell) pneumonia, progressive encephalitis beginning weeks to months after initial infection, and (in HIV-infected patients) progression to AIDS.

MEASLES IN ADULTS Measles is naturally a disease of childhood and, like many other viral infections, is more severe in adults than in children. About 3% of young adults with measles develop primary viral pneumonia and require hospitalization. Hepatitis and bronchospasm are more common among adults with measles than among children, and the rash is more severe and more confluent in adults. Bacterial superinfection is more common among adults, more than one-third of whom develop respiratory complications such as otitis media, sinusitis, and pneumonia. Adults may develop measles because they were never immunized or (more rarely) because their vaccine-induced immunity has waned. Very low titers of antibody to measles virus have been associated with lack of protection.

LABORATORY FINDINGS Lymphopenia and neutropenia are common in measles and may be due to invasion of leukocytes by the virus, with subsequent cell death. Leukocytosis may herald a bacterial superinfection. Patients with measles encephalitis usually have an elevated protein concentration in CSF as well as lymphocytosis.

DIAGNOSIS A specific diagnosis of measles can be made quickly by immunofluorescent staining of a smear of respiratory secretions for measles antigen; monoclonal antibodies conjugated to fluorescein are commercially available for this purpose. Secretions can also be examined microscopically for multinucleated giant cells. Measles virus can be isolated from respiratory secretions or urine and rapidly identified in tissue culture with fluorescein-labeled monoclonal antibodies. The presence of measles virus RNA has been demonstrated by diagnostic reverse-transcription polymerase chain reaction. A number of serologic tests are available for the diagnosis of measles; however, a serologic diagnosis cannot necessarily be made quickly because both acute- and convalescent-phase sera are usually tested, ideally at the same time. The older hemagglutination inhibition test has been re-

FIGURE 176-3 Petechial lesions in a patient with atypical measles. *(Photo courtesy of Stephen E. Gellis, MD.)*

placed by enzyme immunoassay (EIA), which is more sensitive and simpler to perform. EIA can be used to measure specific IgM and thus to diagnose measles on the basis of an acute-phase serum sample alone. Specific IgM antibodies are detectable within 1 to 2 days after the appearance of rash, and the IgG titer rises significantly after 10 days. As already mentioned, atypical measles and SSPE are associated with extremely high titers of antibody.

DIFFERENTIAL DIAGNOSIS Classic measles—with Koplik's spots, cough, coryza, conjunctivitis, and a rash beginning on the head—is easily diagnosed on clinical grounds. Modified measles is more difficult to diagnose clinically because one or more characteristic signs may be lacking. The differential diagnosis of measles includes Kawasaki disease, scarlet fever, infectious mononucleosis, toxoplasmosis, drug eruption, and *Mycoplasma pneumoniae* infection. Most of these conditions can be identified by either culture or serologic assay. In the differential diagnosis of measles, attention should be paid to the current epidemiology of the disease in the community and to the patient's history of measles vaccination and foreign travel.

PREVENTION The development of live attenuated measles vaccine by Enders and colleagues was a milestone in American medicine. This vaccine, used in the United States for the routine immunization of children since 1963, induces seroconversion in about 95% of recipients and probably confers lifelong protection. Waning immunity to measles after immunization has been documented only on rare occasions. For the past three decades, measles vaccine has been available as the combination vaccine measles-mumps-rubella (MMR); MMR vaccine should be administered to children between the ages of 12 and 15 months. (Vaccination at 12 months is preferred for infants whose mothers were immunized against measles in childhood. These mothers have lower antibody titers than women who have had natural measles, and their infants correspondingly have transplacental antibodies of lower titer and shorter duration.) A second dose of MMR vaccine is recommended for school-age children at 4 to 12 years of age. This two-dose policy was developed in the late 1980s in response to measles outbreaks in the United States. Since the institution of the two-dose regimen and the increased effort to immunize all children, measles has again become an unusual disease in the United States. Regional guidelines that reflect the current local epidemiology of measles should be followed.

Older susceptible persons should also be immunized. Individuals should be considered susceptible to measles unless they have documentation of physician-diagnosed measles or of the receipt of two doses of vaccine, have laboratory evidence of measles immunity, or were born before 1957. Rarely, individuals born before 1957 develop measles, and those who are at risk of exposure to measles (e.g., health care workers, teachers, and international travelers) should be tested for measles antibody and immunized if necessary. Approximately 10% of healthy vaccinees develop a fever, with temperatures up to 39.4°C (103°F), 5 to 7 days after vaccination; this fever lasts 1 to 5 days and is accompanied by a transient rash. Individuals previously immunized only with killed vaccine are considered susceptible and should receive at least one dose—preferably two doses—of MMR vaccine. Transient adverse reactions in these individuals include fever, malaise, and redness and swelling at the injection site.

Because of the severity of measles in this group and the lack of reported problems following vaccination, children with asymptomatic HIV infection should receive MMR vaccine; those with severe immunosuppression (<15% CD4 lymphocytes) should not. A case of fatal measles due to vaccine-type virus was reported in a college student with AIDS. Measles vaccine is contraindicated for persons with impaired cell-mediated immunity, for pregnant women, and for persons with a history of anaphylaxis due to egg protein or neomycin. Minor illnesses, with or without fever and a history of convulsions, are not contraindications to vaccination. Vaccination should be deferred for 6 to 11 months after the receipt of immune globulin or of blood products containing antibodies and for at least 3 months after the discontinuation of immunosuppressive treatment. Vaccine failures

have been ascribed to faulty storage of the preparation used, immunization of infants with preexisting (maternally derived) antibodies, and simultaneous administration of measles vaccine and immune globulin.

The only temporally related apparent complications of measles vaccination that are thought to be causal are febrile seizures, which rarely have long-term sequelae; thrombocytopenia, which is self-limited; and anaphylaxis, which is very rare. An exhaustive analysis conducted in 2000 by a number of official committees, including those of the American Academy of Pediatrics and the Institute of Medicine, found no causal relationship between MMR vaccination and development of autism.

Children and adults who are susceptible to measles and are exposed to the disease should receive postexposure prophylaxis. Standard immune globulin, given intramuscularly within 6 days of exposure, can exert a protective or modifying effect; the earlier it is given, the better the outcome. The dose is 0.25 mL/kg for healthy persons and 0.5 mL/kg for immunocompromised persons, with a maximum dose of 15 mL. Immune globulin is particularly strongly indicated for susceptible household contacts, especially those <1 year of age, and for immunocompromised persons. HIV-infected persons, particularly those with severe immunosuppression, should be given immune globulin after exposure, regardless of their measles immune status and whether or not they are receiving intravenous immune globulin. Vaccination within 72 h of exposure may also provide protection against clinical measles, but this strategy is contraindicated as postexposure prophylaxis for immunocompromised individuals. Vaccine and immune globulin should not be given concurrently.

℞ TREATMENT

Therapy for measles is largely supportive and symptom based. Patients with otitis media and pneumonia should be given standard antibiotics. Patients with encephalitis need supportive care, including observation for increased intracranial pressure. Controlled trials suggest clinical benefit from high doses of vitamin A in severe or potentially severe measles, especially in children under the age of 2 years who are or may be malnourished. On the basis of limited data, a dose of 50,000 IU is used for infants 1 to 6 months old; a dose of 100,000 IU is recommended for infants 7 to 12 months old; and a dose of 200,000 IU is recommended for children >1 year old. A single dose is administered on two consecutive days. In the United States, vitamin A treatment is recommended for young children hospitalized for measles and for pediatric measles patients with immunodeficiency, clinical evidence of vitamin A deficiency, impaired intestinal absorption, moderate to severe malnutrition, or recent immigration from an area where there is high mortality from measles. Transient vomiting and headache may be associated with the administration of vitamin A. Ribavirin is effective against measles virus in vitro and may be considered for use in immunocompromised individuals.

FURTHER READING

CENTERS FOR DISEASE CONTROL AND PREVENTION: Measles, mumps, and rubella—vaccine use and strategies for elimination of measles, rubella, and congenital rubella syndrome and control of mumps. MMWR 47:1, 1998

D'SOUZA RM, D'SOUZA R: Vitamin A for preventing secondary infections in children with measles—a systematic review. J Trop Pediatr 48:72, 2002

FOMBONE E et al: No evidence for a new variant of MMR-induced autism. Pediatrics 108:E58, 2001

FORNI AL et al: Severe measles pneumonitis in adults: Evaluation of clinical characteristics and therapy with intravenous ribavirin. Clin Infect Dis 19:454, 1994

KAPLAN LJ et al: Severe measles in immunocompromised patients. JAMA 267:1237, 1992

PELTOLA H et al: The elimination of indigenous measles, mumps, and rubella from Finland by a 12-year, two-dose vaccination program. N Engl J Med 331:1397, 1994

STALKUP JR: A review of measles virus. Dermatol Clin 20:209, 2002

DEFINITION Rubella is an acute viral infection of children and adults that characteristically includes rash, fever, and lymphadenopathy and has a broad spectrum of other possible manifestations. However, a high percentage of rubella infections in both children and adults are subclinical. In addition, the illness can resemble a mild attack of measles (rubeola) and can cause arthritis, especially in adults. Rubella was formerly known as *German measles* because it was first described clinically as distinct from rubeola in Germany, where it generated much medical interest in the mid-eighteenth and early nineteenth centuries. Rubella during pregnancy can lead to fetal infection, with the production of a significant constellation of malformations (*congenital rubella syndrome*) in a high proportion of infected fetuses. Rubella virus was first isolated in cell culture just before the last pandemic of the disease began in 1962. Since the licensing of rubella vaccine in the United States in 1969, there have been no further epidemics in this country.

ETIOLOGIC AGENT Rubella virus, a togavirus, is the only member of the *Rubivirus* genus and is closely related to the alphaviruses. Unlike these agents, however, it does not require a vector for transmission. Moreover, there is no RNA sequence homology between rubella virus and the alphaviruses.

The rubella virion is composed of an inner icosahedral capsid of RNA and protein that is surrounded by a lipid-containing envelope with glycoprotein spikes and a diameter of about 60 nm. The structural proteins associated with rubella virus are E1 and E2 (transmembrane envelope glycoproteins) and C (the capsid protein that surrounds the viral RNA). Only one serotype has been identified.

EPIDEMIOLOGY In the United States during the prevaccine era, rubella was most common in the spring and most often affected school-age children; only 80 to 90% of adults were immune; and major epidemics occurred every 6 to 9 years. The most recent epidemic in the United States occurred in 1964 to 1965, when more than 12 million cases of postnatal rubella and more than 20,000 cases of the congenital rubella syndrome were reported. Although there have been no epidemics since the introduction of live attenuated rubella vaccine in 1969, limited outbreaks have been reported in settings where susceptible individuals come into close contact with one another (e.g., schools and workplaces). In 2001, only 23 cases of postnatally acquired rubella—most of them in young adults—and 3 confirmed cases of congenital rubella syndrome were reported to the Centers for Disease Control and Prevention (CDC).

Whether symptomatic or subclinical, rubella is contagious, albeit less so than measles. Its incubation period is 18 days on average, with a range of 12 to 23 days. The virus, which is spread in droplets shed in respiratory secretions, infects the respiratory tract and then the bloodstream. In postnatally acquired infections, rubella virus is shed during the prodromal phase of the illness, and shedding from the pharynx can continue for about a week after onset. Despite high titers of specific neutralizing antibodies, infants with congenital rubella may excrete rubella virus from the respiratory tract and in the urine until the age of 2 years. This excretion raises important issues related to infection control in hospital and day-care settings. Persons recently immunized with live attenuated rubella vaccine do not transmit the vaccine virus to others, although low titers of rubella virus may be detected transiently in the pharynx.

After an attack of rubella, specific antibodies and cell-mediated immunity develop and probably play a significant role in protection against future disease. Asymptomatic reinfection at the level of the respiratory tract is common upon re-exposure to the virus but is rarely, if ever, associated with viremia.

Rubella virus has been cultured from respiratory secretions during reinfection. Fetal infection may occur during maternal reinfection but is acknowledged to be extremely rare because of the absence of maternal viremia under these circumstances. Viremia following reinfection of individuals immunized against rubella is also rare. Thus the current level of congenital rubella in the United States is exceedingly low. Recently, however, it has been observed that young immigrants to the United States from countries in Latin America and the Caribbean, where rubella vaccine is not routinely given to children, are at increased risk for rubella susceptibility. Because infants with the congenital rubella syndrome have been born to immigrant Hispanic women, increasing efforts are being made to identify and vaccinate such women before they become pregnant.

PATHOGENESIS AND PATHOLOGY Little is known about the microscopic pathology of postnatally acquired rubella because the disease is invariably self-limited. Like that of measles, the rash of rubella is immunologically mediated; its onset coincides with the development of specific antibodies. Viremia can be demonstrated for about a week before and ends within a few days after the onset of rash.

The cause of the damage to cells and organs in congenital rubella is not well understood. Proposed mechanisms of fetal damage include mitotic arrest of cells, tissue necrosis without inflammation, and chromosomal damage. The growth of the fetus may be retarded. Other findings may include decreased numbers of megakaryocytes in the bone marrow, extramedullary hematopoiesis, and interstitial pneumonia.

CLINICAL MANIFESTATIONS ■ Postnatally Acquired Rubella Infection acquired after birth usually results in an extremely mild or subclinical illness. A prodromal phase is uncommon in children; adults may have more severe disease, with a brief prodrome of malaise, fever, and anorexia. The foremost symptoms of postnatally acquired rubella include posterior auricular, cervical, and suboccipital lymphadenopathy; fever; and rash. The rash often begins on the face (Fig. 177-1) and spreads down the body. It is maculopapular but not confluent, is sometimes accompanied by mild coryza and conjunctivitis, and generally lasts for 3 to 5 days. A petechial enanthem on the soft palate, designated *Forschheimer spots*, may occur but is not specific for rubella. Fever may be absent entirely or may be present for only several days in the early phase of the illness.

Complications of postnatally acquired rubella are uncommon; bacterial superinfection is rare. One particularly troublesome complication

FIGURE 177-1 In rubella, an erythematous exanthem spreads from the hairline downward and clears as it spreads. (*Photo courtesy of Stephen E. Gellis, MD.*)

is seen almost exclusively in women: arthritis, most frequently involving the fingers, wrists, and/or knees. Arthritis develops as the rash is appearing and may take several weeks to resolve. Chronic arthritis resulting from rubella is extremely rare. Rubella virus has been isolated from joint fluid during acute rubella arthritis and from peripheral blood in chronic rubella arthritis.

Another complication of postnatally acquired rubella is hemorrhage due to both thrombocytopenia and vascular damage; this complication occurs in 1 of every 3000 patients. Thrombocytopenia may last for weeks or months; it can have long-term consequences if there is bleeding into organs such as the eye or the brain.

Both children and adults may develop encephalitis after rubella; the incidence is about five times lower than that of encephalitis following measles. Adults are more likely than children to develop encephalitis; the mortality rate from this complication is 20 to 50%. Mild hepatitis is an unusual complication. Immunosuppressed patients are not at increased risk for rubella as they are for measles.

Congenital Rubella   Maternal infection in early pregnancy can lead to fetal infection, with resultant congenital rubella. The classic signs of congenital rubella are cataract, heart disease, deafness, and myriad other defects (Table 177-1). The most important factor in the pathogenicity of rubella virus for the fetus is gestational age at the time of infection. Maternal infection during the first trimester leads to fetal infection in about 50% of cases; maternal infection early in the second trimester leads to fetal infection in about one-third of cases. Fetal malformations not only are more common after maternal infection in the first trimester but also tend to be more severe and to involve more organ systems. Whereas a fetus infected in the fourth week of gestation may develop many problems, one infected later (e.g., in the twentieth week) may have isolated deafness as the only symptom.

DIAGNOSIS   Because postnatally acquired rubella is often a mild disease and because many cases are subclinical, diagnosis on clinical grounds can be difficult. Other diseases that may mimic rubella include toxoplasmosis, scarlet fever, modified measles, roseola, fifth disease (erythema infectiosum due to parvovirus B19), and enteroviral infection. Routine laboratory tests usually reveal leukopenia and atypical lymphocytes.

The isolation of rubella virus in cell cultures of throat samples, urine, or other secretions is difficult and expensive but is sometimes undertaken. This technique is most useful when congenital rubella is suspected. A laboratory diagnosis is more often made serologically. The most commonly used test is an enzyme-linked immunosorbent assay (ELISA) for IgG and IgM antibodies. Acute rubella is diagnosed by the documentation of a fourfold or greater rise in the titer of IgG antibodies in paired acute- and convalescent-phase serum specimens or by the detection of rubella-specific IgM antibodies in one serum specimen. However, false-negative and false-positive IgM reactions are sometimes obtained. Moreover, true-positive IgM reactions can occur in both primary infection and reinfection. Congenital rubella is diagnosed by the isolation of rubella virus, the detection of IgM antibodies in a single serum sample, and/or the documentation of either the persistence of rubella antibodies in serum beyond 1 year of age or a rising antibody titer anytime during infancy in an unvaccinated child. Biopsied tissues and/or blood and cerebrospinal fluid have also been used for the demonstration of rubella antigens with monoclonal antibodies and for the detection of rubella RNA by in situ hybridization and polymerase chain reaction.

PREVENTION   Live attenuated rubella vaccine was licensed in 1969, 7 years after the virus was first isolated in culture. This vaccine was developed as a strategy to prevent congenital rubella by ensuring that very few pregnant women would be susceptible and that there would be little circulating wild-type virus. Rubella vaccine induces seroconversion in more than 95% of recipients. Since its licensure, there have been no major epidemics in the United States, and the number of cases has declined by 98%. The vaccine currently licensed in the United States, RA 27/3, is propagated in human diploid cells and is more immunogenic (particularly with regard to the stimulation of secretory immunity) than previously licensed vaccines. The present vaccination strategy, developed in part when measles was not being adequately controlled, is to immunize all infants at 12 to 15 months of age with measles-mumps-rubella (MMR) vaccine and to administer a second dose in early childhood. Rubella vaccine may also be administered to anyone who is thought to be susceptible to the infection and is not pregnant; it is particularly important that hospital workers of either sex be immune to rubella so that nosocomial transmission is avoided. Although there has been little change in the prevalence of immunity to rubella among women of childbearing age (about 80%), the incidence of congenital rubella is extremely low—fewer than 10 cases annually. It is likely that, although antibody may be undetectable years after immunization, protection against infection—possibly due to cell-mediated immunity—is the rule. At present, there is little if any evidence of significant waning of clinically important immunity to rubella with time.

On occasion, rubella vaccine may cause arthralgia or arthritis, especially in young women. Very rarely, rubella vaccination results in chronic arthritis; however, even cases of frank arthritis in vaccinees are self-limited, lasting only about 1 week.

After investigation of a series of more than 400 women who were inadvertently immunized during pregnancy and who carried their infants to term, the CDC has concluded that vaccine-type rubella virus either does not cause the congenital rubella syndrome at all or does so at an incidence too low to be detected. Nonetheless, rubella vaccine is contraindicated for use in pregnant women, and it is recommended that pregnancy be avoided for at least 3 months after rubella vaccination. It is acceptable for rubella-susceptible children whose mothers are also susceptible to be immunized, as vaccinated individuals do not shed rubella virus or transmit it to susceptible individuals. Although it is recommended that rubella vaccine not be given to immunosuppressed persons, the vaccine is given to children infected with HIV. No adverse effects of rubella vaccine have been reported in immunocompromised patients.

℞ **TREATMENT**

There is no specific therapy for rubella. At one time, immune globulin was used in an effort to prevent congenital rubella when pregnant women became infected. However, because administration of immune globulin did not prevent maternal viremia, this approach was discarded. Symptom-based treatment is given for manifestations such as fever, arthralgia, and arthritis.

TABLE 177-1 *Clinical Problems Associated with the Congenital Rubella Syndrome*

Transient Signs/Symptoms (at Birth Only)	Permanent Signs/Symptoms (Developmental)
Bony abnormalities	Autism
Cloudy cornea	Behavioral disorders
Hemolytic anemia	Congenital heart disease (patent ductus arteriosus, pulmonic stenosis)
Hepatitis	
Hepatosplenomegaly	Cryptorchidism
Jaundice	Deafness
Low birth weight	Degenerative brain disease
Lymphadenopathy	Diabetes mellitus
Meningoencephalitis	Glaucoma
Rubella viral pneumonia	Inguinal hernia
Thrombocytopenic purpura	Mental retardation
	Microcephaly
	Myopia
	Precocious puberty
	Retinopathy
	Seizures
	Spastic diplegia
	Thyroid disorders

FURTHER READING

CENTERS FOR DISEASE CONTROL AND PREVENTION: Measles, mumps, and rubella—vaccine use and strategies for elimination of measles, rubella, and congenital rubella syndrome and control of mumps. MMWR 47:1, 1998

———: Control and prevention of rubella: Evaluation and management of suspected outbreaks, rubella in pregnant women, and surveillance for congenital rubella syndrome. MMWR 50:1, 2001

DANAVARO-HOLLIDAY MC et al: A large rubella outbreak with spread from the workplace to the community. JAMA 284:2733, 2000

DYKEWICZ C et al: Rubella seropositivity in the United States, 1988–1994. Clin Infect Dis 233:1279, 2001

MELLINGER AK et al: High incidence of congenital rubella syndrome after a rubella outbreak. Pediatr Infect Dis J 14:573, 1995

REEF SE et al: The changing epidemiology of rubella in the 1990s: On the verge of elimination and new challenges for control and prevention. JAMA 287:464, 2002

SHERIDAN E: Congenital rubella syndrome: A risk in immigrant populations. Lancet 359:674, 2002

178   MUMPS
Anne Gershon

DEFINITION   Mumps is an acute, systemic, communicable viral infection whose most distinctive feature is swelling of one or both parotid glands. Involvement of other salivary glands, the meninges, the pancreas, and the gonads is also common.

ETIOLOGIC AGENT   Mumps virus, a paramyxovirus, is pleomorphic and has a diameter ranging from 100 to 300 nm. The virion is composed of RNA and seven proteins. The RNA is surrounded by an envelope with glycoprotein projections. There are two envelope glycoproteins—a hemagglutinin-neuraminidase (HN) and a hemolysis cell fusion antigen (F)—as well as a matrix envelope protein (M). A fourth protein (SH) may also be membrane-associated. There are three internal components: a nucleocapsid protein (NP), a phosphoprotein (P), and a large protein (L). There is only one antigenic type of mumps virus. The polymerase chain reaction (PCR) has detected geographic differences among mumps viruses from different locales.

EPIDEMIOLOGY   After the introduction of mumps vaccine in 1967, the incidence of clinical mumps declined significantly in the United States. In 1968 (before widespread immunization), 185,691 cases of mumps were reported in this country. The 266 cases reported in 2001 represent a reduction in the number of cases by >99% from prevaccine levels; this is the lowest number of cases ever reported in a year. Before widespread vaccination, the incidence of mumps was highest in the winter and spring, with epidemics every 2 to 5 years. At that time, mumps was principally a disease of childhood, although today more than 50% of cases occur in young adults. Epidemics tended to occur in confined populations, such as those in schools and the military services.

The incubation period of mumps generally ranges from 14 to 18 days, with extremes of 7 and 23 days. However, because a contact may be shedding virus before the onset of clinical disease or (like one-third of patients) may have subclinical infection, the incubation period in individual cases is often uncertain. One attack of mumps usually confers lifelong immunity. Long-term immunity is also associated with immunization.

PATHOGENESIS   Mumps virus is transmitted by droplet nuclei, saliva, and fomites. Replication of the virus in the epithelium of the upper respiratory tract leads to viremia, which is followed by infection of glandular tissues and/or the central nervous system (CNS).

Little is known of the pathology of mumps since the disease is rarely fatal. The affected glands contain perivascular and interstitial mononuclear cell infiltrates with prominent edema. Necrosis of acinar and epithelial duct cells is evident in the salivary glands and in the germinal epithelium of the seminiferous tubules.

CLINICAL MANIFESTATIONS   The prodrome of mumps consists of fever, malaise, myalgia, and anorexia. Parotitis, if it develops, usually does so within the next 24 h but may be delayed for as long as a week; it is generally bilateral, although the onset on the two sides may not be synchronous and at times only one side is affected. The submaxillary and sublingual glands are involved less often than the parotid and are almost never involved alone. Swelling of the parotid is accompanied by tenderness and obliteration of the space between the ear lobe and the angle of the mandible. The patient frequently reports an earache and finds it difficult to eat, swallow, or talk. Glandular swelling increases for a few days and then gradually subsides, disappearing within a week. The orifice of Stensen's duct is commonly red and swollen. Presternal pitting edema has been described in about 5% of mumps cases, often in association with submandibular adenitis.

Other than parotitis, orchitis is the most common manifestation of mumps among postpubertal males, developing in about 20% of cases. The testis is painful and tender and is enlarged to several times its normal size; accompanying fever is common. Later, testicular atrophy develops in half of the affected men. Since orchitis is bilateral in fewer than 15% of cases, sterility after mumps is rare. Oophoritis in women—far less common than orchitis in men—may cause lower abdominal pain but does not lead to sterility.

Aseptic meningitis, which may develop before, during, after, or in the absence of parotitis, is a common manifestation of mumps in both children and adults. Symptoms include stiff neck, headache, and drowsiness. Pleocytosis of the cerebrospinal fluid (CSF), with up to 1000 cells/μL, may develop in up to 50% of cases of clinical mumps, but clinical signs of meningeal irritation are documented in only 5 to 25% of cases. Within the first 24 h, polymorphonuclear leukocytes may predominate in CSF, but by the second day nearly all the cells are lymphocytes. The glucose level in CSF may be abnormally low, and this finding may arouse suspicion of bacterial meningitis. Aseptic meningitis due to mumps without parotitis is indistinguishable clinically from that caused by other viruses. Mumps meningitis is almost invariably self-limited, although cranial nerve palsies have occasionally led to permanent sequelae, particularly deafness. More rarely, mumps virus may cause encephalitis, which presents as high fever with marked changes in the level of consciousness and frequently results in permanent sequelae in survivors. Other CNS problems occasionally associated with mumps include cerebellar ataxia, facial palsy, transverse myelitis, Guillain-Barré syndrome, and aqueductal stenosis leading to hydrocephalus.

Mumps pancreatitis, which may present as abdominal pain, is difficult to diagnose because an elevated serum amylase level can be associated with either parotitis or pancreatitis. Other unusual complications of mumps include myocarditis, mastitis, thyroiditis, nephritis, arthritis, and thrombocytopenic purpura. An excessive number of spontaneous abortions are associated with gestational mumps when the disease occurs during the first trimester. Mumps in pregnancy does not lead to premature birth or fetal malformations.

DIFFERENTIAL DIAGNOSIS   The diagnosis of mumps is made easily in patients with acute bilateral parotitis and a history of recent exposure, but mumps is currently a rare disease in the United States due to widespread vaccination. When parotitis is unilateral or absent or when sites other than the parotid gland are involved, laboratory diagnosis may be required. The differential diagnosis of parotitis is presented in Table 178-1.

Other entities should be considered when manifestations consistent with mumps appear in organs other than the parotid. Testicular torsion may produce a painful scrotal mass resembling that seen in mumps

TABLE 178-1 *Differential Diagnosis of Parotitis*

Etiology	Comments
SYSTEMIC INFECTIONS	
Mumps	Rare in countries with vaccination programs
Coxsackievirus infection	Particularly likely in children
HIV infection	In HIV-positive children receiving no antiretroviral therapy; additional disease manifestations likely
Parainfluenza virus type 3 infection	Particularly likely in children, associated with acute respiratory tract symptoms
Influenza A virus infection	Seasonal (winter, spring), associated with acute respiratory tract symptoms
Cat-scratch disease	Unusual but described
Epstein-Barr virus infection	Unusual but described
SYSTEMIC NONINFECTIOUS CAUSES	
Sarcoidosis	Additional manifestations of disease likely
Sjögren's syndrome	Additional manifestations of disease likely
Uremia	Additional manifestations of disease likely
Diabetes mellitus	Additional manifestations of disease likely
Drugs	Phenylbutazone, thiouracil
UNILATERAL PAROTITIS	
Ductal obstruction due to stones or strictures	Unilateral, gradual onset, suppurative
Parotid cyst	Unilateral, gradual onset
Parotid tumor	Unilateral, gradual onset
ACUTE SUPPURATIVE PAROTITIS	
Staphylococcus aureus, *Streptococcus* species, and (rarely) gram-negative bacteria, anaerobes	

orchitis. Other viruses (e.g., enteroviruses) may cause aseptic meningitis that is clinically indistinguishable from that due to mumps virus.

Myocarditis as a severe but usually self-limited complication of mumps has been described. Molecular diagnostic assays have implicated mumps virus in some cases of endocardial fibroelastosis following myocarditis.

LABORATORY DIAGNOSIS Mumps virus is readily isolated after inoculation of appropriate clinical specimens into a variety of host systems, such as rhesus monkey kidney cells and human embryonic lung fibroblasts. The virus can be rapidly identified by inoculation of cells grown in shell vials and subsequent staining with fluorescein-labeled monoclonal antibodies to detect viral growth. Mumps virus may be recovered from saliva, throat, and urine during the first few days of illness and from the CSF of patients with mumps meningitis. Shedding of virus in the urine may persist for as long as 2 weeks. PCR is also used to detect mumps virus in clinical specimens. No particular peripheral blood cell count is characteristic of mumps.

Highly sensitive enzyme-linked immunosorbent assays are useful for serologic diagnosis of mumps and for determination of susceptibility to the disease. Acute mumps can be diagnosed either by the examination of acute- and convalescent-phase sera for a significant increase in IgG antibody titer or by the demonstration of specific IgM in one serum specimen. Use of a skin-test antigen to assess immunity to mumps has been replaced by serologic testing.

PREVENTION Live attenuated mumps vaccine (Jeryl Lynn strain) induces antibodies that protect the recipient against infection in more than 95% of cases. The subcutaneously administered vaccine may be given to children older than 1 year but is not recommended for younger infants because of the potential for interference by passive maternal antibodies. Mumps vaccine is usually administered as part of the measles-mumps-rubella (MMR) vaccine at the age of 12 to 15 months and again at 4 to 12 years of age. This MMR vaccine is also recommended for susceptible older children, adolescents, and adults, particularly adolescent males who have not had mumps. For these patients, either MMR or monovalent mumps vaccine may be given; two doses are preferred. Inadvertent immunization of individuals who are already immune is not associated with significant adverse reactions. Mumps vaccine is not recommended for pregnant women, for patients receiving glucocorticoids, or for other immunocompromised hosts. However, children with HIV infection who are not severely immunocompromised can safely be immunized against mumps; MMR vaccine is usually used for this purpose (Chap. 107). Occasionally, febrile reactions and parotitis have been reported soon after mumps vaccination. Allergic reactions after vaccination, such as rash and pruritus, occur uncommonly and are usually mild and self-limited. In the United States, the incidence of encephalitis during the month after mumps vaccination is no greater than the background incidence rate of encephalitis in the population.

℞ TREATMENT

Therapy for parotitis and other manifestations of mumps is symptom-based. The administration of analgesics and the application of warm or cold compresses to the parotid area may be helpful. Mumps immune globulin is of no value in prophylaxis or treatment of established disease. Testicular pain may be minimized by the local application of cold compresses and gentle support for the scrotum. Anesthetic blocks may also be used. Neither the administration of glucocorticoids nor incision of the tunica albuginea is of proven value for the treatment of severe orchitis. Anecdotal information on a small number of patients with orchitis suggests that administration of interferon α may be helpful.

FURTHER READING

BRISS PA et al: Sustained transmission of mumps in a highly vaccinated population: Assessment of primary vaccine failure and waning vaccine-induced immunity. J Infect Dis 169:77, 1994

CENTERS FOR DISEASE CONTROL AND PREVENTION: Notice to readers: Final 2001 reports of notifiable diseases. MMWR 51:710, 2002

———: Measles, mumps, and rubella—vaccine use and strategies for elimination of measles, rubella, and congenital rubella syndrome and control of mumps. MMWR 47:1, 1998

CHAUDARY S et al: Fulminant mumps myocarditis. Ann Intern Med 110:569, 1989

GUT JP et al: Symptomatic mumps reinfections. J Med Virol 45:17, 1995

MCDONALD JC et al: Clinical and epidemiologic features of mumps encephalitis and possible causes of vaccine-related disease. Pediatr Infect Dis J 8: 751, 1989

SWIERKOSZ EM et al: Mumps, in *Manual of Clinical Virology*, 8th ed, PR Murray (ed). Washington, DC, ASM Press, 2002 (in press)

179 RABIES VIRUS AND OTHER RHABDOVIRUSES
Cathleen A. Hanlon, Lawrence Corey

RABIES VIRUS

DEFINITION Rabies is an invariably lethal, acute viral disease of the central nervous system (CNS) that affects all mammals and that is transmitted by infected secretions. Most commonly, transmission to humans takes place through exposure to saliva during a bite by an infected animal.

ETIOLOGY The rabies and rabies-related viruses are in the family Rhabdoviridae, with at least seven distinct types within the genus *Lyssa-*

virus. Isolates of rabies virus from different animal species and locales differ in their antigenic and biologic properties. These variations may account for differences in virulence between isolates. The bullet-shaped, enveloped viruses are single-strand RNA viruses of negative polarity. The rabies virus genome encodes five proteins: the nucleoprotein, the matrix protein, the glycoprotein, the phosphorylated protein, and a large polymerase protein. In immunofluorescence and complement fixation studies, broadly cross-reacting antigenic sites on the nucleoprotein are used to determine placement within the genus. The relatedness of a viral isolate to rabies and rabies-related viruses is determined by the comparison of specific antigenic sites or, more recently, by examination of RNA sequences. Cross-neutralization by rabies virus antisera ranges from moderate to very low. Only one serogroup is recognized within the genus. Recently, four new lyssaviruses have been described that expand current knowledge, classification, and taxonomy of rabies and rabies-related viruses.

EPIDEMIOLOGY An understanding of the epizootiology of rabies is necessary in evaluating the risk of exposure and the need for rabies postexposure prophylaxis (PEP) in humans. Rabies is found in mammals in all regions of the world except Antarctica. The susceptibility of mammals varies greatly and most likely is related to differences in cell surface receptor characteristics (e.g., type and abundance) and the impact of these differences on receptor-virus interactions. Rabies exists in two forms: *urban rabies*, propagated chiefly by unimmunized domestic dogs, and *sylvatic rabies*, propagated by skunks, foxes, raccoons, mongooses, wolves, and bats. Infection in domestic animals usually represents a "spillover" from sylvatic reservoirs of infection. Human infection occurs through contact with unimmunized domestic animals or from exposure to wild animals in locales where rabies is enzootic or epizootic. The worldwide incidence of human rabies is estimated at more than 30,000 cases per year. Southeast Asia, the Philippines, Africa, the Indian subcontinent, and tropical South America are areas where the disease is especially common. In some endemic areas, 1 to 2% of autopsies yield evidence of rabies. Increased travel of humans, along with intentional and unintentional translocation of animals (including known potential rabies-reservoir species), has made the recognition of clinical rabies and its prevention of increasing importance.

Although there are island countries and whole continents that consider themselves rabies-free, the designation is relative and should take into account potential animal translocation events, the capacity of rabies reservoir hosts (e.g., bats) for long-distance flight, the lack of adequate rabies diagnostic capacity and expertise, and the reluctance of national authorities to change official designations despite the identification of lyssaviruses among volant hosts (i.e., those capable of flight) and the identification of associated human rabies deaths.

The main reservoir of rabies throughout the world is the domestic dog. In developed countries, control of stray dogs and mandatory vaccination of owned dogs have resulted in the virtual elimination of this problem across large geographic areas (e.g., most of North America). With the virtual elimination of dog rabies in the United States since the 1960s, a dog bite now poses a dramatically reduced risk of rabies exposure that is appropriately managed by a 10-day observation of the dog. Tremendous advances in the control of dog rabies have recently been made in Latin and South American countries. However, dog rabies remains largely uncontrolled in most of Asia and Africa.

In addition to rabies in dogs, diverse rabies virus variants occur among other mammalian hosts. For example, the disease is found in the several species of mongoose in Asia and Africa and has been translocated to several Caribbean Islands. In Canada, rabies occurs among skunks and foxes, and raccoon rabies has invaded Ontario from New York. In Eastern Europe, rabies occurs among raccoon dogs. Coyotes, jackals, and other wild canids may serve as reservoirs or vectors in North America, Asia, and Africa. The major rabies virus variants in the United States occur among raccoons, skunks, red and gray foxes,

coyotes, and multiple insectivorous bat species. The most recent outbreak—and the most intense to date—affects raccoons in the eastern states from Florida to Maine and westward to the Appalachians and eastern Ohio. At the epizootic front in Ohio, New York, Pennsylvania, and West Virginia, the largest evaluation of oral rabies vaccination of free-ranging raccoons is in progress and represents an attempt to contain the westward spread of raccoon rabies. The vaccine, which is contained in baits and distributed primarily by air, is a vaccinia-rabies glycoprotein recombinant virus. Although highly attenuated by the lack of a critical enzyme (thymidine kinase), the vaccine is a live vaccinia virus and can infect humans, as demonstrated by at least one accidental human infection. In the United States, the domestic animal most commonly infected with rabies is the cat (~300 cases per year vs. ~100 cases in dogs). All other domestic animals combined (i.e., cattle, horses, sheep, goats, and pigs) account for a total of 150 to 200 cases per year.

Rabies in insectivorous bats occurs in the United States, Canada, Europe, Asia, Australia, and Africa—i.e., in essentially every locality where these bats are found. The epidemiology of rabies in bats is not well understood. In the United States, multiple rabies virus variants are generally associated with particular bat species, but variants may infect bat species other than their primary reservoir and may also infect terrestrial mammals, including other wildlife, domestic animals, and humans. Because migratory bat species travel widely and aggregate in large numbers, the rabies virus variants associated with these species are relatively homogeneous. In contrast, variants associated with nonmigratory bat species may demonstrate more genetic variation, such that isolates from particular geographic areas form distinct lineages. In general, the rate of rabies among seemingly healthy captured bats is low (1 in 100 to 1000). However, the rate of rabies among dead and dying bats in high-density colonies may be >50%. Rabies cannot be ruled out definitively in an individual bat or in any other animal except by direct fluorescent antibody testing of brain tissue.

The "bat" category in rabies surveillance reports includes a wide variety of species as well as many individual bats whose species is never identified. For surveillance purposes, it is uninformative to lump all bats together by order, as is the current practice in many states. Nevertheless, the total of rabid bats is second only to the number of rabid raccoons and skunks. In contrast to a single human case due to the raccoon rabies virus variant, a single human case of skunk-associated rabies, and two human cases of dog/coyote-associated rabies since 1980, the 30 human rabies cases due to bats account for >90% of all human rabies cases in the United States since that date. It is intriguing that a particular bat-associated rabies virus is implicated in most human cases: Ln/Ps, which is associated with silver-haired and eastern pipistrelle bats. Several factors may be involved in this observation. One possibility is that the teeth of these bats are so small that a bite may be dismissed (e.g., if the victim is unaware of the potential for rabies in these animals) or even go unrecognized (e.g., if the victim is asleep or under the influence of drugs or alcohol). Another possibility is that this virus variant may be better than others at replicating in cells of epidermal origin and at cooler temperatures. Perhaps a unique viral adaptation coupled with a relatively nontraumatic bite introduction is facilitating the emergence of this source of rabies in humans in the United States.

Human rabies is rare in the United States. The disease can be prevented if the exposure is recognized and appropriate local wound care and human rabies PEP are administered. From 1980 to 2002, most human rabies cases in the United States were acquired indigenously, with no apparent geographic trends. Two indigenously acquired human cases were associated with a localized outbreak of rabies among coyotes and dogs at the U.S.–Mexico border; however, this was a small outbreak in terms of relative animal case numbers.

A comparison of the epidemiology of animal rabies, human rabies PEP, and human rabies cases in the United States presents an interesting conundrum. Raccoons are the leading rabies reservoir, but only one human death from the raccoon-associated rabies virus variant has been documented. Since human rabies PEP is not reportable, there are few epidemiologic data on exposure to this reservoir. However, according to limited studies, most human rabies PEP is administered because of potential exposure to domestic cats and dogs in which rabies is suspected rather than because of direct exposure to raccoons or skunks—the first and second most commonly rabid animals in the United States.

PATHOGENESIS The first event in rabies is the inoculation of virus through the skin, usually through a bite that delivers virus-laden saliva. Initial viral replication appears to occur within striated muscle cells at the site of inoculation. The peripheral nervous system is exposed at the neuromuscular and/or neurotendinous spindles of unmyelinated sensory nerve cell endings, with neurotransmitter receptors such as acetylcholine implicated in viral attachment and internalization. The virus then spreads centripetally up the nerve to the CNS, probably via peripheral nerve axoplasm, at a rate of ~3 mm/h. Viremia has been documented in experimental conditions but is not thought to play a role in naturally acquired disease. Once the virus reaches the CNS, it replicates almost exclusively within the gray matter and then passes centrifugally along autonomic nerves to other tissues—the salivary glands, adrenal medulla, kidneys, lungs, liver, skeletal muscles, skin, and heart. Passage of the virus into the salivary glands and viral replication in mucinogenic acinar cells facilitate further transmission via infected saliva. The incubation period of rabies is exceedingly variable, ranging from 7 days to >1 year (mean, 1 to 2 months) and apparently depending on the amount of virus introduced, the amount of tissue involved, host defense mechanisms, and the actual distance that the virus has to travel from the site of inoculation to the CNS. Rates of infection and mortality are highest from bites on the face, intermediate from bites on the hands and arms, and lowest from bites on the legs. Cases of human rabies with an extended incubation period (2 to 7 years) have been reported, but they are rare. Host immune responses and viral strains also influence disease expression.

The neuropathology of rabies resembles that of other viral diseases of the CNS: hyperemia, varying degrees of chromatolysis, nuclear pyknosis, and neuronophagia of the nerve cells; infiltration by lymphocytes and plasma cells of the Virchow-Robin space; microglial infiltration; and parenchymal areas of nerve cell destruction. In experimental animal models, adenohypophyseal infection with rabies virus, with reduction in growth hormone and vasopressin release, is common. The most characteristic pathologic finding of rabies in the CNS is the formation of cytoplasmic inclusions called *Negri bodies* within neurons. Each eosinophilic mass measures ~10 nm and is made up of a finely fibrillar matrix and rabies virus particles. Negri bodies are distributed throughout the brain, particularly in Ammon's horn, the cerebral cortex, the brainstem, the hypothalamus, the Purkinje cells of the cerebellum, and the dorsal spinal ganglia. Negri bodies are not demonstrated in at least 20% of cases of rabies, and their absence from brain material does not rule out the diagnosis.

CLINICAL MANIFESTATIONS (See also Table 179-1) The clinical manifestations of rabies can be divided into four stages: (1) a nonspecific prodrome; (2) an acute encephalitis similar to other viral encephalitides; (3) a profound dysfunction of brainstem centers that produces the classic features of rabies encephalitis; and (4) death or, in rare cases, recovery.

The prodromal period usually lasts 1 to 4 days and is marked by fever, headache, malaise, myalgias, increased fatigability, anorexia, nausea and vomiting, sore throat, and a nonproductive cough. The prodromal symptom suggestive of rabies is the complaint of paresthesia and/or fasciculations at or around the site of inoculation of virus. These sensations, which may be related to the multiplication of virus in the dorsal root ganglion of the sensory nerve supplying the area of the bite, are reported by 50 to 80% of patients.

The encephalitic phase is usually ushered in by periods of excessive motor activity, excitation, and agitation. Confusion, hallucinations, combativeness, bizarre aberrations of thought, muscle spasms, meningismus, opisthotonic posturing, seizures, and focal paralysis soon appear. Characteristically, the periods of mental aberration are inter-

TABLE 179-1 *General Clinical Course of Human Rabies*

Phase	Duration	Features/Comments
Exposure	—	Often unrecognized, particularly if of bat origin
Incubation period	3–4 weeks to 3–4 months in 95% of cases; 1–7 years in 1% of cases	—
Prodrome	1–2 days to 1 week	Fever, headache, anorexia, nausea, vomiting, malaise, lethargy, focal pain, paresthesia, anxiety, agitation, depression
Acute neurologic (encephalitic) phase	1–2 days to <1 week	Confusion, delirium, hallucinations, dysphagia, hypersalivation, aphasia, incoordination, marked hyperactivity, pharyngeal spasms, hydrophobia, aerophobia, hyperventilation, hypoxia, seizures
Coma, death	Several days to 1 week	Autonomic instability, hypoventilation, apnea, respiratory arrest, hypo-/hyperthermia, hypotension, pituitary dysfunction, rhabdomyolysis, cardiac arrhythmia, cardiac arrest

spersed with completely lucid periods, but as the disease progresses the lucid periods get shorter until the patient lapses into coma. Hyperesthesia, with excessive sensitivity to bright light, loud noise, touch, and even gentle breezes, is very common. On physical examination, the temperature may be found to be as high as 40.6°C (105°F). Abnormalities of the autonomic nervous system include dilated irregular pupils; increased lacrimation, salivation, and perspiration; and postural hypotension. Evidence of upper motor neuron paralysis, with weakness, increased deep tendon reflexes, and extensor plantar responses, is the rule. Paralysis of the vocal cords is common. Unfortunately, the presenting signs and symptoms of rabies are indistinguishable from those of other viral and neurologic diseases. Thus delays in diagnosis are frequent. The presence of hydrophobia or aerophobia (seen in about two-thirds of recent cases) increases the likelihood of antemortem diagnosis.

The manifestations of brainstem dysfunction begin shortly after the onset of the encephalitic phase. Cranial nerve involvement causes diplopia, facial palsies, optic neuritis, and the characteristic difficulty with deglutition. The combination of excessive salivation and difficulty in swallowing produces the traditional picture of "foaming at the mouth." Hydrophobia—the painful, violent, involuntary contraction of the diaphragmatic, accessory respiratory, pharyngeal, and laryngeal muscles initiated by swallowing liquids—is seen in ~50% of cases. Involvement of the amygdaloid nucleus may result in priapism and spontaneous ejaculation. The patient lapses into coma, and involvement of the respiratory center produces an apneic death. The prominence of early brainstem dysfunction distinguishes rabies from other viral encephalitides and accounts for the rapid downhill course. The median period of survival after the onset of symptoms is 4 days, with a maximum of 20 days, unless artificial supportive measures are instituted.

If intensive respiratory support is used, a number of late complications may appear. These include inappropriate secretion of antidiuretic hormone, diabetes insipidus, cardiac arrhythmias, vascular instability, adult respiratory distress syndrome, gastrointestinal bleeding, thrombocytopenia, and paralytic ileus. Recovery is very rare and, when it occurs, gradual.

Rabies may also present as an ascending paralysis resembling the Landry/Guillain-Barré syndrome (dumb rabies, *rage tranquille*). Initially, this clinical pattern was reported most frequently among persons given PEP after being bitten by vampire bats. Paralytic rabies also occurs in Southeast Asia among persons with canine exposures. The difficulty of diagnosing rabies associated with ascending paralysis is illustrated by cases of person-to-person transmission of the virus by tissue transplantation. Corneal transplants from donors who died of presumed Landry/Guillain-Barré syndrome produced clinical rabies in and caused the deaths of the recipients. Retrospective pathologic examinations of the brains of recipients demonstrated Negri bodies, and rabies virus was subsequently isolated from each donor's frozen eye.

LABORATORY FINDINGS   During the early clinical period of rabies infection, laboratory findings—like signs and symptoms—are nonspecific. Complete blood cell counts and differentials are compatible with an acute viral illness. As with encephalitis or meningitis of any viral etiology, there is mild pleocytosis (>5 cells/μL) in the cerebrospinal fluid (CSF), with lymphocytosis. The CSF protein level may be mildly elevated, but the glucose level is generally normal. A decreased level of glucose in the CSF suggests the possibility of fungal, tuberculous, parasitic, leptospiral, syphilitic, sarcoid, or neoplastic meningitis. Severe pleocytosis (>1000 cells/μL) is compatible with nonviral and other inflammatory etiologies. The presence of large numbers of polymorphonuclear cells is indicative of bacterial infection, leptospirosis, amebic infection, and some noninfectious processes.

The most critical laboratory findings in suspected cases of human rabies are those that permit the exclusion of other etiologies (i.e., the most common sources of encephalitis) and that document a rapidly deteriorating clinical course compatible with rabies (see "Differential Diagnosis," below). Antemortem diagnosis of human rabies can be arranged through consultation with the relevant state health department and the Centers for Disease Control and Prevention (CDC). Such a diagnosis requires samples of the patient's CSF and serum (preferably paired), fresh saliva, and a full-thickness skin biopsy sample from the nape of the neck. If a patient dies during the effort to rule out rabies, fresh brain material is the optimal sample for a definitive postmortem diagnosis.

Rabies Virus–Specific Antibodies in Serum and CSF   Since rabies virus remains in the "immunologically privileged" CNS (with no viremia), the infection is largely undetected by the immune system until late in the clinical course. Once encephalitis develops, immune surveillance within the CNS is substantially heightened and viral antigen is widespread, resulting in the development of an antibody response and the influx of cytotoxic T cells. Thus, rabies virus–specific antibodies in serum and CSF develop relatively late in the clinical course and, when the patient dies during the acute phase, may be undetectable.

Two laboratory methods are commonly used to detect rabies virus–specific antibodies. The *indirect fluorescent antibody test* involves the addition of dilutions of test serum to plates with wells containing rabies virus–infected cells. If rabies antigen–specific antibodies are present in the serum, they bind to infected cells. The bound antibody is then detected with fluorescein-tagged antihuman antibodies. This rapid test predominantly detects antibodies to the rabies virus nucleoprotein. The *rapid fluorescent focus inhibition test* (RFFIT) is a valuable but labor-intensive method that takes 1 day to complete. The RFFIT requires that a fixed amount of live rabies virus and dilutions of test serum be added to cell monolayers and allowed to incubate for 20 h. If neutralizing antibodies to the rabies virus glycoprotein are present in the patient's serum, few or no infected foci are seen when the direct fluorescent antibody (DFA) test is applied to the cell monolayer, because the viral particles will have been neutralized by antibodies and prevented from infecting cells. Rabies virus–specific antibodies may be found in serum as a result of previous vaccination against rabies. In contrast, the occurrence of rabies virus antibodies in the CSF is diagnostic for rabies (or, in extremely rare cases, indicative of previous exposure to and survival of rabies virus), since antibodies from vaccination do not cross an intact blood-brain barrier.

Reverse-Transcription Polymerase Chain Reaction (RT-PCR) on Fresh Saliva   Viral shedding in the saliva directly precedes and accompanies the development of clinical signs in animals and probably in humans as well. During early CNS infection, the host may appear normal, but virus may already be present in the saliva as a result of centrifugal spread. With the exquisitely sensitive RT-PCR, the presence of rabies virus nucleic acid in fresh saliva can be confirmed or ruled out. If testing is performed very early in the clinical course, additional samples may need to be evaluated, because viral shedding may be intermittent at this time.

DFA Testing and RT-PCR on a Skin Biopsy Sample   As a result of wide centrifugal spread, the rabies virus genome and antigen may be detectable in a skin biopsy from the nape of the patient's neck during the clinical course of suspected rabies. With the DFA test, viral antigen may be demonstrated in peripheral nerves associated with hair follicles in the skin sample. RT-PCR has shown greater sensitivity for detection of rabies genomic material in skin samples.

Other Tests   Although patients with encephalitis are invariably evaluated with advanced tests (e.g., magnetic resonance imaging, computed tomography, electroencephalography, evoked response studies, electromyography, and nerve conduction studies), the results are nondiagnostic for rabies.

DIFFERENTIAL DIAGNOSIS   The differential diagnosis in a case of suspected human rabies may initially include any cause of encephalitis, particularly infection with viruses such as herpesviruses, enteroviruses, and arboviruses (e.g., West Nile virus). The most important viruses to rule out are herpes simplex virus type 1, varicella-zoster virus, and (less commonly) enteroviruses, including coxsackieviruses, echoviruses, polioviruses, and human enteroviruses 68 to 71. A specific diagnosis may be made by a variety of diagnostic techniques, including CSF PCR testing, culture, and serology. In addition, consideration should be given to the local epidemiology of encephalitis caused by arboviruses belonging to several taxonomic groups, including eastern and western equine encephalitis viruses, St. Louis encephalitis virus, Powassan virus, the California encephalitis virus serogroup, and La Crosse virus.

New causes of viral encephalitis are also possible, as was evidenced by the recent outbreak in Malaysia of ~300 cases of encephalitis (mortality rate, 40%) caused by Nipah virus, a new paramyxovirus. Similarly, well-known viruses may be introduced into new locations, as is illustrated by the recent outbreak of encephalitis due to West Nile virus in the eastern United States. Epidemiologic factors (e.g., season, geographic location, and the patient's age, travel history, and possible exposure to animal bites, rodents, and ticks) may help direct the diagnostic workup.

℞ **TREATMENT**

There is no specific treatment for clinical rabies. Death is virtually inevitable once clinical signs develop. Medical management is supportive and palliative.

POSTEXPOSURE PROPHYLAXIS   When an exposure to rabies is recognized, immediate and thorough wound cleansing and the prompt administration of PEP (Table 179-2) are extremely effective in preventing infection. With regard to the prevention of human rabies in developed countries, recognition of a potential exposure and its distinction from circumstances in which no exposure has occurred are key steps in the judicious administration of rabies biologics. In developing countries, the prevention of rabies is hindered by economic conditions and inadequate access to modern biologics.

Unprovoked bites, especially if severe and multiple, by a confirmed rabid animal constitute the most obvious and highest-risk route of exposure to rabies. As stated in the recommendations of the Advisory Committee on Immunization Practices (ACIP, Table 179-2), simply touching a rabid animal (or person) does not constitute an exposure to rabies. Rabies virus forms an infectious aerosol only under intentional

TABLE 179-2 *Rabies Postexposure Prophylaxis Guide—United States*

Animal Type	Evaluation and Disposition of Animal	Postexposure Prophylaxis Recommendations
Dogs, cats, and ferrets	Healthy and available for 10 days observation	No treatment is necessary unless animal develops clinical signs of rabies.[a]
	Rabid or suspected rabid	Begin PEP.
	Unknown (e.g., escaped)	Consult public health officials.
Skunks, raccoons, foxes, and most other carnivores; bats	Regarded as rabid unless animal proven negative by laboratory tests[b]	Consider immediate vaccination.
Livestock, small rodents, lagomorphs (rabbits and hares), large rodents (woodchucks and beavers), and other mammals	Consider individually	Consult public health officials. Bites of squirrels, hamsters, guinea pigs, gerbils, chipmunks, rats, mice, other small rodents, small rodents, rabbits, and hares almost never require antirabies postexposure prophylaxis.

[a] During the 10-day observation period, begin postexposure prophylaxis at the first sign of rabies in a dog, cat, or ferret that has bitten someone. If the animal exhibits clinical signs of rabies, it should be euthanized immediately and tested.

[b] The animal should be euthanized and tested as soon as possible. Holding for observation is not recommended. Discontinue vaccine if immunofluorescence test results of the animal are negative.

Source: Human rabies prevention—United States, 1999. Recommendations of the Advisory Committee on Immunization Practices (ACIP). MMWR Recomm Rep 48(RR-1): 1-21, 1999; erratum in MMWR 48(1):16, 1999; MMWR 49(32):737, 2000.

or highly unnatural conditions. The only cases in which the aerosol route has been implicated are laboratory accidents and the Frio cave incidents of 50 years ago; in the latter situation, other routes of exposure for the bat biologists (e.g., bat bites or—in one person—contamination of an excoriated area of eczema) could not be ruled out. Contamination of mucous membranes with infectious material is considered an exposure to rabies because of observations in various species of occasional rabies cases resulting from intentional oral or intranasal exposure to high titers of virus; however, the majority of animals so exposed are unaffected, and a few such animals even develop immunity to rabies. Limited laboratory experiments with direct ocular exposure to rabies in one animal species did not result in viral infection; nevertheless, ocular contact with potentially contaminated material is considered an exposure because of the historic occurrence of human rabies cases after the transplantation of corneas from donors retrospectively diagnosed with rabies. Contamination of a fresh wound with infectious material (brain, salivary gland, or other innervated tissue from a rabid animal) constitutes an exposure to rabies.

Once the possibility of exposure has been identified, the wound should be thoroughly scrubbed with soap and then flushed with water. Both mechanical cleansing and chemical cleansing are important. Quaternary ammonium compounds such as 1 to 4% benzalkonium chloride, 1% cetrimonium bromide, or povidone-iodine solutions should be used. Tetanus toxoid and antibiotic prophylaxis should be administered as needed.

With an established exposure, the decision to administer human rabies biologics is straightforward if the animal is available for rabies diagnosis (i.e., euthanasia, brain removal, and laboratory testing). In dogs, cats, and ferrets in the United States, the potential shedding period indicates the adequacy of observation of the animal for 10 days after a bite to a human. If the animal remains clinically normal, laboratory and epidemiologic data indicate no risk of rabies exposure through the bite (although clearly, if unvaccinated, the animal may develop rabies in the future). If the animal develops signs suggestive

of rabies, it should be euthanized and tested immediately, and the human victim should be treated according to the laboratory test result. If the animal is unavailable, the decision to treat depends upon the risk of rabies in the individual animal, the local epizootiology of rabies and the consequent risk to the individual animal, the potential route of exposure (i.e., multiple severe bites vs. potential contamination of mucous membranes with infectious material), and other factors. This decision may best be made in consultation with local, state, and federal public health professionals who have specialized knowledge of these variables.

Human rabies PEP consists of five doses of a modern cell culture vaccine, of which two types are commonly available for use in the United States (Table 179-3). The current cell culture vaccines are virtually equivalent in their unfailing potency and relative paucity of adverse effects. A reaction compatible with delayed-type hypersensitivity may occur in up to 12% of patients receiving human diploid cell vaccine; continuation of the pre- or postexposure series with an alternative vaccine may be sufficient for the resolution of this reaction. Doses are administered on a schedule of 0, 3, 7, 14, and 28 days. In addition to vaccine on day 0, one dose of human rabies immune globulin (20 IU/kg) should be given; as much of the dose as is anatomically feasible should be administered at the site of the bite, with any excess administered intramuscularly at a distant site—e.g., in the deltoid opposite the vaccine site. Periodically, human rabies immune globulin is in short supply. If it is not immediately available, the vaccine series should be initiated and the rabies immune globulin may be added at any point through day 7. After day 7, it is not necessary to add rabies immune globulin to the patient's regimen because endogenous antibodies are being produced and exogenous antibodies may actually be counterproductive. If a patient presents at a long interval after a potential exposure, it is not too late to initiate full human PEP unless clinical signs are present.

PREEXPOSURE RABIES VACCINATION Preexposure rabies vaccination is available to persons at risk of rabies exposure. The ACIP recommends a series of 1-mL doses of modern cell culture vaccine administered intramuscularly on days 0, 7, and 21 or 28. Once immunized against rabies with potent vaccines, individuals are primed against rabies for the rest of their lives. If an exposure occurs, a previously immunized

TABLE 179-3 *Commonly Available Human Rabies Biologics*

Vaccine Type	Product	Source
AVAILABLE IN UNITED STATES		
Human rabies vaccine		
Rabies vaccine, human diploid cell (HDCV), IM	Imovax Rabies	Aventis-Pasteur[a]
Rabies vaccine, purified chick embryo cell (PCEC), IM	RabAvert	Chiron Behring GmbH[b]
Rabies immune globulin, human (RIG)	Imogam Rabies-HT	Aventis-Pasteur[a]
	BayRab	Bayer Corporation Pharmaceutical Division[c]
CELL CULTURE RABIES VACCINES WIDELY AVAILABLE OUTSIDE UNITED STATES		
Purified chick embryo cell vaccine (PCEC)	Rabipur	
Purified Vero cell vaccine (PVRV)	Verorab Imovax-Rabies Vero TRC Verorab	
Human diploid cell vaccine (HDCV)	Rabivac	
Purified duck embryo vaccine (PDEV)	Lyssavac N	

[a] Phone: 1-800-VACCINE.
[b] Phone: 1-800-CHIRON8.
[c] Phone: 1-800-288-8370.

person should receive postexposure boosters consisting of two doses 3 days apart. Persons in the high-risk and moderate-risk rabies exposure categories should have their rabies virus–neutralizing antibody titers monitored every 6 months and every 2 years, respectively. Persons in the low-exposure category do not require serologic monitoring but, like all previously immunized persons, must receive the two booster vaccinations upon exposure to rabies. Moreover, appropriate wound care (i.e., copious flushing and the use of soap or detergent) remains critical.

MOKOLA VIRUS

Mokola virus was first isolated from wild shrews captured in Nigeria and was shown to be related morphologically and serologically to rabies virus. The subsequent isolation of the virus from cats in South Africa suggested a wider prevalence of the agent than had previously been expected. Only two cases of clinical infection have been reported; both were in children. One patient had a nonfatal illness characterized by fever, pharyngitis, and convulsions; Mokola virus was recovered from CSF. In the second patient, fever with cough and vomiting was followed within several days by drowsiness, confusion, and generalized flaccid weakness. The CSF was normal. The patient progressed to deep coma and died within 10 days of onset. Mokola virus was isolated from the brain, and examination of histopathologic sections revealed finely granular cytoplasmic inclusions that were distinguishable from Negri bodies in many neurons.

VESICULAR STOMATITIS VIRUS

Vesicular stomatitis is a viral illness of animals that occasionally affects humans. It presents as an acute, self-limited, influenza-like disease. The disease in animals is found in the United States and South America and affects chiefly domestic cattle, horses, swine, wild deer, raccoons, skunks, and bobcats.

In animals, vesicular stomatitis is characterized by the development of vesicles on the oral mucosa, particularly the tongue; the udders; and the heels. The mode of spread is probably by direct contact; however, epidemics tend to occur in warm weather, and isolation of the virus from *Phlebotomus* sandflies in Panama and *Aedes* mosquitoes in New Mexico suggests that these insects may be vectors. Two distinct types, New Jersey and Indiana, have been recognized, and most outbreaks in North America have been attributed to the New Jersey strain.

In humans, vesicular stomatitis is most common among laboratory workers. In one report, three-fourths of laboratory personnel handling experimentally infected animals or manipulating the virus developed neutralizing antibodies. The disease is also transmissible, however, under natural conditions among workers having direct contact with infected animals, especially cattle. An incubation period ranging from 1 to 6 days is followed by the sudden onset of fever [with temperatures of up to 40°C (104°F)], chills, profuse sweating, myalgias, malaise, headache, and pain on ocular movement. One-third to one-half of patients have a sore throat and cervical and/or submandibular adenopathy. Small raised vesicular lesions may appear on the buccal mucosa. Conjunctivitis and coryza are evident in ~20% of cases. Small subcorneal, intraepithelial vesicles occasionally appear on the fingers, usually in association with direct inoculation of the virus. Symptoms generally last 3 to 4 days, but occasionally the course is diphasic. Inapparent infection is common: among laboratory workers with serologic evidence of infection, only about one-half report symptoms. In some areas of Panama, 17 to 35% of the population have neutralizing antibodies to vesicular stomatitis virus.

The differential diagnosis includes hand-foot-and-mouth disease, herpangina, primary herpetic pharyngitis and other mucocutaneous syndromes, and influenza. The virus is not commonly isolated from patients. However, a rise in titer of complement-fixation and/or neutralizing antibody to vesicular stomatitis virus between acute- and convalescent-phase sera helps to confirm the diagnosis. Treatment is nonspecific.

FURTHER READING

CENTERS FOR DISEASE CONTROL AND PREVENTION: Human rabies—Iowa, 2002. MMWR 52:47, 2003

————: First human rabies case associated with raccoon rabies—Virginia, 2003. MMWR 52:1102, 2003

————: Human rabies prevention—United States, 1999: Recommendations of the Advisory Committee on Immunization Practices (ACIP). MMWR 48(RR-1), 1999

CONSTANTINE DG: Geographic translocation of bats: Known and potential problems. Emerg Infect Dis 9:17, 2003

JACKSON AC et al: Management of rabies in humans. Clin Infect Dis 36:60, 2003

KREBS JW et al: Rabies surveillance in the United States during 2002. J Am Vet Med Assoc 223:1736, 2003

KUZMIN IV et al: Bat lyssaviruses (Aravan and Khujand) from Central Asia: Phylogenetic relationships according to N, P, and G gene sequences. Virus Res 97:65, 2003

———— et al: Novel lyssaviruses isolated from bats in Russia. Emerg Infect Dis 9:1623, 2003

MESSENGER SL et al: Emerging epidemiology of bat-associated cryptic cases of rabies in the United States. Clin Infect Dis 35:738, 2002

NOAH DL et al: Epidemiology of human rabies in the United States, 1980 to 1996. Ann Intern Med 128:922, 1998

Some viruses are transmitted in nature without regard to humans and only incidentally infect and produce disease in humans; in addition, a few agents are regularly spread among humans by arthropods. Most of these viruses either are maintained by arthropods or chronically infect rodents. Obviously, the mode of transmission is not a rational basis for taxonomic classification. Indeed, zoonotic viruses from at least seven virus families act as significant human pathogens (Table 180-1). The virus families differ fundamentally from one another in terms of morphology, replication mechanisms, and genetics. Information on a virus's membership in a family or genus is enlightening with regard to maintenance strategies, sensitivity to antivirals, and some aspects of pathogenesis but does not necessarily predict which clinical syndromes—if any—the virus will cause in humans.

FAMILIES OF ARTHROPOD- AND RODENT-BORNE VIRUSES (Table 180-1)

■ **The Arenaviridae** The Arenaviridae are spherical, 110- to 130-nm particles that bud from the cell's plasma membrane and utilize ambisense RNA genomes with two segments for replication. There are two main phylogenetic branches of Arenaviridae: the Old World viruses, such as Lassa fever and lymphocytic choriomeningitis (LCM) viruses, and the New World viruses, including those causing the South American hemorrhagic fevers (HFs). Arenaviruses persist in nature by chronically infecting rodents with a striking one-virus–one-rodent species relationship. These rodent infections result in long-term virus excretion and perhaps in lifelong viremia; vertical infection is common with some arenaviruses. Humans become infected through the inhalation of aerosols containing arenaviruses, which are then deposited in the terminal air passages, and probably also through close contact with

rodents and their excreta, which results in the contamination of mucous membranes or breaks in the skin.

The Bunyaviridae The family Bunyaviridae includes four medically significant genera. All of these spherical viruses have three negative-sense RNA segments maturing into 90- to 120-nm particles in the Golgi complex and exiting the cell by exocytosis. Viruses of the genus *Bunyavirus* are largely mosquito-borne and have a viremic vertebrate intermediate host; many are also transovarially transmitted in their specific mosquito host. One serologic group also uses biting midges as vectors. Sandflies or mosquitoes are the vectors for the genus *Phlebovirus* (named after phlebotomus fever or sandfly fever, the best-known disease associated with the genus), while ticks serve as vectors for the genus *Nairovirus*. Viruses of both of these genera are also associated with vertical transmission in the arthropod host and with horizontal spread through viremic vertebrate hosts. The genus *Hantavirus* is unique among the Bunyaviridae in that it is not transmitted by arthropods but is maintained in nature by rodent hosts that chronically shed virus. Like the arenaviruses, the hantaviruses usually display striking virus-rodent species specificity. Hantaviruses do not cause chronic viremia in their rodent hosts and are transmitted only horizontally from rodent to rodent.

Other Families The Flaviviridae are positive-sense, single-strand RNA viruses that form particles of 40 to 50 nm in the endoplasmic reticulum. The flaviviruses discussed here are from the genus *Flavivirus* and make up two phylogenetically and antigenically distinct divisions transmitted among vertebrates by mosquitoes and ticks, respectively.

TABLE 180-1 *Major Zoonotic Virus Families and Some Characteristics of Typical Members*

Family	Genus or Group	Syndrome(s): Typical Viruses	Maintenance Strategy
Arenaviridae	Old World complex	FM, E: Lymphocytic choriomeningitis virus HF: Lassa fever virus	Chronic infection of rodents, often with persistent viremia; vertical transmission common
	New World or Tacaribe complex	HF: South American HF viruses (Machupo, Junin, Guanarito, Sabia)	Chronic infection of rodents, sometimes with persistent viremia; vertical infection may occur
Bunyaviridae	*Bunyavirus*	E: California serogroup viruses (La Crosse, Jamestown Canyon, California encephalitis) FM: Bunyamwera, group C, Tahyna viruses	Mosquito-vertebrate cycle; transovarial transmission in mosquito common
		FM: Oropouche virus	Transmitted by *Culicoides*
	Phlebovirus	FM: Sandfly fever, Toscana viruses FM: Punta Toro virus	Sandfly transmission between vertebrates, with prominent transovarial component in sandfly
		HF, FM, E: Rift Valley fever virus	Mosquito-vertebrate transmission, with transovarial component in mosquito
	Nairovirus	HF: Crimean-Congo HF virus	Tick-vertebrate, with transovarial transmission in tick
	Hantavirus	HF: Hantaan, Dobrava, Puumala viruses	Rodent reservoir; chronic virus shedding, but chronic viremia unknown
		HF: Sin Nombre and related hantaviruses	Sigmodontine rodent reservoir
Filoviridae[a]		HF: Marburg viruses, Ebola viruses (4 subtypes)	Unknown
Flaviviridae	*Flavivirus* (mosquito-borne)	HF: Yellow fever virus FM, HF: Dengue viruses (4 subtypes) E: St. Louis, Japanese, West Nile, and Murray Valley encephalitis viruses; Rocio viruses	Mosquito-vertebrate; transovarial rare
	Flavivirus (tick-borne)	E: Central European tick-borne encephalitis, Russian spring-summer encephalitis, Powassan viruses HF: Omsk HF, Kyasanur Forest disease viruses	Tick-vertebrate
Reoviridae	*Coltivirus*	FM, E: Colorado tick fever virus	Tick-vertebrate
	Orbivirus	FM, E: Orungo, Kemerova viruses	Arthropod-vertebrate
Rhabdoviridae[b]	*Vesiculovirus*	FM: Vesicular stomatitis virus (Indiana, New Jersey); Chandipura, Piry viruses	Sandfly-vertebrate, with prominent transovarial component in sandfly
Togaviridae	*Alphavirus*	AR: Sindbis, chikungunya, Mayaro, Ross River, Barmah Forest viruses	Mosquito-vertebrate
		E: Eastern, western, and Venezuelan equine encephalitis viruses	

[a] The Filoviridae are discussed in Chap. 181.
[b] The Rhabdoviridae are discussed in Chap. 179.

Note: Abbreviations refer to the disease syndrome most commonly associated with the virus: FM, fever, myalgia; AR, arthritis, rash; E, encephalitis; HF, hemorrhagic fever.

The mosquito-borne viruses fall into phylogenetic groups that include yellow fever virus, the four dengue viruses, and encephalitis viruses, while the tick-borne group encompasses a geographically varied spectrum of species, some of which are responsible for encephalitis or for hemorrhagic disease with encephalitis. The Reoviridae are double-strand RNA viruses with multisegmented genomes. These 80-nm particles are the only viruses discussed in this chapter that do not have a lipid envelope and thus are insensitive to detergents. The Togaviridae have a single positive-strand RNA genome and bud particles of ~60 to 70 nm from the plasma membrane. The togaviruses discussed here are all members of the genus *Alphavirus* and are transmitted among vertebrates by mosquitoes in their natural cycle. →*The Filoviridae and the Rhabdoviridae are discussed in Chaps. 181 and 179, respectively.*

PROMINENT FEATURES OF ARTHROPOD- AND RODENT-BORNE VIRUSES Although this chapter discusses the major features of selected arthropod- and rodent-borne viruses, it does not deal with >500 other distinct recognized zoonotic viruses, about one-fourth of which infect humans. Zoonotic viruses are undergoing genetic evolution, "new" zoonotic viruses are being discovered, and the epidemiology of zoonotic viruses is continuing to evolve through environmental changes affecting vectors, reservoirs, and humans. These zoonotic viruses are most numerous in the tropics but are also found in temperate and frigid climates. Their distribution and seasonal activity may be variable and often depend largely on ecologic conditions such as rainfall and temperature, which in turn affect the density of vectors and reservoirs and the development of infection therein.

Maintenance and Transmission Arthropod-borne viruses infect their vectors after the ingestion of a blood meal from a viremic vertebrate. The vectors then develop chronic, systemic infection as the viruses penetrate the gut and spread throughout the body. The viruses eventually reach the salivary glands during a period that is referred to as *extrinsic incubation* and that typically lasts 1 to 3 weeks in mosquitoes. At this point an arthropod is competent to continue the chain of transmission by infecting another vertebrate when a subsequent blood meal is taken.

The arthropod generally is unharmed by the infection, and the natural vertebrate partner usually has only transient viremia with no overt disease. An alternative mechanism for virus maintenance in its arthropod host is transovarial transmission, which is common among members of the family Bunyaviridae.

Rodent-borne viruses such as the hantaviruses and arenaviruses are maintained in nature by chronic infection transmitted between rodents. As in arthropod-borne virus cycles, there is usually a high degree of rodent-virus specificity, and there is no overt disease in the reservoir/vector.

Epidemiology The distribution of arthropod- and rodent-borne viruses is restricted by the areas inhabited by their reservoir/vectors and provides an important clue in the differential diagnosis. Table 180-2 shows the approximate geographic distribution of the most important of these viruses. Members of each family, each genus, and even each serologically related group usually occur in each area but may not be pathogenic in all areas or may not be a commonly recognized cause of disease in all areas and so may not be included in the table.

Most of these diseases are acquired in a rural setting; a few have urban vectors. Seoul, sandfly fever, and Oropouche viruses are examples of urban viruses, but the most notable are yellow fever, dengue, and chikungunya viruses. A history of mosquito bite has little diagnostic significance in the individual; a history of tick bite is more diagnostically specific. Rodent exposure is often reported by persons infected with an arenavirus or a hantavirus but again has little specificity. Indeed, aerosols may infect persons who have no recollection of having even seen rodents.

Syndromes Human disease caused by arthropod- and rodent-borne viruses is often subclinical. The spectrum of possible responses to infection is wide, and our knowledge of the outcome of most of these infections is limited. The usual disease syndromes associated with these viruses have been grouped into four categories: fever and myalgia, arthritis and rash, encephalitis, and hemorrhagic fever. Although for the purposes of this discussion most viruses have been placed in a single group, the categories often overlap. For example, West Nile and Venezuelan equine encephalitis viruses are discussed as encephalitis viruses, but during epidemics they may cause many cases of milder

TABLE 180-2 *Geographic Distribution of Some Important and Commonly Encountered Human Zoonotic Viral Diseases*

Area	Arenaviridae	Bunyaviridae	Flaviviridae	Rhabdoviridae	Togaviridae
North America	Lymphocytic choriomeningitis	La Crosse, Jamestown Canyon, California encephalitis; hantavirus pulmonary syndrome	St. Louis, Powassan, West Nile encephalitis; dengue	Vesicular stomatitis	Eastern, western equine encephalitis
South America	Bolivian, Argentine, Venezuelan, and Brazilian HF; lymphocytic choriomeningitis	Oropouche, group C, Punta Toro infection; hantavirus pulmonary syndrome	Yellow fever, dengue, Rocio virus infection	Vesicular stomatitis, Piry virus infection	Mayaro virus infection, Venezuelan equine encephalitis
Europe	Lymphocytic choriomeningitis	Tahyna, Toscana, sandfly fever, HF with renal syndrome	West Nile, Central European tick-borne, Russian spring-summer encephalitis	—	Sindbis virus infection
Middle East	—	Sandfly fever, Crimean-Congo HF	West Nile encephalitis, dengue	—	—
Eastern Asia	—	Sandfly fever; Hantaan, Seoul virus infection	Dengue; Japanese, Russian spring-summer encephalitis; Omsk HF	Chandipura virus infection	—
Southwestern Asia	—	Sandfly fever, Crimean-Congo HF	West Nile, Japanese encephalitis; dengue; Kyasanur Forest disease	—	Chikungunya
Southeast Asia	—	Seoul virus infection	Japanese encephalitis, dengue	—	Chikungunya
Africa	Lassa fever	Bunyamwera virus infection, Rift Valley fever	Yellow fever, dengue	—	Sindbis virus infection, chikungunya
Australia	—	—	Murray Valley encephalitis, dengue	—	Ross River, Barmah Forest virus infection

Note: HF, hemorrhagic fever.

febrile syndromes and relatively uncommon cases of encephalitis. Similarly, Rift Valley fever virus is best known as a cause of HF, but the attack rates for febrile disease are far higher, and encephalitis is occasionally seen as well. LCM virus is classified as a cause of fever and myalgia because this syndrome is its most common disease manifestation and because, even when central nervous system (CNS) disease occurs, it is usually mild and is preceded by fever and myalgia. Dengue virus infection is considered as a cause of fever and myalgia (dengue fever) because this is by far the most common manifestation worldwide and is the syndrome most likely to be seen in the United States; however, dengue HF is also discussed in the HF section because of its complicated pathogenesis and importance in pediatric practice in certain areas of the world.

Diagnosis Laboratory diagnosis is required in any given case, although epidemics occasionally provide clinical and epidemiologic clues on which an educated guess as to etiology can be based. For most arthropod- and rodent-borne viruses, acute-phase serum samples (collected within 3 or 4 days of onset) have yielded isolates, and paired sera have been used to demonstrate rising antibody titers by a variety of tests. Intensive efforts to develop rapid tests for HF have resulted in an antigen-detection enzyme-linked immunosorbent assay (ELISA) and an IgM-capture ELISA that can provide a diagnosis based on a single serum sample within a few hours and are particularly useful in severe cases. More sensitive reverse-transcription polymerase chain reaction (RT-PCR) tests may yield diagnoses based on samples without detectable antigen and may also provide useful genetic information about the virus. Hantavirus infections differ from others discussed here in that severe acute disease is immunopathologic; patients present with serum IgM that serves as the basis for a sensitive and specific test.

At diagnosis, patients with encephalitis are generally no longer viremic or antigenemic and usually do not have virus in cerebrospinal fluid (CSF). In this situation, the value of serologic methods and RT-PCR is being validated. IgM capture is increasingly being used for the simultaneous testing of serum and CSF. IgG ELISA or classic serology is useful in the evaluation of past exposure to the viruses, many of which circulate in areas with a minimal medical infrastructure and sometimes cause mild or subclinical infection.

The remainder of this chapter offers general descriptions of the broad syndromes caused by arthropod- and rodent-borne viruses. Most of the diseases under consideration have not been studied in detail with modern medical approaches; thus available data may be incomplete or biased.

FEVER AND MYALGIA

Fever and myalgia constitute the syndrome most commonly associated with zoonotic virus infection. Many of the numerous viruses belonging to the families listed in Table 180-1 probably cause this syndrome, but several viruses have been selected for inclusion in the table because of their prominent associations with the syndrome and their biomedical importance.

The syndrome typically begins with the abrupt onset of fever, chills, intense myalgia, and malaise. Patients may also report joint pains, but no true arthritis is detectable. Anorexia is characteristic and may be accompanied by nausea or even vomiting. Headache is common and may be severe, with photophobia and retroorbital pain. Physical findings are minimal and are usually confined to conjunctival injection with pain on palpation of muscles or the epigastrium. The duration of symptoms is quite variable but generally is 2 to 5 days, with a biphasic course in some instances. The spectrum of disease varies from subclinical to temporarily incapacitating.

Less constant findings include a maculopapular rash. Epistaxis may occur but does not necessarily indicate a bleeding diathesis. A minority of the cases caused by some viruses are known or suspected to include aseptic meningitis, but this diagnosis is difficult in remote areas, given the patients' photophobia and myalgia as well as the lack of opportunity to examine the CSF. Although pharyngitis may be noted or radiographic evidence of pulmonary infiltrates found in some cases,

these viruses are not primary respiratory pathogens. The differential diagnosis includes anicteric leptospirosis, rickettsial diseases, and the early stages of other syndromes discussed in this chapter. These diseases are often described as "flulike," but the usual absence of cough and coryza makes influenza an unlikely confounder except at the earliest stages.

Complete recovery is generally the outcome in this syndrome, although prolonged asthenia and nonspecific symptoms have been described in some cases, particularly after infection with LCM or dengue virus. Treatment is supportive, with aspirin avoided because of the potential for exacerbated bleeding and Reye's syndrome. Efforts at prevention are best based on vector control, which, however, may be expensive or impossible. For mosquito control, destruction of breeding sites is generally the most economically and environmentally sound approach. Measures taken by the individual to avoid the vector can be valuable. Avoiding the vector's habitat and times of peak activity, preventing the vector from entering dwellings by using screens or other barriers, judiciously applying arthropod repellents such as diethyltoluamide (DEET) to the skin, and wearing permethrin-impregnated clothing are all possible approaches, depending on the vector and its habits.

LYMPHOCYTIC CHORIOMENINGITIS LCM is transmitted from the common house mouse (*Mus musculus*) to humans by aerosols of excreta and secreta. LCM virus, an arenavirus, is maintained in the mouse mainly by vertical transmission from infected dams. The vertically infected mouse remains viremic for life, with high concentrations of virus in all tissues. Infected colonies of pet hamsters have also served as a link to humans. LCM virus is widely used in immunology laboratories as a model of T cell function and can silently infect cell cultures and passaged tumor lines, resulting in infections among scientists and animal caretakers. Patients with LCM may have a history of residence in rodent-infested housing or other exposure to rodents. An antibody prevalence of ~5 to 10% has been reported among adults from the United States, Argentina, and endemic areas of Germany.

LCM differs from the general syndrome of fever and myalgia in that its onset is gradual. Among the conditions occasionally associated with LCM are orchitis, transient alopecia, arthritis, pharyngitis, cough, and maculopapular rash. An estimated one-fourth of patients or fewer suffer a febrile phase of 3 to 6 days and then, after a brief remission, develop renewed fever accompanied by severe headache, nausea and vomiting, and meningeal signs lasting for about a week. These patients virtually always recover fully, as do the uncommon patients with clear-cut signs of encephalitis. Recovery may be delayed by transient hydrocephalus.

During the initial febrile phase, leukopenia and thrombocytopenia are common and virus can usually be isolated from blood. During the CNS phase of the illness, virus may be found in the CSF, but antibodies are present in blood. The pathogenesis of LCM is thought to resemble that following direct intracranial inoculation of the virus into adult mice; the onset of the immune response leads to T cell–mediated immunopathologic meningitis. During the meningeal phase, CSF mononuclear-cell counts range from the hundreds to the low thousands per microliter, and hypoglycorrhachia is found in one-third of cases. The IgM-capture ELISA of serum and CSF is usually positive; RT-PCR assays have been developed for application to CSF.

Infection with LCM virus should be suspected in acutely ill febrile patients with marked leukopenia and thrombocytopenia. In cases of aseptic meningitis, any of the following should suggest LCM: well-marked febrile prodrome, adult age, autumn seasonality, low CSF glucose levels, or CSF mononuclear cell counts of $>1000/\mu L$.

In pregnant women, LCM virus infection may lead to fetal invasion with consequent congenital hydrocephalus and chorioretinitis. Since the maternal infection may be mild, consisting of only a short febrile illness, antibodies to the virus should be sought in both the mother and the fetus in suspicious circumstances, particularly TORCH-negative neonatal hydrocephalus. [TORCH is a battery of tests encompassing *t*oxoplasmosis, *o*ther conditions (congenital syphilis and viruses), *ru*bella, *c*ytomegalovirus, and *h*erpes simplex virus.]

SANDFLY FEVER The sandfly *Phlebotomus papatasi* transmits sandfly fever. Female sandflies may be infected by the oral route as they take a blood meal and may transmit the virus to offspring when they lay their eggs after a second blood meal. This prominent transovarial pattern was the first to be recognized among dipterans and complicates virus control. A previous designation for sandfly fever, "3-day fever," instructively describes the brief, debilitating course associated with this essentially benign infection. There is neither a rash nor CNS involvement, and complete recovery is the rule.

Sandfly fever is found in the circum-Mediterranean area, extending to the east through the Balkans into China as well as into the Middle East and southwestern Asia. The vector is found in both rural and urban settings and is known for its small size, which enables it to penetrate standard mosquito screens and netting, and for its short flight range. Epidemics have been described in the wake of natural disasters and wars. In parts of Europe, sandfly populations and virus transmission were greatly reduced by the extensive residual spraying conducted after World War II to control malaria, and the incidence continues to be low. A common pattern of disease in endemic areas consists of high attack rates among travelers and military personnel with little or no disease in the local population, who are protected after childhood infection. More than 30 related phleboviruses are transmitted by sandflies and mosquitoes, but most are of unknown significance in terms of human health.

DENGUE FEVER All four distinct dengue viruses (dengue 1–4) have *Aedes aegypti* as their principal vector, and all cause a similar clinical syndrome. In rare cases, second infection with a serotype of dengue virus different from that involved in the primary infection leads to dengue HF with severe shock (see below). Sporadic cases are seen in the settings of endemic transmission and epidemic disease. Year-round transmission between latitudes 25°N and 25°S has been established, and seasonal forays of the viruses to points as far north as Philadelphia are thought to have taken place in the United States. Dengue fever is seen in the Caribbean region, including Puerto Rico. With increasing spread of the vector mosquito throughout the tropics and subtropics, large areas of the world have become vulnerable to the introduction of dengue viruses, particularly through air travel by infected humans, and both dengue fever and the related dengue HF are becoming increasingly common. Conditions favorable to dengue transmission exist in the southern United States, and bursts of dengue fever activity are to be expected in this region, particularly along the Mexican border, where water may be stored in containers and *A. aegypti* numbers may therefore be greatest: this mosquito, which is also an efficient vector of the yellow fever and chikungunya viruses, typically breeds near human habitation, using relatively fresh water from sources such as water jars, vases, discarded containers, coconut husks, and old tires. *A. aegypti* usually inhabits dwellings and bites during the day.

After an incubation period of 2 to 7 days, the typical patient experiences the sudden onset of fever, headache, retroorbital pain, and back pain along with the severe myalgia that gave rise to the colloquial designation "break-bone fever." There is often a macular rash on the first day as well as adenopathy, palatal vesicles, and scleral injection. The illness may last a week, with additional symptoms usually including anorexia, nausea or vomiting, marked cutaneous hypersensitivity, and—near the time of defervescence—a maculopapular rash beginning on the trunk and spreading to the extremities and the face. Epistaxis and scattered petechiae are often noted in uncomplicated dengue, and preexisting gastrointestinal lesions may bleed during the acute illness.

Laboratory findings include leukopenia, thrombocytopenia, and, in many cases, serum aminotransferase elevations. The diagnosis is made by IgM ELISA or paired serology during recovery or by antigen-detection ELISA or RT-PCR during the acute phase. Virus is readily isolated from blood in the acute phase if mosquito inoculation or mosquito cell culture is used.

COLORADO TICK FEVER Several hundred cases of Colorado tick fever are reported annually in the United States. The infection is acquired between March and November through the bite of an infected *Dermacentor andersoni* tick in mountainous western regions at altitudes of 1200 to 3000 m (4000 to 10,000 ft). Small mammals serve as the amplifying host. The most common presentation consists of fever and myalgia; meningoencephalitis is not uncommon, and hemorrhagic disease, pericarditis, myocarditis, orchitis, and pulmonary presentations are also reported. Rash develops in a substantial minority of cases. The disease usually lasts 7 to 10 days and is often biphasic. The most important differential diagnostic considerations since the beginning of the twentieth century have been Rocky Mountain spotted fever and tularemia. In Colorado, Colorado tick fever is much more common than Rocky Mountain spotted fever.

Infection of erythroblasts and other marrow cells by Colorado tick fever virus results in the appearance and persistence (for several weeks) of erythrocytes containing the virus. This feature, detected in smears stained by immunofluorescence, can be diagnostically helpful. The clinical laboratory detects leukopenia and thrombocytopenia.

OTHER VIRUSES CAUSING FEVER AND MYALGIA For a discussion of additional zoonotic viral infections presenting with fever and myalgia, see Chap. 180 in *Harrison's Online* (*www.harrisonsonline.com*).

ENCEPHALITIS

Arboviral encephalitis is a seasonal disease, commonly occurring in the warmer months. Its incidence varies markedly with time and place, depending on ecologic factors. The causative viruses differ substantially in terms of case-infection ratio (i.e., the ratio of clinical to subclinical infections), mortality, and residua (Table 180-3). Humans are not an important amplifier of these viruses.

All the viral encephalitides discussed in this section have a similar pathogenesis as far as is known. An infected arthropod ingests a blood meal from a human and infects the host. The initial period of viremia is thought to originate most commonly from the lymphoid system. Viremia leads to CNS invasion, presumably through infection of olfactory neuroepithelium with passage through the cribriform plate or through infection of brain capillaries and multifocal entry into the CNS. During the viremic phase, there may be little or no recognized disease except in the case of tick-borne flaviviral encephalitis, in which there may be a clearly delineated phase of fever and systemic illness. The disease process in the CNS arises partly from direct neuronal infection and subsequent damage and partly from edema, inflammation, and other indirect effects. The usual pathologic picture is one of focal necrosis of neurons, inflammatory glial nodules, and perivascular lymphoid cuffing; the severity and distribution of these abnormalities vary with the infecting virus. Involved areas display the "luxury perfusion" phenomenon, with normal or increased total blood flow and low oxygen extraction.

The typical patient presents with a prodrome of nonspecific constitutional symptoms, including fever, abdominal pain, vertigo, sore throat, and respiratory symptoms. Headache, meningeal signs, photophobia, and vomiting follow quickly. Involvement of deeper structures may be signaled by lethargy, somnolence, and intellectual deficit (as disclosed by the mental status examination or failure at serial 7 subtraction); more severely affected patients will be obviously disoriented and may be comatose. Tremors, loss of abdominal reflexes, cranial nerve palsies, hemiparesis, monoparesis, difficulty in swallowing, and frontal lobe signs are all common. Spinal and motor neuron diseases are documented with West Nile and Japanese encephalitis viruses. Convulsions and focal signs may be evident early or may appear during the course of the disease. Some patients present with an abrupt onset of fever, convulsions, and other signs of CNS involvement. The results of human infection range from no significant symptoms through febrile headache to aseptic meningitis and finally to

TABLE 180-3 *Prominent Features of Arboviral Encephalitis*

Virus	Natural Cycle	Incubation Period, Days	Annual No. of Cases	Case-to-Infection Ratio	Age of Cases	Case-Fatality Rate, %	Residua
La Crosse	*Aedes triseriatus–*chipmunk (transovarial component in mosquito also important)	~3–7	70 (U.S.)	<1:1000	<15 years	<0.5	Recurrent seizures in ~10%; severe deficits in rare cases; decreased school performance and behavioral change suspected in small proportion
St. Louis	*Culex tarsalis, C. pipiens, C. quinquefasciatus–*birds	4–21	85, with hundreds to thousands in epidemic years (U.S.)	<1:200	Milder cases in the young; more severe cases in adults >40 years old, particularly the elderly	7	Common in the elderly
Japanese	*Culex tritaeniorhyncus–*birds	5–15	>25,000	1:200–300	All ages; children in highly endemic areas	20–50	Common (approximately half of cases); may be severe
West Nile	*Culex* mosquitoes–birds	3–6	?	Very low	Mainly the elderly	5–10	Uncommon
Central European	*Ixodes ricinus–*rodents, insectivores	7–14	Thousands	1:12	All ages; milder in children	1–5	20%
Russian spring-summer	*I. persulcatus–*rodents, insectivores	7–14	Hundreds	—	All ages; milder in children	20	Approximately half of cases; often severe; limb-girdle paralysis
Powassan	*I. cookei–*wild mammals	~10	~1 (U.S.)	—	All ages; some predilection for children	~10	Common (approximately half of cases)
Eastern equine	*Culiseta melanura–*birds	~5–10	5 (U.S.)	1:40 adult 1:17 child	All ages; predilection for children	50–75	Common
Western equine	*Culex tarsalis–*birds	~5–10	~20 (U.S.)	1:1000 adult 1:50 child 1:1 infant	All ages; predilection for children <2 years old (increased mortality in elderly)	3–7	Common only among infants <1 year old
Venezuelan equine (epidemic)	Unknown (multiple mosquito species and horses in epidemics)	1–5	?	1:250 adult 1:25 child (approximate)	All ages; predilection for children	~10	—

full-blown encephalitis; the proportions and severity of these manifestations vary with the infecting virus.

The acute encephalitis usually lasts from a few days to as long as 2 to 3 weeks, but recovery may be slow, with weeks or months required for the return of maximal recoupable function. Common complaints during recovery include difficulty concentrating, fatigability, tremors, and personality changes. The acute illness requires management of a comatose patient who may have intracranial pressure elevations, inappropriate secretion of antidiuretic hormone, respiratory failure, and convulsions. There is no specific therapy for these viral encephalitides. The only practical preventive measures are vector management and personal protection against the arthropod transmitting the virus; for Japanese encephalitis or tick-borne encephalitis, vaccination should be considered in certain circumstances (see relevant sections below).

The diagnosis of arboviral encephalitis depends on the careful evaluation of a febrile patient with CNS disease, with rapid identification of treatable herpes simplex encephalitis, ruling out of brain abscess, exclusion of bacterial meningitis by serial CSF examination, and performance of laboratory studies to define the viral etiology. Leptospirosis, neurosyphilis, Lyme disease, cat-scratch fever, and newer viral encephalitides such as Nipah virus infection from Malaysia should be considered. The CSF examination usually shows a modest cell count—in the tens or hundreds or perhaps a few thousand. Early in the process, a significant proportion of these cells may be polymorphonuclear leukocytes, but usually there is a mononuclear cell predominance. CSF glucose levels are usually normal. There are exceptions to this pattern of findings. In eastern equine encephalitis, for example, polymorphonuclear leukocytes may predominate during the first 72 h of disease and hypoglycorrhachia may be detected. In LCM, lymphocyte counts may be in the thousands, and the glucose concen-

tration may be diminished. Experience with imaging studies is still evolving; clearly, however, both computed tomography (CT) and magnetic resonance imaging (MRI) may be normal, except for evidence of preexisting conditions, or sometimes may suggest diffuse edema. Several patients with eastern equine encephalitis have had focal abnormalities, and individuals with severe Japanese encephalitis have presented with bilateral thalamic lesions that have often been hemorrhagic. Electroencephalography usually shows diffuse abnormalities and is not directly helpful.

A humoral immune response is usually detectable at or near the onset of disease. Both serum and CSF should be examined for IgM antibodies. Virus generally cannot be isolated from blood or CSF, although Japanese encephalitis virus has been recovered from CSF in severe cases. Virus can be obtained from and viral antigen is present in brain tissue, although its distribution may be focal.

CALIFORNIA, LA CROSSE, AND JAMESTOWN CANYON VIRUS ENCEPHALITIS The isolation of California encephalitis virus established the California serogroup of viruses as a cause of encephalitis, and its use as a diagnostic antigen led to the description of many cases of "California encephalitis." In fact, however, this virus has been implicated in only a few cases of encephalitis, and the serologically related La Crosse virus is the major cause of encephalitis among viruses in the California serogroup. "California encephalitis" due to La Crosse virus infection is most commonly reported from the upper Midwest but is also found in other areas of the central and eastern United States, most often in West Virginia, Tennessee, North Carolina, and Georgia. The serogroup includes 13 other viruses, some of which may also be involved in human disease that is misattributed because of the complexity of the group's serology; these viruses include the Jamestown Canyon, snowshoe hare, Inkoo, and Trivittatus viruses, all of which have *Aedes* mosquitoes as their vector and all of which have a strong element of transovarial transmission in their natural cycles.

The mosquito vector of La Crosse virus is *A. triseriatus*. In addition to a prominent transovarial component of transmission, a mosquito can also become infected through feeding on viremic chipmunks and other mammals as well as through venereal transmission from another mosquito. The mosquito breeds in sites such as tree holes and abandoned tires and bites during daylight hours; these findings correlate with the risk factors for cases: recreation in forested areas, residence at the forest's edge, and the presence of abandoned tires around the home. Intensive environmental modification based on these findings has reduced the incidence of disease in a highly endemic area in the Midwest. Most cases occur from July through September. The Asian tiger mosquito, *A. albopictus*, efficiently transmits the virus to mice and also transmits the agent transovarially in the laboratory; this aggressive anthropophilic mosquito has the capacity to urbanize, and its possible impact on transmission to humans is of concern.

An antibody prevalence of ≥20% in endemic areas indicates that infection is common, but CNS disease has been recognized primarily in children <15 years of age. The illness varies from a picture of aseptic meningitis accompanied by confusion to severe and occasionally fatal encephalitis. Although there may be prodromal symptoms, the onset of CNS disease is sudden, with fever, headache, and lethargy often joined by nausea and vomiting, convulsions (in one-half of patients), and coma (in one-third of patients). Focal seizures, hemiparesis, tremor, aphasia, chorea, Babinski's sign, and other evidence of significant neurologic dysfunction are common, but residua are not. Perhaps 10% of patients have recurrent seizures in the succeeding months. Other serious sequelae are rare, although a decrease in scholastic standing has been reported and mild personality change has occasionally been suggested. Treatment is supportive over a 1- to 2-week acute phase during which status epilepticus, cerebral edema, and inappropriate secretion of antidiuretic hormone are important concerns. Ribavirin has been used in severe cases, and a clinical trial of this drug is under way.

The blood leukocyte count is commonly elevated, sometimes reaching levels of 20,000/μL, and there is usually a left shift. CSF cell counts are typically 30 to 500/μL with a mononuclear cell predominance (although 25 to 90% of cells are polymorphonuclear in some cases). The protein level is normal or slightly increased, and the glucose level is normal. Specific virologic diagnosis based on IgM-capture assays of serum and CSF is efficient. The only human anatomical site from which virus has been isolated is the brain.

Jamestown Canyon virus has been implicated in several cases of encephalitis in adults; in these cases the disease was usually associated with a significant respiratory illness at onset. Human infection with this virus has been documented in New York, Wisconsin, Ohio, Michigan, Ontario, and other areas of North America where the vector mosquito, *A. stimulans*, feeds on its main host, the white-tailed deer.

ST. LOUIS ENCEPHALITIS St. Louis encephalitis virus is transmitted between *Culex* mosquitoes and birds. This virus causes low-level endemic infection among rural residents of the western and central United States, where *C. tarsalis* is the vector (see "Western Equine Encephalitis," below), but the more urbanized mosquito species *C. pipiens* and *C. quinquefasciatus* have been responsible for epidemics resulting in hundreds or even thousands of cases in cities of the central and eastern United States. Most cases occur in June through October. The urban mosquitoes breed in accumulations of stagnant water and sewage with high organic content and readily bite humans in and around houses at dusk. The elimination of open sewers and trash-filled drainage systems is expensive and may not be possible, but screening of houses and implementation of personal protective measures may be an effective approach for individuals. The rural vector is most active at dusk and outdoors; its bites can be avoided by modification of activities and use of repellents.

Disease severity increases with age: infections that result in aseptic meningitis or mild encephalitis are concentrated in children and young adults, while severe and fatal cases primarily affect the elderly. Infection rates are similar in all age groups; thus the greater susceptibility of older persons to disease is a biologic consequence of aging. The disease has an abrupt onset, sometimes following a prodrome, and begins with fever, lethargy, confusion, and headache. In addition, nuchal rigidity, hypotonia, hyperreflexia, myoclonus, and tremor are common. Severe cases can include cranial nerve palsies, hemiparesis, and convulsions. Patients often complain of dysuria and may have viral antigen in urine as well as pyuria. The overall mortality is generally ~7% but may reach 20% among patients over the age of 60. Recovery is slow. Emotional lability, difficulties in concentration and memory, asthenia, and tremor are commonly prolonged in older patients.

The CSF of patients with St. Louis encephalitis usually contains tens to hundreds of cells, with a lymphocytic predominance and a normal glucose level. Leukocytosis with a left shift is often documented.

JAPANESE ENCEPHALITIS Japanese encephalitis virus is found throughout Asia, including far eastern Russia, Japan, China, India, Pakistan, and Southeast Asia, and causes occasional epidemics on western Pacific islands. The virus has been detected in the Torres Strait islands, and a human encephalitis case has been identified on the nearby Australian mainland. This flavivirus is particularly common in areas where irrigated rice fields attract the natural avian vertebrate hosts and provide abundant breeding sites for mosquitoes such as *C. tritaeniorhyncus*, which transmit the virus to humans. Additional amplification by pigs, which suffer abortion, and horses, which develop encephalitis, may be significant as well. Vaccination of these additional amplifying hosts may reduce the transmission of the virus. An effective, formalin-inactivated vaccine purified from mouse brain is produced in Japan and licensed for human use in the United States. It is given on days 0, 7, and 30 or—with some sacrifice in serum neutralizing titer—on days 0, 7, and 14. Vaccination is indicated for summer travelers to rural Asia, where the risk of clinical disease may be 0.05 to 2.1/10,000 per week (Table 107-5). The severe and often fatal disease reported in expatriates must be balanced against the 0.1 to 1% chance of a late systemic or cutaneous allergic reaction. These reactions are rarely fatal but may be severe and have been known to begin 1 to 9 days after vaccination, with associated pruritus, urticaria, and angioedema. Live attenuated vaccines are being used in China but are not recommended in the United States at this time.

WEST NILE VIRUS INFECTION West Nile virus is transmitted among wild birds by *Culex* mosquitoes in Africa, the Middle East, southern Europe, and Asia. It is a frequent cause of febrile disease without CNS involvement, but it occasionally causes aseptic meningitis and severe encephalitis; these serious infections are particularly common among the elderly. The febrile-myalgic syndrome caused by West Nile virus differs from many others by the frequent appearance of a maculopapular rash concentrated on the trunk and lymphadenopathy. Headache, ocular pain, sore throat, nausea and vomiting, and arthralgia (but not arthritis) are common accompaniments. In addition, the virus has been implicated in severe and fatal hepatic necrosis in Africa.

In 1996 West Nile virus caused >300 cases of CNS disease, with 10% mortality, in the Danube flood plain, including Bucharest. In 1999 the virus appeared in New York City and other areas of the northeastern United States, causing >60 cases of aseptic meningitis or encephalitis among humans as well as die-offs among crows, exotic zoo birds, and other avians. The encephalitis was most severe among the elderly and was often associated with notable muscle weakness and even with flaccid paralysis. The virus, thought to have been transmitted in New York City by the ubiquitous *C. pipiens* mosquito, spread as far west as Minnesota and Texas as well as north into Canada by 2002. It seems likely that further spread will occur, and involvement of new vectors may enhance transmission to humans.

West Nile virus falls into the same phylogenetic group of flaviviruses as St. Louis and Japanese encephalitis viruses, as do Murray

Valley and Rocio viruses. The latter two viruses are both maintained in mosquitoes and birds and produce a clinical picture resembling that of Japanese encephalitis. Murray Valley virus has caused occasional epidemics and sporadic cases in Australia. Rocio virus caused recurrent epidemics in a focal area of Brazil in 1975 to 1977 and then virtually disappeared.

CENTRAL EUROPEAN TICK-BORNE ENCEPHALITIS AND RUSSIAN SPRING-SUMMER ENCEPHALITIS A spectrum of tick-borne flaviviruses has been identified across the Eurasian land mass. Many are known mainly as agricultural pathogens (e.g., louping ill virus in the United Kingdom). From Scandinavia to the Urals, central European tick-borne encephalitis is transmitted by *Ixodes ricinus*. Human cases occur between April and October, with a peak in June and July. A related and more virulent virus is that of Russian spring-summer encephalitis, which is associated with *I. persulcatus* and is distributed from Europe across the Urals to the Pacific Ocean. The ticks transmit the disease primarily in the spring and early summer, with a lower rate of transmission later in summer. Small mammals are the vertebrate amplifiers for both viruses. The risk varies by geographic area and can be highly localized within a given area; human cases usually follow outdoor activities or consumption of raw milk from infected goats or other infected animals.

After an incubation period of 7 to 14 days or perhaps longer, the central European viruses classically result in a febrile-myalgic phase that lasts for 2 to 4 days and is thought to correlate with viremia. A subsequent remission for several days is followed by the recurrence of fever and the onset of meningeal signs. The CNS phase varies from mild aseptic meningitis, which is more common among younger patients, to severe encephalitis with coma, convulsions, tremors, and motor signs lasting for 7 to 10 days before improvement begins. Spinal and medullary involvement can lead to typical limb-girdle paralysis and to respiratory paralysis. Most patients recover, only a minority with significant deficits. Infections with the far eastern viruses generally run a more abrupt course. The encephalitic syndrome caused by these viruses sometimes begins without a remission and has more severe manifestations than the European syndrome. Mortality is high, and major sequelae—most notably, lower motor neuron paralyses of the proximal muscles of the extremities, trunk, and neck—are common.

In the early stage of the illness, virus may be isolated from the blood. In the CNS phase, IgM antibodies are detectable in serum and/or CSF. Thrombocytopenia sometimes develops during the initial febrile illness, which resembles the early hemorrhagic phase of some other tick-borne flaviviral infections, such as Kyasanur Forest disease. Other tick-borne flaviviruses are less common causes of encephalitis, including louping ill virus in the United Kingdom and Powassan virus.

There is no specific therapy for infection with these viruses. However, effective alum-adjuvanted, formalin-inactivated vaccines are produced in Austria, Germany, and Russia. Two doses of the Austrian vaccine separated by an interval of 1 to 3 months appear to be effective in the field, and antibody responses are similar when vaccine is given on days 0 and 14. Other vaccines have elicited similar neutralizing antibody titers. Since rare cases of postvaccination Guillain-Barré syndrome have been reported, vaccination should be reserved for persons likely to experience rural exposure in an endemic area during the season of transmission. Cross-neutralization for the central European and far eastern strains has been established, but there are no published field studies on cross-protection of formalin-inactivated vaccines. Because 0.2 to 4% of ticks in endemic areas may be infected, tick bites raise the issue of immunoglobulin prophylaxis. Prompt administration of high-titered specific preparations should probably be undertaken, although no controlled data are available to prove the efficacy of this measure. Immunoglobulin should not be administered late because of the risk of antibody-mediated enhancement.

POWASSAN ENCEPHALITIS Powassan virus is a member of the tick-borne encephalitis virus complex and is transmitted by *I. cookei* among small mammals in eastern Canada and the United States, where it has been responsible for 20 recognized cases of human disease. Other ticks may

transmit the virus in a wider geographic area, and there is some concern that *I. scapularis* (also called *I. dammini*), a competent vector in the laboratory, may become involved as it becomes more prominent in the United States. Patients with Powassan encephalitis—often children—present in May through December after outdoor exposure and an incubation period thought to be ~1 week. Powassan encephalitis is severe, and sequelae are common.

EASTERN EQUINE ENCEPHALITIS Eastern equine encephalitis is found primarily within endemic swampy foci along the eastern coast of the United States, with a few inland foci as far removed as Michigan. Human cases present from June through October, when the bird–*Culiseta* mosquito cycle spills over into other mosquito species such as *A. sollicitans* or *A. vexans*, which are more likely to bite mammals. There is concern over the potential role of the introduced anthropophilic mosquito species *A. albopictus*, which has been found to be naturally infected and is an effective vector in the laboratory. Horses are a common target for the virus; contact with unvaccinated horses may be associated with human disease, but horses probably do not play a significant role in amplification of the virus.

Eastern equine encephalitis is one of the most destructive of the arboviral conditions, with a brusque onset, rapid progression, high mortality, and frequent residua. This severity is reflected in the extensive necrotic lesions and polymorphonuclear infiltrates found at postmortem examination of the brain and the acute polymorphonuclear CSF pleocytosis often occurring during the first 1 to 3 days of disease. In addition, leukocytosis with a left shift is a common feature. A formalin-inactivated vaccine has been used to protect laboratory workers but is not generally available or applicable.

WESTERN EQUINE ENCEPHALITIS The primary maintenance cycle for western equine encephalitis virus in the United States is between *C. tarsalis* and birds, principally sparrows and finches. Equines and humans become infected, and both species suffer encephalitis without amplifying the virus in nature. St. Louis encephalitis is transmitted in a similar cycle in the same region but causes human disease about a month earlier than the period (July through October) in which western equine encephalitis virus is active. Large epidemics of western equine encephalitis took place in the western and central United States and Canada during the 1930s to 1950s, but in recent years the disease has been uncommon. There were 41 reported cases in the United States in 1987 but only 5 reported cases from 1988 to 2001. This decline in incidence may reflect in part the integrated approach to mosquito management that has been employed in irrigation projects and the increasing use of agricultural pesticides; it almost certainly reflects the increased tendency for humans to be indoors behind closed windows at dusk, the peak period of biting by the major vector.

Western equine encephalitis virus causes a typical diffuse viral encephalitis with an increased attack rate and increased morbidity in the young, particularly children <2 years old. In addition, mortality is high among the young and the very elderly. One-third of individuals who have convulsions during the acute illness have subsequent seizure activity. Infants <1 year old—particularly those in the first months of life—are at serious risk of motor and intellectual damage. Twice as many males as females develop clinical encephalitis after 5 to 9 years of age; this difference may be related to greater outdoor exposure of boys to the vector but is also likely to be due in part to biologic differences. A formalin-inactivated vaccine has been used to protect laboratory workers but is not generally available or applicable.

VENEZUELAN EQUINE ENCEPHALITIS There are six known types of virus in the Venezuelan equine encephalitis complex. An important distinction is between the "epizootic" viruses (subtypes IAB and IC) and the "enzootic" viruses (subtypes ID to IF and types II to VI). The epizootic viruses have an unknown natural cycle but periodically cause extensive epidemics in equines and humans in the Americas. These epidemics rely on the high-level viremia in horses and mules that results in the infection of several species of mosquitoes, which in turn infect humans and perpetuate virus transmission. Humans also have high-level viremia but probably are not important in virus transmission. Enzootic viruses are found primarily in humid tropical forest habitats and are maintained between *Culex* mosquitoes and rodents; these viruses cause human disease but are not pathogenic for horses and do not cause epizootics.

Epizootics of Venezuelan equine encephalitis occurred repeatedly in Venezuela, Colombia, Ecuador, Peru, and other South American countries at intervals of ≤10 years from the 1930s until 1969, when a massive epizootic spread throughout Central America and Mexico, reaching southern Texas in 1972. Genetic sequencing of the virus from the 1969 to 1972 outbreak suggested that it originated from residual "un-inactivated" virus in veterinary vaccines. The outbreak was terminated in Texas with the use of a live attenuated vaccine (TC-83) originally developed for human use by the U.S. Army; this virus was then used for further production of inactivated veterinary vaccines. No further epizootic disease was identified until 1995 and subsequently, when additional epizootics took place in Colombia, Venezuela, and Mexico. The viruses involved in these epizootics as well as previously epizootic subtype IC viruses have been shown to be close phylogenetic relatives of known enzootic subtype ID viruses. This finding suggests that active evolution and selection of epizootic viruses are under way in northern South America.

During epizootics, extensive human infection is the rule, with clinical disease in 10 to 60% of infected individuals. Most infections result in notable acute febrile disease, while relatively few result in encephalitis. A low rate of CNS invasion is supported by the absence of encephalitis among the many infections resulting from exposure to aerosols in the laboratory or from vaccine accidents. The most recent large epizootic of Venezuelan equine encephalitis occurred in Colombia and Venezuela in 1995; of the >85,000 clinical cases, 4% (with a higher proportion among children than adults) included neurologic symptoms and 300 ended in death.

Enzootic strains of Venezuelan equine encephalitis virus are common causes of acute febrile disease, particularly in areas such as the Florida Everglades and the humid Atlantic coast of Central America. Encephalitis has been documented only in the Florida infections; the three cases were caused by type II enzootic virus, also called *Everglades virus*. All three patients had preexisting cerebral disease. Extrapolation from the rate of genetic change suggests that Everglades virus may have been introduced into Florida <200 years ago and that it is most closely related to the ID subtypes that appear to have given evolutionary rise to the epizootic strains active in South America.

The prevention of epizootic Venezuelan equine encephalitis depends on vaccination of horses with the attenuated TC-83 vaccine or with an inactivated vaccine prepared from that strain. Humans can be protected with similar vaccines, but the use of such products is restricted to laboratory personnel because of reactogenicity and limited availability. In addition, wild-type virus and perhaps TC-83 vaccine may have some degree of fetal pathogenicity. Enzootic viruses are genetically and antigenically different from epizootic viruses, and protection against the former with vaccines prepared from the latter is relatively ineffective.

ARTHRITIS AND RASH

True arthritis is a common accompaniment of several viral diseases, such as rubella (caused by a non-alphavirus togavirus), parvovirus B19 infection, and hepatitis B; it is an occasional accompaniment of infection due to mumps virus, enteroviruses, herpesviruses, and adenoviruses. It is not generally appreciated that the alphaviruses are also common causes of arthritis. In fact, the alphaviruses discussed below all cause acute febrile diseases accompanied by the development of true arthritis and a maculopapular rash. Rheumatic involvement includes arthralgia alone, periarticular swelling, and (less commonly) joint effusions. Most of these diseases are less severe and have fewer articular manifestations in children than in adults. In temperate cli-

mates, these are summer diseases. No specific therapy or licensed vaccines exist.

SINDBIS VIRUS INFECTION   Sindbis virus is transmitted among birds by mosquitoes. Infections with the northern European strains of this virus (which cause, for example, Pogosta disease in Finland, Karelian fever in the independent states of the former Soviet Union, and Okelbo disease in Sweden) and with the genetically related southern African strains are particularly likely to result in the arthritis-rash syndrome. Exposure to a rural environment is commonly associated with this infection, which has an incubation period of <1 week.

The disease begins with rash and arthralgia. Constitutional symptoms are not marked, and fever is modest or lacking altogether. The rash, which lasts about a week, begins on the trunk, spreads to the extremities, and evolves from macules to papules that often vesiculate. The arthritis of this condition is multiarticular, migratory, and incapacitating, with resolution of the acute phase in a few days. Wrists, ankles, phalangeal joints, knees, elbows, and—to a much lesser extent—proximal and axial joints are involved. Persistence of joint pains and occasionally of arthritis is a major problem and may go on for months or even years despite a lack of deformity.

CHIKUNGUNYA VIRUS INFECTION   It is likely that chikungunya virus ("that which bends up") is of African origin and is maintained among nonhuman primates on that continent by *Aedes* mosquitoes of the subgenus *Stegomyia* in a fashion similar to yellow fever virus. Like yellow fever virus, chikungunya virus is readily transmitted among humans in urban areas by *A. aegypti*. The *A. aegypti*–chikungunya virus transmission cycle has also been introduced into Asia, where it poses a prominent health problem. The disease is endemic in rural areas of Africa, and intermittent epidemics take place in towns and cities of Africa and Asia. Chikungunya is one more reason (in addition to dengue and yellow fever) that *A. aegypti* must be controlled.

Full-blown disease is most common among adults, in whom the clinical picture may be dramatic. The abrupt onset follows an incubation period of 2 to 3 days. Fever and severe arthralgia are accompanied by chills and constitutional symptoms such as headache, photophobia, conjunctival injection, anorexia, nausea, and abdominal pain. Migratory polyarthritis mainly affects the small joints of the hands, wrists, ankles, and feet, with lesser involvement of the larger joints. Rash may appear at the outset or several days into the illness; its development often coincides with defervescence, which takes place around day 2 or day 3 of disease. The rash is most intense on the trunk and limbs and may desquamate. Petechiae are occasionally seen, and epistaxis is not uncommon, but this virus is not a regular cause of the HF syndrome, even in children. A few patients develop leukopenia. Elevated levels of aspartate aminotransferase (AST) and C-reactive protein have been described, as have mildly decreased platelet counts. Recovery may require weeks. Some older patients continue to suffer from stiffness, joint pain, and recurrent effusions for several years; this persistence may be especially common in HLA-B27 patients. An investigational live attenuated vaccine has been developed but requires further testing.

A related virus, O'nyong-nyong, caused a major epidemic of arthritis and rash involving at least 2 million people as it moved across eastern and central Africa in the 1960s. After its mysterious emergence, the virus virtually disappeared, leaving only occasional evidence of its persistence in Kenya until a transient resurgence of epidemic activity in 1997.

EPIDEMIC POLYARTHRITIS (ROSS RIVER VIRUS INFECTION)   Ross River virus has caused epidemics of distinctive clinical disease in Australia since the beginning of the twentieth century and continues to be responsible for thousands of cases in rural and suburban areas annually. The virus is transmitted by *A. vigilax* and other mosquitoes, and its persistence is thought to involve transovarial transmission. No definitive vertebrate host has been identified, but several mammalian species, including wallabies, have been suggested. Endemic transmission has also been documented in New Guinea, and in 1979 the virus swept through the eastern Pacific Islands, causing hundreds of thousands of illnesses.

The virus was carried from island to island by infected humans and was believed to have been transmitted among humans by *A. polynesiensis* and *A. aegypti.*

The incubation period is 7 to 11 days long, and the onset of illness is sudden, with joint pain usually ushering in the disease. The rash generally develops coincidentally or follows shortly but in some cases precedes joint pains by several days. Constitutional symptoms such as low-grade fever, asthenia, myalgia, headache, and nausea are not prominent and indeed are absent in many cases. Most patients are incapacitated for considerable periods by joint involvement, which interferes with sleeping, walking, and grasping. Wrist, ankle, metacarpophalangeal, interphalangeal, and knee joints are the most commonly involved, although toes, shoulders, and elbows may be affected with some frequency. Periarticular swelling and tenosynovitis are common, and one-third of patients have true arthritis. Only half of all arthritis patients can resume normal activities within 4 weeks, and 10% still must limit their activity at 3 months. Occasional patients are symptomatic for 1 to 3 years but without progressive arthropathy. Aspirin and nonsteroidal anti-inflammatory drugs are effective for the treatment of symptoms.

Clinical laboratory values are normal or variable in Ross River virus infection. Tests for rheumatoid factor and antinuclear antibodies are negative, and the erythrocyte sedimentation rate is acutely elevated. Joint fluid contains 1000 to 60,000 mononuclear cells per microliter, and Ross River virus antigen is demonstrable in macrophages. IgM antibodies are valuable in the diagnosis of this infection, although they occasionally persist for years. The isolation of the virus from blood by mosquito inoculation or mosquito cell culture is possible early in the illness. Because of the great economic impact of annual epidemics in Australia, an inactivated vaccine is being developed and has been found to be protective in mice.

Perhaps because of the local interest in arboviruses in general and in Ross River virus in particular, other arthritogenic arboviruses have been identified in Australia, including Gan Gan virus, a member of the family Bunyaviridae; Kokobera virus, a flavivirus; and Barmah Forest virus, an alphavirus. The last virus is a common cause of infection and must be differentiated from Ross River virus by specific testing.

HEMORRHAGIC FEVERS

The viral HF syndrome is a constellation of findings based on vascular instability and decreased vascular integrity. An assault, direct or indirect, on the microvasculature leads to increased permeability and (particularly when platelet function is decreased) to actual disruption and local hemorrhage. Blood pressure is decreased, and in severe cases shock supervenes. Cutaneous flushing and conjunctival suffusion are examples of common, observable abnormalities in the control of local circulation. The hemorrhage is inconstant and is in most cases an indication of widespread vascular damage rather than a life-threatening loss of blood volume. Disseminated intravascular coagulation (DIC) is occasionally found in any severely ill patient with HF but is thought to occur regularly only in the early phases of HF with renal syndrome, Crimean-Congo HF, and perhaps some cases of filovirus HF. In some viral HF syndromes, specific organs may be particularly impaired, such as the kidney in HF with renal syndrome, the lung in hantavirus pulmonary syndrome, or the liver in yellow fever, but in all these diseases the generalized circulatory disturbance is critically important.

The pathogenesis of HF is poorly understood and varies among the viruses regularly implicated in the syndrome, which number more than a dozen. In some cases direct damage to the vascular system or even to parenchymal cells of target organs is important, whereas in others soluble mediators are thought to play the major role. The acute phase in most cases of HF is associated with ongoing virus replication and viremia. Exceptions are the hantavirus diseases and dengue HF/dengue shock syndrome (DHF/DSS), in which the immune response plays a major pathogenic role.

The HF syndromes all begin with fever and myalgia, usually of abrupt onset. Within a few days the patient presents for medical atten-

tion because of increasing prostration that is often accompanied by severe headache, dizziness, photophobia, hyperesthesia, abdominal or chest pain, anorexia, nausea or vomiting, and other gastrointestinal disturbances. Initial examination often reveals only an acutely ill patient with conjunctival suffusion, tenderness to palpation of muscles or abdomen, and borderline hypotension or postural hypotension, perhaps with tachycardia. Petechiae (often best visualized in the axillae), flushing of the head and thorax, periorbital edema, and proteinuria are common. Levels of AST are usually elevated at presentation or within a day or two thereafter. Hemoconcentration from vascular leakage, which is usually evident, is most marked in hantavirus diseases and in DHF/DSS. The seriously ill patient progresses to more severe symptoms and develops shock and other findings typical of the causative virus. Shock, multifocal bleeding, and CNS involvement (encephalopathy, coma, convulsions) are all poor prognostic signs.

One of the major diagnostic clues is travel to an endemic area within the incubation period for a given syndrome (Table 180-4). Except for Seoul, dengue, and yellow fever virus infections, which have urban vectors, travel to a rural setting is especially suggestive of a diagnosis of HF.

Early recognition is important because of the need for virus-specific therapy and supportive measures, including prompt, atraumatic hospitalization; judicious fluid therapy that takes into account the patient's increased capillary permeability; administration of cardiotonic drugs; use of pressors to maintain blood pressure at levels that will support renal perfusion; treatment of the relatively common secondary bacterial infections; replacement of clotting factors and platelets as indicated; and the usual precautionary measures used in the treatment of patients with hemorrhagic diatheses. DIC should be treated only if clear laboratory evidence of its existence is found and if laboratory monitoring of therapy is feasible; there is no proven benefit of such therapy. The available evidence suggests that HF patients have a decreased cardiac output and will respond poorly to fluid loading as it is often practiced in the treatment of shock associated with bacterial sepsis. Specific therapy is available for several of the HF syndromes. In addition, several diseases considered in the differential diagnosis—malaria, shigellosis, typhoid, leptospirosis, relapsing fever, and rickettsial disease—are treatable and potentially lethal. Strict barrier nursing and other precautions against infection of medical staff and visitors are indicated in HF except that due to hantaviruses, yellow fever, Rift Valley fever, and dengue.

LASSA FEVER Lassa virus is known to cause endemic and epidemic disease in Nigeria, Sierra Leone, Guinea, and Liberia, although it is probably more widely distributed in West Africa. This virus and its relatives exist elsewhere in Africa, but their health significance is unknown. Like other arenaviruses, Lassa virus is spread to humans by small-particle aerosols from chronically infected rodents and may also be acquired during the capture or eating of these animals. It can be transmitted by close person-to-person contact. The virus is often present in urine during convalescence and is suspected to be present in seminal fluid early in recovery. Nosocomial spread has occurred but is uncommon if proper sterile parenteral techniques are used. Individuals of all ages and both sexes are affected; the incidence of disease is highest in the dry season, but transmission takes place yearround. In countries where Lassa virus is endemic, Lassa fever can be a prominent cause of febrile disease. For example, in one hospital in Sierra Leone, laboratory-confirmed Lassa fever is consistently responsible for one-fifth of admissions to the medical wards. There are probably tens of thousands of Lassa fever cases annually in West Africa alone.

The average case has a gradual onset (among the HF agents, only the arenaviruses are typically associated with a gradual onset) that gives way to more severe constitutional symptoms and prostration. Bleeding is seen in only ~15 to 30% of cases. A maculopapular rash is often noted in light-skinned Lassa patients. Effusions are common,

TABLE 180-4 *Viral Hemorrhagic Fever (HF) Syndromes and Their Distribution*

Disease	Incubation Period, Days	Case-Infection Ratio	Case-Fatality Rate, %	Geographic Range	Target Population
Lassa fever	5–16	Mild infections probably common	15	West Africa	All ages, both sexes
South American HF	7–14	Most infections (more than half) result in disease	15–30	Selected rural areas of Bolivia, Argentina, Venezuela, and Brazil	Bolivia: Men in countryside; all ages, both sexes in villages. Argentina: All ages, both sexes; excess exposure and disease in men. Venezuela: All ages, both sexes
Rift Valley fever	2–5	~1:100[a]	~50	Sub-Saharan Africa, Madagascar, Egypt	All ages, both sexes; more often diagnosed in men; preexisting liver disease may predispose
Crimean-Congo HF	3–12	≥1:5	15–30	Africa, Middle East, Balkans, southern region of former Soviet Union, western China	All ages, both sexes; men more exposed in some settings
HF with renal syndrome	9–35	Hantaan, >1:1.25; Puumala, 1:20	5–15, Hantaan; <1, Puumala	Worldwide, depending on rodent reservoir	Excess of male patients (partly due to greater exposure); mainly adults
Hantavirus pulmonary syndrome	~7–28	Very high	40–50	Americas	Excess of male patients due to some occupational exposure; mainly adults
Marburg or Ebola HF	3–16	High	25–90	Sub-Saharan Africa	All ages, both sexes; children less exposed
Yellow fever	3–6	1:2–1:20	20	Africa, South America	All ages, both sexes; adults more exposed in jungle setting; preexisting flavivirus immunity may cross-protect
Dengue HF/dengue shock syndrome	2–7	1:10,000, nonimmune; 1:100, heterologous immune	<1 with supportive treatment	Tropics and subtropics worldwide	Predominantly children; previous heterologous dengue infection predisposes to HF
Kyasanur Forest/ Omsk HF	3–8	Variable	0.5–10	Mysore State, India/ western Siberia	Variable

[a] Figure is for HF cases only. Most infections with Rift Valley fever virus result in fever and myalgia rather than HF.

and male-dominant pericarditis may develop late. The fetal death rate is 92% in the last trimester, when maternal mortality is also increased from the usual 15% to 30%; these figures suggest that interruption of the pregnancy of infected women should be considered. White blood cell counts are normal or slightly elevated, and platelet counts are normal or somewhat low. Deafness coincides with clinical improvement in ~20% of cases and is permanent and bilateral in some. Reinfection may occur but has not been associated with severe disease.

High-level viremia or a high serum concentration of AST statistically predicts a fatal outcome. Thus patients with an AST level of >150 IU/mL should be treated with intravenous ribavirin. This antiviral nucleoside analogue appears to be effective in reducing mortality from rates among retrospective controls, and its only major side effect is reversible anemia that usually does not require transfusion. The drug should be given by slow intravenous infusion in a dose of 32 mg/kg; this dose should be followed by 16 mg/kg every 6 h for 4 days and then by 8 mg/kg every 8 h for 6 days.

SOUTH AMERICAN HF SYNDROMES (ARGENTINE, BOLIVIAN, VENEZUELAN, AND BRAZILIAN) These diseases are similar to one another clinically, but their epidemiology differs with the habits of their rodent reservoirs and the interactions of these animals with humans (Table 180-4). Person-to-person or nosocomial transmission is rare but has occurred.

The basic disease resembles Lassa fever, with two marked differ-

ences. First, thrombocytopenia—often marked—is the rule, and bleeding is quite common. Second, CNS dysfunction is much more common than in Lassa fever and is often manifest by marked confusion, tremors of the upper extremities and tongue, and cerebellar signs. Some cases follow a predominantly neurologic course, with a poor prognosis. The clinical laboratory is helpful in diagnosis since thrombocytopenia, leukopenia, and proteinuria are typical findings.

Argentine HF is readily treated with convalescent-phase plasma given within the first 8 days of illness. In the absence of passive antibody therapy, intravenous ribavirin in the dose recommended for Lassa fever is likely to be effective in all the South American HF syndromes. The transmission of the disease from men convalescing from Argentine HF to their wives suggests the need for counseling of arenavirus HF patients concerning the avoidance of intimate contacts for several weeks after recovery. A safe, effective, live attenuated vaccine exists for Argentine HF. In experimental animals, this vaccine is cross-protective against the Bolivian HF virus.

RIFT VALLEY FEVER The mosquito-borne Rift Valley fever virus is also a pathogen of domestic animals such as sheep, cattle, and goats. It is maintained in nature by transovarial transmission in floodwater *Aedes* mosquitoes and presumably also has a vertebrate amplifier. Epizootics and epidemics occur when sheep or cattle become infected during particularly heavy rains; developing high-level viremia, these animals infect many different species of mosquitoes. Remote sensing via satellite can detect the ecologic changes associated with high rainfall that predict the likelihood of Rift Valley fever transmission; it can also detect the special depressions from which the floodwater *Aedes* mosquito vectors emerge. In addition, the virus is infectious when transmitted by contact with blood or aerosols from domestic animals or their abortuses. The slaughtered meat is not infectious; anaerobic glycolysis in postmortem tissues results in an acidic environment that rapidly inactivates Bunyaviridae such as Rift Valley fever virus and Crimean-Congo HF virus. The natural range of Rift Valley fever virus is confined to sub-Saharan Africa, where its circulation is markedly enhanced by substantial rainfall such as that which occurred during the El Niño phenomenon of 1997; subsequent spread to the Arabian Peninsula caused epidemic disease in 2000. The virus has also been found in Madagascar and has been introduced into Egypt, where it caused major epidemics in 1977 to 1979, 1993, and subsequently. Neither person-to-person nor nosocomial transmission has been documented.

Rift Valley fever virus is unusual in that it causes at least four different clinical syndromes. Most infections are manifested as the febrile-myalgic syndrome. A small proportion result in HF with especially prominent liver involvement. Perhaps 10% of otherwise mild infections lead to retinal vasculitis; funduscopic examination reveals edema, hemorrhages, and infarction, and some patients have permanently impaired vision. A small proportion of cases (<1 in 200) are followed by typical viral encephalitis. One of the complicated syndromes does not appear to predispose to another.

There is no proven therapy for any of the syndromes described above. The sensitivity of animal models of Rift Valley fever to antibody or ribavirin therapy suggests that either could be given intravenously to persons with HF. Both retinal disease and encephalitis occur after the acute febrile syndrome has ended and serum neutralizing antibody has developed—events suggesting that only supportive care need be given. Epidemic disease is best prevented by vaccination of livestock. The established ability of this virus to propagate after an introduction into Egypt suggests that other potentially receptive areas, including the United States, should have a response ready for such an eventuality. It seems likely that this disease, like Venezuelan equine encephalitis, can be controlled only with adequate stocks of an effective live attenuated vaccine, and there are no such global stocks. A formalin-inactivated vaccine confers immunity to humans, but quantities are limited and three injections are required; this vaccine is recommended for exposed laboratory workers and for veterinarians working in sub-Saharan Africa.

CRIMEAN-CONGO HF This severe HF syndrome has a wide geographic distribution, potentially being found wherever ticks of the genus *Hyalomma* occur (Table 180-4). The propensity of these ticks to feed on domestic livestock and certain wild mammals means that veterinary serosurveys are the most effective mechanism for the surveillance of virus circulation in a region. Human infection is acquired via a tick bite or during the crushing of infected ticks. Domestic animals do not become ill but do develop viremia; thus there is danger of infection at the time of slaughter and for a brief interval thereafter (through contact with hides or carcasses). Cases have followed sheep shearing. An epidemic in South Africa was associated with slaughter of tick-infested ostriches. Nosocomial epidemics are common and are usually related to extensive blood exposure or needle sticks.

Although generally similar to other HF syndromes, Crimean-Congo HF causes extensive liver damage, resulting in jaundice in some cases. Clinical laboratory values indicate DIC and show elevations in AST, creatine phosphokinase, and bilirubin. Patients with fatal cases generally have more marked changes, even in the early days of illness, and also develop leukocytosis rather than leukopenia. Thrombocytopenia is also more marked and develops earlier in cases with a fatal outcome.

No controlled trials have been performed with intravenous ribavirin, but clinical experience and retrospective comparison of patients with ominous clinical laboratory values suggest that ribavirin is efficacious and should be given. No human or veterinary vaccines are recommended.

HF WITH RENAL SYNDROME This disease, the first to be identified as an HF, is widely distributed over Europe and Asia; the major causative viruses and their rodent reservoirs on these two continents are Puumala virus (bank vole, *Clethrionomys glareolus*) and Hantaan virus (striped field mouse, *Apodemus agrarius*), respectively. Other potential causative viruses exist, including Dobrava virus (yellow-necked field mouse, *A. flavicollus*), which causes severe HF with renal syndrome in the Balkans. Seoul virus is associated with the Norway or sewer rat, *Rattus norvegicus*, and has a worldwide distribution through the migration of the rodent; it is associated with mild or moderate HF with renal syndrome in Asia, but in many areas of the world the human disease has been difficult to identify. Most cases occur in rural residents or vacationers; the exception is Seoul virus disease, which may be acquired in an urban or rural setting or from contaminated laboratory rat colonies. Classic Hantaan disease in Korea (Korean HF) and in rural China (epidemic HF) is most common in spring and fall and is related to rodent density and agricultural practices. Human infection is acquired primarily through aerosols of rodent urine, although virus is also present in saliva and feces. Patients with hantavirus diseases are not infectious. HF with renal syndrome is the most important form of HF today, with >100,000 cases of severe disease in Asia annually and milder Puumala infections numbering in the thousands as well.

Severe cases of HF with renal syndrome caused by Hantaan virus evolve in identifiable stages: the febrile stage with myalgia, lasting 3 to 4 days; the hypotensive stage, often associated with shock and lasting from a few hours to 48 h; the oliguric stage with renal failure, lasting 3 to 10 days; and the polyuric stage with diuresis and hyposthenuria.

The *febrile period* is initiated by the abrupt onset of fever, headache, severe myalgia, thirst, anorexia, and often nausea and vomiting. Photophobia, retroorbital pain, and pain on ocular movement are common, and the vision may become blurred with ciliary body inflammation. Flushing over the face, the V area of the neck, and the back are characteristic, as are pharyngeal injection, periorbital edema, and conjunctival suffusion. Petechiae often develop in areas of pressure, the conjunctivae, and the axillae. Back pain and tenderness to percussion at the costovertebral angle reflect massive retroperitoneal edema. Laboratory evidence of mild to moderate DIC is present. Other laboratory findings include proteinuria and an active urinary sediment.

The *hypotensive phase* is ushered in by falling blood pressure and sometimes by shock. The relative bradycardia typical of the febrile phase is replaced by tachycardia. Kinin activation is marked. The rising hematocrit reflects increasing vascular leakage. Leukocytosis with a left shift develops, and thrombocytopenia continues. Atypical lymphocytes—which in fact are activated CD8+ and to a lesser extent CD4+ T cells—circulate. Proteinuria is marked, and the urine's specific gravity falls to 1.010. The renal circulation is congested and compromised from local and systemic circulatory changes resulting in necrosis of tubules, particularly at the corticomedullary junction, and oliguria.

During the *oliguric phase*, hemorrhagic tendencies continue, probably in large part because of uremic bleeding defects. The oliguria persists for 3 to 10 days before renal function returns and marks the onset of the *polyuric stage*, which carries the danger of dehydration and electrolyte abnormalities.

Mild cases of HF with renal syndrome may be much less stereotypical. The presentation may include only fever, gastrointestinal abnormalities, and transient oliguria followed by hyposthenuria.

HF with renal syndrome should be suspected in patients with rural exposure in an endemic area. Prompt recognition of the disease will permit rapid hospitalization and expectant management of shock and renal failure. Useful clinical laboratory parameters include leukocytosis, which may be leukemoid and is associated with a left shift; thrombocytopenia; and proteinuria. Mainstays of therapy are the management of shock, reliance on pressors, modest crystalloid infusion, intravenous use of human serum albumin, and treatment of renal failure with prompt dialysis for the usual indications. Hydration may result in pulmonary edema, and hypertension should be avoided because of the possibility of intracranial hemorrhage. Use of intravenous ribavirin has reduced mortality and morbidity in severe cases provided treatment is begun within the first 4 days of illness. The case-fatality ratio may be as high as 15% but with proper therapy should be <5%. Sequelae have not been definitely established, but there is a correlation in the United States between chronic hypertensive renal failure and the presence of antibodies to Seoul virus.

Infections with Puumala virus, the most common cause of HF with renal syndrome in Europe, result in a much attenuated picture but the same general presentation. The syndrome may be referred to by its former name, *nephropathia epidemica*. Bleeding manifestations are found in only 10% of cases, hypotension rather than shock is usually seen, and oliguria is present in only about half of patients. The dominant features may be fever, abdominal pain, proteinuria, mild oliguria, and sometimes blurred vision or glaucoma followed by polyuria and hyposthenuria in recovery. Mortality is <1%.

The diagnosis is readily made by IgM-capture ELISA, which should be positive at admission or within 24 to 48 h thereafter. The isolation of virus is difficult, but RT-PCR of a blood clot collected early in the clinical course or of tissues obtained postmortem will give positive results. Such testing is usually undertaken only if definitive identification of the infecting viral species is required or if molecular epidemiologic questions exist.

HANTAVIRUS PULMONARY SYNDROME Hantavirus pulmonary syndrome was discovered in 1993, but retrospective identification of cases by immunohistochemistry (1978) and serology (1959) support the idea that it is a recently discovered rather than a truly new disease. The causative viruses are hantaviruses of a distinct phylogenetic lineage that is associated with the rodent subfamily Sigmodontinae. Sin Nombre virus chronically infects the deer mouse (*Peromyscus maniculatus*) and is the most important virus causing hantavirus pulmonary syndrome in the United States. The disease is also caused by a Sin Nombre virus variant from the white-footed mouse (*P. leucopus*), by Black Creek Canal virus (*Sigmodon hispidus*, the cotton rat), and by Bayou virus (*Oryzomys palustris*, the rice rat). Several other related viruses cause the disease in South America, but Andes virus is unusual in that it, alone among hantaviruses, has been implicated in human-to-human transmission. The disease is linked to rodent exposure and particularly affects rural residents living in dwellings permeable to rodent entry or working at occupations that pose a risk of rodent exposure. Each rodent species has its own particular habits; in the case of the deer mouse, these behaviors include living in and around human habitation.

The disease begins with a prodrome of about 3 to 4 days (range, 1 to 11 days) comprising fever, myalgia, malaise, and often gastrointestinal disturbances such as nausea, vomiting, and abdominal pain. Dizziness is common and vertigo occasional. Severe prodromal symptoms bring some individuals to medical attention, but patients are usually recognized as the cardiopulmonary phase begins. Typically, there is slightly lowered blood pressure, tachycardia, tachypnea, mild hypoxemia, and early radiographic signs of pulmonary edema. Physical findings in the chest are often surprisingly scant. The conjunctival and cutaneous signs of vascular involvement seen in other types of HF are absent. During the next few hours, decompensation may progress rapidly to severe hypoxemia and respiratory failure. Most patients surviving the first 48 h of hospitalization are extubated and discharged within a few days, with no apparent residua.

Management during the first few hours after presentation is critical. The goal is to prevent severe hypoxemia by oxygen therapy and, if needed, intubation and intensive respiratory management. During this period, hypotension and shock with increasing hematocrit invite aggressive fluid administration, but this intervention should be undertaken with great caution. Because of low cardiac output with myocardial depression and increased pulmonary vascular permeability, shock should be managed expectantly with pressors and modest infusion of fluid guided by the pulmonary capillary wedge pressure. Mild cases can be managed by frequent monitoring and oxygen administration without intubation. Many patients require intubation to manage hypoxemia and also develop shock. Mortality remains at ~30 to 40% with good management. The antiviral drug ribavirin inhibits the virus in vitro but did not have a marked effect on patients treated in an open-label study.

During the prodrome, the differential diagnosis of hantavirus pulmonary syndrome is difficult, but by the time of presentation or within 24 h thereafter, a number of diagnostically helpful clinical features become apparent. Cough is not usually present at the outset but may develop later. Interstitial edema is evident on the chest x-ray. Later, bilateral alveolar edema with a central distribution develops in the setting of a normal-sized heart; occasionally, the edema is initially unilateral. Pleural effusions are often visualized. Thrombocytopenia, circulating atypical lymphocytes, and a left shift (often with leukocytosis) are almost always evident; thrombocytopenia has been a particularly important early clue. Hemoconcentration, proteinuria, and hypoalbuminemia should also be sought. Although thrombocytopenia virtually always develops and prolongation of the partial thromboplastin time is the rule, clinical evidence for coagulopathy or laboratory indications of DIC are found in only a minority of cases, usually in severely ill patients. Severely ill patients also have acidosis and elevated serum levels of lactate. Mildly increased values in renal function tests are common, but patients with severe cases often have markedly elevated concentrations of serum creatinine; some of the viruses other than Sin Nombre virus have been associated with more kidney involvement, but few such cases have been studied. The differential diagnosis includes abdominal surgical conditions and pyelonephritis as well as rickettsial disease, sepsis, meningococcemia, plague, tularemia, influenza, and relapsing fever.

A specific diagnosis is best made by IgM testing of acute-phase serum, which has yielded positive results even in the prodrome. Tests using a Sin Nombre virus antigen detect the related hantaviruses causing the pulmonary syndrome in the Americas. Occasionally, heterologous viruses will react only in the IgG ELISA, but this finding is highly suspicious given the very low seroprevalence of these viruses in normal populations. RT-PCR is usually positive when used to test blood clots obtained in the first 7 to 9 days of illness as well as tissues; this test is useful in identifying the infecting virus in areas outside the home range of the deer mouse and in atypical cases.

YELLOW FEVER Yellow fever virus caused major epidemics in the Americas, Africa, and Europe before the discovery of mosquito transmission in 1900 led to its control through attacks on its urban vector, *A. aegypti*. Only then was it found that a jungle cycle also existed in Africa, involving other *Aedes* mosquitoes and monkeys, and that colonization of the New World with *A. aegypti*, originally an African species, had established urban yellow fever as well as an independent sylvatic yellow fever cycle in American jungles involving *Haemagogus* mosquitoes and New World monkeys. Today, urban yellow fever transmission occurs only in some African cities, but the threat exists in the great cities of South America, where reinfestation by *A. aegypti* has taken place and dengue transmission by the same mosquito is common. As late as 1905, New Orleans suffered >3000 cases with 452 deaths from "yellow jack." Despite the existence of a highly effective and safe vaccine, several hundred jungle yellow fever cases occur annually in South America, and thousands of jungle and urban cases occur each year in Africa.

Yellow fever is a typical HF accompanied by prominent hepatic necrosis. A period of viremia, typically lasting 3 or 4 days, is followed by a period of "intoxication." During the latter phase in severe cases, the characteristic jaundice, hemorrhages, black vomit, anuria, and terminal delirium occur, perhaps related in part to extensive hepatic involvement. Blood leukocyte counts may be normal or reduced and are often high in terminal stages. Albuminuria is usually noted and may be marked; as renal function fails in terminal or severe cases, the level of blood urea nitrogen rises proportionally. Abnormalities detected in liver function tests range from modest elevations of AST levels in mild cases to severe derangement.

Urban yellow fever can be prevented by the control of *A. aegypti*. The continuing sylvatic cycle requires vaccination of all visitors to areas of potential transmission. With few exceptions (in the very young and the elderly), reactions to vaccine are minimal; immunity is provided within 10 days and lasts for at least 10 years. An egg allergy dictates caution in vaccine administration. Although there are no documented harmful effects of the vaccine on the fetus, pregnant women should be immunized only if they are definitely at risk of yellow fever exposure. Since vaccination has been associated with several cases of encephalitis in children <6 months of age, it should be delayed until after 12 months of age unless the risk of exposure is very high. Timely information on changes in yellow fever distribution and yellow fever vaccine requirements can be obtained from Health Information for Travelers, Centers for Disease Control and Prevention, Atlanta, GA 30333; by fax request (404-332-4565; document number 220022#); by phone (404-332-4559); or via the Internet (*www.cdc.gov*).

DENGUE HEMORRHAGIC FEVER/DENGUE SHOCK SYNDROME A syndrome of HF noted in the 1950s among children in the Philippines and Southeast Asia was soon associated with dengue virus infections, particularly those occurring against a background of previous exposure to another serotype. The transient heterotypic protection after dengue virus infection is replaced within several weeks by the potential for heterotypic infection resulting in typical dengue fever (see above) or—uncommonly—for enhanced disease (secondary DHF/DSS). In rare instances, primary dengue infections lead to an HF syndrome, but much less is known about pathogenesis in this situation. In the past 20 years, *A. aegypti* has progressively reinvaded Latin America and other areas, and frequent travel by infected individuals has introduced multiple strains of dengue virus from many geographic areas. Thus the pattern of hyperendemic transmission of multiple dengue serotypes has now been established in the Americas and the Caribbean and has led to the emergence of DHF/DSS as a major problem there as well. Millions of dengue infections, including many thousands of cases of DHF/DSS, occur annually. The severe syndrome is unlikely to be seen in U.S. citizens since few children have the dengue antibodies that can trigger the pathogenetic cascade when a second infection is acquired.

Macrophage/monocyte infection is central to the pathogenesis of dengue fever and to the origin of DHF/DSS. Previous infection with a heterologous dengue-virus serotype may result in the production of nonprotective antiviral antibodies that nevertheless bind to the virion's surface and through interaction with the Fc receptor focus secondary dengue viruses on the target cell, the result being enhanced infection. The host is also primed for a secondary antibody response when viral antigens are released and immune complexes lead to activation of the classic complement pathway, with consequent phlogistic effects. Cross-reactivity at the T cell level results in the release of physiologically active cytokines, including interferon γ and tumor necrosis factor α. The induction of vascular permeability and shock depends on multiple factors, including the following:

1. *Presence of enhancing and nonneutralizing antibodies*—Transplacental maternal antibody may be present in infants <9 months old, or antibody elicited by previous heterologous dengue infection may be present in older individuals. T cell reactivity is also intimately involved.
2. *Age*—Susceptibility to DHF/DSS drops considerably after 12 years of age.
3. *Sex*—Females are more often affected than males.

4. *Race*—Caucasians are more often affected than blacks.
5. *Nutritional status*—Malnutrition is protective.
6. *Sequence of infection*—For example, serotype 1 followed by serotype 2 seems to be more dangerous than serotype 4 followed by serotype 2.
7. *Infecting serotype*—Type 2 is apparently more dangerous than other serotypes.

In addition, there is considerable variation among strains of a given serotype, with Southeast Asian serotype 2 strains having more potential to cause DHF/DSS than others.

Dengue HF is identified by the detection of bleeding tendencies (tourniquet test, petechiae) or overt bleeding in the absence of underlying causes such as preexisting gastrointestinal lesions. Dengue shock syndrome, usually accompanied by hemorrhagic signs, is much more serious and results from increased vascular permeability leading to shock. In mild DHF/DSS, restlessness, lethargy, thrombocytopenia (<100,000/μL), and hemoconcentration are detected 2 to 5 days after the onset of typical dengue fever, usually at the time of defervescence. The maculopapular rash that often develops in dengue fever may also appear in DHF/DSS. In more severe cases, frank shock is apparent, with low pulse pressure, cyanosis, hepatomegaly, pleural effusions, ascites, and in some cases severe ecchymoses and gastrointestinal bleeding. The period of shock lasts only 1 or 2 days, and most patients respond promptly to close monitoring, oxygen administration, and infusion of crystalloid or—in severe cases—colloid. The case-fatality rates reported vary greatly with case ascertainment and the quality of treatment; however, most DHF/DSS patients respond well to supportive therapy, and overall mortality in an experienced center in the tropics is probably as low as 1%.

A virologic diagnosis can be made by the usual means, although multiple flavivirus infections lead to a broad immune response to several members of the group, and this situation may result in a lack of virus specificity of the IgM and IgG immune responses. A secondary antibody response can be sought with tests against several flavivirus antigens to demonstrate the characteristic wide spectrum of reactivity.

The key to control of both dengue fever and DHF/DSS is the control of *A. aegypti*, which also reduces the risk of urban yellow fever and chikungunya virus circulation. Control efforts have been handicapped by the presence of nondegradable tires and long-lived plastic containers in trash repositories, insecticide resistance, urban poverty, and an inability of the public health community to mobilize the populace to respond to the need to eliminate mosquito breeding sites. Live attenuated dengue vaccines are in the late stages of development and have produced promising results in early tests. Whether vaccines can provide safe, durable immunity to an immunopathologic disease such as DHF/DSS in endemic areas is an issue that will have to be tested, but it is hoped that vaccination will reduce transmission to negligible levels.

KYASANUR FOREST DISEASE AND OMSK HEMORRHAGIC FEVER See Chap. 180 in *Harrison's Online (www.harrisonsonline.com)*.

FILOVIRUS HEMORRHAGIC FEVER See Chap. 181.

FURTHER READING

Bruno P et al: The protean manifestations of hemorrhagic fever with renal syndrome. A retrospective review of 26 cases from Korea. Ann Intern Med 113:385, 1990

Calisher CH: Medically important arboviruses of the United States and Canada. Clin Microbiol Rev 7:89, 1994

Centers for Disease Control and Prevention: Update: Management of patients with suspected viral hemorrhagic fever—United States. MMWR 44:475, 1995 (*http://www.cdc.gov/mmwr/preview/mmwrhtml/00038033.htm*)

DERESIEWICZ RL et al: Clinical and neuroradiographic manifestations of eastern equine encephalitis. N Engl J Med 336:1867, 1997

ENRIA D et al: Arenaviruses, in *Tropical Infectious Diseases: Principles, Pathogens, & Practice*, RL Guerrant et al (eds). New York, Saunders, 1999, pp 1189–1212

PETERS CJ, KHAN AS: Hantavirus pulmonary syndrome: The new American hemorrhagic fever. Clin Infect Dis 34:1224, 2002

RIVAS F et al: Epidemic Venezuelan equine encephalitis in La Guajira, Colombia, 1995. J Infect Dis 175:828, 1997

SOLOMON SR, VAUGHN DW: Pathogenesis and clinical features of Japanese encephalitis and West Nile virus infections. Curr Top Microbiol Immunol 267:171, 2002

SOLOMON T et al: West Nile encephalitis. BMJ 326:865, 2003

WURTZ R, PALEOLOGOS N: La Crosse encephalitis presenting like herpes simplex encephalitis in an immunocompromised adult. Clin Infect Dis 31: 1113, 2000

181 EBOLA AND MARBURG VIRUSES
Clarence J. Peters

DEFINITION   Both Marburg virus and Ebola virus cause an acute febrile illness associated with high mortality. This illness is characterized by multisystem involvement that begins with the abrupt onset of headache, myalgias, and fever and proceeds to prostration, rash, and shock and often to bleeding manifestations. Epidemics usually begin with a single case acquired from an unknown reservoir in nature and spread mainly through close contact with sick persons or their body fluids, either in the home or at the hospital.

ETIOLOGY   The family Filoviridae comprises two antigenically and genetically distinct viruses: Marburg virus and Ebola virus. Ebola virus has four readily distinguishable subtypes named for their original sites of recognition (Zaire, Sudan, Cote d'Ivoire, and Reston). Except for Ebola virus subtype Reston, all the Filoviridae are African viruses that cause severe and often fatal disease in humans. The Reston virus, which has been exported from the Philippines on several occasions, has caused fatal infections in monkeys but only subclinical infections in humans. Different isolates of the four Ebola subtypes made over time and space exhibit remarkable sequence conservation, indicating marked genetic stability in their selective niche. Typical filovirus particles contain a single linear, negative-sense, single-stranded RNA arranged in a helical nucleocapsid. The virions are 790 to 970 nm in length; they may also appear in elongated, contorted forms. The lipid envelope confers sensitivity to lipid solvents and common detergents. The viruses are largely destroyed by heat (60°C, 30 min) and by acidity but may persist for weeks in blood at room temperature. The surface glycoprotein self-associates to form the virion surface spikes, which presumably mediate attachment to cells and fusion. The glycoprotein's high sugar content may contribute to its low capacity to elicit neutralizing antibodies. A smaller form of the glycoprotein, bearing many of its antigenic determinants, is produced by in vitro–infected cells and is found in the circulation in human disease; it has been speculated that this circulating soluble protein may suppress the immune response to the virion surface protein or block antiviral effector mechanisms. Both Marburg virus and Ebola virus are biosafety level 4 pathogens because of their high associated mortality rate and aerosol infectivity.

EPIDEMIOLOGY   Marburg virus was first identified in Germany in 1967, when infected African green monkeys (*Cercopithecus aethiops*) imported from Uganda transmitted the agent to vaccine-laboratory workers. Of the 25 human cases acquired from monkeys, 7 ended in death. The six secondary cases were associated with close contact or parenteral exposure. Secondary spread to the wife of one patient was documented, and virus was isolated from the husband's semen despite the presence of circulating antibodies. Subsequently, isolated cases of Marburg virus infection have been reported from eastern and southern Africa, with limited spread.

In 1999, repeated transmission of Marburg virus to workers in a gold mine in eastern Democratic Republic of Congo was documented. The secondary spread of the virus among patients' families was more extensive than previously noted, resembling that of Ebola virus and emphasizing the importance of hygiene and proper barrier nursing in the epidemiology of these viruses in Africa.

In 1976, epidemics of severe hemorrhagic fever (550 human cases) occurred simultaneously in Zaire and Sudan, and Ebola virus was found to be the etiologic agent. Later, it was shown that different subtypes of virus—associated with 90 and 50% mortality, respectively—caused the two epidemics. Both epidemics were associated with interhuman spread (particularly in the hospital setting) and the use of unsterilized needles and syringes, a common practice in developing-country hospitals. The epidemics dwindled as the clinics were closed and people in the endemic area increasingly shunned affected persons and avoided traditional burial practices.

The Zaire subtype of Ebola virus recurred in a major epidemic (317 cases, 88% mortality) in Democratic Republic of Congo in 1995 and in smaller epidemics in Gabon in 1994–1996. Mortality was high, transmission to caregivers and others who had direct contact with body fluids was common, and poor hygiene in hospitals exacerbated spread. In the Congo epidemic, an index case was infected in Kikwit in January 1995. The epidemic smoldered until April, when intense nosocomial transmission forced closure of the hospitals; samples were finally sent to the laboratory for Ebola testing, which yielded positive results within a few hours. International assistance, with barrier nursing instruction and materials, was provided; nosocomial transmission ceased, hospitals reopened, and patients were segregated to prevent intrafamilial spread. The last case was reported in June 1995.

Separate emergences of Ebola virus (subtype Zaire) were detected in Gabon from 1994 through 2003, usually in association with deep forest exposure and subsequent familial and nosocomial transmission. Nonhuman primates sometimes exhibited die-offs, and Ebola infection was confirmed in at least some animals. In a 1996 episode, a physician exposed to Ebola-infected patients traveled to South Africa with a fever; a nurse who assisted in a cutdown on the physician developed Ebola hemorrhagic fever and died despite intensive care. The index patient was identified retrospectively on the basis of serum antibodies and virus isolation from semen. Thus, distant transport of Ebola virus is an established risk, but limited nosocomial spread occurs under proper hygienic conditions.

In 2000–2001, an indolent outbreak of the Sudan subtype claimed the lives of 224 (53%) of 425 patients with presumptive cases in Uganda.

The Reston subtype of Ebola virus was first seen in the United States in 1989, when it caused a fatal, highly transmissible disease among cynomolgus macaques imported from the Philippines and quarantined in Reston, VA, pending distribution to biomedical researchers. This and other appearances of the Reston virus have been traced to a single export facility in the Philippines, but no source in nature has been established.

Epidemiologic studies (including a specific search in the Kikwit epidemic) have failed to yield evidence for an important role of airborne particles in human disease. This lack of epidemiologic evidence is surprising and seems to conflict with the viruses' classification as biosafety level 4 pathogens based in part on their aerosol infectivity and with formal laboratory assessments showing a high degree of aerosol infectivity for monkeys. Sick humans apparently do not usually generate sufficient amounts of infectious aerosols to pose a significant hazard to those around them.

Available evidence points to a nonprimate reservoir for these viruses, but an intensive search has failed to elucidate what this reservoir might be. Speculation has centered on a possible role for bats, but that hypothesis has risen in part merely because of the ubiquity of bats when sought in affected areas and the frustration of researchers in identifying a source of virus.

PATHOLOGY AND PATHOGENESIS   In humans and in animal models, Ebola and Marburg viruses replicate well in virtually all cell types, including endothelial cells, macrophages, and parenchymal cells of multiple organs. The earliest involvement is that of the mononuclear phagocyte system, and this is responsible for initiation of the disease process. Viral replication is associated with cellular necrosis both in vivo and in vitro. Significant findings at the light-microscopic level include liver necrosis with Councilman bodies (intracellular inclusions that correlate with extensive collections of viral nucleocapsids), interstitial pneumonitis, cerebral glial nodules, and small infarcts. Antigen and virions are abundant in fibroblasts, interstitium, and (to a lesser extent) the appendages of the subcutaneous tissues in fatal cases; escape through small breaks in the skin or possibly through sweat glands may occur and, if so, may be correlated with the established epidemiologic risk of close contact with patients and the touching of the deceased. Inflammatory cells are not prominent, even in necrotic areas.

In addition to sustaining direct damage from viral infection, patients infected with Ebola virus (Zaire subtype) have high circulating levels of proinflammatory cytokines, which presumably contribute to the severity of the illness. In fact, the virus interacts intimately with the cellular cytokine system. It is resistant to the antiviral effects of interferon α, although this mediator is amply induced. Viral infection of endothelial cells selectively inhibits the expression of MHC class I molecules and blocks the induction of several genes by the interferons. In addition, glycoprotein expression inhibits αV integrin expression, an effect that has been shown in vitro to lead to detachment and subsequent death of endothelial cells.

Acute infection is associated with high levels of circulating virus and viral antigen. Clinical improvement takes place when viral titers decrease concomitantly with the onset of a virus-specific immune response, as detected by enzyme-linked immunosorbent assay (ELISA) or fluorescent antibody test. In fatal cases, there is usually little evidence of an antibody response and there is extensive depletion of spleen and lymph nodes. Recovery is apparently mediated by the cellular immune response: convalescent-phase plasma has little in vitro virus-neutralizing capacity and is not protective in passive transfer experiments in monkey and guinea pig models.

CLINICAL MANIFESTATIONS   After an incubation period of ~7 to 10 days (range, 3 to 16 days), the patient abruptly develops fever, severe headache, malaise, myalgia, nausea, and vomiting. Continued fever is joined by diarrhea (often severe), chest pain (accompanied by cough), prostration, and depressed mentation. In light-skinned patients (and less often in dark-skinned individuals), a maculopapular rash appears around day 5 to 7 and is followed by desquamation. Bleeding may begin about this time and is apparent from any mucosal site and into the skin. In some epidemics, fewer than half of patients have had overt bleeding, and this manifestation has been absent even in some fatal cases. Additional findings include edema of the face, neck, and/or scrotum; hepatomegaly; flushing; conjunctival injection; and pharyngitis. Around 10 to 12 days after the onset of disease, the sustained fever may break, with improvement and eventual recovery of the patient. Recrudescence of fever may be associated with secondary bacterial infections or possibly with localized virus persistence. Late hepatitis, uveitis, and orchitis have been reported, with isolation of virus from semen or detection of polymerase chain reaction (PCR) products in vaginal secretions for several weeks.

LABORATORY FINDINGS   Leukopenia is common early on; neutrophilia has its onset later. Platelet counts fall below (sometimes much below) 50,000/μL. Laboratory evidence of disseminated intravascular coagulation may be found, but its clinical significance and the need for therapy are controversial. Serum levels of alanine and aspartate aminotransferases (particularly the latter) rise progressively, and jaundice develops in some cases. The serum amylase level may be elevated, and this elevation may be associated with abdominal pain suggesting pancreatitis. Proteinuria is usual; decreased kidney function is proportional to shock.

DIAGNOSIS   Most patients acutely ill as a result of infection with Ebola or Marburg viruses have high concentrations of virus in blood. Antigen-detection ELISA is a sensitive, robust diagnostic modality. Virus isolation and reverse-transcriptase PCR are also effective and provide additional sensitivity in some cases. Patients who are recovering develop IgM and IgG antibodies that are best detected by ELISA but are also reactive in the less specific fluorescent antibody test. Skin biopsies are an extremely useful adjunct in postmortem diagnosis of Ebola (and, to a lesser extent, Marburg) virus infections because of the presence of large amounts of viral antigen, the relative safety of obtaining the sample, and the freedom from cold-chain requirements for formalin-fixed tissues.

℞ TREATMENT

No virus-specific therapy is available, and, given the extensive viral involvement in fatal cases, supportive treatment may not be as useful as was once hoped. However, recent studies in rhesus monkeys have shown improved survival among animals treated with an inhibitor of factor VIIa/tissue factor. Vigorous treatment of shock should take into account the likelihood of vascular leak in the pulmonary and systemic circulation and of myocardial functional compromise. The membrane fusion mechanism of Ebola resembles that of retroviruses, and the identification of "fusogenic" sequences suggests that inhibitors of cell entry may be developed. Despite the poor neutralizing capacity of polyclonal convalescent-phase sera, phage display of immunoglobulin mRNA from convalescent bone marrow has produced monoclonal antibodies that have in vitro neutralizing capacity and mediate protection in guinea pig—but, unfortunately, not in monkey—models.

PREVENTION   No vaccine or antiviral drug is currently available, but barrier nursing precautions in African hospitals can greatly decrease the spread of the virus beyond the index case and thus prevent epidemics of filoviruses and other agents as well. An adenovirus-vectored Ebola glycoprotein gene has proved protective in nonhuman primates and is undergoing phase 1 trials in humans.

FURTHER READING

CENTERS FOR DISEASE CONTROL AND PREVENTION: Outbreak of Ebola hemorrhagic fever—Uganda, August 2000–January 2001. JAMA 285: 1010, 2001

GEISBERT TW et al: Treatment of Ebola virus infection with a recombinant inhibitor of factor VIIa/tissue factor: A study in rhesus monkeys. Lancet 362:1953, 2003

PETERS CJ, LEDUC JW: An introduction to Ebola: The virus and the disease. J Infect Dis 179(Suppl 1):ix, 1999 (Also available at *www.journals.uchicago.edu/ JID/*)

SULLIVAN NT: Accelerated vaccination for Ebola virus haemorrhagic fever in non-human primates. Nature 424:681, 2003

WORLD HEALTH ORGANIZATION: Outbreak(s) of Ebola haemorrhagic fever in the Republic of the Congo, January–April 2003. Wkly Epidemiol Rec 78:285, 2003

182 | DIAGNOSIS AND TREATMENT OF FUNGAL INFECTIONS
John E. Bennett

MYCOLOGY FUNDAMENTALS

Fungi can appear microscopically as either rounded, budding forms (yeastlike organisms) or hyphae (molds). Yeastlike colonies are smooth, while mold colonies are fuzzy; fungi that grow as yeasts include species of *Candida* and *Cryptococcus*, while fungi that grow as molds include species of *Aspergillus*, *Rhizopus*, and dermatophytes (ringworm fungi). The fungi that cause histoplasmosis, blastomycosis, sporotrichosis, coccidioidomycosis, and paracoccidioidomycosis are called *dimorphic* ("having two forms") because they are spherical in tissue but grow like molds when cultured at room temperature. *Candida* species other than *Candida glabrata* appear in tissue as both budding yeasts and tubular elements called *pseudohyphae*. Pseudohyphae, unlike true hyphae, have constrictions in the cell wall where septa are located and have septa at branching points. *Pneumocystis* (Chap. 191) is closer to fungi than to parasites by ribosomal sequences. Because the drugs used to treat *Pneumocystis* pneumonia are also used to treat parasitic or bacterial infections (see Chaps. 118 and 193), those drugs will not be discussed in this chapter.

Many fungi can form two different types of spores and are given different names, depending on the spore-bearing structures. When the spores are produced by mitosis, the fungus is said to be an *anamorph*, or to be in the imperfect state. Many fungi can have different sporulating structures in which genetic recombination occurs, often as a result of coculture with a strain of the opposite mating type. A fungus producing those distinctive spores is said to be a *teleomorph*, or to be in the perfect state. Diagnostic laboratories usually use the name of the anamorph because they do not use culture conditions that would produce the teleomorph. One exception is *Scedosporium apiospermum*, which is often observed as a teleomorph in the diagnostic laboratory and identified as *Pseudallescheria boydii*.

Most fungi that are pathogenic for humans are saprophytes in nature; they cause infection when airborne spores reach the lung or paranasal sinus or when hyphae or spores are accidentally inoculated into the skin or cornea. Acquisition of infection from another person or an animal has been reported in the case of ringworm but is very rare in other mycoses. Thus, hospitalized patients with fungal infections do not require special isolation. Most fungi infect hosts preferentially by one route and only infrequently by other routes. For example, the agents of ringworm, pityriasis versicolor, and piedra infect the epidermis and its appendages. Sporotrichosis and mycetoma usually arise from subcutaneous inoculation. Inhalation is the route of inoculation for the agents of most deep mycoses. Ingestion of fungi rarely causes infection; *Candida albicans*, a normal commensal in the mouth and intestine, reaches deeper tissues only when mucosal or cutaneous barriers are breached by disease, surgery, trauma, or catheterization. Histoplasmosis, blastomycosis, coccidioidomycosis, and paracoccidioidomycosis have been called "endemic" mycoses to emphasize their restricted geographic distribution. Some fungi, such as *Aspergillus* and *Fusarium*, are said to be opportunists in that they usually infect hosts with compromised immunity. This distinction is relative, not absolute.

Immunity after exposure to fungi may confer partial protection against reinfection. Residents of areas in which mycoses are endemic are less subject to infection than are newcomers. Predisposing factors are helpful in defining host defense. Immunoglobulin deficiencies do not appear to predispose to any mycosis, whereas neutropenia is common among patients who develop invasive mold infections or deep candidiasis. Cell-mediated immunity appears to be of paramount importance in cryptococcosis, histoplasmosis, and coccidioidomycosis.

DIAGNOSIS

Many fungi can be identified to the genus or even the species level by microscopic examination of smears or biopsy specimens. Calcofluor white staining with fluorescence microscopy is a sensitive technique for smears of sputum, bronchoalveolar lavage fluid, or pus. India ink smear remains the method of choice for detecting cryptococci in cerebrospinal fluid (CSF). *Candida* yeast cells and pseudohyphae are the only fungi that are usually gram-positive on smears. For other fungi, Gram's staining is distinctly suboptimal. For histopathology slides, Gomori methenamine silver and a neutral counterstain are preferred.

The method used has a marked effect on the rapidity and sensitivity of blood cultures for fungi except in the case of *Candida* species, which are relatively easy to grow. For most other fungi, concentration of the blood by lysis centrifugation and culture on solid medium constitute the optimal technique. Commercially available nucleic acid hybridization techniques can speed the identification of slow-growing molds, such as *Histoplasma capsulatum* and *Coccidioides immitis*. Serology has limited value, but testing of serum or CSF for cryptococcal antigen or antibody to *C. immitis* can be diagnostic. Detection of *Histoplasma* antigen in urine or serum is helpful in diagnosis and in following the results of treatment for disseminated histoplasmosis. Skin testing with fungal antigens is not useful in detecting active infection.

ANTIFUNGAL THERAPY

TOPICAL AGENTS ■ Imidazoles and Triazoles (See also "Systemic Antifungals") These synthetic compounds act by inhibiting ergosterol synthesis in the fungal cell wall and, when given topically, may cause direct damage to the fungal cytoplasmic membrane. The imidazoles available for cutaneous application include clotrimazole, econazole, ketoconazole, sulconazole, oxiconazole, and miconazole. Vaginal formulations include four imidazoles (miconazole, clotrimazole, tioconazole, and butoconazole) and one triazole (terconazole). As yet, no substantial differences in the efficacy of or local intolerance to the various topical azoles have become apparent. All are effective in the treatment of cutaneous candidiasis, tinea (pityriasis) versicolor, and mild to moderately severe ringworm of the glabrous skin. Vaginal formulations are effective for vulvovaginal candidiasis. Clotrimazole is poorly absorbed from the gastrointestinal tract, but the oral troche is useful as a topical treatment for oral and esophageal candidiasis.

Polyene Macrolide Antibiotics These broad-spectrum antifungal agents combine with sterol in the fungal cytoplasmic membrane, increasing membrane permeability. Topically, they are not active against ringworm but are effective against candidiasis of the skin and mucous membranes. Nystatin and amphotericin B suspensions are effective in oral thrush, and vaginal troches are effective in vulvovaginal candidiasis. Both nystatin and amphotericin B are available in topical preparations for cutaneous candidiasis.

Other Topical Antifungals Ciclopirox olamine, haloprogin, terbinafine, and naftifine have the same clinical spectrum among the cutaneous mycoses as the imidazoles. Tolnaftate and undecylenic acid are effective against ringworm but not candidiasis. Keratolytic agents, such as salicylic acid, are helpful as accessory drugs for some hyperkeratotic skin lesions.

SYSTEMIC ANTIFUNGALS ■ Griseofulvin Griseofulvin is a useful drug in the treatment of certain kinds of ringworm; however, it is ineffective in the treatment of candidiasis. The microcrystalline and ultramicrocrystalline preparations differ in dose but not in efficacy. Absorption of both is enhanced when the drug is ingested with fat-containing foods. Griseofulvin interacts with phenobarbital and warfarin.

Terbinafine   Oral terbinafine (250 mg once daily) is at least as effective as itraconazole and more effective than griseofulvin in onychomycosis and ringworm. Treatment duration ranges from 3 months for fingernails to 6 months for toenails. Gastrointestinal distress is the most common side effect. Rash, hepatitis, and pancytopenia have occurred, but serious adverse effects have been uncommon. Terbinafine decreases cyclosporine levels. Cimetidine increases and rifampin decreases terbinafine levels in blood.

Imidazoles and Triazoles ■ *GENERAL FEATURES*   The azole antifungals include imidazoles and triazoles. Fluconazole, itraconazole, voriconazole, and the investigational azoles posaconazole and ravuconazole are all triazoles, so named because they have three nitrogens in the ring structure. This class has less impact on human hormonal synthesis and less hepatotoxicity than the only widely used systemic imidazole, ketoconazole. Itraconazole has many structural features in common with ketoconazole; however, it has a broader spectrum of activity and has largely replaced ketoconazole.

Interactions between azoles and other drugs can increase the plasma concentrations of the other drugs to toxic levels or decrease the azole plasma concentrations to subtherapeutic levels. A few drugs can increase the plasma concentrations of azoles, but the effect is modest. Drug-drug interactions are most numerous with itraconazole and ketoconazole; some drugs are contraindicated for concomitant use with these agents. Azole interactions with any one class of drugs, such as benzodiazepines, HMG-CoA reductase inhibitors, or drugs that decrease gastric acidity, should be considered to apply to all drugs of that class until proven otherwise. Fluconazole differs substantially from itraconazole: unlike that of itraconazole, the absorption of fluconazole is independent of food or gastric acid, and fluconazole has much less effect on the hepatic metabolism of other drugs than does itraconazole. High fluconazole blood levels engendered by azotemia or by dosages above those used in pharmacologic studies may lead to new and profound drug interactions.

All azoles have the potential for embryotoxicity and teratogenicity. In fact, it seems likely that azoles should not be given during pregnancy without a discussion of the serious risks and possible benefits with the mother. Four infants born to mothers taking at least 400 mg of fluconazole daily for coccidioidal meningitis have had severe bone, craniofacial, or cardiac abnormalities. Similarity of these abnormalities to those in pregnant animals given fluconazole suggests that fluconazole caused the defects.

ITRACONAZOLE   Itraconazole is useful in the treatment of blastomycosis, histoplasmosis, cutaneous candidiasis, coccidioidomycosis, sporotrichosis, pseudallescheriasis, onychomycosis, ringworm, tinea versicolor, and indolent cases of aspergillosis. The drug is metabolized in the liver, with the hydroxy metabolite accounting for at least half of the antifungal activity in serum. The sum of the blood levels of the native drug and its hydroxylated metabolite is usually at least 2 μg/mL a few hours after oral administration. Almost no bioactive drug appears in urine or CSF.

Itraconazole is available as a 100-mg capsule, an oral solution, and an intravenous formulation. Although itraconazole capsules are less expensive and cause less gastrointestinal distress than the oral solution, their absorption is sometimes problematic. Cyclodextrin, which is used to formulate both the oral solution and the intravenous formulation, is renally excreted but is not absorbed from the gastrointestinal tract. Food increases the absorption of itraconazole capsules by about threefold but substantially reduces the absorption of the cyclodextrin suspension.

The oral solution is effective in oropharyngeal and esophageal candidiasis at a dose of 100 mg (10 mL) twice daily and has also been used at twice that dose for the treatment of deep mycoses in patients who absorb itraconazole capsules poorly. The efficacy of itraconazole in mycoses of the central nervous system has been modest at best, given the drug's inability to reach the CSF. For deep infections, itraconazole capsules are given at an initial dosage of 600 to 800 mg daily for 3 days and a subsequent dosage of 200 to 400 mg once daily

continued for 6 to 12 months. Itraconazole blood levels (see above) are helpful in documenting absorption when the oral drug is used for the treatment of deep mycoses. The commercially available intravenous formulation should be considered for initial therapy in hospitalized patients whose itraconazole absorption from the gastrointestinal tract may be suboptimal and whose creatinine clearance rate exceeds 30 mL/min. The dose is 200 mg twice daily for four doses followed by 200 mg daily for up to 2 weeks. Intravenous itraconazole, followed by the oral solution, is approved for the treatment of fever of unknown origin in neutropenic patients not responding to at least 96 h of therapy with antibacterial antibiotics.

Except for gastrointestinal distress from the oral solution, the toxicity of itraconazole is generally low, although life-threatening hepatotoxicity, congestive heart failure, edema, cardiac dysrhythmias, and peripheral neuropathy have been reported.

FLUCONAZOLE   This triazole can be administered in tablet form, as a suspension, or as an intravenous infusion. With a half-life of about 31 h, fluconazole can be given once a day. Approximately 80% of the drug is excreted unchanged in the urine. Patients with creatinine clearance rates of 21 to 50 mL/min and 11 to 20 mL/min should have their fluconazole doses reduced by 50 and 75%, respectively. The drug penetrates the CSF and other body fluids very well.

Nausea and abdominal distress are the most common forms of dose-limiting fluconazole toxicity. An allergic rash may develop and is particularly common among patients infected with HIV. Fatal cases of Stevens-Johnson syndrome have been described in the HIV-infected population. Alopecia commonly follows prolonged administration of $\geq$400 mg daily but resolves when therapy is discontinued. Rare cases of anaphylaxis, hepatic necrosis, and neutropenia have been described.

Fluconazole is useful in the treatment of oropharyngeal and esophageal candidiasis in adults. A single 150-mg tablet is effective in vulvovaginal candidiasis. Catheter-acquired candidemia in the immunocompetent host responds to 400 mg of fluconazole daily in conjunction with the removal of the infected catheter. Treatment should be continued for 10 to 14 days after the patient has become afebrile. Fluconazole is also effective in initial and maintenance therapy for cryptococcal meningitis in patients with AIDS, although most of these patients should initially receive a 2-week course of intravenous amphotericin B. Fluconazole is the drug of choice for coccidioidal meningitis.

The incidence of deep candidiasis among recipients of allogeneic bone marrow transplants can be reduced by the administration of fluconazole (400 mg daily) for 75 days after initiation of the transplantation-preparative regimen. Prophylaxis in other neutropenic patients has not appeared useful. Fluconazole (200 mg daily) reduced the incidence of cryptococcosis and mucosal candidiasis among AIDS patients whose CD4+ cell counts were $<200/\mu L$ and was particularly effective among those with counts of $<50/\mu L$. However, this regimen is not recommended because it does not reduce mortality, is expensive, and can lead to drug resistance.

Fluconazole is less effective than itraconazole in blastomycosis, histoplasmosis, and sporotrichosis. The drug is not active in aspergillosis, pseudallescheriasis, or mucormycosis.

VORICONAZOLE   This recently marketed triazole is available as 50- and 200-mg tablets and as vials of 200 mg for intravenous administration. The average-sized adult is given 6 mg/kg intravenously every 12 h for two doses followed by maintenance doses of 4 mg/kg intravenously every 12 h. In patients whose condition is improving, the regimen can be changed to 200 mg twice daily by mouth. Up to 300 mg twice daily by mouth can be given to patients who do not respond adequately to the lower dose.

Voriconazole is well absorbed from the gastrointestinal tract and is metabolized completely by the liver by way of CYP2C9, CYP2C19, and CYP3A4. Genetic polymorphisms in CYP2C19 activity cause substantial variation in voriconazole metabolism. Dose adjustment for azotemia is not necessary, but the dose should be reduced by half in patients with moderate liver disease. Because the cyclodextrin used in the intravenous formulation is renally excreted, oral—not intravenous—voriconazole should be used in patients with creatinine clearance rates below 50 mL/min. Penetration into the CSF is good. Concurrent use of sirolimus is contraindicated because its serum levels are markedly increased in the presence of voriconazole. Until more complete data are available, the drug interactions for voriconazole should be considered to be similar to those for itraconazole. The toxic effects of voriconazole include transient visual disturbances (color changes, blurring) in 30% of patients, hepatotoxicity in 10%, and rash in 5%.

The spectrum of voriconazole includes all the fungi against which itraconazole and fluconazole are active. Voriconazole is indicated for initial treatment of invasive aspergillosis, pseudallescheriasis, and fusariosis. The drug is also useful as empirical therapy in febrile neutropenic patients who do not respond to at least 96 h of treatment with antibacterial antibiotics and who are at high risk of invasive mold infections.

INVESTIGATIONAL TRIAZOLES Posaconazole and ravuconazole, which are undergoing early clinical trials, have antifungal spectra similar to that of voriconazole. Ravuconazole is notable for a half-life of ~1 week.

Echinocandins One echinocandin (caspofungin) is on the market, and two others (micafungin and anidulafungin) are being assessed in clinical trials. All are administered intravenously and act by inhibiting synthesis of $(1,3)\beta$-D-glucan in the cell wall. The in vitro activity of these drugs against nearly all *Candida* species is similar and is independent of azole resistance. The possible exception is *Candida parapsilosis*, a species whose susceptibility varies with the isolate and the particular echinocandin. Activity against *Aspergillus* species is more obvious in experimentally infected animals than in vitro, where changes in hyphal shape are more obvious than decreased growth. The recommended regimen is a 70-mg loading dose followed by 50 mg daily. Toxicity is low and includes histamine-like acute infusion reactions and hepatotoxicity. Cyclosporine elevates caspofungin blood levels, but other drug-drug interactions have been minor so far. No dosage adjustment is needed in patients with azotemia or hemodialysis, but the dose should be reduced for moderate hepatic insufficiency. Penetration into CSF is negligible. On the basis of an open trial in 63 patients, caspofungin has been approved for salvage therapy in aspergillosis. Data on candidemia in nonneutropenic patients indicate an efficacy equivalent to that of fluconazole or amphotericin B.

Amphotericin B A colloidal deoxycholate complex of the polyene drug amphotericin B is available for intravenous or intrathecal administration. The catabolism of amphotericin B is extremely slow and is not influenced by renal failure, hepatic failure, or hemodialysis. The drug's penetration into CSF and vitreous humor is poor; however, the concentrations in pleural, peritoneal, and articular exudates are adequate for many mycoses. Histoplasmosis, blastomycosis, paracoccidioidomycosis, candidiasis, and cryptococcosis are the most responsive mycoses; coccidioidomycosis, extraarticular sporotrichosis, aspergillosis, and mucormycosis are less responsive; and chromoblastomycosis, mycetoma, and pseudallescheriasis respond little, if at all. The usual course is 0.5 to 0.7 mg/kg daily for 8 to 10 weeks. Infusions are generally given in 5% dextrose over 2 to 4 h.

Initial doses of amphotericin B occasionally cause marked febrile reactions that may be poorly tolerated by adult patients with limited cardiac or pulmonary function. It may be prudent to give such patients an initial 1-mg test dose followed by rapidly escalating doses, depending on tolerance. Premedication with aspirin or acetaminophen or the addition of hydrocortisone (25 mg) to the infusion decreases chills and fever. Azotemia during treatment is usual, the extent depending on the daily dose, underlying renal disease, and concomitant nephrotoxic agents. Saline infusions have been advocated to reduce azotemia. Continuous amphotericin B infusions may reduce nephrotoxicity, but the impact on efficacy is unknown. Other side effects include anemia, hypokalemia, renal tubular acidosis, nausea, anorexia, weight loss, phlebitis, and occasionally hypomagnesemia. Intrathecal amphotericin B has been used in coccidioidal meningitis and refractory cryptococcal meningitis, although this therapy is associated with transient fever, headache, nausea, and vomiting.

Three lipid formulations of intravenous amphotericin B are commercially available in the United States. These formulations and their usual once-daily doses are amphotericin B lipid complex (ABLC), 5 mg/kg; amphotericin B colloidal dispersion (ABCD), 6 mg/kg; and liposomal amphotericin B (L-AB), 4–5 mg/kg. The most nephrotoxic lipid formulation is ABLC; ABCD causes less azotemia; and L-AB is the least nephrotoxic. Acute, febrile, infusion-related reactions occur with all amphotericin B formulations; their degree of severity is greatest with ABCD and lesser with ABLC and L-AB. The recommended duration for initial infusions of ABCD is 6 h for 6 mg/kg, slower than the 2-h duration of ABLC or L-AB infusions. Infusions of ABCD given more rapidly than 1 mg/kg per hour have caused severe reactions with fever and hypoxia. Use of these remarkably expensive formulations should be restricted to patients who cannot tolerate the nephrotoxicity of the deoxycholate formulation (ABD). Although the lipid formulations are also approved for patients with mycoses failing to respond to ABD, there is no indication that these formulations are more effective than ABD for any mycosis. ABLC and L-AB are probably equivalent in efficacy to ABD for most mycoses. Data on the efficacy of ABCD are largely confined to aspergillosis, in which the efficacy of this lipid formulation was equivalent to that of conventional amphotericin B.

Flucytosine Flucytosine (5-fluorocytosine) is a synthetic oral drug useful in cryptococcosis, candidiasis, and chromoblastomycosis. Within the fungal cell, flucytosine is converted to the antimetabolite 5-fluorouracil. Drug resistance appears rather rapidly when flucytosine is used alone. For this reason, the drug is generally used in combination with amphotericin B. The usual dose of flucytosine is 25 to 37.5 mg/kg every 6 h. Flucytosine is well absorbed from the gastrointestinal tract. The drug penetrates well into the CSF and is excreted unchanged in the urine. Even modest reductions in renal function may elevate flucytosine blood levels into the toxic range (≥100 to 125 μg/mL). Elevated levels are associated with a significant incidence of neutropenia and thrombocytopenia and also seem to predispose to colitis, the other major toxic effect of this drug. Hepatotoxicity is idiosyncratic and uncommon. An allergic rash may develop.

FURTHER READING

BOWDEN R et al: A double-blind, randomized, controlled trial of amphotericin B colloidal dispersion versus amphotericin B for treatment of invasive aspergillosis in immunocompromised patients. Clin Infect Dis 35:359, 2002

HERBRECHT R et al: Voriconazole versus amphotericin B for primary therapy of invasive aspergillosis. N Engl J Med 347:408, 2002

HOSPENTHAL DR et al: Flucytosine monotherapy for cryptococcosis. Clin Infect Dis 27:260, 1998

MANGINO JE, PAPPAS PG: Itraconazole for the treatment of histoplasmosis and blastomycosis. Int J Antimicrob Agents 5:219, 1995

MORA-DUARTE J et al: Comparison of caspofungin and amphotericin B in invasive candidiasis. N Engl J Med 347:2070, 2002

SOBEL JD: Practice guidelines for the treatment of fungal infections. Clin Infect Dis 30:652, 2000

VAN DER HORST CM et al: Treatment of cryptococcal meningitis associated with the acquired immunodeficiency syndrome. N Engl J Med 337:15, 1997

VILLANUEVA A et al: A randomized double-blind study of caspofungin versus amphotericin for the treatment of candidal esophagitis. Clin Infect Dis 33:1529, 2001

WALSH TJ et al: Voriconazole compared with liposomal amphotericin B for empirical antifungal therapy in patients with neutropenia and persistent fever. N Engl J Med 346:225, 2002

——— et al: Liposomal amphotericin B for empirical therapy in patients with persistent fever and neutropenia. N Engl J Med 340:764, 1999

WINGARD J et al: A randomized, double-blind comparative trial evaluating the safety of liposomal amphotericin B versus amphotericin B lipid complex in the empirical treatment of febrile neutropenia. LAmph/ABLC Collaborative Study Group. Clin Infect Dis 31:1155, 2000

183 | HISTOPLASMOSIS
John E. Bennett

ETIOLOGIC AGENT *Histoplasma capsulatum* var. *capsulatum* is a dimorphic fungus that grows as a mold in nature or on Sabouraud's agar at room temperature. Hyphae bear both large and small spores, which are used for identification. Nucleic acid hybridization can also be used to identify the organism in culture. *H. capsulatum* var. *capsulatum* grows as a small budding yeast in host tissue and on enriched agar, such as blood cysteine glucose, at 37°C. Despite its name, the fungus is unencapsulated. Coculture of isolates with opposite mating types can produce different sporulating structures in which genetic recombination occurs. When these structures, referred to as a *teleomorph* or the *perfect state*, are seen in culture, the name *Ajellomyces capsulatus* is used. *H. capsulatum* var. *duboisii* is a rare cause of infection, with most cases originating in Africa. The yeast cells of the *duboisii* variant are larger than those of *H. capsulatum* var. *capsulatum*, but the mold forms of the two appear identical.

EPIDEMIOLOGY Infection with *H. capsulatum* has been encountered in many areas of the world but is much more frequent in certain areas. Within the United States, infection is most common in the southeastern, mid-Atlantic, and central states. Infection has been reported in travelers returning from Latin America and other endemic areas overseas. Endemicity is contingent on the availability of proper conditions in nature for growth of the fungus. *H. capsulatum* prefers moist surface soil, particularly soil enriched by droppings of certain birds and bats. The fungus persists in contaminated soil for years and becomes airborne when the soil is disturbed. Acute infection is usually recognized as case clusters occurring 5 to 18 days after the exposure of groups of people to dust while (for example) cleaning dirt-floored chicken coops; raking or rototilling soil; exploring caves; and cleaning, remodeling, or demolishing old buildings. Skin-test reactivity in many endemic areas indicates that ≥80% of residents over age 16 have been exposed.

PATHOGENESIS AND PATHOLOGY Microconidia, or small spores, of *H. capsulatum* are small enough to reach the alveoli on inhalation and are transformed there to budding forms. With time, an intense granulomatous reaction occurs. Caseation necrosis or calcification may mimic tuberculosis. In children, the primary infection usually heals completely but may leave spotty calcification in the hilar nodes or lung. Transient dissemination may leave calcified granulomas in the spleen. In adults, a rounded mass of scar tissue, with or without central calcification, may remain in the lung. This mass has been called a *histoplasmoma*. Previous exposure is thought to confer some protection against reinfection, but infection in persons with prior positive skin tests clearly has occurred.

In a small proportion of patients, histoplasmosis becomes a progressive, potentially fatal infection. The disease occurs either as chronic fibrocavitary pneumonia or, less commonly, as disseminated infection. Patients with either form lack a history of acute primary pulmonary histoplasmosis. Chronic pulmonary infection favors otherwise-healthy males over the age of 40. A history of cigarette use or the presence of emphysema is elicited from nearly all patients with chronic progressive pulmonary histoplasmosis. An acute, rapidly fatal disseminated infection is most likely to be encountered among young children and immunosuppressed patients, including those with AIDS. Use of tumor necrosis factor α antagonists, particularly infliximab, also appears to predispose to severe disseminated histoplasmosis. A more chronic but equally lethal disseminated infection is more common among previously healthy adults.

CLINICAL MANIFESTATIONS The vast majority of infections are either asymptomatic or mild, and the diagnosis is elusive. Cough, fever, malaise, and chest x-ray findings of hilar adenopathy with or without one or more areas of pneumonitis are typical features. Erythema nodosum and erythema multiforme have been reported in a few outbreaks. Hilar adenopathy may cause temporary compression of the right-middle-lobe bronchus in children and young adults. Subacute pericarditis may develop, probably by extension from contiguous lymph nodes. Rarely, hilar nodes undergo a caseous, granulomatous reaction with perinodal fibrosis. Mediastinal structures become encased by progressive fibrosis, and compression of the pulmonary veins, superior vena cava, pulmonary arteries, and esophagus may take place over many years. Late in mediastinal disease, only rare nonviable *Histoplasma* cells can be found in caseous residua of lymph nodes.

Chronic pulmonary histoplasmosis is characterized by a gradual onset (over weeks or months) of increasing productive cough, weight loss, and sometimes night sweats. Chest x-ray reveals uni- or bilateral fibronodular apical infiltrates. Approximately one-third of cases stabilize or improve spontaneously early in the course. The remainder progress insidiously. Retraction and cavitation of the upper lobes occur, with spread to the apex of the lower lobes and other areas of the lung. Emphysema and bulla formation further compromise pulmonary function. Death from cor pulmonale, bacterial pneumonia, or histoplasmosis occurs after months or years.

Disseminated histoplasmosis has many features in common with hematogenously disseminated tuberculosis (Chap. 150). Common findings include fever, emaciation, hepatosplenomegaly, lymphadenopathy, abnormal liver function, anemia, leukopenia, and thrombocytopenia. Although skin lesions are uncommon in histoplasmosis, patients with far-advanced HIV infection may present with one or more discrete erythematous skin papules. Diffuse pulmonary disease may be mistaken for *Pneumocystis* pneumonia in patients infected with HIV. HIV-infected patients responding to highly active antiretroviral therapy may experience a return of the symptoms of histoplasmosis as a result of immune reconstitution. Previously normal patients usually have a much more indolent disease that progresses over weeks or months. Disease tends to be more focal, with one or more indurated ulcers of the mouth, tongue, nose, or larynx in about one-fourth of cases. Other focal findings include granulomatous hepatitis, Addison's disease, gastrointestinal ulcers, endocarditis, and chronic meningitis. Chest x-ray abnormalities are evident in half of cases and characteristically have a miliary pattern.

Infection with *H. capsulatum* var. *duboisii* is rare but should be considered in previous residents of Africa. Clinical manifestations resemble those of blastomycosis more than those of histoplasmosis in that skin and bone lesions are very common.

Presumed ocular histoplasmosis syndrome (POHS) is a clinical syndrome characterized by discrete atrophic choroidal scars in the macula or midperiphery, peripapillary atrophy, and choroidal neovascularization. These changes lead to a severe loss of central vision. It is unclear whether POHS represents an immune response to prior histoplasmosis, but there is no evidence of active infection. Susceptibility may be correlated with certain HLA types.

DIAGNOSIS Culture of the etiologic organism is the preferred method for diagnosis of histoplasmosis but is often difficult. Blood cultures are best performed by the lysis-centrifugation technique, with plates held at 30°C for at least 2 weeks. Approximately 15 mL of blood should be cultured from adults. Routine blood cultures in broth are generally unsuitable. Cultures of bone marrow, mucosal lesions, liver, and bronchoalveolar lavage fluid are diagnostically useful in disseminated histoplasmosis. Sputum culture is the preferred method for the diagnosis of chronic pulmonary histoplasmosis. However, growth may require 2 to 4 weeks to become visible, and other organisms may overgrow the plate. Diagnosis based on Giemsa-stained smears of blood or bronchoalveolar lavage fluid or on methenamine silver staining of infected lung, bone marrow, lymph node, or mucosal lesions requires considerable expertise, although these techniques yield results rapidly and provide specimens that can easily be sent to a referral laboratory. Organisms may be very scanty in lesions with marked caseous necrosis. An assay for *Histoplasma* antigen in blood or urine is commercially available and is useful both for diagnosis and for monitoring the response to therapy in patients with disseminated infection.

Antigen is detected occasionally in acute pulmonary histoplasmosis but rarely in chronic pulmonary disease. Diagnosis by antigen detection requires confirmation by culture or histopathology because false-positive results have occasionally been obtained. Tests for antibody to *H. capsulatum* have been of limited value in diagnosis. Histoplasmin skin testing has proven useful in epidemiologic studies but is no longer commercially available.

℞ TREATMENT

See also Table 183-1. Acute pulmonary histoplasmosis requires no therapy. Oral itraconazole (200 mg/d) can be given in the hope of shortening the course of illness, although this effect has not been proven. Patients with mediastinal fibrosis may benefit from vascular stent placement, but their ultimate prognosis is poor. All patients with disseminated or chronic pulmonary histoplasmosis should receive antifungal therapy. Intravenous amphotericin B (conventional or lipid formulation) is the drug of choice for the initial treatment of patients with disseminated histoplasmosis who are severely ill or immunosuppressed or whose infection involves the central nervous system; the regimen can be changed to itraconazole (200 mg twice daily) once clinical improvement is evident, and the latter regimen can be used as the initial therapy in less severely ill patients. Fluconazole at doses up to 400 mg/d has been less effective. Patients with AIDS whose disseminated histoplasmosis has responded to 10 weeks of therapy should receive itraconazole (200 mg/d) for life to prevent relapse. Lifelong maintenance therapy may not be necessary for HIV-infected patients who have received prolonged itraconazole treatment, have had a sustained response to highly active antiretroviral therapy, and no longer have detectable *Histoplasma* antigen in serum.

Immunocompetent patients with disseminated or chronic pulmonary histoplasmosis are given itraconazole (200 mg twice daily) and are generally treated for 6 to 12 months. Alternatively, immunocompetent patients can be given a 10-week course of amphotericin B (0.5 mg/kg daily).

Long-term maintenance therapy with an azole is not recommended for patients other than those with AIDS. However, relapse of chronic pulmonary and disseminated histoplasmosis is not rare and warrants careful follow-up for 1 year after therapy.

TABLE 183-1 *Treatment of Histoplasmosis[a]*

Type of Disease	Preferred Treatment	Alternatives
Acute pulmonary	None	. . .
Chronic pulmonary	Itraconazole	Amphotericin B
Disseminated		
Immunocompetent patient, less severe illness	Itraconazole	Amphotericin B
Rapid progression, severe illness, CNS involvement, HIV infection or other immunocompromise	Amphotericin B	Switch to itraconazole after 2 weeks if patient is improved and clinically stable.

[a] Amphotericin B is given as 0.5 mg/kg daily for 10 to 12 weeks. Liposomal amphotericin B (3–5 mg/kg daily) can also be used. Itraconazole is given as 200 mg twice daily for 6 to 12 months except in AIDS patients, in whom therapy is lifelong.

FURTHER READING

CANO MV et al: The epidemiology of histoplasmosis. A review. Semin Respir Infect 16:109, 2001

HECHT FM et al: Itraconazole maintenance treatment for histoplasmosis in AIDS: A prospective, multicenter trial. J Acquir Immune Defic Syndr 16: 100, 1997

LEE JH et al: Life-threatening histoplasmosis complicating immunotherapy with tumor necrosis factor alpha antagonists infliximab and etanercept. Arthritis Rheum 46:2565, 2002

ONGKOSUWITO JV et al: Amino acid residue 67 (isoleucine) of HLA-DRB is associated with POHS. Invest Ophthalmol Vis Sci 43:1725, 2002

WHEAT J et al: Antigen clearance during treatment of disseminated histoplasmosis with itraconazole versus fluconazole in patients with AIDS. Antimicrob Agents Chemother 46:248, 2002

——— et al: Practice guidelines for the management of patients with histoplasmosis. Clin Infect Dis 30:688, 2000

———: Histoplasmosis. Experience during outbreaks in Indianapolis and review of the literature. Medicine (Baltimore) 76:339, 1997

——— et al: Disseminated histoplasmosis in the acquired immune deficiency syndrome: Clinical findings, diagnosis and treatment, and review of the literature. Medicine 69:361, 1990

184 COCCIDIOIDOMYCOSIS
John E. Bennett

ETIOLOGIC AGENT *Coccidioides immitis* has two forms, growing as a white fluffy mold on most culture media but as a nonbudding spherical form (a spherule) in host tissue or under special conditions. Solely on the basis of DNA evidence, isolates from outside the San Joaquin Valley of California have been designated *Coccidioides posadasii* by some authorities. *C. immitis* reproduces in host tissue by forming small endospores within mature spherules. After rupture of the spherule, the released endospores enlarge, become spherules, and repeat the cycle. The fungus is identified by its appearance and by the formation of thick-walled, barrel-shaped spores, called *arthrospores*, in the hyphae of the mold form. Nucleic acid hybridization is a highly accurate and relatively safe way to identify this biohazard level 3 fungus.

EPIDEMIOLOGY, PATHOGENESIS, AND PATHOLOGY *C. immitis* is a soil saprophyte found in certain arid regions of the United States, Mexico, Central America, and South America. Within the United States, most cases of infection with *C. immitis* are acquired in California, Arizona, and western Texas (Fig. 184-1). A few cases are acquired by exposure to fomites from endemic areas (e.g., in cotton bales). Use of *C. immitis* by bioterrorists should be kept in mind should large outbreaks occur (Chap. 205).

Infection in humans and animals results from inhalation of wind-borne arthrospores from soil sites. This primary pulmonary infection is symptomatic in only 40% of cases, with symptoms ranging from a mild influenza-like illness to severe pneumonia. Mild self-limited infections may come to medical attention because of case clusters or hypersensitivity reactions: erythema nodosum, erythema multiforme, toxic erythema, arthralgia, arthritis, conjunctivitis, or episcleritis. Case clusters occur 10 to 14 days after a group of susceptible individuals is exposed to dust in an endemic area through such activities as archaeologic excavation, rock hunting, military maneuvers, model airplane contests, or construction work. Windstorms can carry spores to adjacent nonendemic areas and cause case clusters. The usual course of primary pneumonia is complete healing, although an area of pneumonitis (detected on radiographs) may heal by the formation of a coin-like lesion called a *coccidioidoma*. Less commonly, a single thin-walled cavity remains as a chronic sequela in the area of consolidation. Alternatively, an area of consolidation may persist as chronic pneumonia or progress to fibronodular cavitary disease.

Pleural effusion may be the only manifestation of primary infection. Spontaneous healing of this form is common.

An uncommon but dreaded complication of coccidioidomycosis is dissemination beyond the lung and hilar lymph nodes. Dissemination is especially frequent among blacks, Filipinos, Native Americans, Mexican Americans, pregnant women, and immunosuppressed patients, including those with AIDS.

C. immitis incites a chronic pyogranuloma in host tissue, often with areas of caseation necrosis. Lung and hilar node lesions may show

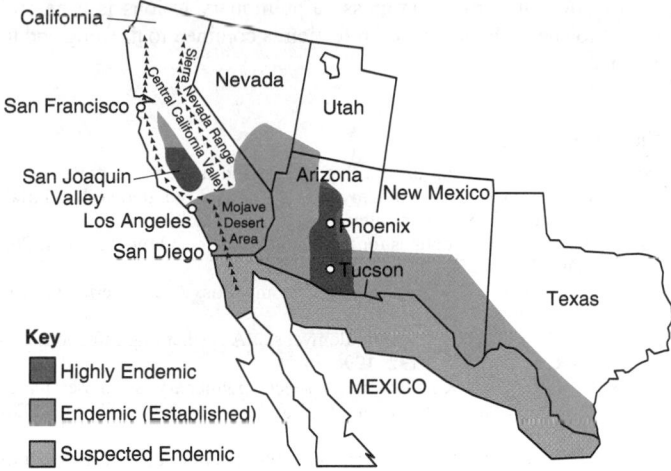

FIGURE 184-1 Geographic distribution of coccidioidomycosis. (*From Emerg Infect Dis 2:192, 1996*)

Key
■ Highly Endemic
▨ Endemic (Established)
▥ Suspected Endemic

calcification. Both IgM and IgG antibodies to *C. immitis* are induced by infection, but neither type of antibody appears to be protective. The amount of specific IgG antibody is a rough measure of the antigenic mass (i.e., of the intensity of infection), and a high titer is a poor prognostic sign. Appearance of delayed hypersensitivity to antigens of *C. immitis* is most common in clinical forms of disease with a good prognosis, such as self-limited primary pulmonary disease.

CLINICAL MANIFESTATIONS Symptomatic primary pulmonary infection begins 10 to 14 days after exposure and is manifested by fever, cough, chest pain, malaise, and sometimes the hypersensitivity reactions listed above. Chest radiographs may show an infiltrate, hilar adenopathy, or pleural effusion. Mild peripheral-blood eosinophilia may be found. Spontaneous improvement begins after several days to 2 weeks of illness and usually culminates in complete recovery.

The symptoms of a chronic thin-walled cavity include cough or hemoptysis in half of cases; the other half are asymptomatic. The cavity contracts to a nodule during the first year in about half of cases. Chronic fibrocavitary pulmonary coccidioidomycosis causes cough, sputum production, variable degrees of fever, and weight loss. The first indications of dissemination usually appear during primary infection. Reactivation with dissemination in later years occurs occasionally, especially if Hodgkin's disease, non-Hodgkin's lymphoma, renal transplantation, AIDS, or immunosuppression of some other etiology has supervened. Dissemination should be suspected when fever, malaise, hilar or paratracheal lymphadenopathy, elevated sedimentation rate, and high complement fixation titers signal abnormal persistence in patients with primary pulmonary coccidioidomycosis. With time, lesions appear in the bone, skin, subcutaneous tissue, meninges, joints, and other sites. Chronic meningitis presents as headache of indolent onset, with or without other signs of disseminated coccidioidomycosis. Cultures and smears of cerebrospinal fluid (CSF) are most often negative, but antibody is usually detectable in CSF by complement fixation. Skin lesions are indolent and maculopapular. Soft tissue and bony lesions contain pus and may present as a draining sinus. Without treatment, disseminated coccidioidomycosis progresses to death over weeks to years.

Disseminated coccidioidomycosis can progress rapidly in patients with advanced HIV infection. Fever with skin

or bone lesions may be the first sign. Those who present with diffuse pulmonary infiltrates have a poor prognosis. Blood cultures are positive late in the disease, if at all.

DIAGNOSIS When coccidioidomycosis is suspected, sputum, urine, and pus should be examined for *C. immitis* by wet smear and culture. *The laboratory request should indicate clearly that coccidioidomycosis is suspected, because the mold form must be handled with extreme care to prevent infection of laboratory personnel.* On biopsy, smaller spherules must be distinguished from nonbudding forms of *Blastomyces* and *Cryptococcus*, but the appearance of the mature spherule is diagnostic.

Serologic tests are very helpful in the diagnosis of coccidioidomycosis. Latex agglutination and agar gel diffusion tests are useful in screening sera for antibody to *Coccidioides*. The complement fixation test is used for CSF determinations and for the confirmation and quantitation of serum antibody detected by screening tests. The number of cases with a positive complement fixation test depends on the severity of disease and on the laboratory performing the test. Positive tests are least common among patients with solitary pulmonary cavities or primary pulmonary infection, while sera from patients with disseminated disease in multiple organs are nearly all positive. Seroconversion is helpful in diagnosing primary pulmonary coccidioidomycosis but may not occur for up to 8 weeks after onset. A positive complement fixation test of unconcentrated CSF is diagnostic of meningitis. Rarely, a parameningeal focus causes a positive complement fixation test of CSF.

Conversion of the skin test from negative to positive ($\geq$5 mm of induration at 24 or 48 h) with spherulin may take place between days 3 and 21 of symptoms in primary pulmonary coccidioidomycosis. Spherulin is not currently available commercially, but skin testing can be helpful in epidemiologic studies, such as investigations of case clusters or the definition of endemic areas. The utility of skin testing as a diagnostic tool is limited by the persistence of positive tests resulting from remote exposures to *Coccidioides* and by the frequency of negative skin tests among patients with either thin-walled cavities or disseminated coccidioidomycosis. A positive skin test has not predicted dissemination in HIV-infected patients. The presence of complement-fixing antibody to *C. immitis* in AIDS patients should prompt a search for active infection.

℞ TREATMENT

See also Table 184-1. Primary pulmonary coccidioidomycosis usually resolves spontaneously. Some physicians give a few weeks of treatment with intravenous amphotericin B followed by oral itracon-

TABLE 184-1 *Treatment of Coccidioidomycosis*

Type of Disease	Preferred Treatment	Alternatives
Asymptomatic pulmonary nodule	None	. . .
Solitary pulmonary cavity	None; excision with persistence for >1 year	Itraconazole or fluconazole
Chronic fibrocavitary pneumonia	Itraconazole or fluconazole[a]	Amphotericin B[b]; excision if refractory
Acute pneumonia		
No risk factors[c]	Itraconazole or fluconazole	Observation
Risk factors, severe illness, rapid progression, or diffuse pulmonary infiltrates	Amphotericin B	Switch to itraconazole or fluconazole after 2–3 months if patient's condition improves.
Chronic dissemination (no CNS disease)	Itraconazole or fluconazole[d]	Amphotericin B
Meningitis	Fluconazole[e]	Intrathecal amphotericin B

[a] Itraconazole is given as 200 mg twice daily by mouth and fluconazole as 400 mg/d by mouth.
[b] Amphotericin B is given as 0.5–0.7 mg/kg daily or as a lipid formulation (5 mg/kg daily).
[c] Risk factors include HIV infection, organ transplantation, treatment with high-dose glucocorticoids, and pregnancy.
[d] The optimal duration of therapy for disseminated infection is unclear but should probably be lifelong in both immunocompetent and immunocompromised patients.
[e] Patients in whom fluconazole therapy fails at the 400-mg dose may be advanced to 600 or 800 mg daily. Lifelong therapy for meningitis is recommended.

azole or fluconazole to patients with unusually severe or protracted primary infection in the hope of aborting disseminated or chronic pulmonary disease. Solitary pulmonary cavities that do not close spontaneously over the first year can be excised electively, particularly if complicated by hemoptysis or recurrent bacterial infection. Response to systemic antifungal therapy is poor.

Patients with severe or rapidly progressing disseminated coccidioidomycosis are first given intravenous amphotericin B at a dose of 0.5 to 0.7 mg/kg daily. Patients whose condition improves after 2 to 3 months of amphotericin B treatment or who have more indolent disseminated infection are given itraconazole (200 mg twice daily) or fluconazole (400 mg/d). These oral agents are useful for long-term suppression of infection, and treatment should be continued for years. Patients with coccidioidal meningitis usually are initially given fluconazole (400 to 800 mg/d) but may require intrathecal amphotericin B. Hydrocephalus is a frequent complication of uncontrolled meningitis. Surgical debridement of bone lesions or drainage of abscesses can be helpful. The prognosis for ultimate cure of disseminated coccidioidomycosis is guarded.

Resection of chronic progressive pulmonary lesions is a helpful adjunct to chemotherapy when infection is confined to the lung and to one lobe.

FURTHER READING

GALGIANI JN: Comparison of oral fluconazole and itraconazole for progressive, nonmeningeal coccidioidomycosis. A randomized, double-blind trial. Mycoses Study Group. Ann Intern Med 133:676, 2000

———— et al: Practice guidelines for the treatment of coccidioidomycosis. Clin Infect Dis 30:658, 2000

HOLLEY K et al: *Coccidioides immitis* osteomyelitis: A case series review. Orthopedics 25:827, 2002

KIRKLAND TN, FIERER J: Coccidioidomycosis: A reemerging infectious disease. Emerg Infect Dis 2:192, 1996

ROSENSTEIN NE et al: Risk factors for severe pulmonary and disseminated coccidioidomycosis: Kern County, California, 1995–1996. Clin Infect Dis 32:708, 2001

STEVENS DA, SHATSKY SA: Intrathecal amphotericin in the management of coccidioidal meningitis. Semin Respir Infect 16:263, 2001

WHEAT LJ et al: State-of-the-art review of pulmonary fungal infections. Semin Respir Infect 17:158, 2002

185   BLASTOMYCOSIS
John E. Bennett

ETIOLOGIC AGENT   *Blastomyces dermatitidis* is a dimorphic fungus that grows at room temperature as a white or tan mold but grows within the host or at 37°C as budding, round yeastlike cells. The fungus can be identified on the basis of its appearance, its dimorphism, the small spores borne on hyphae of the mold form, or the results of nucleic acid hybridization. When isolates of the two opposite mating types are grown close together on special culture medium, such as yeast extract or soil extract agar, sporulating structures that characterize the perfect state (*teleomorph*), called *Ajellomyces dermatitidis*, appear.

EPIDEMIOLOGY   The infection is restricted by geography and age. Blastomycosis is uncommon in any locality, but most cases occur in the southeastern, central, and mid-Atlantic areas of the United States and in the Canadian provinces of Ontario and Manitoba. Mississippi, Kentucky, Arkansas, Tennessee, North Carolina, Wisconsin, and Illinois typically report the most cases. Cases have also been encountered in Africa, Mexico, Central America, and (rarely) South America. Most patients are between 20 and 69 years old. The male-to-female ratio is about 10:1. There is no occupational predisposition to the development of blastomycosis.

PATHOGENESIS AND PATHOLOGY   Infection with *B. dermatitidis* appears to be acquired by inhalation of the fungus from soil, decomposed vegetation, or rotting wood. Several case clusters have resulted from participation in recreational activities in wooded areas along waterways. Infection is not transmissible from person to person. The initial pulmonary infection may either heal spontaneously or become chronic. Spread to other portions of the lung, cavitation, or endobronchial lesions may be found in patients with chronic disease. Whether or not the lung lesion resolves spontaneously, infection commonly spreads hematogenously to the skin, subcutaneous tissue, bone, prostate, epididymis, or mucosa of the nose, mouth, or larynx. Less commonly, infection spreads to the brain, meninges, liver, lymph nodes, or spleen. Dissemination may not be evident for weeks or years after the appearance of the lung lesion. Progressive infection is only rarely attributable to an underlying disease, to HIV infection, or to immunosuppressive treatment. The inflammatory response includes lymphocytes, giant cells, and neutrophils. Pseudoepitheliomatous hyperplasia may be striking and may lead to a mistaken diagnosis of squamous cell carcinoma of the skin, lung, or larynx.

CLINICAL MANIFESTATIONS   A few patients have acute, self-limited pneumonia. Fever, productive cough, myalgia, and malaise usually resolve within a month. Pulmonary infiltrates clear slowly as *B. dermatitidis* disappears from the sputum.

In the vast majority of patients, blastomycosis has an indolent onset and a chronically progressive course. Fever, cough, weight loss, lassitude, skin lesions, and chest ache are common. Skin lesions favor exposed areas and enlarge over many weeks from pimples to well-circumscribed, verrucous, crusted, or ulcerated lesions. Pain and regional lymphadenopathy are minimal. Large chronic lesions may undergo central healing with scarring and contracture. Mucous membrane and laryngeal lesions present as an indurated, nontender, sharply circumscribed hypertrophic plaque, often mistaken for squamous cell carcinoma. Chest x-ray findings are abnormal in two-thirds of patients, with one or more densely consolidated areas of pneumonia or nodular infiltrates that occasionally include areas of cavitation. Pleural thickening or small pleural effusions develop occasionally, but large pleural effusions are rare, as is calcification of the lung or hilar nodes. Patients may present with an acute respiratory distress syndrome (ARDS), although indolent symptoms usually precede this syndrome. The lungs of ARDS patients are filled with myriad organisms, and the patient often dies within a few days of admission to the hospital. Calcification, hilar adenopathy, and large pleural effusions are rare. Osteolytic lesions occur in one-fourth of patients and may involve nearly any bone. Osseous lesions, which appear radiologically as circumscribed osteolytic areas, present clinically as a cold abscess or a draining sinus or extend to a contiguous joint and cause an indolent arthritis yielding pus on aspiration. Prostatic and epididymal lesions present as an indurated nontender mass. Hydrocele or a draining sinus may accompany blastomycotic epididymitis.

DIAGNOSIS   The diagnosis of blastomycosis is made by demonstration of the fungus in a culture of sputum, pus, or urine. An expert can diagnose blastomycosis by the appearance of the organism in wet smear or histopathologic section. The fungus may be visible in a sputum cytology smear but is easily overlooked.

℞ TREATMENT

See also Table 185-1. A few patients have developed only transitory lung lesions, but no guidelines are known to distinguish these patients from those whose disease will progress locally or disseminate. Therefore, every patient should receive treatment. Intravenous amphotericin B is the drug of choice for patients with rapidly progressive infections, severe illness, or central nervous system lesions. Because the clinical

TABLE 185-1 *Treatment of Blastomycosis*

Type of Disease	Preferred Treatment[a]	Alternatives
Rapid progression or severe illness	Amphotericin B for 10–12 weeks	Switch to itraconazole (400 mg/d) when condition stabilizes; continue for 6–12 months.
CNS disease	Amphotericin B for 10–12 weeks	Give fluconazole (800 mg/d) if patient improves and cannot tolerate amphotericin B; continue for 6–12 months.
Indolent infection, mild to moderate illness, no CNS disease	Itraconazole (400 mg/d) for 6–12 months	. . .

[a] See text for dosage of amphotericin B.

response to amphotericin B is more rapid than that to an azole, intravenous itraconazole is less appropriate. However, therapy may be switched to itraconazole when the patient's condition stabilizes. Skin and noncavitary lung lesions should be treated for about 8 to 10 weeks when amphotericin B alone is used. The recommended total dose for an adult is ~2 g. Cavitary lung disease or infection extending beyond the lung and skin is more likely to relapse after 10 weeks of amphotericin B administration at this total dose; thus it should be treated for about 10 to 12 weeks with a total dose of ≥2.5 g, or the patient should be switched to itraconazole for prolonged therapy. Experience with lipid amphotericin B formulations is limited, but they are likely to prove effective.

Oral itraconazole (200 mg twice daily with food) is the drug of choice for the treatment of patients who have indolent nonmeningeal blastomycosis of mild to moderate severity and who take the drug reliably. Therapy with itraconazole is continued for 6 to 12 months, whether given initially or after a short course of amphotericin B. HIV-infected patients should probably receive lifelong therapy, but relevant experience is limited. Fluconazole is less effective than itraconazole; however, because of its good penetration into the central nervous system, treatment with 400 to 800 mg daily may be considered to follow amphotericin B therapy in CNS blastomycosis. The mortality rate in appropriately treated cases of blastomycosis is ≤15% but exceeds 50% in cases presenting as ARDS.

FURTHER READING

BAUMGARDNER DJ et al: Epidemiology of blastomycosis in a region of high endemicity in north-central Wisconsin. Clin Infect Dis 15:629, 1992

CHAPMAN SW et al: Endemic blastomycosis in Mississippi: Epidemiological and clinical studies. Semin Respir Infect 12:219, 1997

CRAMPTON TL et al: Epidemiology and clinical spectrum of blastomycosis diagnosed at Manitoba hospitals. Clin Infect Dis 34:1310, 2002

LEMOS LB et al: Acute respiratory distress syndrome and blastomycosis: Presentation of nine cases and review of the literature. Ann Diagn Pathol 5:1, 2001

MANGINO JE, PAPPAS PG: Itraconazole for the treatment of histoplasmosis and blastomycosis. Int J Antimicrob Agents 5:219, 1995

PAPPAS PG et al: Blastomycosis in immunocompromised patients. Medicine 72:311, 1993

SACCENTE M et al: Vertebral blastomycosis with paravertebral abscess: Report of eight cases and review of the literature. Clin Infect Dis 26:413, 1998

WINER-MURAM HT et al: Blastomycosis of the lung: CT features. Radiology 182:829, 1992

186 CRYPTOCOCCOSIS
John E. Bennett

ETIOLOGIC AGENT Cryptococcosis is an infection caused by the yeastlike fungus *Cryptococcus neoformans*. This fungus reproduces by budding and forms round, yeastlike cells. Within the host and on certain culture media, a large polysaccharide capsule surrounds each yeast cell. The fungus grows well in smooth, creamy-white colonies on Sabouraud's or other simple media at 20° to 37°C. Identification of the organism is based on gross and microscopic appearance, biochemical test results, and growth at 37°C. The results of nucleic acid hybridization or the formation of brown pigment on Niger seed agar can also be used for identification.

The fungus has four capsular serotypes, designated A, B, C, and D. There are also two mating types. Coculture of opposite mating types creates a transient diploid state called *Filobasidiella neoformans* var. *neoformans* for serotypes A and D and *F. neoformans* var. *bacillispora* for serotypes B and C. Organisms not cultured under mating conditions are designated *C. neoformans* var. *neoformans* for serotypes A and D and *C. neoformans* var. *gattii* for serotypes B and C; a simple color medium distinguishes the two varieties. Some authorities have called serotype A *C. neoformans* var. *grubii*.

EPIDEMIOLOGY Weathered pigeon droppings commonly contain serotype A or D (*C. neoformans* var. *neoformans*). *C. neoformans* var. *gattii* has been isolated from the litter around trees of the species *Eucalyptus camaldulensis* and *E. tereticornis*. Eucalyptus isolates have so far typed as serotype B. The distribution of these eucalyptus species in Australia corresponds to the distribution of infections due to *C. neoformans* var. *gattii* in that country. The high prevalence of these trees in other subtropical climates has been postulated to explain the relative restriction of such infections to warm climates. A notable exception is the cluster of clinical cases and environmental isolates *not* from eucalyptus trees on the eastern coast of Vancouver Island in British Columbia, Canada.

The most common predisposing factor to cryptococcosis worldwide is currently AIDS. CD4+ cell counts are usually below 200/μL in AIDS patients who develop cryptococcal infection. The incidence of cryptococcosis has been declining in the United States since the advent of highly active antiretroviral therapy (HAART). More than half of non-AIDS patients with cryptococcosis have been receiving glucocorticoids or other immunosuppressive drugs prior to the onset of the fungal infection. Solid organ transplantation, lymphoma, sarcoidosis, and idiopathic CD4+ lymphocytopenia also predispose to infection by *C. neoformans* var. *neoformans*. Most infections in immunocompromised patients are caused by serotype A, although serotype D occurs in up to 20% of cases in Western Europe. Infections with var. *gattii* have been rare among AIDS patients and other immunocompromised patients, even in subtropical climates where var. *gattii* infection occurs in previously healthy individuals.

Animals, particularly cats, can acquire cryptococcosis but have not been known to transmit the infection to other animals or to humans. The source from which humans acquire the infection is unknown, with the rare exception of cases acquired through a transplanted cornea, kidney, or other solid organ. Cryptococcosis is rare before puberty.

PATHOGENESIS AND PATHOLOGY Cryptococcal infection is thought to be acquired by inhalation of the fungus into the lungs, although rare cases of cutaneous cryptococcosis appear to arise by minor trauma. Pulmonary infection has a tendency toward spontaneous resolution and is frequently asymptomatic. Silent hematogenous spread to the brain leads to clusters of cryptococci in the perivascular areas of cortical gray matter, in the basal ganglia, and, to a lesser extent, in other areas of the central nervous system. The inflammatory response around these foci is usually scant. In the more chronic cases, a dense basilar arachnoiditis is typical. Lung lesions are characterized by intense granulomatous inflammation. Cryptococci are best seen in tissue by staining with methenamine silver or periodic acid–Schiff. Although a strongly positive result on mucicarmine staining of tissue is diagnostic, staining varies from intense to absent.

CLINICAL MANIFESTATIONS   Most patients have *meningoencephalitis* at the time of diagnosis. This form of cryptococcosis is invariably fatal without appropriate therapy; death occurs anytime from 2 weeks to several years after the onset of symptoms. Early manifestations include headache, nausea, staggering gait, dementia, irritability, confusion, and blurred vision. Both fever and nuchal rigidity are often mild or lacking. Papilledema is evident in one-third of cases at the time of diagnosis. Rapid and permanent loss of vision may occur, leaving a central scotoma or optic atrophy. Cranial nerve palsies, typically asymmetric, occur in about one-fourth of cases. Other lateralized signs are rare. With progression of the infection, deepening coma and signs of brainstem compression appear. Autopsy often reveals cerebral edema in more acute cases and hydrocephalus in more chronic cases. Neuroimaging is most often normal. Focal lesions called *cryptococcomas* are more common in previously normal patients, particularly those with var. *gattii* infections, than in immunosuppressed patients. These lesions are commonly located in the basal ganglia or the head of the caudate nucleus. Cryptococcomas are best seen on magnetic resonance imaging (MRI) with T2 or FLARE imaging and gadolinium enhancement. Edema around the mass disappears with successful therapy, but the cryptococcoma can persist for years.

Pulmonary cryptococcosis causes chest pain in ~40% of patients and cough in ~20%. Fever is modest or absent. The chest x-ray shows one or more dense infiltrates, which are often well circumscribed. Cavitation, pleural effusions, and hilar adenopathy are infrequent. Calcification is not evident, and fibrotic stranding is rarely noticeable.

Some 10% of patients with cryptococcosis have skin lesions, and the vast majority of patients with skin lesions have disseminated infection (Fig. 186-1). One or a few asymptomatic tiny papular lesions appear and slowly enlarge; they display a tendency toward central softening leading to ulceration. Osteolytic lesions occur in 4% of cases and usually present as a cold abscess. Rare manifestations of cryptococcosis include prostatitis, endophthalmitis, hepatitis, pericarditis, endocarditis, and renal abscess.

Cryptococcosis in AIDS patients is notable for the relative paucity of symptoms and signs, even in severe disease. Headache is present in ~90% of cases and fever in ~75%. Blurred vision, cranial nerve

palsies, lethargy, and confusion signal advanced infection. Cerebrospinal fluid (CSF) abnormalities in protein and glucose levels and in cell count are modest (see "Diagnosis"). A CSF leukocyte count of $<10/\mu L$ and an opening pressure of >250 mm are bad prognostic signs. Immune reconstitution during a response to HAART can lead to a return of fever and headache, suppuration of mediastinal lymph nodes, or meningeal enhancement on MRI.

DIAGNOSIS   Fever and headache in a patient with AIDS or with risk factors for HIV infection suggest the possibility of cryptococcosis, toxoplasmosis, or central nervous system lymphoma. Evidence of a focal lesion on MRI is unusual in cryptococcosis. Most cryptococcal cerebral mass lesions occur in patients infected with *C. neoformans* var. *gattii* who also have meningitis. In patients without AIDS, meningitis due to *C. neoformans* resembles that due to *Mycobacterium tuberculosis*, *Histoplasma capsulatum*, *Coccidioides immitis*, or metastatic cancer. Lumbar puncture is the single most useful diagnostic test. An india ink smear of centrifuged CSF sediment reveals encapsulated yeast in more than half of cases, although artifacts can cause confusion. In patients without AIDS, levels of glucose in CSF are reduced in half of all cases; protein levels are usually increased; and lymphocytic pleocytosis is usually found. CSF abnormalities are less pronounced in patients with AIDS, although india ink smear and serum antigen tests are more often positive.

Approximately 90% of patients with cryptococcal meningoencephalitis, including all those with a positive CSF smear and nearly all AIDS patients, have capsular antigen detectable in CSF or serum by latex agglutination. An enzyme immunoassay for cryptococcal antigen does not offer useful quantitative results but more clearly establishes positivity. Occasional false-positive results in both antigen tests make culture the definitive diagnostic test and have prevented serum antigen from being a useful screening test in asymptomatic patients with AIDS. Testing for serum antigen in AIDS patients with headache or fever is helpful. *C. neoformans* can often be cultured from the urine of patients with meningoencephalitis. Fungemia occurs in 10 to 30% of non-AIDS patients and in 60% of AIDS patients.

Pulmonary cryptococcosis appears on computed tomography (CT) as nodules with smooth or relatively undefined margins and homogeneous attenuation. In rare instances, ground-glass opacification is seen. Sputum culture is positive in only 10% of cases, and serum antigen tests are positive in only one-third. Occasionally, *C. neoformans* appears in one or more sputum specimens as an endobronchial saprophyte. Biopsy is usually required for diagnosis.

Cutaneous cryptococcosis may be mistaken for a comedo, basal cell carcinoma, or sarcoidosis. In patients with AIDS, skin lesions may be numerous and are sometimes mistaken for molluscum contagiosum (as shown for a liver transplant recipient in Fig. 186-1). Biopsy reveals myriad cryptococci. Osseous cryptococcosis is diagnosed by examination of bone or an adjacent soft tissue abscess.

FIGURE 186-1   Disseminated fungal infection. A liver transplant recipient developed six cutaneous lesions similar to the one shown. Biopsy and serum antigen testing demonstrated *Cryptococcus*. Important features of the lesion include a benign-appearing fleshy papule with central umbilication resembling molluscum contagiosum. (*Photo courtesy of Dr. Lindsey Baden.*)

℞ **TREATMENT**

See also Table 186-1. Patients with AIDS and cryptococcosis are treated initially with intravenous amphotericin B (0.7 to 1.0 mg/kg daily) for at least 2 weeks and until their clinical condition is stable; thereafter, they receive fluconazole. The addition of flucytosine (25 mg/kg every 6 h) to amphotericin B for 2 weeks has minimal impact on morbidity and mortality. After treatment with amphotericin B, fluconazole (400 mg) is given once daily; daily doses of 800 mg have been used with marginal changes in toxicity or efficacy. The addition of flucytosine to fluconazole increases gastrointestinal intolerance. Serum and CSF antigen have not been helpful in determining the efficacy of therapy, but CSF cultures should convert to negative. After at least 10 weeks of treatment and when the patient is asymptomatic, treatment with fluconazole (200 mg/d) is continued indefinitely. Itraconazole is less effective than fluconazole in cryptococcal meningitis but can be used. Patients with incapacitating symptoms of immune reconstitution improve with glucocorticoid therapy; it is unclear whether amphotericin B should be restarted until the glucocorticoid dose has been tapered. AIDS patients who have negative antigen and fungal cultures of CSF after prolonged fluconazole treatment and who have a sustained ($\geq$6-month) CD4+ response to HAART (with counts of at least 100 to 200/μL) may be candidates for discontinuation of maintenance therapy. Should CD4+ cell counts fall again, resumption of maintenance therapy would be reasonable.

In patients without AIDS, the therapeutic goal is to cure cryptococcal meningitis, not merely to control its symptoms. A single intensive course of amphotericin B is given for at least 10 weeks until cultures from all previously positive sites (particularly CSF) become convincingly negative. Normalization of the glucose level in lumbar CSF is important. The CSF antigen titer should fall by the end of therapy, but complete clearance of CSF or serum antigen during therapy is not essential. Amphotericin B (0.6 to 0.7 mg/kg daily for 10 weeks) is the best-studied regimen, but liposomal amphotericin B (4 to 5 mg/kg daily) is probably equivalent. Amphotericin B lipid complex and amphotericin B colloidal dispersion are not recommended pending further study. Flucytosine has been added to amphotericin B to accelerate the culture response, but grave toxicity can result unless flucytosine blood levels are kept below 100 μg/mL. Fluconazole (400 mg daily), given initially or begun after a course of amphotericin B, has cured cryptococcal meningitis or pulmonary cryptococcosis in some less immunosuppressed patients. Useful parameters for deciding when to discontinue therapy are unknown, but culture conversion, normalization of CSF glucose levels, and a fall in CSF antigen titer are minimal end points. A 6- to 12-month course of treatment is often used. Routine follow-up CSF cultures for the next year are useful in detecting relapse before symptoms supervene. Lung lesions on CT may take 6 weeks to improve and many months to resolve, if they ever do. Some immunosuppressed patients are treated as described above for AIDS patients, with indefinite fluconazole maintenance therapy.

Hydrocephalus may be the presenting manifestation or a later complication of cryptococcosis. Blindness, dementia, and personality change are among the other sequelae. Cerebral edema (in the absence of a cryptococcoma) causing headache, confusion, or blurred vision should be treated by daily lumbar puncture or CSF shunting to avert blindness. The shunt does not act as a nidus of persistent infection.

TABLE 186-1 *Treatment of Cryptococcosis*

Type of Disease	Preferred Treatment	Alternatives
Disease in AIDS patient	Amphotericin B (0.7–1.0 mg/kg daily) or liposomal amphotericin B (4–5 mg/kg daily) for 2 weeks and until symptoms improve; then fluconazole (400 mg/d) for 8 weeks; then fluconazole (200 mg/d) for life	Itraconazole (400 mg/d) for 8 weeks after amphotericin B; then 200 mg/d maintenance
Disease in non-AIDS patient		
Meningitis	Amphotericin B (0.6–0.7 mg/kg daily) or liposomal amphotericin B (4–5 mg/kg daily) for 10 weeks[a]	Switch to fluconazole (400 mg/d) when patient's condition has improved; continue for 6–12 months
Pulmonary disease	Treat immunosuppressed patients as for meningitis; previously normal patients may respond to fluconazole (400 mg/d) for 6–12 months.	Itraconazole (400 mg/d) for previously normal patients

[a] CSF culture should be negative, antigen titer falling, and glucose level normal.

PROPHYLAXIS Fluconazole (200 mg/d) has been shown to decrease the incidence of cryptococcosis in HIV-infected patients with CD4+ cell counts of <200/μL and particularly in those with counts of <50/μL. Weekly fluconazole has not provided this protection. Daily fluconazole has not conferred a survival advantage; in light of its cost and the currently low incidence of cryptococcosis in patients with AIDS in the United States, prophylaxis is strongly discouraged.

FURTHER READING

HOSPENTHAL DR, BENNETT JE: Persistence of cryptococcomas on neuroimaging. Clin Infect Dis 31:1303, 2000

KIRK O et al: Safe interruption of maintenance therapy against previous infection with four common HIV-associated opportunistic infections during potent antiretroviral therapy. Ann Intern Med 137:239, 2002

LILIANG P et al: Use of ventriculoperitoneal shunts to treat uncontrollable intracranial hypertension in patients who have cryptococcal meningitis without hydrocephalus. Clin Infect Dis 34:E64, 2002

MASUR H et al: Guidelines for preventing opportunistic infections among HIV-infected persons—2002. Ann Intern Med 137:435, 2002

NEWTON PN et al: A randomized, double-blind, placebo-controlled trial of acetazolamide for the treatment of elevated intracranial pressure in cryptococcal meningitis. Clin Infect Dis 35:769, 2002

SAAG MS et al: Practice guidelines for the management of cryptococcal disease. Clin Infect Dis 30:710, 2000

———— et al: A comparison of itraconazole versus fluconazole as maintenance therapy for AIDS-associated cryptococcal meningitis. Clin Infect Dis 28:291, 1999

ZINCK SE et al: Pulmonary cryptococcosis: CT and pathologic findings. J Comput Assist Tomogr 26:330, 2002

187 CANDIDIASIS
John E. Bennett

ETIOLOGIC AGENTS *Candida albicans* is the most common cause of mucosal candidiasis and is responsible for about half of all cases of candidemia in hospitalized patients. A small proportion of isolates previously identified as *C. albicans* have been transferred to a new species, *C. dubliniensis. C. tropicalis, C. parapsilosis, C. guilliermondii, C. glabrata* (formerly *Torulopsis glabrata*), *C. krusei*, and a few other *Candida* species account for the other half of candidemia cases; all can cause potentially lethal septic shock. The majority of these non-*albicans* species enter the bloodstream through intravascular catheters. *Candida* species, taken together, are the fourth or fifth most common cause of nosocomial bloodstream infections in the United States.

All *Candida* species pathogenic for humans are also encountered as commensals of humans, particularly in the mouth, stool, and vagina. These species grow rapidly at 25° to 37°C on simple media as oval, budding cells. In tissue, both yeasts and pseudohyphae are present. The latter are elongated branching structures with constrictions at the septae. Budding yeasts may be seen as separate structures or as projections from pseudohyphae. *C. glabrata* differs from other members of the genus in that it forms no true hyphae or pseudohyphae in vitro or in infected tissue. *C. albicans* and *C. dubliniensis* can be identified preliminarily by their ability to form germ tubes in serum—a test that requires only a few hours. These two species can be more accurately identified by the formation in special culture medium of thick-walled large spores called *chlamydospores*. Culture media now available for primary inoculation allow preliminary identification of *Candida* species by colony color. Accurate identification of *Candida* species other than *C. albicans* requires biochemical tests.

PATHOGENESIS Deeply invasive candidiasis is often preceded by increased colonization of the mouth, vagina, and stool with *Candida* due to broad-spectrum antibiotic therapy. Additional local and systemic factors favor infection. Oropharyngeal thrush is particularly likely to occur in neonates and in patients with diabetes mellitus, HIV infection, or dentures. Vulvovaginal candidiasis (Chap. 115) is especially common in the third trimester of pregnancy. *Candida* from the perineum can enter the urinary tract via an indwelling bladder catheter. Cutaneous candidiasis most often involves macerated skin, such as that in the diapered area of infants, under pendulous breasts, or on hands constantly in water or covered by occlusive gloves. *Candida* can pass from the colonized surface into deep tissue when the integrity of the mucosa or skin is violated, as, for example, by perforation of the gastrointestinal tract through trauma, surgery, or peptic ulceration or by mucosal damage due to cytotoxic agents used for cancer chemotherapy. Although *Candida* is not normally a resident of the skin, secretions from the mouth, rectum, or vagina as well as drainage from surgical wounds or tracheostomy sites can contaminate the hub or skin site of a catheter in an umbilical or central vein. Intravenous drug abuse or third-degree burns can also provide a skin portal for *Candida* that can lead to deep candidiasis. Once *Candida* has passed the integumentary barrier, very low birth weight (in neonates) and neutropenia or glucocorticoid therapy (in any patient) markedly compromise host defense. Hematogenous seeding is particularly evident in the retina, kidney, spleen, and liver.

CLINICAL MANIFESTATIONS ■ Mucocutaneous Candidiasis *Oral thrush* presents as discrete and confluent adherent white plaques on the oral and pharyngeal mucosa, particularly in the mouth and on the tongue. These lesions are usually painless, but fissuring at the corners of the mouth can be painful. Unexplained oropharyngeal thrush raises the possibility of HIV infection. Oral thrush is common in acute HIV infection and becomes increasingly common late in disease as the CD4+ cell count falls. At CD4+ counts of <50/μL, esophageal thrush also becomes common. HIV infection appears not to be an independent risk factor for vulvovaginal thrush.

Cutaneous candidiasis presents as red macerated intertriginous areas, paronychia, balanitis, or pruritus ani. Candidiasis of the perineal and scrotal skin may be accompanied by discrete pustular lesions on the inner aspects of the thighs. *Chronic mucocutaneous candidiasis* (*CMC*) or *candidal granuloma* typically presents as circumscribed hyperkeratotic skin lesions, crumbling dystrophic nails, partial alopecia in areas of scalp lesions, and both oral and vaginal thrush. Other findings may include chronic ringworm, dental dysplasia, and hypofunction of the parathyroid, adrenal, or thyroid gland. CMC is a major component of the immune polyendocrinopathy syndrome caused by a mutation in the autoimmune regulator gene (*AIRE*) on chromosome 21q22,3 (Chap. 330). CMC can begin in childhood as an autosomal dominant or recessive disorder or in association with Job's syndrome and can occur in adults in association with thymoma. Systemic infection is very rare in CMC, but permanent alopecia and disfigurement of the face and hands can be severe. Vulvovaginal thrush (Chap. 115) causes pruritus, discharge, and sometimes pain on intercourse or urination. Speculum examination reveals an inflamed mucosa and a thin exudate, often with white curds. Excessive colonization of the gastrointestinal tract has been associated with diarrhea and with chronic fatigue syndrome, but the linkage is unconvincing.

Esophageal candidiasis is often asymptomatic but can cause substernal pain or a sense of obstruction on swallowing. The pain of esophageal candidiasis may be mistaken for pain of cardiac origin. Most lesions are in the distal third of the esophagus and appear on endoscopy as areas of redness and edema, focal white patches, or ulcers. Biopsy or brushing is required for diagnosis and for detection of concomitant infections, particularly herpes simplex in patients with hematologic malignancies and cytomegalovirus infection in AIDS patients. *Candida* esophagitis can cause bleeding and impaired alimentation. Hematogenous dissemination from the esophagus probably occurs in some neutropenic patients but is rarely reported in HIV-infected patients.

Deeply Invasive Candidiasis In the obstructed *urinary tract*, *Candida* can cause cystitis, pyelitis, or renal papillary necrosis. When a colonized urinary tract is operated on or instrumented, candidemia may result. However, most patients with *Candida* cultured from the urine simply have bladder colonization from a Foley catheter or a sizable volume

of residual urine. Contamination of a voided midstream specimen by vaginal *Candida* is also common.

Candidemia originating from an intravascular catheter may clear in the immunocompetent patient when the catheter is removed. Focal seeding of the retina can take place even if candidemia clears and the patient becomes afebrile. Unilateral or bilateral small white retinal exudates appear within 2 weeks of the onset of candidemia. Lesions may regress spontaneously or enlarge slowly. The vitreous humor becomes cloudy, and the patient notices blurring, ocular pain, or a scotoma. Retinal detachment, vitreous abscess, and extension to the anterior chamber can occur over the ensuing weeks. These retinal lesions, present in ~10% of nonneutropenic patients with candidemia, are the principal reason that systemic antifungal therapy is recommended for all patients with candidemia. Funduscopy should be performed to ensure that retinal lesions, if present, resolve completely. Most cases with ocular involvement have occurred in nonneutropenic patients. In contrast, so-called *hepatosplenic candidiasis* is usually recognized in patients with acute leukemia who are recovering from profound neutropenia. This entity, better called *chronic disseminated candidiasis*, originates from intestinal seeding of the portal and venous circulation. Fever, modestly elevated serum concentrations of alkaline phosphatase, and multiple small abscesses evident on ultrasonography, magnetic resonance imaging, or computed tomography (CT) of the liver, spleen, or kidney suggest the diagnosis. During acute candidemia in neutropenic patients, small erythematous papules may appear anywhere on the skin (Fig. 187-1). If the patient does not expire promptly from disseminated candidiasis, the lesions will develop a necrotic center. Painful muscle lesions may also be found. Punch biopsy of a skin lesion helps distinguish this extremely grave condition from *Malassezia* folliculitis, a similar-appearing but benign condition that can involve the cape area of the chest or the extremities of a sweaty febrile patient.

Hematogenous seeding in the neutropenic patient is occasionally visible radiologically as tiny pulmonary nodules. *Candida pneumonia*, apart from hematogenous candidiasis, is very rare. *Candida endocarditis* can be caused by any *Candida* species and favors previously damaged or prosthetic heart valves. The source is often an intravascular catheter or contaminated equipment used for illicit intravenous drug injection. An interval of weeks or even months between candidemia and discovery of endocarditis is common. Emboli to large arteries, such as the iliac or femoral artery, are characteristic. Intravenous injection of impure brown heroin has caused a clinical syndrome consisting of *Candida endophthalmitis* and purulent *folliculitis*, sometimes accompanied by vertebral *osteomyelitis*.

Candida can cause indolent *arthritis*, most commonly of the knee, in patients who have received glucocorticoid injections into the joint, in patients who are immunosuppressed, and in low-birth-weight neonates. Prosthetic joints may become infected during implantation. Scanty growth of *Candida* from joint fluid can cause the laboratory to

FIGURE 187-1 Disseminated candidiasis. Tender, erythematous, nodular lesions developed in a neutropenic patient with leukemia who was undergoing induction chemotherapy. (Photo courtesy of *Dr. Lindsey Baden*.)

incorrectly dismiss the organism as a contaminant. *Candida* can cause subacute *peritonitis* arising either from a perforated viscus or from a peritoneal dialysis catheter.

Hematogenous dissemination can lead to *brain abscess* or chronic *meningitis*. Diagnosis of infections of ventriculoperitoneal shunts is difficult because symptoms are indolent and cultures of lumbar fluid are usually sterile.

DIAGNOSIS Demonstration of pseudohyphae on wet smear with confirmation by culture is the procedure of choice for diagnosing superficial candidiasis. Scrapings for the smear may be obtained from skin, nails, and oral and vaginal mucosa. A culture of urine, sputum, existing abdominal drains, endotracheal aspirates, or the vagina is not diagnostic; however, recovery of *Candida* species from multiple superficial sites has been identified as a risk factor for deeply invasive candidiasis in some studies of patients with prolonged neutropenia or complicated abdominal surgery.

Deeper lesions due to *Candida* may be diagnosed by histologic section of biopsies or by culture of cerebrospinal fluid, blood, joint fluid, CT-guided needle aspirates, or surgical specimens. Blood cultures are useful in the diagnosis of *Candida* endocarditis and intravenous catheter–induced sepsis but are positive less often in other forms of disseminated disease. Serologic tests for antibody or antigen are not useful.

TABLE 187-1	Treatment of Candidiasis	
Type of Disease	**Preferred Treatment[a]**	**Alternatives**
Mucocutaneous		
Cutaneous	Topical azole	Topical nystatin
Vulvovaginal	Azole cream or suppository or oral fluconazole (150 mg)	Nystatin suppository
Oropharyngeal	Clotrimazole troche or fluconazole tablet (100 mg/d) or itraconazole solution (200 mg/d)	Nystatin suspension; for azole-unresponsive disease: caspofungin (50 mg/d) or amphotericin B (0.3–0.5 mg/kg daily)
Esophageal	Fluconazole tablet (100–200 mg/d) or itraconazole solution (200 mg/d)	For azole-unresponsive disease: caspofungin (70 mg once, then 50 mg/d) or amphotericin B (0.3–0.5 mg/kg daily)
Deeply invasive		
Nonneutropenic	Fluconazole (400 mg/d) or amphotericin B[b] or caspofungin (70 mg once, then 50 mg/d)	
Neutropenic	Amphotericin B[b]	

[a] Removal of foreign bodies is critical, including plastic catheters for intravenous fluids, peritoneal dialysis or cerebrospinal fluid shunts, prosthetic cardiac valves, and prosthetic joints.

[b] The dosage of amphotericin B for deeply invasive candidiasis is 0.5 mg/kg daily, although initial doses of 0.7–1.0 mg/kg daily may be appropriate for severely immunosuppressed patients. Amphotericin B lipid complex and liposomal amphotericin B are given as 5 mg/kg daily.

℞ TREATMENT

(See also Table 187-1.) Cutaneous candidiasis of macerated areas responds to measures that reduce moisture and chafing plus topical application of an antifungal agent in a nonocclusive base. Nystatin powder or a cream containing ciclopirox or an azole is useful. Clotrimazole, miconazole, econazole, ketoconazole, sulconazole, and oxiconazole are available as creams or lotions. *Candida* vulvovaginitis responds better to an azole than to nystatin suppositories. There is little difference in efficacy among miconazole, clotrimazole, tioconazole, butoconazole, and terconazole vaginal formulations. Systemic treatment of *Candida* vulvovaginitis with a single 150-mg capsule of fluconazole is more convenient than topical treatment; however, this option is contraindicated in pregnancy, is less effective in patients with multiple relapses, and poses a higher risk of adverse effects. Clotrimazole troches, used five times a day, are more effective in oral candidiasis than nystatin suspension and are approximately as effective as oral fluconazole (100 mg daily). Oral fluconazole (100 to 200 mg once daily) is more convenient and more effective in esophagitis than clotrimazole troches. Esophagitis not responding to fluconazole may warrant repeat endoscopy to exclude other conditions. Itraconazole suspension (100 mg twice daily) alleviates *Candida* esophagitis in some patients in whom fluconazole treatment fails. Nearly all patients with azole-resistant oropharyngeal or esophageal candidiasis respond to a 2-week course of intravenous amphotericin B (0.3 to 0.5 mg/kg daily) or caspofungin (70 mg for one dose, then 50 mg daily). Relapse is usual.

Management of recurrent oropharyngeal candidiasis in the HIV-infected patient presents special problems. Patients with CD4+ cell counts of <100/μL who have received prolonged fluconazole therapy are at risk of developing azole resistance, requiring an increased dose to mount a response, relapsing early, and eventually failing to respond well to any dose of fluconazole. The increasing azole resistance in this population suggests that HIV-infected patients with oropharyngeal or esophageal candidiasis should be treated for each individual episode

and that only when episodes become intolerably frequent or severe should prophylaxis be given.

Bladder thrush responds to bladder irrigations with amphotericin B (50 μg/mL for 5 days). If no bladder catheter is in place, oral fluconazole can be used to control candiduria. Most patients with candiduria do not have unrelieved urinary tract obstruction and do not benefit from therapy.

Intravenous amphotericin B is the drug of choice for deeply invasive candidiasis in neutropenic or seriously immunosuppressed patients. The deoxycholate formulation is usually given at a dosage of 0.5 to 0.7 mg/kg daily. Open, noncomparative studies of amphotericin B lipid complex and liposomal amphotericin B indicate that either preparation is effective in deeply invasive candidiasis. The usual dose of either formulation is 5 mg/kg daily by the intravenous route.

Candida endocarditis on prosthetic or native valves usually relapses unless the valve is replaced. Long-term fluconazole administration has been used to prevent recurrence after valve replacement.

In immunocompetent patients with intravenous catheter–acquired *C. albicans* fungemia, the catheter should be removed in conjunction with the administration of fluconazole (400 mg/d), amphotericin B (0.5 mg/kg daily), or caspofungin (one 70-mg dose followed by 50 mg daily by the intravenous route). Amphotericin B (0.7 to 1.0 mg/kg daily) may be appropriate as initial therapy in severely neutropenic patients. Candidemia from suppurative phlebitis of a peripheral vein may not respond until the infected portion of the vein is excised. Therapy for candidemia is continued for 2 weeks after the patient becomes afebrile. The *Candida* species involved should be considered in choosing a drug for candidemia. *C. krusei* and *C. inconspicua* are rare causes of candidemia but are resistant to fluconazole in vitro. *C. glabrata* exhibits intermediate susceptibility to fluconazole. Thus either increasing the daily fluconazole dose to 800 mg or using amphotericin B or caspofungin may be appropriate. Caspofungin displays approximately equal activity in vitro against all *Candida* species, including azole-resistant strains. Strains of *C. lusitaniae* resistant to amphotericin B but susceptible to azoles or caspofungin have been encountered. Intravenous amphotericin B, with or without flucytosine, is the preferred treatment for *Candida* endophthalmitis, although cures have been reported with fluconazole. Pars plana vitrectomy may facilitate diagnosis and cure when a *Candida* vitreous abscess is present. Injection of amphotericin B into the vitreous humor can also be helpful.

Because amphotericin B and fluconazole penetrate reasonably well into an infected joint, the pleural cavity, and the peritoneum, local injection is not indicated. Removal of prostheses (including prosthetic joints and cardiac valves), peritoneal dialysis catheters, and central venous catheters is usually essential. Debridement, along with antifungal therapy, is beneficial in *Candida* osteomyelitis. All collections of pus, such as those in the postoperative abdomen, need to be drained surgically or by percutaneous, CT-guided catheterization; an exception relates to the numerous small abscesses in liver, spleen, or kidney in chronic disseminated candidiasis, which cannot be drained effectively and require prolonged antifungal therapy. In general, treatment should continue until the patient with chronic disseminated candidiasis has been afebrile and nonneutropenic for at least 2 weeks. Defects may persist on imaging studies long after cure. Relapse during another episode of neutropenia is common unless the patient is receiving amphotericin B. Repeat cytotoxic therapy or even bone marrow transplantation can be undertaken in patients with prior chronic disseminated candidiasis, but amphotericin B should be given empirically during neutropenia.

PROPHYLAXIS   Fluconazole can decrease the incidence of deeply invasive candidiasis in recipients of allogeneic bone marrow transplants when 400 mg is given daily. Some centers continue such prophylaxis for 70 days; others discontinue it after engraftment. Studies of leukemic and other neutropenic patients have found no significant reduction in the incidence of deeply invasive candidiasis associated with prophylactic use of fluconazole or itraconazole oral suspension, although this topic remains controversial. Prophylaxis against recurrent oropharyngeal or esophageal candidiasis in HIV-infected patients is no longer recommended unless recurrences are very frequent or severe. Fluconazole (3 to 6 mg/kg) or itraconazole solution (5 mg/kg) is the recommended daily oral dose. Fluconazole prophylaxis at 400 mg daily may be useful in preventing deeply invasive candidiasis in some high-risk postoperative patients. Definition of groups at sufficient risk to benefit from fluconazole depends on the intensive care unit but likely includes patients undergoing repeat, complicated abdominal surgery and patients who are both heavily colonized with *Candida* and immunosuppressed at the time of complicated surgery. The presence of intravenous catheters, prolonged stays in the intensive care unit, and renal failure increase the risk of candidemia.

FURTHER READING

BENOIT D et al: Management of candidal thrombophlebitis of the central veins: Case report and review. Clin Infect Dis 26:393, 1998

MARR KA et al: Prolonged fluconazole prophylaxis is associated with persistent protection against candidiasis-related death in allogeneic marrow transplant recipients: Long-term follow-up of a randomized, placebo-controlled trial. Blood 96:2055, 2000

MASUR H et al: Guidelines for preventing opportunistic infections among HIV-infected persons—2002. Recommendations of the U.S. Public Health Service and the Infectious Diseases Society of America. Ann Intern Med 137: 435, 2002

MELGAR GR et al: Fungal prosthetic valve endocarditis in 16 patients. An 11-year experience in a tertiary care hospital. Medicine 76:94, 1997

PELZ RK et al: Double-blind placebo-controlled trial of fluconazole to prevent candidal infections in critically ill surgical patients. Ann Surg 233:542, 2001

REX JH et al: Practice guidelines for the treatment of candidiasis. Clin Infect Dis 30:662, 2000

ZUCCARELLO D et al: Familial chronic nail candidiasis with ICAM-1 deficiency: A new form of chronic mucocutaneous candidiasis. J Med Genet 39:671, 2002

188   ASPERGILLOSIS
John E. Bennett

ETIOLOGIC AGENTS   *Aspergillus fumigatus* is the most common cause of aspergillosis, but *A. flavus*, *A. niger*, *A. nidulans*, *A. terreus*, and several other species can also cause disease. *Aspergillus* is a mold with septate branching hyphae ~2 to 4 μm in diameter. The fungus is identified by its gross and microscopic appearance in culture.

PATHOGENESIS AND PATHOLOGY   All the common species of *Aspergillus* that cause disease in humans are ubiquitous in the environment, growing on dead leaves, stored grain, compost piles, hay, and other decaying vegetation. The fungus can also be isolated from potable water, although the clinical significance of this observation is unknown. Inhalation of *Aspergillus* spores must be extremely common, but disease is rare. Invasion of lung tissue is confined almost entirely to immunosuppressed patients, in roughly 90% of whom two of the following three conditions will be operative: a granulocyte count in peripheral blood of <500/μL, treatment with supraphysiologic doses of adrenal glucocorticoids, and a history of treatment with other immunosuppressive drugs such as cyclosporine. Invasive aspergillosis is an occasional complication of AIDS. *Aspergillus* infection in the neutropenic patient is characterized by hyphal invasion of blood vessels, thrombosis, necrosis, and hemorrhagic infarction. Chronic granulomatous disease of childhood also predisposes to invasive pulmonary aspergillosis, but in that situation the inflammatory response is a pyogranuloma and blood vessel invasion is rare.

Massive inhalation of *Aspergillus* spores by healthy persons can lead to acute, diffuse, self-limited pneumonitis. Epithelioid granulomas with giant cells and central pyogenic areas containing hyphae are detected in these cases. Spontaneous recovery taking several weeks is the usual course. Such patients should be tested for underlying chronic granulomatous disease.

Aspergillus can colonize the damaged bronchial tree, pulmonary cysts, or cavities of patients with underlying lung disease. Balls of hyphae within cysts or cavities (aspergillomas), usually in the upper lobe, may reach several centimeters in diameter and may be visible on chest x-ray. Tissue invasion does not occur.

CLINICAL MANIFESTATIONS   *Allergic bronchopulmonary aspergillosis* occurs in patients with preexisting asthma (particularly glucocorticoid-dependent asthma) or cystic fibrosis and causes intermittent episodes of wheezing, pulmonary infiltrates from transient bronchial plugging, sputum and blood eosinophilia, low-grade fever, and brownish or greenish flecks in the sputum. These flecks contain *Aspergillus* hyphae, thick mucus, eosinophils, and Charcot-Leyden crystals. Some patients with repeated exacerbations develop central bronchiectasis and progressive loss of pulmonary function.

Endobronchial saprophytic pulmonary aspergillosis presents as chronic productive cough, often with hemoptysis, in a patient with prior chronic lung disease, such as tuberculosis, sarcoidosis, bronchiectasis, or histoplasmosis. *Aspergillus* may be spread from its endocavitary or endobronchial site to the pleura during the course of bacterial lung abscess or surgery. Patients reported to have chronic necrotizing *Aspergillus* pneumonia appear in most instances to have had saprophytic endobronchial colonization and a pulmonary process attributable to another disease, with or without superimposed bacterial infections. Patients with chronic pneumonia and *Aspergillus* in the sputum should be assumed to have either pneumonia of a different etiology (e.g., histoplasmosis) or *Aspergillus* pneumonia with underlying immunosuppression (e.g., chronic granulomatous disease or infection with HIV).

Invasive aspergillosis in the immunocompromised host presents as an acute, rapidly progressive, densely consolidated pulmonary infiltrate and is most common among patients with acute leukemia and recipients of tissue transplants. Infection progresses by direct extension across tissue planes and by hematogenous dissemination to lung, brain, and other organs. Computed tomography (CT) has been particularly valuable in suggesting the diagnosis of invasive pulmonary aspergillosis in patients with neutropenia. The earliest CT finding is one or more small pulmonary nodules. As a nodule enlarges, the dense central core of infarcted tissue becomes surrounded by edema or hemorrhage, forming a hazy rim called the *halo sign*. This rim disappears in a few days as the dense core enlarges. When bone marrow function recovers, the infarcted central core cavitates, creating the *crescent sign*. *Aspergillus* may invade immunosuppressed patients through the skin at a site of minor trauma or through the upper airway mucosa. Early lesions in the nose should be sought in patients with neutropenia who have fever and minimal epistaxis. Scarlet-red patches of the mucosa rapidly become necrotic and white, then black. Rapid extension into the adjacent paranasal sinus, orbit, or face is usual, with or without the appearance of lung lesions.

Aspergillus sinusitis in immunocompetent patients may take three forms. A ball of hyphae may form in a chronically obstructed paranasal sinus, without tissue invasion. Much less commonly, a chronic, fibrosing granulomatous inflammation associated with *Aspergillus* hyphae within tissue may begin in the sinus and spread slowly to the orbit and the brain. *Aspergillus* is also a cause of allergic fungal sinusitis, but dark-walled fungi (e.g., *Curvularia*, *Alternaria*) are more common in this setting. Patients usually have a history of chronic allergic rhinitis, sometimes with nasal polyps, but are otherwise healthy, presenting with painless proptosis, nasal obstruction, or dull aching pain. On CT or magnetic resonance imaging, a solid soft-tissue mass pushing out the lateral wall of the ethmoid sinus or the medial wall of the maxillary sinus may be detected. On sinus exploration, the mucosa is found to be thickened and inflamed but intact. Within the sinus cavity, sticky mucopus with strands of neutrophils, eosinophils, Charcot-Leyden crystals, and occasional hyphae can be found.

Aspergillosis in HIV-infected patients most commonly involves the lung, presenting as fever, cough, and dyspnea. Typically, the CD4+ cell count is $<50/\mu L$. Roughly half of these patients have neutropenia or have recently been treated with glucocorticoids. Bilateral diffuse or focal pulmonary infiltrates with a tendency to cavitate constitute the most common radiologic manifestation. Well-localized, white, necrotic pseudomembranes full of hyphae or ulcers may develop in the trachea or the major bronchi. Progression of bronchitis to pneumonia is usual, but hematogenous dissemination is uncommon. Either allergic or invasive *Aspergillus* sinusitis can occur in HIV-infected patients; the allergic form can develop even at CD4+ cell counts of $>50/\mu L$.

The growth of *Aspergillus* on cerumen and detritus within the external auditory canal is termed *otomycosis*. Trauma to the cornea may cause *Aspergillus* keratitis. Endophthalmitis follows the introduction of *Aspergillus* into the globe by trauma or surgery. *Aspergillus* may infect intracardiac or intravascular prostheses.

DIAGNOSIS The repeated isolation of *Aspergillus* from sputum or the demonstration of hyphae in sputum or bronchoalveolar lavage fluid suggests endobronchial colonization or infection. Even a single isolation of *Aspergillus* from the sputum of a neutropenic patient or a hematopoietic stem-cell transplant recipient with pneumonia, particularly a child or a nonsmoker, suggests the diagnosis of invasive aspergillosis. In patients with advanced AIDS, fever, and cough, the isolation of *Aspergillus* from respiratory secretions raises the possibility of aspergillosis and thus should prompt bronchoscopy. Fungus ball of the lung is usually detectable by chest x-ray. IgG antibody to *Aspergillus* antigens is demonstrable in the serum of many colonized patients and of virtually all patients with fungus ball. Patients with allergic bronchopulmonary aspergillosis have specific serum IgE antibody to *Aspergillus* antigens and often have IgG antibody as well. No standardized test for these antibodies exists. Serum IgE concentrations are often >1000 ng/mL.

Biopsy is usually required for the diagnosis of invasive aspergillosis of the lung, nose, paranasal sinus, bronchi, or sites of dissemination. Blood cultures are rarely positive, even in patients with infected cardiac valves (native or prosthetic). Detection of galactomannan an-

tigen in serum suggests the diagnosis, but sensitivity is low early in the disease and false-positive results occur, particularly in children. *Aspergillus* hyphae can be identified presumptively by histology, but culture is required for confirmation and for identification of the species. Only culture can reliably distinguish aspergillosis from pseudallescheriasis; drug therapy for these two diseases differs.

℞ TREATMENT

(See also Table 188-1.) Patients with severe hemoptysis due to fungus ball of the lung may benefit from lobectomy. Poor pulmonary function in residual lung and dense pleural adhesions around the lesion can complicate the resection. Bead embolization directed to the bronchial arterial supply has been used as a temporizing measure. Systemic chemotherapy is of no value in endobronchial or endocavitary aspergillosis. Short courses of oral adrenal glucocorticoids have been used to treat acute bronchial plugging in patients with allergic bronchopulmonary aspergillosis. Two small studies have indicated that patients with allergic bronchopulmonary aspergillosis require less glucocorticoid therapy and have fewer exacerbations when given prophylaxis with oral itraconazole (200 mg twice daily). Itraconazole has also been used with glucocorticoids to treat exacerbations.

Treatment with intravenous amphotericin B (1.0 to 1.5 mg/kg daily) has elicited a response in 30 to 40% of patients with invasive aspergillosis. Intravenous voriconazole (6 mg/kg every 12 h for two doses, then 4 mg/kg every 12 h) is better tolerated and more efficacious than a regimen starting with conventional amphotericin B. Once the patient has begun to respond, voriconazole can be given orally as 200 mg twice daily. Liposomal amphotericin B at daily doses of 5 mg/kg is probably comparable to voriconazole, but no comparative study is available. Compared with conventional amphotericin B, amphotericin B colloidal dispersion shows equivalent efficacy in aspergillosis, is less nephrotoxic, and more often causes infusion-related chills and fever. Itraconazole (200 mg twice daily) is useful in some less immunosuppressed patients with indolent or slowly progressive invasive aspergillosis. Over the first 2 weeks, itraconazole can be given intravenously as 200 mg twice daily for four doses and then 200 mg daily to patients who are unable to take or unlikely to absorb oral itraconazole. The intravenous formulation is contraindicated in patients with a creatinine clearance rate of <30 mL/min. Itraconazole capsules are given as 200 mg twice daily. Intravenous caspofungin (70 mg once, then 50 mg daily) can be considered for patients in whom therapy with other drugs fails. Surgery is the only treatment needed for fungus ball of the sinus and for allergic fungal sinusitis. Antifungal therapy has little effect on either entity if used alone, but chronic suppressive therapy has been begun postoperatively for relapse of allergic fungal si-

TABLE 188-1 *Treatment of Aspergillosis*

Type of Disease	Preferred Treatment	Alternatives
Fungus ball of the lung	Surgical resection	Bead embolization for hemoptysis
Allergic bronchopulmonary aspergillosis	Short courses of glucocorticoids	Itraconazole prophylaxis
Invasive aspergillosis[a]	Voriconazole, liposomal or conventional amphotericin B	Amphotericin B colloidal dispersion or lipid complex, itraconazole, or caspofungin

[a] Voriconazole dose: 6 mg/kg twice daily for two doses; then 4 mg/kg twice daily; for later oral administration, 200 mg twice daily. Liposomal amphotericin B dose: 5 mg/kg daily. Conventional amphotericin B dose: 1.0 to 1.5 mg/kg daily. Amphotericin B colloidal dispersion dose: 6 mg/kg daily. Amphotericin B lipid complex dose: 5 mg/kg daily. Intravenous itraconazole dose: 200 mg twice daily for four doses, then 200 mg daily. Intravenous caspofungin dose: 70 mg once, then 50 mg daily.

nusitis. The prognosis for cure of invasive aspergillosis in the paranasal sinus is very poor when the patient has profound and unremitting neutropenia. The prognosis is better in less immunosuppressed patients.

FURTHER READING

BOWDEN R et al: A double-blind, randomized, controlled trial of amphotericin B colloidal dispersion versus amphotericin B for treatment of invasive aspergillosis in immunocompromised patients. Clin Infect Dis 35:359, 2002

CAILLOT D et al: Increasing volume and changing characteristics of invasive pulmonary aspergillosis on sequential thoracic computed tomography scans in patients with neutropenia. J Clin Oncol 19:253, 2001

DENNING DW: Invasive aspergillosis. Clin Infect Dis 26:781, 1998

HERBRECHT R et al: Voriconazole versus amphotericin B for primary therapy of invasive aspergillosis. N Engl J Med 347:408, 2002

MAERTENS J et al: Use of circulating galactomannan screening for early diagnosis of invasive aspergillosis in allogeneic stem cell transplant recipients. J Infect Dis 186:1297, 2002

MARR KA: Invasive aspergillosis in allogeneic stem cell transplant recipients: Changes in epidemiology and risk factors. Blood 102:827, 2003

MOSS RB: Allergic bronchopulmonary aspergillosis. Clin Rev Allergy Immunol 23:87, 2002

SHIRAKUSA T et al: Surgical treatment of pulmonary aspergilloma and *Aspergillus* empyema. Ann Thorac Surg 48:779, 1989

STEVENS DA et al: Practice guidelines for diseases caused by *Aspergillus*. Clin Infect Dis 30:696, 2000

189 MUCORMYCOSIS
John E. Bennett

ETIOLOGIC AGENTS Species of *Rhizopus*, *Rhizomucor*, and *Cunninghamella* are the most common causes of mucormycosis, but species of *Apophysomyces*, *Saksenaea*, *Mucor*, and *Absidia* also are occasionally responsible for this infection. The etiologic organism in tissue is composed of broad, rarely septate hyphae of uneven diameter (6 to 15 μm). The organisms are inexplicably difficult to grow from infected tissue. When growth does take place, it is rapid and profuse on most media at room temperature. Identification is based on the gross and microscopic appearance of the mold.

Zygomycosis is a term that includes mucormycosis and entomophthoramycosis. The latter is a tropical infection of the subcutaneous tissue or paranasal sinuses caused by species of *Basidiobolus* and *Conidiobolus*, respectively.

EPIDEMIOLOGY AND PATHOLOGY *Rhizopus* and *Rhizomucor* species are ubiquitous, appearing on decaying vegetation, dung, and foods of high sugar content. Mucormycosis is uncommon and is largely confined to patients with serious preexisting diseases. Mucormycosis originating in the paranasal sinuses and nose predominantly affects patients with poorly controlled diabetes mellitus. Patients who have undergone organ transplantation, who have a hematologic malignancy, or who are receiving long-term deferoxamine therapy are predisposed to mucormycosis of either sinus or lung. Deferoxamine chelates iron in a form that the fungus can utilize. Gastrointestinal mucormycosis occurs in a variety of conditions, including uremia, severe malnutrition, and diarrheal diseases. The infection is acquired from nature, with no person-to-person spread. In all forms of mucormycosis, vascular invasion by hyphae is a prominent feature. Ischemic or hemorrhagic necrosis is the foremost histologic finding.

CLINICAL MANIFESTATIONS Mucormycosis originating in the nose and paranasal sinuses produces a characteristic clinical picture. Low-grade fever, dull sinus pain, and sometimes nasal congestion or a thin, bloody nasal discharge are followed in a few days by double vision, increasing fever, and obtundation. Examination reveals a unilateral generalized reduction of ocular motion, chemosis, and proptosis. The nasal turbinates on the involved side may be dusky red or necrotic. A sharply delineated area of necrosis, strictly respecting the midline, may appear in the hard palate. Facial skin adjacent to paranasal sinuses may be invaded by direct extension, turning progressively red, purple, and black. Fungal invasion of the globe or ophthalmic artery leads to blindness. Opacification of one or more sinuses is detected by computed tomography (CT) or magnetic resonance imaging (MRI). Magnetic resonance angiography (MRA) with gadolinium enhancement may show invasion or obstruction of the carotid siphon. Coma is due to direct invasion of the frontal lobe. Early symptoms mimic those of bacterial sinusitis. Clouding of the sensorium may be attributed to diabetic acidosis. Cavernous sinus thrombosis may be considered when orbital invasion occurs. Without treatment, the patient may die after an interval ranging from a few days to a few weeks.

Pulmonary mucormycosis manifests as progressive severe pneumonia accompanied by high fever and toxicity. The necrotic center of large infiltrates may cavitate. Fatal hemoptysis may occur from cavities formed near the hilum. Hematogenous spread to other areas of the lung, as well as to the brain and other organs, is common. Survival beyond 2 weeks is unusual. Gastrointestinal invasion presents as one or more ulcers that tend to perforate. Hematogenous dissemination can originate from the gastrointestinal tract, lung, or paranasal sinuses. Sometimes no portal of entry can be found. Primary cutaneous inoculation is uncommon but occurs in burn eschars, underneath occlusive dressings, and at sites of minor trauma in immunocompromised adults and low-birth-weight neonates. Several reported infections with *Apophysomyces elegans* have manifested as cellulitis in diabetics or previously normal patients.

DIAGNOSIS CT or MRI is very helpful in assessing the extent of sinusitis before surgery and in evaluating the patient afterward. CT is better for detecting bony erosion; MRI better visualizes extension into the frontal lobe or carotid artery in the siphon. Lesions of the lung and craniofacial structures are best diagnosed by biopsy and histologic section. Cultural confirmation should be attempted. Wet smear of crushed tissue can provide a rapid diagnosis. Cultures of blood and cerebrospinal fluid are negative. Smear and culture of sputum may be positive during cavitation of a lung lesion.

Rx TREATMENT

Regulation of diabetes mellitus and a decrease in the dose of immunosuppressive drugs facilitate the treatment of mucormycosis. Extensive debridement of craniofacial lesions appears to be very important. Orbital exenteration may be required. Intravenous amphotericin B is clearly of value in craniofacial mucormycosis and should be employed in the other forms of mucormycosis as well. The maximal tolerated doses are given until progression is halted. Endoscopic examination of paranasal sinuses can help assess progression. With the deoxycholate formulation, a dosage of 1 to 1.5 mg/kg daily is indicated. Amphotericin B lipid complex or liposomal amphotericin B, each at 5 mg/kg daily, appears to be as effective as and less toxic than conventional amphotericin B. Therapy is continued for a total of 10 to 12 weeks. Voriconazole and itraconazole are of no value. Results of hyperbaric oxygen therapy have been unimpressive. Appropriate management results in cure of about half of craniofacial infections. Primary cutaneous lesions benefit from debridement; extensive plastic surgical repair may be required, but the prognosis is good. Survival is rare among patients who have received deferoxamine and among those with pulmonary, gastrointestinal, or disseminated mucormycosis.

BLAIR JE et al: Locally invasive cutaneous *Apophysomyces elegans* infection acquired from snapdragon patch test. A review. Mayo Clin Proc 77:717, 2002

HOLLAND J: Emerging zygomycoses of humans: *Saksenaea vasiformis* and *Apophysomyces elegans*. Curr Top Med Mycol 8:27, 1997

MCADAMS HP et al: Pulmonary mucormycosis: Radiologic findings in 32 cases. Am J Radiol 168:1541, 1997

OH D, NOTRICA D: Primary cutaneous mucormycosis in infants and neonates: Case report and review of the literature. J Pediatr Surg 37:1607, 2002

RICKERTS V et al: Cluster of pulmonary infections caused by *Cunninghamella bertholletiae* in immunocompromised patients. Clin Infect Dis 31:910, 2000

TEDDER M et al: Pulmonary mucormycosis: Results of medical and surgical therapy. Ann Thorac Surg 57:1044, 1994

WARWAR RE, BULLOCK JD: Rhino-orbital-cerebral mucormycosis: A review. Orbit 17:237, 1998

190 MISCELLANEOUS MYCOSES AND ALGAL INFECTIONS
John E. Bennett

CHROMOBLASTOMYCOSIS (CHROMOMYCOSIS) This chronic subcutaneous mycosis, rarely seen in the United States, presents as nodular or verrucoid, ulcerated, or crusted skin lesions on exposed areas of skin, particularly on the lower extremities. Over months and years, lesions extend to contiguous skin; they may be tender or itchy. Pain is not a prominent symptom. The disease, which in fact causes few symptoms, follows the introduction of any of several fungi into subcutaneous tissue by thorns or bits of vegetation. The appearance of thick-walled, dark-colored, rounded forms ("copper pennies") in a histopathologic section of the dermis is diagnostic. Dark-walled hyphae may be seen in the stratum corneum. Surgical excision is the treatment of choice for small lesions. Cryotherapy and itraconazole with or without flucytosine have ameliorated larger lesions. Repeated treatments may be necessary.

DERMATOPHYTOSIS ■ Definition Dermatophytosis, also known as ringworm or tinea, is a chronic fungal infection of the skin, hair, or nails.

Etiology Species of *Trichophyton*, *Microsporum*, and *Epidermophyton* are called *dermatophytes*. These organisms grow in and remain confined to the keratinous structures of the body. Other mycoses, such as candidiasis, pityriasis versicolor, and tinea nigra, may include fungal invasion of keratinous structures but traditionally are not called dermatophytoses.

Pathology and Pathogenesis Dermatophyte species are referred to as *anthropophilic*, *zoophilic*, or *geophilic*, depending on whether their usual reservoir in nature appears to be humans, animals, or soil, respectively. The infectivity of organisms from all these sources is low, and outbreaks are largely confined to occasional clusters of cases of scalp infection in children. Acquisition of a dermatophytosis appears to be favored by minor trauma (including that incurred during wrestling), maceration, and poor hygiene of the skin. Infection does not seem to confer solid immunity: repeated infection with the same species is common, particularly with anthropophilic species. The infrequency of scalp infection among adults has been attributed to local factors rather than immunity.

Invasion of the stratum corneum by dermatophytes may cause inflammation that is either mild or (particularly with zoophilic fungi) intense. Shedding of the stratum corneum is increased by inflammation. To the extent that fungal growth cannot keep up with shedding, inflammation may help terminate infection. Conversely, infection is probably favored when shedding is reduced by treatment with glucocorticoids and cytotoxic drugs. Antifungal drugs interfere with the ability of fungal growth to keep up with shedding.

Clinical Manifestations The disease varies with the site of infection and the fungal species involved. Foot infection (athlete's foot, tinea pedis) may present as fissuring of the toe webs, scaling of the plantar surfaces, or vesicles around the toe webs and soles. Interdigital lesions may be pruritic or, when bacterial superinfection occurs, may be painful. Hand infection is less common but resembles foot infection.

Scalp dermatophytosis (tinea capitis) is characterized by areas of alopecia and scaling. In so-called endothrix infection, the hair shaft breaks off at the skin surface, leaving the hairs visible as black dots in the scalp. Some forms of scalp infection include an area of intense boggy suppuration called a *kerion*.

Dermatophytosis of the glabrous skin (Fig. 190-1) presents as circumscribed lesions with a wide variety of appearances, including scales, vesicles, and pustules. Inflammation may be minimal or intense. Central healing of less inflamed lesions may take place. The serpiginous border of inflammation is the source of the name *ringworm*.

Dermatophytosis of the bearded area (tinea barbae) appears as a pustular folliculitis. Onychomycosis (tinea unguium) presents as a white discoloration of the nails or as thickening, chalkiness, and crumbling of the nails. Peeling and fissuring of paronychial nail folds or keratotic debris under the nail edge also may be evident.

Diagnosis Discolored hairs, scales, and keratotic debris under infected nails should be collected for KOH or calcofluor smear and culture. In the scraping of skin lesions, a drop of water on the skin site may keep the removed scales from flying off and thus may aid in their collection. Culture is important in distinguishing dermatophytes from *Candida* and fungal saprophytes growing in keratinaceous debris.

℞ TREATMENT

Noninflammatory lesions of the trunk, groin, hands, and feet usually respond to twice-daily applications of clotrimazole, miconazole, ketoconazole, econazole, naftifine, terbinafine, or ciclopirox olamine cream. Hyperkeratotic lesions of the palms and soles respond slowly to these agents and may benefit from the initial application of Whitfield's ointment to thin the keratin. Ointment should not be used between the toes, in the groin, or in the gluteal crease because maceration promotes bacterial infection.

Ringworm that is moderately severe, that is unresponsive to topical

FIGURE 190-1 Tinea corporis is a superficial fungal infection, seen here as an erythematous annular scaly plaque with central clearing.

therapy, or that involves the scalp, nails, or bearded area should be treated systemically. Once-daily therapy with itraconazole (200 mg), terbinafine (250 mg), microcrystalline griseofulvin (500 mg), or ultramicrocrystalline griseofulvin (375 mg) is effective. Treatment must be continued until all infected keratin is gone. Cutting off infected hair and cleansing interdigital webs can expedite cure. Secondary bacterial infection of the foot may require soaks or antibacterial agents. The likelihood of relapse of dermatophyte foot infections may be decreased by keeping the feet clean and dry. For nail infections, itraconazole or terbinafine is preferred. In distal subungual onychomycosis, a single course of either drug results in initial improvement in half of patients, of whom half relapse. Results are better with fingernails than with toenails and for more distal rather than proximal nail involvement. To save money, itraconazole can be given as a double dose (400 mg) for 1 week each month with only marginal loss of efficacy. The rare but life-threatening complications of itraconazole must be weighed against the patient's desire to have normal-appearing nails. The duration of therapy with itraconazole or terbinafine is 2 to 3 months for fingernails and 4 to 6 months for toenails.

PROTOTHECOSIS *Prototheca* species are ubiquitous achlorophyllic algae that enter exposed areas of skin through contaminated wounds and cause localized infections in the skin, olecranon bursa, and, rarely, tendon sheaths or deeper tissue. Diagnosis is based on culture or histopathologic demonstration of morula-like sporangia containing endospores in tissue. *Prototheca wickerhamii*, the usual agent, grows readily on fungal culture medium. Surgical debridement and treatment with itraconazole or intravenous amphotericin B are useful.

FUSARIOSIS *Fusarium* species can cause localized or hematogenously disseminated infection. Indolent cellulitis or soft-tissue necrosis can occur in immunocompetent patients at the site of trauma (including burns) or adjacent to onychomycosis. Immunocompromised patients may develop skin lesions at the site of minor trauma or, more often, as a result of hematogenous dissemination. Two-thirds of patients with disseminated infection who are severely immunosuppressed, particularly those who are profoundly neutropenic, develop skin lesions. One or more tender erythematous papules enlarge rapidly, may develop a surrounding rim of erythema, and may become necrotic or ulcerated in the center. A portal of infection is not usually apparent. Blood cultures have been positive in 59% of cases. The presence of a mold growing in a culture of blood from a neutropenic patient suggests fusariosis. Blood cultures are rarely positive in aspergillosis or mucormycosis. Voriconazole or amphotericin B is the drug of choice for fusariosis, but survival from disseminated infection depends on the diminution of neutropenia. Debridement of localized lesions in immunocompetent patients is useful.

MALASSEZIA INFECTION (PITYRIASIS) *Malassezia furfur* is part of the normal flora of the human skin but can cause tinea (pityriasis) versicolor or catheter-acquired sepsis. Tinea versicolor appears as asymptomatic, well-delineated, hyperpigmented or hypopigmented macules centered on the upper trunk and upper arms. Confluent lesions may cover large areas, making the border difficult to find. A fine "branny" scale or folliculitis is sometimes visible. When examined microscopically by KOH mount, skin sections are seen to contain characteristic round and elongated cells. On inspection with Wood's light, lesions either do not fluoresce or appear yellow-green. *Erythrasma* resembles tinea versicolor but is characterized by gram-positive bacilli on smear and coral-red fluorescence. Azole creams are effective for the treatment of small areas of tinea versicolor; however, the application of selenium sulfide shampoo (Selsun) for 10 min daily, followed by showering to remove the shampoo, is more practical for large areas. Itraconazole is also effective. Catheter-acquired sepsis due to *M. furfur* develops in patients (particularly neonates) receiving intravenous lipid. The organism requires special culture conditions for growth, and the infection is cured by catheter removal.

mycetes of the genera *Nocardia* (Chap. 146), *Nocardiopsis*, *Streptomyces*, and *Actinomadura*. *Eumycetoma* is caused by true fungi of many different genera. The predominant agent varies with the locality.

Pathogenesis and Pathology The pathogens live in the soil and enter the skin through minor trauma. The most common site of infection is the foot. The infection runs a relentless course over many years, with destruction of contiguous bone and fascia. Grains are found in purulent foci surrounded by fibrosis and a mononuclear cell inflammatory response.

Clinical Manifestations Mycetoma is a chronic suppurative infection originating in subcutaneous tissue and characterized by the presence of grains, which are tightly clumped colonies of the causative agent. The infected site is characterized by painless swelling, woody induration, and sinus tracts that discharge pus intermittently. Systemic symptoms do not develop, and spread to distant sites in the body does not take place.

Diagnosis Although the clinical picture is characteristic, mycetoma is sometimes confused with chronic osteomyelitis or botryomycosis. The diagnosis requires demonstration of grains in pus from the draining sinus or in biopsy sections. Many histologic sections may need to be examined to locate a grain.

 TREATMENT

Actinomycetoma may respond to prolonged combination chemotherapy—e.g., with streptomycin and either dapsone or trimethoprim-sulfamethoxazole. Eumycetoma rarely responds to chemotherapy; some cases caused by *Madurella mycetomatis* have appeared to respond to ketoconazole or itraconazole.

PARACOCCIDIOIDOMYCOSIS ■ **Etiology** Formerly called *South American blastomycosis*, this mycosis is caused by *Paracoccidioides brasiliensis*. A dimorphic fungus, *P. brasiliensis* grows as a budding yeast in tissue and as either a yeast or a mold on culture medium. The organism is identified by its gross and microscopic appearance.

Pathogenesis and Pathology Infection is thought to be acquired by inhalation of spores from environmental sources, possibly soil. Pulmonary infection produces few symptoms initially. Hematogenous spread to the mucous membranes of the mouth and nose, the lymph nodes, and other sites causes patients to seek medical attention. In fatal cases, the infection spreads to the adrenals, the gastrointestinal tract, and many other viscera.

Clinical Manifestations Common signs include indurated ulcers of the mouth, oropharynx, larynx, and nose; enlarged and draining lymph nodes; lesions of the skin and genitalia; and productive cough, weight loss, dyspnea, and sometimes fever. Paracoccidioidomycosis is acquired only in South America, Central America, and Mexico, but its extreme indolence may delay its recognition until many years after the patient has left the endemic area. Chest radiography most often shows bilateral patchy pneumonia.

Diagnosis Cultures of sputum, pus, and mucosal lesions are often diagnostic. The diagnosis can be made by smear or histologic section, although confirmation by culture is preferable. Serologic tests are useful in suggesting the diagnosis and monitoring the response to therapy.

 TREATMENT

Relatively mild cases of paracoccidioidomycosis may be cured by 1 year of treatment with oral itraconazole (200 to 400 mg daily). More advanced cases are treated with intravenous amphotericin B followed by itraconazole.

PENICILLIOSIS MARNEFFEI *Penicillium marneffei* has emerged as a leading cause of opportunistic infection in patients in the late stages of HIV infection in Southeast Asia—notably, northern Thailand and southern China. Infection is probably acquired by the inhalation of spores from an unknown site in nature. At the time of diagnosis, infection has usually disseminated to bone marrow, liver, spleen, skin, or bone. Clinical manifestations and histopathologic findings resemble those of histoplasmosis. Both *P. marneffei* and *Histoplasma* are dimorphic fungi, appearing as small yeast cells in tissue and as a mold in culture. Unlike *Histoplasma*, the yeastlike cells of *P. marneffei* do not bud but divide by longitudinal fission. During growth as a mold, a red pigment forming in the agar underneath *P. marneffei* colonies can aid in the organism's identification. Treatment consists of amphotericin B administration for 2 weeks or until improvement is documented, with subsequent administration of itraconazole (400 mg daily for 8 weeks, then 200 mg daily as maintenance therapy). A few patients with a sustained response to highly active antiretroviral therapy and prolonged maintenance therapy have had itraconazole discontinued, with no subsequent relapse.

PHAEOHYPHOMYCOSIS This is the name given to infections caused by fungi with dark-walled hyphae, excluding those given conventional names like chromoblastomycosis. Although an extraordinary variety of fungi and clinical syndromes are encompassed by this definition, most patients have brain abscess, subcutaneous abscess, or allergic fungal sinusitis. Most of the brain abscesses are due to *Cladophialophora bantiana*, *Ochroconis gallopavum*, *Exophiala dermatitidis*, *Bipolaris* species, and *Ramichloridium mackenziei (obovoideum)*. Patients are previously healthy. Subcutaneous abscesses are usually single, arise at the site of minor trauma, and occur in both immunosuppressed and immunocompetent individuals. A large number of dematiaceous (dark-walled) mold species cause subcutaneous phaeohyphomycosis as well as allergic fungal sinusitis. The latter entity develops in patients with allergic rhinitis and presents as an expanding mucoid mass in one or more paranasal sinuses. The tenacious mucus contains eosinophils, Charcot-Leyden crystals, and occasional hyphae. Surgical excision of phaeohyphomycotic lesions is important. Antifungal therapy may retard recurrences but is of little value without surgical excision.

PSEUDALLESCHERIASIS ■ **Etiology** Also called *Petriellidium boydii*, *Pseudallescheria boydii* is a mold frequently found in soil. When isolated in the imperfect state, the anamorph is called *Scedosporium apiospermum*. *Scedosporium prolificans* is a closely related species.

Pathogenesis and Pathology Wind-borne spores of *P. boydii*, arising from the soil, are the presumed source of infection. The fungus grows as a mold within tissue, causing necrosis and abscess formation.

Clinical Manifestations *P. boydii* resembles *Aspergillus* in its ability to colonize the endobronchial tree, to form fungus balls in the lungs or paranasal sinuses, and to invade the cornea or globe of the eye, the soft tissues, the joints, or the bones after trauma or surgery and in its propensity to invade the lungs and paranasal sinuses of immunosuppressed hosts, including patients with AIDS. Hematogenous dissemination to the eye, brain, soft tissues, and other sites is common. Severe pneumonia, often with hematogenous dissemination and brain abscesses, has followed near-drowning in stagnant water. Hyphae of *P. boydii* in tissue may be difficult to distinguish from those of *Aspergillus*. Intravascular hyphae, a hallmark of invasive aspergillosis, are also found in pseudallescheriasis in neutropenic patients.

S. prolificans has caused infections in bones, joints, and soft tissue, usually after trauma.

Diagnosis Demonstration of hyphae in tissue and culture confirmation are required for diagnosis.

℞ TREATMENT

Soft-tissue infections in previously normal patients respond well to surgical debridement and treatment with itraconazole or voriconazole. Immunosuppressed patients respond poorly, and those with disseminated infection usually die. Surgical drainage is useful in brain abscesses. Voriconazole is the drug of choice for immunosuppressed individuals, and itraconazole is a suitable alternative. *P. boydii* appears to be unresponsive to systemic amphotericin B therapy, although injection of amphotericin B into an infected joint has been helpful in a few cases. In previously normal patients with *S. prolificans* soft-tissue infection, surgical debridement has been useful. The response to all antifungal agents has been poor in immunosuppressed patients, but voriconazole treatment has resulted in cure in a few cases.

SPOROTRICHOSIS ■ **Etiology** *Sporothrix schenckii* lives as a saprophyte on plants in many areas of the world. In nature and on culture at room temperature, the fungus grows as a mold; within host tissue or at 37°C on enriched media, it grows as a budding yeast. It is identified by its appearance in mold and yeast forms.

Pathogenesis and Pathology Infection results from the inoculation of *S. schenckii* into subcutaneous tissue through minor trauma. Nursery workers, florists, and gardeners acquire the illness from roses, sphagnum moss, and other plants. Infection may be limited to the site of inoculation (plaque sporotrichosis) or extend along proximal lymphatic channels (lymphangitic sporotrichosis). Spread beyond an extremity—the usual site of infection—is rare, and hematogenous dissemination from the skin remains unproven. The portal for osteoarticular, pulmonary, and other extracutaneous forms of sporotrichosis is unknown but is probably the lung. Untreated sporotrichosis persists for months. The inflammatory response includes neutrophil clustering and a marked granulomatous response with epithelioid and giant cells.

Clinical Manifestations In lymphangitic sporotrichosis, which is by far the most common manifestation, a nearly painless red papule forms at the site of inoculation. Over the next several weeks, similar nodules form along proximal lymphatic channels. The nodules intermittently discharge small amounts of pus. Ulceration may occur. The proximal extension of these lesions, often with skip areas, is quite distinctive but may be mimicked by lesions of *Nocardia brasiliensis*, *Mycobacterium marinum*, or (in rare cases) *Leishmania brasiliensis* or *Mycobacterium kansasii*.

Plaque sporotrichosis manifests as a nontender red maculopapular granuloma confined to the site of inoculation. Osteoarticular sporotrichosis presents as mono- or polyarticular arthritis of indolent onset and progression over months or years, involving the elbows, knees, wrists, ankles, and (rarely) smaller joints of the extremities. Periarticular bone develops areas of demineralization detectable on x-ray, and draining sinuses may appear over joints and bursae. Hematogenous spread to the skin may take place during polyarticular disease, but none of the skin lesions shows lymphangitic spread. Immunosuppression, including that due to advanced infection with HIV, predisposes to hematogenous spread. Pulmonary sporotrichosis usually presents as a single chronic cavitary upper-lobe lung lesion. Chronic meningitis can develop in the absence of skin or lung lesions. *S. schenckii* is difficult to recover from cerebrospinal fluid.

Diagnosis Culture of pus, joint fluid, sputum, or a skin biopsy specimen is preferred. The appearance of *S. schenckii* in tissue is variable. In skin lesions, the organisms are hard to find.

℞ TREATMENT

Itraconazole (100 to 200 mg daily) is the drug of choice for the treatment of cutaneous sporotrichosis. A saturated solution of potassium iodide given orally is also effective, but side effects often prevent the effective use of this regimen. Therapy should be continued for 1 month after the resolution of all lesions. Fluconazole is less effective. Extracutaneous sporotrichosis may be cured by itraconazole (200 mg twice daily), but the response is slow and may be incomplete. Prolonged courses of intravenous amphotericin B are more effective. Cavitary pulmonary sporotrichosis may require resection for cure.

TRICHOSPORONOSIS A change in the taxonomy of the genus *Trichosporon* moved most of the agents causing deep infections from *T. beigelii* into the species *T. asahii*, with a few categorized as *T. mucoides*. White piedra of the scalp is caused by *T. ovoides* and that of the pubic hair by *T. inkin*. *T. cutaneum* and *T. asteroides* cause superficial infections. Most of what is currently known about *Trichosporon* infections is not species specific, so the following description refers to *T. beigelii*. *T. capitatum*, which causes disseminated infection in patients with neutropenia, was previously reclassified as *Blastoschizomyces capitatus* and will not be covered here.

T. beigelii can be isolated from soil, the human gastrointestinal tract, and skin. The organism can enter the bloodstream of patients with severe neutropenia through an inapparent source. Hematogenously disseminated infection is manifested by fever and often by the development of several erythematous or purpuric tender papules anywhere on the body. Lesions can form large, tense hemorrhagic bullae. In some patients, native or prosthetic cardiac valves become infected. In tissue, hyphae and yeastlike cells are seen. Amphotericin B is probably the drug of choice for treatment, but recovery depends on the return of bone marrow function.

PFIESTERIA INFECTION   See Chap. 378.

FURTHER READING

BONIFAZ A et al: Chromoblastomycosis: Clinical and mycologic experience of 51 cases. Mycoses 44:1, 2001

CASTIGLIONI B et al: *Pseudallescheria boydii* (anamorph *Scedosporium apiospermum*). Infection in solid organ transplant recipients in a tertiary medical center and review of the literature. Medicine 81:333, 2002

CHAO SC et al: Cutaneous protothecosis: Report of five cases. Br J Dermatol 146:688, 2002

HAUGH M et al: Terbinafine in fungal infections of the nails: A meta-analysis of randomized clinical trials. Br J Dermatol 47:118, 2002

KAUFFMAN CA et al: Practice guidelines for the management of patients with sporotrichosis. Clin Infect Dis 30:684, 2000

MELLINGHOFF IK et al: Treatment of *Scedosporium apiospermum* brain abscesses with posaconazole. Clin Infect Dis 34:1648, 2002

NUCCI M, ANAISSIE E: Cutaneous infection by *Fusarium* species in healthy and immunocompromised hosts: Implications for diagnosis and management. Clin Infect Dis 35:909, 2002

SUPPARATPINYO K et al: A controlled trial of itraconazole to prevent relapse of *Penicillium marneffei* infection in patients infected with the human immunodeficiency virus. N Engl J Med 339:1739, 1998

191 PNEUMOCYSTIS INFECTION
Peter D. Walzer

DEFINITION AND DESCRIPTION   *Pneumocystis* is an opportunistic fungal pulmonary pathogen that is an important cause of pneumonia (pneumocystosis) in the immunocompromised host. The taxonomic classification of *Pneumocystis* as a fungus is based on factors such as analysis of gene sequences for ribosomal RNA, mitochondrial proteins, and major enzymes; the presence of β-1,3 glucan in the cell wall; and the efficacy of antifungal drugs that inhibit β-glucan synthesis in animal models. However, in contrast to most fungi, *Pneumocystis* lacks ergosterol and is not susceptible to antifungal drugs that inhibit ergosterol synthesis.

Although *Pneumocystis* organisms obtained from different sources are morphologically very similar, they are genetically diverse and host specific. New nomenclature, which is still evolving, has established that organisms derived from rats and humans are separate species termed *P. carinii* and termed *P. jiroveci*, respectively. For the purpose of clarity, only the genus designation, *Pneumocystis*, will be used in this chapter.

Research on *Pneumocystis* has been limited by the lack of a reliable in vitro culture system. Developmental stages of the organism include the small (1- to 4-μm) pleomorphic trophic form; the 5- to 8-μm cyst, which has a thick cell wall and contains up to eight intracystic bodies; and the precyst, an intermediate stage. The life cycle of *Pneumocystis* probably involves sexual and asexual reproduction. *Pneumocystis* contains several different antigen groups, the most prominent of which is the 95- to 140-kDa major surface glycoprotein (MSG). MSG represents a multigene family of proteins, and the ability of MSG to undergo antigenic variation may represent a mechanism by which *Pneumocystis* evades host defenses. MSG is highly immunogenic, contains protective epitopes, and facilitates adherence of the organism to host cells via extracellular matrix proteins, surfactant proteins, and the mannose receptor.

EPIDEMIOLOGY   Serologic surveys have demonstrated that *Pneumocystis* has a worldwide distribution and that most healthy children have been exposed to the organism by 3 to 4 years of age. Airborne transmission of *Pneumocystis* has been documented in animal studies; person-to-person transmission has been suggested by hospital outbreaks of pneumocystosis and by molecular analysis of isolates from patients and their close contacts. Geography has also emerged as a contributory factor in the epidemiology of *Pneumocystis* infection.

PATHOGENESIS AND PATHOLOGY   The host factors that predispose to the development of pneumocystosis include defects in cellular and humoral immunity. The risk of developing *Pneumocystis* pneumonia among HIV patients rises markedly when circulating CD4+ cell counts fall below 200/μL. The frequency of serum antibodies to a specific segment of MSG is significantly higher in HIV patients who have recovered from an episode of pneumocystosis than in HIV patients who have never had the disease. Other persons at risk for *Pneumocystis* pneumonia are patients receiving immunosuppressive therapy (particularly glucocorticoids) for cancer, organ transplantation, and other disorders; children with primary immunodeficiency diseases; and premature malnourished infants.

The principal host effector cells against *Pneumocystis* are alveolar macrophages, which ingest and kill the organism, releasing a variety of inflammatory mediators. Tumor necrosis factor α and interleukin (IL) 1, interferon γ, and granulocyte-macrophage colony-stimulating factor contribute to host defenses against *Pneumocystis*. HIV reduces the mannose receptor–mediated binding and phagocytosis of *Pneumocystis* and alters the cytokine responses to the organism.

After being inhaled, *Pneumocystis* takes up residence in the alveoli, where it attaches tightly to type I cells but maintains an extracellular existence. It was formerly thought that the organism remains latent in the host for long periods, but more recent data suggest that pneumonia can arise from a new bout of infection. As the immune system of the host becomes compromised, *Pneumocystis* organisms propagate and gradually fill the alveoli. This scenario is accompanied by a complex series of events that result in increased alveolar-capillary permeability and damage to alveolar type I cells. Surfactant abnormalities include a fall in bronchoalveolar lavage (BAL) fluid phospholipids and an increase in surfactant proteins A and D. Contributions of the host inflammatory response to lung injury are suggested by the correlation of increased IL-8 levels and neutrophil counts in BAL fluid from patients with severe disease. In addition, immune reconstitution with the start of highly potent anti-HIV drugs and treatment of pneumocystosis is sometimes associated with new pulmonary infiltrates.

On lung sections stained with hematoxylin and eosin, the alveoli are filled with a typical foamy, vacuolated exudate. Severe disease may include interstitial edema, fibrosis, and hyaline membrane formation. The host inflammatory changes usually consist of hypertrophy of alveolar type II cells, a typical reparative response, and a mild mononuclear cell interstitial infiltrate. Malnourished infants display an intense plasma cell infiltrate that gave the disease its early name: interstitial plasma cell pneumonia.

CLINICAL FEATURES   Patients with pneumocystosis develop dyspnea, fever, and nonproductive cough. Symptoms in non-HIV-infected patients often begin after the glucocorticoid dose has been tapered and typically last 1 to 2 weeks. HIV-infected patients are usually ill for several weeks or longer and have relatively subtle manifestations. The clinical picture in individual patients is variable. A high index of suspicion and a thorough history are key factors in early detection.

Physical findings include tachypnea, tachycardia, and cyanosis, but lung auscultation reveals few abnormalities. The white blood cell count is variable and is usually governed by the patient's underlying disease. Reduced arterial oxygen pressure (Pa_{O_2}), increased alveolar-arterial oxygen gradient ($PA_{O_2} - Pa_{O_2}$), and respiratory alkalosis are evident. There also may be changes in pulmonary function test values (diffusing capacity) and heightened uptake with nonspecific nuclear imaging techniques (gallium scan). Elevated serum concentrations of lactate dehydrogenase (LDH) have been reported; the increase probably reflects lung parenchymal damage but is not specific to *Pneumocystis* infection. In general, laboratory abnormalities are less severe in HIV-infected patients than in non-HIV-infected patients.

The classic findings on chest radiography consist of bilateral diffuse infiltrates beginning in the perihilar regions (Fig. 191-1), but various atypical manifestations (nodular densities, cavitary lesions) have also been reported. Patients who receive aerosolized pentamidine have an increased frequency of upper-lobe infiltrates. Pneumothorax also occurs, and management is often difficult. Early in the course of pneumocystosis, the chest radiograph may be normal.

Although *Pneumocystis* usually remains confined to the lungs, cases of disseminated infection have occurred in both HIV-infected and non-HIV-infected patients. One risk factor for extrapulmonary spread in patients with HIV is the administration of aerosolized pentamidine. The most common sites of involvement are the lymph nodes, spleen, liver, and bone marrow. Eye lesions (choroiditis) also occur and must be distinguished from retinitis caused by cytomegalovirus. Clinical manifestations range from incidental findings at autopsy to specific organ involvement. Histopathologic examination reveals *Pneumocystis* and the characteristic associated foamy material.

DIAGNOSIS Because the clinical picture of *Pneumocystis* infection can be produced by many other infectious and noninfectious agents, the diagnosis must be based on specific identification of the organism. A definitive diagnosis is made by histopathologic staining. Traditional stains have included reagents such as methenamine silver, toluidine blue, and cresyl echt violet, which selectively stain the wall of *Pneumocystis* cysts, and reagents such as Wright-Giemsa, which stain the nuclei of all developmental stages. Other reagents include nonspecific fluorochrome stains (calcofluor white) and Papanicolaou's stain. Immunofluorescence with monoclonal antibodies is more sensitive than histologic staining but is also more expensive. DNA amplification by the polymerase chain reaction (PCR) is most sensitive and should be part of routine diagnosis if commercial kits become available.

The successful diagnosis of pneumocystosis depends upon the collection of proper specimens. In general, the yield from different diagnostic procedures is higher in HIV-infected patients than in non-HIV-infected patients because of the higher organism burden in the former group. Sputum induction has gained popularity as a simple, noninvasive technique; this procedure requires trained and dedicated personnel, and its success has varied at different institutions. Oral washes, combined with PCR, have also shown promise. Fiberoptic bronchoscopy with BAL, which is more sensitive than sputum induction, remains the mainstay of *Pneumocystis* diagnosis. This procedure also provides information about the organism burden, the host inflammatory response, and the presence of other opportunistic infections. Transbronchial biopsy and open lung biopsy, the most invasive procedures, are used only when a diagnosis cannot be made by BAL.

COURSE AND PROGNOSIS In the typical case of untreated *Pneumocystis* pneumonia, progressive respiratory embarrassment leads to death. Therapy is most effective when instituted early in the course of the disease, before there is extensive alveolar damage. If induced sputum is nondiagnostic and BAL cannot be performed in a timely manner, it is reasonable to begin empirical therapy with drugs active against *Pneumocystis*. However, this practice does not obviate a specific etiologic diagnosis. With improved management of HIV and its complications, mortality from pneumocystosis is 15 to 20% at 1 month and 50 to 55% at 1 year. Rates of early death remain high among people who require mechanical ventilation (60%) and among non-HIV patients (40%). The most widely used prognostic factor is the degree of hypoxemia. Other factors include pneumocystosis history, age, CD4+ count, neutrophil and IL-8 levels in BAL fluid, albumin and LDH levels in serum, and the degree of expertise with which HIV infection is managed.

℞ TREATMENT

For decisions about therapy (see also Chaps. 118 and 193), pneumocystosis has been classified as mild (a Pa_{O_2} of >70 mmHg or a $PA_{O_2} - Pa_{O_2}$ of <35 mmHg) or as moderate to severe (a Pa_{O_2} of ≤70 mmHg or a $PA_{O_2} - Pa_{O_2}$ of ≥35 mmHg) on breathing room air. Trimethoprim-sulfamethoxazole (TMP-SMX), which acts by inhibiting folic acid synthesis, is considered the drug of choice for all forms of pneumocystosis (Table 191-1). Treatment for extrapulmonary disease is the same as that for pneumonia. Therapy is continued for 14 days in non-HIV-infected patients and for 21 days in persons infected with HIV. Since HIV-infected patients respond more slowly than non-HIV-infected patients, it is prudent to wait at least 7 days after the initiation of treatment before concluding that therapy has failed. Adding drugs to an existing regimen is no more effective than switching regimens and may increase the risk of toxicity. TMP-SMX is well tolerated by non-HIV-infected patients, whereas more than half of HIV-infected patients experience serious adverse reactions.

Several alternative regimens are available for the treatment of mild to moderate cases of pneumocystosis. TMP plus dapsone and clindamycin plus primaquine are about as effective as TMP-SMX. Dapsone and primaquine should not be used in patients with glucose-6-phosphate dehydrogenase (G6PD) deficiency. Atovaquone is less effective than TMP-SMX but is better tolerated. Atovaquone should be given with food to enhance absorption.

One alternative regimen for the treatment of moderate to severe *Pneumocystis* pneumonia is parenteral pentamidine. Pentamidine is about as effective as TMP-SMX but is highly toxic to both HIV-infected and non-HIV-infected patients. Other regimens include parenteral clindamycin plus primaquine and trimetrexate plus leucovorin (with leucovorin administered to prevent bone marrow suppression).

In recent years, molecular evidence of resistance to sulfonamides—and, to a lesser extent, atovaquone—has emerged among human *Pneumocystis* isolates. Although prior sulfonamide exposure has been a risk factor, this resistance has also occurred in HIV-infected patients who never used sulfonamides. Some studies have found an association of sulfonamide resistance with a poor response to therapy, whereas other studies have not.

Patients infected with HIV frequently experience deterioration in respiratory function shortly after receiving anti-*Pneumocystis* drugs. The adjunctive administration of tapering doses of glucocorticoids to patients with HIV infection and moderate to severe pneumocystosis can prevent this problem and improve the rate of survival (Table 191-1). For maximal benefit, this adjunctive therapy should be started early in the course of the illness (usually when antimicrobial drugs are begun). This regimen has generally proved to be safe despite concern about its effects on other opportunistic infections. The use of steroids as adjunctive therapy in HIV-infected patients with mild pneumocystosis or in non-HIV-infected patients remains to be evaluated.

PREVENTION Primary prophylaxis is indicated for HIV-infected patients with CD4+ cell counts of <200/μL or a history of oropharyngeal candidiasis. Primary prophylaxis guidelines for other immunocompromised hosts are less clear. Secondary prophylaxis is indicated for both HIV-infected and non-HIV-infected patients who have recovered from pneumocystosis. Primary and secondary prophylaxis may be discontinued in HIV-infected persons once CD4+ counts have risen to >200/μL and remained at that level for ≥3 months.

TABLE 191-1   *Treatment of Pneumocystosis*

Drug(s), Dose, Route	Adverse Effects
FIRST CHOICE[a]	
TMP-SMX (5 mg/kg TMP, 25 mg/kg SMX[b]) q6–8 h PO or IV	Fever, rash, cytopenias, hepatitis, hyperkalemia, GI disturbances
OTHER AGENTS[a]	
TMP, 5 mg/kg q6–8h, plus dapsone, 100 mg qd PO	Hemolysis (G6PD deficiency), methemoglobinemia, fever, rash, GI disturbances
Atovaquone, 750 mg bid PO	Rash, fever, GI and hepatic disturbances
Clindamycin, 300–450 mg q6h PO or 600 mg q6–8h IV, plus primaquine, 15–30 mg qd PO	Hemolysis (G6PD deficiency), methemoglobinemia, rash, colitis, neutropenia
Pentamidine, 3–4 mg/kg qd IV	Hypotension, azotemia, cardiac arrhythmias, pancreatitis, dysglycemias, hypocalcemia, neutropenia, hepatitis
Trimetrexate, 45 mg/m² qd IV, plus leucovorin[c], 20 mg/kg q6h PO or IV	Cytopenias, peripheral neuropathy, hepatic disturbances
ADJUNCTIVE AGENT	
Prednisone, 40 mg bid × 5 d, 40 mg qd × 5 d, 20 mg qd × 11 d; PO or IV	Immunosuppression, peptic ulcer, hyperglycemia, mood changes, hypertension

[a] Therapy is administered for 14 days to non-HIV-infected patients and for 21 days to HIV-infected patients.
[b] Equivalent of 2 double-strength (DS) tablets. (One DS tablet contains 160 mg of TMP and 800 mg of SMX.)
[c] Leucovorin prevents bone marrow toxicity from trimetrexate.
Note: GI, gastrointestinal; G6PD, glucose-6-phosphate dehydrogenase; TMP-SMX, trimethoprim-sulfamethoxazole.

TABLE 191-2   *Prophylaxis of Pneumocystosis*[a]

Drug, Dose, Route	Comments
FIRST CHOICE	
TMP-SMX, 1 DS tablet or 1 SS tablet qd PO[b]	TMP-SMX can be safely reintroduced in some patients who have experienced mild to moderate side effects.
OTHER AGENTS	
Dapsone, 50 mg bid or 100 mg qd PO	—
Dapsone, 50 mg qd PO, plus pyrimethamine, 50 mg weekly PO, plus leucovorin, 25 mg weekly PO	Leucovorin prevents bone marrow toxicity from pyrimethamine.
Dapsone, 200 mg weekly PO, plus pyrimethamine, 75 mg weekly PO, plus leucovorin, 25 mg weekly PO	Leucovorin prevents bone marrow toxicity from pyrimethamine.
Pentamidine, 300 mg monthly via Respirgard II nebulizer	Adverse reactions include cough, bronchospasm.
Atovaquone, 1500 mg qd PO	—
TMP-SMX, 1 DS tablet three times weekly PO	TMP-SMX can be safely reintroduced in some patients who have experienced mild to moderate side effects.

[a] For list of adverse effects, see Table 191-1.
[b] One DS tablet contains 160 mg of TMP and 800 mg of SMX.
Note: DS, double-strength; SS, single-strength; TMP-SMX, trimethoprim-sulfamethoxazole.

TMP-SMX is the drug of choice for primary and secondary prophylaxis (Table 191-2). This agent also provides protection against toxoplasmosis and some bacterial infections. Alternative regimens include dapsone, dapsone plus pyrimethamine plus leucovorin, aerosolized pentamidine, and atovaquone. Although there are no specific recommendations for preventing the spread of *Pneumocystis* infection in health care facilities, it seems prudent to prevent direct contact between patients with pneumocystosis and other susceptible hosts.

FURTHER READING

BARRY SM et al: *Pneumocystis carinii* pneumonia: A review of current issues in diagnosis and management. HIV Medicine 2:123, 2001

CENTERS FOR DISEASE CONTROL AND PREVENTION: Guidelines for preventing opportunistic infections among HIV-infected persons—2002 recommendations of the U.S. Public Health Service and the Infectious Diseases Society of America. MMWR 51(RR-8):1, 2002

DWORKIN MS et al: Survival of patients with AIDS, after diagnosis of *Pneumocystis carinii* pneumonia, in the United States. J Infect Dis 183:1409, 2001

LEOUNG GS et al: Trimethoprim-sulfamethoxazole (TMP-SMX) dose escalation versus direct rechallenge for *Pneumocystis carinii* pneumonia prophylaxis in human immunodeficiency virus–infected patients with previous adverse reaction to TMP-SMX. J Infect Dis 184:992, 2001

STRINGER JR et al: A new name (*Pneumocystis jiroveci*) for *Pneumocystis* from humans. Emerg Infect Dis 8:891, 2002

WALZER PD: Immunological features of *Pneumocystis carinii* infection in humans. Clin Diagn Lab Immunol 6:149, 1999

192 | LABORATORY DIAGNOSIS OF PARASITIC INFECTIONS
Charles E. Davis

The cornerstone for the diagnosis of parasitic infections is a thorough history of the patient's illness. Epidemiologic aspects of the illness are especially important because the risks of acquiring many parasites are closely related to occupation, recreation, or travel to areas of high endemicity. Without a basic knowledge of the epidemiology and life cycles of the major parasites, it is difficult to approach the diagnosis of parasitic infections systematically. Accordingly, the medical classification of important human parasites in this chapter emphasizes their

TABLE 192-1 *Flatworm Infections*

Parasite	Geographic Distribution	Intermediate (Transmission)	Definitive	Parasite Stage	Body Fluid or Tissue	Serologic Tests	Other
TAPEWORMS (CESTODES)							
Intestinal tapeworms							
Taenia saginata (beef tapeworm)	Worldwide	Beef	Humans	Ova, segments	Feces	—	Motile segments
Hymenolepis nana (dwarf tapeworm)	Worldwide	Grain beetles	Humans, mice[a]	Ova	Feces	—	—
Diphyllobothrium latum (fish tapeworm)	Worldwide	Copepods–fish[c]	Humans, other mammals	Ova, segments	Feces	—	Megaloblastic anemia in 1%
T. solium[b] (pork tapeworm)	Worldwide	Swine	Humans	Ova, segments	Feces	WB	Especially Mexico, Central and South America, Africa
Somatic tapeworms							
Echinococcus granulosus (hydatid disease)	Sheep-raising and hunting areas	Sheep, camels, humans, others	Dogs	Hydatid	Lung, liver	WB, EIA	Chest radiography, CT, MRI
E. multilocularis (hydatid disease)	Subarctic areas	Rodents, humans	Foxes, dogs, cats	Hydatid	Liver	—	May resemble cholangio-cellular carcinoma
T. solium[b] (pork tapeworm)	Worldwide	Swine, humans	Humans	Cysticercus	Muscles, CNS	WB	CT, MRI, radiography
FLUKES (TREMATODES)							
Intestinal flukes							
Fasciolopsis buski	China, India	Snails–water chestnuts	Humans	Ova	Feces	—	—
Heterophyes heterophyes	Far East, India	Snails–fish	Humans	Ova	Feces	—	—
Metagonimus yokogawai	Focal in Europe and North Africa	Snails–fish	Humans	Ova	Feces	—	—
Liver flukes							
Clonorchis sinensis	China, Southeast Asia	Snails–fish	Humans	Ova	Feces, bile	—	Recurrent bacterial cholangitis
Fasciola hepatica	Sheep-raising areas	Snails–watercress	Humans, sheep	Ova	Feces,[d] bile	EIA	Cirrhosis, portal hypertension
Lung flukes							
Paragonimus spp.	Orient, Africa, South America	Snails–crabs/crayfish	Humans, other mammals	Adults, ova	Lung, sputum, feces	WB	Chest radiography, CT, MRI
Blood flukes							
Schistosoma mansoni	Africa, Central and South America, West Indies	Snails	Humans	Ova, adults	Feces	EIA, WB	Rectal snips, liver biopsy
S. haematobium	Africa	Snails	Humans	Ova, adults	Urine	WB	Liver, urine, or bladder biopsy
S. japonicum	Far East	Snails	Humans	Ova, adults	Feces	WB	Liver biopsy

[a] Larvae also can mature in intestinal villi of humans and mice.
[b] *T. solium* can cause either intestinal infections or cysticercosis. Its ova are identical to those of *T. saginata*; scolices and segments of the two species differ.
[c] When there are two intermediate hosts, the first is separated from the second by a dash. Definitive hosts are infected by the second intermediate host.

[d] Ova seldom reach the fecal stream during acute disease.

Note: WB, western blot; CT, computed tomography; MRI, magnetic resonance imaging; CNS, central nervous system; EIA, enzyme immunoassay. Serologic tests listed in Tables 192-1, 192-2, and 192-3 are available commercially or from the Centers for Disease Control and Prevention, Atlanta, GA.

TABLE 192-2 *Roundworm Infections*

| Parasite | Geographic Distribution | Life-Cycle Hosts | | Diagnosis | | | |
		Intermediate (Transmission)	Definitive	Parasite Stage	Body Fluid or Tissue	Serologic Tests	Other
INTESTINAL ROUNDWORMS							
Enterobius vermicularis (pinworm)	Temperate and tropical zones	Fecal-oral	Humans	Ova	Perianal skin	—	"Scotch tape" test
Trichuris trichiura (whipworm)	Temperate and tropical zones	Soil, fecal-oral	Humans	Ova	Feces	—	Rectal prolapse
Ascaris lumbricoides (roundworm of humans)	Temperate and tropical zones	Soil, fecal-oral	Humans	Ova	Feces	—	Sx of pulmonary migration
Ancylostoma duodenale (Old World hookworm)	Eurasia, Africa, Pacific	Soil→skin	Humans	Ova/larvae	Feces	—	Sx of pulmonary migration, anemia
Necator americanus (New World hookworm)	U.S., Africa, worldwide	Soil→skin	Humans	Ova/larvae	Feces	—	Sx of pulmonary migration, anemia
Strongyloides stercoralis (strongyloidiasis)	Moist tropics and subtropics	Soil→skin	Humans	Larvae	Feces, sputum, duodenal fluid	EIA	Dissemination in immunodeficiency
TISSUE ROUNDWORMS							
Trichinella spiralis (trichinosis)	Worldwide	Swine/humans	Swine/humans	Larvae	Muscle	EIA	Muscle biopsy
Wuchereria bancrofti (filariasis)	Coastal areas in tropics and subtropics	Mosquitoes	Humans	Microfilariae	Blood, lymph nodes	EIA	Nocturnal periodicity[a]
Brugia malayi (filariasis)	Asia, Indian subcontinent	Mosquitoes	Humans	Microfilariae	Blood	EIA	Nocturnal
Loa loa (African eye worm)	West and Central Africa	Mango flies (*Chrysops*)	Humans	Microfilariae	Blood	—	May be visible in eye, diurnal
Onchocerca volvulus (river blindness)	Africa, Mexico, Central and South America	Blackflies	Humans	Adults/larvae	Skin/eye	—	Examine nodules or skin snips
Dracunculus medinensis (guinea worm)	Africa	*Cyclops*	Humans	Adults/larvae	Skin	—	May be visible in lesion
LARVA MIGRANS SYNDROMES							
Ancylostoma braziliense (creeping eruption)	Tropical and temperate zones	Soil→skin	Dogs/cats, humans	Larvae	Skin	—	Dog and cat hookworm
Toxocara canis and *cati* (visceral larva migrans)	Tropical and temperate zones	Soil, fecal-oral	Dogs/cats, humans	Larvae	Viscera, CNS, eye	EIA[b]	Also caused by roundworms of other species

[a] Blood should be drawn at midnight, except for infection acquired in the South Pacific.
[b] The presence of hemagglutinins is a useful clue.

Note: Sx, signs/symptoms; EIA, enzyme immunoassay; CNS, central nervous system.

geographic distribution, their transmission, and the anatomic location and stages of their life cycle in humans. The text and tables are intended to serve as a guide to the correct diagnostic procedures for the major parasitic infections and to direct the reader to other chapters that contain more comprehensive information about each infection. Tables 192-1, 192-2, and 192-3 summarize the geographic distributions, the anatomic locations, and the methods employed for the diagnosis of flatworm, roundworm, and protozoal infections, respectively.

In addition to selecting the correct diagnostic procedures, physicians must counsel their patients to ensure that specimens are collected properly and arrive at the laboratory promptly. For example, the diagnosis of bancroftian filariasis is unlikely to be confirmed by the laboratory unless blood is drawn near midnight, when the nocturnal microfilariae are active. Laboratory personnel and surgical pathologists should be notified in advance when a parasitic infection is suspected. Continuing interaction with the laboratory staff and the sur-

gical pathologists increases the likelihood that parasites in body fluids or biopsy specimens will be examined carefully by the most capable individuals.

INTESTINAL PARASITES Most helminths and protozoa exit the body in the fecal stream. The patient should be instructed to collect feces in a clean cardboard container and to record the time of collection on the container. Contamination with water (which could contain free-living protozoa) or with urine should be avoided. Fecal samples should be collected before ingestion of barium or other contrast agents for radiologic procedures and before treatment with antidiarrheal agents and antacids, because these substances change the consistency of the feces and interfere with microscopic detection of parasites. Because of the cyclic shedding of most parasites in the feces, a minimum of three samples collected on alternate days should be examined. When delays in transport to the laboratory are unavoidable, fecal samples should be kept in polyvinyl alcohol to preserve protozoal trophozoites. Refrig-

TABLE 192-3 Protozoal Infections

Parasite	Geographic Distribution	Life-Cycle Hosts Intermediate (Transmission)	Definitive	Parasite Stage	Body Fluid or Tissue	Serologic Tests	Other
INTESTINAL PROTOZOANS							
Entamoeba histolytica (amebiasis)	Worldwide, especially tropics	Fecal-oral	Humans	Troph, cyst	Feces, liver	EIA, antigen detection	Ultrasound, liver CT, PCR
Giardia lamblia (giardiasis)	Worldwide	Fecal-oral	Humans	Troph, cyst	Feces	Antigen detection	String test
Isospora belli	Worldwide	Fecal-oral	Humans	Oocyst	Feces	—	Acid-fast
Cryptosporidium	Worldwide	Fecal-oral	Humans, other animals	Oocyst	Feces	Antigen detection	Acid-fast, biopsy, PCR
Cyclospora cayetanensis	Worldwide?	Fecal-oral	Humans, other animals?	Oocyst	Feces	—	Modified safranin, epifluorescence, PCR
Enterocytozoon bieneusi (microsporidiosis)	Worldwide?	?	Animals, humans	Spore	Feces	—	Modified trichrome, biopsy, PCR
FREE-LIVING AMEBAS							
Naegleria	Worldwide	Warm water	Humans	Troph, cyst	CNS, nares	—	Biopsy, nasal swab
Acanthamoeba	Worldwide	Soil, water	Humans	Troph, cyst	CNS, skin, cornea	—	Biopsy, scrapings
BLOOD AND TISSUE PROTOZOANS							
Plasmodium spp. (malaria)	Subtropics and tropics	Mosquitoes	Humans	Asexual	Blood	Limited use	PCR
Babesia microti (babesiosis)	U.S., especially New England	Ticks	Rodents, humans	Asexual	Blood	IIF	Animal spp. in asplenia, PCR
Trypanosoma rhodesiense (African sleeping sickness)	Sub-Saharan East Africa	Tsetse flies	Humans, herbivores	Tryp	Blood, CSF	Card agglutination, IIF[a]	Also chancre, lymph nodes
T. gambiense (African sleeping sickness)	Sub-Saharan West Africa	Tsetse flies	Humans, swine	Tryp	Blood, CSF	Card agglutination, IIF[a]	Also chancre, lymph nodes
T. cruzi (Chagas' disease)	Mexico→South America	Reduviid bugs (triatomes)	Humans, dogs, wild animals	Amastigote, tryp	Multiple organs/blood	IIF, EIA	Reactivation in immunosuppression
Leishmania tropica, etc.	Widespread in tropics and subtropics	Sandflies (*Phlebotomus*)	Humans, dogs, rodents	Amastigote	Skin	IFA, EIA[b]	Biopsy, scraping, culture
L. braziliensis (mucocutaneous)	Mexico→South America	Sandflies (*Lutzomyia*)	Humans, dogs, rodents	Amastigote	Skin, mucous membranes	IFA[b], EIA	Biopsy, scraping, culture
L. donovani (kala-azar)	Widespread in tropics and subtropics	Sandflies (*Phlebotomus*)	Humans, dogs, wild animals	Amastigote	RE system	IFA[b], EIA	Biopsy, culture, PCR
Toxoplasma gondii (toxoplasmosis)	Worldwide	Humans, other mammals	Cats	Cyst, troph	CNS, eye, muscles, other	EIA, IIF	PCR

[a] Card agglutination provided to endemic countries by the World Health Organization; contact the CDC at 770-488-7760.
[b] Limited specificity. Most sensitive for *L. donovani* (kala-azar).
Note: CT, computed tomography; troph, trophozoite; tryp, trypomastigote form; IIF, in-direct immunofluorescence; RE, reticuloendothelial; PCR, polymerase chain reaction; EIA, enzyme immunoassay; CNS, central nervous system; IFA, indirect fluorescent antibody; CSF, cerebrospinal fluid.

eration will also preserve trophozoites for a few hours and protozoal cysts and helminthic ova for several days.

Analysis of fecal samples consists of both a macroscopic and a microscopic examination. Watery or loose stools are more likely to contain protozoal trophozoites, but protozoal cysts and all stages of helminths may be found in formed feces. If adult worms or tapeworm segments are observed, they should be transported promptly to the laboratory or washed and preserved in fixative for later examination. The only tapeworm with motile segments is *Taenia saginata*, the beef tapeworm, which patients sometimes bring to the physician. Motility is an important distinguishing characteristic, because the ova of *T. saginata* and *Taenia solium*, the cause of cysticercosis, are morphologically indistinguishable.

Microscopic examination of feces (Table 192-4) is not complete until direct wet mounts have been evaluated and concentration techniques as well as permanent stains have been applied. Before accepting a report of negativity for ova and parasites as final, the physician should insist that the laboratory undertake each of these procedures. Some intestinal parasites are more readily detected in material other than feces. For example, use of the string test to sample duodenal contents is sometimes necessary to detect *Giardia lamblia*, *Cryptosporidium*, and *Strongyloides* larvae. Use of the "Scotch tape" technique to detect pinworm ova on the perianal skin sometimes also reveals ova of *T. saginata* deposited perianally when the motile segments disintegrate (Table 192-4).

Two routine solutions are used to make wet mounts for the identification of the various life stages of helminths and protozoa: physiologic saline for trophozoites, cysts, ova, and larvae and dilute iodine solution for protozoal cysts and ova. Iodine solution must never be used to examine specimens for trophozoites because it kills the parasites and thus eliminates their characteristic motility.

The two most common concentration procedures for detecting small numbers of cysts and ova are formalin-ether sedimentation and zinc sulfate flotation. The formalin-ether technique is preferable, be-

TABLE 192-4 *Alternative Procedures for Laboratory Diagnosis of Parasites Found in Feces[a]*

Parasites and Fecal Stages	Alternative Diagnostic Procedures
TAPEWORMS (CESTODES)	
Taenia saginata ova and segments	Perianal "Scotch tape" test for ova
T. solium ova and segments	Serology; brain biopsy for neurocysticercosis
FLUKES (TREMATODES)	
Clonorchis (Opisthorchis) sinensis ova	Examination of bile for ova and adults in cholangitis
Fasciola hepatica ova	Examination of bile for ova and adults in cholangitis
Paragonimus spp. ova	Serology; sputum; biopsy of lung or brain for ova
Schistosoma ova	Serology for all; rectal snips (especially for *S. mansoni*), urine (*S. haematobium*), liver biopsy and liver ultrasound
ROUNDWORMS	
Enterobius vermicularis ova and adults	Perianal "Scotch tape" test for ova and adults
Trichuris trichiura ova	None
Ascaris lumbricoides ova and adults	Examination of sputum for larvae in lung disease
Hookworm ova and occasional larvae	Examination of sputum for larvae in lung disease
Strongyloides larvae	Duodenal aspirate or jejunal biopsy; serology, sputum or lung biopsy for filariform larvae in disseminated disease
PROTOZOANS	
Entamoeba histolytica trophozoites and cysts	Serology; liver biopsy for trophozoites
Giardia lamblia trophozoites and cysts	Duodenal aspirate or jejunal biopsy[b]
Isospora belli oocysts	Duodenal aspirate or jejunal biopsy[b]
Cryptosporidium oocysts	Duodenal aspirate or jejunal biopsy[b]
Enterocytozoon bieneusi spores	Duodenal aspirate or jejunal biopsy[b]

[a] Stains and concentration techniques are discussed in the text.
[b] Commercial string test is satisfactory; *Isospora* and *Cryptosporidium* are acid-fast.

cause all parasites sediment but not all float. Slides permanently stained for trophozoites should be prepared before concentration. Additional slides stained for cysts and ova may be made from the concentrate.

In many instances, especially in the differentiation of *Entamoeba histolytica* from other amebas, identification of parasites from wet mounts or concentrates must be considered tentative. Permanently stained smears allow study of the cellular detail necessary for definitive identification. The iron-hematoxylin stain is excellent for critical work, but trichrome staining, which can be completed in 1 h, is a satisfactory alternative that also reveals parasites in specimens preserved in polyvinyl alcohol fixative.

BLOOD AND TISSUE PARASITES Invasion of tissue by protozoa and helminths renders the choice of diagnostic techniques more difficult. For example, physicians must understand that aspiration of an amebic liver abscess rarely reveals *E. histolytica* because the trophozoites are located primarily in the abscess wall. They must remember that the urine sediment offers the best opportunity to detect *Schistosoma haematobium* in the Ethiopian youngster or the American traveler who returns from Africa with hematuria (Table 192-5). Tables 192-1, 192-2, and 192-3, which offer a quick guide to the geographic distribution and anatomic locations of the major tissue parasites, should help the physician to select the appropriate body fluid or biopsy site for microscopic examination. Tables 192-5 and 192-6 provide additional information about the identification of parasites in samples from specific anatomic locations. The laboratory procedures for detection of parasites in other body fluids are similar to those used in the examination of feces. The physician should insist on wet mounts, concentration techniques, and permanent stains for all body fluids. The trichrome or iron-hematoxylin stain is satisfactory for all tissue helminths in body fluids other than blood, but microfilarial worms and blood protozoa are more easily visualized when stained with Giemsa or Wright's stain.

The most common parasites detected in Giemsa-stained blood smears are the plasmodia, microfilariae, and African trypanosomes (Table 192-5). Most patients with Chagas' disease present in the chronic phase, when *Trypanosoma cruzi* is no longer microscopically detectable in blood smears. Wet mounts are sometimes more sensitive than stained smears for the detection of microfilariae and African trypanosomes because these active parasites cause noticeable movement of the erythrocytes in the microscopic field. Nuclepore filtration of blood facilitates the detection of microfilariae. The intracellular amastigote forms of *Leishmania* spp. and *T. cruzi* can sometimes be visualized in stained smears of peripheral blood, but aspirates of the bone marrow, liver, and spleen are the best sources for microscopic detection and culture of *Leishmania* in kala-azar and of *T. cruzi* in chronic Chagas' disease. The diagnosis of malaria and the critical distinction among the various *Plasmodium* species are made by microscopic examination of stained thick and thin blood films (Chap. 195).

TABLE 192-5 *Identification of Parasites in Blood and Other Body Fluids*

Body Fluid, Parasite	Enrichment/Stain	Culture Technique
BLOOD		
Plasmodium spp.	Thick and thin smears/Giemsa or Wright's	Not useful for diagnosis
Leishmania spp.	Buffy coat/Giemsa	Media available from CDC
African trypanosomes[a]	Buffy coat, anion column/wet mount and Giemsa	Mouse or rat inoculation[b]
Trypanosoma cruzi[c]	As for African species	As above and xenodiagnosis
Toxoplasma gondii	Buffy coat/Giemsa	Fibroblast cell lines
Microfilariae[d]	Nuclepore filtration/wet mount and Giemsa	None
URINE		
Schistosoma haematobium	Centrifugation/wet mount	None
Microfilariae (in chyluria)	As for blood	None
SPINAL FLUID		
African trypanosomes	Centrifugation, anion column/wet mount and Giemsa	As for blood
Naegleria fowleri	Centrifugation/wet mount and Giemsa or trichrome	Nonnutrient agar overlaid with *Escherichia coli*

[a] *Trypanosoma rhodesiense* and *T. gambiense*.
[b] Inject mice intraperitoneally with 0.2 mL of whole heparinized blood (0.5 mL for rats). After 5 days, tail blood should be checked daily for trypanosomes as described above.
[c] Detectable in blood by conventional techniques only during acute disease. Xenodiagnosis is successful in ~ 50% of patients with chronic Chagas' disease.
[d] Day (1000–1400 h) and night (2200–0200 h) blood should be drawn to maximize the chance of detecting *Wuchereria* (nocturnal except for Pacific strains), *Brugia* (nocturnal), and *Loa loa* (diurnal).

Although most tissue parasites stain with the traditional hematoxylin and eosin, surgical biopsy specimens should also be stained with appropriate special stains. The surgical pathologist who is accustomed to applying silver stains for *Pneumocystis carinii* to induced sputum and transbronchial biopsies may have to be reminded to examine wet mounts and iron-hematoxylin–stained preparations of pulmonary specimens for helminthic ova and *E. histolytica*. The clinician should also be able to advise the surgeon and pathologist about optimal techniques for the identification of parasites in specimens obtained by certain specialized minor procedures (Table 192-6). For example, the excision of skin snips for the diagnosis of onchocerciasis, the collection of rectal snips for the diagnosis of schistosomiasis, and punch biopsy of skin lesions for the identification and culture of cutaneous and mucocutaneous species of *Leishmania* are simple procedures, but the diagnosis can be missed if the specimens are improperly obtained or processed.

TABLE 192-6 *Minor Procedures for Diagnosis of Parasitic Infections*

Parasite(s) and Stage	Procedure
Onchocerca volvulus and *Mansonella streptocerca* microfilariae	*Skin snips:* Lift skin with a needle and excise ~ 1 mg to a depth of 0.5 mm from several sites. Weigh each sample, place it in 0.5 mL of saline for 4 h, and examine wet mounts and Giemsa stains of the saline either directly or after filtration. Count microfilariae.[a]
Loa loa adults and *O. volvulus* adults and microfilariae	*Biopsies of subcutaneous nodules:* Stain routine histopathologic sections and impression smears with Giemsa.
Trichinella spiralis larvae (and perhaps *Taenia solium* cysticerci)	*Muscle biopsies:* Excise about 1.0 g of deltoid or gastrocnemius muscle and squash between two glass slides for direct microscopic examination.
Schistosoma ova of all species, but especially *S. mansoni*	*Rectal snips:* From four areas of mucosa, take 2-mg snips, tease onto a glass slide, and flatten with a second slide before examining directly at 10×. Preparations may be fixed in alcohol or stained.
Trypanosoma gambiense and *T. rhodesiense* trypomastigotes	*Aspirate of chancre or lymph node[b]:* Aspirate center with 18-gauge needle, place a drop on a slide, and examine for motile forms. An otherwise insufficient volume of material may be stained with Giemsa.
Acanthamoeba spp. trophozoites or cysts	*Corneal scrapings:* Obtain sample from ophthalmologist for immediate Giemsa staining and culture on nutrient agar overlaid with *Escherichia coli*.
Cutaneous and mucocutaneous *Leishmania* spp.	*Swabs, aspirates, or punch biopsies of skin lesions:* Obtain specimen from margin of lesion for Giemsa staining of impression smears, and section and culture on special media from CDC.

[a] Counts of >100/mg are associated with significant risk of complications.
[b] Lymph node aspiration is contraindicated in some infections and should be used judiciously.

NONSPECIFIC TESTS Eosinophilia is a common accompaniment of infections with most of the tissue helminths; absolute numbers of eosinophils may be high in trichinosis and the migratory phases of filariasis (Table 192-7). Intestinal helminths provoke eosinophilia only during pulmonary migration of the larval stages. Eosinophilia is not a manifestation of protozoal infections, with the possible exceptions of those due to *Isospora* and *Dientamoeba fragilis*.

Like the hypochromic, microcytic anemia of heavy hookworm infections, other nonspecific laboratory abnormalities may suggest parasitic infection in patients with appropriate geographic and/or environmental exposures. Biochemical evidence of cirrhosis or an abnormal urine sediment in an African immigrant certainly raises the possibility of schistosomiasis, and anemia and thrombocytopenia in a febrile traveler or immigrant are among the hallmarks of malaria. Computed tomography and magnetic resonance imaging also contribute to the diagnosis of infections with many tissue parasites and have become invaluable adjuncts in the diagnosis of neurocysticercosis and cerebral toxoplasmosis.

ANTIBODY AND ANTIGEN DETECTION Useful antibody assays for many of the important tissue parasites are available; most of those listed in Table 192-8 can be obtained from the Centers for Disease Control and Prevention (CDC) in Atlanta. The results of serologic tests not listed in the tables should be interpreted with caution.

The value of antibody assays is limited by several factors. For example, the preparation of thick and thin blood smears remains the procedure of choice for the diagnosis of malaria in individual patients because diagnostic titers to plasmodia develop slowly. Filarial antigens cross-react with those from other nematodes; as in assays for antibody to most parasites, the presence of antibody in the filarial assay fails to distinguish between past and current infection. Despite these specific limitations, the restricted geographic distribution of many tropical parasites increases the diagnostic usefulness of both the presence and the absence of antibody in travelers from industrialized countries. In contrast, a large proportion of the world's population has been exposed to *Toxoplasma gondii*, and the presence of IgG antibody to *T. gondii* does not constitute proof of active disease.

Fewer antibody assays are available for the diagnosis of infection with intestinal parasites. *E. histolytica* is the major exception. Sensitive, specific serologic tests are invaluable in the diagnosis of amebiasis. Commercial kits for the detection of antigen by enzyme-linked immunosorbent assay or of whole organisms by fluorescent antibody assay are now available for several protozoan parasites (Table 192-8).

MOLECULAR TECHNIQUES DNA hybridization with probes that are repeated many times in the genome of a specific parasite and amplifi-

TABLE 192-7 *Parasites Frequently Associated with Eosinophilia[a]*

Parasite	Comment
TAPEWORMS (CESTODES)	
Echinococcus granulosus	When hydatid cyst leaks
Taenia solium	During muscle encystation and in CSF with neurocysticercosis
FLUKES (TREMATODES)	
Paragonimus spp.	Uniformly high in acute stage
Fasciola hepatica	May be high in acute stage
Clonorchis (Opisthorchis) sinensis	Variable
Schistosoma mansoni	50% of infected travelers
S. haematobium	25% of infected travelers
S. japonicum	Up to 6000/μL in acute infection
ROUNDWORMS	
Ascaris lumbricoides	During larval migration
Hookworm species	During larval migration
Strongyloides stercoralis	Profound during migration and early years of infection
Trichinella spiralis	Up to 7000/μL
Filarial species[b]	Varies but can reach 5000 to 8000/μL
Toxocara spp.	>3000/μL
Ancylostoma braziliense	With extensive cutaneous eruption
Gnathostoma spinigerum	In visceral larva migrans and eosinophilic meningitis
Angiostrongylus cantonensis	In eosinophilic meningitis
A. costaricensis	During larval migration in mesenteric vessels

[a] Virtually every helminth has been associated with eosinophilia. This table includes both common and uncommon parasites that frequently elicit eosinophilia during infection.
[b] *Wuchereria bancrofti*, *Brugia* spp., *Loa loa*, and *Onchocerca volvulus*.

TABLE 192-8 *Serologic and Molecular Tests for Parasitic Infections*

Parasite, Infection	Antibody	Antigen or DNA/RNA
TAPEWORMS		
Echinococcosis	WB, EIA	
Cysticercosis	WB	
FLUKES		
Paragonimiasis	WB, EIA	
Schistosomiasis	EIA, WB	
Fascioliasis	EIA[a]	
ROUNDWORMS		
Strongyloidiasis	EIA	
Trichinellosis	EIA	
Toxocariasis	EIA	
Filariasis	EIA[b]	
PROTOZOANS		
Amebiasis	EIA	EIA, PCR
Giardiasis	—	EIA, IIF, DFA
Cryptosporidiosis	—	IIF, EIA, DFA, PCR
Malaria (all species)	IIF[c]	PCR
Babesiosis	IIF	PCR
Chagas' disease	IIF, EIA	PCR
Leishmaniasis	IIF, EIA	PCR
Toxoplasmosis	IIF, EIA (IgM)	PCR
Microsporidiosis		PCR
Cyclosporiasis	—	PCR

[a] Commercial laboratories only.
[b] Available at the NIH (301-496-5398) and commercially.
[c] Of limited use for management of acute disease.
Note: WB, western blot; EIA, enzyme immunoassay; IIF, indirect immunofluorescence; DFA, direct fluorescent antibody; PCR, polymerase chain reaction. Unless specified, antibody tests listed are available from the CDC. Antigen and parasite detection kits are available commercially. The PCRs listed are available in commercial or research laboratories. The CDC currently uses PCRs as research tools and in selected diagnostic situations (contact Dr. Alexandre da Silva 770-488-4072).

cation of a specific DNA fragment by the polymerase chain reaction (PCR) are promising techniques for the diagnosis of parasitic infections. Although molecular techniques for the detection of many parasites are already being used in insect vectors, animal models, and human trials, relatively few are available for routine use in patients at this time. Several commercial laboratories now perform PCRs for detection of the nucleic acid of a few specific parasites in stool, biopsy, bronchoalveolar lavage, and blood samples (Table 192-8). Because their roles in the diagnosis and management of individual patients are still being defined, the CDC currently uses PCRs as research tools and in selected diagnostic situations (contact Dr. Alexandre da Silva, 770-488-4072).

FURTHER READING

FLECK SL, MOODY AH: *Diagnostic Techniques in Medical Parasitology.* London, Wright, 1988

GARCIA LS: Laboratory identification of the microsporidia. J Clin Microbiol 40:1892, 2002

——— et al: Algorithms for detection and identification of parasites, in *Manual of Clinical Microbiology*, 7th ed, PR Murray et al (eds). Washington, DC, ASM Press, 1999, pp. 1336–1354

HAQUE R et al: Comparison of PCR, isoenzyme analysis, and antigen detection for diagnosis of *Entamoeba histolytica* infection. J Clin Microbiol 36:449, 1998

HERWALDT BL: *Cyclospora cayetanensis*: A review, focusing on the outbreaks of cyclosporiasis in the 1990s. Clin Infect Dis 31:1040, 2000

SHULTE C (ed): et al: Diagnostic significance of blood eosinophilia in returning travelers. Clin Infect Dis 34:407, 2002

WILSON M et al: Evaluation of six commercial kits for detection of human immunoglobulin M antibodies to *Toxoplasma gondii*. J Clin Microbiol 35:3112, 1997

——— et al: Clinical immunoparasitology, in *Manual of Clinical Laboratory Immunology*, 6th ed, NR Rose et al (eds). Washington, DC, ASM Press, 2002, pp. 547–558

---

193 AGENTS USED TO TREAT INFECTIONS DUE TO PARASITES AND *PNEUMOCYSTIS*
Thomas A. Moore

Parasitic infections afflict more than half of the world's population and impose a substantial health burden, particularly in underdeveloped nations, where they are most prevalent. The remarkable success of global campaigns aimed at controlling or eliminating ancient scourges such as dracunculiasis and onchocerciasis has been offset by the spread of other diseases such as trypanosomiasis due to crumbling infrastructures in settings of HIV infection, civil war, and unstable government. The reach of some parasitic diseases, including malaria, has expanded over the past few decades as a result of factors such as deforestation, population shifts, global warming, and other climatic events. Despite major efforts at vaccine development, chemotherapy remains the single most effective means of controlling parasitic infections. However, efforts to combat the spread of some diseases are hindered by the development and spread of drug resistance and the limited introduction of new antiparasitic agents. Since the last edition of this text was published, new and significant obstacles have arisen. The most serious problems include the discontinued production of inexpensive agents that appear on the essential medicine list of the World Health Organization (WHO)—e.g., amphotericin B deoxycholate, eflornithine, metrifonate, and praziquantel—and the introduction in some areas of counterfeit antiparasitic agents.

Significant advances toward the reduction of the burden of parasitic disease have nevertheless been made. The continued generous donation of ivermectin and albendazole for global eradication programs has improved the health of countless individuals and offers the promise of

eradication of some diseases (e.g., the filariases). Shortages of some drugs have prompted a fresh look at currently available agents (e.g., high-dose metronidazole for schistosomiasis). The broader use of newer agents, either alone (e.g., fumagillin, metrifonate, nitazoxanide) or in combination (e.g., lumefantrine with artemether), also appears promising.

This chapter deals exclusively with the agents used to treat infections due to parasites and the fungus *Pneumocystis* (Chap. 191). Specific treatment recommendations for the parasitic diseases of humans are listed in subsequent chapters. Table 193-1 presents a brief overview of each agent (including some that are not discussed in the text but are covered in other chapters), along with its major toxicities, spectrum of activity, and safety for use during pregnancy and lactation. Many of the agents are approved by the U.S. Food and Drug Administration (FDA) but are considered investigational for the treatment of certain infections; these drugs are marked accordingly in Table 193-1. Drugs marked in the text with an asterisk (*) are available only through the Centers for Disease Control and Prevention (CDC) Drug Service (telephone: 404-639-3670 or 404-639-2888; *www.cdc.gov/ncidod/dpd/professional/drug_service.htm*). Other drugs, marked with a dagger (†), are available only through their manufacturers; contact information for these manufacturers may be available from the CDC.

Albendazole　Like all benzimidazoles, albendazole acts by binding to free β-tubulin, inhibiting the polymerization of tubulin and the microtubule-dependent uptake of glucose. This fundamental disruption of

Drug	Infection(s)	Adverse Effects	Major Drug Interactions	Pregnancy Class[a]	Breast Milk
Albendazole	Ascariasis, capillariasis, clonorchiasis, cutaneous larva migrans, cysticercosis,[b] echinococcosis,[b] enterobiasis, eosinophilic enterocolitis, gnathostomiasis, hookworm, microsporidiosis, strongyloidiasis, trichinellosis, trichostrongyliasis, trichuriasis, visceral larva migrans	Occasional: nausea, vomiting, abdominal pain, headache, reversible alopecia, elevated aminotransferases. Rare: leukopenia, rash	Dexamethasone, praziquantel: increase plasma level of albendazole sulfoxide by ~50%	C	Yes[c]
Amphotericin B [amphotericin B deoxycholate, Amphotec (InterMune), amphotericin B lipid complex (ABLC, Abelcet), liposomal amphotericin B (AmBisome)]	Leishmaniasis,[d] amebic meningoencephalitis	Frequent: fever, chills, hypokalemia, hypomagnesemia, nephrotoxicity. Occasional: vomiting, dyspnea, hypotension	Antineoplastic agents: renal toxicity, bronchospasm, hypotension Glucocorticoids, ACTH, digitalis: hypokalemia Zidovudine: increased myelo- and nephrotoxicity (ABLC only)	B	No information
Antimonials [pentavalent antimony (Pentostam), meglumine antimonate (Glucantime)]	Leishmaniasis	Frequent: arthralgias/myalgias, pancreatitis, ECG changes (QT prolongation, T wave flattening or inversion)	Antiarrhythmics and tricyclic antidepressants: increased risk of cardiotoxicity (meglumine antimonate only)	Not assigned	Yes (pentavalent antimony); unknown (meglumine antimonate)
Artemisinin derivatives	Malaria	Occasional: neurotoxicity (ataxia, convulsions), nausea, vomiting, anorexia, contact dermatitis	Mefloquine: levels decreased and clearance accelerated by artesunate	Not assigned	Yes
Atovaquone	Malaria,[b] pneumocystosis,[b] babesiosis	Frequent: nausea, vomiting. Occasional: abdominal pain, headache	Plasma levels decreased by rifampin, tetracycline; bioavailability decreased by metoclopramide	C	No information
Azithromycin	Babesiosis	Occasional: nausea, vomiting, diarrhea, abdominal pain. Rare: angioedema, cholestatic jaundice	Cyclosporine and digoxin: levels increased by azithromycin. Nelfinavir: increases levels of azithromycin	B	
Azoles (fluconazole, itraconazole, ketoconazole)	Leishmaniasis	Occasional: hepatotoxicity. Rare: exfoliative skin disorders, anaphylaxis	Warfarin, oral hypoglycemics, phenytoin, cyclosporine, theophylline, digoxin, dofetilide, quinidine, carbamazepine, rifabutin, busulfan, docetaxel, vinca alkaloids, pimozide, alprazolam, diazepam, midazolam, triazolam, verapamil, atorvastatin, cerivastatin, lovastatin, simvastatin, tacrolimus, sirolimus, indinavir, ritonavir, saquinavir, alfentanil, buspirone, methylprednisolone, trimetrexate: plasma levels increased by azoles. Carbamazepine, phenobarbital, phenytoin, isoniazid, rifabutin, rifampin, antacids, H2-receptor antagonists, proton pump inhibitors, nevirapine: decrease plasma levels of azoles. Clarithromycin, erythromycin, indinavir, ritonavir: increase plasma levels of azoles	C	Yes
Benznidazole	Chagas' disease	Frequent: rash, pruritus, nausea, leukopenia, paresthesias	No major interactions	Not assigned	No information

(continued)

Drug	Infection(s)	Adverse Effects	Major Drug Interactions	Pregnancy Class[a]	Breast Milk
Chloroquine	Malaria[b]	Occasional: pruritus, nausea, vomiting, headache, hair depigmentation, exfoliative dermatitis, reversible corneal opacity. Rare: irreversible retinal injury, nail discoloration, blood dyscrasias	Antacids and kaolin: reduce absorption of chloroquine. Ampicillin: bioavailability reduced by chloroquine. Cimetidine: increases serum levels of chloroquine. Cyclosporine: serum levels increased by chloroquine	Not assigned[e]	Yes
Ciprofloxacin	Cyclosporiasis, isosporiasis	Occasional: nausea, diarrhea, vomiting, abdominal pain/discomfort, headache, restlessness, rash. Rare: myalgias/arthralgias, tendon rupture, CNS symptoms (nervousness, agitation, insomnia, anxiety, nightmares, or paranoia), convulsions	Probenecid: increases serum levels of ciprofloxacin. Theophylline, warfarin: serum levels increased by ciprofloxacin	C	Yes
Clindamycin	Babesiosis, malaria, toxoplasmosis, pneumocystosis	Occasional: pseudomembranous colitis, abdominal pain, diarrhea, nausea/vomiting. Rare: pruritus, skin rashes	No major interactions	B	Yes[c]
Dapsone	Leishmaniasis, malaria, pneumocystosis, toxoplasmosis	Frequent: rash, anorexia. Occasional: hemolysis, methemoglobinemia, neuropathy, allergic dermatitis, anorexia, nausea, vomiting, tachycardia, headache, insomnia, psychosis, hepatitis. Rare: agranulocytosis	Rifampin: lowers plasma levels of dapsone	C	Yes
Diethylcarbamazine	Lymphatic filariasis, loiasis	Frequent: dose-related nausea, vomiting. Rare: fever, chills, arthralgias, headaches	None reported	Not assigned[e]	No information
Diloxanide furoate	Amebiasis	Frequent: flatulence. Occasional: nausea, vomiting, diarrhea. Rare: pruritus	None reported	Contraindicated	No information
Eflornithine (difluoromethylornithine, DFMO)	Trypanosomiasis	Frequent: pancytopenia. Occasional: diarrhea, seizures. Rare: transient hearing loss	No major interactions	Contraindicated	No information
Fumagillin	Microsporidiosis	Rare: neutropenia, thrombocytopenia	None reported	No information	No information
Furazolidone	Giardiasis	Frequent: nausea/vomiting, brown urine. Occasional: rectal itching, headache. Rare: hemolytic anemia, disulfiram-like reactions, MAO-inhibitor interactions	Risk of hypertensive crisis when administered >5 days with MAO inhibitors	No information	No information
Halofantrine	Malaria[b]	Frequent: abdominal pain, diarrhea. Occasional: ECG disturbances (dose-related prolongation of QTc and PR interval), nausea, pruritus. Contraindicated in persons who have cardiac disease or who have taken mefloquine in preceding 3 weeks	Concomitant use of agents that prolong QTc interval contraindicated	C	No information
Iodoquinol	Amebiasis,[b] balantidiasis, *Dientamoeba fragilis* infection	Occasional: headache, rash, pruritus, thyrotoxicosis, nausea, vomiting, abdominal pain, diarrhea. Rare: optic neuritis, peripheral neuropathy, seizures, encephalopathy	No major interactions	No information	No information
Ivermectin	Ascariasis, cutaneous larva migrans, enterobiasis, gnathostomiasis, loiasis, lymphatic filariasis, onchocerciasis,[b] scabies, strongyloidiasis[b]	Occasional: fever, pruritus, headache, myalgias. Rare: hypotension	No major interactions	C	Yes[c]

(continued)

TABLE 193-1—(Continued)

Drug	Infection(s)	Adverse Effects	Major Drug Interactions	Pregnancy Class[a]	Breast Milk
Lumefantrine	Malaria	Occasional: nausea, vomiting, diarrhea, abdominal pain, anorexia, headache, dizziness	No major interactions	Not assigned	No information
Mebendazole	Ascariasis,[b] capillariasis, eosinophilic enterocolitis, enterobiasis,[b] hookworm,[b] trichinellosis, trichostrongyliasis, trichuriasis,[b] visceral larva migrans	Occasional: diarrhea, abdominal pain, elevated aminotransferases. Rare: agranulocytosis, thrombocytopenia, alopecia	Cimetidine: inhibits mebendazole metabolism	C	No information
Mefloquine	Malaria[b]	Frequent: light-headedness, nausea, headache. Occasional: confusion, nightmares, insomnia, visual disturbances, transient and clinically silent ECG abnormalities (including sinus bradycardia, sinus arrhythmia, first-degree AV block, prolongation of QTc interval, and abnormal T waves). Rare: psychosis, convulsions, hypotension	Administration of halofantrine <3 weeks after mefloquine use may produce fatal QTc prolongation. Mefloquine may lower plasma levels of anticonvulsants. Mefloquine levels decreased and clearance accelerated by artesunate	C	Yes
Melarsoprol	Trypanosomiasis	Frequent: myocardial injury, encephalopathy, peripheral neuropathy, hypertension. Occasional: G6PD-induced hemolysis, erythema nodosum leprosum. Rare: hypotension	No major interactions	Not assigned	No information
Metrifonate	Schistosomiasis	Frequent: abdominal pain, nausea, vomiting, diarrhea, headache, vertigo, bronchospasm. Rare: cholinergic symptoms	No major interactions	Not assigned	No information
Metronidazole	Amebiasis,[b] balantidiasis, dracunculiasis, giardiasis, trichomoniasis,[b] D. fragilis infection	Frequent: nausea, headache, anorexia, metallic aftertaste. Occasional: vomiting, insomnia, vertigo, paresthesias, disulfiram-like effects. Rare: seizures, peripheral neuropathy	Warfarin: effect enhanced by metronidazole. Disulfiram: psychotic reaction. Phenobarbital, phenytoin: accelerate elimination of metronidazole. Lithium: serum levels elevated by metronidazole. Cimetidine: prolongs half-life of metronidazole	B	Yes
Miltefosine	Leishmaniasis	Frequent: mild and transient (1-2 days) gastrointestinal disturbances within first 2 weeks of therapy (resolve after treatment completion), motion sickness. Occasional: reversible elevations of creatinine and aminotransferases	No major interactions	Not assigned	No information
Niclosamide	Intestinal cestodes[b]	Occasional: nausea, vomiting, dizziness, pruritus	No major interactions	Not assigned	No information
Nifurtimox	Chagas' disease	Frequent: nausea, vomiting, abdominal pain, insomnia, paresthesias, weakness, tremors. Rare: seizures. All effects reversible and dose-related	No major interactions	Not assigned	No information
Nitazoxanide	Cryptosporidiosis,[b] giardiasis[b]	Occasional: abdominal pain, diarrhea. Rare: vomiting, headache	No major interactions	B	No information
Oxamniquine	Schistosomiasis	Occasional: dizziness, drowsiness, headache, orange urine, elevated aminotransferases. Rare: seizures	No major interactions	Not assigned	No information

(continued)

Drug	Infection(s)	Adverse Effects	Major Drug Interactions	Pregnancy Class[a]	Breast Milk
Paromomycin	Amebiasis,[b] D. fragilis infection, giardiasis, leishmaniasis	Frequent: gastrointestinal disturbances (oral dosing only). Occasional: nephrotoxicity, ototoxicity, vestibular toxicity (parenteral dosing only)	No major interactions	Not assigned[e]	No information
Pentamidine isethionate	Pneumocystosis,[b] leishmaniasis, trypanosomiasis	Frequent: hypotension, hypoglycemia, pancreatitis, sterile abscesses at intramuscular injection sites, gastrointestinal disturbances, reversible renal failure. Occasional: hepatotoxicity, cardiotoxicity, delirium. Rare: pancreatitis, anaphylaxis	No major interactions	C	No information
Praziquantel	Clonorchiasis,[b] cysticercosis, diphyllobothriasis, hymenolepiasis, taeniasis, opisthorchiasis, intestinal trematodes, paragonimiasis, schistosomiasis[b]	Frequent: abdominal pain, diarrhea, dizziness, headache, malaise. Occasional: fever, nausea. Rare: pruritus, singultus	No major interactions	B	Yes
Primaquine phosphate	Malaria,[b] pneumocystosis	Frequent: hemolytic anemia in patients with G6PD deficiency. Occasional: methemoglobinemia, gastrointestinal disturbances. Rare: CNS symptoms	Quinacrine: potentiates toxicity of primaquine	Contraindicated	No information
Proguanil (chloroguanide)	Malaria	Occasional: urticaria. Rare: hematuria, gastrointestinal disturbances	No major interactions	C	Yes
Pyrantel pamoate	Ascariasis, eosinophilic enterocolitis, enterobiasis,[b] hookworm, trichostrongyliasis	Occasional: gastrointestinal disturbances, headache, dizziness, elevated aminotransferases	No major interactions	C	No information
Pyrimethamine	Malaria,[b] pneumocystosis, toxoplasmosis[b]	Occasional: folate deficiency. Rare: rash, seizures, severe skin reactions (toxic epidermal necrolysis, erythema multiforme, Stevens-Johnson syndrome)	Sulfonamides, proguanil, zidovudine: increased risk of bone marrow suppression when used concomitantly	C	Yes
Quinacrine	Giardiasis[b]	Frequent: headache, nausea, vomiting, bitter taste. Occasional: yellow-orange discoloration of skin, sclerae, urine (begins after 1 week of treatment and lasts up to 4 months after drug discontinuation). Rare: psychosis, exfoliative dermatitis, retinopathy, G6PD-induced hemolysis, exacerbation of psoriasis, disulfiram-like effects	Primaquine: toxicity potentiated by quinacrine	Contraindicated	No information
Quinine and quinidine	Malaria, babesiosis	Frequent: cinchonism (tinnitus, high-tone deafness, headache, dysphoria, nausea, vomiting, abdominal pain, visual disturbances, postural hypotension), hyperinsulinemia resulting in life-threatening hypoglycemia. Occasional: deafness, hemolytic anemia, arrhythmias, hypotension due to rapid intravenous infusion	Carbonic-anhydrase inhibitors, thiazide diuretics: reduce renal elimination of quinidine. Amiodarone, cimetidine: increase quinidine levels. Nifedipine: decreases quinidine levels; quinidine slows metabolism of nifedipine. Phenobarbital, phenytoin, rifampin: accelerate hepatic elimination of quinidine. Verapamil: reduces hepatic clearance of quinidine. Diltiazem: decreases clearance of quinidine	X	Yes[c]

(continued)

TABLE 193-1— (Continued)

Drug	Infection(s)	Adverse Effects	Major Drug Interactions	Pregnancy Class[a]	Breast Milk
Spiramycin	Toxoplasmosis	Occasional: gastrointestinal disturbances, transient skin eruptions. Rare: thrombocytopenia, QT prolongation in an infant, cholestatic hepatitis	No major interactions	Not assigned[e]	Yes[c]
Sulfonamides	Malaria,[b] pneumocystosis,[b] toxoplasmosis[b]	Frequent: gastrointestinal disturbances, allergic skin reactions. Rare: severe skin reactions (toxic epidermal necrolysis, erythema multiforme, Stevens-Johnson syndrome), agranulocytosis, aplastic anemia, hypersensitivity of respiratory tract, hepatitis, interstitial nephritis, hypoglycemia, aseptic meningitis	Thiazide diuretics: increased risk of thrombocytopenia in elderly patients. Warfarin: effect prolonged by sulfonamides. Methotrexate: levels increased by sulfonamides. Phenytoin: metabolism impaired by sulfonamides	B	Yes
Suramin	Trypanosomiasis	Frequent, immediate: fever, urticaria, nausea, vomiting, hypotension. Frequent, delayed (up to 24 h): exfoliative dermatitis, stomatitis, paresthesias, photophobia, renal dysfunction. Occasional: nephrotoxicity, adrenal toxicity, optic atrophy, anaphylaxis	No major interactions	Not assigned	No information
Tetracyclines	Balantidiasis, *D. fragilis* infection, malaria	Frequent: gastrointestinal disturbances. Occasional: photosensitivity dermatitis. Rare: exfoliative dermatitis, esophagitis, hepatotoxicity	Warfarin: effect prolonged by tetracyclines	D	Yes
Thiabendazole	Strongyloidiasis,[b] cutaneous larva migrans,[b] visceral larva migrans[b]	Frequent: anorexia, nausea, vomiting, diarrhea, headache, dizziness, asparagus-like urine odor. Occasional: drowsiness, giddiness, crystalluria, elevated aminotransferases, psychosis. Rare: hepatitis, seizures, angioneurotic edema, Stevens-Johnson syndrome, tinnitus	Theophylline: serum levels increased by thiabendazole	C	No information
Tinidazole	Amebiasis,[b] giardiasis, trichomoniasis	Occasional: nausea, vomiting, metallic taste	See metronidazole	Not assigned	No information
Triclabendazole	Fascioliasis, paragonimiasis	Occasional: abdominal cramps, diarrhea, biliary colic, transient headache	No information	Not assigned	Yes
Trimethoprim-sulfamethoxazole	Cyclosporiasis, isosporiasis, pneumocystosis	See sulfonamides	See sulfonamides	C	Yes

[a] Based on U.S. Food and Drug Administration (FDA) pregnancy categories A through D and X.
[b] Approved by the FDA for this indication.
[c] Not believed to be harmful.
[d] Only AmBisome has been approved for this indication.
[e] Use in pregnancy is recommended by international organizations outside the United States.

Abbreviations: ACTH, adrenocorticotropic hormone; AV, atrioventricular; CNS, central nervous system; ECG, electrocardiogram; G6PD, glucose 6-phosphate dehydrogenase; MAO, monoamine oxidase.

cellular metabolism offers treatment for a wide range of parasitic diseases.

Albendazole is poorly absorbed from the gastrointestinal tract. Administration with a fatty meal increases its absorption by two- to sixfold. While poor absorption may be advantageous for the treatment of intestinal helminths, successful treatment of tissue helminth infections such as hydatid disease or neurocysticercosis requires that a sufficient quantity of active drug reach the site of infection. The metabolite albendazole sulfoxide is responsible for the drug's therapeutic effect outside the gut lumen. Significant quantities of this metabolite are measurable in lung and liver tissues and in hydatid cyst fluid obtained at surgery. Cyst concentrations are considerably higher than those obtained with mebendazole. Albendazole sulfoxide crosses the blood-brain barrier, reaching a level significantly higher than that achieved in plasma. The high concentrations of albendazole sulfoxide attained in cerebrospinal fluid (CSF) probably explain the efficacy of albendazole in the treatment of neurocysticercosis.

Albendazole is extensively metabolized in the liver, but there are few data regarding the drug's use in patients with significant hepatocellular disease. Prolonged therapy with full-dose albendazole (800 mg/d) should be approached cautiously in patients also receiving drugs with known effects on the cytochrome P450 system. A single dose of 400 mg is generally recommended for clearance of gastrointestinal nematode infection in both adults and children >2 years of age.

Single-dose albendazole therapy in humans is largely without side effects (overall frequency, ≤1%). More prolonged courses (e.g., as administered for cystic and alveolar echinococcal disease) have been associated with liver function abnormalities and bone marrow toxicity. Thus, when prolonged use is anticipated, the drug should be administered in treatment cycles of 28 days interrupted by 14 days off therapy.

Amphotericin B See Table 193-1 and Chap. 182.

Antimonials* Despite associated adverse reactions and the need for prolonged parenteral treatment, the pentavalent antimonial compounds (designated Sb^v) have remained the first-line therapy for all forms of leishmaniasis throughout the world, primarily because they are affordable, are effective, and have survived the test of time. Although they have been used for almost 100 years, their mechanism of action against *Leishmania* spp. remains unknown. Presumably, the compounds interfere with parasite metabolism. The drugs are taken up by the reticuloendothelial system, and their activity against *Leishmania* spp. may be enhanced by this localization. Sodium stibogluconate is the only pentavalent antimonial available in the United States; meglumine antimonate is principally used in francophone countries.

Resistance is a major problem in some areas. Although low-level unresponsiveness to Sb^v was identified in India in the 1970s, incremental increases in both the recommended daily dosage (to 20 mg/kg) and the duration of treatment (to 28 days) satisfactorily compensated for the growing resistance until around 1990. Since that time, there has been steady erosion in the capacity of Sb^v to induce long-term cure in patients with kala-azar who live in eastern India. Foremost among the many factors that have probably contributed to this failure is the provision of suboptimal treatment for years, which led to the development of drug resistance among parasites. Co-infection with HIV impairs the response to therapy.

Sodium stibogluconate is available in aqueous solution and is administered parenterally. Antimony appears to have two elimination phases. When administered intravenously, the mean half-life of the first phase is <2 h; the mean half-life of the terminal elimination phase is nearly 36 h. This slower phase may be due to conversion of pentavalent antimony to a trivalent form that is the likely cause of the side effects often seen with prolonged therapy.

Artemisinin Derivatives Artesunate, artemether, arteether, and the parent compound artemisinin are sesquiterpene lactones derived from the wormwood plant *Artemisia annua*. These agents are at least ten-fold more potent in vivo than other antimalarial drugs and presently show no cross-resistance with known antimalarials; thus they have become first-line treatments for severe falciparum malaria in some areas where multidrug resistance is a major problem. They are rapidly effective against the asexual blood forms of *Plasmodium* spp., including multidrug-resistant *Plasmodium falciparum*, but they are not active against intrahepatic forms. A combined formulation of artemether and lumefantrine has been developed for the treatment of acute uncomplicated falciparum malaria in areas where *P. falciparum* is resistant to chloroquine and antifolates. Artemether appears to be effective for the treatment of schistosomiasis and is being evaluated for community-based treatment programs.

The antimalarial effect of artemisinin compounds results primarily from dihydroartemisinin, a compound to which artemether and artesunate are both converted. In the presence of antiparasitic iron, dihydroartemisinin produces superoxide radicals, resulting in damage to parasite proteins. Long treatment courses are required. When these agents are used alone, recrudescence may occur. The compounds are available for oral, rectal, intravenous, or intramuscular administration, depending on the derivative. Artemisinin and its derivatives are cleared rapidly from the circulation. Their short half-lives limit their value for prophylaxis. These drugs are not available in the United States.

Atovaquone Atovaquone is a hydroxynaphthoquinone that exerts broad-spectrum antiprotozoal activity via selective inhibition of parasite mitochondrial electron transport. Atovaquone is an alternative to trimethoprim-sulfamethoxazole for the treatment of *Pneumocystis* pneumonia. This agent exhibits potent activity against toxoplasmosis when used with pyrimethamine. It is active against the erythrocytic and exoerythrocytic stages of *Plasmodium* spp.; when combined with proguanil or doxycycline, it is effective for both treatment and prophylaxis of malaria. Malarone is a fixed-dose combination of atovaquone and proguanil used for malaria prophylaxis as well as for the treatment of acute, uncomplicated *P. falciparum* malaria. Malarone has been shown to be effective in regions with multidrug-resistant *P. falciparum*. Resistance to atovaquone has yet to be reported, although strains of *P. falciparum* with diminished susceptibility to atovaquone alone can be selected both in vitro and in vivo. The drug does not eradicate hypnozoites from the liver; thus patients with *P. vivax* or *P. ovale* infections must be given radical prophylaxis.

The bioavailability of atovaquone varies considerably. Absorption after a single oral dose is slow, increases two- to three-fold with a fatty meal, and is dose-limited above 750 mg. The elimination half-life is increased in patients with moderate hepatic impairment. Because of the potential for drug accumulation, the use of atovaquone is contraindicated in persons with severe renal impairment (creatinine clearance rate <30 mL/min). No dosage adjustments are needed in patients with mild to moderate renal impairment. It is unknown if atovaquone is dialyzable.

Azithromycin See Table 193-1 and Chap. 118.

Azoles See Table 193-1 and Chap. 182.

Benznidazole This oral nitroimidazole derivative is used to treat Chagas' disease, with cure rates of 80 to 90% recorded in acute infections. Benznidazole exerts its trypanocidal effects by generating oxygen radicals to which the parasite is more sensitive than mammalian cells because of a relative deficiency in antioxidant enzymes. Benznidazole also appears to alter the balance between pro- and anti-inflammatory mediators by downregulating the synthesis of nitrite, interleukin (IL) 6, and IL-10 in macrophages.

Benznidazole is highly lipophilic and readily absorbed. The drug is extensively metabolized; only 5% of the dose is excreted unchanged in the urine. Benznidazole is currently unavailable in the United States.

Chloroquine This 4-aminoquinoline has marked, rapid schizontocidal and gametocidal activity against blood forms of *P. ovale* and *Plasmodium malariae* and against susceptible strains of *P. vivax* and *P. falciparum*. It is not active against intrahepatic forms (*P. vivax* and *P. ovale*). Chloroquine is concentrated in the acidic food vacuoles of intraerythrocytic parasites, reaching levels at this site that are 600-fold higher than plasma levels. The drug inhibits a parasite heme polymerase; as a result, the parasite is effectively killed with its own metabolic waste. Compared with susceptible strains, chloroquine-resistant plasmodia transport chloroquine out of intraparasitic compartments more rapidly and maintain lower chloroquine concentrations in their acid vesicles. Hydroxychloroquine, a congener of chloroquine, is equivalent to chloroquine in its antimalarial efficacy but is preferred to chloroquine for the treatment of autoimmune disorders because it produces less ocular toxicity when used in high doses.

Chloroquine is well absorbed. However, because it exhibits extensive tissue binding, a loading dose is required to yield effective plasma concentrations. A therapeutic drug level in plasma is reached 2 to 3 h after oral administration (the preferred route). Chloroquine can be administered intravenously, but excessively rapid parenteral administration can result in seizures and death from cardiovascular collapse. The mean half-life of chloroquine is 4 days, but the rate of excretion decreases as plasma levels decline, making once-weekly administration possible for prophylaxis in areas with sensitive strains. About half of the parent drug is excreted in urine, but the dose should not be reduced for persons with acute malaria and renal insufficiency.

Ciprofloxacin See Table 193-1 and Chap. 118.

Clindamycin See Table 193-1 and Chap. 118.

Dapsone See Table 193-1 and Chap. 149.

Diethylcarbamazine[*] A derivative of the antihelminthic agent piperazine with a long history of successful use, diethylcarbamazine (DEC) remains the treatment of choice for lymphatic filariasis and loiasis and has also been used for visceral larva migrans. While piperazine itself has no antifilarial activity, the piperazine ring of DEC is essential for activity of the drug. DEC exerts various effects on helminths, including immobilization due to a decrease in muscle activity, disruption of microtubule formation, and alteration of helminthic surface membrancs resulting in enhanced killing by the host's immune system. In addition, this agent enhances adherence properties of eosinophils. The development of resistance under drug pressure (i.e., a progressive decrease in efficacy when the drug is used widely in human populations) has not been observed, although the drug's effect is variable when administered to persons with filariasis. Monthly administration provides effective prophylaxis against both bancroftian filariasis and loiasis.

DEC is well absorbed after oral administration, with peak plasma concentrations reached within 1 to 2 h. No parenteral form is available. The drug is eliminated largely by renal excretion, with <5% found in feces. If more than one dose is to be administered to an individual with renal dysfunction, the dose should be reduced commensurate with the reduction in creatinine clearance rate. Alkalinization of the urine prevents renal excretion and increases the half-life of the drug. Use in patients with onchocerciasis can precipitate a Mazzotti reaction, with pruritus, fever, and arthralgias.

Diloxanide Furoate Diloxanide furoate, a substituted acetanilide, is a luminally active agent used to eradicate the cysts of *Entamoeba histolytica*. After ingestion, diloxanide furoate is hydrolyzed by enzymes in the lumen or mucosa of the intestine, releasing furoic acid and the ester diloxanide, the latter of which acts directly as an amebicide.

Diloxanide furoate is given alone in asymptomatic cyst passers. For patients with active amebic infections, diloxanide is generally administered in combination with a 5-nitroimidazole such as metronidazole or tinidazole. Diloxanide furoate is rapidly absorbed after oral administration. When coadministered with a 5-nitroimidazole, only diloxanide appears in the systemic circulation; levels peak within 1 h and disappear within 6 h. About 90% of an oral dose is excreted in the urine within 48 h, chiefly as the glucuronide metabolite. Diloxanide furoate is contraindicated in pregnant and breast-feeding women and in children <2 years of age. The drug is not currently available in the United States.

Eflornithine[†] Eflornithine (difluoromethylornithine, or DFMO) is a fluorinated analogue of the amino acid ornithine. Although originally designed as an antineoplastic agent, eflornithine has proven effective against some trypanosomatids as well as *Pneumocystis*. At one point, the production of this effective agent ceased despite the increasing incidence of human African trypanosomiasis; however, production resumed after eflornithine was discovered to be an effective cosmetic depilatory agent.

Eflornithine has specific activity against all stages of infection with *Trypanosoma brucei gambiense*; however, it is inactive against *T. b. rhodesiense*. The drug acts by irreversibly inhibiting ornithine decarboxylase—an enzyme critical to the formation of polyamines, which are essential to the growth, differentiation, and replication of the trypanosomatids. The diminished effectiveness of eflornithine against *T. b. rhodesiense* appears to be due to the parasite's ability to replace the inhibited enzyme more rapidly than *T. b. gambiense*. Eflornithine is less toxic but more costly than conventional therapy. Supplies of the drug are very limited due to the aforementioned halt in production.

Eflornithine HCl can be administered intravenously or orally; however, its bioavailability after oral administration is only 54%. Eflornithine readily crosses the blood-brain barrier; CSF levels are highest in persons with the most severe central nervous system involvement.

The kidney excretes >80% of the drug; therefore, the dosage should be reduced in patients with renal failure.

Fumagillin Fumagillin, an antibiotic derived from the fungus *Aspergillus fumigatus*, has been used to treat microsporidiosis in honeybees and has been effective against other microsporidia in vitro. This agent was used >40 years ago for the treatment of intestinal amebiasis, and it is effective when used topically in the treatment of microsporidial keratoconjunctivitis.

Fumagillin is being investigated as an angiogenesis inhibitor for the treatment of solid tumors.

Fumagillin exerts its antineoplastic action by inhibiting endothelial cell proliferation and angiogenesis. However, the mechanisms by which fumagillin inhibits microsporidial replication are poorly understood. Fumagillin is not yet available in the United States.

Furazolidone This nitrofuran derivative is an effective alternative agent for the treatment of giardiasis and exhibits activity against *Isospora belli*. Like other nitrofurans, it acts by damaging DNA. Since it is the only agent active against *Giardia* that is available in liquid form, it is often used to treat young children. Although furazolidone had been thought to be largely unabsorbed when administered orally, the occurrence of systemic adverse reactions indicates that this is not the case. More than 65% of the drug can be recovered from the urine as colored metabolites.

Furazolidone is a monoamine oxidase (MAO) inhibitor; thus caution should be used in its concomitant administration with other drugs (especially indirectly acting sympathomimetic amines) and in the consumption of food and drink containing tyramine during treatment. However, hypertensive crises have not been reported in patients receiving furazolidone, and it has been suggested that—since furazolidone inhibits MAO gradually over several days—the risks are small if treatment is limited to a 5-day course. Because hemolytic anemia can occur in patients with glucose-6-phosphate dehydrogenase (G6PD) deficiency and glutathione instability, furazolidone treatment is contraindicated in mothers who are breast-feeding and in neonates.

Halofantrine This 9-phenanthrenemethanol is one of three classes of arylaminoalcohols first identified as potential antimalarial agents by the World War II Malaria Chemotherapy Program. Its activity is believed to be similar to that of chloroquine, although it is an oral alternative for the treatment of malaria due to chloroquine-resistant *P. falciparum*. The mechanism of action is poorly understood.

Halofantrine exhibits erratic bioavailability, but its absorption is significantly enhanced when it is taken with a fatty meal. The elimination half-life of halofantrine is 1 to 2 days; it is excreted mainly in feces. Halofantrine is metabolized into *N*-debutyl-halofantrine by the cytochrome P450 enzyme CYP3A4. Grapefruit juice should be avoided during treatment because it increases both halofantrine's bioavailability and halofantrine-induced QT interval prolongation by inhibiting CYP3A4 at the enterocyte level. Halofantrine is currently unavailable in the United States.

Iodoquinol Iodoquinol (diiodohydroxyquin), a hydroxyquinoline, is an effective luminal agent for the treatment of amebiasis, balantidiasis, and infection with *Dientamoeba fragilis*. Its mechanism of action is unknown. It is poorly absorbed. Because the drug contains 64% organically bound iodine, it should be used with caution in patients with thyroid disease. Iodine dermatitis occurs occasionally during iodoquinol treatment. Protein-bound serum iodine levels may be increased during treatment and can interfere with certain tests of thyroid function. These effects may persist for as long as 6 months after discontinuation of therapy. Iodoquinol is contraindicated in patients with liver disease. Most serious are the reactions related to prolonged high-dose therapy (optic neuritis, peripheral neuropathy), which should not occur if the recommended dosage regimens are followed.

Ivermectin Ivermectin (22,23 dihydroavermectin) is a derivative of the macrocyclic lactone avermectin produced by the soil-dwelling actinomycete *Streptomyces avermitilis*. Ivermectin is active at low doses against a wide range of helminths and ectoparasites. It is the drug of choice for the treatment of onchocerciasis, strongyloidiasis, cutaneous larva migrans, and scabies. Ivermectin is highly active against microfilariae of the lymphatic filariases but has no macrofilaricidal activity. When ivermectin is used in combination with other agents such as diethylcarbamazine or albendazole for treatment of lymphatic filariasis, synergistic activity is seen. While active against the intestinal helminths *Ascaris lumbricoides* and *Enterobius vermicularis*, ivermectin is only variably effective in trichuriasis and is ineffective against hookworms. Widespread use of ivermectin for treatment of intestinal nematode infections in sheep and goats has led to the emergence of drug resistance in veterinary practice; this development may portend problems in human medical use.

Recent data suggest that ivermectin acts by opening the neuromuscular membrane-associated, glutamate-dependent chloride channels that are unique to nematodes and arthropods. In this proposed scenario, the result is an influx of chloride ions followed by worm paralysis and subsequent death (via immune or other mechanisms).

Because of its low water solubility, ivermectin is available only as an oral formulation. The drug is highly protein bound; it is almost completely excreted in feces. The effect of food on bioavailability is unknown. Ivermectin is distributed widely throughout the body; animal studies indicate that it accumulates at the highest concentration in adipose tissue and liver, with little accumulation in the brain. Few data exist to guide therapy in hosts with conditions that may influence drug pharmacokinetics.

Ivermectin is generally administered as a single dose of 150 to 200 μg/kg. In the absence of parasitic infection, the adverse effects of ivermectin in therapeutic doses are minimal. Adverse effects in patients with filarial infections include fever, myalgia, malaise, lightheadedness, and (occasionally) postural hypotension. The severity of such side effects is related to the intensity of parasite infection, with more symptoms in individuals with a heavy parasite burden. In onchocerciasis, skin edema, pruritus, and mild eye irritation may also occur. The adverse effects are generally self-limiting and only occasionally require symptom-based treatment with antipyretics or antihistamines. More severe complications of ivermectin therapy for onchocerciasis include encephalopathy in patients heavily infected with *Loa loa*. This reaction has led to the suspension of ivermectin distribution for this indication in regions where the two filarial infections are coendemic.

Lumefantrine   Lumefantrine (benflumetol), a fluorene (benzindene) derivative synthesized in the 1970s by the Chinese Academy of Military Medical Sciences (Beijing), has marked blood schizontocidal activity against a wide range of plasmodia. This agent conforms structurally and in mode of action to the arylaminoalcohol group of antimalarial drugs, including quinine, mefloquine, and halofantrine. Lumefantrine exerts its antimalarial effect as a consequence of its interaction with heme, a degradation product of hemoglobin metabolism. Its antimalarial activity is slower than that of the artemisinin-based drugs, but at the recommended dose regimen the recrudescence rate with lumefantrine is lower. The pharmacokinetic properties of lumefantrine are reminiscent of those of halofantrine, with variable oral bioavailability, considerable augmentation of oral bioavailability by concomitant fat intake, and a terminal elimination half-life of ~4 to 5 days in patients with malaria.

Artemether and lumefantrine have synergistic activity, and clinical studies in China on several hundred patients show the combination to be safe and well tolerated. The combined formulation of artemether and lumefantrine has been developed for the treatment of falciparum malaria in areas where *P. falciparum* is resistant to chloroquine and antifolates. Neither drug is available in the United States.

Mebendazole   This benzimidazole is a broad-spectrum antiparasitic agent widely used to treat intestinal helminthiases. Its mechanism of action is similar to that of albendazole.

Mebendazole is available only in oral form but is poorly absorbed from the gastrointestinal tract; only 5 to 10% of a standard dose is measurable in plasma. The proportion absorbed from the gastrointestinal tract is extensively metabolized in the liver. Metabolites appear in the urine and bile; impaired liver or biliary function results in higher plasma mebendazole levels in treated patients. No dose reduction is warranted in patients with renal function impairment. Because mebendazole is poorly absorbed, its incidence of side effects is low. Transient abdominal pain and diarrhea sometimes occur, usually in persons with massive parasite burdens.

Mefloquine   Like quinine and chloroquine, this quinoline is active only against the asexual erythrocytic stages of malarial parasites. It is the preferred drug for prophylaxis of chloroquine-resistant malaria; high doses can be used for treatment. Despite the recent development of drug-resistant strains of *P. falciparum* in parts of Africa and Southeast Asia, mefloquine is an effective drug throughout most of the world. Cross-resistance of mefloquine with halofantrine and with quinine has been documented in limited areas. Mefloquine's mode of action is similar to that of chloroquine, but mefloquine is not concentrated so extensively in the food vacuole and may act on alternative targets in the parasite.

Mefloquine HCl is available as 250-mg tablets (equivalent to 228.0 mg of the free base). The presence of food significantly enhances the rate and extent of absorption. About 98% of the drug binds to protein. Mefloquine is excreted mainly in the bile and feces; therefore, no dose adjustment is needed in persons with renal insufficiency. The drug and its main metabolite are not appreciably removed by hemodialysis. No special chemoprophylactic dosage adjustments are indicated for dialysis patients to achieve plasma concentrations similar to those in healthy persons. Pharmacokinetic differences have been detected between various ethnic populations. In practice, however, these are of minor importance compared with host immune status and parasite sensitivity. In patients with impaired liver function, the elimination of mefloquine may be prolonged, leading to higher plasma levels.

Mefloquine should be used with caution in individuals participating in activities requiring alertness and fine-motor coordination (e.g., driving, piloting aircraft, operating machinery, and deep-sea diving). If the drug is to be administered for a prolonged period, periodic evaluations are recommended, including liver function tests and ophthalmic examinations. Sleep abnormalities (insomnia, abnormal dreams) have occasionally been reported. Psychosis and seizures occur rarely; mefloquine should not be prescribed to patients with neuropsychiatric conditions, including depression, generalized anxiety disorder, psychosis, schizophrenia, and seizure disorder. If acute anxiety, depression, restlessness, or confusion develops during prophylaxis, these psychiatric symptoms may be considered prodromal to a more serious event, and the drug should be discontinued.

Concomitant use of quinine, quinidine, or drugs producing β-adrenergic blockade may cause significant electrocardiographic abnormalities or cardiac arrest. Halofantrine must not be given simultaneously with or <3 weeks after mefloquine because a potentially fatal prolongation of the QTc interval on electrocardiography may occur. No data exist on mefloquine use after halofantrine use. Administration of mefloquine with quinine or chloroquine may increase the risk of convulsions. Mefloquine may lower plasma levels of anticonvulsants. Caution should be exercised with regard to concomitant antiretroviral therapy, since mefloquine has been shown to exert variable effects on ritonavir pharmacokinetics that are not explained by hepatic CYP3A4 activity or ritonavir protein binding. Vaccinations with attenuated live bacteria should be completed at least 3 days before the first dose of mefloquine.

Women of childbearing age who are traveling to areas where malaria is endemic should be warned against becoming pregnant and encouraged to practice contraception during malaria prophylaxis with mefloquine and for up to 3 months thereafter. However, in the case of unplanned pregnancy, use of mefloquine is not considered an indication for pregnancy termination.

Melarsoprol* This trivalent arsenical compound has been used outside the United States since 1949 for the treatment of human African trypanosomiasis (HAT). It is considered investigational in the United States and is indicated for the treatment of HAT with neurologic involvement and for the treatment of early HAT that is resistant to suramin or pentamidine. The drug enters the parasite via an adenosine transporter; resistant strains lack this transport system. Arsenicals react avidly with sulfhydryl groups on proteins, inhibiting their function. This is the likely mechanism of action and the cause of the severe adverse reactions that commonly occur. Resistance to melarsoprol is attributed to the expression of an unusual purine transporter, resulting in altered drug uptake.

Melarsoprol is always administered intravenously. The most common treatment protocol consists of three or four series of three or four injections each (one intravenous injection per day) separated by rest periods. A recently proposed alternative protocol for *T. b. gambiense* HAT appears to be similarly efficacious and consists of 10 consecutive injections of 2.2 mg/kg per day. A small but therapeutically significant amount of the drug enters the CSF. The compound is excreted rapidly, with ~80% of the arsenic found in feces.

Melarsoprol is highly toxic. The most serious adverse reaction is reactive encephalopathy, which affects 6% of treated individuals and usually develops within 4 days of the start of therapy, with an average case-fatality rate of 50%. Glucocorticoids are administered with melarsoprol to prevent this development. Because melarsoprol is intensely irritating, care must be taken to avoid infiltration of the drug.

Metrifonate This organophosphorous compound has selective activity against *Schistosoma haematobium*. Metrifonate is a prodrug; it is converted nonenzymatically to dichlorvos (2,2-dichlorovinyl dimethylphosphate, DDVP), a highly active chemical that irreversibly inhibits the acetylcholinesterase enzyme. Schistosomal cholinesterase is more susceptible to dichlorvos than is the corresponding human enzyme. The exact mechanism of action of metrifonate is uncertain, but it is believed to inhibit tegumental acetylcholine receptors that mediate glucose transport.

Metrifonate is administered in a series of three doses at 2-week intervals. After a single oral dose, metrifonate produces a 95% decrease in plasma cholinesterase activity within 6 h, with a fairly rapid return to normal. However, 2.5 months are required for erythrocyte cholinesterase levels to return to normal. Treated persons should not be exposed to neuromuscular blocking agents or organophosphate insecticides for at least 48 h after treatment. Metrifonate is currently unavailable in the United States.

Metronidazole and Other Nitroimidazoles See Table 193-1 and Chap. 118.

Miltefosine Miltefosine (hexadecylphosphocholine), originally developed as an antineoplastic agent, was discovered to have significant antiproliferative activity against *Leishmania* spp., *Trypanosoma cruzi*, and *T. brucei* parasites in vitro and in experimental animal models in the early 1990s. In 1995, Tropical Disease Research, a program sponsored by the WHO and other international groups, entered into an agreement with the company now known as ASTA Medica/Zentaris to develop miltefosine for the treatment of visceral leishmaniasis in India. Miltefosine is the first oral drug that has proved to be highly effective and comparable to amphotericin B against visceral leishmaniasis in India, where antimonial-resistant cases are now prevalent. Miltefosine exerts activity in both previously untreated and pentavalent antimonial–unresponsive visceral infections. A recently concluded study in Colombia demonstrated miltefosine cure rates comparable to those for antimony against cutaneous leishmaniasis.

The activity of miltefosine is attributed to interaction with cell signal transduction pathways and inhibition of phospholipid and sterol biosynthesis.

Resistance to miltefosine has not been observed clinically.

Miltefosine is readily absorbed from the gastrointestinal tract, is widely distributed, and accumulates in several tissues. The efficacy of a 28-day treatment course in Indian visceral leishmaniasis is equivalent to that of amphotericin B therapy; however, it appears that a shortened course of 21 days may be equally efficacious.

General recommendations for the use of miltefosine are limited by the exclusion of specific groups from the published clinical trials: persons <12 or >65 years of age, persons with the most advanced disease, breast-feeding women, HIV-infected patients, and individuals with significant renal or hepatic insufficiency. Miltefosine is currently unavailable in the United States.

Niclosamide Niclosamide is active against a wide variety of adult tapeworms but not against tissue cestodes. It is also a molluscacide and is used in snail-control programs. The drug acts by inhibiting oxidative phosphorylation in worm mitochondria, with consequent energy depletion. Use of the drug is limited by side effects, necessary duration of therapy, the recommended use of purgatives, and—most important—limited availability (i.e., availability on a named-patient basis from the manufacturer).

Niclosamide is poorly absorbed. Tablets are given on an empty stomach in the morning after a liquid meal the night before, and this dose is followed by another 1 h later. For treatment of hymenolepiasis, the drug is administered for 7 days. A second course is often prescribed. The scolex and proximal segments of the tapeworms are killed on contact with niclosamide and may be digested in the gut. However, disintegration of the adult tapeworm results in the release of viable ova, which theoretically can result in autoinfection. Although fears of the development of cysticercosis in patients with *Taenia solium* infections have proved unfounded, it is still recommended that a brisk purgative be given 2 h after the first dose. Niclosamide is no longer approved for use in the United States.

Nifurtimox* This nitrofuran compound is a cheap and effective oral agent for the treatment of acute Chagas' disease. Intracellular reduction followed by auto-oxidation yielding oxygen radicals has been suggested as the mode of action of nifurtimox on *T. cruzi* and as the basis of the drug's toxicity to humans. Prolonged use is required, but the course may have to be interrupted because of drug toxicity, which develops in 40 to 70% of recipients.

Nifurtimox is well absorbed and undergoes rapid and extensive biotransformation: <0.5% of the original drug is excreted in urine.

Nitazoxanide† Nitazoxanide is a 5-nitrothiazole compound used for the treatment of cryptosporidiosis and giardiasis; it is active against other intestinal protozoa as well. The drug is approved for use in children 1 through 11 years of age.

The antiprotozoal activity of nitazoxanide is believed to be due to interference with the pyruvate-ferredoxin oxidoreductase (PFOR) enzyme–dependent electron transfer reaction that is essential to anaerobic energy metabolism. Studies have shown that the PFOR enzyme from *Giardia lamblia* directly reduces nitazoxanide by transfer of electrons in the absence of ferredoxin. The DNA-derived PFOR protein sequence of *Cryptosporidium parvum* appears to be similar to that of *G. lamblia*. Interference with the PFOR enzyme–dependent electron transfer reaction may not be the only pathway by which nitazoxanide exerts antiprotozoal activity.

Nitazoxanide is currently available only as an oral suspension. After oral administration, nitazoxanide is rapidly hydrolyzed to an active metabolite, tizoxanide (desacetyl-nitazoxanide). Tizoxanide then undergoes conjugation, primarily by glucuronidation. It is recommended that nitazoxanide be taken with food; however, no studies have been conducted to determine whether the pharmacokinetics of tizoxanide and tizoxanide glucuronide differ in fasted versus fed subjects. Tizoxanide is excreted in urine, bile, and feces, and tizoxanide glucuronide is excreted in urine and bile. The pharmacokinetics of nitazoxanide in patients with impaired hepatic and/or renal function have not been studied. Tizoxanide is highly bound to plasma protein (>99.9%). Therefore, caution should be used when administering this agent concurrently with other highly plasma protein–bound drugs with narrow therapeutic indices, as competition for binding sites may occur.

Oxamniquine This tetrahydroquinoline derivative is an effective alternative agent for the treatment of *Schistosoma mansoni*, although susceptibility to this drug exhibits regional variation. Oxamniquine exhibits anticholinergic properties, but its primary mode of action seems to rely on ATP-dependent enzymatic drug activation generating an intermediate that alkylates essential macromolecules, including DNA. In treated adult schistosomes, oxamniquine produces marked tegumental alterations similar to those seen with praziquantel but developing less rapidly (i.e., evident 4 to 8 days after treatment).

Oxamniquine is administered orally as a single dose and is well absorbed. Food retards absorption and reduces bioavailability. About 70% of an administered dose is excreted in urine as a mixture of pharmacologically inactive metabolites. Patients should be warned that their urine might have an intense orange-red color. Side effects are uncommon and usually mild, although hallucinations and seizures have been reported. Oxamniquine remains unavailable in the United States.

Paromomycin (Aminosidine) First isolated in 1956, this aminoglycoside is an effective oral agent for the treatment of infections due to intestinal protozoa. Parenteral paromomycin appears to be effective against visceral leishmaniasis in India.

Paromomycin inhibits protozoan protein synthesis by binding to the 30S ribosomal RNA in the aminoacyl-tRNA site, causing misreading of mRNA codons. Paromomycin is less active against *G. lamblia* than standard agents; however, like other aminoglycosides, paromomycin is poorly absorbed from the intestinal lumen, and the high levels of drug in the gut compensate for this relatively weak activity. If absorbed or administered systemically, paromomycin can cause ototoxicity and nephrotoxicity. However, systemic absorption is very limited, and toxicity should not be a concern in persons with normal kidneys. Topical formulations are not generally available.

Pentamidine Isethionate This diamidine is an effective alternative agent for *Pneumocystis* pneumonia and for some forms of leishmaniasis and trypanosomiasis. It is available for parenteral and aerosolized administration. While its mechanism of action remains undefined, it is known to exert a wide range of effects, including interaction with trypanosomal kinetoplast DNA; interference with polyamine synthesis by a decrease in the activity of ornithine decarboxylase; and inhibition of RNA polymerase, ribosomal function, and the synthesis of nucleic acids and proteins.

Pentamidine isethionate is well absorbed, is highly tissue bound, and is excreted slowly over several weeks, with an elimination half-life of 12 days. No steady-state plasma concentration is attained in persons given daily injections; the result is extensive accumulation of pentamidine in tissues, primarily the liver, kidney, adrenal, and spleen. Pentamidine does not penetrate well into the central nervous system. Pulmonary concentrations of pentamidine are increased when delivered in aerosolized form.

Praziquantel This heterocyclic pyrazinoisoquinoline derivative is highly active against a broad spectrum of trematodes and cestodes. It is the mainstay of treatment for schistosomiasis and is a critical part of community-based control programs.

All of the effects of praziquantel can be attributed either directly or indirectly to an alteration of intracellular calcium concentrations. Although the exact mechanism of action remains unclear, the major mechanism is disruption of the parasite tegument, causing tetanic contractures with loss of adherence to host tissues and, ultimately, disintegration or expulsion. Praziquantel induces changes in the antigenicity of the parasite by causing the exposure of concealed antigens. Praziquantel also produces alterations in schistosomal glucose metabolism, including decreases in glucose uptake, lactate release, glycogen content, and ATP levels.

Praziquantel exerts its parasitic effects directly and does not need to be metabolized to be effective. It is well absorbed but undergoes extensive first-pass hepatic clearance. Levels of the drug are increased when it is taken with food, particularly carbohydrates, or with cimetidine. Serum levels are reduced by glucocorticoids, chloroquine, carbamazepine, and phenytoin. Praziquantel is completely metabolized in humans, with 80% of the dose recovered as metabolites in urine within 4 days. It is not known to what extent praziquantel crosses the placenta.

Patients with schistosomiasis who have heavy parasite burdens may develop abdominal discomfort, nausea, headache, dizziness, and drowsiness. Symptoms begin 30 min after ingestion, may require spasmolytics for relief, and usually disappear spontaneously after a few hours.

Primaquine Phosphate This drug is the only agent available for eradication of the hepatic stage of malarial parasites. Primaquine must be metabolized by the host to be effective. It is, in fact, rapidly metabolized; only a small fraction of the dose of the parent drug is excreted unchanged. Although the parasiticidal activity of the three oxidative metabolites remains unclear, they are believed to affect both pyrimidine synthesis and the mitochondrial electron transport chain. The metabolites appear to have significantly less antimalarial activity than primaquine; however, their hemolytic activity is greater than that of the parent drug.

Primaquine causes marked hypotension after parenteral administration and therefore is given only by the oral route. It is rapidly and almost completely absorbed from the gastrointestinal tract.

Patients should be tested for G6PD deficiency before they receive primaquine. Primaquine is otherwise well tolerated.

Proguanil (Chloroguanide) Proguanil inhibits plasmodial dihydrofolate reductase and is used with atovaquone for oral treatment of uncomplicated malaria or with chloroquine for malaria prophylaxis in parts of Africa without widespread chloroquine-resistant *P. falciparum*.

Proguanil primarily exerts its effect by means of the metabolite cycloguanil, whose inhibition of dihydrofolate reductase in the parasite disrupts deoxythymidylate synthesis, thus interfering with a key pathway involved in the biosynthesis of pyrimidines required for nucleic acid replication. There are no clinical data indicating that folate supplementation diminishes drug efficacy; women of childbearing age for whom atovaquone/proguanil is prescribed should continue taking folate supplements to prevent neural-tube birth defects.

Proguanil is extensively absorbed regardless of food intake. The drug is 75% protein-bound. The main routes of elimination are hepatic biotransformation and renal excretion. Between 40 and 60% of proguanil is excreted by the kidneys. Drug levels are increased and elimination is impaired in patients with hepatic impairment. Proguanil is not available in the United States.

Pyrantel Pamoate Pyrantel is a tetrahydropyrimidine formulated as pamoate. This safe, well-tolerated, inexpensive drug is used to treat a variety of intestinal nematode infections but is ineffective in trichuriasis. Pyrantel pamoate is usually effective in a single dose. It depolarizes the neuromuscular junctions of most intestinal nematodes, resulting in their irreversible paralysis and allowing natural expulsion of the worms with the host's feces.

Pyrantel pamoate is poorly absorbed from the intestine; >85% of the dose is passed unaltered in feces. The absorbed portion is metabolized and excreted in urine. Piperazine, which produces hyperpolarization of muscle cells in intestinal helminths, is antagonistic to pyrantel pamoate and should not be used concomitantly.

Pyrantel pamoate has minimal toxicity at the oral doses used to treat intestinal helminthic infection. It is not recommended for pregnant women or children <12 months old.

Pyrimethamine When combined with short-acting sulfonamides, this diaminopyrimidine is effective in malaria, toxoplasmosis, and isosporiasis. Unlike mammalian cells, the parasites that cause these infections cannot utilize preformed pyrimidines obtained through salvage pathways but rather rely completely on de novo pyrimidine synthesis, for which folate derivatives are essential cofactors. The efficacy of pyrimethamine is increasingly limited by the development of resistant strains of *P. falciparum* and *P. vivax*. Single amino acid substitutions to parasite dihydrofolate reductase confer resistance to pyrimethamine by decreasing the enzyme's binding affinity for the drug.

Pyrimethamine is well absorbed; the drug is 87% bound to human plasma proteins. In healthy volunteers, drug concentrations remain at therapeutic levels for up to 2 weeks; drug levels are lower in patients with malaria. Pyrimethamine is extensively metabolized; <3% is excreted unchanged in urine.

At the usual dosage, pyrimethamine alone causes little toxicity except for occasional skin rashes and blood dyscrasias. Bone marrow suppression sometimes occurs at the higher doses used for toxoplasmosis; at these doses, the drug should be administered with folinic acid.

Quinacrine* First introduced as an antimalarial agent in 1930, quinacrine is the only drug approved by the FDA for the treatment of giardiasis. Its production was discontinued in 1992. Although not commercially available, quinacrine can be obtained from alternative sources through the CDC Drug Service. The antiprotozoal mechanism of quinacrine has not been fully elucidated. Quinacrine, a substituted acridine, intercalates into parasite DNA, and it is this interaction that is thought to cause an inhibition of nucleic acid synthesis. The drug inhibits NADH oxidase—the same enzyme that activates furazolidone. The differing relative quinacrine uptake rate between human cells and *G. lamblia* may explain the selective toxicity of the drug. Resistance correlates with decreased drug uptake.

Quinacrine is rapidly absorbed from the intestinal tract and is widely distributed in body tissues. Alcohol is best avoided due to a disulfiram-like effect.

Quinine and Quinidine When combined with another agent, the cinchona alkaloid quinine is effective for the oral treatment of both uncomplicated, chloroquine-resistant malaria and babesiosis. Quinine acts rapidly against the asexual blood stages of all forms of human malaria. For severe malaria, only quinidine (the dextroisomer of quinine) is available in the United States. Quinine concentrates in the acidic food vacuoles of *Plasmodium* spp. The drug inhibits the nonenzymatic polymerization of the highly reactive, toxic heme molecule into a nontoxic polymer pigment called *hemozoin*.

Quinine is readily absorbed when given orally. In patients with malaria, the elimination half-life of quinine increases according to the severity of the infection. However, toxicity is avoided by an increase in the concentration of plasma glycoproteins. The cinchona alkaloids are extensively metabolized, particularly by CYP3A4; only 20% of the dose is excreted unchanged in urine. The drug's metabolites are also excreted in urine and may be responsible for toxicity in patients with renal failure. Renal excretion of quinine is decreased when cimetidine is taken and increased when the urine is acidic. The drug readily crosses the placenta.

Quinidine is both more potent as an antimalarial and more toxic than quinine. Its use requires cardiac monitoring. Dose reduction is necessary in persons with severe renal impairment.

Spiramycin† This macrolide is used to treat acute toxoplasmosis in pregnancy and congenital toxoplasmosis. While the mechanism of action is similar to that of other macrolides, the efficacy of spiramycin in toxoplasmosis appears to stem from its rapid and extensive intracellular penetration, resulting in macrophage drug concentrations 10 to 20 times greater than serum concentrations.

Spiramycin is rapidly and widely distributed throughout the body and reaches concentrations in the placenta up to five times those in serum. This agent is excreted mainly in bile. Indeed, in humans, the urinary excretion of active compounds represents only 20% of the administered dose.

Serious reactions to spiramycin are rare. Of the available macrolides, spiramycin appears to have the lowest risk of drug interactions. Complications of treatment are rare but, in neonates, can include life-threatening ventricular arrhythmias that disappear with drug discontinuation. Although not yet licensed in the United States, spiramycin is available through the FDA.

Sulfonamides See Table 193-1 and Chap. 118.

Suramin* This derivative of urea is the drug of choice for the early stage of African trypanosomiasis. The drug is polyanionic and acts by forming stable complexes with proteins, inhibiting multiple enzymes essential to parasite energy metabolism.

Suramin is parenterally administered. It binds to plasma proteins and persists at low levels for several weeks after infusion. Its metabolism is negligible. This drug does not penetrate the central nervous system.

Tetracyclines See Table 193-1 and Chap. 118.

Thiabendazole Discovered in 1961, thiabendazole remains one of the most potent of the numerous benzimidazole derivatives. However, its use has declined significantly because of a higher frequency of adverse effects than is seen with other, equally effective agents.

Thiabendazole is available in tablet form and as an oral suspension. The drug is rapidly absorbed from the gastrointestinal tract but can also be absorbed through the skin. Thiabendazole should be taken after meals. This agent is extensively metabolized in the liver before ultimately being excreted, principally as glucuronide or sulfate conjugates of 5-hydroxythiabendazole. Within 48 h, 87% of an oral dose of thiabendazole is excreted in urine, and 5% is excreted in feces; most of the dose is excreted within the first 24 h. The usual dose of thiabendazole is determined by the patient's weight, but some treatment regimens are parasite-specific. No specific adjustments are recommended in patients with renal or hepatic failure; only cautious use is advised.

Thiabendazole is active against most intestinal nematodes that infect humans. Although the exact mechanism of its antihelminthic activity has not been fully elucidated, it is likely to be similar to that of other benzimidazole drugs: namely, inhibition of polymerization of parasite β-tubulin. The drug also inhibits the helminth-specific enzyme fumarate reductase. In animals, thiabendazole has anti-inflammatory, antipyretic, and analgesic effects, which may explain its usefulness in dracunculiasis and trichinosis. Thiabendazole also suppresses egg and/or larval production by some nematodes and may inhibit the subsequent development of eggs or larvae passed in feces. Despite the emergence and global spread of thiabendazole-resistant trichostrongyliasis among sheep, there have been no reports of drug resistance in humans.

Coadministration of thiabendazole in patients taking theophylline can result in an increase in theophylline levels by >50%. Therefore, serum levels of theophylline should be monitored closely in this situation.

Tinidazole This nitroimidazole is effective for the treatment of amebiasis, giardiasis, and trichomoniasis. Its mechanism of action and side effects are similar to those of metronidazole, but adverse events appear to be less frequent and severe with tinidazole. In addition, the significantly longer half-life of tinidazole (>12 h) offers potential cure with a single dose. This agent is currently unavailable in the United States.

Triclabendazole This narrow-spectrum benzimidazole is effective against paragonimiasis and all stages of *Fasciola hepatica*, a trematode with inherent resistance to praziquantel. Triclabendazole was originally introduced into veterinary practice in 1983 for the treatment of fascioliasis and was first used in humans in Iran in 1989 during an epidemic of fascioliasis near the Caspian Sea. In 1990, the WHO Division of Control of Tropical Diseases and the pharmaceutical company Ciba-Geigy (now Novartis) agreed to conduct additional clinical trials of triclabendazole for the treatment of fascioliasis and paragonimiasis. In light of the remarkable success of these trials, the WHO Expert Committee on the Use of Essential Drugs recommended in 1997 that the drug be put on the essential drug list. The manufacturer has initiated the process of registering triclabendazole for human use in countries where fascioliasis is endemic. The FDA has not yet approved triclabendazole for use in humans.

While most benzimidazoles have broad-spectrum antihelminthic activity, they exhibit minimal or no activity against *F. hepatica*. In contrast, the antihelminthic activity of triclabendazole is highly specific for *Fasciola* spp. and *Paragonimus* spp., with little activity against nematodes, cestodes, and other trematodes. Triclabendazole is effective against all stages of *Fasciola* spp. The active sulfoxide metabolite of triclabendazole binds to fluke tubulin by assuming a unique nonplanar configuration and disrupts microtubule-based processes. Resistance to triclabendazole in veterinary use has been reported in Australia and Europe; however, no resistance has been documented in humans.

Triclabendazole is rapidly absorbed after oral ingestion and undergoes extensive first-pass metabolism in the liver. Its administration with food enhances its absorption and shortens the elimination half-life of the active metabolite. Both the sulfoxide and sulfone metabolites are highly protein-bound (>99%). Treatment with triclabendazole is typically given in one or two doses. No clinical data are available regarding dose adjustment in renal or hepatic insufficiency; however,

given the short course of therapy and extensive hepatic metabolism of triclabendazole, dose adjustment is unlikely to be necessary. No information exists on drug interactions. Triclabendazole is currently unavailable in the United States.

Trimethoprim-Sulfamethoxazole See Table 193-1 and Chap. 118.

FURTHER READING

ABRAMOWICZ M (ed): Drugs for parasitic infections. Med Lett Drugs Ther 40:1, 2000

MOORE TA, NASH TE: Tissue nematodes, in *Current Therapy of Infectious Disease*, 2d ed, D Schlossberg (ed). St. Louis, Mosby, 2000, pp 660–665

ROSENBLATT JE: Antiparasitic agents. Mayo Clin Proc 74:1161, 1999

TRACY JW, WEBSTER LT: Drugs used in the chemotherapy of protozoal infections: Malaria, in *Goodman and Gilman's The Pharmacological Basis of Therapeutics*, 10th ed, JG Hardman, LE Limbird (eds). New York, McGraw-Hill, 2001, pp 1069–1140

WORLD HEALTH ORGANIZATION: *Model Prescribing Information: Drugs Used in Parasitic Diseases*, 2d ed. Geneva, WHO, 1995

Section 18 Protozoal Infections

194 AMEBIASIS AND INFECTION WITH FREE-LIVING AMEBAS
Sharon L. Reed

AMEBIASIS

DEFINITION Amebiasis is an infection with the intestinal protozoan *Entamoeba histolytica*. About 90% of infections are asymptomatic, and the remaining 10% produce a spectrum of clinical syndromes ranging from dysentery to abscesses of the liver or other organs.

LIFE CYCLE AND TRANSMISSION *E. histolytica* is acquired by ingestion of viable cysts from fecally contaminated water, food, or hands. Foodborne exposure is most prevalent and is particularly likely when food handlers are shedding cysts or food is being grown with feces-contaminated soil, fertilizer, or water. Less common means of transmission include contaminated water, oral and anal sexual practices, and—in rare instances—direct rectal inoculation through colonic irrigation devices. Motile trophozoites are released from cysts in the small intestine and, in most patients, remain as harmless commensals in the large bowel. After encystation, infectious cysts are shed in the stool and can survive for several weeks in a moist environment. In some patients, the trophozoites invade either the bowel mucosa, causing symptomatic colitis, or the bloodstream, causing distant abscesses of the liver, lungs, or brain. The trophozoites may not encyst in patients with active dysentery, and motile hematophagous trophozoites are frequently present in fresh stools. Trophozoites are rapidly killed by exposure to air or stomach acid, however, and therefore cannot cause infection.

EPIDEMIOLOGY About 10% of the world's population is infected with *Entamoeba*, the majority with noninvasive *Entamoeba dispar*. Amebiasis results from infection with *E. histolytica* and is the third most common cause of death from parasitic disease (after schistosomiasis and malaria). Areas of highest incidence (due to inadequate sanitation and crowding) include most developing countries in the tropics, particularly Mexico, India, and nations of Central and South America, tropical Asia, and Africa. The main groups at risk in developed countries are travelers, recent immigrants, homosexual men, and inmates of institutions.

The wide spectrum of clinical disease is caused in part by infection with the two different species of *Entamoeba*. Isolates of *E. histolytica* from patients with invasive amebiasis have unique isoenzymes, surface antigens, DNA markers, and virulence properties and now are recognized as a distinct species from the noninvasive *E. dispar* (Table 194-1).

TABLE 194-1 *E. histolytica and E. dispar, Compared and Contrasted*

SIMILARITIES

1. Both species are spread through ingestion of infectious cysts.
2. Cysts of the two species are morphologically identical.
3. Both species colonize the large intestine.

DIFFERENCES

1. Only *E. histolytica* causes invasive disease.
2. Only *E. histolytica* infections elicit a positive amebic serology.
3. The two species have distinct rRNA sequences.
4. The two species have distinct surface antigens and isoenzyme markers.
5. Gal/GalNAc lectin can be used to differentiate the two species in stool ELISA.

Note: ELISA, enzyme-linked immunosorbent assay; Gal/GalNAc, galactose *N*-acetylgalactosamine. See text.

Most asymptomatic carriers, including homosexual men and AIDS patients, harbor *E. dispar* and have self-limited infections. These observations suggest that *E. dispar* is incapable of causing invasive disease, since *Cryptosporidium* and *Isospora belli*, which also cause only self-limited illnesses in immunocompetent people, cause devastating diarrhea in patients with AIDS. However, host factors play a role as well. In one study, 10% of asymptomatic patients who were colonized with *E. histolytica* went on to develop amebic colitis, while the rest remained asymptomatic and cleared the infection within 1 year.

PATHOGENESIS AND PATHOLOGY Both trophozoites (Fig. 194-1) and cysts (Fig. 194-2) are found in the intestinal lumen, but only trophozoites of *E. histolytica* invade tissue. The trophozoite is 20 to 60 μm in diameter and contains vacuoles and a nucleus with a characteristic central nucleolus. In animals, depletion of intestinal mucus, diffuse inflammation, and disruption of the epithelial barrier occur before trophozoites actually come into contact with the colonic mucosa. Trophozoites attach to colonic mucus and epithelial cells by galactose *N*-acetylgalactosamine (Gal/GalNAc) lectin. The earliest intestinal lesions are microulcerations of the mucosa of the cecum, sigmoid colon, or rectum that release erythrocytes, inflammatory cells, and epithelial cells. Proctoscopy reveals small ulcers with heaped up margins and normal intervening mucosa. Submucosal extension of ulcerations under viable-appearing surface mucosa causes the classic "flask-shaped"

FIGURE 194-1 Trophozoite of *E. histolytica* demonstrating a single nucleus with a central, dotlike nucleolus (trichrome stain).

ulcer containing trophozoites at the margins of dead and viable tissues. Although neutrophilic infiltrates may accompany the early lesions in animals, human intestinal infection is marked by a paucity of inflammatory cells, probably in part because of the killing of neutrophils by trophozoites. Treated ulcers characteristically heal with little or no scarring. Occasionally, however, full-thickness necrosis and perforation occur.

Rarely, intestinal infection results in the formation of a mass lesion, or *ameboma*, in the bowel lumen. The overlying mucosa is usually thin and ulcerated, while other layers of the wall are thickened, edematous, and hemorrhagic; this condition results in exuberant formation of granulation tissue with little fibrous-tissue response.

A number of virulence factors have been linked to the ability of *E. histolytica* to invade through the interglandular epithelium. One consists of the extracellular cysteine proteinases that degrade collagen, elastin, IgA, IgG, and the anaphylatoxins C3a and C5a. Other enzymes may disrupt glycoprotein bonds between mucosal epithelial cells in the gut. Amebas can lyse neutrophils, monocytes, lymphocytes, and cells of colonic and hepatic cell lines. The cytolytic effect of amebas appears to require direct contact with target cells and may be linked to the release of phospholipase A and pore-forming peptides.

Liver abscesses are always preceded by intestinal colonization, which may be asymptomatic. Blood vessels may be compromised early by lysis of the wall and thrombus formation. Trophozoites invade veins to reach the liver through the portal venous system. *E. histolytica* is resistant to complement-mediated lysis, a property critical to survival in the bloodstream. In contrast, *E. dispar* is rapidly lysed by complement and is thus restricted to the bowel lumen. Inoculation of amebas into the portal system of hamsters results in an acute cellular infiltrate consisting predominantly of neutrophils. Later, the neutro-

phils are lysed by contact with amebas, and the release of neutrophil toxins may contribute to necrosis of hepatocytes. The liver parenchyma is replaced by necrotic material that is surrounded by a thin rim of congested liver tissue. The necrotic contents of a liver abscess are classically described as "anchovy paste," although the fluid is variable in color and is composed of bacteriologically sterile granular debris with few or no cells. Amebas, if seen, tend to be found near the capsule of the abscess.

A recent study in Bangladeshi schoolchildren revealed that an intestinal IgA response to the Gal/GalNAc lectin reduced the risk of new *E. histolytica* infection by 64%. Serum IgG antibody is not protective; titers correlate with the length of illness rather than with the severity of disease. Indeed, Bangladeshi children with a serum IgG response were more likely than those without such a response to develop new *E. histolytica* infection. Studies of animals suggest that cell-mediated immunity may be important for protection, although patients with AIDS appear not to be predisposed to more severe disease.

CLINICAL SYNDROMES ■ Intestinal Amebiasis The most common type of amebic infection is asymptomatic cyst passage. Even in highly endemic areas, most patients harbor *E. dispar*.

Symptomatic amebic colitis develops 2 to 6 weeks after the ingestion of infectious cysts. Lower abdominal pain and mild diarrhea develop gradually and are followed by malaise, weight loss, and diffuse lower abdominal or back pain. Cecal involvement may mimic acute appendicitis. Patients with full-blown dysentery may pass 10 to 12 stools per day. The stools contain little fecal material and consist mainly of blood and mucus. In contrast to those with bacterial diarrhea, fewer than 40% of patients with amebic dysentery are febrile. Virtually all patients have heme-positive stools.

More fulminant intestinal infection, with severe abdominal pain, high fever, and profuse diarrhea, is rare and occurs predominantly in children. Patients may develop toxic megacolon, in which there is severe bowel dilation with intramural air. Patients receiving glucocorticoids are at risk for severe amebiasis. Uncommonly, patients develop a chronic form of amebic colitis, which can be confused with inflammatory bowel disease. The association between severe amebiasis complications and glucocorticoid therapy emphasizes the importance of excluding amebiasis when inflammatory bowel disease is suspected. An occasional patient presents with only an asymptomatic or tender abdominal mass caused by an ameboma, which is easily confused with cancer on barium studies. A positive serologic test or biopsy can prevent unnecessary surgery in this setting. The syndrome of postamebic colitis—persistent diarrhea following documented cure of amebic colitis—is controversial; no evidence of recurrent amebic infection can be found, and re-treatment usually has no effect.

Amebic Liver Abscess Extraintestinal infection by *E. histolytica* most often involves the liver. Of travelers who develop an amebic liver abscess after leaving an endemic area, 95% do so within 5 months. Young patients with an amebic liver abscess are more likely than older patients to present in the acute phase with prominent symptoms of <10 days' duration. Most patients are febrile and have right-upper-quadrant pain, which may be dull or pleuritic in nature and radiate to the shoulder. Point tenderness over the liver and right-sided pleural effusion are common. Jaundice is rare. Although the initial site of infection is the colon, fewer than one-third of patients with an amebic abscess have active diarrhea. Older patients from endemic areas are more likely to have a subacute course lasting 6 months, with weight loss and hepatomegaly. About one-third of patients with chronic presentations are febrile. Thus, the clinical diagnosis of an amebic liver abscess may be difficult to establish because the symptoms and signs are often nonspecific. Since 10 to 15% of patients present only with fever, amebic liver abscess must be considered in the differential diagnosis of fever of unknown origin (Chap. 18).

Complications of Amebic Liver Abscess Pleuropulmonary involvement, which is reported in 20 to 30% of patients, is the most frequent com-

FIGURE 194-2 Cyst of *E. histolytica* showing three of the four nuclei (trichrome stain).

plication of amebic liver abscess. Manifestations include sterile effusions, contiguous spread from the liver, and rupture into the pleural space. Sterile effusions and contiguous spread usually resolve with medical therapy, but frank rupture into the pleural space requires drainage. A hepatobronchial fistula may cause cough productive of large amounts of necrotic material that may contain amebas. This dramatic complication carries a good prognosis. Abscesses that rupture into the peritoneum may present as an indolent leak or an acute abdomen and require both percutaneous catheter drainage and medical therapy. Rupture into the pericardium, usually from abscesses of the left lobe of the liver, carries the gravest prognosis; it can occur during medical therapy and requires surgical drainage.

Other Extraintestinal Sites   The genitourinary tract may become involved by direct extension of amebiasis from the colon or by hematogenous spread of the infection. Painful genital ulcers, characterized by a punched-out appearance and profuse discharge, may develop secondary to extension from either the intestine or the liver. Both these conditions respond well to medical therapy. Cerebral involvement has been reported in fewer than 0.1% of patients in large clinical series. Symptoms and prognosis depend on the size and location of the lesion.

DIAGNOSTIC TESTS ■ Laboratory Diagnosis   Stool examinations, serologic tests, and noninvasive imaging of the liver are the most important procedures in the diagnosis of amebiasis. Fecal findings suggestive of amebic colitis include a positive test for heme, a paucity of neutrophils, and amebic cysts or trophozoites. The definitive diagnosis of amebic colitis is made by the demonstration of hematophagous trophozoites of *E. histolytica* (Fig. 194-1). Because trophozoites are killed rapidly by water, drying, or barium, it is important to examine at least three fresh stool specimens. Examination of a combination of wet mounts, iodine-stained concentrates, and trichrome-stained preparations of fresh stool and concentrates for cysts (Fig. 194-2) or trophozoites (Fig. 194-1) confirms the diagnosis in 75 to 95% of cases. Cultures of amebas are more sensitive but are not routinely available. If stool examinations are negative, sigmoidoscopy with biopsy of the edge of ulcers may increase the yield, but this procedure is dangerous during fulminant colitis because of the risk of perforation. Trophozoites in a biopsy specimen from a colonic mass confirm the diagnosis of ameboma, but trophozoites are rare in liver aspirates because they are found in the abscess capsule and not in the readily aspirated necrotic center. Accurate diagnosis requires experience, since the trophozoites may be confused with neutrophils and the cysts must be differentiated morphologically from *Entamoeba hartmanni*, *Entamoeba coli*, and *Endolimax nana*, which do not cause clinical disease and do not warrant therapy. Unfortunately, the cysts of *E. histolytica* cannot be distinguished microscopically from those of *E. dispar*. Therefore, the microscopic diagnosis of *E. histolytica* can be made only by the detection of *Entamoeba* trophozoites that have ingested erythrocytes (Fig. 194-1). In terms of sensitivity, stool diagnostic tests based on the detection of the Gal/GalNAc lectin of *E. histolytica* compare favorably with the polymerase chain reaction and with isolation in culture followed by isoenzyme analysis.

Serology is an important addition to the methods used for the parasitologic diagnosis of invasive amebiasis. Enzyme-linked immunosorbent assays (ELISAs) and agar gel diffusion assays are positive in more than 90% of patients with colitis, amebomas, or liver abscess. Positive results in conjunction with the appropriate clinical syndrome suggest active disease because serologic findings usually revert to negative within 6 to 12 months. Even in highly endemic areas such as South Africa, fewer than 10% of asymptomatic individuals have a positive amebic serology. The interpretation of the indirect hemagglutination test is more difficult because titers may remain positive for as long as 10 years.

Up to 10% of patients with acute amebic liver abscess may have negative serologic findings; in suspected cases with an initially negative result, testing should be repeated in a week. In contrast to carriers

of *E. dispar*, most asymptomatic carriers of *E. histolytica* develop antibodies. Thus, serologic tests are helpful in assessing the risk of invasive amebiasis in asymptomatic, cyst-passing individuals in nonendemic areas. Serologic tests also should be performed in patients with ulcerative colitis before the institution of glucocorticoid therapy to prevent the development of severe colitis or toxic megacolon owing to unsuspected amebiasis.

Routine hematology and chemistry tests usually are not very helpful in the diagnosis of invasive amebiasis. About three-fourths of patients with an amebic liver abscess have leukocytosis ($>10,000$ cells/μL); this condition is particularly likely if symptoms are acute or complications have developed. Invasive amebiasis does not elicit eosinophilia. Anemia, if present, is usually multifactorial. Even with large liver abscesses, liver enzyme levels are normal or minimally elevated. The alkaline phosphatase level is most often elevated and may remain so for months. Aminotransferase elevations suggest acute disease or a complication.

Radiographic Studies   Radiographic barium studies are potentially dangerous in acute amebic colitis. Amebomas are usually identified first by a barium enema, but biopsy is necessary for differentiation from carcinoma.

Radiographic techniques such as ultrasonography, computed tomography (CT) (Fig. 194-3), and magnetic resonance imaging are all useful for detection of the round or oval hypoechoic cyst. More than 80% of patients who have had symptoms for >10 days have a single abscess of the right lobe of the liver. Approximately 50% of patients who have had symptoms for <10 days have multiple abscesses. Findings associated with complications include large abscesses (>10 cm) in the superior part of the right lobe, which may rupture into the pleural space; multiple lesions, which must be differentiated from pyogenic abscesses; and lesions of the left lobe, which may rupture into the pericardium. Because abscesses resolve slowly and may increase in size in patients who are responding clinically to therapy, frequent follow-up ultrasonography may prove confusing. Complete resolution of a liver abscess within 6 months can be anticipated in two-thirds of patients, but 10% may have persistent abnormalities for a year.

DIFFERENTIAL DIAGNOSIS   The differential diagnosis of intestinal amebiasis includes bacterial diarrheas caused by *Campylobacter*; enteroinvasive *Escherichia coli*; and *Shigella*, *Salmonella*, and *Vibrio* species. Although the typical patient with amebic colitis has less prominent fever than in these other conditions as well as heme-positive stools with few neutrophils, correct diagnosis requires bacterial cultures, microscopic examination of stools, and amebic serologic testing. As has already been mentioned, amebiasis must be ruled out in any patient thought to have inflammatory bowel disease.

FIGURE 194-3   Abdominal computed tomography scan of a large amebic abscess of the right lobe of the liver. (*Courtesy of the Department of Radiology, UCSD Medical Center, San Diego.*)

liver abscess can easily be confused with pulmonary or gallbladder disease or with any febrile illness with few localizing signs, such as malaria or typhoid fever. The diagnosis should be considered in members of high-risk groups who have recently traveled outside the United States and in inmates of institutions. Once radiographic studies have identified an abscess in the liver, the most important differential diagnosis is between amebic and pyogenic abscess. Patients with pyogenic abscess typically are older and have a history of underlying bowel disease or recent surgery. Amebic serology is helpful, but aspiration of the abscess, with Gram's staining and culture of the material, may be required for differentiation of the two diseases.

℞ TREATMENT

Intestinal Disease The drugs used to treat amebiasis can be classified according to their primary site of action. Luminal amebicides are poorly absorbed and reach high concentrations in the bowel, but their activity is limited to cysts and trophozoites close to the mucosa. Only two luminal drugs are available in the United States: iodoquinol and paromomycin (Table 194-2). Indications for the use of luminal agents include eradication of cysts in patients with colitis or a liver abscess and treatment of asymptomatic carriers. The majority of asymptomatic individuals who pass cysts are colonized with *E. dispar*, which does not warrant specific therapy. However, it is prudent to treat asymptomatic individuals who pass cysts unless *E. dispar* colonization can be definitively demonstrated by specific antigen-detection tests.

Tissue amebicides reach high concentrations in the blood and tissue after oral or parenteral administration. The development of nitroimidazole compounds, especially metronidazole, was a major advance in the treatment of invasive amebiasis. Patients with amebic colitis should be treated with intravenous or oral metronidazole (750 mg three times daily for 5 to 10 days). Side effects include nausea, vomiting, abdominal discomfort, and a disulfiram-like reaction. Other imidazole compounds, such as tinidazole and ornidazole, are as effective but are not available in the United States. All patients should also receive a full course of therapy with a luminal agent, since metronidazole does not eradicate cysts. Resistance to metronidazole has not been identified. Relapses are not uncommon and probably represent reinfection or failure to eradicate amebas from the bowel because of an inadequate dosage or duration of therapy.

Amebic Liver Abscess Metronidazole is the drug of choice for amebic liver abscess. Longer-acting nitroimidazoles (tinidazole and ornidazole) have been shown to be effective as single-dose therapy in developing countries. With early diagnosis and therapy, mortality from uncomplicated amebic liver abscess is <1%. The second-line therapeutic agents emetine and chloroquine should be avoided if possible because of the potential cardiovascular and gastrointestinal side effects of the former and the higher relapse rates with the latter. There is no

evidence that combined therapy with two drugs is more effective than the single-drug regimen. Studies of South Africans with liver abscesses demonstrated that 72% of patients without intestinal symptoms had bowel infection with *E. histolytica*; thus, all treatment regimens should include a luminal agent to eradicate cysts and prevent further transmission. Amebic liver abscess recurs rarely.

Aspiration of Liver Abscesses More than 90% of patients respond dramatically to metronidazole therapy with decreases in both pain and fever within 72 h. Indications for aspiration of liver abscesses are (1) the need to rule out a pyogenic abscess, particularly in patients with multiple lesions; (2) the failure to respond clinically in 3 to 5 days; (3) the threat of imminent rupture; and (4) the prevention of rupture of left-lobe abscesses into the pericardium. There is no evidence that aspiration, even of large abscesses (up to 10 cm), accelerates healing. Percutaneous drainage may be successful even if the liver abscess has already ruptured. Surgery should be reserved for instances of bowel perforation and rupture into the pericardium.

PREVENTION Amebic infection is spread by ingestion of food or water contaminated with cysts. Since an asymptomatic carrier may excrete up to 15 million cysts per day, prevention of infection requires adequate sanitation and eradication of cyst carriage. In high-risk areas, infection can be minimized by the avoidance of unpeeled fruits and vegetables and the use of bottled water. Because cysts are resistant to readily attainable levels of chlorine, disinfection by iodination (tetraglycine hydroperiodide) is recommended. There is no effective prophylaxis.

INFECTION WITH FREE-LIVING AMEBAS

EPIDEMIOLOGY Free-living amebas of the genera *Acanthamoeba*, *Naegleria*, and *Balamuthia* are distributed throughout the world and have been isolated from a wide variety of fresh and brackish water, including that from lakes, taps, hot springs, swimming pools, and heating and air-conditioning units, and even from the nasal passages of healthy children. Encystation may protect the protozoa from desiccation and food deprivation. The persistence of *Legionella pneumophila* in water supplies may be attributable in part to chronic infection of free-living amebas, particularly *Naegleria*.

NAEGLERIA INFECTIONS Primary amebic meningoencephalitis caused by *Naegleria fowleri* follows the aspiration of water contaminated with trophozoites or cysts or the inhalation of contaminated dust, leading to invasion of the olfactory neuroepithelium. After an incubation period of 2 to 15 days, severe headache, high fever, nausea, vomiting, and meningismus develop. Photophobia and palsies of the third, fourth, and sixth cranial nerves are common. Rapid progression to seizures and coma may follow, and most patients die within a week. Infection is most common in otherwise-healthy children or young adults, who often report recent swimming in lakes or heated swimming pools.

Diagnosis depends on the detection of motile trophozoites in wet mounts of fresh spinal fluid. Other laboratory findings resemble those for fulminant bacterial meningitis, with elevated intracranial pressure, high white blood cell counts (up to 20,000 cells/μL), and elevated protein concentrations and low glucose levels in cerebrospinal fluid. The diagnosis should be considered in any patient who has purulent meningitis without evidence of bacteria on Gram's staining, antigen detection assay, and culture. The prognosis is uniformly poor. Only a few survivors, treated with high-dose amphotericin B and rifampin, have been reported. Antibodies to *Naegleria* spp. have been detected in normal adults; serologic testing is not useful in the diagnosis of acute infection.

ACANTHAMOEBA INFECTIONS ■ **Granulomatous Amebic Encephalitis** Infection with *Acanthamoeba* species follows a more indolent course and occurs typically in chronically ill or debilitated patients. Risk factors include lymphoproliferative disorders, chemotherapy, glucocorticoid

TABLE 194-2 *Drug Therapy for Amebiasis*	
Drug	Dosage
ASYMPTOMATIC CARRIER (LUMINAL AGENTS)	
Iodoquinol (650-mg tablets)	650 mg tid for 20 days
Paromomycin (250-mg tablets)	500 mg tid for 10 days
ACUTE COLITIS	
Metronidazole (250- or 500-mg tablets) *plus* Luminal agent as above	750 mg PO or IV tid for 5 to 10 days
AMEBIC LIVER ABSCESS	
Metronidazole	750 mg PO or IV tid for 5 to 10 days
Tinidazole[a]	2 g PO
Ornidazole[a] *plus* Luminal agent as above	2 g PO

[a] Not available in the United States.

therapy, lupus erythematosus, and AIDS. Infection usually reaches the central nervous system hematogenously from a primary focus in the sinuses, skin, or lungs. In the central nervous system, the onset is insidious, and the syndrome often mimics a space-occupying lesion. Altered mental status, headache, and stiff neck may be accompanied by focal findings such as cranial nerve palsies, ataxia, and hemiparesis. Cutaneous ulcers or hard nodules containing amebas are frequently detected in AIDS patients with disseminated *Acanthamoeba* infection.

Examination of the cerebrospinal fluid for trophozoites may be diagnostically helpful, but lumbar puncture may be contraindicated because of increased intracerebral pressure. CT frequently reveals cortical and subcortical lesions of decreased density consistent with embolic infarcts. In other patients, multiple enhancing lesions with edema may mimic the computed tomographic appearance of toxoplasmosis. Demonstration of the trophozoites and cysts of *Acanthamoeba* on wet mounts or in biopsy specimens establishes the diagnosis. Culture on nonnutrient agar plates seeded with *Escherichia coli* may also be helpful. Fluorescein-labeled antiserum is available from the Centers for Disease Control and Prevention (CDC) for the detection of protozoa in biopsy specimens. Granulomatous amebic encephalitis in patients with AIDS may have an accelerated course (with survival for only 3 to 40 days) because of the difficulty these individuals have in forming granulomas. Although studies in animals suggest that rifampin may be useful, the infection is almost uniformly fatal.

Keratitis   The incidence of keratitis caused by *Acanthamoeba* has increased in the past 20 years, in part as a result of improved diagnosis. The first of these infections to be recognized were associated with trauma to the eye and exposure to contaminated water. At present, most infections are linked to extended-wear contact lenses. Risk factors include the use of homemade saline, the wearing of lenses while swimming, and inadequate disinfection. Since contact lenses presumably cause microscopic trauma, the early corneal findings may be nonspecific. The first symptoms usually include tearing and the painful sensation of a foreign body. Once infection is established, progression is rapid; the characteristic clinical sign is an annular, paracentral corneal ring representing a corneal abscess. Deeper corneal invasion and loss of vision may follow.

The differential diagnosis includes bacterial, mycobacterial, and herpetic infection. The irregular polygonal cysts of *Acanthamoeba* (Fig. 194-4) may be identified in corneal scrapings or biopsy material, and trophozoites can be grown on special media. Cysts are resistant to available drugs, and the results of medical therapy have been disappointing. Some reports have suggested partial responses to propamidine isethionate eyedrops. Severe infections usually require keratoplasty.

BALAMUTHIA INFECTIONS   *Balamuthia mandrillaris*, a free-living ameba previously referred to as a leptomyxid ameba, is an important etiologic agent of amebic meningoencephalitis in immunocompetent hosts. The course is typically subacute, with focal neurologic signs, fever, sei-

FIGURE 194-4   Double-walled cyst of *Acanthamoeba castellani*, as seen by phase-contrast microscopy. [*From DJ Krogstad et al, in A Balows et al (eds): Manual of Clinical Microbiology, 5th ed. Washington, DC, American Society for Microbiology, 1991.*]

zures, and headaches leading to death within 1 week to several months after onset. Examination of cerebrospinal fluid reveals mononuclear pleocytosis, elevated protein levels, and normal to low glucose concentrations. Multiple hypodense lesions are usually detected with imaging studies. The diagnosis is almost always made post-mortem, and specific identification may require immunofluorescence with antibodies from the CDC to differentiate the trophozoites from *Acanthamoeba*.

FURTHER READING

DENNEY CF et al: Amebic meningoencephalitis caused by *Balamuthia mandrillaris*: Case report and review. Clin Infect Dis 25:1354, 1997

HAQUE R et al: Innate and acquired resistance to amebiasis in Bangladeshi children. J Infect Dis 186:547, 2002

———— et al: Comparison of PCR, isoenzyme analysis, and antigen detection for diagnosis of *Entamoeba histolytica* infection. J Clin Microbiol 36:449, 1998

KUMAR R, LLOYD D: Recent advances in the treatment of *Acanthamoeba* keratitis. Clin Infect Dis 35:434, 2002

MARTINEZ AJ, VISVESVARA GS: Free-living, amphizoic and opportunistic amebas. Brain Pathol 7:583, 1997

PETRI WA et al: The bittersweet interface of parasite and host lectin-carbohydrate interactions during human invasion by the parasite *Entamoeba histolytica*. Annu Rev Microbiol 56:39, 2002

————, SINGH U: Diagnosis and management of amebiasis. Clin Infect Dis 29:1117, 1999

QUE X, REED SL: Cysteine proteinases and the pathogenesis of amebiasis. Clin Microbiol Rev 13:196, 2002

SISON P et al: Disseminated acanthamoeba infection in patients with AIDS: Case reports and review. Clin Infect Dis 20:1207, 1995

STANLEY SL, REED SL: Microbes and microbial toxins: Paradigms for microbial-mucosal interactions. VI. *Entamoeba histolytica*: Parasite-host interactions. Am J Physiol Gastrointest Liver Physiol 280:G1049, 2001

————: Protective immunity to amebiasis: New insights and new challenges. J Infect Dis 184:504, 2001

---

195   MALARIA AND BABESIOSIS: DISEASES CAUSED BY RED BLOOD CELL PARASITES
Nicholas J. White, Joel G. Breman

"Humanity has but three great enemies: Fever, famine and war; of these by far the greatest, by far the most terrible, is fever."

William Osler

MALARIA

Malaria is a protozoan disease transmitted by the bite of infected *Anopheles* mosquitoes. It is the most important of the parasitic diseases of humans, with transmission in 103 countries affecting >1 billion people and causing between 1 and 3 million deaths each year. Malaria

has now been eliminated from North America, Europe, and Russia but, despite enormous control efforts, has resurged in many parts of the tropics. Added to this resurgence are the increasing problems of drug resistance of the parasite and insecticide resistance of the vectors. Occasional local transmission following importation of malaria has occurred recently in several southern and eastern areas of the United States and in Europe, indicating the continual danger to nonmalarious countries. Malaria remains today, as it has been for centuries, a heavy burden on tropical communities, a threat to nonendemic countries, and a danger to travelers.

ETIOLOGY AND PATHOGENESIS Four species of the genus *Plasmodium* cause nearly all malarial infections in humans (although rare infections involve species normally affecting other primates). These are *P. falciparum*, *P. vivax*, *P. ovale*, and *P. malariae* (Table 195-1). Almost all deaths are caused by falciparum malaria. Human infection begins when a female anopheline mosquito inoculates plasmodial *sporozoites* from its salivary gland during a blood meal (Fig. 195-1). These microscopic motile forms of the malarial parasite are carried rapidly via the bloodstream to the liver, where they invade hepatic parenchymal cells and begin a period of asexual reproduction. By this amplification process (known as intrahepatic or preerythrocytic *schizogony* or *merogony*), a single sporozoite eventually may produce 10,000 to >30,000 daughter merozoites. The swollen liver cell eventually bursts, discharging motile *merozoites* into the

TABLE 195-1 Characteristics of Plasmodium Species Infecting Humans[a]

Characteristic	Finding for Indicated Species			
	P. falciparum	*P. vivax*	*P. ovale*	*P. malariae*
Duration of intrahepatic phase (days)	5.5	8	9	15
Number of merozoites released per infected hepatocyte	30,000	10,000	15,000	15,000
Duration of erythrocytic cycle (hours)	48	48	50	72
Red cell preference	Younger cells (but can invade cells of all ages)	Red cells up to 14 days old	Reticulocytes	Older cells
Morphology	Usually only ring forms; banana-shaped gametocytes	Irregularly shaped large rings and trophozoites; enlarged erythrocytes; Schüffner's dots	Infected erythrocytes, enlarged and oval with tufted ends; Schüffner's dots	Band or rectangular forms of trophozoites common
Pigment color	Black	Yellow-brown	Dark brown	Brown-black
Ability to cause relapses	No	Yes	Yes	No

[a] Parasitemias of >2% are suggestive of *P. falciparum* infection.

bloodstream. These then invade the red blood cells (RBCs) and multiply 6- to 20-fold every 48 to 72 h. When the parasites reach densities of ~50/μL of blood, the symptomatic stage of the infection begins. In *P. vivax* and *P. ovale* infections, a proportion of the intrahepatic forms do not divide immediately but remain dormant for a period ranging from 3 weeks to a year or longer before reproduction begins. These dormant forms, or *hypnozoites*, are the cause of the relapses that characterize infection with these two species.

After entry into the bloodstream, merozoites rapidly invade erythrocytes and become *trophozoites*. Attachment is mediated via a specific erythrocyte surface receptor. In the case of *P. vivax*, this receptor is related to the Duffy blood-group antigen Fy^a or Fy^b. Most West Africans and people with origins in that region carry the Duffy-negative FyFy phenotype and are therefore resistant to *P. vivax* malaria. During the early stage of intraerythrocytic development, the small "ring forms" of the four parasitic species appear similar under light microscopy. As the trophozoites enlarge, species-specific characteristics become evident, pigment becomes visible, and the parasite assumes an irregular or ameboid shape. By the end of the 48-h intraerythrocytic life cycle (72 h for *P. malariae*), the parasite has consumed nearly all the hemoglobin and grown to occupy most of the RBC. It is now called a *schizont*. Multiple nuclear divisions have taken place (*shizogony* or *merogony*), and the RBC ruptures to release 6 to 30 daughter merozoites, each potentially capable of invading a new RBC and repeating the cycle. The disease in human beings is caused by the direct effects of RBC invasion and destruction by the asexual parasite and the host's reaction. After a series of asexual cycles (*P. falciparum*) or immediately after release from the liver (*P. vivax*, *P. ovale*, *P. malariae*), some of the parasites develop into morphologically distinct, long-lived sexual forms (*gametocytes*) that can transmit malaria.

After being ingested in the blood meal of a biting female anopheline mosquito, the male and female gametocytes form a zygote in the insect's midgut. This zygote matures into an ookinete, which penetrates and encysts in the mosquito's gut wall. The resulting oocyst expands by asexual division until it bursts to liberate myriad motile sporozoites, which then migrate in the hemolymph to the salivary gland of the mosquito to await inoculation into another human at the next feeding.

EPIDEMIOLOGY Malaria occurs throughout most of the tropical regions of the world (Fig. 195-2). *P. falciparum* predominates in Africa, New Guinea, and Haiti; *P. vivax* is more common in Central America and the Indian subcontinent. The prevalence of these two species is approximately equal in South America, eastern Asia, and Oceania. *P. malariae* is found in most endemic areas, especially throughout sub-Saharan Africa, but is much less common. *P. ovale* is relatively unusual outside of Africa and, where it is found, comprises <1% of isolates.

The epidemiology of malaria is complex and may vary considerably even within relatively small geographic areas. Endemicity tradi-

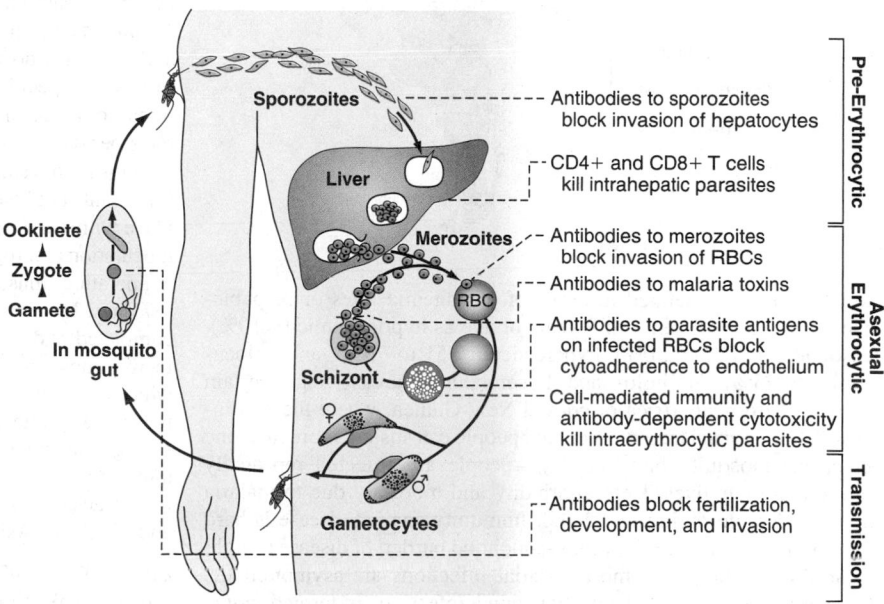

FIGURE 195-1 The malaria transmission cycle from mosquito to human. RBC, red blood cell.

FIGURE 195-2 Malaria-endemic countries in the Americas (*bottom*) and in Africa, the Middle East, Asia, and the South Pacific (*top*), 2002.

Malaria-Endemic Areas
- ⬤ Chloroquine-resistant
- ⬤ Chloroquine-sensitive
- ◯ None

tionally has been defined in terms of parasitemia rates or palpable-spleen rates in children 2 to 9 years of age as hypoendemic (<10%), mesoendemic (11 to 50%), hyperendemic (51 to 75%), and holoendemic (>75%). In holo- and hyperendemic areas—e.g., certain regions of tropical Africa or coastal New Guinea, where there is intense *P. falciparum* transmission and people can sustain more than one infectious mosquito bite per day—people are infected repeatedly throughout their lives. Here, morbidity and mortality due to malaria are considerable during childhood. Immunity against disease is hard won in these areas, and the young-childhood burden of disease is high; by adulthood, however, most malarial infections are asymptomatic. This situation, with frequent year-round infection, is termed *stable transmission*. In areas where transmission is low, erratic, or focal, full

protective immunity is not acquired, and symptomatic disease may occur at all ages. This situation usually exists in hypoendemic areas and is termed *unstable transmission*. Even in areas with stable transmission, there is often an increased incidence of symptomatic malaria coinciding with increased mosquito breeding and transmission during the rainy season. Malaria behaves like an epidemic disease in some areas, particularly those with unstable malaria, such as northern India, Sri Lanka, Southeast Asia, Ethiopia, southern Africa, and Madagascar. An epidemic can develop when there are changes in environmental, economic, or social conditions, such as heavy rains following drought or migrations (usually of refugees or workers) from a nonmalarious region to an area of high transmission; a breakdown in malaria control and prevention services can intensify epidemic conditions. This situation usually results in considerable mortality among all age groups.

The principal determinants of the epidemiology of malaria are the number (density), the human-biting habits, and the longevity of the anopheline mosquito vectors. Not all anophelines can transmit malaria, and those that do vary considerably in their efficiency as malaria vectors. More specifically, the transmission of malaria is directly proportional to the density of the vector, the square of the number of human bites per day per mosquito, and the tenth power of the probability of the mosquito's surviving for 1 day. Mosquito longevity is particularly important, because the portion of the parasite's life cycle that takes place within the mosquito—from gametocyte ingestion to subsequent inoculation (sporogony)—lasts for 8 to 30 days, depending on ambient temperature; thus, to transmit malaria, the mosquito must survive for >7 days. In general, at temperatures <16° to 18°C, sporogony is not completed and transmission does not occur. Therefore, the most effective mosquito vectors of malaria are those such as *A. gambiae*, which are long-lived, occur in high densities in tropical climates, breed readily, and bite humans in preference to other animals. The entomologic inoculation rate—the number of sporozoite-positive mosquito bites per person per year—is the most common measure of malarial transmission and varies from <1 in some parts of Latin America and Southeast Asia to >300 in parts of tropical Africa.

ERYTHROCYTE CHANGES IN MALARIA After invading an erythrocyte, the growing malarial parasite progressively consumes and degrades intracellular proteins, principally hemoglobin. The potentially toxic heme is polymerized to biologically inert hemozoin, or malaria pigment. The parasite also alters the RBC membrane by changing its transport properties, exposing cryptic surface antigens, and inserting new parasite-derived proteins. The RBC becomes more irregular in shape, more antigenic, and less deformable.

In *P. falciparum* infections, membrane protuberances appear on the erythrocyte's surface toward the end of the first 24 h of the asexual cycle. These "knobs" extrude a high-molecular-weight, antigenically variant, strain-specific, adhesive protein (PfEMP1) that mediates attachment to receptors on venular and capillary endothelium—an event termed *cytoadherence*. Several vascular receptors have been identified, of which intercellular adhesion molecule 1 is probably the most important in the brain, chondroitin sulfate B in the placenta, and CD36 in most other organs. Thus the infected erythrocytes stick inside the small blood vessels. At the same stage, these *P. falciparum*–infected RBCs may also adhere to uninfected RBCs to form rosettes and to other parasitized erythrocytes (agglutination). The processes of cytoadherence, rosetting, and agglutination are central to the pathogenesis of falciparum malaria. They result in the sequestration of RBCs containing mature forms of the parasite in vital organs (particularly the brain), where they interfere with microcirculatory flow and metabolism. Sequestered parasites continue to develop out of reach of the principal host defense mechanism: splenic processing and filtration. As a consequence, only the younger ring forms of the asexual parasites are seen circulating in the peripheral blood in falciparum malaria, and the level of peripheral parasitemia underestimates the true number of parasites within the body. Severe malaria is also associated with reduced deformability of the uninfected erythrocytes, which compromises their passage through the partially obstructed capillaries and venules and shortens RBC survival.

In the other three ("benign") malarias, sequestration does not occur, and all stages of the parasite's development are evident on peripheral blood smears. Whereas *P. vivax*, *P. ovale*, and *P. malariae* show a marked predilection for either young RBCs (*P. vivax*, *P. ovale*) or old cells (*P. malariae*) and produce a level of parasitemia seldom >2%, *P. falciparum* can invade erythrocytes of all ages and may be associated with very high levels of parasitemia.

HOST RESPONSE   Initially, the host responds to plasmodial infection by activating nonspecific defense mechanisms. Splenic immunologic and filtrative clearance functions are augmented in malaria, and the removal of both parasitized and uninfected erythrocytes is accelerated. The parasitized cells escaping splenic removal are destroyed when the schizont ruptures. The material released induces the activation of macrophages and the release of proinflammatory mononuclear cell–derived cytokines, which cause fever and exert other pathologic effects. Temperatures of ≥40°C damage mature parasites; in untreated infections, the effect of such temperatures is to further synchronize the parasitic cycle, with eventual production of the regular fever spikes and rigors that originally served to characterize the different malarias. These regular fever patterns (tertian, every 2 days; quartan, every 3 days) are seldom seen today in patients who receive prompt and effective antimalarial treatment.

The geographic distributions of sickle cell disease, thalassemia, and glucose-6-phosphate dehydrogenase (G6PD) deficiency closely resemble that of malaria before the introduction of control measures. This observation suggests that these genetic disorders confer protection against death from falciparum malaria. For example, HbA/S heterozygotes (sickle cell trait) have a sixfold reduction in the risk of dying from severe falciparum malaria. This decrease in risk appears to be related to impaired parasite growth at low oxygen tensions. Parasite multiplication in HbA/E heterozygotes is reduced at high parasite densities. In Melanesia, children with α-thalassemia appear to have more frequent malaria (both vivax and falciparum) in the early years of life, and this pattern of infection appears to protect against severe disease. In Melanesian ovalocytosis, rigid erythrocytes resist merozoite invasion, and the intraerythrocytic milieu is hostile.

The specific immune response to malaria eventually controls the infection and, with exposure to sufficient strains, confers protection from high-level parasitemia and disease but not from infection. As a result of this state of infection without illness (*premunition*), asymptomatic parasitemia is common among adults and older children living in regions with stable and intense transmission (i.e., holo- or hyperendemic areas). Immunity is mainly specific for both the species and the strain of infecting malarial parasite. Both humoral immunity and cellular immunity are necessary for protection, but the mechanisms of each are incompletely understood (Fig. 195-1). Immune individuals have a polyclonal increase in serum levels of IgM, IgG, and IgA, although much of this antibody is unrelated to protection. Antibodies to a variety of parasitic antigens presumably act in concert to limit in vivo replication of the parasite. In the case of falciparum malaria, the most important of these antigens is the variant protein PfEMP1 mentioned above. Passively transferred IgG from immune adults has been shown to reduce levels of parasitemia in children, and passive transfer of maternal antibody contributes to the relative protection of infants from severe malaria in the first months of life. This complex immunity to disease declines when a person lives outside an endemic area for several months or longer.

Several factors retard the development of cellular immunity to malaria. These factors include the absence of major histocompatibility antigens on the surface of infected RBCs, which precludes direct T cell recognition; malaria antigen–specific immune unresponsiveness; and the enormous strain diversity of malarial parasites along with the ability of the parasites to express variant immunodominant antigens on the erythrocyte surface that change during the period of infection. Strain diversity also has an impact on the heterogeneity of the humoral antibody response. Immunity to all strains is never achieved. Parasites may persist in the blood for months (or, in the case of *P. malariae*, for many years) if treatment is not given. The complexity of the immune response in malaria, the sophistication of the parasites' evasion mechanisms, and the lack of a good in vitro correlate with clinical immunity have all slowed progress toward an effective vaccine.

CLINICAL FEATURES   Malaria is a very common cause of fever in tropical countries. The first symptoms of malaria are nonspecific; the lack of a sense of well-being, headache, fatigue, abdominal discomfort, and muscle aches followed by fever are all similar to the symptoms of a minor viral illness. In some instances, a prominence of headache, chest pain, abdominal pain, arthralgia, myalgia, or diarrhea may suggest another diagnosis. Although headache may be severe in malaria, there is no neck stiffness or photophobia resembling that in meningitis. While myalgia may be prominent, it is not usually as severe as in dengue fever, and the muscles are not tender as in leptospirosis or typhus. Nausea, vomiting, and orthostatic hypotension are common. The classic malarial paroxysms, in which fever spikes, chills, and rigors occur at regular intervals, are relatively unusual and suggest infection with *P. vivax* or *P. ovale*. The fever is irregular at first (that of falciparum malaria may never become regular); the temperature of nonimmune individuals and children often rises above 40°C in conjunction with tachycardia and sometimes delirium. Although childhood febrile convulsions may occur with any of the malarias, generalized seizures are specifically associated with falciparum malaria and may herald the development of cerebral disease. Many clinical abnormalities have been described in acute malaria, but most patients with uncomplicated infections have few abnormal physical findings other than fever, malaise, mild anemia, and (in some cases) a palpable spleen. Anemia is quite common among young children living in areas with stable transmission, particularly where there is parasite resistance to chloroquine or other drugs. Splenic enlargement is very common among otherwise-healthy individuals in malaria-endemic areas and reflects repeated infections; however, in nonimmune individuals with malaria, the spleen takes several days to become palpable. Slight enlargement of the liver is also common, particularly among young children. Mild jaundice is common among adults; it may develop in patients with otherwise-uncomplicated falciparum malaria and usually resolves over 1 to 3 weeks. Malaria is not associated with a rash like those seen in meningococcal septicemia, typhus, enteric fever, viral exanthems, and drug reactions. Petechial hemorrhages in the skin or mucous membranes—features of viral hemorrhagic fevers and leptospirosis—develop only rarely in severe falciparum malaria.

Severe Falciparum Malaria Appropriately treated, uncomplicated falciparum malaria carries a mortality rate of ~0.1%. However, once vital-organ dysfunction occurs or the proportion of erythrocytes infected increases to >3%, mortality rises steeply. The major manifestations of severe falciparum malaria are shown in Table 195-2, and features indicating a poor prognosis are listed in Table 195-3.

CEREBRAL MALARIA Coma is a characteristic and ominous feature of falciparum malaria and, despite treatment, is associated with death rates of ~20% among adults and 15% among children. Lesser degrees of obtundation, delirium, and abnormal behavior should also be taken very seriously. The onset may be gradual or sudden following a convulsion.

Cerebral malaria manifests as diffuse symmetric encephalopathy; focal neurologic signs are unusual. Although some passive resistance to head flexion may be detected, signs of meningeal irritation are lack-

TABLE 195-2 *Manifestations of Severe Falciparum Malaria*

Signs	Manifestations
Major	
Unarousable coma/ cerebral malaria	Failure to localize or respond appropriately to noxious stimuli; coma persisting for >30 min after generalized convulsion
Acidemia/acidosis	Arterial pH <7.25 or plasma bicarbonate level of <15 mmol/L; venous lactate level of >5 mmol/L manifests as labored deep breathing, often termed "respiratory distress"
Severe normochromic, normocytic anemia	Hematocrit of <15% or hemoglobin level of <50 g/L (<5 g/dL) with parasitemia of >100,000/μL
Renal failure	Urine output (24 h) of <400 mL in adults or <12 mL/kg in children; no improvement with rehydration; serum creatinine level of >265 μmol/L (>3.0 mg/dL)
Pulmonary edema/ adult respiratory distress syndrome	Noncardiogenic pulmonary edema, often aggravated by overhydration
Hypoglycemia	Plasma glucose level of <2.2 mmol/L (<40 mg/dL)
Hypotension/shock	Systolic blood pressure of <50 mmHg in children 1–5 years or <80 mmHg in adults; core/skin temperature difference of >10°C
Bleeding/ disseminated intravascular coagulation	Significant bleeding and hemorrhage from the gums, nose, and gastrointestinal tract and/or evidence of disseminated intravascular coagulation
Convulsions	More than two generalized seizures in 24 h
Hemoglobinuria[a]	Macroscopic black, brown, or red urine; not associated with effects of oxidant drugs and red blood cell enzyme defects (such as G6PD deficiency)
Other	
Impaired consciousness	Obtunded but arousable
Extreme weakness	Prostration; inability to sit unaided[b]
Hyperparasitemia	Parasitemia level of >5% in nonimmune patients (>20% in any patient)
Jaundice	Serum bilirubin level of >50 mmol/L (>3.0 mg/dL) if combined with other evidence of vital-organ dysfunction

[a] Hemoglobinuria may occur in uncomplicated malaria.
[b] In a child who is normally able to sit.
Note: G6PD, glucose-6-phosphate dehydrogenase.

TABLE 195-3 *Features Indicating a Poor Prognosis in Severe Falciparum Malaria*

Clinical
  Marked agitation
  Hyperventilation (respiratory distress)
  Hypothermia (<36.5°C)
  Bleeding
  Deep coma
  Repeated convulsions
  Anuria
  Shock
Laboratory
  Biochemistry
    Hypoglycemia (<2.2 mmol/L)
    Hyperlactatemia (>5 mmol/L)
    Acidosis (arterial pH <7.3, serum HCO₃ <15 mmol/L)
    Elevated serum creatinine (>265 μmol/L)
    Elevated total bilirubin (>50 μmol/L)
    Elevated liver enzymes (AST/ALT 3 times upper limit of normal, 5-nucleotidase ↑)
    Elevated muscle enzymes (CPK ↑, myoglobin ↑)
    Elevated urate (>600 μmol/L)
  Hematology
    Leukocytosis (>12,000/μL)
    Severe anemia (PCV <15%)
    Coagulopathy
      Decreased platelet count (<50,000/μL)
      Prolonged prothrombin time (>3 s)
      Prolonged partial thromboplastin time
      Decreased fibrinogen (<200 mg/dL)
  Parasitology
    Hyperparasitemia
      Increased mortality at >100,000/μL
      High mortality at >500,000/μL
      >20% of parasites identified as pigment-containing trophozoites and schizonts
      >5% of neutrophils with visible pigment

Note: ALT, alanine aminotransferase; AST, aspartate aminotransferase; CPK, creatine phosphokinase; PCV, packed cell volume.

ing. The eyes may be divergent and a pout reflex is common, but other primitive reflexes are usually absent. The corneal reflexes are preserved except in deep coma. Muscle tone may be either increased or decreased. The tendon reflexes are variable, and the plantar reflexes may be flexor or extensor; the abdominal and cremasteric reflexes are absent. Flexor or extensor posturing may be documented. Approximately 15% of patients have retinal hemorrhages; with pupillary dilatation and indirect ophthalmoscopy, this figure increases to 30 to 40%. Other funduscopic abnormalities include discrete spots of retinal opacification (30 to 60%), papilledema (8% among children, rare among adults), cotton wool spots (<5%), and decolorization of a retinal vessel or segment of vessel (occasional cases). Convulsions, usually generalized and often repeated, occur in up to 50% of children with cerebral malaria. More covert seizure activity is also common, particularly among children, and may manifest as repetitive tonic-clonic eye movements. Whereas adults rarely (i.e., in <3% of cases) suffer neurologic sequelae, ~15% of children surviving cerebral malaria—especially those with hypoglycemia, severe anemia, repeated seizures, and deep coma—have some residual neurologic deficit when they regain consciousness; hemiplegia, cerebral palsy, cortical blindness, deafness, and impaired cognition and learning—all of varying duration—have been reported.

HYPOGLYCEMIA An important and common complication of severe malaria, hypoglycemia is associated with a poor prognosis and is particularly problematic in children and pregnant women. Hypoglycemia in malaria results from a failure of hepatic gluconeogenesis and an increase in the consumption of glucose by both host and—to a lesser extent—the malaria parasites. To compound the situation, quinine and quinidine—drugs commonly used for the treatment of severe chloroquine-resistant malaria—are powerful stimulants of pancreatic insulin secretion. Hyperinsulinemic hypoglycemia is especially troublesome in pregnant women receiving quinine treatment. In severe disease, the clinical diagnosis of hypoglycemia is difficult: the usual physical signs (sweating, gooseflesh, tachycardia) are absent, and the neurologic impairment caused by hypoglycemia cannot be distinguished from that caused by malaria.

LACTIC ACIDOSIS Lactic acidosis commonly coexists with hypoglycemia and is an important contributor to death from severe malaria. In adults, coexisting renal impairment often compounds the acidosis; in children, ketoacidosis may also contribute. Acidotic breathing, sometimes called respiratory distress, is a sign of poor prognosis. It is often followed by circulatory failure refractory to volume expansion or inotropic drugs or by respiratory arrest. The plasma concentrations of bicarbonate or lactate are the best biochemical prognosticators in severe malaria. Lactic acidosis is caused by the combination of anaerobic glycolysis in tissues where sequestered parasites interfere with microcirculatory flow, hypovolemia, lactate production by the parasites, and a failure of hepatic and renal lactate clearance. The prognosis of severe lactic acidosis is poor.

NONCARDIOGENIC PULMONARY EDEMA Adults with severe falciparum malaria may develop noncardiogenic pulmonary edema even after several days of antimalarial therapy. The pathogenesis of this variant of the adult respiratory distress syndrome is unclear. The mortality rate is >80%. This condition can be aggravated by overly vigorous administration of intravenous fluid. Noncardiogenic pulmonary edema can also develop in otherwise uncomplicated vivax malaria, where recovery is usual.

RENAL IMPAIRMENT Renal impairment is common among adults with severe falciparum malaria but rare among children. The pathogenesis of renal failure is unclear but may be related to erythrocyte sequestration interfering with renal microcirculatory flow and metabolism. Clinically and pathologically, this syndrome manifests as acute tubular necrosis, although renal cortical necrosis never develops. Acute renal failure may occur simultaneously with other vital-organ dysfunction (in which case mortality is high) or may progress as other disease manifestations resolve. In survivors, urine flow resumes in a median of 4 days, and serum creatinine levels return to normal in a mean of 17 days (Chap. 260). Early dialysis or hemofiltration considerably enhances the likelihood of a patient's survival, particularly in acute hypercatabolic renal failure.

HEMATOLOGIC ABNORMALITIES Anemia results from accelerated RBC destruction and removal by the spleen in conjunction with ineffective erythropoiesis. In severe malaria, both infected and uninfected RBCs show reduced deformability, which correlates with prognosis and development of anemia. Splenic clearance of RBCs is increased. In nonimmune individuals and in areas with unstable transmission, anemia can develop rapidly and transfusion is often required. As a consequence of repeated malarial infections, children in many areas of Africa may develop severe anemia resulting from both shortened RBC survival and masked dyserythropoiesis. Anemia is a common consequence of antimalarial drug resistance, which results in repeated or continued infection.

Slight coagulation abnormalities are common in falciparum malaria, and mild thrombocytopenia is usual. As mentioned above, <5% of patients with severe malaria have significant bleeding with evidence of disseminated intravascular coagulation. Hematemesis from stress ulceration or acute gastric erosions may also occur.

LIVER DYSFUNCTION Mild hemolytic jaundice is common in malaria. Severe jaundice is associated with *P. falciparum* infections, is more common among adults than among children, and results from hemolysis, hepatocyte injury, and cholestasis. When accompanied by other vital-organ dysfunction (often renal impairment), liver dysfunction carries a poor prognosis. Hepatic dysfunction contributes to hypoglycemia, lactic acidosis, and impaired drug metabolism. Occasional patients with falciparum malaria may develop deep jaundice (with hemolytic, hepatitic, and cholestatic components) without evidence of other vital-organ dysfunction.

TABLE 195-4 *Relative Incidence of Severe Complications of Falciparum Malaria*

Complication	Nonpregnant Adults	Pregnant Women	Children
Anemia	+	+ +	+ + +
Convulsions	+	+	+ + +
Hypoglycemia	+	+ + +	+ + +
Jaundice	+ + +	+ + +	+
Renal failure	+ + +	+ + +	−
Pulmonary edema	+ +	+ + +	+

Key: −, rare; +, infrequent; + +, frequent; + + +, very frequent.

OTHER COMPLICATIONS Aspiration pneumonia following convulsions is an important cause of death in cerebral malaria. Chest infections and catheter-induced urinary tract infections are common among patients who are unconscious for >3 days. Septicemia may complicate severe malaria, particularly in children; in endemic areas, *Salmonella* bacteremia has been associated specifically with *P. falciparum* infections. The frequency of complications of severe falciparum malaria is summarized in Table 195-4.

Malaria in Pregnancy In hyper- and holoendemic areas, falciparum malaria in primi- and secundigravid women is associated with low birth weight (average reduction, ~170 g) and consequently increased infant and childhood mortality. In general, infected mothers in areas of stable transmission remain asymptomatic despite intense accumulation of parasitized erythrocytes in the placental microcirculation. Maternal HIV infection predisposes pregnant women to malaria and predisposes their newborns to congenital malaria infection and low birth weight.

In areas with unstable transmission of malaria, pregnant women are prone to severe infections and are particularly vulnerable to high-level parasitemia with anemia, hypoglycemia, and acute pulmonary edema. Fetal distress, premature labor, and stillbirth or low birth weight are common results. Fetal death is usual in severe malaria. Congenital malaria occurs in <5% of newborns whose mothers are infected and is related directly to the parasite density in maternal blood and in the placenta. *P. vivax* malaria in pregnancy is also associated with a reduction in birth weight (average, 100 g), but, in contrast to the situation in falciparum malaria, this effect is more pronounced in multigravid than in primigravid women.

Malaria in Children Most of the estimated 1 to 3 million persons who die of falciparum malaria each year are young African children. Convulsions, coma, hypoglycemia, metabolic acidosis, and severe anemia are relatively common among children with severe malaria, whereas deep jaundice, acute renal failure, and acute pulmonary edema are unusual. Severely anemic children may present with labored deep breathing, which in the past has been attributed incorrectly to "anemic congestive cardiac failure" but in fact is usually caused by metabolic acidosis, often compounded by hypovolemia. In general, children tolerate antimalarial drugs well and respond rapidly to treatment.

Transfusion Malaria Malaria can be transmitted by blood transfusion, needle-stick injury, sharing of needles by infected drug addicts, or organ transplantation. The incubation period in these settings is often short because there is no preerythrocytic stage of development. The clinical features and management of these cases are the same as for naturally acquired infections. Radical chemotherapy with primaquine is unnecessary for transfusion-transmitted *P. vivax* and *P. ovale* infections.

CHRONIC COMPLICATIONS OF MALARIA ■ **Tropical Splenomegaly (Hyperreactive Malarial Splenomegaly)** Chronic or repeated malarial infections produce hypergammaglobulinemia; normochromic, normocytic anemia; and, in certain situations, splenomegaly. Some residents of malaria-endemic areas in tropical Africa and Asia exhibit an abnormal immunologic response to repeated infections that is characterized by massive splenomegaly, hepatomegaly, marked elevations in serum titers of IgM and malarial antibody, hepatic sinusoidal lymphocytosis, and (in Af-

FIGURE 195-3 Thin blood films of *Plasmodium falciparum*. *A.* Young trophozoites. *B.* Old trophozoites. *C.* Pigment in polymorphonuclear cells and trophozoites. *D.* Mature schizonts. *E.* Female gametocytes. *F.* Male gametocytes. (*Reproduced from Benchaids for the Diagnosis of Malaria Infections, 2d ed, with the permission of the World Health Organization.*)

rica) peripheral B cell lymphocytosis. This syndrome has been associated with the production of cytotoxic IgM antibodies to CD8+ T lymphocytes, antibodies to CD5+ T lymphocytes, and an increase in the ratio of CD4+ T cells to CD8+ T cells. These events may lead to uninhibited B cell production of IgM and the formation of cryoglob-

FIGURE 195-4 Thin blood films of *Plasmodium vivax*. *A.* Young trophozoites. *B.* Old trophozoites. *C.* Mature schizonts. *D.* Female gametocytes. *E.* Male gametocytes. (*Reproduced from Benchaids for the Diagnosis of Malaria Infections, 2d ed, with the permission of the World Health Organization.*)

ulins (IgM aggregates and immune complexes). This immunologic process stimulates reticuloendothelial hyperplasia and clearance activity and eventually produces splenomegaly. Patients with hyperreactive malarial splenomegaly (HMS) present with an abdominal mass or a dragging sensation in the abdomen and occasional sharp abdominal pains suggesting perisplenitis. Anemia and some degree of pancytopenia are usually evident, but in many cases malarial parasites cannot be found in peripheral-blood smears. Vulnerability to respiratory and skin infections is increased; many patients die of overwhelming sepsis. Persons with HMS who are living in endemic areas should receive antimalarial chemoprophylaxis: the results are usually good. In nonendemic areas, antimalarial treatment is advised. In some cases refractory to therapy, clonal lymphoproliferation may develop and then evolve into a malignant lymphoproliferative disorder.

Quartan Malarial Nephropathy Chronic or repeated infections with *P. malariae* (and possibly with other malarial species) may cause soluble immune-complex injury to the renal glomeruli, resulting in the nephrotic syndrome. Other, unidentified factors must contribute to this process since only a very small proportion of infected patients develop renal disease. The histologic appearance is that of focal or segmental glomerulonephritis with splitting of the capillary basement membrane. Subendothelial dense deposits are seen on electron microscopy, and immunofluorescence reveals deposits of complement and immunoglobulins; in samples of renal tissue from children, *P. malariae* antigens are often visible. A coarse-granular pattern of basement-membrane immunofluorescent deposits (predominantly IgG3) with selective proteinuria carries a better prognosis than a fine-granular, predominantly IgG2 pattern with nonselective proteinuria. Quartan nephropathy usually responds poorly to treatment with either antimalarial agents or glucocorticoids and cytotoxic drugs.

Burkitt's Lymphoma and Epstein-Barr Virus Infection It is possible that malaria-related immunosuppression provokes infection with lymphoma viruses. Burkitt's lymphoma is strongly associated with Epstein-Barr virus. The prevalence of this childhood tumor is high in malarious areas of Africa.

DIAGNOSIS ■ **Demonstration of the Parasite**
The diagnosis of malaria rests on the demonstration of asexual forms of the parasite in stained peripheral-blood smears. After a negative blood smear, repeat smears should be made if there is a high degree of suspicion. Of the Romanowsky stains, Giemsa at pH 7.2 is preferred; Wright's, Field's, or Leishman's stain can also be used. Both thin (Fig. 195-3 through Fig. 195-6) and thick (Fig. 195-7 through Fig. 195-10) blood smears should be examined.

The thin blood smear should be rapidly

FIGURE 195-5   Thin blood films of *Plasmodium ovale*. *A.* Old trophozoites. *B.* Mature schizonts. *C.* Male gametocytes. *D.* Female gametocytes. *(Reproduced from Benchaids for the Diagnosis of Malaria Infections, 2d ed, with the permission of the World Health Organization.)*

FIGURE 195-6   Thin blood films of *Plasmodium malariae*. *A.* Old trophozoites. *B.* Mature schizonts. *C.* Male gametocytes. *D.* Female gametocytes. *(Reproduced from Benchaids for the Diagnosis of Malaria Infections, 2d ed, with the permission of the World Health Organization.)*

air-dried, fixed in anhydrous methanol, and stained, and the RBCs in the tail of the film should then be examined under oil immersion ($\times 1000$ magnification). The level of parasitemia is expressed as the number of parasitized erythrocytes per 1000 RBCs, or per 200 white blood cells (WBCs), and this figure is converted to the number of parasitized erythrocytes per microliter. In high-transmission areas, the presence of up to 10,000 parasites per microliter of blood may be tolerated without symptoms or signs in partially immune individuals. Rapid, simple, sensitive, and specific antibody-based diagnostic stick or card tests that detect *P. falciparum*–specific, histidine-rich protein 2 (PfHRP2) or lactate dehydrogenase antigens in finger-prick blood samples have been introduced (Table 195-5). Some of these tests carry a second antibody, which allows falciparum malaria to be distinguished from the less dangerous malarias. PfHRP2-based tests may remain positive for several weeks after acute infection. This feature is a disadvantage in high-transmission areas where infections are frequent but is of value in the diagnosis of severe malaria in patients who have taken antimalarial drugs and cleared peripheral parasitemia (but in whom the PfHRP2 test remains strongly positive) or where malaria is alleged to have been eliminated. The relationship between parasitemia and prognosis is complex; in general, patients with $>10^5$ parasites per microliter are at increased risk of dying, but nonimmune patients may die with much lower counts, and semi-immune persons may tolerate parasitemia levels many times higher with only minor symptoms. In severe malaria, a poor prognosis is indicated by a predominance of more mature *P. falciparum* parasites (i.e., >20% of parasites with visible pigment) in the peripheral blood film or by the presence of phagocytosed malarial pigment in >5% of neutrophils. In *P. falciparum* infections, gametocytemia peaks 1 week after the peak of asexual parasites. Because the mature gametocytes of *P. falciparum* are not affected by most antimalarial drugs, their persistence does not constitute evidence of drug resistance.

The thick blood film should be of uneven thickness. The smear should be dried thoroughly and stained without fixing. As many layers

of erythrocytes overlie one another and are lysed during the staining procedure, the thick film has the advantage of concentrating the parasites (by 20- to 40-fold compared with a thin blood film) and thus increasing diagnostic sensitivity. Both parasites and WBCs are counted, and the number of parasites per unit volume is calculated from the total leukocyte count. Alternatively, a WBC count of 8000/ μL is assumed. A minimum of 200 WBCs should be counted under oil immersion. Interpretation of blood smear films requires some experience because artifacts are common. Before a thick smear is judged to be negative, 100 to 200 fields should be examined under oil immersion. Phagocytosed malarial pigment is sometimes seen inside peripheral-blood monocytes or polymorphonuclear leukocytes and may provide a clue to recent infection if malaria parasites are not detectable. After the clearance of the parasites, this intraphagocytic malarial pigment is often evident for several days in the peripheral blood or for longer in bone marrow aspirates or smears of fluid expressed after

FIGURE 195-7   Thick blood films of *Plasmodium falciparum*. *A.* Trophozoites. *B.* Gametocytes. *(Reproduced from Benchaids for the Diagnosis of Malaria Infections, 2d ed, with the permission of the World Health Organization.)*

FIGURE 195-8 Thick blood films of *Plasmodium vivax.* A. Trophozoites. B. Schizonts. C. Gametocytes. (*Reproduced from Benchaids for the Diagnosis of Malaria Infections, 2d ed, with the permission of the World Health Organization.*)

FIGURE 195-9 Thick blood films of *Plasmodium ovale.* A. Trophozoites. B. Schizonts. C. Gametocytes. (*Reproduced from Benchaids for the Diagnosis of Malaria Infections, 2d ed, with the permission of the World Health Organization.*)

FIGURE 195-10 Thick blood films of *Plasmodium malariae.* A. Trophozoites. B. Schizonts. C. Gametocytes. (*Reproduced from Benchaids for the Diagnosis of Malaria Infections, 2d ed, with the permission of the World Health Organization.*)

℞ TREATMENT (Table 195-6)

When a patient in or from a malarious area presents with fever, thick and thin blood smears should be prepared and examined immediately to confirm the diagnosis and identify the species of infecting parasite (Figs. 195-3 through 195-10). Repeat blood smears should be performed at least every 12 to 24 h for 2 days if the first smears are negative. Alternatively, a rapid antigen detection card or stick test should be performed. Patients with severe malaria or those unable to take oral drugs should receive parenteral antimalarial therapy. If there is any doubt about the resistance status of the infecting organism, it should be considered resistant. Antimalarial susceptibility testing can be performed but is not generally available and yields results too slowly to influence choice of treatment. Several drugs are available for oral treatment, and the choice of drug depends on the likely sensitivity of the infecting parasites. Despite recent evidence of chloroquine resistance in *P. vivax* (from parts of Indonesia, Oceania, and Central and South America), chloroquine remains the treatment of choice for the "benign" human malarias (*P. vivax, P. ovale, P. malariae*). Characteristics of various antimalarial agents are shown in Table 195-7, and drug regimens approved by the U.S. Food and Drug Administration are detailed in Table 195-6. The availability of antimalarial drugs varies considerably between countries. Many of the drugs used to treat malaria in endemic areas are not available in temperate countries such as the United States. Fake or adulterated drugs, including antimalarial agents, are being sold in many low-income countries; thus careful attention is required at purchase, especially when the patient fails to respond as expected.

intradermal puncture. Staining of parasites with the fluorescent dye acridine orange allows more rapid diagnosis of malaria (but not speciation of the infection) in patients with low-level parasitemia.

Laboratory Findings Normochromic, normocytic anemia is usual. The leukocyte count is generally normal, although it may be raised in very severe infections. The erythrocyte sedimentation rate, plasma viscosity, and levels of C-reactive protein and other acute-phase proteins are high. The platelet count is usually reduced to ~$10^5/\mu L$. Severe infections may be accompanied by prolonged prothrombin and partial thromboplastin times and by more severe thrombocytopenia. Levels of antithrombin III are reduced even in mild infection. In uncomplicated malaria, plasma concentrations of electrolytes, blood urea nitrogen (BUN), and creatinine are usually normal. Findings in severe malaria may include metabolic acidosis, with low plasma concentrations of glucose, sodium, bicarbonate, calcium, phosphate, and albumin together with elevations in lactate, blood urea nitrogen, creatinine, urate, muscle and liver enzymes, and conjugated and unconjugated bilirubin. Hypergammaglobulinemia is usual in immune and semi-immune subjects. Urinalysis generally gives normal results. In adults and children with cerebral malaria, the mean opening pressure at lumbar puncture is ~160 mm of cerebrospinal fluid (CSF); usually the CSF is normal or has a slightly elevated total protein level [<1.0 g/L (<100 mg/dL)] and cell count (<20/μL).

Severe Malaria Because of resistance, chloroquine can no longer be relied upon in most countries for the treatment of severe malaria. The antiarrhythmic quinidine gluconate is as effective as quinine and, as it is more readily available, has replaced quinine for the treatment of malaria in the United States. The administration of quinidine must be closely monitored if dysrrhythmias and hypotension are to be avoided. Total plasma levels >8 μg/mL, a QT_c interval >0.6 s, or QRS widening beyond 25% of baseline are indications for slowing infusion rates. If arrhythmia or saline-unresponsive hypotension develops, treatment with this drug should be discontinued. Quinine is safer than quinidine; cardiovascular monitoring is not required except when the recipient has cardiac disease. Quinine is the most widely used drug for the treatment of severe malaria worldwide. In some areas, the Chinese drugs derived from artemisinin (artemether and artesunate) have become first-line treatments for severe malaria. These agents are rapidly effective against multidrug-resistant falciparum malaria and are at least as effective as and considerably safer than quinine or quinidine. Artesunate, a water-soluble derivative, can be given by intravenous or intramuscular injection or in a rectal formulation for use primarily in the rural tropics. Artemether and the closely related drug arteether are oil-based formulations given by intramuscular injection. They are not yet available in the United States.

Severe falciparum malaria constitutes a medical emergency re-

TABLE 195-5 *Methods for the Diagnosis of Malaria[a]*

Method	Procedure	Advantages	Disadvantages
Thick blood film[b]	Blood should be uneven in thickness but sufficiently thin to read watch hands through part of the spot. Stain dried, unfixed blood spot with Giemsa, Field's, or other Romanowsky stain. Count number of asexual parasites per 200 WBCs (or per 500 at low densities). Count gametocytes separately.[c]	Sensitive (0.001% parasitemia); species specific; inexpensive	Requires experience (artifacts may be misinterpreted as low-level parasitemia); underestimates true count
Thin blood film[d]	Stain fixed smear with Giemsa, Field's, or other Romanowsky stain. Count number of RBCs containing asexual parasites per 1000 RBCs. In severe malaria, assess stage of parasite development and count neutrophils containing malaria pigment.[e] Count gametocytes separately.[c]	Rapid; species specific; inexpensive; in severe malaria, provides prognostic information[e]	Insensitive (>0.05% parasitemia); uneven distribution of *P. vivax*, as enlarged infected red cells concentrate at leading edge
PfHRP2 dipstick or card test	A drop of blood is placed on the stick or card, which is then immersed in washing solutions. Monoclonal antibody captures the parasite antigen and reads out as a colored band.	Rapid; sensitivity similar to or slightly lower than that of thick films (~0.001% parasitemia)	Detects only *Plasmodium falciparum*; remains positive for weeks after infection[f]; does not quantitate *P. falciparum* parasitemia
Plasmodium LDH dipstick or card test	A drop of blood is placed on the stick or card, which is then immersed in washing solutions. Monoclonal antibodies capture the parasites and read out as colored bands. One band is genus specific (all malarias), and the other is specific for *P. falciparum*.	Rapid; sensitivity similar to or slightly lower than that of thick films for *P. falciparum* (~0.001% parasitemia); provides less sensitive diagnosis for other malarias (*P. vivax, P. ovale, P. malariae*) and does not speciate these organisms	Slightly more difficult preparation than PfHRP2 tests; may miss low-level parasitemia with *P. vivax, P. ovale,* and *P. malariae*; does not quantitate *P. falciparum* parasitemia
Microtube concentration methods with acridine orange staining	Blood is collected in a specialized tube containing acridine orange, anticoagulant, and a float. After centrifugation, which concentrates the parasitized cells around the float, fluorescence microscopy is performed.	Sensitivity similar or superior to that of thick films (~0.001% parasitemia); ideal for processing large numbers of samples rapidly	Does not speciate or quantitate; requires fluorescence microscopy

[a] Malaria cannot be diagnosed clinically with accuracy, but treatment should be started on clinical grounds if the laboratory confirmation is likely to be delayed. In areas of the world where malaria is endemic and transmission is high, low-level asymptomatic parasitemia is common in otherwise-healthy people. Thus malaria may not be the cause of a fever, although in this context the presence of >10,000 parasites/µL (~0.2%) *does* indicate that malaria is the cause. Antibody and polymerase chain reaction tests have no role in the diagnosis of malaria.

[b] Asexual parasites/200 WBCs × 40 = parasite count/µL (assumes a WBC count of 8000/µL). See Figs. 195-7 through 195-10.

[c] Gametocytemia may persist for days or weeks after clearance of asexual parasites. Gametocytemia without asexual parasitemia does not indicate active infection.

[d] Parasitized RBCs (%) × hematocrit × 1256 = parasite count/µL. See Figs. 195-3 through 195-6.

[e] The presence of >100,000 parasites/µL (~2%) is associated with an increased risk of severe malaria, but some patients have severe malaria with lower counts. At any level of parasitemia, the finding that >50% of parasites are tiny rings (cytoplasm width less than half of nucleus width) carries a relatively good prognosis. The presence of visible pigment in >20% of parasites or in >5% of polymorphonuclear leukocytes (indicating massive recent schizogony) carries a worse prognosis.

[f] Persistence of PfHRP2 is a disadvantage in high-transmission settings, where many asymptomatic people have positive tests, but can be used to diagnostic advantage in low-transmission settings when a sick patient has received previous unknown treatment (which, in endemic areas, often consists of antimalarial drugs). A positive PfHRP2 test indicates that the illness is falciparum malaria, even if the blood smear is negative.

Note: LDH, lactate dehydrogenase; PfHRP2, *P. falciparum* histidine-rich protein 2; RBCs, red blood cells; WBCs, white blood cells.

quiring intensive nursing care and careful management. The patient should be weighed and, if comatose, placed on his or her side or prone. Frequent evaluation of the patient's condition is essential. Ancillary drugs such as high-dose glucocorticoids, urea, heparin, dextran, desferrioxamine, antibody to tumor necrosis factor α, and high-dose phenobarbital (20 mg/kg) have proved either ineffective or harmful in clinical trials and should not be used. In acute renal failure or severe metabolic acidosis, hemofiltration or hemodialysis should be started as early as possible.

Parenteral antimalarial treatment should be started as soon as possible. An initial loading dose must be given so that therapeutic concentrations are reached as soon as possible. Both quinine and quinidine will cause dangerous hypotension if injected rapidly; when given intravenously, they must be administered carefully by rate-controlled infusion only. The optimal therapeutic range for quinine and quinidine in severe malaria is not known with certainty, but total plasma concentrations of 8 to 15 mg/mL for quinine and 3.5 to 8.0 mg/mL for quinidine are effective and do not cause serious toxicity. The systemic clearance and apparent volume of distribution of these alkaloids are markedly reduced and plasma protein binding is increased in severe malaria, so that the blood concentrations attained with a given dose are higher. If the patient remains seriously ill or in acute renal failure for >2 days, the maintenance doses of quinine or quinidine should be reduced by 30 to 50% to prevent toxic accumulation of the drugs. The initial doses should never be reduced. If one of the artemisinin derivatives or chloroquine is given, dose reductions are unnecessary, even in renal failure. Exchange transfusion should be considered for severely ill patients, although the precise indications for this procedure have not been agreed upon. It has been recommended that—if safe and feasible—exchange should be considered for patients with severe malaria and parasitemia levels of 5 to 15% and is indicated for parasitemia levels of >15%. The role of prophylactic anticonvulsants is uncertain. If respiratory support is not available, then a full loading dose of phenobarbital (20 mg/kg) to prevent convulsions should not be given as it may cause respiratory arrest.

When the patient is unconscious, the blood glucose level should be measured every 4 to 6 h, and values <2.2 mmol/L (40 mg/dL) should mandate treatment with intravenous dextrose. All patients treated with intravenous quinine or quinidine should receive a continuous infusion of 5 to 10% dextrose. The parasite count and hematocrit level should be measured every 6 to 12 h. Anemia develops rapidly; if the hematocrit falls to <20%, then whole blood (preferably fresh) or packed cells should be transfused slowly, with careful attention to circulatory status. Renal function should be checked daily. Children presenting with severe anemia and acidotic breathing are often hypovolemic; in this situation, resuscitation with crystalloids or blood is

TABLE 195-6 *Recommended Therapeutic Doses of Antimalarial Drugs*

Drug	Uncomplicated Malaria (Oral)	Severe Malaria[a] (Parenteral)
Chloroquine[b]	10 mg of base/kg followed by 10 mg/kg at 24 h and 5 mg/kg at 48 h *or* by 5 mg/kg at 12, 24, and 36 h (total dose, 25 mg/kg); for *P. vivax* or *P. ovale*, primaquine (0.25 mg of base/kg per day for 14 days[d]) added for radical cure	10 mg of base/kg by constant-rate infusion over 8 h followed by 15 mg/kg over 24 h *or* by 3.5 mg of base/kg by IM or SC injection every 6 h (total dose, 25 mg/kg)[c]
Amodiaquine[b]	15 mg of base/kg followed by 10 mg/kg per day at 24 and 48 h (total dose, 35 mg/kg)	—
Sulfadoxine/ pyrimethamine[b]	25/1.25 mg/kg, single oral dose (3 tablets for adults)	—
Mefloquine[b]	15 mg/kg followed 8–12 h later by second dose of 10 mg/kg	—
Quinine	10 mg of salt/kg q8h for 7 days combined with tetracycline[e] (4 mg/kg qid) or doxycycline (3 mg/kg once daily) or clindamycin (10 mg/kg bid) for 7 days	20 mg of salt/kg by IV infusion over 4 h[f] followed by 10 mg/kg infused over 2–8 h every 8 h
Quinidine gluconate	—	10 mg of base/kg by constant-rate infusion over 1–2 h followed by 0.02 mg/kg per min, with ECG monitoring[g]
Artesunate	In combination with 25 mg of mefloquine/kg, 12 mg/kg given in divided doses over 3–5 days (e.g., 4 mg/kg for 3 days or 4 mg/kg followed by 2 mg/kg per day for 4 days); if used alone or in combination with clindamycin or doxycycline, give for 7 days (usually 4 mg/kg initially followed by 2 mg/kg daily)	2.4 mg/kg IV or IM stat followed by 1.2 mg/kg at 12 and 24 h and then daily (or 2.4 mg/kg once daily)
Artemether	Same regimen as for artesunate	3.2 mg/kg IM stat followed by 1.6 mg/kg per day
Atovaquone-proguanil (Malarone)	For adults >40 kg, each dose comprises 4 tablets (each tablet containing atovaquone 250 mg and proguanil 100 mg) taken once daily for 3 days with food	—
Artemether-lumefantrine	For adults ≥35 kg, each dose comprises 4 tablets (each tablet containing artemether 20 mg and lumefantrine 120 mg) at 0, 8, 24, 36, 48, and 60 h, taken after food	—

[a] Oral treatment should be substituted for parenteral therapy as soon as the patient can take tablets by mouth.

[b] These drugs should be combined with either artesunate or artemether when used to treat falciparum malaria. Where there is full susceptibility to both drugs, chloroquine or amodiaquine can be combined with sulfadoxine/pyrimethamine.

[c] Chloroquine-resistant *P. falciparum* is now very widespread, so this regimen should not be used unless there is confirmed full susceptibility in the area.

[d] In Oceania and Southeast Asia, the dose should be 0.33 to 0.5 mg of base/kg. This regimen should not be used in patients with severe variants of G6PD deficiency.

[e] Neither tetracycline nor doxycycline should be given to pregnant women or to children <8 years old.

[f] Alternatively, infusion of 7 mg of salt/kg over 30 min can be followed by 10 mg of salt/kg over 4 h.

[g] Some authorities recommend a lower dose of intravenous quinidine: 6.2 mg of base/kg over 1–2 h followed by 0.0125 mg/kg per min.

Note: In severe malaria, quinine or quinidine should be used if there is any doubt about the infecting strain's sensitivity to chloroquine.

Abbreviations: IM, intramuscular; SC, subcutaneous; IV, intravenous; ECG, electrocardiogram; G6PD, glucose-6-phosphate dehydrogenase.

or to children <8 years of age. Oral quinine is extremely bitter and regularly produces cinchonism comprising tinnitus, high-tone deafness, nausea, vomiting, and dysphoria. Compliance is poor with the required 5- to 7-day regimens of this drug. Mefloquine should be given at a total dosage of 25 mg/kg (15 mg/kg followed 8 to 12 h later by 10 mg/kg) and, where available and approved for use, combined with artesunate or artemether (4 mg/kg per day for 3 days). Although significant resistance to mefloquine has been documented in Thailand, Myanmar, Vietnam, and Cambodia (Fig. 195-11), mefloquine is usually effective against multidrug-resistant strains of *P. falciparum* outside these areas. Artemether-lumefantrine and atovaquone-proguanil (Malarone) are recently introduced, well-tolerated antimalarial drugs used in 3-day regimens. They are both highly effective against multidrug-resistant falciparum malaria.

Patients should be monitored for vomiting for 1 h after the administration of any oral antimalarial drug. If there is vomiting, the dose should be repeated. Symptom-based treatment, with tepid sponging and acetaminophen administration, lowers fever and thereby reduces the patient's propensity to vomit these drugs. Minor central nervous system reactions (nausea, dizziness, sleep disturbances) are common. The incidence of serious adverse neuropsychiatric reactions to mefloquine treatment is ~1 in 1000 in Asia but may be as high as 1 in 200 among Africans and Caucasians. All the antimalarial quinolines (chloroquine, mefloquine, and quinine) exacerbate the orthostatic hypotension associated with malaria, and all are tolerated better by children than by adults. Pregnant women, young children, patients unable to tolerate oral therapy, and nonimmune subjects (e.g., travelers) with suspected malaria should be evaluated carefully and hospitalization considered. If there is any doubt as to the identity of the infecting malarial species, treatment for falciparum malaria should be given. A negative blood smear does not rule out malaria; thick blood films should be checked 1 and 2 days later to exclude the diagnosis. Nonimmune subjects receiving treatment for malaria should have daily parasite counts performed until negative thick films indicate clearance of the parasite. If the level of parasitemia does not fall below 25% of the admission value in 48 h or if parasitemia has not cleared by 7 days (and adherence is assured), drug resistance is likely and the regimen should be changed. If treatment failures occur with commonly used antimalarial agents, alternative drugs should be used (Table 195-8).

To eradicate persistent liver stages and prevent relapse (radical treatment), primaquine (0.3 mg of base/kg; 15 mg of base, adult dose) should be given daily for 14 days to patients with *P. vivax* or *P. ovale* infections after laboratory tests for G6PD deficiency have proved negative. A dose of 22.5 to 30 mg for an adult is recommended for infections acquired in Southeast Asia and Oceania. If the patient has a mild variant of G6PD deficiency, primaquine can be given in a dose of 0.6 mg of base/kg (45 mg maximum) once weekly for 8 weeks.

PREVENTING DRUG RESISTANCE In much of the tropics, drug-resistant *P. falciparum* is increasing in distribution, frequency, and intensity.

indicated. Accurate assessment is vital. Management of fluid balance is difficult in severe malaria, particularly in adults, because of the thin dividing line between overhydration (leading to pulmonary edema) and underhydration (contributing to renal impairment). If necessary, pulmonary artery occlusion pressures should be measured and maintained in the low-normal range. As soon as the patient can take fluids, oral therapy should be substituted for parenteral treatment.

Uncomplicated Malaria Infections due to *P. vivax*, *P. malariae*, *P. ovale*, and known sensitive strains of *P. falciparum* should be treated with oral chloroquine (total dose, 25 mg of base/kg). Chloroquine-resistant *P. falciparum* is now widespread. Chloroquine-resistant strains may be sensitive to sulfadoxine/pyrimethamine in some areas. Where there is resistance to the latter combination, either (1) quinine plus tetracycline or doxycycline (or clindamycin) or (2) mefloquine should be used; tetracycline and doxycycline cannot be given to pregnant women

TABLE 195-7 *Properties of Antimalarial Drugs*

Drug(s)	Pharmacokinetic Properties	Antimalarial Activity	Minor Toxicity	Major Toxicity
Quinine, quinidine	Good oral and IM absorption (quinine); Cl and V_d reduced, but plasma protein binding (principally to $\propto 1$ acid glycoprotein) increased (90%) in malaria; quinine $t_{1/2}$: 16 h in malaria, 11 h in healthy persons; quinidine $t_{1/2}$: 13 h in malaria, 8 h in healthy persons	Acts mainly on trophozoite blood stage; kills gametocytes of *P. vivax*, *P. ovale*, and *P. malariae* (but not *P. falciparum*); no action on liver stages	*Common:* "Cinchonism": tinnitus, high-tone hearing loss, nausea, vomiting, dysphoria, postural hypotension; ECG QT_c interval prolongation (quinine usually by <10% but quinidine by up to 25%) *Rare:* Diarrhea, visual disturbance, rashes *Note:* Very bitter taste	*Common:* Hypoglycemia *Rare:* Hypotension, blindness, deafness, cardiac arrhythmias, thrombocytopenia, hemolysis, hemolytic-uremic syndrome, vasculitis, cholestatic hepatitis, neuromuscular paralysis *Note:* Quinidine more cardiotoxic
Chloroquine	Good oral absorption, very rapid IM and SC absorption; complex pharmacokinetics; enormous Cl and V_d (unaffected by malaria); blood concentration profile determined by distribution processes in malaria; $t_{1/2}$: 1–2 months	As for quinine but acts slightly earlier in asexual cycle	*Common:* Nausea, dysphoria, pruritus in dark-skinned patients, postural hypotension *Rare:* Accommodation difficulties, keratopathy, rash *Note:* Bitter taste, well tolerated	*Acute:* Hypotensive shock (parenteral), cardiac arrhythmias, neuropsychiatric reactions *Chronic:* Retinopathy (cumulative dose, >100 g), skeletal and cardiac myopathy
Amodiaquine	Good oral absorption; largely converted to active metabolite desethylamodiaquine	As for chloroquine	Nausea (tastes better than chloroquine)	Agranulocytosis; hepatitis, mainly with prophylactic use
Mefloquine	Adequate oral absorption; no parenteral preparation; $t_{1/2}$: 14–20 days (shorter in malaria)	As for quinine	Nausea, giddiness, dysphoria, fuzzy thinking, sleeplessness, nightmares, sense of dissociation	Neuropsychiatric reactions, convulsions, encephalopathy
Tetracycline, doxycycline[a]	Excellent absorption; $t_{1/2}$: 8 h for tetracycline, 18 h for doxycycline	Weak antimalarial activity; should not be used alone for treatment	Gastrointestinal intolerance, deposition in growing bones and teeth, photosensitivity, moniliasis, benign intracranial hypertension	Renal failure in patients with impaired renal function (tetracycline)
Halofantrine[b]	Highly variable absorption related to fat intake; $t_{1/2}$: 1–3 days (active desbutyl metabolite $t_{1/2}$: 3–7 days)	As for quinine	Diarrhea	Cardiac conduction disturbances; atrioventricular block; ECG QT_c interval prolongation; potentially lethal ventricular tachyarrhythmias
Artemisinin and derivatives (artemether, artesunate)	Good oral absorption, slow and variable absorption of IM artemether; artesunate and artemether biotransformed to active metabolite dihydroartemisinin; all drugs eliminated very rapidly; $t_{1/2}$: <1 h	Broader stage specificity and more rapid than other drugs; no action on liver stages; kills all but fully mature gametocytes of *P. falciparum*	Reduction in reticulocyte count (but not anemia)	Anaphylaxis, urticaria, fever
Pyrimethamine	Good oral absorption, variable IM absorption; $t_{1/2}$: 4 days	For blood stages, acts mainly on mature forms; causal prophylactic	Well tolerated	Megaloblastic anemia, pancytopenia, pulmonary infiltration
Proguanil (chloroguanide)	Good oral absorption; biotransformed to active metabolite cycloguanil; $t_{1/2}$: 16 h; biotransformation reduced by oral contraceptive use and in pregnancy	Causal prophylactic; not used alone for treatment	Well tolerated; mouth ulcers and rare alopecia	Megaloblastic anemia in renal failure
Primaquine	Complete oral absorption; active compound not known; $t_{1/2}$: 7 h	Radical cure; eradicates hepatic forms of *P. vivax* and *P. ovale*; kills all stages of gametocyte development of *P. falciparum*	Nausea, vomiting, diarrhea, abdominal pain, hemolysis, methemoglobinemia	Massive hemolysis in subjects with severe G6PD deficiency
Atovaquone	Highly variable absorption related to fat intake; $t_{1/2}$: 30–70 h	Acts mainly on trophozoite blood stage	None identified	None identified
Lumefantrine	Highly variable absorption related to fat intake; $t_{1/2}$: 3–4 days	As for quinine	None identified	None identified

[a] Tetracycline and doxycycline should not be given to pregnant women or to children <8 years of age.

[b] Halofantrine should not be used by patients with long ECG QT_c intervals or known conduction disturbances or by those taking drugs that may affect ventricular repolarization, e.g., quinidine, quinine, mefloquine, chloroquine, neuroleptics, antiarrhythmics, tricyclic antidepressants, terfenadine, or astemizole.

Abbreviations: Cl, systemic clearance; V_d, total apparent volume of distribution; IM, intramuscular; SC, subcutaneous; ECG, electrocardiogram; G6PD, glucose-6-phosphate dehydrogenase.

FIGURE 195-11 Mefloquine resistance in *Plasmodium falciparum* in Southeast Asia: high-level mefloquine resistance (*brown*), low-level mefloquine resistance (*red*), and mefloquine sensitivity (failure rate, <20%; *green*). There is insufficient information for the other areas.

There is a growing belief among malariologists that, to prevent resistance, falciparum malaria should be treated with drug combinations and should no longer be treated with single drugs in endemic areas; the same rationale has been applied successfully in the treatment of tuberculosis and HIV/AIDS. This combination strategy is based upon simultaneous use of two or more drugs with different modes of action: one, usually an artemisinin derivative (artesunate, artemether, or dihydroartemisinin), given for 3 days; and the other, a slower-acting antimalarial to which *P. falciparum* is sensitive. Where the malaria parasites are fully sensitive, either amodiaquine or sulfadoxine/pyrimethamine can be used in combination with the artemisinin derivative, or amodiaquine can be combined with sulfadoxine/pyrimethamine. Where there is also resistance to sulfadoxine/pyrimethamine or amodiaquine, a combination of artesunate plus mefloquine, artemether plus lumefantrine, or quinine plus tetracycline or clindamycin can be considered (although tetracycline cannot be given to pregnant women or to children <8 years of age). Atovaquone-proguanil, which is also effective against drug-resistant malaria, can also be combined with artesunate to prevent the emergence of resistance. While there is significant resistance to mefloquine in parts of Southeast Asia, the mefloquine/artesunate combinations are still reliably effective in these areas. The artemisinin derivatives and lumefantrine (all unlicensed in the United States) as well as atovaquone-proguanil are all very well tolerated, with no significant adverse effects.

COMPLICATIONS ■ Acute Renal Failure   If the level of BUN or creatinine rises despite adequate rehydration, fluid administration should be restricted to prevent volume overload. As in other forms of hypercatabolic acute renal failure, renal replacement is best performed early (Chap. 260). Hemofiltration and hemodialysis are more effective than peritoneal dialysis and are associated with lower mortality. Some patients with renal impairment pass small volumes of urine sufficient to allow control of fluid balance; these cases can be managed conservatively if other indications for dialysis do not arise. Renal function usually improves within days, but full recovery may take weeks.

Acute Pulmonary Edema   Patients should be positioned at 45° and given oxygen and intravenous diuretics. Pulmonary artery occlusion pres-

sures may be normal, indicating increased pulmonary capillary permeability. Positive-pressure ventilation should be started early if the immediate measures fail (Chap. 217).

Hypoglycemia   An initial slow injection of 50% dextrose (0.5 g/kg) should be followed by an infusion of 10% dextrose (0.10 g/kg per hour). The blood glucose level should be checked regularly thereafter, as recurrent hypoglycemia is common, particularly in patients receiving quinine or quinidine. In severely ill patients, hypoglycemia commonly occurs together with metabolic (lactic) acidosis and carries a poor prognosis.

Other Complications   Patients who develop spontaneous bleeding should be given fresh blood and intravenous vitamin K. Convulsions should be treated with intravenous or rectal benzodiazepines and, if necessary, respiratory support. Aspiration pneumonia should be suspected in any unconscious patient with convulsions, particularly with persistent hyperventilation; intravenous antimicrobial agents and oxygen should be administered, and pulmonary toilet should be undertaken. Hypoglycemia or gram-negative septicemia should be suspected when the condition of any patient suddenly deteriorates for no obvious reason during antimalarial treatment. Systemic *Salmonella* infections are common complications among African children with falciparum malaria.

PREVENTION   In most of the tropics, the eradication of malaria is not yet feasible because of the widespread distribution of *Anopheles* breeding sites; the great number of infected persons; the use of ineffective antimalarial drugs; and inadequacies in resources, infrastructure, and control programs. Malaria may be contained by judicious use of insecticides to kill the mosquito vector, rapid diagnosis and appropriate patient management, and—where effective and feasible—administration of chemoprophylaxis to high-risk groups. Malaria researchers are intensifying their efforts to understand parasite-human-mosquito interactions better and to develop more effective control and prevention interventions. Despite the enormous investment in efforts to develop a malaria vaccine, no safe, effective, long-lasting vaccine is likely to be available for general use in the near future (Chap. 107). While there is promise for one or more malaria vaccines on the more distant horizon, prevention and control measures continue to rely on antivector and drug use strategies.

Personal Protection Against Malaria   Simple measures to reduce the frequency of mosquito bites in malarious areas are very important. These measures include the avoidance of exposure to mosquitoes at their peak feeding times (usually dusk and dawn), but also throughout the night and the use of insect repellents containing DEET (10 to 35%), suitable clothing, and insecticide-impregnated bed nets or other materials. Widespread use of bed nets treated with residual pyrethroids reduces the incidence of malaria in areas where vectors bite indoors at night and has been shown to reduce mortality in western and eastern Africa.

Chemoprophylaxis (Table 195-9)   Few areas of therapeutics are as controversial as antimalarial drug prophylaxis. Recommendations for prophylaxis depend on knowledge of local patterns of plasmodial drug sensitivity and the likelihood of acquiring malarial infection. When there is uncertainty, drugs effective against resistant *P. falciparum* should be used [mefloquine, atovaquone-proguanil (Malarone), doxy-

TABLE 195-8 *Alternative Drugs for Use When Initial Malaria Treatment Fails*

Drug Used Initially	Drug Used to Treat Recrudescence
Chloroquine	→ Sulfadoxine/pyrimethamine[a] ↘
Sulfadoxine/pyrimethamine	→ Artesunate-mefloquine[a]
Mefloquine ± artesunate	→ Quinine ± tetracycline (or doxycycline) for 7 days ↘ Artesunate + doxycycline or clindamycin for 7 days

[a] Or artemether-lumefantrine.

cycline, or primaquine]. Chemoprophylaxis is never entirely reliable, and malaria should always be considered in the differential diagnosis of fever in patients who have traveled to endemic areas, even if they are taking prophylactic antimalarial drugs.

Pregnant women traveling to malarious areas should be warned about the potential risks. All pregnant women at risk in endemic areas should be encouraged to attend regular antenatal clinics and should receive either prophylaxis with chloroquine (300 mg of base weekly) alone or with proguanil (chloroguanide, 200 mg daily) or intermittent preventive treatment (IPT) with sulfadoxine/pyrimethamine, provided there is not high-level resistance to these drugs. The safety of other prophylactic antimalarial agents in pregnancy has not been established. In addition, antimalarial prophylaxis should be considered for children between the ages of 3 months and 4 years in areas where malaria causes high childhood mortality; such prophylaxis may not be logistically or economically feasible in many countries. Research on IPT for infants and young children shows promise for more widespread use. Children born to nonimmune mothers in endemic areas (usually expatriates moving to these areas) should receive prophylaxis from birth.

Travelers should start taking antimalarial drugs at least 1 week before departure so that any untoward reactions can be detected and therapeutic antimalarial blood concentrations will be present when needed. Antimalarial prophylaxis should continue for 4 weeks after the traveler has left the endemic area, except if atovaquone-proguanil or primaquine has been taken; these drugs have significant activities against the liver stage of the infection (causal prophylaxis) and can be discontinued 1 week after departure from the endemic area.

Mefloquine (250 mg of salt weekly, adult dose) has been the antimalarial

TABLE 195-9	Prophylaxis and Self-Treatment for Malaria			
Drug	Usage	Adult Dosage	Child Dosage
Prophylaxis			
Mefloquine	Used in areas where chloroquine-resistant malaria has been reported	228 mg of base (250 mg of salt) orally, once/week[a]	<15 kg: 4.6 mg of base/kg (5 mg of salt/kg) 15–19 kg: ¼ tablet/week 20–30 kg: ½ tablet/week 31–45 kg: ¾ tablet/week >45 kg: 1 tablet/week
Doxycycline[b]	Used as alternative to mefloquine or atovaquone-proguanil	100 mg orally, once/day	>8 years of age: 2 mg/kg per day orally; maximum dose, 100 mg/d
Atovaquone-proguanil (Malarone)[c]	Used as alternative to mefloquine or doxycycline	250/100 mg orally once/day	11–20 kg: 62.5 mg/25 mg 21–30 kg: 125 mg/50 mg 31–40 kg: 187.5 mg/75 mg >40 kg: 250 mg/100 mg
Chloroquine	Used in areas where chloroquine-resistant malaria has *not* been reported	300 mg of base (500 mg of salt) orally, once/week	5 mg of base/kg (8.3 mg of salt/kg) orally, once/week; maximum dose, 300 mg of base
Proguanil (not available in U.S.)	Used simultaneously *with* chloroquine as alternative to mefloquine or doxycycline	200 mg orally, once/day, in combination with weekly chloroquine	<2 years: 50 mg/d 2–6 years: 100 mg/d 7–10 years: 150 mg/d >10 years: 200 mg/d
Primaquine[c]	Used for travelers only after testing for G6PD deficiency; postexposure prevention for relapsing malaria or prophylaxis	Postexposure: 15 mg of base (26.3 mg of salt) orally, once/day for 14 days Prophylaxis: 30 mg of base daily	0.3 mg of base/kg (0.5 mg of salt/kg) orally, once/day for 14 days
Self-treatment			
Atovaquone-proguanil (Malarone)[d]	In areas with chloroquine-resistant malaria, should be carried during travel to very remote areas by persons taking mefloquine or doxycycline	4 tablets (1000 mg of atovaquone and 400 mg of proguanil) orally, as a single daily dose for 3 consecutive days	11–20 kg: 1 adult tablet 21–30 kg: 2 adult tablets 31–40 kg: 3 adult tablets >40 kg: 4 adult tablets
Sulfadoxine/pyrimethamine[e]	Used as alternative to atovaquone-proguanil for self-treatment	3 tablets (75 mg of pyrimethamine and 1500 mg of sulfadoxine) orally, as a single dose	5–10 kg: ½ tablet 11–20 kg: 1 tablet 21–30 kg: 1½ tablets 31–45 kg: 2 tablets >45 kg: 3 tablets

[a] Tablets manufactured outside the United States contain 250 mg of base.

[b] Not in pregnant women or children <8 years old.

[c] Primaquine and atovaquone-proguanil have both proved safe and effective for antimalarial chemoprophylaxis in areas with chloroquine-resistant falciparum malaria, but more data are needed, particularly in children. These drugs should not be used in pregnancy.

[d] Not for patients on atovaquone-proguanil prophylaxis.

[e] Regimen is used for treatment only (*not* prophylaxis) in areas with known susceptibility.

prophylactic agent of choice for much of the tropics because it is usually effective against multidrug-resistant falciparum malaria and is reasonably well tolerated. Mild nausea, dizziness, fuzzy thinking, disturbed sleep patterns, vivid dreams, and malaise are relatively common. Approximately 1 in every 10,000 recipients develops an acute reversible neuropsychiatric reaction manifested by confusion, psychosis, convulsions, or encephalopathy. The role of mefloquine prophylaxis during pregnancy remains uncertain; in studies in Africa, mefloquine prophylaxis was found to be effective and safe during pregnancy. However, in one study from Thailand, treatment of malaria with mefloquine was associated with an increased risk of stillbirth.

Atovaquone-proguanil (Malarone; 3.75/1.5 mg per kg or 250/100 mg, daily adult dose) is a fixed-combination once-daily prophylactic agent that is very well tolerated by adults and children, with fewer adverse gastrointestinal effects than chloroquine-proguanil and fewer adverse central nervous system effects than mefloquine. It is proguanil itself, rather than the antifolate metabolite cycloguanil, that acts syn-

ergistically with atovaquone. This combination is effective against all types of malaria, including multidrug-resistant falciparum malaria, and, because of its causal activity, may be discontinued 1 week after departure from the endemic area. Atovaquone-proguanil is best taken with food or a milky drink to optimize absorption. There are insufficient data on the safety of this regimen in pregnancy.

Daily administration of doxycycline (100 mg daily, adult dose) is an effective alternative to mefloquine. Doxycycline is generally well tolerated but may cause vulvovaginal thrush, diarrhea, and photosensitivity and cannot be used by children <8 years old or by pregnant women.

Chloroquine remains the drug of choice for the prevention of infection with drug-sensitive *P. falciparum* and with the other human malarial species (although chloroquine-resistant *P. vivax* has been reported from parts of eastern Asia, Oceania, and Central and South America). Unfortunately, there are now few areas of the world with chloroquine-sensitive *P. falciparum*. Chloroquine is generally well tolerated, although some patients are unable to take the drug because of malaise, headache, visual symptoms (from reversible keratopathy), gastrointestinal intolerance, or (in dark-skinned patients) pruritus. A concomitant filarial infection may provoke or aggravate chloroquine-induced pruritus. Chloroquine is considered safe in pregnancy. With chronic administration for >5 years, a characteristic dose-related retinopathy may develop, but this condition is rare at the doses used for antimalarial prophylaxis. Idiosyncratic or allergic reactions are also rare. Skeletal and cardiac myopathy are potential problems with protracted prophylactic use; they are more likely to occur with the high doses used in the treatment of rheumatoid arthritis. Neuropsychiatric reactions and skin rashes are unusual. When used continuously, amodiaquine, a related aminoquinoline, is associated with a high risk of agranulocytosis (~1 person in 2000) and also hepatotoxicity (~1 person in 16,000) and should not be used for prophylaxis.

Primaquine (0.5 mg of base/kg or 30 mg, daily adult dose) has proved safe and effective in the prevention of drug-resistant falciparum and vivax malaria in adults. Abdominal pain and oxidant hemolysis, the principal adverse effects, are not common as long as the drug is taken with food and is not given to G6PD-deficient persons. Primaquine should not be given to pregnant women or neonates.

In the past, the dihydrofolate reductase inhibitors pyrimethamine and proguanil (chloroguanide) have been administered widely, but the rapid selection of resistance in both *P. falciparum* and *P. vivax* has limited their use. Whereas antimalarial quinolines such as chloroquine act on the erythrocyte stage of parasitic development, the dihydrofolate reductase inhibitors also inhibit preerythrocytic growth in the liver (causal prophylaxis) and development in the mosquito (sporontocidal activity). Proguanil is safe and well tolerated, although mouth ulceration occurs in ~8% of persons using this drug; it is considered safe for antimalarial prophylaxis in pregnancy. The prophylactic use of the combination of pyrimethamine and sulfadoxine is not recommended because of an unacceptable incidence of severe toxicity, principally exfoliative dermatitis and other skin rashes, agranulocytosis, hepatitis, and pulmonary eosinophilia (incidence, 1:7000; fatal reactions, 1:18,000). The combination of pyrimethamine with dapsone (0.2/1.5 mg/kg weekly; 12.5/100 mg, adult dose) is a second-line alternative available in some countries. Dapsone may cause methemoglobinemia and allergic reactions and (at higher doses) may pose a significant risk of agranulocytosis. Proguanil and the pyrimethamine-dapsone combination are not available in the United States.

Because of the increasing spread and intensity of antimalarial drug resistance (Figs. 195-2 and 195-11), the Centers for Disease Control and Prevention (CDC; *www.cdc.gov/travel/index.htm*), which recommends a weekly dose of mefloquine for all travelers, maintains an updated 24-h travel and malaria information audiotape that can be accessed by touch-tone telephone (888-232-3228). Regional and disease-specific documents may be requested from the CDC Fax Information Service (888-232-3299). Consultation for the evaluation of prophylaxis failures or treatment of malaria can be obtained from state and local health departments and the CDC Malaria Hotline (770-488-7788).

BABESIOSIS

Babesiosis is a worldwide protozoan disease of animals that is transmitted by ticks; humans are infected incidentally and initially develop a nonspecific febrile illness that can lead to hemolytic anemia. *Babesia* organisms enter RBCs and resemble malarial parasites morphologically, thus posing a diagnostic problem.

ETIOLOGY AND NATURAL CYCLE   Of the >100 species of *Babesia*, *B. microti* and *B. divergens* are the two that cause most human infections. *Babesia* species infect many mammalian hosts. The majority of species are from rodents and birds; however, almost any mammal serving as a host for *Babesia*-infected ticks can be a reservoir. Ixodid (hard-bodied) ticks, in particular *Ixodes scapularis* (*I. dammini*) and *I. ricinus*,

are the vectors of the parasite. Ticks ingest *Babesia* while feeding, and the parasite multiplies within the tick's gut wall. The organisms then spread to the salivary glands; their inoculation into a vertebrate host by a tick larva, nymph, or adult completes the cycle of transmission. Asexual reproduction of *Babesia* within RBCs produces two or four parasites.

EPIDEMIOLOGY   While *Babesia* infections in wild and domestic animals are distributed globally, almost all of the >300 *B. microti* infections in the United States have occurred along the northeastern coast, including Nantucket Island, Martha's Vineyard, and Cape Cod in Massachusetts; Block Island in Rhode Island; Long Island, Shelter Island, and Fire Island in New York; and the nearby mainland, including eastern Connecticut and areas of Westchester County in New York. In Nantucket, 60% of deer mice are infected with *B. microti*. Cases have also been reported from Wisconsin, Minnesota, Virginia, Maryland, Georgia, and Mexico. *Babesia* isolates from patients in Washington (WA-1) and California (CA-1) are structurally similar but genetically and antigenically distinct from *B. microti*. A strain isolated in Japan and another in Missouri (MO-1) differ from these isolates, suggesting that babesiosis may be an "emerging infection." The vast majority of *Babesia* infections are not clinically apparent. The deer tick, *I. scapularis*, is the vector associated with *B. microti*. In Europe, *B. divergens* has been responsible for the majority of the 30 reported cases of babesiosis; Yugoslavia, Russia, France, the United Kingdom, and Ireland have accounted for most of these infections.

Transfusions are another source of babesiosis. In the >20 transfusion-associated cases reported, parasites were uncommonly detected in blood donors, but serologic testing of their blood for *Babesia* gave positive results.

Infections with *B. divergens* have occurred sporadically in previously splenectomized patients in several countries in Europe. *I. ricinus* is probably the vector in these cases, as it is for the transmission of this organism among cattle. The infected persons were predisposed to illness by their asplenic status.

I. scapularis feeds on rodents as a larva and a nymph and on deer as an adult; nymphs are abundant during the spring and summer and feed on humans readily. In some endemic areas, the seroprevalence in the human population may be >2%; residents of Shelter Island and Nantucket have had a 4 to 7% seroconversion rate. These figures indicate that asymptomatic infection is more frequent than is generally thought and that *Babesia* can be a peril for persons being transfused.

CLINICAL PRESENTATION   The incubation period for *B. microti* infection is ~1 to 4 weeks. Immunosuppressed patients, splenectomized individuals, and the elderly have the most severe illness. The clinical presentation varies widely and resembles malaria or rickettsiosis; symptoms and signs include a gradual onset of irregular fever, chills, sweating, muscle pain, and fatigue. Mild hepatosplenomegaly and mild hemolytic anemia may develop, but a rash is not present. The level of parasitemia may range from 1 to 50%. The illness may continue for weeks or months, particularly in patients with HIV infection or AIDS.

Patients infected with *B. divergens* have usually been splenectomized and have a more severe illness, with a rapid onset of chills,

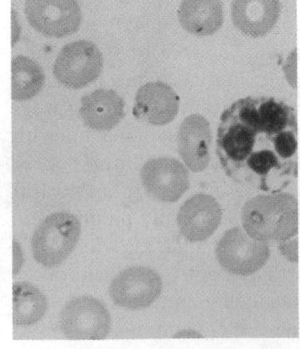

FIGURE 195-12 Thin blood film showing trophozoites of *Babesia*. (*Reproduced from Benchaids for the Diagnosis of Malaria Infections, 2d ed, with the permission of the World Health Organization.*)

fever, nausea, vomiting, and hemolytic anemia progressing to jaundice, hemoglobinemia, and renal failure. *B. divergens* infections are often fatal.

DIAGNOSIS Whether or not they have a history of exposure to ticks or tick bites, febrile persons living in endemic areas should have Giemsa-stained thick and thin blood films (Fig. 195-12) examined for small intraerythrocytic parasites. *B. microti* appears as a small ring form resembling *P. falciparum*. Unlike infection with *Plasmodium*, however, that with *Babesia* does not cause the production of pigment in parasites, nor are schizonts or gametocytes formed. Dividing within RBCs, *B. microti* can form four daughter parasites attached by strands of cytoplasm; these "tetrad" forms are seen infrequently in human blood films but are a distinguishing feature. A sensitive and specific indirect immunofluorescence antibody test is useful for the diagnosis of infection with *B. microti* and exists for *B. divergens* and WA-1 but does not replace the blood smear. The serum antibody titer rises 2 to 4 weeks after the onset of illness and then wanes over 6 to 12 months; cross-reactions can occur with other species of *Babesia* and with *Plasmodium*. A species-specific polymerase chain reaction test using the RNA gene has been used to show parasite persistence when the blood smear is negative.

About 50% of patients infected with *B. microti* have antibody to *Borrelia burgdorferi*, the agent of Lyme disease (Chap. 157); this figure varies with the geographic area. The occurrence of mixed infections is not surprising since both organisms are transmitted by *I. scapularis*. This tick species is also a potential vector of human granulocytotropic ehrlichiosis; the same tick may carry more than one tick-borne disease. Intraperitoneal inoculation of blood from patients with babesiosis into hamsters or gerbils results in detectable parasitemia within 2 to 4 weeks.

Rx TREATMENT (See Table 195-10)

B. microti infections in patients with intact spleens are often self-limiting without treatment, although symptoms may persist for months with or without treatment. Because silent parasitemia may have prolonged symptoms and signs, treatment is advised for all patients infected with *Babesia*. Patients infected with *B. divergens* or other *Babesia* species (including MO-1, WA-1, and CA-1) should receive quinine, clindamycin, and atovaquone; in addition, exchange transfusion or apheresis should be strongly considered. Treatment with the combination of quinine sulfate (650 mg of salt orally three times daily) plus clindamycin (600 mg orally three times daily or 1.2 g parenterally twice daily) for 7 to 10 days is usually effective but may not always eliminate parasites. Especially severe infections with high-level *B. microti* parasitemia in asplenic patients have been successfully treated with exchange transfusions in addition to quinine and clindamycin. The current view is that the combination of atovaquone (750 mg twice daily for adults) and azithromycin (600 mg/d for adults) for 7 to 10 days offers optimal therapy.

TABLE 195-10 *Treatment of Babesiosis*

Organism	Adults	Children
Babesia microti	Atovaquone 750 mg bid PO *plus* azithromycin 600 mg/d PO *or* Quinine 650 mg tid PO *plus* clindamycin 1200 mg bid IV (or 600 mg tid PO)	Atovaquone 40 mg/kg/d PO *plus* azithromycin 12 mg/kg/d PO *or* Quinine 25 mg/kg tid PO *plus* clindamycin 20–40 mg/kg tid PO
Babesia divergens and other *Babesia* species, including MO-1, WA-1, and CA-1	Quinine 650 mg tid PO *plus* clindamycin 1200 mg bid IV (or 600 mg tid PO) *plus* atovaquone 750 mg bid PO[a]	Quinine 25 mg/kg tid PO *plus* clindamycin 20–40 mg/kg tid PO *plus* atovaquone 40 mg/kg per day PO[a]

[a] Consider exchange transfusion or apheresis.

FURTHER READING

ARTEMETHER–QUININE META-ANALYSIS STUDY GROUP: A meta-analysis using individual patient data of trials comparing artemether with quinine in the treatment of severe falciparum malaria. Trans R Soc Trop Med Hyg 95:637, 2001

CENTERS FOR DISEASE CONTROL AND PREVENTION: *Health Information for International Travel, 1999–2000*. Atlanta, Department of Health and Human Services, 2000

GUERIN PJ et al: Malaria: Current status of control, diagnosis, treatment, and a proposed agenda for research and development. Lancet Infect Dis 2:564, 2002

HOGH B: Atovaquone-proguanil versus chloroquine-proguanil for malaria prophylaxis in non-immune travellers: A randomised, double-blind study. Lancet 356:1888, 2000

NEWTON P, WHITE NJ: Malaria: New developments in treatment and prevention. Annu Rev Med 50:179, 1999

PHU NH et al: Hemofiltration and peritoneal dialysis in infection-associated acute renal failure in Vietnam. N Engl J Med 347:895, 2002

VAN VUGT M et al: Treatment of uncomplicated multidrug-resistant falciparum malaria with artesunate-atovaquone-proguanil. Clin Infect Dis 35:1498, 2002

WEISS LM: Babesiosis in humans: A treatment review. Expert Opin Pharmacother 3:1109, 2002

WHITE NJ: The assessment of antimalarial drug efficacy. Trends Parasitol 18:865, 2002

WORLD HEALTH ORGANIZATION: Severe falciparum malaria. Trans R Soc Trop Med Hyg 94(Suppl 1):51, 2000

196 LEISHMANIASIS
Barbara L. Herwaldt

OVERVIEW

DEFINITION The term *leishmaniasis* refers collectively to various clinical syndromes caused by obligate intracellular protozoa of the genus *Leishmania* (order Kinetoplastida). Leishmaniasis is endemic in diverse ecologic settings in the tropics, the subtropics, and southern Europe that range from deserts to rain forests and from rural to periurban areas. It is typically a vector-borne zoonosis, with rodents and canids as common reservoir hosts and humans as incidental hosts. In humans, visceral, cutaneous, and mucosal leishmaniasis result from infection of macrophages throughout the reticuloendothelial system, in the skin, and in the naso-oropharyngeal mucosa, respectively. Current challenges include the emergence of leishmaniasis in new geographic areas and host populations (e.g., visceral leishmaniasis in persons infected with HIV) as well as the need for field-applicable, rapid diagnostic tests and for effective, safe, and affordable oral therapics, control measures, and vaccines.

ETIOLOGY The organisms that cause the various forms of leishmaniasis in humans (Table 196-1) are in the subgenus *Leishmania* or the subgenus *Viannia*. Visceral leishmaniasis is typically but not exclusively caused by organisms of the *Leishmania donovani* complex; Old World cutaneous leishmaniasis by *L. tropica*, *L. major*, and *L. aethiopica*; and New World (or American) cutaneous leishmaniasis by organisms of the *L. mexicana* complex and the *Viannia* subgenus. Mucosal leishmaniasis is caused primarily by some organisms in the *Viannia* subgenus and also by *L. amazonensis*.

LIFE CYCLE *Leishmania* parasites are transmitted by the bite of female phlebotomine sandflies [genus *Phlebotomus* (Old World) or *Lutzomyia* (New World)]. As the flies attempt to feed, they regurgitate the para-

TABLE 196-1 *Major* Leishmania *Species That Cause Disease in Humans*

Species[a]	Clinical Syndrome[b]	Geographic Distribution
SUBGENUS LEISHMANIA		
L. donovani complex		
L. donovani sensu stricto	VL (PKDL, OWCL)	China, Indian subcontinent, southwestern Asia, Ethiopia,[c] Kenya, Sudan, Uganda; possibly sporadic in sub-Saharan Africa
L. infantum sensu stricto[d]	VL (OWCL)	China, central and southwestern Asia, Middle East, southern Europe, North Africa, Ethiopia,[c] Sudan; sporadic in sub-Saharan Africa
L. chagasi[d]	VL (NWCL)	Central and South America
L. mexicana complex		
L. mexicana	NWCL (DCL)	Texas, Mexico, Central and South America
L. amazonensis	NWCL (ML, DCL, VL)	Panama and South America
L. tropica	OWCL (VL)[e]	Central Asia, India, Pakistan, southwestern Asia, Middle East, Turkey, Greece, North Africa, Ethiopia,[c] Kenya, Namibia
L. major	OWCL[f]	Central Asia, India, Pakistan, southwestern Asia, Middle East, Turkey, North Africa, Sahel region of north-central Africa, Ethiopia,[c] Sudan, Kenya
L. aethiopica	OWCL (DCL, ML)	Ethiopia,[c] Kenya, Uganda
SUBGENUS VIANNIA		
L. (V.) braziliensis	NWCL (ML)	Central and South America
L. (V.) guyanensis	NWCL (ML)	South America
L. (V.) panamensis	NWCL (ML)	Central America, Venezuela, Colombia, Ecuador, Peru
L. (V.) peruviana	NWCL[g]	Peru (western slopes of Andes)

[a] Species other than those listed here have been reported to infect humans.

[b] **Abbreviations**: VL, visceral leishmaniasis; PKDL, post–kala-azar dermal leishmaniasis; OWCL, Old World cutaneous leishmaniasis; NWCL, New World (American) cutaneous leishmaniasis; DCL, diffuse cutaneous leishmaniasis; ML, mucosal leishmaniasis. Clinical syndromes less frequently associated with the various species are shown in parentheses.

[c] Cutaneous and visceral leishmaniasis also are endemic in parts of Eritrea, but the causative species have not been well established.

[d] "*L. infantum*" and "*L. chagasi*" are synonymous.

[e] *L. tropica* also causes leishmaniasis recidivans and viscerotropic leishmaniasis.

[f] *L. major*–like organisms also cause New World cutaneous leishmaniasis.

[g] The cutaneous leishmaniasis syndrome caused by this species is called *uta*.

site's flagellated promastigote stage into the skin of mammalian hosts. Components of sandfly saliva can affect the host's response to the parasite. Promastigotes attach to receptors on macrophages, are phagocytized, and transform within phagolysosomes into the nonflagellated amastigote stage, which multiplies by binary fission. After rupture of infected macrophages, amastigotes are phagocytized by other macrophages. If ingested by feeding sandflies, amastigotes transform back into promastigotes, which require at least 7 days to become infective.

IMMUNOLOGY Advances in the understanding of the immunology of leishmaniasis have made this parasitic disease the paradigm for studies of the T cell subsets and cytokines that govern resistance and susceptibility to intracellular pathogens. The paradigm is best demonstrated in murine *L. major* infection. In inbred mice, production of interferon γ (IFN-γ) by T_H1 and natural killer cells confers resistance. Interleukin (IL)12 induces naive T cells to differentiate into T_H1 cells and induces T cells and natural killer cells to produce IFN-γ. In contrast, expansion of IL-4-producing T_H2 cells and IL-10 mediate susceptibility.

Not all aspects of leishmaniasis in mice, whose susceptibility to leishmanial infection is genetically determined, apply to human infection, for which the genetic determinants are being investigated. However, a consistent principle is that healing and resistance to reinfection are associated with an intact T_H1 cell response, production of IFN-γ, and activation of macrophages to kill intracellular amastigotes. In human visceral leishmaniasis, IL-10, which deactivates the T_H1 cell response, appears particularly important in the progression of disease.

GENERAL DIAGNOSTIC PRINCIPLES Definitive diagnosis of leishmaniasis requires demonstration of the parasite. To identify amastigotes by light-microscopic examination, the specimen obtained from an infected site (e.g., thin smear, histologic section) should be stained with Giemsa or another Romanovsky stain and presumptive amastigotes (2 to 4 μm in diameter) examined under oil immersion for the presence of a nucleus and a rod-shaped kinetoplast (Fig. 196-1); the latter is a specialized mitochondrial structure that contains extranuclear DNA. Other means of parasitologic confirmation include in vitro culture (e.g., on Novy-MacNeal-Nicolle medium), animal inoculation, and use of investigational molecular techniques [e.g., polymerase chain reaction (PCR)].

The *Leishmania* species that infect humans are morphologically similar. They can be distinguished by isoenzyme analysis of cultured promastigotes, determination of monoclonal antibody specificity, or various molecular methods.

Indirect immunologic methods for diagnosis include serologic assays and tests for *Leishmania*-specific cell-mediated immunity (e.g., skin testing for delayed-type hypersensitivity reactions). The usefulness of such methods depends in part on the clinical syndrome (see below). Traditional serologic assays (e.g., indirect fluorescent antibody testing) do not reliably distinguish past from current infection, and no leishmanin skin test preparation has been approved for use in the United States. Advances in molecular methods (e.g., production of recombinant/synthetic antigens) are leading to the development of better diagnostic techniques.

GENERAL THERAPEUTIC PRINCIPLES For a given case of leishmaniasis, it is important to consider whether the patient's illness could result in substantial morbidity or in death and therefore requires expeditious treatment with a regimen that generally is highly effective. For more than half a century, the pentavalent antimonial (Sb^V) compounds sodium stibogluconate and meglumine antimonate have been the mainstays of antileishmanial therapy (Table 196-2). Toxicity (such as myalgia, arthralgia, fatigue,

FIGURE 196-1 Amastigotes (the tissue form of the *Leishmania* parasite) in a bone marrow specimen from a patient with visceral leishmaniasis. Each amastigote has a nucleus and kinetoplast. Visualization of the kinetoplast is essential in differentiating leishmaniasis from diseases such as histoplasmosis. The extracellular amastigotes probably were released from mononuclear phagocytes during specimen collection and processing. (*Photograph courtesy of Dr. R. Hamill.*)

TABLE 196-2 *Parenteral and Oral Drug Regimens for Treatment of Leishmaniasis*[a]

Clinical Syndrome, Drug	Route of Administration	Regimen
VISCERAL LEISHMANIASIS		
First-line therapy		
Pentavalent antimony[b]	IV, IM	20 mg Sb^V/kg qd for 28 days
Amphotericin B, lipid formulation[c]	IV	2–5 mg/kg qd (total: usually ~15–21 mg/kg)
Alternatives		
Amphotericin B (deoxycholate)	IV	0.5–1 mg/kg qod or qd (total: usually ~15–20 mg/kg)
Paromomycin sulfate[d]	IV, IM	15–20 mg/kg qd for ~21 days
Pentamidine isethionate	IV, IM	4 mg/kg qod or thrice weekly for ~15–30 doses
Miltefosine	PO	See text
CUTANEOUS LEISHMANIASIS		
First-line therapy		
Pentavalent antimony[b]	IV, IM	20 mg Sb^V/kg qd for 10–20 days (standard recommendation is 20 days)
Parenteral alternatives		
Pentamidine isethionate	IV, IM	3 mg/kg qod for 4 doses or 2 mg/kg qod for 7 doses
Amphotericin B (deoxycholate)	IV	0.5–1 mg/kg qod or qd (total: up to ~20 mg/kg)[e]
Oral alternatives		
Fluconazole	PO	200 mg qd or bid for 6 weeks[f]
Ketoconazole	PO	600 mg/d for 28 days[f]
Itraconazole	PO	200 mg bid for 28 days[f]
Dapsone	PO	100 mg bid for 6 weeks[f]
MUCOSAL LEISHMANIASIS		
First-line therapy		
Pentavalent antimony[b]	IV, IM	20 mg Sb^V/kg qd for 28 days
Amphotericin B (deoxycholate)	IV	1 mg/kg qod or qd (total: usually ~20–40 mg/kg)
Alternative		
Pentamidine isethionate	IV, IM	2–4 mg/kg qod or thrice weekly for ≥15 doses

[a] See text for additional details. Some of the listed drugs are effective only against certain *Leishmania* species and only in certain areas of the world. To maximize effectiveness and minimize toxicity, the listed regimens should be individualized according to the particularities of the case and in consultation with an expert. Children may need different dosage regimens. Except for liposomal amphotericin B (see footnote[c]), none of the drugs listed are licensed by the U.S. Food and Drug Administration (FDA) for the treatment of leishmaniasis per se.

[b] The Centers for Disease Control and Prevention (CDC) provides the pentavalent antimonial (Sb^V) compound sodium stibogluconate (Pentostam; GlaxoSmithKline Export Limited, Middlesex, United Kingdom; 100 mg Sb^V/mL) to U.S.-licensed physicians through the CDC Drug Service (404-639-3670) under an IND mechanism with the FDA. The other widely used pentavalent antimonial compound, meglumine antimonate (Glucantime; Aventis Pharma Venezuela, Caracas; 85 mg Sb^V/mL), is available primarily in Spanish- and French-speaking areas of the world. Locally made Sb^V preparations may have different Sb^V concentrations and may vary in quality and safety.

[c] The lipid formulations of amphotericin B include liposomal amphotericin B and amphotericin B lipid complex. The FDA has approved the following regimen of liposomal amphotericin B for immunocompetent patients: 3 mg/kg qd on days 1–5, 14, and 21, for a total of 21 mg/kg. For immunosuppressed patients, the approved regimen is 4 mg/kg qd on days 1–5, 10, 17, 24, 31, and 38, for a total of 40 mg/kg. Alternative regimens that have been proposed for immunocompetent patients include treatment on days 1–5 and 10 with 3–4 mg/kg qd for cases from Europe or Brazil, with 3 mg/kg qd for cases from Africa, and with 2–3 mg/kg qd for cases from India.

[d] Not commercially available as of this writing.

[e] No dosage regimen has been established for use of this drug to treat cutaneous leishmaniasis.

[f] Adult dosage.

elevated aminotransferase levels, chemical pancreatitis, and electrocardiographic abnormalities) becomes increasingly common as the course of treatment progresses but usually does not limit therapy and is reversible.

The traditional parenteral alternatives to Sb^V—amphotericin B and pentamidine isethionate—are generally considered more apt to induce serious or irreversible toxicity (e.g., nephrotoxicity or diabetes). However, these agents, especially amphotericin B, are being advocated for use in some situations (see below; Table 196-2), in part because of the benefits of new formulations (e.g., lipid formulations of amphotericin B) and the decreasing effectiveness of Sb^V in some settings. Many other agents have been touted as alternatives or adjuncts to Sb^V, often on the basis of suboptimal data. Some of these agents may be useful in certain situations, with the caveat that even the results of well-conducted clinical trials are not always generalizable to the treatment of patients infected with other leishmanial species acquired in other settings. With the apparent exception of miltefosine, the other oral agents evaluated to date typically have at best modest activity against some of the *Leishmania* species.

PREVENTION AND CONTROL The transmission of *Leishmania* species typically is focal, in part because of the limited flight range of sandflies; these insects usually remain within a few hundred meters of their breeding site. They rest in dark, moist places in habitats ranging from deserts to rain forests; peridomestic sandflies rest in debris or rubble near buildings. Vector control may be useful in some settings.

Personal protective measures include avoiding outdoor activities when sandflies are most active (dusk to dawn); using mechanical barriers such as screens and bed-nets that keep out sandflies, which typically are about one-third the size of mosquitoes; wearing protective clothing; and applying insect repellent to exposed skin. Impregnating clothing, bed-nets, and screens with permethrin may also be useful, as may spraying dwellings with residual-action insecticide, if transmission of infection is intra- or peridomiciliary. If dogs are important reservoir hosts, use of insecticide-impregnated dog collars might be helpful. Vaccine strategies are being investigated. Treating human cases is an effective control measure only where humans are the primary reservoir hosts of infection (e.g., of *L. donovani* infection in India).

VISCERAL LEISHMANIASIS

More than 90% of the world's cases of visceral leishmaniasis occur in Bangladesh, northeastern India (particularly Bihar State), Nepal, Sudan, and northeastern Brazil. The causative species typically are those of the *L. donovani* complex (Table 196-1). The organisms can be transmitted not only by sandflies but also congenitally and parenterally (e.g., through blood transfusions or needle sharing). Infection begins in macrophages at the inoculation site (e.g., in dermal macrophages at the site of a sandfly bite) and disseminates throughout the reticuloendothelial system.

CLINICAL MANIFESTATIONS Visceral infection often remains subclinical but can become symptomatic, with an acute, subacute, or chronic course. In some settings, inapparent infections far outnumber clinically apparent ones; malnutrition is among the risk factors for the development of disease. The incubation period usually ranges from weeks to months but can be as long as years. Whereas the general term *visceral leishmaniasis* covers a broad spectrum of severity and manifestations, the term *kala-azar* (Hindi for "black fever," indicating that the skin of some patients turns gray) generally conjures up the classic image of profoundly cachectic, febrile patients who are heavily infected with parasites and have life-threatening disease. Splenomegaly (with the spleen most often soft and nontender) typically is more impressive than hepatomegaly, and the spleen can be massive. Peripheral lymphadenopathy is common in some settings, including Sudan.

The abnormal laboratory findings associated with advanced disease include pancytopenia—anemia, leukopenia (neutropenia, marked eosinopenia, relative lymphocytosis and monocytosis), and thrombocytopenia—as well as hypergammaglobulinemia (chiefly involving IgG, from polyclonal B cell activation) and hypoalbuminemia. Causes of anemia can include bone-marrow infiltration, hypersplenism, autoimmune hemolysis, and bleeding.

Some patients develop post-kala-azar dermal leishmaniasis. This syndrome is manifested by skin lesions (including macules, papules, nodules, and patches) that typically are most prominent on the face. These lesions can develop during therapy or within a few months thereafter (e.g., in East Africa) or can develop years later (e.g., in India); relapse of visceral infection can occur. Persons in India (i.e., in areas where humans are the primary reservoir hosts of infection) who have persistent skin lesions can serve as reservoir hosts who maintain transmission of infection.

Viscerotropic leishmaniasis caused by *L. tropica*, which is thought typically to be dermotropic, was parasitologically confirmed in 12 U.S. soldiers who participated in Operation Desert Storm in the Persian Gulf in the early 1990s. The affected persons had light parasite burdens and nonspecific manifestations of visceral infection (e.g., fatigue, fever, and gastrointestinal symptoms).

DIAGNOSIS Although molecular techniques are under investigation, parasitologic diagnosis of visceral leishmaniasis has traditionally been accomplished by demonstration of the parasite on stained slides (Fig. 196-1) or in cultures of a tissue aspirate or a biopsy specimen (e.g., of spleen, liver, bone marrow, or lymph node). The diagnostic yield is highest for splenic aspiration (specifically, as high as 98% vs. <90% for other specimens), but this procedure can cause hemorrhage.

Patients with florid kala-azar commonly have relatively heavy parasite burdens, develop high titers of antibody to *Leishmania* (diagnostically useful but not protective), and have undetectable *Leishmania*-specific cell-mediated immunity. (Leishmanin skin-test reactivity as well as lymphocyte proliferation and IFN-γ responses to leishmanial antigens develop after recovery.) Promising noninvasive serologic methods for diagnosing kala-azar use recombinant leishmanial antigens or synthetic peptides (e.g., K39); these techniques are being field-tested.

DIFFERENTIAL DIAGNOSIS The differential diagnosis of visceral leishmaniasis includes other tropical and infectious diseases that cause fever or organomegaly (e.g., typhoid fever, miliary tuberculosis, brucellosis, histoplasmosis, malaria, tropical splenomegaly syndrome, and schistosomiasis) as well as diseases such as leukemia and lymphoma. Post-kala-azar dermal leishmaniasis should be differentiated from syphilis, yaws, and leprosy.

℞ TREATMENT (Table 196-2)

Because persons who have kala-azar generally die if not appropriately treated, highly effective therapy is essential, as is close monitoring for bleeding and intercurrent infectious conditions such as pneumonia and diarrhea. Outside of India, treatment with a pentavalent antimonial compound still is usually effective. The use of an alternative parenteral agent should be considered even for first-line therapy if unresponsiveness to Sb^V therapy is prevalent, as it is in India, or if nonantimonial therapy would be advantageous for other reasons (e.g., toxicity profile or duration of therapy).

A major advance has been the advent of lipid formulations of amphotericin B, in which various lipids have replaced deoxycholate. These formulations, which passively target amphotericin to macrophage-rich organs, are much more costly than conventional amphotericin B (cost-prohibitive in poor countries) but are associated with less nephrotoxicity and can be given in considerably shorter courses. Other parenteral alternatives that have merit in some settings include the aminoglycoside paromomycin (identical to aminosidine; not commercially available at present), which has been used as monotherapy (in India) or as an adjunct to Sb^V, and pentamidine. As judged by clinical trials in India, miltefosine (not currently available in the United States) is the first highly effective oral agent for this infection. In the phase 3 trial, the dosage regimen for adults was 50 or 100 mg (~2.5 mg/kg) daily for 28 days. Sitamaquine, another oral agent, is also being field-tested.

VISCERAL LEISHMANIASIS IN PERSONS INFECTED WITH HIV Visceral leishmaniasis is an important opportunistic infection among persons in-

fected with HIV-1 in geographic areas in which both infections are endemic. Although most dual infections have been reported from southern Europe, where *L. infantum* (of the *L. donovani* complex) is endemic, co-infection is becoming increasingly common elsewhere. Most (95%) of the co-infected cases reported to the World Health Organization have been cases of visceral leishmaniasis. (The remaining 5% have been cases of cutaneous disease.) In patients infected with HIV, even relatively avirulent *Leishmania* strains can disseminate to the viscera. Clinical leishmaniasis in co-infected patients can represent newly acquired or reactivated infection; most co-infected patients with clinically evident leishmaniasis have fewer than 200 CD4+ T lymphocytes per microliter. The use of highly active antiretroviral therapy (HAART) decreases the incidence of clinical leishmaniasis. The diagnosis of visceral leishmaniasis should be considered for HIV-infected patients who have ever been in leishmaniasis-endemic areas and who have manifestations such as unexplained fever, organomegaly, anemia, or pancytopenia. Co-infected patients can develop unusual manifestations of visceral leishmaniasis, in part because of atypical localization of the parasite (e.g., in the gastrointestinal tract).

The diagnostic sensitivity of classic serologic methods is lower in co-infected than in immunocompetent patients (~50% vs. >90%), especially if the HIV infection preceded the leishmanial infection. However, parasitologic diagnosis by noninvasive means is easier in co-infected patients. Parasites are more commonly found in the circulating blood monocytes of these patients; the sensitivities are ~50% for a Giemsa-stained peripheral-blood smear and ~70% for culture of a buffy-coat preparation. Invasive methods of parasitologic diagnosis (e.g., microscopic examination or culture of a bone marrow aspirate) typically are highly sensitive, especially for previously untreated patients, who commonly have heavy parasite burdens.

Co-infected patients may initially respond well to standard antileishmanial therapy, albeit with more drug toxicity than is experienced by most immunocompetent persons. However, relapses are common and can occur despite the use of HAART. No standard approach to secondary prophylaxis has been established. Various drug regimens are being evaluated.

CUTANEOUS LEISHMANIASIS

Cutaneous leishmaniasis has traditionally been classified as New World (American) or Old World disease. More than 90% of the world's cases of cutaneous leishmaniasis occur in Afghanistan (Fig. 196-2), Algeria, Iran, Iraq, Saudi Arabia, Syria, Brazil, and Peru. In the Americas, the leishmaniasis-endemic area extends from southern Texas to northern Argentina; the etiologic agents typically are those of the *L. mexicana* complex and the *Viannia* subgenus (Table 196-1) but also include *L. major*–like organisms and *L. chagasi* (which is synonymous with *L. infantum*). Old World cutaneous leishmaniasis is caused by *L. tropica*, *L. major*, and *L. aethiopica* as well as by *L. infantum* and *L. donovani*.

CLINICAL MANIFESTATIONS The incubation period for clinically evident disease typically ranges from weeks to months. The first manifestation is usually a papule at the site of the sandfly bite but can be regional lymphadenopathy (sometimes bubonic) in *L. (V.) braziliensis* infection. Most skin lesions evolve from papular to nodular to ulcerative, with a central depression (which can be several centimeters in diameter) surrounded by a raised indurated border (Fig. 196-2). Some lesions persist as nodules or plaques. The skin lesions can cause considerable morbidity (Fig. 196-3). Multiple primary lesions, satellite lesions, regional adenopathy, sporotrichoid subcutaneous nodules, lesion pain or pruritus, and secondary bacterial infection are variably present. The infecting species, the location of the lesion, and the host's immune response are among the determinants of the clinical manifestations and chronicity of untreated lesions. For example, in the New World, lesions caused by *L. mexicana* tend to be smaller and less chronic than those caused by *L. (V.) braziliensis*; in the Old World, *L. major* tends to cause "wet" exudative lesions that are less chronic than

FIGURE 196-2 Ulcerative skin lesions with raised outer borders on the arm of a patient with New World (American) cutaneous leishmaniasis acquired in Costa Rica. (*Photograph courtesy of Dr. A. Wright.*)

the "dry" lesions with central crusting caused by *L. tropica*. The spontaneous resolution of lesions does not preclude reactivation or reinfection.

The polyparasitic and oligoparasitic ends of the spectrum of cutaneous leishmaniasis are respectively represented by the rare syndromes of diffuse cutaneous leishmaniasis (DCL) and leishmaniasis recidivans, both of which are notoriously difficult to treat. DCL, caused by *L. aethiopica* (Old World) or by the *L. mexicana* complex (New World), develops in the context of *Leishmania*-specific anergy and is manifested by chronic, disseminated, nonulcerative skin lesions; on histopathologic examination of specimens from these lesions, abundant parasites but few lymphocytes are noted. Leishmaniasis recidivans, a hyperergic variant with scarce parasites, is usually caused by *L. tropica* and manifested by a chronic solitary lesion on the cheek that expands slowly despite central healing.

DIAGNOSIS Although examination of histologic sections of biopsy specimens with special stains can help exclude other diagnoses (see below), amastigotes appear larger and are more easily recognizable on Giemsa-stained thin smears (e.g., smears of dermal scrapings, touch preparations of biopsy specimens). Aspirates of skin lesions and lymph nodes are useful for in vitro culture, and biopsy specimens are useful for histologic examination, culture, and PCR. As lesions age, amastigotes become scarcer, and parasitologic confirmation becomes more difficult. Species identification (see above) can be important in guiding therapy.

Serologic testing currently is an insensitive means for diagnosing cutaneous leishmaniasis; antibody titers usually are at most minimally elevated except in patients who have DCL. In contrast, leishmanin skin-test reactivity usually develops during active infection in persons who have simple cutaneous leishmaniasis or leishmaniasis recidivans but not in those who have DCL.

DIFFERENTIAL DIAGNOSIS Cutaneous leishmaniasis is frequently confused with tropical, traumatic, and venous-stasis ulcers; foreign-body reactions; superinfected insect bites; myiasis; impetigo; fungal infections (e.g., sporotrichosis); mycobacterial infections; and other diseases (e.g., sarcoidosis, neoplasms). DCL and leishmaniasis recidivans should be differentiated from lepromatous leprosy and lupus vulgaris, respectively.

℞ TREATMENT (Table 196-2)

Decisions about whether and how to treat cutaneous leishmaniasis should take into account the species, if known, and therefore whether mucosal dissemination is possible (as it is to variable degrees in the Americas with some organisms in the *Viannia* subgenus; Table 196-1) as well as the likelihood of rapid self-healing and the location (e.g., on the face), number, size, evolution, and chronicity of the cutaneous

lesions. When optimal effectiveness is important, intravenous or intramuscular Sb^V therapy is generally recommended. In studies in Colombia (predominantly with the *Viannia* subgenus), relatively short courses of treatment with pentamidine were effective (cure rate, 96%) and quite well tolerated. However, preliminary data from a clinical trial in Peru with *L. (V.) braziliensis* are not looking as promising. No controlled clinical trials have been conducted for cutaneous leishmaniasis with conventional or lipid formulations of amphotericin B. Some data suggest that conventional amphotericin B is likely to be effective. The data for the lipid formulations are too few and too conflicting for this therapy to be recommended at this time. In general, the clinical response to antileishmanial therapy begins with lessening induration; the process of healing often continues after the end of therapy. Relapse typically is manifested by clinical reactivation at the margin of the lesion.

Although many oral agents have been touted for treatment of leishmaniasis, even those that are the most effective typically are moderately active at best and are effective only against some *Leishmania* species or strains. The oral agent miltefosine is being evaluated. In the New World, ketoconazole has some activity against *L. mexicana* and *L. (V.) panamensis* and may be more active than itraconazole (at least against the *Viannia* subgenus), which is better tolerated. Fluconazole led to more rapid healing of *L. major* infection in a clinical trial in Saudi Arabia. Dapsone has looked promising in India but not in Colombia. Adjunctive immunotherapy remains highly investigational. Local or topical therapy can be considered for some cases of infection without risk for mucosal dissemination (e.g., for relatively benign lesions caused by *L. mexicana* or *L. major*). Examples of local approaches include the application of an ointment containing paromomycin and methylbenzethonium chloride (not licensed in the United States), the intralesional administration of Sb^V, heat therapy, and cryotherapy.

FIGURE 196-3 People in Kabul, Afghanistan, infected with *Leishmania tropica*, standing in line for hours on a bitterly cold day in February 1997 at a treatment center for cutaneous leishmaniasis. [*Photograph courtesy of Dr. R. Ashford and reprinted with permission from Elsevier Science (Lancet 354:1193, 1999).*]

MUCOSAL LEISHMANIASIS

Clinically evident leishmanial infection of the naso-oropharyngeal mucosa is a relatively rare but potentially disfiguring metastatic complication of cutaneous leishmaniasis. Mucosal disease develops despite antileishmanial cell-mediated immunity; most commonly is caused by organisms of the *Viannia* subgenus, typically *L. (V.) braziliensis* but also *L. (V.) panamensis* and occasionally *L. (V.) guyanensis*; and is more common in South America than in Central America. Although mucosal disease usually becomes clinically evident within several years after the healing of the original cutaneous lesions, cutaneous and mucosal lesions can coexist or appear decades apart; the potential for long delay is one of the reasons that the risk for mucosal leishmaniasis in particular settings is so difficult to determine. Typically, the original cutaneous lesions of patients who develop mucosal disease were not treated or were suboptimally treated.

Mucosal involvement generally is manifested first by persistent unusual nasal symptoms (e.g., epistaxis), with erythema and edema of the nasal mucosa, and then by progressive, ulcerative, naso-oropharyngeal destruction. Supportive laboratory data (e.g., a positive serologic or PCR result) are useful, but the scarcity of amastigotes makes parasitologic confirmation difficult. The differential diagnosis includes sarcoidosis, neoplasms, midline granuloma, rhinoscleroma, paracoccidioidomycosis, histoplasmosis, leprosy, syphilis, and tertiary yaws.

℞ TREATMENT (Table 196-2)

Treatment with a pentavalent antimonial compound is moderately effective for mild mucosal disease, whereas advanced disease may not respond to such treatment or may relapse repeatedly. Amphotericin B (deoxycholate) can also be considered first-line therapy. Conflicting and limited data have been obtained for lipid formulations of amphotericin B, which therefore are not generally recommended at this time. Patients who develop respiratory compromise after initiation of therapy (e.g., because of an inflammatory reaction) may benefit from the concomitant administration of glucocorticoids.

FURTHER READING

BERMAN JD: Human leishmaniasis: Clinical, diagnostic, and chemotherapeutic developments in the last 10 years. Clin Infect Dis 24:684, 1997

DAVIES CR et al: Leishmaniasis: New approaches to disease control. BMJ 326:377, 2003

DE LA ROSA R et al: Incidence of and risk factors for symptomatic visceral leishmaniasis among human immunodeficiency virus type 1–infected patients from Spain in the era of highly active antiretroviral therapy. J Clin Microbiol 40:762, 2002

HERWALDT BL: Leishmaniasis. Lancet 354:1191, 1999

———, BERMAN JD: Recommendations for treating leishmaniasis with sodium stibogluconate (Pentostam) and review of pertinent clinical studies. Am J Trop Med Hyg 46:296, 1992

MURRAY HW: Clinical and experimental advances in treatment of visceral leishmaniasis. Antimicrob Agents Chemother 45:2185, 2001

SUNDAR S, RAI M: Laboratory diagnosis of viseral leishmaniasis. Clin Diagn Lab Immunol 9:951, 2002

——— et al: Oral miltefosine for Indian visceral leishmaniasis. N Engl J Med 347:1739, 2002

WEIGLE K, SARAVIA NG: Natural history, clinical evolution, and the host-parasite interaction in New World cutaneous leishmaniasis. Clin Dermatol 14:433, 1996

---

197 TRYPANOSOMIASIS
Louis V. Kirchhoff

The genus *Trypanosoma* contains many species of protozoans. *Trypanosoma cruzi*, the cause of Chagas' disease in the Americas, and the two trypanosome subspecies that cause human African trypanosomiasis, *Trypanosoma brucei gambiense* and *T. brucei rhodesiense*, are the only members of the genus that cause disease in humans.

CHAGAS' DISEASE

DEFINITION Chagas' disease, or American trypanosomiasis, is a zoonosis caused by the protozoan parasite *T. cruzi*. Acute Chagas' disease is usually a mild febrile illness that results from initial infection with the organism. After spontaneous resolution of the acute illness, most infected persons remain for life in the indeterminate phase of chronic Chagas' disease, which is characterized by subpatent parasitemia, easily detectable antibodies to *T. cruzi*, and an absence of symptoms. In a minority of chronically infected patients, cardiac and gastrointestinal lesions develop that can result in serious morbidity and even death.

LIFE CYCLE AND TRANSMISSION *T. cruzi* is transmitted among its mammalian hosts by hematophagous triatomine insects, often called *reduviid bugs*. The insects become infected by sucking blood from animals or humans who have circulating parasites. Ingested organisms multiply in the gut of the triatomines, and infective forms are discharged with the feces at the time of subsequent blood meals. Transmission to a second vertebrate host occurs when breaks in the skin, mucous membranes, or conjunctivae become contaminated with bug feces that contain infective parasites. *T. cruzi* can also be transmitted by the transfusion of blood donated by infected persons, by organ transplantation, from mother to fetus, and in laboratory accidents.

PATHOLOGY An indurated inflammatory lesion called a *chagoma* often appears at the parasites' portal of entry. Local histologic changes include the presence of parasites within leukocytes and cells of subcutaneous tissues and the development of interstitial edema, lymphocytic infiltration, and reactive hyperplasia of adjacent lymph nodes. After dissemination of the organisms through the lymphatics and the bloodstream, muscles (including the myocardium) may become heavily parasitized. The characteristic pseudocysts present in sections of infected tissues are intracellular aggregates of multiplying parasites.

In the minority of persons with chronic *T. cruzi* infections who develop related clinical manifestations, the heart is the organ most commonly affected. Changes include thinning of the ventricular walls, biventricular enlargement, apical aneurysms, and mural thrombi. Widespread lymphocytic infiltration, diffuse interstitial fibrosis, and atrophy of myocardial cells are often apparent, but parasites are difficult to find in myocardial tissue. Conduction-system involvement often affects the right branch and the left anterior branch of the bundle of His. In chronic Chagas' disease of the gastrointestinal tract (megadisease), the esophagus and colon may exhibit varying degrees of dilatation. On microscopic examination, focal inflammatory lesions with lymphocytic infiltration are seen, and the number of neurons in the myenteric plexus may be markedly reduced. Accumulating experimental evidence implicates the persistence of parasites and the accompanying chronic inflammation—rather than autoimmune mechanisms—as the basis for the pathology in patients with chronic *T. cruzi* infection.

EPIDEMIOLOGY *T. cruzi* is found only in the Americas. Wild and domestic mammals harboring *T. cruzi* and infected triatomines are found in spotty distributions from the southern United States to southern Argentina. Humans become involved in the cycle of transmission when infected vectors take up residence in the primitive wood, adobe, and stone houses common in much of Latin America. Thus human *T. cruzi* infection is a health problem primarily among the poor in rural areas of Mexico and Central and South America. Most new *T. cruzi* infections in rural settings occur in children, but the incidence is unknown because most cases go undiagnosed. Historically, transfusion-associated transmission of *T. cruzi* has been a serious public health problem in many endemic countries. However, with some notable exceptions, transmission by this route has been markedly reduced as effective programs for the screening of donated blood have been implemented. Several dozen patients with HIV and chronic *T. cruzi* infections who underwent acute recrudescence of the latter have been described. These patients generally presented with *T. cruzi* brain abscesses, a manifestation of the illness that does not occur in immunocompetent persons. Currently, it is estimated that 16 to 18 million people are chronically infected with *T. cruzi* and that 45,000 deaths due to the illness occur each year. Of chronically infected persons, 10 to 30% eventually develop symptomatic cardiac lesions or gastrointestinal disease. The resulting morbidity and mortality make Chagas' disease the most important parasitic disease burden in Latin America.

In recent years, the rate of *T. cruzi* transmission has decreased markedly in several endemic countries as a result of successful programs involving vector control, blood-bank screening, and education of at-risk populations. A major program begun in 1991 in the "southern cone" nations of South America (Uruguay, Paraguay, Bolivia, Brazil, Chile, and Argentina) has provided the framework for much of this progress. Uruguay and Chile were certified transmission-free in the late 1990s, and Argentina and Brazil are expected to follow suit shortly. Similar control programs have been initiated in the countries of northern South America and in the Central American nations.

Acute Chagas' disease is rare in the United States. Five cases of autochthonous transmission and six instances of transmission by blood transfusion have been reported. *T. cruzi* was recently transmitted to three recipients of organs from a single *T. cruzi*–infected donor from Central America. In the past 30 years, more than a dozen instances of laboratory-acquired infection and imported cases of acute Chagas' disease were reported to the Centers for Disease Control and Prevention (CDC). Acute Chagas' disease has not been reported in tourists returning to the United States from Latin America. In contrast, the prevalence of chronic *T. cruzi* infections in the United States has increased considerably in recent years. Data from the 2000 census indicate that >12 million immigrants from Chagas'-endemic countries currently live in the United States, ~8 million of whom are Mexicans. The prevalence of *T. cruzi* infection in Mexico is 0.5 to 1.0%, and most of the 4 million immigrants from Chagas'-endemic nations who are not Mexicans come from countries in which the prevalence of *T. cruzi* infection is greater than it is in Mexico. The total number of *T. cruzi*–infected persons living in the United States can be estimated reasonably to be 80,000 to 120,000. The number of instances of transfusion-associated transmission in this country is likely to be considerably greater than the number reported.

CLINICAL COURSE The first signs of acute Chagas' disease develop at least 1 week after invasion by the parasites. When the organisms enter through a break in the skin, an indurated area of erythema and swelling (the chagoma), accompanied by local lymphadenopathy, may appear. *Romaña's sign*—the classic finding in acute Chagas' disease, which consists of unilateral painless edema of the palpebrae and periocular tissues—can result when the conjunctiva is the portal of entry (Fig. 197-1). These initial local signs may be followed by malaise, fever, anorexia, and edema of the face and lower extremities. A morbilliform rash may also appear. Generalized lymphadenopathy and hepatosplenomegaly may develop. Severe myocarditis develops rarely; most deaths in acute Chagas' disease are due to heart failure. Neurologic signs are not common, but meningoencephalitis occurs occasionally. The acute symptoms resolve spontaneously in virtually all patients, who then enter the asymptomatic or indeterminate phase of chronic *T. cruzi* infection.

Symptomatic chronic Chagas' disease becomes apparent years or even decades after the initial infection. The heart is commonly involved, and symptoms are caused by rhythm disturbances, dilated cardiomyopathy, and thromboembolism. Right bundle-branch block is a common electrocardiographic abnormality, but other types of atrioventricular block, premature ventricular contractions, and tachy- and bradyarrhythmias occur frequently. Cardiomyopathy often results in right-sided or biventricular heart failure. Embolization of mural

FIGURE 197-1 Romaña's sign in an Argentinean patient with acute *T. cruzi* infection. (*Courtesy of Dr. Humberto Lugones, Centro de Chagas, Santiago del Estero, Argentina.*)

thrombi to the brain or other areas may take place. Patients with megaesophagus suffer from dysphagia, odynophagia, chest pain, and regurgitation. Aspiration can occur (especially during sleep) in patients with severe esophageal dysfunction, and repeated episodes of aspiration pneumonitis are common. Weight loss, cachexia, and pulmonary infection can result in death. Patients with megacolon are plagued by abdominal pain and chronic constipation, and advanced megacolon can cause obstruction, volvulus, septicemia, and death.

DIAGNOSIS The diagnosis of acute Chagas' disease requires the detection of parasites. Microscopic examination of fresh anticoagulated blood or of the buffy coat is the simplest way to see the motile organisms. Parasites also can be seen in Giemsa-stained thin and thick blood smears. Microhematocrit tubes containing acridine orange as a stain can be used for the same purpose. When repeated attempts to visualize the organisms are unsuccessful, polymerase chain reaction (PCR) or hemoculture in specialized media can be performed. When used by experienced personnel, all of these methods yield positive results in a high proportion of patients with acute Chagas' disease. Hemoculture has the disadvantage of taking several weeks to give positive results. Serologic testing plays no role in diagnosing acute Chagas' disease.

Chronic Chagas' disease is diagnosed by the detection of specific antibodies that bind to *T. cruzi* antigens. Demonstration of the parasite is not of primary importance. In Latin America, ~20 assays are commercially available, including several based on recombinant antigens. Unfortunately, these tests have varying levels of sensitivity and specificity, and false-positive reactions are a particular problem—typically with samples from patients who have other infectious and parasitic diseases or autoimmune disorders. In addition, confirmatory testing has presented a persistent challenge. For these reasons, it is generally recommended that specimens be tested in at least two assays and that well-characterized positive and negative comparison samples be included in each run. A highly sensitive and specific confirmatory method for detecting antibodies to *T. cruzi* [approved under the Clinical Laboratory Improvement Amendment (CLIA) and available in the author's laboratory] employs immunoprecipitation of radiolabeled *T. cruzi* antigens and electrophoresis. The use of PCR assays to detect *T. cruzi* DNA in chronically infected persons has been studied extensively. The sensitivity of this approach has not been shown to be reliably greater than that of serology, and no PCR assays are commercially available.

Rx TREATMENT

Therapy for Chagas' disease is unsatisfactory. For many years, only two drugs—nifurtimox and benznidazole—have been available for this purpose. Unfortunately, both drugs lack efficacy and often cause severe side effects.

In acute Chagas' disease, nifurtimox markedly reduces the duration of symptoms and parasitemia and decreases the mortality rate. Nevertheless, limited studies have shown that only ~70% of acute infections are cured parasitologically by a full course of treatment. Despite its limitations, treatment with nifurtimox should be initiated as early as possible in acute Chagas' disease. Moreover, when laboratory accidents occur in which it appears likely that *T. cruzi* infection could become established, nifurtimox therapy should be initiated without waiting for clinical or parasitologic indications of infection.

Common adverse effects of nifurtimox include abdominal pain, anorexia, nausea, vomiting, and weight loss. Neurologic reactions to the drug may include restlessness, disorientation, insomnia, twitching, paresthesia, polyneuritis, and seizures. These symptoms usually disappear when the dosage is reduced or treatment is discontinued. The recommended daily dosage is 8 to 10 mg/kg for adults, 12.5 to 15 mg/kg for adolescents, and 15 to 20 mg/kg for children 1 to 10 years of age. The drug should be given orally in four divided doses each day, and therapy should be continued for 90 to 120 days. Nifurtimox is available from the Drug Service of the CDC in Atlanta (telephone number, 770-639-3670).

The efficacy of benznidazole is similar to that of nifurtimox; a cure rate of 90% among congenitally infected infants treated before their first birthday has been reported. Adverse effects include peripheral neuropathy, rash, and granulocytopenia. The recommended oral dosage is 5 mg/kg per day for 60 days. Benznidazole is generally considered the drug of choice in Latin America.

The question of whether patients in the indeterminate or chronic symptomatic phase of Chagas' disease should be treated with nifurtimox or benznidazole has been debated for years. The fact that parasitologic cure rates in chronically infected persons are <20% is central to this controversy. Limited studies of *T. cruzi*–infected laboratory animals and humans suggest that elimination of the parasites reduces the appearance or progression of cardiac pathology. In view of these findings, an international panel of experts recommended that all patients infected with *T. cruzi* be treated with one drug or the other, regardless of their clinical status or the duration of infection. Considerable debate has followed this recommendation, and the issue remains unresolved.

The usefulness of allopurinol, fluconazole, and itraconazole for the treatment of acute Chagas' disease has been studied in laboratory animals and to a lesser extent in humans. None of these drugs has exhibited a level of anti–*T. cruzi* activity that warrants its use in patients. Several newer antifungal azoles have shown promise in animal studies but have not yet been tested in humans. Studies in mice have shown that recombinant interferon γ decreases the duration and severity of acute *T. cruzi* infection; however, its usefulness in persons with acute Chagas' disease has not been evaluated systematically.

Patients who develop cardiac and/or gastrointestinal disease in association with *T. cruzi* infection should be referred to appropriate subspecialists for further evaluation and treatment. Cardiac transplantation is an option for patients with end-stage chagasic cardiopathies, and >100 such transplantations have been done in Brazil and the United States. The survival rate among Chagas' disease cardiac transplant recipients is higher than that among persons receiving cardiac transplants for other reasons. This better outcome may be due to the fact that lesions are limited to the heart in most patients with symptomatic chronic Chagas' disease.

PREVENTION Since drug therapy is unsatisfactory and vaccines are not available, the control of *T. cruzi* transmission in endemic countries must depend on reduction of domiciliary vector populations by spraying of insecticides, improvements in housing, and education of at-risk persons. As noted above, these measures, coupled with serologic screening of blood donors, have markedly reduced transmission of the parasite in many endemic countries. Tourists would be wise to avoid sleeping in dilapidated houses in rural areas in endemic countries. Mosquito nets and insect repellent provide additional protection.

The question of whether blood donated in the United States should be screened for antibodies to *T. cruzi* has been considered by both public and private blood banking authorities for more than a decade. Since no assay for this purpose has been cleared by the U.S. Food and Drug Administration (FDA), serologic testing is not yet an option. Some blood-donor centers currently use a questionnaire to identify and defer donors at high risk for *T. cruzi* infection. The efficacy of this approach has not been assessed specifically, and it is important to bear in mind that approaches based solely on questionnaires have not been entirely successful at eliminating transfusion-associated transmission of other infectious agents.

In view of the possibly serious consequences of chronic *T. cruzi* infection, it would be prudent for all immigrants from endemic regions living in the United States to be tested for evidence of infection. Identification of persons harboring the parasite would permit periodic electrocardiographic monitoring, which can be important because pacemakers benefit some patients who develop ominous rhythm disturbances. The possibility of congenital transmission is yet another justification for screening.

Laboratory personnel should wear gloves and eye protection when working with *T. cruzi* and infected vectors.

SLEEPING SICKNESS

DEFINITION Sleeping sickness, or human African trypanosomiasis (HAT), is caused by flagellated protozoan parasites that belong to the *T. brucei* complex and are transmitted to humans by tsetse flies. In untreated patients, the trypanosomes first cause a febrile illness that is followed months or years later by progressive neurologic impairment and death.

THE PARASITES AND THEIR TRANSMISSION The East African (*rhodesiense*) and the West African (*gambiense*) forms of sleeping sickness are caused, respectively, by two trypanosome subspecies: *T. brucei rhodesiense* and *T. brucei gambiense*. These subspecies are morphologically indistinguishable but cause illnesses that are epidemiologically and clinically distinct (Table 197-1). The parasites are transmitted by blood-sucking tsetse flies of the genus *Glossina*. The insects acquire the infection when they ingest blood from infected mammalian hosts. After many cycles of multiplication in the midgut of the vector, the

TABLE 197-1 *Comparison of West African and East African Trypanosomiases*

Point of Comparison	West African (Gambiense)	East African (Rhodesiense)
Organism	*T. b. gambiense*	*T. b. rhodesiense*
Vectors	Tsetse flies (palpalis group)	Tsetse flies (morsitans group)
Primary reservoir	Humans	Antelope and cattle
Human illness	Chronic (late CNS disease)	Acute (early CNS disease)
Duration of illness	Months to years	<9 months
Lymphadenopathy	Prominent	Minimal
Parasitemia	Low	High
Diagnosis by rodent inoculation	No	Yes
Epidemiology	Rural populations	Workers in wild areas, rural populations, tourists in game parks

Abbreviation: CNS, central nervous system.
Source: Reprinted with permission from LV Kirchhoff in GL Mandell et al (eds): *Principles and Practice of Infectious Diseases*, 5th ed. Philadelphia, Churchill Livingstone, 2000.

parasites migrate to the salivary glands. Their transmission takes place when they are inoculated into a mammalian host during a subsequent blood meal. The injected trypanosomes multiply in the blood and other extracellular spaces and evade immune destruction for long periods by undergoing antigenic variation, a process whereby the antigenic structure of their surface coat of glycoproteins changes periodically.

PATHOGENESIS AND PATHOLOGY A self-limited inflammatory lesion (trypanosomal chancre) may appear a week or so after the bite of an infected tsetse fly. A systemic febrile illness then evolves as the parasites are disseminated through the lymphatics and bloodstream. Systemic HAT without central nervous system (CNS) involvement is generally referred to as *stage I disease*. In this stage, widespread lymphadenopathy and splenomegaly reflect marked lymphocytic and histiocytic proliferation and invasion of morular cells, which are plasmacytes that may be involved in the production of IgM. Endarteritis, with perivascular infiltration of both parasites and lymphocytes, may develop in lymph nodes and spleen. Myocarditis develops frequently in patients with stage I disease and is especially common in *T. b. rhodesiense* infections.

Hematologic manifestations that accompany stage I HAT include moderate leukocytosis, thrombocytopenia, and anemia. High levels of immunoglobulins, consisting primarily of polyclonal IgM, are a constant feature, and heterophile antibodies, antibodies to DNA, and rheumatoid factor are often detected. High levels of antigen-antibody complexes may play a role in the tissue damage and increased vascular permeability that facilitate dissemination of the parasites.

Stage II disease involves invasion of the CNS. The presence of trypanosomes in perivascular areas is accompanied by intense infiltration of mononuclear cells. Abnormalities in cerebrospinal fluid (CSF) include increased pressure, elevated total protein concentration, and pleocytosis. In addition, trypanosomes are frequently found in CSF.

EPIDEMIOLOGY The trypanosomes that cause sleeping sickness are found only in Africa. Approximately 50 million persons are at risk of acquiring HAT, and tens of thousands of new cases occur every year. Precise data are not available because health statistics are often incomplete in the developing countries where HAT is endemic. Sleeping sickness has undergone a resurgence in recent years, with major epidemics in the Sudan, Ivory Coast, Chad, the Central African Republic, and several other endemic countries.

Humans are the only reservoir of *T. b. gambiense*, which occurs in widely distributed foci in tropical rain forests of Central and West Africa. *Gambiense* trypanosomiasis is primarily a problem in rural populations; tourists rarely become infected. Trypanotolerant antelope species in savanna and woodland areas of Central and East Africa are the principal reservoir of *T. b. rhodesiense*. Cattle can also be infected with *T. b. rhodesiense* and other trypanosome species but generally succumb to the infection. Since risk results for the most part from contact with tsetse flies that feed on wild animals, humans acquire *T. b. rhodesiense* infection only incidentally, usually while visiting or working in areas where infected game and vectors are present. Roughly one or two patients with HAT acquired in East African game parks (and typically caused by *T. b. rhodesiense*) are reported to the CDC each year.

CLINICAL COURSE A painful trypanosomal chancre appears in some patients at the site of inoculation of the parasite. Hematogenous and lymphatic dissemination (stage I disease) is marked by the onset of fever. Typically, bouts of high temperatures lasting several days are separated by afebrile periods. Lymphadenopathy is prominent in *T. b. gambiense* trypanosomiasis. The nodes are discrete, movable, rubbery, and nontender. Cervical nodes are often visible, and enlargement of the nodes of the posterior cervical triangle, or *Winterbottom's sign*, is a classic finding. Pruritus and maculopapular rashes are common. Inconstant findings include malaise, headache, arthralgias, weight loss, edema, hepatosplenomegaly, and tachycardia. The differential diagnosis of stage I HAT includes many diseases that are common in the tropics and are associated with fevers. HIV infection, malaria, and typhoid fever are common in populations at risk for HAT and need to be considered.

CNS invasion (stage II disease) is characterized by the insidious development of protean neurologic manifestations that are accompanied by progressive abnormalities in the CSF. A picture of progressive indifference and daytime somnolence develops (hence the designation "sleeping sickness"), sometimes alternating with restlessness and insomnia at night. A listless gaze accompanies a loss of spontaneity, and speech may become halting and indistinct. Extrapyramidal signs may include choreiform movements, tremors, and fasciculations. Ataxia is frequent, and the patient may appear to have Parkinson's disease, with a shuffling gait, hypertonia, and tremors. In the final phase, progressive neurologic impairment ends in coma and death.

The most striking difference between the West African and East African trypanosomiases is that the latter illness tends to follow a more acute course. Typically, in tourists with *T. b. rhodesiense* disease, systemic signs of infection, such as fever, malaise, and headache, appear before the end of the trip or shortly after the return home. Persistent tachycardia unrelated to fever is common early in the course of *T. b. rhodesiense* trypanosomiasis, and death may result from arrhythmias and congestive heart failure before CNS disease develops. In general, untreated *T. b. rhodesiense* trypanosomiasis leads to death in a matter of weeks to months, often without a clear distinction between the hemolymphatic and CNS stages. In contrast, *T. b. gambiense* disease can smolder for many months or even for years.

DIAGNOSIS A definitive diagnosis of HAT requires detection of the parasite. If a chancre is present, fluid should be expressed and examined directly by light microscopy for the highly motile trypanosomes. The fluid also should be fixed and stained with Giemsa. Material obtained by needle aspiration of lymph nodes early in the illness should be examined similarly. Examination of wet preparations and Giemsa-stained thin and thick films of serial blood samples is also useful. If parasites are not seen initially in blood, efforts should be made to concentrate the organisms; the simplest method involves the use of microhematocrit tubes containing acridine orange. In these tubes the parasites are separated from blood cells by centrifugation and are easily seen under light microscopy because of the stain. Alternatively, the buffy coat from 10 to 15 mL of anticoagulated blood can be examined directly under a microscope. The likelihood of finding parasites in blood is higher in stage I than in stage II disease and in patients infected with *T. b. rhodesiense* rather than *T. b. gambiense*. Trypanosomes may also be seen in material aspirated from the bone marrow; the aspirate can be inoculated into liquid culture medium, as can blood, buffy coat, lymph node aspirates, and CSF. Finally, *T. b. rhodesiense* infection can be detected by inoculation of these specimens into mice or rats, which—when positive—results in patent parasitemias in a week or two. Although this method is highly sensitive for the detection of *T. b. rhodesiense*, it does not detect *T. b. gambiense* because of host specificity.

It is essential to examine CSF from all patients in whom HAT is suspected. Abnormalities in the CSF that may be associated with stage II disease include an increase in the CSF mononuclear cell count as well as increases in opening pressure and in levels of total protein and IgM. Trypanosomes may be seen in the sediment of centrifuged CSF. Any CSF abnormality in a patient in whom trypanosomes have been found at other sites must be viewed as pathognomonic for CNS involvement and thus must prompt specific treatment for CNS disease. In patients with CSF pleocytosis in whom parasites are not found, tuberculous meningitis and HIV-associated CNS infections such as cryptococcosis should be considered in the differential diagnosis.

A number of serologic assays are available to aid in the diagnosis of HAT, but their variable sensitivity and specificity mandate that decisions about treatment be based on demonstration of the parasite. These tests are of value for epidemiologic surveys. PCR assays for detecting African trypanosomes in humans have been developed, but none is commercially available.

℞ TREATMENT

The drugs traditionally used for treatment of HAT are suramin, pentamidine, and organic arsenicals. An addition to this list is eflornithine (difluoromethylornithine), which was approved by the FDA in November 1990 for the treatment of West African trypanosomiasis. In the United States these drugs can be obtained from the CDC. Therapy for HAT must be individualized on the basis of the infecting subspecies, the presence or absence of CNS disease, adverse reactions, and occasionally drug resistance. The choices of drugs for the treatment of HAT are summarized in Table 197-2.

Suramin is highly effective against stage I disease. However, it can cause serious adverse effects and must be administered under the close supervision of a physician. A 100- to 200-mg intravenous test dose should be administered to detect hypersensitivity. The dosage for adults is 1 g on days 1, 3, 7, 14, and 21. The regimen for children is 20 mg/kg (maximum, 1 g) on days 1, 3, 7, 14, and 21. The drug is given by slow intravenous infusion of a freshly prepared 10% aqueous solution. Approximately 1 patient in 20,000 has an immediate, severe, and potentially fatal reaction to the drug, developing nausea, vomiting, shock, and seizures. Less severe reactions include fever, photophobia, pruritus, arthralgias, and skin eruptions. Renal damage is the most common important adverse effect of suramin. Transient proteinuria often appears during treatment. A urinalysis should be done before each dose, and treatment should be discontinued if proteinuria increases or if casts and red cells appear in the sediment. Suramin should not be given to patients with renal insufficiency.

Eflornithine is highly effective for treatment of both stages of West African trypanosomiasis. In the trials on which the FDA based its approval, this agent cured >90% of 600 patients with stage II disease. The recommended treatment schedule is 400 mg/kg per day, given intravenously in four divided doses, for 2 weeks. Adverse reactions include diarrhea, anemia, thrombocytopenia, seizures, and hearing loss. The high dosage and duration of therapy required are disadvantages that make widespread use of eflornithine difficult.

Pentamidine is the alternative drug for patients with stage I HAT, although some *T. b. rhodesiense* infections are unresponsive to this agent. The dose for both adults and children is 4 mg/kg per day, given intramuscularly or intravenously, for 10 days. Frequent, immediate adverse reactions include nausea, vomiting, tachycardia, and hypotension. These reactions are usually transient and do not warrant cessation of therapy. Other adverse reactions include nephrotoxicity, abnormal liver function tests, neutropenia, rashes, hypoglycemia, and sterile abscesses.

The arsenical melarsoprol is the drug of choice for the treatment of East African trypanosomiasis with CNS involvement. Melarsoprol cures both stages of the disease and therefore is also indicated for the treatment of stage I disease in patients who fail to respond to or cannot

tolerate suramin and/or pentamidine. However, because of its relatively high toxicity, melarsoprol is never the first choice for the treatment of stage I disease. The drug should be given to adults in three courses of 3 days each. The dosage is 2 to 3.6 mg/kg per day, given intravenously in three divided doses for 3 days, followed 1 week later by 3.6 mg/kg per day, also in three divided doses and for 3 days. The latter course is repeated 10 to 21 days later. In debilitated patients, suramin is administered for 2 to 4 days before therapy with melarsoprol is initiated; an 18-mg initial dose of the latter drug, followed by progressive increases to the standard dose, has been recommended. For children, a total of 18 to 25 mg/kg should be given over 1 month. An intravenous starting dose of 0.36 mg/kg should be increased gradually to a maximum of 3.6 mg/kg at 1- to 5-day intervals, for a total of 9 or 10 doses.

Melarsoprol is highly toxic and should be administered with great care. The incidence of reactive encephalopathy has been reported to be as high as 18% in some series. Clinical manifestations of reactive encephalopathy include high fever, headache, tremor, impaired speech, seizures, and even coma and death. Treatment with melarsoprol should be discontinued at the first sign of encephalopathy but may be restarted cautiously at lower doses a few days after signs have resolved. Extravasation of the drug results in intense local reactions. Vomiting, abdominal pain, nephrotoxicity, and myocardial damage can occur.

The treatment of patients with stage II East African disease who cannot tolerate melarsoprol is problematic. The combination of the arsenical tryparsamide and suramin is one possible approach, but its efficacy is limited because suramin does not penetrate the CNS well and tryparsamide is much less effective against *T. b. rhodesiense* than it is against *T. b. gambiense*. The schedule for tryparsamide therapy is 30 mg/kg (maximum, 2 g) in a single intravenous dose every 5 days for a total of 12 doses; that for suramin treatment is 10 mg/kg intravenously every 5 days, also for a total of 12 injections. Tryparsamide can cause encephalopathy, fever, vomiting, abdominal pain, rash, tinnitus, and a variety of ocular symptoms. Alternatively, eflornithine can be administered as outlined above to patients who cannot tolerate melarsoprol; however, the effectiveness of eflornithine against *T. b. rhodesiense* is variable.

PREVENTION HAT poses complex public-health and epizootic problems in Africa. Considerable progress has been made in some areas through control programs that focus on eradication of vectors and drug treatment of infected humans; however, there is no consensus on the best approach to solving the overall problem, and major epidemics continue to occur. Individuals can reduce their risk of acquiring trypanosomiasis by avoiding areas known to harbor infected insects, by wearing protective clothing, and by using insect repellent. Chemoprophylaxis is not recommended, and no vaccine is available to prevent transmission of the parasites.

FURTHER READING

BOCCHI EA, FIORELLI A: The paradox of survival results after heart transplantation for cardiomyopathy caused by *Trypanosoma cruzi*. First Guidelines Group for Heart Transplantation of the Brazilian Society of Cardiology. Ann Thorac Surg 71:1833, 2001

HUTCHINSON OC et al: Lessons learned from the emergence of a new *Trypanosoma brucei rhodesiense* sleeping sickness focus in Uganda. Lancet Infect Dis 3:42, 2003

JELINEK T et al: Cluster of African trypanosomiasis in travelers to Tanzanian national parks. Emerg Infect Dis 8:634, 2002

KIERSZENBAUM F: Views on the autoimmunity hypothesis for Chagas' disease pathogenesis. FEMS Immunol Med Microbiol 37:1, 2003

KIRCHHOFF LV et al: Transfusion-associated Chagas' disease (American trypanosomiasis) in Mexico: Implications for transfusion medicine in the United States. Submitted 2004

SARTORI AM et al: Exacerbation of HIV viral load simultaneous with asymptomatic reactivation of chronic Chagas' disease. Am J Trop Med Hyg 67:521, 2002

TABLE 197-2	Treatment of Human African Trypanosomiases[a]	
	Clinical Stage	
Causative Organism	I (Normal CSF)	II (Abnormal CSF)
T. brucei gambiense (West African)	Suramin or eflornithine Alternative: Pentamidine	Eflornithine Alternative: Tryparsamide plus suramin
T. brucei rhodesiense (East African)	Suramin Alternative: Pentamidine	Melarsoprol

[a] For doses and duration, see text.
Note: CSF, cerebrospinal fluid.

DEFINITION   Toxoplasmosis is the disease caused by infection with the obligate intracellular parasite *Toxoplasma gondii*. Acute infection acquired after birth may be asymptomatic but frequently results in the chronic persistence of cysts within the tissues of the host. Both acute and chronic toxoplasmosis are conditions in which the parasite is responsible for the development of clinically evident disease, including lymphadenopathy, encephalitis, myocarditis, and pneumonitis. Congenital toxoplasmosis is an infection of newborns that results from the transplacental passage of parasites from an infected mother to the fetus. These infants usually are asymptomatic at birth but later manifest a wide range of signs and symptoms, including chorioretinitis, strabismus, epilepsy, and psychomotor retardation.

ETIOLOGY   *T. gondii* is an intracellular coccidian that infects both birds and mammals. There are two distinct stages in the life cycle of *T. gondii*: the nonfeline and feline stages (Fig. 198-1). In the nonfeline stage, tissue cysts that contain bradyzoites or sporulated oocysts are ingested by an intermediate host (e.g., a human, mouse, sheep, or pig). The cyst is rapidly digested by the acidic-pH gastric secretions. Bradyzoites or sporozoites are released, enter the small-intestinal epithelium, and transform into rapidly dividing tachyzoites. The tachyzoites can infect and replicate in all mammalian cells except red blood cells. Once attached to the host cell, the parasite penetrates the cell and forms a parasitophorous vacuole within which it divides. Parasite replication continues until the number of parasites within the cell approaches a

FIGURE 198-1   Life cycle of *Toxoplasma gondii*. The cat is the definitive host in which the sexual phase of the cycle is completed. Oocysts shed in cat feces can infect a wide range of animals, including birds, rodents, grazing domestic animals, and humans. The bradyzoites found in the muscle of food animals may infect humans who eat insufficiently cooked meat products, particularly lamb and pork. Although human disease can take many forms, congenital infection and encephalitis from reactivation of latent infection in the brains of immunosuppressed persons are the most important manifestations. CNS, central nervous system. (*Courtesy of Dominique Buzoni-Gatel, Institut Pasteur, Paris.*)

critical mass and the cell ruptures, releasing parasites that infect adjoining cells.

As a result of this process, an infected organ soon shows evidence of cytopathology. Most tachyzoites are eliminated by means of the host's humoral and cell-mediated immune responses. Tissue cysts containing many bradyzoites develop 7 to 10 days after the systemic tachyzoite infection. These tissue cysts occur in a variety of host organs but persist principally within the central nervous system (CNS) and muscle. The development of this chronic stage completes the nonfeline portion of the life cycle. Active infection in the immunocompromised host is most likely due to the spontaneous release of encysted parasites that undergo rapid transformation into tachyzoites within the CNS.

The principal stage in the life cycle of the parasite takes place in the cat (the definitive host) and its prey. The parasite's sexual phase is defined by the formation of oocysts within the feline host. This enteroepithelial cycle begins with the ingestion of the bradyzoite tissue cysts and culminates after several intermediate stages in the production of gametes. Gamete fusion produces a zygote, which envelops itself in a rigid wall and is secreted in the feces as an unsporulated oocyst. After 2 to 3 days of exposure to air at ambient temperature, the non-infectious oocyst sporulates to produce eight sporozoite progeny. The sporulated oocyst can be ingested by an intermediate host, such as a person emptying a cat's litter box, a pig rummaging in a barnyard, or perhaps a mouse. It is in the intermediate host that the parasite completes its life cycle.

EPIDEMIOLOGY   *T. gondii* infects a wide range of mammals and birds. Its seroprevalence depends on the locale and the age of the population. Generally, hot arid climatic conditions are associated with a low prevalence of infection. In the United States and most European countries, the prevalence of seroconversion increases with age and exposure. For example, in the United States, 5 to 30% of individuals 10 to 19 years old and 10 to 67% of those over the age of 50 years show serologic evidence of exposure; seroprevalence increases by ~1% per year. In Central America, France, Turkey, and Brazil, the seroprevalence is higher. There may be as many as 2100 cases of toxoplasmic encephalitis each year in the United States.

TRANSMISSION   ■ **Oral Transmission**   The principal source of human *Toxoplasma* infection remains uncertain. Transmission usually takes place by the oral route and can be attributable to ingestion of either sporulated oocysts from contaminated soil or bradyzoites from undercooked meat. During acute feline infection, a cat may excrete as many as 100 million parasites per day. These very stable sporozoite-containing oocysts are highly infectious and may remain viable for many years in the soil. Humans infected during a well-documented outbreak of oocyst-transmitted infection develop stage-specific antibodies to the oocyst/sporozoite.

Children and adults also can acquire infection from tissue cysts containing bradyzoites. The ingestion of a single cyst is all that is required for human infection. Undercooking or insufficient freezing of meat is an important source of infection in the developed world. In the United States, 10 to 20% of lamb products and 25 to 35% of pork products show evidence of cysts that contain bradyzoites. The incidence in beef is much lower—perhaps as low as 1%. Direct ingestion of bradyzoite cysts in these various meat products leads to acute infection.

Transmission via Blood or Organs   In addition to oral transmission, direct transmission of the parasite by blood or organ products during transplantation takes place at a low rate. Viable parasites can be cultured from refrigerated anticoagulated blood, which may be a source of infection in individuals receiving blood transfusions. *T. gondii* infection also has been reported in kidney and heart transplant recipients who were uninfected before transplantation.

Transplacental Transmission   About one-third of all women who acquire infection with *T. gondii* during pregnancy transmit the parasite to the fetus; the remainder give birth to normal, uninfected babies. Of the various factors that influence fetal outcome, gestational age at the time of infection is the most critical (see below). Few data support a role for recrudescent maternal infection as the source of congenital disease. Thus, women who are seropositive before pregnancy usually are protected against acute infection and do not give birth to congenitally infected neonates.

The following general guidelines can be used to evaluate congenital infection. There is essentially no risk if the mother becomes infected ≥6 months before conception. If infection is acquired <6 months before conception, the likelihood of transplacental infection increases as the interval between infection and conception decreases. In pregnancy, if the mother becomes infected during the first trimester, the incidence of transplacental infection is lowest (~15%), but the disease in the neonate is most severe. If maternal infection occurs during the third trimester, the incidence of transplacental infection is greatest (65%), but the infant is usually asymptomatic at birth. Infected infants who are normal at birth may have a higher incidence of learning disabilities and chronic neurologic sequelae than uninfected children. Only a small proportion (20%) of women infected with *T. gondii* develop clinical signs of infection. Often the diagnosis is first appreciated when routine postconception serologic tests show evidence of specific antibody.

PATHOGENESIS   Upon the host's ingestion of either tissue cysts containing bradyzoites or oocysts containing sporozoites, the parasites are released from the cysts by a digestive process. Bradyzoites are resistant to the effect of pepsin and invade the host's gastrointestinal tract. Within enterocytes (or other gut-associated cells), the parasites undergo morphologic transformation, giving rise to invasive tachyzoites. These tachyzoites induce a parasite-specific secretory IgA response. From the gastrointestinal tract, parasites are disseminated to a variety of organs, particularly lymphatic tissue, skeletal muscle, myocardium, retina, placenta, and the CNS. At these sites, the parasite infects host cells, replicates, and invades the adjoining cells. In this fashion, the hallmarks of the infection develop: cell death and focal necrosis surrounded by an acute inflammatory response.

In the normal immune host, both the humoral and the cellular immune responses control infection; parasite virulence and tissue tropism may be strain specific. Tachyzoites are sequestered by a variety of immune mechanisms, including induction of parasiticidal antibody, activation of macrophages with radical intermediates, production of interferon γ (IFN-γ), and stimulation of cytotoxic T lymphocytes of the CD8+ phenotype. These antigen-specific lymphocytes are capable of killing both extracellular parasites and target cells infected with parasites. As tachyzoites are cleared from the acutely infected host, tissue cysts containing bradyzoites begin to appear, usually within the CNS and the retina. In the immunocompromised or fetal host, the immune factors necessary to control the spread of tachyzoite infection are lacking. This altered immune state allows the persistence of tachyzoites and gives rise to the progressive focal destruction that results in organ failure (i.e., necrotizing encephalitis, pneumonia, and myocarditis).

Persistence of infection with cysts containing bradyzoites is common in the immunocompetent host. This lifelong infection usually remains subclinical. Although bradyzoites are in a slow metabolic phase, cysts do degenerate and rupture within the CNS. This degenerative process, with the development of new bradyzoite-containing cysts, is the most probable source of recrudescent infection in immunocompromised individuals and the most likely stimulus for the persistence of antibody titers in the immunocompetent host.

PATHOLOGY   Cell death and focal necrosis due to replicating tachyzoites induce an intense mononuclear inflammatory response in any tissue or cell type infected. Tachyzoites rarely can be visualized by routine histopathologic staining of these inflammatory lesions. However, immunofluorescence staining with parasitic antigen-specific antibodies

can reveal either the organism itself or evidence of antigen. In contrast to this inflammatory process caused by tachyzoites, bradyzoite-containing cysts cause inflammation only at the early stages of development, and even this inflammation may be a response to the presence of tachyzoite antigens. Once the cysts reach maturity, the inflammatory process can no longer be detected, and the cysts remain immunologically quiescent within the brain matrix until they rupture.

Lymph Nodes   During acute infection, lymph node biopsy demonstrates characteristic findings, including follicular hyperplasia and irregular clusters of tissue macrophages with eosinophilic cytoplasm. Granulomas rarely are evident in these specimens. Although tachyzoites are not usually visible, they can be sought either by subinoculation of infected tissue into mice, with resultant disease, or by polymerase chain reaction (PCR). PCR amplification of DNA fragments representing either p30 (SAG-1) or p22 (SAG-2) surface antigen or B1 antigen is an effective and sensitive assay for establishing infection of lymph node tissue by tachyzoites.

Eyes   In the eye, infiltrates of monocytes, lymphocytes, and plasma cells may produce uni- or multifocal lesions. Granulomatous lesions and chorioretinitis can be observed in the posterior chamber following acute necrotizing retinitis. Other ocular complications of infection include iridocyclitis, cataracts, and glaucoma.

Central Nervous System   During CNS involvement, both focal and diffuse meningoencephalitis can be documented, with evidence of necrosis and microglial nodules. Necrotizing encephalitis in patients without AIDS is characterized by small diffuse lesions with perivascular cuffing in contiguous areas. In the AIDS population, polymorphonuclear leukocytes may be present in addition to monocytes, lymphocytes, and plasma cells. Cysts containing bradyzoites frequently are found contiguous with the necrotic tissue border. It is estimated that there are as many as 2100 cases of *Toxoplasma* encephalitis (TE) in the United States each year.

Lungs   Among patients with AIDS who die of toxoplasmosis, 40 to 70% have involvement of the heart and lung. Interstitial pneumonitis can develop in the neonate and the immunocompromised patient. Thickened and edematous alveolar septa infiltrated with mononuclear and plasma cells are apparent. This inflammation may extend to the endothelial walls. Tachyzoites and bradyzoite-containing cysts have been observed within the alveolar membrane. Superimposed bronchopneumonia can be caused by other microbial agents.

Heart   Cysts and aggregates of parasites in cardiac muscle tissue are evident in patients with AIDS who die of toxoplasmosis. Focal necrosis surrounded by inflammatory cells is associated with hyaline necrosis and disrupted myocardial cells. Pericarditis is associated with toxoplasmosis in some patients.

Gastrointestinal Tract   Acute infection in certain strains of inbred mice (B6) results in the development of lethal ileitis within 7 to 9 days. This inflammatory bowel disease has been recognized in several mammalian species, including pigs and nonhuman primates. The association between human inflammatory bowel disease and either acute or recurrent *Toxoplasma* infection has not been established.

Other Sites   Pathologic changes during disseminated infection are similar to those described for the lymph nodes, eyes, and CNS. In patients with AIDS, the skeletal muscle, pancreas, stomach, and kidneys can be involved, with necrosis, invasion by inflammatory cells, and (rarely) the presence of tachyzoites detectable by routine staining. Large necrotic lesions may cause direct tissue destruction. In addition, secondary effects from acute infection of these various organs, including pancreatitis, myositis, and glomerulonephritis, have been reported.

HOST IMMUNE RESPONSE   Acute *Toxoplasma* infection evokes a cascade of protective immune responses in the normal host. *Toxoplasma* enters the host at the gut mucosal level and evokes a mucosal immune response that includes the production of antigen-specific secretory IgA. Titers of serum IgA antibody directed at p30 (SAG-1) have been shown to be a useful marker of congenital and acute toxoplasmosis. Milk-whey IgA from acutely infected mothers contains a high titer of antibody to *T. gondii* and can block infection of enterocytes in vitro. In mice, IgA intestinal secretions directed at the parasite are abundant and are associated with the induction of mucosal T cells.

Within the host, *T. gondii* rapidly induces detectable levels of both IgM and IgG serum antibodies. Monoclonal gammopathy of the IgG class can occur in congenitally infected infants. IgM levels may be increased in newborns with congenital infection. The polyclonal IgG antibodies evoked by infection are parasiticidal in vitro in the presence of serum complement and are the basis for the Sabin-Feldman dye test. However, cell-mediated immunity is the major protective response evoked by the parasite during host infection. Macrophages are activated following phagocytosis of antibody-opsonized parasites. This activation can lead to death of the parasite by either an oxygen-dependent or an oxygen-independent process. If the parasite is not phagocytosed and enters the macrophage by active penetration, it continues to replicate, and this replication may represent the mechanism for transport and dissemination to distant organs. *Toxoplasma* stimulates a robust interleukin (IL) 12 response by human dendritic cells. The requirement for costimulation via CD40/154 has been established. The CD4+ and CD8+ T cell responses are antigen-specific and further stimulate the production of a variety of important lymphokines that expand the T cell and natural killer cell repertoire. *T. gondii* is a potent inducer of a T_H1 phenotype, with IL-12 and IFN-γ playing an essential role in the control of the parasites' growth in the host. Regulation of the inflammatory response is at least partially under the control of a T_H2 response that includes the production of IL-4 and IL-10 in seropositive individuals. Both asymptomatic patients and those with active infection may show a depression in the ratio of CD4+ to CD8+ lymphocytes. This shift may be correlated with a disease syndrome but is not necessarily correlated with disease outcome. Human T cell clones of both the CD4+ and the CD8+ phenotypes are cytolytic against parasite-infected macrophages. These T cell clones produce cytokines that are "microbistatic." IL-18, IL-7, and IL-15 upregulate the production of IFN-γ and may be important during acute and chronic infection. The effect of IFN-γ may be paradoxical, with stimulation of a host downregulatory response as well.

Although in patients with AIDS *T. gondii* infection is believed to be recrudescent, determination of antibody titers is not helpful in establishing reactivation. Because of the severe depletion in CD4+ T cells, quite frequently there is no observed increase in antibody titer during exacerbation of infection. T cells from AIDS patients with reactivation of toxoplasmosis fail to secrete both IFN-γ and IL-2. This alteration in the production of these critical immune cytokines contributes to the persistence of infection. *Toxoplasma* infection frequently develops late in the course of AIDS, when the loss of T cell–dependent protective mechanisms, particularly CD8+ T cells, becomes most pronounced.

CLINICAL MANIFESTATIONS In persons whose immune systems are intact, acute toxoplasmosis is usually asymptomatic and self-limited. This condition can go unrecognized in 80 to 90% of adults and children with acquired infection. The asymptomatic nature of this infection makes diagnosis difficult in mothers infected during pregnancy. In contrast, the wide range of clinical manifestations in congenitally infected children includes severe neurologic complications such as hydrocephalus, microcephaly, mental retardation, and chorioretinitis. If prenatal infection is severe, multiorgan failure and subsequent intrauterine fetal death can occur. In children and adults, chronic infection can persist throughout life, with little consequence to the immunocompetent host.

FIGURE 198-2 Toxoplasmic encephalitis in a 36-year-old patient with AIDS. The multiple lesions are demonstrated by magnetic resonance scanning (T_1 weighted with gadolinium enhancement). (*Courtesy of Clifford Eskey, Dartmouth Hitchcock Medical Center, Hanover, NH.*)

Toxoplasmosis in Immunocompetent Patients The most common manifestation of acute toxoplasmosis is cervical lymphadenopathy. The nodes may be single or multiple, are usually nontender, are discrete, and vary in firmness. Lymphadenopathy also may be found in suboccipital, supraclavicular, inguinal, and mediastinal areas. Generalized lymphadenopathy occurs in 20 to 30% of symptomatic patients. Between 20 and 40% of patients with lymphadenopathy also have headache, malaise, fatigue, and fever [usually with a temperature of <40°C (<104°F)]. A smaller proportion of symptomatic individuals have myalgia, sore throat, abdominal pain, maculopapular rash, meningoencephalitis, and confusion. Rare complications associated with infection in the normal immune host include pneumonia, myocarditis, encephalopathy, pericarditis, and polymyositis. Symptoms associated with acute infection usually resolve within several weeks, although the lymphadenopathy may persist for some months. In one epidemic, toxoplasmosis was diagnosed correctly in only 3 of the 25 patients who consulted physicians. If toxoplasmosis is considered in the differential diagnosis, routine laboratory and serologic screening should be performed before node biopsy.

The results of routine laboratory studies are usually unremarkable except for minimal lymphocytosis, an elevated sedimentation rate, and a nominal increase in liver aminotransferases. Evaluation of cerebrospinal fluid (CSF) in cases with evidence of encephalopathy or meningoencephalitis shows an elevation of intracranial pressure, mononuclear pleocytosis (10 to 50 cells/mL), a slight increase in protein concentration, and (occasionally) an increase in the gamma globulin level. PCR amplification of the *Toxoplasma* DNA target sequence in the CSF may be beneficial. The CSF of chronically infected individuals is normal.

Infection of Immunocompromised Patients Patients with AIDS and those receiving immunosuppressive therapy for lymphoproliferative disorders are at greatest risk for developing acute toxoplasmosis. This predilection may be due either to reactivation of latent infection or to acquisition of parasites from exogenous sources such as blood or transplanted organs. In individuals with AIDS, more than 95% of cases of TE are believed to be due to recrudescent infection. In most of these cases, encephalitis develops when the CD4+ cell count falls below $100/\mu L$. In the immunocompromised individual, the disease may be rapidly fatal if untreated. Thus accurate diagnosis and initiation of appropriate therapy are necessary to prevent fulminant infection.

Toxoplasmosis is a principal opportunistic infection of the CNS in persons with AIDS. Although geographic origin may be related to frequency of infection, it has no correlation with the severity of disease in the immunocompromised host. Individuals with AIDS who are seropositive for *T. gondii* are at a very high risk for developing encephalitis. In the United States, about one-third of the 15 to 40% of adult patients with AIDS who are latently infected with the parasite develop TE.

The signs and symptoms of acute toxoplasmosis in the immunocompromised patient principally involve the CNS (Fig. 198-2). More than 50% of patients with clinical manifestations have intracerebral involvement. Clinical findings at the time of presentation range from nonfocal to focal dysfunction. CNS findings include encephalopathy, meningoencephalitis, and mass lesions. Patients may present with altered mental status (75%), fever (10 to 72%), seizures (33%), headaches (56%), and focal neurologic findings (60%), including motor deficits, cranial nerve palsies, movement disorders, dysmetria, visual-field loss, and aphasia. Patients who present with evidence of diffuse cortical dysfunction develop evidence of focal neurologic disease as the infection progresses. This altered condition is due not only to the necrotizing encephalitis caused by direct invasion of the parasite but also to secondary effects, including vasculitis, edema, and hemorrhage. The onset of infection can range from an insidious process over several weeks to an acute confusional state with fulminant focal deficits, including hemiparesis, hemiplegia, visual-field defects, localized headache, and focal seizures.

Although lesions can occur anywhere within the CNS, the areas most involved appear to be the brainstem, basal ganglia, pituitary gland, and corticomedullary junction. Brainstem involvement gives rise to a variety of neurologic dysfunctions, including cranial nerve palsy, dysmetria, and ataxia. With basal ganglionic infection, patients may develop hydrocephalus, choreiform movements, and choreoathetosis. Because *Toxoplasma* usually causes encephalitis, meningeal involvement is uncommon, and thus CSF findings may be unremarkable or may include a modest increase in cell count and in protein—but not glucose—concentration.

Cerebral toxoplasmosis needs to be differentiated from other opportunistic infections or tumors within the CNS of those afflicted with AIDS. The differential diagnosis includes herpes simplex encephalitis, cryptococcal meningitis, progressive multifocal leukoencephalopathy, and primary CNS lymphoma. Involvement of the pituitary gland can give rise to panhypopituitarism and hyponatremia from inappropriate secretion of vasopressin (antidiuretic hormone). AIDS-dementia complex may present as cognitive impairment, attention loss, and altered memory. Brain biopsy in those patients who have been treated for TE but who continue to exhibit neurologic dysfunction often fails to identify organisms.

Autopsies of patients infected with *Toxoplasma* have demonstrated the involvement of multiple organs, including the lungs, gastrointestinal tract, pancreas, skin, eyes, heart, and liver. *Toxoplasma* pneumonia can occur and can be confused with *Pneumocystis carinii* infection. Respiratory involvement usually presents as dyspnea, fever, and a nonproductive cough and may rapidly progress to acute respiratory failure with hemoptysis, metabolic acidosis, hypotension, and (occasionally) disseminated intravascular coagulation. Histopathologic studies demonstrate necrosis and a mixed cellular infiltrate. The presence of organisms is a helpful diagnostic indicator, but organisms can also be found in healthy tissue. Infection of the heart is usually asymptomatic but can be associated with cardiac tamponade or biventricular failure. Infections of the gastrointestinal tract and the liver have been documented.

Congenital Toxoplasmosis   Between 400 and 4000 infants born each year in the United States are affected by congenital toxoplasmosis. Infection of the placenta leads to hematogenous infection of the fetus. As has already been stated, the proportion of fetuses that become infected increases but the clinical severity of the infection declines as gestation proceeds. Persistence of the parasite can ultimately result in reactivation and further damage decades later. Factors associated with relatively severe disabilities include delayed diagnosis and initiation of therapy, neonatal hypoxia and hypoglycemia, profound visual impairment (see "Ocular Infection," below), uncorrected hydrocephalus, and increased intracranial pressure. If treated appropriately, upwards of 70% of children have normal developmental, neurologic, and ophthalmologic findings at follow-up evaluations. Treatment for 1 year with pyrimethamine and a sulfonamide is tolerated with minimal toxicity (see "Treatment," below).

Ocular Infection   Infection with *T. gondii* is estimated to cause 35% of all cases of chorioretinitis in the United States and Europe. Most ocular involvement is believed to be due to congenital infection, with a very low incidence following acquired infection. Between 1 and 3% of all patients with AIDS develop debilitating chorioretinitis due to *T. gondii*. A variety of ocular manifestations are documented, including blurred vision, scotoma, photophobia, and eye pain. Macular involvement occurs with loss of central vision, and nystagmus is secondary to poor fixation. Involvement of the extraocular muscles may lead to disorders of convergence and to strabismus. Ophthalmologic examination should be undertaken in newborns with suspected congenital infection. As the inflammation resolves, vision improves, but episodic flare-ups of chorioretinitis, which progressively destroy retinal tissue and lead to glaucoma, are common.

The ophthalmologic examination reveals yellow-white, cotton-like patches with indistinct margins of hyperemia. As the lesions age, white plaques with distinct borders and black spots within the retinal pigment become more apparent. Lesions usually are located near the posterior pole of the retina; they may be single but are more commonly multiple. Congenital lesions may be unilateral or bilateral and show evidence of massive chorioretinal degeneration with extensive fibrosis. Surrounding these areas of involvement are a normal retina and vasculature. In patients with AIDS, retinal lesions are often large, with diffuse retinal necrosis, and include both free tachyzoites and cysts containing bradyzoites. Toxoplasmic chorioretinitis may be a prodrome to the development of encephalitis.

DIAGNOSIS ■ Tissue and Body Fluids   The differential diagnosis of acute toxoplasmosis can be made by appropriate culture, serologic testing, and PCR (Table 198-1). Although difficult, the isolation of *T. gondii* from blood or other body fluids can be accomplished after subinoculation of the sample into the peritoneal cavity of mice. Mice should be tested for organisms in the peritoneal fluid 6 to 10 days after inoculation. If no parasites are found in the mouse's peritoneal fluid, its anti-*Toxoplasma* serum titer can be evaluated 4 to 6 weeks after inoculation. Isolation of *T. gondii* from the patient's body fluids reflects acute infection, whereas isolation from biopsied tissue is an indication only of the presence of tissue cysts and should not be misinterpreted as evidence of acute toxoplasmosis. Persistent parasitemia in patients with latent, asymptomatic infection is rare. Histologic examination of lymph nodes may suggest the characteristic changes described above.

TABLE 198-1   *Differential Laboratory Diagnosis of Toxoplasmosis*

Clinical Setting	Alternative Diagnosis	Distinguishing Characteristics
Mononucleosis syndrome	Epstein-Barr virus	Serologic test
	Cytomegalovirus	Serologic test
	HIV	Serologic test
Congenital infection	Cytomegalovirus	Viral culture
	Herpes simplex virus	Viral culture
	Rubella virus	Viral culture/serologic test
	Syphilis	Serologic test
	Listeriosis	Bacterial culture
Retinochoroiditis in immunocompetent individual	Tuberculosis	Bacterial culture
	Syphilis	Serologic test
	Histoplasmosis	Serologic test/culture
Retinochoroiditis in AIDS	Cytomegalovirus	Viral culture/PCR
	Syphilis	Serologic test
	Herpes simplex virus	Viral culture/PCR
	Varicella-zoster virus	Viral culture/PCR
	Fungal infection	Culture
CNS lesions in AIDS	Lymphoma or metastatic tumor	Tissue biopsy
	Brain abscess	Bacterial culture
	Progressive multifocal leukoencephalopathy	PCR
	Fungal/mycobacterial infection	Biopsy and culture

Source: Adapted from Schwartzman JD: Toxoplasmosis, in *Principles and Practice of Clinical Parasitology*. Hoboken, Wiley, 2001.

Demonstration of tachyzoites in lymph nodes establishes the diagnosis of acute toxoplasmosis. Like subinoculation into mice, histologic demonstration of cysts containing bradyzoites confirms prior infection with *T. gondii* but is nondiagnostic for acute infection.

Serology   The procedures just described have great diagnostic value but are limited by difficulties encountered either in the growth of parasites in vivo or in the identification of tachyzoites by histochemical methods. Serologic testing has become the routine method of diagnosis. A wide range of serologic tests that can be used to measure antibody to *T. gondii* are available commercially.

Diagnosis of acute infection with *T. gondii* can be established by detection of the simultaneous presence of IgG and IgM antibody to *Toxoplasma* in serum. The presence of circulating IgA favors the diagnosis of an acute infection. The Sabin-Feldman dye test, the indirect fluorescent antibody test, and the enzyme-linked immunosorbent assay (ELISA) all satisfactorily measure circulating IgG antibody to *Toxoplasma*. Positive IgG titers (>1:10) can be detected as early as 2 to 3 weeks after infection. These titers usually peak at 6 to 8 weeks and decline slowly to a new baseline level that persists for life. It is necessary to measure the serum IgM titer in concert with the IgG titer to better establish the time of infection. The methods currently available for this determination are the double-sandwich IgM-ELISA and the IgM-immunosorbent assay (IgM-ISAGA). Both of these assays are specific and sensitive, and their use precludes the false-positive results associated with tests for rheumatoid factor and antinuclear antibody. The double-sandwich IgA-ELISA is more sensitive than the IgM-ELISA for detecting congenital infection in the fetus and newborn.

Recently, the results obtained with PCR have suggested high sensitivity, specificity, and clinical utility in the diagnosis of TE in a resource-poor setting.

The Immunocompetent Adult or Child   For the patient who presents with lymphadenopathy only, a positive IgM titer is an indication of acute infection—and an indication for therapy, if that is clinically warranted (see "Treatment," below). The serum IgM titer should be determined again in 3 weeks. An elevation in the IgG titer without an increase in the IgM titer suggests that infection is present but that it is not acute. If there is a borderline increase in either IgG or IgM, the titers should be assessed again in 3 to 4 weeks.

The Immunocompromised Host   A presumptive clinical diagnosis of TE in patients with AIDS is based on clinical presentation, history of exposure as evidenced by positive serology, and radiologic evaluation. To detect latent infection with *T. gondii*, HIV-infected persons should be tested for IgG antibody to *Toxoplasma* soon after the diagnosis of HIV infection. When these criteria are used, the predictive value is as high as 80%. More than 97% of patients with AIDS and toxoplasmosis have IgG antibody to the parasite in their sera. IgM serum antibody is usually not demonstrable. Attempts to evaluate rising IgG titers or to determine whether IgM is present are not productive. Serologic evidence of infection virtually always precedes the development of TE. It is therefore important to determine the *Toxoplasma* antibody status of all patients infected with HIV. Antibody titers may range from negative to 1:1024 in patients with AIDS and TE. Fewer than 3% of patients have no demonstrable antibody to *Toxoplasma* at the time of diagnosis. Intrathecal antibody to *T. gondii* may be present; determination of the intrathecal antibody titer may be useful in identifying prior infection.

Patients with TE have focal or multifocal abnormalities demonstrable by computed tomography (CT) or magnetic resonance imaging (MRI). Neuroradiologic evaluation should include double-dose contrast CT of the head. By this test, single and frequently multiple contrast-enhancing lesions (<2 cm) may be identified. MRI usually demonstrates multiple lesions located in both hemispheres, with the basal ganglia and corticomedullary junction most commonly involved; MRI provides a more sensitive evaluation of the efficacy of therapy than does CT (Fig. 198-2). These findings are not pathognomonic of *Toxoplasma* infection since 40% of CNS lymphomas are multifocal and 50% are ring-enhancing. For both MRI and CT scans, the rate of false-negative results is ~10%. The finding of a single lesion on an MRI scan increases the suspicion of primary CNS lymphoma (in which solitary lesions are four times more likely than in TE) and strengthens the argument for the performance of a brain biopsy. A therapeutic trial of anti-*Toxoplasma* medications is frequently used to assess the diagnosis. Treatment of presumptive TE with pyrimethamine clindamycin results in quantifiable clinical improvement in more than 50% of patients by day 3. By day 7, more than 90% of treated patients show evidence of improvement. In contrast, if patients fail to respond or have lymphoma, clinical signs and symptoms worsen by day 7. Patients in this category require brain biopsy with or without a change in therapy. This procedure can now be performed by a stereotactic CT-guided method that reduces the potential for complications. Brain biopsy for *T. gondii* identifies organisms in 50 to 75% of cases. PCR amplification of genetic material of the parasite found in the CSF may prove diagnostically beneficial in the future.

Now used in some centers, single photon emission CT (SPECT) has been touted as a definitive means of detecting or ruling out *Toxoplasma* infection when a CNS lesion is suspected. In the future, SPECT may well be widely used for this purpose.

As in other conditions, the radiologic response may lag behind the clinical response. Resolution of lesions may take from 3 weeks to 6 months. Some patients show clinical improvement despite worsening radiographic findings.

Congenital Infection   The issue of concern when a pregnant woman has evidence of recent *T. gondii* infection is obviously whether the fetus is infected. PCR of the amniotic fluid to detect the B1 gene of the parasite has replaced fetal blood sampling. Serologic diagnosis is based on the persistence of IgG antibody or a positive IgM titer after the first week of life (a time frame that excludes placental leak). The IgG determination should be repeated every 2 months. An increase in IgM beyond the first week of life is indicative of acute infection. However, up to 25% of infected newborns may be seronegative and have normal routine physical examinations. Thus assessment of the eye and the brain, with ophthalmologic testing, CSF evaluation, and radiologic studies, is important in establishing the diagnosis.

Ocular Toxoplasmosis   Because of the congenital nature of ocular toxoplasmosis, the serum antibody titer may not correlate with the presence of active lesions in the fundus. In general, a positive IgG titer (measured in undiluted serum if necessary) in conjunction with typical lesions establishes the diagnosis. If lesions are atypical and the titer is in the low-positive range, the diagnosis is presumptive. The parasitic antigen-specific polyclonal IgG assay as well as the parasitic antigen-specific PCR may facilitate the diagnosis.

℞ TREATMENT

Congenital Infection   Congenitally infected neonates are treated with daily oral pyrimethamine (0.5 to 1 mg/kg) and sulfadiazine (100 mg/kg) for 1 year. In addition, therapy with spiramycin (100 mg/kg per day) plus prednisone (1 mg/kg per day) has been shown to be efficacious for congenital infection.

Infection in Immunocompetent Patients   Immunologically competent adults and older children who have only lymphadenopathy do not require specific therapy unless they have persistent, severe symptoms. Patients with ocular toxoplasmosis should be treated for 1 month with pyrimethamine plus either sulfadiazine or clindamycin. Prenatal antibiotic therapy can reduce the number of infants severely affected by *Toxoplasma* infection.

Infection in Immunocompromised Patients ■ *PRIMARY PROPHYLAXIS*   Patients with AIDS should be treated for acute toxoplasmosis; in the immunocompromised patient, toxoplasmosis is rapidly fatal if untreated. AIDS patients who are seropositive for *T. gondii* and have a CD4+ T lymphocyte count of <100/μL should receive prophylaxis against TE. The daily dose of trimethoprim-sulfamethoxazole (TMP-SMX) recommended as the preferred regimen for *P. carinii* pneumonia (PCP) prophylaxis (one double-strength tablet) is effective against TE. If patients cannot tolerate TMP-SMX, the recommended alternative is dapsone-pyrimethamine, which is also effective against PCP. Atovaquone with or without pyrimethamine also can be considered. Prophylactic monotherapy with dapsone, pyrimethamine, azithromycin, clarithromycin, or aerosolized pentamidine is probably insufficient. AIDS patients who are seronegative for *Toxoplasma* and are not receiving prophylactic medication for PCP should be retested for IgG antibody to *Toxoplasma* if their CD4+ T cell count drops to <100/μL. If seroconversion has taken place, then the patient should be given prophylactic medication as described above.

DISCONTINUING PRIMARY PROPHYLAXIS   Some current studies indicate that prophylaxis against TE can be discontinued in patients who have responded to highly active antiretroviral therapy (HAART) and whose CD4+ T lymphocyte count has been >200/μL for 3 months. Although patients with CD4+ T lymphocyte counts of <100/μL are at greatest risk for developing TE, the risk that this condition will develop when the CD4+ T lymphocyte count has increased to 100–200/μL has not been established. Thus, prophylaxis should be discontinued only when the CD4+ T cell count has increased to >200/μL. Continued prophylaxis when the CD4+ count is >200/μL has only a limited preventive effect against TE. Discontinuation of therapy reduces pill burden, potential for drug toxicity, drug interaction, selection of drug-resistant pathogens, and cost. Prophylaxis should be reintroduced if the CD4+ T lymphocyte count decreases to <100–200/μL.

Individuals who have completed initial therapy for TE should continue treatment indefinitely unless immune reconstitution, with a CD4+ T cell count of >200/μL, occurs as a consequence of HAART. Combination therapy with pyrimethamine plus sulfadiazine plus leucovorin is effective for this purpose. An alternative to sulfadiazine in this regimen is clindamycin. Unfortunately, only the combination of pyrimethamine plus sulfadiazine provides protection against PCP as well.

DISCONTINUING SECONDARY PROPHYLAXIS (CHRONIC MAINTENANCE THERAPY)   Patients receiving secondary prophylaxis for TE are at low risk for recurrence when they have completed initial therapy for TE, remain asymptomatic, and have a CD4+ T lymphocyte count of >200/μL for at least 6 months after HAART. This recommendation is based on limited patient assessment and is consistent with more extensive data indicating the safety of discontinuing secondary prophylaxis for other opportunistic infections during advanced HIV disease. Discontinuation of chronic maintenance therapy among these patients appears rea-

sonable. A repeat MRI scan of the brain is recommended to determine whether discontinuing therapy is appropriate. Secondary prophylaxis should be reintroduced if the CD4+ T lymphocyte count decreases to <200/μL.

PREVENTION   All HIV-infected persons, including those who lack IgG antibody to *Toxoplasma*, should be counseled regarding sources of *Toxoplasma* infection. The chances of primary infection with *Toxoplasma* can be reduced by not eating undercooked meat and by avoiding oocyst-contaminated material (i.e., a cat's litter box). Specifically, lamb, beef, and pork should be cooked to an internal temperature of 165° to 170°F; from a more practical perspective, meat cooked until it is no longer pink inside usually satisfies this requirement. Hands should be washed thoroughly after work in the garden, and all fruits and vegetables should be washed. If the patient owns a cat, the litter box should be cleaned or changed daily, preferably by an HIV-negative, nonpregnant person; alternatively, patients should wash their hands thoroughly after changing the litter box. Patients should be encouraged to keep their cats inside and not to adopt or handle stray cats. Cats should be fed only canned or dried commercial food or well-cooked table food, not raw or undercooked meats. Patients need not be advised to part with their cats or to have their cats tested for toxoplasmosis. Blood intended for transfusion into *Toxoplasma*-seronegative immunocompromised individuals should be screened for antibody to *T. gondii*. Although such serologic screening is not routinely performed, seronegative women should be screened for evidence of infection several times during pregnancy if they are exposed to environmental conditions that put them at risk for infection with *T. gondii*. HIV-positive individuals should adhere closely to these preventive measures.

FURTHER READING

DWORKIN MS et al: Risk for preventable opportunistic infections in persons with AIDS after antiretroviral therapy increases CD4+ T lymphocyte counts above prophylaxis thresholds. J Infect Dis 182:611, 2000

FOULON W et al: Treatment of toxoplasmosis during pregnancy. Am J Obstet Gynecol 180:410, 1999

FURRER H et al: Stopping primary prophylaxis in HIV-1-infected patients at high risk of *toxoplasma* encephalitis. Swiss HIV Cohort Study (letter). Lancet 355:2217, 2000

MASUR H et al: Guidelines for preventing opportunistic infections among HIV-infected persons—2002. Ann Intern Med 137:435, 2002

MUSSINI C et al: Discontinuation of primary prophylaxis for *Pneumocystis carinii* pneumonia and toxoplasmic encephalitis in human immunodeficiency virus type I–infected patients: The Changes in Opportunistic Prophylaxis Study. J Infect Dis 181:1635, 2000

VILLENA I et al: Pyrimethamine-sulfadoxine treatment of congenital toxoplasmosis. Scand J Infect Dis 30:295, 1999

199   PROTOZOAL INTESTINAL INFECTIONS AND TRICHOMONIASIS
Peter F. Weller

PROTOZOAL INFECTIONS

GIARDIASIS   *Giardia lamblia* (also known as *G. intestinalis*) is a cosmopolitan protozoal parasite that inhabits the small intestines of humans and other mammals. Giardiasis is one of the most common parasitic diseases worldwide and causes both endemic and epidemic intestinal disease and diarrhea.

Life Cycle and Epidemiology (Fig. 199-1)   Infection follows the ingestion of the environmentally hardy cysts, which excyst in the small intestine, releasing flagellated trophozoites (Fig. 199-2) that multiply by binary fission. *Giardia* remains a pathogen of the proximal small bowel and does not disseminate hematogenously. Trophozoites remain free in the lumen or attach to the mucosal epithelium by means of a ventral sucking disk. As a trophozoite encounters altered conditions, it forms a morphologically distinct cyst, which is the stage of the parasite usually found in the feces. Trophozoites may be present and even predominate in loose or watery stools, but it is the resistant cyst that survives outside the body and is responsible for transmission. Cysts do not tolerate heating, desiccation, or continued exposure to feces but do remain viable for months in cold fresh water. The number of cysts excreted varies widely but can approach 10^7 per gram of stool.

Giardia infections are common in both developed and developing countries. Ingestion of as few as 10 cysts is sufficient to cause infection in humans. Because cysts are infectious when excreted or shortly thereafter, person-to-person transmission occurs where fecal hygiene is poor. Giardiasis, as a symptomatic or an asymptomatic infection, is especially prevalent in day-care centers; person-to-person spread also takes place in other institutional settings with poor fecal hygiene and during anal-oral contact. If food is contaminated with *Giardia* cysts after cooking or preparation, food-borne transmission can occur. Wa-

Excystation follows exposure to stomach acid and intestinal proteases releasing trophozoite forms that multiply by binary fission and reside in the upper small bowel adherent to enterocytes

Causes: Asymptomatic infection, acute diarrhea, or chronic diarrhea and malabsorption
Small bowel may demonstrate villous blunting, crypt hypertrophy, and mucosal inflammation

Encystation occurs under conditions of bile salt concentration changes and alkaline pH
Smooth-walled cysts can contain two trophozoites

Cysts ingested (≥10–25 cysts) in contaminated water or food or by direct fecal-oral transmission (as in day-care centers)

Cysts and trophozoites passed in the stool into the environment

Cysts can survive in the environment (up to several weeks in cold water)
May also infect non-human mammalian species

FIGURE 199-1   Life cycle of *Giardia*. (*Reprinted from RL Guerrant et al: Essentials of Tropical Infectious Diseases, 2001, p 330, with permission from Elsevier Science.*)

terborne transmission accounts for episodic infections (e.g., in campers and other travelers) and for massive epidemics in metropolitan areas. Surface water, ranging from mountain streams to large municipal reservoirs, can become contaminated with fecally derived *Giardia* cysts; outmoded water systems are subject to cross-contamination from leaking sewer lines. The efficacy of water as a means of transmission is enhanced by the small infectious inoculum of *Giardia*, the prolonged

FIGURE 199-2   Flagellated, binucleate *Giardia* trophozoite.

survival of cysts in cold water, and the resistance of cysts to killing by routine chlorination methods that are adequate for controlling bacteria. Viable cysts can be eradicated from water by either boiling or filtration. In the United States, *Giardia* is a common agent identified in waterborne epidemics of gastroenteritis; it is also common in developing countries.

The importance of animal reservoirs as sources of infection for humans is unclear. *Giardia* parasites morphologically similar to those in humans are found in a large number of mammals, including beavers from reservoirs implicated in epidemics, dogs, cats, and ruminants.

Giardiasis, like cryptosporidiosis (see below), creates a significant economic burden because of the costs incurred in the installation of water filtration systems required to prevent waterborne epidemics, in the management of epidemics that involve large communities, and in the evaluation and treatment of endemic infections.

Pathophysiology   The reasons that some, but not all, infected patients develop clinical manifestations and the mechanisms by which *Giardia* causes alterations in small-bowel function are largely unknown. Although trophozoites adhere to the epithelium, they do not cause invasive or locally destructive alterations. The lactose intolerance and significant malabsorption that develop in a minority of infected adults and children are clinical signs of the loss of brush border enzyme activities. In most infections the morphology of the bowel is unaltered, but in a few cases—usually in chronically infected, symptomatic patients—the histopathologic findings (including flattened villi) and the clinical manifestations resemble those of tropical sprue and gluten-sensitive enteropathy. The pathogenesis of diarrhea in giardiasis is not known.

The natural history of *Giardia* infection varies markedly. Infections may be aborted, transient, recurrent, or chronic. Parasite as well as host factors may be important in determining the course of infection and disease. Both cellular and humoral responses develop in human infections, but their precise roles in the control of infection and/or disease are unknown. Because patients with hypogammaglobulinemia commonly suffer from prolonged, severe infections that are poorly responsive to treatment, humoral immune responses appear to be important. The greater susceptibility of the young than of the old and of newly exposed persons than of chronically exposed populations also suggests that at least partial protective immunity may develop. Although no strains of the parasite that are clearly nonpathogenic have been identified, *Giardia* isolates vary genotypically, biochemically, and biologically. The marked biochemical differences among some isolates may help account for the different courses of infection in experimentally infected humans and animals.

Clinical Manifestations   Disease manifestations of giardiasis range from asymptomatic carriage to fulminant diarrhea and malabsorption. Most infected persons are asymptomatic, but in epidemics the proportion of symptomatic cases may be higher. Symptoms may develop suddenly or gradually. In persons with acute giardiasis, symptoms develop after an incubation period that lasts at least 5 to 6 days and usually 1 to 3 weeks. Prominent early symptoms include diarrhea, abdominal pain, bloating, belching, flatus, nausea, and vomiting. Although diarrhea is common, upper intestinal manifestations such as nausea, vomiting, bloating, and abdominal pain may predominate. The duration of acute giardiasis is usually >1 week, although diarrhea often subsides. Individuals with chronic giardiasis may present with or without having experienced an antecedent acute symptomatic episode. Diarrhea is not necessarily prominent, but increased flatus, loose stools, sulfurous burping, and (in some instances) weight loss occur. Symptoms may be continual or episodic and can persist for years. Some persons who have relatively mild symptoms for long periods recognize the extent of their discomfort only in retrospect. Fever, the presence of blood and/or mucus in the stools, and other signs and symptoms of colitis are uncommon and suggest a different diagnosis or a concomitant illness. Symptoms tend to be intermittent yet recurring and gradually debilitating, in contrast with the acute disabling symptoms associated with many enteric bacterial infections. Because of the less severe illness and the propensity for chronic infections, patients may seek medical advice late in the course of the illness; however, disease can be severe, resulting in malabsorption, weight loss, growth retardation, dehydration, and (in rare cases) death. A number of extraintestinal manifestations have been described, such as urticaria, anterior uveitis, and arthritis; whether these are caused by giardiasis or concomitant processes is unclear.

Giardiasis can be life-threatening in patients with hypogammaglobulinemia and is typically difficult to treat and eradicate. *Giardia* infections can complicate other preexisting intestinal diseases, such as cystic fibrosis. Although *Giardia* can cause enteric illness in patients with AIDS, neither the course of infection nor the response to treatment differs for patients with and without AIDS.

Diagnosis   Giardiasis is diagnosed by the detection of parasite antigen in the feces or by the identification of cysts in the feces or of trophozoites in the feces or small intestines. Cysts are oval, measure 8 to 12 μm $\times$ 7 to 10 μm, and characteristically contain four nuclei. Trophozoites are pear-shaped, dorsally convex, flattened parasites with two nuclei and four pairs of flagella. The diagnosis is sometimes difficult to establish. Direct examination of fresh or properly preserved stools as well as concentration methods should be used. Because cyst excretion is variable and may be undetectable at times, repeated examination of stool, sampling of duodenal fluid, and biopsy of the small intestine may be required to detect the parasite. Tests for parasitic antigen in stool are at least as sensitive and specific as good microscopic examinations and are easier to perform. All of these methods occasionally yield false-negative results.

R_x TREATMENT

Cure rates with metronidazole (250 mg thrice daily for 5 days) are usually >90%. Alternatively, quinacrine (100 mg thrice daily for 5 days) is effective but is available from only a limited number of compounding pharmacies. Tinidazole, which is not available in the United States, is more effective than metronidazole or quinacrine. Furazolidone (6 mg/kg daily in four doses for 7 to 10 days) is used principally for children because it is available as a palatable elixir that is not bitter. Nitazoxanide, currently available in the United States as an oral suspension, is approved by the U.S. Food and Drug Administration (FDA) for the treatment of giardiasis in children. Paromomycin, an oral aminoglycoside that is not well absorbed, can be given to symptomatic pregnant patients, although information is limited on how effectively this agent eradicates infection.

Patients in whom initial treatment fails can be re-treated with a longer course. Almost all patients respond to therapy and are cured, although some with chronic giardiasis experience delayed resolution of symptoms after eradication of *Giardia*. Those who remain infected after repeated treatments should be evaluated for reinfection through family members, close personal contacts, and environmental sources as well as for hypogammaglobulinemia. In cases refractory to multiple treatment courses, prolonged therapy with metronidazole (750 mg thrice daily for 21 days), alone or in combination with quinacrine, has been successful. When children attending day-care centers infect an entire family, treatment of all infected family members, including asymptomatic carriers, may be required to prevent reinfection.

Prevention   Although *Giardia* is extremely infectious, disease can be prevented by the exclusive consumption of noncontaminated food and water. Cooking food adequately and boiling or filtering potentially contaminated water prevent infection.

CRYPTOSPORIDIOSIS   The coccidian parasite *Cryptosporidium* causes diarrheal disease that is self-limited in immunocompetent human hosts but can be severe in persons with AIDS or other forms of immunodeficiency. Two distinct genotypes of *Cryptosporidium parvum* cause most human infections, although other *Cryptosporidium* species have been identified in immunocompromised patients.

Life Cycle and Epidemiology   Cryptosporidiosis is acquired by the consumption of oocysts (50% infectious dose: ~132 oocysts in nonimmune individuals), which excyst to liberate sporozoites that in turn enter and infect intestinal epithelial cells. The parasite's further development involves both asexual and sexual cycles, which produce forms capable of infecting other epithelial cells and of generating oocysts that are passed in the feces. *Cryptosporidium* species infect a number of animals and can spread from infected animals to humans. Since oocysts are immediately infectious when passed in feces, person-to-person transmission takes place in child day-care centers and among household contacts and medical providers. Waterborne transmission accounts for infections in travelers and for common-source epidemics. Oocysts are quite hardy and resist killing by routine chlorination. Both drinking water and recreational water (e.g., pools, waterslides) have been increasingly recognized as sources of infection.

Pathophysiology   Although intestinal epithelial cells harbor the parasite in an intracellular vacuole, the means by which secretory diarrhea is elicited remain uncertain. No characteristic pathologic changes are found by biopsy. The distribution of infection can be spotty within the principal site of infection, the small bowel. Cryptosporidia are found in some patients in the pharynx, stomach, and large bowel and at times in the respiratory tract. Especially in patients with AIDS, involvement of the biliary tract can cause papillary stenosis, sclerosing cholangitis, or cholecystitis.

Clinical Manifestations   Asymptomatic infections can occur in both immunocompetent and immunocompromised hosts. In immunocompetent persons, symptoms develop after an incubation period of about a week and consist principally of watery nonbloody diarrhea, sometimes in conjunction with abdominal pain, nausea, anorexia, fever, and/or weight loss. In these hosts, the illness usually subsides after 1 to 2 weeks, whereas in immunocompromised hosts, especially those with AIDS and CD4+ cell counts <100/μL, diarrhea can be chronic, persistent, and remarkably profuse, causing clinically significant fluid and electrolyte depletion. Stool volumes may range from 1 to 25 L/d. Weight loss, wasting, and abdominal pain may be severe. Biliary tract involvement can manifest as midepigastric or right upper quadrant pain.

Diagnosis   Evaluation usually starts with fecal examination for small oocysts, which are 4 to 5 μm in diameter and are smaller than the fecal stages of most other parasites. Because conventional stool examination for ova and parasites will not detect *Cryptosporidium*, specific testing must be requested. Detection is enhanced by evaluation of stools (obtained on multiple days) by several techniques, including modified acid-fast and direct immunofluorescent stains and enzyme immunoassays. Cryptosporidia also can be identified by light and electron microscopy at the apical surfaces of intestinal epithelium from biopsy specimens of the small bowel and, less frequently, the large bowel.

R_x TREATMENT

Until recently, no chemotherapeutic agents effective against *Cryptosporidium* had been identified, although paromomycin (500 to 750 mg four times daily) was thought to be partially effective for some patients infected with HIV. Nitazoxanide, currently available in the United States as an oral suspension, is FDA-approved for the treatment of cryptosporidiosis in children. In addition, improvement in immune status with antiretroviral therapy often leads to amelioration of cryptosporidiosis. Otherwise, treatment includes supportive care with replacement of fluids and electrolytes and administration of antidiarrheal agents. Biliary tract obstruction may require papillotomy or T-tube placement. Prevention requires minimizing exposure to infectious oocysts in human or animal feces. Use of submicron water filters may minimize acquisition of infection from drinking water.

ISOSPORIASIS The coccidian parasite *Isospora belli* causes human intestinal disease. Infection is acquired by the consumption of oocysts, after which the parasite invades intestinal epithelial cells and undergoes both sexual and asexual cycles of development. Oocysts excreted in stool are not immediately infectious but must undergo further maturation. Although *I. belli* infects many animals, little is known about the epidemiology or prevalence of this parasite in humans. It appears to be most common in tropical and subtropical countries. Acute infections can begin abruptly with fever, abdominal pain, and watery nonbloody diarrhea and can last for weeks or months. In patients who have AIDS or are immunocompromised for other reasons, infections often are not self-limited but rather resemble cryptosporidiosis, with chronic, profuse watery diarrhea. Eosinophilia, which is not found in other enteric protozoan infections, may be detectable. The diagnosis is usually made by detection of the large (~25-μm) oocysts in stool by modified acid-fast staining. Oocyst excretion may be low-level and intermittent; if repeated stool examinations are unrevealing, sampling of duodenal contents by aspiration or small-bowel biopsy (often with electron-microscopic examination) may be necessary.

℞ **TREATMENT**

In contrast to cryptosporidiosis, isosporiasis responds to chemotherapy. Trimethoprim-sulfamethoxazole (160/800 mg four times daily for 10 days and then three times daily for 3 weeks) has been effective; for patients intolerant of sulfonamides, pyrimethamine (50 to 75 mg/d) or ciprofloxacin (500 mg twice daily for 7 days) can be used. Relapses can occur in persons with AIDS and necessitate maintenance therapy with trimethoprim-sulfamethoxazole (160/800 mg three times a week) or combined sulfadoxine (500 mg) and pyrimethamine (25 mg) once weekly.

CYCLOSPORIASIS Coccidian parasites of the genus *Cyclospora* have been identified as the causative organisms in diarrheal illness formerly ascribed to blue-green algae or *Cyanobacteria*-like forms. This parasite is globally distributed: illness due to *Cyclospora cayetanensis* has been reported in the United States, Asia, Africa, Latin America, and Europe. The epidemiology of this parasite has not yet been fully defined, but waterborne transmission and food-borne transmission by basil and imported raspberries have been recognized. The full spectrum of illness attributable to *Cyclospora* has not been delineated. Some patients may harbor the infection without symptoms, but many with cyclosporiasis have diarrhea, flulike symptoms, and flatulence and burping. The illness can be self-limited, can wax and wane, or (in many cases) can involve prolonged diarrhea, anorexia, and upper gastrointestinal symptoms, with sustained fatigue and weight loss in some instances. Diarrheal illness may persist for longer than a month. *Cyclospora* can cause enteric illness in patients infected with HIV, albeit at an unknown frequency.

The parasite is detectable in epithelial cells of small-bowel biopsy samples and elicits secretory diarrhea by an unknown means. The absence of fecal blood and leukocytes indicates that disease due to *Cyclospora* is not caused by destruction of the small-bowel mucosa. The diagnosis can be made by detection of spherical 8- to 10-μm oocysts in the stool, although routine stool O and P examinations are not sufficient. Specific fecal examinations must be requested to detect the oocysts, which are variably acid-fast and are fluorescent when viewed with ultraviolet light microscopy. Cyclosporiasis should be considered in the differential diagnosis of prolonged diarrhea, with or without a history of travel by the patient to other countries.

℞ **TREATMENT**

Cyclosporiasis is effectively treated with trimethoprim-sulfamethoxazole (160/800 mg twice daily for 7 days). For patients intolerant of sulfonamides, ciprofloxacin (500 mg twice daily for 7 days) may be used. Patients infected with HIV, however, may experience relapses after such treatment and thus may require longer-term suppressive maintenance therapy.

MICROSPORIDIOSIS Microsporidia are obligate intracellular spore-forming protozoa that infect many animals and cause disease in humans, especially as opportunistic pathogens in AIDS. Microsporidia are members of a distinct phylum, Microspora, which contains dozens of genera and hundreds of species. The various microsporidia are differentiated by their developmental life cycles, by ultrastructural features, and by molecular taxonomy based on ribosomal RNA. The complex life cycles of the organisms result in the production of infectious spores. Currently, seven genera of microsporidia—*Encephalitozoon*, *Pleistophora*, *Nosema*, *Vittaforma*, *Trachipleistophora*, *Brachiola*, and *Enterocytozoon*—are recognized as causes of human disease; an eighth genus—*Microsporidium*, which includes organisms of uncertain taxonomic status—also causes disease in humans. Although some microsporidia are probably prevalent causes of self-limited or asymptomatic infections in immunocompetent patients, little is known of how microsporidiosis is acquired.

Microsporidiosis is most common among patients with AIDS, less common among patients with other types of immunocompromise, and rare among immunocompetent hosts. In patients with AIDS, intestinal infections with *Enterocytozoon bieneusi* and *Encephalitozoon* (formerly *Septata*) *intestinalis* are increasingly recognized to contribute to chronic diarrhea and wasting; these infections are found in 10 to 40% of patients with chronic diarrhea. Both organisms have been found in the biliary tracts of patients with cholecystitis. *E. intestinalis* may also disseminate to cause fever, diarrhea, sinusitis, cholangitis, and bronchiolitis. In patients with AIDS, *Encephalitozoon hellem* has caused superficial keratoconjunctivitis as well as sinusitis, respiratory tract disease, and disseminated infection. Myositis due to *Pleistophora* has been documented. *Nosema*, *Vittaforma*, and *Microsporidium* have caused stromal keratitis associated with trauma in immunocompetent patients.

Microsporidia are small gram-positive organisms with mature spores measuring 0.5 to 2 μm $\times$ 1 to 4 μm. Diagnosis of microsporidial infections in tissue often requires electron microscopy, although intracellular spores can be visualized by light microscopy with hematoxylin and eosin, Giemsa, or tissue Gram's stains. For the diagnosis of intestinal microsporidiosis, modified trichrome or chromotrope 2R-based staining and Uvitex 2B or calcofluor fluorescent staining reveal spores in smears of feces or duodenal aspirates. Definitive therapies for microsporidial infections remain to be established. For superficial keratoconjunctivitis due to *E. hellem*, topical therapy with fumagillin suspension has shown promise (Chap. 193). For enteric infections with *E. bieneusi* and *E. intestinalis* in HIV-infected patients, therapy with albendazole may be efficacious (Chap. 193).

OTHER INTESTINAL PROTOZOA ■ **Balantidiasis** *Balantidium coli* is a large ciliated protozoal parasite that can produce a spectrum of large-intestinal disease analogous to amebiasis. The parasite is widely distributed in the world. Since it infects pigs, cases in humans are more common where pigs are raised; in Muslim countries, rodents may be important carriers. Infective cysts can be transmitted from person to person and through water, but many cases are due to the ingestion of cysts derived from porcine feces in association with slaughtering, with use of pig feces for fertilizer, or with contamination of water supplies by pig feces.

Ingested cysts liberate trophozoites, which reside and replicate in the large bowel. Many patients remain asymptomatic, but some have persisting intermittent diarrhea, and a few develop more fulminant dysentery. In symptomatic individuals, the pathology in the bowel—both gross and microscopic—is similar to that seen in amebiasis, with varying degrees of mucosal invasion, focal necrosis, and ulceration. Balantidiasis, unlike amebiasis, does not spread hematogenously to other organs. The diagnosis is usually made by detection of the trophozoite stage in stool or sampled colonic tissue. Tetracycline (500 mg four times daily for 10 days) is an effective therapeutic agent.

***Blastocystis hominis* Infection** *B. hominis*, long considered a nonpathogenic yeast, is believed by some to be a protozoan capable of causing intestinal disease, although its taxonomy and inherent pathogenicity remain uncertain. Some patients who pass *B. hominis* in their stools are asymptomatic, whereas others have diarrhea and associated intestinal symptoms. Diligent evaluation reveals other potential bacterial, viral, or protozoal causes of diarrhea in some but not all patients with symptoms. Because the pathogenicity of *B. hominis* is uncertain and because therapy for *Blastocystis* infection is neither specific nor uniformly effective, patients with prominent intestinal symptoms should be fully evaluated for other infectious causes of diarrhea. If diarrheal symptoms associated with *Blastocystis* are prominent, either metronidazole (750 mg thrice daily for 10 days) or iodoquinol (650 mg thrice daily for 20 days) can be used.

***Dientamoeba fragilis* Infection**   *D. fragilis* is unique among intestinal protozoa in that it has a trophozoite stage but not a cyst stage. How trophozoites survive to transmit infection is not known, but the unusually high prevalence of *D. fragilis* infection among persons with pinworm infection raises the possibility that eggs or larvae of *Enterobius* facilitate the transmission of *D. fragilis*. When symptoms develop in patients with *D. fragilis* infection, they are generally mild and include intermittent diarrhea, abdominal pain, and anorexia. The diagnosis is made by the detection of trophozoites in stool; the lability of these forms accounts for the greater yield when fecal samples are preserved immediately after collection. Since fecal excretion rates vary, examination of several samples obtained on alternate days increases the rate of detection. Iodoquinol (650 mg three times daily for 20 days), paromomycin (25 to 30 mg/kg per day in three doses for 7 days), metronidazole (500 to 750 mg three times daily for 10 days), or tetracycline (500 mg four times daily for 10 days) is appropriate for treatment.

Sarcosporidiosis   Various *Sarcocystis* species of coccidian parasites are widely distributed agents of infection in numerous animals. These parasites have an obligatory cycle of development involving two hosts. Sexual reproduction occurs in the intestine, with sporocysts passed in the feces; asexual multiplication leads to the development of muscle cysts. Humans can develop intestinal infections—although they apparently do so infrequently—by ingesting muscle-stage cysts in undercooked pork or beef. While the full spectrum of the intestinal disease is not defined, a diarrheal illness can ensue, and sporocysts are found in the stool. Alternatively, ingestion of fecally derived sporocysts can lead to the development of cysts in striated or cardiac muscle. Some patients experience muscle pain and swelling, but the frequency and nature of symptoms elicited by muscle involvement are not clear, and these cysts, measuring 100 to 325 μm, also have been found incidentally in muscle specimens. Muscle-stage infections are not followed by further spread in humans. No specific therapy exists for either intestinal or muscle-stage *Sarcocystis* infections in humans.

TRICHOMONIASIS

Various species of trichomonads can be found in the mouth (in association with periodontitis) and occasionally in the gastrointestinal tract. *Trichomonas vaginalis*—one of the most prevalent protozoal parasites in the United States—is a pathogen of the genitourinary tract and a major cause of symptomatic vaginitis.

Life Cycle and Epidemiology   *T. vaginalis* is a pear-shaped, actively motile organism that measures about 10 by 7 μm, replicates by binary fission, and inhabits the lower genital tract of females and the urethra and prostate of males. In the United States, it accounts for ~3 million infections per year in women. While the organism can survive for a few hours in moist environments and could be acquired by direct contact, person-to-person venereal transmission accounts for virtually all cases of trichomoniasis. Its prevalence is greatest among persons with multiple sexual partners and among those with other sexually transmitted diseases (Chap. 115).

Clinical Manifestations   Most men infected with *T. vaginalis* are asymptomatic, although some develop urethritis and a few have epididymitis or prostatitis. In contrast, infection in women, which has an incubation period of 5 to 28 days, is usually symptomatic and manifests with malodorous vaginal discharge (often yellow), vulvar erythema and itching, dysuria or urinary frequency (in 30 to 50% of patients), and dyspareunia. These manifestations, however, do not clearly distinguish trichomoniasis from other types of infectious vaginitis.

Diagnosis   Detection of motile trichomonads by microscopy of wet mounts of vaginal or prostatic secretions has been the conventional means of diagnosis. Although such microscopy provides an immediate diagnosis, its sensitivity for the detection of *T. vaginalis* is only ~50 to 60% in routine evaluations of vaginal secretions. Direct immunofluorescent antibody staining is more sensitive (70 to 90%) than wet-mount examinations. *T. vaginalis* can be recovered from the urethra of both males and females and is detectable in males after prostatic massage. Culture of the parasite is the most sensitive means of detection; however, the facilities for culture are not generally available, and detection of the organism takes 3 to 7 days.

R̶x̶ TREATMENT

Metronidazole is the mainstay of treatment and may be given either as a single 2-g dose or as 500 mg twice daily for 7 days. Tinidazole (a single 2-g dose or 500 mg twice daily) is also effective but is not available in the United States. All sexual partners must be treated concurrently to prevent reinfection, especially from asymptomatic males. In males with persistent symptomatic urethritis after therapy for nongonococcal urethritis, metronidazole therapy should be considered for possible trichomoniasis. Alternatives to metronidazole for treatment during pregnancy are not readily available, although use of 100-mg clotrimazole vaginal suppositories nightly for 2 weeks may cure some infections in pregnant women. Reinfection often accounts for apparent treatment failures, but strains of *T. vaginalis* exhibiting high-level resistance to metronidazole have been encountered. Treatment of these resistant infections with higher oral doses, parenteral doses, or concurrent oral and vaginal doses of metronidazole has been successful.

FURTHER READING

CHEX XM et al: Cryptosporidiosis. N Engl J Med 346:1723, 2002

FURNESS BW et al: Giardiasis surveillance—United States, 1992–1997. MMWR Surveill Summ 49(SS-07):1, 2000

GARNER TB, HILL DR: Treatment of giardiasis. Clin Microbiol Rev 14:114, 2001

HO AY et al: Outbreak of cyclosporiasis associated with imported raspberries, Philadelphia, Pennsylvania, 2000. Emerg Infect Dis 8:783, 2002

KAPLAN JE et al: Guidelines for preventing opportunistic infections among HIV-infected persons—2002. Recommendations of the U.S. Public Health Service and the Infectious Diseases Society of America, MMWR Recomm Rep 51(RR-8):1, 2002

LEE SH et al: Surveillance for waterborne-disease outbreaks—United States, 1999–2000. MMWR Surveill Summ 51(SS-8):1, 2002

NASH TE et al: Treatment of patients with refractory giardiasis. Clin Infect Dis 33:22, 2001

VERDIER RI et al: Trimethoprim-sulfamethoxazole compared with ciprofloxacin for treatment and prophylaxis of *Isospora belli* and *Cyclospora cayetanensis* infection in HIV-infected patients. A randomized, controlled trial. Ann Intern Med 132:885, 2000

200 | TRICHINELLA AND OTHER TISSUE NEMATODES
Peter F. Weller

Nematodes are elongated, symmetric roundworms. Parasitic nematodes of medical significance may be broadly classified as either predominantly intestinal or tissue nematodes. This chapter covers trichinellosis, visceral and ocular larva migrans, cutaneous larva migrans, cerebral angiostrongyliasis, and gnathostomiasis. All are zoonotic infections caused by incidental exposure to infectious nematodes. The clinical symptoms of these infections are due largely to invasive larval stages that (except in the case of *Trichinella*) do not reach maturity in humans.

TRICHINELLOSIS   Trichinellosis develops after the ingestion of meat containing cysts of *Trichinella*—for example, pork or other meat from a carnivore. Although most infections are mild and asymptomatic, heavy infections can cause severe enteritis, periorbital edema, myositis, and (infrequently) death.

Life Cycle and Epidemiology   Seven species of *Trichinella* are now recognized as causes of infection in humans. Two species are distributed worldwide: *T. spiralis*, which is found in a great variety of carnivorous and omnivorous animals, and *T. pseudospiralis*, which is found in mammals and birds. *T. nativa* is present in Arctic regions and infects bears; *T. nelsoni* is found in equatorial Africa, where it is common among felid predators and scavengers such as hyenas and bush pigs; and *T. britovi* is found in temperate areas of Europe and western Asia among carnivores but not among domestic swine. *T. murrelli* is present in North American game animals, and *T. papuae* is found in pigs and game animals in Papua New Guinea.

After the consumption of trichinous meat by the host, encysted larvae are liberated by digestive acid and pepsin (Fig. 200-1). The larvae invade the small-bowel mucosa and mature rapidly into adult worms. After ~1 week, female worms release newborn larvae that migrate via the circulation to striated muscle. The larvae of all species except *T. pseudospiralis* and *T. papuae* then encyst by inducing a radical transformation in the muscle cell architecture. Although host immune responses may help to expel adult worms, they have little effect on muscle-dwelling larvae.

Human trichinellosis is most often caused by the ingestion of infected pork products and thus can occur in almost any location where the meat of domestic or wild swine is eaten. Human trichinellosis also may be acquired from the meat of other animals, including dogs (in parts of Asia and Africa), horses (in Italy and France), and bears and walruses (in northern regions). Although cattle (being herbivores) are not natural hosts of *Trichinella*, beef has been implicated in outbreaks when contaminated or adulterated with trichinous pork. Laws that prohibit the feeding of uncooked garbage to pigs have greatly reduced the transmission of trichinellosis in the United States. About 40 cases of trichinellosis are reported annually in this country, but most mild cases probably remain undiagnosed. Recent U.S. outbreaks have been attributable to undercooked ethnic pork dishes, homemade and commercial sausage, wild boar meat, and walrus meat.

Pathogenesis and Clinical Features   Clinical symptoms of trichinellosis arise from the successive phases of parasite enteric invasion, larval migration, and muscle encystment (Fig. 200-1). Most light infections (those with <10 larvae per gram of muscle) are asymptomatic, whereas heavy infections (which can involve >50 larvae per gram of muscle) can be life-threatening. Invasion of the gut by large numbers of parasites occasionally provokes diarrhea during the first week after infection. Abdominal pain, constipation, nausea, or vomiting also may be prominent.

Symptoms due to larval migration and muscle invasion begin to appear in the second week after infection. The migrating *Trichinella* larvae provoke a marked local and systemic hypersensitivity reaction, with fever and hypereosinophilia. Periorbital and facial edema is common, as are hemorrhages in the subconjunctivae, retina, and nail beds ("splinter" hemorrhages). A maculopapular rash, headache, cough, dyspnea, or dysphagia sometimes develops. Myocarditis with tachyarrhythmias or heart failure—and, less commonly, encephalitis or pneumonitis—may develop and accounts for most deaths of patients with trichinellosis.

Upon onset of larval encystment in muscle 2 to 3 weeks after in-

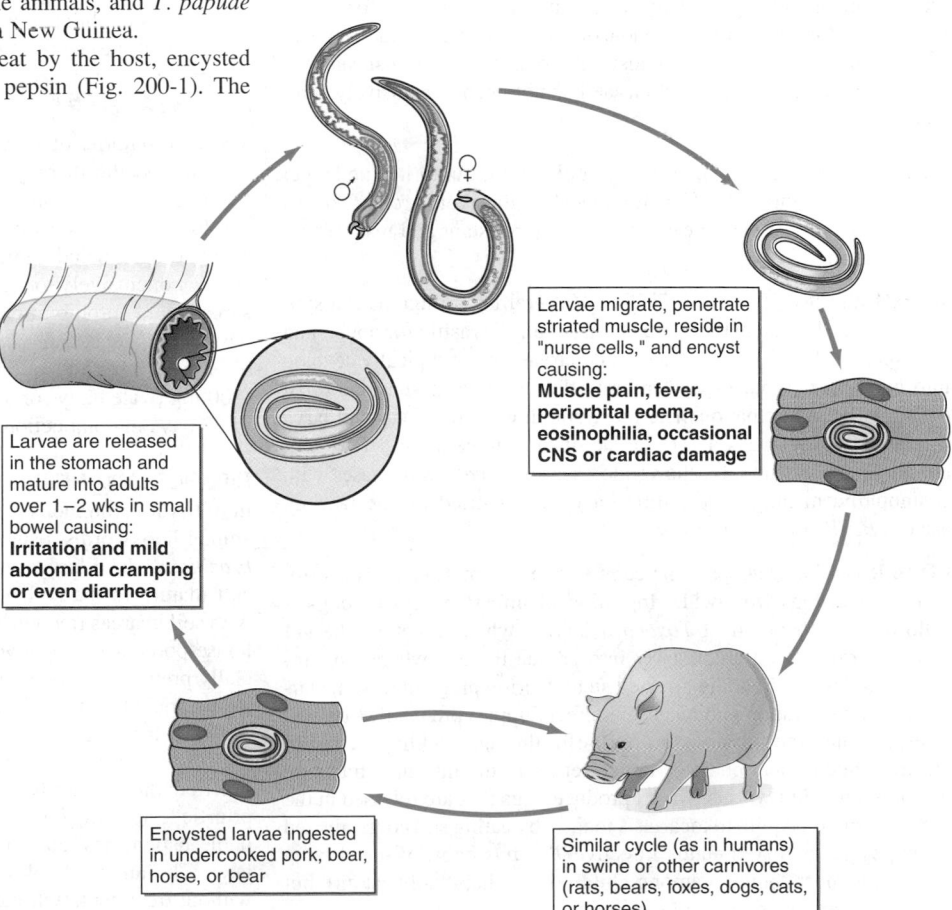

Larvae migrate, penetrate striated muscle, reside in "nurse cells," and encyst causing:
Muscle pain, fever, periorbital edema, eosinophilia, occasional CNS or cardiac damage

Larvae are released in the stomach and mature into adults over 1–2 wks in small bowel causing:
Irritation and mild abdominal cramping or even diarrhea

Encysted larvae ingested in undercooked pork, boar, horse, or bear

Similar cycle (as in humans) in swine or other carnivores (rats, bears, foxes, dogs, cats, or horses)

FIGURE 200-1   Life cycle of *Trichinella spiralis* (cosmopolitan); *nelsoni* (Africa); *britovi* (S. Europe); *nativa* (Arctic); and *pseudospiralis* (New Zealand). (*Reprinted from Guerrant RL et al: Essentials of Tropical Infectious Diseases, p 434. © 2001, with permission from Elsevier Science.*)

fection, symptoms of myositis with myalgias, muscle edema, and weakness develop, usually overlapping with the inflammatory reactions to migrating larvae. The most commonly involved muscle groups include the extraocular muscles; the biceps; and the muscles of the jaw, neck, lower back, and diaphragm. Peaking ~3 weeks after infection, symptoms subside only gradually during a prolonged convalescence.

Laboratory Findings and Diagnosis   Blood eosinophilia develops in >90% of patients with symptomatic trichinellosis and may peak at a level of >50% between 2 and 4 weeks after infection. Serum levels of IgE and muscle enzymes, including creatine phosphokinase, are elevated in most symptomatic patients. Patients should be questioned thoroughly about their consumption of pork or wild-animal meat and about illness in other individuals who ate the same meat. A presumptive clinical diagnosis can be based on fevers, eosinophilia, periorbital edema, and myalgias after a suspect meal. A rise in the titer of parasite-specific antibody, which usually does not occur until after the third week of infection, confirms the diagnosis. Alternatively, a definitive diagnosis requires surgical biopsy of at least 1 g of involved muscle; the yields are highest near tendon insertions. The fresh muscle tissue should be compressed between glass slides and examined microscopically, because larvae may be overlooked by examination of routine histopathologic sections alone.

℞ TREATMENT

Current anthelmintic drugs are ineffective against *Trichinella* larvae in muscle. Fortunately, most lightly infected patients recover uneventfully with bed rest, antipyretics, and analgesics. Glucocorticoids like prednisone (1 mg/kg daily for 5 days) are beneficial for severe myositis and myocarditis. Mebendazole and albendazole, like thiabendazole, appear to be active against enteric stages of the parasite, but their efficacy against encysted larvae has not been conclusively demonstrated.

Prevention   Larvae may be killed by cooking pork until it is no longer pink or by freezing it at −15°C for 3 weeks. However, Arctic *T. nativa* larvae in walrus or bear meat are relatively resistant and may remain viable despite freezing.

VISCERAL AND OCULAR LARVA MIGRANS   Visceral larva migrans is a syndrome caused by nematodes that are normally parasitic for nonhuman host species. In humans, the nematode larvae do not typically develop into adult worms but instead migrate through host tissues and elicit eosinophilic inflammation. The most common form of visceral larva migrans is toxocariasis due to larvae of the canine ascarid *Toxocara canis* or, less commonly, the feline ascarid *T. cati*. Rare cases with eosinophilic meningoencephalitis have been caused by the raccoon ascarid *Baylisascaris procyonis*.

Life Cycle and Epidemiology   The canine roundworm *T. canis* is distributed among dogs worldwide. Ingestion of infective eggs by dogs is followed by liberation of *Toxocara* larvae, which penetrate the gut wall and migrate intravascularly into canine tissues, where most remain in a developmentally arrested state. During pregnancy, some larvae resume migration in bitches and infect puppies prenatally (through transplacental transmission) or after birth (through suckling). Thus, in lactating bitches and puppies, larvae return to the intestinal tract and develop into adult worms, which produce eggs that are released in the feces. Humans acquire toxocariasis mainly by eating soil contaminated by puppy feces that contains infective *T. canis* eggs. Visceral larva migrans is most common among children who habitually eat dirt, but most toxocaral infections are subclinical.

Pathogenesis and Clinical Features   Clinical disease most commonly afflicts preschool children. After humans ingest *Toxocara* eggs, the larvae hatch and penetrate the intestinal mucosa, from which they are carried by the circulation to a wide variety of organs and tissues. The larvae invade the liver, lungs, central nervous system, and other sites, releasing toxic products and provoking intense local eosinophilic granulomatous responses. The degree of clinical illness depends on larval number and tissue distribution, reinfection, and host immune responses. Most light infections are asymptomatic and may be manifest only by blood eosinophilia. Characteristic symptoms of visceral larva migrans include fever, malaise, anorexia and weight loss, cough, wheezing, and rashes. Hepatosplenomegaly is common. These features are often accompanied by extraordinary peripheral eosinophilia, which may approach 90%. Uncommonly, seizures or behavioral disorders develop. Rare deaths are due to severe neurologic, pneumonic, or myocardial involvement.

The ocular form of the larva migrans syndrome occurs when *Toxocara* larvae invade the eye. An eosinophilic granulomatous mass, most commonly in the posterior pole of the retina, develops around the entrapped larva. The retinal lesion can mimic retinoblastoma in appearance, and mistaken diagnosis of the latter condition can lead to unnecessary enucleation. The spectrum of eye involvement also includes endophthalmitis, uveitis, and chorioretinitis. Unilateral visual disturbances, strabismus, and eye pain are the most common presenting symptoms. In contrast to visceral larva migrans, ocular toxocariasis usually develops in older children or young adults with no history of pica; these patients seldom have eosinophilia or visceral manifestations.

Diagnosis   In addition to eosinophilia, leukocytosis and hypergammaglobulinemia may be evident. Transient pulmonary infiltrates are apparent on chest x-rays of about half of patients with symptoms of pneumonitis. The clinical diagnosis can be confirmed by an enzyme-linked immunosorbent assay for toxocaral antibodies. Stool examination for parasite eggs, while important in the evaluation of unexplained eosinophilia, is worthless for toxocariasis, since the larvae do not develop into egg-producing adults in humans.

℞ TREATMENT

The vast majority of *Toxocara* infections are self-limited and resolve without specific therapy. In patients with severe myocardial, central nervous system, or pulmonary involvement, glucocorticoids may be employed to reduce inflammatory complications. Available anthelmintic drugs, including mebendazole, and albendazole, have not been shown conclusively to alter the course of larva migrans. Control measures include prohibiting dog excreta in public parks and playgrounds, deworming dogs, and preventing pica in children. Treatment of ocular disease is not fully defined, but the administration of albendazole (800 mg twice daily for adults; 400 mg twice daily for children) for 5 to 20 days in conjunction with glucocorticoids has been effective.

CUTANEOUS LARVA MIGRANS   Cutaneous larva migrans ("creeping eruption") is a serpiginous skin eruption caused by burrowing larvae of animal hookworms, usually the dog and cat hookworm *Ancylostoma braziliense*. The larvae hatch from eggs passed in dog and cat feces and mature in the soil. Humans become infected after skin contact with soil in areas frequented by dogs and cats, such as areas underneath house porches or scrub vegetation. Cutaneous larva migrans is especially prevalent among children and in regions with warm humid climates, including the southeastern United States.

After larvae penetrate the skin, erythematous lesions form along the tortuous tracts of their migration through the dermal-epidermal junction; the larvae advance several centimeters in a day. The intensely pruritic lesions may occur anywhere on the body and can be numerous if the patient has lain on the ground. Vesicles and bullae may form later. The animal hookworm larvae do not mature in humans and, without treatment, will die out after several weeks, with resolution of skin lesions. The diagnosis is made readily on clinical grounds, and a skin biopsy only rarely yields diagnostic parasite material. Symptoms can be alleviated by ivermectin (a single dose of 200 µg/kg) or albendazole (200 mg twice daily for 3 days).

ANGIOSTRONGYLUS CANTONENSIS INFECTION *A. cantonensis*, the rat lungworm, is the most common cause of human eosinophilic meningitis (Fig. 200-2).

Life Cycle and Epidemiology This infection occurs principally in Southeast Asia and the Pacific Basin but has spread to other areas of the world. *A. cantonensis* larvae produced by adult worms in the rat lung migrate to the gastrointestinal tract and are expelled with the feces. They develop into infective larvae in land snails and slugs. Humans acquire the infection by ingesting raw infected mollusks; vegetables contaminated by mollusk slime; or crabs, freshwater shrimp, and certain marine fish that have themselves eaten infected mollusks. The larvae then migrate to the brain.

Pathogenesis and Clinical Features The parasites eventually die in the central nervous system, but not before initiating pathologic consequences that, in heavy infections, can result in permanent neurologic sequelae or death. Migrating larvae cause proteolytic damage and marked local eosinophilic inflammation and hemorrhage, with subsequent necrosis and granuloma formation around dying worms. Clinical symptoms develop between 2 and 35 days after the ingestion of larvae. Patients usually present with an insidious or abrupt excruciating frontal, occipital, or bitemporal headache. Neck stiffness, nausea and vomiting, and paresthesias are also common. Fever, cranial and extraocular nerve palsies, seizures, paralysis, and lethargy are uncommon.

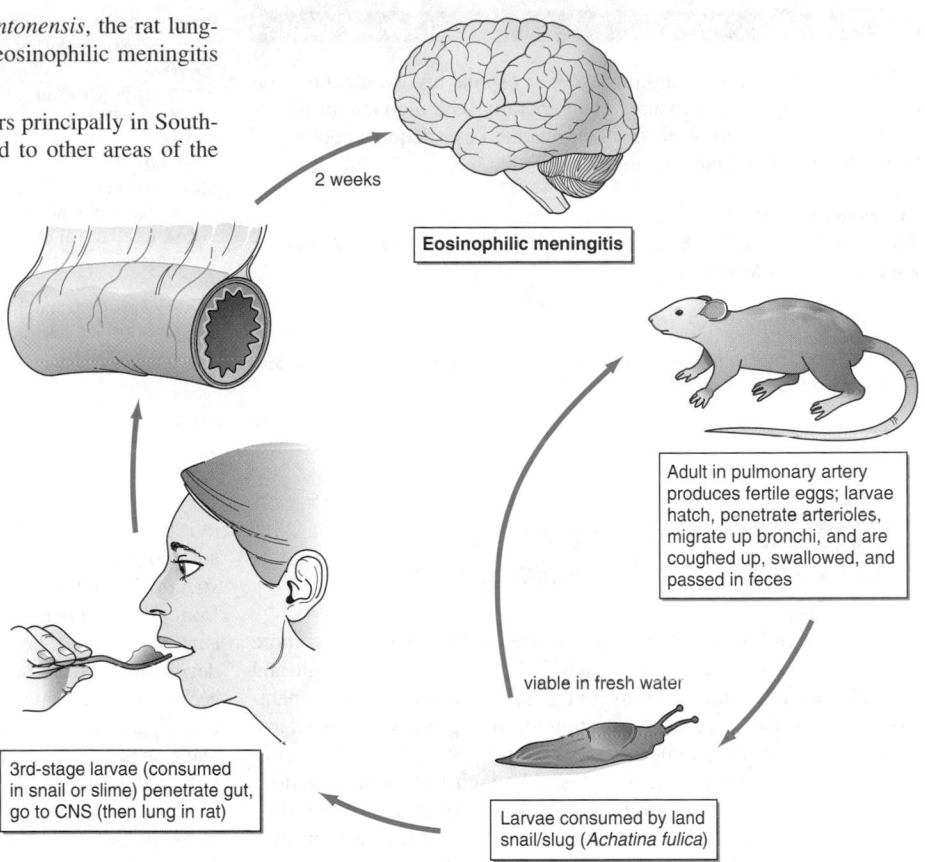

FIGURE 200-2 Life cycle of *Angiostrongylus cantonensis* (rat lung worm). Also found in Southeast Asia, Pacific Islands, and in U.S. ports, Cuba, Australia, Japan, China, and Mauritius. (*Reprinted from Guerrant RL et al: Essentials of Tropical Infectious Diseases, p 439. © 2001, with permission from Elsevier Science.*)

Labels in figure: 2 weeks — Eosinophilic meningitis — Adult in pulmonary artery produces fertile eggs; larvae hatch, penetrate arterioles, migrate up bronchi, and are coughed up, swallowed, and passed in feces — viable in fresh water — Larvae consumed by land snail/slug (*Achatina fulica*) — 3rd-stage larvae (consumed in snail or slime) penetrate gut, go to CNS (then lung in rat)

Laboratory Findings Examination of the cerebrospinal fluid is mandatory in suspected cases and usually reveals an elevated opening pressure, a white blood cell count of 150 to 2000/μL, and an eosinophilic pleocytosis of >20%. The protein concentration is usually elevated and the glucose level normal. The motile larvae of *A. cantonensis* are only rarely seen in the cerebrospinal fluid. Peripheral-blood eosinophilia may be mild. The diagnosis is generally based on the clinical presentation of eosinophilic meningitis together with a compatible epidemiologic history.

Rx TREATMENT

Specific chemotherapy is not of benefit in angiostrongyliasis; larvicidal agents may actually exacerbate inflammatory brain lesions. Management consists of supportive measures, including the administration of analgesics, sedatives, and—in severe cases—glucocorticoids. In most patients, cerebral angiostrongyliasis has a self-limited course, and recovery is complete. The infection may be prevented by adequately cooking snails, crabs, and prawns and inspecting vegetables for mollusk infestation. Other parasitic or fungal causes of eosinophilic meningitis in endemic areas may include gnathostomiasis, paragonimiasis, schistosomiasis, neurocysticercosis, and coccidioidomycosis.

GNATHOSTOMIASIS Infection of human tissues with larvae of *Gnathostoma spinigerum* can cause eosinophilic meningoencephalitis, migratory cutaneous swellings, or invasive masses of the eye and visceral organs.

Life Cycle and Epidemiology Human gnathostomiasis occurs in many countries and is notably endemic in Southeast Asia and parts of China and Japan. In nature, the mature adult worms parasitize the gastrointestinal tract of dogs and cats. First-stage larvae hatch from eggs passed into water and are ingested by *Cyclops* species (water fleas). Infective third-stage larvae develop in the flesh of many animal species (including fish, frogs, eels, snakes, chickens, and ducks) that have eaten either infected *Cyclops* or another infected second intermediate host. Humans typically acquire the infection by eating raw or undercooked fish or poultry. Raw fish dishes, such as *somfak* in Thailand and *sashimi* in Japan, account for many cases of human gnathostomiasis. Some cases in Thailand result from the local practice of applying frog or snake flesh as a poultice.

Pathogenesis and Clinical Features Clinical symptoms are due to the aberrant migration of a single larva into cutaneous, visceral, neural, or ocular tissues. After invasion, larval migration may cause local inflammation, with pain, cough, or hematuria accompanied by fever and eosinophilia. Painful, itchy, migratory swellings may develop in the skin, particularly in the distal extremities or periorbital area. Cutaneous swellings usually last about a week but often recur intermittently over many years. Larval invasion of the eye can provoke a sight-threatening inflammatory response. Finally, invasion of the central nervous system results in eosinophilic meningitis with myeloencephalitis, a serious complication due to ascending larval migration along a large nerve track. Patients characteristically present with agonizing radicular pain and paresthesias in the trunk or a limb, which are followed shortly by paraplegia. Cerebral involvement, with focal hemorrhages and tissue destruction, is often fatal.

Diagnosis and Treatment Cutaneous migratory swellings with marked peripheral eosinophilia, supported by an appropriate geographic and dietary history, generally constitute an adequate basis for a clinical diagnosis of gnathostomiasis. However, patients may present with ocular or cerebrospinal involvement without antecedent cutaneous swellings. In the latter case, eosinophilic pleocytosis is demonstrable (usually along with hemorrhagic or xanthochromic cerebrospinal fluid), but worms are almost never recovered from the cerebrospinal fluid. Surgical removal of the parasite from subcutaneous or ocular tissue, though rarely feasible, is both diagnostic and therapeutic. Albendazole (400 mg twice daily for 21 days) or ivermectin (200 μg/kg daily for

2 days) may be helpful. At present, cerebrospinal involvement is managed with supportive measures and generally with a course of glucocorticoids. Gnathostomiasis can be prevented by adequate cooking of fish and poultry in endemic areas.

ACKNOWLEDGMENT

The contributions of Leo X. Liu, M.D., to earlier editions of this chapter are gratefully acknowledged.

FURTHER READING

BARISANI-ASENBAUER T et al: Treatment of ocular toxocariasis with albendazole. J Ocul Pharmacol Ther 17:287, 2001

BOUCHARD O et al: Cutaneous larva migrans in travelers: A prospective study, with assessment of therapy with ivermectin. Clin Infect Dis 31:493, 2000

BRUSCHI F, MURRELL KD: New aspects of human trichinellosis: The impact of new *Trichinella* species. Postgrad Med J 78:15, 2002

CAUMES E: Treatment of cutaneous larva migrans. Clin Infect Dis 30:811, 2000

MOOREHEAD A et al: Trichinellosis in the United States, 1991–1996: Declining but not gone. Am J Trop Med Hyg 60:66, 1999

SLOM TJ et al: An outbreak of eosinophilic meningitis caused by *Angiostrongylus cantonensis* in travelers returning from the Caribbean. N Engl J Med 346:668, 2002

TSAI HC et al: Eosinophilic meningitis caused by *Angiostrongylus cantonensis*: Report of 17 cases. Am J Med 111:109, 2001

201 INTESTINAL NEMATODES
Peter F. Weller, Thomas B. Nutman

More than a billion people worldwide are infected with one or more species of intestinal nematodes. Table 201-1 summarizes biologic and clinical features of infections due to the major intestinal parasitic nematodes. These parasites are most common in regions with poor fecal sanitation, particularly in developing countries in the tropics and subtropics but also in the United States. Although nematode infections are not usually fatal, they contribute to malnutrition and diminished work capacity. An interesting point is that these same infections may protect some individuals from allergic disease. Humans may on occasion be infected with nematode parasites that ordinarily infect animals; these zoonotic infections include trichostrongyliasis, anisakiasis, capillariasis, and abdominal angiostrongyliasis.

Intestinal nematodes are roundworms; they range in length from 1 mm to many centimeters when mature (Table 201-1). Their life cycles are complex and highly varied; some species, including *Strongyloides stercoralis* and *Enterobius vermicularis*, can be transmitted directly from person to person, while others, such as *Ascaris lumbricoides*, *Necator americanus*, and *Ancylostoma duodenale*, require a soil phase for development. Because most helminth parasites do not self-replicate, the acquisition of a heavy burden of adult worms requires repeated exposure to the parasite in its infectious stage, whether larva or egg. Hence, clinical disease, as opposed to asymptomatic infection, generally develops only with prolonged residence in an endemic area. In persons with marginal nutrition, intestinal helminth infections may impair growth and development. Eosinophilia and elevated serum IgE levels are features of many helminthic infections and, when unexplained, should always prompt a search for occult helminthiasis. Significant protective immunity to intestinal nematodes appears not to develop in humans, although mechanisms of parasite immune evasion and host immune responses to these infections have not been elucidated in detail.

TABLE 201-1 *Major Human Intestinal Parasitic Nematodes*

Feature	Ascaris lumbricoides (Roundworm)	Necator americanus, Ancylostoma duodenale (Hookworm)	Strongyloides stercoralis	Trichuris trichiura (Whipworm)	Enterobius vermicularis (Pinworm)
Global prevalence in humans (millions)	1273	1277	50	902	300
Endemic areas	Worldwide	Hot, humid regions	Hot, humid regions	Worldwide	Worldwide
Infective stage	Egg	Filariform larva	Filariform larva	Egg	Egg
Route of infection	Oral	Percutaneous	Percutaneous or autoinfection	Oral	Oral
Gastrointestinal location of worms	Jejunal lumen	Jejunal mucosa	Small-bowel mucosa	Cecum, colonic mucosa	Cecum, appendix
Adult worm size	15–40 cm	7–12 mm	2 mm	30–50 mm	8–13 mm (female)
Pulmonary passage of larvae	Yes	Yes	Yes	No	No
Incubation period[a] (days)	60–75	40–100	17–28	70–90	35–45
Longevity	1 y	N. americanus: 2–5 y A. duodenale: 6–8 y	Decades (owing to autoinfection)	5 y	2 months
Fecundity (eggs/day/worm)	240,000	N. americanus: 4000–10,000 A. duodenale: 10,000–25,000	5000–10,000	3000–7000	2000
Principal symptoms	Rarely gastrointestinal or biliary obstruction	Iron-deficiency anemia in heavy infection	Gastrointestinal symptoms; malabsorption or sepsis in hyperinfection	Gastrointestinal symptoms, anemia	Perianal pruritus
Diagnostic stage	Eggs in stool	Eggs in fresh stool, larvae in old stool	Larvae in stool or duodenal aspirate; sputum in hyperinfection	Eggs in stool	Eggs from perianal skin on cellulose acetate tape
Treatment	Mebendazole Albendazole Pyrantel pamoate	Mebendazole Pyrantel pamoate Albendazole	1. Ivermectin 2. Albendazole 3. Thiabendazole	Mebendazole Albendazole	Mebendazole Pyrantel pamoate Albendazole

[a] Time from infection to egg production by mature female worm.

ASCARIASIS *A. lumbricoides* is the largest intestinal nematode parasite of humans, reaching up to 40 cm in length. Most infected individuals have low worm burdens and are asymptomatic. Clinical disease arises from larval migration in the lungs or effects of the adult worms in the intestines.

Life Cycle Adult worms live in the lumen of the small intestine. Mature female *Ascaris* worms are extraordinarily fecund, each producing up to 240,000 eggs a day, which pass with the feces. Ascarid eggs, which are remarkably resistant to environmental stresses, become infective after several weeks of maturation in the soil and can remain infective for years. After infective eggs are swallowed, larvae hatched in the intestine invade the mucosa, migrate through the circulation to the lungs, break into the alveoli, ascend the bronchial tree, and return via swallowing to the small intestine, where they develop into adult worms. Between 2 and 3 months elapse between initial infection and egg production. The adult worms live for 1 to 2 years.

Epidemiology *Ascaris* is widely distributed in tropical and subtropical regions as well as in other humid areas, including the rural southeastern United States. Transmission typically occurs through fecally contaminated soil and is due either to a lack of sanitary facilities or to the use of human manure ("night soil") as fertilizer. With their propensity for hand-to-mouth fecal carriage, younger children in impoverished rural areas are most affected. Infection outside endemic areas, though uncommon, can occur from eggs borne on transported vegetables.

Clinical Features During the lung phase of larval migration, about 9 to 12 days after egg ingestion, patients may develop an irritating nonproductive cough and burning substernal discomfort that is aggravated by coughing or deep inspiration. Dyspnea and blood-tinged sputum are less common. Fever is usually reported, with temperatures sometimes exceeding 38.5°C (101.3°F). Eosinophilia develops during this symptomatic phase and subsides slowly over weeks. Chest x-rays may reveal evidence of eosinophilic pneumonitis (Löffler's syndrome), with round or oval infiltrates a few millimeters to several centimeters in size. These infiltrates may be transient and intermittent, clearing after several weeks. Where there is seasonal transmission of the parasite, seasonal pneumonitis with eosinophilia may develop in previously infected and sensitized hosts.

In established infections, adult worms in the small intestine usually cause no symptoms. In heavy infections, particularly in children, a large bolus of entangled worms can cause pain and small-bowel obstruction, sometimes complicated by perforation, intussusception, or volvulus. Single worms may cause disease when they migrate into aberrant sites. A large worm can enter and occlude the biliary tree, causing biliary colic, cholecystitis, cholangitis, pancreatitis, or (rarely) intrahepatic abscesses. Migration of an adult worm up the esophagus can provoke coughing and oral expulsion of the worm. In highly endemic areas, intestinal and biliary ascariasis can rival acute appendicitis and gallstones as causes of surgical acute abdomen.

Laboratory Findings Most cases of ascariasis can be diagnosed by the microscopic detection of characteristic mamillated *Ascaris* eggs (65 by 45 μm) in fecal samples. Occasionally, patients present after passing an adult worm—identifiable by its large size and smooth cream-colored surface—in the stool or through the mouth or nose. During the early transpulmonary migratory phase, when eosinophilic pneumonitis occurs, larvae can be found in sputum or gastric aspirates before diagnostic eggs appear in the stool. The eosinophilia that is prominent during this early stage usually decreases to minimal levels in established infection. The large adult worms may be visualized, occasionally serendipitously, on contrast studies of the gastrointestinal tract. A plain abdominal film may reveal masses of worms in gas-filled loops of bowel in patients with intestinal obstruction. Pancreaticobiliary worms can be detected by ultrasound and endoscopic retrograde cholangiopancreatography; the latter method also has been used to extract biliary *Ascaris* worms.

℞ TREATMENT

Ascariasis should always be treated to prevent potentially serious complications. Albendazole (400 mg once), which is considered an investigational drug by the Food and Drug Administration for this indication, or mebendazole (500 mg once) is effective. These benzimidazoles are contraindicated in pregnancy, however. Pyrantel pamoate (11 mg/kg once; maximum, 1 g) is safe in pregnancy. Mild diarrhea and abdominal pain are uncommon side effects of these agents. Partial intestinal obstruction should be managed with nasogastric suction, intravenous fluid administration, and instillation of piperazine through the nasogastric tube, but complete obstruction and its severe complications require immediate surgical intervention.

HOOKWORM One-fourth of the world's population is infected with one of the two hookworm species (*A. duodenale* and *N. americanus*). Most infected individuals are asymptomatic. Hookworm disease develops from a combination of factors—a heavy worm burden, a prolonged duration of infection, and an inadequate iron intake—and results in iron-deficiency anemia and, on occasion, hypoproteinemia.

Life Cycle Adult hookworms, which are ~1 cm long, use buccal teeth (*Ancylostoma*) or cutting plates (*Necator*) to attach to the small-bowel mucosa and suck blood (0.2 mL/d per *Ancylostoma* adult) and interstitial fluid. The adult hookworms produce thousands of eggs daily. The eggs are deposited with feces in soil, where rhabditiform larvae hatch and develop over a 1-week period into infectious filariform larvae. Infective larvae penetrate the skin and reach the lungs by way of the bloodstream. There they invade alveoli and ascend the airways before being swallowed and reaching the small intestine. The prepatent period from skin invasion to appearance of eggs in the feces is about 6 to 8 weeks, but it may be longer with *A. duodenale*. Larvae of *A. duodenale*, if swallowed, can survive and develop directly in the intestinal mucosa. Adult hookworms may survive over a decade but usually live about 6 to 8 years for *A. duodenale* and 2 to 5 years for *N. americanus*.

Epidemiology *A. duodenale* is prevalent in southern Europe, North Africa, and northern Asia, and *N. americanus* is the predominant species in the western hemisphere and equatorial Africa. The two species overlap in many tropical regions, particularly Southeast Asia. In most areas, older children have the greatest incidence and intensity of hookworm infection. In rural areas where fields are fertilized with night soil, older working adults also may be heavily affected.

Clinical Features Most hookworm infections are asymptomatic. Infective larvae may provoke pruritic maculopapular dermatitis ("ground itch") at the site of skin penetration as well as serpiginous tracks of subcutaneous migration (similar to cutaneous larva migrans) in previously sensitized hosts. Larvae migrating through the lungs occasionally cause mild transient pneumonitis, but this condition develops less frequently in hookworm infection than in ascariasis. In the early intestinal phase, infected persons may develop epigastric pain (often with postprandial accentuation), inflammatory diarrhea, or other abdominal symptoms accompanied by eosinophilia. The major consequence of chronic hookworm infection is iron deficiency. Symptoms are minimal if iron intake is adequate, but marginally nourished individuals develop symptoms of progressive iron-deficiency anemia and hypoproteinemia, including weakness, shortness of breath, and skin depigmentation.

Laboratory Findings The diagnosis is established by the finding of characteristic 40- by 60-μm oval hookworm eggs in the feces. Stool-concentration procedures may be required to detect light infections. Eggs of the two species are indistinguishable by light microscopy. In a stool sample that is not fresh, the eggs may have hatched to release rhabditiform larvae, which need to be differentiated from those of *S. ster-*

coralis. Hypochromic microcytic anemia, occasionally with eosinophilia or hypoalbuminemia, is characteristic of hookworm disease.

℞ TREATMENT

Hookworm infection can be eradicated with several safe and highly effective anthelmintic drugs, including albendazole (400 mg once), mebendazole (500 mg once), and pyrantel pamoate (11 mg/kg for 3 days). Mild iron-deficiency anemia can often be treated with oral iron alone. Severe hookworm disease with protein loss and malabsorption necessitates nutritional support and oral iron replacement along with deworming.

Ancylostoma caninum* and *Ancylostoma braziliense   *A. caninum*, the canine hookworm, has been identified as a cause of human eosinophilic enteritis, especially in northeastern Australia. In this zoonotic infection, adult hookworms attach to the small intestine (where they may be visualized by endoscopy) and elicit abdominal pain and intense local eosinophilia. Treatment with mebendazole (100 mg twice daily for 3 days) or albendazole (400 mg once) is effective. Both of these animal hookworm species can cause cutaneous larva migrans ("creeping eruption"; Chap. 200).

STRONGYLOIDIASIS   *S. stercoralis* is distinguished by its ability—unusual among helminths—to replicate in the human host. This capacity permits ongoing cycles of autoinfection as infective larvae are internally produced. Strongyloidiasis can thus persist for decades without further exposure of the host to exogenous infective larvae. In immunocompromised hosts, large numbers of invasive *Strongyloides* larvae can disseminate widely and can be fatal.

Life Cycle   In addition to a parasitic cycle of development, *Strongyloides* can undergo a free-living cycle of development in the soil. This adaptability facilitates the parasite's survival in the absence of mammalian hosts. Rhabditiform larvae passed in feces can transform into infectious filariform larvae either directly or after a free-living phase of development. Humans acquire strongyloidiasis when filariform larvae in fecally contaminated soil penetrate the skin or mucous membranes. The larvae then travel through the bloodstream to the lungs, where they break into the alveolar spaces, ascend the bronchial tree, are swallowed, and thereby reach the small intestine. There the larvae mature into adult worms that penetrate the mucosa of the proximal small bowel. The minute (2-mm-long) parasitic adult female worms reproduce by parthenogenesis; parasitic adult males do not exist. Eggs hatch locally in the intestinal mucosa, releasing rhabditiform larvae that migrate to the lumen and pass with the feces into soil. Alternatively, rhabditiform larvae in the bowel can develop directly into filariform larvae that penetrate the colonic wall or perianal skin and enter the circulation to repeat the migration that establishes ongoing internal reinfection. This autoinfection cycle allows strongyloidiasis to persist for decades after the host has left an endemic area.

Epidemiology   *S. stercoralis* is spottily distributed in tropical areas and other hot, humid regions and is particularly common in Southeast Asia, sub-Saharan Africa, and Brazil. In the United States, the parasite is endemic in parts of the South and is found in institutionalized patients who practice poor hygiene and in immigrants and military veterans who have lived in endemic areas abroad.

Clinical Features   In uncomplicated strongyloidiasis, many patients are asymptomatic or have mild cutaneous and/or abdominal symptoms. Recurrent urticaria, often involving the buttocks and wrists, is the most common cutaneous manifestation. Migrating larvae can elicit a pathognomonic serpiginous eruption, *larva currens* ("running larva")—a pruritic, raised, erythematous lesion that advances as rapidly as 10 cm/h along the course of larval migration. Adult parasites burrow into the duodenojejunal mucosa and can cause abdominal (usually midepigastric) pain, which resembles peptic ulcer pain except that it is aggravated by food ingestion. Nausea, diarrhea, gastrointestinal bleeding, mild chronic colitis, and weight loss can occur. Small-bowel obstruction may develop with early, heavy infection. Pulmonary symptoms are rare in uncomplicated strongyloidiasis. Eosinophilia is common, with levels fluctuating over time.

The ongoing autoinfection cycle of strongyloidiasis is normally contained by unknown factors of the host's immune system. Abrogation of host immunity, especially with glucocorticoid therapy and much less commonly with other immunosuppressive medications, leads to hyperinfection, with the generation of large numbers of filariform larvae. Colitis, enteritis, or malabsorption may develop. In disseminated strongyloidiasis, larvae may invade not only gastrointestinal tissues and the lungs but also the central nervous system, peritoneum, liver, and kidney. Moreover, bacteremia may develop because of the entry of enteric flora through disrupted mucosal barriers. Gram-negative sepsis, pneumonia, or meningitis may complicate or dominate the clinical course. Eosinophilia is often absent in severely infected patients. Disseminated strongyloidiasis, particularly in patients with unsuspected infection who are given glucocorticoids, can be fatal. Strongyloidiasis is a frequent complication of infection with human T cell lymphotropic virus type I, but disseminated strongyloidiasis is not common among patients infected with HIV.

Diagnosis   In uncomplicated strongyloidiasis, the finding of rhabditiform larvae in feces is diagnostic. The eggs are almost never detectable because they hatch in the intestine. Rhabditiform larvae are 200 to 250 μm long, with a short buccal cavity that distinguishes them from hookworm rhabditiform larvae. Single stool examinations detect only about one-third of uncomplicated infections, in which few larvae are passed. Serial examinations and the use of the agar plate detection method improve the sensitivity of stool diagnosis. In uncomplicated—but not hyperinfection—strongyloidiasis, stool examinations may be repeatedly negative. If stool examinations are negative, *Strongyloides* can be assayed by sampling of the duodenojejunal contents by aspiration or biopsy. An enzyme-linked immunosorbent assay for antibodies to excretory-secretory or somatic antigens of *Strongyloides* is a sensitive method of diagnosing uncomplicated infections. In disseminated strongyloidiasis, filariform larvae (550 μm long) should be sought in stool as well as in samples obtained from sites of potential larval migration, including sputum, bronchoalveolar lavage fluid, or surgical drainage fluid.

℞ TREATMENT

Even in the asymptomatic state, strongyloidiasis must be treated because of the potential for fatal hyperinfection. Ivermectin (200 μg/kg daily for 1 or 2 days) is more effective than albendazole (400 mg daily for 3 days, repeated at 2 weeks) and is better tolerated than thiabendazole (25 mg/kg twice daily for 2 days), whose common adverse effects include nausea, vomiting, diarrhea, dizziness, and neuropsychiatric disturbances. Because thiabendazole is not uniformly effective, stool examinations, eosinophil counts, and monitoring of clinical symptoms should be continued after treatment. For disseminated strongyloidiasis, treatment with ivermectin should be extended for at least 5 to 7 days or until the parasites are eradicated.

Strongyloides fülleborni   This unusual species, which has been encountered in Africa and Papua New Guinea, is thought to be transmitted from person to person and through maternal milk. *S. fülleborni* releases membranous sacs filled with eggs into the stool. Most commonly affected are infants and young children, who present with abdominal distention, respiratory distress, vomiting, or diarrhea.

TRICHURIASIS   Most infections with the whipworm *Trichuris trichiura* are asymptomatic, but heavy infections may cause gastrointestinal symptoms. Like the other soil-transmitted helminths, whipworm is distributed globally in the tropics and subtropics and is most common among poor children.

Life Cycle   A broad posterior section and a thin anterior portion give *Trichuris* its characteristic whiplike shape. The adult worms reside in the colon and cecum, the anterior portions threaded into the superficial mucosa. Thousands of eggs laid daily by adult female worms pass with the feces and mature in the soil. After ingestion, infective eggs hatch in the duodenum, releasing larvae that mature before migrating to the large bowel. The entire cycle takes about 3 months, and adult worms may live for several years.

Clinical Features Tissue reactions to whipworms are mild. Most infected individuals have no symptoms or eosinophilia. Heavy infections may result in abdominal pain, anorexia, and bloody or mucoid diarrhea resembling inflammatory bowel disease. Rectal prolapse can result from massive infections in children, who often suffer from malnourishment and other diarrheal illnesses. Moderately heavy whipworm burdens also contribute to growth retardation.

Diagnosis and Treatment The characteristic 50- by 20-μm lemon-shaped whipworm eggs are readily detected on stool examination. Adult worms, which are 3 to 5 cm long, occasionally can be seen on proctoscopy. Mebendazole (500 mg once) or albendazole (400 mg daily for 3 doses) is safe and effective for treatment.

ENTEROBIASIS (PINWORM) *E. vermicularis* is more common in temperate countries than in the tropics. In the United States, >40 million people are estimated to be infected with pinworms; schoolchildren account for a disproportionate number of cases.

Life Cycle and Epidemiology *Enterobius* adult worms are ~1 cm long and dwell in the bowel lumen. The gravid female worm migrates nocturnally out into the perianal region and releases up to 10,000 immature eggs. The eggs become infective within hours and are transmitted by hand-to-mouth passage. The larvae hatch and mature entirely within the intestine. This life cycle takes ~1 month, and adult worms survive for ~2 months. Self-infection results from perianal scratching and transport of infective eggs on the hands or under the nails to the mouth. Because of the ease of person-to-person spread, pinworm infections are common among family members and institutionalized populations.

Clinical Features Most pinworm infections are asymptomatic. Perianal pruritus is the cardinal symptom. The itching, which is often worse at night as a result of the nocturnal migration of the female worms, may lead to excoriation and bacterial superinfection. Heavy infections have been claimed to cause abdominal pain and weight loss. On rare occasions, pinworms invade the female genital tract, causing vulvovaginitis and pelvic or peritoneal granulomas. Eosinophilia or elevated levels of serum IgE are rare.

Diagnosis Since pinworm eggs are not usually released in the bowel, the diagnosis cannot be made by looking for eggs in the feces. Instead, eggs deposited in the perianal region are detected by the application of clear cellulose acetate tape to the perianal region in the morning. After the tape is transferred to a microscope slide, low-power examination will reveal the characteristic pinworm eggs, which are oval, measure 55 by 25 μm, and are flattened along one side.

℞ TREATMENT

All affected individuals should be given a dose of mebendazole (100 mg once), albendazole (400 mg once), or pyrantel pamoate (11 mg/kg base once; maximum, 1 g), with the same treatment repeated after 10 to 14 days. Treatment of household members is also advocated to eliminate asymptomatic reservoirs of potential reinfection.

TRICHOSTRONGYLIASIS *Trichostrongylus* species, which are normally parasites of herbivorous animals, occasionally infect humans, particularly in Asia and Africa. This parasite has been termed *pseudohookworm* because of similarities to the hookworms in life cycle and egg morphology. Humans acquire the infection by accidentally ingesting *Trichostrongylus* larvae on contaminated leafy vegetables. The larvae do not migrate in humans but mature directly into adult worms in the small bowel. These worms ingest far less blood than hookworms; most infected people are asymptomatic, but heavy infections may give rise to mild anemia and eosinophilia. *Trichostrongylus* eggs encountered

on stool examination resemble those of hookworms but are larger (85 by 115 μm). Appropriate treatment consists of mebendazole or albendazole (Chap. 193).

ANISAKIASIS Anisakiasis is a gastrointestinal infection caused by the accidental ingestion in uncooked saltwater fish of nematode larvae belonging to the family Anisakidae. The incidence of anisakiasis in the United States has increased as a result of the growing popularity of raw fish dishes. Most cases occur in Japan, the Netherlands, and Chile, where raw fish—sushi, pickled green herring, and seviche, respectively—are national culinary staples. Anisakid nematodes parasitize large sea mammals such as whales, dolphins, and seals. As part of a complex parasitic life cycle involving marine food chains, infectious larvae migrate to the musculature of a variety of fish. Both *Anisakis simplex* and *Pseudoterranova decipiens* have been implicated in human anisakiasis, but an identical gastric syndrome may be caused by the red larvae of eustrongylid parasites of fish-eating birds.

When humans consume infected raw fish, live larvae may be coughed up within 48 h. Alternatively, larvae may immediately penetrate the mucosa of the stomach. Within hours, violent upper abdominal pain accompanied by nausea and occasionally vomiting ensues, mimicking an acute abdomen. The diagnosis can be established by direct visualization on upper endoscopy, outlining of the worm by contrast radiographic studies, or histopathologic examination of extracted tissue. In experienced hands, the first technique is preferable because extraction of the burrowing larvae by endoscopic technique is curative. In addition, larvae may pass to the small bowel, where they penetrate the mucosa and provoke a vigorous eosinophilic granulomatous response. Symptoms may appear 1 or 2 weeks after the infective meal, with intermittent abdominal pain, diarrhea, nausea, and fever resembling the manifestations of Crohn's disease. The diagnosis may be suggested by barium studies and confirmed by curative surgical resection of a granuloma in which the worm is embedded. Anisakid eggs are not found in the stool, since the larvae do not mature in humans. Anisakid larvae in saltwater fish are killed by cooking to 60°C, freezing at −20°C for 3 days, or commercial blast freezing, but not usually by salting, marinating, or cold smoking. No medical treatment is available; if possible, surgical or endoscopic removal should be undertaken.

CAPILLARIASIS Intestinal capillariasis is caused by ingestion of raw fish infected with *Capillaria philippinensis*. Subsequent autoinfection can lead to a severe wasting syndrome. The disease occurs in the Philippines and Thailand and, on occasion, elsewhere in Asia. The natural cycle of *C. philippinensis* involves fish from fresh and brackish water. When humans eat infected raw fish, the larvae mature in the intestine into adult worms, which produce invasive larvae that cause intestinal inflammation and villus loss. Capillariasis has an insidious onset with nonspecific abdominal pain and watery diarrhea. If untreated, progressive autoinfection can lead to protein-losing enteropathy and severe malabsorption and ultimately to death from cachexia, cardiac failure, or superinfection. The diagnosis is established by identification of the characteristic peanut-shaped (20- by 40-μm) eggs on stool examination. Severely ill patients require hospitalization and supportive therapy in addition to prolonged anthelmintic treatment with mebendazole or albendazole (Chap. 193).

ABDOMINAL ANGIOSTRONGYLIASIS Abdominal angiostrongyliasis is found in Latin America and Africa. The zoonotic parasite *Angiostrongylus costaricensis* causes eosinophilic ileocolitis after the ingestion of contaminated vegetation. *A. costaricensis* normally parasitizes the cotton rat and other rodents, with slugs and snails serving as intermediate hosts. Humans become infected by accidentally ingesting infective larvae in mollusk slime deposited on fruits and vegetables; children are at highest risk. The larvae penetrate the gut wall and migrate to the mesenteric artery, where they develop into adult worms. Eggs deposited in the gut wall provoke an intense eosinophilic granulomatous reaction, and adult worms may cause mesenteric arteritis, thrombosis, or frank bowel infarction. Symptoms may mimic those of appendicitis, including abdominal pain and tenderness, fever, vomiting, and a palpable mass in the right iliac fossa. Leukocytosis and eosinophilia are prominent. A barium enema may reveal ileocecal filling defects, but a definitive diagnosis is usually made surgically with partial bowel resection. Pathologic study reveals a thickened bowel wall with eosinophilic granulomas surrounding the *Angiostrongylus* eggs. In nonsurgical cases, the diagnosis rests solely on clinical grounds because larvae and eggs cannot be detected in the stool. Medical therapy for abdominal angiostrongyliasis (thiabendazole; Chap. 193) is of uncertain efficacy. Careful observation and surgical resection for severe symptoms are the mainstays of treatment.

FURTHER READING

BECKINGHAM IJ et al: Management of hepatobiliary and pancreatic *Ascaris* infestation in adults after failed medical treatment. Br J Surg 85:907, 1998

COWDEN J et al: Mebendazole and albendazole treatment of geohelminth infections in children and pregnant women. Pediatr Infect Dis J 19:659, 2000

CROESE J et al: Human enteric infection with canine hookworms. Ann Intern Med 120:369, 1994

CROSS JH: Intestinal capillariasis. Clin Microbiol Rev 5:120, 1992

GOTUZZO E et al: *Strongyloides stercoralis* hyperinfection associated with human T cell lymphotropic virus type-1 infection in Peru. Am J Trop Med Hyg 60:146, 1999

HORTON J: Albendazole: A broad spectrum anthelminthic for treatment of individuals and populations. Curr Opin Infect Dis 15:599, 2002

KEISER PB et al: *Strongyloides stercoralis* in the immunocompromised population. Clin Microbiol Rev (in press)

REEDER MM: The radiological and ultrasound evaluation of ascariasis of the gastrointestinal, biliary, and respiratory tracts. Semin Roentgenol 33:57, 1998

202 FILARIAL AND RELATED INFECTIONS
Thomas B. Nutman, Peter F. Weller

Filarial worms are nematodes that dwell in the subcutaneous tissues and the lymphatics. Eight filarial species infect humans (Table 202-1); of these, four—*Wuchereria bancrofti*, *Brugia malayi*, *Onchocerca volvulus*, and *Loa loa*—are responsible for most serious filarial infections. Filarial parasites, which infect an estimated 170 million persons worldwide, are transmitted by specific species of mosquitoes or other arthropods and have a complex life cycle including infective larval stages carried by insects and adult worms that reside in either lymphatic or subcutaneous tissues of humans. The offspring of adults are microfilariae, which, depending on their species, are 200 to 250 μm long and 5 to 7 μm wide, may or may not be enveloped in a loose sheath, and either circulate in the blood or migrate through the skin (Table 202-1). To complete the life cycle, microfilariae are ingested by the arthropod vector and develop over 1 to 2 weeks into new infective larvae. Adult worms live for many years, whereas microfilariae survive from 3 to 36 months. There has been a resurgence of interest in the rickettsia-like endosymbiont of *Wolbachia* that has been found intracellularly in all stages of *Brugia*, *Wuchereria*, *Mansonella*, and *Onchocerca*. These intracellular bacteria have recently been viewed as possible targets for antifilarial chemotherapy.

Usually, infection is established only with repeated and prolonged exposures to infective larvae. Since the clinical manifestations of filarial diseases develop relatively slowly, these infections should be considered chronic diseases with possible long-term debilitating effects. In terms of the nature, severity, and timing of clinical manifestations, patients with filarial infections who are native to endemic areas and undergo lifelong exposure may differ significantly from those who are travelers or who have recently moved to these areas. Characteristically, the disease is more acute and intense in newly exposed individuals than in natives of endemic areas.

LYMPHATIC FILARIASIS

Lymphatic filariasis is caused by *W. bancrofti*, *B. malayi*, or *B. timori*. The threadlike adult parasites reside in lymphatic channels or lymph nodes, where they may remain viable for more than two decades.

EPIDEMIOLOGY *W. bancrofti*, the most widely distributed human filarial parasite, affects an estimated 115 million people and is found throughout the tropics and subtropics, including Asia and the Pacific Islands, Africa, areas of South America, and the Caribbean basin. Humans are the only definitive host for the parasite. Generally, the subperiodic form is found only in the Pacific Islands; elsewhere, *W. bancrofti* is nocturnally periodic. (Nocturnally periodic forms of microfilariae are scarce in peripheral blood by day and increase at night, whereas sub-

TABLE 202-1 *Characteristics of the Filariae*

Organism	Periodicity	Distribution	Vector	Location of Adult	Microfilarial Location	Sheath
Wuchereria bancrofti	Nocturnal	Cosmopolitan areas worldwide, including South America and Africa	*Culex* (mosquitoes)	Lymphatic tissue	Blood	+
		Mainly India	*Anopheles* (mosquitoes)			
		China, Indonesia	*Aedes* (mosquitoes)			
	Subperiodic	Eastern Pacific	*Aedes* (mosquitoes)	Lymphatic tissue	Blood	+
Brugia malayi	Nocturnal	Southeast Asia, Indonesia, India	*Mansonia, Anopheles* (mosquitoes)	Lymphatic tissue	Blood	+
	Subperiodic	Indonesia, Southeast Asia	*Coquillettidia, Mansonia* (mosquitoes)	Lymphatic tissue	Blood	+
B. timori	Nocturnal	Indonesia	*Anopheles* (mosquitoes)	Lymphatic tissue	Blood	+
Loa loa	Diurnal	West and Central Africa	*Chrysops* (deerflies)	Subcutaneous tissue	Blood	+
Onchocerca volvulus	None	South and Central America, Africa	*Simulium* (blackflies)	Subcutaneous tissue	Skin, eye	−
Mansonella ozzardi	None	South and Central America Caribbean	*Culicoides* (midges) *Simulium* (blackflies)	Undetermined site	Blood	−
M. perstans	None	South and Central America, Africa	*Culicoides* (midges)	Body cavities, mesentery, perirenal tissue	Blood	−
M. streptocerca	None	West and Central Africa	*Culicoides* (midges)	Subcutaneous tissue	Skin	

periodic forms are present in peripheral blood at all times and reach maximal levels in the afternoon.) Natural vectors for *W. bancrofti* are *Culex fatigans* mosquitoes in urban settings and anopheline or aedean mosquitoes in rural areas.

Brugian filariasis due to *B. malayi* occurs primarily in China, India, Indonesia, Korea, Japan, Malaysia, and the Philippines. *B. malayi* also has two forms distinguished by the periodicity of microfilaremia. The more common nocturnal form is transmitted in areas of coastal rice fields, while the subperiodic form is found in forests. *B. malayi* naturally infects cats as well as humans. *B. timori* exists only on islands of the Indonesian archipelago.

PATHOLOGY The principal pathologic changes result from inflammatory damage to the lymphatics, which is caused by adult worms and not by microfilariae. Adult worms live in afferent lymphatics or sinuses of lymph nodes and cause lymphatic dilatation and thickening of the vessel walls. The infiltration of plasma cells, eosinophils, and macrophages in and around the infected vessels, along with endothelial and connective tissue proliferation, leads to tortuosity of the lymphatics and damaged or incompetent lymph valves. Lymphedema and chronic-stasis changes with hard or brawny edema develop in the overlying skin. These consequences of filariasis are due both to direct effects of the worms and to the inflammatory response of the host to the parasite. These inflammatory responses are believed to cause the granulomatous and proliferative processes that precede total lymphatic obstruction. It is thought that the lymphatic vessel remains patent as long as the worm remains viable and that death of the worm leads to enhanced granulomatous reaction and fibrosis. Lymphatic obstruction results, and, despite collateralization of the lymphatics, lymphatic function is compromised.

CLINICAL FEATURES The most common presentations of the lymphatic filariases are asymptomatic (or subclinical) microfilaremia, hydrocele (Fig. 202-1), acute adenolymphangitis (ADL), and chronic lymphatic disease. In areas where *W. bancrofti* or *B. malayi* is endemic, the overwhelming majority of infected individuals have few overt clinical manifestations of filarial infection despite large numbers of circulating microfilariae in the peripheral blood. Although they may be clinically asymptomatic, virtually all persons with *W. bancrofti* or *B. malayi* microfilaremia have some degree of subclinical disease that includes microscopic hematuria and/or proteinuria, dilated (and tortuous) lymphatics (visualized by imaging), and—in men—scrotal lymphangiectasia (detectable by ultrasound). In spite of these findings, the majority of individuals appear to remain clinically asymptomatic for years; relatively few progress to the acute and chronic stages of infection.

ADL is characterized by high fever, lymphatic inflammation (lymphangitis and lymphadenitis), and transient local edema. The lymphangitis is retrograde, extending peripherally from the lymph node draining the area where the adult parasites reside. Regional lymph nodes are often enlarged, and the entire lymphatic channel can become indurated and inflamed. Concomitant local thrombophlebitis can occur as well. In brugian filariasis, a single local abscess may form along the involved lymphatic tract and subsequently rupture to the surface. The lymphadenitis and lymphangitis can involve both the upper and lower extremities in both bancroftian and brugian filariasis, but involvement of the genital lymphatics occurs almost exclusively with *W. bancrofti* infection. This genital involvement can be manifested by funiculitis, epididymitis, and scrotal pain and tenderness. In endemic areas, another type of acute disease—dermatolymphangioadenitis (DLA)—is recognized as a syndrome that includes high fever, chills, myalgias, and headache. Edematous inflammatory plaques clearly demarcated from normal skin are seen. Vesicles, ulcers, and hyperpigmentation may also be noted. There is often a history of trauma, burns, radiation, insect bites, punctiform lesions, or chemical injury. Entry lesions, especially in the interdigital area, are common. DLA is often diagnosed as cellulitis.

If lymphatic damage progresses, transient lymphedema can develop into lymphatic obstruction and the permanent changes associated with elephantiasis (Fig. 202-2). Brawny edema follows early pitting edema, and thickening of the subcutaneous tissues and hyperkeratosis occur. Fissuring of the skin develops, as do hyperplastic changes. Superinfection of these poorly vascularized tissues becomes a problem. In bancroftian filariasis, in which genital involvement is common, hydroceles may develop; in advanced stages, this condition may evolve into scrotal lymphedema and scrotal elephantiasis. Furthermore, if there is obstruction of the retroperitoneal lymphatics, the increased renal lymphatic pressure leads to rupture of the renal lymphatics and the development of chyluria, which is usually intermittent and most prominent in the morning.

FIGURE 202-1 Hydrocele associated with *Wuchereria bancrofti* infection.

FIGURE 202-2 Elephantiasis of the lower extremity associated with *Wuchereria bancrofti* infection.

The clinical manifestations of filarial infections in travelers or transmigrants who have recently entered an endemic region are distinctive. Given a sufficient number of bites by infected vectors, usually over a 3- to 6-month period, recently exposed patients can develop acute lymphatic or scrotal inflammation with or without urticaria and localized angioedema. Lymphadenitis of epitrochlear, axillary, femoral, or inguinal lymph nodes is often followed by retrogradely evolving lymphangitis. Acute attacks are short-lived and, in contrast to filarial fevers in patients native to endemic areas, are usually not accompanied by fever. With prolonged exposure to infected mosquitoes, these attacks, if untreated, become more severe and lead to permanent lymphatic inflammation and obstruction.

DIAGNOSIS A definitive diagnosis can be made only by detection of the parasites and hence can be difficult. Adult worms localized in lymphatic vessels or nodes are largely inaccessible. Microfilariae can be found in blood, in hydrocele fluid, or (occasionally) in other body fluids. Such fluids can be examined microscopically, either directly or—for greater sensitivity—after concentration of the parasites by the passage of fluid through a polycarbonate cylindrical pore filter (pore size, 3 μm) or by the centrifugation of fluid fixed in 2% formalin (Knott's concentration technique). The timing of blood collection is critical and should be based on the periodicity of the microfilariae in the endemic region involved. Many infected individuals do not have microfilaremia, and definitive diagnosis in such cases can be difficult. Assays for circulating antigens of *W. bancrofti* permit the diagnosis of microfilaremic and cryptic (amicrofilaremic) infection. Two tests are commercially available: one is an enzyme-linked immunosorbent assay (ELISA) and the other a rapid-format immunochromatographic card test. Both assays have sensitivities that range from 96 to 100% and specificities that approach 100%. There are currently no tests for circulating antigens in brugian filariasis.

Polymerase chain reaction (PCR)–based assays for DNA of *W. bancrofti* and *B. malayi* in blood have been developed. A number of studies indicate that this diagnostic method is of equivalent or greater sensitivity compared with parasitologic methods, detecting patent infection in almost all infected subjects.

In cases of suspected lymphatic filariasis, examination of the scrotum or the female breast using high-frequency ultrasound in conjunction with Doppler techniques may result in the identification of motile adult worms within dilated lymphatics. Worms may be visualized in the lymphatics of the spermatic cord in up to 80% of infected men. Live adult worms have a distinctive pattern of movement within the lymphatic vessels (termed the *filaria dance sign*). Radionuclide lymphoscintigraphic imaging of the limbs reliably demonstrates widespread lymphatic abnormalities in both asymptomatic microfilaremic persons and those with clinical manifestations of lymphatic pathology. While of potential utility in the delineation of anatomic changes associated with infection, lymphoscintigraphy is unlikely to assume primacy in the diagnostic evaluation of individuals with suspected infection; it is principally a research tool, although it has been used more widely for assessment of lymphedema of all causes. Eosinophilia and elevated serum concentrations of IgE and antifilarial antibody support the diagnosis of lymphatic filariasis. There is, however, extensive cross-reactivity between filarial antigens and antigens of other helminths, including the common intestinal roundworms; thus, interpretations of serologic findings can be difficult. In addition, residents of endemic areas can become sensitized to filarial antigens through exposure to infected mosquitoes without having patent filarial infections.

In acute episodes, lymphatic filariasis must be distinguished from thrombophlebitis, infection, and trauma. Retrogradely evolving lymphangitis is a characteristic feature that helps distinguish filarial lymphangitis from typically ascending bacterial lymphangitis. Chronic filarial lymphedema must be distinguished from the lymphedema of malignancy, postoperative scarring, trauma, chronic edematous states, and congenital lymphatic system abnormalities.

℞ TREATMENT

With newer definitions of clinical syndromes in lymphatic filariasis and new tools to assess clinical status (e.g., ultrasound, lymphoscintigraphy, circulating filarial antigen assays, PCR), approaches to treatment based on infection status can be considered. Diethylcarbamazine (DEC, 6 mg/kg daily for 12 days), which has both macro- and microfilaricidal properties, remains the treatment of choice for the individual with active lymphatic filariasis (microfilaremia, antigen positivity, or adult worms on ultrasound), although albendazole (400 mg twice daily for 21 days) has also demonstrated macrofilaricidal efficacy.

As has already been mentioned, a growing body of evidence indicates that, although they may be asymptomatic, virtually all persons with *W. bancrofti* or *B. malayi* microfilaremia have some degree of subclinical disease (hematuria, proteinuria, abnormalities on lymphoscintigraphy). Thus, early treatment of asymptomatic persons is recommended to prevent further lymphatic damage. For ADL, supportive treatment (including the administration of antipyretics and analgesics) is recommended, as is antibiotic therapy if secondary bacterial infection is likely. Similarly, because lymphatic disease is associated with the presence of adult worms, treatment with DEC is recommended for microfilaria-negative adult-worm carriers.

In persons with chronic manifestations of lymphatic filariasis, treatment regimens that emphasize hygiene, prevention of secondary bacterial infections, and physiotherapy have gained wide acceptance for morbidity control. These regimens are similar to those recommended for lymphedema of most nonfilarial causes and known by a variety of names, including *complex decongestive physiotherapy* and *complex lymphedema therapy*. Hydroceles can be drained repeatedly or managed surgically. With chronic manifestations of lymphatic filariasis, drug treatment should be reserved for individuals with evidence of active infection; therapy has been associated with clinical improvement and, in some cases, reversal of lymphedema.

The recommended course of DEC treatment (12 days; total dose, 72 mg/kg) has remained standard for many years; however, data indicate that single-dose DEC treatment with 6 mg/kg may be equally efficacious. The 12-day course provides more rapid short-term microfilarial suppression. Regimens that utilize single-dose DEC or ivermectin or combinations of single doses of albendazole and either DEC or ivermectin have all been demonstrated to have a sustained microfilaricidal effect.

Side effects of DEC treatment include fever, chills, arthralgias, headaches, nausea, and vomiting. Both the development and the severity of these reactions are directly related to the number of microfilariae circulating in the bloodstream and may represent either an acute hypersensitivity reaction to the antigens being released by dead and dying parasites or an inflammatory reaction induced by lipopolysaccharides from the intracellular *Wolbachia* endosymbionts freed from their intracellular niche. Ivermectin has a side effect profile similar to that of DEC when used in lymphatic filariasis.

PREVENTION AND CONTROL Avoidance of mosquito bites is usually not feasible for residents of endemic areas, but visitors should make use of insect repellent and mosquito nets. Impregnated bednets have been shown to have a salutary effect. DEC can kill developing forms of filarial parasites and has been shown to be useful as a prophylactic agent in humans.

Community-based intervention is the current approach to elimination of lymphatic filariasis as a public health problem. The underlying tenet of this approach is that mass annual distribution of antimicrofilarial chemotherapy—albendazole with either DEC (for all areas except those where onchocerciasis is coendemic) or ivermectin—will profoundly suppress microfilaremia. If the suppression is sustained, then transmission can be interrupted. As an added benefit, these combinations have secondary effects on gastrointestinal helminths. An alternative approach to the control of lymphatic filariasis is the use of salt fortified with DEC. Community use of DEC-fortified salt dramatically reduces microfilarial density with no apparent adverse reactions. Community education and clinical care for persons already suffering from the chronic sequelae of lymphatic filariasis are important components of filariasis control and elimination programs.

TROPICAL PULMONARY EOSINOPHILIA

Tropical pulmonary eosinophilia (TPE) is a distinct syndrome that develops in some individuals infected with lymphatic filarial species. This syndrome affects males and females in a ratio of 4:1, often during the third decade of life. The majority of cases have been reported from India, Pakistan, Sri Lanka, Brazil, Guyana, and Southeast Asia.

CLINICAL FEATURES The main features include a history of residence in filarial-endemic regions, paroxysmal cough and wheezing that are usually nocturnal (and probably related to the nocturnal periodicity of microfilariae), weight loss, low-grade fever, adenopathy, and pronounced blood eosinophilia (>3000 eosinophils/μL). Chest x-rays may be normal but generally show increased bronchovascular markings; diffuse miliary lesions or mottled opacities may be present in the middle and lower lung fields. Tests of pulmonary function show restrictive abnormalities in most cases and obstructive defects in half. Total serum IgE levels (10,000 to 100,000 ng/mL) and antifilarial antibody titers are characteristically elevated.

PATHOLOGY In TPE there is rapid clearance of microfilariae and parasite antigens from the bloodstream by the lungs, and the clinical symptoms result from allergic and inflammatory reactions elicited by the cleared parasites. In some patients, trapping of microfilariae in other reticuloendothelial organs can cause hepatomegaly, splenomegaly, or lymphadenopathy. A prominent, eosinophil-enriched, intraalveolar infiltrate is often reported, and with it comes the release of cytotoxic proinflammatory granular proteins that may mediate some of the pathology seen in TPE. In the absence of successful treatment, interstitial fibrosis can lead to progressive pulmonary damage.

DIFFERENTIAL DIAGNOSIS TPE must be distinguished from asthma, Löffler's syndrome, allergic bronchopulmonary aspergillosis, allergic granulomatosis with angiitis (Churg-Strauss syndrome), the systemic vasculitides (most notably periarteritis nodosa and Wegener's granulomatosis), chronic eosinophilic pneumonia, and the idiopathic hypereosinophilic syndrome. In addition to a geographic history of filarial exposure, useful features for distinguishing TPE include wheezing that is solely nocturnal, very high levels of antifilarial antibodies, and a rapid initial response to treatment with DEC.

℞ TREATMENT

DEC is used at a dosage of 4 to 6 mg/kg of body weight per day for 14 days. Symptoms usually resolve within 3 to 7 days after the initiation of therapy. Relapse, which occurs in ~12 to 25% of cases (sometimes after an interval of years), requires re-treatment.

ONCHOCERCIASIS

Onchocerciasis ("river blindness") is caused by the filarial nematode *O. volvulus*, which infects an estimated 13 million individuals. The majority of individuals infected with *O. volvulus* live in the equatorial region of Africa extending from the Atlantic coast to the Red Sea. About 70,000 persons are infected in Guatemala and Mexico, with smaller foci in Venezuela, Colombia, Brazil, Ecuador, Yemen, and Saudi Arabia. Onchocerciasis is the second leading cause of infectious blindness worldwide.

ETIOLOGY AND EPIDEMIOLOGY Infection in humans begins with the deposition of infective larvae on the skin by the bite of an infected blackfly. The larvae develop into adults, which are typically found in subcutaneous nodules. About 7 months to 3 years after infection, the gravid female releases microfilariae that migrate out of the nodule and throughout the tissues, concentrating in the dermis. Infection is transmitted to other persons when a female fly ingests microfilariae from the host's skin and these microfilariae then develop into infective lar-

vae. Adult *O. volvulus* females and males are about 40 to 60 cm and 3 to 6 cm in length, respectively. The life span of adults can be as long as 18 years, with an average of ~9 years. Because the blackfly vector breeds along free-flowing rivers and streams (particularly in rapids) and generally restricts its flight to an area within several kilometers of these breeding sites, both biting and disease transmission are most intense in these locations.

PATHOLOGY Onchocerciasis affects primarily the skin, eyes, and lymph nodes. In contrast to that in lymphatic filariasis, the damage in onchocerciasis is elicited by microfilariae and not by adult parasites. In the skin, there are mild but chronic inflammatory changes that can result in loss of elastic fibers, atrophy, and fibrosis. The subcutaneous nodules, or onchocercomata, consist primarily of fibrous tissues surrounding the adult worm, often with a peripheral ring of inflammatory cells. In the eye, neovascularization and corneal scarring lead to corneal opacities and blindness. Inflammation in the anterior and posterior chambers frequently results in anterior uveitis, chorioretinitis, and optic atrophy. Although punctate opacities are due to an inflammatory reaction surrounding dead or dying microfilariae, the pathogenesis of most manifestations of onchocerciasis is still unclear.

CLINICAL FEATURES ■ Skin Pruritus and rash are the most frequent manifestations of onchocerciasis. The pruritus can be incapacitating; the rash is typically a papular eruption (Fig. 202-3) that is generalized rather than localized to a particular region of the body. Long-term infection results in exaggerated and premature wrinkling of the skin, loss of elastic fibers, and epidermal atrophy that can lead to loose, redundant skin and hypo- or hyperpigmentation. Localized eczematoid dermatitis can cause hyperkeratosis, scaling, and pigmentary changes. Such lesions are often seen in the lower extremities but can be distributed more extensively.

Onchocercomata These subcutaneous nodules, which can be palpable and/or visible, contain the adult worm. In African patients, they are common over the coccyx and sacrum, the trochanter of the femur, the lateral anterior crest, and other bony prominences; in Latin American patients, nodules tend to develop preferentially in the upper part of the body, particularly on the head, neck, and shoulders. Nodules vary in size and characteristically are firm and not tender. It has been estimated that, for every palpable nodule, there are four deeper nonpalpable ones.

Ocular Tissue Visual impairment is the most serious complication of onchocerciasis and usually affects only those persons with moderate or heavy infections. Lesions may develop in all parts of the eye. The most common early finding is conjunctivitis with photophobia. In the

FIGURE 202-3 Papular eruption as a consequence of onchocerciasis.

cornea, punctate keratitis—consisting of acute inflammatory reactions surrounding dying microfilariae manifested as "snowflake" opacities—is frequent in younger patients and resolves without apparent complications. Sclerosing keratitis occurs in 1 to 5% of infected persons and is the leading cause of onchocercal blindness in Africa. Anterior uveitis and iridocyclitis develop in ~5% of infected persons in Africa. In Latin America, complications of the anterior uveal tract (pupillary deformity) may cause secondary glaucoma. Characteristic chorioretinal lesions develop as a result of atrophy and hyperpigmentation of the retinal pigment epithelium. Constriction of the visual field and frank optic atrophy may occur.

Lymph Nodes   Mild to moderate lymphadenopathy is frequent, particularly in the inguinal and femoral areas, where the enlarged nodes may hang down in response to gravity ("hanging groin"), sometimes predisposing to inguinal and femoral hernias.

Systemic Manifestations   Some heavily infected individuals develop cachexia with loss of adipose tissue and muscle mass. Among adults who become blind, there is a three- to fourfold increase in the mortality rate.

DIAGNOSIS   Definitive diagnosis depends on the detection of an adult worm in an excised nodule or, more commonly, of microfilariae in a skin snip. Skin snips are obtained with a corneal-scleral punch, which collects a blood-free skin biopsy sample extending to just below the epidermis, or by lifting of the skin with the tip of a needle and excision of a small (1- to 3-mm) piece with a sterile scalpel blade. The biopsy tissue is incubated in tissue culture medium or in saline on a glass slide or flat-bottomed microtiter plate. After incubation for 2 to 4 h (or occasionally overnight in light infections), microfilariae emergent from the skin can be visualized by low-power microscopy.

Eosinophilia and elevated serum IgE levels are common but, because they occur in many parasitic infections, are not diagnostic in themselves. Assays to detect specific antibodies to *Onchocerca* and PCR to detect onchocercal DNA in skin snips are now in use in specialized laboratories and are highly sensitive and specific.

The *Mazzotti test* is a provocative technique that can be used in cases where the diagnosis of onchocerciasis is still in doubt (i.e., when skin snips and ocular examination reveal no microfilariae). A small dose of DEC (0.5 to 1.0 mg/kg) is given orally; the development or exacerbation of pruritus or dermatitis within hours is highly suggestive of onchocerciasis.

℞ TREATMENT

The main goals of therapy are to prevent the development of irreversible lesions and to alleviate symptoms. Surgical excision is recommended when nodules are located on the head (because of the proximity of microfilaria-producing adult worms to the eye), but chemotherapy is the mainstay of management. Ivermectin, a semisynthetic macrocyclic lactone active against microfilariae, is the first-line agent for the treatment of onchocerciasis. It is given orally in a single dose of 150 μg/kg, either yearly or semiannually. Recently, more frequent ivermectin administration (every 3 months) has been suggested to ameliorate pruritus and skin disease; moreover, quadrennial administration of ivermectin has been demonstrated to have some macrofilaricidal activity. After treatment, most individuals have few or no reactions. Pruritus, cutaneous edema, and/or maculopapular rash occurs in ~1 to 10% of treated individuals. In areas of Africa coendemic for *O. volvulus* and *L. loa*, however, ivermectin is contraindicated (as it is for pregnant or breastfeeding women) because of severe posttreatment encephalopathy seen in patients, especially children, who are heavily microfilaremic for *L. loa* (2000 to 5000 microfilariae per milliliter). Although ivermectin treatment results in a marked drop in microfilarial density, its effect can be short-lived (<3 months in some cases). Thus, it is occasionally necessary to give ivermectin more frequently for persistent symptoms. A 6-week course of doxycycline has

been demonstrated to be macrofilaristatic (rendering the female adult worms sterile for long periods). Because this regimen targets the *Wolbachia* endosymbiont of the filarial parasite, new options for definitive treatment may become available.

PREVENTION   Vector control has been beneficial in highly endemic areas in which breeding sites are vulnerable to insecticide spraying, but most areas endemic for onchocerciasis are not suited to this type of control. Community-based administration of ivermectin every 6 to 12 months is now being used to interrupt transmission in endemic areas. This measure, in conjunction with vector control, has already helped reduce the prevalence of disease in endemic foci in Africa and Latin America. No drug has proven useful for prophylaxis of *O. volvulus* infection.

LOIASIS

ETIOLOGY AND EPIDEMIOLOGY   Loiasis is caused by *L. loa* (the African eye worm), which is present in the rain forests of West and Central Africa. Adult parasites (females, 50 to 70 mm long and 0.5 mm wide; males, 25 to 35 mm long and 0.25 mm wide) live in subcutaneous tissues; microfilariae circulate in the blood with a diurnal periodicity that peaks between 12:00 noon and 2:00 P.M.

CLINICAL FEATURES   Manifestations of loiasis in natives of endemic areas may differ from those in temporary residents or visitors. Among the indigenous population, loiasis is often an asymptomatic infection with microfilaremia. Infection may be recognized only after subconjunctival migration of an adult worm (Fig. 202-4) or may be manifested by episodic Calabar swellings—evanescent localized areas of angioedema and erythema developing on the extremities and less frequently at other sites. Nephropathy, encephalopathy, and cardiomyopathy are rare. In patients who are not residents of endemic areas, allergic symptoms predominate, episodes of Calabar swelling tend to be more frequent and debilitating, microfilaremia is rare, and eosinophilia and increased levels of antifilarial antibodies are characteristic.

PATHOLOGY   The pathogenesis of the manifestations of loiasis is poorly understood. Calabar swellings are thought to result from a hypersensitivity reaction to the adult worm.

DIAGNOSIS   Definitive diagnosis of loiasis requires the detection of microfilariae in the peripheral blood or the isolation of the adult worm from the eye or from a subconjunctival biopsy specimen from a site of swelling developing after treatment. PCR-based assays for the detection of *L. loa* DNA in blood are now available in specialized laboratories and are highly sensitive and specific. In practice, the diagnosis must often be based on a characteristic history and clinical presentation, blood eosinophilia, and elevated levels of antifilarial antibodies,

FIGURE 202-4   Adult *Loa loa* in the process of surgical removal after its subconjunctival migration.

particularly in travelers to an endemic region, who are usually amicrofilaremic. Other clinical findings in the latter individuals include hypergammaglobulinemia, elevated levels of serum IgE, and elevated leukocyte and eosinophil counts.

 TREATMENT

DEC (8 to 10 mg/kg per day for 21 days) is effective against both the adult and the microfilarial forms of *L. loa*, but multiple courses are frequently necessary before the disease resolves completely. In cases of heavy microfilaremia, allergic or other inflammatory reactions can take place during treatment, including central nervous system involvement with coma and encephalitis. Heavy infections can be treated initially with apheresis to remove the microfilariae and with glucocorticoids (40 to 60 mg of prednisone per day) followed by doses of DEC (0.5 mg/kg per day). If antifilarial treatment has no adverse effects, the prednisone dose can be rapidly tapered and the dose of DEC gradually increased to 8 to 10 mg/kg per day.

Albendazole or ivermectin (although neither is approved for this use by the Food and Drug Administration) has been shown to be effective in reducing microfilarial loads. DEC (300 mg weekly) is an effective prophylactic regimen for loiasis.

STREPTOCERCIASIS

Mansonella streptocerca, found mainly in the tropical forest belt of Africa from Ghana to Zaire, is transmitted by biting midges. The major clinical manifestations involve the skin and include pruritus, papular rashes, and pigmentation changes. Many infected individuals have inguinal adenopathy, although most are asymptomatic. The diagnosis is made by detection of the characteristic microfilariae in skin snips. DEC (6 mg/kg per day in divided doses for 14 to 21 days) is effective in killing both microfilariae and adult worms. As in onchocerciasis, treatment is sometimes accompanied by urticaria, arthralgias, myalgias, headaches, and abdominal discomfort. Ivermectin at a single dose of 150 μg/kg leads to sustained suppression of microfilariae in the skin and is likely to assume primacy in the treatment of streptocerciasis.

MANSONELLA PERSTANS INFECTION

Mansonella perstans, distributed across the center of Africa and in northeastern South America, is transmitted by midges. Adult worms reside in serous cavities—pericardial, pleural, and peritoneal—as well as in the mesentery and the perirenal and retroperitoneal tissues. Microfilariae circulate in the blood without periodicity. The clinical and pathologic features of the infection are poorly defined. Most patients appear to be asymptomatic, but manifestations may include transient angioedema and pruritus of the arms, face, or other parts of the body (analogous to the Calabar swellings of loiasis); fever; headache; arthralgias; and right-upper-quadrant pain. Occasionally, pericarditis and hepatitis occur. The diagnosis is based on the demonstration of microfilariae in blood or serosal effusions. Perstans filariasis is often associated with peripheral-blood eosinophilia and antifilarial antibody elevations. Although DEC (8 to 10 mg/kg per day for 21 days) is the standard therapeutic agent, there is little evidence that it is effective. Cure is indicated by the disappearance of symptoms and eosinophilia; multiple courses of therapy are usually required. Ivermectin, used in frequent repeated doses, has been shown to be capable of reducing blood microfilarial levels. Both mebendazole (100 mg twice daily for 30 days) and albendazole (400 mg twice daily for 10 days) have been reported occasionally to be effective.

MANSONELLA OZZARDI INFECTION

The distribution of *Mansonella ozzardi* is restricted to Central and South America and certain Caribbean islands. Adult worms are rarely recovered from humans. Microfilariae circulate in the blood without periodicity. Although this organism has often been considered nonpathogenic, headache, articular pain, fever, pulmonary symptoms, adenopathy, hepatomegaly, pruritus, and eosinophilia have been ascribed to *M. ozzardi* infection. Diagnosis is made by the detection of micro-

filariae in peripheral blood. Ivermectin (a single dose of 6 mg) has been shown to be effective in treating this infection.

DRACUNCULIASIS (GUINEA WORM INFECTION)

ETIOLOGY AND EPIDEMIOLOGY Dracunculiasis, caused by *Dracunculus medinensis*, is a parasitic infection whose incidence has declined dramatically because of global eradication efforts. Current estimates suggest that there are 56,000 cases worldwide, the majority in Sudan. Humans acquire this infection when they ingest water containing infective larvae derived from *Cyclops*, a crustacean that is the intermediate host. Larvae penetrate the stomach or intestinal wall, mate, and mature. The adult male probably dies; the female *Dracunculus* develops over a year and migrates to subcutaneous tissues, usually in the lower extremity. As the thin female *Dracunculus*, ranging in length from 300 cm to 1 m, approaches the skin, a blister forms that, over days, breaks down and forms an ulcer. When the blister opens, large numbers of motile, rhabditiform larvae can be released into stagnant water; ingestion by *Cyclops* completes the life cycle.

CLINICAL FEATURES Few or no clinical manifestations of dracunculiasis are evident until just before the blister forms, when there is an onset of fever and generalized allergic symptoms, including periorbital edema, wheezing, and urticaria. The emergence of the worm is associated with local pain and swelling. When the blister ruptures (usually as a result of immersion in water), the adult worm releases larva-rich fluid, and this release is associated with a relief of symptoms. The shallow ulcer surrounding the emerging adult worm heals over weeks to months. Such ulcers, however, can become secondarily infected, the result being cellulitis, local inflammation, abscess formation, or (uncommonly) tetanus. Occasionally, the adult worm does not emerge but becomes encapsulated and calcified.

DIAGNOSIS The diagnosis is based on the findings developing with the emergence of the adult worm, as described above.

 TREATMENT

Gradual extraction of the worm by winding of a few centimeters on a stick each day remains the common and effective practice. Worms may be excised surgically. The administration of metronidazole (250 mg three times daily for 10 days) may relieve symptoms but has no proven activity against the worm.

PREVENTION Prevention, which remains the only real control measure, depends on the provision of safe drinking water.

ZOONOTIC FILARIAL INFECTIONS

Dirofilariae that affect primarily dogs, cats, and raccoons occasionally infect humans incidentally, as do *Brugia* and *Onchocerca* parasites that affect small mammals. Because humans are an abnormal host, the parasites never develop fully. Pulmonary dirofilarial infection caused by the canine heartworm *Dirofilaria immitis* generally presents in humans as a solitary pulmonary nodule. Chest pain, hemoptysis, and cough are uncommon. Infections with *D. repens* (from dogs) or *D. tenuis* (from raccoons) can cause local subcutaneous nodules in humans. Zoonotic *Brugia* infection can produce isolated lymph node enlargement, whereas zoonotic *Onchocerca* can cause subconjunctival masses. Eosinophilia levels and antifilarial antibody titers are not commonly elevated. Excisional biopsy is both diagnostic and curative; these infections usually do not respond to chemotherapy.

FURTHER READING

ADDISS DA, DREYER G: Treatment of lymphatic filariasis, in *Lymphatic Filariasis*, TB Nutman (ed). London, Imperial College Press, 1999, pp 151–199

BOCKARIE MJ et al: Mass treatment to eliminate filariasis in Papua New Guinea. N Engl J Med 347:1841, 2002

DREYER G et al: Acute attacks in the extremities of persons living in an area endemic for bancroftian filariasis: Differentiation of two syndromes. Trans R Soc Trop Med Hyg 93:413, 1999

GARDON J et al: Serious reactions after mass treatment of onchocerciasis with ivermectin in an area endemic for *Loa loa* infection. Lancet 350:18, 1997

——— et al: Effects of standard and high doses of ivermectin on adult worms of *Onchocerca volvulus*: A randomised controlled trial. Lancet 360:203, 2002

HOERAUF A et al: Depletion of *Wolbachia* endobacteria in *Onchocerca vol-*

vulus by doxycycline and microfilaridermia after ivermectin treatment. Lancet 357:1415, 2001

——— et al: Onchocerciasis. BMJ 326:207, 2003

HOPKINS DR et al: Dracunculiasis eradication: And now, Sudan. Am J Trop Med Hyg 67:415, 2002

MCCARTHY JS: Diagnosis of lymphatic filarial infections, in *Lymphatic Filariasis*, TB Nutman (ed). London, Imperial College Press, 1999, pp 127–149

WHO EXPERT COMMITTEE ON ONCHOCERCIASIS: Onchocerciasis and its control: Fourth report. Tech Rep Ser No 852. Geneva, World Health Organization, 1995

203   SCHISTOSOMIASIS AND OTHER TREMATODE INFECTIONS
Adel A.F. Mahmoud

Trematodes, or flatworms, are a group of morphologically and biologically heterogeneous organisms that belong to the phylum Platyhelminthes. Human infection with trematodes occurs in many geographic areas and can cause considerable morbidity and mortality. For clinical purposes, the significant trematode infections of humans may be divided according to the tissues invaded by adult flukes: blood, biliary tree, intestines, and lungs (Table 203-1).

Trematodes share some common morphologic features, including macroscopic size (from 1 cm to several cm); dorsoventral, flattened, bilaterally symmetric bodies (adult worms); and the prominence of two suckers. Except for the schistosomes, all trematodes that parasitize humans are hermaphroditic. The life cycle of trematodes involves a definitive host (mammalian/human), in which adult worms initiate sexual reproduction, and an intermediate host (snails), in which asexual multiplication of the larval forms occurs. More than one intermediate host may be necessary for some species of trematodes. Human infection is initiated either by direct penetration of intact skin or by ingestion. Upon maturation within the human host, adult flukes initiate sexual reproduction that results in egg production. Helminth ova leave the definitive host in excreta or sputum and, upon reaching suitable environmental conditions, they hatch, releasing free-living miracidia that must find a specific snail intermediate host. After asexual reproduction, cercariae are released from infected snails; these organisms either infect humans or must find another intermediate host to allow encystment into metacercariae—the infective stage in these species.

The host-parasite relationship in trematode infections is a product of the biologic features of these organisms: they are multicellular, undergo several developmental changes within the host, and usually result in chronic infections. In general, the distribution of worm infections in human populations is *overdispersed*; i.e., it follows a negative binomial mathematical relationship in which most infected individuals harbor low worm burdens while a small percentage are heavily infected. It is the heavily infected minority who are particularly prone to disease sequelae and who constitute an epidemiologically significant reservoir of infection in endemic areas. It is also important to appreciate that worms do not multiply within the definitive host and that they have a relatively long life span, ranging from a few months to a few years. Morbidity and mortality due to trematode infections reflect a multifactorial process that results from the tipping of a delicate balance based on the intensity of infection and the host reactions that initiate and modulate pathologic outcome. Furthermore, the genetics of the parasite and the human host contribute to the outcome of infection and disease. Infections with trematodes that migrate through or reside in host tissues are associated with a moderate to high degree of peripheral blood eosinophilia; this association is of significance in protective and immunopathologic sequelae and is a useful clinical indicator of infection.

APPROACH TO THE PATIENT

The approach to individuals with suspected trematode infection begins with a question: Where have you been? Details of geo-

graphic history, exposure to freshwater bodies, and indulgence in local eating habits without ensuring safety of food and drink are all essential elements in the history. The workup plan must include a detailed physical examination and tests appropriate for the suspected infection. Diagnosis is based either on detection of the relevant stage of the parasite in excreta, sputum, or (rarely) tissue samples or on sensitive and specific serologic tests. Consultation with physicians familiar with these infections or with the U.S. Centers for Disease Control and Prevention (CDC) is helpful in guiding diagnosis and selecting therapy.

BLOOD FLUKES: SCHISTOSOMIASIS

Human schistosomiasis is caused by five species of this parasitic trematode: the intestinal species *Schistosoma mansoni*, *S. japonicum*, *S. mekongi*, and *S. intercalatum* and the urinary species *S. haematobium*. Infection may cause considerable morbidity in the intestines, liver, and urinary tract, and a proportion of affected individuals die. Other schistosome species (e.g., avian species) may invade human skin but then die in subcutaneous tissue, producing only self-limiting cutaneous manifestations.

Information on the prevalence and geographic distribution of human schistosomiasis is inexact. The five species are estimated to infect 200 to 300 million people in South America, the Caribbean, Africa, the Middle East, and Southeast Asia. The total population living under conditions favoring transmission approximates double or triple that number—a fact reflecting the public health significance of schistosomiasis.

ETIOLOGY Human infection is initiated by penetration of intact skin with infective cercariae. These organisms are released from infected snails in freshwater bodies; they measure ~2 mm in length and possess an anterior and a ventral sucker that attach to the skin surface and facilitate penetration. Once in the subcutaneous tissue, the organism transforms into the next stage: the schistosomula. This transformation involves morphologic, membrane, and immunologic changes, prominent among which is the transformation of the cercarial outer membrane from a trilaminar to a heptalaminar membrane that is then maintained throughout the life span of the worms in humans. The transformation to a heptalaminar structure is thought to be the schistosome's main adaptive mechanism for survival in humans. Schistosomulae begin their migration within 2 to 4 days via venous or lymphatic vessels, reaching the lungs and finally the liver parenchyma. Sexually mature worms descend into the venous system at specific anatomical locations: intestinal veins (*S. mansoni*, *S. japonicum*, *S. mekongi*, and *S. intercalatum*) and vesical veins (*S. haematobium*). After mating, adult gravid females travel against venous blood flow to small tributaries, where they deposit their ova intravascularly. Schistosome ova (Fig. 203-1) have specific morphologic features that can be used to differentiate species. Aided by enzymatic secretions through minipores in eggshells, ova move through the venous wall, traversing host tissues to reach the lumen of the intestinal or urinary tract, and are voided with stools or urine. Approximately 50% of ova are retained in host tissues locally (intestines or urinary tract) or are carried by venous blood flow to the liver and other organs. Schistosome ova that reach freshwater bodies hatch, releasing free-living miracidia that seek the snail intermediate host to undergo several asexual multiplication cycles. Finally, infective cercariae are shed from snails.

Adult schistosome worms measure ~1 to 2 cm in length. The male is slightly shorter, with a flattened body; its edges curve anteriorly to form the gynecophoral canal, in which mature adult females are usually held. The females are longer, slender, and rounded in cross-section. The precise nature of biochemical and reproductive exchanges between the two sexes is unknown, as are the regulatory mechanisms for pairing. Adult schistosomes parasitize specific sites in the host venous system. What guides adult intestinal schistosomes to branches of the superior or inferior mesenteric veins or adult *S. haematobium* worms to the vesical plexus is unknown. In addition, the evasion mechanisms by which adult worms inhibit the coagulation cascade and the effector arms of the host immune responses are not fully understood. The genome of schistosomes is made of 16 chromosomes; its DNA sequence is currently being determined.

EPIDEMIOLOGY The distribution of schistosome infection and related disease syndromes in human populations (Fig. 203-2) is dependent on both parasite and host factors. In endemic areas, the rate of yearly onset of new infection, or incidence, is generally low. Prevalence, on the other hand, starts to be appreciable by the age of 3 to 4 years and builds to a maximum that varies by endemic region (up to 100%) in the 15- to 20-year age group. Prevalence then stabilizes or decreases slightly in older age groups (>40 years). Intensity of infection (as measured by fecal or urinary egg counts, which correlate with adult worm burdens in most circumstances) follows the increase in prevalence up to the age of 15 to 20 years and then declines markedly in older age groups. This decline may reflect acquisition of resistance, or it may be due to changes in water contact patterns, since older people are exposed less. Furthermore, the unique distribution of schistosomes in human populations (i.e., an overdispersed distribution) may be due to the heterogeneity of worm populations, with some more invasive than others; alternatively, it may be due to differences in the genetic susceptibility of host populations, as has recently been demonstrated.

Disease due to schistosome infection is the outcome of parasitologic, host, and additional infectious, nutritional, and environmental factors. Most of the disease syndromes relate to the presence of one or more of the parasite stages in the human host. The distribution of disease manifestations in the populations of endemic areas correlates, in general, with the intensity and duration of infection as well as with the age and genetic susceptibility of the host. Overall, disease manifestations are clinically relevant in only a small proportion of persons infected with any of the intestinal schistosomes. In contrast, urinary schistosomiasis manifests clinically in most infected individuals.

Patients with both HIV infection and schistosomiasis have been found to excrete far fewer eggs in their stools than those infected with *S. mansoni* alone; the mechanism underlying this difference is unknown. The two groups, however, respond equally to treatment with praziquantel.

PATHOGENESIS AND IMMUNITY During the invasive stage, cercaria-associated dermatitis reflects dermal and subdermal inflammatory responses—both humoral and cell-mediated. As the parasites approach

TABLE 203-1	*Major Human Trematode Infections*	
Trematode	Transmission	Endemic Area(s)
BLOOD FLUKES		
Schistosoma mansoni	Skin penetration by cercariae released from snails	Africa, South America, Middle East
S. japonicum	Skin penetration by cercariae released from snails	China, Philippines, Indonesia
S. intercalatum	Skin penetration by cercariae released from snails	West Africa
S. mekongi	Skin penetration by cercariae released from snails	Southeast Asia
S. haematobium	Skin penetration by cercariae released from snails	Africa, Middle East
BILIARY (HEPATIC) FLUKES		
Clonorchis sinensis	Ingestion of metacercariae in freshwater fish	Far East
Opisthorchis viverrini	Ingestion of metacercariae in freshwater fish	Far East, Thailand
O. felineus	Ingestion of metacercariae in freshwater fish	Far East, Europe
Fasciola hepatica	Ingestion of metacercariae on aquatic plants or in water	Worldwide
F. gigantica	Ingestion of metacercariae on aquatic plants or in water	Sporadic, Africa
INTESTINAL FLUKES		
Fasciolopsis buski	Ingestion of metacercariae on aquatic plants	Southeast Asia
Heterophyes heterophyes	Ingestion of metacercariae in freshwater or brackish-water fish	Far East, North Africa
LUNG FLUKES		
Paragonimus westermani	Ingestion of metacercariae in crayfish or crabs	Global except North America and Europe

sexual maturity and the commencement of oviposition, acute schistosomiasis or Katayama fever (a serum sickness–like illness; see "Clinical Features," below) may occur. The associated antigen excess results in the formation of soluble immune complexes, which may be deposited in several tissues, initiating the sequence of pathologic events. In chronic schistosomiasis, most disease manifestations are due to eggs retained in host tissues. The granulomatous response around these ova is cell-mediated and is regulated both positively and negatively by a cascade of cytokine, cellular, and humoral responses. Granuloma formation begins with recruitment of a host of inflammatory cells in response to antigens secreted by the living organism within the ova. Cells recruited initially include phagocytes, antigen-specific T cells, and eosinophils. Fibroblasts, giant cells, and B lymphocytes predominate later. Once activated, T cells produce cytokines [such as tumor necrosis factor α (TNF-α), interleukin (IL) 2, IL-4, and IL-5, which in turn activate endothelial cells] as well as specific chemokines [such as monocyte chemotactic protein 1 (MCP-1)]. The result is recruitment of the cellular elements that organize in the form of granulomas around parasite eggs. These lesions reach a size many times that of the eggs, thus inducing organomegaly and obstruction. Immunomodulation or downregulation of host responses to schistosome eggs plays a significant role in limiting the extent of the granulomatous lesions—and consequently disease—in chronically infected experimental animals or humans. The underlying mechanisms involve another cascade of regulatory cytokines (IL-10, IL-12) and idiotypic antibodies. Subsequent to the granulomatous response, fibrosis sets in, resulting in more permanent disease sequelae. Because schistosomiasis is a chronic infection, the accumulation of antigen-antibody complexes results in deposits in renal glomeruli and may cause significant kidney disease.

The better-studied pathologic sequelae in schistosomiasis are those observed in liver disease. Ova that are carried by portal blood embolize to the liver. Because of their size (~150 × 60 μm in the case of *S. mansoni*), they lodge at presinusoidal sites, where granulomas are formed. The granulomas contribute to the liver enlargement observed in infected individuals. Schistosomal hepatomegaly is also associated

FIGURE 203-1 Morphology of schistosome eggs, the diagnostic stage of the parasite's life cycle. *A. S. haematobium* egg found in urine sample. Egg is large (~140 μm long), with a terminal spine. *B. S. mansoni* egg found in feces. Egg is large (~150 μm long), with a thin shell and lateral spine. *C. S. japonicum* egg found in feces. Egg is smaller than that of *S. mansoni* (~90 μm long), with a small spine or hooklike structure. *D. S. mekongi* egg found in feces. Egg is similar to that of *S. japonicum* but smaller (~65 μm long). *E. S. intercalatum* egg found in feces. Egg is larger than that of *S. haematobium* (~190 μm long), with a longer, sharply pointed spine. (*From LR Ash, TC Orihel: Atlas of Human Parasitology, 3d ed. Chicago, ASCP Press, 1990; with permission.*)

with certain class I and class II human leukocyte antigen (HLA) markers; its genetic basis appears to be multigenic. Presinusoidal portal blockage causes several hemodynamic changes, including portal hypertension and associated development of portosystemic collaterals at the esophagogastric junction and other sites. Esophageal varices are most likely to break and cause repeated episodes of hematemesis. Because changes in liver hemodynamics in schistosomiasis are slow, compensatory arterialization of blood flow through the liver is established. While this compensatory mechanism may be associated with certain metabolic side effects, the retention of hepatocyte perfusion permits the maintenance of normal liver function for several years.

After granuloma formation, the second most significant pathologic change in the liver relates to the onset of fibrosis. It is characteristically periportal (Symmers' clay pipe–stem fibrosis) but may be diffuse. Fibrosis, when diffuse, may be seen in areas of egg deposition and granuloma formation, but it is also seen in distant locations such as portal tracts. Schistosomiasis alone results in pure fibrotic lesions in the liver; cirrhosis occurs when other nutritional or infectious agents (e.g., hepatitis B or C virus) are involved. In recent years, it has been recognized that deposition of fibrotic tissue in the extracellular matrix

results from the interaction of T lymphocytes with cells of the fibroblast series; several cytokines, such as IL-2, IL-4, IL-1, and transforming growth factor β (TGF-β), are known to stimulate fibrogenesis. The process may be dependent on the genetic constitution of the host. Furthermore, regulatory cytokines that can suppress fibrogenesis, such as interferon γ (IFN-γ) or IL-12, may play a role in modulating the response.

While the above description focuses on granuloma formation and fibrosis of the liver, similar processes occur in urinary schistosomiasis. Granuloma formation at the lower end of the ureters obstructs urinary flow, with subsequent development of hydroureter and hydronephrosis. Similar lesions in the urinary bladder cause the protrusion of papillomatous structures into its cavity; these may ulcerate and/or bleed. The chronic stage of infection is associated with scarring and deposition of calcium in the bladder wall.

Immunomodulation is an essential mechanism in shaping the clinical and pathologic outcome of schistosomiasis. While most detailed immunologic analyses have been performed in experimental animals, enough evidence exists from studies in humans to delineate the suppression of T cell responses in association with active infections and a regulatory role for IL-10.

FIGURE 203-2 Global distribution of schistosomiasis. *A. S. mansoni* infection (*dark blue*) is endemic in Africa, the Middle East, South America, and a few Caribbean countries. *S. intercalatum* infection (*green*) is endemic in sporadic foci in West and Central Africa. *B. S. haematobium* infection (*purple*) is endemic in Africa and the Middle East. The major endemic countries for *S. japonicum* infection (*green*) are China, the Philippines, and Indonesia. *S. mekongi* infection (*red*) is endemic in sporadic foci in Southeast Asia.

Studies on immunity to schistosomiasis, whether innate or acquired, have expanded our knowledge of the components of these responses and the target antigens. The concept of innate immunity is illustrated by the inability of avian schistosomes, which cause swimmers' itch, to reach maturity in humans. The critical question, however, is whether humans acquire immunity to schistosomes. Epidemiologic evidence suggests the onset of acquired immunity during the course of infection in young adults. Curative treatment of infection divides populations in endemic areas into those who acquire reinfection rapidly (susceptible) and those who follow a protracted course (resistant). This difference may be explained by differences in transmission, immunologic response, or genetic susceptibility. The mechanism of acquired immunity involves antibodies, complement, and several effector cells, particularly eosinophils. Furthermore, the intensity of schistosome infection has been correlated with a region in chromosome 5. In several recent studies, a few protective schistosome antigens have been identified as vaccine candidates, but none has been evaluated in human populations to date.

CLINICAL FEATURES In general, disease manifestations of schistosomiasis occur in three stages, which vary not only by species but also by intensity of infection and other host factors, such as age and genetics. During the phase of cercarial invasion, a form of dermatitis may be observed. This so-called swimmers' itch occurs most often with *S. mansoni* and *S. japonicum* infections, manifesting 2 or 3 days after invasion as an itchy maculopapular rash on the affected areas of the skin. The condition is particularly severe when humans are exposed to avian schistosomes. This form of cercarial dermatitis is seen around the freshwater lakes in the northern United States, particularly in the spring. Cercarial dermatitis is a self-limiting clinical entity. During worm maturation and at the beginning of oviposition (i.e., 4 to 8 weeks after skin invasion), acute schistosomiasis or Katayama fever—a serum sickness–like syndrome with fever, generalized lymphadenopathy, and hepatosplenomegaly—may develop. Individuals suffering from acute schistosomiasis show a high degree of peripheral blood eosinophilia. Parasite-specific antibodies may be detected before schistosome eggs are identified in excreta. Acute schistosomiasis has become an important clinical entity worldwide because of increased travel to endemic areas. Travelers are exposed to parasites while swimming or wading in freshwater bodies and upon their return present with the acute manifestations. The course of acute schistosomiasis is generally benign, but deaths are occasionally reported in association with heavy exposure to schistosomes.

The main clinical manifestations of chronic schistosomiasis are species-dependent. Intestinal species (*S. mansoni*, *S. japonicum*, *S. mekongi*, and *S. intercalatum*) cause intestinal and hepatosplenic disease as well as several manifestations associated with portal hypertension. During the intestinal phase, which may begin a few months after infection and may last for years, symptomatic patients characteristically have colicky abdominal pain and bloody diarrhea. Patients may also report fatigue and an inability to perform daily routine functions and may show evidence of growth retardation. The severity of intestinal schistosomiasis is often related to the intensity of the worm burden. The disease runs a chronic course but rarely progresses to a functional level (e.g., malabsorption) or to anatomical lesions of the gut. The exception is colonic polyposis, which has been seen in some endemic areas, such as Egypt.

The hepatosplenic phase of disease manifests early (during the first year of infection, particularly in children) with enlargement of the liver due to parasite-induced granulomatous lesions. Hepatomegaly is seen in ~15 to 20% of infected individuals; it correlates roughly with intensity of infection, occurs more often in children, and may be related to specific HLA haplotypes. In subsequent phases of infection, presinusoidal blockage of blood flow leads to portal hypertension and splenomegaly. Moreover, portal hypertension may lead to varices at the lower end of the esophagus and at other sites. Patients with schistosomal liver disease may have right-upper-quadrant "dragging" pain during the hepatomegaly phase, and this pain may move to the left upper quadrant as splenomegaly progresses. Bleeding from esophageal varices may, however, be the first clinical manifestation of this phase. Patients may experience repeated bleeding but seem to tolerate its impact, since an adequate total hepatic blood flow permits normal liver function for a considerable period in schistosomal hepatomegaly. In late-stage disease, typical fibrotic changes occur along with liver function deterioration and the onset of ascites, hypoalbuminemia, and defects in coagulation. Intercurrent viral infections of the liver (especially hepatitis B and C) or nutritional deficiencies may well accelerate or exacerbate the deterioration of hepatic function.

The extent and severity of intestinal and hepatic disease in schistosomiasis mansoni and japonica have been well described. While it was originally thought that *S. japonicum* might induce more severe disease manifestations because the adult worms can produce ten times more eggs than *S. mansoni*, subsequent field studies have not supported this claim. Clinical observations of individuals infected with *S. mekongi* or *S. intercalatum* have been less detailed, partly because of the far more limited geographic distribution of these organisms.

The clinical manifestations of *S. haematobium* infection occur relatively early and involve a relatively high percentage of individuals. Up to 80% of children infected with *S. haematobium* have dysuria, frequency, and hematuria, which may be terminal. Urine examination reveals blood and albumin as well as an unusually high frequency of bacterial urinary tract infection and urinary sediment cellular metaplasia. These manifestations correlate with intensity of infection, the presence of urinary bladder granulomas, and subsequent ulceration. Along with the local effects of granuloma formation in the urinary bladder, obstruction of the lower end of the ureters results in hydroureter and hydronephrosis, which can be seen in 25 to 50% of infected children. As infection progresses, bladder granulomas undergo fibrosis; the result is the presence of typical sandy patches visible on cystoscopy. In many endemic areas, an association between squamous cell carcinoma of the bladder and *S. haematobium* infection has been observed. Such malignancy is detected in a younger age group than is transitional cell carcinoma. In fact, *S. haematobium* has now been classified as a human carcinogen.

Significant disease may occur in other organs during chronic schistosomiasis. Most important is disease in the lungs and central nervous system (CNS); other locations, such as the skin and the genital organs, are far less frequently affected. In pulmonary schistosomiasis, embolized eggs lodge in small arterioles, producing acute necrotizing arteriolitis and granuloma formation. During *S. mansoni* and *S. japonicum* infection, schistosome eggs reach the lungs after the development of portosystemic collateral circulation; in *S. haematobium* infection, ova may reach the lungs directly via connections between the vesical and systemic circulation. After the development of arteriolitis and granuloma formation, fibrous tissue deposition is detected and leads to endarteritis obliterans, pulmonary hypertension, and cor pulmonale. This clinical entity is an uncommon presentation during chronic schistosomiasis. The most frequent symptoms are cough, fever, and dyspnea; ascites and hemoptysis are less frequently encountered. Cor pulmonale may be diagnosed radiologically on the basis of prominent right side of the heart and dilation of the pulmonary artery. Frank evidence of right-sided heart failure may be seen in late cases.

CNS schistosomiasis is important but less common than pulmonary schistosomiasis. It characteristically occurs as cerebral disease due to *S. japonicum* infection. Migratory worms deposit eggs in the brain and induce a granulomatous response. The frequency of this manifestation among infected individuals in some endemic areas (e.g., the Philippines) is calculated at 2 to 4%. Jacksonian epilepsy due to *S. japonicum* infection is the second most common cause of epilepsy in these areas. *S. mansoni* and *S. haematobium* infections have been associated with transverse myelitis. This syndrome is thought to be due to eggs traveling to the venous plexus around the spinal cord. In schistosomiasis mansoni, transverse myelitis is usually seen in the chronic stage after the development of portal hypertension and portosystemic shunts, which allow ova to travel to the spinal cord veins. This proposed sequence of events has been challenged because of a few reports of transverse myelitis occurring early in the course of *S. mansoni* infection. More information is needed to confirm these observations. During schistosomiasis haematobia, ova may travel through communication between vesical and systemic veins, resulting in spinal cord disease that may be detected at any stage of infection. Pathologic study of lesions in schistosomal transverse myelitis may reveal eggs along with necrotic or granulomatous lesions. Patients usually present with acute or rapidly progressing lower-leg weakness accompanied by sphincter dysfunction.

DIAGNOSIS Physicians in areas not endemic for schistosomiasis face considerable diagnostic challenges. In the most common clinical presentation, a traveler returns with symptoms and signs of acute syndromes of schistosomiasis—namely, cercarial dermatitis or Katayama fever. Central to correct diagnosis is a thorough inquiry into travel history and exposure to freshwater bodies, whether slow or fast running. Differential diagnosis of fever in returned travelers includes a spectrum of infections whose etiologies are viral (e.g., Dengue fever), bacterial (e.g., enteric fever, leptospirosis), rickettsial, or protozoal (e.g., malaria). In cases of Katayama fever, prompt diagnosis is essential and is based on clinical presentation, high-level peripheral blood eosinophilia, and a positive serologic assay for schistosomal antibodies. Two tests are available at the CDC: the Falcon assay screening test/enzyme-linked immunosorbent assay (FAST-ELISA) and the confirmatory enzyme-linked immunoelectrotransfer blot (EITB). Both tests are highly sensitive and ~96% specific. In some instances, examination of stool or urine for ova may yield positive results.

Individuals with established infection are diagnosed by a combination of geographic history, characteristic clinical presentation, and presence of schistosome ova in excreta. The diagnosis may also be established with the serologic assays mentioned above or with those that detect circulating schistosome antigens. These assays can be applied either to blood or to other body fluids (e.g., cerebrospinal fluid). For stool examination, the Kato thick smear or any other concentration method generally identifies all but the most lightly infected individuals. Urine may be examined by microscopy of sediment or by filtration of a known volume through Nuclepore filters. Kato thick smear and Nuclepore filtration provide quantitative data on the intensity of infection, which is of value in assessing the degree of tissue damage and in monitoring the effect of chemotherapy. Finally, schistosome infection may be diagnosed by examination of tissue samples, typically rectal biopsies; other biopsy procedures (e.g., liver biopsy) are not needed, except in special circumstances.

Differential diagnosis of schistosomal hepatomegaly must include viral hepatitis of all etiologies, miliary tuberculosis, malaria, visceral leishmaniasis, ethanol abuse, and causes of hepatic and portal vein obstruction. Of patients with these conditions, only a few may present with organomegaly and relatively intact liver function. The differential diagnosis of hematuria in *S. haematobium* infection includes bacterial cystitis, tuberculosis, urinary stones, and malignancy.

℞ TREATMENT

Treatment of schistosomiasis depends on the stage of infection and the clinical presentation. Other than topical dermatologic applications for relief of itching, no specific treatment is indicated for cercarial dermatitis caused by avian schistosomes. Therapy for acute schistosomiasis or Katayama fever needs to be adjusted appropriately for each case. While antischistosomal chemotherapy is indicated, it does not address immediate pathologic changes. In severe acute schistosomiasis, management in an acute-care setting is necessary, with supportive measures and consideration of glucocorticoid treatment. Once the acute critical phase is over, specific chemotherapy is indicated. For all individuals with infection established by either the demonstration of schistosome eggs or positive serology, treatment to eradicate the parasite should be administered. The drug of choice is praziquantel, which—depending on the infecting species (Table 203-2)—is administered orally as 40 or 60 mg/kg in two or three doses over a single day. Praziquantel treatment results in parasitologic cure in ~85% of cases and reduces egg counts by >90%. Few side effects have been encountered, and those that do develop usually do not interfere with completion of treatment. The dependence on a single chemotherapeutic agent has raised the possibility of the development of resistance in the schistosomes; to date, such resistance does not seem to be clinically significant. Other antischistosomal chemotherapeutic agents are cur-

TABLE 203-2 *Drug Therapy for Human Trematode Infections*

Infection	Drug of Choice	Adult Dose and Duration
BLOOD FLUKES		
S. mansoni, S. intercalatum, S. haematobium	Praziquantel	20 mg/kg, 2 doses in 1 day
S. japonicum, S. mekongi	Praziquantel	20 mg/kg, 3 doses in 1 day
BILIARY (HEPATIC) FLUKES		
C. sinensis, O. viverrini, O. felineus	Praziquantel	25 mg/kg, 3 doses in 1 day
F. hepatica, F. gigantica	Triclabendazole	10 mg/kg once
INTESTINAL FLUKES		
F. buski, H. heterophyes	Praziquantel	25 mg/kg, 3 doses in 1 day
LUNG FLUKES		
P. westermani	Praziquantel	25 mg/kg, 3 doses per day for 2 days

rently considered only as alternatives when praziquantel is unavailable. The effect of antischistosomal treatment on disease manifestations varies by stage. Early hepatomegaly and bladder lesions are known to resolve following chemotherapy, but the late established manifestations, such as fibrosis, do not change. Additional management modalities are needed for individuals with other manifestations, such as hepatocellular failure or recurrent hematemesis. The use of these interventions is guided by general medical and surgical principles.

PREVENTION AND CONTROL Since transmission of schistosomiasis is dependent on human behavior, it is theoretically possible to devise an effective preventive strategy. The geographic distribution of infections in endemic regions of the world is not clearly demarcated. It is therefore prudent for travelers to avoid contact with all freshwater bodies, irrespective of the speed of water flow or unsubstantiated claims of safety. Some topical agents, when applied to the skin, may conceivably inhibit cercarial penetration, but none of these agents is currently available. If exposure occurs, a follow-up visit with a health care provider is strongly recommended. Prevention of infection in inhabitants of endemic areas is a significant challenge. People of these regions use freshwater bodies for sanitary, domestic, recreational, and agricultural purposes. Several control measures have been used, including application of molluscicides, provision of sanitary water and means for sewage disposal, chemotherapy, and health education. Current recommendations to countries endemic for schistosomiasis emphasize the use of multiple approaches. Particularly with the advent of an oral, safe, and effective antischistosomal agent, chemotherapy has been most successful in reducing the intensity of infection and reversing disease. The duration of this positive impact depends on transmission dynamics of the parasite in any specific endemic region. The ultimate goal of research on prevention and control is the development of a vaccine. Although there are a few promising leads, this goal is probably not within reach during the next decade or so.

LIVER (BILIARY) FLUKES

Several species of biliary fluke infecting humans are particularly common in Southeast Asia and Russia. Other species are transmitted in Europe, Africa, and the Americas. On the basis of their migratory pathway in humans, these infections may be divided into the *Clonorchis* and *Fasciola* groups (Table 203-1).

CLONORCHIASIS AND OPISTHORCHIASIS Infection with *Clonorchis sinensis*, the Chinese or oriental fluke, is endemic among fish-eating mammals in Southeast Asia. Humans are an incidental host; the prevalence of human infection is highest in China, Vietnam, and Korea. Infection with *Opisthorchis viverrini* and *O. felineus* is zoonotic in cats and dogs. Transmission to humans occurs occasionally, particularly in Thailand (*O. viverrini*) and in Southeast Asia and eastern Europe (*O. felineus*). Data on the exact geographic distribution of these infectious agents in human populations are rudimentary.

Infection with any of these three species is established by ingestion of raw or inadequately cooked freshwater fish harboring metacercariae. These organisms excyst in the duodenum, releasing larvae that travel through the ampulla of Vater and mature into adult worms in the bile canaliculi. Mature flukes are flat and elongated, measuring 1 to 2 cm in length. The hermaphroditic worms reproduce by releasing small operculated eggs, which pass with bile into the intestines and are voided with stools. The life cycle is completed in the environment in specific freshwater snails (the first intermediate host) and encystment of metacercariae in freshwater fish.

Except for late sequelae, the exact clinical syndromes caused by clonorchiasis and opisthorchiasis are not well defined. Since most infected individuals harbor a low worm burden, many are asymptomatic. Moderate to heavy infection may be associated with vague right-upper-quadrant pain. In contrast, chronic or repeated infection is associated with manifestations such as cholangitis, cholangiohepatitis, and biliary obstruction. Cholangiocarcinoma is epidemiologically related to *C. sinensis* infection in China and to *O. viverrini* infection in northeastern Thailand. This association has resulted in the classification of these infectious agents as human carcinogens.

FASCIOLIASIS Infections with *Fasciola hepatica* and *F. gigantica* are worldwide zoonoses that are particularly endemic in sheep-raising countries. Human cases have been reported in South America, Europe, Africa, Australia, and the Far East. Recent estimates indicate a worldwide prevalence of 17 million cases. High endemicity has been reported in certain areas of Peru and Bolivia. In most endemic areas the predominant species is *F. hepatica*, but in Asia and Africa a varying degree of overlap with *F. gigantica* has been observed.

Humans acquire fascioliasis by ingestion of metacercariae attached to certain aquatic plants, such as watercress. Infection may also be acquired by consumption of contaminated water or ingestion of food items washed with such water. Acquisition of human infection through consumption of freshly prepared raw liver containing immature flukes has been reported. Infection is initiated when metacercariae excyst, penetrate the gut wall, and travel through the peritoneal cavity to invade the liver capsule. Adult worms finally reach the bile ducts, where they produce large operculated eggs, which are voided in the bile and through the gastrointestinal tract to the outside environment. The flukes' life cycle is completed in specific snails (the first intermediate host) and encystment on aquatic plants.

The clinical features of fascioliasis relate to the stage and intensity of infection. Acute disease develops during the parasites' migration (1 to 2 weeks after infection) and includes fever, right-upper-quadrant pain, hepatomegaly, and eosinophilia. Computed tomography of the liver may show migratory tracks. Symptoms and signs usually subside as the parasites reach their final habitat. In individuals with chronic infection, bile duct obstruction and biliary cirrhosis are infrequently demonstrated. No relation to hepatic malignancy has been ascribed to fascioliasis.

DIAGNOSIS The diagnosis of infection with any of the biliary flukes depends on a high degree of suspicion, the elicitation of an appropriate geographic history, and stool examination for the characteristically shaped parasite ova. Additional evidence may be obtained by documenting peripheral blood eosinophilia or imaging the liver. Serologic testing is helpful, particularly in lightly infected individuals.

℞ **TREATMENT**

Drug therapy (praziquantel or triclabendazole) is summarized in Table 203-2. Patients with anatomical lesions in the biliary tract or malignancy are managed according to general medical guidelines.

INTESTINAL FLUKES

Two species of intestinal flukes cause human infection in defined geographic areas worldwide (Table 203-1). The large *Fasciolopsis buski* (adults measure 2 by 7 cm) is endemic in Southeast Asia, while the smaller *Heterophyes heterophyes* is found in the Nile Delta of Egypt and in the Far East. Infection is initiated by ingestion of metacercariae attached to aquatic plants (*F. buski*) or encysted in freshwater or brackish-water fish (*H. heterophyes*). Flukes mature in human intestines, and eggs are passed with stools. Most individuals infected with intestinal flukes are asymptomatic. In heavy *F. buski* infection, diarrhea, abdominal pain, and malabsorption may be encountered. Heavy infection with *H. heterophyes* may be associated with abdominal pain and mucous diarrhea. The diagnosis is established by detection of the characteristically shaped ova in stool samples. The drug of choice for treatment is praziquantel (Table 203-2).

LUNG FLUKES

Infection with the lung fluke *Paragonimus westermani* (Table 203-1) and related species (e.g., *P. africanus*) is endemic in many parts of the world, excluding North America and Europe. Endemicity is particularly noticeable in West Africa, Central and South America, and Asia. In nature, the reservoir hosts of *P. westermani* are wild and domestic felines. In Africa, *P. africanus* has been found in other species, such as dogs. Adult lung flukes, which are 7 to 12 mm in length, are found encapsulated in the lungs of infected persons. In rare circumstances, flukes are found encysted in the CNS (cerebral paragonimiasis) or abdominal cavity. Humans acquire lung fluke infection by ingesting infective metacercariae encysted in the muscles and viscera of crayfish and freshwater crabs. In endemic areas, these crustaceans are consumed either raw or pickled. Once the organisms reach the duodenum, they excyst, penetrate the gut wall, and travel through the peritoneal cavity, diaphragm, and pleural space to reach the lungs. Mature flukes are found in the bronchioles surrounded by cystic lesions. Parasite eggs are either expectorated with sputum or swallowed and passed to the outside environment with feces. The life cycle is completed in snails and freshwater crustacea.

When maturing flukes lodge in lung tissues, they cause hemorrhage and necrosis, resulting in cyst formation. The adjacent lung parenchyma shows evidence of inflammatory infiltration, predominantly by eosinophils. Cysts usually measure 1 to 2 cm in diameter and may contain 1 or 2 worms each. With the onset of oviposition, cysts usually rupture in adjacent bronchioles—an event allowing ova to exit from the human host. Older cysts develop thickened walls, which may undergo calcification. During the active phase of paragonimiasis, lung tissues surrounding parasite cysts may contain evidence of pneumonia, bronchitis, bronchiectasis, and fibrosis.

Pulmonary paragonimiasis is particularly symptomatic in persons with moderate to heavy infection. Productive cough with brownish sputum or frank hemoptysis associated with peripheral blood eosinophilia is usually the presenting feature. Chest examination may reveal signs of pleurisy. In chronic cases, bronchitis or bronchiectasis may predominate, but these conditions rarely proceed to lung abscess. Imaging of the lungs demonstrates characteristic features, including patchy densities, cavities, pleural effusion, and ring shadows. Cerebral paragonimiasis presents as either space-occupying lesions or epilepsy.

DIAGNOSIS   Pulmonary paragonimiasis is diagnosed by the detection of parasite ova in sputum and/or stools. Serology is of considerable help in egg-negative cases and in cerebral paragonimiasis.

Rx TREATMENT

The drug of choice for treatment is praziquantel (Table 203-2). Other medical or surgical management may be needed for pulmonary or cerebral lesions.

CONTROL AND PREVENTION OF TISSUE FLUKES

For residents of nonendemic areas who are visiting an endemic region, the only effective preventive measure is to avoid ingestion of local plants, fish, or crustaceans; if their ingestion is necessary, these items should be washed or cooked thoroughly. Instruction on water and food preparation and consumption should be included in physicians' advice to travelers (Chap. 108). Interruption of transmission among residents of endemic areas depends on avoiding ingestion of the infective stage of the helminths and appropriate disposal of feces and sputum to prevent the hatching of eggs in the environment. These two approaches rely greatly on socioeconomic development and health education. In countries where economic progress has resulted in financial and social improvements, transmission has decreased. The third approach to control in endemic communities entails selective use of chemotherapy for individuals posing the highest risk of transmission—i.e., those with heavy infections. The availability of praziquantel—a broad-spectrum, safe, and effective anthelmintic agent—provides a means for reducing the reservoirs of infection in human populations. However, the existence of most of these helminths as zoonoses in several animal species complicates control efforts.

FURTHER READING

CHAN HH et al: The clinical and cholangiographic picture of hepatic clonorchiasis. J Clin Gastroenterol 34:183, 2002

DOENHOFF MJ et al: Resistance of *Schistosoma mansoni* to praziquantel: Is there a problem? Trans R Soc Trop Med Hyg 96:465, 2002

DRUGS FOR PARASITIC INFECTIONS. Med Lett Drugs Ther 1:44, 2002

JUKES MC et al: Heavy schistosomiasis associated with poor school term memory and slower reaction times in Tanzanian school children. Top Med Int Health 2:104, 2002

LIU LX, HARINASUTA KT: Liver and intestinal flukes. Gastroenterol Clin North Am 25:627, 1996

MAHMOUD AAFM (ed): Schistosomiasis, in *Tropical Medicine: Science and Practice*, G Pasvol and S Hoffman (eds). London, Imperial College Press, 2001, pp 1–510

MAS-COMA MS et al: Epidemiology of human fascioliasis: A review and proposed new classification. Bull World Health Organ 77:340, 1999

ROSS AG et al: Schistosomiasis. N Engl J Med 346:1212, 2002

QUINNELL RJ: Genetics of susceptibility to human helminth infection. Int J Parasitol 33:1219, 2003

WORLD HEALTH ORGANIZATION: Prevention and control of schistosomiasis and soil-transmitted helminthiasis. Technical report series 912. Geneva, World Health Organization, 2002, pp 1–57

204 CESTODES
A. Clinton White, Jr., Peter F. Weller

Cestodes, or tapeworms, are segmented worms. The adults reside in the gastrointestinal tract, but the larvae can be found in almost any organ. Human tapeworm infections can be divided into two major clinical groups. In one group, humans are the definitive hosts, with the adult tapeworms living in the gastrointestinal tract (*Taenia saginata*, *Diphyllobothrium*, *Hymenolepis*, and *Dipylidium caninum*). In the other, humans are intermediate hosts, with larval-stage parasites present in the tissues. Diseases in this category include echinococcosis, sparganosis, and coenurosis. For *Taenia solium*, the human may be either the definitive or the intermediate host.

The ribbon-shaped tapeworm attaches to the intestinal mucosa by means of sucking cups or hooks located on the scolex. Behind the scolex is a short, narrow neck from which proglottids (segments) form. As each proglottid matures, it is displaced further back from the neck by the formation of new, less mature segments. The progressively elongating chain of attached proglottids, called the *strobila*, constitutes the bulk of the tapeworm. The length varies among species. In some, the tapeworm may consist of more than 1000 proglottids and may be several meters long. The mature proglottids are hermaphroditic and produce eggs, which are intermittently released. Since eggs of the different *Taenia* species are morphologically identical, differences in the morphology of the scolex or proglottids provide the basis for diagnostic identification to the species level. Most human tapeworms require at least one intermediate host for complete larval development. After ingestion of the eggs or proglottids by an intermediate host, the larval oncospheres are activated, escape the egg, and penetrate the intestinal mucosa. The oncosphere migrates to tissues and develops into an encysted form known as a *cysticercus* (single scolex), a *coenurus* (multiple scolices), or a *hydatid* (cyst with daughter cysts, each containing several protoscolices). Ingestion by the definitive host of tissues containing a cyst enables a scolex to develop into a tapeworm.

TAENIASIS SAGINATA The beef tapeworm *T. saginata* occurs in all countries where raw or undercooked beef is eaten. It is most prevalent in sub-Saharan African and Middle Eastern countries. *T. saginata asiatica* is a variant of *T. saginata* that is found in Asia and for which pigs are the intermediate host.

Etiology and Pathogenesis Humans are the only definitive host for the adult stage of *T. saginata*. This tapeworm, which can reach 8 m in length, inhabits the upper jejunum and has a scolex with four prominent suckers and 1000 to 2000 proglottids. Each gravid segment has 15 to 30 uterine branches (in contrast to 8 to 12 for *T. solium*). The eggs are indistinguishable from those of *T. solium*; they measure 30 to 40 μm, contain the oncosphere, and have a thick brown striated shell. Eggs deposited on vegetation can live for months to years until they are ingested by cattle or other herbivores. The embryo released after ingestion invades the intestinal wall and is carried to striated muscle, where it transforms into a cysticercus. When ingested in raw or undercooked beef, this form can infect humans. After the cysticercus is ingested, it takes ~2 months for the mature adult worm to develop.

Clinical Manifestations Patients become aware of the infection most commonly by noting passage of proglottids in their feces. The proglottids are often motile, and patients may experience perianal discomfort when proglottids are discharged. Mild abdominal pain or discomfort, nausea, change in appetite, weakness, and weight loss can occur with *T. saginata* infection.

Diagnosis The diagnosis is made by the detection of eggs or proglottids in the stool. Eggs may also be present in the perianal area; thus, if proglottids or eggs are not found in the stool, the perianal region should be examined with use of a cellophane-tape swab (as in pinworm infection; Chap. 201). Distinguishing *T. saginata* from *T. solium* requires examination of mature proglottids or the scolex. Serologic tests are not helpful diagnostically. Eosinophilia and elevated levels of serum IgE may be detected.

℞ TREATMENT

A single dose of praziquantel (10 mg/kg) is highly effective.

Prevention The major method of preventing infection is the adequate cooking of beef; exposure to temperatures as low as 56°C for 5 min will destroy cysticerci. Refrigeration or salting for long periods or freezing at −10°C for 9 days also kills cysticerci in beef. General preventive measures include inspection of beef and proper disposal of human feces.

TAENIASIS SOLIUM AND CYSTICERCOSIS The pork tapeworm *T. solium* can cause two distinct forms of infection. The form that develops depends on whether humans are infected with adult tapeworms in the intestine or with larval forms in the tissues (cysticercosis). Humans are the only definitive hosts for *T. solium*; pigs are the usual intermediate hosts, although other animals may harbor the larval forms. *T. solium* exists worldwide but is most prevalent in Latin America, sub-Saharan Africa,

China, southern and Southeast Asia, and eastern Europe. Cysticercosis occurs in industrialized nations largely as a result of the immigration of infected persons from endemic areas.

Etiology and Pathogenesis The adult tapeworm generally resides in the upper jejunum. The scolex attaches by both sucking disks and two rows of hooklets. Often only one adult worm is present, but that worm may live for years. The tapeworm, usually about 3 m in length, may have as many as 1000 proglottids, each of which produces up to 50,000 eggs. Groups of three to five proglottids are generally released and excreted into the feces, and the eggs in these proglottids are infective for both humans and animals. The eggs may survive in the environment for several months. After ingestion of eggs by the intermediate host, the larvae are activated, escape the egg, penetrate the intestinal wall, and are carried to many tissues, with a predilection for striated muscle of the neck, tongue, and trunk. Within 60 to 90 days, the encysted larval stage develops. These cysticerci can survive for months to years. Humans acquire infections that lead to intestinal tapeworms by ingesting undercooked pork containing cysticerci. Infections that cause human cysticercosis follow the ingestion of *T. solium* eggs, usually from close contact with a tapeworm carrier. Autoinfection may occur if an individual with an egg-producing tapeworm ingests eggs derived from his or her own feces.

Clinical Manifestations Intestinal infections with *T. solium* may be asymptomatic. Epigastric discomfort, nausea, a sensation of hunger, weight loss, and diarrhea are infrequent. Fecal passage of proglottids may be noted by patients.

In cysticercosis, the clinical manifestations are variable. Cysticerci can be found anywhere in the body but are most commonly detected in the brain, skeletal muscle, subcutaneous tissue, or eye. The clinical presentation of cysticercosis depends on the number and location of cysticerci as well as the extent of associated inflammatory responses or scarring. Neurologic manifestations are the most common (Fig. 204-1). Seizures are associated with inflammation surrounding cysticerci in the brain parenchyma. These seizures may be generalized, focal, or Jacksonian. Hydrocephalus results from obstruction of cerebrospinal fluid (CSF) flow by cysticerci and accompanying inflammation or by CSF outflow obstruction from arachnoiditis. Signs of increased intracranial pressure, including headache, nausea, vomiting, changes in vision, dizziness, ataxia, or confusion, are often evident. Patients with hydrocephalus may develop papilledema or display altered mental status. When cysticerci develop at the base of the brain or in the subarachnoid space, they may cause chronic meningitis or arachnoiditis, communicating hydrocephalus, or strokes.

Diagnosis The diagnosis of intestinal *T. solium* infection is made by the detection of eggs or proglottids, as described for *T. saginata*. In cysticercosis, diagnosis can be difficult. A consensus conference has proposed absolute, major, minor, and epidemiologic criteria for diagnosis (Table 204-1). Diagnostic certainty is possible only with definite demonstration of the parasite (absolute criteria). This task can be accomplished by histologic observation of the parasite in excised tissue, by funduscopic visualization of the parasite in the eye (in the anterior chamber, vitreous, or subretinal spaces), or by neuroimaging studies demonstrating cystic lesions containing a characteristic scolex. In most cases, diagnostic certainty is not possible. Instead, a clinical diagnosis is made on the basis of a combination of clinical presentation, radiographic studies, serologic tests, and exposure history.

Neuroimaging findings suggestive of neurocysticercosis constitute the primary major diagnostic criterion. These findings include cystic lesions with or without enhancement (e.g., ring enhancement), one or more nodular calcifications (which may also have associated enhancement), or focal enhancing lesions. Cysticerci in the brain parenchyma are usually 5 to 20 mm in diameter and rounded. Cystic lesions in the subarachnoid space or fissures may enlarge up to 6 cm in diameter and may be lobulated. For cysticerci within the subarachnoid space or ventricles, the walls may be very thin and the cyst fluid is often isodense

FIGURE 204-1 Neurocysticercosis is caused by *Taenia solium*. Neurologic infection can be classified on the basis of the location and viability of the parasites. When the parasites are in the ventricles, they often cause obstructive hydrocephalus. *Left*: MRI scan showing a cysticercus in the lateral ventricle, with resultant hydrocephalus. The arrow points to the scolex within the cystic parasite. *Center*: CT scan showing a parenchymal cysticercus, with enhancement of the cyst wall and an internal scolex (*arrow*). *Right*: Multiple cysticerci, including calcified lesions from prior infection (*arrowheads*), viable cysticerci in the basilar cisterns (*white arrow*), and a large degenerating cysticercus in the Sylvian fissure (*black arrow*). (*Modified with permission from JC Bandres et al: Clin Infect Dis 15:799, 1992.*)

with CSF. Thus, obstructive hydrocephalus or enhancement of the basilar meninges may be the only finding on computed tomography (CT) in extraparenchymal neurocysticercosis. Cysticerci in the ventricles or subarachnoid space are usually visible to an experienced neuroradiologist on magnetic resonance imaging (MRI) or on CT with intraventricular contrast injection. CT is more sensitive than MRI in identifying calcified lesions, whereas MRI is better for identifying cystic lesions and enhancement.

The second major diagnostic criterion is detection of specific antibodies to cysticerci. While most tests employing unfractionated antigen have high rates of false-positive and false-negative results, this problem can be overcome by using the more specific immunoblot assay. An immunoblot assay using lentil-lectin purified glycoproteins has >99% specificity and is highly sensitive. However, patients with single intracranial lesions or with calcifications may be seronegative. With this assay, serum samples provide greater diagnostic sensitivity than CSF. CSF may be useful when only unfractionated antigens are used. Antigen detection assays, especially those detecting antigen in the spinal fluid, may also improve diagnosis. However, these assays are not widely available, and the number of publications on their use is limited.

Studies have demonstrated that clinical criteria can aid in the diagnosis in selected cases. In patients from endemic areas who had single enhancing lesions presenting with seizures, a normal physical examination, and no evidence of systemic disease (e.g., no fever, adenopathy, or abnormal chest radiograph), the constellation of rounded CT lesions 5 to 20 mm in diameter with no midline shift was almost always caused by neurocysticercosis. Finally, spontaneous resolution or resolution after therapy with albendazole alone is consistent with neurocysticercosis.

Minor diagnostic criteria include neuroimaging findings consistent with but less characteristic of cysticercosis, clinical manifestations suggestive of neurocysticercosis (e.g., seizures, hydrocephalus, or altered mental status), evidence of cysticercosis outside the central nervous system (e.g., cigar-shaped soft tissue calcifications), or antibody in CSF detected by enzyme-linked immunosorbent assay (ELISA). Epidemiologic criteria include exposure to a tapeworm carrier or household member infected with *T. solium*, current or prior residence in an endemic area, and frequent travel to an endemic area.

Diagnosis is confirmed in patients with either one absolute criterion or a combination of two major criteria, one minor criterion, and one epidemiologic criterion (Table 204-1). A probable diagnosis is supported by the fulfillment of (1) one major criterion plus two minor criteria; (2) one major criterion plus one minor criterion and one epidemiologic criterion; or (3) three minor criteria plus one epidemiologic criterion. While the CSF is usually abnormal in neurocysticercosis, CSF abnormalities are not pathognomonic. Patients may have CSF

pleocytosis with a predominance of lymphocytes, neutrophils, or eosinophils. The protein level in CSF may be elevated; the glucose concentration is usually normal but may be depressed.

℞ TREATMENT

Intestinal *T. solium* infection is treated with a single dose of praziquantel (10 mg/kg). However, praziquantel can evoke an inflammatory response in the central nervous system if concomitant cryptic cysticercosis is present. Niclosamide (2 g) is also effective but is not widely available.

The management of neurocysticercosis focuses primarily on symptom-based treatment of seizures or hydrocephalus. Seizures can usually be controlled with antiepileptics. If parenchymal lesions resolve without development of calcifications and patients remain free of seizures, antiepileptic therapy can usually be discontinued after 2 years. Five placebo-controlled trials failed to identify any clinical advantage of antiparasitic drugs for parenchymal neurocysticercosis. However, trends toward faster resolution of neuroradiologic abnormalities were observed. Thus, some authorities favor use of antiparasitic drugs, including praziquantel (50 to 60 mg/kg daily in three divided doses for 15 days or 100 mg/kg in three doses given over a single day) or albendazole (15 mg/kg per day for 8 to 28 days). Both agents may exacerbate the inflammatory response around the dying parasite, exacerbating seizures or hydrocephalus. Thus, patients receiving these drugs should be carefully monitored. High-dose glucocorticoids can be used during treatment or if symptoms worsen. Since glucocorticoids induce first-pass metabolism of praziquantel and may decrease its antiparasitic effect, cimetidine should be coadministered to inhibit praziquantel metabolism.

For patients with hydrocephalus, the emergent reduction of intracranial pressure is the mainstay of therapy. In the case of obstructive hydrocephalus, the preferred approach is removal of the cysticercus via endoscopic surgery. However, this intervention is not always possible. An alternative approach is initially to perform a diverting procedure, such as ventriculoperitoneal shunting. Historically, shunts

TABLE 204-1 *Proposed Diagnostic Criteria for Human Cysticercosis, 2001*

1. Absolute criteria
   a. Demonstration of cysticerci by histologic or microscopic examination of biopsy material
   b. Visualization of the parasite in the eye by funduscopy
   c. Neuroradiologic demonstration of cystic lesions containing a characteristic scolex
2. Major criteria
   a. Neuroradiologic lesions suggestive of neurocysticercosis
   b. Demonstration of antibodies to cysticerci in serum by enzyme-linked immunoelectrotransfer blot
   c. Resolution of intracranial cystic lesions spontaneously or after therapy with albendazole or praziquantel alone
3. Minor criteria
   a. Lesions compatible with neurocysticercosis detected by neuroimaging studies
   b. Clinical manifestations suggestive of neurocysticercosis
   c. Demonstration of antibodies to cysticerci or cysticercal antigen in cerebrospinal fluid by ELISA
   d. Evidence of cysticercosis outside the central nervous system (e.g., cigar-shaped soft tissue calcifications)
4. Epidemiologic criteria
   a. Residence in a cysticercosis-endemic area
   b. Frequent travel to a cysticercosis-endemic area
   c. Household contact with an individual infected with *Taenia solium*

Note: ELISA, enzyme-linked immunosorbent assay.
Source: Modified from Del Brutto et al.

have usually failed, but low failure rates have recently been attained with treatment with antiparasitic drugs, chronic administration of glucocorticoids, or use of flow-sensitive shunts. Open craniotomy to remove the cysticerci is now required only infrequently. For patients with subarachnoid cysts or giant cysticerci, glucocorticoids are needed to reduce arachnoiditis and accompanying vasculitis. Most authorities recommend prolonged courses of antiparasitic drugs and shunting when hydrocephalus is present. In patients with cerebral edema and elevated intracranial pressure due to multiple inflamed lesions, glucocorticoids are the mainstay of therapy, and antiparasitic drugs should be avoided. For ocular and spinal medullary lesions, drug-induced inflammation may cause irreversible damage. Most patients should be managed surgically, although case reports have described cures with medical therapy.

Prevention Measures for the prevention of intestinal *T. solium* infection consist of the application to pork of precautions similar to those described above for beef with regard to *T. saginata* infection. The prevention of cysticercosis involves minimizing the opportunities for ingestion of fecally derived eggs by means of good personal hygiene, effective fecal disposal, and treatment and prevention of human intestinal infections.

ECHINOCOCCOSIS Echinococcosis is an infection caused in humans by the larval stage of *Echinococcus granulosus*, *E. multilocularis*, or *E. vogeli*. *E. granulosus*, which produces unilocular cystic lesions, is prevalent in areas where livestock is raised in association with dogs. This tapeworm species is found in Australia, Argentina, Chile, Africa, eastern Europe, the Middle East, New Zealand, and the Mediterranean region, particularly Lebanon and Greece. Molecular evidence suggests that *E. granulosus* strains may actually belong to more than one species; specifically, strains from sheep, cattle, pigs, horses, and camels probably represent separate species. *E. multilocularis*, which causes multilocular alveolar lesions that are locally invasive, is found in Alpine, sub-Arctic, or Arctic regions, including Canada, the United States, and central and northern Europe and Asia. *E. vogeli* causes polycystic hydatid disease and is found only in Central and South America. Like other cestodes, echinococcal species have both intermediate and definitive hosts. The definitive hosts are dogs that pass eggs in their feces. Cysts develop in the intermediate hosts—sheep, cattle, humans, goats, camels, and horses for *E. granulosus* and mice and other rodents for *E. multilocularis*—after the ingestion of eggs. When a dog ingests beef or lamb containing cysts, the life cycle is completed.

Etiology The small (5 mm long) adult *E. granulosus* worm, which lives for 5 to 20 months in the jejunum of dogs, has only three proglottids—one immature, one mature, and one gravid. The gravid segment splits to release eggs that are morphologically similar to *Taenia* eggs and are extremely hardy. After humans ingest the eggs, embryos escape from the eggs, penetrate the intestinal mucosa, enter the portal circulation, and are carried to various organs, most commonly the liver and lungs. Larvae develop into fluid-filled unilocular hydatid cysts that consist of an external membrane and an inner germinal layer. Daughter cysts develop from the inner aspect of the germinal layer, as do germinating cystic structures called *brood capsules*. New larvae, called *protoscolices*, develop in large numbers within the brood capsule. The cysts expand slowly over a period of years.

The life cycle of *E. multilocularis* is similar except that small rodents serve as the intermediate hosts. The larval form of *E. multilocularis*, however, is quite different in that it remains in the proliferative phase, the parasite is always multilocular, and vesicles without brood capsule or protoscolices progressively invade the host tissue by peripheral extension of processes from the germinal layer.

Clinical Manifestations Slowly enlarging echinococcal cysts generally remain asymptomatic until their expanding size or their space-occupying effect in an involved organ elicits symptoms. The liver and the lungs are the most common sites of these cysts. The liver is involved in about two-thirds of *E. granulosus* infections and in nearly all *E. multilocularis* infections. Since a period of years elapses before cysts enlarge sufficiently to cause symptoms, they may be discovered incidentally on a routine x-ray or ultrasound study.

Patients with hepatic echinococcosis who are symptomatic most often present with abdominal pain or a palpable mass in the right upper quadrant. Compression of a bile duct or leakage of cyst fluid into the biliary tree may mimic recurrent cholelithiasis, and biliary obstruction can result in jaundice. Rupture of or episodic leakage from a hydatid cyst may produce fever, pruritus, urticaria, eosinophilia, or anaphylaxis. Pulmonary hydatid cysts may rupture into the bronchial tree or peritoneal cavity and produce cough, chest pain, or hemoptysis. Rupture of hydatid cysts may lead to multifocal dissemination of protoscolices, which can form additional cysts. Rupture can occur spontaneously or at surgery. Other presentations are due to the involvement of bone (invasion of the medullary cavity with slow bone erosion producing pathologic fractures), the central nervous system (space-occupying lesions), the heart (conduction defects, pericarditis), and the pelvis (pelvic mass).

The larval forms of *E. multilocularis* characteristically present as a slowly growing hepatic tumor, with progressive destruction of the liver and extension into vital structures. Patients commonly complain of upper quadrant and epigastric pain, and obstructive jaundice may be apparent. The lesions may infiltrate adjoining organs (e.g., diaphragm, kidneys, or lungs) or may metastasize to the spleen, lungs, or brain.

Diagnosis Radiographic and related imaging studies are important in detecting and evaluating echinococcal cysts. Plain films will define pulmonary cysts of *E. granulosus*—usually as rounded masses of uniform density—but may miss cysts in other organs unless there is cyst wall calcification (as occurs in the liver). MRI, CT, and ultrasound reveal well-defined cysts with thick or thin walls. When older cysts contain a layer of hydatid sand that is rich in accumulated scolices, these imaging methods may detect this fluid layer of different density. However, the most pathognomonic finding, if demonstrable, is that of daughter cysts within the larger cyst. This finding, like eggshell or mural calcification on CT, is indicative of *E. granulosus* infection and helps to distinguish the cyst from carcinomas, bacterial or amebic liver abscesses, or hemangiomas. In contrast, ultrasound or CT of alveolar hydatid cysts reveals indistinct solid masses with central necrosis and plaquelike calcifications.

A specific diagnosis of *E. granulosus* infection can be made by the examination of aspirated fluids for protoscolices or hooklets, but diagnostic aspiration is not usually recommended because of the risk of fluid leakage resulting in either dissemination of infection or anaphylactic reactions. Serodiagnostic assays can be useful, although a negative test does not exclude the diagnosis of echinococcosis. Cysts in the liver elicit positive antibody responses in ~90% of cases, whereas up to 50% of individuals with cysts in the lungs are seronegative. Detection of antibody to specific echinococcal antigens by immunoblotting has the highest degree of specificity.

℞ TREATMENT

Therapy for cystic echinococcosis is based on considerations of the size, location, and manifestations of cysts and the overall health of the patient. Surgery has traditionally been the principal definitive method of treatment. Currently, ultrasound staging is recommended for *E. granulosus* infections (Fig. 204-2). For uncomplicated CE1 lesions and for some CE2 and CE3 lesions, PAIR (*p*ercutaneous *a*spiration, *i*nfusion of scolicidal agents, and *r*easpiration) is now recommended instead of surgery. PAIR is contraindicated for superficially located cysts (because of the risk of rupture), for cysts with multiple thick internal septal divisions (honeycombing pattern), and for cysts communicating with the biliary tree. For prophylaxis of secondary peritoneal echinococcosis due to inadvertent spillage of fluid during PAIR, the administration of albendazole (15 mg/kg daily in two divided

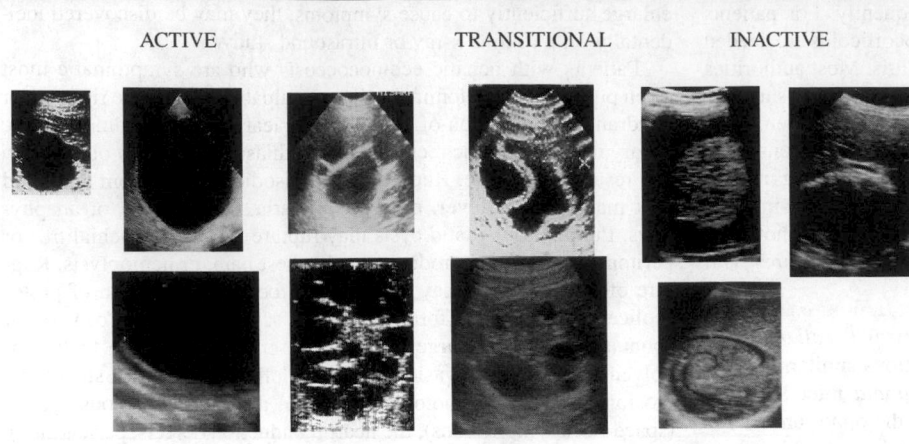

TYPE OF CYST

CL	CE1	CE2	CE3	CE4	CE5

ACTIVE TRANSITIONAL INACTIVE

FIGURE 204-2 Management of cystic hydatid disease caused by *Echinococcus granulosus* should be based on viability of the parasite, which can be estimated from radiographic appearance. The ultrasound appearance includes lesions classified as active, transitional, and inactive. *Active* cysts include types CL (with a cystic lesion and no visible cyst wall), CE1 [with a visible cyst wall and internal echoes (snowflake sign)], and CE2 (with a visible cyst wall and internal septation). *Transitional cysts* (CE3) may have detached laminar membranes or may be partially collapsed. *Inactive* cysts include types CE4 (a nonhomogeneous mass) and CE5 (a cyst with a thick calcified wall).

doses) should be initiated at least 4 days before the procedure and continued for at least 4 weeks afterward. Ultrasound- or CT-guided aspiration allows confirmation of the diagnosis by demonstration of protoscolices in the aspirate. After aspiration, contrast material should be injected to detect occult communications with the biliary tract. Alternatively, the fluid should be checked for bile staining by dipstick. If no bile is found and no communication visualized, the contrast material is reaspirated, with subsequent infusion of scolicidal agents (usually either alcohol or hypertonic saline). Daughter cysts within the primary cyst may need to be punctured separately. In experienced hands, this approach yields rates of cure and relapse equivalent to those following surgery, with less perioperative morbidity and shorter hospitalization.

Surgery remains the treatment of choice for complicated *E. granulosus* cysts (e.g., those communicating with the biliary tract) or for areas where PAIR is not possible. For *E. granulosus*, the preferred surgical approach is pericystectomy, in which the entire cyst and the surrounding fibrous tissue are removed. The risks posed by leakage of fluid during surgery or PAIR include anaphylaxis and dissemination of infectious protoscolices. The latter complication has been minimized by careful attention to the prevention of spillage of the cyst and by soaking of the drapes with hypertonic saline. Infusion of scolicidal agents is no longer recommended because of problems with hypernatremia, intoxication, or sclerosing cholangitis. Albendazole, which is active against *Echinococcus*, should be administered adjunctively, beginning several days before resection and continuing for several weeks for *E. granulosus*. Praziquantel (50 mg/kg daily for 2 weeks), may hasten the death of the protoscolices. Medical therapy with albendazole alone for 12 weeks to 6 months results in cure in ~30% of cases and improvement in another 50%. In many instances of treatment failure, *E. granulosus* infections are subsequently treated successfully with PAIR or additional courses of medical therapy. Response to treatment is best assessed by serial imaging studies, with attention to cyst size and consistency.

Surgical resection remains the treatment of choice for *E. multilocularis* infection. Complete removal of the parasite continues to offer the best chance for cure. Ongoing therapy with albendazole for at least 2 years after presumptively curative surgery is recommended. Most cases are diagnosed at a stage at which complete resection is not possible; in these cases, albendazole treatment should be continued indefinitely, with careful monitoring. In some cases, liver transplantation has been used because of the size of the necessary liver resection.

However, continuous immunosuppression favors the proliferation of *E. multilocularis* larvae and reinfection of the transplant. Thus, indefinite treatment with albendazole is required.

Prevention In endemic areas, echinococcosis can be prevented by administering praziquantel to infected dogs, by denying dogs access to infected animals, or by vaccinating sheep. Limitation of the number of stray dogs is helpful in reducing the prevalence of infection among humans.

HYMENOLEPIASIS NANA Infection with *Hymenolepis nana*, the dwarf tapeworm, is the most common of all the cestode infections. *H. nana* is endemic in both temperate and tropical regions of the world. Infection is spread by fecal/oral contamination and is common among institutionalized children.

Etiology and Pathogenesis *H. nana* is the only cestode of humans that does not require an intermediate host. Both the larval and adult phases take place in the human. The adult—the smallest tapeworm parasitizing humans—is ~2 cm long and dwells in the proximal ileum. Proglottids, which are quite small and are rarely seen in the stool, release spherical eggs 30 to 44 μm in diameter, each of which contains an oncosphere with six hooklets. The eggs are immediately infective and are unable to survive for >10 days in the external environment. *H. nana* can also be acquired by the ingestion of infected insects (especially larval meal-worms and larval fleas). When the egg is ingested by a new host, the oncosphere is freed and penetrates the intestinal villi, becoming a cysticercoid larva. Larvae migrate back into the intestinal lumen, attach to the mucosa, and mature into adult worms over 10 to 12 days. Eggs may also hatch before passing into the stool, causing internal autoinfection with increasing numbers of intestinal worms. Although the life span of adult *H. nana* is only ~4 to 10 weeks, the autoinfection cycle perpetuates the infection.

Clinical Manifestations *H. nana* infection, even with many intestinal worms, is usually asymptomatic. When infection is intense, anorexia, abdominal pain, and diarrhea develop.

Diagnosis Infection is diagnosed by the finding of eggs in the stool.

℞ TREATMENT

Praziquantel (25 mg/kg once) is the treatment of choice, since it acts against both the adult worms and the cysticercoids in the intestinal villi.

Prevention Good personal hygiene and improved sanitation can eradicate the disease. Epidemics have been controlled by mass chemotherapy coupled with improved hygiene.

HYMENOLEPIASIS DIMINUTA *Hymenolepis diminuta*, a cestode of rodents, occasionally infects small children, who ingest the larvae in uncooked cereal foods contaminated by fleas and other insects in which larvae develop. Infection is usually asymptomatic and is diagnosed by the detection of eggs in the stool. Treatment with praziquantel results in cure in most cases.

DIPHYLLOBOTHRIASIS *Diphyllobothrium latum* and other *Diphyllobothrium* species are found in the lakes, rivers, and deltas of the northern hemisphere, Central Africa, and Chile.

Etiology and Pathogenesis The adult worm—the longest tapeworm (up to 25 m)—attaches to the ileal and occasionally to the jejunal mucosa by its suckers, which are located on its elongated scolex. The adult worm has 3000 to 4000 proglottids, which release ~1 million eggs daily into the feces. If an egg reaches water, it hatches and releases a free-swimming embryo that can be eaten by small freshwater crustaceans (*Cyclops* or *Diaptomus* species). After an infected crustacean containing a developed procercoid is swallowed by a fish, the larva migrates into the fish's flesh and grows into a plerocercoid, or sparganum larva. Humans acquire the infection by ingesting infected raw fish. Within 3 to 5 weeks, the tapeworm matures into an adult in the human intestine.

Clinical Manifestations Most *D. latum* infections are asymptomatic, although manifestations may include transient abdominal discomfort, diarrhea, vomiting, weakness, and weight loss. Occasionally, infection can cause acute abdominal pain and intestinal obstruction; in rare cases, cholangitis or cholecystitis may be produced by migrating proglottids. Because the tapeworm absorbs large quantities of vitamin B_{12} and interferes with ileal B_{12} absorption, vitamin B_{12} deficiency can develop. Up to 2% of infected patients, especially the elderly, have megaloblastic anemia resembling pernicious anemia and may exhibit neurologic sequelae of B_{12} deficiency.

Diagnosis The diagnosis is made readily by the detection of the characteristic eggs in the stool. The eggs possess a single shell with an operculum at one end and a knob at the other. Mild to moderate eosinophilia may be detected.

℞ TREATMENT

Praziquantel (5 to 10 mg/kg once) is highly effective. Parenteral vitamin B_{12} should be given if B_{12} deficiency is manifest.

Prevention Infection can be prevented by heating fish to 54°C for 5 min or by freezing it at −18°C for 24 h. Placing fish in brine with a high salt concentration for long periods kills the eggs.

DIPYLIDIASIS *Dipylidium caninum*, a common tapeworm of dogs and cats, may accidentally infect humans. Dogs, cats, and occasionally humans become infected by ingesting fleas harboring cysticercoids. Children are more likely to become infected than adults. Most infections are asymptomatic, but abdominal pain, diarrhea, anal pruritus, urticaria, eosinophilia, or passage of segments in the stool may occur. The diagnosis is made by the detection of proglottids in the stool. As in *D. latum* infection, therapy consists of praziquantel. Prevention requires anthelmintic treatment and flea control for pet dogs or cats.

SPARGANOSIS Humans can be infected by the sparganum, or plerocercoid larva, of a diphyllobothrid tapeworm of the genus *Spirometra*. Infection can be acquired by the consumption of water containing infected *Cyclops*; by the ingestion of infected snakes, birds, or mammals; or by the application of infected flesh as poultices. The worm migrates slowly in tissues, and infection commonly presents as a subcutaneous swelling. Periorbital tissues can be involved, and ocular sparganosis may destroy the eye. Surgical excision is used to treat localized sparganosis.

COENUROSIS This rare infection of humans by the larval stage (coenurus) of the dog tapeworm *Taenia multiceps* or *T. serialis* results in a space-occupying cystic lesion. As in cysticercosis, involvement of the central nervous system and subcutaneous tissue is most common. Both definitive diagnosis and treatment require surgical excision of the lesion. Chemotherapeutic agents generally are not effective.

FURTHER READING

DEL BRUTTO OH et al: Proposed diagnostic criteria for neurocysticercosis. Neurology 57:177, 2001

GARCIA HH et al: Current consensus guidelines for treatment of neurocysticercosis. Clin Microbiol Rev 15:747, 2002

KELLY R et al: Characteristics of ventricular shunt malfunctions among patients with neurocysticercosis. Neurosurgery 50:757, 2002

KERN P et al: European echinococcosis registry: Human alveolar echinococcosis, Europe, 1982–2000. Emerg Infect Dis 9:343, 2003

MENEZES DA SILVA A: Hydatid cyst of the liver—criteria for the selection of appropriate treatment. Acta Tropica 85:237, 2003

PAWLOWSKI ZS et al: Echinococcosis in humans: Clinical aspects, diagnosis, and treatment, in J Eckert et al (eds): *WHO/OIE Manual on Echinococcosis in Humans and Animals: A Public Health Problem of Global Concern.* World Organization for Animal Health, Paris, 2001

SINGH G, PRABHAKAR S: *Taenia solium Cysticercosis: From Basic Science to Clinical Science.* CABI Publishing, Wallingford, Oxon, UK, 2002

WORLD HEALTH ORGANIZATION INFORMAL WORKING GROUP ON ECHINOCOCCOSIS: Guidelines for treatment of cystic and alveolar echinococcosis in humans. Bull World Health Organ 74:231, 1996

——— PAIR puncture, aspiration, injection, re-aspiration: An option for the treatment of cystic echinococcosis. WHO/CDS/CSR/APH/2001.6. WHO, Geneva, 2001

205 | MICROBIAL BIOTERRORISM
H. Clifford Lane, Anthony S. Fauci

Descriptions of the use of microbial pathogens as potential weapons of war or terrorism date from ancient times. Among the most frequently cited of such episodes are the poisoning of water supplies in the sixth century B.C. with the fungus *Calviceps purpurea* (rye ergot) by the Assyrians, the hurling of the dead bodies of plague victims over the walls of the city of Kaffa by the Tartar army in 1346, and the spreading of smallpox via contaminated blankets by the British to the native American population loyal to the French in 1767. Although the use of chemical weapons in wartime took place in the not-too-distant past (Chap. 206), the tragic events of September 11, 2001, followed closely by the anthrax attacks through the U.S. Postal System, dramatically changed the mindset of the American public regarding both our vulnerability to microbial bioterrorist attacks and the seriousness and intent of the Federal government to protect its citizens against future attacks.

Although the potential impact of a bioterrorist attack can be enormous, leading to thousands of deaths and extensive morbidity, acts of bioterrorism typically have their greatest impact through the fear and terror they generate. In contrast to biowarfare, where the primary goal is destruction of the enemy through mass casualties, an important goal of bioterrorism is to destroy the morale of a society through fear and uncertainty. While the actual biologic impact of a single act may be small, the degree of disruption created by the realization that such an attack is possible may be enormous. This was readily apparent with the impact on the U.S. Postal System and the functional interruption of the activities of the legislative branch of government following the anthrax attacks noted above. Thus, the key to the defense against these attacks is a highly functioning system of public health surveillance and education so that attacks can be quickly recognized and effectively contained. This is complemented by the availability of appropriate countermeasures in the form of diagnostics, therapeutics, and vaccines, both in response to and in anticipation of bioterrorist attacks.

The Working Group for Civilian Biodefense has put together a list of key features that characterize the elements of biologic agents that make them particularly effective as weapons (Table 205-1). Included among these are the ease of spread and transmission of the agent as well as the presence of an adequate database to allow newcomers to the field to quickly apply the good science of others to bad intentions of their own. Agents of bioterrorism may be used in their naturally occurring forms or they can be deliberately modified to provide maximal impact. Among the approaches to maximizing the deleterious effects of biologic agents are the genetic modification of microbes for the purposes of antimicrobial resistance or evasion by the immune system, creation of fine-particle aerosols, chemical treatment to stabilize and prolong infectivity, and alteration of host range through changes in surface proteins. Certain of these approaches fall under the category of *weaponization*, which is a term generally used to describe the processing of microbes or toxins in a manner that would ensure a devastating effect of a release. For example, weaponization of anthrax by the Soviets comprised the production of vast amounts of spores in a form that maintained aerosolization for prolonged periods of time; the spores were of sufficient size to enter the lower respiratory tract easily and could be delivered in a massive release, such as via a bomblet.

The U.S. Centers for Disease Control and Prevention (CDC) classifies potential biologic threats into three categories: A, B, and C (Table 205-2). Category A agents are the highest-priority pathogens. They pose the greatest risk to national security because they (1) can be easily disseminated or transmitted from person to person, (2) result in high mortality rates and have the potential for major public health impact, (3) might cause public panic and social disruption, and (4) require special action for public health preparedness. Category B agents are the second highest priority pathogens and include those that are moderately easy to disseminate, result in moderate morbidity rates and low mortality rates, and require specifically enhanced diagnostic capacity. Category C agents are the third highest priority. These include emerging pathogens, to which the general population lacks immunity, that could be engineered for mass dissemination in the future because of availability, ease of production, ease of dissemination, potential for high morbidity and mortality, and major public health impact. The recent emergence of a novel human coronavirus leading to outbreaks of severe acute respiratory syndrome (SARS) is one example of such an agent. It should be pointed out, however, that these designations are empirical, and, depending on evolving circumstances such as threat assessments, the priority rating of any given microbe or toxin could change.

TABLE 205-1 *Key Features of Biologic Agents Used as Bioweapons*

1. High morbidity and mortality
2. Potential for person-to-person spread
3. Low infective dose and highly infectious by aerosol
4. Lack of rapid diagnostic capability
5. Lack of universally available effective vaccine
6. Potential to cause anxiety
7. Availability of pathogen and feasibility of production
8. Environmental stability
9. Database of prior research and development
10. Potential to be "weaponized"

Source: From L Borio et al: JAMA 287:2391, 2002; with permission.

TABLE 205-2 *CDC Category A, B, and C Agents*

Category A
Anthrax (*Bacillus anthracis*)
Botulism (*Clostridium botulinum* toxin)
Plague (*Yersinia pestis*)
Smallpox (*Variola major*)
Tularemia (*Francisella tularensis*)
Viral hemorrhagic fevers
  Arenaviruses: Lassa, New World (Machupo, Junin, Guanarito, and Sabia)
  Bunyaviridae: Crimean Congo, Rift Valley
  Filoviridae: Ebola, Marburg
  Flaviviridae: Yellow fever; Omsk fever; Kyasanur Forest

Category B
Brucellosis (*Brucella* spp.)
Epsilon toxin of *Clostridium perfringens*
Food safety threats (e.g., *Salmonella* spp., *Escherichia coli* 0157:H7, *Shigella*)
Glanders (*Burkholderia mallei*)
Melioidosis (*B. pseudomallei*)
Psittacosis (*Chlamydia psittaci*)
Q fever (*Coxiella burnetii*)
Ricin toxin from *Ricinus communis* (castor beans)
Staphylococcal enterotoxin B
Typhus fever (*Rickettsia prowazekii*)
Viral encephalitis [alphaviruses (e.g., Venezuelan, eastern, and western equine encephalitis)]
Water safety threats (e.g., *Vibrio cholerae*, *Cryptosporidium parvum*)

Category C
Emerging infectious diseases threats such as Nipah, hantavirus, and SARS coronavirus.

Source: Centers for Disease Control and Prevention and the National Institute of Allergy and Infectious Diseases.

CATEGORY A AGENTS

ANTHRAX (*BACILLUS ANTHRACIS*) (See also Chap. 122) ■ **Anthrax as a Bioweapon** Anthrax may be the prototypic disease of bioterrorism. Although rarely spread from person to person, it contains the other features of an ideal bioweapon outlined in Table 205-1. U.S. and British government scientists studied anthrax as a biologic weapon beginning approximately at the time of World War II (WWII). Offensive bioweapons activity including bioweapons research on microbes and toxins in the United States ceased in 1969 as a result of two executive orders by President Richard M. Nixon. The 1972 Biological and Toxin Weapons Convention Treaty outlawed research of this type worldwide. Clearly, the Soviet Union was in direct violation of this treaty until at least the dissolution of the Soviet Union in the late 1980s. It is well documented that during this post-treaty period, the Soviets produced and stored hundreds of tons of anthrax spores for potential use as a bioweapon. At present there is suspicion that research on anthrax as an agent of bioterrorism is ongoing by several nations and extremist groups. One example of this is the release of anthrax spores by the Aum Shrinrikyo cult in Tokyo in 1993. Fortunately, there were no casualties associated with this episode because of the inadvertent use of a nonpathogenic strain of anthrax by the terrorists.

The potential impact of anthrax spores as a bioweapon was clearly demonstrated in 1979 following the accidental release of spores into the atmosphere from a Soviet Union bioweapons facility in Sverdlosk, Russia. While actual figures are not known, at least 77 cases of anthrax were diagnosed with certainty, of which 66 were fatal. These victims appeared to have been exposed in an area within 4 km downwind of the facility. Deaths due to anthrax were also noted in livestock up to 50 km away from the facility. The interval between probable exposure and development of clinical illness ranged from 2 to 43 days. The majority of cases were within the first 2 weeks. Death typically occurred within 1 to 4 days following the onset of symptoms. It is likely that the widespread use of penicillin prophylaxis limited the total number of cases. The extended period of time between exposure and disease in some individuals supports the data from nonhuman primate studies suggesting the anthrax spores can lie dormant in the respiratory tract for at least 4 to 6 weeks. This extended period of microbiologic latency following exposure poses a significant challenge for management of victims in the postexposure period.

In September 2001, the American public was exposed to anthrax spores as a bioweapon delivered through the U.S. Postal System. The CDC identified 22 confirmed or suspected cases of anthrax as a consequence of this attack. These included 11 patients with inhalational anthrax, of whom 5 died, and 11 patients with cutaneous anthrax (7 confirmed), all of whom survived (Fig. 205-1). Cases occurred in individuals who opened contaminated letters as well as in postal workers involved in the processing of mail. A minimum of five letters mailed from Trenton, NJ, served as the vehicles for these attacks. One of these letters was reported to contain 2 g of material, equivalent to 100 billion to 1 trillion weapon-grade spores. This is an inoculum with a theoretical potential under optimal conditions of infecting up to 50 million individuals when one considers an LD_{50} of 10,000 spores. The strain used in this attack was the Ames strain. Although it was noted to have an inducible β-lactamase and to constitutively express a cephalosporinase, it was susceptible to all antibiotics standard for *B. anthracis*.

Microbiology and Clinical Features Anthrax is caused by *B. anthracis*, a gram-positive, nonmotile, spore-forming rod that is found in soil and predominantly causes disease in herbivores such as cattle, goats, and sheep. The long-lived spores of this organism can also be found in soil, and their stability makes them an ideal bioweapon. Anthrax spores can remain viable for decades, and their destruction in decontamination activities can be a challenge. Naturally occurring human infection is generally the result of contact with anthrax-infected animals or animal products such as goat hair. Studies performed in the 1950s using monkeys exposed to aerosolized anthrax suggested that ~10,000 spores were required to produce lethal disease in 50% of animals exposed to this dose (the LD_{50}). However, it has also been suggested that as few as one to three spores may be adequate to cause disease in some settings. Advanced technology is likely to be necessary to generate spores of the optimal size (1 to 5 μm) to travel to the alveolar spaces as a bioweapon.

The three major clinical forms of anthrax are gastrointestinal, cutaneous, and inhalational. *Gastrointestinal anthrax* is rarely seen and is unlikely to be the result of a bioterrorism event. The lesion of *cutaneous anthrax* typically begins as a papule following the introduction of spores through an opening in the skin. This papule then evolves to a painless vesicular stage followed by the development of a coal-black, necrotic eschar. It is the Greek word for coal (*anthrax*) that gives the organism and the disease its name. Cutaneous anthrax was ~20% fatal prior to the availability of antibiotics. *Inhalational anthrax* is the form most likely to be responsible for death in the setting of a bioterrorist attack. It occurs following the inhalation of spores that become de-

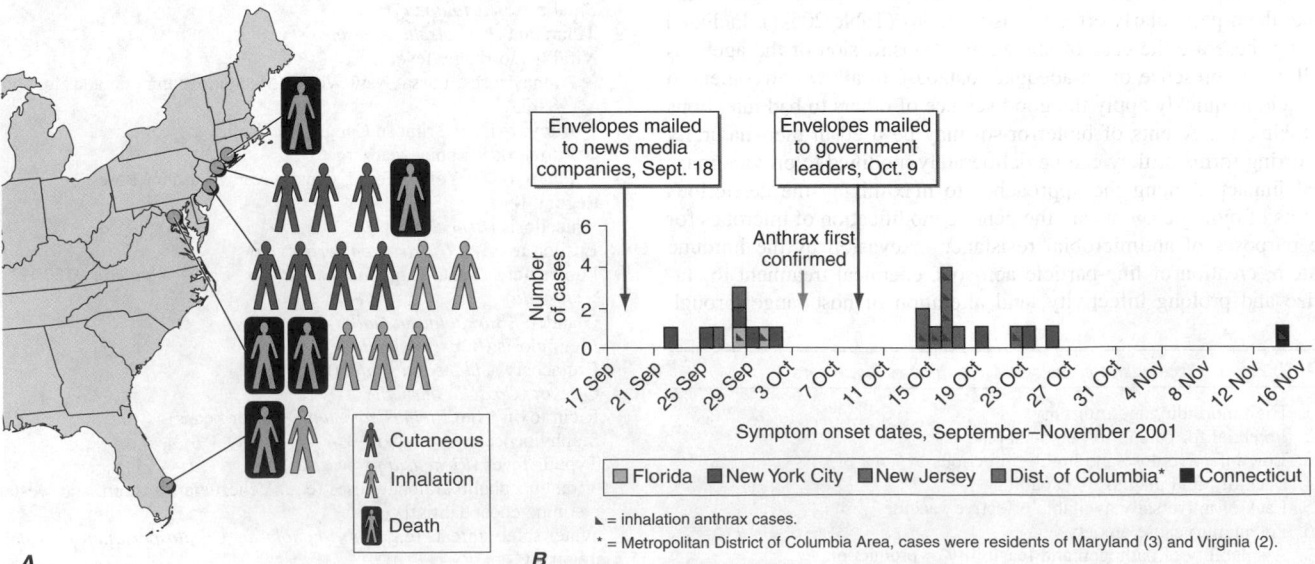

FIGURE 205-1 Confirmed anthrax cases associated with bioterrorism: United States, 2001. *A.* Geographic location, clinical manifestation, and outcome of the 11 cases of confirmed inhalational and 7 cases of confirmed cutaneous anthrax. *B.* Epidemic curve for the 18 confirmed cases of inhalational and cutaneous anthrax and additional 4 cases of suspected cutaneous anthrax. (*From DB Jernigan et al: Investigation of bioterrorism-related anthrax, US 2001: Epidemiologic findings. Emerg Infect Dis 8:1019, 2002; with permission.*)

posited in the alveolar spaces. These spores are phagocytosed by macrophages and transported to the mediastinal and peribronchial lymph nodes where they germinate, leading to active bacterial growth and elaboration of the bacterial products edema toxin and lethal toxin. Subsequent hematogenous spread of bacteria is accompanied by cardiovascular collapse and death. The earliest symptoms are typically a viral-like prodrome with fever, malaise, and abdominal and/or chest symptoms that rapidly progress to a moribund state. A characteristic finding is mediastinal widening and pleural effusions on chest x-ray (Fig. 205-2). While initially thought to be 100% fatal, the experiences at Sverdlosk in 1979 and in the United States in 2001 (see below) indicate that with prompt initiation of antibiotic therapy survival is possible. The characteristics of the 11 cases of inhalational anthrax diagnosed in the United States in 2001 following exposure to contaminated letters postmarked September 18 or October 9, 2001, are detailed in Table 205-3. These cases followed the classic pattern established for this illness, with patients presenting with a rapidly progressive course characterized by fever, fatigue or malaise, nausea or vomiting, cough, and shortness of breath. At presentation, the total white blood cell counts were ~10,000 cells/μL; transaminases tended to be elevated, and all 11 had abnormal findings on chest x-ray and computed tomography (CT). Pulmonary findings included infiltrates, mediastinal widening, and hemorrhagic pleural effusions. For cases in which the dates of exposure were known, symptoms appeared within 4 to 6 days. Death occurred within 7 days of diagnosis in the five fatal

cases (overall mortality rate 55%). Rapid diagnosis and prompt initiation of antibiotic therapy were key to survival.

R_X TREATMENT

Anthrax can be successfully treated if the disease is promptly recognized and appropriate therapy is initiated early. While penicillin, ciprofloxacin, and doxycycline are the currently licensed antibiotics for this indication, clindamycin and rifampin have in vitro activity against the organism and have been used as part of treatment regimens. Until sensitivity results are known, suspected cases are best managed with a combination of widely active agents (Table 205-4). Patients with inhalational anthrax are not contagious and do not require special isolation procedures.

Vaccination and Prevention The first successful vaccine for anthrax was developed for animals by Louis Pasteur in 1881. At present, the single vaccine licensed for human use is a product produced from the cell-free culture supernatant of an attenuated, nonencapsulated strain of *B. anthracis* (Stern strain), referred to as *anthrax vaccine adsorbed* (AVA). Clinical trials for safety in humans and efficacy in animals are currently under way to evaluate the role of recombinant protective antigen (one of the major components, along with lethal factor and edema factor, of *B. anthracis* toxins) as an alternative to AVA. Since

FIGURE 205-2 Progression of chest x-ray findings in a patient (Table 205-3, Patient 9) with inhalational anthrax. Findings evolved from subtle hilar prominence and right perihilar infiltrate to a progressively widened mediastinum, marked perihilar infiltrates, peribronchial cuffing, and air bronchograms. (*From L Borio et al: Death due to bioterrorism-related inhalational anthrax. JAMA 286:2554, 2001; with permission.*)

Case	Age/Sex	Location	Occupation	Initial Symptoms	Radiograph Findings CXR/CT	Initial WBC	Time Interval from 1st Symptom to Death, Days	Treatment[a]
FATAL CASES								
1	63 y/o man	FL	Photo editor, media company	Fever, malaise, fatigue, altered mental state	Widened upper mediastinum, pleural effusion	9400	8	Cefotaxime, ceftazidime, gentamicin, metronidazole, doxycycline, ampicillin, trimethoprim-sulfamethoxazole, penicillin G, levofloxacin, clindamycin
2	55 y/o man	DC	Postal worker	Fever, fatigue, myalgia, cough	Infiltrate, perihilar fullness, pleural effusion	10,300	5	Levofloxacin, diltiazem, insulin, mechanical ventilation
3	47 y/o man	DC	Postal worker	Nausea, vomiting, abdominal pain, syncope, cough	Perihilar infiltrate, mediastinal adenopathy, pleural effusion	13,300	6	Penicillin, ceftriaxone, rifampin, levofloxacin, mechanical ventilation
4	61 y/o woman	NY	Hospital worker	Malaise, myalgia, cough, chest pain, dyspnea, fatigue	Mediastinal adenopathy, pleural effusions	11,400	6	Levofloxacin, rifampin, gentamicin, nafcillin, ciprofloxacin, clindamycin, ceftazidime, mechanical ventilation, chest tubes
5	94 y/o woman	CT	Retired	Fever, fatigue, loss of appetite, cough, myalgia	Perihilar fullness, pleural effusion	8100	8	Vancomycin, ceftazidime, ampicillin, sulbactam, ciprofloxacin, clindamycin, thoracentesis, mechanical ventilation
NONFATAL CASES								
6	73 y/o man	FL	Mail handler, media company	Fever, fatigue, abdominal pain, vomiting, cough, dyspnea, conjunctivitis	Consolidation, pleural effusion	9900		Azithromycin, cefotaxime, ciprofloxacin
7	56 y/o woman	NJ	Postal worker	Fever, vomiting, diarrhea, cough, chest pain, dyspnea	Bibasilar infiltrates, mediastinal adenopathy, pleural effusion	8100		Levofloxacin, rifampin, ciprofloxacin, vancomycin, thoracentesis, chest tube
8	43 y/o woman	NJ	Postal worker	Fever, myalgia, vomiting, fatigue, cough, chest pain, dyspnea, headache	Perihilar consolidation, mediastinal adenopathy, pleural effusion	11,200		Levofloxacin, azithromycin, ciprofloxacin, clindamycin, ceftriaxone, doxycycline, thoracentesis X2
9	56 y/o man	DC	Postal worker	Fever, headache, malaise, sore throat, cough, dyspnea, nausea, vomiting	Bilateral hilar adenopathy, widened mediastinum, pleural effusion	7500		Ciprofloxacin, rifampin, clindamycin, diuretics, glucocorticoids, thoracentesis X3
10	56 y/o man	DC	Postal worker	Fever, headache, malaise, sore throat, nausea, photophobia, cough, dyspnea, chest pain	Widened mediastinum, bilateral hilar adenopathy, airspace disease, pleural effusion	9700		Ciprofloxacin, rifampin, clindamycin, glucocorticoids thoracentesis X2
11	59 y/o man	VA	Postal worker	Fever, sweats, myalgia, fatigue, headache, nausea, vomiting, abdominal pain, cough, chest pain	Mediastinal widening, mediastinal adenopathy, pleural effusion	9700		Ciprofloxacin, penicillin, rifampin, vancomycin, thoracentesis

[a] At anytime during the illness.
Note: CT, computed tomography; CXR, chest x-ray; WBC, white blood cell count.

the efficacy of AVA in a postexposure setting in humans has not been established, the current recommendation for postexposure prophylaxis is 60 days of antibiotics. Given the potential for *B. anthracis* to be engineered to express penicillin resistance, the empirical regimen of choice in this setting is either ciprofloxacin or doxycycline.

PLAGUE (*YERSINIA PESTIS*) (See also Chap. 143) ■ **Plague as a Bioweapon** Although it lacks the environmental stability of anthrax, the highly contagious nature and high mortality of plague make it a close to ideal agent of bioterrorism, particularly if delivered in a weaponized form. Occupying a unique place in history, plague has been alleged to have been used as a biologic weapon for centuries. The catapulting of plague-infected corpses into besieged fortresses is a practice that was first noted in 1346 during the assault of the city of Kaffa by the Tartars. There are some who believe this may have played a role in the start

TABLE 205-4 *Clinical Syndromes, Prevention, and Treatment Strategies for Diseases Caused by Category A Agents*

Agent	Clinical Syndrome	Incubation Period	Diagnosis	Treatment	Prophylaxis
Bacillus anthracis (anthrax)	Cutaneous lesion: Papule to eschar Inhalational disease: Fever, malaise, chest and abdominal discomfort Pleural effusion, widened mediastinum on chest x-ray	1–12 days 1–60 days	Culture, Gram stain, PCR, Wright stain of peripheral smear	*Postexposure:* Ciprofloxacin, 500 mg, PO bid × 60 d *or* Doxycycline, 100 mg PO bid ×60 d Amoxicillin, 500 mg PO q8h, likely to be effective if strain penicillin sensitive *Active disease:* Ciprofloxacin, 400 mg IV q12h *or* Doxycycline, 100 mg IV q12 *plus* Clindamycin, 900 mg IV q8h and/or rifampin, 300 mg IV q12h; switch to PO when stable ×60 d total *Antitoxin strategies:* Neutralizing monoclonal antibodies are under study	Anthrax vaccine adsorbed Recombinant protective antigen vaccines are under study
Yersinia pestis (pneumonic plague)	Fever, cough, dyspnea, hemoptysis Infiltrates and consolidation on chest x-ray	1–6 days	Culture, Gram stain, direct fluorescent antibody, PCR	Gentamicin, 2.0 mg/kg IV loading then 1.7 mg/kg q8h IV *or* Streptomycin, 1.0 g q12h IM or IV Alternatives include doxycycline, 100 mg bid PO or IV; chloramphenicol 500 mg bid PO or IV	Doxycycline, 100 mg PO bid (ciprofloxacin may also be active) Formalin-fixed vaccine (FDA licensed; not available)
Variola major (smallpox)	Fever, malaise, headache, backache, emesis Maculopapular to vesicular to pustular skin lesions	7–17 days	Culture, PCR, electron microscopy	Supportive measures; consideration for cidofovir, antivaccinia immunoglobulin	Vaccinia immunization
Francisella tularensis (tularemia)	Fever, chills, malaise, myalgia, chest discomfort, dyspnea, headache, skin rash, pharyngitis, conjunctivitis Hilar adenopathy on chest x-ray	1–14 days	Gram stain, culture, immunohistochemistry, PCR	Streptomycin, 1 g IM bid *or* Gentamicin, 5 mg/kg per day div q8h IV for 14 days *or* Doxycycline, 100 mg IV bid *or* Chlorphenid, 15 mg/kg IV qid *or* Ciprofloxacin, 400 mg IV bid	Doxycycline, 100 mg PO bid × 14 days *or* Ciprofloxacin, 500 mg PO bid × 14 days
Viral hemorrhagic fevers	Fever, myalgia, rash, encephalitis, prostration	2–21 days	RT-PCR, serologic testing for antigen or antibody Viral isolation by CDC or U.S. Army Medical Institute of Infectious Diseases (USAMRIID)	Supportive measures Ribavirin 30 mg/kg up to 2 g × 1, followed by 16 mg/kg IV up to 1 g q6h for 4 days, followed by 8 mg/kg IV up to 0.5 g q8h × 6 days	No known chemoprophylaxis Consideration for ribavirin in high-risk situations Vaccine exists for yellow fever
Botulinum toxin (*Clostridium botulinum*)	Dry mouth, blurred vision, ptosis, weakness, dysarthria, dysphagia, dizziness, respiratory failure, progressive paralysis, dilated pupils	12–72 h	Mouse bioassay, toxin immunoassay	Supportive measures including ventilation 5000–9000 IU equine antitoxin	Administration of antitoxin

Note: CDC, U.S. Centers for Disease Control and Prevention; FDA, U.S. Food and Drug Administration; PCR, polymerase chain reaction; RT-PCR, reverse transcriptase PCR.

of the Black Death pandemic of the fourteenth and fifteenth centuries in Europe. Given that plague was already moving across Asia toward Europe at this time, it is unclear whether such an allegation is accurate. During WWII, the infamous Unit 731 of the Japanese army was reported to have repeatedly dropped plague-infested fleas over parts of China, including Manchuria. These drops were associated with subsequent outbreaks of plague in the targeted areas. Following WWII, the United States and the Soviet Union conducted programs of research on how to create direct aerosols containing *Y. pestis* that could be used as a direct bioweapon leading to primary pneumonic plague. As mentioned above, plague was thought to be an excellent bioweapon due to the fact that in addition to causing infection in those inhaling the aerosol, significant numbers of secondary cases of primary pneumonic plague would likely occur due to the contagious nature of the disease and person-to-person transmission via respiratory aerosol. Secondary reports of research conducted during that time suggest that organisms remain viable for up to 1 h and can be dispersed for distances up to 10 km. While the offensive bioweapons program in the United States was terminated prior to production of sufficient quantities of plague organisms for use as a weapon, it is believed that Soviet scientists did manufacture quantities sufficient for such a purpose. It has also been reported that more than 10 Soviet Institutes and over 1000 scientists were working with plague as a biologic weapon. Of concern is the fact that in 1995 a microbiologist in Ohio was arrested for having obtained *Y. pestis* in the mail from the American Type Culture Collection, using a credit card and a false letterhead. In the wake of this incident, the U.S. Congress passed a law in 1997 requiring that anyone intending to send or receive any of 42 different agents that could potentially be used as bioweapons first register with the CDC.

Microbiology and Clinical Features   Plague is caused by *Y. pestis*, a nonmotile, gram-negative bacillus that exhibits bipolar, or "safety pin," staining with Wright, Giemsa, or Wayson stains. It has had a major impact on the course of history, thus adding to the element of fear evoked by its mention. The earliest reported plague epidemic was in 224 B.C. in China. The most infamous pandemic began in Europe in the fourteenth century, during which time one-third to one-half of the entire population of Europe was killed. During a plague outbreak in India in 1994, it is estimated that 500,000 individuals fled their homes in fear of this disease.

The clinical syndromes of plague generally reflect the mode of infection. *Bubonic plague* is the consequence of an insect bite; primary *pneumonic plague* arises through the inhalation of bacteria. Most of the plague seen in the world today is bubonic plague and is the result of a bite by a plague-infected flea. Plague infection of rodents exists widely in nature, and each year thousands of cases of plague occur worldwide through contact with infected animals or fleas. Following inoculation of regurgitated bacteria into the skin by a flea bite, organisms travel through the lymphatics to regional lymph nodes, where they are phagocytized but not destroyed. Inside the cell, they multiply rapidly leading to inflammation, painful lymphadenopathy with necrosis, fever, bacteremia, septicemia, and death. The characteristic enlarged nodes, or *buboes*, give this form of plague its name. In some instances, patients may develop bacteremia without lymphadenopathy following infection, a condition referred to as *primary septicemic plague*. Extensive ecchymoses may develop due to disseminated intravascular coagulation, and gangrene of the digits and/or nose may develop in patients with advanced septicemic plague. It is thought that this appearance of some patients gave rise to the term *Black Death* in reference to the plague epidemic of the fourteenth and fifteenth centuries. Some patients may develop pneumonia (secondary pneumonic plague) as a complication of bubonic or septicemic plague. These patients may then transmit the agent to others via the respiratory route, causing cases of primary pneumonic plague. Primary pneumonic plague is the manifestation most likely to occur as the result of a bioterrorist attack, with an aerosol of bacteria spread over a wide area or a particular environment that is densely populated. In this setting patients would be expected to develop fever, cough with hemoptysis, dyspnea, and gastrointestinal symptoms 1 to 6 days following exposure. Clinical features of pneumonia would be accompanied by pulmonary infiltrates and consolidation on chest x-ray. In the absence of antibiotics, the mortality of this disease is on the order of 85%, and death usually occurs within 2 to 6 days.

℞ TREATMENT

Streptomycin, tetracycline, and doxycycline are licensed by the U.S. Food and Drug Administration (FDA) for the treatment of plague. Multiple additional antibiotics licensed for other infections are commonly used and are likely effective. Among these are aminoglycosides such as gentamicin, cephalosporins, trimethoprim/sulfamethoxazole, chloramphenicol, and ciprofloxacin (Table 205-4). A multidrug resistant strain of *Y. pestis* was identified in 1995 from a patient with bu-

bonic plague in Madagascar. While this organism was resistant to streptomycin, ampicillin, chloramphenicol, sulfonamides, and tetracycline, it retained its susceptibility to other aminoglycosides and cephalosporins. Given the subsequent identification of a similar organism in 1997 coupled with the fact that this resistance is plasmid-mediated, it seems likely that genetically modifying *Y. pestis* to a multidrug resistant form is possible. Unlike patients with inhalational anthrax (see above), patients with pulmonary plague should be cared for under conditions of strict respiratory isolation comparable to that used for multidrug resistant tuberculosis.

Vaccination and Prevention   A formalin-fixed, whole-organism vaccine was licensed by the FDA for the prevention of plague. That vaccine is no longer being manufactured, but its potential value as a current countermeasure against bioterrorism would likely have been modest at best as it was ineffective against primary pneumonic plague in animal studies. Efforts are under way to develop a second generation of vaccines that will protect against aerosol challenge. Among the candidates being tested are recombinant forms of the F1 and V antigens of *Y. pestis*. It is likely that doxycycline or ciprofloxacin would provide coverage in a chemoprophylaxis setting. Unlike the case with anthrax, in which one has to be concerned about the presence of spores, the duration of prophylaxis against plague need only extend to 7 days following exposure.

SMALLPOX (*VARIOLA MAJOR* AND *V. MINOR*) (See also Chap. 167)

■ Smallpox as a Bioweapon   Given that an effective vaccine exists for smallpox, it would not have been considered a good candidate as a bioweapon 30 years ago. However, with the cessation of immunization programs in the United States in 1972 and throughout the world in 1980 due to the successful global eradication of smallpox, close to 50% of the U.S. population is fully susceptible to smallpox today. Given its infectious nature and the 10 to 30% mortality in unimmunized individuals, the deliberate spread of this virus could have a devastating effect on our society and unleash a previously conquered deadly disease. It is estimated that an initial infection of 50 to 100 persons in a first-generation of cases could expand by a factor of 10 to 20 with each succeeding generation in the absence of any effective containment measures.

At the time that the World Health Organization (WHO) recommended that all immunization programs be terminated in 1980, it also recommended that remaining stocks of virus be destroyed and that samples be transferred to only two locations: one at the CDC in Atlanta, GA, in the United States and the other at the Institute of Virus Preparations in the Soviet Union. Several years later, it was recommended that these remaining two stocks be destroyed. However, these latter recommendations were reversed in the wake of increased concerns on the use of *Variola* as a biologic weapon and thus the need to maintain an active program of defensive research. Many of these concerns were based upon allegations made by former Soviet officials that extensive programs had been in place in that country for the production and weaponization of large quantities of smallpox virus. The dismantling of these programs with the fall of the Soviet Union led to fears that stocks of *V. major* may have made their way to other countries. In addition, accounts that efforts had been taken to produce recombinant strains of *Variola* that would be more virulent and more contagious than the wild-type virus have led to an increase in the need to be vigilant for the reemergence of this often fatal infectious disease.

Microbiology and Clinical Features   Smallpox is caused by one of two closely related viruses, *V. major* and *V. minor*. Both are double-strand DNA viruses and members of the Orthopoxvirus genus of the Poxviridae family. Infections with *V. minor* are generally less severe, with milder constitutional symptoms and lower mortality rates; thus *V. major* is the only one considered to be a viable bioweapon. Infection with *V. major* typically occurs following contact with an infected person from the time that a maculopapular rash occurs through the appearance of scabbing of the pustular lesions. Infection is thought to occur from inhalation of saliva droplets containing virus from the oropharyngeal exanthem. Contaminated clothing or linen can also spread infection.

Several days after exposure, a primary viremia is believed to occur that results in dissemination of virus to lymphoid tissues. A secondary viremia occurs ~4 days later that leads to localization of infection in the dermis. Approximately 12 to 14 days following the initial exposure the patient develops high fever, malaise, vomiting, headache, backache, and a maculopapular rash that begins on the face and extremities and spreads to the trunk (centripetal). The lesions are initially maculopapular and evolve to vesicles that eventually become pustules and then scabs. The oral mucosa also develops maculopapular lesions that evolve to ulcers. The lesions appear over a period of 1 to 2 days and evolve at the same rate. Although virus can be isolated from the scabs on the skin, the conventional thinking is that once the scabs have formed the patient is no longer contagious. Smallpox is associated with a 10 to 30% mortality, with patients typically dying of severe systemic illness during the second week of symptoms. Historically, ~5 to 10% of naturally occurring smallpox cases take either of two highly virulent atypical forms, classified as *hemorrhagic* and *malignant*. These are difficult to recognize because of their atypical presentations. The hemorrhagic form is uniformly fatal and begins with the relatively abrupt onset of a severely prostrating illness characterized by high fevers and severe headache and back and abdominal pain. Cutaneous erythema develops accompanied by petechiae and hemorrhages into the skin and mucous membranes. Death usually occurs within 5 to 6 days. The malignant form is frequently fatal and has an onset similar to the hemorrhagic form, but with confluent lesions developing more slowly and never progressing to the pustular stage.

℞ TREATMENT

Given the highly infectious nature of smallpox and the extreme vulnerability of contemporary society, patients who are suspected cases should be handled with strict isolation procedures. While laboratory confirmation of a suspected case by culture and electron microscopy is essential, it is equally important that appropriate precautions be employed when obtaining samples for culture and laboratory testing. All health care and laboratory workers caring for patients should have been recently immunized with vaccinia, and all samples should be transported in doubly sealed containers. Patients should be cared for in negative-pressure rooms with strict isolation precautions.

There is no licensed specific therapy for smallpox, and historic treatments have focused solely on supportive care. While several antiviral agents, including cidofovir, that are licensed for other diseases have in vitro activity against *V. major*, they have never been tested in the setting of human disease. For this reason it is difficult to predict whether or not they would be effective in cases of smallpox and, if effective, whether or not they would be of value in patients with advanced disease. Research programs studying the efficacy of new antiviral compounds against *V. major* are currently under way.

Vaccination and Prevention In 1796 Edward Jenner demonstrated that deliberate infection with cowpox could prevent subsequent infection with smallpox. Today, smallpox is a preventable disease following immunization with vaccinia. The current dilemma facing our society regarding assessment of the risk and/or benefit of smallpox vaccination is that the degree of risk that someone will deliberately and effectively release smallpox into our society is unknown. As a prudent first step in preparedness for a smallpox attack, virtually all members of the U.S. armed services have received primary or booster immunizations with vaccinia. In addition, tens of thousands of civilian health care workers who comprise smallpox-response teams at the state and local public health level have been vaccinated. The voluntary vaccination of other civilian first responders continues as part of a broader smallpox preparedness program.

Initial fears regarding the immunization of a segment of the American population with vaccinia when there are more individuals receiving immunosuppressive drugs and other immunocompromised patients than ever before have largely been dispelled as data are generated from the current military and civilian immunization campaigns. Adverse event rates for the first 450,000 immunizations are similar to

and, in certain categories of adverse events, even lower than those from historic data (Table 205-5). In addition, 11 patients with early stage HIV infection have been inadvertently immunized without problem. One significant concern during the recent immunization campaign, however, has been the description of a syndrome of myopericarditis, which was not appreciated during prior immunization campaigns with vaccinia.

TULAREMIA (*FRANCISELLA TULARENSIS*) (See also Chap. 142) ■ **Tularemia as a Bioweapon** Tularemia has been studied as an agent of bioterrorism since the mid-twentieth century, and it has been suggested that the outbreak of tularemia among German and Soviet soldiers during fighting on the Eastern Front during WWII might have been the consequence of a deliberate release. Unit 731 of the Japanese Army studied the use of tularemia as a bioweapon during WWII. Large quantities of *F. tularensis* were grown by the United States and were reportedly grown by the Soviet Union in the mid-1950s. It has also been suggested that the Soviet program extended into the era of molecular biology and that some strains were engineered to be resistant to common antibiotics. *F. tularensis* is an extremely infectious organism, and human infections have occurred from merely examining an uncovered petri dish streaked with colonies. Given these facts, it is reasonable to conclude that this organism might be utilized as a bioweapon through either an aerosol or contamination of food or drinking water.

Microbiology and Clinical Features While similar in many ways to anthrax and plague, tularemia, also referred to as rabbit fever or deer fly fever, is neither as lethal nor as fulminant as either of these other two category A bacterial infections. It is, however, extremely infectious, and as few as 10 organisms can lead to establishment of infection. Despite this fact, it is not spread from person to person. Tularemia is caused by *F. tularensis*, a small, nonmotile, gram-negative coccobacillus. Although it is not a spore-forming organism, it is a hardy bacterium that can survive for weeks in the environment. Infection typically comes from insect bites or contact with organisms in the environment. Large waterborne outbreaks have been recorded.

Humans can become infected through a variety of environmental sources. Infection is most common in rural areas where a variety of small mammals may serve as reservoirs. Human infections in the summer are often the result of insect bites from ticks, flies, or mosquitoes that have bitten infected animals. In colder months infections are most likely the result of direct contact with infected mammals and are most common in hunters. In these settings infection typically presents as a systemic illness with an area of inflammation and necrosis at the site

TABLE 205-5 *Complications from 438,134 Administrations of Vaccinia During the United States Department of Defense (DoD) Smallpox Immunization Campaign Initiated in December 2002*

Complication	Number of Cases	DoD Rate per Million Vaccinees (95% Confidence Interval)	Historic Rate Per Million Vaccinees
Mild or temporary:			
Generalized vaccinia, mild	35	67 (52, 85)	45 to 212[a]
Inadvertent inoculation, self	62	119 (98, 142)	606[a]
Vaccinia transfer to contact	28	53 (40, 69)	8 to 27[a]
Moderate or serious:			
Encephalitis	1	2.2 (0.6, 7.2)	2.6 to 8.7[a]
Acute myopericarditis	69	131 (110, 155)	100[b]
Eczema vaccinatum	0	0 (0, 3.7)	2 to 35[a]
Progressive vaccinia	0	0 (0, 3.7)	1 to 7[a]
Death	1	1.9 (0.2, 5.6)	1 to 2[a]

[a] Based on adolescent and adult smallpox vaccinations from 1968 studies, both primary and revaccinations.
[b] Based on case series in Finnish military recruits given the Finnish strain of smallpox vaccine.
[c] Potentially attributable to vaccination; after lupus-like illness.
Source: From Grabenstein and Winkenwerder. *http://www.smallpox.mil/event/SPSafetySum.asp*

of tissue entry of the infection. Drinking of contaminated water may lead to an oropharyngeal form of tularemia characterized by pharyngitis with cervical and/or retropharyngeal lymphadenopathy (Chap. 142). The most likely mode of dissemination of tularemia as a biologic weapon would be as an aerosol. Approximately 1 to 14 days following exposure by this route one would expect to see inflammation of the airways with pharyngitis, pleuritis, and bronchopneumonia. Typical symptoms would include the abrupt onset of fever, fatigue, chills, headache, and malaise (Table 205-3). Some patients might experience conjunctivitis with ulceration, pharyngitis, and/or cutaneous exanthems. A pulse-temperature dissociation might be present. Approximately 50% of patients would show a pulmonary infiltrate on chest x-ray. Hilar adenopathy might also be present, and a small percent of patients could have adenopathy without infiltrates. Diagnosis is made by immunohistochemistry or culture of infected tissues or blood. Untreated, mortality rates range from 5 to 15% for cutaneous routes of infection and 30 to 60% for infection by inhalation. Since the advent of antibiotic therapy, these rates have dropped to <2%.

℞ TREATMENT

Both streptomycin and doxycycline are licensed for treatment of tularemia. Other agents likely to be effective include gentamicin, chloramphenicol, and ciprofloxacin (Table 205-4). Given the potential for genetic modification of this organism to yield antibiotic-resistant strains, broad-spectrum coverage should be the rule until sensitivities have been determined. As mentioned above, special isolation procedures are not required.

Vaccination and Prevention There are no vaccines currently licensed for the prevention of infection with *F. tularensis*. While a live, attenuated strain of the organism has been used in the past with some reported success, there are inadequate data to support its widespread use at this time. Development of a vaccine for this agent is an important part of the current biodefense research agenda. In the absence of an effective vaccine, chemoprophylaxis with either doxycycline or ciprofloxacin appears to be a reasonable approach in individuals who have been exposed (Table 205-4).

VIRAL HEMORRHAGIC FEVERS (See also Chaps. 180 and 181) ■ **Hemorrhagic Fever Viruses as Bioweapons** Several of the hemorrhagic fever viruses have been reported to have been weaponized by the Soviet Union and the United States. Nonhuman primate studies indicate that infection can be established with very few virions and that infectious aerosol preparations can be produced. Under the guise of wanting to aid victims of the latest Ebola outbreak, members of the Aum Shrinrikyo cult in Japan were reported to have traveled to central Africa in 1992 in an attempt to obtain Ebola virus for use in a bioterrorist attack. Thus, while there has been no evidence that these agents have ever been used in a biologic attack, there is clear interest in their potential for this purpose.

Microbiology and Clinical Features The viral hemorrhagic fevers are a group of illnesses caused by any one of a number of similar viruses (Table 205-2). These viruses are all enveloped, single-strand RNA viruses that are thought to depend upon a rodent or insect host reservoir for long-term survival. They tend to be geographically restricted according to the migration patterns of their hosts. It is felt that Ebola has been responsible for the deaths of significant numbers of apes in sub-Saharan Africa. While humans are not a reservoir for these viruses, humans can become infected with them if they come into contact with an infected host or other infected animals. Person-to-person transmission has been documented for Ebola, Marburg, Lassa, and New World arenaviruses. While the modes of transmission for naturally occurring infections are largely unknown, these viruses have been shown in animal models to be highly infectious by the aerosol route. This, coupled with mortality rates as high as 90%, makes them excellent candidate agents of bioterrorism.

The clinical features of the viral hemorrhagic fevers may vary depending upon the particular agent (Table 205-4). Initial signs and symptoms typically include fever, myalgia, prostration, and diffuse intravascular coagulation with thrombocytopenia and capillary hemorrhage. A variety of different maculopapular or erythematous rashes may be seen. Leukopenia, temperature-pulse dissociation, renal failure, and seizures may also be part of the clinical presentation. Outbreaks of most of these diseases are sporadic and unpredictable. As a consequence it has been very difficult to study the pathogenesis and epidemiology in any detail. The diagnosis should be suspected in anyone with temperature >38.3°C for <3 weeks who also exhibits at least two of the following: hemorrhagic or purpuric rash, epistaxis, hematemesis, hemoptysis, or hematochezia in the absence of any other identifiable cause. In this setting, samples of blood should be sent to the CDC or the U.S. Army Medical Research Institute of Infectious Diseases (USAMRIID) for serologic testing for antigen and antibody as well as reverse transcriptase polymerase chain reaction (RT-PCR) testing for hemorrhagic fever viruses. All samples should be handled with double-bagging. Given how little is known regarding the human-to-human transmission of these viruses, appropriate isolation measures would include full barrier precautions with negative-pressure rooms and use of N95 masks or powered air-purifying respirators (PAPRs). Unprotected skin contact with cadavers has been implicated in the transmission of certain hemorrhagic fever viruses such as Ebola, so it is recommended that autopsies be performed using the strictest measures for protection and that burial or cremation be performed promptly without embalming.

℞ TREATMENT

There are no approved and effective antiviral therapies for this class of viruses (Table 205-4). While there are anecdotal reports of the efficacy of ribavirin, interferon α, or hyperimmune immunoglobulin, definitive data are lacking. The best data for ribavirin are in arenavirus (Lassa and New World) infections. In some animal models specific immunoglobulin has been reported to enhance disease progression, and thus these potential treatments must be approached with caution.

Vaccination and Prevention A live attenuated virus vaccine is available in limited quantities for prevention of yellow fever. There are no other licensed and effective vaccines for these agents. Studies are currently under way examining the potential role of DNA, recombinant viruses, and attenuated viruses as vaccines for several of these infections. Among the most promising at present are vaccines for Argentine, Ebola, Rift Valley, and Kayasanur Forest viruses. Vaccines for Marburg and Lassa viruses are in preclinical testing.

BOTULISM TOXIN (*CLOSTRIDIUM BOTULINUM*) (See also Chap. 126) ■ **Botulism Toxin as a Bioweapon** In a bioterrorist attack, botulinum toxin would likely be dispersed as an aerosol or as contamination of a food supply. While contamination of a water supply is possible, it is likely that any toxin would be rapidly inactivated by the chlorine used to purify drinking water. Similarly, toxin can be inactivated by heating any food to >85°C for >5 min. Without external facilitation, the environmental decay rate is estimated at 1% per minute, and thus the time interval between deposition and ingestion or inhalation needs to be rather short. The Japanese biologic warfare group, Unit 731, is reported to have conducted experiments on botulism poisoning in prisoners in the 1930s. The United States and the Soviet Union both acknowledged producing botulinum toxin, and there is some evidence that the Soviet Union attempted to create recombinant bacteria containing the gene for botulinum toxin. In records submitted to the United Nations, Iraq admitted to having produced 19,000 L of concentrated toxin—enough toxin to kill the entire population of the world three times over. By many accounts, botulinum toxin was the primary focus of the pre-1991 Iraqi bioweapons program. In addition to these examples of state-supported research into the use of botulinum toxin as a bioweapon, the Aum Shrinrikyo cult has unsuccessfully attempted on a least three occasions to disperse botulism toxin into the civilian population of Tokyo.

Microbiology and Clinical Features Unique among the category A agents for not being a live microorganism, botulinum toxin is one of the most potent toxins ever described and is thought by some to be the most poisonous substance in existence. It is estimated that 1 g of botulinum toxin would be sufficient to kill 1 million individuals if adequately dispersed. Botulinum toxin is produced by the gram-positive, spore-forming anaerobe *C. botulinum* (Chap. 126). Its natural habitat is soil. There are seven antigenically distinct forms of botulinum toxin, designated A to G. The majority of naturally occurring human cases are of types A, B, and E. Antitoxin directed toward one of these will have little to no activity against the others. The toxin is a 150-kDa zinc-containing protease that prevents the intracellular fusion of acetylcholine vesicles with the motor neuron membrane, thus preventing the release of acetylcholine. In the absence of acetylcholine-dependent triggering of muscle fibers, a flaccid paralysis develops. Although person-to-person spread does not occur, the ease of production of botulinum toxin coupled with its high morbidity and 60 to 100% mortality make it a close to ideal bioweapon.

Botulism can result from the presence of *C. botulinum* infection in a wound or the intestine, the ingestion of contaminated food, or the inhalation of aerosolized toxin. The latter two forms are the most likely modes of transmission for bioterrorism. Once toxin is absorbed into the bloodstream it binds to the neuronal cell membrane, enters the cell, and cleaves one of the proteins required for the intracellular binding of the synaptic vesicle to the cell membrane, thus preventing release of the neurotransmitter to the membrane of the adjacent muscle cell. Patients initially develop multiple cranial nerve palsies that are followed by a flaccid paralysis. The extent of the neuromuscular compromise is dependent upon the level of toxemia. The majority of patients experience diploplia, dysphagia, dysathria, dry mouth, ptosis, dilated pupils, fatigue, and extremity weakness. There are minimal true central nervous system effects, and patients rarely show significant alterations in mental status. Severe cases can involve complete muscular collapse, loss of the gag reflex, and respiratory failure. Recovery requires the regeneration of new motor neuron synapses with the muscle cell, a process that can take weeks to months. In the absence of secondary infections, which may be common during the protracted recovery phase of this illness, patients remain afebrile. The diagnosis is suspected on clinical grounds and confirmed by a mouse bioassay or toxin immunoassay.

℞ TREATMENT

Treatment for botulism is mainly supportive and may require intubation, mechanical ventilation, and parenteral nutrition (Table 205-4). If diagnosed early enough, administration of equine antitoxin may lead to a decrease in the level of nerve damage and severity of disease. At present antitoxins are available on a limited basis as a licensed bivalent product with activity against toxin types A and B and as an experimental product with activity against toxin type E. In the event of attack with another toxin type, an investigational antitoxin with activity against all seven toxin types is also available through the U.S. Army. A single dose of antitoxin is usually adequate to neutralize any circulating toxin. Given that these preparations are all derived from horse serum, one needs to be vigilant for hypersensitivity reactions, including serum sickness and anaphylaxis following their administration. Once the damage to the nerve axon has been done, however, there is little possible in the way of specific therapy, and vigilance for secondary complications during recovery is of the utmost importance. During the protracted recovery phase of botulism, patients may experience secondary infections. Due to their ability to worsen neuromuscular blockade, aminoglycosides and clindamycin should be avoided in the treatment of these infections.

Vaccination and Prevention A botulinum toxoid preparation has been used as a vaccine for laboratory workers at high risk of exposure and

in certain military situations; however, it is not currently available in quantities that could be used for the general population. At present, early recognition of the clinical syndrome and use of appropriate equine antitoxin is the mainstay of prevention of full-blown disease in exposed individuals. The development of human monoclonal antibodies as a replacement for equine antitoxin antibodies is an area of active research interest.

CATEGORY B AND C AGENTS

The category B agents include those that are moderately easy to disseminate and result in moderate morbidity and low mortality rates. A listing of the current category B agents is provided in Table 205-2. As can be seen, it includes a wide array of microorganisms and products of microorganisms. Several of these agents have been used in bioterrorist attacks, although never with the impact of the agents described above. Among the more notorious of these was the contamination of salad bars in Oregon in 1984 with *Salmonella typhimurium* by the Indian religious cult Rajneeshee. In this outbreak, which many consider to be the first bioterrorist attack against U.S. citizens, >750 individuals were poisoned and 40 were hospitalized in an effort to influence a local election.

Category C agents are the third highest priority agents in the biodefense agenda. These agents include emerging pathogens to which little or no immunity exists in the general population, such as the SARS coronavirus, that could potentially be engineered for mass dissemination in the future because of their availability in nature. These agents are characterized as being relatively easy to produce and disseminate and as having high morbidity and mortality rates as well as a major public health impact. There is no running list of category C agents at the present time.

PREVENTION AND PREPAREDNESS

As noted above, a numerous and diverse array of agents have the potential to be used in a bioterrorist attack. In contrast to the military situation with biowarfare, where the primary objective is to inflict mass casualties on a healthy and prepared militia, the objectives of bioterrorism are to harm civilians as well as to create fear and disruption among the civilian population. While the military needs only to prepare their troops to deal with the limited number of agents that pose a legitimate threat of biowarfare, the public health system needs to prepare the entire civilian population to deal with the multitude of agents and settings that could be utilized in a bioterrorism attack. This includes anticipating issues specific to the very young and the very old, the pregnant patient, and the immunocompromised individual. The challenges in this regard are enormous and immediate. While military preparedness emphasizes vaccines toward a limited number of agents, civilian preparedness needs to rely upon rapid diagnosis and treatment of a wide array of conditions.

The medical profession must maintain a high index of suspicion that unusual clinical presentations or clustering of rare disease may not be a chance occurrence but rather the first sign of a bioterrorist event. This is particularly true when such diseases occur in traditionally healthy populations, when surprisingly large numbers of rare conditions occur, and when diseases commonly seen in rural settings appear in urban populations. Given the importance of rapid diagnosis and early treatment for many of these conditions, it is important that the medical care team report any suspected cases of bioterrorism immediately to local and state health authorities and/or to the CDC (888-246-2675). Recent enhancements have been made to the public health surveillance network to facilitate the rapid sharing of information among public health agencies.

At present a series of efforts are taking place to ensure the biomedical security of the civilian population in the United States. The Public Health Service is moving toward a larger, more highly trained, fully deployable force. A National Pharmaceutical Stockpile (NPSP) has been created by the CDC to provide rapid access to quantities of pharmaceuticals, antidotes, vaccines, and other medical supplies that may be of value in the event of a biologic or biochemical terrorist event. The NPSP has two basic components. The first of these consists of eight 50-ton (45,360-kg) "push packages" that can be deployed anywhere in the United States within 12 h. These push packages are a preassembled set of supplies, pharmaceuticals, and medical equipment ready for immediate delivery to the field. They provide treatment for a variety of conditions given the fact that an actual threat may not have been precisely identified at the time of stockpile deployment. The contents of the push packs are constantly updated to ensure that they reflect current needs as determined by national security threat assessments; they include antibiotics for treatment of anthrax, plague, and tularemia as well as a cache of vaccine to deal with a smallpox threat. The second component of the NPSP comprises inventories managed by specific vendors and consists of the provision of additional pharmaceuticals, supplies, and/or products tailored to the specific attack.

The number of FDA-approved and -licensed drugs and vaccines for category A and B agents is currently limited and not reflective of the pharmacy of today. In an effort to speed the licensure of additional drugs and vaccines for these diseases, the FDA has proposed a new rule for the licensure of such countermeasures against agents of bioterror when adequate and well-controlled clinical efficacy studies cannot be ethically conducted in humans. Thus, for indications in which field trials of naturally occurring disease are not feasible, the FDA is proposing to rely on evidence solely from animal studies. For this rule to apply it must be shown that (1) there are reasonably well-understood pathophysiologic mechanisms for the condition and its treatment; (2) the effect of the intervention is independently substantiated in multiple animal species, including species expected to react with a response predictive for humans; (3) the animal study end point is clearly related predictive for humans; and (4) the data in animals allow selection of an effective dose in humans.

Finally, an initiative referred to as Project BioShield has been established to facilitate biodefense research within the federal government, create a stable source of funding for the purchase of countermeasures against agents of bioterrorism, and create a category of "emergency use authorization" to allow the FDA to approve the use of unlicensed treatments during times of extraordinary unmet needs as might be present in the context of a bioterrorist attack.

While the prospect of a deliberate attack on civilians with disease-producing agents may seem to be an act of incomprehensible evil, history shows us that it is something that has been done in the past and will likely be done again in the future. It is the responsibility of health care providers to be aware of this possibility, to be able to recognize early signs of a potential bioterrorist attack and alert the public health system, and to respond quickly to provide care to the individual patient. Among the web sites with current information on microbial bioterrorism are *www.bt.cdc.gov*, *www.niaid.nih.gov*, *www.hopkinsbiodefense.org*, and *www.cns.miis.edu/research/cbw/index.htm*.

FURTHER READING

ALIBEK K, HANDELMAN S: *Biohazard: The Chilling True Story of the Largest Covert Biological Weapons in the World, Told from the Inside by the Man who Ran it*. New York, Random House, 1999

CRODDY E (with C Perey-Armendariz and J Hart): *Chemical and Biological Warfare: A Comprehensive Survey for the Concerned Citizen*. New York, Copernicus Books, 2001

GRABENSTEIN JD, WINKENWERDER W: United States military smallpox vaccination program experience. JAMA 289:3278, 2003

HENDERSON DA et al (eds): *Bioterrorism: Guidelines for Medical and Public Health Management*. JAMA and Archives Journals, AMA press, 2002

JERNIGAN JA et al: Bioterrorism-related inhalational anthrax: The first 10 cases reported in the United States. Emerg Infect Dis 7:933,2001

206   CHEMICAL BIOTERRORISM

Charles G. Hurst, Jonathan Newmark, James A. Romano

The use of chemical warfare agents (CWAs) as weapons of terror against civilian populations is a potential reality that must be addressed by public health officials and by the medical profession. The use of sulfur mustard and nerve agents by Iraq against the Iranian military and Kurdish civilians, the sarin attacks in 1994–1995 in Japan, and the terrorist strikes of September 11, 2001, followed by the anthrax attacks in Florida, New York, and Washington, D.C., underscore this threat.

Many of the World War I (WWI) chemical agents, including chlorine, phosgene, and cyanide, are used in large amounts in industry. They are produced in chemical plants, stockpiled in large tanks, and travel up and down highways and railways in large tanker cars. The rupture of any of these by accident or purposefully could cause many injuries and deaths. Hazardous materials (HAZMATs), not used on the battlefield, can also be used as terrorist weapons. Some of these, including insecticides and ammonia, could wreak as much damage and injury as the weaponized chemical agents.

Military planners consider the WWI blistering agent, sulfur mustard, and the organophosphorus nerve agents as the most likely agents to be used on the battlefield. In a civilian or terrorist scenario, the choice widens considerably. Cyanide, a common chemical, causes symptoms within seconds and death in 5 to 10 min if not treated rapidly. Chlorine and phosgene have no specific antidotes but can require intensive care for weeks to months. Many believe these agents or one of the industrial HAZMATs will be the likely choice of terrorists.

Many mistakenly believe that chemical attacks will always be so severe that little can be done except to bury the dead. History proves the opposite. Even in WWI, when intravenous fluids, endotracheal tubes, and antibiotics were unavailable, the mortality rate in U.S. forces on the battlefield from chemical warfare agents, chiefly sulfur mustard and the pulmonary intoxicants, was only 1.9%. This was far less than the mortality rate from conventional wounds (7%). In the 1995 Tokyo subway sarin incident, of the 5500 patients who sought medical attention at hospitals, 80% of whom were not actually symptomatic, only 12 died. Thus, it is prudent to attempt to understand the pathophysiology of the syndromes that these agents cause, with a view to treating all patients who present for care expeditiously and with an expectation of saving the vast majority. As we prepare to defend our civilian population from the effects of chemical terrorism, we must also consider that the concept of terrorism can itself produce sequelae in some individuals—physiologic and/or psychological effects that may resemble the effects of nonlethal exposures to CWAs. These effects are due to a general fear of chemicals, fear of decontamination, fear of protective ensemble, or other phobic reactions.

There may be difficulty in differentiating between stress reactions and nerve agent–induced organic brain syndromes. Knowledge of the behavioral effects of CWAs and their medical countermeasures is imperative in order to ensure that military and civilian medical and mental health organizations can deal with possible incidents involving weapons of mass destruction.

The agents of chemical terrorism together with their North Atlantic Treaty Organization (NATO) codes, their unique characteristics, and initial effects are summarized in Table 206-1. An outline of the approaches to decontamination and treatment of the agents of chemical terrorism is shown in Table 206-2. This chapter will restrict its discussion to vesicants and nerve agents, which are considered as a priority based on threat assessments and prior experiences in chemical warfare. For a more comprehensive listing and discussion of agents of

Agent	Agent Name	Unique Characteristics	Initial Effects
Nerve	Cyclohexyl sarin (GF) Sarin (GB) Soman (GD) Tabun (GA) VX	Miosis (pinpoint pupils) Copious secretions Muscle twitching/fasciculations	Miosis (pinpoint pupils) Blurred/dim vision Headache Nausea, vomiting, diarrhea Copious secretions/sweating Muscle twitching/fasciculations Breathing difficulty Seizures
Asphyxiant/blood	Arsine Cyanogen chloride Hydrogen cyanide	Possible cherry red skin Possible cyanosis Possible frostbite[a]	Confusion Nausea Patients may gasp for air, similar to asphyxiation but more abrupt onset Seizures prior to death
Choking/pulmonary-damaging	Chlorine Hydrogen chloride Nitrogen oxides Phosgene	Chlorine is a greenish-yellow gas with pungent odor Phosgene gas smells like newly mown hay or grass Possible frostbite[a]	Eye and skin irritation Airway irritation Dyspnea, cough Sore throat Chest tightness
Blistering/vesicant	Mustard/Sulfur mustard (HD, H) Mustard gas (H) Nitrogen mustard (HN-1, HN-2, HN-3) Lewisite (L) Phosgene oxime (CX)	Mustard (HD) has an odor like burning garlic or horseradish Lewisite (L) has an odor like penetrating geranium Phosgene oxime (CX) has a pepperish or pungent odor	Severe irritation Redness and blisters of the skin Tearing, conjunctivitis, corneal damage Mild respiratory distress to marked airway damage May cause death
Incapacitating/behavior-altering	Agent 15/BZ	May appear as mass drug intoxication with erratic behaviors, shared realistic and distinct hallucinations, disrobing and confusion Hyperthermia Mydriasis (dilated pupils)	Dry mouth and skin Initial tachycardia Altered consciousness, delusions, denial of illness, belligerence Hyperthermia Ataxia (lack of coordination) Hallucinations Mydriasis (dilated pupils)

[a] Frostbite may occur from skin contact with liquid arsine, cyanogen chloride, or phosgene.   **Source**: State of New York, Department of Health.

chemical terrorism, the reader is referred to Tables 206-1 and 206-2 as well as to the Centers for Disease Control and Prevention website at http://www.bt.cdc.gov/agent/agentlistchem.asp. Also, the antidote recommendations for exposure to cyanide are given in Table 206-3.

VESICANTS

SULFUR MUSTARD, NITROGEN MUSTARD, LEWISITE Sulfur mustard has been a military threat since it first appeared on the battlefield in Belgium during WWI. In modern times it remains a threat on the battlefield as well as a potential terrorist threat because of simplicity of manufacture and extreme effectiveness. Sulfur mustard accounted for 70% of the 1.3 million chemical casualties in WWI. Only sulfur mustard will be discussed here due to space constraints and because it is the prototypical vesicant or blistering agent (Table 206-1).

Mechanism Sulfur mustard constitutes both a vapor and a liquid threat to all exposed epithelial surfaces. Mustard's effects are delayed, appearing hours after exposure. Organs most commonly affected are the skin (with erythema and vesicles), eyes (ranging from mild conjunctivitis to severe eye damage), and airways (ranging from mild upper airway irritation, to severe bronchiolar damage). Following exposure to large quantities of mustard, precursor cells of the bone marrow are damaged, leading to pancytopenia and secondary infection. The gastrointestinal mucosa may be damaged, and there are sometimes central nervous system (CNS) signs of unknown mechanism. No specific antidotes exist; management is entirely supportive.

Mustard dissolves slowly in aqueous media, such as sweat, but once dissolved, it rapidly forms extremely reactive cyclic ethylene sulfonium ions, which reacts with cell proteins, cell membranes, and especially DNA in rapidly dividing cells. Mustard's ability to react with and alkylate DNA gives rise to the effects by which it has been characterized as "radiomimetic," similar to radiation injury. Mustard has many biological actions, but their actual mechanism of action is largely unknown. Much of the biological damage from mustard results from DNA alkylation and cross-linking in rapidly dividing cells: cor-

neal epithelium, basal keratinocytes, bronchial mucosal epithelium, gastrointestinal mucosal epithelium, and bone marrow precursor cells. This may lead to cellular death and inflammatory reactions. In the skin, proteolytic digestion of anchoring filaments at the epidermal-dermal junction may be the major mechanism of action resulting in blister formation. Mustard also possesses mild cholinergic activity, which may be responsible for effects such as early gastrointestinal and CNS symptoms.

Mustard reacts with tissue within minutes of entering the body. Its circulating half-life in unaltered form is extremely brief.

Clinical Features Topical effects of mustard occur in the skin, airways, and eyes, with the latter being most sensitive, followed by the airways. Absorbed mustard may produce effects in the bone marrow, gastrointestinal tract, and CNS. Direct injury to the gastrointestinal tract may also occur following ingestion of the compound through contamination of water or food.

Erythema is the mildest and earliest form of mustard skin injury (Table 206-1). It resembles sunburn and is associated with pruritus, burning, or stinging pain. Erythema begins to appear within 2 h to 2 days after vapor exposure. Time of onset depends on the severity of exposure, ambient temperature and humidity, and type of skin. The most sensitive sites are the warm moist locations and thin delicate skin, such as the perineum, external genitalia, axillae, antecubital fossae, and neck.

Within the erythematous areas, small vesicles can develop, which may later coalesce to form bullae. The typical bulla is large, dome-shaped, flaccid, thin-walled, translucent, and surrounded by erythema. The blister fluid, a transudate, is clear to straw-colored, which becomes yellow, tending to coagulate. The fluid does not contain mustard and is not itself a vesicant. Lesions from high-dose liquid exposure may develop a central zone of coagulation necrosis with blister formation at the periphery. These lesions take longer to heal and are more prone to secondary infection than the uncomplicated lesions seen at lower exposure levels. Severe lesions may require skin grafting.

TABLE 206-2 Decontamination and Treatment of Chemical Terrorism

Agent	Decontamination	First Aid	Other Patient Considerations
Nerve	Remove clothing immediately Gently wash skin with soap and water Do not abrade skin For eyes, flush with plenty of water or normal saline	Atropine before other measures Pralidoxime (2-PAM) chloride	Onset of symptoms from dermal contact with liquid forms may be delayed Repeated antidote administration may be necessary
Asphyxiant/blood	Remove clothing immediately if no frostbite* Gently wash skin with soap and water Do not abrade skin For eyes, flush with plenty of water or normal saline	Rapid treatment with oxygen For cyanide, use antidotes (sodium nitrate and then sodium thiosulfate)	Arsine and cyanogen chloride may cause delayed pulmonary edema
Choking/pulmonary-damaging	Remove clothing immediately if no frostbite* Gently wash skin with soap and water Do not abrade skin For eyes, flush with plenty of water or normal saline	Fresh air, forced rest Semi-upright position If signs of respiratory distress are present, oxygen with or without positive airway pressure may be needed Other supportive therapy, as needed	May cause delayed pulmonary edema, even following a symptom-free period that varies in duration with the amount inhaled
Blistering/vesicant	Immediate decontamination is essential to minimize damage Remove clothing immediately Gently wash skin with soap and water Do not abrade skin For eyes, flush with plenty of water or normal saline	Immediately decontaminate skin Flush eyes with water or normal saline for 10–15 minutes If breathing difficulty, give oxygen Supportive care	Mustard has an asymptomatic latent period There is no antidote or treatment for mustard Lewisite has immediate burning pain, blisters later Specific antidote British Anti-Lewisite (BAL) may decrease systemic effects of Lewisite Phosgene oxime causes immediate pain Possible pulmonary edema
Incapacitating/behavior-altering	Remove clothing immediately Gently wash skin with water or soap and water Do not abrade skin	Remove heavy clothing Evaluate mental status Use restraints as needed Monitor core temperature carefully Supportive care	Hyperthermia and self-injury are largest risks Hard to detect because it is an odorless and non-irritating substance Possible serious arrhythmias Specific antidote (physostigmine) may be available

a For frostbite areas, do NOT remove any adhering clothing. Wash area with plenty of warm water to release clothing.
Source: State of New York, Department of Health.

The primary airway lesion is necrosis of the mucosa with possible damage to underlying smooth muscle. The damage begins in the upper airways and descends to the lower airways in a dose-dependent manner. Usually, the terminal airways and alveoli are affected only as a terminal event. Pulmonary edema is not usually present unless the damage is very severe; in this case, it often becomes hemorrhagic.

The earliest effects from mustard, perhaps the only effects from a low concentration, involve the nose, sinuses, and pharynx. There may be irritation or burning of the nares, epistaxis, sinus pain, and pharyngeal pain. As the concentration increases, laryngitis, voice changes, and nonproductive cough develop. Damage to the trachea and upper bronchi leads to a productive cough. Lower airway involvement causes dyspnea, severe cough, and increasing quantities of sputum. Terminally, there may be necrosis of the smaller airways with hemorrhagic edema into the surrounding alveoli. Hemorrhagic pulmonary edema is rare.

Necrosis of airway mucosa causes "pseudomembrane" formation. These membranes may cause obstruction of the bronchi. During WWI, high-dose mustard exposure caused acute death via this mechanism in a small minority of cases.

The eyes are the organs most sensitive to mustard vapor injury. The latent period is shorter for eye injury than for skin injury and is also exposure concentration–dependent. After low-dose vapor exposure, irritation evidenced by reddening of the eyes may be the only effect. As the dose increases, the injury includes progressively more severe conjunctivitis, photophobia, blepharospasm, pain, and corneal damage (Fig. 206-1).

Ninety percent of eye casualties heal in 2 weeks to 2 months without sequelae. Scarring between the iris and lens may follow severe effects; this scarring may restrict pupillary movements and may predispose victims to glaucoma. The most severe damage is caused by liquid mustard. After extensive eye exposure, severe corneal damage with possible perforation of the cornea and loss of the eye can occur. In some individuals, chronic eye irritation, sometimes associated with corneal ulcerations, has been described 10 to 20 years after exposure.

The mucosa of the gastrointestinal tract is susceptible to mustard damage, either from systemic absorption or ingestion of the agent. Mustard exposure in small amounts will cause nausea and possible vomiting lasting up to 24 h. The mechanism of the nausea and vomiting is not understood, but mustard does have a cholinergic-like effect. The CNS effects of mustard, likewise, remain poorly defined. Large exposures can cause seizures in animals. Reports from WWI and Iran described the behavior of persons exposed to small amounts of mustard as sluggish, apathetic, and lethargic. These reports suggest that minor psychological problems could linger for a year or longer.

The causes of death in the majority of mustard poisoning cases are sepsis and respiratory failure. Mechanical obstruction via pseudomembrane formation and agent-induced laryngospasm is important in the first 24 h, but only in cases of severe exposure. From the third through the fifth day after exposure, a secondary bacterial pneumonia can be expected due to invasion of denuded necrotic mucosa. The third wave of death is caused by agent-induced bone marrow suppression, which peaks 7 to 21 days after exposure and causes death via sepsis.

℞ TREATMENT

A patient severely ill from mustard poisoning requires the general supportive care provided for any severely ill patient as well as the specific care given to a burn patient. Liberal use of systemic analgesics, maintenance of fluid and electrolyte balance and nutrition, use of appropriate antibiotics, and other supportive measures are necessary (Table 206-2).

The management of a patient exposed to mustard may range from simple, as in the provision of symptomatic care for a sunburn-like erythema, to complex, as in the provision of total management for a severely ill patient with burns, immunosuppression, and multisystem involvement. Before raw denuded areas of skin develop, especially with less severe exposures, topical cortisone creams or lotions may be of benefit. Some very basic research data point to the early use of anti-inflammatory preparations. Small blisters (<1 to 2 cm) should be left intact. Because larger bullae will eventually break, they should be carefully unroofed. Denuded areas should be irrigated three to four times daily with saline, other sterile solutions, or soapy water and then liberally covered with the topical antibiotic of choice, such as silver sulfadiazine or mafenide acetate, to a thickness of 1 to 2 mm. Some advocate sterile needle drainage of large blisters, collapsing the blister roof to form a sterile dressing. Mustard blister fluid does not contain sulfur mustard, only sterile tissue fluid. Health care staff should not fear possible contamination. If an antibiotic cream is not available, sterile petrolatum is useful. Modified Dakins solution (sodium hypochlorite 0.5%) was used both in WWI and in Iranian casualties (1984–1987) for field-expedient irrigation and antisepsis. Large areas of vesication require hospitalization, intravenous therapy, and whirlpool bath irrigation.

Systemic analgesics should be used liberally, particularly before manipulation of the patient. Monitoring of fluids and electrolytes is important in any sick patient, but it must be recognized that fluid loss is usually not of the magnitude seen with thermal burns. This may be because mustard burns, in general, are more superficial than thermal burns (no definitive data exist to support this supposition). Overly rigorous hydration seems to have precipitated pulmonary edema in a few Iranian casualties sent to European hospitals.

Conjunctival irritation from a low vapor exposure will respond to any of a number of available ophthalmic solutions after the eyes are thoroughly irrigated. A topical antibiotic applied several times a day will reduce the incidence and severity of infection. Animal laboratory data have shown remarkable results with commercially available topical antibiotic/glucocorticoid ophthalmologic ointments applied early. Topical glucocorticoids alone are not of proven value, but their use during the first few hours or days may significantly reduce inflammation and subsequent damage. Further use should be relegated to an ophthalmologist, who should be consulted in any case.

Vaseline or a similar substance should be applied regularly to the edges of the lids to prevent them from sticking together. Although topical analgesics may be useful initially if blepharospasm is too severe to permit an adequate examination, they have limited value.

A productive cough and dyspnea accompanied by fever and leukocytosis occurring within 12 to 24 h is indicative of a chemical pneumonitis. The clinician must resist the urge to use prophylactic antibiotics for this process. Infection often occurs on the third to fifth day and is signaled by an increased fever, pulmonary infiltrate, and an increase in sputum production with a change in color. Initial antibiotic therapy should await evidence of infection from Gram stain of sputum;

TABLE 206-3 *Antidote Recommendations Following Exposure to Cyanide*

Patient	Mild (Conscious)	Severe (Unconscious)	Other Treatment
Child	If patient is conscious and has no other signs or symptoms, antidotes may not be necessary.	Sodium nitrate[a]: 0.12–0.33 mL/kg, not to exceed 10 mL of 3% solution[b] slow IV over no less than 5 min, or slower if hypotension develops *and* Sodium thiosulfate: 1.65 mL/kg of 25% solution IV over 10–20 min	For sodium nitrite–induced orthostatic hypotension, normal saline infusion and supine position are recommended. If still apneic after antidote administration, consider sodium bicarbonate for severe acidosis.
Adult	If patient is conscious and has no other signs or symptoms, antidotes may not be necessary.	Sodium nitrite[a]: 10–20 mL of 3% solution[b] slow IV over no less than 5 min, or slower if hypotension develops *and* Sodium thiosulfate: 50 mL of 25% solution IV over 10–20 min	

[a] If sodium nitrite is unavailable, administer amyl nitrite by inhalation from crushable ampules.
[b] Available in Pasadena Cyanide Antidote Kit, formerly Lilly Cyanide Kit.
Note: Victims whose clothing or skin is contaminated with hydrogen cyanide liquid or solution can secondarily contaminate response personnel by direct contact or through off-gassing vapors. Avoid dermal contact with cyanide-contaminated victims or with gastric contents of victims who may have ingested cyanide-containing materials. Victims exposed only to hydrogen cyanide gas do not pose contamination risks to rescuers. *If the patient is a victim of recent smoke inhalation (may have high carboxyhemoglobin levels), administer only sodium thiosulfate.*
Source: State of New York, Department of Health.

regimens can then be changed, if appropriate according to the results of sputum culture and sensitivity.

Intubation may be necessary if laryngeal spasm or edema makes it difficult or becomes life-threatening. Intubation permits better ventilation and facilitates suction of the necrotic and inflammatory debris. Early use of positive end-expiratory pressure (PEEP) or continuous positive airway pressure (CPAP) may be beneficial. Pseudomembrane formation may require fiberoptic bronchoscopy for suctioning of the necrotic debris.

Bronchodilators are of benefit for bronchospasm. If additional relief of bronchospasm is needed, glucocorticoids should be used. There is little evidence that the routine use of glucocorticoids is beneficial, except for additional relief of bronchospasm.

Leukopenia begins around day 3 with major systemic absorption. Marrow suppression peaks at 7 to 14 days. In the Iran-Iraq war, a white blood count of ≤200/μL usually resulted in death of the patient. Sterilization of the gut by nonabsorbable antibiotics should be considered to reduce the possibility of sepsis from enteric organisms. Cellular

FIGURE 206-1 World War I photograph of troops exposed to sulfur mustard vapor. The vast majority of these troops survived with no long-term damage to the eyes; however, they were effectively rendered blind for days to weeks.

replacement (bone marrow transplants or transfusions) may be successful. In one study, granulocyte colony-stimulating factor produced a 50% reduction in the time for the bone marrow to recover in non-human primates exposed to sulfur mustard and should be considered in the case of human exposure. Medication for nausea and vomiting may be necessary for gastrointestinal side effects.

Excellent assessments of the contributions of DNA alkylation, inflammation, activation of proteolytic enzymes, or lipid peroxidation to the mustard injury have been developed in the past 15 years. Examples include (1) the demonstration up to 75% reduction of inflammation and tissue damage in the mouse ear swelling test by vanilloid compounds, and (2) the demonstration of 50 to 60% protection by N-acetylcysteine in the generation of free radicals within guinea pig lung exposed to mustard. In many cases, the demonstration of protection is dependent on the availability of sufficient amounts of drug with adequate half-lives. Strategies to enhance bioavailability include attachment of polyethylene glycol to the antioxidant drug/enzyme or delivery of the drug/enzyme in a liposome (or both).

NERVE AGENTS

The organophosphorus nerve agents are the deadliest of the chemical warfare agents. They work by inhibition of tissue synaptic acetylcholinesterase, creating an acute cholinergic crisis. Death ensues because of respiratory depression and can occur within seconds to minutes (Table 206-1).

The "classic" nerve agents include tabun (GA), sarin (GB), soman (GD), cyclosarin (GF), and VX. VR, similar to VX, was manufactured in the former Soviet Union (Table 206-1). The two-letter codes are a NATO international convention and convey no clinical implications. All of the nerve agents are organophosphorus compounds, which are liquid at standard temperature and pressure. The "G" agents evaporate at about the rate of water, except for GF, which is oily, and thus will probably have evaporated within 24 h after deposition on the ground. Their high volatility thus makes a spill of any amount a serious vapor hazard. In the Tokyo subway attack where sarin was used (see below), 100% of the symptomatic patients inhaled sarin vapor that spilled out on the floor of the subway cars. VX, an oily liquid, is the exception. Its low vapor pressure makes it much less of a vapor hazard but potentially a greater environmental hazard because it persists in the environment far longer.

The nerve agents tabun and sarin were first used on the battlefield by Iraq against Iran during the first Persian Gulf war, 1984–1987. Estimates of casualties from these agents range from 20,000 to 100,000. In 1994 and 1995, the Japanese cult Aum Shinrikyo used sarin in two terrorist attacks in Matsumoto and Tokyo.

Mechanism Acetylcholinesterase inhibition accounts for the major life-threatening effects of nerve agent poisoning. Reversal of this inhibition by antidotal therapy is effective, proving that this is the primary toxic action of these poisons. At cholinergic synapses, acetylcholinesterase, bound to the postsynaptic membrane, functions as a turn-off switch to regulate cholinergic transmission. Inhibition of acetylcholinesterases causes the released neurotransmitter, acetylcholine, to accumulate abnormally. End-organ overstimulation, recognized by clinicians as cholinergic crisis, ensues (Fig. 206-2).

Clinical Features Clinical effects of nerve agent exposure are identical for vapor and liquid exposure routes if the dose is sufficiently large. The speed and order of symptom onset will differ (Table 206-1).

Exposure of a patient to nerve agent vapor, overwhelmingly the more likely route of exposure in both battlefield and terrorist scenarios, will cause cholinergic symptoms in the order that the toxin encounters cholinergic synapses. The most exposed synapses on the integument of the human are in the pupillary muscles. Nerve agent vapor easily crosses the cornea, interacts with these synapses, and produces miosis, described by Tokyo subway victims as "the world going black." Rarely, this can also cause eye pain and nausea. Exocrine glands lo-

FIGURE 206-2 Schematic diagram of the pathophysiology of nerve agent exposure. Nerve agent (◆) binds to the active site of acetylcholinesterase (AChE), which is shown as floating free in space but is in reality a postsynaptic membrane-bound enzyme. As a result, acetylcholine (○), which is normally released from presynaptic membrane but not normally degraded, accumulates, and this leads (↯) to organ overstimulation and cholinergic crisis.

cated in the nose, mouth, and pharynx next become exposed to the vapor, and cholinergic overload here causes increased secretions, rhinorrhea, excess salivation, and drooling. Next, toxin interacts with exocrine glands in the upper airway, causing bronchorrhea, and with bronchial smooth muscle, causing bronchospasm, the combination of which can cause hypoxia.

Once the victim has inhaled, vapor can passively cross the alveolar-capillary membrane, enter the bloodstream, and, incidentally and asymptomatically, inhibit circulating cholinesterases, particularly free butyrylcholinesterase and erythrocyte acetylcholinesterase, both of which can be assayed. Unfortunately, the assay may not be easily interpreted without a baseline, since cholinesterase levels vary enormously between persons and over time in an individual healthy patient.

Usually the first organ system to become symptomatic from blood-borne nerve agent exposure is the gastrointestinal tract, where cholinergic overload causes abdominal cramping and pain, nausea, vomiting, and diarrhea. After the gastrointestinal tract is involved, nerve agents affect the heart, distant exocrine glands, muscles, and brain. Because there are cholinergic synapses on both the vagal (parasympathetic) and sympathetic sides of the autonomic input to the heart, one cannot predict how heart rate and blood pressure will change. Remote exocrine activity will include oversecretion in the salivary, nasal, respiratory, and sweat glands—the patient will be "wet all over." Bloodborne nerve agents overstimulate neuromuscular junctions in skeletal muscles, causing fasciculations followed by frank twitching. If the process goes on long enough, ATP in muscle will eventually be depleted and flaccid paralysis will ensue, although this is never the first sign.

In the brain, since the cholinergic system is so widely distributed, bloodborne nerve agents, in sufficient doses, cause rapid loss of consciousness, seizures, and central apnea, leading to death within minutes. If respiration is supported, status epilepticus, which does not respond to usual anticonvulsants, may ensue (Chap. 349). If status persists, neuronal death and permanent brain dysfunction may occur. Even in mild nerve agent intoxication, patients may recover but experience weeks of irritability, sleep disturbance, and nonspecific neurobehavioral symptoms.

The time from exposure to development of the full-blown cholinergic crisis from nerve agent vapor inhalation can be minutes or even seconds; however, there is no depot effect. Since nerve agents have a short circulating half-life, improvement should be rapid with no subsequent deterioration if the patient is supported and, ideally, treated with antidotes.

Liquid exposure to nerve agents differs in speed and order of symptom onset. A nerve agent on intact skin will partially evaporate and partially begin to travel through the skin, causing localized sweating and then localized fasciculations when it encounters neuromuscular junctions. Once in muscle, it will cross into the circulation and cause gastrointestinal discomfort, respiratory distress, heart rate changes, generalized fasciculations and twitching, loss of consciousness, seizures, and central apnea. The time course will be much longer than with vapor inhalation; even a large, lethal droplet can take up to 30 min to have effect, and a small, sublethal dose could continue to take effect over 18 h. Clinical worsening that occurs hours after treatment has started is far more likely with liquid than with vapor exposure.

Additionally, miosis, practically unavoidable with vapor exposure, is not always present with liquid exposure and may be the last symptom to present in this situation. This is due to the relative insulation of the pupillary muscle from the systemic circulation.

Unless a nerve agent is removed by specific therapy (oximes), its binding to cholinesterase is essentially irreversible. Erythrocyte acetylcholinesterase activity recovers at about 1% per day. Plasma butyrylcholinesterase recovers more quickly and is a better guide to recovery of tissue enzyme activity.

℞ TREATMENT

Acute nerve agent poisoning is treated by decontamination, respiratory support, and three antidotes—an anticholinergic, an oxime, and an anticonvulsant (Tables 206-2 and 206-4). In acute cases, all of these forms of therapy may be given simultaneously.

Decontamination Decontamination of a vapor is theoretically not necessary, but in the Tokyo subway attack, sarin vapor trapped in the patients' clothing caused miosis in 10% of emergency personnel. Removal of clothing would have avoided most of this. Decontamination of liquid is accomplished in the military using the M291 skin decontamination kit, containing an active carbon impregnated with ion exchange resins (Ambergard) capable of absorbing liquid off the skin. Civilian agencies now stockpile this product, which is approved by the U.S. Food and Drug Administration (FDA). At hospitals, soap and copious amounts of water should suffice. Physical removal of the agent trumps all known decontamination solutions and lotions. In any even, decontamination must be accomplished before the patient enters the hospital facility to avoid contaminating the facility and its staff. In patients with contaminated wounds, extract from the wound potentially contaminated clothing and other foreign material that may serve as a depot for liquid agent.

Respiratory Support Death from nerve agent poisoning is almost always respiratory. Ventilation will be complicated by increased resistance and secretions. Atropine should be given before ventilation or as it begins as it will make ventilation far easier.

Antidotal Therapy ■ ATROPINE In theory, any anticholinergic could be used to treat nerve agent poisoning, but worldwide the choice is invariably atropine because of its wide temperature stability and rapid effectiveness, either intramuscularly or intravenously, and because inadvertent administration of this drug usually causes little CNS dysfunction (Table 206-4). Atropine rapidly reverses cholinergic overload at muscarinic synapses but has little effect at nicotinic synapses. Practically, this implies that atropine can quickly treat the life-threatening respiratory effects of nerve agents but will probably not help neuromuscular and possibly sympathetic effects. In the field, military personnel are given MARK I kits (Fig. 206-3A), which contain 2 mg atropine in autoinjector form for use intramuscularly. Civilian agencies are now stockpiling this FDA-approved product as well. One can only give full autoinjector doses and not divide them. The field-loading dose is 2, 4, or 6 mg, with retreatment every 5 to 10 min until the patient's breathing and secretions improve. The Iranians used larger doses initially during the Iran-Iraq war, in which oximes were in short supply. When the patient reaches a level of medical care where drugs can be given intravenously, this is the preferred route; in small children, this may be the preferred initial route of administration of atropine therapy. There is no upper bound to atropine therapy in a patient either intra-

muscularly or intravenously; however, a total average adult dose for a severely afflicted patient would usually be 20 to 30 mg.

In a mildly afflicted patient with miosis and no other systemic symptoms, atropine or homatropine eye drops may suffice for therapy. This will produce roughly 24 h of mydriasis. Frank miosis or imperfect accommodation may persist for weeks or even months after all other signs and symptoms have resolved.

TABLE 206-4	Antidote Recommendations Following Exposure to Nerve Agents		
	Antidotes		
Patient Age	Mild/Moderate Effects[a]	Severe Effects[b]	Other Treatment
Infants (0–2 yrs)	Atropine: 0.05 mg/kg IM, or 0.02 mg/kg IV; and 2-PAM chloride: 15 mg/kg IM or IV slowly	Atropine: 0.1 mg/kg IM, or 0.02 mg/kg IV; and 2-PAM chloride: 25 mg/kg IM, or 15 mg/kg IV slowly	Assisted ventilation after antidotes for severe exposure. Repeat atropine (2 mg IM, or 1 mg IM for infants) at 5- to 10-min intervals until secretions have diminished and breathing is comfortable or airway resistance has returned to near normal. Phentolamine for 2-PAM-induced hypertension: (5 mg IV for adults; 1 mg IV for children). Diazepam for convulsions: (0.2 to 0.5 mg IV for infants <5 years: 1 mg IV for children >5 years; 5 mg IV for adults).
Child (2–10 yrs)	Atropine: 1 mg IM, or 0.02 mg/kg IV; and 2-PAM chloride[c]: 15 mg/kg IM or IV slowly	Atropine: 2 mg IM, or 0.02 mg/kg IV; and 2-PAM chloride[c]: 25 mg/kg IM, or 15 mg/kg IV slowly	
Adolescent (>10 yrs)	Atropine: 2 mg IM, or 0.02 mg/kg IV; and 2-PAM chloride[c]: 15 mg/kg IM or IV slowly	Atropine: 4 mg IM, or 0.02 mg/kg IV; and 2-PAM chloride[c]: 25 mg/kg IM, or 15 mg/kg IV slowly	
Adult	Atropine: 2 to 4 mg IM or IV; and 2-PAM chloride: 600 mg IM, or 15 mg/kg IV slowly	Atropine: 6 mg IM; and 2-PAM chloride: 1800 mg IM, or 15 mg/kg IV slowly	
Elderly, frail	Atropine: 1 mg IM; and 2-PAM chloride: 10 mg/kg IM, or 5 to 10 mg/kg IV slowly	Atropine: 2 to 4 mg IM; and 2-PAM chloride: 25 mg/kg IM, or 5 to 10 mg/kg IV slowly	

[a] Mild/moderate effects include localized sweating, muscle fasciculations, nausea, vomiting, weakness, dyspnea.
[b] Severe effects include unconsciousness, convulsions, apnea, flaccid paralysis.
[c] If calculated dose exceeds the adult IM dose, adjust accordingly.
Note: 2-PAM chloride is pralidoxime chloride or protopam chloride.
Source: State of New York, Department of Health.

A

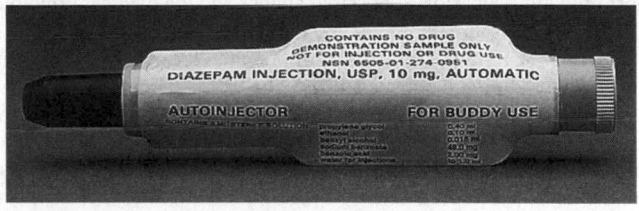

B

FIGURE 206-3 Antidotes to nerve agents. *A.* MARK I autoinjector set containing one 600-mg dose of 2-pralidoxime chloride and one 2-mg dose of atropine. Such sets are carried by all U.S. military forces in a potentially chemical battlefield and are now being stockpiled by civilian first responders. *B.* Diazepam 10-mg autoinjector. These are carried by all U.S. military forces in a potential chemical battlefield and are being stockpiled by civilian first responders.

OXIME THERAPY Oximes are nucleophiles that reactivate the cholinesterase whose active site has been occupied and bound to nerve agent (Table 206-4). Therapy with oximes therefore restores normal enzyme function. Oxime therapy is limited by a second side reaction, called *aging*, in which a side chain on nerve agents falls off the complex at a characteristic rate. "Aged" complexes are negatively charged, and oximes cannot reactivate negatively charged complexes. The practical effect of this differs from one nerve agent to another since each ages at a characteristic rate. VX, for practical purposes, never ages, sarin ages in 3 to 5 h, and tabun ages over a longer period. All of these are so much longer than the patient's expected lifespan after untreated acute nerve agent toxicity that they may be ignored. Soman, on the other hand, ages in 2 min. Thus, after only a few minutes following exposure, oximes are useless in treating soman poisoning. The oxime used varies by country; the United States has approved and fielded 2-pralidoxime chloride (2-PAM Cl). MARK I kits (Fig. 206-3A) contain autoinjectors of 600 mg of 2-PAM Cl. Initial field loading doses are 600, 1200, or 1800 mg. Since blood pressure elevation may occur after administration of 45 mg/kg in adults, field use of 2-PAM Cl is restricted to 1800 mg, intramuscularly, per hour. During the time when more oxime cannot be given, atropine alone is recommended. In the hospital setting, 2.5 to 25 mg/kg of 2-PAM Cl intravenously has been found to reactive 50% of inhibited cholinesterase. The usual recommendation is 1000 mg through slow intravenous drip over 20 to 30 min, with no more than 2500 mg over a period of 1 to 1.5 h.

ANTICONVULSANT Nerve agent–induced seizures do not respond to the usual anticonvulsants used for status epilepticus, including phenytoin, phenobarbital, carbamazepine, valproic acid, and lamotrigine (Chap. 349). The only class of anticonvulsants that has been shown to stop this form of status are the benzodiazepines. Diazepam is the only benzodiazepine approved for seizures in humans, although other FDA-approved benzodiazepines work well against nerve agent–induced seizures in animal models. Diazepam, therefore, is manufactured in 10-mg injectors for intramuscular use and given to U.S. forces for this purpose (Fig. 206-3B). Civilian agencies are stockpiling this field product (convulsive antidote for nerve agent, "CANA"), which is not generally used in hospital practice. Extrapolation from animal studies indicates that adults will probably require 30 to 40 mg diazepam, intramuscularly, to stop nerve agent–induced status epilepticus. In the hospital, or in a small child unable to receive the autoinjector, intravenous diazepam may be used at similar doses. The clinician may confuse seizures with the neuromuscular signs of nerve agent poisoning. In the hospital, early electroencephalography is recommended in order to distinguish between nonconvulsive status epilepticus, actual seizures, and postictal paralysis. Recent studies have shown that the most effective benzodiazepine in this situation is midazolam, which is not FDA-approved for seizures.

Peripheral neuropathy and the so-called intermediate syndrome, prominent long-term effects of insecticide poisoning, are not described in nerve agent survivors.

Recent research has explored approaches leading to a transient "immunity" or drugs that would provide protection against lethal nerve agents yet be devoid of side effects. A novel approach is to use enzymes to scavenge these highly toxic nerve agents before they attack their intended targets. The total body of studies has shown that if a scavenger is present at the time of nerve agent exposure, rapid reduction of toxicant levels is observed. This reduction is so rapid and profound that the need to administer a host of pharmacologically active drugs as antidotes is, in theory, eliminated.

FURTHER READING

AGENCY FOR TOXIC SUBSTANCES AND DISEASE REGISTRY (ATSDR): Managing Hazardous Materials Incidents, Vols I–III. Atlanta, GA, US Department of Health and Human Services, 2001

BROOMFIELD CA et al: Progress on the road to new nerve agent treatments. J Appl Toxicol 21:S43, 2001

KARALLIEDDE L et al: Possible immediate and long-term health effects following exposure to chemical warfare agents. Public Health 114:238, 2000

SIDELL FR: Clinical considerations in nerve agent intoxication, in *Chemical Warfare Agents*, SM Somani (ed). San Diego, California, Academic Press, 1992, pp 156–194

——— et al (eds): *Medical Aspects of Chemical and Biological Warfare, Vol I of Textbook of Military Medicine*. Washington, DC, Walter Reed Army Medical Center, Borden Institute, 1997. [Available on the website: *http://ccc.apgea.army.mil*]

SMITH WJ: Vesicant agents and antivesicant medical countermeasures: Clinical toxicology and psychological implications. Mil Psychol 14:145, 2002

STATE OF NEW YORK, DEPARTMENT OF HEALTH. *Chemical Terrorism Preparedness and Response Card*, #7002. August, 2002

US ARMY EDGEWOOD RESEARCH, DEVELOPMENT AND ENGINEERING CENTER: Technician EMS Course. Domestic Preparedness Training Program, Version 8.0. Aberdeen Proving Ground, Maryland, 1999

US ARMY MEDICAL RESEARCH INSTITUTE OF CHEMICAL DEFENSE, CHEMICAL CASUALTY CARE DIVISION: *Medical Management of Chemical Casualties Handbook*, 3d ed. Aberdeen Proving Ground, Maryland, 1999. [Available on the website: *http://ccc.apgea.army.mil*]

---

207 RADIATION BIOTERRORISM
Zelig A. Tochner, Ofer Lehavi, Eli Glatstein

Terror attacks using nuclear or radiation-related devices are an unequivocal threat in the twenty-first century and are capable of unique medical and psychological effects. In this chapter we will focus on the most probable scenarios of possible attacks and the medical principles of handling such threats.

There are two major categories of potential terrorist incidents with widespread radiologic consequences. The first is the use of radiologic dispersal devices. This could cause a purposeful dissemination of radioactive material without nuclear detonation by using conventional explosives with radionuclides, attacking fixed nuclear facilities, or attacking nuclear powered surface vessels or submarines. Malfunctioning nuclear weapons that are detonated with no nuclear yield (nuclear "duds") and/or installation of radionuclides in food or water are also a possible means of generating a terror attack. The second, and less probable, scenario is the actual use of nuclear weapons. Each scenario has its own medical aspects, including "conventional" blast or thermal injury, introduction to a radiation field, and exposure to either external or internal contamination from a radioactive explosion.

TYPES OF RADIOISOTOPIC RADIATION

Isotopes of atoms with uneven numbers of protons and/or neutrons are typically unstable; such isotopes discharge particles or energy to matter, a process that we define as *radiation*. The main radiation types are alpha, beta, gamma, and neutrons.

Alpha (α) radiation consists of heavy, positively charged particles containing two protons and two neutrons. Alpha particles are usually emitted from isotopes with an atomic number of ≥82, such as uranium or plutonium. Due to their large size, alpha particles have limited penetrating power. Fine obstacles such as cloth or human skin can usually stop them from penetrating into the body, and they represent a small risk to external exposure due to their limited penetration. If they somehow are internalized, then alpha particles can cause significant cellular damage within their immediate proximity.

Beta (β) radiation consists of electrons, which are small, light, negatively charged particles (about 1/2000 the mass of a neutron or proton). They can travel only a short finite distance in tissue, depending on their energy. Exposure to beta particles is common in many radiation accidents. Radioactive iodine, released in nuclear plant accidents, is the best known member of this group. Plastic layers and clothing can stop most beta particles, and their penetration is measured to be a few millimeters. A large quantum of energy to the basal stratum of the skin can cause a burn that is similar to a thermal burn and is treated as such.

Gamma (γ) rays and *x-rays* (both photons) are similar. Gamma rays are uncharged electromagnetic radiation discharged from a nucleus as a wave or photons of energy. X-rays are the result of abrupt mechanical deceleration of electrons striking a heavy target such as tungsten. Gamma and x-rays have similar properties, i.e., no charge and no mass, just energy. Both travel easily through matter, sometimes called *penetrating radiation*, and are the principal type of radiation to cause total-body exposure.

Neutrons (η) particles are heavy and uncharged, often emitted during nuclear detonation. They possess a wide energy range; their ability to penetrate tissues is variable, depending upon their energy. They are less likely to be present in most scenarios of radiation bioterrorism.

The ionization resulting from protons, electrons, and gamma rays is either a direct or indirect (i.e., mediated through water) effect of particles or photons on DNA. Ionization of DNA resulting from neutrons is secondary to the neutrons knocking electrons out of their atomic orbit and the formation of free radicals, which can also damage DNA directly.

The commonly used units of radiation are the rad and the gray (Gy). The rad (radiation absorbed dose) is energy deposited within living matter and is equal to 100 ergs/g of tissue. It is a simple concept but difficult to measure directly. The traditional rad has been replaced by the Système Internationale (SI) unit of the gray; 100 rad ⁻ 1 Gy.

TYPES OF EXPOSURE

Whole-body exposure represents deposition of radiation energy over the entire body. Alpha and beta particles have limited penetration and do not cause significant noncutaneous injury unless emission results from an internalized source. Whole-body exposure from gamma rays, x-rays, or neutrons, which can penetrate through the body (depending on their energy), can result in damage to multiple tissues and organs. The tissue damage is proportional to the radiation exposure of that organ or tissue.

External contamination is a result of fallout of radioactive particles that land on the body surface, clothing, skin, and hair. This is the dominant element to consider in the mass casualty situation resulting from a radioactive terrorist strike. The common contaminants will primarily emit alpha and beta radiation. Alpha particles do not penetrate beyond the skin and thus have minimal systemic effects. Beta emitters can cause significant cutaneous burns and scarring. Gamma emitters may not only cause local damage but can also cause whole-body radiation exposures and injury. The medical treatment is primarily decontamination of the body, including wounds and burns, to prevent the contamination from becoming internalized. Removing the contaminated clothing reduces the contamination significantly and is a first step in the decontamination process. Generally patients will not constitute a significant radiation hazard to health care providers, and life-saving treatment should not be delayed for fear of secondary contamination of the medical team. Any damage to health care personnel will depend directly on the duration of exposure and will be inversely proportional to the square of the distance from any radioactive source. Gowns that can be removed are essential to protect health-care personnel.

Internal contamination will occur when radioactive material is inhaled, ingested, or able to enter the body through open wounds or burns or via skin absorption. In principle, any externally contaminated casualty should be evaluated for internal contamination. Some isotopes may have toxic effects on specific target organs due to their chemical properties, in addition to radiologic injury. The respiratory system is the main portal of entrance for internal contamination, and the lung is the organ at greatest risk. Aerosol particles <5 μm can reach the alveoli, whereas larger particles will remain in proximal airways. The tiny particles can be absorbed by the lymphatic system or the bloodstream, continuing to irradiate (depending on their biologically active half-life) until being exhaled. Bronchial lavage is often helpful treat-

ment in this situation. Radioactive material entering the gastrointestinal (GI) tract will be absorbed according to its chemical structure and solubility. The insoluble radionuclides may affect the lower GI tract. Intact skin is normally a good barrier to most radionuclides. Penetration through the skin usually takes place when wounds or burns have altered the skin barriers. Therefore, any skin erosion should be cleaned and decontaminated promptly.

Absorbed radioactive materials will travel throughout the body. Liver, kidney, adipose tissue, and bone tend to bind and retain the radioactive material more than other tissues. The medical treatment includes preventing absorption, reducing incorporation, and enhancing elimination (see below).

Localized exposure means close contact between a highly radioactive source and a part of the body, causing discrete damage to the skin and deeper tissues, similar to a thermal burn. Later signs include epilation, erythema, moist desquamation, ulceration, blistering, or necrosis in proportion to exposure. Alopecia, transient or permanent, is dose-related and starts at cutaneous doses >3 Gy. Overt tissue damage can take weeks and even months to develop; the healing process can also be very slow and last for months. Long-term cutaneous changes, including keratosis, fibrosis, and telangiectasias, may appear years after the exposure. Treatment is based on analgesia and infection prophylaxis. Nevertheless, severe burns can often require grafting or even amputation. Long-term radiation effects are characterized by cell loss and cell death.

RADIOLOGIC DISPERSAL EVENTS

Radiologic dispersal incidents are generally of two types resulting from: (1) small, usually localized sources; or (2) wide dispersals over large areas. The radioactive materials can take the form of solid state, aerosol, gas, or liquid. They can be put into food or water, released from vehicles, or be spread by explosion. The principal route of exposure is usually by direct contact between the victim's skin and the radioactive particles, although internal contamination could occur if the material were inhaled or ingested. The radiation field is also a potential source of whole-body exposure. The psychosocial effects that accompany such an event are significant and are beyond the scope of this chapter. A list of radioactive materials, including information on their major properties and medical treatment, is shown in Table 207-1.

In a localized event, the amount and spread of the radioactive materials are usually limited and can be treated like a spill of hazardous material. Protective clothing prevents or minimizes the contamination of emergency responders.

The use of explosives coupled with a large amount of radioactive materials can result in wide dispersion of radiation, which is of far greater concern. Other potential sources of radiation are nuclear reactors, spent nuclear fuel, and transport vehicles. Less probable but still possible is the use of a large source of penetrating radiation without explosion. It is expected that most exposures would be low, and the principal health and psychosocial effects would be similar to the former scenario but on a larger scale.

Whenever an explosion is involved, conventional life-saving treatment should be given first priority. Only then should decontamination and specific treatment be given for the radiation exposure.

Silent exposure represents a scenario in which a powerful radiologic source could be hidden in a crowded place or radiologic materials spread without any awareness or announcement. It might take a long time to recognize the event and the source of exposure. One of the major clues to this situation is the appearance of unusual clinical manifestations in many individuals; such manifestations are often nonspecific and include symptoms of acute radiation sickness (see below) such as headache, fatigue, malaise, and opportunistic infections. GI phenomena such as diarrhea, nausea, vomiting, and anorexia may occur. Dermatologic symptoms (burns, ulceration, and epilation) and hematopoietic manifestations such as bleeding tendency, thrombocy-

Isotope Name	Symbol	Common Usage	Radiation Type $t_{1/2}$ Radiologic $t_{1/2}$ Biologic, days	Exposure Type	Mode of Contamination	Focal Accumulation in Body	Treatment
Manganese	Mn-56	Reactors, research laboratories	β, γ 2.6 h 5.7	External, internal	N/A	Liver	N/A
Cobalt	Co-60	Medical radiotherapy devices, commercial food irradiators	β, γ 5.26 y 9.5	External, internal	Lungs	Liver	Gastric lavage, purgatives; penicillamine in severe cases
Strontium	Sr-90	Fission product of uranium	β 28 y 18,000	Internal	Moderate GI tract	Bones—similar to calcium	Strontium, calcium, ammonium chloride
Molybdenum	Mo-99	Hospitals—scans	β, γ 66.7 h 3	External, internal	N/A	Kidneys	N/A
Technetium	Tc-99m	Hospitals—scans	β, γ 6.049 h 1	External, internal	IV administration	Kidneys, total body	Potassium perchlorate to reduce thyroid dose
Cesium	Cs-137	Medical radiotherapy devices	β, γ 30 y 70	External, internal	Lungs, GI tract, wounds, follows potassium	Renal excretion	Ion-exchange resins, Prussian blue
Gadolinium	Gd-153	Hospitals	β, γ 242 d 1000	External, internal	N/A	N/A	N/A
Iridium	Ir-192	Commercial radiography	β, γ 74 d 50	External, internal	N/A	Spleen	N/A
Radium	Ra-226	Instrument illumination, industrial applications, old medical equipment, former Soviet Union military equipment	α, β, γ 1602 y 16,400	External, internal	GI tract	Bones	$MgSO_4$ lavage, ammonium chloride, calcium alginates
Tritium	H-3	Luminescent gun sights, muzzle-velocity detectors, nuclear weapons	β 12.5 y 12	Internal	Inhalation, GI tract, wounds	Total body	Dilution with controlled water intake, diuretics
Iodine	I-131	Reactor accidents, thyroid ablators	β, γ 8.1 d 138	Internal	Inhalation, GI tract, wounds	Thyroid	Potassium/sodium iodide, propylthiouracil, methimazole
Uranium	U-235	Depleted uranium, natural uranium, fuel rods, weapons-grade material	α, (α, β, γ) 7.1×10^8 y 15	Internal	GI tract	Kidneys, bones	$NaHCO_3$, chelation with EDTA
Plutonium	Pu-239	Produced from uranium in reactors, nuclear weapons	α 2.2×10^4 y 73,000	Internal	Limited lung absorption, high retention	Lungs, bones, bone marrow, liver, gonads	Chelating with DTPA or EDTA
Americium	Am-241	Smoke detectors, nuclear weapon detonation fallout	α 458 y 73,000	Internal	Inhalation, skin wounds	Lungs, liver, bones, bone marrow	Chelating with DTPA or EDTA
Polonium	Po-210	Calibration source	α 138.4 d 60	Internal	Inhalation, wounds	Spleen, kidneys	Lavage, dimercaprol
Thallium	Th-232	Calibration source	α 1.41×10^{10} y 73,000	Internal	N/A	N/A	N/A
Phosphorus	P-32	Research laboratories, medical facilities	β 14.3 d 1155	Internal	Inhalation, GI tract, wounds	Bones, bone marrow, rapidly replicating cells	Lavage, aluminum hydroxide, phosphate

Note: N/A, not available; h, hours; y, years; GI, gastrointestinal

topenia, purpura, lymphopenia, or neutropenia are also possible and dose-related. Careful epidemiologic studies may be necessary to identify the source of such exposure.

NUCLEAR WEAPONS

The most likely scenario of nuclear terror would be the detonation of a single low-yield device. The estimated yield of such device is anywhere between 0.01 and 10 kiloton of TNT, although the probability would more likely be toward the lower yield. Coping with such an event is certainly possible. The effects of such an explosion are a combination of several components: ground shock, air blast, thermal radiation, initial nuclear radiation, residual nuclear radiation, crater formation, and radioactive fallout.

The nuclear detonation, like a conventional explosion, will produce a shock wave that can further damage structures and cause many casualties. In addition, the detonation can produce an extremely hot fireball that can ignite materials and cause severe burns. The detonation also releases an intense pulse of ionizing radiation, mainly gamma rays and neutrons. The radiation produced in the first minute is termed *initial radiation*, while the ongoing radiation due to fallout is termed *residual radiation*. Both types of radiation can cause acute radiation sickness (ARS; see below). The $LD_{50/30}$ (i.e., a dose that causes 50% mortality at 30 days) is ~4 Gy for whole-body exposure without medical support; with medical support, the $LD_{50/30}$ ranges between 8 and 10 Gy. Winds can carry fallout and contaminate large areas.

On top of its effects, a massive blast forms a crater in the soil and usually produces a ground shock compounding the damage and number of casualties. Inhalation of large amounts of radioactive dust causes pneumonitis that can lead to pulmonary fibrosis. Use of a mask covering the mouth and nose can be very helpful. The intense flash of infrared and visible light can cause either temporary or permanent blindness. Cataracts can develop months to years later among those who survive.

ACUTE RADIATION SICKNESS

Radiation interactions with atoms can result in ionization and the formation of free radicals that damage tissue by disrupting chemical bonds and molecular structures in the cell, including DNA. Radiation damage can lead to cell death; those cells that recover may be mutated and at higher risk for subsequent cancer. Cell sensitivity increases as the replication rate increases and the cell differentiation decreases. Bone marrow and mucosal surfaces of the GI tract, which have vast mitotic activity, are significantly more sensitive to radiation than slowly dividing tissues such as bones and muscles. Following exposure of either all or most of the human body to ionizing radiation, ARS can develop. The clinical manifestations of ARS reflect the dose and type of radiation as well as the part of the body exposed.

CLINICAL MANIFESTATIONS ARS manifests as three major groups of signs and symptoms: gastrointestinal, hematopoietic, and neurovascular. There are four major stages in ARS: prodrome, latent phase, illness, and either recovery or death. The higher the radiation doses, the shorter and more severe each stage. The prodrome appears a few hours to 4 days postexposure; lasts between a few hours to a few days; and can include nausea, vomiting, anorexia, and diarrhea. At the end of the prodrome, ARS progresses to the latent phase. Minimal or no symptoms are present during the latent phase, which commonly lasts up to 2.5 weeks, but can last up to 6 weeks. The duration depends on the radiation dose, the health of the patient, and the coexisting illness or injury. Following the latent phase, the exposed person manifests illness that may eventuate in recovery or lead to death.

With exposure to doses <1 Gy, ARS is generally mild. At this dose symptoms can be minimal or nonexistent, even if the entire body is exposed to penetrating radiation. The clinical picture will mainly be transient depression of bone marrow that lasts up to 2 to 3 weeks and then recovers.

ARS is significantly more acute and severe with exposure to very high doses—>30 Gy. At this dose the prodrome appears in minutes and is followed by 5 to 6 h of latency before a cardiovascular collapse occurs secondary to irreversible damage to the microcirculation.

The type and dose of radiation and the part of the body exposed will determine not only the timing of the different stages of ARS but also the dominant clinical picture. At low radiation doses of 0.7 to 4 Gy, hematopoietic depression due to bone marrow suppression takes place and constitutes the main illness. The patient may develop infections and bleeding secondary to low leukocyte and platelet counts, respectively. The bone marrow will eventually recover in almost all patients if they are supported with transfusions and fluids; antibiotics are often needed in addition. With exposure to 6 to 8 Gy, the clinical picture is significantly more complicated. At these doses the bone marrow will not always recover and death may ensue. A GI syndrome may also accompany the hematopoietic manifestations and further worsen the patient's condition. Compromise of the absorptive layer of the gut alters absorption of fluids, electrolytes, and nutrients. GI injury can lead to diarrhea, hemorrhage, sepsis, and electrolyte and fluid imbalance in a patient whose blood counts are compromised for a period of weeks, often leading to death. Whole-body exposure to doses >9 to 10 Gy is almost always fatal. Crucial elements of the bone marrow simply will not recover. In addition to the GI syndrome associated with very large exposures, patients may develop a neurovascular syndrome; the latter dominates with whole-body doses >20 Gy. Vascular collapse, seizures, and death are usually seen. In this variant the prodrome and latent phase both shorten to a few hours.

Rx TREATMENT

The treatment of ARS is focused on maintaining homeostasis, giving damaged organs the chance to recover. Aggressive support is given to every damaged system. Treatment for the hematopoietic system includes mainly therapy for neutropenia and infection, transfusion and blood products as needed, and hematopoietic growth factors. The value of bone marrow transplantation in this situation is questionable. None of the transplants that were performed among the victims of the nuclear reactor accident in Chernobyl proved successful. Another major component of the treatment of ARS is partial or total parenteral nutrition, to bypass the damaged GI system. For blast and thermal injuries, standard therapy for trauma is given. Psychological support is essential in many cases.

MEDICAL MANAGEMENT OF RADIATION BIOTERRORISM

Victims of radiation bioterrorism can suffer from conventional thermal or blast injuries, exposure to radiation, and contamination by radioactive materials. Many will have combinations of the above, which can be synergistic and cause higher morbidity and mortality than when they occur alone. The number of casualties will be the major factor in determining the response of the medical system to an act of radiation bioterrorism. If only a few people are affected, then no significant changes and adaptation of the system are needed to treat the victims. However, if a terror attack results in a large number (hundreds or more) of casualties, then an organized disaster plan at the local and state levels must be invoked to deal with the crisis properly. Medical personnel should have a prior assignment and be prepared to function in a scenario with which they are familiar. Stockpiles of specific equipment and medications have to be preplanned (see the Centers for Disease Control and Prevention website—*http://www.bt.cdc.gov*). One needs to recognize that one of the goals of terrorists is to overwhelm medical facilities and to minimize the salvage of casualties.

Initial management consists of *primary triage and transportation* of the wounded to emergency rooms for treatment. The rationale behind the triage is to sort patients into classes according to the severity of injury, for the purpose of expediting clinical care and maximizing the use of the available clinical services and facilities. Triage requires determination of the level of emergency care needed. The higher the number and range of casualties, the more complex and difficult triage becomes. The mildly wounded and victims of contamination only can be sent to evacuation, registration with disaster response teams, and decontamination and treatment centers. In this way, the hospitals themselves can avoid being directly overwhelmed, and those who are severely wounded can receive better treatment. Emergency treatment will be administered initially according to the presence of conventional injuries such as wounds, trauma, and thermal or chemical burns. Individuals with such injuries should be stabilized, if possible, and immediately transported to a medical facility. Removing the victim's clothes and wrapping him or her in clean blankets or nylon sheets reduces both the exposure of the patient and the contamination risk to the staff. However, the possibility of contamination needs to be determined. Less severely injured victims should receive a preliminary decontamination before or during evacuation to a hospital.

One must remember that radionuclide contamination of the skin is commonly not an acute life-threatening situation to the patient or the personnel who care for the patient. Only powerful gamma emitters are likely to cause real damage from contamination. It is important to emphasize that exposure to a radiation field alone does not necessarily create any contamination. The exposed person, if not contaminated, is not radioactive and does not directly emit any radiation.

In order to protect the staff, protective gear (gowns, gloves, masks, and caps) should be used. NBC masks with filters and chemically pro-

FIGURE 207-1 Flow chart of hospital triage. O.R., operating room.

Legend:
- ▲ Radioactivity detection
- ⊕ Medical staff
- Decontamination
- ☢ Radioactive

tective overgarments provide excellent protection from contamination. Waterproof shoe covers are also important. Remaining in the contaminated area and dealing with life-saving procedures should take place according to the "ALARA" principle: as low as reasonably achievable. It is better to send many people for short exposure times than to send a few people for longer periods of time to do the same job.

Decontamination of victims should take place in the field prior to their arrival at medical facilities, but radiologic decontamination should never interfere with medical care. Removal of outer clothing and shoes will usually reduce the patient's contamination by 80 to 90%. Contaminated clothes should be carefully removed by rolling them over themselves, placing them in marked plastic bags, and removing them to a predefined area for contaminated clothes and equipment. A radiation detector should then be used to check for the presence of any residual radiologic contamination on the patient's body. In order to prevent internalization of the radioactive materials, one should cover open wounds prior to decontamination. Showering or washing of the entire skin and hair is very important. The skin is dried and reassessed for residual contamination until no radiation is found. Contamination-removing chemical agents are more than sufficient to remove radiologic contamination.

Wound decontamination should be as conservative as possible. The main goal is to prevent both extensive local damage and internal contamination through lacerated skin. The bandages should be removed and the wounds flushed. The wound should then be dried and assessed for radiation. This procedure can be repeated again and again until contamination is undetectable. Excision of contaminated wounds should be attempted only when surgically necessary.

In the hospital, staff can wear normal hospital barrier clothing, including two pairs of gloves, a gown, shoe covers, a head cover, and a face mask. Eye protection is recommended. Decontamination of medical personnel is obligatory following emergency treatment and decontamination of the patient. All protective clothing should be placed after use in a designated container for contaminated clothing.

Radiation intensity decays rapidly with the square of the distance from the source, and increasing the distance from the source and decreasing the time spent near it are basic principles of radiation safety.

Shielding with lead can be used as protection from small radioactive gamma sources. Geiger counters can detect gamma and beta radiation. Pocket chamber (pencil) dosimeters, film badges, and thermoluminescent dosimeters can measure accumulated exposure to gamma radiation. All of these detectors are in common use in medical facilities and should be used to help and define the level of contamination. Alpha radiation is harder to detect due to its poor penetration. An alpha scintillation counter, which is capable of detecting alpha radiation, is not commonly used in medical facilities.

GUIDELINES FOR HOSPITAL MANAGEMENT

Figure 207-1 illustrates a model for hospital arrangement for triage. Persons contaminated either externally or internally should be identified, externally decontaminated, and, if needed, treated immediately and specifically for internal contamination. In all other cases, the need for treatment of radiation injuries does not constitute a medical emergency. Early actions, such as blood sampling both for assessing the degree of severity of the exposure and for blood type and cross-matching for possible transfusion, need to be promptly taken if ARS is evident.

In the hospital entrance, a distinct decontamination area should be set up promptly. Separation between clean and contaminated areas is essential. Medical personnel in this area should wear protective gear as noted above. They also should be rotated in their assignments every 1 to 2 h to ensure minimal exposure to radiation. If patients are critically wounded and require either surgery or resuscitation, they need to pass directly to "contaminated" operating rooms or resuscitation sites for life-saving procedures. Once such patients are stable, they should then be decontaminated. It is important to obtain details concerning the exposure, to look for prodromal signs of radiation sickness, and to do a physical examination. One of the best ways to estimate exposure clinically is to measure the time of prodromal appearance. The earlier the prodromal signs and symptoms appear, the higher the dose of radiation exposure. A few laboratory tests need to be routinely taken, such as blood count and urinalysis. If internal contamination is suspected, specific treatment should be given, as outlined below.

℞ TREATMENT

Treatment for internal radionuclide contamination should begin within hours of exposure. The goal is to leave the smallest amount of radionuclides as possible in the body. Treatment is given in order to reduce absorption and to enhance elimination and excretion. Many of the drugs for these indications are not approved by the U.S. Food and Drug Administration and are used as investigational drugs.

Clearance of the GI tract may be achieved by stomach lavage, emetics (such as apomorphine, 5 to 10 mg, or ipecac, 1- to 2-g capsules or 15 mL in syrup), or by using purgatives, laxatives, ion exchangers, and aluminum antacids. Prussian blue, 1 g tid for ≥3 weeks, is an ion exchanger used to treat cesium 137 internal contamination. Aluminum antacids (such as aluminum phosphate gel, 100 mL) may reduce strontium uptake in the gut if given immediately after exposure. Aluminum hydroxide, 60 to 100 mL, is less effective.

Prevention or reversal of radionuclide interaction with tissues can be done by blocking, diluting, mobilizing, and chelating agents. *Blocking agents* prevent entrance of radioactive materials. A good example is potassium iodide (KI), which blocks the uptake of radioactive iodine (^{131}I) by the thyroid. KI is most effective if taken within the first hour after exposure and is still effective 6 h after exposure. The effectiveness subsequently declines until 24 h after exposure; however, it is recommended that KI be taken up to 48 h postexposure. The KI dose is based on age, predicted thyroid exposure, and pregnancy and lactation status. Adults between the ages of 18 to 40 should receive 130 mg/d for 7 to 14 days if exposed to ≥10 cGy of radioactive iodine. Other thyroid-blocking agents include prophylthiouracil, 100 mg tid for 8 days, or methimazole, 10 mg tid for 2 days followed by 5 mg tid for 6 days, but they are somewhat less effective.

Diluting agents decrease the absorption of the radionuclide; for example, water may be used as a diluting agent in the treatment for tritium (^{3}H) contamination. The recommended amount is 3 to 4 L/d for at least 3 weeks.

Mobilizing agents are most effective when given immediately; however, they may be effective for up to 2 weeks after exposure. These include antithyroid drugs, parathyroid extract, glucocorticoids, ammonium chloride, diuretics, expectorants, and inhalants. All of them should induce the release of radionuclides from tissues.

Chelating agents can bind many radioactive materials, after which the complexes are excreted from the human body. In this regard, diethylenetriaminepentaacetic acid (DTPA) is superior to ethylenediamine tetraacetic acid (EDTA); it chelates plutonium, berkelium, californium, americium, curium, or any material with an atomic number >92. The dose is 1 g of Ca-DTPA or Zn-DTPA, dissolved in 250 mL of normal saline or 5% glucose, given intravenously over 1 hour daily for up to 5 days. DTPA can also be administered by inhalation; 1 g is given in 1:1 dilution with water or saline over 15 to 20 min. Treating uranium contamination with DTPA is contraindicated, due to its synergistic damage to the kidneys.

Lung lavage can reduce radiation-induced pneumonitis and is indicated only when a large amount of radionuclide enters the lungs and has the potential for acute radiation injury. The procedure requires anesthesia. Table 207-2 summarizes the common treatment regimens for internal radionuclide contamination.

TABLE 207-2 *Common Drugs^a for Treatment of Internal Contamination*

Medication	Administered for Radionuclides	Route of Administration	Dosage	Duration	Mechanism of Action
KI	Iodine-131	PO	130 mg/d for adults >40 with thyroid exposure >500 cGy 130 mg/d for adults 18–40 with thyroid exposure >10 cGy 130 mg/d for pregnant or lactating women with thyroid exposure >5 cGy 65 mg/d for children and adolescents 3–18 with thyroid exposure >5 cGy 32.5 mg/d for infants 1 month to 3 years with thyroid exposure >5 cGy 16 mg/d for neonates from birth to 1 month with thyroid exposure >5 cGy	7–14 days	Blocking agent
Zn-DTPA	Plutonium, trans-plutonium, yttrium, americium, curium	IV	1 g in 250 mL NS or 5% glucose, given in 1–2 h, *or* bolus over 3–4 min	Up to 5 days	Chelating agent
		Inhalation	1 g in 1:1 dilution with water or NS over 15–20 min		
		IM	1 g; not recommended because of pain		
Ca-DTPA	Plutonium, *trans*-plutonium, yttrium, americium, curium	IV	1 g in 250 mL NS or 5% glucose, given in 1–2 h, *or* bolus over 3–4 min	Up to 5 days	Chelating agent
		Inhalation	1 g in 1:1 dilution with water or NS over 15–20 min		
		IM	1 g; not recommended because of pain		
Bicarbonate	Uranium	IV	2 ampules sodium bicarbonate (44.3 meq each, 7.5%) in 1000 mL NS, 125 mL/L, *or* 1 ampule of sodium bicarbonate (44.3 meq, 7.5%) in 500 mL NS, 500 mL/h	Usually IV for the first 24 h, PO for additional 2 days; continuation of treatment for >3 days is rare and can be done according to titration of uranium amounts in the body	Increased excretion via the kidneys
		PO	2 tablets every 4 h until urine pH = 7–8, *or* 4 g (8 tablets) 3 tid		
Prussian blue	Cesium-137	PO	1 g tid with 100–200 mL water, up to 10 g/d	≥3 weeks titrated by urine and fecal bioassay and whole-body counting	Ion exchanger
Water	Tritium (H-3)	PO	>3–4 L per day	3 weeks	Excretion of water
Aluminum phosphate gel	Strontium	PO	100 mL immediately after exposure	Once	Decreased gut absorption
Aluminum hydroxide		PO	60–100 mL	Once	Decreased gut absorption

^{a} Excluding KI, these drugs have not been approved for this purpose by the U.S. Food and Drug Administration at the time of publication.
Note: NS, normal saline

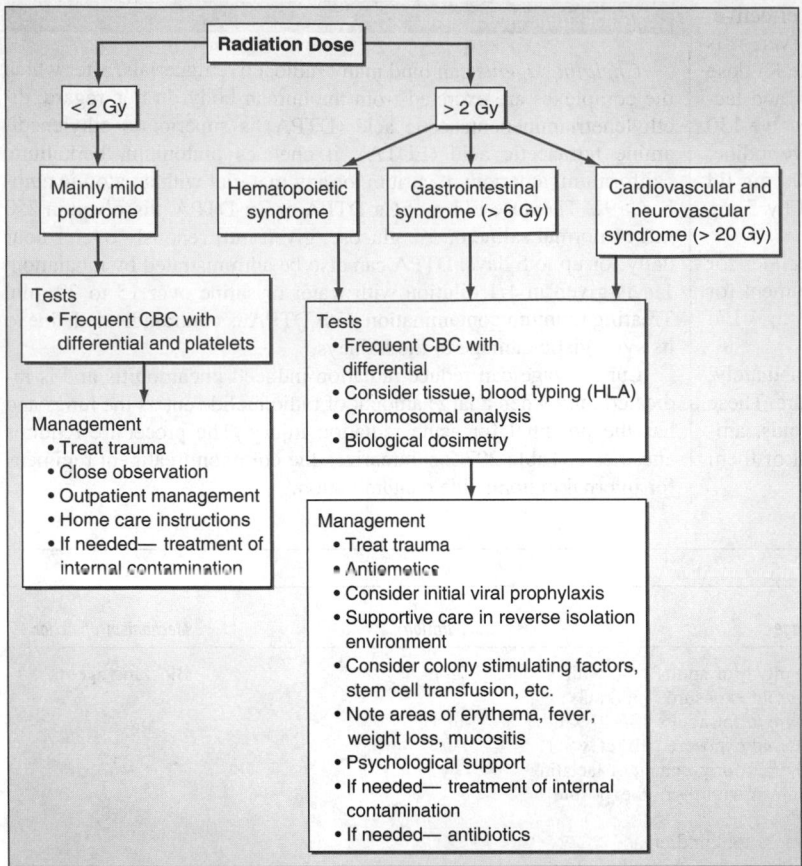

FIGURE 207-2 General guidelines for treatment of radiation casualties. CBC, complete blood count.

MEDICAL ASSAY OF THE RADIATION-EXPOSED PATIENT

One of the major difficulties in treating victims exposed to radiation is the determination of the amount of exposure. Clinical assessment of the patient is the best approach. Appearance of an early prodrome indicates high exposure to radiation. Victims who arrive at the hospital complaining of severe weakness, nausea, vomiting, diarrhea, or seizures probably will not survive despite support measures. Decontamination and the use of radiation-detection equipment are both very important. Few tests can be performed in order to estimate the radiation exposure and the contamination. Baseline laboratory tests should include a complete blood count with differential and platelet count, renal evaluation, and determination of electrolytes. Urine and stool samples should be obtained if internal contamination is suspected. Baseline samples should be taken and repeated every 24 h. Nasal swabs should be taken from each nostril for determination of inhalation of radionuclides. After exhalation, each swab is labeled and sealed in a plastic bag and sent for analysis to appropriate laboratories.

Follow-up complete blood counts including platelets are important on a daily basis as they reflect the bone marrow status. Patients exposed to 0.7 to 4 Gy will develop pancytopenia from as early as 10 days to as long 8 weeks postexposure. Lymphocytes show the most rapid decline, while other leukocytes and platelets decline less rapidly. Erythrocytes are the least vulnerable blood elements.

Absolute lymphocyte counts should be taken every 12 h for 3 days; they are the most valuable early indicator because they are recognized to be a sensitive marker for radiation damage and correlate with both the exposure and prognosis. A 50% drop in absolute lymphocyte count within the first 24 h indicates a significant injury. HLA typing is necessary whenever there is suspicion of irreversible bone marrow damage. Lymphocyte chromosomal analysis can detect radiation exposure as low as 0.03 to 0.06 Gy, and 15 mL of blood should be drawn early as possible in a heparinized collection tube and kept cool. Radiation-induced chromosomal aberrations in peripheral blood lymphocytes include dicentric chromosomes that last for a few weeks. By calibrating a dose-response curve, the radiation dose can be assessed.

Another method for estimating exposure is the micronucleus (MN/Mni) scoring, which is simple and fast but still empirical. An algorithm for the treatment of radiation casualties is provided in Figure 207-2.

FOLLOW-UP

It is desirable to continue follow-up in some circumstances, such as in cases of internal contamination, especially with exposure from uranium with its nephrotoxic properties; in cases of radiation exposure to distinct organs; and in cases where there is risk for carcinogenicity.

FURTHER READING

DAINIAK N: Hematologic consequences of exposure to ionizing radiation. Exp Hematol 30:513, 2002

Guidance for radiation accident management, Oak Ridge–associated universities. *http://www.orau.gov/reacts/guidance.htm*, updated 03/22/2002

JARRETT D et al (eds): *Medical Management of Radiation Casualties: Handbook*. AFRRI special publication 99-2. Bethesda, Md., Armed Forces Radiobiology Research Institute, 1999 (also available at *http://www.afrri.usuhs.mil*.)

Management of Terrorist Events Involving Radioactive Material. NCRP report no. 138. Bethesda, Md, National Council on Radiation Protection, 2001

METTLER FA JR, VOELZ GL: Major radiation exposure—what to expect and how to respond. N Engl J Med 346:1554, 2002

MOULDER JE: Report on an interagency workshop on the radiobiology of nuclear terrorism. Molecular and Cellular Biology of Moderate Dose (1–10 Sv) Radiation and Potential Mechanisms of Radiation Protection (Bethesda, Md, December 17–18, 2001). Radiat Res 158: 118, 2002

208 APPROACH TO THE PATIENT WITH CARDIOVASCULAR DISEASE
Eugene Braunwald

THE MAGNITUDE OF THE PROBLEM

Cardiovascular diseases comprise the most prevalent serious disorders in the developed nations. The American Heart Association has reported that in 2002, 62 million Americans—32 million females and 30 million males (i.e., more than one in five persons)—had a cardiovascular disease (including hypertension). The prevalence rises progressively with age from 5% at age 20 to 75% at age >75 years.

Discharges from U.S. hospitals for cardiovascular disorders have been rising steadily and now exceed 6 million per year. Despite substantial progress in the primary and secondary prevention of coronary heart disease, approximately 6.5 million Americans suffer from angina pectoris and more than 1 million experience a myocardial infarction each year. About 4.8 million Americans have congestive heart failure and more than half a million new cases occur each year. Hospitalizations for heart failure have risen from 400,000 to 950,000 per year in the past 20 years. More than 1.4 million patients undergo cardiac catheterization each year, and approximately 1.2 million undergo revascularization (either percutaneous coronary intervention or coronary artery bypass grafting). There are approximately 1 million Americans with congenital heart disease now alive, and 40,000 babies with congenital heart disease are born each year. The annual total costs of cardiovascular diseases are estimated at $280 billion—$170 billion in direct costs and $110 billion in indirect costs in lost productivity.

Although age-adjusted death rates for coronary heart disease have declined by two-thirds from their peak in 1965, cardiovascular diseases remain the most common causes of death, responsible for 40% of all deaths, almost 1 million deaths each year. Approximately one-fourth of these deaths are sudden. Among developed nations, death rates from cardiovascular diseases are highest in the nations of the former Soviet Union, are intermediate in the United States and Western Europe, and lowest in Japan. The prevalence of cardiovascular disease, especially coronary artery disease, is rising alarmingly in China, India, Pakistan, and the Middle East, as nutritional and infectious causes of death decline in these regions. It has been projected that by 2020 cardiovascular diseases will be the leading causes of death worldwide.

CARDIAC SYMPTOMS

The symptoms caused by heart disease result most commonly from myocardial ischemia, from disturbance of the contraction and/or relaxation of the myocardium, from obstruction to blood flow, or from an abnormal cardiac rhythm or rate. Ischemia is manifest most frequently as chest discomfort, while reduction of the pumping ability of the heart commonly leads to fatigability and shortness of breath or, when severe, produces cyanosis, hypotension, syncope, and elevated intravascular pressure behind a failing ventricle. The latter results in abnormal fluid accumulation, which in turn leads to dyspnea, orthopnea, and systemic or pulmonary edema. Obstruction to blood flow, as in valvular stenosis, can cause symptoms resembling those resulting from congestive heart failure. Cardiac arrhythmias often develop suddenly, and the resulting signs and symptoms—palpitation, dyspnea, hypotension, presyncope, and syncope—generally occur abruptly and may disappear as rapidly as they develop. Ischemic heart disease, by far the most common form of heart disease in adults, may present with chest discomfort but also as heart failure, tachyarrhythmia, and sudden cardiac death.

Myocardial or coronary function that may be adequate at rest may be inadequate during exertion. Thus chest discomfort and/or dyspnea that appear only during activity are characteristic of heart disease, while the opposite pattern, i.e., the appearance of these symptoms at rest and their remission during exertion, is rarely observed in patients with organic heart disease.

Many patients with cardiocirculatory disease may also be asymptomatic, both at rest and during exertion, but may present an abnormal physical finding, such as a heart murmur, elevated arterial pressure, or an abnormality of the electrocardiogram (ECG) or of the cardiac silhouette on the chest roentgenogram. Patients may exhibit asymptomatic ischemia on an exercise stress test. In some asymptomatic patients the first clinical event may be catastrophic—sudden cardiac death, acute myocardial infarction, or stroke.

FEAR OF HEART DISEASE

Diseases of the heart and circulation are so common and the laity is so well acquainted with the major symptoms resulting from these disorders that patients, and occasionally physicians, erroneously attribute many noncardiac complaints to cardiovascular disease. The combination of the widespread fear of heart disease with the deep-seated emotional connotations concerning this organ's function results in the frequent development of symptoms that mimic those of organic disease in persons with normal cardiovascular systems. The unraveling of symptoms and signs due to organic heart disease from those not directly related is an important and challenging task in such patients.

Patients in whom heart disease has been confirmed, especially those who have experienced a major cardiovascular event such as a myocardial infarction or a serious arrhythmia, are often frightened and anxious about hospital discharge and resuming normal activity, including sexual relations. Attention to these matters is vital in the care of cardiac patients.

Dyspnea, one of the cardinal manifestations of heart failure, is not limited to patients with heart disease but is also observed in conditions as diverse as pulmonary disease, marked obesity, and anxiety (Chap. 29). Similarly, chest discomfort may result from a variety of causes other than myocardial ischemia (Chap. 12). Whether heart disease is responsible for these symptoms can frequently be determined by carrying out a careful clinical examination. Noninvasive testing using electrocardiography at rest and during exercise (Chap. 210), echocardiography (Chap. 211), roentgenography, and myocardial imaging usually provides important additional information to permit the correct interpretation of symptoms; more specialized invasive examinations (catheterization and angiography; Chap. 212) are occasionally necessary.

DIAGNOSIS

As outlined by the New York Heart Association, the elements of a complete cardiac diagnosis include consideration of the following:

1. *The underlying etiology.* Is the disease congenital, infectious, hypertensive, or ischemic in origin?

2. *The anatomic abnormalities.* Which chambers are involved? Are they hypertrophied, dilated, or both? Which valves are affected? Are they regurgitant and/or stenotic? Is there pericardial involvement? Has there been a myocardial infarction?

3. *The physiologic disturbances.* Is an arrhythmia present? Is there evidence of congestive heart failure or of myocardial ischemia?

4. *Functional disability.* How strenuous is the physical activity

required to elicit symptoms? The classification provided by the New York Heart Association has been found to be useful in describing functional disability (Table 208-1).

One example may serve to illustrate the importance of establishing a complete diagnosis. In a patient who presents with exertional chest pain, the identification of myocardial ischemia as the etiology is of great clinical importance. However, the simple recognition of ischemia is insufficient to formulate a therapeutic strategy or prognosis until the underlying anatomic abnormalities responsible for the myocardial ischemia, e.g., coronary atherosclerosis or aortic stenosis, are identified and a judgment made as to whether other physiologic disturbances that cause an imbalance between myocardial oxygen supply and demand, such as severe anemia, thyrotoxicosis, or supraventricular tachycardia, play a contributory role. Finally, the severity of the disability will govern the extent and tempo of the workup and strongly influence the therapeutic strategy that is selected.

The establishment of a correct and complete cardiac diagnosis often commences with the history and physical examination (Chap. 209). Indeed, the clinical examination remains the basis for the diagnosis of a wide variety of disorders (Table 208-2). The clinical examination may then be supplemented by four types of laboratory tests: (1) ECG (Chap. 210); (2) chest roentgenogram; (3) noninvasive graphic examinations (echocardiogram, radionuclide and imaging techniques; Chap. 211); and occasionally (4) specialized invasive examinations, i.e., cardiac catheterization, angiocardiography, and coronary angiography (Chap. 212).

THE DIAGNOSTIC PROCESS   In the diagnostic process, the results obtained from each of these several modalities should be analyzed independently of one another as well as together. Only in this way can one avoid overlooking a subtle, though important, finding. For example, an ECG should be obtained in every patient suspected of heart disease. It may provide the critical clue in establishing the correct diagnosis, e.g., the finding of a mild atrioventricular conduction disturbance in a patient with unexplained syncope, even when all other methods of examination reveal no abnormal findings, can be the clue that advanced heart block and asystole might be the cause and can dictate electrophysiologic testing. On the other hand, when combined intelligently with the results of other methods of examination, the ECG may provide essential confirmatory data. Thus, the knowledge that a patient has an apical diastolic rumbling murmur may direct particular attention to the P waves, and the recognition of electrocardiographic left atrial enlargement supports the suggestion that the murmur is caused by mitral stenosis. The diagnosis can then be confirmed by echocardiography, a technique that can also determine the severity of the obstruction and its effects on pulmonary artery pressure and on right and left ventricular function.

FAMILY HISTORY   In eliciting the history of a patient with known or suspected cardiovascular disease, particular attention should be directed to the family history. Familial clustering is common in many forms of heart disease. Mendelian transmission of single-gene defects may occur, as in hypertrophic cardiomyopathy (Chap. 221), the Marfan syndrome (Chap. 342), and sudden death associated with a pro-

TABLE 208-2 *Conditions in Which Clinical Examination Is an Important Determinant of Diagnosis: Confirmation by Echocardiography Is Often Useful*

Mitral valve prolapse	Tricuspid regurgitation
Congestive heart failure	Aortic stenosis
Cardiac tamponade	Acute pulmonary hypertension
Hypertension	Chronic pulmonary hypertension
Mitral stenosis	High-output states
Chronic mitral regurgitation	Atrial septal defect
Chronic aortic regurgitation	Anginal syndrome

longed QT syndrome (Chap. 214). Essential hypertension or coronary atherosclerosis are often polygenic disorders. While familial transmission may be less obvious than in the single-gene disorders, it is also helpful in assessing risk and prognosis. Familial clustering of cardiovascular diseases may occur not only on a genetic basis but may also be related to familial dietary or behavior patterns, such as excessive ingestion of salt or calories or cigarette smoking.

ASSESSMENT OF FUNCTIONAL IMPAIRMENT   When an attempt is made to determine the severity of functional impairment in a patient with heart disease, it is helpful to ascertain with as much precision as possible the level of activity and the rate at which it is performed before symptoms develop. Thus, it is not sufficient to state that the patient complains of dyspnea. The breathlessness that occurs after running up two long flights of stairs denotes far less functional impairment than similar symptoms occurring after taking a few steps on the level. Also, the degree of customary physical activity at work and during recreation should be considered. The development of two-flight dyspnea in a well-conditioned marathon runner may be far more significant than the development of one-flight dyspnea in a previously sedentary person. Similarly, the history must include a detailed consideration of the patient's therapeutic regimen. For example, the persistence or development of edema, breathlessness, and other manifestations of heart failure in a patient whose diet is rigidly restricted in sodium content and who is receiving optimal doses of diuretics is far more grave than are similar manifestations in the absence of these measures. In an effort to determine the progression of symptoms, and thereby the severity of the underlying illness, it may be useful to ascertain what, if any, specific tasks the patient could carry out 1 year earlier that he or she cannot carry out at present.

THE PATIENT WITH A HEART MURMUR (Fig. 208-1)   The cause of a heart murmur can often be readily elucidated from a systematic evaluation of its major attributes: timing, duration, intensity, quality, frequency, configuration, location, radiation, and response to maneuvers when considered in the light of the history, general physical examination, and other features of the cardiac examination, as described in Chap. 209.

The majority of heart murmurs are midsystolic and soft (grades I to II/VI). When such a murmur occurs in an asymptomatic child or young adult *without* other evidence of heart disease on clinical examination, it is usually benign and echocardiography is not generally required. On the other hand, two-dimensional and Doppler echocardiography (Chap. 211) are indicated in patients with loud systolic murmurs (grades ≥III/VI), especially those that are holosystolic or late systolic; in most patients with diastolic or continuous murmurs; and in patients with additional unexplained abnormal physical findings on cardiac examination.

ELECTROCARDIOGRAM (See also Chap. 210)   Although an ECG should be recorded in every patient with known or suspected heart disease, with the exception of the identification of arrhythmias and of acute myocardial infarction, it rarely permits establishment of a specific diagnosis. The range of normal electrocardiographic findings is wide, and the tracing can be affected significantly by many noncardiac factors, such as age, body habitus, and serum electrolyte concentrations. In the absence of other abnormal findings, electrocardiographic changes must not be overinterpreted.

TABLE 208-1 *New York Heart Association Functional Classification*

Class I	**Class III**
No limitation of physical activity	Marked limitation of physical activity
No symptoms with ordinary exertion	Less than ordinary activity causes symptoms
Class II	Asymptomatic at rest
Slight limitation of physical activity	**Class IV**
Ordinary activity causes symptoms	Inability to carry out any physical activity without discomfort
	Symptoms at rest

Source: Modified from The Criteria Committee of the New York Heart Association.

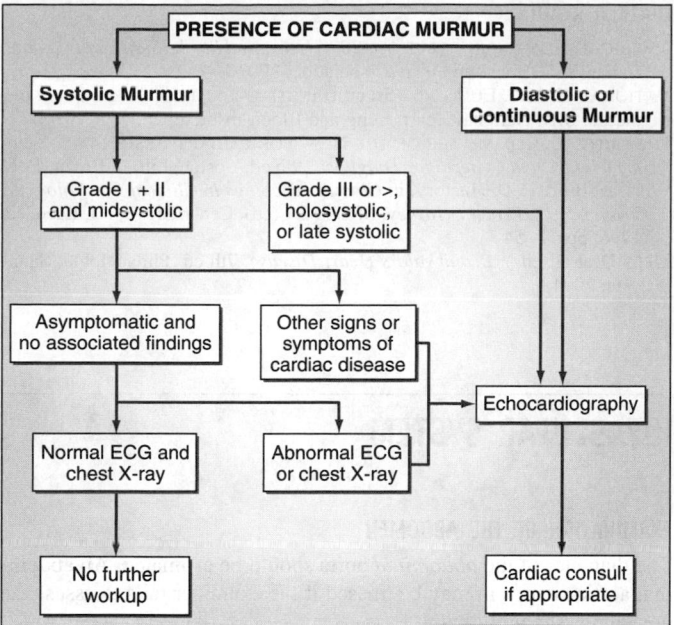

FIGURE 208-1 An alternative "echocardiography first" approach to the evaluation of a heart murmur that also uses the results of the electrocardiogram (ECG) and chest x-ray in asymptomatic patients with soft midsystolic murmurs and no other physical findings. This algorithm is useful to patients over age 40 years in whom the prevalence of coronary artery disease and aortic stenosis increases as the cause of systolic murmur. [From RA O'Rourke, in E Braunwald, L Goldman (eds): Primary Cardiology, 2d ed. Philadelphia, Saunders, 2003.]

NATURAL HISTORY Cardiovascular disorders often present acutely, as in a previously asymptomatic patient with extensive coronary atherosclerosis who develops an acute myocardial infarction (Chap. 228) or the previously asymptomatic patient with hypertrophic cardiomyopathy (Chap. 221) whose first clinical manifestation is syncope or even sudden death. However, in both instances, the alert physician may recognize the patient at risk of these complications long before they occur and can often take measures to prevent their occurrence. For example, the patient with acute myocardial infarction may well have had risk factors for atherosclerosis for many years. Had these been recognized, their elimination or reduction might have delayed or even prevented the infarction. Similarly, the patient with hypertrophic cardiomyopathy may have had a heart murmur for years, and a positive family history might have led to an echocardiographic examination and the recognition of the condition and appropriate therapy long before the acute manifestations.

PITFALLS IN CARDIOVASCULAR MEDICINE

Increasing subspecialization in internal medicine and the perfection of advanced diagnostic techniques in cardiology can lead to several undesirable consequences. Examples include:

1. Failure by the *noncardiologist* to recognize important cardiac manifestations of systemic illnesses. Examples of the latter are (a) stroke (secondary to atrial fibrillation or mitral stenosis); (b) skeletal muscular dystrophies (associated with cardiomyopathy); (c) hemochromatosis (associated with myocardial infiltration and restrictive cardiomyopathy); (d) congenital deafness (associated with prolonged QT interval and serious cardiac arrhythmias); (e) Raynaud's disease (associated with primary pulmonary hypertension and coronary vasospasm); (f) connective tissue disorders, e.g., the Marfan syndrome (aortic dilatation and aneurysm, prolapsed mitral valve); (g) hyperthyroidism (heart failure, atrial fibrillation); (h) hypothyroidism (pericardial effusion, coronary artery disease); (i) rheumatoid arthritis (pericarditis, aortic valve disease); (j) scleroderma (cor pulmonale, myocardial fibrosis, pericarditis); (k) systemic lupus erythematosus (valvulitis, myocarditis, pericarditis); and (l) sarcoidosis (arrhythmias, cardiomyopathy). In patients with these and other systemic disorders,

a cardiovascular examination should be carried out to identify and estimate the severity of cardiovascular involvement.

2. Failure by the cardiologist to recognize underlying systemic disorders, such as those listed above, in patients with a cardiac disorder. Patients with heart disease should be assessed for the frequent *noncardiac* manifestations of systemic disorders with cardiovascular manifestations. For example, hyperthyroidism should be considered in an elderly patient with unexplained heart failure and atrial fibrillation. Similarly, Lyme disease should be considered in patients with unexplained fluctuating atrioventricular block. A cardiovascular abnormality may provide the clue critical to the recognition of some systemic disorders. For instance, unexplained atrial fibrillation may provide the first clue to the diagnosis of thyrotoxicosis.

3. Overreliance on and overutilization of laboratory tests, particularly invasive techniques for the examination of the cardiovascular system. Cardiac catheterization and coronary arteriography (Chap. 212) provide precise diagnostic information under many circumstances. For example, they aid in establishing a specific anatomic diagnosis, which, in turn, may be critical to developing a therapeutic plan in patients with known or suspected ischemic heart disease. Although a great deal of attention has been lavished on these expensive examinations, it should be recognized that they serve to *supplement*, not *supplant*, a careful examination carried out by clinical and noninvasive techniques. A coronary arteriogram should not be carried out in lieu of a careful history in patients with chest pain suspected of having ischemic heart disease. Although coronary arteriography may establish whether the coronary arteries are obstructed, the results often do not provide a definite answer to the question of whether a patient's complaint of chest pain is attributable to coronary arteriosclerosis. Catheterization of the left side of the heart is all too frequently employed to assess patients with valvular heart disease when echocardiographic examination would actually provide more useful information.

Despite the enormous value of these invasive tests in certain circumstances, they entail some small risk to the patient, involve discomfort and substantial cost, and place a strain on medical facilities. Therefore, they should be carried out only if, after clinical examination and assessment by noninvasive tests, the results of the invasive examination can be expected to modify the patient's management.

MANAGEMENT

After a complete diagnosis has been established, a number of management options are usually available. Several examples may be used to demonstrate some of the principles of cardiovascular therapeutics:

1. In the absence of evidence of heart disease, a clear, definitive statement to that effect should be made and the patient should *not* be asked to return at intervals for repeated examinations. If there is no evidence for disease, such continued attention may lead to the patient developing inappropriate anxiety and fixation on the heart.

2. If there is no evidence of cardiovascular disease but the patient has one or more risk factors for the development of ischemic heart disease (Chap. 224), a plan for their reduction should be developed and the patient should be retested at intervals to assess that he or she is complying and that these risk factors are in fact being reduced.

3. Asymptomatic or mildly symptomatic patients with valvular heart disease that is anatomically severe should be evaluated periodically, every 6 to 12 months, by clinical and noninvasive examinations. Early signs of deterioration of ventricular function can be detected in this manner and in appropriate patients may signify the need for surgical treatment before the development of disabling symptoms, irreversible myocardial damage, and excessive risk of surgical treatment (Chap. 219).

4. It is critical to establish clear criteria for deciding on the form of treatment (medical, percutaneous coronary intervention, or surgical revascularization) in patients with ischemic heart disease (Chap. 226). Mechanical revascularization, i.e., the latter two modalities, is proba-

bly being employed too frequently in the United States; the mere presence of angina pectoris and/or the demonstration of critical coronary arterial narrowing at angiography should not reflexly evoke a decision to treat the patient by revascularization. Instead, this approach should be limited to those patients with ischemic heart disease whose angina has not responded adequately to medical treatment or in whom revascularization has been shown to improve the natural history (e.g., acute coronary syndrome, or multivessel coronary artery disease with left ventricular dysfunction).

FURTHER READING

AMERICAN HEART ASSOCIATION: *2004 Heart and Stroke Statistical Update*. Dallas, TX, American Heart Association, 2003

NATIONAL HEART, LUNG AND BLOOD INSTITUTE: *FY 2003 Fact Book*. Bethesda, MD, National Heart, Lung and Blood Institute, 2004

THE CRITERIA COMMITTEE OF THE NEW YORK HEART ASSOCIATION: *Nomenclature and Criteria for Diagnosis*, 9th ed. Boston, Little, Brown, 1994

VANDEN BELT J: The history, in *Classic Teachings in Clinical Cardiology: A Tribute to W. Proctor Harvey*, M Chizner (ed). Cedar Grove, NJ, Laennec, 1996, pp 41–54

ZIPES D et al (eds): *Braunwald's Heart Disease*, 7th ed. Philadelphia, Saunders, 2004

209 PHYSICAL EXAMINATION OF THE CARDIOVASCULAR SYSTEM
Robert A. O'Rourke, Eugene Braunwald

A meticulous physical examination is an often inadequately utilized low-cost method for assessing the cardiovascular system and frequently provides important information for the appropriate selection of additional tests. First, the general physical appearance should be evaluated. The patient may appear tired because of a chronic low cardiac output; the respiratory rate may be rapid in cases of pulmonary venous congestion. Central cyanosis, often associated with clubbing of the fingers and toes, indicates right-to-left cardiac or extracardiac shunting or inadequate oxygenation of blood by the lungs. Cyanosis in the distal extremities, cool skin, and increased sweating result from vasoconstriction in patients with severe heart failure (Chap. 31). Noncardiovascular details can be equally important. For example, infective endocarditis is the likely diagnosis in patients with petechiae, Osler's nodes, and Janeway lesions (Chap. 109).

The blood pressure should be taken in both arms and with the patient supine and upright; the heart rate should be timed for 30 s. Orthostatic hypotension and tachycardia may indicate a reduced blood volume, while resting tachycardia may be due to heart failure.

EXAMINATION OF THE RETINA

Inspection of the smaller vessels of the body is possible in the retina. The optic disc should be observed first, with a search for evidence of edema and blurred margins and for cupping with sharp contours. Neovascularization or the pallor of optic atrophy should be ruled out. Next, the examiner should scan along the superior temporal arcade, inspecting the arteries carefully for embolic plaques at each bifurcation and noting the arteriovenous crossing for evidence of obscuration of the vein and for pronounced nicking and banking of the vessels.

Early diabetic microaneurysms, a manifestation of diabetic microvascular disease, are found just temporal to the fovea, along the horizontal raphe, and cotton-wool infarcts are found circularly around the disc (see Fig. 323-9). Thus, the retina can be searched efficiently for evidence of cardiovascular disease.

Variations in the caliber of a single vessel are more important than determinations of arteriovenous ratios. These changes may take the form of focal narrowing, sometimes called *beading*, and are seen in hypercholesterolemia or spasm. In severe hypertension, hypertensive retinopathy with scattered flame-shaped hemorrhages, very constricted arterioles, and cotton-wool spots are evident (see Fig. 25-8).

Retinal emboli have particular cardiovascular significance. Of these, platelet emboli are both the most common and the most evanescent. Hollenhorst cholesterol plaques may be identified at the same bifurcations for months to years after the embolic shower. Platelet emboli, Hollenhorst plaques, and calcium emboli are usually seen along the course of a retinal artery, and their appearance indicates that a patient is shedding from the heart, aorta, great vessels, or carotid arteries (see Fig. 25-6). Roth spots and fat emboli may not appear to be intravascular and may not be associated with a vessel that is ophthalmoscopically visible.

EXAMINATION OF THE ABDOMEN

The diameter of the *abdominal* aorta should be estimated. An abdominal aortic aneurysm may be missed if the examiner fails to assess the area above the umbilicus.

Specific abnormalities of the abdomen may be secondary to heart disease. A large, tender liver is common in patients with heart failure or constrictive pericarditis. Systolic hepatic pulsations are frequent in patients with tricuspid regurgitation. A palpable spleen is a late sign in patients with severe heart failure and is also often present in patients with infective endocarditis.

Ascites may occur with heart failure alone, although it is less common with the use of diuretic therapy. Severe tricuspid regurgitation often results in an enlarged pulsating liver and ascites. Constrictive pericarditis should be considered when the ascites is out of proportion to peripheral edema. When there is an arteriovenous fistula, a continuous murmur may be heard over the abdomen. Fistulas due to trauma and surgery may occur.

A systolic bruit heard over the kidney areas may signify renal artery stenosis in patients with systemic hypertension.

EXAMINATION OF THE EXTREMITIES

Examination of the upper and lower extremities may provide important diagnostic information. Palpation of the peripheral arterial pulses in the upper and lower extremities is necessary to define the adequacy of systemic blood flow and to detect the presence of occlusive arterial lesions. Atherosclerosis of the peripheral arteries may produce intermittent claudication of the buttock, calf, thigh, or foot, with severe disease resulting in tissue damage of the toes. Peripheral atherosclerosis is an important risk factor for coincident ischemic heart disease.

Thrombophlebitis often causes pain (in the calf or thigh) or edema, and when present, pulmonary emboli should be considered as well. Edema is a late sign of heart failure; it frequently involves the right leg prior to the left. However, edema of the lower extremities may be secondary to local factors, such as varicose veins or thrombophlebitis, or to the removal of veins at coronary artery bypass surgery. Under such circumstances, the edema is often unilateral.

ARTERIAL PRESSURE PULSE

The normal central aortic pulse wave is characterized by a fairly rapid rise to a somewhat rounded peak (Fig. 209-1). The anacrotic shoulder, present on the ascending limb, occurs at the time of peak rate of aortic flow just before maximum pressure is reached. The less steep descending limb is interrupted by a sharp downward deflection, coincident with aortic valve closure, called the *incisura*. As the pulse wave is transmitted peripherally, the initial upstroke becomes steeper, the anacrotic shoulder becomes less apparent, and the incisura is replaced by the smoother dicrotic notch. Accordingly, palpation of a peripheral arterial pulse (e.g., the radial pulse) frequently gives less information than examination of a more central pulse (e.g., the carotid pulse) re-

FIGURE 209-1 *A.* Schematic representation of electrocardiogram, aortic pressure pulse (AOP), phonocardiogram recorded at the apex, and apex cardiogram (ACG). On the phonocardiogram, S_1, S_2, S_3, and S_4 represent the first through fourth heart sounds; OS represents the opening snap of the mitral valve, which occurs coincident with the 0 point of the apex cardiogram. S_3 occurs coincident with the termination of the rapid-filling wave (RFW) of the ACG, while S_4 occurs coincident with the *a* wave of the ACG. *B.* Simultaneous recording of electrocardiogram, indirect carotid pulse (CP), phonocardiogram along the left sternal border (LSB), and indirect jugular venous pulse (JVP). ES, ejection sound; SC, systolic click.

garding alterations in left ventricular ejection or aortic valve function. However, certain findings, such as the bisferiens pulse of aortic regurgitation or pulsus alternans, are more evident in peripheral arteries (Fig. 209-2).

The carotid pulse is best examined with the sternocleidomastoid muscle relaxed and with the patient's head rotated slightly toward the examiner. In palpating the brachial arterial pulse, the examiner can support the patient's relaxed elbow with the right arm while compressing the brachial pulse with the thumb. The usual technique is to compress the artery with the thumb or forefinger until the maximum pulse is sensed. Varying degrees of pressure should then be applied while concentrating on the separate phases of the pulse wave. This method, known as *trisection*, is useful for assessing the sharpness of the upstroke, systolic peak, and diastolic slope of the arterial pulse. In most normal persons, a dicrotic wave is not palpable.

A small weak pulse, *pulsus parvus*, is common in conditions with a diminished left ventricular stroke volume, a narrow pulse pressure, and increased peripheral vascular resistance (Fig. 209-2). A *hypokinetic* pulse may be due to hypovolemia, to left ventricular failure, to restrictive pericardial disease, or to mitral valve stenosis. In aortic valve stenosis, the delayed systolic peak, *pulsus tardus*, results from obstruction to left ventricular ejection. In contrast, a large, bounding (*hyperkinetic*) pulse is usually associated with an increased ventricular stroke volume, a wide pulse pressure, and a decrease in pe-

ripheral vascular resistance. This pattern occurs characteristically in patients with an elevated stroke volume, as in complete heart block; with hyperkinetic circulation due to anxiety, anemia, exercise, or fever; or with a rapid runoff of blood from the arterial system (as caused by a patent ductus arteriosus or peripheral arteriovenous fistula). Patients with mitral regurgitation or a ventricular septal defect may also have a bounding pulse, since vigorous left ventricular ejection produces a rapid upstroke in the arterial pulse, even though the duration of systole and the forward stroke volume may be reduced. In aortic regurgitation, the rapidly rising, bounding arterial pulse results from an increased left ventricular stroke volume and an increased rate of ventricular ejection.

The *bisferiens pulse*, which has two systolic peaks, is characteristic of aortic regurgitation (with or without accompanying stenosis) and of hypertrophic cardiomyopathy (Chap. 221). In the latter condition, the pulse wave upstroke rises rapidly and forcefully, producing the first systolic peak ("percussion wave"). A brief decline in pressure follows because of the sudden midsystolic decrease in the rate of left ventricular ejection, when severe obstruction often develops. This pressure trough is followed by a smaller and more slowly rising positive pulse wave ("tidal wave") produced by continued ventricular ejection and by reflected waves from the periphery. The *dicrotic pulse* has two palpable waves, one in systole and one in diastole. It usually denotes a very low stroke volume, particularly in patients with dilated cardiomyopathy.

Pulsus alternans is a pattern in which there is regular alteration of the pressure pulse amplitude, despite a regular rhythm (Fig. 209-2). It is due to alternating left ventricular contractile force, usually indicates severe impairment of left ventricular function, and commonly occurs in patients who also have a loud third heart sound. Pulsus alternans may also occur during or following paroxysmal tachycardia or for several beats following a premature beat in patients without heart disease. In *pulsus bigeminus*, there is also a regular alteration of pressure pulse amplitude, but it is caused by a premature ventricular contraction that follows each regular beat. In *pulsus paradoxus*, the decrease in systolic arterial pressure that normally accompanies the reduction in arterial pulse amplitude during inspiration is accentuated. In patients with pericardial tamponade (Chap. 222), airway obstruction, or superior vena cava obstruction, the decrease in systolic arterial pressure frequently exceeds the normal decrease of 10 mmHg and the peripheral pulse may disappear completely during inspiration.

Simultaneous palpation of the radial and femoral arterial pulses, which normally are virtually coincident, is important to rule out aortic coarctation, in which the latter pulse is weakened and delayed (Chap. 218).

JUGULAR VENOUS PULSE (JVP)

The two main objectives of the examination of the neck veins are inspection of their waveform and estimation of the central venous pressure (CVP). In most patients, the right internal jugular vein is best for both purposes. Usually, the pulsation of the internal jugular vein is greatest when the trunk is inclined by less than 30°. In patients with elevated venous pressure, it may be necessary to elevate the trunk further, sometimes to as much as 90°. When the neck muscles are relaxed, shining a beam of light tangentially across the skin overlying the vein exposes the pulsations of the internal jugular vein. Simultaneous palpation of the left carotid artery aids the examiner in deciding which pulsations are venous and in relating the venous pulsations to their timing in the cardiac cycle.

The normal JVP reflects phasic pressure changes in the right atrium and consists of two or sometimes three positive waves and two negative troughs (Fig. 209-1). The positive presystolic *a* wave is produced by venous distention due to right atrial contraction and is the dominant wave in the JVP, particularly during inspiration. Large *a* waves indicate that the right atrium is contracting against an increased resistance (Fig. 209-3), such as occurs with tricuspid stenosis or more commonly

FIGURE 209-2 Schematic representation of arterial pulse waveforms that occur with alterations in cardiac hemodynamics, which may result from normal physiologic responses or may be due to cardiac disease. S, systole; D, diastole. [*Modified from RA O'Rourke, in Hurst's The Heart, 10th ed, V Fuster et al (eds). New York, McGraw-Hill, 2001, with permission.*]

FIGURE 209-3 Abnormal jugular venous pulse waveforms commonly present in patients with cardiac disease and/or arrhythmias. See text. [*Modified from RA O'Rourke, in Hurst's The Heart, 10th ed, V Fuster et al (eds). New York, McGraw-Hill, 2001, with permission.*]

with increased resistance to right ventricular filling (pulmonary hypertension or pulmonic stenosis). Large *a* waves also occur during arrhythmias whenever the right atrium contracts while the tricuspid valve is closed by right ventricular systole. Such "cannon" *a* waves may occur regularly (as during junctional rhythm) or irregularly (as in atrioventricular dissociation with ventricular tachycardia or complete heart block). The *a* wave is absent in patients with atrial fibrillation, and there is an increased delay between the *a* wave and the carotid arterial pulse in patients with first-degree atrioventricular block.

The *c* wave, often observed in the JVP, is a positive wave produced by the bulging of the tricuspid valve into the right atrium during right ventricular isovolumetric systole and by the impact of the carotid artery adjacent to the jugular vein. The *x* descent is due both to atrial relaxation and to the downward displacement of the tricuspid valve during ventricular systole. The *x* descent wave during systole is often accentuated in patients with constrictive pericarditis (Fig. 209-3), but the nadir of this wave is reduced with right ventricular dilation and is often reversed in tricuspid regurgitation. The positive, late systolic *v* wave results from the increasing volume of blood in the right atrium during ventricular systole when the tricuspid valve is closed. Tricuspid regurgitation causes the *v* wave to be more prominent; when tricuspid regurgitation becomes severe, the combination of a prominent *v* wave and obliteration of the *x* descent results in a single large positive systolic wave. After the *v* wave peaks, the right atrial pressure falls because of the decreased bulging of the tricuspid valve into the right atrium as right ventricular pressure declines and the tricuspid valve opens (Fig. 209-3).

This negative descending limb—the *y* descent of the JVP—is produced mainly by the opening of the tricuspid valve and the subsequent rapid inflow of blood into the right ventricle. A rapid, deep *y* descent in early diastole occurs with severe tricuspid regurgitation. A venous pulse characterized by a sharp *y* descent, a deep *y* trough, and a rapid ascent to the baseline is seen in patients with constrictive pericarditis or with severe right-sided heart failure and a high venous pressure. A slow *y* descent in the JVP suggests an obstruction to right ventricular filling, as occurs with tricuspid stenosis or right atrial myxoma.

The right internal jugular is the best vein to use for accurate estimation of the CVP. The sternal angle is used as the reference point, because the center of the right atrium lies approximately 5 cm below the sternal angle in the average patient, regardless of body position. The patient is examined at the optimal degree of trunk elevation for visualization of venous pulsations. The vertical distance between the top of the oscillating venous column and the level of the sternal angle is determined; generally it is less than 3 cm (3 cm + 5 cm = 8 cm blood). The most common cause of a high venous pressure is an elevated right ventricular diastolic pressure.

In patients suspected of having right ventricular failure who have a normal CVP at rest, the *abdominojugular reflux test* may be helpful. The palm of the examiner's hand is placed over the abdomen, and firm pressure is applied for 10 s or more. In normal persons, this maneuver

does not alter the jugular venous pressure significantly, but when right heart function is impaired, the upper level of venous pulsation usually increases. A positive abdominojugular test is best defined as an increase in JVP during 10 s of firm midabdominal compression followed by a rapid drop in pressure of 4 cm blood on release of the compression. The most common cause of a positive test is right-sided heart failure secondary to elevated left heart filling pressures. Also, abdominal compression may elicit the JVP pattern typical of tricuspid regurgitation when the resting pulse wave is normal. *Kussmaul's sign*—an increase rather than the normal decrease in the CVP during inspiration—is most often caused by severe right-sided heart failure; it is a frequent finding in patients with constrictive pericarditis or right ventricular infarction.

PRECORDIAL PALPATION

The location, amplitude, duration, and direction of the cardiac impulse usually can be best appreciated with the fingertips. The normal left ventricular apex impulse is located at or medial to the left midclavicular line in the fourth or fifth intercostal space and is a tapping, early systolic outward thrust localized to a point usually less than 2.5 cm in diameter. It is due primarily to recoil of the heart as blood is ejected and should be evaluated with the patient supine and in the left lateral position. Left ventricular hypertrophy results in exaggeration of the amplitude, duration, and often size of the normal left ventricular thrust. The impulse may be displaced laterally and downward into the sixth or seventh intercostal space, particularly in patients with a left ventricular volume load such as occurs in cases of aortic regurgitation or dilated cardiomyopathy.

Additional abnormal features that are detectable at the left ventricular apex include (1) marked presystolic distention of the left ventricle, usually accompanied by a fourth heart sound in patients with an excessive left ventricular pressure load or myocardial ischemia/infarction; and (2) a prominent early diastolic rapid-filling wave, often accompanied by a third heart sound in patients with left ventricular failure or mitral valve regurgitation (Fig. 209-1). A double systolic apical impulse is palpable in many patients with hypertrophic cardiomyopathy.

Right ventricular hypertrophy often results in a sustained systolic lift at the lower left parasternal area, which starts in early systole and is synchronous with the left ventricular apical impulse.

Abnormal precordial pulsations occur during systole in patients with left ventricular dyssynergy due to ischemic heart disease or to diffuse myocardial disease from some other cause. These pulsations often occur in patients with a recent myocardial infarction and may be present in some patients only during episodes of angina. They are most commonly felt in the left midprecordium one or two interspaces above and/or 1 to 2 cm medial to the left ventricular apex. A systolic bulge occurring in the region of the apex is difficult to distinguish from the impulse of left ventricular hypertrophy.

A left parasternal lift is frequently present in patients with severe mitral regurgitation. This pulsation occurs distinctly later than the left ventricular apical impulse, is synchronous with the *v* wave in the left atrial pressure curve, and is due to anterior displacement of the right ventricle by an enlarged, expanding left atrium. A similar impulse occurs to the right of the sternum in some patients with severe tricuspid regurgitation and a giant right atrium. Pulsation of the right sternoclavicular joint may indicate a right-sided aortic arch or aneurysmal dilation of the ascending aorta. Pulmonary artery pulsation is often visible and palpable in the second left intercostal space. While it may be normal in children or thin young adults, this pulsation usually denotes pulmonary hypertension, increased pulmonary blood flow, or poststenotic pulmonary artery dilation.

Thrills are palpable, low-frequency vibrations associated with heart murmurs. The systolic murmur of mitral regurgitation may be palpated at the cardiac apex. When the palm of the hand is placed over the precordium, the thrill of aortic stenosis crosses the palm toward the right side of the neck, while the thrill of pulmonic stenosis radiates more often to the left side of the neck. The thrill due to a ventricular septal defect is usually located in the third and fourth intercostal spaces near the left sternal border.

Percussion should be performed in each patient to identify normal or abnormal position of the heart, stomach, and liver. However, in patients with a normal cardiac situs, percussion adds little to careful inspection and palpation in the recognition of cardiac enlargement.

CARDIAC AUSCULTATION

To obtain the most information from cardiac auscultation, the observer should keep in mind several principles: (1) Auscultation should be performed in a quiet room to avoid the distracting noises of normal activity. (2) For optimal auscultation, attention must be focused on the phase of the cardiac cycle during which the auscultatory event is expected to occur. (3) The timing of a heart sound or murmur can be determined accurately from its relation to other observable events in the cardiac cycle—the carotid arterial pulse, the apical impulse, or the JVP. (4) To define the significance of a cardiac sound or murmur, it is often necessary to observe alterations in its timing or intensity during various physiologic and/or pharmacologic interventions (Table 209-1).

HEART SOUNDS

The major components of heart sounds are vibrations associated with the abrupt acceleration or deceleration of blood in the cardiovascular system. Studies using simultaneous echocardiographic-phonocardiographic recordings indicate that the first and second heart sounds are produced primarily by the closure of the atrioventricular (AV) and semilunar valves and the events that accompany these closures. The intensity of the *first heart sound* (S_1) is influenced by (1) the position

of the mitral leaflets at the onset of ventricular systole; (2) the rate of rise of the left ventricular pressure pulse; (3) the presence or absence of structural disease of the mitral valve; and (4) the amount of tissue, air, or fluid between the heart and the stethoscope. S_1 is louder if diastole is shortened because of tachycardia, if AV flow is increased because of high cardiac output or prolonged because of mitral stenosis, or if atrial contraction precedes ventricular contraction by an unusually short interval, reflected in a short PR interval. The loud S_1 in mitral stenosis usually signifies that the valve is pliable and that it remains open at the onset of isovolumetric contraction because of the elevated left atrial pressure. A soft S_1 may be due to poor conduction of sound through the chest wall, a slow rise of the left ventricular pressure pulse, a long PR interval, or imperfect closure due to reduced valve substance, as in mitral regurgitation. S_1 is also soft when the anterior mitral leaflet is immobile because of rigidity and calcification, even in the presence of predominant mitral stenosis.

Splitting of the two high-pitched components of S_1 by 10 to 30 ms is a normal phenomenon (Fig. 209-1). The first component of S_1 is usually attributed to mitral valve closure, and the second to tricuspid valve closure. Widening of the S_1 is due most often to complete right bundle branch block and the resulting delay in onset of the right ventricular pressure pulse. Reversed splitting of the S_1, in which the mitral component follows the tricuspid component, may be present in patients with severe mitral stenosis, left atrial myxoma, and left bundle branch block.

SPLITTING OF THE *SECOND HEART SOUND* This sound (S_2) normally splits into audibly distinct aortic (A_2) and pulmonic (P_2) components during inspiration, when the augmented inflow into the right ventricle increases its stroke volume and ejection period and thus delays closure of the pulmonic valve. P_2 is coincident with the incisura of the pulmonary artery pressure curve, which is separated from the right ventricular pressure tracing by an interval termed the *hangout time*. The absolute value of this interval reflects the resistance to pulmonary blood flow and the impedance characteristics of the pulmonary vascular bed. This interval is prolonged, and physiologic splitting of S_2 is accentuated, in conditions associated with right ventricular volume overload and a distensible pulmonary vascular bed. However, in patients with an increase in pulmonary vascular resistance, the hangout time is markedly reduced, and narrow splitting of S_2 is present. Splitting that persists with expiration (heard best at the pulmonic area or left sternal border) is usually abnormal when the patient is in the upright position. Such splitting may be due to many causes: delayed activation of the right ventricle (right bundle branch block); left ventricular ectopic beats; a left ventricular pacemaker; prolongation of right ventricular contraction with an increased right ventricular pressure load (pulmonary embolism or pulmonic stenosis); or delayed pulmonic valve closure because of right ventricular volume overload associated with right ventricular failure or diminished impedance of the pulmonary vascular bed and a prolonged hangout time (atrial septal defect).

In pulmonary hypertension, P_2 is loud, and splitting of the second heart sound may be diminished, normal, or accentuated, depending on the cause of the pulmonary hypertension, the pulmonary vascular resistance, and the presence or absence of right ventricular decompensation. Early aortic valve closure, occurring with mitral regurgitation or a ventricular septal defect, may also produce splitting that persists during expiration. It may also occur with constrictive pericarditis. In patients with an atrial septal defect, the proportion of right atrial filling contributed by the left atrium and the venae cavae varies reciprocally during the respiratory cycle, so that right atrial inflow remains relatively constant. Therefore, the volume and duration of right ventricular ejection are not significantly increased by inspiration, and there is little inspiratory exaggeration of the splitting of S_2. This phenomenon, termed *fixed splitting* of the second heart sound, is of considerable diagnostic value.

TABLE 209-1 *Effects of Physiologic and Pharmacologic Interventions on the Intensity of Heart Murmurs and Sounds*

Respiration Systolic murmurs due to TR or pulmonic blood flow through a normal or stenotic valve and diastolic murmurs of TS or PR generally increase with inspiration, as do right-sided S_3 and S_4. Left-sided murmurs and sounds usually are louder during expiration.

Valsalva maneuver Most murmurs decrease in length and intensity. Two exceptions are the systolic murmur of HCM, which usually becomes much louder, and that of MVP, which becomes longer and often louder. Following release of the Valsalva maneuver, right-sided murmurs tend to return to control intensity earlier than left-sided murmurs.

After VPB or AF Murmurs originating at normal or stenotic semilunar valves increase in the cardiac cycle following a VPB or in the cycle after a long cycle length in AF. By contrast, systolic murmurs due to AV valve regurgitation either do not change, diminish (papillary muscle dysfunction), or become shorter (MVP).

Positional changes With *standing*, most murmurs diminish, two exceptions being the murmur of HCM, which becomes louder, and that of MVP, which lengthens and often is intensified. With *squatting*, most murmurs become louder, but those of HCM and MVP usually soften and may disappear. Passive leg raising usually produces the same results.

Exercise Murmurs due to blood flow across normal or obstructed valves (e.g., PS, MS) become louder with both isotonic and submaximal isometric (handgrip) exercise. Murmurs of MR, VSD, and AR also increase with handgrip exercise. However, the murmur of HCM often decreases with near maximum handgrip exercise. Left-sided S_4 and S_3 are often accentuated by exercise, particularly when due to ischemic heart disease.

Pharmacologic interventions During the initial relative hypotension following amyl nitrite inhalation, murmurs of MR, VSD, and AR decrease, while murmurs of aortic stenosis or sclerosis increase. During the later tachycardia phase, murmurs of MS and right-sided lesions also increase. The response in MVP often is biphasic (first softer and then louder than control). The arterial constrictor phenylephrine tends to produce the opposite effects.

Transient arterial occlusion Transient external compression of both arms by bilateral cuff inflation to 20 mmHg over peak systolic pressure augments the murmurs of MR, VSD, and AR, but not murmurs due to other causes.

Note: TR, tricuspid regurgitation; TS, tricuspid stenosis; PR, pulmonic regurgitation; HCM, hypertrophic cardiomyopathy; MVP, mitral valve prolapse; PS, pulmonic stenosis; MS, mitral stenosis; MR, mitral regurgitation; VSD, ventricular septal defect; AR, aortic regurgitation; VPB, ventricular premature beat; and AF, atrial fibrillation.

A delay in aortic valve closure causing P_2 to precede A_2 results in so-called reversed (paradoxic) splitting of S_2. Splitting is then maximal in expiration and decreases during inspiration with the normal delay of pulmonic valve closure. The most common causes of reversed splitting of S_2 are left bundle branch block and delayed excitation of the left ventricle from a right ventricular ectopic beat. Mechanical prolongation of left ventricular systole, resulting in reversed splitting of S_2, may also be caused by severe aortic outflow obstruction, a large aorta-to-pulmonary artery shunt, systolic hypertension, and ischemic heart disease or cardiomyopathy with left ventricular failure. P_2 is normally softer than A_2 in the second left intercostal space; a P_2 that is greater than A_2 in this area suggests pulmonary hypertension, except in patients with atrial septal defect.

SYSTOLIC SOUNDS   The *ejection sound* is a sharp, high-pitched event occurring in early systole and closely following the first heart sound. Ejection sounds occur in the presence of semilunar valve stenosis and in conditions associated with dilation of the aorta or pulmonary artery. The aortic ejection sound is usually heard best at the left ventricular apex and the second right intercostal space; the pulmonary ejection sound is loudest at the upper left sternal border. The latter, unlike most other right-sided acoustical events, is heard better during expiration.

Nonejection clicks, or *midsystolic clicks*, occurring with or without a late systolic murmur, often denote prolapse of one or both leaflets of the mitral valve (Chap. 219). They also may be caused by tricuspid valve prolapse. They probably result from chordae tendineae that are functionally unequal in length on either or both AV valves and are heard best along the lower left sternal border and at the left ventricular apex. Systolic clicks may be single or multiple, and they may occur at any time in systole but are usually later than the systolic ejection sound.

DIASTOLIC SOUNDS   The *opening snap* (OS) is a brief, high-pitched, early diastolic sound, which is usually due to stenosis of an AV valve, most often the mitral valve. It is generally heard best at the lower left sternal border and radiates well to the base of the heart. The A_2-OS interval is inversely related to the height of the mean left atrial pressure and ranges from 0.04 to 0.12 s. In the second intercostal space, an OS is often confused with P_2. However, careful auscultation will reveal both components of S_2, followed by the OS. The OS of tricuspid stenosis occurs later in diastole than the mitral OS and is often overlooked in patients with more prominent mitral valve disease.

The *third heart sound* (S_3) is a low-pitched sound produced in the ventricle 0.14 to 0.16 s after A_2, at the termination of rapid filling. This sound is frequent in normal children and in patients with high cardiac output. However, in patients over 40 years old, an S_3 usually indicates impairment of ventricular function, AV valve regurgitation, or other conditions that increase the rate or volume of ventricular filling. The left-sided S_3 is best heard with the bell piece of the stethoscope at the left ventricular apex during expiration and with the patient in the left lateral position. The right-sided S_3 is best heard at the left sternal border or just beneath the xiphoid and is usually louder with inspiration. Often it is accompanied by the systolic murmur of functional tricuspid regurgitation. Third heart sounds often disappear with treatment of heart failure.

An S_3 that is earlier (0.10 to 0.12 s after A_2) and higher-pitched than normal (a pericardial knock) often occurs in patients with constrictive pericarditis (Chap. 222); its presence depends on the restrictive effect of the adherent pericardium, which abruptly halts diastolic filling.

The *fourth heart sound* (S_4) is a low-pitched, presystolic sound produced in the ventricle during ventricular filling; it is associated with an effective atrial contraction and is best heard with the bell piece of the stethoscope. The sound is absent in patients with atrial fibrillation. The S_4 occurs when diminished ventricular compliance increases the resistance to ventricular filling, and it is frequently present in patients with systemic hypertension, aortic stenosis, hypertrophic cardiomyopathy, ischemic heart disease, and acute mitral regurgitation. Most patients with an acute myocardial infarction and sinus rhythm have an audible S_4. The fourth heart sound is frequently accompanied by visible and palpable presystolic distention of the left ventricle. It is loudest at the left ventricular apex when the patient is in the left lateral position and is accentuated by mild isotonic or isometric exercise in the supine position. The right-sided S_4 is present in patients with right ventricular hypertrophy secondary to either pulmonic stenosis or pulmonary hypertension and frequently accompanies a prominent presystolic *a* wave in the JVP.

An S_4 frequently accompanies delayed AV conduction even in the absence of clinically detectable heart disease. The incidence of an audible S_4 increases with increasing age. Whether an audible S_4 in adults without other evidence of cardiac disease is abnormal remains controversial. Both left-sided S_3 and S_4 sounds increase with isometric exercise and both may radiate to the subclavian and carotid arteries.

HEART MURMURS

Cardiac murmurs result from vibrations set up in the bloodstream and the surrounding heart and great vessels as a result of turbulent blood flow, the formation of eddies, and cavitation (bubble formation as a result of sudden decrease in pressure).

The evaluation of the patient with a heart murmur may vary greatly depending on many of the considerations discussed below. These include the intensity of the cardiac murmur, its timing in the cardiac cycle, its location and radiation, and its response to various physiologic maneuvers. Also of importance are the presence or absence of cardiac and noncardiac symptoms and whether other cardiac or noncardiac physical findings suggest that the cardiac murmur is clinically significant. The skill and confidence of the cardiac auscultator, the relative costs of various diagnostic approaches, and the accuracy and reliability of additional tests in the laboratory where they are performed are also important factors.

The intensity (loudness) of murmurs may be graded from I to VI. A grade I murmur is so faint that it can be heard only with special effort; a grade IV murmur is commonly accompanied by a thrill; and a grade VI murmur is audible with the stethoscope removed from contact with the chest. The configuration of a murmur may be crescendo, decrescendo, crescendo-decrescendo (diamond-shaped), or plateau (Fig. 209-4). The precise time of onset and time of cessation of a murmur depend on the instant in the cardiac cycle at which an adequate pressure difference between two chambers arises and disappears (Fig. 209-5).

The location on the chest wall where the murmur is best heard and the areas to which it radiates can aid in identifying the cardiac structure from which the murmur originates. For example, the murmur of aortic valve stenosis is usually loudest in the second right intercostal space and radiates to the carotid arteries. By contrast, the murmur of mitral regurgitation is most often loudest at the cardiac apex. It may radiate to the left sternal border and base of the heart when the posterior mitral leaflet is predominantly involved or to the axilla and back when the anterior leaflet is more severely affected. In the latter case, the regurgitant blood is directed toward the posterior left atrial wall.

EFFECTS OF PHYSIOLOGIC INTERVENTIONS   It is often difficult to classify a cardiac murmur with certainty on the basis of its timing, configuration, location, radiation, pitch, or intensity. However, by noting changes in the characteristics of the murmur during maneuvers that alter cardiac hemodynamics, the auscultator can often identify its correct origin and significance (Table 209-1).

Accentuation of a murmur during inspiration (a maneuver that augments systemic venous return) implies that it originates on the right side of the circulation; expiratory exaggeration has less significance. Prolonged expiratory pressure against a closed glottis (i.e., the Valsalva maneuver) reduces the intensity of most murmurs by diminishing both right and left ventricular filling (i.e., ventricular preload). The systolic murmur associated with *hypertrophic cardiomyopathy* and the late systolic murmur due to *mitral valve prolapse* are exceptions and may be paradoxically accentuated during the Valsalva maneuver. Mur-

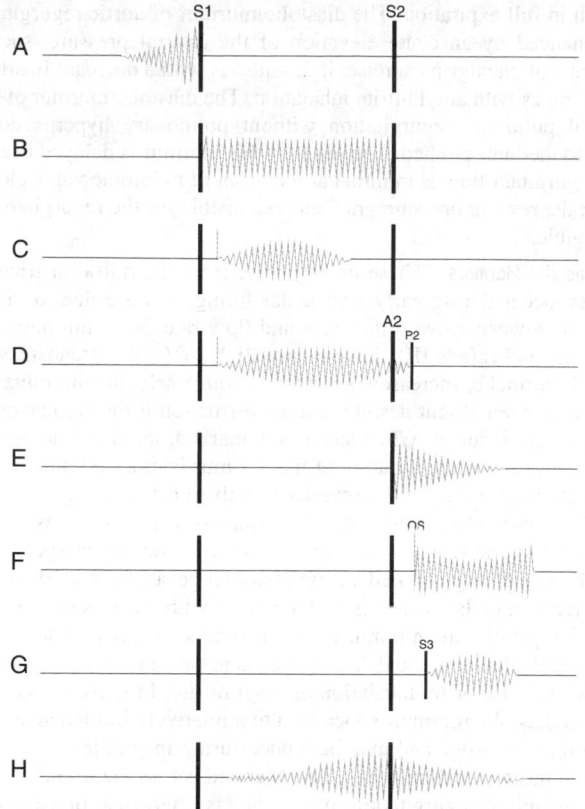

FIGURE 209-4 Diagram depicting principal heart murmurs. *A.* Presystolic murmur of mitral or tricuspid stenosis. *B.* Holosystolic (pansystolic) murmur of mitral or tricuspid regurgitation or of ventricular septal defect. *C.* Aortic ejection murmur beginning with an ejection click and fading before the second heart sound. *D.* Systolic murmur in pulmonic stenosis spilling through the aortic second sound, pulmonic valve closure being delayed. *E.* Aortic or pulmonary diastolic murmur. *F.* Long diastolic murmur of mitral stenosis following the opening snap. *G.* Short middiastolic inflow murmur following a third heart sound. *H.* Continuous murmur of patent ductus arteriosus *(Adapted by P O'Gara from P Wood, Diseases of the Heart and Circulation. Philadelphia, Lippincott, 1968, with permission.)*

murs due to flow across a normal or obstructed semilunar valve increase in intensity in the cycle following a premature ventricular beat or a long RR interval in atrial fibrillation. In contrast, murmurs due to AV valve regurgitation or a ventricular septal defect do not change appreciably during the beat following a prolonged diastole. Standing, which decreases left ventricular volume, accentuates the murmur of hypertrophic cardiomyopathy and occasionally the murmur due to mitral valve prolapse. Squatting, which increases both venous return and systemic arterial resistance and thus ventricular afterload, increases most murmurs, except those due to hypertrophic cardiomyopathy and mitral regurgitation due to a prolapsed mitral valve, which often decrease. In the patient who cannot squat, jackknifing the legs will produce the same response. Sustained handgrip exercise, which increases systemic arterial pressure and heart rate, often accentuates the murmurs of mitral regurgitation, aortic regurgitation, and mitral stenosis but usually diminishes those due to aortic stenosis or hypertrophic cardiomyopathy.

SYSTOLIC MURMURS ■ Holosystolic (Pansystolic) Murmurs

These are generated when there is flow between two chambers that have widely different pressures throughout systole, such as the left ventricle and either the left atrium or the right ventricle (Fig. 209-5). The pressure gradient occurs early in contraction and lasts until relaxation is almost complete. Therefore, holosystolic murmurs begin before aortic ejection, and at the area of maximal intensity they begin with S_1 and end after S_2 (Fig. 209-4B). Holosystolic murmurs accompany mitral or tricuspid regurgitation, ventricular septal defect, and, under certain circumstances, aortopulmonary shunts. Although the typical high-pitched murmur of mitral regurgitation usually continues throughout systole,

the shape of the murmur may vary considerably. The holosystolic murmurs of mitral regurgitation and ventricular septal defect are augmented by transient exercise.

The murmur of tricuspid regurgitation associated with pulmonary hypertension is holosystolic and frequently increases during inspiration. Not all patients with mitral or tricuspid regurgitation or ventricular septal defect have holosystolic murmurs. Often, a mild valvular regurgitant jet, detected by color flow Doppler techniques (Chap. 211), is not associated with an audible murmur despite optimal auscultation. Such regurgitant jets usually do not indicate clinical heart disease. Trivial mitral regurgitation can be detected by Doppler in up to 45% of normal individuals; tricuspid regurgitation in up to 70%; and pulmonic regurgitation in up to 88%. Aortic regurgitation is encountered much less frequently in normal persons, and its incidence increases with advancing age. An overinterpretation of the significance of mild regurgitation by echocardiographers often results in a misdiagnosis of "echocardiographic heart disease," resulting in unnecessary patient anxiety and infective endocarditis prophylaxis.

Midsystolic Murmurs These also called *systolic ejection murmurs,* which are often crescendo-decrescendo in shape, and occur when blood is ejected across the aortic or pulmonic outflow tracts (Figs. 209-4C and 209-5). The murmur starts shortly after S_1, when the ventricular pressure becomes high enough to open the semilunar valve. As the velocity of ejection increases, the murmur gets louder; as ejection declines, it diminishes. The murmur ends before the ventricular pressure falls enough to permit closure of the aortic or pulmonic leaflets. When the semilunar valves are normal, an increased flow rate (as occurs in states of elevated cardiac output), ejection into a dilated vessel beyond the valve, or increased transmission of sound through a thin chest wall may be responsible for this murmur. Most benign, functional murmurs are midsystolic and originate from the pulmonary outflow tract. Valvular or subvalvular obstruction of either ventricle may also cause such a midsystolic murmur, the intensity being related to the flow rate.

The murmur of aortic stenosis is the prototype of the left-sided midsystolic murmur. The location and radiation of this murmur are influenced by the direction of the high-velocity jet within the aortic

FIGURE 209-5 *A.* Schematic representation of ECG, aortic pressure (AOP), left ventricular pressure (LVP), and left atrial pressure (LAP). The shaded areas indicate a transvalvular pressure difference during systole. HSM, holosystolic murmur; MSM, midsystolic murmur. *B.* Graphic representation of ECG, aortic pressure (AOP), left ventricular pressure (LVP), and left atrial pressure (LAP) with shaded areas indicating transvalvular diastolic pressure difference. EDM, early diastolic murmur; PSM, presystolic murmur; MDM, middiastolic murmur.

root. In *valvular aortic stenosis*, the murmur is usually maximal in the second right intercostal space, with radiation into the neck. In *supravalvular aortic stenosis*, the murmur is occasionally loudest even higher, with disproportionate radiation into the right carotid artery. In hypertrophic cardiomyopathy, the midsystolic murmur originates in the left ventricular cavity and is usually maximal at the lower left sternal edge and apex, with relatively little radiation to the carotids. When the aortic valve is immobile (calcified), the aortic closure sound (A_2) may be soft and inaudible so that the length and configuration of the murmur are difficult to determine. Midsystolic murmurs also occur in patients with mitral regurgitation or, less frequently, tricuspid regurgitation resulting from papillary muscle dysfunction. Such murmurs due to mitral regurgitation are often confused with those originating in the aorta, particularly in elderly patients.

The patient's age and the area of maximal intensity aid in determining the significance of midsystolic murmurs. Thus, in a young adult with a thin chest and a high velocity of blood flow, a faint or moderate midsystolic murmur heard only in the pulmonic area is usually without clinical significance, while a somewhat louder murmur in the aortic area may indicate congenital aortic stenosis. In elderly patients, pulmonic flow murmurs are rare, while aortic systolic murmurs are common and may be due to aortic dilation, to a significant degree of valvular aortic stenosis, or to nonstenotic thickening of the aortic valve leaflets. Midsystolic aortic and pulmonic murmurs are intensified after amyl nitrite inhalation and during the cardiac cycle following a premature ventricular beat, while those due to mitral regurgitation are unchanged or softer. Aortic systolic murmurs are diminished by interventions that increase aortic impedance, such as transient arterial occlusion. Echocardiography or cardiac catheterization may be necessary to separate a prominent and exaggerated functional murmur from one due to congenital or acquired semilunar valve stenosis.

Early Systolic Murmurs These murmurs begin with the first heart sound and end in midsystole. In *large ventricular septal defects with pulmonary hypertension*, the shunting at the end of systole may be small or absent, resulting in an early systolic murmur. A similar murmur may occur with very small *muscular ventricular septal defects*, the shunt being interrupted in late systole. An early systolic murmur is a feature of *tricuspid regurgitation occurring in the absence of pulmonary hypertension*. This lesion is common in narcotics abusers with infective endocarditis, in whom a tall regurgitant right atrial *v* wave reaches the level of the normal right ventricular pressure in late systole, confining the murmur to early systole. Patients with acute mitral regurgitation into a noncompliant left atrium and a large *v* wave often have a loud early systolic murmur that diminishes as the pressure gradient between the left ventricle and left atrium decreases in late systole (Chap. 219).

Late Systolic Murmurs These murmurs are faint or moderately loud, high-pitched apical murmurs that start well after ejection and do not mask either heart sound. They are probably related to papillary muscle dysfunction caused by infarction or ischemia of these muscles or to their distortion by left ventricular dilation. They may appear only during angina but are common in patients with myocardial infarction or diffuse myocardial disease. Late systolic murmurs following midsystolic clicks are due to late systolic mitral regurgitation caused by prolapse of the mitral valve into the left atrium (Chap. 219).

DIASTOLIC MURMURS ■ **Early Diastolic Murmurs** (Figs. 209-4*E*, 209-5) These murmurs begin with or shortly after S_2, as soon as the corresponding ventricular pressure falls enough below that in the aorta or pulmonary artery. The high-pitched murmurs of aortic regurgitation or of pulmonic regurgitation due to pulmonary hypertension are generally decrescendo, since there is a progressive decline in the volume or rate of regurgitation during diastole. Faint, high-pitched murmurs of aortic regurgitation are difficult to hear unless they are specifically sought by applying firm pressure with the diaphragm over the left midsternal border while the patient sits leaning forward and holds a

breath in full expiration. The diastolic murmur of aortic regurgitation is enhanced by an acute elevation of the arterial pressure, such as occurs with handgrip exercise; it diminishes with a decrease in arterial pressure, as with amyl nitrite inhalation. The diastolic murmur of congenital pulmonic regurgitation without pulmonary hypertension is low- to medium-pitched. The onset of this murmur is delayed because the regurgitant flow is minimal at the onset of pulmonic valve closure when the reverse pressure gradient responsible for the regurgitation is negligible.

Middiastolic Murmurs These usually arise from the mitral or tricuspid valves, occur during early ventricular filling, and are due to disproportion between valve orifice size and flow rate. Such murmurs may be quite loud (grade III), despite only slight AV valve stenosis, when there is normal or increased blood flow. Conversely, the murmurs may be soft or even absent despite severe obstruction if the cardiac output is markedly reduced. When stenosis is marked, the diastolic murmur is prolonged, and the duration of the murmur is more reliable than its intensity as an index of the severity of valve obstruction.

The low-pitched, middiastolic murmur of mitral stenosis characteristically follows the OS (Fig. 209-4*F*). It should be specifically sought by placing the bell of the stethoscope at the site of the left ventricular impulse, which is best localized with the patient on the left side. Frequently, the murmur of mitral stenosis is present only at the left ventricular apex, and it may be increased in intensity by mild supine exercise or by inhalation of amyl nitrite. In tricuspid stenosis, the middiastolic murmur is localized to a relatively limited area along the left sternal edge and may be louder during inspiration.

Middiastolic murmurs may be generated across the mitral valve in cases of mitral regurgitation, patent ductus arteriosus, or ventricular septal defect, and across the tricuspid valve in cases of tricuspid regurgitation or atrial septal defect. These murmurs are related to the very rapid flow across an AV valve, usually follow an S_3 (Fig. 209-4*G*), and tend to occur with large left-to-right shunts or severe AV valve regurgitation. A soft middiastolic murmur may sometimes be heard in patients with acute rheumatic fever (Carey-Coombs murmur). It has been attributed to inflammation of the mitral valve cusps or excessive left atrial blood flow as a consequence of mitral regurgitation.

In acute, severe aortic regurgitation, the left ventricular diastolic pressure may exceed the left atrial pressure, resulting in a middiastolic murmur due to "diastolic mitral regurgitation." In severe, chronic aortic regurgitation, a murmur is frequently present that may be either middiastolic or presystolic (Austin-Flint murmur). This murmur appears to originate at the anterior mitral valve leaflet when blood enters the left ventricle simultaneously from both the aortic root and the left atrium.

Presystolic Murmurs (Fig. 209-4*A*) These murmurs begin during the period of ventricular filling that follows atrial contraction and therefore occur in sinus rhythm. They are usually due to AV valve stenosis and have the same quality as the middiastolic filling rumble, but they are usually crescendo, reaching peak intensity at the time of a loud S_1. The presystolic murmur corresponds to the AV valve gradient, which may be minimal until the moment of right or left atrial contraction. It is the presystolic murmur that is most characteristic of tricuspid stenosis and sinus rhythm. A right or left *atrial myxoma* may occasionally cause either middiastolic or presystolic murmurs that resemble the murmurs of mitral or tricuspid stenosis.

CONTINUOUS MURMURS These begin in systole, peak near S_2, and continue into all or part of diastole (Fig. 209-4*H*). These murmurs result from continuous flow due to a communication between high- and low-pressure areas that persists through the end of systole and the beginning of diastole. A *patent ductus arteriosus* causes a continuous murmur as long as the pressure in the pulmonary artery is much below that in the aorta. The murmur is intensified by elevation of the systemic arterial pressure. When pulmonary hypertension is present, the diastolic portion may disappear, leaving the murmur confined to systole. A continuous murmur is uncommon in cases of aortopulmonary septal defect, which usually is associated with severe pulmonary hypertension. Surgically produced connections and the subclavian–pulmonary artery anastomosis result in murmurs similar to that of a patent ductus.

Continuous murmurs may result from congenital or acquired *systemic arteriovenous fistula, coronary arteriovenous fistula*, anomalous origin of the left coronary artery from the pulmonary artery, and *communications between the sinus of Valsalva and the right side of the heart*. Continuous murmurs may also occur in patients with a small atrial septal defect with a high left atrial pressure. Murmurs associated with *pulmonary arteriovenous fistulas* may be continuous but are usually only systolic. Continuous murmurs may also be due to disturbances of flow pattern in constricted systemic (e.g., renal) or pulmonary arteries when marked pressure differences between the two sides of the narrow segment persist; a continuous murmur in the back may be present in *coarctation of the aorta*; *pulmonary embolism* may cause continuous murmurs in partially occluded vessels.

In nonconstricted arteries, continuous murmurs may be due to rapid flow through a tortuous bed. Such murmurs typically occur within the bronchial arterial collateral circulation in cyanotic patients with severe pulmonary outflow obstruction. The "mammary souffle," an innocent murmur heard over the breasts during late pregnancy and in the early postpartum period, may be systolic or continuous. The innocent cervical venous hum is a continuous murmur usually audible over the medial aspect of the right supraclavicular fossa with the patient upright. The hum is usually louder during diastole and can be abolished instantaneously by digital compression of the ipsilateral internal jugular vein. Transmission of a loud venous hum to the area below the clavicles may result in a mistaken diagnosis of patent ductus arteriosus.

PERICARDIAL FRICTION RUB These adventitious sounds may have presystolic, systolic, and early diastolic scratchy components and may be confused with a murmur or extracardiac sound when heard only in systole. A pericardial friction rub is best appreciated with the patient upright and leaning forward and may be accentuated during inspiration.

FURTHER READING

ABRAMS J: *Synopsis of Cardiac Physical Diagnosis*, 2d ed. Boston, Butterworth, 2001

BRAUNWALD E: The clinical examination, in *Primary Cardiology*, 2d ed, E Braunwald, L Goldman (eds). Philadelphia, Saunders, 2003

CHISNER MA: The diagnosis of heart disease by clinical assessment alone. Curr Probl Cardiol 26:285, 2001

CHOONG CY et al: Prevalence of valvular regurgitation by Doppler echocardiography in patients with structurally normal hearts by 2-dimensional echocardiography. Am Heart J 117:636, 1989

CLEMENT DL, COHN JN: Salvaging the history, physical examination and doctor-patient relationship in a technological cardiology environment. J Am Coll Cardiol 33:892, 1999

O'ROURKE RA: Approach to a patient with a heart murmur, in *Primary Cardiology*, 2d ed, E Braunwald, L Goldman (eds). Philadelphia, Saunders, 2003

PERLOFF JK (ed): *Physical Examination of the Heart and Circulation*, 3d ed. Philadelphia, Saunders, 2000

VLACHOPOULOUS C, O'ROURKE RA: Genesis of the normal and abnormal arterial pulse. Curr Probl Cardiol 25:297, 2000

210 ELECTROCARDIOGRAPHY
Ary L. Goldberger

The electrocardiogram (ECG or EKG) is a graphic recording of electric potentials generated by the heart. The signals are detected by means of metal electrodes attached to the extremities and chest wall and are then amplified and recorded by the electrocardiograph. ECG *leads* actually display the instantaneous *differences* in potential between these electrodes.

The clinical utility of the ECG derives from its immediate availability as a noninvasive, inexpensive, and highly versatile test. In addition to its use in detecting arrhythmias, conduction disturbances, and myocardial ischemia, electrocardiography may reveal other findings related to life-threatening metabolic disturbances (e.g., hyperkalemia) or increased susceptibility to sudden cardiac death (e.g., QT prolongation syndromes). The advent of coronary thrombolysis or angioplasty in the early therapy of acute myocardial infarction (Chap. 228) has refocused particular attention on the sensitivity and specificity of ECG signs of myocardial ischemia.

ELECTROPHYSIOLOGY (See also Chaps. 213 and 214)

Depolarization of the heart is the initiating event for cardiac contraction. The electric currents that spread through the heart are produced by three components: cardiac pacemaker cells, specialized conduction tissue, and the heart muscle itself. The ECG, however, records only the depolarization (stimulation) and repolarization (recovery) potentials generated by the atrial and ventricular myocardium.

The depolarization stimulus for the normal heartbeat originates in the *sinoatrial* (SA) *node* (Fig. 210-1), or *sinus node*, a collection of *pacemaker cells*. These cells fire spontaneously; that is, they exhibit *automaticity*. The first phase of cardiac electrical activation is the spread of the depolarization wave through the right and left atria, followed by atrial contraction. Next, the impulse stimulates pacemaker and specialized conduction tissues in the atrioventricular (AV) nodal and His-bundle areas; together, these two regions constitute the AV junction. The bundle of His bifurcates into two main branches, the right and left bundles, which rapidly transmit depolarization wavefronts to the right and left ventricular myocardium by way of Purkinje fibers. The main left bundle bifurcates into two primary subdivisions, a left anterior fascicle and a left posterior fascicle. The depolarization wavefronts then spread through the ventricular wall, from endocardium to epicardium, triggering ventricular contraction.

Since the cardiac depolarization and repolarization waves have direction and magnitude, they can be represented by vectors. *Vectorcardiograms* that measure and display these instantaneous potentials are no longer used much in clinical practice. However, the general principles of vector analysis remain fundamental to understanding the genesis of normal and pathologic ECG waveforms. Vector analysis illustrates a central concept of electrocardiography—that the ECG re-

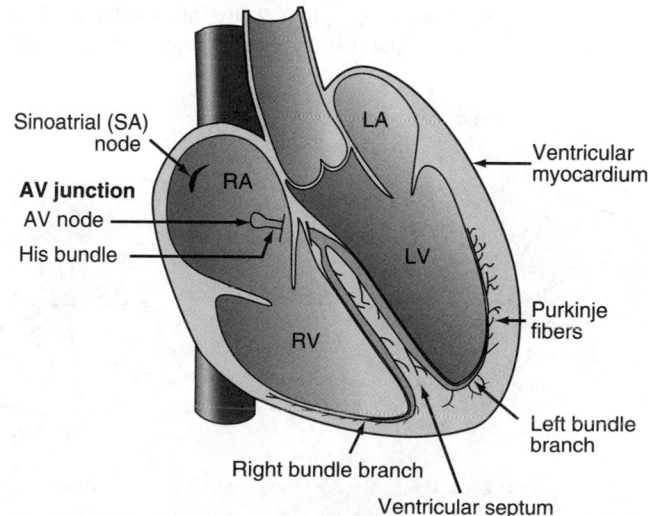

FIGURE 210-1 Schematic of the cardiac conduction system.

FIGURE 210-2 Basic ECG waveforms and intervals. Not shown is the R-R interval, the time between consecutive QRS complexes.

cords the complex spatial and temporal summation of electrical potentials from multiple myocardial fibers conducted to the surface of the body. This principle accounts for inherent limitations in both ECG *sensitivity* (activity from certain cardiac regions may be canceled out or may be too weak to be recorded) and *specificity* (the same vectorial sum can result from either a selective gain or a loss of forces in opposite directions).

ECG WAVEFORMS AND INTERVALS

The ECG waveforms are labeled alphabetically, beginning with the P wave, which represents atrial depolarization (Fig. 210-2). The QRS complex represents ventricular depolarization, and the ST-T-U complex (ST segment, T wave, and U wave) represents ventricular repolarization. The J point is the junction between the end of the QRS complex and the beginning of the ST segment. Atrial repolarization is usually too low in amplitude to be detected, but it may become apparent in such conditions as acute pericarditis or atrial infarction.

The QRS-T waveforms of the surface ECG correspond in a general way with the different phases of simultaneously obtained ventricular *action potentials*, the intracellular recordings from single myocardial fibers (see Fig. 213-2). The rapid upstroke (phase 0) of the action potential corresponds to the onset of QRS. The plateau (phase 2) corresponds to the isoelectric ST segment, and active repolarization (phase 3) to the inscription of the T wave. Factors that decrease the slope of phase 0 by impairing the influx of Na^+ (e.g., drugs such as flecainide or procainamide, or hyperkalemia) tend to increase QRS duration. Conditions that prolong phase 2 (use of amiodarone, hypocalcemia) increase the QT interval. In contrast, shortening of ventric-

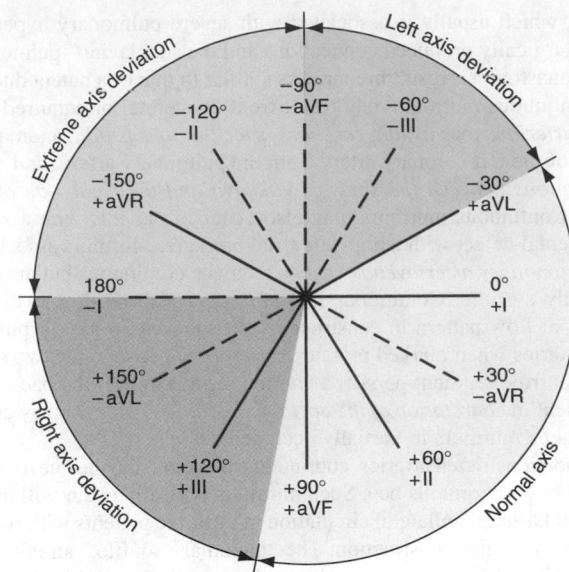

FIGURE 210-4 The frontal plane (extremity or limb) leads are represented on a hexaxial diagram. Each ECG lead has a specific spatial orientation and polarity. The positive pole of each lead axis (*solid line*) and negative pole (*hatched line*) are designated by their angular position relative to the positive pole of lead I (0°). The mean electrical axis of the QRS complex is measured with respect to this display.

ular repolarization (phase 2), as by digitalis administration or hypercalcemia, abbreviates the ST segment.

The electrocardiogram is ordinarily recorded on special graph paper which is divided into 1-mm² gridlike boxes. Since the ECG paper speed is generally 25 mm/s, the smallest (1 mm) horizontal divisions correspond to 0.04 s (40 ms), with heavier lines at intervals of 0.20 s (200 ms). Vertically, the ECG graph measures the amplitude of a given wave or deflection (1 mV = 10 mm with standard calibration; the voltage criteria for hypertrophy mentioned below are given in millimeters). There are four major ECG intervals: R-R, PR, QRS, and QT (Fig. 210-2). The heart rate (beats per minute) can be readily computed from the interbeat (R-R) interval by dividing the number of large (0.20 s) time units between consecutive R waves into 300 or the number of small (0.04 s) units into 1500. The PR interval measures the time (normally 120 to 200 ms) between atrial and ventricular depolarization, which includes the physiologic delay imposed by stimulation of cells in the AV junction area. The QRS interval (normally 100 ms or less) reflects the duration of ventricular depolarization. The QT interval includes both ventricular depolarization and repolarization times and varies inversely with the heart rate. A rate-related ("corrected") QT interval, QT_c, can be calculated as $QT/\sqrt{R\text{-}R}$ and normally is ≤0.44 s.

The QRS complex is subdivided into specific deflections or waves. If the initial QRS deflection in a given lead is negative, it is termed a *Q wave*; the first positive deflection is termed an *R wave*. A negative deflection after an R wave is an *S wave*. Subsequent positive or negative waves are labeled R′ and S′, respectively. Lowercase letters (qrs) are used for waves of relatively small amplitude. An entirely negative QRS complex is termed a *QS wave*.

ECG LEADS

The 12 conventional ECG leads record the difference in potential between electrodes placed on the surface of the body. These leads are divided into two groups: six extremity (limb) leads and six chest (precordial) leads. The extremity leads record potentials transmitted onto the *frontal plane* (Fig. 210-3A), and the chest leads record potentials transmitted onto the *horizontal plane* (Fig. 210-3B). The six extremity leads are further subdivided into three *bipolar leads* (I, II, and III) and three *unipolar*

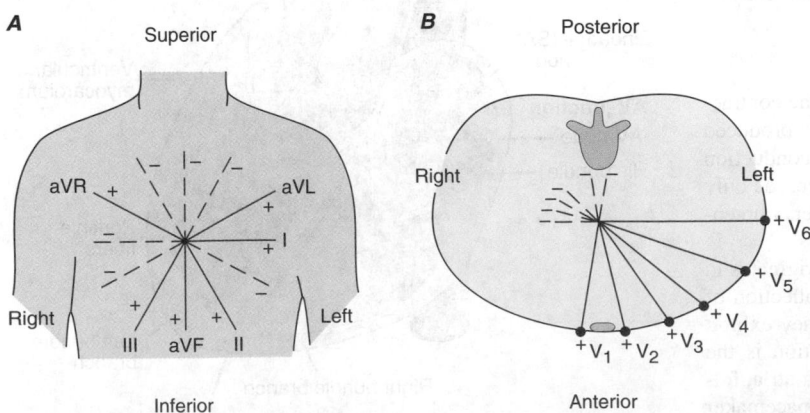

FIGURE 210-3 The six frontal plane (*A*) and six horizontal plane (*B*) leads provide a three-dimensional representation of cardiac electrical activity.

FIGURE 210-5 The horizontal plane (chest or precordial) leads are obtained with electrodes in the locations shown.

leads (aVR, aVL, and aVF). Each bipolar lead measures the difference in potential between electrodes at two extremities: lead I = left arm − right arm voltages, lead II = left leg − right arm, and lead III = left leg − left arm. The unipolar leads measure the voltage (V) at one locus relative to an electrode (called the *central terminal* or *indifferent electrode*) that has approximately zero potential. Thus, aVR = right arm, aVL = left arm, and aVF = left leg (foot). The lowercase *a* indicates that these unipolar potentials are electrically augmented by 50%. The right leg electrode functions as a ground. The spatial orientation and polarity of the six frontal plane leads is represented on the hexaxial diagram (Fig. 210-4).

The six chest leads (Fig. 210-5) are unipolar recordings obtained by electrodes in the following positions: lead V_1, fourth intercostal space, just to the right of the sternum; lead V_2, fourth intercostal space, just to the left of the sternum; lead V_3, midway between V_2 and V_4; lead V_4, midclavicular line, fifth intercostal space; lead V_5, anterior axillary line, same level as V_4; and lead V_6, midaxillary line, same level as V_4 and V_5.

Together, the frontal and horizontal plane electrodes provide a three-dimensional representation of cardiac electrical activity. Each lead can be likened to a different camera angle "looking" at the same events—atrial and ventricular depolarization and repolarization—from different spatial orientations. The conventional 12-lead ECG can be supplemented with additional leads under special circumstances. For example, right precordial leads V_3R, V_4R, etc. are useful in detecting evidence of acute right ventricular ischemia. Bedside monitors and ambulatory ECG (Holter) recordings usually employ only one or two modified leads. →*Intracardiac electrocardiography and electrophysiologic testing are discussed in Chaps. 213 and 214.*

The ECG leads are configured so that a positive (upright) deflection is recorded in a lead if a wave of depolarization spreads toward the positive pole of that lead, and a negative deflection if the wave spreads toward the negative pole. If the mean orientation of the depolarization vector is at right angles to a given lead axis, a biphasic (equally positive and negative) deflection will be recorded.

GENESIS OF THE NORMAL ECG

P WAVE

The normal atrial depolarization vector is oriented downward and toward the subject's left, reflecting the spread of depolarization from the sinus node to the right and then the left atrial myocardium. Since this vector points toward the positive pole of lead II and toward the negative pole of lead aVR, the normal P wave will be positive in lead II and negative in lead aVR. By contrast, activation of the atria from an ectopic pacemaker in the lower part of either atrium or in the AV junction region may produce retrograde P waves (negative in lead II, positive in lead aVR).

QRS COMPLEX

Normal ventricular depolarization proceeds as a rapid, continuous spread of activation wavefronts. This complex process can be divided into two major, sequential phases, and each phase can be represented by a mean vector (Fig. 210-6). The first phase is depolarization of the interventricular septum from the left to the right and anteriorly (vector 1). The second results from the simultaneous depolarization of the right and left ventricles; it is normally dominated by the more massive left ventricle, so that vector 2 points leftward and posteriorly. Therefore, a right precordial lead (V_1) will record this biphasic depolarization process with a small positive deflection (septal r wave) followed by a larger negative deflection (S wave). A left precordial lead, e.g., V_6, will record the same sequence with a small negative deflection (septal q wave) followed by a relatively tall positive deflection (R wave). Intermediate leads show a relative increase in R-wave amplitude (normal R-wave progression) and a decrease in S-wave amplitude progressing across the chest from the right to left. The precordial lead where the R and S waves are of approximately equal amplitude is referred to as the *transition zone* (usually V_3 or V_4) (Fig. 210-7).

The QRS pattern in the extremity leads may vary considerably from one normal subject to another depending on the *electrical axis* of the QRS, which describes the mean orientation of the QRS vector with reference to the six frontal plane leads. Normally, the QRS axis ranges from −30° to +100° (Fig. 210-4). An axis more negative than −30° is referred to as *left axis deviation*, while an axis more positive than +100° is referred to as *right axis deviation*. Left axis deviation may

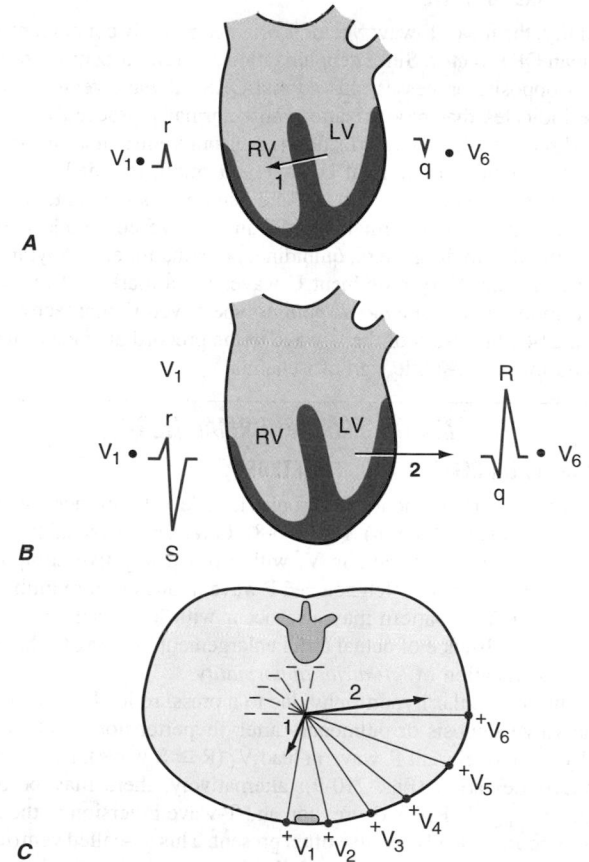

FIGURE 210-6 Ventricular depolarization can be divided into two major phases, each represented by a vector. *A.* The first phase (*arrow 1*) denotes depolarization of the ventricular septum, beginning on the left side and spreading to the right. This process is represented by a small "septal" r wave in lead V_1 and a small septal q wave in lead V_6. *B.* Simultaneous depolarization of the left and right ventricles (LV and RV) constitutes the second phase. Vector 2 is oriented to the left and posteriorly, reflecting the electrical predominance of the LV. *C.* Vectors (*arrows*) representing these two phases are shown in reference to the horizontal plane leads. (*After Goldberger, 1999.*)

FIGURE 210-7 Normal electrocardiogram from a healthy subject. Sinus rhythm is present with a heart rate of 75 beats per minute. PR interval is 0.16 s; QRS interval (duration) is 0.08 s; QT interval is 0.36 s; the mean QRS axis is about +70°. The precordial leads show normal R-wave progression with the transition zone (R wave = S wave) in lead V_3.

occur as a normal variant but is more commonly associated with left ventricular hypertrophy, a block in the anterior fascicle of the left bundle system (left anterior fascicular block or hemiblock), or inferior myocardial infarction. Right axis deviation may also occur as a normal variant (particularly in children and young adults); as a spurious finding due to reversal of the left and right arm electrodes; or in conditions such as right ventricular overload (acute or chronic), infarction of the lateral wall of the left ventricle, dextrocardia, left pneumothorax, or left posterior fascicular block.

T WAVE AND U WAVE

Normally, the mean T-wave vector is oriented roughly concordant with the mean QRS vector. Since depolarization and repolarization are electrically opposite processes, this normal QRS–T-wave vector concordance indicates that repolarization must normally proceed in the reverse direction from depolarization (i.e., from ventricular epicardium to endocardium). The normal U wave is a small, rounded deflection (≤1 mm) that follows the T wave and usually has the same polarity as the T wave. An abnormal increase in U-wave amplitude is most commonly due to drugs (e.g., quinidine, procainamide, disopyramide) or hypokalemia. Very prominent U waves are a marker of increased susceptibility to the *torsades de pointes* type of ventricular tachycardia (Chap. 214). Inversion of the U wave in the precordial leads is abnormal and may be a subtle sign of ischemia.

MAJOR ECG ABNORMALITIES

CARDIAC ENLARGEMENT AND HYPERTROPHY

Right atrial overload (acute or chronic) may lead to an increase in P-wave amplitude (≥2.5 mm) (Fig. 210-8). Left atrial overload typically produces a biphasic P wave in V_1 with a broad negative component or a broad (≥120 ms), often notched P wave in one or more limb leads (Fig. 210-8). This pattern may also occur with left atrial conduction delays in the absence of actual atrial enlargement, leading to the more general designation of *left atrial abnormality*.

Right ventricular hypertrophy due to a pressure load (as from pulmonic valve stenosis or pulmonary artery hypertension) is characterized by a relatively tall R wave in lead V_1 (R ≥ S wave), usually with right axis deviation (Fig. 210-9); alternatively, there may be a qR pattern in V_1 or V_3R. ST depression and T-wave inversion in the right to midprecordial leads are also often present. This so-called ventricular strain pattern is attributed to repolarization abnormalities in hypertrophied muscle. Right ventricular hypertrophy due to ostium secundum–type atrial septal defects, with the accompanying right ventricular volume overload, is commonly associated with an incomplete or complete right bundle branch block pattern with a rightward QRS axis.

Acute cor pulmonale due to pulmonary embolism (Chap. 244), for example, may be associated with a normal ECG or a variety of abnormalities. Sinus tachycardia is the most common arrhythmia, al-

though other tachyarrhythmias, such as atrial fibrillation or flutter, may occur. The QRS axis may shift to the right, sometimes in concert with the so-called $S_1Q_3T_3$ pattern (prominence of the S wave in lead I, Q wave in lead III, with T-wave inversion in lead III). Acute right ventricular dilation may also be associated with poor R-wave progression and T-wave inversions in V_1 to V_4 (right ventricular "strain") simulating acute anterior infarction. A right ventricular conduction disturbance may appear.

Chronic cor pulmonale due to obstructive lung disease (Chap. 220) usually does not produce the classic ECG patterns of right ventricular hypertrophy noted above. Instead of tall right precordial R waves, chronic lung disease more typically is associated with small R waves in right to midprecordial leads (poor R-wave progression) due in part to downward displacement of the diaphragm and the heart. Low-voltage complexes are commonly present, owing to hyperaeration of the lungs.

A number of different voltage criteria for *left ventricular hypertrophy* (Fig. 210-9) have been proposed on the basis of the presence of tall left precordial R waves and deep right precordial S waves [e.g., $SV_1 + (RV_5$ or $RV_6) ≥ 35$ mm; or $(RV_5$ or $RV_6) ≥ 25$ mm]. Repolarization abnormalities (ST depression with T-wave inversions) may

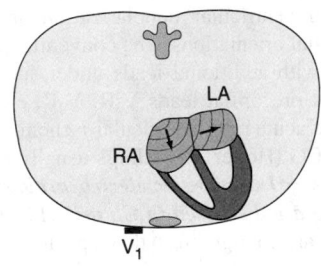

	Normal	Right	Left
II	RA ↘ ↙ LA	RA ∧ LA ↘	RA ↗ ∧∧ LA
V_1	RA ⌒ LA	RA ∧ LA	RA ⌒ LA

FIGURE 210-8 Right atrial (RA) overload may cause tall, peaked P waves in the limb or precordial leads. Left atrial (LA) abnormality may cause broad, often notched P waves in the limb leads and a biphasic P wave in lead V_1 with a prominent negative component representing delayed depolarization of the LA. (*After MK Park, WG Guntheroth: How to Read Pediatric ECGs, 3d ed. St. Louis, Mosby–Year Book, 1992.*)

QRS in hypertrophy   **Main QRS vector**

V$_1$ V$_6$

Normal

LVH

RVH   or   or

V$_6$

V$_1$

FIGURE 210-9 Left ventricular hypertrophy (LVH) increases the amplitude of electrical forces directed to the left and posteriorly. In addition, repolarization abnormalities may cause ST segment depression and T-wave inversion in leads with a prominent R wave ("strain" pattern). Right ventricular hypertrophy (RVH) may shift the QRS vector to the right; this effect usually is associated with an R, RS, or qR complex in lead V$_1$. T-wave inversions may be present in right precordial leads ("strain" pattern).

also appear (left ventricular "strain" pattern) in leads with prominent R waves. However, prominent precordial voltages may occur as a normal variant, especially in athletic or young individuals. Left ventricular hypertrophy may increase limb lead voltage (e.g., RaVL $\geq$ 11 to 13 mm, RaVF $\geq$ 20 mm; R$_1$ + S$_{III}$ $\geq$ 25 mm) with or without increased precordial voltage. The presence of left atrial abnormality increases the likelihood of underlying left ventricular hypertrophy in cases with borderline voltage criteria. Left ventricular hypertrophy often progresses to incomplete or complete left bundle branch block. The sensitivity of conventional voltage criteria for left ventricular hypertrophy is decreased in obese persons and in smokers. ECG evidence for left ventricular hypertrophy is a major noninvasive marker of increased risk of cardiovascular morbidity and mortality, including sudden cardiac death. However, because of false-positive and false-negative diagnoses, the ECG is of limited utility in diagnosing atrial or ventricular enlargement. More definitive information is provided by echocardiography (Chap. 211).

BUNDLE BRANCH BLOCKS

Intrinsic impairment of conduction in either the right or left bundle system (intraventricular conduction disturbances) leads to prolongation of the QRS interval. With complete bundle branch blocks the QRS interval is $\geq$120 ms in duration; with incomplete blocks the QRS interval is between 100 and 120 ms. The QRS vector is usually oriented in the direction of the myocardial region where depolarization is delayed (Fig. 210-10). Thus, with right bundle branch block, the terminal QRS vector is oriented anteriorly and to the right (rSR' in V$_1$ and qRS in V$_6$, typically). Left bundle branch block alters both early and later phases of ventricular depolarization. The major QRS vector is directed to the left and posteriorly. In addition, the normal early left-to-right pattern of septal activation is disrupted such that septal depolarization proceeds from right to left as well. As a result, left bundle branch block generates wide, predominantly negative (QS) complexes in lead V$_1$ and entirely positive (R) complexes in lead V$_6$. A pattern identical to that of left bundle branch block, preceded by a sharp spike,

is seen in most cases of electronic right ventricular pacing because of the relative delay in left ventricular activation.

Bundle branch block may occur in a variety of conditions. In subjects without structural heart disease, right bundle branch block is seen more commonly than left bundle branch block. Right bundle branch block also occurs with heart disease, both congenital (e.g., atrial septal defect) and acquired (e.g., valvular, ischemic). Left bundle branch block is often a marker of one of four underlying conditions: coronary heart disease (often with impaired left ventricular function), hypertensive heart disease, aortic valve disease, and cardiomyopathy. Bundle branch blocks may be chronic or intermittent. A bundle branch block may be rate-related; for example, it often occurs when the heart rate exceeds some critical value.

Bundle branch blocks and depolarization abnormalities secondary to artificial pacemakers not only affect ventricular depolarization (QRS) but are also characteristically associated with *secondary repolarization* (ST-T) abnormalities. With bundle branch blocks, the T wave is typically opposite in polarity to the last deflection of the QRS (Fig. 210-10). This discordance of the QRS–T-wave vectors is caused by the altered sequence of repolarization that occurs secondary to altered depolarization. In contrast, *primary repolarization* abnormalities are independent of QRS changes and are related instead to actual alterations in the electrical properties of the myocardial fibers themselves (e.g., in the resting membrane potential or action potential duration), not just to changes in the sequence of repolarization. Ischemia, electrolyte imbalance, and drugs such as digitalis all cause such primary ST–T-wave changes. Primary and secondary T-wave changes may coexist. For example, T-wave inversions in the right precordial leads with left bundle branch block or in the left precordial leads with right bundle branch block may be important markers of underlying ischemia or other abnormalities.

Partial blocks ("hemiblocks") in the left bundle system (left anterior or posterior fascicular blocks) generally do not prolong the QRS duration substantially but instead are associated with shifts in the frontal plane QRS axis (leftward or rightward, respectively). More complex combinations of fascicular and bundle branch blocks may occur involving the left and right bundle system. Examples of *bifascicular*

FIGURE 210-10 Comparison of typical QRS-T patterns in right bundle branch block (RBBB) and left bundle branch block (LBBB) with the normal pattern in leads V$_1$ and V$_6$. Note the secondary T-wave inversions (*arrows*) in leads with an rSR' complex with RBBB and in leads with a wide R wave with LBBB.

FIGURE 210-11 Acute ischemia causes a current of injury. With predominant subendocardial ischemia (*A*), the resultant ST vector will be directed toward the inner layer of the affected ventricle and the ventricular cavity. Overlying leads therefore will record ST depression. With ischemia involving the outer ventricular layer (*B*) (transmural or epicardial injury), the ST vector will be directed outward. Overlying leads will record ST elevation.

block include right bundle branch block and left posterior fascicular block, right bundle branch block with left anterior fascicular block, and complete left bundle branch block. Chronic bifascicular block in an asymptomatic individual is associated with a relatively low risk of progression to high-degree AV heart block. In contrast, new bifascicular block with acute anterior myocardial infarction carries a much greater risk of complete heart block. Alternation of right and left bundle branch block is a sign of *trifascicular disease*. However, the presence of a prolonged PR interval and bifascicular block does not necessarily indicate trifascicular involvement, since this combination may arise with AV node disease and bifascicular block. Intraventricular conduction delays can also be caused by extrinsic (toxic) factors that slow ventricular conduction, particularly hyperkalemia or drugs (class 1 antiarrhythmic agents, tricyclic antidepressants, phenothiazines).

Prolongation of QRS duration does not necessarily indicate a conduction delay but may be due to *preexcitation* of the ventricles via a bypass tract, as in the Wolff-Parkinson-White (WPW) syndrome (Chap. 214) and related variants. The diagnostic triad of WPW consists of a wide QRS complex associated with a relatively short PR interval and slurring of the initial part of the QRS (delta wave), the latter effect due to aberrant activation of ventricular myocardium. The presence of a bypass tract predisposes to reentrant supraventricular tachyarrhythmias.

MYOCARDIAL ISCHEMIA AND INFARCTION (See also Chap. 228)

The ECG is a cornerstone in the diagnosis of acute and chronic ischemic heart disease. The findings depend on several key factors: the nature of the process [reversible (i.e., ischemia) versus irreversible (i.e., infarction)], the duration (acute versus chronic), extent (transmural versus subendocardial), and localization (anterior versus inferoposterior), as well as the presence of other underlying abnormalities (ventricular hypertrophy, conduction defects).

Ischemia exerts complex time-dependent effects on the electrical properties of myocardial cells. Severe, acute ischemia lowers the resting membrane potential and shortens the duration of the action potential. Such changes cause a voltage gradient between normal and ischemic zones. As a consequence, current flows between these regions. These currents of injury are represented on the surface ECG by deviation of the ST segment (Fig. 210-11). When the acute ischemia is *transmural*, the ST vector is usually shifted in the direction of the outer (epicardial) layers, producing ST elevations and sometimes, in the earliest stages of ischemia, tall, positive so-called hyperacute T waves over the ischemic zone. With ischemia confined primarily to the *subendocardium*, the ST vector typically shifts toward the subendocardium and ventricular cavity, so that overlying (e.g., anterior precordial) leads show ST-segment depression (with ST elevation in lead aVR). Multiple factors affect the amplitude of acute ischemic ST deviations. Profound ST elevation or depression in multiple leads usually indicates very severe ischemia. From a clinical viewpoint, the division of acute myocardial infarction into ST segment elevation and non-ST elevation types is useful since the efficacy of acute reperfusion therapy is limited to the former group.

The ECG leads are more helpful in localizing regions of ST elevation than non-ST elevation ischemia. For example, acute transmural anterior (including apical and lateral) wall ischemia is reflected by ST

elevations or increased T-wave positivity (Fig. 210-12) in one or more of the precordial leads (V_1 to V_6) and leads I and aVL. Inferior wall ischemia produces changes in leads II, III, and aVF. Posterior wall ischemia may be indirectly recognized by *reciprocal* ST depressions in leads V_1 to V_3. Prominent reciprocal ST depressions in these leads also occur with certain inferior wall infarcts, particularly those with posterior or lateral wall extension. Right ventricular ischemia usually produces ST elevations in right-sided chest leads (Fig. 210-5). When ischemic ST elevations occur as the earliest sign of acute infarction, they are typically followed within a period ranging from hours to days by evolving T-wave inversions and often by Q waves occurring in the same lead distribution. (T-wave inversions due to evolving or chronic ischemia correlate with prolongation of repolarization and are often associated with QT lengthening.) Reversible transmural ischemia, for example, due to coronary vasospasm (Prinzmetal's variant angina), may cause transient ST-segment elevations without development of Q waves. Depending on the severity and duration of such ischemia, the ST elevations may either resolve completely in minutes or be followed by T-wave inversions that persist for hours or even days. Patients with ischemic chest pain who present with deep T-wave inversions in multiple precordial leads (e.g., V_1 to V_4) with or without cardiac enzyme elevations typically have severe obstruction in the left anterior descending coronary artery system (Fig. 210-13). In contrast, patients whose baseline ECG already shows abnormal T-wave inversions may develop T-wave normalization (pseudonormalization) during episodes of acute transmural ischemia.

With infarction, depolarization (QRS) changes often accompany repolarization (ST-T) abnormalities. Necrosis of sufficient myocardial tissue may lead to decreased R-wave amplitude or abnormal Q waves in the anterior or inferior leads (Fig. 210-14). Previously, abnormal Q waves were considered to be markers of transmural myocardial in-

FIGURE 210-12 Hyperacute phase of anteroseptal myocardial infarction (MI). Note the tall positive T waves (V_2 to V_3) along with ST-segment elevations and Q waves (V_1 to V_3).

FIGURE 210-13 Severe anterior wall ischemia (with or without infarction) may cause prominent T-wave inversions in the precordial leads. This pattern is usually associated with a high-grade stenosis of the left anterior descending coronary artery.

farction, while subendocardial infarcts were thought not to produce Q waves. However, careful ECG-pathology correlative studies have indicated that transmural infarcts may occur without Q waves and that subendocardial (nontransmural) infarcts may sometimes be associated with Q waves. Therefore, infarcts are more appropriately classified as "Q-wave" or "non-Q-wave." The major acute ECG changes in syndromes of ischemic heart disease are schematically summarized in Fig. 210-15. Loss of depolarization forces due to posterior or lateral infarction may cause reciprocal increases in R-wave amplitude in leads V_1 and V_2 without diagnostic Q waves in any of the conventional leads. Atrial infarction may be associated with PR-segment deviations due to an atrial current of injury, changes in P-wave morphology, or atrial arrhythmias. In the weeks and months following infarction, these ECG changes may persist or begin to resolve. Complete normalization of the ECG following Q-wave infarction is uncommon but may occur, particularly with smaller infarcts. In contrast, ST-segment elevations that persist for several weeks or more after a Q-wave infarct usually correlate with a severe underlying wall motion disorder (akinetic or dyskinetic zone), although not necessarily a frank ventricular aneurysm.

ECG changes due to ischemia may occur spontaneously or may be provoked by various exercise protocols (stress electrocardiography) (Chap. 226). In patients with severe ischemic heart disease, exercise testing is most likely to elicit signs of subendocardial ischemia (horizontal or downsloping ST depression in multiple leads). ST-segment elevation during exercise is most often observed after a Q-wave infarct. This repolarization change does not necessarily indicate active ischemia but correlates strongly with the presence of an underlying ventricular wall motion abnormality. However, in patients *without* prior

infarction, transient ST-segment elevation with exercise is a reliable sign of transmural ischemia.

The ECG has important limitations in both sensitivity and specificity in the diagnosis of ischemic heart disease. Although a single normal ECG does not exclude ischemia or even acute infarction, a normal ECG *throughout* the course of an acute infarct is distinctly uncommon. Prolonged chest pain without diagnostic ECG changes, therefore, should always prompt a careful search for other noncoronary causes of chest pain (Chap. 12). Furthermore, the diagnostic changes of acute or evolving ischemia are often masked by the presence of left bundle branch block, electronic ventricular pacemaker patterns, and WPW preexcitation. On the other hand, clinicians may overdiagnose ischemia or infarction based on the presence of ST-segment elevations or depressions, T-wave inversions, tall positive T waves, or Q waves *not* related to ischemic heart disease (pseudoinfarct patterns). For example, ST-segment elevations simulating ischemia may occur with acute pericarditis (Fig. 210-16) or myocarditis, as a normal variant ("early repolarization" pattern), or in a variety of other conditions (Table 210-1). Similarly, tall, positive T waves do not invariably represent hyperacute ischemic changes but may also be caused by normal variants, hyperkalemia, cerebrovascular injury, and left ventricular volume overload due to mitral or aortic regurgitation, among other causes. ST-segment elevations and tall, positive T waves are common findings in leads V_1 and V_2 in left bundle branch block or left ventricular hypertrophy in the absence of ischemia. The differential diagnosis of Q waves (Table 210-2) includes physiologic or positional variants, ventricular hypertrophy, acute or chronic noncoronary myocardial injury, hypertrophic cardiomyopathy, and ventricular conduction disorders. Digitalis, ventricular hypertrophy, hypokalemia, and a variety of other

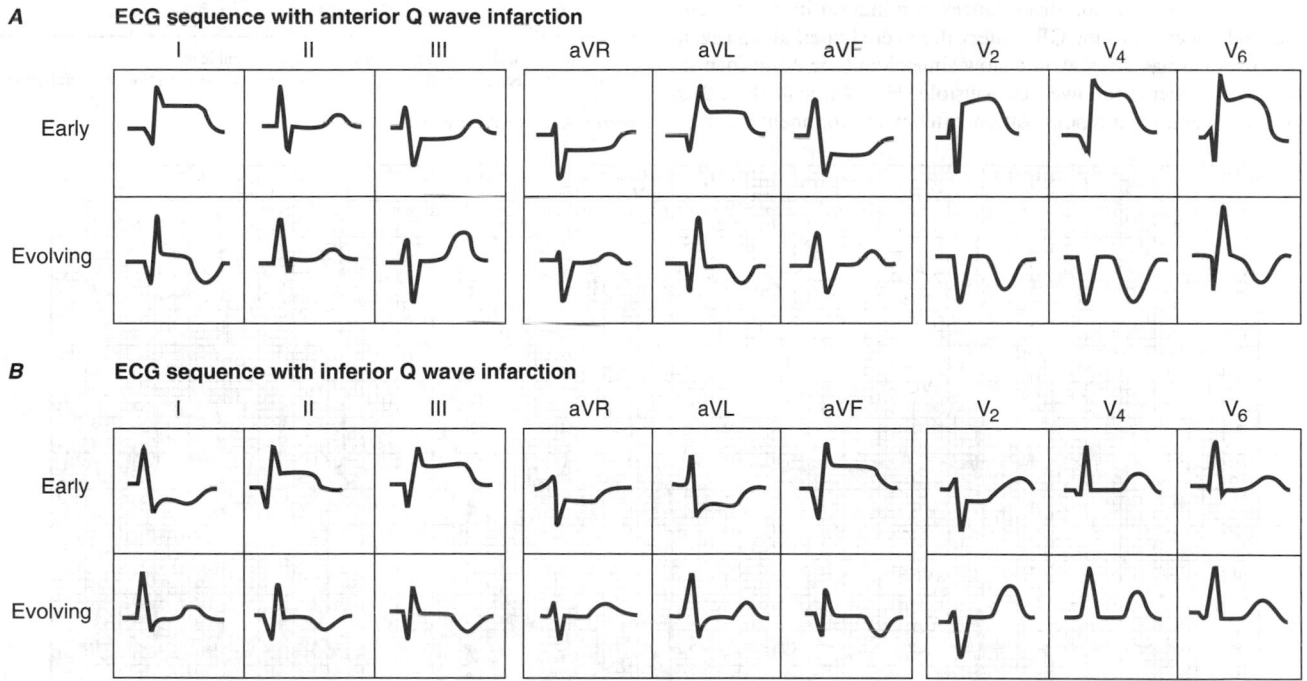

FIGURE 210-14 54Sequence of depolarization and repolarization changes with (*A*) acute anterior and (*B*) acute inferior wall Q-wave infarctions. With anterior infarcts, ST elevation in leads I, aVL, and the precordial leads may be accompanied by reciprocal ST depressions in leads II, III, and aVF. Conversely, acute inferior (or posterior) infarcts may be associated with reciprocal ST depressions in leads V_1 to V_3. (*After Goldberger, 1999.*)

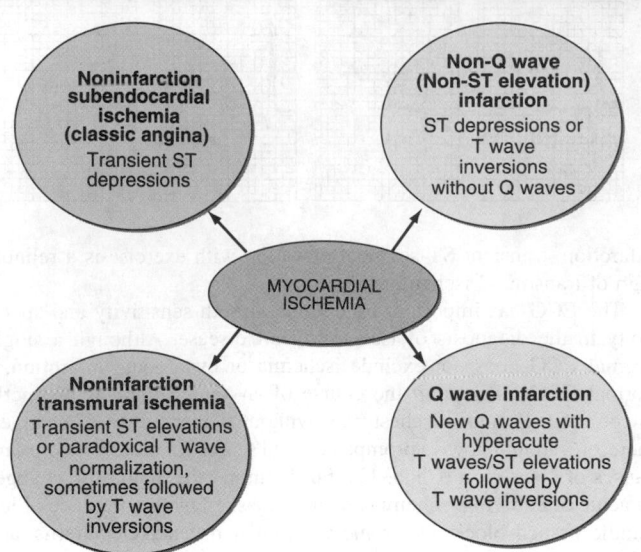

FIGURE 210-15 Variability of ECG patterns with acute myocardial ischemia. The ECG also may be normal or nonspecifically abnormal. Furthermore, these categorizations are not mutually exclusive. For example, a non-ST elevation infarct may evolve into a Q-wave infarct; ST elevations may be followed by a non-Q-wave infarct; or ST depressions and T-wave inversions may be followed by a Q-wave infarct. (*After Goldberger, 1991.*)

factors may cause ST-segment depression mimicking subendocardial ischemia. Prominent T-wave inversion may occur with ventricular hypertrophy, cardiomyopathy, myocarditis, and cerebrovascular injury (particularly intracranial bleeds; Fig. 210-17), among many other conditions.

METABOLIC FACTORS AND DRUG EFFECTS

A variety of metabolic and pharmacologic agents alter the ECG and, in particular, cause changes in repolarization (ST-T-U) and sometimes QRS prolongation. Certain life-threatening electrolyte disturbances may be diagnosed initially and monitored from the ECG. *Hyperkalemia* produces a sequence of changes usually beginning with narrowing and peaking (tenting) of the T waves. Further elevation of extracellular K^+ leads to AV conduction disturbances, diminution in P-wave amplitude, and widening of the QRS interval. Severe hyperkalemia eventually causes cardiac arrest with a slow sinusoidal type of mechanism ("sine-wave" pattern) followed by asystole. *Hypokalemia* (Fig. 210-17) prolongs ventricular repolarization, often with prominent U waves.

TABLE 210-1 *Differential Diagnosis of ST Segment Elevations*

Ischemia/myocardial infarction
    Noninfarction, transmural ischemia (Prinzmetal's angina pattern)
    Acute myocardial infarction
    Postmyocardial infarction (ventricular aneurysm pattern)
Acute pericarditis
Normal variant ("early repolarization" pattern)
Left ventricular hypertrophy/left bundle branch block[a]
Other (rarer)
    Brugada syndrome (right bundle branch block-like pattern with ST elevations in right precordial leads)[a]
    Class 1C antiarrhythmic drugs[a]
    DC cardioversion
    Hypercalcemia[a]
    Hyperkalemia[a]
    Hypothermia (J wave/Osborn wave)
    Myocardial injury
        Myocarditis
        Tumor invading left ventricle
        Trauma to ventricles

[a] Usually localized to V_1-V_2 or V_3
Source: Modified from Goldberger, 1999.

TABLE 210-2 *Differential Diagnosis of Q Waves (with Selected Examples)*

Physiologic or positional factors
1. Normal variant "septal" q waves
2. Normal variant Q waves in V_1 to V_2, aVL, III, and aVF
3. Left pneumothorax or dextrocardia: loss of lateral R-wave progression
Myocardial injury or infiltration
1. Acute processes: myocardial ischemia or infarction, myocarditis, hyperkalemia
2. Chronic processes: myocardial infarction, idiopathic cardiomyopathy, myocarditis, amyloid, tumor, sarcoid, scleroderma, Chagas' disease, echinococcus cyst
Ventricular hypertrophy/enlargement
1. Left ventricular (poor R-wave progression[a])
2. Right ventricular (reversed R-wave progression[b] or poor R-wave progression[a], particularly with chronic obstructive lung disease)
3. Hypertrophic cardiomyopathy (may simulate anterior, inferior, posterior, or lateral infarcts)
Conduction abnormalities
1. Left bundle branch block (poor R-wave progression[a])
2. Wolff-Parkinson-White patterns

[a] Small or absent R waves in the right to midprecordial leads.
[b] Progressive decrease in R-wave amplitude from V_1 to the mid- or lateral precordial leads.
Source: After Goldberger, 1991.

FIGURE 210-16 Acute pericarditis often produces diffuse ST-segment elevations (in this case in leads I, II, aVF, and V_2 to V_6) due to a ventricular current of injury. Note the characteristic PR-segment deviation (opposite in polarity to the ST segment) due to a concomitant atrial injury current.

Prolongation of the QT interval (Fig. 210-17) is also seen with drugs that increase the duration of the ventricular action potential—class 1A antiarrhythmic agents and related drugs (e.g., quinidine, disopyramide, procainamide, tricyclic antidepressants, phenothiazines) and class III agents (amiodarone, sotalol, ibutilide). Marked QT prolongation, sometimes with deep, wide T-wave inversions, may occur with intracranial bleeds, particularly subarachnoid hemorrhage ("CVA T-wave" pattern) (Fig. 210-17). Systemic *hypothermia* (Fig. 210-17) also prolongs repolarization, usually with a distinctive convex elevation of the J point (Osborn wave). *Hypocalcemia* typically prolongs the QT interval (ST portion), while *hypercalcemia* shortens it (Fig. 210-18). Digitalis glycosides also shorten the QT interval, often with a characteristic "scooping" of the ST–T-wave complex (*digitalis effect*).

Many other factors are associated with ECG changes, particularly alterations in ventricular repolarization. T-wave flattening, minimal T-wave inversions, or slight ST-segment depression ("nonspecific ST–T-wave changes") may occur with a variety of electrolyte and acid-base disturbances, a variety of infectious processes, central nervous system disorders, endocrine abnormalities, many drugs, ischemia, hypoxia, and virtually any type of cardiopulmonary abnormality. While subtle ST–T-wave changes may be markers of ischemia, transient nonspecific repolarization changes may also occur following a meal or with postural (orthostatic) change, hyperventilation, or exercise in healthy individuals.

ELECTRICAL ALTERNANS

Electrical alternans—a beat-to-beat alternation in one or more components of the ECG signal—is a common type of nonlinear cardiovascular response to a variety of hemodynamic and electrophysiologic perturbations. Total electrical alternans (P-QRS-T) with sinus tachycardia is a relatively specific sign of pericardial effusion, usually with cardiac tamponade. The mechanism relates to a periodic swinging motion of the heart in the effusion at a frequency exactly one-half the heart rate. Repolarization (ST-T) alternans is a sign of electrical instability and may precede ventricular tachyarrhythmias.

CLINICAL INTERPRETATION OF THE ECG

Accurate analysis of ECGs requires thoroughness and care. The patient's age, gender, and clinical status should always be taken into account. For example, T-wave inversions in leads V_1 to V_3 are more

Hypokalemia   **Hypothermia**   **Quinidine excess**

Tricyclic overdose   **Subarachnoid hemorrhage**

FIGURE 210-17 A variety of metabolic derangements, drug effects, and other factors may prolong ventricular repolarization with QT prolongation or prominent U waves. Repolarization prolongation, particularly if due to hypokalemia or pharmacologic agents, indicates increased susceptibility to *torsades de pointes* type ventricular tachycardia. Hypothermia is associated with a distinctive convex "hump" at the J point (Osborn wave, *arrow*). Note QRS and QT prolongation along with sinus tachycardia in the case of tricyclic antidepressant overdose.

likely to represent a normal variant in a healthy young adult woman ("persistent juvenile T-wave pattern") than in an elderly man with chest discomfort. Similarly, the likelihood that ST-segment depression during exercise testing represents ischemia depends partly on the prior probability of coronary artery disease.

Many mistakes in ECG interpretation are errors of omission. Therefore, a systematic approach is desirable. The following 14 points should be analyzed carefully in every ECG: (1) standardization (calibration) and technical features (including lead placement and artifacts); (2) heart rate; (3) rhythm; (4) PR interval; (5) QRS interval; (6) QT interval; (7) mean QRS electrical axis; (8) P waves; (9) QRS voltages; (10) precordial R-wave progression; (11) abnormal Q waves; (12) ST segments; (13) T waves; (14) U waves.

Only after analyzing all these points should the interpretation be formulated. Where appropriate, important clinical correlates or inferences should be mentioned. For example, the combination of left atrial abnormality (enlargement) and signs of right ventricular hypertrophy suggests mitral stenosis. Low voltage with sinus tachycardia raises the possibility of pericardial tamponade or chronic obstructive lung disease. Sinus tachycardia with QRS and QT (U) prolongation suggests tricyclic antidepressant overdose (Fig. 210-17). Comparison with previous ECGs is essential. →*The diagnosis and management of specific cardiac arrhythmias and conduction disturbances are discussed in Chaps. 213 and 214.*

COMPUTERIZED ELECTROCARDIOGRAPHY

Computerized ECG systems are widely used. Digital systems provide for convenient storage and immediate retrieval of thousands of ECG records. Despite advances, computer interpretation of ECGs has important limitations. Incomplete or inaccurate readings are most likely with arrhythmias and complex abnormalities. Therefore, computerized interpretation (including measurements of basic ECG intervals) should not be accepted without careful physician review.

FURTHER READING

ASHLEY EA et al: An evidence-based review of the resting electrocardiogram as a screening technique for heart disease. Prog Cardiovasc Dis 44:55, 2001

GOLDBERGER AL: *Clinical Electrocardiography: A Simplified Approach*, 6th ed. St. Louis, Mosby, 1999

——— AL: *Myocardial Infarction: Electrocardiographic Differential Diagnosis*, 4th ed. St. Louis, Mosby–Year Book, 1991

SURAWICZ B, KNILANS TK: *Chou's Electrocardiography in Clinical Practice*, 5th ed. Philadelphia, Saunders, 2001

Hypocalcemia   **Normal**   **Hypercalcemia**

QT 0.48 s   QT 0.36 s   QT 0.26 s
QT$_c$ 0.52   QT$_c$ 0.41   QT$_c$ 0.36

FIGURE 210-18 Prolongation of the Q-T interval (ST-segment portion) is typical of hypocalcemia. Hypercalcemia may cause abbreviation of the ST segment and shortening of the QT interval.

Cardiovascular imaging has significantly enhanced the practice of cardiology over the past few decades. Two-dimensional (2D) echocardiography is able to visualize the heart directly in real time using ultrasound, providing instantaneous assessment of the myocardium, cardiac chambers, valves, pericardium, and great vessels. Doppler echocardiography measures the velocity of moving red blood cells and has become a noninvasive alternative to cardiac catheterization for assessment of hemodynamics. Transesophageal echocardiography (TEE) provides a unique window for high-resolution imaging of posterior structures of the heart, particularly the left atrium, mitral valve, and aorta. Nuclear cardiology uses isotopes to assess myocardial perfusion and function and has contributed greatly to the evaluation of patients with ischemic heart disease. Cardiac magnetic resonance imaging (MRI) and computed tomography (CT) can delineate cardiac structure and function with high resolution. They are particularly useful in the examination of cardiac masses, the pericardium, and the great vessels and there is growing interest in their utility in patients with suspected coronary artery disease (CAD). This chapter provides an overview of the basic concepts of these cardiac imaging modalities, as well as the clinical indications for each procedure.

ECHOCARDIOGRAPHY

TWO-DIMENSIONAL ECHOCARDIOGRAPHY ■ **Basic Principles** 2D echocardiography uses the principle of ultrasound reflection off cardiac structures to produce images of the heart (Table 211-1). The imaging is performed from multiple acoustic windows with different transducer rotations so that the entire heart and great vessels can be displayed in real time and in various 2D planes. Most information from a study is obtained from a visual analysis of the 2D images, although objective measurements of cardiac dimensions can be obtained. For a transthoracic echocardiogram (TTE), the imaging is performed with a handheld transducer placed directly on the chest wall. In selected patients, a TEE may be performed, in which an ultrasound transducer is mounted on the tip of an endoscope placed in the esophagus and directed toward the cardiac structures, so that high-resolution images of the posterior structures are obtained.

Current echocardiographic machines are portable; they can be wheeled directly to the patient's bedside. Thus, a major advantage of echocardiography over other imaging modalities is the ability to obtain instantaneous images of the cardiac structures for immediate interpretation, even in emergency or trauma units or in critical care settings.

"Handheld" echocardiographic units weighing less than 6 lb have now become available, further enhancing the ease and portability of echocardiography. These units can easily be carried to the bedside of the patient. Although prototype instruments had only 2D echocardiographic capabilities, there are now units that can also perform pulsed Doppler, continuous-wave Doppler, and color-flow Doppler imaging. As these units become smaller and more functional, they may soon become an essential part of the physical examination.

A limitation of a 2D echocardiogram performed via a transthoracic approach is the inability to obtain high-quality images in all patients, especially those with a thick chest wall or severe lung disease. Ultrasound waves are poorly transmitted through lung parenchyma. The diagnostic accuracy of an echocardiogram is highly dependent on both the operator of the echocardiographic equipment and the interpreter of the study.

Chamber Size and Function 2D echocardiography is an ideal imaging modality for assessing left ventricular (LV) size and function (Fig. 211-1). A qualitative assessment of the cavity size of the ventricle and systolic function can be made directly from the 2D image by experienced observers (Fig. 211-2). Quantitative assessment of LV size and function can be made by electronic calipers (measuring systolic and diastolic dimensions of the short axis of the LV) or quantitative 2D echocardiography. With quantitative 2D echocardiography, endocardial outlines of the LV cavity are traced in systole and diastole and the LV cavity areas are then fitted to computer models of the LV to obtain systolic and diastolic volumes. The presence or absence of regional wall motion abnormalities can be visually assessed by examining endocardial motion as well as wall thickening. 2D echocardiography is useful in the diagnosis of LV hypertrophy, seen as an

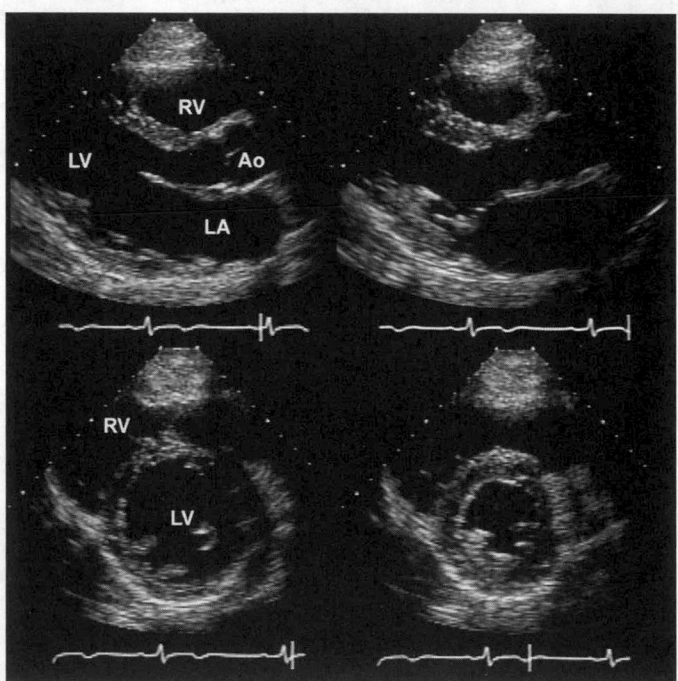

FIGURE 211-1 Two-dimensional echocardiographic still-frame images from a normal patient with a normal heart. *Upper:* Parasternal long axis view during systole and diastole (*left*) and systole (*right*). During systole, there is thickening of the myocardium and reduction in the size of the left ventricle (LV). The valve leaflets are thin and open widely. *Lower:* Parasternal short axis view during diastole (*left*) and systole (*right*) demonstrating a decrease in the left ventricular cavity size during systole as well as an increase in wall thickening. LA, left atrium; RV, right ventricle; Ao, aorta.

TABLE 211-1 Clinical Uses of Echocardiography	
Two-Dimensional Echocardiography	**Doppler Echocardiography**
Cardiac chambers	Valve stenosis
Chamber size	Gradient
Left ventricular	Valve area
Hypertrophy	Valve regurgitation
Regional wall motion abnormalities	Semiquantitation
Valve	Intracardiac pressures
Morphology and motion	Volumetric flow
Pericardium	Diastolic filling
Effusion	Intracardiac shunts
Tamponade	**Transesophageal Echocardiography**
Masses	Inadequate transthoracic images
Great vessels	Aortic disease
Stress Echocardiography	Infective endocarditis
Two-dimensional	Source of embolism
Myocardial ischemia	Valve prosthesis
Viable myocardium	Intraoperative
Doppler	
Valve disease	

FIGURE 211-2 Apical four-chamber view from a patient with a dilated cardiomyopathy. The left ventricle (LV) is dilated, and there is little change in the LV cavity size from diastole (*left*) to systole (*right*). RV, right ventricle; RA, right atrium; LA, left atrium.

increase in wall thickness. Other chamber sizes are assessed by visual analysis, including the left atrium and right-sided chambers. There is no method for quantitative analysis of right ventricular size and function by 2D echocardiography, due to the complex geometry of the right ventricle.

Valve Abnormalities (See also Chap. 219)   2D echocardiography is the gold standard for imaging valve morphology and motion (Fig. 211-1). Leaflet thickness and mobility, valve calcification, and the appearance of subvalvular and supravalvular structures can be assessed. Valve stenosis is reliably diagnosed by the thickening and decreased mobility of the valve. 2D echocardiography is the gold standard for the diagnosis of mitral stenosis, which produces typical tethering and diastolic doming. The severity of the stenosis can be obtained from a direct planimeter measurement of the mitral valve orifice from the short axis view. The presence and etiology of stenosis of the semilunar valves can be made by 2D echocardiography. Estimating the severity of the stenosis by 2D echocardiography alone is less reliable and requires Doppler echocardiography. The diagnosis of valvular regurgitation must be made by Doppler echocardiography, but 2D echocardiography is valuable for determining the etiology of the regurgitation. Annular dilatation, prolapse, flail leaflets, vegetation, and rheumatic involvement can be diagnosed and the LV response to volume overload can be assessed by 2D echocardiography.

Pericardial Effusion (See also Chap. 222)   2D echocardiography is the imaging modality of choice for the detection of pericardial effusion, which is easily visualized as a black echolucent ovoid structure surrounding the heart. In the hemodynamically unstable patient with pericardial tamponade, typical echo findings of right ventricular collapse, right atrial collapse, and a dilated inferior vena cava are seen (see Fig. 222-2). In patients with subclinical tamponade, these 2D echocardiographic features may not be present, but the diagnosis of elevated pericardial pressure can be made by Doppler findings of variations of inflow velocities with respiration (see Fig. 222-3). Echocardiographically guided pericardiocentesis has now become a standard of care. A 2D echocardiogram can directly visualize the location of the pericardial fluid in relationship to the entry point, and this technique has led to a low complication rate. Increased thickness of the pericardium is difficult to assess by 2D echocardiography. Subtle clues to pericardial constriction can be seen on 2D echocardiography from enhanced ventricular interaction, but Doppler imaging is required for confirmation of this diagnosis.

Intracardiac Masses (See also Chap. 223)   Intracardiac masses can be visualized on 2D echocardiography, provided that image quality is adequate. Solid masses appear as echo-dense structures, which can be located inside the cardiac chambers or infiltrating into the myocardium or pericardium (see Fig. 223-1). Although an echocardiographic examination cannot provide pathologic confirmation of the etiology of a mass, there are several instances in which the diagnosis of the mass can be suspected from its appearance, mobility, attachments, and the concomitant abnormalities seen. *LV* thrombus appears as an echo-dense structure, usually in the apical region associated with regional wall motion abnormalities. The appearance and mobility of the thrombus are predictive of embolic events. *Atrial myxoma* can be diagnosed by the appearance of a well-circumscribed mobile mass with attachments to the atrial septum. Prominent benign structures, such as *lipomatous infiltration of the atrial septum* and a *calcified mitral annulus*, may appear as cardiac masses. The high-resolution images provided by TEE may be required for further delineation of myocardial masses.

Aortic Disease (See also Chap. 231)   2D echocardiography can provide extremely useful information on diseases of the aorta. The proximal ascending aorta, the arch, and the distal descending aorta can usually be visualized via the transthoracic approach. For patients in whom a dilated aorta is well visualized, 2D echocardiography can be used for serial follow-up. Aortic dissection can be diagnosed when an intimal flap is visualized on a TTE. However, the definitive diagnosis of an aortic dissection usually requires a TEE.

DOPPLER ECHOCARDIOGRAPHY ■ Basic Principles   Doppler echocardiography uses ultrasound reflecting off moving red blood cells to measure the velocity of blood flow across valves, within cardiac chambers, and through the great vessels. Normal and abnormal blood flow patterns can be assessed noninvasively. Color-flow Doppler imaging (Fig. 211-3) displays the blood velocities in real time superimposed upon a 2D echocardiographic image. The different colors indicate the direction of blood flow (blue toward and red away from the transducer), with green superimposed when there is turbulent flow. Thus regurgitant lesions and shunts may be assessed by color-flow Doppler. Pulsed-wave Doppler measures the blood flow velocity in a specific location on the 2D echocardiographic image and displays the velocities in a spectral pattern using time as the x-axis. Continuous-wave Doppler

FIGURE 211-3 *Left:* Transesophageal echocardiographic view of a patient with severe mitral regurgitation due to a flail posterior leaflet. The arrow points to the portion of the posterior leaflet that is unsupported and moves into the left atrium during systole. *Right:* Color-flow imaging demonstrating a large mosaic jet of mitral regurgitation during systole. LA, left atrium; LV, left ventricle; AV, aortic valve.

echocardiography can measure high velocities of blood flow directed along the line of the Doppler beam, such as occur in the presence of valve stenosis, valve regurgitation, or intracardiac shunts. These high velocities can be used to determine intracardiac pressure gradients by a modified Bernoulli equation:

$$\text{Pressure change} = 4 \times (\text{velocity})^2$$

The derived pressure gradient can be used to determine intracardiac pressures and stenosis severity.

Tissue Doppler echocardiography measures the velocity of the myocardium. The velocity of myocardium is several magnitudes lower than the velocity of moving red blood cells. Analysis of specific myocardial motion allows for quantification of regional myocardial contraction and relaxation.

Valve Gradients (See also Chap. 219)   In the presence of valvular stenosis, there is an increase in the velocity of blood flow across the stenotic valve. A continuous-wave Doppler beam can be placed into this jet of blood, and the measured velocity used to determine an instantaneous gradient across the valve by applying the modified Bernoulli equation. Integration of this velocity over time provides an accurate measurement of the mean gradient across the valve. Since the valve gradient is dependent upon transvalvular flow, a calculated "valve area" is of clinical benefit and can be derived noninvasively

Valvular Regurgitation (See also Chap. 219)   Valvular regurgitation is diagnosed by Doppler echocardiography when there is an abnormal retrograde flow across the valve. Color-flow imaging is the Doppler method used most frequently to detect valve regurgitation by visualization of a high-velocity turbulent jet in the chamber proximal to the regurgitant valve. The sensitivity of Doppler echocardiography for the detection of regurgitant lesions is high, and even trivial or mild regurgitation in the absence of clinical auscultatory evidence of a regurgitant murmur may be detected. The size and extent of the color-flow jet into the receiving cardiac chamber provide a semiqualitative estimate of the severity of regurgitation, but there are many limitations to using color jet size alone.

Intracardiac Pressures   These can be calculated from the peak continuous-wave Doppler signal of a regurgitant lesion. The Bernoulli equation is applied to the peak velocity to obtain the pressure gradient between two cardiac chambers. This is commonly applied to a tricuspid regurgitant jet, from which the systolic pressure gradient between the right atrium and right ventricle can be calculated. Adding an assumed right atrial pressure to this gradient will give a derived right ventricular systolic pressure, which provides the pulmonary artery systolic pressure in the absence of right ventricular outflow tract obstruction. Change in pressure over time during isovolumic contraction can be derived from a mitral regurgitation signal. This measurement provides an index of systolic contractility.

Cardiac Output   Volume flow rates can be reliably measured noninvasively from Doppler echocardiography. Using the hydrodynamic principle of flow through a rigid tube, the volume of flow can be calculated from the area of an orifice through which blood flows multiplied by the time of the velocity. The most accurate site for this measurement is through the LV outflow tract. The product of the outflow area and velocity provides a beat-to-beat measurement of stroke volume, which, when multiplied by heart rate, provides a measurement of cardiac output.

Diastolic Filling (See also Chap. 215)   Doppler echocardiography allows noninvasive evaluation of ventricular diastolic filling. The transmitral velocity curves reflect the relative pressure gradients between the left atrium and LV throughout the diastolic filling period. They are influenced by the rate of ventricular relaxation, the driving force across the valve, and the compliance of the LV. There is a progression of diastolic dysfunction in disease states, which can be assessed by Doppler flow velocity curves (Fig. 211-4). In the early phase of diastolic

Abnormal Relaxation   **Restriction**

LVEDP 6 mmHg   LVEDP 34 mmHg

FIGURE 211-4   High-fidelity left ventricular pressure curve superimposed on a mitral inflow velocity curve obtained by Doppler echocardiography. The ratio of early and late diastolic flows is termed an *E:A ratio*. *Left*: In early stages of diastolic dysfunction, there is an abnormality of relaxation. There is a decrease in the early diastolic filling and an increase with filling at atrial contraction, resulting in a low E:A ratio of 0.5, with deceleration time (DT) of 280 ms. In this instance, the left ventricular end-diastolic pressure (LVEDP) is low at 6 mmHg. *Right*: As diastolic dysfunction progresses, there is a restriction to filling, in which there is a high early diastolic velocity and low velocity at atrial contraction resulting in a high E:A ratio of 3.0, with DT of 120 ms. In this instance, the LVEDP is markedly elevated to 34 mmHg. The DT reflects the rate of decline of the early velocity and is a measure of the effective operative compliance of the left ventricle. (See text for explanation.)

dysfunction there is primarily an abnormality of relaxation, with decreased early transmitral flow and a compensatory increase in flow during atrial contraction. As disease progresses, there is a higher left atrial pressure and reduced compliance of the LV, resulting in a higher early transmitral velocity and shortening of the deceleration of flow in early diastole, termed *restriction to filling*. These transmitral flow curves can be used to estimate ventricular filling pressures and to determine prognosis in certain disease entities. The addition of Doppler interrogation of pulmonary venous flow, analysis of Doppler tissue velocities of annular motion, and right-sided chamber flow velocities provides further information concerning the diastolic properties. Grading of the severity of diastolic dysfunction is now possible based on the Doppler velocities (Grades I–IV).

Congenital Heart Disease (See also Chap. 218)   Doppler echocardiography has been useful in the evaluation of patients with congenital heart disease. Congenital stenotic or regurgitant valve lesions can be assessed. The detection and semiquantitation of intracardiac shunts is possible by Doppler echocardiography. Patency of surgical shunts and conduits can be determined.

STRESS ECHOCARDIOGRAPHY (See also Chap. 226)   2D and Doppler echocardiography are usually performed in the resting state. Further information can be obtained by reimaging during either exercise or pharmacologic stress. The primary indications for stress echocardiography are to confirm the suspicion of CAD and estimate its severity. Stress echocardiography using both 2D echocardiography and Doppler echocardiography provides additional information for the patient with valvular heart disease.

The response of the myocardium to ischemia consists of a cascade of events. A decrease in systolic contraction of the ischemic area, termed a *regional wall motion abnormality*, occurs before symptoms or electrocardiographic changes. During a stress echocardiogram, 2D echocardiographic images at rest and during stress are digitized and displayed in a side-by-side format so that induced regional wall motion abnormalities may be detected. Changes in overall systolic function as well as end-systolic volume are also assessed. New regional wall motion abnormalities, a decline in ejection fraction, and an increase in end-systolic volume with stress are all indicators of myocardial ischemia (Fig. 211-5).

FIGURE 211-5   Stress echocardiographic images in a patient with known coronary artery disease. *Left*: The systolic views from a patient in the resting state is shown. The upper frame is taken from a four-chamber view and the lower frame is taken from a two-chamber view. *Right*: The systolic views are shown immediately after exercise. The arrows point to the appearance of a regional wall motion abnormality in the anterior and apical segments. LV, left ventricle; RV, right ventricle. (*From JK Oh et al, The Echo Manual, 2d ed. Philadelphia, Lippincott, Williams & Wilkins, 1999; with permission.*)

Exercise stress testing is usually done with exercise protocols using either upright treadmill or bicycle exercise. The echocardiographic imaging is done at baseline and then immediately after exercise. In patients who are not able to exercise, pharmacologic testing can be performed by infusion of dobutamine to increase myocardial oxygen demand. Dobutamine echocardiography has also been used to assess myocardial viability in patients with poor systolic function and concomitant CAD. In this type of study, dobutamine is started at a low dose of 5 to 10 μg/kg per min and then incrementally increased every few minutes. In the presence of viable myocardium, an increase in the systolic contraction of the myocardium is evident at low doses of dobutamine, and is followed by an ischemic response at higher doses.

It is important that the images be obtained as soon as possible after exercise is stopped since regional wall motion abnormalities may dissipate rapidly with time. Interpretation of the images is highly operator-dependent, and thus this technique requires an experienced echocardiographer.

Doppler echocardiography can be used at rest and during exercise in patients with valvular heart disease to determine the hemodynamic response to stress. Gradients across stenotic valves can be measured at rest and immediately after exercise; this provides information previously obtained by right heart catheterization during exercise. Pulmonary pressures can be obtained from the tricuspid regurgitation velocities at rest and during exercise.

TRANSESOPHAGEAL ECHOCARDIOGRAPHY   This technique has provided an additional window to the heart (see Fig. 211-3). Because of the close proximity of the esophagus to the heart, high-resolution images of posterior structures are consistently obtained. TEE should be performed when further information is required after comprehensive 2D and Doppler transthoracic echocardiograms. Diseases of the aorta, such as aortic dissection, can be readily diagnosed and quantitated by TEE (Fig. 211-6; Chap. 231). Defining the source of embolism is a common indication for TEE, as abnormalities such as atrial thrombi, patent foramen ovale, and aortic debris can be detected. Other masses, particularly those in the atria, can be visualized. The presence of vegetations for the diagnosis of infective endocarditis and its compli-

cations can be assessed by TEE (Chap. 109). The evaluation of suspected abnormalities of a mitral prosthesis is an indication for TEE, as the posterior imaging window will avoid the problems of acoustic reflection caused by the prosthetic valve seen with TTE. TEE can be used during cardiac surgery to guide various operations, such as mitral valve repair and septal myectomy. When limited information is obtained from a TTE due to poor imaging windows, TEE can be useful.

Patients presenting with atrial fibrillation of indeterminate duration pose a difficult therapeutic challenge. Cardioversion may be the preferred treatment modality for these patients but if the time of onset of the atrial fibrillation is either greater than 48 h or unclear, there may be a higher risk of an embolic event at the time of cardioversion. In this situation, TEE has been used before cardioversion to look for a thrombus in the left atrium or left atrial appendage. If no thrombus is present, cardioversion can be safely performed emergently, as long as there is full dose anticoagulation before, during, and after the procedure.

EMERGENCY ECHOCARDIOGRAPHY   A major advantage of echocardiography is the ability to obtain instantaneous images of the cardiac structures for immediate interpretation at the patient's bedside. Thus, echocardiography has become an ideal imaging modality for cardiac emergencies.

Unstable Hemodynamics   For the patient with unstable hemodynamics, echocardiography can determine left ventricular size and function, right ventricular size and function, and the presence of acute valvular regurgitation and pericardial tamponade. Echocardiography is especially useful in the hemodynamically unstable patient following myocardial infarction, where acute mechanical complications (e.g., papillary muscle rupture, ventricular septal defect, myocardial perforation with tamponade, and right ventricular infarction) can be diagnosed and need to be differentiated from severe left ventricular systolic dysfunction. An enlarged right ventricle in a hemodynamically unstable patient can indicate the presence of acute right ventricular pressure overload, which is seen in acute pulmonary embolism. Echocardiography is the imaging modality of choice for the diagnosis of pericardial tamponade. 2D echocardiography can also be used to guide emergency pericardiocentesis.

Chest Pain Syndromes   (See also Chap. 12)   Echocardiography can be useful in selected patients with chest pain syndromes. For those patients who have an equivocal electrocardiogram, the presence of regional wall motion abnormalities on an echocardiogram can lead to the diagnosis of myocardial ischemia as an etiology for the pain. Other

FIGURE 211-6   Transesophageal echocardiographic view of a patient with a dilated aorta, aortic dissection, and severe aortic regurgitation. The arrow points to the intimal flap that is seen in the dilated ascending aorta. *Left*: The long axis apex down view of the black and white two-dimensional image in diastole. *Right*: Color-flow imaging that demonstrates a large mosaic jet of aortic regurgitation. Ao, aorta; RV, right ventricle; AR, aortic regurgitation.

etiologies of chest pain, such as acute dissection or pericarditis with effusion, can also be diagnosed by echocardiography.

NUCLEAR CARDIOLOGY

BASIC PRINCIPLES OF NUCLEAR CARDIOLOGY All nuclear cardiology studies depend on the injection into the patient of an isotope that emits photons, generally gamma rays generated during radioactive decay when the nucleus of an isotope changes from one energy level to a lower one. Radionuclide imaging uses a special camera that images these photons. A common problem with all nuclear studies is that photons are emitted in all directions from the point of origin, and scattering, attenuation, and absorption of the photons can occur. The higher the energy of the isotope, the less chance for scatter or absorption. The two most commonly used isotopes are technetium 99m (^{99m}Tc) and thallium 201 (^{201}Tl).

ASSESSMENT OF VENTRICULAR FUNCTION Equilibrium radionuclide angiography, also known as *multiple-gated blood pool imaging*, is useful for the noninvasive assessment of ventricular function. It involves the imaging of ^{99m}Tc-labeled albumin or red cells that are uniformly distributed throughout the blood volume. Resting images of the blood pool of isotopes within the cardiac chambers are obtained by electrocardiographic gating through multiple cycles, so that sufficient counts can be detected to obtain an image. This requires that the heart rate be reasonably constant without significant arrhythmia. It provides an accurate, reproducible method for assessment of LV function. Other clinical variables that can be obtained include size and function of the right ventricle, size of atrial chambers and great vessels, diastolic filling parameters, and the severity of valvular regurgitation.

First-pass radionuclide angiography is an alternative method for the noninvasive assessment of ventricular function that involves the recording of the movement of a bolus of radionuclide during its "first pass" through the central circulation. This does not require labeling of red blood cells. ^{99m}Tc is utilized because of its low cost and short half-life. During this testing, the passage of the radioisotope through the right atrium, right ventricle, pulmonary circulation, left atrium, left ventricle, and aorta is recorded with a high-count (usually multicrystal) camera. The high count rates allow temporal definition of the passage of the bolus. The disadvantage of first-pass radionuclide angiography compared to equilibrium testing is its poorer resolution of ventricular wall motion.

Gated single-photon emission computed tomography (SPECT) can also be used to assess ejection fraction and regional wall motion (usually poststress) by gating the acquisition of SPECT myocardial perfusion images (see below). Although this can potentially be done using ^{201}Tl, ^{99m}Tc- labeled compounds are preferable because of their higher count rates. An automated technique determines the endocardial borders of the LV cavity and a geometric model is used to calculate the ejection fraction. As for equilibrium radionuclide angiography, the heart rhythm should be regular without significant arrhythmia.

ASSESSMENT OF MYOCARDIAL PERFUSION Myocardial perfusion imaging by nuclear techniques is now widely applied for the evaluation of ischemic heart disease (Chap. 226). Injection of radioisotopes at rest and during stress is performed to produce images of myocardial regional uptake proportional to regional blood flow. With maximal exercise, myocardial blood flow is increased up to fivefold above the resting condition. In the presence of a fixed coronary stenosis, there is an inability to increase myocardial perfusion in the territory supplied by the stenosis, creating a flow differential and inhomogeneous distribution of the isotope. In patients who are unable to exercise, pharmacologic agents are used to increase blood flow and create similar inhomogeneities. The preferred pharmacologic agents are adenosine or dipyridamole, which increase blood flow to a similar degree as exercise. In patients with bronchospastic lung disease, which is a contraindication to the use of adenosine or dipyridamole, dobutamine may

be used as an alternative, although it does not increase blood flow to the same extent.

^{201}Tl is a potassium analogue and is avidly taken up by viable myocardial cells. The degree of uptake is related directly to the coronary blood flow. An initial injection is usually performed at peak exercise, and hypoperfused myocardium will have less thallium uptake than a region of normal perfusion. Over the next several hours, a complex process occurs that is known as "redistribution." There is a continuous input of thallium into the myocardium from a large reservoir of thallium in the blood pool. At the same time, thallium continuously washes out of portions of the myocardium at a rate that is dependent on local myocardial perfusion. The final result is that a region of ischemia that initially appears as an area of reduced uptake becomes apparently normal over time; this redistribution is seen on delayed imaging. In regions of fibrosis (infarction), there will be no redistribution on delayed imaging. A "reinjection" of additional thallium before acquisition of the delayed images enhances the detection of ischemia. The presence of redistribution in areas of hypokinesia has been associated with recovery of LV function after revascularization.

Other findings on thallium imaging may be of considerable clinical importance. Increased lung uptake of thallium may be seen immediately after stress and assessed either quantitatively or qualitatively. This finding reflects increased pulmonary capillary wedge pressure during stress. It occurs in the presence of severe CAD and/or LV dysfunction. It provides important adverse prognostic information that is incremental to other clinical, stress, and coronary angiographic variables. Thallium images may also show evidence of transient poststress LV dilatation. This finding is also associated with severe CAD and/or LV dysfunction as well as with an adverse prognosis.

^{99m}Tc-labeled compounds have a higher photon energy and shorter half-life than ^{201}Tl, permitting the injection of larger doses (Fig. 211-7). As a result, these compounds generally provide higher quality scans with fewer artifacts. Three technetium-labeled agents have been approved for general use: teboroxime, tetrofosmin, and sestamibi. The last is the best studied of these agents and is currently used most frequently. Like thallium, sestamibi distributes to the myocardium in relation to blood flow, and its uptake requires a viable myocardial cell and an intact cell membrane. It is transported through the cytoplasm and bound to the mitochondria in a nearly irreversible fashion. Compared to thallium, there is far less redistribution. As a result, the agent must generally be injected twice—once at rest and once during stress.

COMPARISON OF THALLIUM AND TECHNETIUM Both ^{201}Tl- and ^{99m}Tc-labeled compounds provide clinically useful myocardial perfusion images in the majority of patients. The choice between the two is often dictated by local experience and economics. However, in selected patients, there may be factors that suggest a clear advantage for one or the other. The relative advantages of both agents are listed in Table 211-2.

POSITRON EMISSION TOMOGRAPHY The underlying physics of positron emission tomography (PET) scanning is quite different from that involved in the standard radionuclide techniques described above. The annihilation of the positron leads to the simultaneous emission of two very high energy (511 keV) photons in opposite directions. These can then be imaged by a series of detectors placed in a ring around the patient. The very high energy of the photons results in far less scatter and attenuation than with conventional nuclear cardiology techniques. PET cameras are considerably more expensive than conventional nuclear cardiology cameras. The radiopharmaceuticals involved require a cyclotron for production and generally have half-lives that are so short that transportation beyond the immediate local region is not feasible. Although the initial availability of PET was limited, the increasing role of PET imaging in oncology has increased its availability for cardiac imaging.

Positron emitters can be employed to study both myocardial blood flow and myocardial metabolism. Nitrogen-13 ammonia, oxygen-15 water, and rubidium-82 have all been employed to assess myocardial blood flow. They permit measurement of absolute regional blood flows, in contrast to the relative blood flows that are assessed with

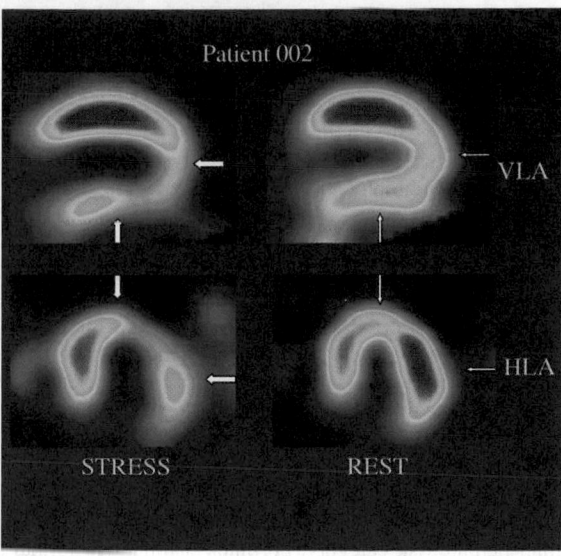

FIGURE 211-7 *A.* Exercise sestamibi study on a 71-year-old, white female with atypical angina. *Left:* Stress images; *right:* rest images. The images are normal. There is even sestamibi update throughout the myocardium at rest and during stress. *B.* Exercise sestamibi study on a 75-year-old male with a history of typical angina. *Left:* Stress images; *right:* rest images. The stress images show a large defect involving the apex, lateral, and inferior walls (thick arrows), which improves at rest (thin arrows). Subsequent coronary angiography demonstrates severe three-vessel coronary artery disease. SA, short axis; Mid, middle of the left ventricle; VLA, vertical long axis; HLA, horizontal long axis.

^{201}Tl- or ^{99m}Tc-labeled compounds. This advantage has been utilized for research purposes but has not yet been exploited clinically. Myocardial metabolism is most often assessed using fluorine-18 deoxyglucose. This agent permits the detection and quantification of exogenous glucose utilization in areas of hypoperfused myocardium.

The clinical application of PET scanning that has been most well studied is the assessment of myocardial viability. The pattern of enhanced fluorodeoxyglucose uptake in regions of decreased perfusion (termed *glucose/blood flow "mismatch"*) indicates the presence of ischemic myocardium that has preferentially shifted its metabolic substrate toward glucose rather than fatty acid or lactate. This pattern identifies regions of ischemic or hibernating myocardium that are likely to improve in function after revascularization (Chap. 226).

Careful studies have consistently shown the ability of PET to identify ischemic or hibernating myocardium in 10 to 20% of regions that would be classified as fibrotic (infarcted) by ^{201}Tl- or ^{99m}Tc-labeled compounds. For that reason, this technique is generally regarded as the gold standard for the assessment of myocardial viability. When large fixed defects (infarcts) are detected by ^{201}Tl- or ^{99m}Tc-labeled-compounds in patients who are candidates for coronary revascularization, PET imaging can suggest if the risk of revascularization is justified by the potential benefit.

Within the past few years, specially modified conventional gamma cameras have been employed to image fluorodeoxyglucose in an attempt to avoid the expense related to cameras dedicated to PET. The limited evidence available suggests that this approach is inferior to standard PET.

TABLE 211-2 *Relative Advantages of Thallium 201 and Technetium 99m Sestamibi*

THALLIUM

Lower radiopharmaceutical cost
Measurement of increased pulmonary uptake
Detection of resting ischemia (hibernating myocardium)

SESTAMIBI

Better image quality (particularly in obese patients or female patients with breast attenuation)
Ventricular function assessment (first-pass or gated SPECT)
Shorter imaging times (lower cost)
Shorter imaging protocols (patient/scheduling convenience)
Acute imaging in myocardial infarction (myocardium at risk) and unstable angina (chest pain triage)
Superior quantification, particularly of resting perfusion defect (infarct size)

Note: SPECT, single-photon emission computed tomography.

OVERVIEW OF STRESS TESTING

CHOOSING THE APPROPRIATE INITIAL STRESS TEST The choice of an initial stress testing modality should be based on the evaluation of the patient's resting electrocardiogram, the physical ability to perform exercise, and the local expertise and technology available in an institution. For the standard risk assessment of CAD, the exercise electrocardiographic test (Chap. 226) should be the initial mode of stress testing in patients with a normal electrocardiogram who are not taking digoxin and who are able to exercise. If there are resting electrocardiographic abnormalities (ST depression >1 mm, LV hypertrophy, bundle branch block, paced rhythm, pre-excitation) or the patient is taking digoxin or has had a prior coronary revascularization, an imaging modality (either nuclear imaging or echocardiography) should be used for initial evaluation. Pharmacologic stress testing with imaging should be used in patients who are unable to exercise.

When an imaging modality is appropriate, the decision as to whether to use an echocardiographic or a nuclear test is dependent not only on the patient's situation but also on the local expertise and technology available in the institution. Both echocardiography and nuclear imaging require expertise in the performance and interpretation of the tests and the best information is obtained from the imaging modality in which there is most expertise and experience. There are, however, certain situations in which one imaging modality has an advantage over the other.

Echocardiography provides additional structural information. Therefore, if there is a question of concomitant valve disease, pericardial disease, or aortic disease, echocardiography is able to provide information regarding these issues. The major limitation of echocardiography is the inability to obtain diagnostic images in all patients, especially those with chronic obstructive pulmonary disease or severe obesity. Tissue harmonic imaging and contrast injection may help in further delineating endocardial motion in these patients. However, if there is inadequate definition of endocardial motion on the resting echocardiogram, stress echocardiography should not be performed. If the patient has had a previous infarction and one needs to determine whether a specific area of the myocardium is ischemic, nuclear imaging is the preferred modality. Nuclear imaging using ^{99m}Tc-labeled compounds is preferred in obese patients and those with severe lung disease. Nuclear imaging is more sensitive and less specific than echocardiography for the detection of myocardial ischemia.

There are certain instances in which there are false-positives with imaging stress testing. In patients with left bundle branch block, exercise may provoke abnormalities in regional perfusion and regional ventricular function in the absence of CAD. Therefore, the modality of choice in these patients is pharmacologic perfusion imaging.

STRESS TESTING FOR PROGNOSIS Exercise electrocardiography, stress nuclear imaging, and stress echocardiography can all provide important information regarding diagnosis and the patient's subsequent risk for cardiac death. The results are often pivotal in defining the need for coronary angiography and coronary revascularization. For the exercise electrocardiogram, the Duke treadmill score is a well-validated index that is useful for both diagnosis and prognosis. Patients who exercise for > 5 min on the treadmill using a Bruce protocol without angina or ST segment changes have a low risk of subsequent cardiac death (< 1% annual mortality). In contrast, patients with markedly abnormal stress tests are at high risk for subsequent death (> 3% annual mortality); coronary angiography and possible revascularization are appropriate. For the exercise electrocardiogram, a high-risk Duke score consists of a low exercise workload with angina and early ST segment changes.

The imaging tests can add further prognostic information, especially when the results of an exercise electrocardiogram fall into an intermediate risk category. For nuclear imaging, normal stress (exercise) or pharmacologic myocardial perfusion scans (p. 1325) are highly predictive of the absence of significant coronary disease and a low risk of subsequent cardiac death. For stress (exercise or dobutamine) echocardiography, an increase in ejection fraction and a decrease in end-systolic volume at a high workload predict the absence of significant coronary disease and a low risk of subsequent cardiac death. For nuclear imaging, large stress-induced defects, multiple stress-induced defects of moderate size, or a large fixed defect with LV dilatation or increased ^{201}Tl lung uptake are high-risk findings. For stress echocardiography, patients with a drop in ejection fraction, the appearance of multiple regional wall motion abnormalities, and an increase in end-systolic volume are at high risk.

MRI AND CT IMAGING

MRI MRI is a technique based on the magnetic properties of hydrogen nuclei. In the presence of a large magnetic field, nuclear spin transitions from the ground state to excited states can be induced, and as the nuclei relax and return to their ground state, they release energy in the form of electromagnetic radiation that is detected and processed into an image. Contrast agents are frequently employed in MRI to provide magnetic resonance angiograms (MRAs). These provide enhanced soft-tissue contrast as well as the opportunity to obtain rapid angiographic images during the first pass of contrast through the vascular system. Cardiac MRI is particularly challenging because of the rapid physiologic motion of the heart and coronary arteries. Both static and cine images can be obtained using electrocardiographic triggering, often within a short breath-hold of 10 to 15 s (Fig. 211-8). Cine images can be acquired in any plane with excellent blood-myocardial contrast, and these images can be used to quantify ejection fraction, end-systolic and end-diastolic volumes, and cardiac mass with high accuracy and reliability.

Clinical Utility The multiplanar capabilities of MRI, coupled with excellent contrast and spatial resolution, are often valuable in defining anatomic relationships in patients with complex congenital heart disease. Cardiac masses can be characterized and their relationship to normal anatomic structures defined. Likewise, MRI is often the examination of choice to determine whether a mediastinal or pulmonary mass has invaded the pericardium or heart. The entire pericardium can be visualized in multiple planes, and MRI has proved useful in characterization of pericardial effusions, pericardial thickening, and constrictive pericarditis in patients with indeterminate results on echocardiography. MRI is an important technique for evaluation of patients with suspected arrhythmogenic right ventricular dysplasia, where fatty infiltration of the right ventricular free wall can be identified, as can right ventricular dilatation and dyskinesis.

MRA is a standard technique for imaging the aorta and large vessels of the chest and abdomen, with results essentially identical to

FIGURE 211-8 Axial dark-blood MRI from a patient with aortic stenosis and dilatation of the ascending aorta (arrows). Image was acquired in approximately 10 s during suspended respiration.

conventional catheter-based angiography. MRA of the coronary arteries is a much more difficult challenge, both because of the small size of these vessels and because of their rapid and complex motion during the cardiac cycle. Although promising results have been achieved, coronary MRA is not yet an accurate and reliable clinical technique.

MRI is a promising technology for the evaluation of myocardial perfusion. Myocardial perfusion is evaluated by injecting a bolus of contrast and then continuously scanning the heart as the contrast passes through the cardiac chambers and into the myocardium. Relative perfusion deficits are reflected as regions of low signal intensity within the myocardium. Myocardial viability may be determined by imaging the heart 10 to 20 min after contrast injection, as infarcted tissue retains contrast by virtue of its larger extracellular volume. Specialized pulse sequences have been designed to measure the velocity of blood in each pixel of the image, so that flow across valves and within blood vessels may be accurately determined. These techniques may allow characterization of the severity of valvular disease as well as quantification of shunt volumes.

Cardiac MRI has several limitations. Absolute contraindications include the presence of pacemakers, internal defibrillators, or cerebral aneurysm clips. A small percentage of patients are claustrophobic and unable to tolerate the examination within the relatively confined quarters of the magnet bore. Examination of clinically unstable patients is problematic, since close monitoring is difficult.

CT IMAGING CT is fast, simple, and noninvasive, and it provides images with excellent spatial resolution and good soft-tissue contrast. Imaging the heart is a more difficult problem, however, because image acquisition times for conventional CT have until recently been on the order of 1 s, far too long to freeze cardiac motion.

Electron-beam CT employs a fixed detector array and radiation source. The x-rays are generated by an electron beam sweeping continuously across the target anode ring. This is accomplished very rapidly, on the order of 50 to 100 ms. The electron beam can be triggered by the electrocardiogram trace, and single static images or cine images are generated with excellent temporal resolution.

Clinical Applications Cardiac CT has several clinical applications. Pericardial calcification is an important sign of constrictive pericarditis and is easily detected by CT. CT is useful in characterizing cardiac masses, particularly those containing fat or calcium. The ability to detect small amounts of fat with high spatial resolution makes CT an

FIGURE 211-9 Noncontrast image from electron-beam CT revealing small foci of calcification in the left anterior descending coronary artery (arrow).

attractive technique for imaging patients with suspected arrhythmogenic right ventricular dysplasia. Cine images can be used to evaluate wall motion and determine ejection fraction, end-diastolic and end-systolic volumes, and cardiac mass.

CT angiography (CTA) has demonstrated accuracy similar to MRA in imaging the aorta and great vessels, and CTA is rapidly becoming the examination of choice in the evaluation of patients with suspected pulmonary embolus. Coronary CTA with multidetector spiral CT is in the developmental stage. Both CT and MRI are valuable in delineating the presence and course of anomalous coronary vessels; however, the clinical utility of either technique in detecting and grading coronary artery stenoses has not been widely demonstrated.

Coronary Calcification Calcium in the coronary arteries occurs in atherosclerosis and is absent in the normal coronary artery. CT is very sensitive for the detection of coronary artery calcification and is being promoted as a noninvasive modality for the screening and diagnosis of CAD (Fig. 211-9). The amount of coronary calcification (coronary calcium score) is related to the severity of coronary disease. However, although CT has a very high sensitivity for the detection of CAD, it has a low specificity. The overall predictive accuracy for angiographic obstructive coronary disease in a typical CAD patient population is similar to other imaging modalities, such as SPECT. Due to its low specificity, CT should not be used for the diagnosis of obstructive coronary disease. However, in asymptomatic patients, more severe coronary atherosclerosis (and thus a higher calcium score) is associated with a higher risk of future cardiac events. Nonetheless, there are no data to show that the information from CT is additive to standard clinical assessment of the risk of CAD and coronary events. The results of properly designed outcomes research studies are required for determination of the ultimate clinical role of CT scanning in patients with known or suspected CAD.

Limitations of CT Limitations of CT include ionizing radiation and the need for iodinated contrast, which is problematic in patients with renal insufficiency or contrast allergy. Radiation doses tend to increase as the spatial and temporal resolution improve; however, the dose for cardiac CT is almost always significantly lower than the dose delivered during cardiac catheterization.

FURTHER READING

DUTKA DP et al: The contribution of positron emission tomography to the study of ischemic heart failure. Prog Cardiovasc Dis 43:399, 2001

GIBBONS RJ et al: ACC/AHA guideline update for exercise testing: A report of the American College of Cardiology/American Heart Association Task Force on Practice Guidelines Circulation 106:1883, 2002

GIBBONS RJ: Myocardial perfusion imaging. Heart 83:355, 2000

HABERL R et al: Correlation of coronary calcification and angiographically documented stenoses in patients with suspected coronary artery disease: Results of 1,764 patients. J Am Coll Cardiol 37:451, 2001

KIMURA BJ et al: Screening cardiac ultrasonographic examination in patients with suspected cardiac disease in the emergency department. Am Heart J 142:324, 2001

MAZUR W: Myocardial viability: Recent developments in detection and clinical significance. Curr Opin Cardiol 16:277, 2001

MULVAGH SL et al: Contrast echocardiography: Current and future applications. J Am Soc Echocardiogr 13:331, 2000

TRAMBAIOLO P et al: New insights into regional systolic and diastolic left ventricular function with tissue Doppler echocardiography: From qualitative analysis to a quantitative approach. J Am Soc Echocardiogr 14:85, 2001

212 DIAGNOSTIC CARDIAC CATHETERIZATION AND ANGIOGRAPHY
Donald S. Baim, William Grossman

Despite progressive improvements in noninvasive techniques, cardiac catheterization remains a key clinical tool for assessing the anatomy and physiology of the heart and its associated vasculature. It involves the insertion of small (diameter, 2 to 3 mm), hollow plastic tubes or catheters into a peripheral artery or vein under local anesthesia, and passage of their tips into the heart for pressure measurement or for the injection of a liquid radiographic contrast agent. The findings of diagnostic cardiac catheterization characterize the extent and severity of cardiac disease and thereby help in deciding on the most appropriate plan for medical, surgical, or catheter-based treatment. While the majority of patients with coronary artery disease (CAD) or valvular disease can be managed using only clinical and noninvasive data, more than 2 million cardiac catheterization and angiographic procedures are performed each year for diagnostic or interventional purposes, or both. This chapter focuses on the uses of cardiac catheterization as a diagnostic tool. →*For further discussion of catheter-based interventions, see Chap. 229.*

INDICATIONS, CONTRAINDICATIONS, AND COMPLICATIONS

INDICATIONS Given the expense and small, but real, risks of cardiac catheterization, its performance is not routine whenever cardiac disease is diagnosed or suspected. Instead, cardiac catheterization is recommended only when there is a need to confirm the presence of a clinically suspected condition, define its anatomic and physiologic severity, and determine whether important associated conditions are present. This need most commonly arises when a patient is experiencing limiting or escalating symptoms of cardiac dysfunction (Chap. 216) or myocardial ischemia (Chap. 226) or when objective measures (such as exercise testing or echocardiography) suggest that the patient has a high risk of progressing to rapid functional deterioration, myocardial infarction, or other adverse events. Under these circumstances, catheterization may serve as a checkpoint prior to treatment by cardiac surgery or a catheter-based intervention. While cardiac catheterization was previously considered mandatory in *all* patients being considered for cardiac surgery, currently many patients with congenital or valvular

TABLE 212-1 *Relative Contraindications to Cardiac Catheterization and Angiography*

Uncontrolled ventricular irritability: increased risk of ventricular tachycardia and fibrillation during catheterization if ventricular irritability is uncontrolled

Uncorrected hypokalemia or digitalis toxicity

Uncorrected hypertension: predisposes to myocardial ischemia and/or heart failure during angiography

Intercurrent febrile illness

Decompensated heart failure: especially acute pulmonary edema, unless catheterization can be done with patient sitting up

Anticoagulated state: prothrombin time >18 s

Severe allergy to radiographic contrast agent

Severe renal insufficiency and/or anuria: unless dialysis is planned to remove fluid and radiographic contrast load

heart disease undergo surgical correction based solely on clinical and noninvasive test data. Cardiac catheterization and coronary arteriography still remain, however, the only way to define *coronary anatomy* with sufficient precision to inform decisions regarding coronary surgery or catheter-based interventions in patients with CAD. In patients with other forms of heart disease (e.g., dilated cardiomyopathy, valvular heart disease), cardiac catheterization can provide hemodynamic characterization essential for the design of an appropriate medical regimen, or to assess prognosis.

CONTRAINDICATIONS When there is a clinical "need to know," there are very few absolute contraindications to diagnostic cardiac catheterization in a patient who understands and accepts the associated risks. Some relative contraindications to cardiac catheterization, however, are listed in Table 212-1. Most center on factors that increase the risk of the procedure above the baseline mortality risk of roughly 1 in 1000 for clinically stable patients. For example, risk is increased more than tenfold in patients with severe symptoms, certain types of coronary anatomy, valve disease, left ventricular dysfunction, or severe noncardiac disease, as outlined in Table 212-2.

COMPLICATIONS Beyond the mortality risk, cardiac catheterization carries a 1 in 1000 risk of stroke or myocardial infarction. Other problems, such as transient tachy- or bradyarrhythmias or bruising or bleeding at the catheter insertion site, occur in fewer than 1% of patients and respond to drug therapy, countershock, or vascular surgical repair, without long-term sequelae. Although serious, problems such as cardiac perforation or arterial dissection are very rare in the modern era of cardiac catheterization.

Some patients, however, are intolerant of the iodinated contrast agents used for angiography, which may produce transient deterioration in renal function (particularly in patients with baseline renal dys-

TABLE 212-2 *Patient Characteristics Associated with Increased Mortality from Cardiac Catheterization*

Age Infants (<1 month old) and the elderly (>85 years old) are at increased risk of death during cardiac catheterization. Elderly women appear to be at higher risk than elderly men.

Functional class Mortality in class IV patients is more than 10 times greater than in class I–II patients.

Severity of coronary obstruction Mortality for patients with left main coronary artery disease is more than 10 times greater than in patients with one- or two-vessel disease.

Valvular heart disease Especially when severe and combined with coronary disease, is associated with a higher risk of death at cardiac catheterization than coronary artery disease alone.

Left ventricular dysfunction Mortality in patients with a left ventricular ejection fraction <30% is more than 10 times greater than in patients with an ejection fraction ≥50%.

Severe noncardiac disease Patients with renal insufficiency, insulin-requiring diabetes, advanced cerebrovascular and/or peripheral vascular disease, or severe pulmonary insufficiency have an increased incidence of death and other major complications from cardiac catheterization.

function or proteinuria who are not adequately prehydrated) or *allergic reactions* ranging from urticaria to frank anaphylaxis in sensitive patients. These allergic reactions can be suppressed by pretreatment with glucocorticoids (prednisone, 20 to 40 mg every 6 h), conventional antihistamines (e.g., diphenhydramine, 25 mg every 6 h), and H_2 antagonists (cimetidine, 300 mg every 6 h), starting 18 to 24 h prior to the procedure. Despite these precautions, anaphylactic reactions during radiographic contrast angiography may require emergency treatment with intravenous epinephrine. In contemporary practice, however, use of newer nonionic contrast agents has almost eliminated these severe allergic reactions. Compared to the original high-osmolar agents, the newer contrast agents also have a lesser myocardial depressant effect and produce fewer side effects (hypotension, nausea, bradycardia, or a sensation of marked warmth following injection).

TECHNIQUES

Cardiac catheterization is performed with the patient in the fasting state and awake but lightly sedated. Typical preprocedure sedatives include diazepam (Valium, 5 to 10 mg orally) or midazolam (Versed, 1 mg intravenously). Although cardiac catheterization was previously performed exclusively as an inpatient procedure, current practice is to perform most elective procedures on an *outpatient* basis, with the patient discharged 2 to 4 h after the procedure is completed. Since cardiac catheterization is a sterile procedure, prophylactic antibiotics are not necessary. To minimize the risks of bleeding at the local catheter insertion site, patients who have been anticoagulated chronically with warfarin should have this agent discontinued at least 48 h prior to the procedure, so that the INR falls below 2. Oral aspirin (325 mg per day) is recommended in patients undergoing diagnostic catheterization for suspected coronary disease, since aspirin pretreatment is required if a coronary intervention is to be performed.

Most (>95%) cardiac catheterizations are performed by the percutaneous femoral technique, in which a needle puncture is performed in the femoral artery (for left heart catheterization) and the femoral vein (for right heart catheterization). A flexible guidewire is inserted through this needle, over which a vascular access sheath is placed, through which the desired catheters can be advanced. This percutaneous technique has been modified for other sites, including the brachial and radial artery. The brachial or radial approach has an advantage in the patient with peripheral vascular disease involving the abdominal aorta and iliac or femoral arteries or in whom immediate postprocedure ambulation is desired, but it involves some limitations in the range of devices that can be used if the diagnostic procedure evolves into a catheter-based intervention. With these alternatives, the original cut-down, or Sones, technique of cardiac catheterization by direct exposure of the brachial artery and vein in the antecubital fossa is rarely used.

Cardiac catheterization may include a variety of different measurements of pressure and flow (hemodynamics) as well as a variety of different contrast injections recorded as x-ray movies (angiography). The exact types of testing performed in any given procedure depend on the nature of the clinical problem being evaluated. In patients with CAD, the procedure may include only left ventriculography and coronary angiography, while in patients with valvular heart disease, full left and right heart hemodynamic studies may be performed.

RIGHT HEART CATHETERIZATION

Measurement of the pressures in the right side of the heart was once a routine part of each cardiac catheterization, but it is now used in fewer than 25% of procedures since it adds little to the evaluation of the patient with CAD. It is still useful, however, when significant left and/or right ventricular dysfunction, valve disease, myopericardial disease, or intracardiac shunting is suspected. The right heart catheterization procedure is similar to the placement of a Swan-Ganz catheter at the bedside in the intensive care unit, except that it is performed under fluoroscopic guidance. A balloon flotation catheter is advanced from a suitable vein (femoral, brachial, subclavian, or internal jugular) into the superior vena cava, where blood is sampled for oximetry. The catheter is then positioned in the right atrium, where pressure is measured. The balloon is inflated with air (or carbon dioxide, if intracardiac shunting is suspected) and advanced sequentially into the right ventricle, pulmonary artery, and pulmonary artery wedge position. Pressure is recorded at each of these locations, with normal values for pressures measured during cardiac catheterization summarized in Table 212-3. After recording the pulmonary wedge pressure (which approximates left atrial pressure), the balloon is deflated so that pulmonary artery pressure can be monitored and blood samples obtained for oximetry. Comparison of oxygen saturations in the superior and inferior vena cava, the chambers of the right heart, and pulmonary artery permits assessment of the presence of a left-to-right shunt at the atrial, ventricular, or pulmonary artery level, which will be manifested as an increase ("step-up") in oxygen saturation of blood as it traverses these vessels and chambers.

MEASUREMENT OF CARDIAC OUTPUT   Measurements of the pulmonary artery and aortic oxygen content and oxygen consumption allow calculation of the cardiac output by the Fick principle, which states that

$$Q \text{ (L/min)} = \frac{O_2 \text{ consumption (mL/min)}}{\text{arteriovenous } O_2 \text{ difference (mL/L)}}$$

In order to compare individuals of different body weights and sizes, cardiac output (Q) is commonly divided by body surface area to yield the cardiac index (CI). Normal values for O_2 consumption and cardiac output are given in Table 212-3. It should be noted, however, that dividing the O_2 consumption by the arteriovenous O_2 difference across the lungs (estimated pulmonary venous–pulmonary arterial O_2 content) actually measures the *pulmonary* blood flow (Q_p). In patients with an intracardiac left-to-right shunt at the atrial, ventricular, or pulmonary artery levels, this calculated pulmonary blood flow overestimates systemic blood flow by the amount flowing through the shunt. In such cases, calculation of systemic blood flow (Q_s) requires dividing O_2 consumption by the *systemic* arteriovenous O_2 difference, estimated as the systemic arterial blood O_2 content minus the mixed venous blood O_2 content derived from the chamber immediately proximal to the level of the shunt. The Fick method is most dependable when the cardiac output is low and a large arteriovenous oxygen difference can be measured.

Another approach to the measurement of cardiac output during right heart catheterization is the thermodilution technique, in which a thermistor is mounted on the tip of a balloon flotation catheter and positioned in the pulmonary artery. An aliquot (10 mL) of room tem-

FIGURE 212-1   Left ventricular (LV), radial artery, and pulmonary capillary wedge (PCW) pressures in a patient with normal cardiovascular function. Note the absence of a pressure gradient between the LV and radial artery in systole and between the LV and PCW in diastole.

perature or chilled intravenous solution is then injected into the vena cava or right atrium via a proximal port on the catheter. The resulting change in temperature at the thermistor is monitored, and the integral of temperature drop at the thermistor is calculated electronically. By conservation of heat, this temperature integral is inversely proportional to the volume flow rate past the thermistor, allowing calculation of the

TABLE 212-3 *Normal Values for Hemodynamic Parameters*	
Pressures (mmHg)	
Systemic arterial	
Peak systolic/end-diastolic	100–140/60–90
Mean	70–105
Left ventricle	
Peak systolic/end-diastolic	100–140/3–12
Left atrium (or pulmonary capillary wedge)	
Mean	2–10
a wave	3–15
v wave	3–15
Pulmonary artery	
Peak systolic/end-diastolic	15–30/4–12
Mean	9–18
Right ventricle	
Peak systolic/end-diastolic	15–30/2–8
Right atrium	
Mean	2–8
a wave	2–10
v wave	2–10
Resistances [(dyn·s)/cm⁵]	
Systemic vascular resistance	700–1600
Pulmonary vascular resistance	20–130
Cardiac index [(L/min)/m²]	2.6–4.2
Oxygen consumption index [(L/min)/m²]	110–150
Arteriovenous oxygen difference (mL/L)	30–50

FIGURE 212-2   Pulmonary capillary wedge (PCW) and left ventricular (LV) pressure tracings in a 40-year-old woman with mitral stenosis. This patient also had systemic hypertension and significant elevation of her LV diastolic pressure. *[From BA Carabello, W Grossman, in Grossman's Cardiac Catheterization, Angiography, and Intervention, 6th ed, DS Baim, W Grossman (eds). Baltimore, Lippincott Williams & Wilkins, 2000.]*

FIGURE 212-3 Hemodynamic findings at rest and during exercise in a patient with mitral regurgitation. Left ventricular (LV), pulmonary capillary wedge (PCW), and radial artery pressure tracings are shown before (*left*) and during (*right*) the sixth minute of supine bicycle exercise. PCW mean pressure and *v* wave increase substantially with exercise. [*From BH Lorell, W Grossman, in Grossman's Cardiac Catheterization, Angiography, and Intervention, 6th ed, DS Baim, W Grossman (eds). Baltimore, Lippincott Williams & Wilkins, 2000.*]

corresponding pulmonary blood flow. In contrast to the Fick method, the indicator-dilution method is least reliable when the cardiac output is low and transit of the cold bolus through the right heart is delayed.

LEFT HEART CATHETERIZATION

Whether performed using the femoral, brachial, or radial approach, the left heart catheter is advanced under fluoroscopic guidance into the central aorta, where pressure is measured and recorded. Next, the catheter is advanced in retrograde fashion across the aortic valve into the left ventricle, where pressure is measured. If a right heart catheter is in place, this is an appropriate time for simultaneous measurement and recording of left heart, right heart, and peripheral arterial pressures together with a determination of cardiac output by either thermodilution or the Fick method. This hemodynamic "snap-shot" allows assessment of possible pressure gradients across the mitral and aortic valves and calculation of systemic and pulmonary vascular resistances. The resistance to blood flow through the systemic vascular bed is

$$SVR = 80(MAP - RA)/SBF$$

where *SVR* is systemic vascular resistance [(dyn·s)/cm⁵], *MAP* and *RA*

where SVR is systemic vascular resistance [(dyn·s)/cm^5], MAP and RA

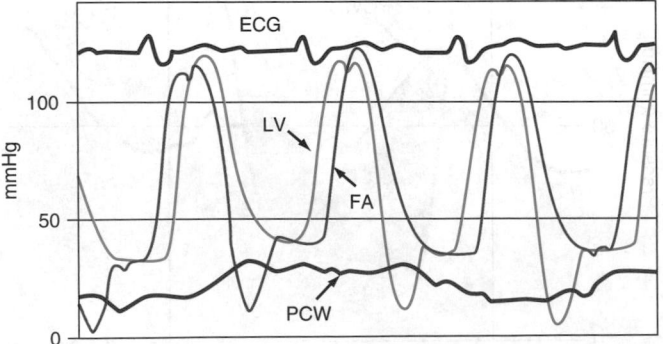

FIGURE 212-4 Severe aortic regurgitation. There is equilibration between the left ventricular (LV) and aortic or femoral artery (FA) pressures in diastole. Also, LV diastolic pressure exceeds pulmonary capillary wedge (PCW) pressure early in diastole, indicating premature closure of the mitral valve (a characteristic feature of severe aortic regurgitation). [*From W Grossman, in Grossman's Cardiac Catheterization, Angiography, and Intervention, 6th ed, DS Baim, W Grossman (eds). Baltimore, Lippincott Williams & Wilkins, 2000.*]

are mean aortic and right atrial pressures (mmHg), 80 is a constant for converting to metric units, and *SBF* is systemic blood flow (L/min). Resistance to blood flow through the pulmonary vascular bed is

$$PVR = 80(PA - PCW \text{ or } LA)/PBF$$

where *PVR* is pulmonary vascular resistance [(dyn·s)/cm⁵]; *PA*, *PCW*, and *LA* are pulmonary artery, pulmonary capillary wedge, and left atrial mean pressures, respectively (mmHg); and *PBF* is pulmonary blood flow (L/min). Normal values for pulmonary and systemic vascular resistances are given in Table 212-3.

When valvular stenosis is present, the measurements of the upstream and downstream pressures and flow allow calculation of the valve orifice using the Gorlin formula

$$A = flow/K\sqrt{\Delta P}$$

where *A* is the valve orifice area (cm²), *flow* is the blood flow (mL/s) across the stenotic valve; Δ*P* is the mean pressure gradient (mmHg) during the period of blood flow; and *K* is a constant (44.3 for the aortic valve and 37.7 for the mitral valve).

In the normal heart, left ventricular and aortic pressures should be essentially equal during systole, while left atrial (pulmonary capillary wedge) and left ventricular pressures should be equal during diastole, as seen in Fig. 212-1. The presence of a systolic pressure gradient between the left ventricle and aorta indicates obstruction at the level of the aortic valve (e.g., calcific *aortic stenosis*) or at subaortic level (e.g., *hypertrophic obstructive cardiomyopathy*). Similarly, the presence of a diastolic pressure gradient between the left atrium (or pulmonary capillary wedge pressure) and the left ventricle generally indicates *mitral stenosis*, although it may also be seen in rare conditions such as cor triatriatum and left atrial myxoma. An example of a large diastolic pressure gradient in a patient with mitral stenosis is seen in Fig. 212-2. As seen in Fig. 212-3, patients with significant mitral regurgitation may have a prominent *v* wave in the pulmonary capillary wedge pressure, which often increases substantially during modest exercise. Severe *aortic regurgitation* produces a widening of the aortic pulse pressure, with equilibration of aortic and left ventricular pressures in diastole (Fig. 212-4). In the presence of valvular heart disease affecting the tricuspid or pulmonic valves, right-sided pressures exhibit characteristic deformities. In patients with severe *tricuspid regurgitation*, the right atrial pressure resembles the right ventricular pressure closely in appearance. Mean right atrial pressure and right ventricular end-diastolic pressure are both elevated in tricuspid regurgitation. In *tricuspid stenosis*, there is a pressure gradient between the right atrium and ventricle during diastole.

In *cardiac tamponade* or *pericardial constriction* (Chap. 222), there is equalization of left and right ventricular diastolic pressures. In pericardial tamponade, diastolic pressures continue to increase gradually throughout diastole, but in constrictive pericarditis ventricular filling ceases shortly after mitral and tricuspid valve opening. This produces an abrupt rise in ventricular diastolic pressure with a mid- and late-ventricular pressure plateau, giving the so-called square root sign (Fig. 212-5).

Congestive heart failure due to myocardial contractile dysfunction is associated with characteristic alterations in the ventricular pressure waveforms seen at cardiac catheterization. Neither the rise nor the decline in isovolumic pressure is as steep as in the normal heart. The reduced slopes of pressure rise and decline are associated with an abbreviated ejection period, giving the left ventricular pressure tracing a triangular appearance (Fig. 212-6). Also, the pressure decline does not continue to zero, so the minimal left ventricular pressure may be elevated. This hemodynamic finding correlates with an increased ventricular end-systolic volume, which is a sign of depressed contractile function of the left ventricular myocardium.

CARDIAC ANGIOGRAPHY

LEFT VENTRICULOGRAPHY

Following the measurement of cardiac pressures, the angiographic portion of the cardiac catheterization usually begins with left ventriculography—the injection of radiographic contrast material directly into the left ventricular cavity. A power injector is used to inject 30 to 45 mL of radiographic contrast material into the left ventricular chamber at a rate of 10 to 12 mL/s. The resulting radiographic images are recorded, and the left ventricular silhouette is defined at end-diastole and end-systole. This permits calculation of the left ventricular chamber volumes and ejection fraction, as well as qualitative assessment of regional wall motion abnormalities. The normal left ventricle ejects 50 to 80% of its end-diastolic volume with each beat; i.e., its *ejection fraction* is 0.50 to 0.80. In adults, normal values for left ventricular volumes are, for end-diastolic volume, 72 ± 15 mL/m² (mean $\pm$ standard deviation) and, for end-systolic volume, 20 ± 8 mL/m². Regional abnormalities of wall motion are illustrated in Fig. 212-7 and include diminished inward motion of a myocardial segment (*hypokinesis*), absence of inward movement of a myocardial segment (*akinesis*), and paradoxical systolic expansion of a regional myocardial segment (*dyskinesis*).

Performing left ventriculography in the right anterior oblique projection allows assessment of the mitral and aortic valves. Mitral regurgitation is easily visualized as the leakage of radiographic contrast material back into the left atrium during left ventricular systole. Its severity can be estimated qualitatively using a grading system of 1+ (mild; radiographic contrast material clears with each beat and never opacifies the entire left atrium) to 4+ (severe; opacification of the

FIGURE 212-5 Left ventricular (LV), right ventricular (RV), and pulmonary capillary wedge (PCW) pressure tracings in a patient with severe constrictive pericarditis. Note the diastolic dip and plateau ("square root sign") pattern for left and right ventricular diastolic pressures (*left*). The wedge pressure (*right*) shows early systolic and early diastolic dips.

entire left atrium occurs within one beat, and contrast material can be seen refluxing into the pulmonary veins).

On occasion, left ventriculography may also be performed in the *left* anterior oblique projection to evaluate contraction of the septal or lateral walls or to detect abnormal communications such as ventricular septal defect (Chap. 218). In the most common form of hypertrophic cardiomyopathy (idiopathic hypertrophic subaortic stenosis; Chap. 221), left ventriculography in this projection shows anterior motion of the anterior leaflet of the mitral valve during systole and bulging of the interventricular septum into the left ventricular cavity, especially in the subaortic region. Mural thrombi within the left ventricular chamber may be well visualized during left ventriculography; they occur most commonly in the left ventricular apex.

It should be pointed out, however, that many of these findings could

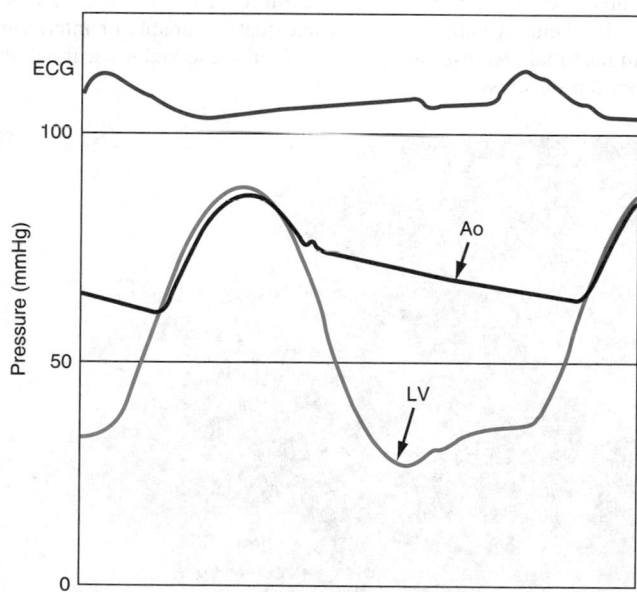

FIGURE 212-6 Left ventricular (LV) and aortic (Ao) pressures in a patient with advanced dilated cardiomyopathy. Marked slowing of the rates of LV pressure rise and fall (impairment of contractility and relaxation) give the LV pressure pulse a triangular appearance. Also, the minimal value for LV diastolic pressure is markedly elevated, suggesting an increased end-systolic volume and a reduced LV ejection fraction. [*From W Grossman, in Grossman's Cardiac Catheterization, Angiography, and Intervention, 6th ed, DS Baim, W Grossman (eds). Baltimore, Lippincott Williams & Wilkins, 2000.*]

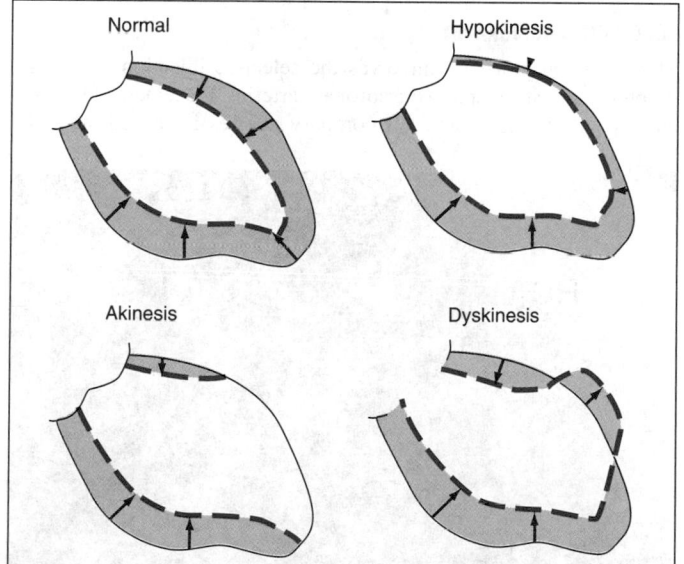

FIGURE 212-7 Diagrammatic representation of end-diastolic (*solid line*) and end-systolic (*dashed line*) silhouettes of left ventricular cineangiograms in various forms of localized wall motion disorder in patients with coronary heart disease. Normal wall motion is symmetric; a patient with *hypokinesis* exhibits reduced contraction, seen here over the anterior and apical surfaces; a patient with *akinesis* exhibits absent wall motion, seen here over the anteroapical surface; a patient with *dyskinesis* exhibits paradoxic bulging of a small portion of the anterior wall with systole.

FIGURE 212-8 Representation of coronary anatomy relative to the interventricular and atrioventricular valve planes. Coronary branches are indicated as L Main (left main), LAD (left anterior descending), D (diagonal), S (septal), CX (circumflex), OM (obtuse marginal), RCA (right coronary artery), CB (conus branch), SN (sinus node), AcM (acute marginal), PD (posterior descending), PL (posterolateral left ventricular). RAO, right anterior oblique, LAO, left anterior oblique. *[From DS Baim, W Grossman, in Grossman's Cardiac Catheterization, Angiography, and Intervention, 6th ed, DS Baim, W Grossman (eds). Baltimore, Lippincott Williams & Wilkins, 2000.]*

also be evaluated using either cardiac echo or cardiac magnetic resonance imaging. This allows avoidance of left ventriculography in patients where a reduction in total contrast load is desired.

AORTOGRAPHY

Rapid injection of radiographic contrast material into the ascending aorta allows detection of abnormalities that involve the aorta and aortic valve. When suspected clinically, aortography permits detection and qualitative assessment of the severity of abnormalities such as aortic regurgitation, which is graded using a 1+ to 4+ scale, as for mitral regurgitation. Abnormal communications between the aorta and right side of the heart, such as a patent ductus arteriosus or ruptured aneurysm of a sinus of Valsalva, may be visualized. Aortography can permit identification of aortic aneurysm and of aortic dissection (Chap. 231) by visualizing an intimal flap within the aortic lumen.

CORONARY ANGIOGRAPHY

This common procedure involves the selective injection of a radiographic contrast agent into the coronary arteries. Placement of the catheter tip into the right and left coronary arteries is carried out under fluoroscopic guidance, and contrast agent is injected by hand during recording of the radiographic image. Each coronary artery is usually viewed in several projections to permit assessment of the severity of stenosis and to minimize the overlap of adjacent vessels. In addition to the detection of coronary artery stenoses, coronary angiography evaluates the rapidity of coronary flow, the blush of capillary filling in the myocardium, the presence of congenital abnormalities of the coronary circulation, and patency of any coronary artery bypass grafts. Examples of normal and abnormal coronary anatomy are shown in Figs. 212-8 and 212-9. The location, severity, and morphology of the stenotic lesions can be analyzed in great detail, and the resulting information is essential to planning either bypass surgery or catheter-based intervention (Fig. 212-10). This is usually done by visual estimation of percent diameter stenosis of each lesion relative to the "uninvolved" adjacent reference segment, with stenosis > 50% taken as being hemodynamically significant (that is capable of interfering with maximal increases in perfusion of the subserved myocardial territory during stress).

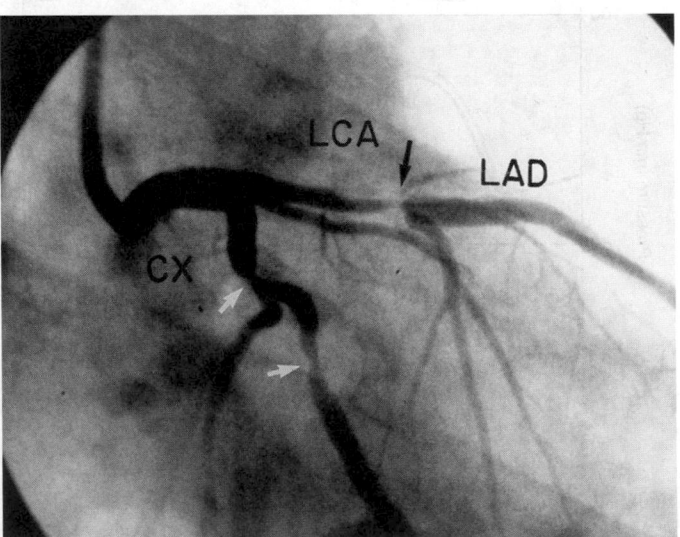

FIGURE 212-9 Coronary angiogram showing a right coronary artery (RCA) with a severe (95%) stenosis at its midpoint (*arrow*).

FIGURE 212-10 Coronary angiogram of a left coronary artery (LCA) with a tight stenosis in the proximal left anterior descending (LAD) artery (*black arrow*) immediately prior to the origin of a large septal branch. The circumflex artery (CX) has two moderately severe stenoses (*white arrows*).

POSTPROCEDURE CARE

The average diagnostic cardiac catheterization procedure takes roughly 30 min. Intravenous heparin (2000 to 3000 IU) may be given at the time of catheter insertion and reversed with intravenous protamine at the conclusion, but increasingly diagnostic catheterization is being performed without anticoagulant administration. The vascular sheaths are removed at the end of the procedure, and hemostasis is achieved by applying local pressure over the puncture site for 10 to 15 min, followed by a 2- to 4-h period of bed rest before ambulation and discharge. Alternatively, a variety of devices are now available for sealing the arterial puncture site, to allow a shorter period of bed rest and earlier ambulation. Most patients with suitable anatomy, however, now undergo a catheter-based intervention during the same procedure as the diagnostic cardiac catheterization, entailing an overnight hospital stay (Chap. 229).

FURTHER READING

BAIM DS, GROSSMAN W (eds): *Grossman's Cardiac Catheterization, Angiography, and Intervention*, 6th ed. Baltimore, Lippincott Williams & Wilkins, 2000

DAVIDSON CJ et al: Cardiac catheterization, in *Braunwald's Heart Disease*, 7th ed, D Zipes et al (eds). Philadelphia, Saunders, 2004

KERN MJ et al: Interpretation of cardiac pathophysiology from pressure waveform analysis: Simultaneous left and right ventricular pressure measurements. Cathet Cardiovasc Diagn 28:51, 1993

RYAN TJ: The coronary angiogram and its seminal contributions to cardiovascular medicine over five decades. Circulation 106:752, 2002

SCANLON PJ et al: AHA/ACC guidelines for coronary angiography—executive summary and recommendations. Circulation 99:2345, 1999

Section 2   Disorders of Rhythm

213 THE BRADYARRHYTHMIAS: DISORDERS OF SINUS NODE FUNCTION AND AV CONDUCTION DISTURBANCES
Mark E. Josephson, Peter Zimetbaum

ANATOMY OF THE CONDUCTING SYSTEM Under normal conditions, the pacemaker function of the heart resides in the sinoatrial (SA) node, which lies at the junction of the right atrium and superior vena cava. The SA node is approximately 1.5 cm long and 2 to 3 mm wide and is supplied by the sinus node artery, which arises from either the right coronary artery (60%) or the left circumflex coronary artery (40%). Once the impulse exits the sinus node and perinodal tissue, it traverses the atrium until it reaches the atrioventricular (AV) node. The blood supply of the AV node is derived from the posterior descending coronary artery (90%). The AV node lies at the base of the interatrial septum just above the tricuspid annulus and anterior to the coronary sinus. The electrophysiologic properties of the AV node result in slow conduction, which is responsible for the normal delay in AV conduction, i.e., the PR interval.

The bundle of His emerges from the AV node, enters the fibrous skeleton of the heart, and courses anteriorly across the membranous interventricular septum. It has a dual blood supply from the AV nodal artery and a branch of the anterior descending coronary artery. The branching (distal) portion of the bundle of His gives rise to a broad sheet of fibers that course over the left side of the interventricular septum to form the left bundle branch and a narrow cable-like structure on the right side that forms the right bundle branch. The arborization of both the right and left bundle branches gives rise to the distal His-Purkinje system, which ultimately extends throughout the endocardium of the right and left ventricles.

The SA node, atrium, and AV node are significantly influenced by autonomic tone. Vagal influences depress automaticity of the SA node, depress conduction, and prolong refractoriness in the tissue surrounding the SA node; inhomogeneously decrease atrial refractoriness and slow atrial conduction; and prolong AV nodal conduction and refractoriness. Sympathetic influences exert the opposite effect.

ELECTROPHYSIOLOGIC PRINCIPLES

In the resting state, the interior of most cardiac cells, with the exception of the SA and AV nodes, is approximately −80 to −90 mV, negative with respect to a reference extracellular electrode. The resting membrane potential is determined primarily by the concentration gradient of potassium across the cell membrane. Activation of cardiac cells results from movement of ions across the cell membrane, causing a transient depolarization known as the *action potential*. The ionic species responsible for the action potential varies among the cardiac tissues, and the configuration of the action potential is therefore unique to each tissue (Fig. 213-1).

The action potential of the His-Purkinje system has five phases (Fig. 213-2). The rapid depolarizing current (phase 0) is mainly determined by an influx of sodium into myocardial cells followed by a secondary (slower) influx of calcium, which produces a slow inward current. The repolarization phases of the action potential (phases 1 to 3) are primarily related to outward flux of potassium. The resting membrane potential is phase 4. Recent studies have demonstrated hetero-

FIGURE 213-1   Action potential configurations in different regions of the mammalian heart. (*From AM Katz, Physiology of the Heart, 2d ed. New York, Raven, 1992, with permission.*)

FIGURE 213-2 Schematic representation of the action potential in normal ventricle depicting the direction, strength, and period of flow of the ionic currents underlying the action potential. The arrow's direction and size indicate whether current is inward- or outward-directed and the approximate current strength of the ion identified at the arrow's base. The horizontal position of the arrow corresponds to the same moment in the time course of action potential (see text). The five phases of the action potential are indicated by the numerals placed along the waveform *(From Ten Eick et al, Prog Cardiovasc Dis 24:157, 1981, with permission.)*

geneity of action potentials in the epicardium, mid-myocardium, and endocardium as well as between right and left ventricles. These differences are due to different ion currents in different layers.

The bradyarrhythmias result from abnormalities either of impulse formation, i.e., automaticity, or of conduction. *Automaticity*, which is normally observed in the sinus node, the specialized fibers of the His-Purkinje system, and some specialized atrial fibers, is the property of a cardiac cell that causes it to depolarize spontaneously during phase 4 of the action potential, leading to the generation of an impulse. To exhibit automaticity, the resting membrane potential must decrease spontaneously until threshold potential is reached and an all-or-none regenerative response occurs. The ionic currents producing spontaneous diastolic depolarization appear to involve the inward currents of sodium and/or calcium and a decreasing outward potassium current.

The velocity of *conduction*, i.e., impulse propagation through cardiac tissues, depends on the magnitude of inward current, which is directly related to the rate of rise and amplitude of phase 0 of the action potential. The more positive the threshold potential and the slower the rate of depolarization toward threshold, the lower is the rate of rise and amplitude of phase 0 of the action potential and the slower is the conduction velocity. Disease states or drugs may result in lower rates of rise of phase 0 at any given membrane potential. Passive membrane properties (e.g., intracellular resistance and intercellular coupling) can also affect impulse propagation. Propagation is more rapid parallel to fiber orientation than transverse to it, a property termed *anisotropic conduction*.

Refractoriness is a property of cardiac cells that defines the period of recovery that cells require after being discharged before they can be reexcited by a stimulus. The *absolute refractory period* is defined by that portion of the action potential during which no stimulus, regardless of its strength, can evoke another response. The *effective refractory period* is that part of the action potential during which a stimulus can evoke only a local, nonpropagated response. The *relative refractory period* extends from the end of the effective refractory period to the time that the tissue is fully recovered. During this time, a stimulus of greater than threshold strength is required to evoke a response, which is propagated more slowly than normal. In the normal His-Purkinje system or ventricular myocytes, excitability is recovered following completion of the action potential, and evoked responses

have characteristics similar to the spontaneous normal response. In the AV node, recovery of excitability occurs well after completion of the action potential.

INTRACARDIAC RECORDINGS OF THE SPECIALIZED CONDUCTING SYSTEM Electrode catheters allow the recording of activation of portions of the specialized conducting system, including the bundle of His. To obtain a recording from the bundle of His, the electrode catheter is positioned across the tricuspid valve (Fig. 213-3). The interval from local atrial depolarization in the His bundle recording to the onset of depolarization of the His bundle deflection is called the *AH interval* (normal = 60 to 125 ms) and represents an indirect method of assessing AV nodal conduction time. The interval from the beginning of the His bundle deflection to the earliest onset of ventricular activation, as measured from any of multiple-surface electrocardiogram (ECG) leads or the intracardiac ventricular electrogram, is called the *HV interval* (normal = 35 to 55 ms) and represents conduction time through the His-Purkinje system. Electrode catheters can be positioned in the area of the sinus node to record high right atrial activity. Left atrial activity may be recorded directly via a catheter placed across a patent foramen ovale or indirectly using a catheter inserted into the coronary sinus. The atrial activation sequence may be "mapped," and sites of intra- and interatrial conduction abnormalities may be ascertained.

FIGURE 213-3 *(Top)* Schema relating the surface electrocardiogram with intracardiac conduction. The normal AV nodal conduction time (AH interval) is 60–125 ms and normal His-Purkinje conduction time (HV interval) is 35–55 ms. Surface ECG leads I, II, and V₁ are displayed with intracardiac ECGs from the high right atrium (HRA), left atrium from the coronary sinus (CS), and AV junction to obtain a His bundle electrogram (HBE). T, time lines; A, atrial activation; H, His bundle activation; V, ventricular activation. Atrial activation begins in the HRA and spreads inferiorly to the low atrial septum, as recorded in the HBE, and the left atrium, as recorded in the CS. The AH and HV intervals represent AV nodal and His-Purkinje conduction times, respectively. *(Bottom)* Normal intracardiac recording. Normal atrioventricular conduction. Vertical lines at bottom = 0.10 s. *(From ME Josephson, Clinical Cardiac Electrophysiology: Techniques and Interpretations, 3d ed. Philadelphia, Lippincott Williams & Wilkins 2002, with permission.)*

SINUS NODE DYSFUNCTION

The SA node is normally the dominant cardiac pacemaker because its intrinsic discharge rate is the highest of all potential cardiac pacemakers. Its responsiveness to alterations in autonomic nervous system tone is responsible for the normal acceleration of heart rate during exercise and the slowing that occurs during rest and sleep. Increases in sinus rate normally result from an increase in parasympathetic tone acting

FIGURE 213-4 Tachycardia-bradycardia syndrome. Rhythm strip of ECG lead II showing spontaneous cessation of supraventricular tachycardia followed by a 6-s pause prior to resumption of sinus activity. The patient was asymptomatic during supraventricular tachycardia, but the sinus pause caused severe light-headedness.

via muscarinic receptors and/or an increase in sympathetic tone acting via β-adrenergic receptors. Slowing of the heart rate is normally due to opposite alterations. In adults, the normal sinus rate under basal conditions is 60 to 100 beats/min. *Sinus bradycardia* is said to exist when the sinus rate is <60 beats/min, and *sinus tachycardia* when it is >100 beats/min. However, there is wide variation among individuals, and rates <60 beats/min do not necessarily indicate pathologic states. For example, trained athletes often exhibit resting rates <50 beats/min due to increases in vagal tone. Normal elderly individuals may also show marked sinus bradycardia at rest.

ETIOLOGY SA node dysfunction is most often found in the elderly as an isolated phenomenon. Although interruption of the blood supply to the SA node may produce dysfunction, the correlation between obstruction of the sinus node artery and clinical evidence of SA node dysfunction is poor. Specific disease states associated with SA node dysfunction include senile amyloidosis and other conditions associated with infiltration of the atrial myocardium. Sinus bradycardia is associated with hypothyroidism, advanced liver disease, hypothermia, typhoid fever, and brucellosis; it occurs during episodes of hypervagotonia (vasovagal syncope), severe hypoxia, hypercapnia, acidemia, and acute hypertension. However, most cases of SA node dysfunction are due to idiopathic degeneration or are secondary to pharmacologic agents.

MANIFESTATIONS Although marked and/or inappropriate (≤50 beats/min) sinus bradycardia may cause fatigue and other symptoms due to inadequate cardiac output, more commonly sinus node dysfunction is manifest as paroxysmal dizziness, presyncope, or syncope. These symptoms usually result from abrupt, prolonged sinus pauses caused by failure of sinus impulse formation (sinus arrest) or block of conduction of sinus impulses to the surrounding atrial tissue (sinus exit block). In either case, the ECG manifestation is a prolonged period (3 s) of atrial asystole. In some patients, SA node dysfunction is accompanied by abnormalities in AV conduction. In addition to the absence of atrial activity, lower pacemakers fail to emerge during the sinus pauses, resulting in periods of ventricular asystole and syncope. Occasionally, SA node dysfunction is manifested by an inadequate acceleration in sinus rate in response to a stress such as exercise or fever. In some patients, SA node dysfunction may become manifest only in the presence of certain cardioactive drugs: cardiac glycosides, β-adrenergic blocking drugs, calcium channel blockers, amiodarone, and other antiarrhythmic agents. These agents, which do not usually cause sinus node dysfunction in normal individuals, may unmask evidence of sinus node dysfunction in susceptible individuals.

The *sick sinus syndrome* refers to a combination of symptoms (dizziness, confusion, fatigue, syncope, and congestive heart failure) caused by SA node dysfunction and manifested by marked sinus bradycardia, sinoatrial block, or sinus arrest. Because these symptoms are nonspecific, and because ECG manifestations of sinus node dysfunction are often intermittent, it may be difficult to prove that such symptoms are actually caused by SA node dysfunction.

Atrial tachyarrhythmias such as atrial fibrillation, atrial flutter, or atrial tachycardia may be accompanied by SA node dysfunction. The *bradycardia-tachycardia syndrome* refers to paroxysmal atrial arrhythmia that upon termination is followed by prolonged sinus pauses

(Fig. 213-4) or in which there are alternating periods of tachyarrhythmia and bradyarrhythmia. Syncope or presyncope may result from failure of the sinus node to recover function following suppression of automaticity by atrial tachyarrhythmia.

DIAGNOSIS *First-degree sinoatrial exit block* denotes a prolonged conduction time from the SA node to the surrounding atrial tissue. It cannot be recognized on a standard (surface) ECG but requires invasive intracardiac recordings, which can detect this condition indirectly, by measuring the sinus response to atrial premature beats, or directly, by recording SA node electrograms. *Second-degree sinoatrial exit block* denotes the intermittent failure of conduction of sinus impulses to the surrounding atrial tissue; it is manifested as the intermittent absence of P waves (Fig. 213-5). *Third-degree*, or *complete, sinoatrial block* is characterized by a lack of atrial activity or by the presence of an ectopic subsidiary atrial pacemaker. On the standard ECG it cannot be distinguished from sinus arrest, but direct intracardiac recordings of SA node activity permit this distinction. The bradycardia-tachycardia syndrome is manifested on the standard ECG as tachyarrhythmias (Fig. 213-4). Most often these are atrial flutter or fibrillation, although any tachycardia during which the atria are activated may cause overdrive suppression of the sinus node, resulting in clinical appearance of this syndrome.

The most important step in the diagnosis of sick sinus syndrome is to correlate symptoms with ECG evidence of SA node dysfunction. While ambulatory ECG (Holter) monitoring remains a mainstay in evaluating sinus node function, most episodes of syncope are paroxysmal and unpredictable. Single and even multiple 24-h Holter monitor recordings may fail to include a symptomatic episode. Caution must be taken in interpreting the Holter monitor results. For instance, a pause during sleep is often a normal finding associated with heightened vagal tone. This should not be interpreted as sinus node dysfunction requiring pacemaker implantation. Continuous-loop event records represent a more specific diagnostic tool. These devices may be worn for prolonged periods of time and allow close correlation between electrocardiographic findings and symptoms. They do require the patient's ability to activate the monitor at the time of symptoms. More recently, an implantable event recorder, which can be interrogated like a pacemaker, has been developed for patients with rare events.

The response to carotid sinus pressure and pharmacologic autonomic "denervation" of the heart may be helpful. Carotid sinus pressure can be particularly useful in patients in whom paroxysmal dizziness or syncope is compatible with the hypersensitive carotid si-

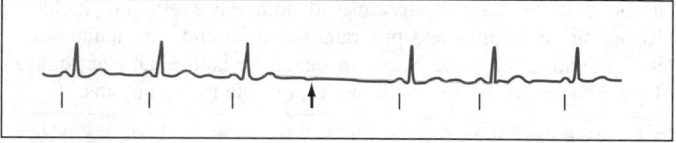

FIGURE 213-5 Second-degree sinoatrial exit block. Surface ECG denoting abrupt absence of P wave during sinus rhythm. Prior to the pause, the sinus rate is regular. The interval of the pause is exactly twice the basal sinus cycle length. The arrow marks the appropriate location for the absent P wave. SA exit block can be 2:1 as above or longer, as shown in Fig. 213-6.

nus syndrome (Chap. 20). In such patients, the response can be dramatic, and sinus pauses in excess of 5 s may occur. Although pauses in excess of 3 s are considered abnormal, in elderly, asymptomatic patients such pauses are common and do not require therapy. This is a major limitation of the use of carotid sinus pressure as a diagnostic test in the elderly. The other noninvasive test of SA node function involves the use of pharmacologic agents to manipulate the autonomic nervous system and assess the balance of parasympathetic and sympathetic activity on the sinus node. Physiologic or pharmacologic maneuvers that are vagomimetic (Valsalva maneuver or phenylephrine-induced hypertension), vagolytic (atropine), sympathomimetic (isoproterenol or hypotension by nitroprusside), or sympatholytic (β-adrenergic blocking agents) can be utilized, singly and in combination. These studies are designed to test the response of the sinus node to autonomic stimulation and inhibition and thereby characterize the status of autonomic regulation of the sinus node. Abnormalities of the autonomic control of sinus function are particularly common in patients in whom asymptomatic sinus bradycardia is documented.

Intrinsic Heart Rate This is a manifestation of the primary activity of the SA node, and its determination requires chemical autonomic blockade of the heart with a combination of atropine and a beta blocker. Normal values of intrinsic heart rate (in beats per minute) are calculated by the formula $118.1 - (0.57 \times age)$. The use of autonomic blockade can separate patients with asymptomatic sinus bradycardia into a group with primary sinus node dysfunction (slow intrinsic heart rate) and a group with autonomic imbalance (normal intrinsic heart rate). Autonomic blockade is particularly useful when combined with invasive assessment of sinus node function. Autonomic blockade may depress conduction in patients with intrinsic disease of the conduction system and should be carried out only in a setting where arrhythmias can be monitored and treated rapidly.

EVALUATION The invasive electrophysiologic investigation of SA node dysfunction should be undertaken in patients who have had symptoms compatible with SA node dysfunction and in whom no documentation of the arrhythmia responsible for these symptoms has been obtained by prolonged monitoring. Asymptomatic patients with sinus bradycardia need not be tested, since no therapy is indicated. Similarly, symptomatic patients with ECG documentation of asystole, sinoatrial block or arrest, or the bradycardia-tachycardia syndrome do not require electrophysiologic tests for diagnosis. However, in symptomatic patients without documentation of an arrhythmia, electrophysiologic assessment of SA node function can yield information that may be used to guide appropriate therapy. The tools most commonly employed are the sinus node recovery time (a response to overdrive atrial pacing) and sinoatrial conduction time calculated indirectly by response to atrial premature complexes or recorded directly by a sinus node electrogram.

The results of electrophysiologic tests of sinus node function must be interpreted with caution. SA node dysfunction coexists frequently with other disorders such as AV conduction disturbances, which may cause symptoms such as syncope. Electrophysiologic evaluation of patients with symptoms such as undiagnosed syncope must not stop with the demonstration of abnormalities of SA node dysfunction or carotid sinus hypersensitivity. Instead, complete evaluation, including His bundle recordings and programmed atrial and ventricular stimulation (Chap. 214), is necessary to search for additional electrophysiologic abnormalities that could be responsible for symptoms.

℞ TREATMENT

Permanent pacemakers (p. 1339) are the mainstay of therapy for patients with symptomatic SA node dysfunction. Patients with intermittent paroxysms of bradycardia or sinus arrest and with the cardioinhibitory form of the hypersensitive carotid sinus syndrome are usually adequately treated by demand ventricular pacemakers. These devices are reliable, relatively inexpensive, and suffice to prevent episodic symptoms due to abrupt bradycardia. Although an atrial demand pacemaker should be adequate for patients with SA node dysfunction, the frequent accompaniment of dysfunction in other portions of the cardiac conduction system mandates placement of a pacemaker also capable of ventricular pacing. Whether dual-chamber pacing offers any advantages to ventricular pacing in such circumstances remains uncertain. Patients with symptomatic chronic sinus bradycardia or frequent prolonged episodes of sinus node dysfunction do better with dual-chamber pacemakers that preserve the normal AV activation sequence. Recent studies suggest that AV sequential pacing may also be useful in preventing atrial fibrillation, an important component of the bradycardia-tachycardia syndrome, and stroke, a known complication of atrial fibrillation.

AV CONDUCTION DISTURBANCES

The specialized cardiac conducting system normally ensures synchronous conduction of each sinus impulse from the atria to the ventricles. Abnormalities of conduction of the sinus impulse to the ventricles may portend the development of heart block, which can ultimately lead to syncope or cardiac arrest. In order to evaluate the clinical significance of conduction abnormalities, the physician must assess (1) the site of conduction disturbance, (2) the risk of progression to complete block, and (3) the probability that a subsidiary escape rhythm arising distal to the site of block will be electrophysiologically and hemodynamically stable. This latter point is perhaps the most important, since the rate and stability of the escape pacemaker determine what symptoms result from heart block. The escape pacemaker following AV nodal block is usually in the His bundle, which generally has a stable rate of 40 to 60 beats/min and is associated with a QRS complex of normal duration (in the absence of a preexisting intraventricular conduction defect). This contrasts with escape rhythms arising in the distal His-Purkinje system, which have lower intrinsic rates (25 to 45 beats/min), manifest wide QRS complexes with prolonged duration, and are unstable. Thus, the most important issue is to assess the risk of infra- or intra-His block (which always mandates a pacemaker) or AV nodal block in which the frequency of the escape pacemaker is not sufficient to meet hemodynamic requirements (Table 213-1). Although prolonged QRS complexes are invariable when the distal His-Purkinje pacemakers form the escape mechanism, wide QRS complexes can also coexist with AV nodal block and a His bundle rhythm. Therefore, QRS morphology alone may not be adequate to identify the site of block.

ETIOLOGY The AV node is supplied by the parasympathetic and sympathetic nervous systems and is sensitive to variations in autonomic tone. Chronic slowing of AV nodal conduction may be seen in highly trained athletes who have hypervagotonia at rest. A variety of diseases and drugs can also influence AV nodal conduction. These include acute processes such as myocardial infarction (particularly inferior); coronary spasm (usually of the right coronary artery); digitalis intoxication; excesses of beta and/or calcium blockers; acute infections such as viral myocarditis, acute rheumatic fever, infectious mononucleosis; and miscellaneous disorders such as Lyme disease, sarcoidosis, amyloidosis, and neoplasms, particularly cardiac mesotheliomas. AV nodal block may also be congenital.

TABLE 213-1 Atrioventricular Conduction Evaluation

1. Atrial activation times: Measurement of intraatrial conduction times. Prolonged activation times may be associated with atrial flutter or fibrillation.
2. Measurement of AH and HV intervals: Prolongation of AH interval (>125 ms) or prolongation of the HV interval (>55 ms) may help localize the site of delay.
3. Incremental atrial pacing: To determine the cycle length at which block occurs in the AV node and/or His-Purkinje system. Block below the His bundle at rates of <150 beats per minute portends the development of infra-His block.

Two degenerative diseases are commonly responsible for damage to the specialized conducting system and produce AV block usually associated with bundle branch block (Chap. 210). In *Lev's disease*, there are calcification and sclerosis of the fibrous cardiac skeleton, which frequently involve the aortic and mitral valves, the central fibrous body, and the summit of the ventricular septum. *Lenegre's disease* appears to be a primary sclerodegenerative disease of the conducting system with no involvement of the myocardium or the fibrous skeleton of the heart. These two diseases are probably the most common causes of isolated chronic heart block in adults. Hypertension and aortic and/or mitral stenosis are specific disorders that either accelerate the degeneration of the conducting system or have a direct effect by calcification and fibrosis involving the conducting system.

First-degree AV block, more properly termed *prolonged AV conduction*, is classically characterized by a PR interval >0.20 s, but use of this value may be misleading in terms of clinical significance. Since the PR interval is determined by atrial, AV nodal, and His-Purkinje activation, delay in any one or more of these structures can contribute to a prolonged PR interval. In the presence of a QRS complex of normal duration, a PR interval >0.24 s almost invariably is due to a delay within the AV node. If the QRS is prolonged, delays may be present at any of the levels mentioned above. Delay within the His-Purkinje system is always accompanied by a prolonged QRS duration but can occur with a relatively normal PR interval (Fig. 213-6). However, as indicated below, it is only with intracardiac recordings that the exact site of delay can be determined.

Second-degree heart block (intermittent AV block) is present when some atrial impulses fail to conduct to the ventricles. Mobitz type I second-degree AV block (AV Wenckebach block) is characterized by progressive PR interval prolongation prior to block of an atrial impulse (Fig. 213-7A). The pause that follows is less than fully compensatory (i.e., is less than two normal sinus intervals), and the PR interval of the first conducted impulse is shorter than the last conducted atrial impulse prior to the blocked P wave. Usually the difference between the longest and shortest PR intervals exceeds 100 ms. This type of block is almost always localized to the AV node and associated with a normal QRS duration, although bundle branch block may be present. It is seen most often as a transient abnormality with inferior wall infarction or with drug intoxication, particularly digitalis, beta blockers, and occasionally calcium channel antagonists. This type of block can

also be observed in normal individuals with heightened vagal tone. Although Mobitz type I block can progress to complete heart block, this is uncommon, except in the setting of acute inferior wall myocardial infarction. Even when it does, however, the heart block is usually well tolerated because the escape pacemaker usually arises in the proximal His bundle and provides a stable rhythm. As a result, the presence of Mobitz type I second-degree AV block rarely mandates aggressive therapy. Therapeutic decisions depend on the ventricular response and the symptoms of the patient. If the ventricular rate is adequate and the patient is asymptomatic, observation is sufficient.

In Mobitz type II second-degree AV block, conduction fails suddenly and unexpectedly without a preceding change in PR intervals (Fig. 213-7B). It is generally due to disease of the His-Purkinje system and is most often associated with a prolonged QRS duration. When Mobitz type II block occurs with a normal QRS duration, an intra-His site of block should be expected. It is important to recognize this type of block because it has a high incidence of progression to complete heart block with an unstable, slow, lower escape pacemaker. Therefore, pacemaker implantation is necessary in this condition. Mobitz type II block may occur in the setting of anteroseptal infarction or in the primary or secondary sclerodegenerative or calcific disorders of the fibrous skeleton of the heart. In so-called high-degree AV block there are periods of two or more consecutively blocked P waves, but intermittent conduction can be demonstrated. Block is usually in the His-Purkinje system, but simultaneous block in the AV node may also be present. Regardless of the site of origin of the escape rhythm, if it is slow and the patient is symptomatic, a cardiac pacemaker is mandatory.

Third-degree AV block is present when no atrial impulse propagates to the ventricles. If the QRS complex of the escape rhythm is of normal duration, occurs at a rate of 40 to 55 beats/min, and increases with atropine or exercise, AV nodal block is probable. Congenital complete AV block is usually localized to the AV node. If the block is within the His bundle, the escape pacemaker is usually less responsive to these perturbations. If the escape rhythm of the QRS is wide and associated with rates ≤40 beats/min, block is usually localized in, or distal to, the His bundle and mandates a pacemaker, since the escape rhythm in this setting is unreliable (Fig. 213-8). Some patients with infra-His bundle block are capable of retrograde conduction. In such patients, a "pacemaker syndrome" (see below) may develop if a simple ventricular pacemaker is used. Dual-chamber pacemakers eliminate this potential problem.

AV DISSOCIATION AV dissociation exists whenever the atria and ventricles are under the control of two separate pacemakers and, while present in complete AV block, can occur in the absence of a primary conduction disturbance. AV dissociation unrelated to heart block may occur under two circumstances: First, it may develop with an AV junctional rhythm in response to severe sinus bradycardia. When the sinus rate and the escape rate are similar and the P waves occur just before, in, or following the QRS complex, isorhythmic AV dissociation is said to be present. Treatment usually consists of removal of the offending cause of sinus bradycardia (i.e., discontinuation of digitalis, beta blockers, or calcium antagonists), accelerating the sinus node by vagolytic agents, or insertion of a pacemaker if the escape rhythm is slow and results in symptoms. Second, AV dissociation can be caused by an enhanced lower (junctional or ventricular) pacemaker that competes with normal sinus rhythm and frequently exceeds it. This has been called *interference AV dissociation* because the rapid lower pacemaker results in bombardment of the AV node in a retrograde fashion, rendering it refractory to the normal sinus impulses. Thus failure of antegrade conduction is a physiologic response in this circumstance. Interference dissociation commonly occurs during ventricular tachycardia, accelerated junctional or ventricular rhythms seen with digitalis intoxication, myocardial ischemia and/or infarction, or local irritation following cardiac surgery. The accelerated rhythm should be treated

FIGURE 213-6 Example of marked His-Purkinje system disease with a relatively normal PR interval. Surface leads I, aVF, and V₁ are shown with electrograms from the high right atrium (HRA), His bundle electrogram (HBE), and time lines (T). The QRS shows right bundle branch block and left anterior hemiblock; the PR interval is minimally elevated at 205 ms, but the HV interval exceeds 100 ms. Such a prolonged HV interval mandates a pacemaker.

FIGURE 213-7 *A.* Mobitz type I second-degree AV block. Intracardiac recordings demonstrate that the PR prolongation (320, 615 ms) is localized to the AV node (AH 240, 535 ms, respectively). HBE, His bundle electrogram; A, atrium; H, His; V, ventricle. Time lines (T) = 100 ms. *B.* Mobitz type II second-degree AV block. Intracardiac recordings document block below the His bundle. During sinus rhythm right bundle branch block is present. AV nodal conduction is normal (AH, 85 ms), but His-Purkinje conduction is markedly prolonged (HV, 95 ms). The third sinus P wave suddenly blocks below the recorded His deflection without any preceeding change in AV conduction. *(From ME Josephson, Clinical Cardiac Electrophysiology: Techniques and Interpretations, 3d ed. Philadelphia, Lippincott Williams & Wilkins 2002, with permission.)*

with either antiarrhythmic drugs (Chap. 214), removal of an offending drug, or correction of the metabolic abnormality or ischemia.

INTRACARDIAC ELECTROCARDIOGRAPHIC RECORDINGS IN DIAGNOSIS AND MANAGEMENT

The main therapeutic decision in patients with AV conduction disturbance is whether or not a permanent pacemaker is required, and a number of circumstances exist in which His bundle electrocardiography can be a useful diagnostic tool upon which to base

FIGURE 213-8 Third-degree AV block. The figure shows surface leads 1, aVF, V_1, and an intracardiac His bundle recording (HBE). Complete heart block is evident on the surface leads. The intracardiac recording demonstrates an absence of QRS deflection (V) after a His bundle (H) spike. This indicates block below the His bundle. Note that following the second QRS complex (V), there is an atrial (A) deflection indicating retrograde conduction. Retrograde conduction is often present when block is in the His-Purkinje system but is virtually never present when block is in the AV node. *(From ME Josephson, Clinical Cardiac Electrophysiology: Techniques and Interpretations, 3d ed. Philadelphia, Lippincott Williams & Wilkins, 2002, with permission.)*

this decision. It is unquestionable that patients with symptomatic second- or third-degree AV block should be paced, and therefore these patients do not require electrophysiologic study. However, intracardiac ECG recordings can be useful in at least the following four groups of patients:

1. *Patients with syncope and bundle branch or bifascicular block without documentation of AV block.* In such patients, the demonstration of marked infra-His bundle conduction disturbances, i.e., a prolonged HV interval (>100 ms), may usually be taken as an indication of the need for the insertion of the permanent pacemaker. Complete electrophysiologic evaluation, including atrial and ventricular programmed stimulation, is indicated to help identify other possible cardiac etiologies for the syncope. Since the incidence of significant advanced AV block is low in asymptomatic patients who have bifascicular block, electrophysiologic evaluation or permanent pacemakers are not cost-effective. In this group, observation appears most reasonable.

2. *Patients with 2:1 AV conduction.* Intracardiac recordings are necessary to ascertain the site of the conduction disturbance because the typical ECG features of Mobitz type I or Mobitz type II block cannot be discerned during a 2:1 pattern of AV conduction on the surface ECG. Intracardiac recordings may demonstrate that AV nodal block, intra-His bundle block, infra-His bundle block, or combinations of block may be responsible (Figs. 213-7 and 213-8). A surface ECG finding that suggests an infra-His bundle lesion is the presence of alternating bundle branch block associated with changing PR intervals. Intracardiac recordings in such patients confirm that the block is almost always in the His-Purkinje system. Increasing block with exercise or following atropine suggests intra- or infra-His block (Table 213-2). The finding of infra- or intra-His bundle block in patients with asymptomatic second-degree AV block mandates pacemaker therapy because of the high likelihood of the development of symptomatic high-grade AV block and syncope.

3. *Patients with Wenckebach block in the presence of bundle branch block.* This situation, particularly when the maximal change in PR interval is 50 ms, can suggest intra- or infra-His Wenckebach block, in which case a pacemaker is mandated. Intracardiac recordings are necessary to make this diagnosis.

4. *Asymptomatic patients with third-degree AV block.* In such patients, electrophysiologic studies may be useful in assessing the stability of the junctional pacemaker. Pacing is indicated when the His bundle escape pacemaker is shown to be unstable by an inadequate response to exercise, atropine, or isoproterenol or by a prolonged junctional recovery time following ventricular pacing.

GENETIC CONSIDERATIONS A number of congenital and familial syndromes involving the cardiac conduction system have been described. An example of a congenital condition that is transmitted but not genetic is congenital complete heart block associated with maternal systemic lupus erythematosus. This disorder is associated with maternal IgG autoantibodies to several ribonucleoproteins that are transplacentally transmitted to the fetus and damage the fetal AV node. The fetal conduction disease is generally clinically evident by the second trimester and is associated with significant fetal mortality and neonatal requirement of cardiac pacing.

The embryonic development of the cardiac septa and conduction system occur together, and clinical disorders have been described, including the *Holt-Oram syndrome*, an autosomal dominant disorder including upper limb dysplasia and atrial septal defect, often with conduction disturbances in the AV node. Studies of families with a high incidence of congenital heart disease, including ostium secundum atrial septal defect and conduction disorders in the AV node, have

TABLE 213-2 Site of 2:1 Atrioventricular Block

Characteristic	Observation—Site of Block
1. QRS width	BBB—anywhere
	Normal QRS—in AV node or His bundle
2. PR interval of conducted P wave	>0.30 s—in AV node
	≤0.16 s—in HPS or His bundle[a]
3. Atropine or exercise	Improve conduction—in AV node
	Worsen conduction—in HPS or His bundle[a]
4. CSP	Worsen conduction—in AV node
	Improve conduction—in HPS or His bundle[a]
5. Retrograde conduction	Present—in HPS or His bundle[a]
	Absent—may be anywhere

[a] Use of a pacemaker is indicated.
Note: BBB, bundle branch block; HPS, His-Purkinje system; CSP, carotid sinus pressure.

identified the gene NKX2-5 on chromosome 5q35 as important in the regulation of septation and in the development and function of the AV node. A familial syndrome of progressive complete heart block has also long been recognized. The gene for this disorder has been mapped to a region on chromosome 19q13. Familial disorders of SA node function have also been described, but specific details of abnormal genetic sites are not available.

℞ TREATMENT

Pharmacologic Therapy Pharmacologic therapy is usually reserved for acute situations. Atropine (0.5 to 2.0 mg intravenously) and isoproterenol (1 to 4 µg/min intravenously) are useful in increasing heart rate and decreasing symptoms in patients with sinus bradycardia or AV block localized to the AV node. They have an insignificant effect on lower pacemakers. In patients with neurocardiac syncope, beta blockers and disopyramide have been suggested as methods to depress left ventricular function and decrease mechanoreceptor-related reflexes. Mineralocorticoids, midodrine, ephedrine, and theophylline have also been reported to be of benefit to occasional patients. Unfortunately, no controlled study has shown that any of these pharmacologic modalities works in a predictable fashion in all patients. Recently, serotonin-reuptake inhibitors have been shown to benefit some patients. Further work on delineating different mechanisms in different patient groups may allow us to apply pharmacologic agents more appropriately. Long-term therapy of bradyarrhythmias is best accomplished by pacemakers.

Pacemakers External energy sources can be used to stimulate the heart when disorders in impulse formation and/or transmission lead to symptomatic bradyarrhythmias. Pacer stimuli can be applied to the atria and/or ventricles. Indications for pacemaker insertion are listed in the guidelines summarized on p. 1340.

TEMPORARY PACING This is usually instituted to provide immediate stabilization prior to permanent pacemaker placement or to provide pacemaker support when a bradycardia is precipitated by what is presumed to be a transient event such as ischemia or drug toxicity. Temporary pacing is usually achieved by the transvenous insertion of an electrode catheter with the catheter positioned in the right ventricular apex and attached to an external generator. This procedure is associated with a small risk of cardiac perforation, infection at the insertion site, and thromboembolism; the risk of the latter two complications increases markedly if the pacing wire is left in place for >48 h. The development of an entirely external transthoracic cardiac pacing system may preclude the need for transvenous pacing in selected patients. However, occasional failure of ventricular capture and significant discomfort related to the large current required for effective transthoracic ventricular stimulation preclude the uniform use of this approach.

PERMANENT PACING This mode of pacing is instituted for persistent or intermittent symptomatic bradycardia not related to a self-limiting precipitating factor or for documented infranodal second- or third-degree AV block. Permanent pacing leads are usually inserted transvenously through the subclavian or cephalic vein with the leads positioned in the right atrial appendage for atrial pacing and the right ventricular apex for ventricular pacing. The leads are then attached to the pulse generator, which is inserted into a subcutaneous pocket below the clavicle. Epicardial lead placement is used when (1) transvenous access cannot be obtained; (2) the chest is already open, i.e., in the course of a cardiac operation; and (3) adequate endocardial lead placement cannot be achieved. Most pacemaker generators are powered by lithium batteries. The life expectancy of the generator is related to (1) voltage output required for capture, (2) requirement for incessant or intermittent pacing, and (3) number of cardiac chambers paced. Life expectancy of the simple ventricular demand pacemaker can exceed 10 years.

PACING CODE A code consisting of three to five letters has been developed for describing pacemaker type and function (Table 213-3). The first letter indicates the chamber(s) paced and is designated V for ventricular pacing, A for atrial pacing, or D for dual-chamber (both atrial and ventricular) pacing. The second letter indicates the chamber in which electrical activity is sensed and is also indicated by A, V, or D. An additional designation, O, has been used when pacemaker discharge is not dependent on a sensed electrical activity. The third letter refers to the response to a sensed electric signal. The letter O represents no response to an underlying electric signal, usually related to the absence of associated sensing function; I represents inhibition of pacing function; T represents triggering of pacing function; and D indicates a dual response, i.e., spontaneous atrial and ventricular activity inhibiting atrial and ventricular pacing and atrial activity triggering a ventricular response. Additional fourth and fifth letters of the pacing code have been recommended to indicate whether the pacemaker is programmable and has rate modulation (fourth) and whether special antitachycardia functions are available (i.e., antitachycardia pacing, T, and delivery of high- or low-energy shocks). In the fourth category, M represents multiprogrammability and R represents rate response ("physiologic") pacing.

It follows from the described code that the standard VVIR (ventricular demand pacemaker) paces the ventricle, senses the ventricle, is inhibited by sensed spontaneous ventricular activity, and has rate modulation, while the DDDR pulse generator is capable of sensing and pacing both the atria and ventricles and has a dual response to the sensed atrial and ventricular activity as described above (Fig. 213-9). Both pacemakers have rate modulation (R). "Physiologic" pacemakers use sensors (muscular activity, respiratory rate, temperature, O_2 saturation, QT interval, etc.) as methods to allow the pacemaker to increase the heart rate in response to physiologic demands, i.e., exercise. These pacemakers are essential when chronotropic incompetence is present and an increase in heart rate is required to enhance physiologic performance. Studies have shown that such "physiologic" pacemakers improve exercise tolerance and relieve symptoms to a greater degree than fixed-rate pacemakers.

Selection of the appropriate pacemaker and pacing mode depends on the clinical condition and the type of bradyarrhythmia being treated. The two most common pacing mode selections are DDD and VVI. DDD provides AV sequential pacing, which is ideally suited for the relatively young and active patient who has intact sinus node function or intermittent dysfunction and high-grade persistent or intermittent AV block. The DDD mode will allow for physiologic atrial sensed and ventricular paced rates and improve exercise tolerance. AV synchrony and dual-chamber pacing may also be desirable in patients with borderline hemodynamic reserve who are dependent on atrial contribution to cardiac output and in those patients who develop the pacemaker syndrome (see below) in response to ventricular demand pacing.

Rate-responsive DDD (i.e., DDDR) pacing is indicated when chronotropic incompetence is present in a patient who requires AV synchrony. The DDD pacing mode is contraindicated in chronic atrial

Acquired AV Block in Adults

Class I

1. Third-degree and advanced second-degree AV block, associated with any one of the following:
   a. Symptomatic bradycardia
   b. Arrhythmias and other conditions that require drugs that result in symptomatic bradycardia
   c. Documented periods of asystole ≥ 3.0 s or any escape rate less than 40 beats/min
   d. After catheter ablation of the AV junction
   e. Postoperative AV block that is not expected to resolve
   f. Neuromuscular diseases

Class IIa

1. Asymptomatic third-degree block with average awake ventricular rates of ≥ 40 beats/min
2. Asymptomatic type II second-degree AV block with a narrow QRS
3. Asymptomatic type I second-degree AV block at intra- or infra-His levels
4. First- or second-degree AV block with symptoms similar to those of pacemaker syndrome

Class IIb

1. Marked first-degree AV block (> 0.3 s) in patients with LV dysfunction in whom a shorter AV interval results in hemodynamic improvement, presumably by decreasing left atrial filling pressure

Class III

1. Intermittent third-degree AV block
2. Asymptomatic type I second-degree AV block at the AV node
3. AV block expected to resolve

Chronic Bifascicular and Trifascicular Block

Class I

1. Intermittent third-degree AV block
2. Type II second-degree AV block
3. Alternating bundle-branch block

Class IIa

1. Syncope when other likely causes have been excluded
2. Incidental finding at EP study of HV interval ≥ 100 ms
3. Incidental finding at EP study

Class IIb

1. Neuromuscular diseases

Class III

1. Fascicular block without AV block or symptoms
2. Fascicular block with first-degree AV block without symptoms

After Acute Myocardial Infarction

Class I

1. Persistent second-degree AV block in the His-Purkinje system with bilateral bundle branch block or third-degree AV block
2. Transient advanced (second- or third-degree) infranodal AV block and associated bundle branch block
3. Persistent and symptomatic second- or third-degree AV block

Class IIb

1. Persistent second- or third-degree AV nodal block

Class III

1. Transient AV block in the absence of intraventricular conduction defects
2. Transient AV block in the presence of isolated left anterior fascicular block
3. Acquired left anterior fascicular block in absence of AV block
4. Persistent first-degree AV block in the presence of old bundle branch block

Sinus Node Dysfunction

Class I

1. With documented symptomatic bradycardia
2. Symptomatic chronotropic incompetence

Class IIa

1. With heart rate < 40 beats/min not associated with symptoms
2. With syncope of unexplained origin

Class IIb

1. With minimal symptoms

Class III

1. Asymptomatic patients
2. In patients with symptoms documented as not associated with a slow heart rate
3. With symptomatic bradycardia due to nonessential drug therapy

Pacemakers That Automatically Detect and Pace to Terminate Tachycardias

Class I

1. Symptomatic recurrent supraventricular tachycardia that is reducibly terminated by pacing after drugs and catheter ablation failure
2. Symptomatic recurrent sustained VT as part of an automatic defibrillator system

Pacing Recommendations to Prevent Tachycardia

Class I

1. Sustained pause-dependent VT

Class IIa

1. High-risk patients with congenital long-QT syndrome

Class IIb

1. AV reentrant or AV node reentrant supraventricular tachycardia not responsive to therapy
2. Prevention of symptomatic, drug-refractory, recurrent atrial fibrillation

Hypersensitive Carotid Sinus Syndrome and Neurocardiogenic Syncope

Class I

1. Recurrent syncope caused by carotid sinus stimulation
2. Minimal carotid sinus pressure induces ventricular asystole of >3 s duration in the absence of any medication that depresses the sinus node or AV conduction

Class IIa

1. Recurrent syncope without clear, provocative events and with a hypersensitive cardioinhibitory response
2. Syncope of unexplained origin when major abnormalities of sinus node function or AV conduction are discovered or provoked in EP studies
3. Significantly symptomatic and recurrent neurocardiogenic syncope associated with bradycardia documented spontaneously or at the time of tilt-table testing

Class IIb

1. Neurally mediated syncope with significant bradycardia reproduced by a head-up tilt

Class III

1. Hyperactive cardioinhibitory response to carotid sinus stimulation in the absence of symptoms
2. Recurrent syncope, lightheadedness, or dizziness in the absence of a hyperactive cardioinhibitory response

---

Note: Class I: Evidence that procedure/treatment is indicated; Class IIa: Conflicting evidence but weight of evidence in favor; Class IIb: Efficacy less well established; Class III: Evidence that procedure/treatment is not effective; EP: electrophysiologic.

Source: Adapted from the American College of Cardiology/American Heart Association: J Am Coll Cardiol 31:1175, 1998, and incorporating new recommendations from G Gregoratas: Circulation 106:2145, 2002.

---

fibrillation or flutter, because rapid and irregular ventricular pacing will occur to the upper rate limit. In some cases this will produce a more rapid ventricular rate than the patient's own rate in the absence of a pacemaker. DDD pacemakers must either automatically switch (i.e., mode-switching function) or be reprogrammed to the VVI mode. Almost all such pacemakers are now combined with some form of rate responsiveness so that when the device functions in the VVI mode, it also will respond to physiologic demands (VVIR).

Chronotropic insufficiency (i.e., the inability of the sinus rate to accelerate) is a contraindication for a DDD pacemaker, since such a pacemaker will act as a "fixed-rate" pacemaker at the programmed lower rate. In these situations, a rate-adaptive or "physiologic" pace-maker is indicated (VVIR or DDDR). In patients with impaired sinus node function or chronic atrial fibrillation, a sensor-driven, rate-adaptive pacemaker must be implanted. As mentioned earlier, these pacemakers automatically adjust ventricular pacing rates to a sensed indicator of exertion. The DDD pacing mode may also be contraindicated in patients with intermittent or persistent ventriculoatrial conduction, who may develop pacemaker-mediated tachycardia (see below).

Specific pacemaker programming is often effective for the management of vasovagal syncope. These algorithms result in rapid pacing (≥100 beats/min) following the detection of an abrupt and significant drop in sinus rates. Biventricular pacing is a new therapy for class 3

TABLE 213-3 *The NASPE/BPEG Generic Pacemaker Code*

Position Category	I — Chamber(s) Paced	II — Chamber(s) Sensed	III — Response to Sensing	IV — Programmability, Rate Modulation	V — Antitachyarrhythmia Function(s)
	O, None	O, None	O, None	O, None	O, None
	A, Atrium	A, Atrium	T, Triggered	P, Simple programmable	P, Pacing (antitachyarrhythmia)
	V, Ventricle	V, Ventricle	I, Inhibited	M, Multiprogrammable	S, Shock
	D, Dual (A + V)	D, Dual (A + V)	D, Dual (T + I)	C, Communicating	D, Dual (P + S)
				R, Rate modulation	
Manufacturer's designation	S, Single (A or V)	S, (A or V)			

Source: From DP Zipes, in *Braunwald's Heart Disease: A Textbook of Cardiovascular Medicine,* 7th ed. Philadelphia, Saunders, 2005.

and 4 heart failure with QRS prolongation (Chap. 216). This technique involves the addition of a lead placed in the coronary sinus to pace the posterolateral aspect of the left ventricle. The synchronized activation of the lateral (coronary sinus lead) and septal (right ventricular lead) aspects of the left ventricle results in improved hemodynamic function in some patients.

PROGRAMMABILITY OF PACEMAKERS This allows for modification of pacing function after implantation and for adaptation to changes in clinical needs. Pacemaker programming is accomplished by activation of the programming head positioned over the implanted pulse generator after making the desired changes in programmable parameters (Table 213-3). A radio frequency system is routinely used to communicate the program to the pacemaker. A high degree of sophistication is required to recognize the presence and causes of pacemaker malfunction and their treatment.

COMPLICATIONS Adverse effects of permanent pacing are usually associated with failure or malfunction of the pacing system. These problems are usually secondary to over- or undersensing, output failure, and/or lead fracture or displacement. Two other problems may occur. The *pacemaker syndrome* consists of fatigue, dizziness, syncope, and distressing pulsations in the neck and chest and can be associated with adverse hemodynamic effects. The pathophysiologic contributors to the pacemaker syndrome include (1) loss of atrial contribution to ventricular systole; (2) vasodepressor reflex initiated by cannon *a* waves, which are caused by atrial contractions against a closed tricuspid valve and observed in the jugular venous pulse (Chap. 209); and (3) systemic and pulmonary venous regurgitation due to atrial contraction against a closed AV valve. The symptoms associated with the pacemaker syndrome can be prevented by maintaining AV synchrony by dual-chamber pacing or, in the case of a ventricular demand pacemaker, by programming an escape rate 15 to 20 beats/min below that of the paced rate (i.e., hysteresis). As a result of this programming, sinus activity and thus atrial contraction will be less likely to occur at the same time as ventricular pacing and ventricular contraction. The second major problem peculiar to dual-chamber pacemakers is the development of *pacemaker-mediated tachycardia*. In this instance, retrograde depolarization of the atria, resulting from a premature ventricular depolarization or a paced ventricular complex, is sensed and leads to subsequent triggering of ventricular pacing. This, in turn, can result in repetition of the phenomenon of ventriculoatrial conduction with the development of an endless-loop, pacemaker-mediated tachycardia. It may be corrected by reprogramming the atrial refractory period.

FURTHER READING

ABRAHAM WT et al: Cardiac resynchronization in chronic heart failure. N Engl J Med 346:1845, 2002

BRINK P et al: Gene for progressive familial heart block type 1 maps to chromosome 19q13. Circulation 91:1633, 1995

BUYON J et al: Autoimmune associated congenital heart block: Demographics, mortality, morbidity and recurrence rates obtained from a national neonatal lupus registry. J Am Coll Cardiol 31:1685, 1998

ELLENBOGEN KA et al: New insights into pacemaker syndrome gained from hemodynamic, humoral and vascular responses during ventriculo-atrial pacing. Am J Cardiol 65:53, 1990

GREGORATAS G: ACC/AHA/NASPE 2002 Guideline for implantation of cardiac pacemakers and antiarrhythmia devices: Summary article. Circulation 106:2145, 2002

HAYES DL, ZIPES DP: Cardiac pacemakers, in *Braunwald's Heart Disease: A Textbook of Cardiovascular Medicine,* 7th ed, D Zipes et al (eds). Philadelphia, Saunders, 2005

HUANG SK et al: Carotid sinus hypersensitivity in patients with unexplained syncope: Clinical, electrophysiologic and long-term follow-up observations. Am Heart J 116:989, 1988

JOSEPHSON ME: *Clinical Cardiac Electrophysiology: Techniques and Interpretations,* 3d ed. Philadelphia, Lippincott Williams & Wilkins, 2002, Chaps 3,4,5,11

MENDES LA, DAVIDOFF R: Cardiogenic seizure with bradyarrhythmia: Documentation of the mechanism during asystole. Am Heart J 125:1786, 1993

SCHOTT J et al: Congenital heart disease caused by mutations in the transcription factor NKX2-5. Science, 1998; 281:108−111

WALLER BF et al: Anatomy, histology and pathology of the cardiac conduction system: Part II. Clin Cardiol 16:347, 1993

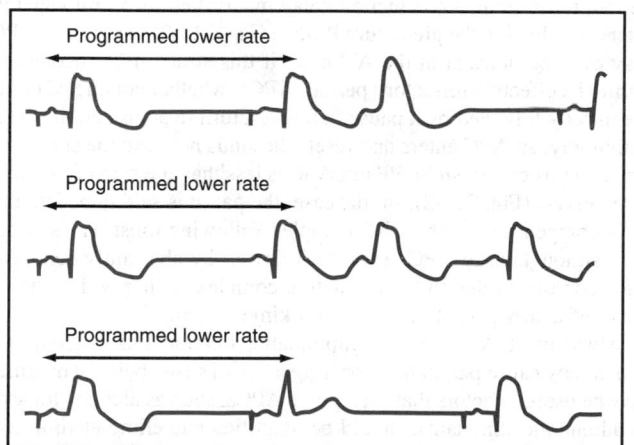

FIGURE 213-9 Normally functioning DDD pacemaker. All three panels show a lead II rhythm strip at 50 mm/s. The programmed lower rate is approximately 55 beats/min. (*Top*) AV sequential pacing with a paced AV interval of 160 ms is shown for the first two complexes. A ventricular premature complex occurs and is sensed, resetting the cycle. (*Middle*) The first beat is AV paced, but spontaneous sinus P waves and atrial premature complex trigger a ventricular paced complex with a sensed P to QRS of 120 ms. (*Bottom*) After the first AV paced complex, a paced atrial complex conducts to the ventricle with a PR of 120 ms, inhibiting the ventricular pacemaker.

THE TACHYARRHYTHMIAS
Mark E. Josephson, Peter Zimetbaum

MECHANISMS OF TACHYARRHYTHMIAS

Tachyarrhythmias may be divided into disorders of impulse propagation and disorders of impulse formation.

REENTRY Disorders of impulse propagation (reentry) are generally considered to be the most common mechanism of sustained paroxysmal tachyarrhythmia. The requirements for initiating reentry include (1) electrophysiologic inhomogeneity (i.e., differences in conduction and/or refractoriness) in two or more regions of the heart connected with each other to form a potentially closed loop; (2) unidirectional block in one pathway; (3) slow conduction over an alternative pathway, allowing time for the initially blocked pathway to recover excitability; and (4) reexcitation of the initially blocked pathway to complete a loop of activation (Fig. 214-1). Repetitive circulation of the impulse over this loop can produce a sustained tachyarrhythmia. While anatomic obstacles may underlie reentry and provide an inexcitable center around which the impulse can circulate, they are not essential. Reentrant arrhythmias can be reproducibly initiated and terminated by premature complexes and rapid stimulation. The response of these arrhythmias to stimulation can help distinguish them from arrhythmias caused by triggered activity.

ENHANCED AUTOMATICITY Disorders of impulse formation can be subdivided into tachyarrhythmias caused by enhanced automaticity and those caused by triggered activity. In addition to the sinus node, automatic pacemaker activity can be observed in specialized atrial fibers, fibers of the atrioventricular (AV) junction, and Purkinje fibers (Chap. 213). Myocardial cells do not normally possess pacemaker activity. Enhancement of normal automaticity in latent pacemaker fibers or the development of abnormal automaticity due to partial depolarization of the resting membrane occurs as a consequence of a variety of pathophysiologic states, which include (1) increased endogenous or exogenous catecholamines, (2) electrolyte disturbances (e.g., hypokalemia), (3) hypoxia or ischemia, (4) mechanical effects (e.g., stretch), and (5) drugs (e.g., digitalis). Tachycardia caused by automaticity cannot be started or stopped by pacing.

TRIGGERED ACTIVITY Rhythms due to triggered activity are events that do not occur spontaneously but require a change in cardiac electrical frequency as a trigger. Triggered activity may be caused by early afterdepolarizations, which occur during phases 2 and 3 of the action potential, or delayed afterdepolarizations, which occur following completion of phase 3 of the action potential (Fig. 213-2). Triggered activity has been observed in atrial, ventricular, and His-Purkinje tissue under conditions such as increased local catecholamine concentration, hypercalcemia, and digitalis intoxication (delayed afterdepolariza-

tions) or during bradycardia, hypokalemia, or other situations prolonging action potential duration (early afterdepolarizations). All of these conditions produce an accumulation of intracellular calcium. With increasing amplitude of the afterdepolarizations, threshold can be reached and repetitive activity produced. The exact role of triggered activity in spontaneous clinical arrhythmias is unknown, but tachyarrhythmias associated with digitalis intoxication, accelerated idioventricular rhythm in acute infarction and/or reperfusion, and exercise-induced ventricular tachycardia (VT) are believed to be caused by triggered activity due to delayed afterdepolarizations. *Torsades de pointes* ("twisting of the points"; polymorphic VT associated with long QT intervals) may be caused by triggered activity due to early afterdepolarizations, although reentry may also be operative.

The use of electrophysiologic studies, i.e., intracardiac recordings and programmed stimulation, has greatly expanded the understanding of the mechanisms of tachyarrhythmias. In addition to helping diagnose arrhythmias, these techniques may be of value in determining the most appropriate types of therapy because they allow the physician to observe the hemodynamic and symptomatic consequences of the arrhythmia in the presence or absence of therapy. Electrophysiologic studies of tachycardias require the positioning of multiple electrode catheters at critical areas within the heart. These electrodes must be capable of both stimulating and recording from multiple sites in the atria and/or ventricles.

PREMATURE COMPLEXES

ATRIAL PREMATURE COMPLEXES (APCs) APCs can be found on 24-h Holter monitoring in over 60% of normal adults. APCs are usually asymptomatic and benign, although at times they may be associated with palpitations. In susceptible patients, they can initiate paroxysmal supraventricular tachycardias (PSVTs). APCs may originate from any location in either atrium, and they are recognized on the electrocardiogram (ECG) as early P waves with a morphology that differs from the sinus P wave (Fig. 214-2). While APCs usually conduct to the ventricles when they occur late in the cardiac cycle, early APCs may reach the AV conduction system while it is still in its relative refractory period, resulting in a conduction delay manifested by a prolonged PR interval following the premature P wave (Fig. 214-2). Very early APCs may even be blocked in the AV node if this structure is encountered during its effective refractory period. APCs, whether conducted or not, are usually followed by a pause before a return to sinus activity. Most commonly, an APC enters and resets the sinus node, so the sum of the pre- and postextrasystolic PP intervals is less than the sum of two sinus PP intervals (Fig. 214-2). In this case, the pause is said to be less than fully compensatory. The QRS complex following most APCs is normal, although early APCs may be followed by aberrantly conducted QRS complexes due to the premature complex falling within the relative refractory period of the His-Purkinje system.

Since most APCs are asymptomatic, treatment is not required. When they cause palpitations or trigger PSVTs (see below), treatment may be useful. Factors that precipitate APCs, such as alcohol, tobacco, or adrenergic stimulants, should be identified and eliminated; in their absence, mild sedation or the use of a beta blocker may be tried.

AV JUNCTIONAL COMPLEXES The site of origin of these complexes is thought to be in the bundle of His, since the normal AV node in vivo possesses no automaticity. AV junctional complexes are less common than either atrial or ventricular premature complexes and are more often associated with cardiac disease or digitalis intoxication. Junctional premature impulses can conduct both antegradely to the ventricles and retrogradely to the atrium and, on rare occasions, may fail to conduct in either direction. Premature AV junctional complexes can be recognized by normal-appearing QRS complexes that are not preceded by a P wave. Retrograde P waves (inverted in leads II, III, and aVF) may be observed after the QRS complex.

While often asymptomatic, junctional premature complexes may be associated with palpitations and cause cannon *a* waves, which may

FIGURE 214-1 Schema of reentry. Y branching of the Purkinje system to ventricular muscle is shown in panels *A* through *C*. The right limb (*blue*) of the Purkinje system has a longer refractory period than the left. *A.* During a slow stimulated rate (S_1), conduction proceeds normally over both Purkinje fibers, resulting in collision in the ventricular muscle. *B.* An early premature stimulus (S_2) results in block in the Purkinje fiber on the right and slow conduction down the left. The impulse conducts through the ventricle and attempts to reenter the initial site of block but fails because this site has not fully recovered excitability. *C.* An earlier stimulus (S_3) again results in block on the left. The resulting slower propagation down the left fiber provides enough time for the initial site of block to recur and allows the impulse to conduct through it to produce a reentrant circuit.

result in distressing pulsations in the neck. When symptomatic, they should be treated like APCs.

VENTRICULAR PREMATURE COMPLEXES (VPCs)

These are among the most common arrhythmias and occur in patients with and without heart disease. Of adult males, ≥60% will exhibit VPCs during a 24-h Holter monitoring. In patients without heart disease, VPCs have not been shown to be associated with any increased incidence in mortality or morbidity. VPCs may occur in up to 80% of patients with previous myocardial infarction, and in this setting, if frequent (>10 per hour) and/or complex (occurring in couplets), they have been associated

FIGURE 214-2 ECG lead II. Sinus rhythm with one atrial premature complex (*arrow*). Note the difference in P-wave configuration between sinus and the premature atrial complexes. In addition, note that the PR interval of the premature complex is prolonged, due to slowed conduction of the premature impulse through the AV conduction system.

with increased mortality. However, cardiac mortality in such patients usually occurs in association with significantly impaired ventricular function. While frequent and complex ventricular ectopy is an independent risk factor, it is not as strong a risk factor as is impaired ventricular function. Moreover, even though VT and/or ventricular fibrillation (VF) may be the basis for the sudden death in these patients, this does not a priori establish a cause-and-effect relation between spontaneous ectopy and life-threatening VT or VF. Very early cycle (R-on-T) VPCs have been stated by some to increase the risk of sudden death. Although this has been observed during acute ischemia and in the setting of QT prolongation, frequently, VT or VF is precipitated by VPCs that occur after the T wave of the prior beat.

VPCs are recognized by wide (usually >0.14 s), bizarre QRS complexes that are not preceded by P waves (Fig. 214-3A). However, when they arise in the specialized conduction system (e.g., fascicles) they may be <0.12 s in duration. They may bear a relatively fixed relationship to the preceding sinus complex (i.e., fixed coupled VPCs). When fixed coupling is not present and the interval between VPCs has a common denominator, *ventricular parasystole* is said to be present (Fig. 214-4). Under these circumstances, the VPCs are a manifestation of abnormal automaticity of a protected ventricular focus. Because this focus is not penetrated by sinus impulses, it is not reset by them, and the interectopic intervals remain relatively fixed (≤120 ms variation of mean RR cycle length).

VPCs may occur singly; in patterns of bigeminy, in which every sinus beat is followed by a VPC; in trigeminy, in which two sinus beats are followed by a VPC; in quadrigeminy, etc. Two successive VPCs are termed *pairs* or *couplets*, while three or more consecutive VPCs are termed *ventricular tachycardia* when the rate exceeds 100 beats/min (Fig. 214-3B). VPCs may have similar morphologies (monomorphic, or uniform) or different morphologies (polymorphic, or multiformed).

Most commonly, VPCs are not conducted retrogradely to the atrium to reset the sinoatrial node. Thus they result in a fully compensatory pause, i.e., the interval between conducted sinus beats that bracket the VPC equals two basic RR intervals. Ventricular impulses may also manifest retrograde conduction to the atrium and cause inverted P waves in leads II, III, and aVF. This retrograde atrial activation can reset the sinus node, and the pause that results may therefore be less than compensatory. In many instances, the VPC will not be associated with retrograde ventriculoatrial (VA) conduction but may block retrogradely

in the AV node. This renders the AV node refractory to the subsequent sinus beat and causes slowed conduction (i.e., prolonged PR interval) or block of the next sinus P wave. This prolonged PR interval is said to be a manifestation of concealed retrograde conduction of the ventricular impulse into the AV node. A VPC that does not produce any manifestation of retrograde concealed conduction and fails to influence the oncoming sinus impulse is termed an *interpolated VPC*.

VPCs can cause palpitations or neck pulsations secondary to either the occurrence of cannon *a* waves or the increased force of contraction due to postextrasystolic potentiation of ventricular contractility. Patients with frequent VPCs or bigeminy may rarely develop syncope or lightheadedness because the VPCs do not result in an adequate stroke volume and the cardiac output is reduced by the "halving" of the heart rate.

℞ TREATMENT

In the absence of cardiac disease, isolated asymptomatic VPCs, regardless of configuration and frequency, need no treatment. When arrhythmias are symptomatic, the symptoms should first be addressed by either allaying the patient's anxiety or, if this is not successful, reducing the frequency of the VPCs with antiarrhythmic agents. β-Adrenergic blockers may be successful in managing VPCs that occur primarily in the daytime or under stressful situations and in specific settings such as mitral valve prolapse and thyrotoxicosis. While other antiarrhythmic agents may be tried should this be unsuccessful, their risk may outweigh any benefits. In patients with cardiac disease, fre-

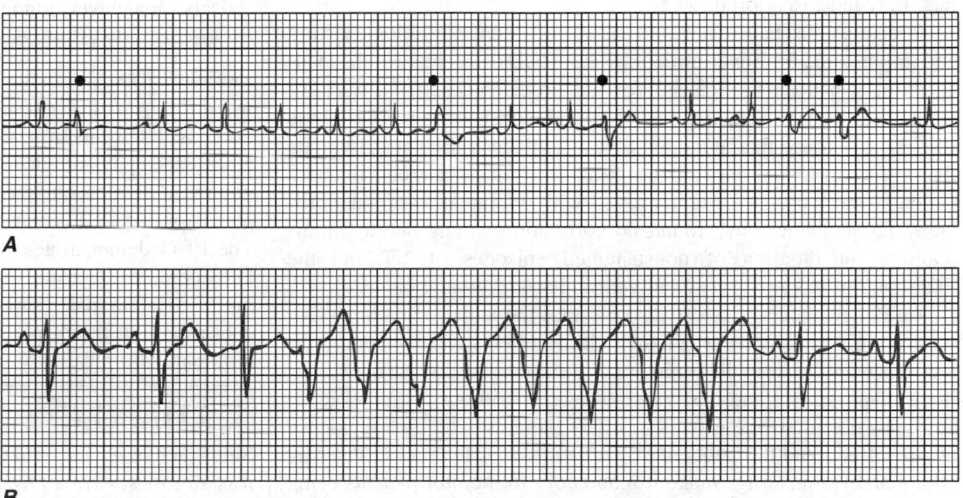

A

B

FIGURE 214-3 A. Single ventricular ectopy. During sinus rhythm, five premature ventricular complexes (*filled circles*) occur. Note that the QRS configuration is bizarre and different from that during sinus rhythm. The premature ventricular complexes are not preceded by P waves. The QRS widths of the premature complexes are 120–160 ms and multiple morphologies are present. The pause following the premature complexes is fully compensatory, the sinus beat after the premature complex occurring on time. B. Nonsustained ventricular tachycardia (VT). Following two sinus beats, an atrial premature contraction with long PR interval initiates an 8-beat run of wide complex tachycardia. Atrial activity can be seen following the fourth and seventh beats. The greater number of QRS complexes compared with P waves confirms the diagnosis of VT.

FIGURE 214-4 Ventricular parasystole. At varying sinus cycle lengths during exercise, interectopic intervals remain constant at 1620 to 1640 ms. However, the coupling intervals between sinus and ectopic complexes vary between 510 and 310 ms.

quent VPCs are associated with an increased risk of sudden and nonsudden cardiac death, and many physicians have attempted to eliminate or reduce the frequency of these VPCs in an attempt to reduce this risk. However, the cause-and-effect relationship of the VPCs to fatal events has never been established.

The ability of pharmacologic antiarrhythmic therapy guided by continuous ECG monitoring to reduce the risk of sudden death in postmyocardial infarction patients with frequent (≥ 6 per minute) VPCs was tested by the Cardiac Arrhythmia Suppression Trial (CAST). This study compared mortality in patients whose ectopy was suppressed by one of three agents (encainide, flecainide, or moricizine) and then randomized to treatment with either the "effective" drug or placebo. After a mean follow-up of 2 years, the study was discontinued because both the sudden death and overall mortality rate were significantly increased in patients receiving antiarrhythmic agents (encainide, flecainide). This study has shown that in patients having the characteristics of the study population, abolition of ventricular ectopy by pharmacologic therapy cannot be used as a marker to define reduction of the risk of sudden death after myocardial infarction and, in fact, may increase mortality.

Recent studies have evaluated the use of electrophysiologic testing and implantable cardioverter/defibrillator (ICD) placement in the management of patients at high risk for sudden death (i.e., those with left ventricular ejection fractions <40% and nonsustained VT). These studies have found that induction of a sustained ventricular arrhythmia through programmed electrical stimulation selects a group of these patients whose prognosis is improved with implantation of a defibrillator. These studies have found no correlation among the rate, morphology, or duration of nonsustained episodes of VT and the likelihood of having a sustained ventricular arrhythmia induced.

Antiarrhythmic agents can also produce the lethal arrhythmias that they are given to prevent (proarrhythmic effects). Thus therapy directed toward VPCs in the setting of chronic cardiac disease may result in an inappropriate and costly use of agents without proven efficacy and with potential side effects in many patients. The high incidence of side effects and the frequent exacerbation of arrhythmias caused by all antiarrhythmic drugs make it mandatory to monitor patients being treated with such agents. Congestive heart failure (CHF) is the most important risk factor for proarrhythmia.

In acute myocardial infarction, the greatest incidence of primary VF occurs within the first 24 h (Chap. 228). Temporary prophylactic antiarrhythmic therapy with lidocaine or procainamide was formerly recommended for all patients with acute infarction, regardless of the presence or degree of spontaneous ectopy. However, failure to improve

overall survival and drug toxicity have led most physicians to recommend prophylactic antiarrhythmic therapy only to young patients with complicated infarctions, where a favorable risk-benefit ratio may be obtained. Other studies have shown that intravenous beta blockers may also reduce the incidence of primary VF.

TACHYCARDIAS

Tachycardias refer to arrhythmias with three or more complexes at rates exceeding 100 beats/min; they occur more often in structurally diseased than in normal hearts. Those paroxysmal tachycardias that are initiated by APCs or VPCs are considered to be due to reentry, except some of the digitalis-induced tachyarrhythmias, which are probably due to triggered activity (see below).

If the patient is hemodynamically stable, an attempt should be made to determine the mechanism and origin of the tachycardia, since this will usually lead to an appropriate therapeutic decision. Information to be obtained from the ECG includes (1) the presence, frequency, morphology, and regularity of P waves and QRS complexes; (2) the relationship between atrial and ventricular activity; (3) a comparison of the QRS morphology during sinus rhythm and during the tachycardia; and (4) the response to carotid sinus massage or other vagal maneuvers. It is useful first to compare a 12-lead ECG during the tachycardia with one recorded during sinus rhythm. One can also utilize the electrodes situated at the end of a flexible pacing catheter inserted into the esophagus behind the left atrium to record atrial activity.

Observation of the jugular venous pulse can provide clues to the presence of atrial activity and its relationship to ventricular ectopy. Intermittent cannon *a* waves suggest AV dissociation, while persistent cannon *a* waves suggest 1:1 VA conduction. Flutter waves may be seen or no atrial activity may be apparent, as in the presence of atrial flutter and atrial fibrillation (AF), respectively. The arterial pulse may also manifest AV dissociation or AF by demonstrating variations in amplitude. A first heart sound of variable intensity during a regular rhythm also suggests AV dissociation or AF.

Carotid sinus pressure should be applied only while the patient is electrocardiographically monitored with resuscitative equipment available to manage the rare episode of asystole and/or VF associated with this procedure. Carotid sinus massage should not be performed in patients with carotid arterial bruits. The patient should be positioned flat with the neck extended. Massage of one carotid bulb at a time should be performed by applying firm pressure just underneath the angle of the jaw for up to 5 s. Alternative vagomimetic maneuvers include the Valsalva maneuver, immersion of the face in cold water, and administration of 5 to 10 mg edrophonium.

SINUS TACHYCARDIA   In the adult, sinus tachycardia is said to be present when the heart rate exceeds 100 beats/min. Sinus tachycardia rarely exceeds 200 beats/min and is not a primary arrhythmia; instead, it represents a physiologic response to a variety of stresses, such as fever, volume depletion, anxiety, exercise, thyrotoxicosis, hypoxemia, hypotension, or CHF. Sinus tachycardia has a gradual onset and offset. The ECG demonstrates P waves with sinus contour preceding each QRS complex. Carotid sinus pressure usually produces modest slowing with a gradual return to the previous rate upon cessation. This contrasts with the response of PSVTs, which may slow slightly and terminate abruptly.

℞ TREATMENT

Sinus tachycardia should not be treated as a primary arrhythmia, since it is almost always a physiologic response to a demand placed on the heart. As such, therapy should be directed to the primary disorder. However, in the setting of CHF, enhanced sympathetic activity has detrimental effects on myocardial function and merits treatment. Use of beta blockers in this situation decreases the effects of neurohormonal activation that leads to worsening CHF. Angiotensin-converting enzyme (ACE) inhibitors and angiotensin receptor blockers are additional drugs affecting neurohormonal activation in heart failure whose use improves outcomes. The other situations in which sinus tachycardia is a consequence (listed above) can all be readily treated.

ATRIAL FIBRILLATION AF is a common arrhythmia that may occur in paroxysmal and persistent forms. It may be seen in normal individuals, particularly during emotional stress or following surgery, exercise, acute alcoholic intoxication, or a prominent surge of vagal tone (i.e., vasovagal response). It may also occur in patients with heart or lung disease who develop acute hypoxia, hypercapnia, or metabolic or hemodynamic derangements. Persistent AF usually occurs in patients with cardiovascular disease, most commonly rheumatic heart disease, nonrheumatic mitral valve disease, hypertensive cardiovascular disease, chronic lung disease, atrial septal defect, and a variety of miscellaneous cardiac abnormalities. AF may be the presenting finding in thyrotoxicosis. So-called lone AF, which occurs in patients without underlying heart disease, often represents the tachycardia phase of the tachycardia-bradycardia syndrome.

The morbidity associated with AF is related to (1) excessive ventricular rate, which in turn may lead to hypotension, pulmonary congestion, or angina pectoris in susceptible individuals, and in some patients can produce a tachycardia-mediated cardiomyopathy; (2) the pause following cessation of AF, which can cause syncope; (3) systemic embolization, which occurs most commonly in patients with rheumatic heart disease (Table 214-1); (4) loss of the contribution of atrial contraction to cardiac output, which may cause fatigue; and (5) anxiety secondary to palpitations. In patients with severe cardiac dysfunction, particularly those with hypertrophied, noncompliant ventricles, the combination of the loss of the atrial contribution to ventricular filling and the abbreviated filling period due to the rapid ventricular rate in AF can produce marked hemodynamic instability, resulting in hypotension, syncope, or heart failure. In patients with mitral stenosis, in whom ventricular filling time is critical, development of AF with a rapid ventricular rate may precipitate pulmonary edema (Chap. 219). AF may also cause a cardiomyopathy related to persistent rapid rates (so-called tachycardia-induced cardiomyopathy).

AF is characterized by disorganized atrial activity without discrete P waves on the surface ECG (Fig. 214-5A). Atrial activation is manifested by an undulating baseline or by more sharply inscribed atrial deflections of varying amplitude and frequency ranging from 350 to 600 beats/min. The ventricular response is irregularly irregular. This results from the large number of atrial impulses that penetrate the AV node, making it partially refractory to subsequent impulses. This effect of nonconducted atrial impulses to influence the response to subsequent atrial impulses is termed *concealed conduction*. As a result, the ventricular response is relatively slow, considering the actual atrial rate. AF may convert to atrial flutter, especially in response to antiarrhythmic drugs such as quinidine or flecainide. If AF converts to atrial flutter, which has a slower atrial rate, the effect of concealed conduction may be diminished, and a paradoxical increase in the ventricular response may occur. The main factor determining the rate of the ventricular response is the functional refractory period of the AV node or the most rapid paced rate at which 1:1 conduction through the AV node can be observed.

If, in the presence of AF, the ventricular rhythm becomes regular and slow (e.g., 30 to 60 beats/min), complete heart block is suggested,

---

TABLE 214-1 *Factors Associated with High Risk of Stroke in Patients with Atrial Fibrillation*

1. Age >65
2. Hypertension
3. Rheumatic heart disease
4. Prior stroke or transient ischemic attack
5. Diabetes mellitus
6. Congestive heart failure
7. Transesophageal echocardiographic characteristics
   Spontaneous echo contrast in left atrium
   Left atrial appendage velocity <20 cm/s
   Complex aortic atheroma

FIGURE 214-5 Atrial fibrillation and atrial flutter. *A.* Lead V_1 demonstrating an irregular ventricular rhythm associated with poorly defined irregular atrial activity consistent with atrial fibrillation. *B.* Lead II demonstrates atrial flutter, identified by the regular "sawtooth-like" activity (*arrows*) at an atrial rate of 300 beats/min with 2:1 ventricular response.

and if the ventricular rhythm is regular and rapid (e.g., ≥100 beats/min), a tachycardia arising in the AV junction or ventricle should be suspected. Digitalis intoxication is a common cause of both phenomena.

Patients with AF exhibit a loss of *a* waves in the jugular venous pulse and variable pulse pressures in the carotid arterial pulse. The first heart sound usually varies in intensity. On echocardiography, the left atrium is frequently enlarged, and in patients in whom the left atrial diameter >4.5 cm, it may be difficult to convert AF to sinus rhythm and/or maintain the latter, despite therapy.

℞ TREATMENT

In acute AF, a precipitating factor such as fever, pneumonia, alcoholic intoxication, thyrotoxicosis, pulmonary emboli, CHF, or pericarditis should be sought. When such a factor is present, therapy should be directed toward the primary abnormality. If the patient's clinical status is severely compromised, electrical cardioversion is the treatment of choice. In the absence of severe cardiovascular compromise, slowing of the ventricular rate becomes the initial therapeutic goal. This may be most rapidly accomplished with β-adrenergic blockers and/or calcium channel antagonists. Both prolong the refractory period of the AV node and slow conduction within it. When catecholamine levels or sympathetic nervous system tone are likely to be elevated, beta blockers may be favored. Digitalis preparations are less effective, take longer to act, and are associated with more toxicity. Conversion to sinus rhythm may then be attempted. Prior to cardioversion, precautions must be taken to reduce the risk of systemic embolization. Patients should be anticoagulated to an INR of at least 1.8 for the prior 3 consecutive weeks or have had AF for <48 h. Alternatively, for those patients with AF for >48 h who are not anticoagulated, a transesophageal echocardiogram can exclude the presence of left atrial thrombus and allow safe cardioversion. Following cardioversion, anticoagulation must be maintained for at least 4 weeks until atrial mechanical function returns to normal.

Antiarrhythmic medications in either oral or intravenous form may be employed but are only modestly effective in restoring sinus rhythm. When antiarrhythmic agents such as the quinidine-like drugs (class IA) or the flecainide-like agents (class IC) are used (Table 214-2), it is important to increase AV node refractoriness prior to administering

TABLE 214-2 *Classification of Antiarrhythmic Drugs*

Class I	Drugs that reduce maximal velocity of phase of depolarization (V_{max}) due to block of inward Na^+ current in tissue with fast response action potentials
IA	↓ V_{max} at all heart rates and ↑ action potential duration, e.g., quinidine, procainamide, disopyramide
IB	Little effect at slow rates on V_{max} in normal tissue; ↓ V_{max} in partially depolarized cells with fast response action potentials Effects increased at faster rates No change or ↓ in action potential duration, e.g., lidocaine, phenytoin, tocainide, mexiletine
IC	↓ V_{max} at normal rates in normal tissue Minimal effect on action potential duration, e.g., flecainide, propafenone, moricizine
Class II	Antisympathetic agents, e.g., propranolol and other β-adrenergic blockers: ↓ SA nodal automaticity, ↑ AV nodal refractoriness, and ↓ AV nodal conduction velocity
Class III	Agents that prolong action potential duration in tissue with fast-response action potentials, e.g., bretylium, amiodarone, sotalol, ibutilide, dofetilide
Class IV	Calcium (slow) channel blocking agents: ↓ conduction velocity and ↑ refractoriness in tissue with slow-response action potentials, e.g., verapamil, diltiazem
Drugs that cannot be classified by this schema: Digitalis, Adenosine	

Note: SA, sinoatrial; AV, atrioventricular.

such drugs because their vagolytic effect and/or their ability to convert AF to atrial flutter may reduce the concealed conduction in the AV node and lead to an excessively rapid ventricular response. β-Adrenergic blockers are especially useful in this regard. Intravenous ibutilide, a class III agent, is reasonably effective in converting new-onset AF to sinus rhythm.

Direct-current (DC) electrical cardioversion is a highly effective method to restore sinus rhythm, either as a primary method of therapy or following the failure of antiarrhythmic medications. DC cardioversion is accomplished through the delivery of at least 200 W·s of energy between electrodes placed to the right of the sternum and the cardiac apex or to the left of the scapula. New methods of cardioversion using biphasic waveforms have increased the efficacy of transthoracic cardioversion to >90%. If external cardioversion is unsuccessful, internal cardioversion with energy delivered between two catheters inside the heart or one inside and a patch outside the heart may prove effective. Recent studies suggest pretreatment with ibutilide can facilitate cardioversion.

It is unlikely that patients with chronic AF will convert to and remain in sinus rhythm in the presence of long-standing rheumatic heart disease and/or when the atria are markedly enlarged. The goal of therapy in patients in whom AF cannot be converted to sinus rhythm is control of the ventricular response. This can usually be accomplished by beta blockers, calcium channel blockers, or digitalis, singly or in combination. In occasional patients, the ventricular response cannot be controlled by pharmacologic therapy alone. In such patients, the creation of complete heart block by radiofrequency catheter ablation of the AV junction followed by permanent pacemaker implantation is appropriate.

If sinus rhythm is restored electrically or pharmacologically, quinidine or related agents as well as the class IC agents (e.g., flecainide or propafenone), sotalol, dofetilide, or amiodarone may be used to prevent recurrence. In patients in whom cardioversion is unsuccessful or in whom AF has recurred or is likely to recur despite antiarrhythmic therapy, it is probably wisest to allow the patient to remain in AF and to control the ventricular response with calcium antagonists, β-adrenergic blockers, or digitalis glycosides. Since such patients are always at risk of systemic embolization, particularly in the presence of organic heart disease, chronic anticoagulation must be considered (Table 214-3). Chronic anticoagulation is particularly important in the elderly, where the attributable risk of AF for stroke approaches 30%. Several

TABLE 214-3 *Recommendations for Long-Term Anticoagulation in Patients with Chronic Atrial Fibrillation*

Age, years	Risk Factors[a]	Recommendations
<65	Absent	Aspirin
	Present	Warfarin [target INR 2.5 (range 2.0–3.0)]
65–75	Absent	Aspirin or warfarin
	Present	Warfarin [target INR 2.5 (range 2.0–3.0)]
>75	All patients	Warfarin [target INR 2.5 (range 2.5–3.0)]

[a] Risk factors are prior transient ischemic attack, systemic embolus or stroke, hypertension, poor left ventricular function, rheumatic mitral valve disease, prosthetic heart valve, congestive heart failure.

Source: From ACC/AHA/ESC.

studies have now demonstrated conclusively that the incidence of embolization in patients with AF not associated with valvular heart disease is reduced by chronic anticoagulation with warfarin-like agents. Recommendation for chronic anticoagulation should be instituted based on clinical risk factors for stroke regardless of whether or not an antiarrhythmic medication is utilized. Studies have demonstrated that antiarrhythmic drugs are not associated with stroke reduction perhaps because of asymptomatic (unrecognized) recurrences. Aspirin also may be effective for this purpose in patients who are not at high risk for stroke. Although anticoagulation may be associated with hemorrhagic complications, the risk is largely associated with INRs above the recommended range of 2.0 to 3.0. Recommendations for the selection of antiarrhythmic medications to prevent the recurrence of AF are shown in Fig. 214-6.

Ablation therapy for cure of AF is an active area of investigation. This therapy is generally employed for patients with paroxysmal AF. This type of AF is often triggered by automatic foci located in the pulmonary veins. Ablation around the pulmonary veins to prevent electrical transit of impulses from the pulmonary veins to and from the left atrium may be curative. While ablation or isolation of these foci is possible, the procedure can result in pulmonary vein stenosis, pulmonary hypertension, and stroke. The MAZE procedure is a surgical approach to cure AF through the creation of multiple scars in the right and left atria to compartmentalize the electrical conduction in these chambers and disallow the propagation of fibrillatory waves. The

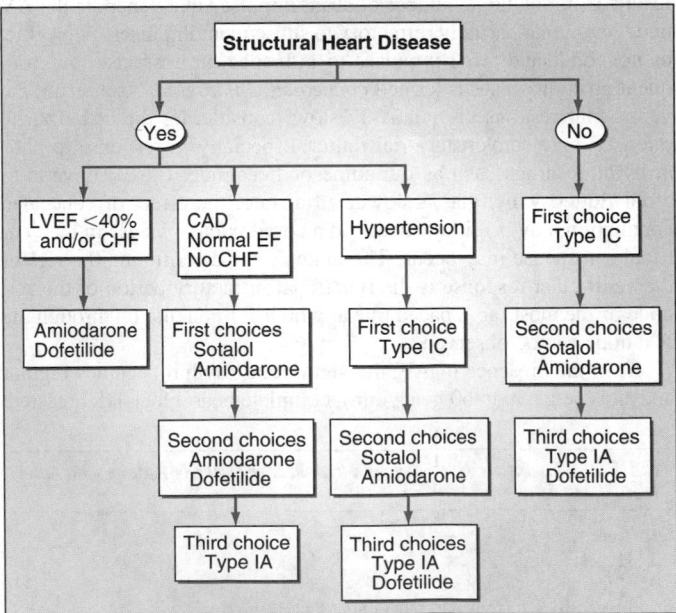

FIGURE 214-6 Recommendations for the selection of antiarrhythmic medications to prevent the recurrence of atrial fibrillation. See Tables 214-2 and 214-4 for definition of class IA and IC drugs. An atrioventricular nodal blocking agent (i.e., beta blocker, calcium channel blocker, or digoxin) should be added to all class IC and IA agents as well as to dofetilide. LVEF, left ventricular ejection fraction; CHF, congestive heart failure; CAD, coronary artery disease; EF, ejection fraction.

morbidity, mortality, and success rate of such catheter-based procedures render them experimental at this time.

ATRIAL FLUTTER

This arrhythmia occurs most often in patients with organic heart disease. Flutter may be paroxysmal, in which case there is usually a precipitating factor, such as pericarditis or acute respiratory failure, or it may be persistent. Atrial flutter (as well as AF) is very common during the first week following open-heart surgery. Atrial flutter is usually less long-lived than is AF, although on occasion it may persist for months to years. Often, if it lasts for more than a week, atrial flutter will convert to AF. Systemic embolization is less common in atrial flutter than in AF.

Atrial flutter is characterized by an atrial rate between 250 and 350 beats/min. Typically, the ventricular rate is half the atrial rate, i.e., ~150 beats/min because of 2:1 block in the AV node. If the atrial rate is slowed to <220 beats/min by antiarrhythmic agents such as quinidine, which also possess vagolytic properties, the ventricular rate may rise suddenly because of the development of 1:1 AV conduction. Classically, flutter waves are seen as regular sawtooth-like atrial activity, most prominent in the inferior leads (Fig. 214-5D). When the ventricular response is regular and not a simple fraction of the atrial rate, complete AV block is present, which may be a manifestation of digitalis toxicity. Activation mapping suggests that atrial flutter is a form of atrial reentry localized to the right atrium.

℞ TREATMENT

The most effective treatment of atrial flutter is DC cardioversion, which can be accomplished at low energy (25 to 50 W·s) under mild sedation. Higher energies (100 to 200 W·s) are often used because they are less likely to cause AF, which not infrequently occurs following lower energy delivery. Although atrial flutter is associated with a slightly lower risk of embolization than AF, the same precautions should be followed in regard to anticoagulation as are used with AF. The reason for the increased risk of emboli in atrial flutter is uncertain, but the coexistence of AF is common. In patients who develop atrial flutter following open-heart surgery or recurrent flutter in the setting of acute myocardial infarction, particularly if they are being treated with digitalis, atrial pacing (using temporary pacing wires implanted at the time of operation or a pacing lead inserted into the atrium pervenously) at rates of 115 to 130% of the atrial flutter rate can usually convert the atrial flutter to sinus rhythm. Atrial pacing may also result in the conversion of atrial flutter to AF, which allows for easier control of the ventricular response.

If immediate conversion of atrial flutter is not mandated by the patient's clinical status, the ventricular response should first be slowed by blocking the AV node with a beta blocker, calcium antagonist, or digitalis. Digitalis is the least effective and occasionally converts atrial flutter into AF. Once AV nodal conduction is slowed with any of these drugs, an attempt to convert flutter to sinus rhythm using a class I (A or C) agent or amiodarone should be made. Increasing doses of the drug selected are administered until the rhythm converts or side effects occur. Ibutilide is a new antiarrhythmic agent that is administered intravenously and appears to be particularly effective for conversion of atrial flutter to sinus rhythm.

Quinidine, other class IA drugs, flecainide, propafenone, sotalol, dofetilide, and amiodarone (Table 214-4) may be useful in preventing recurrences of atrial flutter. Radiofrequency ablation is a highly effective treatment for patients with the most typical forms of atrial flutter, which are due to reentry around the tricuspid valve in a counterclockwise or clockwise fashion. The coronary sinus and inferior vena cava cause the wavefront of activation to pass between them and the tricuspid valve. Ablation of the narrowed isthmus using radiofrequency energy can cure flutter in >85% of cases. This is far more successful than the response to drugs. As such, ablation is considered by many to be the therapy of choice for recurrent atrial flutter.

PAROXYSMAL SUPRAVENTRICULAR TACHYCARDIAS (Fig. 214-7)

In most cases, functional differences in conduction and refractoriness in the

AV node or the presence of an AV bypass tract provide the substrate for the development of PSVT (previously termed *paroxysmal atrial tachycardia*). Electrophysiologic studies have demonstrated that reentry is responsible for the vast majority of cases of PSVT. Reentry has been localized to the sinus node, atrium, AV node, or a macro-reentrant circuit involving conduction in the antegrade direction through the AV node and retrograde through an AV bypass tract (Fig. 214-8). Such a bypass tract may also conduct antegradely, in which case the Wolff-Parkinson-White (WPW) syndrome is said to be present. When the bypass tract manifests only retrograde conduction, it is termed a *concealed bypass tract* (Fig. 214-7B). In these cases, the QRS complex during sinus rhythm is normal. In the absence of the WPW syndrome, reentry through the AV node or through a concealed bypass tract makes up nearly 90% of all PSVTs. Atrial tachycardias due to automaticity are not paroxysmal and often present as an incessant arrhythmia.

AV NODAL REENTRANT TACHYCARDIA

There is no age or disease predisposition for the development of AV nodal reentrant tachycardia, the most common cause of supraventricular tachycardia. It is, however, more commonly observed in women. It usually presents as a regular narrow QRS complex tachycardia at rates of 120 to 250 beats/min. APCs that initiate the arrhythmia are almost always associated with a prolonged PR interval. Retrograde P waves may be absent, buried in the QRS complex, or appear as distortions at the terminal parts of the QRS complex (Fig. 214-7A).

AV nodal reentrant PSVT (Fig. 214-7A) can be reproducibly initiated and terminated by appropriately timed atrial premature stimuli. The onset of the tachycardia is almost always associated with prolongation of the PR interval due to marked AV nodal conduction delay (prolonged AH interval) following the APC that is critical for the genesis of the arrhythmia. The sudden prolongation of the AH interval is consistent with the concept of dual AV nodal pathways: a *fast pathway*, which exhibits rapid conduction and a long refractory period, and a *slow pathway*, which has a short refractory period but conducts slowly. During sinus rhythm, only conduction over the fast pathway is manifest, resulting in a normal PR interval (Fig. 214-8). Atrial extrastimuli at a critical coupling interval are blocked in the fast pathway because of its longer refractory period and are conducted slowly through the slow pathway. If conduction down the slow pathway is slow enough to allow the previously refractory fast pathway time to recover excitability, a single atrial (echo) reentrant beat or sustained tachycardia ensues. A critical balance between conduction velocity and refractoriness within the node is required to sustain AV nodal reentry. Retrograde atrial and antegrade ventricular activation occur simultaneously, explaining why P waves may not be apparent on the surface ECG.

Clinical Features   AV nodal reentry may produce palpitations, syncope, and heart failure depending on the rate and duration of the arrhythmia and the presence and severity of any underlying heart disease. Hypotension and syncope may occur due to both the sudden loss of the atrial contribution to ventricular filling and a reflex baroreceptor response to simultaneous atrial and ventricular contraction, which produce high atrial pressures. This situation can also result in acute pulmonary edema.

℞ TREATMENT

In patients without hypotension, vagal maneuvers, particularly carotid sinus massage, can terminate the arrhythmia in 80% of cases. If these maneuvers are unsuccessful, adenosine (12 mg intravenously) is the agent of choice. Beta blockers may also be used to slow or terminate the tachycardia but are agents of second choice. Digitalis glycosides have a slower onset of action and should *not* be used for acute therapy. When these drugs fail to terminate the tachycardia, or when the tachycardia is recurrent, atrial or ventricular pacing via a temporary pacemaker inserted pervenously may be used to terminate the arrhythmia.

TABLE 214-4 *Drugs Used to Treat Cardiac Tachyarrhythmias*

Drug	Mode of Administration	$t_{1/2}$ (oral), h	Route of Metabolism	Clinical Effects and/or Indications for Use
Digoxin	IV, 0.25–1.5 mg Oral, 0.75–1.5 mg loading dose over 12–24 h Maintenance, 0.23–0.50 mg/kg	36	Renal	Slowing of ventricular rate during AF, flutter, and other atrial tachycardias in the absence of preexcitation; slowing, termination, and/or prevention of SVT due to AV nodal reentry and AV reentry utilizing bypass tracts; may terminate or prevent intraatrial reentrant tachycardias; ineffective in prevention of automatic atrial tachycardias
Adenosine	IV bolus, 6–12 mg	<10s		Acute termination of regular reentrant SVT involving the AV node
Quinidine (class IA)	Oral, 200–400 mg q6h	8–9	Hepatic, 80% Renal, 20%	Atrial and ventricular tachyarrhythmias; all types of SVT; control of ventricular rate in patients with preexcitation and AF and flutter
Procainamide (class IA)	IV, 40–50 mg/min to total of 10–20 mg/kg Oral, 500–1000 mg q6h (sustained-release forms)	3–5	Hepatic, 50% Renal, 50%	Same as quinidine
Disopyramide (class IA)	Oral, 100–300 mg q6h	8–9	Hepatic, 50% Renal, 50%	Same as quinidine
Lidocaine (class IB)	IV, 20–50 mg/min to total of 5 mg/kg loading dose, followed by 1–4 mg/kg	1–2	Hepatic	VT and VF, especially during acute ischemia and myocardial infarction
Phenytoin (class IB)	IV, 20 mg/kg to total dose of 1000 mg Oral, 1000-mg loading dose over 24 h Maintenance, 100–400 mg/d	18–36	Hepatic	Tachyarrhythmias induced by digitalis; occasionally effective for ventricular tachyarrhythmias not induced by digitalis alone or in combination with other antiarrhythmic agents; polymorphic VT associated with increased QT interval
Mexiletine (class IB)	Oral, 100–300 mg q6–8h	9–12	Hepatic	Ventricular tachyarrhythmias; secondary agent in combination with other class I medication
Flecainide (class IC)	Oral, begin at 50–100 mg bid, increase by ≤50 mg in 4-day intervals to a maximum of mg daily	7–23	Hepatic, 75% Renal, 25%	Supraventricular tachyarrhythmias including atrial fibrillation and flutter; also ventricular arrhythmias refractory to other medications or radiofrequency ablation
Propafenone (class IC)	Oral, 150–300 mg q8h	5–8	Hepatic	Same as flecainide
Moricizine (class IC)	Oral, 200–400 mg q8h	2–6	Hepatic	Same as flecainide
Beta blockers (class II) e.g., metoprolol	IV, load with 5–10 mg q5min for 3 doses, then 3 mg q6h Oral, 25–100 mg bid	3–4	Hepatic	Slowing of ventricular rate during AF, atrial flutter, and other atrial tachyarrhythmias in the absence of preexcitation; SVT due to AV nodal reentry; reentry utilizing bypass tracts; arrhythmias (e.g., VT) induced by exercise or occurring in the presence of hyperthyroidism; polymorphic VT associated with congenital long QT syndrome
Bretylium (class III)	IV, 1–2 mg/kg per min to total load, 5–10 mg/kg Maintenance, 0.5–2 mg/kg	8–14	Renal	Refractory VT and VF, especially due to acute ischemia
Amiodarone (class III)	IV, 5–10 mg/kg load over 20 min, then 1 g/24 h Oral, load 800–1600 mg/d for 1 week, then 400–600 mg/d for 3 weeks, then 200–400 mg/d thereafter	13–103	Hepatic	Sustained VT and VF AF and atrial flutter, other types of SVT, VT, VF
Sotalol (class III)	Oral, 80–320 mg q12h	10–20	Renal, 90% Hepatic, 10%	Atrial and ventricular tachyarrhythmias
Ibutilide (class III)	IV, <60 kg: 0.01 mg/kg over 10 min IV, ≥60 kg: 1 mg over 10 min, repeat after 10 min if no effect	2–6	Hepatic	AF, atrial flutter, and other SVTs including preexcitation tachycardias
Dofetilide	125–250 mg PO bid	8–12	Renal	AF, atrial flutter, and other SVTs
Calcium channel blockers (class IV) e.g., verapamil	IV, 2.5–10 mg over 1–2 min to total of 0.15 mg/kg Oral, 240–480 qd	6–24	Hepatic	Slowing of ventricular rate during AF and flutter, and other SVTs in the absence of preexcitation; idiopathic VT
Diltiazem	IV, load with 0.25 mg/kg over 2 min; if needed, repeat after 15 min with 0.35 mg over 2 min Maintenance, 10–15 mg/h		Hepatic	Same as verapamil

Note: AF, atrial fibrillation; AV, atrioventricular; SVT, supraventricular tachycardia; VF, ventricular fibrillation; VT, ventricular tachycardia.

FIGURE 214-7 Examples of supraventricular tachycardia (SVT). Arrows indicate P waves. *A.* AV nodal reentry. Upright P waves are visible at the end of the QRS complex. *B.* AV reentry using a concealed bypass tract. Inverted retrograde P waves are superimposed on the T waves. *C.* Automatic atrial tachycardia. Inverted P waves follow the T waves and precede the QRS complex.

However, if severe ischemia and/or hypotension is caused by the tachycardia, (DC) cardioversion should be considered.

AV nodal reentry can usually be prevented by the use of drugs that act primarily on the antegrade slow pathway (such as digitalis, beta blockers, or calcium channel antagonists) or on the fast pathway (class IA or IC; Table 214-4). We favor initial therapy with beta blockers, calcium channel antagonists, or digoxin because the risk-benefit ratio associated with treatment with these agents is more favorable than that of IA or IC agents. Drugs most likely to avert recurrences prevent induction of the arrhythmias by programmed stimulation. This technique utilizes temporary pacemaker catheters connected to a physiologic stimulator capable of variable rate pacing and stimulation with one or more precisely timed premature impulses. In the past decade it has been recognized that in symptomatic patients who require chronic therapy, radiofrequency catheter modification of the AV node should be considered the treatment of choice. This technique can cure AV nodal reentry in >95% of cases and has been proven to be safe, although a 1 to 2% risk of AV block requiring a permanent pacemaker exists.

AV REENTRANT TACHYCARDIA PSVT due to AV reentry incorporates a concealed AV bypass tract as part of the tachycardia circuit. Thus the impulse passes antegradely from the atria through the AV node and His-Purkinje system to the ventricles and then retrogradely through the (concealed) bypass tract back to

the atrium. Patients with this disorder manifest the same type of PSVT as do patients with the WPW syndrome (see below), but the bypass tract cannot conduct in an antegrade direction during sinus rhythm or other atrial tachyarrhythmias.

AV reentrant tachycardia can be initiated and terminated by either APCs or VPCs. Initiation of PSVT by a VPC is virtually diagnostic of AV reentry. Alternation of the QRS complexes occurs in approximately one-third of such tachycardias. Since atrial activation must follow ventricular activation during AV reentry, the P wave usually occurs after the QRS complex (Fig. 214-7*B*).

Atrial activation mapping is of major value in evaluating the origin of these tachycardias. Most concealed bypass tracts are left-sided. Thus, during PSVT or during ventricular pacing, the earliest activation sequence is recorded in the left atrium, usually via a catheter in the coronary sinus. This eccentric atrial activation is quite distinct from the normal retrograde activation sequence in which the earliest activation of the atria is in the area of the AV junction. The ability of a ventricular stimulus to conduct to the atrium at a time when the bundle of His is refractory or more specifically terminate the tachycardia without depolarizing the atria is diagnostic of retrograde conduction over a concealed bypass tract.

℞ TREATMENT

This is similar to the treatment for AV nodal reentry tachycardia. Although pharmacologic agents may be used, patients who require chronic therapy should be considered candidates for radiofrequency catheter ablation of the bypass tract. This requires detailed electrophysiologic study to exclude other arrhythmias that may be responsible for patients' symptoms and to determine the location of the bypass tract(s). The efficacy of this procedure exceeds 90%, with minimal risks. In the remaining small number of patients failing catheter ablation, surgical ablation or pharmacologic therapy can be used.

SINUS NODE REENTRY AND OTHER ATRIAL TACHYCARDIAS Reentry in the region of the sinus node or within the atria is invariably initiated by APCs. These arrhythmias are less common than AV nodal or AV

FIGURE 214-8 Mechanism of AV nodal reentry: The atrium, AV node (AVN), and His bundle are shown schematically. The AV node is longitudinally dissociated into two pathways, slow and fast, with different functional properties (see text). In each panel of this diagram, red lines denote excitation in the AV node, which is manifest on the surface electrocardiogram (ECG), while black lines denote conduction that is concealed and not apparent on the surface electrocardiogram. *A.* During sinus rhythm (NSR) the impulse from the atrium conducts down both pathways. However, only conduction over the fast pathway is manifest on the surface ECG, producing a normal PR interval of 0.16 s. *B.* An atrial premature depolarization (APD) blocks in the fast pathway. The impulse conducts over the slow pathway to the His bundle and ventricles, producing a PR interval of 0.24 s. Because the impulse is premature, conduction over the slow pathway occurs more slowly than it would during sinus rhythm. *C.* A more premature atrial impulse blocks in the fast pathway, conducting with increased delay in the slow pathway, producing a PR interval of 0.28 s. The impulse conducts retrogradely up the fast pathway producing a single atrial echo. Sustained reentry is prevented by subsequent block in the slow pathway. *D.* A still more premature atrial impulse blocks initially in the fast pathway, conducting over the slow pathway with increasing delay, producing a PR interval of 0.36 s. Retrograde conduction occurs over the fast pathway and reentry occurs, producing a sustained tachycardia (SVT). *(After ME Josephson: Clinical Cardiac Electrophysiology, 2d ed. Phildelphia, Lea & Febiger, 2002; with permission.)*

FIGURE 214-9 Multifocal atrial tachycardia. A lead I rhythm strip demonstrates a multifocal atrial tachycardia defined by ≥3 consecutive P waves of variable morphology and rate >100 beats/min (*arrows*).

reentry and are more often associated with underlying cardiac disease. During sinus node reentry, the P-wave morphology is identical to that occurring in sinus rhythm, but the PR interval is prolonged. This is in contrast to sinus tachycardia, in which the PR interval tends to shorten. With intraatrial reentry, the P-wave configuration differs from that during sinus rhythm, and the PR interval is prolonged.

℞ TREATMENT

Sinus node and atrial reentrant arrhythmias are managed like other reentrant PSVTs, except that catheter ablation is less successful because multiple foci may be present.

NONREENTRANT ATRIAL TACHYCARDIAS These may be a manifestation of digitalis intoxication or may be associated with severe pulmonary or cardiac disease, with hypokalemia, or with the administration of theophylline or adrenergic drugs. Multifocal atrial tachycardia (MAT) (Fig. 214-9) is particularly common following theophylline administration. By definition, MAT requires three or more consecutive P waves of different morphologies at rates greater than 100 beats/min. MAT usually has an irregular ventricular rate because of varying AV conduction. There is a high incidence of AF (50 to 70%) in patients with MAT.

℞ TREATMENT

Treatment should be directed at the underlying disorder. The digitalis-induced arrhythmias are caused by triggered activity. In such atrial tachycardias with AV block secondary to digitalis intoxication, the atrial rate rarely exceeds 180 beats/min, and 2:1 block is typically present. Atrial arrhythmias precipitated by digitalis can usually be treated by withdrawal of the drug.

Automatic atrial tachycardias not caused by digitalis are difficult to terminate, and in such cases the main goal of therapy should be to control the ventricular response, either by drugs that affect the AV node, such as digitalis, beta blockers, or calcium channel antagonists, or by ablation techniques. Catheter ablation and surgery have been employed to eradicate the arrhythmia's focus or create heart block for rate control. Catheter ablation can cure incessant atrial tachycardia in <75% of cases and reverse tachycardia-mediated cardiomyopathy. Ablation should be considered for all patients with incessant atrial tachycardia.

PREEXCITATION (WPW) SYNDROME The most frequently encountered type of ventricular preexcitation is that associated with AV bypass tracts. These connections are composed of strands of atrial-like muscle, which may occur almost anywhere around the AV rings. The term *Wolff-Parkinson-White syndrome* is applied to patients with both preexcitation on the ECG and paroxysmal tachycardias. AV bypass tracts can be associated with certain congenital abnormalities, the most important of which is Ebstein's anomaly.

AV bypass tracts that conduct in an antegrade direction produce a typical ECG pattern of a short PR interval (<0.12 s), a slurred upstroke of the QRS complex (delta wave), and a wide QRS complex. This pattern results from a fusion of activation of the ventricles over both the bypass tract and the AV nodal His-Purkinje system (Fig. 214-10). The relative contribution of activation over each system determines the amount of preexcitation.

During PSVT in WPW, the impulse is usually conducted antegradely over the normal AV system and retrogradely through the bypass tract. The characteristics are identical to those described on p. 1347. Rarely (~5%), tachycardias occurring in patients with WPW will exhibit a reverse pattern with antegrade conduction through the bypass tract and retrograde conduction through the normal AV system. This produces a tachycardia with a wide QRS complex in which the ventricles are totally activated by the bypass tract. Atrial flutter and AF also occur commonly in patients with WPW syndrome. Since the bypass tract does not have the same decremental conducting properties as the AV node, the ventricular responses during atrial flutter or fibrillation may be unusually rapid and may cause VF.

The goals of electrophysiologic evaluation in patients suspected of having the WPW syndrome are (1) to confirm the diagnosis, (2) to localize the bypass tract and determine how many

FIGURE 214-10 ECG in Wolff-Parkinson-White syndrome. There is a short PR interval (0.11 s), a wide QRS complex (0.12 s), and slurring on the upstroke of the QRS produced by early ventricular activation over the bypass tract (delta wave, d in lead I). The negative delta waves in V₁ are diagnostic of a right-sided bypass tract. Note the Q wave (negative delta wave) in lead III, mimicking myocardial infarction.

bypass tracts are present, (3) to demonstrate the role of the bypass tract in the genesis of the arrhythmias, (4) to determine the potential for the development of possibly life-threatening rates during atrial flutter or fibrillation, and (5) to evaluate therapeutic options.

℞ TREATMENT

Pharmacologic therapy is aimed at altering the electrophysiologic properties (i.e., refractoriness or conduction velocity) of one or more components of the reentrant circuit. This is most often accomplished by agents such as beta blockers or calcium channel blockers that slow conduction and increase refractoriness of the AV node or by agents such as quinidine or flecainide that slow conduction and increase refractoriness primarily in the bypass tract. Some drugs may affect multiple sites.

Acute management of episodes of PSVT in patients with WPW syndrome is similar to that of PSVT in patients with concealed bypass tracts.

In patients with the WPW syndrome and AF, DC cardioversion should be carried out if there is a life threatening, rapid ventricular response. In non-life-threatening situations, lidocaine (3 to 5 mg/kg) or procainamide (15 mg/kg) administered intravenously over 15 to 20 min will usually slow the ventricular response. More recently, ibutilide has become available as an alternative therapy for preexcitation tachycardia. Caution should be employed when using digitalis or intravenous verapamil in patients with the WPW syndrome and AF, since these drugs can shorten the refractory period of the accessory pathway and can increase the ventricular rate, thereby placing the patient at increased risk for VF. Chronic oral therapy with verapamil is not associated with this risk. In addition to these drugs, beta-blocking agents are of no utility in controlling the ventricular response during AF when conduction proceeds over the bypass tract. Although atrial or ventricular pacing can almost always terminate PSVT in patients with the WPW syndrome, they can induce AF. As such, chronic pacemaker therapy is to be discouraged.

While surgical ablation of bypass tracts offers a permanent cure of supraventricular tachycardia (SVT) and most AFs associated with SVT, the advent of radiofrequency catheter ablation has virtually eliminated the need for surgery. Catheter ablation of bypass tracts is possible in >90% of patients and is the treatment of choice in patients with symptomatic arrhythmias. It is safer, more cost-effective, and just as successful as surgery. Nevertheless, surgical ablation may be required in the occasional patient in whom catheter ablation fails.

NONPAROXYSMAL JUNCTIONAL TACHYCARDIA This rhythm usually results from conditions that produce enhanced automaticity or triggered activity in the AV junction and is most commonly due to digitalis intoxication, inferior wall myocardial infarction, myocarditis, endogenous or exogenous catecholamine excess, acute rheumatic fever, or valve surgery.

The onset of nonparoxysmal junctional tachycardia is usually gradual, with a "warm-up" period prior to stabilization of the rate, which can range from 70 to 150 beats/min, faster rates usually being associated with digitalis intoxication. Nonparoxysmal junctional tachycardia is recognized by a QRS complex identical to that of sinus rhythm. The rate can be influenced by autonomic tone and can be increased by catecholamines, vagolytic agents, or exercise and slowed somewhat by carotid sinus pressure. When this rhythm is due to digitalis intoxication, it usually is associated with AV block and/or dissociation. Soon after cardiac surgery, retrograde conduction is more likely to be present because of the heightened sympathetic state.

℞ TREATMENT

This is directed toward elimination of the underlying etiologic factors. Since digitalis is the most common cause of this rhythm, discontinuation of this drug is indicated. If the rhythm is associated with other serious manifestations of digitalis intoxication, such as ventricular or atrial irritability, active intervention with lidocaine or a beta blocker

may be useful, and in some instances use of digitalis antibodies (Fab fragments) should be considered. Cardioversion of this rhythm should not be attempted, particularly in the setting of digitalis intoxication. When AV conduction is intact, atrial pacing can capture and override the junctional focus and provide the AV synchrony necessary to maximize cardiac output. Nonparoxysmal junctional tachycardia is usually not a chronic, recurrent problem, and attention to the acute precipitating events can often resolve the tachycardia.

VENTRICULAR TACHYCARDIA *Sustained ventricular tachycardia* is defined as VT that persists for >30 s or requires termination because of hemodynamic collapse. VT generally accompanies some form of structural heart disease, most commonly chronic ischemic heart disease associated with a prior myocardial infarction. Sustained VT may also be associated with nonischemic cardiomyopathies, metabolic disorders, drug toxicity, or prolonged QT syndrome, and it occurs occasionally in the absence of heart disease or other predisposing factors. *Nonsustained VT* (three beats to 30 s) is also associated with cardiac disease but occurs in its absence more often than the sustained arrhythmia. While nonsustained VT usually does not produce symptoms, sustained VT is almost always symptomatic and is often associated with marked hemodynamic compromise and/or the development of myocardial ischemia. A fixed anatomic substrate, not acute ischemia, is responsible for most recurrent episodes of sustained uniform VT. Acute ischemia appears to have little role in the genesis of sustained uniform VT associated with chronic infarction but may play a role in the degeneration of stable VT into VF or initiation of polymorphic VT. Most episodes of VF begin with VT.

The ECG diagnosis of VT is suggested by a wide-complex QRS tachycardia at a rate exceeding 100 beats/min. The QRS configuration during any episode of VT may be uniform (monomorphic) or it may vary from beat to beat (polymorphic). *Bidirectional tachycardia* refers to VT that shows an alternation in QRS axis. Typically this appears as a QRS with a right bundle branch block pattern with alternating superior (leftward) and inferior axes (rightward). While the rhythm is usually quite regular, slight irregularity may exist. Atrial activity may be dissociated from ventricular activity, or the atria may be depolarized retrogradely. The onset of the tachycardia is generally abrupt, but in nonparoxysmal tachycardias it can be gradual. Paroxysmal VT is usually initiated by a VPC.

It is important to distinguish SVT with aberration of intraventricular conduction from VT because the clinical implications and management of these two arrhythmias are totally different. The most important clinical predictor of VT is the presence of structural heart disease. The observation of intermittent cannon *a* waves and varying first heart sounds suggests AV dissociation and is diagnostic of VT. In a majority of cases, the diagnosis can and should be made by close examination of the 12-lead ECG. Pharmacologic maneuvers, such as administration of intravenous verapamil or adenosine, can be hazardous and should be avoided. It is always useful to have a 12-lead ECG recorded during sinus rhythm for comparison with that during tachycardia. When the tracing obtained during sinus rhythm demonstrates the same morphologic features as those during the tachycardia, the diagnosis of PSVT with aberration is favored. An infarction pattern on the sinus rhythm tracing suggests the potential presence of the anatomic substrate necessary for VT.

Characteristics of the 12-lead ECG during the tachycardia that suggest a ventricular origin for the arrhythmia are (1) a QRS complex >0.14 s in the absence of antiarrhythmic therapy, (2) AV dissociation (with or without fusion or captured beats) or variable retrograde conduction (Fig. 214-11), (3) a superior QRS axis in the presence of a right bundle branch block pattern, (4) concordance of the QRS pattern in all precordial leads (i.e., all positive or all negative deflections), and (5) other QRS patterns (morphology) with prolonged duration that are inconsistent with typical right or left bundle branch block patterns (Table 214-5). A wide, complex, bizarre tachycardia that is very ir-

FIGURE 214-11 Ventricular tachycardia with AV dissociation. P waves are dissociated from the underlying wide complex rhythm (best seen on lead V₁).

have a threefold greater risk of death than a comparable group of patients without this arrhythmia. However, a cause-and-effect relationship between the nonsustained tachycardia and subsequent sudden death has not been established. Patients without heart disease who have uniform VT have a good prognosis and an extremely low risk of sudden death.

℞ TREATMENT

The risk-benefit ratio of treating each specific type of VT should be considered before beginning therapy. This is important because antiarrhythmic agents can produce or exacerbate the very arrhythmias that they are given to prevent. In general, patients with VT but without organic heart disease have a benign course; such patients with asymptomatic, nonsustained VT need not be treated because their prognosis will not be affected. An exception is the patient with congenital long QT syndrome. Such patients have recurrent polymorphic VT and a high mortality from sudden death if untreated. Patients with sustained VT in the absence of heart disease usually require therapy because the arrhythmia causes symptoms. These tachycardias may respond to beta blockers; verapamil; class IA, IC, or III agents; or amiodarone.

In patients with VT and organic heart disease, if marked hemodynamic compromise is present or if there is evidence of ischemia, CHF, or central nervous system hypoperfusion, the rhythm should be promptly terminated by (DC) cardioversion (see below). If the patient with organic heart disease tolerates the VT well, pharmacologic therapy may be tried. Procainamide is probably the most effective agent

regular suggests AF with conduction over an AV bypass tract. Similarly, a QRS complex in excess of 0.20 s is uncommon during VT in the absence of drug therapy and is more common with preexcitation. Intravenous verapamil will stop most recalcitrant SVTs involving the AV junction, but it is rarely effective for VT. Because of this property, verapamil has been utilized to attempt to differentiate SVT with aberrant conduction from VT. However, this is extremely hazardous, since intravenous verapamil can precipitate cardiac arrest in patients with VT. A similar caveat can be made for use of adenosine. This agent can produce a coronary stent in patients with multivessel disease and produce a cardiac arrest.

It has been possible to replicate sustained uniform VT in >95% of patients with this arrhythmia using programmed electrical stimulation. In most patients the tachycardia is initiated with ventricular premature stimuli. A sustained monomorphic VT with a morphology identical to that of the spontaneous arrhythmia is the rule. The clinical significance of polymorphic VT initiated by programmed stimulation is not clear, since more aggressive stimulation (i.e., the use of three or four extrastimuli) can induce polymorphic VT and even VF in some normal subjects and in patients who have never had a clinical arrhythmia.

Sustained uniform VT can be terminated by programmed stimulation or rapid pacing in at least 75% of patients; the remainder require cardioversion. The ability to reproducibly initiate and terminate a sustained, uniform VT permits assessment of pharmacologic and electrical therapy of these arrhythmias.

The reproducible termination of VT by programmed stimulation permits evaluation of the effectiveness of antitachycardia pacemakers for long-term therapy of paroxysmal episodes of arrhythmia. Unfortunately, rapid pacing, the most effective form of therapy, can accelerate the tachycardia and/or produce VF. Therefore, antitachycardia pacing is a viable form of therapy only when the pacing device includes backup defibrillation capabilities.

Clinical Features Symptoms resulting from VT depend on the ventricular rate, duration of the tachycardia, and presence and extent of underlying cardiac disease. When the tachycardia is rapid and associated with severe myocardial dysfunction and cerebrovascular disease, hypotension and syncope are common. However, the presence of hemodynamic stability does not preclude a diagnosis of VT. The rate, loss of the atrial contribution to ventricular filling, and abnormal sequence of ventricular activation are important factors producing a decreased cardiac output during VT.

The *prognosis* of VT depends on the underlying disease state. If sustained VT develops within the first 6 weeks following acute myocardial infarction, the prognosis is poor, with a 75% mortality rate at 1 year. Patients with nonsustained VT following myocardial infarction

---

TABLE 214-5 *Wide Complex Tachycardia*

ECG CRITERIA THAT FAVOR VENTRICULAR TACHYCARDIA

1. AV dissociation
2. QRS width: >0.14 s with RBBB configuration
   >0.16 s with LBBB configuration
3. QRS axis: Left axis deviation with RBBB morphology
   Extreme left axis deviation (northwest axis) with LBBB morphology
4. Concordance of QRS in precordial leads
5. Morphologic patterns of the QRS complex
   RBBB: Mono- or biphasic complex in V₁
   RS (*only with left axis deviation*) or QS in V₆

LBBB: Broad R wave in V₁ or V₂ ≥0.04 s
   Onset of QRS to nadir of S wave in V₁ or V₂ of ≥0.07 s
   Notched downslope of S wave in V₁ or V₂
   Q wave in V₆

Note: AV, atrioventricular; BBB, bundle branch block.

for acute therapy. It may or may not terminate the tachycardia but almost always slows the rate. In stable patients in whom these drugs do not terminate the arrhythmia, a pacing catheter can be inserted pervenously into the right ventricular apex, and the tachycardia can be terminated by overdrive pacing.

Although programmed stimulation has been used to select the appropriate antiarrhythmic agent to prevent recurrent, sustained VT, recent data suggest ICD implantation is more effective. As such, drugs are used in patients in whom ICDs are contraindicated or according to patient preference. These drugs may also be used as adjunctive therapy with ICDs to suppress recurrent ventricular or coexisting supraventricular arrhythmias.

Antitachycardia pacing has been used as a means to terminate tachycardias that have been reproducibly terminated by pacing in the electrophysiology laboratory. Automatic antitachycardia pacing devices are not used alone because pacing during VT may accelerate tachycardia, converting a stable arrhythmia into an unstable one and resulting in severe hemodynamic compromise. However, devices combining antitachycardia pacing with an ICD (see below) afford a "backup" means of terminating unstable arrhythmias.

The advent of endocardial catheter and intraoperative mapping led to the development of surgical techniques for the management of VT. Even though most patients with VT and ischemic heart disease have markedly impaired left ventricular function and multivessel coronary artery disease, the operative mortality rate has ranged between 8 and 15%. Following operation, >90% of survivors are controlled either off (two-thirds of patients) or on (one-third) antiarrhythmic agents that were previously ineffective in controlling these rhythms. With the development of radiofrequency ablation and refinement of mapping criteria to locate the critical sites of the VT circuit precisely, catheter ablation can be performed as a curative procedure in selected patients. In experienced centers, cure of VT in these *selected* patients approaches 75%.

Specific Types of VT *Torsades de pointes* (Fig. 214-12) refers to VT characterized by polymorphic QRS complexes that change in amplitude and cycle length, giving the appearance of oscillations around the baseline. This rhythm is, by definition, associated with QT prolongation. The latter may result from electrolyte disturbances (particularly hypokalemia and hypomagnesemia), use of a variety of antiarrhythmic drugs (especially quinidine), phenothiazines and tricyclic antidepressants, liquid protein diets, intracranial events, and bradyarrhythmias, particularly third-degree AV block. It may also occur as a congenital anomaly that most often presents with torsades de pointes (syncope or sudden death) at a young age.

The electrocardiographic hallmark is polymorphic VT preceded by marked QT prolongation, often in excess of 0.60 s. These patients often have multiple episodes of nonsustained polymorphic VT associated with recurrent syncope, but they may also develop VF and sudden cardiac death.

℞ TREATMENT

This should be directed at removing the precipitating factors, i.e., correcting metabolic abnormalities and removing drugs that have induced the prolonged QT interval. In the setting of drug-induced torsades de pointes, atrial or ventricular overdrive pacing and the administration of magnesium have also been useful in terminating and preventing the arrhythmia. For patients with the congenital prolonged QT interval syndrome, β-adrenergic blocking agents have been the mainstay of therapy; agents that shorten the QT interval may also be useful (e.g., phenytoin). Cervicothoracic sympathectomy has been proposed as a form of therapy for congenital prolonged QT syndrome, but it is not often effective as the sole therapy. Pacing in combination with beta blockers and sympathectomy has been used by some investigators when beta blockers fail, but it is not uniformly successful and results in a Horner's syndrome. ICDs with dual-chambered pacing capability and beta blockers have become the treatment of choice for patients with recurrent episodes despite beta blockers.

Polymorphic tachycardias associated with normal QT intervals in patients with ischemic heart disease that are initiated by "R-on-T" VPCs are probably caused by reentry, and their treatment is totally different. They should not be considered torsades de pointes. In such cases, class I or III agents may be the most effective form of therapy and should be administered in full antiarrhythmic doses. However, these arrhythmias may also result from acute, severe ischemia and will only respond to abolition of the ischemia, usually by revascularization. Another group of patients has recently been defined who have polymorphic VT initiated by short coupled VPCs during exercise or other catecholamine states due to triggered activity associated with release of Ca^{2+} from the sarcoplasmic reticulum. This is a lethal syndrome requiring an implantable defibrillator.

Accelerated idioventricular rhythm, also termed *slow VT*, with a rate that ranges from 60 to 120 beats/min, usually occurs in acute myocardial infarction, often during reperfusion. It may also be seen following cardiac operations; in patients with cardiomyopathy, rheumatic fever, or digitalis intoxication; and in patients with no evidence of heart disease. The rhythm is usually transient and rarely causes significant hemodynamic compromise or symptoms. Treatment is rarely necessary and should usually be considered only if symptoms arise due to impaired hemodynamics, most commonly due to AV dissociation. In most cases, atropine can accelerate the sinus rate to overdrive the ventricular rhythm.

FIGURE 214-12   Rhythm strips of patients with drug (disopyramide)-induced torsades de pointes. The polymorphic ventricular tachycardia is associated with very long QT intervals.

FIGURE 214-13 Ventricular fibrillation. In a patient with coronary disease, ventricular fibrillation is initiated by an early ventricular premature complex that produces a rapid polymorphic ventricular tachycardia, which rapidly degenerates to ventricular fibrillation (note the undulating baseline with indistinguishable systole and diastole).

VENTRICULAR FLUTTER AND VENTRICULAR FIBRILLATION (Fig. 214-13; see also Chap. 256) These arrhythmias occur most often in patients with ischemic heart disease. They also occur following administration of antiarrhythmic drugs, particularly those that induce prolonged QT intervals and torsades de pointes (see above), in patients with severe hypoxia or ischemia, and in those with WPW syndrome who develop AF with an extremely rapid ventricular response (p. 1345). Electrical accidents frequently cause cardiac arrest due to the development of VF. The onset of these arrhythmias is rapidly followed by loss of consciousness and, if untreated, death. Episodes of cardiac arrest recorded during Holter monitoring reveal that approximately three-fourths of the sudden deaths are due to VT or VF.

In patients with nonischemic VF, the onset usually begins with a short run of rapid VT, which is initiated by a relatively late coupled VPC. In patients with acute myocardial infarction or ischemia, however, VF is usually precipitated by a single early ventricular complex beat falling on the T wave (the vulnerable period), which produces a rapid VT that degenerates into VF (Fig. 214-13).

The clinical setting in which VF occurs is important. Most patients who have primary VF within the first 48 h of the onset of acute infarction have a good long-term prognosis, with a very low rate of recurrence or sudden cardiac death. Their short-term mortality may, however, be slightly increased. In contrast, patients who experience VF unassociated with the development of acute myocardial infarction have a recurrence rate of 20 to 30% in the year following the event (Chap. 256).

Ventricular flutter usually appears as a sine wave with a rate between 150 and 300 beats/min. These oscillations make it impossible to assign a specific morphology to the arrhythmia and in some cases to distinguish it from rapid VT. VF is recognized by grossly irregular undulations of varying amplitudes, contours, and rates (Fig. 214-13). Electrophysiologic studies have demonstrated that regardless of the apparent gross irregularity on the surface ECG, VF usually starts out with a rapid repetitive sequence of VT that ultimately breaks down into multiple wavelets of reentry.

Electrophysiologic studies have been useful in patients who have been resuscitated from cardiac arrest. In approximately 70% of patients with prior infarction, programmed stimulation can reproducibly initiate a sustained VT. Ablation may be possible in some of these patients, particularly if the VT can be slowed so that it can be mapped. Several recent secondary prevention trials have demonstrated superior survival (3 years) in patients treated with ICDs versus amiodarone (Table 214-6). However, in patients with ejection fractions >35% or <20%, survival was comparable.

GENETIC CONSIDERATIONS Many advances have been made in the identification of genes responsible for syndromes associated with VTs and sudden cardiac death. Specific examples include the congenital long QT syndrome (LQTS), hypertrophic obstructive cardiomyopathy (Chap. 221), arrhythmogenic right ventricular dysplasia, catecholamine-related VT/VF, and the *Brugada syndrome* (Table 214-7). The latter is a recently described disorder characterized by the electrocardiographic profile of a pseudo right bundle branch block pattern with ST elevation and terminal T-wave inversion in leads V_1-V_3 (Fig. 214-14). The clinical presentation is VF in patients with structurally normal hearts. A mutation in the cardiac sodium channel, SCN 5A, is believed to be responsible. While the same gene is responsible for the LQTS, the mutation is different in the two syndromes.

TREATMENT

PHARMACOLOGIC ANTIARRHYTHMIC THERAPY Prior to initiation of pharmacologic antiarrhythmic therapy, potential aggravating factors such as transient metabolic abnormalities, CHF, or acute ischemia must be corrected; in some cases this may suffice to control arrhythmias. In addition, the potential role of drugs as a cause or exacerbating factor in the development of the arrhythmia must be considered. It must be recognized that we do not have a good understanding of the effects of antiarrhythmic agents on the spontaneous onset of tachyarrhythmias. In some cases, they may facilitate the onset.

Antiarrhythmic drugs are used in three principal situations: (1) to terminate an acute arrhythmia, (2) to prevent recurrence of an

TABLE 214-6 *Trials of ICD Therapy for Secondary Prevention in VT/VF Patients*

	AVID			CIDS	CASH
Protocol	ICD vs. empiric amiodarone or sotolol (mainly amiodarone)			ICD vs. empiric amiodarone	ICD vs. empiric amiodarone, metoprolol, and propafenone[a]
Sample size	$n = 1016$ AAD = 509 ICD = 507			$n = 659$ Amiodarone = 331 ICD = 328	$n = 346$ Amiodarone = 92 Metoprolol = 97 Propafenone[a] = 58 ICD = 99
Patient inclusion criteria	Survivors of VF VT with syncope VT with EF $\leq$ 40%			Survivors of VF VT with syncope VT with EF $\leq$ 35% and cycle length $\leq$ 400 ms	Survivors of VF (no EF requirement)
Mortality in "drug" or "control" arm	17.7% 1 year	25.3% 2 years	35.9% 3 years	30% 3 years	19.6% 2 years
Mortality in ICD arm	10.7% 1 year	18.4% 2 years	24.6% 3 years	25% 3 years	12.1% 2 years
Reduction in mortality with ICD	39% 1 year	27% 2 years	31% 3 years	20% 3 years	37% 2 years

[a] Following an interim analysis in March, 1992, enrollment in propafenone arm was discontinued because mortality was increased significantly over mortality in the ICD arm.
Note: EF, ejection fraction; ICD, implanted cardioverter/defibrillator; VF, ventricular fibrillation; VT, ventricular tachycardia.
Sources: AVID Investigators: N Engl J Med 337(22):1576, 1997; K Kuck, S Connolly: ACC NewsOnline, 1998.

arrhythmia, and (3) to prevent a life-threatening arrhythmia for which the patient is perceived to be at risk but which has never occurred.

Most currently available antiarrhythmic agents (Table 214-4) have a relatively low toxic/therapeutic ratio; all can exert proarrhythmic effects (Table 214-8) and therefore may exacerbate underlying arrhythmias. Serum levels can be determined for most currently available antiarrhythmic agents. Standards for therapeutic and toxic levels can serve only as a rough guide for selecting the appropriate dose in any individual patient. In the final analysis, the therapeutic level in a given patient is the concentration that achieves the desired antiarrhythmic effect, and the toxic level for each patient is the concentration at which undesirable side effects occur. Since many adverse effects are directly related to drug concentrations, the lowest serum level that achieves an effective antiarrhythmic response should be chosen.

In order to determine the therapeutic level for a patient, one must have a standard to judge drug efficacy. For a patient with an incessant arrhythmia, antiarrhythmic drugs may be administered empirically until the arrhythmia is suppressed. If a reproducible precipitating factor such as exercise can be identified, serial drug testing during such a provocative maneuver may be performed. Unfortunately, most arrhythmias are sporadic and occur unpredictably without identifiable precipitating factors. In these cases, if one waits to observe spontaneous recurrences on each antiarrhythmic drug, assessment of drug efficacy may require months. This type of assessment of efficacy may be adequate for arrhythmias that are not life-threatening such as AF or SVT. In the current era, most patients with ventricular arrhythmia have ICDs, and recurrence can be monitored through ICD arrhythmic logs. However, this mode of assessment is inadequate for arrhythmias that compromise hemodynamic stability, result in syncope, or cause cardiac arrest.

CLASSIFICATION OF ANTIARRHYTHMIC DRUGS A number of classifications of antiarrhythmic drugs have been proposed; the most frequently used is a modification of one proposed by Vaughan-Williams (Table 214-2). This classification is based in part on the ability of antiarrhythmic drugs to modify the cardiac cellular (1) excitatory currents (Na^+ or Ca^{2+}), (2) action potential duration, and (3) automaticity (phase 4 depolarization). These effects of the drugs on isolated cardiac cells are thought to account for some of the antiarrhythmic properties of the drugs. Thus depression of excitatory currents by class I and class IV antiarrhythmics results in slowing of conduction velocity and may interrupt arrhythmias by blocking conduction in areas of marginal excitability, where conduction velocity is already slow. Class III antiarrhythmics allegedly exert their action by increasing refractoriness through prolongation of the action potential duration. However, this classification has a number of limitations. The electrophysiologic effects of these drugs in vivo may differ from their effects on isolated cells. Also, the effects of heart rate and fiber geometry are not considered. Not all drugs (e.g., adenosine) fit into the classifications. Finally, some drugs (e.g., amiodarone) exhibit properties consistent with multiple classes. The uses, actions, and toxic actions of currently available antiarrhythmic drugs are summarized in Tables 214-4 and 214-7.

ELECTRICAL THERAPY OF TACHYARRHYTHMIAS ■ Pacemakers Cardiac pacing can be used to terminate and, in selected cases, prevent recurrent supraventricular and ventricular arrhythmias. Because many tachyarrhythmias appear to be due to a reentrant mechanism with the impulse traveling in a circuit, a properly timed paced impulse can penetrate and prematurely depolarize part of the circuit, rendering it refractory to the next circulating wavefront and thereby interrupting the circus movement. Pacing therapy for arrhythmias is generally reserved for patients whose arrhythmias are refractory to drug therapy and who remain hemodynamically stable during the tachycardia. All forms of pacing therapy require repeated demonstration of their effectiveness and reliability in terminating the arrhythmias during electrophysiologic testing prior to implantation of the pacing device.

The type of pacing device and modality selected for arrhythmia termination depend on (1) the rate of the tachycardia (rates >160 beats/min are rarely terminated by a single premature stimulus), (2) the type of arrhythmia (atrial flutter and VT are rarely terminated by single extrastimuli), and (3) concomitant drug therapy.

Because many tachycardias cannot be terminated by single premature stimuli, pacemakers have been developed that allow for multiple extrastimuli (burst pacing) to be introduced. In the current era, antitachycardia pacing is used almost exclusively for ventricular arrhythmias because of the success of radiofrequency ablative therapy for supraventricular arrhythmias.

Cardiac pacing has also been used to prevent ventricular tachyarrhythmias. Polymorphic VT associated with a long QT interval and bradycardia (torsades de pointes, p. 1351) is most likely to respond. Pacing the atrium and/or ventricle at rates between 90 and 120 beats/min appears to increase the homogeneity of electrical recovery and markedly reduces the propensity for a recurrence of arrhythmias.

FIGURE 214-14 Brugada syndrome. Note ST elevation with terminal T wave inversion in leads V_1–V_3 mimicking right bundle branch block.

TABLE 214-7 Genetically Determined Arrhythmia Syndromes

Disease	Inheritance	Involved Gene	Protein
LQT	Autosomal dominant	KVLQT 1	I_{K3} K channel
		HERG	I_{Kr} K channel
		SCN5A	I_{Na} Na channel
		LQT 4	Unknown
		minK	I_{KS} K channel
		MiRP1	I_{Kr} K channel
	Autosomal recessive (with neural deafness)	KVLQT 1	I_{KS} K channel
		MinK	I_{KS} K channel
	Drug-induced	HERG	I_{Kr} K channel
		MiRP1	I_{Kr} K channel
Brugada syndrome	Autosomal dominant	SNC5A	I_{Na} Na channel
Catecholamine VT	Autosomal dominant	RyR2	Ryanodine receptor
	Autosomal recessive	CASQ2	Calsequestran receptor
Arrhythmogenic RV dysplasia	Autosomal dominant	Unknown genes	
Hypertrophic cardiomyopathy	Autosomal dominant	Multiple cardiac sarcomeric genes (troponin T, troponin I, myosin heavy chain, myosin binding protein C, α tropomyosin)	

TABLE 214-8 *Toxicity of Most Frequently Used Antiarrhythmic Agents*

Drug	Nonarrhythmic Toxicity	Proarrhythmic Toxicity			
		TDP[a]	A Flutter 1:1	VT/VF	Bradycardia
Digoxin	Anorexia, nausea, vomiting, visual changes	Atrial tachycardia, VT, AV nodal block, accelerated junctional rhythms, atrial and ventricular premature depolarizations; acceleration of ventricular rate during atrial fibrillation or flutter in the presence of preexcitation			
Quinidine[b]	Anorexia, nausea, vomiting, diarrhea, cinchonism, tinnitus, hearing and visual changes, thrombocytopenia, hemolytic anemia, rash, potentiation of digoxin levels	2%	++	++	+
Procainamide[b]	Lupus erythematosus–like syndrome, anorexia, nausea	2%	+	++	+
Disopyramide[b]	Anticholinergic actions: dry mouth, urinary retention, visual disturbances (avoid in narrow-angle glaucoma) constipation, congestive heart failure	2%	+	++	+
Lidocaine	Dizziness, confusion, delirium, seizures, coma; side effects potentiated by liver and heart failure	—	—	—	+[b]
Mexiletine	Ataxia, tremor, gait disturbances, rash, vomiting	—	—	—	—
Flecainide	Dizziness, nausea	Rare	+++	++	++
Propafenone[c]	Taste disturbance, bronchospasm	Rare	+++	++	++
Amiodarone	Pulmonary infiltrates and fibrosis, hepatitis, hypo- and hyperthyroidism, photosensitivity, peripheral neuropathy, tremor	Rare	+++	+++	+++
Sotalol	Bronchospasm	+++	+	+	+++

[a] TDP (torsades de pointes) occurs most often in the setting of slow heart rates, QT prolongation, and hypokalemia or hypomagnesemia and at the time of conversion from atrial fibrillation to sinus rhythm. QT prolongation and torsades de pointes are not dose-related phenomena. QRS prolongation is a dose-related phenomenon also and will occur at toxic concentrations. QT and WRS intervals should be monitored and dose reductions made for interval prolongations.

[b] May suppress sinus node function in patients with underlying sinus node dysfunction. May suppress escape foci in patients with complete heart block.

[c] Avoid in patients with prior myocardial infarction and depressed left ventricular function. Use in combination with AV nodal blocking agent to limit risk of atrial flutter with 1:1 conduction.

Note: A flutter 1:1, atrial flutter with 1:1 atrioventricular (AV) conduction; VT/VF, ventricular tachycardia/ventricular fibrillation.

Pacemakers may be self-contained or energized by an external radiofrequency source. The self-contained pacemaker may function automatically [i.e., it incorporates an arrhythmia-recognition program (circuit)], or it may be activated by an external magnet. The major advantage of a fully automatic system is that there is no need for the patient to recognize the arrhythmia in order for termination to occur. The advantages of the externally activated system (rarely used today) include (1) the decreased risk of unnecessary treatment because of faulty sensing, and (2) the opportunity to initiate monitoring at the time of attempted termination of arrhythmia. This type of monitoring is frequently helpful if pacing techniques are employed to terminate VT, given the risk of acceleration of the arrhythmia by pacing.

The limitations of pacing therapy are primarily related to (1) the changes in the characteristics of the arrhythmia over time such that programmed pacing parameters no longer terminate the tachycardia; (2) the risk of acceleration of the tachycardia with the development of AF when stimulating the atrium and the development of rapid VT and VF when stimulating the ventricles; and (3) inappropriate recognition of supraventricular tachyarrhythmias as VTs, leading to delivery of therapy unnecessarily, which can initiate VT or VF. Future pacing generators that can perform cardioversion and defibrillation will increase the applicability of pacing therapy for the treatment of arrhythmias (see below).

Cardioversion and Defibrillation Electrical cardioversion and defibrillation remain the most reliable methods for terminating arrhythmias. By depolarizing all or at least a large portion of excitable myocardium in a near homogeneous fashion, the electrical shock can interrupt reentrant arrhythmias. External cardioversion is routinely performed by placing two paddles 12 cm in diameter in firm contact with the chest wall, with one paddle usually located to the right of the sternum at the level of the second rib and the other in the left anterior axillary line in the fifth intercostal space. If the patient is conscious, a short-acting anesthetic or an amnesic drug should be administered to prevent patient discomfort. A person skilled in maintaining an airway should be present.

Energy is delivered synchronously with the QRS complex for all arrhythmias except ventricular flutter and VF, since asynchronous shocks can produce VF. The amount of energy used will vary with the type of tachycardia being treated. With the exception of AF, SVTs can frequently be terminated with energy levels in the range of 25 to 50 W·s, while AF usually requires ≥100 W·s for termination. For terminating VT, energy levels ≥100 W·s should probably be employed. While energies as low as 25 W·s may be used successfully, they also have a higher incidence of producing VF or AF. At least 200 W·s of energy should be used for initial attempts at terminating VF. If the initial shock fails, all repeated attempts at defibrillation should be with the maximum energy that the defibrillator is capable of delivering (320 to 400 W·s). As noted earlier, biphasic cardioversion has proven more effective with lower energy requirements than monophasic cardioversion.

Indications for cardioversion depend on the clinical setting and the patient's general condition. Any tachycardia (except sinus tachycardia) that produces hypotension, myocardial ischemia, or heart failure warrants consideration of prompt termination using external cardioversion. Arrhythmias that fail to terminate with pharmacologic therapy may also be terminated by electrical cardioversion. Transient bradycardias and supraventricular and ventricular irritability following cardioversion are common and usually do not warrant antiarrhythmic intervention.

Implanted Cardioverter/Defibrillator ICD devices have been developed that will promptly recognize and terminate life-threatening ventricular arrhythmias. These devices can deliver <1 to 40 W·s, the amount of which can be programmed. Current devices have antitachycardia pacing capabilities such that VT can be sensed and terminated without resorting to a painful shock. In such devices, high-energy shocks are reserved for hypotensive VT, acceleration of VT, or failure to terminate VT after a programmed duration (Fig. 214-15). ICDs are generally implanted transvenously, in a manner similar to pacemakers. Clinical trials testing the function of these devices in patients with drug-refractory ventricular arrhythmias have demonstrated survival from sudden death at 1 year ranging between 92 and 100%. Currently, ICDs

FIGURE 214-15 Normally functioning implantable defibrillators. A continuous Holter monitoring tracing is shown. On the top strip, a rapid polymorphic tachycardia is initiated which beats more uniformly. The automatic implantable cardioverter/defibrillator (ICD) senses the rhythm and delivers a shock which restores sinus rhythm.

should be considered for patients with VT that is not hemodynamically tolerated. As mentioned earlier, recent randomized trials suggest that ICDs confer improved mortality over amiodarone in patients with hemodynamically untolerated VT and a cardiac arrest not due to reversible causes (Table 214-9). Finally, they are indicated for patients with depressed left ventricular function, prior myocardial infarction, and nonsustained and sustained VT at electrophysiologic study (Table 214-9). A more recent study has defined a mortality benefit conferred by ICDs in patients with coronary artery disease and severely depressed ventricular function, regardless of the presence of nonsustained VT in electrophysiologic study results. Guidelines for their use are given in Table 214-10.

The most frequent problem with the ICD has been its inappropriate discharge in the absence of sustained ventricular arrhythmias. Additional potential problems include an increase in defibrillation threshold and decrease in tachycardia rates below the rate cut-off of the device in response to many antiarrhythmic drugs. Permanently implanted ventricular pacemakers may interfere with the device's ability to sense VF. This can be avoided by using committed bipolar pacing systems that are better able to sense local ventricular activity. Diagnostic fea-

tures of newer, all-in-one devices are able to identify the probable cause of an inappropriate ICD discharge (e.g., AF, SVT, fractured lead) and to adjust pharmacologic therapy or reprogram the device to avoid such inappropriate shocks. These newer devices have the capability to take a "second look" prior to shock delivery and thus may abort delivery for self-terminating arrhythmias. In addition, the range of candidates suitable for implantation will be expanded because the newer devices have the capability of shock therapy for patients whose arrhythmias do not cause loss of consciousness.

Newer generations of ICDs are smaller and frequently allow placement of a second lead in the right atrium. This lead senses atrial activity and provides enhanced discrimination of atrial from ventricular electrical activity. This enhanced discrimination of SVT from VT prevents inappropriate shocks for SVT that may be misinterpreted as VT and allows the device to switch from a dual-chamber to a single-chamber device should an SVT-like AF develop. These dual-chamber devices also allow AV sequential pacing.

DEVICES FOR HEART FAILURE MANAGEMENT (See also Chap. 216) The addition of a lead in the coronary sinus to pace the left ventricle at the same time that the right ventricle is being paced is called *cardiac resynchronization*. This technique has proven complementary to standard pharmacologic management of CHF. Resynchronization with biventricular pacing can be instituted with a pacemaker or ICD.

Ablative Therapy for Arrhythmias Catheter-based mapping techniques have provided a nonoperative approach to the identification and cure of a variety of arrhythmias. In fact, catheter ablation techniques are now the procedures of choice for symptomatic patients with (1) concealed or manifest (WPW) bypass tracts; (2) AV nodal reentrant SVT; (3) typical atrial flutter; and (4) poorly controlled ventricular responses to atrial arrhythmias, most commonly AF. Successful ablation of bypass tracts and modifications of the AV node by radiofrequency energy are extremely successful and cost-effective and are the procedure of choice for patients with recurrent episodes. The creation of AV block with implantation of a pacemaker is the method of choice in managing patients with AF and poorly controlled ventricular response. Idiopathic VTs and some VTs that are associated with coronary artery disease are also amenable to ablation, but the result is less successful than for ablation of SVTs.

Surgical therapy is now relegated to cases of sustained VT associated with coronary artery disease when operative intervention is needed for coronary bypass surgery and/or aneurysmectomy or VT associated with specific structural abnormalities [e.g., idiopathic left ventricle aneurysm, status post (s/p) surgery for tetralogy of Fallot]. It may also be undertaken for the unusual instances of failed catheter ablation for SVTs associated with bypass tracts and for AF.

TABLE 214-9 *Trials of ICD Therapy for Primary Prevention of Sudden Cardiac Death*

	MADIT	MUSTT	MADIT II
Protocol	ICD vs conventional (AAD, primary empirical amiodarone)	EP-guided Rx (AAD, ICD) vs. control	ICD vs. conventional drug therapy (beta blockers), ACD inhibitor
Sample size	n = 196 Conventional = 101 ICD = 95	n = 704 EP-guided Rx = 351 Control = 353	n = 1232 ICD = 742 Conventional drug therapy = 490
Patient inclusion	S/P MI, EF ≤ 35% NSVT, inducible sustained VT not suppressible by procainamide	CAD, EF ≤ 40%, NSVT, inducible sustained VT	S/P MI, LVEF ≤ 30%
Total mortality	Conventional = 39% ICD = 16% (27 months)	Control = 48% EP-guided Rx = 42% AAD = 55% ICD = 24% (60 months)	Conventional = 19.6% ICD = 14.2% (23 months)

Note: AAD, antiarrhythmic drug; CAD, coronary artery disease; EF, ejection fraction; EP, electrophysiology; ICD, implantable cardioverter/defibrillator; MADIT, Multicenter Automatic Defibrillator Trial; MUSTT, Multicenter Unsustained Tachycardia Trial; NSVT, nonsustained ventricular tachycardia; Rx, therapy; S/P MI, status post–myocardial infarction; VT, ventricular tachycardia.
Source: From Buxton et al; Moss et al.

TABLE 214-10 *Guidelines for ICD Implantation*

CLASS 1[a]

1. Cardiac arrest due to VF or VT not due to a transient or reversible cause.
2. Spontaneous sustained VT in association with structural heart disease.
3. Syncope of undetermined origin with clinically relevant, hemodynamically significantly sustained VT or VF induced at EP study when drug therapy is ineffective, not tolerated, or not preferred.
4. Nonsustained VT in patients with coronary disease, prior myocardial infarction, LV dysfunction, and inducible VT or sustained VT at electrophysiological study that is not suppressible by a class I antiarrhythmic drug.
5. Spontaneous sustained VT in patients who do not have structured heart disease that is not amenable to other treatments.

CLASS 2[a]

1. Patients with LV ejection fraction ≤30%, at least 1 month post-MI and 3 months post-coronary artery revascularization.*

CLASS 2[b]

1. Cardiac arrest presumed to be due to VF when EP testing is precluded by other medical conditions.
2. Severe symptoms (e.g., syncope) attributable to ventricular tachyarrhythmia in patients awaiting cardiac transplantation.
3. Familial or inherited conditions with a high risk for life-threatening ventricular tachyarrhythmias such as long QT syndrome or hypertrophic cardiomyopathy.
4. Nonsustained VT with coronary artery disease, prior MI, and LV dysfunction, and inducible sustained VT or VF at EP study.
5. Recurrent syncope of undetermined etiology in the presence of ventricular dysfunction and inducible ventricular arrhythmias at EP study, when other causes of syncope have been excluded.
6. Syncope of unexplained etiology or family history of unexplained death in association with typical or atypical right bundle branch block and ST-segment elevations (Brugada syndrome).

CLASS 3[c]

1. Syncope of undetermined cause in a patient without inducible ventricular tachyarrhythmias and without structural heart disease.
2. Incessant VT or VF.
3. VF or VT resulting from arrhythmias amenable to surgical or catheter ablation; e.g., atrial arrhythmias associated with the Wolff-Parkinson-White syndrome, right ventricular outflow tract VT, idiopathic LV tachycardia, or fascicular VT.
4. Ventricular tachyarrhythmias due to a transient or reversible disorder when correction of the disorder is considered feasible and likely to substantially reduce the risk of recurrent arrhythmia.

[a] Evidence and/or agreement that procedure is indicated.
[b] Divergence in evidence opinion that procedure is indicated.
[c] Evidence/agreement that procedure is not indicated or is harmful.
Note: EP, electrophysiology; ICD, implantable cardioverter/defibrillator; LV, left ventricular; MI, myocardial infarction; VF, ventricular fibrillation, VT, ventricular tachycardia.

Sources: Adapted from American College of Cardiology/American Heart Association: J Am Coll Cardiol 31:1175, 1998, and incorporating new recommendations from G Gregoratas: Circulation 106:2145, 2002, with permission.
*The benefit of an ICD is greatest in this subgroup when the QRS duration is greater than 0.12 seconds.

FURTHER READING

ACC/AHA/ESC: Guidelines for the management of patients with atrial fibrillation. Executive Summary. J Am Coll Cardiol 38:1231, 2001

BUXTON AE et al: A randomized study of the prevention of sudden death in patients with coronary artery disease. N Engl J Med 341:1882, 1999

CLANCY CE, RUDY Y: Na$^{(+)}$ channel mutation that causes both Brugada and long QT syndrome phenotypes: A simulation study of mechanism. Circulation 105:1208, 2002

JOSEPHSON ME: *Clinical Cardiac Electrophysiology: Techniques and Interpretations*, 3d ed. Philadelphia, Lippincott Williams & Wilkins, 2002

KEATING MJ, SANGUINETTI MC: Molecular and cellular mechanisms of cardiac arrhythmia. Cell 104:569, 2001

MOSS AJ et al. Prophylactic implantation of a defibrillator in patients with myocardial infarction and reduced ejection fraction. N Engl J Med 346:877, 2002

OZCAN C et al: Long-term survival after ablation of the atrioventricular node and implantation of a permanent pacemaker in patients with atrial fibrillation. N Engl J Med 377:1043, 2001

TANG W et al: A comparision of biphasic and monophasic waveform defibrillation after prolonged ventricular fibrillation. Chest 120:948, 2001

THE ATRIAL FIBRILLATION FOLLOW-UP INVESTIGATION OF RHYTHM MANAGEMENT (AFFIRM) Investigators: A comparison of rate control and rhythm control in patients with atrial fibrillation. N Engl J Med 347:1825, 2002

ZIPES DP: Specific arrhythmias: Diagnosis and treatment, in *Braunwald's Heart Disease: A Textbook of Cardiovascular Medicine*, 7th ed, DP Zipes et al (eds). Philadelphia, Saunders, 2005

Section 3   Disorders of the Heart

215 NORMAL AND ABNORMAL MYOCARDIAL FUNCTION
Eugene Braunwald

CELLULAR BASIS OF CARDIAC CONTRACTION

THE CARDIAC ULTRASTRUCTURE

About three-fourths of the ventricular *myocardium* is composed of individual striated muscle cells (myocytes), normally 60 to 140 μm in length and 17 to 25 μm in diameter (Fig. 215-1*A*). Each fiber contains multiple, rodlike cross-banded strands (myofibrils) that run the length of the fiber and are, in turn, composed of serially repeating structures, the sarcomeres. The cytoplasm between the myofibrils contains other cell constituents (Fig. 215-1*B*), such as the single centrally-located nucleus, numerous mitochondria, and the intracellular membrane system, the sarcoplasmic reticulum.

The *sarcomere*, the structural and functional unit of contraction, is delimited by two adjacent dark lines, the Z lines (Fig. 215-1*C*). The distance between Z lines varies with the degree of contraction or stretch of the muscle and ranges between 1.6 and 2.2 μm. Within the confines of the sarcomere are alternating light and dark bands, giving the myocardial fibers their striated appearance under the light microscope. At the center of the sarcomere is a dark band of constant length (1.5 μm), the A band, which is flanked by two lighter bands, the I bands, which are of variable length. The sarcomere of heart muscle, like that of skeletal muscle, is made up of two sets of interdigitating myofilaments (Fig. 215-1D). Thicker filaments, composed principally of the protein myosin, traverse the A band. They are about 10 nm (100 Å) in diameter, with tapered ends, and measure 1.5 to 1.6 μm in length. Thinner filaments, composed primarily of actin, course from the Z line through the I band into the A band. They are approximately 5 nm (50 Å) in diameter and 1.0 μm in length. Thus there is overlapping of thick and thin filaments only within the A band, while the I band contains only thin filaments (Fig. 215-1C). On electron-microscopic (EM) examination, bridges may be seen to extend between the thick and thin filaments within the A band.

THE CONTRACTILE PROCESS

The sliding model for muscle contraction rests on the fundamental observation that the thick and thin filaments are constant in overall length during both contraction and relaxation. With activation, the actin filaments are propelled further into the A band. In the process, the A band remains constant in length, whereas the I band shortens and the Z lines move toward one another.

The *myosin* molecule is a complex, asymmetric fibrous protein with a molecular weight of about 500,000; it has a rodlike portion that is about 150 nm (1500 Å) in length with a globular portion at its end (Fig. 215-1D). This globular portion of the myosin forms the bridges between the myosin and actin and is the site of ATPase activity. In forming the thick myofilament, which is composed of ~300 longitudinally stacked myosin molecules, the rodlike segments of the myosin molecules are laid down in an orderly, polarized manner, leaving the globular portions projecting outward so that they can interact with actin to generate force and shortening (Fig. 215-2).

Actin has a molecular weight of about 47,000. The thin filament is composed of a double helix of two chains of actin molecules wound about each other on a larger molecule, tropomyosin, which serves as a "backbone" to the thin filament. A group of these regulatory proteins, troponins C, I, and T, are spaced at regular intervals on this filament (Fig. 215-3). In contrast to myosin, actin has no intrinsic enzymatic activity, but it has the ability to combine reversibly with myosin in the presence of ATP and Ca^{2+}. The latter activates the myosin ATPase, which in turn breaks down ATP, the energy source for contraction. In relaxed muscle this interaction is inhibited by tropomyosin. *Titin* (Fig. 215-1D) is a large, flexible, myofibrillar protein that connects myosin to the Z line. Its stretching is believed to contribute to the elasticity of the heart.

During activation of the myocyte, Ca^{2+} becomes attached to troponin C, which results in a conformational change in the regulatory protein tropomyosin; the latter in turn exposes the actin cross-bridge interaction sites. Repetitive interaction between myosin heads and actin filaments is termed *cross-bridge cycling*, which results in sliding of the actin along the myosin filaments, ultimately causing muscle shortening and/or the development of tension. The splitting of ATP, which is synthesized in the mitochondria, then dissociates the myosin cross-bridge from the actin. In the presence of ATP (Fig. 215-2), linkages between actin and myosin filaments are made and broken cyclically as long as sufficient Ca^{2+} is present; these linkages cease when [Ca^{2+}] falls below a critical level, and the troponin-tropomyosin complex once more prevents interactions between the myosin cross-bridges and the actin filaments. Intracytoplasmic Ca^{2+} is a principal mediator of the inotropic state of the heart. The fundamental action of most positive inotropic drugs, including the digitalis glycosides, β-

FIGURE 215-1 *A.* Microscopic evidence of heart muscle. *B.* Cardiac contraction and relaxation result from changing concentrations of Ca^{2+} ions in the myocardial cytosol. Ca^{2+} ions are shown schematically as entering via the calcium channel, which opens in response to the wave of depolarization that travels along the sarcolemma. These Ca^{2+} ions "trigger" the release of more calcium from the sarcoplasmic reticulum (SR) and thereby initiate a contraction-relaxation cycle. Eventually, the small amount of calcium that has entered the cell leaves, predominantly by a Na$^+$-Ca^{2+} exchanger with a lesser role for the sarcolemmal calcium pump. *C.* The varying actin-myosin overlap is shown for systole and diastole. *D.* The myosin heads, attached to the thick filaments, interact with the thin actin filaments. (*Copyright 2001 LH Opie. Reprinted with permission.*)

adrenergic agonists, and phosphodiesterase inhibitors, is to raise the [Ca^{2+}] in the vicinity of the myofilaments.

The *sarcoplasmic reticulum* (SR) (Fig. 215-1B) is a complex network of anastomosing intracellular channels that invests the myofibrils. Its longitudinally disposed membrane-lined tubules are closely applied to the surfaces of individual sarcomeres but have no direct continuity with the outside of the cell. However, closely related to the SR, both structurally and functionally, are the transverse tubules, or T system, formed by tubelike invaginations of the sarcolemma that extend into the myocardial fiber along the Z lines, i.e., the ends of the sarcomeres.

CARDIAC ACTIVATION

In the inactive state, the cardiac cell is polarized, i.e., the interior has a negative charge relative to the outside of the cell, with a transmembrane potential of -80 to -100 mV (Chap. 213). The sarcolemma, which in the resting state is largely impermeable to Na$^+$, has a Na$^+$-

FIGURE 215-2 Four steps in cardiac muscle contraction and relaxation. In relaxed muscle (*upper left*), ATP bound to the myosin cross-bridge dissociates the thick and thin filaments. *Step 1:* Hydrolysis of myosin-bound ATP by the ATPase site on the myosin head transfers the chemical energy of the nucleotide to the activated cross-bridge (*upper right*). When cytosolic Ca²⁺ concentration is low, as in relaxed muscle, the reaction cannot proceed because tropomyosin and the troponin complex on the thin filament do not allow the active sites on actin to interact with the cross-bridges. Therefore, even though the cross-bridges are energized, they cannot interact with actin. *Step 2:* When Ca²⁺ binding to troponin C has exposed active sites on the thin filament, actin interacts with the myosin cross-bridges to form an active complex (lower right) in which the energy derived from ATP is retained in the actin-bound cross-bridge, whose orientation has not yet shifted. *Step 3:* The muscle contracts when ADP dissociates from the cross-bridge; this step leads to the formation of the low-energy rigor complex (lower left), in which the chemical energy derived from ATP hydrolysis has been expended to perform mechanical work (the "rowing" motion of the cross-bridge). *Step 4:* The muscle returns to its resting state, and the cycle ends when a new molecule of ATP binds to the rigor complex and dissociates the cross-bridge from the thin filament. This cycle continues until calcium is dissociated from troponin C in the thin filament, which causes the contractile proteins to return to the resting state with the cross-bridge in the energized state. [*From AM Katz, in WS Colucci (ed): Heart Failure: Cardiac Function and Dysfunction, in Atlas of Heart Diseases, 3d ed, E Braunwald (series ed). Philadelphia, Current Medicine, 2002. Reprinted with permission.*]

and K⁺-stimulating pump energized by ATP that extrudes Na⁺ from the cell; this pump plays a critical role in establishing the resting potential. Thus, on the inside of the cell [K⁺] is relatively high and [Na⁺] is far lower, while in the extracellular milieu [Na⁺] is high and [K⁺] is low. At the same time, in the resting state, the extracellular [Ca²⁺] greatly exceeds the free intracellular [Ca²⁺]. →*The four phases of the action potential are discussed and illustrated in Chapter 213.*

During the plateau of the action potential (phase 2) there is a slow inward current through L-type Ca²⁺ channels in the sarcolemma (Fig. 215-4). The absolute quantity of Ca²⁺ that crosses the surface membrane is relatively small and itself appears to be insufficient to bring about full activation of the contractile apparatus. The depolarizing current not only extends across the surface of the cell but penetrates deeply into the cell by way of the ramifying T system; this Ca²⁺ current triggers the release of much larger quantities of Ca²⁺ from the SR, a process termed *Ca²⁺-induced Ca²⁺ release.*

The Ca²⁺ released from the SR then diffuses toward the myofibrils, where, as already described, it combines with troponin C. By repressing this inhibitor of contraction, Ca²⁺ activates the myofilaments to shorten. During repolarization the activity of the Ca²⁺ pump in the SR reaccumulates Ca²⁺ against a concentration gradient, and the Ca²⁺ is stored by its attachment to a protein *calsequestrin.* This is an energy-requiring process that lowers the [Ca²⁺] in the vicinity of the myofibrils to a level that inhibits the actin-myosin interaction responsible for contraction and in this manner leads to relaxation. Also, there is an exchange of Ca²⁺ for Na⁺ at the sarcolemma, reducing the cytoplasmic [Ca²⁺]. Thus, the combination of the cell membrane, transverse tubules, and SR, with their ability to transmit the action potential, to release, and then to reaccumulate Ca²⁺, appears to play a fundamental role in the rhythmic contraction and relaxation of heart muscle.

The ATP formed from substrate oxidation is the principal source of energy for almost all of the mechanical work of contraction performed by the myocardial cell. The high-energy phosphate stores in ATP are in equilibrium with those in creatine phosphate. The activity of myosin ATPase determines the rate of forming and breaking of the actin-myosin cross-bridges and ultimately the velocity of muscle contraction.

THE ROLE OF MUSCLE LENGTH

In cardiac muscle, indeed in all striated muscle, the force of contraction depends on initial muscle length. The sarcomere length associated with the most forceful contraction is approximately 2.2 μm. At this length the two sets of myofilaments of the sarcomere are configured so as to provide the greatest area for their interaction (Fig. 215-1). The length of the sarcomere also regulates the extent of activation of the contractile system, i.e., its sensitivity to Ca²⁺. According to this concept, termed *length-dependent activation*, at the optimal sarcomere length of 2.2 μm, the myofilament sensitivity to Ca²⁺ is also maximal.

The relation between the initial length of the muscle fibers and the developed force is of prime importance for the function of heart muscle. This forms the basis of the Frank-Starling relation (Starling's law of the heart), which states that, within limits, the force of ventricular contraction is a function of the end-diastolic length of the cardiac muscle; in the intact heart the latter is closely related to the ventricular end-diastolic volume.

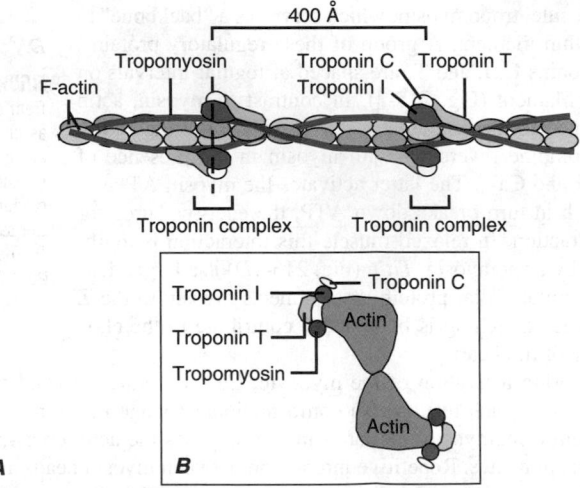

FIGURE 215-3 Structure of the thin filament. *A.* The "backbone" of the thin filament, seen in a longitudinal view, is F-actin, which contains two strands of actin monomers (blue and white). Troponin complexes, made up of one molecule each of troponin C, troponin I, and troponin T, are distributed at approximately 40 nm (400 Å) intervals along the thin filament. Elongated tropomyosin molecules (solid line in the grooves between the two actin strands). *B.* A cross-section of the thin filament at the level where the troponin complexes are located shows probable relationships between actin, tropomyosin, and the three components of the troponin complex. The strength of the bond linking troponin I and actin varies, depending on whether Ca²⁺ is bound to troponin C. [*Adapted from AM Katz, Molecular and cellular basis of contraction, in WS Colucci (ed): Heart Failure: Cardiac Function and Dysfunction, in Atlas of Heart Diseases, 3d ed, E Braunwald (series ed). Philadelphia, Current Medicine, 2002. Reprinted with permission.*]

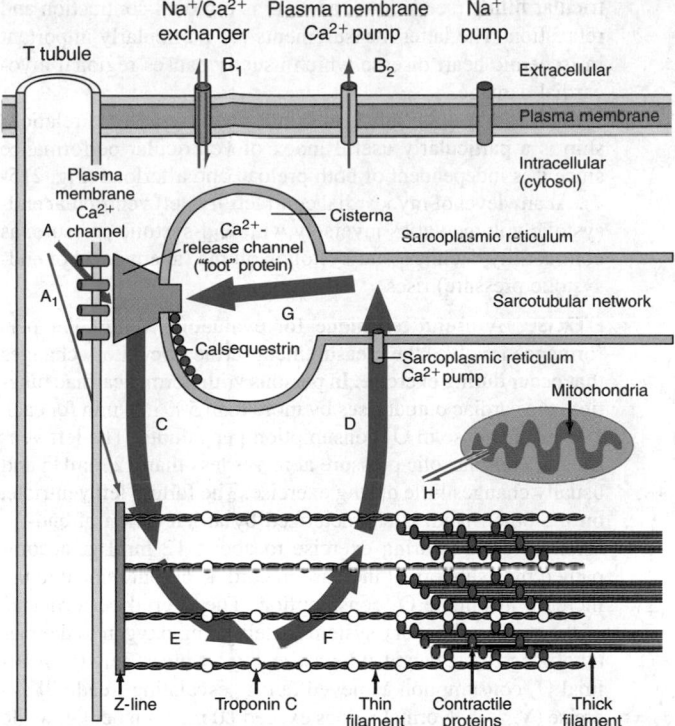

FIGURE 215-4 The Ca²⁺ fluxes and key structures involved in cardiac excitation-contraction coupling. The *arrows* denote the direction of Ca²⁺ fluxes. The thickness of each arrow indicates the magnitude of the calcium flux. Two Ca²⁺ cycles regulate excitation-contraction coupling and relaxation. The larger cycle is entirely intracellular and involves Ca²⁺ fluxes into and out of the sarcoplasmic reticulum, and Ca²⁺ binding to and release from troponin C. The smaller extracellular Ca²⁺ cycle occurs when this cation moves into and out of the cell. The action potential opens plasma membrane Ca²⁺ channels to allow passive entry of Ca²⁺ into the cell from the extracellular fluid (*arrow A*). Only a small portion of the Ca²⁺ that enters the cell directly activates the contractile proteins (*arrow A₁*). The extracellular cycle is completed when Ca²⁺ is actively transported back out to the extracellular fluid by way of two plasma membrane fluxes mediated by the sodium-calcium exchanger (*arrow B₁*) and the plasma membrane calcium pump (*arrow B₂*). In the intracellular Ca²⁺ cycle, passive Ca²⁺ release occurs through channels in the cisternae (*arrow C*) and initiates contraction, and active Ca²⁺ uptake by the Ca²⁺ pump of the sarcotubular network (*arrow D*) relaxes the heart. Diffusion of Ca²⁺ within the sarcoplasmic reticulum (*arrow G*) returns this activator cation to the cisternae, where it is stored in a complex with calsequestrin and other calcium-binding proteins. Ca²⁺ released from the sarcoplasmic reticulum initiates systole when it binds to troponin C (*arrow E*). Lowering of cytosolic [Ca²⁺] by the SR cause this ion to dissociate from troponin (*arrow F*) and relaxes the heart. Ca²⁺ may also move between mitochondria and cytoplasm (H). (*Adapted from Katz, with permission.*)

MYOCARDIAL MECHANICS AND CARDIAC FUNCTION

THE FORCE-VELOCITY CURVE

The mechanical activity of cardiac muscle may be expressed externally in two ways: shortening and tension development. In both skeletal and cardiac muscle the velocity of shortening is inversely related to the development of tension, an expression of the so-called force-velocity relation. Expressed simply, the greater the load the muscle is called upon to lift, the lower its velocity (and extent) of shortening, and vice versa. However, the contractile activity of cardiac muscle is readily altered under physiologic conditions by changes in resting fiber length and by changes in the contractility, both of which shift the myocardial force-velocity curve.

VENTRICULAR EJECTION

Analysis of the heart as a pump has classically centered on the relation between the end-diastolic volume of the ventricle (which is related to the length of the muscle fibers) and its stroke volume (the Frank-Starling relation). The end-diastolic or "filling" pressure of the ventricle is sometimes used as a surrogate for the end-diastolic volume. In the heart-lung preparation the stroke volume varies directly with the

diastolic fiber length (preload) and inversely with the arterial resistance (afterload), and as the heart fails it delivers a progressively smaller stroke volume from a normal or even elevated end-diastolic volume. The relation between the ventricular end-diastolic pressure and the stroke work of the ventricle (the ventricular function curve) provides a useful definition of the level of *contractility* of the intact heart. An increase in ventricular contractility is accompanied by a shift of the ventricular function curve upward and to the left [greater stroke work at any level of ventricular end-diastolic pressure (or volume), or lower end-diastolic pressure at any level of stroke work], while depression of contractility is characterized by a shift downward and to the right (Fig. 215-5).

Increased impulse traffic in the cardiac adrenergic nerves stimulates ventricular function as a consequence of the release of norepinephrine from adrenergic nerve endings in the heart. Norepinephrine activates myocardial β receptors and through the Gs-stimulated guanine nucleotide binding protein activates the enzyme adenylate cyclase, which leads to the formation of the intracellular second messenger cyclic AMP from ATP (Fig. 215-6). Cyclic AMP, in turn, activates protein kinase, which causes a more rapid, forceful contraction by phosphorylating the Ca²⁺ channel in the myocardial sarcolemma, thereby enhancing the influx of Ca²⁺ into the myocyte. Ca²⁺ acts on the contractile apparatus, as described on p. 1359. Cyclic AMP also phosphorylates the SR protein phospholamban, which increases the uptake of Ca²⁺ by the SR, increasing the rate of relaxation and providing larger quantities of Ca²⁺ in the SR to be released by subsequent depolarization and thereby further stimulating contraction. Adrenergic activation is evidenced by tachycardia, increased rates of ejection and filling, and a reduction in cardiac dimensions.

ASSESSMENT OF CARDIAC FUNCTION

Several techniques are available for defining impaired cardiac function. The cardiac output and stroke volume may be depressed in the presence of heart failure (HF), but not uncommonly these variables are within normal limits. A more sensitive index is the ejection fraction, i.e., the ratio of stroke volume to end-diastolic volume (normal

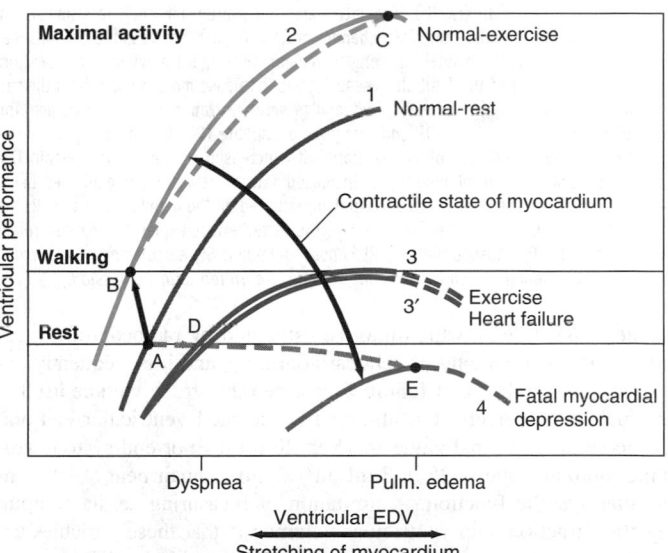

FIGURE 215-5 Diagram showing the interrelations among influences on ventricular end-diastolic volume (EDV) through stretching of the myocardium and the contractile state of the myocardium. Levels of ventricular EDV associated with filling pressures that result in dyspnea and pulmonary edema are shown on the abscissa. Levels of ventricular performance required when the subject is at rest, while walking, and during maximal activity are designated on the ordinate. The broken lines are the descending limbs of the ventricular-performance curves, which are rarely seen during life but which show the level of ventricular performance if end-diastolic volume could be elevated to very high levels. For further explanation see text. (*Modified from E Braunwald et al: Mechanisms of Contraction of the Normal and Failing Heart. Boston, Little, Brown, 1976.*)

FIGURE 215-6 Signal systems involved in positive intropic and lusitropic (enhanced relaxation) effects of β-adrenergic stimulation. When the β-adrenergic agonist interacts with the β receptor, a series of G protein-mediated changes leads to activation of adenylate cyclase and formation of cyclic AMP (cAMP). The latter acts via protein kinase A to stimulate metabolism (left) and to phosphorylate the Ca²⁺ channel protein (right). The result is an enhanced opening probability of the Ca²⁺ channel, thereby increasing the inward movement of Ca²⁺ ions through the sarcolemma (SL) of the T tubule. These Ca²⁺ ions release more calcium from the sarcoplasmic reticulum (SR) to increase cytosolic Ca²⁺ and to activate troponin C. Ca²⁺ ions also increase the rate of breakdown of ATP to ADP and inorganic phosphate (Pᵢ). Enhanced myosin ATPase activity explains the increased rate of contraction, with increased activation of troponin C explaining increased peak force development. An increased rate of relaxation is explained because cyclic AMP also activates the protein phospholamban, situated on the membrane of the SR, that controls the rate of uptake of calcium into the SR. The latter effect explains enhanced relaxation (lusitropic effect). P, phosphorylation; PL, phospholamban; SL, sarcolemma; SR, sarcoplasmic reticulum; TnI, troponin I. *(Copyright 2001, L Opie. Reprinted with permission.)*

value = 67 ± 8%), which may be estimated by radiocontrast or radionuclide angiography or echocardiography, and it is frequently depressed in systolic heart failure even when the stroke volume itself is normal. Alternatively, the abnormally elevated ventricular end-diastolic volume (normal value = 75 ± 20 mL/m²) or end-systolic volume (normal value = 25 ± 7 mL/m²) signify impairment of left ventricular systolic function. A limitation of measuring cardiac output, ejection fraction, and ventricular volumes is that these variables are influenced strongly by ventricular loading conditions. Thus, a depressed ejection fraction and lowered cardiac output may be observed in patients with normal ventricular function but reduced preload, as occurs in hypovolemia, or with increased afterload, as occurs in acutely elevated arterial pressure.

Noninvasive techniques, particularly echocardiography and radionuclide angiography (Chap. 211), are of great value in the clinical assessment of myocardial function. They provide measurements of end-diastolic and end-systolic volumes, global ejection fraction, and systolic shortening rate and they allow assessment of ven-

tricular filling (see below), as well as regional contraction and relaxation. The latter measurements are particularly important in ischemic heart disease which usually causes regional myocardial damage.

The end-systolic left ventricular pressure-volume relationship is a particularly useful index of ventricular performance since it is independent of both preload and afterload (Fig. 215-7). At any level of myocardial contractility, left ventricular end-systolic volume varies inversely with end-systolic pressure; as contractility declines, end-systolic volume (at any level of end-systolic pressure) rises.

EXERCISE A useful technique for evaluating ventricular performance involves the measurement of the circulatory changes that occur during exercise. In persons with normal cardiac function, the cardiac output rises by more than 500 mL/min for each 100 mL increase in O₂ consumption per minute. The left ventricular end-diastolic pressure at rest is less than 12 mmHg and usually changes little during exercise. The failing left ventricle, on the other hand, is characterized by an elevation of end-diastolic pressure during exercise to above 12 mmHg, accompanied by a subnormal increase in cardiac output related to the increase in minute O₂ consumption. The overall performance of the cardiopulmonary system in delivering oxygen to the metabolizing tissue can also be estimated by measuring the maximal O₂ consumption achieved during escalating treadmill exercise ($\dot{V}_{maxO_2}$). Normal values exceed 20 mL/min per kg, while values under 10 mL/min per kg represent severe impairment of function, usually seen in patients with severe heart failure and a poor prognosis.

The potential value of stressing the left ventricle to assess its performance is emphasized by the fact that the normal ranges of left ventricular end-diastolic pressure, cardiac index, and ventricular stroke work in the resting state are wide, with values that frequently overlap those seen in patients with ventricular dysfunction.

DIASTOLIC FUNCTION (Fig. 215-8)

This important variable is best assessed by continuously measuring the flow velocity across the mitral valve using Doppler echocardiography. Normally, the velocity of inflow is more rapid in early diastole than during atrial systole; with impaired relaxation the rate of early diastolic filling declines, while the rate of presystolic filling rises. With severe impairment of filling the pattern is "pseudo-normalized" and early ventricular filling becomes more rapid as left atrial pressure upstream to the stiff left ventricle rises (Fig. 211-4).

CONTROL OF CARDIAC PERFORMANCE AND OUTPUT

The extent of shortening of heart muscle and, therefore, the stroke volume of the intact ventricle are determined by three major influences: (1) the length of the muscle at the onset of contraction, i.e., the preload; (2) the contractility of the muscle, i.e., the position of its force-velocity-length relation; and (3) the tension that the muscle is called upon to develop during contraction, i.e., the afterload. Ventricular filling is influenced by the extent and speed of myocardial relaxation, which in turn is determined by the rate of uptake of Ca²⁺ by the SR; the latter may be enhanced by adrenergic activation and reduced by ischemia. Filling may also be impeded by the stiffness of the ventricular wall, which may be increased by ventricular hypertrophy and conditions that infiltrate the ventricle, such as amyloid, or by an extrinsic constraint (e.g., pericardial compression) (Fig. 215-8).

VENTRICULAR END-DIASTOLIC VOLUME (PRELOAD)

At any level of contractility, the performance of the myocardium is influenced profoundly by ventricular end-diastolic fiber length and therefore by diastolic ventricular volume, i.e., by operation of the

FIGURE 215-7 The responses of the left ventricle to increased afterload, increased preload, and increased and reduced contractility are shown in the pressure-volume plane. ESPVR, end-systolic pressure-volume relation; E_{ES}, the slope of the end-systolic pressure-volume relation. *Left.* Effects of increases in preload and afterload on the pressure-volume loop. Since there has been no change in contractility, ESPVR is unchanged. With an increase in afterload, stroke volume falls (1 → 2); with an increase in preload, stroke volume rises (1 → 3). *Right.* With increased myocardial contractility, the normal ESPVR moves to the left of the normal line (lower end-systolic volume at any end-systolic pressure) and stroke volume rises (1 → 3). With reduced myocardial contractility, the ESPVR moves to the right; end-systolic volume is increased and stroke volume falls (1 → 2).

Frank-Starling mechanism (Fig. 215-5). The following are the major determinants of ventricular preload in the intact organism:

TOTAL BLOOD VOLUME When blood volume is depleted, as in hemorrhage or dehydration (Chap. 253), venous return to the heart declines and ventricular end-diastolic volume (preload) falls, as does ventricular performance, as reflected in stroke volume, cardiac output, and ventricular work.

DISTRIBUTION OF BLOOD VOLUME The ventricular end-diastolic volume is influenced by the distribution of blood volume between the intra- and extrathoracic compartments. This distribution in turn is influenced by the following:

1. *Body position.* Gravitational forces pool blood in dependent portions of the body; upright posture augments extrathoracic at the expense of intrathoracic blood volume and reduces ventricular work.

2. *Intrathoracic pressure.* Normally, mean intrathoracic pressure is negative, which increases thoracic blood volume and enhances the return of blood to the heart, particularly when this pressure becomes more negative during inspiration. Elevation of intrathoracic pressure, as occurs during the Valsalva maneuver, prolonged bouts of coughing, or positive-pressure ventilation, has the opposite effect.

3. *Intrapericardial pressure.* When this pressure is elevated, as in pericardial tamponade (Chap. 222), there is interference with cardiac

filling, and the resultant reduction in ventricular diastolic volume reduces stroke volume and ventricular work.

4. *Venous tone.* The venous system is not a simple system of passive conduits between the systemic capillary bed and the right atrium. Instead, the smooth muscle in the walls of the venules and veins responds to a variety of neural and humoral stimuli. Venoconstriction occurs during muscular exercise, deep respiration, fright, or hypovolemic shock, enhancing venous return to the heart and thereby effecting ventricular performance.

5. *The pumping action of skeletal muscle.* During muscular exercise the contracting skeletal muscles squeeze blood out of the venous bed and, with the aid of the venous valves, displace it centrally, thereby increasing intrathoracic blood volume, ventricular end-diastolic volume, and ventricular work.

ATRIAL CONTRACTION Vigorous, appropriately-timed atrial contraction augments ventricular filling and end-diastolic volume. The atrial contribution to ventricular filling, the so-called "atrial kick," is of particular importance in patients with concentric ventricular hypertrophy. In such patients, the loss of atrial systole (as occurs with the development of atrial fibrillation) reduces ventricular end-diastolic pressure and volume, ultimately lowering myocardial performance.

MYOCARDIAL CONTRACTILITY

A number of factors determine the level of ventricular performance at any given ventricular end-diastolic volume, i.e., the position of the ventricular function curve (Fig. 215-5) as well as the position of the left ventricular end-systolic pressure-volume relation (Fig. 215-7). These influences may be considered to operate by modifying myocardial force-velocity relations. In the final analysis, most of these influences act by altering the $[Ca^{2+}]$ in the vicinity of the myofilaments, which in turn trigger cross-bridge cycling (p. 1359).

ADRENERGIC NERVE ACTIVITY The quantity of norepinephrine released by adrenergic nerve endings in the heart is determined by the adrenergic nerve impulse traffic; norepinephrine acts on the β-adrenergic receptors in the myocardium. This mechanism is the most important one that acutely modifies myocardial contractility under physiologic conditions.

CIRCULATING CATECHOLAMINES When it is stimulated by adrenergic nerve impulses, the adrenal medulla releases catecholamines, which augment both heart rate and myocardial contractility when they reach the heart.

FORCE-FREQUENCY RELATION Myocardial contractility is also influenced by the rate and rhythm of cardiac contraction. The contractility of the normal (but to a lesser extent the failing) heart is augmented by an increase in frequency of contraction, and ventricular extrasystoles result in post-extrasystolic potentiation, presumably by increasing the quantity of Ca^{2+} that enters the cardiac cell.

EXOGENOUSLY ADMINISTERED INOTROPIC AGENTS Isoproterenol, dopamine, dobutamine, and other sympathomimetic agents, cardiac glycosides, Ca^{2+}, and the phosphodiesterase inhibitors amrinone and milrinone all

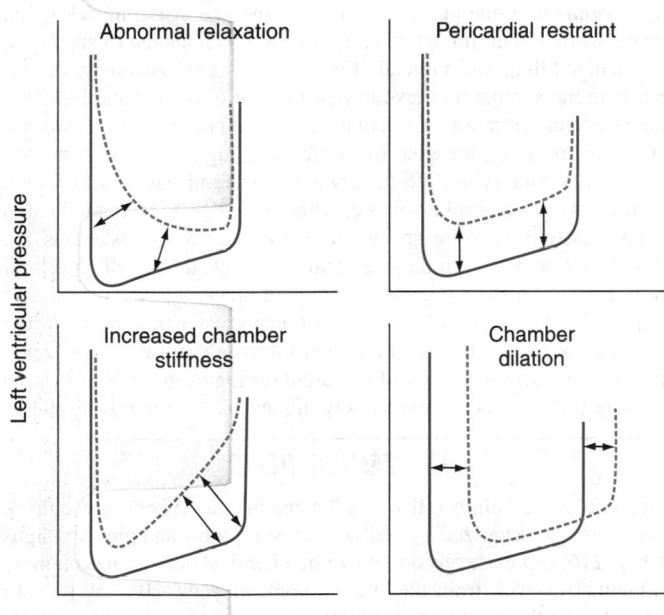

FIGURE 215-8 Mechanisms that cause diastolic dysfunction reflected in the pressure-volume relation. The bottom half of the pressure-volume loop is depicted. Solid lines represent normal subjects; dashed lines represent patients with diastolic dysfunction. *(From MR Zile: Diastolic dysfunction: detection, consequences, and treatment: II. Diagnosis and treatment of diastolic function. Mod Concepts Cardiovasc Dis 59:1, 1990. Reprinted with permission.)*

improve the contractility and therefore may be used to stimulate ventricular performance.

PHYSIOLOGIC DEPRESSANTS   Included among these are severe myocardial hypoxia, ischemia, and acidosis. Acting either singly or in combination, these conditions depress myocardial contractility and left ventricular work at any given ventricular end-diastolic volume.

PHARMACOLOGIC DEPRESSANTS   These include many antiarrhythmic drugs such as procainamide and disopyramide; calcium antagonists such as verapamil; β-adrenergic blockers; and large doses of barbiturates, alcohol, and general anesthetics as well as many other drugs.

MYOCARDIAL DEPRESSION   Although the fundamental mechanisms responsible for depression of myocardial contractility in most cases of chronic congestive heart failure secondary to prolonged ventricular overload or cardiomyopathy remain to be elucidated it is now apparent that in this condition the inotropic state of individual myocytes is depressed, and as a consequence the ventricular performance at any ventricular preload and afterload is lowered.

VENTRICULAR AFTERLOAD

The stroke volume is ultimately a function of the extent of ventricular fiber shortening. In the intact heart, as in isolated cardiac muscle, the extent (and velocity) of shortening of ventricular muscle fibers at any level of preload and of myocardial contractility are inversely related to the afterload, i.e., the load that opposes shortening. In the intact heart the afterload may be defined as the tension or stress developed in the ventricular wall during ejection. It is determined by the aortic pressure as well as by the volume and thickness of the ventricular cavity. Laplace's law indicates that the tension of the myocardial fiber is a function of the product of the intracavitary ventricular pressure and ventricular radius divided by the wall thickness. Therefore, at any given level of aortic pressure, the afterload on a dilated left ventricle of normal thickness is higher than that on a normal-sized ventricle. Conversely, at the same aortic pressure and ventricular diastolic volume, the afterload of a hypertrophied ventricle is lower than of a normal chamber. The aortic pressure, in turn, is determined by the peripheral vascular resistance, the physical characteristics of the arterial tree, and the volume of blood it contains at the onset of ejection.

The critical role played by the ventricular afterload in cardiovascular regulation is shown in Fig. 215-9. As already noted, elevations of both preload and contractility increase myocardial fiber shortening, while increases in afterload reduce it. The extent of myocardial fiber shortening and left ventricular size are the determinants of stroke volume. Arterial pressure, in turn, is related to the product of cardiac output and systemic vascular resistance, while afterload is a function of left ventricular volume, wall thickness, and arterial pressure. An increase in arterial pressure induced by vasoconstriction, for example, augments afterload, which opposes myocardial fiber shortening, reducing stroke volume. This in turn tends to limit the increase in pressure.

When myocardial contractility becomes impaired and the ventricle dilates, afterload rises and limits cardiac output. Increased afterload may result from neural and humoral stimuli that occur in response to a fall in cardiac output. This increased afterload may reduce cardiac output further while increasing myocardial O_2 requirements, and can initiate a vicious circle in patients with ischemic heart disease and limited myocardial O_2 supply. Treatment with vasodilators has the opposite effect; by reducing afterload, cardiac output rises (Chap. 216).

Under normal circumstances, the various influences acting on cardiac performance enumerated above interact in a complex fashion to maintain cardiac output at a level appropriate to the requirements of the metabolizing tissues; interference with a single mechanism may not influence the cardiac output. For example, a moderate reduction of blood volume or the loss of the atrial contribution to ventricular contraction can ordinarily be sustained without a reduction in the car-

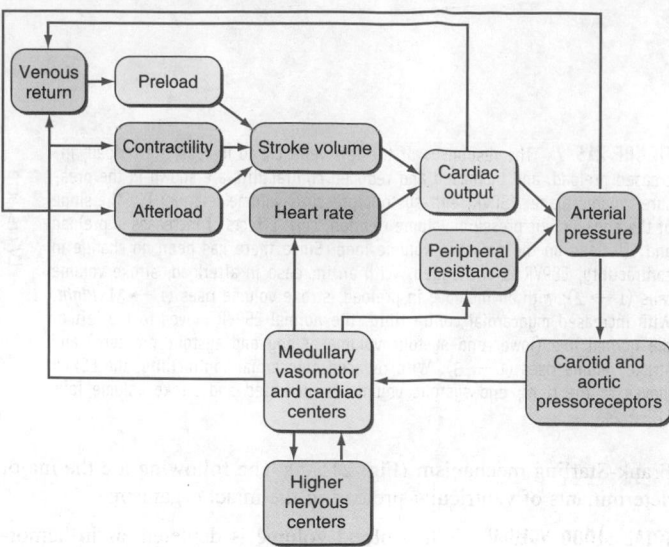

FIGURE 215-9   Interactions in the intact circulation of preload, contractility and afterload in producing stroke volume. Stroke volume combined with heart rate determines cardiac output, which, in turn, when combined with peripheral vascular resistance, determines arterial pressure for tissue perfusion. The characteristics of the arterial system also contribute to afterload, an increase of which reduces stroke volume. The interaction of these components with carotid and aortic arch baroreceptors provides a feedback mechanism to higher medullary and vasomotor cardiac centers and to higher levels in the central nervous system to affect a modulating influence on heart rate, peripheral vascular resistance, venous return, and contractility. *[From MR Starling: Physiology of myocardial contraction, in WS Colucci and E Braunwald (eds). Atlas of Heart Failure: Cardiac Function and Dysfunction, 3d ed, Philadelphia: Current Medicine, 2002, pp 19–35. Adapted from FR Badke and RA O'Rourke: Cardiovascular physiology, in JH Stein (ed): Internal Medicine, ed 1. Boston: Little, Brown and Co. 1983:407–423.]*

diac output at rest. Under these circumstances, other factors, such as increases in the frequency of adrenergic nerve impulses to the heart, in heart rate, and in venous tone will, in a normal individual, serve as compensatory mechanisms and sustain cardiac output.

EXERCISE

Hyperventilation, the pumping action of the exercising muscles, and venoconstriction during exercise all augment venous return and hence ventricular filling and preload (Fig. 215-5). Simultaneously, the increase in the adrenergic nerve impulse traffic to the myocardium, the increased concentration of circulating catecholamines, and the tachycardia that occur during exercise combine to augment the contractility of the myocardium (Fig. 215-5, curves 1 and 2) and lead to an elevation of stroke work and stroke volume, without change or even a reduction of end-diastolic pressure and volume (Fig. 215-5, points A and B). Vasodilatation occurs in the exercising muscles, thus tending to limit the increase in arterial pressure that would otherwise occur as cardiac output rises to levels as high as five times greater than basal during maximal exercise. This vasodilatation ultimately allows the achievement of a greatly elevated cardiac output during exercise, at an arterial pressure (afterload) only moderately higher than in the resting state.

THE FAILING HEART

Although heart failure (HF) may be readily described as a clinical syndrome, characterized by well-known symptoms and physical signs (Chap. 216), a precise physiologic or biochemical definition is far more difficult. However, from the clinical point of view, HF may be considered to be the condition in which *an abnormality of cardiac structure or function is responsible for the inability of the heart to fill with or eject blood at a rate commensurate with the requirements of the metabolizing tissues.*

Abnormalities during systole and/or diastole may be present in HF. In so-called *systolic heart failure* (p. 1369), an impairment of myocardial contractility causes weakened systolic contraction, which leads,

FIGURE 215-10   Mechanisms responsible for diastolic dysfunction in hypertrophic and ischemic heart disease. These factors, alone or in combination, contribute to the increased left ventricular chamber stiffness and impaired myocardial relaxation. As a result, left ventricular diastolic pressures are increased and filling is impaired. *[From WH Gaasch, EC Schick: Heart failure with normal left ventricular ejection fraction: A manifestation of diastolic dysfunction, in MH Crawford et al (eds). Cardiology. London, Mosby, 2001, pp 6.1–6.8. Reprinted with permission.]*

ultimately, to a reduction in stroke volume and cardiac output, inadequate ventricular emptying, cardiac dilatation, and often elevation of ventricular diastolic pressure. Idiopathic dilated cardiomyopathy (Chap. 221) and cardiogenic shock secondary to acute myocardial infarction (Chap. 255) are the prototypes of chronic and acute systolic HF, respectively.

In *diastolic heart failure* (p. 1369), the principal abnormality is impaired relaxation and filling of the ventricle, which leads to an elevation of ventricular diastolic pressure at any given diastolic volume (Fig. 215-8). Failure of relaxation can be functional and transient, as during ischemia, which reduces the ATP required for the SR pump to lower cytoplasmic $[Ca^{2+}]$. Chronically impaired ventricular filling can be caused by a stiffened, thickened ventricle and a number of conditions illustrated in Fig. 215-10. Typical conditions in which diastolic HF occurs are restrictive cardiomyopathy secondary to infiltrative conditions, such as amyloidosis or hemochromatosis, and hypertrophic cardiomyopathy (Chap. 221). The concentric hypertrophy associated with chronic hypertension can also impair ventricular filling. In many patients with cardiac hypertrophy and dilatation, systolic and diastolic HF coexist; the left ventricle both empties and fills abnormally.

MECHANISMS OF HEART FAILURE

ADAPTIVE AND MALADAPTIVE MECHANISMS
A number of mechanisms aid the heart faced with an increased hemodynamic burden (such as pressure or volume overload) or one that has sustained loss of myocardium or contractility. On a short-term basis many of these responses are adaptive (beneficial). However, on a long-term basis these responses are often maladaptive (deleterious) (Table 215-1).

1. The *Frank-Starling mechanism* operates through an increase in preload (p. 1361). As outlined above, an increase in the end-diastolic volume of the ventricle is associated with stretching of the sarcomeres, which increases the interaction between actin and myosin filaments and their sensitivity to Ca^{2+},

thereby enhancing contraction. However, ventricular dilatation may become maladaptive when it becomes excessive, as may occur in severe valvular regurgitation, dilatation increases wall stress through the operation of Laplace's law and thereby reduces shortening.

2. *Compensatory hypertrophy* occurs in hemodynamic overload, which in turn restores elevated ventricular wall stress to normal (Fig. 216-1). If the hypertrophy is insufficient to restore wall stress to normal, the ventricle dilates and this increases wall stress further, leading to a vicious circle. Also, severe ventricular hypertrophy may impair ventricular filling and cause myocardial ischemia.

3. In *ventricular remodeling* there are changes in the size, mass, and configuration of the ventricle as a consequence of hemodynamic changes following mechanical overload, hypertension, cardiomyopathy, and myocardial infarction. Remodeling is triggered by myocyte growth, interstitial fibrosis and apoptosis (Table 215-2), ischemia, vasoactive peptides, and fibrosis. A change to a more spherical shape, which decreases the effectiveness of ejection, is common in the remodeled ventricle.

4. *Redistribution of a subnormal cardiac output* away from the skin, skeletal muscle, and kidneys with maintenance of blood flow to the most vital organs, i.e., the brain and the heart, occurs. The vasoconstriction, however, may increase afterload, thereby reducing cardiac output further.

REDUCTION IN CARDIAC EFFICIENCY   The common forms of low-output systolic HF, secondary to coronary atherosclerosis, hypertension, cardiomyopathy, and certain valvular and congenital lesions, are characterized by a reduction in the external work performed by the heart, while myocardial oxygen consumption remains normal or nearly so. Therefore, the external efficiency, i.e., the ratio of external work performed to energy consumed, is often depressed.

ALTERATIONS IN ENERGY METABOLISM   When HF occurs in the presence of acute or chronic ischemia, it can be attributed to reduced supply of oxygen with a resultant reduction of ATP generation. Severe ventricular hypertrophy and/or dilatation from any etiology can contribute to ischemia, especially in the subendocardium, and this can impair both ventricular contraction and filling. In some forms of HF without ischemia, myocardial energy stores in the form of creatine phosphate are decreased, as is the activity of the enzyme creatine kinase required for the shuttling of high-energy phosphate between creatine phosphate and ADP, suggesting that reductions in myocardial energy reserves may play a role in nonischemic conditions as well.

ALTERATIONS IN SARCOMERIC PROTEINS   Hemodynamic overload, neurohormonal and/or cytokine stimulation and gene mutations in familial cardiomyopathies may all reinduce the expression of fetal sarcomeric

TABLE 215-1   *Short-Term and Long-Term Responses to Impaired Cardiac Performance*

Response	Short-term Effects (mainly adaptive; hemorrhage, acute heart failure)	Long-term Effects (mainly deleterious; chronic heart failure)
Salt and water retention	Augments preload	Pulmonary congestion, anasarca
Vasoconstriction	Maintains pressure for perfusion of vital organs (brain, heart)	Exacerbates pump dysfunction, increases cardiac energy expenditure
Sympathetic stimulation	Increases heart rate and ejection	Increases energy expenditure
Cytokine activation	Vasodilatation	Skeletal muscle catabolism, deterioration of endothelial function, impaired contraction, LV remodeling.
Hypertrophy	Unloads individual muscle fibers	Deterioration and death of cardiac cells: cardiomyopathy of overload
Increased collagen	May reduce dilatation	Impairs relaxation

LV, left ventricle.
Source: From H Drexler, G Hasenfuss: Physiology of the normal and failing heart, in MH Crawford and JP DeMarco et al (eds): *Cardiology*. London, Mosby, 2001, pp 1.1–1.16, Modified from AM Katz: Cardiomyopathy of overload. A major determinant of prognosis in congestive heart failure. N Engl J Med 322:100, 1990

TABLE 215-2 *Factors that Lead to the Progressive Remodeling of the Left Ventricle*

Mechanism of Progressive Remodeling and Heart Failure			
Cell Growth	Fibrosis	Apoptosis	Counter-regulatory Factors
Angiotensin II	Angiotensin II	TNF-α	ANP
Catecholamines	Endothelin	*Fas* ligand	Bradykinin
Endothelin	Aldosterone		Nitric oxide
TNF-α	TGF-β		BNP
Growth hormone			
IGF			
Cardiotrophin-1			
Mechanical stretch			

Growth of cardiac myocytes is a primary feature and is due to a number of growth factors, including neurohormones and cytokines as well as mechanical stretch. Fibrosis is promoted by activation of the renin-angiotensin-aldosterone axis and through activation of endothelin and TGF-β. Apoptosis regulation is altered via changes in the expression of *p53*, *Bcl-2*, and *Bax* genes, perhaps as a consequence of increases in TNF-α acting to stimulate the *Fas* ligand. Programmed cell death is enhanced, producing cell drop-out. Counter-regulatory forces, including atrial natriuretic peptide (ANP) and brain natriuretic peptide (BNP) are activated. Nitric oxide, driven by bradykinin and ANP, may have antigrowth properties and hold uncontrolled growth in check to some extent; however, on balance, cardiac myocytes elongate, which contributes to left ventricular remodeling. IGF, insulin-like growth factor.
Source: G. Francis: Changing the remodeling process in heart failure: basic mechanisms and laboratory results. Curr Opin Cardiol 13:156, 1998

proteins whose contractility is depressed. It has been postulated that these alterations in sarcomeric proteins cause systolic HF. A reduction of myosin ATPase activity, which may be caused by an alteration in the expression of troponin T and/or of myosin light chain kinase 2, may also lower the rate of interaction between myosin and actin myofilaments and impair muscle shortening.

MYOCARDIAL CELL DEATH When a sufficiently large portion of ventricular myocardium becomes nonfunctional or necrotic, as occurs transiently during ischemia (Chap. 226) and permanently in myocardial infarction (Chap. 228), total ventricular performance at any given level of end-diastolic volume becomes depressed. Apoptosis of myocytes, like the reinduction of fetal sarcomeric proteins, can be caused by hemodynamic overload, excessive neurohormone and/or cytokine stimulation, as well as by severe ischemia. As a consequence of cell death, whatever the mechanism, the load on surviving myocytes is increased, setting the stage for a vicious circle of repeated cell death.

ABNORMALITIES OF EXCITATION-CONTRACTION COUPLING Substantial evidence supports the view that in many forms of heart failure the delivery of Ca^{2+} to the contractile sites is disturbed, thereby impairing cardiac performance. However, the molecular basis of this abnormality—indeed of the subcellular structures involved, i.e., the sarcolemma, T tubules, and/or SR—has yet to be defined. There is, however, evidence for a reduction in the activity of the Ca^{2+} release (ryanodine) channel in the SR and of messenger RNAs of the proteins regulating Ca^{2+} movements. The latter include the sarcolemmal Na^{+}-Ca^{2+} channels, and the activity of the SR Ca^{2+} uptake pump (SERCa-2a), which play critical roles in the movement of Ca^{2+} between the SR and the cytoplasm. Impaired expression of the genes encoding these proteins can impair both myocardial contraction and relaxation and thereby contribute to the development of HF.

NEUROHUMORAL AND CYTOKINE ADJUSTMENTS

A reduction in cardiac performance evokes a series of neurohumoral adjustments, which may at different times be adaptive or maladaptive (Table 215-1). These adjustments are adaptive when they maintain arterial perfusion pressure in the face of a sudden reduction of cardiac output. However, they are maladaptive when they increase the hemodynamic burden and oxygen requirements of the failing ventricle and when they exacerbate myocardial injury (Fig. 215-11).

THE ADRENERGIC NERVOUS SYSTEM In patients with HF the levels of circulating norepinephrine may be markedly elevated, reflecting the increased activity of the adrenergic nervous system. This increased activity supports ventricular contractility in acute HF that is intensified when large doses of β-adrenergic blocking agents are administered acutely, providing evidence for the protective action of adrenergic nervous activation. However, the chronic adrenergic stimulation that occurs in HF may increase afterload by raising vascular resistance, cause cardiac arrhythmias, and may damage myocytes further, perhaps by increasing myocardial energy expenditures and Ca^{2+} overload. Gradually increasing doses of β blockers are of benefit in patients with chronic HF (Chap. 216).

The density of β_1 adrenergic receptors, their coupling to G proteins, and the concentration of cardiac norepinephrine stores are all reduced in chronic, severe HF. These changes are accompanied by a reduction in the activity of adenylate cyclase, which may lower the intracellular concentration of cyclic AMP (Fig. 215-6). The reduction in turn depresses the activation of protein kinase, the phosphorylation of Ca^{2+} channels and transarcolemmal Ca^{2+} entry. It also reduces the phosphorylation of phospholamban, a protein in the SR, which in its unphosphorylated state inhibits the reuptake of Ca^{2+} by the SR. Changes in the G proteins, which couple the β receptor to adenylate cyclase (which is responsible for the production of cyclic AMP), may also occur in HF, with increased activity of the inhibitory subunit of the proteins.

THE RENIN-ANGIOTENSIN-ALDOSTERONE SYSTEM When cardiac output declines, the renin-angiotensin-aldosterone system (Chap. 321) is activated. Concentrations of both circulating angiotensin II and aldosterone are increased, the former contributing to excess vasoconstriction and the latter to the retention of salt and water and perhaps to cardiac fibrosis (Table 215-1). The local (tissue) renin-angiotensin system is also activated in HF and angiotensin II exerts a local cardiotoxic effect by stimulating G$_q$ proteins that activate phospholipase C, which in turn activates protein kinase C. The latter stimulates cardiac hypertrophy and causes ventricular remodeling. Patients with HF are usually improved by blocking this system with angiotensin-converting enzyme (ACE) inhibitors, angiotensin II receptor blockers, and aldosterone antagonists (Chap. 216).

ENDOTHELIN AND TUMOR NECROSIS FACTOR α The concentration of circulating endothelin, a polypeptide that is a very powerful vasoconstrictor, is increased in HF and it contributes to the excessive afterload. The overexpression of a number of cytokines also appears to play a

FIGURE 215-11 Interplay between cardiac function and neurohumoral and cytokine systems. Myocardial injury, of many etiologies, can depress cardiac function, which in turn causes activation of the sympathoadrenal system (SAS) and the renin-angiotensin-aldosterone system (RAAS) and the elaboration of endothelin, arginine vasopressin (AVP), and cytokines such as tumor necrosis factor (TNF) α. In acute heart failure (*left*), these are adaptive and tend to maintain arterial pressure and cardiac function. In chronic heart failure (*right*) they cause maladaptive hypertrophic remodeling and apoptosis, which cause further myocardial injury and impairment of cardiac function. The horizontal line on the right (*) shows that chronic maladaptive influences can be inhibited by angiotensin converting enzyme inhibitors, β-adrenergic blockers, angiotensin type I receptor blockers, and aldosterone antagonists.

prominent role in the pathogenesis of HF. It has now been well established that patients with HF exhibit elevated levels of TNF-α, both in the circulation and in cardiac muscle; the pathophysiologic significance of this finding is just unfolding. Transgenic mice with overexpressed cardiac TNF-α exhibit systolic dysfunction, myocarditis, ventricular dilatation, HF, and shortened survival. The infusion of TNF-α impairs ventricular function. However, thus far, blockade of endothelin and TNF-α have not been shown to improve the outcome of patients with HF.

VASODILATOR PEPTIDES A number of vasodilator peptides are released by the dilated heart. Best known are the natriuretic peptides atrial natriuretic peptide (ANP) and brain natriuretic peptide (BNP). When stretch receptors in the atria (site of ANP and BNP stores) and ventricles (site of BNP stores) are stimulated, these hormones (or their prohormones) are released and act on specific natriuretic peptide receptors, which increase the concentrations of cyclic GMP in the kidney, adrenal glomerulosa, vascular smooth muscle, and platelets. Urine volume and sodium excretion are augmented, vascular resistance is reduced, and the release of renin and the secretion of aldosterone are reduced. These effects, while beneficial, are not sufficiently powerful to neutralize the sodium-retaining and vasoconstrictor influences of the aforementioned neurohumoral systems activated in HF. Elevated circulating concentrations of ANP and particularly BNP correlate with a poor prognosis in HF. The direct administration of recombinant BNP in acute pulmonary edema is promising.

Figure 215-11 illustrates current concepts of neurohumoral-cytokine activation in HF. The activation of the adrenergic nervous system and the renin-angiotensin-aldosterone system and the enhanced elaboration of endothelin and arginine vasopressin appear to be adaptive in *acute*, severe HF. However, they all appear to exert a maladaptive response in chronic HF. Inflammatory cytokines and oxidative stress are emerging as potent noxious stimuli as well. Together they result in a vicious circle, causing myocyte hypertrophy, remodeling, and cell death, the latter often due to myocardial apoptosis (see below), all resulting in further impairment of cardiac function and myocardial injury. Agents that interfere with the adverse effects of these stimuli on cardiac function, especially β-adrenergic blockers, ACE inhibitors, angiotensin receptor blockers, aldosterone receptor blockers, and perhaps arginine vasopressin blockers appear to be capable of blocking this vicious circle.

ABNORMALITIES OF THE INTERNAL AND EXTERNAL SKELETONS Both hemodynamic overload and mutations of genes encoding cytoskeletal proteins interfere with the regulation of myocyte architecture and thereby interfere with contraction and relaxation. Proliferation of the *extracellular matrix* occurs in myocardial infarction, longstanding hypertension, and a variety of cardiomyopathic disorders. Since this matrix forms the extracellular "skeleton" of the heart, its excessive proliferation can interfere with both systolic shortening and diastolic lengthening. Thus abnormalities of both the internal and external skeleton can contribute to the progression of HF.

HEART FAILURE—A DISTURBANCE OF THE MYOCARDIAL PUMP
(See also Chap. 216)

In the final analysis, in systolic HF the basic problem is depression of the myocardial force-velocity relationship and of the length–active tension curve, reflecting reductions in myocardial contractility (Fig. 215-5, curves 1 to 3, Fig. 215-7, right). In diastolic HF there is upward displacement of the diastolic pressure–volume relation (Fig. 215-8). In many instances, cardiac output and external ventricular performance at rest are within normal limits but are maintained at these levels only by an increased end-diastolic fiber length and an elevated ventricular end-diastolic volume, i.e., through the operation of the Frank-Starling mechanism (Fig. 215-5, points A to D). The elevation of left ventricular preload is associated with increases in the pulmonary capillary pressure, contributing to the dyspnea experienced by patients with HF, while elevation of right ventricular preload raises systemic venous pressure and contributes to the development of edema. The improvement of contractility that normally accompanies augmented adrenergic activity during exercise is attenuated or even prevented by norepinephrine depletion and downregulation of myocardial β receptors, which occur in severe HF (Fig. 215-5, curves 3 and 3').

The factors that augment ventricular filling during exercise in the normal individual push the failing myocardium along its flattened length–active tension curve. Although the function of left ventricle may be improved at this higher diastolic volume, through the operation of the Frank-Starling mechanism, this improvement occurs only as a consequence of an inordinate elevation of ventricular end-diastolic volume and pressure and, therefore, of the pulmonary capillary pressure. The latter intensifies dyspnea and limits the intensity of exercise that the patient can perform. Left ventricular failure becomes fatal when the myocardial length–active tension curve is depressed (Fig. 215-5, curve 4) to the point at which cardiac performance fails to satisfy the requirements of the peripheral tissues even at rest, and/or the left ventricular end-diastolic and pulmonary capillary pressures are elevated to levels that result in pulmonary edema (Fig. 215-5, point E).

FURTHER READING

ALPERT NR et al: The failing human heart. Cardiovasc Res 54:1, 2002

ANVERSA P et al: Myocyte death in heart failure. Curr Opin Cardiol 11:245, 1996

BRAUNWALD E: Congestive heart failure: A half century perspective. The Denolin lecture. Eur Heart J 22:825, 2001

COLUCCI WS (ed): Heart failure: Cardiac function and dysfunction, in *Atlas of Heart Diseases*, 3d ed, E Braunwald (series ed). Philadelphia, Current Medicine, 2002

KATZ AM: *Heart Failure*, New York, Raven, 2000, pp 381

CARROLL J, HESS O: Assessment of cardiac function, in *Braunwald's Heart Disease*, 7th ed, D Zipes et al (eds). Philadelphia, Saunders, 2005

OPIE LH: Mechanisms of cardiac contraction and relaxation, in *Heart Disease*, 6th ed, E Braunwald et al (ed). Philadelphia, Saunders, 2001

SCHWARTZ K, MERCADIER J-J: Molecular and cellular biology of heart failure. Curr Opin Cardiol 11:227, 1996

216 HEART FAILURE AND COR PULMONALE
Eugene Braunwald

HEART FAILURE

Heart failure (HF) is a clinical syndrome in which an abnormality of cardiac structure or function is responsible for the inability of the heart to eject or fill with blood at a rate commensurate with the requirements of the metabolizing tissues. HF results in a constellation of clinical manifestations, including, in various combinations, circulatory congestion, dyspnea, fatigue, and weakness. The severity of the clinical manifestations are commonly described according to criteria developed by the New York Heart Association.

HF is a major public health problem in industrialized nations. It appears to be the only common cardiovascular condition that is increasing in prevalence and incidence in North America and Europe. In the United States, HF is responsible for almost 1 million hospital admissions and 50,000 deaths annually. Since HF is more common in the elderly, its prevalence is likely to continue to increase as the population ages.

HF is frequently, but not always, caused by a defect in myocardial contraction, and then the term *myocardial failure* is appropriate. The latter may result from a primary abnormality in heart muscle, as occurs in the cardiomyopathies, or in viral myocarditis (Chap. 221). HF also results commonly from coronary atherosclerosis, which interferes with cardiac contraction by causing myocardial infarction and ischemia. HF may also occur in congenital, valvular, and hypertensive heart disease in which the myocardium is damaged by the long-standing hemodynamic overload. In other patients with HF, however, a similar clinical syndrome is present but without any detectable abnormality of *myocardial* function. In some cases the normal heart is suddenly presented with a mechanical load that exceeds its capacity, such as an acute hypertensive crisis, rupture of an aortic valve leaflet, in endocarditis or with a massive pulmonary embolism. HF in the presence of normal systolic function also occurs in chronic conditions in which there is impaired filling of the ventricles due to a mechanical abnormality such as tricuspid and/or mitral stenosis without myocardial involvement, endocardial fibrosis, and some forms of hypertrophic cardiomyopathy (see Fig. 215-8).

CAUSES OF HEART FAILURE

UNDERLYING CAUSES Although HF may occur as a consequence of most forms of heart disease, in the United States and Western Europe, ischemic heart disease is responsible for about three-quarters of all cases. Cardiomyopathies are second in frequency, while congenital, valvular, and hypertensive heart disease are less common causes. It is important to identify potentially treatable underlying causes of HF, such as the latter three groups of disorders.

PRECIPITATING CAUSES In evaluating patients with HF, it is important to identify not only the *underlying* but also the *precipitating cause*. Frequently, clinical manifestations of HF are seen for the first time in the course of an acute disturbance that places an additional load on a myocardium that is chronically excessively burdened. Such a heart may be adequately compensated under normal circumstances but have little additional reserve, the additional load imposed by a precipitating cause results in further deterioration of cardiac function. The ten most common precipitating causes are described below.

1. *Infection*. Patients with pulmonary vascular congestion due to left ventricular failure are more susceptible to pulmonary infection than are normal persons; however, any infection may precipitate HF. The resulting fever, tachycardia, hypoxemia, and the increased metabolic demands may place a further burden on an overloaded, but compensated, myocardium of a patient with chronic heart disease.

2. *Arrhythmias*. These are among the most frequent precipitating causes of HF. They exert a deleterious effect on cardiac function through a variety of mechanisms: (a) Tachyarrhythmias reduce the time available for ventricular filling, contributing especially to diastolic HF; they may also cause ischemic myocardial dysfunction in patients with ischemic heart disease. (b) The dissociation between atrial and ventricular contractions characteristic of many brady- and tachyarrhythmias results in the loss of the atrial booster pump mechanism, i.e., the "atrial kick," thereby raising atrial pressures. (c) Cardiac performance may become further impaired because of the loss of normally synchronized ventricular contraction in any arrhythmia associated with abnormal intraventricular conduction (see resynchronization therapy below). (d) Slowing of the heart rate associated with complete atrioventricular block or other severe bradyarrhythmias reduces cardiac output unless stroke volume rises reciprocally; this compensatory response is limited in myocardial dysfunction, even in the absence of overt HF.

3. *Physical, Dietary, Fluid, Environmental, and Emotional Excesses*. The sudden augmentation of sodium intake as with a large holiday meal, the inappropriate discontinuation of drugs or other therapy for HF, blood transfusions, physical overexertion, excessive environmental heat or humidity, and emotional crises all may precipitate HF in patients who were previously compensated.

4. *Myocardial Infarction*. In patients with chronic but compen-

sated ischemic heart disease, a new infarct, sometimes otherwise silent clinically, may further impair ventricular function and precipitate HF (Chap. 228).

5. *Pulmonary Embolism*. Physically inactive patients with low cardiac output are at increased risk of developing thrombi in the veins of the lower extremities or the pelvis. Pulmonary emboli may result in further elevation of pulmonary arterial pressure, which in turn may produce or intensify ventricular failure. In the presence of pulmonary vascular congestion, such emboli also may cause pulmonary infarction (Chap. 244).

6. *Anemia*. In the presence of anemia, the oxygen needs of the metabolizing tissues can be met only by an increase in the cardiac output (Chap. 52). Such an increase may be sustained by a normal heart. However, a diseased, overloaded, but otherwise compensated heart may be unable to augment sufficiently the volume of blood that it delivers to the periphery. In this manner, the combination of anemia and previously compensated heart disease can precipitate HF and lead to inadequate delivery of oxygen to the periphery.

7. *Thyrotoxicosis and Pregnancy*. Similar to anemia and fever, thyrotoxicosis and pregnancy are also high cardiac output states. The development or intensification of HF in a patient with previously compensated heart disease may actually be one of the first clinical manifestations of hyperthyroidism (Chap. 320). Similarly, HF may occur for the first time during pregnancy in women with rheumatic valvular disease, in whom cardiac compensation may return following delivery (Chap. 6).

8. *Aggravation of Hypertension*. Rapid elevation of arterial pressure, as may occur in some instances of renal hypertension or upon abrupt discontinuation of antihypertensive medication in patients with essential hypertension, may result in cardiac decompensation.

9. *Rheumatic, Viral, and Other Forms of Myocarditis*. Acute rheumatic fever and a variety of other inflammatory or infectious processes affecting the myocardium may precipitate HF in patients with or without preexisting heart disease (Chaps. 221 and 302).

10. *Infective Endocarditis*. The additional valvular damage, anemia, fever, and myocarditis that often occur as a consequence of infective endocarditis may, singly or in combination, precipitate HF (Chap. 109).

A systematic search for these precipitating causes should be made in every patient with the new development or recent intensification of HF. If properly recognized, the precipitating cause of HF usually can be treated effectively. Therefore, the prognosis in patients with HF in whom a precipitating cause can be identified, treated, and eliminated is more favorable than in patients in whom the underlying disease process has progressed to the point of producing HF without a detectable precipitating cause.

HF resembles but should be distinguished from (1) conditions in which there is circulatory congestion secondary to abnormal salt and water retention but in which there is no disturbance of cardiac function *per se*, as occurs in renal failure; and (2) noncardiac causes of inadequate cardiac output, such as hypovolemic shock (Chap. 253).

The ventricles respond to chronic hemodynamic overload with the development of hypertrophy (Fig. 216-1). When the ventricle is called on to deliver an elevated cardiac output for prolonged periods, as in valvular regurgitation, it develops *eccentric hypertrophy*, i.e., cavity dilatation, with an increase in muscle mass so that the ratio between wall thickness and ventricular cavity diameter remains relatively constant early in the process. With chronic pressure overload, as in valvular aortic stenosis or untreated hypertension, *concentric ventricular hypertrophy* develops; in this condition the ratio between wall thickness and ventricular cavity size increases. In both eccentric and concentric hypertrophy, wall tension is initially maintained at a normal level and cardiac function may remain stable for many years. However, myocardial function may ultimately deteriorate, leading to HF. Often at this time, the ventricle dilates and the ratio between wall thickness and cavity size declines, leading to increased stress on each unit of myocardium, further dilatation, and a vicious cycle is initiated. Remodeling of the ventricle occurs with a change to a more spherical

FIGURE 216-1 Patterns of ventricular hypertrophy. Specific patterns of ventricular remodeling occur in response to the imposed augmentation in work load. A pattern of hypertrophic growth characterized as concentric, in which increased mass is out of proportion to chamber volume, is particularly effective in reducing systolic wall stress (σ) under conditions of heightened pressure load. In contrast, in volume overload conditions, in which the major stimulus is diastolic loading, a predominant finding is a great increase in the cavity size or volume. Although there can be extensive increases in mass, the relationship between mass and volume is either preserved or, in severe cases, reduced. The fundamental response is generated by cellular hypertrophy. However, the configuration of the new contractile tissue is specific and offsets the mechanical stimulus. [Modified from W Grossman et al in NR Alpert (ed): Perspectives in Cardiovascular Research. Myocardial Hypertrophy and Failure, vol 7. New York, Raven Press, 1993, with permission.]

shape, which increases the hemodynamic stresses on the wall and may cause or intensify mitral regurgitation. Activation of endogenous neurohormonal systems and cytokines (Chap. 215) appears to be involved in ventricular remodeling and thereby the progression of HF. Remodeling is particularly prominent in patients with transmural myocardial infarction, in whom the infarcted area stretches and the remaining viable portion of the ventricle dilates.

FORMS OF HEART FAILURE

HF may be described as *systolic* or *diastolic*, *high-output* or *low-output*, *acute* or *chronic*, *right-sided* or *left-sided*, and *forward* or *backward*. These descriptors are often useful in a clinical setting, particularly early in the patient's course, but the differences often become blurred late in the course of chronic HF.

SYSTOLIC VERSUS DIASTOLIC FAILURE The distinction between these two forms of HF relates to whether the principal abnormality is the inability of the ventricle to contract normally and expel sufficient blood (systolic failure) or to relax and fill normally (diastolic failure). The manifestations of systolic failure relate to an inadequate cardiac output with weakness, fatigue, reduced exercise tolerance, and other symptoms of hypoperfusion, while in diastolic HF the manifestations relate principally to the elevation of filling pressures in the left and/or right ventricles. Diastolic HF is usually defined as HF in patients with an ejection fraction >50%.

Diastolic HF (see Fig. 215-8) may be caused by increased resistance to ventricular inflow and reduced ventricular diastolic capacity (constrictive pericarditis and restrictive, hypertensive, and hypertrophic cardiomyopathy), impaired ventricular relaxation (acute myocardial ischemia), and myocardial fibrosis and infiltration (restrictive cardiomyopathy). Diastolic HF occurs more frequently in women than men, especially elderly women with hypertension. In most patients with HF, abnormalities both of contraction and relaxation coexist.

LOW-OUTPUT VERSUS HIGH-OUTPUT HEART FAILURE *Low-output HF* occurs secondary to ischemic heart disease, hypertension, dilated cardiomyopathy, and valvular and pericardial disease, while *high-output HF* occurs in patients with reduced systemic vascular resistance, i.e., hyperthyroidism, anemia, pregnancy, arteriovenous fistulas, beriberi, and Paget's disease. In clinical practice, however, low-output and high-output HF cannot always be readily distinguished. The normal range of cardiac output is wide (2.2 to 3.5 L/min per m²); in many patients with low-output HF, the cardiac output may actually be just above the lower limit of normal range at rest (although lower than it had been previously), but fails to rise normally during exertion. On the other hand, in patients with so-called high-output HF, the output may not exceed the upper limits of normal (although it would have been abnormally elevated had it been measured before HF supervened); instead, it may have fallen to within normal limits with HF.

The hemodynamic burden placed on the myocardium by many forms of high-output heart failure resembles that produced by chronic aortic regurgitation. In addition, thyrotoxicosis and beriberi may also impair myocardial metabolism directly, while very severe anemia may interfere with myocardial function by producing myocardial anoxia, especially in the subendocardium and in the presence of underlying obstructive coronary artery disease.

ACUTE VERSUS CHRONIC HEART FAILURE An example of causes of *acute HF* are the sudden rupture of a cardiac valve leaflet secondary to trauma or infective endocarditis or a massive myocardial infarction in a patient who previously had no cardiac dysfunction. In acute HF the sudden reduction in cardiac output often results in systemic hypotension without peripheral edema. *Chronic HF* is typically observed in patients with dilated cardiomyopathy or multivalvular heart disease and develops or progresses slowly. Vascular congestion is common in chronic HF, but arterial pressure is ordinarily well maintained until very late.

RIGHT-SIDED VERSUS LEFT-SIDED HEART FAILURE Many of the clinical manifestations of HF result from the accumulation of fluid upstream to (behind) the ventricles that is initially affected. For example, patients in whom the left ventricle is hemodynamically overloaded (e.g., aortic regurgitation) or weakened due to myocyte loss (e.g., postmyocardial infarction) develop dyspnea and orthopnea as a result of pulmonary congestion, a condition referred to as *left-sided HF*. When the underlying abnormality affects the right ventricle primarily (e.g., primary pulmonary hypertension secondary to chronic pulmonary thromboembolism), symptoms resulting from pulmonary congestion are uncommon, and edema, congestive hepatomegaly, and systemic venous distention, i.e., clinical manifestations of *right-sided HF*, are prominent. The muscle bundles composing both ventricles are continuous, and both ventricles share a common wall, the interventricular septum. The biochemical changes that occur in the myocardium in HF (Chap. 215) usually occur in the myocardium of *both* ventricles. Therefore, when HF has existed for months or years, localization of excess fluid behind one ventricle may no longer exist.

BACKWARD VERSUS FORWARD HEART FAILURE A controversy has revolved around the mechanism of the clinical manifestations resulting from HF. The concept of *backward HF* contends that in HF, one or the other ventricle fails to discharge its contents or fails to fill normally. As a consequence, the pressures in the atrium and venous system behind (upstream to) the failing ventricle rise, and retention of sodium and water occurs as a consequence of the elevation of systemic venous and capillary pressures and the resultant transudation of fluid into the pulmonary or systemic interstitial space. On the other hand, proponents of the *forward HF* hypothesis maintain that the clinical manifestations of HF result directly from an inadequate discharge of blood into the arterial system. According to this concept, salt and water retention is a consequence of diminished renal perfusion and excessive proximal and distal tubular reabsorption of sodium, the latter through activation of the renin-angiotensin-aldosterone system (RAAS) (Chap. 32).

The rate of onset of HF often influences the clinical manifestations. For example, when a large portion of the left ventricle is suddenly destroyed, as in myocardial infarction, the patient may succumb to acute pulmonary edema, a manifestation of *backward failure*. If the patient survives the acute insult, clinical manifestations resulting from a chronically depressed cardiac output, including the abnormal retention of fluid within the systemic vascular bed, may develop, which is a manifestation of *forward failure*.

SALT AND WATER RETENTION (See also Chap. 32) When the volume of blood pumped by the left ventricle into the systemic vascular bed is reduced, a complex sequence of adjustments occurs that ultimately results in the abnormal accumulation of fluid. This may be considered a two-edged sword. Many of the troubling clinical manifestations of HF, such as pulmonary congestion and edema, are secondary to this excessive retention of fluid (see Fig. 32-1). However, this abnormal fluid accumulation and the expansion of blood volume that accompanies it also constitute an important compensatory mechanism that tends to maintain cardiac output and therefore perfusion of the vital organs. Except in the terminal stages of HF, the ventricle operates on an ascending, albeit depressed and flattened, function curve (see Fig. 215-5), and the augmented ventricular end-diastolic volume characteristic of HF must be regarded as helping to maintain the reduced cardiac output, despite causing pulmonary and/or systemic venous congestion.

CLINICAL MANIFESTATIONS OF HEART FAILURE

RESPIRATORY DISTURBANCES ■ Dyspnea (Chap. 29) In early HF, dyspnea is observed only during exertion, when it may simply represent an aggravation of the breathlessness that occurs normally. As HF advances, dyspnea occurs with progressively less strenuous activity and ultimately it is present even at rest. The principal difference between exertional dyspnea in normal persons and in patients with HF is the degree of exertion necessary to induce this symptom. Cardiac dyspnea is observed most frequently in patients with elevations of pulmonary venous and capillary pressures who have engorged pulmonary vessels and interstitial accumulation of interstitial fluid. The activation of receptors in the lungs results in the rapid, shallow breathing characteristic of cardiac dyspnea. The oxygen cost of breathing is increased by the excessive work of the respiratory muscles required to move air into and out of the congested lungs. This is coupled with the diminished delivery of oxygen to these muscles, a consequence of a reduced cardiac output. This imbalance may contribute to fatigue of the respiratory muscles and the sensation of shortness of breath.

Orthopnea This symptom, i.e., dyspnea in the recumbent position, is usually a later manifestation of HF than exertional dyspnea. Orthopnea results from the redistribution of fluid from the abdomen and lower extremities into the chest during recumbency, which increases the pulmonary capillary pressure, combined with elevation of the diaphragm. Patients with orthopnea must elevate their head on several pillows at night and frequently awaken short of breath and/or coughing if their head slips off the pillows. Orthopnea is usually relieved by sitting upright, and some patients report that they find relief from sitting in front of an open window. In advanced HF, patients cannot lie down at all and must spend the entire night in a sitting position.

Paroxysmal (Nocturnal) Dyspnea This term refers to attacks of severe shortness of breath and coughing that generally occur at night, usually

awaken the patient from sleep, and may be quite frightening. Though simple orthopnea may be relieved by sitting upright at the side of the bed with legs dependent, in the patient with paroxysmal nocturnal dyspnea, coughing and wheezing often persist even in this position. Paroxysmal nocturnal dyspnea may be caused in part by the depression of the respiratory center during sleep, which may reduce ventilation sufficiently to lower arterial oxygen tension, particularly in patients with interstitial lung edema and reduced pulmonary compliance. *Cardiac asthma* is closely related to paroxysmal nocturnal dyspnea and nocturnal cough and is characterized by wheezing secondary to bronchospasm—most prominent at night. *Acute pulmonary edema* (Chaps. 29 and 255) is a severe form of cardiac asthma due to marked elevation of pulmonary capillary pressure leading to alveolar edema, associated with extreme shortness of breath, rales over the lung fields, and the expectoration of blood-tinged fluid. If not treated promptly, acute pulmonary edema may be fatal.

Cheyne-Stokes Respiration Also known as *periodic respiration* or *cyclic respiration*, Cheyne-Stokes respiration is characterized by diminished sensitivity of the respiratory center to arterial P_{CO_2}. There is an apneic phase, during which the arterial P_{O_2} falls and the arterial P_{CO_2} rises. These changes in the arterial blood stimulate the depressed respiratory center, resulting in hyperventilation and hypocapnia, followed in turn by recurrence of apnea. Cheyne-Stokes respiration occurs most often in patients with cerebral atherosclerosis and other cerebral lesions, but the prolongation of the circulation time from the lung to the brain that occurs in HF, particularly in patients with hypertension and coronary artery disease, also appears to contribute to this form of disordered breathing.

OTHER SYMPTOMS ■ Fatigue and Weakness These nonspecific but common symptoms of HF are related to the reduction of skeletal muscle perfusion. Exercise capacity is reduced by the limited ability of the failing heart to increase its output and deliver oxygen to the exercising muscles.

Abdominal Symptoms Anorexia and nausea associated with abdominal pain and fullness are frequent complaints and may be related to the congested liver and portal venous system.

Cerebral Symptoms Patients with severe HF, particularly elderly patients with cerebral arteriosclerosis, reduced cerebral perfusion, and arterial hypoxemia, may develop alterations in the mental state characterized by confusion, difficulty in concentration, impairment of memory, headache, insomnia, and anxiety. *Nocturia* is common in HF and may contribute to insomnia.

PHYSICAL FINDINGS (See Chap. 209) In mild or moderately severe HF, the patient appears in no distress at rest except feeling uncomfortable when lying flat for more than a few minutes. In severe HF, the pulse pressure may be diminished, reflecting a reduction in stroke volume, and the diastolic arterial pressure may be elevated as a consequence of generalized vasoconstriction. In severe acute HF, systolic hypotension may be present, with cool, diaphoretic extremities, and Cheyne-Stokes respiration. There may be cyanosis of the lips and nail beds (Chap. 31) and sinus tachycardia. *Systemic venous pressure* is often abnormally elevated, and this may be reflected in distention of the jugular veins. In the early stages of HF, the venous pressure may be normal at rest but may become abnormally elevated, with sustained pressure on the abdomen (positive abdominojugular reflux).

Third and fourth heart sounds are often audible but are not specific for HF, and *pulsus alternans*, i.e., a regular rhythm with alternation of strong and weak cardiac contractions and therefore alternation in the strength of the peripheral pulses, may be present. This sign of severe HF may be detected by sphygmomanometry and in more severe cases even by palpation; it frequently follows an extrasystole and is observed most commonly in patients with cardiomyopathy, hypertensive, or ischemic heart disease.

Pulmonary Rales Moist, inspiratory, crepitant rales and dullness to percussion over the lung bases are common in patients with HF and elevated pulmonary venous and capillary pressures. In patients with pulmonary edema, rales may be heard widely over both lung fields; they are frequently coarse and sibilant and may be accompanied by expiratory wheezing. Rales may, however, be caused by many conditions other than left ventricular failure. Some patients with longstanding HF and elevated pulmonary vascular pressures have no rales because of increased lymphatic drainage of alveolar fluid.

Cardiac Edema (See Chap. 32) This is usually symmetric and dependent in HF, occurring in the legs, particularly in the ankles and pretibial region in ambulatory patients, in whom it is most prominent in the evening. In patients who are bedridden, cardiac edema occurs in the sacral region.

Hydrothorax and Ascites Pleural effusion in HF (hydrothorax) results from the elevation of pleural capillary pressure and the resultant transudation of fluid into the pleural cavities. Since the pleural veins drain into *both* the systemic and pulmonary veins, hydrothorax occurs most commonly with marked elevation of pressure in both venous systems but may also be seen with marked elevation of pressure in either venous bed. It occurs more frequently in the right pleural cavity than in the left. *Ascites* also occurs as a consequence of transudation and results from increased pressure in the hepatic veins and the veins draining the peritoneum (Chap. 39). Among patients with HF, ascites occurs most frequently in those with constrictive pericarditis and those with tricuspid valve disease.

Congestive Hepatomegaly Like edema, an enlarged, tender, pulsating liver also accompanies systemic venous hypertension. With prolonged, severe hepatomegaly, as in patients with tricuspid valve disease or chronic constrictive pericarditis, enlargement of the spleen, i.e., congestive splenomegaly, may also occur.

Jaundice This is a late finding in HF and is associated with elevations of both direct and indirect bilirubin. It results from impairment of hepatic function secondary to hepatic congestion and the hepatocellular hypoxia associated with central lobular atrophy. Hepatic enzymes are frequently elevated. If hepatic congestion occurs acutely, the jaundice may be severe and the enzymes strikingly elevated.

Cardiac Cachexia With severe chronic HF there may be marked weight loss and cachexia because of: (1) elevation of the metabolic rate, which results in part from the extra work performed by the respiratory muscles, the increased O_2 needs of the hypertrophied heart, and/or the discomfort associated with severe HF; (2) anorexia, nausea, and vomiting due to congestive hepatomegaly and abdominal fullness and/or digitalis intoxication (see below); (3) impairment of intestinal absorption due to congestion of the intestinal veins; (4) elevation of circulating concentrations of cytokines such as tumor necrosis factor; and (5) rarely, due to protein-losing enteropathy in patients with particularly severe failure of the right side of the heart.

Other Manifestations With reduction of blood flow, the skin, especially in the extremities, may be cold, pale, and diaphoretic. Urine flow is depressed, contains albumin, has a high specific gravity, and a low concentration of sodium. In addition, prerenal azotemia may be present. In patients with long-standing severe HF, depression and sexual dysfunction are common.

DIFFERENTIAL DIAGNOSIS The diagnosis of congestive HF may be established by observing some combination of the clinical manifestations of HF described above, together with the findings characteristic of one of the underlying forms of heart disease. Table 216-1 shows the Framingham criteria, which are useful in the diagnosis of HF. Since chronic HF is often associated with cardiac enlargement, the diagnosis should be questioned, but is by no means excluded, when all chambers are normal in size. HF is sometimes difficult to distinguish from *pulmonary disease*, and the differential diagnosis is discussed in Chap. 29. *Pulmonary embolism* also presents many of the manifestations of HF, but hemoptysis, pleuritic chest pain, a right ventricular lift, and the characteristic mismatch between ventilation and perfusion on lung scan should point to this diagnosis (Chap. 244).

TABLE 216-1 *Framingham Criteria for Diagnosis of Congestive Heart Failure*[a]

MAJOR CRITERIA

Paroxysmal nocturnal dyspnea
Neck vein distention
Rales
Cardiomegaly
Acute pulmonary edema
S_3 gallop
Increased venous pressure (>16 cmH_2O)
Positive hepatojugular reflux

MINOR CRITERIA

Extremity edema
Night cough
Dyspnea on exertion
Hepatomegaly
Pleural effusion
Vital capacity reduced by one-third from normal
Tachycardia (≥ 120 bpm)

MAJOR OR MINOR

Weight loss ≥ 4.5 kg over 5 days' treatment

[a] To establish a clinical diagnosis of congestive heart failure by these criteria, at least one major and two minor criteria are required.
Source: KKL Ho et al, Circulation 88:107, 1993.

Ankle edema may be due to varicose veins, cyclic edema, or gravitational effects (Chap. 32), but in patients with these conditions, there is no jugular venous hypertension at rest or with pressure over the abdomen. Edema secondary to *renal disease* can usually be recognized by appropriate renal function tests and urinalysis and it is rarely associated with elevation of venous pressure. Enlargement of the liver and ascites occur in patients with *hepatic cirrhosis* and also may be distinguished from HF by normal jugular venous pressure and the absence of a positive abdominojugular reflux.

BRAIN NATRIURETIC PEPTIDE (BNP) Pre pro-BNP is formed in the ventricles and, with myocyte stretch, is broken down to N-terminal-pro-BNP (NT-pro-BNP) and BNP. These hormones are highly accurate for identifying or excluding HF with high sensitivity and specificity and add significant independent predictive power when added to the chemical features. BNP is particularly valuable in differentiating cardiac from pulmonary causes of dyspnea. The availability of a bedside assay makes BNP useful in evaluating patients in the Emergency Department.

APPROACH TO THE PATIENT

In addition to a detailed clinical examination, a two-dimensional echocardiogram with Doppler flow studies is of critical importance in determining the underlying causes of HF and in assessing the severity of ventricular systolic and/or diastolic dysfunction, as well as valvular dysfunction. Such ultrasound studies are part of the workup of all patients in whom the diagnosis of HF is considered. The electrocardiogram is rarely normal in systolic HF. The chest roentgenogram is helpful in detecting cardiomegaly and pulmonary congestion. BNP is extremely useful in diagnosis, prognosis, and monitoring therapy.

℞ TREATMENT

A simple rule for the treatment of all patients with HF cannot be formulated because of its varied etiologies, hemodynamic features, clinical manifestations, and severity. The treatment of HF may be divided into five components: (1) general measures; (2) correction of the underlying cause; (3) removal of the precipitating cause; (4) prevention of deterioration of cardiac function; and (5) control of the congestive HF state. An example of correction of the underlying course is the surgical repair or replacement of a deformed valve. An example of removal of a precipitating cause is the restoration of sinus rhythm in a patient with atrial fibrillation and a rapid ventricular rate. An approach that applies to many patients is shown in Table 216-2 and Fig. 216-2.

GENERAL MEASURES   Every effort should be made to prevent HF, not only by treating hypertension and other coronary risk factors (Chap. 225) but also by the administration of angiotensin-converting enzyme (ACE) inhibitors (or, in patients who are intolerant of them, angiotensin receptor blockers, ARBs), even in asymptomatic patients with a history of atherosclerotic vascular disease, diabetes mellitus, or hypertension.

General measures in patients with HF include moderate dietary Na⁺ restriction (see below), daily measurement of weight to aid in the adjustment of diuretic dosage, as well as immunization with influenza and pneumococcal vaccines to prevent respiratory infection. Education of the patient and family about the condition and the critical importance of close attention to compliance with the medical regimen and supervision of outpatient care by a specially trained nurse or physician assistant have all been found to be helpful. Excessive alcohol, temperature extremes, and tiring trips should be avoided.

Activity   In acute, severe HF, meals should be small in quantity, but more frequent, and every effort should be made to diminish anxiety; sometimes drugs such as diazepam (2 to 5 mg tid) for several days are useful. Physical and emotional rest tends to lower arterial pressure and reduce the load on the myocardium by diminishing the requirements for cardiac output. Reduced physical exertion should be continued for several days after the patient's condition has stabilized. The hazards of phlebothrombosis and pulmonary embolism which occur with bed rest may be reduced with anticoagulants, leg exercises, and elastic stockings. *Absolute* bed rest is rarely required or advisable, and even the patient with severe HF should ordinarily be encouraged to sit in a chair. In ambulatory patients with chronic, moderately severe HF, additional periods of rest on weekends frequently allow continuation of gainful employment. A scheduled nap or rest following lunch and the avoidance of particularly strenuous exertion are often helpful.

Once the patient has become compensated, regular isotonic exercise such as walking or riding a stationary-bicycle ergometer as tolerated should be strongly encouraged. Some trials of exercise training have led to encouraging results with reduced symptoms, increased exercise capacity, and improved quality of life. Weight reduction by restriction of caloric intake in obese patients with HF also diminishes cardiac work load and is an essential component of the therapeutic program.

CONTROL OF EXCESSIVE FLUID   Many of the clinical manifestations of HF result from expansion of the extracellular fluid volume. A negative Na⁺ balance can be achieved in such patients by reducing the dietary intake and increasing the urinary excretion of this ion with the aid of diuretics. Rarely, in severe HF, mechanical removal of extracellular fluid by means of thoracentesis and paracentesis may be necessary.

Diet   In patients with mild HF, symptomatic improvement may result simply from reducing the sodium intake. The normal diet contains approximately 6 to 10 g NaCl per day; this intake can be reduced in half simply by excluding salt-rich foods and salt added at the table. Further reduction of the ordinary dietary intake of NaCl to approximately one-fourth of normal may be achieved if, in addition, NaCl is omitted from cooking. In patients with severe HF who have fluid accumulation despite vigorous diuretic therapy (see below), the dietary intake of NaCl should be reduced to 1 g/d. In order to achieve this, milk, cheese, bread, cereals, canned vegetables and soups, some salted cuts of meat, and some fresh vegetables (including spinach, celery, and beets) must be eliminated. A variety of fresh fruit, green vegeta-

---

TABLE 216-2   *Stages in the Evolution of Heart Failure/Recommended Therapy by Stage*

Stage A ⟶		Stage B ⟶		Stage C ⟶		Stage D
At high risk for heart failure but without structural heart disease or symptoms of HF		Structural heart disease but without symptoms of HF		Structural heart disease with prior or current symptoms of HF		Refractory HF requiring specialized interventions
Patients with hypertension coronary artery disease diabetes mellitus *or* Patients using cardiotoxins with FHx CM	Structural heart disease	Patients with previous MI LV systolic dysfunction asymptomatic valvular disease	Symptoms of HF develop	Patients with known structural heart disease shortness of breath and fatigue, reduced exercise tolerance	Refractory symptoms of HF at rest	Patients who have marked symptoms at rest despite maximal medical therapy (e.g., those who are recurrently hospitalized or cannot be safely discharged from the hospital without specialized interventions)
THERAPY						
Treat hypertension Encourage smoking cessation Treat lipid disorders Encourage regular exercise Discourage alcohol intake, illicit drug use ACE inhibition		All measures under stage A ACE inhibitors in appropriate patients Beta-blockers		All measures under stage A Drugs for routine use: Diuretics ACE inhibitors Beta-blockers Digitalis Dietary Salt restriction		All measures under stages A, B, and C Mechanical assist devices Heart transplantation Continuous (not intermittent) IV inotropic infusions for palliation Hospice care

Abbreviations: HF, heart failure, FHxCM, family history of cardiomyopathy; ACE, angiotensin-converting enzyme; MI, myocardial infarction; LV, left ventricular; IV, intravenous.

Source: Modified from S Hunt: J Am Coll Cardiology, 38:2101, 2001, with permission.

Stepped Therapy for Heart Failure

Disease Severity

Asymptomatic   Symptomatic   Advanced   Refractory

Salt and Fluid Intake
Consider 2000 mL fluid restriction

◄---- No added salt   2 g Na⁺

Aerobic Activity

◄---- As tolerated   Exercise training   Rest

Medications

ACE inhibitor or angiotensin II receptor blocker if not tolerated

◄-----β-Blockers-----►

Digoxin for persistent symptoms -------------►

Diurotics to treat fluid retention ---------------►

Add spironolactone if normal potassium-handling --------►

Reevaluate diagnosis and therapy to relieve persistent congestion: More diuresis? Nitrates ± hydralazine?

◄------- Heart failure disease --------►? Hospice management programs

Transplantation/mechanical assist devices

FIGURE 216-2   The step diagram demonstrates addition of therapies in relation to the clinical severity of heart failure with reduced left ventricular ejection fraction. Angiotensin-converting enzyme (ACE) inhibitors are prescribed at every level of disease severity. Angiotensin receptor-blocking agents (ARBs) are a reasonable alternative for patients who cannot tolerate ACE inhibitors due to angioedema or severe cough. β-Adrenergic blocking agents are prescribed for patient with mild to moderate symptoms of heart failure, but they are not initiated in patients with severe symptoms of heart failure unresponsive to stabilization with other therapies. Diuretics are prescribed to maintain fluid balance, with spironolactone added in patients with severely symptomatic disease when renal function and potassium handling are preserved. When severe symptoms persist, patients may benefit from addition of nitrates with or without hydralazine. Transplantation and mechanical assist devices are relevant to only a very small population with advanced heart failure. Restriction of sodium and fluid intake is increasingly required as heart failure becomes more severe. Heart failure management programs are most cost-effective in patients at high risk for repeated heart failure hospitalization. *(From A Nohria et al, 2002, with permission.)*

bles, specially processed breads and milk, and NaCl substitutes are permissible. Late in the course of HF, dilutional hyponatremia may develop in patients who are unable to excrete an H_2O load, sometimes because of excessive secretion of antidiuretic hormone. In such cases, both H_2O and NaCl must be restricted.

Diuretics   (See also Chap. 230)   These agents should be given to achieve euvolemia and reduce or prevent edema and jugular venous distention. A variety of diuretics is available (Tables 216-3 and 230-8), and almost all are effective in patients with mild HF. However, in the more severe forms of HF, the selection of diuretics is more difficult, and abnormalities in serum electrolytes must be watched for. On the other hand, overtreatment with diuretics must be avoided, since the resultant hypovolemia may reduce cardiac output, interfere with renal function, and produce profound weakness and lethargy.

THIAZIDE DIURETICS   These agents are useful by themselves in patients with mild HF and in combination with other diuretics in patients with severe HF. In patients with chronic mild HF, the continued administration of a thiazide diuretic abolishes or diminishes the need for *rigid* dietary Na⁺ restriction, although salty foods and table salt still should be avoided. Thiazide diuretics reduce the reabsorption of Na⁺ and Cl⁻ in the first half of the distal convoluted tubule and a portion of the cortical ascending limb of the loop of Henle, and H_2O follows the unreabsorbed salt. However, thiazides can cause excretion of a hypertonic urine and contribute to dilutional hyponatremia. As a conse-

quence of increased delivery of Na⁺ to the distal nephron, Na⁺-K⁺ exchange is enhanced, and kaliuresis results.

K⁺ depletion and metabolic alkalosis (the latter due to increased H⁺ secretion as a substitute for the depleted intracellular stores of K⁺) are the chief adverse metabolic effects following prolonged administration of the thiazides, and also of metolazone, and of the loop diuretics. Hypokalemia may seriously enhance the dangers of digitalis intoxication (see below), and induce fatigue and lethargy; it may be prevented by oral supplementation with KCl or preferably by the addition of a K⁺-retaining diuretic. Other side effects of thiazides include reduction of the excretion of uric acid, which may lead to hyperuricemia, and impaired glucose tolerance. Skin rashes, thrombocytopenia, and granulocytopenia have also been reported.

Thiazide diuretics are effective and useful in the treatment of HF as long as the glomerular filtration rate exceeds approximately one half of normal. Chlorothiazide (25 to 50 mg/d) is especially useful since it may be administered once daily.

METOLAZONE   This quinethazone derivative has a site of action and potency similar to the thiazides but is effective in the presence of moderate renal failure. Both metolazone and thiazides potentiate the diuretic efficacy of intravenous loop diuretics.

FUROSEMIDE, BUMETANIDE, AND TORSEMIDE   These "loop" diuretics are similar physiologically but differ chemically from one another. They reversibly inhibit the reabsorption of Na⁺, K⁺, and Cl⁻ in the thick ascending limb of Henle's loop, apparently by blocking a cotransport system in the luminal membrane. They may induce renal cortical vasodilatation and can produce rates of urine formation that may be as high as one-fourth of the glomerular filtration rate. Metabolic alkalosis may be caused by a large increase in the urinary excretion of Cl⁻, H⁺, and K⁺. Hypokalemia, hyperuricemia, and hyperglycemia are observed occasionally, as with thiazide diuretics. The reabsorption of free H_2O is decreased. These three drugs are usually effective both intravenously and by mouth, and are excreted in the bile and urine. Weakness, nausea, and dizziness may complicate the administration of all loop diuretics.

These powerful diuretics are useful in all forms of HF, particularly in patients with otherwise refractory HF and pulmonary edema. They have been shown to be effective in patients with hypoalbuminemia, hyponatremia, hypochloremia, and with reductions in glomerular filtration rate, and to produce a diuresis in patients in whom thiazide diuretics and potassium-sparing diuretics, alone and in combination, are ineffective. In patients with refractory HF, the action of loop diuretics may be potentiated by intravenous administration and by the addition of other diuretics, i.e., thiazides, metozalone, and the potassium-sparing diuretics.

POTASSIUM-SPARING DIURETICS   These agents act on the distal tubule and cortical collecting ducts, are relatively weak, and therefore are rarely indicated as sole agents. Spironolactone resemble aldosterone structurally and acts by competitive inhibition of aldosterone, thereby blocking the exchange between Na⁺ and both K⁺ and H⁺ in the distal tubules and collecting ducts. Amiloride and triamterene have a similar effect but act directly on the distal tubule/collecting duct. These agents produce a Na⁺ diuresis, and in contrast to the thiazides, metolazone and the thiazides result in K⁺ *retention*.

Potassium-sparing diuretics are most effective when administered in combination with loop and/or thiazide diuretics. The opposing action of these drugs on urine and serum potassium makes possible a sodium diuresis without either hyper- or hypokalemia when spironolactone and one of these other agents are administered in combination. Also, since potassium-sparing diuretics act on the distal tubule, they are particularly effective when used in combination with one of the other diuretics that act more proximally. Spironolactone, triamterene, and amiloride should *not* be administered to patients with serum K⁺ > 5 mmol/L, renal failure, or hyponatremia. Reported complications include nausea, epigastric distress, mental confusion, drowsiness,

TABLE 216-3 Common Medications for Heart Failure

Medication	Initial Dose	Maximum Dose
Loop diuretics		
Furosemide	20–40 mg 1–2 times daily PO; 20 mg IV	400 mg/d; 80 mg IV
Bumetanide	0.5–1.0 mg 1–2 times daily PO; 0.5 mg IV	10 mg/d; 2 mg IV
Torsemide	10 mg 1–2 times daily PO; 5 mg IV	200 mg/d; 20 mg IV
Supplemental thiazides		
Metolazone	2.5 mg 1–2 times daily	10 mg/d
Hydrochlorathiazide	25 mg/d	100 mg/d
Chlorthalidone	50 mg/d	100 mg/d
Spironolactone (only with loop diuretics)	25 mg/d or every other day	25 mg twice daily, occasionally higher for refractory hypokalemia
Angiotensin-converting enzyme inhibitors		
Captopril	6.25 mg/d or every other day	50–100 mg 4 times daily
Enalapril maleate	2.5 mg twice daily	10–20 mg twice daily
Fosinopril sodium	5–10 mg/d	40 mg/d
Lisinopril	2.5–5.0 mg/d	20–40 mg/d
Quinapril hydrochloride	10 mg twice daily	40 mg twice daily
Ramipril	1.25–2.5 mg/d	10 mg/d
β-Blockers		
Bisoprolol	1.25 mg/d	10 mg/d
Carvedilol	3.125 mg twice daily	25–50 mg twice daily
Metoprolol tartrate	6.25 mg twice daily	75 mg twice daily
Metoprolol CR/XL*	12.5–25 mg/d	200 mg/d
Digoxin	0.125 mg every other day to 0.25 mg	0.50 mg/d to avoid toxic effects
Other vasodilators		
Isosorbide dinitrate	10 mg 3 times daily	80 mg 3 times daily
Sublingual isosorbide	2.5 mg as occasion requires or prior to exercise to decrease dyspnea	
Hydralazine	25 mg 3 times daily	150 mg 4 times daily

* CR/XL indicates controlled-release extended release metoprolol succinate
Source: Modified from Nohria A et al, 2002; data adapted from Hunt et al: ACC/AHA Guidelines for the Evaluation and Management of Chronic Heart Failure in the Adult. *J Am Coll Cardiol*. 38:2101, 2001

gynecomastia, and erythematous eruptions. As mentioned below, a lower dose of spironolactone (25 mg/d), which exerts little if any diuretic effect, has been shown to prolong life in patients with advanced HF (Table 216-3).

Triamterene and *amiloride* exert renal effects similar to those of spironolactone. However, their action does not depend on the presence of aldosterone. The effective dose of triamterene is 100 to 200 mg/d, and that of amiloride is 5 to 10 mg/d. Side effects include nausea, vomiting, diarrhea, headache, granulocytopenia, eosinophilia, and skin rash. Combination therapy, e.g., spironolactone and hydrochlorothiazide in a single tablet (e.g. Aldactazide) have proved popular.

When *choosing a diuretic*, an orally administered loop diuretic, thiazide or metolazone are the agents of choice in the treatment of chronic cardiac edema of mild to moderate degree in patients without hyperglycemia, hyperuricemia, or hypokalemia. Spironolactone, triamterene, and amiloride potentiate the thiazide and loop diuretics. In severe HF, the combination of a loop diuretic, a thiazide, and a potassium-sparing diuretic is required. In acute HF, especially pulmonary edema, intravenous loop diuretics are often effective.

PREVENTION OF DETERIORATION OF MYOCARDIAL INFARCTION *Chronic* activation of the renin-angiotensin-aldosterone system (RAAS) and of the adrenergic nervous systems in HF cause ventricular remodeling, further deterioration of cardiac function and/or potentially fatal arrhythmias (Chap. 215). Drugs that block these two systems have been found to be useful in the management of HF (Tables 216-2 and 216-3).

Angiotensin-Converting Enzyme (ACE) Inhibitors ACE inhibitors play a central role in the prevention and treatment of HF at almost all stages.

In addition to slowing maladaptive remodeling of the injured or abnormally burdened ventricle, ACE inhibitors reduce the impedance to left ventricular ejection. These drugs may be particularly helpful in (but are by no means limited to) patients with systolic HF due to myocardial infarction, hypertension, and valvular regurgitation. In patients with systolic HF who are treated with ACE inhibitors, cardiac output rises, the pulmonary wedge pressure falls, the signs and symptoms of HF are relieved, and a new steady state is achieved in which cardiac output is higher and afterload lower with no or only mild reduction of arterial pressure.

The administration of ACE inhibitors has been shown to prevent or retard the development of HF in patients with left ventricular dysfunction without HF, to reduce symptoms, enhance exercise performance, and to reduce long-term mortality and the need for rehospitalization in patients with HF, in patients shortly after acute myocardial infarction as well as in patients with vascular disease who are at high risk for recurrent events. These beneficial effects are related only in part to the salutary hemodynamic effects, i.e., the reduction of preload and afterload. The major effect of ACE inhibitors appears to be on inhibition of local (tissue) renin-angiotensin systems. Once begun and an optimal dose has been reached (Table 216-3) an ACE inhibitor should be maintained indefinitely. However, ACE inhibition should *not* be used in hypotensive patients.

Angiotensin Receptor Blockers In patients who cannot tolerate ACE inhibitors because of cough, angioneurotic edema, leukopenia, an angiotensin II receptor blocker (type AT1) antagonist may be used instead and appears to be equally effective.

Aldosterone Antagonist The activation of the RAAS in HF increases not only the circulating and tissue angiotensin II but also aldosterone. The latter, in addition to causing Na$^+$ retention and worsening edema (Chaps. 32 and 321), causes sympathetic activation, myocardial, vascular, and perivascular fibrosis, and reduces arterial compliance. In one large multicenter trial in patients with HF with recent or current class IV symptoms and reduced ejection fraction who were receiving ACE inhibitors, diuretics and digoxin, the addition of spironolactone, 25 mg/d reduced total mortality, as well as sudden death and death from pump failure. Since spironolactone is also a useful, albeit weak, diuretic (see above), its widespread use in severe systolic HF should be considered.

Beta-Adrenoceptor Blockers While the abrupt administration of large doses of beta-adrenergic receptor blockers can intensify HF, especially acute HF, the administration of gradually escalating doses has been reported to improve the symptoms of HF, and to reduce all-cause death, cardiovascular death, sudden death, rehospitalization for HF, and pump failure death in patients with chronic heart failure already receiving ACE inhibitors (Table 216-3). These drugs are indicated in patients with moderately severe HF (classes II and III), but are not indicated with unstable HF, in hypotensive patients (systolic pressure < 90 mmHg), in patients with severe fluid overload, in patients who have required recent treatment with an intravenous inotropic agent, and in patients with sinus bradycardia, atrioventricular block, or a bronchospastic disorder.

Three beta-adrenergic blockers (metoprolol, bisoprolol and carvedilol) have been shown to improve survival in patients with HF. The first two are selective and block only β_1 receptors, while the third blocks both β_1 and β_2 receptors as well as α receptors, thereby causing mild vasodilation. Carvedilol also appears to exert antioxidant activity.

Before commencing beta-blocker therapy, patients should be stabilized on an ACE inhibitor, diuretics and possibly digoxin. They should be begun in very low doses, e.g., carvedilol 3.125 mg bid or metoprolol XL 12.5 mg qd and titrated upward slowly every 2 to 4 weeks. During titration, the patients should be observed closely for hypertension, bradycardia, and worsening HF. Approximately 15% of patients cannot tolerate beta blockade, and an equal number cannot tolerate target doses (carvedilol 25 mg bid and metoprolol XL 200 mg). In the latter, low-dose beta-blocker therapy is preferred to no therapy.

Once a maintenance dose has been achieved, administration of the beta blocker should be continued indefinitely. If treatment of a patient on a beta blocker with a positive inotropic agent is required, a phosphodiesterase III inhibitor (see below) should be used.

ENHANCEMENT OF MYOCARDIAL CONTRACTILITY ■ Digitalis

The improvement of myocardial contractility by means of cardiac glycosides is useful in the control of HF. Cardiac glycosides inhibit the monovalent cation transport enzyme–coupled Na$^+$, K$^+$-ATPase and increase intracellular [Na$^+$]; the latter, in turn, increases intracellular [Ca^{2+}] through a Na$^+$-Ca^{2+} exchange carrier mechanism. The increased myocardial [Ca^{2+}] augments Ca^{2+} released to the myofilaments during excitation and, therefore, invokes a positive inotropic response (Chap. 215). Cardiac glycosides causes increased automaticity and ectopic impulse activity. They also prolong the effective refractory period of the atrioventricular node and thereby slow ventricular rate in atrial flutter and fibrillation.

Digitalis is effective in patients with systolic HF complicated by atrial flutter and fibrillation and a rapid ventricular rate, who benefit both from slowing of the ventricular rate and from the positive inotropic effect. Although digitalis does not improve survival in patients with systolic HF and sinus rhythm, it reduces symptoms of HF and the need for hospitalization. Digitalis is of *little* or *no* value in patients with HF, sinus rhythm, and the following conditions: hypertrophic cardiomyopathy, myocarditis, mitral stenosis, chronic constrictive pericarditis, and any form of diastolic HF.

Digoxin, which has a half-life of 1.6 days, is filtered in the glomeruli and secreted by the renal tubules. Significant reductions of the glomerular filtration rate reduce the elimination of digoxin and, therefore, may prolong digoxin's effect, allowing it to accumulate to toxic levels, unless the dose is reduced.

DIGITALIS INTOXICATION This is a serious and potentially fatal complication. Advanced age, hypokalemia, hypomagnesemia, hypoxemia, renal insufficiency, hypercalcemia, and acute myocardial infarction all may reduce tolerance to digitalis. Chronic digitalis intoxication may be insidious in onset and is characterized by anorexia, nausea, and vomiting, exacerbations of HF, weight loss, cachexia, neuralgias, gynecomastia, yellow vision, and delirium.

The most frequent disturbances of cardiac rhythm are ventricular premature beats, bigeminy, ventricular tachycardia, and, rarely, ventricular fibrillation. Atrioventricular block and nonparoxysmal atrial tachycardia with variable atrioventricular block are characteristic of digitalis intoxication; withdrawal of the drug and treatment with β-adrenoceptor blocker or lidocaine are indicated. If hypokalemia is present, potassium should be administered cautiously by the oral route. Fab fragments of purified, intact digitalis antibodies are a potentially lifesaving approach to the treatment of severe intoxication.

The administration of quinidine, verapamil, amiodarone, and propafenone to patients receiving digoxin raises the serum concentration of the latter, increasing the propensity to digitalis intoxication. The dose of digitalis should be reduced by half in patients receiving these drugs.

Sympathomimetic Amines

Two sympathomimetic amines that act largely on β-adrenergic receptors—dopamine and dobutamine—improve myocardial contractility and are effective in the management of severe, acute HF. They must be administered by constant intravenous infusion and can be given for several days to patients with intractable, severe HF, particularly those with a reversible component, such as exists in patients who have undergone cardiac surgery, as well as to patients with acute myocardial infarction and shock or pulmonary edema (Chap. 255), and they may be used in patients with refractory HF as a "bridge" to cardiac transplantation. The administration of sympathomimetic amines should be accompanied by careful and continuous monitoring of the electrocardiogram, arterial pressure, and, if possible, pulmonary artery wedge pressure.

Dopamine is a naturally occurring, immediate precursor of norepinephrine and has a combination of actions that makes it particularly useful in the treatment of a variety of hypotensive states and HF. At very low doses (i.e., 1 to 2 μg/kg per min), it dilates renal and mesenteric blood vessels through stimulation of specific dopaminergic receptors, thereby augmenting renal and mesenteric blood flow and sodium excretion. In the range of 2 to 10 μg/kg per min, dopamine stimulates myocardial β_1 receptors but induces relatively little tachycardia, while at higher doses it also stimulates α-adrenergic receptors and elevates arterial pressure.

Dobutamine is a synthetic sympathomimetic agent that acts on β_1, β_2, and α_1 receptors. It exerts a potent inotropic action, has only a modest cardio accelerating effect, and lowers peripheral vascular resistance. Since it simultaneously raises cardiac output, it may not lower systemic arterial pressure in patients with severe HF. Dobutamine, given in continuous infusions of 2.5 to 10 μg/kg per min, is useful in the treatment of acute HF without hypotension.

A major problem with all sympathomimetics is the loss of responsiveness, apparently due to "downregulation" of adrenergic receptors, which becomes evident within 8 h of continuous administration. This problem may be managed by intermittent therapy.

Phosphodiesterase Inhibitors

These bipyridines, amrinone and milrinone, are noncatecholamine, nonglycoside agents that exert both *positive* inotropic and vasodilator actions by inhibiting phosphodiesterase III, an enzyme that breaks down intracytoplasmic cyclic AMP, the second messenger which is critical to adrenergic stimulation. These agents are administered intravenously; by simultaneously stimulating cardiac contractility and dilating the systemic vascular bed they reverse the major hemodynamic abnormalities associated with HF. Amrinone and milrinone may be administered for the same conditions in which dopamine or dobutamine are useful; they may be employed together with and potentiate the sympathomimetics.

VASODILATORS

Direct vasodilators may be useful in patients with severe, acute HF who demonstrate systemic vasoconstriction despite ACE inhibitor therapy. The ideal vasodilator for the treatment of *acute* HF should have a rapid onset and brief duration of action when administered by intravenous infusion; sodium nitroprusside (0.1 to 3.0 μg/kg per min) qualifies as such a drug, but its use requires careful monitoring of the arterial pressure and, if possible, of the pulmonary artery wedge pressure. Intravenous nitroglycerin (beginning at 20 μg/min and titrated upwards to achieve the desired result or a maximum of 400 μg/min) and nesiritide (recombinant BNP, I.V. bolus = 2 μg/kg followed by 0.01 μg/kg per min) are effective vasodilators. The combination of hydralazine (up to 100 mg tid orally) and isosorbide dinitrate (up to 60 mg tid orally) may be useful for chronic oral administration.

VENTRICULAR RESYNCHRONIZATION

Intraventricular conduction is depressed in about one-fourth of patients with chronic HF. This depression is manifest in prolongation of the QRS complex to more than 120 ms, leading to dyssynchrony of cardiac contraction, which further impairs cardiac contraction and thereby aggravates HF. "Resynchronization" with a device that has three pacing leads (right atrium, right ventricle, and cardiac vein, which provides left ventricular stimulation) has been shown to improve performance in patients with HF. This device, which has been approved by the FDA, has been demonstrated to increase ejection fraction as well as the distance walked in 6 min, improved functional New York Heart Association class, and the quality of life. Hospitalization for worsening HF and/or requiring use of intravenous medication were reduced in half. Device placement was not possible or complications occurred in 8% of patients. Devices that incorporate the ability to achieve resynchronization and internal cardioversion-defibrillation are now also available and may simultaneously improve contraction and prevent sudden death due to ventricular fibrillation in patients with HF (see below).

MANAGEMENT OF ARRHYTHMIAS   Premature ventricular contractions and episodes of asymptomatic ventricular tachycardia are common in advanced HF. Sudden death, presumably due to ventricular fibrillation, is responsible for about one-half of all deaths in this condition. The remainder are due to failure of the cardiac pump. The management of arrhythmias should commence with correction of electrolyte and acid-base disturbances (Chaps. 41 and 42), especially diuretic-induced hypokalemia, as well as digitalis intoxication (see above). Treatment with class I antiarrhythmics such as quinidine, procainamide, or flecainide (Chap. 214) is *contraindicated* because these drugs are proarrhythmic in patients with HF. Amiodarone, a class III antiarrhythmic, on the other hand, is well tolerated and is the drug of choice for patients with HF and atrial fibrillation.

Patients who have been resuscitated from sudden death, those with syncope or presyncope due to ventricular arrhythmias, and those with asymptomatic ventricular tachyarrhythmias in whom ventricular tachycardia can be induced during electrophysiologic testing should be strongly considered for the implantable automatic defibrillator (ICD). The MADIT II trial showed a 30% reduction in all-cause mortality in patients with a prior myocardial infarction and a left ventricular ejection fraction ≤30% in whom an ICD had been implanted. Although the societal costs of treating the majority of all such patients with a prophylactic ICD will be immense, this may soon become the treatment of choice in patients with severe systolic HF. The addition to the device of the capacity for "back-up pacing" may prevent sudden death due to bradyarrhythmias. (See also Chap. 214.)

Anticoagulants   Patients with severe HF are at increased risk of pulmonary emboli secondary to venous thrombosis and of systemic emboli secondary to intracardiac thrombi and should be treated with warfarin. Patients with HF and atrial fibrillation, previous venous thrombosis, and pulmonary or systemic emboli are at especially high risk and should receive heparin followed by warfarin.

DIASTOLIC HEART FAILURE   The major goal in the treatment of this condition is to eliminate or reduce the causes of diastolic dysfunction, such as ventricular hypertrophy, fibrosis, or ischemia. The second goal is to reduce pulmonary and/or systemic venous congestion, a major consequence of diastolic dysfunction. Dietary Na^+ restriction and diuretics are useful for this purpose. Slowing of heart rate with beta blockers or nondihydropyridine calcium antagonists is also important since it provides more time for ventricular filling.

REFRACTORY HEART FAILURE   When the response to ordinary treatment as described above is inadequate, HF is considered to be refractory. Before assuming that this condition simply reflects terminal myocardial depression, careful consideration must be given to several possibilities: (1) an underlying or precipitating cause that may be amenable to specific surgical or medical therapy, such as infective endocarditis, thyrotoxicosis, or silent aortic or mitral stenosis has been overlooked; and (2) complications of overly vigorous therapy, such as digitalis intoxication, hypovolemia, or electrolyte imbalance. Recognition and proper treatment of the aforementioned problems, if they exist, are likely to restore responsiveness to therapy.

Patients with refractory HF ordinarily require hospital management (Table 216-4). The combination of an intravenously administered vasodilator such as nitroglycerin, niseritide, *or.* of a phosphodiesterase inhibitor (amrinone or milrinone), together with a sympathomimetic

TABLE 216-4   Therapeutic Options for Patients with Refractory Heart Failure

Combination diuretics	Left ventricular or biventricular pacing
Additional vasodilators	Novel cardiac surgery
Positive inotropic agents	Ventricular remodeling surgery
Mechanical circulatory support	Dynamic cardiomyoplasty
Cardiac transplantation	Mitral valve repair

Source: From MM Givertz, JN Cohn in EM Antman (ed): *Cardiovascular Therapeutics*, 2d ed. Philadelphia, Saunders, 2002, with permission.

amine (dopamine or dobutamine) often results in additive effects, raising cardiac output and lowering filling pressure further.

In hospitalized patients with refractory HF, therapy guided by hemodynamic measurements provided by a balloon flotation (Swan-Ganz) catheter may be helpful. The goal of manipulating diuretics, inotropic agents, and vasodilators is to achieve a pulmonary capillary wedge pressure of 15 to 18 mmHg, a right atrial pressure of 5 to 8 mmHg, a cardiac index >2.2 L/min per m², and a systemic vascular resistance of 800 to 1200 dyne · s/cm⁵. Once these values are achieved, an attempt should be made to convert the patient from intravenous to oral vasodilator therapy.

ASSISTED CIRCULATION/CARDIAC TRANSPLANTATION   When patients with HF become unresponsive to a combination of all the aforementioned therapeutic measures, are in New York Heart Association class IV, and are deemed unlikely to survive one year, they should be considered for assisted circulation and/or cardiac transplantation (see Chap. 217). Prolonged left ventricular assistance may be used as a "bridge to transplantation." In a small (~10%) of patients receiving this therapy, there is sufficient improvement in cardiac function after two or three months to allow recovery after withdrawal of the device.

Treatment of Acute Pulmonary Edema   →*Cardiogenic pulmonary edema is described in Chap. 29. Its management is described in Chap. 255.*

PROGNOSIS

The prognosis in patients with HF depends primarily on the nature of the underlying heart disease and on the presence or absence of a precipitating factor that can be treated. When one of the latter can be identified and removed, the outlook for immediate survival is far better than if HF occurs without any obvious precipitating cause. The long-term prognosis is more favorable when the underlying forms of heart disease, e.g., valvular heart disease, can be treated effectively. When this is not possible, the prognosis can be estimated by observing the response to treatment. When patients can be rendered free of congestion, survival may be 80% at two years. Survival may be as low as 50% at six months in patients with refractory symptoms (Fig. 216-3).

Other factors that have been shown to be associated with a poor

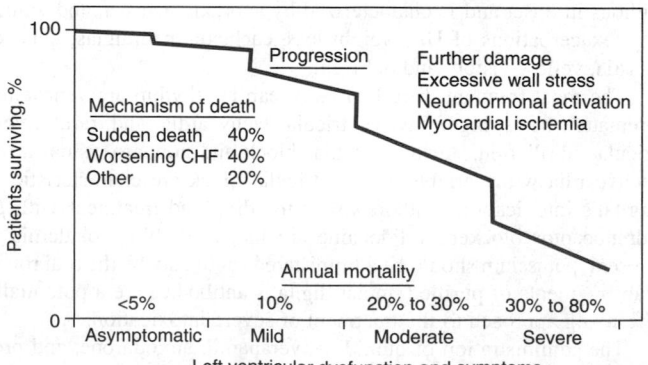

FIGURE 216-3   The natural history of congestive heart failure (CHF). Once left ventricular systolic dysfunction is present, it usually progresses, albeit not predictably. As left ventricular dysfunction progresses and symptoms increase, mortality rate increases and the process becomes inexorable. Myocyte loss and fibrosis become irreversible. An effective preventive measure must be introduced before onset or early in the course of progressive left ventricular dysfunction. (*From BM Massie, NH Shah: Curr Opin Cardiol 11:221, 1996; with permission.*)

prognosis include a severely depressed ejection fraction (<15%), a reduced maximal O_2 uptake (<10 mL/kg per min), the inability to walk on a level and at a normal pace for more than 3 min, reduced serum Na^+ concentration (<133 mEq/L), reduced serum K^+ (<3 meq/ L), a markedly elevated (>500 pg/mL) BNP, as well as frequent ventricular extrasystoles. If sudden cardiac death is prevented by implantation of an ICD, patients may later go on to develop and succumb to pump failure and the number of such patients is likely to grow. When all available therapeutic measures have been exhausted, comfort care, sometimes in a hospice, with continued infusions of inotropic agents, diuretics, and the administration of anxiolytics and analgesics should be considered.

COR PULMONALE

Cor pulmonale is defined as enlargement of the right ventricle (RV) secondary to abnormalities of the lungs, thorax, pulmonary ventilation, or circulation. It sometimes leads to RV failure, with an elevation of transmural RV end-diastolic pressure.

NORMAL FUNCTION OF THE PULMONARY CIRCULATION

PATHOPHYSIOLOGY The stroke volume of the RV, as of the left, is regulated by its preload, contractility, and afterload (Chap. 215). Since the RV is a relatively thin, compliant reservoir, acute changes in venous return (e.g., an increase with inhalation and decline with exhalation) can occur with little change in transmural RV pressure. However, the ability of the RV to increase its systolic pressure is limited. Normally, the RV afterload, which is closely related to the pulmonary artery pressure, is low. The pulmonary artery pressure normally rises slightly when blood is displaced into the chest at the start of exercise; on assuming recumbency; or with cold, anxiety, or pain. A driving pressure of only about 5 cmH_2O between the pulmonary artery (15 cmH_2O) and the left atrium (10 cmH_2O) normally propels the entire cardiac output of approximately 5 L/min at rest through the lungs, and only a modest increase in pressure is necessary to drive a flow of up to 25 L/min through the pulmonary capillary bed during maximal exercise.

The severity of RV enlargement in cor pulmonale is a function of the increase in afterload. When the pulmonary vascular resistance is elevated and relatively fixed, as in pulmonary vascular or severe parenchymal lung disease, an elevation in cardiac output, as occurs with physical exertion, can elevate pulmonary artery pressure markedly. RV afterload may be augmented when the lungs are hyperinflated, as in chronic obstructive lung disease (COLD), due to the compression of the alveolar capillaries and the lengthening of the pulmonary vessels (Chap. 242). RV afterload can also increase when lung volume is reduced following extensive pulmonary resection, as well as in restrictive lung diseases in which pulmonary vessels are compressed and distorted. RV afterload rises with hypoxic pulmonary vasoconstriction caused by hypoxia or acidosis, which are important causes of pulmonary hypertension (Chap. 220).

The elevation of RV afterload responsible for cor pulmonale is caused principally by pulmonary vascular or parenchymal disease.

PULMONARY VASCULAR DISEASES
In these conditions the RV afterload is elevated as a consequence of restriction to pulmonary blood flow. In cor pulmonale secondary to pulmonary vascular disease, pulmonary hypertension is usually more severe than in pulmonary parenchymal disease. Chronic cor pulmonale secondary to pulmonary vascular disease may result from repeated pulmonary emboli, pulmonary vasculitis, pulmonary vasoconstriction secondary to high altitude, congenital heart disease with left-to-right shunting (e.g., atrial or ventricular septal defect, patent ductus arteriosus; Chap. 218), as well as pulmonary venoocclusive disease. When the cause of elevated pulmonary vascular resistance responsible for cor pulmonale cannot be defined, the condition is referred to as *primary pulmonary hypertension* (Chap. 220).

COR PULMONALE DUE TO PULMONARY EMBOLI
This condition is associated with two distinct syndromes.

Acute Cor Pulmonale It has been estimated that in the United States about 50,000 people die each year from pulmonary thromboembolism

(Chap. 244). Probably half die within the first hour from acute right heart failure due to massive or multiple emboli. A sudden, large embolic burden causes a low-output state resulting from the RV's inability to generate the pressure necessary to drive blood through the acutely compromised pulmonary vascular bed. Depression of cardiac output can also occur with a moderate-sized embolism if the pulmonary circulation has been critically compromised by previous pulmonary vascular or parenchymal disease. The RV begins to fail when systolic pressure is forced to double acutely, i.e., to exceed approximately 50 mmHg. Acute RV failure secondary to pulmonary embolism is suggested by the history of the sudden onset of severe dyspnea and cardiovascular collapse in a patient with, or predisposed to, venous thrombosis.

Clinical Manifestations Acute RV failure causes pallor, sweating, hypotension, and a rapid pulse of small amplitude. The neck veins are distended and often exhibit prominent *v* waves secondary to tricuspid regurgitation. The liver may be pulsatile, distended, and tender. A systolic murmur of tricuspid regurgitation along the left sternal border may be accompanied by a presystolic (S_4) gallop sound. Arterial blood gas frequently shows reduced Pa_{O_2} due to ventilation/perfusion mismatching and a low Pa_{CO_2} due to hyperventilation.

℞ TREATMENT

The treatment of pulmonary embolism is described in Chap. 244. In acute cor pulmonale [and in RV failure due to acute RV infarction (Chap. 228)], an increase in RV preload can be achieved by a cautious expansion of blood volume, which helps to maintain cardiac output. When hypoxic pulmonary vasoconstriction contributes to pulmonary hypertension, inhalation of 100% O_2 reduces RV afterload.

CHRONIC COR PULMONALE SECONDARY TO PULMONARY VASCULAR DISEASE In contrast to acute, massive thromboembolism, when the elevation in pulmonary vascular resistance and the RV hypertrophy develop gradually, higher pulmonary vascular pressures, sometimes even approaching systemic arterial levels, may be generated. Chronic cor pulmonale can be caused by recurrent, medium-sized emboli that fail to lyse, but organize, resulting in chronic thromboembolic pulmonary hypertension. Particles from intravenous drug abuse, parasites, or tumor tissue that embolizes into the pulmonary vascular bed may also cause persistent pulmonary hypertension. Chronic cor pulmonale can also be caused by *primary pulmonary hypertension* (Chap. 220) or any chronic widespread vasculitis, such as occurs in association with collagen vascular disorders and that may affect the pulmonary vascular bed, particularly the CREST syndrome (Chap. 303).

Clinical Manifestations Dyspnea and tachypnea are characteristic features of pulmonary hypertension secondary to pulmonary vascular disease. They may be distressing during mild exertion or even at rest and are *not* relieved by sitting upright. An unproductive cough is another frequent complaint. Anterior chest pain, due to acute dilation of the root of the pulmonary artery or RV ischemia, can occur. The elevation in systemic venous pressure can cause hepatomegaly and ankle edema.

Occasionally there is cyanosis due to arterial hypoxemia and low cardiac output. An RV heave may be palpable along the left sternal border or in the epigastrium, and a high-pitched pulmonary ejection click may be audible to the left of the upper sternum. The second (pulmonary) component of the second heart sound is intensified and may be palpable; fixed, narrow splitting of the second heart sound and a right ventricular protodiastolic gallop (S_3) that may increase during inspiration can be present. A systolic murmur of tricuspid regurgitation, which is augmented by inspiration, is often audible; occasionally, a diastolic murmur of pulmonary regurgitation is also heard. Prominent *a* (and sometimes also *v*) waves in the jugular venous pulse are evident. The onset of RV failure is reflected by an increase of venous pressure, the development of larger *v* waves associated with increasing tricuspid regurgitation, a positive hepatojugular reflux, and a gallop rhythm with both third and fourth heart sounds. These physical findings of RV failure can disappear rapidly when pulmonary artery pressure is reduced by relief of hypoxemia.

Laboratory Examination On *radiologic examination* the pulmonary trunk and hilar vessels are enlarged, as is the descending right pulmonary artery. Ventilation and perfusion lung scans and systemic venography showing deep vein thrombosis in the lower extremities are helpful in confirming the diagnosis of embolic pulmonary vascular disease. In the presence of severe pulmonary hypertension, the *electrocardiogram* (ECG) shows P pulmonale, right axis deviation, and RV hypertrophy (Chap. 210).

Echocardiography allows measurement of the thickness of the RV wall and may show enlargement of the RV cavity in relation to the left. The interventricular septum may be displaced leftward and may move paradoxically during the cardiac cycle. Pulmonary artery and RV systolic pressure can be estimated from measurement of the peak tricuspid regurgitant flow and pulmonic regurgitant flow with Doppler echocardiography.

Magnetic resonance imaging is useful for measuring RV mass, wall thickness, cavity volume, and ejection fraction.

Cardiac catheterization provides precise measurement of pulmonary vascular pressures, calculation of pulmonary vascular resistance, and their responses to oxygen and vasodilators. Catheterization is sometimes helpful in patients with cor pulmonale to exclude congenital and left heart diseases, and it allows pulmonary angiography to be carried out to confirm the nature of the pulmonary vascular obstruction. Measurements of pulmonary vascular pressure and flow during exercise may reveal abnormal pressure increments of pulmonary artery systolic and diastolic and RV diastolic pressures and an inadequate response to cardiac output.

Lung biopsy can be useful in demonstrating vasculitis in some types of pulmonary vascular disease such as the collagen vascular diseases, rheumatoid arthritis, and Wegener's granulomatosis.

PARENCHYMAL PULMONARY DISEASES Cor pulmonale may be caused by both obstructive and restrictive lung diseases, more frequently the former. In these conditions there are usually only modest elevations of pulmonary artery pressure. The development of cor pulmonale confers a poor prognosis on patients with respiratory disease, not because RV failure cannot be treated, but because it reflects the seriousness of the underlying pulmonary disease.

℞ TREATMENT (See Chap. 242)

Acute respiratory infection, often the precipitant of RV failure, must be treated promptly and vigorously. Alveolar hypoxia at rest and dur-

ing exertion and sleep should be corrected by improving alveolar ventilation through relieving the airflow obstruction and by judiciously increasing the inspired O_2 concentration. Long-term O_2 therapy is helpful in patients with severe COLD and reduces pulmonary artery pressure and pulmonary vascular resistance. Bronchodilators and antibiotics lessen airflow obstruction, and diuretics relieve the edema. Loop diuretics must be used with care since they may cause a metabolic alkalosis and thereby blunt the respiratory drive. Digitalis should be used cautiously in the presence of overt RV failure, and small phlebotomies should be considered when the hematocrit exceeds 55 to 60%. Inhalation of nitric oxide and infusion of prostacyclin are undergoing evaluation as agents to reduce pulmonary hypertension.

FURTHER READING

ABRAHAM WT et al: Cardiac resynchronization in chronic heart failure. N Engl J Med 346:1845, 2002

ACC/AHA Guidelines for the Evaluation and Management of Chronic Heart Failure in the Adult—Executive Summary. J Am Coll Cardiol 38:2101, 2001. Full report found at www.acc.org/clinical/guidelines/failure/hf_index.htm; www.americanheart.org/presenter

ASHER CR, KLEIN AL: Diastolic heart failure: Restrictive cardiomyopathy, constrictive pericarditis and cardiac tamponade: Clinical and echocardiographic evaluation. Card Review 10:218, 2002

BRAUNWALD E, BRISTOW MR: Congestive heart failure: Fifty years of progress. Circulation 102:IV-14, 2000

GARG R, YUSUF S: Overview of randomized trials of angiotensin-converting enzyme inhibitors on mortality and morbidity in patients with heart failure. Collaborative Group on ACE Inhibitor Trials. JAMA 274:462, 1995

KITZMAN DW et al. Pathophysiological characterization of isolated diastolic heart failure in comparison to systolic heart failure. JAMA 288:2144, 2002

MAISEL AS et al: Rapid measurement of B-type natriuretic peptide in the emergency diagnosis of heart failure. N Engl J Med 347:161, 2002

McCULLOUGH PA et al: Uncovering heart failure in patients with a history of pulmonary disease: Rationale for the early use of B-type natriuretic peptide in the emergency department. Acad Emerg Med 10:275, 2003

MOSS AJ et al: Prophylactic implantation of a defibrillator in patients with myocardial infarction and reduced ejection fraction. N Engl J Med 346:877, 2002

NOHRIA A et al: Medical management of advanced heart failure. JAMA 287:628, 2002

PITT B et al: The effect of spironolactone on morbidity and mortality in patients with severe heart failure. N Engl J Med 341:709, 1999

PUBLICATION COMMITTEE FOR THE VMAC INVESTIGATORS: Intravenous nesiritide vs. nitroglycerin for treatment of decompensated congestive heart failure: A randomized controlled trial. JAMA 287:1531, 2002

RAPAPORT E: Cor pulmonale, in *Textbooks of Respiratory Medicine*, JF Murray, JA Nadel (eds). Philadelphia, Saunders, 2000

RICH S: Pulmonary hypertension and cor pulmonale, in *Braunwald's Heart Disease*, 7th ed, D Zipes et al (eds). Philadelphia, Saunders, 2005

WEITZENBLUM E: Chronic cor pulmonale. Heart 89:225, 2003

WILCOX CS: Diuretics, in *The Kidney*, 7th ed, BM Brenner (ed). Philadelphia, Saunders, 2004

217 CARDIAC TRANSPLANTATION AND PROLONGED ASSISTED CIRCULATION
Sharon A. Hunt

Advanced or end-stage heart failure is an increasingly frequent sequela as progressively more effective palliation for the earlier stages of heart disease and prevention of sudden death associated with heart disease become more widely recognized and employed (Chap. 216). When patients with end-stage or refractory heart failure are identified, the physician is faced with the decision of advising compassionate end-of-life care or choosing to recommend extraordinary life-extending measures. For the occasional patient who is relatively young and without serious comorbidities, the latter may represent a reasonable option. Current therapeutic options are limited to cardiac transplantation (with the option of mechanical cardiac assistance as a "bridge" to transplantation), but the option of permanent mechanical assistance of the circulation is not far off.

CARDIAC TRANSPLANTATION

Surgical techniques for orthotopic transplantation of the heart were devised in the 1960s and taken into the clinical arena in 1967. The procedure did not gain widespread clinical acceptance until the introduction of "modern" and more effective immunosuppression in the early 1980s. By the 1990s the demand for transplantable hearts met, and then exceeded, the available donor supply and peaked at 4400 annually worldwide in the early 1990s and declined to about 3000 in 2002.

SURGICAL TECHNIQUE Donor and recipient hearts are excised in virtually identical operations with incisions made across the atria and atrial septa at the midatrial level (leaving the posterior of the atria in place)

and across the great vessels just above the semilunar valves. The donor heart is generally "harvested" in an anatomically identical manner by a separate surgical team and transported from the donor hospital in a bag of iced saline solution and then is reanastomosed into the waiting recipient in the orthotopic or normal anatomical position. The only change in surgical technique since this method was first described has been a movement in recent years to move the right atrial anastamosis back to the level of the superior and inferior vena cavae in order to better preserve right atrial geometry and prevent atrial arrhythmias. This method of implantation leaves the recipient with a surgically denervated heart that does not respond to any direct sympathetic or parasympathetic stimuli but does respond to circulating catecholamines. The physiologic responses of the denervated heart to the demands of exercise are atypical but quite adequate to carry on normal physical activity.

DONOR ALLOCATION SYSTEM In the United States the allocation of donor organs is accomplished under the supervision of the United Network for Organ Sharing (UNOS), a private organization under contract to the federal government. The United States is divided geographically into eleven regions for donor heart allocation. Allocation of donor hearts within a region is decided according to a system of priority that takes into account (1) the severity of illness, (2) geographic distance from the donor, and (3) patient time on the waiting list. A physiologic limit of approximately 3 h of "ischemic" (out of body) time for hearts precludes a national sharing of hearts. This allocation system design is reissued annually and is responsive to input from a variety of constituencies, including donor families and transplant professionals.

At the current time, higher priority according to severity of illness is assigned only to patients requiring hospitalization for intravenous inotropic support either with a pulmonary artery catheter in place for hemodynamic monitoring or without hemodynamic monitoring. All other patients have priority according to their time on the waiting list, and matching is achieved only according to ABO blood group compatibility and gross body size compatibility.

INDICATIONS/CONTRAINDICATIONS Heart failure is an increasingly common cause of death, particularly in the elderly. Most patients who reach what has recently been categorized as stage D, or refractory end-stage heart failure, are appropriately treated with compassionate end-of-life care. A subset of such patients who are younger and without significant comorbidities can be considered as candidates for heart transplantation. Exact criteria vary in different centers but generally take into consideration the patient's physiologic age and the existence of comorbidities such as peripheral or cerebrovascular disease, obesity, diabetes, cancer, or chronic infection.

RESULTS A registry organized by the International Society for Heart and Heart-Lung Transplantation has tracked worldwide and U.S. survival rates after heart transplantation since 1982. The most recent update reveals 83% and 76% survival 1 and 3 years posttransplant or a posttransplant "half-life" of 9.3 years (Fig. 217-1). The quality of life in these patients is generally excellent, with well over 90% of patients in the registry returning to normal and unrestricted function following transplantation.

IMMUNOSUPPRESSION Medical regimens employed to provide suppression of the normal immune response to a solid organ allograft vary from center to center and are in a constant state of evolution as more effective agents with improved side-effect profiles and less toxicity are introduced. All currently used regimens are nonspecific, providing general hyporeactivity to foreign antigens rather than donor-specific hyporeactivity and the attendant, and unwanted, susceptibility to infections and malignancy. Most cardiac transplant programs currently use a three-drug regimen including a calcineurin inhibitor (cyclosporine or tacrolimus), an inhibitor of T cell proliferation or differentiation (azathioprine, mycophenolate mofetil, or sirolimus), and at least a short initial course of glucocorticoids. Many programs also include an initial "induction" course of polyclonal or monoclonal anti-T cell antibodies in the perioperative period to decrease the frequency or severity of early posttransplant rejection. Most recently introduced have been monoclonal antibodies (daclizumab and basiliximab), which

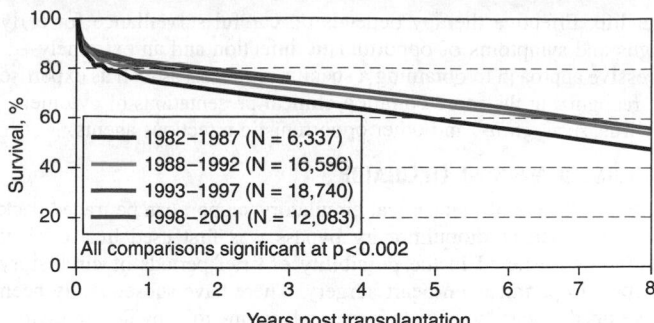

FIGURE 217-1 Actuarial survival for heart transplants performed between 1982 and 2001 by era of transplantation. (*Data by permission from United Network for Organ Sharing/International Society for Heart and Heart-Lung Transplantation Registry.*)

block the interleukin 2 receptor and may provide prevention of allograft rejection without additional global immunosuppression.

Diagnosis of cardiac allograft rejection is usually made with the use of endomyocardial biopsy, either done on a surveillance basis or in response to clinical deterioration. Therapy consists of augmentation of immunosuppression, the intensity and duration of which is dictated by the severity of the rejection.

LATE POSTTRANSPLANT MANAGEMENT ISSUES Increasing numbers of heart transplant patients are surviving for years following transplantation and constitute a population of patients with long-term management issues.

Allograft Coronary Artery Disease Despite having young donor hearts, cardiac allograft recipients are prone to develop coronary artery disease (CAD). This CAD is generally a diffuse, concentric, and longitudinal process that is quite different from "ordinary" atherosclerotic CAD, which is more focal and often eccentric. The underlying etiology is most likely primarily immunologic injury of the vascular endothelium, but a variety of risk factors influence its existence and progression. It is hoped that newer and improved immunosuppressive modalities will reduce the incidence and impact of these devastating complications, which currently account for the majority of late posttransplant deaths. Palliation of the disease with percutaneous interventions is probably safe and effective in the short term. Because of the denervated status of the organ, patients rarely experience angina pectoris, even with advanced stages of the disease.

Retransplantation is the only definitive form of therapy for advanced allograft CAD, but inferior survival rates after retransplantation and the scarcity of donor hearts make the decision to pursue retransplantation a difficult one in an individual patient, as well as a difficult ethical issue.

Malignancy The occurrence of an increased incidence of malignancy is a well-recognized sequela of any program of chronic immunosuppression, and organ transplantation is no exception. Lymphoproliferative disorders are among the most frequent posttransplant complications and, in most cases, seem to be driven by the Epstein-Barr virus. Effective therapy includes reduction of immunosuppression (a clear "double-edged sword" in the setting of a life-sustaining organ), antiviral agents, and traditional chemo- and radiotherapy. Most recently, specific antilymphocyte (CD20) therapy has shown great promise. Cutaneous malignancies (both basal cell and squamous cell carcinomas) also occur with increased frequency in transplant recipients and can pursue very aggressive courses. The role of decreasing immunosuppression for treatment of these cancers is much less clear.

Infections The use of currently available nonspecific immunosuppressive modalities to prevent allograft rejection naturally results in an increased susceptibility to infectious complications in transplant recipients. Although their incidence has decreased since the introduction of cyclosporine, infections with unusual and opportunistic organisms remain the major cause of death during the first postoperative year and remain a threat to the chronically immunosuppressed patient throughout life. Effective therapy depends on careful surveillance for early signs and symptoms of opportunistic infection and an extremely aggressive approach to obtaining a specific diagnosis as well as expertise in recognizing the more common clinical presentations of cytomegalovirus, *Aspergillus*, and other opportunistic infectious agents.

PROLONGED ASSISTED CIRCULATON

The modern era of mechanical circulatory support can be traced back to 1953 when cardiopulmonary bypass was first used in a clinical setting and ushered in the possibility of brief periods of circulatory support to permit open heart surgery. There have subsequently been developed a variety of extracorporeal pumps to provide circulatory support for brief periods of time. The use of a mechanical device to support the circulation for more than a few hours got off to a slow start in the 1980s when the first artificial hearts were introduced with much publicity but failed to produce the hoped-for treatment of end-stage heart disease. Subsequently, technology evolved to provide mechanical assistance to (rather than replacement of) the failing ventricle, although newer versions of the total artificial heart are now once again in preliminary clinical trials.

Although conceived of initially as alternatives to biologic replacement of the heart, left ventricular assist devices (LVADs) were introduced as, and are still employed primarily as, temporary "bridges" to heart transplantation in candidates who begin to fail medical therapy before a donor heart becomes available. Several devices are approved by the U.S. Food and Drug Administration (FDA) and are currently in widespread use. Those that are implantable within the body are compatible with hospital discharge and offer the patient chance for life at home while waiting for a donor heart. However successful such "bridging" is for the individual patient, it does nothing to alleviate the scarcity of donor hearts, and the ultimate goal in the field remains that of providing a reasonable alternative to biologic replacement of the heart—one that is widely and easily available and cost effective.

AVAILABLE DEVICES   In the United States there are currently three FDA-approved devices that are used as bridges to transplantation. None as yet are totally implantable, and, because of this need for transcutaneous connections, all share a common problem with infectious complications. Likewise, all share some tendency to thromboembolic complications as well as the expected possibility of mechanical device failure common to any man-made machine.

The Thoratec LVAD (Thoratec Corp., Pleasanton, CA) is an extracorporeal pump that takes blood from a large cannula placed in the left ventricular apex and propels it forward through an outflow cannula inserted into the ascending aorta. The pump itself sits in the paracorporeal position on the abdomen and is attached to a device console cart with wheels, allowing for limited ambulation. The extracorporeal nature of this pump allows it to be used for small adults for whom the intracorporeal pumps would be too large.

The Novacor LVAD (WorldHeart Inc., Oakland, CA) also takes blood from the left ventricular apex through a cannula and propels it into the ascending aorta through a second cannula. With this device the pump itself is placed in a surgically created pocket in the preperitoneal fascia in the abdomen. A drive line that connects to the power source is tunneled subcutaneously and usually exits in the right upper quadrant of the abdomen.

The HeartMate LVAD (Thoratec Corp., Pleasanton, CA) uses a configuration identical to that of the Novacor device (Fig. 217-2). Differences between the two have to do with the materials used and the tendency for thromboembolic complications. Both commonly lead to hospital discharge and an outpatient wait for a donor heart.

RESULTS   The use of these devices in the United States is limited mainly to patients with postcardiac surgery shock and those who are "bridged" to transplantation. Approximately 6000 patients per year receive support devices after cardiac surgery, with hospital survival

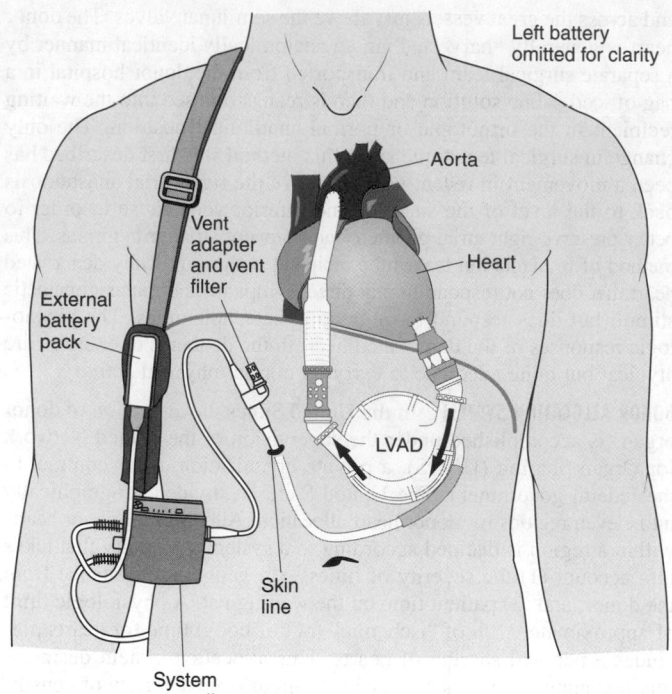

FIGURE 217-2   Diagram of HeartMate left ventricular assist device. (*Reprinted with permission from Thoratec Corp., Pleasanton, CA.*)

rates between 20 and 40%. Approximately 300 to 400 patients per year have devices placed as bridges to transplantation, with an overall discharge rate of 50 to 70% from implantation through transplantation.

GOALS   Future developments in this field can be expected in two directions. First, newer generations of the pumps will likely be smaller and simpler mechanically and, most important, totally implantable. Several much smaller devices, which use a mechanical propeller to provide axial, or non-pulsatile, flow of blood, are already in clinical trials. Second, use of the pumps as "permanent" (destination) therapy in patients with end-stage heart failure who are not considered eligible for transplantation will likely happen in the near future. In a randomized trial of long-term circulatory support with the HeartMate device in such patients, survival with the device was superior to continued medical management. FDA approval of the HeartMate device as permanent circulatory support for patients not eligible for transplantation was granted in 2002. Eventually it is hoped that improved assist devices will be accepted as valid alternatives to biologic replacement of the heart even in transplant-eligible patients and help to modify the supply/demand mismatch for cardiac replacement therapy.

FURTHER READING

BENIAMINOVITZ A et al: Prevention of rejection in cardiac transplantation by blockade of the interleukin-2 receptor with a monoclonal antibody. N Engl J Med 342:613, 2000

GARNIER JL et al: Treatment of post-transplant lymphomas with anti-B-cell monoclonal antibodies. Recent Results Cancer Res 159:113, 2002

HERTZ MI et al: The registry of the International Society for Heart and Lung Transplantation: Nineteenth official report—2002. J Heart Lung Transplant 21:950, 2002

HUNT SA et al: ACC/AHA Practice Guidelines: ACC/AHA Guidelines for the Evaluation and Management of Chronic Heart Failure in the Adult: A report of the American College of Cardiology/American Heart Association Task Force on Practice Guidelines. J Am Coll Cardiol 38:2101, 2001

ROSE EA et al: Long-term use of a left ventricular assist device for end-stage heart failure. N Engl J Med 345:1435, 2001

SCHNETZLER B et al: The role of percutaneous transluminal coronary angioplasty in heart transplant recipients. J Heart Lung Transplant 19:557, 2000

STEVENSON LW, KORMOS RL: Mechanical cardiac support 2000: Current applications and future trial design. Circulation 103:337, 2001

Congenital heart disease complicates ~1% of all live births. It occurs in about 4% of offspring of women with congenital heart disease. Substantial numbers of affected infants reach adulthood because of successful medical and/or surgical management, or because the alteration caused in cardiovascular physiology is well tolerated.

ETIOLOGY Congenital cardiovascular malformations are generally the result of aberrant embryonic development of a normal structure, or failure of such a structure to progress beyond an early stage of embryonic or fetal development. Malformations are due to complex multifactorial genetic and environmental causes. Recognized chromosomal aberrations and mutations of single genes account for <10% of all cardiac malformations (Table 218-1).

The presence of a cardiac malformation as one component of the multiple system involvement in Down's, Turner's, and the trisomy 13-15(D1) and 17-18 (E) syndromes may be anticipated in occasional pregnancies by detection of abnormal chromosomes in fetal cells obtained from amniotic fluid or chorionic villus biopsy. Identification in such cells of the enzyme disorders characteristic of Hurler's syndrome, homocystinuria, or type II glycogen storage disease may also allow one to predict cardiac disease.

PATHOPHYSIOLOGY The anatomic and physiologic changes in the heart and circulation due to any specific congenital cardiocirculatory lesion are not static but rather progress from prenatal life to adulthood. Thus, malformations that are benign or escape detection in childhood may become clinically significant in the adult. For example, the functionally normal, congenitally bicuspid aortic valve may thicken and calcify with time, resulting in significant aortic stenosis; or the well-tolerated left-to-right shunt of an atrial septal defect may not result in cardiac decompensation, with or without pulmonary hypertension, until the fourth or fifth decade.

Pulmonary Hypertension This is a common companion of many congenital cardiac lesions, and the status of the pulmonary vascular bed is often the principal determinant of the clinical manifestations, the course, and the feasibility of surgical repair. Increases in pulmonary arterial pressure result from elevation of pulmonary blood flow and/or resistance, the latter due sometimes to an increase in vascular tone but usually the result of obstructive, obliterative structural changes within the pulmonary vascular bed. Because pulmonary vascular obstructive disease can be the determining factor in assessing the advisability of operation, it is important to quantitate and compare pulmonary to systemic flows and resistances in patients with severe pulmonary hypertension. The causes of pulmonary vascular obstructive disease are unknown, although increased pulmonary blood flow, increased pulmonary arterial blood pressure, elevated pulmonary venous pressure, erythrocytosis, systemic hypoxemia, acidosis, and the bronchial circulation have been implicated. The designation *Eisenmenger syndrome* is applied to patients with a large communication between the two circulations at the aortopulmonary, ventricular, or atrial levels and bidirectional or predominantly right-to-left shunts because of high-resistance and obstructive pulmonary hypertension. No specific treatment has proved beneficial for obstructive pulmonary vascular disease, although newer pulmonary vasodilators and both single lung transplantation with intracardiac defect repair and total heart-lung transplantation are under investigation (Chaps. 217 and 248).

Erythrocytosis The chronic hypoxemia in cyanotic congenital heart disease results in *erythrocytosis* due to increased erythropoietin production (Chap. 31). The commonly used term *polycythemia* is a misnomer because white cell counts are normal and platelet counts are normal to decreased. Cyanotic patients with erythrocytosis may have compensated or decompensated hematocrits. Compensated erythrocytosis with iron-replete equilibrium hematocrits rarely result in symp-

toms of hyperviscosity at hematocrits <65% and occasionally not even with hematocrits ≥70%. Therapeutic phlebotomy is rarely required in compensated erythrocytosis. In contrast, patients with decompensated erythrocytosis fail to establish equilibrium with unstable, rising hematocrits and recurrent hyperviscosity symptoms. Therapeutic phlebotomy, a two-edged sword, allows temporary relief of symptoms but begets instability of the hematocrit and compounds the problem by iron depletion. Iron-deficiency symptoms are usually indistinguishable from those of hyperviscosity; progressive symptoms after recurrent phlebotomy are usually due to iron depletion with hypochromic microcytosis. Iron depletion results in a larger number of smaller (microcytic) hypochromic red cells that are less capable of carrying oxygen and less deformable in the microcirculation. Because these microcytes are less deformable in the microcirculation and there are more of them relative to the plasma volume, the viscosity is greater than for an equivalent hematocrit with fewer, larger, iron-replete, deformable cells. As such, iron-depleted erythrocytosis results in increasing symptoms due to decreased oxygen delivery to the tissues.

Hemostasis is abnormal in cyanotic congenital heart disease, due in part to the increased blood volume and engorged capillaries, abnormalities in platelet function and sensitivity to aspirin or nonsteroidal anti-inflammatory agents, and abnormalities of the extrinsic and intrinsic coagulation system. Oral contraceptives are contraindicated for cyanotic women because of the enhanced risk of vascular thrombosis.

The risk of stroke is greatest in children <4 years with cyanotic heart disease and iron deficiency, often with dehydration as an aggravating cause. In contrast, adults with cyanotic congenital heart disease do not appear to be at increased risk for stroke, unless there are excessive injudicious phlebotomies, inappropriate use of aspirin or anticoagulants, or the presence of atrial arrhythmias or infective endocarditis.

Symptoms of hyperviscosity can be produced in any cyanotic patient with erythrocytosis if dehydration causes a reduction of plasma volume. Phlebotomy, when required for symptoms of hyperviscosity not due to dehydration or iron deficiency, is a simple outpatient removal of 500 mL of blood over 45 min with isovolumetric replacement with isotonic saline (5% dextrose if congestive heart failure exists). Acute phlebotomy without volume replacement is contraindicated. Iron repletion in decompensated iron-depleted erythrocytosis ameliorates iron-deficiency symptoms but must be done gradually to avoid a sudden excessive rise in hematocrit and resultant hyperviscosity.

Pregnancy The physiologic alterations during normal gestation (Chap. 6) can create symptoms and physical findings that may be attributed erroneously to heart disease. Dyspnea due to the hormonal influence of progesterone and elevation of the diaphragm in association with peripheral edema and fatigability may be attributed inappropriately to heart failure. The jugular venous pulsations normally become more apparent after the twentieth week. Elevation of the diaphragm can cause basal rales (which disappear with deep breathing). Both ventricles are more easily palpated due to the normal increase in ventricular volumes and elevation of the diaphragm. Third heart sounds, already relatively frequent in normal nongravid young women, increase in frequency and intensity with pregnancy because of increased heart rate and volume of flow across the mitral and tricuspid valves. Midsystolic murmurs across the pulmonary outflow tract and supraclavicular systolic murmurs are caused by increased cardiac output. Venous hums and mammary souffles are usual during pregnancy.

These normal circulatory changes may impinge upon the woman's cardiac reserve. The mother is most at risk if she has a cardiovascular lesion associated with pulmonary vascular disease and pulmonary hypertension (e.g., Eisenmenger's physiology or mitral stenosis) or left

TABLE 218-1 *Syndromes with Associated Cardiovascular Involvement*

Syndrome (Genetic Locus)	Major Cardiovascular Manifestations	Major Noncardiac Abnormalities
HERITABLE AND POSSIBLY HERITABLE		
Ellis–van Creveld	Single atrium or atrial septal defect	Chondrodystrophic dwarfism, nail dysplasia, polydactyly
TAR (thrombocytopenia-absent radius)	Atrial septal defect, tetralogy of Fallot	Radial aplasia or hypoplasia, thrombocytopenia
Holt-Oram (12q21–q3)	Atrial septal defect (other defects common)	Skeletal upper limb defect, hypoplasia of clavicles
Kartagener	Dextrocardia	Situs inversus, sinusitis, bronchiectasis
Laurence-Moon-Biedl-Bardet	Variable defects	Retinal pigmentation, obesity, polydactyly
Noonan (12q24)	Pulmonic valve dysplasia, cardiomyopathy (usually hypertrophic)	Webbed neck, pectus excavatum, cryptorchidism
Tuberous sclerosis (type 1—4q); type 2—16p)	Rhabdomyoma, cardiomyopathy	Phakomatosis, bone lesions, hamartomatous skin lesions
Multiple lentigines (LEOPARD) syndrome	Pulmonic stenosis	Basal cell nevi, broad facies, rib anomalies, deafness
Rubenstein-Taybi (16p13.3)	Patent ductus arteriosus (others)	Broad thumbs and toes, hypoplastic maxilla, slanted palpebral fissures
Familial deafness	Arrhythmias, sudden death	Sensorineural deafness
Weber-Osler-Rendu (9q33)	Arteriovenous fistulas (lung, liver, mucous membranes)	Multiple telangiectasias
Apert (10q26)	Ventricular septal defect	Craniosynostosis, midfacial hypoplasia, syndactyly
Crouzon (10q26, 4p16.3)	Patent ductus arteriosus, aortic coarctation	Ptosis with shallow orbits, craniosynostosis, maxillary hypoplasia
Hypertrophic cardiomyopathy (locus heterogeneity, 14q11.2–12, 1q32, 15q22, 11p11.2, etc.)	Asymmetric septal hypertrophy	Family history of sudden death
Incontinentia pigmenti	Patent ductus arteriosus	Irregular pigmented skin lesions, patchy alopecia, hypodontia
Alagille (arteriohepatic dysplasia) (20p12)	Peripheral pulmonic stenosis, pulmonic stenosis	Biliary hypoplasia, vertebral anomalies, prominent forehead, deep-set eyes
Catch-22 (DiGeorge) (22q11)	Interrupted aortic arch, tetralogy of Fallot, truncus arteriosus	Thymic hypoplasia or aplasia, parathyroid aplasia or hypoplasia, abnormal facies
Shprintzen (velocardiofacial) (22q11.2)	Ventricular septal defect, tetralogy of Fallot, right aortic arch	Cleft palate, prominent nose, slender hands, learning disability
Williams (7q11.23)	Supravalvular aortic stenosis, peripheral pulmonic stenosis	Mental deficiency, elfin facies, loquacious personality, hoarse voice
Long QT (Jervell and Lange-Nielsen, Romano-Ward) (11p15.5, 7q35, 3p21, 21q22)	Long QT interval, ventricular arrhythmias	Family history of sudden death, congenital deafness (not in Romano-Ward)
Friedreich's ataxia (9q)	Hypertrophic or dilated cardiomyopathy; conduction defects	Ataxia, speech defect, degeneration of spinal cord dorsal columns
Muscular dystrophy	Cardiomyopathy	Pseudohypertrophy of calf muscles, weakness of trunk and proximal limb muscles
Cystic fibrosis (7q)	Cor pulmonale	Pancreatic insufficiency, malabsorption, chronic lung disease
Sickle cell anemia	Cardiomyopathy, mitral regurgitation	Hemoglobin SS
Conradi-Hunermann	Ventricular septal defect, patent ductus arteriosus	Asymmetrical limb shortness, early punctate mineralization, large skin pores
Cockayne	Accelerated atherosclerosis	Cachectic dwarfism, retinal pigment abnormalities, photosensitivity dermatitis
Progeria	Accelerated atherosclerosis	Premature aging, alopecia, atrophy of subcutaneous fat, skeletal hypoplasia
CONNECTIVE TISSUE DISORDERS		
Cutis laxa	Peripheral pulmonic stenosis	Generalized disruption of elastic fibers, diminished skin resilience, hernias
Ehlers-Danlos (2q31)	Arterial dilatation and rupture, mitral regurgitation	Hyperextensible joints, hyperelastic and friable
Marfan (15q21.1)	Aortic dilatation, aortic and mitral incompetence	Gracile habitus, arachnodactyly with hyperextensibility, lens subluxation
Osteogenesis imperfecta (4.17)	Aortic incompetence	Fragile bones, blue sclerae
Pseudoxanthoma elasticum	Peripheral and coronary arterial disease	Degeneration of elastic fibers in skin, retinal angioid streaks
INBORN ERRORS OF METABOLISM		
Pompe disease	Glycogen storage disease of heart	Acid maltase deficiency, muscular weakness
Homocystinuria	Aortic and pulmonary arterial dilatation, intravascular thrombosis	Cystathionine synthetase deficiency, lens subluxation, osteoporosis
Mucopolysaccharidoses: Hurler; Hunter	Multivalvular and coronary and great artery disease, cardiomyopathy	Hurler: Deficiency of α-L-iduronidase, corneal clouding, coarse features, growth and mental retardation Hunter: Deficiency of L-iduranosulfate sulfatase, coarse facies, clear cornea, growth and mental retardation

(continued)

TABLE 218-1—(Continued)

Syndrome (Genetic Locus)	Major Cardiovascular Manifestations	Major Noncardiac Abnormalities
Morquio; Scheie; Maroteaux-Lamy	Aortic regurgitation	Morquio: Deficiency of *N*-acetylhexosamine sulfate sulfatase, cloudy cornea, severe bone changes involving vertebrae and epiphyses Scheie: Deficiency of α-L-iduronidase, cloudy cornea, normal intelligence, peculiar facies Maroteaux-Lamy: Deficiency of arylsulfatase B, cloudy cornea, osseous changes
CHROMOSOMAL ABNORMALITIES		
Trisomy 21 (Down syndrome)	Endocardial cushion defect, atrial or ventricular septal defect, tetralogy of Fallot	Hypotonia, hyperextensible joints, mongoloid facies, mental retardation
Trisomy 13 (D)	Ventricular septal defect, patent ductus arteriosus, double-outlet right ventricle	Single midline intracerebral ventricle with midfacial defects, polydactyly, nail changes, mental retardation
Trisomy 18 (E)	Congenital polyvalvular dysplasia, ventricular septal defect, patent ductus	Clenched hand, short sternum, low arch dermal ridge pattern on fingertips, mental retardation
Cri du chat (short-arm deletion-5)	Ventricular septal defect	Cat cry, microcephaly, antimongoloid slant of palpebral fissures, mental retardation
XO (Turner)	Coarctation of aorta, bicuspid aortic valve, aortic dilatation	Short female, broad chest, lymphedema, webbed neck
XXXY and XXXXX	Patent ductus arteriosus	XXXY: Hypogenitalism, mental retardation, radial-ulnar synostosis XXXXX: Small hands, incurving of fifth fingers, mental retardation
SPORADIC DISORDERS		
VATER association	Ventricular septal defect	Vertebral anomalies, anal atresia, tracheo-esophageal fistula, radial and renal anomalies
CHARGE association	Tetralogy of Fallot (other defects common)	Colobomas, choanal atresia, mental and growth deficiency, genital and ear anomalies
Cornelia de Lange	Ventricular septal defect	Micromelia, synophrys, mental and growth deficiency
TERATOGENIC DISORDERS		
Rubella	Patent ductus arteriosus, pulmonic valvular and/or arterial stenosis, atrial septal defect	Cataracts, deafness, microcephaly
Alcohol	Ventricular septal defect (other defects)	Microcephaly, growth and mental deficiency, short palpebral fissures, smooth philtrum, thin upper lip
Dilantin	Pulmonic stenosis, aortic stenosis, coarctation, patent ductus arteriosus	Hypertelorism, growth and mental deficiency, short phalanges, bowed upper lip
Thalidomide	Variable	Phocomelia
Lithium	Ebstein's anomaly, tricuspid atresia	None

Source: Modified from WF Friedman and N Silverman: Congenital heart disease in infancy and childhood, in E Braunwald et al (eds), *Heart Disease*, 6th ed. Philadelphia, Saunders, 1998; with permission.

ventricular (LV) outflow tract obstruction (e.g., aortic stenosis) but also risks death with any malformation that may cause heart failure or a hemodynamically important arrhythmia (Table 218-2). The fetus is most at risk in the presence of maternal cyanosis, heart failure, or pulmonary hypertension. Women with aortic coarctation or Marfan's syndrome are at risk for aortic dissection. Patients with cyanotic heart disease, pulmonary hypertension, or Marfan's syndrome should not become pregnant; those with correctable lesions should be counseled about the risks of pregnancy with an uncorrected malformation versus repair and later pregnancy. The effect of pregnancy in postoperative patients depends on the outcome of the repair including the presence and severity of residua, sequelae, or complications. Contraception is an important topic with such patients. Tubal ligation should be considered in those in whom pregnancy is strictly contraindicated.

INFECTIVE ENDOCARDITIS (See also Chap. 109) Routine antimicrobial prophylaxis is recommended for most patients with congenital heart disease whether operated on or not. Antibiotic prophylaxis is not uniformly effective. Nonetheless, it is recommended for all dental procedures, gastrointestinal and genitourinary surgery, and diagnostic procedures such as proctosigmoidoscopy and cystoscopy. The clinical and bacteriologic profile of infective endocarditis in patients with congenital heart disease has changed with the advent of intracardiac surgery and of prosthetic devices. Two major predisposing causes of infective endocarditis are a susceptible cardiovascular substrate and a source of bacteremia. Prophylaxis includes both chemotherapeutic (antimicrobial) and nonchemotherapeutic (hygienic) measures. Meticulous dental and skin care is required.

TABLE 218-2 *Tolerance of Pregnancy by Patients with Various Congenital Cardiac Malformations*

Well Tolerated	Intermediate Effect	Poorly Tolerated
NYHA class I	NYHA class II–III	NHYA class IV
Left-right shunts without PHTN	Repaired transposition of the great arteries	Right-left shunt, unrepaired cyanotic heart disease
Aortic or mitral valvular regurgitation (mild-moderate)	Fontan repairs	PHTN and/or pulmonary vascular disease (e.g., Eisenmenger's, "primary PHTN")
Pulmonic or tricuspid regurgitation (if low pressure, even severe)	Aortic or mitral stenosis (moderate)	Aortic or mitral stenosis (severe)
Pulmonic stenosis (mild-moderate)	Ebstein's anomaly	Pulmonic stenosis (severe)
Well-repaired tetralogy of Fallot		Marfan's or aortic coarctation

Note: NYHA, New York Heart Association; PHTN, pulmonary hypertension.

EXERCISE Advice on athletics and exercise is governed by the nature of the exercise and by the type and severity of the congenital cardiovascular lesion. Patients with lesions characterized by LV outflow tract obstruction, if more than mild to moderate, or pulmonary vascular disease, risk syncope or even sudden death. In Fallot's tetralogy, isotonic exercise–induced decrease in systemic vascular resistance relative to the right ventricular (RV) outflow obstruction augments the right-to-left shunt, increases hypoxemia, and causes an increase in subjective breathlessness due to the response of the respiratory center to the changes in blood gases and pH.

INSURABILITY AND EMPLOYABILITY Most patients with congenital heart disease must pay significantly more than standard life insurance rates, assuming their anomaly places them in a category that companies have determined is eligible for insurance. A paucity of actuarial survival data beyond adolescence for persons with most congenital cardiac lesions that have undergone operative repair has made it difficult to convince insurance companies to offer reasonable cost insurance even to individual patients whose long-term prognosis is quite good.

Employment is affected by the patient's physical capacity relative to the type of job sought. Job discrimination exists, often because the employer is reluctant to accept health insurance responsibilities. Eligibility for some occupations is governed by public safety regulations, e.g., airline pilots, bus drivers.

SPECIFIC CARDIAC DEFECTS

Table 218-3 provides a classification of cardiac anomalies that recognizes the general categories of clinical presentation, functional consequences, and site of origin of congenital defects.

Categorizing the defect(s) in an individual patient requires an answer to a number of basic questions. Is the patient acyanotic or cyanotic? Is pulmonary arterial blood flow increased or not? Does the malformation originate in the left or right side of the heart? Which is the dominant ventricle? Is pulmonary hypertension present or not? With the above information as a foundation, the use of more refined

---

TABLE 218-3 *Classification of Congenital Heart Disease*

ACYANOTIC WITH LEFT-TO-RIGHT SHUNT

I. Atrial level shunt
   A. Atrial septal defect
      1. Ostium primum
      2. Ostium secundum
      3. Sinus venosus
   B. Atrial septal defect with mitral stenosis (Lutembacher's syndrome)
   C. Partial anomalous pulmonary venous connection
II. Ventricular level shunt
   A. Ventricular septal defect
      1. Inlet septum
      2. Muscular septum
      3. Perimembranous septum
      4. Infundibular septum
   B. Ventricular septal defect with aortic regurgitation
   C. Ventricular septal defect with left ventricular to right atrial shunt

III. Aortic root to right heart shunt
   A. Ruptured sinus of Valsalva aneurysm
   B. Coronary arteriovenous fistula
   C. Anomalous origin of the left coronary artery from the pulmonary trunk
IV. Aortopulmonary level shunt
   A. Aortopulmonary window
   B. Patent ductus arteriosus
V. Multiple level shunts
   A. Complete common atrioventricular canal
   B. Ventricular septal defect with atrial septal defect
   C. Ventricular septal defect with patent ductus arteriosus

ACYANOTIC WITHOUT A SHUNT

I. Left heart malformations
   A. Congenital obstruction to left atrial inflow
      1. Pulmonary vein stenosis
      2. Mitral stenosis
      3. Cor triatriatum
   B. Mitral regurgitation
      1. Atrioventricular septal (endocardial cushion)
      2. Congenitally corrected transposition of the great arteries
      3. Anomalous origin of the left coronary artery from the pulmonary trunk
      4. Miscellaneous (double-orifice mitral valve, congenital perforations, accessory commissures with anomalous chordal insertion, congenitally short or absent chordae, cleft posterior leaflet, parachute mitral valve, etc.)
   C. Primary dilated endocardial fibroelastosis

   D. Aortic stenosis
      1. Discrete subvalvular
      2. Valvular
      3. Supravalvular
   E. Aortic valve regurgitation
   F. Coarctation of the aorta
II. Right heart malformations
   A. Acyanotic Ebstein's anomaly of the tricuspid valve
   B. Pulmonic stenosis
      1. Subinfundibular
      2. Infundibular
      3. Valvular
      4. Supravalvular (stenosis of pulmonary artery and its branches)
   C. Congenital pulmonary valve regurgitation
   D. Idiopathic dilatation of the pulmonary trunk

CYANOTIC

I. Increased pulmonary blood flow
   A. Complete transposition of the great arteries
   B. Double-outlet right ventricle of the Taussig-Bing type
   C. Truncus arteriosus
   D. Total anomalous pulmonary venous connection
   E. Single ventricle without pulmonic stenosis
   F. Common atrium
   G. Tetralogy of Fallot with pulmonary atresia and increased collateral arterial flow
   H. Tricuspid atresia with large ventricular septal defect and no pulmonic stenosis
   I. Hypoplastic left heart (aortic atresia, mitral atresia)

II. Normal or decreased pulmonary blood flow
   A. Tricuspid atresia
   B. Ebstein's anomaly with right-to-left atrial shunt
   C. Pulmonary atresia with intact ventricular septum
   D. Pulmonic stenosis or atresia with ventricular septal defect (tetralogy of Fallot)
   E. Pulmonic stenosis with right-to-left atrial shunt
   F. Complete transposition of the great arteries with pulmonic stenosis
   G. Double-outlet right ventricle with pulmonic stenosis
   H. Single ventricle with pulmonic stenosis
   I. Pulmonary arteriovenous fistula
   J. Vena caval to left atrial communication

OTHER

I. Congenitally corrected transposition of the great arteries
II. The cardiac malpositions

III. Congenital complete heart block

Source: Modified from JK Perloff, *The Clinical Recognition of Congenital Heart Disease*, Philadelphia, Saunders, 1991.

diagnostic techniques such as transthoracic (precordial) and trans-esophageal echocardiography and Doppler imaging, magnetic resonance imaging, and/or hemodynamic study and angiocardiography leads to a precise anatomic and functional assessment.

ACYANOTIC CONGENITAL HEART DISEASE WITH A LEFT-TO-RIGHT SHUNT

ATRIAL SEPTAL DEFECT This common cardiac anomaly in adults occurs more frequently in females. The *sinus venosus* type occurs high in the atrial septum near the entry of the superior vena cava and is associated frequently with anomalous connection of pulmonary veins from the right lung to the junction of the superior vena cava and right atrium. *Ostium primum* anomalies are a form of atrioventricular septal defect that lie immediately adjacent to the atrioventricular valves, either of which may be deformed and incompetent. Ostium primum defects occur commonly in patients with Down's syndrome, although the more complex atrioventricular septal defects with a common atrioventricular valve and a posterior defect of the basal portion of the interventricular septum are more characteristic of this chromosomal defect. The most common atrial septal defect involves the fossa ovalis, is midseptal in location, and is of the *ostium secundum type*. This type of defect should not be confused with a *patent foramen ovale*. Anatomic obliteration of the foramen ovale ordinarily follows its functional closure soon after birth, but residual "probe patency" is a normal variant; atrial septal defect denotes a true deficiency of the atrial septum and implies functional and anatomic patency.

The magnitude of the left-to-right shunt through an atrial septal defect depends on the defect size, the diastolic properties of both ventricles, and the relative impedance in the pulmonary and systemic circulations. The left-to-right shunt causes diastolic overloading of the right ventricle and increased pulmonary blood flow.

Patients with atrial septal defect are usually asymptomatic in early life, although there may be some physical underdevelopment and an increased tendency for respiratory infections; cardiorespiratory symptoms occur in many older patients. Beyond the fourth decade, a significant number of patients develop atrial arrhythmias, pulmonary arterial hypertension, bidirectional and then right-to-left shunting of blood, and cardiac failure. Patients exposed to the chronic environmental hypoxia of high altitude tend to develop pulmonary hypertension at younger ages. In some older patients, left-to-right shunting across the defect increases as progressive systemic hypertension and/or coronary artery disease result in reduced compliance of the left ventricle.

Physical Examination Examination usually reveals a prominent right ventricular impulse and palpable pulmonary artery pulsation. The first heart sound is normal or split, with accentuation of the tricuspid valve closure sound. Increased flow across the pulmonic valve is responsible for a midsystolic pulmonary outflow murmur. The second heart sound is widely split and is relatively fixed in relation to respiration. A mid-diastolic rumbling murmur, loudest at the fourth intercostal space and along the left sternal border, reflects increased flow across the tricuspid valve. In patients with ostium primum defects, an apical thrill and holosystolic murmur indicate associated mitral or tricuspid incompetence or a ventricular septal defect.

The physical findings are altered when an increase in the pulmonary vascular resistance results in diminution of the left-to-right shunt. Both the pulmonary and tricuspid murmurs decrease in intensity, the pulmonic component of the second heart sound and a systolic ejection sound are accentuated, the two components of the second heart sound may fuse, and a diastolic murmur of pulmonic regurgitation appears. Cyanosis and clubbing accompany the development of a right-to-left shunt.

In adults with an atrial septal defect and atrial fibrillation, the physical findings may be confused with the findings of mitral stenosis with pulmonary hypertension because the tricuspid flow murmur and widely split second heart sound may be mistakenly thought to represent the diastolic murmur of mitral stenosis and the mitral "opening snap," respectively.

Electrocardiogram In patients with an ostium secundum defect, the electrocardiogram (ECG) usually shows right axis deviation and an rSr' pattern in the right precordial leads representing delayed posterobasal activation of the ventricular septum and enlargement of the RV outflow tract. An ectopic atrial pacemaker or first-degree heart block occurs occasionally in patients with defects of the sinus venosus type. In patients with an ostium primum defect, the RV conduction defect is characteristically accompanied by left axis deviation and by superior orientation and counterclockwise rotation of the QRS loop in the frontal plane. Varying degrees of RV and right atrial (RA) hypertrophy may occur with each type of defect, depending on the height of the pulmonary artery pressure. *Chest roentgenograms* reveal enlargement of the right atrium and right ventricle, dilatation of the pulmonary artery and its branches, and increased pulmonary vascular markings.

Echocardiogram This test shows pulmonary arterial and RV dilatation, and anterior systolic (paradoxical) or flat interventricular septal motion if a significant RV volume overload is present. The defect may be visualized directly from subcostal, right parasternal, or apical echocardiographic windows. In most institutions, two-dimensional echocardiography, supplemented by conventional or color Doppler flow examination, has supplanted cardiac catheterization as the confirmatory test for atrial septal defect. Transesophageal echocardiography is indicated if the transthoracic echocardiogram is ambiguous, which is often the case with sinus venosus defects. Cardiac catheterization is then performed if inconsistencies exist in the clinical data, if significant pulmonary hypertension or associated malformations are suspected, or if coronary artery disease is a possibility.

℞ TREATMENT

Operative repair, usually with a patch of pericardium or of prosthetic material, or percutaneous transcatheter device closure, ideally in children ages 3 to 6, should be advised for all patients with uncomplicated secundum atrial septal defects in whom there is significant left-to-right shunting, i.e., pulmonary-to-systemic flow ratios ~2.0:1.0. Excellent results may be anticipated, at low risk, even in patients >40 years, in the absence of pulmonary hypertension. Patients with ostium primum defects, cleft, deformed, and incompetent valves require repair in addition to patch closure of the atrial defect. Intraoperative transesophageal echocardiography is used to monitor the surgical results of atrioventricular valve repair. Closure should not be carried out in patients with small defects and trivial left-to-right shunts or in those with severe pulmonary vascular disease without a significant left-to-right shunt.

Patients with atrial septal defect of the sinus venosus or ostium secundum types rarely die before the fifth decade. During the fifth and sixth decades the incidence of progressive symptoms, often leading to severe disability, increases substantially. Medical management should include prompt treatment of respiratory tract infections, antiarrhythmic medications for atrial fibrillation or supraventricular tachycardia, and the usual measures for hypertension, coronary disease, or heart failure (Chap. 216), if these complications occur. The risk of infective endocarditis is quite low unless the defect is complicated by valvular regurgitation or has recently been repaired with a patch (Chap. 109).

VENTRICULAR SEPTAL DEFECT Defects of the ventricular septum are common as isolated defects and as one component of a combination of anomalies. The opening is usually single and situated in the membranous portion of the septum. The functional disturbance is dependent primarily on its size and on the status of the pulmonary vascular bed, rather than on the location of the defect. Only small or moderate-size defects are usually seen initially in adulthood as most patients with isolated large defects come to medical and, often, surgical attention very early in life.

A wide spectrum exists in the natural history of ventricular septal defect, ranging from spontaneous closure to congestive cardiac failure and death in early infancy. Within this spectrum is the possible development of pulmonary vascular obstruction, RV outflow tract obstruction, aortic regurgitation, and infective endocarditis. Spontaneous closure is more common in patients born with a small ventricular septal defect and occurs in early childhood in most patients.

Patients with large ventricular septal defects and pulmonary hypertension are those at greatest risk for developing pulmonary vascular obstruction. Thus, large defects should be corrected surgically early in life when pulmonary vascular disease is still reversible or not yet developed. In patients with severe pulmonary vascular obstruction (Eisenmenger syndrome), symptoms in adult life consist of exertional dyspnea, chest pain, syncope, and hemoptysis. The right-to-left shunt leads to cyanosis, clubbing, and erythrocytosis. In all patients, the degree to which pulmonary vascular resistance is elevated before operation is a critical factor determining prognosis. If the pulmonary vascular resistance is one-third or less of the systemic value, progression of pulmonary vascular disease after operation is unusual. However, if a moderate to severe increase in pulmonary vascular resistance exists preoperatively, either no change or a progression of pulmonary vascular disease is common postoperatively.

RV outflow tract obstruction develops in ~5 to 10% of patients who present in infancy with a moderate to large left-to-right shunt. With time, as subvalvular RV outflow tract obstruction progresses, the findings in these patients begin to resemble more closely those of the cyanotic tetralogy of Fallot.

In ~5% of patients, incompetence of the aortic valve results from insufficient cusp tissue or prolapse of the cusp through the interventricular defect; the aortic regurgitation then complicates and usually dominates the clinical course.

Two-dimensional *echocardiography* with conventional or color Doppler examination can usually define the number and location of defects in the ventricular septum and detect associated anomalies. Hemodynamic and angiographic study may be employed to assess the status of the pulmonary vascular bed and clarify details of the altered anatomy.

℞ TREATMENT

Surgery is not recommended for patients with normal pulmonary arterial pressures with small shunts (pulmonary-to-systemic flow ratios of <1.5 to 2.0:1.0). Operative correction is indicated when there is a moderate to large left-to-right shunt with a pulmonary-to-systemic flow ratio >1.5:1.0 or 2.0:1.0, in the absence of prohibitively high levels of pulmonary vascular resistance.

PATENT DUCTUS ARTERIOSUS The ductus arteriosus is a vessel leading from the bifurcation of the pulmonary artery to the aorta just distal to the left subclavian artery. Normally, the vascular channel is open in the fetus but closes immediately after birth. The flow across the ductus is determined by the pressure and resistance relationships between the systemic and pulmonary circulations and by the cross-sectional area and length of the ductus. In most adults with this anomaly, pulmonary pressures are normal and a gradient and shunt from aorta to pulmonary artery persist throughout the cardiac cycle, resulting in a characteristic thrill and a continuous "machinery" murmur with a late systolic accentuation at the upper left sternal edge. In adults who were born with a large left-to-right shunt through the ductus arteriosus, pulmonary vascular obstruction (Eisenmenger syndrome) with pulmonary hypertension, right-to-left shunting, and cyanosis have usually developed. Severe pulmonary vascular disease results in reversal of flow through the ductus; unoxygenated blood is shunted to the descending aorta; and the toes, but not the fingers, become cyanotic and clubbed, a finding termed *differential cyanosis*. The leading causes of death in adults with patent ductus are cardiac failure and infective endocarditis; occasionally severe pulmonary vascular obstruction may cause aneurysmal dilatation, calcification, and rupture of the ductus.

℞ TREATMENT

In the absence of severe pulmonary vascular disease and predominant left-to-right shunting of blood, the patent ductus should be surgically ligated or divided. Transcatheter closure using coils, buttons, plugs, and umbrellas has become commonplace for appropriately shaped defects. Thoracoscopic surgical approaches are considered experimental. Operation should be deferred for several months in patients treated successfully for infective endocarditis, because the ductus may remain somewhat edematous and friable.

AORTIC ROOT TO RIGHT HEART SHUNTS The three most common causes of aortic root to right heart shunts are congenital aneurysm of an aortic sinus of Valsalva with fistula, coronary arteriovenous fistula, and anomalous origin of the left coronary artery from the pulmonary trunk. *Aneurysm of an aortic sinus of Valsalva* consists of a separation or lack of fusion between the media of the aorta and the annulus of the aortic valve. Rupture usually occurs in the third or fourth decade of life; most often the aorticocardiac fistula is between the right coronary cusp and the right ventricle, but occasionally, when the noncoronary cusp is involved, the fistula drains into the right atrium. Abrupt rupture causes chest pain, bounding pulses, a continuous murmur accentuated in diastole, and volume overload of the heart. Diagnosis is confirmed by two-dimensional and Doppler echocardiographic studies; cardiac catheterization quantitates the left-to-right shunt, and thoracic aortography visualizes the fistula. Medical management is directed at cardiac failure, arrhythmias, or endocarditis. At operation, the aneurysm is closed and amputated, and the aortic wall is reunited with the heart, either by direct suture or with a prosthesis.

Coronary arteriovenous fistula, an unusual anomaly, consists of a communication between a coronary artery and another cardiac chamber, usually the coronary sinus, right atrium, or right ventricle. The shunt is usually of small magnitude, and myocardial blood flow is not usually compromised. Potential complications include infective endocarditis, thrombus formation with occlusion or distal embolization, rupture of an aneurysmal fistula, and rarely, pulmonary hypertension and congestive failure. A loud, superficial, continuous murmur at the lower or midsternal border usually prompts a further evaluation of asymptomatic patients. Doppler echocardiography demonstrates the site of drainage; if the site of origin is proximal, it may be detectable by two-dimensional echocardiography. Retrograde thoracic aortography or coronary arteriography permits identification of the size and anatomic features of the fistulous tract, which may be closed by suture or transcatheter obliteration.

The third anomaly causing a shunt from the aortic root to the right heart is *anomalous origin of the left coronary artery from the pulmonary artery*. Myocardial infarction and fibrosis commonly lead to death within the first year, though up to 20% of patients survive to adolescence and beyond without surgical correction. The diagnosis is supported by the ECG findings of an anterolateral myocardial infarction. Operative management of adults consists of coronary artery bypass with an internal mammary artery graft or saphenous vein–coronary artery graft.

ACYANOTIC CONGENITAL HEART DISEASE WITHOUT A SHUNT

CONGENITAL AORTIC STENOSIS Malformations that cause obstruction to LV outflow include congenital valvular aortic stenosis, discrete subaortic stenosis, supravalvular aortic stenosis, and hypertrophic obstructive cardiomyopathy (Chap. 221).

Valvular Aortic Stenosis This malformation occurs three to four times more often in males than in females. The congenital bicuspid aortic valve, which is not necessarily stenotic, is one of the most common congenital malformations of the heart, although it may go undetected in early life. Because bicuspid valves may become stenotic with time or be the site of the infective endocarditis, the lesion may be difficult to distinguish in adults from acquired rheumatic or degenerative calcific aortic stenosis.

The dynamics of blood flow associated with a congenitally deformed, rigid aortic valve commonly lead to thickening of the cusps and, in later life, to calcification. Hemodynamically significant obstruction causes concentric hypertrophy of the LV wall. The ascending aorta is often dilated, misnamed "poststenotic" dilatation; this is due to histologic abnormalities similar to those in Marfan syndrome, and may result in aortic dissection. →*The clinical manifestations and hemodynamic abnormalities are discussed in Chap. 219.*

℞ TREATMENT

The medical management of congenital valvular aortic stenosis includes prophylaxis against infective endocarditis and, in patients with diminished cardiac reserve, the administration of digitalis and diuretics and sodium restriction while awaiting operation. A dilated aortic root may require beta blockers. If severe aortic stenosis is present, strenuous physical activity should be avoided even when the patient is asymptomatic, and participation in competitive sports should probably be restricted in patients with milder degrees of obstruction. Aortic valve replacement is indicated in adults with critical obstruction, i.e., with an aortic valve area <0.5 cm^2/m^2, with symptoms secondary to LV dysfunction or myocardial ischemia, or with hemodynamic evidence of LV dysfunction. In asymptomatic children or adolescents or young adults with critical aortic stenosis without valvular calcification or these features, aortic balloon valvuloplasty is often useful (Chap. 229). If surgery is contraindicated in older patients because of a complicating medical problem such as malignancy or renal or hepatic failure, balloon valvuloplasty may provide short-term improvement. It may serve as a bridge to aortic valve replacement in patients with severe heart failure.

Subaortic Stenosis The most common form of subaortic stenosis is the *idiopathic hypertrophic* variety, also termed *hypertrophic cardiomyopathy*, which is present at birth in about one-third of the patients and is discussed in Chap. 221. In contrast, both clinically and physiologically, the *discrete* form of subaortic stenosis resembles valvular aortic stenosis. The lesion usually consists of a membranous diaphragm or fibrous ring encircling the LV outflow tract just beneath the base of the aortic valve. Echocardiography demonstrates the subaortic obstruction; Doppler studies show turbulence proximal to the aortic valve and also detect and quantitate the pressure gradient and severity of aortic regurgitation. Treatment consists of excision of the membrane or fibrous ridge.

Supravalvular Aortic Stenosis This anomaly consists of a localized or diffuse narrowing of the ascending aorta originating just above the level of the coronary arteries at the superior margin of the sinuses of Valsalva. In contrast to other forms of aortic stenosis, the coronary arteries are subjected to elevated systolic pressures from the left ventricle, are often dilated and tortuous, and are susceptible to premature atherosclerosis. In most patients a genetic defect for the anomaly is located in the same chromosomal subunit as elastin on chromosome 7.

COARCTATION OF THE AORTA Narrowing or constriction of the lumen of the aorta may occur anywhere along its length but is most common distal to the origin of the left subclavian artery near the insertion of the ligamentum arteriosum. Coarctation occurs in ~7% of patients with congenital heart disease, is twice as common in males as in females, and is most frequent in patients with gonadal dysgenesis. Clinical manifestations depend on the site and extent of obstruction and the presence of associated cardiac anomalies, most commonly a bicuspid aortic valve. Aneurysmal arterial dilatation of the circle of Willis produces a high risk of sudden rupture and death.

Most children and young adults with isolated, discrete coarctation are asymptomatic. Headache, epistaxis, cold extremities, and claudication with exercise may occur, and attention is usually directed to the cardiovascular system when a heart murmur or hypertension in the upper extremities and absence, marked diminution, or delayed pulsations in the femoral arteries are detected on physical examination.

Enlarged and pulsatile collateral vessels may be palpated in the intercostal spaces anteriorly, in the axillae, or posteriorly in the interscapular area. The upper extremities and thorax may be more developed than the lower extremities. A midsystolic murmur over the anterior part of the chest, back, and spinous processes may become continuous if the lumen is narrowed sufficiently to result in a high-velocity jet across the lesion throughout the cardiac cycle. Additional systolic and continuous murmurs over the lateral thoracic wall may reflect increased flow through dilated and tortuous collateral vessels. The ECG usually reveals LV hypertrophy. Roentgenograms may show a dilated left subclavian artery high on the left mediastinal border and a dilated ascending aorta. Indentation of the aorta at the site of coarctation and pre- and poststenotic dilatation (the "3" sign) along the left paramediastinal shadow are almost pathognomonic. Notching of the ribs, an important radiographic sign, is due to erosion by dilated collateral vessels. Two-dimensional echocardiography from para- or suprasternal windows identifies the site and length of coarctation, while Doppler studies record and quantitate the pressure gradient. Transesophageal echocardiography and magnetic resonance imaging or three-dimensional computed tomography allow visualization of the length and severity of the obstruction and the associated collateral arteries. In adults, cardiac catheterization is indicated primarily to evaluate the coronary arteries.

The chief hazards result from severe hypertension and include the development of cerebral aneurysms and hemorrhage, dissection and/or rupture of the aorta, premature coronary arteriosclerosis, LV failure, and infective endocarditis.

℞ TREATMENT

Treatment is usually surgical; resection and end-to-end anastomosis or subclavian flap angioplasty are used commonly, although it may be necessary to use a tubular graft, patch, or bypass conduit if the narrowed segment is long. Systemic hypertension postoperatively, in the absence of residual coarctation, appears to be related to the duration of preoperative hypertension. Percutaneous balloon dilatation is controversial in native unoperated aortic coarctation but commonly successful for postsurgical recoarctation, often with deployment of a stent.

PULMONARY STENOSIS WITH INTACT VENTRICULAR SEPTUM Obstruction to RV outflow may be localized to the supravalvular, valvular, or subvalvular levels or occur at a combination of these sites. Multiple sites of narrowing of the peripheral pulmonary arteries are a feature of *rubella embryopathy* and may occur with both the familial and sporadic forms of supravalvular aortic stenosis. Valvular pulmonic stenosis is the most common form of isolated RV obstruction.

The severity of the obstructing lesion, rather than the site of narrowing, is the most important determinant of the clinical course. In the presence of a normal cardiac output, a peak systolic transvalvular pressure gradient between 50 and 80 mmHg is considered to be moderate stenosis; levels below and above that range are classified as mild and severe, respectively. Patients with mild pulmonic stenosis are generally asymptomatic and demonstrate little or no progression in the severity of obstruction with age. In patients with more significant stenosis, the severity may increase with time. Symptoms vary with the degree of obstruction. Fatigue, dyspnea, RV failure, and syncope may limit the activity of older patients, in whom moderate or severe obstruction may prevent an augmentation of cardiac output with exercise. In patients with severe obstruction, the systolic pressure in the right ventricle may exceed that in the left ventricle, since the ventricular septum is intact. RV ejection is prolonged with moderate or severe stenosis, and the sound of pulmonary valve closure is delayed and soft. RV hypertrophy reduces the compliance of that chamber, and a forceful RA contraction is necessary to augment RV filling.

A fourth heart sound, prominent *a* waves in the jugular venous pulse, and, occasionally, presystolic pulsations of the liver reflect vigorous atrial contraction. The clinical diagnosis is supported by a left parasternal lift and harsh systolic crescendo-decrescendo murmur and thrill at the upper left sternal border, typically preceded by a systolic ejection sound, if the obstruction is valvular. The holosystolic decrescendo murmur of tricuspid regurgitation may accompany severe pulmonic stenosis, especially in the presence of congestive heart failure. Cyanosis usually reflects right-to-left shunting through a patent foramen ovale or atrial septal defect. In patients with supravalvular or peripheral pulmonary arterial stenosis, the murmur is systolic or continuous and is best heard over the area of narrowing, with radiation to the peripheral lung fields.

The ECG may be helpful in assessing the degree of RV obstruction. In mild cases, the ECG is often normal, whereas moderate and severe stenoses are associated with right axis deviation and RV hypertrophy. A ventricular strain pattern, as well as high-amplitude P waves in leads II and V_1, indicating RA enlargement, are associated with severe stenosis. The chest roentgenogram with mild or moderate pulmonic stenosis often shows a heart of normal size and normal vascularity of the lungs. In the presence of valvular stenosis, dilatation of the main and left pulmonary arteries may be evident, in part poststenotic and in part due to intrinsic tissue weakness. With severe obstruction and resultant RV failure, RA and RV enlargement are generally evident. The pulmonary vascularity may be reduced with severe stenosis, RV failure, and/or a right-to-left shunt at the atrial level. Two-dimensional echocardiography visualizes pulmonary valve morphology; the outflow tract pressure gradient can be estimated by Doppler ultrasonography.

℞ TREATMENT

The cardiac catheter technique of balloon valvuloplasty (Chap. 212) is usually effective. Direct surgical relief of moderate and severe obstruction may be accomplished at a low risk. Multiple stenoses of the peripheral pulmonary arteries are usually inoperable, but narrowing of a single branch or at the bifurcation of the main pulmonary trunk may be surgically corrected or undergo balloon dilatation and stenting.

CYANOTIC CONGENITAL HEART DISEASE WITH INCREASED PULMONARY BLOOD FLOW

COMPLETE TRANSPOSITION OF THE GREAT ARTERIES In this condition the aorta arises from the right ventricle to the right of and anterior to the pulmonary artery, which emerges from the left ventricle (Fig. 218-1, *left panel*). This results in two separate and parallel circulations, and some communication between them must exist after birth to sustain life. Most patients have an interatrial communication, two-thirds have a patent ductus arteriosus, and about one-third have an associated ven-

FIGURE 218-1 Complete transposition of the great arteries is depicted in the left panel. The aorta arises from the right ventricle and the pulmonary artery from the left ventricle. The only mixing between the two circulations occurs across a patent foramen ovale. In the right panel, the tetralogy of Fallot drawing illustrates the two most important anatomic findings, a large ventricular septal defect and RV outflow tract obstruction. A right-to-left shunt is shown across the ventricular septum.

tricular septal defect. Transposition is more common in males and accounts for ~10% of cyanotic heart disease.

The course is determined by the degree of tissue hypoxia, the ability of each ventricle to sustain an increased work load in the presence of reduced coronary arterial oxygenation, the nature of the associated cardiovascular anomalies, and the status of the pulmonary vascular bed. Pulmonary vascular obstruction develops by 1 to 2 years of age in patients with an associated large ventricular septal defect or large patent ductus arteriosus in the absence of obstruction to LV outflow.

℞ TREATMENT

The balloon or blade catheter or surgical creation or enlargement of an interatrial communication in the neonate is the simplest procedure for providing increased intracardiac mixing of systemic and pulmonary venous blood. Systemic–pulmonary artery anastomosis may be indicated in the patient with severe obstruction to LV outflow and diminished pulmonary blood flow. Intracardiac repair may be accomplished by rearranging the venous returns (intraatrial switch, i.e., Mustard or Senning operation) so that the systemic venous blood is directed to the mitral valve and thence to the left ventricle and pulmonary artery, while the pulmonary venous blood is diverted through the tricuspid valve and right ventricle to the aorta. The late survival after these repairs is good, but late sudden death is the most worrisome feature. Preferably, this malformation is corrected in infancy by transposing both coronary arteries to the posterior artery and transecting, contraposing, and anastomosing the aorta and pulmonary arteries (arterial switch operation). For those patients with a ventricular septal defect in whom it is necessary to bypass a severely obstructed LV outflow tract, corrective operation employs an intracardiac ventricular baffle and extracardiac prosthetic conduit to replace the pulmonary artery (Rastelli procedure).

SINGLE VENTRICLE This is a family of complex lesions with both atrioventricular valves or a common atrioventricular valve opening to a single ventricular chamber. Associated anomalies include abnormal great artery positional relationships, pulmonic valvular or subvalvular stenosis, and subaortic stenosis.

Survival to adulthood depends on a relatively normal pulmonary blood flow, yet normal pulmonary resistance, and good ventricular function. Modifications of the Fontan approach are generally applied to carefully selected patients with creation of a pathway(s) from the systemic veins to the pulmonary arteries.

CYANOTIC CONGENITAL HEART DISEASE WITH DECREASED PULMONARY BLOOD FLOW

TRICUSPID ATRESIA This malformation is characterized by atresia of the tricuspid valve, an interatrial communication, and, frequently, hypoplasia of the right ventricle and pulmonary artery. The clinical picture is usually dominated by severe cyanosis due to obligatory admixture of systemic and pulmonary venous blood in the left ventricle. The ECG characteristically shows RA enlargement, left axis deviation, and LV hypertrophy.

Atrial septostomy and palliative operations to increase pulmonary blood flow, often by anastomosis of a systemic artery or vein to a pulmonary artery, may allow survival to the second or third decade. A Fontan atriopulmonary or total cavopulmonary connection may then allow functional correction in those patients with normal or low pulmonary arterial resistance pressure and good LV function.

EBSTEIN'S ANOMALY Characterized by a downward displacement of the tricuspid valve into the right ventricle, due to anomalous attachment of the tricuspid leaflets, the Ebstein tricuspid valve tissue is dysplastic and results in tricuspid regurgitation. The abnormally situated tricuspid orifice produces an "atrialized" portion of the right ventricle lying between the atrioventricular ring and the origin of the valve, which is continuous with the RA chamber. Often the right ventricle is hypoplastic. Although the clinical manifestations are variable, some patients come to initial attention because of progressive cyanosis from right-to-left atrial shunting, or symptoms due to tricuspid regurgitation and RV dysfunction, or paroxysmal atrial tachyarrhythmias with or without atrioventricular bypass tracts ("WPW" syndrome). Diagnostic findings by two-dimensional echocardiography include the abnormal positional relation between the tricuspid and mitral valves with apical displacement of the septal tricuspid leaflet. Tricuspid regurgitation is quantitated by Doppler examination. Surgical approaches include prosthetic replacement of the tricuspid valve when the leaflets are tethered or repair of the native valve.

TETRALOGY OF FALLOT The four components of the tetralogy of Fallot are malaligned ventricular septal defect, obstruction to RV outflow, aortic override of the ventricular septal defect, and RV hypertrophy (Fig. 218-1, *right panel*).

The severity of RV outflow obstruction determines the clinical presentation. The severity of hypoplasia of the RV outflow tract varies from mild to complete (pulmonary atresia). Pulmonary valve stenosis and supravalvular and peripheral pulmonary arterial obstruction may coexist; rarely there is unilateral absence of a pulmonary artery (usually the left). A right-sided aortic arch and descending aorta occur in ~25% of patients with tetralogy.

The relationship between the resistance of blood flow from the ventricles into the aorta and into the pulmonary vessels plays a major role in determining the hemodynamic and clinical picture. Thus, the severity of obstruction to RV outflow is of fundamental significance. When the obstruction is severe, the pulmonary blood flow is reduced markedly, and a large volume of desaturated systemic venous blood is shunted from right to left across the ventricular septal defect. Severe cyanosis and erythrocytosis occur, and symptoms and sequelae of systemic hypoxemia are prominent. In many infants and children the obstruction is mild but progressive.

The ECG ordinarily shows RV and, less often, RA hypertrophy. Radiologic examination characteristically reveals a normal-sized, boot-shaped heart (*coeur en sabot*) with prominence of the right ventricle and a concavity in the region of the pulmonary conus. The pulmonary vascular markings are typically diminished, and the aortic arch and knob may be on the right side. Two-dimensional echocardiography from the parasternal or subcostal windows demonstrates the malalignment of the ventricular septal defect and the subpulmonary stenosis. Selective angiocardiography with RV injection provides architectural details of the RV outflow tract, pulmonary valve and annulus, and caliber of the main branches of the pulmonary artery; coronary arteriography identifies the anatomy and course of the coronary arteries.

℞ TREATMENT

Factors that may complicate the treatment of patients with tetralogy of Fallot include infective endocarditis, paradoxic embolism, excessive erythrocytosis, coagulation defects, and cerebral infarction or abscess. Corrective operation is advisable at some point for almost all patients with this anomaly. Successful correction avoids progressive infundibular obstruction, delayed growth, and complications due to hypoxemia and excessive erythrocytosis. The size of the pulmonary arteries rather than the age or size of the infant or child is the most important determinant in establishing candidacy for primary repair. Pronounced hypoplasia of the pulmonary arteries is a relative contraindication for an early corrective surgical procedure. When this problem is present, a palliative operation, such as creation of a systemic arterial–pulmonary arterial shunt, is carried out and is usually followed by complete correction, which can be carried out at a lower risk later in childhood.

OTHER FORMS OF CONGENITAL HEART DISEASES
CONGENITALLY CORRECTED TRANSPOSITION The two fundamental anatomic abnormalities in this malformation are transposition of the ascending aorta and pulmonary trunk and inversion of the ventricles. This arrangement results in desaturated systemic venous blood passing from the right atrium through the mitral valve to the left ventricle and into

the pulmonary trunk, whereas oxygenated pulmonary venous blood flows from the left atrium through the tricuspid valve to the right ventricle and into the aorta. Thus, the circulation is corrected functionally. The clinical presentation, course, and prognosis of patients with congenitally corrected transposition vary depending on the nature and severity of any complicating intracardiac anomalies and of development of dysfunction of the systemic subaortic RV. Ebstein-type anomalies of the left-side tricuspid atrioventricular valve, with progressive regurgitation, ventricular septal defect, obstruction to outflow from the venous ventricle, and congenital heart block are often associated with corrected transposition. The diagnosis of the malformation and associated lesions can be established by two-dimensional echocardiography and Doppler examination.

MALPOSITIONS OF THE HEART Positional anomalies refer to conditions in which the cardiac apex is in the right side of the chest (*dextrocardia*), or at the midline (*mesocardia*), or in which there is a normal location of the heart in the left side of the chest but abnormal position of the viscera (*isolated levocardia*). Knowledge of the position of the abdominal organs and of the branching pattern of the main stem bronchi is important in categorizing these malpositions. When dextrocardia occurs without situs inversus, when the visceral situs is indeterminate, or if isolated levocardia is present, associated, often complex, multiple cardiac anomalies are usually present. In contrast, mirror-image dextrocardia is usually observed with complete situs inversus, which occurs most frequently in individuals whose hearts are otherwise normal.

SURGICALLY MODIFIED CONGENITAL HEART DISEASE

Because of the enormous strides in cardiovascular surgical techniques that have occurred in the past 20 years, a large number of long-term survivors of corrective operations in infancy and childhood have reached adulthood. These patients are often challenging because of the diversity of anatomic, hemodynamic, and electrophysiologic residua and sequelae of cardiac operations.

The proper care of the survivor of operation for congenital heart disease requires that the clinician understand the details of the malformation before operation; pay meticulous attention to the details of the operative procedure; and recognize the postoperative residua (conditions left totally or partially uncorrected), the sequelae (conditions caused by surgery), and the complications that may have resulted from the operation. With the exception of ligation and division of an uncomplicated patent ductus arteriosus, almost every other surgical repair of an anomaly leaves behind or causes some abnormality of the heart and circulation that may range from trivial to serious. Intraoperative transesophageal echocardiography assists in detecting unsuspected lesions, in monitoring the repair, and in verifying a satisfactory result or directing further repair. Thus, even with results that are considered clinically to be good to excellent, continued long-term postoperative follow-up is advisable.

Table 218-4 lists the categories of common late postoperative problems. Cardiac operations importantly involving the atria, such as closure of atrial septal defect, repair of total or partial anomalous pulmonary venous return, or venous switch corrections of complete transposition of the great arteries (the Mustard or Senning operations), may be followed years later by sinus node or atrioventricular node dysfunction or by atrial arrhythmias. Intraventricular surgery may also result in electrophysiologic consequences, including complete heart block necessitating pacemaker insertion to avoid sudden death. In ad-

TABLE 218-4 Potential Late Postoperative Problems

Residual shunts	Arrhythmias and conduction
Residual ventricular outflow	defects
obstruction	Myocardial dysfunction
Residual valvular anomalies	Prosthetic valve malfunction
Systemic arterial hypertension	Prosthetic conduit obstruction
Pulmonary vascular obstruction	Infective endocarditis

dition, valvular problems may arise late after initial cardiac operation. An example is the progressive stenosis of an initially nonobstructive bicuspid aortic valve in the patient who underwent aortic coarctation repair. Such aortic valves may also be the site of infective endocarditis. After repair of the ostium primum atrial septal defect, the cleft mitral valve may become progressively incompetent. Tricuspid regurgitation may also be progressive in the postoperative patient with tetralogy of Fallot if RV outflow tract obstruction was not relieved adequately at initial surgery. In many patients with surgically modified congenital heart disease, inadequate relief of an obstructive lesion, or a residual regurgitant lesion, or a residual shunt will cause or hasten the onset of clinical signs and symptoms of myocardial dysfunction. Despite a good hemodynamic repair, many patients with a subaortic right ventricle develop RV decompensation and signs of "left heart failure." In many patients, particularly those who were cyanotic for many years before operation, a preexisting compromise in ventricular performance is due to the original underlying malformation.

A final category of postoperative problems involves the use of prosthetic valves, patches, or conduits in the operative repair. The special risks include infective endocarditis, thrombus formation, and prema-

ture degeneration and calcification of the prosthetic materials. There are many patients in whom extracardiac conduits are required to correct the circulation functionally and often to carry blood to the lungs from the right atrium or right ventricle. These conduits may develop intraluminal obstruction, and, if they include a prosthetic valve, it may show progressive calcification and thickening.

FURTHER READING

BRICKNER ME et al: Congenital heart disease in adults (2 parts). N Engl J Med 342:256, and 334, 2000

GERSONY WM, ROSENBAUM MS: *Congenital Heart Disease in the Adult.* New York, McGraw-Hill, 2002

PERLOFF JK: *Clinical Recognition of Congenital Heart Disease*, 5th ed. Philadelphia, Saunders, 2003

——, WARNES CA: Challenges posed by adults with repaired congenital heart disease. Circulation 103:2637, 2001

SIU SC et al: Prospective multicenter study of pregnancy outcomes in women with heart disease. Circulation 104:515, 2001

WEBB G, REDINGTON A: Congenital heart disease in children and adults, in *Braunwald's Heart Disease*, 7th ed, DP Zipes et al (eds). Philadelphia, Saunders, 2005

ZHONG-DONG D et al: Comparison between transcatheter and surgical closure of secundum atrial septal defect in children and adults. Results of a multicenter nonrandomized trial. J Am Coll Cardiol 39:1836, 2002

219 | VALVULAR HEART DISEASE
Eugene Braunwald

The role of physical examination in the evaluation of patients with valvular disease is also considered in Chap. 209; of electrocardiography (ECG) in Chap. 210; of echocardiography in Chap. 211; and of cardiac catheterization and angiography in Chap. 212.

MITRAL STENOSIS

ETIOLOGY AND PATHOLOGY   Two-thirds of all patients with mitral stenosis (MS) are female. MS and mixed MS and mitral regurgitation (MR) are generally rheumatic in origin; very rarely, MS is congenital. Pure or predominant MS occurs in approximately 40% of all patients with rheumatic heart disease. In other patients with rheumatic heart disease, lesser degrees of MS may accompany MR and aortic valve lesions. With reductions in the incidence of acute rheumatic fever, particularly in temperate climates and developed nations, the incidence of MS is declining. However, it remains a major problem in developing nations, especially in tropical and semitropical climates.

In rheumatic stenosis the valve leaflets are diffusely thickened by fibrous tissue and/or calcific deposits. The mitral commissures fuse, the chordae tendineae fuse and shorten, the valvular cusps become rigid, and these changes, in turn, lead to narrowing at the apex of the funnel-shaped ("fish-mouth") valve. Although the initial insult to the mitral valve is rheumatic, the later changes may be a nonspecific process resulting from trauma to the valve caused by altered flow patterns due to the initial deformity. Calcification of the stenotic mitral valve immobilizes the leaflets and narrows the orifice further. Thrombus formation and arterial embolization may arise from the calcific valve itself, but more frequently arise from the dilated left atrium (LA) in patients with atrial fibrillation (AF).

PATHOPHYSIOLOGY   In normal adults the mitral valve orifice is 4 to 6 cm². In the presence of significant obstruction, i.e., when the orifice is less than approximately 2 cm², blood can flow from the LA to the left ventricle (LV) only if propelled by an abnormally elevated left atrioventricular pressure gradient (see Fig. 212-2), the hemodynamic hallmark of MS. When the mitral valve opening is reduced to 1 cm², often referred to as "critical" MS, a LA pressure of approximately 25 mmHg is required to maintain a normal cardiac output (CO). The elevated pulmonary venous and pulmonary arterial (PA) wedge pressures re-

duce pulmonary compliance, contributing to exertional dyspnea. The first bouts of dyspnea are usually precipitated by clinical events that increase the rate of blood flow across the mitral orifice, resulting in further elevation of the LA pressure (see below). To assess the severity of obstruction, both the transvalvular pressure gradient and the flow rate must be measured (Chap. 212). The latter depends not only on the CO but on the heart rate as well. An increase in heart rate shortens diastole proportionately more than systole and diminishes the time available for flow across the mitral valve. Therefore, at any given level of CO, tachycardia including that resulting from atrial fibrillation augments the transvalvular gradient and elevates further the LA pressure. Similar considerations apply to the tricuspid stenosis.

The LV diastolic pressure and ejection fraction (EF) are normal in isolated MS. In MS and sinus rhythm, the elevated LA and PA wedge pressures exhibit a prominent atrial contraction (*a* wave) and a gradual pressure decline after mitral valve opening (*y* descent) (see Fig. 212-2). In severe MS and whenever pulmonary vascular resistance is significantly increased, the pulmonary arterial pressure (PAP) is elevated at rest and rises further during exercise, often causing secondary elevations of right ventricle (RV) end-diastolic pressure and volume.

Cardiac Output   In patients with moderately severe MS (mitral valve orifice 1.2 cm² to 1.7 cm²), the CO is normal or almost so at rest but rises subnormally during exertion. In patients with critical MS, particularly those in whom pulmonary vascular resistance is strikingly elevated, the CO is subnormal at rest and may fail to rise or may even decline during activity.

Pulmonary Hypertension   The clinical and hemodynamic features of MS are influenced importantly by the level of the PAP. Pulmonary hypertension results from (1) passive backward transmission of the elevated LA pressure; (2) pulmonary arteriolar constriction, which presumably is triggered by LA and pulmonary venous hypertension (reactive pulmonary hypertension); (3) interstitial edema in the walls of the small pulmonary vessels; and (4) organic obliterative changes in the pulmonary vascular bed. Severe pulmonary hypertension results in tricuspid regurgitation (TR) and pulmonary incompetence as well as right-sided heart failure.

SYMPTOMS   In temperate climates the latent period between the initial attack of rheumatic carditis (in the increasingly rare circumstances in which a history of one can be elicited) and the development of symptoms due to MS is generally about two decades; most patients begin to experience disability in the fourth decade of life. Studies carried out before the development of mitral valvotomy revealed that once a patient with MS became seriously symptomatic, the disease progressed continuously to death within 2 to 5 years. In economically deprived areas, in tropical and subtropical climates, particularly on the Indian subcontinent, in Central America, and in the Middle East, MS tends to progress more rapidly and frequently causes serious symptoms in patients less than 20 years of age. In contrast, slowly progressive MS in the elderly is being recognized with increasing frequency in the United States and Western Europe.

When valvular obstruction is mild, the physical signs of MS may be present without symptoms. However, even in patients whose mitral orifices are large enough to accommodate a normal blood flow with only mild elevations of LA pressure, marked elevations of this pressure leading to dyspnea and cough may be precipitated by severe exertion, excitement, fever, severe anemia, paroxysmal atrial fibrillation and other tachycardias, sexual intercourse, pregnancy, and thyrotoxicosis. As MS progresses, lesser stresses precipitate dyspnea, and the patient becomes limited in daily activities. The redistribution of blood from the dependent portions of the body to the lungs, which occurs when the recumbent position is assumed, leads to orthopnea and paroxysmal nocturnal dyspnea. *Pulmonary edema* develops when there is a sudden surge in flow across a markedly narrowed mitral orifice. When moderately severe MS has existed for several years, *atrial arrhythmias* occur with increasing frequency. The development of permanent AF often marks a turning point in the patient's course and is generally associated with acceleration of the rate at which symptoms progress.

Hemoptysis (Chap. 30) results from rupture of pulmonary-bronchial venous connections secondary to pulmonary venous hypertension. It occurs most frequently in patients who have elevated LA pressures without markedly elevated pulmonary vascular resistances and is almost never fatal. *Recurrent pulmonary emboli* (Chap. 244), sometimes with infarction, are an important cause of morbidity and mortality late in the course of MS. *Pulmonary infections*, i.e., bronchitis, bronchopneumonia, and lobar pneumonia, commonly complicate untreated MS. *Infective endocarditis* (Chap. 109) is rare in isolated MS.

Pulmonary Changes In addition to the aforementioned changes in the pulmonary vascular bed, fibrous thickening of the walls of the alveoli and pulmonary capillaries occurs commonly in MS. The vital capacity, total lung capacity, maximal breathing capacity, and oxygen uptake per unit of ventilation are reduced (Chap. 234), and the latter fails to rise normally during exertion. Pulmonary compliance falls further as pulmonary capillary pressure rises during exercise. In some patients, airway resistance is abnormally increased and the diffusing capacity may be reduced. These changes in the lungs are due, in part, to increased transudation of fluid from the pulmonary capillaries into the interstitial and alveolar spaces. However, the increased capacity of the pulmonary lymphatic system to drain excess fluid retards the development of alveolar edema.

Thrombi and Emboli *Thrombi* may form in the left atria, particularly in the enlarged atrial appendages of patients with MS. Embolization occurs much more frequently in patients with AF, in older patients, and in those with a reduced cardiac output (CO). However, systemic embolization may be the presenting complaint in otherwise asymptomatic patients with mild MS. Rarely, a large pedunculated or a freefloating thrombus may suddenly obstruct the stenotic mitral orifice and cause syncope, angina, and changing auscultatory signs with alterations in position.

PHYSICAL FINDINGS (See also Chap. 209) ■ **Inspection and Palpation** In patients with severe MS, there may be a malar flush with pinched and blue facies. In patients with sinus rhythm and severe pulmonary hypertension or associated tricuspid stenosis (TS), the jugular venous pulse reveals prominent *a* waves due to vigorous right atrial systole. The systemic arterial pressure is usually normal or slightly low. An RV tap along the left sternal border signifies an enlarged RV. A dia-stolic thrill is frequently present at the cardiac apex, with the patient in the left lateral recumbent position.

Auscultation The first heart sound (S_1) is generally accentuated and snapping, and slightly delayed. The pulmonary component of the second heart sound (P_2) is often accentuated, and the two components of the second heart sound (S_2) are closely split or fixed. A pulmonary systolic ejection click may be heard in patients with severe pulmonary hypertension. The opening snap (OS) of the mitral valve is most readily audible in expiration at, or just medial to the cardiac apex. This sound generally follows the sound of aortic valve closure (A_2) by 0.05 to 0.12 s. The time interval between A_2 and OS varies inversely with the severity of the MS. The OS is followed by a low-pitched, rumbling, diastolic murmur, heard best at the apex with the patient in the left lateral recumbent position (see Fig. 209-5B). It is accentuated by mild exercise (e.g., a few rapid situps) carried out just before auscultation. In general, the duration of this murmur correlates with the severity of the stenosis. In patients with sinus rhythm, the murmur often reappears or becomes reaccentuated during atrial systole. Soft grade I or II/VI systolic murmurs are commonly heard at the apex or along the left sternal border in patients with pure MS and do not necessarily signify the presence of MR. Hepatomegaly, ankle edema, ascites, and pleural effusion, particularly in the right pleural cavity, may occur in patients with MS and RV failure.

Associated Lesions With severe pulmonary hypertension, a pansystolic murmur produced by functional TR may be audible along the left sternal border. Characteristically, this murmur is accentuated by inspiration and diminishes during forced expiration (Carvallo's sign); it should not be confused with the apical pansystolic murmur of MR. When the S_1 and/or the OS are soft or absent in a patient with mitral valve disease who also has an apical systolic murmur, it is likely that significant MR and/or serious calcification of the deformed mitral valve leaflets are present. When the CO is markedly reduced in MS, the typical auscultatory findings, including the diastolic rumbling murmur, may not be detectable (silent MS), but they may reappear as compensation is restored. The *Graham Steell murmur* of pulmonary regurgitation (PR), a high-pitched, diastolic, decrescendo blowing murmur along the left sternal border, results from dilatation of the pulmonary valve ring and occurs in patients with mitral valve disease and severe pulmonary hypertension. This murmur may be indistinguishable from the more common murmur produced by aortic regurgitation (AR).

LABORATORY EXAMINATION ■ EKG In MS and sinus rhythm, the P wave usually suggests LA enlargement (see Fig. 210-8). It may become tall and peaked in lead II and upright in lead V_1 when severe pulmonary hypertension or TS complicates MS and right atrial (RA) enlargement occurs. The QRS complex is usually normal. However, with severe pulmonary hypertension, right axis deviation and RV hypertrophy are often present.

Echocardiogram (See also Chap. 211) This is the most sensitive and specific noninvasive method for diagnosing MS. Transthoracic two-dimensional color flow Doppler echocardiographic imaging and Doppler ultrasound provide critical information, including an estimate of the transvalvular gradient and of mitral orifice size, the presence and severity of accompanying MR, the extent of restriction of valve leaflets, their thickness, the degree of distortion of the subvalvular apparatus, and the anatomic suitability for balloon mitral valvotomy (see below). In addition, echocardiography provides an assessment of the size of the cardiac chambers, an estimation of the LV function, an estimation of the PAP, and an indication of the presence and severity of associated valvular lesions. Transesophageal echocardiography provides superior images and should be employed when transthoracic imaging is inadequate for guiding therapy.

TABLE 219-1 Summary of Useful Medical Treatments in Valvular Heart Disease

Lesion	Symptom Control	Secondary Prevention and Natural History
Mitral stenosis	Diuretics for heart failure; Digoxin, β blockers, and rate-limiting calcium antagonists for rate control in atrial fibrillation	Penicillin prophylaxis against recurrent episodes of rheumatic fever; Anticoagulants to prevent systemic thromboembolism.
Mitral regurgitation	Diuretics and vasodilators (usually ACE inhibitors) for heart failure	No proven treatment
Aortic stenosis	Diuretics for heart failure; nitrates and β blockers for angina	No proven treatment but lipid lowering therapy may slow progression of calcific aortic stenosis
Aortic regurgitation	Diuretics and vasodilators (usually ACE inhibitors) for heart failure	Vasodilators (nifedipine or ACE inhibitors) to protect the left ventricular myocardium and delay the need for surgery

Source: NA Boon, P Bloomfield: The medical management of valvular heart disease. Heart 87:395, 2002, with permission

Roentgenogram The earliest changes are straightening of the left border of the cardiac silhouette, prominence of the main pulmonary arteries, dilatation of the upper lobe pulmonary veins, and backward displacement of the esophagus by an enlarged LA. In severe MS, however, all chambers and vessels upstream to the narrowed valve are prominent. Kerley B lines are fine, dense, opaque, horizontal lines that are most prominent in the lower and midlung fields and that result from distention of interlobular septa and lymphatics with edema when the resting mean LA pressure exceeds approximately 20 mmHg.

DIFFERENTIAL DIAGNOSIS Like MS, significant MR may also be associated with a prominent diastolic murmur at the apex, but in MR this diastolic murmur commences slightly later than in patients with MS, and there is often clear-cut evidence of LV enlargement. An apical pansystolic murmur of at least grade III/VI intensity as well as an S_3 suggests significant associated MR. Similarly, the apical middiastolic murmur associated with AR (*Austin Flint murmur*) may be mistaken for MS. TS, which occurs rarely in the absence of MS, may mask many of the clinical features of MS.

Atrial septal defect (Chap. 218) may be mistaken for MS; in both conditions there is often clinical, EKG, and roentgenographic evidence of RV enlargement and accentuation of the pulmonary vascularity. The widely split S_2 of atrial septal defect may be confused with the mitral OS, and the diastolic flow murmur across the tricuspid valve may be mistaken for the mitral diastolic murmur. However, the absence of LA enlargement and of Kerley B lines and the demonstration of fixed splitting of S_2 all favor atrial septal defect over MS.

Left atrial myxoma (Chap. 223) may obstruct LA emptying, causing dyspnea, a diastolic murmur, and hemodynamic changes resembling those of MS. However, patients with an LA myxoma often have features suggestive of a systemic disease, such as weight loss, fever, anemia, systemic emboli, and elevated serum IgG concentrations. The auscultatory findings may change markedly with body position. The diagnosis can be established by the demonstration of a characteristic echo-producing mass in the LA with two-dimensional echocardiography.

CARDIAC CATHETERIZATION AND ANGIOCARDIOGRAPHY

Left heart catheterization is useful when there is a discrepancy between clinical and echocardiographic findings. It is helpful in assessing associated lesions such as aortic stenosis (AS) and aortic regurgitation (AR). Catheterization and coronary arteriography are not usually necessary to aid in the decision about surgery in younger patients with typical findings of severe obstruction on clinical examination and echocardiography. In males over 45 years of age, females over 55 years of age, and younger patients with coronary risk factors, especially those with positive noninvasive stress tests for myocardial ischemia, coronary angiography is usually advisable preoperatively to detect patients with critical coronary obstructions that should be bypassed at the time of operation. Catheterization and LV angiography are also indicated in most patients who have undergone balloon mitral valvot-

omy or previous mitral valve operations and who have redeveloped serious symptoms.

Rx TREATMENT

Penicillin prophylaxis of β-hemolytic streptococcal infections (Chap. 302) to prevent rheumatic fever and prophylaxis for infective endocarditis (Chap. 109) are important for all patients (Table 219-1). In symptomatic patients, some improvement usually occurs with restriction of sodium intake and maintenance doses of oral diuretics. Digitalis glycosides usually do not benefit patients with MS and sinus rhythm but are helpful in slowing the ventricular rate of patients with AF. Beta blockers or nondihydropyridine calcium antagonists (e.g., verapamil or diltiazem) are useful in this regard. Warfarin to an INR of 2-3:1 should be administered for at least 1 year to patients with MS who have suffered systemic and/or pulmonary embolization and permanently to those with AF.

If AF is of relatively recent origin in a patient whose MS is not severe enough to warrant balloon mitral valvotomy or surgical valvotomy, reversion to sinus rhythm pharmacologically or by means of electrical countershock is indicated. Usually this reversion should be undertaken after the patient has had 3 weeks of anticoagulant treatment. Conversion to sinus rhythm is rarely helpful in patients with severe MS, particularly those in whom the LA is especially enlarged or in whom AF has been present for more than 1 year, since sinus rhythm is rarely sustained in such patients.

Mitral Valvotomy Unless there is a contraindication, mitral valvotomy is indicated in symptomatic patients with isolated MS whose effective orifice is less than approximately $1.0 \text{ cm}^2/\text{m}^2$ body surface area, or $<1.7 \text{ cm}^2$ in normal-sized adults. Mitral valvotomy can be carried out by two techniques: percutaneous balloon mitral valvotomy and surgical valvotomy. In balloon mitral valvotomy (Figs. 219-1 and 219-2), a catheter is directed into the LA after transseptal puncture and a single or double balloon (Inoue balloon) is directed across the valve and inflated in the valvular orifice. Ideal patients have relatively mobile, thin leaflets with no or little calcium, without extensive subvalvular thickening and with no or mild MR. The short- and long-term results of this procedure in appropriate patients are similar to those of surgical valvotomy, but with less morbidity and a lower mortality rate. Therefore, balloon valvotomy has become the procedure of choice for such patients. Transthoracic echocardiography is helpful in identifying patients for the percutaneous procedure (Fig. 219-3).

In patients in whom percutaneous valvotomy is not possible, unsuccessful, or in those with restenosis, an "open" valvotomy using cardiopulmonary bypass is necessary. In addition to opening the valve

FIGURE 219-1 Technique of double balloon mitral valvuloplasty. *A.* The position of the guidewire in the left atrium after left atrial puncture using the Brockenbrough needle. *B.* The position of the guidewire as it is advanced into the left ventricle across the stenotic mitral valve. *C.* Partial inflation of a balloon catheter across the stenotic mitral valve. [*From JP Srebro, TA Ports, Catheter-balloon valvuloplasty, in K Chatterjee et al (eds): Cardiology: An Illustrated Text. Philadelphia, Lippincott, 1991.*]

PREDILATATION

ECG

Mean mitral gradient 15 mmHg
Cardiac output 3.0 L/min
Mitral valve area 0.6 cm²

POSTDILATATION

ECG

Mean mitral gradient 3 mmHg
Cardiac output 3.8 L/min
Mitral valve area 1.8 cm²

FIGURE 219-2 Simultaneous left atrial (LA) and left ventricular (LV) pressure before and after balloon mitral valvuloplasty in a patient with severe mitral stenosis. *(Courtesy of Raymond G. McKay, MD).*

commissures, it is important to loosen any subvalvular fusion of papillary muscles and chordae tendineae and to remove large deposits of calcium, thereby improving valvular function, as well as to remove atrial thrombi. The mortality rate is approximately 2%.

Successful valvotomy, whether balloon or surgical, usually results in striking symptomatic and hemodynamic improvement and prolongs survival. However, there is no evidence that the procedure improves the prognosis of patients with slight or no functional impairment. Therefore, unless recurrent systemic embolization or severe pulmonary hypertension has occurred, valvotomy is *not* recommended for patients who are entirely asymptomatic. When there is little symptomatic improvement after valvotomy, it is likely that the procedure was ineffective, that it induced MR, or that associated valvular or myocardial disease was present. About half of all patients undergoing mitral valvotomy require reoperation by 10 years. In the pregnant patient with MS, valvotomy should be carried out if pulmonary congestion occurs despite intensive medical treatment.

Mitral valve replacement (MVR) is necessary in patients with MS and significant associated MR, those in whom the valve has been severely distorted by previous transcatheter or operative manipulation, or those in whom the surgeon does not find it possible to improve

FIGURE 219-3 Event-free survival following percutaneous balloon mitral valvuloplasty. The echo score is derived from examining leaflet rigidity, thickening, calcification and the extent of subvalvular disease and grading each from 1 (not detectable) to 4 (very severe) and calculating the total. The minimum score is 4 and the maximum is 16. Event-free survival is survival without mitral valve replacement or repeat balloon valvuloplasty. *(From Palacios et al 2002.)*

TABLE 219-2 *Mortality Rates After Valve Replacement and Repair*

Operative Category	Number	Operative Mortality (%)
AVR (isolated)	26,317	4.3
MVR (isolated)	13,936	6.4
Multiple valve replacement	3,840	9.6
AVR + CAB	22,713	8.0
MVR + CAB	8,788	15.3
Multiple valve replacement + CAB	1,424	18.8
AVR + any valve repair	938	7.4
MVR + any valve repair	1,266	12.5
Aortic valve repair	597	5.9
Mitral valve repair	4,167	3.0
Tricuspid valve repair	144	13.9

Note: AVR, aortic valve replacement; CAB, coronary artery bypass; MVR, mitral valve replacement.
Source: Modified from Jamieson et al.

valve function significantly. Since the operative mortality rate of isolated MVR is still approximately 6% (Table 219-2), and since there are long-term complications of valve replacement, patients in whom preoperative evaluation suggests the possibility that MVR may be required should be operated on only if they have critical MS, i.e., an orifice ≤1 cm² area and are in New York Heart Association class III, i.e., symptomatic with ordinary activity despite optimal medical therapy. The overall 10-year survival of surgical survivors is approximately 70%. Long-term prognosis is worse in older patients and those with marked disability and striking depression of the cardiac index preoperatively.

MITRAL REGURGITATION

ETIOLOGY Chronic rheumatic heart disease is the cause of severe MR in only about one-third of cases and occurs more frequently in males. The rheumatic process produces rigidity, deformity, and retraction of the valve cusps and commissural fusion, as well as shortening, contraction, and fusion of the chordae tendineae. MR may occur as a congenital anomaly (Chap. 218), most commonly as a defect of the endocardial cushions (atrioventricular cushion defects). MR is frequently secondary to ischemia. Thus, it may occur as a consequence of ventricular remodeling or with fibrosis of a papillary muscle in patients with healed myocardial infarction. It may develop acutely in patients with acute infarction involving the base of a papillary muscle. Transient MR also may occur during periods of ischemia involving a papillary muscle or the adjacent myocardium and may accompany bouts of angina pectoris. MR may occur with marked LV enlargement of any cause in which dilatation of the mitral annulus and lateral displacement of the papillary muscles interfere with coaptation of the valve leaflets, most commonly ischemia. In hypertrophic cardiomyopathy, the anterior leaflet of the mitral valve is displaced anteriorly during systole, causing MR (Chap. 221). Calcification of the mitral annulus of unknown cause, presumably degenerative, which occurs most commonly in elderly women, also can be responsible for significant MR. Acute MR may occur secondary to infective endocarditis involving the valve leaflets or chordae tendineae, or as a consequence of trauma. Mitral valve prolapse (MVP), an important cause of MR, is considered in the next section.

Irrespective of cause, severe MR is often progressive, since enlargement of the LA places tension on the posterior mitral leaflet, pulling it away from the mitral orifice and thereby aggravating the valvular dysfunction. Similarly, LV dilatation increases the regurgitation, which in turn enlarges the LA and LV further, causing chordal rupture and resulting in a vicious circle; hence the aphorism, "mitral regurgitation begets mitral regurgitation."

PATHOPHYSIOLOGY The resistance to LV emptying is reduced in patients with MR. As a consequence, the LV is decompressed into the LA during ejection, and with the reduction in LV size during systole, there is a rapid decline in LV tension. The initial compensation to acute MR is more complete LV emptying. However, LV volume increases progressively as the severity of the regurgitation increases and as LV function deteriorates. This increase in LV volume is often accompanied by a reduced forward CO. The regurgitant volume varies directly with the LV systolic pressure and the size of the regurgitant orifice; as mentioned above, the latter, in turn, is influenced profoundly by the extent of LV dilatation. Since ejection fraction (EF) rises in severe MR in the presence of normal LV function, even a modest reduction in this parameter (<60%) reflects significant dysfunction.

The v wave in the LA pressure pulse is usually prominent (see Fig. 212-3). During early diastole, as the distended LA empties, there is a particularly rapid y descent (as long as there is no associated MS). In chronic MR, there is often an increase in LV compliance, so that LV volume rises with little elevation in LV diastolic pressure. The effective (forward) CO is usually reduced in seriously symptomatic patients. A brief, early diastolic atrioventricular pressure gradient (often accompanying a murmur) may occur in patients with pure MR as a result of the very rapid flow of blood across a normal-sized mitral orifice.

The prompt appearance of contrast material in the LA after its injection into the LV signifies the presence of MR. The regurgitant volume can be measured by determining the difference between the total LV stroke volume, estimated angiocardiographically, and the effective forward stroke volume determined by the Fick method (Chap. 212). In severe cases, as much as 50% of the total LV stroke volume regurgitates with each beat. Qualitative, but clinically useful, estimates of the severity of regurgitation may be made by observation on cineangiograms of the degree of LA opacification after the injection of contrast material into the LV. Color flow Doppler imaging is most commonly used for this purpose (see below).

Left ventricular contractility becomes reduced, sometimes irreversibly, with longstanding MR. The compliance, i.e., the pressure-volume relationship of the LA and pulmonary venous bed affects the clinical picture. Patients with acute MR usually have *normal or reduced LA compliance*, with little enlargement of the LA, but marked elevation of the LA pressure, particularly of the v wave. Severe pulmonary congestion and pulmonary edema are common in this group. Patients with a *marked increase in LA compliance* are at the opposite end of the spectrum, having longstanding, severe MR, marked enlargement of the LA, and normal or only slightly elevated LA and PA pressures. These patients usually complain of severe fatigue and exhaustion secondary to a low CO, while symptoms resulting from pulmonary congestion are less prominent; AF is almost invariably present. Most common are patients whose clinical and hemodynamic features are intermediate between those in the two aforementioned groups.

SYMPTOMS Fatigue, exertional dyspnea, and orthopnea are the most prominent complaints in patients with chronic, severe MR. Systemic embolism occurs less frequently than in MS. Right-sided heart failure, with painful hepatic congestion, ankle edema, distended neck veins, ascites, and TR, occur in patients with MR who have associated pulmonary vascular disease and marked pulmonary hypertension. In patients with acute, severe MR, LV failure with acute pulmonary edema is common.

PHYSICAL FINDINGS The arterial pressure is usually normal, and in patients with severe MR the arterial pulse may show a sharp upstroke. The jugular venous pulse shows abnormally prominent a waves in patients with sinus rhythm and marked pulmonary hypertension and prominent v waves in those with accompanying severe TR. A systolic thrill is often palpable at the cardiac apex, the LV is hyperdynamic with a brisk systolic impulse and a palpable rapid-filling wave, and the apex beat is often displaced laterally. An RV tap and the shock of pulmonary valve closure may be palpable in patients with marked pulmonary hypertension.

Auscultation The S_1 is generally absent, soft, or buried in the systolic murmur. In patients with severe MR, the aortic valve may close prematurely, resulting in wide splitting of the S_2. An OS indicates associated MS but does not exclude predominant regurgitation. A low-pitched S_3 occurring 0.12 to 0.17 s after the aortic valve closure sound, i.e., at the completion of the rapid-filling phase of the LV, is believed to be caused by the sudden tensing of the papillary muscles, chordae tendineae, and valve leaflets and is an important auscultatory feature of severe MR. The S_3 may be followed by a short, rumbling, diastolic murmur, even in the absence of MS. A fourth heart sound is often audible in patients with acute, severe MR of recent onset who are in sinus rhythm. A presystolic murmur is not ordinarily heard with isolated MR but is present in patients with sinus rhythm and associated MS.

A systolic murmur of at least grade III/VI intensity, is the most characteristic auscultatory finding in severe MR. It is usually holosystolic (see Figs. 209-4 and 209-5A), but it may be decrescendo and cease in late systole in patients with acute, severe MR. In MR due to papillary muscle dysfunction or MVP, the systolic murmur commences in midsystole (see below). The systolic murmur is usually most prominent at the apex and radiates to the axilla. However, in patients with ruptured chordae tendineae or primary involvement of the posterior mitral leaflet, the regurgitant jet strikes the LA wall adjacent to the aortic root. In this situation, the systolic murmur is transmitted to the base of the heart and therefore may be confused with the murmur of AS. In patients with ruptured chordae tendineae the systolic murmur may have a cooing or "sea gull" quality, while a flail leaflet may cause a murmur with a musical quality. The systolic murmur of MR is intensified by isometric strain but is reduced during the Valsalva maneuver.

LABORATORY EXAMINATION ■ Electrocardiogram In patients with sinus rhythm there is evidence of LA enlargement, but RA enlargement also may be present when pulmonary hypertension is severe. Chronic, severe MR is generally associated with AF. In many patients there is no clear-cut electrocardiographic evidence of enlargement of either ventricle. In others, the signs of LV hypertrophy are present.

Echocardiogram Color flow Doppler imaging is the most accurate noninvasive technique for the detection and estimation of MR. Two-dimensional echocardiography is useful for assessing the cause of MR and for estimating LV function from end-systolic and end-diastolic volumes and EF. The LA is usually enlarged and/or exhibits increased pulsation while the LV may be hyperdynamic. Findings that help to determine the etiology of MR, such as mitral annular calcification and LV dyskinesis in ischemic MR, can often be identified by two-dimensional echocardiography. With ruptured chordae tendineae or a flail leaflet, coarse, erratic motion of the involved leaflets may be noted. Vegetations associated with infective endocarditis, incomplete coaptation of the anterior and posterior mitral leaflets, and annular calcification, as well as MR secondary to LV dilatation, aneurysm, or dyskinesis may be recognized. Transesophageal imaging provides greater detail than transthoracic imaging (see Fig. 211-3). The echocardiogram in patients with MVP is described in the next section.

Roentgenogram The LA and LV are the dominant chambers; late in the course of the disease, the former may be massively enlarged and forms the right border of the cardiac silhouette. Pulmonary venous congestion, interstitial edema, and Kerley B lines are sometimes noted. Marked calcification of the mitral leaflets occurs commonly in patients with longstanding combined MR and MS. Calcification of the mitral annulus may be visualized.

℞ TREATMENT

MEDICAL (Table 219-1) The nonsurgical management of patients with severe MR begins with restricting those physical activities that regularly produce dyspnea and excessive fatigue, reducing sodium intake, and enhancing sodium excretion with the appropriate use of diuretics (Chap. 216). Vasodilators and digitalis glycosides increase the forward output of the failing LV. Intravenous nitroprusside or nitroglycerin reduce afterload and thereby the volume of regurgitant flow and are useful in stabilizing patients with acute and/or severe MR. Angiotensin-converting enzyme (ACE) inhibitors are useful in the treatment of chronic MR. The same considerations as in patients with MS apply to the reversion of AF to sinus rhythm. In the late stages of heart failure anticoagulants and leg binders are used to diminish the likelihood of venous thrombi and pulmonary emboli. Endocarditis prophylaxis is important. In patients with severe MR secondary to dilated cardiomyopathy, intensive medial therapy can reduce the severity of MR.

SURGICAL In the selection of patients with severe MR for surgical treatment, the chronic, often slowly progressive nature of the condition must be balanced against the immediate and long-term risks associated with the operation. Patients with MR who are asymptomatic or who are limited only during strenuous exertion and whose LV functions are normal are not considered to be candidates for surgical treatment, since their condition may remain stable for years. By contrast, unless there are contraindications, surgical treatment should be offered to patients with severe MR whose limitations do not allow fulltime employment or the performance of normal household activities despite optimal medical management. Surgical treatment of severe MR should be considered even in asymptomatic patients or those with mild symptoms when LV dysfunction is progressive, with LV EF declining below 60% and/or end-systolic cavity dimension on echocardiography rising above 45 mm. In patients with impaired LV function, the risk of surgery rises, the recovery of LV performance is incomplete, and the long-term survival is reduced (Fig. 219-4). However, conservative management has little to offer these patients, so operative treatment may be indicated and occasionally, the clinical and hemodynamic improvement that follows surgical treatment of patients with advanced disease is dramatic. However, unless chordal continuity can be preserved, operation is contraindicated in patients whose LV ejection fraction has declined to below 30%. Though most patients who survive surgery appear to be greatly improved, some degree of myocardial dysfunction often persists.

When surgical treatment is contemplated, left-sided heart catheterization and angiocardiography may be helpful in confirming the presence of severe MR in patients in whom there is a discrepancy between the clinical picture and the echocardiographic findings; these procedures may also aid in detecting and assessing the severity of associated valve lesions. Importantly, coronary arteriography identifies patients who require concomitant coronary revascularization.

Surgical treatment of MR, especially that caused by valves that are markedly deformed, with shrunken, calcified leaflets secondary to rheumatic fever, requires MVR with a prosthesis. However, in an increasing number of patients, particularly those with severe annular dilatation, flail leaflets, MVP, ruptured chordae, or infective endocarditis, reconstruction of the mitral valve apparatus (mitral valvuloplasty) and/or mitral annuloplasty with an annuloplasty ring may be successful. Valve reconstruction should be carried out whenever fea-

sible since the operative risk is about half (~3%) of that associated with MVR (Table 219-1). Also, reconstruction spares the patient the long-term adverse consequences of valve replacement, i.e., thromboembolic and hemorrhagic complications in the case of mechanical prostheses and late valve failure necessitating repeat valve replacement in the case of bioprostheses. In addition, by preserving the integrity of the papillary muscles, subvalvular apparatus and chordae tendinae, mitral repair and valvuloplasty maintains LV function. In asymptomatic patients with preserved left ventricular function, surgical treatment can be considered as long as mitral repair seems feasible and pulmonary hypertension or recent atrial fibrillation are present.

MITRAL VALVE PROLAPSE

MVP, also variously termed the *systolic click-murmur syndrome, Barlow's syndrome, floppy-valve syndrome*, and *billowing mitral leaflet syndrome*, is a relatively common, but highly variable clinical syndrome resulting from diverse pathogenic mechanisms of the mitral valve apparatus. Among these are excessive or redundant mitral leaflet tissue, which is commonly associated with myxomatous degeneration and greatly increased concentrations of acid mucopolysaccharide. MVP is a frequent finding in patients with heritable disorders of connective tissue, including the Marfan syndrome (Chap. 342), osteogenesis imperfecta, and the Ehler-Danlos syndrome. In most patients with MVP, however, myxomatous degeneration is confined to the mitral (or less commonly the tricuspid or aortic) valves without other clinical or pathologic manifestations of disease. The posterior leaflet is usually more affected than the anterior, and the mitral valve annulus is often greatly dilated. In many patients, elongated redundant chordae tendineae cause or contribute to the regurgitation.

In most patients with MVP, the cause is unknown, but in some it appears to be a genetically determined collagen tissue disorder. A reduction in the production of type III collagen has been incriminated, and electron microscopy has revealed fragmentation of collagen fibrils. MVP may be associated with thoracic skeletal deformities similar to but not as severe as those in the Marfan syndrome, including a high-arched palate and alterations of the chest and thoracic spine, including the so-called straight back syndrome. MVP also may occur as a sequel of acute rheumatic fever, in ischemic heart disease, and in cardiomyopathies, as well as in 20% of patients with ostium secundum atrial septal defect.

MVP may lead to excessive stress on the papillary muscles, which in turn leads to dysfunction and ischemia of the papillary muscles and the subjacent ventricular myocardium. Rupture of chordae tendineae and progressive annular dilatation and calcification also contribute to valvular regurgitation, which then places more stress on the diseased mitral valve apparatus, thereby creating a vicious circle. The electrocardiographic changes (see below) and ventricular arrhythmias appear to result from regional ventricular dysfunction related to increased stress placed on the papillary muscles.

CLINICAL FEATURES MVP is more common in females. It affects individuals in a wide age range but most commonly those between the ages of 14 and 30 years. The clinical course is often benign. MVP may also be observed in older (>50 years) patients, often males, and in them MR is more often severe and requires surgical treatment. There is an increased familial incidence for some patients, suggesting an autosomal dominant form of inheritance. MVP encompasses a broad spectrum of severities, ranging from only a systolic click and murmur and mild prolapse of the posterior leaflet of the mitral valve to severe MR due to chordal rupture and massive prolapse of both leaflets. In many patients, this condition progresses over years or decades.

Most patients are asymptomatic and remain so for their entire lives. However, MVP is now the most common cause of isolated severe MR requiring surgical treatment in North America. Arrhythmias, most commonly ventricular premature contractions and paroxysmal supraventricular and ventricular tachycardia, have been reported and may

FIGURE 219-4 Late survival rates of patients surviving surgical correction of MR according to preoperative echocardiographic ejection fraction (EF). *(From M Enriquez-Sarano et al: Echocardiographic prediction of survival after surgical correction of organic mitral regurgitation. Circulation 90:833, 1994, with permission.)*

cause palpitations, light-headedness, and syncope. Sudden death is a very rare complication. Many patients have chest pain that is difficult to evaluate. It is often substernal, prolonged, poorly related to exertion, and rarely resembles angina pectoris. Transient cerebral ischemic attacks secondary to emboli from the mitral valve due to endothelial disruption have been reported. Infective endocarditis may occur in patients with MR associated with MVP.

Auscultation   The most important finding is the mid- or late (nonejection) systolic click, which occurs 0.14 s or more after the S_1 and is thought to be generated by the sudden tensing of slack, elongated chordae tendineae or by the prolapsing mitral leaflet when it reaches its maximum excursion. Systolic clicks may be multiple and may be followed by a high-pitched, late systolic crescendo-decrescendo murmur, which occasionally is "whooping" or "honking," and is heard best at the apex. The click and murmur occur earlier with standing, during the strain of the Valsalva maneuver, and with any intervention that decreases LV volume, exaggerating the propensity of mitral leaflet prolapse. Conversely, squatting and isometric exercise, which increase LV volume, diminish MVP, and the click-murmur complex is delayed and may even disappear. Some patients have a midsystolic click without the murmur; others have the murmur without a click. Still others have both sounds at different times.

LABORATORY EXAMINATION   The ECG most commonly is normal but may show biphasic or inverted T waves in leads II, III, and aVF, and occasionally supraventricular or ventricular premature contractions. *Two-dimensional echocardiography* is particularly effective in identifying the abnormal position and prolapse of the mitral valve leaflets. A useful echocardiographic definition of MVP is systolic displacement (in the parasternal view) of the mitral valve leaflets by at least 2 mm into the LA superior to the plane of the mitral annulus. Thickening of the mitral valve leaflets identifies a subgroup of patients at higher risk of infective endocarditis and the development of severe MR. Prolapse of the tricuspid and/or aortic valve may be found. *Color-imaging* and *Doppler studies* are helpful in revealing and evaluating accompanying MR. *Angiocardiography* generally shows prolapse of the posterior and sometimes of both mitral valve leaflets.

℞ TREATMENT

The management of patients with MVP consists of the asymptomatic patient without severe MR or arrhythmias and the prevention of infective endocarditis with antibiotic prophylaxis in patients with a systolic murmur and/or thickening of mitral valve leaflets on endocardiography. Beta blockers sometimes relieve chest pain. If symptomatic tachyarrhythmias have occurred, antiarrhythmic agents as dictated by electrophysiologic studies should be administered. If the patient is symptomatic from severe MR, mitral valve repair (or rarely, replacement) is indicated. Antiplatelet aggregation agents such as aspirin should be given to patients with transient ischemic attacks, and if these are not effective, anticoagulants should be used.

AORTIC STENOSIS

AS occurs in about one-fourth of all patients with chronic valvular heart disease; approximately 80% of adult patients with symptomatic valvular AS are male.

ETIOLOGY   AS in adults may be due to degenerative calcification of the aortic cusps. It may be congenital in origin or it may be secondary to rheumatic inflammation. *Age-related degenerative calcific AS* (also known as senile or sclerocalcific AS) is now the most common cause of AS in adults in North America and Western Europe. About 30% of persons >65 years exhibit aortic valve sclerosis, many of whom have a systolic murmur of AS but without obstruction, while an additional 2% exhibit frank stenosis. On histologic examination these valves frequently exhibit inflammatory changes similar to those seen in athero-

sclerotic vessels. Interestingly, risk factors for atherosclerosis, such as age, male sex, smoking, diabetes mellitus, hypertension, increased LDL, reduced HDL cholesterol, and elevated C-reactive protein are all risk factors for aortic valve calcification.

The *congenitally affected valve* may be stenotic at birth (Chap. 218) and may become progressively more fibrotic, calcified, and stenotic. In other cases the valve may be congenitally deformed, usually bicuspid, without serious narrowing of the aortic orifice during childhood; its abnormal architecture makes its leaflets susceptible to otherwise ordinary hemodynamic stresses, which ultimately lead to valvular thickening, calcification, increased rigidity, and narrowing of the aortic orifice.

Rheumatic endocarditis of the aortic leaflets produces commissural fusion, sometimes resulting in a bicuspid valve. This condition in turn, makes the leaflets more susceptible to trauma and ultimately leads to fibrosis, calcification, and further narrowing. By the time the obstruction to LV outflow causes serious clinical disability, the valve is usually a rigid calcified mass, and careful examination may make it difficult or even impossible to determine the etiology of the underlying process. Rheumatic AS is almost always associated with involvement of the mitral valve and by associated severe AR.

OTHER FORMS OF OBSTRUCTION TO LEFT VENTRICULAR OUTFLOW   Besides valvular AS, three other lesions may be responsible for obstruction to LV outflow.

1. *Hypertrophic cardiomyopathy* (Chap. 221). This condition is characterized by marked hypertrophy of the LV and involves in particular the interventricular septum; it may cause subaortic obstruction.

2. *Discrete congenital subvalvular AS* (Chap. 218). This congenital anomaly is produced by either a membranous diaphragm or a fibrous ridge just below the aortic valve.

3. *Supravalvular AS* (Chap. 218). This uncommon congenital anomaly is produced by narrowing of the ascending aorta or by a fibrous diaphragm with a small opening just above the aortic valve.

PATHOPHYSIOLOGY   The obstruction to LV outflow produces a systolic pressure gradient between the LV and aorta. When severe obstruction is suddenly produced experimentally, the LV responds by dilatation and reduction of stroke volume. However, in patients the obstruction may be present at birth and/or increase gradually over the course of many years, and LV output is maintained by the presence of concentric LV hypertrophy. This serves as a useful compensatory mechanism because it reduces toward normal the systolic stress developed by the myocardium. A large transaortic valvular pressure gradient may exist for many years without a reduction of CO or LV dilatation; ultimately, however, these changes occur.

A peak systolic pressure gradient >50 mmHg in the face of a normal cardiac output or an effective aortic orifice less than approximately 1.0 cm² or <0.6 cm²/m² body surface area, i.e., less than approximately one-third of the normal orifice, is generally considered to represent severe obstruction to LV outflow. The elevated LV end-diastolic pressure observed in many patients with severe AS signifies the presence of LV dilatation and/or diminished compliance of the hypertrophied LV wall. A large *a* wave in the LA pressure pulse is usually present. Although the CO at rest is within normal limits in most patients with severe AS, it usually fails to rise normally during exercise. Loss of an appropriately timed, vigorous atrial contraction, as occurs in AF or atrioventricular dissociation, may cause a rapid progression of symptoms. Late in the course the CO and LV–aortic pressure gradient decline, and the mean LA, PA, and RV pressures rise.

The hypertrophied LV muscle mass elevates myocardial oxygen requirements. In addition, even in the absence of obstructive coronary artery disease, there may be interference with coronary blood flow. This is because the pressure compressing the coronary arteries exceeds the coronary perfusion pressure, often causing ischemia, especially in the subendocardium, and during tachycardia, both in the presence and in the absence of coronary arterial narrowing.

SYMPTOMS AS is rarely of clinical importance until the valve orifice has narrowed to approximately 0.5 cm²/m² body surface area in adults. Even severe AS may exist for many years without producing any symptoms because of the ability of the hypertrophied LV to generate the elevated intraventricular pressures required for a normal stroke volume.

Most patients with pure or predominant AS have gradually increasing obstruction for years but do not become symptomatic until the sixth to eighth decades. Exertional dyspnea, angina pectoris, and syncope are the three cardinal symptoms. Often there is a history of insidious progression of fatigue and dyspnea associated with gradual curtailment of activities. *Dyspnea* results primarily from elevation of the pulmonary capillary pressure caused by elevations of LV diastolic pressures secondary to reduced compliance. *Angina pectoris* usually develops somewhat later and reflects an imbalance between the augmented myocardial oxygen requirements and reduced oxygen availability; the former results from the increased myocardial mass and intraventricular pressure, while the latter may result from accompanying coronary artery disease, which is not uncommon in patients with AS, as well as from compression of the coronary vessels by the hypertrophied myocardium. Therefore, angina may occur in severe AS even without obstructive epicardial coronary artery disease. *Exertional syncope* may result from a decline in arterial pressure caused by vasodilatation in the exercising muscles and inadequate vasoconstriction in nonexercising muscles in the face of a fixed CO, or from a sudden fall in CO produced by an arrhythmia.

Since the CO at rest is usually well maintained until late in the course, marked fatigability, weakness, peripheral cyanosis, and other clinical manifestations of a low CO are usually not prominent until this stage is reached. Orthopnea, paroxysmal nocturnal dyspnea, and pulmonary edema, i.e., symptoms of LV failure, also occur only in the advanced stages of the disease. Severe pulmonary hypertension leading to RV failure and systemic venous hypertension, hepatomegaly, AF, and TR are usually late findings in patients with isolated, severe AS.

When AS and MS coexist, the reduction of cardiac output induced by MS lowers the pressure gradient across the aortic valve and thereby masks many of the clinical findings produced by AS. Left heart catheterization is helpful in defining the relative importance of each valvular abnormality.

PHYSICAL FINDINGS The rhythm is generally regular until very late in the course; at other times, AF should suggest the possibility of associated mitral valve disease. The systemic arterial pressure is usually within normal limits. In the late stages, however, when stroke volume declines, the systolic pressure may fall and the pulse pressure narrow. Systemic hypertension is unusual in patients with severe AS. The peripheral arterial pulse, as palpated in the carotid or brachial arteries, rises slowly to a delayed sustained peak (pulsus parvus et tardus) (see Fig. 209-2). In the elderly, the stiffening of the arterial wall may mask this important physical sign. A palpable double systolic arterial pulse, the so-called bisferiens pulse, excludes pure or predominant AS and signifies dominant AR. In the late stages of AS, when the pulse pressure is reduced, the pulse amplitude may be so small that the anacrotic nature of the pulse and the delay in its upstroke may become difficult to appreciate. In many patients the *a* wave in the jugular venous pulse is accentuated. This results from the diminished distensibility of the RV cavity caused by the bulging, hypertrophied intraventricular septum.

The LV impulse is usually active and displaced laterally, reflecting the presence of LV hypertrophy. A double apical impulse may be recognized, particularly with the patient in the left lateral recumbent position. A systolic thrill is generally present at the base of the heart, in the jugular notch, and along the carotid arteries. In patients who do not have marked pulmonary emphysema, a thick chest wall, thoracic deformity, or heart failure, the absence of a systolic thrill suggests that the AS is relatively mild.

Auscultation An early systolic ejection sound, actually the OS of the aortic valve, is frequently audible in children and adolescents with congenital noncalcific valvular AS. This sound usually disappears when the valve becomes calcified and rigid. As AS increases in severity, LV systole may become prolonged so that the aortic valve closure sound no longer precedes the pulmonic valve closure sound, and the two components may become synchronous, or aortic valve closure may even follow pulmonic valve closure, causing paradoxic splitting of the S₂ (Chap. 209). The sound of aortic valve closure can be heard most frequently in patients with AS who have pliable valves, and calcification diminishes the intensity of this sound. Frequently, an S₄ is audible at the apex and reflects the presence of LV hypertrophy and an elevated LV end-diastolic pressure; an S₃ generally occurs when the LV dilates.

The murmur of AS is characteristically an ejection (mid) systolic murmur that commences shortly after the S₁, increases in intensity to reach a peak toward the middle of ejection, and ends just before aortic valve closure (see Figs. 209-4 and 209-5A). It is characteristically low pitched, rough and rasping in character, and loudest at the base of the heart, most commonly in the second right intercostal space. It is transmitted upward along the carotid arteries. Occasionally, it is transmitted downward and to the apex where it may be confused with the systolic murmur of MR. In almost all patients with severe obstruction, the murmur is at least grade III/VI. In patients with mild degrees of obstruction or in those with severe stenosis with heart failure in whom the stroke volume and therefore the transvalvular flow rate are reduced, the murmur may be relatively soft and brief.

LABORATORY EXAMINATION ■ Electrocardiogram In most patients with severe AS there is LV hypertrophy (see Fig. 210-9). In advanced cases, ST-segment depression and T-wave inversion (LV "strain") in standard leads I and aVL and in the left precordial leads are evident. However, there is no close correlation between the ECG and the hemodynamic severity of obstruction, and the absence of ECG signs of LV hypertrophy does not exclude severe obstruction.

The key findings are LV hypertrophy and, in patients with valvular calcification (i.e., most adult patients with symptomatic AS), multiple, bright, thick, echoes from within the aortic root. Eccentricity of the aortic valve cusps is characteristic of congenitally bicuspid valves. Transesophageal imaging usually displays the obstructed orifice extremely well. The transaortic valvular gradient can be estimated by Doppler echocardiography. LV dilatation and reduced systolic shortening reflect impairment of LV function. Echocardiography is also useful for identifying valvular abnormalities such as MS and AR, which sometimes accompany AS, and for differentiating valvular AS from obstructive hypertrophic cardiomyopathy.

Roentgenogram The chest roentgenogram may show no or little overall cardiac enlargement for many years, since the development of concentric LV hypertrophy is the initial response to obstruction to LV outflow. Hypertrophy without dilatation may produce some rounding of the cardiac apex in the frontal projection and slight backward displacement in the lateral view; critical AS is often associated with poststenotic dilatation of the ascending aorta (Fig. 211-5). Aortic calcification is usually readily apparent on fluoroscopic examination or by echocardiography; the absence of valvular calcification in an adult suggests that severe valvular AS is not present. In later stages of the disease as the LV dilates, there is increasing roentgenographic evidence of LV enlargement; pulmonary congestion; and enlargement of the LA, PA, and right side of the heart.

Catheterization Catheterization of the left side of the heart and coronary arteriography should generally be carried out in patients suspected of having severe AS who are being considered for operative treatment. These investigations are especially indicated in the following:

1. *Patients with clinical signs of AS and symptoms of myocardial ischemia*, in whom associated coronary artery disease is suspected. An

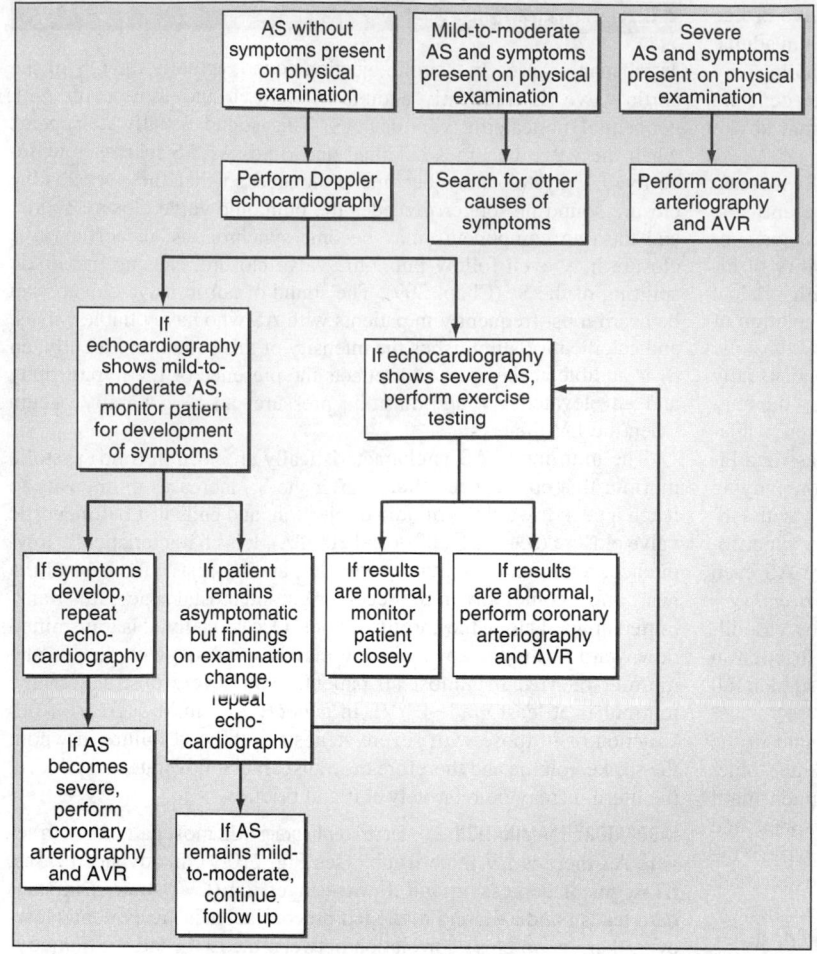

FIGURE 219-5 Algorithm for the management of aortic stenosis. AS, aortic stenosis; AVR, aortic valve replacement. *(From Carabello, 2002.)*

effort should be made to determine whether AS or coronary atherosclerosis is primarily responsible for the symptoms. Coronary arteriography should be carried out to identify patients who require coronary bypass grafting at the time of aortic valve surgery.

2. *Patients with multivalvular disease*, in whom the role played by each valvular deformity should be defined to aid in the planning of definitive operative treatment.

3. *Young, asymptomatic patients with noncalcific congenital AS*, to define with precision the severity of obstruction to LV outflow, since operation [which does not usually require aortic valve replacement (AVR)] or balloon valvotomy may be indicated if severe AS is present, even in the absence of symptoms. Balloon valvotomy may follow left heart catheterization immediately.

4. *Patients in whom it is suspected that the obstruction to LV outflow may not be at the aortic valve* but rather in the sub- or supravalvular regions.

NATURAL HISTORY Death in patients with severe AS occurs most commonly in the seventh and eighth decades. Based on data obtained at postmortem examination in patients before surgical treatment became widely available, the average time to death after the onset of various symptoms was as follows: angina pectoris, 3 years; syncope, 3 years; dyspnea, 2 years; and congestive heart failure, 1.5 to 2 years. Moreover, in >80% of patients who died with AS, symptoms had existed for <4 years. Congestive heart failure was considered to be the cause of death in one-half to two-thirds of patients. Among adults dying with valvular AS, sudden death, which presumably resulted from an arrhythmia, occurred in 10 to 20% and at an average age of 60 years. However, most sudden deaths occur in patients who had previously been symptomatic; thus sudden death is very uncommon (3 per 1000 patient years) in asymptomatic patients with severe AS. Obstructive

calcific AS is a progressive disease, with an annual reduction in valve area of approximately 0.1 mm²/year.

℞ TREATMENT

Medical Treatment (Fig. 219-5, Table 219-1) In patients with severe AS (<0.5 cm²/m²), strenuous physical activity should be avoided, even in the asymptomatic stage. Sodium restriction, the cautious administration of diuretics and digitalis glycosides are indicated in the treatment of congestive heart failure, but care must be taken to avoid volume depletion since this may cause a marked reduction of CO. Nitroglycerin is helpful in relieving angina pectoris. Retrospective studies have shown that patients with degenerative calcific AS who receive HMG-CoA reductase inhibitors ("statins") exhibit slower progression of leaflet calcification and aortic valve area reduction than those who do not. Treatment with these relatively safe agents should be considered while the results of clinical trials are awaited.

Surgical Treatment The most critical decision in the management of AS concerns the advisability of surgical treatment which, in most adults with calcific AS and severe obstruction consists of AVR. However, these patients should be followed carefully for the development of symptoms and by serial echocardiograms for evidence of deteriorating LV function. Operation is generally indicated in patients with severe AS (valve area <1.0 cm² or 0.6 cm²/m² body surface area) who are symptomatic, those who exhibit LV dysfunction, as well as those with an expanding poststenotic aortic root, even if they are asymptomatic. In patients without heart failure, the operative risk of AVR is approximately 4% (Table 219-2). In most instances, it is prudent to postpone operation in patients with severe calcific AS who are asymptomatic and who exhibit normal LV function, i.e., EF >50%, since they may continue to do well for many years. The risk of surgical mortality exceeds that of sudden death in asymptomatic patients. However, AVR can be carried out in asymptomatic patients with severe stenosis who undergo coronary artery bypass grafting.

Operation should, if possible, be carried out before frank LV failure develops; at this late stage, the aortic valve pressure gradient declines as the stroke volume and ejection fraction decline. In such patients, the operative risk is high (15 to 20%), and evidence of myocardial disease may persist even when the operation is technically successful. Furthermore, long-term postoperative survival also correlates inversely with preoperative LV dysfunction. Nonetheless, in view of the even worse prognosis of such patients when they are treated medically, there is usually little choice but to advise surgical treatment, especially in patients in whom contractile reserve can be demonstrated by dobutamine echocardiography. In patients in whom severe AS and coronary artery disease coexist, relief of the AS and revascularization of the myocardium by means of aortocoronary bypass grafting may result in striking clinical and hemodynamic improvement.

Because many patients with calcific AS are elderly, particular attention must be directed to the adequacy of hepatic, renal, and pulmonary function before AVR is recommended. The mortality rate depends to a substantial extent on the patient's preoperative clinical and hemodynamic state. The 10-year survival rate of patients with AVR is approximately 60%. Approximately 30% of bioprosthetic valves evidence primary valve failure in 10 years, requiring rereplacement, and an approximately equal percentage of patients with mechanical prostheses develop significant hemorrhagic complications as a consequence of treatment with anticoagulants.

Percutaneous Balloon Aortic Valvuloplasty This procedure is preferable to operation in children and young adults with congenital, noncalcific AS. It is not commonly used in adults with severe calcific AS because of a high restenosis rate, but has on occasion been used successfully in patients as a "bridge to operation" in patients with severe LV dysfunction who are too ill to tolerate surgery.

AORTIC REGURGITATION

ETIOLOGY   AR may be caused by primary valve disease or by primary aortic root disease.

Primary Valve Disease   Approximately three-fourths of patients with pure or predominant valvular AR are males; females predominate among patients with primary valvular AR who have associated mitral valve disease. In approximately two-thirds of patients with AR the disease is rheumatic in origin, resulting in thickening, deformity, and shortening of the individual aortic valve cusps, changes that prevent their proper opening during systole and closure during diastole. A rheumatic origin is less common in patients with isolated AR. Patients with congenital membranous subaortic stenosis often develop thickening of the aortic valve leaflets, which makes the valves particularly susceptible to endocarditis. AR also may occur in patients with rheumatoid spondylitis and in patients with congenital bicuspid aortic valves. Prolapse of an aortic cusp, resulting in progressive chronic AR, occurs in approximately 15% of patients with ventricular septal defect (Chap. 218). Congenital fenestrations of the aortic valve occasionally produce mild AR.

Acute AR may result from infective endocarditis, which can develop on a valve previously affected by rheumatic disease, a congenitally deformed valve, or, rarely, on a normal aortic valve, and perforate or erode one or more of the leaflets. Although traumatic rupture of the aortic valve is an uncommon cause of acute AR, it does represent the most frequent serious lesion in patients surviving nonpenetrating cardiac injuries. The coexistence of hemodynamically significant AS with AR usually excludes all the rarer forms of AR because it occurs almost exclusively in patients with rheumatic or congenital AR. In patients with AR due to primary valvular disease, dilatation of the aortic annulus may occur secondarily and intensify the regurgitation.

Primary Aortic Root Disease   AR, both acute and chronic, also may be due entirely to marked aortic dilatation, i.e., aortic root disease, without primary involvement of the valve leaflets; widening of the aortic annulus and separation of the aortic leaflets are responsible for the AR (Chap. 231). Cystic medial necrosis of the ascending aorta, which may or may not be associated with other manifestations of the Marfan syndrome, idiopathic dilatation of the aorta, osteogenesis imperfecta, and severe hypertension all may widen the aortic annulus and lead to progressive AR. Occasionally, AR is caused by retrograde dissection of the aorta involving the aortic annulus. Syphilis and rheumatoid ankylosing spondylitis may be associated with cellular infiltration and scarring of the media of the thoracic aorta, leading to aortic dilatation, aneurysm formation, and severe regurgitation. In syphilis of the aorta, now a very rare condition (Chap. 153), the involvement of the intima may narrow the coronary ostia, which in turn may be responsible for myocardial ischemia.

PATHOPHYSIOLOGY   The total stroke volume ejected by the LV (i.e., the sum of the effective forward stroke volume and the volume of blood that regurgitates back into the LV) is increased in patients with AR. In patients with wide-open (free) AR, the volume of regurgitant flow may equal the effective forward stroke volume. In contrast to MR, in which a fraction of the LV stroke volume is delivered into the low-pressure LA, in AR the entire LV stroke volume is ejected into a high-pressure zone, the aorta. An increase in the LV end-diastolic volume (increased preload) constitutes the major hemodynamic compensation for AR. The dilatation and eccentric hypertrophy of the LV allows this chamber to eject a larger stroke volume without requiring any increase in the relative shortening of each myofibril. Therefore, severe AR may occur with a normal effective forward stroke volume and a normal left ventricular EF [total (forward plus regurgitant) stroke volume/end-diastolic volume], together with an elevated LV end-diastolic pressure and volume. However, through the operation of Laplace's law (which

holds that myocardial wall tension is the product of intracavitary pressure and LV radius), LV dilatation increases the LV systolic tension required to develop any given level of systolic pressure. Ultimately, these adaptive measures fail. As LV function deteriorates, the end-diastolic volume rises further and the forward stroke volume and EF decline. Deterioration of LV function often precedes the development of symptoms. Considerable thickening of the LV wall also occurs with chronic AR, and at autopsy the hearts of these patients may be among the largest encountered, sometimes weighing >1000 g.

The reverse pressure gradient from aorta to LV, which drives the AR flow, falls progressively during diastole (see Fig. 212-4), accounting for the decrescendo nature of the diastolic murmur. Equilibration between aortic and LV pressures may occur toward the end of diastole in patients with severe AR, particularly when the heart rate is slow, and the LV end-diastolic pressure may be elevated, occasionally to extremely high levels (>40 mmHg). Rarely, in acute, severe AR, the LV pressure exceeds the LA pressure toward the end of diastole, and this reversed pressure gradient closes the mitral valve prematurely or causes diastolic MR.

In patients with severe AR, the effective forward CO usually is normal or only slightly reduced at rest, but often it fails to rise normally during exertion. Early signs of LV dysfunction include reduction in the EF, determined by echocardiography or radionuclide angiography. In advanced stages there may be considerable elevation of the LA, PA wedge, PA, and RV pressures and lowering of the forward CO at rest.

Myocardial ischemia may occur in patients with AR because myocardial oxygen requirements are elevated by both LV dilatation and elevated LV systolic tension. However, a large fraction of coronary blood flow occurs during diastole, when arterial pressure is subnormal, thereby reducing coronary perfusion pressure. This combination of increased oxygen demand and reduced supply may cause myocardial ischemia, particularly of the subendocardium, even in the absence of concomitant coronary artery disease.

HISTORY   A family history may frequently be elicited from patients with AR associated with the Marfan syndrome. A history compatible with infective endocarditis may sometimes be elicited from patients with rheumatic or congenital involvement of the aortic valve, and the infection often precipitates or seriously aggravates preexisting symptoms. Ankylosing spondylitis is usually self evident.

In patients with *acute, severe AR*, as may occur in infective endocarditis or trauma, the LV cannot dilate sufficiently to maintain stroke volume, and LV diastolic pressure rises rapidly with associated elevations of LA and PA wedge pressures. Pulmonary edema and/or cardiogenic shock may develop rapidly.

Chronic, severe AR may have a long latent period, and patients may remain relatively asymptomatic for as long as 10 to 15 years. However, uncomfortable awareness of the heartbeat, especially on lying down, may be an early complaint. Sinus tachycardia during exertion or with emotion, or premature ventricular contractions may produce particularly uncomfortable palpitations, as well as head pounding. These complaints may persist for many years before the development of exertional dyspnea, usually the first symptom of diminished cardiac reserve. The dyspnea is followed by orthopnea, paroxysmal nocturnal dyspnea, and excessive diaphoresis. Anginal chest pain occurs frequently in patients with severe AR, even in younger patients, and it is not necessary to invoke the presence of coronary artery disease to explain this symptom in patients with severe AR. Anginal pain may develop at rest as well as during exertion. Nocturnal angina may be a particularly troublesome symptom, and it may be accompanied by marked diaphoresis. The anginal episodes can be prolonged and often do not respond satisfactorily to sublingual nitroglycerin. Systemic fluid accumulation, including congestive hepatomegaly and ankle edema, may develop late in the course of the disease.

PHYSICAL FINDINGS   In severe AR, the jarring of the entire body and the bobbing motion of the head with each systole can be appreciated, and

FIGURE 219-6 Transesophageal echocardiographic view of a patient with a dilated aorta, aortic dissection, and severe aortic regurgitation. The *arrow* points to the intimal flap that is seen in the dilated ascending aorta. *Left:* the long axis apex down view of the black and white two-dimensional image in diastole. *Right:* color flow imaging that demonstrates a large mosaic jet of aortic regurgitation. AO, aorta; RV, right ventricle; AR, aortic regurgitation.

the abrupt distention and collapse of the larger arteries are easily visible. The examination should be directed toward the detection of conditions predisposing to AR, such as the Marfan syndrome, rheumatoid ankylosing spondylitis, and ventricular septal defect.

Arterial Pulse A rapidly rising "water-hammer" pulse, which collapses suddenly as arterial pressure falls rapidly during late systole and diastole (Corrigan's pulse), and capillary pulsations, an alternate flushing and paling of the skin at the root of the nail while pressure is applied to the tip of the nail (Quincke's pulse), are characteristic of free AR. A booming, "pistol-shot" sound can be heard over the femoral arteries (Traube's sign), and a to-and-fro murmur (Duroziez's sign) is audible if the femoral artery is lightly compressed with a stethoscope.

The arterial pulse pressure is widened, with an elevation of the systolic pressure, sometimes to as high as 300 mmHg, and a depression of the diastolic pressure. The measurement of arterial diastolic pressure with a sphygmomanometer may be complicated by the fact that systolic sounds are frequently heard with the cuff completely deflated. However, the level of cuff pressure at the time of muffling of the Korotkoff sounds (Phase IV) generally corresponds fairly closely to the true intraarterial diastolic pressure. The severity of AR does not always correlate directly with the arterial pulse pressure, and severe regurgitation may exist in patients with arterial pressures in the range of 140/60 mmHg. As the disease progresses and the LV end-diastolic pressure rises markedly, the arterial diastolic pressure may actually rise also, since the aortic diastolic pressure cannot fall below the LV end-diastolic pressure. For the same reason, *severe, acute* AR may also be accompanied by only light widening of the pulse pressure.

Palpation The LV impulse is heaving and displaced laterally and inferiorly. The systolic expansion and diastolic retraction of the apex are prominent and contrast with the sustained systolic thrust characteristic of severe AS. A diastolic thrill is often palpable along the left sternal border, and a prominent systolic thrill may be palpable in the jugular notch and transmitted upward along the carotid arteries. This systolic thrill and the accompanying murmur are due to the markedly increased blood flow across the aortic orifice and do not necessarily signify the coexistence of AS. In many patients with pure AR or with combined AS and AR, the carotid arterial pulse is bisferiens, i.e., with two systolic waves separated by a trough.

Auscultation In patients with severe AR, the aortic valve closure sound (A_2) is usually absent. An S_3 and systolic ejection sound are frequently audible, and occasionally, an S_4 also may be heard. The murmur of chronic AR is typically a high-pitched, blowing, decrescendo diastolic murmur, heard best in the third intercostal space along the left sternal border (see Fig. 209-5B). In patients with mild AR, this murmur is

brief, but as the severity increases, generally becomes louder and longer, indeed holodiastolic. When the murmur is soft, it can be heard best with the diaphragm of the stethoscope and with the patient sitting up, leaning forward, and with the breath held in forced expiration. In patients in whom the AR is caused by primary valvular disease, the diastolic murmur is usually louder along the left than the right sternal border. However, when the murmur is heard best along the right sternal border, it suggests that the AR is caused by aneurysmal dilatation of the aortic root. "Cooing" or musical diastolic murmurs suggest eversion of an aortic cusp vibrating in the regurgitant stream.

A midsystolic ejection murmur is frequently audible in AR. It is generally heard best at the base of the heart and is transmitted along the carotid vessels. This murmur may be quite loud without signifying aortic obstruction; it is often higher pitched, shorter, and less rasping in quality than the ejection systolic murmur heard in patients with predominant AS. A third murmur frequently heard in patients with severe AR is the *Austin Flint murmur*, a soft, low-pitched, rumbling middiastolic bruit. It is probably produced by the diastolic displacement of the anterior leaflet of the mitral valve by the AR stream but does not appear to be associated with hemodynamically significant mitral obstruction and, in contrast to the diastolic murmur of MS, it is not accompanied by an OS or loud S_1. The auscultatory features of AR are intensified by isometric exercise such as strenuous handgrip, which augments systemic resistance, and reduced by inhalation of amyl nitrite.

In *severe, acute* AR, the elevation of LV end-diastolic pressure may lead to early closure of the mitral valve, an associated middiastolic sound, a soft or absent S_1, a pulse pressure that is not particularly wide, and a soft, short diastolic murmur of AR.

LABORATORY EXAMINATION ■ EKG In patients with severe, chronic AR, the EKG signs of LV hypertrophy become manifest (Chap. 210). In addition, these patients frequently exhibit ST-segment depression and T-wave inversion in leads I, aVL, V_5, and V_6 ("LV strain"). Left axis deviation and/or QRS prolongation denote diffuse myocardial disease, generally associated with patchy fibrosis, and usually signify a poor prognosis.

Echocardiogram The extent and velocity of wall motion are normal or even supernormal, until myocardial contractility declines. A rapid, high-frequency fluttering of the anterior mitral leaflet produced by the impact of the regurgitant jet is a characteristic finding. The echocardiogram is also useful in determining the cause of AR, by detecting dilatation of the aortic annulus (Fig. 219-6). Thickening and failure of coaptation of the leaflets also may be noted. Color flow Doppler echocardiographic imaging is very sensitive in the detection of AR, and Doppler echocardiography is helpful in assessing its severity. Serial two-dimensional echocardiography is valuable in assessing LV performance and in detecting progressive myocardial dysfunction.

Roentgenogram In severe chronic AR, the apex is displaced downward and to the left in the frontal projection, and frequently the cardiac shadow extends below the left diaphragm. LV enlargement also may be apparent in the left anterior oblique and lateral projections, in which the LV is displaced posteriorly and encroaches on the spine. In patients in whom primary valvular disease is responsible for the AR, the ascending aorta and aortic knob may be moderately dilated. When AR is caused by primary disease of the aortic wall, aneurysmal dilatation of the aorta may be noted, and the aorta may fill the retrosternal space in the lateral view.

Cardiac Catheterization and Angiography In addition to providing accurate confirmation of the magnitude of regurgitation and the status of

LV function, the condition of the coronary arterial bed should ordinarily be evaluated preoperatively.

℞ TREATMENT

Medical Treatment (Table 219-1) Although operation constitutes the definitive treatment of AR and should be carried out before the development of heart failure, the latter usually responds briefly to treatment with digitalis glycosides, salt restriction, diuretics, and vasodilators, especially ACE inhibitors. Digitalis also may be indicated in patients with severe regurgitation and dilated left ventricles without frank LV failure. Cardiac arrhythmias and infections are poorly tolerated in patients with severe AR and must be treated promptly and vigorously. Although nitroglycerin and long-acting nitrates are not as helpful in relieving anginal pain as they are in patients with ischemic heart disease, they are worth a trial. Long-acting nifedipine has been found to delay the need for operation. Patients with syphilitic aortitis should receive a full course of penicillin therapy (Chap. 153).

Surgical Treatment In deciding on the advisability and proper timing of surgical treatment, two points should be kept in mind: (1) patients with chronic AR usually do not become symptomatic until *after* the development of myocardial dysfunction, and (2) when delayed too long, surgical treatment often does not restore normal LV function. Therefore, in patients with severe AR, careful clinical follow-up and noninvasive testing with echocardiography at approximately 6-month intervals are necessary if operation is to be undertaken at the optimal time, i.e., *after* the onset of LV dysfunction but *prior* to the development of severe symptoms. Operation can be deferred as long as the patient both remains asymptomatic and retains normal LV function. In general, operation should be carried out even in asymptomatic patients with progressive LV dysfunction and a left ventricular ejection fraction (LVEF) <55% or a LV end-systolic volume >55 mL/m². These parameters have been referred to as the "55/55 rule."

AVR with a suitable mechanical or tissue prosthesis is generally necessary in patients with rheumatic AR and in many patients with other forms of regurgitation. Rarely, when a leaflet has been perforated during infective endocarditis or torn from its attachments to the aortic annulus by thoracic trauma, surgical repair may be possible. When AR is due to aneurysmal dilatation of the annulus and ascending aorta rather than to primary valvular involvement, it may be possible to reduce the regurgitation by narrowing the annulus or by excising a portion of the aortic root without replacing the valve. More frequently, however, regurgitation can be eliminated only by replacing the aortic valve, excising the dilated or aneurysmal ascending aorta responsible for the regurgitation, and replacing it with a graft. This formidable procedure entails a higher risk than isolated AVR.

As in patients with other valvular abnormalities, both the operative risk and the late mortality are largely dependent on the stage of the disease and on myocardial function at the time of operation. The overall operative mortality for isolated AVR is 4.3% (Table 219-2). However, patients with marked cardiac enlargement and prolonged LV dysfunction experience an operative mortality rate of approximately 10% and a late mortality rate of approximately 5% per year due to LV failure despite a technically satisfactory operation. Nonetheless, because of the very poor prognosis with medical management, even patients with LV failure should be considered for operation.

Patients with acute, severe AR require prompt surgical treatment, which may be lifesaving.

TRICUSPID STENOSIS

TS, a relatively uncommon valvular lesion in North America and Western Europe, is more common in tropical and subtropical climates, especially in southern Asia and in Latin America. It is generally rheumatic in origin and is more common in females than in males. It does not occur as an isolated lesion and is usually associated with MS. Hemodynamically significant TS occurs in 5 to 10% of patients with severe MS; rheumatic TS is commonly associated with some degree of TR.

PATHOPHYSIOLOGY A diastolic pressure gradient between the RA and RV can be recorded with a double-lumen cardiac catheter. It is augmented when the transvalvular blood flow increases during inspiration and declines during expiration. A mean diastolic pressure gradient of 4 mmHg is usually sufficient to elevate the mean RA pressure to levels that result in systemic venous congestion. Unless sodium intake has been restricted and diuretics administered, this venous congestion is associated with ascites and edema, sometimes severe. In patients with sinus rhythm, the RA *a* wave may be extremely tall and may even approach the level of the RV systolic pressure. The CO at rest is usually depressed and it fails to rise during exercise. The low CO is responsible for the normal or only slightly elevated LA, PA, and RV systolic pressures despite the presence of MS. Thus, the presence of TS can mask the hemodynamic and clinical features of the MS which usually accompanies it.

SYMPTOMS Since the development of MS generally precedes that of TS, many patients initially have symptoms of pulmonary congestion. Amelioration of these symptoms should raise the possibility that TS may be developing. Characteristically, patients complain of relatively little dyspnea for the degree of hepatomegaly, ascites, and edema that they have. However, fatigue secondary to a low CO and discomfort due to refractory edema, ascites, and marked hepatomegaly are common in patients with TS and/or TR. In some patients, TS may be suspected for the first time when symptoms of RV failure persist after an adequate mitral valvotomy.

PHYSICAL FINDINGS

Since TS usually occurs in the presence of other obvious valvular disease, the diagnosis may be missed unless it is specifically searched for. Severe TS is associated with marked hepatic congestion, often resulting in cirrhosis, jaundice, serious malnutrition, anasarca, and ascites. Congestive hepatomegaly and, in cases of severe tricuspid valve disease, splenomegaly are present. The jugular veins are distended, and in patients with sinus rhythm there may be giant *a* waves. The *v* waves are less conspicuous, and since tricuspid obstruction impedes RA emptying during diastole, there is a slow *y* descent. In patients with sinus rhythm there may be prominent presystolic pulsations of the enlarged liver as well.

On auscultation, the pulmonic valve closure sound is not accentuated, and occasionally, an OS of the tricuspid valve may be heard approximately 0.06 s after pulmonic valve closure. The diastolic murmur of TS has many of the qualities of the diastolic murmur of MS, and since TS almost always occurs in the presence of MS, the less common valvular lesion may be missed. However, the tricuspid murmur is generally heard best along the left lower sternal margin and over the xiphoid process and is most prominent during presystole in patients with sinus rhythm. The diastolic murmur is reduced in amplitude as the stethoscope is inched laterally, only to intensify or reappear as the mitral murmur at the apex. The murmur of TS is augmented during inspiration, and it is reduced during expiration and particularly during the strain of Valsalva maneuver, when tricuspid blood flow is reduced.

LABORATORY EXAMINATION The ECG features of RA enlargement (Chap. 210) include tall, peaked P waves in lead II, as well as prominent, upright P waves in lead V_1. The *absence* of ECG evidence of right ventricular hypertrophy (RVH) in a patient with right-sided heart failure who is believed to have MS should suggest associated tricuspid valve disease. The chest roentgenogram in patients with combined TS and MS shows particular prominence of the RA and superior vena cava without much enlargement of the PA and with less evidence of pulmonary vascular congestion than occurs in patients with isolated MS. On echocardiographic examination, the tricuspid valve is usually thickened; the transvalvular gradient can be estimated by Doppler echocardiography.

℞ TREATMENT

Patients with TS generally exhibit marked systemic venous congestion; intensive salt restriction and diuretic therapy are required during the preoperative period. Such a preparatory period may diminish hepatic congestion and thereby improve hepatic function sufficiently so that the risks of operation are diminished. Surgical relief of the TS should be carried out, preferably at the time of surgical mitral valvotomy or MVR, in patients with moderate or severe TS who have mean diastolic pressure gradients exceeding approximately 4 mmHg and tricuspid orifices less than 1.5 to 2.0 cm^2. TS is almost always accompanied by significant TR. Open-heart repair may permit substantial improvement of tricuspid valve function. If this cannot be accomplished, the tricuspid valve may have to be replaced with a prosthesis, preferably a large bioprosthetic valve.

TRICUSPID REGURGITATION

Most commonly, TR is functional and secondary to marked dilatation of the tricuspid annulus. Functional TR may complicate RV enlargement of any cause, including inferior wall infarcts that involve the RV. It is commonly seen in the late stages of heart failure due to rheumatic or congenital heart disease with severe pulmonary hypertension, as well as in ischemic heart disease, cardiomyopathy, and cor pulmonale. It is in part reversible if pulmonary hypertension is relieved. Rheumatic fever may produce organic TR, often associated with TS. Infarction of RV papillary muscles, tricuspid valve prolapse, carcinoid heart disease, endomyocardial fibrosis, infective endocarditis, and trauma all may produce TR. Less commonly, TR results from congenitally deformed tricuspid valves, and it occurs with defects of the atrioventricular canal as well as with Ebstein's malformation of the tricuspid valve (Chap. 218).

As is the case for TS, the clinical features of TR result primarily from systemic venous congestion and reduction of CO. With the onset of TR in patients with pulmonary hypertension, symptoms of pulmonary congestion diminish, but the clinical manifestations of right-sided heart failure become intensified. The neck veins are distended with prominent *v* waves; and marked hepatomegaly, ascites, pleural effusions, edema, systolic pulsations of the liver, and a positive hepatojugular reflux are common. A prominent RV pulsation along the left parasternal region and a blowing holosystolic murmur along the lower left sternal margin, which may be intensified during inspiration and reduced during expiration or the strain of the Valsalva maneuver, are characteristic findings; AF is usually present.

The ECG usually shows changes characteristic of the lesion responsible for the enlargement of the RV that leads to TR, e.g., inferior wall myocardial infarction or severe RVH. Echocardiography may be helpful by demonstrating RV dilatation and prolapsing or flail tricuspid leaflets; the diagnosis of TR can be made by color flow Doppler echocardiography, and the severity estimated by Doppler examination. The latter is also useful in estimating PA pressure. Roentgenographic examination usually reveals enlargement of both the RA and RV.

In patients with severe TR, the CO is usually markedly reduced, and the RA pressure pulse may exhibit no *x* descent during early systole but a prominent *c-v* wave with a rapid *y* descent. The mean RA and the RV end-diastolic pressures are often elevated.

℞ TREATMENT

Isolated TR, in the absence of pulmonary hypertension, such as that occurring as a consequence of infective endocarditis or trauma, is usually well tolerated and does not require operation. Indeed, even total excision of an infected tricuspid valve may be well tolerated for several years if the PA pressure is normal. Treatment of the underlying cause of heart failure usually reduces the severity of functional TR by reducing the size of the tricuspid annulus. In patients with mitral valve disease and TR secondary to pulmonary hypertension and massive RV

enlargement, effective surgical correction of the mitral valvular abnormality results in lowering of the PA pressures and gradual reduction or disappearance of the TR without direct treatment of the tricuspid valve. However, recovery may be much more rapid in patients with severe secondary TR if, at the time of mitral valve surgery, tricuspid annuloplasty (generally with the insertion of a plastic ring), open tricuspid valve repair, or, in the rare instance of severe organic tricuspid valve disease, tricuspid valve replacement is performed. Surgical treatment of the TR also should be carried out in patients with severe regurgitation secondary to deformity of the tricuspid valve due to rheumatic fever, particularly those *without* severe pulmonary hypertension.

PULMONIC VALVE DISEASE

The pulmonic valve is affected by rheumatic fever far less frequently than are the other valves, and it is uncommonly the seat of infective endocarditis. The most common *acquired* abnormality affecting the pulmonic valve is regurgitation secondary to dilatation of the pulmonic valve ring as a consequence of severe pulmonary hypertension. This produces the *Graham Steell murmur*, a high-pitched, decrescendo, diastolic blowing murmur along the left sternal border, which is difficult to differentiate from the far more common murmur produced by AR. It is usually of little hemodynamic significance; indeed, surgical removal or destruction of the pulmonic valve by infective endocarditis does not produce heart failure unless serious pulmonary hypertension is also present. The *carcinoid syndrome* may cause pulmonic stenosis and/or regurgitation. ➔*Congenital pulmonic stenosis is discussed in Chap. 218.*

VALVE REPLACEMENT

The results of replacement of any valve are dependent primarily on (1) the patient's myocardial function and general medical condition at the time of operation; (2) the technical abilities of the operative team and the quality of the postoperative care; and (3) the durability, hemodynamic characteristics, and thrombogenicity of the prosthesis. Increased operative mortality is associated with advanced age, comorbidity (e.g., pulmonary or renal disease, the need for nonvalvular cardiovascular surgery, diabetes mellitus) as well as with higher levels of preoperative functional disability and pulmonary hypertension. Late complications of valve replacement include paravalvular leakage, thromboemboli, bleeding due to anticoagulants, mechanical dysfunction of the prosthesis, and infective endocarditis.

The considerations involved in the choice between a bioprosthetic (tissue) and artificial mechanical valve are similar in the mitral and aortic sites and in the treatment of stenotic, regurgitant, or mixed lesions. All patients who have undergone replacement of any valve with a mechanical prosthesis are at risk of thromboembolic complications and must be maintained permanently on anticoagulants, a treatment that imposes a hazard of hemorrhage. The primary advantage of bioprostheses over mechanical prostheses is the virtual absence of thromboembolic complications 3 months after implantation, and except for patients with chronic AF, few such instances have been associated with their use. The major disadvantage of bioprosthetic valves is their mechanical deterioration, the incidence of which is inversely proportional to the patient's age. This results in the need to replace the prosthesis in 30% of patients by 10 years and in 50% by 15 years. Because this complication is age-related, bioprostheses are ordinarily not used in patients under 65 years but are particularly useful in the elderly (>70 years), in whom there is more concern about chronic anticoagulation than about long-term (>20 years) valve durability. Patients between 65 and 70 years should be evaluated on a case-by-case basis as to the use of a bioprosthetic or mechanical valve. Bioprosthetic valves are also indicated in women who expect to become pregnant, as well as others in whom anticoagulation may be contraindicated. Alternative bioprostheses are xenografts [i.e., porcine aortic valves; cryopreserved, mounted bovine pericardium; homograft (allograft) aortic valves obtained from cadavers as well as pulmonary autografts transplanted into the aortic position.]

In patients without contraindications to anticoagulants, particularly those under 65 years, a mechanical prosthesis may be preferable. Many surgeons now select the St. Jude prosthesis, a double-disk tilting prosthesis, for replacement of both aortic and mitral valves because of favorable hemodynamic characteristics and possible association with lower thrombogenicity.

FURTHER READING

BONOW RO et al: ACC/AHA Guidelines for the management of patients with valvular heart disease. J Am Coll Cardiol 32:1486, 1998

BONOW RD, BRAUNWALD E: Valvular heart disease, in D Zipes et al (eds): *Braunwald's Heart Disease*, 7th ed. Philadelphia, Saunders, 2005

CANNEGIETER SC et al: Oral anticoagulant treatment in patients with mechanical heart valves: How to reduce the risk of thromboembolic and bleeding complications. J Intern Med 245:369, 1999

CARABELLO BA: Aortic stenosis. N Engl J Med 346:677, 2002

ENRIQUEZ-SARANO M: Timing of mitral valve surgery. Heart 87:79, 2002

FANN JI, BURDON TA: Are the indications for tissue valves different in 2001 and how do we communicate these changes to our cardiology colleagues? Curr Opin Cardiol 16:126, 2001

HA JW et al: Tricuspid stenosis and regurgitation: Doppler and color flow echocardiography and cardiac catheterization findings. Clin Cardiol 23:51, 2000

HUNG L, RAHIMTOOLA SH: Prosthetic heart valves and pregnancy. Circulation 107:1240, 2003

JAMIESON WRE et al: Risk stratification for cardiac valve replacement. National Cardiac Surgery Database. Ann Thorac Surg 67:943, 1999

NOVARO GM et al: Effect of hydroxymethylglutaryl coenzyme A reductase inhibitors on the progression of calcific aortic stenosis. Circulation 104:2205, 2001

PALACIOS IF et al: Which patients benefit from percutaneous mitral balloon valvuloplasty? Prevalvuloplasty and postvalvuloplasty variables that predict long-term outcome. Circulation 105:1465, 2002

PEREIRA JJ et al: Survival after aortic valve replacement for severe aortic stenosis with low transvalvular gradients and severe left ventricular dysfunction. J Am Coll Cardiol 39:1356, 2002

220 | PULMONARY HYPERTENSION
Stuart Rich

Pulmonary hypertension, an abnormal elevation in pulmonary artery pressure, may reflect an increase in left heart filling pressure in the presence of normal pulmonary vascular resistance, pulmonary vascular or parenchymal disease with an elevation in pulmonary vascular resistance, or a combination of these initiating factors. Whether the pulmonary hypertension arises from cardiac, pulmonary, or intrinsic vascular disease, it generally is a feature of advanced disease. Because the causes of pulmonary hypertension are so diverse, it is essential that the etiology underlying the pulmonary hypertension be clearly determined before embarking on treatment. Recent data suggest that mild increases in pulmonary artery pressure also occur with age as the pulmonary circulation becomes less compliant.

Cor pulmonale (Chap. 216) is a term used to indicate right ventricular (RV) enlargement secondary to any underlying cardiac or pulmonary disease. Pulmonary hypertension is the most common cause of cor pulmonale. Advanced cor pulmonale is associated with the development of RV failure.

PATHOPHYSIOLOGY The right ventricle responds to an increase in resistance within the pulmonary circulation by increasing RV systolic pressure as necessary to preserve cardiac output. The increase in pulmonary vascular resistance may be attributed to excessive production of vascular growth factors, mechanical obstruction of the pulmonary arteries, hypoxia, or other stimuli. Over time, chronic changes occur in the pulmonary circulation resulting in remodeling of the vasculature, which can sustain or promote pulmonary hypertension even if the initiating factor is removed.

On occasion a patient may have marked elevations in pulmonary artery pressure in association with obstructive or interstitial lung disease, essential hypertension, ischemic heart disease, or valvular heart disease. Although it may appear that the pulmonary hypertension is out of proportion to the underlying associated condition, it likely represents a pulmonary vasoconstrictor response to the associated condition, which serves as a trigger of the pulmonary arteriopathy. The distinction is important because the treatment of pulmonary hypertension should include treating the underlying associated cause whenever possible.

The ability of the right ventricle to adapt to increased vascular resistance is influenced by several factors including age and the rapidity of the development of pulmonary hypertension. For example, a large acute pulmonary thromboembolism can result in RV failure and shock, whereas chronic thromboembolic disease of equal severity may result in only mild exercise intolerance. Coexisting hypoxemia from lung disease or myocardial ischemia from coronary artery disease can impair the ability of the ventricle to compensate. The onset of clinical RV failure, usually manifest by peripheral edema, is associated with a poor outcome.

DIAGNOSIS A thorough diagnostic evaluation of all potential causes of pulmonary hypertension should be undertaken (Fig. 220-1). The most

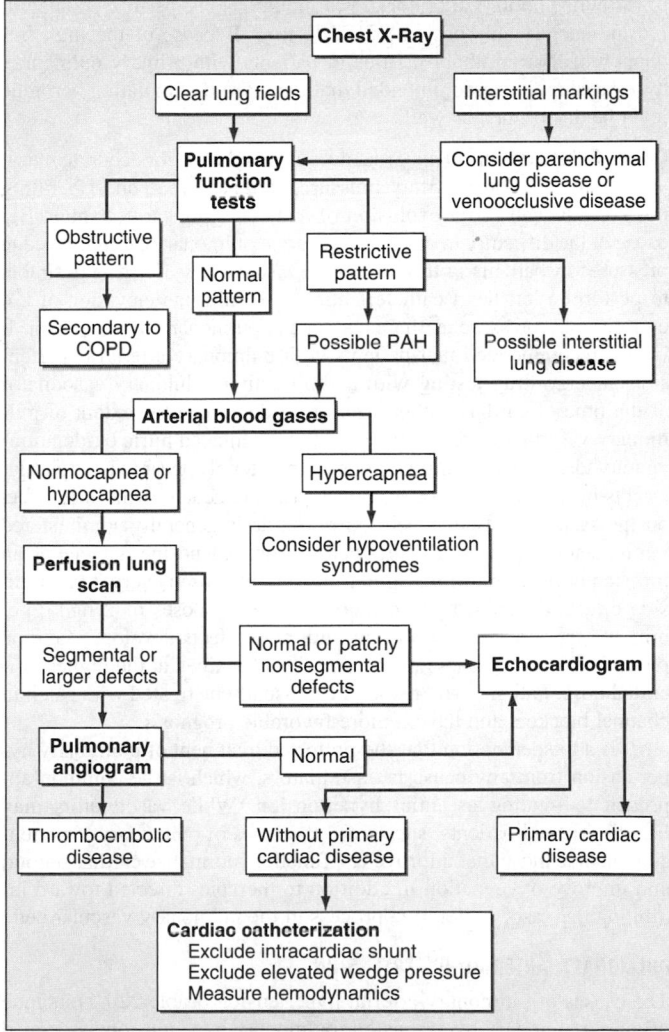

FIGURE 220-1 An algorithm for the workup of a patient with unexplained pulmonary hypertension. (*Adapted with permission from Rich.*)

common symptom attributable to pulmonary hypertension is exertional dyspnea. Other common symptoms are fatigue, angina pectoris that may represent RV ischemia, syncope, near syncope, and peripheral edema.

The physical examination typically reveals increased jugular venous pressure, a reduced carotid pulse, and a palpable RV lift. Most patients have an increased pulmonic component of the second heart sound and a right-sided fourth heart sound (Chap. 209). Tricuspid regurgitation is a clinical feature of RV failure. Peripheral cyanosis and/or edema tend to occur in later stages of the disease. The presence of clubbing can be a clinical clue that the patient has underlying congenital heart disease or hypoxemic lung disease.

Laboratory Findings   The chest x-ray generally shows enlarged central pulmonary arteries. The lung fields may or may not reveal other pathology. The electrocardiogram usually reveals right axis deviation and RV hypertrophy. The echocardiogram commonly demonstrates RV and right atrial enlargement, a reduction in left ventricular (LV) cavity size, and a tricuspid regurgitant jet that can be used to estimate RV systolic pressure. Pulmonary function tests are helpful in documenting underlying obstructive airways disease or severe restrictive lung disease. Hypoxemia and an abnormal diffusing capacity for carbon monoxide are common findings of pulmonary hypertension of most causes. A perfusion lung scan is almost always abnormal in patients with thromboembolic pulmonary hypertension (Chap. 244). However, diffuse patchy filling defects of a nonsegmental nature can often be seen in longstanding pulmonary hypertension in the absence of thromboemboli. Laboratory tests should also be performed, including antinuclear antibody and HIV testing. Because of the high frequency of thyroid abnormalities in patients with primary pulmonary hypertension, it is recommended that the thyroid-stimulating hormone level be determined as well.

Cardiac Catheterization   This procedure is mandatory for accurate measurement of pulmonary artery pressure, cardiac output, and LV filling pressure, as well as for exclusion of an underlying cardiac shunt. Because of the difficulty in obtaining accurate pulmonary capillary wedge pressures in patients with pulmonary vascular disease, it is desirable to perform a left heart catheterization to identify an elevation of LV end-diastolic pressure as the cause of the pulmonary hypertension. It is also recommended that patients with pulmonary arterial hypertension undergo drug testing with a short-acting pulmonary vasodilator at the time of cardiac catheterization to determine the extent of pulmonary vasodilator reactivity (Fig. 220-2). Inhaled nitric oxide, intravenous adenosine, and intravenous epoprostenol appear to have similar effects in reducing pulmonary artery pressure acutely with little effect on the systemic vascular bed. Nitric oxide is generally administered via inhalation in 10 to 20 parts per million. Adenosine is given as an infusion of doses of 50 μg/kg per min and increased every 2 min until side effects develop. Epoprostenol is given in doses of 2 ng/kg per min and increased every 30 min until side effects develop. Maximal physiologic effectiveness of the drug is determined at the highest tolerated dose. Patients who respond can usually be treated with calcium channel blockers and have a more favorable prognosis.

It is a misperception that the preferred treatment of pulmonary hypertension from any cause is vasodilators, which is the common approach to treating essential hypertension. While vasodilators may benefit selected patients, successful therapies of pulmonary hypertension include those that improve RV function, normalize cardiac output, and improve oxygenation in addition to therapies directed toward inhibiting the vasoproliferative process in the pulmonary vascular bed.

PULMONARY ARTERIAL HYPERTENSION

The causes of pulmonary arterial hypertension (Table 220-1) include primary pulmonary hypertension, pulmonary hypertension associated with the collagen vascular diseases, congenital systemic to pulmonary shunts, portal hypertension, HIV infection, anorexigen use, and per-

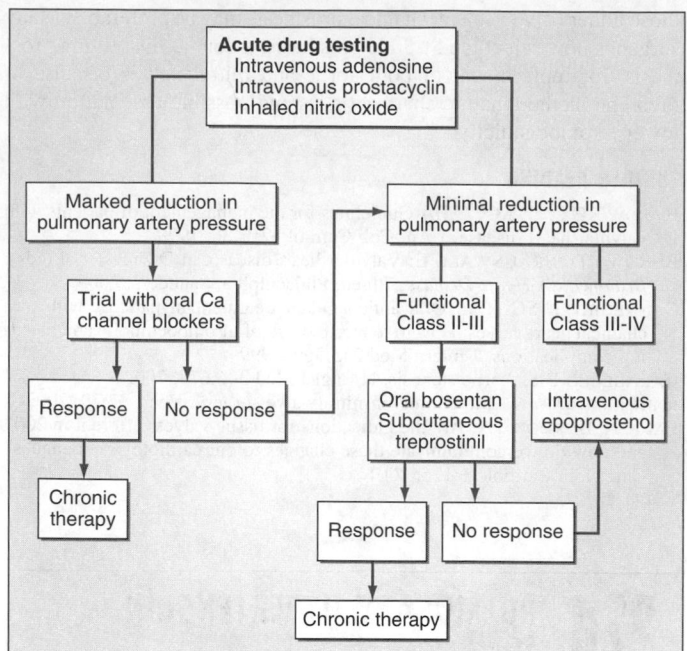

FIGURE 220-2   An algorithm for the selection of optimal drug treatment of a patient with pulmonary arterial hypertension. (*Adapted with permission from Rich.*)

sistent pulmonary hypertension of the newborn. These patients share a common histopathology that includes pulmonary vascular abnormalities involving the endothelium, smooth-muscle cells, and extracellular matrix. The most common features are medial hypertrophy, eccentric and concentric intimal fibrosis, recanalized thrombi appearing as fibrous webs, and plexiform lesions.

Pathobiology   There are likely several pathobiologic processes that result in pulmonary arterial hypertension as a final common pathway. These include inhibition of the voltage-regulated potassium channel producing vasoconstriction of the pulmonary artery smooth-muscle cells, reduced expression of nitric oxide synthase in the endothelium of the pulmonary arterial bed, increased expression of endothelin and basic fibroblast growth factor, and thrombin deposition related to a procoagulant state. The types of abnormalities that occur are likely influenced by the patient's genotype and exposure to risk factors that serve to trigger these processes.

TABLE 220-1   *Additional Diagnostic Tests to Evaluate the Suspected Cause of Pulmonary Hypertension*

Cause	Diagnostic Test
Collagen vascular disease	Serologic and immunogenetic studies
Congenital heart disease	Transesophageal echocardiography with contrast
Portal hypertension	Ultrasonography, computed tomography (CT)
Human immunodeficiency virus	HIV serologic test
Left ventricular diastolic dysfunction	Left ventricular end-diastolic pressure or left atrial pressure measurement
Mitral valve disease	Echocardiography with Doppler
Mediastinal fibrosis	CT, magnetic resonance imaging
Chronic obstructive lung disease	Pulmonary function tests
Obstructive sleep apnea	Sleep apnea study
Pulmonary fibrosis	High-resolution chest CT
Interstitial pneumonitis	Transbronchial or open-lung biopsy
Pulmonary thromboembolic disease	Perfusion lung scan, contrast-enhanced
	Spiral CT, pulmonary angiography
Sarcoidosis	Lung or lymph node biopsy

PRIMARY PULMONARY HYPERTENSION

Primary pulmonary hypertension (PPH) is uncommon, with an estimated incidence of 2 cases per million. There is a strong female predominance, with most patients presenting in the fourth and fifth decades, although the age range is from infancy to >60 years.

GENETIC CONSIDERATIONS Familial PPH accounts for 12 to 20% of cases of PPH and is characterized by autosomal dominant inheritance, variable age of onset, and incomplete penetrance. The clinical and pathologic features of familial and sporadic PPH are identical. Heterozygous germline mutations that involve the gene coding the type II bone morphogenetic protein receptor (BMPR II), a member of the transforming growth factor β superfamily, have been found to underlie many cases of familial PPH. This gene, which is located on chromosome 2q31, has been designated as the PPH I gene. An interruption in the BMP-mediated signaling pathway predisposes the cells within the small pulmonary arteries to proliferation rather than apoptosis. These observations support the concept that PPH is a result of abnormal proliferation of pulmonary vascular endothelial and smooth-muscle cells.

NATURAL HISTORY The natural history of PPH is uncertain because initially the disease can be asymptomatic. Because the predominant symptom is dyspnea, which can have an insidious onset, the disease is typically diagnosed late in its course. Prior to current therapies, a mean survival of 2 to 3 years from the time of diagnosis was reported. It appears that the survival of patients with pulmonary hypertension secondary to congenital heart disease is longer than for patients with PPH, while the survival of patients with pulmonary hypertension secondary to scleroderma is shorter. Functional class remains a strong predictor of survival, with patients who are in New York Heart Association (NYHA) functional class IV having a mean survival of <6 months. The cause of death is usually RV failure, which is manifest by progressive hypoxemia, tachycardia, hypotension, and edema.

℞ TREATMENT

Because the pulmonary artery pressure in PPH increases dramatically with exercise, patients should be cautioned against participating in activities that demand increased physical stress. Digoxin may increase cardiac output and lower circulating levels of norepinephrine. Diuretic therapy relieves peripheral edema and may be useful in reducing RV volume overload in the presence of tricuspid regurgitation. Resting and exercise pulse oximetry should be obtained, as oxygen supplementation helps to alleviate dyspnea and RV ischemia in patients whose arterial oxygen saturation is reduced. Anticoagulant therapy is advocated for all patients with PPH since thrombin deposition occurs in the pulmonary circulation; thrombin can serve as a growth factor to promote the disease process. One retrospective study and one prospective study demonstrated that the anticoagulant warfarin increases survival of patients with PPH. The dose of warfarin is generally titrated to achieve an INR of two to three times control.

Calcium Channel Blockers Patients who have substantial reductions in pulmonary arterial pressure in response to short-acting vasodilators at the time of cardiac catheterization may be candidates for oral calcium channel blockers. Typically, patients require high doses (e.g., nifedipine, 240 mg/d, or amlodipine, 20 mg/d[1]). Patients who respond favorably usually have dramatic reductions in pulmonary artery pressure and pulmonary vascular resistance associated with improved symptoms, regression of RV hypertrophy, and improved survival with chronic therapy. However, <20% of patients respond to calcium channel blockers in the long term. These drugs can be particularly hazardous when given to patients who are unresponsive, as they can result in hypotension, hypoxemia, tachycardia, and worsening right heart failure.

Prostacyclins *Epoprostenol* is the best characterized approved treatment of pulmonary arterial hypertension for patients who are NYHA functional class III or IV and unresponsive to other therapies. Clinical trials have demonstrated an improvement in symptoms, exercise tolerance, and survival even if no acute hemodynamic response to drug challenge occurs. Recent reports have documented sustained benefits for >10 years in some patients. The drug can only be administered intravenously and requires placement of a permanent central venous catheter and infusion through an ambulatory infusion pump system. It generally takes several months to titrate the dose gradually upwards to optimal clinical efficacy, which is usually between 25 and 50 ng/kg per min. Side effects include flushing, jaw pain, and diarrhea, which are generally tolerated by most patients. The major problem with this therapy is infection related to the venous catheter, which requires close monitoring and diligence on behalf of the patient.

Recently, *treprostinil* has been approved for patients with PPH who are NYHA functional classes II to IV and who are unresponsive to conventional therapy, defined as anticoagulation, diuretics, and calcium blockers. An analogue of epoprostenol, treprostinil has a longer half-life and is stable at room temperature, allowing it to be administered subcutaneously through a small infusion pump that was originally developed for insulin. Short-term clinical trials have demonstrated an increase in exercise capacity and a reduction of dyspnea. The major problem with this treatment has been local pain at the infusion site, which has caused patients to discontinue therapy.

Endothelin Receptor Antagonists The nonselective endothelin receptor antagonist *bosentan* was recently approved as an oral treatment of PPH for patients who are NYHA functional classes III and IV and who are unresponsive to conventional therapy. In randomized clinical trials, bosentan was shown to improve exercise tolerance as measured by an increase in 6-min walk distance, improve functional class, and extend time until clinical worsening versus placebo. Therapy is initiated at 62.5 mg bid for the first month and then increased to 125 mg bid thereafter. Because of the high frequency of abnormal hepatic function tests associated with drug use, primarily an increase in transaminases, it is recommended that liver function be monitored monthly throughout the duration of use. Bosentan is also contraindicated in patients who are currently on cyclosporine or glyburide. There are no data to support the use of bosentan for other forms of pulmonary hypertension.

Sildenafil There have been several case reports on the use of sildenafil (Viagra), an oral phosphodiesterase-5 inhibitor, in the treatment of pulmonary hypertension. Phosphodiesterase-5 is responsible for the hydrolysis of cyclic GMP in pulmonary vascular smooth muscles, the mediator through which nitric oxide lowers pulmonary artery pressure and inhibits pulmonary vascular growth. These reports suggest that oral sildenafil has a similar efficacy to inhaled nitric oxide. Large randomized clinical trials using sildenafil as a treatment of pulmonary hypertension are under consideration.

Lung Transplantation (See also Chap. 248) Lung transplantation is considered for patients who, while on epoprostenol, continue to manifest right heart failure. Acceptable results have been achieved with heart-lung, bilateral lung, and single lung transplant. The availability of donor organs often influences the choice of procedure. The recurrence of PPH has never been reported in a patient who has undergone lung transplantation.

CONDITIONS ASSOCIATED WITH PULMONARY HYPERTENSION

COLLAGEN VASCULAR DISEASE All of the collagen vascular diseases may be associated with pulmonary arterial hypertension. This complication occurs commonly with the CREST syndrome (calcinosis, Raynaud's phenomenon, esophageal involvement, sclerodactyly, and telangiectasia) and in scleroderma (Chap. 303), and less frequently in systemic lupus erythematosus (Chap. 300), Sjögrens syndrome (Chap. 304), dermatomyositis, polymyositis (Chap. 306), and rheumatoid arthritis (Chap. 301). It is usual for these patients to have some element of coexistent interstitial pulmonary fibrosis even though it may not be apparent on chest x-ray, computed tomography, or pulmonary function tests. Consequently, these patients tend to have hypoxemia as an important clinical feature, along with the other classic findings of pulmonary hypertension.

Treatment for these patients is identical to that for patients with PPH (see above) but is less effective. It is rare for these patients to respond to calcium channel blockers. Bosentan, treprostinil, and epoprostenol have been effective in clinical trials. The treatment of the pulmonary hypertension, however, does not affect the natural history of the underlying collagen vascular disease.

CONGENITAL SYSTEMIC TO PULMONARY SHUNTS It is common for large post-tricuspid cardiac shunts (e.g., ventricular septal defect, patent ductus arteriosus) to produce severe pulmonary hypertension (Chap. 218), which, although less common, may also occur in pre-tricuspid shunts (e.g., atrial septal defect, anomalous pulmonary venous drainage). In patients with uncorrected shunts, the clinical features include those associated with right-to-left shunting such as hypoxemia and peripheral cyanosis, which worsen dramatically with exertion (Chap. 31). Pulmonary arterial hypertension may occur years or even decades after surgical correction of these lesions, in which case there will be no associated right-to-left shunting. These patients present similarly to patients with PPH but tend to have better long-term survival. This has been attributed to the more slowly progressive nature of the underlying vascular disease. The treatments are similar to those for PPH.

PORTAL HYPERTENSION Portal hypertension is associated with pulmonary arterial hypertension, but the mechanism remains unknown. The risk is not related to the severity of underlying liver disease. Patients with advanced cirrhosis can have the combined features of a high-output cardiac state in association with the features of pulmonary hypertension and RV failure. Thus, a normal cardiac output may actually reflect a marked impairment of RV function. The etiology of ascites and edema can be confusing in these patients since it can have both cardiac and hepatic causes. Venous congestion from right heart failure, however, is poorly tolerated by cirrhotic livers. Patients with mild pulmonary hypertension who have a favorable response to epoprostenol have undergone successful liver transplantation with improvement of the pulmonary vascular disease.

HIV INFECTION The mechanism by which HIV infection produces pulmonary hypertension remains unknown (Chap. 173). The evaluation and treatment are identical to those for PPH. Treatment of the HIV infection does not appear to affect the severity or natural history of the underlying pulmonary hypertension.

ANOREXIGENS A causal relationship has been established between exposure to several anorexigens, including aminorex and the fenfluramines, and the development of pulmonary arterial hypertension. Although the fenfluramines were removed from the world markets in 1997, there are still patients who were exposed prior to that time who are now developing pulmonary hypertension. While the clinical features are identical to those of PPH, the patients appear to be less responsive to medical treatments and have a poorer prognosis.

PULMONARY VENOOCCLUSIVE DISEASE Pulmonary venoocclusive disease is a rare and distinct pathologic entity found in <10% of patients who present with the diagnosis of unexplained pulmonary hypertension. Histologically it is manifest by widespread intimal proliferation and fibrosis of the intrapulmonary veins and venules, occasionally extending to the arteriolar bed. The pulmonary venous obstruction explains the increase in pulmonary capillary wedge pressure observed in patients with advanced disease. These patients may develop orthopnea that can mimic LV failure. The therapy of this condition is not established.

PULMONARY CAPILLARY HEMANGIOMATOSIS Pulmonary capillary hemangiomatosis is a very rare form of pulmonary hypertension. Histologically it is characterized by the presence of infiltrating thin-walled blood vessels throughout the pulmonary interstitium and walls of the pulmonary arteries and veins. The presenting symptoms are usually those of PPH but often with hemoptysis as a clinical feature. The diagnosis can be made with pulmonary angiography. The clinical course is usually one of progressive deterioration leading to severe pulmonary hypertension, right-sided heart failure, and death. There is no established therapy.

PULMONARY VENOUS HYPERTENSION

Pulmonary hypertension occurs as a result of increased resistance to pulmonary venous drainage. It is often associated with diastolic dysfunction of the left ventricle; diseases affecting the pericardium or mitral or aortic valves; or rare entities such as cor triatriatum, left atrial myxoma, extrinsic compression of the central pulmonary veins from fibrosing mediastinitis, and pulmonary venoocclusive disease. Pulmonary venous hypertension affects the pulmonary veins and venules, producing arterialization of the external elastic lamina, medial hypertrophy, and focal eccentric intimal fibrosis. Microcirculatory lesions include capillary congestion, focal alveolar edema, and dilatation of the interstitial lymphatics. Although these lesions are potentially reversible, regression may take years after the underlying cause is removed. In some patients pulmonary venous hypertension triggers reactive vasoconstriction in the pulmonary arterial bed and results in proliferative changes of the intima and media that can produce severe elevations in pulmonary artery pressure. Clinically it may be confusing and appear as if two separate disease processes are occurring simultaneously.

LEFT VENTRICULAR DIASTOLIC DYSFUNCTION Pulmonary hypertension as a result of LV diastolic failure is common but often unrecognized (Chap. 216). It can occur with or without LV systolic failure. The most common causes are hypertensive heart disease; coronary artery disease; or impaired LV compliance related to age, diabetes, and hypoxemia. Symptoms of orthopnea and paroxysmal nocturnal dyspnea are prominent. Many patients improve considerably if LV end-diastolic pressure is lowered.

MITRAL VALVE DISEASE Mitral stenosis and mitral regurgitation represent important causes of pulmonary hypertension (Chap. 219). These patients often have superimposed pulmonary vasoconstriction resulting in marked elevations in pulmonary artery pressures. An echocardiogram usually shows abnormalities such as thickened mitral valve leaflets with reduced mobility or severe mitral regurgitation documented by Doppler echocardiography (Chap. 211). At cardiac catheterization a pressure gradient between the pulmonary capillary wedge pressure and LV end-diastolic pressure is diagnostic of mitral stenosis.

In patients with mitral stenosis corrective surgery of the mitral valve or mitral balloon valvuloplasty predictably results in a reduction in pulmonary artery pressure and pulmonary vascular resistance. Patients with mitral regurgitation, however, may not have as dramatic a response from surgery due to persistent elevations in LV end-diastolic pressure.

PULMONARY HYPERTENSION ASSOCIATED WITH LUNG DISEASE AND HYPOXEMIA

The mechanism of hypoxic pulmonary vasoconstriction involves the inhibition of potassium currents and membrane depolarization of pulmonary vascular smooth muscle as a result of the change in membrane sulfhydryl redox status. Increased calcium entry into the vascular smooth-muscle cells mediates hypoxic pulmonary vasoconstriction. Pulmonary vascular remodeling in response to chronic hypoxia is also mediated by a reduction in nitric oxide production; an increase in endothelin 1; and increased expression of platelet-derived growth factors, vascular endothelial growth factor, and angiotensin II. Chronic hypoxia results in muscularization of the arterioles with minimal effects on the intima. When it occurs as an isolated entity, the changes produced are potentially reversible.

Although chronic hypoxia is an established cause of pulmonary hypertension, it rarely leads to an increase in the mean pulmonary artery pressure >40 mmHg. Polycythemia in response to the hypoxemia is a characteristic finding. Hypoxia may also occur in conjunction with other causes of pulmonary hypertension associated with more extensive vascular changes. Clinically, the hypoxia will tend to have an added adverse affect. Patients with chronic hypoxia who have a marked elevation in pulmonary pressure should be evaluated for other causes of the pulmonary hypertension.

CHRONIC OBSTRUCTIVE LUNG DISEASE Chronic obstructive lung disease (COLD) is a common cause of pulmonary hypertension in the advanced stages (Chap. 242). Pulmonary hypertension has been attributed to multiple factors, including hypoxic pulmonary vasoconstriction, acidemia, hypercapnia, the mechanical effects of high lung volume on pulmonary vessels, the loss of small vessels in the vascular bed, and regions of emphysematous lung destruction.

Although the elevation of pulmonary artery pressure associated with COLD tends to be mild, the presence of pulmonary hypertension confers a worse outcome. The only effective therapy is supplemental oxygen. Several large clinical trials have documented that continuous oxygen therapy relieves some of the pulmonary vasoconstriction, relieves chronic ischemia throughout the systemic and pulmonary vascular beds, and improves survival. Long-term oxygen therapy is indicated if the resting arterial P_{O_2} remains <55 mmHg.

INTERSTITIAL LUNG DISEASE Pulmonary hypertension from interstitial lung disease is often associated with obliteration of the pulmonary vascular bed by lung destruction and fibrosis (Chap. 243). In addition, hypoxemia and pulmonary vasculopathy can be contributory factors. A large number of patients have pulmonary fibrosis of unknown etiology. Interstitial lung disease is often associated with the collagen vascular diseases. Patients are commonly older than 50 years and report an insidious onset of progressive dyspnea and cough for months to years. A definitive diagnosis requires an open-lung biopsy to rule out other diseases such as bronchiolitis obliterans, nonspecific interstitial pneumonia, and hypersensitivity pneumonitis. Management of these disorders is discussed in Chap. 243. None of the medical treatments developed for pulmonary arterial hypertension have been shown to be effective in these patients.

SLEEP-DISORDERED BREATHING *Sleep apnea*, defined as repeated episodes of obstructive apnea and hypopnea during sleep together with daytime somnolence and altered cardiopulmonary function, is a common condition (Chap. 247). The incidence of pulmonary hypertension in the setting of obstructive sleep apnea appears to be <20% and is generally mild. Therapeutic strategies for patients with sleep apnea should be directed towards establishing normal nocturnal oxygenation and ventilation, abolishing snoring, eliminating disruption of sleep due to upper airway closure, and avoiding factors that tend to aggravate the condition such as alcohol, sedatives, and hypnotic agents. The most important advance in medical treatment has been positive airway pressure delivered through a face mask during sleep.

When mild pulmonary hypertension is associated with sleep apnea, the treatments directed towards the sleep apnea are often effective in reducing pulmonary arterial pressure. Some patients, however, will present with severe pulmonary hypertension in conjunction with sleep apnea, which may or may not be related. In these cases it is recommended that the patients be treated for sleep apnea for a minimum of 3 months before treating the pulmonary arterial hypertension as a separate entity.

ALVEOLAR HYPOVENTILATION Pulmonary hypertension can occur in patients with chronic hypoventilation and hypoxia secondary to thoracovertebral deformities. Symptoms are slowly progressive and related to hypoxemia (Chap. 246). In patients with advanced disease, intermittent positive-pressure breathing and supplemental oxygen have been used successfully.

Pulmonary hypertension secondary to hypoxemia has been reported in patients with neuromuscular disease as a result of generalized weakness of the respiratory muscles and in patients with diaphragmatic paralysis. Diaphragmatic paralysis is generally a result of trauma to the phrenic nerve. Patients with nontraumatic bilateral diaphragmatic paralysis may go unrecognized until they present with either respiratory failure or pulmonary hypertension.

PULMONARY HYPERTENSION DUE TO THROMBOEMBOLIC DISEASE

ACUTE PULMONARY THROMBOEMBOLISM See Chap. 244

CHRONIC THROMBOEMBOLIC PULMONARY HYPERTENSION Patients appropriately treated for acute pulmonary thromboembolism with intravenous heparin and chronic oral warfarin therapy rarely develop chronic pulmonary hypertension. However, there is a subset of patients with impaired fibrinolytic resolution of the thromboembolism, which leads to organization and incomplete recanalization and chronic obstruction of the pulmonary vascular bed. The entity of chronic thromboembolic pulmonary hypertension has been well characterized and often mimics PPH. In many patients, the initial pulmonary thromboembolism was undetected or untreated.

Diagnosis The physical examination is typical of pulmonary hypertension but may include bruits heard over areas of the lung, representing blood flow through vessels with partial occlusion. A perfusion lung scan or contrast-enhanced spiral computed tomography scan usually reveals underlying thromboemboli. However, pulmonary angiography is necessary to determine the precise location and proximal extent of the thromboemboli, and hence the potential for operability.

℞ TREATMENT

Pulmonary thromboendarterectomy is an established surgical treatment in patients whose thrombi are accessible to surgical removal. The operative mortality is fairly high, at ~12% in experienced centers. Postoperative survivors who have a good result can expect to realize an improvement in functional class and exercise tolerance. Life-long anticoagulation using warfarin is mandatory. Thrombolytic therapy is rarely of help in patients with chronic thromboembolic pulmonary hypertension and may expose these patients to the increased risk of bleeding without potential benefit. Patients who are not surgical candidates have a poor outcome.

SICKLE CELL DISEASE Cardiovascular system abnormalities are prominent in the clinical spectrum of sickle cell disease, and pulmonary hypertension has been reported to occur in 20% of patients (Chap. 91). The pulmonary hypertension can usually be attributed to LV diastolic dysfunction. Although patients with sickle cell disease have an increased risk of thromboembolism, sickle cell disease rarely produces pulmonary arterial hypertension.

OTHER DISORDERS DIRECTLY AFFECTING PULMONARY VASCULATURE

SARCOIDOSIS Sarcoidosis can produce severe pulmonary hypertension as a result of chronic severe fibrocystic lung involvement (Chap. 309). In addition, direct cardiovascular involvement can coexist. Consequently, patients with sarcoidosis who present with progressive dyspnea and clinical features of pulmonary hypertension need a thorough evaluation. There is a subset of patients with sarcoidosis who present with severe pulmonary hypertension believed to be due to direct pulmonary vascular involvement. Many of these patients exhibit a favorable response to intravenous epoprostenol therapy.

SCHISTOSOMIASIS Although extremely rare in North America, schistosomiasis is the most common cause of pulmonary hypertension worldwide (Chap. 203). The development of pulmonary hypertension almost always occurs in the setting of hepatosplenic disease and portal hypertension. Schistosome ova can embolize from the liver to the lungs, where they result in an inflammatory pulmonary vascular reaction and chronic changes. The diagnosis is confirmed by finding the parasite ova in the urine or stools of patients with symptoms, which can be difficult. The efficacy of therapies directed towards pulmonary hypertension in these patients is unknown.

FURTHER READING

ARCHER S, RICH S: Primary pulmonary hypertension: A vascular biology and translational research "Work in Progress." Circulation 102:2781, 2000

HUMBERT M, TREMBATH RC: Genetics of pulmonary hypertension: From bench to bedside. Eur Respir J 20:741, 2002

MCLAUGHLIN WV, SHILLINGTON A et al: Survival in primary pulmonary hypertension: The impact of epoprostenol therapy. Circulation 106:1477, 2002

MICHELAKIS E et al: Oral sildenafil is an effective and specific pulmonary vasodilator in patients with pulmonary arterial hypertension. Circulation 105:2398, 2002

RICH S: Primary pulmonary hypertension, in *World Symposium—Primary Pulmonary Hypertension*, S Rich (ed). 1998. Also available from the World Health Organization via the Internet (*http://www.who.int/ncd/cvd/pph.html*)

RUBIN L et al: Bosentan therapy for pulmonary arterial hypertension. N Engl J Med 346:896, 2002

SIMONNEAU G et al: Continuous subcutaneous infusion of treprostinil, a prostacyclin analogue, in patients with pulmonary arterial hypertension: A double-blind, randomized, placebo-controlled trial. Am J Respir Crit Care Med 165:800, 2002

221 | CARDIOMYOPATHY AND MYOCARDITIS
Joshua Wynne, Eugene Braunwald

The cardiomyopathies are a group of diseases that affect the heart muscle itself and are not the result of hypertension or congenital or acquired valvular, coronary, or pericardial abnormalities. The diffuse myocardial fibrosis that accompanies multiple myocardial scars produced by extensive coronary artery disease can impair left ventricular function and is frequently referred to as *ischemic cardiomyopathy*. This colloquial use of the term should be avoided; the term *cardiomyopathy* should be restricted to a condition *primarily* involving the myocardium. When the cardiomyopathies are classified on an etiologic basis, two fundamental forms are recognized: (1) a primary type, consisting of heart muscle disease of unknown cause; and (2) a secondary type, consisting of myocardial disease of known cause or associated with a disease involving other organ systems (Table 221-1). (In the World Health Organization classification, the term *specific cardiomyopathy* is used to describe heart muscle diseases associated with certain systemic or cardiac disorders; examples include hypertensive and metabolic cardiomyopathy.) In many cases, however, it is not possible to arrive at a specific etiologic diagnosis, and thus it is often more desirable to classify the cardiomyopathies into one of three types

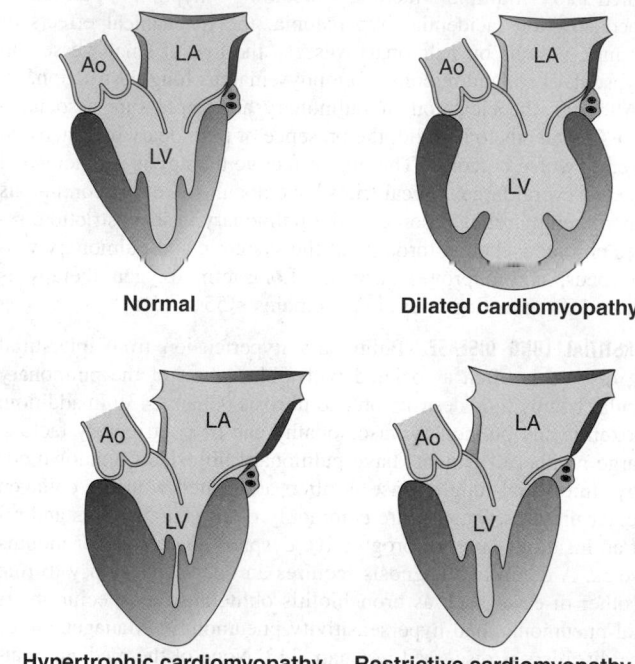

FIGURE 221-1 Drawing comparing the three broad classes of cardiomyopathies. Ao, aorta; LA, left atrium; LV, left ventricle. *(From BF Waller: J Am Soc Echocardiogr 1:4, 1988.)*

(dilated, restrictive, hypertrophic) on the basis of differences in their pathophysiology and clinical presentation (Fig. 221-1; Tables 221-2 and 221-3).

DILATED CARDIOMYOPATHY

About one in three cases of congestive heart failure (CHF) is due to dilated cardiomyopathy, with the remainder the consequence of coronary artery disease. Left and/or right ventricular systolic pump function is impaired, leading to progressive cardiac enlargement and hypertrophy, a process called *remodeling*. Symptoms of CHF typically appear only after remodeling has been ongoing for some time (months or even years). There is, however, no close correlation between the degree of contractile dysfunction and the severity of symptoms.

Although no cause is apparent in many cases, dilated cardiomyopathy is probably the end result of myocardial damage produced by

---

TABLE 221-1 *Etiologic Classification of Cardiomyopathies*

PRIMARY MYOCARDIAL INVOLVEMENT

Idiopathic (D,R,H)
Familial (D,R,H)
Eosinophilic endomyocardial disease (R)
Endomyocardial fibrosis (R)

SECONDARY MYOCARDIAL INVOLVEMENT

Infective (D)	Connective tissue disorders (D)
Viral myocarditis	Systemic lupus erythematosus
Bacterial myocarditis	Polyarteritis nodosa
Fungal myocarditis	Rheumatoid arthritis
Protozoal myocarditis	Progressive systemic sclerosis
Metazoal myocarditis	Dermatomyositis
Spirochetal	Infiltrations and granulomas (R,D)
Rickettsial	Amyloidosis
Metabolic (D)	Sarcoidosis
Familial storage disease (D,R)	Malignancy
Glycogen storage disease	Neuromuscular (D)
Mucopolysaccharidoses	Muscular dystrophy
Hemochromatosis	Myotonic dystrophy
Fabry's disease	Friedreich's ataxia (H,D)
Deficiency (D)	Sensitivity and toxic reactions (D)
Electrolytes	Alcohol
Nutritional	Radiation
	Drugs
	Peripartum heart disease (D)

Note: The principal clinical manifestation(s) of each etiologic grouping is denoted by D (dilated), R (restrictive), or H (hypertrophic) cardiomyopathy.
Source: Adapted from the WHO/ISFC task force report on the definition and classification of cardiomyopathies, 1980.

TABLE 221-2 *Clinical Classification of Cardiomyopathies*

1. Dilated: Left and/or right ventricular enlargement, impaired systolic function, congestive heart failure, arrhythmias, emboli
2. Restrictive: Endomyocardial scarring or myocardial infiltration resulting in restriction to left and/or right ventricular filling
3. Hypertrophic: Disproportionate left ventricular hypertrophy, typically involving septum more than free wall, with or without an intraventricular systolic pressure gradient; usually of a nondilated left ventricular cavity

a variety of toxic, metabolic, or infectious agents. Dilated cardiomyopathy may be the late sequel of acute viral myocarditis, possibly mediated through an immunologic mechanism. Although it may occur in any patient population, it is most commonly a disease of middle-aged men and is more common in African Americans than in whites. The prevalence of this condition is increasing. A reversible form of dilated cardiomyopathy may be found with alcohol abuse, pregnancy, thyroid disease, cocaine use, and chronic uncontrolled tachycardia. Obesity increases the risk of developing heart failure, as does sleep apnea. At least 20% (and perhaps as many as 40%) of patients have familial forms of the disease, with mutations of genes encoding cytoskeletal (such as the dystrophin and desmin genes), contractile, nuclear membrane (such as the lamin A/C gene), and other proteins. The disease is genetically heterogeneous but most commonly autosomal dominant in transmission; autosomal recessive, mitochondrial (especially in children), and X-linked inheritance is found as well.

Right ventricular dysplasia is a unique familial cardiomyopathy marked by progressive replacement of the right ventricular wall with adipose tissue. Often associated with ventricular arrhythmias, the clinical course is variable, but sudden death is a constant threat. Catheter ablation of arrhythmia sites and insertion of an implantable cardioverter-defibrillator are often employed.

CLINICAL MANIFESTATIONS Symptoms of left- and right-sided congestive failure develop gradually in most patients (Chap. 216). Some patients have left ventricular dilatation for months or even years before becoming symptomatic. Although vague chest pain may be present, typical angina pectoris is unusual and suggests the presence of concomitant ischemic heart disease. Syncope due to arrhythmias and systemic embolism (often emanating from a ventricular thrombus) may occur.

PHYSICAL EXAMINATION Variable degrees of cardiac enlargement and findings of CHF are noted. In patients with advanced disease, the pulse pressure is narrow and the jugular venous pressure is elevated. Third and fourth heart sounds are common, and mitral or tricuspid regurgitation may occur.

LABORATORY EXAMINATIONS The chest roentgenogram demonstrates enlargement of the cardiac silhouette due to left ventricular dilatation, although generalized cardiomegaly is often seen. The lung fields may demonstrate evidence of pulmonary venous hypertension and interstitial or alveolar edema. The electrocardiogram often shows sinus tachycardia or atrial fibrillation, ventricular arrhythmias, left atrial abnormality, diffuse nonspecific ST-T-wave abnormalities, and sometimes intraventricular conduction defects and low voltage. Echocardiography and radionuclide ventriculography show left ventricular dilatation, with normal, minimally thickened, or thinned walls, and systolic dysfunction (reduced ejection fraction). The detection of elevated circulating levels of brain natriuretic peptide (Chaps. 32 and 216) may help clarify which patients with dyspnea of uncertain etiology actually have heart failure rather than pulmonary disease as the cause of their symptoms, and indentifies patients at increased risk of sudden death.

Cardiac catheterization and coronary angiography are often performed to exclude ischemic heart disease, and bedside hemodynamic monitoring may be helpful in the management of the acutely decompensated patient. Angiography reveals a dilated, diffusely hypokinetic left ventricle, often with some degree of mitral regurgitation. Transvenous endomyocardial biopsy is usually not necessary in idiopathic or familial dilated cardiomyopathy. However, it may be helpful in the recognition of secondary cardiomyopathies, such as amyloidosis and acute myocarditis.

TABLE 221-3 *Laboratory Evaluation of the Cardiomyopathies*

	Dilated	Restrictive	Hypertrophic
Chest roentgenogram	Moderate to marked cardiac silhouette enlargement Pulmonary venous hypertension	Mild cardiac silhouette enlargement	Mild to moderate cardiac silhouette enlargement
Electrocardiogram	ST-segment and T-wave abnormalities	Low voltage, conduction defects	ST-segment and T-wave abnormalities Left ventricular hypertrophy Abnormal Q waves
Echocardiogram	Left ventricular dilatation and dysfunction	Increased left ventricular wall thickness Normal or mildly reduced systolic function	Asymmetric septal hypertrophy (ASH) Systolic anterior motion (SAM) of the mitral valve
Radionuclide studies	Left ventricular dilatation and dysfunction (RVG)	Normal or mildly reduced systolic function (RVG)	Vigorous systolic function (RVG) Perfusion defect (^{201}Tl)
Cardiac catheterization	Left ventricular dilatation and dysfunction Elevated left- and often right-sided filling pressures Diminished cardiac output	Normal or mildly reduced systolic function Elevated left- and right-sided filling pressures	Vigorous systolic function Dynamic left ventricular outflow obstruction Elevated left- and right-sided filling pressures

Note: RVG, radionuclide ventriculogram; ^{201}Tl, thallium 201.

 TREATMENT

Most patients pursue an inexorably downhill course, and the majority, particularly those >55 years, die within 3 years of the onset of symptoms. African Americans are more likely to suffer progressive heart failure and death than Caucasians. Spontaneous improvement or stabilization occurs in about a quarter of patients. Death is due to either CHF or ventricular tachy- or bradyarrhythmia; sudden death is a constant threat. Systemic embolization is a concern, and patients should be considered for chronic anticoagulation. Standard therapy of heart failure with salt restriction, angiotensin-converting enzyme (ACE) inhibitors, diuretics, and digitalis produces symptomatic improvement (Chap. 216). An angiotensin II receptor blocker may be substituted in ACE-intolerant patients. Most patients should be treated with a β-adrenergic blocker. Spironolactone should be added for most patients with recent or current advanced heart failure. Some patients with dilated cardiomyopathy who have biopsy evidence of myocardial inflammation have been treated with immunosuppressive therapy, but long-term evidence of efficacy is lacking. Alcohol should be avoided because of its cardiac toxic effects, as should calcium channel blockers and nonsteroidal anti-inflammatory drugs. Antiarrhythmic agents are best avoided for fear of proarrhythmia, unless they are needed to treat symptomatic or serious arrhythmias. For the one in three patients with an intraventricular conduction delay (such as right or left bundle branch block), biventricular pacing (termed *resynchronization therapy*) improves symptoms, reduces hospitalizations, and perhaps reduces mortality. Insertion of an implantable cardioverter-defibrillator is useful in patients with symptomatic ventricular arrhythmias, and its use in other patients is evolving. In patients with advanced disease who are refractory to medical therapy, cardiac transplantation should be considered (Chap. 217).

ALCOHOLIC CARDIOMYOPATHY Individuals who consume large quantities of alcohol over many years may develop a clinical picture identical to idiopathic dilated cardiomyopathy. The risk of developing cardiomyopathy is partially genetically determined. Reducing or ceasing alcohol consumption before severe heart failure has developed may halt the progression or even reverse the course of this disease. Alcoholic patients with advanced heart failure have a poor prognosis, particularly if they continue to drink; fewer than one-quarter survive 3 years.

A second presentation of alcoholic cardiotoxicity may be found in individuals without overt heart failure and consists of recurrent supraventricular or ventricular tachyarrhythmias. Termed the *holiday heart syndrome*, it typically appears after a drinking binge; atrial fibrillation is seen most frequently, followed by atrial flutter and ventricular premature depolarizations.

PERIPARTUM CARDIOMYOPATHY (See also Chap. 6)   Cardiac dilatation and CHF of unexplained cause may develop during the last trimester of pregnancy or within 6 months after delivery; most women develop symptoms in the month before or immediately after delivery. The patient who develops peripartum cardiomyopathy typically is multiparous, African American, and over the age of 30, although the disease may be found in a wide spectrum of patients. The symptoms, signs, and treatment are similar to those in patients with idiopathic dilated cardiomyopathy. The mortality rate is around 10 to 20%. The prognosis in these patients appears to be related to whether the heart size returns to normal after the first episode of CHF. If it does, subsequent pregnancies may sometimes be tolerated, albeit with an increased risk of recurrent heart failure; if the heart remains enlarged, however, further pregnancies frequently produce additional myocardial damage, ultimately leading to refractory CHF and death. Those who recover should be encouraged to avoid further pregnancies, particularly if cardiomegaly persists.

NEUROMUSCULAR DISEASE (See also Chap. 367)   Cardiac involvement is common in many of the muscular dystrophies. In *Duchenne's progressive muscular dystrophy*, mutations in a gene that encodes a cardiac structural protein (*dystrophin*) lead to myocyte death. Myocardial involvement is most frequently indicated by a distinctive and unique electrocardiographic pattern consisting of tall R waves in right precordial leads with an R/S ratio >1.0, often associated with deep Q waves in the limb and lateral precordial leads. A variety of supraventricular and ventricular arrhythmias are frequently found. Rapidly progressive CHF may develop despite extended periods of apparent circulatory stability during which the only detectable abnormalities are in the electrocardiogram. *Myotonic dystrophy* is characterized by a variety of electrocardiographic abnormalities, especially disorders of impulse formation and conduction, but other overt clinical evidence of heart disease is uncommon. Because of these abnormalities, syncope and sudden death are major hazards; in appropriate patients, insertion of a permanent pacemaker may be effective. Involvement of the heart is very common in *Friedreich's ataxia* (manifested by abnormal electrocardiographic or echocardiographic findings), with as many as half the patients developing cardiac symptoms. The electrocardiogram most commonly demonstrates ST-segment and T-wave abnormalities. The echocardiogram may demonstrate left ventricular hypertrophy, with either symmetric or asymmetric hypertrophy of the left ventricular septum compared with the free wall. Although morphologically similar to some cases of hypertrophic cardiomyopathy, cellular disarray is lacking.

DRUGS   A variety of pharmacologic agents may damage the myocardium acutely, producing a pattern of inflammation (myocarditis), or they may lead to chronic damage of the type seen with idiopathic dilated cardiomyopathy. Certain drugs produce only electrocardiographic abnormalities, while others may precipitate fulminant CHF and death.

The anthracycline derivatives, particularly doxorubicin (Adriamycin), are powerful antineoplastic agents that, when given in high doses (>550 mg/m² for doxorubicin), may produce fatal heart failure. The incidence of heart failure is related not only to the dose of the drug but also to the presence or absence of several risk factors (cardiac irradiation, age >70 years, underlying heart disease, hypertension, treatment with cyclophosphamide); at any dose of doxorubicin, patients with these risk factors have an eight- to tenfold greater frequency

of developing heart failure than do patients lacking them. Radionuclide ventriculography and echocardiography, usually combined with exercise stress, may document preclinical deterioration of left ventricular function and allow appropriate dose adjustments. By monitoring left ventricular function, it is often possible to continue doxorubicin even in patients at high risk for developing heart failure. Efforts to modify the dose schedule by giving the drug more slowly, along with the selective use of potentially cardioprotective agents such as the iron-chelator dexrazoxone, have further reduced the risk of cardiotoxicity. Some patients with CHF, even those with severe depression of left ventricular function, have demonstrated recovery of cardiac function with aggressive management with ACE inhibitors and diuretics. In others, late asymptomatic contractile dysfunction may occur, even in those without initial cardiotoxicity.

High-dose *cyclophosphamide* may produce CHF acutely or within 2 weeks of administration; a characteristic histopathologic feature is myocardial edema and hemorrhagic necrosis. Electrocardiographic changes and arrhythmias may result from treatment with tricyclic antidepressants, the phenothiazines, emetine, lithium, and various aerosol propellants. *Cocaine abuse* is associated with a variety of life-threatening cardiac complications, including sudden death, myocarditis, dilated cardiomyopathy, and acute myocardial infarction (resulting from coronary spasm and/or thrombosis with or without underlying coronary artery stenosis). Nitrates, calcium channel blockers, and benzodiazepines have been used to treat cocaine-induced cardiotoxicities; β-adrenergic blockers should be avoided.

HYPERTROPHIC CARDIOMYOPATHY

Hypertrophic cardiomyopathy (HCM) is characterized by left ventricular hypertrophy, typically of a nondilated chamber, without obvious cause such as hypertension or aortic stenosis. It is found in about 1 in 500 of the general population. Two features of HCM have attracted the greatest attention: (1) asymmetric left ventricular hypertrophy, often with preferential hypertrophy of the interventricular septum; and (2) a dynamic left ventricular outflow tract pressure gradient, related to a narrowing of the subaortic area as a consequence of the midsystolic apposition of the anterior mitral valve leaflet against the hypertrophied septum, i.e., systolic anterior motion (SAM) of the mitral valve. Initial studies of this disease emphasized the dynamic "obstructive" features, and it has been termed *idiopathic hypertrophic subaortic stenosis* and *hypertrophic obstructive cardiomyopathy*. It has become clear, however, that only about one-quarter of patients with HCM demonstrate an outflow tract pressure gradient. The ubiquitous pathophysiologic abnormality is not systolic but rather *diastolic* dysfunction (Chap. 215), characterized by increased stiffness of the hypertrophied muscle. This results in elevated diastolic filling pressures and is present despite a hyperdynamic left ventricle.

The pattern of hypertrophy is distinctive in HCM and differs from that seen in secondary hypertrophy (as in hypertension). Most patients have striking regional variations in the extent of hypertrophy in different portions of the left ventricle, and the majority demonstrate a ventricular septum whose thickness is disproportionately increased when compared with the free wall. Other patients may demonstrate disproportionate involvement of the apex or left ventricular free wall; 10% or more of patients have concentric involvement of the ventricle. A bizarre and disorganized arrangement of cardiac muscle cells in the septum occurs, with disorganization of the myofibrillar architecture, along with a variable degree of myocardial fibrosis and thickening of the small intramural coronary arteries. In some children, systolic compression of an intramyocardial segment of a coronary artery may lead to ischemia and death.

GENETIC CONSIDERATIONS   About half of all patients with HCM have a positive family history compatible with autosomal-dominant transmission. More than 150 different mutations of 10 different genes that encode sarcomeric proteins have been identified. About 40% of these are associated with mutations of the cardiac β-myosin heavy chain gene on chromosome 14, with certain mutations associated with more malignant prognoses. About 15% have a mutation of the cardiac troponin T gene on chromosome 1, 20% a mutation of myosin-binding protein C (chromosome 11), and ~5% a mutation of the α-tropomyosin gene. The remainder of familial cases are due to mutations of other genes such as the gene for troponin I. Echocardiographic studies have confirmed that about one-third of the first-degree relatives of patients with familial HCM have evidence of the disease, although in many of these patients the extent of hypertrophy is mild, no outflow tract pressure gradient is present, and symptoms are not prominent. Since the hypertrophic characteristics may not be apparent in childhood and often appear first in adolescence, a single normal echocardiogram in a child does not exclude the presence of the disease. Many sporadic cases of HCM probably represent spontaneous mutations.

CLINICAL FEATURES   The clinical course of HCM is highly variable. Many patients are asymptomatic or mildly symptomatic and may be relatives of patients with known disease. Unfortunately, the first clinical manifestation of the disease may be sudden death, frequently occurring in children and young adults, often during or after physical exertion. In symptomatic patients, the most common complaint is dyspnea, largely due to increased stiffness of the left ventricular walls, which impairs ventricular filling and leads to elevated left ventricular diastolic and left atrial pressures. Other symptoms include angina pectoris, fatigue, and syncope. Symptoms are not closely related to the presence or severity of an outflow pressure gradient. Most patients with gradients demonstrate a double or triple apical precordial impulse, a rapidly rising carotid arterial pulse, and a fourth heart sound. The hallmark of obstructive HCM is a systolic murmur, which is typically harsh, diamond-shaped, and usually begins well after the first heart sound, since ejection is unimpeded early in systole. The murmur is best heard at the lower left sternal border as well as at the apex, where it is often more holosystolic and blowing in quality, no doubt due to the mitral regurgitation that usually accompanies obstructive HCM.

HEMODYNAMICS   In contrast to the obstruction produced by a fixed narrowed orifice, such as valvular aortic stenosis, the pressure gradient in HCM, when present, is dynamic and may change between examinations and even from beat to beat. Obstruction appears to result from further narrowing of an already small left ventricular outflow tract by SAM of the mitral valve against the hypertrophied septum. While SAM is occasionally found in a variety of conditions besides HCM, it is *always* found when obstruction is present in HCM. Three basic mechanisms are involved in the production and intensification of the dynamic pressure gradient: (1) increased left ventricular contractility, (2) decreased ventricular volume (preload), and (3) decreased aortic impedance and pressure (afterload). Interventions that increase myocardial contractility, such as exercise, sympathomimetic amines, and digitalis glycosides, and those that reduce ventricular volume, such as the Valsalva maneuver, sudden standing, nitroglycerin, amyl nitrite, or tachycardia, may all cause an increase in the gradient and the murmur. Conversely, elevation of arterial pressure by phenylephrine, squatting, sustained handgrip, augmentation of venous return by passive leg raising, and expansion of the blood volume all increase ventricular volume and ameliorate the gradient and murmur.

LABORATORY EVALUATION   The *electrocardiogram* commonly shows left ventricular hypertrophy and widespread, deep, broad Q waves that suggest an old myocardial infarction. Many patients demonstrate arrhythmias, both atrial (supraventricular tachycardia or atrial fibrillation) and ventricular (ventricular tachycardia), during ambulatory (Holter) monitoring. *Chest roentgenography* may be normal, although a mild to moderate increase in the cardiac silhouette is common. The mainstay of the diagnosis of HCM is the *echocardiogram*, which demonstrates left ventricular hypertrophy, often with the septum 1.3 or more times the thickness of the high posterior left ventricular free wall. The septum may demonstrate an unusual "ground-glass" appearance, probably related to its abnormal cellular architecture and myocardial fibrosis. SAM of the mitral valve is found in patients with pressure

gradients. The left ventricular cavity typically is small in HCM, with vigorous posterior wall motion but reduced septal excursion. A rare form of HCM, characterized by apical hypertrophy, is often associated with giant negative T waves on the electrocardiogram and a "spade-shaped" left ventricular cavity on angiography; it usually has a benign clinical course. *Radionuclide scintigraphy* with thallium 201 frequently reveals evidence of myocardial perfusion defects even in asymptomatic patients.

Although cardiac catheterization is not required to diagnose HCM, the two typical *hemodynamic* features are an elevated left ventricular diastolic pressure due to diminished left ventricular compliance and, when obstruction is present, a systolic pressure gradient between the body of the left ventricle and the subaortic region. When a gradient is not present, it can be induced in some patients by provocative maneuvers such as infusion of isoproterenol, inhalation of amyl nitrite, or the Valsalva maneuver.

℞ TREATMENT

Since sudden death often occurs during or just after physical exertion, competitive sports and probably strenuous activity should be proscribed. Dehydration should be avoided, and diuretics should be used with caution. β-Adrenergic blockers are often used and ameliorate angina pectoris and syncope in one-third to one-half of patients. Resting intraventricular pressure gradients are usually unchanged, although these drugs may limit the increase in the gradient that occurs during exercise. It does not appear that β-adrenergic blockers offer any protection against sudden death. Amiodarone appears to be effective in reducing the frequency of supraventricular as well as life-threatening ventricular arrhythmias, and anecdotal data suggest that it may reduce the risk of sudden death. Verapamil and diltiazem may reduce the stiffness of the ventricle, reduce the elevated diastolic pressures, increase exercise tolerance, and, in some instances, reduce the severity of outflow tract pressure gradients, although adverse side effects occur in about one-quarter of patients. Nifedipine should be avoided. Disopyramide has been used in some patients to reduce left ventricular contractility and the outflow pressure gradient.

If atrial fibrillation occurs, a strenuous effort should be made to restore and then maintain sinus rhythm. Dual-chamber permanent pacing with a short PR interval has been reported to improve symptoms and reduce the outflow gradient in some patients with severe symptoms, presumably by altering the pattern of ventricular depolarization and contraction, although much of the putative benefit has been attributed to a placebo effect. Infarction of the interventricular septum induced by ethanol injections into the septal artery has also been reported to reduce obstruction. A surgical myotomy/myectomy of the hypertrophied septum may result in lasting symptomatic improvement in about three-quarters of severely symptomatic patients with large pressure gradients who are unresponsive to medical management. Digitalis, diuretics, nitrates, vasodilators, and β-adrenergic agonists are best avoided if possible, particularly in patients with known left ventricular outflow tract pressure gradients. Even social alcohol ingestion may produce sufficient vasodilatation to exacerbate an outflow pressure gradient. First-degree relatives of patients with HCM should be screened by echocardiography. The insertion of an implantable cardioverter defibrillator should be considered in patients (Chap. 214) with a high-risk profile for sudden cardiac death (see below).

PROGNOSIS   The natural history of HCM is variable, although many patients never exhibit any clinical manifestations. Atrial fibrillation is common late in the course of the disease; its onset often leads to an increase in symptoms in two out of three patients, due to loss of the atrial contribution to filling of the thickened ventricle. Infective endocarditis occurs in <10% of patients, but endocarditis prophylaxis is indicated, particularly in patients with resting obstruction and mitral regurgitation. Progression of HCM to left ventricular dilatation and dysfunction with wall thinning without an outflow pressure gradient occurs in about 5 to 10% of patients. The major cause of mortality in HCM is sudden death, which may occur in asymptomatic patients or interrupt an otherwise stable course in symptomatic ones. The annual risk of dying from HCM is about 1% per year, similar to the normal adult population. Patients at higher risk of sudden death include those with a history of resuscitation from sudden cardiac death, ventricular tachycardia on ambulatory monitoring or at electrophysiologic testing, marked ventricular hypertrophy, (ventricular septal thickness >30 mm), syncope (especially in children), genetic mutations associated with an increased risk, an abnormal blood pressure response to exercise, and a family history of sudden death. There is no correlation between the risk of sudden death and the severity of symptoms, but there is an increased risk of death in patients with outflow gradients.

RESTRICTIVE CARDIOMYOPATHY

The hallmark of the restrictive cardiomyopathies is abnormal diastolic function (Chap. 215); the ventricular walls are excessively rigid and impede ventricular filling. Myocardial fibrosis, hypertrophy, or infiltration due to a variety of causes is usually responsible. The infiltrative diseases, which represent important causes for secondary restrictive cardiomyopathy, may also show some impairment of systolic function. Myocardial involvement with *amyloid* is a common cause of secondary restrictive cardiomyopathy, although restriction is also seen in hemochromatosis, glycogen deposition, endomyocardial fibrosis, sarcoidosis, Fabry's disease, the eosinophilias, and scleroderma; in the transplanted heart and following mediastinal irradiation; and in neoplastic infiltration and myocardial fibrosis of diverse causes. In many of these conditions, particularly those with substantial concomitant endocardial involvement, partial obliteration of the ventricular cavity by fibrous tissue and thrombus contributes to the abnormally increased resistance to ventricular filling. Thromboembolic complications ensue in about a third of patients.

The inability of the ventricle to fill limits cardiac output and raises filling pressure. Therefore, exercise intolerance and dyspnea are usually the most prominent symptoms. As a result of persistently elevated venous pressure, these patients commonly have dependent edema, ascites, and an enlarged, tender, and often pulsatile liver. The jugular venous pressure is elevated and does not fall normally, or it may rise with inspiration (Kussmaul's sign). The heart sounds may be distant, and third and fourth heart sounds are common. In contrast to constrictive pericarditis, which the restrictive cardiomyopathies resemble in many respects, the apex impulse is usually easily palpable, and mitral regurgitation is more common. The electrocardiogram often shows low-voltage, nonspecific ST-T-wave changes and various arrhythmias. Pericardial calcification on x-ray, which occurs in constrictive pericarditis, is absent. Echocardiography typically reveals symmetrically thickened left ventricular walls and normal or slightly reduced ventricular volumes and systolic function. Cardiac catheterization shows a decreased cardiac output, elevation of the right and left ventricular end-diastolic pressures, and a dip-and-plateau configuration of the diastolic portion of the ventricular pressure pulse resembling that seen in constrictive pericarditis.

Differentiation from constrictive pericarditis may be challenging (Chap. 222). This distinction is of importance because the latter condition is potentially curable by operation. Helpful in the differentiation of these two diseases are right ventricular transvenous endomyocardial biopsy (by revealing myocardial infiltration or fibrosis in restrictive cardiomyopathy) and computed tomography or magnetic resonance imaging (by demonstrating a thickened pericardium in constrictive pericarditis). Treatment is usually disappointing, except for hemochromatosis (where deferoxamine has been helpful in reducing myocardial iron content), and Fabry's disease (where infusion of galactose stimulates the activity of the deficient enzyme with attendant improvement in cardiac function). Chronic anticoagulation is often recommended to reduce the risk of embolization from the heart.

ENDOMYOCARDIAL FIBROSIS This is a progressive disease of unknown cause that occurs most commonly in children and young adults residing in tropical and subtropical Africa, particularly Uganda and Nigeria. Endomyocardial fibrosis is a frequent cause of heart failure in Africa, accounting for up to one-quarter of deaths due to heart disease. The condition is characterized by fibrous endocardial lesions of the inflow portion of the right or left ventricle (or both) and often involves the atrioventricular valves, producing valvular regurgitation. The apex of the ventricles may be obliterated by a mass of thrombus and fibrous tissue. In some ways this disease resembles eosinophilic endomyocardial disease (see below), although they occur in quite different geographic areas and age groups and generally are felt to be different diseases.

The clinical picture depends on which ventricle and atrioventricular valve show predominant involvement; left-sided involvement results in symptoms of pulmonary congestion, while predominant right-sided disease presents features of a restrictive cardiomyopathy. Medical treatment is often disappointing, and surgical excision of the fibrotic endocardium and replacement of the involved atrioventricular valve have led to substantial symptomatic improvement in some patients.

EOSINOPHILIC ENDOMYOCARDIAL DISEASE Also called *Loeffler's endocarditis* and *fibroplastic endocarditis*, this disease appears to be a subcategory of the hypereosinophilic syndrome in which the heart is predominantly involved, with cardiac damage the apparent result of the toxic effects of eosinophilic proteins. Typically, the endocardium of either or both ventricles thickens markedly, with involvement of the underlying myocardium. Large mural thrombi may develop in either ventricle, thereby compromising the size of the ventricular cavity and serving as a source of pulmonary and systemic emboli. Hepatosplenomegaly and localized eosinophilic infiltration of other organs are usually present. Management usually includes diuretics, afterload-reducing agents, and anticoagulation. The use of glucocorticoids and cytotoxic drugs (hydroxyurea in particular) appears to have improved survival substantially. Surgical treatment, as for endomyocardial fibrosis, may be helpful in selected patients.

DIFFERENTIAL DIAGNOSIS Involvement of the heart is the most frequent cause of death in *primary amyloidosis* (Chap. 310), while clinically significant cardiac involvement is uncommon in the secondary form. Focal deposits of amyloid in elderly patients (*senile cardiac amyloidosis*) are common and usually clinically insignificant. Aspiration of abdominal fat or biopsy of the myocardium or other organs permits the diagnosis to be made before death in over three-quarters of cases. The heart is firm, rubbery, and noncompliant, and four clinical presentations (alone or in combination) are seen: (1) diastolic dysfunction (restrictive cardiomyopathy), (2) systolic dysfunction, (3) arrhythmias and conduction disturbances, and (4) orthostatic hypotension. The two-dimensional echocardiogram may be helpful in making the diagnosis of amyloidosis and may show a thickened myocardial wall with a distinctive "speckled" appearance. Chemotherapy, often with alkylating agents, appears to have improved survival in specific cases, and heart transplantion (often combined with bone marrow transplantation, or liver or kidney transplantation for hereditary amyloidosis) may help selected patients, but the overall prognosis is poor, especially in the primary form with advanced cardiac involvement.

Hemochromatosis (Chap. 336) is often the result of multiple transfusions or a hemoglobinopathy; the familial (autosomal recessive) form should be suspected if cardiomyopathy occurs in the setting of diabetes mellitus, hepatic cirrhosis, and increased skin pigmentation. The diagnosis may be confirmed by endomyocardial biopsy. Phlebotomy may be of some benefit if employed early in the course of the disease. Continuous subcutaneous administration of deferoxamine may reduce body iron stores and result in clinical improvement.

Myocardial *sarcoidosis* (Chap. 309) is generally associated with other manifestations of systemic disease and may cause restrictive as well as congestive features, since cardiac infiltration by sarcoid granulomas results not only in increased stiffness of the myocardium but also in diminished systolic contractile function. A variety of arrhythmias, including high-grade atrioventricular block, have been noted. A common cardiac manifestation of systemic sarcoidosis is right heart overload due to pulmonary artery hypertension as a result of parenchymal pulmonary involvement. Many patients are treated empirically with glucocorticoids. The *carcinoid syndrome* results in endocardial fibrosis and stenosis and/or regurgitation of the tricuspid and/or pulmonary valve (Chap. 219); morphologically similar lesions have been seen with the use of the anorexic agents fenfluramine and phentermine.

MYOCARDITIS

Myocarditis, i.e., cardiac inflammation, is most commonly the result of an infectious process. Myocarditis may also result from a hypersensitivity to drugs or may be caused by radiation, chemicals, or physical agents. In an unknown number of cases, acute myocarditis progresses to chronic dilated cardiomyopathy. While almost every infectious agent is capable of producing myocarditis (Table 221-1), clinically significant acute myocarditis in the United States is caused most commonly by viruses, especially coxsackievirus B. The clinical manifestations range from an asymptomatic state, with the presence of myocarditis inferred only by the finding of transient electrocardiographic ST-T-wave abnormalities, to a fulminant condition with arrhythmias, heart failure, and death. In some patients, myocarditis simulates acute myocardial infarction, with chest pain, electrocardiographic changes, and elevated serum levels of myocardial enzymes. Patients with myocarditis and pulmonary hypertension are at a particularly high risk of death.

The physical examination is often normal, although more severe cases may show a muffled first heart sound, along with a third heart sound and a murmur of mitral regurgitation. A pericardial friction rub may be audible in patients with associated pericarditis.

Though viral myocarditis is most often self-limited and without sequelae, severe involvement may recur, and it is likely that acute viral myocarditis occasionally progresses to a chronic form and to dilated cardiomyopathy. Patients with viral myocarditis often give a history of a preceding upper respiratory febrile illness or a flulike syndrome, and viral nasopharyngitis or tonsillitis may be evident clinically. The isolation of virus from the stool, pharyngeal washings, or other body fluids and changes in specific antibody titers are helpful clinically. Endomyocardial biopsy, carried out early in the illness, may show round-cell infiltration and necrosis of adjacent myocytes.

Exercise may be deleterious in patients with viral myocarditis, and strenuous activity should be proscribed until the electrocardiogram has returned to normal. Patients who develop CHF respond to the usual measures (ACE inhibitors, diuretics, and salt restriction), but they appear to be unusually sensitive to digitalis. Arrhythmias are common and are occasionally difficult to manage. Deaths attributed to heart failure, tachyarrhythmias, and heart block have been reported, and it seems prudent to monitor the electrocardiogram of patients with arrhythmias, especially during the acute illness. Patients with fulminant myocarditis may require mechanical cardiopulmonary support or cardiac transplantation, but the majority survive and many demonstrate substantial recovery of ventricular function.

HIV MYOCARDITIS (See also Chap. 173) Many HIV-infected patients have subclinical cardiac involvement, including pericardial effusion, right-sided chamber enlargement, and neoplastic involvement. Overt clinical involvement is seen in 10% of HIV patients, and the most common finding is left ventricular dysfunction that in some cases appears to be due to infiltration of the myocardium by the virus itself. In other patients, the heart is affected by any of the various opportunistic infections common in AIDS, such as toxoplasmosis, as well as by cardiac metastases in Kaposi's sarcoma. The clinical manifestations of cardiac involvement may be incorrectly attributed to concurrent noncardiac problems such as pneumonia. This is unfortunate, since the dilated cardiomyopathy of HIV infection may respond at least transiently to standard therapy with digitalis, diuretics, and ACE inhibitors.

BACTERIAL MYOCARDITIS Bacterial involvement of the heart is uncommon, but when it does occur, it is usually as a complication of endocarditis. Myocardial abscess formation may involve the valve rings and interventricular septum. *Diphtheritic myocarditis* develops in over one-quarter of the patients with diphtheria, is one of the most serious complications, and is the most common cause of death (Chap. 122). Cardiac damage is due to the liberation of a toxin that inhibits protein synthesis and leads to a dilated, flabby, hypocontractile heart; the conduction system is frequently involved as well. Cardiomegaly and severe CHF typically appear after the first week of illness. Prompt therapy with antitoxin is crucial; antibiotic therapy is also indicated but is of less urgency.

CHAGAS DISEASE Chagas disease, caused by the protozoan *Trypanosoma cruzi* and transmitted by an insect vector (Chap. 197), produces an extensive myocarditis that typically becomes evident years after the initial infection. It is one of the most common causes of heart disease encountered in Central and South America; in rural endemic areas 20 to 75% of the population may be affected. An increasing number of cases are found in the United States as patients migrate from endemic areas; in rare cases, it has been transmitted by transfusion and organ donation. Although only about 1% of infected individuals have an acute illness, which may include acute myocarditis, upwards of one-third develop chronic myocardial damage many years later. The chronic form is characterized by dilatation of several cardiac chambers, fibrosis and thinning of the ventricular wall, aneurysm formation (especially at the left ventricular apex), and mural thrombi. Chronic progressive heart failure is the rule and is associated with poor survival. The electrocardiogram is abnormal in most patients with cardiac involvement and typically shows right bundle branch block and left anterior hemiblock, which may progress to complete atrioventricular block. The *echocardiogram* may reveal a unique pattern of hypokinesis of the posterior left ventricular wall and relatively preserved septal motion. Ventricular arrhythmias are common and are seen especially during and after exertion; oral amiodarone appears to be particularly effective in treating ventricular tachyarrhythmias. The cause of death is either intractable CHF or an arrhythmia, with a minority of patients dying from embolic phenomena.

℞ TREATMENT

Therapy is directed toward amelioration of the CHF and arrhythmias; progressive conduction system disease and heart block may require implantation of a pacemaker. Anticoagulation (if feasible) may reduce the risk of thromboembolism. Medical therapy is often unsatisfactory or unavailable (especially in poor rural areas), however, and a more promising tactic in endemic areas has been the use of insecticides to eliminate the vector.

GIANT CELL MYOCARDITIS This rare myocarditis of unknown cause is characterized by rapidly fatal CHF and arrhythmia in young to middle-aged adults. At necropsy, the distinctive features include cardiac enlargement, ventricular thrombi, grossly visible serpiginous areas of myocardial necrosis in both ventricles, and microscopic evidence of giant cells within an extensive inflammatory infiltrate. The cause of giant cell myocarditis remains obscure, although it occurs in association with thymoma, systemic lupus erythematosus, and thyrotoxicosis. While treatment with immunosuppressive therapy may help some patients, cardiac transplantation is the treatment of choice.

LYME CARDITIS (See also Chap. 157) Lyme disease is caused by a tick-borne spirochete and is most common in the Northeast, upper Midwest, and Pacific Coastal regions of the United States during the summer months. About 10% of patients develop symptomatic cardiac involvement during the acute phase of the disease. Conduction abnormalities are the most common manifestations of involvement and may lead to syncope. Concomitant myopericarditis is not uncommon, and mild asymptomatic left ventricular dysfunction may occur. Intravenous ceftriaxone or penicillin is used in all but the mildest forms of Lyme carditis, in which case oral amoxicillin or doxycycline is employed. Hospitalization with electrocardiographic monitoring is indicated in patients with second- or third-degree atrioventricular block. A temporary pacemaker may be needed for symptomatic heart block, but permanent pacing is rarely required. The utility of glucocorticoids in reversing heart block is uncertain, but they are often employed. Long-term cardiac manifestations of Lyme disease are uncommon.

FURTHER READING

BANSCH D et al: Primary prevention of sudden cardiac death in idiopathic dilated cardiomyopathy: The Cardiomyopathy Trial (CAT). Circulation 105:1453, 2002

ELKAYAM U et al: Maternal and fetal outcomes of subsequent pregnancies in women with peripartum cardiomyopathy. N Engl J Med 344:1567, 2001

LANGE RA, HILLIS LD: Cardiovascular complications of cocaine use. N Engl J Med 345:351, 2001

LOWES BD et al: Myocardial gene expression in dilated cardiomyopathy treated with beta-blocking agents. N Engl J Med 346:1357, 2002

MARON MS et al: Effect of left ventricular outflow tract obstruction on clinical outcome in hypertrophic cardiomyopathy. N Engl J Med 348:295, 2003

MCCARTHY RE 3rd et al: Long-term outcome of fulminant myocarditis as compared with acute (nonfulminant) myocarditis. N Engl J Med 342:690, 2000

NICOLAS JM et al: The effect of controlled drinking in alcoholic cardiomyopathy. Ann Intern Med 136:192, 2002

WYNNE J: Stirred, not shaken. Ann Intern Med 136:247, 2002

———, BRAUNWALD E: The cardiomyopathies, in *Braunwald's Heart Disease*, 7th ed, D Zipes et al (eds). Philadelphia, Saunders, 2005

YAZAKI Y et al: Prognostic determinants of long-term survival in Japanese patients with cardiac sarcoidosis treated with prednisone. Am J Cardiol 88:1006, 2001

222 PERICARDIAL DISEASE
Eugene Braunwald

NORMAL FUNCTIONS OF THE PERICARDIUM The visceral pericardium is a serous membrane that is separated by a small quantity (15 to 50 mL) of fluid, an ultrafiltrate of plasma from a fibrous sac, the parietal pericardium. The pericardium normally prevents sudden dilatation of the cardiac chambers during exercise and with hypervolemia. The pericardium also restricts the anatomic position of the heart, minimizes friction between the heart and surrounding structures, prevents displacement of the heart and kinking of the great vessels, and probably retards the spread of infections from the lungs and pleural cavities to the heart. Notwithstanding the foregoing, total absence of the pericardium does not produce obvious clinical disease. In partial left pericardial defects, the main pulmonary artery and left atrium may bulge through the defect; very rarely, herniation and subsequent strangulation of the left atrium may cause sudden death.

ACUTE PERICARDITIS

Acute pericarditis, by far the most common pathologic process involving the pericardium, may be classified both clinically and etiologically (Table 222-1). Pain, a pericardial friction rub, electrocardiographic changes, and pericardial effusion with cardiac tamponade and paradoxical pulse are cardinal manifestations of many forms of acute pericarditis.

Chest pain is an important but not invariable symptom in various forms of acute pericarditis (Chap. 12); it is usually present in the acute infectious types and in many of the forms presumed to be related to hypersensitivity or autoimmunity. Pain is often absent in a slowly developing tuberculous, postirradiation, neoplastic, or uremic pericarditis. The pain of pericarditis is often severe, retrosternal and left precordial, and referred to the back and the left trapezius ridge. Often the pain is pleuritic consequent to accompanying pleural inflammation, i.e., sharp and aggravated by inspiration, coughing, and changes in body position, but sometimes it is a steady, constricting pain that radiates into either arm or both arms and resembles that of myocardial ischemia; therefore, confusion with acute myocardial infarction (AMI) is common. Characteristically, however, pericardial pain may be relieved by sitting up and leaning forward and is intensified by lying supine. The differentiation of AMI from acute pericarditis becomes perplexing when, with acute pericarditis, serum biomarkers of myocardial damage such as creatine kinase and troponin rise, presumably because of concomitant involvement of the epicardium. However, these elevations, if they occur, are quite modest, given the extensive electrocardiographic ST-segment elevation in pericarditis.

The *pericardial friction rub,* the most important physical sign of acute pericarditis, may have up to three components per cardiac cycle and is high-pitched, scratching, and grating, as described in Chap. 209; it can sometimes be elicited only when firm pressure with the diaphragm of the stethoscope is applied to the chest wall at the left lower sternal border. It is heard most frequently during expiration with the patient in the sitting position. The rub is often inconstant, and the loud to-and-fro leathery sound may disappear within a few hours, possibly to reappear the following day.

The *electrocardiogram* (ECG) in acute pericarditis without massive effusion usually displays changes secondary to acute subepicardial inflammation (see Fig. 210-16). There is widespread elevation of the ST segments, often with upward concavity, involving two or three standard limb leads and V_2 to V_6, with reciprocal depressions only in aVR and sometimes V_1. Usually there are no significant changes in QRS complexes, except for some reduction in voltage in patients with large pericardial effusions. After several days, the ST segments return to normal, and only then do the T waves become inverted. In contrast, in AMI, ST elevations are convex, and reciprocal depression is usually more prominent; QRS changes occur, particularly the development of Q waves, as well as notching and loss of R-wave amplitude; and T-wave inversions are usually seen within hours *before* the ST segments have become isoelectric. Sequential ECGs are useful in distinguishing acute pericarditis from AMI. In the latter, elevated ST segments return to normal within hours. Early repolarization is a normal variant and may also cause widespread ST-segment elevation, most prominent in left precordial leads. However, in this condition the T waves are usually tall and the ST/T ratio is <0.25, but this ratio is higher in acute pericarditis. Depression of the PR segment (below the TP segment) is also common and reflects atrial involvement.

PERICARDIAL EFFUSION In acute pericarditis, effusion is usually associated with pain and/or the above-mentioned ECG changes characteristic of pericarditis and an enlargement of the cardiac silhouette. Pericardial effusion is especially important clinically when it develops within a relatively short time, since it may lead to cardiac tamponade (see below). Differentiation from cardiac enlargement may be difficult on physical examination, but heart sounds tend to become faint with pericardial effusion; the friction rub may disappear, and the apex impulse may vanish, but sometimes it remains palpable, albeit medial to the left border of cardiac dullness. The base of the left lung may be compressed by pericardial fluid, producing Ewart's sign, a patch of dullness beneath the angle of the left scapula. The chest roentgenogram may show a "water bottle" configuration of the cardiac silhouette (Fig. 222-1) but may also be normal or almost so. Lucent pericardial fat lines may be seen deep within the cardiopericardial silhouette. Fluoroscopic examination may show the ventricular pulsations to be diminished.

Diagnosis *Echocardiography* (Chap. 211) is the most effective imaging technique available, since it is sensitive, specific, simple, non-

TABLE 222-1 Classification of Pericarditis

CLINICAL CLASSIFICATION

I. Acute pericarditis (<6 weeks)
   A. Fibrinous
   B. Effusive (serous or sanguineous)
II. Subacute pericarditis (6 weeks to 6 months)
   A. Effusive-constrictive
   B. Constrictive
III. Chronic pericarditis (<6 months)
   A. Constrictive
   B. Effusive
   C. Adhesive (nonconstrictive)

ETIOLOGIC CLASSIFICATION

I. Infectious pericarditis
   A. Viral (coxsackievirus A and B, echovirus, mumps, adenovirus, hepatitis, HIV)
   B. Pyogenic (pneumococcus, streptococcus, staphylococcus, *Neisseria, Legionella*)
   C. Tuberculous
   D. Fungal (histoplasmosis, coccidioidomycosis, *Candida,* blastomycosis)
   E. Other infections (syphilitic, protozoal, parasitic)
II. Noninfectious pericarditis
   A. Acute myocardial infarction
   B. Uremia
   C. Neoplasia
     1. Primary tumors (benign or malignant, mesothelioma)
     2. Tumors metastatic to pericardium (lung and breast cancer, lymphoma, leukemia)
   D. Myxedema
   E. Cholesterol
   F. Chylopericardium
   G. Trauma
     1. Penetrating chest wall
     2. Nonpenetrating
   H. Aortic dissection (with leakage into pericardial sac)
   I. Postirradiation
   J. Familial Mediterranean fever
   K. Familial pericarditis
     1. Mulibrey nanism[a]
   L. Acute idiopathic
   M. Whipple's disease
   N. Sarcoidosis
III. Pericarditis presumably related to hypersensitivity or autoimmunity
   A. Rheumatic fever
   B. Collagen vascular disease (SLE, rheumatoid arthritis, ankylosing spondylitis, scleroderma, acute rheumatic fever, Wegener's granulomatosis)
   C. Drug-induced (e.g., procainamide, hydralazine, phenytoin, isoniazide, minoxidil, anticoagulants, methysergide)
   D. Postcardiac injury
     1. Postmyocardial infarction (Dressler's syndrome)
     2. Postpericardiotomy
     3. Posttraumatic

[a] An autosomal recessive syndrome, characterized by growth failure, muscle hypotonia, hepatomegaly, ocular changes, enlarged cerebral ventricles, mental retardation, and chronic constrictive pericarditis.

invasive, may be performed at the bedside, and can identify accompanying cardiac tamponade (see below) (Fig. 222-2). The presence of pericardial fluid is recorded by two-dimensional transthoracic echocardiography as a relatively echo-free space between the posterior pericardium and left ventricular epicardium in patients with small effusions and as a space between the anterior right ventricle and the parietal pericardium just beneath the anterior chest wall in those with larger effusions. In the latter the heart may swing freely within the pericardial sac; when severe, the extent of this motion alternates and may be associated with electrical alternans. Echocardiography allows localization and estimation of the quantity of pericardial fluid. The diagnosis of pericardial fluid or thickening may be confirmed by computed tomography (CT) or magnetic resonance imaging (MRI); these techniques may be superior to echocardiography in detecting loculated pericardial effusions and pericardial thickening.

FIGURE 222-1 Chest radiogram from a patient with a pericardial effusion showing typical "water bottle" heart. There is also a right pleural effusion. [*From SS Kabbani, M LeWinter, in MH Crawford et al (eds): Cardiology. London, Mosby, 2001.*]

Pericardiocentesis When pericardial fluid is removed for diagnostic and/or therapeutic purposes, a needle attached to a properly grounded ECG lead is inserted into the pericardial space, usually through a subxiphoid approach, and, if possible, using echocardiographic control. Intrapericardial pressure should be measured before fluid is withdrawn. Pericardial effusion nearly always has the physical characteristics of an exudate. Bloody fluid is commonly due to tuberculosis or neoplasm but may also be found in the effusion of rheumatic fever, post-cardiac injury, and post-myocardial infarction (MI) and in uremic pericarditis. Transudative pericardial effusions may occur in heart failure.

CARDIAC TAMPONADE The accumulation of fluid in the pericardium in a quantity sufficient to cause serious obstruction to the inflow of blood

FIGURE 222-2 Large pericardial effusion (PE) with tamponade. Arrow indicates right ventricular (RV) collapse. LV, left ventricle. (*From LeWinter, with permission.*)

Characteristic	Tamponade	Constrictive Pericarditis	Restrictive Cardiomyopathy	RVMI
Clinical				
Pulsus paradoxus	Common	Usually absent	Rare	Rare
Jugular veins				
Prominent y descent	Absent	Usually present	Rare	Rare
Prominent x descent	Present	Usually present	Present	Rare
Kussmaul's sign	Absent	Present	Absent	Absent
Third heart sound	Absent	Absent	Rare	May be present
Pericardial knock	Absent	Often present	Absent	Absent
Electrocardiogram				
Low ECG voltage	May be present	May be present	May be present	Absent
Electrical alternans	May be present	Absent	Absent	Absent
Echocardiography				
Thickened pericardium	Absent	Present	Absent	Absent
Pericardial calcification	Absent	Often present	Absent	Absent
Pericardial effusion	Present	Absent	Absent	Absent
RV size	Usually small	Usually normal	Usually normal	Enlarged
Myocardial thickness	Normal	Normal	Usually increased	Normal
Right atrial collapse and RVDC	Present	Absent	Absent	Absent
Increased early filling, ↑ mitral flow velocity	Absent	Present	Present	May be present
Exaggerated respiratory variation in flow velocity	Present	Present	Absent	Absent
CT/MRI				
Thickened/calcific pericardium	Absent	Present	Absent	Absent
Cardiac catheterization				
Equalization of diastolic pressures	Usually present	Usually present	Usually absent	Absent or present
Cardiac biopsy helpful?	No	No	Sometimes	No

Abbreviations: RV, right ventricle; RVMI, right ventricular myocardial infarction; RVDC, right ventricular diastolic collapse; ECG, electrocardiograph.
Source: From GM Brockington et al, Cardiol Clin 8:645, 1990, with permission.

to the ventricles results in cardiac tamponade. This complication may be fatal if it is not recognized and treated promptly. The three most common causes of tamponade are neoplastic disease, idiopathic pericarditis, and uremia. Tamponade may also result from bleeding into the pericardial space either following cardiac operations and trauma (including cardiac perforation during cardiac catheterization or insertion of pacemaker wires) or from tuberculosis and hemopericardium. The latter may occur when a patient with any form of acute pericarditis is treated with anticoagulants.

The three principal features of tamponade are elevation of intracardiac pressures, limitation of ventricular filling, and reduction of cardiac output. The quantity of fluid necessary to produce this critical state may be as small as 200 mL when the fluid develops rapidly or >2000 mL in slowly developing effusions when the pericardium has had the opportunity to stretch and adapt to an increasing volume. The volume of fluid required to produce tamponade also varies directly with the thickness of the ventricular myocardium and inversely with the thickness of the parietal pericardium.

Table 222-2 lists the features that distinguish cardiac tamponade from constrictive pericarditis. The classic findings of falling arterial pressure, rising venous pressure, and faint heart sounds usually occur only with severe, acute tamponade, as occurs with cardiac trauma or rupture. Tamponade may also develop more slowly, and under these circumstances the clinical manifestations may resemble those of heart failure, including dyspnea, orthopnea, hepatic engorgement, and jugular venous hypertension. A high index of suspicion for cardiac tamponade is required, since, in many instances, no obvious cause for pericardial disease is apparent. Tamponade should be considered in any patient with hypotension and elevation of jugular venous pressure with a prominent *x* descent and a diminutive or absent *y* descent. In contrast, in constrictive pericarditis, the *y* descent is prominent (Chap. 209). A positive Kussmaul sign (see below) is rare in cardiac tamponade, as is a pericardial knock. Their presence suggests that an organizing process and epicardial constriction are present in addition to effusion. A widening of the area of flatness to percussion across the anterior aspect of the chest wall, a paradoxical pulse (see below), hypotension, relatively clear lung fields, diminished pulsations of the cardiac silhouette on fluoroscopy, enlargement of the cardiac silhouette (especially in subacute or chronic tamponade), reduction in amplitude of the QRS complexes, and *electrical alternans* of the P, QRS, and T waves should raise the suspicion of cardiac tamponade.

Paradoxical Pulse This important clue to the presence of cardiac tamponade consists of *a greater than normal (10 mmHg) inspiratory decline in systolic arterial pressure.* When severe, it may be detected by palpating weakness or disappearance of the arterial pulse during inspiration, but usually sphygmomanometric measurement of systolic pressure during slow respiration is required.

Since both ventricles share a tight incompressible covering, i.e., the pericardial sac, the inspiratory enlargement of the right ventricle in cardiac tamponade compresses and reduces left ventricular volume; leftward bulging of the interventricular septum further reduces the left ventricular cavity as the right ventricle enlarges during inspiration. Thus, in cardiac tamponade the normal inspiratory augmentation of right ventricular volume causes an exaggerated reciprocal reduction in left ventricular volume. Also, respiratory distress increases the fluctuations in intrathoracic pressure, which exaggerates the mechanism just described. Right ventricular infarction (Chap. 228) may resemble cardiac tamponade with hypotension, elevated jugular venous pressure, an absent *y* descent in the jugular venous pulse, and occasionally pulsus paradoxus. The differences between these two conditions are shown in Table 222-2.

Paradoxical pulse occurs not only in cardiac tamponade but also in approximately one-third of patients with constrictive pericarditis. This physical finding is not pathognomonic of pericardial disease because it may be observed in some cases of hypovolemic shock, acute and chronic obstructive airways disease, and pulmonary embolus.

Low-pressure tamponade refers to mild tamponade in which the intrapericardial pressure is increased from its slightly subatmospheric levels to +5 to +10 mmHg; in some instances hypovolemia coexists. As a consequence, the central venous pressure is normal or only slightly elevated, while arterial pressure is unaffected and there is no paradoxical pulse. The patients are asymptomatic or complain of mild weakness and dyspnea. The diagnosis is aided by echocardiography, and both hemodynamic and clinical manifestations improve following pericardiocentesis.

Diagnosis Since immediate treatment of cardiac tamponade may be lifesaving, prompt measures to establish the diagnosis by echocardiography should be undertaken (Fig. 222-2). When pericardial effusion causes tamponade, Doppler ultrasound shows that tricuspid and pulmonic valve flow velocities increase markedly during inspiration, while pulmonic vein, mitral, and aortic flow velocities diminish (Fig. 222-3). Often the right ventricular cavity is reduced in diameter, and there is late diastolic inward motion (collapse) of the right ventricular free wall and of the right atrium. Transesophageal echocardiography may be necessary to diagnose a loculated effusion or hemorrhage responsible for cardiac tamponade.

℞ TREATMENT

Patients with acute pericarditis should be observed frequently for the development of an effusion; if a large effusion is present, the patient should be hospitalized and watched closely for signs of tamponade. In the presence of an effusion, arterial and venous pressures and heart rate should be monitored or followed carefully and serial echocardiograms obtained. If manifestations of tamponade appear, pericardiocentesis must be carried out at once, since relief of the intrapericardial pressure may be lifesaving. Intravenous saline may be administered as the patient is being readied. It is helpful, though not essential, to carry this out in the catheterization laboratory with hemodynamic and fluoroscopic monitoring. A small, multiholed catheter advanced over the needle inserted into the pericardial cavity may be left in place to allow draining of the pericardial space if fluid reaccumulates. When a *diagnostic* pericardiocentesis of a large effusion is carried out, an attempt should be made to remove as much fluid as possible. Surgical drainage through a limited (subxiphoid) thoracotomy may be required in recurrent tamponade, when it is necessary to remove loculated effusions, and/or when it is necessary to obtain tissue for diagnosis.

VIRAL OR IDIOPATHIC FORM OF ACUTE PERICARDITIS In some cases of this common disorder, an A or B coxsackievirus or the virus of influenza, echovirus, mumps, herpes simplex, chickenpox, adenovirus, or Epstein-Barr has been isolated from pericardial fluid and/or appropriate elevations in viral antibody titers have been noted. In many instances, acute pericarditis occurs in association with illnesses of known viral origin and, presumably, are caused by the same agent. Commonly, there is an antecedent infection of the respiratory tract, but in many patients such an association is not evident and viral isolation and serologic studies are negative. Most frequently, a viral causation cannot be established; the term *acute idiopathic pericarditis* is then appropriate. Pericardial effusion is the most common cardiac manifestation of HIV; it is usually secondary to infection (often mycobacterial) or neoplasm—most frequently lymphoma or Kaposi's sarcoma. Approx-

imately 80% are asymptomatic, while dyspnea or chest pain occur in the remainder. Pericardial effusion in full-blown AIDS is associated with a shortened survival (Chap. 173).

Acute pericarditis occurs at all ages but is more frequent in young adults and is often associated with pleural effusions and pneumonitis. The almost simultaneous development of fever and precordial pain, often 10 to 12 days after a presumed viral illness, constitutes an important feature in the differentiation of acute pericarditis from AMI, in which pain precedes fever. The constitutional symptoms are usually mild to moderate, and a pericardial friction rub is often audible. The disease ordinarily runs its course in a few days to 4 weeks, but one or more recurrences occur in about one-fourth of patients. Although accumulation of some pericardial fluid is common, tamponade is unusual, and constrictive pericarditis is a possible complication. The ST-segment alterations in the ECG usually disappear after 1 or more weeks, but the abnormal T waves may persist for several years and be a source of confusion in persons without a clear history of pericarditis. Pleuritis and pneumonitis frequently accompany pericarditis. Granulocytosis followed by lymphocytosis is common.

℞ TREATMENT

There is no specific therapy, but bed rest and anti-inflammatory treatment with aspirin may be given. If this is ineffective, one of the nonsteroidal anti-inflammatory agents, such as indomethacin (25 to 75 mg qid), or a glucocorticoid (e.g., prednisone, 40 to 80 mg daily) usually suppresses the clinical manifestations of the acute illness and may be useful in patients in whom the purulent and tuberculous forms of pericarditis have been excluded. Anticoagulants should be avoided. After the patient has been asymptomatic and afebrile for about a week, the dose of the anti-inflammatory agent is gradually tapered. Colchicine may prevent recurrences, but when recurrences are multiple, frequent, disabling, and continue beyond 2 years, pericardiectomy may be effective in terminating the illness.

POST-CARDIAC INJURY SYNDROME Acute pericarditis may appear under a variety of circumstances that have one common feature: previous injury to the myocardium, with blood in the pericardial cavity. The syndrome may develop after a cardiac operation (postpericardiotomy syndrome); after cardiac trauma (Chap. 223), e.g., a stab wound, contusions after a nonpenetrating blow to the chest; or after perforation of the heart with a catheter. Rarely, it follows AMI.

The clinical picture mimics acute viral or idiopathic pericarditis. The principal symptom is the pain of acute pericarditis, which usually develops 1 to 4 weeks following the cardiac injury but sometimes appears only after an interval of months. Recurrences are common and may occur up to 2 years or more after the injury. Fever with temperature up to 40°C, pericarditis, pleuritis, and pneumonitis are the outstanding features, and the bout of illness usually subsides in 1 or 2 weeks. The pericarditis may be of the fibrinous variety or it may be a pericardial effusion, which is often serosanguineous, and may be accompanied by arthralgias, but rarely causes tamponade. Leukocytosis, an increased sedimentation rate, and electrocardiographic changes typical of acute pericarditis may also occur.

The mechanisms responsible for this syndrome have not been identified, but they are probably the result of a hypersensitivity reaction in which the antigen originates from injured myocardial tissue and/or pericardium; the suggested designation of *post-cardiac injury syndrome* for this group of disorders implies that they may have a common pathogenetic mechanism. Circulating autoantibodies to myocardium occur frequently, but their precise role has not been defined. Viral infection may also play an etiologic role, since antiviral antibodies are often elevated in patients who develop this syndrome following cardiac surgery.

Often no treatment is necessary aside from aspirin and analgesics. The management of pericardial effusion and tamponade has already been discussed. When the illness is followed by a series of disabling

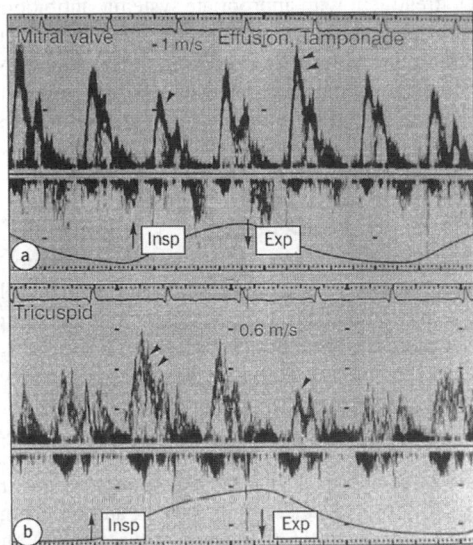

FIGURE 222-3 Doppler tracing of (*A*) mitral and (*B*) tricuspid inflow velocities in a patient with cardiac tamponade. Note the marked respiratory variation from inspiration (Insp) to (exp) expiration. (*From JJ Schultzman et al. Am J Cardiol 70:1353, 1992; with permission.*)

recurrences, therapy with a nonsteroidal anti-inflammatory agent or a glucocorticoid is usually effective.

DIFFERENTIAL DIAGNOSIS Since there is no specific test for *acute idiopathic pericarditis*, the diagnosis is one of exclusion. Consequently, all other disorders that may be associated with acute fibrinous pericarditis must be considered. A common diagnostic error is mistaking acute viral or idiopathic pericarditis for AMI and vice versa. When acute fibrinous pericarditis is associated with AMI, it may be confused with acute viral or idiopathic pericarditis; this complication of infarction, described in Chap. 228, is characterized by fever, pain, and a friction rub in the first 4 days following the development of the infarct. ECG abnormalities (such as the appearance of Q waves, brief ST-segment elevations with reciprocal changes, and earlier T-wave changes in MI) and the extent of the elevations of myocardial enzymes are helpful in differentiating pericarditis from AMI.

Pericarditis secondary to post-cardiac injury is differentiated from acute idiopathic pericarditis chiefly by timing. If it occurs within a few weeks of an MI or a chest blow, it may be justified to conclude that the two are probably related. If the infarct has been silent or the chest blow forgotten, the relationship to the pericarditis may not be recognized.

It is important to distinguish *pericarditis due to collagen vascular disease* from acute idiopathic pericarditis. Most important in the differential diagnosis is the pericarditis due to systemic lupus erythematosus (SLE; Chap. 300) or drug-induced (procainamide or hydralazine) lupus. Pain is often present in pericarditis due to collagen vascular disease. Sometimes in SLE the pericarditis appears as an asymptomatic effusion and, rarely, tamponade develops. When pericarditis occurs in the absence of any obvious underlying disorder, the diagnosis may be made on discovery of LE cells or a rise in the titer of antinuclear antibodies. Acute pericarditis may complicate the viral, pyogenic, mycobacterial, and fungal infections that occur in AIDS. Acute pericarditis is an occasional complication of *rheumatoid arthritis, scleroderma,* and *polyarteritis nodosa,* and other evidence of these diseases is usually obvious. Asymptomatic pericardial effusion is also frequent in these disorders. It is important to question every patient with acute pericarditis about the ingestion of procainamide, hydralazine, isoniazid, cromolyn, and minoxidil, since these drugs can cause this syndrome.

The pericarditis of *acute rheumatic fever* is generally associated with evidence of severe pancarditis and with cardiac murmurs (Chap. 302). *Pyogenic (purulent) pericarditis* is usually secondary to cardiothoracic operations, immunosuppressive therapy, rupture of the esophagus into the pericardial sac, or rupture of a ring abscess in a patient with infective endocarditis and with septicemia complicating aseptic pericarditis. It is accompanied by fever, chills, septicemia, and evidence of infection elsewhere.

Uremic pericarditis (Chap. 261) occurs in up to one-third of patients with chronic uremia and is seen most frequently in patients undergoing chronic hemodialysis. It may be fibrinous and is generally associated with an effusion that may be sanguineous. A friction rub is common, but pain is usually absent. Treatment with an anti-inflammatory agent and intensification of hemodialysis is usually adequate. Pericardial instillation of glucocorticoids may be helpful. Occasionally, tamponade occurs and pericardiocentesis is required. When uremic pericarditis is recurrent or persistent, pericardiectomy may be necessary. Pericarditis due to *neoplastic diseases* results from extension or invasion of metastatic tumors (most commonly carcinoma of the lung and breast, malignant melanoma, lymphoma, and leukemia) to the pericardium; pain, atrial arrhythmias, and tamponade are complications that occur occasionally. *Mediastinal irradiation* for neoplasm may cause acute pericarditis and/or chronic constrictive pericarditis after eradication of the tumor. Unusual causes of acute pericarditis include syphilis, fungal infection (histoplasmosis, blastomycosis, aspergillosis, and candidiasis), and parasitic infestation (amebiasis, toxoplasmosis, echinococcosis, trichinosis).

CHRONIC PERICARDIAL EFFUSIONS Chronic pericardial effusions are sometimes encountered in patients without an antecedent history of acute pericarditis. They may cause few symptoms per se, and their presence may be detected by finding an enlarged cardiac silhouette on chest roentgenogram.

Tuberculosis This is a common cause of chronic pericardial effusion, although less so in the United States than in other parts of the world (Chap. 150). The clinical picture is that of a chronic, systemic illness in a patient with pericardial effusion. It is important to consider this condition in a middle-aged or elderly person with fever and enlargement of the cardiac silhouette of undetermined origin, with or without elevation of venous pressure. Weight loss, fever, and fatigability are sometimes observed. Inasmuch as treatment is quite effective, overlooking a tuberculous pericardial effusion may have serious consequences. If the etiology of chronic pericardial effusion remains obscure, a pericardial biopsy, preferably by a limited thoracotomy, should be performed. If definitive evidence is then still lacking but the specimen shows caseation necrosis, antituberculous chemotherapy is indicated. If the biopsy specimen shows a thickened pericardium, pericardiectomy should be carried out in order to prevent the development of constriction.

Other Causes *Myxedema* may be responsible for a pericardial effusion that is sometimes massive but rarely, if ever, causes cardiac tamponade. The cardiac silhouette is markedly enlarged, and an echocardiogram is necessary to distinguish cardiomegaly from pericardial effusion. The diagnosis of myxedema is frequently overlooked. It is important, therefore, to carry out appropriate tests for thyroid function (Chap. 320) as well as echocardiography in patients with an enlarged cardiac outline of undetermined origin. Myxedematous pericardial effusion responds to thyroid hormone replacement. *Cholesterol pericardial disease* is sometimes associated with myxedema. It is characterized by large pericardial effusions with a high cholesterol content, which may induce an inflammatory response and constrictive pericarditis.

Neoplasms, SLE, rheumatoid arthritis, mycotic infections, radiation therapy, pyogenic infections, severe chronic anemia, and chylopericardium may also cause chronic pericardial effusion and should be considered and specifically looked for in such patients.

Aspiration and analysis of the pericardial fluid are often helpful in diagnosis, especially in patients with chronic large effusions that are nonresponsive to nonsteroidal anti-inflammatory drugs. Fluid should be sent for hematocrit, cell count, protein, culture, and cytology. In infections the organism can often be identified by smear or culture and should lead to treatment with appropriate systemic antibiotics. Grossly sanguineous pericardial fluid results most commonly from a neoplasm, tuberculosis, uremia, or slow leakage from an aortic aneurysm. Pericardiocentesis may resolve large effusions, but pericardiectomy may be required with recurrence. Intrapericardial instillation of sclerosing agents or anti-neoplastc agents (e.g., bleomycin) may be used to prevent reaccumulation of fluid.

CHRONIC CONSTRICTIVE PERICARDITIS

This disorder results when the healing of an acute fibrinous or serofibrinous pericarditis or a chronic pericardial effusion is followed by obliteration of the pericardial cavity with the formation of granulation tissue. The latter gradually contracts and forms a firm scar, encasing the heart and interfering with filling of the ventricles. In some reports, a high percentage of cases has been of tuberculous origin, but in North America, tuberculosis is now an infrequent cause. Chronic constrictive pericarditis may also follow trauma, cardiac operation of any type, mediastinal irradiation, purulent infection, histoplasmosis, neoplastic disease (especially breast cancer, lung cancer, and lymphoma), acute viral or idiopathic pericarditis, rheumatoid arthritis, SLE, and chronic renal failure with uremia treated by chronic dialysis. In many patients the cause of the pericardial disease is undetermined, and in them an asymptomatic or forgotten bout of viral pericarditis, acute or idiopathic, may have been the inciting event. The heart may also be constricted and compressed by malignant tumors or organized blood clot in the pericardial cavity.

The basic physiologic abnormality in symptomatic patients with chronic constrictive pericarditis, as in those with cardiac tamponade, is the inability of the ventricles to fill because of the limitations imposed by the rigid, thickened pericardium or the tense pericardial fluid. In constrictive pericarditis, ventricular filling is unimpeded during early diastole but is reduced abruptly when the elastic limit of the pericardium is reached, while in cardiac tamponade, ventricular filling is impeded throughout diastole. In chronic constrictive pericarditis, ventricular end-diastolic and stroke volumes are reduced and the end-diastolic pressures in both ventricles and the mean pressures in the atria, pulmonary veins, and systemic veins are all elevated to similar levels, i.e., within 5 mmHg of one another. The fibrotic process may extend into the myocardium and cause myocardial scarring, and venous congestion may then be due to the combined effects of the myocardial and pericardial lesions. Despite these hemodynamic changes, myocardial function may be normal or only slightly impaired.

In constrictive pericarditis, the central venous and right and left atrial pressure pulses display an M-shaped contour, with prominent *x* and *y* descents; the *y* descent, which is absent or diminished in cardiac tamponade, is the most prominent deflection in constrictive pericarditis and is interrupted by a rapid rise in pressure during early diastole, when ventricular filling is impeded by the constricting pericardium. These characteristic changes are transmitted to the jugular veins, where they may be recognized by inspection. In constrictive pericarditis, the ventricular pressure pulses in both ventricles exhibit characteristic "square root" signs during diastole (Fig. 222-4). These hemodynamic changes, although characteristic, are not pathognomonic of constrictive pericarditis but may also be observed in cardiomyopathies characterized by restriction of ventricular filling (Chap. 221).

CLINICAL AND LABORATORY FINDINGS (Table 222-2) Weakness, fatigue, weight gain, increased abdominal girth, abdominal discomfort, and edema are common. The patient often appears chronically ill with decreased skeletal muscle mass and a protuberant abdomen. Exertional dyspnea is common, and orthopnea may occur, although it is usually not severe. Acute left ventricular failure (acute pulmonary edema) is very uncommon. The cervical veins are distended and may remain so even after intensive diuretic treatment, and venous pressure may fail to decline during inspiration (Kussmaul's sign). The latter is frequent in chronic pericarditis but may also occur in tricuspid stenosis, right ventricular infarction, and restrictive cardiomyopathy. The pulse pressure is normal or reduced. In about one-third of the cases a paradoxical pulse can be detected. Congestive hepatomegaly is pronounced and may impair hepatic function; ascites is common and is usually more prominent than dependent edema. In about half of patients the heart is normal in size. The apical pulse is reduced and retracts in systole.

FIGURE 222-4 Pressure recording in a patient with constrictive pericarditis. *A.* Simultaneous right ventricular (RV) and left ventricular (LV) pressure tracings with equalization of diastolic pressure as well as "dip and plateau" morphology. *B.* Simultaneous right atrial (RA) and LV pressure with equalization of RA and LV diastolic pressure. Note the prominent *y* descent. (*From P Vaitkus et al: Circulation 93:834, 1996; with permission.*)

The heart sounds may be distant; an early third heart sound, i.e., a pericardial knock, occurring 0.09 to 0.12 s after aortic valve closure is often conspicuous. Protein-losing enteropathy is a rare complication.

The *ECG* frequently displays low voltage of the QRS complex and diffuse flattening or inversion of the T waves. Atrial fibrillation is present in about one-third of patients. The *chest roentgenogram* shows a normal or slightly enlarged heart, sometimes with pericardial calcification.

Inasmuch as the usual physical signs of cardiac disease (murmurs, cardiac enlargement) may be inconspicuous or absent in chronic constrictive pericarditis, hepatic enlargement and dysfunction associated with intractable ascites may lead to a mistaken diagnosis of cirrhosis of the liver. This error can be avoided if the neck veins are inspected carefully in patients with ascites and hepatomegaly. *Given a clinical picture resembling hepatic cirrhosis, but with the added feature of distended neck veins, careful search for calcification of the pericardium by chest roentgenography and CT or MRI should be carried out and may disclose this curable or remediable form of heart disease.*

The echocardiogram typically shows pericardial thickening, atrial enlargement, dilatation of the inferior vena cava and hepatic veins, and a sharp halt in ventricular filling in early diastole, with normal ventricular systolic function and flattening of the left ventricular posterior wall endocardium. There is a distinctive pattern of transvalvular flow velocity on Doppler echocardiography, with an exaggerated reduction in blood flow velocity in the pulmonary veins and across the mitral valve during inspiration, and the opposite occurring during expiration. Diastolic flow velocity in the vena cavae into the right atrium and across the tricuspid valve increases in an exaggerated manner during inspiration and declines during expiration. However, echocardiography cannot definitively exclude the diagnosis. MRI and CT scanning, especially the latter, are more accurate than echocardiography in establishing or excluding the presence of a thickened pericardium. Pericardial thickening and even pericardial calcification, however, are not synonymous with constrictive pericarditis since they may occur without seriously impairing ventricular filling.

DIFFERENTIAL DIAGNOSIS Like cor pulmonale (Chap. 216), chronic constrictive pericarditis may be associated with severe systemic venous hypertension but little pulmonary congestion; the heart is usually not enlarged, and a paradoxical pulse may be present. However, in cor pulmonale advanced parenchymal pulmonary disease is usually obvious and venous pressure *falls* during inspiration, i.e., Kussmaul's sign is negative. *Tricuspid stenosis* (Chap. 219) may also simulate chronic constrictive pericarditis; congestive hepatomegaly, splenomegaly, ascites, and venous distention may be equally prominent, and the manifestations of left-sided heart failure may be inconspicuous. However, in tricuspid stenosis, a characteristic murmur as well as mitral stenosis are usually present. In tricuspid stenosis, a paradoxical pulse and a steep, deep *y* descent in the jugular venous pulse do not occur, serving to differentiate it from chronic constrictive pericarditis.

Because constrictive pericarditis can be corrected surgically, it is important, though often difficult, to distinguish chronic constrictive pericarditis from restrictive cardiomyopathy (Chap. 221), which has a similar physiologic abnormality, i.e., restriction of ventricular filling. In many of these patients the ventricular wall is thickened on echocardiographic examination (Table 222-2). The features favoring the diagnosis of restrictive cardiomyopathy over chronic constrictive pericarditis include a well-defined apex beat, cardiac enlargement, and pronounced orthopnea with attacks of acute left ventricular failure, left ventricular hypertrophy, gallop sounds (in place of a pericardial knock), bundle branch block, and in some cases abnormal Q waves on the ECG. The echocardiogram in chronic constrictive pericarditis characteristically shows pericardial thickening, i.e., a distinct echo posterior to the left ventricular wall, and paradoxical septal motion.

The left ventricular wall moves sharply outward in early diastole on Doppler myocardial imaging. Marked respiratory variations in atrioventricular flow velocities on Doppler echocardiography are also characteristic of constrictive pericarditis but not restrictive cardiomyopathy (Fig. 222-4). The definitive diagnosis of restrictive cardiomyopathy, when it is due to an infiltrative disease such as amyloidosis, can often be established by endomyocardial biopsy. CT scanning and MRI are very useful in distinguishing between restrictive cardiomyopathy and chronic constrictive pericarditis. In the former, the ventricular walls are hypertrophied, while in the latter the pericardium is thickened and sometimes calcified.

When a patient has progressive, disabling, and unresponsive congestive failure and displays any of the features of constrictive heart disease, the most careful and detailed clinical and laboratory studies must be carried out in order to detect or exclude constrictive pericarditis, since the latter is usually curable.

℞ TREATMENT

Pericardial resection is the only definitive treatment of constrictive pericarditis, but dietary sodium restriction and diuretics are useful during preoperative preparation. The benefits derived from cardiac decortication are often striking, and the improvement, though slight at first, is usually progressive over a period of months. The risk of this operation depends on the extent of penetration of the myocardium by the calcific process, by the severity of myocardial atrophy, by the extent of secondary impairment of hepatic and/or renal function, and by the patient's general condition. Operative mortality is in the range of 5 to 15%; the patients with the most severe and/or advanced disease are at highest risk. Therefore, surgical treatment should be carried out relatively early in the course.

Many cases of constrictive pericarditis are of tuberculous origin. Antituberculous therapy during the phase of effusion may prevent the development of constriction, and such therapy should be carried out before and after operation if a tuberculous origin can be diagnosed or suspected (Chap. 150).

Subacute Effusive-Constrictive Pericarditis This form of pericardial disease is characterized by the combination of a tense effusion in the pericardial space and constriction of the heart by thickened pericardium. It shares a number of features both with chronic pericardial effusion producing cardiac compression and with pericardial constric-

tion. It may be caused by tuberculosis, multiple attacks of acute idiopathic pericarditis, radiation, traumatic pericarditis, uremia, and scleroderma. The heart is generally enlarged, and a paradoxical pulse and a prominent x descent (without a prominent y descent) are present in the atrial and jugular venous pressure pulses. Following pericardiocentesis, the physiologic findings may change from those of cardiac tamponade to those of pericardial constriction, with a "square root" sign in the ventricular pressure pulse and a prominent y descent in the atrial and jugular venous pressure pulses. Furthermore, the intrapericardial pressure and the central venous pressure may decline, but not to normal. In many patients the condition progresses to the chronic constrictive form of the disease. Wide excision of both the visceral and parietal pericardium is usually effective.

OTHER DISORDERS OF THE PERICARDIUM

Pericardial cysts appear as rounded or lobulated deformities of the cardiac silhouette, most commonly at the right cardiophrenic angle. They do not cause symptoms, and their major clinical significance lies in the possibility of confusion with a tumor, ventricular aneurysm, or massive cardiomegaly. *Tumors* involving the pericardium are most commonly secondary to malignant neoplasms originating in or invading the mediastinum, including carcinoma of the bronchus and breast, lymphoma, and melanoma. The most common *primary* malignant tumor is the mesothelioma. The usual clinical picture of malignant pericardial tumor is an insidiously developing, often bloody, pericardial effusion. Surgical exploration is required to establish a definitive diagnosis and to carry out definitive or, more commonly, palliative treatment.

FURTHER READING

HOIT BD: Management of effusive and constrictive pericardial heart disease. Circulation 105:2939, 2002

LEWINTER M: Pericardial diseases, in D Zipes et al (eds): *Braunwald's Heart Disease*, 7th ed. Philadelphia, Saunders, 2005

LING LH et al: Constrictive pericarditis in the modern era: Evolving clinical spectrum and impact on outcome after pericardiectomy. Circulation 100: 1380, 1999

OH JK et al: Diagnostic role of Doppler echocardiography in constrictive pericarditis. J Am Coll Cardiol 23:154, 1994

RAJAGOPALAN N et al: Comparison of new Doppler echocardiographic methods to differentiate constrictive pericardial heart disease and restrictive cardiomyopathy. Am J Cardiol 87:86, 2001

SAGRISTA A et al: Long-term follow-up of idiopathic chronic pericardial effusions. N Engl J Med 341:2054, 1999

223 CARDIAC TUMORS, CARDIAC MANIFESTATIONS OF SYSTEMIC DISEASES, AND TRAUMATIC CARDIAC INJURY
Wilson S. Colucci, Daniel T. Price

TUMORS OF THE HEART

PRIMARY TUMORS

Primary tumors of the heart are rare. Approximately three-quarters are histologically benign, and the remainder, which in almost all cases are sarcomas, are malignant (Table 223-1). Because all cardiac tumors have the potential to cause life-threatening complications, and many are now curable by surgery, it is important that the diagnosis be made whenever possible.

CLINICAL PRESENTATION
Cardiac tumors may present with a wide array of cardiac and noncardiac manifestations. The location and the size of the tumor are the major determinants of the specific signs and symptoms, many of which are present in more common forms of heart disease, such as chest pain, syncope, heart failure, murmurs, arrhyth-

mias, conduction disturbances, and pericardial effusion with or without tamponade.

MYXOMA
Myxomas are the most common type of primary cardiac tumor in all age groups, accounting for one-third to one-half of all cases at postmortem and for about three-quarters of the tumors treated surgically. They occur at all ages, most commonly in the third through sixth decades, with a female predilection. Although most myxomas are sporadic, some are familial with autosomal dominant transmission or are part of a syndrome that involves a complex of abnormalities including lentigines or pigmented nevi, primary nodular adrenal cortical disease with or without Cushing's syndrome, myxomatous mammary fibroadenomas, testicular tumors, and/or pituitary adenomas with gigantism or acromegaly. Patients with Carney complex have spotty skin pigmentation, myxomas, endocrine overactivity, and schwanno-

TABLE 223-1 *Relative Incidence of Primary Tumors of the Heart*

Type	Number	Percent
Benign	199	58.0
Myxoma	114	33.2
Rhabdomyoma	20	5.8
Fibroma	20	5.8
Hemangioma	17	5.0
Atrioventricular nodal	10	2.9
Granular cell	4	1.2
Lipoma	2	0.6
Paraganglioma	2	0.6
Myocytic hamartoma	2	0.6
Histiocytoid cardiomyopathy	2	0.6
Inflammatory psuedotumor	2	0.6
Other benign tumors	4	1.2
Malignant	144	42.0
Sarcoma	137	39.9
Lymphoma	7	2.1

Source: Modified from A Burke, R Virmani: *Atlas of Tumor Pathology. Tumors of the Heart and Great Vessels.* Washington, DC, Armed Forces Institute of Pathology 1996, p 231; with permission.

FIGURE 223-1 Transthoracic echocardiogram during diastole demonstrating a large myocardial mass, which is an atrial myxoma (Myx) that prolapses into the left ventricle (LV). LA, left atrium; RA, right atrium; RV, right ventricle. *(Courtesy of Dr. Rick Nishimura.)*

mas that are due to mutations of the gene encoding the protein kinase A type I-α regulatory subunit. Certain constellations of findings have been referred to as the *NAME* syndrome (nevi, atrial myxoma, myxoid neurofibroma, and ephelides) or the *LAMB* syndrome (lentigines, atrial myxoma, and blue nevi). Approximately 7% of cardiac myxomas are familial or part of the myxoma syndrome with the complex of abnormalities described above.

Pathologically, myxomas are gelatinous structures consisting of myxoma cells imbedded in a stroma rich in glycosaminoglycans. Most are pedunculated on a fibrovascular stalk and average 4 to 8 cm in diameter. Most are solitary and located in the atria, particularly the left, where they arise from the interatrial septum in the vicinity of the fossa ovalis. In contrast to sporadic tumors, familial or myxoma syndrome tumors tend to occur in younger individuals, be multiple or ventricular in location, and have more postoperative recurrences, probably reflecting their multicentric nature.

Myxomas commonly present with obstructive, embolic, or constitutional signs and symptoms. The most common clinical presentation mimics that of mitral valve disease—either stenosis due to tumor prolapse into the mitral orifice, or regurgitation due to tumor-induced valvular trauma. Ventricular myxomas may cause outflow obstruction similar to that caused by subaortic or subpulmonic stenosis. The symptoms and signs of myxoma may be of sudden onset or positional in nature, reflecting changes in tumor position due to gravity. An auscultatory finding, termed a "tumor plop," is a characteristic low-pitched sound that may be audible during early or mid-diastole and is thought to result from the tumor abruptly stopping as it strikes the ventricular wall. Myxomas may also present with peripheral or pulmonary emboli, or constitutional signs and symptoms including fever, weight loss, cachexia, malaise, arthralgias, rash, clubbing, Raynaud's phenomenon, hypergammaglobulinemia, anemia, polycythemia, leukocytosis, elevated erythrocyte sedimentation rate, thrombocytopenia, or thrombocytosis. Not surprisingly, myxomas are frequently misdiagnosed as endocarditis, collagen vascular disease, or noncardiac tumor.

Two-dimensional transthoracic or transesophageal echocardiography is useful in the diagnosis of cardiac myxoma and allows determination of the site of tumor attachment and tumor size, which are important considerations in the planning of surgical excision (Fig. 223-1). Computed tomography (CT) and particularly magnetic resonance imaging (MRI) may provide important information regarding size, shape, composition, and surface characteristics of the tumor. Because myxomas may be familial, echocardiographic screening of first-degree relatives is appropriate, particularly if the patient is young and has multiple tumors or evidence of myxoma syndrome. Although cardiac catheterization and angiography have previously been performed rou-

tinely before surgery, catheterization of the chamber from which the tumor arises carries the risk of tumor emboli. Catheterization is no longer considered mandatory when adequate noninvasive information is available and other cardiac diseases (e.g., coronary artery disease) are not considered likely.

℞ TREATMENT

Surgical excision utilizing cardiopulmonary bypass is indicated and is generally curative. Myxomas recur in approximately 12 to 22% of familial cases and in about 1 to 2% of sporadic cases. Tumor recurrence is most likely due to multifocal lesions in the former and inadequate resection in the latter.

OTHER BENIGN TUMORS Cardiac *lipomas*, although relatively common, are usually incidental findings at postmortem examination. However, they may grow as large as 15 cm and may present with symptoms due to mechanical interference with cardiac function, arrhythmias, or conduction disturbances, or as an abnormality of the cardiac silhouette on chest x-ray. *Papillary fibroelastomas*, similarly, are relatively common findings on cardiac valves or the adjacent endothelium at postmortem, but seldom result in clinical symptoms. Occasionally, these growths may cause mechanical interference with valve function. *Rhabdomyomas* and *fibromas*, the most frequent tumors in infants and children, most commonly occur in the ventricles and therefore produce signs and symptoms by mechanical obstruction that may mimic valvular stenosis, congestive heart failure, restrictive or hypertrophic cardiomyopathy, and pericardial constriction. Rhabdomyomas are probably hamartomatous growths; are multiple in 90% of cases; and may be associated with tuberous sclerosis, adenoma sebaceum, and benign kidney tumors in approximately 30% of patients. Calcification of a cardiac tumor strongly suggests that it is a fibroma, although myxomas and sarcomas also may be calcified. *Hemangiomas* and *mesotheliomas* are generally small tumors, most often intramyocardial in location, and may cause atrioventricular (AV) conduction disturbances and even sudden death as a result of their predilection for the region of the AV node. Other benign tumors arising from the heart include *teratoma*, *chemodectoma*, *neurilemoma*, *granular cell myoblastoma*, and *bronchogenic cysts*.

SARCOMA Almost all primary cardiac malignancies are sarcomas, which may be of several histologic types. In general, these tumors are characterized by a rapidly downhill course leading to the patient's death in weeks to months from the time of presentation as a result of hemodynamic compromise, local invasion, or distant metastases. Sarcomas commonly involve the right side of the heart, and because of their rapid growth, invasion of the pericardial space and obstruction of the cardiac chambers or vena cavae are common. Sarcomas can also occur on the left side of the heart and may be mistaken for myxomas.

℞ TREATMENT

At the time of presentation these tumors have often spread too extensively for surgical excision. Although scattered reports exist of palliation with surgery, radiotherapy, and/or chemotherapy, the overall experience with cardiac sarcomas is poor. The one exception appears to be cardiac lymphosarcomas, which may respond to a combination of chemo- and radiotherapy.

TUMORS METASTATIC TO THE HEART

Tumors metastatic to the heart are much more common than primary tumors, and their incidence is likely to increase as the life expectancy of patients with various forms of malignant neoplasms is extended by more effective therapy. Although cardiac metastases occur in 1 to 20% of all tumor types, the relative incidence is especially high in malignant melanoma and, to a somewhat lesser extent, in leukemia and lymphoma. In absolute numbers, the most common primary originating sites of cardiac metastases are carcinoma of the breast and lung, reflecting the high incidence of these cancers. Cardiac metastases almost always occur in the setting of widespread primary disease, and most often either primary or metastatic disease exists elsewhere in the thoracic cavity. Nevertheless, a cardiac metastasis may occasionally be the initial presentation of a tumor elsewhere in the body.

Cardiac metastases reach the heart from the blood stream, the lymphatics, or by direct invasion. They generally are small, firm nodules. Diffuse infiltration may also occur, especially with sarcomas or hematologic neoplasms. The pericardium is most often involved, followed by myocardial involvement of any chamber, and, rarely, by involvement of the endocardium or cardiac valves.

Cardiac metastases result in clinical manifestations only about 10% of the time and rarely are the cause of death. In most instances the metastases are not the cause of the presenting clinical features but occur in the setting of a previously recognized malignant neoplasm. Although cardiac metastases may present with a large number of nonspecific signs and symptoms, the most common are dyspnea, signs of acute pericarditis, cardiac tamponade, a rapid increase in the cardiac silhouette on chest x-ray, new onset of ectopic tachyarrhythmia or AV block, and congestive heart failure. As with primary cardiac tumors, the clinical presentation is more closely related to the location and size of the tumor than to histologic type. Many of these signs and symptoms also occur with myocarditis, pericarditis, or cardiomyopathy resulting from radiotherapy or chemotherapy.

Electrocardiographic (ECG) findings are nonspecific. On chest x-ray the cardiac silhouette is most often normal but may reveal a pericardial effusion or bizarre contour. Echocardiography is useful for the diagnosis of pericardial effusion and the visualization of larger metastases. Computed tomography (CT), MRI, and radionuclide imaging with gallium or thallium may provide useful anatomic information. Angiography may delineate discrete lesions, and pericardiocentesis can allow a specific cytologic diagnosis.

℞ TREATMENT

Because most patients with cardiac metastases have widespread disease, therapy generally consists of treatment of the primary tumor. Symptomatic malignant effusions are treated by removal of fluid by pericardiocentesis, with or without concomitant instillation of a sclerosing agent (e.g., tetracycline), or placement of a pericardial window for drainage to the pleural space, to palliate symptoms, and to delay or prevent reaccumulation of the effusion.

CARDIAC EFFECTS OF CANCER THERAPY See Chap. 221

CARDIOVASCULAR MANIFESTATIONS OF SYSTEMIC DISEASES

DIABETES MELLITUS (See also Chap. 323)

There is an increased incidence of large-vessel atherosclerosis and myocardial infarction in patients with both insulin- and noninsulin-dependent diabetes mellitus. Coronary artery disease is the most common cause of death in adults with diabetes mellitus. Diabetes mellitus is an independent risk factor for coronary artery disease (Chap. 224), and the incidence of coronary artery disease is related to the duration of diabetes. In patients with diabetes mellitus, myocardial infarctions are not only more frequent but also tend to be larger in size and more likely to result in complications such as heart failure, shock, and death. Patients with diabetes mellitus are more likely to have an abnormal or absent pain response to myocardial ischemia, probably as a result of generalized autonomic nervous system dysfunction. Ambulatory ECG monitoring has shown that up to 90% of episodes of ischemia are silent in diabetic patients with coronary artery disease; the presentation of their ischemia may be exertional or episodic dyspnea, flash pulmonary edema, arrhythmias, heart block, or syncope. Since coronary artery disease is more common in patients with diabetes mellitus and often is not associated with typical anginal symptoms, the threshold for the diagnosis should be low, particularly when the duration of disease is long and concomitant risk factors for coronary artery disease (e.g., hypertension, smoking, hyperlipidemia) are present.

Patients with diabetes mellitus may also have myocardial dysfunction characteristic of a restrictive cardiomyopathy in the absence of large-vessel (epicardial) coronary artery disease, with abnormal relaxation of the myocardium, and evidenced clinically by elevated left ventricular filling pressures. Histologically, these patients have interstitial fibrosis with increased amounts of collagen, glycoprotein, triglycerides, and cholesterol in the myocardial interstitium. In some cases intimal thickening, hyaline deposition, and inflammatory changes have been observed in small intramural arteries. Patients with diabetes mellitus have an increased risk of developing clinical heart failure, even after correction for the presence of coronary artery disease, hypertension, and obesity, and it is likely that diabetic cardiomyopathy contributes to excessive cardiovascular morbidity and mortality in these patients. There is some evidence that insulin therapy results in an amelioration of the myocardial dysfunction.

MALNUTRITION AND VITAMIN DEFICIENCY MALNUTRITION (See also Chap. 62)

In patients whose intake of protein, calories, or both is severely deficient, the heart may become thin, pale, and flabby with myofibrillar atrophy and interstitial edema. The systolic pressure and cardiac output are low, and the pulse pressure is narrow. Generalized edema is common and is due to a combination of factors, including reduced serum oncotic pressure and myocardial dysfunction. Such profound states of malnutrition, termed *marasmus* in the case of caloric deficiency and *kwashiorkor* in the case of relative protein deficiency, are most common in underdeveloped countries. However, significant nutritional heart disease may also occur in developed nations, particularly in patients with chronic diseases such as AIDS, in patients with anorexia nervosa, and in patients with severe cardiac failure in whom gastrointestinal hypoperfusion and venous congestion may lead to anorexia and malabsorption. Open-heart surgery poses increased risk in malnourished patients, and they may benefit from preoperative hyperalimentation.

THIAMINE DEFICIENCY (BERIBERI) (See also Chap. 61)
In many cases, malnutrition is accompanied by thiamine deficiency, although this hypovitaminosis may also occur in the presence of an adequate protein and caloric intake, particularly in the Far East, where polished rice deficient in thiamine may be a major dietary component. In Western nations, the widespread use of thiamine-enriched flour limits the presence of deficiency primarily to alcoholics and food faddists. The meas-

urement of the thiamine-pyrophosphate effect (TPPE) can biochemically quantitate thiamine stores. An elevated TPPE, indicative of thiamine deficiency, has been found in 20 to 90% of patients with chronic heart failure. The deficiency appears to result from both reduced dietary intake and a diuretic-induced increase in the urinary excretion of thiamine. The acute administration of thiamine to these patients increases the left ventricular ejection fraction and the excretion of salt and water.

Clinically, there is usually evidence of generalized malnutrition, peripheral neuropathy, glossitis, and anemia. The characteristic cardiovascular syndrome is heart failure with increased cardiac output, tachycardia, and often elevated filling pressures in the left and right sides of the heart. The major cause of the high-output cardiac state is vasomotor depression, the precise mechanism of which is not understood but which leads to a reduced systemic vascular resistance. The cardiac examination reveals a wide pulse pressure, tachycardia, a third heart sound, and, frequently, an apical systolic murmur. The ECG may show decreased voltage, a prolonged QT interval, and T-wave abnormalities. The chest x-ray generally shows a large heart with signs of congestive heart failure. The response to thiamine is often dramatic, with an increase in systemic vascular resistance, decrease in cardiac output, clearing of pulmonary congestion, and a reduction in heart size often occurring in 12 to 48 h. Although the response to digitalis and diuretics may be poor before thiamine therapy, these agents may be important *after* thiamine is given, since the left ventricle may not be capable of dealing with the increased work load presented by the return of vascular tone.

VITAMIN B₆, B₁₂, AND FOLATE DEFICIENCY (See also Chap. 61) These vitamin cofactors in the metabolism of homocysteine probably contribute to the majority of cases of hyperhomocysteinemia in the general population. Hyperhomocysteinemia is associated with increased risk of atherosclerosis. Supplementation of these vitamins has reduced the incidence of hyperhomocysteinemia in the United States. The clinical benefit of normalizing elevated homocysteine levels, however, remains unproven.

OBESITY (See also Chap. 64)

Severe obesity, particularly when it occurs in an upper-body distribution, is associated with an increase in cardiovascular morbidity and mortality. Although obesity itself is not considered a disease, there is clearly an increased prevalence of hypertension, glucose intolerance, and atherosclerotic coronary artery disease in obese patients. In addition, these patients have a distinct abnormality of the cardiovascular system characterized by increases in total and central blood volumes, cardiac output, and left ventricular filling pressure. The elevated cardiac output appears to be required to support the metabolic needs of the excessive adipose tissue. Left ventricular filling pressure is often at the upper limits of normal and rises excessively with exercise. As a result of chronic volume overload, eccentric cardiac hypertrophy with cardiac dilatation and abnormal ventricular function may develop. Pathologically, there are left and, in some cases, right ventricular hypertrophy and generalized cardiac dilatation, which is not due simply to fatty infiltration of the myocardium. Although these patients may develop pulmonary congestion, peripheral edema, and exercise intolerance, the recognition of these findings may be difficult in massively obese patients.

Weight reduction is the most effective therapy and results in reduction in blood volume and in the return of cardiac output toward normal. However, rapid weight reduction may be dangerous, as cardiac arrhythmias and sudden death due to electrolyte imbalance have been described. Digitalis, sodium restriction, and diuretics may also be useful. This form of heart disease should be distinguished from the Pickwickian syndrome (Chap. 246), which may share several of the cardiovascular features of heart disease secondary to severe obesity but, in addition, frequently has components of central apnea, hypoxemia, pulmonary hypertension, and cor pulmonale.

THYROID DISEASE (See also Chap. 320)

Thyroid hormone exerts a major influence on the cardiovascular system by a number of direct and indirect mechanisms, and not surprisingly, cardiovascular effects are prominent in both hypo- and hyperthyroidism. Thyroid hormone causes increases in total-body metabolism and oxygen consumption that indirectly place an increased work load on the heart. In addition, although the exact mechanism has not been defined, thyroid hormone exerts direct inotropic, chronotropic, and dromotropic effects that are similar to those seen with adrenergic stimulation (e.g., tachycardia, increased cardiac output). Thyroid hormone increases the synthesis of myosin and of Na⁺,K⁺-ATPase, as well as the density of myocardial β-adrenergic receptors.

HYPERTHYROIDISM Cardiovascular presentations of hyperthyroidism include palpitations, systolic hypertension, fatigue, or, in patients with underlying heart disease, angina or heart failure. Sinus tachycardia is found in about 40% of patients and atrial fibrillation in about 15%. Other findings include a hyperdynamic precordium, a widened pulse pressure, an increase in the intensity of the first heart sound and the pulmonic component of the second heart sound, and a third heart sound. An increased incidence of mitral valve prolapse has been associated with hyperthyroidism, and in some cases there may be a midsystolic murmur heard best at the left sternal border with or without a systolic ejection click. A *Means-Lerman scratch* is a systolic scratchy sound, heard at the left second intercostal space during expiration; it is thought to result from the rubbing of the hyperdynamic pericardium against the pleura.

Elderly patients with hyperthyroidism, so-called apathetic hyperthyroidism, may present with only the cardiovascular manifestations of thyrotoxicosis, such as atrial fibrillation, which may be resistant to therapy until the hyperthyroidism is controlled. Angina pectoris and congestive heart failure are unusual unless there is coexistent underlying heart disease, and in many cases symptoms resolve with treatment of the hyperthyroidism.

HYPOTHYROIDISM Cardiac manifestations of hypothyroidism include a reduction in cardiac output, stroke volume, heart rate, blood pressure, and pulse pressure. In about one-third of patients there is a pericardial effusion which only rarely results in tamponade. Increased capillary permeability results in pleural and pericardial effusions. Other clinical signs include cardiomegaly, bradycardia, weak arterial pulses, and distant heart sounds. Although the signs and symptoms of myxedema may suggest the diagnosis of congestive heart failure, in the absence of other cardiac disease, myocardial failure is uncommon. The ECG generally shows sinus bradycardia and low voltage and may show prolongation of the QT interval, decreased P-wave voltage, prolonged AV conduction time, intraventricular conduction disturbances, and nonspecific ST-T wave abnormalities. Chest x-ray may show cardiomegaly, often with a "water bottle" configuration, pleural effusions, and, in some cases, evidence of congestive heart failure. Pathologically, the heart is pale, dilated, and flabby, often with myofibrillar swelling, loss of striations, and interstitial fibrosis.

Patients with hypothyroidism frequently have elevations of cholesterol and triglycerides, and severe atherosclerotic coronary artery disease. Before treatment with thyroid hormone, patients with hypothyroidism frequently do not have angina pectoris, presumably because of the low metabolic demands caused by their condition. However, angina and myocardial infarction may be precipitated during initiation of thyroid hormone replacement, especially in elderly patients with underlying heart disease. Therefore, replacement should be done with care, starting with low doses that are increased gradually.

MALIGNANT CARCINOID (See also Chap. 329)

These tumors elaborate a variety of vasoactive amines (e.g., serotonin), kinins, indoles, and other substances believed to be responsible for the diarrhea, flushing, and labile blood pressure in these patients. The cardiac lesions due to gastrointestinal carcinoids are almost exclusively in the right side of the heart and occur only when there are hepatic metastases, suggesting that the substance responsible for the cardiac lesions is inactivated by passage through the liver and lungs. Similar lesions occur in the left side of the heart when there exists a right-to-left shunt or when the tumor is located in the lungs. These lesions are fibrous plaques on the endothelium of the cardiac chambers, valves, and great vessels. These plaques, which result in distortion of the cardiac valves, consist of smooth-muscle cells embedded in a stroma of acid mucopolysaccharide and collagen and presumably result from healing of endothelial injury.

The clinical syndrome is most often that of tricuspid regurgitation, pulmonic stenosis, or both. In some cases a high-output cardiac state may occur, presumably as a result of a decrease in systemic vascular resistance due to a vasoactive substance released by the tumor. Progression of the cardiac lesions does not appear to be affected by treatment with serotonin antagonists, and, in some severely symptomatic patients, valve replacement is indicated. Coronary artery spasm, presumably due to a circulating vasoactive substance, may occur in patients with carcinoid syndrome.

PHEOCHROMOCYTOMA (See also Chap. 322)

In addition to causing labile or sustained hypertension, the high circulating levels of catecholamines as a result of the pheochromocytoma may also cause direct myocardial injury. Focal myocardial necrosis and inflammatory cell infiltration are present in about 50% of patients who die with pheochromocytoma and may contribute to clinically significant left ventricular failure and pulmonary edema. In addition, hypertension results in left ventricular hypertrophy. Left ventricular function and congestive heart failure may resolve after removal of the tumor.

ACROMEGALY (See also Chap. 318)

The effect of excessive growth hormone on cardiac function results in congestive heart failure that may be due to high cardiac output, diastolic dysfunction due to ventricular hypertrophy (with increased left ventricular chamber size or wall thickness), or global systolic dysfunction. Hypertension occurs in up to one-third of patients and is characterized by suppression of the renin-aldosterone axis and increases in total body sodium and plasma volume. Cardiac disease occurs in about one-third of patients with acromegaly, and is associated with a doubling in the risk of death from heart disease.

RHEUMATOID ARTHRITIS AND THE COLLAGEN VASCULAR DISEASES

RHEUMATOID ARTHRITIS (See also Chap. 301)   There may be inflammation of any or all anatomical parts of the heart in patients with rheumatoid arthritis. Pericarditis is the most common cause of clinically apparent disease and may be found by echocardiography in 10 to 50% of all patients with rheumatoid arthritis, particularly those with subcutaneous nodules. However, only a small fraction of these patients have clinical evidence of pericarditis, which usually follows a benign course but occasionally may progress to cardiac tamponade or constrictive pericarditis. The pericardial fluid is generally an exudate, with decreased concentrations of complement and glucose, and elevated cholesterol. Coronary arteritis with intimal inflammation and edema is present in about 20% of cases but only rarely results in angina pectoris or myocardial infarction. The cardiac valves, most often the mitral and aortic, may be involved by inflammation and granuloma formation that in some cases may cause clinically significant regurgitation due to valve deformity. Myocarditis rarely results in cardiac dysfunction.

Treatment is directed at the underlying rheumatoid arthritis and may include glucocorticoids. Pericardiectomy is usually required in cases of tamponade or persistent effusion.

SERONEGATIVE ARTHROPATHIES (See also Chap. 305)   The seronegative arthropathies, ankylosing spondylitis, Reiter's syndrome, psoriatic ar-

thritis, and the arthritides associated with ulcerative colitis and regional enteritis all may be accompanied by a pancarditis and proximal aortitis; the latter may result in aortic regurgitation and may extend into the anterior mitral valve ring and/or AV node. Conduction disturbances are common, occurring in up to one-third of patients; they are more common in patients with aortic valve disease and appear to be associated with the presence of the HLA-B27 antigen. Both aortic regurgitation and AV block are more common in patients with peripheral joint involvement and longstanding disease; treatment with aortic valve replacement and permanent pacemaker placement may be required. Up to one-fifth of patients with peripheral joint involvement and disease for more than 30 years have significant aortic regurgitation. Occasionally, aortic regurgitation precedes the onset of arthritis, and, therefore, the diagnosis of a seronegative arthritis should be considered in young males with isolated aortic regurgitation.

SYSTEMIC LUPUS ERYTHEMATOSUS (SLE) (See also Chap. 300)   Pericarditis is common, occurring in about two-thirds of patients, and generally follows a benign course, although rarely tamponade or constriction may result. The characteristic *endocardial lesions* of SLE, described by Libman and Sacks, consist of wartlike lesions most often located at the angles of the AV valves or on the ventricular surface of the mitral valve. Hemodynamically important valvular regurgitation is rare. Patients with the antiphospholipid syndrome have a higher incidence of cardiovascular abnormalities, including valvular disease (particularly regurgitant lesions), a variety of thrombotic disorders (venous and arterial thrombosis, thrombocytopenia, premature stroke), myocardial infarction, pulmonary hypertension, and cardiomyopathy. Myocarditis generally parallels the activity of the disease and, although common histologically, seldom results in clinical heart failure unless associated with hypertension. Although arteritis of large coronary arteries may rarely result in myocardial ischemia, there is also an increased frequency of coronary atherosclerosis that may be related to hypertension or glucocorticoid therapy.

TRAUMATIC CARDIAC INJURY

Traumatic cardiac damage may be due to either penetrating or nonpenetrating injuries. The most frequent cause of a *nonpenetrating injury* is the impact of the chest against the steering wheel of an automobile. The absence of external signs of thoracic trauma does not exclude serious injury of the heart. Although the most common injury is myocardial contusion, any structure of the heart may be affected by the trauma.

Myocardial contusions are often not immediately recognized in trauma patients due to focus on more obvious injuries. Myocardial contusion may cause arrhythmias, bundle branch block, or ECG abnormalities resembling those of infarction or pericarditis; hence, it is important to consider trauma as a cause of otherwise unexplained ECG changes. Serum creatine kinase (CK-MB) isoenzyme levels are increased in about 20% of patients, but false-positive elevations of MB may occur in the presence of massive injuries associated with large increases in total CK. Cardiac troponin levels may have a greater diagnostic value than CK-MB levels. Echocardiography can detect abnormal wall motion and the presence of pericardial effusion, in addition to aiding in diagnosis of other forms of cardiac trauma. Myocardial contusion may produce positive radionuclide scans and regional impairment of ventricular function, as occurs in myocardial infarction (Chap. 228). Pericardial effusion may occur weeks or even months after the accident. In these cases, the pericardial effusion is a manifestation of the postcardiac injury syndrome, which resembles the post-pericardiotomy syndrome (Chap. 222).

Rupture of the heart valves or the supporting structures leads to acute valvular incompetence. The presence of a loud heart murmur followed by the development of rapidly progressive heart failure after trauma heralds this diagnosis, which can be made by either transthoracic or transesophageal echocardiography.

The most serious consequence of nonpenetrating injury is myocardial rupture, leading to tamponade or intracardiac shunting. Although it is generally immediately fatal, up to 40% of patients with cardiac rupture have been reported to survive long enough to reach a specialized trauma center. Hemopericardium may also follow tearing of a pericardial vessel or coronary artery.

Rupture of the aorta is a common consequence of nonpenetrating chest trauma. Indeed, rupture of the aorta at the isthmus or just above the aortic valve is the most common vascular deceleration injury. The clinical presentation is similar to that of aortic dissection (Chap. 231). The arterial pressure and pulse amplitude may be increased in the upper extremities and decreased in the lower extremities, and on chest x-ray there may be widening of the mediastinum. Occasionally, aortic rupture is limited by the aortic adventitia and results in a silent false aneurysm that may be discovered months or years after the injury.

Penetrating injuries of the heart, produced by bullets or stab wounds, usually result in immediate or very rapid death because of hemopericardium or massive hemorrhage. However, up to half of such patients may survive if they are resuscitated and/or survive long enough to reach a specialized trauma center. Perforation complicating the placement of an intravenous intracardiac catheter or pacemaker lead is another common cause of penetrating injuries to the heart and great vessels.

When great vessel rupture is due to a penetrating injury, there is usually a hemothorax and, less often, a hemopericardium. Hematoma formation may compress major vessels, and AV fistulae may form, sometimes resulting in high-output congestive heart failure.

Patients who suffer penetrating injuries of the heart should be carefully examined several weeks after the event to rule out a ventricular septal defect or mitral regurgitation that may have gone undetected at the time of emergency surgery. Sometimes the patient survives the acute incident and presents with a cardiac murmur and congestive heart failure. A left-to-right shunt due to traumatic ventricular septal defect, aortopulmonary artery fistula, or coronary AV fistula may be suspected and confirmed by cardiac catheterization and angiocardiography.

Rx TREATMENT

The treatment of an uncomplicated myocardial contusion, with or without myocardial infarction, is similar to that for a myocardial infarction, except that anticoagulation is contraindicated, and should include monitoring for the development of complications such as arrhythmia and cardiac rupture (Chap. 228). Acute myocardial failure resulting from the rupture of a valve usually requires operative correction. Immediate thoracotomy should be carried out for most cases of penetrating injury, or if there is evidence of cardiac tamponade and/or shock regardless of the type of trauma. Pericardiocentesis may be helpful in patients with tamponade, but usually only as a temporizing maneuver on the way to the operating room. Pericardial hemorrhage often leads to constriction, which must be treated by decortication.

FURTHER READING

KENCHAIAH S et al: Obesity and the risk of heart failure. N Engl J Med 347: 305, 2002

KLEIN I, OJAMAA K: Thyroid hormone and the cardiovascular system. N Engl J Med 344:501, 2001

KLUKE MH, MAYER RJ: Carcinoid tumors. N Engl J Med 340:858, 1999

MATTOX KL: Traumatic heart disease, in *Braunwald's Heart Disease*, 7th ed, DP Zipes et al (eds). Philadelphia, Saunders, 2005

REYMAN K: Cardiac myxomas. N Engl J Med 333:1610, 1995

RHEE PM et al: Penetrating cardiac injuries: A population-based study. J Trauma 45:366, 1998

SABATINE M, SCHOEN F: Primary tumors of the heart, in *Braunwald's Heart Disease*, 7th ed, DP Zipes et al (eds). Philadelphia, Saunders, 2005

SOWERS JR: Diabetes mellitus and cardiovascular disease in women. Arch Intern Med 158:617, 1998

VAUGHAN CJ et al: Tumors and the heart: Molecular genetic advances. Curr Opin Cardiol 16:195, 2001

Section 4   Vascular Disease

224 THE PATHOGENESIS OF ATHEROSCLEROSIS
Peter Libby

Atherosclerosis is the leading cause of death and disability in the developed world. Despite our familiarity with this disease, some of its fundamental characteristics remain poorly recognized and understood. Although many generalized or systemic risk factors predispose to its development, atherosclerosis affects various regions of the circulation preferentially and yields distinct clinical manifestations depending on the particular circulatory bed affected. Atherosclerosis of the coronary arteries commonly causes myocardial infarction (Chap. 228) and angina pectoris (Chap. 226). Atherosclerosis of the arteries supplying the central nervous system frequently provokes strokes and transient cerebral ischemia (Chap. 349). In the peripheral circulation, atherosclerosis causes intermittent claudication and gangrene and can jeopardize limb viability. Involvement of the splanchnic circulation can cause mesenteric ischemia. Atherosclerosis can affect the kidneys either directly (e.g., renal artery stenosis) or as a frequent site of atheroembolic disease (Chap. 231).

Even within a given arterial bed, atherosclerosis tends to occur focally, typically in certain predisposed regions. In the coronary circulation, for example, the proximal left anterior descending coronary artery exhibits a particular predilection for developing atherosclerotic occlusive disease. Likewise, atherosclerosis preferentially affects the proximal portions of the renal arteries and, in the extracranial circulation to the brain, the carotid bifurcation. Indeed, atherosclerotic lesions often form at branching points of arteries, regions of disturbed blood flow. Not all manifestations of atherosclerosis result from stenotic, occlusive disease. Ectasia and development of aneurysmal disease, for example, frequently occur in the aorta (Chap. 231). The mechanisms that underlie this discontinuous anatomic distribution of atherosclerosis remain uncertain.

Atherosclerosis manifests itself focally not only in space, as just described, but in time as well. Atherogenesis in humans typically occurs over a period of many years, usually many decades. Growth of atherosclerotic plaques probably does not occur in a smooth linear fashion, but rather discontinuously, with periods of relative quiescence punctuated by periods of rapid evolution. After a generally prolonged "silent" period, atherosclerosis may become clinically manifest. The clinical expressions of atherosclerosis may be *chronic*, as in the development of stable, effort-induced angina pectoris or of predictable and reproducible intermittent claudication. Alternatively, a much more dramatic *acute* clinical event such as myocardial infarction, a cerebrovascular accident, or sudden cardiac death may first herald the presence of atherosclerosis. Other individuals may never experience clinical manifestations of arterial disease despite the presence of widespread atherosclerosis demonstrated post mortem.

INITIATION OF ATHEROSCLEROSIS

FATTY STREAK FORMATION An integrated view of experimental results in animals and study of human atherosclerosis suggests that the "fatty streak" represents the initial lesion of atherosclerosis. The formation of these early lesions of atherosclerosis most often seems to arise from focal increases in the content of lipoproteins within regions of the intima. This accumulation of lipoprotein particles may not result simply from an increased permeability, or "leakiness," of the overlying endothelium (Fig. 224-1). Rather, these lipoproteins may collect in the intima of arteries because they bind to constituents of the extracellular matrix, increasing the residence time of the lipid-rich particles within the arterial wall. Lipoproteins that accumulate in the extracellular space of the intima of arteries often associate with proteoglycan molecules of the arterial extracellular matrix, an interaction that may promote the retention of lipoprotein particles by binding them and slowing their egress from the intima.

Lipoprotein particles in the extracellular space of the intima, particularly those bound to matrix macromolecules, may undergo chem-

ical modifications. Accumulating evidence supports a pathogenic role for such modifications of lipoproteins in atherogenesis. Two types of such alterations in lipoproteins bear particular interest in the context of understanding how risk factors actually promote atherogenesis: oxidation and nonenzymatic glycation.

Lipoprotein Oxidation   Lipoproteins sequestered from plasma antioxidants in the extracellular space of the intima become susceptible to oxidative modification. Oxidatively modified low-density lipoprotein (LDL), rather than being a defined homogenous entity, actually comprises a variable and incompletely defined mixture. Both the lipid and protein moieties of these particles can participate in oxidative modification. Modifications of the lipids may include formation of hydroperoxides, lysophospholipids, oxysterols, and aldehydic breakdown products of fatty acids. Modifications of the apoprotein moieties may include breaks in the peptide backbone as well as derivatization of certain amino acid residues. A more recently recognized modification may result from local hypochlorous acid production by inflammatory cells within the plaque, giving rise to chlorinated species such as chlorotyrosyl moieties. Considerable evidence supports the presence of such oxidation products in atherosclerotic lesions.

Nonenzymatic Glycation   In diabetic patients with sustained hyperglycemia, nonenzymatic glycation of apolipoproteins and other arterial proteins likely occurs that may alter their function and propensity to accelerate atherogenesis. A good deal of experimental work suggests that both oxidatively modified and glycated lipoproteins or their constituents can contribute to many of the subsequent cellular events of lesion development.

LEUKOCYTE RECRUITMENT   After the accumulation of extracellular lipid, recruitment of leukocytes occurs as a second step in the formation of the fatty streak (Fig. 224-1). The white blood cell types typically found in the evolving atheroma include primarily cells of the mononuclear lineage: monocytes and lymphocytes. A number of adhesion molecules or receptors for leukocytes expressed on the surface of the arterial endothelial cell likely participate in the recruitment of leukocytes to the nascent fatty streak. Constituents of oxidatively modified LDL can augment expression of leukocyte adhesion molecules. This example illustrates how the accumulation of lipoproteins in the arterial intima may link mechanistically with leukocyte recruitment and subsequent events in lesion formation.

Laminar shear forces, such as those encountered in most regions of normal arteries, can also suppress the expression of leukocyte adhesion molecules. Sites of predilection for forming atherosclerotic lesions (e.g., branch points) often have disturbed laminar flow. Ordered laminar shear of normal blood flow augments the production of nitric oxide by endothelial cells. This molecule, in addition to its vasodilator properties, can act at the low levels constitutively produced by arterial endothelium as a local anti-inflammatory autacoid, for example, limiting local adhesion molecule expression. These examples indicate how hemodynamic forces may influence the cellular events that underlie atherosclerotic lesion initiation and provide a potential explanation for the focal distribution of atherosclerotic lesions at certain sites predetermined by altered flow patterns.

FIGURE 224-1   Cross-sectional view of an artery depicting steps in development of an atheroma, from left to right. The *upper panel* shows a detail of the boxed area below. The endothelial monolayer overlying the intima contacts blood. Hypercholesterolemia promotes accumulation of LDL particles (light spheres) in the intima. The lipoprotein particles often associate with constituents of the extracellular matrix, notably proteoglycans. Sequestration within the intima separates lipoproteins from some plasma antioxidants and favors oxidative modification. Such modified lipoprotein particles (darker spheres) may trigger a local inflammatory response responsible for signaling subsequent steps in lesion formation. The augmented expression of various adhesion molecules for leukocytes recruits monocytes to the site of a nascent arterial lesion.

Once adherent, some white blood cells will migrate into the intima. The directed migration of leukocytes probably depends on chemoattractant factors including modified lipoprotein particles themselves and chemoattractant cytokines depicted by the smaller spheres, such as the chemokine macrophage chemoattractant protein 1 produced by vascular wall cells in response to modified lipoproteins. Leukocytes in the evolving fatty streak can divide and exhibit augmented expression of receptors for modified lipoproteins (scavenger receptors). These mononuclear phagocytes ingest lipids and become foam cells, represented by a cytoplasm filled with lipid droplets. As the fatty streak evolves into a more complicated atherosclerotic lesion, smooth-muscle cells migrate from the media (*bottom of lower panel*), through the internal elastic membrane (*solid wavy line*), and accumulate within the expanding intima where they lay down extracellular matrix that forms the bulk of the advanced lesion (*bottom panel, right-hand side*).

Once adherent to the surface of the arterial endothelial cell via interaction with adhesion receptors, the monocytes and lymphocytes penetrate the endothelial layer and take up residence in the intima. In addition to products of modified lipoproteins, cytokines (a class of protein mediators of inflammation) can regulate the expression of adhesion molecules involved in leukocyte recruitment. For example, the cytokines interleukin 1 (IL-1) or tumor necrosis factor α (TNF-α) induce or augment the expression of leukocyte adhesion molecules on endothelial cells. Because modified lipoproteins can induce cytokine release from vascular wall cells, this pathway may provide an additional link between accumulation and modification of lipoproteins and leukocyte recruitment. The directed migration of leukocytes into the arterial wall may also result from the actions of modified lipoprotein. For example, oxidized LDL may promote the chemotaxis of leukocytes. Also, oxidatively modified lipoproteins can elicit the production by vascular wall cells of chemoattractant cytokines such as monocyte chemoattractant protein 1.

FOAM CELL FORMATION Once resident within the intima, the mononuclear phagocytes differentiate into macrophages and transform into lipid-laden foam cells. The conversion of mononuclear phagocytes into foam cells requires the uptake of lipoprotein particles by receptor-mediated endocytosis. One might suppose that the well-recognized "classical" receptor for LDL mediates this lipid uptake. Patients or animals lacking effective LDL receptors due to genetic alterations (e.g., familial hypercholesterolemia), however, have abundant arterial lesions and extraarterial xanthomata rich in macrophage-derived foam cells. Also, the exogenous cholesterol suppresses expression of the LDL receptor, such that under hypercholesterolemic conditions the level of this cell-surface receptor for LDL decreases. Candidates for alternative receptors that can mediate lipid-loading of foam cells include a growing number of macrophage "scavenger" receptors, which preferentially endocytose modified lipoproteins, and other receptors for oxidized LDL or β-VLDL (very low density lipoprotein), a type of lipoprotein commonly encountered in certain hypercholesterolemic states (Chap. 335). By ingesting lipids from the extracellular space, the mononuclear phagocytes bearing such scavenger receptors may remove lipoproteins from the developing lesion. Some lipid-loaded macrophages may leave the artery wall, functioning to clear lipid from the artery. Lipid accumulation, and hence propensity to form atheroma, ensues if the amount of lipid entering the artery wall exceeds that exported by mononuclear phagocytes or other pathways. Macrophages may thus play a vital role in the dynamic economy of lipid accumulation in the arterial wall during atherogenesis. Some lipid-laden foam cells within the expanding intimal lesion perish. Some foam cells may die as a result of programmed cell death known as *apoptosis*. This death of mononuclear phagocytes results in formation of the lipid-rich center, often called the *necrotic core*, of more complicated atherosclerotic plaques.

Macrophages taking up modified lipoproteins, much like intrinsic vascular wall cells, may elaborate cytokines and growth factors that can further signal some of the cellular events in lesion complication. A number of growth factors or cytokines elaborated by mononuclear phagocytes can stimulate smooth-muscle cell proliferation and production of extracellular matrix, which accumulates in atherosclerotic plaques. Cytokines found in the plaque, including IL-1 or TNF-α, can induce local production of growth factors such as forms of platelet-derived growth factor (PDGF), fibroblast growth factor, and others that may contribute to plaque evolution and complication. Other cytokines, notably interferon γ (IFN-γ) derived from activated T cells within lesions, can inhibit smooth-muscle proliferation and synthesis of interstitial forms of collagen. These examples illustrate how atherogenesis likely depends on a complex balance between mediators that can promote lesion formation and other pathways that can mitigate the atherogenic process.

FACTORS THAT MODULATE INHIBITION OF ATHEROMA

Elaboration of small molecules by activated mononuclear phagocytes and vascular wall cells in the evolving lesion may also modulate atherogenesis. Notably, reactive oxygen species can modulate growth of smooth-muscle cells, activate inflammatory gene expression via the nuclear factor kappa B (NFκB) transcriptional control system, and annihilate NO radicals, decreasing the effect of this endogenous vasodilator. However, the macrophage in the lesion may be activated to express the inducible form of the enzyme that can synthesize NO, known as inducible NO synthase. This high-capacity form of the enzyme can produce relatively large, potentially cytotoxic amounts of NO radicals. While at the low concentrations of NO produced by the constitutive NO synthase in endothelial cells, this radical may produce beneficial effects; when overproduced by activated phagocytes, however, it may prove deleterious.

Export by phagocytes may constitute one response to local lipid overload in the evolving lesion. Another mechanism, reverse cholesterol transport mediated by high-density lipoproteins (HDL), may provide an independent pathway for lipid removal from atheroma. This transfer of cholesterol from the cell to the HDL particle involves specialized cell surface molecules such as the ATP binding cassette transporter (ABCA1) (the gene mutated in Tangier disease, a condition characterized by very low HDL levels) and a family of scavenger receptors (the "B" family). Such "reverse cholesterol transport" explains part of HDL's antiatherogenic action.

Although clear evidence supports lipoprotein disorders as predisposing factors for atheroma formation, other etiologies may contribute to or modulate atherogenesis (see Table 225-1). For example, hypertension constitutes an independent risk factor for coronary events. Male gender and the postmenopausal state also augment the risk of developing coronary artery disease. Premenopausal women have increased HDL levels compared to age-matched men. However, a favorable lipoprotein pattern only partially accounts for the protection against atherosclerosis conferred by the premenopausal state. Although laboratory studies suggest that estrogens have direct beneficial effects on the arterial wall, clinical trials have not shown that estrogen replacement therapy prevents recurrent myocardial infarction in postmenopausal women. Indeed, treatment with a combination of estrogen and progesterone appears to augment cardiovascular events in women with or without prior myocardial infarction.

Diabetes mellitus aggravates atherogenesis. In addition to the well-known microvascular complications of diabetes (Chap. 323), macrovascular disease such as atherosclerosis causes a great deal of excess mortality in the diabetic population. Diabetes-associated dyslipidemias strongly promote atherogenesis. In particular, the constellation of insulin resistance, high triglycerides, and low HDL, often in association with the central adiposity and hypertension frequently seen in type 2 diabetic patients, seems to accelerate atherogenesis potently. As noted above, hyperglycemia may promote the nonenzymatic glycation of LDL. LDL modified in this manner, like oxidatively modified LDL, may signal many of the initial events in atherogenesis. Triglyceride-rich lipoprotein particles, often elevated in poorly controlled diabetic patients, also accentuate atherogenesis.

Lp(a) (often pronounced "lipoprotein little a" to distinguish it from apolipoprotein AI and others found in HDL) provides a potential link between hemostasis and blood lipids. The Lp(a) particle consists of an apoprotein (a) molecule bound by a sulfhydryl link to the apolipoprotein B moiety of an LDL particle. Apoprotein (a) has homology with plasminogen and may inhibit fibrinolysis by competing with plasminogen. Other risk factors for atherosclerosis related to blood clotting include elevated levels of fibrinogen or of the inhibitor of fibrinolysis, plasminogen-activator inhibitor 1 (PAI-1). Another nonlipid risk factor for coronary events, elevated levels of *homocysteine*, may act by promoting thrombosis, although the pathophysiology of this association is uncertain at present. Although individuals with marked elevations of Lp(a) or homocysteine do appear to have heightened risk of coronary thrombosis, in the population at large these factors show a much weaker correlation with vascular events than LDL, HDL, or the global inflammatory marker C-reactive protein (CRP).

The relationship between *tobacco use* and atherosclerosis also remains poorly understood. The rapid reduction in risk for cardiac events after cessation of cigarette smoking implies that tobacco may promote thrombosis or some other determinant of plaque stability as well as contribute to the evolution of the atherosclerotic lesion itself. For example, tobacco smokers have elevated fibrinogen levels, a variable associated with increased atherosclerosis and acute cardiovascular events.

INFLAMMATION In other situations, antecedent inflammatory states may predispose toward atherosclerosis. For example, *Kawasaki disease* in childhood may promote development of vascular lesions in the arteries of adults. Infectious agents continue to be proposed as instigators or potentiators of atherogenesis. However, in humans, an atherogenic role for viral or microbial pathogens (e.g., Herpesviridiae, including cytomegalovirus, or *Chlamydia*) remains speculative. In some patients, immune or autoimmune reactions may contribute to atherogenesis. In the particular example of the accelerated form of coronary arteriopathy that plagues heart transplant recipients, immunologic factors may contribute importantly to the pathogenesis.

Known monogenic defects in lipoprotein metabolism account for only a fraction of the familial risk for coronary artery disease. Thus, other as yet undefined and perhaps multiple genetic factors may contribute to coronary risk. Mechanisms of disease susceptibility involving the arterial wall might account for some of the genetic predisposition to atherosclerosis unexplained by lipoprotein disorders. Application of molecular genetic techniques may identify new polymorphisms linked to coronary risk and may eventually shed light on new pathophysiologic mechanisms. For example, some data suggest a link between certain alleles of the genes encoding angiotensin-converting enzyme, the cytokine lymphotoxin, or PAI-1 with increased risk of myocardial infarction. Application of genomic technologies may aid identification of "modifier" genes that modulate individual responses to established risk factors. Large studies currently in progress should clarify these and other potential genetic factors that influence atherosclerosis.

ATHEROMA EVOLUTION AND COMPLICATIONS

INVOLVEMENT OF ARTERIAL SMOOTH-MUSCLE CELLS Although the fatty streak commonly precedes the development of a more advanced atherosclerotic plaque, not all fatty streaks progress to form complex atheromas. Why do some fatty streaks progress to fibrous lesions while others do not? By what mechanisms do fatty streaks evolve into more complex lesions? While accumulation of lipid-laden macrophages is the hallmark of the fatty streaks, accumulation of fibrous tissue typifies the more advanced atherosclerotic lesion. The smooth-muscle cell synthesizes the bulk of the extracellular matrix of the complex atherosclerotic lesion. Hence, arrival of smooth-muscle cells and their elaboration of extracellular matrix probably provides a critical transition, yielding a fibrofatty lesion in place of a simple accumulation of macrophage-derived foam cells.

Recent research has provided insight into the mechanisms that may trigger migration and proliferation of smooth-muscle cells into and within the evolving intimal lesion and signal the accumulation of extracellular matrix. Cytokines and growth factors elicited by modified lipoproteins or other agents from both vascular wall cells and infiltrating leukocytes can modulate functions of the smooth-muscle cell (Fig. 224-1). For example, PDGF elaborated by activated endothelial cells can stimulate the migration of smooth-muscle cells. In this manner, smooth-muscle cells resident in the tunica media may migrate into the intima. Various growth factors produced locally can stimulate the proliferation of both resident smooth-muscle cells in the intima and those that have migrated from the media. Transforming growth factor β (TGF-β), among other mediators, potently stimulates interstitial collagen production by smooth-muscle cells. These mediators may arise not only from neighboring vascular cells or leukocytes (a "paracrine" pathway) but also, in some instances, from the same cell that responds to the factor (an "autocrine" pathway). Together, these alterations in smooth-muscle cells, signaled by these mediators acting at short distances, can hasten transformation of the fatty streak into a more fibrous smooth-muscle cell and extracellular matrix-rich lesion.

BLOOD COAGULATION In addition to locally produced mediators, atherogenic risk factor signals related to blood coagulation and thrombosis likely contribute to atheroma evolution and complication. Current evidence suggests that fatty streak formation begins underneath a morphologically intact endothelium. In advanced fatty streaks, however, microscopic breaches in endothelial integrity may occur. Microthrombi rich in platelets can form at such sites of limited endothelial denudation, due to exposure of the highly thrombogenic extracellular

matrix of underlying basement membrane. Activated platelets release numerous factors that can promote the fibrotic response. In addition to PDGF and TGF-β, low-molecular-weight mediators such as serotonin can also alter smooth-muscle function. Most of these microthrombi probably resolve without clinical manifestation by a process of local fibrinolysis, resorption, and endothelial repair.

MICROVESSELS As atherosclerotic lesions advance, abundant plexi of microvessels develop in connection with the artery's vasa vasorum. These newly developing microvascular networks may contribute to lesion complication in several ways. These blood vessels provide an abundant surface area for leukocyte trafficking and may serve as the portal of entry and exit of white blood cells from the established atheroma. The plaques' microvessels may also furnish foci for intraplaque hemorrhage. Like the neovessels in the diabetic retina, microvessels of the plaque may be friable and prone to rupture and produce focal hemorrhage. Such a vascular leak leads to thrombosis in situ and thrombin generation from prothrombin. In addition to its role in blood coagulation, thrombin can modulate many aspects of vascular cell function including stimulation of proliferation and cytokine release from smooth-muscle cells and production of growth factors such as PDGF from endothelial cells. Atherosclerotic plaques often contain fibrin and hemosiderin, indicating episodes of intraplaque hemorrhage as an element in plaque complication.

As they advance, atherosclerotic plaques also accumulate *calcium*. Proteins that are usually associated with bone also occur in atherosclerotic lesions. For example, osteocalcin, osteopontin, and bone morphogenetic proteins localize in atherosclerotic plaques. In fact, mineralization of the atherosclerotic plaque recapitulates many aspects of bone formation.

PLAQUE EVOLUTION Traditionally, atherosclerosis research has focused much attention on proliferation of smooth-muscle cells, yet these cells actually replicate rather slowly in complicated atherosclerotic lesions. Estimates of the rate of smooth-muscle cell division in such lesions at a given time show a replicative rate below 1%. Such observations do not exclude bursts of proliferative activity at certain junctures in the history of an atheroma, perhaps in association with local thrombin generation due to microvascular hemorrhage or formation of a microthrombus at a site of localized endothelial denudation, as discussed above. On the other hand, cell death has been recognized as a component of atherogenesis since the time of Virchow in the mid-nineteenth century. Indeed, complex atheroma often have a primarily fibrous character lacking the hypercellular appearance of less advanced lesions and actually exhibiting a paucity of smooth-muscle cells. This relative lack of smooth-muscle cells in advanced atheroma may result from the ultimate predominance of cytostatic mediators such as TGF-β or IFN-γ, which can inhibit smooth-muscle cell proliferation. Also, smooth-muscle cells as well as macrophages in advanced atherosclerotic lesions can undergo programmed cell death, or apoptosis. Some of the same cytokines that activate atherogenic functions of vascular wall cells can also trigger apoptosis in these cells.

Thus, during the evolution of the atherosclerotic plaque, a complex balance between entry and egress of lipoproteins and leukocytes, cell proliferation and cell death, extracellular matrix production and remodeling, as well as calcification and neovascularization contribute to lesion formation. Multiple and often competing signals trigger these various cellular events. Increasingly, we appreciate links between atherogenic risk factors and the altered behavior of intrinsic vascular wall cells and infiltrating leukocytes that underlie the complex pathogenesis of these lesions.

CLINICAL SYNDROMES OF ATHEROSCLEROSIS

Atherosclerotic lesions occur ubiquitously in Western societies. Most atheroma produce no symptoms, and many never cause clinical manifestations. Numerous patients with diffuse atherosclerosis may succumb to unrelated illnesses without ever having experienced a clinically significant manifestation of atherosclerosis. What accounts for this variability in the clinical expression of atherosclerotic disease?

FIGURE 224-2 Plaque rupture, thrombosis, and healing. *A.* Arterial remodeling during atherogenesis. During the initial part of the life history of an atheroma, growth is often outward, preserving the caliber of lumen. This phenomenon of "compensatory enlargement" accounts in part for the tendency of coronary arteriography to underestimate the degree of atherosclerosis. *B.* Rupture of the plaque's fibrous cap causes thrombosis. Physical disruption of the atherosclerotic plaque commonly causes arterial thrombosis by allowing blood coagulant factors to contact thrombogenic collagen found in the arterial extracellular matrix and tissue factor produced by macrophage-derived foam cells in the lipid core of lesions. In this manner, sites of plaque rupture form the nidus for thrombi. The normal artery wall possesses several fibrinolytic or antithrombotic mechanisms that tend to resist thrombosis and lyse clots that begin to form in situ. Such antithrombotic or thrombolytic molecules include thrombomodulin, tissue and urokinase-type plasminogen activators, heparan sulfate proteoglycans, prostacyclin, and nitric oxide. *C.* When the clot overwhelms the endogenous fibrinolytic mechanisms, it may propagate and lead to arterial occlusion. The consequences of this occlusion depend on the degree of existing collateral vessels. In a patient with chronic multivessel, occlusive coronary artery disease, collateral channels have often formed. In such circumstances, even a total arterial occlusion may not lead to myocardial infarction, or it may produce an unexpectedly modest or a non-ST segment elevation infarct because of collateral flow. In the patient with less advanced disease and without substantial stenotic lesions to provide a stimulus to collateral vessel formation, sudden plaque rupture and arterial occlusion commonly produces ST-segment elevation infarction. These are the types of patients who may present with myocardial infarction or sudden death as a first manifestation of coronary atherosclerosis. In some cases, the thrombus may lyse or organize into a mural thrombus without occluding the vessel. Such instances may be clinically silent. *D.* The subsequent thrombin-induced fibrosis and healing causes a fibroproliferative response that can lead to a more fibrous lesion, one that can produce an eccentric plaque that causes a hemodynamically significant stenosis. In this way, a nonocclusive mural thrombus, even if clinically silent or causing unstable angina rather than infarction, can provoke a healing response that can promote lesion fibrosis and luminal encroachment. Such a sequence of events may convert a "vulnerable" atheroma with a thin fibrous cap prone to rupture into a more "stable" fibrous plaque with a reinforced cap. Angioplasty of unstable coronary lesions may "stabilize" the lesions by a similar mechanism, producing a wound followed by healing.

Arterial remodeling during atheroma formation (Fig. 224-2*A*) represents a frequently overlooked but clinically important feature of lesion evolution. During the initial phases of atheroma development, the plaque usually grows outward, in an abluminal direction. Vessels affected by atherogenesis tend to increase in diameter, a phenomenon known as *compensatory enlargement*, a type of vascular remodeling. The growing atheroma does not encroach upon the arterial lumen until the burden of atherosclerotic plaque exceeds approximately 40% of the area encompassed by the internal elastic lamina. Thus, during much of its life history, an atheroma will not cause stenosis that can limit tissue perfusion.

Flow-limiting stenoses commonly form later in the history of the plaque. Many such plaques cause stable syndromes such as demand-induced angina pectoris or intermittent claudication in the extremities. In the coronary and other circulations, even occlusion due to atheroma does not invariably lead to infarction. The hypoxic stimulus of repeated bouts of ischemia characteristically induces formation of collateral vessels in the myocardium, mitigating the consequences of an acute occlusion of an epicardial coronary artery. On the other hand, we now appreciate that many lesions that cause acute or unstable atherosclerotic syndromes, particularly in the coronary circulation, may arise from atherosclerotic plaques that do not produce a flow-limiting stenosis. Such lesions may produce only minimal luminal irregularities on traditional angiograms and often do not meet the traditional criteria for "significance" by arteriography. Instability of such nonocclusive stenoses may explain the frequency of myocardial infarction as an initial manifestation of coronary artery disease (in at least a third of cases) in patients who report no prior history of angina pectoris, a syndrome usually caused by flow-limiting stenoses.

PLAQUE INSTABILITY AND RUPTURE Pathologic studies afford considerable insight into the microanatomic substrate underlying the "instability" of plaques that are not critically stenotic. A superficial erosion of the endothelium or a frank plaque rupture or fissure usually produces the thrombus that causes episodes of unstable angina pectoris or the occlusive and relatively persistent thrombus that causes acute myocardial infarction (Fig. 224-2*B*). In the case of carotid atheroma, a deeper ulceration that provides a nidus for formation of platelet thrombi may underlie the unstable syndromes that cause transient ischemic attacks.

Rupture of the plaque's fibrous cap (Fig. 224-2*C*) permits contact between coagulation factors in the blood with highly thrombogenic tissue factor expressed by macrophage foam cells in the plaque's lipid-rich core. If the ensuing thrombus is nonocclusive or transient, the episode of plaque disruption may not cause symptoms or may result in ischemic symptoms such as rest angina. Occlusive thrombi that endure will often cause acute myocardial infarction, particularly in the absence of a well-developed collateral circulation supplying the affected territory. Repetitive episodes of plaque disruption and healing provide one likely mechanism of transition of the fatty streak to a more complex fibrous lesion (Fig. 224-2*D*). The healing process in arteries, as in skin wounds, involves the laying down of new extracellular matrix and fibrosis.

Not all atheroma exhibit the same propensity to rupture. Pathologic studies of culprit lesions that have caused acute myocardial infarction reveal several characteristic features. Plaques that have proved vulnerable tend to have thin fibrous caps, relatively large lipid cores, and a high content of macrophages. Morphometric studies of such culprit lesions show that macrophages and T lymphocytes predominate at the site of plaque rupture. On the other hand, sites of plaque rupture contain relatively few smooth-muscle cells. The cells that concentrate at sites of plaque rupture bear markers of inflammatory activation. The presence of the transplantation, or histocompatibility, antigen HLA-DR provides one convenient gauge of the degree of inflammation in cells in atheroma. Resting cells in normal arteries seldom express this transplantation antigen. However, macrophages and smooth-muscle cells at sites of human coronary artery plaque disruption do bear this inducible cell-surface marker. Therefore, the presence of HLA-DR-positive macrophages and T cells indicates an ongoing inflammatory response at sites of plaque rupture.

Inflammatory mediators may actually regulate processes that govern the integrity of the plaque's fibrous cap and hence its propensity to rupture. For example, the T cell–derived cytokine IFN-γ, found in atherosclerotic plaques and required to induce the HLA-DR present at sites of rupture, can inhibit growth and collagen synthesis of smooth-muscle cells. Cytokines derived from activated macrophages such as TNF-α or IL-1 in addition to T cell–derived IFN-γ can elicit the expression of genes that encode proteolytic enzymes that can degrade the extracellular matrix of the plaque's fibrous cap. Thus, inflammatory mediators can impair collagen synthesis required for maintenance and repair of the fibrous cap and trigger degradation of extracellular matrix macromolecules, processes that weaken the plaque's fibrous cap and enhance its vulnerability to rupture. In contrast to vulnerable plaques, those with a dense extracellular matrix and relatively thick fibrous cap without substantial tissue factor-rich lipid cores seem generally resistant to rupture and unlikely to provoke thrombosis.

CONCLUSION

We now appreciate that features of the biology of the atheromatous plaque in addition to its degree of luminal encroachment influence the clinical manifestations of this disease. This enhanced understanding of plaque biology provides insight into the diverse ways in which atherosclerosis can present clinically and why the disease may remain silent or stable for prolonged periods, punctuated by acute complications at certain times. Increased understanding of atherogenesis provides new insight into the ways in which current therapies may improve outcomes and also suggests new targets for future intervention.

FURTHER READING

GLASS CK, WITZTUM JL: Atherosclerosis. The road ahead. Cell 104:503, 2001
LIBBY P: Current concepts of the pathogenesis of the acute coronary syndromes. Circulation 104:365, 2001
———— et al: Inflammation and atherosclerosis. Circulation 105:1135, 2002
LUSIS AJ: Atherosclerosis. Nature 407:233, 2000
VIRMANI R et al: Pathology of the unstable plaque. Prog Cardiovasc Dis 44: 349, 2002

225   PREVENTION AND TREATMENT OF ATHEROSCLEROSIS
Peter Libby

Atherosclerosis remains the major cause of death and premature disability in developed societies. Moreover, current predictions estimate that by the year 2020 cardiovascular diseases, notably atherosclerosis, will become the leading global cause of total disease burden, defined as the years subtracted from healthy life by disability or premature death. Substantial success has been achieved in recent years in reducing morbidity and mortality due to acute coronary events. However, the treatment of the underlying disease process, atherosclerosis, and preventing its acute complications presents an enormous challenge and opportunity simultaneously.

THE CONCEPT OF ATHEROSCLEROTIC RISK FACTORS

During the first half of the twentieth century, animal experiments and clinical observation linked certain variables, such as hypercholesterolemia, to the risk of atherosclerotic events. The systematic study of risk factors in humans, however, began approximately mid-century. The prospective, community-based Framingham Heart Study provided rigorous support for the concept that hypercholesterolemia, hypertension, and other factors correlated with cardiovascular risk. Similar observational studies performed in the United States and abroad provided independent support for the concept of "risk factors" for cardiovascular disease. Numerous data suggested a link between dietary habits and cardiovascular risk based upon population surveys.

From a practical viewpoint, the cardiovascular risk factors that have emerged from such studies fall into two categories: those modifiable by lifestyle and/or pharmacotherapy and those that are essentially unmodifiable. The weight of evidence supporting various risk factors differs. For example, hypercholesterolemia and hypertension certainly predict coronary risk, but other so-called nontraditional risk factors, such as levels of homocysteine, lipoprotein (a) [Lp(a)], or infection, remain controversial. One must further distinguish factors that actually participate in atherogenesis from those that may merely serve as markers of risk without direct involvement in pathogenesis. Table 225-1 lists the risk factors recognized by the current National Cholesterol Education Project Adult Treatment Panel III (ATP III). The sections below will consider some of these risk factors and approaches to their modification.

LIPID DISORDERS   Abnormalities in plasma lipoproteins and derangements in lipid metabolism rank as the most firmly established and best understood risk factors for atherosclerosis. Chap. 335 describes the lipoprotein classes and provides a detailed discussion of lipoprotein metabolism. Chap. 224 considers the mechanisms by which lipoproteins may influence atherogenesis. Therefore, this section will focus on preventive aspects of the treatment of lipid disorders.

Current ATP III guidelines recommend cholesterol screening in all adults >20 years. The screen should include a fasting lipid profile [total cholesterol, triglycerides, low-density lipoprotein (LDL) cholesterol, and high-density lipoprotein (HDL) cholesterol] repeated every 5 years. The ATP III guidelines strive to match the intensity of treatment to an individual's risk. A quantitative estimate of risk places individuals in one of three treatment strata (Table 225-2). The first step in applying these guidelines is to count an individual's risk factors (Table 225-1). Individuals with fewer than two risk factors fall into the lowest treatment intensity stratum [LDL goal <4.1 mmol/L (< 160 mg/dL)]. In those with two or more of these risk factors, the next step involves a simple calculation of an estimate of the 10-year risk of developing coronary heart disease (CHD) (Table 225-1); (see also *http://www.nhlbi.nih.gov/guidelines/cholesterol/* for the algorithm and a downloadable risk calculator). Those with a 10-year risk ≤ 20% fall into the intermediate stratum [LDL goal <3.4 mmol/L (< 130 mg/

TABLE 225-1   Major Risk Factors (Exclusive of LDL Cholesterol) That Modify LDL Goals

Cigarette smoking
Hypertension (BP ≥ 140/90 mmHg or on antihypertensive medication)
Low HDL cholesterol[a] [<1.0 mmol/L (<40 mg/dL)]
Diabetes mellitus
Family history of premature CHD
   CHD in male first-degree relative <55 years
   CHD in female first-degree relative <65 years
Age (men ≥45 years; women ≥55 years)
Lifestyle risk factors
   Obesity (BMI ≥ 30 kg/m²)
   Physical inactivity
   Atherogenic diet
Emerging risk factors
   Lipoprotein(a)
   Homocysteine
   Prothrombotic factors
   Proinflammatory factors
   Impaired fasting glucose
   Subclinical atherogenesis

[a] HDL cholesterol ≥1.6 mmol/L (≥60 mg/dL) counts as a "negative" risk factor; its presence removes one risk factor from the total count.
Note: LDL, low-density lipoprotein; BP, blood pressure; HDL, high-density lipoprotein; CHD, coronary heart disease; BMI, body-mass index.
Source: Modified from Expert Panel on Detection, Evaluation, and Treatment of High Blood Cholesterol in Adults (Adult Treatment Panel III). JAMA 285:2486, 2001.

dL)]. Those with a calculated 10-year CHD risk of > 20%, any evidence of established atherosclerosis, or diabetes (now considered a CHD risk-equivalent) fall into the most intensive treatment group [LDL goal <2.6 mmol/L (< 100 mg/dL)]. The first maneuver to achieve the LDL goal involves therapeutic lifestyle changes (TLC), including specific diet and exercise recommendations established by the guidelines. According to ATP III criteria, those with LDL levels exceeding goal for their risk group by >0.8 mmol/L (> 30 mg/dL) merit consideration for drug therapy. In patients with triglycerides >2.6 mmol/L (>200 mg/dL), ATP III guidelines specify a secondary goal for therapy, "non-HDL cholesterol" (simply the HDL cholesterol level subtracted from the total cholesterol). Cutpoints for therapeutic decision for non-HDL cholesterol are 0.8 mmol/L (30 mg/dL) more than those for LDL. A robust body of clinical trial evidence now supports the effectiveness of aggressive management of dyslipidemia. Addition of drug therapy to dietary and other nonpharmacologic measures reduces cardiovascular risk in patients with established coronary atherosclerosis and in individuals who have not previously suffered CHD events as well (Fig. 225-1). As guidelines inevitably lag the emerging clinical trial evidence base, the practitioner may elect to exercise clinical judgement in making therapeutic decisions in individual patients.

Lipid-lowering therapies do not appear to exert their beneficial effect on cardiovascular events by causing a marked "regression" of obstructive coronary lesions. Angiographically monitored studies of lipid lowering have shown at best a modest reduction in coronary artery stenoses over the duration of study. Yet these same studies consistently show substantial decreases in coronary events. These results suggest that the beneficial mechanism of lipid lowering does not require a substantial reduction in the fixed stenoses. Rather, the benefit may derive from "stabilization" of atherosclerotic lesions without decreased stenosis. Such stabilization of atherosclerotic lesions and the attendant decrease in coronary events may result from the egress of lipids or by favorably influencing aspects of the biology of atherogenesis discussed in Chap. 224. In addition, as sizeable lesions may protrude abluminally rather than into the lumen, shrinkage of such plaques might not be apparent on angiograms.

The benefit of LDL lowering by HMG-CoA reductase inhibitor (statin) therapy on cardiovascular events seems to require 6 to 24 months of treatment. Improvement of vasomotor responses to endothelial-dependent vasodilators occurs much more rapidly, requiring ≤6 months. Thus, HMG-CoA reductase inhibitors may act by two or more mechanisms on the arteries of hypercholesterolemic individuals. The relatively rapid improvement in endothelial-dependent vasomotion may reflect enhanced production or reduced destruction of the endogenous vasodilator nitric oxide at the level of the arterial endothelium. Reduction in the thrombotic complications of atherosclerosis, such as myocardial infarction or unstable angina, probably requires more prolonged treatment to effect removal of lipid from deeper within the atheroma, yielding improvements in the biology underlying plaque destabilization described in Chap. 224. In addition to their potent beneficial effects on the lipid profile, statins may have direct actions on the biology of the atheroma independent of lipid lowering.

In addition to statins, clinical trials have shown reductions in CHD events in certain populations with drugs that affect the lipoprotein profile, including fibric acid derivatives and nicotinic acid. New classes of lipid-lowering medications, including cholesterol absorption inhibitors, may prove useful adjuncts to current therapies; however, clinical trial evidence demonstrating benefits for CHD outcomes are not yet available.

Current understanding of the mechanism by which elevated LDL levels promote atherogenesis relates to oxidative modification of these particles within the artery wall, promoting formation of macrophage-derived foam cells and providing a stimulus for inflammation (Chap. 224). These concepts stimulated interest in the possibility that anti-

oxidants, either dietary or pharmacologic, might reduce CHD events. Both experimental and observational clinical studies supported this notion. However, rigorous and well-controlled clinical trials have consistently shown that antioxidant vitamin therapy does *not* improve CHD outcomes. Therefore, the current evidence base does *not* support the use of antioxidant vitamins for this indication.

HYPERTENSION (See also Chap. 230)   A wealth of epidemiologic data support a relationship between hypertension and atherosclerotic risk, and extensive clinical trial evidence has established that pharmacologic treatment of hypertension can reduce the risk of stroke and heart failure. More recent studies also show a reduction in CHD risk by antihypertensive therapy, particularly interruption of the renin-angiotensin system.

DIABETES MELLITUS, INSULIN RESISTANCE, AND THE METABOLIC SYNDROME (See also Chap. 323)   Diabetes mellitus is a CHD risk equivalent; most patients with diabetes mellitus die of atherosclerosis and its complications. Aging and rampant obesity in the U.S. population underlie a current epidemic of type 2 (non-insulin-dependent) diabetes mellitus. The abnormal lipoprotein profile associated with insulin resistance, known as *diabetic dyslipidemia*, accounts for part of the elevated cardiovascular risk in patients with type 2 diabetes. While diabetic patients often have LDL cholesterol levels near average, the LDL particles tend to be smaller and denser and thus more atherogenic (Chap. 335). Other features of diabetic dyslipidemia include low HDL and elevated triglyceride levels. Hypertension also frequently accompanies

TABLE 225-2 *LDL Cholesterol Goals and Cutpoints for Therapeutic Lifestyle Changes (TLC) and Drug Therapy in Different Risk Categories*

Risk Category	LDL Goal, mmol/L (mg/dL)	LDL Level at which to Initiate TLC, mmol/L (mg/dL)	LDL Level at which to Consider Drug Therapy, mmol/L (mg/dL)
CHD or CHD risk equivalents[a] (10-year risk >20%)	<2.6 (<100)	≥2.6 (≥100)	≥3.4 (≥130) [drug optional between 2.6 and 3.3 (100 and 129)]
2+ Risk factors (10-year risk ≤20%)	<3.4 (<130)	≥3.4 (≥130)	10-Year risk 10–20%: ≥3.4 (≥130) 10-Year risk 10%: ≥4.1 (≥160)
0–2 Risk factors	<4.1 (<160)	≥4.1 (≥160)	≥4.9 (≥190) [drug optional between 4.1 and 4.9 (160 and 189)]

[a] Diabetes mellitus is a CHD risk equivalent.
Note: LDL, low-density lipoprotein; CHD, coronary heart disease.

FIGURE 225-1   Lipid lowering reduces coronary events, as reflected on this graph showing the reduction percentages for onset of the acute coronary syndromes achieved by participants in six major clinical studies. 4S, Scandinavian Simvastatin Survival Study (patients with coronary heart disease and elevated cholesterol); CARE, Cholesterol and Recurrent Events (patients with coronary heart disease and average cholesterol); LIPID, Long-Term Intervention with Pravastatin in Ischemic Disease (patients with coronary heart disease and average cholesterol); WOSCOPS, West of Scotland Coronary Prevention Study (normal patients with elevated cholesterol); AFCAPS/TexCAPS, Air Force Coronary Atherosclerosis Prevention Study/Texas Coronary Atherosclerosis Prevention Study (normal patients with average cholesterol); HPS, Heart Protection Study (patients with coronary heart disease, or at high risk, with a wide range of cholesterol).

obesity, insulin resistance, and dyslipidemia. Indeed, the ATP III guidelines now recognize this cluster of risk factors and provide criteria for diagnosis of the "metabolic syndrome" (Table 225-3).

Therapeutic objectives for intervention in these patients include addressing the underlying causes, including obesity and low physical activity, by initiating TLC. The ATP III guidelines provide an explicit step-by-step plan for implementing TLC. Treatment of the component risk factors should accompany TLC. Establishing that strict glycemic control reduces the risk of macrovascular complications of diabetes has proved much more elusive than the established beneficial effects on microvascular complications such as retinopathy or renal disease. In the absence of clear-cut evidence that tight glycemic control reduces coronary risk in diabetic patients, attention to other aspects of risk in this patient population assumes even greater importance. In this regard, multiple clinical trials have demonstrated unequivocal benefit of HMG-CoA reductase inhibitor therapy in diabetic patients over all ranges of LDL cholesterol levels. The Veterans Affairs HDL Intervention Trial showed that gemfibrozil, a fibric acid derivative, reduced CHD and stroke in a population of men, many of whom had features of the metabolic syndrome. Diabetic populations appear to derive particular benefit from antihypertensive strategies that block the action of angiotensin II. Thus, the antihypertensive regimen for patients with the metabolic syndrome should include angiotensin-converting enzyme inhibitors or angiotensin receptor blockers when possible. Most of these individuals will require more than one antihypertensive agent to achieve the current American Diabetes Association blood pressure goal of 130/85 mmHg.

MALE GENDER/POSTMENOPAUSAL STATE Decades of observational studies have verified excess coronary risk in men compared with premenopausal women. After menopause, however, coronary risk accelerates in women. At least part of the apparent protection against CHD in premenopausal women derives from their relatively higher HDL levels compared with those of men. After menopause, HDL values fall in concert with increased coronary risk. Estrogen therapy lowers LDL cholesterol and raises HDL cholesterol, changes that should decrease coronary risk.

Multiple observational and experimental studies suggested that estrogen therapy (ET) might reduce coronary risk. However, several recent clinical trials have failed to demonstrate a net benefit of estrogen when combined with progestin on CHD outcomes. In the Heart and Estrogen/Progestin Replacement Study, postmenopausal female survivors of acute myocardial infarction were randomized to an estrogen/progestin combination or to placebo. This study showed no overall reduction in recurrent coronary events in the active treatment arm. Indeed, early in the 5-year course of this trial, there was a trend toward an actual increase in vascular events in the treated women. Extended follow-up of this cohort did not disclose an accrual of benefit in the treatment group. The Women's Health Initiative (WHI) study arm using a similar ET plus progesterone regimen was halted because of a small but significant hazard of cardiovascular events, stroke, and breast cancer. The excess cardiovascular events may result from an increase in thromboembolism (Chap. 327).

These clinical trials do not exclude a potential CHD benefit of estrogen alone or selective estrogen receptor modulator regimens; the estrogen *without progestin* arm of the WHI continues and should prove informative in this regard. Physicians should work with women to provide information and help weigh the small but evident CHD risk of estrogen/progestin vs. the benefits on postmenopausal symptoms and osteoporosis, taking personal preferences into account. The current disappointment surrounding estrogen/progestin therapy as a means of reducing cardiovascular risk highlights the need for redoubled attention to known modifiable risk factors in women. In the recent clinical trials with HMG-CoA reductase inhibitors, women, when included, have derived benefits at least commensurate with those seen in men.

DYSREGULATED COAGULATION OR FIBRINOLYSIS Thrombosis ultimately causes the gravest complications of atherosclerosis. The propensity to form thrombi and/or to lyse clots once they form clearly influences the manifestations of atherosclerosis. Thrombosis provoked by atheroma rupture and subsequent healing may promote plaque growth (Chap. 224). Certain individual characteristics can influence thrombosis or fibrinolysis and have received attention as potential coronary risk factors. For example, fibrinogen levels correlate with coronary risk and provide information regarding coronary risk independent of the lipoprotein profile. Elevated fibrinogen levels might promote a thrombotic diathesis. Alternatively, fibrinogen, an acute-phase reactant, may serve as a marker of inflammation rather than directly participating in the pathogenesis of coronary events.

The stability of an arterial thrombus depends on the balance between fibrinolytic factors, such as plasmin, and inhibitors of the fibrinolytic system, such as plasminogen activator inhibitor (PAI) 1. However, the levels of tissue plasminogen activator and PAI-1 in plasma have not proven to add information beyond the lipid profile to assessment of cardiovascular risk. Lp(a) (Chap. 335) may modulate fibrinolysis, and although individuals with elevated Lp(a) levels have increased CHD risk, Lp(a) levels do not potently predict risk in the population at large.

Aspirin reduces CHD events in several contexts. Chap. 226 discusses aspirin therapy in stable ischemic heart disease, Chap. 227 reviews recommendations for aspirin treatment in acute coronary syndromes, and Chap. 349 describes aspirin's role in preventing recurrent ischemic stroke. In primary prevention, pooled trial data show that low-dose aspirin treatment (81 mg qd to 325 mg qod) can reduce risk of first myocardial infarction in men. Individuals with CHD risk factors, and especially men > 45 years old, should take aspirin in the absence of contraindications.

HOMOCYSTEINE A large body of literature suggests a relationship between hyperhomocysteinemia and coronary events. Several mutations in the enzymes involved in homocysteine accumulation correlate with thrombosis and, in some studies, coronary risk. Prospective studies have not shown a robust utility of hyperhomocysteinemia in CHD risk stratification, and there are no clinical trial data showing that intervention to lower homocysteine levels reduces CHD events. Fortification of the U.S. diet with folic acid to reduce neural tube defects has lowered homocysteine levels in the population at large. Measurement of homocysteine levels should be reserved for individuals with atherosclerosis at a young age or out of proportion to established risk factors. Physicians who advise consumption of supplements containing folic acid should consider that this treatment might mask pernicious anemia.

INFLAMMATION/INFECTION An accumulation of clinical evidence shows that markers of inflammation correlate with coronary risk. For example, variations of plasma levels of C-reactive protein (CRP), as mea-

TABLE 225-3 *Clinical Identification of the Metabolic Syndrome—Any Three Risk Factors*

Risk Factor	Defining Level
Abdominal obesity[a]	
Men (waist circumference)[b]	>102 cm (>40 in.)
Women	>88 cm (>35 in.)
Triglycerides	>1.7 mmol/L (>150 mg/dL)
HDL cholesterol	
Men	<1.0 mmol/L (<40 mg/dL)
Women	<1.3 mmol/L (<50 mg/dL)
Blood pressure	≥130/≥85 mmHg
Fasting glucose	>6.1 mmol/L (>110 mg/dL)

[a] Overweight and obesity are associated with insulin resistance and the metabolic syndrome. However, the presence of abdominal obesity is more highly correlated with the metabolic risk factors than is an elevated body-mass index (BMI). Therefore, the simple measure of waist circumference is recommended to identify the BMI component of the metabolic syndrome.

[b] Some male patients can develop multiple metabolic risk factors when the waist circumference is only marginally increased, e.g., 94–102 cm (37–39 in.). Such patients may have a strong genetic contribution to insulin resistance. They should benefit from lifestyle changes, similarly to men with categorical increases in waist circumference.

sured by a high-sensitivity assay, can prospectively predict risk of myocardial infarction. CRP levels also correlate with outcome of patients with acute coronary syndromes. In contrast to several other novel risk factors, CRP adds predictive information to that derived from established risk factors such as cholesterol (Fig. 225-2). Elevated levels of the acute-phase reactant CRP may merely reflect ongoing inflammation rather than a direct etiologic role for CRP in coronary artery disease. Elevations in acute-phase reactants such as fibrinogen or CRP could reflect overall atherosclerotic burden and/or extravascular inflammation that could potentiate atherosclerosis or its complications. In all likelihood, both factors contribute to elevation of inflammatory markers in patients at risk for coronary events. Indeed, lipid-lowering therapy may reduce coronary events in part by reducing the inflammatory aspects of the pathogenesis of atherosclerosis.

One source of inflammatory stimulus could arise from infectious agents. Interest has resurged in the possibility that infections may cause or contribute to atherosclerosis. A spate of recent publications has furnished evidence that supports a role of *Chlamydia pneumoniae*, cytomegalovirus, or other infectious agents in atherosclerosis and restenosis following coronary intervention. Some microorganisms exist in human atherosclerotic plaques. However, prospective and well-controlled seroepidemiologic studies show little or no association between infection with various agents and atherosclerosis. At present no sufficiently powered clinical trial supports the use of antibiotics to reduce CHD risk.

LIFESTYLE MODIFICATION The prevention of atherosclerosis presents a long-term challenge to all health care professionals and for public health policy as well. Both individual practitioners and organizations providing health care should strive to help patients optimize their risk factor profile long before atherosclerotic disease becomes manifest. The care plan for all patients seen by internists should include measures to assess and minimize cardiovascular risk. Physicians must counsel patients regarding the health risks of tobacco use and provide guidance regarding smoking cessation. Likewise, physicians should advise all patients about prudent dietary and exercise habits for maintaining ideal body weight. The recent National Institutes of Health Consensus Panel on Physical Activity and Cardiovascular Health established a goal of accumulating at least 30 min of moderate-intensity physical activity on a daily basis. Obesity, particularly the male pattern of centripetal or visceral fat accumulation, can contribute to the elements of the metabolic syndrome (Table 225-3). Physicians should encourage their patients to take responsibility for behavior related to modifiable risk factors for development of premature atherosclerotic disease. Conscientious counseling and patient education may forestall the need for pharmacologic measures intended to reduce coronary risk.

ISSUES IN RISK ASSESSMENT A growing panel of markers of coronary risk presents a perplexing array to the practitioner. Markers measured in peripheral blood include size fractions of LDL particles and concentrations of homocysteine, Lp(a), fibrinogen, CRP, and PAI-1

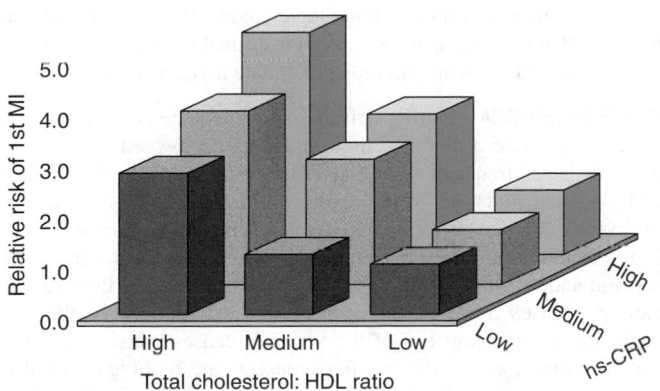

FIGURE 225-2 Measurement of C-reactive protein (CRP) level adds predictive value to TC:HDL ratio in determining risk of first MI among apparently healthy men. TC, total cholesterol; HDL, high-density lipoprotein; MI, myocardial infarction; hs-CRP, high-sensitivity measurement of CRP. (*Adapted from PM Ridker et al: Circulation 97:2007, 1998*).

among others. In general, such specialized tests add little to the information available from a careful history and physical examination combined with measurement of a plasma lipoprotein profile and fasting blood sugar. The high-sensitivity CRP measurement may well prove an exception in view of its robustness in risk prediction, its ease of reproducible and standardized measurement, its relative stability in individuals over time, and, most importantly, its ability to add to the risk information disclosed by standard measurements such as the lipid profile. Given the utility of high-sensitivity CRP measurement in predicting a gamut of important cardiovascular outcomes, this simple blood test may prove useful in the future in guiding therapy, particularly in primary prevention. Current guidelines, however, recommend the use of this test only in individuals with intermediate risk of a CHD event (10–20%, 10-year risk).

Similar concerns pertain to the use of specialized radiographic estimations of coronary artery calcification. Accumulating information indicates that the amount of calcium determined by such techniques as electron beam computed tomography correlates with coronary risk. However, the utility of using such estimates of coronary artery calcium content as a guide to therapy remains unproven, particularly in asymptomatic individuals. Inappropriate use of such imaging modalities might promote excessive invasive diagnostic and therapeutic procedures. Widespread application of such modalities for screening should await proof that clinical benefit derives from their application.

THE CHALLENGE OF IMPLEMENTATION: CHANGING PHYSICIAN AND PATIENT BEHAVIOR

Despite declining age-adjusted rates of coronary death, cardiovascular mortality is on the rise due to the aging of the population overall. There is a powerful global trend toward increased atherosclerotic disease. Enormous challenges remain regarding translation of the current evidence base into practice. We must learn how to help individuals adopt a healthy lifestyle and learn to deploy our increasingly powerful pharmacologic tools most economically and effectively. The obstacles to implementation of current evidence-based prevention and treatment of atherosclerosis include economics, education, physician awareness, and patient adherence to recommended regimens. Future goals in the field of treatment of atherosclerosis should include application of the current knowledge regarding risk-factor management and, when appropriate, drug therapy.

FURTHER READING

BECKMAN JA et al: Diabetes and atherosclerosis: Epidemiology, pathophysiology, and management. JAMA 287:2570, 2002

GAZIANO JM et al: Primary and secondary prevention of coronary heart disease, in *Braunwald's Heart Disease: A Textbook of Cardiovascular Medicine*. 7th ed, D Zipes et al (eds). Philadelphia, Saunders, 2005

GRADY D et al: Cardiovascular disease outcomes during 6.8 years of hormone therapy: Heart and Estrogen/Progestin Replacement Study follow-up (HERS II). JAMA 288:49, 2002

MRC/BHF HEART PROTECTION STUDY OF ANTIOXIDANT VITAMIN SUPPLEMENTATION IN 20,536 HIGH-RISK INDIVIDUALS: A randomised placebo-controlled trial. Lancet 360:23, 2002

THE NATIONAL CHOLESTEROL EDUCATION PROGRAM: Executive summary of the third report of the NCEP expert panel on detection, evaluation, and treatment of high blood cholesterol in adults (Adult Treatment Panel). JAMA 285:2486, 2001

PEARSON TA et al: Markers of inflammation and cardiovascular disease: Application to clinical and public health practice. A statement for healthcare professionals from the Centers for Disease Control and Prevention and The American Heart Association. Circulation 107:499, 2003

RIDKER PM: Role of inflammatory biomarkers in prediction of coronary heart disease. Lancet 358:946, 2001

WOMEN'S HEALTH INITIATIVE RANDOMIZED CONTROLLED TRIAL: Principal results on the risks and benefits of estrogen plus progestin in healthy postmenopausal women. JAMA 288:321, 2002

YUSUF S et al: Effects of an angiotensin-converting-enzyme inhibitor, ramipril, on cardiovascular events in high-risk patients. The Heart Outcomes Prevention Evaluation Study Investigators. N Engl J Med 342:145, 2000

Ischemia refers to a lack of oxygen due to inadequate perfusion of the myocardium, which causes an imbalance between oxygen supply and demand. The most common cause of myocardial ischemia is obstructive atherosclerotic disease of epicardial coronary arteries.

EPIDEMIOLOGY Ischemic heart disease (IHD) causes more deaths and disability and incurs greater economic costs than any other illness in the developed world. IHD is the most common, serious, chronic, life-threatening illness in the United States, where >12 million persons have IHD, >6 millon have angina pectoris, and >7 million have sustained a myocardial infarction. A high-fat and energy-rich diet, smoking, and a sedentary life-style are associated with the emergence of IHD (Chap. 225). In the United States and western Europe, it is growing amongst the poor rather than the rich (who are adopting more healthful life-styles), while primary prevention has delayed the disease to later in life in all socioeconomic groups. Obesity, insulin resistance, and type 2 diabetes mellitus are increasing and are powerful risk factors for IHD. With urbanization in the developing world, the prevalence of risk factors for IHD is increasing rapidly in these regions. Large increases in IHD throughout the world are projected, and IHD is likely to become the most common cause of death worldwide by 2020.

PATHOPHYSIOLOGY Although the large epicardial coronary arteries are capable of constriction and relaxation, in healthy persons they serve as conduits and are referred to as *conductance vessels*, while the intramyocardial arterioles normally exhibit changes in tone and are therefore referred to as *resistance vessels*. Abnormal constriction of the conductance vessels can cause severe ischemia in Prinzmetal's angina (Chap. 227). Abnormal constriction or failure of normal dilation of the coronary resistance vessels can also cause ischemia. When it causes angina this condition is referred to as *microvascular angina*.

The normal coronary circulation is dominated and controlled by the heart's requirements for oxygen. This need is met by the ability of the coronary vascular bed to vary its resistance (and therefore blood flow) considerably while the myocardium extracts a high and relatively fixed percentage of oxygen. Normally, intramyocardial resistance vessels demonstrate an immense capacity for dilation. For example, the changing oxygen needs of the heart with exercise and emotional stress affect coronary vascular resistance and in this manner regulate the supply of oxygen and substrate to the myocardium (*metabolic regulation*). The coronary resistance vessels also adapt to physiologic alterations in blood pressure in order to maintain coronary blood flow at levels appropriate to myocardial needs (*autoregulation*).

By reducing the lumen of the coronary arteries, atherosclerosis limits appropriate increases in perfusion when the demand for flow is augmented, as occurs during exertion or excitement. When the luminal reduction is severe, myocardial perfusion in the basal state is reduced. Coronary blood flow can also be limited by spasm, arterial thrombi, and, rarely, coronary emboli as well as by ostial narrowing due to luetic aortitis. Congenital abnormalities, such as origin of the left anterior descending coronary artery from the pulmonary artery, may cause myocardial ischemia and infarction in infancy, but this cause is very rare in adults. Myocardial ischemia can also occur if myocardial oxygen demands are markedly increased, and when coronary blood flow may be limited, as occurs in severe left ventricular hypertrophy due to aortic stenosis. The latter can present with angina that is indistinguishable from that caused by coronary atherosclerosis (Chap. 219). A reduction in the oxygen-carrying capacity of the blood, as in extremely severe anemia or in the presence of carboxyhemoglobin, rarely causes myocardial ischemia by itself but it may lower the threshold for ischemia in patients with moderate coronary obstruction. Not infrequently, two or more causes of ischemia coexist, such as an increase in oxygen demand due to left ventricular hypertrophy secondary to hypertension and a reduction in oxygen supply secondary to coronary atherosclerosis and anemia.

CORONARY ATHEROSCLEROSIS Epicardial coronary arteries are the major site of atherosclerotic disease. The major risk factors for atherosclerosis [high plasma low-density lipoprotein (LDL), low plasma high-density lipoprotein (HDL), cigarette smoking, hypertension, and diabetes mellitus (Chaps. 224 and 225)] disturb the normal functions of the vascular endothelium. These functions include local control of vascular tone, maintenance of an anticoagulant surface, and defense against inflammatory cells. The loss of these defenses leads to inappropriate constriction, luminal clot formation, and abnormal interactions with blood monocytes and platelets. The latter results in the subintimal collections of fat, smooth-muscle cells, fibroblasts, and intercellular matrix (i.e., atherosclerotic plaques), which develop at irregular rates in different segments of the epicardial coronary tree and lead eventually to segmental reductions in cross-sectional area. When a stenosis reduces the cross-sectional area by ~75%, a full range of increases in flow to meet increased myocardial demand is not possible. When the luminal area is reduced by ≥80%, blood flow at rest may be reduced, and further minor decreases in the stenotic orifice can reduce coronary flow dramatically and cause myocardial ischemia.

Segmental atherosclerotic narrowing of epicardial coronary arteries is caused most commonly by the formation of a plaque, which is subject to fissuring, erosion, hemorrhage, and thrombosis. Any of these events can temporarily worsen the obstruction, reduce coronary blood flow, and cause clinical manifestations of myocardial ischemia, as described below. The location of the obstruction influences the quantity of myocardium rendered ischemic and determines the severity of the clinical manifestations. Thus, critical obstructions in vessels such as the left main coronary artery or the proximal left anterior descending coronary artery are particularly hazardous. Severe coronary narrowing and myocardial ischemia are frequently accompanied by the development of collateral vessels, especially when the narrowing develops gradually. When well developed, such vessels can, by themselves, provide sufficient blood flow to sustain the viability of the myocardium at rest but not during conditions of increased demand.

Once stenosis of a proximal epicardial artery has reduced the cross-sectional area by ≥70%, the distal resistance vessels (when they function normally) dilate to reduce vascular resistance and maintain coronary blood flow. A pressure gradient develops across the proximal stenosis, and poststenotic pressure falls. When the resistance vessels are maximally dilated, myocardial blood flow becomes dependent on the pressure in the coronary artery distal to the obstruction. In these circumstances ischemia, manifest clinically by angina or electrocardiographically by ST-segment depression, can be precipitated by increases in myocardial oxygen demands caused by physical activity, emotional stress, and/or tachycardia. Changes in the caliber of the stenosed coronary artery due to physiologic vasomotion, loss of endothelial control of dilation, pathologic spasm (Prinzmetal's angina), or small platelet plugs can also upset the critical balance between oxygen supply and demand and thus precipitate myocardial ischemia.

EFFECTS OF ISCHEMIA During episodes of inadequate perfusion caused by coronary atherosclerosis, myocardial tissue oxygen tension falls and may cause transient disturbances of the mechanical, biochemical, and electrical functions of the myocardium. The abrupt development of severe ischemia, as occurs with total or subtotal coronary occlusion, is associated with almost instantaneous failure of normal muscle contraction and relaxation. The relatively poor perfusion of the subendocardium causes more intense ischemia of this portion of the wall. Ischemia of large portions of the ventricle causes transient left ventricular failure, and if the papillary muscles are involved, mitral regurgitation can complicate this event. When ischemia is transient, it may be associated with angina pectoris; when it is prolonged, it can lead to myocardial necrosis and scarring with or without the clinical picture of acute myocardial infarction (Chap. 228). Coronary atherosclerosis is a focal process that usually causes nonuniform ischemia.

Regional disturbances of ventricular contractility cause segmental akinesis or, in severe cases, bulging (dyskinesia), which can greatly reduce myocardial pump function.

A wide range of abnormalities in cell metabolism, function, and structure underlie these mechanical disturbances during ischemia. The normal myocardium metabolizes fatty acids and glucose to carbon dioxide and water. With severe oxygen deprivation, fatty acids cannot be oxidized, and glucose is broken down to lactate; intracellular pH is reduced, as are the myocardial stores of high-energy phosphates, i.e., ATP and creatine phosphate. Impaired cell membrane function leads to the leakage of potassium and the uptake of sodium by myocytes. The severity and duration of the imbalance between myocardial oxygen supply and demand determine whether the damage is reversible ($\leq$20 min for total occlusion in the absence of collaterals) or whether it is permanent, with subsequent myocardial necrosis (>20 min).

Ischemia also causes characteristic changes in the electrocardiogram (ECG) such as repolarization abnormalities, as evidenced by inversion of T waves and, when more severe, by displacement of ST segments (Chap. 210). Transient ST-segment depression often reflects subendocardial ischemia, while ST-segment elevation is thought to be caused by more severe transmural ischemia. Another important consequence of myocardial ischemia is electrical instability, which may lead to ventricular tachycardia or ventricular fibrillation (Chap. 214). Most patients who die suddenly from IHD do so as a result of ischemia-induced ventricular tachyarrhythmias (Chap. 256).

ASYMPTOMATIC VERSUS SYMPTOMATIC IHD Postmortem studies on accident victims and military casualties in western countries have shown that coronary atherosclerosis often begins to develop prior to age 20 and is widespread even among adults who were asymptomatic during life. Exercise stress tests in asymptomatic persons may show evidence of silent myocardial ischemia, i.e., exercise-induced ECG changes not accompanied by angina pectoris; coronary angiographic studies of such persons may reveal coronary artery obstruction (Chap. 212)]. Postmortem examination of patients with such obstruction without a history of clinical manifestations of myocardial ischemia often shows macroscopic scars secondary to myocardial infarction in regions supplied by diseased coronary arteries. According to population studies, ~25% of patients who survive acute myocardial infarction may not reach medical attention, and these patients carry the same adverse prognosis as those who present with the classic clinical syndrome (Chap. 228). Sudden death may be unheralded and is a common presenting manifestation of IHD (Chap. 256). Patients with IHD can also present with cardiomegaly and heart failure secondary to ischemic damage of the left ventricular myocardium that may have caused no symptoms prior to the development of heart failure; this condition is referred to as *ischemic cardiomyopathy*. In contrast to the asymptomatic phase of IHD, the symptomatic phase is characterized by chest discomfort due to either angina pectoris or acute myocardial infarction (Chap. 228). Having entered the symptomatic phase, the patient may exhibit a stable or progressive course, revert to the asymptomatic stage, or suddenly die.

STABLE ANGINA PECTORIS

This episodic clinical syndrome is due to transient myocardial ischemia. Various diseases that cause myocardial ischemia as well as the numerous forms of discomfort with which it may be confused are discussed in Chap. 12. Males constitute ~70% of all patients with angina pectoris and an even greater fraction of those <50 years.

HISTORY The typical patient with angina is a man >50 years or a woman >60 years who complains of chest discomfort, usually described as heaviness, pressure, squeezing, smothering, or choking and only rarely as frank pain. When the patient is asked to localize the sensation, he or she will typically press on the sternum, sometimes with a clenched fist, to indicate a squeezing, central, substernal discomfort (Levine's sign). Angina is usually crescendo-decrescendo in nature, typically lasts 2 to 5 min, and can radiate to the left shoulder and to both arms, especially to the ulnar surfaces of the forearm and

hand. It can also arise in or radiate to the back, interscapular region, root of the neck, jaw, teeth, and epigastrium. Angina is rarely localized below the umbilicus or above the mandible.

Although episodes of angina are typically caused by exertion (e.g., exercise, hurrying, or sexual activity) or emotion (e.g., stress, anger, fright, or frustration) and are relieved by rest, they may also occur at rest [see "Unstable Angina Pectoris," (Chap. 227)] and at night while the patient is recumbent (angina decubitus). The patient may be awakened at night distressed by typical chest discomfort and dyspnea. Nocturnal angina may be due to episodic tachycardia or to the expansion of the intrathoracic blood volume that occurs with recumbency; the latter causes an increase in cardiac size and myocardial oxygen demand that lead to ischemia and transient left ventricular failure.

The threshold for the development of angina pectoris may vary by time of day and emotional state. Many patients report a fixed threshold for angina, which occurs predictably at a certain level of activity, such as climbing two flights of stairs at a normal pace. In these patients coronary stenosis and myocardial oxygen supply are fixed and ischemia is precipitated by an increase in myocardial oxygen demand. In other patients the threshold for angina may vary considerably within any given day and from day to day. In such patients variations in myocardial oxygen supply, most likely due to changes in coronary vascular tone, may play an important role. A patient may report symptoms upon minor exertion in the morning (a short walk or shaving) yet by midday may be capable of much greater effort without symptoms. Angina may also be precipitated by unfamiliar tasks, a heavy meal, exposure to cold, or a combination. Exertional angina is typically relieved by rest in 1 to 5 min and even more rapidly by rest and sublingual nitroglycerin (see below). Indeed, the diagnosis of angina should be suspect if it does not respond to the combination of these two measures. The severity of angina can be expressed by the Canadian Cardiac Society functional classification (Table 226-1).

Sharp, fleeting chest pain or prolonged, dull aches localized to the left submammary area are rarely due to myocardial ischemia. However, angina pectoris may be atypical in location and not strictly related to provoking factors. In addition, this symptom may exacerbate and remit over days, weeks, or months. Its occurrence can be seasonal, being more frequent in the winter in temperate climates. Anginal "equivalents" are symptoms of myocardial ischemia other than angina. These include dyspnea, fatigue, and faintness and are more common in the elderly and in diabetic patients.

TABLE 226-1	Grading of Angina Pectoris According to CCS Classification
Class	Description of Stage
I	"Ordinary physical activity does not cause . . . angina," such as walking or climbing stairs. Angina occurs with strenuous, rapid, or prolonged exertion at work or recreation.
II	"Slight limitation of ordinary activity." Angina occurs on walking or climbing stairs rapidly; walking uphill; walking or stair climbing after meals; in cold, in wind, or under emotional stress; or only during the few hours after awakening. Angina occurs on walking >2 blocks on the level and climbing >1 flight of ordinary stairs at a normal pace and under normal conditions.
III	"Marked limitations of ordinary physical activity." Angina occurs on walking 1 to 2 blocks on the level and climbing 1 flight of stairs under normal conditions and at a normal pace.
IV	"Inability to carry on any physical activity without discomfort—anginal symptoms may be present at rest."

Note: CCS, Canadian Cardiovascular Society.
Source: Braunwald E et al. ACC/AHA guidelines for the management of patients with unstable angina-non-ST segment elevation myocardial infarction: A report of the American College of Cardiology/American Heart Association Task Force on Practice Guidelines (Committee on the Management of Patients with Unstable Angina). J Am Coll Cardiol 36: 970, 2000. Adapted with permission from L Campeau: Grading of angina pectoris (letter). Circulation 54:522, 1976, with permission, American Heart Association, Inc.

Systematic questioning of the patient with suspected IHD is important to uncover the features of an unstable syndrome associated with increased risk, such as angina occurring at rest or awakening the patient from sleep. Since coronary atherosclerosis is often accompanied by similar diseases in other arteries, the patient with angina should be questioned and examined for peripheral arterial disease (intermittent claudication, Chap. 232), stroke, or transient ischemic attacks (Chap. 349). It is also important to uncover a family history of premature IHD (<45 years in first-degree male relatives and <55 in female relatives) and the presence of diabetes mellitus, hyperlipidemia, hypertension, cigarette smoking, and other risk factors for coronary atherosclerosis (Chap. 224). The history of typical angina pectoris establishes the diagnosis of IHD until proven otherwise. In patients with atypical angina (Chap. 12), the coexistence of advanced age, male gender, the postmenopausal state, and risk factors for atherosclerosis increase the likelihood of important coronary disease.

PHYSICAL EXAMINATION   This is often normal in patients with stable angina, but it may reveal evidence of atherosclerotic disease at other sites, such as an abdominal aortic aneurysm, carotid arterial bruits, and diminished arterial pulse in the lower extremities, or of risk factors for atherosclerosis, such as xanthelasma and xanthomas (Chap. 224). Examination of the fundi may reveal increased light reflexes and arteriovenous nicking as evidence of hypertension. There may also be signs of anemia, thyroid disease, and nicotine stains on the fingertips from cigarette smoking. Palpation may reveal cardiac enlargement and abnormal contraction of the cardiac impulse (left ventricular akinesia or dyskinesia). Auscultation can uncover arterial bruits, a third and/or fourth heart sound, and, if acute ischemia or previous infarction has impaired papillary muscle function, an apical systolic murmur due to mitral regurgitation. These auscultatory signs are best appreciated with the patient in the left decubitus position. Aortic stenosis, aortic regurgitation (Chap. 219), pulmonary hypertension (Chap. 220), and hypertrophic cardiomyopathy (Chap. 221) must be excluded, since these disorders may cause angina in the absence of coronary atherosclerosis. Examination during an anginal attack is useful, since ischemia can cause transient left ventricular failure with the appearance of a third and/or fourth heart sound, a dyskinetic cardiac apex, mitral regurgitation, and even pulmonary edema. Tenderness of the chest wall or reproduction of the pain with palpation of the chest discomfort makes it unlikely that it is caused by angina.

LABORATORY EXAMINATION   Although the diagnosis of IHD can be made with confidence from the clinical examination, a number of simple laboratory tests can be helpful. The urine should be examined for evidence of diabetes mellitus and renal disease (including microalbuminuria) since these conditions accelerate atherosclerosis. Similarly, examination of the blood should include measurements of lipids (cholesterol—total, LDL, HDL—and triglycerides), glucose, creatinine, hematocrit, and, if indicated based on the physical examination, thyroid function. A chest x-ray is important, since it may show the consequences of IHD, i.e., cardiac enlargement, ventricular aneurysm, or signs of heart failure. These signs can support the diagnosis of IHD and are important in assessing the degree of cardiac damage.

ELECTROCARDIOGRAM   A 12-lead ECG recorded at rest is normal in about half the patients with typical angina pectoris, but there may be signs of an old myocardial infarction (Chap. 210). Although repolarization abnormalities, i.e., ST-segment and T-wave changes as well as left ventricular hypertrophy and intraventricular conduction disturbances, are suggestive of IHD, they are nonspecific, since they can also occur in pericardial, myocardial, and valvular heart disease or, in the case of the former, transiently with anxiety, changes in posture, drugs, or esophageal disease. Typical ST-segment and T-wave changes that accompany episodes of angina pectoris and disappear thereafter are more specific.

STRESS TESTING ■ Electrocardiographic   The most widely used test for both the diagnosis of IHD and estimating the prognosis involves recording the 12-lead ECG before, during, and after exercise, usually on a treadmill. The test consists of a standardized incremental increase in external workload while the symptoms, ECG, and arm blood pressure are monitored. Performance is usually symptom-limited, and the test is discontinued upon evidence of chest discomfort, severe shortness of breath, dizziness, severe fatigue, ST-segment depression > 0.2 mV (2 mm), a fall in systolic blood pressure >10 mmHg, or the development of a ventricular tachyarrhythmia. This test seeks to discover any limitation in exercise performance, to detect typical ECG signs of myocardial ischemia, and to establish their relationship to chest discomfort. The ischemic ST-segment response is generally defined as flat depression of the ST segment >0.1 mV below baseline (i.e., the PR segment) and lasting longer than 0.08 s (Fig. 226-1). Upsloping or junctional ST-segment changes are not considered characteristic of ischemia and do not constitute a positive test. Although T-wave abnormalities, conduction disturbances, and ventricular arrhythmias that develop during exercise should be noted, they are also not diagnostic. Negative exercise tests in which the target heart rate (85% of maximal heart rate for age and sex) is not achieved are considered to be nondiagnostic.

When interpreting ECG stress tests, the probability that coronary artery disease (CAD) exists in the patient or population under study (i.e., pretest probability) should be considered (Fig. 2-2). Overall, false-positive or false-negative results occur in one-third of cases. However, a positive result on exercise indicates that the likelihood of CAD is 98% in males >50 years with a history of typical angina pectoris and who develop chest discomfort during the test. The likelihood decreases if the patient has atypical or no chest pain by history and/or during the test. The incidence of false-positive tests is significantly increased in patients with low probabilities of IHD, such as asymptomatic men under the age of 40 or in premenopausal women with no risk factors for premature atherosclerosis. It is also increased in patients taking cardioactive drugs, such as digitalis and quinidine, or in those with intraventricular conduction disturbances, resting ST-segment and T-wave abnormalities, ventricular hypertrophy, or abnormal serum potassium levels. Obstructive disease limited to the circumflex coronary artery may result in a false-negative stress test since the posterior portion of the heart which this vessel supplies is not well represented on the surface 12-lead ECG. Since the overall sensitivity of exercise stress electrocardiography is only ~75%, a negative result does not exclude CAD, although it makes the likelihood of three-vessel or left main CAD extremely unlikely.

FIGURE 226-1   Lead V_4 at rest (*top*) and after 4½ min of exercise (*bottom*). There is 3 mm (0.3 mV) of horizontal ST-segment depression, indicating a positive test for ischemia. [*Modified from BR Chaitman, in E Braunwald et al (eds): Heart Disease, 6th ed, Philadelphia, Saunders, 2001.*]

The physician should be present throughout the exercise test, and it is important to measure total duration of exercise, the times to the onset of ischemic ST-segment change and chest discomfort, the external work performed (generally expressed as the stage of exercise), and the internal cardiac work performed, i.e., by the heart rate–blood pressure product. The depth of the ST-segment depression and the time needed for recovery of these ECG changes are also important. Because the risks of exercise testing are small but real—estimated at one fatality and two nonfatal complications per 10,000 tests—equipment for resuscitation should be available. Modified (heart rate–limited rather than symptom-limited) exercise tests can be performed safely in patients as early as 6 days after uncomplicated myocardial infarction. Contraindications to exercise stress testing include rest angina within 48 h, unstable rhythm, severe aortic stenosis, acute myocarditis, uncontrolled heart failure, and active infective endocarditis.

The normal response to graded exercise includes progressive increases in heart rate and blood pressure. Failure of the blood pressure to increase or an actual decrease with signs of ischemia during the test is an important adverse prognostic sign, since it may reflect ischemia-induced global left ventricular dysfunction. The development of angina and/or severe (>0.2 mV) ST-segment depression at a low workload, i.e., before completion of stage II of the Bruce protocol, and/or ST-segment depression that persists for >5 min after the termination of exercise increases the specificity of the test and suggests severe IHD and a high risk of future adverse events.

Cardiac Imaging (See also Chap. 211) When the resting ECG is abnormal (e.g., Wolff-Parkinson-White syndrome, >1 mm of resting ST-segment depression, left bundle branch block, paced ventricular rhythm), information gained from an exercise test can be enhanced by stress myocardial perfusion imaging after the intravenous administration of thallium 201 or technetium 99m sestamibi during exercise (or a pharmacologic) stress; the imaging is carried out both immediately after cessation of exercise to detect regional ischemia and 4 h later to confirm reversible ischemia and regions of persistent absent uptake that signify infarction.

A sizable fraction of patients who need noninvasive stress testing to identify myocardial ischemia and increased risk of coronary events cannot exercise because of peripheral vascular or musculoskeletal disease, exertional dyspnea, or deconditioning. In these circumstances intravenous dipyridamole or adenosine can be used in place of exercise. The development of a transient perfusion defect with a tracer such as radioactive thallium or technetium 99m sestamibi is used to detect myocardial ischemia. Ambulatory monitoring of the ECG can assess myocardial ischemia as episodes of ST-segment depression. These techniques are sensitive and capable of identifying patients with ischemia who are at increased risk of coronary events.

Two-dimensional echocardiography can assess both global and regional wall motion abnormalities of the left ventricle due to myocardial infarction or persistent ischemia. Stress (exercise or dobutamine) echocardiography may cause the emergence of regions of akinesis or dyskinesis not present at rest. Stress echocardiography, like stress myocardial perfusion imaging, is more sensitive than exercise electrocardiography in the diagnosis of IHD. The relative advantages of stress echocardiography and stress radionuclide perfusion imaging in the diagnosis of IHD are shown in Table 226-2.

Echocardiography or radionuclide angiography should be carried out to assess left ventricular function in patients with chronic stable angina and in patients with a history of a prior myocardial infarction, pathologic Q waves, or clinical evidence of heart failure.

CORONARY ARTERIOGRAPHY (See also Chap. 212) This diagnostic method outlines the lumina of the coronary arteries and can be used to detect or exclude serious coronary obstruction. However, coronary arteriography provides no information regarding the arterial wall, and severe atherosclerosis that does not encroach on the lumen may go undetected.

Indications Coronary arteriography is indicated in (1) patients with chronic stable angina pectoris who are severely symptomatic despite medical therapy and who are being considered for revascularization, i.e., a percutaneous coronary intervention (PCI) or coronary artery bypass grafting (CABG); (2) patients with troublesome symptoms that present diagnostic difficulties in whom there is need to confirm or rule out the diagnosis of IHD; (3) patients with known or possible angina pectoris who have survived cardiac arrest; (4) patients with angina or evidence of ischemia on noninvasive testing with clinical or laboratory evidence of ventricular dysfunction; and (5) patients judged to be at high risk of sustaining coronary events based on signs of severe ischemia on noninvasive testing, regardless of the presence or severity of symptoms (see below).

Examples of other indications include:

1. Patients with chest discomfort suggestive of angina pectoris but a negative or nondiagnostic stress test who require a definitive diagnosis for guiding medical management, alleviating psychological stress, career or family planning, or insurance purposes.
2. Patients who have been admitted repeatedly to the hospital for suspected acute coronary syndromes (acute myocardial infarction or unstable angina) but in whom this diagnosis has not been established and in whom the presence or absence of CAD should be determined.
3. Patients with careers that involve the safety of others (e.g., pilots, fire fighters, police) who have questionable symptoms, suspicious or positive noninvasive tests, and in whom there are reasonable doubts about the state of the coronary arteries.
4. Patients with aortic stenosis or hypertrophic cardiomyopathy and angina in whom the chest pain could be due to IHD.
5. Male patients >45 and females >55 years who are to undergo a cardiac operation, such as valve replacement or repair, and who may or may not have clinical evidence of myocardial ischemia.
6. Patients who are at high risk after myocardial infarction because of the recurrence of angina or the presence of heart failure, frequent ventricular premature contractions, or signs of ischemia on the stress test.
7. Patients with angina pectoris, regardless of severity, in whom noninvasive testing indicates a high risk of coronary events.
8. Patients in whom coronary spasm or another nonatherosclerotic cause of myocardial ischemia (e.g., coronary artery anomaly, Kawasaki's disease) is suspected.

PROGNOSIS The principal prognostic indicators in patients known to have IHD are age, the functional state of the left ventricle, the location(s) and severity of coronary artery narrowing, and the severity or activity of myocardial ischemia. Angina pectoris of recent onset, unstable angina (Chap. 227), early post-myocardial infarction angina, angina that is unresponsive or poorly responsive to medical therapy or is accompanied by symptoms of congestive heart failure all indicate an increased risk for adverse coronary events. The same is true for the

---

TABLE 226-2 *Comparative Advantages of Stress Echocardiography and Stress Radionuclide Perfusion Imaging in Diagnosis of CAD*

Advantages of stress echocardiography
1. Higher specificity
2. Versatility—more extensive evaluation of cardiac anatomy and function
3. Greater convenience/efficacy/availability
4. Lower cost

Advantages of stress perfusion imaging
1. Higher technical success rate
2. Higher sensitivity—especially for single vessel coronary disease involving the left circumflex
3. Better accuracy in evaluating possible ischemia when multiple resting LV wall motion abnormalities are present
4. More extensive published data base—especially in evaluation of prognosis

Note: CAD, coronary artery disease; LV, left ventricular.
Source: From Gibbons RJ et al, 1999, with permission.

physical signs of heart failure, episodes of pulmonary edema, transient third heart sounds, or mitral regurgitation, and for echocardiographic or radioisotopic (or roentgenographic) evidence of cardiac enlargement and reduced (<0.40) ejection fraction. Most importantly, any of the following signs during noninvasive testing indicate a high risk for coronary events: inability to exercise for 6 minutes, i.e., stage II (Bruce protocol) of the exercise test; a strongly positive exercise test showing onset of myocardial ischemia at low workloads (≥0.1 mV ST-segment depression before completion of stage II; ≥0.2 mV ST depression at any stage; ST depression for >5 min following the cessation of exercise; a decline in systolic pressure >10 mmHg during exercise; the development of ventricular tachyarrhythmias during exercise); the development of large or multiple perfusion defects or increased lung uptake during stress radioisotope perfusion imaging; and a decrease in left ventricular ejection fraction during exercise on radionuclide ventriculography or during stress echocardiography. Conversely, patients who can complete stage III of the Bruce exercise protocol and have a normal stress perfusion scan or negative stress echocardiographic evaluation are at very low risk of future coronary events.

On cardiac catheterization, elevations of left ventricular end-diastolic pressure and ventricular volume and reduced ejection fraction are the most important signs of left ventricular dysfunction and are associated with a poor prognosis. Patients with chest discomfort but normal left ventricular function and normal coronary arteries have an excellent prognosis. In patients with normal left ventricular function and mild angina but with critical stenoses (≥70% luminal diameter) of one, two, or three epicardial coronary arteries, the 5-year mortality rates are approximately 2, 8, and 11%, respectively. Obstructive lesions of the left anterior descending coronary artery proximal to the origin of the first septal artery are associated with a greater risk than are lesions of the right or left circumflex coronary artery, since the former vessel usually perfuses a greater quantity of myocardium. Stenosis (>50% luminal diameter) of the left main coronary artery is associated with a mortality rate of about 15% per year. The segmental atherosclerotic plaques in epicardial arteries with fissuring or filling defects indicates increased risk. These lesions go through phases of inflammatory cellular activity, degeneration, endothelial instability, abnormal vasomotion, platelet aggregation, and fissuring or hemorrhage. These factors can temporarily worsen the stenosis and cause abnormal reactivity of the vessel wall, thus exacerbating the manifestations of ischemia. The recent onset of symptoms, the development of severe ischemia during stress testing (see above), and unstable angina pectoris (Chap. 227) all reflect episodes of rapid progression in coronary lesions.

With any degree of obstructive CAD, mortality is greatly increased when left ventricular function is impaired; conversely, at any level of left ventricular function, the prognosis is influenced importantly by the quantity of myocardium perfused by critically obstructed vessels. Therefore, it is useful to collect all the evidence substantiating past myocardial damage (evidence of myocardial infarction on ECG, echocardiography, radioisotope imagine, or left ventriculography), residual left ventricular function (ejection fraction and wall motion), and risk of future damage from coronary events (extent of coronary disease and severity of ischemia defined by noninvasive stress testing). The larger the quantity of established myocardial necrosis, the less the heart is able to withstand additional damage and the poorer the prognosis. All the above signs of past damage plus the risk of future damage should be considered indicators of risk.

The plasma level of C-reactive protein is an indicator of inflammation and risk of future adverse coronary events in populations with atherosclerosis (Chap. 225). Similarly, electron beam computed tomography to measure coronary calcification and ultrasound measures of carotid intimal thickening can be used for the same purpose. The presence of other risk factors for coronary atherosclerosis [advanced age (>75 years), diabetes, morbid obesity, accompanying peripheral and/or cerebrovascular disease, previous myocardial infarction] worsen the prognosis of angina.

Rx TREATMENT

Each patient must be evaluated individually with respect to his or her expectations and goals, control of symptoms, and prevention of adverse clinical outcomes such as myocardial infarction and premature death. The degree of disability as well as the physical and emotional stress that precipitate angina must be carefully recorded in order to set treatment goals. The management plan should include the following components: (1) explanation and reassurance, (2) identification and treatment of aggravating conditions, (3) adaptation of activity, (4) treatment of risk factors that will decrease the occurrence of adverse coronary outcomes, (5) drug therapy for angina, and (6) consideration of mechanical revascularization (Table 226-3).

Explanation and Reassurance   Patients with IHD need to understand their condition as best they can and to realize that a long and useful life is possible even though they suffer from angina pectoris or have experienced and recovered from an acute myocardial infarction. Offering case histories of persons in public life who have lived with coronary disease as well as results of national studies showing improved outcomes can be of great value when encouraging patients to resume or maintain activity and return to their occupation. A planned program of rehabilitation can encourage patients to lose weight, improve exercise tolerance, and control risk factors with more confidence.

Identification and Treatment of Aggravating Conditions   A number of conditions may either increase oxygen demand or decrease oxygen supply to the myocardium and may precipitate or exacerbate angina in patients with IHD. Aortic valve disease and hypertrophic cardiomyopathy may cause or contribute to angina and should be excluded or treated. Obesity, hypertension, and hyperthyroidism should be treated aggressively in order to reduce the frequency and severity of anginal episodes. Decreased myocardial oxygen supply may be due to reduced oxygenation of the arterial blood (e.g., in pulmonary disease or, when carboxyhemoglobin is present, due to cigarette or cigar smoking) or decreased oxygen-carrying capacity (e.g., in anemia). Correction of these abnormalities, if present, may reduce or even eliminate angina pectoris.

Adaptation of Activity   Myocardial ischemia is caused by a discrepancy between the demand of the heart muscle for oxygen and the ability of the coronary circulation to meet this demand. Most patients can be helped to understand this concept and utilize it in the rational programming of activity. Many tasks that ordinarily evoke angina may be accomplished without symptoms simply by reducing the speed at which they are performed. Patients must appreciate the diurnal variation in their tolerance of certain activities and should reduce their energy requirements in the morning, immediately after meals, and in cold or inclement weather.

It may be necessary to recommend a change in employment or residence to avoid physical stress. However, with the exception of manual laborers, most patients with IHD can continue to function merely by allowing more time to complete each task. In some patients, anger and frustration may be the most important factors precipitating myocardial ischemia. If these cannot be avoided, training in stress management may be useful. A treadmill exercise test to determine the approximate heart rate at which ischemic ECG changes or symptoms develop may be helpful in the development of a specific exercise program.

Physical conditioning usually improves the exercise tolerance of patients with angina and exerts substantial psychological benefits. It may also improve the chances of surviving a myocardial infarction. A regular program of isotonic exercise within the limits of each patient's threshold for the development of angina pectoris and that does not exceed 80% of the heart rate associated with ischemia on exercise testing should be strongly encouraged.

TABLE 226-3 *Guidelines for the Treatment of Chronic Stable Angina*

Treatment of Symptoms

Class I[a]

1. Aspirin
2. β-blockers—particularly with a prior history of MI
3. Calcium antagonists as initial therapy
   a. If β-blockers are contraindicated
   b. With β-blockers to control symptom
   c. When β-blockers are stopped due to side effects
4. Sublingual nitroglycerin (tablets or spray) for relief of symptoms
5. Lipid lowering; LDL <2.6 mmol/L (100 mg/dL)
6. Health-promoting behaviors including smoking cessation, treatment of obesity, low-fat diet, supervised exercise program

Class IIa[b]

1. Clopidogrel when aspirin is contraindicated
2. Long-acting nondihydropyridine calcium antagonists (not short-acting) instead of β-blockers as initial therapy
3. Add long-acting nitrates and β-blockers or calcium antagonists for symptoms as needed

Class III[d]

1. Dypiridamole
2. Chelation therapy

Treatment of Risk Factors to Improve Outcomes

Class I

1. Smoking cessation
2. Treatment of dyslipidemia; LDL ≤2.6 mmol/L (100 mg/dL)
3. Angiotensin-converting enzyme inhibitor
4. Treatment of hypertension
5. Ideal weight and supervised exercise program
6. Low-fat diet
7. Treatment of diabetes using ADA National Guidelines

Class IIb[c]

1. Folate therapy for elevated homocysteine
2. Interventions directed at psychosocial stress

Class III

1. Hormone replacement therapy in postmenopausal women
2. Vitamins E and C
3. Treatment of depression
4. Chelation therapy
5. Herbal remedies and acupuncture

Treatment Using Revascularization

Class I

1. Coronary artery bypass surgery (CABG) for significant left main disease
2. CABG for 3-vessel coronary disease and reduced (≤50%) left ventricular function
3. CABG for 2-vessel CAD including LAD disease and reduced LV function
4. CABG for 3-vessel CAD plus high risk for percutaneous coronary intervention (PCI), abnormal (high risk) stress test, or diabetes
5. CABG in patients with prior CABG or PCI, recurrent restenosis, and high risk on noninvasive testing
6. PCI for 1- to 3-vessel CAD, normal LV function, no diabetes, lesions suitable (low risk) for PCI
7. PCI or CABG for failed medical therapy and acceptable risk with either modality

Class IIa

1. Repeat CABG for multiple vein graft stenoses, particularly including the LAD
2. PCI for simple focal vein graft stenosis
3. PCI or CABG for 1- or 2-vessel disease and moderate ischemia on noninvasive testing, including disease of the LAD

Class IIb

1. PCI instead of CABG in 2- or 3-vessel CAD (including the LAD) with controlled diabetes and lesions suitable (low risk) for PCI
2. PCI for technically suitable left main disease when CABG is not possible
3. PCI instead of CABG in 1- to 3-vessel CAD when each lesion is suitable (low risk) but the patient exhibits reduced LV function, treated diabetes, history of malignant arrhythmia, survived sudden death

Class III

1. PCI in left main disease or 3-vessel CAD with diabetes or poor LV function in patients who are candidates for CABG surgery
2. PCI or CABG in patients with mild symptoms, no evidence of ischemia in noninvasive testing, and not yet given an adequate trial of medical therapy
3. Baseline coronary stenoses (≤ 60%) and no signs of ischemia on noninvasive testing

Follow-up—Monitoring Disease, Testing, and Therapies

Class I

1. Chest x-ray with new evidence of congestive heart failure (CHF)
2. LV function testing for new evidence of CHF or MI
3. Echocardiogram for worsening of valvular disease
4. Treadmill testing for any change in clinical state
5. Stress imaging for any change in clinical state if the ECG cannot be interpreted or patient cannot exercise
6. Stress imaging for patients with prior revascularization and any change in clinical state
7. Coronary angiography in patients with obvious change in clinical state and limitations in daily activity despite medical therapy

Class IIb

1. Repeat annual treadmill exercise testing in patients with no change in clinical state, who can exercise, have no ECG abnormalities at rest, with an estimated morality of ≤ 1% per year

Class III

1. Echo or nuclear stress imaging for LV function and ischemia with no change in symptoms, normal ECG, no MI, and no CHF
2. Repeat treadmill stress test in ≤ 3 years in stable patients with estimated annual mortality ≤1% on an initial evaluation shown by:
   a. Low-risk Duke treadmill score
   b. Negative imaging study
   c. Normal LV function and no obstructive CAD
3. Stress imaging if stable, can exercise, normal resting ECG
4. Repeat coronary arteriogram with no change in clinical state, exercise testing, or stress imaging or insignificant CAD on initial examination

[a] Class I, therapies supported by evidence of efficacy.
[b] Class IIa, weight of evidence in favor of a therapy.
[c] Class IIb, evidence of efficacy less well established.
[d] Class III, therapies that are not useful and can be harmful.

Note: MI, myocardial infarction; LDL, low-density lipoprotein; ADA, American Diabetes Association; CAD, coronary artery disease; LAD, left anterior descending (coronary artery); LV, left ventricular; ECG, electrocardiogram.
Source: Adapted from Gibbons et al., 1999.

Treatment of Risk Factors A *family history* of premature IHD is an important indicator of increased risk and should trigger a search for treatable risk factors such as hyperlipidemia, hypertension, and diabetes. *Obesity* impairs the treatment of other risk factors and increases the risk of adverse coronary events. In addition, obesity is often accompanied by three other risk factors—diabetes mellitus, hypertension, and hyperlipidemia. The treatment of obesity and these accompanying risk factors is an important component of any management plan. A diet low in saturated fatty acids and a caloric intake to achieve optimal body weight is a cornerstone in the management of chronic IHD. Small controlled trials have shown that the combination of a 10% fat vegetarian diet, aerobic exercise, stress management training, smoking cessation, and psychosocial support can reduce the progression of coronary obstructive lesions, reduce angina, and result in fewer coronary events.

Cigarette smoking accelerates coronary atherosclerosis in both sexes and at all ages and increases the risk of thrombosis, plaque instability, myocardial infarction, and death (Chap. 225). Also, by increasing myocardial oxygen needs and reducing oxygen supply, it aggravates angina. Smoking cessation studies have demonstrated important benefits with a significant decline in the occurrence of these adverse outcomes. The physician's message must be clear and strong and supported by programs that achieve and monitor abstinence (Chap. 375). *Hypertension* (Chap. 230) is associated with increased risk of adverse clinical events from coronary atherosclerosis as well as stroke. In addition, the left ventricular hypertrophy that results from sustained

TABLE 226-4 Drugs Commonly Used for Angina Pectoris

Drug	Usual Dose	Side Effects	Contraindications
NITRATES			
Sublingual NTG	0.3–0.6 mg	Flushing, headache	Intolerance of side effects
Isosorbide dinitrate SR			
Oral	10–60 mg q8h	Flushing, headache, tolerance after 24 h	As above, worsening ischemia on withdrawal
Sublingual	2.5–10 mg q4–6h		
Transdermal NTG patch	0.4–1.2 mg/h for 12–14 h	Flushing, headache, tolerance after 24 h	As above, worsening ischemia on withdrawal
Isosorbide-5-monitrate			
Oral	20–30 mg bid	Flushing, headache, tolerance after 24 h	As above, worsening ischemia on withdrawal
Oral SR	60–240 mg once daily		
BETA BLOCKERS			
Propranolol	20–80 mg qid	Depression, constipation, impotence, bronchospasm, heart failure, bradycardia	Asthma, AV conduction block, heart failure
Metoprolol	25–200 mg bid	As above	As above
Atenolol	50–150 mg once daily	As above	As above
CALCIUM CHANNEL BLOCKING DRUGS			
Nifedipine XL	30–90 mg daily	Hypotension, flushing, edema, worsening angina	Hypotension, intolerance of side effects
Diltiazem SR	60–120 mg bid	Constipation, AV conduction block, worsening heart failure	AV conduction block, impaired LV function, bradycardia
Verapamil SR	180–240 mg daily	Constipation, AV conduction block, worsening heart failure	AV conduction delay, impaired LV function, bradycardia
Amlodipine	5–10 mg daily	Edema	Intolerance of side effects

Note: NTG, nitroglycerin; SR, slow release; XL, slow release preparation.

hypertension aggravates ischemia. There is evidence that long-term, effective treatment of hypertension can decrease the occurrence of adverse coronary events. *Diabetes mellitus* (Chap. 323) accelerates coronary and peripheral atherosclerosis and is frequently associated with dyslipidemias and increases in the risk of angina, myocardial infarction, and sudden coronary death. Strict control of the dyslipidemia and hypertension that are frequently found in diabetic patients is essential, as described below.

Dyslipidemia The treatment of dyslipidemia is central when aiming for long-term relief from angina, reduced need for revascularization, and reduction in myocardial infarction and death. Epidemiologic observations, angiographic trials, and controlled trials have shown that (1) men >45 years and women >55 years with two risk factors (family history of premature IHD, cigarette smoking, hypertension), diabetes mellitus, or evidence of atherosclerotic disease should have a total cholesterol $\leq$ 5.17 mmol/L ($\leq$200 mg/dL), LDL $\leq$ 2.58 mmol/L ($\leq$100 mg/dL), and HDL $\geq$ 1.03 mmol/L ($\geq$40 mg/dL). The control of lipids can be achieved by the combination of a diet low in saturated fatty acids, exercise, and weight loss. Frequently, HMG-CoA reductase inhibitors (statins) are required and can lower LDL cholesterol (25 to 50%), raise HDL cholesterol (5 to 9%), and lower triglycerides (5 to 30%). Niacin or fibrates can be used to raise HDL cholesterol and lower triglycerides (Chaps. 225 and 335). Controlled trials with lipid-regulating regimens have shown equal proportional benefit for men, women, the elderly, diabetics, and even smokers.

Risk Reduction in Women with IHD The incidence of clinical IHD in premenopausal women is very low. However, following the menopause, the atherogenic risk factors increase (e.g., increased LDL, reduced HDL) and the rate of clinical coronary events accelerates to the levels observed in men. Women have not given up cigarette smoking as effectively as have men. Diabetes mellitus, which is more common in women, greatly increases the occurrence of clinical IHD and amplifies the deleterious effects of hypertension, hyperlipidemia, and

smoking. Cardiac catheterization and coronary revascularization are often applied more sparingly in women and at a later, and more severe, stage of the disease than in men. When cholesterol lowering, beta blockers after myocardial infarction, and coronary artery bypass grafting (CABG) are applied in the appropriate patient groups, women enjoy the same benefits of improved outcome as do men.

Compliance with regard to the health-promoting behaviors listed above is generally very poor, and the conscientious physician must not underestimate the major effort required to meet this challenge. Fewer than one-half of patients in the United States discharged from the hospital with proven coronary disease receive treatment for dyslipidemia. Given the proof that treating dyslipidemia brings major benefits, physicians need to secure treatment pathways, monitor compliance, and follow up.

Drug Therapy The commonly used drugs for the treatment of angina pectoris are summarized in Table 226-4.

NITRATES This valuable class of drugs in the management of angina pectoris acts by causing systemic venodilation, thereby reducing myocardial wall tension and oxygen requirements, and by dilating the epicardial coronary vessels and increasing blood flow in collateral vessels. The nitrates likely bind to guanylate cyclase in vascular smooth-muscle cells, oxidize sulfhydryl groups, and are converted to S-nitrosothiols. This leads to an increase in cyclic guanosine monophosphate, which causes relaxation of vascular smooth muscle. The absorption of these agents is most rapid and complete through the mucous membranes. For this reason, nitroglycerin is most commonly administered sublingually in tablets of 0.4 or 0.6 mg. Patients with angina should be instructed to take the medication both to relieve angina and also approximately 5 min before stress that is likely to induce an episode. The value of this prophylactic use of the drug cannot be overemphasized.

A pulsating feeling in the head or headache is the most common side effect of nitroglycerin and fortunately is only rarely disturbing at the doses usually required to relieve or prevent angina. Postural dizziness has also been reported. Nitroglycerin deteriorates with exposure to air, moisture, and sunlight, so that if the drug neither relieves discomfort nor produces a slight sensation of burning at the sublingual site of absorption, the preparation may be inactive and a fresh supply should be obtained. If relief is not achieved by rest and within 2 or 3 min after nitroglycerin, a second or third dose may be given at 5-min intervals. If discomfort continues despite treatment, the patient should consult a physician or report promptly to a hospital emergency room for evaluation of possible unstable angina or acute myocardial infarction (Chap. 228).

Nitrates improve exercise tolerance in patients with chronic angina and relieve ischemia in patients with unstable angina as well as in patients with Prinzmetal's variant angina (Chap. 227). A diary of angina and nitroglycerin use may be valuable for detecting changes in the frequency, severity, or threshold for discomfort that may signify the development of unstable angina pectoris and/or herald an impending myocardial infarction.

Long-Acting Nitrates None of the long-acting nitrates is as effective as sublingual nitroglycerin for the acute relief of angina. These preparations can be swallowed, chewed, or administered as a patch or paste by the transdermal route. They can provide effective plasma levels for up to 24 h, but the therapeutic response is highly variable. Different preparations and/or administration during the daytime should be tried only to prevent discomfort while avoiding side effects such as headache and dizziness. Individual dose titration is important in order to prevent side effects. Useful preparations include isosorbide dinitrate (10 to 60 mg orally bid or tid), nitroglycerin ointment (0.5 to 2.0 in. qid), or sustained-release transdermal patches (5 to 25 mg/d). Tolerance with loss of efficacy develops with 12 to 24 h of continuous exposure to all of the long-acting nitrates due to depletion of sulfhydryl groups, decreased benefit through increased generation of oxygen free radicals, and to counterregulatory alterations in intravascular fluid balance with fluid retention. In order to minimize the effects of tolerance, the minimum effective dose should be used and a minimum of 8 h each day kept free of the drug so as to restore any useful response(s).

β-ADRENERGIC BLOCKERS These drugs represent an important component of the pharmacologic treatment of angina pectoris. They reduce myocardial oxygen demand by inhibiting the increases in heart rate, arterial pressure, and myocardial contractility caused by adrenergic activation. Beta blockade reduces these variables most strikingly during exercise while causing only small reductions at rest. Long-acting beta-blocking drugs (e.g., atenolol, 50 to 100 mg/d, or nadolol, 40 to 80 mg/d) offer the advantage of once-a-day dosage (Table 226-4). The therapeutic aims include relief of angina and ischemia. These drugs can also reduce mortality and reinfarction in patients after myocardial infarction and are moderately effective antihypertensive agents. Relative contraindications include asthma and reversible airway obstruction in patients with chronic lung disease, atrioventricular conduction disturbances, severe bradycardia, Raynaud's phenomenon, and a history of mental depression. Side effects include fatigue, reduced exercise tolerance, nightmares, impotence, cold extremities, intermittent claudication, bradycardia (sometimes severe), impaired atrioventricular conduction, left ventricular failure, bronchial asthma, worsening claudication, and intensification of the hypoglycemia produced by oral hypoglycemic agents and insulin. Reducing the dose or even discontinuation may be necessary if these side effects develop and persist. Since sudden discontinuation can intensify ischemia, the doses should be tapered over 2 weeks.

Beta blockers with relative β_1-receptor specificity, such as metoprolol and atenolol, may be preferable in patients with mild bronchial obstruction, insulin-requiring diabetes mellitus, or intermittent claudication.

CALCIUM ANTAGONISTS Slow-release nifedipine (30 to 90 mg once daily), verapamil (80 to 120 mg tid), diltiazem (30 to 90 mg qid), amlodipine (2.5 to 10 mg daily), and other calcium antagonists are coronary vasodilators that produce variable and dose-dependent reductions in myocardial oxygen demand, contractility, and arterial pressure. These combined pharmacologic effects are advantageous and make these agents as effective as beta blockers in the treatment of angina pectoris. They are indicated when beta blockers are contraindicated, poorly tolerated, or ineffective. Verapamil and diltiazem may produce symptomatic disturbances in cardiac conduction and bradyarrhythmias. They also exert negative inotropic actions and are more likely to aggravate left ventricular failure, particularly when used in patients with left ventricular dysfunction, especially if they are also receiving beta blockers. Although useful effects are usually achieved when calcium antagonists are combined with beta blockers and nitrates, careful individual titrations of the doses are essential with these combinations. Variant (Prinzmetal's) angina responds particularly well to calcium antagonists, supplemented when necessary by nitrates (Chap. 227). Nifedipine as well as other calcium antagonists are formulated as long-acting preparations, including diltiazem (60 to 120 mg twice daily) and verapamil (180 to 240 mg once daily).

Verapamil should not ordinarily be combined with beta blockers because of the combined effects on heart rate and contractility. Diltiazem can be combined with beta blockers with caution in patients with normal ventricular function and no conduction disturbances. Amlodipine and beta blockers have complementary actions on coronary blood supply and myocardial oxygen demands. While the former decreases blood pressure and dilates coronary arteries, the latter slows heart rate and decreases contractility. Amlodipine and the other second-generation dihydropyridine calcium antagonists (nicardipine, isradipine, long-acting nifedipine, and felodipine) are potent vasodilators and useful in the simultaneous treatment of angina and hypertension. Short-acting dihydropyridines should be avoided because of the risk of precipitating infarction, particularly in the absence of beta blockers.

CHOICE BETWEEN BETA BLOCKERS AND CALCIUM ANTAGONISTS FOR INITIAL THERAPY Since beta blockers have been shown to improve life expectancy following acute myocardial infarction (Chap. 228) while calcium antagonists have not, the former may also be preferable in patients with chronic IHD. However, calcium antagonists are indicated in patients with the following: (1) inadequate responsiveness to the combination of beta blockers and nitrates; many such patients do well with a combination of a beta blocker and a dihydropyridine calcium antagonist; (2) adverse reactions to beta blockers such as depression, sexual disturbances, and fatigue; (3) angina and a history of asthma or chronic obstructive pulmonary disease; (4) sick-sinus syndrome or significant atrioventricular conduction disturbances; (5) Prinzmetal's angina; or (6) symptomatic peripheral arterial disease.

ANTIPLATELET DRUGS Aspirin is an irreversible inhibitor of platelet cyclooxygenase activity and thereby interferes with platelet activation. Chronic administration of 75 to 325 mg orally per day has been shown to reduce coronary events in asymptomatic adult men, patients with chronic stable angina, and patients with or who have survived unstable angina and myocardial infarction. Administration of this drug should be considered in all patients with IHD in the absence of gastrointestinal bleeding, allergy, or dyspepsia. Clopidogrel (300 mg loading and 75 mg/d) is an oral agent that blocks ADP receptor–mediated platelet aggregation. It provides the same benefits as aspirin, if not better, particularly if aspirin causes the side effects listed above. Clopidogrel with aspirin can improve coronary outcomes when given to patients for 1 year after an episode of unstable angina but with some increase in the risk of bleeding (Chap. 227). This increased risk is improved when the dose of aspirin is reduced.

Other Therapies The angiotensin-converting enzyme inhibitors have become widely used in the treatment of survivors of myocardial infarction, patients with hypertension or chronic IHD including angina pectoris, and those at high risk of vascular disease, such as diabetes. A large clinical trial (the Heart Outcomes Prevention Evaluation Study) has shown that up to 10 mg/d of ramipril can result in the reduction of major adverse events (death, myocardial infarction, and stroke), angina, and the need for revascularization in a group of high-risk patients with atherosclerotic cardiovascular disease (including chronic IHD) and normal left ventricular function. →*The dosing and side effects of these agents are discussed in Chaps. 216, 228, and 230.*

Enhanced external counterpulsation utilizes pneumatic cuffs on the lower extremities to provide diastolic augmentation and systolic unloading of blood pressure in order to decrease cardiac work and oxygen consumption while enhancing coronary blood flow. Recent trials have shown that regular application improves angina, exercise capacity, and regional myocardial perfusion.

In summary, a regimen of diet, exercise, smoking cessation, together with treatment of hypertension and dyslipidemia and use of aspirin and beta blockers form a treatment plan that reduces angina, the need for revascularization, myocardial infarction, and coronary death. ACE inhibitors should be used in patients with angina, particularly those with hypertension and/or diabetes.

ANGINA AND HEART FAILURE Transient left ventricular failure with angina can be controlled by the use of nitrates. For patients with established congestive heart failure the increased left ventricular wall tension raises myocardial oxygen demand. Treatment of congestive heart failure with an angiotensin-converting enzyme inhibitor, diuretic, and digitalis (Chap. 216) reduces heart size, wall tension, and myocardial oxygen demand, which, in turn, helps to control angina and ischemia. If the symptoms and signs of heart failure are controlled, every effort should be made to cautiously use beta blockers not only for angina but because trials in heart failure have shown significant improvement in survival. Nocturnal angina can often be relieved by the treatment of heart failure. Nitrates are useful and can simultaneously improve the disturbed hemodynamics of congestive heart failure by vasodilatation, thereby reducing preload, and relieve angina by preventing or reversing myocardial ischemia. The combination of congestive heart failure and angina in patients with IHD usually indicates a poor prognosis and warrants serious consideration of cardiac catheterization and coronary revascularization.

CORONARY REVASCULARIZATION

While the basic management of patients with IHD is medical, as described above, many patients are improved by coronary revascularization procedures. These interventions should be employed in conjunction with but do not replace the continuing need to modify risk factors and medical therapy.

PERCUTANEOUS CORONARY INTERVENTION (See also Chap. 229 and Table 226-5) PCI, most commonly percutaneous transluminal coronary angioplasty with stenting, is widely used to achieve revascularization of the myocardium in patients with symptomatic IHD and suitable stenoses of epicardial coronary arteries. Whereas patients with stenosis of the left main coronary artery and those with three-vessel IHD (especially with diabetes and/or impaired left ventricular function) who require revascularization are best treated with CABG, PCI is widely employed in patients with symptoms and evidence of ischemia due to stenoses of one or two vessels, and even in selected patients with three-vessel disease, and may offer many advantages over surgery.

Indications and Patient Selection The most common clinical indication for PCI is angina pectoris, despite medical therapy, accompanied by

evidence of ischemia during a stress test. PCI is more effective than medical therapy for the relief of angina. Whereas PCI improves outcomes in patients with unstable angina and myocardial infarction, the value of this procedure in reducing the occurrence of coronary death and myocardial infarction in patients with chronic stable angina has not been established. PCI can be used to treat stenoses in native coronary arteries as well as in bypass grafts in patients who have recurrent angina following CABG. This is an important indication when the technical difficulties and the increased mortality that accompanies reoperation are considered. PCI has also been carried out in patients with recent total occlusion (within 3 months) of a coronary artery and angina; in this group the primary success rate is slightly decreased.

Risks When coronary stenoses are discrete and symmetric, two and even three vessels can be dilated in sequence. However, case selection is essential in order to avoid a prohibitive risk of complications, which are usually due to dissection or thrombosis with vessel occlusion, uncontrolled ischemia, and ventricular failure. Oral aspirin, clopidogrel, and intravenous heparin are given to reduce coronary thrombus formation. In unstable angina and when intracoronary thrombus is seen, the use of specific platelet glycoprotein receptor (GpIIb/IIIa) antagonists further reduces thrombotic complications and increases success. In experienced hands, the overall mortality rate is <0.5%, the need for emergency coronary surgery <1%, and the occurrence of clinical myocardial infarction <2%. Minor complications occur in 5 to 10% of patients and include occlusion of a branch of a coronary artery, myocardial infarction manifest only by release of CK-MB into the circulation, and complications of arterial catheterization. Left main coronary artery stenosis is generally regarded as a contraindication to PCI; such patients should be treated with CABG.

Efficacy Primary success, i.e., adequate dilation (an increase in luminal diameter >20% to a residual diameter obstruction <50%) with relief of angina, is achieved in >95% of cases. Recurrent stenosis of the dilated vessels occurs in ~20% of cases within 6 months of PCI with base metal stents, and angina will recur within 6 months in 10% of cases. Restenosis is more common in patients with diabetes mellitus, arteries with small caliber, incomplete dilation of the stenosis, occluded vessels, obstructed vein grafts, dilation of the left anterior descending coronary artery, and stenoses containing thrombi. It is usual clinical practice to administer aspirin for months after the procedure. Although aspirin and the antiplatelet drug clopidogrel may help prevent acute coronary thrombosis during and shortly following PCI with stenting, there is no evidence that these medications reduce the incidence of restenosis. Controlled trials have shown that the catheter-based local delivery of beta irradiation can significantly reduce the recurrence of in-stent restenosis. In diseased vein grafts procedural success has been improved by the use of capture devices or filters that prevent embolization, ischemia, and infarction. Moreover, the use of stents that locally deliver antiproliferative drugs such as rapamycin can reduce restenosis to near zero within the stent and 3 to 7% at the edges. These significant advances are extending the use of PCI.

Successful PCI produces effective relief of angina in >95% of cases and has been shown to be more effective than medical therapy for up to 2 years. More than one-half of patients with symptomatic IHD who require revascularization can be treated initially by PCI. Successful PCI is less invasive and expensive than CABG, usually requires only 1 to 2 days in the hospital, and permits considerable savings in the initial cost of care. Successful PCI also allows earlier return to work and the resumption of an active life. However, this economic benefit is reduced over time because of the greater need for follow-up and for repeat procedures. Clinical trials in patients after PCI have shown improvements in outcome with statin treatment.

CORONARY ARTERY BYPASS GRAFTING (See Table 226-5) Anastomosis of one or both of the internal mammary arteries or a radial artery to the coronary artery distal to the obstructive lesion is carried out. For additional obstructions that cannot be bypassed by an artery, a section of a vein (usually the saphenous) is used to form a connection between the aorta and the coronary artery distal to the obstructive lesion.

TABLE 226-5 *Comparison of Revascularization Procedures in Multivessel Disease*

Procedure	Advantages	Disadvantages
Percutaneous coronary intervention (PCI)	Less invasive Shorter hospital stay Lower initial cost Easily repeated Effective in relieving symptoms	Restenosis High incidence of incomplete revascularization Unknown effect on outcomes in patients with severe left ventricular dysfunction Limited to specific anatomic subsets Poor outcome in diabetics with 2- or 3-vessel coronary disease
Coronary artery bypass grafting (CABG)	Effective in relieving symptoms Improved survival in certain subsets Ability to achieve complete revascularization	Cost Increased risk of a repeat procedure due to late graft closure Morbidity and mortality of major surgery

Source: Modified from DP Faxon, in GA Beller (ed), *Chronic Ischemic Heart Disease*, in E Braunwald (series ed), *Atlas of Heart Diseases*, Philadelphia, Current Medicine, 1995.

Although some indications for CABG are controversial, certain areas of agreement exist:

1. The operation is relatively safe, with mortality rates <1% in patients without serious comorbid disease and normal left ventricular function, and when the procedure is performed by an experienced surgical team.

2. Intraoperative and postoperative mortality increase with the severity of ventricular dysfunction, comorbidities, age >80 years, and lack of surgical experience. The effectiveness and risk of CABG vary widely depending on case selection and the skill and experience of the surgical team.

3. Occlusion of *venous* grafts is observed in 10 to 20% of patients during the first postoperative year and in approximately 2% per year during 3- to 7-year follow-up and 4% per year thereafter. Long-term patency rates are considerably higher for internal mammary and radial artery implantations than saphenous vein grafts. In patients with left anterior descending coronary artery obstruction, survival is better when coronary bypass involves the internal mammary artery rather than a saphenous vein. Graft patency and outcomes are improved by meticulous treatment of risk factors, particularly dyslipidemia.

4. Angina is abolished or greatly reduced in ~90% of patients following complete revascularization. Although this is usually associated with graft patency and restoration of blood flow, the pain may also have been alleviated as a result of infarction of the ischemic segment or a placebo effect. Within 3 years, angina recurs in about one-fourth of patients but is rarely severe.

5. Survival may be improved by operation in patients with stenosis of the left main coronary artery as well as in patients with three- or two-vessel disease with significant obstruction of the proximal left anterior descending coronary artery. The survival benefit is greater in patients with abnormal left ventricular function (ejection fraction < 50%). Survival *may* also be improved in the following patients: (1) with obstructive CAD who have survived sudden cardiac death or sustained ventricular tachycardia; (2) who have undergone previous CABG and who have multiple saphenous vein graft stenoses, especially of a graft supplying the left anterior descending coronary artery; and (3) with recurrent stenosis following PCI, and high-risk criteria on noninvasive testing.

6. Minimally invasive CABG through a small thoracotomy and/or off-pump surgery can reduce morbidity and shorten convalescence in suitable patients.

Indications for CABG are usually based on the severity of symptoms, coronary anatomy, and ventricular function. The ideal candidate is male, <80 years of age, has no other complicating disease, has troublesome or disabling angina that is not adequately controlled by medical therapy or does not tolerate medical therapy and wishes to lead a more active life, and has severe stenoses of two or three epicardial coronary arteries with objective evidence of myocardial ischemia as a cause of the chest discomfort. Great symptomatic benefit can be anticipated in such patients. Congestive heart failure and/or left ventricular dysfunction, advanced age (>80 years), reoperation, urgent need for surgery, and the presence of diabetes mellitus are all associated with a higher perioperative mortality.

Left ventricular dysfunction can be due to noncontractile segments that are viable (hibernating myocardium). These can be detected by using radionuclide scans of myocardial perfusion and metabolism, positron emission tomography, or delayed scanning with thallium-201 or by improvement of regional functional impairment, provoked by low-dose dobutamine. In such patients, revascularization can return function and improve survival.

	One-vessel	One-vessel ≥95%	Two-vessel	Two-vessel ≥95%	One-vessel ≥95% Proximal LAD / Two-vessel ≥95%	Two-vessel ≥95% Proximal LAD / Three-vessel	Three-vessel ≥95%	Three-vessel Proximal LAD	Three-vessel ≥95% Proximal LAD
PTCA (n)	194	891	255	91	363	119	135	22	41
CABG (n)	45	222	235	148	481	333	898	276	530

FIGURE 226-2   Results from the Duke database comparing percutaneous transluminal coronary angioplasty (PTCA) and coronary artery bypass grafting (CABG). The preferred method of therapy depends on the extent and severity of coronary disease. PTCA seems to be superior in patients with less extensive disease, whereas CABG is more advantageous for patients with more extensive coronary disease. LAD, left anterior descending [*Modified from RH Jones et al. J Thorac Cardiovasc Surg III: 1013, 1996; with permission.*]

The Choice between PCI and CABG (Table 226-5; Fig. 226-2)   A number of randomized clinical trials have compared PCI and CABG in patients with multivessel CAD who were suitable technically for both procedures. The redevelopment of angina requiring repeat coronary angiography and repeat revascularization due to restenosis was higher in the PCI groups. (This disadvantage of PCI may be abolished by the use of drug-eluting stents.) However, the occurrence of death or myocardial infarction has been found to be similar between both groups for up to 5 years. In patients with diabetes mellitus as well as obstruction of two or more coronary arteries, CABG results in significantly better outcomes and survival and should be the revascularization technique of choice.

Based on these trials and observational studies, it is now recommended that patients with an unacceptable level of angina despite optimal medical management be considered for coronary revascularization. Patients with single- or two-vessel disease with normal left ventricular function and anatomically suitable lesions are ordinarily advised to undergo PCI (Chap. 229). Patients with three-vessel disease (or two-vessel disease that includes the proximal left descending coronary artery) and impaired global left ventricular function (left ventricular ejection fraction < 50%) or diabetes mellitus or those with left main coronary artery disease or other lesions unsuitable for catheter-based procedures should be considered for CABG as the initial method of revascularization (Table 226-3, Table 226-5, and Fig. 226-2).

ASYMPTOMATIC (SILENT) ISCHEMIA

Obstructive CAD, acute myocardial infarction, and transient myocardial ischemia are frequently asymptomatic. During continuous ambulatory ECG monitoring, the majority of ambulatory patients with typical chronic stable angina are found to have objective evidence of myocardial ischemia (ST-segment depression) during episodes of chest discomfort while they are active outside the hospital, but many of these patients have more frequent episodes of asymptomatic ischemia. In addition, there is a large (but as yet unknown) number of totally asymptomatic persons with severe coronary atherosclerosis who exhibit ST-segment changes during activity. Some of these patients exhibit higher thresholds to electrically induced pain, others show higher endorphin levels, and still others may be diabetics with autonomic dysfunction.

Frequent episodes of ischemia (symptomatic and asymptomatic) during daily life appear to be associated with an increased likelihood of adverse coronary events (death and myocardial infarction). In addition, patients with asymptomatic ischemia after suffering a myocardial infarction are at greater risk for a second coronary event. The widespread use of exercise ECG during routine examinations has also identified some of these heretofore unrecognized patients with asymptomatic CAD. Longitudinal studies have demonstrated an increased incidence of coronary events in asymptomatic patients with positive exercise tests.

℞ TREATMENT

The management of patients with asymptomatic ischemia must be individualized. Thus, the physician should consider the following: (1) the degree of positivity of the stress test, particularly the stage of exercise at which ECG signs of ischemia appear, the magnitude and number of the perfusion defect(s) on thallium scintigraphy, and the change in left ventricular ejection fraction which occurs on radionuclide ventriculography or echocardiography during ischemia and/or during exercise; (2) the ECG leads showing a positive response, with changes in the anterior precordial leads indicating a less favorable prognosis than changes in the inferior leads; and (3) the patient's age, occupation, and general medical condition. Most would agree that an asymptomatic 45-year-old commercial airline pilot with 0.4-mV ST-segment depression in leads V_1 to V_4 during mild exercise should undergo coronary arteriography, whereas the asymptomatic, sedentary 75 year old retiree with 0.1-mV ST-segment depression in leads II and III during maximal activity need not. However, there is no consensus about the appropriate procedure in the large majority of patients for whom the situation is less extreme. Asymptomatic patients with silent ischemia, three-vessel CAD, and impaired left ventricular function may be considered appropriate candidates for CABG.

The treatment of risk factors, particularly lipid lowering as described above, and the use of aspirin and beta blockers have been shown to reduce events and improve outcomes in asymptomatic as well as symptomatic patients with ischemia and proven CAD. While the incidence of asymptomatic ischemia can be reduced by treatment with beta blockers, calcium channel antagonists, and long-acting nitrates, it is not clear whether this is necessary or desirable in patients who have not suffered a myocardial infarction. However, there is evidence that β-adrenoceptor blockade begun 7 to 35 days after acute myocardial infarction improves survival (Chap. 228).

FURTHER READING

BLUMENTHAL RS et al: Medical therapy versus coronary angioplasty in stable coronary artery disease: A critical review of the literature. J Am Coll Cardiol 36:668, 2000

CLEEMAN JI et al: Executive summary of the Third Report of the National Cholesterol Education Program (NCEP) Expert Panel on Detection, Evaluation, and Treatment of High Blood Cholesterol in Adults (Adult Treatment Panel III). JAMA 285:2486, 2001

DEFEYTER PJ et al: Bypass surgery versus stenting for the treatment of multivessel disease in patients with unstable angina compared with stable angina. Circulation 105:2367, 2002

GIBBONS RJ et al: ACC/AHA/ACP-ASIM Guidelines for the Management of Patients with Chronic Stable Angina: Executive summary and recommendations. A report of the American College of Cardiology/American Heart Association Task Force on Practice Guidelines (Committee on Management of Patients with Chronic Stable Angina). Circulation 99:2829, 1999

KIM MC et al: Refractory angina pectoris. Mechanism and therapeutic options. J Am Coll Cardiol 39:923, 2002

LEE TH et al: Noninvasive tests in patients with stable coronary artery disease. N Engl J Med 344:1840, 2001

MORROW D et al: Chronic ischemic heart disease, in *Braunwald's Heart Disease*, 7th ed, D Zipes et al (eds). Philadelphia, Saunders, 2005

VAN DEN BRAND MJBM et al: The effect of completeness of revascularization on event-free survival at one year in the ARTS trial. J Am Coll Cardiol 39:559, 2002

YUSUF S et al: Effects of an angiotensin-converting enzyme inhibitor, ramipril, on cardiovascular events in high-risk patients. The Heart Outcomes Prevention Evaluation Study Investigators. N Engl J Med 342:145, 2000

227 UNSTABLE ANGINA AND NON-ST-ELEVATION MYOCARDIAL INFARCTION
Christopher P. Cannon, Eugene Braunwald

Patients with ischemic heart disease fall into two large groups: patients with stable angina secondary to chronic coronary artery disease (Chap. 226) and patients with acute coronary syndromes (ACS). The latter group, in turn, is composed of patients with acute myocardial infarction (MI) with ST-segment elevation on their presenting electrocardiogram (STEMI; Chap. 228) and those with unstable angina (UA) and non-ST-segment elevation MI (UA/NSTEMI; Fig. 228-1). Every year in the United States, ~1.4 million patients are admitted to hospitals with UA/NSTEMI as compared with 400,000 patients with acute STEMI.

DEFINITION   The diagnosis of UA is based largely on the clinical presentation. *Stable* angina pectoris is characterized by chest or arm discomfort that is rarely described as pain, but that is reproducibly associated with physical exertion or stress and is relieved within 5 to 10 min by rest and/or sublingual nitroglycerin (Chaps. 12 and 226). UA is defined as angina pectoris or equivalent ischemic discomfort with at least one of three features: (1) it occurs at rest (or with minimal exertion) usually lasting > 10 min, (2) it is severe and of new onset (i.e., within the prior 4 to 6 weeks), and/or (3) it occurs with a crescendo pattern (i.e., distinctly more severe, prolonged, or frequent than previously). The diagnosis of NSTEMI is established if a patient with the clinical features of UA develops evidence of myocardial necrosis, as reflected in elevated cardiac biomarkers.

PATHOPHYSIOLOGY   UA/NSTEMI can be caused by a reduction in oxygen supply and/or by an increase in myocardial oxygen demand (e.g., by tachycardia or severe anemia) superimposed on a coronary obstruction. Four pathophysiologic processes that may contribute to the development of UA have been identified: (1) plaque rupture or erosion with superimposed nonocclusive thrombus, believed to be the most common cause; (2) dynamic obstruction [e.g., coronary spasm, as in Prinzmetal's variant angina (p. 1448)]; (3) progressive mechanical obstruction [e.g., rapidly advancing coronary atherosclerosis or restenosis following percutaneous coronary intervention (PCI)]; and (4) secondary UA related to increased myocardial oxygen demand and/or decreased supply (e.g., anemia). More than one of these processes may be involved in many patients.

Among patients with UA/NSTEMI studied at angiography, ~5% have left main stenosis, 15% have three-vessel coronary artery disease, 30% have two-vessel disease, 40% have single-vessel disease, and 10% have no critical coronary stenosis; some of the latter have Prinzmetal's variant angina (see below). The "culprit lesion" on angiography may show an eccentric stenosis with scalloped or overhanging edges and a narrow neck. Angioscopy may reveal "white" (platelet-rich) thrombi, as opposed to "red" thrombi, more often seen in patients with acute STEMI.

CLINICAL PRESENTATION ■ History and Physical Examination   The clinical hallmark of UA/NSTEMI is chest pain, typically located in the substernal region or sometimes in the epigastrium, that frequently radiates to the neck, left shoulder, and left arm (Chap. 12). This discomfort is usually severe enough to be considered painful. Anginal "equivalents" such as dyspnea and epigastric discomfort may also occur. The examination resembles that in patients with stable angina (Chap. 226) and may be unremarkable. If the patient has a large area of myocardial ischemia or a large NSTEMI, the physical findings can include diaphoresis, pale cool skin, sinus tachycardia, a third and/or fourth heart sound, basilar rales, and sometimes hypotension, resembling the findings of large STEMI.

Electrocardiogram   In UA, ST-segment depression, transient ST-segment elevation, and/or T-wave inversion occur in 30 to 50% of patients, depending on the severity of the clinical presentation. In patients with the clinical features of UA, the presence of new ST-segment deviation, even of only 0.05 mV, is an important predictor of adverse outcome. T-wave changes are sensitive for ischemia but are less specific, unless they are new, deep T-wave inversions (≥0.3 mV).

Cardiac Biomarkers   Patients with UA who have elevated biomarkers of necrosis, such as CK-MB and troponin (a much more specific marker of myocardial necrosis), are at increased risk for death or recurrent MI. Elevated levels of these markers distinguish patients with NSTEMI from those with UA. There is a direct relationship between the degree of troponin elevation and mortality. However, in patients *without* a clear clinical history of myocardial ischemia, minor troponin elevations have been reported and can be caused by congestive heart failure, myocarditis, or pulmonary embolism or may be false-positive readings. Thus, in patients with an *unclear* history, small troponin elevations may not be diagnostic of an ACS.

DIAGNOSTIC EVALUATION (See also Chap. 12)   Approximately 6 to 7 million persons per year in the United States present to hospital emergency departments (EDs) with a complaint of chest pain or other symptoms suggestive of ACS. A diagnosis of an ACS is established in 20 to 25% of such patients. The first step in evaluating patients with possible UA/NSTEMI is to determine the *likelihood* that coronary artery disease is the cause of the presenting symptoms. The 2002 American College of Cardiology/American Heart Association (ACC/AHA) Guidelines include, among the factors associated with a high likelihood of ACS, a clinical history typical of ischemic discomfort, a history of established coronary artery disease by angiography, prior MI, congestive heart failure, new electrocardiographic (ECG) changes, or elevated cardiac biomarkers. Factors associated with an intermediate likelihood of ACS in patients with the clinical features of this condition are: age >70 years, male gender, diabetes mellitus, known peripheral arterial or cerebrovascular disease, and old ECG abnormalities.

Diagnostic Pathways   There are four major diagnostic tools used in the diagnosis of UA/NSTEMI in the ED—the clinical history, the ECG, cardiac markers, and stress testing. The goals are to: (1) recognize or exclude MI (using cardiac markers), (2) evaluate for rest ischemia (chest pain at rest, serial or continuous ECGs), and (3) evaluate for significant coronary artery disease (using provocative stress testing). Typical pathways begin with assessment of the likelihood that the presenting symptoms are due to ischemia. Patients with a low likelihood of ischemia are usually managed with an ED-based critical pathway (which in some institutions is carried out in a "chest pain unit" (Fig. 227-1). Evaluation of such patients includes clinical monitoring for recurrent ischemic discomfort, serial ECGs, and cardiac markers, typically performed at baseline and at 4 to 6 h and 12 h after presentation. If new elevations in cardiac markers (currently CK-MB and troponin) or ECG changes are noted, the patient is admitted to the hospital. If the patient remains pain free and the markers are negative, the patient may go on to stress testing. This may be performed as early as 6 h after presentation in the ED or chest pain center, or on an outpatient basis within 72 h. For most patients, standard treadmill ECG stress testing is used, but for patients with fixed abnormalities on the ECG (e.g., left bundle branch block), perfusion or echocardiographic imaging is used. For patients who cannot walk, pharmacologic stress is used. By demonstrating normal myocardial perfusion, sestamibi or thallium imaging (Chap. 211) can reduce unnecessary hospitalizations by excluding acute ischemia.

RISK STRATIFICATION AND PROGNOSIS   Patients with documented UA/NSTEMI exhibit a wide spectrum of early (30 day) risk, ranging from ~2 to 10%, and of new or recurrent infarction of 3 to 10%. Assessment of "global risk" can be accomplished by clinical risk scoring systems

Critical Pathway for ED Evaluation of Chest Pain/ "Rule Out MI"

FIGURE 227-1   Diagnostic evaluation of patients presenting with suspected UA/NSTEMI. The first step is to assess the likelihood of coronary artery disease. Patients at high or intermediate likelihood are admitted to the hospital. Those with clearly atypical chest pain are discharged home. Patients with a *low* likelihood of ischemia enter the pathway and are observed in a monitored bed in the emergency department (ED) or observation unit over a period of 6 h and 12-lead electrocardiograms are performed if the patient has recurrent chest discomfort. A panel of cardiac markers (e.g., troponin and CK-MB) are drawn at baseline and 6 h later. If the patient develops recurrent pain, has ST-segment or T-wave changes, or had positive cardiac markers, he/she is admitted to the hospital and treated for UA/NSTEMI. If the patient has negative markers and no recurrence of pain, he/she is sent for exercise treadmill testing, with imaging reserved for patients with abnormal baseline electrocardiograms (e.g., left bundle branch block or left ventricular hypertrophy). If positive, the patient is admitted; if negative, the patient is discharged home with follow-up to his/her primary physician. (CAD, coronary artery disease; ECG, electrocardiogram; E.D., emergency department; ETT, exercise tolerance test; MI, myocardial infarction; OBS, observation unit.) [*Adapted from CP Cannon, E Braunwald, in E Braunwald et al (eds): Heart Disease: A Textbook of Cardiovascular Medicine, 6th ed. Philadelphia, Saunders, 2001.*]

such as that used in the Thrombolysis in Myocardial Ischemia Trial (TIMI), which includes seven independent risk factors: age > 65 years, three or more risk factors for coronary artery disease, documented coronary artery disease at catheterization, development of UA/NSTEMI while on aspirin, more than two episodes of angina within the preceeding 24 h, ST deviation ≥ 0.5 mm, and an elevated cardiac marker (Fig. 227-2).

Early risk assessment (especially using troponin, ST-segment changes, and/or a global risk scoring system) is useful both in predicting the risk of recurrent cardiac events and in identifying those patients who would derive the greatest benefit from the newer and more potent antithrombotic therapies, such as low-molecular-weight heparin (LMWH) and glycoprotein (GP)IIb/IIIa inhibitors, and from an early invasive strategy. For example, in the TACTICS-TIMI 18 Trial, an early invasive strategy conferred a 40% reduction in recurrent cardiac events in patients with a positive troponin level, whereas no benefit was observed in those with a negative troponin level.

Among other cardiac biomarkers under intensive investigation are C-reactive protein, B-type natriuretic peptide, and CD-40 ligand, all of which correlate independently with increased mortality and recurrent cardiac events in patients presenting with UA/NSTEMI. Multimarker strategies are now gaining favor both to define the pathophysiologic mechanisms underlying a given patient's presentation more fully and to stratify the patient's risk further.

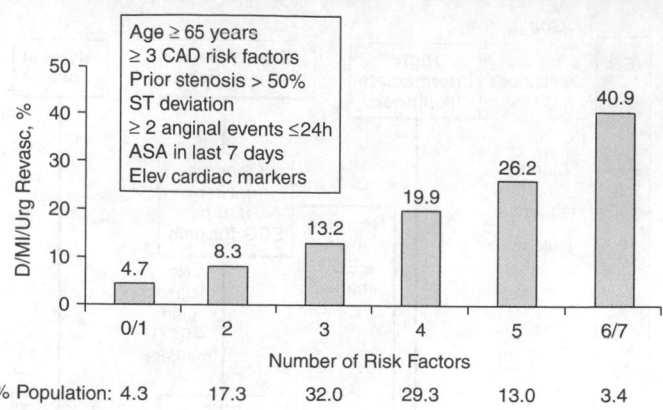

FIGURE 227-2 The TIMI Risk Score for UA/NSTEMI, a simple but comprehensive clinical risk stratification score to identify increasing risk of death, myocardial infarction, or urgent revascularization to day 14. (*Adapted from Antman et al.*)

℞ TREATMENT

Medical Treatment   Patients with UA/NSTEMI should be placed at bed rest with continuous ECG monitoring for ST-segment deviation and cardiac rhythm. Ambulation is permitted if the patient shows no recurrence of ischemia (discomfort or ECG changes) and does not develop a biomarker of necrosis for 12 to 24 h. Medical therapy involves simultaneous anti-ischemic treatment and antithrombotic treatment.

Anti-Ischemic Treatment (Table 227-1)   In order to provide relief and prevention of recurrence of chest pain, initial treatment should include nitrates and beta blockers.

NITRATES   Nitrates should first be given sublingually or by buccal spray (0.3 to 0.6 mg) if the patient is experiencing ischemic pain. If pain persists after three doses given 5 min apart, intravenous nitroglycerin (5 to 10 μg/min using nonabsorbing tubing) is recommended. The rate of the infusion may be increased by 10 μg/min every 3 to 5 min until symptoms are relieved or systolic arterial pressure falls to <100 mmHg. Topical or oral nitrates (Chap. 226) can be used once the pain has resolved, or they may replace intravenous nitroglycerin when the

---

TABLE 227-1   *Drugs Commonly Used in Intensive Medical Management of Patients with Unstable Angina and Non-ST Elevation MI*

Drug Category	Clinical Condition	When to Avoid[a]	Dosage
Nitrates	Symptoms are not fully relieved with three sublingual nitroglycerin tablets and initiation of beta-blocker therapy	Hypotension	5–10 μg/min by continuous infusion Titrated up to 75–100 μg/min until relief of symptoms or limiting side effects (headache or hypotension with a systolic blood pressure <90 mmHg or more than 30% below starting mean arterial pressure levels if significant hypertension is present) Topical, oral, or buccal nitrates are acceptable alternatives for patients without ongoing or refractory symptoms

Beta blockers[b]	Unstable angina	PR interval (ECG) >0.24 s
		2° or 3° atrioventricular block
		Heart rate <60 beats/min
		Blood pressure <90 mmHg
		Shock
		Left ventricular failure with congestive heart failure
		Severe reactive airway disease
			Metoprolol[c]
			  5-mg increments by slow (over 1–2 min IV administration
			  Repeated every 5 min for a total initial dose of 15 mg
			  Followed in 1–2 h by 25–50 mg by mouth every 6 h
			  If a very conservative regimen is desired, initial doses can be reduced to 1–2 mg
			Esmolol[c]
			  Starting maintenance dose of 0.1 mg/kg per min IV
			  Titration in increments of 0.05 mg/kg per min every 10–15 min as tolerated by blood pressure until the desired therapeutic response has been obtained, limiting symptoms develop, or a dose of 0.20 mg/kg per min is reached
			  Optional loading dose of 0.5 mg/kg may be given by slow IV administration (2–5 min) for more rapid onset of action

Calcium channel blockers	Patients whose symptoms are not relieved by adequate doses of nitrates and beta blockers or in patients unable to tolerate adequate doses of one or both of these agents or in patients with variant angina	Pulmonary edema Evidence of left ventricular dysfunction (for diltiazem or verapamil)	Dependent on specific agent
Morphine sulfate	Patients whose symptoms are not relieved after three serial sublingual nitroglycerin tablets or whose symptoms recur with adequate anti-ischemic therapy	Hypotension Respiratory depression Confusion Obtundation	2–5 mg IV dose May be repeated every 5–30 min as needed to relieve symptoms and maintain patient comfort

[a] Allergy or prior intolerance is a contraindication for all categories of drugs listed in this chart.
[b] Choice of the specific agent is not as important as ensuring that appropriate candidates receive this therapy. If there are concerns about patient intolerance owing to existing pulmonary disease, especially asthma, left ventricular dysfunction, or risk of hypotension or severe bradycardia, initial selection should favor a short-acting agent, such as propranolol or metoprolol or the ultra-short-acting agent esmolol. Mild wheezing or a history of chronic obstructive pulmonary disease should prompt a trial of a short-acting agent at a reduced dose (e.g., 2.5 mg IV metoprolol, 12.5 mg oral metoprolol, or 25 μg/kg per min esmolol as initial doses) rather than complete avoidance of beta-blocker therapy.

[c] Metoprolol and esmolol are two of several beta blockers that may be employed.
Note: Some of the recommendations in this guide suggest the use of agents for purposes or in doses other than those specified by the U.S. Food and Drug Adminstration. Such recommendations are made after consideration of concerns regarding nonapproved indications. Where made such recommendations are based on more recent clinical trials or expert consensus.
IV, intravenous; aPTT, activated partial thromboplastin time; ECG, electrocardiogram; 2°, second-degree, 3°, third-degree.
Source: Modified from E Braunwald et al: Circulation 1994;90:613–622.

patient has been pain free for 12 to 24 h. The only absolute contraindications to the use of nitrates are hypotension or the use of sildenafil (Viagra) or other drugs in that class within the previous 24 h.

β-ADRENERGIC BLOCKADE These agents are the other mainstay of anti-ischemic treatment. Intravenous beta blockade followed by oral beta blockade targeted to a heart rate of 50 to 60 beats/min is recommended. Heart rate slowing calcium channel blockers, e.g., verapamil or diltiazem, are recommended in patients who have persistent or recurrent symptoms after treatment with full-dose nitrates and beta blockers and in patients with contraindications to beta blockade. Additional medical therapy includes angiotensin-converting enzyme (ACE) inhibition and HMG-CoA reductase inhibitors (statins) for long-term secondary prevention.

If pain persists despite intravenous nitroglycerin and beta blockade, morphine sulfate, 1 to 5 mg intravenously, can be administered every 5 to 30 min as needed.

Antithrombotic Therapy (Table 227-2) This is the other main component of treatment for UA/NSTEMI. Initial treatment should begin with the platelet cyclooxygenase inhibitor aspirin (Fig. 227-3). The thienopyridine clopidogrel, which blocks the platelet adenosine receptor (in combination with aspirin), was shown in the CURE trial to confer a 20% relative reduction in cardiovascular death, MI, or stroke compared with aspirin alone in both low- and high-risk patients with UA/NSTEMI, but to be associated with a moderate (absolute 1%) increase in serious bleeding, which is more marked in patients who undergo coronary artery bypass grafting. Pretreatment with clopidogrel has also been shown to reduce adverse outcomes associated with and following PCI (Chap. 229). Continued benefit of long-term (~1 year) treatment with the combination of clopidogrel and aspirin has been observed both in patients treated conservatively and in those who underwent a PCI. This combination is recommended for all patients with UA/NSTEMI who are not at excessive risk for bleeding.

Unfractionated heparin (UFH) or LMWH should be added to aspirin and clopidogrel. Based on several randomized trials showing the superiority of the LMWH enoxaparin to UFH in reducing recurrent cardiac events, the 2002 ACC/AHA UA/NSTEMI guidelines favor enoxaparin as the preferred antithrombin. Direct thrombin inhibitors and factor Xa inhibitors are being studied as replacements for heparin.

Intravenous GP IIb/IIIa inhibitors have also been shown to be beneficial in treating UA/NSTEMI (Fig. 227-3). For "upstream" manage-

FIGURE 227-3 Platelets initiate thrombosis at the site of a ruptured plaque: *platelet adhesion* occurs via: (1) the GP 1b receptor in conjunction with von Willebrand factor. This is followed by *platelet activation* (2), which leads to a shape change in the platelet, degranulation of the alpha and dense granules, and expression of glycoprotein IIb/IIIa receptors on the platelet surface with activation of the receptor, such that it can bind fibrinogen. The final step is *platelet aggregation* (3), in which fibrinogen (or von Willebrand factor) binds to the activated GP IIb/IIIa receptors. Aspirin (ASA) and clopidogrel act to decrease platelet activation, whereas the glycoprotein IIb/IIIa inhibitors inhibit the final step of platelet aggregation. [*From CP Cannon, E Braunwald, in E Braunwald et al (eds): Heart Disease: A Textbook of Cardiovascular Medicine, 6th ed. Philadelphia, Saunders, 2001.*]

ment of high-risk patients in whom an invasive management is intended (i.e., initiating therapy when the patient first presents to the hospital), the small molecule inhibitors eptifibatide and tirofiban show benefit, while the monoclonal antibody abciximab appears not to be effective in patients treated conservatively, (i.e., in those not undergoing coronary angiography or PCI). However, abciximab has been shown to be beneficial in patients with UA/NSTEMI undergoing PCI. As with all antithrombotic agents, bleeding is the most important adverse effect of these drugs. Thus, patients with a history of bleeding must be screened carefully and given fewer antithrombotic agents.

INVASIVE VERSUS CONSERVATIVE STRATEGY Multiple clinical trials have shown the benefit of an early invasive strategy in high-risk patients, i.e., patients with multiple clinical risk factors, ST-segment deviation, and/or positive biomarkers (Table 227-3). In this strategy, following treatment with anti-ischemic and antithrombotic agents, coronary arteriography is carried out within ~48 h of admission, followed by coronary revascularization (PCI or coronary artery bypass grafting), depending on the coronary anatomy.

Such a strategy is quite cost-effective in high-risk patients. In low-risk patients, the outcomes from an invasive strategy are similar to those obtained from a conservative strategy, which consists of anti

---

TABLE 227-2 *Clinical Use of Antithrombotic Therapy*

ORAL ANTIPLATELET THERAPY

Aspirin	Initial dose of 162–325 mg nonenteric formulation followed by 75–160 mg/d of an enteric or a nonenteric formulation
Clopidogrel (Plavix)	Loading dose of 300 mg followed by 75 mg/d

HEPARINS[a]

Dalteparin (Fragmin)	120 IU/kg SC every 12 h (maximum 10,000 IU twice daily)
Enoxaparin (Lovenox)	1 mg/kg SC every 12 h; the first dose may be preceded by a 30-mg IV bolus
Heparin (UFH)	Bolus 60–70 U/kg (maximum 5000 U) IV followed by infusion of 12–15 U/kg per h (initial maximum 1000 U/h) titrated to a PTT 1.5–2.5 times control

INTRAVENOUS ANTIPLATELET THERAPY

Abciximab (ReoPro)	0.25 mg/kg bolus followed by infusion of 0.125 μg/kg per min (maximum 10 μg/min) for 12 to 24 h
Eptifibatide (Integrilin)	180 μg/kg bolus followed by infusion of 2.0 μg/kg per min for 72 to 96 h
Tirofiban (Aggrastat)	0.4 μg/kg per min for 30 min followed by infusion of 0.1 μg/kg per min for 48 to 96 h

[a] Other LMWH exist beyond those listed.
Note: IV, intravenous; SC, subcutaneously; UFH, unfractionated heparin.
Source: Modified from E Braunwald et al: J Am Coll Cardiol 2000;36:970–1056.

TABLE 227-3 *Class I Recommendations for Use of an Early Invasive Strategy[a]*

Class I (level of evidence: A) indications
Recurrent angina at rest/low-level activity despite Rx
Elevated TnT or TnI
New ST-segment depression
Rec. angina/ischemia with CHF symptoms, rales, MR
Positive stress test
EF < 0.40
Decreased BP
Sustained VT
PCI < 6 mos, prior CABG

[a] Any one of the high-risk indicators.
Abbreviations: TnT, troponin T; TnI, troponin I; CHF, congestive heart failure; MR, mitral regurgitation; EF, ejection fraction; BP, blood pressure; VT, ventricular tachycardia; PCI, percutaneous coronary intervention; CABG, coronary artery bypass grafting.
Source: From E Braunwald et al: Circulation 106:1893, 2002.

ischemic and antithrombotic therapy followed by "watchful waiting," in which coronary arteriography is carried out only if rest pain or ST-segment changes recur or there is evidence of ischemia on a stress test.

LONG-TERM MANAGEMENT   The time of hospital discharge is a "teachable moment" for the patient, when the physician can review and optimize the medical regimen. Risk factor modification is key, and the physician should discuss with the patient the importance of smoking cessation, achieving optimal weight, daily exercise, following an appropriate diet, blood pressure control, tight control of hyperglycemia (for diabetic patients), and lipid management, as recommended for patients with chronic stable angina (Chap. 225).

There is evidence of benefit with long-term therapy with five classes of drugs that are directed at different components of the atherothrombotic process. Beta blockers are appropriate anti-ischemic therapy and may help decrease triggers for MI. Statins and ACE inhibitors are recommended for long-term plaque stabilization. Antiplatelet therapy, now recommended to be the combination of aspirin and clopidogrel for at least 9 to 12 months, with aspirin continued thereafter, prevents or reduces the severity of any thrombosis that would occur if a plaque does rupture. Thus, a multifactorial approach to long-term medical therapy is directed at preventing the various components of atherothrombosis

PRINZMETAL'S VARIANT ANGINA

In 1959, Prinzmetal et al. described a syndrome of ischemic pain that occurs at rest but not usually with exertion and is associated with transient ST-segment elevation. This syndrome is due to focal spasm of an epicardial coronary artery, leading to severe myocardial ischemia. Although it is frequently thought that the spasm occurs in arteries without stenosis, many Prinzmetal patients have spasm adjacent to atheromatous plaques. The exact cause of the spasm is not well defined, but it may be related to hypercontractility of vascular smooth muscle due to vasoconstrictor mitogens, leukotrienes, or serotonin. In some patients it is a manifestation of a vasospastic disorder and is associated with migraine, Raynaud's phenomenon, or aspirin-induced asthma.

CLINICAL AND ANGIOGRAPHIC MANIFESTATIONS   Patients with variant angina are younger and have fewer coronary risk factors (with the exception of cigarette smoking) than patients with UA secondary to coronary atherosclerosis. The anginal discomfort is often extremely severe and has usually not progressed from a period of chronic stable angina. Cardiac examination is usually normal in the absence of ischemia.

The clinical diagnosis of variant angina is made with the detection of transient ST-segment *elevation* with rest pain. Many patients also exhibit multiple episodes of asymptomatic ST-segment elevation (*silent ischemia*). Small elevations of CK-MB may occur in patients with prolonged attacks of variant angina. Exercise testing in patients with variant angina is of limited value because the patients can demonstrate ST elevation, depression, or no ST changes.

Coronary angiography demonstrates transient coronary spasm as the diagnostic hallmark of Prinzmetal's angina. Significant proximal coronary stenosis of at least one major vessel occurs in the majority of patients, and in them spasm usually occurs within 1 cm of the obstruction. Focal spasm is most common in the right coronary artery, and it may occur at one or more sites in one artery or in multiple arteries simultaneously. Ergonovine, acetylcholine, other vasoconstrictor medications, and hyperventilation have been used to provoke and demonstrate focal coronary stenosis to establish the diagnosis. Hyperventilation has also been used to provoke rest angina, ST-segment elevation, and spasm on coronary arteriography.

℞ TREATMENT

Nitrates and calcium channel blockers are the main treatments for patients with variant angina. Sublingual or intravenous nitroglycerin often abolishes episodes of variant angina promptly, and long-acting nitrates are useful in preventing recurrences. Calcium antagonists are extremely effective in preventing the coronary artery spasm of variant angina, and they should be prescribed in maximally tolerated doses. Similar efficacy rates have been noted among the various types of calcium antagonists. Prazosin, a selective α-adrenoreceptor blocker, has also been found to be of value in some patients, while aspirin may actually increase the severity of ischemic episodes. The response to beta blockers is variable. Coronary revascularization may be helpful in patients with variant angina who also have discrete, proximal fixed obstructive lesions.

PROGNOSIS   Many patients with Prinzmetal's angina pass through an acute, active phase, with frequent episodes of angina and cardiac events during the first 6 months after presentation. Long-term survival at 5 years is excellent (~90 to 95%). Patients with no or mild fixed coronary obstruction tend to experience a more benign course than do patients with associated severe obstructive lesions. Nonfatal MI occurs in up to 20% of patients by 5 years. Patients with variant angina who develop serious arrhythmias during spontaneous episodes of pain are at a higher risk for sudden death. In most patients who survive an infarction or the initial 3- to 6-month period of frequent episodes, the condition stabilizes and there is a tendency for symptoms and cardiac events to diminish with time.

FURTHER READING

ANTMAN EM et al: The TIMI risk score for unstable angina/non-ST elevation MI: A method for prognostication and therapeutic decision making. JAMA 284:835, 2000

BOERSMA E et al: Platelet glycoprotein IIb/IIIa inhibitors in acute coronary syndromes: A meta-analysis of all major randomised clinical trials. Lancet 359:189, 2002

BRAUNWALD E: Unstable angina: A classification. Circulation 80:410, 1989
——— et al: ACC/AHA guideline update for the management of patients with unstable angina and non-ST segment elevation myocardial infarction: A report of the American College of Cardiology/American Heart Association Task Force on Practice Guidelines (Committee on the Management of Unstable Angina). *www.acc.org* 2002; accessed 3/15/2002

CANNON CP, BRAUNWALD E: Unstable angina, in *Braunwald's Heart Disease*, 7th ed, DP Zipes et al (eds). Philadelphia, Saunders, 2005
——— et al: Comparison of early invasive and conservative strategies in patients with unstable coronary syndromes treated with the glycoprotein IIb/IIIa inhibitor tirofiban. N Engl J Med 344:1879, 2001

CLOPIDOGREL IN UNSTABLE ANGINA TO PREVENT RECURRENT EVENTS TRIAL INVESTIGATORS: Effects of clopidogrel in addition to aspirin in patients with acute coronary syndromes without ST-segment elevation. N Engl J Med 345:494, 2001

228   ST-SEGMENT ELEVATION MYOCARDIAL INFARCTION
Elliott M. Antman, Eugene Braunwald

Acute myocardial infarction (AMI) is one of the most common diagnoses in hospitalized patients in industrialized countries. In the United States, approximately 650,000 patients experience a new AMI and 450,000 experience a recurrent AMI each year. The early (30-day) mortality rate from AMI is ~30%, with more than half of these deaths occurring before the stricken individual reaches the hospital. Although the mortality rate after admission for AMI has declined by ~30% over the past two decades, approximately 1 of every 25 patients who survives the initial hospitalization dies in the first year after AMI. Survival is markedly reduced in elderly patients (over age 75).

FIGURE 228-1 Acute coronary syndromes. Following disruption of a vulnerable plaque, patients experience ischemic discomfort resulting from a reduction of flow through the affected epicardial coronary artery. The flow reduction may be caused by a completely occlusive thrombus (right) or subtotally occlusive thrombus (left). Patients with ischemic discomfort may present with or without ST-segment elevation. Of patients with ST-segment elevation, the majority (*large red arrow*) ultimately develop a Q-wave MI (QwMI), while a minority (*small red arrow*) develop a non-Q-wave MI (NQMI). Patients who present with ST-segment elevation are suffering from either unstable angina or a non-ST-segment elevation MI (NSTEMI) (*large green arrows*), a distinction that is ultimately made on the presence or absence of a serum cardiac marker such as CKMB or a cardiac troponin detected in the blood. The majority presenting with NSTEMI ultimately develop a NQMI on the ECG; a minority develop a QwMI (*small green arrow*). (Adapted from CW Hamm et al: Lancet 358:1533, 2001, and MJ Davies: Heart 83:361, 2000.)

When patients with acute ischemic discomfort are first seen, the working diagnosis is that they are suffering from an acute coronary syndrome (Fig. 228-1). The 12-lead electrocardiogram (ECG) is at the center of the decision pathway for management since it permits distinction of those patients presenting with ST-segment elevation from those presenting without ST-segment elevation. Serum cardiac biomarkers are obtained to distinguish unstable angina from non-ST-segment MI (NSTEMI) (Chap. 227) and to assess the magnitude of an ST-segment elevation MI (STEMI).

PATHOPHYSIOLOGY: ROLE OF ACUTE PLAQUE RUPTURE

STEMI generally occurs when coronary blood flow decreases abruptly after a thrombotic occlusion of a coronary artery previously affected by atherosclerosis. Slowly developing, high-grade coronary artery stenoses do not usually precipitate STEMI because of the development of a rich collateral network over time. Instead, STEMI occurs when a coronary artery thrombus develops rapidly at a site of vascular injury. This injury is produced or facilitated by factors such as cigarette smoking, hypertension, and lipid accumulation. In most cases, infarction occurs when an atherosclerotic plaque fissures, ruptures, or ulcerates and when conditions (local or systemic) favor thrombogenesis, so that a mural thrombus forms at the site of rupture and leads to coronary artery occlusion. Histologic studies indicate that the coronary plaques prone to rupture are those with a rich lipid core and a thin fibrous cap (Chap. 224). After an initial platelet monolayer forms at the site of the ruptured plaque, various agonists (collagen, ADP, epinephrine, serotonin) promote platelet activation. After agonist stimulation of platelets, there are production and release of thromboxane A_2 (a potent local vasoconstrictor), further platelet activation, and potential resistance to thrombolysis.

In addition to the generation of thromboxane A_2, activation of platelets by agonists promotes a conformational change in the glycoprotein IIb/IIIa receptor (Chap. 101). Once converted to its functional state, this receptor develops a high affinity for amino acid sequences on soluble adhesive proteins (i.e., integrins) such as von Willebrand factor (vWF) and fibrinogen. Since vWF and fibrinogen are multiva-

lent molecules, they can bind to two different platelets simultaneously, resulting in platelet cross-linking and aggregation.

The coagulation cascade is activated on exposure of tissue factor in damaged endothelial cells at the site of the ruptured plaque. Factors VII and X are activated, ultimately leading to the conversion of prothrombin to thrombin, which then converts fibrinogen to fibrin (Chap. 102). Fluid-phase and clot-bound thrombin participate in an autoamplification reaction that leads to further activation of the coagulation cascade. The culprit coronary artery eventually becomes occluded by a thrombus containing platelet aggregates and fibrin strands.

In rare cases, STEMI may be due to coronary artery occlusion caused by coronary emboli, congenital abnormalities, coronary spasm, and a wide variety of systemic—particularly inflammatory—diseases. The amount of myocardial damage caused by coronary occlusion depends on (1) the territory supplied by the affected vessel, (2) whether or not the vessel becomes totally occluded, (3) the duration of coronary occlusion, (4) the quantity of blood supplied by collateral vessels to the affected tissue, (5) the demand for oxygen of the myocardium whose blood supply has been suddenly limited, (6) native factors that can produce early spontaneous lysis of the occlusive thrombus, and (7) the adequacy of myocardial perfusion in the infarct zone when flow is restored in the occluded epicardial coronary artery.

Patients at increased risk of developing STEMI include those with multiple coronary risk factors (Chap. 224) and those with unstable angina or Prinzmetal's variant angina (Chap. 227). Less common underlying medical conditions predisposing patients to STEMI include hypercoagulability, collagen vascular disease, cocaine abuse, and intracardiac thrombi or masses that can produce coronary emboli.

CLINICAL PRESENTATION

In up to one-half of cases, a precipitating factor appears to be present before STEMI, such as vigorous physical exercise, emotional stress, or a medical or surgical illness. Although STEMI may commence at any time of the day or night, circadian variations have been reported such that clusters are seen in the morning within a few hours of awakening.

Pain is the most common presenting complaint in patients with STEMI. The pain is deep and visceral; adjectives commonly used to describe it are *heavy*, *squeezing*, and *crushing*, although occasionally it is described as stabbing or burning (Chap. 12). It is similar in character to the discomfort of angina pectoris (Chap. 226) but is usually more severe and lasts longer. Typically the pain involves the central portion of the chest and/or the epigastrium, and on occasion it radiates to the arms. Less common sites of radiation include the abdomen, back, lower jaw, and neck. The frequent location of the pain beneath the xiphoid and patients' denial that they may be suffering a heart attack are chiefly responsible for the common mistaken impression of indigestion. The pain of STEMI may radiate as high as the occipital area but not below the umbilicus. It is often accompanied by weakness, sweating, nausea, vomiting, anxiety, and a sense of impending doom. The pain may commence when the patient is at rest, but when it begins during a period of exertion, it does not usually subside with cessation of activity, in contrast to angina pectoris.

The pain of STEMI can simulate pain from acute pericarditis (Chap. 222), pulmonary embolism (Chap. 244), acute aortic dissection (Chap. 231), costochondritis, and gastrointestinal disorders. These conditions should therefore be considered in the differential diagnosis. Radiation of discomfort to the trapezius is not seen in patients with STEMI and may be a useful distinguishing feature that suggests pericarditis is the correct diagnosis. However, *pain is not uniformly present in patients with STEMI*. The proportion of painless STEMIs is greater in patients with diabetes mellitus, and it increases with age. In the elderly, STEMI may present as sudden-onset breathlessness, which may progress to pulmonary edema. Other less common presentations, with or without pain, include sudden loss of consciousness, a confusional state, a sensation of profound weakness, the appearance of an arrhythmia, evidence of peripheral embolism, or merely an un-explained drop in arterial pressure.

PHYSICAL FINDINGS Most patients are anxious and restless, attempting unsuccessfully to relieve the pain by moving about in bed, altering their position, and stretching. Pallor associated with perspiration and coolness of the extremities occurs commonly. The combination of sub-sternal chest pain persisting for >30 min and diaphoresis strongly suggests STEMI. Although many patients have a normal pulse rate and blood pressure within the first hour of STEMI, about one-fourth of patients with anterior infarction have manifestations of sympathetic nervous system hyperactivity (tachycardia and/or hypertension), and up to one-half with inferior infarction show evidence of parasympathetic hyperactivity (bradycardia and/or hypotension).

The precordium is usually quiet, and the apical impulse may be difficult to palpate. In patients with anterior wall infarction, an abnormal systolic pulsation caused by dyskinetic bulging of infarcted myocardium may develop in the periapical area within the first days of the illness and then may resolve. Other physical signs of ventricular dysfunction include fourth (S_4) and third (S_3) heart sounds, decreased intensity of the first heart sound, and paradoxical splitting of the second heart sound (Chap. 209). A transient midsystolic or late systolic apical systolic murmur due to dysfunction of the mitral valve apparatus may be present. A pericardial friction rub is heard in many patients with transmural STEMI at some time in the course of the disease, if they are examined frequently. The carotid pulse is often decreased in volume, reflecting reduced stroke volume. Temperature elevations up to 38°C may be observed during the first week after STEMI. The arterial pressure is variable; in most patients with transmural infarction, systolic pressure declines by approximately 10 to 15 mmHg from the preinfarction state.

LABORATORY FINDINGS

Myocardial infarction (MI) progresses through the following temporal stages: (1) acute (first few hours to 7 days), (2) healing (7 to 28 days), and (3) healed (≥29 days). When evaluating the results of diagnostic tests for STEMI, the temporal phase of the infarction process must be considered. The laboratory tests of value in confirming the diagnosis may be divided into four groups: (1) ECG, (2) serum cardiac biomarkers, (3) cardiac imaging, and (4) nonspecific indexes of tissue necrosis and inflammation.

ELECTROCARDIOGRAM The electrocardiographic manifestations of STEMI are described in Chap. 210. During the initial stage of the acute phase of MI, total occlusion of an epicardial artery produces ST-segment elevation. Most patients initially presenting with ST-segment elevation evolve Q waves on the ECG and are ultimately diagnosed as having sustained a Q-wave MI (Fig. 228-1). A small proportion may sustain only a non-Q-wave MI. When the obstructing thrombus is not totally occlusive, obstruction is transient, or if a rich collateral network is present, no ST-segment elevation is seen. Such patients are initially considered to be experiencing either unstable angina or NSTEMI (Chap. 227). Among patients presenting *without* ST-segment elevation, if a serum cardiac biomarker of necrosis (see below) is detected and no Q wave develops, the diagnosis of non-Q-wave MI is ultimately made (Fig. 228-1). A minority of patients who present initially without ST-segment elevation may develop a Q-wave MI. Previously it was believed that transmural MI is present if the ECG demonstrates Q waves or loss of R waves, and nontransmural MI may be present if the ECG shows only transient ST-segment and T-wave changes. However, electrocardiographic-pathologic correlations are far from perfect; therefore a more rational nomenclature for designating electrocardiographic infarction is now commonly in use, with the terms *Q-wave MI* and *non-Q-wave MI* replacing the terms *transmural MI* and *nontransmural MI*, respectively (Fig. 228-1).

SERUM CARDIAC BIOMARKERS Certain proteins, called serum cardiac markers, are released into the blood in large quantities from necrotic

heart muscle after STEMI. The rate of liberation of specific proteins differs depending on their intracellular location and molecular weight and the local blood and lymphatic flow. The temporal pattern of protein release is of diagnostic importance, but contemporary urgent reperfusion strategies necessitate making a decision (based largely on a combination of clinical and ECG findings) before the results of blood tests have returned from the central laboratory. Rapid whole-blood bedside assays for serum cardiac markers are now available and may facilitate management decisions, particularly in patients with nondiagnostic ECGs.

Creatine phosphokinase (CK) rises within 4 to 8 h and generally returns to normal by 48 to 72 h (Fig. 228-2). An important drawback of total CK measurement is its lack of specificity for STEMI, as CK may be elevated with skeletal muscle trauma. A two- to threefold elevation of total CK may follow an intramuscular injection, for example. This ambiguity may lead to the erroneous diagnosis of STEMI in a patient who has been given an intramuscular injection of a narcotic for chest pain of noncardiac origin. Other potential sources of total CK elevation are (1) skeletal muscular diseases, including muscular dystrophy, myopathies, and polymyositis; (2) electrical cardioversion; (3) hypothyroidism; (4) stroke; (5) surgery; and (6) skeletal muscle damage secondary to trauma, convulsions, and prolonged immobilization.

The MB isoenzyme of CK has the advantage over total CK that it is not present in significant concentrations in extracardiac tissue and therefore is considerably more specific. However, cardiac surgery, myocarditis, and electrical cardioversion often result in elevated serum levels of the MB isoenzyme. A ratio (relative index) of CKMB mass: CK activity ≥2.5 suggests but is not diagnostic of a myocardial rather than a skeletal muscle source for the CKMB elevation. This ratio is less useful when levels of total CK are high owing to skeletal muscle injury or when the total CK level is within the normal range but CKMB is elevated.

Cardiac-specific troponin T (cTnT) and *cardiac-specific troponin I* (cTnI) have amino acid sequences different from those of the skeletal muscle forms of these proteins. These differences permitted the development of quantitative assays for cTnT and cTnI with highly specific monoclonal antibodies. Since cTnT and cTnI are not normally detectable in the blood of healthy individuals but may increase after

FIGURE 228-2 Typical cardiac biomarkers that are used to evaluate patients with STEMI include the MB isoenzyme of CK (CKMB) and cardiac-specific troponins. The white horizontal line depicts the upper reference limit (URL) for the cardiac biomarker in the clinical chemistry laboratory. The kinetics of release of CKMB and cardiac troponin in patients who do not undergo reperfusion are shown in the solid green and red curves as multiples of the URL. When patients with STEMI undergo reperfusion, as depicted in the dashed green and red curves, the cardiac biomarkers are detected sooner, rise to a higher peak value, but decline more rapidly, resulting in a smaller area under the curve and limitation of infarct size. (*Adapted from JS Alpert et al: J Am Coll Cardiol 36:959, 2000, and AH Wu et al. Clin Chem 45:1104, 1999.*)

STEMI to levels >20 times higher than the upper reference limit, the noise level of the assay), the measurement of cTnT or cTnI is of considerable diagnostic usefulness, and they are now the preferred biochemical markers for MI (Fig. 228-2). The cardiac troponins are particularly valuable when there is clinical suspicion of either skeletal muscle injury or a small MI that may be below the detection limit for CK and CKMB measurements. Levels of cTnI and cTnT may remain elevated for 7 to 10 days after STEMI.

Myoglobin is released into the blood within only a few hours of the onset of STEMI. Although myoglobin is one of the first serum cardiac markers that rises above the normal range after STEMI, it lacks cardiac specificity, and it is rapidly excreted in the urine, so that blood levels return to the normal range within 24 h of the onset of infarction.

Many hospitals are using cTnT or cTnI rather than CKMB as the routine serum cardiac marker for diagnosis of STEMI, although any of these analytes remains clinically acceptable. It is *not* cost-effective to measure both a cardiac-specific troponin and CKMB at all time points in every patient. However, in view of the prolonged elevation of cardiac-specific troponins (>1 week), episodes of recurrent ischemic discomfort and suspected recurrent MI are more readily diagnosed with a serum cardiac marker that remains elevated in the blood more briefly, such as CKMB or myoglobin.

While it has long been recognized that the total quantity of protein released correlates with the size of the infarct, the peak protein concentration correlates only weakly with infarct size. Recanalization of a coronary artery occlusion (either spontaneously or by mechanical or pharmacologic means) in the early hours of STEMI causes earlier and higher peaking (at about 8 to 12 h after reperfusion) of serum cardiac markers (Fig. 228-2).

For the purposes of confirming the diagnosis of MI, serum cardiac markers should be measured on admission, 6 to 9 h after admission, and 12 to 24 h after admission if the diagnosis remains uncertain.

The *nonspecific reaction* to myocardial injury is associated with polymorphonuclear leukocytosis, which appears within a few hours after the onset of pain and persists for 3 to 7 days; the white blood cell count often reaches levels of 12,000 to 15,000/μL. The erythrocyte sedimentation rate rises more slowly than the white blood cell count, peaking during the first week and sometimes remaining elevated for 1 or 2 weeks.

CARDIAC IMAGING Abnormalities of wall motion on *two-dimensional echocardiography* (Chap. 211) are almost universally present. Although acute STEMI cannot be distinguished from an old myocardial scar or from acute severe ischemia by echocardiography, the ease and safety of the procedure make its use appealing as a screening tool. In the emergency department setting, early detection of the presence or absence of wall motion abnormalities by echocardiography can aid in management decisions, such as whether the patient should receive reperfusion therapy [e.g., fibrinolysis or a percutaneous coronary intervention (PCI)]. Echocardiographic estimation of left ventricular (LV) function is useful prognostically; detection of reduced function serves as an indication for therapy with an angiotensin-converting enzyme (ACE) inhibitor (see "Angiotensin-Converting Enzyme Inhibitors," below). Echocardiography may also identify the presence of right ventricular (RV) infarction, ventricular aneurysm, pericardial effusion, and LV thrombus. In addition, Doppler echocardiography is useful in the detection and quantitation of a ventricular septal defect and mitral regurgitation, two serious complications of STEMI (see below).

Several *radionuclide imaging techniques* (Chap. 211) are available for evaluating patients with suspected STEMI. However, these imag-

FIGURE 228-3 Major components of time delay between onset of symptoms from STEMI and restoration of flow in the infarct-related artery. Plotted sequentially from left to right are shown the times for patients to recognize symptoms and seek medical attention, transportation to the hospital, in-hospital decision-making, implementation of reperfusion strategy, and restoration of flow once the reperfusion strategy has been initiated. The time to initiate fibrinolytic therapy is the "door-to-needle" (D-N) time; this is followed by the period of time required for pharmacologic restoration of flow. More time is required to move the patient to the catheterization laboratory for a percutaneous coronary interventional (PCI) procedure, referred to as the "door-to-balloon" (D-B) time, but restoration of flow in the epicardial infarct-related artery occurs promptly after PCI. At the bottom are shown a variety of methods for speeding the time to reperfusion along with the goals for the time intervals for the various components of the time delay. *(Adapted from CP Cannon et al: J Thromb Thrombol 1:27, 1994.)*

ing modalities are used less often than echocardiography because they are more cumbersome and lack sensitivity and specificity in many clinical circumstances. Myocardial perfusion imaging with ^{201}Tl or ^{99m}Tc-sestamibi, which are distributed in proportion to myocardial blood flow and concentrated by viable myocardium (Chap. 226), reveal a defect ("cold spot") in most patients during the first few hours after development of a transmural infarct. However, although perfusion scanning is extremely sensitive, it cannot distinguish acute infarcts from chronic scars and thus is not specific for the diagnosis of *acute* MI. Radionuclide ventriculography, carried out with ^{99m}Tc-labeled red blood cells, frequently demonstrates wall motion disorders and reduction in the ventricular ejection fraction in patients with STEMI. While of value in assessing the hemodynamic consequences of infarction and in aiding in the diagnosis of RV infarction when the RV ejection fraction is depressed, this technique is nonspecific, as many cardiac abnormalities other than MI alter the radionuclide ventriculogram.

INITIAL MANAGEMENT

PREHOSPITAL CARE The prognosis in STEMI is largely related to the occurrence of two general classes of complications: (1) electrical complications (arrhythmias) and (2) mechanical complications ("pump failure"). Most out-of-hospital deaths from STEMI are due to the sudden development of ventricular fibrillation. The vast majority of deaths due to ventricular fibrillation occur within the first 24 h of the onset of symptoms, and, of these, over half occur in the first hour. Therefore, the major elements of prehospital care of patients with suspected STEMI include (1) recognition of symptoms by the patient and prompt seeking of medical attention; (2) rapid deployment of an emergency medical team capable of performing resuscitative maneuvers, including defibrillation; (3) expeditious transportation of the patient to a hospital facility that is continuously staffed by physicians and nurses skilled in managing arrhythmias and providing advanced cardiac life support; and (4) expeditious implementation of reperfusion therapy (Fig. 228-3). The biggest delay usually occurs not during transportation to the hospital but rather between the onset of pain and the patient's decision to call for help. This delay can best be reduced by education of the public by health care professionals concerning the significance of chest pain and the importance of seeking early medical attention. Increasingly, monitoring and treatment are carried out by trained personnel in the ambulance, further shortening the time between the onset of the infarction and appropriate treatment. General guidelines for initiation of fibrinolysis in the prehospital setting include the ability to transmit 12-lead ECGs to confirm the diagnosis, the presence of paramedics in the ambulance, training of paramedics in the interpretation of ECGs and management of STEMI, and online medical command and control that can authorize the initiation of treatment in the field.

MANAGEMENT IN THE EMERGENCY DEPARTMENT In the emergency department, the goals for the management of patients with suspected STEMI include control of cardiac pain, rapid identification of patients who are candidates for urgent reperfusion therapy, triage of lower-risk patients to the appropriate location in the hospital, and avoidance of inappropriate discharge of patients with STEMI. Many aspects of the treatment of STEMI are initiated in the emergency department and then continued during the in-hospital phase of management.

Aspirin is essential in the management of patients with suspected STEMI and is effective across the entire spectrum of acute coronary syndromes (Fig. 228-1). Rapid inhibition of cyclooxygenase in platelets followed by a reduction of thromboxane A_2 levels is achieved by buccal absorption of a chewed 160- to 325-mg tablet in the emergency department. This measure should be followed by daily oral administration of aspirin in a dose of 75 to 162 mg.

In patients whose arterial oxygen saturation is normal as estimated by pulse oximetry or measured by an arterial blood gas specimen, supplemental oxygen is of limited if any clinical benefit and therefore is not cost-effective. However, when hypoxemia is present, oxygen should be administered by nasal prongs or face mask (2 to 4 L/min) for the first 6 to 12 h after infarction; the patient should then be reassessed to determine if there is a continued need for such treatment.

Control of Pain Sublingual *nitroglycerin* can be given safely to most patients with STEMI. Up to three doses of 0.4 mg should be administered at about 5-min intervals. In addition to diminishing or abolishing chest discomfort, nitroglycerin may be capable of both decreasing myocardial oxygen demand (by lowering preload) and increasing myocardial oxygen supply (by dilating infarct-related coronary vessels or collateral vessels). In patients whose initially favorable response to sublingual nitroglycerin is followed by the return of chest pain, particularly if accompanied by other evidence of ongoing ischemia such as further ST-segment or T-wave shifts, the use of intravenous nitroglycerin should be considered. Therapy with nitrates should be avoided in patients who present with low systolic arterial pressure (<90 mmHg) or in whom there is clinical suspicion of RV infarction (inferior infarction on ECG, elevated jugular venous pressure, clear lungs, and hypotension). Nitrates should not be administered to patients who have taken the phosphodiesterase-5 inhibitor sildenafil for erectile dysfunction within the preceding 24 h since it may potentiate the hypotensive effects of nitrates. An idiosyncratic reaction to nitrates, consisting of sudden marked hypotension, sometimes occurs but can usually be reversed promptly by the rapid administration of intravenous atropine.

Morphine is a very effective analgesic for the pain associated with STEMI. However, it may reduce sympathetically mediated arteriolar and venous constriction, and the resulting venous pooling may reduce cardiac output and arterial pressure. These hemodynamic disturbances usually respond promptly to elevation of the legs, but in some patients volume expansion with intravenous saline is required. The patient may experience diaphoresis and nausea, but these events usually pass and are replaced by a feeling of well-being associated with the relief of pain. Morphine also has a vagotonic effect and may cause bradycardia or advanced degrees of heart block, particularly in patients with pos-

teroinferior infarction. These side effects usually respond to atropine (0.5 mg intravenously). Morphine is routinely administered by repetitive (every 5 min) intravenous injection of small doses (2 to 4 mg) rather than by the subcutaneous administration of a larger quantity, because absorption may be unpredictable by the latter route.

Intravenous *beta blockers* are also useful in the control of the pain of STEMI. These drugs control pain effectively in some patients, presumably by diminishing myocardial oxygen demand and hence ischemia. More important, there is evidence that intravenous beta blockers reduce in-hospital mortality, particularly in high-risk patients (see "Beta-Adrenoceptor Blockers," below). A commonly employed regimen is metoprolol, 5 mg every 2 to 5 min for a total of three doses, provided the patient has a heart rate > 60 beats per minute (bpm), systolic pressure > 100 mmHg, a PR interval < 0.24 s, and rales that are no higher than 10 cm up from the diaphragm. Fifteen minutes after the last intravenous dose, an oral regimen is initiated of 50 mg every 6 h for 48 h, followed by 100 mg every 12 h.

Unlike beta blockers, calcium antagonists are of little value in the acute setting, and there is evidence that short-acting dihydropyridines may be associated with an increased mortality risk.

Management Strategies The primary tool for screening patients and making triage decisions is the initial 12-lead ECG. When ST-segment elevation of at least 2 mm in two contiguous precordial leads and 1 mm in two limb leads is present, a patient should be considered a candidate for *reperfusion therapy* (Fig. 228-4). The process of selecting patients for fibrinolysis versus primary PCI (angioplasty, or stenting; Chap. 229) is discussed below. In the absence of ST-segment elevation, fibrinolysis is not helpful, and evidence exists suggesting that it may be harmful.

Limitation of Infarct Size The quantity of myocardium that becomes necrotic as a consequence of a coronary artery occlusion is determined by factors other than just the site of occlusion. While the central zone of the infarct contains necrotic tissue that is irretrievably lost, the fate of the surrounding ischemic myocardium may be improved by timely restoration of coronary perfusion, reduction of myocardial oxygen demands, prevention of the accumulation of noxious metabolites, and blunting of the impact of mediators of reperfusion injury (e.g., calcium overload and oxygen-derived free radicals). Up to one-third of patients with STEMI may achieve *spontaneous* reperfusion of the infarct-related coronary artery within 24 h and experience improved healing of infarcted tissue. Reperfusion either pharmacologically (by fibrinolysis)

FIGURE 228-4 Reperfusion strategies for STEMI. Following the onset of symptoms of STEMI, the patient is transported to the hospital where reperfusion options are assessed. If the hospital is not capable of performing percutaneous coronary intervention (PCI), the patient is treated with fibrinolytic therapy; if the hospital is capable of performing PCI, reperfusion is implemented in the form of primary PCI. Patients who receive fibrinolytic therapy should undergo noninvasive risk stratification (Noninv. Risk Strat.). Patients with continued chest pain or failure to resolve ST-segment elevation by about 90 min should be referred for rescue PCI; if spontaneous recurrent ischemia or provoked ischemia is detected on noninvasive testing later in the hospital, patients should be referred for PCI or coronary artery bypass graft (CABG) surgery. All patients should receive therapies for secondary prevention of STEMI. (*Adapted from PW Armstrong, D Collen, EM Antman: Circulation 107:2533, 2003, with permission.*)

or by PCI accelerates the occluded infarct-related artery in those patients in whom spontaneous thrombolysis ultimately would have occurred and also greatly increases the number of patients in whom restoration of flow in the infarct-related artery is accomplished. Timely restoration of flow in the epicardial infarct–related artery combined with improved perfusion of the downstream zone of infarcted myocardium results in a limitation of infarct size. Protection of the ischemic myocardium by the maintenance of an optimal balance between myocardial oxygen supply and demand through pain control, treatment of congestive heart failure (CHF), and minimization of tachycardia and hypertension extends the "window" of time for the salvage of myocardium by reperfusion strategies.

Glucocorticoids and nonsteroidal anti-inflammatory agents, with the exception of aspirin, should be avoided in the setting of STEMI. They can impair infarct healing and increase the risk of myocardial rupture, and their use may result in a larger infarct scar. In addition, they can increase coronary vascular resistance, thereby potentially reducing flow to ischemic myocardium.

Primary Percutaneous Coronary Intervention (See also Chap. 229) PCI, usually angioplasty and/or stenting without preceding fibrinolysis, referred to as *primary PCI*, is effective in restoring perfusion in STEMI when carried out on an emergency basis in the first few hours of MI. It has the advantage of being applicable to patients who have contraindications to fibrinolytic therapy but otherwise are considered appropriate candidates for reperfusion. It appears to be more effective than fibrinolysis in opening occluded coronary arteries and, *when performed by experienced operators [≥75 PCI cases (not necessarily primary) per year] in dedicated medical centers (≥36 primary PCI cases per year)*, is associated with better short-term and long-term clinical outcomes. Compared with fibrinolysis, primary PCI is generally preferred when the diagnosis is in doubt, cardiogenic shock is present (especially in patients <75 years), bleeding risk is increased, or symptoms have been present for at least 2 to 3 h when the clot is more mature and less easily lysed by fibrinolytic drugs. However, PCI is expensive in terms of personnel and facilities, and its applicability is limited by its availability, around the clock, in only a minority of hospitals.

Fibrinolysis If no contraindications are present (see below), fibrinolytic therapy should ideally be initiated within 30 min of presentation (i.e., door-to-needle time ≤30 min). The principal goal of fibrinolysis is prompt restoration of full coronary arterial patency. The fibrinolytic agents tissue plasminogen activator (tPA), streptokinase, tenecteplase (TNK), and reteplase (rPA) have been approved by the U.S. Food and Drug Administration for intravenous use in the setting of STEMI. These drugs all act by promoting the conversion of plasminogen to plasmin, which subsequently lyses fibrin thrombi. Although considerable emphasis was first placed on a distinction between more fibrin-specific agents, such as tPA, and non-fibrin-specific agents, such as streptokinase, it is now recognized that these differences are only relative, as some degree of systemic fibrinolysis occurs with tPA. TNK and rPA are referred to as *bolus fibrinolytics* since their administration does not require a prolonged intravenous infusion.

When assessed angiographically, flow in the culprit coronary artery is described by a simple qualitative scale called the *thrombolysis in myocardial infarction (TIMI) grading system*: grade 0 indicates complete occlusion of the infarct-related artery; grade 1 indicates some penetration of the contrast material beyond the point of obstruction but without perfusion of the distal coronary bed; grade 2 indicates perfusion of the entire infarct vessel into the distal bed but with flow that is delayed compared with that of a normal artery; and grade 3 indicates full perfusion of the infarct vessel with normal flow. Early reports frequently lumped TIMI grades 2 and 3 under the general category of *patency*, but it is now recognized that grade 3 flow is the goal of reperfusion therapy, because full perfusion of the infarct-related coronary artery yields far better results in terms of limiting infarct size, maintenance of LV function, and reduction of both short- and long-term mortality rates. Relatively new methods of angiographic assessment of the efficacy of fibrinolysis include counting the number of frames on the cine film required for dye to flow from the origin of the infarct-related artery to a landmark in the distal vascular bed (*TIMI frame count*) and determining the rate of entry and exit of contrast dye from the microvasculature in the myocardial infarct zone (*TIMI myocardial perfusion grade*).

Fibrinolytic therapy can reduce the relative risk of in-hospital death by up to 50% when administered within the first hour of the onset of symptoms of STEMI, and much of this benefit is maintained for at least 10 years. Appropriately used fibrinolytic therapy appears to reduce infarct size, limit LV dysfunction, and reduce the incidence of serious complications such as septal rupture, cardiogenic shock, and malignant ventricular arrhythmias. Since myocardium can be salvaged only before it has been irreversibly injured, the timing of reperfusion therapy, by fibrinolysis or a catheter-based approach, is of extreme importance in achieving maximum benefit. While the upper time limit depends on specific factors in individual patients, it is clear that "every minute counts" and that patients treated within 1 to 3 h of the onset of symptoms generally benefit most. Although reduction of the mortality rate is more modest, the therapy remains of benefit for many patients seen 3 to 6 h after the onset of infarction, and some benefit appears to be possible up to 12 h, especially if chest discomfort is still present and ST segments remain elevated in ECG leads that do not yet demonstrate new Q waves. Compared with PCI for STEMI (primary PCI), fibrinolysis is generally the preferred reperfusion strategy for patients presenting in the first hour of symptoms, if there are logistical concerns about transportation of the patient to a suitable PCI center (experienced operator and team with a track record for a "door-to-balloon" time of < 2 h), or there is an anticipated delay of at least 1 h between the time that fibrinolysis could be started versus implementation of PCI. Although patients <75 years achieve a greater relative reduction in the mortality rate with fibrinolytic therapy than do older patients, the higher *absolute* mortality rate (15 to 25%) in the latter results in similar absolute reductions in the mortality rates for both age groups.

tPA and the other relatively fibrin-specific plasminogen activators rPA and TNK are more effective than streptokinase at restoring full perfusion—i.e., TIMI grade 3 coronary flow—and have a small edge in improving survival as well. The current recommended regimen of tPA consists of a 15-mg bolus followed by 50 mg intravenously over the first 30 min, followed by 35 mg over the next 60 min. Streptokinase is administered as 1.5 million units (MU) intravenously over 1 h. rPA is administered in a double-bolus regimen consisting of a 10-MU bolus given over 2 to 3 min followed by a second 10-MU bolus 30 min later. TNK is given as a single weight-based intravenous bolus of 0.53 mg/kg over 10 s. In addition to the fibrinolytic agents discussed above, pharmacologic reperfusion typically involves adjunctive antiplatelet and antithrombotic drugs, as discussed subsequently.

Alternative pharmacologic regimens for reperfusion combine an intravenous glycoprotein IIb/IIIa inhibitor with a reduced dose of a fibrinolytic agent. Compared with fibrinolytic agents that involve a prolonged infusion (e.g., tPA) such combination reperfusion regimens facilitate the rate and extent of fibrinolysis by inhibiting platelet aggregation, weakening the clot structure, and allowing penetration of the thrombolytic agent deeper into the clot. However, combination reperfusion regimens have similar efficacy as compared with bolus fibrinolytics (e.g., rPA) and are associated with an increased risk of bleeding, especially in patients >75 years. Therefore, combination reperfusion regimens have not been approved for use but remain under active investigation to determine if they are helpful for preparing patients who are referred promptly for PCI—an experimental strategy called *facilitated PCI*.

CONTRAINDICATIONS AND COMPLICATIONS Clear contraindications to the use of fibrinolytic agents include a history of cerebrovascular hemorrhage at any time, a nonhemorrhagic stroke or other cerebrovascular event within the past year, marked hypertension (a reliably determined systolic arterial pressure > 180 mmHg and/or a diastolic pressure > 110 mmHg) at any time during the acute presentation, suspicion of aortic dissection, and active internal bleeding (excluding menses). While advanced age is associated with an increase in hemorrhagic complications, the benefit of fibrinolytic therapy in the elderly appears to justify its use if no other contraindications are present and the amount of myocardium in jeopardy appears to be substantial.

Relative contraindications to fibrinolytic therapy, which require assessment of the risk:benefit ratio, include current use of anticoagulants (international normalized ratio ≥ 2), a recent (<2 weeks) invasive or surgical procedure or prolonged (>10 min) cardiopulmonary resuscitation, known bleeding diathesis, pregnancy, a hemorrhagic ophthalmic condition (e.g., hemorrhagic diabetic retinopathy), active peptic ulcer disease, and a history of severe hypertension that is currently adequately controlled. Because of the risk of an allergic reaction, patients should not receive streptokinase if that agent had been received within the preceding 5 days to 2 years.

Allergic reactions to streptokinase occur in ~2% of patients who receive it. While a minor degree of hypotension occurs in 4 to 10% of patients given this agent, marked hypotension occurs, although rarely, in association with severe allergic reactions.

Hemorrhage is the most frequent and potentially the most serious complication. Because bleeding episodes that require transfusion are more common when patients require invasive procedures, unnecessary venous or arterial interventions should be avoided in patients receiving thrombolytic agents. Hemorrhagic stroke is the most serious complication and occurs in ~0.5 to 0.9% of patients being treated with these agents. This rate increases with advancing age, with patients >70 years experiencing roughly twice the rate of intracranial hemorrhage as those <65 years. Large-scale intervention trials have suggested that the rate of intracranial hemorrhage with tPA or rPA is slightly higher than with streptokinase.

Cardiac catheterization and coronary angiography should be carried out after fibrinolytic therapy if there is evidence of either (1) failure of reperfusion (persistent chest pain and ST-segment elevation >90 min), in which case a *rescue PCI* should be considered; or (2) coronary artery reocclusion (reelevation of ST segments and/or recurrent chest pain) or the development of recurrent ischemia (such as recurrent angina in the early hospital course or a positive exercise stress test before discharge), in which case an *elective PCI* should be considered. The potential benefits of routine angiography after PCI even in asymptomatic patients following administration of fibrinolytic therapy are controversial, but such an approach may have merit given the numerous technological advances that have occurred in the catheterization laboratory and the increasing number of skilled interventionalists. Coronary artery bypass surgery should be reserved for patients whose coronary anatomy is unsuited to angioplasty but in whom revascularization appears to be advisable because of extensive jeopardized myocardium or recurrent ischemia.

HOSPITAL PHASE MANAGEMENT

CORONARY CARE UNITS These units are routinely equipped with a system that permits continuous monitoring of the cardiac rhythm of each patient and hemodynamic monitoring in selected patients. Defibrillators, respirators, noninvasive transthoracic pacemakers, and facilities for introducing pacing catheters and flow-directed balloon-tipped catheters are also usually available. Equally important is the organization of a highly trained team of nurses who can recognize arrhythmias; adjust the dosage of antiarrhythmic, vasoactive, and anticoagulant drugs; and perform cardiac resuscitation, including electroshock, when necessary.

Patients should be admitted to a coronary care unit early in their illness when it is expected that they will derive benefit from the sophisticated and expensive care provided. The availability of electrocardiographic monitoring and trained personnel outside the coronary care unit has made it possible to admit lower-risk patients (e.g., those not hemodynamically compromised and without active arrhythmias) to "intermediate care units."

The duration of stay in the coronary care unit is dictated by the ongoing need for intensive care. If STEMI has been ruled out (ideally within 8 to 12 h) and symptoms are controlled with oral therapy, patients may be transferred out of the coronary care unit. Also, patients who have a confirmed STEMI but who are considered to be at low risk (no prior infarction and no persistent chest discomfort, CHF, hypotension, or cardiac arrhythmias) may be safely transferred out of the coronary care unit within 24 h.

Activity Factors that increase the work of the heart during the initial hours of infarction may increase the size of the infarct. Therefore, patients with STEMI should be kept at bed rest for the first 12 h. However, in the absence of complications, patients should be encouraged, under supervision, to resume an upright posture by dangling their feet over the side of the bed and sitting in a chair within the first 24 h. This practice is psychologically beneficial and usually results in a reduction in the pulmonary capillary wedge pressure. In the absence of hypotension and other complications, by the second or third day patients typically are ambulating in their room with increasing duration and frequency, and they may shower or stand at the sink to bathe. By day 3 after infarction, patients should be increasing their ambulation progressively to a goal of 185 m (600 ft) at least three times a day.

Diet Because of the risk of emesis and aspiration soon after MI, patients should receive either nothing or only clear liquids by mouth for the first 4 to 12 h. The typical coronary care unit diet should provide $\leq 30\%$ of total calories as fat and have a cholesterol content of ≤ 300 mg/d. Complex carbohydrates should make up 50 to 55% of total calories. Portions should not be unusually large, and the menu should be enriched with foods that are high in potassium, magnesium, and fiber but low in sodium. Diabetes mellitus and hypertriglyceridemia are managed by restriction of concentrated sweets in the diet.

Bowels Bed rest and the effect of the narcotics used for the relief of pain often lead to constipation. A bedside commode rather than a bedpan, a diet rich in bulk, and the routine use of a stool softener such as dioctyl sodium sulfosuccinate (200 mg/d) are recommended. If the patient remains constipated despite these measures, a laxative can be prescribed. Contrary to prior belief, it is safe to perform a gentle rectal examination on patients with STEMI.

Sedation Many patients require sedation during hospitalization to withstand the period of enforced inactivity with tranquillity. Diazepam (5 mg), oxazepam (15 to 30 mg), or lorazepam (0.5 to 2 mg), given three or four times daily, is usually effective. An additional dose of any of the above medications may be given at night to ensure adequate sleep. Attention to this problem is especially important during the first few days in the coronary care unit, where the atmosphere of 24-h vigilance may interfere with the patient's sleep. However, sedation is no substitute for reassuring, quiet surroundings. Many drugs used in the coronary care unit, such as atropine, H_2 blockers, and narcotics, can produce delirium, particularly in the elderly. This effect should not be confused with agitation, and it is wise to conduct a thorough review of the patient's medications before arbitrarily prescribing additional doses of anxiolytics.

PHARMACOTHERAPY

ANTITHROMBOTIC AGENTS The use of antiplatelet and antithrombin therapy during the initial phase of STEMI is based on extensive laboratory and clinical evidence that thrombosis plays an important role in the pathogenesis of this condition. The primary goal of treatment with antiplatelet and antithrombin agents is to establish and maintain patency of the infarct-related artery. A secondary goal is to reduce the patient's tendency to thrombosis and thus the likelihood of mural thrombus formation or deep venous thrombosis, either of which could result in pulmonary embolization. The degree to which antiplatelet and antithrombin therapy achieves these goals partly determines how effectively it reduces the risk of mortality from STEMI.

As noted previously (see "Management in the Emergency Department," above), aspirin is the standard antiplatelet agent for patients with STEMI. The most compelling evidence for the benefits of anti-platelet therapy (mainly with aspirin) in STEMI is found in the comprehensive overview by the Antiplatelet Trialists' Collaboration. Data from nearly 20,000 patients with MI enrolled in 15 randomized trials were pooled and revealed a relative reduction of 27% in the mortality rate, from 14.2% in control patients to 10.4% in patients receiving antiplatelet agents.

The glycoprotein IIb/IIIa receptor is the focus of intense investigation (Chaps. 101 and 103). Glycoprotein inhibitors appear useful for preventing thrombotic complications in patients with STEMI undergoing PCI.

The standard antithrombin agent used in clinical practice is unfractionated heparin (UFH). Despite numerous clinical trials, the precise role of heparin in patients treated with fibrinolytic agents remains uncertain. The available data fail to show any convincing benefit of UFH with respect to either coronary arterial patency or mortality rate when UFH is added to a regimen of aspirin and a non-fibrin-specific thrombolytic agent such as streptokinase. Although not conclusively proven, it appears that the immediate administration of intravenous UFH, in addition to a regimen of aspirin and relatively fibrin-specific fibrinolytic agents (tPA, rPA, or TNK), helps to facilitate thrombolysis and to establish and maintain patency of the infarct-related artery. This effect is achieved at the cost of a small increased risk of bleeding. The recommended dose of UFH is an initial bolus of 60 U/kg (maximum 4000 U) followed by an initial infusion of 12 U/kg per hour (maximum 1000 U/h). The activated partial thromboplastin time during maintenance therapy should be 1.5 to 2 times the control value.

An alternative to UFH for anticoagulation of patients with STEMI that is being used with increased frequency in patients with unstable angina/NSTEMI (Chap. 227) are the low-molecular-weight heparin (LMWH) preparations, which are formed by enzymatic or chemical depolymerization to produce saccharide chains of varying length but with a mean molecular weight of about 5000 Da. The risks and benefits of LMWHs for management of patients with STEMI are under investigation.

Patients with an anterior location of the infarction, severe LV dysfunction, CHF, a history of embolism, two-dimensional echocardiographic evidence of mural thrombus, or atrial fibrillation are at increased risk of systemic or pulmonary thromboembolism. Such individuals should receive full therapeutic levels of antithrombin therapy (UFH or LMWHs) while hospitalized, followed by at least 3 months of warfarin therapy.

BETA-ADRENOCEPTOR BLOCKERS The benefits of beta blockers in patients with STEMI can be divided into those that occur immediately when the drug is given acutely and those that accrue over the long term when the drug is given for secondary prevention after an infarction. Acute intravenous beta blockade improves the myocardial oxygen supply-demand relationship, decreases pain, reduces infarct size, and decreases the incidence of serious ventricular arrhythmias. An overview of the data from 27,000 patients enrolled in nine randomized trials in the prethrombolytic era indicates that intravenous followed by oral beta blockade is associated with a 15% relative reduction in mortality, nonfatal reinfarction, and nonfatal cardiac arrest. In patients who undergo fibrinolysis soon after the onset of chest pain, no incremental reduction in mortality rate is seen with beta blockers, but recurrent ischemia and reinfarction are reduced.

Thus, beta blocker therapy after STEMI is useful for most patients (including those treated with an ACE inhibitor) except those in whom it is specifically contraindicated (patients with heart failure or severely compromised LV function, heart block, orthostatic hypotension, or a history of asthma) and perhaps those whose excellent long-term prognosis (defined as an expected mortality rate of <1% per year) markedly diminishes any potential benefit (patients <55 years with normal ventricular function, no complex ventricular ectopy, and no angina).

ANGIOTENSIN-CONVERTING ENZYME INHIBITORS ACE inhibitors reduce the mortality rate after STEMI, and the mortality benefits are additive to those achieved with aspirin and beta blockers. The maximum benefit is seen in high-risk patients (those who are elderly or who have an anterior infarction, a prior infarction, and/or globally depressed LV

function), but evidence suggests that a short-term benefit occurs when ACE inhibitors are prescribed unselectively to all hemodynamically stable patients with STEMI (i.e., those with a systolic pressure > 100 mmHg). The mechanism involves a reduction in ventricular remodeling after infarction (see "Ventricular Dysfunction," below) with a subsequent reduction in the risk of CHF. The rate of recurrent infarction may also be lower in patients treated chronically with ACE inhibitors after infarction.

ACE inhibitors should be prescribed within 24 h to all patients with STEMI. Before hospital discharge, LV function should be assessed with an imaging study. ACE inhibitors should be continued indefinitely in patients who have clinically evident CHF, in patients in whom an imaging study shows a reduction in global LV function or a large regional wall motion abnormality, or in those who are hypertensive. The use of angiotensin receptor blockers (ARBs) has not been as thoroughly explored as ACE inhibitors in STEMI patients. However, clinical experience in the management of patients with heart failure as well as data from clinical trials in STEMI patients suggest that ARBs may be useful in patients with depressed LV function or with clinical heart failure who are intolerant of an ACE inhibitor.

OTHER AGENTS Although the actual impact on the mortality rate is slight (three to four lives saved per 1000 patients treated), *nitrates* (intravenous or oral) may be useful in the relief of pain associated with STEMI. Favorable effects on the ischemic process and ventricular remodeling (see below) previously led many physicians to routinely use *intravenous nitroglycerin* (5 to 10 μg/min initial dose and up to 200 μg/min as long as hemodynamic stability is maintained) for the first 24 to 48 h after the onset of infarction. However, the benefits of routine use of intravenous nitroglycerin are less in the contemporary era where beta-adrenoceptor blockers and ACE inhibitors are routinely prescribed for patients with STEMI.

Results of multiple trials of different calcium antagonists have failed to establish a role for these agents in the treatment of most patients with STEMI, in contrast to the more consistent data that exist for other drugs (e.g., beta blockers, aspirin, fibrinolytic agents). The routine use of calcium antagonists cannot be recommended. Strict control of blood glucose in diabetic patients with STEMI has been shown to reduce the mortality rate. Serum magnesium should be measured in all patients on admission, and any demonstrated deficits should be corrected to minimize the risk of arrhythmias.

COMPLICATIONS AND THEIR MANAGEMENT

VENTRICULAR DYSFUNCTION After STEMI, the left ventricle undergoes a series of changes in shape, size, and thickness in both the infarcted and noninfarcted segments. This process is referred to as *ventricular remodeling* and generally precedes the development of clinically evident CHF in the months to years after infarction. Soon after STEMI, the left ventricle begins to dilate. Acutely, this results from expansion of the infarct, i.e., slippage of muscle bundles, disruption of normal myocardial cells, and tissue loss within the necrotic zone, resulting in disproportionate thinning and elongation of the infarct zone. Later, lengthening of the noninfarcted segments occurs as well. The overall chamber enlargement that occurs is related to the size and location of the infarct, with greater dilation following infarction of the apex of the left ventricle and causing more marked hemodynamic impairment, more frequent heart failure, and a poorer prognosis. Progressive dilation and its clinical consequences may be ameliorated by therapy with ACE inhibitors and other vasodilators (e.g., nitrates). In patients with an ejection fraction <40%, regardless of whether or not heart failure is present, ACE inhibitors should be prescribed.

HEMODYNAMIC ASSESSMENT Pump failure is now the primary cause of in-hospital death from STEMI. The extent of ischemic necrosis correlates well with the degree of pump failure and with mortality, both early (within 10 days of infarction) and later. The most common clinical signs are pulmonary rales and S_3 and S_4 gallop sounds. Pulmonary congestion is also frequently seen on the chest roentgenogram. Elevated LV filling pressure and elevated pulmonary artery pressure are the characteristic hemodynamic findings, but these findings may result from a reduction of ventricular compliance (diastolic failure) and/or a reduction of stroke volume with secondary cardiac dilation (systolic failure) (Chap. 215).

A classification originally proposed by Killip divides patients into four groups: class I, no signs of pulmonary or venous congestion; class II, moderate heart failure as evidenced by rales at the lung bases, S_3 gallop, tachypnea, or signs of failure of the right side of the heart, including venous and hepatic congestion; class III, severe heart failure, pulmonary edema; and class IV, shock with systolic pressure < 90 mmHg and evidence of peripheral vasoconstriction, peripheral cyanosis, mental confusion, and oliguria. When this classification was established in 1967, the expected hospital mortality rate of patients in these classes was as follows: class I, 0 to 5%; class II, 10 to 20%; class III, 35 to 45%; and class IV, 85 to 95%. With advances in management, the mortality rate in each class has fallen, perhaps by as much as one-third to one-half.

Hemodynamic evidence of abnormal LV function appears when contraction is seriously impaired in 20 to 25% of the left ventricle. Infarction of $\geq 40\%$ of the left ventricle usually results in cardiogenic shock (Chap. 255). Positioning of a balloon flotation catheter in the pulmonary artery permits monitoring of LV filling pressure; this technique is useful in patients who exhibit hypotension and/or clinical evidence of CHF. Cardiac output can also be determined with a pulmonary artery catheter. With the addition of intraarterial pressure monitoring, systemic vascular resistance can be calculated as a guide to adjusting vasopressor and vasodilator therapy. Some patients with STEMI have markedly elevated LV filling pressures (>22 mmHg) and normal cardiac indexes [>2.6 and >3.6 L/(min/m²)], while others have relatively low LV filling pressures (<15 mmHg) and reduced cardiac indexes. The former patients usually benefit from diuresis, while the latter may respond to volume expansion by means of intravenous administration of colloid-containing solutions.

Hypovolemia   This is an easily corrected condition that may contribute to the hypotension and vascular collapse associated with STEMI in some patients. It may be secondary to previous diuretic use, to reduced fluid intake during the early stages of the illness, and/or to vomiting associated with pain or medications. Consequently, hypovolemia should be identified and corrected in patients with STEMI and hypotension before more vigorous forms of therapy are begun. Central venous pressure reflects RV rather than LV filling pressure and is an inadequate guide for adjustment of blood volume, since LV function is almost always affected much more adversely than RV function in patients with STEMI. The optimal LV filling or pulmonary artery wedge pressure may vary considerably among patients. Each patient's ideal level (generally ~20 mmHg) is reached by cautious fluid administration during careful monitoring of oxygenation and cardiac output. Eventually, the cardiac output level plateaus, and further increases in LV filling pressure only increase congestive symptoms and decrease systemic oxygenation without raising arterial pressure.

℞ TREATMENT

The management of CHF in association with STEMI is similar to that of acute heart failure secondary to other forms of heart disease (avoidance of hypoxemia, diuresis, afterload reduction, inotropic support) (Chap. 216), except that the benefits of digitalis administration to patients with STEMI are unimpressive. By contrast, diuretic agents are extremely effective, as they diminish pulmonary congestion in the presence of systolic and/or diastolic heart failure (Chap. 255). LV filling pressure falls and orthopnea and dyspnea improve after the intravenous administration of furosemide or other loop diuretics. These drugs should be used with caution, however, as they can result in a massive diuresis with associated decreases in plasma volume, cardiac output, systemic blood pressure, and hence coronary perfusion. Nitrates in various forms may be used to decrease preload and congestive

symptoms. Oral isosorbide dinitrate, topical nitroglycerin ointment, or intravenous nitroglycerin all have the advantage over a diuretic of lowering preload through venodilation without decreasing the total plasma volume. In addition, nitrates may improve ventricular compliance if ischemia is present, as ischemia causes an elevation of LV filling pressure. Vasodilators must be used with caution to prevent serious hypotension. As noted earlier, ACE inhibitors are an ideal class of drugs for management of ventricular dysfunction after STEMI, especially for the long term.

CARDIOGENIC SHOCK   Efforts to reduce infarct size and prompt treatment of ongoing ischemia and other complications of MI appear to have reduced the incidence of cardiogenic shock from 20% to about 7%. Only 10% of patients with this condition present with it on admission, while 90% develop it during hospitalization. Typically, patients who develop cardiogenic shock have severe multivessel coronary artery disease with evidence of "piecemeal" necrosis extending outward from the original infarct zone. →*The evaluation and management of cardiogenic shock and severe power failure after STEMI are discussed in detail in Chap. 255.*

RIGHT VENTRICULAR INFARCTION   Approximately one-third of patients with inferoposterior infarction demonstrate at least a minor degree of RV necrosis. An occasional patient with inferoposterior LV infarction also has extensive RV infarction, and rare patients present with infarction limited primarily to the right ventricle. Clinically significant RV infarction causes signs of severe RV failure [jugular venous distention, Kussmaul's sign (Chap. 209), hepatomegaly] with or without hypotension. ST-segment elevations of right-sided precordial ECG leads, particularly lead V_4R, are frequently present in the first 24 h in patients with RV infarction. Two-dimensional echocardiography is helpful in determining the degree of RV dysfunction. Catheterization of the right side of the heart often reveals a distinctive hemodynamic pattern resembling cardiac tamponade or constrictive pericarditis (steep right atrial "y" descent and an early diastolic dip and plateau in RV waveforms) (Chap. 222). Therapy consists of volume expansion to maintain adequate RV preload and efforts to improve LV performance with attendant reduction in pulmonary capillary wedge and pulmonary arterial pressures.

ARRHYTHMIAS   (See also Chaps. 213 and 214)   The incidence of arrhythmias after STEMI is higher in patients seen early after the onset of symptoms. The mechanisms responsible for infarction-related arrhythmias include autonomic nervous system imbalance, electrolyte disturbances, ischemia, and slowed conduction in zones of ischemic myocardium. An arrhythmia can usually be managed successfully if trained personnel and appropriate equipment are available when it develops. Since most deaths from arrhythmia occur during the first few hours after infarction, the effectiveness of treatment relates directly to the speed with which patients come under medical observation. The prompt management of arrhythmias constitutes a significant advance in the treatment of STEMI.

Ventricular Premature Beats   Infrequent, sporadic ventricular premature depolarizations occur in almost all patients with STEMI and do not require therapy. Whereas in the past, frequent, multifocal, or early diastolic ventricular extrasystoles (so-called warning arrhythmias) were routinely treated with antiarrhythmic drugs to reduce the risk of development of ventricular tachycardia and ventricular fibrillation, pharmacologic therapy is now reserved for patients with sustained ventricular arrhythmias. Prophylactic antiarrhythmic therapy (either intravenous lidocaine early or oral agents later) is contraindicated for ventricular premature beats in the absence of clinically important ventricular tachyarrhythmias, as such therapy may actually increase the mortality rate. Beta-adrenoceptor blocking agents are effective in abolishing ventricular ectopic activity in patients with STEMI and in the prevention of ventricular fibrillation. As described above (see "Beta-Adrenoceptor Blockers"), they should be used routinely in patients without contraindications. In addition, hypokalemia and hypomagnesemia are risk factors for ventricular fibrillation in patients with

STEMI; the serum potassium concentration should be adjusted to approximately 4.5 mmol/L and magnesium to about 2.0 mmol/L.

Ventricular Tachycardia and Fibrillation Within the first 24 h of STEMI, ventricular tachycardia and fibrillation can occur without prior warning arrhythmias. The occurrence of ventricular fibrillation can be reduced by prophylactic administration of intravenous lidocaine. However, prophylactic use of lidocaine has not been shown to reduce overall mortality from STEMI. In fact, in addition to causing possible noncardiac complications, lidocaine may predispose to an excess risk of bradycardia and asystole. For these reasons, and with earlier treatment of active ischemia, more frequent use of beta-blocking agents, and the nearly universal success of electrical cardioversion or defibrillation, routine prophylactic antiarrhythmic drug therapy *is no longer recommended*. It should be reserved for patients who cannot reach a hospital or for those treated in hospitals that lack the constant presence in the coronary care unit of a physician or nurse trained in the recognition and treatment of ventricular fibrillation.

Sustained ventricular tachycardia that is well tolerated hemodynamically should be treated with an intravenous regimen of amiodarone (bolus of 150 mg over 10 min, followed by infusion of 1.0 mg/min for 6 h and then 0.5 mg/min); or procainamide (bolus of 15 mg/kg over 20 to 30 min; infusion of 1 to 4 mg/min); if it does not stop promptly, electroversion should be used (Chap. 214). An unsynchronized discharge of 200 to 300 J (defibrillation) is used immediately in patients with ventricular fibrillation or when ventricular tachycardia causes hemodynamic deterioration. Ventricular tachycardia or fibrillation that is refractory to electroshock may be more responsive after the patient is treated with epinephrine (1 mg intravenously or 10 mL of a 1:10,000 solution via the intracardiac route), bretylium (a 5-mg/kg bolus), or amiodarone (a 75- to 150-mg bolus).

Ventricular arrhythmias, including the unusual form of ventricular tachycardia known as *torsades de pointes* (Chap. 214), may occur in patients with STEMI as a consequence of other concurrent problems (such as hypoxia, hypokalemia, or other electrolyte disturbances) or of the toxic effects of an agent being administered to the patient (such as digoxin or quinidine). A search for such secondary causes should always be undertaken.

Although the in-hospital mortality rate is increased, the long-term survival is good in patients who survive to hospital discharge after *primary* ventricular fibrillation, i.e., ventricular fibrillation that is a primary response to acute ischemia and is not associated with predisposing factors such as CHF, shock, bundle branch block, or ventricular aneurysm. This result is in sharp contrast to the poor prognosis for patients who develop ventricular fibrillation *secondary* to severe pump failure. For patients who develop ventricular tachycardia or ventricular fibrillation late in their hospital course (i.e., after the first 48 h), the mortality rate is increased both in-hospital and during long-term follow-up. Such patients should be considered for electrophysiologic study and implantation of a cardioverter/defibrillator (Fig. 228-5) (Chap. 214).

Accelerated Idioventricular Rhythm Accelerated idioventricular rhythm (AIVR, "slow ventricular tachycardia"), a ventricular rhythm with a rate of 60 to 100 bpm, occurs in 25% of patients with STEMI. It often occurs transiently during fibrinolytic therapy at the time of reperfusion. The rate of AIVR is usually similar to that of the sinus rhythm that precedes and follows it, and this similarity of rate plus the relatively minor hemodynamic effects make this rhythm more difficult to detect except by electrocardiographic monitoring. For the most part, AIVR is benign and does not presage the development of classic ventricular tachycardia. Most episodes of AIVR do not require treatment if the patient is monitored carefully, as degeneration into a more serious arrhythmia is rare, and, if it occurs, AIVR can generally be treated readily with a drug that increases the sinus rate (atropine).

Supraventricular Arrhythmias Sinus tachycardia is the most common supraventricular arrhythmia. If it occurs secondary to another cause (such as anemia, fever, heart failure, or a metabolic derangement), the primary problem should be treated first. However, if it appears to be due

FIGURE 228-5 Algorithm for assessment of need for electrophysiologic study and implantation of a cardioverter/defibrillator. The appropriate management path is selected based upon the timing of and measurement of left ventricular ejection fraction (table at top of figure). In path A, patients with markedly depressed left ventricular function at least 1 month post-STEMI are referred for insertion of an implantable cardioverter/defibrillator (ICD). Path B illustrates the management of patients in an intermediate-risk category who require further evaluation with an electrophysiology study (EPS). If the EPS reveals inducible ventricular tachycardia/ventricular fibrillation, an ICD is implanted; if the EPS is negative, no ICD is implanted and the patient receives medical therapy post-STEMI. Path C illustrates the management of patients with preserved left ventricular function who do not receive an ICD and are treated with medical therapy post-STEMI. (*Adapted from EM Antman et al: ACC/AHA guidelines for the management of patients with ST elevation myocardial infarction. Circulation and JACC, 2004, in press; with permission.*)

to sympathetic overstimulation (e.g., as part of a hyperdynamic state), then treatment with a beta blocker is indicated. Other common arrhythmias in this group are atrial flutter and atrial fibrillation, which are often secondary to LV failure. Digoxin is usually the treatment of choice for supraventricular arrhythmias if heart failure is present. If heart failure is absent, beta blockers, verapamil, or diltiazem are suitable alternatives for controlling the ventricular rate, as they may also help to control ischemia. If the abnormal rhythm persists for >2 h with a ventricular rate >120 bpm or if tachycardia induces heart failure, shock, or ischemia (as manifested by recurrent pain or ECG changes), a synchronized electroshock (100 to 200 J) should be used.

Accelerated junctional rhythms have diverse causes but may occur in patients with inferoposterior infarction. Digitalis excess must be ruled out. In some patients with severely compromised LV function, the loss of appropriately timed atrial systole results in a marked decrease in cardiac output. Right atrial or coronary sinus pacing is indicated in such instances.

Sinus Bradycardia Treatment of sinus bradycardia is indicated if hemodynamic compromise results from the slow heart rate. Atropine is the most useful drug for increasing heart rate and should be given intravenously in doses of 0.5 mg initially. If the rate remains <50 to 60 bpm, additional doses of 0.2 mg, up to a total of 2.0 mg, may be given. Persistent bradycardia (<40 bpm) despite atropine may be treated with electrical pacing. Isoproterenol should be avoided.

Atrioventricular and Intraventricular Conduction Disturbances (See also Chap. 213) Both the in-hospital mortality rate and the post-discharge mortality rate of patients who have complete atrioventricular (AV) block in association with anterior infarction are markedly higher than those of patients who develop AV block with inferior infarction. This difference is related to the fact that heart block in inferior infarction is commonly a result of increased vagal tone and/or the release of adenosine and therefore is transient. In anterior wall infarction, heart block is usually related to ischemic malfunction of the conduction system, which is commonly associated with extensive myocardial necrosis.

Temporary electrical pacing provides an effective means of increasing the heart rate of patients with bradycardia due to AV block. However, acceleration of the heart rate may have only a limited impact on prognosis in patients with anterior wall infarction and complete heart block in whom the large size of the infarct is the major factor determining outcome. It should be carried out if it improves hemodynamics, however. Pacing does appear to be beneficial in patients with inferoposterior infarction who have complete heart block associated with heart failure, hypotension, marked bradycardia, or significant ventricular ectopic activity. A subgroup of these patients, those with RV infarction, often respond poorly to ventricular pacing because of the loss of the atrial contribution to ventricular filling. In such patients, dual-chamber AV sequential pacing may be required.

External noninvasive pacing electrodes should be positioned in a "demand" mode for patients with sinus bradycardia (rate < 50 bpm) that is unresponsive to drug therapy, Mobitz II second-degree AV block, third-degree heart block, or bilateral bundle branch block (e.g., right bundle branch block plus left anterior fascicular block). Retrospective studies suggest that permanent pacing may reduce the long-term risk of sudden death due to bradyarrhythmias in the rare patient who develops combined persistent bifascicular and transient third-degree heart block during the acute phase of MI.

OTHER COMPLICATIONS ■ Recurrent Chest Discomfort Recurrent angina develops in ~25% of patients hospitalized for STEMI. This percentage is even higher in patients who undergo successful thrombolysis. Since recurrent or persistent ischemia often heralds extension of the original infarct or reinfarction in a new myocardial zone and is associated with a doubling of risk after STEMI, patients with these symptoms should be referred for prompt coronary arteriography and mechanical revascularization. Repeat administration of a fibrinolytic agent is an alternative to early mechanical revascularization.

Pericarditis (See also Chap. 222)   Pericardial friction rubs and/or pericardial pain are frequently encountered in patients with transmural STEMI. This complication can usually be managed with aspirin (650 mg qid). It is important to diagnose the chest pain of pericarditis accurately, since failure to recognize it may lead to the erroneous diagnosis of recurrent ischemic pain and/or infarct extension, with resulting inappropriate use of anticoagulants, nitrates, beta blockers, or coronary arteriography. When it occurs, complaints of pain radiating to either trapezius muscle is helpful since such a pattern of discomfort is typical of pericarditis but rarely occurs with ischemic discomfort. Anticoagulants potentially could cause tamponade in the presence of acute pericarditis (as manifested by either pain or persistent rub) and therefore should not be used unless there is a compelling indication.

Thromboembolism   Clinically apparent thromboembolism complicates STEMI in ~10% of cases, but embolic lesions are found in 20% of patients in necropsy series, suggesting that thromboembolism is often clinically silent. Thromboembolism is considered to be an important contributing cause of death in 25% of patients with STEMI who die after admission to the hospital. Arterial emboli originate from LV mural thrombi, while most pulmonary emboli arise in the leg veins.

Thromboembolism typically occurs in association with large infarcts (especially anterior), CHF, and a LV thrombus detected by echocardiography. The incidence of arterial embolism from a clot originating in the ventricle at the site of an infarction is small but real. Two-dimensional echocardiography reveals LV thrombi in about one-third of patients with anterior wall infarction but in few patients with inferior or posterior infarction. Arterial embolism often presents as a major complication, such as hemiparesis when the cerebral circulation is involved or hypertension if the renal circulation is compromised. When a thrombus has been clearly demonstrated by echocardiographic or other techniques or when a large area of regional wall motion abnormality is seen even in the absence of a detectable mural thrombus, systemic anticoagulation should be undertaken (in the absence of contraindications), as the incidence of embolic complications appears to

be markedly lowered by such therapy. The appropriate duration of therapy is unknown, but 3 to 6 months is probably prudent.

Left Ventricular Aneurysm   The term *ventricular aneurysm* is usually used to describe *dyskinesis* or local expansile paradoxical wall motion. Normally functioning myocardial fibers must shorten more if stroke volume and cardiac output are to be maintained in patients with ventricular aneurysm; if they cannot, overall ventricular function is impaired. True aneurysms are composed of scar tissue and neither predispose to nor are associated with cardiac rupture.

The complications of LV aneurysm do not usually occur for weeks to months after STEMI; they include CHF, arterial embolism, and ventricular arrhythmias. Apical aneurysms are the most common and the most easily detected by clinical examination. The physical finding of greatest value is a double, diffuse, or displaced apical impulse. Ventricular aneurysms are readily detected by two-dimensional echocardiography, which may also reveal a mural thrombus in an aneurysm.

Rarely, myocardial rupture may be contained by a local area of pericardium, along with organizing thrombus and hematoma. Over time, this *pseudoaneurysm* enlarges, maintaining communication with the LV cavity through a narrow neck. Because a pseudoaneurysm often ruptures spontaneously, it should be surgically repaired if recognized.

POSTINFARCTION RISK STRATIFICATION AND MANAGEMENT

Many clinical factors have been identified that are associated with an increase in cardiovascular risk after initial recovery from STEMI. Some of the most important factors include persistent ischemia (spontaneous or provoked), depressed LV ejection fraction (<40%), rales above the lung bases on physical examination or congestion on chest radiograph, and symptomatic ventricular arrhythmias. Other features associated with increased risk include a history of previous MI, age >75, diabetes mellitus, prolonged sinus tachycardia, hypotension, ST-segment changes at rest without angina ("silent ischemia"), an abnormal signal-averaged ECG, nonpatency of the infarct-related coronary artery (if angiography is undertaken), and persistent advanced heart block or a new intraventricular conduction abnormality on the ECG. Therapy must be individualized on the basis of the relative importance of the risk(s) present.

The goal of preventing reinfarction and death after recovery from STEMI has led to strategies to evaluate risk after infarction. In stable patients, submaximal exercise stress testing may be carried out before hospital discharge to detect residual ischemia and ventricular ectopy and to provide the patient with a guideline for exercise in the early recovery period. Alternatively, or in addition, a maximal (symptom-limited) exercise stress test may be carried out 4 to 6 weeks after infarction. Evaluation of LV function is usually warranted as well. Recognition of a depressed LV ejection fraction by echocardiography or radionuclide ventriculography identifies patients who should receive ACE inhibitors (see "Angiotensin-Converting Enzyme Inhibitors," above). Patients in whom angina is induced at relatively low workloads, those who have a large reversible defect on perfusion imaging or a depressed ejection fraction, those with demonstrable ischemia, and those in whom exercise provokes symptomatic ventricular arrhythmias should be considered at high risk for recurrent MI or death from arrhythmia (Fig. 228-5). Cardiac catheterization with coronary angiography and/or invasive electrophysiologic evaluation is advised.

Exercise tests also aid in formulating an individualized exercise prescription, which can be much more vigorous in patients who tolerate exercise without any of the above-mentioned adverse signs. Additionally, predischarge stress testing may provide an important psychological benefit, building the patient's confidence by demonstrating a reasonable exercise tolerance. Furthermore, particularly when no arrhythmias or signs of ischemia are identified, the patient benefits by the physician's reassurance that objective evidence suggests no immediate jeopardy.

In many hospitals a cardiac rehabilitation program with progressive exercise is initiated in the hospital and continued after discharge. Ideally, such programs should include an educational component that informs patients about their disease and its risk factors.

The usual duration of hospitalization for an uncomplicated STEMI is about 5 days. The remainder of the convalescent phase may be accomplished at home. During the first 1 to 2 weeks, the patient should be encouraged to increase activity by walking about the house and outdoors in good weather. Normal sexual activity may be resumed during this period. After 2 weeks, the physician must regulate the patient's activity on the basis of exercise tolerance. Most patients will be able to return to work within 2 to 4 weeks.

SECONDARY PREVENTION

Various secondary preventive measures are at least partly responsible for the improvement in the long-term mortality and morbidity rates after STEMI. Long-term treatment with an antiplatelet agent (usually aspirin) after STEMI is associated with a 25% reduction in the risk of recurrent infarction, stroke, or cardiovascular mortality (36 fewer events for every 1000 patients treated). In addition, in patients taking aspirin chronically, STEMIs tend to be smaller and are more likely to be non-Q-wave in nature. An alternative antiplatelet agent that may be used for secondary prevention in patients intolerant of aspirin is the ADP receptor antagonist clopidogrel (75 mg orally daily). ACE inhibitors should be used indefinitely by patients with clinically evident heart failure, a moderate decrease in global ejection fraction, or a large regional wall motion abnormality to prevent late ventricular remodeling and recurrent ischemic events.

The chronic routine use of oral beta-adrenoceptor blockers for at least 2 years after STEMI is supported by well-conducted, placebo-controlled trials that have convincingly demonstrated reductions in the rates of total mortality, sudden death, and, in some instances, reinfarction. In contrast, calcium antagonists are not recommended for routine secondary prevention.

Evidence suggests that warfarin lowers the risk of late mortality and the incidence of reinfarction after STEMI. Most physicians prescribe aspirin routinely for all patients without contraindications and add warfarin for patients at increased risk of embolism (see "Thromboembolism," above). Several studies suggest that in patients <75 years a low dose of aspirin (75 to 81 mg/d) in combination with warfarin administered to achieve an INR > 2.0 is more effective than aspirin alone for preventing recurrent MI and embolic cerebrovascular accident. However, there is an increased risk of bleeding and a high rate of discontinuation of warfarin that has limited clinical acceptance of combination antithrombotic therapy. Combination antiplatelet therapy with aspirin and clopidogrel has been established as an important treatment strategy for reducing the risk of death and recurrent ischemic events in the year following presentation with unstable angina/NSTEMI. Trials are underway to assess whether such combined antiplatelet therapy is also effective and safe in patients recovering from STEMI.

Finally, risk factors for *atherosclerosis* (Chap. 224) should be discussed with the patient, and, when possible, favorably modified. In particular, efforts should be made to ensure the cessation of smoking and the control of hypertension and hyperlipidemia [the target low-density lipoprotein level is <2.6 mmol/L (<100 mg/dL)]. In addition, regular physical exercise and reduction of emotional stress should be encouraged. Hormone replacement therapy prevention of coronary events should not be given de novo to postmenopausal women after STEMI. Postmenopausal women already taking estrogen plus progestin at the time of STEMI may continue that therapy.

FURTHER READING

AMERICAN HEART ASSOCIATION: *Heart and Stroke Facts: 2002 Statistical Supplement*. Dallas, American Heart Association, 2003

ANTMAN EM, BRAUNWALD E: Acute myocardial infarction, in *Braunwald's Heart Disease*, 7th ed, DP Zipes et al. (eds). Philadelphia, Saunders, 2005

—— et al: ACC/AHA guidelines for the management of patients with ST elevation myocardial infarction. Circulation and JACC, 2004, in press; www.acc.org/clinical/guidelines/stemi/index.htm

BOERSMA E et al: Acute myocardial infarction. Lancet 361:847, 2003

FALK E et al: Coronary plaque disruption. Circulation 92:657, 1995

FIBRINOLYTIC THERAPY TRIALISTS (FTT) COLLABORATIVE GROUP: Indications for fibrinolytic therapy in suspected acute myocardial infarction: Collaborative overview of early mortality and major morbidity results from all randomised trials of more than 1000 patients. Lancet 343:311, 1994

GOTTLIEB SS et al: Effect of beta-blockade on mortality among high-risk and low-risk patients after myocardial infarction. N Engl J Med 339:489, 1998

MICHAELS AD, GOLDSCHLAGER N: Risk stratification after acute myocardial infarction in the reperfusion era. Prog Cardiovasc Dis 42:273, 2000

MONTALESCOT G et al: Platelet glycoprotein IIb/IIIa inhibition with coronary stenting for acute myocardial infarction. N Engl J Med 344:1895, 2001

TOPOL EJ: Acute myocardial infarction: Thrombolysis. Heart 83:122, 2000

229 PERCUTANEOUS CORONARY REVASCULARIZATION
Donald S. Baim

While bypass surgery was once the only means of coronary revascularization, in 1977 Andreas Gruntzig introduced a form of catheter-based coronary revascularization that he termed *percutaneous transluminal coronary angioplasty (PTCA)*. Given the limitations of his early equipment, fewer than 1000 PTCA procedures were performed worldwide each year. By the mid-1980s, progressive improvements in the balloon angioplasty equipment led to improved results, expanded indications for use, and explosive growth in the numbers of PTCA procedures; the annual number of PTCA procedures (~300,000) then roughly matched the number of surgical bypass operations. During the 1990s, a number of newer devices (including stents and atherectomy devices) were introduced that further improved the acute success, safety, and long-term durability and allowed the number of percutaneous coronary revascularizations (PCRs), or percutaneous coronary interventions (PCIs), to grow further (from 800,000 to 1 million procedures annually), more than double the annual number of coronary bypass operations (~400,000). This dominant role of catheter-based intervention in the treatment of coronary artery disease has led to creation of a separate area within the field of cardiovascular diseases known as *interventional cardiology*, with incremental fellowship requirements and Board certification based on training, ongoing experience (75 procedures per year), and a written examination.

All catheter-based coronary interventions are derivatives of diagnostic cardiac catheterization (Chap. 212), in which catheters are introduced into the arterial circulation by needle puncture, advanced into the heart under fluoroscopic guidance, and used for pressure measurements or injections of radiopaque liquid contrast agents. Interventional procedures differ in that the catheter placed into the ostium of the narrowed coronary artery has a slightly larger lumen diameter to allow passage of a flexible, steerable guidewire (diameter <0.5 mm) down the coronary artery lumen, through the narrowing, and into the vessel beyond. This guidewire then serves as the rail over which angioplasty balloons or other therapeutic devices are advanced and used to enlarge the narrowed segment of coronary artery (Fig. 229-1). Because PCR is performed with local anesthesia and requires only a short (1-day) hospitalization, its use in suitable patients can greatly decrease recovery time and expense compared to coronary bypass surgery. While not all types of coronary narrowing are well suited to catheter-based intervention, PCR is the treatment of choice for roughly 70% of patients with symptomatic single-vessel disease and roughly 20% of patients with symptomatic three-vessel disease. Selection of suitable cases for PCR versus bypass surgery takes into account the anatomic restrictions of PCR (in dealing with diffuse disease, bifurcation lesions, etc.). Both patient and physician need to be aware that while catheter-based in-

FIGURE 229-1 Focal discrete stenosis of the mid-right coronary angioplasty in a patient with unstable angina, shown before (*left panel*) and after (*right panel*) inflation of the PTCA balloon catheter. The lesion is typical of the straightforward lesion anatomy treated by early (pre-1985) coronary angioplasty.

tervention is done under anesthesia and has a lower elective mortality rate than bypass surgery (0.4 to 1.0%, compared to a rate of 1 to 3%), it is still an invasive procedure whose risks and benefits need to be weighed carefully for each individual patient. To decide which patients should undergo revascularization (rather than continued medical management), and to select which patients should undergo catheter-based rather than surgical revascularization, a detailed understanding of both clinical and coronary angiographic factors, as well as the applicability of various interventional techniques, is required.

INDICATIONS

The fundamental indication for PCR is the presence of one or more coronary stenoses that are approachable by catheter-based techniques and are thought to be responsible for a clinical syndrome that warrants revascularization. Moreover, the risks and benefits of revascularization by PCR for the individual patient should compare favorably with those of surgery. In patients with significant narrowing of a single coronary artery, the main benefit of revascularization lies in relief of anginal symptoms rather than in increasing their already good prognosis with medical therapy. By contrast, for the patient with significant left main stenosis or multivessel disease, revascularization may both relieve angina *and* improve long-term survival. For most patients with multivessel coronary disease, the current choice is surgical rather than catheter-based revascularization, particularly when one or more vessels supplying significant areas of viable myocardium are not well suited to PCR due to unfavorable anatomic features. In patients for whom either PCR or bypass surgery is a possible treatment for multivessel coronary artery disease, randomized trials have suggested that the two procedures are essentially equivalent in terms of in-hospital and 3- to 5-year mortality rates, except for patients with diabetes mellitus and multivessel coronary artery disease where surgical treatment appears to offer improved 5- to 7-year survival compared to PCR. However, patients who undergo PCR are more likely to need a second revascularization procedure (generally repeat PCR to treat restenosis) to maintain an equivalent level of symptom relief at 5 years. Repeat procedures will thus be needed in 50% of patients undergoing PTCA and in 20% of patients undergoing stenting, compared to 7 to 10% for patients undergoing bypass surgery, for multivessel disease.

The current clinical indications for PCR cover the spectrum of ischemic heart disease, from patients with unstable angina or acute infarction to patients with silent ischemia, as summarized in the recent ACC/AHA guidelines. One clear indication is *moderately severe, chronic, stable angina*, which persists despite medical antianginal therapy (Chap. 226). Occasionally, PCR is offered to patients with objective evidence of ischemia on noninvasive testing (i.e., an abnormal exercise test) and suitable coronary lesions, even though they have comparatively mild anginal symptoms. At the other extreme, many patients undergo PCR for more pressing indications, including unstable angina or acute myocardial infarction (MI) (with or without prior thrombolytic therapy). An aggressive approach to the treatment of unstable angina is now favored. It involves initial stabilization with beta blockers, nitrates, heparin, and antiplatelet agents (aspirin and frequently a platelet glycoprotein IIb/IIIa receptor blocker), followed by prompt diagnostic catheterization and same-procedure PCR of the culprit blockage. This approach offers the patient a more rapid return to work, fewer readmissions and late revascularizations, and potentially a reduction in late events compared to more prolonged initial trials of medical stabilization before proceeding with invasive evaluation and treatment.

In the early 1980s the introduction of intravenous fibrinolytic agents to reopen the occluded infarct-related vessel represented a major advance in the treatment of acute MI (Chap. 228). While use of immediate PCR would be expected to improve the results of fibrinolytic therapy further (by treating the underlying atherosclerotic stenosis), randomized trials showed that routine PCR after thrombolytic administration had no benefit compared to "watchful waiting," reserving PCR for patients who exhibited spontaneous or exercise-induced ischemia. In contrast, there is now strong evidence that *primary* or direct PCR (that is, PCR used instead of fibrinolytic therapy) can reduce the in-hospital mortality rate (from roughly 7 to 4%) when performed promptly by a skilled operator (Fig. 229-2). Another advantage of PCR is that it can be performed even in acute MI patients who have relative contraindications to fibrinolytic therapy (advanced age, hypertension, prior stroke, recent surgery, etc.).

FIGURE 229-2 Left coronary angiogram in a patient with acute anterior myocardial infarction and cardiogenic shock shows occlusion of the proximal left anterior descending coronary artery (*top panel, arrow*) with only faint filling beyond the obstructing thrombus. After initial PTCA (*lower left panel*), there is restored antegrade flow with residual stenosis. After stent placement (*lower right panel*), there is no residual stenosis and brisk flow. This improvement was associated with reversal of shock hemodynamics, including normalization of severe lactic acidosis.

As the clinical indications for PCR have broadened, so have its anatomic capabilities. Largely through the introduction of newer interventional devices such as stents, PCR has advanced well beyond the treatment of proximal, discrete, subtotal, concentric, noncalcified lesions. Calcified, complex, or diffuse disease lesions respond well to coronary stent placement, sometimes after pretreatment with rotational atherectomy. Even totally occluded coronary arteries (particularly ones that have been occluded for <6 months) can be crossed and dilated effectively, although the success rate remains lower than for subtotal lesions (60% versus 90% for subtotal stenotic lesions). In addition to lesions in the native coronary tree, obstructions in the saphenous vein (Fig. 229-3) or internal mammary artery bypass grafts can also be dilated successfully to treat postbypass angina. If multiple lesions are responsible for the clinical syndrome, they generally can be dilated during a single procedure. When the severity of some individual lesions is unclear based on prior stress testing and angiography, special guidewires can be used to measure their physiologic severity during maximal coronary flow induced by adenosine infusion.

FIGURE 229-3 Stent placement in a diseased saphenous vein graft. *Left*: Severe eccentric stenosis in an 8-year-old saphenous vein graft to the left anterior descending coronary artery. *Middle*: After balloon angioplasty, the lumen remains stenotic due to elastic recoil of the vessel wall and disruption (dissection) of the plaque. *Right*: After placement of a coronary stent, both recoil and dissection have been overcome, providing a large smooth lumen.

NONBALLOON TECHNIQUES

While conventional balloon angioplasty (PTCA) offered anatomic versatility and acceptable short- and long-term results, it was limited when used to approach certain anatomic lesion types (e.g., calcified eccentric, ostial, thrombus-containing, or bifurcation lesions). It was also plagued by the problems of intimal dissection (which led to abrupt closure of the dilated segment in 3% of cases, requiring emergency bypass surgery) and restenosis of 30 to 40% of the dilated segments within 6 months of initially successful treatment. These problems motivated the development of a number of newer, nonballoon techniques that entered routine clinical practice during the early 1990s. These include atherectomy and stent placement, the latter of which now dominates current PCR (see below). In parallel, improvements in adjunctive pharmacotherapy (especially thienopyridines and platelet glycoprotein IIb/IIIa receptor blockers) has helped produce significant improvements in the success, safety, and long-term results. While most newer PCR procedures have higher in-hospital cost than conventional balloon angioplasty, much of this incremental cost can be recouped by the reduction in acute complications and the treatment of subsequent restenosis.

STENTS These are metallic scaffolds that are inserted into a diseased vessel segment in their collapsed form and are then deployed by balloon inflation or self-expansion (after removal of an external constraining membrane) (Fig. 229-4). They overcome two of the principal limitations of balloon dilatation—local dissection of the plaque and the tendency for elastic recoil of the vessel wall—allowing stents consistently to establish a normal-appearing vessel lumen. Since 1994, when the first two balloon-expandable stent designs were approved by the U.S. Food and Drug Administration (FDA), a number of second- and third-generation stent designs have been developed that offer easier delivery of a wider variety of sizes and lengths, into tortuous or distal lesions. Other refinements in stent design include optional membranous coverings (to seal aneurysms or perforations) and drug-eluting coatings (to suppress stent thrombosis and in-stent proliferation).

In the early experience, metallic stents proved prone to thrombotic occlusion, either acute (<24 h) or subacute (1 to 14 days with a peak at 6 days), requiring an aggressive anticoagulation regimen (aspirin, dipyridamole, and warfarin) to reduce such thromboses to ~3%. This aggressive anticoagulant regimen prolonged hospitalization and increased the incidence of local vascular complications at the femoral arterial entry site. Many of these thrombotic complications were the result of incomplete stent expansion, and greater attention to full initial deployment allowed even more favorable thrombosis rates (<1%), with only antiplatelet drugs (aspirin plus the platelet ADP-receptor blockers, ticlopidine or clopidogrel). This rapid evolution in devices, concomitant medications, and indications has led to the dominance of stent placement in catheter-based coronary revascularization, with placement of one or more stents in 85% of all procedures.

In addition to controlling complications related to abrupt vessel closure, the fact that stenting provides a large acute luminal area compared to PTCA alone has reduced the incidence of subsequent restenosis (e.g., angiographic restenosis rates of 20% versus 33%, and clinical restenosis rates of 10% versus 16 to 20%). When in-stent restenosis does occur, it is the consequence of excessive neointimal hyperplasia within the stent (Fig. 229-5). This can be treated by balloon dilatation, followed by catheter-delivered local β or γ radiation to suppress subsequent neointimal regrowth. Since such radiation treatment also inhibits endothelialization, placement of new stents at the time of radiation should be avoided or they should be protected by prolonging antiplatelet therapy to 9 to 12 months. More recent research has demonstrated that stents can be coated to elute antiproliferative agents such as rapamycin or taxol that inhibit excessive proliferation. Local release of these agents has further decreased angiographic restenosis rates (to <10%) and clinical restenosis rates (to roughly 5%)—benefits that have broadened the use of stents and PCR following their release in early 2003.

FIGURE 229-4 Second-generation stent. *Left*: The flexibility typical of second-generation stents is shown in bending the collapsed stent on its delivery balloon. *Right*: The same stent design is shown in its balloon-expanded configuration, in some of the available lengths [32 mm (*top*), 16 mm, and 9 mm]. The availability of a variety of second-generation stents since 1997 has helped make stent placement a part of more than 85% of all PCRs.

FIGURE 229-5 Short- and long-term results in a long lesion in the right coronary artery. *Left*: A long (~50 mm) area of disease (*arrows*) is present in the right coronary artery. *Middle*: Contrast injection after placement of two long second-generation stents (25 and 35 mm long) shows excellent patency throughout the proximal- and mid-portions of the vessel. *Right*: Follow-up angiogram 6 months after stent placement shows mild lumen reduction throughout the stented segment due to neointimal hyperplasia within the stent (note the separation between the stent shadows and the contrast-filled lumen). Mild degrees of proliferative narrowing are benign and common within stents (particularly long stents such as this one). Had the degree of lumen reduction been greater and associated with recurrent symptoms or an abnormal exercise test, however, re-intervention would have been performed, possibly followed by local radiation delivery (brachytherapy) to inhibit excessive subsequent tissue regrowth. Use of a drug-eluting stent would have virtually eliminated this in-stent neointimal hyperplasia.

ATHERECTOMY Whereas both balloon angioplasty and stent placement enlarge the coronary lumen by displacing plaque, atherectomy catheters enlarge the lumen by removing plaque mass from the treated lesion. Several mechanical atherectomy devices were developed in the 1990s, including directional, rotational, extraction, and laser atherectomy. Although each has certain applications, the greater technical difficulty and procedural complication profile of atherectomy compared to stenting has relegated these devices to niche roles in current PCR. Suction thrombectomy devices may be useful when large intracoronary thrombi are present (e.g., acute MI), and embolic protection devices (distal filters or occlusion/aspiration devices) may be useful adjuncts during the treatment of saphenous vein graft or other lesions prone to the liberation of debris that may compromise the distal myocardial microcirculation.

RESULTS

The success rate for PCR—defined as leaving a residual diameter stenosis <50% (<30% when a stent has been used), without producing an associated complication—now exceeds 97%. Failures may result from inability to cross the target lesion with the guidewire or balloon catheter, particularly when that target lesion is a chronic total occlusion, or failure to dilate a rigid calcified stenosis (now treated by rotational atherectomy). Before the advent of stents, some local dissection was present in virtually all successful balloon dilatation procedures, and more extensive dissection led to abrupt closure of the dilated segment soon after withdrawal of the balloon catheter, necessitating emergency bypass surgery in approximately 3% of cases. In the stent era, however, the incidence of emergency bypass surgery is now <0.3%. The main remaining hazards of PCR are thrombosis and vessel perforation, each of which is well below 1%.

Since PCR causes local endothelial injury and leaves metallic foreign bodies (stents) in the vessel lumen, platelet activation and thrombosis are expected potential complications. All PCRs are thus performed under systemic anticoagulation (heparin, 7000 to 10,000 units, or a direct-acting thrombin inhibitor), to maintain an activated clotting time of 250 to 300, and antiplatelet therapy (aspirin, 325 mg/d starting at least 24 h before PCR and continued for at least 3 to 6 months after the procedure). If a coronary stent has been placed, aspirin is supplemented by a blocker of the platelet ADP receptor, clopidogrel, to reduce the likelihood of stent thrombosis. Intravenous antiplatelet agents (blockers of the platelet glycoprotein IIb/IIIa receptors) may reduce

further the incidence of ischemic complications (especially postprocedural elevation of cardiac enzymes). They are used prophylactically in what are perceived to be high-risk interventions or provisionally in interventions that have left behind an imperfect mechanical result (e.g., a nonstented distal dissection).

Perforation of a coronary artery was an extremely rare complication of conventional balloon angioplasty but may occur in up to 1% of patients undergoing more aggressive atherectomy procedures. Even small perforations of the distal vessel by the angioplasty guidewire may lead to significant hemopericardium requiring urgent pericardiocentesis in the setting of intense anticoagulant and antiplatelet therapy. Finally, catheter-based interventions are subject to all of the complications of diagnostic catheterization, including adverse reactions to iodinated contrast agents and groin hematoma. For most patients, however, catheter-based coronary revascularization offers a safe and effective alternative to surgical revascularization.

FOLLOW-UP

After successful PCR of all "culprit" lesions, marked improvement or complete resolution of the presenting ischemic syndrome should be evident. In approximately 20% of patients, however, evidence of recurrent ischemia develops within 6 months, reflecting restenosis of the dilated segment in response to the local injury of PCR. When recurrent ischemia develops later than 6 months after PCR, it tends to reflect progression of disease at another site, rather than restenosis of a previous treatment site. Whether due to restenosis or disease progression, most post-PCR ischemia can be treated by repeat PCR, so that only about 10% of patients require bypass surgery during the 5 years after a successful procedure. Since all post-PCR patients have provided evidence of severe obstructive coronary atherosclerosis requiring revascularization, an aggressive program to reduce atherosclerotic risk factors and thereby slow the pace of development of new lesions should be part of any post-PCR regimen. This should include control of hypertension, hyperlipidemia, and smoking cessation (Chap. 226).

SUMMARY

Over the past 25 years, the development of new techniques (such as stent placement), new drug regimens, and refinements in practice driven by "evidence-based" medicine, catheter-based revascularization (PCR) has developed from a procedural curiosity to what is now the dominant form of coronary revascularization. As short- and long-term results have improved and the number of procedures has continued to grow, the pace of development continues to accelerate.

FURTHER READING

BAIM DS: Coronary angioplasty, in *Cardiac Catheterization, Angiography and Intervention*, 6th ed, D Baim, W Grossman (eds). Philadelphia, Lippincott Williams & Wilkins, 2000

BERGER PB et al: Survival following coronary angioplasty versus coronary artery bypass in anatomic subsets in which coronary artery bypass improves survival compared with medical therapy—results from the Bypass Angioplasty Revascularization Investigation (BARI). J Am Coll Cardiol 38:1440, 2001

BROWN DL et al: Meta-analysis of effectiveness and safety of abciximab versus eptifibatide or tirofiban in percutaneous coronary intervention. Am J Cardiol 87:537, 2001

CUTLIP DE et al: Stent thrombosis in the modern era—a pooled analysis of multicenter stent clinical trials. Circulation 103:1967, 2001

DE FEYTER PJ et al: Bypass surgery versus stenting for the treatment of multivessel disease in patients with unstable angina compared with stable angina. Circulation 105:2367, 2002

LEON MD et al: Localized intracoronary gamma radiation therapy to inhibit the recurrence of restenosis after stenting. N Engl J Med 344:250, 2001

MORRICE MC et al: A randomized comparison of a sirolimus-eluting stent with a standard stent for coronary revascularization. N Engl J Med 346:1773, 2002

SMITH SC et al: ACC/AHA guidelines of percutaneous coronary interventions. J Am Coll Cardiol 37:2215, 2001

VAN DE WERF F et al: Reperfusion for ST-elevation myocardial infarction—an overview of current treatment options. Circulation 105:2813, 2002

An elevated arterial pressure is probably the most important public health problem in developed countries. It is common, asymptomatic, readily detectable, usually easily treatable, and often leads to lethal complications if left untreated. As a result of extensive educational programs in the late 1960s and 1970s by both private and government agencies, the number of undiagnosed and/or untreated patients was reduced significantly by the late 1980s to a level of ~25%, with a concomitant decline in cardiovascular mortality. Unfortunately, by the mid-1990s, this beneficial trend began to wane. The number of undiagnosed patients with hypertension increased to nearly 33%, the decline in cardiovascular mortality flattened, and the number of individuals with chronic diseases with untreated or poorly treated hypertension increased. For example, the prevalence of end-stage renal disease per million population increased from <100 in 1982 to >250 in 1995, and the prevalence of congestive heart failure from ages 55 to 75 more than doubled between 1976 to 1980 and 1988 to 1991. Thus, although our understanding of the pathophysiology of elevated arterial pressure has increased, in 90 to 95% of cases the etiology (and thus potentially the means of prevention or cure) is still largely unknown. As a consequence, in most cases the hypertension is treated nonspecifically, resulting in a large number of minor side effects and a relatively high (50 to 60%) noncompliance rate.

PREVALENCE   The prevalence of hypertension depends on both the racial composition of the population studied and the criteria used to define the condition. In a white suburban population like that in the Framingham Study, nearly one-fifth of individuals have blood pressures >160/95 mmHg, while almost one-half have pressures >140/90 mmHg. An even higher prevalence has been documented in the nonwhite population. In females the prevalence is closely related to age, with a substantial increase occurring after age 50. This increase is presumably related to the hormonal changes of menopause, although the mechanism is unclear. Thus, the ratio of hypertension frequency in women versus men increases from 0.6 to 0.7 at age 30 to 1.1 to 1.2 at age 65.

The prevalence of various forms of secondary hypertension depends on the nature of the population studied and on how extensive the evaluation is. There are no available data to define the frequency of secondary hypertension in the general population, although in middle-aged males it has been reported to be 6%. On the other hand, in referral centers where patients undergo an extensive evaluation, it has been reported to be as high as 35%. The various forms of hypertension are outlined in Table 230-1, and their relative frequencies are given in Table 230-2.

ESSENTIAL HYPERTENSION

Patients with arterial hypertension and no definable cause are said to have *primary*, *essential*, or *idiopathic hypertension*. Undoubtedly, the primary difficulty in uncovering the responsible mechanisms in these patients is attributable to the variety of systems that are involved in the regulation of arterial pressure: peripheral and/or central adrenergic, renal, hormonal, and vascular. In addition, these systems are interrelated in a complex fashion, with input from multiple genes (see below). Several abnormalities have been described in patients with essential hypertension, often with a claim that one or more of them are primarily responsible for the hypertension. While it is still uncertain whether these individual abnormalities are primary or secondary, varying expressions of a single disease process, or reflective of separate disease entities, the accumulating data increasingly support the latter hypothesis. Therefore, just as pneumonia is caused by a variety of infectious agents, even though the clinical picture observed may be similar, so essential hypertension likely has a number of distinct causes. Thus, the distinction between primary and secondary hypertension has become blurred, and the approach to both the diagnosis and therapy of

hypertensive patients has been modified. For example, when a group of patients with essential hypertension is separated into a distinct subset (e.g., low-renin essential hypertension), the patients have not been reclassified as having a form of secondary hypertension but rather remain in the essential hypertensive group. In this chapter, individuals in whom a specific structural organ or gene defect is responsible for hypertension are defined as having a *secondary* form of hypertension. In contrast, individuals in whom generalized or functional abnormalities may be the cause of hypertension, even if the abnormalities are discrete, are defined as having *essential* hypertension.

ENVIRONMENT   A number of environmental factors have been implicated in the development of hypertension, including salt intake, obesity, occupation, alcohol intake, family size, and crowding. These factors have all been assumed to be important in the increase in blood pressure with age in more affluent societies, in contrast to the decline in blood pressure with age in less affluent groups.

SALT SENSITIVITY   The environmental factor that has received the greatest attention is salt intake. Even this factor illustrates the heterogeneous nature of the essential hypertensive population, in that the blood pressure is particularly responsive to the level of sodium intake in only ~60% of hypertensives. The cause of this special sensitivity to salt

---

TABLE 230-1   Classification of Arterial Hypertension

SYSTOLIC HYPERTENSION WITH WIDE PULSE PRESSURE

  I. Decreased compliance of aorta (arteriosclerosis)
 II. Increased stroke volume
    A. Aortic regurgitation
    B. Thyrotoxicosis
    C. Hyperkinetic heart syndrome
    D. Fever
    E. Arteriovenous fistula
    F. Patent ductus arteriosus

SYSTOLIC AND DIASTOLIC HYPERTENSION (INCREASED PERIPHERAL VASCULAR RESISTANCE)

  I. Renal
    A. Chronic pyelonephritis
    B. Acute and chronic glomerulonephritis
    C. Polycystic renal disease
    D. Renovascular stenosis or renal infarction
    E. Most other severe renal diseases (arteriolar nephrosclerosis, diabetic nephropathy, etc.)
    F. Renin-producing tumors
 II. Endocrine
    A. Oral contraceptives
    B. Adrenocortical hyperfunction
      1. Cushing's disease and syndrome
      2. Primary hyperaldosteronism
      3. Congenital or hereditary adrenogenital syndromes (17α-hydroxylase and 11β-hydroxylase defects)
    C. Pheochromocytoma
    D. Myxedema
    E. Acromegaly
 III. Neurogenic
    A. Psychogenic
    B. Diencephalic syndrome
    C. Familial dysautonomia (Riley-Day)
    D. Polyneuritis (acute porphyria, lead poisoning)
    E. Increased intracranial pressure (acute)
    F. Spinal cord section (acute)
 IV. Miscellaneous
    A. Coarctation of aorta
    B. Increased intravascular volume (excessive transfusion, polycythemia vera)
    C. Polyarteritis nodosa
    D. Hypercalcemia
    E. Medications, e.g., glucocorticoids, cyclosporine
  V. Unknown etiology
    A. Essential hypertension (>90% of all cases of hypertension)
    B. Toxemia of pregnancy
    C. Acute intermittent porphyria

TABLE 230-2 *Prevalence of Various Forms of Hypertension in the General Population and in Specialized Referral Clinics*[a]

Diagnosis	General Population, %	Specialty Clinic, %
Essential hypertension	92–94	65–85
Renal hypertension:		
Parenchymal	2–3	4–5
Renovascular	1–2	4–16
Endocrine hypertension:		
Primary aldosteronism	0.3	0.5–12
Cushing's syndrome	<0.1	0.2
Pheochromocytoma	<0.1	0.2
Oral contraceptive–induced	0.5–1	1–2
Miscellaneous	0.2	1

[a] Estimates based on a number of reports in the literature.

varies, with primary aldosteronism, bilateral renal artery stenosis, renal parenchymal disease, and low-renin essential hypertension accounting for about half the patients. In the remainder, the pathophysiology is still uncertain, but postulated contributing factors include chloride intake, calcium intake, a generalized cellular membrane defect, insulin resistance, and "nonmodulation" (see below).

ROLE OF RENIN Renin is an enzyme secreted by the juxtaglomerular cells of the kidney and linked with aldosterone in a negative feedback loop (Chap. 321). While a variety of factors can modify its rate of secretion, the primary determinant is the volume status of the individual, particularly as related to changes in dietary sodium intake. The end product of the action of renin on its substrate is the generation of the peptide angiotensin II. The response of target tissues to this peptide is uniquely determined by the prior dietary electrolyte intake. For example, sodium intake normally modulates adrenal and renal vascular responses to angiotensin II. With sodium restriction, adrenal responses are enhanced and the renal vascular responses reduced. Sodium loading has the opposite effect. The range of plasma renin activities observed in hypertensive subjects is broader than in normotensive individuals. In consequence, some hypertensive patients have been defined as having *low-renin* and others as having *high-renin* essential hypertension.

Low-Renin Essential Hypertension Approximately 20% of patients who by all other criteria have essential hypertension have suppressed plasma renin activity. Low-renin essential hypertension describes a widely recognized classification validated by clinical features, including salt-sensitivity of blood pressure and diuretic responsiveness. This situation is more common in individuals of African descent than in white patients, and in diabetics and the elderly. Though these patients are not hypokalemic, they have been reported to have expanded extracellular fluid volumes, and one unproven suggestion is that they have sodium retention and renin suppression due to excessive production of an unidentified mineralocorticoid. There are data to suggest that the low-renin state confers a beneficial natural history compared to that in patients with normal- or high-renin hypertension.

Nonmodulating Essential Hypertension Another subset of hypertensive patients who are also salt-sensitive has a reduced adrenal response to sodium restriction. In these individuals, sodium intake does not modulate either adrenal or renal vascular responses to angiotensin II. Hypertensives in this subset have been termed *nonmodulators* because of the absence of the sodium-mediated modulation of target tissue responses to angiotensin II. These individuals make up 25 to 30% of the hypertensive population, have plasma renin activity levels that are normal to high if measured when the patient is on a low-salt diet, and have hypertension that is salt-sensitive because of a defect in the kidney's ability to excrete sodium appropriately. They also are more insulin-resistant than other hypertensive patients, and the pathophysiologic characteristics can be corrected by the administration of an angiotensin-converting enzyme (ACE) inhibitor. Nonmodulation is

much more frequent among males and postmenopausal females. Furthermore, the nonmodulation characteristic appears to be genetically determined (associated with a certain allele of the angiotensinogen gene). Thus, nonmodulators are probably the most completely characterized intermediate phenotype in the hypertensive population.

High-Renin Essential Hypertension Approximately 15% of patients with essential hypertension have plasma renin activity levels above the normal range. It has been suggested that plasma renin plays an important role in the pathogenesis of the elevated arterial pressure in these patients. However, most studies have found that saralasin (a substance that, like losartan, acts as a competitive antagonist of angiotensin II) significantly reduces blood pressure in fewer than half of these patients. This finding has led some investigators to postulate that the elevated renin levels and blood pressure may both be secondary to an increase in adrenergic system activity. It has been proposed that in patients with angiotensin-dependent high-renin hypertension whose arterial pressures are lowered by an angiotensin II antagonist, the mechanism responsible for the increase in renin and, therefore, for the hypertension is the nonmodulating defect.

SODIUM ION VERSUS CHLORIDE OR CALCIUM Most studies assessing the role of salt in the hypertensive process have assumed that it is the sodium ion that is important. However, some investigators have suggested that the chloride ion may be equally important. This suggestion is based on the observation that feeding chloride-free sodium salts to salt-sensitive hypertensive animals fails to increase arterial pressure. Calcium has also been implicated in the pathogenesis of some forms of essential hypertension. A low-calcium intake has been associated with an increase in blood pressure in epidemiologic studies; an increase in leukocyte cytosolic calcium levels has been reported in some hypertensives. Finally, calcium entry blockers are effective antihypertensive agents. Several studies have reported a potential link between the salt-sensitive forms of hypertension and calcium. It has been postulated that salt loading in combination with a defect in the kidney's ability to excrete salt may lead to a secondary increase in circulating natriuretic factors. One of these factors, the so-called digitalis-like natriuretic factor, inhibits ouabain-sensitive Na^+,K^+-ATPase and thereby leads to intracellular calcium accumulation and a hyperreactive vascular smooth muscle.

CELL MEMBRANE DEFECT Another postulated explanation for salt-sensitive hypertension is a generalized cell membrane defect. This hypothesis derives most of its data from studies on circulating blood elements, particularly red blood cells, in which abnormalities in the transport of sodium across the cell membrane have been documented. Since both increases and decreases in the activity of different transport systems have been reported, it is likely that some abnormalities are primary and some are secondary. It has been assumed that an abnormality in sodium transport reflects an undefined alteration in the cell membrane and that this defect occurs in many, perhaps all, cells of the body, particularly the vascular smooth-muscle cells. The defect leads to an abnormal accumulation of calcium in vascular smooth muscle, resulting in a heightened vascular responsiveness to vasoconstrictor agents. This defect has been proposed to be present in 35 to 50% of essential hypertensive persons on the basis of studies using red cells. Other studies suggest that the abnormality in red cell sodium transport is not fixed but can be modified by environmental factors.

The common final pathway in all these hypotheses is an increase in cytosolic calcium resulting in increased vascular reactivity. However, as described above, several mechanisms might produce this calcium accumulation.

INSULIN RESISTANCE Insulin resistance and/or hyperinsulinemia have been suggested as being responsible for the increased arterial pressure in some patients with hypertension. This feature is now widely recognized as part of syndrome X, or the metabolic syndrome (Chap. 225), marked also by central obesity, dyslipidemia (especially elevated triglycerides), and high blood pressure. While it is clear that a substantial fraction of the hypertensive population has insulin resistance and hyperinsulinemia, it is less certain that this is more than an association. Insulin resistance is common in patients with diabetes mellitus type 2 and in obesity; both of these conditions are more common in hypertensive than in normotensive subjects. However, several studies have found that hyperinsulinemia and insulin resistance are present even in lean hypertensive patients without type 2 diabetes, suggesting that this relationship is more than a coincidence. As noted earlier, these individuals seem to be concentrated in the nonmodulation phenotype.

Hyperinsulinemia can increase arterial pressure by one or more of four mechanisms. An underlying assumption in each case is that some, but not all, of the target tissues of insulin are resistant to its effects. Specifically, tissues involved in glucose homeostasis are resistant (thereby producing the hyperinsulinemia), while tissues involved in the hypertensive process are not. First, hyperinsulinemia produces renal sodium retention (at least acutely) and increases sympathetic activity. Either or both of these effects could lead to an increase in arterial pressure. Another mechanism is vascular smooth-muscle hypertrophy secondary to the mitogenic action of insulin. Third, insulin also modifies ion transport across the cell membrane, thereby potentially increasing the cytosolic calcium levels of insulin-sensitive vascular or renal tissues. This mechanism would increase arterial pressure for reasons similar to those described above for the membrane-defect hypothesis. Finally, insulin resistance may be a marker for another pathologic process, e.g., nonmodulation, which could be the primary mechanism increasing blood pressure. It is important to point out, however, that the role of insulin in controlling arterial pressure is only vaguely understood, and, therefore, its potential as a pathogenic factor in hypertension remains unclear.

Few of the features of hypertension discussed above remain constant in a given patient. Some may be a reflection of the current metabolic and hormonal status of the patient rather than a permanent feature of the disease process. For example, at one point a patient might have insulin resistance secondary to obesity, which could lead to sodium retention, intravascular volume expansion, and renin suppression. This patient would be labeled as having "low-renin essential hypertension." If the patient lost weight, however, the salt-retaining tendency would be reversed. If the blood pressure did not normalize, the patient might then have "normal- or high-renin essential hypertension." Thus, the features reviewed above should not be considered mutually exclusive or permanent characteristics in a given patient with hypertension.

GENETIC CONSIDERATIONS Hypertension is one of the most common complex genetic disorders, with genetic heritability averaging ~30%. Data supporting this view emerge from animal studies as well as in population studies in humans. One approach has been to assess the correlation of blood pressure in families (familial aggregation). From these studies, the minimum size of the genetic factor can be expressed by a correlation coefficient of ~0.2. However, the variation in the size of the genetic factor in different studies reemphasizes the probably heterogeneous nature of the essential hypertensive population. In addition, most studies support the concept that the inheritance is probably multifactorial or that a number of different genetic defects each have an elevated blood pressure as one of their phenotypic expressions.

However, genes responsible for three distinct but rare monogenic hypertensive syndromes have been identified, two of which are inherited in a dominant fashion. Patients with *glucocorticoid-remediable hypertension* (GRA) have characteristically early-onset hypertension with increased frequency of strokes and evidence of hyperaldosteronism. Plasma aldosterone concentrates are high, plasma renin activity is low, and hypokalemia is frequent. A chimeric gene containing the promoter of the 11β-hydroxylase gene and the coding sequence for the aldosterone synthase gene has been identified in these patients, resulting in the ectopic production of aldosterone, which is corticotropin-dependent. The second dominant form is also a rare familial syndrome in which patients also *appear* to have elevated aldosterone

activity, with suppressed plasma renin activity and hypokalemia. In these patients, however, plasma aldosterone is normal. Mutations in the epithelial amiloride-sensitive sodium channel located in the collecting cortical tubule are responsible. The third monogenic syndrome is also a low-renin state, termed the *syndrome of apparent mineralocorticoid excess* (AME), caused by a defect in renal 11β-hydroxysteroid dehydrogenase. In these patients, the protective conversion of cortisol to the inactive cortisone does not occur, and local cortisol binds to the renal mineralocorticoid receptor.

In addition to these monogenic syndromes, susceptibility genes have now been reported which have as one of their consequences an increased arterial pressure (see below and Chap. 321). The most promising of these is the gene for renin substrate, angiotensinogen, in which a substitution of threonine for methionine at codon 235 has been associated with hypertension. Also, in patients with low-renin essential hypertension, an association with the G460W polymorphism of the α-adducin gene has been demonstrated. One of the hints of the genetic heritability of the low-renin state has emerged from studies revealing the familial aggregation of low-renin hypertension.

More than 50 genes have been examined in association studies with hypertension, and the number is constantly growing. As can be seen in Table 230-3, most studies of likely genes have failed to document linkage or consistent association with hypertension. However, uncertainty exists as to the validity of these negative conclusions. A positive relationship between hypertension and a gene could be obscured by the high probability of a false-negative result because of the heterogeneity of the hypertensive population. Thus, intermediate phenotypes in the hypertensive population need to be identified to differentiate patients into more homogeneous subgroups; the role of a specific candidate gene can then be more readily assessed. Such an approach is illustrated in Table 230-4.

TABLE 230-3 *Genesis Hypothesized to be Involved in Essential Hypertension*

Gene	Statistical Approach[a]	
	Linkage +/−	Association +/−
Renin-angiotensin-aldosterone system/sodium-volume		
Angiotensin-converting enzyme	0/1	12/14
Angiotensinogen	3/4	12/9
Aldosterone synthase	1/1	5/7
α-Adducin	0/1	5/3
AT1 receptor		4/6
Atrial natriuretic peptide		2/5
Human natriuretic peptide receptor (A)		1/1
Human natriuretic peptide receptor (B)		1/2
Renin	3/2	2/2
Adrenergic		
β₂-Adrenergic receptor		3/4
β₃-Adrenergic receptor		3/1
Dopamine D₂ receptor		2/0
α₂-Adrenergic receptor		1/1
Vascular		
Endothelin-1		3/1
Nitric oxide synthase, endothelial (NOS3)	0/2	5/10
Nitric oxide synthase, inducible (NOS2A)		1/1
Metabolic		
Glycogen synthase		1/1
Insulin receptor	0/1	3/0
Lipoprotein lipase		1/2
Apolipoprotein C-III		1/1
Miscellaneous		
G protein β₃ subunit		3/5

[a] Number of pertinent positive (+) and negative (−) published studies in humans.

TABLE 230-4   Role of Intermediate Phenotypes in Genetic Analysis

Gene	Phenotype	
	Intermediate	Distant
Converting enzyme ⎱ Angiotensinogen ⎰	Angiotensin II effect on kidney	Increases BP Increases BP
Aldo synthase	Increases 18-OH cortisol	Increases BP
Kallikrein	Decreases urine kallikrein	Increases BP
Na⁺/H⁺ exchanger	Increases Na/Li CTT	Increases BP
α-adducin	Low-renin hypertension	Increases BP
11 HSD₂	↑Cortisol/cortisone	Increases BP
ENaC	↓Renin, ↓aldosterone, ↓K⁺	Increases BP

Note: BP, blood pressure; OH, hydroxy; CTT, countertransport; HSD, hydroxy steroid-dehydrogenase; eNac, epithelial sodium channel.

FACTORS THAT MODIFY THE COURSE OF ESSENTIAL HYPERTENSION   Age, race, sex, smoking, alcohol intake, serum cholesterol, glucose intolerance, and weight all may alter the prognosis of this disease. The younger the patient when hypertension is first noted, the greater is the reduction in life expectancy if the hypertension is left untreated. In the United States, urban blacks have about twice the prevalence of hypertension as whites and more than four times the hypertension-induced morbidity rate. At all ages and in both white and nonwhite populations, females with hypertension fare better than males up to the age of 65, and the prevalence of hypertension in premenopausal females is substantially less than that in age-matched males or postmenopausal women. Yet, compared with their normotensive counterparts, females with hypertension run the same relative risk of a morbid cardiovascular event as do males. Accelerated atherosclerosis is an invariable companion of hypertension. Thus, it is not surprising that independent risk factors associated with the development of atherosclerosis, such as an elevated serum cholesterol, glucose intolerance, and/or cigarette smoking, significantly enhance the effect of hypertension on mortality rate regardless of age, sex, or race (Chap. 224). There is also no question that a positive correlation exists between obesity and arterial pressure. A gain in weight is associated with an increased frequency of hypertension in persons with previously normal blood pressure, and weight loss in obese persons with hypertension lowers their arterial pressure and, if they are being treated for hypertension, the intensity of therapy required to keep them normotensive. Whether these changes are mediated by changes in insulin resistance is unknown.

NATURAL HISTORY   Because essential hypertension is a heterogeneous disorder, variables other than the arterial pressure modify its course. Thus, the probability of developing a morbid cardiovascular event with a given arterial pressure may vary as much as 20-fold depending on whether associated risk factors are present (Table 230-5). Although exceptions have been reported, most untreated adults with hypertension will develop further increases in arterial pressure with time. Furthermore, it has been demonstrated from both actuarial data and experience in the era prior to effective therapy that untreated hypertension is associated with a shortening of life by 10 to 20 years, usually related to an acceleration of the atherosclerotic process, with the rate of acceleration in part related to the severity of the hypertension. Even individuals who have relatively mild disease—i.e., without evidence of end-organ damage—that is left untreated for 7 to 10 years have a high risk of developing significant complications. Nearly 30% will exhibit atherosclerotic complications, and >50% will have end-organ damage related to the hypertension itself, such as cardiomegaly, congestive heart failure, retinopathy, a cerebrovascular accident, and/or renal insufficiency. Thus, even in its mild forms, hypertension is a progressive and lethal disease if left untreated.

SECONDARY HYPERTENSION

As noted earlier, in only a small minority of patients with elevated arterial pressure can a specific cause be identified. Yet these patients should not be ignored for at least two reasons: (1) correction of the

TABLE 230-5   Risk Factors for An Adverse Prognosis in Hypertension

Black race
Youth
Male sex
Persistent diastolic pressure >115 mmHg
Smoking
Diabetes mellitus
Hypercholesterolemia
Obesity
Excess alcohol intake
Evidence of end organ damage
1. Cardiac
   a. Cardiac enlargement
   b. Electrocardiographic signs of ischemia or left ventricular strain
   c. Myocardial infarction
   d. Congestive heart failure
2. Eyes
   a. Retinal exudates and hemorrhages
   b. Papilledema
3. Renal: impaired renal function
4. Nervous system: cerebrovascular accident

cause may cure their hypertension, and (2) these secondary forms of the disease may provide insight into the etiology of essential hypertension. Nearly all the secondary forms of hypertension are related to an alteration in hormone secretion and/or renal function and are discussed in detail in other chapters.

RENAL HYPERTENSION (See also Chap. 267)   Hypertension produced by renal disease is the result of either (1) an alteration in renal secretion of vasoactive materials resulting in a systemic or local change in arteriolar tone, or (2) a derangement in the renal handling of sodium and fluids leading to volume expansion. The main subdivisions of renal hypertension are renovascular hypertension, including preeclampsia and eclampsia, and renal parenchymal hypertension. A simple explanation for *renal vascular hypertension* is that decreased perfusion of renal tissue due to stenosis of a main or branch renal artery activates the renin-angiotensin system, described in Chap. 321. Circulating angiotensin II elevates arterial pressure by directly causing vasoconstriction, by stimulating aldosterone secretion with resulting sodium retention, and/or by stimulating the adrenergic nervous system. In practice, only about one-half of patients with renovascular hypertension have an absolute elevation in renin activity in peripheral plasma, although when renin measurements are referenced against an index of sodium balance, a much higher fraction have inappropriately high values.

Activation of the renin-angiotensin system has also been offered as an explanation for the hypertension in both acute and chronic *renal parenchymal disease*. In this formulation, the only difference between renovascular and renal parenchymal hypertension is that the decreased perfusion of renal tissue in the latter case results from inflammatory and fibrotic changes involving multiple small intrarenal vessels. There are enough differences between the two conditions, however, to suggest that other mechanisms are active in renal parenchymal disease. Specifically, (1) peripheral plasma renin activity is elevated far less frequently in renal parenchymal than in renovascular hypertension; (2) cardiac output is said to be normal in renal parenchymal hypertension (unless uremia and anemia are present) but slightly elevated in renovascular hypertension; (3) circulatory responses to tilting and to the Valsalva maneuver are exaggerated in the latter condition; and (4) blood volume tends to be high in patients with severe renal parenchymal disease and low in patients with severe unilateral renovascular hypertension. Alternative explanations for the hypertension in renal parenchymal disease include the possibilities that the damaged kidneys (1) produce an unidentified vasopressor substance other than renin, (2) fail to produce a necessary humoral vasodilator substance (perhaps prostaglandin or bradykinin), (3) fail to inactivate circulating vasopressor substances, and/or (4) are ineffective in disposing of sodium. In the last case, the retained sodium would be responsible for the hypertension as outlined earlier.

Although all of these explanations, including participation of the renin-angiotensin system, probably have some validity in individual patients, the hypothesis involving sodium retention is particularly attractive. It is supported by the observation that those patients with chronic pyelonephritis or polycystic renal disease who are salt wasters do not develop hypertension and by the observation that removal of salt and water by dialysis or diuretics is effective in controlling arterial pressure in most patients with renal parenchymal disease.

A rare form of renal hypertension results from the excess secretion of renin by juxtaglomerular cell tumors or nephroblastomas. The initial presentation is similar to that of hyperaldosteronism, with hypertension, hypokalemia, and overproduction of aldosterone. However, in contrast to primary aldosteronism, peripheral renin activity is *elevated instead of subnormal*. This disease can be distinguished from other forms of secondary aldosteronism by the presence of normal renal function and unilateral increases in renal vein renin concentration without a renal artery lesion.

ENDOCRINE HYPERTENSION ■ Adrenal Hypertension Hypertension is a feature of a variety of adrenal cortical abnormalities. In *primary aldosteronism* (Chap. 321), there is a clear relationship between the aldosterone-induced sodium retention and the hypertension. Normal individuals given aldosterone develop hypertension only if they also ingest sodium. Since aldosterone causes sodium retention by stimulating renal tubular exchange of sodium for potassium, hypokalemia is a prominent feature in most patients with primary aldosteronism, and, therefore, the measurement of serum potassium provides a simple screening test. The effect of sodium retention and volume expansion in chronically suppressing plasma renin activity is critical for the definitive diagnosis. In most clinical situations, plasma renin activity and plasma or urinary aldosterone levels parallel each other, but in patients with primary aldosteronism, aldosterone levels are high and relatively fixed because of autonomous aldosterone secretion, whereas plasma renin activity levels are suppressed and respond sluggishly to sodium depletion. Primary aldosteronism may be secondary to either a tumor or bilateral adrenal hyperplasia. It is important to distinguish between these two conditions preoperatively, since the hypertension in the latter case is usually not modified by operation.

The sodium-retaining effect of large amounts of glucocorticoids (perhaps resulting in part from saturation of the 11β-hydroxysteroid hydrogenase enzyme system in the kidney by the increased concentration of cortisol) also offers an explanation for the hypertension in severe cases of Cushing's syndrome (Chap. 321). Moreover, increased production of mineralocorticoids has also been documented in some patients with Cushing's syndrome. However, the hypertension in many cases of Cushing's syndrome does not seem volume-dependent, leading investigators to speculate that it may be secondary to glucocorticoid-induced production of renin substrate (angiotensin-mediated hypertension). In the forms of the adrenogenital syndrome due to C-11 or C-17 hydroxylase deficiency (Chap. 321), deoxycorticosterone accounts for the sodium retention and the resulting hypertension, which is accompanied by suppression of plasma renin activity.

In patients with pheochromocytoma (Chap. 322), increased secretion of epinephrine and norepinephrine by a tumor (most often located in the adrenal medulla) causes excessive stimulation of adrenergic receptors, which results in peripheral vasoconstriction and cardiac stimulation. This diagnosis is confirmed by demonstrating increased urinary excretion of epinephrine and norepinephrine and/or their metabolites.

Acromegaly (See also Chap. 318) Hypertension, coronary atherosclerosis, and cardiac hypertrophy are frequent complications of this condition.

Hypercalcemia (See also Chap. 331) The hypertension that occurs in up to one-third of patients with hyperparathyroidism ordinarily can be attributed to renal parenchymal damage due to nephrolithiasis and nephrocalcinosis. However, increased calcium levels can also have a direct vasoconstrictive effect. In some cases, the hypertension disappears when the hypercalcemia is corrected. Thus, paradoxically, the increased serum calcium level in hyperparathyroidism raises blood pressure, while epidemiologic studies suggest that a high calcium intake lowers blood pressure. To confuse the issue further, calcium entry-blocking agents are effective antihypertensive agents. Additional studies are needed to resolve these seemingly conflicting observations.

COARCTATION OF THE AORTA (See also Chap. 218) The hypertension associated with coarctation may be caused by the constriction itself or perhaps by the changes in the renal circulation, which result in an unusual form of renal arterial hypertension. The diagnosis of coarctation is usually evident from physical examination and routine x-ray findings.

EFFECTS OF HYPERTENSION

Patients with hypertension die prematurely; the most common cause of death is heart disease, with stroke and renal failure also frequent, particularly in patients with significant retinopathy.

EFFECTS ON THE HEART Cardiac compensation for the excessive workload imposed by increased systemic pressure is at first sustained by concentric left ventricular hypertrophy, characterized by an increase in wall thickness. Ultimately, the function of this chamber deteriorates, the cavity dilates, and the symptoms and signs of heart failure appear (Chap. 215). Angina pectoris may also occur because of the combination of accelerated coronary arterial disease and increased myocardial oxygen requirements as a consequence of the increased myocardial mass (Chap. 226). On physical examination, the heart is enlarged and has a prominent left ventricular impulse. The sound of aortic closure is accentuated, and there may be a faint murmur of aortic regurgitation. Presystolic (atrial, fourth) heart sounds appear frequently in hypertensive heart disease, and a protodiastolic (ventricular, third) heart sound or summation gallop rhythm may be present. Electrocardiographic changes of left ventricular hypertrophy (Chap. 210) may occur, but the electrocardiogram substantially underestimates the frequency of cardiac hypertrophy compared with that observed with the echocardiogram. Evidence of ischemia or infarction may be observed late in the disease. Most deaths due to hypertension result from myocardial infarction or congestive heart failure. Recent data suggest that some of the myocardial damage may be mediated by aldosterone in the presence of a normal/high salt intake rather than just the increased blood pressure or an increase in angiotensin II levels per se.

NEUROLOGIC EFFECTS The neurologic effects of long-standing hypertension may be divided into retinal and central nervous system changes. Because the retina is the only tissue in which the arteries and arterioles can be examined directly, repeated ophthalmoscopic examination provides the opportunity to observe the progress of the vascular effects of hypertension. The Keith-Wagener-Barker classification of the *retinal changes* in hypertension has provided a simple and excellent means for serial evaluation of hypertensive patients (see Fig. 25-1).

Central nervous system dysfunction also occurs frequently in patients with hypertension. Occipital headaches, most often occurring in the morning, are among the most prominent early symptoms of hypertension. Dizziness, light-headedness, vertigo, tinnitus, and dimmed vision or syncope may also be observed, but the more serious manifestations are due to vascular occlusion, hemorrhage, or encephalopathy (Chap. 349). The pathogeneses of the former two disorders are quite different. *Cerebral infarction* is secondary to the increased atherosclerosis observed in hypertensive patients, whereas *cerebral hemorrhage* is the result of both the elevated arterial pressure and the development of cerebral vascular microaneurysms (Charcot-Bouchard aneurysms). Only age and arterial pressure are known to influence the development of the microaneurysms. Thus, it is not surprising that arterial pressure shows a better association with cerebral hemorrhage than with either cerebral or myocardial infarction.

Hypertensive encephalopathy (see p. 1480) consists of the following symptom complex: severe hypertension, disordered consciousness, increased intracranial pressure, retinopathy with papilledema, and seizures. The pathogenesis is uncertain but is probably not related to arteriolar spasm or cerebral edema. Focal neurologic signs are infrequent and, if present, suggest that infarction, hemorrhage, or transient ischemic attacks are more likely diagnoses. Although some investigators have suggested that prompt lowering of arterial pressure in these patients may adversely affect cerebral blood flow, most studies indicate that this is not the case.

EFFECTS ON THE KIDNEY (See also Chap. 267) Arteriosclerotic lesions of the afferent and efferent arterioles and the glomerular capillary tufts are the most common renal vascular lesions in hypertension and result in a decreased glomerular filtration rate and tubular dysfunction. Proteinuria and microscopic hematuria occur because of glomerular lesions, and ~10% of the deaths caused by hypertension result from renal failure. Blood loss in hypertension occurs not only from renal lesions; epistaxis, hemoptysis, and metrorrhagia also occur frequently in these patients.

APPROACH TO THE PATIENT

DEFINITION Since there is no dividing line between normal and high blood pressure, arbitrary levels have been established to define persons who have an increased risk of developing a morbid cardiovascular event and/or will benefit from medical therapy. These should be based upon not only the level of diastolic pressure but also systolic pressure, age, sex, race, and concomitant diseases. For example, patients with a diastolic pressure >90 mmHg have a significant reduction in morbidity and mortality rate if they receive adequate therapy. These, then, are patients who have hypertension and who should be considered for treatment.

The level of *systolic* pressure is very important in assessing the influence of arterial pressure on cardiovascular morbidity. Data increasingly suggest that it may be more important than diastolic pressure, especially in those over the age of 50. For example, males with normal diastolic pressures (<82 mmHg) but elevated systolic pressures (>158 mmHg) have a cardiovascular mortality rate 2.5 times higher than individuals who have similar diastolic pressures but whose systolic pressures clearly are normal (<130 mmHg). A reduction in mortality and morbidity with treatment, specifically in the elderly, has been documented in these patients. This beneficial effect results mainly from a reduction in strokes and occurs in women as well. Other significant demographic factors that modify the influence of blood pressure on the frequency of morbid cardiovascular events are age, race, and sex, with young black males being most adversely affected by hypertension.

When hypertension is suspected, blood pressure should be measured at least twice during two separate examinations after the initial screening. In adults, a *diastolic* pressure <85 mmHg is considered to be normal; one between 85 and 89 mmHg is high normal; one of 90 to 99 mmHg represents stage 1 or mild hypertension; one of 100 to 109 mmHg represents stage 2 or moderate hypertension; and one of ≥110 mmHg represents stage 3 or severe hypertension. A *systolic* pressure <130 mmHg indicates normal blood pressure; one between 130 and 139 mmHg indicates high normal; one between 140 and 159 mmHg indicates stage 1 or mild hypertension; one between 160 and 179 mmHg indicates stage 2 or moderate hypertension; and one ≥180 mmHg indicates stage 3 or severe hypertension. Isolated systolic hypertension, common among the elderly, is defined by systolic pressure <140 mmHg together with a normal diastolic pressure. *White coat hypertension* describes a significant percentage of individuals whose blood pressure, measured in the office by a professional, is persistently higher than when measured at home or under casual circumstances. Current estimates are that 10 to 20% of patients declared hypertensive in their doctors' offices are normotensive outside it; this diagnosis is relatively more common among the elderly and pregnant women.

Increasing use of ambulatory blood pressure monitoring (ABPM) may provide additional useful information in patients who are difficult to classify. These devices measure blood pressure over a 12- or 24-h period as patients perform normal activities and during sleep. However, normal values for this procedure and its usefulness in relation to therapeutic outcomes are not currently known. A useful classification of hypertension derived from the 2003 European Society of Hypertension Guidelines is shown in Table 230-6. Of note, the Seventh US Joint National Committee on Prevention, Detection, Evaluation, and Treatment of High Blood Pressure (JNC 7) published a new classification in 2003 which limited normal blood pressure to <120 mmHg systolic and <80 mmHg diastolic, and added a new category of "prehypertension" defined by systolic pressure between 120 and 139 or diastolic blood pressure between 80 and 89 mm. Prevention strategies are recommended for this population.

Arterial pressure fluctuates in most persons, whether they are normotensive or hypertensive. Patients who are classified as having *labile hypertension* are those who sometimes, but not always, have arterial pressures in the hypertensive range. These patients are often considered to have borderline hypertension. Sustained hypertension can become accelerated or enter a malignant phase (p. 1480), although that is unusual in treated patients. *Accelerated hypertension* is defined as a significant recent increase over previous hypertensive levels associated with evidence of vascular damage on funduscopic examination but without papilledema.

PATIENT EVALUATION In evaluating patients with hypertension, the initial history, physical examination, and laboratory tests should be directed at (1) uncovering correctable secondary forms of hypertension (see below), (2) establishing a pretreatment baseline, (3) assessing factors that may influence the type of therapy or be changed adversely by therapy, (4) determining if target organ damage is present, and (5) determining whether other risk factors for the development of arteriosclerotic cardiovascular disease are present (Table 230-5).

Symptoms and Signs Most patients with hypertension have no specific symptoms referable to their blood pressure elevation and are identified only in the course of a physical examination. When symptoms do bring the patient to the physician, they fall into three categories. They are related to (1) the elevated pressure itself, (2) the hypertensive vascular disease, and (3) the underlying disease, in the case of secondary hypertension. Though popularly considered a symptom of elevated arterial pressure, headache is characteristic of only severe hypertension; most commonly such headaches are localized to the occipital region and are present when the patient awakens in the morning but subside spontaneously after several hours. Other complaints that may be related to elevated blood pressure include dizziness, palpitations, easy fatigability, and

TABLE 230-6 *Classification of Blood Pressure for Adults ≥18 Years Old*

Category	Systolic Pressure, mmHg	Diastolic Pressure, mmHg
Optimal	<120	<80
Normal	<130	<85
High normal	130–139	85–89
Hypertension[a]		
Stage 1 (mild)	140–159	90–99
Stage 2 (moderate)	160–179	100–109
Stage 3 (severe)	≥180	≥110
Isolated systolic hypertension	≥140	<90

[a] Based on the average of ≥2 readings taken at each of two or more visits after an initial screening.

Note: Classification of blood pressure for adults aged 18 years and older not taking antihypertensive drugs and not acutely ill. When systolic and diastolic pressures fall into different categories, the higher category should be selected to classify the individual's blood pressure status.

Source: 2003 European Society of Hypertension—European Society of Cardiology guidelines for the management of arterial hypertension.

impotence. Complaints referable to vascular disease include epistaxis, hematuria, blurring of vision owing to retinal changes, episodes of weakness or dizziness due to transient cerebral ischemia, angina pectoris, and dyspnea due to cardiac failure. Pain due to dissection of the aorta or to a leaking aneurysm is a rare presenting symptom.

Examples of symptoms related to the underlying disease in secondary hypertension are polyuria, polydipsia, and muscle weakness secondary to hypokalemia in patients with primary aldosteronism or weight gain, and emotional lability in patients with Cushing's syndrome. The patient with a pheochromocytoma may present with episodic headaches, palpitations, diaphoresis, and postural dizziness.

History A strong family history of hypertension, along with the reported finding of intermittent pressure elevation in the past, favors the diagnosis of essential hypertension. Secondary hypertension often develops before the age of 35 years or after 55. A history of repeated urinary tract infections suggests chronic pyelonephritis, although this condition may occur in the absence of symptoms. A history of weight gain is compatible with Cushing's syndrome, and one of weight loss is compatible with pheochromocytoma. A number of aspects of the history aid in determining whether vascular disease has progressed to a dangerous stage. These include angina pectoris and symptoms of cerebrovascular insufficiency, congestive heart failure, and/or peripheral vascular insufficiency. Other risk factors that should be asked about include cigarette smoking, diabetes mellitus, lipid disorders, and a family history of early deaths due to cardiovascular disease. Finally, aspects of the patient's lifestyle that could contribute to the hypertension or affect its treatment should be assessed, including diet, physical activity, family status, work, and educational level.

Physical Examination The physical examination starts with the patient's general appearance. For instance, are the round face and truncal obesity of Cushing's syndrome present? Is muscular development in the upper extremities out of proportion to that in the lower extremities, suggesting coarctation of the aorta? The next step is to compare the blood pressures and pulses in the two upper extremities and in the supine and standing positions (for at least 2 min). A rise in diastolic pressure when the patient goes from the supine to the standing position is most compatible with essential hypertension; a fall, in the absence of antihypertensive medications, suggests secondary forms of hypertension. Funduscopic findings provide one of the best indications of the duration of hypertension and of prognosis. A useful guide is the Keith-Wagener-Barker classification of funduscopic changes, in which classification from normal through grade IV retinopathy is based upon the presence of arteriolar light reflex, arteriovenous crossing defects, hemmorhages and exudates; the specific changes in each fundus should be recorded and a grade assigned (see Fig. 25-8). Palpation and auscultation of the carotid arteries for evidence of stenosis or occlusion should be carried out. In examination of the heart and lungs, evidence of left ventricular hypertrophy and cardiac decompensation should be sought. Is there a left ventricular lift? Are third and fourth heart sounds present? Are there pulmonary rales? A third heart sound and pulmonary rales are unusual in uncomplicated hypertension. Their presence suggests ventricular dysfunction. Chest examination also includes a search for extracardiac murmurs and palpable collateral vessels that may result from coarctation of the aorta.

The most important part of the abdominal examination is auscultation for bruits originating in stenotic renal arteries. Bruits due to renal arterial narrowing nearly always have a diastolic component or may be continuous and are best heard just to the right or left of the midline above the umbilicus or in the flanks. The abdomen should also be palpated for an abdominal aneurysm and for the enlarged kidneys of polycystic renal disease. The femoral pulses should be felt, and, if they are decreased and/or delayed in

comparison with the radial pulse, the blood pressure in the lower extremities must be measured. Even if the femoral pulse is normal to palpation, arterial pressure in the lower extremities should be recorded at least once in patients in whom hypertension is discovered before the age of 30 years.

Laboratory Investigation The *basic* laboratory studies that should be performed in all patients are described in Table 230-7. Renal status is evaluated by assessing the presence of protein, blood, and glucose in the urine and measuring serum creatinine and/or blood urea nitrogen. Microscopic examination of the urine is also helpful. The serum potassium level should be measured both as a screen for mineralocorticoid-induced hypertension and to provide a baseline before diuretic therapy is begun. A blood glucose determination is helpful both because diabetes mellitus may be associated with accelerated arteriosclerosis, renal vascular disease, and diabetic nephropathy in patients with hypertension and because primary aldosteronism, Cushing's syndrome, and pheochromocytoma may all be associated with hyperglycemia. The possibility of hypercalcemia may also be investigated. Serum cholesterol, high-density lipoprotein cholesterol, and triglyceride levels identify other factors that predispose to the development of arteriosclerosis.

An electrocardiogram should be obtained in all cases. The echocardiogram is more sensitive than either the electrocardiogram or physical examination in determining whether cardiac hypertrophy is present and may be a useful addition to the *baseline* evaluation of a hypertensive patient, particularly as left ventricular hypertrophy is an independent cardiovascular risk factor and its presence indicates the need for vigorous antihypertensive therapy. Because of the cost of an echocardiogram and the uncertainty as to whether the resultant information would modify therapy, it is unclear that routine *follow-up* echocardiograms during therapy are justified. The chest roentgenogram may also be helpful by providing the opportunity to identify aortic dilation or elongation and the rib notching that occurs in coarctation of the aorta.

Most patients do not require ABPM, but readings are useful in diagnosing white coat hypertension and also in evaluating refractory hypertension, circadian patterns of blood pressure, and relation

---

TABLE 230-7 *Laboratory Tests for Evalution of Hypertension*

BASIC TESTS FOR INITIAL EVALUATION

1. Always included
   a. Urine for protein, blood, and glucose
   b. Microscopic urinalysis
   c. Hematocrit
   d. Serum potassium
   e. Serum creatinine and/or blood urea nitrogen
   f. Fasting glucose
   g. Total cholesterol
   h. Electrocardiogram
2. Usually included, depending on cost and other factors
   a. Thyroid-stimulating hormone
   b. White blood cell count
   c. HDL and LDL cholesterol and triglycerides
   d. Serum calcium and phosphate
   e. Chest x-ray; limited echocardiogram

SPECIAL STUDIES TO SCREEN FOR SECONDARY HYPERTENSION

1. Renovascular disease: angiotensin-converting enzyme inhibitor radionuclide renal scan, renal duplex Doppler flow studies, and MRI angiography
2. Pheochromocytoma: 24-h urine assay for creatinine, metanephrines, and catecholamines
3. Cushing's syndrome: overnight dexamethasone suppression test or 24-h urine cortisol and creatinine
4. Primary aldosteronism: plasma aldosterone: renin activity ratio

Note: HDL, high-density lipoprotein; LDL, low-density lipoprotein; MRI, magnetic resonance imaging.

of blood pressure to symptoms like dizziness and visual changes. ABPM readings are good predictors of future cardiovascular events. Mean 24-h systolic pressure ≥ 135 mmHg has been associated with a nearly double cardiovascular risk. When the normal nocturnal decline in blood pressure ("dipping") is absent, readings correlate well with the prevalence and extent of target organ damage in hypertensive individuals.

DIAGNOSIS OF SECONDARY HYPERTENSION   The abrupt onset of severe hypertension and/or the onset of hypertension of any severity in a patient under the age of 35 or over the age of 55 should lead to laboratory tests to exclude renovascular hypertension and pheochromocytoma, and the finding on physical examination of bilateral upper abdominal masses consistent with polycystic renal disease should lead to the performance of an abdominal ultrasound. An elevated creatinine or blood urea nitrogen level, associated with proteinuria and hematuria, should prompt a detailed workup for renal insufficiency (Chap. 259). A familial history of hypertension, particularly with early age of onset, should spark consideration of a genetic form. Special studies for secondary hypertension are also indicated if there is therapeutic failure with the initial drug program. The specific diagnostic measures depend on the most likely causes of secondary hypertension.

Pheochromocytoma (See also Chap. 322)   A history of headaches, palpitations, anxiety attacks, unusual sweating, hyperglycemia, and weight loss should also lead to tests to exclude pheochromocytoma. The easiest and best screening procedure for pheochromocytoma is the measurement of catecholamines and their metabolites in a 24-h urine sample collected while the patient is hypertensive. Measurement of plasma catecholamine levels may also be useful, while the assay of plasma-free metanephrines holds promise for heightened sensitivity. These tests may be indicated even in patients who do not have episodic hypertension, since over half the patients with pheochromocytoma have fixed hypertension. Provocative tests are seldom, if ever, indicated, although occasionally a suppressive test may be useful.

Cushing's Syndrome (See also Chap. 321)   A 24-h urine test for cortisol and creatinine or the administration of 1 mg of dexamethasone at bedtime, followed by the measurement of plasma cortisol at 7 to 10 A.M., is the best test to screen for the presence of Cushing's syndrome. A urine cortisol level of <2750 nmol (100 μg) or suppression of the plasma cortisol level to <140 nmol/L (5 μg/dL) effectively rules out Cushing's syndrome.

Renovascular Hypertension (See also Chap. 267)   The presence of an abdominal bruit should lead to a workup for renovascular hypertension. Suspicion for this form of hypertension should also be especially high in patients with deterioration of renal function after institution of ACE inhibitor therapy or in older patients with atherosclerotic disease. Over the past decades the standard approach to screen for renovascular hypertension has progressed from the rapid-sequence intravenous pyelogram to one of three noninvasive techniques: the captopril-enhanced radionuclide renal scan (the preferred choice), a duplex Doppler flow study, or magnetic resonance (MR) angiography with gadolinium enhancements. Perhaps the most sensitive and specific screening test, the spiral computed tomography (CT) scan, which gives a three-dimensional view, also requires giving an intravenous contrast agent.

The definitive test for surgically correctable renal disease is the combination of a renal angiogram and renal vein renin determinations. The renal arteriogram both establishes the presence of a renal arterial lesion and aids in the determination of whether the lesion is due to atherosclerosis or to one of the fibrous or fibromuscular dysplasias. It does not, however, prove that the lesion is responsible for the hypertension, nor does it permit prediction of the chances of surgical cure. It must be noted that (1) renal artery stenosis is a frequent finding by angiography and at postmortem in normotensive individuals, and (2) essential hypertension is a common condition and may occur in combination with renal arterial stenosis that is not responsible for the hypertension. Bilateral renal vein catheterization for measurement of plasma renin activity is therefore used to assess the functional significance of any lesion noted on arteriography. When one kidney is ischemic and the other is normal, all the renin released comes from the involved kidney. In the most straightforward situation, the ischemic kidney has a significantly higher venous plasma renin activity than the normal kidney, by a factor of ≥ 1.5. Moreover, the renal venous blood draining the uninvolved kidney exhibits levels similar to those in the inferior vena cava below the entrance of the renal veins.

Significant benefit from operative correction may be anticipated in at least 80% of patients with the findings described above if care is taken to prepare the patient properly before renal vein blood sampling, i.e., by discontinuing renin-suppressing drugs, such as beta blockers, for at least 10 days; restricting the patient to a low-sodium intake for 4 days; and/or giving a converting-enzyme inhibitor for 24 h. When obstructing lesions in the *branches* of the renal arteries are demonstrated by arteriography, an attempt to obtain blood samples from the *main branches* of the renal vein should be made in an effort to identify a localized intrarenal arterial lesion responsible for the hypertension.

Primary Aldosteronism (See also Chap. 321)   These patients usually exhibit hypokalemia. Diuretic therapy often complicates the picture when the hypokalemia is first observed and needs to be assessed. Given the presence of hypokalemia, the relation between plasma renin activity and the aldosterone level becomes the key to the diagnosis of primary aldosteronism. The aldosterone concentration or excretion rate is high and plasma renin activity is low in primary aldosteronism, and these levels are relatively unaffected by changes in sodium balance. Thus, the aldosterone:renin ratio is high. A critical part of the evaluation after primary aldosteronism has been established is to determine whether disease is unilateral or bilateral, because surgical removal of the lesion usually reduces arterial pressure only in patients with unilateral disease.

Rx TREATMENT

INDICATIONS FOR THERAPY   Patients with a diastolic pressure repeatedly >90 mmHg or systolic pressure >140 mmHg should be treated unless specific contraindications exist. Patients with isolated *systolic* hypertension (levels >160 mmHg with diastolic pressure <89 mmHg) should also be treated if they are over age 65 (Fig. 230-1). Patients with labile hypertension or isolated systolic hypertension who are not treated should have regular follow-up examinations at 6-month intervals because of the frequent development of progressive and/or sustained hypertension. Finally, patients with atherosclerotic vascular disease or diabetes mellitus and diastolic blood pressures between 85 and 90 mmHg should also receive antihypertensive therapy (Fig. 230-2).

Appropriate therapy for patients with white coat hypertension is debated, largely because the ultimate risk of cardiovascular events in these patients is still unknown. Some believe that subjects whose blood pressure is susceptible to apprehension and anxiety in the doctor's office are likely to have elevations during other periods of stress in their lives. Others hold white coat hypertension to be a tightly circumscribed phenomenon. In either case, these individuals would clearly benefit from life-style modifications to reduce progression to sustained hypertension. At present, there are insufficient data to warrant treatment with antihypertensive therapy unless other risk factors are present.

What should the blood pressure goal be? Previously it was assumed that 140/90 mmHg was the desired level. This still seems reasonable for nondiabetic patients since the Hypertension Optimal Treatment (HOT) study did not detect a significant difference in cardiovascular risk between nondiabetic patients treated to goal diastolic blood pressures of 90 versus 80 mmHg. However, in patients with

FIGURE 230-1 Initiation of treatment in patients with hypertension. See Table 230-11 for listing of classes of agents to use initially. In the initial evaluation, patients are stratified for cardiovascular risk using: level of blood pressure; the presence of risk factors—smoking, obesity, male gender, etc.—which vary from 0 factors (low risk) to three or more factors (high risk equivalent to having diabetes mellitus), target organ damage (TOD, i.e., clinical cardiovascular or renal disease) or diabetes (both high risk if present regardless of other risk factors). SBP, systolic blood pressure; DBP, diastolic blood pressure

diabetes this is not the case. In the U.K. Prospective Diabetes Study (UKPDS), patients reaching a blood pressure of 144/82 mmHg had a substantially lower risk compared to those with a blood pressure of 154/87 mmHg. The HOT study investigators documented a similar finding in their diabetic subset. Importantly, these studies have failed to document the existence of a "J" or "U" curve, indicating no increased risk of excessive blood pressure reduction. Thus, it is reasonable to target a blood pressure well within the normal range for diabetic patients, at most 130/85 mmHg. Newer studies may force this recommended goal even lower (see "Diabetes Mellitus," below). While not definitively proven, it seems prudent to use the same goal in patients with target organ damage, and in young and middle-aged patients, depending on what other cardiovascular risk factors are present. For elderly individuals, a goal of 140/90 mmHg is appropriate. Importantly, how aggressive one should be in achieving these blood pressure goals depends on the number and severity of other risk factors present.

Probably fewer than one-third of hypertensive patients in the United States are being treated effectively. Only a small number of these failures are related to drug unresponsiveness. Most are related to (1) failure to detect hypertension, (2) failure to institute effective treatment of an asymptomatic hypertensive patient, and (3) failure of the asymptomatic hypertensive patient to adhere to therapy. To help with the latter problem, patients must be educated to continue treatment once an effective regimen has been identified. Side effects and inconveniences of treatment must be minimized or counteracted in order to obtain the patient's continued cooperation.

The identification of an operable form of secondary hypertension does not automatically mean that surgical treatment is indicated. The decision depends on the age and general health of the patient, the natural history of the lesion, and the response of the arterial pressure to drug therapy. In patients with renovascular hypertension, the feasibility of renal angioplasty, the advantages of surgical repair versus nephrectomy, and the degree of overall renal functional impairment must be considered. Age and general health are important in patients with renovascular hypertension due to arteriosclerosis, because there is no evidence that repair of the stenosis increases life expectancy in the elderly patient with other evidence of vascular disease. Knowledge of the natural history of the disease is especially important when making a decision in the case of a young patient with renal artery stenosis due to fibrous dysplasia. If the arteriographic appearance suggests that the stenosis is due to intimal or subadventitial fibroplasia, the lesion may be expected to progress, and operation or angioplasty is required. Medial fibroplasia, on the other hand, often remains stable, and operation or angioplasty may not be necessary if pressure can be controlled by drug therapy.

The decision regarding operation should also be considered carefully in patients with primary aldosteronism when neither abdominal CT nor bilateral adrenal venous sampling for aldosterone demonstrates a tumor, because such patients may prove to have multinodular hyperplasia. In that case, bilateral adrenalectomy would be required to eliminate the aldosterone excess, and, even then, hypertension would usually persist. If hypokalemia can be controlled by an aldosterone receptor antagonist, e.g., spironolactone, or other drug therapy and arterial pressure lowered with antihypertensive agents, then it is reasonable to withhold operative treatment.

GENERAL MEASURES Nondrug therapeutic intervention is probably indicated in all patients with sustained hypertension and probably in most with labile hypertension. The general measures employed include (1) relief of stress, (2) dietary management, (3) regular aerobic exercise, (4) weight reduction (if needed), and (5) control of other risk factors contributing to the development of arteriosclerosis. Though it

FIGURE 230-2 Approach to the hypertensive patient after initiating antihypertensive drug treatment. See Fig. 230-1 for initial steps and definition of risk and Table 230-11 for initial choice of agents.

is usually impossible to extricate the hypertensive patient from all internal and external stresses, he or she should be advised to avoid unnecessary tensions. In rare instances, it may be appropriate to recommend a change of job or of life-style. It has been suggested that relaxation techniques may also lower arterial pressure.

Dietary management has three aspects:

1. Because of the documented efficacy of sodium restriction and volume contraction in lowering blood pressure, patients previously were instructed to curtail sodium intake drastically. Some investigators have suggested that this is not necessary. They base their conclusion on two observations: (1) In many patients the blood pressure is not sensitive to the level of sodium intake, and (2) diuretics provide another method of decreasing body sodium stores in individuals whose blood pressure is sodium-sensitive. However, meta-analyses of previous diet studies have documented a 5-mmHg reduction in systolic pressure and a 2.6-mmHg reduction in diastolic pressure when sodium intake is reduced by ~75 meq/d. In addition, several reports have documented that, while mild sodium restriction has little if any direct action on blood pressure, it significantly potentiates the efficacy of nearly all antihypertensive agents. Thus, by making it possible to control blood pressure with lower doses of drugs, sodium restriction leads to a reduction in side effects. In addition, it is quite clear that some hypertensive patients are salt-sensitive (p. 1463), and the level of sodium intake does influence the blood pressure. Thus, since there is no apparent risk to mild sodium restriction, the most practical approach is to advise mild dietary sodium restriction (up to 5 g NaCl per day), which can be achieved by eliminating all additions of salt to food that is prepared normally. Some studies have also reported a lowering of arterial pressure related to an *increase* in potassium and/or calcium intake. For example, in one meta-analysis, dietary potassium supplements of 50 to 120 meq/d reduced blood pressure by about the same amount as salt restriction (by 6 mmHg systolic and 3.4 mmHg diastolic). While the advisability of these forms of dietary alteration is still controversial, the fact that a moderately high calcium intake (1.5 g elemental calcium daily) probably also reduces the extent of age-related osteoporosis, combined with the results of the potassium supplementation studies, indicate that they are probably useful adjuncts. A particularly useful approach is the DASH (Dietary Approaches to Stop Hypertension) diet, which uses natural foods that are high in potassium and low in saturated and total fat, emphasizing fruits, vegetables, and low-fat dairy products. This diet significantly lowered blood pressure in borderline and stage 1 hypertensive subjects (11.4/5.5 mm Hg)(see Table 230-6 for definitions). The sequel DASH-sodium trial found that coupling the DASH diet with moderate sodium restriction led to greater falls in pressure than dietary manipulation alone, although the gain was modest. While salt restriction has been shown to lower blood pressure, no study has yet examined whether cardiovascular outcomes are reduced.

2. Caloric restriction should be urged for hypertensive patients who are overweight. Some obese patients will show a significant reduction in blood pressure simply as a consequence of weight loss. In the Trial of Antihypertensive Interventions and Management (TAIM) study, weight reduction (average 4.4 kg over 6 months) lowered blood pressure by 2.5 mmHg.

3. A restriction in the intake of cholesterol and saturated fats is recommended, as this diet modification may diminish the incidence of arteriosclerotic complications. Reducing alcohol intake to <15 mL daily is also beneficial. Regular exercise is indicated within the limits of the patient's cardiovascular status. Not only is exercise helpful in controlling weight, but there is also evidence that physical conditioning itself may lower arterial pressure. Isotonic exercises (jogging, swimming) are better than isometric exercises (weight lifting) since the latter, if anything, raises arterial pressure. The dietary management outlined above is aimed at the control of other risk factors. Probably the most significant additional step that could be taken in this area would be to convince the smoker to give up cigarettes.

DRUG THERAPY FOR HYPERTENSION (Table 230-8)

To make rational use of antihypertensive drugs, the sites and mechanisms of their action must be understood. In general, there are seven classes of drugs: diuretics, ACE inhibitors, angiotensin receptor antagonists, calcium channel antagonists; antiadrenergic agents, vasodilators, and mineralocorticoid receptor antagonists.

Diuretics (See also Chap. 216) The thiazides are the most frequently used and most extensively investigated members of this group, and their early effect is related to sodium diuresis and volume depletion. A reduction in peripheral vascular resistance has also been reported by some workers to be important in the long term. Traditionally, thiazide diuretics have formed the cornerstone of most therapeutic programs designed to lower arterial pressure, and they are usually effective within 3 to 4 days. Furthermore, they have been shown to reduce mortality and morbidity in long-term trials. Resistance to their routine use arose primarily because of their adverse metabolic effects, which include hypokalemia due to renal potassium loss, hyperuricemia due to uric acid retention, carbohydrate intolerance, and hyperlipidemia. These effects are minimized if the dose is kept below the equivalent of 25 mg/d of hydrochlorothiazide. The more potent loop-acting diuretics furosemide and bumetanide have also been shown to be antihypertensive but have been used less extensively for this indication, primarily because of their shorter duration of action. Triamterene and amiloride also impede sodium reabsorption, although triamterene has little intrinsic antihypertensive effect. Their major disadvantage is that they can produce hyperkalemia, particularly in patients with impaired renal function. Any of the potassium-sparing diuretics can also be given along with thiazide diuretics to minimize renal potassium loss.

ACE Inhibitors Drugs in this group inhibit the enzyme converting angiotensin I into angiotensin II—ACE. These agents are an increasingly popular choice for initial therapy. They are useful because they not only inhibit the generation of a potent vasoconstrictor (angiotensin II) but also retard the degradation of a potent vasodilator (bradykinin), alter prostaglandin production, and can modify the activity of the adrenergic nervous system. They are especially useful in renal or renovascular hypertension and in diabetic patients, as well as in accelerated and malignant hypertension. They are also as effective in mild, uncomplicated hypertension as beta blockers and thiazides—and have fewer side effects, particularly ones that adversely affect the patient's quality of life, such as fatigue, impotence, and forgetfulness. Ten ACE inhibitors are currently available in the United States. As a group they can cause the adverse effects of cough in 5 to 10% of patients, hyperkalemia in patients with renal insufficiency, and the idiosyncratic reaction of angioedema.

Usually, diuretics are stopped 2 to 3 days before administration of an ACE inhibitor is begun and are added back later if needed. These drugs should be used with caution when the renin system is activated (e.g., by severe heart failure, prior diuretic therapy, or substantial salt restriction) to avoid profound hypotension. In patients with bilateral renal artery stenosis, rapid deterioration of renal function may occur.

It is now well-established than activation of the renin-angiotensin system is responsible for detrimental effects on the cardiovascular and renal systems, and that blockade with ACE inhibitors is effective against these end-organ changes, even in patients without hypertension. The HOPE (Heart Outcomes Prevention Evaluation) trial demonstrated a significant reduction in the rates of death, myocardial infarction, and stroke in a broad range of high-risk patients given ramipril.

Angiotensin Receptor Antagonists (ARBs) These drugs are the most selective blockers of the renin-angiotensin system currently available. They have effects similar to those of ACE inhibitors. However, instead of blocking the production of angiotensin II, they competitively inhibit its binding to the angiotensin II AT_1 receptor subtype. It is not yet known what the long-term effects, in any, will be from exposure of the angiotensin II receptors to chronic increased circulating concentrations of angiotensin II. The utility, efficacy, and tolerability of ARBs are similar to those of the ACE inhibitors, but they appear to cause

Site of Action	Drug	Dosage	Indications	Contraindications/Cautions	Frequent or Peculiar Side Effects
DIURETICS					
Renal tubule	Thiazides: e.g., hydrochloro-thiazide	Depends on specific drug Oral: 12.5–25 mg daily	Mild hypertension; as adjunct in treatment of moderate to severe hypertension	Diabetes mellitus, hyperuricemia, primary aldosteronism	Potassium depletion, hyperglycemia, hyperuricemia, hypercholesterolemia, dermatitis, purpura, depression, hypercalcemia
	Loop-acting: e.g., furosemide	Oral: 20–80 mg 2 or 3 times a day	Mild hypertension; as adjunct in severe or malignant hypertension, particularly with renal failure	Hyperuricemia, primary aldosteronism	Potassium depletion, hyperuricemia, hyperglycemia, hypocalcemia, blood dyscrasias, rash, nausea, vomiting, diarrhea
	Potassium-sparing: Spironolactone	Oral: 25 mg 2 to 4 times daily	Hypertension due to hypermineralocorti-coidism; as adjunct to thiazide therapy	Renal failure	Hyperkalemia, diarrhea, gynecomastia, menstrual irregularities
	Triamterene	Oral: 25–100 mg daily			Hyperkalemia, nausea, vomiting, leg cramps, nephrolithiasis, GI disturbances
	Amiloride	Oral: 5–10 mg daily			
ANTIADRENERGIC AGENTS					
Central	Clonidine	Oral: 0.05–0.6 mg twice daily	Mild to moderate hypertension, renal disease with hypertension		Postural hypotension, drowsiness, dry mouth, rebound hypertension after abrupt withdrawal, insomnia
	Guanabenz	Oral: 4–16 mg twice daily			
	Guanfacine	Oral: 1–3 mg daily			
	Methyldopa (also acts by blocking sympathetic nerves)	Oral: 250–1000 mg twice daily IV: 250–1000 mg every 4–6 h (tolerance may develop)	Mild to moderate hypertension (oral), malignant hypertension (IV)	Pheochromocytoma, active hepatic disease (IV), during MAO inhibitor administration	Postural hypotension, sedation, fatigue, diarrhea, impaired ejaculation, fever, gynecomastia, lactation, positive Coombs' tests (occasionally associated with hemolysis), chronic hepatitis, acute ulcerative colitis, lupus-like syndrome
Autonomic ganglia	Trimethaphan	IV: 1–6 mg/min	Severe or malignant hypertension	Severe coronary artery disease, cerebrovascular insufficiency, diabetes mellitus (on hypoglycemic therapy), glaucoma, prostatism	Postural hypotension, visual symptoms, dry mouth, constipation, urinary retention, impotence
Nerve endings	Guanethidine	Oral: 10–150 mg daily	Moderate to severe hypertension	Pheochromocytoma, severe coronary artery disease, cerebrovascular insufficiency, during MAO inhibitor administration	Postural hypotension, bradycardia, dry mouth, diarrhea, impaired ejaculation, fluid retention, asthma
	Guanadrel	Oral: 5–50 mg twice daily			
α Receptors	Phentolamine	IV: 1–5 mg bolus	Suspected or proved pheochromocytoma	Severe coronary artery disease	Tachycardia, weakness, dizziness, flushing
	Phenoxybenzamine	Oral: 10–50 mg once or twice daily (tolerance may develop)	Proved pheochromocytoma		Postural hypotension, tachycardia, miosis, nasal congestion, dry mouth
	Prazosin	Oral: 1–10 mg twice daily	Mild to moderate hypertension	Use with caution in the elderly	Sudden syncope, headache, sedation, dizziness, tachycardia, anticholinergic effect, fluid retention
	Terazosin	Oral: 1–20 mg daily			
	Doxazosin	Oral: 1–16 mg daily			
β Receptors	Propranolol	Oral: 10–120 mg 2 to 4 times daily	Mild to moderate hypertension (especially with evidence of hyperdynamic circulation); as adjunct to hydralazine therapy	Congestive heart failure, asthma, diabetes mellitus (on hypoglycemic therapy), during MAO inhibitor administration, COPD, sick sinus syndrome, 2d or 3d degree heart block	Dizziness, depression, bronchospasm, nausea, vomiting, diarrhea, constipation, heart failure, fatigue, Raynaud's phenomenon, hallucinations, hypertriglyceridemia, hypercholesterolemia, psoriasis; sudden withdrawal may precipitate angina or myocardial injury in patients with heart disease
	Metoprolol	Oral: 25–150 mg twice daily			
	Nadolol	Oral: 20–120 mg daily			
	Atenolol	Oral: 25–100 mg daily			
	Timolol	Oral: 5–15 mg twice daily			

(continued)

Site of Action	Drug	Dosage	Indications	Contraindications/Cautions	Frequent or Peculiar Side Effects
α/β Receptors	Betaxolol	Oral: 10–20 mg daily			
	Carteolol	Oral: 2.5–10 mg daily			
	Pindolol	Oral: 5–30 mg twice daily			Less resting bradycardia than other beta blockers
	Acebutolol	Oral: 200–600 mg twice daily			
	Labetalol	Oral: 100–600 mg twice daily IV: 2 mg/min			Similar to beta blockers with more postural effects
	Carvediol	Oral: 12.5–50 mg daily or in divided doses			

VASODILATORS

Site of Action	Drug	Dosage	Indications	Contraindications/Cautions	Frequent or Peculiar Side Effects
Vascular smooth muscle	Hydralazine	Oral: 10–75 mg 4 times daily IV or IM: 10–50 mg every 6 h (tolerance may develop)	As adjunct in treatment of moderate to severe hypertension (oral), malignant hypertension (IV or IM), renal disease with hypertension	Lupus erythematosus, severe coronary artery disease	Headache, tachycardia, angina pectoris, anorexia, nausea, vomiting, diarrhea, lupus-like syndrome, rash, fluid retention
	Minoxidil	Oral: 2.5–40 mg twice daily	Severe hypertension	Severe coronary artery disease	Tachycardia, aggravates angina, marked fluid retention, hair growth on face and body, coarsening of facial features, possible pericardial effusions
	Diazoxide	IV: 1–3 mg/kg up to 150 mg rapidly	Severe or malignant hypertension	Diabetes mellitus, hyperuricemia, congestive heart failure	Hyperglycemia, hyperuricemia, sodium retention
	Nitroprusside	IV: 0.5–8 (μg/kg)/min	Malignant hypertension		Apprehension, weakness, diaphoresis, nausea, vomiting, muscle twitching, cyanide toxicity

ANGIOTENSIN-CONVERTING ENZYME INHIBITORS

Site of Action	Drug	Dosage	Indications	Contraindications/Cautions	Frequent or Peculiar Side Effects
Converting enzyme	Captopril	Oral: 12.5–75 mg twice daily	Mild to severe hypertension, renal artery stenosis	Renal failure (reduction of dose), bilateral renal artery stenosis, pregnancy	Leukopenia, pancytopenia, hypotension, cough, angioedema, urticarial rash, fever, loss of taste, acute renal failure in bilateral renal artery stenosis, hyperkalemia
	Benazepril	Oral: 5–40 mg daily			Same as captopril, but little evidence for leukopenia, but perhaps increased frequency of cough and angioedema. All can be given once daily, but side effects are reduced if one-half dose is given twice daily. Fosinopril is excreted more in bile than the others.
	Enalapril	Oral: 2.5–40 mg daily			
	Enalaprilat	IV: 0.625–1.25 mg over 5 min every 6–8 h			
	Fosinopril	Oral: 10–40 mg daily			
	Lisinopril	Oral: 5–40 mg daily			
	Quinapril	Oral: 5–80 mg daily			
	Ramipril	Oral: 1.25–20 mg daily			
	Trandolapril	Oral: 1–4 mg daily			

ANGIOTENSIN RECEPTOR ANTAGONISTS

Site of Action	Drug	Dosage	Indications	Contraindications/Cautions	Frequent or Peculiar Side Effects
	Losartan	Oral: 25–50 mg once or twice daily	Mild to severe hypertension, renal artery stenosis	Pregnancy, bilateral renal artery stenosis	Hypotension, acute renal failure in bilateral renal artery stenosis, hyperkalemia
	Valsartan	Oral: 80–320 mg			
	Irbesartan	Oral: 150–300 mg daily			

(continued)

TABLE 230-8— (Continued)

Site of Action	Drug	Dosage	Indications	Contraindications/Cautions	Frequent or Peculiar Side Effects
CALCIUM CHANNEL ANTAGONISTS					
Vascular smooth muscle	Dihydropyridines: Nifedipine XL Amlodipine	Oral: 30–90 mg daily Oral: 2.5–10 mg daily	Mild to moderate hypertension	Heart failure, 2d or 3d degree heart block	Tachycardia, flushing, gastrointestinal disturbances, hyperkalemia, edema, headache
	Felodipine XL	Oral: 5–10 mg daily			
	Isradipine	Oral: 2.5–10 mg daily			
	Nicardipine	Oral: 20–40 mg 3 times daily			
	Benzothiazepines: Diltiazem	Oral: 30–90 mg 4 times daily or as CD form 180–300 mg daily	Mild to moderate hypertension	Heart failure, 2d or 3d degree heart block	Same as amlodipine, except no tachycardia or edema, but can cause heart block, constipation, and liver dysfunction
	Phenylalkylamine: Verapamil	Oral: 30–120 mg 4 times daily or as SR form 120–480 mg daily	Mild to moderate hypertension	Heart failure, 2d or 3d degree heart block	
MINERALOCORTICOID RECEPTOR ANTAGONISTS					
Renal tubule	Spironolactone	Oral: 25–50 mg 2 to 4 times daily	Hypertension due to hypermineralo-corticoidism; as adjunct to thiazide therapy	Renal failure	Hyperkalemia, diarrhea, menstrual irregularities, gynecomastia
	Eplerenone	50–100 mg daily	Hypertension due to hypermineralo-corticoidism; as adjunct to thiazide therapy	Renal failure, diabetic nephropathy	Hyperkalemia, no anti-androgenic or progesterone side effects

Note: MAO, monoamine oxidase; COPD, chronic obstructive pulmonary disease; XL, CD, SR are long-acting or sustained-release formulations.

fewer side effects. Specifically, they do not cause excessive cough or angioedema. There appears to be variation within the class in terms of antihypertensive efficacy. No studies are available to allow comparison of efficacy between ACE inhibitors and ARBs, and their joint use, while already in clinical practice, awaits more substantiating data.

A number of large-scale prospective studies are under way to investigate the effects of ARBs on mortality and morbidity in patients with cardiovascular disease. The Losartan Intervention for Endpoint Reduction in Hypertension (LIFE) study has shown that losartan-based antihypertensive treatment was superior to atenolol in reducing cardiovascular mortality and morbidity, especially stroke and regression of left ventricular hypertrophy (Table 230-9). Three studies have demonstrated that irbesartan and losartan significantly reduce the progression on diabetic nephropathy in patients with type 2 diabetes mellitus.

Calcium Channel Antagonists There are three subclasses of calcium channel antagonists: the phenylalkylamine derivatives (e.g., verapamil), the benzothiazepines (e.g., diltiazem), and the dihydropyridines (e.g., amlodipine). To date, there is only one therapeutic agent in each of the first two classes but a number of agents in the third class. All three subclasses modify calcium entry into cells by interacting with specific binding sites on the α_1 subunit of the L-type voltage-dependent calcium channel. Thus, since there are other calcium channels (e.g., the T and N types), the actions of these drugs only partially modify total calcium transport into cells. The relative specificity of each agent stems from the fact that each class has a unique binding site on the α_1 subunit, and these sites are variably expressed in different tissues. Thus, while agents from all three subclasses cause vasodilation, usually only the dihydropyridines produce reflex tachycardia. Diltiazem and verapamil can both slow atrioventricular conduction—a feature not observed with the dihydropyridines. While calcium channel antagonists are also useful in angina pectoris (Chap. 226), because of their negative inotropic actions, they should be used with caution in hypertensive patients with heart failure.

Considerable controversy has surrounded the use of calcium channel antagonists in the treatment of hypertension. In part the controversy was secondary to the inadequacy of the data and the confusion between the use of short-acting agents (e.g., nifedipine) and long-acting agents. Several facts have helped partially to resolve this controversy. First has been the general recognition that despite its previously frequent use as an antihypertensive agent, short-acting nifedipine rarely, if ever, should be used to treat hypertension, since it has been reported to increase the incidence of acute coronary events. Second, the results of the SYST-EUR (Systolic Hypertension in Europe) trial documented, in patients over the age of 60 with isolated systolic hypertension, that a long-acting dihydropyridine calcium channel antagonist reduced cardiovascular morbidity and mortality to an extent equivalent to that previously reported for diuretics and beta blockers. The effect was greater among diabetics. Thus, long-acting calcium channel antagonists are often used as first-line hypertension therapy.

Antiadrenergic Agents ■ *β-ADRENERGIC RECEPTOR BLOCKERS* (See also Chap. 226) A number of effective β-adrenergic receptor blocking agents are available that block sympathetic effects on the heart and are most effective in reducing cardiac output and in lowering arterial pressure when there is increased cardiac sympathetic nerve activity. These agents are also often used as first-line therapy. In addition, they block the adrenergic nerve–mediated release of renin from the renal juxtaglomerular cells. This action may be an important component of their blood pressure–lowering action. β-Adrenergic blockers are particularly useful when employed in conjunction with vasodilators, which tend to evoke a reflex increase in heart rate, and with diuretics, the administration of which often results in an elevation of circulating renin activity. In practice, beta blockers appear to be effective even when there is no evidence of increased sympathetic tone, with about one-half or more of all hypertensive patients showing a fall in pressure. Furthermore, like diuretics, they have been shown to reduce morbidity and mortality in long-term clinical trials. However, these agents can precipitate congestive heart failure and asthma in susceptible individuals, and they must be used with caution in diabetic patients receiving

TABLE 230-9 *Randomized Clinical Trials in Hypertension*

Trial Reference	Patient Number and Characteristics	Trial Arms	Endpoints	Results	Conclusion
SYST-EUR, JA Staessen et al, Lancet 350: 757, 1997	4695, >60 years old 2 years' follow-up	Nitrendipine/ enalapril or HTZ Placebo	Primary: Death, all cardiovascular events, strokes	Active treatment reduced total stroke rate 42% ($p = .003$); nonfatal stroke decreased 44% ($p = .007$). All fatal and nonfatal cardiac endpoints declined 26% ($p = .03$). Cardiovascular mortality decreased 27% ($p = .07$).	Among elderly patients with isolated systolic hypertension, nitrendipine reduced cardiovascular complications; treatment of 1000 patients for 5 years with this regimen may prevent 29 strokes and/or 53 major cardiovascular endpoints
SYST-EUR, J Tuomilehto et al, N Engl J Med 341:372, 1999	4695 (diabetic = 492) >60 years old 2 years' follow-up	Nitrendipine/enalapril or HTZ Placebo	Primary: Death, all cardiovascular events, strokes	In diabetics total mortality reduced 55%; mortality from cardiovascular disease by 76%; all cardiovascular events combined by 69%; nonfatal stroke by 73% Reductions in mortality and all cardiovascular events were significantly larger among diabetic than nondiabetic patients ($p = .04$ to .01).	Calcium channel antagonist significantly reduces cardiovascular morbidity and mortality in elder hypertensive patients; the effect is greater in diabetic than nondiabetic subjects
CAPPP Trial, L Hansson et al, Lancet 353: 611, 1999	10,985, age 25–66, diastolic BP ≥ 100 mmHg 2–3 years' follow-up	Captopril Diuretics/beta blocker	Primary: Composite of fatal and nonfatal myocardial infarction, stroke, and other cardiovascular deaths	Primary endpoint relative risk 1.05, $p = .52$; Cardiovascular mortality was lower with captopril, relative risk (RR) 0.77, $p = .092$ Fatal and nonfatal stroke was more common with captopril, RR 1.25, $p = .044$	Captopril and conventional treatment did not differ in preventing cardiovascular morbidity and mortality
HOT Study, Hansson et al, Lancet 351: 1755, 1998	18,790, 50–80 years with diastolic BP 100–115 mmHg 3–4 years' follow-up	Felodipine plus four other agents to reduce diastolic BP to 90 mmHg or 85 mmHg or 80 mmHg	Major cardiovascular events	Lowest cardiovascular mortality occurred at 86.5 mmHg; further reduction below these BPs was safe but no further reduction in risk; in patients with diabetes, a 51% reduction in cardiovascular events in target group = 80 mmHg compared with target group = 90 mmHg (p for trend = .006)	Intensive lowering of BP was associated with a low rate of cardiovascular events down to a diastolic BP of 82.6 mmHg
DASH Trial, LJ Appel et al, N Engl J Med 336:1117, 1997	459 with diastolic blood pressure 80–95 mmHg; 8 wks. Sodium intake and body weight were maintained constant.	Diet rich in fruits and vegetables Diet rich in fruits, vegetables, and low-fat dairy products Control (average U.S. diet)	Blood pressure	Combination diet reduced systolic and diastolic BP by 5.5 and 3.0 mmHg more than the control diet ($p < .001$); the fruit and vegetable diet had an intermediate effect	A diet rich in fruits, vegetables, and low-fat dairy food can substantially lower BP
FG Messerli et al, JAMA 279: 1903, 1998	Meta-analysis of efficacy of beta blockers vs. diuretics as first-line therapy for elderly patients (>60 years) with hypertension Approximate mean of 5 years' follow-up	Diuretics, 8 trials Beta blockers, 2 trials	Cerebrovascular events, coronary heart disease, stroke mortality, cardiovascular mortality, all-cause mortality	Diuretics significantly reduced cerebrovascular events odds ratio (0.61), coronary heart disease odds ratio (0.74), stroke mortality odds ratio (0.67), cardiovascular mortality odds ratio (0.75), and all-cause mortality odds ratio (0.86); beta blockers significantly reduced only cerebrovascular events odds ratio (0.74)	In elderly patients with hypertension, first-line diuretics reduced morbidity and mortality better than beta blockers

(continued)

TABLE 230-9—(Continued)

Trial Reference	Patient Number and Characteristics	Trial Arms	Endpoints	Results	Conclusion
HOPE, S Yusuf et al, 2000	9297 high-risk patients (≥55 years old) with vascular disease or diabetes plus one other cardiovascular risk factor	Ramipril vs. placebo for a mean of 5 years	Primary: Composite of myocardial infarction, stroke, or death from cardiovascular causes	Ramipril significantly reduced the rates of death from cardiovascular causes (RR 0.74), MI (RR 0.80), stroke (RR 0.68), cardiac arrest (RR 0.62), heart failure (RR 0.77), and complications related to diabetes (RR 0.84).	Ramipril significantly reduced the rates of death, MI, and stroke in high-risk patients not known to have a low ejection fraction or heart failure.
LIFE, B Dahlof et al, Lancet 359: 995, 2002	9193, age 55–80, with essential hypertension and LVH by ECG	Once daily losartan-based or atenolol-based antihypertensive treatment for at least 4 years and until 1040 patients had primary cardiovascular event	Primary cardiovascular event (death, MI, or stroke)	BP fell by 30.2/16.6 (SD 18.5/10.1) and 29.1/16.8 mmHg (19.2/10.1) in the losartan vs. atenolol groups. The primary composite endpoint occurred in 508 losartan and 588 atenolol patients (RR 0.87). New-onset diabetes was less frequent with losartan	Losartan prevented more cardiovascular morbidity and death than atenolol for similar reduction in BP
ALLHAT, ALLHAT Collaborative Research Group, 2002	42,419 high-risk hypertensives ≥ 55 years	Chlorthalidone vs. lisinopril vs. amlodipine vs. doxazosin	Fatal coronary heart disease and nonfatal MI	Doxazosin arm stopped after 3 years because of increased rate of heart failure	No difference in primary endpoints or in all-cause mortality between ACE inhibition, calcium channel blockade, and diuretics

Note: HTZ, hydrochlorothiazine; BP, blood pressure; MI, myocardial infarction; LVH, left ventricular hypertrophy; ECG, electrocardiogram.

hypoglycemic therapy because they inhibit the usual sympathetic responses to hypoglycemia.

Cardioselective beta-blocking agents (so-called beta$_1$ blockers, e.g., metoprolol, atenolol) have been developed and may be superior to nonselective beta blockers such as propranolol and timolol in patients with bronchospasm. Nadolol, a nonselective beta blocker, unlike other drugs of this class, is excreted unchanged in the urine and has a half-life of 14 to 20 h; only one dose a day is required. Atenolol also usually needs to be given only once a day. Pindolol and acebutolol are nonselective beta blockers that have partial agonist activity and, therefore, produce less bradycardia. Labetalol exerts both α- and β-adrenergic blocking actions. Thus, it lowers arterial pressure not only by the same complex actions as do beta blockers but also directly by reducing systemic vascular resistance. Usually it has a more rapid onset of action but produces more postural symptoms and sexual dysfunction than the other beta blockers. It is usually not used as first-line therapy as there is no mortality study in which it has been tested.

Centrally acting agents include clonidine and methyldopa. These drugs and their metabolites stimulate α$_2$ receptors in the vasomotor centers of the brain, thereby reducing sympathetic outflow and arterial pressure. Usually a fall in cardiac output and heart rate also occurs. Since the baroreceptor reflex is intact, postural symptoms are absent. However, rebound hypertension may occur rarely when clonidine is stopped. This effect is probably secondary to an increase in norepinephrine release, which is inhibited by these agents owing to their agonist effect on presynaptic α receptors. They are usually not used as first-line therapy.

α-ADRENERGIC RECEPTOR BLOCKERS These agents are also not usually used as first-line therapy. Phentolamine and phenoxybenzamine block the action of norepinephrine at α-adrenergic receptor sites. These two compounds block both presynaptic (α$_2$) and postsynaptic (α$_1$) α receptors, and the former action accounts for the tolerance that develops. Prazosin, terazosin, and doxazosin are more effective because they selectively block only *postsynaptic* α receptors, i.e., α$_1$ receptors. Thus, presynaptic α activity remains, suppressing norepinephrine release, and tolerance occurs only infrequently. Accordingly, these three agents can produce substantial hypotension following the first dose. Their use has decreased with a report of their association with an increase in cardiovascular events. The doxazosin arm of the Antihypertensive and Lipid Lowering Treatment to Prevent Heart Attack Trial (ALLHAT) was terminated prematurely because of a significant increase in the risk of congestive heart failure.

Vasodilators These agents are usually not used for initial therapy. Hydralazine is the most versatile of the drugs that cause direct relaxation of vascular smooth muscle; it acts mainly on arterial resistance. Unfortunately, the effect of hydralazine on peripheral resistance is partly negated by a reflex increase in sympathetic discharge that raises heart rate and cardiac output, limiting the usefulness of hydralazine, especially in patients with severe coronary artery disease. Minoxidil is even more potent than hydralazine but unfortunately produces significant hypertrichosis and fluid retention and, therefore, is mainly limited to patients with severe hypertension and renal insufficiency.

Diazoxide is restricted in its application to acute situations. It begins to act immediately to lower blood pressure, and its effects may last for several hours. Nitroprusside given intravenously also acts as a direct vasodilator, with onset and offset of actions that are almost immediate. Nitroglycerin is a third direct-acting vasodilator useful as an intravenous agent. These latter three drugs are useful only for the treatment of hypertensive emergencies (Table 230-10).

Mineralocorticoid Receptor Antagonists In addition to its classic hormonal effects on the kidney causing sodium retention and potassium excretion, aldosterone is now recognized as a paracrine hormone that can act locally not only in the kidneys but also in the heart and blood vessels, contributing to fibrosis and hypertrophy. Aldosterone antagonists are emerging as agents that may counter these detrimental ef-

TABLE 230-10 *Therapeutic Agents Used to Treat Malignant Hypertension*

Drug	Route	Starting Dose	Onset	Peak	Duration	Oral Preparation Available
			Time Course of Action			
IMMEDIATE ONSET						
Nitroprusside	Continuous IV	0.25 μg/kg per min	<1 min	1–2 min	2–5 min	No
Nitroglycerin	Continuous IV	5 μg/min	1–5 min	2–6 min	3–10 min	No
Diazoxide	IV bolus	50 mg q5–10min up to 600 mg	1–5 min	2–4 min	4–12 h	No
Fenoldopan	Continuous IV	0.1–0.3 μg/kg per min	<5 min	5–10 min	30 min	No
Esmolol	Continuous IV	250–500 μg/min × 1 min; then 50–100 μg/kg per min × 4 min	1–2 min	2–3 min	10–20 min	No
DELAYED ONSET						
Enalaprilat	IV	1.25 mg q6h	10–15 min	3–4 h	6–24 h	Yes
Hydralazine	IV, IM	5–10 mg q20min × 3	10–20 min	20–40 min	4–12 h	Yes
Labetalol	IV	20–80 mg q10min up to 300 mg	5 min	20–30 min	3–6 h	Yes
Nicardipine	IV	5–15 mg/h	5–10 min	20–40 min	1–4 h	Yes

fects of aldosterone, including but not limited to hypertension. Spironolactone causes renal sodium loss by blocking the effect of mineralocorticoids, and it was initially employed as more effective management in hypertensive patients whose mineralocorticoid levels are excessive, such as patients with primary or secondary aldosteronism. However, the Randomized Aldactone Evaluation Study (RALES) clinical trial in heart failure using low doses of spironolactone achieved a 30% reduction in mortality, suggesting that an aldosterone receptor antagonist may be beneficial even when aldosterone levels are relatively normal (Chap. 216). Eplerenone is a new, selective mineralocorticoid receptor antagonist without clinically significant androgen receptor blocking or progesterone receptor stimulating activities, which translates into absence of gynecomastia and impotence in men and of menstrual irregularity in women. Both agents, like ACE inhibitors and angiotensin II receptor antagonists, can increase potassium levels significantly in patients with renal insufficiency. Initial close monitoring of serum potassium levels in patients with compromised renal function is, therefore, advised.

APPROACH TO DRUG THERAPY The aim of drug therapy is to use the agents described, alone or in combination, to return arterial pressure to normal levels with minimal side effects. Ideally, one would choose a therapeutic program that specifically corrects the underlying defect resulting in the elevated blood pressure, e.g., treatment with spironolactone or eplerenone for patients with primary aldosteronism. As our knowledge of the mechanisms underlying the hypertension in individual patients increases, more specific drug programs will become available. Such programs presumably will result in normalization of blood pressure with fewer side effects. In the absence of this information, an empirical approach is used, which takes into consideration efficacy, safety, impact on the quality of life, compliance, ease of administration, and cost. When used in combination, drugs are chosen for their different sites of action. Three major trials of anti-hypertensive agents have been reported recently. The mammoth ALLHAT trial resulted in no difference in either combined fatal coronary heart disease or nonfatal myocardial infarction between patients started on treatment with an ACE inhibitor, diuretic, or calcium channel blocker. In an Australian randomized trial of >6000 elderly hypertensives, in contrast, treatment with ACE inhibitors resulted in fewer cardiovascular events than treatment with diuretic agents, despite similar reductions of blood pressure. Guidelines for the initiation of antihypertensive therapy should be based upon two criteria: level of systolic and diastolic blood pressure and the total level of cardiovascular risk.

Since many effective antihypertensive agents are available, a number of useful therapeutic regimens have been developed. There are two major authoritative groups that have published treatment guidelines in 2003: The US Joint National Committee (JNC) and the European Society of Hypertension (ESH) and the European Society of Cardiology (ESC). In the absence of specific therapy, their approaches are similar in many respects, relying heavily on the results of randomized clinical trials (Table 230-9), except for which drugs should be used to initiate therapy. JNC7 recommends starting with diuretics because mortality trials have demonstrated a positive effect of treatment with these agents. The ESH/ESC guidelines recommend initiating therapy with any of five classes of agents (Table 230-11), or with a combination; recent study results from ALLHAT have made it advisable to remove alpha blockade from this list (see below). The different rec-

TABLE 230-11 *Guidelines for Selecting Initial Drug Treatment of Hypertension*

Class of Drug	Compelling Indications	Possible Indications	Compelling Contraindications	Possible Contraindications
Diuretics	Heart failure Elderly patients Systolic hypertension	Diabetes	Gout	Dyslipidemia Sexually active males
β-Blockers	Angina After myocardial infarct Tachyarrhythmias	Heart failure Pregnancy Diabetes	Asthma and COPD Heart block[a]	Dyslipidemia Athletes and physically active patients Peripheral vascular disease
ACE inhibitors	Heart failure Left ventricular dysfunction After myocardial infarct Diabetic nephropathy		Pregnancy Hyperkalemia Bilateral renal artery stenosis	
Calcium antagonists	Angina Elderly patients Systolic hypertension	Peripheral vascular disease	Heart block[b]	Congestive heart failure[c]
Angiotensin II antagonists	ACE inhibitor cough	Heart failure	Pregnancy Bilateral renal artery stenosis Hyperkalemia	

[a] Grade 2 or 3 atrioventricular block.
[b] Grade 2 or 3 atrioventricular block with verapamil or diltiazem.
[c] Verapamil or diltiazem.

Note: COPD, chronic obstructive pulmonary disease; ACE, angiotensin-converting enzyme.
Source: Adapted with permission from 1999 WHO.

ommendations, in part, reflect the fact that European committees reviewed more recent data from mortality clinical trials that, in one case, documented reductions in morbidity and mortality with a long-acting calcium channel antagonist versus placebo similar to previous reports for diuretics and beta blockers; in another case, ACE inhibitors were shown to be as effective as beta blockers and diuretics in reducing mortality. Practically, it has become less important which agent is chosen as "initial therapy" since the majority of hypertensive patients will require more than one agent to reach goal blood pressure.

There are several critical caveats common to both the JNC 7 and ESH/ESC approaches:

1. Start with an agent that may also treat and/or not harm a coexisting condition.
2. Start with an agent that the patient is likely to tolerate best; long-term compliance is related to tolerability and efficacy of the first agent used.
3. For low- or medium-risk patients, start with a low dose of an agent and, if blood pressure is not controlled, increase only moderately.
4. Add an additional agent from a different, complementary class if blood pressure is not controlled with a moderate dose of the first agent.
5. Use a diuretic when two agents are used, in nearly all cases.
6. Use thiazide diuretics only at low doses, i.e., ≤25 mg/d of hydrochlorothiazide or its equivalent, unless some pressing reason exists.
7. For medium- to high-risk patients, strongly consider low-dose combination therapy as initial therapy:
   a. A diuretic with a beta blocker, ACE inhibitor, or angiotensin II antagonist;
   b. A calcium channel blocker with an ACE inhibitor or a beta blocker.

If therapy with low doses of two drugs does not achieve blood pressure control, the primary agent should be increased to full dose, e.g., 20 mg of enalapril or 360 mg of diltiazem. If the blood pressure is still not controlled, then a detailed search for a secondary cause of hypertension, as outlined above, is indicated, with lower levels of suspicion in diabetics and the elderly. If none is found, then a dietary assessment will often reveal a high sodium intake. With reduction in salt intake to ≤5 g/d, blood pressure is often controlled. If the blood pressure is still not controlled, a third agent should be added. Caution should be used with the addition of an ACE inhibitor, as administration of such an agent to a patient who is already taking a diuretic occasionally may lead to profound hypotension.

If the blood pressure is controlled, then a stepwise reduction in the dose and/or withdrawal of some of the agents should be carried out to determine the minimal therapeutic program that will maintain the blood pressure at ≤140/90 mmHg. Fewer than 5% of patients will still be hypertensive at this point. For these, one first should consider the reasons for therapeutic failure, as shown in Table 230-12. If none can be identified, then one of the other agents listed in Table 230-11 should be added. If blood pressure is still not controlled, then consideration should be given to an alternate class as listed in Table 230-8. If blood

TABLE 230-12 *Reasons for Poor Therapeutic Response in Patients with Hypertension*

Inadequate patient compliance
Volume expansion
   Caused by excessive sodium intake
   Caused by nondiuretic antihypertensive agent
   Caused by renal damage
Excessive weight gain
Inadequate doses
Drug antagonism
Cold remedies
Sympathomimetics
Oral contraceptives (estrogens)
Adrenal steroids
Secondary forms of hypertension

pressure is controlled, previous drugs are withdrawn sequentially to determine the minimal therapeutic program that will maintain a normal blood pressure.

While the recommendations outlined above are satisfactory for a large majority of patients, it is important to use a flexible approach, because individual patients may respond differently to individual drugs and drug combinations. For those patients requiring multiple drugs, once the appropriate combination has been found, the use of a single formulation with the appropriate combination of drugs may simplify the regimen and thereby increase compliance. Every effort should be made to reduce the number of times each day the patients must interrupt their schedules for the medication. Pharmacologic treatment of essential hypertension is usually lifelong, and since most patients are asymptomatic, compliance with a complex regimen may be a serious problem, particularly if the therapeutic regimen has a negative impact on the quality of the patient's life. Finally, it is uncertain what level of arterial pressure should be accepted as representing adequate control. It is clear that reducing diastolic blood pressure to <90 mmHg is appropriate and reduces morbidity and/or mortality.

SPECIAL CONSIDERATIONS Five groups of patients with hypertension require special consideration because of associated conditions: those with renal disease, coronary artery disease, or diabetes mellitus; women of reproductive age; and the elderly. These groups are considered in the following sections.

Renal Disease Reduction of arterial pressure in hypertensive patients with impaired renal function is often accompanied initially by an increase in serum creatinine. This change does not represent further structural renal damage and should not deter the physician from continuing the therapy, since achievement of blood pressure control may eventually reduce the value toward normal. However, if serum creatinine increases in a patient treated with an ACE inhibitor, care needs to be exercised, because these patients may have bilateral renal artery disease. Their renal function will continue to deteriorate as long as the ACE inhibitor is given. Thus, ACE inhibitors should be used cautiously in patients with impaired renal function, and renal function should be assessed frequently (every 4 to 5 days) for the first 3 weeks. While these drugs are contraindicated in patients with bilateral renal artery stenosis, together with angiotensin receptor blockers they are the drugs of choice in patients with unilateral renal artery stenosis and a normally functioning contralateral kidney and probably also in patients with chronic renal failure with or without diabetes mellitus.

Coronary Artery Disease Beta blockers, important in reducing mortality after myocardial infarction and in the treatment of angina, are useful antihypertensive agents in patients with coronary artery disease. ACE inhibitors are useful in these patients as well, especially those with hypertension and left ventricular dysfunction.

Diabetes Mellitus The diabetic patient with hypertension is particularly challenging to treat because multiple agents are usually needed to achieve goal blood pressure and because many of the agents used to lower blood pressure can affect glucose metabolism adversely. ACE inhibitors or angiotensin receptor blockers should be first-line therapy in hypertensive individuals with type 2 diabetes. They have no known adverse effects on glucose or lipid metabolism and minimize the development of diabetic nephropathy by reducing renal vascular resistance and renal perfusion pressure—the primary factor underlying renal deterioration in these patients (Chap. 323). Meta-analyses of clinical studies have demonstrated that setting a lower blood pressure goal in diabetic patients is ideal to prevent progression of end-organ disease, with current recommendations shifting from 130/85 mmHg downward to 130/80. The average hypertensive diabetic patient will require at least three medications to achieve appropriate control.

Women of Reproductive Age ■ *ORAL CONTRACEPTIVES* Several years ago, a common cause of endocrine hypertension was the use of estrogen-containing oral contraceptives. However, more recent studies have suggested that this is no longer true, probably owing to the lower estrogen content of modern oral contraceptives. In patients receiving these agents who do become hypertensive, the mechanism is likely to be activation of the renin-angiotensin-aldosterone system. The estrogen component of oral contraceptive agents stimulates the hepatic synthesis of the renin substrate angiotensinogen, which in turn favors the increased production of angiotensin II and secondary aldosteronism. However, only a small number of women taking oral contraceptives actually have an increase in arterial pressure to a level >140/90mmHg, and in about half of these, the hypertension will remit within 6 months of stopping the drug. Why some women taking oral contraceptives develop hypertension and others do not is unclear but may be related to (1) increased vascular sensitivity to angiotensin II, (2) the presence of mild renal disease, (3) familial factors (>50% have a positive family history for hypertension), (4) age (hypertension is significantly more prevalent in women over age 35), (5) the estrogen content of the contraceptive, and/or (6) obesity. Indeed, some investigators have suggested that oral contraceptives simply unmask women with essential hypertension.

PREGNANCY (See also Chap. 6) The patient who is pregnant and hypertensive or who develops hypertension during pregnancy (pregnancy-induced hypertension, preeclampsia, eclampsia) is particularly difficult to treat. Because it is uncertain whether autoregulation of uterine blood flow occurs, lowering blood pressure in the pregnant hypertensive patient may result in reduced placental and fetal perfusion. Thus, a conservative approach to lowering blood pressure is usually indicated. In the second and third trimesters, antihypertensive agents are often not indicated unless the diastolic pressure exceeds 95 mmHg. In general, severe salt restriction and/or diuretics are not used because of the associated increase in fetal wastage. Beta blockers need to be used cautiously for similar reasons. Methyldopa and hydralazine, and to a lesser extent calcium channel antagonists, are the antihypertensive agents used most often, because they have no known adverse effects on the fetus. Little is known about the safety of other antihypertensive agents in pregnancy, except that nitroprusside, ACE inhibitors, and angiotensin receptor blockers may cause adverse effects on the fetus and are contraindicated.

Elderly Patients Hypertensive patients who are over age 65, and particularly those over age 75, offer substantial challenges to the physician. Several studies have reported that healthy elderly patients, whether male or female, who are treated with relatively modest doses of antihypertensive agents show a substantial reduction in strokes and stroke-related deaths. This is true whether the patient has systolic and diastolic hypertension or isolated systolic hypertension. What is not clear from these studies is how broadly the results can be extrapolated, since the studies were performed in healthy elderly patients, while many such patients have other diseases. Thus, in the elderly hypertensive patient, individualization of therapy is warranted.

MALIGNANT HYPERTENSION

In addition to marked blood pressure elevation (usually diastolic blood pressure > 130 mmHg) in association with papilledema and retinal hemorrhages and exudates, the full-blown medical emergency of malignant hypertension may include manifestations of hypertensive encephalopathy, such as severe headache, vomiting, visual disturbances (including transient blindness), transient paralyses, convulsions, stupor, and coma. These manifestations have been attributed to spasm of cerebral vessels and to cerebral edema. In some patients who have died, multiple small thrombi have been found in the cerebral vessels. Cardiac decompensation and rapidly declining renal function are other critical features of malignant hypertension. Oliguria may, in fact, be the presenting feature. The vascular lesion characteristic of malignant hypertension is fibrinoid necrosis of the walls of small arteries and arterioles, and this development can be reversed by effective antihypertensive therapy.

The pathogenesis of malignant hypertension is unknown. However, at least two independent processes—dilation of cerebral arteries and generalized arteriolar fibrinoid necrosis—contribute to the associated signs and symptoms. The cerebral arteries dilate because the normal autoregulation of cerebral blood flow decompensates as a result of the markedly elevated arterial pressure. Cerebral blood flow therefore is excessive, producing the encephalopathy associated with malignant hypertension. Many patients also show evidence of a microangiopathic hemolytic anemia; this secondary phenomenon could contribute to the deterioration of renal function. Most patients also have elevated levels of peripheral plasma renin activity and increased aldosterone production, and these effects may be involved in causing vascular damage.

Perhaps <1% of hypertensive patients develop the malignant phase, which can occur in the course of both essential and secondary hypertension. Rarely, it is the first recognized manifestation of hypertension, and it is unusual for it to occur in patients under treatment. The average age at diagnosis is 40, and men are affected more often than women. Prior to the availability of effective therapy, the life expectancy after diagnosis of malignant hypertension was <2 years, with most deaths being due to renal failure, cerebral hemorrhage, or congestive heart failure. With the advent of effective antihypertensive therapy, at least half the patients survive for >5 years.

℞ TREATMENT

Malignant hypertension is a medical emergency that requires immediate therapy. However, it needs to be distinguished from severe hypertension, in which overly aggressive therapy could result in a potentially hazardous reduction in myocardial and cerebral perfusion. The initial aims of therapy should be (1) correction of medical complications, and (2) reduction of diastolic pressure by one-third, but not to a level <95 mmHg. The drugs available for treatment of malignant hypertension can be divided into two groups on the basis of time of onset of action (Table 230-9). If the patient has hypertensive encephalopathy or pulmonary edema, and if arterial pressure must be reduced rapidly, then one from the immediate-acting group should be used, but they are not satisfactory for long-term management.

Furosemide is an important adjunct to the therapy just discussed. Given either orally or intravenously, it serves to maintain sodium diuresis in the face of a falling arterial pressure and thus will speed recovery from encephalopathy and congestive heart failure as well as maintain the sensitivity to the primary antihypertensive drug. Digitalis (Chap. 216) may also be indicated if there is evidence of cardiac decompensation.

In patients with malignant hypertension in whom the existence of pheochromocytoma is suspected, urine should be collected for measurement of the products of catecholamine metabolism, and drugs that might release additional catecholamines, such as methyldopa, reserpine, and guanethidine, must be avoided. The parenteral drug of choice in these patients is phentolamine, administered with care to avoid a precipitous reduction in arterial pressure.

FURTHER READING

ALLHAT COLLABORATIVE RESEARCH GROUP: The Antihypertensive and Lipid Lowering Treatment to Prevent Heart Attack Trial (ALLHAT). Major outcomes in high-risk hypertensive patients randomized to angiotensin converting enzyme inhibitor or calcium channel blocker vs. diuretic. JAMA 288:2981, 2002

CHOBANIAN AV et al: The Seventh Report of the Joint National Committee on Prevention Detection, Evaluation, and Treatment of High Blood Pressure: The JNC 7 report. JAMA 289:2560, 2003

CLEMENT DL et al: Prognostic value of ambulatory blood-pressure recordings in patients with treated hypertension. N Engl J Med 348:2407, 2003

DOMINICZAK AF et al: Genes and hypertension: From gene mapping in experimental models to vascular gene transfer strategies. Hypertension 35: 164, 2000

GUIDELINES COMMITTEE. 2003 European Society of Hypertension—European Society of Cardiology guidelines for the management of arterial hypertension. J Hypertens 21:1011, 2003

KAPLAN N: Systemic hypertension: Mechanisms and diagnosis, in *Braunwald's Heart Disease*, 7th ed, D Zipes et al (eds). Philadelphia, Saunders, 2005

MORTENSEN RM, WILLIAMS GH: Aldosterone action (physiology), in *Endocrinology*, 4th ed, LJ DeGroot et al (eds). Philadelphia, Saunders, 2000

O'BRIEN E et al: Use and interpretation of ambulatory blood pressure monitoring: Recommendations of the British Hypertension Society. BMJ 320: 1128, 2000

PRISANT LM, MOSER M: Hypertension in the elderly: Can we improve results of therapy? Arch Intern Med 160:283, 2000

REEVES RA: Does this patient have hypertension? How to measure blood pressure. JAMA 273:1211, 1995

SACKS FM et al: Effects on blood pressure of reduced dietary sodium and the Dietary Approaches to Stop Hypertension (DASH) diet. N Engl J Med 344: 3, 2001

WING LM et al: SA comparison of outcomes with angiotensin-converting enzyme inhibitors and diuretics for hypertension in the elderly. N Engl J Med 13:583, 2003

1999 WORLD HEALTH ORGANIZATION–INTERNATIONAL SOCIETY OF HYPERTENSION GUIDELINES FOR THE MANAGEMENT OF HYPERTENSION. J Hypertens 17:151, 1999

YUSUF S et al: Effects of an angiotensin-converting-enzyme inhibitor, ramipril, on cardiovascular events in high-risk patients. The Heart Outcomes Prevention Evaluation Study Investigators. N Engl J Med 342:145, 2000

231 DISEASES OF THE AORTA
Victor J. Dzau, Mark A. Creager

The aorta is the conduit through which the blood ejected from the left ventricle is delivered to the systemic arterial bed. In adults, its diameter is approximately 3 cm at the origin, 2.5 cm in the descending portion in the thorax, and 1.8 to 2 cm in the abdomen. The aortic wall consists of a thin intima composed of endothelium, subendothelial connective tissue, and an internal elastic lamina; a thick tunica media composed of smooth-muscle cells and extracellular matrix; and an adventitia composed primarily of connective tissue enclosing the vasa vasorum and nervi vascularis. In addition to its conduit function, the viscoelastic and compliant properties of the aorta also subserve a buffering function. The aorta is distended during systole to enable a portion of the stroke volume to be stored, and it recoils during diastole so that blood continues to flow to the periphery. Because of its continuous exposure to high pulsatile pressure and shear stress, the aorta is particularly prone to injury and disease resulting from mechanical trauma (Table 231-1). The aorta is also more prone to rupture than any other vessel, especially with the development of aneurysmal dilatation, since its wall tension, as governed by Laplace's law (i.e., proportional to the product of pressure and radius), would be increased.

AORTIC ANEURYSM

An *aneurysm* is defined as a pathologic dilatation of a segment of a blood vessel. A *true aneurysm* involves all three layers of the vessel wall and is distinguished from a *pseudoaneurysm*, in which the intimal and medial layers are disrupted and the dilatation is lined by adventitia only and sometimes by perivascular clot. Aneurysms may also be classified according to their gross appearance. A *fusiform aneurysm* affects the entire circumference of a segment of the vessel, resulting in a diffusely dilated lesion. In contrast, a *saccular aneurysm* involves only a portion of the circumference, resulting in an outpouching of the vessel wall. Aortic aneurysms are also classified according to location, i.e., abdominal versus thoracic. Aneurysms of the descending thoracic aorta are usually contiguous with infradiaphragmatic aneurysms and are referred to as *thoracoabdominal aortic aneurysms*.

TABLE 231-1 Diseases of the Aorta: Etiology and Associated Factors

Aortic aneurysm	Aortic occlusion
Atherosclerosis	Atherosclerosis
Cystic medial necrosis	Thromboembolism
Tuberculosis	Aortitis
Syphilitic infection	Syphilitic aortitis
Mycotic infection	Rheumatic aortitis
Rheumatic aortitis	Takayasu's arteritis
Trauma	Giant cell arteritis
Aortic dissection	
Cystic medial necrosis	
Systemic hypertension	
Atherosclerosis	
Takayasu's arteritis	
Giant cell arteritis	

ETIOLOGY The most common pathologic condition associated with aortic aneurysm is *atherosclerosis*. It is controversial whether atherosclerosis itself actually causes aortic aneurysms or whether atherosclerosis develops as a secondary event in the dilated aorta. Causality is implied by studies that have shown that many patients with aortic aneurysms have coexisting risk factors for atherosclerosis (Chap. 224), particularly cigarette smoking, as well as atherosclerosis in other blood vessels. Seventy-five percent of atherosclerotic aneurysms are located in the distal abdominal aorta, below the renal arteries.

Cystic medial necrosis is the term used to describe the degeneration of collagen and elastic fibers in the tunica media of the aorta, as well as the loss of medial cells that are replaced by multiple clefts of mucoid material. Cystic medial necrosis characteristically affects the proximal aorta, results in circumferential weakness and dilatation, and leads to development of fusiform aneurysms involving the ascending aorta and the sinuses of Valsalva. This condition is particularly prevalent in patients with Marfan syndrome and Ehlers-Danlos syndrome type IV (Chap. 342) but also occurs in pregnant women, in patients with hypertension, and in those with valvular heart disease. Sometimes it appears as an isolated condition in patients without any other apparent disease. Familial clusterings of aortic aneurysms occur in 20% of patients, suggesting a hereditary basis of the disease. Mutations of the genes encoding fibrillin-1 and type III procollagen have been implicated in some cases. Linkage analysis has identified loci on chromosomes 5q13-14 and 11q23.3-q24 in several families, although the specific culprit genes have not been described. *Syphilis* (Chap. 153) is a relatively uncommon cause of aortic aneurysm. Syphilitic periaortitis and mesoaortitis damage elastic fibers, resulting in thickening and weakening of the aortic wall. Approximately 90% of syphilitic aneurysms are located in the ascending aorta or aortic arch. *Tuberculous aneurysms* (Chap. 150) typically affect the thoracic aorta and result from direct extension of infection from hilar lymph nodes or contiguous abscesses or from bacterial seeding. Loss of aortic wall elasticity results from granulomatous destruction of the medial layer. A *mycotic aneurysm* is a rare condition that develops as a result of staphylococcal, streptococcal, or salmonella infections of the aorta, usually at an atherosclerotic plaque. These aneurysms are usually saccular. Blood cultures are often positive and reveal the nature of the infecting agent.

Vasculitides associated with aortic aneurysm include Takayasu's arteritis and giant cell arteritis, which may cause aneurysms of the aortic arch and descending thoracic aorta. Spondyloarthropathies such as ankylosing spondylitis, rheumatoid arthritis, psoriatic arthritis, relapsing polychondritis and Reiter's syndrome are associated with dilatation of the ascending aorta. Behçet's disease (Chap. 307) causes thoracic and abdominal aortic aneurysms. *Traumatic aneurysms* may develop after penetrating or nonpenetrating chest trauma and most commonly affect the descending thoracic aorta just beyond the site of insertion of the ligamentum arteriosum. *Congenital aortic aneurysms* may be primary or associated with anomalies such as a bicuspid aortic valve or aortic coarctation.

THORACIC AORTIC ANEURYSMS The clinical manifestations and natural history of thoracic aortic aneurysms depend on their location. Cystic medial necrosis is the most common cause of ascending aortic aneurysms, whereas atherosclerosis is the condition most frequently associated with aneurysms of the aortic arch and descending thoracic aorta. The average growth rate of thoracic aneurysms is 0.1 to 0.4 cm per year. The risk of rupture is related to the size of the aneurysm and the presence of symptoms; it increases substantially for ascending aortic aneurysms >6 cm and descending thoracic aneurysms >7 cm. Most thoracic aortic aneurysms are asymptomatic. However, compression or erosion of adjacent tissue by aneurysms may cause symptoms such as chest pain, shortness of breath, cough, hoarseness, or dysphagia. Aneurysmal dilatation of the ascending aorta may cause congestive heart failure as a consequence of aortic regurgitation; and compression of the superior vena cava may produce congestion of the head, neck, and upper extremities.

A chest x-ray may be the first test to suggest the diagnosis of a thoracic aortic aneurysm (Fig. 231-1). Findings include widening of the mediastinal shadow and displacement or compression of the trachea or left mainstem bronchus. Two-dimensional echocardiography, and particularly transesophageal echocardiography, can be used to assess the proximal ascending aorta and descending thoracic aorta. Both contrast-enhanced computed tomography (CT) and magnetic resonance imaging (MRI) are sensitive and specific tests for assessment of aneurysms of the thoracic aorta. In asymptomatic patients whose aneurysms are too small to justify surgery, noninvasive testing with either contrast-enhanced CT or MRI should be performed at least every 6 to 12 months to monitor expansion. Contrast aortography is frequently required preoperatively to assess the length of the aneurysm and involvement of branch vessels (Fig. 231-2).

Patients with thoracic aortic aneurysms, and particularly patients with Marfan syndrome who have evidence of aortic root dilatation, should receive long-term beta-blocker therapy. Additional medical therapy should be given, as necessary, to control hypertension. Operative repair with placement of a prosthetic graft is indicated in patients with symptomatic thoracic aortic aneurysms, and in those in whom the aortic diameter is >6 cm or has increased by >1 cm per year. In patients with Marfan syndrome, thoracic aortic aneurysms >5 cm should be considered for surgery.

ABDOMINAL AORTIC ANEURYSMS Abdominal aortic aneurysms occur more frequently in males than in females, and the incidence increases with age. Abdominal aortic aneurysms may affect 1 to 2% of men older than 50 years. At least 90% of all abdominal aortic aneurysms >4.0 cm are affected by atherosclerosis, and most of these aneurysms are below the level of the renal arteries. Prognosis is related to both the size of the aneurysm and the severity of coexisting coronary artery and cerebrovascular disease. The risk of rupture increases with the size of the aneurysm. The 5-year risk of rupture for aneurysms <5 cm is 1 to 2%, whereas it is 20 to 40% for aneurysms >5 cm in diameter. The formation of mural thrombi within the aneurysm may predispose to peripheral embolization.

An abdominal aortic aneurysm commonly produces no symptoms. It is usually detected on routine examination as a palpable, pulsatile, and nontender mass, or it is an incidental finding during an abdominal x-ray or ultrasound performed for other reasons. However, as abdominal aortic aneurysms expand, they may become painful. Some patients complain of strong pulsations in the abdomen; others experience pain in the chest, lower back, or scrotum. Aneurysmal pain is usually a harbinger of rupture and represents a medical emergency. More often, acute rupture occurs without any prior warning, and this complication is always life-threatening. Rarely, there is leakage of the aneurysm with severe pain and tenderness. Acute pain and hypotension occur with rupture of the aneurysm, which requires emergency operation.

Abdominal radiography may demonstrate the calcified outline of the aneurysm. However, about 25% of aneurysms are not calcified and cannot be visualized by plain x-ray. An abdominal ultrasound can delineate the transverse and longitudinal dimensions of an abdominal aortic aneurysm and may detect mural thrombus. Abdominal ultra-

FIGURE 231-1 A chest x-ray of a patient with a thoracic aortic aneurysm.

sound is useful for serial documentation of aneurysm size and can be used to screen patients at risk for developing aortic aneurysm, such as those with affected siblings, peripheral atherosclerosis, or peripheral artery aneurysms. In one larger study, ultrasound screening of men aged 65 to 74 years was associated with a risk reduction in aneurysm-related death by 42%. CT with contrast and MRI are accurate, noninvasive tests to determine the location and size of abdominal aortic aneurysms (Fig. 231-3). Contrast aortography is used for the evaluation of patients with aneurysms before surgery, but the procedure carries a small risk of complications, such as bleeding, allergic reactions, and atheroembolism. This technique is useful in documenting the length of the aneurysm, especially its upper and lower limits, and the extent of associated atherosclerotic vascular disease. However, since the presence of mural clots may reduce the luminal size, aortography may underestimate the diameter of an aneurysm.

7.8 cm

FIGURE 231-2 An aortogram demonstrating a large fusiform aneurysm of the descending thoracic aorta.

FIGURE 231-3 A computed tomographic angiogram (CTA) depicting a fusiform abdominal aortic aneurysm that has been treated with a bifurcated stent graft.

℞ TREATMENT

Operative repair of the aneurysm and insertion of a prosthetic graft is indicated for abdominal aortic aneurysms of any size that are expanding rapidly or are associated with symptoms. For asymptomatic aneurysms, operation is indicated if the diameter is >5.5 cm. Operation may be recommended in patients with aneurysm diameters of 4 to 5 cm, except for patients with exceptionally high operative risk. However, in recent randomized trials of patients with abdominal aortic aneurysms <5.5 cm, there was no difference in the long-term (5- to 8-year) mortality rate between those followed with ultrasound surveillance and those undergoing elective aneurysm repair. Thus, serial noninvasive follow-up of smaller aneurysms (<5 cm) is an alternative to immediate surgery. Percutaneous placement of endovascular stent grafts (Fig. 231-3) for treatment of infrarenal abdominal aortic aneurysms is currently available for selected patients, and initial reports have been favorable.

In surgical candidates, careful preoperative cardiac and general medical evaluations (followed by appropriate therapy of complicating conditions) are essential. Preexisting coronary artery disease, congestive heart failure, pulmonary disease, diabetes, and advanced age add to the risk of surgery. Perioperative management should include the placement of a Swan-Ganz catheter and arterial line to monitor and optimize left ventricular filling pressure, cardiac output, and arterial pressure, especially during clamping and unclamping of the aorta, as well as during the immediate postoperative period. With careful preoperative cardiac evaluation and postoperative care, the operative mortality rate approximates 1 to 2%. After acute rupture, the mortality rate of emergent operation generally exceeds 50%.

AORTIC DISSECTION

Aortic dissection is caused by a circumferential or, less frequently, transverse tear of the intima. It often occurs along the right lateral wall of the ascending aorta where the hydraulic shear stress is high. Another common site is the descending thoracic aorta just below the ligamentum arteriosum. The initiating event is either a primary intimal tear with secondary dissection into the media or a medial hemorrhage that dissects into and disrupts the intima. The pulsatile aortic flow then dissects along the elastic lamellar plates of the aorta and creates a false lumen. The dissection usually propagates distally down the descending aorta and into its major branches, but it may also propagate proximally. In some cases, a secondary distal intimal disruption occurs, resulting in the reentry of blood from the false to the true lumen.

There are at least two important pathologic and radiologic variants: intramural hematoma without an intimal flap and penetrating atherosclerotic ulcer. The clinical picture and therapeutic management of intramural hematoma are similar to those for classic aortic dissection. By contrast, penetrating ulcers are usually localized and are not associated with extensive propagation. They are primarily found in the mid and distal portions of the descending thoracic aorta and are associated with extensive atherosclerotic disease. The ulcer can erode beyond the intimal border, leading to medial hematoma, and may progress to false aneurysm formation or rupture.

DeBakey and coworkers initially classified aortic dissections as type I, in which an intimal tear occurs in the ascending aorta but which involves the descending aorta as well; type II, in which the dissection is limited to the ascending aorta; and type III, in which the intimal tear is located in the descending area with distal propagation of the dissection (Fig. 231-4). Another classification (Stanford) is that of type A, in which the dissection involves the ascending aorta (proximal dissection), and type B, in which it is limited to the descending aorta (distal dissection). From a management standpoint, classification into type A or B is more practical and useful, since DeBakey types I and II are managed in a similar manner.

The factors that predispose to aortic dissection include systemic hypertension, a coexisting condition in 70% of patients, and cystic medial necrosis. Aortic dissection is the major cause of morbidity and mortality in patients with Marfan syndrome (Chap. 342) and similarly may affect patients with Ehlers-Danlos syndrome. The incidence is

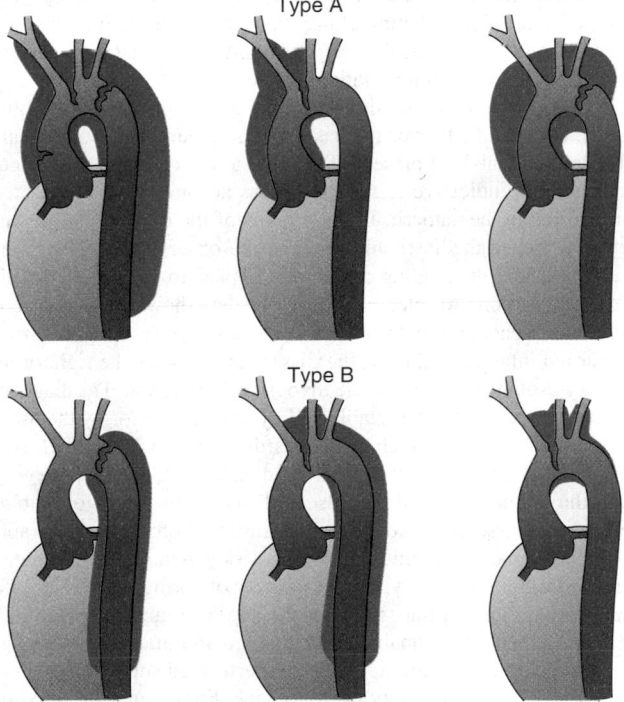

FIGURE 231-4 Classification of aortic dissections. Stanford classification: Type A dissections (*top panels*) involve the ascending aorta independent of site of tear and distal extension; type B dissections (*bottom panels*) involve transverse and/or descending aorta without involvement of the ascending aorta. DeBakey classification: Type I dissection involves ascending to descending aorta (*top left*); type II dissection is limited to ascending or transverse aorta, without descending aorta (*top center + top right*); type III dissection involves descending aorta only (*bottom left*). [*From DC Miller, in RM Doroghazi, EE Slater (eds): Aortic Dissection. New York, McGraw-Hill, 1983, with permission.*]

also increased in patients with inflammatory aortitis (i.e., Takayasu's arteritis, giant cell arteritis), congenital aortic valve anomalies (e.g., bicuspid valve), in those with coarctation of the aorta, and in otherwise normal women during the third trimester of pregnancy.

CLINICAL MANIFESTATIONS   The peak incidence is in the sixth and seventh decades. Men are more affected than women by a ratio of 2:1. The presentations of aortic dissection and its variants are the consequences of intimal tear, dissecting hematoma, occlusion of involved arteries, and compression of adjacent tissues. Acute aortic dissection presents with the sudden onset of pain (Chap. 12), which is often described as very severe and tearing and is associated with diaphoresis. The pain may be localized to the front or back of the chest, often the interscapular region, and typically migrates with propagation of the dissection. Other symptoms include syncope, dyspnea, and weakness. Physical findings may include hypertension or hypotension, loss of pulses, aortic regurgitation, pulmonary edema, and neurologic findings due to carotid artery obstruction (hemiplegia, hemianesthesia) or spinal cord ischemia (paraplegia). Bowel ischemia, hematuria, and myocardial ischemia have all been observed. These clinical manifestations reflect complications resulting from the dissection occluding the major arteries. Furthermore, clinical manifestations may result from the compression of adjacent structures (e.g., superior cervical ganglia, superior vena cava, bronchus, esophagus) by the expanding dissection causing aneurysmal dilatation, and include Horner's syndrome, superior vena caval syndrome, hoarseness, dysphagia, and airway compromise. Hemopericardium and cardiac tamponade may complicate a type A lesion with retrograde dissection. Acute aortic regurgitation is an important and common (>50%) complication of proximal dissection. It is the outcome of either a circumferential tear that widens the aortic root or a disruption of the annulus by dissecting hematoma that tears a leaflet(s) or displaces it below the line of closure. Signs of aortic regurgitation include bounding pulses, a wide pulse pressure, a diastolic murmur often radiating along the right sternal border, and evidence of congestive heart failure. The clinical manifestation depends on the severity of the regurgitation.

In dissections involving the ascending aorta, the chest x-ray often reveals a widened superior mediastinum. A pleural effusion (usually left-sided) may also be present. This effusion is typically serosanguineous and not indicative of rupture unless accompanied by hypotension and falling hematocrit. In dissections of the descending thoracic aorta, a widened mediastinum may also be observed on chest x-ray. In addition, the descending aorta may appear to be wider than the ascending portion. An electrocardiogram that shows no evidence of myocardial ischemia is helpful in distinguishing aortic dissection from myocardial infarction. Rarely, the dissection involves the right or left coronary ostium and causes acute myocardial infarction. The diagnosis of aortic dissection can be established by aortography or by the use of noninvasive techniques such as echocardiography, CT, or MRI. Aortography may be used to document the diagnosis; to identify the entry point, the intimal flap, and the false and true lumina; and to establish the extent of dissection into the major arteries. Coronary angiography may be performed concomitantly in high-risk patients in the evaluation and preparation for surgery. The sensitivity of aortography is 70% for visualizing an intimal flap, 56% for the site of intimal tear, and 87% for false lumen. It is unable to recognize intramural hemorrhage. Transthoracic echocardiography can be performed simply and rapidly and has an overall sensitivity of 60 to 85%. For diagnosing proximal ascending aortic dissections, its sensitivity exceeds 80%; it is less useful for detecting dissection of the arch and descending thoracic aorta. Transesophageal echocardiography requires greater skill and patient cooperation but is very accurate in identifying dissections of the ascending and descending thoracic aorta, but not the arch, achieving 98% sensitivity and approximately 90% specificity. Echocardiography also provides important information regarding the presence and severity of aortic regurgitation and pericardial effusion. CT and MRI are both

highly accurate in identifying the intimal flap and the extent of the dissection; each has a sensitivity and specificity >90%. They are useful in recognizing intramural hemorrhage and penetrating ulcers. MRI can also detect blood flow, which may be useful in characterizing antegrade versus retrograde dissection. Transesophageal echocardiography, CT, and MRI are the diagnostic procedures of choice over contrast aortography. Their relative utility depends on the availability and expertise in individual institutions as well as on the hemodynamic stability of the patient, with CT and MRI obviously less suitable for unstable patients.

℞ TREATMENT

Medical therapy should be initiated as soon as the diagnosis is considered. The patient should be admitted to an intensive care unit for monitoring hemodynamics and urine output. Unless hypotension is present, therapy should be aimed at reducing cardiac contractility and systemic arterial pressure, and thereby shear stress. For acute dissection, unless contraindicated, β-adrenergic blockers should be administered parenterally, using intravenous propranolol, metoprolol, or the short-acting esmolol to achieve a heart rate of approximately 60 beats/ min. This should be accompanied by sodium nitroprusside infusion to lower systolic blood pressure to ≤120 mmHg. Labetalol (Chap. 230), a drug with both β- and α-adrenergic blocking properties, is also used as a parenteral agent in the acute therapy of dissection.

The calcium channel antagonists, verapamil and diltiazem, may be used intravenously if nitroprusside or labetalol cannot be employed. The addition of a parenteral angiotensin-converting enzyme (ACE) inhibitor, such as enalaprilat, to a β-adrenergic blocker may also be considered. Isolated use of direct vasodilators, such as diazoxide and hydralazine, is contraindicated because these agents can increase hydraulic shear and may propagate dissection.

Emergent or urgent surgical correction is the preferred treatment for ascending aortic dissections (type A) and complicated type B dissections including those characterized by propagation, compromise of major aortic branches, impending rupture, or continued pain. Surgery involves excision of the intimal flap, obliteration of the false lumen, and placement of an interposition graft. A composite valve-graft conduit is used if the aortic valve is disrupted. The overall in-hospital mortality rate after surgical treatment of patients with aortic dissection is reported to be 15 to 25%. The major causes of perioperative mortality and morbidity include myocardial infarction, paraplegia, renal failure, tamponade, hemorrhage, and sepsis. Reports of the use of endoluminal stent grafts in selected patients with type B dissection are encouraging. Other transcatheter techniques, such as fenestration of the intimal flaps and stenting of narrowed branch vessels to increase flow to compromised organs, are also under investigation. For uncomplicated and stable distal dissection (type B), medical therapy is the preferred treatment. The in-hospital mortality rate of medically treated patients with type B dissection is 10 to 20%. Long-term therapy for patients with aortic dissection (with or without surgery) consists of the control of hypertension and reduction of cardiac contractility with the use of beta blockers plus other antihypertensive agents such as ACE inhibitors or calcium antagonists. Patients with chronic type B dissection should be followed on an outpatient basis every 6 to 12 months by contrast-enhanced CT or MRI to detect propagation or expansion. Patients with Marfan syndrome are at high risk for postdissection complications. The long-term prognosis for patients with treated dissections is generally good with careful follow-up; the 10-year survival rate is approximately 60%.

AORTIC OCCLUSION

CHRONIC ATHEROSCLEROTIC OCCLUSIVE DISEASE   Atherosclerosis may affect the thoracic and abdominal aorta. Occlusive aortic disease caused by atherosclerosis is usually confined to the distal abdominal aorta below the renal arteries. Frequently the disease extends to the iliac arteries (Chap. 232). Claudication characteristically involves the lower back, buttocks, and thighs and may be associated with impotence in males

(Leriche syndrome). The severity of the symptoms depends on the adequacy of collaterals. With sufficient collateral blood flow, a complete occlusion of the abdominal aorta may occur without the development of ischemic symptoms. The physical findings include absence of femoral and other distal pulses bilaterally and the detection of an audible bruit over the abdomen (usually at or below the umbilicus) and the common femoral arteries. Atrophic skin, loss of hair, and coolness of the lower extremities are usually observed. In advanced ischemia, rubor on dependency and pallor on elevation can be seen.

The diagnosis is usually established by the physical examination and noninvasive testing, including leg pressure measurements, Doppler velocity analysis, pulse volume recordings, and duplex ultrasonography. The anatomy may be defined by MRI, CT or conventional aortography before revascularization. Operative treatment is indicated in patients with debilitating symptoms and/or with the development of leg ischemia.

ACUTE OCCLUSION Acute occlusion in the distal abdominal aorta represents a medical emergency because it threatens the viability of the lower extremities. It usually results from an occlusive embolus that almost always originates from the heart. Rarely, acute occlusion may occur as the result of in situ thrombosis in a preexisting severely narrowed segment of the aorta or plaque rupture and hemorrhage into such an area.

The clinical picture is one of acute ischemia of the lower extremities. Severe rest pain, coolness, and pallor of the lower extremities and the absence of distal pulses bilaterally are the usual manifestations. Diagnosis should be established rapidly by aortography. Emergency thrombectomy or revascularization is indicated.

AORTITIS

Aortitis frequently affects the thoracic aorta and may result in aneurysmal dilatation and aortic regurgitation; it occasionally obstructs branch vessels of the aorta.

SYPHILITIC AORTITIS This late manifestation of luetic infection (Chap. 153) usually affects the proximal ascending aorta, particularly the aortic root, resulting in aortic dilatation and aneurysm formation. Syphilitic aortitis may occasionally involve the aortic arch or the descending aorta. The aneurysms may be saccular or fusiform and are usually asymptomatic, but compression of and erosion into adjacent structures may result in symptoms; rupture may also occur.

The initial lesion is an obliterative endarteritis of the vasa vasorum, especially in the adventitia. This is an inflammatory response to the invasion of the adventitia by the spirochetes. Destruction of the aortic media occurs as the spirochetes spread into this layer, usually via the lymphatics accompanying the vasa vasorum. Destruction of collagen and elastic tissues leads to dilation of the aorta, scar formation, and calcification. These changes account for the characteristic radiographic appearance of a calcified ascending aortic aneurysm.

The disease typically presents as an incidental chest radiographic finding 15 to 30 years after initial infection. Symptoms may result from aortic regurgitation, narrowing of coronary ostia due to syphilitic aortitis, compression of adjacent structures (e.g., esophagus), or rupture. Diagnosis is established by a positive serologic test, i.e., rapid plasmin reagin (RPR) or fluorescent treponemal antibody. Treatment includes penicillin and surgical excision and repair.

RHEUMATIC AORTITIS Rheumatoid arthritis (Chap. 301), ankylosing spondylitis (Chap. 305), psoriatic arthritis (Chap. 305), Reiter's syndrome (Chap. 305), relapsing polychondritis, and inflammatory bowel disorders may all be associated with aortitis involving the ascending aorta. The inflammatory lesions usually involve the ascending aorta and may extend to the sinuses of Valsalva, the mitral valve leaflets, and adjacent myocardium. The clinical manifestations are aneurysm,

aortic regurgitation, and involvement of the cardiac conduction system.

TAKAYASU'S ARTERITIS This inflammatory disease often affects the ascending aorta and aortic arch causing obstruction of the aorta and its major arteries. Takayasu's arteritis is also termed *pulseless disease* because of the frequent occlusion of the large arteries originating from the aorta. It may also involve the descending thoracic and abdominal aorta and occlude large branches such as the renal arteries. Aortic aneurysms may also occur. The pathology is a panarteritis, characterized by mononuclear cells and occasionally giant cells, with marked intimal hyperplasia, medial and adventitial thickening, and, in chronic form, fibrotic occlusion. The disease is most prevalent in young females of Asian descent but does occur in women of other geographic and ethnic origins and also in young men. During the acute stage, fever, malaise, weight loss, and other systemic symptoms may be evident. An elevation of the erythrocyte sedimentation rate is common. The chronic stages of the disease present with symptoms related to large artery occlusion, such as upper extremity claudication, cerebral ischemia, and syncope. The chronic disease is intermittently active. Since the process is progressive and there is no definitive therapy, the prognosis is usually poor. Glucocorticoids and immunosuppressive agents have been reported to be effective in some patients during the acute phase. Occasionally, anticoagulation prevents thrombosis and complete occlusion of a large artery. Surgical bypass or endovascular intervention of a critically stenotic artery may be necessary.

GIANT CELL ARTERITIS (See also Chap. 306) This vasculitis occurs in older individuals and affects women more often than men. Primarily large and medium-sized arteries are affected. The pathology is that of focal granulomatous lesions involving the entire arterial wall. It may be associated with polymyalgia rheumatica. Obstruction of medium-sized arteries (e.g., temporal and ophthalmic arteries) and of major branches of the aorta and the development of aortitis and aortic regurgitation are some of the complications of the disease. High-dose glucocorticoid therapy may be effective when given early.

FURTHER READING

THE ANEURYSM DETECTION AND MANAGEMENT VETERANS AFFAIRS COOPERATIVE STUDY GROUP: Immediate repair compared with surveillance of small abdominal aortic aneurysms. N Engl J Med 346:1437, 2002

GANAHA F et al: Prognosis of aortic intramural hematoma with and without penetrating atherosclerotic ulcer. A clinical and radiological analysis. Circulation 106:342, 2002

GUO D et al: Familial thoracic aortic aneurysms and dissections: Genetic heterogeneity with a major locus mapping to 5q13-14. Circulation 103:2461, 2001

HAGAN PG et al: The International Registry of Acute Aortic Dissection (IRAD): New insights into an old disease. JAMA 283:897, 2000

HASHIMOTO H: Takayasu's arteritis and giant cell (temporal or cranial) arteritis. Intern Med 39:4, 2000

ISSELBACHER EM et al: Diseases of the aorta, in *Braunwald's Heart Disease: A Textbook of Cardiovascular Medicine,* 7th ed, DP Zipes et al (eds). Philadelphia, Saunders, 2005

THE MULTICENTRE ANEURYSM SCREENING STUDY GROUP: The Multicentre Aneurysm Screening Study (MASS) into the effect of abdominal aortic aneurysm screening on mortality in men: A randomized controlled trial. Lancet 360:1531, 2002

PARODI JC et al: Endovascular treatment of aneurysmal disease. Cardiol Clin 20:579, 2002

THE UK SMALL ANEURYSM TRIAL PARTICIPANTS: Long-term outcomes of immediate repair compared with surveillance of small abdominal aortic aneurysms. N Engl J Med 346:1445, 2002

VAUGHAN CJ et al: Identification of a chromosome 11q23.2-q24 locus for familial aortic aneurysm disease, a genetically heterogeneous disorder. Circulation 103:2469, 2001

ARTERIAL DISORDERS

PERIPHERAL ARTERIAL DISEASE Atherosclerosis is the leading cause of occlusive arterial disease of the extremities in patients over 40 years old; the highest incidence occurs in the sixth and seventh decades of life. As in patients with atherosclerosis of the coronary and cerebral vasculature, there is an increased prevalence of peripheral atherosclerotic disease in individuals with diabetes mellitus, hypercholesterolemia, hypertension, or hyperhomocysteinemia and in cigarette smokers.

Pathology (See also Chap. 224) Segmental lesions causing stenosis or occlusion are usually localized in large and medium-sized vessels. The pathology of the lesions includes atherosclerotic plaques with calcium deposition, thinning of the media, patchy destruction of muscle and elastic fibers, fragmentation of the internal elastic lamina, and thrombi composed of platelets and fibrin. The primary sites of involvement are the abdominal aorta and iliac arteries (30% of symptomatic patients), the femoral and popliteal arteries (80 to 90% of patients), and the more distal vessels, including the tibial and peroneal arteries (40 to 50% of patients). Atherosclerotic lesions occur preferentially at arterial branch points, sites of increased turbulence, altered shear stress, and intimal injury. Involvement of the distal vasculature is most common in elderly individuals and patients with diabetes mellitus.

Clinical Evaluation Fewer than 50% of patients with peripheral arterial disease (PAD) are symptomatic, though many have a slow or impaired gait. The most common *symptom* is intermittent claudication, which is defined as a pain, ache, cramp, numbness, or a sense of fatigue in the muscles; it occurs during exercise and is relieved by rest. The site of claudication is distal to the location of the occlusive lesion. For example, buttock, hip, and thigh discomfort occur in patients with aortoiliac disease (Leriche syndrome), whereas calf claudication develops in patients with femoral-popliteal disease. Symptoms are far more common in the lower than in the upper extremities because of the higher incidence of obstructive lesions in the former region. In patients with severe arterial occlusive disease, critical limb ischemia may develop. Patients will complain of rest pain or a feeling of cold or numbness in the foot and toes. Frequently, these symptoms occur at night when the legs are horizontal and improve when the legs are in a dependent position. With severe ischemia, rest pain may be persistent.

Important *physical findings* of PAD include decreased or absent pulses distal to the obstruction, the presence of bruits over the narrowed artery, and muscle atrophy. With more severe disease, hair loss, thickened nails, smooth and shiny skin, reduced skin temperature, and pallor or cyanosis are frequent physical signs. In addition, ulcers or gangrene may occur. Elevation of the legs and repeated flexing of the calf muscles produce pallor of the soles of the feet, whereas rubor, secondary to reactive hyperemia, may develop when the legs are dependent. The time required for rubor to develop or for the veins in the foot to fill when the patient's legs are transferred from an elevated to a dependent position is related to the severity of the ischemia and the presence of collateral vessels. Patients with severe ischemia may develop peripheral edema because they keep their legs in a dependent position much of the time. Ischemic neuritis can result in numbness and hyporeflexia.

Noninvasive Testing The history and physical examination are usually sufficient to establish the diagnosis of PAD. An objective assessment of the severity of disease is obtained by noninvasive techniques. These include digital pulse volume recordings, Doppler flow velocity waveform analysis, duplex ultrasonography (which combines B-mode imaging and pulse-wave Doppler examination), segmental pressure measurements, transcutaneous oximetry, stress testing (usually using a treadmill), and tests of reactive hyperemia. In the presence of significant PAD, the volume displacement in the leg is decreased with each pulse, and the Doppler velocity contour becomes progressively flatter. Duplex ultrasonography is often useful in detecting stenotic lesions in native arteries and bypass grafts.

Arterial pressure can be recorded noninvasively along the legs by serial placement of sphygmomanometric cuffs and use of a Doppler device to auscultate or record blood flow. Normally, systolic blood pressure in the legs and arms is similar. Indeed, ankle pressure may be slightly higher than arm pressure due to pulse-wave reflection. In the presence of hemodynamically significant stenoses, the systolic blood pressure in the leg is decreased. Thus, if one were to obtain a ratio of the ankle and brachial artery pressures (termed the *ankle:brachial index*, or ABI), it would be ≥1.0 in normal individuals and <1.0 in patients with peripheral arterial disease. A ratio of <0.5 is consistent with severe ischemia.

Treadmill testing allows the physician to assess functional limitations objectively. Decline of the ankle-brachial systolic pressure ratio immediately after exercise may provide further support for the diagnosis of PAD in patients with equivocal symptoms and findings on examination. Exercise testing also allows simultaneous evaluation for the presence of coronary artery disease.

Magnetic resonance angiography and conventional contrast angiography should not be used for routine diagnostic testing but are performed prior to potential revascularization. Either test is useful in defining the anatomy to assist operative planning and is also indicated if nonsurgical interventions are being considered, such as percutaneous transluminal angioplasty (PTA) or thrombolysis. Studies have suggested that magnetic resonance angiography has diagnostic accuracy comparable to that of contrast angiography.

Prognosis The natural history of patients with PAD is influenced primarily by the extent of coexisting coronary artery and cerebral vascular disease. Studies using coronary angiography have estimated that approximately one-half of patients with symptomatic PAD also have significant coronary artery disease. Life-table analysis has indicated that patients with claudication have a 70% 5-year and a 50% 10-year survival rate. Most deaths are either sudden or secondary to myocardial infarction. The likelihood of symptomatic progression of PAD appears less than the chance of succumbing to coronary artery disease. Approximately 75% of nondiabetic patients who present with mild to moderate claudication remain symptomatically stable or improve. Deterioration is likely to occur in the remainder, with approximately 5% of the group ultimately undergoing amputation. The prognosis is worse in patients who continue to smoke cigarettes or who have diabetes mellitus.

℞ TREATMENT

Therapeutic options include supportive measures, pharmacologic treatment, nonoperative interventions, and surgery. Supportive measures include meticulous care of the feet, which should be kept clean and protected against excessive drying with moisturizing creams. Well-fitting and protective shoes are advised to reduce trauma. Sandals and shoes made of synthetic materials that do not "breathe" should be avoided. Elastic support hose should be avoided, as they reduce blood flow to the skin. In patients with ischemia at rest, shock blocks under the head of the bed together with a canopy over the feet may improve perfusion pressure and ameliorate some of the rest pain.

Treatment of associated factors that contribute to the development of atherosclerosis should be initiated. The importance of discontinuing cigarette smoking cannot be overemphasized. The physician must assume a major role in this life-style modification. It is important to control blood pressure in hypertensive patients but to avoid hypotensive levels. Treatment of hypercholesterolemia is advocated, although reduction in cholesterol levels has not been shown unequivocally to reverse peripheral atherosclerotic lesions. However, it has been shown to prevent or to slow progression of the disease and to improve survival in patients with atherosclerosis. Patients with claudication should also be encouraged to exercise regularly and at progressively more strenuous levels. Supervised exercise training programs may improve muscle efficiency and prolong walking distance. Patients also should be advised to walk for 30 to 45 min daily, stopping at the onset of claudication and resting until the symptoms resolve before resuming ambulation.

Pharmacologic Management This form of treatment of patients with PAD has not been as successful as the medical treatment of coronary artery disease (Chap. 226). In particular, vasodilators as a class have not proved to be beneficial. During exercise, peripheral vasodilation occurs distal to sites of significant arterial stenoses. As a result, perfusion pressure falls, often to levels less than that generated in the interstitial tissue by the exercising muscle. Drugs such as α-adrenergic blocking agents, calcium channel antagonists, papaverine, and other vasodilators have not been shown to be effective in patients with PAD. Pentoxifylline, a substituted xanthine derivative, has been reported to decrease blood viscosity and to increase red cell flexibility, thereby increasing blood flow to the microcirculation and enhancing tissue oxygenation. Several placebo-controlled studies have found that pentoxifylline increased the duration of exercise in patients with claudication, but its efficacy has not been confirmed in all clinical trials.

Cilostazol, a phosphodiesterase inhibitor with vasodilator and antiplatelet properties, has been reported to increase claudication distance in multiple trials. Several studies have suggested that long-term parenteral administration of vasodilator prostaglandins decreases pain and facilitates healing of ulcers in patients with severe limb ischemia. Clinical trials with angiogenic growth factors such as vascular endothelial growth factor (VEGF) and basic fibroblast growth factor (bFGF) are proceeding. One placebo-controlled trial reported that intraarterial administration of recombinant bFGF modestly increased walking time in patients with claudication. Intramuscular gene transfer of DNA encoding VEGF or bFGF may promote collateral blood vessel growth in patients with critical limb ischemia, but evidence documenting clinical efficacy is not available and awaits the outcome of ongoing trials.

Platelet inhibitors, particularly aspirin, reduce the risk of adverse cardiovascular events in patients with peripheral atherosclerosis. Clopidogrel, a drug that inhibits platelet aggregation via its effect on ADP-dependent platelet-fibrinogen binding, appears to be more effective than aspirin in reducing cardiovascular morbidity and mortality in patients with PAD. The anticoagulants heparin and warfarin have not been shown to be effective in patients with chronic PAD but may be useful in acute arterial obstruction secondary to thrombosis or systemic embolism. Similarly, thrombolytic intervention using drugs such as streptokinase, urokinase, or recombinant tissue plasminogen activator (tPA) (alteplase) may have a role in the treatment of acute thrombotic arterial occlusion but is not effective in patients with chronic arterial occlusion secondary to atherosclerosis.

Revascularization Revascularization procedures, including nonoperative as well as operative interventions, are usually reserved for patients with progressive, severe, or disabling symptoms and ischemia at rest, as well as for individuals who must be symptom-free because of their occupation. Angiography should be performed mainly in patients who are being considered for a revascularization procedure. Nonoperative interventions include PTA, stent placement, and atherectomy (Chap. 229). PTA of the iliac artery is associated with a higher success rate than PTA of the femoral and popliteal arteries. Approximately 90 to 95% of iliac PTAs are initially successful, and the 3-year patency rate is >75%. Patency rates may be higher if a stent is placed in the iliac artery. The initial success rate for femoral-popliteal PTA is approximately 80%, with a 60% 3-year patency rate. Patency rates are influenced by the severity of pretreatment stenoses; the prognosis of

total occlusive lesions is worse than that of nonocclusive stenotic lesions.

Several operative procedures are available for treating patients with aortoiliac and femoral-popliteal artery disease. The preferred operative procedure depends on the location and extent of the obstruction(s) and general medical condition of the patient. Operative procedures for aortoiliac disease include aortobifemoral bypass, axillofemoral bypass, femoral-femoral bypass, and aortoiliac endarterectomy. The most frequently used procedure is the aortobifemoral bypass using knitted Dacron grafts. Immediate graft patency approaches 99%, and 5- and 10-year graft patency in survivors is >90 and 80%, respectively. Operative complications include myocardial infarction and stroke, infection of the graft, peripheral embolization, and sexual dysfunction from interruption of autonomic nerves in the pelvis. Operative mortality ranges from 1 to 3%, mostly due to ischemic heart disease.

Operative therapy for femoral-popliteal artery disease includes in situ and reverse autogenous saphenous vein bypass grafts, placement of polytetrafluoroethylene (PTFE) or other synthetic grafts, and thromboendarterectomy. Operative mortality ranges from 1 to 3%. The long-term patency rate depends on the type of graft used, the location of the distal anastomosis, and the patency of runoff vessels beyond the anastomosis. Patency rates of femoral-popliteal saphenous vein bypass grafts at 1 year approach 90% and at 5 years, 70 to 80%. Five-year patency rates of infrapopliteal saphenous vein bypass grafts are 60 to 70%. In contrast, 5-year patency rates of infrapopliteal PTFE grafts are <30%. Lumbar sympathectomy alone or as an adjunct to aortofemoral reconstruction has fallen into disfavor.

Preoperative cardiac risk assessment may identify individuals especially likely to experience an adverse cardiac event during the perioperative period. Patients with angina, prior myocardial infarction, ventricular ectopy, heart failure, or diabetes are among those at increased risk. Noninvasive tests, such as treadmill testing (if feasible), dipyridamole or adenosine radionuclide myocardial perfusion imaging, dobutamine echocardiography, and ambulatory ischemia monitoring permit further stratification of patient risk (Chap. 229). Patients with abnormal test results require close supervision and adjunctive management with anti-ischemic medications. β-Adrenergic blockers reduce the risk of postoperative cardiovascular complications. It is not known whether coronary angiography and coronary arterial revascularization reduce overall perioperative mortality in high-risk patients undergoing peripheral vascular surgery, but cardiac catheterization should be considered in patients suspected of having left main or three-vessel coronary artery disease.

FIBROMUSCULAR DYSPLASIA This is a hyperplastic disorder affecting medium-sized and small arteries. It occurs predominantly in females and usually involves renal and carotid arteries but can affect extremity vessels such as the iliac and subclavian arteries. The histologic classification includes intimal, medial, and periadventitial dysplasia. Medial dysplasia is the most common type and is characterized by hyperplasia of the media with or without fibrosis of the elastic membrane. It is identified angiographically by a "string of beads" appearance caused by thickened fibromuscular ridges contiguous with thin, less involved portions of the arterial wall. When limb vessels are involved, clinical manifestations are similar to those for atherosclerosis, including claudication and rest pain. PTA and surgical reconstruction have been beneficial in patients with debilitating symptoms or threatened limbs.

THROMBOANGIITIS OBLITERANS Thromboangiitis obliterans (Buerger's disease) is an inflammatory occlusive vascular disorder involving small and medium-sized arteries and veins in the distal upper and lower extremities. Cerebral, visceral, and coronary vessels may also be affected. This disorder develops most frequently in men under age 40. The prevalence is higher in Asians and individuals of eastern European descent. While the cause of thromboangiitis obliterans is not known, there is a definite relationship to cigarette smoking in patients with this disorder.

In the initial stages of thromboangiitis obliterans, polymorphonuclear leukocytes infiltrate the walls of the small and medium-sized arteries and veins. The internal elastic lamina is preserved, and thrombus may develop in the vascular lumen. As the disease progresses, mononuclear cells, fibroblasts, and giant cells replace the neutrophils. Later stages are characterized by perivascular fibrosis and recanalization.

The clinical features of thromboangiitis obliterans often include a triad of claudication of the affected extremity, Raynaud's phenomenon (p. 1489), and migratory superficial vein thrombophlebitis. Claudication is usually confined to the calves and feet or the forearms and hands, because this disorder primarily affects distal vessels. In the presence of severe digital ischemia, trophic nail changes, painful ulcerations, and gangrene may develop at the tips of the fingers or toes. The physical examination shows normal brachial and popliteal pulses but reduced or absent radial, ulnar, and/or tibial pulses. Arteriography is helpful in making the diagnosis. Smooth, tapering segmental lesions in the distal vessels are characteristic, as are collateral vessels at sites of vascular occlusion. Proximal atherosclerotic disease is usually absent. The diagnosis can be confirmed by excisional biopsy and pathologic examination of an involved vessel.

There is no specific treatment except abstention from tobacco. The prognosis is worse in individuals who continue to smoke, but results are discouraging even in those who do stop smoking. Arterial bypass of the larger vessels may be used in selected instances, as well as local debridement, depending on the symptoms and severity of ischemia. Antibiotics may be useful; anticoagulants and glucocorticoids are not helpful. If these measures fail, amputation may be required.

VASCULITIS   Other vasculitides may affect the arteries supplying the upper and lower extremities. →*Takayasu's arteritis and giant cell (temporal) arteritis are discussed in Chap. 306.*

ACUTE ARTERIAL OCCLUSION   This results in the sudden cessation of blood flow to an extremity. The severity of ischemia and the viability of the extremity depend on the location and extent of the occlusion and the presence and subsequent development of collateral blood vessels. There are two principal causes of acute arterial occlusion: embolism and thrombus in situ.

The most common sources of arterial emboli are the heart, aorta, and large arteries. Cardiac disorders that cause thromboembolism include atrial fibrillation, both chronic and paroxysmal; acute myocardial infarction; ventricular aneurysm; cardiomyopathy; infectious and marantic endocarditis; prosthetic heart valves; and atrial myxoma. Emboli to the distal vessels may also originate from proximal sites of atherosclerosis and aneurysms of the aorta and large vessels. Less frequently, an arterial occlusion results paradoxically from a venous thrombus that has entered the systemic circulation via a patent foramen ovale or other septal defect. Arterial emboli tend to lodge at vessel bifurcations because the vessel caliber decreases at these sites; in the lower extremities, emboli lodge most frequently in the femoral artery, followed by the iliac artery, aorta, and popliteal and tibioperoneal arteries.

Acute arterial thrombosis in situ occurs most frequently in atherosclerotic vessels at the site of an atherosclerotic plaque or aneurysm and in arterial bypass grafts. Trauma to an artery may also result in the formation of an acute arterial thrombus. Arterial occlusion may complicate arterial punctures and placement of catheters. Less frequent causes include the thoracic outlet compression syndrome, which causes subclavian artery occlusion, and entrapment of the popliteal artery by abnormal placement of the medial head of the gastrocnemius muscle. Polycythemia and hypercoagulable disorders (Chaps. 95 and 103) are also associated with acute arterial thrombosis.

Clinical Features   The symptoms of an acute arterial occlusion depend on the location, duration, and severity of the obstruction. Often, severe pain, paresthesia, numbness, and coldness develop in the involved ex

tremity within 1 h. Paralysis may occur with severe and persistent ischemia. Physical findings include loss of pulses distal to the occlusion, cyanosis or pallor, mottling, decreased skin temperature, muscle stiffening, loss of sensation, weakness, and/or absent deep tendon reflexes. If acute arterial occlusion occurs in the presence of an adequate collateral circulation, as is often the case in acute graft occlusion, the symptoms and findings may be less impressive. In this situation, the patient complains about an abrupt decrease in the distance walked before claudication occurs or of modest pain and paresthesia. Pallor and coolness are evident, but sensory and motor functions are generally preserved. The diagnosis of acute arterial occlusion is usually apparent from the clinical presentation. Arteriography is useful for confirming the diagnosis and demonstrating the location and extent of occlusion.

℞ TREATMENT

Once the diagnosis is made, the patient should be anticoagulated with intravenous heparin to prevent propagation of the clot. In cases of severe ischemia of recent onset, and particularly when limb viability is jeopardized, immediate intervention to ensure reperfusion is indicated. Endovascular or surgical thromboembolectomy or arterial bypass procedures are used to restore blood flow to the ischemic extremity promptly, particularly when a large proximal vessel is occluded.

Intraarterial thrombolytic therapy is effective when acute arterial occlusion is caused by a thrombus in an atherosclerotic vessel or arterial bypass graft. Thrombolytic therapy may also be indicated when the patient's overall condition contraindicates surgical intervention or when smaller distal vessels are occluded, thus preventing surgical access. One approach for administering intraarterial urokinase is to give 240,000 IU/h for 4 h, followed by 120,000 IU/h for a maximum of 48 h. Intraarterial recombinant tPA may be administered at infusion rates of 1 mg/h or 0.05 mg/kg per hour. Meticulous observation for hemorrhagic complications is required during intraarterial thrombolytic therapy.

If the limb is not in jeopardy, a more conservative approach that includes observation and administration of anticoagulants may be taken. Anticoagulation prevents recurrent embolism and reduces the likelihood of thrombus propagation. It can be initiated with intravenous heparin and followed by oral warfarin. Recommended dosages are the same as those used for deep vein thrombosis (see below). Emboli resulting from infectious endocarditis, the presence of prosthetic heart valves, or atrial myxoma often require surgical intervention to remove the cause.

ATHEROEMBOLISM   Atheroembolism constitutes a subset of acute arterial occlusion. In this condition, multiple small deposits of fibrin, platelet, and cholesterol debris embolize from proximal atherosclerotic lesions or aneurysmal sites. Large protruding aortic atheromas are a source of emboli that may lead to stroke and renal insufficiency as well as limb ischemia. Atheroembolism may occur after intraarterial procedures. Since the emboli tend to lodge in the small vessels of the muscle and skin and may not occlude the large vessels, distal pulses usually remain palpable. Patients complain of acute pain and tenderness at the site of embolization. Digital vascular occlusion may result in ischemia and the "blue toe" syndrome; digital necrosis and gangrene may develop (Fig. 232-1). Localized areas of tenderness, pallor, and livedo reticularis (see below) occur at sites of emboli. Skin or muscle biopsy may demonstrate cholesterol crystals.

Ischemia resulting from atheroemboli is notoriously difficult to treat. Usually neither surgical revascularization procedures nor thrombolytic therapy is helpful because of the multiplicity, composition, and distal location of the emboli. Some evidence suggests that platelet inhibitors prevent atheroembolism. Surgical intervention to remove or bypass the atherosclerotic vessel or aneurysm that causes the recurrent atheroemboli may be necessary.

THORACIC OUTLET COMPRESSION SYNDROME   This is a symptom complex resulting from compression of the neurovascular bundle (artery, vein,

FIGURE 232-1 Atheroembolism causing cyanotic discoloration and impending necrosis of the toes (blue toe syndrome).

or nerves) at the thoracic outlet as it courses through the neck and shoulder. Cervical ribs, abnormalities of the scalenus anticus muscle, proximity of the clavicle to the first rib, or abnormal insertion of the pectoralis minor muscle may compress the subclavian artery and brachial plexus as these structures pass from the thorax to the arm. Patients may develop shoulder and arm pain, weakness, paresthesia, claudication, Raynaud's phenomenon, and even ischemic tissue loss and gangrene. Examination is often normal unless provocative maneuvers are performed. Occasionally, distal pulses are decreased or absent and digital cyanosis and ischemia may be evident. Tenderness may be present in the supraclavicular fossa. Abducting the affected arm by 90° and externally rotating the shoulder may precipitate symptoms. Several additional maneuvers are used to confirm the diagnosis of vascular compression and to suggest the location of the abnormality. These include the scalene maneuver (extension of the neck and rotation of the head to the side of the symptoms), the costoclavicular maneuver (posterior rotation of shoulders), and the hyperabduction maneuver (raising the arm 180°), which may cause subclavian bruits and loss of pulses in the arm. A chest x-ray will indicate the presence of cervical ribs. The electromyogram will be abnormal if the brachial plexus is involved.

℞ TREATMENT

Most patients can be managed conservatively. They should be advised to avoid the positions that cause symptoms. Many patients benefit from shoulder girdle exercises. Surgical procedures such as removal of the first rib or resection of the scalenus anticus muscle are necessary occasionally for relief of symptoms or treatment of ischemia.

ARTERIOVENOUS FISTULA Abnormal communications between an artery and a vein, bypassing the capillary bed, may be congenital or acquired. Congenital arteriovenous fistulas are the result of persistent embryonic vessels that fail to differentiate into arteries and veins; they may be associated with birthmarks, can be located in almost any organ of the body, and frequently occur in the extremities. Acquired arteriovenous fistulas are either created to provide vascular access for hemodialysis or occur as a result of a penetrating injury such as a gunshot or knife wound or as complications of arterial catheterization or surgical dissection. An infrequent cause of arteriovenous fistula is rupture of an arterial aneurysm into a vein.

The clinical features depend on the location and size of the fistula. Frequently, a pulsatile mass is palpable, and a thrill and bruit lasting throughout systole and diastole are present over the fistula. With long-standing fistulas, clinical manifestations of chronic venous insufficiency, including peripheral edema, large, tortuous varicose veins, and stasis pigmentation become apparent because of the high venous pressure. Evidence of ischemia may occur in the distal portion of the extremity. Skin temperature is higher over the arteriovenous fistula.

Large arteriovenous fistulas may result in an increased cardiac output with consequent cardiomegaly and high-output heart failure (Chap. 216).

Diagnosis The diagnosis is often evident from the physical examination. Compression of a large arteriovenous fistula may cause reflex slowing of the heart rate (Nicoladoni-Branham sign). Arteriography can confirm the diagnosis and is useful in demonstrating the site and size of the arteriovenous fistula.

℞ TREATMENT

Management of arteriovenous fistulas may involve surgery, radiotherapy, or embolization. Congenital arteriovenous fistulas are often difficult to treat because the communications may be numerous and extensive, and new ones frequently develop after ligation of the most obvious ones. Many of these lesions are best treated conservatively using elastic support hose to reduce the consequences of venous hypertension. Occasionally, embolization with autologous material, such as fat or muscle, or with hemostatic agents, such as gelatin sponges or silicon spheres, is used to obliterate the fistula. Acquired arteriovenous fistulas are usually amenable to surgical treatment that involves division or excision of the fistula. Occasionally, autogenous or synthetic grafting is necessary to reestablish continuity of the artery and vein.

RAYNAUD'S PHENOMENON Raynaud's phenomenon is characterized by episodic digital ischemia, manifested clinically by the sequential development of digital blanching, cyanosis, and rubor of the fingers or toes following cold exposure and subsequent rewarming. Emotional stress may also precipitate Raynaud's phenomenon. The color changes are usually well demarcated and are confined to the fingers or toes. Typically, one or more digits will appear white when the patient is exposed to a cold environment or touches a cold object. The blanching, or pallor, represents the ischemic phase of the phenomenon and results from vasospasm of digital arteries. During the ischemic phase, capillaries and venules dilate, and cyanosis results from the deoxygenated blood that is present in these vessels. A sensation of cold or numbness or paresthesia of the digits often accompanies the phases of pallor and cyanosis.

With rewarming, the digital vasospasm resolves, and blood flow into the dilated arterioles and capillaries increases dramatically. This "reactive hyperemia" imparts a bright red color to the digits. In addition to rubor and warmth, patients often experience a throbbing, painful sensation during the hyperemic phase. Although the triphasic color response is typical of Raynaud's phenomenon, some patients may develop only pallor and cyanosis; others may experience only cyanosis.

Pathophysiology Raynaud originally proposed that cold-induced episodic digital ischemia was secondary to exaggerated reflex sympathetic vasoconstriction. This theory is supported by the fact that α-adrenergic blocking drugs as well as sympathectomy decrease the frequency and severity of Raynaud's phenomenon in some patients. An alternative hypothesis is that the digital vascular responsiveness to cold or to normal sympathetic stimuli is enhanced. It is also possible that normal reflex sympathetic vasoconstriction is superimposed on local digital vascular disease or that there is enhanced adrenergic neuroeffector activity.

Raynaud's phenomenon is broadly separated into two categories: the idiopathic variety, termed *Raynaud's disease*, and the secondary variety, which is associated with other disease states or known causes of vasospasm (Table 232-1).

Raynaud's Disease This appellation is applied when the secondary causes of Raynaud's phenomenon have been excluded. Over 50% of patients with Raynaud's phenomenon have Raynaud's disease. Women are affected about five times more often than men, and the age of presentation is usually between 20 and 40 years. The fingers

TABLE 232-1　Classification of Raynaud's Phenomenon

Primary or idiopathic Raynaud's phenomenon: Raynaud's disease
Secondary Raynaud's phenomenon
　Collagen vascular diseases: scleroderma, systemic lupus
　　erythematosus, rheumatoid arthritis, dermatomyositis, polymyositis
　Arterial occlusive diseases: atherosclerosis of the extremities,
　　thromboangiitis obliterans, acute arterial occlusion, thoracic outlet
　　syndrome
　Pulmonary hypertension
　Neurologic disorders: intervertebral disk disease, syringomyelia, spinal
　　cord tumors, stroke, poliomyelitis, carpal tunnel syndrome
　Blood dyscrasias: cold agglutinins, cryoglobulinemia,
　　cryofibrinogenemia, myeloproliferative disorders, Waldenström's
　　macroglobulinemia
　Trauma: vibration injury, hammer hand syndrome, electric shock, cold
　　injury, typing, piano playing
　Drugs: ergot derivatives, methysergide, β-adrenergic receptor
　　blockers, bleomycin, vinblastine, cisplatin

are involved more frequently than the toes. Initial episodes may involve only one or two fingertips, but subsequent attacks may involve the entire finger and may include all the fingers. The toes are affected in 40% of patients. Although vasospasm of the toes usually occurs in patients with symptoms in the fingers, it may happen alone. Rarely, the earlobes and the tip of the nose are involved. Raynaud's phenomenon occurs frequently in patients who also have migraine headaches or variant angina. These associations suggest that there may be a common predisposing cause for the vasospasm.

Results of physical examination are often entirely normal; the radial, ulnar, and pedal pulses are normal. The fingers and toes may be cool between attacks and may perspire excessively. Thickening and tightening of the digital subcutaneous tissue (*sclerodactyly*) develop in 10% of patients. Angiography of the digits for diagnostic purposes is not indicated.

In general, patients with Raynaud's disease appear to have the milder forms of Raynaud's phenomenon. Fewer than 1% of these patients lose a part of a digit. After the diagnosis is made, the disease improves spontaneously in approximately 15% of patients and progresses in about 30%.

Secondary Causes of Raynaud's Phenomenon　Raynaud's phenomenon occurs in 80 to 90% of patients with systemic sclerosis (scleroderma) and is the presenting symptom in 30% (Chap. 303). It may be the only symptom of scleroderma for many years. Abnormalities of the digital vessels may contribute to the development of Raynaud's phenomenon in this disorder. Ischemic fingertip ulcers may develop and progress to gangrene and autoamputation. About 20% of patients with systemic lupus erythematosus (SLE) have Raynaud's phenomenon (Chap. 300). Occasionally, persistent digital ischemia develops and may result in ulcers or gangrene. In most severe cases, the small vessels are occluded by a proliferative endarteritis. Raynaud's phenomenon occurs in about 30% of patients with dermatomyositis or polymyositis (Chap. 369). It frequently develops in patients with rheumatoid arthritis and may be related to the intimal proliferation that occurs in the digital arteries.

Atherosclerosis of the extremities is a frequent cause of Raynaud's phenomenon in men over age 50. Thromboangiitis obliterans is an uncommon cause of Raynaud's phenomenon but should be considered in young men, particularly in those who are cigarette smokers. The development of cold-induced pallor in these disorders may be confined to one or two digits of the involved extremity. Occasionally, Raynaud's phenomenon may follow acute occlusion of large and medium-sized arteries by a thrombus or embolus. Embolization of atheroembolic debris may cause digital ischemia. The latter situation often involves one or two digits and should not be confused with Raynaud's phenomenon. In patients with the thoracic outlet syndrome, Raynaud's phenomenon may result from diminished intravascular pressure, stimulation of sympathetic fibers in the brachial plexus, or a combination

of both. Raynaud's phenomenon occurs in patients with primary pulmonary hypertension (Chap. 220); this is more than coincidental and may reflect a neurohumoral abnormality that affects both the pulmonary and digital circulations.

A variety of blood dyscrasias may be associated with Raynaud's phenomenon. Cold-induced precipitation of plasma proteins, hyperviscosity, and aggregation of red cells and platelets may occur in patients with cold agglutinins, cryoglobulinemia, or cryofibrinogenemia. Hyperviscosity syndromes that accompany myeloproliferative disorders and Waldenström's macroglobulinemia should also be considered in the initial evaluation of patients with Raynaud's phenomenon.

Raynaud's phenomenon occurs often in patients whose vocations require the use of vibrating hand tools, such as chain saws or jackhammers. The frequency of Raynaud's phenomenon also seems to be increased in pianists and keyboard operators. Electric shock injury to the hands or frostbite may lead to the later development of Raynaud's phenomenon.

Several drugs have been causally implicated in Raynaud's phenomenon. These include ergot preparations; methysergide; β-adrenergic receptor antagonists; and the chemotherapeutic agents bleomycin, vinblastine, and cisplatin.

℞ TREATMENT

Most patients with Raynaud's phenomenon experience only mild and infrequent episodes. These patients need reassurance and should be instructed to dress warmly and avoid unnecessary cold exposure. In addition to gloves and mittens, patients should protect the trunk, head, and feet with warm clothing to prevent cold-induced reflex vasoconstriction. Tobacco use is contraindicated.

Drug treatment should be reserved for the severe cases. The calcium channel antagonists, especially nifedipine and diltiazem, decrease the frequency and severity of Raynaud's phenomenon. Adrenergic blocking agents, such as reserpine, have been shown to increase nutritional blood flow to the fingers. The postsynaptic α_1-adrenergic antagonist prazosin has been used with favorable responses. Doxazosin and terazosin may also be effective. Other sympatholytic agents, such as methyldopa, guanethidine, and phenoxybenzamine, may be useful in some patients. Surgical sympathectomy is helpful in some patients who are unresponsive to medical therapy, but benefit is often transient.

ACROCYANOSIS　In this condition, there is arterial vasoconstriction and secondary dilation of the capillaries and venules with resulting persistent cyanosis of the hands and, less frequently, the feet. Cyanosis may be intensified by exposure to a cold environment. Women are affected much more frequently than men, and the age of onset is usually <30 years. Generally, patients are asymptomatic but seek medical attention because of the discoloration. Examination reveals normal pulses, peripheral cyanosis, and moist palms. Trophic skin changes and ulcerations do *not* occur. The disorder can be distinguished from Raynaud's phenomenon because it is persistent and not episodic, the discoloration extends proximally from the digits, and blanching does not occur. Ischemia secondary to arterial occlusive disease can usually be excluded by the presence of normal pulses. Central cyanosis and decreased arterial oxygen saturation are not present. Patients should be reassured and advised to dress warmly and avoid cold exposure. Pharmacologic intervention is not indicated.

LIVEDO RETICULARIS　In this condition, localized areas of the extremities develop a mottled or netlike appearance of reddish to blue discoloration. The mottled appearance may be more prominent following cold exposure. The idiopathic form of this disorder occurs equally in men and women, and the most common age of onset is in the third decade. Patients with the idiopathic form are usually asymptomatic and seek attention for cosmetic reasons. Livedo reticularis can also occur following atheroembolism (see above). Rarely, skin ulcerations develop. Patients should be reassured and advised to avoid cold environments. No drug treatment is indicated.

PERNIO (CHILBLAINS) This is a vasculitic disorder associated with exposure to cold; acute forms have been described. Raised erythematous lesions develop on the lower part of the legs and feet in cold weather. These are associated with pruritus and a burning sensation, and they may blister and ulcerate. Pathologic examination demonstrates angiitis characterized by intimal proliferation and perivascular infiltration of mononuclear and polymorphonuclear leukocytes. Giant cells may be present in the subcutaneous tissue. Patients should avoid exposure to cold, and ulcers should be kept clean and protected with sterile dressings. Sympatholytic drugs may be effective in some patients.

ERYTHROMELALGIA (ERYTHERMALGIA) This disorder is characterized by burning pain and erythema of the extremities. The feet are involved more frequently than the hands, and males are affected more frequently than females. Erythromelalgia may occur at any age but is most common in middle age. It may be primary or secondary to myeloproliferative disorders such as polycythemia vera and essential thrombocytosis, or it may occur as an adverse effect of drugs such as nifedipine or bromocriptine. Patients complain of burning in the extremities that is precipitated by exposure to a warm environment and aggravated by a dependent position. The symptoms are relieved by exposing the affected area to cool air or water or by elevation. Erythromelalgia can be distinguished from ischemia secondary to peripheral arterial disorders and peripheral neuropathy because the peripheral pulses are present and the neurologic examination is normal. There is no specific treatment; aspirin may produce relief in patients with erythromelalgia secondary to myeloproliferative disease. Treatment of associated disorders in secondary erythromelalgia may be helpful.

FROSTBITE In this condition, tissue damage results from severe environmental cold exposure or from direct contact with a very cold object. Tissue injury results from both freezing and vasoconstriction. Frostbite usually affects the distal aspects of the extremities or exposed parts of the face, such as the ears, nose, chin, and cheeks. Superficial frostbite involves the skin and subcutaneous tissue. Patients experience pain or paresthesia, and the skin appears white and waxy. After rewarming, there is cyanosis and erythema, wheal-and-flare formation, edema, and superficial blisters. Deep frostbite involves muscle, nerves, and deeper blood vessels. It may result in edema of the hand or foot, vesicles and bullae, tissue necrosis, and gangrene.

Initial treatment is rewarming, performed in an environment where reexposure to freezing conditions will not occur. Rewarming is accomplished by immersion of the affected part in a water bath at temperatures of 40 to 44°C (104 to 111°F). Massage, application of ice water, and extreme heat are contraindicated. The injured area should be cleansed with soap or antiseptic and sterile dressings applied. Analgesics are often required during rewarming. Antibiotics are used if there is evidence of infection. The efficacy of sympathetic blocking drugs is not established. Following recovery, the affected extremity may exhibit increased sensitivity to cold.

DISORDERS OF THE VEINS AND LYMPHATICS

VENOUS DISORDERS

Veins in the extremities can be broadly classified as either superficial or deep. In the lower extremity, the superficial venous system includes the greater and lesser saphenous veins and their tributaries. The deep veins of the leg accompany the major arteries. Perforating veins connect the superficial and deep systems at multiple locations. Bicuspid valves are present throughout the venous system to direct the flow of venous blood centrally.

VENOUS THROMBOSIS The presence of thrombus within a superficial or deep vein and the accompanying inflammatory response in the vessel wall is termed *venous thrombosis* or *thrombophlebitis*. Initially, the thrombus is composed principally of platelets and fibrin. Red cells become interspersed with fibrin, and the thrombus tends to propagate in the direction of blood flow. The inflammatory response in the vessel wall may be minimal or characterized by granulocyte infiltration, loss of endothelium, and edema.

TABLE 232-2 *Conditions Associated with an Increased Risk for Development of Venous Thrombosis*

Surgery
  Orthopedic, thoracic, abdominal, and genitourinary procedures
Neoplasms
  Pancreas, lung, ovary, testes, urinary tract, breast, stomach
Trauma
  Fractures of spine, pelvis, femur, or tibia; spinal cord injuries
Immobilization
  Acute myocardial infarction, congestive heart failure, stroke, postoperative convalescence
Pregnancy
Estrogen use (for replacement or contraception)
Hypercoagulable states
  Resistance to activated protein C; deficiencies of antithrombin III, protein C, or protein S; antiphospholipid antibodies; myeloproliferative diseases; dysfibrinogenemia; disseminated intravascular coagulation
Venulitis
  Thromboangiitis obliterans, Behçet's disease, homocysteinuria
Previous deep vein thrombosis

The factors that predispose to venous thrombosis were initially described by Virchow in 1856 and include stasis, vascular damage, and hypercoagulability. Accordingly, a variety of clinical situations are associated with increased risk of venous thrombosis (Table 232-2). Venous thrombosis may occur in >50% of patients having orthopedic surgical procedures, particularly those involving the hip or knee, and in 10 to 40% of patients who undergo abdominal or thoracic operations. The prevalence of venous thrombosis is particularly high in patients with cancer of the pancreas, lungs, genitourinary tract, stomach, and breast. Approximately 10 to 20% of patients with idiopathic deep vein thrombosis have or develop clinically overt cancer; there is no consensus on whether these individuals should be subjected to intensive diagnostic workup to search for occult malignancy.

The risk of thrombosis is increased following trauma, such as fractures of the spine, pelvis, femur, and tibia. Immobilization, regardless of the underlying disease, is a major predisposing cause of venous thrombosis. This fact may account for the relatively high incidence in patients with acute myocardial infarction or congestive heart failure. The incidence of venous thrombosis is increased during pregnancy, particularly in the third trimester and in the first month postpartum, and in individuals who use oral contraceptives or receive postmenopausal hormone replacement therapy. A variety of clinical disorders that produce systemic hypercoagulability, including resistance to activated protein C (factor V Leiden); prothrombin G20210A gene mutation; antithrombin III, protein C, and protein S deficiencies; antiphospholipid syndrome; hyperhomocysteinemia; SLE; myeloproliferative diseases; dysfibrinogenemia; and disseminated intravascular coagulation, are associated with venous thrombosis. Venulitis occurring in thromboangiitis obliterans, Behçet's disease, and homocysteinuria may also cause venous thrombosis.

DEEP VENOUS THROMBOSIS (DVT) The most important consequences of this disorder are pulmonary embolism (Chap. 244) and the syndrome of chronic venous insufficiency. DVT of the iliac, femoral, or popliteal veins is suggested by unilateral leg swelling, warmth, and erythema. Tenderness may be present along the course of the involved veins, and a cord may be palpable. There may be increased tissue turgor, distention of superficial veins, and the appearance of prominent venous collaterals. In some patients, deoxygenated hemoglobin in stagnant veins imparts a cyanotic hue to the limb, a condition called *phlegmasia cerulea dolens*. In markedly edematous legs, the interstitial tissue pressure may exceed the capillary perfusion pressure, causing pallor, a condition designated *phlegmasia alba dolens*.

The diagnosis of DVT of the calf is often difficult to make at the bedside. This is so because only one of multiple veins may be involved, allowing adequate venous return through the remaining patent vessels. The most common complaint is calf pain. Examination may reveal posterior calf tenderness, warmth, increased tissue turgor or modest swelling, and, rarely, a cord. Increased resistance or pain during dorsiflexion of the foot (Homans' sign) is an unreliable diagnostic sign.

DVT occurs less frequently in the upper extremity than in the lower extremity, but the incidence is increasing because of greater utilization of indwelling central venous catheters. The clinical features and complications are similar to those described for the leg.

Diagnosis D-Dimer, a degradation product of cross-linked fibrin, is often elevated in patients with venous thrombosis. It is a sensitive, but not specific, test for venous thrombosis. The noninvasive test used most often to diagnose DVT is duplex venous ultrasonography (B-mode, i.e., two-dimensional, imaging, and pulse-wave Doppler interrogation). By imaging the deep veins, thrombus can be detected either by direct visualization or by inference when the vein does not collapse on compressive maneuvers. The Doppler ultrasound measures the velocity of blood flow in veins. This velocity is normally affected by respiration and by manual compression of the foot or calf. Flow abnormalities occur when deep venous obstruction is present. The sensitivity of duplex venous ultrasonography approaches 95% for proximal DVT and 75% for symptomatic calf vein thrombosis.

Magnetic resonance imaging (MRI) is another noninvasive means to detect DVT. Its diagnostic accuracy for assessing proximal DVT is similar to that of duplex ultrasonography. It is useful in patients with suspected thrombosis of the superior and inferior venae cavae or pelvic veins.

DVT can also be diagnosed by venography. Contrast medium is injected into a superficial vein of the foot and directed to the deep system by the application of tourniquets. The presence of a filling defect or absence of filling of the deep veins is required to make the diagnosis.

DVT must be differentiated from a variety of disorders that cause unilateral leg pain or swelling, including muscle rupture, trauma, or hemorrhage; a ruptured popliteal cyst; and lymphedema. It may be difficult to distinguish swelling caused by the postphlebitic syndrome from that due to acute recurrent DVT. Leg pain may also result from nerve compression, arthritis, tendinitis, fractures, and arterial occlusive disorders. A careful history and physical examination can usually determine the cause of these symptoms.

℞ TREATMENT

Anticoagulants (See also Chap. 244) Prevention of pulmonary embolism is the most important reason for treating patients with DVT, since in the early stages the thrombus may be loose and poorly adherent to the vessel wall. Patients should be placed in bed, and the affected extremity should be elevated above the level of the heart until the edema and tenderness subside. Anticoagulants prevent thrombus propagation and allow the endogenous lytic system to operate. Initial therapy should include either unfractionated heparin or low-molecular-weight heparin. Unfractionated heparin should be administered intravenously as an initial bolus of 7500 to 10,000 IU, followed by a continuous infusion of 1000 to 1500 IU/h. The rate of the heparin infusion should be adjusted so that the activated partial thromboplastin time (aPTT) is approximately twice the control value. Subcutaneous injection of heparin has been used as an alternative form of therapy. In <5% of patients, heparin therapy may cause thrombocytopenia (heparin-induced thrombocytopenia, HIT). Infrequently, these patients develop arterial thrombosis and ischemia.

Low-molecular-weight (4000 to 6000 Da) heparins are as effective as or better than conventional, unfractionated heparin in preventing extension or recurrence of venous thrombosis. Depending on the specific preparation, low-molecular-weight heparin is administered subcutaneously, in fixed doses, once or twice daily; for example, the dose of enoxaparin is 1 mg/kg subcutaneously bid. The incidence of throm-

bocytopenia is less with low-molecular-weight heparin than with conventional preparations. A direct thrombin inhibitor, such as lepirudin or argatroban, may be used as initial anticoagulant therapy for patients in whom heparin is contraindicated because of HIT. Warfarin is administered during the first week of treatment with heparin and may be started as early as the first day of heparin treatment if the aPTT is therapeutic. It is important to overlap heparin treatment with oral anticoagulant therapy for at least 4 to 5 days because the full anticoagulant effect of warfarin is delayed. The dose of warfarin should be adjusted to maintain the prothrombin time at an international normalized ratio (INR) of 2.0 to 3.0.

Anticoagulant treatment is indicated for patients with proximal DVT, since pulmonary embolism may occur in ~50% of untreated individuals. The use of anticoagulants for isolated DVT of the calf is controversial. However, approximately 20 to 30% of calf thrombi propagate to the thigh, thereby increasing the risk of pulmonary embolism. The overall incidence of pulmonary embolism in patients presenting initially with deep calf vein thrombosis is 5 to 20%. Also, isolated calf vein thrombosis has been identified as a cause of embolic stroke via a patent foramen ovale.

Therefore, patients with calf vein thrombosis should either receive anticoagulants or be followed with serial noninvasive tests to determine whether proximal propagation has occurred. Anticoagulant treatment should be continued for at least 3 to 6 months for patients with acute idiopathic DVT and for those with a temporary risk factor for venous thrombosis to decrease the chance of recurrence. In a recent study of patients with idiopathic venous thromboembolism, long-term management with low-intensity warfarin using a targeted INR of 1.5 to 2.0, following at least 3 months of therapy with full-dose anticoagulation, reduced the risk of recurrent DVT and pulmonary embolism. The duration of treatment is indefinite for patients with recurrent DVT and for those in whom associated causes, such as malignancy or hypercoagulability, have not been eliminated. If treatment with anticoagulants is contraindicated because of a bleeding diathesis or risk of hemorrhage, protection from pulmonary embolism can be achieved by mechanically interrupting the flow of blood through the inferior vena cava. Inferior vena cava plication generally has been replaced by percutaneous insertion of a filter.

Thrombolytics Thrombolytic drugs such as streptokinase, urokinase, and tPA may also be used, but there is no evidence that thrombolytic therapy is more effective than anticoagulants in preventing pulmonary embolism. However, early administration of thrombolytic drugs may accelerate clot lysis, preserve venous valves, and decrease the potential for developing postphlebitic syndrome.

Prophylaxis Prophylaxis should be considered in clinical situations where the risk of DVT is high. Low-dose unfractionated heparin (5000 units 2 h prior to surgery and then 5000 units every 8 to 12 h postoperatively), warfarin, and external pneumatic compression are all useful. Low-dose heparin reduces the risk of DVT associated with thoracic and abdominal surgery and with prolonged bed rest. Low-molecular-weight heparins have been shown to prevent DVT in patients undergoing general or orthopedic surgery and in acutely ill medical patients. They are said to be more effective than conventional heparin and to cause an equal or lower incidence of bleeding. Danaparoid, a low-molecular-weight heparinoid, may be used for prophylaxis in patients undergoing hip surgery. Fondaparinux, a synthetic pentasaccharide capable of catalysing antithrombin-mediated inhibition of factor Xa, may be used for prophylaxis in patients undergoing major orthopedic surgery. Warfarin in a dose that yields a prothrombin time equivalent to an INR of 2.0 to 3.0 is effective in preventing DVT associated with bone fractures and orthopedic surgery. Warfarin is started the night before surgery and continued throughout the convalescent period. External pneumatic compression devices applied to the legs are used to prevent DVT when even low doses of heparin or warfarin might cause serious bleeding, as during neurosurgery or transurethral resection of the prostate.

SUPERFICIAL VEIN THROMBOSIS   Thrombosis of the greater or lesser saphenous veins or their tributaries—i.e., superficial vein thrombosis—does not result in pulmonary embolism. It is associated with intravenous catheters and infusions, occurs in varicose veins, and may develop in association with DVT. Migrating superficial vein thrombosis is often a marker for a carcinoma and may also occur in patients with vasculitides, such as thromboangiitis obliterans. The clinical features of superficial vein thrombosis are easily distinguished from those of DVT. Patients complain of pain localized to the site of the thrombus. Examination reveals a reddened, warm, and tender cord extending along a superficial vein. The surrounding area may be red and edematous.

℞ TREATMENT

Treatment is primarily supportive. Initially, patients can be placed at bed rest with leg elevation and application of warm compresses. Nonsteroidal anti-inflammatory drugs may provide analgesia but may also obscure clinical evidence of thrombus propagation. If a thrombosis of the greater saphenous vein develops in the thigh and extends toward the saphenofemoral vein junction, it is reasonable to consider anticoagulant therapy to prevent extension of the thrombus into the deep system and a possible pulmonary embolism.

VARICOSE VEINS   Varicose veins are dilated, tortuous superficial veins that result from defective structure and function of the valves of the saphenous veins, from intrinsic weakness of the vein wall, from high intraluminal pressure, or, rarely, from arteriovenous fistulas. Varicose veins can be categorized as primary or secondary. Primary varicose veins originate in the superficial system and occur two to three times as frequently in women as in men. Approximately half of patients have a family history of varicose veins. Secondary varicose veins result from deep venous insufficiency and incompetent perforating veins or from deep venous occlusion causing enlargement of superficial veins that are serving as collaterals.

Patients with venous varicosities are often concerned about the cosmetic appearance of their legs. Symptoms consist of a dull ache or pressure sensation in the legs after prolonged standing; it is relieved with leg elevation. The legs feel heavy, and mild ankle edema develops occasionally. Extensive venous varicosities may cause skin ulcerations near the ankle. Superficial venous thrombosis may be a recurring problem, and, rarely, a varicosity ruptures and bleeds. Visual inspection of the legs in the dependent position usually confirms the presence of varicose veins.

Varicose veins can usually be treated with conservative measures. Symptoms often decrease when the legs are elevated periodically, when prolonged standing is avoided, and when elastic support hose are worn. External compression stockings provide a counterbalance to the hydrostatic pressure in the veins. Small symptomatic varicose veins can be treated with sclerotherapy, in which a sclerosing solution is injected into the involved varicose vein and a compression bandage is applied. Surgical therapy usually involves extensive ligation and stripping of the greater and lesser saphenous veins and should be reserved for patients who are very symptomatic, suffer recurrent superficial vein thrombosis, and/or develop skin ulceration. Surgical therapy may also be indicated for cosmetic reasons.

CHRONIC VENOUS INSUFFICIENCY   Chronic venous insufficiency may result from DVT and/or valvular incompetence. Following DVT, the delicate valve leaflets become thickened and contracted so that they cannot prevent retrograde flow of blood; the vein becomes rigid and thick-walled. Although most veins recanalize after an episode of thrombosis, the large proximal veins may remain occluded. Secondary incompetence develops in distal valves because high pressures distend the vein and separate the leaflets. Primary deep venous valvular dysfunction may also occur without previous thrombosis. Patients with venous insufficiency often complain of a dull ache in the leg that worsens with prolonged standing and resolves with leg elevation. Examination demonstrates increased leg circumference, edema, and superficial varicose veins. Erythema, dermatitis, and hyperpigmentation develop along the distal aspect of the leg, and skin ulceration may occur near the medial and lateral malleoli. Cellulitis may be a recurring problem. Patients should be advised to avoid prolonged standing or sitting; frequent leg elevation is helpful. Graduated compression stockings should be worn during the day. These efforts should be intensified if skin ulcers develop. Ulcers should be treated with applications of wet to dry dressings and, occasionally, dilute topical antibiotic solutions. Commercially available dressings comprising antiseptic solutions and compressive bandages may be applied and should be changed weekly until healing occurs. Recurrent ulceration and severe edema may be treated by surgical interruption of incompetent communicating veins. Rarely, surgical valvuloplasty and bypass of venous occlusions are employed.

LYMPHATIC DISORDERS

Lymphatic capillaries are blind-ended tubes formed by a single layer of endothelial cells. The absent or widely fenestrated basement membrane of lymphatic capillaries allows access to interstitial proteins and particles. Lymphatic capillaries merge to form larger vessels that contain smooth muscle and are capable of vasomotion. Small and medium-sized lymphatic vessels empty into progressively larger channels, most of which drain into the thoracic duct. The lymphatic circulation is involved in the absorption of interstitial fluid and in the response to infection.

LYMPHEDEMA   Lymphedema may be categorized as primary or secondary (Table 232-3). The prevalence of primary lymphedema is approximately 1 per 10,000 individuals. Primary lymphedema may be secondary to agenesis, hypoplasia, or obstruction of the lymphatic vessels. It may be associated with Turner syndrome, Klinefelter syndrome, Noonan syndrome, the yellow nail syndrome, the intestinal lymphangiectasia syndrome, and lymphangiomyomatosis. Women are affected more frequently than men. There are three clinical subtypes: congenital lymphedema, which appears shortly after birth; lymphedema praecox, which has its onset at the time of puberty; and lymphedema tarda, which usually begins after age 35. Familial forms of congenital lymphedema (Milroy's disease) and lymphedema praecox (Meige's disease) may be inherited in an autosomal dominant manner with variable penetrance; autosomal or sex-linked recessive forms are less common.

Secondary lymphedema is an acquired condition resulting from damage to or obstruction of previously normal lymphatic channels (Table 232-3). Recurrent episodes of bacterial lymphangitis, usually caused by streptococci, are a very common cause of lymphedema. The most common cause of secondary lymphedema worldwide is filariasis (Chap. 202). Tumors, such as prostate cancer and lymphoma, can also obstruct lymphatic vessels. Both surgery and radiation therapy for breast carcinoma may cause lymphedema of the upper extremity. Less common causes include tuberculosis, contact dermatitis, lymphogranuloma venereum, rheumatoid arthritis, pregnancy, and self-induced or factitious lymphedema following application of tourniquets.

Lymphedema is generally a painless condition, but patients may experience a chronic dull, heavy sensation in the leg, and most often

---

TABLE 232-3   Causes of Lymphedema

Primary
    Congenital (includes Milroy's disease)
    Lymphedema praecox (includes Meige's disease)
    Lymphedema tarda
Secondary
    Recurrent lymphangitis
    Filariasis
    Tuberculosis
    Neoplasm
    Surgery
    Radiation therapy

they are concerned about the appearance of the leg. Lymphedema of the lower extremity, initially involving the foot, gradually progresses up the leg so that the entire limb becomes edematous. In the early stages, the edema is soft and pits easily with pressure. In the chronic stages, the limb has a woody texture, and the tissues become indurated and fibrotic. At this point the edema may no longer be pitting. The limb loses its normal contour, and the toes appear square. Lymphedema should be distinguished from other disorders that cause unilateral leg swelling, such as DVT and chronic venous insufficiency. In the latter condition, the edema is softer, and there is often evidence of a stasis dermatitis, hyperpigmentation, and superficial venous varicosities.

The evaluation of patients with lymphedema should include diagnostic studies to clarify the cause. Abdominal and pelvic ultrasound and computed tomography can be used to detect obstructing lesions such as neoplasms. MRI may reveal edema in the epifascial compartment and identify lymph nodes and enlarged lymphatic channels. Lymphoscintigraphy and lymphangiography are rarely indicated, but either can be used to confirm the diagnosis or to differentiate primary from secondary lymphedema. Lymphoscintigraphy involves the injection of radioactively labeled technetium-containing colloid into the distal subcutaneous tissue of the affected extremity. In lymphangiography, contrast material is injected into a distal lymphatic vessel that has been isolated and cannulated. In primary lymphedema, lymphatic channels are absent, hypoplastic, or ectatic. In secondary lymphedema, lymphatic channels are usually dilated, and it may be possible to determine the level of obstruction.

℞ TREATMENT

Patients with lymphedema of the lower extremities must be instructed to take meticulous care of their feet to prevent recurrent lymphangitis. Skin hygiene is important, and emollients can be used to prevent drying. Prophylactic antibiotics are often helpful, and fungal infection

should be treated aggressively. Patients should be encouraged to participate in physical activity; frequent leg elevation can reduce the amount of edema. Physical therapy, including massage to facilitate lymphatic drainage, may be helpful. Patients can be fitted with graduated compression hose to reduce the amount of lymphedema that develops with upright posture. Occasionally, intermittent pneumatic compression devices can be applied at home to facilitate reduction of the edema. Diuretics are contraindicated and may cause depletion of intravascular volume and metabolic abnormalities. Microsurgical lymphatico-venous anastomotic procedures have been performed to rechannel lymph flow from obstructed lymphatic vessels into the venous system.

FURTHER READING

AGNELLI G: Three months versus one year of oral anticoagulant therapy for idiopathic deep venous thrombosis. Warfarin Optimal Duration Italian Trial Investigators. N Engl J Med 345:165, 2001

BOUNAMEAUX H, PERNEGER T: Fondaparinux: A new synthetic pentasaccharide for thrombosis prevention. Lancet 359:1710, 2002

HIATT WR: Medical treatment of peripheral arterial disease and claudication. N Engl J Med 344:1608, 2001

KEARON C et al: Management of suspected deep venous thrombosis in outpatients by using clinical assessment and D-dimer testing. Ann Intern Med 135:108, 2001

McDERMOTT MM et al: The ankle brachial index is associated with leg function and physical activity: The Walking and Leg Circulation Study. Ann Intern Med 136:873, 2002

MILLER J et al: Postmenopausal estrogen replacement and risk for venous thromboembolism: A systematic review and meta-analysis for the U.S. Preventive Services Task Force. Ann Intern Med 136:680, 2002

OLIN JW: Thromboangiitis obliterans (Buerger's disease). N Engl J Med 343:864, 2000

RIDKER PM et al, on behalf of the Prevention of Recurrent Venous Thromboembolism (PREVENT) Investigators: Long-term, low-intensity warfarin therapy for the prevention of recurrent venous thromboembolism: A randomized, double-blind, placebo-controlled trial. N Engl J Med 348:1425, 2003

WIGLEY FM: Clinical practice. Raynaud's phenomenon. N Engl J Med 347:1001, 2002

233 | APPROACH TO THE PATIENT WITH DISEASE OF THE RESPIRATORY SYSTEM
Jeffrey M. Drazen, Steven E. Weinberger

Patients with disease of the respiratory system generally present because of symptoms, an abnormality on a chest radiograph, or both. These findings often lead to a set of diagnostic possibilities; the differential diagnosis is then refined on the basis of additional information gleaned from physical examination, pulmonary function testing, additional imaging studies, and bronchoscopic examination. This chapter will consider the approach to the patient based on the major patterns of presentation, focusing on the history, the physical examination, and the chest radiograph. →*For further discussion of pulmonary function testing, see Chap. 234, and of other diagnostic studies, see Chap. 235.*

CLINICAL PRESENTATION

HISTORY   Dyspnea (shortness of breath) and cough are common presenting symptoms for patients with respiratory system disease. Less common symptoms include hemoptysis (the coughing up of blood) and chest pain, often with a pleuritic quality.

Dyspnea (See also Chap. 29)   When evaluating a patient with shortness of breath, one should first determine the time course over which the symptom has become manifest. Patients who were well previously and developed *acute* shortness of breath (over a period of hours to days) can have acute disease affecting the airways (an acute attack of asthma), the pulmonary parenchyma (acute pulmonary edema or an acute infectious process such as a bacterial pneumonia), the pleural space (a pneumothorax), or the pulmonary vasculature (a pulmonary embolus). A *subacute* presentation (over days to weeks) can suggest an exacerbation of preexisting airways disease (asthma or chronic bronchitis), an indolent parenchymal infection (*Pneumocystis carinii* pneumonia in a patient with AIDS, mycobacterial or fungal pneumonia), a noninfectious inflammatory process that proceeds at a relatively slow pace (Wegener's granulomatosis, eosinophilic pneumonia, bronchiolitis obliterans with organizing pneumonia, and many others), neuromuscular disease (Guillain-Barré syndrome, myasthenia gravis), pleural disease (pleural effusion from a variety of possible causes), or chronic cardiac disease (congestive heart failure). A *chronic* presentation (over months to years) often indicates chronic obstructive lung disease, chronic interstitial lung disease, or chronic cardiac disease. Chronic diseases of airways (not only chronic obstructive lung disease but also asthma) are characterized by exacerbations and remissions. Patients often have periods when they are severely limited by shortness of breath, but these may be interspersed with periods in which symptoms are minimal or absent. In contrast, many of the diseases of pulmonary parenchyma are characterized by a slow but inexorable progression.

Other Respiratory Symptoms   *Cough* (Chap. 30) may indicate the presence of lung disease, but cough per se is not useful for the differential diagnosis. The presence of sputum accompanying the cough often suggests airway disease and may be seen in asthma, chronic bronchitis, or bronchiectasis.

Hemoptysis (Chap. 30) can originate from disease of the airways, the pulmonary parenchyma, or the vasculature. Diseases of the airways can be inflammatory (acute or chronic bronchitis, bronchiectasis, or cystic fibrosis) or neoplastic (bronchogenic carcinoma or bronchial carcinoid tumors). Parenchymal diseases causing hemoptysis may be either localized (pneumonia, lung abscess, tuberculosis, or infection with *Aspergillus*) or diffuse (Goodpasture's syndrome, idiopathic pul-

monary hemosiderosis). Vascular diseases potentially associated with hemoptysis include pulmonary thromboembolic disease and pulmonary arteriovenous malformations.

Chest pain (Chap. 12) caused by diseases of the respiratory system usually originates from involvement of the parietal pleura. As a result, the pain is accentuated by respiratory motion and is often referred to as *pleuritic*. Common examples include primary pleural disorders, such as neoplasm or inflammatory disorders involving the pleura, or pulmonary parenchymal disorders that extend to the pleural surface, such as pneumonia or pulmonary infarction.

Additional Historic Information   Information about risk factors for lung disease should be explicitly explored to assure a complete basis of historic data. A history of current and past smoking, especially of cigarettes, should be sought from all patients. The smoking history should include the number of years of smoking, the intensity (i.e., number of packs per day), and, if the patient no longer smokes, the interval since smoking cessation. The risk of lung cancer falls progressively in the decade following discontinuation of smoking, and loss of lung function above the expected age-related decline ceases with the discontinuation of smoking. Even though chronic obstructive lung disease and neoplasia are the two most important respiratory complications of smoking, other respiratory disorders (e.g., spontaneous pneumothorax, respiratory bronchiolitis–interstitial lung disease, eosinophilic granuloma of the lung, and pulmonary hemorrhage with Goodpasture's syndrome) are also associated with smoking. A history of significant secondhand (passive) exposure to smoke, whether in the home or at the workplace, should also be sought as it may be a risk factor for neoplasia or an exacerbating factor for airways disease.

The patient may have been exposed to other inhaled agents associated with lung disease, which act either via direct toxicity or through immune mechanisms (Chaps. 237 and 238). Such exposures can be either occupational or avocational, indicating the importance of detailed occupational and personal histories, the latter stressing exposures related to hobbies or the home environment. Important agents include the inorganic dusts associated with pneumoconiosis (especially asbestos and silica dusts) and organic antigens associated with hypersensitivity pneumonitis (especially antigens from molds and animal proteins). Asthma, which is more common in women than men, is often exacerbated by exposure to environmental allergens (dust mites, pet dander, or cockroach allergens in the home or allergens in the outdoor environment such as pollen and ragweed) or may be caused by occupational exposures (diisocyanates). Exposure to particular infectious agents can be suggested by contacts with individuals with known respiratory infections (especially tuberculosis) or by residence in an area with endemic pathogens (histoplasmosis, coccidioidomycosis, blastomycosis).

A history of coexisting nonrespiratory disease or of risk factors for or previous treatment of such diseases should be sought, as they may predispose a patient to both infectious and noninfectious respiratory system complications. Common examples include systemic rheumatic diseases that are associated with pleural or parenchymal lung disease (Chap. 301), metastatic neoplastic disease in the lung, or impaired host defense mechanisms and secondary infection, which occur in the case of hematologic and lymph node malignancies. Risk factors for AIDS should be sought, as the lungs are not only the most common site of AIDS-defining infection but can also be involved by noninfectious complications of AIDS (Chap. 173). Treatment of nonrespiratory dis-

TABLE 233-1 *Typical Chest Examination Findings in Selected Clinical Conditions*

Condition	Percussion	Fremitus	Breath Sounds	Voice Transmission	Adventitious Sounds
Normal	Resonant	Normal	Vesicular (at lung bases)	Normal	Absent
Consolidation or atelectasis (with patent airway)	Dull	Increased	Bronchial	Bronchophony, whispered pectoriloquy, egophony	Crackles
Consolidation or atelectasis (with blocked airway)	Dull	Decreased	Decreased	Decreased	Absent
Asthma	Resonant	Normal	Vesicular	Normal	Wheezing
Interstitial lung disease	Resonant	Normal	Vesicular	Normal	Crackles
Emphysema	Hyperresonant	Decreased	Decreased	Decreased	Absent or wheezing
Pneumothorax	Hyperresonant	Decreased	Decreased	Decreased	Absent
Pleural effusion	Dull	Decreased	Decreased[a]	Decreased[a]	Absent or pleural friction rub

[a] May be altered by collapse of underlying lung, which will increase transmission of sound.
Source: Adapted from Weinberger.

ease can be associated with respiratory complications, either because of effects on host defense mechanisms (immunosuppressive agents, cancer chemotherapy) with resulting infection or because of direct effects on the pulmonary parenchyma (cancer chemotherapy, radiation therapy, or treatment with other agents, such as amiodarone) or on the airways (β-blocking agents causing airflow obstruction, angiotensin-converting enzyme inhibitors causing cough) (Chap. 237).

Family history is important for evaluating diseases that have a genetic component. These include disorders such as cystic fibrosis, α_1-antitrypsin deficiency, pulmonary hypertension, pulmonary fibrosis, and asthma.

PHYSICAL EXAMINATION The general principles of inspection, palpation, percussion, and auscultation apply to the examination of the respiratory system. However, the physical examination should be directed not only toward ascertaining abnormalities of the lungs and thorax but also toward recognizing other findings that may reflect underlying lung disease.

On *inspection*, the rate and pattern of breathing as well as the depth and symmetry of lung expansion are observed. Breathing that is unusually rapid, labored, or associated with the use of accessory muscles of respiration generally indicates either augmented respiratory demands or an increased work of breathing. Asymmetric expansion of the chest is usually due to an asymmetric process affecting the lungs, such as endobronchial obstruction of a large airway, unilateral parenchymal or pleural disease, or unilateral phrenic nerve paralysis. Visible abnormalities of the thoracic cage include kyphoscoliosis and ankylosing spondylitis, either of which can alter compliance of the thorax, increase the work of breathing, and cause dyspnea.

On *palpation*, the symmetry of lung expansion can be assessed, generally confirming the findings observed by inspection. Vibration produced by spoken sounds is transmitted to the chest wall and is assessed by the presence or absence and symmetry of tactile fremitus. Transmission of vibration is decreased or absent if pleural liquid is interposed between the lung and the chest wall or if an endobronchial obstruction alters sound transmission. In contrast, transmitted vibration may increase over an area of underlying pulmonary consolidation. Palpation may also reveal focal tenderness, as seen with costochondritis or rib fracture.

The relative resonance or dullness of the tissue underlying the chest wall is assessed by *percussion*. The normal sound of underlying air-containing lung is resonant. In contrast, consolidated lung or a pleural effusion sounds dull, while emphysema or air in the pleural space results in a hyperresonant percussion note.

On *auscultation* of the lungs, the examiner listens for both the quality and intensity of the breath sounds and for the presence of extra, or adventitious, sounds. Normal breath sounds heard through the stethoscope at the periphery of the lung are described as *vesicular breath sounds*, in which inspiration is louder and longer than expiration. If sound transmission is impaired by endobronchial obstruction or by air or liquid in the pleural space, breath sounds are diminished in intensity or absent. When sound transmission is improved through consolidated lung, the resulting *bronchial breath sounds* have a more tubular quality and a more pronounced expiratory phase. Sound transmission can also be assessed by listening to spoken or whispered sounds; when these are transmitted through consolidated lung, *bronchophony* and *whispered pectoriloquy*, respectively, are present. The sound of a spoken E becomes more like an **A**, though with a nasal or bleating quality, a finding that is termed *egophony*.

The primary adventitious (abnormal) sounds that can be heard include crackles (rales), wheezes, and rhonchi. *Crackles* are the discontinuous, typically inspiratory, sound created when alveoli and small airways open and close with respiration. They are often associated with interstitial lung disease, microatelectasis, or filling of alveoli by liquid. *Wheezes*, which are generally more prominent during expiration than inspiration, reflect the oscillation of airway walls that occurs when there is airflow limitation, as may be produced by bronchospasm, airway edema or collapse, or intraluminal obstruction by neoplasm or secretions. *Rhonchi* is the term applied to the sounds created when there is free liquid in the airway lumen; the viscous interaction between the free liquid and the moving air creates a low-pitched vibratory sound. Other adventitious sounds include pleural friction rubs and stridor. The gritty sound of a *pleural friction rub* indicates inflamed pleural surfaces rubbing against each other, often during both inspiratory and expiratory phases of the respiratory cycle. *Stridor*, which occurs primarily during inspiration, represents flow through a narrowed upper airway, as occurs in an infant with croup.

A summary of the patterns of physical findings on pulmonary examination in common types of respiratory system disease is shown in Table 233-1.

A meticulous *general physical examination* is mandatory in patients with disorders of the respiratory system. Enlarged lymph nodes in the cervical and supraclavicular regions should be sought. Disturbances of mentation or even coma can occur in patients with acute carbon dioxide retention and hypoxemia. Telltale stains on the fingers point to heavy cigarette smoking; infected teeth and gums may occur in patients with aspiration pneumonitis and lung abscess.

Clubbing of the digits can be found in lung cancer, interstitial lung disease, and chronic infections in the thorax, such as bronchiectasis, lung abscess, and empyema. Clubbing can also be seen with congenital heart disease associated with right-to-left shunting and with a variety of chronic inflammatory or infectious diseases, such as inflammatory bowel disease and endocarditis. A number of systemic diseases, such as systemic lupus erythematosus, scleroderma, and rheumatoid arthritis, may be associated with pulmonary complications, even though their primary clinical manifestations and physical findings are not primarily related to the lungs. Conversely, other diseases that most commonly affect the respiratory system, such as sarcoidosis, can have findings on physical examination not related to the respiratory system, including ocular findings (uveitis, conjunctival granulomas) and skin findings (erythema nodosum, cutaneous granulomas).

FIGURE 233-1 Posteroanterior (PA) chest radiograph of a patient with diffuse interstitial lung disease due to idiopathic pulmonary fibrosis. (*From Weinberger, with permission.*)

CHEST RADIOGRAPHY

Chest radiography is often the initial diagnostic study performed to evaluate patients with respiratory symptoms, but it can also provide the initial evidence of disease in patients who are free of symptoms. Perhaps the most common example of the latter situation is the finding of one or more nodules or masses when the radiograph is performed for a reason other than evaluation of respiratory symptoms.

A number of diagnostic possibilities are often suggested by the radiographic pattern (Figs. 233-1 and 233-2). A localized region of opacification involving the pulmonary parenchyma can be described as a nodule (usually <3 cm in diameter), a mass (usually ≥3 cm in diameter), or an infiltrate. Diffuse disease with increased opacification is usually characterized as having an alveolar, an interstitial, or a nodular pattern. In contrast, increased radiolucency can be localized, as seen with a cyst or bulla, or generalized, as occurs with emphysema. The chest radiograph is also particularly useful for the detection of pleural disease, especially if manifested by the presence of air or liquid in the pleural space. An abnormal appearance of the hila and/or the mediastinum can suggest a mass or enlargement of lymph nodes.

FIGURE 233-2 Anteroposterior (AP) chest radiograph demonstrating a diffuse alveolar filling pattern due to the acute respiratory distress syndrome (ARDS).

A summary of representative diagnoses suggested by these common radiographic patterns is presented in Table 233-2.

ADDITIONAL DIAGNOSTIC EVALUATION Further information for clarification of radiographic abnormalities is frequently obtained with computed tomographic scanning of the chest (see Figs. 235-1, -2; 243-1, -2; 251-3). This technique is more sensitive than plain radiography in detecting subtle abnormalities and can suggest specific diagnoses based on the pattern of abnormality. →*For further discussion of the use of other imaging studies, including magnetic resonance imaging, scintigraphic studies, ultrasound, and angiography, see Chap. 235.*

Alteration in the function of the lungs as a result of respiratory system disease is assessed objectively by pulmonary function tests, and effects on gas exchange are evaluated by measurement of arterial blood gases or by oximetry (Chap. 234). As part of pulmonary function testing, quantitation of forced expiratory flow assesses the presence of obstructive physiology, which is consistent with diseases affecting the structure or function of the airways, such as asthma and chronic obstructive lung disease. Measurement of lung volumes assesses the presence of restrictive disorders, seen with diseases of the pulmonary parenchyma or respiratory pump and with space-occupying processes within the pleura.

Bronchoscopy is useful in some settings for visualizing abnormalities of the airways and for obtaining a variety of samples from either the airway or the pulmonary parenchyma (Chap. 235).

INTEGRATION OF THE PRESENTING CLINICAL PATTERN AND DIAGNOSTIC STUDIES

Patients with respiratory symptoms but a normal chest radiograph most commonly have diseases affecting the airways, such as asthma or chronic obstructive pulmonary disease. However, the latter diagnosis

TABLE 233-2 *Major Respiratory Diagnoses with Common Chest Radiographic Patterns*

Solitary circumscribed density—nodule (<3 cm) or mass (≥3 cm)
  Primary or metastatic neoplasm
  Localized infection (bacterial abscess, mycobacterial or fungal infection)
  Wegener's granulomatosis (one or several nodules)
  Rheumatoid nodule (one or several nodules)
  Vascular malformation
  Bronchogenic cyst

Localized opacification (infiltrate)
  Pneumonia (bacterial, atypical, mycobacterial, or fungal infection)
  Neoplasm
  Radiation pneumonitis
  Bronchiolitis obliterans with organizing pneumonia
  Bronchocentric granulomatosis
  Pulmonary infarction

Diffuse interstitial disease
  Idiopathic pulmonary fibrosis
  Pulmonary fibrosis with systemic rheumatic disease
  Sarcoidosis
  Drug-induced lung disease
  Pneumoconiosis
  Hypersensitivity pneumonitis
  Infection (*Pneumocystis*, viral pneumonia)
  Eosinophilic granuloma

Diffuse alveolar disease
  Cardiogenic pulmonary edema
  Acute respiratory distress syndrome
  Diffuse alveolar hemorrhage
  Infection (*Pneumocystis*, viral or bacterial pneumonia)
  Sarcoidosis

Diffuse nodular disease
  Metastatic neoplasm
  Hematogenous spread of infection (bacterial, mycobacterial, fungal)
  Pneumoconiosis
  Eosinophilic granuloma

is also commonly associated with radiographic abnormalities, such as diaphragmatic flattening and attenuation of vascular markings. Other disorders of the respiratory system for which the chest radiograph is normal include disorders of the respiratory pump (either the chest wall or the neuromuscular apparatus controlling the chest wall) or pulmonary circulation and occasionally interstitial lung disease. Chest examination and pulmonary function tests are generally helpful in sorting out these diagnostic possibilities. Obstructive diseases associated with a normal or relatively normal chest radiograph are often characterized by findings on physical examination and pulmonary function testing that are typical for these conditions. Similarly, diseases of the respiratory pump or interstitial diseases may also be suggested by findings on physical examination or by particular patterns of restrictive disease seen on pulmonary function testing.

When respiratory symptoms are accompanied by radiographic abnormalities, diseases of the pulmonary parenchyma or the pleura are usually present. Either diffuse or localized parenchymal lung disease

is generally visualized well on the radiograph, and both air and liquid in the pleural space (pneumothorax and pleural effusion, respectively) are usually readily detected by radiography.

Radiographic findings in the absence of respiratory symptoms often indicate localized disease affecting the airways or the pulmonary parenchyma. One or more nodules or masses can suggest intrathoracic malignancy, but they can also be the manifestation of a current or previous infectious process. Patients with diffuse parenchymal lung disease on radiographic examination may be free of symptoms, as is sometimes the case with pulmonary sarcoidosis.

FURTHER READING

ALBERT RK et al (eds): *Comprehensive Respiratory Medicine.* St. Louis, Mosby, 1999

IRWIN RS, MADISON JM: The diagnosis and treatment of cough. N Engl J Med 343:1715, 2000

PATZ EF et al: Screening for lung cancer. N Engl J Med 343:1627, 2000

WEINBERGER SE: *Principles of Pulmonary Medicine,* 3d ed. Philadelphia, Saunders, 1998

234 DISTURBANCES OF RESPIRATORY FUNCTION
Steven E. Weinberger, Jeffrey M. Drazen

The respiratory system includes the lungs, the central nervous system (CNS), the chest wall (with the diaphragm and intercostal muscles), and the pulmonary circulation. The CNS controls the activity of the muscles of the chest wall, which constitute the pump of the respiratory system. Because these components of the respiratory system act in concert to achieve gas exchange, malfunction of an individual component or alteration of the relationships among components can lead to disturbances in function. In this chapter we consider three major aspects of disturbed respiratory function: (1) disturbances in ventilatory function, (2) disturbances in the pulmonary circulation, and (3) disturbances in gas exchange. →*For further discussion of disorders relating to CNS control of ventilation, see Chap. 246.*

DISTURBANCES IN VENTILATORY FUNCTION

Ventilation is the process whereby the lungs replenish the gas in the alveoli. Measurements of ventilatory function in common diagnostic use consist of quantification of the gas volume contained in the lungs under certain circumstances and the rate at which gas can be expelled from the lungs. The two measurements of lung volume commonly used for respiratory diagnosis are (1) total lung capacity (TLC), the volume of gas contained in the lungs after a maximal inspiration; and (2) residual volume (RV), the volume of gas remaining in the lungs at the end of a maximal expiration. The volume of gas that is exhaled from

the lungs in going from TLC to RV is the *vital capacity* (VC) (Fig. 234-1).

Common clinical measurements of airflow are obtained from maneuvers in which the subject inspires to TLC and then forcibly exhales to RV. Three measurements are commonly made from a recording of forced exhaled volume versus time—i.e., a *spirogram*: (1) the volume of gas exhaled during the first second of expiration [forced expiratory volume (FEV) in 1 s, or FEV_1], (2) the total volume exhaled [forced vital capacity (FVC)], and (3) the average expiratory flow rate during the middle 50% of the VC [forced expiratory flow (FEF) between 25 and 75% of the VC, or $FEF_{25-75\%}$, also called the maximal midexpiratory flow rate (MMFR)] (Fig. 234-2).

PHYSIOLOGIC FEATURES

The lungs are elastic structures, containing collagen and elastic fibers that resist expansion. For normal lungs to contain air, they must be distended either by a positive internal pressure—i.e., by a pressure in

FIGURE 234-1   Lung volumes, shown by block diagrams *(left)* and by a spirographic tracing *(right)*. TLC, total lung capacity; VC, vital capacity; RV, residual volume; IC, inspiratory capacity; ERV, expiratory reserve volume; FRC, functional residual capacity; V_T, tidal volume *(From Weinberger, with permission.)*

FIGURE 234-2   Spirographic tracings of forced expiration, comparing a normal tracing *(A)* and tracings in obstructive *(B)* and parenchymal restrictive *(C)* disease. Calculations of FVC, FEV_1, and $FEF_{25-75\%}$ are shown only for the normal tracing. Since there is no measure of absolute starting volume with spirometry, the curves are artificially positioned to show the relative starting lung volumes in the different conditions.

FIGURE 234-3 *A.* Pressure-volume curve of the lungs. *B.* Pressure-volume curve of the chest wall. *C.* Pressure-volume curve of the respiratory system, showing the superimposed component curves of the lungs and the chest wall. RV, residual volume; FRC, functional residual capacity; TLC, total lung capacity. *(From Weinberger, with permission.)*

the airways and alveolar spaces—or by a negative external pressure—i.e., by a pressure outside the lung. The relationship between the volume of gas contained in the lungs and the distending pressure (the *transpulmonary pressure*, or P_{TP}, defined as alveolar pressure minus pleural pressure) is described by the pressure-volume curve of the lungs (Fig. 234-3*A*).

The chest wall is also an elastic structure, with properties similar to those of an expandable and compressible spring. The relationship between the volume enclosed by the chest wall and the distending pressure for the chest wall is described by the pressure-volume curve of the chest wall (Fig. 234-3*B*). For the chest wall to assume a volume different from its resting volume, the internal or external pressures acting on it must be altered.

At functional residual capacity (FRC), defined as the volume of gas in the lungs at the end of a normal exhalation, the lungs are partially inflated, so their elastic recoil exerts a force tending to empty the lungs. At the same time, chest wall volume is such that its elastic recoil promotes outward expansion. FRC occurs at the lung volume at which the tendency of the lungs to contract is opposed by the equal and opposite tendency of the chest wall to expand (Fig. 234-3*C*).

For the lungs and the chest wall to achieve a volume other than the resting volume (FRC), either the pressures acting on them must be changed passively—e.g., by a mechanical ventilator that delivers positive pressure to the airways and alveoli—or the respiratory muscles must actively oppose the tendency of the lungs and the chest wall to return to FRC. During inhalation to volumes above FRC, the inspiratory muscles actively overcome the tendency of the respiratory system to decrease volume back to FRC. During active exhalation to volumes below FRC, expiratory muscle activity must overcome the tendency of the respiratory system to increase volume back to FRC.

At TLC, the maximal force applied by the inspiratory muscles to expand the lungs is opposed mainly by the inward recoil of the lungs. As a consequence, the major determinants of TLC are the stiffness of the lungs and inspiratory muscle strength. If the lungs become stiffer—

i.e., less compliant—TLC is decreased. If the lungs become less stiff (more compliant), TLC is increased. If the inspiratory muscles are significantly weakened, they are less able to overcome the inward elastic recoil of the lungs, and TLC is lowered.

At RV, the force exerted by the expiratory muscles to decrease lung volume further is balanced by the outward recoil of the chest wall, which becomes extremely stiff at low lung volumes. Two factors influence the volume of gas contained in the lungs at RV. The first is the ability of the subject to exert a prolonged expiratory effort, which is related to muscle strength and the ability to overcome sensory stimuli from the chest wall. The second is the ability of the lungs to empty to a small volume. In normal lungs, as P_{TP} is lowered, lung volume decreases. In lungs with diseased airways, as P_{TP} is lowered, flow limitation or airway closure may limit the amount of gas that can be expired. Consequently, either weak expiratory muscles or intrinsic airways disease can result in an elevation in measured RV.

Dynamic measurements of ventilatory function are made by having the subject inhale to TLC and then perform a forced expiration to RV. If a subject performs a series of such expiratory maneuvers using increasing muscular intensity, expiratory flow rates will increase until a certain level of effort is reached. Beyond this level, additional effort at any given lung volume will not increase the forced expiratory flow rate; this phenomenon is known as the *effort independence* of forced expiratory flow. The physiologic mechanisms determining the flow rates during this effort-independent phase of forced expiratory flow have been shown to be the elastic recoil of the lung, the airflow resistance of the airways between the alveolar zone and the physical site of flow limitation, and the airway wall compliance up to the site of flow limitation. Physical processes that decrease elastic recoil, increase airflow resistance, or increase airway wall compliance decrease the flow rate that can be achieved at any given lung volume. Conversely, processes that increase elastic recoil, decrease resistance, or stiffen airway walls increase the flow rate that can be achieved at any given lung volume.

MEASUREMENT OF VENTILATORY FUNCTION

Ventilatory function is measured under static conditions for determination of lung volumes and under dynamic conditions for determination of forced expiratory flow rates. VC, expiratory reserve volume (ERV), and inspiratory capacity (IC) (Fig. 234-1) are measured by having the patient breathe into and out of a spirometer, a device capable of measuring expired or inspired gas volume while plotting volume as a function of time. Other volumes—specifically, RV, FRC, and TLC—cannot be measured in this way because they include the volume of gas present in the lungs even after a maximal expiration. Two techniques are commonly used to measure these volumes: helium dilution and body plethysmography. In the helium dilution method, the subject repeatedly breathes in and out from a reservoir with a known volume of gas containing a trace amount of helium. The helium is diluted by the gas previously present in the lungs and very little is absorbed into the pulmonary circulation. From knowledge of the reservoir volume and the initial and final helium concentrations, the volume of gas present in the lungs can be calculated. The helium dilution method may underestimate the volume of gas in the lungs if there are slowly communicating airspaces, such as bullae. In this situation, lung volumes can be measured more accurately with a body plethysmograph, a sealed box in which the patient sits while panting against a closed mouthpiece. Because there is no airflow into or out of the plethysmograph, the pressure changes in the thorax during panting cause compression and rarefaction of gas in the lungs and simultaneous rarefaction and compression of gas in the plethysmograph. By measuring the pressure changes in the plethysmograph and at the mouthpiece, the volume of gas in the thorax can be calculated using Boyle's law.

Lung volumes and measurements made during forced expiration are interpreted by comparing the values measured with the values expected given the age, height, sex, and weight of the patient (Appendix

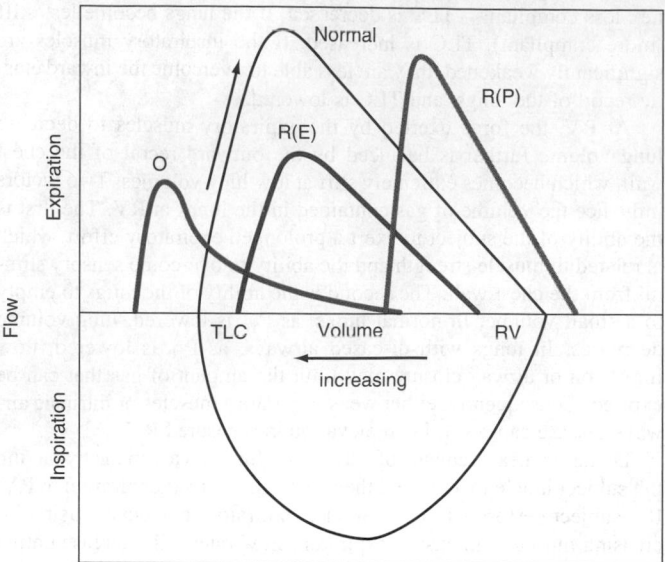

FIGURE 234-4   Flow-volume curves in different conditions: O, obstructive disease; R(P), parenchymal restrictive disease; R(F), extraparenchymal restrictive disease with limitation in inspiration and expiration. Forced expiration is plotted in all conditions; forced inspiration is shown only for the normal curve. TLC, total lung capacity; RV, residual volume. By convention, lung volume increases to the left on the abscissa. The arrow alongside the normal curve indicates the direction of expiration from TLC to RV.

Table C-4). Regression curves have been constructed on the basis of data obtained from large numbers of normal, nonsmoking individuals without evidence of lung disease. Predicted values for a given patient can then be obtained by using the patient's age and height in the appropriate regression equation; different equations are used depending on the patient's race and sex. Because there is some variability among normal individuals, values between 80 and 120% of the predicted value have traditionally been considered normal. Increasingly, calculated percentiles are used in determining normality. Specifically, values of individual measurements falling below the fifth percentile are considered to be below normal.

The normal value for the ratio FEV_1/FVC is approximately 0.75 to 0.80, although this value does fall somewhat with advancing age. The $FEF_{25-75\%}$ is often considered a more sensitive measurement of early airflow obstruction, particularly in small airways. However, this measurement must be interpreted cautiously in patients with abnormally small lungs (low TLC and VC). These patients exhale less air during forced expiration, and the $FEF_{25-75\%}$ may appear abnormal relative to the usual predicted value, even though it is normal relative to the size of the patient's lungs.

It is also a common practice to plot expiratory flow rates against lung volume (rather than against time); the close linkage of flow rates to lung volumes produces a typical *flow-volume curve* (Fig. 234-4). In addition, the spirometric values mentioned above can be calculated from the flow-volume curve. Commonly, flow rates during a maximal inspiratory effort performed as rapidly as possible are plotted as well,

making the flow-volume curve into a *flow-volume loop*. At TLC, before expiratory flow starts, the flow rate is zero; once forced expiration has begun, a high peak flow rate is rapidly achieved. As expiration continues and lung volume approaches RV, the flow rate falls progressively, in a nearly linear fashion as a function of lung volume for a person with normal lung function. During maximal inspiration from RV to TLC, inspiratory flow is most rapid at the midpoint of inspiration, so the inspiratory portion of the loop is U-shaped or saddle-shaped. The flow rates achieved during maximal expiration can be analyzed quantitatively by comparing the flow rates at specified lung volumes with the predicted values, or qualitatively by analyzing the shape of the descending limb of the expiratory curve.

Assessing the strength of respiratory muscles is an additional part of the overall evaluation of some patients with respiratory dysfunction. When a patient exhales completely to RV and then tries to inspire maximally against an occluded airway, the pressure that can be generated is called the *maximal inspiratory pressure* (MIP). On the other hand, when a patient inhales to TLC and then tries to expire maximally against an occluded airway, the pressure generated is called the *maximal expiratory pressure* (MEP). In the proper clinical setting, these studies may provide useful information regarding the cause of abnormal lung volumes and the possibility that respiratory muscle weakness may be causally related to the lung volume abnormalities.

PATTERNS OF ABNORMAL FUNCTION

The two major patterns of abnormal ventilatory function, as measured by static lung volumes and spirometry, are restrictive and obstructive patterns. In the *obstructive pattern*, the hallmark is a decrease in expiratory flow rates. With fully established disease, the ratio FEV_1/FVC is decreased, as is the $FEF_{25-75\%}$ (Fig. 234-2, line *B*). The expiratory portion of the flow-volume loop demonstrates decreased flow rates for any given lung volume. Nonuniform emptying of airways is reflected by a coved (scooped) configuration of the descending part of the expiratory curve (Fig. 234-4). With early obstructive disease, which originates in the small airways, FEV_1/FVC may be normal; the only abnormalities noted on routine testing of pulmonary function may be a depression in $FEF_{25-75\%}$ and an abnormal, i.e., coved, configuration in the terminal portion of the forced expiratory flow-volume curve.

In *obstructive* disease, the TLC is normal or increased. When helium equilibration tests are used to measure lung volumes, the measured volume may be less than the actual volume if helium was not well distributed to all regions of the lung. Residual volume is elevated as a result of airway closure during expiration, and the ratio RV/TLC is increased. VC is frequently decreased in obstructive disease because of the striking elevations in RV with only minor changes in TLC.

The hallmark of a *restrictive pattern* is a decrease in lung volumes, primarily TLC and VC. Disorders resulting in a restrictive pattern can be broadly divided into two subgroups, depending on the location of the pathology: pulmonary parenchymal and extraparenchymal. In pulmonary parenchymal disease, RV is also generally decreased, and forced expiratory flow rates are preserved. In fact, when FEV_1 is considered as a percentage of the FVC, the flow rates are often supranormal, i.e., disproportionately high relative to the size of the lungs (Fig. 234-2, line *C*). The flow-volume curve may graphically demonstrate this disproportionate relationship between flow rates and lung volumes, since the expiratory portion of the curve appears relatively tall (preserved flow rates) but narrow (decreased lung volumes), as shown in Fig. 234-4.

With extraparenchymal disease, dysfunction can be predominantly in inspiration or in both inspiration and expiration (Table 234-1). In the extraparenchymal pattern characterized by *inspiratory dysfunction*, caused by either inspiratory muscle weakness or a stiff chest wall, inadequate distending forces are exerted on an otherwise nor-

TABLE 234-1 *Alterations in Ventilatory Function*						
	TLC	*RV*	*VC*	*FEV₁/FVC*	*MIP*	*MEP*
Obstructive	N to ↑	↑	↓	↓[a]	N	N
Restrictive						
Pulmonary parenchymal	↓	↓	↓	N to ↑	N	N
Extraparenchymal—inspiratory	↓	N to ↓	↓	N	↓/N[b]	N
Extraparenchymal—inspiratory + expiratory	↓	↑	↓	Variable	↓/N[b]	↓/N[b]

[a] Mild obstructive (small airways) disease may have decreased $FEF_{25-75\%}$ with normal (N) FEV_1/FVC.
[b] Reduced if due to respiratory muscle weakness; normal if due to chest wall stiffness.
Note: N, normal; for other abbreviations, see text.

TABLE 234-2 *Common Respiratory Diseases by Diagnostic Categories*

Obstructive
    Asthma
    Chronic obstructive lung disease (chronic bronchitis, emphysema)
    Bronchiectasis
    Cystic fibrosis
    Bronchiolitis
Restrictive—Parenchymal
    Sarcoidosis
    Idiopathic pulmonary fibrosis
    Pneumoconiosis
    Drug- or radiation-induced interstitial lung disease
Restrictive—Extraparenchymal

Neuromuscular	Chest wall
Diaphragmatic weakness/paralysis	Kyphoscoliosis
Myasthenia gravis[a]	Obesity
Guillain-Barré syndrome[a]	Ankylosing spondylitis[a]
Muscular dystrophies[a]	
Cervical spine injury[a]	

[a] Can have inspiratory and expiratory limitation (see text).

mal lung. As a result, TLC values are less than predicted, RV is often not significantly affected, and expiratory flow rates are preserved. If inspiratory muscle weakness is the cause of this pattern, then MIP is decreased. In the extraparenchymal pattern characterized by *inspiratory and expiratory dysfunction*, the ability to expire to a normal RV is also limited, because of either expiratory muscle weakness or a deformed chest wall that is abnormally rigid at volumes below FRC. Consequently, RV is often elevated, unlike the pattern observed in the other restrictive subcategories. The ratio FEV$_1$/FVC is variable and depends on expiratory muscle strength. If expiratory muscle strength is significantly decreased, then MEP is decreased, the ability to expire rapidly is impaired, and FEV$_1$/FVC may be decreased even though there is no airflow obstruction. If expiratory muscle strength is normal but the chest wall is abnormally stiff below FRC, then FEV$_1$/FVC is normal or increased.

CLINICAL CORRELATIONS

Table 234-1 summarizes the typical patterns of altered ventilatory function as indicated by pulmonary function testing. This information can then be useful in diagnosis, as outlined in Table 234-2.

DISTURBANCES IN THE PULMONARY CIRCULATION

PHYSIOLOGIC FEATURES

The pulmonary vasculature must handle the entire output of the right ventricle, approximately 5 L/min in a normal adult at rest. The comparatively thin-walled vessels of the pulmonary arterial system provide relatively little resistance to flow and are capable of handling this large volume of blood at perfusion pressures that are low compared with those of the systemic circulation. The normal mean pulmonary artery pressure is 15 mmHg, as compared to approximately 95 mmHg for the normal mean aortic pressure. Regional blood flow in the lung is dependent on vascular geometry and on hydrostatic forces. In an upright person, perfusion is least at the apex of the lung and greatest at the base. When cardiac output increases, as occurs during exercise, the pulmonary vasculature is capable of recruiting previously unperfused vessels and distending underperfused vessels, thus responding to the increase in flow with a decrease in pulmonary vascular resistance. In consequence, the increase in mean pulmonary arterial pressure (PAP), even with a three- to fourfold increase in cardiac output, is small.

METHODS OF MEASUREMENT

Assessment of circulatory function in the pulmonary vasculature depends on measuring pulmonary vascular pressures and cardiac output. Clinically, these measurements are commonly made in intensive care units capable of invasive monitoring and in cardiac catheterization laboratories. With a flow-directed pulmonary arterial (Swan-Ganz) catheter, PAP and pulmonary capillary wedge pressure can be mea-

sured directly, and cardiac output can be obtained by the thermodilution method. Pulmonary vascular resistance (PVR) can then be calculated according to the equation

$$PVR = 80(PAP - PCW)/CO$$

where PVR = pulmonary vascular resistance (dyn·s/cm^5); PAP = mean pulmonary arterial pressure (mmHg); PCW = pulmonary capillary wedge pressure (mmHg); and CO = cardiac output (L/min).

The normal value for pulmonary vascular resistance is approximately 50 to 150 dyn·s/cm^5.

MECHANISMS OF ABNORMAL FUNCTION (See also Chap. 220)

PVR may increase by a variety of mechanisms. Pulmonary arterial and arteriolar vasoconstriction is a prominent response to alveolar hypoxia. PVR also increases if intraluminal thrombi or proliferation of smooth muscle in vessel walls diminishes the luminal cross-sectional area. If small pulmonary vessels are destroyed, either by scarring or by loss of alveolar walls, the total cross-sectional area of the pulmonary vascular bed diminishes, and PVR increases. When PVR is elevated, either PAP rises to maintain normal cardiac output or cardiac output falls if PAP does not increase.

CLINICAL CORRELATIONS

Disturbances in the function of the pulmonary vasculature as a result of primary cardiac disease, either congenital heart disease or conditions that elevate left atrial pressure, such as mitral stenosis, are beyond the scope of this chapter and are discussed in Chaps. 218 and 219, respectively. Instead, the focus will be on the pulmonary vasculature as its function is affected by diseases primarily involving the respiratory system, including the pulmonary vessels themselves.

All diseases of the respiratory system causing hypoxemia are potentially capable of increasing PVR, since alveolar hypoxia is a very potent stimulus for pulmonary vasoconstriction. The more prolonged and intense the hypoxic stimulus, the more likely it is that a significant increase in PVR producing pulmonary hypertension will result. In practice, patients with hypoxemia caused by chronic obstructive lung disease, interstitial lung disease, chest wall disease, and the obesity hypoventilation–sleep apnea syndrome are particularly prone to developing pulmonary hypertension. If there are additional structural changes in the pulmonary vasculature secondary to the underlying process, these will increase the likelihood of developing pulmonary hypertension.

With diseases directly affecting the pulmonary vessels, a decrease in the cross-sectional area of the pulmonary vascular bed is primarily responsible for increased PVR, while hypoxemia generally plays a lesser role. In the case of recurrent pulmonary emboli, parts of the pulmonary arterial system are occluded by intraluminal thrombi originating in the systemic venous system. With primary pulmonary hypertension (Chap. 220) or with pulmonary vascular disease secondary to scleroderma, the small pulmonary arteries and arterioles are affected by a generalized obliterative process that narrows and occludes these vessels. PVR increases, and significant pulmonary hypertension often results.

DISTURBANCES IN GAS EXCHANGE

PHYSIOLOGIC FEATURES

The primary functions of the respiratory system are to remove the appropriate amount of CO_2 from blood entering the pulmonary circulation and to provide adequate O_2 to blood leaving the pulmonary circulation. For these functions to be carried out properly, there must be adequate provision of fresh air to the alveoli for delivery of O_2 and removal of CO_2 (ventilation), adequate circulation of blood through the pulmonary vasculature (perfusion), adequate movement of gas between alveoli and pulmonary capillaries (diffusion), and appropriate contact between alveolar gas and pulmonary capillary blood (ventilation-perfusion matching).

A normal individual at rest inspires approximately 12 to 16 times per minute, each breath having a tidal volume of approximately 500 mL. A portion (approximately 30%) of the fresh air inspired with each breath does not reach the alveoli but remains in the conducting airways of the lung. This component of each breath, which is not generally available for gas exchange, is called the *anatomic dead space component*. The remaining 70% reaches the alveolar zone, mixes rapidly with the gas already there, and can participate in gas exchange. In this example, the total ventilation each minute is approximately 7 L, composed of 2 L/min of dead space ventilation and 5 L/min of alveolar ventilation. In certain diseases, some alveoli are ventilated but not perfused, so that some ventilation in addition to the anatomic dead space component is wasted. If total dead space ventilation is increased but total minute ventilation is unchanged, then alveolar ventilation must fall correspondingly.

Gas exchange is dependent on alveolar ventilation rather than total minute ventilation, as outlined below. The partial pressure of CO_2 in arterial blood (Pa_{CO_2}) is directly proportional to the amount of CO_2 produced per minute ($\dot{V}_{CO_2}$) and inversely proportional to alveolar ventilation ($\dot{V}A$), according to the relationship

$$Pa_{CO_2} = 0.863 \times \dot{V}_{CO_2}/\dot{V}A$$

where $\dot{V}_{CO_2}$ is expressed in mL/min, $\dot{V}A$ in L/min, and Pa_{CO_2} in mmHg. At fixed $\dot{V}_{CO_2}$, when alveolar ventilation increases, Pa_{CO_2} falls, and when alveolar ventilation decreases, Pa_{CO_2} rises. Maintaining a normal level of O_2 in the alveoli (and consequently in arterial blood) also depends on provision of adequate alveolar ventilation to replenish alveolar O_2. This principle will become more apparent from consideration of the alveolar gas equation below.

DIFFUSION OF O_2 AND CO_2   Both O_2 and CO_2 diffuse readily down their respective concentration gradients through the alveolar wall and pulmonary capillary endothelium. Under normal circumstances, this process is rapid, and equilibration of both gases is complete within one-third of the transit time of erythrocytes through the pulmonary capillary bed. Even in disease states in which diffusion of gases is impaired, the impairment is unlikely to be severe enough to prevent equilibration of CO_2 and O_2. Consequently, a diffusion abnormality rarely results in arterial hypoxemia at rest. If erythrocyte transit time in the pulmonary circulation is shortened, as occurs with exercise, and diffusion is impaired, then diffusion limitation may contribute to hypoxemia. Exercise testing can often demonstrate such physiologically significant abnormalities due to impaired diffusion. Even though diffusion limitation rarely makes a clinically significant contribution to resting hypoxemia, clinical measurements of what is known as *diffusing capacity* (see below) can be a useful measure of the integrity of the alveolar-capillary membrane.

VENTILATION-PERFUSION MATCHING   In addition to the absolute levels of alveolar ventilation and perfusion, gas exchange depends critically on the proper matching of ventilation and perfusion. The spectrum of possible ventilation-perfusion ($\dot{V}/\dot{Q}$) ratios in an alveolar-capillary unit ranges from zero, in which ventilation is totally absent and the unit behaves as a shunt, to infinity, in which perfusion is totally absent and the unit behaves as dead space. The P_{O_2} and P_{CO_2} of blood leaving each alveolar-capillary unit depend on the gas tension (of blood and air) entering that unit and on the particular $\dot{V}/\dot{Q}$ ratio of the unit. At one extreme, when an alveolar-capillary unit has a $\dot{V}/\dot{Q}$ ratio of 0 and behaves as a shunt, blood leaving the unit has the composition of mixed venous blood entering the pulmonary capillaries, i.e., $P\bar{v}_{O_2} \approx$ 40 mmHg and $P\bar{v}_{CO_2} \approx 46$ mmHg. At the other extreme, when an alveolar-capillary unit has a high $\dot{V}/\dot{Q}$ ratio, it behaves almost like dead space, and the small amount of blood leaving the unit has partial pressures of O_2 and CO_2 ($P_{O_2} \approx 150$ mmHg, $P_{CO_2} \approx 0$ mmHg while breathing room air) approaching the composition of inspired gas.

In the ideal situation, all alveolar-capillary units have equal matching of ventilation and perfusion, i.e., a ratio of approximately 1 when each is expressed in L/min. However, even in the normal individual, some $\dot{V}/\dot{Q}$ mismatching is present, since there is normally a gradient of blood flow from the apices to the bases of the lungs. There is a similar gradient of ventilation from the apices to the bases, but it is less marked than the perfusion gradient. As a result, ventilation-perfusion ratios are higher at the lung apices than at the lung bases. Therefore, blood coming from the apices has a higher P_{O_2} and lower P_{CO_2} than blood coming from the bases. The net P_{O_2} and P_{CO_2} of the blood mixture coming from all areas of the lung is a flow-weighted average of the individual components, which reflects both the relative amount of blood from each unit and the O_2 and CO_2 *content* of the blood coming from each unit. Because of the sigmoid shape of the oxyhemoglobin dissociation curve (see Fig. 91-2), it is important to distinguish between the partial pressure and the content of O_2 in blood. Hemoglobin is almost fully (~90%) saturated at a P_{O_2} of 60 mmHg, and little additional O_2 is carried by hemoglobin even with a substantial elevation of P_{O_2} above 60 mmHg. On the other hand, significant O_2 desaturation of hemoglobin occurs once P_{O_2} falls below 60 mmHg and onto the steep descending limb of the curve. As a result, blood coming from regions of the lung with a high $\dot{V}/\dot{Q}$ ratio and a high P_{O_2} has only a small elevation in O_2 content and cannot compensate for blood coming from regions with a low $\dot{V}/\dot{Q}$ ratio and a low P_{O_2}, which has a significantly decreased O_2 content. Although $\dot{V}/\dot{Q}$ mismatching can influence P_{CO_2}, this effect is less marked and is often overcome by an increase in overall minute ventilation.

MEASUREMENT OF GAS EXCHANGE

ARTERIAL BLOOD GASES   The most commonly used measures of gas exchange are the partial pressures of O_2 and CO_2 in arterial blood, i.e., Pa_{O_2} and Pa_{CO_2}, respectively. These partial pressures do not measure directly the quantity of O_2 and CO_2 in blood but rather the driving pressure for the gas in blood. The actual quantity or content of a gas in blood also depends on the solubility of the gas in plasma and the ability of any component of blood to react with or bind the gas of interest. Since hemoglobin is capable of binding large amounts of O_2, oxygenated hemoglobin is the primary form in which O_2 is transported in blood. The actual content of O_2 in blood therefore depends both on the hemoglobin concentration and on the Pa_{O_2}. The Pa_{O_2} determines what percentage of hemoglobin is saturated with O_2, based on the position on the oxyhemoglobin dissociation curve. Oxygen content in normal blood (at 37°C, pH 7.4) can be determined by adding the amount of O_2 dissolved in plasma to the amount bound to hemoglobin, according to the equation

$$O_2 \text{ content} = 1.34 \times [\text{hemoglobin}] \times \text{saturation} + 0.0031 \times P_{O_2}$$

since each gram of hemoglobin is capable of carrying 1.34 mL O_2 when fully saturated, and the amount of O_2 that can be dissolved in plasma is proportional to the P_{O_2}, with 0.0031 mL O_2 dissolved per deciliter of blood per mmHg P_{O_2}. In arterial blood, the amount of O_2 transported dissolved in plasma (approximately 0.3 mL O_2 per deciliter of blood) is trivial compared with the amount bound to hemoglobin (approximately 20 mL O_2 per deciliter of blood).

Most commonly, P_{O_2} is the measurement used to assess the effect of respiratory disease on the oxygenation of arterial blood. Direct measurement of O_2 saturation in arterial blood by oximetry is also important in selected clinical conditions. For example, in patients with carbon monoxide intoxication, carbon monoxide preferentially displaces O_2 from hemoglobin, essentially making a portion of hemoglobin unavailable for binding to O_2. In this circumstance, carbon monoxide saturation is high and O_2 saturation is low, even though the driving pressure for O_2 to bind to hemoglobin, reflected by P_{O_2}, is normal. Measurement of O_2 saturation is also important for the determination of O_2 content when mixed venous blood is sampled from a pulmonary arterial catheter to calculate cardiac output by the Fick technique. In mixed venous blood, the P_{O_2} is normally about 40 mmHg, but small changes in P_{O_2} may reflect relatively large changes in O_2 saturation.

A useful calculation in the assessment of oxygenation is the alveolar-arterial O_2 difference ($PA_{O_2} - Pa_{O_2}$), commonly called the *alveolar-arterial O_2* gradient (or A − a gradient). This calculation takes into account the fact that alveolar and, hence, arterial P_{O_2} can be expected to change depending on the level of alveolar ventilation, reflected by the arterial P_{CO_2}. When a patient hyperventilates and has a low P_{CO_2} in arterial blood and alveolar gas, alveolar and arterial P_{O_2} will rise; conversely, hypoventilation and a high P_{CO_2} are accompanied by a decrease in alveolar and arterial P_{O_2}. These changes in arterial P_{O_2} are independent of abnormalities in O_2 transfer at the alveolar-capillary level and reflect only the dependence of alveolar P_{O_2} on the level of alveolar ventilation.

In order to determine the alveolar-arterial O_2 difference, the alveolar P_{O_2} (PA_{O_2}) must first be calculated. The equation most commonly used for this purpose, a simplified form of the alveolar gas equation, is

$$PA_{O_2} = FI_{O_2} \times (P_B - P_{H_2O}) - Pa_{CO_2}/R$$

where FI_{O_2} = fractional concentration of inspired O_2 (≈ 0.21 when breathing room air); P_B = barometric pressure (approximately 760 mmHg at sea level); P_{H_2O} = water vapor pressure (47 mmHg when air is fully saturated at 37°C); and R = respiratory quotient (the ratio of CO_2 production to O_2 consumption, usually assumed to be 0.8). If the preceding values are substituted into the equation for the patient breathing air at sea level, the equation becomes

$$PA_{O_2} = 150 - 1.25 \times Pa_{CO_2}$$

The alveolar-arterial O_2 difference can then be calculated by subtracting measured Pa_{O_2} from calculated PA_{O_2}. In a healthy young person breathing room air, the $PA_{O_2} - Pa_{O_2}$ is normally less than 15 mmHg; this value increases with age and may be as high as 30 mmHg in elderly patients.

The adequacy of CO_2 elimination is measured by the partial pressure of CO_2 in arterial blood, i.e., Pa_{CO_2}. A more complete understanding of the mechanisms and chronicity of abnormal levels of P_{CO_2} also requires measurement of pH and/or bicarbonate (HCO_3^-), since P_{CO_2} and the patient's acid-base status are so closely intertwined (Chap. 42).

PULSE OXIMETRY Because measurement of Pa_{O_2} requires arterial puncture, it is not ideal either for office use or for routine or frequent measurement in the inpatient setting. Additionally, because it provides intermittent rather than continuous data about the patient's oxygenation, it is not ideal for close monitoring of unstable patients. Pulse oximetry, an alternative method for assessing oxygenation, is readily available in many clinical settings. Using a probe usually clipped over a patient's finger, the pulse oximeter calculates oxygen saturation (rather than Pa_{O_2}) based on measurements of absorption of two wavelengths of light by hemoglobin in pulsatile, cutaneous arterial blood. Because of differential absorption of the two wavelengths of light by oxygenated and nonoxygenated hemoglobin, the percentage of hemoglobin that is saturated with oxygen, i.e., the Sa_{O_2}, can be calculated and displayed instantaneously.

Although the pulse oximeter has been a major advance in the noninvasive, continuous monitoring of oxygenation, there are several issues and potential problems concerning its use. First, the clinician must be aware of the relationship between oxygen saturation and tension as shown by the oxyhemoglobin dissociation curve (see Fig. 91-2). Because the curve becomes relatively flat above an arterial P_{O_2} of 60 mmHg (corresponding to Sa_{O_2} = 90%), the oximeter is relatively insensitive to changes in Pa_{O_2} above this level. In addition, the position of the curve and therefore the specific relationship between Pa_{O_2} and Sa_{O_2} may change depending on factors such as temperature, pH, and the erythrocyte concentration of 2,3-diphosphoglycerate. Second, when cutaneous perfusion is decreased, e.g., owing to low cardiac output or the use of vasoconstrictors, the signal from the oximeter may be less reliable or even unobtainable. Third, other forms of hemoglobin, such as carboxyhemoglobin and methemoglobin, are not distinguishable from oxyhemoglobin when only two wavelengths of light are used. The Sa_{O_2} values reported by the pulse oximeter are not reliable in the presence of significant amounts of either of these forms of hemoglobin. In contrast, the device used to measure oxygen saturation in samples of arterial blood, called the CO-oximeter, uses at least four wavelengths of light and is capable of distinguishing oxyhemoglobin, deoxygenated hemoglobin, carboxyhemoglobin, and methemoglobin. Finally, the clinician must remember that the often-used goal of $Sa_{O_2} \geq 90\%$ does not indicate anything about CO_2 elimination and therefore does not ensure a clinically acceptable P_{CO_2}.

DIFFUSING CAPACITY The ability of gas to diffuse across the alveolar-capillary membrane is ordinarily assessed by the diffusing capacity of the lung for carbon monoxide (DL_{CO}). In this test, a small concentration of carbon monoxide (0.3%) is inhaled, usually in a single breath that is held for approximately 10 s. The carbon monoxide is diluted by the gas already present in the alveoli and is also taken up by hemoglobin as the erythrocytes course through the pulmonary capillary system. The concentration of carbon monoxide in exhaled gas is measured, and DL_{CO} is calculated as the quantity of carbon monoxide absorbed per minute per mmHg pressure gradient from the alveoli to the pulmonary capillaries. The value obtained for DL_{CO} depends on the alveolar-capillary surface area available for gas exchange and on the pulmonary capillary blood volume. In addition, the thickness of the alveolar-capillary membrane, the degree of $\dot{V}/\dot{Q}$ mismatching, and the patient's hemoglobin level will affect the measurement. Because of this effect of hemoglobin levels on DL_{CO}, the measured DL_{CO} is frequently corrected to take the patient's hemoglobin level into account. The value for DL_{CO}, ideally corrected for hemoglobin, can then be compared with a predicted value, based either on age, height, and gender or on the alveolar volume (VA) at which the value was obtained. Alternatively, the DL_{CO} can be divided by VA and the resulting value for DL_{CO}/VA compared with a predicted value.

APPROACH TO THE PATIENT

ARTERIAL BLOOD GASES Hypoxemia is a common manifestation of a variety of diseases affecting the lungs or other parts of the respiratory system. The broad clinical problem of hypoxemia is often best characterized according to the underlying mechanism. The four basic, and not mutually exclusive, mechanisms of hypoxemia are (1) a decrease in inspired P_{O_2}, (2) hypoventilation, (3) shunting, and (4) $\dot{V}/\dot{Q}$ mismatching. Hypoxemia due to decreased diffusion occurs only under selected clinical circumstances and is not usually included among the general categories of hypoxemia. Determining the underlying mechanism for hypoxemia depends on measurement of the Pa_{CO_2}, calculation of $PA_{O_2} - Pa_{O_2}$, and knowledge of the response to supplemental O_2. A flowchart summarizing the approach to the hypoxemic patient is given in Fig. 234-5. →*See also Chap. 31.*

A decrease in the inspired P_{O_2} and hypoventilation both cause hypoxemia by lowering PA_{O_2} and therefore Pa_{O_2}. In each case, gas exchange at the alveolar-capillary level occurs normally, and $PA_{O_2} - Pa_{O_2}$ is not elevated. Hypoxemia due to decreased inspired P_{O_2} can be diagnosed from knowledge of the clinical situation. Inspired P_{O_2} is lowered either because the patient is at a high altitude, where barometric pressure is low, or, much less commonly, because the patient is breathing a gas mixture containing less than 21% O_2. The hallmark of hypoventilation as a cause of hypoxemia is an elevation in Pa_{CO_2}. This is associated with an increase in PA_{CO_2} and a fall in PA_{O_2}. When hypoxemia is due purely to a low inspired P_{O_2} or to alveolar hypoventilation, $PA_{O_2} - Pa_{O_2}$ is normal. If $PA_{O_2} - Pa_{O_2}$ and Pa_{CO_2} are both elevated, then an additional mechanism, such as $\dot{V}/\dot{Q}$ mismatching or shunting, is contributing to hypoxemia.

Shunting is a cause of hypoxemia when desaturated blood effectively bypasses oxygenation at the alveolar-capillary level. This situation occurs either because a structural problem allows desaturated blood to bypass the normal site of gas exchange or because

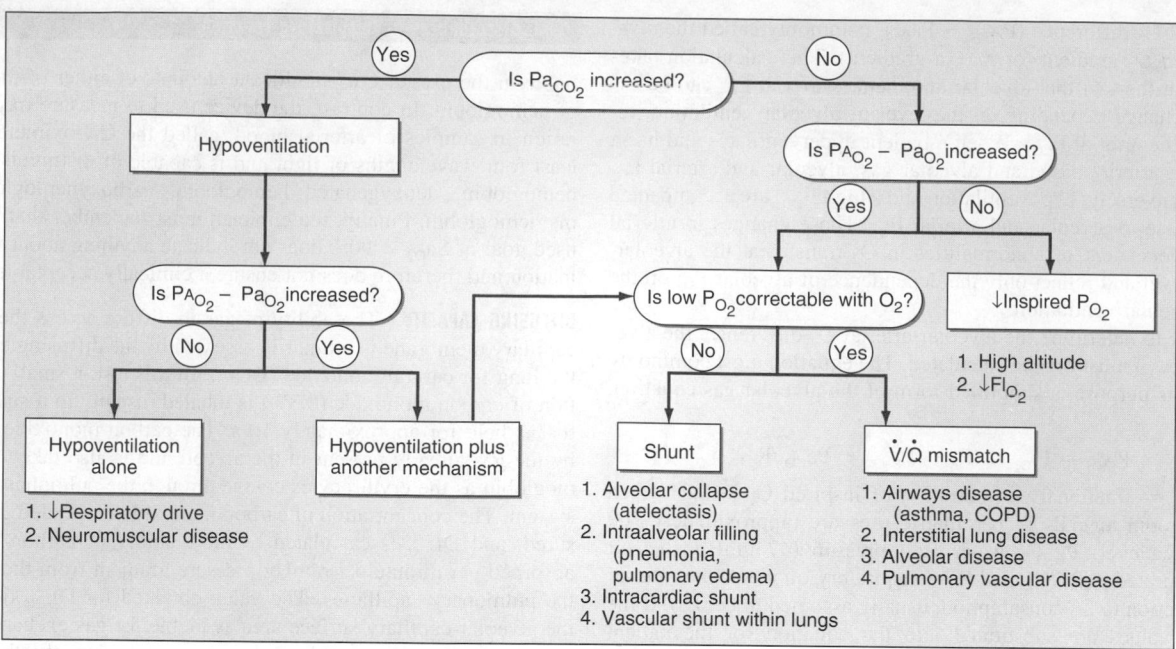

FIGURE 234-5 Flow diagram outlining the diagnostic approach to the patient with hypoxemia (Pa_{O_2} < 80 mmHg). PA_{O_2} – Pa_{O_2} is usually < 15 mmHg for subjects ≤30 years old and increases by ~3 mmHg per decade after age 30. COPD, chronic obstructive pulmonary disease.

perfused alveoli are not ventilated. Shunting is associated with an elevation in the PA_{O_2} – Pa_{O_2} value. When shunting is an important contributing factor to hypoxemia, the lowered Pa_{O_2} is relatively refractory to improvement by supplemental O_2.

Finally, the largest clinical category of hypoxemia is $\dot{V}/\dot{Q}$ mismatching. With $\dot{V}/\dot{Q}$ mismatching, regions with low $\dot{V}/\dot{Q}$ ratios contribute blood with a low P_{O_2} and a low O_2 content. Corresponding regions with high $\dot{V}/\dot{Q}$ ratios contribute blood with a high P_{O_2}. However, because blood is already almost fully saturated at a normal P_{O_2}, elevation of the P_{O_2} to a high value does not significantly increase O_2 saturation or content and therefore cannot compensate for the reduction of O_2 saturation and content in blood coming from regions with a low $\dot{V}/\dot{Q}$ ratio. When $\dot{V}/\dot{Q}$ mismatch is the primary cause of hypoxemia, PA_{O_2} – Pa_{O_2} is elevated, and P_{CO_2} generally is normal. Supplemental O_2 corrects the hypoxemia by raising the P_{O_2} in blood coming from regions with a low $\dot{V}/\dot{Q}$ ratio; this response distinguishes hypoxemia due to $\dot{V}/\dot{Q}$ mismatching from that due to true shunt.

The essential mechanism underlying all cases of hypercapnia is alveolar ventilation that is inadequate for the amount of CO_2 produced. It is conceptually useful to characterize CO_2 retention further, based on a more detailed examination of the potential contributing factors. These include (1) increased CO_2 production; (2) decreased ventilatory drive ("won't breathe"); (3) malfunction of the respiratory pump or increased airways resistance, which makes it more difficult to sustain adequate ventilation ("can't breathe"); and (4) inefficiency of gas exchange (increased dead space or $\dot{V}/\dot{Q}$ mismatch) necessitating a compensatory increase in overall minute ventilation. In practice, more than one of these mechanisms is commonly responsible for hypercapnia, since increased minute ventilation is capable of compensating for increased CO_2 production and for inefficiencies of gas exchange.

DIFFUSING CAPACITY Although abnormalities in diffusion are rarely responsible for hypoxemia, clinical measurement of diffusing capacity is frequently used to assess the functional integrity of the alveolar-capillary membrane, which includes the pulmonary capillary bed. Diseases that affect solely the airways generally do not lower DL_{CO}, whereas diseases that affect the alveolar walls or the pulmonary capillary bed will have an effect on DL_{CO}. Even though DL_{CO} is a useful marker for assessing whether disease affecting the alveolar-capillary bed is present, an abnormal DL_{CO} does not nec-

essarily imply that diffusion limitation is responsible for hypoxemia in a particular patient.

CLINICAL CORRELATIONS

Useful clinical correlations can be made with the mechanisms underlying hypoxemia (Fig. 234-5). A lowered inspired P_{O_2} contributes to hypoxemia if either the patient is at high altitude or the concentration of inspired O_2 is less than 21%. The latter problem occurs if a patient receiving anesthesia or ventilatory support is inadvertently given a gas mixture to breathe containing less than 21% O_2 or if O_2 is consumed from the ambient gas, as can occur during smoke inhalation from a fire. The primary feature of hypoventilation as a cause of hypoxemia is an elevation in arterial P_{CO_2}. →*For further discussion of the clinical correlations with hypoventilation, see Chap. 246.*

Shunting as a cause of hypoxemia can reflect transfer of blood from the right to the left side of the heart without passage through the pulmonary circulation, as occurs with an intracardiac shunt. This problem is most common in the setting of cyanotic congenital heart disease, when an interatrial or interventricular septal defect is associated with pulmonary hypertension so that shunting is in the right-to-left rather than the left-to-right direction. Shunting of blood through the pulmonary parenchyma is most frequently due to disease causing absence of ventilation to perfused alveoli. This can occur if the alveoli are atelectatic or if they are filled with fluid, as in pulmonary edema (both cardiogenic and noncardiogenic), or with extensive intraalveolar exudation of fluid due to pneumonia. Less commonly, vascular anomalies with arteriovenous shunting in the lung can cause hypoxemia. These anomalies can be hereditary, as found with hereditary hemorrhagic telangiectasia (Osler-Rendu-Weber syndrome), or acquired, as in pulmonary vascular malformations secondary to hepatic cirrhosis, which are similar to the commonly recognized cutaneous vascular malformations ("spider hemangiomas").

Ventilation-perfusion mismatch is the most common cause of hypoxemia clinically. Most of the processes affecting either the airways or the pulmonary parenchyma are distributed unevenly throughout the lungs and do not necessarily affect ventilation and perfusion equally. Some areas of lung may have good perfusion and poor ventilation, whereas others may have poor perfusion and relatively good ventilation. Important examples of airways diseases in which $\dot{V}/\dot{Q}$ mismatch causes hypoxemia are asthma and chronic obstructive lung disease.

Parenchymal lung diseases causing $\dot{V}/\dot{Q}$ mismatch and hypoxemia include interstitial lung disease and pneumonia.

Clinically important alterations in CO_2 elimination range from excessive ventilation and hypocapnia to inadequate CO_2 elimination and hypercapnia. →*For further discussion of these clinical problems, see Chap. 246.*

DIFFUSING CAPACITY   Measurement of DL_{CO} may be useful for assessing disease affecting the alveolar-capillary bed or the pulmonary vasculature. In practice, three main categories of disease are associated with lowered DL_{CO}: interstitial lung disease, emphysema, and pulmonary vascular disease. With interstitial lung disease, scarring of alveolar-capillary units diminishes the area of the alveolar-capillary bed as well as pulmonary blood volume. With emphysema, alveolar walls are destroyed, so the surface area of the alveolar-capillary bed is again diminished. In patients with disease causing a decrease in the cross-sectional area and volume of the pulmonary vascular bed, such as recurrent pulmonary emboli or primary pulmonary hypertension, DL_{CO} is commonly diminished.

Diffusing capacity may be elevated if pulmonary blood volume is increased, as may be seen in congestive heart failure. However, once interstitial and alveolar edema ensue, the net DL_{CO} depends on the opposing influences of increased pulmonary capillary blood volume elevating DL_{CO} and pulmonary edema decreasing it. Finding an elevated DL_{CO} may be useful in the diagnosis of alveolar hemorrhage, as in Goodpasture's syndrome. Hemoglobin contained in erythrocytes in the alveolar lumen is capable of binding carbon monoxide, so the exhaled carbon monoxide concentration is diminished and the measured DL_{CO} is increased.

FURTHER READING

AMERICAN THORACIC SOCIETY: Lung function testing: Selection of reference values and interpretative strategies. Am Rev Respir Dis 144:1202, 1991

CELLI BR: The importance of spirometry in COPD and asthma: Effect on approach to management. Chest 117:15S, 2000

CHUPP GL (ed): Pulmonary function testing. Clin Chest Med 22:599, 2001

LAFFEY JG, KAVANAGH BP: Hypocapnia. N Engl J Med 347:43, 2002

LEVITZKY MG: *Pulmonary Physiology,* 5th ed. New York, McGraw-Hill, 1999

WEINBERGER SE: *Principles of Pulmonary Medicine,* 3d ed. Philadelphia, Saunders, 1998

235 DIAGNOSTIC PROCEDURES IN RESPIRATORY DISEASE
Steven E. Weinberger, Jeffrey M. Drazen

The diagnostic modalities available for assessing the patient with suspected or known respiratory system disease include imaging studies and techniques for acquiring biologic specimens, some of which involve direct visualization of part of the respiratory system. →*Methods used to characterize the functional changes developing as a result of disease, including pulmonary function tests and measurements of gas exchange, are discussed in Chap. 234.*

IMAGING STUDIES

ROUTINE RADIOGRAPHY   Routine chest radiography, which generally includes both posteroanterior and lateral views, is an integral part of the diagnostic evaluation of diseases involving the pulmonary parenchyma, the pleura, and, to a lesser extent, the airways and the mediastinum (see Figs. 233-1 and 233-2). Lateral decubitus views are often useful for determining whether pleural abnormalities represent freely flowing fluid, whereas apical lordotic views can often visualize disease at the lung apices better than the standard posteroanterior view. Portable equipment, which is often used for acutely ill patients who either cannot be transported to a radiology suite or cannot stand up for posteroanterior and lateral views, generally yields just a single radiograph taken in the anteroposterior direction. →*Common radiographic patterns and their clinical correlates are reviewed in Chap. 233.*

COMPUTED TOMOGRAPHY   Computed tomography (CT) offers several advantages over routine chest radiography (Figs. 235-1, -2; 243-1, -2; 251-3). First, the use of cross-sectional images often makes it possible to distinguish between densities that would be superimposed on plain radiographs. Second, CT is far better than routine radiographic studies at characterizing tissue density, distinguishing subtle differences in density between adjacent structures, and providing accurate size assessment of lesions. As a result, CT is particularly valuable in assessing hilar and mediastinal disease (which is often poorly characterized by plain radiography), in identifying and characterizing disease adjacent to the chest wall or spine (including pleural disease), and in identifying areas of fat density or calcification in pulmonary nodules (Fig. 235-1). Its utility in the assessment of mediastinal disease has made CT an important tool in the staging of lung cancer (Chap. 75), as an assessment of tumor involvement of mediastinal lymph nodes is critical to proper staging. With the additional use of contrast material, CT also makes it possible to distinguish vascular from nonvascular structures, which is particularly important in distinguishing lymph nodes and masses from vascular structures.

Helical CT scanning allows the collection of continuous data over a larger volume of lung during a single breath-holding maneuver than is possible with conventional CT. With CT angiography, in which intravenous contrast is administered and images are acquired rapidly by helical scanning, pulmonary emboli can be detected in segmental and larger pulmonary arteries. With high-resolution CT (HRCT), the thickness of individual cross-sectional images is approximately 1 to 2 mm, rather than the usual 7 to 10 mm, and the images are reconstructed using high-spatial-resolution algorithms. The detail that can be seen on HRCT scans allows better recognition of subtle parenchymal and airway disease, such as bronchiectasis, emphysema, and diffuse parenchymal disease (Fig. 235-2). Certain nearly pathognomonic patterns have now been recognized for many of the interstitial lung diseases, such as lymphangitic carcinoma, idiopathic pulmonary fibrosis, sarcoidosis, and eosinophilic granuloma; however, it is not yet

FIGURE 235-1   CT scan demonstrating a mediastinal mass of heterogeneous density (*arrow*). CT is superior to plain radiography for the detection of abnormal mediastinal densities and the distinction of masses from adjacent vascular structures.

FIGURE 235-2 High-resolution CT scan from a patient with idiopathic pulmonary fibrosis. There are scattered reticular densities (arrows point to examples) that are especially prominent at the periphery of the lungs. This particular cross-section is from the base of the lungs, where the findings in idiopathic pulmonary fibrosis tend to be most marked.

clear in what settings these patterns obviate the need for obtaining lung tissue.

Recent advances in computer processing of the data acquired by helical scanning have allowed images to be presented in novel ways. For example, images may be displayed in views and planes other than the traditional cross-sectional view, and sophisticated three-dimensional reconstructions produce images (called *virtual bronchoscopy*) that mimic those seen by direct visualization through a bronchoscope.

MAGNETIC RESONANCE IMAGING The role of magnetic resonance (MR) imaging in the evaluation of respiratory system disease is less well defined than that of CT. Because MR generally provides a less detailed view of the pulmonary parenchyma as well as poorer spatial resolution, its usefulness in the evaluation of parenchymal lung disease is limited at present. However, MR images can be reconstructed in sagittal and coronal as well as transverse planes, so that the technique is well suited for imaging abnormalities near the lung apex, the spine, and the thoracoabdominal junction. MR images are dependent on tissue characteristics other than tissue density, unlike CT scanning. Therefore, in selected circumstances, MR images can better suggest the nature of abnormal tissue than can density-determined CT images. Finally, MR can be used to evaluate cardiac and vascular pathology within the thorax and to distinguish vascular from nonvascular structures without the need for contrast. Flowing blood does not produce a signal on MR imaging, so vessels appear as hollow tubular structures. This feature can be useful in determining whether abnormal hilar or mediastinal densities are vascular in origin and in defining aortic lesions such as aneurysms or dissection. In addition, gadolinium can be used as an intravascular contrast agent for MR angiography.

SCINTIGRAPHIC IMAGING Radioactive isotopes, administered by either intravenous or inhaled routes, allow the lungs to be imaged with a gamma camera. The most common use of such imaging is ventilation-perfusion lung scanning performed for evaluation of pulmonary embolism. When injected intravenously, albumin macroaggregates labeled with technetium 99m become lodged in pulmonary capillaries; therefore, the distribution of the trapped radioisotope follows the distribution of blood flow. When inhaled, radiolabeled xenon gas can be used to demonstrate the distribution of ventilation. For example, pulmonary thromboembolism usually produces one or more regions of ventilation-perfusion mismatch—that is, regions in which there is a

defect in perfusion that follows the distribution of a vessel and that is not accompanied by a corresponding defect in ventilation (Chap. 244). Another common use of such radioisotope scans is in a patient with impaired lung function who is being considered for lung resection. The distribution of the isotope(s) can be used to assess the regional distribution of blood flow and ventilation, allowing the physician to estimate the level of postoperative lung function.

POSITRON EMISSION TOMOGRAPHIC SCANNING Positron emission tomographic (PET) scanning is increasingly being used to identify malignant lesions in the lung based on their increased uptake and metabolism of glucose. The technique involves injection of a radiolabeled glucose analogue, ^{18}F-fluoro-2-deoxyglucose (FDG), which is taken up by metabolically active malignant cells. However, FDG is trapped within the cell following phosphorylation, and the unstable fluorine 18 decays by emission of positrons, which can be detected by a specialized PET camera or by a gamma camera that has been adapted for imaging of positron-emitting radionuclides. This technique has been used in the evaluation of solitary pulmonary nodules and as an aid to staging lung cancer, through identification of mediastinal lymph node involvement by malignancy.

PULMONARY ANGIOGRAPHY The pulmonary arterial system can be visualized by pulmonary angiography, in which radiopaque contrast medium is injected through a catheter previously threaded into the pulmonary artery. When performed in cases of pulmonary embolism, pulmonary angiography demonstrates the consequences of an intravascular clot—either a defect in the lumen of a vessel (a "filling defect") or an abrupt termination ("cutoff") of the vessel. Other, less common indications for pulmonary angiography include visualization of a suspected pulmonary arteriovenous malformation and assessment of pulmonary arterial invasion by a neoplasm. However, with advances in CT scanning, traditional pulmonary angiography is increasingly being replaced by CT angiography. The latter allows rapid acquisition of images with a less invasive procedure, since the radiocontrast material is injected intravenously rather than into a pulmonary artery.

ULTRASOUND Because ultrasound energy is rapidly dissipated in air, ultrasound imaging is not useful for evaluation of the pulmonary parenchyma. However, it is helpful in the detection and localization of pleural abnormalities and is often used as a guide to placement of a needle for sampling of pleural liquid (i.e., for thoracentesis).

TECHNIQUES FOR OBTAINING BIOLOGIC SPECIMENS

COLLECTION OF SPUTUM Sputum can be collected either by spontaneous expectoration or after inhalation of an irritating aerosol, such as hypertonic saline. The latter method, called *sputum induction*, is commonly used to obtain sputum for diagnostic studies, either because sputum is not spontaneously being produced or because of an expected higher yield of certain types of findings. Knowledge of the appearance and quality of the sputum specimen obtained is especially important when one is interested in Gram's staining and culture. Because sputum consists mainly of secretions from the tracheobronchial tree rather than the upper airway, the finding of alveolar macrophages and other inflammatory cells is consistent with a lower respiratory tract origin of the sample, whereas the presence of squamous epithelial cells in a "sputum" sample indicates contamination by secretions from the upper airways.

Besides processing for routine bacterial pathogens by Gram's staining and culture, sputum can be processed for a variety of other pathogens, including staining and culture for mycobacteria or fungi, culture for viruses, and staining for *Pneumocystis carinii*. In the specific case of sputum obtained for evaluation of *P. carinii* pneumonia in a patient infected with HIV, for example, sputum should be collected by induction, rather than spontaneous expectoration, and an immunofluorescent stain should be used to detect the organisms. Cytologic staining of sputum for malignant cells, using the traditional Papanicolaou method, allows noninvasive evaluation for suspected lung cancer. Traditional stains and cultures are now also being supplemented in some cases by immunologic techniques and by molecular biologic methods, including the use of polymerase chain reaction amplification and DNA probes.

PERCUTANEOUS NEEDLE ASPIRATION   A needle can be inserted through the chest wall into a pulmonary lesion for the purpose of aspirating material for analysis by cytologic or microbiologic techniques. The procedure is usually carried out under CT guidance, which assists in the positioning of the needle and assures that it is localized in the lesion. Although the potential risks of this procedure include intrapulmonary bleeding and creation of a pneumothorax with collapse of the underlying lung, the low risk of complication in experienced hands is usually worth the information obtained. However, a limitation of the technique is sampling error due to the small amount of material obtained. Thus, findings other than a specific cytologic or microbiologic diagnosis are of limited clinical value.

THORACENTESIS   Sampling of pleural liquid by thoracentesis is commonly performed for diagnostic purposes or, in the case of a large effusion, for palliation of dyspnea. Diagnostic sampling, either by blind needle aspiration or after localization by ultrasound, allows the collection of liquid for microbiologic and cytologic studies. Analysis of the fluid obtained for its cellular composition and chemical constituents, including glucose, protein, and lactate dehydrogenase, allows the effusion to be classified as either exudative or transudative (Chap. 245).

BRONCHOSCOPY   Bronchoscopy is the process of direct visualization of the tracheobronchial tree. Although bronchoscopy is now performed almost exclusively with flexible fiberoptic instruments, rigid bronchoscopy, generally performed in an operating room on a patient under general anesthesia, still has a role in selected circumstances, primarily because of a larger suction channel and the fact that the patient can be ventilated through the bronchoscope channel. These situations include the retrieval of a foreign body and the suctioning of a massive hemorrhage, for which the small suction channel of the bronchoscope may be insufficient.

Flexible Fiberoptic Bronchoscopy   This is an outpatient procedure that is usually performed in an awake but sedated patient. The bronchoscope is passed through either the mouth or the nose, between the vocal cords, and into the trachea. The ability to flex the scope makes it possible to visualize virtually all airways to the level of subsegmental bronchi. The bronchoscopist is able to identify endobronchial pathology, including tumors, granulomas, bronchitis, foreign bodies, and sites of bleeding. Samples from airway lesions can be taken by several methods, including washing, brushing, and biopsy. Washing involves instillation of sterile saline through a channel of the bronchoscope and onto the surface of a lesion. A portion of the liquid is collected by suctioning through the bronchoscope, and the recovered material can be analyzed for cells (cytology) or organisms (by standard stains and cultures). Brushing or biopsy of the surface of the lesion, using a small brush or biopsy forceps at the end of a long cable inserted through a channel of the bronchoscope, allows recovery of cellular material or tissue for analysis by standard cytologic and histopathologic methods.

The bronchoscope can be used to sample material not only from the regions that can be directly visualized (i.e., the airways) but also from the more distal pulmonary parenchyma. With the bronchoscope wedged into a subsegmental airway, aliquots of sterile saline can be instilled through the scope, allowing sampling of cells and organisms even from alveolar spaces. This procedure, called *bronchoalveolar lavage*, has been particularly useful for the recovery of organisms such as *P. carinii* in patients with HIV infection.

Brushing and biopsy of the distal lung parenchyma can also be performed with the same instruments that are used for endobronchial sampling. These instruments can be passed through the scope into small airways, where they penetrate the airway wall, allowing biopsy of peribronchial alveolar tissue. This procedure, called *transbronchial biopsy*, is used when there is either relatively diffuse disease or a localized lesion of adequate size. With the aid of fluoroscopic imaging,

the bronchoscopist is able to determine not only whether and when the instrument is in the area of abnormality, but also the proximity of the instrument to the pleural surface. If the forceps are too close to the pleural surface, there is a risk of violating the visceral pleura and creating a pneumothorax; the other potential complication of transbronchial biopsy is pulmonary hemorrhage. The incidence of these complications is less than several percent.

Another procedure involves use of a hollow-bore needle passed through the bronchoscope for sampling of tissue adjacent to the trachea or a large bronchus. The needle is passed through the airway wall, and cellular material can be aspirated from mass lesions or enlarged lymph nodes, generally in a search for malignant cells. This procedure can facilitate the staging of lung cancer by identifying mediastinal lymph node involvement and in some cases obviates the need for a more invasive procedure. Other new techniques that are not yet widely available include fluorescence bronchoscopy (to detect early endobronchial malignancy) and endobronchial ultrasound (to identify and localize mediastinal pathology).

The bronchoscope may provide the opportunity for treatment as well as diagnosis. For example, an aspirated foreign body may be retrieved with an instrument passed through the scope, and bleeding may be controlled with a balloon catheter similarly introduced. Newer interventional techniques performed through a bronchoscope include methods for achieving and maintaining patency of airways that are partially or completely occluded, especially by tumors. These techniques include laser therapy, cryotherapy, electrocautery, and stent placement.

VIDEO-ASSISTED THORACIC SURGERY   Recent advances in video technology have allowed the development of thoracoscopy, or video-assisted thoracic surgery (VATS), for the diagnosis and management of pleural as well as parenchymal lung disease. This procedure involves the passage of a rigid scope with a distal lens through a trocar inserted into the pleura. A high-quality image is shown on a monitor screen, allowing the operator to manipulate instruments passed into the pleural space through separate small intercostal incisions. With these instruments, the operator can biopsy lesions of the pleura under direct vision. In addition, this procedure is now used commonly to biopsy peripheral lung tissue or to remove peripheral nodules, for both diagnostic and therapeutic purposes. Because this procedure is much less invasive than the traditional thoracotomy performed for lung biopsy, it has largely supplanted "open lung biopsy."

THORACOTOMY   Although frequently replaced by VATS, thoracotomy remains an option for the diagnostic sampling of lung tissue. It provides the largest amount of material, and it can be used to biopsy and/or excise lesions that are too deep or too close to vital structures for removal by VATS. The choice between VATS and thoracotomy needs to be made on a case-by-case basis, and the relative indications for each are still evolving as more experience is being gained with VATS.

MEDIASTINOSCOPY AND MEDIASTINOTOMY   Tissue biopsy is often critical for the diagnosis of mediastinal masses or enlarged mediastinal lymph nodes. Although CT and PET scanning are useful for determining the size and nature of mediastinal lymph nodes as part of the staging of lung cancer, confirmation that enlarged lymph nodes are actually involved with tumor generally requires biopsy and histopathologic examination. The two major procedures used to obtain specimens from masses or nodes in the mediastinum are mediastinoscopy (via a suprasternal approach) and mediastinotomy (via a parasternal approach). Both procedures are performed under general anesthesia by a qualified surgeon. In the case of suprasternal mediastinoscopy, a rigid mediastinoscope is inserted at the suprasternal notch and passed into the mediastinum along a pathway just anterior to the trachea. Tissue can be obtained with biopsy forceps passed through the scope, sampling masses or nodes that are in a paratracheal or pretracheal position. Left paratracheal and aortopulmonary lymph nodes are not accessible by this route and thus are commonly sampled by parasternal mediastinotomy (the Chamberlain procedure). This approach involves either a right or left parasternal incision and dissection directly down to a mass or node that requires biopsy.

FURTHER READING

BOLLIGER CT, MATHUR PN: ERS/ATS statement on interventional pulmonology. Eur Respir J 19:356, 2002

GOULD MK et al: Accuracy of positron emission tomography for diagnosis of pulmonary nodules and mass lesions. A meta-analysis. JAMA 285:914, 2001

MEHTA AC (ed): Flexible bronchoscopy update. Clin Chest Med 22:225, 2001

MÜLLER NL: Computed tomography and magnetic resonance imaging: Past, present and future. Eur Respir J 19(suppl 35):3s, 2002

RYU JH et al: Diagnosis of pulmonary embolism with use of computed tomographic angiography. Mayo Clin Proc 76:59, 2001

SEIJO LM, STERMAN DH: Interventional pulmonology. N Engl J Med 344:740, 2001

WEINBERGER SE: *Principles of Pulmonary Medicine*, 3d ed. Philadelphia, Saunders, 1998

Section 2 Diseases of the Respiratory System

236 ASTHMA
E. R. McFadden, Jr.

Asthma is defined as a chronic inflammatory disease of airways that is characterized by increased responsiveness of the tracheobronchial tree to a multiplicity of stimuli. It is manifested physiologically by a widespread narrowing of the air passages, which may be relieved spontaneously or as a result of therapy, and clinically by paroxysms of dyspnea, cough, and wheezing. Asthma is an episodic disease, with acute exacerbations interspersed with symptom-free periods. Typically, most attacks are short-lived, lasting minutes to hours, and clinically the patient seems to recover completely after an attack. However, there can be a phase in which the patient experiences some degree of airway obstruction daily. This phase can be mild, with or without superimposed severe episodes, or much more serious, with severe obstruction persisting for days or weeks; the latter condition is known as *status asthmaticus*. In unusual circumstances, acute episodes can cause death.

PREVALENCE AND ETIOLOGY Asthma is a very common disease with immense social impact. The prevalence of asthma is rising in many parts of the world, but it is unclear whether this is due to an actual increase in incidence or merely to the fact that the size of the overall population is growing. It is estimated that 4 to 5% of the population of the United States is affected. Data from the Centers for Disease Control and Prevention suggest that 10 to 11 million persons had acute attacks in 1998, which resulted in 13.9 million outpatient visits, 2 million requests for urgent care, and 423,000 hospitalizations, with a total cost >$6 billion. The impact of the disease appears to fall more heavily on minorities and inner-city African-American and Hispanic persons.

Bronchial asthma occurs at all ages but predominantly in early life. About one-half of cases develop before age 10, and another third occur before age 40. In childhood, there is a 2:1 male/female preponderance, but the sex ratio equalizes by age 30. From an etiologic standpoint, asthma is a heterogeneous disease and genetic (atopic) and environmental factors, such as viruses, occupational exposures, and allergens, contribute to its initiation and continuance.

Atopy is the single largest risk factor for the development of asthma. *Allergic asthma* is often associated with a personal and/or family history of allergic diseases such as rhinitis, urticaria, and eczema; with positive wheal-and-flare skin reactions to intradermal injection of extracts of airborne antigens; with increased levels of IgE in the serum; and/or with a positive response to provocation tests involving the inhalation of specific antigen.

A significant fraction of patients with asthma present with no personal or family history of allergy, with negative skin tests, and with normal serum levels of IgE, and therefore have disease that cannot be classified on the basis of currently defined immunologic mechanisms. These patients are said to have *idiosyncratic asthma* or *nonatopic asthma*. Many patients have disease that does not fit clearly into either of the preceding categories but instead falls into a mixed group with features of each. In general, asthma that has its onset in early life tends to have a strong allergic component, whereas asthma that develops late tends to be nonallergic or to have a mixed etiology.

PATHOGENESIS (See also Chap. 298) Asthma results from a state of persistent subacute inflammation of the airways. Even in asymptomatic patients, the airways can be edematous and infiltrated with eosinophils, neutrophils, and lymphocytes, with or without an increase in the collagen content of the epithelial basement membrane. Overall, there is a generalized increase in cellularity associated with an elevated capillary density. There may also be glandular hypertrophy and denudation of the epithelium. These changes may persist despite treatment and often do not relate to the severity of the disease.

The physiologic and clinical features of asthma derive from an interaction among the resident and infiltrating inflammatory cells in the airway surface epithelium, inflammatory mediators, and cytokines. The cells thought to play important parts in the inflammatory response are mast cells, eosinophils, lymphocytes, and airway epithelial cells. The roles of neutrophils, macrophages, and other cellular constituents of the airways are less well defined. Each of the major cell types can contribute mediators and cytokines to initiate and amplify both acute inflammation and the long-term pathologic changes described (Fig. 236-1). The mediators released produce an intense, immediate inflammatory reaction involving bronchoconstriction, vascular congestion, edema formation, increased mucus production, and impaired mucociliary transport. This intense local event can then be followed by a more chronic one. Other elaborated chemotactic factors (eosinophil and neutrophil chemotactic factors of anaphylaxis and leukotriene B_4) also bring eosinophils, platelets, and polymorphonuclear leukocytes to the site of the reaction. The airway epithelium is both the target of, and a contributor to, the inflammatory cascade. This tissue both amplifies bronchoconstriction and promotes vasodilatation through the release of the compounds shown in Fig. 236-2.

FIGURE 236-1 Cellular sources of inflammatory mediators and their physiologic effects. PAF, platelet-activating factor; AHR, antihyaluronidase reaction. [*From PJ Barnes, in E Middleton et al (eds): Allergy Principles and Practice, 5th ed. St. Louis, Mosby, 1998, with permission.*]

FIGURE 236-2 Inflammatory mediators derived from epithelial sources. NO, nitrous oxide; PGE₂, prostaglandin E₂; GM-CSF, granulocyte-macrophage colony-stimulating factor; IL, interleukin; RANTES, regulated on activation, T cell expressed and secreted; EGF, epidermal growth factor; IGF, insulin-like growth factor; PDGF, platelet-derived growth factor. [*From PJ Barnes, in E Middleton et al (eds): Allergy Principles and Practice, 5th ed. St. Louis, Mosby, 1998, with permission.*]

The eosinophil appears to play an important part in the infiltrative component. Interleukin (IL) 5 stimulates the release of these cells into the circulation and extends their survival. Once activated, these cells are a rich source of leukotrienes, and the granular proteins released (major basic protein and eosinophilic cationic protein) and oxygen-derived free radicals are capable of destroying the airway epithelium, which then is sloughed into the bronchial lumen in the form of Creola bodies. Besides resulting in a loss of barrier and secretory function, such damage elicits the production of chemotactic cytokines, leading to further inflammation. In theory, it can also expose sensory nerve endings, thus initiating neurogenic inflammatory pathways. That, in turn, could convert a primary local event into a generalized reaction via a reflex mechanism. Although an important element in inflammation, the role that the eosinophil plays in establishing and maintaining airway hyperresponsiveness is undergoing reevaluation. Studies using antibodies against IL-5 show a disassociation between the inflammatory and physiologic events following an antigen challenge and blood and sputum eosinophilia. The cytokine network possibly involved in asthma is shown in Fig. 236-3.

T lymphocytes also appear to be important in the inflammatory response. Activated T$_H$2 cells are present in increased numbers in asthmatic airways and produce cytokines such as IL-4 that initiate humoral (IgE) immune responses. They also elaborate IL-5 with its effect on eosinophils. Data are accumulating that asthma may be related to an imbalance between T$_H$1 and T$_H$2 immune responses, but firm conclusions are not yet available.

GENETIC CONSIDERATIONS Although there is little doubt that asthma has a strong familial component, the identification of the genetic mechanisms underlying the illness has proven difficult for such fundamental reasons as a lack of uniform agreement on the definition of the disease, the inability to define a single phenotype, non-Mendelian modes of inheritance, and an incomplete understanding of how environmental factors modify genetic expression. Screening families for candidate genes has identified multiple chromosomal regions that relate to atopy, elevated IgE levels, and airway hyperresponsiveness. Evidence for genetic linkage of high total serum IgE levels and atopy has been observed on chromosomes 5q, 11q, and 12q in a number of populations scattered throughout the world. Regions of the genome demonstrating evidence for linkage to bronchial hyperreactivity also typically show evidence for linkage to elevated total serum IgE levels. Excellent candidate genes exist for specific abnormalities in asthma within the regions that were identified in the linkage studies. For example, chromosome 5q contains cytokine clusters including IL-4, IL-5, IL-9, and IL-13. Other regions on chromosome 5q also contain the β-adrenergic receptors and the glucocorticoid receptors. Chromosome 6p contains regions that are important in antigen presentation and me-

diation of the inflammatory response. Chromosome 12q contains two genes that could influence atopy and airway hyperresponsiveness, including nitric oxide synthase.

STIMULI THAT INCITE ASTHMA The stimuli that incite acute episodes of asthma can be grouped into seven major categories: allergenic, pharmacologic, environmental, occupational, infectious, exercise-related, and emotional.

Allergens Allergic asthma is dependent on an IgE response controlled by T and B lymphocytes and activated by the interaction of antigen with mast cell–bound IgE molecules. The airway epithelium and submucosa contain dendritic cells that capture and process antigen. After taking up an immunogen, these cells migrate to the local lymph nodes where they present the material to T cell receptors. In the appropriate genetic setting, the interaction of antigen with a naïve T cell T$_H$0 in the presence of IL-4 leads to the differentiation of the cell to a T$_H$2 subset. This process not only helps facilitate the inflammation of asthma but also causes B lymphocytes to switch their antibody production from IgG and IgM to IgE.

Once synthesized and released by B cells, IgE circulates in the blood until it attaches to high-affinity receptors on mast cells and low-affinity receptors on basophils. Most of the allergens that provoke asthma are airborne, and to induce a state of sensitivity they must be reasonably abundant for considerable periods of time. Once sensitization has occurred, however, the patient can exhibit exquisite responsivity, so that minute amounts of the offending agent can produce significant exacerbations of the disease. Immune mechanisms appear to be causally related to the development of asthma in 25 to 35% of all cases and to be contributory in perhaps another third. Higher prev-

FIGURE 236-3 Cytokine network in allergic asthma. IL, interleukin; GM-CSF, granulocyte-macrophage colony-stimulating factor; RANTES, regulated on activation, T cell expressed and secreted; TNF, tumor necrosis factor; SCS, stem cell factor. [*From PJ Barnes, in E Middleton et al (eds): Allergy Principles and Practice, 5th ed. St. Louis, Mosby, 1998, with permission.*]

alences have been suggested, but it is difficult to know how to interpret the data because of confounding factors. Allergic asthma is frequently seasonal, and it is most often observed in children and young adults. A nonseasonal form may result from allergy to feathers, animal danders, dust mites, molds, and other environmental antigens that are present continuously. Exposure to antigen typically produces an immediate response in which airway obstruction develops in minutes and then resolves. In 30 to 50% of patients, a second wave of bronchoconstriction, the so-called late reaction, develops 6 to 10 h later. In a minority, only a late reaction occurs. It was formerly thought that the late reaction was essential to the development of the increase in airway reactivity that follows antigen exposure. This is now known not to be the case.

The mechanism by which an inhaled allergen provokes an acute episode of asthma depends in part on antigen-antibody interactions on the surface of pulmonary mast cells, with the subsequent generation and release of the mediators of immediate hypersensitivity. Current hypotheses hold that very small antigenic particles penetrate the lung's defenses and come in contact with mast cells that interdigitate with the epithelium at the luminal surface of the central airways. The subsequent elaboration of mediators and cytokines then produces the sequence outlined above.

Pharmacologic Stimuli   The drugs most commonly associated with the induction of acute episodes of asthma are aspirin, coloring agents such as tartrazine, β-adrenergic antagonists, and sulfiting agents. It is important to recognize drug-induced bronchial narrowing because its presence is often associated with great morbidity. Furthermore, death sometimes has followed the ingestion of aspirin (or other nonsteroidal anti-inflammatory agents) or β-adrenergic antagonists. The typical aspirin-sensitive respiratory syndrome primarily affects adults, although the condition may occur in childhood. This problem usually begins with perennial vasomotor rhinitis that is followed by a hyperplastic rhinosinusitis with nasal polyps. Progressive asthma then appears. On exposure to even very small quantities of aspirin, affected individuals typically develop ocular and nasal congestion and acute, often severe episodes of airways obstruction.

The prevalence of aspirin sensitivity in patients with asthma varies from study to study, but many authorities feel that 10% is a reasonable figure. There is a great deal of cross-reactivity between aspirin and other nonsteroidal anti-inflammatory compounds that inhibit prostaglandin G/H synthase 1 (cyclooxygenase type 1). Indomethacin, fenoprofen, naproxen, zomepirac sodium, ibuprofen, mefenamic acid, and phenylbutazone are particularly important in this regard. However, acetaminophen, sodium salicylate, choline salicylate, salicylamide, and propoxyphene are well tolerated. The exact frequency of cross-reactivity to tartrazine and other dyes in aspirin-sensitive individuals with asthma is also controversial; again, 10% is the commonly accepted figure. This peculiar complication of aspirin-sensitive asthma is particularly insidious, however, in that tartrazine and other potentially troublesome dyes are widely present in the environment and may be unknowingly ingested by sensitive patients.

Patients with aspirin sensitivity can be desensitized by daily administration of the drug. After this form of therapy, cross-tolerance also develops to other nonsteroidal anti-inflammatory agents. The mechanism by which aspirin and other such drugs produce bronchospasm appears to be a chronic overexcretion of cysteinyl leukotrienes, which activate mast cells. The adverse reaction to aspirin can be inhibited with the use of leukotriene synthesis blockers or receptor antagonists.

β-Adrenergic antagonists regularly obstruct the airways in individuals with asthma as well as in others with heightened airway reactivity and should be avoided by such individuals. Even the selective beta$_1$ agents have this propensity, particularly at higher doses. In fact, the local use of beta$_1$ blockers in the eye for the treatment of glaucoma has been associated with worsening asthma.

Sulfiting agents, such as potassium metabisulfite, potassium and sodium bisulfite, sodium sulfite, and sulfur dioxide, which are widely used in the food and pharmaceutical industries as sanitizing and preserving agents, can also produce acute airway obstruction in sensitive individuals. Exposure usually follows ingestion of food or beverages containing these compounds, e.g., salads, fresh fruit, potatoes, shellfish, and wine. Exacerbation of asthma has been reported after the use of sulfite-containing topical ophthalmic solutions, intravenous glucocorticoids, and some inhalational bronchodilator solutions. The incidence and mechanism of action of this phenomenon are unknown. When suspected, the diagnosis can be confirmed by either oral or inhalational provocations.

Environment and Air Pollution   (See also Chap. 238)   Environmental causes of asthma are usually related to climatic conditions that promote the concentration of atmospheric pollutants and antigens. These conditions tend to develop in heavily industrial or densely populated urban areas and are frequently associated with thermal inversions or other situations creating stagnant air masses. In these circumstances, although the general population can develop respiratory symptoms, patients with asthma and other respiratory diseases tend to be more severely affected. The air pollutants known to have this effect are ozone, nitrogen dioxide, and sulfur dioxide. All produce greater effects during periods of high ventilation. In some regions of North America, seasonal concentrations of airborne antigens such as pollen can rise high enough to result in epidemics of asthma admissions to hospitals and an increase in the death rate. These events may be ameliorated by treating patients prophylactically with anti-inflammatory drugs before the allergy season begins.

Occupational Factors   (See also Chap. 238)   Occupation-related asthma is a significant health problem, and acute and chronic airway obstruction have been reported to follow exposure to a large number of compounds used in many types of industrial processes. In general, the agents can be classified into high-molecular-weight compounds, which are believed to induce asthma through immunologic mechanisms, and low-molecular-weight agents, which serve as haptines or can release bronchoconstrictor substances. High-molecular-weight compounds of importance are *wood and vegetable dusts* (e.g., those of oak, grain, flour, castor bean, green coffee bean, mako, gum acacia, karay, gum, and tragacanth), *pharmaceutical agents* (e.g., antibiotics, piperazine, and cimetidine), *biologic enzymes* (e.g., laundry detergents, pancreatic enzymes, and *Bacillus subtilis*), and *animal and insect dusts, serums, and secretions* (e.g., laboratory animals, chickens, crabs, prawns, oysters, flys, bees, and moths). Troublesome low-molecular-weight compounds are *metal salts* (e.g., platinum, chrome, vanadium, and nickel) and *industrial chemicals and plastics* (e.g., toluene diisocyanate, phthalic acid anhydride, trimellitic anhydride, persulfates, ethylenediamine, *p*-phenylenediamine, western red cedar, azidrocarbonamide, and various dyes). Formaldehyde and urea formaldehyde also fall into this group. It is important to recognize that exposure to sensitizing chemicals, particularly those used in paints, solvents, and plastics, can also occur during leisure or non-work-related activities.

If the occupational agent causes an immediate or dual immunologic reaction, the history is similar to that which occurs with exposure to other antigens. Often, however, patients will give a characteristic cyclic history. They are well when they arrive at work, and symptoms develop toward the end of the shift, progress after the work site is left, and then regress. Absence from work during weekends or vacations brings about remission. Frequently, there are similar symptoms in fellow employees.

Infections   Respiratory infections are the most common of the stimuli that evoke acute exacerbations of asthma. Respiratory viruses and not bacteria or allergy to microorganisms are the major etiologic factors. In young children, the most important infectious agents are respiratory syncytial virus and parainfluenza virus. In older children and adults, rhinovirus and influenza virus predominate as pathogens. Simple colonization of the tracheobronchial tree is insufficient to evoke acute episodes of bronchospasm, and attacks of asthma occur only when symptoms of an ongoing respiratory tract infection are, or have been, present. Viral infections can actively and chronically destabilize asthma, and they are perhaps the only stimuli that can produce constant symptoms for weeks. The mechanism by which viruses induce exacerbations of asthma may be related to the production of T cell–derived cytokines that potentiate the infiltration of inflammatory cells into already susceptible airways.

Exercise Exercise is a very common precipitant of acute episodes of asthma. This stimulus differs from other naturally occurring provocations, such as antigens, viral infections, and air pollutants, in that it does not evoke any long-term sequelae, nor does it increase airway reactivity. Typically the attacks follow exertion and do not occur during it. The critical variables that determine the severity of the postexertional airway obstruction are the levels of ventilation achieved and the temperature and humidity of the inspired air. The higher the ventilation and the lower the heat content of the air, the greater the response. For the same inspired air conditions, running produces a more severe attack of asthma than walking because of its greater ventilatory cost. Conversely, for a given task, the inhalation of cold air markedly enhances the response, while warm, humid air blunts or abolishes it. Consequently, activities such as ice hockey, cross-country skiing, and ice skating (high ventilations of cold air) are more provocative than is swimming in an indoor, heated pool (relatively low ventilation of humid air). The mechanism by which exercise produces obstruction may be related to a thermally produced hyperemia and capillary leakage in the airway wall.

Emotional Stress Psychological factors can worsen or ameliorate asthma. Changes in airway caliber seem to be mediated through modification of vagal efferent activity, but endorphins may also play a role. The extent to which psychological factors participate in the induction and/or continuation of any given acute exacerbation is not established but probably varies from patient to patient and in the same patient from episode to episode.

PATHOLOGY In a patient who has died of acute asthma, the most striking feature of the lungs at necropsy is their gross overdistention and failure to collapse when the pleural cavities are opened. When the lungs are cut, numerous gelatinous plugs of exudate are found in most of the bronchial branches down to the terminal bronchioles. Histologic examination shows hypertrophy of the bronchial smooth muscle, hyperplasia of mucosal and submucosal vessels, mucosal edema, denudation of the surface epithelium, pronounced thickening of the basement membrane, and eosinophilic infiltrates in the bronchial wall. There is an absence of any of the well-recognized forms of destructive emphysema.

PATHOPHYSIOLOGY The pathophysiologic hallmark of asthma is a reduction in airway diameter brought about by contraction of smooth muscle, vascular congestion, edema of the bronchial wall, and thick, tenacious secretions. The net result is an increase in airway resistance, a decrease in forced expiratory volumes and flow rates, hyperinflation of the lungs and thorax, increased work of breathing, alterations in respiratory muscle function, changes in elastic recoil, abnormal distribution of both ventilation and pulmonary blood flow with mismatched ratios, and altered arterial blood gas concentrations. Thus, although asthma is considered to be primarily a disease of airways, virtually all aspects of pulmonary function are compromised during an acute attack. In addition, in very symptomatic patients there frequently is electrocardiographic evidence of right ventricular hypertrophy and pulmonary hypertension. When a patient presents for therapy, the 1-s forced expiratory volume (FEV_1) or peak expiratory flow rate (PEFR) is typically <40% of predicted. In keeping with the alterations in mechanics, the associated air trapping is substantial. In acutely ill patients, residual volume frequently approaches 400% of normal, while functional residual capacity doubles.

Hypoxia is a universal finding during acute exacerbations, but frank ventilatory failure is relatively uncommon, being observed in 10 to 15% of patients presenting for therapy. Most individuals with asthma

have hypocapnia and a respiratory alkalosis. In acutely ill patients, the finding of a normal arterial carbon dioxide tension tends to be associated with quite severe levels of obstruction. Consequently, when found in a symptomatic individual, it should be viewed as representing impending respiratory failure, and the patient should be treated accordingly. Equally, the presence of metabolic acidosis in the setting of acute asthma signifies severe obstruction. Cyanosis is a very late sign. Trying to judge the state of an acutely ill patient's ventilatory status on clinical grounds alone can be extremely hazardous, and clinical indicators should not be relied on with any confidence. Therefore, in patients with suspected alveolar hypoventilation, arterial blood gas tensions must be measured.

CLINICAL FEATURES The symptoms of asthma consist of a triad of dyspnea, cough, and wheezing, the last often being regarded as the sine qua non. In its most typical form, all three symptoms coexist. At the onset of an attack, patients experience a sense of constriction in the chest, often with a nonproductive cough. Respiration becomes audibly harsh; wheezing in both phases of respiration becomes prominent; expiration becomes prolonged; and patients frequently have tachypnea, tachycardia, and mild systolic hypertension. The lungs rapidly become overinflated, and the anteroposterior diameter of the thorax increases. If the attack is severe or prolonged, there may be a loss of adventitial breath sounds, and wheezing becomes very high pitched. Furthermore, the accessory muscles become visibly active, and a paradoxical pulse often develops. These two signs are extremely valuable in indicating the severity of the obstruction. In the presence of either, pulmonary function tends to be significantly more impaired than in their absence. It is important to note that the development of a paradoxical pulse depends on the generation of large negative intrathoracic pressures. Thus, if the patient's breathing is shallow, this sign and/or the use of accessory muscles could be absent even though obstruction is quite severe. The other signs and symptoms of asthma only imperfectly reflect the physiologic alterations that are present. Indeed, if the disappearance of subjective complaints or even of wheezing is used as the end point at which therapy for an acute attack is terminated, an enormous reservoir of residual disease will be missed.

The end of an episode is frequently marked by a cough that produces thick, stringy mucus, which often takes the form of casts of the distal airways (Curschmann's spirals) and, when examined microscopically, often shows eosinophils and Charcot-Leyden crystals. In extreme situations, wheezing may lessen markedly or even disappear, cough may become extremely ineffective, and the patient may begin a gasping type of respiratory pattern. These findings imply extensive mucus plugging and impending suffocation. Ventilatory assistance by mechanical means may be required. Atelectasis due to inspissated secretions occasionally occurs with asthmatic attacks. Spontaneous pneumothorax and/or pneumomediastinum occur but are rare.

Less typically, a patient with asthma may complain of intermittent episodes of nonproductive cough or exertional dyspnea. Unlike other individuals with asthma, when these patients are examined during symptomatic periods, they tend to have normal breath sounds but may wheeze after repeated forced exhalations and/or may show ventilatory impairments when tested in the laboratory. In the absence of both these signs, a bronchoprovocation test may be required to make the diagnosis.

DIFFERENTIAL DIAGNOSIS The differentiation of asthma from other diseases associated with dyspnea and wheezing is usually not difficult, particularly if the patient is seen during an acute episode. The physical findings and symptoms listed above and the history of periodic attacks are quite characteristic. A personal or family history of allergic diseases such as eczema, rhinitis, or urticaria is valuable contributory evidence. An extremely common feature of asthma is nocturnal awakening with dyspnea and/or wheezing. In fact, this phenomenon is so prevalent that its absence raises doubt about the diagnosis.

Upper airway obstruction by tumor or *laryngeal edema* can occa-

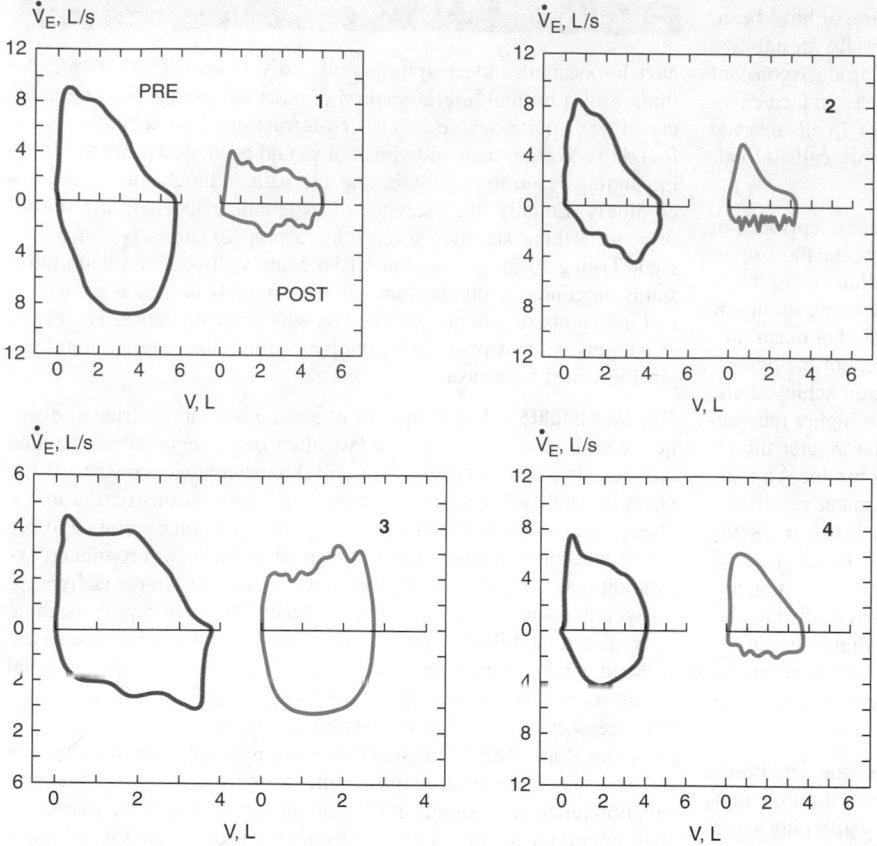

FIGURE 236-4 Representative examples of glottic dysfunction in four patients. The left-hand panels show normal flow-volume curves (red). The right-hand panels (green) represent the development of glottic dysfunction after exercise challenges (green). Note the variable waveforms that can exist. When the patients' attacks ended, the post provocation flow-volume curves returned to normal. $\dot{V}_E$, ventilation; L/s, liters/second; V, L, lung volume in liters.

sionally be confused with asthma. Typically, a patient with such a condition will present with stridor, and the harsh respiratory sounds can be localized to the area of the trachea. Representative flow–volume curves are shown in Fig. 236-4. Diffuse wheezing throughout both lung fields is usually absent. However, differentiation can sometimes be difficult, and indirect laryngoscopy or bronchoscopy may be required. Asthma-like symptoms have been described in patients with glottic dysfunction. These individuals narrow their glottis during inspiration and expiration, producing episodic attacks of severe airway obstruction. Occasionally, carbon dioxide retention develops. However, unlike in asthma, the arterial oxygen tension is well preserved, and the alveolar-arterial gradient for oxygen narrows during the episode, instead of widening as with lower airway obstruction. To establish the diagnosis of glottic dysfunction, the glottis should be examined when the patient is symptomatic. Normal findings at such a time exclude the diagnosis; normal findings during asymptomatic periods do not.

Persistent wheezing localized to one area of the chest in association with paroxysms of coughing indicates *endobronchial disease* such as foreign-body aspiration, a neoplasm, or bronchial stenosis.

The signs and symptoms of *acute left ventricular failure* occasionally mimic asthma, but the findings of moist basilar rales, gallop rhythms, blood-tinged sputum, and other signs of heart failure (Chap. 216) allow the appropriate diagnosis to be reached.

Recurrent episodes of bronchospasm can occur with *carcinoid tumors* (Chap. 329), *recurrent pulmonary emboli* (Chap. 244), and *chronic bronchitis* (Chap. 242). In chronic bronchitis there are no true symptom-free periods, and one can usually obtain a history of chronic cough and sputum production as a background on which acute attacks of wheezing are superimposed. Recurrent emboli can be very difficult to separate from asthma. Frequently, patients with this condition present with episodes of breathlessness, particularly on exertion, and

they sometimes wheeze. Lung scans may not be diagnostic because of the ventilation-perfusion abnormalities characteristic of asthma, and pulmonary angiography may be necessary to establish the correct diagnosis.

Eosinophilic pneumonias (Chap. 237) are often associated with asthmatic symptoms, as are various chemical pneumonias and exposures to insecticides and cholinergic drugs. Bronchospasm is occasionally a manifestation of *systemic vasculitis* with pulmonary involvement.

DIAGNOSIS The diagnosis of asthma is established by demonstrating reversible airway obstruction. *Reversibility* is traditionally defined as a $\geq 15\%$ increase in FEV_1 after two puffs of a β-adrenergic agonist. When the spirometry results are normal at presentation, the diagnosis can be made by showing heightened airway responsiveness to challenges with histamine, methacholine, or isocapnic hyperventilation of cold air. Once the diagnosis is confirmed, the course of the illness and the effectiveness of therapy can be followed by measuring PEFRs at home and/or the FEV_1 in the office or laboratory. Positive wheal-and-flare reactions to skin tests can be demonstrated to various allergens, but such findings do not necessarily correlate with the intrapulmonary events. Sputum and blood eosinophilia and measurement of serum IgE levels are also helpful but are not specific for asthma. Chest roentgenograms showing hyperinflation are also nondiagnostic.

℞ TREATMENT

Elimination of the causative agent(s) from the environment of an allergic individual with asthma is the most successful means available for treating this condition (for details on avoidance, see Chap. 298). Desensitization or immunotherapy with extracts of the suspected allergens has enjoyed widespread favor, but controlled studies are limited and have not proved to be highly effective.

DRUG TREATMENT The available agents for treating asthma can be divided into two general categories: drugs that inhibit smooth-muscle contraction, i.e., the so-called "quick relief medications" (β-adrenergic agonists, methylxanthines, and anticholinergics) and agents that prevent and/or reverse inflammation, i.e., the "long-term control medications" (glucocorticoids, long-acting β_2-agonists, combined medications, mast cell–stabilizing agents, leukotriene modifiers, and methylxanthines (Table 236-1).

Quick Relief Medications ■ *ADRENERGIC STIMULANTS* The drugs in this category consist of the catecholamines, resorcinols, and saligenins. These agents produce airway dilation through stimulation of β-adrenergic receptors and activation of G proteins with the resultant formation of cyclic adenosine monophosphate (AMP). They also decrease release of mediators and improve mucociliary transport. The catecholamines (epinephrine, isoproterenol, and isoetharine) are short-acting (30 to 90 min) and are effective only when administered by inhalational or parenteral routes. Their use has been superceded by the longer acting selective β_2-agonists terbutaline, fenoterol (a resorcinol), and albuterol (a saligenin). The resorcinols and saligenins are highly selective for the respiratory tract and are virtually devoid of significant cardiac effects except at high doses.

Their major side effect is tremor. They are active by all routes of administration and are relatively long-lasting (4 to 6 h). Inhalation is the preferred route because it allows maximal bronchodilation with fewer side effects. In treating episodes of severe asthma, intravenous administration offers no advantages over the inhaled route.

Very long lasting compounds (salmeterol and formoterol) are available and provide sustained effects for 9 to 12 h (Table 236-1). They are particularly helpful for conditions such as nocturnal and exercise-induced asthma. Salmeterol is not recommended for the treatment of acute episodes because of its relatively slow onset of action (~30 min), nor is it intended as a rescue drug for breakthrough symptoms. In addition, its long half-life means that administration of extra doses can cause cumulative side effects. The limits to the use of formoterol are not yet fully established. These compounds are now thought of as long-term controller medications by some, presumably because of their anti-inflammatory activities. The clinical significance of this aspect of their pharmacology has yet to be completely elucidated.

METHYLXANTHINES Theophylline and its various salts are medium-potency bronchodilators with questionable anti-inflammatory properties. The therapeutic plasma concentrations of theophylline lie between 5 and 15 $\mu g/mL$. The dose required to achieve the desired level varies widely from patient to patient owing to differences in the metabolism of the drug. Clearance falls with age and the concurrent use of erythromycin and other macrolide antibiotics, the quinolone antibiotics, and troleandomycin, allopurinol, cimetidine, and propranolol. It rises with use of cigarettes, marijuana, phenobarbital, phenytoin, or any other drug that is capable of inducing hepatic microsomal enzymes.

For maintenance therapy, long-acting theophylline compounds are available and are usually given once or twice daily. The dose is adjusted on the basis of the clinical response with the aid of serum theophylline measurements. Single-dose administration in the evening reduces nocturnal symptoms and helps keep the patient complaint-free during the day. However, the methylxanthines can disrupt sleep architecture. They are now considered second-line therapy, and as such they are rarely used in acute situations and infrequently in chronic ones. There is minimal evidence for additional benefit when used with optimal doses of β-adrenergics. There are some data that the methylxanthines can decrease inflammation, but as with the long-acting β_2-agonists, the effect is not large and its clinical impact is undefined. Nonetheless, some authorities now place these compounds in the "controller" class (Fig. 236-1). The most common side effects are nervousness, nausea, vomiting, anorexia, and headache. At plasma levels >30 $\mu g/mL$ there is a risk of seizures and cardiac arrhythmias.

ANTICHOLINERGICS Anticholinergic drugs such as ipratropium bromide have been found to be both effective and free of untoward effects. They may be of particular benefit for patients with coexistent heart disease, in whom the use of methylxanthines and β-adrenergic stimulants may be dangerous. The major disadvantages of the anticholinergics are that they are slow to act (60 to 90 min may be required before peak bronchodilation is achieved) and they are of only modest potency.

Long-Term Controller Medications (Table 236-1) ■ *GLUCOCORTICOIDS* Glucocorticoids are the most potent and most effective anti-inflammatory medications available. Systemic or oral steroids are most beneficial in acute illness, when severe airway obstruction is not resolving or

is worsening despite intense optimal bronchodilator therapy, and in chronic disease, when there has been failure of a previously optimal regimen with frequent recurrences of symptoms of increasing severity. Inhaled glucocorticoids are used in the long-term control of asthma.

Glucocorticoids are not bronchodilators, and the correct dose to use in acute situations is a matter of debate. In the United States, the recommended starting dose is 120 to 180 mg of methylprednisolone intravenously every 6 h. Since intravenous and oral administration produce the same effects, prednisone, 60 mg every 6 h, can be substituted. Clinical impressions suggest that smaller quantities may work as effectively, but there are no confirmatory data. In the United Kingdom and elsewhere, acute asthma both in and out of hospital is frequently treated with doses of prednisolone ranging from 30 to 40 mg given once daily. It should be emphasized that the effects of steroids in acute asthma are not immediate and may not be seen for ≥6 h after the initial administration. Consequently, it is mandatory to continue vigorous bronchodilator therapy during this interval.

Some believe that glucocorticoids should be given to all acutely ill patients upon presentation because of their long delay to peak effect. While there is some merit to this argument, glucocorticoids are often not necessary; the symptoms of ~80% of patients seen in emergency departments resolve rapidly with only inhaled β-agonists. Those who need steroids can be rapidly identified by monitoring their PEFR. Irrespective of the regimen chosen, it is important to appreciate that rapid tapering of glucocorticoids frequently results in recurrent obstruction. Most authorities recommend reducing the dose by one half every third to fifth day, over 10 to 12 days, after an acute episode. Beyond this point, the drug can be abruptly stopped. In situations in which it appears that continued steroid therapy is needed, an alternate-day schedule should be instituted to minimize side effects. This is particularly important in children, since continuous glucocorticoid administration interrupts growth. Long-acting preparations such as dexamethasone should not be used in this approach, for they defeat the purpose of alternate-day schedules by causing prolonged suppression of the pituitary-adrenal axis. The availability of inhaled agents has all but eliminated the need for this form of therapy. The usual doses of

TABLE 236-1 *Usual Dosages for Long-Term-Control Medications*

Medication	Dosage Form	Adult Dose
Inhaled glucocorticoids	(See Table 236-2)	
Systemic glucocorticoids	*(Applies to all three formulations)*	
Methylprednisolone	2-, 4-, 8-, 16-, 32-mg tablets	7.5–60 mg daily in a single dose in A.M. or qod as needed for control
Prednisolone	5-mg tablets, 5 mg/5 mL, 15 mg/5 mL	Short-course "burst" to achieve control: 40–60 mg/d as single or 2 divided doses for 3–10 days
Prednisone	1, 2.5, 5, 10, 20, 50 mg tablets; 5 mg/mL, 5 mg/5 mL	
Long-acting inhaled β_2-agonists *(Should not be used for symptom relief or for exacerbations. Use with inhaled glucocorticoids.)*		
Salmeterol	MDI 21 μg/puff	2 puffs q 12 h
	DPI 50 μg/blister	1 blister q 12 h
Formoterol	DPI 12 μg/single-use capsule	1 capsule q 12 h
Combined medication		
Fluticasone/salmeterol	DPI 100, 250, or 500 μg/50 μg	1 inhalation bid; dose depends on severity of asthma
Cromolyn and Nedocromil		
Cromolyn	MDI 1 mg/puff	2–4 puffs tid-qid
	Nebulizer 20 mg/ampule	1 ampule tid-qid
Nedocromil	MDI 1.75 mg/puff	2–4 puffs bid-qid
Leukotriene modifiers		
Montelukast	4- or 5-mg chewable tablet, 10-mg tablet	10 mg qhs
Zafirlukast	10- or 20-mg tablet	40 mg daily (20-mg tablet bid)
Zileuton	300- or 600-mg tablet	2400 mg daily (given tablets qid)
Methylxanthines *[Serum monitoring is important (serum concentration of 5–15 $\mu g/mL$ at steady state)].*		
Theophylline	Liquids, sustained-release tablets, and capsules	Starting dose 10 mg/kg per day up to 300 mg max; usual max, 800 mg/d

Note: MDI, metered-dose inhaler; DPI, daily permissible intake.

TABLE 236-2   Comparative Daily Doses for Inhaled Steroids

Drug	How Supplied	Dose Range		
		Low	Medium	High
Beclomethasone		168–540 μg	504–840 μg	>840 μg
	42 μg/puff	4–12 puffs	10–12 puffs	>20 puffs
	84 μg/puff	2–6 puffs	6–10 puffs	>10 puffs
Budesonide		200–400 μg	400–600 μg	>600 μg
	200 μg/dose	1–2 inhalations	2–3 inhalations	>3 inhalations
Flunisolide		500–1000 μg	1000–2000 μg	>2000 μg
	250 μg/dose	2–4 puffs	4–8 puffs	>8 puffs
Fluticasone		88–264 μg	264–660 μg	>660 μg
	MDI: 44,110, 220 μg/puff	2–6 puffs (44 μg) 2 puffs (110 μg)	2–6 puffs (110 μg)	>6 puffs (110 μg)
	DPI: 50,100, 250 μg/puff	2–6 inhalations (50 μg)	3–6 inhalations (100 μg)	>6 inhalations (100 μg)
Triamcinolone		400–1000 μg	1000–2000 μg	>2000 μg
	100 μg/puff	4–10 puffs	10–20 puffs	>20 puffs

Note: MDI, metered-dose inhaler; DPI, daily permissible intake.

oral glucocorticoids for nonemergent episodes of asthma are summarized in Table 236-1.

Inhaled Glucocorticoids   These drugs are indicated in patients with persistent symptoms. The agents currently available in the United States and their comparative doses are presented in Table 236-2. These drugs share the ability to control inflammation, facilitate the long-term prevention of symptoms, reduce the need for oral glucocorticoids, minimize acute occurrences, and prevent hospitalizations.

There is no fixed dose of inhaled steroid that works for all patients. Requirements are dictated by the response of the individual and wax and wane in concert with progression of the disease. Generally, the worse the patient's condition, the more inhaled steroid is needed to gain control. Once achieved, however, remission can often be maintained with quantities as low as one or two puffs/day. Inhaled steroids can take up to a week or more to produce improvements; consequently, in rapidly deteriorating situations, it is best to prescribe oral preparations and initiate inhaled drugs as the dose of the former is reduced. In less emergent circumstances, the quantity of inhaled drug can be increased up to 2 to 2.5 times the recommended starting doses. The side effects increase in proportion to the dose-time product. In addition to thrush and dysphonia, the increased systemic absorption that accompanies larger doses of inhaled steroids has been reported to produce adrenal suppression, cataract formation, decreased growth in children, interference with bone metabolism, and purpura. As is the case with oral agents, suppression of inflammation, per se, cannot be relied upon to provide optimal results. It is essential to continue adrenergic or methylxanthine bronchodilators if the patient's disease is unstable. The combination of a long acting β-agonist and inhaled steroid seems particularly efficacious in patients with mild to moderate disease.

COMBINED MEDICATIONS   The combination of an inhaled steroid and a long-acting β_2 agonist is gaining popularity. The only such combination available in the United States at present is fluticasone and salmeterol. Other combinations are being tested but are not yet available. There is little question that combinations of agents add a significant degree of convenience in the care of chronic asthma. They tend to work best in patients with milder disease. It has been suggested that the combination provides better pharmacologic activity than the individual drugs given alone.

MAST CELL–STABILIZING AGENTS   Cromolyn sodium and nedocromil sodium do not influence airway tone. Their major therapeutic effect is to inhibit the degranulation of mast cells, thereby preventing the release of the chemical mediators of anaphylaxis.

Cromolyn sodium and nedocromil sodium, like the inhaled steroids, improve lung function, reduce symptoms, and lower airway reactivity in persons with asthma. They are most effective in atopic patients who have either seasonal disease or perennial airway stimulation. A therapeutic trial of two puffs four times daily for 4 to 6 weeks is frequently necessary before the beneficial effects of the drug appear. Unlike steroids, nedocromil and cromolyn sodium, when given prophylactically, block the acute obstructive effects of exposure to antigen, industrial chemicals, exercise, or cold air. With antigen, the late response is also abolished. Therefore, a patient who has intermittent exposure to either antigenic or nonantigenic stimuli that provoke acute episodes of asthma need not use these drugs continuously but instead can obtain protection by taking the drug only 15 to 20 min before contact with the precipitant.

LEUKOTRIENE MODIFIERS   As mentioned earlier, the cysteinyl leukotrienes (LTC$_4$, LTD$_4$, and LTE$_4$) produce many of the critical elements of asthma, and drugs have been developed that either reduce the synthesis of all of the leukotrienes by inhibiting 5-lipoxygenase (5-LO), the enzyme involved in their production, or competitively antagonize the principal moiety (LTD$_4$). Zileuton is the only 5-LO synthesis inhibitor that is available in the United States. It is a modest bronchodilator that reduces asthma morbidity, provides protection against exercise-induced asthma, and diminishes nocturnal symptoms, but it has limited effectiveness against allergens. Hepatic enzyme levels can be elevated after its use, and there are significant interactions with other drugs metabolized in the liver. The LTD$_4$ receptor antagonists (zafirlukast and montelukast) have therapeutic and toxicologic profiles similar to that of zileuton but are long acting and permit twice- to once-daily dose schedules.

This class of drugs does not appear to be uniformly effective in all patients with asthma. Although precise figures are lacking, most authorities put the number of positive responders at <50%. As yet, there is no way of determining prospectively who will benefit, so clinical trials are required. Typically, if there is no improvement after 1 month, treatment can be discontinued. The leukotriene blockers have been associated with uncovering of Churg-Strauss syndrome (Chap. 306).

Miscellaneous Agents   It has been suggested that steroid-dependent patients might benefit from the use of immunosuppressant agents such as methotrexate, gold salts, or colchicine. The effects of these agents on steroid dosage and disease activity are minor, and side effects can be considerable. Opiates, sedatives, and tranquilizers should be absolutely avoided in the acutely ill patient with asthma because the risk of depressing alveolar ventilation is great, and respiratory arrest has been reported to occur shortly after their use. Admittedly, most individuals are anxious and frightened, but experience has shown that they can be calmed equally well by the physician's presence and reassurances. β-Adrenergic blockers and parasympathetic agonists are contraindicated because they can cause marked deterioration in lung function.

Expectorants and mucolytic agents have enjoyed great vogue in the past, but they do not add significantly to the treatment of the acute or chronic phases of this disease. The use of intravenous fluids in the treatment of acute asthma has also been advocated. There is little evidence that this adjunct hastens recovery. Nonstandard bronchodilators, such as intravenous magnesium sulfate, for the treatment of acute asthma attacks are not yet warranted in clinical practice because of the controversy surrounding their efficacy.

Special Instructions   The treatment of patients with asthma who have coexisting conditions such as heart disease or pregnancy does not differ materially from that outlined above. Therapy with inhaled β_2-selective and anti-inflammatory agents is the mainstay. The lowest doses of adrenergics that produce the desired effects should be used.

Framework for Management ■ *EMERGENCY SITUATIONS* The most effective treatment for acute episodes of asthma requires a systematic approach based on the aggressive use of sympathomimetic agents and serial objective monitoring of key indices of improvement. Reliance on empiricism and subjective assessment is no longer acceptable. Multiple inhalations of a short-acting sympathomimetic, such as albuterol, are the cornerstone of most regimens. These drugs provide three to four times more relief than does intravenous aminophylline. Anticholinergic drugs are not first-line therapy because of their long lag time to onset (~30 to 40 min) and their relatively modest bronchodilator properties. In emergency situations, β_2-agonists can be given every 20 min by handheld nebulizer for 2 to 3 doses. The optimum cumulative dose of albuterol appears to lie between 5 and 10 mg. It does not matter how the adrenergic agonists are inhaled. Treatment with albuterol administered by jet nebulizer, metered dose inhaler, or dry powder inhaler all provide equal resolution in acute situations when the doses are matched. Continuous nebulization of β_2-agonists has also been employed, but it is unclear if it is materially better than the other forms of treatment. Ipratropium can be added to the regimen in an attempt to speed resolution. The benefits on lung function are small, but the need for admission has decreased in some studies. There are no hard and fast rules as to who should be admitted.

Acute episodes of bronchial asthma are one of the most common respiratory emergencies, and it is essential that the physician recognize which episodes of airway obstruction are life-threatening and which patients demand what level of care. These distinctions can be made readily by assessing selected clinical parameters in combination with measures of expiratory flow and gas exchange. The presence of a paradoxical pulse, use of accessory muscles, and marked hyperinflation of the thorax signify severe airways obstruction, and failure of these signs to remit promptly after aggressive therapy mandates objective monitoring of the patient with measurements of arterial blood gases and PEFR or FEV_1. Although pulse and respiratory rates are commonly recorded, there is no relationship between these variables and the severity of the obstruction or the outcome of treatment.

Patients with the most impairment typically require the most extensive therapy for resolution. If the PEFR or FEV_1 is ≤20% of predicted on presentation and does not double within an hour of receiving the preceding therapy, the patient is likely to require extensive treatment, including glucocorticoids, before the obstruction dissipates. This group represents ~20% of all the patients who present for acute care. They generally require inpatient treatment before becoming asymptomatic. In such patients, if the clinical signs of a paradoxical pulse and accessory muscle use are diminishing and/or the PEFR is increasing, there is no need to change medications or doses, but the patient needs to be followed closely. However, if the PEFR falls by >20% of its previous value or if the magnitude of the pulsus paradoxicus is increasing, serial measures of arterial blood gases are required, as well as a reconsideration of the therapeutic modalities being employed. If the patient has hypocarbia, one can afford to continue the current approaches a while longer. On the other hand, if the Pa_{CO_2} is within the normal range or is elevated, the patient should be monitored in an intensive care setting, and therapy should be intensified to reverse or arrest the patient's respiratory failure.

Treatment with 70 to 80% helium (balance oxygen) may be beneficial in patients with severe airway obstruction. This gas mixture reduces airway resistance and improves the effect of aerosolized bronchodilators. This form of treatment should be considered in patients whose airway obstruction and gas exchange are worsening despite aggressive therapy. However, there are no large-scale clinical trials comparing this approach with other forms of treatment. The criteria for intubation and ventilatory support have not been standardized. The decision to use this therapy should be made by physicians with the most experience in caring for severely ill asthmatic patients.

Chronic Treatment The goal of chronic therapy is to achieve a stable, asymptomatic state with the best pulmonary function possible using the least amount of medication. The specific recommendations from consensus guidelines are to promote a state of health encompassing the following: (1) minimal or absent daytime or nocturnal chronic symptoms, (2) minimal or absent exacerbations, (3) no limitation on activities, (4) no absences from school or work, (5) maintenance of normal or near-normal pulmonary functions, (6) the minimal use of short-acting β_2-agonists (< once per day, <1 canister/month), (7) and minimal or absent adverse effects from medications. A primary step is to educate patients to function as partners in their management. The severity of the illness needs to be assessed and monitored with objective measures of lung function. Asthma triggers should be avoided or controlled, and plans should be made for both chronic management and treatment of exacerbations. Regular follow-up care is mandatory.

A stepwise pharmacologic approach recommended by the National Asthma Education and Prevention Program is presented in Table 236-3. The purpose of this schema is to assist and not replace the clinical decision-making required to meet individual patient needs. In general, the simplest approach works best. Infrequent symptoms (step 1) require only the use of an inhaled sympathomimetic on an "as-needed" basis. When the disease worsens to a persistent state (step 2), as manifested by nocturnal awakenings and daytime symptoms, inhaled steroids, mast cell–stabilizing agents, and/or leukotriene modifiers should be added. Methylxanthines can also be employed. If symptoms do not abate (step 3), the dose of inhaled steroids can be increased. An upper limit has not yet been established, but side effects of glucocorticoid excess begin to appear more frequently when the dose exceeds 2.0 mg/kg per d. Persistent asthma complaints can be treated with low- to medium-dose inhaled glucocorticoids and long-acting inhaled β_2-agonists. Alternative treatments include leukotriene modifiers or sustained-release theophylline. In patients with recurrent or perennial symptoms and unstable lung function (step 4), the preferred treatment is high-dose inhaled glucocorticoids and long-acting inhaled β_2-agonists. If needed, oral glucocorticoids in a single daily dose are added to the regimen. Acute symptoms are treated with short-acting rescue medications such as albuterol alone or in combination with a parasympatholytic.

Once control is reached and sustained for several weeks, a step-down reduction in therapy should be undertaken, beginning with the most toxic drug, to find the minimum amount of medication required to keep the patient well. During this process, the PEFR should be monitored and medication adjustments should be based on objective changes in lung function as well as on the patient's symptoms. The recommendations in the step-down mode are that treatment be reviewed every 1 to 6 months. In many instances, shorter periods can be employed. We have found that 2 to 4 weeks are a reasonable period. When a patient's asthma is destabilizing, frequent assessments are required. It is important to gain control as quickly as possible and then step down to the least medication necessary to maintain control. If there are difficulties in achieving this goal, then referral to an asthma specialist should be considered. Prior to increasing treatment, an important component is to review patients' inhaler technique, their adherence to therapeutic recommendations, and environment control.

PROGNOSIS AND CLINICAL COURSE The mortality rate from asthma is small. The most recent figures for the United States indicate fewer than 6000 deaths per year out of a population of ~10 million patients at risk. Death rates, however, appear to be rising in inner-city areas where there is limited availability of health care. Even so, only 0.09 to 0.25% of admissions to hospital are at risk of an untoward event.

Information on the clinical course of asthma suggests a good prognosis, particularly for those whose disease is mild and develops in childhood. The number of children who still have asthma 7 to 10 years after the initial diagnosis varies from 26 to 78%, averaging 46%; how-

TABLE 236-3 *Stepwise Approach for Managing Asthma in Adults*

Classify Severity: Clinical Features Before Treatment or Adequate Control

	Symptoms		PEFR or FEV₁	
	Day	**Night**	**(PEFR Variability)**	*Daily Medications to Maintain Long-Term Control*
Step 1: Mild intermittent	≤2 days/week	≤ 2 nights/month	≥80% (< 20%)	No daily medication needed. Severe exacerbations may occur, separated by long periods of normal lung function and no symptoms. A course of systemic glucocorticoids is recommended.
Step 2: Mild persistent	> 2 days/week but <1 per day	>2 nights/months	≥ 80% (20–30%)	Low-dose inhaled glucocorticoids Alternative treatment (listed alphabetically): cromolyn, leukotriene modifier, nedocromil, *or* sustained-release theophylline to serum concentration of 5–15 μg/mL.
Step 3: Moderate persistent	Daily	> 1 night/week	> 60%–< 80% (>30%)	Low- to medium-dose inhaled glucocorticoids and long-acting inhaled β_2-agonists. Alternative treatment: leukotriene modifier or theophylline instead of β_2 agents
Step 4: Severe persistent	Continual	Frequent	≤60% (> 30%)	High-dose inhaled glucocorticoids *and* Long-acting inhaled β_2-agonists *and,* if needed, Glucocorticoid tablets or syrup long term (2mg/kg per day, generally do not exceed 60 mg/d). (Make repeat attempts to reduce systemic glucocorticoids and maintain control with high-dose inhaled glucocorticoids.)
Quick relief for all patients				Short-acting bronchodilator: 2–4 puffs short-acting inhaled β_2-agonists as needed for symptoms. Intensity of treatment will depend on severity of exacerbation; up to 3 treatments at 20-min intervals or a single nebulizer treatment as needed. Course of systemic glucocorticoids may be needed. Use of short-acting β_2-agonists >2 times a week in intermittent asthma (daily, or increasing use in persistent asthma) may indicate the need to initiate (increase) long-term control therapy.

Note: PEFR, peak expiratory flow rate; FEV₁, forced expiratory volume in 1 s.　　*Source*: Modified from National Asthma Education and Prevention Program.

ever, the percentage who continue to have severe disease is relatively low (6 to 19%).

Although there are reports of patients with asthma developing irreversible changes in lung function, these individuals frequently have comorbid stimuli such as cigarette smoking that could account for these findings. Even when untreated, individuals with asthma do not continuously move from mild to severe disease with time. Rather, their clinical course is characterized by exacerbations and remissions. Some studies suggest that spontaneous remissions occur in approximately 20% of those who develop the disease as adults, and that ~40% can be expected to experience improvement, with less frequent and severe attacks, as they grow older.

FURTHER READING

BEASLEY DM et al: Prevalence and etiology of asthma. J Allergy Clin Immunol 105:S466, 2000

BUSSE WW: Anti-immunoglobulin E (omalizumab) therapy in allergic asthma. Am J Respir Crit Care Med 164:S12, 2001

———, LEMANSKE RF: Asthma. N Engl J Med 344:350, 2001

FITZGERALD M: Acute asthma. BMJ 323:841, 2001

HALL JB: Concise review: Contemporary management of status asthmaticus. New York: McGraw-Hill, www.harrisonsonline.com

ISRAEL E et al: The effect of polymorphisms of the beta2-adrenergic receptor on the response to regular use of albuterol in asthma. Am J Respir Crit Care Med 162:75, 2000

LAZARUS SC et al: Long-acting β_2-agonist monotherapy vs continued therapy with inhaled corticosteroids in patients with persistent asthma: A randomized controlled trial. JAMA 285:2583, 2001

MARTIN RJ et al: Systemic effect comparisons of six inhaled corticosteroid preparations. Am J Respir Crit Care Med 165:1377, 2002

THE NAEPP EXPERT PANEL REPORT: *Guidelines for the Diagnosis and Management of Asthma—Update on Selected Topics, 2002.* NIH publication no. 02-5075

O'BYRNE PM et al: Low dose inhaled budesonide and formoterol in mild persistent asthma: The OPTIMA randomized trial. Am J Respir Crit Care Med 164:1392, 2001

SZCZEKLIK A, STEVENSON DD: Aspirin-induced asthma: Advances in pathogenesis, diagnosis, and management. J Allergy Clin Immunol 111:913, 2003

TOGIAS A: Rhinitis and asthma: evidence for respiratory system integration. J Allergy Clin Immunol 111:1171, 2003

237 HYPERSENSITIVITY PNEUMONITIS AND PULMONARY INFILTRATES WITH EOSINOPHILIA
Joel N. Kline, Gary W. Hunninghake

HYPERSENSITIVITY PNEUMONITIS

First described in 1874, hypersensitivity pneumonitis (HP), or extrinsic allergic alveolitis, is an inflammatory disorder of the lung, involving alveolar walls and terminal airways, that is induced by repeated inhalation of a variety of organic agents by a susceptible host. Factors responsible for the expression of HP include both those related to the host (susceptibility) and the inciting agent. Causes of HP are typically designated with colorful names denoting the occupational or avocational risk associated with the disease; "farmer's lung" is the term most commonly used for HP due to inhalation of antigens present in moldy hay, such as thermophilic actinomyces, *Micropolyspora faeni*, and As-

pergillus species. The frequency of HP is unknown but varies with the environmental exposure and the specific antigen involved. The prevalence of farmer's lung among Wisconsin dairy farmers has been reported as 4.2 per 1000 and a Finnish cohort study demonstrated an annual incidence of 5 per 10,000 farmers. The diagnosis of HP requires a constellation of clinical, radiographic, physiologic, pathologic, and immunologic criteria, each of which is rarely pathognomonic alone, and the preferred treatment is avoidance of the causative antigen.

ETIOLOGY Agents implicated as causes of HP are diverse and include those listed in Table 237-1. Many cases of HP occurring in various occupations involve exposure to similar agents, particularly the thermophilic actinomycetes. In the United States, the most common types of HP are farmer's lung, bird fancier's lung, and chemical worker's lung. In *farmer's lung*, inhalation of proteins such as thermophilic bacteria and fungal spores that are present in moldy bedding and feed are most commonly responsible for the development of HP. These antigens are probably also responsible for the etiology of *mushroom worker's disease* (moldy composted growth medium is the source of the proteins) and *bagassosis* (moldy sugar cane is the source). *Bird fancier's lung* (and the related disorders of duck fever, turkey handler's lung, and dove pillow's lung) is a response to inhalation of proteins from feathers and droppings. *Chemical worker's lung* is an example of how simple chemicals, such as isocyanates, may also cause immune-mediated diseases. In this case, antihapten antibodies may be responsible for the development of HP. Although HP requires an immunologic response to the inciting agent, such a response alone does not ensure the development of disease. Environmental factors such as ambient humidity and temperature play an important role in the development of disease, as do the concentration, frequency, and duration of exposure as well as the nature and size of the antigen particles. In some cases, the responsible exposure environment (for example, metalworking fluid) may be identified without implicating a specific antigen. Finally, personal habits may alter the apperance and course of disease: smokers appear more likely to present with chronic rather than acute HP, suggesting that smoking may inhibit antibody production.

PATHOGENESIS The finding that precipitating antibodies against extracts of moldy hay were demonstrable in most patients with farmer's lung led to the early conclusion that HP was an immune complex–mediated reaction. Sub-

TABLE 237-1 Selected Examples of Hypersensitivity Pneumonitis (HP)

Disease	Antigen	Source of Antigen
Bagassosis	Thermophilic actinomycetes[a]	"Moldy" bagasse (sugar cane)
Bird fancier's, breeder's, or handler's lung[b]	Parakeet, pigeon, chicken, turkey proteins	Avian droppings or feathers
Cephalosporium HP	Contaminated basement (sewage)	*Cephalosporium*
Cheese washer's lung	*Penicillium casei*	Moldy cheese
Chemical worker's lung[a]	Isocyanates	Polyurethane foam, varnishes, lacquer
Coffee worker's lung	Coffee bean dust	Coffee beans
Compost lung	*Aspergillus*	Compost
Detergent worker's disease	*Bacillus subtilis* enzymes (subtilisins)	Detergent
Familial HP	*Bacillus subtilis*	Contaminated wood dust in walls
Farmer's lung[a]	Thermophilic actinomycetes[b]	"Moldy" hay, grain, silage
Fish food lung	Unknown	Fish food
Fish meal worker's lung	Fish meal dust	Fish meal
Furrier's lung	Animal fur dust	Animal pelts
Hot tub lung	*Cladosporium* sp.	Mold on ceiling
Humidifier or air-conditioner lung (ventilation pneumonitis)	*Aureobasidium pullulans, Candida albicans,* other microorganisms	Contaminated water in humidification or forced-air air-conditioning systems
Japanese summer-type HP	*Trichosporon cutaneum, asahii,* and *mucoides*	House dust? Bird droppings
Laboratory worker's HP	Male rat urine	Laboratory rat
Lycoperdonosis	*Lycoperdon* puffballs	Puffball spores
Malt worker's lung	*Aspergillus fumigatus* or *A. clavatus*	Moldy barley
Maple bark disease	*Cryptostroma corticale*	Maple bark
Miller's lung	*Sitophilus granarius* (wheat weevil)	Infested wheat flour
Miscellaneous medication	Amiodarone, bleomycin, efavrienz, hydralazine, hydroxyurea, iosoniazid, methotrexate, paclitaxel, penicillin, procarbazine, propanolol, sulfasalazine	Medication
Mushroom worker's lung	Thermophilic actinomycetes,[b] *Hypsizigus marmoreus,* others	Mushroom compost
Pituitary snuff taker's lung	Animal proteins	Heterologous pituitary snuff
Potato riddler's lung	Thermophilic actinomycetes,[a] *Aspergillus*	"Moldy" hay around potatoes
Sauna taker's lung	*Aureobasidium* sp., other	Contaminated sauna water
Sausage worker's lung	*Penicillium nalgiovense*	Dry sausage mold
Sequoiosis	*Aureobasidium, Graphium* sp.	Redwood sawdust
Streptomyces albus HP	*Streptomyces albus*	Contaminated fertilizer
Suberosis	Cork dust mold	Cork dust
Tap water lung	Unknown	Contaminated tap water
Thatched roof disease	*Saccharomonospora viridis*	Dried grasses and leaves
Tobacco worker's disease	*Aspergillus* sp.	Mold on tobacco
Winegrower's lung	*Botrytis cinerea*	Mold on grapes
Wood trimmer's disease	*Rhizopus* sp., *Mucor* sp.	Contaminated wood trimmings
Woodman's disease	*Penicillium* sp.	Oak and maple trees
Woodworker's lung	Wood dust, *Alternaria*	Oak, cedar, pine, and mahogany dusts

[a] Thermophilic actinomycetes species include *Micropolyspora faeni, Thermoactinomyces vulgaris, T. saccharrii, T. viridis,* and *T. candidus.*
[b] Most common causes of hypersensitivity pneumonitis in the United States.

sequent investigations of HP in human beings and animal models provided evidence for the importance of cell-mediated hypersensitivity. The very early (acute) reaction is characterized by an increase in polymorphonuclear leukocytes in the alveoli and small airways. This early lesion is followed by an influx of mononuclear cells into the lung and the formation of granulomas that appear to be the result of a classic delayed (T cell mediated) hypersensitivity reaction to repeated inhalation of antigen and adjuvant-active materials. Studies in animal models suggest that the disease is a T_H1-mediated immune response to antigen, with both interferon-α and interleukin (IL) 12 contributing to disease expression. Most likely, multiple cytokines [including also IL-1β, transforming growth factor (TGF) β, tumor necrosis factor (TNF) α and others] interact to promote HP; their source includes both alveolar macrophages and T lymphocytes in the lung. Observations support a genetic predisposition to the development of HP; certain polymorphisms of the TNF-α promoter region reportedly confer an enhanced susceptibility to pigeon breeder's disease.

The attraction and accumulation of inflammatory cells in the lung

may be due to one or more of the following mechanisms: induction of the adhesion molecules L-selectin and E-selectin; elaboration by dendritic cells of CC chemokine 1 [dendritic cell–derived chemokine-1 (DC-CK-1)/cysteine-cysteine chemokine 18 (CCL18)]; and increased levels of Fas protein and FasL in the lung. Bronchoalveolar lavage (BAL) in patients with HP consistently demonstrates an increase in T lymphocytes in lavage fluid (a finding that is also observed in patients with other granulomatous lung disorders). Patients with recent or continual exposure to antigen may have an increase in polymorphonuclear leukocytes in lavage fluid; this has been associated with lung fibrosis. A role for oxidant injury has been proposed in HP, which is supported by the finding that BAL levels of the antioxidant glutathione are reduced following airway challenge in patients with HP, whereas they are increased in asymptomatic controls. In most patients examined during recovery from acute disease, the T lymphocytes in lavage fluid are predominantly the CD8+ T cell subset. In patients with very recent exposure to antigen, however, the numbers of CD4+ T cells may increase in lavage fluid. These observations and

1517

others in animal models suggest that there is an active modulation of granuloma formation in the lung by immunoregulatory T cells and associated cytokines in this disorder.

CLINICAL PRESENTATION The clinical picture is that of an interstitial pneumonitis, which varies from patient to patient and seems related to the frequency and intensity of exposure to the causative antigen and perhaps other host factors. The presentation can be *acute, subacute,* or *chronic*. In the *acute form,* symptoms such as cough, fever, chills, malaise, and dyspnea may occur 6 to 8 h after exposure to the antigen and usually clear within a few days if there is no further exposure to antigen. The *subacute form* often appears insidiously over a period of weeks marked by cough and dyspnea and may progress to cyanosis and severe dyspnea requiring hospitalization. In some patients, a subacute form of the disease may persist after an acute presentation of the disorder, especially if there is continued exposure to antigen. In most patients with the acute or subacute form of HP, the symptoms, signs, and other manifestations of HP disappear within days, weeks, or months if the causative agent is no longer inhaled. Transformation to a chronic form of the disease may occur in patients with continued antigen exposure, but the frequency of such progression is uncertain. The *chronic form* of HP may be clinically indistinguishable from pulmonary fibrosis due to a wide variety of causes. Physical examination may reveal clubbing. This stage may progressively worsen, resulting in dependence on supplemental oxygen, pulmonary hypertension, and death from respiratory failure. An indolent, gradually progressive form of the disease can be associated with cough and exertional dyspnea without a prior history consistent with acute or subacute manifestations. Such a gradual onset frequently occurs with low-dose exposure to the antigen.

As strict definitions of acute, subacute, and chronic stages of hypersensitivity pneumonitis have not been generally agreed on, interpretation of epidemiologic and clinical studies can be difficult. Because of this, it has been proposed that hypersensitivity pneumonitis be described as recently diagnosed, recurrent or progressive, or residual disease. For these categories, required diagnostic criteria include the history of symptoms following an exposure to a putative HP agent and symptoms associated with re-exposure; compatible radiologic findings; if performed, lymphocytic alveolitis on BAL; and, if performed, compatible histopathology on biopsy. Supportive criteria include bibasilar crackles, diminished carbon monoxide diffusion capacity, and hypoxemia.

DIAGNOSIS Following acute exposure to antigen, neutrophilia and lymphopenia are frequently present. Eosinophilia is not a feature. All forms of the disease may be associated with elevations in erythrocyte sedimentation rate, C-reactive protein, rheumatoid factor, and serum immunoglobulins. Antinuclear antibodies are rarely present and appear to have no pathogenic role. Examination for *serum precipitins* against suspected antigens, such as those listed in Table 237-1, is an important part of the diagnostic workup and should be performed on any patient with interstitial lung disease, especially if a suggestive exposure history is elicited. If found, precipitins indicate sufficient exposure to the causative agent for generation of an immunologic response. The diagnosis of HP is not established solely by the presence of precipitins, however, as precipitins are found in sera of many individuals exposed to appropriate antigens who demonstrate no other evidence of HP. False-negative results may occur because of poor-quality antigens or an inappropriate choice of antigens. Extraction of antigens from the suspected source may at times be helpful.

Chest x-ray shows no specific or distinctive changes in HP. It can be normal even in symptomatic patients. The acute or subacute phase may be associated with poorly defined, patchy, or diffuse infiltrates or with discrete, nodular infiltrates. In the chronic phase, the chest x-ray usually shows a diffuse reticulonodular infiltrate. Honeycombing may eventually develop as the condition progresses. Apical sparing is common, suggesting that disease severity correlates with inhaled antigen

load, but no particular distribution or pattern is classic for HP. Abnormalities rarely seen in HP include pleural effusion or thickening, and hilar adenopathy. High-resolution chest computed tomography (CT) has become the procedure of choice for imaging of HP, and a consensus is developing as to the typical appearance of the disease. Although pathognomonic features have not been identified, ground grass changes predominate in the lower lobes, especially in acute disease; this pattern is more common in workers whose exposure to antigen continues rather than those in whom removal from antigen exposure has occurred. Centrilobular nodules are also commonly seen. In chronic HP, patchy emphysema is seen more often than interstitial fibrosis, although neither predominates in the lower lobes; CT is far more sensitive than plain films at detecting these changes. Hilar or mediastinal adenopathy is not associated with HP, but its presence has no diagnostic significance (Fig. 237-1). Although not currently clinically used, *radionuclide studies* may have a role in the future diagnosis of HP: several case reports have inadvertently demonstrated rapid pulmonary uptake of radionuclides associated with a lymphocytic alveolitis in acute HP.

Pulmonary function studies in all forms of HP may show a restrictive or obstructive pattern with loss of lung volumes, impaired diffusion capacity, decreased compliance, and an exercise-induced hypoxemia. A resting hypoxemia may also be found. Bronchospasm and bronchial hyperreactivity are sometimes found in acute hypersensitivity pneumonitis. With antigen avoidance, the pulmonary function abnormalities are usually reversible, but they may gradually increase in severity or may occur rapidly following acute or subacute exposure to antigen.

Bronchoalveolar lavage is used in some centers to aid in diagnostic evaluation. A marked lymphocytic alveolitis on (BAL) is almost universal, although not pathognomonic. Lymphocytes typically have a decreased helper/suppressor ratio, and are activated. Alveolar neutrophilia is also prominent acutely, but tends to fade in the absence of recurrent exposure. Bronchoalveolar mastocytosis may correlate with disease activity. *Lung biopsy,* obtained through flexible bronchoscopy, open-lung procedures, or thoracoscopy, may be diagnostic. Although the histopathology is distinctive, it may not be pathognomonic of HP (Fig. 237-2). When the biopsy is taken during the active phase of disease, typical findings include an interstitial alveolar infiltrate consisting of plasma cells, lymphocytes, and occasional eosinophils and neutrophils, usually with accompanying loose, noncaseating peribronchial granulomas. Interstitial fibrosis may be present but most often is mild in earlier stages of the disease. Some degree of bronchiolitis is found in about half the cases, whereas vasculitis is not a feature of the

FIGURE 237-1 Chest CT scan of a case of acute hypersensitivity pneumonitis in which scattered regions of ground glass and nodular infiltrates are seen bilaterally. *(Courtesy of IS Wilson.)*

FIGURE 237-2 Open lung biopsy of a case of acute hypersensitivity pneumonitis demonstrating loose, nonnecrotizing granulomas and thickened interstitium with an associated interstitial inflammatory response. (*Courtesy of B DeYoung.*)

disorder. Rarely, bronchiolitis obliterans with organizing pneumonia (BOOP) can be seen. The triad of mononuclear bronchiolitis; interstitial infiltrates of lymphocytes and plasma cells; and single, nonnecrotizing, and randomly scattered parenchymal granulomas without mural vascular involvement is consistent with but not specific for HP.

Inhalation challenge studies have been described as useful to differentiate between HP and other interstitial lung diseases; a positive response to inhaled antigen may include fever, chills, dyspnea, diminished oxygen saturation, transient airflow obstruction, and peripheral and bronchoalveolar leukocytosis. These tests should be performed in a center that specializes in provocation testing for reasons of both safety and accuracy. Moreover, as the antigens used for provocation testing are not standardized, interpretation of these tests is difficult. In general, these tests may be used to support a diagnosis of HP, but they are not sufficiently accepted to either confirm or deny the diagnosis. The lack of standardized, nonirritating antigens and of proven controlled protocols makes *skin testing* useful only for research purposes. Similarly, in vitro tests of cell-mediated (delayed) hypersensitivity have not consistently been shown to correlate with clinical HP and have no place in the routine diagnostic workup.

In summary, the diagnosis in most cases is established by (1) consistent history, physical findings, pulmonary function tests, and chest x-ray; (2) exposure to a recognized antigen; and (3) finding an antibody to that antigen. In a few circumstances, (BAL) and/or lung biopsy may be needed. Provocation tests may be useful but are not essential. The most important tool in diagnosing HP may, in fact, be a high index of suspicion.

DIFFERENTIAL DIAGNOSIS Chronic HP may often be difficult to distinguish from a number of other interstitial lung disorders such as idiopathic pulmonary fibrosis, sarcoidosis, interstitial lung disease associated with a collagen vascular disorder, and drug-induced lung diseases. A negative history for use of relevant drugs and no evidence of a systemic disorder usually exclude the presence of drug-induced lung disease or a collagen vascular disorder. BAL often shows predominance of neutrophils in idiopathic pulmonary fibrosis and a predominance of CD4+ lymphocytes in sarcoidosis. Hilar/paratracheal lymphadenopathy or evidence of multisystem involvement also favors the diagnosis of sarcoidosis. In some patients, a lung biopsy may be required to differentiate chronic HP from other interstitial diseases. The lung disease associated with acute or subacute HP may clinically resemble other disorders that present with systemic symptoms and recurrent pulmonary infiltrates, including the allergic bronchopulmonary mycoses and other eosinophilic pneumonias.

Eosinophilic pneumonia is often associated with asthma and is typified by peripheral eosinophilia; neither of these is a feature of HP.

Allergic bronchopulmonary aspergillosis (ABPA) is the most common example of the allergic bronchopulmonary mycoses and is sometimes confused with HP because of the presence of precipitating antibodies to *Aspergillus fumigatus*. ABPA is associated with allergic (atopic) asthma. Acute HP may be confused with *organic dust toxic syndrome* (ODTS), a condition that is more common than HP. ODTS follows heavy exposure to organic dusts and is characterized by transient fever and muscle aches, with or without dyspnea and cough. Serum precipitins are absent and the chest x-ray is usually normal. Studies have shown no immunologic basis for ODTS, and endotoxin is suspected to be involved in its pathogenesis. This distinction is important, as ODTS is a self-limited disorder without significant long-term sequelae, whereas continued antigen exposure in HP can result in permanent disability. Massive exposure to moldy silage may result in a syndrome termed *pulmonary mycotoxicosis*, with fever, chills, and cough and the presence of pulmonary infiltrates within a few hours of exposure. No previous sensitization is required, and precipitins are absent to *Aspergillus*, the suspected causative agent.

℞ TREATMENT

Because effective treatment depends largely on avoiding the antigen, identification of the causative agent and its source is essential. This is usually possible if the physician takes a careful environmental and occupational history or, if necessary, visits the patient's environment. The simplest way to avoid the incriminated agent is to remove the patient from the environment or the source of the agent from the patient's environment. This recommendation cannot be taken lightly when it completely changes the lifestyle or livelihood of the patient. In many cases, however, the source of exposure (birds, humidifiers) can easily be removed. If occupational exposure is involved, an initial attempt can be made at antigen avoidance maneuvers least disruptive to the patient's livelihood, which usually means avoiding areas associated with heavy exposure and wearing an appropriate mask. This will not suffice for small-molecular-weight agents such as isocyanates, which require more elaborate respiratory systems. Pollen masks, personal dust respirators, airstream helmets, and ventilated helmets with a supply of fresh air are increasingly efficient means of purifying inhaled air. If symptoms recur or physiologic abnormalities progress in spite of these measures, then more effective measures to avoid antigen exposure must be pursued. Compromises with environmental control pertain primarily to the acute, recurrent, transient clinical form of HP and must be accompanied by careful follow-up. Subacute forms are ordinarily the result of a heavy, sustained exposure. The chronic form typically results from low-grade or recurrent exposure over many months to years, and the lung disease may already be partially or completely irreversible. These patients are usually advised to avoid all possible contact with the offending agent, although follow-up studies of farmer's lung and bird fancier's lung have found resolution of the disease despite continued exposure in some patients.

Patients with the *acute*, recurrent form of HP usually recover without need for glucocorticoids. *Subacute* HP may be associated with severe symptoms and marked physiologic impairment and may continue to progress for several days despite hospitalization. Urgent establishment of the diagnosis and prompt institution of glucocorticoid treatment are indicated in such patients. Such therapy may also hasten recovery in patients with lesser involvement. Prednisone at a dosage of 1 mg/kg per day or its equivalent is continued for 7 to 14 days and then tapered over the ensuing 2 to 6 weeks at a rate that depends on the patient's clinical status. Patients with *chronic* HP may gradually recover without therapy following environmental control. In many patients, however, a trial of prednisone may be useful to obtain maximal reversibility of the lung disease. Following initial prednisone therapy (1 mg/kg per day for 2 to 4 weeks), the drug is tapered to the lowest dosage that will maintain the functional status of the patient. Many patients will not require or benefit from long-term therapy if there is no further exposure to antigen. Available studies report no effect of glucocorticoid therapy on long-term prognosis of farmer's lung.

PULMONARY INFILTRATES WITH EOSINOPHILIA

Pulmonary infiltrates with eosinophilia (PIE, eosinophilic pneumonias) include distinct individual syndromes characterized by eosinophilic pulmonary infiltrates and, commonly, peripheral blood eosinophilia. Since Loeffler's initial description of a transient, benign syndrome of migratory pulmonary infiltrates and peripheral blood eosinophilia of unknown cause, this group of disorders has been enlarged to include several diseases of both known and unknown etiology (Table 237-2). These diseases may be considered as immunologically mediated lung diseases, but are not to be confused with HP, in which eosinophilia is not a feature. When an eosinophilic pneumonia is associated with bronchial asthma, it is important to determine if the patient has atopic asthma and has wheal-and-flare skin reactivity to *Aspergillus* or other relevant fungal antigens. If so, other criteria should be sought for diagnosis of ABPA (Table 237-3) or other, rarer examples of allergic bronchopulmonary mycosis such as those caused by *Penicillium*, *Candida*, *Curvularia*, or *Helminthosporium* spp. *A. fumigatus* is the most common cause of ABPA, although other *Aspergillus* species have also been implicated. ABPA has been reported to complicate cystic fibrosis. The chest roentgenogram in ABPA may show transient, recurrent infiltrates or may suggest the presence of proximal bronchiectasis. High-resolution chest CT is a sensitive, noninvasive technique for the recognition of proximal bronchiectasis. The bronchial asthma of ABPA likely involves an IgE-mediated hypersensitivity, whereas the bronchiectasis associated with this disorder is thought to result from a deposition of immune complexes in proximal airways. Adequate treatment usually requires the long-term use of systemic glucocorticoids.

Tropical eosinophilia is usually caused by filarial infection; however, eosinophilic pneumonias also occur with other parasites such as *Ascaris*, *Ancyclostoma* sp., *Toxocara* sp., and *Strongyloides stercoralis*. Tropical eosinophilia due to *Wuchereria bancrofti* or *W. malayi* occurs most commonly in southern Asia, Africa, and South America, and is treated successfully with diethylcarbamazine.

Drug-induced eosinophilic pneumonias are exemplified by acute reactions to nitrofurantoin, which may begin 2 h to 10 days after nitrofurantoin is started, with symptoms of dry cough, fever, chills, and dyspnea; an eosinophilic pleural effusion accompanying patchy or diffuse pulmonary infiltrates may also occur. Other drugs associated with eosinophilic pneumonias include sulfonamides, penicillin, chlorpropamide, thiazides, tricyclic antidepressants, hydralazine, mephenesin, mecamylamine, nickel carbonyl vapor, gold salts, isoniazid, para-amnosalicylic acid, indomethacin, and others. One recent report has identified anti-TNF-α monoclonal antibody therapy as a cause of eosinophilic pneumonitis. Treatment consists of withdrawal of the incriminated drugs and the use of glucocorticoids, if necessary. The eosinophilia-myalgia syndrome, caused by dietary supplements of impure L-tryptophan, is occasionally associated with pulmonary infiltrates.

TABLE 237-2 Pulmonary Infiltrates with Eosinophilia

ETIOLOGY KNOWN

Allergic bronchopulmonary mycoses
Parasitic infestations
Drug reactions
Eosinophilia-myalgia syndrome

IDIOPATHIC

Loeffler's syndrome
Acute eosinophilic pneumonia
Chronic eosinophilic pneumonia
Allergic granulomatosis of Churg and Strauss
Hypereosinophilic syndrome

TABLE 237-3 Diagnostic Features of Allergic Bronchopulmonary Aspergillosis (ABPA)

MAIN DIAGNOSTIC CRITERIA

Bronchial asthma
Pulmonary infiltrates
Peripheral eosinophilia ($>1000/\mu L$)
Immediate wheal-and-flare response to *A. fumigatus*
Serum precipitins to *A. fumigatus*
Elevated serum IgE
Central bronchiectasis

OTHER DIAGNOSTIC FEATURES

History of brownish plugs in sputum
Culture of *A. fumigatus* from sputum
Elevated IgE (and IgG) class antibodies specific for *A. fumigatus*

The group of idiopathic eosinophilic pneumonias consists of diseases of varying severity. *Loeffler's syndrome* was originally reported as a benign, acute eosinophilic pneumonia of unknown cause characterized by migrating pulmonary infiltrates and minimal clinical manifestations. In some patients, these clinical characteristics may prove to be secondary to parasites or drugs. *Acute eosinophilic pneumonia* has been described as an idiopathic acute febrile illness of less than 7 days' duration with severe hypoxemia, pulmonary infiltrates, and no history of asthma. *Chronic eosinophilic pneumonia* presents with significant systemic symptoms including fever, chills, night sweats, cough, anorexia, and weight loss of several weeks' to months' duration. The chest x-ray classically shows peripheral infiltrates resembling a photographic negative of pulmonary edema. Some patients also have bronchial asthma of the intrinsic or nonallergic type. Dramatic clearing of symptoms and chest x-rays is often noted within 48 h after initiation of glucocorticoid therapy.

Allergic angiitis and granulomatosis of Churg and Strauss is a multisystem vasculitic disorder that frequently involves the skin, kidney, and nervous system in addition to the lung. The disorder may occur at any age and is almost invariably found in patients with a history of bronchial asthma. The asthma often is progressive until the onset of fever and exaggerated eosinophilia, at which time the symptoms of asthma may ease. The illness may be fulminating and the prognosis grave unless treated aggressively with glucocorticoids and, at times, immunosuppressive therapy. The use of leukotriene-modifying agents (zafirlukast, zyleuton, and montelukast) has been associated with Churg-Strauss syndrome, but it remains uncertain whether the drugs cause the disease or rather unmask previously undiagnosed vasculitis, perhaps suppressed by the use of inhaled or systemic glucocorticoids.

The *hypereosinophilic syndrome* is characterized by the presence of over 1500 eosinophils per microliter of peripheral blood for 6 months or longer; lack of evidence for parasitic, allergic, or other known causes of eosinophilia; and signs or symptoms of multisystem organ dysfunction. Consistent features are blood and bone marrow eosinophilia with tissue infiltration by relatively mature eosinophils. The heart may be involved with tricuspid valve abnormalities or endomyocardial fibrosis and a restrictive, biventricular cardiomyopathy. Other organs affected typically include the lungs, liver, spleen, skin, and nervous system. Therapy of the disorder consists of glucocorticoids and/or hydroxyurea, plus therapy as needed for cardiac dysfunction, which is frequently responsible for much of the morbidity and mortality in this syndrome. Pulmonary eosinophilia has also been associated with T cell lymphoma, and has been reported following lung and bone marrow transplantation.

FURTHER READING

CORMIER Y et al: High-resolution computed tomographic characteristics in acute farmer's lung and in its follow-up. Eur Respir J 16:56, 2000

GLAZER CS et al: Acute eosinophilic pneumonia in AIDS. Chest 120:1732, 2001

JOHKOH T et al: Eosinophilic lung diseases: Diagnostic accuracy of thin-section CT in 111 patients. Radiology 216:773, 2000

KATZENSTEIN AL: Diagnostic features and differential diagnosis of Churg-Strauss syndrome in the lung. A review. Am J Clin Pathol 114:767, 2000

KAZUYOSHI K et al: Expression of FasL and Fas protein and their soluble form in patients with hypersensitivity pneumonitis. Int Arch Allergy Immunol 122:209, 2000

NAVARRO C et al: Up-regulation of L-selectin and E-selectin in hypersensitivity pneumonitis. Chest 121:354, 2002

OHTANI Y et al: Inhalation provocation tests in chronic bird fancier's lung. Chest 118:1382, 2000

PARDO A et al: Increase of lung neutrophils in hypersensitivity pneumonitis is associated with lung fibrosis. Am J Respir Crit Care Med 161:1698, 2000

PATEL AM et al: Hypersensitivity pneumonitis: Current concepts and future questions. J Allergy Clin Immunol 108:661, 2001

ROSENOW EC III et al: Drug-induced pulmonary disease. An update. Chest 102:239, 1992

ZACHARISEN MC et al: The long-term outcome in acute, subacute, and chronic forms of pigeon breeder's disease hypersensitivity pneumonitis. Ann Allergy Asthma Immunol 88:175, 2002

238 ENVIRONMENTAL LUNG DISEASES
Frank E. Speizer

This chapter provides perspectives on ways to assess pulmonary diseases for which environmental or occupational causes are suspected. This assessment is important because removal of the patient from harmful exposure is often the only intervention that might prevent further significant deterioration or lead to improvement in a patient's condition. Furthermore, the identification of an environment-associated disease in a single patient may lead to primary preventive strategies affecting other similarly exposed people who have not yet developed disease.

The exact magnitude of the problem is unknown, but there is no question that large numbers of individuals are at risk for developing serious respiratory disease as a result of occupational or environmental exposures. For example, recent estimates suggest that approximately 2.4 million workers in the United States have been exposed to crystalline silica or asbestos dust in mining and nonmining industries. Even if only 5% of these workers (a conservative estimate) are to suffer from respiratory disease as a result of their exposure, this figure represents more than 100,000 individuals.

HISTORY AND PHYSICAL EXAMINATION

The patient's history is of paramount importance in assessing any potential occupational or environmental exposure. Inquiry into specific work practices should include questions about specific contaminants involved, the availability and use of personal respiratory protection devices, the size and ventilation of workspaces, and whether coworkers have similar complaints. The temporal association of exposure at work and symptoms may provide clues to occupation-related disease. In addition, the patient must be questioned about alternative sources for potentially toxic exposures, including hobbies or other environmental exposures at home. Short-term exposures to potential toxic agents in the distant past must also be considered (Chap. 376).

Many people are aware of the potential hazards in their workplaces, and many states require that employees be informed about potentially hazardous exposures. These requirements include the provision of specific educational materials (including Material Safety Data Sheets), personal protective equipment and instructions in its use, and information on environmental control procedures. Reminders posted in the workplace may warn workers about hazardous substances. Protective clothing, lockers, and shower facilities may be considered necessary parts of the job. However, even in these more progressive industries, the introduction of new processes, particularly when related to the use of new chemical compounds, may change exposure significantly, and often only the employee on the production line is aware of the change. For the physician who regularly sees patients from a particular industry, a visit to the work site can be very instructive. Alternatively, physicians can request inspections by appropriate federal and/or state authorities.

The physical examination of patients with environment-related lung diseases may help to determine the nature and severity of the pulmonary condition. Unfortunately, the pulmonary response to most injurious agents is the development of a limited number of nonspecific physical signs. These findings do not point to the specific causative agent, and other types of information must be used to arrive at an etiologic diagnosis.

PULMONARY FUNCTION TESTS AND CHEST RADIOGRAPHY

Many mineral dusts produce characteristic alterations in the mechanics of breathing and lung volumes that clearly indicate a restrictive pattern (Chaps. 234 and 243). Exposures to a number of organic dusts or chemical agents capable of producing occupational asthma result in pronounced obstructive patterns of pulmonary dysfunction that may be reversible (Chap. 236). Measurement of change in forced expiratory volume (FEV_1) before and after a working shift can be used to detect an acute inflammatory or bronchoconstrictive response. An acute decrement of FEV_1 over the first work shift of the week is a characteristic feature of cotton textile workers with byssinosis.

The chest radiograph is useful in detecting and monitoring the pulmonary response to mineral dusts. The International Labour Organisation (ILO) International Classification of Radiographs of Pneumoconioses classifies chest radiographs according to the nature and size of opacities seen and the extent of involvement of the parenchyma. In general, opacities may be round or irregular, small (<10 mm in diameter) or large. They may be few in number, with visible normal lung markings, partially obscure normal markings, or totally obscure normal markings. Although useful for screening large numbers of workers, the ILO system lacks specificity and may over- or underestimate the functional impact of pneumoconiosis. With dusts causing rounded, regular opacities like those evident in coal worker's pneumoconiosis, the degree of involvement on the chest radiograph may be extensive, while pulmonary function may be only minimally impaired. In contrast, in pneumoconiosis causing linear, irregular opacities like those seen in asbestosis, the radiograph may lead to underestimation of the severity of the impairment until relatively late in the disease. For the individual patient with a history of exposure, conventional computed tomography (CT) and high-resolution computed tomography (HRCT) have improved the sensitivity of identifying diffuse parenchymal abnormalities of the lung. The procedures have been shown to provide earlier detection of silicosis and asbestosis.

Other diagnostic procedures of use in identifying environment-induced lung disease include evaluation of heavy metal concentrations in urine (arsenic in smelter workers, cadmium in battery plant workers); bacteriologic studies (tuberculosis in medical care personnel, anthrax in wool sorters); fungal studies (coccidioidomycosis in southwestern farm workers, histoplasmosis in poultry or pigeon handlers); and serologic studies (psittacosis in pet shop workers or owners of sick birds, Q fever in tanners or slaughterhouse workers). Ultimately, a lung biopsy may be required both for morphologic diagnosis of the underlying pulmonary disease and for attempted identification of the specific etiologic agent.

MEASUREMENT OF EXPOSURE

If reliable environmental sampling data are available, this information should be used in assessing a patient's exposure. Since many of the chronic diseases result from exposure over many years, current environmental measurements should be combined with work histories to arrive at estimates of past exposure.

In situations where individual exposure to specific agents—either in a work setting or via ambient air pollutants—has been determined, transport of these agents through the airways may be an important factor affecting dose. Highly soluble gases such as sulfur dioxide are absorbed in the upper airway and presumably produce their effects by reflex response of sensitive neural fibrils in the trachea or larger airways. In contrast, nitrogen dioxide, which is less soluble, may reach the bronchioles and alveoli in sufficient quantities to result in an acute life-threatening disease in farmers exposed even briefly to the gas evolved from moldy hay in silos (silo-filler's disease).

Particle size and chemistry of air contaminants must also be considered. Particles above 10 to 15 μm in diameter, because of their settling velocities in air, do not penetrate beyond the upper airways. These larger particles are often referred to as "fugitive dusts" and include pollens, other windblown dusts, and dusts resulting from mechanical industrial processes. They have little or no role in chronic respiratory disease except perhaps as related to cancer (see below).

Particles below 10 μm in size are created by the burning of fossil fuels or high-temperature industrial processes resulting in condensation products from gases, fumes, or vapors. These particles are divided into three size fractions on the basis of their size characteristics and sources. Particles of approximately 2.5 to 10 μm (coarse-mode fraction) contain crustal elements, such as silica, aluminum, and iron. These particles mostly deposit relatively high in the tracheobronchial tree. Although the total mass of an ambient sample is dominated by these larger respirable particles, the number of particles, and therefore the surface area on which potential toxic agents can deposit and be carried to the lower airways, is dominated by particles smaller than 2.5 μm (fine-mode fraction or accumulation mode). The smallest particles, those less than 0.1 μm in size, represent the ultrafine fraction and make up the largest number of particles, which tend to remain in the airstream and deposit in the lung only on a random basis as they come into contact with the alveolar walls.

Besides the size characteristics of particles and the solubility of gases, the actual chemical composition, mechanical properties, and immunogenicity or infectivity of inhaled material determine in large part the nature of the diseases found among exposed persons.

OCCUPATIONAL EXPOSURES AND PULMONARY DISEASE

Table 238-1 provides broad categories of exposure in the workplace and diseases associated with chronic exposure in these industries.

ASBESTOSIS

Except in localized regions with single industrial exposures, such as coal-mining or granite-quarrying regions, the most frequent inorganic dust-related chronic pulmonary diseases are associated with industries using *asbestiform fibers*. *Asbestos* is a generic term for several different mineral silicates, including chrysolite, amosite, anthophyllite, and crocidolite. Besides workers involved in the mining, milling, and manufacturing of asbestos products, workers in the building trades, including pipe fitters and boilermakers, were exposed to asbestos, which was widely used in construction because of its exceptional thermal and electric insulation properties. In addition, asbestos was used in the manufacture of fire-smothering blankets and safety garments, as filler for plastic materials, in cement and floor tiles, and in friction materials, such as brake and clutch linings.

Exposure to asbestos is not limited to persons who directly handle the material. Cases of asbestos-related diseases have been encountered in individuals with only moderate exposure, such as the painter or electrician who works alongside the insulation worker in a shipyard or the housewife who does no more than shake out and wash her husband's work clothes. Community exposure has probably resulted from the use of asbestos-containing material sprayed on steel girders in many large buildings as a safety feature to prevent buckling in case of fire.

Asbestos was first used extensively in the 1940s. Starting in 1975 it was mostly replaced with synthetic mineral fibers, such as fiberglass or slag wool, but it continues to be used increasingly in the developing world. Despite current regulations mandating adequate training for any worker potentially exposed to asbestos, exposure probably continues among inexperienced demolition workers. The major health effects from exposure to asbestos are pulmonary fibrosis (asbestosis) and cancers of the respiratory tract, the pleura, and (in rare cases) the peritoneum.

Asbestosis is a diffuse interstitial fibrosing disease of the lung that is directly related to the intensity and duration of exposure. Except for its association with a history of exposure to asbestos (generally in a work setting), asbestosis resembles the other forms of diffuse interstitial fibrosis (Chap. 243). Usually, moderate to severe exposure has taken place for at least 10 years before the disease becomes manifest.

Physiologic studies reveal a restrictive pattern with a decrease in lung volumes. Flow rates are commonly reduced less than would be predicted on the basis of the volume reduction. An early sign of severe disease may be a reduction in diffusing capacity.

Pulmonary fibrosis may occur following sufficient exposure to any of the asbestiform fiber types. The fibrotic lesions result from proinflammatory effects of reactive oxygen species released from phagocytes reacting with transition metals on the surface of the fibers. The clinical manifestations are typical of those physical findings in any patient with pulmonary fibrosis (Chap. 243).

DIAGNOSIS The chest radiograph can be used to detect a number of manifestations of asbestos exposure as well as to identify specific lesions. Past exposure is specifically indicated by pleural plaques, which are characterized by either thickening or calcification along the parietal pleura, particularly along the lower lung fields, the diaphragm, and the cardiac border. Without additional manifestations, pleural plaques imply only exposure, not pulmonary impairment. Benign pleural effusions may occur, particularly in patients with asbestosis, but are not necessarily restricted to those with overt disease. The fluid is sterile but may be a serous or blood-stained exudate and may occur bilaterally. The effusion may be slowly progressive or may resolve spontaneously.

The radiographic diagnosis of asbestosis depends on the presence of irregular or linear opacities, usually first noted in the lower lung fields and spreading into the middle and upper lung fields as the disease progresses. An indistinct heart border or a "ground glass" appearance in the lung fields is seen in some cases. In cases in which the x-ray changes are less obvious, HRCT may show distinct changes of subpleural curvilinear lines 5 to 10 cm in length that appear to be parallel to the pleural surface.

In general, newly diagnosed cases will have resulted from exposure levels that were present many years before and, in spite of the patients' having left the industry, are attributable to that former exposure. Since the patient may be eligible for compensation within a specific time frame after the diagnosis of an asbestos-related disease is made, the physician making the diagnosis should be certain to inform the patient promptly. On occasion, the physician may have reason to suspect ongoing exposure from a patient's current job description or actual monitoring data. In such cases, federal or state health authorities may need to be notified.

Casual, nonoccupational exposure to undisturbed sources of asbestos-containing materials—e.g., in walls of schools or other buildings—represents little if any hazard to people who inhabit or work in such buildings. Because the association of smoking and asbestos exposure increases the risk of developing lung cancer (see below), it is extremely important to advise patients with a history of exposure to asbestos to stop smoking. No specific therapy is available in the management of patients with asbestosis. The supportive care is the same as that given to any patient with diffuse interstitial fibrosis from any cause.

Lung cancer (Chap. 75), either squamous cell carcinoma or adenocarcinoma, is the most frequent cancer associated with asbestos ex-

Occupational Exposures	Estimated Number of Workers Exposed	Nature of Respiratory Responses
Inorganic dusts		
Asbestos: mining	~250,000	Fibrosis (asbestosis), COPD, cancer, mesothelioma
Processing, nonagricultural	4.20×10^6	
Silica: mining, stone cutting, construction, quarrying	2.3×10^6	Fibrosis (silicosis), PMF, silicotuberculosis
Coal dust: mining	200,000	Fibrosis, pneumoconiosis
Beryllium: processing alloys for high tech industries	800,000	Acute pneumonitis, chronic granulomatous disease
Other metals: aluminum, chromium, cobalt, nickel, titanium, tungsten	~500,000	Wide variety of conditions from acute pneumonitis to lung cancer and asthma
Organic dusts		
Cotton dust: milling, processing	>800,000	Chronic bronchitis, reduced pulmonary function, byssinosis
Grain dust: elevator agents, dock workers, milling, bakers	>500,000	Asthma, chronic phlegm production, obstructive airways disease
Other agricultural dusts: fungal spores, vegetable product, insect fragments, animal dander, bird and rodent feces, endotoxins, microorganisms, pollens	$~5 \times 10^6$	Hypersensitivity pneumonitis (farmers' lung), asthma, chronic bronchitis
Toxic chemicals: wide variety of industries—see Table 238-3	$>9 \times 10^6$ (does not include firefighters)	See Table 238-2
Other respiratory environmental carcinogens (proven or highly suspect): uranium and radon daughters, environmental tobacco smoke, nickel compounds, chromium salts, polycyclic hydrocarbons, mustard gas, diesel exhaust, welding fumes, woods or wood finishing products	Essentially unknowable, but a major fraction of U.S. population is exposed to low environmental levels of one or more of these agents	Estimates vary from ~3% to <10% of all lung cancers

Note: COPD, chronic obstructive pulmonary disease; PMF, progressive massive fibrosis.

posure. The excess frequency of lung cancer in asbestos workers is associated with a minimum lapse of 15 to 19 years between first exposure and development of the disease. Persons with more exposure are at greater risk of disease. In addition, there appears to be a significant multiplicative effect that leads to a far greater risk of lung cancer in persons who are cigarette smokers and have asbestos exposure than would be expected from the additive risk of each factor. To date, efforts to consider these high-risk individuals for special surveillance studies, including sputum cytologic examinations and repeated chest x rays as frequently as every 4 to 6 months, have resulted in neither significant early detection nor prolonged survival once the lung cancer is found. The use of HRCT in such at-risk subjects is currently under investigation.

Mesotheliomas (Chap. 245), both pleural and peritoneal, are also associated with asbestos exposure. In contrast to lung cancers, these tumors do not appear to be associated with smoking. Relatively short-term asbestos exposures of 1 to 2 years or less occurring some 20 to 25 years in the past have been associated with the development of mesotheliomas (an observation that emphasizes the importance of obtaining a complete environmental exposure history). The risk for this type of tumor peaks 30 to 35 years after initial exposure. Since maximum exposure took place in the United States between 1930 and 1960, peak incidence of disease in men occurred in 1997, with a total of 2300 cases. Incidence is expected to decline over the next 30+ years to about 500 cases per year.

Although approximately 50% of mesotheliomas metastasize, the tumor generally is locally invasive, and death usually results from local extension. Most patients present with effusions that may obscure the underlying pleural tumor. In contrast to the findings in effusion due to other causes, because of the restriction placed on the chest wall, no shift of mediastinal structures toward the opposite side of the chest will be seen. The major diagnostic problem is differentiation from peripherally spreading pulmonary adenocarcinoma or from adenocarcinoma metastasized to pleura from an extrathoracic primary site. Although a needle biopsy may be diagnostic, an open biopsy is often necessary, and even the latter procedure may not provide a definitive diagnosis of the origin of the tumor.

Since epidemiologic studies have shown that more than 80% of mesotheliomas may be associated with asbestos exposure, documented mesothelioma in a worker with occupational exposure to asbestos may be compensable in many parts of the United States.

SILICOSIS

In spite of the technical adequacy of existing protective equipment, *free silica* (SiO_2), or crystalline quartz, is still a major occupational hazard. In the United States, estimates of potential numbers of exposed workers range between 1.2 and 3 million persons. The major occupational exposures include: mining; stonecutting; employment in abrasive industries, such as stone, clay, glass, and cement manufacturing; foundry work; packing of silica flour; and quarrying, particularly of granite. Most often, progressive pulmonary fibrosis (silicosis) occurs in a dose-response fashion after many years of exposure.

Workers exposed through sandblasting in confined spaces, tunneling through rock with high quartz content (15 to 25%), or the manufacture of abrasive soaps may develop acute silicosis with as little as 10 months' exposure. The disease may be rapidly fatal in less than 2 years, despite the discontinuation of exposure. A radiographic picture of profuse miliary infiltration or consolidation is characteristic of acute silicosis.

In long-term, less intense exposure, small rounded opacities in the upper lobes, with retraction and hilar adenopathy, classically appear on the radiograph after 15 to 20 years. Calcification of hilar nodes may occur in as many as 20% of cases and produces the characteristic "eggshell" pattern. These changes may be preceded by or associated with a reticular pattern of irregular densities that are uniformly present throughout the upper lung zones.

The nodular fibrosis may be progressive in the absence of further exposure, with coalescence and formation of nonsegmental conglomerates of irregular masses in excess of 1 cm in diameter. These masses become quite large and are characteristic of progressive massive fibrosis (PMF). Significant functional impairment with both restrictive and obstructive components may be associated with this form of silicosis. In the late stages of the disease, ventilatory failure may develop. In more subtle cases, CT may be helpful both in identifying nodules, which are preferentially located in the posterior aspect of the upper lobes, as well as in identifying larger opacities and more coalescence than might be noted on regular chest x-rays. Patients with silicosis are at greater risk of acquiring *Mycobacterium tuberculosis* infections (silicotuberculosis) and atypical mycobacterial infections. Because the frequency with which tuberculosis has been found at autopsy in patients with PMF exceeds considerably the frequency of premorbid diagnosis, treatment for tuberculosis is indicated in any patient with silicosis and a positive tuberculin test.

Other less hazardous silicates include Fuller's earth, kaolin, mica, diatomaceous earths, silica gel, soapstone, carbonate dusts, and cement dusts. The production of fibrosis in workers exposed to these agents is believed to be related either to the free silica content of these dusts or, for substances that contain no free silica, to the potentially large dust loads to which these workers may be exposed.

Other silicates, including *talc dusts*, may be contaminated with asbestos and/or free silica. Accidental exposure to significant quantities of talc may result in an acute syndrome with cough, cyanosis, and labored breathing (acute talcosis). Severe progressive fibrosis with respiratory failure may ensue within a few years. Fibrosis and/or pleural or lung cancer have been associated with chronic exposure to commercial talc. Pure talc does not produce fibrosis; thus, it is difficult to sort out whether the effects are due to the contamination of commercial talc by asbestos or by free silica.

COAL WORKER'S PNEUMOCONIOSIS (CWP)

Coal dust is associated with CWP, which has enormous social, economic, and medical significance in every nation in which coal mining is an important industry. Simple radiographically identified CWP is seen in 12% of all miners and in as many as 50% of anthracite miners with more than 20 years' work on the coal face. The prevalence of disease is lower in workers in bituminous coal mines. Since much western U.S. coal is bituminous, CWP is less prevalent in that region.

Much of the symptomatology associated with simple CWP appears to be similar and additive to the effects of cigarette smoking on the development of chronic bronchitis and obstructive lung disease (Chap. 242). In the early stages of simple CWP, radiographic abnormalities consist of small, irregular opacities (reticular pattern). With prolonged exposure, one sees small, rounded, regular opacities, 1 to 5 mm in diameter (nodular pattern). Calcification is generally not seen, although approximately 10% of older anthracite miners have calcified nodules.

Complicated CWP is manifested by the appearance on the chest radiograph of nodules ranging from 1 cm in diameter to the size of an entire lobe, generally confined to the upper half of the lungs. This condition, considered a form of PMF, is accompanied by a significant reduction in diffusing capacity and is associated with premature mortality.

Caplan's syndrome (Chap. 301), first described in coal miners but subsequently found in patients with a variety of pneumoconioses, includes seropositive rheumatoid arthritis with characteristic PMF. The syndrome suggests an immunopathologic mechanism. Over the past decade, the mechanisms by which the chronic inhalation of mineral dusts produce an increase in inflammatory cells (including macrophages and neutrophils), which in turn causes PMF, have been explored. All of these inorganic dusts can: (1) be directly cytotoxic; (2) stimulate reactive oxygen species; (3) activate macrophages to produce cytokines and enhance production of (anti)fibrogenic factors such as tumor necrosis factor-α; (4) increase protease activity; and (5) increase inactivation of α_1-antitrypsin and leukocyte elastase activity. The final pathologic pathway may be fibrosis resulting from the interactions of a variety of these mechanisms.

BERYLLIOSIS

Beryllium may produce an acute pneumonitis or, far more commonly, a chronic granulomatous disease. Unless one inquires specifically about occupational exposures to beryllium in the manufacture of alloys, ceramics, high-technology electronics, and (before the 1950s) the production of fluorescent lights, one may miss entirely the etiologic relationship to an occupational exposure. Nonspecific pulmonary function tests may be normal or may indicate evidence of restrictive disease. Between 2 and 15 years of exposure, depending on its intensity, are required for the disease to become manifest. On open lung biopsy, granulomatous formation similar to that seen in sarcoidosis (Chap. 309) may make differentiation impossible unless tissue levels of be-

ryllium are measured. Recent studies have identified T cell clones in the lungs of affected patients that suggest a gene-by-environment interaction that is necessary for the disease to become manifest.

Other hard metals, including aluminum powders, chromium, cobalt, titanium dioxide, and tungsten, may produce an interstitial pneumonitis, but this is rare.

OTHER INORGANIC DUSTS

Other dusts are considered *nuisance dusts* because their major environmental and health effects seem to be reduction in visibility and irritation of eyes, ears, nasal passages, and other mucous membranes, respectively. If they penetrate to the lower airways, these dusts do not affect the architecture of the terminal bronchioles or acinar spaces nor do they destroy collagen. Generally, clinical effects are reversible. Pulmonary function tests are usually normal unless another disease process coexists. If the dusts are radiodense, macular collections may produce striking radiographic pictures that are so characteristic that patients with a history of significant exposure are easily diagnosed as having the condition that bears the name reflecting the nature of the dust. Examples of radiodense dusts include iron and iron oxides from welding or silver finishing (*siderosis*); tin oxide used in metallurgy, color stabilization, printing, and the manufacture of porcelain, glass, and fabric (*stannosis*); and barium sulfate used as a catalyst for organic reactions, drilling mud components, and electroplating (*baritosis*). Other metal dusts producing similar radiodense pictures include *cerium dioxide* and *antimony salts*.

Most of the inorganic dusts discussed thus far are associated with the production of either dust macules or interstitial fibrotic changes in the lung. Another set of dusts (Table 238-2), along with some of the dusts previously discussed, is associated with chronic mucous hypersecretion (chronic bronchitis), with or without reduction of expiratory flow rates. These conditions are caused by cigarette smoking, and any effort to attribute some component of the disease to occupational and environmental exposures must take cigarette smoking into account. Most studies suggest an additive effect of dust exposure and smoking. The pattern of the effect is similar to that of cigarette smoking, suggesting that small airway inflammation may be the initial site of pathologic response in those cases associated with the development of obstructive lung disease. Cigarette smoke is usually the more noxious agent, and dust effects may be discernible only in nonsmokers.

ORGANIC DUSTS

Some of the specific diseases associated with organic dusts are discussed in detail in the chapters on asthma (Chap. 236) and hypersensitivity pneumonitis (Chap. 237). Many of these diseases are named for the specific setting in which they are found, e.g., farmer's lung, malt worker's disease, or mushroom worker's disease. Often the temporal relation of symptoms to exposure furnishes the best evidence for the diagnosis. Three occupational groups are singled out for discussion because they represent the largest proportion of people affected by the diseases resulting from organic dusts.

COTTON DUST (BYSSINOSIS) Estimates of the number of exposed persons in the United States vary, but probably over 800,000 persons are exposed occupationally to cotton, flax, or hemp in the production of yarns for cotton, linen, and rope making. Although this discussion focuses on cotton, the same syndrome—albeit somewhat less severe—has been reported in association with exposure to flax, hemp, and jute.

Exposure occurs throughout the manufacturing process but is most pronounced in those portions of the factory involved with the treatment of the cotton prior to spinning—i.e., blowing, mixing, and carding (straightening of fibers). Attempts to control dust levels by use of exhaust hoods, general increases in ventilation, and wetting procedures in some settings have been highly successful. However, respiratory protective equipment appears to be required during certain operations to prevent workers from being exposed to levels of dust that exceed the current U.S. cotton dust standard.

TABLE 238-2 *Selected Occupational Dusts Believed to Be Associated with Mucous Hypersecretion and/or Obstructive Airway Disease and Other Respiratory Diseases[a]*

Agent (Exposure)	Mucous Hypersecretion	Obstruction	Other Conditions[b]
INORGANIC DUSTS			
Antimony (storage batteries, solder, ceramics, glass, plastics)	X		P
Arsenic (manufacture of pesticides, pigments, glass, alloys)	X		C
Barium and compounds including BaO, BaSO$_4$, BaCO$_3$ (catalysts, drilling mud, electroplating)	X		P
Cadmium dust (electroplating, battery manufacture, welding, smelting, aluminum soldering)	X	X	P
Cement dust (construction trades, manufacture of cement blocks)	X	X	
Chromium and CrO$_3$, CrF$_2$ (corrosion inhibitor pigment, metallurgy, electroplating)	X		C
Coal dust (mining)	X		P
Coke oven emissions (retort house, coke ovens)	X	X	P, C
Graphite (steelmaking, lubricants, pencils, paints, stove polish)	X	X	P
Iron dust (steel and nonferrous foundry workers, welding)	X		P
Mica (insulation, roofing shingles, oil refining, rubber manufacturing)	X		P
Phosphorus, elemental chlorides, sulfides (manufacture of fireworks, agricultural chemicals, insecticides, pesticides)	X	X	
Rock dusts (miners, tunnelers, quarry workers)	X		P
Vanadium pentoxide (welding electrodes, additive to steel, by product in ash from oil burning)	X	X	
ORGANIC DUSTS (SEE CHAP. 237)			
Cotton dust, flax, hemp (manufacture of yarns for linen, rope, cotton; ginning, cottonseed crushing; waste fiber processing)	X	X	
Grain dusts (farmers, workers in grain elevators, barge and grain ship crew members)	X	X	
Moldy hay (farmers, other animal attendants)	X		HP

[a] The table excludes agents associated with asthma as the primary disease (see Chap. 236).
[b] Other conditions include hypersensitivity pneumonitis (HP), pneumoconiosis (P), and cancers (C).
Note: X indicates that mucous hypersecretion or obstruction is associated with exposure.

Byssinosis is characterized clinically as occasional (early stage) and then regular (late stage) chest tightness toward the end of the first day of the workweek ("Monday chest tightness"). In epidemiologic studies, depending on the level of exposure via the carding room air, up to 80% of employees may show a significant drop in their FEV_1 over the course of a Monday shift.

Initially the symptoms do not recur on subsequent days of the week. However, in 10 to 25% of workers, the disease may be progressive, with chest tightness recurring or persisting throughout the workweek. After more than 10 years of exposure, workers with recurrent symptoms are more likely to have an obstructive pattern on pulmonary function testing. There is an additive effect of cotton dust exposure plus cigarette smoking. The highest grades of impairment are generally seen in smokers.

Treatment in the early stages of the disease is directed toward reversing the bronchospasm with bronchodilators; however, the chest tightness appears to relate, at least in part, to histamine release, and antihistamines have been shown to lessen the anticipated fall in FEV_1 the first day of the week. Clearly, reduction of dust exposure is of primary importance. All workers with persistent symptoms or significantly reduced levels of pulmonary function should be moved to areas of lower risk of exposure. Regular surveillance of pulmonary function in the industry has made it easier to identify affected persons. Persons with reduced pulmonary function, a personal history of respiratory allergy, and a history of continued cigarette smoking should be considered at increased risk of developing byssinosis in association with work in the cotton industry.

GRAIN DUST Although the exact number of workers at risk in the United States is not known, at least 500,000 people work in grain elevators, and over 2 million farmers are potentially exposed to grain dust. The presentation of disease in grain elevator employees or in workers in flour or feed mills is virtually identical to the characteristic findings in cigarette smokers, i.e., persistent cough, mucous hypersecretion, wheeze and dyspnea on exertion, and reduced FEV_1 and FEV_1/FVC ratio (Chap. 234).

Dust concentrations in grain elevators vary greatly but appear to be in excess of 10,000 $\mu g/m^3$; approximately one-third of the particles, by weight, are in the respirable range. The effect of grain dust exposure is additive to that of cigarette smoking, with approximately 50% of workers who smoke having symptoms. Among nonsmoking grain elevator operators, approximately one-quarter have mucous hypersecretion, about five times the number that would be expected in unexposed nonsmokers. However, evidence of obstruction on pulmonary function studies is observed only in workers who smoke.

FARMER'S LUNG This condition results from exposure to moldy hay containing spores of thermophilic actinomycetes that produce a hypersensitivity pneumonitis (Chap. 237). There are few good population-based estimates of the frequency of occurrence of this condition in the United States. However, among farmers in Great Britain, the rate of disease ranges from approximately 10 to 50 per 1000. The prevalence of disease varies in association with rainfall, which determines the amount of fungal growth, and with differences in agricultural practices related to turning and stacking hay.

The patient with acute farmer's lung presents 4 to 8 h after exposure with fever, chills, malaise, cough, and dyspnea without wheezing. The history of exposure is obviously essential to distinguish this disease from influenza or pneumonia with similar symptoms. In the chronic form of the disease, the history of repeated attacks after similar exposure is important in differentiating this syndrome from other causes of patchy fibrosis (e.g., sarcoidosis).

A wide variety of other organic dusts are associated with the occurrence of hypersensitivity pneumonitis (Chap. 237). For those patients who present with hypersensitivity pneumonitis, specific and careful inquiry about occupations, hobbies, or other home environmental exposures will, in most cases, reveal the source of the etiologic agent.

TOXIC CHEMICALS

Exposure to toxic chemicals affecting the lung generally involves gases and vapors. A common accident is one in which the victim is trapped in a confined space where the chemicals have accumulated to toxic levels. In addition to the specific toxic effects of the chemical, the victim will often sustain considerable anoxia, which can play a dominant role in determining whether the individual survives.

Table 238-3 lists a variety of toxic agents that can produce acute and sometimes life-threatening reactions in the lung. All these agents in sufficient concentrations have been demonstrated, at least in animal studies, to affect the lower airways and disrupt alveolar architecture, either acutely or as a result of chronic exposure. Some of these agents may be generated acutely in the environment. For example, when plastics burn, a number of compounds, including hydrogen cyanide and hydrochloric acid, may be formed and released.

Firefighters and fire victims are at risk of *smoke inhalation*, a numerically important cause of acute cardiorespiratory failure. Smoke inhalation kills more fire victims than does thermal injury. Carbon monoxide poisoning with resulting significant hypoxemia can be life-threatening (Chap. 377). The use of synthetic materials (plastic, polyurethanes), which, when burned, may release a variety of other toxic agents (such as cyanide or hydrochloric acid), must be considered when evaluating smoke inhalation victims. Exposed victims may suffer some degree of lower respiratory tract inflammation and/or pulmonary edema.

Firefighters and victims may also be exposed to large quantities of particulate smoke. Significant long-term effects are not clearly associated with this particulate exposure except as related to the production of irritating effects on the upper airways; however, increased airway responsiveness in firefighters with repeated episodes of smoke inhalation has been demonstrated.

Some agents used in the manufacture of synthetic materials have resulted in some workers' being sensitized to extremely low levels of *isocyanates*, *aromatic amines*, or *aldehydes*. Repeated exposure to these agents causes some workers to develop chronic cough and sputum production, asthma, or episodes of low-grade fever and malaise.

Fluoropolymers, which at normal temperatures produce no reaction, upon heating become volatilized. The inhaled agents cause a characteristic syndrome of fever, chills, malaise, and occasionally mild wheezing leading to the diagnosis of *polymer fume fever* or, in the

---

TABLE 238-3   Selected Common Toxic Chemical Agents Affecting the Lung

Agent(s)	Selected Exposures	Acute Effects from High or Accidental Exposure	Chronic Effects from Relatively Low Exposure
Acid fumes: H_2SO_4, HNO_3	Manufacture of fertilizers, chlorinated organic compounds, dyes, explosives, rubber products, metal etching, plastics	Mucous membrane irritation, followed by chemical pneumonitis 2–3 days later	Bronchitis and suggestion of mildly reduced pulmonary function in children with lifelong residential exposure to high levels; clinical significance unknown
Ammonia	Refrigeration; petroleum refining; manufacture of fertilizers, explosives, plastics, and other chemicals	Same as for acid fumes	Chronic bronchitis
Cyanides	Electroplating; extraction of gold or silver; manufacture of mirrors, fumigants, photo supplies	Increase in respiratory rate followed by respiratory arrest, lactic acidosis, pulmonary edema, death	No data
Diazomethane	Methylating agent for acid compounds; laboratory workers	Violent coughing, dyspnea, wheezing, pulmonary edema	No data
Formaldehyde	Manufacture of resins, leathers, rubber, metals, and woods; laboratory workers, embalmers; emission from urethane foam insulation	Same as for acid fumes	Cancers in one species; no data on humans
Halides (Cl, Br, F)	Bleaching in pulp, paper, textile industry; manufacture of chemical compounds; synthetic rubber, plastics, disinfectant, rocket fuel, gasoline	Mucous membrane irritation, pulmonary edema; possible reduced FVC 1–2 yrs after exposure	Dryness of mucous membrane, epistaxis, dental fluorosis, tracheobronchitis
Hydrogen sulfide	By-product of many industrial processes, oil, other petroleum processes and storage	Respiratory paralysis similar to cyanides	Conjunctival irritation, chronic bronchitis, recurrent pneumonitis
Isocyanates (TDI, HDI, MDI)	Production of polyurethane foams, plastics, adhesives, surface coatings	Mucous membrane irritation, dyspnea, cough, wheeze, pulmonary edema	Upper respiratory tract irritation, cough, asthma, allergic alveolitis
Nitrogen dioxide	Silage, metal etching, explosives, rocket fuels, welding, by-product of burning fossil fuels	Cough, dyspnea, pulmonary edema may be delayed 4–12 h; possible result from acute exposure: bronchiolitis obliterans in 2–6 wks	Emphysema in animals, ?chronic bronchitis, associated with reduced lung function in children with lifelong residential exposure, clinical significance unknown
Ozone	Arc welding, flour bleaching, deodorizing, emissions from copying equipment, photochemical air pollutant	Mucous membrane irritant, pulmonary hemorrhage and edema, reduced pulmonary function transiently in children and adults exposed to summer haze	Chronic eye irritation
Phosgene	Organic compound, metallurgy, volatilization of chlorine-containing compounds	Delayed onset of bronchiolitis and pulmonary edema	Chronic bronchitis
Phthalic anhydride	Manufacture of resin esters, polyester resins, thermoactivated adhesives	Nasal irritation, cough	Asthma, chronic bronchitis
Sulfur dioxide	Manufacture of sulfuric acid, bleaches, coating of nonferrous metals, food processing, refrigerant, burning of fossil fuels, wood pulp industry	Mucous membrane irritant, epistaxis	?Chronic bronchitis

meat industry, *meat wrappers' asthma*. A similar self-limited, influenza-like syndrome—*metal fume fever*—results from acute exposure to fumes or smoke of zinc, copper, magnesium, and other volatilized metals. The syndrome may begin several hours after work and resolves within 24 h, only to return on repeated exposure. A proper occupational history should make the diagnosis evident.

ENVIRONMENTAL RESPIRATORY CARCINOGENS

Historically, it has been the astute clinician who has recognized a higher incidence of malignant tumors associated with certain environmental exposures. When these observations are linked to an occupational setting, they must be pursued by epidemiologic studies of relatively large groups of both current and former workers. Often the concentration and/or exact nature of the substances involved in the putative exposures cannot be determined. Rarely, the possibility that a substance can play an etiologic role in cancer is supported by observing that a few cases of a very rare tumor in a particular group represent "an epidemic." Examples are nasal sinus and lung cancer in nickel workers, angiosarcomas of the liver in vinyl chloride workers, and adenocarcinomas of the nose in woodworkers.

In addition to asbestos exposures, other occupational exposures associated with either proven or suspected respiratory carcinogens include those to acrylonitrile, arsenic compounds, beryllium (animal studies only), bis(chloromethyl) ether, chromium, polycyclic hydrocarbons (through coke oven emissions), iron oxide, isopropyl oil (nasal sinuses), mustard gas, the various ores used to produce pure nickel, talc (possible asbestos contamination in both mining and milling), vinyl chloride, welding materials, wood used in woodworking (nasal cancer only), and uranium. The occurrence of excess cancers in uranium miners raises the possibility that a large number of workers are at risk by virtue of exposure to similar radiation hazards. This number includes not only workers involved in processing uranium but also workers exposed in underground mining operations where radon daughters may be emitted from rock formations.

ASSESSMENT OF DISABILITY

Most commonly the need for disability assessment comes about because of the patient's complaint of shortness of breath. Pathophysiologically, dyspnea most often results from cardiac, respiratory, or neuromuscular diseases. With regard to respiratory diseases, the complaint most often relates to asthma. It is the physician's task to assess both the degree to which the symptoms are related to work or other environmental exposures and the severity of the symptoms, which result in the disability that may prevent the individual from performing his or her normal work tasks. Evaluating relation to work exposure requires a detailed work history, as previously discussed in this chapter. Objective assessment of severity of symptoms can generally be measured with pulmonary function tests including simple spirometry, lung volume measures, and diffusing capacity. In cases where these tests are normal, repeated measures of spirometry, airways hyperactivity, or degree of oxygen desaturation after modest exercise may be sufficient to demonstrate impairment. Occasionally, challenge to the putative work environment with repeated pulmonary function measures may be required.

With these data the physician should be able to make a judgment about the degree of impairment and its relation to exposure. How this information is formally used is often beyond the physician's control. Administrative panels, legal authorities, and sometimes confrontational employer/employee relations, as in a worker's compensation case, may have alternative reasons for collecting and using such data. Different authorities may have different guidelines and rules for setting levels of disability. What the physician may consider significant impairment may not be considered a disability for a worker with a sedentary job. Nevertheless, the treating physician is often asked for an opinion and must respond as objectively as possible. When this is being done for the physician's own patient, he or she needs to indicate to the patient what his or her specific role is and that most often the physician is not in the position of making the adjudicating decision.

If the physician is operating as an independent medical examiner, he or she should make clear to the agency that hires him or her that, from a medical-ethical perspective, the patient will be informed of all findings.

GENERAL ENVIRONMENTAL EXPOSURES

AIR POLLUTION

Dramatic and disastrous episodes of air pollution inversion have been documented in many industrialized centers in the world. Each of these episodes has been associated with excess acute mortality in the very old, the very young, and those with chronic cardiopulmonary diseases. The most dramatic event was the London fog of 1952, in which approximately 4000 excess deaths occurred over a 2-week period following 5 days of severe cold and dense fog. Similar episodes in the United States, although less dramatic in terms of total deaths, occurred in Donora, Pennsylvania, in 1948 and in New York City in the 1960s. In these episodes, which were generally associated with cold temperature and air stagnation, patients with underlying cardiopulmonary disease were most severely affected.

In addition to significant excess mortality during these episodes, a large number of people required medical care for cardiorespiratory complaints. Subsequent follow-up studies failed to implicate these episodic disasters in the etiology of chronic respiratory disease in adults. On the other hand, many epidemiologic studies of both international and regional differences in the prevalences of chronic respiratory disease suggest that long-term exposures in polluted areas in the early to middle part of the twentieth century were associated with excess chronic respiratory disease.

In 1970, the U.S. government established air quality standards for several pollutants believed to be responsible for excess cardiorespiratory diseases. Primary standards regulated by the Environmental Protection Agency (EPA) designed to protect the public health with an adequate margin of safety exist for sulfur dioxide, particulates <10 μm in size, nitrogen dioxide, ozone, lead, and carbon monoxide. Standards for each of these pollutants are updated regularly through an extensive review process conducted by the EPA. In 1997, a new standard was added for particles less than 2.5 μm; however, up through 2002 that new standard has not been implemented.

Pollutants are generated from both stationary sources (power plants and industrial complexes) and mobile sources (automobiles), and none of the pollutants occurs in isolation. Thus, except for the change in carboxyhemoglobin from carbon monoxide exposure, it becomes extremely difficult to relate any specific health effect to any single pollutant. Furthermore, pollutants may be changed by chemical reactions after being emitted. For example, reducing agents, such as sulfur dioxide and particulate matter from a power plant stack, may react in air to produce acid sulfates and aerosols, which can be transported long distances in the atmosphere. Oxidizing substances, such as oxides of nitrogen and oxidants from automobile exhaust, may react with sunlight to produce ozone. Although originally a problem confined to the southwestern part of the United States, in recent years, at least during the summertime, elevated ozone and acid aerosol levels have been documented throughout the United States. Both acute and chronic effects of these exposures have also been documented.

The symptoms and diseases associated with air pollution are the same as the nononcogenic conditions commonly associated with cigarette smoking. In addition, respiratory illness in early childhood has been associated with chronic exposure to only modestly elevated levels of traffic-related gases and respirable particles. Recent population-based studies comparing cities that have relatively high levels of particulate exposures with less polluted communities suggest excess morbidity and mortality from cardiorespiratory conditions in long-term residents of the former communities. This finding, in part, has led to greater emphasis on publicizing pollution alert levels. One can only advise individuals with significant cardiopulmonary impairment to stay indoors during periods when pollution exceeds current standards.

INDOOR EXPOSURE

Over the past 15 years, greater attention has been given to the effects of *passive cigarette smoking* (Chap. 375). Several studies have shown that the respirable particulate load in any household is directly proportional to the number of cigarette smokers living in the home. Increases in prevalence of respiratory illnesses and reduced levels of pulmonary function measured with simple spirometry have been found in children of smoking parents in a number of studies.

Evidence from numerous case-control and cohort studies shows modest excess disease associations for cardiopulmonary diseases and lung cancer. Because most of these excess relative risks appear to be below 50%, it is virtually impossible for any one of the studies to be considered definitive. Thus, the techniques of meta-analysis have been used effectively to combine data from the best of these studies. The most recent meta-analyses for lung cancer, cardiac disease, and respiratory disease in terms of excess mortality suggest an approximately 25% increase for each condition, even after adjustment for major potential confounders. According to measures of plasma cotinine, a metabolite of nicotine, a nonsmoker living with a smoker is exposed to approximately 1% of the level of tobacco smoke to which a smoker of 20 cigarettes a day is exposed. In spite of some prominent detractors, these combined relative risks appear to be consistent with the estimated exposure levels and suggest a consensus that the associations are causal.

Radon gas is believed to be a risk factor for lung cancer. The main radon product (radon 222) is a gas that results from the decay series of uranium 238, with the immediate precursor being radium 226. The amount of radium in earth materials determines how much radon gas will be emitted. Outdoors, the concentrations are trivial. Indoors, levels are dependent on the ventilation rate and the size of the space into which the gas is emitted. Levels associated with excess lung cancer risk may be present in as many as 10% of the houses in the United States. When smokers reside in the household, the problem is potentially greater, since the molecular size of radon particles allows them to readily attach to smoke particles that are inhaled. Fortunately, technology is available for assessing and reducing the level of exposure.

Other indoor exposures associated with an increased risk of atopy and asthma include those to such specific recognized putative biologic agents as cockroach antigen, dust mites, and pet danders. Other indoor chemical agents include formaldehyde, perfumes, and latex particles. Nonspecific responses associated with "tight-building syndrome," in which no particular agent has been implicated, have included a wide variety of complaints, among them respiratory symptoms, that are relieved only by avoiding exposure in the building in question. The degree to which "smells" or other sensory stimuli are involved in the triggering of potentially incapacitating psychological or physical responses has yet to be determined, and the long-term consequences of such environmental exposures are as yet unknown.

PORTAL OF ENTRY

The lung is a primary point of entry into the body for a number of toxic agents that affect other organ systems. For example, the lung is a route of entry for benzene (bone marrow), carbon disulfide (cardiovascular and nervous systems), cadmium (kidney), and metallic mercury (kidney, central nervous system). Thus, in any disease state of obscure origin, it is important to consider the possibility of inhaled environmental agents. Such consideration can sometimes furnish the clue needed to identify a specific external cause for a disorder that might otherwise be labeled "idiopathic."

FURTHER READING

BLANC PD: Acute pulmonary responses to toxic exposures, in *Textbook of Respiratory Medicine*, 3d ed, JF Murray, JA Nadel (eds). Philadelphia, Saunders, 2000, pp 1903–1914

CASTRANOVA V, VALLYATHAN V: Silicosis and coal workers' pneumoconiosis. Environ Health Perspect 108 (Suppl 4):675, 2000

CHAN-YEUNG M, MALO J-L: Occupational asthma. N Engl J Med 333: 107, 1995

CHEN R et al: Environmental tobacco smoke and lung function in employees who never smoked: The Scottish MONICA Study. Occup Environ Med 58: 563, 2001

MAIER LA et al: Angiotensin-1 converting enzyme polymorphisms in chronic beryllium disease. Am J Respir Crit Care Med 159:1342, 1999

MANNING CV et al: Diseases caused by asbestos: Mechanisms of injury and disease development. Int Immunopharmacol 2:191, 2002

PARKES WR: *Occupational Lung Disorders*, 3d ed. Oxford, Butterworth-Heinemann, 1994

SCHINS RP, BORM PJ: Mechanisms and mediators in coal dust–induced toxicity: A review. Ann Occup Hyg 43:7, 1999

YCESOY B et al: Association of tumor necrosis factor-α and interleukin-1 gene polymorphism with silicosis. Toxicol Appl Pharmacol 172:75, 2001

239 PNEUMONIA

Thomas J. Marrie, G. Douglas Campbell, David H. Walker, Donald E. Low

To the pathologist, pneumonia is an infection of the alveoli, distal airways, and interstitium of the lung that is manifested by increased weight of the lungs, replacement of the normal lung's sponginess by consolidation, and alveoli filled with white blood cells, red blood cells, and fibrin. To the clinician, pneumonia is a constellation of symptoms and signs (fever, chills, cough, pleuritic chest pain, sputum production, hyper- or hypothermia, increased respiratory rate, dullness to percussion, bronchial breathing, egophony, crackles, wheezes, pleural friction rub) in combination with at least one opacity on chest radiography. There is often a degree of uncertainty about the clinical diagnosis of pneumonia, since a number of noninfectious disorders may mimic this entity.

Pneumonia can be broadly categorized as community-acquired or hospital-acquired (nosocomial). When pneumonia occurs in residents of long-term-care facilities (LTCFs), it is treated as community-acquired by some physicians and as nosocomial by others. It is also useful to subdivide cases of community-acquired pneumonia (CAP) into those that can be treated in an ambulatory setting and those that are severe enough to require admission to the hospital. Similarly, nosocomial pneumonia can be categorized as ventilator-associated or non-ventilator-associated. These categories provide a rough guide as to likely pathogens and disease severity.

HOST DEFENSES PROTECTING THE LUNGS   With a surface area of ~ 70 m^2 that is exposed to the external environment, the lungs are protected by an elegant defense system aimed at preventing potential pathogens from reaching this site and at containing and eliminating the organisms that do gain entry. The pulmonary host defenses can be classified as innate (nonspecific) and acquired (specific).

Anatomical features of the upper airway constitute the first line of innate defense. The nasal turbinates and the sharp angular turn from the naso- and anterior oropharynx into the posterior pharynx act as baffles where inhaled particulate matter can impact. The mucociliary transport system includes ciliated cells of the trachea, bronchi, and terminal bronchioles as well as the overlying mucus layer. The ciliated cells move a mucus layer (produced by goblet cells and submucosal glands), which "floats" on a solute layer to the back of the throat and is swallowed. Mucus consists of complex glycoproteins called *mucins* that trap microorganisms. To prevent pathogens from attaching to and colonizing upper respiratory tract surfaces, binding is inhibited by a decreased mucosal pH, the presence of naturally occurring bacterial and epithelial cell binding analogues, secretory IgA, and the constant desquamation of epithelial cells. In addition, the naso-oropharynx is colonized with nonpathogenic bacteria that can interfere with attachment of pathogens to host cells by a variety of mechanisms.

The entry to the lower respiratory tract is protected by the glottis. If secretions do enter the lower respiratory tract, they can be cleared readily by coughing. In the lower respiratory tract, nonspecific defenses include macrophages, fibronectin, lysozymes, lactoferrin, IgG, defensins, cathelicidins, collectins (including surfactant proteins A and D), and complement. Surfactant is bactericidal to certain pathogens and, along with IgG and fibronectin, can opsonize bacteria. Alveolar macrophages (present at a density of one per alveolus) play a role in both innate and acquired immunity. Their long life span (20 to 80 days) and their ability to phagocytose multiple times are characteristics that particularly suit their role as primary lung phagocytes in innate immunity. As components of acquired immunity, alveolar macrophages present antigens to T cells and produce many regulatory cytokines and mediators. If, however, the concentration of organisms is great (e.g., with gross aspiration) or if especially virulent pathogens are present, the macrophages recruit polymorphonuclear leukocytes (PMNs), and a more intense inflammatory process ensues.

The epithelial cells act as a barrier to dissemination of microorganisms and serve an important immune function. Throughout the lower respiratory tract, these cells produce antimicrobial molecules and participate in the upregulation of inflammation by recruiting phagocytic cells and by producing certain chemokines, including interleukin (IL) 8, macrophage-inflammatory protein 2, granulocyte-macrophage colony-stimulating factor, and by-products of the arachidonic acid cascade. In addition, epithelial cells regulate the expression of endothelial adhesion molecules, thereby targeting the recruitment of PMNs to the lung.

The advantages of the specific host defenses, which require T cell activation, are that they specifically target the offending pathogen, further upregulate the inflammatory response, and result in lifelong immunity to the offending antigen. Lymphocytes and mononuclear phagocytes are present throughout the respiratory tract, from the submucosa of the nasopharynx to the interstitial and alveolar spaces of the pulmonary parenchyma; their presence ensures a fast response of immunoreactive cells to events in the respiratory tract. →*Specific host defenses are discussed in detail in Chap. 295.*

FACTORS IN PATHOGENESIS ■ Routes of Infection For pneumonia to occur, a potential pathogen must reach the lower respiratory tract in sufficient numbers or with sufficient virulence to overwhelm host defenses. Possible routes include gross aspiration, microaspiration, aerosolization, hematogenous spread from a distant infected site, and direct spread from a contiguous infected site. By far the most common route for bacterial pneumonia is microaspiration of oropharyngeal secretions colonized with pathogenic microorganisms. Oropharyngeal colonization by *Streptococcus pneumoniae* and by *Haemophilus influenzae* may occur among healthy individuals (with persistence for weeks) but is more likely with significant comorbidities, antibiotic therapy, or physiologic stress (e.g., due to surgery). Gross aspiration can occur postoperatively and in patients with central nervous system disorders that affect swallowing (seizures, strokes); common pathogens include anaerobic organisms and gram-negative bacilli. Hematogenous spread can take place in the setting of endocarditis, intravenous catheter infections, or infections at other sites, such as the urinary tract. *Staphylococcus aureus* (including methicillin-resistant *S. aureus*, or MRSA) frequently infects the lungs in association with intravascular catheter–related infections, in endocarditis, and with a decreased level of consciousness following head trauma. *Escherichia coli* commonly originates from urinary tract infections. Aerosolization is the route by which *Mycobacterium tuberculosis*, endemic fungi (*Coccidioides immitis*, *Blastomyces dermatitidis*, *Histoplasma capsulatum*), *Legionella* spp., *Coxiella burnetii*, and many respiratory viruses (especially influenza viruses A and B) reach the lungs.

Microbial Factors Pathogenic microorganisms have developed a variety of mechanisms to counteract host defenses. *Chlamydia pneumoniae* produces a ciliostatic factor; *Mycoplasma pneumoniae* can shear off cilia; influenza virus infection markedly reduces tracheal mucus velocity within hours of onset and for up to 12 weeks afterward. *S. pneumoniae* and *Neisseria meningitidis* produce proteases that can split secretory IgA. *Mycobacterium*, *Nocardia*, and *Legionella* spp. are resistant to the microbicidal activity of phagocytes. The pneumococcal capsule inhibits phagocytosis. Another virulence factor produced by all pneumococci is the 53-kDa polypeptide pneumolysin, a thiol-activated cytolysin that interacts with any cell whose membrane contains cholesterol. Pneumococci also produce neuraminidase, hyaluronidase, and IgA1 protease.

Host Factors Pneumonia is more common when host defense is impaired, as it is in severe underlying illness. Hypogammaglobulinemia, defects in phagocytosis or ciliary function, neutropenia, functional or anatomical asplenia, or a reduction in CD4+ T lymphocyte counts are all host defense deficits that can result in increased frequency or severity of pneumonia. Viral infection of alveolar macrophages may explain in part the very high rate of pneumococcal disease in the HIV-infected population. Anatomical defects such as obstructed bronchus, bronchiectasis, or sequestration of a pulmonary segment all lead to recurrent pneumonia or the failure of pneumonia to resolve.

A number of polymorphisms in or near the tumor necrosis factor α (TNF-α) gene are associated with variability in TNF-α production and with outcomes in pneumonia. In patients with CAP, the TNF-α 238 GA genotype is an independent risk factor for a fatal outcome, the lymphotoxin-α (LT-α) +250 AA genotype is a risk factor for septic shock, and the TNF α 308:LT-α +250 GC haplotype is protective against septic shock. Patients with the DRB1*1501/DQB1*0602 haplotype have been found to mount significantly reduced responses to invasive group A streptococcal pulmonary infection and to be less likely to develop severe disease. In one study, 50% of patients with bacteremic pneumococcal pneumonia—but only 29% of uninfected controls—were homozygous for FcγRIIa-R31, which binds weakly to IgG2; this difference suggested that genetic factors may also be important risk factors for bacteremic pneumococcal pneumonia.

Functional or anatomical asplenia is an important risk factor for pneumonia presenting as overwhelming infection, with 80% of cases due to *S. pneumoniae*. Such overwhelming infection has a mortality rate of ~45%.

PATHOPHYSIOLOGY Vital capacity, lung compliance, functional residual capacity, and total lung capacity are below normal in patients with pneumonia. Ventilation-perfusion mismatch and intrapulmonary shunting are responsible for the hypoxemia that occurs in many patients with pneumonia.

PATHOLOGY The pathology of pneumonia manifests as four general patterns: lobar pneumonia, bronchopneumonia, interstitial pneumonia, and miliary pneumonia.

Lobar Pneumonia *Lobar pneumonia* classically involves an entire lung lobe relatively homogeneously, although in some patients a small portion of the lobe may be unaffected or at an earlier stage of involvement. Four stages of lobar pneumonia may exist simultaneously in the same lung, as the tendency of the progression to be synchronous is not absolute.

The first stage—*congestion*—occurs during the first 24 h and is characterized grossly by redness and a doughy consistency and microscopically by vascular congestion and alveolar edema. At this stage, many bacteria are present and are swept by the rapid expansion of edema fluid throughout the lobe via the pores of Kohn. Only a few neutrophils are seen at this stage. The second stage—termed *red hepatization* because of the color of the lung and the similarity of its airless, noncrepitant firmness to the consistency of liver—is characterized microscopically by the presence of many erythrocytes, neutrophils, desquamated epithelial cells, and fibrin in the alveolar spaces. In the third stage—*gray hepatization*—the lung is dry, friable, and gray-brown to yellow as a consequence of a persistent fibrinopurulent exudate, a progressive disintegration of red blood cells, and the variable presence of hemosiderin. The exudate contains macrophages as well as neutrophils, but bacteria are seldom visible. The second and third stages last for 2 to 3 days each, with a 2- to 6-day duration of maximal consolidation. The final stage—*resolution*—is characterized by enzymatic digestion of the alveolar exudate; resorption, phagocytosis, or coughing up of the residual debris; and restoration of the pulmonary architecture. Fibrinous inflammation may extend to and across the pleural space, causing a rub heard by auscultation, and may lead to resolution or to organization and pleural adhesions.

Bronchopneumonia *Bronchopneumonia*, a patchy consolidation involving one or several lobes, usually involves the dependent lower and posterior portions of the lung—a pattern attributable to the distribution of aspirated oropharyngeal contents by gravity. The consolidated areas are usually poorly demarcated, although in some cases there is an abrupt delimitation of the pneumonia at interlobular septa. The neutrophilic exudate is centered in bronchi and bronchioles, with centrifugal spread to the adjacent alveoli and diminishing cellular exudate; often there is only edema in the periphery of the lesion.

Interstitial Pneumonia *Interstitial pneumonia* is defined by histopathologic identification of an inflammatory process predominantly involving the interstitium, including the alveolar walls and the connective tissue around the bronchovascular tree. The inflammation may be patchy or diffuse. The alveolar septa contain an infiltration of lymphocytes, macrophages, and plasma cells. The alveoli do not contain a significant exudate, but protein-rich hyaline membranes similar to those found in adult respiratory distress syndrome (ARDS) may line the alveolar spaces. Some viruses with tropism for epithelial cells of the airways and alveoli may cause necrosis of the epithelium. In some instances, there may be a significant inflammatory exudate, with extensive degradation of inflammatory cells. Bacterial superinfection of viral pneumonia can also produce a mixed pattern of interstitial and alveolar airspace inflammation.

Miliary Pneumonia The original description of miliary pneumonia was based on the resemblance of the diffusely distributed 2- to 3-mm lesions of hematogenous tuberculosis to millet seeds. The current concept of *miliary pneumonia* is based on its numerous discrete lesions resulting from the spread of the pathogen to the lungs via the bloodstream. The varying degrees of immunocompromise in miliary tuberculosis, histoplasmosis, and coccidioidomycosis manifest as variations in the tissue reaction (from granulomas with caseous necrosis to foci of necrosis); the fibrinous exudate; and the weak, poorly formed cellular reaction. Miliary herpesvirus, cytomegalovirus, or varicella-zoster virus infection in severely immunocompromised patients results in numerous acute necrotizing hemorrhagic lesions.

PULMONARY COMPLICATIONS OF PNEUMONIA Uncontrolled infection by particular agents may lead to necrotizing pneumonia, formation of abscesses, vascular invasion with infarction, cavitation, and extension to the pleura with empyema or bronchopleural fistula. Complications of mechanical ventilation and supplemental oxygen administration include interstitial emphysema, pneumothorax, and ARDS. In patients with severe damage, tissue repair may lead to fibrosis with various anatomical distributions, such as organizing pneumonia, bronchiolitis obliterans, and pleural adhesions.

COMMUNITY-ACQUIRED PNEUMONIA

EPIDEMIOLOGY   With an annual cost of $9.7 billion, CAP affects 4 million adults per year in the United States, ~20% of whom are admitted to a hospital for treatment. The overall rate of pneumonia ranges from 8 to 15 per 1000 persons per year, with the highest rates at the extremes of age and during the winter months. Rates of pneumonia are higher for men than for women and for black than for white persons.

Independent risk factors for CAP include alcoholism [RR (relative risk) 9], asthma (RR 4.2), immunosuppression (RR 1.9), and an age of >70 years (RR 1.5 vs. an age of 60 to 69 years). Dementia, seizures, congestive heart failure, cerebrovascular disease, tobacco smoking, alcoholism, and chronic obstructive pulmonary disease (COPD) are risk factors for pneumococcal pneumonia. Independent risk factors for invasive pneumococcal disease include male gender, black race, chronic illness, current tobacco smoking, and passive exposure to tobacco smoke. Cigarette smoking is the strongest independent predictor of invasive pneumococcal disease among immunocompetent young adults. The rate of pneumococcal pneumonia is up to 40 times higher among HIV-infected patients than among age-matched patients not infected with HIV. Risk factors for Legionnaires' disease include male gender, current tobacco smoking, diabetes, hematologic malignancy, cancer, end-stage renal disease, and HIV infection. Probable aspiration, previous hospital admission, previous antimicrobial treatment, and bronchiectasis are predictive of pneumonia due to gram-negative bacteria, including *Pseudomonas aeruginosa*. Heavy drinkers (i.e., those consuming >100 g of ethanol per day for the preceding 2 years) have a higher incidence of gram-negative bacterial pneumonia, experience worse clinical symptoms, and require longer courses of intravenous antibiotic therapy than do nondrinkers. More prolonged fever, slower resolution, and a higher rate of empyema have been noted in pneumococcal pneumonia patients with chronic alcoholism than in their nondrinking counterparts. The clinical entity designated ALPS—alcoholism, leukopenia, and pneumococcal sepsis—is associated with a mortality rate of 80%. In addition, excessive alcohol use is an independent risk factor for the development of ARDS.

ETIOLOGY   The organism causing pneumonia may be identified from cultures of blood, sputum, pleural fluid, pulmonary tissue, or endobronchial secretions obtained with a bronchial brush or via lavage. Other methods for determining the etiology of pneumonia include the detection of an IgM response or a fourfold rise in the titer of antibody to an antigen of a particular microorganism and the detection of an antigen in urine, serum, or pleural fluid. In some instances, amplification of DNA or RNA of a respiratory pathogen from one of the above specimens or from material collected with a nasopharyngeal swab can be used for this purpose.

Identification of an etiologic agent in a case of pneumonia should be categorized as definite, probable, or possible, depending on the source of the microorganism or the test used to detect it (Table 239-1). Such diagnostic categorization is useful not only in comparative studies of pneumonia etiology but also in the approach to the patient with pneumonia.

The past 30 years have seen the identification of new etiologic agents of CAP, often during the detailed investigation of dramatic outbreaks. Thus *Legionella pneumophila* was isolated during the investigation of an outbreak of pneumonia at a convention of the American Legion in Philadelphia in 1976. Other etiologic agents identified during this period include *C. pneumoniae*, hantavirus, Nipah virus, Hendra virus, and metapneumovirus. Investigations of an outbreak of severe acute respiratory syndrome (SARS) originating in China and Hong Kong during the winter of 2003 and subsequently found to be caused by a novel coronavirus are ongoing.

The >100 documented microbial causes of CAP include bacteria, fungi, viruses, and parasites. Fortunately, most cases of pneumonia are caused by a few common respiratory pathogens, including *S. pneumoniae*, *H. influenzae*, *S. aureus*, *M. pneumoniae*, *C. pneumoniae*, *Moraxella catarrhalis*, *Legionella* spp., aerobic gram-negative bacteria, influenza viruses, adenoviruses, and respiratory syncytial virus. The relative frequency of these pathogens differs with the age of the patient and the severity of the pneumonia (Table 239-2). Overall, *S. pneumoniae* accounts for ~50% of all cases of CAP requiring admission to the hospital, although in everyday practice the etiology of CAP is unknown in up to 70% of patients.

Determination of the etiology of pneumonia starts with the gathering of clues from the history and physical examination (Table 239-3)

TABLE 239-1 Categories Reflecting the Certainty of an Etiologic Diagnosis of Pneumonia

Category	Definition
Definite	Pathogen recovered from blood, pleural fluid, or lung tissue Isolation of *Legionella* spp. or *Mycobacterium tuberculosis* from sputum Positive urinary antigen test for *Legionella*
Probable	Isolation from a purulent sputum specimen of any of the following microorganisms, with a morphologically compatible organism seen in moderate or large numbers on Gram's staining: *Staphylococcus aureus, Streptococcus pneumoniae, Haemophilus influenzae, Moraxella catarrhalis, Pseudomonas aeruginosa* Fourfold or greater rise in titer of antibody to a respiratory pathogen between acute- and convalescent-phase serum samples Positive urinary antigen test for *S. pneumoniae* in adults[a]
Possible	1. Gram's stain of an acceptable sputum specimen[b] showing a predominance of gram-positive diplococci (*S. pneumoniae*), gram-positive cocci in clusters (*S. aureus*), or gram-negative coccobacilli (*H. influenzae*) 2. Isolation of a pathogen from a purulent sputum specimen in the absence of a compatible Gram's stain 3. High single or static titer of antibody to *Legionella pneumophila* (≥1:1024) or *Mycoplasma pneumoniae* (≥1:64)

[a] Nasopharyngeal carriage of *S. pneumoniae* may be associated with a positive test in children.
[b] An acceptable sputum specimen is one with >25 white blood cells and <10 squamous epithelial cells per low-power field.

and proceeds to a diagnostic workup tailored to the severity of the pneumonia or to other circumstances, such as the setting of an outbreak. All patients with pneumonia who are admitted to the hospital should have blood cultured, and sputum should be cultured when the patient has a productive cough. This basic workup should be supplemented with more aggressive diagnostic methods (such as bronchoscopy with bronchoalveolar lavage or bronchial brush specimens) for patients admitted to intensive care units (ICUs).

TABLE 239-2 Frequency of Most Common Pathogens Causing Community-Acquired Pneumonia, According to Severity of Illness

Severity of Pneumonia	Rank Order of Pathogens
Ambulatory	1. *Streptococcus pneumoniae* 2. *Mycoplasma pneumoniae* 3. *Chlamydia pneumoniae* 4. *Haemophilus influenzae* 5. Influenza viruses 6. *Pneumocystis*
Treated on hospital ward	1. *S. pneumoniae* 2. Mixed etiology 3. Viruses 4. *H. influenzae* 5. *C. pneumoniae* 6. *Legionella* spp. 7. *M. pneumoniae* 8. *Staphylococcus aureus* 9. *Moraxella catarrhalis* 10. Aerobic gram-negative bacilli 11. *Mycobacterium tuberculosis* 12. *Pneumocystis*
Treated in intensive care unit	1. *S. pneumoniae* 2. *S. aureus* 3. Viruses 4. Mixed etiology 5. Aerobic gram-negative bacilli 6. *Legionella* spp. 7. *M. pneumoniae* 8. *Pneumocystis* 9. *H. influenzae*

TABLE 239-3 Clues to the Etiology of Pneumonia from History and Physical Examination

Factor	Possible Agent(s)
OCCUPATIONAL HISTORY	
Health care worker	*Mycobacterium tuberculosis*
Veterinarian, farmer, abattoir worker	*Coxiella burnetii*
Cooling tower maintenance worker	*Legionella* spp.
HOST FACTOR	
Diabetic ketoacidosis	*Streptococcus pneumoniae, Staphylococcus aureus*
Alcoholism	*S. pneumoniae, Klebsiella pneumoniae, S. aureus*, oral anaerobes, *Acinetobacter* spp.
Chronic obstructive pulmonary disease	*S. pneumoniae, Haemophilus influenzae, Moraxella catarrhalis*
Solid organ transplantation	*S. pneumoniae, H. influenzae, Legionella* spp., *Pneumocystis*, cytomegalovirus, *Strongyloides stercoralis*
Sickle cell disease	*S. pneumoniae*
HIV infection and CD4+ lymphocyte count of <200/μL	*S. pneumoniae, Pneumocystis, H. influenzae, Cryptococcus neoformans, M. tuberculosis, Rhodococcus equi*
Dementia, stroke, altered level of consciousness	Agents of aspiration pneumonitis (see text)
Structural lung disease (bronchiectasis)	*Pseudomonas aeruginosa*
TRAVEL AND OTHER ENVIRONMENTAL FACTORS	
Travel to Southeast Asia	*Burkholderia pseudomallei,[a] M. tuberculosis*
Travel to China, Taiwan, Toronto (Canada)[b]	Coronavirus causing severe acute respiratory syndrome (SARS)
Travel to many countries	*M. tuberculosis*
Travel to Arizona, parts of California	*Coccidioides immitis*
Travel to Ohio and St. Lawrence river valleys	*Histoplasma capsulatum*
Exposure to contaminated air-conditioning cooling towers, hot tub, grocery store mist machine; recent stay in a hotel; visit to or recent stay in a hospital with Legionellaceae-contaminated drinking water	*Legionella pneumophila*, other Legionellaceae
Exposure to mouse droppings in an endemic area	Hantavirus
Exposure to windstorm in an endemic area	*C. immitis, C. burnetii*
Pneumonia outbreak in shelter for homeless men or in jail	*S. pneumoniae, M. tuberculosis*
Pneumonia outbreak in military training camp	*S. pneumoniae, Chlamydia pneumoniae*, adenovirus
Pneumonia outbreak in nursing home	*C. pneumoniae, S. pneumoniae*, respiratory syncytial virus, influenza A virus, *M. tuberculosis*
Lawn mowing in an endemic area	*Francisella tularensis*
Exposure to bats, excavation or residence in an endemic area[c]	*H. capsulatum*
Exposure to parturient cats in an endemic area	*C. burnetii*
Sleeping in a rose garden	*Sporothrix schenckii*
Camping, cutting down trees in an endemic area	*Blastomyces dermatitidis*
Exposure to Vancouver Island (camping, residence)	*C. neoformans* var. *gattii*

[a] Agent of melioidosis.
[b] In 2003.
[c] Ohio and Mississippi river valleys.

TABLE 239-4 *British Thoracic Society Rule for Definition of Severe Community-Acquired Pneumonia (Acronym: CURB)*

Confusion
Urea[a]: >7 mmol/L
Respiratory rate: >30/min
Blood pressure: diastolic <60 mmHg or systolic <90 mmHg

[a] Blood urea nitrogen (BUN).

CLINICAL MANIFESTATIONS Pneumonia can range in severity from mild to fulminant and fatal, with serious disease developing even in previously healthy persons. The onset may be sudden and dramatic or insidious. Fever, cough (nonproductive or productive of purulent or rust-colored sputum), pleuritic chest pain, chills or rigors, and shortness of breath are typical—albeit nonspecific—manifestations of pneumonia. Symptoms reported with some frequency include headache, nausea, vomiting, diarrhea, myalgia, arthralgia, and/or fatigue. Falls and new-onset or worsening confusion may be important manifestations in an elderly person. The physical signs associated with pneumonia are tachypnea, dullness to percussion, increased tactile and vocal fremitus, egophony, whispering pectoriloquy, crackles, and pleural friction rub. In two studies, patients with a respiratory rate of >25/min had a pneumonia likelihood ratio of 1.5 to 3.4. In another study, patients with a heart rate of ≤100/min, a temperature of ≤37.8°C, and a respiratory rate of ≤20/min were five times less likely to have pneumonia than patients who had all of these abnormal parameters. A diagnosis of pneumonia based on physical examination has a sensitivity of 47 to 69% and a specificity of 58 to 75%; thus a clinical diagnosis of pneumonia should be confirmed by chest radiography. For patients who have pneumonia clinically diagnosed in an office setting, the physician must decide whether or not to obtain a chest radiograph. Even if the clinical assessment suggests mild disease, all patients with pneumonia who have an oral temperature of >38.5°C or who have pleuritic chest pain should have a chest radiograph. Pulmonary embolus is always a consideration with pleuritic chest pain, and further investigations are warranted if the chest radiograph is normal in this setting. If pneumonia is extensive in a patient with this degree of fever, further evaluation and perhaps hospitalization are necessary.

The single most useful clinical sign of the severity of pneumonia is a respiratory rate of >30/min in a person without underlying lung disease. Of the several measures of pneumonia severity, the simplest is the British Thoracic Society rule, which relies on three clinical findings and one laboratory finding (Table 239-4). If none of these features is present, the mortality rate is 2.4%; with one feature, the mortality rate is 8%; with two, 23%; with three, 33%; and with all four, 83%. The American Thoracic Society criteria for severe pneumonia are given in Table 239-5. To derive a scoring system for classifying pneumonia cases across the spectrum from mild to severe, the Pneumonia Patient Outcomes Research Team (PORT) assigned points to each of 20 items associated with mortality (Table 239-6). The resulting PORT score allowed categorization of patients with pneumonia into five risk groups (Table 239-7). Although this system was developed as a mortality prediction tool and is no substitute for clinical judgment, it is often used in making site-of-treatment decisions (see "Treatment," below).

Certain causes of pneumonia and organisms within a species are

TABLE 239-5 *American Thoracic Society Definition of Severe Pneumonia*

Category	Criteria
Major	Need for mechanical ventilation
	Requirement for vasopressors: >4 h
Minor	Systolic blood pressure: <90 mmHg
	Pa_{O_2}/Fi_{O_2}: <250
	Multilobar involvement

TABLE 239-6 *Severity-of-Illness Scoring System Based on Pneumonia Patient Outcomes Research Team (PORT) Cohort Study Data*

Patient Characteristic	No. of Points
Age	
Men	Age, years
Women	Age, years −10
Nursing home residents	Age, years +10
Coexisting illnesses	
Neoplastic disease[a]	30
Liver disease[b]	20
Congestive heart failure[c]	10
Cerebrovascular disease[d]	10
Renal disease[e]	10
Physical examination findings	
Altered mental status[f]	20
Respiratory rate >30/min	20
Systolic blood pressure <90 mmHg	20
Temperature <35°C (<95°F) or >40°C (>104°F)	15
Pulse rate >125/min	10
Laboratory and radiographic findings	
Arterial pH < 7.35	30
Blood urea nitrogen >30 mg/dL (>11 mmol/L)	20
Sodium <130 mmol/L	20
Glucose >250 mg/dL (>14 mmol/L)	10
Hematocrit <30%	10
Partial pressure of arterial oxygen <60 mmHg	10
Pleural effusion	10

[a] Any cancer (except basal or squamous cell carcinoma of the skin) active at presentation or within 1 year of presentation with community-acquired pneumonia.
[b] Clinical or histologic cirrhosis or chronic active hepatitis.
[c] Diagnosis documented by history or by findings on physical examination, chest radiography, echocardiography, multiple gated acquisition scan, or left ventriculography.
[d] Clinical diagnosis of stroke or transient ischemic attack; stroke documented by magnetic resonance imaging or computed tomography.
[e] History of chronic renal disease or abnormal blood urea nitrogen and creatinine concentrations documented in medical record.
[f] Disorientation as to person, place, or time that is not known to be chronic; stupor or coma.

associated with a high mortality rate. The mortality rate is highest (>50%) for pneumonia due to *P. aeruginosa*, followed by the rates for *Klebsiella* spp., *E. coli*, *S. aureus*, and *Acinetobacter* spp. (all 30 to 35%). The capsular serotype 3 pneumococcus is associated with a much higher mortality rate than serotype 1, as are M serotypes 1 and 3 of group A *Streptococcus* (compared with other serotypes).

Young, otherwise healthy adults who develop pneumonia and who are treated as outpatients usually feel well enough to return to work in 4 or 5 days, and almost all will have recovered in 2 weeks. However, those with relatively severe symptoms may require longer to recover. About 2 to 4% of those who are treated as outpatients experience a progression of symptoms and require admission to the hospital. In general, those admitted during the first week after the initial visit are admitted because pneumonia has worsened, while those admitted later are often admitted because of worsening of comorbid illnesses (e.g., diabetes mellitus, congestive heart failure, asthma, or ischemic heart disease). Currently, up to 25% of persons treated for pneumonia as outpatients are >65 years old, and the natural history of ambulatory

TABLE 239-7 *Mortality Rate at 30 Days among Patients with Community-Acquired Pneumonia, According to PORT Risk Class[a]*

Risk Class	Criteria	% Mortality Outpatient	% Mortality Inpatient
I	Age <50 years	0	0.5
	No existing illnesses or vital-sign abnormalities		
II	70 points	0.4	0.9
III	71–90 points	0	1.25
IV	91–130 points	12.5	9.0
V	131 points	NA	27.1
Mean		0.6	8.0

[a] PORT, Pneumonia Patient Outcomes Research Team.

pneumonia in this group is probably different from that in younger patients.

Among patients admitted to the hospital for the treatment of pneumonia, clinical stability is usually attained in 3 to 7 days, depending on the definition used. In one study, a median of 2 days was required to achieve a heart rate of ≤100/min and 3 days to achieve a respiratory rate of ≤24/min, an oxygen saturation of ≥90%, and a temperature of ≤37.2°C. Once stability is attained, clinical deterioration is uncommon.

Since most patients admitted to the hospital with pneumonia are elderly and have multiple comorbid conditions, it is not uncommon for complications to occur during the hospital stay. The most common complications are respiratory failure, congestive heart failure, shock, atrial dysrhythmias, myocardial infarction, gastrointestinal bleeding, and renal insufficiency. Indeed, only ~30% of patients hospitalized for the treatment of pneumonia have no complications.

The in-hospital mortality rate from pneumonia is ~8%. The most common immediate causes of death among patients with pneumonia are respiratory failure, heart disease, and infections. About half of deaths are related to pneumonia, and the other half are due to comorbid illnesses. Pneumonia-related deaths are much more likely to occur during the first week of hospitalization. Factors independently associated with pneumonia-unrelated mortality include dementia, immunosuppression, active cancer, systolic hypotension, male gender, and multilobar pulmonary infiltrates. Increasing age and evidence of aspiration independently predict both pneumonia-related and comorbidity-related mortality.

DIAGNOSIS The usual standard for the diagnosis of pneumonia is chest radiography, which, however, is not 100% sensitive. High-resolution computed tomography (CT) occasionally detects pulmonary opacities in patients with symptoms and signs suggestive of pneumonia in whom chest radiographs are reported as not showing pneumonia. CT is also more likely than chest radiography to show bilateral involvement. If pneumonia is strongly suspected on clinical grounds and no opacity is seen on the initial chest radiograph, it is useful to repeat the radiograph in 24 to 48 h or to perform CT. It is important to remember that an opacity visible on chest radiograph may not be due to pneumonia; many other disease processes can result in opacities. Furthermore, there is variability among radiologists in the interpretation of chest radiographs; most commonly, subsegmental lower-lobe opacities in patients with suboptimal chest radiographs may be reported as atelectasis by one radiologist and as pneumonia by another. Occasionally, an etiologic diagnosis is suggested by the findings on chest radiography. For example, a cavitating upper-lobe lesion raises the likelihood of tuberculosis, and pneumatoceles suggest *S. aureus* pneumonia. An air-fluid level suggests a pulmonary abscess, which is often polymicrobial. In the immunocompromised host, a crescent (meniscus) sign suggests aspergillosis. In most instances, however, no etiologic inference can be made from radiographic findings.

Concomitant diseases (such as congestive heart failure or pulmonary fibrosis) may make both the clinical and the radiologic diagnosis of pneumonia difficult. However, serial clinical and radiographic observations usually allow the clinician to determine whether there are two diseases or just one and to identify which one is causing the clinical and radiographic findings.

Etiologic Diagnosis ■ *BLOOD CULTURE* Blood should be obtained for culture from patients to be treated on an ambulatory basis if they have been receiving antibiotic therapy and have presented because of any of the following: hyperthermia (temperature >38.5°C), hypothermia (temperature <36°C), homelessness, or alcohol abuse. All patients who are admitted to the hospital for CAP should have two sets of blood cultures done before initiation of antibiotic therapy (positivity rate: 6 to 20%). The most common isolates, in descending order, are *S. pneumoniae* (~60%), *S. aureus*, and *E. coli*.

SPUTUM STAINS AND CULTURE Gram's stain is used to screen a sputum sample for suitability for culture and to make a presumptive etiologic diagnosis. A sputum sample with >25 white blood cells and <10 squamous epithelial cells per low-power field is suitable for culture. There is a great deal of interobserver variability in the interpretation of gram-stained sputum smears. The presence of any gram-positive diplococci has a sensitivity of 100% but a specificity of 0 for a diagnosis of pneumococcal infection. The presence of >10 gram-positive diplococci per oil-immersion field has a sensitivity of 55% and a specificity of 85% for this diagnosis. Culture results should always be correlated with those of Gram's staining. If an organism is isolated from sputum and its morphologic correlate is not seen on Gram's staining, the isolate may be colonizing the upper airway. Certain microorganisms, if isolated from sputum, should always be considered pathogens. These include *M. tuberculosis*, *Legionella* spp., *B. dermatitidis*, *H. capsulatum*, and *C. immitis*. In practice, only about one-third of elderly patients admitted with CAP produce sputum suitable for culture, and one-third of these specimens fail to yield a pathogen.

Other types of sputum staining are also useful for determining the etiology of CAP. A variety of stains for acid-fast bacilli are used to diagnose tuberculosis; *Pneumocystis* pneumonia can be diagnosed with monoclonal antibody staining; and special stains for fungi are useful in selected patients, as are cytologic stains.

DETECTION OF ANTIGENS OF PULMONARY PATHOGENS IN URINE *L. pneumophila* serogroup 1 antigen can be detected in the urine of patients with Legionnaires' disease due to this organism by means of an enzyme-linked immunosorbent assay (ELISA). The sensitivity of this assay is 69 to 72% on average, 88 to 100% in severe disease, and 40 to 53% in mild disease. The assay's sensitivity is low in nosocomial Legionnaires' disease. The results may be negative early in the illness, and antigen excretion can be prolonged. The test should be used in patients in whom Legionnaires' disease is strongly suspected, including those with rapidly progressive pneumonia. The urine antigen test is now the most frequently used diagnostic method for Legionnaires' disease. A critical point, however, is that infection with *Legionella* spp. other than *L. pneumophila* serogroup 1 gives a negative test result.

S. pneumoniae urinary antigen detection by ELISA has a sensitivity of 80% and a specificity of 97 to 100% in patients with bacteremic pneumococcal pneumonia. The antigen may be detected for up to 1 month after the onset of pneumonia, and the results can be available in 15 min. In children, nasopharyngeal carriage of *S. pneumoniae* can result in a positive urinary antigen test.

SEROLOGY The detection of IgM antibody or the demonstration of a fourfold rise in the titer of antibody to a particular agent between acute and convalescent-phase serum samples is generally considered good evidence that this agent is the cause of the pneumonia. The following etiologic agents are often diagnosed serologically: *M. pneumoniae*, *C. pneumoniae*, *Chlamydia psittaci*, *Legionella* spp., *C. burnetii*, adenovirus, parainfluenza viruses, and influenza virus A. The various serologic tests include complement fixation, indirect immunofluorescence, and ELISA. Separate IgM and IgG antibody detection tests can be performed with the latter two assays. One difficulty in relying on serology is that a polyclonal antibody response to one agent may result in a fourfold rise in antibody titer to others; thus the results may be nonspecific. Serologic testing is not recommended for routine use; however, if agents such as *C. burnetii* are suspected, such testing is necessary. Serology is also a useful part of the workup of outbreaks of pneumonia associated with negative blood and sputum cultures.

POLYMERASE CHAIN REACTION Amplification of the DNA or RNA of microorganisms that are not part of the pharyngeal flora (from microbial cells collected by throat swab) has been used to infer that the implicated microorganism is the cause of pneumonia. A multiplex polymerase chain reaction allows detection of DNA of *Legionella* spp., *M. pneumoniae*, and *C. pneumoniae*. This test is expensive and is not routinely available.

℞ TREATMENT

Successful treatment of CAP involves all the elements listed in Tables 239-8, 239-9, and 239-10.

Site of Care As described above, the PORT score (based on a pneumonia-specific severity-of-illness scoring system; Tables 239-6 and 239-7) has been advocated as a tool to guide the decision regarding the site of care (home vs. hospital). Because of the low mortality rates in risk classes I and II, it is recommended that these patients be treated at home, while patients in risk classes IV and V require hospital admission. Patients in class III may benefit from a period of observation in the emergency room before a decision is made regarding the site of care. Reliance on this or any other such system as the sole criterion for this decision has several limitations: (1) These systems are mortality prediction tools only and do not take into account psychosocial reasons for admission. (2) Although illness is dynamic, scoring systems capture events at a single point in time. (3) A physician's judgment is often the most critical element in decision-making and should override any scoring system. For example, some patients in classes I to III may have a complicated hospital course and may even require admission to an ICU, although the scoring system would dictate that they should be sent home. In practice, a physician should use a number of approaches in deciding on the site of care—intuition, specific assessment of the severity of illness, and the parameters given in Table 239-10. When a patient with pneumonia is sent home from the emergency room or the physician's office, it is advisable to follow up with a telephone call within 48 h. In our experience, most patients have begun to feel better by this time, ~10% are unchanged, and ~5% are worse; this last group of patients should be reassessed by a physician. Patients who are treated on an ambulatory basis should be given written information about the warning signs of pneumonia exacerbation, such as shortness of breath while walking on level ground (for those who have no underlying lung disease), a temperature of >38.5°C after 72 h of antibiotic therapy, or a new onset of confusion or pleuritic chest pain. In addition, patients should be advised to report hemoptysis to their physicians.

TABLE 239-8   *Approach to the Patient with Community-Acquired Pneumonia*

1. Assess pneumonia severity. Pay attention to vital signs, including oxygen saturation. Always count the respiratory rate yourself for 1 min.
2. Ensure adequate oxygenation and support of circulation.
3. Perform etiologic workup (dictated by pneumonia severity).
4. Determine site of treatment: home, hospital (ward or intensive care unit), or long-term-care facility.
5. Institute empirical antibiotic therapy.
6. Rule out empyema in all patients with a pleural effusion of >1 cm on lateral decubitus chest radiography.
7. Never forget tuberculosis and *Pneumocystis* infection as possible etiologies. Check your hospital policy regarding the isolation of patients with CAP. In some centers where tuberculosis is common, all patients with CAP are isolated until sputum smears are found to be negative for acid-fast bacilli.
8. Consider pulmonary embolus in all patients with pleuritic chest pain.
9. Consider end-of-life decision-making.
10. Monitor and treat comorbid illnesses.
11. Monitor for achievement of stability of selected physiologic parameters.
12. Assess ability to perform activities of daily living.
13. Assess mental status.
14. Consider preventive measures:
    a. Smoking cessation counseling (if appropriate)
    b. Assessment of pneumococcal and influenza vaccination status, with vaccine administration as necessary
    c. Assessment of risk of aspiration and institution of preventive measures
15. Follow up to ensure radiographic clearance of pneumonia. All patients >40 years old and all tobacco smokers should have a follow-up chest radiograph to document pneumonia resolution.

Antibiotic Therapy ■ *EMPIRICAL TREATMENT AND DRUG RESISTANCE* Since the etiology of pneumonia is frequently unknown, initial antibiotic therapy is often empirical. There are currently three sets of North American guidelines for empirical antibiotic treatment of CAP: those developed under the auspices of the Infectious Diseases Society of America, the American Thoracic Society, and the Canadian Infectious Diseases and Canadian Thoracic Societies. Table 239-9 combines various elements of these guidelines with the opinions of the authors.

There are no data from randomized clinical trials to indicate that one antibiotic or combination of antibiotics is better than another for the empirical treatment of CAP. A retrospective review of 12,945 Medicare patients (all >65 years old) indicated that treatment with a macrolide plus a second-generation or nonpseudomonal third-generation cephalosporin was associated with a significantly lower mortality rate than treatment with a second- or third-generation cephalosporin alone. Use of a fluoroquinolone alone was likewise associated with a significantly lower mortality rate, while the combination of an aminoglycoside and any other antibiotic resulted in a significantly higher mortality rate. Data from the Medicare study also indicated that timely administration is important: Patients who received antibiotics within 8 h after arrival at the emergency room had a lower mortality rate than those who received the first dose >8 h afterward. Data from a retrospective review of bacteremic pneumococcal pneumonia indicated that therapy with a single antimicrobial agent was not as effective as therapy with two or more agents effective against *S. pneumoniae*; data from randomized clinical trials must confirm or refute this observation.

In the selection of empirical antibiotic therapy, risk factors for drug-resistant *S. pneumoniae* must be considered (Table 239-9). Before 1980, strains of *S. pneumoniae* were almost universally susceptible to penicillin and other antimicrobial drugs. [The current National Committee for Clinical Laboratory Standards interpretive breakpoints for the minimal inhibitory concentration (MIC) of penicillin are ≤0.06 μg/mL (susceptible), 0.12 to 1.0 μg/mL (intermediate), and ≥2.0 μg/mL (resistant). Isolates classified as either intermediately resistant or resistant are considered nonsusceptible. Isolates resistant to three or more classes of drugs are termed multidrug-resistant.] In the late 1980s, the prevalence of penicillin-nonsusceptible *S. pneumoniae* in the United States was 4.0%; less than a decade later, it was 35%. In the United States, a multicenter national surveillance study conducted from November 1999 through April 2000 found that 35% of pneumococci were nonsusceptible to penicillin, with 60% of these isolates resistant. Resistance to non-β-lactam antibiotics also emerged among North American *S. pneumoniae* strains during the 1990s. In 1999 to 2000, the rate of resistance among U.S. isolates of *S. pneumoniae* was 25.9% for macrolides, 8.8% for clindamycin, 16.4% for tetracyclines, 8.4% for chloramphenicol, and 30.3% for trimethoprim-sulfamethoxazole. Furthermore, 22.5% of clinical isolates of *S. pneumoniae* were multidrug-resistant. The dominant factor in the emergence of drug-resistant *S. pneumoniae* in North America has been human-to-human spread of relatively few clonal groups that harbor resistance determinants to multiple classes of antibiotics. Serotypes 6A, 6B, 9V, 14, 19F, and 23F accounted for 92.3% of penicillin-resistant pneumococcal isolates in one study.

Emergence of pneumococcal resistance to quinolones has been described in Canada, Spain, Hong Kong, Eastern and Central Europe, and (to a lesser extent) the United States. In Canada, the prevalence of ciprofloxacin-resistant pneumococci (MIC ≥ 4 μg/mL) increased from 0 in 1993 to 1.7% in 1997 to 1998 ($p = .01$); the figures for adults were 0 in 1993 and 3.7% in 1998. The Active Bacterial Core Surveillance program carried out by the U.S. Centers for Disease Control and Prevention during 1995 to 1999 reported levofloxacin nonsusceptibility rates of 0.2%. The emergence of quinolone resistance has been documented in two pandemic multidrug-resistant pneumococcal clones, Spain 23F-1 and Spain 9V-3. Strains of the Spain 23F-1 clone have been found to be resistant to quinolones in the United States, Europe, and Hong Kong.

The rapid increase in drug resistance has not been accompanied by clear evidence of therapy failure among patients with pneumococcal

CAP. There have been only a few controlled studies on the impact of pneumococcal resistance to penicillin on CAP outcomes. Overall, the results from these studies suggest that mortality is not higher among patients with penicillin-nonsusceptible pneumococcal isolates than among patients with susceptible isolates, particularly when an isolate's MIC is ≤ 2 $\mu g/$ mL. Two case-control studies have reported adverse outcomes among patients with CAP due to penicillin-nonsusceptible pneumococci. In one study, after the exclusion of deaths occurring during the first 4 days of hospitalization, there was a significant risk of death among patients whose pneumococcal isolates had a penicillin MIC of at least 4 $\mu g/mL$ or a cefotaxime MIC of at least 2 $\mu g/mL$. While the risk of death was not elevated among patients with penicillin-nonsusceptible pneumococcal pneumonia, the risk of suppurative complications was greater than that among patients with penicillin-susceptible infections.

Given their excellent activity against *S. pneumoniae* as well as against the so-called atypical pathogens *M. pneumoniae*, *C. pneumoniae*, and *Legionella* spp., macrolide antibiotics (either alone or combined with β-lactams) have been widely used to treat CAP. Despite the rapid escalation of macrolide resistance in *S. pneumoniae*, there is little evidence of therapy failures, especially among nonbacteremic patients treated in the community. However, there is now evidence of breakthrough bacteremia during macrolide or azalide treatment of patients infected with erythromycin-resistant *S. pneumoniae*. Doxycycline, which is active against penicillin-susceptible *S. pneumoniae* and against the atypical pathogens, is underused for the treatment of CAP in an ambulatory setting.

Although anecdotal, a number of reports have described failures of quinolone therapy for CAP due to *S. pneumoniae* resistant to the specific agent used. Among the risk factors that identify patients likely to be colonized or infected with quinolone-resistant pneumococci are an age of >64 years and a history of COPD and/or quinolone exposure. Indeed, patients with pneumonia who have been treated with a quinolone in the past 3 months should receive treatment with another class of antibiotics.

If there is clinical evidence of meningitis in a patient with CAP, vancomycin and ceftriaxone should be used (Table 239-9) to ensure that potentially drug-resistant *S. pneumoniae* is adequately treated.

SWITCH FROM INTRAVENOUS TO ORAL ANTIBIOTIC THERAPY Switching from intravenous to oral antibiotics can be done safely when (1) the white blood cell count is returning toward normal, (2) there are two normal temperature readings (<37.5°C) 16 h apart, and (3) there is improvement in cough and shortness of breath. Some antibiotics, such as amoxicillin and respiratory quinolones (moxifloxacin, gatifloxacin, and levofloxacin), are so well absorbed from the gastrointestinal tract that intravenous therapy is necessary only when the patient is hypotensive, is nauseated, and/or is vomiting.

TABLE 239-9 Initial Empirical Antibiotic Therapy for Community-Acquired Pneumonia

Treatment Setting; Patient's Condition	Regimen[a]
Outpatient; no cardiopulmonary disease, no risk factors for DRSP infection[b]	Macrolide (e.g., clarithromycin 500 mg bid PO × 10 days; or azithromycin 500 mg PO once, then 250 mg/d × 4 days) *or* Doxycycline 100 mg bid PO × 10 days
Outpatient; cardiopulmonary disease and/or (1) risk factors for DRSP infection or (2) high DRSP prevalence in community	Quinolone with enhanced activity against *Streptococcus pneumoniae*—e.g., levofloxacin 500 mg/d PO (or, with C_{cr} <50 mL/min, 250 mg/d), moxifloxacin 400 mg/d PO, or gatifloxacin 400 mg/d PO *or* β-Lactam (cefpodoxime 200 mg bid, cefuroxime axetil 750 mg tid, or amoxicillin 1000 mg tid, PO; amoxicillin/clavulanic acid 875/175 mg tid) plus macrolide or doxycycline *or* Telithromycin 800 mg q24h × 10 days
Hospital ward	Cefuroxime 750 mg q8h IV or ceftriaxone 1 g/d IV or cefotaxime 2 g q6h IV or ampicillin/ sulbactam 1.5–3 g q6h IV *plus* Azithromycin 1 g/d IV followed by 500 mg/d IV *or* Quinolone with enhanced activity against *S. pneumoniae* (see above)[c]
Intensive care unit; no risk factors for *Pseudomonas aeruginosa* infection	Azithromycin 1 g IV, then start 500 mg IV 24 h later *plus* Ceftriaxone 1 g q12h IV *or* Cefotaxime 2 g q6h IV *or* Quinolone IV
Intensive care unit; risk factors for *P. aeruginosa*[b]	Imipenem (or meropenem) 500 mg q6h IV *or* Piperacillin/tazobactam 3.375 g q6h IV *plus* Ciprofloxacin 750 mg q8h IV
Nursing home[d]	Amoxicillin/clavulanic acid 875/125 mg tid PO *plus* Macrolide PO (see above) *or* Quinolone PO with enhanced activity against *S. pneumoniae* (see above) *or* Ceftriaxone 500–1000 mg/d IM or cefotaxime 500 mg IM q12h *plus* Macrolide (see above)
Aspiration pneumonitis (presumed to be due to effects of gastric acid or other irritants)	Wait 24 h; if symptoms persist, give antibiotic therapy delineated below for aspiration pneumonia
Aspiration pneumonia; poor dental hygiene or putrid sputum, alcoholism (anaerobic infection suspected)	Metronidazole 500 mg q12h PO[e] *or* Piperacillin/tazobactam 3.375 g q6h IV *or* Imipenem 500 mg q6h IV *plus* One of the following: levofloxacin 500 mg/d IV or PO, moxifloxacin 400 mg/d PO, gatifloxacin 400 mg/d IV or PO, ceftriaxone, or cefotaxime
Aspiration pneumonia; community-acquired	Levofloxacin, moxifloxacin, gatifloxacin, ceftriaxone, or cefotaxime (see above)
Concomitant meningitis (suspected pneumococcal)	Vancomycin 1 g q12h IV *plus* Ceftriaxone 2 g q12h IV

[a] The optimal duration of therapy for CAP is unknown. With the exception of azithromycin (which has a long half-life), a 7- to 10-day course is usually recommended. Pneumonia due to *Legionella* spp., *P. aeruginosa*, or Enterobacteriaceae usually requires therapy of longer duration (often up to 21 days).

[b] Risk factors: (1) For penicillin-resistant *S. pneumoniae*: Previous use (within 3 months) of β-lactam antibiotics, alcoholism, age <5 years or >65 years, and (in some areas) residence in a nursing home. (2) For macrolide-resistant *S. pneumoniae*: Age <5 years or nosocomial acquisition of infection. (3) For quinolone-resistant *S. pneumoniae*: Older age, nursing home residence, chronic obstructive pulmonary disease, previous exposure to quinolones (especially ciprofloxacin in patients with chronic obstructive pulmonary disease) in the past 3 months, multiple hospitalizations, and β-lactam use. (4) For *P. aeruginosa*: Bronchiectasis, malnutrition, treatment with >10 mg of prednisone/d, previously undiagnosed HIV infection, and broad-spectrum antibiotic therapy for >7 days in the past month.

[c] Some authorities suggest that a β-lactam be added if a quinolone is chosen as empirical therapy until it is clear that quinolone-resistant pneumococci are not involved.

[d] For nursing home residents transferred to the hospital for treatment, see appropriate hospital/intensive care unit recommendations.

[e] Clindamycin could be used, but, because of the increased rate of *Clostridium difficile*–associated diarrhea associated with this drug, metronidazole is preferred.

Note: DRSP, drug-resistant *S. pneumoniae*.

DURATION OF ANTIBIOTIC THERAPY The standard duration of treatment for most patients with CAP is 10 to 14 days. However, no data from randomized clinical trials indicate the optimal duration. Patients treated on an ambulatory basis with an antibiotic with a long half-life

TABLE 239-10 *Criteria for Hospital Admission of an Adult with Community-Acquired Pneumonia*[a]

1. Respiratory rate >28/min
2. Systolic blood pressure <90 mmHg or 30 mmHg below baseline
3. New-onset confusion or impaired level of consciousness
4. Hypoxemia: P_{O_2} <60 mmHg while breathing room air or oxygen saturation <90%
5. Unstable comorbid illness (e.g., decompensated congestive heart failure, uncontrolled diabetes mellitus, alcoholism, immunosuppression)
6. Multilobar pneumonia, if hypoxemia is present
7. Pleural effusion that is >1 cm on lateral decubitus chest radiography and has the characteristics of a complicated parapneumonic effusion on pleural fluid analysis

[a] Patient should be admitted if any of the above criteria applies. Social factors such as homelessness must also be considered in the admission decision.

(e.g., azithromycin) require only 5 days of treatment. Patients with severe Legionnaires' disease require 21 days of therapy, as do those with pneumonia due to *P. aeruginosa* or other aerobic gram-negative bacilli.

Discharge from the Hospital The decision about when to discharge a patient with pneumonia is often a complicated matter. Once physiologic stability is achieved (defined as an oral temperature of <37.5°C for 24 h, a heart rate of <100/min, a respiratory rate of <24/min, a systolic blood pressure of >90 mmHg, an oxygen saturation of >90% while breathing room air, and the ability to eat and drink well enough to maintain hydration), clinical deterioration requiring admission to a critical-care unit or telemetry monitoring has occurred in <1% of patients. Since most patients hospitalized with CAP are elderly, it is necessary to assess functional and mental status before discharge. Comorbid illnesses should be stable, and any complications that have occurred during the hospital stay should have been addressed. Instability at the time of discharge is associated with higher rates of mortality and readmission than have been documented among patients stable at discharge.

In one study, patients with HIV infection and *Pneumocystis* pneumonia who were treated by an experienced medical team had a lower mortality rate than those who were treated by a team that managed such patients infrequently. Patients with pneumonia who were treated by subspecialists working outside their specialty had an 18% longer hospital stay and a slightly higher mortality rate than patients with pneumonia who were treated by general internists. High patient-to-nurse ratios are associated with increased mortality rates on surgical floors, and this association is likely to hold true and to be linked with suboptimal outcomes among patients hospitalized with pneumonia as well.

Failure to Improve When a patient with pneumonia fails to improve despite therapy, an organized approach that considers all the factors listed in Table 239-11 is useful. Many noninfectious conditions may mimic pneumonia, including lung cancer, pulmonary thromboembolic disease with infarction, collagen vascular diseases involving the lungs, and hypersensitivity pneumonitis due to drugs and a variety of antigens. A careful physical examination, with a search for metastatic foci of infection or physical signs suggestive of other diseases (e.g., subconjunctival petechiae, a new cardiac murmur suggestive of endocarditis), should be conducted and should be followed by blood, urine, and sputum cultures and repeat chest radiography. Depending on the results of chest radiography, high-resolution CT of the chest may be the next step. Indeed, CT of the chest in patients who fail to respond to therapy results in new findings not seen on chest radiographs 50% of the time, and these findings frequently lead to a change in therapy. If these investigations are unrewarding and pulmonary infection is still thought to be the most likely diagnosis, bronchoscopy with bronchoalveolar lavage is indicated. The respiratory secretions obtained should

be cultured both aerobically and anaerobically as well as for *M. tuberculosis*, atypical mycobacteria, respiratory viruses, and fungi. Monoclonal antibody staining for *Pneumocystis* should be done. The secretions should also be examined cytologically; although this type of examination is usually undertaken to detect malignant cells, the investigator is occasionally surprised by the finding of *Strongyloides stercoralis* larvae in immunosuppressed patients with hyperinfection syndrome.

FOLLOW-UP Up to 2% of patients hospitalized with CAP are found to have cancer of the lung (with pneumonia distal to an obstructed bronchus). In 50% of these patients, the cancer is evident on the initial chest radiograph; however, in the remaining 50%, the cancer manifests as failure of the pneumonia to resolve radiographically and is evident only when bronchoscopy is performed to determine the reason for delayed pneumonia resolution. The rate of radiographic resolution of pneumonia is influenced by the age of the patient and the underlying lung disease. Thus patients with bacteremic pneumococcal pneumonia who are >60 years old and have COPD require up to 12 weeks for pneumonia resolution. The question, then, is the optimal timing of the follow-up chest radiograph among patients who are clinically well. In elderly patients with COPD, it is reasonable to wait 8 to 12 weeks. Nonsmoking patients <50 years of age who have no underlying lung disease should experience complete resolution of pneumonia within 6 weeks.

PREVENTION All patients with pneumonia who are tobacco smokers should be encouraged to join smoking cessation programs. Influenza and pneumococcal vaccination status should be ascertained and vaccines offered when appropriate. When a patient is prone to aspiration, preventive measures should be taken.

SELECTED COMPLICATIONS OF CAP ■ Complicated Pleural Effusion About 40% of patients hospitalized with CAP have a pleural effusion that can be documented by special techniques, such as CT of the chest. All patients with a pleural effusion should have a lateral decubitus chest radiograph with the affected side down. If the size of the effusion is >1 cm, the fluid should be aspirated. If the fluid has a pH of <7, a glucose level of <2.2 mmol/L, and a lactate dehydrogenase content of >1000 units and is positive on Gram's staining or culture, it should be drained. If frank pus is aspirated, insertion of a chest tube and treatment with intrapleural lytic agents are recommended. Thoracotomy and decortication may be necessary. All patients with a complicated pleural effusion, as defined above, should have a consultation with a thoracic surgeon.

Lung Abscess A lung abscess is a localized area of suppuration within lung tissue that leads to parenchymal destruction and is manifest radiographically as a cavity with an air-fluid level. Lung abscesses are currently uncommon, with an incidence of 4 to 5 cases per 10,000 hospital admissions. Risk factors for lung abscess include conditions associated with impaired cough reflex and/or aspiration, such as al-

TABLE 239-11 *Possibilities to Consider When a Patient with Community-Acquired Pneumonia Fails to Improve Despite Treatment*

1. Reconsider the diagnosis. Is this another illness presenting as pneumonia? Collagen vascular diseases involving the lung are frequently diagnosed at first as pneumonia.
2. Are you treating the wrong pathogen? For example, if you are treating conventional bacterial causes of pneumonia, is this case actually due to *Mycobacterium tuberculosis*, *Pneumocystis*, or another fungus?
3. Are you treating the right pathogen with the wrong drug? For example, if you are using nafcillin or cloxacillin to treat *Staphylococcus aureus* and your patient is infected with methicillin-resistant *S. aureus*, you should be using vancomycin or linezolid.
4. Is there a mechanical reason for the patient's failure to improve (e.g., obstructed bronchus due to carcinoma or sequestration of a segment of lung)?
5. Have you overlooked an undrained or metastatic pyogenic focus (e.g., empyema, brain abscess, endocarditis, splenic abscess, osteomyelitis)?
6. Does the patient have drug-associated fever?

coholism, anesthesia, drug abuse, epilepsy, and stroke. Dental caries, bronchiectasis, bronchial carcinoma, and pulmonary infarction are also risk factors. Most aspiration-associated lung abscesses are due to a combination of aerobic and anaerobic bacteria, with an average of six or seven bacterial species identified in an individual case. The implicated anaerobic bacteria include the *Bacteroides fragilis* group, *Bacteroides gracilis, Prevotella intermedia, Prevotella denticola, Prevotella melaninogenicus, Prevotella oralis, Fusobacterium nucleatum, Peptostreptococcus micros, Peptostreptococcus anaerobius,* and *Peptostreptococcus magnus. Streptococcus milleri* is one of the principal aerobic pathogens; *S. aureus, S. pneumoniae, H. influenzae, P. aeruginosa, E. coli,* and *Klebsiella pneumoniae* are also isolated frequently. Rarely, *S. pneumoniae* alone (usually capsular type 3) can cause a lung abscess. In HIV-infected patients, lung abscesses can be due to *Pneumocystis, Rhodococcus equi,* and *Cryptococcus neoformans* as well as the bacteria noted above.

The clinical presentation is usually indolent, with weight loss, malaise, night sweats, fever, and productive cough. Patients with anaerobic lung abscess have foul-smelling, often foul-tasting sputum. Clubbing of the fingers occurs in ~10% of patients, usually in those who have been symptomatic for >3 weeks.

Spontaneous drainage occurs via bronchial communication and is accompanied by the production of copious amounts of purulent sputum. Percutaneous catheter drainage can be both diagnostic and therapeutic. Antibiotic therapy should be directed at the organisms isolated and should be continued until the abscess has resolved radiographically. The treatment of a lung abscess requires a prolonged duration of therapy (usually 6 to 8 weeks, depending on clinical response). Medical management is unsuccessful in ~10% of cases. When medical management fails or the lung abscess is large, percutaneous drainage or lobectomy should be considered. When empyema is present, closed thoracostomy or open surgical drainage with or without decortication should be performed.

Not all pulmonary cavities are lung abscesses. Cavitating carcinoma, Wegener's granulomatosis, rheumatoid nodules, pulmonary infarcts, tuberculosis, and fungal infections are included in the differential diagnosis.

Recurrent Pneumonia Of patients admitted to the hospital for the treatment of CAP, 10 to 15% have another episode within 2 years. If the recurrence affects the same anatomical location as the previous episode, the most likely cause is an obstructed bronchus due to either a tumor or a foreign body. COPD and repeated macroaspiration are the most common causes of recurrent pneumonia. Persons without COPD, with pneumonia in a different location from the previous episode, and with no risk factors for aspiration should undergo evaluation for immunodeficiency, including HIV testing, immunoglobulin determination, protein electrophoresis, and enumeration of T and B cells. CT of the chest often detects pulmonary anatomical defects such as bronchiectasis that might be the cause of the recurrent pneumonia.

CAP IN LONG-TERM-CARE FACILITIES

EPIDEMIOLOGY About 4% of persons >65 years of age and 15% of those >85 years of age reside in LTCFs. LTCF residents range from healthy, self-sufficient individuals to frail persons who may be bedridden. Pneumonia is the leading cause of infection requiring transfer of nursing home residents to the hospital, accounting for 10 to 18% of all pneumonia admissions in North America. Profound disability (Karnofsky score of <10), bedridden state, urinary incontinence, male gender, difficulty swallowing, and inability to take oral medications are risk factors for pneumonia among LTCF residents, whereas receipt of influenza vaccine is protective. Malnutrition, tube feedings, hyperextended neck, contractures, and use of benzodiazepine and anticholinergic medications are risk factors for aspiration pneumonia in this population.

ETIOLOGY The most common etiologic agents associated with LTCF-acquired pneumonia are *S. aureus* (including MRSA), aerobic gram-negative bacilli, *S. pneumoniae, M. tuberculosis* (~2% of cases), and

the agents of aspiration pneumonitis/pneumonia (about one-third of cases).

CLINICAL PRESENTATION In the frail or functionally impaired LTCF resident, pneumonia may present as an insidious or nonspecific deterioration in general health and/or activity level (e.g., confusion, falls, or sudden exacerbation of—or slow recovery from—an existing primary disease). An increase in respiratory rate to ≥28/min may be the first manifestation of pneumonia and often develops 24 to 48 h before clinical diagnosis. The in-hospital mortality rate can be as high as 30%, and the 1-year mortality rate is >50%.

Rx TREATMENT

Site of Care Nursing homes vary greatly in terms of the facilities and nursing staff available to provide care to very ill patients. Thus decisions about treatment site must be made with knowledge of the available resources as well as the wishes of patients and their families. Criteria helpful in deciding who should be transferred from an LTCF to the hospital for treatment of pneumonia are listed in Table 239-12.

Antibiotic Therapy Suggested regimens for the treatment of pneumonia in LTCF residents—either at the facility or in the hospital—are provided in Table 239-9.

PREVENTION Minimizing the risk of aspiration is a key factor in prevention of LTCF-associated pneumonia. Swallowing should be assessed in at-risk patients. Patients should be positioned upright for meals and during tube feeding. Use of sedatives/hypnotics should be minimized. Attention should be given to oral hygiene and dental care.

All residents should have a two-step Mantoux test at admission to the LTCF, and those with a positive result should be evaluated for evidence of active tuberculosis, with isoniazid treatment or prophylaxis given as needed. Humidifiers should be avoided or used only with sterile water. All LTCF workers should receive influenza vaccine annually.

SEVERE CAP

Severe CAP is generally defined as pneumonia requiring admission to the ICU. The criteria for severe CAP given in Table 239-4 are 100% sensitive and 72.8% specific and have a positive predictive value of 26.4%. Clinical judgment clearly remains paramount in this management decision.

EPIDEMIOLOGY The most common causes of severe CAP are listed in Table 239-2.

VENTILATORY SUPPORT While mechanical ventilation is commonly used to treat the hypoxemia associated with severe CAP, other therapies are also employed. Continuous positive airway pressure is widely used in hypoxemic patients with *Pneumocystis* pneumonia, and early studies suggest that it has the potential to hasten recovery. Hypoxemia is the result of intrapulmonary shunting and ventilation-perfusion mismatch, affecting up to 50% of cardiac output in patients with severe CAP. In patients with unilateral pneumonia, simply positioning the unaffected lung downward may result in improved ventilation-perfusion matching and an increase in Pa_{O_2} of 10 to 15 mmHg. More experimental ap-

TABLE 239-12 *Criteria for Treatment of Pneumonia in a Nursing Home*

1. Respiratory rate <30/min
2. Oxygen saturation ≥92% while breathing room air
3. Pulse rate <90/min
4. Temperature 36.5°C to 38.1°C
5. Systolic and diastolic blood pressure within 10 mmHg of usual readings
6. No feeding tube present
7. Patient conscious
8. Availability of medical and nursing care
9. Wishes of patient and family

proaches include the use of cyclooxygenase inhibitors (e.g., aspirin and indomethacin) to help partially reverse hypoxic pulmonary artery vasoconstriction and the aerosolization of prostacycline (PGI_2) or nitric oxide to reduce intrapulmonary shunting and pulmonary hypertension.

ASPIRATION PNEUMONITIS/PNEUMONIA

Aspiration syndromes refer to the clinical and pathophysiologic effects resulting from the introduction of foreign objects or substances into the lower respiratory tract. The most commonly involved areas—those that are most dependent in the supine position—are the posterior segments of the upper lobes and the superior segments of the lower lobes.

ETIOLOGY The usual causes of aspiration pneumonia in the elderly are Enterobacteriaceae, *S. aureus*, *S. pneumoniae*, and *H. influenzae*.

EPIDEMIOLOGY Aspiration syndromes include two distinct clinical entities. In aspiration pneumonitis, gastric contents (sterile as long as gastric acid is present) are aspirated into the lungs, with a consequent inflammatory response. Pneumonia results from the aspiration of oropharyngeal flora into the lungs, with consequent bacterial infection. The risk factors for aspiration include altered level of consciousness, incompetent gastroesophageal junction, elevated intragastric pressure or volume, and neuromuscular diseases that interfere with glottic closure.

The number of cases of aspiration pneumonia diagnosed in Medicare patients increased by 93.5% between 1991 and 1998. The mortality rate among patients with aspiration pneumonia was 23.1%, compared with 7.6% among those with pneumococcal pneumonia.

CLINICAL FEATURES The manifestations of aspiration pneumonia vary with the volume and nature of the material aspirated. Gastric acid aspiration results in a chemical pneumonitis that can be very severe, requiring assisted ventilation. A pH of <2.5 and a gastric aspirate volume of >0.3 mL/kg (20 to 25 mL in adults) are required for the development of aspiration pneumonitis. There is an acute onset of dyspnea, tachypnea, bronchospasm, and cyanosis, with a chest radiograph often showing diffuse opacities.

Many elderly patients are achlorhydric and so may not fit the typical presentation described above. Indeed, in many of these patients, aspiration pneumonitis is often indistinguishable from pneumonia. A history or a witnessed account of an aspiration event (one or more instances of vomiting, coughing while eating, displacement of a feeding tube, or vomitus or tube feeding on bedclothes or on the patient within 24 h of the diagnosis of pneumonia) is documented in only 40% of definite aspiration events among LTCF residents. Thus the diagnosis of aspiration pneumonitis/pneumonia requires a high index of suspicion. The location of the pneumonia depends on the position of the patient when aspiration occurred. An opacity involving the posterior segment of the upper lobes (especially the right upper lobe) is found in persons who have aspirated in the recumbent position, while aspiration in the upright or semirecumbent position results in involvement of the posterior basal segments of the lower lobes.

In the setting of aspiration of oropharyngeal contents and poor dental hygiene, anaerobic bacteria may be present, and lung abscess is not an uncommon complication. Particulate matter may be aspirated, with consequent mechanical obstruction of the airway.

℞ TREATMENT

Treatment for aspiration occurring in a community setting is outlined in Table 239-9.

PREVENTION Good oral hygiene reduces the risk of aspiration pneumonia among patients with cerebrovascular disease and swallowing impairment. Patients at high risk for aspiration (e.g., those who have had a stroke) should be assessed for aspiration. This evaluation is easily done by having an alert patient sit up and take increasing amounts of water, starting with one spoonful. Water leaking out of the corners of the mouth, coughing, and shortness of breath are all suggestive of aspiration and indicate the need for further evaluation.

CAP IN THE IMMUNOCOMPROMISED HOST

HIV-INFECTED PERSONS See Chap. 173.

TRANSPLANT RECIPIENTS (See also Chap. 117) Organ transplant recipients who develop pneumonia need a comprehensive diagnostic workup (diagnostic yield, 80%) and careful follow-up. Almost all of these patients require admission to the hospital. Newer immunosuppressive regimens and suppressive therapy for cytomegalovirus infection are changing the types and times of onset of opportunistic infections in this population.

An acute onset of symptoms, with presentation to the physician within 24 h, suggests bacterial pneumonia, pulmonary emboli with infarction, or pulmonary hemorrhage. A subacute onset over a few days to a week suggests viral, *Mycoplasma*, or *Pneumocystis* infection. A more chronic course over ≥1 week suggests fungal, nocardial, or tuberculous infection. Bacterial pneumonia is the most common infection in lung transplant recipients, accounting for almost half of the infections in this population. The incidence of pneumonia among these patients peaks in the first 4 to 8 weeks after transplantation and declines by the fourth month.

Nocardia spp., *R. equi*, and *Legionella* spp. are the major opportunistic bacterial pathogens in the lungs of organ transplant recipients; cytomegalovirus, varicella-zoster virus, influenza A and B viruses, respiratory syncytial virus, and adenovirus are the principal viral pathogens; and *Pneumocystis*, *C. neoformans*, *Aspergillus* spp., and Mucoraceae are the major fungal pathogens. *Aspergillus* spp., often in combination with aerobic gram-negative bacilli, is the most common cause of CAP among hematopoietic stem cell transplant recipients with graft-versus-host disease. CT of the chest is particularly useful if aspergillosis is suspected, in that it reveals pulmonary nodules, cavities, and halo or air-crescent signs.

HOSPITAL-ACQUIRED (NOSOCOMIAL) PNEUMONIA

EPIDEMIOLOGY Hospital-acquired pneumonia (HAP) is defined as pneumonia occurring at least 48 h after hospital admission and not incubating at the time of admission (Chap. 116). The incidence of HAP is estimated at 5 to 10 cases per 1000 hospital discharges, with ~300,000 cases annually. HAP is uncommon on obstetrical and psychiatric wards but reportedly develops in 5 to 10% of all hospital discharges on medical and surgical wards. HAP is the second most common nosocomial infection, accounting for up to 30% of all nosocomial infections; it carries the highest morbidity and mortality; it lengthens hospital stay by an average of 7 to 9 days per affected patient; and it increases costs by $2 billion annually. The incidence of HAP is highest among patients in the ICU who are undergoing mechanical ventilation. About 10% of general surgical postoperative patients, 20% of intubated patients, and up to 70% of patients with ARDS develop HAP during their stay in the ICU. A subset of HAP—ventilator-acquired pneumonia (VAP)—has been defined as pneumonia occurring after at least 48 h of mechanical ventilation and not incubating at the time of intubation. Because most patients undergo mechanical ventilation for only a short period, half of all cases of VAP occur within the first 4 days of intubation. The rate of VAP development is 3% for days 1 through 5, 2% for days 6 through 10, and 1% for days 11 through 15 after intubation. Among nonventilated patients, HAP is reported to occur at a median rate of 3.2 cases per 1000 ICU days; the corresponding figure for mechanically ventilated patients is 34.4 cases per 1000 ICU days. The incidence of pneumonia is reported to be 6 to 20 times higher among mechanically ventilated patients than among other hospitalized patients.

Crude mortality rates for HAP range from 30 to 70% and are highest among bacteremic patients, patients infected with high-risk pathogens (e.g., *P. aeruginosa*), and ICU patients. In the ICU setting, risk factors for death include shock, coma, ultimately or rapidly fatal underlying disease, systemic inflammatory response syndrome, a high APACHE score, bilateral pulmonary infiltrates on chest radiography, ARDS, and respiratory failure. Despite high crude mortality rates, not all deaths are due to pneumonia; some patients with HAP die of their underlying illness. The attributable mortality due to HAP (i.e., the percentage of deaths among patients with HAP that would not have occurred in the absence of pneumonia) has been studied and remains controversial, but several studies suggest that one-third to one-half of all HAP deaths are due to infection.

About 1.5% of patients develop pneumonia postoperatively. The mortality rate at 1 month is tenfold higher (21% vs. 2%) among these patients than among those who do not develop postoperative pneumonia. An age of >80 years, poor functional status, recent weight loss, and alcohol use are predictors of postoperative pneumonia. Abdominal aortic aneurysm repair, thoracic surgery, and emergency surgery carry the highest risk for postoperative pneumonia, and general anesthesia carries a higher risk than other types of anesthesia.

PATHOGENESIS In addition to the factors that are important in the pathogenesis of CAP overall, other factors play an important role in the pathogenesis of HAP. Moreover, certain risk factors increase the likelihood of infection by specific pathogens (see below).

The patient's host defense system can be adversely affected by a number of risk factors. Factors that affect upper-respiratory host defenses (nasogastric or endotracheal intubation/reintubation, enteral feedings) increase the risk of both gross aspiration and microaspiration. Endotracheal intubation increases the risk of pneumonia in several ways. The tube serves as a direct conduit for bacterial introduction into the lower respiratory tract, prevents effective coughing to clear lower respiratory secretions, damages the tracheal epithelium, and allows the accumulation of oropharyngeal secretions (which are frequently colonized with bacteria) just above the cuff. Colonization of the endotracheal tube with pathogenic organisms can cause the formation of a biofilm that can be dislodged into the lower respiratory tract during suctioning. Poor infection-control measures and prolonged use of inappropriate antimicrobial agents increase the risk of spread of antimicrobial-resistant and/or especially virulent pathogens.

The presence of nasotracheal or nasogastric tubes increases the risk of nosocomial sinusitis, which occurs in more than half of all patients intubated for >7 days and which is also a risk factor for VAP. In one study, the same organism was isolated by transnasal culture and by protected specimen brushing in 20% of all patients with radiographic evidence of sinusitis. Moreover, the mortality rate was significantly lower when nosocomial sinusitis was identified and aggressively treated with antibiotics and nasal lavage every 8 h.

The role of the stomach as a reservoir for organisms that cause HAP remains controversial. It is accepted that elevation in gastric pH by antacids, H$_2$ antagonists, or enteral gastric feedings often leads to gastric bacterial overgrowth, which could be aspirated into the lower respiratory tract. Patients in the ICU are at high risk of aspiration because of reflux in the supine position, stomach placement of the enteral feeding tube, and large gastric volume.

In mechanically ventilated patients, tracheobronchitis frequently precedes the development of VAP by several days. Tracheobronchitis does not inevitably result in VAP, but bacterial concentrations in the bronchi may reach levels of at least 10^3 colony-forming units (CFU) per milliliter. In addition to fever and purulent sputum, tracheobronchitis may cause a false-positive culture result when lower respiratory tract secretions are sampled with a protected specimen brush (PSB).

ETIOLOGY In a national survey in the United States, 64% of all microorganisms isolated from the lungs of patients with nosocomial pneumonia were gram-negative bacilli, including *P. aeruginosa* (21%), *Acinetobacter* spp. (6%), and traditional enteric pathogens such as *Enterobacter* spp. (9%) and *K. pneumoniae* (8%).

S. aureus is the most common cause of nosocomial pneumonia in the United States. The increasing prevalence of MRSA among nosocomial isolates of *S. aureus* (from 2% in 1974 to as high as 64% in recent surveys) is of great concern in this context. In a comparative study of pneumonia due to MRSA and that due to methicillin-susceptible *S. aureus* (MSSA) in patients in an ICU, MRSA pneumonia resulted in a significantly greater frequency of bacteremia (36.4% vs. 10.5%; RR 3.4) and septic shock (27.3% vs. 7.9%; RR 3.4) and a significantly higher infection-associated mortality rate (54.5% vs. 2.6%; RR 20.7). Mortality rates among patients with MRSA and MSSA pneumonia who are treated with vancomycin are very high, possibly because of the low levels of vancomycin in the lungs 24 h after the initiation of treatment. In some in vitro studies, the bactericidal action of vancomycin against *S. aureus* has been weaker and slower than that of other antimicrobial agents, such as cloxacillin.

The Enterobacteriaceae account for ~30% of cases of ICU-acquired pneumonia. More than one-third of *Enterobacter* strains acquired in this setting are resistant to third-generation cephalosporins. The predominant mechanism of cephalosporin resistance in the Enterobacteriaceae is the production of β-lactamases, of which >300 have been described. The emergence of plasmid-mediated extended-spectrum β-lactamases (ESBLs) in members of the family Enterobacteriaceae has become a worldwide problem. ESBL molecular class A possesses an extended hydrolysis spectrum toward oxyimino-β-lactams and aztreonam but remains susceptible to cefoxitin and β-lactamase inhibitors.

The cephamycins (cefoxitin, cefotetan, and cefmetazole) are structurally different from the true cephalosporins and display enhanced stability in the presence of ESBLs. More than 90% of ESBL-producing organisms are susceptible to cephamycins.

Of major concern is the discovery of plasmid-mediated carbapenemases in Enterobacteriaceae. These enzymes inactivate all carbapenems, cephalosporins, and antipseudomonal penicillins.

Among patients on hospital wards who have no risk factors associated with specific pathogens, the pathogens most frequently causing nosocomial pneumonia include *S. pneumoniae*, *H. influenzae*, *S. aureus*, and enteric gram-negative bacilli (i.e., *E. coli*, *Klebsiella* spp., *Proteus* spp., and *Serratia marcescens*). These organisms have been designated "core pathogens" in the American Thoracic Society's guidelines for the treatment of nosocomial pneumonia.

The spectrum of potential pathogens is increased among patients with mild to moderate HAP if risk factors for specific pathogens are present. If the patient has had recent abdominal surgery or if an aspiration has been witnessed, the involvement of anaerobes should be considered. *S. aureus* (including MRSA) is more common among patients in a coma or with head trauma, diabetes mellitus, or renal failure. In the setting of potable-water contamination by *Legionella* spp., the use of high-dose glucocorticoids increases the risk of infection with this organism.

Among previously healthy patients with severe HAP requiring ICU care, length of stay before the onset of HAP affects the spectrum of pathogens. The most common pathogens among these patients with early-onset HAP or VAP (<5 days after admission) are the core pathogens (see above).

The most important risk factors for HAP due to resistant microorganisms are late onset of infection (>5 days after admission) and recent antibiotic therapy. The most common resistant organisms are MRSA, *Acinetobacter calcoaceticus-baumannii*, *Stenotrophomonas maltophilia*, and ESBL-producing Enterobacteriaceae. In addition, there are risk factors for specific resistant microorganisms. Glucocorticoid therapy, malnutrition, structural lung disease, mechanical ventilation, and underlying fatal medical conditions are risk factors for *P. aeruginosa*. Neurosurgery, head trauma, ARDS, and aspiration are risk factors for *Acinetobacter*. *S. maltophilia* is associated with increased ICU stay, tracheostomy, treatment with cefepime, and severe trauma with lung contusion. Isolation of MRSA has been associated with prior antibiotic therapy (especially with quinolones and macrolides), previous hospitalization, enteral feeding, surgery, and late-onset VAP. ESBL-producing Enterobacteriaceae have been associated with intubation, previous antibiotic therapy, and central venous catheterization. The latter organisms may also be community-acquired and are now a problem in chronic-care facilities.

CLINICAL MANIFESTATIONS The definition of HAP includes the presence of a new or progressive infiltrate on chest radiography plus at least two of the following: fever [>37.8°C (>100°F)], leukocytosis (>10,000 white blood cells/μL), and the production of purulent sputum. Other findings, such as dyspnea, hypoxemia, and pleuritic chest pain, should prompt investigations for nosocomial pneumonia. It is important to exclude noninfectious causes of pulmonary infiltrates when evaluating a patient who presents with possible HAP.

DIAGNOSIS One of the most controversial areas in the management of HAP is how best to ascertain whether pneumonia is present and to determine the most appropriate therapy. Diagnostic accuracy is particularly important in mechanically ventilated patients, in whom VAP is frequently overdiagnosed. Invasive diagnostic testing is generally performed on intubated patients with VAP. The sampling methods used include endotracheal aspiration, PSB or bronchoalveolar lavage (BAL)

sampling via a fiberoptic bronchoscope (FOB), or blinded invasive methods [blinded bronchial sampling (BBS), mini-BAL, and blinded PSB (BPSB)].

Endotracheal aspiration is most sensitive when patients have not received antimicrobial therapy. However, its specificity is low, and the sensitivity and specificity of cultures of endotracheal aspirates vary widely. If the patient has recently received any antibiotics, sensitivity and specificity are further decreased. The reported sensitivity and specificity of quantitative endotracheal aspiration range from 38 to 100% and from 14 to 100%, respectively. Visualization of elastin fibrils on Gram's staining and antibody coating of bacteria are unreliable indicators of infection.

Use of FOB-directed PSB and/or BAL has been advocated by many authorities; when performed at the same time, these studies are generally considered complementary. PSB is considered positive when at least 10^3 CFU of bacteria per brush are obtained, and BAL is considered positive when the recovered lavage fluid contains at least 10^4 CFU of bacteria per milliliter. The sensitivity of PSB ranges from 33 to 100% (median, 67%), and the specificity ranges from 50 to 100% (median, 95%). The sensitivity of BAL ranges from 42 to 93% (median, 73%), while the specificity ranges from 45 to 100% (median,

TABLE 239-13 *Empirical Antibiotic Therapy for Hospital-Acquired Pneumonia (HAP)*

Treatment Setting; Patient's Condition	Risk Factor/Usual Pathogen(s)	Regimen
Hospital ward; mild to moderate HAP, no risk factors for specific pathogens	—	Second-generation cephalosporin (cefuroxime 750 mg q8h IV) *or* Nonpseudomonal third-generation cephalosporin (ceftriaxone 1 g/d IV) *or* β-Lactam/β-lactamase inhibitor combination (piperacillin/tazobactam 3.375 g q6h IV) Penicillin allergy: Respiratory quinolone (levofloxacin 500 mg/d IV, moxifloxacin 400 mg/d IV, or gatifloxacin 400 mg/d IV) *or* Clindamycin plus aztreonam
Hospital ward; mild to moderate HAP with specific risk factors	—	Treat for usual pathogens (enteric gram-negative bacilli, *Staphylococcus aureus, Streptococcus pneumoniae, Haemophilus influenzae*) with cefuroxime, ceftriaxone, or piperacillin/tazobactam (see above) *plus* Treat for other pathogens related to risk factors (see below)
	Witnessed aspiration, recent abdominal surgery/anaerobes	Standard treatment (see above) *plus* Clindamycin 450–900 mg q8h IV *or* β-Lactam/β-lactamase inhibitor combination (piperacillin/tazobactam 3.375 g q6h IV)
	Coma, head trauma, diabetes mellitus, renal failure/*S. aureus*, risk for MRSA	Standard treatment (see above) *plus* Vancomycin 1 g q12h IV
	High-dose glucocorticoids/*Legionella*	Standard treatment (see above) *plus* Macrolide (azithromycin 500 mg/d IV) *or* Respiratory quinolone (see above)
Intensive care unit; severe HAP, early onset, no specific risk factors	—	Second-generation cephalosporin, nonpseudomonal third-generation cephalosporin, or β-lactam/β-lactamase inhibitor combination (see above) Penicillin allergy: Respiratory quinolone (see above)
Intensive care unit; severe HAP, late onset or specific risk factors	—	Treat for usual pathogens (enteric gram-negative bacilli, *S. aureus, S. pneumoniae, H. influenzae*) with cefuroxime, ceftriaxone, or piperacillin/tazobactam (see above) *plus* Treat for other pathogens related to risk factors (see below)
	Malnutrition, structural lung disease, glucocorticoid therapy/*Pseudomonas aeruginosa*; neurosurgery, head trauma, ARDS, aspiration/*Acinetobacter* spp.	Standard treatment (see above) *plus* Aminoglycoside or ciprofloxacin 500 mg q12h IV plus one of the following: antipseudomonal penicillin (piperacillin 4 g q6h IV or piperacillin/tazobactam 4.5 g q6h IV) or cefepime 1–2 g q12h IV or imipenem (or meropenem) 500 mg q8h IV
	Prior antibiotic therapy (especially with quinolones or macrolides), previous hospitalization, enteral feeding/MRSA	Standard treatment (see above) *plus* Vancomycin 1 g q12h IV

Note: ARDS, adult respiratory distress syndrome; MRSA, methicillin-resistant *S. aureus.*

82%). Both procedures require a well-trained, experienced operator and rapid transportation of samples to the laboratory. Because results are not available for at least 18 h, a portion of the BAL fluid should be centrifuged, the pellet stained with Giemsa or Gram's stain, and the stained preparation examined to determine the percentage of white blood cells with intracellular bacteria. Both 1% and 5% of cells containing intracellular bacteria have been used as significant breakpoints for diagnosing pneumonia. The effect of antibiotic therapy on the sensitivity and specificity of PSB and BAL is uncertain.

Blind mini-BAL and BBS have been introduced relatively recently. These tests are easier to perform and are less expensive than FOB-directed BAL. The sensitivity and specificity are 74 to 97% and 74 to 100%, respectively, for BPSB; 63 to 100% and 66 to 96% for mini-BAL; and 58 to 86% and 71 to 100% for blind mini-BAL and BBS. Risks from these procedures appear to be minimal.

℞ TREATMENT

Most initial therapy for HAP is empirical (Table 239-13). The selection of drugs should be guided by an understanding of local patterns of antimicrobial resistance. If MRSA is highly prevalent in the institution and the patient is at risk for MRSA infection, empirical therapy should include vancomycin. Quinupristin-dalfopristin and linezolid can also be used to treat MRSA.

Evaluation of a patient whose condition is not improving or is actually deteriorating despite treatment involves the same considerations in HAP as in CAP (Table 239-11). Broadening the spectrum of antimicrobial therapy should be considered, with administration continued at least until the results of additional tests become available. Lower respiratory tract secretions should be sampled immediately by endotracheal aspiration, FOB-directed PSB or BAL, or a blinded sampling procedure.

PREVENTION   A number of measures can reduce the risk of HAP. Health care providers must adhere strictly to hand-washing protocols. Surveillance of pneumonia rates should be routinely performed and reported. In patients undergoing mechanical ventilation, a concerted effort should be made to extubate rapidly, to minimize ventilator circuit changes, and to ensure careful periodic drainage of tubing condensate. Use of endotracheal tubes with a separate posterior lumen that allows continuous suctioning of subglottic secretions has been reported to decrease the incidence of early-onset VAP; heat-moisture exchanges reportedly reduce the risk of late-onset VAP. When the patient is receiving enteral feedings, a small-bore feeding tube should be placed distal to the pylorus, and large gastric residuals should be avoided. Elevation of the head of the bed by at least 30° lessens the risk of pneumonia, as does the use of kinetic beds. Earlier studies did not support the use of selective decontamination of the digestive tract as a method for preventing HAP. A recent study showed a significant reduction in mortality and colonization with resistant gram-negative aerobic bacteria among critically ill patients admitted to an ICU who underwent selective decontamination.

FURTHER READING

BARTLETT JG et al: Practice guidelines for the management of community-acquired pneumonia in adults. Clin Infect Dis 31:347, 2000

DE JONGE E et al: Effects of selective decontamination of digestive tract in mortality and acquisition of resistant bacteria in intensive care: A randomised controlled trial. Lancet 362:1011, 2003

FILE TM: Community-acquired pneumonia. Lancet 36:1991, 2003

GARAU J: Treatment of drug-resistant pneumococcal pneumonia. Lancet Infect Dis 2:404, 2002

HALM EA et al: Instability on hospital discharge and the risk of adverse outcomes in patients with pneumonia. Arch Intern Med 162:1278, 2002

MANDELL LA et al: Canadian guidelines for the initial management of community-acquired pneumonia: An evidence-based update by the Canadian Infectious Diseases Society and the Canadian Thoracic Society. Clin Infect Dis 31:383, 2000

———— et al: Update of practice guidelines for the management of community-acquired pneumonia in immunocompetent adults. Clin Infect Dis 37:1405, 2003

MEDINA-WALPOLE AM, KATZ PR: Nursing home–acquired pneumonia. J Am Geriatr Soc 47:1005, 1999

METLAY JP, FINE MJ: Testing strategies in the initial management of patients with community-acquired pneumonia. Ann Intern Med 138:109, 2003

MINOGUE MF et al: Patients hospitalized after initial outpatient treatment for community-acquired pneumonia. Ann Emerg Med 31:376, 1998

NEIDERMAN MS et al: Guidelines for the management of adults with community-acquired pneumonia. Diagnosis, assessment of severity, antimicrobial therapy and prevention. Am J Respir Crit Care Med 163:1730, 2001

WHITNEY CG et al: Increasing prevalence of multidrug-resistant *Streptococcus pneumoniae* in the United States. N Engl J Med 343:1917, 2000

240   BRONCHIECTASIS
Steven E. Weinberger

DEFINITION   Bronchiectasis is an abnormal and permanent dilatation of bronchi. It may be either focal, involving airways supplying a limited region of pulmonary parenchyma, or diffuse, involving airways in a more widespread distribution. Although this definition is based on pathologic changes in the bronchi, diagnosis is often suggested by the clinical consequences of chronic or recurrent infection in the dilated airways and the associated secretions that pool within these airways.

PATHOLOGY   The bronchial dilatation of bronchiectasis is associated with destructive and inflammatory changes in the walls of medium-sized airways, often at the level of segmental or subsegmental bronchi. The normal structural components of the wall, including cartilage, muscle, and elastic tissue, are destroyed and may be replaced by fibrous tissue. The dilated airways frequently contain pools of thick, purulent material, while more peripheral airways are often occluded by secretions or obliterated and replaced by fibrous tissue. Additional microscopic features include bronchial and peribronchial inflammation and fibrosis, ulceration of the bronchial wall, squamous metaplasia, and mucous gland hyperplasia. The parenchyma normally supplied by the affected airways is abnormal, containing varying combinations of fibrosis, emphysema, bronchopneumonia, and atelectasis. As a result of the inflammation, vascularity of the bronchial wall increases, with associated enlargement of the bronchial arteries and anastomoses between the bronchial and pulmonary arterial circulations.

Three different patterns of bronchiectasis were described by Reid in 1950. In *cylindrical bronchiectasis* the bronchi appear as uniformly dilated tubes that end abruptly at the point that smaller airways are obstructed by secretions. In *varicose bronchiectasis* the affected bronchi have an irregular or beaded pattern of dilatation resembling varicose veins. In *saccular (cystic) bronchiectasis* the bronchi have a ballooned appearance at the periphery, ending in blind sacs without recognizable bronchial structures distal to the sacs.

ETIOLOGY AND PATHOGENESIS   Bronchiectasis is a consequence of inflammation and destruction of the structural components of the bronchial wall. Infection is the usual cause of the inflammation; microorganisms such as *Pseudomonas aeruginosa* and *Haemophilus influenzae* produce pigments, proteases, and other toxins that injure the respiratory epithelium and impair mucociliary clearance. The host inflammatory response induces epithelial injury, largely as a result of mediators released from neutrophils. As protection against infection is compromised, the dilated airways become more susceptible to colonization and growth of bacteria. Thus, a reinforcing cycle can result, with inflammation producing airway damage, impaired clearance of microorganisms, and further infection, which then completes the cycle by inciting more inflammation.

Infectious Causes   Adenovirus and influenza virus are the main viruses that cause bronchiectasis in association with lower respiratory tract involvement. Virulent bacterial infections, especially with potentially necrotizing organisms such as *Staphylococcus aureus*, *Klebsiella*, and anaerobes, remain important causes of bronchiectasis when antibiotic treatment of a pneumonia is not given or is significantly delayed. Bronchiectasis has been reported in patients with HIV infection, perhaps at least partly due to recurrent bacterial infection. Tuberculosis can produce bronchiectasis by a necrotizing effect on pulmonary parenchyma and airways and indirectly as a consequence of airway obstruction from bronchostenosis or extrinsic compression by lymph nodes. Nontuberculous mycobacteria are frequently cultured from patients with bronchiectasis, often as secondary infections or colonizing organisms. However, it has now also been recognized that these organisms, especially those of the *Mycobacterium avium* complex, can serve as primary pathogens associated with the development and/or progression of bronchiectasis. Mycoplasmal and necrotizing fungal infections are rare causes of bronchiectasis.

Impaired host defense mechanisms are often involved in the predisposition to recurrent infections. The major cause of localized impairment of host defenses is endobronchial obstruction. Bacteria and secretions cannot be cleared adequately from the obstructed airway, which develops recurrent or chronic infection. Slowly growing endobronchial neoplasms such as carcinoid tumors may be associated with bronchiectasis. Foreign-body aspiration is another important cause of endobronchial obstruction, particularly in children. Airway obstruction can also result from bronchostenosis, from impacted secretions, or from extrinsic compression by enlarged lymph nodes.

Generalized impairment of pulmonary defense mechanisms occurs with immunoglobulin deficiency, primary ciliary disorders, or cystic fibrosis. Infections and bronchiectasis are therefore often more diffuse. With panhypogammaglobulinemia, the best described of the immunoglobulin disorders associated with recurrent infection and bronchiectasis, patients often also have a history of sinus or skin infections. Selective deficiency of an IgG subclass, especially IgG2, has also been described in a small number of patients with bronchiectasis.

The primary disorders associated with ciliary dysfunction, termed *primary ciliary dyskinesia*, are responsible for 5 to 10% of cases of bronchiectasis. Numerous defects are encompassed under this category, including structural abnormalities of the dynein arms, radial spokes, and microtubules. The cilia become dyskinetic; their coordinated, propulsive action is diminished, and bacterial clearance is impaired. The clinical effects include recurrent upper and lower respiratory tract infections, such as sinusitis, otitis media, and bronchiectasis. Because normal sperm motility also depends on proper ciliary function, males are generally infertile (Chap. 325). Approximately half of patients with primary ciliary dyskinesia fall into the subgroup of *Kartagener's syndrome*, in which situs inversus accompanies bronchiectasis and sinusitis.

In cystic fibrosis (Chap. 241), the tenacious secretions in the bronchi are associated with impaired bacterial clearance, resulting in colonization and recurrent infection with a variety of organisms, particularly mucoid strains of *P. aeruginosa* but also *S. aureus*, *H. influenzae*, *Escherichia coli*, and *Burkholderia cepacia*.

Noninfectious Causes   Some cases of bronchiectasis are associated with exposure to a toxic substance that incites a severe inflammatory response. Examples include inhalation of a toxic gas such as ammonia or aspiration of acidic gastric contents, though the latter problem is often also complicated by aspiration of bacteria. An immune response in the airway may also trigger inflammation, destructive changes, and bronchial dilatation. This mechanism is presumably important for bronchiectasis with allergic bronchopulmonary aspergillosis (ABPA), which is due at least in part to an immune response to *Aspergillus* organisms that have colonized the airway (Chap. 237). Bronchiectasis accompanying ABPA often involves proximal airways and is associated with mucoid impaction. Bronchiectasis also occurs rarely in ulcerative colitis, rheumatoid arthritis, and Sjögren's syndrome, but it is not known whether an immune response triggers airway inflammation in these patients.

In α_1-antitrypsin deficiency, the usual respiratory complication is the early development of panacinar emphysema, but affected individuals may occasionally have bronchiectasis. In the *yellow nail syndrome*, which is due to hypoplastic lymphatics, the triad of lymphedema, pleural effusion, and yellow discoloration of the nails is accompanied by bronchiectasis in approximately 40% of patients.

CLINICAL MANIFESTATIONS   Patients typically present with persistent or recurrent cough and purulent sputum production. Hemoptysis occurs in 50 to 70% of cases and can be due to bleeding from friable, inflamed airway mucosa. More significant, even massive bleeding is often a consequence of bleeding from hypertrophied bronchial arteries.

When a specific infectious episode initiates bronchiectasis, patients may describe a severe pneumonia followed by chronic cough and sputum production. Alternatively, patients without a dramatic initiating event often describe the insidious onset of symptoms. In some cases, patients are either asymptomatic or have a nonproductive cough, often associated with "dry" bronchiectasis in an upper lobe. Dyspnea or wheezing generally reflects either widespread bronchiectasis or underlying chronic obstructive pulmonary disease. With exacerbations of infection, the amount of sputum increases, it becomes more purulent and often more bloody, and patients may become febrile. Such episodes may be due solely to exacerbations of the airway infection, but associated parenchymal infiltrates sometimes reflect an adjacent pneumonia.

Physical examination of the chest overlying an area of bronchiectasis is quite variable. Any combination of crackles, rhonchi, and wheezes may be heard, all of which reflect the damaged airways containing significant secretions. As with other types of chronic intrathoracic infection, clubbing may be present. Patients with severe, diffuse disease, particularly those with chronic hypoxemia, may have associated cor pulmonale and right ventricular failure. Amyloidosis can result from chronic infection and inflammation but is now seldom seen.

RADIOGRAPHIC AND LABORATORY FINDINGS   Though the chest radiograph is important in the evaluation of suspected bronchiectasis, the findings are often nonspecific. At one extreme, the radiograph may be normal with mild disease. Alternatively, patients with saccular bronchiectasis may have prominent cystic spaces, either with or without air-liquid levels, corresponding to the dilated airways. These may be difficult to distinguish from enlarged airspaces due to bullous emphysema or from regions of honeycombing in patients with severe interstitial lung disease. Other findings are due to dilated airways with thickened walls, which result from peribronchial inflammation. Because of decreased aeration and atelectasis of the associated pulmonary parenchyma, these dilated airways are often crowded together in parallel. When seen longitudinally, the airways appear as "tram tracks"; when seen in cross-section, they produce "ring shadows." Because the dilated airways may be filled with secretions, the lumen may appear dense rather than radiolucent, producing an opaque tubular or branched tubular structure.

Bronchography, which involves coating the airways with a radiopaque, iodinated lipid dye instilled through a catheter or bronchoscope, can provide excellent visualization of bronchiectatic airways. However, this technique has now been replaced by computed tomography (CT), which also provides an excellent view of dilated airways as seen in cross-sectional images (Fig. 240-1). With the advent of high-resolution CT scanning, in which the images are 1.0 to 1.5 mm thick, the sensitivity for detecting bronchiectasis has improved even further. Other features on high-resolution CT scanning can suggest a specific etiology of the bronchiectasis. For example, bronchiectasis of relatively proximal airways suggests ABPA, whereas the presence of multiple small pulmonary nodules (nodular bronchiectasis) suggests infection with *M. avium* complex.

Examination of sputum often reveals an abundance of neutrophils

FIGURE 240-1 High-resolution CT scan of bronchiectasis showing dilated airways in both lower lobes and in the lingula. When seen in cross-section, the dilated airways have a ringlike appearance. *(From SE Weinberger: Principles of Pulmonary Medicine, 3d ed. Philadelphia, Saunders, 1998, with permission).*

and colonization or infection with a variety of possible organisms. Appropriate staining and culturing of sputum often provide a guide to antibiotic therapy.

Additional evaluation is aimed at diagnosing the cause for the bronchiectasis. When bronchiectasis is focal, fiberoptic bronchoscopy may reveal an underlying endobronchial obstruction. In other cases, upper lobe involvement may be suggestive of either tuberculosis or ABPA. With more widespread disease, measurement of sweat chloride levels for cystic fibrosis, structural or functional assessment of nasal or bronchial cilia or sperm for primary ciliary dyskinesia, and quantitative assessment of immunoglobulins may explain recurrent airway infection. In an asthmatic person with proximal bronchiectasis or other historical features to suggest ABPA, skin testing, serology, and sputum culture for *Aspergillus* are helpful in confirming the diagnosis.

Pulmonary function tests may demonstrate airflow obstruction as a consequence of diffuse bronchiectasis or associated chronic obstructive lung disease. Bronchial hyperreactivity, e.g., to methacholine challenge, and some reversibility of the airflow obstruction with inhaled bronchodilators are relatively common.

℞ TREATMENT

Therapy has four major goals: (1) elimination of an identifiable underlying problem; (2) improved clearance of tracheobronchial secretions; (3) control of infection, particularly during acute exacerbations; and (4) reversal of airflow obstruction. Appropriate treatment should be instituted when a treatable cause is found, for example, treatment of hypogammaglobulinemia with immunoglobulin replacement, tuberculosis with antituberculous agents, and ABPA with glucocorticoids.

Secretions are typically copious and thick and contribute to the symptoms. A variety of mechanical methods and devices accompanied by appropriate positioning can facilitate drainage in patients with copious secretions. Mucolytic agents to thin secretions and allow better clearance are controversial. Aerosolized recombinant DNase, which decreases viscosity of sputum by breaking down DNA released from neutrophils, has been shown to improve pulmonary function in cystic fibrosis, but similar benefits have not been found with bronchiectasis due to other etiologies.

Antibiotics have an important role in management. For patients with infrequent exacerbations characterized by an increase in quantity and purulence of the sputum, antibiotics are commonly used only during acute episodes. Although choice of an antibiotic may be guided by Gram's stain and culture of sputum, empiric coverage (e.g., with ampicillin, amoxicillin, trimethoprim-sulfamethoxazole, or cefaclor) is often given initially. When *P. aeruginosa* is present, oral therapy with a quinolone or parenteral therapy with an aminoglycoside or third-generation cephalosporin may be appropriate. In patients with chronic purulent sputum despite short courses of antibiotics, more prolonged courses, e.g., with an oral antibiotic or inhaled aminoglycosides, or intermittent but regular courses of single or rotating antibiotics have been used.

Bronchodilators to improve obstruction and aid clearance of secretions are particularly useful in patients with airway hyperreactivity and reversible airflow obstruction. Although surgical therapy was common in the past, more effective antibiotic and supportive therapy has largely replaced surgery. However, when bronchiectasis is localized and the morbidity is substantial despite adequate medical therapy, surgical resection of the involved region of lung should be considered.

When massive hemoptysis, often originating from the hypertrophied bronchial circulation, does not resolve with conservative therapy, including rest and antibiotics, therapeutic options are either surgical resection or bronchial arterial embolization (Chap. 30). Although resection may be successful if disease is localized, embolization is preferable with widespread disease. In patients with extensive disease, chronic hypoxemia and cor pulmonale may indicate the need for long-term supplemental oxygen. For selected patients who are disabled despite maximal therapy, lung transplantation is a therapeutic option.

FURTHER READING

ANGRILL J et al: Bacterial colonisation in patients with bronchiectasis: microbiologic pattern and risk factors. Thorax 57:15, 2002

BARKER AF: Bronchiectasis. N Engl J Med 346:1383, 2002

KUMAR NA et al: Bronchiectasis: Current clinical and imaging concepts. Semin Roentgenol 36:41, 2001

LILLINGTON GA: Dyskinetic cilia and Kartagener's syndrome. Bronchiectasis with a twist. Clin Rev Allergy Immunol 21:65, 2001

---

241 CYSTIC FIBROSIS
Richard C. Boucher

Cystic fibrosis (CF) is a monogenic disorder that presents as a multisystem disease. The first signs and symptoms typically occur in childhood, but about 7% of patients in the United States are diagnosed as adults. Due to improvements in therapy, >38% of patients are now adults (18 years of age) and 13% are past the age of 30. The median survival is >32 years for males and 29 years for females with CF. Thus, CF is no longer only a pediatric disease, and internists must be prepared to recognize and treat its many complications. This disease is characterized by chronic airways infection that ultimately leads to bronchiectasis and bronchiolectasis, exocrine pancreatic insufficiency and intestinal dysfunction, abnormal sweat gland function, and urogenital dysfunction.

PATHOGENESIS

GENETIC CONSIDERATIONS CF is an autosomal recessive disease resulting from mutations in a gene located on chromosome 7. The prevalence of CF varies with the ethnic origin of a population. CF is detected in approximately 1 in 3000 live births in the Caucasian population of North America and northern Europe, 1 in 17,000 live births of African Americans, and 1 in 90,000 live births of the Asian population of Hawaii. The most common mutation in the CF gene (~70% of CF chromosomes) is a 3-bp deletion that results in an absence of phenylalanine at amino acid position 508 (ΔF_{508}) of the CF gene protein product, known as the CF transmembrane conductance regulator (CFTR). The large number (>1000) of relatively uncommon (<2%) mutations identified in the CF gene makes it difficult to use DNA diagnostic technologies for identifying heterozygotes in populations at large, and no simple physiologic measurements allow heterozygote detection.

CFTR PROTEIN   The CFTR protein is a single polypeptide chain, containing 1480 amino acids, that appears to function both as a cyclic AMP–regulated Cl^- channel and, as its name implies, a regulator of other ion channels. The fully processed form of CFTR is found in the plasma membrane in normal epithelia (Fig. 241-1). Biochemical studies indicate that the ΔF_{508} mutation leads to improper processing and intracellular degradation of the CFTR protein. Thus, absence of CFTR at appropriate cellular sites is often part of the pathophysiology of CF. However, other mutations in the CF gene produce CFTR proteins that are fully processed but are nonfunctional or only partially functional at the appropriate cellular sites.

EPITHELIAL DYSFUNCTION   The epithelia affected by CF exhibit different functions in their native state, i.e., some are volume-absorbing (airways and distal intestinal epithelia), some are salt-absorbing but not volume-absorbing (sweat duct), whereas others are volume-secretory (proximal intestine and pancreas). Given this diverse array of native activities, it should not be surprising that CF produces very different effects on patterns of electrolyte and water transport. However, the unifying concept is that all affected tissues express abnormal ion transport function.

ORGAN-SPECIFIC PATHOPHYSIOLOGY ■ Lung   The diagnostic biophysical hallmark of CF is the raised transepithelial electric potential difference detected in airway epithelia. The transepithelial potential difference reflects components of both the rate of active ion transport and the resistance to ion flow of the superficial epithelium. CF airway epithelia exhibit both raised Na^+ transport rates and decreased Cl^- secretion (Fig. 241-2). The Cl^- secretory defect reflects the absence of cyclic AMP–dependent kinase and protein kinase C–regulated Cl^- transport that is mediated by the Cl^- channel function of CFTR. An important observation is that there is an "alternative" Ca^{2+}-regulated Cl^- channel expressed in airway epithelia. This Cl^- channel is different from CFTR and is regulated by intracellular Ca^{2+} levels. This channel can substitute for CFTR with regard to net Cl^- transport and may be a potential therapeutic target.

Raised Na^+ absorption is a feature of CF airway epithelia. Na^+ transport abnormalities in CF are not a widespread feature of the CF epithelial phenotype and appear confined to volume-absorbing epithelia. Recent studies demonstrate that the increased Na^+ absorption re-

FIGURE 241-1   Cellular metabolism of the cystic fibrosis transmembrane regulator (CFTR) protein conductance (red). In a normal cell (left), CFTR is synthesized in the rough endoplasmic reticulum (RER), is glycosylated in the Golgi apparatus, and functions as a Cl^- channel and regulator of other ion channels when located in the plasma membrane. Two possible outcomes of mutations in the CF gene are shown (right). (1) If a mutation disturbs protein folding, e.g., the ΔF_{508} mutation, CFTR is degraded intracellularly so that no protein is transported to the plasma membrane. (2) With other mutations, the abnormal protein is processed and trafficks to the plasma membrane but functions abnormally at that site.

FIGURE 241-2   Comparison of ion transport properties of normal (top) and CF (bottom) airway epithelia. The vectors describe routes and magnitudes of Na^+ and Cl^- transport that is accompanied by osmotically driven water flow. The normal basal pattern for ion transport is absorption of Na^+ from the lumen via an amiloride-sensitive Na^+ channel. This process is accelerated in CF. The capacity to initiate cyclic AMP–mediated Cl^- secretion is diminished in CF airway epithelia due to absence/dysfunction of the CFTR Cl^- channel. The accelerated Na^+ absorption in CF reflects the absence of CFTR inhibitory effects on Na^+ channels.

flects a second function of CFTR: it acts as a tonic inhibitor of the epithelial Na^+ channel. The molecular mechanism mediating this action of CFTR is still unknown.

Mucus clearance appears to be a primary innate defense mechanism for the airways against infection by inhaled bacteria. Normal airways can vary the rates of active Na^+ absorption and Cl^- secretion to adjust the volume of liquid (water) on airway surfaces for efficient mucus clearance. The central hypothesis of CF airways pathophysiology is that an abnormally high rate of Na^+ absorption and low rate of Cl^- secretion reduce the salt and water content of mucus and deplete the volume of the periciliary liquid. Both the thickening of mucus and the depletion of the periciliary liquid lead to adhesion of mucus to the airway surface. Mucus adhesion leads to a failure to clear mucus normally from the airways by either ciliary or airflow-dependent (cough) mechanisms. Recent data from both human cell culture models and CF mice in vivo support this hypothesis.

The infection that characterizes CF airways involves the mucus layer rather than epithelial or airway wall invasion. The unique predisposition of CF airways to chronic infection by *Staphylococcus aureus* and *Pseudomonas aeruginosa* is consistent with failure to clear mucus, but it has also suggested that as yet undefined abnormalities in airway surface liquid may also contribute to selection of these organisms. Recently, it has been demonstrated that reduced O_2 tension in CF mucus before, and particularly after, infection may in part select for these bacteria and be responsible for their phenotype. Thus, both mucus stasis and mucus hypoxia may contribute to the propensity for *Pseudomonas* to grow in biofilm colonies within mucus plaques adherent to CF airway surfaces.

Gastrointestinal Tract The gastrointestinal effects of CF are diverse. In the exocrine pancreas, the absence of the CFTR Cl^- channel in the apical membrane of pancreatic ductal epithelia limits the function of an apical membrane $Cl^--HCO_3^-$ exchanger to secrete bicarbonate and Na^+ (by a passive process) into the duct. The failure to secrete Na^+ HCO_3^- and water leads to retention of enzymes in the pancreas and ultimately destruction of virtually all pancreatic tissue. The CF intestinal epithelium, because of the lack of Cl^- and water secretion, fails to flush secreted mucins and other macromolecules from intestinal crypts. The diminished CFTR-mediated secretion of liquid may be exacerbated by excessive absorption of liquid, reflecting abnormalities of CFTR-mediated regulation of Na^+ absorption (both mediated by Na^+ channels and possibly other Na^+ transporters, e.g., Na^+-H^+ exchangers). Both dysfunctions lead to dessicated intraluminal contents and obstruction of both the small and large intestine. In the hepatobiliary system, defective hepatic ductal salt (Cl^-) and water secretion causes retention of biliary secretion, focal biliary cirrhosis, and bile duct proliferation in approximately 25 to 30% of patients with CF. The inability of the CF gallbladder epithelium to secrete salt and water can lead to both chronic cholecystitis and cholelithiasis.

Sweat Gland CF patients secrete nearly normal volumes of sweat in the sweat acinus. However, CF patients are not able to absorb NaCl from sweat as it moves through the sweat duct due to the inability to absorb Cl^- across the ductal epithelial cells.

CLINICAL FEATURES

Most patients with CF present with signs and symptoms of the disease in childhood. Approximately 18% of patients present within the first 24 h of life with gastrointestinal obstruction, termed *meconium ileus*. Other common presentations within the first year or two of life include respiratory tract symptoms, most prominently cough and/or recurrent pulmonary infiltrates, and failure to thrive. A significant proportion of patients ($\sim$7%), however, are diagnosed after age 18.

RESPIRATORY TRACT Upper respiratory tract disease is almost universal in patients with CF. Chronic sinusitis is common in childhood and leads to nasal obstruction and rhinorrhea. The occurrence of nasal polyps approaches 25% and often requires surgery.

In the lower respiratory tract, the first symptom of CF is cough. With time, the cough becomes persistent and produces viscous, purulent, often greenish-colored sputum. Inevitably, periods of clinical stability are interrupted by "exacerbations," defined by increased cough, weight loss, increased sputum volume, and decrements in pulmonary function. These exacerbations require aggressive therapy, including frequent postural drainage and oral antibiotics, and often intravenous antibiotics (see below), with the goal being recovery of lung function. Over the course of years, the exacerbations become more frequent and the recovery of lost lung function incomplete, leading to respiratory failure.

CF patients exhibit a characteristic sputum microbiology. *Haemophilus influenzae* and *S. aureus* are often the first organisms recovered from samples of lung secretions in newly diagnosed patients with CF. *P. aeruginosa* is typically cultured from lower respiratory tract secretions thereafter. After repetitive antibiotic exposure, *P. aeruginosa*, often in a mucoid form, is usually the predominant organism recovered from sputum and may be present as several strains with different antibiotic sensitivities. *Burkholderia* (formerly *Pseudomonas*) *cepacia* has been recovered from CF sputum and is also pathogenic. Patient-to-patient spread of certain strains of this organism indicates that strict infection control in the hospital should be practiced. Other gram-negative rods recovered from CF sputum include *Xanthomonas xylosoxidans* and *B. gladioli*, and occasionally mucoid forms of *Proteus*, *Escherichia coli*, and *Klebsiella*. Up to 50% of CF patients have *Aspergillus fumigatus* in their sputum, and up to 10% of these patients exhibit the syndrome of allergic bronchopulmonary aspergillosis. *Mycobacterium tuberculosis* is rare in patients with CF. However, 10 to 20% of adult patients with CF have sputum cultures positive for nontuberculous mycobacteria, and in some patients these microorganisms are associated with disease.

The first lung function abnormalities observed in CF children, increased ratios of residual volume to total lung capacity, suggest that small airways disease is the first functional lung abnormality in CF. As the disease progresses, both reversible and irreversible changes in forced vital capacity and forced expiratory volume in 1 s are noted. The reversible component reflects the accumulation of intraluminal secretions and/or airway reactivity, which occurs in 40 to 60% of patients with CF. The irreversible component reflects chronic destruction of the airway wall and bronchiolitis.

The earliest chest x-ray change in CF lungs is hyperinflation, reflecting small airways obstruction. Later, signs of luminal mucus impaction, bronchial cuffing, and finally bronchiectasis, e.g., ring shadows, are noted. For reasons that are still unknown, the right upper lobe displays the earliest and most severe changes.

CF pulmonary disease is associated with many intermittent complications. Pneumothorax is common ($>$10% of patients). The production of small amounts of blood in sputum is common in CF patients with advanced pulmonary disease and appears to be associated with lung infection. Massive hemoptysis is life-threatening and difficult to localize bronchoscopically. With advanced lung disease, digital clubbing becomes evident in virtually all patients with CF. As late events, respiratory failure and cor pulmonale are prominent features of CF.

GASTROINTESTINAL TRACT The syndrome of meconium ileus in infants presents with abdominal distention, failure to pass stool, and emesis. The abdominal flat plate can be diagnostic, with small-intestinal air-fluid levels, a granular appearance representing meconium, and a small colon. In children and young adults, a syndrome termed *meconium ileus equivalent* or *distal intestinal obstruction syndrome* occurs. The syndrome presents with right lower quadrant pain, loss of appetite, occasionally emesis, and often a palpable mass. The syndrome can be confused with appendicitis, which occurs frequently in CF patients. The characteristic intestinal abnormalities are complicated by exocrine pancreatic insufficiency in $>$90% of patients with CF. Insufficient pancreatic enzyme release yields the typical pattern of protein and fat malabsorption, with frequent, bulky, foul-smelling stools. Signs and symptoms of malabsorption of fat-soluble vitamins, including vitamins E and K, are also noted. Pancreatic beta cells are typically spared, but function decreases with age, causing hyperglycemia and increasing requirements for insulin in older patients with CF.

GENITOURINARY SYSTEM Late onset of puberty is common in both males and females with CF. The delayed maturational pattern is likely secondary to the effects of chronic lung disease and inadequate nutrition on reproductive endocrine function. More than 95% of male patients with CF are azoospermic, reflecting obliteration of the vas deferens that is probably a result of defective liquid secretion. Some 20% of CF women are infertile due to effects of chronic lung disease on the menstrual cycle; thick, tenacious cervical mucus that blocks sperm migration; and possibly fallopian tube/uterine wall abnormalities in liquid transport. More than 90% of completed pregnancies produce viable infants, and women with CF are generally able to breast-feed infants normally.

DIAGNOSIS

Because of the large number of CF mutations, DNA analysis is not used for primary diagnosis. The diagnosis of CF rests on a combination of clinical criteria and analyses of sweat Cl^- values. The values for the Na^+ and Cl^- concentration in sweat vary with age, but typically in adults a Cl^- concentration of $>$70 meq/L discriminates between patients with CF and patients with other lung diseases.

DNA analyses are being performed increasingly in patients with CF. Comprehensive genotype-phenotype relationships have not yet been established sufficiently for prognosis. A relationship between ΔF_{508} homozygosity and pancreatic insufficiency has been established, but no predictive relationship holds for ΔF_{508} homozygosity and lung disease.

Between 1 and 2% of patients with the clinical syndrome of CF have normal sweat Cl⁻ values. In most of these patients, the nasal transepithelial potential difference is raised into the diagnostic range for CF, and sweat acini do not secrete in response to injected β-adrenergic agonists. A single mutation of the CFTR gene, 3849 + 10 kb C→T, is associated with approximately 50% of CF patients with normal sweat Cl⁻ values.

℞ TREATMENT

The major objectives of therapy for CF are to promote clearance of secretions and control infection in the lung, provide adequate nutrition, and prevent intestinal obstruction. Ultimately, gene therapy or therapies that restore the processing of misfolded CFTR may be the treatments of choice.

Lung Disease The principal techniques for clearing pulmonary secretions are breathing exercises, flutter valves, and chest percussion. Regular use of these maneuvers is effective in preserving lung function. There is increasing interest in the use of hypertonic saline (3 to 7%) aerosols to augment the clearance of secretions.

More than 95% of CF patients die of complications resulting from lung infection. Antibiotics are the principal agents available for treating lung infection, and their use should be guided by sputum culture results. Early intervention with antibiotics is useful, and long courses of treatment are the rule. Because of increased total-body clearance and volume of distribution of antibiotics in CF patients, the required doses are higher for patients with CF than for patients with similar chest infections who do not have CF.

Increased cough and mucus production are treated with antibiotics given orally. Typical oral agents used to treat *Staphylococcus* include a semisynthetic penicillin or a cephalosporin. Oral ciprofloxacin may reduce pseudomonal bacterial counts and control symptoms. However, its clinical usefulness may be limited by rapid emergence of resistant organisms, and, accordingly, courses should be intermittent (2 to 3 weeks) and not chronic. More severe exacerbations, or exacerbations associated with bacteria resistant to oral antibiotics, require intravenous antibiotics. Traditionally, intravenous therapy has been given in the hospital, but outpatient intravenous antibiotic administration has gained widespread acceptance. Usually, two drugs with different mechanisms of action (e.g., a cephalosporin and an aminoglycoside) are used to treat *P. aeruginosa* to hinder emergence of resistant organisms. Drug dosage should be monitored so that levels for gentamicin or tobramycin peak at ranges of ~10 μg/mL and exhibit troughs of <2 μg/mL. Cephalosporins (e.g., ceftazidime) and penicillin derivatives also require higher doses. Antibiotics directed at *Staphylococcus* and/or *H. influenzae* are added, depending on the results of the culture. Aerosolized antibiotics also have an important role in treating CF lung infection. Large doses of aminoglycosides, e.g., 300 mg tobramycin twice daily, via aerosol are effective at delaying exacerbations. Aerosol administration also permits other drugs, e.g., colistin, to be utilized that are relatively ineffective by the intravenous route.

A number of pharmacologic agents for increasing mucus clearance are in use. *N*-acetylcysteine, which solubilizes mucous glycoproteins, has not been shown to have clinically significant effects on mucus clearance and/or lung function. Recombinant human DNAse, however, degrades the concentrated DNA in CF sputum, decreases sputum viscosity, and increases airflow during short-term administration. Long-term (6 months) DNAse treatment increases the time between pulmonary exacerbations. Most patients receive a therapeutic trial of DNAse to test for efficacy, and a sizeable minority demonstrate persistent objective benefits. Clinical trials of experimental drugs aimed at restoring salt and water content of secretions are underway. However, these drugs are not yet available clinically.

Inhaled β-adrenergic agonists can be useful to control airways constriction. They achieve a short-term increase in airflow, but long-term benefit has not been shown. Inhaled anticholinergics provide an alternative. Oral glucocorticoids may reduce airways inflammation, but their long-term use has been limited by adverse side effects; however, they may be useful for treating allergic bronchopulmonary aspergillosis.

The chronic damage to airway walls reflects to some extent the destructive activities of inflammatory enzymes generated in part by inflammatory cells. To date, specific therapies with antiproteases have not been successfully developed. However, a subset of adolescents with CF appear to benefit from long-term, high dose nonsteroidal (ibuprofen) therapy.

A number of pulmonary complications require acute interventions. Atelectasis is best treated with chest physiotherapy and antibiotic therapy. Pneumothoraces involving ≤10% of the lung can be observed without intervention. The use of chest tubes to expand collapsed, diseased lung often requires long periods of time, and sclerosing agents should be used with caution because of possible limitations for subsequent lung transplantation. Small-volume hemoptysis requires no specific therapy other than treatment of lung infection and assessment of coagulation and vitamin K status. If massive hemoptysis occurs, bronchial artery embolization can be successful. The most ominous complications of CF are respiratory failure and cor pulmonale. The most effective conventional therapy for these conditions is vigorous medical management of the lung disease and O₂ supplementation. Ultimately, the only effective treatment for respiratory failure in CF is lung transplantation (Chap. 248). The 2-year survival for lung transplantation exceeds 60%, and deaths in transplant patients result principally from graft rejection, often involving obliterative bronchiolitis. The transplanted lungs do not develop a CF-specific phenotype.

Gastrointestinal Disease Maintenance of adequate nutrition is critical for the health of the patient with CF. Most (>90%) of CF patients benefit from pancreatic enzyme replacement. Capsules generally contain between 4000 and 20,000 units of lipase. The dose of enzymes (typically no more than 2500 units/kg per meal) should be adjusted on the basis of weight gain, abdominal symptomatology, and character of stools. Replacement of fat-soluble vitamins, particularly vitamins E and K, is usually required. Hyperglycemia most often becomes manifest in the adult and typically requires insulin treatment.

For treatment of acute obstruction due to distal intestinal obstruction syndrome, megalodiatrizoate or other hypertonic radiocontrast materials delivered by enema to the terminal ileum are utilized. For control of symptoms, adjustment of pancreatic enzymes and the supplementation of intake by salt solutions containing osmotically active agents, e.g., propyleneglycol, are utilized. Persistent symptoms may indicate a diagnosis of gastrointestinal malignancy, which is increased in incidence in patients with CF. Hepatic and gallbladder complications are treated as for patients without CF. End-stage liver disease can be treated by transplantation, which has a 2-year survival rate >50%.

Psychosocial Factors CF imposes a tremendous burden on patients. Health insurance, career options, family planning, and life expectancy become major issues. Thus, assisting patients with the psychosocial adjustments required by CF is critical.

FURTHER READING

BRENNAN AL, GEDDES DM: Cystic fibrosis. Curr Opin Infect Dis 15:175, 2002

GELLER DE et al: Pharmacokinetics and bioavailability of aerosolized tobramycin in cystic fibrosis. Chest 122:219, 2002

GRIESENBACH U et al: Gene therapy progress and prospects: Cystic fibrosis. Gene Ther 9:1344, 2002

HENNEMAN L et al: Evaluation of cystic fibrosis carrier screening programs according to genetic screening criteria. Genet Med 4:241, 2002

MATSUI H et al: Evidence for periciliary liquid layer depletion, not abnormal ion composition, in the pathogenesis of cystic fibrosis airways disease. Cell 95:1005, 1998

PRINCE AS: Biofilms, antimicrobial resistance, and airway infection. N Engl J Med 347:1110, 2002

WORLITSCH D et al: Effects of reduced mucus oxygen concentration in airway pseudomonas infections of cystic fibrosis patients. J Clin Invest 109:317, 2002

Chronic obstructive pulmonary disease (COPD) has been defined by the Global Initiative for Chronic Obstructive Lung Disease (GOLD) as a disease state characterized by airflow limitation that is not fully reversible (http://www.goldcopd.com/). COPD includes *emphysema*, an anatomically defined condition characterized by destruction and enlargement of the lung alveoli; *chronic bronchitis*, a clinically defined condition with chronic cough and phlegm; and *small airways disease*, a condition in which small bronchioles are narrowed. COPD is present only if chronic airflow obstruction occurs; chronic bronchitis *without* chronic airflow obstruction is *not* included within COPD.

COPD is the fourth leading cause of death and affects >16 million persons in the United States. COPD is also a disease of increasing public health importance around the world. GOLD estimates suggest that COPD will rise from the sixth to the third most common cause of death worldwide by 2020.

RISK FACTORS ■ Cigarette Smoking By 1964, the Advisory Committee to the Surgeon General of the United States concluded that cigarette smoking was a major risk factor for mortality from chronic bronchitis and emphysema. Subsequent longitudinal studies have shown accelerated decline in the volume of air exhaled within the first second of the forced expiratory maneuver (FEV_1) in a dose-response relationship to the intensity of cigarette smoking, which is typically expressed as pack-years (average number of packs of cigarettes smoked per day multiplied by the total number of years of smoking). This dose-response relationship between reduced pulmonary function and cigarette smoking intensity accounts for the higher prevalence rates for COPD with increasing age. The historically higher rate of smoking among males is the likely explanation for the higher prevalence of COPD among males; however, the prevalence of COPD among females is increasing as the gender gap in smoking rates has diminished in the past 50 years.

Although the causal relationship between cigarette smoking and the development of COPD has been absolutely proven, there is considerable variability in the response to smoking. Although pack-years of cigarette smoking is the most highly significant predictor of FEV_1 (Fig. 242-1), only 15% of the variability in FEV_1 is explained by pack-years. This finding suggests that additional environmental and/or genetic factors contribute to the impact of smoking on the development of airflow obstruction.

Although cigar and pipe smoking may also be associated with the development of COPD, the evidence supporting such associations is less compelling, likely related to the lower dose of inhaled tobacco byproducts during cigar and pipe smoking.

Airway Responsiveness and COPD A tendency for increased bronchoconstriction in response to a variety of exogenous stimuli, including methacholine and histamine, is one of the defining features of asthma (Chap. 236). However, many patients with COPD also share this feature of airway hyperresponsiveness. The considerable overlap between persons with asthma and those with COPD on airway responsiveness, airflow obstruction, and pulmonary symptoms led to the formulation of the Dutch hypothesis. This suggests that asthma, chronic bronchitis, and emphysema are variations of the same basic disease, which is modulated by environmental and genetic factors to produce these pathologically distinct entities. The alternative British hypothesis contends that asthma and COPD are fundamentally different diseases: Asthma is viewed as largely an allergic phenomenon, while COPD results from smoking-related inflammation and damage. Determination of the validity of the Dutch hypothesis vs. the British hypothesis awaits identification of the genetic predisposing factors for asthma and/or COPD, as well as the interactions between these postulated genetic factors and environmental risk factors.

Longitudinal studies that compared airway responsiveness at the

FIGURE 242-1 Distributions of forced expiratory volume in 1 s (FEV_1) values in a general population sample, stratified by pack-years of smoking. Means, medians, and ± 1 standard deviation of percent predicted FEV_1 are shown for each smoking group. Although a dose-response relationship between smoking intensity and FEV_1 was found, marked variability in pulmonary function was observed among subjects with similar smoking histories. (*From Burrows et al, with permission.*)

beginning of the study to subsequent decline in pulmonary function have demonstrated that increased airway responsiveness is clearly a significant predictor of subsequent decline in pulmonary function. Thus, airways hyperresponsiveness is a risk factor for COPD.

Respiratory Infections These have been studied as potential risk factors for the development and progression of COPD in adults; childhood respiratory infections have also been assessed as potential predisposing factors for the eventual development of COPD. The impact of adult respiratory infections on decline in pulmonary function is controversial, but significant long-term reductions in pulmonary function are not typically seen following an episode of bronchitis or pneumonia. The impact of the effects of childhood respiratory illnesses on the subsequent development of COPD has been difficult to assess due to a lack of adequate longitudinal data. Thus, although respiratory infections are important causes of exacerbations of COPD, the association of both adult and childhood respiratory infections to the development and progression of COPD remains to be proven.

Occupational Exposures Increased respiratory symptoms and airflow obstruction have been suggested as resulting from general exposure to dust at work. Several specific occupational exposures, including coal mining, gold mining, and cotton textile dust, have been suggested as risk factors for chronic airflow obstruction. However, although nonsmokers in these occupations developed some reductions in FEV_1, the importance of dust exposure as a risk factor for COPD, independent of cigarette smoking, is not certain. Among workers exposed to cadmium (a specific chemical fume), FEV_1, FEV_1/FVC, and DL_{CO} were significantly reduced (FVC, forced vital capacity; DL_{CO}, carbon monoxide diffusing capacity of the lung; Chap. 234), consistent with airflow obstruction and emphysema. Although several specific occupational dusts and fumes are likely risk factors for COPD, the magnitude of these effects appears to be substantially less important than the effect of cigarette smoking.

Ambient Air Pollution Some investigators have reported increased respiratory symptoms in those living in urban compared to rural areas, which may relate to increased pollution in the urban settings. However, the relationship of air pollution to chronic airflow obstruction remains unproven. With high rates of COPD reported in nonsmoking women in many developing countries, indoor air pollution, usually associated with cooking, has been suggested as a potential contributor. In most populations, ambient air pollution is a much less important risk factor for COPD than cigarette smoking.

Passive, or Second-Hand, Smoking Exposure Exposure of children to maternal smoking results in significantly reduced lung growth. In utero tobacco smoke exposure also contributes to significant reductions in postnatal pulmonary function. Although passive smoke exposure has been associated with reductions in pulmonary function, the importance of this risk factor in the development of the severe pulmonary function reductions in COPD remains uncertain.

GENETIC CONSIDERATIONS Although cigarette smoking is the major environmental risk factor for the development of COPD, the development of airflow obstruction in smokers is highly variable. Severe α_1 antitrypsin (α_1AT) deficiency is a proven genetic risk factor for COPD; there is increasing evidence that other genetic determinants also exist.

α_1 ANTITRYPSIN DEFICIENCY Many variants of the protease inhibitor (PI) locus that encodes α_1AT have been described. The common M allele is associated with normal α_1AT levels. The S allele, associated with slightly reduced α_1AT levels, and the Z allele, associated with markedly reduced α_1AT levels, also occur with frequencies >1% in most Caucasian populations. Rare individuals inherit null alleles, which lead to the absence of any α_1AT production through a heterogeneous collection of mutations. Individuals with two Z alleles or one Z and one null allele are referred to as Pi^Z, which is the most common form of severe α_1AT deficiency.

Although only 1 to 2% of COPD patients inherit severe α_1AT deficiency, these patients demonstrate that genetic factors can have a profound influence on the susceptibility for developing COPD. Pi^Z individuals often develop early-onset COPD, but the ascertainment bias in the published series of Pi^Z individuals—which have usually included many Pi^Z subjects who were tested for α_1AT deficiency because they had COPD—means that the fraction of Pi^Z individuals who will develop COPD and the age-of-onset distribution for the development of COPD in Pi^Z subjects remain unknown. Approximately 1 in 3000 individuals in the United States inherits severe α_1AT deficiency, but only a small minority of these individuals have been recognized.

A significant percentage of the variability in pulmonary function among Pi^Z individuals is explained by cigarette smoking; cigarette smokers with severe α_1AT deficiency are more likely to develop COPD at early ages. However, the development of COPD in Pi^Z subjects, even among current or ex-smokers, is not absolute. Among Pi^Z nonsmokers, impressive variability has been noted in the development of airflow obstruction. Other genetic and/or environmental factors likely contribute to this variability.

The clinical laboratory test used most frequently to screen for α_1AT deficiency is measurement of the immunologic level of α_1AT in serum (see "Laboratory Findings," below). Specific treatment in the form of α_1AT augmentation therapy is available for severe α_1AT deficiency as a weekly intravenous infusion (see "Treatment" below).

The risk of lung disease in heterozygous Pi^{MZ} individuals, who have intermediate serum levels of α_1AT (~60% of Pi^{MM} levels), is controversial. Although previous general population surveys have not typically shown increased rates of airflow obstruction in Pi^{MZ} com-

pared to Pi^{MM} individuals, case-control studies that compared COPD patients to control subjects have usually found an excess of Pi^{MZ} genotypes in the COPD patient group. Several recent large population studies have suggested that Pi^{MZ} subjects are at slightly increased risk for the development of airflow obstruction, but it remains unclear if all Pi^{MZ} subjects are at slightly increased risk for COPD or if a subset of Pi^{MZ} subjects are at substantially increased risk for COPD due to other genetic or environmental factors.

OTHER GENETIC RISK FACTORS Studies of pulmonary function measurements performed in general population samples have suggested that genetic factors other than PI type influence variation in pulmonary function. Familial aggregation of airflow obstruction within families of COPD patients has also been demonstrated.

Association studies have compared the distribution of variants in genes hypothesized to be involved in the development of COPD in COPD patients and control subjects. However, the results have been quite inconsistent, and no genetic determinants of COPD other than severe α_1AT deficiency have been definitively proven. Recent genome scan linkage analyses of early-onset COPD families have found evidence for linkage of spirometric phenotypes to several chromosomal regions, but the specific genetic determinants in those regions have yet to be identified.

NATURAL HISTORY The effects of cigarette smoking on pulmonary function appear to depend on the intensity of smoking exposure, the timing of smoking exposure during growth, and the baseline lung function of the individual; other environmental factors may have similar effects. Although rare individuals may demonstrate precipitous declines in pulmonary function, most individuals follow a steady trajectory of increasing pulmonary function with growth during childhood and adolescence, followed by a gradual decline with aging. Individuals appear to track in their quartile of pulmonary function based upon environmental and genetic factors that put them on different tracks. The risk of eventual mortality from COPD is closely associated with reduced levels of FEV$_1$. A graphic depiction of the natural history of COPD is shown as a function of the influences on tracking curves of FEV$_1$ in Fig. 242-2. Death or disability from COPD can result from a normal rate of decline after a reduced growth phase (curve B), an early initiation of pulmonary function decline after normal growth (curve C), or an accelerated decline after normal growth (curve D). The rate of decline in pulmonary function can be modified by changing environmental exposures (i.e., quitting smoking), with smoking cessation at an earlier age providing a more beneficial effect than smoking cessation after marked reductions in pulmonary function have already

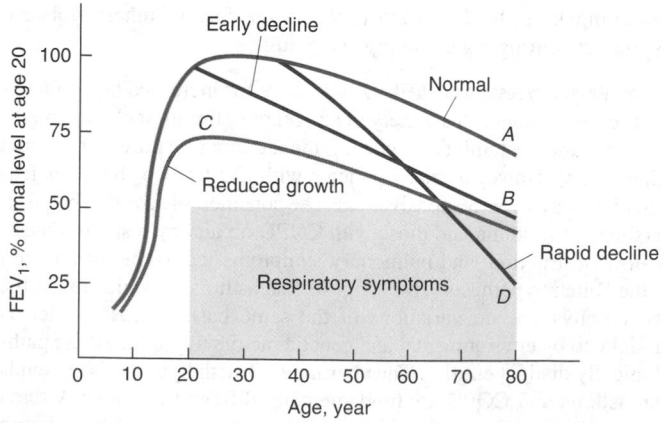

FIGURE 242-2 Hypothetical tracking curves of FEV$_1$ for individuals throughout their lifespans. The normal pattern of growth and decline with age is shown by curve A. Significantly reduced FEV$_1$ (<65% of predicted value at age 20) can develop from a normal rate of decline after a reduced pulmonary function growth phase (curve B), early initiation of pulmonary function decline after normal growth (curve C), or accelerated decline after normal growth (curve D). (*From B Rijcken: Doctoral dissertation, p 133, University of Groningen, 1991; with permission.*)

developed. Genetic factors likely contribute to the level of pulmonary function achieved during growth and to the rate of decline in response to smoking and potentially to other environmental factors as well.

PATHOPHYSIOLOGY Persistent reduction in forced expiratory flow rates is the most typical finding in COPD. Increases in the residual volume and the residual volume/total lung capacity ratio, nonuniform distribution of ventilation, and ventilation-perfusion mismatching also occur.

Airflow Obstruction Airflow limitation, also known as airflow obstruction, is typically determined by spirometry, which involves forced expiratory maneuvers after the subject has inhaled to total lung capacity (Fig. 234-4). Key phenotypes obtained from spirometry include FEV_1 and the total volume of air exhaled during the entire spirometric maneuver (FVC). Patients with airflow obstruction related to COPD have a chronically reduced ratio of FEV_1/FVC. In contrast to asthma, the reduced FEV_1 in COPD seldom shows large responses to inhaled bronchodilators, although improvements up to 15% are common. Asthma patients can also develop chronic (not fully reversible) airflow obstruction. Maximal inspiratory flow can be relatively well preserved in the presence of a markedly reduced FEV_1. Airflow during forced exhalation is the result of the balance between the elastic recoil of the lungs promoting flow and the resistance of the airways limiting flow. In normal lungs, as well as in lungs affected by COPD, maximal expiratory flow diminishes as the lungs empty because the lung parenchyma provides progressively less elastic recoil and because the cross-sectional area of the airways falls, raising the resistance to airflow. The decrease in flow coincident with decreased lung volume is readily apparent on the expiratory limb of a flow-volume curve. In the early stages of COPD, the abnormality in airflow is only evident at lung volumes at or below the functional residual capacity (closer to residual volume), appearing as a scooped-out lower part of the descending limb of the flow-volume curve. In more advanced disease the entire curve has decreased expiratory flow compared to normal.

Hyperinflation Lung volumes are also routinely assessed in pulmonary function testing. In COPD there is often "air trapping" (increased residual volume and increased ratio of residual volume to total lung capacity) and progressive hyperinflation (increased total lung capacity) late in the disease. Hyperinflation of the thorax during tidal breathing preserves maximum expiratory airflow, because as lung volume increases, elastic recoil pressure increases and airways enlarge so that airway resistance decreases. Consequently, hyperinflation helps to compensate for airway obstruction. However, hyperinflation can push the diaphragm into a flattened position with a number of adverse effects. First, by decreasing the zone of apposition between the diaphragm and the abdominal wall, positive abdominal pressure during inspiration is not applied as effectively to the chest wall, hindering rib cage movement and impairing inspiration. Second, because the muscle fibers of the flattened diaphragm are shorter than those of a more normally curved diaphragm they are less capable of generating inspiratory pressures than normal. Third, the flattened diaphragm (with increased radius of curvature, r) must generate greater tension (t) to develop the transpulmonary pressure (p) required to produce tidal breathing. This follows from Laplace's law, $p = 2t/r$. Also, because the thoracic cage is distended beyond its normal resting volume, during tidal breathing the inspiratory muscles must do work to overcome the resistance of the thoracic cage to further inflation instead of gaining the normal assistance from the chest wall recoiling outward towards its resting volume.

Gas Exchange Although there is considerable variability in the relationships between the FEV_1 and other physiologic abnormalities in COPD, certain generalizations may be made. The Pa_{O_2} usually remains near normal until the FEV_1 is decreased to ~50% of predicted, and even much lower FEV_1's can be associated with a normal Pa_{O_2}, at least at rest. An elevation of Pa_{CO_2} is not expected until the FEV_1 is ≤25% of predicted, and even then may not occur. Pulmonary hypertension severe enough to cause cor pulmonale and right ventricular failure due

to COPD occurs only in those individuals who have marked decreases in FEV_1 (<25% of predicted) together with chronic hypoxemia ($Pa_{O_2} < 55$ mmHg), although earlier in the course some elevation of pulmonary artery pressure, particularly with exercise, may occur (Chap. 220).

Nonuniform ventilation and ventilation-perfusion mismatching are characteristic of COPD, reflecting the heterogeneous nature of the disease process within the airways and lung parenchyma. Nitrogen washout while breathing 100% oxygen is delayed due to regions that are poorly ventilated, and the profile of the nitrogen wash-out curve is consistent with multiple parenchymal compartments having different wash-out rates due to regional differences in compliance and airway resistance. Ventilation/perfusion mismatching accounts for essentially all of the reduction in Pa_{O_2} that occurs in COPD; shunting is minimal. This finding explains the effectiveness of modest elevations of inspired oxygen in treating hypoxemia due to COPD and therefore the need to consider problems other than COPD when hypoxemia is difficult to correct with modest levels of supplemental oxygen in the patient with COPD.

PATHOLOGY Cigarette smoke exposure may affect the large airways, small airways (<2 mm diameter), and alveolar space. Changes in large airways cause cough and sputum, while changes in small airways and alveoli are responsible for physiologic alterations. Emphysema and small airway pathology are both present in most persons with COPD, and their relative contributions to obstruction vary from one person to another. Small airway obstruction likely contributes more to initial obstruction, with emphysema predominating later in the course.

Large Airway Cigarette smoking often results in mucous gland enlargement and goblet cell hyperplasia. These changes are proportional to cough and mucus production that define chronic bronchitis, but these abnormalities are not related to airflow limitation. Goblet cells not only increase in number but in extent through the bronchial tree. Bronchi also undergo squamous metaplasia, which not only predisposes to carcinogenesis but also disrupts mucociliary clearance. Although not as prominent as in asthma, patients may have smooth-muscle hypertrophy and bronchial hyperreactivity leading to airflow limitation. Neutrophil influx has been associated with purulent sputum of upper respiratory tract infections that hamper patients with COPD. Independent of its proteolytic activity, neutrophil elastase is among the most potent secretagogues identified.

Small Airways The major site of increased resistance in most individuals with COPD is in airways ≤2 mm diameter. Characteristic cellular changes include goblet cell metaplasia and replacement of surfactant-secreting Clara cells with mucus-secreting and infiltrating mononuclear inflammatory cells. Smooth-muscle hypertrophy may also be present. These abnormalities may cause luminal narrowing by excess mucus, edema, and cellular infiltration. Reduced surfactant may increase surface tension at the air-tissue interface, predisposing to airway narrowing or collapse. Fibrosis in the wall may cause airway narrowing directly or, as in asthma, predispose to hyperreactivity. Respiratory bronchiolitis with mononuclear inflammatory cells collecting in distal airway tissues may cause proteolytic destruction of elastic fibers in the respiratory bronchioles and alveolar ducts where the fibers are concentrated as rings around alveolar entrances. The resulting distortion and narrowing of these structures could be involved in the early airflow obstruction in COPD related to cigarette smoking.

Because small airway patency is maintained by the surrounding lung parenchyma that provides radial traction on bronchioles at points of attachment to alveolar septa, loss of bronchiolar attachments as a result of extracellular matrix destruction may cause airway distortion and narrowing in COPD. Although the significance of alveolar attachments is not resolved, the concept of decreased alveolar attachments leading to small airway obstruction is appealing because it underscores the mechanistic relationship between loss of elastic recoil and increased resistance to airflow in small airways.

Lung Parenchyma Emphysema is characterized by destruction of gas-exchanging airspaces, i.e., the respiratory bronchioles, alveolar ducts, and alveoli. Their walls become perforated and later obliterated with coalescence of small distinct airspaces into abnormal and much larger airspaces. Macrophages accumulate in respiratory bronchioles of young smokers. Bronchoalveolar lavage fluid from such individuals contains roughly five times as many macrophages as lavage from non-smokers. In smokers' lavage fluid, macrophages comprise >95% of the total cell count and neutrophils, nearly absent in nonsmokers' lavage, account for 1 to 2% of the cells. T lymphocytes, particularly CD8+ cells, are also increased in the alveolar space of smokers.

Emphysema is classified into distinct pathologic types, the most important types being centriacinar and panacinar. *Centriacinar emphysema*, the type most frequently associated with cigarette smoking, is characterized by enlarged airspaces found (initially) in association with respiratory bronchioles. Centriacinar emphysema is most prominent in the upper lobes and superior segments of lower lobes and is often quite focal. *Panacinar emphysema* refers to abnormally large airspaces evenly distributed within and across acinar units. Panacinar emphysema is usually observed in patients with α_1AT deficiency, which has a predilection for the lower lobes. Distinctions between centriacinar and panacinar emphysema are interesting and may ultimately be shown to have different mechanisms of pathogenesis. However, garden-variety, smoking-related emphysema is usually mixed, particularly in advanced cases, and these pathologic classifications are not helpful in the care of patients with COPD.

PATHOGENESIS Airflow limitation, the major physiologic change in COPD, can result from both small airway obstruction and emphysema, as discussed above. Pathologic findings that can contribute to small airway obstruction are described above, but their relative importance is unknown. Fibrosis surrounding the small airways appears to be a significant contributor. Mechanisms leading to collagen accumulation around the airways in the face of increased collagenase activity remain an enigma. Although seemingly counterintuitive, there are several potential mechanisms whereby a proteinase can predispose to fibrosis including proteolytic activation of transforming growth factor β, and insulin-like growth factor (IGF) binding protein degradation releasing profibrotic IGF. Largely due to availability of suitable animal models, we know much more about the mechanisms involved in emphysema than in small airway obstruction.

The pathogenesis of emphysema can be dissected into three interrelated events (Fig. 242-3): (1) Chronic exposure to cigarette smoke may lead to inflammatory cell recruitment within the terminal airspaces of the lung, (2) these inflammatory cells release elastolytic proteinases that damage the extracellular matrix of the lung, and (3) ineffective repair of elastin and perhaps other extracellular matrix components results in pulmonary emphysema.

Inflammation Synthesis of existing data regarding inflammatory cell responses in human lungs following cigarette smoke exposure suggests the following sequence of events: (1) Macrophages patrol the lower airspace under normal conditions, and (2) cigarette smoke comes into contact with and activates lung epithelial cells and alveolar macrophages, leading to cytokine/chemokine release followed by acute neutrophil recruitment and subacute accumulation of macrophages in the respiratory bronchioles and alveolar spaces. T cells (CD8+ > CD4+) and perhaps other inflammatory and immune cells are also recruited. Concomitant cigarette smoke–induced loss of cilia in the airway epithelium predisposes to bacterial infection with neutrophilia. Surprisingly, in end-stage lung disease, long after smoking cessation, there remains an exuberant inflammatory response, suggesting that mechanisms of cigarette smoke–induced inflammation that initiate the disease differ from mechanisms that sustain inflammation after smoking cessation. Thus, multiple interacting inflammatory cell types are present and contribute to disease pathogenesis.

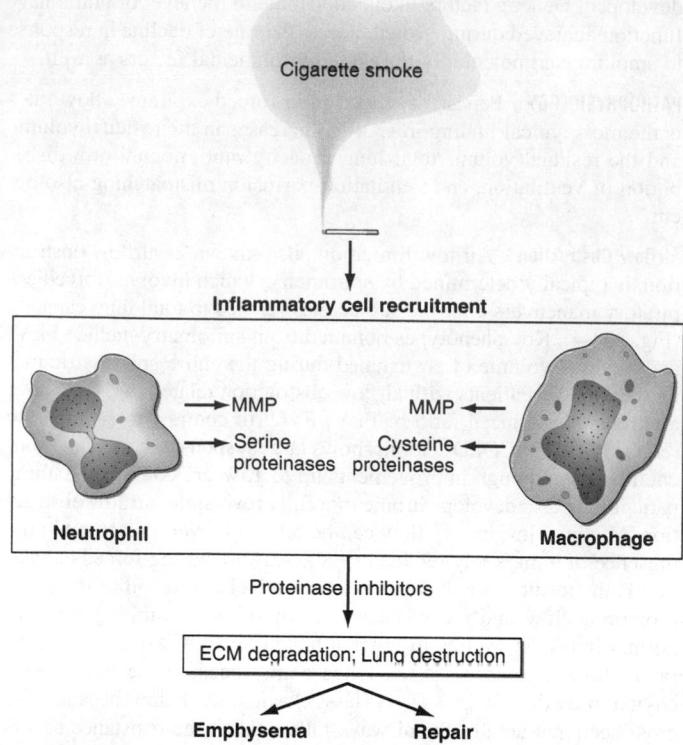

FIGURE 242-3 Pathogenesis of emphysema. Upon long-term exposure to cigarette smoke, inflammatory cells are recruited to the lung; they release proteinases in excess of inhibitors; and, if repair is abnormal, this leads to airspace destruction and enlargement or emphysema.

Extracellular Matrix Proteolysis Elastin, the principal component of elastic fibers, is a highly stable component of the extracellular matrix that is critical to the integrity of both the small airways and the lung parenchyma. The elastase:antielastase hypothesis proposed in the mid-1960s states that the balance of elastin-degrading enzymes and their inhibitors determines the susceptibility of the lung to destruction that results in airspace enlargement. Neutrophil elastase is a potent serine proteinase that clearly plays a major role in emphysema with associated α_1AT deficiency and also contributes to the usual forms of emphysema. The neutrophil also possesses serine proteinase 3 and cathepsin G as well as matrix metalloproteinases (MMPs), neutrophil collagenase (MMP-8), and gelatinase B (MMP-9). The macrophage is becoming recognized as a critical cell, producing several elastolytic MMPs including matrilysin (MMP-7), MMP-9, and macrophage elastase (MMP-12). Macrophages also produce potent cysteine proteinases (cathepsins S, L, and K). Animal models, including gene-targeted mice, suggest that macrophage elastases contribute to cigarette smoke–induced emphysema. Collagen degradation is more complex in that, while there is clearly collagen turnover in COPD, there is a net increase in collagen deposition, particularly around the small airways.

Cell Death Airspace enlargement with loss of alveolar units obviously requires disappearance of both extracellular matrix and cells. Traditional theories suggest that inflammatory cell proteinases degrade lung extracellular matrix as the primary event, with subsequent loss of cell anchoring leading to apoptosis. Recent studies suggest that endothelial and epithelial cell death could be primary events (presumably with secretion of proteinases to dissolve the matrix). Whether these mechanisms play a role in human COPD is unknown; however, it has been shown that there is increased septal cell death associated with reduced lung expression of vascular endothelial growth factor (VEGF) and its receptor VEGFR-2 (KDR/Flk-1) in human emphysematous lungs.

Ineffective Repair The ability of the adult lung to repair damaged alveoli appears limited. Whether the process of septation that is responsible for alveogenesis during lung development can be reinitiated is not clear. In animal models, treatment with all-*trans* retinoic acid results in some repair. Also, lung resection results in compensatory lung growth in the remaining lung in animal models. In addition to restoring cellularity following injury, it appears difficult for an adult to restore completely an appropriate extracellular matrix, particularly functional elastic fibers.

TABLE 242-1 *GOLD Criteria for COPD Severity*

GOLD Stage	Severity	Symptoms	Spirometry
0	At Risk	Chronic cough, sputum production	Normal
I	Mild	With or without chronic cough or sputum production	$FEV_1/FVC < 0.7$ and $FEV_1 \geq 80\%$ predicted
IIA	Moderate	With or without chronic cough or sputum production	$FEV_1/FVC < 0.7$ and $50\% \leq FEV_1 < 80\%$ predicted
III	Severe	With or without chronic cough or sputum production	$FEV_1/FVC < 0.7$ and $30\% \leq FEV_1 < 50\%$ predicted
IV	Very Severe	With or without chronic cough or sputum production	$FEV_1/FVC < 0.7$ and $FEV_1 < 30\%$ predicted *or* $FEV_1 < 50\%$ predicted with respiratory failure or signs of right heart failure

Note: GOLD, Global Initiative for Chronic Obstructive Pulmonary Disease (COPD).
Source: From Pauwels et al.

CLINICAL PRESENTATION ■ History

The three most common symptoms in COPD are cough, sputum production, and exertional dyspnea. Many patients have such symptoms for months or years before seeking medical attention. Although the development of airflow obstruction is a gradual process, many patients date the onset of their disease to an acute illness or exacerbation. A careful history, however, usually reveals the presence of symptoms prior to the acute exacerbation. The development of exertional dyspnea, often described as increased effort to breathe, heaviness, air hunger, or gasping, can be insidious. It is best elicited by a careful history focused on typical physical activities and how the patient's ability to perform them has changed. Activities involving significant arm work, particularly at or above shoulder level, are particularly difficult for patients with COPD. Conversely, activities that allow the patient to brace the arms and use accessory muscles of respiration are better tolerated. Examples of such activities include pushing a shopping cart, walking on a treadmill, or pushing a wheelchair. As COPD advances, the principal feature is worsening dyspnea on exertion with increasing intrusion on the ability to perform vocational or avocational activities. In the most advanced stages, patients are breathless doing simple activities of daily living.

Accompanying worsening airflow obstruction is an increased frequency of exacerbations (described below). Patients may also develop resting hypoxemia and require institution of supplemental oxygen.

Physical Findings In the early stages of COPD, patients may have an entirely normal physical examination. Current smokers may have signs of active smoking, including an odor of smoke or nicotine staining of fingernails. In patients with more severe disease, the physical examination is notable for a prolonged expiratory phase and expiratory wheezing. In addition, signs of hyperinflation include a barrel chest and enlarged lung volumes with poor diaphragmatic excursion as assessed by percussion. Patients with severe airflow obstruction may also exhibit use of accessory muscles of respiration, sitting in the characteristic "tripod" position to facilitate the actions of the sternocleidomastoid, scalene, and intercostal muscles. Patients may develop cyanosis, visible in the lips and nail beds. Patients with predominant emphysema are classically referred to as "pink puffers," a reference to the lack of cyanosis, the use of accessory muscles, and pursed-lip breathing. Such patients also have a dramatic decrease in breath sounds throughout the chest. Patients with a clinical syndrome of chronic bronchitis are classically labeled "blue bloaters," a reference to fluid retention and more marked cyanosis. Typically patients have elements of each and cannot be simply classified. Advanced disease may be accompanied by systemic wasting, with significant weight loss, bitemporal wasting, and diffuse loss of subcutaneous adipose tissue. This syndrome has been associated with both inadequate oral intake and elevated levels of inflammatory cytokines (TNF-α). Such wasting is an independent poor prognostic factor in COPD. Some patients with advanced disease have paradoxical inward movement of the rib cage with inspiration (Hoover's sign), the result of alteration of the vector of diaphragmatic contraction on the rib cage as a result of chronic hyperinflation.

Signs of overt right heart failure, termed *cor pulmonale*, are relatively infrequent since the advent of supplemental oxygen therapy. Prior to the availability of such therapy, patients with advanced disease would develop elevated jugular venous pressures, a right ventricular heave or third heart sound, hepatic congestion, ascites, and peripheral edema as the right ventricle decompensated as a result of chronic pulmonary hypertension.

Clubbing of the digits is not a sign of COPD, and its presence should alert the clinician to initiate an investigation for causes of clubbing. In this population, the development of lung cancer is the most likely explanation for newly developed clubbing.

Laboratory Findings The hallmark of COPD is airflow obstruction (discussed above). Pulmonary function testing shows airflow obstruction with a reduction in FEV_1 and FEV_1/FVC (Chap. 234). With worsening disease severity, lung volumes may increase, resulting in an increase in total lung capacity, functional residual capacity, and residual volume. In patients with emphysema, the diffusing capacity may be reduced, reflecting the parenchymal destruction characteristic of the disease. The degree of airflow obstruction is an important prognostic factor in COPD and is the basis for the GOLD disease classification (Table 242-1).

While arterial blood gases and oximetry are not sensitive (discussed above), they may demonstrate resting or exertional hypoxemia. Arterial blood gases provide additional information about alveolar ventilation and acid-base status by measuring arterial P_{CO_2} and pH. The change in pH with P_{CO_2} is 0.08 units/10 mmHg acutely and 0.03 units/10 mmHg in the chronic state. Knowledge of the arterial pH therefore allows the classification of ventilatory failure, defined as $P_{CO_2} > 45$ mmHg, into acute or chronic conditions (Chap. 250). The arterial blood gas is an important component of the evaluation of patients presenting with symptoms of an exacerbation. An elevated hematocrit suggests the presence of chronic hypoxemia, as does the presence of signs of right ventricular hypertrophy on electrocardiography.

Radiographic studies may assist in the classification of the type of COPD. Obvious bullae, paucity of parenchymal markings, or hyperlucency suggest the presence of emphysema. Increased lung volumes and flattening of the diaphragm suggest hyperinflation, but do not provide information about chronicity of the changes. Computed tomography (CT) scan is the current definitive test for establishing the presence or absence of emphysema. From a practical perspective, the CT scan does little to influence therapy of COPD except in those individuals considering surgical therapy for their disease (described below).

In patients presenting at ≤ 50 years, those with a strong family history, those with predominant basilar disease or those with a minimal smoking history, the serum level of ($\alpha_1 AT$) should be measured. The definitive diagnosis of $\alpha_1 AT$ deficiency requires PI type determination. This is typically performed by isoelectric focusing of serum, which reflects the genotype at the PI locus for the common alleles and many of the rare PI alleles as well. Molecular genotyping can be performed for the common PI alleles (M, S, and Z).

Rx TREATMENT

Stable Phase COPD Only two interventions, smoking cessation and oxygen therapy in chronically hypoxemic patients, have been demonstrated to influence the natural history of patients with COPD. All other current therapies are directed at improving symptoms and decreasing the frequency and severity of exacerbations. The institution of these therapies should involve an assessment of symptoms, potential risks, costs, and benefits of therapy. This should be followed by an assessment of response to therapy, and a decision should be made whether or not to continue treatment.

Pharmacotherapy ■ *SMOKING CESSATION* (See also Chap. 375) It has been shown that middle-aged smokers who were able to successfully stop smoking experienced a significant improvement in the rate of decline in pulmonary function, returning to annual changes similar to that of nonsmoking patients. Thus, all patients with COPD should be strongly urged to quit and educated about the benefits of quitting. An emerging body of evidence demonstrates that combining pharmacotherapy with traditional supportive approaches considerably enhances the chances of successful smoking cessation. There are two principal pharmacologic approaches to the problem: bupropion, originally developed as an antidepressant medication, and nicotine replacement therapy. The latter is available as gum, transdermal patches, inhaler, and nasal spray. Current recommendations from the U.S. Surgeon General are that all smokers considering quitting be offered pharmacotherapy, in the absence of any contraindication to treatment.

BRONCHODILATORS In general, bronchodilators are used for symptomatic benefit in patients with COPD. The inhaled route is preferred for medication delivery as the incidence of side effects is lower than that seen with the use of parenteral medication delivery.

ANTICHOLINERGIC AGENTS While regular use of ipratropium bromide does not appear to influence the rate of decline of lung function, it has been reported to improve symptoms and produce acute improvement in FEV_1. Side effects are minor, and a trial of inhaled anticholinergics is recommended in symptomatic patients with COPD.

BETA AGONISTS These provide symptomatic benefit. The main side effects are tremor and tachycardia. Long-acting inhaled β agonists, such as salmeterol, have benefits comparable to ipratropium bromide. Their use is more convenient than short-acting agents. The addition of a β agonist to inhaled anticholinergic therapy has been demonstrated to provide incremental benefit.

INHALED GLUCOCORTICOIDS Several recent trials have *failed* to find a beneficial effect for the regular use of inhaled glucocorticoids on the rate of decline of lung function, as assessed by FEV_1. Patients studied included those with mild to severe airflow obstruction and current and ex-smokers. Patients with significant acute response to inhaled β agonists were excluded from these trials. Inhaled glucocorticoids were demonstrated to reduce the frequency of exacerbations by 25 to 30%, but their use has been associated with increased rates of oropharyngeal candidiasis and an increased rate of loss of bone density. A trial of inhaled glucocorticoids should be considered in patients with frequent exacerbations, defined as two or more per year, and in patients who demonstrate a significant amount of acute reversibility in response to inhaled bronchodilators.

PARENTERAL CORTICOSTEROIDS The chronic use of oral glucocorticoids for treatment of COPD is not recommended because of an unfavorable benefit/risk ratio. The chronic use of oral glucocorticoids is associated with significant side effects, including osteoporosis, weight gain, cataracts, glucose intolerance, and increased risk of infection. A recent study demonstrated that patients tapered off chronic low-dose prednisone ($\sim$10 mg/d) did not experience any adverse effect on the frequency of exacerbations, health-related quality of life, or lung function. On average, patients lost $\sim$4.5 kg ($\sim$10 lb) when steroids were withdrawn.

THEOPHYLLINE Theophylline produces modest improvements in expiratory flow rates and vital capacity and a slight improvement in arterial oxygen and carbon dioxide levels in patients with moderate to severe COPD. Nausea is a common side effect; tachycardia and tremor have also been reported.

OXYGEN Supplemental O_2 is the only therapy demonstrated to decrease mortality in patients with COPD. For patients with resting hypoxemia (resting O_2 saturation <88% or <90% with signs of pulmonary hypertension or right heart failure), the use of O_2 has been demonstrated to have a significant impact on mortality. The Medical Research Council Trial demonstrated that 12 h per day was superior to no O_2 supplementation. The Nocturnal Oxygen Therapy Trial demonstrated that O_2 use 19 h per day was superior to 12 h per day. Various delivery systems are available, including portable systems that patients may carry to allow mobility outside the home.

Supplemental O_2 is commonly prescribed for patients with exertional hypoxemia or nocturnal hypoxemia. Although the rationale for supplemental O_2 in these settings is physiologically sound, the benefits of such therapy are not well substantiated.

OTHER AGENTS N-acetyl cysteine has been used in patients with COPD for both its mucolytic and antioxidant properties. The latter aspect of its use is the subject of ongoing clinical trials. Specific treatment in the form of intravenous $\alpha_1 AT$ augmentation therapy is available for individuals with severe $\alpha_1 AT$ deficiency. Despite heat treatment of this product and the absence of reported cases of viral infection from therapy, hepatitis B vaccination is recommended prior to starting augmentation therapy. Although biochemical efficacy of $\alpha_1 AT$ augmentation therapy has been shown, a randomized controlled trial of $\alpha_1 AT$ augmentation therapy has never proven the efficacy of augmentation therapy in reducing decline of pulmonary function. Eligibility for $\alpha_1 AT$ augmentation therapy requires a serum $\alpha_1 AT$ level <11 μ M. Typically, Pi^Z individuals will qualify, although other rare types associated with severe deficiency (e.g., null-null) are also eligible. Since only a fraction of individuals with severe $\alpha_1 AT$ deficiency will develop COPD, $\alpha_1 AT$ augmentation therapy is *not* recommended for severely $\alpha_1 AT$-deficient persons with normal pulmonary function and a normal chest CT scan.

Nonpharmacologic Therapies ■ *GENERAL MEDICAL CARE* Patients with COPD should receive the influenza vaccine annually. Polyvalent pneumococcal vaccine is also recommended, although proof of efficacy in this patient population is not definitive.

PULMONARY REHABILITATION This refers to a treatment program that incorporates education and cardiovascular conditioning. In COPD, pulmonary rehabilitation has been demonstrated to improve health-related quality of life, dyspnea, and exercise capacity. It has also been shown to reduce rates of hospitalization over a 6- to 12-month period.

LUNG VOLUME REDUCTION SURGERY (LVRS) Surgery to reduce the volume of lung in patients with emphysema was first introduced with minimal success in the 1950s and was reintroduced in the 1990s. It has been reported to produce symptomatic and functional benefit in selected patients, particularly those with emphysema, which is predominant in the upper lobes. The operation may be performed via either a median sternotomy or a thoracoscopic approach. Patients are excluded if they have significant pleural disease (a pulmonary artery systolic pressure > 45 mmHg), extreme deconditioning, congestive heart failure, or other severe comorbid conditions. Recent data demonstrate that patients with an FEV_1 < 20% of predicted and either diffusely distributed emphysema on CT scan or DL_{CO} < 20% of predicted have an increased mortality after the procedure and thus are not candidates for LVRS.

The National Emphysema Treatment trial demonstrated that LVRS offers both a mortality benefit and a symptomatic benefit in certain patients with emphysema. The anatomic distribution of emphysema and postrehabilitation exercise capacity are important prognostic characteristics. Patients with upper lobe–predominant emphysema and a low postrehabilitation exercise capacity are most likely to benefit from LVRS.

LUNG TRANSPLANTATION (See also Chap. 248)   COPD is the single leading indication for lung transplantation. Current recommendations are that candidates for lung transplantation should be ≤65 years; have severe disability despite maximal medical therapy; and be free of comorbid conditions such as liver, renal, or cardiac disease. In contrast to LVRS, the anatomic distribution of emphysema and the presence of pulmonary hypertension are not contraindications to lung transplantation. Unresolved issues concerning lung transplantation and COPD include whether single- or double-lung transplant is the preferred procedure.

Exacerbations of COPD   Exacerbations are a prominent feature of the natural history of COPD. Exacerbations are commonly considered to be episodes of increased dyspnea and cough and change in the amount and character of sputum. They may or may not be accompanied by other signs of illness, including fever, myalgias, and sore throat. Self-reported health-related quality of life correlates with frequency of exacerbations more closely than it does with the degree of airflow obstruction. Economic analyses have shown that >70% of COPD-related health care expenditures go to emergency department visits and hospital care; this translates to >$10 billion annually in the United States. The frequency of exacerbations increases as airflow obstruction increases; patients with moderate to severe airflow obstruction [GOLD stages III,IV (Table 242-1)] have one to three episodes per year.

The approach to the patient experiencing an exacerbation includes an assessment of the severity of the patient's illness, both acute and chronic components; an attempt to identify the precipitant of the exacerbation; and the institution of therapy.

PRECIPITATING CAUSES AND STRATEGIES TO REDUCE FREQUENCY OF EXACERBATIONS
A variety of stimuli may result in the final common pathway of airway inflammation and increased symptoms that are characteristic of COPD exacerbations. Bacterial infections play a role in many, but by no means all, episodes. Viral respiratory infections are present in approximately one-third of COPD exacerbations. In a significant minority of instances (20 to 35%), no specific precipitant can be identified.

Despite the frequent implication of bacterial infection, chronic suppressive or "rotating" antibiotics are not beneficial in patients with COPD. This is in contrast to their apparent efficacy in patients with significant bronchiectasis. In patients with bronchiectasis due to cystic fibrosis, suppressive antibiotics have been shown to reduce frequency of hospital admissions.

The role of anti-inflammatory therapy in reducing exacerbation frequency is less well studied. Chronic oral glucocorticoids are not recommended for this purpose. Inhaled glucocorticoids did reduce the frequency of exacerbations by 25 to 30% in large clinical trials. It is important to realize that patients with significant pulmonary function reversibility to inhaled bronchodilators were excluded from these trials. Thus, the use of inhaled glucocorticoids should be considered in patients with frequent exacerbations or those who have an asthmatic component, i.e., significant reversibility on pulmonary function testing or marked symptomatic improvement after inhaled bronchodilators.

PATIENT ASSESSMENT   The practitioner should attempt to establish the severity of the exacerbation as well as the severity of preexisting COPD. The more severe either of these two components, the more likely that the patient will require hospital admission. The history should include quantification of the degree of dyspnea by asking about breathlessness during activities of daily living and typical activities for the patient. The patient should be asked about fever; change in character of sputum; any ill contacts; and associated symptoms such as nausea, vomiting, diarrhea, myalgias, and chills. Inquiring about the frequency and severity of prior exacerbations can provide important information. The physical examination should incorporate an assessment of the degree

of distress of the patient. Specific attention should be focused on tachycardia, tachypnea, use of accessory muscles, signs of perioral or peripheral cyanosis, the ability to speak in complete sentences, and the patient's mental status. The chest examination should establish the presence or absence of focal findings, degree of air movement, presence or absence of wheezing, asymmetry in the chest examination (suggesting large airway obstruction or pneumothorax mimicking an exacerbation), and the presence or absence of paradoxical motion of the abdominal wall.

Patients with severe underlying COPD who are in moderate or severe distress or those with focal findings should have a chest x-ray. Approximately 25% of x-rays in this clinical situation will be abnormal, with the most frequent findings being pneumonia and congestive heart failure. Patients with advanced COPD, those with a history of hypercarbia, those with mental status changes (confusion, sleepiness), or those in significant distress should have an arterial blood gas measurement. The presence of hypercarbia, defined as a $P_{CO_2} > 45$ mmHg, has important implications for treatment (discussed below). In contrast to its utility in the management of exacerbations of asthma, measurement of pulmonary function has not been demonstrated to be helpful in the diagnosis or management of exacerbations of COPD.

There are no definitive guidelines concerning the need for inpatient treatment of exacerbations. Patients with respiratory acidosis and hypercarbia, significant hypoxemia, or severe underlying disease or those whose living situation is not conducive to careful observation and the delivery of prescribed treatment should be admitted to the hospital.

Acute Exacerbations ■ *BRONCHODILATORS*   Typically, patients are treated with an inhaled β agonist, often with the addition of an anticholinergic agent. These may be administered separately or together, and the frequency of administration depends on the severity of the exacerbation. Patients are often treated initially with nebulized therapy, as such treatment is often easier to administer in older patients or to those in respiratory distress. It has been shown, however, that conversion to metered-dose inhalers is effective when accompanied by education and training of patients and staff. This approach has significant economic benefits and also allows an easier transition to outpatient care. The addition of methylxanthines (such as theophylline) to this regimen can be considered, although convincing proof of its efficacy is lacking. If added, serum levels should be monitored in an attempt to minimize toxicity.

ANTIBIOTICS   Patients with COPD are frequently colonized with potential respiratory pathogens and it is often difficult to identify conclusively a specific species of bacteria responsible for a particular clinical event. Bacteria frequently implicated in COPD exacerbations include *Streptococcus pneumoniae*, *Haemophilus influenzae*, and *Moraxella catarrhalis*. In addition, *Mycoplasma pneumoniae* or *Chlamydia pneumoniae* are found in 5 to 10% of exacerbations. The choice of antibiotic should be based on local patterns of antibiotic susceptibility of the above pathogens, as well as the patient's clinical condition. Most practitioners treat patients with moderate or severe exacerbations with antibiotics, even in the absence of data implicating a specific pathogen.

GLUCOCORTICOIDS   Among patients admitted to hospital, the use of glucocorticoids has been demonstrated to reduce the length of stay, hasten recovery, and reduce the chance of subsequent exacerbation or relapse for a period of up to 6 months. A recent study demonstrated that 2 weeks of glucocorticoid therapy produced benefit indistinguishable from 8 weeks of therapy. The GOLD guidelines recommend 30 to 40 mg of oral prednisolone or its equivalent for a period of 10 to 14 days. Hyperglycemia, particularly in patients with preexisting diagnosis of diabetes, is the most frequently reported acute complication of glucocorticoid treatment.

OXYGEN   Supplemental O_2 should be supplied to keep arterial saturations ≥90%. Hypoxic respiratory drive plays a small role in patients with COPD. Studies have demonstrated that in patients with both acute and chronic hypercarbia, the administration of supplemental O_2 does not reduce minute ventilation. It does, in some patients, result in modest increases in arterial P_{CO_2}, chiefly by altering ventilation-perfusion relationships within the lung. This should not deter practitioners from providing the oxygen needed to correct hypoxemia.

MECHANICAL VENTILATORY SUPPORT   Recent studies have demonstrated that the initiation of noninvasive positive pressure ventilation (NIPPV) in patients with respiratory failure, defined as $P_{CO_2} > 45$ mmHg, results in a significant reduction in mortality, need for intubation, complications of therapy, and hospital length of stay. Contraindications to NIPPV include cardiovascular instability, impaired mental status or inability to cooperate, copious secretions or the inability to clear secretions, craniofacial abnormalities or trauma precluding effective fitting of mask, extreme obesity, or significant burns.

Invasive (conventional) mechanical ventilation via an endotracheal tube is indicated for patients with severe respiratory distress despite initial therapy, life-threatening hypoxemia, severe hypercapnia and/or acidosis, markedly impaired mental status, respiratory arrest, hemodynamic instability, or other complications. The goal of mechanical ventilation is to correct the aforementioned conditions. Factors to consider during mechanical ventilatory support include the need to provide sufficient expiratory time in patients with severe airflow

obstruction and the presence of auto-PEEP (positive end-expiratory pressure) which can result in patients having to generate significant respiratory effort to trigger a breath during a demand mode of ventilation. The mortality of patients requiring mechanical ventilatory support is 17 to 30% for that particular hospitalization. For patients aged ≥65 admitted to the intensive care unit for treatment, the mortality doubles over the next year to 60%, regardless of whether mechanical ventilation was required.

FURTHER READING

BURROWS B et al: Quantitative relationships between cigarette smoking and ventilatory function. Am Rev Respir Dis 115:195, 1977

CELLI BR et al: Standards for the diagnosis and care of patients with chronic obstructive pulmonary disease. Official Statement of the American Thoracic Society. Am J Respir Crit Care Med. 152:S77, 1995

FIORE MC et al: Treating Tobacco Use and Dependence, Clinical Practice Guideline. Rockville, MD: U.S. Department of Health and Human Services. Public Health Service, June, 2000

KASAHARA Y et al: Inhibition of VEGF receptors causes lung cell apoptosis and emphysema. J Clin Invest 106:1311, 2000

PAUWELS RA et al: Global strategy for the diagnosis, management, and prevention of chronic obstructive pulmonary disease. NHLBI/WHO Global Initiative for Chronic Obstructive Lung Disease (GOLD) Workshop summary. Am J Respir Crit Care Med 163:1256, 2001

SENIOR RM, SHAPIRO SD: Chronic obstructive pulmonary disease: Epidemiology, pathophysiology, and pathogenesis, in Fishman's Pulmonary Diseases and Disorders, 3d ed, AD Fishman et al (eds). New York, McGraw-Hill, 1998, pp 659–681

243 INTERSTITIAL LUNG DISEASES
Talmadge E. King, Jr.

The interstitial lung diseases (ILDs) represent a large number of conditions that involve the parenchyma of the lung—the alveoli, the alveolar epithelium, the capillary endothelium, and the spaces between these structures, as well as the perivascular and lymphatic tissues. This heterogeneous group of disorders is classified together because of similar clinical, roentgenographic, physiologic, or pathologic manifestations. These disorders are often associated with considerable morbidity and mortality, and there is little consensus regarding the best management of most of them.

ILDs have been difficult to classify because more than 200 known individual diseases are characterized by diffuse parenchymal lung involvement, either as the primary condition or as a significant part of a multiorgan process, as may occur in the connective tissue diseases (CTDs). One useful approach to classification is to separate the ILDs into two groups based on the major underlying histopathology: (1) those associated with predominant inflammation and fibrosis, and (2) those with a predominantly granulomatous reaction in interstitial or vascular areas (Table 243-1). Each of these groups can be further subdivided according to whether the cause is known or unknown. For each ILD there may be an acute phase, and there is usually a chronic one as well. Rarely, some are recurrent, with intervals of subclinical disease.

Sarcoidosis (Chap. 309), idiopathic pulmonary fibrosis (IPF), and pulmonary fibrosis associated with CTDs (Chaps. 300 to 306) are the most common ILDs of unknown etiology. Among the ILDs of known cause, the largest group comprises occupational and environmental exposures, especially the inhalation of inorganic dusts, organic dusts, and various fumes or gases (Chaps. 237 and 238). A clinical diagnosis is possible for many forms of ILD, especially if an occupational and environmental history is aggressively pursued. For other forms, tissue examination, usually obtained by thoracoscopic or open-lung biopsy, is critical to confirmation of the diagnosis. High-resolution computed tomography (HRCT) scanning promises to improve diagnostic accuracy further as histologic-image correlation is perfected.

PATHOGENESIS

The ILDs are nonmalignant disorders and are not caused by identified infectious agents. The precise pathway(s) leading from injury to fibrosis is not known. Although there are multiple initiating agent(s) of injury, the immunopathogenic responses of lung tissue are limited, and the mechanisms of repair have common features. As mentioned above, the two major histopathologic patterns are a granulomatous pattern and a pattern in which inflammation and fibrosis predominate.

GRANULOMATOUS LUNG DISEASE   This process is characterized by an accumulation of T lymphocytes, macrophages, and epithelioid cells organized into discrete structures (granulomas) in the lung parenchyma. The granulomatous lesions can progress to fibrosis. Many patients with granulomatous lung disease remain free of severe impairment of lung function, or, when symptomatic, they improve after treatment. The main differential diagnosis is between sarcoidosis (Chap. 309) and hypersensitivity pneumonitis (Chap. 237).

INFLAMMATION AND FIBROSIS   The initial insult is an injury to the epithelial surface causing inflammation in the air spaces and alveolar walls. If the disease becomes chronic, inflammation spreads to adjacent portions of the interstitium and vasculature and eventually causes interstitial fibrosis. Important histopathologic patterns found in the ILDs include: usual interstitial pneumonia (UIP), nonspecific interstitial pneumonia, respiratory bronchiolitis, organizing pneumonia [bronchiolitis obliterans with organizing pneumonia (BOOP) pattern], diffuse alveolar damage (acute or organizing), desquamative interstitial pneumonia, and lymphocytic interstitial pneumonia. The development of irreversible scarring (fibrosis) of alveolar walls, airways, or vasculature is the most feared outcome in all of these conditions because it is often progressive and leads to significant derangement of ventilatory function and gas exchange.

INITIAL EVALUATION

Patients with ILDs come to medical attention mainly because of the onset of progressive exertional dyspnea or a persistent, nonproductive cough. Hemoptysis, wheezing, and chest pain may be present. Often, the identification of interstitial opacities on chest x-ray focuses the diagnostic approach toward one of the ILDs.

TABLE 243-1 *Major Categories of Alveolar and Interstitial Inflammatory Lung Disease*

Lung Response: Alveolitis, Interstitial Inflammation, and Fibrosis

KNOWN CAUSE

Asbestos	Radiation
Fumes, gases	Aspiration pneumonia
Drugs (antibiotics, amiodarone, gold) and chemotherapy drugs	Residual of adult respiratory distress syndrome

UNKNOWN CAUSE

Idiopathic interstitial pneumonias	Pulmonary alveolar proteinosis
Idiopathic pulmonary fibrosis (usual interstitial pneumonia)	Lymphocytic infiltrative disorders (lymphocytic interstitial pneumonitis associated with connective tissue disease)
Desquamative interstitial pneumonia	
Respiratory bronchiolitis-associated interstitial lung disease	Eosinophilic pneumonias
Acute interstitial pneumonia (diffuse alveolar damage)	Lymphangioleiomyomatosis
	Amyloidosis
Cryptogenic organizing pneumonia (bronchiolitis obliterans with organizing pneumonia)	Inherited diseases
	Tuberous sclerosis, neurofibromatosis, Niemann-Pick disease, Gaucher's disease, Hermansky-Pudlak syndrome
Nonspecific interstitial pneumonia	
Connective tissue diseases	
Systemic lupus erythematosus, rheumatoid arthritis, ankylosing spondylitis, systemic sclerosis, Sjögren's syndrome, polymyositis-dermatomyositis	Gastrointestinal or liver diseases (Crohn's disease, primary biliary cirrhosis, chronic active hepatitis, ulcerative colitis)
Pulmonary hemorrhage syndromes	Graft-vs.-host disease (bone marrow transplantation; solid organ transplantation)
Goodpasture's syndrome, idiopathic pulmonary hemosiderosis, isolated pulmonary capillaritis	

Lung Response: Granulomatous

KNOWN CAUSE

Hypersensitivity pneumonitis (organic dusts)	Inorganic dusts: beryllium silica

UNKNOWN CAUSE

Sarcoidosis	Bronchocentric granulomatosis
Langerhans cell granulomatosis (eosinophilic granuloma of the lung)	Lymphomatoid granulomatosis
Granulomatous vasculitides	
Wegener's granulomatosis, allergic granulomatosis of Churg-Strauss	

HISTORY ■ **Duration of Illness** *Acute presentation* (days to weeks), while unusual, occurs with allergy (drugs, fungi, helminths), acute idiopathic interstitial pneumonia, eosinophilic pneumonia, and hypersensitivity pneumonitis. These conditions may be confused with atypical pneumonias because of diffuse alveolar opacities on chest x-ray. *Subacute presentation* (weeks to months) may occur in all ILDs but is seen especially in sarcoidosis, drug-induced ILDs, the alveolar hemorrhage syndromes, cryptogenic organizing pneumonia (COP), and the acute immunologic pneumonia that complicates systemic lupus erythematosus (SLE) or polymyositis. In most ILDs the symptoms and signs form a *chronic presentation* (months to years). Examples include IPF, sarcoidosis, pulmonary Langerhans cell histiocytosis (PLCH) (also known as Langerhans cell granulomatosis, eosinophilic granuloma, or histiocytosis X), pneumoconioses, and CTDs. *Episodic presentations* are unusual and include eosinophilic pneumonia, hypersensitivity pneumonitis, COP, vasculitides, pulmonary hemorrhage, and Churg-Strauss syndrome.

Age Most patients with sarcoidosis, ILD associated with CTD, lymphangioleiomyomatosis (LAM), PLCH, and inherited forms of ILD (familial IPF, Gaucher's disease, Hermansky-Pudlak syndrome) present between the ages of 20 and 40 years. Most patients with IPF are older than 50 years.

Gender LAM and pulmonary involvement in tuberous sclerosis occur exclusively in premenopausal women. Also, ILD in Hermansky-Pudlak syndrome and in the CTDs is more common in women; an exception is ILD in rheumatoid arthritis (RA), which is more common in men. Because of occupational exposures, pneumoconioses also occur more frequently in men.

Family History Family associations (with an autosomal dominant pattern) have been identified in tuberous sclerosis and neurofibromatosis. An autosomal recessive pattern of inheritance occurs in Niemann-Pick disease, Gaucher's disease, and the Hermansky-Pudlak syndrome. Familial clustering has been increasingly identified in sarcoidosis. Familial lung fibrosis has been associated with mutations in the surfactant protein C gene and is characterized by several patterns of interstitial pneumonia, including nonspecific interstitial pneumonia, desquamative interstitial pneumonia, and UIP.

Smoking History Patients with PLCH, desquamative interstitial pneumonia (DIP), Goodpasture's syndrome, respiratory bronchiolitis, and pulmonary alveolar proteinosis are almost always current or former smokers. Two-thirds to 75% of patients with IPF have a history of smoking.

Occupation and Environmental History A strict chronologic listing of the patient's lifelong employment must be sought, including specific duties and known exposures. In hypersensitivity pneumonitis (see Fig. 237-1), respiratory symptoms, fever, chills, and an abnormal chest roentgenogram are often temporally related to a hobby (pigeon breeder's disease) or to the workplace (farmer's lung) (Chap. 237). Symptoms may diminish or disappear after the patient leaves the site of exposure for several days; similarly, symptoms may reappear on returning to the exposure site.

Other Important Past History Parasitic infections may cause pulmonary eosinophilia, and therefore a travel history should be taken in patients with known or suspected ILD. History of risk factors for HIV infection should be elicited from all patients with ILD because several processes may occur at the time of initial presentation or during the clinical course, e.g., HIV infection, BOOP, acute interstitial pneumonia (AIP), lymphocytic interstitial pneumonitis, or diffuse alveolar hemorrhage.

RESPIRATORY SYMPTOMS AND SIGNS Dyspnea is a common and prominent complaint in patients with ILD, especially the idiopathic interstitial pneumonias, hypersensitivity pneumonitis, COP, sarcoidosis, eosinophilic pneumonias, and PLCH. Some patients, especially patients with sarcoidosis, silicosis, PLCH, hypersensitivity pneumonitis, lipoid pneumonia, or lymphangitis carcinomatosis, may have extensive parenchymal lung disease on chest x-ray without significant dyspnea, especially early in the course of the illness. Wheezing is an uncommon manifestation of ILD but has been described in patients with chronic eosinophilic pneumonia, Churg-Strauss syndrome, respiratory bronchiolitis, and sarcoidosis. Clinically significant chest pain is uncommon in most ILDs. However, substernal discomfort is common in sarcoidosis. Sudden worsening of dyspnea, especially if associated with acute chest pain, may indicate a spontaneous pneumothorax, which occurs in PLCH, tuberous sclerosis, LAM, and neurofibromatosis. Frank hemoptysis and blood-streaked sputum are rarely presenting manifestations of ILD but can be seen in the diffuse alveolar hemorrhage (DAH) syndromes, LAM, tuberous sclerosis, and the granulomatous vasculitides. Fatigue and weight loss are common in all ILDs.

PHYSICAL EXAMINATION The findings are usually not specific. Most commonly, physical examination reveals tachypnea and bibasilar end-inspiratory dry crackles, which are common in most forms of ILD associated with inflammation but are less likely to be heard in the granulomatous lung diseases. Crackles may be present in the absence of radiographic abnormalities on the chest radiograph. Scattered late inspiratory high-pitched rhonchi—so-called inspiratory squeaks—are heard in patients with bronchiolitis. The cardiac examination is usually normal except in the mid or late stages of the disease, when findings of pulmonary hypertension and cor pulmonale may become evident (Chap. 220). Cyanosis and clubbing of the digits occur in some patients with advanced disease.

LABORATORY   Antinuclear antibodies, anti-immunoglobulin antibodies (rheumatoid factors), and circulating immune complexes are identified in some patients, even in the absence of a defined CTD. A raised LDH is a nonspecific finding common to ILDs. Elevation of the serum angiotensin-converting enzyme level is common in sarcoidosis. Serum precipitins confirm exposure when hypersensitivity pneumonitis is suspected, although they are not diagnostic of the process. Antineutrophil cytoplasmic or anti-basement membrane antibodies are useful if vasculitis is suspected. The electrocardiogram is usually normal unless pulmonary hypertension is present; then it demonstrates right-axis deviation, right ventricular hypertrophy, or right atrial enlargement or hypertrophy. Echocardiography also reveals right ventricular dilatation and/or hypertrophy in the presence of pulmonary hypertension.

CHEST IMAGING STUDIES ■ **Chest X-ray**   ILD may be first suspected on the basis of an abnormal chest radiograph, which most commonly reveals a bibasilar reticular pattern. A nodular or mixed pattern of alveolar filling and increased reticular markings may also be present (see Fig. 233-1). A subgroup of ILDs exhibit nodular opacities with a predilection for the upper lung zones [sarcoidosis, PLCH, chronic hypersensitivity pneumonitis, silicosis, berylliosis, RA (necrobiotic nodular form), ankylosing spondylitis]. The chest x-ray correlates poorly with the clinical or histopathologic stage of the disease. The radiographic finding of honeycombing correlates with pathologic findings of small cystic spaces and progressive fibrosis; when present, it portends a poor prognosis. In most cases, the chest radiograph is nonspecific and usually does not allow a specific diagnosis.

Computed Tomography   HRCT is superior to the plain chest x-ray for early detection and confirmation of suspected ILD (Fig. 243-1). Also, HRCT allows better assessment of the extent and distribution of disease, and it is especially useful in the investigation of patients with a normal chest radiograph. Coexisting disease is often best recognized on HRCT scanning, e.g., mediastinal adenopathy, carcinoma, or emphysema. In the appropriate clinical setting HRCT may be sufficiently characteristic to preclude the need for lung biopsy in IPF, sarcoidosis,

FIGURE 243-1   Idiopathic pulmonary fibrosis. High-resolution computed tomographic image shows bibasal, peripheral predominant reticular abnormality with traction bronchiectasis and honeycombing. The lung biopsy showed the typical features of usual interstitial pneumonia.

hypersensitivity pneumonitis, asbestosis, lymphangitic carcinoma, and PLCH. When a lung biopsy is required, HRCT scanning is useful for determining the most appropriate area from which biopsy samples should be taken.

Radionuclide Scanning   Gallium-67 or ^{99m}Tc-diethylenetriamene penta-acetate (DTPA) scanning have limited roles in evaluating the inflammatory component of ILD.

PULMONARY FUNCTION TESTING ■ **Spirometry and Lung Volumes**   Measurement of lung function is important in assessing the extent of pulmonary involvement in patients with ILD. Most forms of ILD produce a restrictive defect with reduced total lung capacity (TLC), functional residual capacity, and residual volume (Chap. 234). Forced expiratory volume in one second (FEV_1) and forced vital capacity (FVC) are reduced, but these changes are related to the decreased TLC. The FEV_1/FVC ratio is usually normal or increased. Lung volumes decrease as lung stiffness worsens with disease progression. A few disorders produce interstitial opacities on chest x-ray and obstructive airflow limitation on lung function testing (uncommon in sarcoidosis and hypersensitivity pneumonitis, while common in tuberous sclerosis and LAM).

Diffusing Capacity   A reduction in the diffusing capacity of the lung for carbon monoxide (DL_{CO}) is a common but nonspecific finding in most ILDs. This decrease is due, in part, to effacement of the alveolar capillary units but, more importantly, to mismatching of ventilation and perfusion ($\dot{V}/\dot{Q}$). Lung regions with reduced compliance due to either fibrosis or cellular infiltration may be poorly ventilated but may still maintain adequate blood flow and the ventilation-perfusion mismatch in these regions acts like true venous admixture. The severity of the reduction in DL_{CO} does not correlate with disease stage.

Arterial Blood Gas   The resting arterial blood gas may be normal or reveal hypoxemia (secondary to a mismatching of ventilation to perfusion) and respiratory alkalosis. A normal arterial O_2 tension (or saturation by oximetry) at rest does not rule out significant hypoxemia during exercise or sleep. CO_2 retention is rare and is usually a manifestation of end-stage disease.

CARDIOPULMONARY EXERCISE TESTING   Because hypoxemia at rest is not always present and because severe exercise-induced hypoxemia may go undetected, it is useful to perform exercise testing with measurement of arterial blood gases to detect abnormalities of gas exchange. Arterial oxygen desaturation, a failure to decrease dead space appropriately with exercise [i.e., a high V_D/V_T ratio (Chap. 234)], and an excessive increase in respiratory rate with a lower-than-expected recruitment of tidal volume provide useful information about physiologic abnormalities and extent of disease. Serial assessment of resting and exercise gas exchange is an excellent method for following disease activity and responsiveness to treatment, especially in patients with IPF.

FIBEROPTIC BRONCHOSCOPY AND BRONCHOALVEOLAR LAVAGE (BAL)   In selected diseases (e.g., sarcoidosis, hypersensitivity pneumonitis, DAH syndrome, cancer, pulmonary alveolar proteinosis), cellular analysis of BAL fluid may be useful in narrowing the differential diagnostic possibilities among various types of ILD. The role for BAL in defining the stage of disease and assessment of disease progression or response to therapy remains poorly understood, and the usefulness of BAL in the clinical assessment and management remains to be established.

TISSUE AND CELLULAR EXAMINATION   Lung biopsy is the most effective method for confirming the diagnosis and assessing disease activity. The findings may identify a more treatable process than originally suspected, particularly chronic hypersensitivity pneumonitis, COP, respiratory bronchiolitis–associated ILD, or sarcoidosis. Biopsy should be obtained before initiation of treatment. A definitive diagnosis avoids confusion and anxiety later in the clinical course if the patient does not respond to therapy or suffers serious side effects from it.

Fiberoptic bronchoscopy with multiple transbronchial lung biop-

sies (four to eight biopsy samples) is often the initial procedure of choice, especially when sarcoidosis, lymphangitic carcinomatosis, eosinophilic pneumonia, Goodpasture's syndrome, or infection are suspected. If a specific diagnosis is not made by transbronchial biopsy, then surgical lung biopsy by video-assisted thoracic surgery or open thoracotomy is indicated. Adequate-sized biopsies from multiple sites, usually from two lobes, should be obtained. Relative contraindications to lung biopsy include serious cardiovascular disease, honeycombing and other roentgenographic evidence of diffuse end-stage disease, severe pulmonary dysfunction, or other major operative risks, especially in the elderly.

℞ TREATMENT

Although the course of ILD is variable, progression is common and often insidious. All treatable possibilities should be carefully considered. Since therapy does not reverse fibrosis, the major goals of treatment are permanent removal of the offending agent, when known, and early identification and aggressive suppression of the acute and chronic inflammatory process, thereby reducing further lung damage.

Hypoxemia ($Pa_{O_2} < 55$ mmHg) at rest and/or with exercise should be managed by supplemental oxygen. If cor pulmonale develops, diuretic therapy and phlebotomy may occasionally be required (Chap. 220).

DRUG THERAPY Glucocorticoids are the mainstay of therapy for suppression of the alveolitis present in ILD, but the success rate is low. There have been no placebo-controlled trials of glucocorticoids in ILD, so there is no direct evidence that steroids improve survival in many of the diseases for which they are commonly used. Glucocorticoid therapy is recommended for symptomatic ILD patients with idiopathic interstitial pneumonias, eosinophilic pneumonias, COP, CTD, sarcoidosis, acute inorganic dust exposures, acute radiation pneumonitis, DAH, and drug-induced ILD. In organic dust disease, glucocorticoids are recommended for both the acute and chronic stages.

The optimal dose and proper length of therapy with glucocorticoids in the treatment of most ILDs are not known. A common starting dose is prednisone, 0.5 to 1 mg/kg in a once-daily oral dose (based on the patient's lean body weight). This dose is continued for 4 to 12 weeks, at which time the patient is reevaluated. If the patient is stable or improved, the dose is tapered to 0.25 to 0.5 mg/kg and is maintained at this level for an additional 4 to 12 weeks depending on the course. Rapid tapering or a shortened course of glucocorticoid treatment can result in recurrence. If the patient's condition continues to decline while on glucocorticoids, a second agent (see below) is often added and the prednisone dose is lowered to or maintained at 0.25 mg/kg per day.

Cyclophosphamide and azathioprine (1 to 2 mg/kg lean body weight per day), with or without glucocorticoids, have been tried with variable success in IPF, vasculitis, and other ILDs. An objective response usually requires at least 8 to 12 weeks to occur. In situations in which these drugs have failed or could not be tolerated, other agents, including methotrexate, colchicine, penicillamine, and cyclosporine, have been tried. However, their role in the treatment of ILDs remains to be determined.

Many cases of ILD are chronic and irreversible despite the therapy discussed above, and lung transplantation may then be considered (Chap. 248).

INDIVIDUAL FORMS OF ILD

IDIOPATHIC PULMONARY FIBROSIS IPF is the most common form of idiopathic interstitial pneumonia. Separating IPF from other forms of lung fibrosis is an important step in the evaluation of all patients presenting with ILD. IPF has a distinctly poor response to therapy and prognosis.

Clinical Manifestations Exertional dyspnea, a nonproductive cough, and inspiratory crackles with or without digital clubbing may be present on physical examination. The HRCT lung scans typically show patchy, predominantly basilar, subpleural reticular opacities, often associated with traction bronchiectasis and honeycombing (Fig. 243-1). Atypical findings that should suggest an alternative diagnosis include: extensive ground-glass abnormality, nodular opacities, upper or mid-zone predominance, and prominent hilar or mediastinal lymphadenopathy. Pulmonary function tests often reveal a restrictive pattern, a reduced DL_{CO}, and arterial hypoxemia that is exaggerated or elicited by exercise.

Histologic Findings Confirmation of the presence of the UIP pattern on histologic examination is essential to confirm this diagnosis. Transbronchial biopsies are not helpful in making the diagnosis of UIP, and surgical biopsy is usually required. The histologic hallmark and chief diagnostic criterion of UIP is a heterogeneous appearance at low magnification with alternating areas of normal lung, interstitial inflammation, foci of proliferating fibroblasts, dense collagen fibrosis, and honeycomb changes. These histologic changes affect the peripheral, subpleural parenchyma most severely. The interstitial inflammation is usually patchy and consists of a lymphoplasmacytic infiltrate in the alveolar septa, associated with hyperplasia of type 2 pneumocytes. The fibrotic zones are composed mainly of dense collagen, although scattered foci of proliferating fibroblasts are a consistent finding. The extent of fibroblastic proliferation is predictive of disease progression. Areas of honeycomb change are composed of cystic fibrotic air spaces that are frequently lined by bronchiolar epithelium and filled with mucin. Smooth-muscle hyperplasia is commonly seen in areas of fibrosis and honeycomb change. Histopathologic examinations during this accelerated phase show a combination of UIP and diffuse alveolar damage. A UIP-like pattern can also be seen with CTDs, pneumoconioses (e.g., asbestosis), radiation injury, certain drug-induced lung diseases (e.g., nitrofurantoin), and chronic aspiration. Also, a fibrotic pattern may be found in the chronic stage of several specific disorders such as sarcoidosis, chronic hypersensitivity pneumonitis, organized chronic eosinophilic pneumonia, and PLCH. Since other histopathologic features are frequently present in these syndromes, the term UIP is used for those patients in whom the lesion is idiopathic and not associated with another condition.

℞ TREATMENT

The clinical course is variable, with a 5-year survival rate of 20 to 40% after diagnosis. Treatment options include glucocorticoids, cytotoxic agents (e.g., azathioprine, cyclophosphamide), and antifibrotic agents (e.g., colchicine, pirfenidone, or interferon gamma-1b), alone or in combination with glucocorticoids. However, there is no firm evidence that any of these treatment approaches improves survival or the quality of life. Because of the poor prognosis in untreated patients, a therapeutic trial may be tried. If therapy is recommended, it should be started at the first identification of clinical or physiologic evidence of impairment of lung function. Lung transplantation should be considered for those patients who experience progressive deterioration despite optimal medical management and who meet the established criteria (Chap. 248).

DESQUAMATIVE INTERSTITIAL PNEUMONIA DIP is a rare but distinct clinical and pathologic entity found exclusively in cigarette smokers. The histologic hallmark is the extensive accumulation of macrophages in intraalveolar spaces with minimal interstitial fibrosis. The peak incidence is in the fourth and fifth decades. Most patients present with dyspnea. Lung function testing shows a restrictive pattern with reduced DL_{CO} and arterial hypoxemia. The chest x-ray and HRCT scans usually shows diffuse hazy opacities. Clinical recognition of DIP is important because the process is associated with a better prognosis (10-year survival rate is ~70%) and a better response to smoking cessation and systemic glucocorticoids than the more common IPF. Respiratory bronchiolitis–associated ILD is considered to be a subset of DIP and is characterized by the accumulation of macrophages in peribronchial alveoli.

ACUTE INTERSTITIAL PNEUMONIA (HAMMAN-RICH SYNDROME) AIP is a rare, fulminant form of lung injury characterized histologically by diffuse alveolar damage on lung biopsy. Most patients are older than 40 years. AIP is similar in presentation to the acute respiratory distress syndrome (ARDS) (Chap. 251) and probably corresponds to the subset of cases of idiopathic ARDS. The onset is usually abrupt in a previously healthy individual. A prodromal illness, usually lasting 7 to 14 days before presentation, is common. Fever, cough, and dyspnea are frequent manifestations at presentation. Diffuse, bilateral, air-space opacification is present on chest radiograph. HRCT scans show bilateral, patchy, symmetric areas of ground-glass attenuation. Bilateral areas of air-space consolidation may also be present. A predominantly subpleural distribution may be seen. The diagnosis of AIP requires the presence of a clinical syndrome of idiopathic ARDS and pathologic confirmation of organizing diffuse alveolar damage. Therefore, lung biopsy is required to confirm the diagnosis. Most patients have moderate to severe hypoxemia and develop respiratory failure. Mechanical ventilation is often required. The mortality rate is high (>60%), with most patients dying within 6 months of presentation. Recurrences have been reported. However, those who recover often have substantial improvement in lung function. The main treatment is supportive. It is not clear that glucocorticoid therapy is effective.

NONSPECIFIC INTERSTITIAL PNEUMONIA (NSIP) This condition defines a subgroup of the idiopathic interstitial pneumonias that can be distinguished clinically and pathologically from UIP, DIP, AIP, and idiopathic BOOP. NSIP is a subacute restrictive process with a presentation similar to IPF but usually at a younger age. It is often associated with a febrile illness and there is a relative lack of clubbing. HRCT shows bilateral, subpleural ground-glass opacities, often associated with lower lobe volume loss (Fig. 243-2). Patchy areas of air-space consolidation and reticular abnormalities may be present, but honeycombing is unusual. Unlike patients with IPF (UIP), the majority of patients with NSIP have a good prognosis with most showing improvement after treatment with glucocorticoids.

ILD ASSOCIATED WITH CONNECTIVE TISSUE DISORDERS Clinical findings suggestive of a CTD (musculoskeletal pain, weakness, fatigue, fever, joint pains or swelling, photosensitivity, Raynaud's phenomenon, pleuritis, dry eyes, dry mouth) should be sought in any patient with ILD. The CTDs may be difficult to rule out since the pulmonary manifestations occasionally precede the more typical systemic manifestations by months or years. The most common form of pulmonary involvement is a chronic interstitial pattern similar to that in patients with IPF. However, determining the precise nature of lung involvement in most of the CTDs is difficult due to the high incidence of lung involvement caused by disease-associated complications of esophageal dysfunction (predisposing to aspiration and secondary infections), respiratory muscle weakness (atelectasis and secondary infections), complications of therapy (opportunistic infections), and associated malignancies.

Progressive Systemic Sclerosis (PSS) (See also Chap. 303) Clinical evidence of ILD is present in about one-half of patients with PSS, and pathologic evidence in three-quarters. Pulmonary function tests show a restrictive pattern and impaired diffusing capacity, often before any clinical or radiographic evidence of lung disease appears. Pulmonary vascular disease alone or in association with pulmonary fibrosis, pleuritis, or recurrent aspiration pneumonitis is strikingly resistant to current modes of therapy.

Rheumatoid Arthritis (See also Chap. 301) ILD associated with RA is more common in men. Pulmonary manifestations of RA include pleurisy with or without effusion, ILD in up to 20% of cases, necrobiotic nodules (nonpneumoconiotic intrapulmonary rheumatoid nodules) with or without cavities, Caplan's syndrome (rheumatoid pneumoconiosis), pulmonary hypertension secondary to rheumatoid pulmonary vasculitis, BOOP, and upper airway obstruction due to arytenoid arthritis.

Systemic Lupus Erythematosus (See also Chap. 300) Lung disease is a common complication in SLE. Pleuritis with or without effusion is the most common pulmonary manifestation. Other lung manifestations include the following: atelectasis, diaphragmatic dysfunction with loss of lung volumes, pulmonary vascular disease, pulmonary hemorrhage, uremic pulmonary edema, infectious pneumonia, and BOOP. Acute lupus pneumonitis characterized by pulmonary capillaritis leading to alveolar hemorrhage is uncommon. Chronic, progressive ILD is uncommon. It is important to exclude pulmonary infection. Although pleuropulmonary involvement may not be evident clinically, pulmonary function testing, particularly DL_{CO}, reveals abnormalities in many patients with SLE.

Polymyositis and Dermatomyositis (PM/DM) (See also Chap. 369) ILD occurs in ~10% of patients with PM/DM, and the clinical features are similar to those of IPF. Diffuse reticular or nodular opacities with or without an alveolar component occur radiographically, with a predilection for the lung bases. ILD occurs more commonly in the subgroup of patients with an anti-Jo-1 antibody that is directed to histidyl tRNA synthetase. Weakness of respiratory muscles contributing to aspiration pneumonia may be present. A rapidly progressive illness characterized by diffuse alveolar damage may cause respiratory failure.

Sjögren's Syndrome (See also Chap. 304) General dryness and lack of airways secretion cause the major problems of hoarseness, cough, and bronchitis. Lymphocytic interstitial pneumonitis, lymphoma, pseudolymphoma, bronchiolitis, and bronchiolitis obliterans are associated with this condition. Lung biopsy is frequently required to establish a precise pulmonary diagnosis. Glucocorticoids have been used in the management of ILD associated with Sjögren's syndrome with some degree of clinical success.

DRUG-INDUCED ILD Many classes of drugs have the potential to induce diffuse ILD, which is manifest most commonly as exertional dyspnea and nonproductive cough. A detailed history of the medications taken by the patient is needed to identify drug-induced disease, including over-the-counter medications, oily nose drops, or petroleum products (mineral oil). In most cases, the pathogenesis is unknown, although a combination of direct toxic effects of the drug (or its metabolite) and indirect inflammatory and immunologic events is likely. The onset of the illness may be abrupt and fulminant, or it may be insidious, extending over weeks to months. The drug may have been taken for several years before a reaction develops (e.g., amiodarone), or the lung

FIGURE 243-2   Nonspecific interstitial pneumonia. High-resolution computed tomography through the lower lung shows volume loss with extensive ground-glass abnormality, reticular abnormality and traction bronchiectasis. There is sparing on the lung immediately adjacent to the pleura. Histology showed a combination of inflammation and mild fibrosis.

disease may occur weeks to years after the drug has been discontinued (e.g., carmustine). The extent and severity of disease are usually dose related. Treatment consists of discontinuation of any possible offending drug and supportive care.

CRYPTOGENIC ORGANIZING PNEUMONIA Also known as idiopathic BOOP, COP is a clinicopathologic syndrome of unknown etiology. The onset is usually in the fifth and sixth decades. The presentation may be of a flulike illness with cough, fever, malaise, fatigue, and weight loss. Inspiratory crackles are frequently present on examination. Pulmonary function is usually impaired, with a restrictive defect and arterial hypoxemia being most common. The roentgenographic manifestations are distinctive, revealing bilateral, patchy, or diffuse alveolar opacities in the presence of normal lung volume. Recurrent and migratory pulmonary opacities are common. HRCT shows areas of air-space consolidation, ground-glass opacities, small nodular opacities, and bronchial wall thickening and dilation. These changes occur more frequently in the periphery of the lung and in the lower lung zone. Lung biopsy shows granulation tissue within small airways, alveolar ducts, and airspaces, with chronic inflammation in the surrounding alveoli. Glucocorticoid therapy induces clinical recovery in two-thirds of patients. A few patients have rapidly progressive courses with fatal outcomes despite glucocorticoids.

Foci of organizing pneumonia (i.e., a "BOOP pattern") is a nonspecific reaction to lung injury found adjacent to other pathologic processes or as a component of other primary pulmonary disorders (e.g., cryptococcosis, Wegener's granulomatosis, lymphoma, hypersensitivity pneumonitis, and eosinophilic pneumonia). Consequently, the clinician must carefully reevaluate any patient found to have this histopathologic lesion to rule out these possibilities.

EOSINOPHILIC PNEUMONIA See Chap. 237

PULMONARY ALVEOLAR PROTEINOSIS Although not strictly an ILD, pulmonary alveolar proteinosis (PAP) resembles and is therefore considered with these conditions. It has been proposed that a defect in macrophage function, more specifically an impaired ability to process surfactant, may play a role in the pathogenesis of PAP. This diffuse disease is characterized by the accumulation of an amorphous, periodic acid–Schiff–positive lipoproteinaceous material in the distal air spaces. There is little or no lung inflammation, and the underlying lung architecture is preserved. Mutant mice lacking the gene for granulocyte-macrophage colony-stimulating factor (GM-CSF) have a similar accumulation of surfactant and surfactant apoprotein in the alveolar spaces. Moreover, reconstitution of the respiratory epithelium of GM-CSF knockout mice with the GM-CSF gene completely corrects the alveolar proteinosis. Data from BAL studies in patients suggest that PAP is an autoimmune disease with neutralizing antibody of immunoglobulin G isotype against GM-CSF. These findings suggest that neutralization of GM-CSF bioactivity by the antibody causes dysfunction of alveolar macrophages, which results in reduced surfactant clearance. There are three distinct classes of PAP: acquired (>90% of all cases), congenital, and secondary. Congenital PAP is transmitted in an autosomal recessive manner and is caused by homozygosity for a frame shift mutation (121ins2) in the SP-B gene, which leads to an unstable SP-B mRNA, reduced protein levels, and secondary disturbances of SP-C processing. Secondary PAP is rare among adults and is caused by lysinuric protein intolerance, acute silicosis and other inhalational syndromes, immunodeficiency disorders, and malignancies (almost exclusively of hematopoietic origin) and hematopoietic disorders.

The typical age of presentation is 30 to 50 years, and males predominate. The clinical presentation is usually insidious and manifested by progressive exertional dyspnea, fatigue, weight loss, and low-grade fever. A nonproductive cough is common, but occasionally expectoration of "chunky" gelatinous material may occur. Polycythemia, hypergammaglobulinemia, and increased LDH levels are frequent. Markedly elevated serum levels of lung surfactant proteins A and D have been found in PAP. Radiographically, bilateral symmetric alveolar opacities located centrally in mid and lower lung zones result in a "bat-wing" distribution. HRCT shows a ground-glass opacification and thickened intralobular structures and interlobular septa. Whole lung lavage(s) through a double-lumen endotracheal tube provides relief to many patients with dyspnea or progressive hypoxemia and also may provide long-term benefit.

PULMONARY LYMPHANGIOLEIOMYOMATOSIS Pulmonary LAM is a rare condition that afflicts premenopausal women and should be suspected in young women with emphysema, recurrent pneumothorax, or chylous pleural effusion. It is often misdiagnosed as asthma or chronic obstructive pulmonary disease. Pathologically, LAM is characterized by the proliferation of atypical pulmonary interstitial smooth muscle and cyst formation. The immature-appearing smooth-muscle cells react with monoclonal antibody HMB45, which recognizes a 100-kDa glycoprotein (gp100) originally found in human melanoma cells. Caucasians are affected much more commonly than members of other racial groups. The disease accelerates during pregnancy and abates after oopherectomy. Common complaints at presentation are dyspnea, cough, and chest pain. Hemoptysis may be life threatening. Spontaneous pneumothorax occurs in 50% of patients; it may be bilateral and necessitate pleurodesis. Meningioma and renal angiomyolipomas (hamartomas), characteristic findings in the genetic disorder tuberous sclerosis, are also common in patients with LAM. Chylothorax, chyloperitonium (chylous ascites), chyluria, and chylopericardium are other complications. Pulmonary function testing usually reveals an obstructive or mixed obstructive-restrictive pattern, and gas exchange is often abnormal. HRCT shows thin-walled cysts surrounded by normal lung without zonal predominance. Progression is common, with a median survival of 8 to 10 years from diagnosis. Oophorectomy, progesterone (10 mg/d), and, more recently, tamoxifen and luteinizing hormone–releasing hormone analogues have been used. Lung transplantation offers the only hope for cure despite reports of recurrent disease in the transplanted lung.

SYNDROMES OF ILD WITH DIFFUSE ALVEOLAR HEMORRHAGE Injury to arterioles, venules, and the alveolar septal (alveolar wall or interstitial) capillaries can result in hemoptysis secondary to disruption of the alveolar-capillary basement membrane. This results in bleeding into the alveolar spaces, which characterizes DAH. Pulmonary capillaritis, characterized by a neutrophilic infiltration of the alveolar septae, may lead to necrosis of these structures, loss of capillary structural integrity, and the pouring of red blood cells into the alveolar space. Fibrinoid necrosis of the interstitium and red blood cells within the interstitial space are sometimes seen. Bland pulmonary hemorrhage (i.e., DAH without inflammation of the alveolar structures) may also occur.

The clinical onset is often abrupt, with cough, fever, and dyspnea. Severe respiratory distress requiring ventilatory support may be evident at initial presentation. Although hemoptysis is expected, it can be absent at the time of presentation in one-third of the cases. For patients without hemoptysis, new alveolar opacities, a falling hemoglobin level, and hemorrhagic BAL fluid point to the diagnosis. The chest radiograph is nonspecific and most commonly shows new patchy or diffuse alveolar opacities. Recurrent episodes of DAH may lead to pulmonary fibrosis, resulting in interstitial opacities on the chest radiograph. An elevated white blood cell count and falling hematocrit are frequent. Evidence for impaired renal function caused by focal segmental necrotizing glomerulonephritis, usually with crescent formation, may also be present.

Varying degrees of hypoxemia may occur and are often severe enough to require ventilatory support. The DL_{CO} may be increased, resulting from the increased hemoglobin within the alveoli compartment. Evaluation of either lung or renal tissue by immunofluorescent techniques indicates an absence of immune complexes (pauci-immune) in Wegener's granulomatosis, microscopic polyangiitis pauci-immune glomerulonephritis, and isolated pulmonary capillaritis. A granular pattern is found in the CTDs, particularly SLE, and a characteristic linear deposition is found in Goodpasture's syndrome. Granular deposition of IgA-containing immune complexes is present in Henoch-Schönlein purpura.

The mainstay of therapy for the DAH associated with systemic vasculitis, CTD, Goodpasture's syndrome, and isolated pulmonary capillaritis is intravenous methylprednisolone, 0.5 to 2.0 g daily in divided doses for up to 5 days, followed by a gradual tapering, and then maintenance on an oral preparation. Prompt initiation of therapy is important, particularly in the face of renal insufficiency, since early initiation of therapy has the best chance of preserving renal function. The decision to start other immunosuppressive therapy (cyclophosphamide or azathioprine) acutely depends on the severity of illness.

Goodpasture's Syndrome   Pulmonary hemorrhage and glomerulonephritis are features in most patients with this disease. Autoantibodies to renal glomerular and lung alveolar basement membranes are present. This syndrome can present and recur as DAH without an associated glomerulonephritis. In such case, circulating anti-basement membrane antibody is often absent, and the only way to establish the diagnosis is by demonstrating linear immunofluorescence in lung tissue. The underlying histology may be bland hemorrhage or DAH associated with capillaritis. Plasmapheresis has been recommended as adjunctive treatment.

INHERITED DISORDERS ASSOCIATED WITH ILD   Pulmonary opacities and respiratory symptoms typical of ILD can develop in related family members and in several inherited diseases. These include the phakomatoses, tuberous sclerosis and neurofibromatosis (Chap. 358), and the lysosomal storage diseases, Niemann-Pick disease and Gaucher's disease (Chap. 340). The Hermansky-Pudlak syndrome (Chap. 101) is an autosomal recessive disorder in which granulomatous colitis and ILD may occur. It is characterized by oculocutaneous albinism, bleeding diathesis secondary to platelet dysfunction, and the accumulation of a chromolipid, lipofuscin material in cells of the reticuloendothelial system. A UIP-like pattern is found on lung biopsy, but the alveolar macrophages may contain cytoplasmic ceroid-like inclusions.

ILD WITH A GRANULOMATOUS RESPONSE IN LUNG TISSUE OR VASCULAR STRUCTURES   Inhalation of organic dusts, which cause hypersensitivity pneumonitis, or of inorganic dust, such as silica, which elicits a granulomatous inflammatory reaction leading to ILD, produces diseases of known etiology (Table 243-1) that are discussed in Chaps. 237 and 238. Sarcoidosis (Chap. 309) is prominent among granulomatous diseases of unknown cause in which ILD is an important feature.

Pulmonary Langerhans Cell Histiocytosis   PLCH is a rare, smoking-related, diffuse lung disease that primarily affects men between the ages of 20 and 40 years. The clinical presentation varies from an asymptomatic state to a rapidly progressive condition. The most common clinical manifestations at presentation are cough, dyspnea, chest pain, weight loss, and fever. Pneumothorax occurs in about 25% of patients. Hemoptysis and diabetes insipidus are rare manifestations. The radiographic features vary with the stage of the disease. The combination of ill-defined or stellate nodules (2 to 10 mm in diameter), reticular or nodular opacities, bizarre-shaped upper zone cysts, preservation of lung volume, and sparing of the costophrenic angles are characteristics of PLCH. HRCT that reveals a combination of nodules and thin-walled cysts is virtually diagnostic of PLCH. The most frequent pulmonary function abnormality is a markedly reduced DL_{CO}, although varying degrees of restrictive disease, airflow limitation, and diminished exercise capacity may occur. Discontinuance of smoking is the key treatment, resulting in clinical improvement in one-third of patients. Most patients with PLCH suffer persistent or progressive disease. Death due to respiratory failure occurs in ~10% of patients.

Granulomatous Vasculitides   (See also Chap. 306)   The granulomatous vasculitides are characterized by pulmonary angiitis (i.e., inflammation and necrosis of blood vessels) with associated granuloma formation (i.e., infiltrates of lymphocytes, plasma cells, epithelioid cells, or his-

tiocytes, with or without the presence of multinucleated giant cells, sometimes with tissue necrosis). The lungs are almost always involved, although any organ system may be affected. Wegener's granulomatosis and allergic angiitis and granulomatosis (Churg-Strauss syndrome) primarily affect the lung but are associated with a systemic vasculitis as well. The granulomatous vasculitides generally limited to the lung include necrotizing sarcoid granulomatosis and benign lymphocytic angiitis and granulomatosis. Granulomatous infection and pulmonary angiitis due to irritating embolic material (e.g., talc) are important known causes of pulmonary vasculitis.

LYMPHOCYTIC INFILTRATIVE DISORDERS   This group of disorders features lymphocyte and plasma cell infiltration of the lung parenchyma. The disorders either are benign or can behave as low-grade lymphomas. Included are angioimmunoblastic lymphadenopathy with dysproteinemia, a rare lymphoproliferative disorder characterized by diffuse lymphadenopathy, fever, hepatosplenomegaly, and hemolytic anemia, with ILD in some cases.

Lymphocytic Interstitial Pneumonitis   This rare form of ILD occurs in adults, some of whom have an autoimmune disease or dysproteinemia. It has been reported in patients with Sjögren's syndrome and HIV infection.

Lymphomatoid Granulomatosis   This multisystem disorder of unknown etiology is an angiocentric malignant (T cell) lymphoma characterized by a polymorphic lymphoid infiltrate, an angiitis, and granulomatosis. Although it may affect virtually any organ, it is most frequently characterized by pulmonary, skin, and central nervous system involvement.

BRONCHOCENTRIC GRANULOMATOSIS   Rather than a specific clinical entity, bronchocentric granulomatosis (BG) is a descriptive histologic term that describes an uncommon and nonspecific pathologic response to a variety of airway injuries. There is evidence that BG is caused by a hypersensitivity reaction to *Aspergillus* or other fungi in patients with asthma. About half of the patients described have chronic asthma with severe wheezing and peripheral blood eosinophilia. In patients with asthma, BG probably represents one pathologic manifestation of allergic bronchopulmonary aspergillosis or another allergic mycosis. In patients without asthma, BG has been associated with RA and a variety of infections, including tuberculosis, echinococcosis, histoplasmosis, coccidioidomycosis, and nocardiosis. The chest roentgenogram reveals irregularly shaped nodular or mass lesions with ill-defined margins, which are usually unilateral and solitary, with an upper-lobe predominance. Glucocorticoids are the treatment of choice, often with excellent outcome, although recurrences may occur as therapy is tapered or stopped.

FURTHER READING

AMERICAN THORACIC SOCIETY/EUROPEAN RESPIRATORY SOCIETY: Idiopathic pulmonary fibrosis: Diagnosis and treatment. International consensus statement. Am J Respir Crit Care Med 161:646, 2000

————: International multidisciplinary consensus classification of the idiopathic interstitial pneumonias. Am J Respir Crit Care Med 165:277, 2002

FREEMER M, KING TE JR: Connective tissue disease, in MI Schwarz, TE King, Jr (eds): *Interstitial Lung Diseases*, 4th ed. Hamilton, Ontario, BC Decker, 2003, pp 535–598

KING TE Jr: Idiopathic interstitial pneumonias, in MI Schwarz, TE King, Jr (eds): *Interstitial Lung Diseases,* 4th ed. Hamilton, Ontario, BC Decker, 2003, pp 701–786

SELMAN M et al: Idiopathic pulmonary fibrosis: Prevailing and evolving hypotheses about its pathogenesis and implications for therapy. Ann Intern Med 134:136, 2001

SEYMOUR JF, PRESNEILL JJ: Pulmonary alveolar proteinosis: Progress in the first 44 years. Am J Respir Crit Care Med 166:215, 2002

SULLIVAN EJ: Lymphangioleiomyomatosis: A review. Chest 114:1689, 1998

THOMAS AQ et al: Heterozygosity for a surfactant protein C gene mutation associated with usual interstitial pneumonitis and cellular nonspecific interstitial pneumonitis in one kindred. Am J Respir Crit Care Med 165:1322, 2002

VASSALLO R et al: Clinical outcomes of pulmonary Langerhans'-cell histiocytosis in adults. N Engl J Med 346:484, 2002

244 | PULMONARY THROMBOEMBOLISM
Samuel Z. Goldhaber

PREDISPOSITION TO PULMONARY THROMBOEMBOLISM

Acquired and genetic factors contribute to the likelihood of venous thromboembolism. Acquired predispositions include long-haul air travel, obesity, cigarette smoking, oral contraceptives, pregnancy, postmenopausal hormone replacement, surgery, trauma, and medical conditions such as antiphospholipid antibody syndrome, cancer, systemic arterial hypertension, and chronic obstructive pulmonary disease. Thrombophilia contributes greatly to the risk of venous thrombosis, often due to an inherited risk factor in combination with an acquired predisposition. The two most common autosomal dominant genetic mutations are the factor V Leiden and the prothrombin gene mutations (Chap. 56). Only a minority of patients with venous thromboembolism has identifiable predisposing genetic factors. Some patients with predisposing genetic factors will never develop clinical evidence of clotting.

PATHOPHYSIOLOGY

EMBOLIZATION When venous thrombi dislodge from their site of formation, they embolize to the pulmonary arterial circulation or, paradoxically, to the arterial circulation through a patent foramen ovale or atrial septal defect. About half of patients with pelvic vein thrombosis or proximal leg deep venous thrombosis (DVT) have pulmonary thromboembolism (PE), which is usually asymptomatic. Isolated calf vein thrombi pose a lower risk of PE, but they are the most common source of paradoxical embolism. With increased use of chronic indwelling central venous catheters for hyperalimentation and chemotherapy, as well as more frequent insertion of permanent pacemakers and internal cardiac defibrillators, upper extremity venous thrombosis is becoming a more common problem. These thrombi may also embolize and cause PE.

PHYSIOLOGY Pulmonary embolism can have the following effects:

1. *Increased pulmonary vascular resistance* due to vascular obstruction or platelet secretion of neurohumoral agents including serotonin
2. *Impaired gas exchange* due to increased alveolar dead space from vascular obstruction, hypoxemia from alveolar hypoventilation relative to perfusion in the nonobstructed lung, right-to-left shunting, and impaired carbon monoxide transfer due to loss of gas exchange surface
3. *Alveolar hyperventilation* due to reflex stimulation of irritant receptors
4. *Increased airway resistance* due to constriction of airways distal to the bronchi
5. *Decreased pulmonary compliance* due to lung edema, lung hemorrhage, or loss of surfactant

Right Ventricular Dysfunction Progressive right heart failure is the usual cause of death from PE. In the International Cooperative Pulmonary Embolism Registry (ICOPER), the presence of right ventricular dysfunction on baseline echocardiography of PE patients was associated with a doubling of the 3-month mortality rate. As pulmonary vascular resistance increases, right ventricular wall tension rises and perpetuates further right ventricular dilatation and dysfunction. Consequently, the interventricular septum bulges into and compresses an intrinsically normal left ventricle. Increased right ventricular wall tension also compresses the right coronary artery and may precipitate myocardial ischemia and right ventricular infarction. Underfilling of the left ventricle may lead to a fall in left ventricular output and systemic arterial pressure, thereby provoking myocardial ischemia due to compromised coronary artery perfusion. Eventually, circulatory collapse and death may ensue.

DIAGNOSIS

The clinical setting, including risk factors such as family history or personal prior history of venous thromboembolism, can help suggest the diagnosis of PE. Semi-quantitative clinical scoring systems such as the Wells Diagnostic Scoring System are beginning to replace "gestalt" estimates of clinical likelihood (Table 244-1).

CLINICAL SYNDROMES Patients with *massive PE* present with systemic arterial hypotension and usually have anatomically widespread thromboembolism. Primary therapy with thrombolysis or embolectomy offers the greatest chance of survival. Those with *moderate to large PE* have right ventricular hypokinesis on echocardiography but normal systemic arterial pressure. Optimal management is controversial; such patients may benefit from thrombolysis or embolectomy rather than anticoagulation alone. Patients with *small to moderate PE* have both normal right heart function and normal systemic arterial pressure. They have a good prognosis with either adequate anticoagulation. The presence of *pulmonary infarction* usually indicates a small PE, but one that is exquisitely painful, because it lodges peripherally, near the innervation of pleural nerves. However, larger, more central PEs can occur concomitantly with peripheral pulmonary infarction.

Nonthrombotic pulmonary embolism may be easily overlooked. Possible etiologies include fat embolism after blunt trauma and long bone fractures, tumor embolism, or air embolism. Intravenous drug users may inject themselves with a wide array of substances, such as hair, talc, or cotton. *Amniotic fluid embolism* occurs when fetal membranes leak or tear at the placental margin. The pulmonary edema seen in this syndrome is probably due primarily to alveolar capillary leakage.

SYMPTOMS AND SIGNS Dyspnea is the most frequent symptom of PE, and tachypnea is its most frequent sign. Whereas dyspnea, syncope, hypotension, or cyanosis indicates a massive PE, pleuritic pain, cough, or hemoptysis often suggests a small embolism located distally near the pleura. On physical examination, young and previously healthy individuals may simply appear anxious but otherwise seem deceptively well, even with an anatomically large PE. They may only have dyspnea with moderate exertion. They often lack "classic" signs such as tachycardia, low-grade fever, neck vein distention, or an accentuated pulmonic component of the second heart sound. Sometimes, a paradoxical bradycardia occurs.

In older patients who complain of vague chest discomfort, the diagnosis of PE may not be apparent unless signs of right heart failure are present. Unfortunately, because acute coronary ischemic syndromes are so common, one may overlook the possibility of life-threatening PE and may inadvertently discharge these patients from the hospital after the exclusion of myocardial infarction with serial blood tests to detect cardiac injury and serial electrocardiograms.

DIFFERENTIAL DIAGNOSIS The differential diagnosis of PE is broad (Table 244-2). Although PE is known as "the great masquerader," quite often other illnesses simulate PE. For example, when the proposed diagnosis of PE is supposedly confirmed with a combination of dysp-

---

TABLE 244-1 *Wells Diagnostic Scoring System[a] for Suspected PE*

	Points
• Clinical signs and symptoms of DVT (minimum of leg swelling and pain with palpation of the deep veins)	3.0
• An alternative diagnosis is less likely than PE	3.0
• Heart rate >100 beats/min	1.5
• Immobilization or surgery in the previous 4 weeks	1.5
• Previous DVT/PE	1.5
• Hemoptysis	1.0
• Malignancy (on treatment, treated in the past 6 months, or palliative)	1.0

[a] The Wells Scoring System has a maximum of 12.5 points. If the score is ≤ 4 points, the likelihood of PE is only 8%.

Note: DVT, deep vein thrombosis; PE, pulmonary thromboembolism.

Source: Adapted with permission from PS Wells et al: Thromb Haemost 83.416, 2000.

TABLE 244-2 *Differential Diagnosis of Pulmonary Thromboembolism*

Acute coronary syndrome, including unstable angina and acute
  myocardial infarction
Pneumonia, bronchitis, exacerbation of asthma or chronic obstructive
  pulmonary disease
Congestive heart failure
Pericarditis
Pleurisy, including "viral syndrome," costochondritis, other
  musculoskeletal discomfort
Rib fracture, pneumothorax
Primary pulmonary hypertension
Anxiety

nea, chest pain, and an abnormal lung scan, the correct diagnosis of pneumonia might become apparent 12 h later when an infiltrate blossoms on chest x-ray, purulent sputum is first produced, and high fever and shaking chills develop.

Some patients have PE and a coexisting illness such as pneumonia or heart failure. In such circumstances, clinical improvement will often fail to occur despite standard medical treatment of the concomitant illness. This situation can serve as a clinical clue to the possible coexistence of PE.

NONIMAGING DIAGNOSTIC MODALITIES   These are generally less expensive but also less specific than diagnostic modalities that employ imaging.

Blood Tests   The quantitative *plasma D-dimer enzyme-linked immunosorbent assay (ELISA)* level is elevated (>500 ng/mL) in more than 90% of patients with PE, reflecting plasmin's breakdown of fibrin and indicating endogenous (though clinically ineffective) thrombolysis. However, the D-dimer assay is not specific and therefore has no useful role among patients who are already hospitalized. Levels increase in patients with myocardial infarction, sepsis, or almost any systemic illness. The plasma D-dimer ELISA has a high negative predictive value and can be used to help exclude PE. In a prospective 1-year evaluation, the Emergency Department at Brigham and Women's Hospital mandated obtaining a D-dimer ELISA in all 1106 patients suspected of PE. It served as an excellent screening test, with a sensitivity of 96.4% and negative predictive value of 99.6%.

Data from the Prospective Investigation of Pulmonary Embolism Diagnosis (PIOPED) indicate that, contrary to classic teaching, *arterial blood gases* lack diagnostic utility for PE, even though the P_{O_2} and P_{CO_2} will often both decrease. Among patients suspected of PE, neither the room air arterial P_{O_2} nor calculation of the alveolar-arterial oxygen gradient can reliably differentiate or triage patients who actually have PE at angiography.

Electrocardiogram   Classic abnormalities include sinus tachycardia; new-onset atrial fibrillation or flutter; and an S wave in lead I, a Q wave in lead III, and an inverted T wave in lead III (Chap. 210). Often, the QRS axis is greater than 90°. T-wave inversion in leads V_1 to V_4, perhaps the most frequent but least publicized change, reflects right ventricular strain.

NONINVASIVE IMAGING MODALITIES ■ Chest Roentgenography   A normal or near-normal chest x-ray in a dyspneic patient suggests PE. Well-established abnormalities include focal oligemia (Westermark's sign), a peripheral wedged-shaped density above the diaphragm (Hampton's hump), or an enlarged right descending pulmonary artery (Palla's sign).

Venous Ultrasonography   Confirmed DVT is usually an adequate surrogate for PE. Ultrasonography of the deep venous system relies upon loss of vein compressibility as the primary criterion for DVT. About one-half of patients with PE have no imaging evidence of DVT, probably because the clot has already embolized to the lung or is in the pelvic veins, where ultrasonography is usually inadequate. Therefore, the workup for PE should continue if there is high clinical suspicion, despite a normal ultrasound examination.

Chest CT   Computed tomography (CT) of the chest with intravenous contrast (ordinarily, 100 mL administered at 3 to 4 mL/s via an antecubital vein) is superseding lung scanning (see below) as the principal imaging test for the diagnosis of PE. Chest CT effectively diagnoses large, central PE (Fig. 244-1). New generation multislice scanners image the entire thorax with 1-mm thin sections during a single 12- to 15-s breath-hold and can detect peripherally located thrombi in fifth order branches. In patients without PE, the lung parenchymal images may establish alternative diagnoses not apparent on chest x-ray that explain the presenting symptoms and signs, such as pneumonia, emphysema, pulmonary fibrosis, pulmonary mass, or aortic pathology.

Lung Scanning   (See also Chap. 235)   Small particulate aggregates of albumin labeled with a gamma-emitting radionuclide are injected intravenously and are trapped in the pulmonary capillary bed. The perfusion scan defect indicates absent or decreased blood flow, possibly due to PE. Ventilation scans, obtained with radiolabeled inhaled gases such as xenon or krypton, improve the specificity of the perfusion scan. Abnormal ventilation scans indicate abnormal nonventilated lung, thereby providing possible explanations for perfusion defects other than acute PE. A high probability scan for PE is defined as having two or more segmental perfusion defects in the presence of normal ventilation (Fig. 244-2).

The diagnosis of PE is very unlikely in patients with normal and near-normal scans but is about 90% certain in patients with high-probability scans. Unfortunately, most patients have nondiagnostic scans, and fewer than half of patients with angiographically confirmed PE have a high-probability scan. Importantly, as many as 40% of patients with high clinical suspicion for PE and "low-probability" scans do, in fact, have PE at angiography.

Magnetic Resonance (MR) (Contrast-Enhanced)   MR pulmonary angiography utilizes gadolinium contrast agent, which unlike iodinated contrast agents used in CT angiography, is not nephrotoxic. The risk of a contrast reaction with gadolinium is very low, and no ionizing radiation is used. When compared with first-generation chest CT scanning, results are similar. MR also assesses right ventricular function, thus making it a promising single test for both diagnosis of PE and assessment of hemodynamic effect.

Echocardiography   More than half of patients with PE will have normal echocardiograms Nevertheless, this imaging test helps with the rapid triage of extremely ill patients who may have PE. Bedside echocardiography can usually reliably differentiate among illnesses that have radically different treatment, including acute myocardial infarction, pericardial tamponade, dissection of the aorta, and PE complicated by right heart failure. McConnell's sign, i.e., right ventricular free wall hypokinesis with normal right ventricular apical motion, appears to be specific for PE. Detection of right ventricular dysfunction due to PE

FIGURE 244-1   Bilateral "saddle" pulmonary thromboembolism computed tomography scan of the chest. The arrows outline the "saddle" *(Courtesy of Philip Costello, MD.)*

helps to stratify the risk, delineate the prognosis, and plan optimal management.

INVASIVE DIAGNOSTIC MODALITIES ■ Pulmonary Angiography Selective pulmonary angiography is the most specific examination available for establishing the definitive diagnosis of PE and can detect emboli as small as 1 to 2 mm. A definitive diagnosis of PE depends upon visualization of an intraluminal filling defect in more than one projection. Secondary signs of PE include abrupt occlusion ("cut-off") of vessels; segmental oligemia or avascularity; a prolonged arterial phase with slow filling; or tortuous, tapering peripheral vessels. Chest CT scanning is replacing diagnostic pulmonary angiography, because it is less invasive. In the current era of chest CT with

FIGURE 244-2 Three views of the pulmonary perfusion scan illustrating multiple segmental perfusion defects in both lung fields. The ventilation scan, which is normal, is not shown. The marked mismatch between normal ventilation and abnormal perfusion makes this lung scan *high probability* for pulmonary thromboembolism. LPO, left posterior oblique; POST, posterior; RPO, right posterior oblique.

contrast, pulmonary angiography is reserved for (1) patients with technically inadequate CT scans, (2) scans performed on older machines that cannot image fourth- and fifth-order pulmonary arteries, and (3) patients who will undergo interventions such as catheter embolectomy or catheter-directed thrombolysis.

Contrast Phlebography Venous ultrasonography has virtually replaced contrast phlebography, which is costly, uncomfortable, and occasionally results in contrast allergy or contrast-induced phlebitis.

INTEGRATED DIAGNOSTIC APPROACH We advocate an integrated diagnostic approach to streamline the workup of PE (Fig. 244-3). This strategy combines the clinical likelihood of PE with the results of noninvasive testing, especially D-dimer ELISA, venous ultrasonography, and chest CT or lung scanning to determine whether pulmonary angiography is warranted.

℞ TREATMENT

Primary Therapy versus Secondary Prevention *Primary therapy* consists of clot dissolution with thrombolysis or removal of PE by embolectomy. Anticoagulation with heparin and warfarin or placement of an inferior vena caval filter constitutes *secondary prevention* of recurrent PE rather than primary therapy.

Risk Stratification Risk stratification is crucial in determining treatment strategy. The presence of hemodynamic instability, right ventricular dysfunction, or elevation of the troponin level due to right ventricular microinfarction can identify high-risk patients.

Primary therapy should be reserved for patients at high risk of an adverse clinical outcome. When right ventricular function remains normal in a hemodynamically stable patient, a good clinical outcome is highly likely with anticoagulation alone (Fig. 244-4).

Adjunctive Therapy Important adjunctive measures include pain relief (especially with nonsteroidal anti-inflammatory agents), supplemental oxygenation, and psychological support. Dobutamine—a β-adrenergic agonist with positive inotropic and pulmonary vasodilating actions—may be effective in the treatment of right heart failure and cardiogenic shock. Volume loading should be undertaken cautiously because increased right ventricular dilatation can lead to even further reductions in left ventricular forward output.

Heparin Heparin binds to and accelerates the activity of antithrombin III, an enzyme that inhibits the coagulation factors thrombin (factor IIa), Xa, IXa, XIa, and XIIa. Heparin thus prevents additional thrombus formation and permits endogenous fibrinolytic mechanisms to lyse clot that has already formed. After 5 to 7 days of heparin, residual thrombus begins to stabilize in the endothelium of the vein or pulmonary artery. However, heparin does *not* directly dissolve thrombus that already exists.

MODIFIED CONSENSUS GUIDELINES FOR THE TREATMENT OF PULMONARY EMBOLISM FROM THE AMERICAN COLLEGE OF CHEST PHYSICIANS

1. Treat DVT or PE with therapeutic levels of unfractionated intravenous heparin, adjusted subcutaneous heparin, or low-molecular-weight heparin for at least 5 days, and overlap with oral anticoagulation for at least 4 to 5 days. Consider a longer course of heparin, approximately 10 days, for massive PE or severe iliofemoral DVT.
2. For most patients, heparin and oral anticoagulation can be started

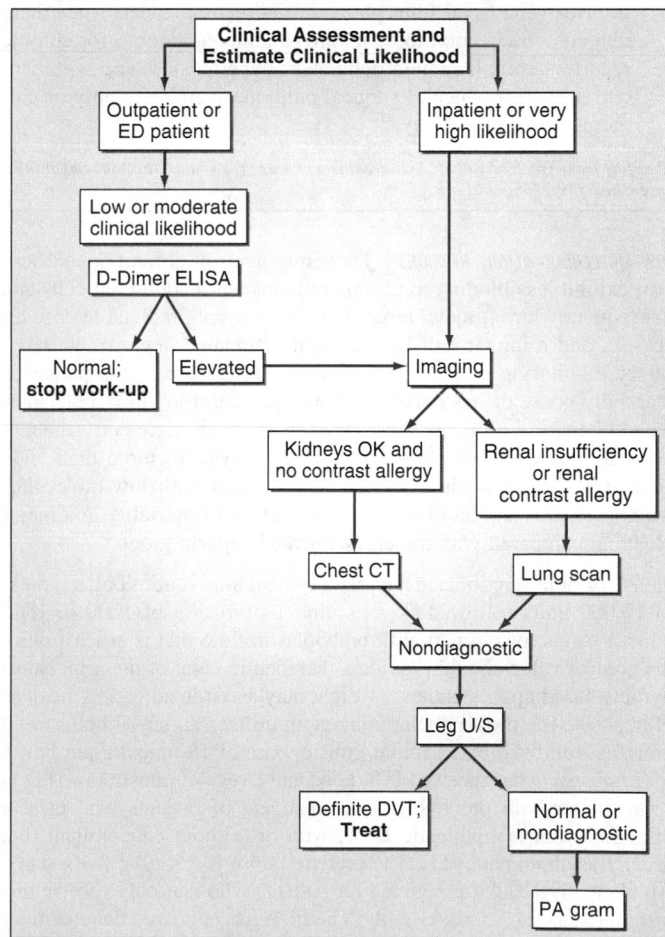

FIGURE 244-3 Diagnosis strategy for pulmonary thromboembolism: An integrated diagnostic approach. ED, emergency department; ELISA, enzyme-linked immunosorbent assay; CT, computed tomography; U/S, ultrasound; DVT, deep vein thrombosis; PA gram, pulmonary arteriogram.

FIGURE 244-4   Acute management of pulmonary thromboembolism: RV, right ventricular; IVC, inferior vena cava.

together and heparin discontinued on day 5 or 6 if the INR has been therapeutic for two consecutive days.

3. Treat patients with reversible or time-limited risk factors for at least 3 months. Patients with a first episode of idiopathic DVT should be treated indefinitely. A proven regimen is warfarin, target INR of 2.0 to 3.0 for 6 months, followed by low-intensity warfarin, target INR of 1.5 to 2.0.
4. The use of thrombolytic agents continues to be highly individualized, and clinicians should have some latitude in using these agents. Patients with hemodynamically unstable PE or massive iliofemoral thrombosis are the best candidates.
5. Inferior vena caval filter placement is recommended when there is a contraindication to or failure of anticoagulation, for chronic recurrent embolism with pulmonary hypertension, and with concurrent performance of surgical pulmonary embolectomy or pulmonary endarterectomy.

Modified from TM Hyers et al: Antithrombotic therapy for venous thromboembolic disease Chest 119:176S, 2001.

LOW-MOLECULAR-WEIGHT HEPARINS   These fragments of unfractionated heparin exhibit less binding to plasma proteins and endothelial cells and consequently have greater bioavailability, a more predictable dose response, and a longer half-life than unfractionated heparin. No laboratory monitoring or dose adjustment is needed unless the patient is markedly obese or has renal insufficiency. Therefore, low-molecular-weight heparins, although more expensive, are far more convenient to use than unfractionated heparin. A meta-analysis of more than 3500 acute DVT patients showed that those treated with low-molecular-weight heparin had an overall 29% reduction in mortality and major bleeding compared with the unfractionated heparin group.

DOSING   For unfractionated heparin, a typical intravenous bolus is 5000 to 10,000 units followed by a continuous infusion of 1000 to 1500 units/h. An activated partial thromboplastin time that is at least twice the control value should provide a therapeutic level of heparin. Nomograms based upon a patient's weight may assist in adjusting the dose of heparin. The most popular nomogram utilizes an initial bolus of 80 units/kg, followed by an initial infusion rate of 18 units/kg per hour.

Enoxaparin has received U.S. Food and Drug Administration (FDA) approval for both prophylaxis and treatment of patients who present primarily with symptomatic DVT, with or without concomitant (but usually asymptomatic) PE. The preferred dose is 1 mg/kg twice daily. An alternative back-up regimen for patients who can only receive one injection daily is 1.5 mg/kg daily. The FDA has approved dalteparin for prophylaxis but not for treatment of venous thromboembolism.

COMPLICATIONS   The most important adverse effect of heparin is hemorrhage. For life-threatening or intracranial hemorrhage, protamine sulfate can be administered. Heparin-induced thrombocytopenia and osteopenia are far less common with low-molecular-weight heparins than with unfractionated heparin. Thrombosis due to heparin-induced thrombocytopenia should be managed with a direct thrombin inhibitor: *argatroban* for patients with renal insufficiency or *hirudin* for patients with hepatic failure. Heparin-associated elevations in transaminase levels occur commonly but are rarely associated with clinical toxicity.

Warfarin   This vitamin K antagonist prevents γ carboxylation activation of coagulation factors II, VII, IX, and X. The full effect of warfarin often requires 5 days, even if the prothrombin time, used for monitoring, becomes elevated more rapidly. When warfarin is initiated during an active thrombotic state, the levels of protein C and S decline, thus creating a paradoxical thrombogenic potential. By overlapping either unfractionated or low-molecular-weight heparin and warfarin for 5 days, the early procoagulant effect of unopposed warfarin can be counteracted. Thus, heparin acts as a "bridge" until the full anticoagulant effect of warfarin is obtained.

DOSING   In an average-sized adult, warfarin is usually initiated in a dose of 5 mg. Doses of 7.5 or 10 mg can be used in obese or large-framed young patients who are otherwise healthy. Patients who are malnourished or who have received prolonged courses of antibiotics are probably deficient in vitamin K and should receive smaller initial doses of warfarin, such as 2.5 mg. An uncommon genetic mutation delays the metabolism of warfarin, resulting in a very low dose requirement, 1 to 2 mg daily, to achieve a therapeutic affect. The prothrombin time is standardized with the INR, which assesses the anticoagulant effect of warfarin (Chap. 103). The target INR is usually 2.5, with a range of 2.0 to 3.0.

COMPLICATIONS   As with heparin, bleeding is the most important and common complication associated with warfarin administration. Life-threatening bleeding can be treated with cryoprecipitate or fresh-frozen plasma (usually 2 units) to achieve immediate hemostasis. Recombinant factor VIIa is an effective, novel therapy for life-threatening bleeding in the setting of excessive warfarin. For less serious bleeding, or an excessively high INR in the absence of bleeding, vitamin K may be administered. Reversing excessive INRs by withholding warfarin and prescribing a low dose of oral vitamin K, such as 2.5 mg, will facilitate reestablishing a stable dose of warfarin.

Warfarin-induced skin necrosis is a rare complication that may be related to warfarin-induced reduction of protein C. It is usually associated with administration of a high initial dose of warfarin during an acute thrombotic state in which heparin is withheld.

During pregnancy, warfarin should be avoided if possible because of warfarin embryopathy, which is most common with exposure during the sixth through twelfth weeks of gestation. However, women can take warfarin postpartum and breast feed safely. Warfarin can also be administered safely during the second trimester.

DURATION OF ANTICOAGULATION   Patients with PE following surgery or trauma ordinarily have a low rate of recurrence after 6 months of anticoagulation. In contrast, among patients with "idiopathic" PE, the recurrence rate is surprisingly high after cessation of anticoagulation. The PREVENT Trial establishes intensive anticoagulation with warfarin for 6 months, target INR of 2.0 to 3.0 followed by an indefinite duration of anticoagulation with low-intensity warfarin, target INR of 1.5 to 2.0.

Inferior Vena Caval Filters   The two principal indications for insertion of an inferior vena caval filter are: (1) active bleeding that precludes anticoagulation, and (2) recurrent venous thrombosis despite intensive anticoagulation. Prevention of recurrent PE in patients with right heart failure who are not candidates for thrombolysis or prophylaxis of extremely high-risk patients are "softer" indications that are being utilized less frequently. The filter itself may fail by permitting the passage of small to medium-sized clots or because large thrombi embolize to the pulmonary arteries via collateral veins that develop. A more common complication is caval thrombosis with marked bilateral leg swelling. Paradoxically, by providing a nidus for clot formation, filters double the DVT rate over the ensuing 2 years following placement.

Thrombolysis Successful thrombolytic therapy rapidly reverses right heart failure and leads to a lower rate of death and recurrent PE. Thrombolysis usually: (1) dissolves much of the anatomically obstructing pulmonary arterial thrombus; (2) prevents the continued release of serotonin and other neurohumoral factors that exacerbate pulmonary hypertension; and (3) dissolves much of the source of the thrombus in the pelvic or deep leg veins, thereby decreasing the likelihood of recurrent PE.

The preferred thrombolytic regimen is 100 mg of recombinant tissue plasminogen activator (tPA) administered as a continuous peripheral intravenous infusion over 2 h. Patients appear to respond to thrombolysis for up to 14 days after the PE has occurred. MAPPET-3 (Management Strategy and Prognosis of Pulmonary Embolism Trial) is the largest randomized trial of thrombolysis (using 100 mg of tPA plus anticoagulation versus anticoagulation alone); 247 patients were enrolled with hemodynamically stable PE. Escalation of therapy (including use of pressors or intubation) was necessary in 24% of those receiving anticoagulation alone compared with 12% of those receiving tPA.

Contraindications to thrombolysis include intracranial disease, recent surgery, or trauma. There is a 1 to 2% risk of intracranial hemorrhage. Careful screening of patients for contraindications to thrombolysis is the best way to minimize bleeding risk.

Embolectomy The risk of intracranial hemorrhage with thrombolysis has prompted reevaluation of surgical embolectomy for acute PE. At Brigham and Women's Hospital, 29 patients with massive PE were operated on in 25 months, with an 89% survival rate. This high survival rate may be attributed to improved surgical technique, rapid diagnosis and triage, and careful patient selection. A possible alternative to open surgical embolectomy is catheter embolectomy.

Pulmonary Thromboendarterectomy Patients who develop chronic pulmonary hypertension due to prior PE may become severely dyspneic at rest or with minimal exertion. They should be considered for pulmonary thromboendarterectomy which, if successful, can markedly reduce and at times even cure pulmonary hypertension (Chap. 220).

PREVENTION

Prophylaxis against PE is of paramount importance because venous thromboembolism is difficult to detect and poses an excessive medical and economic burden. Mechanical and pharmacologic measures often succeed in preventing this complication (Table 244-3). Patients at high risk can receive a combination of mechanical and pharmacologic modalities. Graduated compression stockings and pneumatic compression devices may complement mini-dose unfractionated heparin (5000 units subcutaneously twice or preferably three times daily), low-molecular-weight heparin, a pentasaccharide or warfarin administration. Computerized reminder systems can increase the use of preventive care among these patients. Patients who have undergone total hip replacement, total knee replacement, or cancer surgery will benefit from extended pharmacologic prophylaxis for a total of 4 to 6 weeks, especially with low-molecular-weight heparin.

TABLE 244-3 *Prevention of Pulmonary Thromboembolism*

Condition	Prophylaxis Strategy
High-risk general surgery	Mini-UFH + GCS *or* LMWH + GCS
Thoracic surgery	Mini-UFH + IPC
Cancer surgery, including gynecologic cancer surgery	LMWH, consider 1 month of prophylaxis
Total hip replacement, total knee replacement, hip fracture surgery	LMWH, fondaparinux (a pentasaccharide) 2.5 mg sc, once daily *or* (except for total knee replacement) warfarin (target INR 2.5)
Neurosurgery	GCS + IPC
Neurosurgery for brain tumor	Mini-UFH *or* LMWH, + IPC, + predischarge venous ultrasonography
Benign gynecologic surgery	Mini-UFH + GCS
Medically ill patients	Mini-UFH *or* LMWH
Anticoagulation contraindicated	GCS + IPC
Long-haul air travel	Consider LMWH for very high risk patients

Note: Mini-UFH, minidose unfractionated heparin, 5000 units subcutaneously twice (less effective) or three times daily (more effective); GCS, graduated compression stockings, usually 10–18 mm Hg; LMWH, low-molecular-weight heparin, typically in the United States, enoxaparin, 40 mg once daily, or dalteparin, 2500 or 5000 units once daily; IPC, intermittent pneumatic compression devices.

FURTHER READING

AKLOG L et al: Acute pulmonary embolectomy: A contemporary approach. Circulation 105:1416, 2002

DECOUSUS H et al: A clinical trial of vena caval filters in the prevention of pulmonary embolism in patients with proximal deep-vein thrombosis. N Engl J Med 338:409, 1998

DUNN KL et al: Normal D-dimer levels in emergency department patients suspected of acute pulmonary embolism. J Am Coll Cardiol 40:1475, 2002

GOLDHABER SZ. Echocardiography in the management of pulmonary embolism. Ann Intern Med 136:691, 2002

——— et al: Acute pulmonary embolism: Clinical outcomes in the International Cooperative Pulmonary Embolism Registry (ICOPER). Lancet 353:1386, 1999

——— et al: New onset of venous thromboembolism among hospitalized patients at Brigham and Women's Hospital is caused more often by prophylaxis failure than by withholding treatment. Chest 118:1680, 2000

HIGASHI MK et al: Association between CYP2C9 genetic variants and anticoagulation-related outcomes during warfarin therapy. JAMA 287:1690, 2002

KONSTANTINIDES S et al: Heparin plus alteplase compared with heparin alone in patients with submassive pulmonary embolism. N Engl J Med 347:1143, 2002

LAPOSTOLLE F et al: Severe pulmonary embolism associated with air travel. N Engl J Med 345:779, 2001

RIDKER P et al: Long-term, low-intensity warfarin therapy for the prevention of recurrent venous thromboembolism. N Engl J Med 348:1425, 2003

245 | DISORDERS OF THE PLEURA, MEDIASTINUM, DIAPHRAGM, AND CHEST WALL
Richard W. Light

DISORDERS OF THE PLEURA

PLEURAL EFFUSION The pleural space lies between the lung and chest wall and normally contains a very thin layer of fluid, which serves as a coupling system. A pleural effusion is present when there is an excess quantity of fluid in the pleural space.

Etiology Pleural fluid accumulates when pleural fluid formation exceeds pleural fluid absorption. Normally, fluid enters the pleural space from the capillaries in the parietal pleura and is removed via the lymphatics situated in the parietal pleura. Fluid can also enter the pleural space from the interstitial spaces of the lung via the visceral pleura or from the peritoneal cavity via small holes in the diaphragm. The lymphatics have the capacity to absorb 20 times more fluid than is normally formed. Accordingly, a pleural effusion may develop when there is excess pleural fluid formation (from the interstitial spaces of the lung, the parietal pleura, or the peritoneal cavity) or when there is decreased fluid removal by the lymphatics.

Diagnostic Approach When a patient is found to have a pleural effusion, an effort should be made to determine the cause (Fig. 245-1). The first step is to determine whether the effusion is a transudate or an exudate. A *transudative pleural effusion* occurs when *systemic factors* that in-

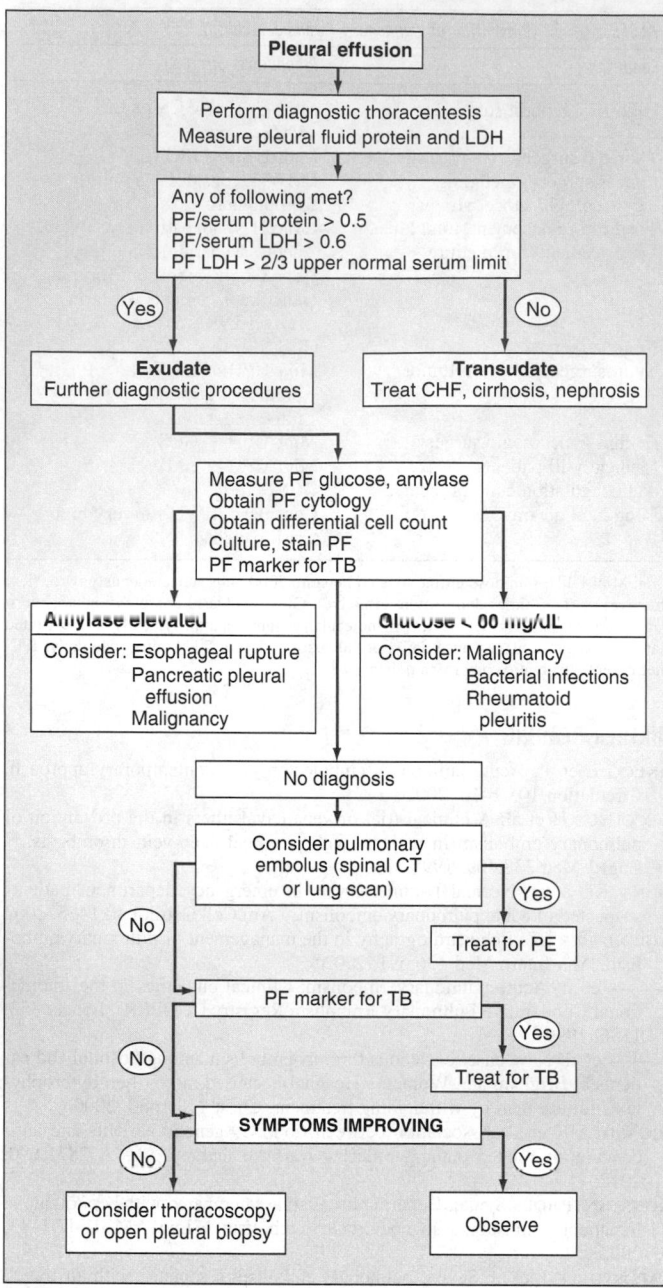

FIGURE 245-1 Approach to the diagnosis of pleural effusions. CHF, congestive heart failure; CT, computed tomography; LDH, lactate dehydrogenase; PE, pulmonary embolism; TB, tuberculosis; PF, pleural fluid.

fluence the formation and absorption of pleural fluid are altered. The leading causes of transudative pleural effusions in the United States are left ventricular failure, pulmonary embolism, and cirrhosis. An *exudative pleural effusion* occurs when *local factors* that influence the formation and absorption of pleural fluid are altered. The leading causes of exudative pleural effusions are bacterial pneumonia, malignancy, viral infection, and pulmonary embolism. The primary reason to make this differentiation is that additional diagnostic procedures are indicated with exudative effusions to define the cause of the local disease.

Transudative and exudative pleural effusions are distinguished by measuring the lactate dehydrogenase (LDH) and protein levels in the pleural fluid. Exudative pleural effusions meet at least one of the following criteria, whereas transudative pleural effusions meet none:

1. pleural fluid protein/serum protein >0.5
2. pleural fluid LDH/serum LDH >0.6
3. pleural fluid LDH more than two-thirds normal upper limit for serum

The above criteria misidentify approximately 25% of transudates as exudates. If one or more of the exudative criteria are met and the patient is clinically thought to have a condition producing a transudative effusion, the difference between the albumin levels in the serum and the pleural fluid should be measured. If this gradient is greater than 12 g/L (1.2 g/dL), the exudative categorization by the above criteria can be ignored because almost all such patients have a transudative pleural effusion.

If a patient has an exudative pleural effusion, the following tests on the pleural fluid should be obtained: description of the fluid, glucose level, differential cell count, microbiologic studies, and cytology.

Effusion due to Heart Failure The most common cause of pleural effusion is left ventricular failure. The effusion occurs because the increased amounts of fluid in the lung interstitial spaces exit in part across the visceral pleura. This overwhelms the capacity of the lymphatics in the parietal pleura to remove fluid. A diagnostic thoracentesis should be performed if the effusions are not bilateral and comparable in size, if the patient is febrile, or if the patient has pleuritic chest pain to verify that the patient has a transudative effusion. Otherwise the patient is best treated with diuretics. If the effusion persists despite diuretic therapy, a diagnostic thoracentesis should be performed.

Hepatic Hydrothorax Pleural effusions occur in approximately 5% of patients with cirrhosis and ascites. The predominant mechanism is the direct movement of peritoneal fluid through small holes in the diaphragm into the pleural space. The effusion is usually right-sided and frequently is large enough to produce severe dyspnea. If medical management does not control the ascites and the effusion, the best treatment is a liver transplant. If the patient is not a candidate for this, the best alternative is insertion of a transjugular intrahepatic portal systemic shunt.

Parapneumonic Effusion Parapneumonic effusions are associated with bacterial pneumonia, lung abscess, or bronchiectasis and are probably the most common exudative pleural effusion in the United States. *Empyema* refers to a grossly purulent effusion.

Patients with aerobic bacterial pneumonia and pleural effusion present with an acute febrile illness consisting of chest pain, sputum production, and leukocytosis. Patients with anaerobic infections present with a subacute illness with weight loss, a brisk leukocytosis, mild anemia, and a history of some factor that predisposes them to aspiration.

The possibility of a parapneumonic effusion should be considered whenever a patient with a bacterial pneumonia is initially evaluated. The presence of free pleural fluid can be demonstrated with a lateral decubitus radiograph, computed tomography (CT) of the chest, or ultrasound. If the free fluid separates the lung from the chest wall by more than 10 mm on one of these examinations, a therapeutic thoracentesis should be performed. Factors indicating the likely need for a procedure more invasive than a thoracentesis (in increasing order of importance) include:

1. loculated pleural fluid
2. pleural fluid pH < 7.20
3. pleural fluid glucose <3.3 mmol/L (<60 mg/dL)
4. positive Gram stain or culture of the pleural fluid
5. the presence of gross pus in the pleural space

If the fluid recurs after the initial therapeutic thoracentesis, a repeat thoracentesis should be performed if any of the above characteristics are present. If the fluid recurs a second time, tube thoracostomy should be performed if any of the poor prognostic factors are present. If the fluid cannot be completely removed with the therapeutic thoracentesis, consideration should be given to inserting a chest tube and instilling a thrombolytic (streptokinase, 250,000 units) or performing thoracoscopy with the breakdown of adhesions. Decortication should be considered when the above are ineffective.

Effusion Secondary to Malignancy Malignant pleural effusions secondary to metastatic disease are the second most common type of exudative pleural effusion. The three tumors that cause approximately 75% of all malignant pleural effusions are lung carcinoma, breast carcinoma, and lymphoma. Most patients complain of dyspnea, which is frequently out of proportion to the size of the effusion. The pleural fluid is an exudate, and its glucose level may be reduced if the tumor burden in the pleural space is high.

The diagnosis is usually made via cytology of the pleural fluid. If the initial cytologic examination is negative, then thoracoscopy is the best next procedure if malignancy is strongly suspected. At the time of thoracoscopy, a procedure such as pleural abrasion should be performed to effect a pleurodesis. If thoracoscopy is unavailable, then needle biopsy of the pleura should be performed.

Patients with a malignant pleural effusion are treated symptomatically for the most part, since the presence of the effusion indicates disseminated disease and most malignancies associated with pleural effusion are not curable with chemotherapy. The only symptom that can be attributed to the effusion itself is dyspnea. If the patient's lifestyle is compromised by dyspnea, and if the dyspnea is relieved with a therapeutic thoracentesis, then one of the following procedures should be considered: (1) tube thoracostomy with the instillation of a sclerosing agent such as doxycycline, 500 mg; or (2) outpatient insertion of a small indwelling catheter.

Mesothelioma Malignant mesotheliomas are primary tumors that arise from the mesothelial cells that line the pleural cavities. Most are related to asbestos exposure. Patients with mesothelioma present with chest pain and shortness of breath. The chest radiograph reveals a pleural effusion, generalized pleural thickening, and a shrunken hemithorax. Thoracoscopy or open pleural biopsy is usually necessary to establish the diagnosis. Various treatment modalities, including radical surgery, chemotherapy, and radiation therapy, have been tried, but none has been proven to be more effective than symptomatic therapy. It is recommended that chest pain be treated with opiates and that shortness of breath be treated with oxygen and/or opiates.

Effusion Secondary to Pulmonary Embolization The diagnosis most commonly overlooked in the differential diagnosis of a patient with an undiagnosed pleural effusion is pulmonary embolism. Dyspnea is the most common symptom. The pleural fluid is usually exudative but can be transudative. The diagnosis is established by spiral CT scan or pulmonary arteriography (Chap. 244). Treatment of the patient with a pleural effusion secondary to pulmonary embolism is the same as for any patient with pulmonary emboli. If the pleural effusion increases in size after anticoagulation, the patient probably has recurrent emboli or another complication such as a hemothorax or a pleural infection.

Tuberculous Pleuritis (See also Chap. 150) In many parts of the world, the most common cause of an exudative pleural effusion is tuberculosis (TB), but this is relatively uncommon in the United States. Tuberculous pleural effusions are thought to be due primarily to a hypersensitivity reaction to tuberculous protein in the pleural space. Patients with tuberculous pleuritis present with fever, weight loss, dyspnea, and/or pleuritic chest pain. The pleural fluid is an exudate with predominantly small lymphocytes. The diagnosis is established by demonstrating high levels of TB markers in the pleural fluid (adenosine deaminase > 45 IU/L, interferon γ > 140 pg/mL, or positive polymerase chain reaction (PCR) for tuberculous DNA). Alternatively, the diagnosis can be established by culture of the pleural fluid, needle biopsy of the pleura, or thoracoscopy. The recommended treatment of pleural and pulmonary tuberculosis is identical (Chap. 150).

Effusion Secondary to Viral Infection Viral infections are probably responsible for a sizable percentage of undiagnosed exudative pleural effusions. In many series, no diagnosis is established for approximately 20% of exudative effusions, and these effusions resolve spontaneously with no long-term residua. The importance of these effusions is that one should not be too aggressive in trying to establish a diagnosis for the undiagnosed effusion, particularly if the patient is improving clinically.

AIDS Pleural effusions are uncommon in such patients. The most common cause is Kaposi's sarcoma, followed by parapneumonic ef-

fusion. Other common causes are TB, cryptococcosis, and primary effusion lymphoma. Pleural effusions are very uncommon with *Pneumocystis carinii* infection.

Chylothorax A chylothorax occurs when the thoracic duct is disrupted and chyle accumulates in the pleural space. The most common cause of chylothorax is trauma, but it also may result from tumors in the mediastinum. Patients with chylothorax present with dyspnea, and a large pleural effusion is present on the chest radiograph. Thoracentesis reveals milky fluid, and biochemical analysis reveals a triglyceride level that exceeds 1.2 mmol/L (110 mg/dL). Patients with chylothorax and no obvious trauma should have a lymphangiogram and a mediastinal CT scan to assess the mediastinum for lymph nodes. The treatment of choice for most chylothoraces is implantation of a pleuroperitoneal shunt. Patients with chylothoraces should not undergo prolonged tube thoracostomy with chest tube drainage because this will lead to malnutrition and immunologic incompetence.

Hemothorax When a diagnostic thoracentesis reveals bloody pleural fluid, a hematocrit should be obtained on the pleural fluid. If the hematocrit is >50% that of the peripheral blood, the patient has a hemothorax. Most hemothoraces are the result of trauma; other causes include rupture of a blood vessel or tumor. Most patients with hemothorax should be treated with tube thoracostomy, which allows continuous quantification of bleeding. If the bleeding emanates from a laceration of the pleura, apposition of the two pleural surfaces is likely to stop the bleeding. If the pleural hemorrhage exceeds 200 mL/h, consideration should be given to thoracotomy.

Miscellaneous Causes of Pleural Effusion There are many other causes of pleural effusion (Table 245-1). Key features of some of these conditions are as follows: If the pleural fluid amylase level is elevated, the diagnosis of esophageal rupture or pancreatic disease is likely. If the

TABLE 245-1 *Differential Diagnoses of Pleural Effusions*

TRANSUDATIVE PLEURAL EFFUSIONS

1. Congestive heart failure
2. Cirrhosis
3. Pulmonary embolization
4. Nephrotic syndrome
5. Peritoneal dialysis
6. Superior vena cava obstruction
7. Myxedema
8. Urinothorax

EXUDATIVE PLEURAL EFFUSIONS

1. Neoplastic diseases
   a. Metastatic disease
   b. Mesothelioma
2. Infectious diseases
   a. Bacterial infections
   b. Tuberculosis
   c. Fungal infections
   d. Viral infections
   e. Parasitic infections
3. Pulmonary embolization
4. Gastrointestinal disease
   a. Esophageal perforation
   b. Pancreatic disease
   c. Intraabdominal abscesses
   d. Diaphragmatic hernia
   e. After abdominal surgery
   f. Endoscopic variceal sclerotherapy
   g. After liver transplant
5. Collagen-vascular diseases
   a. Rheumatoid pleuritis
   b. Systemic lupus erythematosus
   c. Drug-induced lupus
   d. Immunoblastic lymphadenopathy
   e. Sjögren's syndrome
   f. Wegener's granulomatosis
   g. Churg-Strauss syndrome
6. Post-coronary artery bypass surgery
7. Asbestos exposure
8. Sarcoidosis
9. Uremia
10. Meigs' syndrome
11. Yellow nail syndrome
12. Drug-induced pleural disease
    a. Nitrofurantoin
    b. Dantrolene
    c. Methysergide
    d. Bromocriptine
    e. Procarbazine
    f. Amiodarone
13. Trapped lung
14. Radiation therapy
15. Post-cardiac injury syndrome
16. Hemothorax
17. Iatrogenic injury
18. Ovarian hyperstimulation syndrome
19. Pericardial disease
20. Chylothorax

patient is febrile, has predominantly polymorphonuclear cells in the pleural fluid, and has no pulmonary parenchymal abnormalities, an intraabdominal abscess should be considered. The diagnosis of an asbestos pleural effusion is one of exclusion. Benign ovarian tumors can produce ascites and a pleural effusion (Meigs' syndrome), as can the ovarian hyperstimulation syndrome. Several drugs can cause pleural effusion; the associated fluid is usually eosinophilic. Pleural effusions commonly occur following coronary artery bypass surgery. Effusions occurring within the first weeks are typically left-sided and bloody, with large numbers of eosinophils, and respond to one or two therapeutic thoracenteses. Effusions occurring after the first few weeks are typically left-sided and clear yellow, with predominantly small lymphocytes, and tend to recur. Other medical manipulations that induce pleural effusions include abdominal surgery, endoscopic variceal sclerotherapy, radiation therapy, liver or lung transplantation, or the intravascular insertion of central lines.

PNEUMOTHORAX   Pneumothorax is the presence of gas in the pleural space. A *spontaneous pneumothorax* is one that occurs without antecedent trauma to the thorax. A *primary spontaneous pneumothorax* occurs in the absence of underlying lung disease, while a *secondary spontaneous pneumothorax* occurs in its presence. A *traumatic pneumothorax* results from penetrating or nonpenetrating chest injuries. A *tension pneumothorax* is a pneumothorax in which the pressure in the pleural space is positive throughout the respiratory cycle.

Primary Spontaneous Pneumothorax   Primary spontaneous pneumothoraces are usually due to rupture of apical pleural blebs, small cystic spaces that lie within or immediately under the visceral pleura. Primary spontaneous pneumothoraces occur almost exclusively in smokers, which suggests that these patients have subclinical lung disease. Approximately one-half of patients with an initial primary spontaneous pneumothorax will have a recurrence. The initial recommended treatment for primary spontaneous pneumothorax is simple aspiration. If the lung does not expand with aspiration, or if the patient has a recurrent pneumothorax, thoracoscopy with stapling of blebs and pleural abrasion is indicated. Thoracoscopy or thoracotomy with pleural abrasion is almost 100% successful in preventing recurrences.

Secondary Spontaneous Pneumothorax   Most secondary spontaneous pneumothoraces are due to chronic obstructive pulmonary disease, but pneumothoraces have been reported with virtually every lung disease. Pneumothorax in patients with lung disease is more life-threatening than it is in normal individuals because of the lack of pulmonary reserve in these patients. Nearly all patients with secondary spontaneous pneumothorax should be treated with tube thoracostomy and the instillation of a sclerosing agent such as doxycycline. Patients with secondary spontaneous pneumothoraces who have a persistent air leak, an unexpanded lung after 3 days of tube thoracostomy, or a recurrent pneumothorax should be subjected to thoracoscopy with bleb resection and pleural abrasion.

Traumatic Pneumothorax   Traumatic pneumothoraces can result from both penetrating and nonpenetrating chest trauma. Traumatic pneumothoraces should be treated with tube thoracostomy unless they are very small. If a hemopneumothorax is present, one chest tube should be placed in the superior part of the hemithorax to evacuate the air, and another should be placed in the inferior part of the hemithorax to remove the blood. Iatrogenic pneumothorax is a type of traumatic pneumothorax that is becoming more common. The leading causes are transthoracic needle aspiration, thoracentesis, and the insertion of central intravenous catheters. The treatment differs according to the degree of distress and can be observation, supplemental oxygen, aspiration, or tube thoracostomy.

Tension Pneumothorax   This condition usually occurs during mechanical ventilation or resuscitative efforts. The positive pleural pressure is life-threatening both because ventilation is severely compromised and because the positive pressure is transmitted to the mediastinum, which results in decreased venous return to the heart and reduced cardiac output.

Difficulty in ventilation during resuscitation or high peak inspiratory pressures during mechanical ventilation strongly suggests the diagnosis. The diagnosis is made by the finding of an enlarged hemithorax with no breath sounds and shift of the mediastinum to the contralateral side. Tension pneumothorax must be treated as a medical emergency. If the tension in the pleural space is not relieved, the patient is likely to die from inadequate cardiac output or marked hypoxemia. A large-bore needle should be inserted into the pleural space through the second anterior intercostal space. If large amounts of gas escape from the needle after insertion, the diagnosis is confirmed. The needle should be left in place until a thoracostomy tube can be inserted.

DISORDERS OF THE MEDIASTINUM

The mediastinum is the region between the pleural sacs. It is separated into three compartments. The *anterior mediastinum* extends from the sternum anteriorly to the pericardium and brachiocephalic vessels posteriorly. It contains the thymus gland, the anterior mediastinal lymph nodes, and the internal mammary arteries and veins. The *middle mediastinum* lies between the anterior and posterior mediastina and contains the heart; the ascending and transverse arches of the aorta; the venae cavae; the brachiocephalic arteries and veins; the phrenic nerves; the trachea, main bronchi, and their contiguous lymph nodes; and the pulmonary arteries and veins. The *posterior mediastinum* is bounded by the pericardium and trachea anteriorly and the vertebral column posteriorly. It contains the descending thoracic aorta, esophagus, thoracic duct, azygos and hemiazygos veins, and the posterior group of mediastinal lymph nodes.

MEDIASTINAL MASSES   The first step in evaluating a mediastinal mass is to place it in one of the three mediastinal compartments, since each has different characteristic lesions. The most common lesions in the anterior mediastinum are thymomas, lymphomas, teratomatous neoplasms, and thyroid masses. The most common masses in the middle mediastinum are vascular masses, lymph node enlargement from metastases or granulomatous disease, and pleuropericardial and bronchogenic cysts. In the posterior mediastinum, neurogenic tumors, meningoceles, meningomyeloceles, gastroenteric cysts, and esophageal diverticula are commonly found.

CT scanning is the most valuable imaging technique for evaluating mediastinal masses and is the only imaging technique that should be done in most instances. Barium studies of the gastrointestinal tract are indicated in many patients with posterior mediastinal lesions, since hernias, diverticula, and achalasia are readily diagnosed in this manner. An ^{131}I nuclear medicine scan can efficiently establish the diagnosis of intrathoracic goiter.

A definite diagnosis can be obtained with mediastinoscopy or anterior mediastinotomy in many patients with masses in the anterior or middle mediastinal compartments. A diagnosis can be established without thoracotomy via percutaneous fine-needle aspiration biopsy or endoscopic ultrasound-guided biopsy of mediastinal masses. In many cases the diagnosis can be established and the mediastinal mass removed with video-assisted thoracoscopy.

ACUTE MEDIASTINITIS   Most cases of acute mediastinitis either are due to esophageal perforation or occur after median sternotomy for cardiac surgery. Patients with esophageal rupture are acutely ill with chest pain and dyspnea due to the mediastinal infection. The esophageal rupture can occur spontaneously or as a complication of esophagoscopy or the insertion of a Blakemore tube. Appropriate treatment is exploration of the mediastinum with primary repair of the esophageal tear and drainage of the pleural space and the mediastinum.

The incidence of mediastinitis following median sternotomy is 0.4 to 5.0%. Patients most commonly present with wound drainage. Other presentations include sepsis or a widened mediastinum. The diagnosis is usually established with mediastinal needle aspiration. Treatment includes immediate drainage, debridement, and parenteral antibiotic therapy, but the mortality still exceeds 20%.

CHRONIC MEDIASTINITIS The spectrum of chronic mediastinitis ranges from granulomatous inflammation of the lymph nodes in the mediastinum to fibrosing mediastinitis. Most cases are due to TB or histoplasmosis, but sarcoidosis, silicosis, and other fungal diseases are at times causative. Patients with granulomatous mediastinitis are usually asymptomatic. Those with fibrosing mediastinitis usually have signs of compression of some mediastinal structure such as the superior vena cava or large airways, phrenic or recurrent laryngeal nerve paralysis, or obstruction of the pulmonary artery or proximal pulmonary veins. Other than antituberculous therapy for tuberculous mediastinitis, no medical or surgical therapy has been demonstrated to be effective for mediastinal fibrosis.

PNEUMOMEDIASTINUM In this condition, there is gas in the interstices of the mediastinum. The three main causes are: (1) alveolar rupture with dissection of air into the mediastinum; (2) perforation or rupture of the esophagus, trachea, or main bronchi; and (3) dissection of air from the neck or the abdomen into the mediastinum. Typically, there is severe substernal chest pain with or without radiation into the neck and arms. The physical examination usually reveals subcutaneous emphysema in the suprasternal notch and *Hamman's sign*, which is a crunching or clicking noise synchronous with the heartbeat and best heard in the left lateral decubitus position. The diagnosis is confirmed with the chest radiograph. Usually no treatment is required, but the mediastinal air will be absorbed faster if the patient inspires high concentrations of oxygen. If mediastinal structures are compressed, the compression can be relieved with needle aspiration.

DISORDERS OF THE DIAPHRAGM

DIAPHRAGMATIC PARALYSIS The presence of bilateral diaphragmatic paralysis almost always causes severe morbidity in adults. The most common causes include high spinal cord injury, thoracic trauma (including cardiac surgery), multiple sclerosis, anterior horn disease, and muscular dystrophy. Most patients with severe diaphragmatic weakness present with hypercapnic respiratory failure, frequently complicated by cor pulmonale and right ventricular failure, atelectasis, and pneumonia.

The degree of diaphragmatic weakness is best quantitated by measuring transdiaphragmatic pressures. The treatment of choice is assisted ventilation for all or part of each day. This is best accomplished without tracheostomy using nasal intermittent positive airway pressure. If the nerve to the diaphragm is intact, diaphragmatic pacing may be a viable alternative. If the paralysis occurs during open heart surgery, recovery frequently occurs, but it may take 6 months or more.

Unilateral paralysis of the diaphragm is much more common than is bilateral paralysis. The most common cause is nerve invasion from malignancy, usually a bronchogenic carcinoma. If the patient does not have malignancy, then usually no cause for the paralysis is found. The diagnosis is suggested by finding an elevated hemidiaphragm on the chest roentgenogram. Confirmation is best established with the "sniff test." When a patient is observed with fluoroscopy while sniffing, the paralyzed diaphragm will move paradoxically upward due to the negative intrathoracic pressure. Patients with a unilateral paralyzed diaphragm are usually asymptomatic. Their vital capacity and total lung capacity are each reduced about 25%. If a patient has a mediastinal mass in conjunction with the diaphragmatic paralysis, further workup

should be done. However, if the patient is asymptomatic with a normal chest radiograph, no invasive procedures are warranted.

DISORDERS OF THE CHEST WALL

KYPHOSCOLIOSIS Kyphoscoliosis is a combination of excessive anteroposterior and lateral curvature of the thoracic spine. Abnormalities of the spinal curvature are common, occurring in about 3% of the population. However, deformity of a sufficient degree to lead to symptoms and signs referable to the heart or lungs is rare, occurring in fewer than 3% of those with abnormal curvature. The major pathophysiologic effects of severe kyphoscoliosis are restrictive lung disease and ventilation-perfusion imbalances that result in chronic alveolar hypoventilation, hypoxic vasoconstriction, and eventually pulmonary arterial hypertension and cor pulmonale.

The severity of the cardiopulmonary disease correlates roughly with the degree of scoliosis. If the angle of curvature is <60°, ventilatory impairment is rare, while if it is >90°, marked ventilatory abnormalities develop commonly.

Although much effort has been devoted to restoring the normal curvature by either internal fixation or an external device, these efforts result in more improvement in the cosmetic appearance than in pulmonary function. However, the earlier that corrective actions are undertaken, the better the results. Once cardiorespiratory failure has developed, there is a high mortality from operative intervention. Patients with kyphoscoliosis and recurrent episodes of respiratory failure benefit from chronic nocturnal mechanical ventilation or nasal continuous positive airway pressure.

PECTUS EXCAVATUM (FUNNEL CHEST) In this congenital condition, the lower portion of the sternum is displaced posteriorly and the anterior ribs are markedly bowed, which results in a depressed panel in the anterior chest. Respiratory symptoms are uncommon, and pulmonary function tests are nearly normal. Surgical correction is seldom indicated and then only to treat psychological upset resulting from the cosmetic deformity.

PECTUS CARINATUM (PIGEON BREAST) This condition is the reverse of pectus excavatum with the sternum protruding anteriorly. This deformity is associated with congenital atrial or ventricular septal defects and severe prolonged childhood asthma. The deformity itself does not cause symptoms, and surgery is for cosmetic purposes only.

FURTHER READING

BAUMANN MH et al: Management of spontaneous pneumothorax: An American College of Chest Physicians Delphi Consensus Statement. Chest 119: 590, 2001

LARSEN SS et al: Endoscopic ultrasound guided biopsy of mediastinal lesions has a major impact on patient management. Thorax 57:98, 2002

LIGHT RW: *Pleural Diseases*, 4th ed. Philadelphia, Lippincott Williams & Wilkins, 2001

———: Pleural effusion. N Engl J Med 346:1971, 2002

MCCOOL FD, ROCHESTER DF: The lungs and chest wall diseases, in *Textbook of Respiratory Medicine*, JF Murray, JA Nabel (eds). Philadelphia, Saunders, 2000, pp 2357–2376

ZWISCHENBERGER JB et al: Mediastinal transthoracic needle and core lymph node biopsy. Should it replace mediastinoscopy? Chest 121:1165, 2002

246 | DISORDERS OF VENTILATION
Eliot A. Phillipson

HYPOVENTILATION

DEFINITION AND ETIOLOGY Alveolar hypoventilation exists by definition when arterial P_{CO_2} (Pa_{CO_2}) increases above the normal range of 37 to 43 mmHg, but in clinically important hypoventilation syndromes Pa_{CO_2} is generally in the range of 50 to 80 mmHg. Hypoventilation

disorders can be acute or chronic. The acute disorders, which represent life-threatening emergencies, are discussed in Chap. 251; this chapter deals with chronic hypoventilation syndromes.

Chronic hypoventilation can result from numerous disease entities (Table 246-1), but in all cases the underlying mechanism involves a defect in either the metabolic respiratory control system, the respiratory neuromuscular system, or the ventilatory apparatus. Disorders associated with impaired respiratory drive, defects in the respiratory neuromuscular system, some chest wall disorders such as obesity, and

TABLE 246-1   *Chronic Hypoventilation Syndromes*

Mechanism	Site of Defect	Disorder
Impaired respiratory drive	Peripheral and central chemoreceptors	Carotid body dysfunction, trauma Prolonged hypoxia Metabolic alkalosis
	Brainstem respiratory neurons	Bulbar poliomyelitis, encephalitis Brainstem infarction, hemorrhage, trauma Brainstem demyelination, degeneration Chronic drug administration Primary alveolar hypoventilation syndrome
Defective respiratory neuromuscular system	Spinal cord and peripheral nerves	High cervical trauma Poliomyelitis Motor neuron disease Peripheral neuropathy
	Respiratory muscles	Myasthenia gravis Muscular dystrophy Chronic myopathy
Impaired ventilatory apparatus	Chest wall	Kyphoscoliosis Fibrothorax Thoracoplasty Ankylosing spondylitis Obesity hypoventilation
	Airways and lungs	Laryngeal and tracheal stenosis Obstructive sleep apnea Cystic fibrosis Chronic obstructive pulmonary disease

Source: From Phillipson and Slutsky, with permission.

FIGURE 246-1   Physiologic and clinical features of alveolar hypoventilation. Hb, hemoglobin; PA_{CO_2}, alveolar P_{CO_2}; PA_{O_2}, alveolar P_{O_2}. (*After Phillipson and Slutsky.*)

upper airway obstruction produce an increase in Pa_{CO_2}, despite normal lungs, because of a reduction in overall minute volume of ventilation and hence in alveolar ventilation. In contrast, most disorders of the chest wall and disorders of the lower airways and lungs may produce an increase in Pa_{CO_2}, despite a normal or even increased minute volume of ventilation, because of severe ventilation-perfusion mismatching that results in net alveolar hypoventilation.

Several hypoventilation syndromes involve combined disturbances in two elements of the respiratory system. For example, patients with chronic obstructive pulmonary disease may hypoventilate not simply because of impaired ventilatory mechanics but also because of a reduced central respiratory drive, which can be inherent or secondary to a co-existing metabolic alkalosis (related to diuretic and steroid therapy).

PHYSIOLOGIC AND CLINICAL FEATURES   Regardless of cause, the hallmark of all alveolar hypoventilation syndromes is an increase in alveolar P_{CO_2} (PA_{CO_2}) and therefore in Pa_{CO_2} (Fig. 246-1). The resulting respiratory acidosis eventually leads to a compensatory increase in plasma HCO_3^- concentration and a decrease in Cl^- concentration. The increase in PA_{CO_2} produces an obligatory decrease in PA_{O_2}, resulting in hypoxemia. If severe, the hypoxemia manifests clinically as cyanosis and can stimulate erythropoiesis and induce secondary polycythemia. The combination of chronic hypoxemia and hypercapnia may also induce pulmonary vasoconstriction, leading eventually to pulmonary hypertension, right ventricular hypertrophy, and congestive heart failure. The disturbances in arterial blood gases are typically magnified during sleep because of a further reduction in central respiratory drive. The resulting increased nocturnal hypercapnia may cause cerebral vasodilation leading to morning headache; sleep quality may also be severely impaired, resulting in morning fatigue, daytime somnolence, mental confusion, and intellectual impairment. Other clinical features associated with hypoventilation syndromes are related to the specific underlying disease (Table 246-1).

DIAGNOSIS   Investigation of the patient with chronic hypoventilation involves several laboratory tests that will usually localize the disorder

to either the metabolic respiratory control system, the neuromuscular system, or the ventilatory apparatus (Fig. 246-2). Defects in the control system impair responses to chemical stimuli, including ventilatory, occlusion pressure, and diaphragmatic electromyographic (EMG) responses. During sleep, hypoventilation is usually more marked, and central apneas and hypopneas are common. However, because the behavioral respiratory control system (which is anatomically distinct from the metabolic control system), the neuromuscular system, and the ventilatory apparatus are intact, such patients can usually hyperventilate voluntarily, generate normal inspiratory and expiratory muscle pressures (PI_{max}, PE_{max}, respectively) against an occluded airway, generate normal lung volumes and flow rates on routine spirometry, and have normal respiratory system resistance and compliance and a normal alveolar-arterial $P_{O_2}[(A - a)P_{O_2}]$ difference. Patients with defects in the respiratory neuromuscular system also have impaired responses to chemical stimuli but in addition are unable to hyperventilate voluntarily or to generate normal static respiratory muscle pressures, lung volumes, and flow rates. However, at least in the early stages of the disease, the resistance and compliance of the respiratory system and the alveolar-arterial oxygen difference are normal.

In contrast to patients with disorders of the respiratory control or neuromuscular systems, patients with disorders of the chest wall, lungs, and airways typically demonstrate abnormalities of respiratory system resistance and compliance and have a widened $(A - a)P_{O_2}$. Because of the impaired mechanics of breathing, routine spirometric tests are abnormal, as is the ventilatory response to chemical stimuli. However, because the neuromuscular system is intact, tests that are independent of resistance and compliance are usually normal, including tests of respiratory muscle strength and of respiratory control that do not involve airflow.

℞ TREATMENT

The management of chronic hypoventilation must be individualized to the patient's particular disorder, circumstances, and needs and should include measures directed toward the underlying disease. Coexistent metabolic alkalosis should be corrected, including elevations of HCO_3^- that are inappropriately high for the degree of chronic hypercapnia. Administration of supplemental oxygen is effective in attenuating hypoxemia, polycythemia, and pulmonary hypertension but can aggravate CO_2 retention and the associated neurologic symptoms. For this reason, supplemental oxygen must be prescribed judiciously and the results monitored carefully. Pharmacologic agents that stimulate respiration (particularly progesterone) are of benefit in some patients, but generally, results are disappointing.

Site of defect	Responses to CO_2, hypoxia			Sleep studies	Voluntary hyperventil.	PI_{max} PE_{max}	Volume flow rates	Resistance, compliance	$(A - a)\,Po_2$
	Ventil.	P.1	EMGdi						
Metabolic control system (chemoreceptors, brainstem integrating neurons)	↓	↓	↓	↑Hypoventil, central apneas	N	N	N	N	N
Respiratory neuromuscular system (brainstem motoneurons, spinal cord, respiratory nerves, and muscles)	↓	↓	↓	↑Hypoventil, central apneas	↓	↓	↓	N	N
Ventilatory apparatus (chest wall, lungs, airways)	↓	N	N	Variable	↓	N	Abnormal	Abnormal	↑

FIGURE 246-2 Pattern of laboratory test results in alveolar hypoventilation syndromes, based on the site of defect. Ventil, ventilation; P.1, mouth pressure generated after 0.1 s of inspiration against an occluded airway; EMGdi, diaphragmatic EMG; PI_{max}, PE_{max}, maximum inspiratory or expiratory pressure that can be generated against an occluded airway; $(A - a)Po_2$, alveolar-arterial Po_2 difference; N, normal. Defects in the metabolic control system impair central respiratory drive in response to chemical stimuli (CO_2 or hypoxia); therefore responses of EMGdi, P.1, and minute volume of ventilation are reduced and hypoventilation during sleep is aggravated. In contrast, tests of voluntary respiratory control, muscle strength, lung mechanics, and gas exchange $[(A - a)Po_2]$ are normal. Defects in the respiratory neuromuscular system impair muscle strength; therefore all tests dependent on muscular activity (voluntary or in response to metabolic stimuli) are abnormal, but lung resistance, lung compliance, and gas exchange are normal. Defects in the ventilatory apparatus usually impair gas exchange. Because resistance and compliance are also impaired, all tests dependent on ventilation (whether voluntary or in response to chemical stimuli) are abnormal; in contrast, tests of muscle activity or strength that do not involve airflow (i.e., P.1, EMGdi, PI_{max}, PE_{max}) are normal. (After Phillipson and Slutsky.)

Most patients with chronic hypoventilation related to impairment of respiratory drive or neuromuscular disease eventually require mechanical ventilatory assistance for effective management. When hypoventilation is severe, treatment may be required on a 24-h basis, but in most patients ventilatory assistance only during sleep produces dramatic improvement in clinical features and daytime arterial blood gases. In patients with reduced respiratory drive but intact respiratory lower motor neurons, phrenic nerves, and respiratory muscles, diaphragmatic pacing through an implanted phrenic electrode can be very effective. However, for patients with defects in the respiratory nerves and muscles, electrophrenic pacing is contraindicated. Such patients can usually be managed effectively with either intermittent negative-pressure ventilation in a cuirass or intermittent positive-pressure ventilation delivered through a tracheostomy or nose mask. For patients who require ventilatory assistance only during sleep, positive-pressure ventilation through a nose mask is the preferred method because it obviates a tracheostomy and avoids the problem of upper airway occlusion that can arise in a negative-pressure ventilator. Hypoventilation related to restrictive disorders of the chest wall (Table 246-1) can also be managed effectively with nocturnal intermittent positive-pressure ventilation through a nose mask or tracheostomy.

HYPOVENTILATION SYNDROMES

PRIMARY ALVEOLAR HYPOVENTILATION

Primary alveolar hypoventilation (PAH) is a disorder of unknown cause characterized by chronic hypercapnia and hypoxemia in the absence of identifiable neuromuscular disease or mechanical ventilatory impairment. The disorder is thought to arise from a defect in the metabolic respiratory control system, but few neuropathologic studies have been reported in such patients. Studies in animals suggest an important role for genetic factors in the pathogenesis of hypoventilation, and familial cases in humans have been described. Isolated PAH is relatively rare, and although it occurs in all age groups, the majority of reported cases in adults have been in males aged 20 to 50 years. The disorder typically develops insidiously and often first comes to attention when severe respiratory depression follows administration of standard doses of sedatives or anesthetics. As the degree of hypoventilation increases, patients typically develop lethargy, fatigue, daytime somnolence, disturbed sleep, and morning headaches; eventually cyanosis, polycythemia, pulmonary hypertension, and congestive heart failure occur (Fig. 246-1). Despite severe arterial blood gas derangements, dyspnea is uncommon, presumably because of impaired chemoreception and ventilatory drive. If left untreated, PAH is usually progressive over a period of months to years and ultimately fatal.

The key diagnostic finding in PAH is a chronic respiratory acidosis in the absence of respiratory muscle weakness or impaired ventilatory mechanics (Fig. 246-2). Because patients can hyperventilate voluntarily and reduce Pa_{CO_2} to normal or even hypocapnic levels, hypercapnia may not be demonstrable in a single arterial blood sample, but the presence of an elevated plasma HCO_3^- level should draw attention to the underlying chronic disturbance. Despite normal ventilatory mechanics and respiratory muscle strength, ventilatory responses to chemical stimuli are reduced or absent (Fig. 246-2), and breath-holding time may be markedly prolonged without any sensation of dyspnea.

Patients with PAH maintain rhythmic respiration when awake, although the level of ventilation is below normal. However, during sleep, when breathing is critically dependent on the metabolic control system, there is typically a further deterioration in ventilation with frequent episodes of central hypopnea or apnea.

PAH must be distinguished from other central hypoventilation syndromes that are secondary to underlying neurologic disease of the brainstem or chemoreceptors (Table 246-1). This distinction requires a careful neurologic investigation for evidence of brainstem or autonomic disturbances. Unrecognized respiratory neuromuscular disorders, particularly those that produce diaphragmatic weakness, are often misdiagnosed as PAH. However, such disorders can usually be suspected on clinical grounds (see below) and can be confirmed by the finding of reduced voluntary hyperventilation, as well as PI_{max} and PE_{max}.

Some patients with PAH respond favorably to respiratory stimulant medications and to supplemental oxygen. However, the majority eventually require mechanical ventilatory assistance. Excellent long-term benefits can be achieved with diaphragmatic pacing by electrophrenic stimulation or with negative- or positive-pressure mechanical ventilation. The administration of such treatment only during sleep is sufficient in most patients.

RESPIRATORY NEUROMUSCULAR DISORDERS

Several primary disorders of the spinal cord, peripheral respiratory nerves, and respiratory muscles produce a chronic hypoventilation syndrome (Table 246-1). Hypoventilation usually develops gradually over a period of months to years and often first comes to attention when a relatively trivial increase in mechanical ventilatory load (such as mild airways obstruction) produces severe respiratory failure. In some of the disorders (such as motor neuron disease, myasthenia gravis, and muscular dystrophy), involvement of the respiratory nerves or muscles is usually a later feature of a more widespread disease. In other disorders, respiratory involvement can be an early or even isolated feature, and hence the underlying problem is often not suspected. Included in this category are the postpolio syndrome (a form of chronic respiratory insufficiency that develops 20 to 30 years following recovery from poliomyelitis), the myopathy associated with adult acid maltase deficiency, and idiopathic diaphragmatic paralysis.

Generally, respiratory neuromuscular disorders do not result in chronic hypoventilation unless there is significant weakness of the diaphragm. Distinguishing features of bilateral diaphragmatic weakness include orthopnea, paradoxical movement of the abdomen in the supine posture, and paradoxical diaphragmatic movement under fluoroscopy. However, the absence of these features does not exclude diaphragmatic weakness. Important laboratory features are a rapid deterioration of ventilation during a maximum voluntary ventilation maneuver and reduced PI_{max} and PE_{max} (Fig. 246-2). More sophisticated investigations reveal reduced or absent transdiaphragmatic pressures, calculated from simultaneous measurement of esophageal and gastric pressures; reduced diaphragmatic EMG responses (recorded from an esophageal electrode) to transcutaneous phrenic nerve stimulation; and marked hypopnea and arterial oxygen desaturation during rapid eye movement sleep, when there is normally a physiologic inhibition of all nondiaphragmatic respiratory muscles and breathing becomes critically dependent on diaphragmatic activity.

The management of chronic alveolar hypoventilation due to respiratory neuromuscular disease involves treatment of the underlying disorder, where feasible, and mechanical ventilatory assistance as described for the PAH syndrome. However, electrophrenic diaphragmatic pacing is contraindicated in these disorders, except for high cervical spinal cord lesions in which the phrenic lower motor neurons and nerves are intact.

OBESITY-HYPOVENTILATION SYNDROME   Massive obesity represents a mechanical load to the respiratory system because the added weight on the rib cage and abdomen serves to reduce the compliance of the chest wall. As a result, the functional residual capacity (i.e., end-expiratory lung volume) is reduced, particularly in the recumbent posture. An important consequence of breathing at a low lung volume is that some airways, particularly those in the lung bases, may be closed throughout part or even all of each tidal breath, resulting in underventilation of the lung bases and widening of the $(A - a)P_{O_2}$. Nevertheless, in the majority of obese individuals, central respiratory drive is increased sufficiently to maintain a normal Pa_{CO_2}. However, a small proportion of obese patients develop chronic hypercapnia, hypoxemia, and eventually polycythemia, pulmonary hypertension, and right-sided heart failure. Studies in mice demonstrate that genetically obese mice lacking circulating leptin also develop chronic hypoventilation that can be reversed by leptin infusions. In humans with obesity-hypoventilation syndrome, serum leptin levels are elevated, suggesting that leptin resistance may play a role in the pathogenesis of the disorder. In many patients, obstructive sleep apnea is a prominent feature, and even in those patients without sleep apnea, sleep-induced hypoventilation is an important element of the disorder and contributes to its progression. Most patients demonstrate a decrease in central respiratory drive, which may be inherent or acquired, and many have mild to moderate degrees of airflow obstruction, usually related to smoking. Based on these considerations, several therapeutic measures can be of considerable benefit, including weight loss, cessation of smoking, elimination of obstructive sleep apnea, and enhancement of respiratory drive by medications such as progesterone.

HYPERVENTILATION AND ITS SYNDROMES

DEFINITION AND ETIOLOGY   Alveolar hyperventilation exists when Pa_{CO_2} decreases below the normal range of 37 to 43 mmHg. *Hyperventilation* is not synonymous with *hyperpnea*, which refers to an increased minute volume of ventilation without reference to Pa_{CO_2}. Although hyperventilation is frequently associated with dyspnea, patients who are

TABLE 246-2   *Hyperventilation Syndromes*

1. Hypoxemia
   a. High altitude
   b. Pulmonary disease
   c. Cardiac shunts
2. Pulmonary disorders
   a. Pneumonia
   b. Interstitial pneumonitis, fibrosis, edema
   c. Pulmonary emboli, vascular disease
   d. Bronchial asthma
   e. Pneumothorax
   f. Chest wall disorders
3. Cardiovascular disorders
   a. Congestive heart failure
   b. Hypotension
4. Metabolic disorders
   a. Acidosis (diabetic, renal, lactic)
   b. Hepatic failure
5. Neurologic and psychogenic disorders
   a. Psychogenic or anxiety hyperventilation
   b. Central nervous system infection, tumors
6. Drug-induced
   a. Salicylates
   b. Methylxanthine derivatives
   c. β-Adrenergic agonists
   d. Progesterone
7. Miscellaneous
   a. Fever, sepsis
   b. Pain
   c. Pregnancy

hyperventilating do not necessarily complain of shortness of breath; and conversely, patients with dyspnea need not be hyperventilating.

Numerous disease entities can be associated with alveolar hyperventilation (Table 246-2), but in all cases the underlying mechanism involves an increase in respiratory drive that is mediated through either the behavioral or the metabolic respiratory control systems (Fig. 246-3). Thus hypoxemia drives ventilation by stimulating the peripheral chemoreceptors, and several pulmonary disorders and congestive heart failure drive ventilation by stimulating afferent vagal receptors in the lungs and airways. Low cardiac output and hypotension stimulate the peripheral chemoreceptors and inhibit the baroreceptors, both of which increase ventilation. Metabolic acidosis, a potent respiratory stimulant, excites both the peripheral and central chemoreceptors and increases the sensitivity of the peripheral chemoreceptors to coexistent hypoxemia. Hepatic failure can also produce hyperventilation, presumably as a result of metabolic stimuli acting on the peripheral and central chemoreceptors.

Several neurologic and psychological disorders are thought to drive ventilation through the behavioral respiratory control system. Included in this category are psychogenic or anxiety hyperventilation and severe cerebrovascular insufficiency, which may interfere with the inhibitory influence normally exerted by cortical structures on the brainstem respiratory neurons. Rarely, disorders of the midbrain and hypothalamus induce hyperventilation, and it is conceivable that fever and sepsis also cause hyperventilation through effects on these structures. Several drugs cause hyperventilation by stimulating the central or peripheral chemoreceptors or by direct action on the brainstem respiratory neurons. Chronic hyperventilation is a normal feature of pregnancy and

FIGURE 246-3   Schematic diagram of the mechanisms involved in alveolar hyperventilation. *(From Slutsky and Phillipson.)*

results from the effects of progesterone and other hormones acting on the respiratory neurons.

PHYSIOLOGIC AND CLINICAL FEATURES Because hyperventilation is associated with increased respiratory drive, muscle effort, and minute volume of ventilation, the most frequent symptom associated with hyperventilation is dyspnea. However, there is considerable discrepancy between the degree of hyperventilation, as measured by Pa_{CO_2}, and the degree of associated dyspnea. From a physiologic standpoint, hyperventilation is beneficial in patients who are hypoxemic, because the alveolar hypocapnia is associated with an increase in alveolar and arterial P_{O_2}. Conversely, hyperventilation can also be detrimental. In particular, the alkalemia associated with hypocapnia may produce neurologic symptoms, including dizziness, visual impairment, syncope, and seizure activity (secondary to cerebral vasoconstriction); paresthesia, carpopedal spasm, and tetany (secondary to decreased free serum calcium); and muscle weakness (secondary to hypophosphatemia); and may be associated with panic attacks. Severe alkalemia can also induce cardiac arrhythmias and evidence of myocardial ischemia. Patients with a primary respiratory alkalosis are also prone to periodic breathing and central sleep apnea (Chap. 247).

DIAGNOSIS In most patients with a hyperventilation syndrome, the cause is readily apparent on the basis of history, physical examination, and knowledge of coexisting medical disorders (Table 246-2). In patients in whom the cause is not clinically apparent, investigation begins with arterial blood gas analysis, which establishes the presence of alveolar hyperventilation (decreased Pa_{CO_2}) and its severity. Equally important is the arterial pH, which generally allows the disorder to be classified as either a primary respiratory alkalosis (elevated pH) or a primary metabolic acidosis (decreased pH). Also of importance is the Pa_{O_2} and calculation of the $(A - a)P_{O_2}$, since a widened alveolar-arterial oxygen difference suggests a pulmonary disorder as the underlying cause. The finding of a reduced plasma HCO_3^- level establishes the chronic nature of the disorder and points toward an organic cause. Measurements of ventilation and arterial or transcutaneous P_{CO_2} during sleep are very useful in suspected psychogenic hyperventilation, since such patients do not maintain the hyperventilation during sleep.

The disorders that most frequently give rise to unexplained hyperventilation are pulmonary vascular disease (particularly chronic or recurrent thromboembolism) and psychogenic or anxiety hyperventilation. Hyperventilation due to pulmonary vascular disease is associated with exertional dyspnea, a widened $(A - a)P_{O_2}$ and maintenance of hyperventilation during exercise. In contrast, patients with psychogenic hyperventilation typically complain of dyspnea at rest and not during mild exercise and of the need to sigh frequently. They are also more likely to complain of dizziness, sweating, palpitations, and paresthesia. During mild to moderate exercise, their hyperventilation tends to disappear and $(A - a)P_{O_2}$ is normal, but heart rate and cardiac output may be increased relative to metabolic rate.

$R\!\!\!/\,$ TREATMENT

Mild alveolar hyperventilation is usually of relatively minor clinical consequence and therefore is generally managed by appropriate treatment of the underlying cause. In the few patients in whom alkalemia is thought to be inducing significant cerebral vasoconstriction, paresthesia, tetany, or cardiac disturbances, acute inhalation of a low concentration of CO_2 can be very beneficial. For patients with disabling psychogenic hyperventilation, careful explanation of the basis of their symptoms can be reassuring and is often sufficient. Others have benefited from β-adrenergic antagonists or an exercise program. Specific treatment for anxiety may also be indicated.

FURTHER READING

LAFFEY JG, KAVANAGH BP: Hypocapnia. N Engl J Med 347:43, 2002
O'DONNELL CP et al: Leptin prevents respiratory depression in obesity. Am J Respir Crit Care Med 159:1477, 1999
PHILLIPSON EA, SLUTSKY AS: Hypoventilation and hyperventilation syndromes, in *Textbook of Respiratory Medicine*, 3d ed, JF Murray, JA Nadel (eds). Philadelphia, Saunders, 2000, pp 2139–2152
PHIPPS PR: Association of serum leptin with hypoventilation in human obesity. Thorax 57:75, 2002

247 SLEEP APNEA
Eliot A. Phillipson

Sleep apnea is defined as an intermittent cessation of airflow at the nose and mouth during sleep. By convention, apneas of at least 10 s duration have been considered important, but in most patients the apneas are 20 to 30 s in duration and may be as long as 2 to 3 min. *Sleep apnea syndrome* refers to a clinical disorder that arises from recurrent apneas during sleep. The clinical importance of sleep apnea arises from the fact that it is one of the leading causes of excessive daytime sleepiness and contributes to important cardiovascular disorders. Indeed, epidemiologic studies have established a prevalence of clinically important sleep apnea of at least 2% in middle-aged women and 4% in middle-aged men.

Sleep apneas can be central or obstructive in type. In central sleep apnea (CSA) the neural drive to all the respiratory muscles is transiently abolished. In contrast, in obstructive sleep apnea (OSA) airflow ceases despite continuing respiratory drive because of occlusion of the oropharyngeal airway.

OBSTRUCTIVE SLEEP APNEA

PATHOGENESIS The definitive event in OSA is occlusion of the upper airway usually at the level of the oropharynx. The resulting apnea leads to progressive asphyxia until there is a brief arousal from sleep, whereupon airway patency is restored and airflow resumes. The patient then returns to sleep, and the sequence of events is repeated, often up to 400 to 500 times per night, resulting in marked fragmentation of sleep.

The immediate factor leading to collapse of the upper airway in OSA is the generation of a critical subatmospheric pressure during inspiration that exceeds the ability of the airway dilator and abductor muscles to maintain airway stability. During wakefulness, upper airway muscle activity is greater than normal in patients with OSA, presumably to compensate for airway narrowing (see below) and a high upper airway resistance. Sleep plays a permissive but crucial role by reducing the activity of the muscles and their protective reflex response to subatmospheric airway pressures. Alcohol is frequently an important cofactor because of its depressant influence on the upper airway muscles and on the arousal response that terminates each apnea. In most patients the patency of the airway is also compromised structurally and is therefore predisposed to occlusion. In a minority of patients the structural compromise is due to obvious anatomic disturbances, such as adenotonsillar hypertrophy, retrognathia, and macroglossia. However, in the majority of patients the structural defect is simply a subtle reduction in airway size that can often be appreciated clinically as "pharyngeal crowding" and that can usually be demonstrated by imaging techniques. Obesity frequently contributes to the reduction in size of the upper airways, either by increasing fat deposition in the soft tissues of the pharynx or by compressing the pharynx by superficial fat masses in the neck. More sophisticated studies also demonstrate a high airway compliance—i.e., the airway is "floppy" and therefore prone to collapse.

PATHOPHYSIOLOGIC AND CLINICAL FEATURES The narrowing of the upper airways during sleep, which predisposes to OSA, inevitably results in snoring. In most patients, snoring usually antedates the development of obstructive events by several years. However, the majority of snor-

Primary Events	Physiologic Consequences	Clinical Features
Sleep onset	Decreased pleural pressure Increased cardiac afterload	Left heart failure
	Vagal bradycardia Ectopic cardiac beats	"Unexplained" nocturnal death
Apnea	Pulmonary vasoconstriction	Pulmonary hypertension Right heart failure
$\downarrow O_2$, $\uparrow CO_2$ $\downarrow pH$	Systemic vasoconstriction	Systemic hypertension
	Acute CO_2 retention	Chronic hypoventilation
Arousal from sleep	Cerebral dysfunction	Excessive daytime sleepiness Intellectual deterioration Personality changes Behavioral disorders
Resumption of airflow	Loss of deep sleep Sleep fragmentation	
	Excessive motor activity	Restless sleep
Return to sleep		

FIGURE 247-1 The primary sequence of events, physiologic responses, and clinical features of obstructive sleep apnea.

ing individuals do not have an OSA disorder, nor is there definitive evidence that snoring per se is associated with long-term health risks. Hence, in the absence of other symptoms, snoring alone does not warrant an investigation for OSA but does call for preventive counselling, particularly with regard to weight gain and alcohol consumption, and, when habitual, warrants conservative treatment similar to that for mild OSA (see below).

The recurrent episodes of nocturnal asphyxia and of arousal from sleep that characterize OSA lead to a series of secondary physiologic events, which in turn give rise in some patients to the clinical complications of the syndrome (Fig. 247-1). The most common manifestations are cognitive and behavioral disturbances that are thought to arise from the fragmentation of sleep and loss of slow-wave sleep induced by the recurrent arousal responses, and from nocturnal cerebral hypoxia. The most pervasive manifestation is excessive daytime sleepiness. Initially, daytime sleepiness manifests under passive conditions, such as reading or watching television; but as the disorder progresses, sleepiness encroaches into all daily activities and can become disabling and dangerous. Several studies have demonstrated two to seven times more motor vehicle accidents in patients with OSA compared with other drivers. Other related symptoms include intellectual impairment, memory loss, and personality disturbances.

The other major manifestations of OSA are cardiorespiratory in nature and are thought to arise from the recurrent episodes of nocturnal asphyxia and of negative intrathoracic pressure, which increases left ventricular afterload (Fig. 247-1). Many patients demonstrate a cyclical slowing of the heart during the apneas to 30 to 50 beats per minute, followed by a tachycardia of 90 to 120 beats per minute during the ventilatory phase. A small number of patients develop severe bradycardia or dangerous tachyarrhythmias, leading to the notion that OSA may result in sudden death during sleep, but corroborative data are lacking. Unlike in healthy subjects, in patients with OSA systemic blood pressure fails to decrease during sleep. In fact, blood pressure typically rises abruptly at the termination of each obstructive event as a result of sympathetic nervous activation and reflex vasoconstriction. Furthermore, over 50% of patients with OSA have systemic hypertension. Several epidemiologic studies have implicated OSA as a risk factor for the development of systemic hypertension, and studies in an

animal model demonstrate directly that OSA can cause sustained increases in daytime blood pressure. Emerging data also suggest that OSA can precipitate myocardial ischemia in patients with coronary artery disease and can adversely affect left ventricular function, both acutely and chronically, in patients with congestive heart failure. This complication is probably due to the combined effects of increased left ventricular afterload during each obstructive event, secondary to increased negative intrathoracic pressure (Fig. 247-1), recurrent nocturnal hypoxemia, and chronically elevated sympathoadrenal activity. Treatment of OSA in such patients often results in dramatic improvement in left ventricular function and in clinical cardiac status.

DIAGNOSIS Although OSA occurs at any age, and is considerably more prevalent in women than was previously thought, the typical patient is a male aged 30 to 60 years who presents with a history of snoring, excessive daytime sleepiness, nocturnal choking or gasping, witnessed apneas during sleep, moderate obesity and large neck circumference, and often mild to moderate hypertension. In women with OSA, who are typically postmenopausal, the complaint of snoring is less frequent than in men, and daytime fatigue may be more common than outright sleepiness.

The definitive investigation for suspected OSA is polysomnography, a detailed overnight sleep study that includes recording of (1) electrographic variables (electroencephalogram, electrooculogram, and submental electromyogram) that permit the identification of sleep and its various stages, (2) ventilatory variables that permit the identification of apneas and their classification as central or obstructive, (3) arterial O_2 saturation by ear or finger oximetry, and (4) heart rate. Continuous measurement of transcutaneous P_{CO_2} (which reflects arterial P_{CO_2}) can also be very useful, particularly in patients with CSA. The key diagnostic finding in OSA is episodes of airflow cessation or reduction at the nose and mouth despite evidence of continuing respiratory effort. By the time most patients come to clinical attention they have at least 10 to 15 obstructive events per hour of sleep. Although controversial, recent data suggest that a high upper airway resistance during sleep (manifested by snoring) that is accompanied by recurrent arousals from sleep, even in the absence of apneas and hypopneas, can result in a clinically important sleep-related syndrome. Therefore, the absence of outright apneas and hypopneas in a symptomatic patient may not definitely exclude a sleep-related respiratory disorder.

Because polysomnography is a time-consuming and expensive test, there is considerable interest in the role of screening tests and of unattended home sleep-monitoring for the investigation of OSA. However, the predictive value of most screening tests is too low to be clinically definitive, and the role of unattended, simplified sleep studies in routine practice has yet to be established. Nevertheless, in patients with a high probability of OSA (based on a history of habitual snoring, nocturnal choking or gasping, witnessed apneas during sleep, and daytime sleepiness or fatigue), overnight recording of arterial O_2 saturation by oximetry can be used to *confirm* the diagnosis and obviate the need for full polysomnography by demonstrating recurrent episodes of desaturation (at a rate of at least 10 to 15 events per hour). Negative results in such a patient do not exclude the diagnosis and mandate that the patient proceeds to polysomnography. In contrast, when the probability of OSA is low (only occasional snoring, no witnessed apneas, and no daytime sleepiness, fatigue, or other symptoms), the absence of nocturnal desaturation can be used to *exclude* OSA and obviate the need for full polysomnography. Based on these scenarios, it has been

TABLE 247-1 *Management of Obstructive Sleep Apnea (OSA)*

Mechanism	Mild to Moderate OSA	Moderate to Severe OSA
↑ Upper airway muscle tone	Avoidance of alcohol, sedatives	—
↑ Upper airway lumen size	Weight reduction Avoidance of supine posture Oral prosthesis	Uvulopalatopharyngo-plasty
↓ Upper airway subatmospheric pressure	Improved nasal patency	Nasal continuous positive airway pressure
Bypass occlusion		Tracheostomy

Source: From Phillipson, with permission.

estimated that overnight oximetry can obviate the need for polysomnography in about one-third of clinic patients referred for consideration of OSA.

℞ TREATMENT

Several approaches to treatment of OSA have been advocated, based on an understanding of the mechanisms involved ((Table 247-1). In establishing a treatment strategy, defining the severity of the disorder is essential, as indicated by the degree of clinical symptoms (particularly daytime sleepiness and fatigue) and the objective level of nocturnal respiratory and sleep disturbance. In severe OSA (significant daytime sleepiness or >30 obstructive events and arousals per hour of sleep), nasal continuous positive airway pressure (CPAP) is the treatment of choice. Nasal CPAP prevents upper airway occlusion by splinting the pharyngeal airway with a positive pressure delivered through a nasal mask. It is well tolerated and effective in >80% of patients, provided that they have received proper training. The established beneficial effects of CPAP include improvements in sleep quality, reduced daytime sleepiness and driving accidents, and decreased nocturnal hypertension. In patients with ischemic heart disease or congestive heart failure who also have OSA, nasal CPAP is the preferred treatment and the only one demonstrated to have a beneficial effect on cardiac status.

In patients with severe OSA who cannot tolerate nasal CPAP, upper airway surgery can be considered, with uvulopalatopharyngoplasty being the most commonly performed procedure. This operation is designed to increase the pharyngeal lumen by resecting redundant soft tissue. When applied to unselected patients with OSA, the response rate is <50%, but more discriminating selection of patients yields a higher rate of success. Other surgical approaches, including maxillofacial surgery, have variable results, but can be particularly effective in patients with craniofacial skeletal abnormalities.

In patients with mild to moderate OSA, nasal CPAP is superior to more conservative therapy but is often less well tolerated. Such patients can sometimes be managed effectively by modest weight reduction, avoidance of alcohol, improvement of nasal patency, cessation of smoking, and avoidance of sleeping in the supine posture. In addition, intraoral appliances, designed to modify the position of the mandible and tongue, can be effective and often better tolerated than nasal CPAP. Medications are generally ineffective in the management of OSA, except in patients with predominantly rapid eye movement (REM) sleep–related events in whom protriptyline or fluoxetine may be beneficial.

CENTRAL SLEEP APNEA

PATHOGENESIS The definitive event in CSA is transient abolition of central drive to the ventilatory muscles. Several underlying mechanisms can result in CSA (Table 247-2). First are defects in the metabolic respiratory control system and respiratory neuromuscular apparatus. Such defects usually produce a chronic alveolar hypoventilation syndrome (in addition to CSA) that becomes more severe during sleep when the stimulatory effect of wakefulness on breathing is abolished.

TABLE 247-2 *Mechanisms Underlying Central Sleep Apnea*

Underlying Mechanism	Clinical Example
Defects in metabolic control system or respiratory muscles	Primary and secondary central alveolar hypoventilation syndromes Respiratory muscle weakness
Transient instabilities in central respiratory drive	Sleep onset Hyperventilation-induced hypocapnia Idiopathic Hypoxia (high altitude, pulmonary disease) Cardiovascular disease, pulmonary congestion Central nervous system disease Prolonged circulation time

Source: From Phillipson, with permission.

In contrast are CSA disorders that arise from transient instabilities in an otherwise intact respiratory control system. Common to all these disorders is a P_{CO_2} level during sleep that falls transiently below the critical P_{CO_2} required for respiratory rhythm generation. This type of instability is frequent at sleep onset, because the P_{CO_2} level of wakefulness is generally lower than that required for rhythm generation in sleep; hence with loss of the stimulatory effect of wakefulness on breathing (referred to as the *waking neural drive*), an apnea develops at sleep onset until P_{CO_2} rises to the critical level (Fig. 247-2). However, if the central nervous system state fluctuates at sleep onset between "asleep" and "awake," a pattern of periodic breathing with central apneas or hypopneas develops as respiration follows the changes in state.

In most patients with CSA, the tendency to develop periodic breathing and central apneas during sleep is enhanced by some degree of chronic hyperventilation during wakefulness that drives the P_{CO_2} level below the threshold required for rhythm generation during sleep.

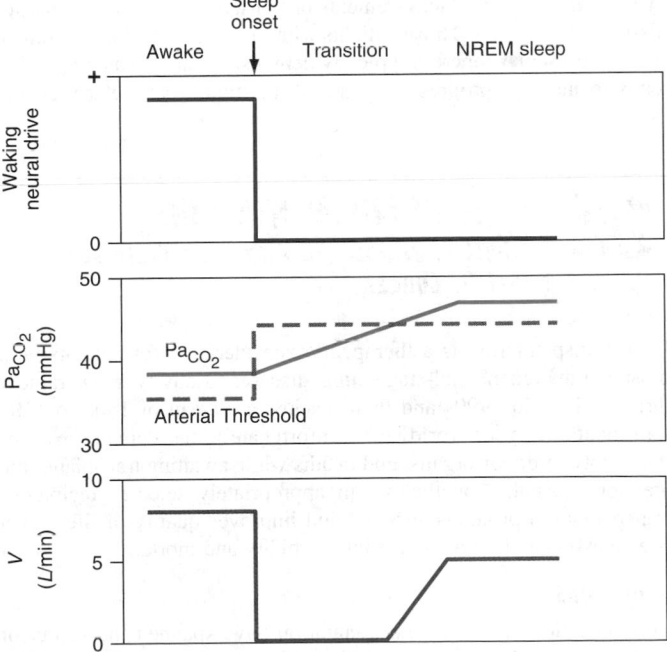

FIGURE 247-2 Schematic diagram of the mechanisms underlying central sleep apnea at sleep onset. With loss of the waking neural drive to breathing, the arterial threshold P_{CO_2} for rhythm generation increases above the Pa_{CO_2} present during wakefulness; ventilation (V) falls to zero and apnea ensues until Pa_{CO_2} rises above the threshold for rhythm generation during sleep. NREM, nonrapid eye movement. (*From TD Bradley, EA Phillipson, Clin Chest Med 13:439, 1992*)

Such hyperventilation is frequently idiopathic in nature. Hypoxia, whether due to high altitude or to underlying cardiorespiratory disease, enhances the tendency to periodic breathing and CSA by a similar mechanism. Periodic breathing and CSA are also common in patients with congestive heart failure, in whom the periodic breathing is characterized by a classic crescendo-decrescendo pattern (Cheyne-Stokes respiration). Patients with heart failure and CSA have a higher left ventricular end-diastolic volume and filling pressure than do heart failure patients without CSA, suggesting that their hyperventilation results, at least in part, from pulmonary congestion and stimulation of pulmonary vagal receptors.

PATHOPHYSIOLOGIC AND CLINICAL FEATURES   In those patients whose CSA is a component of a chronic alveolar hypoventilation syndrome, daytime hypercapnia and hypoxemia are usually evident, and the clinical picture is dominated by a history of recurrent respiratory failure, polycythemia, pulmonary hypertension, and right-sided heart failure. Complaints of sleeping poorly, morning headache, and daytime fatigue and sleepiness are also prominent. In contrast, in patients whose CSA results from an instability in respiratory drive, the clinical picture is dominated by features related to sleep disturbance, including recurrent nocturnal awakenings, morning fatigue, and daytime sleepiness. In patients with congestive heart failure, CSA can be an important (and frequently overlooked) cause of daytime sleepiness and fatigue. In addition, studies indicate a higher mortality rate and higher rate of cardiac transplantation in congestive heart failure patients with CSA than in those without CSA, even when matched for functional class and left ventricular ejection fraction. This outcome probably relates to the fact that CSA can trigger sympathetic nervous activation in patients with heart failure and thereby exert a secondary deleterious effect on the underlying cardiac disorder.

DIAGNOSIS   Initially, many patients with CSA, particularly of the idiopathic type, are suspected clinically of having OSA because of a history of snoring, sleep disturbance, and daytime sleepiness. However, obesity and hypertension are less prominent in CSA than in OSA. Definitive diagnosis of CSA requires a polysomnographic study, with the *key observation being recurrent apneas that are not accompanied by respiratory effort*. Measurements of transcutaneous P_{CO_2} are particularly useful in CSA. Those patients with a defect in respiratory control or neuromuscular function typically demonstrate an elevated P_{CO_2} that tends to increase progressively during the night, particularly during REM sleep. In contrast, patients with instabilities in the respiratory control system typically demonstrate a mild degree of hypocapnia, which is an integral pathogenetic feature of their disorder (see above).

℞ TREATMENT

The management of patients whose CSA is a component of an alveolar hypoventilation syndrome is essentially the same as management of the underlying hypoventilation disorder (Chap. 246). Management of patients whose CSA arises from an instability of respiratory drive is more problematic. Patients with hypoxemia usually respond favorably to nocturnal supplemental oxygen. For those with idiopathic CSA, respiratory stimulation with acetazolamide or central nervous system sedation with triazolam have been advocated, but results are variable and efficacy has not been established. Nasal CPAP (as for OSA) can be effective in idiopathic CSA, although definitive long-term trials are lacking and the treatment is less well tolerated than in patients with OSA. The mechanism by which CPAP abolishes central apneas may involve a small increase in Pa_{CO_2} as a result of the added expiratory mechanical load. In patients whose CSA is secondary to congestive heart failure, CPAP is particularly effective in improving sleep quality and daytime cardiac function. In fact, short-term randomized trials have demonstrated that CPAP has a beneficial effect on several surrogate markers of mortality in patients with congestive heart failure, including left ventricular ejection fraction, functional mitral regurgitation, and norepinephrine concentrations. Small, 5-year follow-up studies in such patients demonstrate that CPAP results in a decreased mortality rate. Larger randomized trials are currently in progress.

FURTHER READING

JAVAHERI S et al: Sleep apnea in 81 ambulatory male patients with stable heart failure. Circulation 97:2154, 1998

KANEKO Y et al: Cardiovascular effects of continuous positive airway pressure in patients with heart failure and obstructive sleep apnea. N Engl J Med 348:1233, 2003

McNICHOLAS WT, PHILLIPSON EA (eds): *Breathing Disorders in Sleep*. London, Saunders, 2002

PHILLIPS BG, SOMERS VK: Neural and humeral mechanisms mediating cardiovascular responses to obstructive sleep apnea. Resp Physiol 119:181, 2000

PHILLIPSON EA: Sleep disorders, in *Textbook of Respiratory Medicine*, 3d ed, JF Murray, JA Nadel (eds). Philadelphia, Saunders, 2000, pp 2153–2170

YOUNG T et al: Population-based study of sleep-disordered breathing as a risk factor for hypertension. Arch Intern Med 157:1746, 1997

---

248   LUNG TRANSPLANTATION
Elbert P. Trulock, G. Alexander Patterson, Joel D. Cooper

Lung transplantation is a therapeutic consideration for patients with most nonmalignant end-stage lung diseases. Activity grew rapidly through the mid-1990s and then reached a plateau of 1400 to 1500 transplants per year worldwide. Unfortunately, the demand exceeds the supply of donor organs, and deaths while awaiting transplantation are not unusual. Nonetheless, in appropriately selected recipients, transplantation prolongs survival and improves quality of life, but it is also associated with significant morbidity and mortality.

INDICATIONS

The indications for lung transplantation have spanned the gamut of lung diseases. The distribution reflects the prevalence and natural history of the various diseases, and the most common indications are shown in Table 248-1. "Other indications" in this table comprise many less prevalent lung diseases. During the past decade the proportion of recipients with primary pulmonary hypertension (PPH) steadily declined from 13% in 1990 to 4% in 2001 as medical therapy improved, and the fraction of recipients with chronic obstructive lung disease (COPD) or α_1-antitrypsin deficiency emphysema increased from 21 to 42%. During the same era, there was a trend toward more bilateral lung transplants, and since 1995 the annual numbers of single and bilateral procedures have been nearly equal.

RECIPIENT SELECTION

Transplantation should be considered when other therapeutic options have been expended and when the patient's prognosis will be improved by the procedure. Survival rates after transplantation can be compared with predictive indices for the underlying disease, but each patient's clinical course must be integrated into the assessment, too. Quality of life is the primary motive for transplantation for many patients, and the prospect of an improved quality-adjusted survival is often attractive to them, even if the survival advantage itself seems marginal.

Disease-specific guidelines for referring patients for transplantation are summarized in Table 248-2. These criteria are derived from prognostic information about the diseases and from clinical experience, and they are intended to identify patients who may benefit from transplantation. Although no randomized trial of transplantation has been carried out, relative risk analyses have demonstrated that transplantation

TABLE 248-1 *Indications for Adult Lung Transplantation (1995–2001)*

Diagnosis	Single Lung Transplantation (n = 4663)		Bilateral Lung Transplantation (n = 4118)		Total (n = 8781)	
Chronic obstructive pulmonary disease	2536	54.4%	926	22.5%	3462	39.4%
Idiopathic pulmonary fibrosis	1110	23.8%	376	9.1%	1486	16.9%
Cystic fibrosis	52	1.1%	1360	33.0%	1412	16.1%
α_1-Antitrypsin deficiency emphysema	408	8.7%	407	9.9%	815	9.3%
Primary pulmonary hypertension	61	1.3%	340	8.3%	401	4.6%
Sarcoidosis	126	2.7%	106	2.6%	232	2.6%
Bronchiectasis	14	0.3%	176	4.3%	190	2.2%
Eisenmenger's syndrome	8	0.2%	95	2.3%	103	1.2%
Lymphoangioleiomyomatosis	42	0.9%	53	1.3%	95	1.1%
Retransplantation	77	1.6%	79	1.9%	156	1.8%
Other indications	229	4.9%	200	4.9%	429	4.9%

Source: Adapted from Hertz et al.

confers a survival advantage in patients with COPD, idiopathic pulmonary fibrosis (IPF), cystic fibrosis (CF), and PPH.

Candidates for lung transplantation are thoroughly screened for any comorbidity that might adversely affect the outcome, and consensus guidelines for selecting potential recipients have been published. In general, suitable candidates should have clinically and physiologically severe lung disease (Table 248-2), but otherwise they must be in reasonably good health. The typical upper age limit is approximately 65 years at most centers. Absolute exclusions include HIV infection, chronic hepatitis B antigenemia or chronic active hepatitis C infection, uncured malignancy, active cigarette smoking, drug or alcohol dependency or abuse, uncontrolled or untreatable pulmonary or extrapulmonary infection, irreversible physical deconditioning, chronic noncompliance with medical care, and significant dysfunction of any vital organ other than the lungs.

Other problems that either increase the risk of complications or will be aggravated by the posttransplantation medical regimen consti-

TABLE 248-2 *Disease-Specific Guidelines for Selecting Candidates for Lung Transplantation*

COPD and α_1-antitrypsin deficiency emphysema
  $FEV_1 < 25\%$ of predicted normal value (post-bronchodilator)
  $Pa_{CO_2} > 55$ mmHg
  Pulmonary arterial hypertension (mean pulmonary artery pressure > 25 mmHg)
Cystic fibrosis/bronchiectasis
  $FEV_1 < 30\%$ of predicted normal value
  $Pa_{CO_2} > 50$ mmHg
  $Pa_{O_2} > 50$ mmHg (on room air)
  Pulmonary arterial hypertension
  Adverse clinical course in spite of optimal medical management
    Increasing hospitalizations
    Recurrent, massive hemoptysis
    Rapidly declining FEV_1
    Cachexia
Idiopathic pulmonary fibrosis
  VC or TLC < 60–70% of predicted normal value
  $DL_{CO} < 50$–60% of predicted normal value
  Pulmonary arterial hypertension
  Hypoxemia ($Pa_{O_2} < 60$ mmHg or $SpO_2 < 90\%$) at rest or with activity (on room air)
  Progressive disease in spite of drug therapy
Primary pulmonary hypertension
  New York Heart Association functional class III or IV in spite of optimal drug therapy
  Unfavorable hemodynamic profile
    Right atrial pressure > 15 mmHg
    Mean pulmonary artery pressure > 55 mmHg
    Cardiac index < 2 (L/min)/m^2

Abbreviations: VC, vital capacity; TLC, total lung capacity; FEV_1, forced expiratory volume in 1 s; DL_{CO}, diffusing capacity for carbon monoxide; Pa_{O_2} and Pa_{CO_2}, partial pressure of oxygen and carbon dioxide, respectively, in arterial blood; SpO_2, oxygen saturation by pulse oximetry.
Source: Modified from International Guidelines for the Selection of Lung Transplant Candidates. Am J Respir Crit Care Med 158:335, 1998; with permission.

tute relative contraindications. Some typical issues are ventilator-dependent respiratory failure, previous thoracic surgical procedures, osteoporosis, systemic hypertension, diabetes mellitus, severe obesity or cachexia, and psychosocial problems. Chronic infection poses a unique concern in patients with bronchiectasis. Infection with antibiotic-resistant *Pseudomonas* species is not unusual after years of treatment, and infection with *Burkholderia* species complicates the course of some patients with CF. In addition, infection with *Aspergillus* species or nontuberculous mycobacteria occurs in some cases. Pretransplantation *Burkholderia* infection has been associated with persistent posttransplantation infection and poor outcomes; however, pretransplantation infection with *Pseudomonas* species that are not panresistant to antibiotics, with *Aspergillus* that is not invasive, and with mycobacteria has not compromised the results of transplantation. The potential impact of these and many other factors have to be judged in their clinical context to determine an individual candidate's suitability for transplantation.

WAITING LIST AND ORGAN ALLOCATION

Suitable candidates for transplantation are placed on a waiting list, but there is a critical shortage of cadaveric donor organs. Organ allocation policies are influenced by ethical, medical, geographic, and political factors, and systems vary from country to country. Under the present lung allocation algorithm in the United States, after matching for body size and blood group compatibility between the donor and patients on the waiting list, donor lungs are assigned to recipients by their seniority on the waiting list. At this time, there is no priority for medical urgency, but the allocation scheme is being reviewed, and modifications may be proposed.

In the United States the median time to transplantation was 1064 days for patients who initially registered on the national waiting list in 1998. Because of the long waiting time, approximately 10% of patients who were at risk have died each year before an organ became available. However, the death rate while waiting has been much higher for patients with IPF, PPH, and CF than for those with COPD or α_1-antitrypsin deficiency emphysema.

TRANSPLANT PROCEDURE

Bilateral transplantation is mandatory for bronchiectasis because the risk of spillover infection from a remaining native lung precludes single lung transplantation. Heart-lung transplantation is obligatory for Eisenmenger's syndrome with complex anomalies that are not readily amenable to surgical repair and for concomitant end-stage lung disease and cardiac disease. However, cardiac replacement is *not* necessary for cor pulmonale because right ventricular function will recover when pulmonary vascular afterload is normalized by lung transplantation.

Either bilateral or single lung transplantation is an acceptable alternative for other diseases unless there are special considerations. However, bilateral transplantation provides more reserve lung function as a buffer against complications, and in recipients with COPD and α_1-antitrypsin deficiency emphysema, survival has been significantly

| Diagnosis | n | Survival Rate, % | | | |
		3 Months	1 Year	3 Years	5 Years
Chronic obstructive pulmonary disease	4643	89	79	61	45
α_1-Antitrypsin deficiency emphysema	1288	85	74	59	50
Cystic fibrosis	1809	87	79	62	52
Idiopathic pulmonary fibrosis	1981	79	66	50	38
Primary pulmonary hypertension	714	81	68	53	48

Source: Data from Hertz et al.

better after bilateral transplantation. Nevertheless, single lung transplantation has been the preponderant procedure for COPD and IPF (Table 248-1). Bilateral transplantation has become the preferable operation for pulmonary vascular disease.

Living donor lobar transplantation has played a limited role in adult lung transplantation. It has been performed predominantly in teenagers or young adults with CF. A right lower lobe is obtained from one living donor and a left lower lobe from another, and these lobes are implanted to replace the right and left lungs, respectively, in the recipient. Since a lobe must replace a whole lung, donor-recipient size considerations are crucial, and the procedure is feasible only in recipients of relatively small stature. The results have been comparable to those with transplantation from cadaveric donors. The usual morbidities associated with a lobectomy have been encountered among the donors, but no deaths have yet been reported. Because of ethical concerns, this approach has been restricted to patients who were unlikely to survive the wait for a cadaveric donor.

POSTTRANSPLANTATION MANAGEMENT

Most recipients are managed with a three-drug maintenance immunosuppressive regimen that includes a calcineurin inhibitor (cyclosporine or tacrolimus), a purine synthesis antagonist (azathioprine or mycophenolate mofetil) and prednisone. Prophylaxis for *Pneumocystis carinii* pneumonia is standard, and prophylaxis against cytomegalovirus (CMV) infection is prescribed in many protocols. The dose of cyclosporine or tacrolimus is adjusted by blood-level monitoring. Both are metabolized by the hepatic cytochrome P450 system, and interactions with other medications that affect the pertinent cytochrome P450 pathways can profoundly alter the clearance and blood levels of these key immunosuppressants.

Routine management is designed to prevent complications or to detect them as soon as possible. The techniques include periodic contact with a transplant nurse coordinator, appointments with a physician, chest radiographs, blood tests, spirometry, and bronchoscopy. Lung function rapidly improves and then stabilizes by 3 to 6 months after transplantation. Subsequently, the coefficient of variation in spirometric measurements is small, and a sustained decline of 10 to 15% or more signals a potentially significant problem.

OUTCOMES

RESULTS Survival results are published regularly from large registries (Table 248-3) and can be accessed via the Internet (www.ishlt.org; www.ustransplant.org).

The main sources of perioperative mortality include technical complications of the operation, primary graft failure that is usually caused by ischemia-reperfusion lung injury, and infections. Although acute rejection and CMV infection are common problems in the first year, they have rarely been fatal. Beyond the first year, chronic rejection and non-CMV infections have caused the majority of deaths.

OUTCOMES Regardless of the pretransplantation diagnosis, successful transplantation has impressively restored cardiopulmonary function. Both overall and health-related quality of life have been enhanced after lung transplantation. With multidimensional profiles, improvements have extended across most domains and have been sustained longitudinally unless a complication such as chronic rejection has developed. However, fewer than one-half of recipients have reported either full- or part-time employment in 1-, 3-, and 5-year posttransplantation surveys.

COST The cost-effectiveness of lung transplantation has not been thoroughly analyzed. In the 1990s transplant hospitalization costs in the range of $160,000 were reported from two centers, but the charge would certainly be higher now. At these centers, the cost per quality-adjusted life-year gained through transplantation was estimated at approximately $155,000 to $175,000. Obviously, as recipients survive longer, the cost per quality-adjusted life-year will decrease, and the cost per quality-adjusted life-year for a 5-year survivor was appraised at $31,494 at one of the centers.

COMPLICATIONS

GRAFT DYSFUNCTION Graft dysfunction is not unusual in the first week after transplantation, and it has been referred to as *reperfusion edema*, *reimplantation response*, and *ischemia-reperfusion injury*. It is a form of acute lung injury with increased vascular permeability, but the severity is variable. Pulmonary venous obstruction and hyperacute rejection can produce a similar clinical picture in the first few days. The treatment is the conventional, supportive paradigm for acute lung injury, but inhaled nitric oxide and extracorporeal membrane oxygenation have been used successfully in severe cases. Most recipients recover, but graft failure is a leading cause of early death.

AIRWAY COMPLICATIONS The bronchial blood supply to the donor lung is disrupted. Consequently, when the lung is implanted in the recipient, the bronchus is dependent on retrograde bronchial blood flow through the pulmonary circulation and is vulnerable to ischemia.

The prevalence of major airway complications—dehiscence, stenosis, and bronchomalacia—has ranged from 4 to 20%, but the associated mortality has been very low. Management depends on the specific features. Laser therapy is effective for removing granulation tissue or fibrous webs. Sometimes, a stricture or stenosis can be managed by dilatation, but stent placement is often necessary for strictures and for bronchomalacia.

ACUTE REJECTION This is an immunologic response to direct or indirect alloantigen recognition, and it is characterized by arteriolar and bronchiolar lymphocytic inflammation. With current immunosuppressive regimens, 50% or more of recipients have at least one episode of acute rejection in the first year. Symptoms and signs can include cough, low-grade fever, dyspnea, hypoxemia, inspiratory crackles, interstitial infiltrates, and declining lung function. The signs and symptoms are nonspecific and overlap with infections like CMV pneumonia, hence the diagnosis should be confirmed by transbronchial biopsy. Treatment usually includes a short course of high-dose steroid therapy and adjustment of the maintenance immunosuppressive regimen.

CHRONIC REJECTION This complication is the main impediment to better medium-term survival rates, and it is the source of substantial morbidity because of its impact on lung function and quality of life. Both alloimmune inflammatory and non-alloimmune fibroproliferative mechanisms are probably important in the pathogenesis.

Clinically, chronic rejection is a form of graft dysfunction that is synonymous with bronchiolitis obliterans syndrome (BOS) (Chap. 243). BOS is characterized primarily by airflow limitation, and a formal diagnosis of BOS requires either a sustained decrement of 20% or more in the FEV_1 or biopsy proof of bronchiolitis obliterans. Clinically, the most useful is the $FEF_{25-75\%}$, which will usually decline before the FEV_1 and may presage BOS.

The prevalence of BOS approaches 50% by 3 years after transplantation. Both antecedent acute rejection and lymphocytic bronchiolitis are risk factors for subsequent BOS, and CMV pneumonitis has been implicated inconsistently. BOS is usually treated with augmented immunosuppression. While immunosuppressive therapy may stabilize lung function, the overall results of treatment have been disappointing, probably because the fibroproliferative process is already well established.

INFECTION The lung allograft is especially susceptible to infection, and infection has been one of the leading causes of death. In addition to a blunted immune response from the immunosuppressive drugs, other normal defenses are breached; the cough reflex is diminished, and mucociliary clearance is impaired in the transplanted lung. The spectrum of infections includes both opportunistic and nonopportunistic pathogens.

Bacterial bronchitis and pneumonia can occur at any time but are almost universal in the early postoperative period. Later, episodes of bronchitis are quite common, especially in recipients with BOS, and *P. aeruginosa* is often the culprit.

CMV is the most frequent viral infection after lung transplantation. Although gastroenteritis, colitis, and hepatitis can occur, CMV viremia and CMV pneumonia are the main illnesses. Most episodes occur in the first 6 months, and treatment with ganciclovir is effective unless resistance develops with repeated exposure. *Aspergillus* species have been the most problematic fungal infection.

OTHER COMPLICATIONS Other potential complications of the transplant operation are phrenic nerve injury with diaphragmatic dysfunction and vagal nerve injury with gastroparesis. Side effects and toxicities of the immunosuppressive drugs can cause new medical problems or aggravate preexisting conditions.

FURTHER READING

ARCASOY SM, KOTLOFF RM: Medical progress: Lung transplantation. N Engl J Med 340:1081, 1999

DEMEESTER J et al: Listing for lung transplantation: Life expectancy and transplant effect, stratified by type of end-stage lung disease, the Eurotransplant experience. J Heart Lung Transplant 20:518, 2001

ESTENNE M et al: Bronchiolitis obliterans syndrome 2001: An update of the diagnostic criteria. J Heart Lung Transplant 21:297, 2002

HERTZ MI et al: The Registry of the International Society for Heart and Lung Transplantation. Nineteenth official report—2002. J Heart Lung Transplant 21:950, 2002

249 | PRINCIPLES OF CRITICAL CARE MEDICINE
John P. Kress, Jesse B. Hall

The care of critically ill patients requires a thorough understanding of pathophysiology and is centered initially around resuscitation of patients at extremes of physiologic deterioration. This resuscitation is often fast-paced and may have to be begun without a detailed awareness of the patient's chronic medical problems. While physiologic stabilization is taking place, intensivists attempt to gather important background medical information to supplement the real-time assessment of the patient's current physiologic conditions. Numerous tools are available to assist intensivists in the accurate assessment of pathophysiology and to support incipient organ failures, thus offering a window of opportunity for diagnosing and treating underlying disease(s) in a stabilized patient. Indeed, the use of invasive interventions such as mechanical ventilation and renal replacement therapy as well as diagnostic tools such as central venous and pulmonary artery catheters are commonplace in the intensive care unit (ICU).

ASSESSMENT OF SEVERITY OF ILLNESS Categorization of a patient's illness into grades of severity occurs frequently in the ICU. There are numerous severity-of-illness scoring systems that have been developed and validated over the past two decades. While these scoring systems have been validated as tools to assess populations of critically ill patients accurately, their utility in predicting individual patient outcomes is not clear.

Severity-of-illness scoring systems are important for defining populations of critically ill patients. This allows effective comparison of groups of patients enrolled in clinical trials. To be assured that a purported benefit of a therapy is real, investigators must be assured that different groups involved in a clinical trial have similar illness severities. These scores are also useful in guiding hospital administrative policies. Allocation of resources, such as nursing and ancillary care, can be directed by such scoring systems. Severity-of-illness scoring systems can also assist in the assessment of quality of ICU care over time.

Currently, the most commonly utilized scoring systems are the APACHE (acute physiology and chronic health evaluation) system, the MPM (mortality probability model), and the SAPS (simplified acute physiology score) system. These were all designed to predict outcomes in critical illness. All of these severity-of-illness scoring systems have common variables. These common threads include age; vital signs; assessments of respiratory, renal, and neurologic function; and an evaluation of chronic medical illnesses.

APACHE II Scoring System (Table 249-1) APACHE II is the most commonly used severity-of-illness scoring system in North America. Age, type of ICU admission (after elective surgery vs. nonsurgical or after emergency surgery), a chronic health problem score, and 12 physiologic variables (the most severely abnormal of each in the first 24 h of ICU admission) are used to derive a score. The predicted hospital mortality is derived from a formula that takes into account the APACHE II score; the need for emergency surgery; and a weighted, disease-specific diagnostic category (Fig. 249-1). The validation of this score is based upon 5815 ICU admissions from 13 different hospitals. Importantly, several studies have reported limitations of scoring systems such as APACHE II in predicting outcomes in specific subgroups of patients, such as postoperative coronary artery bypass graft patients. This is presumably related to the "controlled" temporary physiologic derangements that can occur in such patients (e.g., hypothermia, hypotension). More recently, the APACHE III scoring system has been released. This scoring system is similar to APACHE II, in that it is based upon age, physiologic abnormalities, and chronic medical co-morbidities. Although the APACHE III score can be calculated, conversion of the score to a mortality probability is only available as a proprietary commercial product.

The SAPS II score, used more frequently in Europe, is not disease-specific but rather incorporates three underlying disease variables (AIDS, metastatic cancer, and hematologic malignancy). The MPM can be used to calculate a direct probability of death in patients admitted to the ICU. It has been validated in 19,124 ICU admissions in 12 countries.

Severity-of-illness scoring systems suffer from the problem of inability to predict survival in individual patients. Accordingly, the use of these scoring systems to direct therapy and clinical decision-making cannot be recommended at present. Rather, these tools should be used as important data to complement clinical bedside decision-making. While they can provide valuable statistical probabilities for outcomes in similar groups of patients, they cannot reliably forecast outcomes in individual cases.

SHOCK (See also Chap. 253)

INITIAL EVALUATION Shock is a common condition necessitating admission to the ICU or occurring in the course of critical care. Shock is defined by the presence of multisystem end-organ hypoperfusion. Clinical indicators include reduced mean arterial pressure, tachycardia, tachypnea, cool skin and extremities, acute altered mental status, and oliguria. Hypotension is usually, though not always, present. The end result of multiorgan hypoperfusion is tissue hypoxia, often clinically manifested by lactic acidosis. Since the mean arterial pressure is the product of the cardiac output (CO) and the systemic vascular resistance (SVR), reductions in blood pressure can be categorized by decreased CO and/or decreased SVR. Accordingly, the initial evaluation of a hypotensive patient should evaluate the adequacy of the CO. This should be part of the earliest assessment of the patient by the clinician at the bedside once shock is considered (Fig. 249-2). Clinical evidence of diminished CO includes a narrow pulse pressure (the difference between systolic and diastolic blood pressure—a marker that correlates well with stroke volume) and cool extremities with delayed capillary refill. Signs of increased CO include a widened pulse pressure (particularly with a reduced diastolic pressure), warm extremities with bounding pulses, and rapid capillary refill. If a hypotensive patient has clinical signs of increased CO, it can be inferred that the reduced blood pressure is a result of decreased SVR.

In hypotensive patients with clinical evidence of reduced CO, an assessment of intravascular and cardiac volume status is appropriate. A hypotensive patient with decreased intravascular and cardiac volume status may have a history suggesting hemorrhage or other volume losses (e.g., vomiting, diarrhea, polyuria). The jugular venous pressure is often reduced in such a patient, while the change in pulse pressure as a function of respiration is increased. A hypotensive patient with an increased intravascular and cardiac volume status may have S_3 and/or S_4 gallop sounds on cardiac examination, increased jugular venous pressure, extremity edema, and rales on lung auscultation. The chest x-ray may show cardiomegaly, widening of the vascular pedicle, Kerley B lines, and pulmonary edema. Chest pain and electrocardiographic changes consistent with ischemia may also be noted.

In hypotensive patients with clinical evidence of *increased* CO, a

TABLE 249-1 *Calculation of Acute Physiology and Chronic Health Evaluation II (APACHE II)[a]*

ACUTE PHYSIOLOGY SCORE

Score	4	3	2	1	0	1	2	3	4
Rectal temperature, °C	≥41	39.0–40.9		38.5–38.9	36.0–38.4	34.0–35.9	32.0–33.9	30.0–31.9	≤29.9
Mean blood pressure, mmHg	≥160	130–159	110–129		70–109		50–69		≤49
Heart rate	≥180	140–179	110–139		70–109		55–69	40–54	≤39
Respiratory rate	≥50	35–49		25–34	12–24	10–11	6–9		≤5
Arterial pH	≥7.70	7.60–7.69		7.50–7.59	7.33–7.49		7.25–7.32	7.15–7.24	<7.15
Oxygenation									
If $FI_{O_2} > 0.5$, use $(A-a)D_{O_2}$	≥500	350–499	200–349		<200				
If $FI_{O_2} \leq 0.5$, use Pa_{O_2}					>70	61–70		55–60	<55
Serum sodium, mEq/L	≥180	160–179	155–159	150–154	130–149		120–129	111–119	≤110
Serum potassium, meq/L	≥7.0	6.0–6.9		5.5–5.9	3.5–5.4	3.0–3.4	2.5–2.9		<2.5
Serum creatinine, mg/dL	≥3.5	2.0–3.4	1.5–1.9		0.6–1.4		<0.6		
Hematocrit	≥60		50–59.9	46–49.9	30–45.9		20–29.9		<20
WBC count, 10^3/mL	≥40		20–39.9	15–19.9	3–14.9		1–2.9		<1

GLASGOW COMA SCORE[b,c]

Eye Opening	Verbal (Nonintubated)	Verbal (Intubated)	Motor Activity
4—Spontaneous	5—Oriented and talks	5—Seems able to talk	6—Verbal command
3—Verbal stimuli	4—Disoriented and talks	3—Questionable ability to talk	5—Localizes to pain
2—Painful stimuli	3—Inappropriate words	1—Generally unresponsive	4—Withdraws to pain
1—No response	2—Incomprehensible sounds		3—Decorticate
	1—No response		2—Decerebrate
			1—No response

POINTS ASSIGNED TO AGE AND CHRONIC DISEASE AS PART OF THE APACHE II SCORE

Age, Years	Score
<45	0
45–54	2
55–64	3
65–74	5
≥75	6

Chronic Health (History of Chronic Conditions)[d]	Score
None	0
If patient is admitted after elective surgery	2
If patient is admitted after emergency surgery or for reason other than after elective surgery	5

[a] APACHE II score is the sum of the acute physiology score (vital signs, oxygenation, laboratory values) Glasgow coma score, age, and chronic health points. Worst values during first 24 h in the ICU should be used.

[b] Glasgow coma score (GCS) = eye-opening score + verbal (intubated or nonintubated) score + motor score.

[c] For GCS component of acute physiology score, subtract GCS from 15 to obtain points assigned.

[d] Chronic health conditions: liver, cirrhosis with portal hypertension or encephalopathy; cardiovascular, class IV angina (at rest or with minimal self-care activities); pulmonary, chronic hypoxemia or hypercapnia, polycythemia, ventilator dependent; kidney, chronic peritoneal or hemodialysis; immune, immunocompromised host.

Note: $(A-a)D_{O_2}$, alveolar-arterial oxygen difference; WBC, white blood (cell) count.

search for causes of decreased SVR is appropriate. The most common cause of high CO hypotension is sepsis (Chap. 254). Other causes include liver failure, severe pancreatitis, burns and other trauma that elicit the systemic inflammatory response syndrome (SIRS), anaphylaxis, thyrotoxicosis, and peripheral arteriovenous shunts. In summary, the three most common categories of shock (Table 253-1, p. 1600) are cardiogenic, hypovolemic, and high CO with decreased SVR (high-output hypotension). These categories may overlap and occur simultaneously (e.g., hypovolemic and septic shock, septic and cardiogenic shock).

The initial assessment of a patient in shock as outlined above should take only a few minutes. It is important that aggressive, early resuscitation be instituted based on the initial assessment, particularly since there are recent data suggesting that early resuscitation of septic and cardiogenic shock may improve survival. If the initial bedside assessment yields equivocal or confounding data, more objective assessments such as echocardiography and/or central venous or pulmonary artery catheterization may be useful. The goal of early resuscitation is to reestablish adequate tissue perfusion to prevent or minimize end-organ injury.

MECHANICAL VENTILATORY SUPPORT (See also Chap. 252) During the initial resuscitation of patients in shock, principles of advanced cardiac life support should be followed. Since patients in shock may be obtunded and unable to protect the airway, an early assessment of the patient's airway is mandatory during resuscitation from shock. Early intubation and mechanical ventilation are often required. Reasons for institution of endotracheal intubation and mechanical ventilation include acute hypoxemic respiratory failure and ventilatory failure, which frequently accompany shock. Acute hypoxemic respiratory failure (Chap. 250) may occur in cardiogenic shock (high-pressure pulmonary edema, Chap. 255) and in septic shock (Chap. 254). Ventilatory failure often occurs as a result of an increased load on the respiratory system, which may present in the form of acute metabolic acidosis (often lactic acidosis) or decreased compliance of the lungs ("stiff" lungs) as a result of pulmonary edema. Inadequate perfusion of respiratory muscles in the setting of shock may be another reason for early intubation and mechanical ventilation. Normally, the respiratory muscles receive a very small percentage of the CO. However, in patients who are in shock with respiratory distress for the reasons listed above, the percentage of CO dedicated to respiratory muscles may increase tenfold or more. Lactic acid production from inefficient respiratory muscle activity presents an additional ventilatory load.

Mechanical ventilation may relieve the patient of the work of breathing and allow redistribution of a limited CO to other vital organs,

FIGURE 249-1 APACHE II mortality curve. Blue ■, nonoperative; green, postoperative.

often with an improvement in lactic acidosis. Patients demonstrate signs of respiratory muscle fatigue with a number of clinical signs including inability to speak full sentences, use of accessory respiratory muscles, paradoxical abdominal muscle activity, extreme tachypnea (>40 breaths/min), and decreasing respiratory rate despite an increasing drive to breathe. When patients with shock are treated with mechanical ventilation, a major goal of ventilator settings is to assume all or the majority of the work of breathing, facilitating a state of minimal respiratory muscle work. With the institution of mechanical

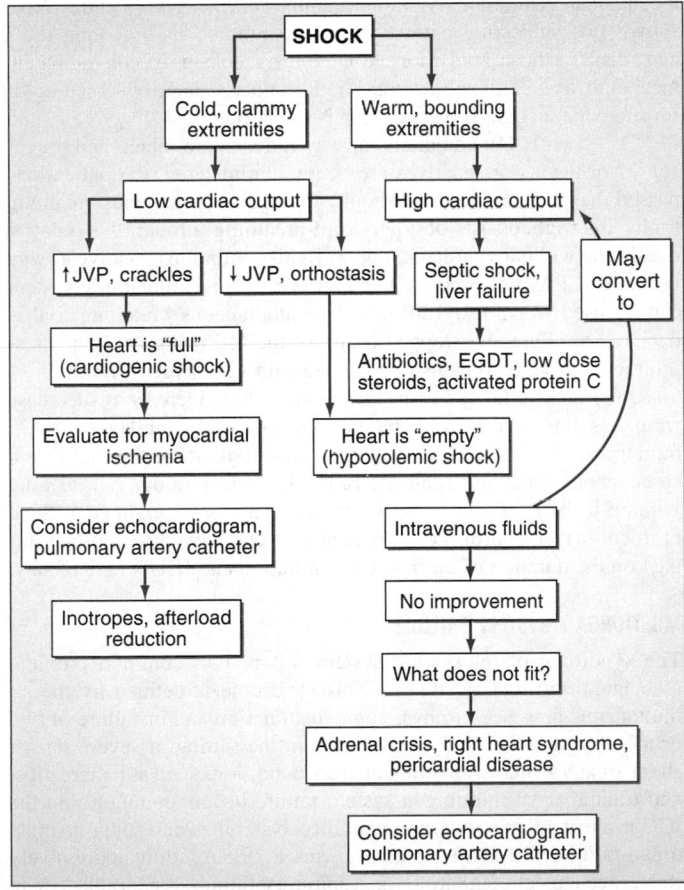

FIGURE 249-2 Approach to the patient in shock. JVP, jugular venous pulse; EGDT, early goal-directed therapy.

ventilation for shock, further worsening of blood pressure is frequently seen. The reasons for this include impedance of venous return with positive-pressure ventilation, reduced endogenous catecholamine secretion once the stress associated with respiratory failure is abated, and drugs used to facilitate endotracheal intubation (e.g., barbiturates, benzodiazepines, opiates), all of which may result in hypotension. Accordingly, hypotension after endotracheal intubation and positive-pressure ventilation should be anticipated. Many of these patients have a component of hypovolemia, which may respond to intravenous volume administration. →*For further discussion of individual forms of shock, see Chap. 253, Chap. 254, and Chap. 255.*

RESPIRATORY FAILURE (See also Chap. 250)

Respiratory failure is one of the most common reasons patients are admitted to the ICU. In some ICU settings, ≥75% of patients require mechanical ventilation during their ICU stay. Respiratory failure can be categorized mechanically, based on pathophysiologic derangements in respiratory function. Accordingly, four different types of respiratory failure can be described, based upon these pathophysiologic derangements.

TYPE I OR ACUTE HYPOXEMIC RESPIRATORY FAILURE This form of respiratory failure occurs when alveolar flooding and subsequent intrapulmonary shunt physiology occur. Alveolar flooding may be a consequence of pulmonary edema, pneumonia, or alveolar hemorrhage. Pulmonary edema can be further categorized as occurring due to elevated intravascular pressures seen in heart failure and intravascular volume overload or to acute lung injury ("low-pressure pulmonary edema") (Chaps. 29 and 255). The acute respiratory distress syndrome (ARDS) describes an extreme degree of lung injury. This syndrome is defined by diffuse bilateral airspace edema seen by chest radiography (Figs. 233-2 and 251-2), the absence of evidence of left atrial hypertension (pulmonary capillary occlusion pressure <18 mmHg), profound shunt physiology with a ratio of Pa_{O_2} to fraction of inspired oxygen (Pa_{O_2}/FI_{O_2}) of <200 (a Pa_{O_2}/FI_{O_2} < 300 is described as *acute lung injury*), and a clinical setting where this syndrome is known to occur. Common clinical settings associated with acute lung injury and ARDS include sepsis, gastric aspiration, pneumonia, near-drowning, multiple blood transfusions, and pancreatitis.

The mortality rate of patients with ARDS was traditionally very high (50 to 70%), but recent changes in ventilator management strategy have led to reports of mortality in the low 30% range (see below). For many years, physicians have suspected that mechanical ventilation of patients with acute lung injury and ARDS may propagate lung injury. Cyclical collapse and reopening of alveoli may be partly responsible for this. As shown in Fig. 249-3, the pressure-volume relationship of the lung in ARDS is not linear. Alveoli may collapse at very low lung volumes. Animal studies have suggested that stretching and overdistention of injured alveoli during mechanical ventilation can further injure the lung.

Concern over this alveolar overdistention, termed *ventilator-induced "volutrauma,"* led to a multicenter, randomized, prospective trial to compare traditional ventilator strategies for acute lung injury and ARDS (large tidal volume—12 mL/kg ideal body weight) to a low tidal volume (6 mL/kg ideal body weight). This study showed a dramatic reduction in mortality in the low tidal volume group (large tidal volume—39.8% mortality—versus low tidal volume—31% mortality) and confirmed that ventilator management could impact outcomes in these patients.

TYPE II RESPIRATORY FAILURE This ventilatory failure occurs as a result of alveolar hypoventilation and results in the inability to effectively eliminate carbon dioxide. Mechanisms by which this occurs are categorized as: (1) impaired central nervous system (CNS) drive to breathe, (2) impaired strength with failure of neuromuscular function in the respiratory system, (3) and increased load(s) on the respiratory system. Reasons for diminished CNS drive to breathe include drug overdose,

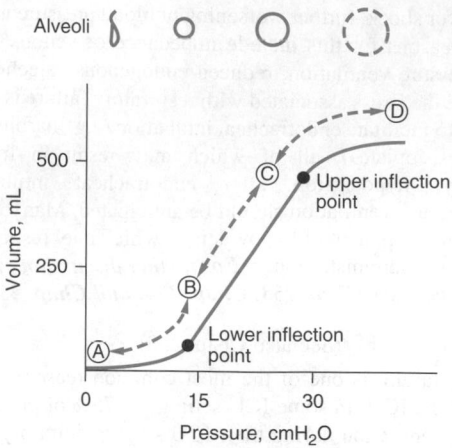

FIGURE 249-3 Pressure-volume relationship of the lungs of a patient with acute respiratory distress syndrome. At the lower inflection point, collapsed alveoli begin to open and the lung compliance changes. At the upper inflection point, alveoli become overdistended. The shape and size of alveoli are illustrated at the top.

brainstem injury, sleep-disordered breathing, and hypothyroidism. Reduced strength can be due to impaired neuromuscular transmission (e.g., myasthenia gravis, Guillain-Barré syndrome, amyotrophic lateral sclerosis, phrenic nerve injury) or respiratory muscle weakness (e.g., myopathy, electrolyte derangements, fatigue).

The overall load on the respiratory system can be classified into: resistive loads (e.g., bronchospasm), loads due to reduced lung compliance [e.g., alveolar edema, atelectasis, intrinsic positive end-expiratory pressure (autoPEEP)—see below], loads due to reduced chest wall compliance (e.g., pneumothorax, pleural effusion, abdominal distention), and loads due to increased minute ventilation requirements (e.g., pulmonary embolus with increased dead space fraction, sepsis).

The mainstays of therapy for type II respiratory failure are treatments directed at reversing the underlying cause(s) of ventilatory failure. Noninvasive positive-pressure ventilation using a mechanical ventilator with a tight-fitting face or nasal mask that avoids endotracheal intubation can often be used to stabilize these patients. This approach has clearly been shown to be beneficial in treating patients with exacerbations of chronic obstructive pulmonary disease. Noninvasive ventilation has been tested less extensively in other types of ventilatory failure but may be attempted nonetheless, in the absence of contraindications (hemodynamic instability, inability to protect airway, respiratory arrest).

TYPE III RESPIRATORY FAILURE This form occurs as a result of lung atelectasis. Because atelectasis occurs so commonly in the perioperative period, this is also called *perioperative respiratory failure*. After general anesthesia, decreases in functional residual capacity lead to collapse of dependent lung units. Such atelectasis can be treated by frequent changes in position, chest physiotherapy, upright positioning, and aggressive control of incisional and/or abdominal pain. Noninvasive positive-pressure ventilation may also be used to reverse regional atelectasis.

TYPE IV RESPIRATORY FAILURE This form occurs because of hypoperfusion of respiratory muscles in patients in shock. Normally, respiratory muscles consume <5% of the total CO and oxygen delivery. Patients in shock often suffer respiratory distress due to pulmonary edema, lactic acidosis, and anemia. In this setting, up to 40% of the CO may be distributed to the respiratory muscles. Intubation and mechanical ventilation can allow redistribution of the CO away from the respiratory muscles and back to vital organs while the shock is treated.

CARE OF THE MECHANICALLY VENTILATED PATIENT Mechanically ventilated patients frequently require sedatives and analgesics. Most patients undergoing mechanical ventilation experience pain, which can be elicited by the presence of the endotracheal tube and endotracheal suctioning. Accordingly, early and aggressive attention to pain control is extremely important. Opiates are the mainstay of therapy for pain control in mechanically ventilated patients. After assuring adequate pain control, additional indications for sedation for mechanically ventilated patients include: anxiolysis; treatment of subjective dyspnea; psychosis; facilitation of nursing care; reduction of autonomic hyperactivity, which may precipitate myocardial ischemia; and reducing global oxygen consumption (V_{O_2}).

Neuromuscular blocking agents are occasionally needed to facilitate mechanical ventilation in patients with profound dyssynchrony with the ventilator despite optimal sedation. The use of neuromuscular blocking agents may result in prolonged weakness—a myopathy known as the *postparalytic syndrome*. As a result, these agents are typically used as a last resort when aggressive sedation fails to achieve patient-ventilator synchrony. Because neuromuscular blocking agents result in pharmacologic paralysis without altering mental status, sedative-induced amnesia is mandatory when such agents are administered. Amnesia can be reliably achieved with benzodiazepines, such as lorazepam or midazolam, or with the intravenous anesthetic agent propofol. Outside of the setting of pharmacologic paralysis, there are few data supporting the idea that amnesia is mandatory in all patients who require intubation and mechanical ventilation. Sedatives and opiates may accumulate in critically ill patients when they are given for prolonged periods of time, since many of these patients have impaired hepatic and renal function. A protocol-driven approach to sedation of mechanically ventilated patients with daily interruption of sedative infusions has been shown to prevent excessive drug accumulation and shorten the duration of mechanical ventilation and length of stay in the ICU.

Weaning from Ventilation While a thorough understanding of the pathophysiology of respiratory failure is essential in order to optimize patient care, recognition of a patient's readiness to be liberated from mechanical ventilation is similarly important. Several studies have shown that subjecting patients to daily spontaneous breathing trials can identify those ready for extubation. Accordingly, all intubated, mechanically ventilated patients should undergo a daily screening of respiratory function. If oxygenation is stable (i.e., $Pa_{O_2}/FI_{O_2} > 200$ and $PEEP \leq 5$ cmH$_2$O), cough and airway reflexes are intact, and no vasopressor agents or sedatives are being administered, the patient has passed the screening test and should undergo a spontaneous breathing trial. This trial consists of a period of breathing through the endotracheal tube without ventilator support [both continuous positive airway pressure (CPAP) of 5 cmH$_2$O and an open T-piece breathing system can be used] for 30 to 120 min. The spontaneous breathing trial is declared a failure and stopped if any of the following occur: (1) respiratory rate > 35 breaths/min for >5 min (2) oxygen saturation < 90%, (3) heart rate > 140 beats/min or a 20% increase or decrease from baseline, (4) systolic blood pressure < 90 mmHg or >180 mmHg, or (5) increased anxiety or diaphoresis. If, at the end of the spontaneous breathing trial, the ratio of the respiratory rate to tidal volume in liters (f/V$_T$) is <105, the patient can be extubated. Such protocol-driven approaches to patient care can have an important impact on the duration of mechanical ventilation and ICU length of stay.

MULTIORGAN SYSTEM FAILURE

The syndrome of multiorgan system failure is a common problem associated with critical illness. This syndrome is defined by the simultaneous presence of physiologic dysfunction and/or failure of two or more organs. Typically, this occurs in the setting of severe sepsis, shock of any kind, severe inflammatory conditions such as pancreatitis, and trauma. That multiorgan system failure occurs commonly in the ICU is a testament to our current ability to stabilize and support single organ failure. The ability to manage single organ failure aggressively (e.g., mechanical ventilation for respiratory failure, renal replacement therapy for acute renal failure) has greatly reduced early mortality in critical illness. As such, it is uncommon for critically ill patients to die in the initial stages of resuscitation. Instead, many patients succumb to critical illness later in the ICU stay, after the initial presenting problem has been stabilized.

While there is debate regarding specific definitions of organ failure, several general principles governing the syndrome of multiorgan system failure apply. First, organ failure, no matter how defined, must persist beyond 24 h. Second, mortality risk increases as patients accrue additional organ failures. Third, prognosis is worsened by increased duration of organ failure. These observations remain true across various critical care settings (e.g., both medical and surgical). SIRS is a common basis for multiorgan system failure. Although infection is a common cause of SIRS, "sterile" triggers such as pancreatitis, trauma, and burns often are responsible for multiorgan system failure.

Gastrointestinal Tract Considerable attention has been directed to the liver and gastrointestinal tract as contributors to the syndrome of multiorgan system failure. Kupffer cells and macrophages in the liver play an important role in the uptake and clearance of endotoxin, cytokines, leukotrienes, and bacteria migrating from the lumen of the bowel to regional lymph nodes and then to the circulation (a process called *translocation*). Since the liver is positioned downstream from the venous drainage of the gastrointestinal tract, it plays a vital role in first-pass clearance of translocated bacteria, endotoxin, and cytokines. Mesenteric hypoperfusion plays a pivotal role in endotoxemia and bacterial translocation from the lumen of the gastrointestinal tract. It appears that mesenteric hypoperfusion leads to loss of integrity of the intestinal mucosa, with subsequent leakage of intact bacteria and endotoxin into mesenteric lymph nodes, mesenteric venous drainage, and the portal venous system. An imbalance favoring a pro-inflammatory state ensues, with overexpression of tumor necrosis factor-α and interleukins (IL), such as IL-1, IL-6, and IL-10. Leukocyte (particularly neutrophil) adherence to endothelial cells and subsequent diapedesis follows, propagating SIRS, which may progress in an unregulated manner.

Lungs While the gastrointestinal tract has received much attention with regard to its role as a nidus for the propagation of multiorgan system failure, other organs may also release inflammatory mediators in an unregulated manner and contribute to the propagation of SIRS and subsequent multiorgan system failure. Recent data suggest that the lungs may be a source of inflammatory cytokines, particularly when patients suffer from acute lung injury or ARDS (Chap. 251). It has been proposed that mechanical ventilation may propagate lung injury and the release of inflammatory cytokines from the lung itself.

MONITORING IN THE ICU

Because respiratory and circulatory failure occur commonly in critically ill patients, monitoring of the respiratory and cardiovascular systems is undertaken frequently in the ICU. Evaluation of respiratory gas exchange is routine in critical illness. The "gold standard" remains arterial blood-gas analysis, where pH, partial pressures of oxygen and carbon dioxide, and oxygen saturation are measured directly. With arterial blood-gas analysis, the two main functions of the lung—oxygenation of arterial blood and elimination of CO_2—can be assessed directly. Importantly, the blood pH, which has a profound effect on the drive to breathe, can only be assessed by sampling of arterial blood. Though sampling of arterial blood is generally safe, it may be painful and cannot provide continuous information for clinicians routinely. Given these limitations, noninvasive monitoring of respiratory function is often employed in the critical care setting.

PULSE OXIMETRY This is the most commonly utilized noninvasive monitor of respiratory function. The technique takes advantage of differences in the absorptive properties of oxygenated and deoxygenated hemoglobin. At wavelengths of 660 nm, oxyhemoglobin reflects light more effectively than does deoxyhemoglobin, whereas the reverse is true in the infrared spectrum (940 nm). A pulse oximeter passes both wavelengths of light through a perfused digit such as a finger, and the relative intensity of light transmission at these two wavelengths is recorded. This allows the derivation of the relative percent of oxyhemoglobin. Since arterial pulsations produce phasic changes in the intensity of transmitted light, the pulse oximeter is designed to detect only light of alternating intensity. This allows distinction of arterial and venous blood saturation.

RESPIRATORY SYSTEM MECHANICS These can be measured during mechanical ventilation (Chap. 252). When volume-controlled modes of mechanical ventilation are used, accompanying airway pressures can be easily measured. The peak airway pressure is determined by two variables—the airways resistance and respiratory system compliance. At the end of inspiration, inspiratory flow can be stopped transiently. This end-inspiratory pause (*plateau pressure*) is a static measurement, impacted only by respiratory system compliance, not airways resistance. The difference between the peak (airways resistance + respiratory system compliance) and plateau (respiratory system compliance only) airway pressure provides a quantitative assessment of airways resistance. Accordingly, during volume-controlled ventilation, patients with increases in airways resistance (e.g., in asthma) typically have increased peak airway pressures as well as an abnormally high gradient between peak and plateau airway pressure (typically >15 cmH$_2$O). In such patients, the use of bronchodilators and/or glucocorticoids may be beneficial.

The plateau airway pressure is a static measurement, determined by the compliance of the respiratory system. Pathophysiologic processes such as pleural effusions, pneumothorax, increased abdominal girth from ascites or obesity all reduce chest wall compliance. Lung compliance may be reduced by pneumonia, pulmonary edema from any cause, or autoPEEP, which occurs when there is insufficient time for emptying of alveoli prior to the next inspiratory cycle. Since the alveoli have not decompressed completely, alveolar pressure remains positive at end-exhalation (functional residual capacity). This phenomenon is caused most commonly by critical narrowing of distal airways in disease processes such as asthma and chronic obstructive pulmonary disease. Modern mechanical ventilators allow breath-to-breath display of pressure and flow, which may allow detection of problems such as patient-ventilator dyssynchrony, airflow obstruction, and autoPEEP.

CIRCULATORY STATUS Monitors to characterize the circulatory status of critically ill patients are used commonly in the ICU. One of the most frequently used is the pulmonary artery catheter, also known as the right heart catheter or Swan-Ganz catheter. This catheter was originally designed as a tool to guide therapy in acute myocardial infarction but is currently used in the ICU for evaluation and treatment of a variety of other conditions such as ARDS, septic shock, congestive heart failure, and acute renal failure. This device has never been validated as a tool associated with reduction in morbidity and mortality.

Pulmonary Artery Catheter (See also Chap. 212) This is inserted via a central vein (jugular, subclavian, femoral) and is sequentially directed to the right atrium, right ventricle, and pulmonary artery after a balloon is inflated to facilitate its flow-directed placement. Waveform pressures in the right atrium, right ventricle, and pulmonary artery can be measured. When the balloon at the end of the pulmonary artery catheter is inflated, the catheter advances into a distal pulmonary artery until it "wedges" into place. Once the catheter is wedged, the measured pressure is transmitted from the "downstream" pulmonary veins and left atrium. Accordingly, the pulmonary capillary occlusion, or wedge, pressure is equal to the left atrial pressure under most circumstances. With a pulmonary artery catheter, the cardiac output can be measured directly using the thermodilution technique. When cool saline is injected into the proximal port of the catheter, the temperature change at the distal port can be measured. The measured temperature change is related to the volume of saline injected (which is known) and the CO. Blood from the pulmonary artery can be obtained from this catheter to measure oxygen saturation. This "mixed" venous saturation allows assessment of the adequacy of whole-body oxygen delivery.

Oxygen delivery is a function of CO and the content of O_2 in the arterial blood. The vast majority of O_2 delivered to tissues is bound to hemoglobin, and the dissolved O_2 contributes very little to O_2 content in arterial blood or O_2 delivery. The normal tissue extraction ratio for O_2 is ~25%. A pulmonary artery catheter allows measurements of O_2 delivery and oxygen extraction ratio.

The mixed venous O_2 saturation allows assessment of global tissue perfusion. A reduced mixed venous O_2 saturation may be caused by inadequate cardiac output, reduced hemoglobin concentration, and/or reduced arterial O_2 saturation. An abnormally high O_2 consumption, which may be caused by a multitude of problems such as fever, agitation, shivering, or thyrotoxicosis, may also lead to a reduced mixed venous O_2 saturation if O_2 delivery is not concomitantly increased.

Pulmonary artery catheters are invasive monitors and may be associated with a number of complications. Since the catheter is inserted via a central vein, all of the complications associated with central venous catheterization are present. These include central venous catheter–related infections, pneumothorax, arterial puncture with or without cannulation, bleeding, air embolism, venous thrombosis, and catheter embolism. The insertion of the pulmonary artery catheter also carries a number of risks, including dysrhythmias, heart block, cardiac perforation, and balloon fragmentation. After the catheter is placed, pulmonary infarction, pulmonary artery rupture, and pulmonic valve insufficiency may occur. Fortunately, most of these complications are quite rare.

Misinterpretation of data derived from the pulmonary artery catheter may be the most common "complication" seen with these monitors. Pressure measurements in various cardiac chambers require careful zeroing of the pressure transducer relative to atmospheric pressure and placement at the proper adjustment, generally 5 cm inferior to the sternal angle in a supine patient. Another potential source of error is the variation in arterial pressure measurements as a function of the respiratory cycle. The atrial chambers are subjected to pleural pressure; therefore, atrial pressure typically falls during inspiration in a spontaneously breathing patient. Conversely, atrial pressure often rises during inspiration in a patient undergoing positive-pressure ventilation. As such, atrial pressure measurements should be made at end-expiration when there is no movement of air in or out of the thorax, often difficult to recognize in patients on mechanical ventilation.

PREVENTION OF COMPLICATIONS OF CRITICAL ILLNESS

SEPSIS IN THE CRITICAL CARE UNIT (See also Chap. 254) Sepsis is a significant problem in the care of critically ill patients. It is the leading cause of death in noncoronary ICUs in the United States. Current estimates suggest that >750,000 patients are affected each year, and these numbers are expected to increase as the population continues to age and a greater percentage of persons vulnerable to infection will likely seek medical care.

Many therapeutic interventions in the ICU are invasive and predispose patients to infectious complications. These interventions include endotracheal intubation, indwelling vascular catheters, nasally placed enteral feeding tubes, transurethral bladder catheters, and other catheters placed into sterile body cavities (e.g., tube thoracostomy, percutaneous intraabdominal drainage catheters). The longer such devices remain in place, the more prone to these infections patients become. For example, ventilator-associated pneumonia correlates strongly with the duration of intubation and mechanical ventilation. Therefore, an important aspect of preventive care is the timely removal of invasive devices as soon as they are no longer needed. Multidrug resistant organisms are commonplace in the ICU.

An important aspect of critical care is infection control in the ICU. Simple measures such as frequent handwashing are effective but underutilized strategies. Protective isolation of patients with colonization or infection by drug-resistant organisms is another frequently used strategy in the critical care setting. Antibiotic-coated vascular catheters or endotracheal tubes with specialized suction ports above the cuff to decrease pooling and aspiration of oral secretions are other strategies

that may be used, with varying degrees of effectiveness reported. Surveillance programs monitoring adherence to infection control practices such as those described here may reduce the incidence of nosocomial infections.

DEEP VENOUS THROMBOSES All ICU patients are at high risk for this complication, given their predilection toward immobility. Therefore, all ICU patients should receive some form of prophylaxis against deep venous thrombosis (DVT). Traditional forms of prophylaxis are subcutaneous low-dose heparin or low-molecular-weight heparin injections and sequential compression devices for the lower extremities. Recently, an observational study reported an alarming incidence of the occurrence of DVTs despite the use of these standard prophylactic regimens. Heparin prophylaxis may result in heparin-induced thrombocytopenia—another relatively common nosocomial complication in critically ill patients. Low-molecular-weight heparins such as enoxaparin are more effective than unfractionated heparin for DVT prophylaxis in high-risk patients, such as those undergoing orthopedic surgery, and they have a lower incidence of heparin-induced thrombocytopenia. Fondaparinux, a selective factor Xa inhibitor, is even more effective than enoxaparin in high-risk orthopedic patients.

STRESS ULCERS Prophylaxis against stress ulcers is frequently administered in most ICUs. Typically, histamine-2 antagonists are administered. Currently available data suggest that high-risk patients, such as those with shock or respiratory failure requiring mechanical ventilation, benefit from such prophylactic treatment. Proton pump inhibitors are also used as agents for prophylaxis against stress ulcers, though outcomes data supporting the benefits of these drugs are largely lacking.

ANEMIA (See also Chap. 52) This is a common problem in critically ill patients. Most suffer from anemia of chronic inflammation. Recent studies have demonstrated that erythropoietin levels are inappropriately reduced in most ICU patients and that exogenous erythropoietin administration may reduce transfusion requirements in the ICU. Phlebotomy contributes significantly to anemia in ICU patients. The hemoglobin level that merits transfusion in critically ill patients has been a long standing area of controversy. A large, multicenter study involving patients in many different ICU settings challenged a conventional notion that a hemoglobin level of 100 g/L (10 g/dL) is needed in critically ill patients. Patients prospectively randomized to red blood cell transfusions only when the hemoglobin level was ≤70 g/L (7 g/dL) had no difference in mortality than those liberally transfused to a target hemoglobin of 100 g/L (10 g/dL). It is noteworthy that even those with risk factors for coronary artery disease did not show increased morbidity or mortality with a restrictive transfusion strategy. Red blood cell transfusion is associated with impairment of immune function, increased risk of infections, acute lung injury, and volume overload—all of which may explain the findings in this study. Accordingly, a conservative transfusion strategy should be the rule in managing critically ill patients who are not actively hemorrhaging.

ACUTE RENAL FAILURE (See also Chap. 260) This complication occurs in a significant percentage of critically ill patients. The most common underlying etiology is acute tubular necrosis, usually precipitated by hypoperfusion and/or nephrotoxic agents. Currently, there are no pharmacologic agents available for prevention of renal injury in critical illness. A recent study showed convincingly that low-dose dopamine is *not* effective in protecting the kidneys from acute injury. Other drugs, such as fenoldapam and vasopressin, have the potential to prove useful as agents for renal protection; however, more data are needed before firm conclusions can be drawn.

MALNUTRITION This is a common problem in the critically ill patient; it may exacerbate respiratory failure, impair wound healing, and debilitate effective immune response. Nutritional support in the management of these patients is of the greatest importance. Early enteral feeding is reasonable, though no data are available to suggest that this improves patient outcome per se. Certainly, enteral feeding, if possible, is preferred over parenteral nutrition, which is associated with numerous complications including hyperglycemia, fatty liver, cholestasis, and sepsis. In addition, enteral feeding may prevent bacterial translocation across the gut mucosa (see "Multiorgan system failure", above). The catabolic state induced by critical illness mandates aggressive nutritional support; these patients often have higher caloric needs than normal patients, and nutrition support teams can play an important role in their management. Another recent study showed a significant mortality benefit when glucose levels were aggressively normalized in a large group of ICU patients, most of whom had recently undergone operations.

NEUROLOGIC DYSFUNCTION IN CRITICALLY ILL PATIENTS

Neurologic dysfunction is common in critically ill patients and a frequent cause of admission to the ICU.

DELIRIUM (See also Chap. 257)   This state is defined by (1) an acute onset of changes or fluctuations in the course of mental status, (2) inattention, (3) disorganized thinking, and (4) an altered level of consciousness (i.e., other than alert). A recent study reported delirium in >80% of patients admitted to the ICU. A rapid test—the Confusion Assessment Method—to assess critically ill patients for delirium is available and has recently been validated. This assessment asks patients to answer simple questions and perform simple tasks and can be completed by the bedside nurse in about 2 min. The differential diagnosis of delirium in the ICU patient is broad and includes infectious etiologies (including sepsis), medications (particularly sedatives and analgesics), drug withdrawal, metabolic/electrolyte derangements, intracranial pathology (e.g., stroke, intracranial hemorrhage), seizures, hypoxia, hypertensive crisis, shock, and vitamin deficiencies (particularly thiamine).

ANOXIC CEREBRAL INJURY (See also Chap. 258)   This condition is common following cardiac arrest and often results in severe and permanent brain injury in patients whose cardiac arrest is resuscitated. Active cooling of patients after cardiac arrest has been shown to improve neurologic outcomes. As such, all patients who present to the ICU after circulatory arrest from ventricular fibrillation or pulseless ventricular tachycardia should be actively cooled with cooling blankets and ice packs if necessary to achieve a core body temperature of 32 to 34°C.

STROKE (See also Chap. 349)   This is a common cause of critical neurologic illness. Hypertension must be managed carefully, since abrupt reductions in blood pressure may be associated with further brain ischemia and injury. Acute ischemic stroke treated with tissue plasminogen activator (tPA) shows improved neurologic outcome when treatment is given within 3 h of onset of symptoms. However, mortality is not improved when tPA is compared to placebo, despite improved neurologic outcome, and cerebral hemorrhage is significantly higher in patients given tPA. A treatment benefit is *not* seen when tPA is given beyond 3 h. Heparin has not been shown to demonstrate improved outcomes convincingly in patients with acute ischemic stroke.

SUBARACHNOID HEMORRHAGE (See also Chap. 349)   This may occur secondary to aneurysm rupture and is often complicated by cerebral vasospasm, rebleeding, and hydrocephalus. Vasospasm can be detected by either transcranial Doppler assessment or cerebral angiography; it is typically treated with the calcium channel blocker nimodipine; aggressive intravenous fluid administration; and therapy aimed at increasing the blood pressure, typically with vasoactive drugs such as phenylephrine. The intravenous fluids and vasoactive drugs (hypertensive hypervolemic therapy) are used to overcome the cerebral vasospasm. Early surgical clipping of aneurysms is advocated to prevent complications related to rebleeding. Hydrocephalus, typically heralded by a decreased level of consciousness, may require ventriculostomy drainage.

STATUS EPILEPTICUS (See also Chap. 348)   Recurrent or relentless seizure activity is a medical emergency. Cessation of seizure activity is required to prevent irreversible neurologic injury. Lorazepam is the most effective benzodiazepine for treating status epilepticus and is the treatment of choice for controlling seizures acutely. Phenytoin or fosphenytoin should be given concomitantly since lorazepam has a short half-life. Other drugs such as gabapentin, carbamazepine, and phenobarbital should be reserved for patients with contraindications to phenytoin (e.g., allergy or pregnancy) or ongoing seizures despite phenytoin.

BRAIN DEATH (See also Chap. 258)   Although critically ill patients usually die from irreversible cessation of circulatory and respiratory function, a diagnosis of death may also be established by irreversible cessation of all functions of the entire brain, including the brainstem, even if circulatory and respiratory functions remain intact as a result of artificial life support. Patients must demonstrate absence of cerebral function (unresponsive to all external stimuli) and brainstem functions [e.g., unreactive pupils, absent ocular movement to head turning or ice water irrigation of ear canals, positive apnea test (no drive to breathe)]. Absence of brain function must have an established cause and be permanent without possibility of recovery (e.g., must confirm the absence of sedative effect, hypothermia, hypoxemia, neuromuscular paralysis, or severe hypotension). If there is uncertainty about the cause of coma, studies of cerebral blood flow and electroencephalography should be performed.

WITHHOLDING AND WITHDRAWING CARE (See also Chap. 9)

The withholding and withdrawing of care occurs commonly in the ICU setting. Concerns about the provision of care deemed futile are occasionally raised during the care of critically ill patients. The Task Force on Ethics of the Society of Critical Care Medicine reported in a consensus statement that it is ethically sound to withhold or withdraw care if a patient or surrogate makes such a request or if the goals of therapy are not achievable according to the physician. Since all medical treatments are justified by their expected benefits, the loss of such an expectation justifies the act of withdrawing or withholding such a treatment. As such, the act of withdrawing care is fundamentally similar to the act of withholding care. An underlying stipulation derived from this task force report is that the informed patient should have his or her wishes respected with regard to life-sustaining therapy. Implicit in this stipulation is the need to ensure that patients are thoroughly and accurately informed regarding the plausibility and expected results of various therapies. The act of informing patients and/or surrogate decision makers is the responsibility of the physician and other health care providers. In the event a patient or surrogate desires therapy deemed futile by the treating physician, the physician is not ethically obligated to provide such treatment. Rather, arrangements may be made to transfer the patient's care to another care provider.

Decisions to withhold or withdraw care should occur only after extensive discussions with the patient (if this is possible), surrogate(s), and other health-care providers, usually in the form of one or more multiple formal meetings. In addition, most institutions have ethics committees to assist in the withholding and withdrawal of care. Though not required routinely, such committees are available to safeguard against patients or surrogates making capricious requests to withhold or withdraw care. In addition, such consultation may be considered in the event that a patient or surrogate does not agree with the physician's impression that care should be withheld or withdrawn.

It is noteworthy that decisions to withhold and withdraw life support from the critically ill are increasing, with recent reports of up to 90% of patients dying in the ICU after care was withheld or withdrawn. Critical care providers should meet regularly with patients and/or surrogates to discuss prognosis when the withholding or withdrawal of care is being considered. After a consensus amongst caregivers has been reached regarding withholding or withdrawal of care, this should be relayed to the patient and/or surrogate decision maker. If a decision to withhold or withdraw life-sustaining care for a patient has been reached, aggressive attention to analgesia and anxiolysis is needed. Opiates and benzodiazepines are typically used to achieve these goals.

Patients may have their death hastened by the aggressive administration of analgesic and anxiolytic drugs; however, if the intent of this therapy is to alleviate suffering and not to hasten death, this "double effect" is ethically acceptable.

FURTHER READING

ELY EW et al: Delirium in mechanically ventilated patients: Validity and reliability of the confusion assessment method for the intensive care unit (CAM-ICU). JAMA 286:2703, 2001

KNAUS WA et al: APACHE II: A severity of disease classification system. Crit Care Med 13:818, 1985

KRESS JP et al: Daily interruption of sedative infusions in critically ill patients undergoing mechanical ventilation. N Engl J Med 342:1471, 2000

RIVERS E et al: Early goal directed therapy in the treatment of severe sepsis and septic shock. N Engl J Med 346:305, 2002

SCHIFFL H et al: Daily hemodialysis and the outcome of acute renal failure. N Engl J Med 346:305, 2002

TASK FORCE ON ETHICS OF THE SOCIETY OF CRITICAL CARE MEDICINE: Consensus report on the ethics of foregoing life-sustaining treatments in the critically ill. Crit Care Med 18:1424, 1990

THE ACUTE RESPIRATORY DISTRESS SYNDROME NETWORK: Ventilation with lower tidal volumes as compared with traditional tidal volumes for acute lung injury and the acute respiratory distress syndrome. N Engl J Med 342:1301, 2000

THE HYPOTHERMIA AFTER CARDIAC ARREST STUDY GROUP: Mild therapeutic hypothermia to improve the neurologic outcome after cardiac arrest. N Engl J Med 346:549, 2002

VAN DEN BERGHE G et al: Intensive insulin therapy in the surgical intensive care unit. N Engl J Med 345:1359, 2001

250   RESPIRATORY FAILURE
Craig Lilly, Edward P. Ingenito, Steven D. Shapiro

DEFINITION AND CLASSIFICATION   Respiratory failure is defined as a failure of gas exchange due to inadequate function of one or more essential components of the respiratory system. Clinically, respiratory failure can be manifest either as hypoxemia ($P_{O_2} < 60$ mmHg at sea level), i.e., inadequate blood oxygenation; hypercarbia ($P_{CO_2} > 45$ mmHg), i.e., excess of circulating carbon dioxide; or frequently, a combination of both types of gas exchange abnormalities. Respiratory failure is classified as hypoxemic, hypercarbic, or combined.

Respiratory failure is also commonly described in terms of its acuity, since it may develop either acutely or chronically. In *acute respiratory failure*, a sudden, catastrophic event leads to life-threatening respiratory insufficiency. In *chronic respiratory failure*, gradual worsening of respiratory function leads to progressive impairment of gas exchange, the metabolic effects of which are partially compensated by adaptations in other systems. In patients with long-standing respiratory disease, compensated *chronic respiratory insufficiency* may exist for many years, resulting in a state in which patients do not have true respiratory failure but have little or no functional respiratory reserve. In such cases, even a mild insult to the respiratory system can precipitate *acute on chronic respiratory failure*.

Independent of cause, as respiratory demand exceeds the functional capacity of the respiratory system, respiratory failure evolves and immediate medical intervention is required.

EPIDEMIOLOGY   Respiratory failure is a common diagnosis among patients in medical intensive care units (ICUs) and is associated with a poor prognosis. The incidence of respiratory failure is 137 cases per 100,000 population, or 360,000 cases per year in the United States, with 36% of these individuals failing to survive the hospitalization. Both the incidence of and mortality from respiratory failure increase exponentially with age and in the presence of other comorbid conditions. Therapeutic advances in both mechanical ventilation and airway management have improved the prognosis for patients with respiratory failure over the past several decades. Even patients with irreversible chronic respiratory failure can now be provided with ventilator support systems that allow an acceptable quality of life and can be managed at home. Lung transplantation is also an option for selected patients with chronic respiratory failure (Chap. 248), although the widespread use of transplantation is limited by both the availability of organ donors and the number of qualified transplant centers.

PHYSIOLOGY   Describing respiratory failure as either hypoxemic or hypercarbic provides some information about the physiologic deficit. However, a better understanding of the underlying pathophysiology and potential treatment strategies can be gained by considering the individual components of the respiratory system that are required for effective function under physiologic conditions. Normal respiration requires the integrated function of five separate components.

1. *Nervous system.* This is the control system, and it comprises the dorsal and ventral nuclei of the medullary respiratory control group and their associated afferent and efferent neural pathways. These act in concert with the cerebral cortex to determine respiratory rate and breathing effort. Respiratory failure due to diseases that cause dysfunction of the central control system can be thought of as *controller dysfunction*, or central apnea.

2. *Musculature* (the pump). The inspiratory muscles of breathing consist primarily of the diaphragm, but accessory muscles also contribute, including the internal intercostals, suprasternal, and sternocleidomastoid, as do supporting structures of the chest wall, which lower the pressure in the pleural space between the chest wall and lung during inspiration, establishing a pressure gradient between the airway opening and alveolar compartment that causes gas to flow into the lung. Respiratory failure due to diseases that cause ineffective function of the respiratory pump can be thought of as *pump dysfunction*. Under normal conditions, only elastic recoil is required for expiration, but during respiratory failure accessory muscles of expiration are required.

3. *Airways* (a complex conduit system for bulk delivery of gases). These consist of the upper airways, cartilaginous bronchi, and small airways distal to the terminal bronchioles capable of conducting gas quickly and evenly into and out of the alveolar compartment where gas exchange can occur. Respiratory failure involving diseases that cause marked obstruction or dysfunction of the air passages can be thought of as *airway system dysfunction*.

4. *Alveolar units* (an efficient, distensible, compact membrane system). This system consists of the respiratory bronchioles, alveolar ducts, and alveoli; these provide sufficient surface area to allow for rapid exchange of gases and sufficient elasticity so that following expansion, the membrane can generate adequate recoil pressure to empty the lung passively during exhalation. Respiratory failure as a result of diseases that cause collapse, flooding, or injury to the alveolar network can be thought of as *alveolar compartment dysfunction*.

5. *Vasculature* (a network of conduits capable of transporting dissolved gases to and from the functioning organs throughout the body). This consists of the pulmonary capillary network, intimately associated with the membrane system, but distinct both in structure and with respect to the types of diseases that can alter its normal function. Respiratory failure as a result of disease involving the pulmonary vasculature can be thought of as *pulmonary vascular dysfunction*.

Failure of any *one* of these essential components or significant dysfunction of more than one essential component can lead to *failure of the integrated system* and produce clinical respiratory failure.

Many diseases cause dysfunction of several of the essential components of the respiratory system, and ultimately this leads to abnormalities in gas exchange. Understanding which components of the respiratory system have failed in a given case provides valuable insight into the underlying disease process that cannot be gained from a simple analysis of the gas exchange abnormalities. For example, a patient with severe asthma, a patient with a large pulmonary embolus, and a patient with pulmonary edema may all present with hypoxemic respiratory failure. In each case, however, the cause and treatment of the respiratory failure are distinct. Developing a clinical approach for evaluating the five different functional components of the respiratory system is essential for identifying the cause of respiratory failure and quickly developing an effective management plan.

CLINICAL EVALUATION ▪ Initial Assessment and Stabilization of Respiratory Failure Initial evaluation of the respiratory system includes an immediate determination of upper airway patency and an examination for central and peripheral cyanosis, followed by measurement of the respiratory rate and observation of the depth and pattern of respiration. One should simultaneously note the presence or absence of signs of respiratory distress including flaring of nostrils, pursed-lip breathing, and use of accessory muscles of respiration. Next, one should assess the configuration of the chest wall and its movement during the respiratory cycle. This is followed by palpation and auscultation over each hemithorax. These observations allow an initial assessment of respiratory drive, pump function, and delivery of gas to the lungs. This examination is supplemented by an estimation of the oxygen and carbon dioxide content of arterial blood determined by arterial blood-gas measurement. Oximetry provides a rapid way to determine blood oxygen content but does not provide information regarding alveolar ventilation and P_{CO_2} levels; an arterial blood-gas measurement is required to assess these parameters.

In contrast to many clinical conditions, the emergent nature of acute respiratory failure and the potential for rapid progression to a life-threatening situation require that initial therapy be implemented before the specific etiology of the respiratory failure is diagnosed and treated. Adequate airway protection, oxygenation, and ventilation should be assured prior to further diagnostic testing. Thus, in concert with the initial assessment one must stabilize the patient with respiratory failure quickly since hypoxemia and hypercarbia can rapidly lead to circulatory failure and death (see "Initial Management," below). Cardiovascular stability must also be rapidly assessed and achieved (see Chap. 253). From the standpoint of respiratory failure, the first priority is to establish adequate oxygenation and ventilation. Administration of supplemental oxygen might be all that is initially required, but if the patient is in distress, artificial ventilation is needed. Initially, ventilation is often administered manually using a bag-valve-mask device followed by use of a mechanical ventilator (Chap. 252). Once an endotracheal tube has been placed and secured, and its position verified, ventilator support can be initiated to help normalize oxygenation and CO_2 elimination. Following stabilization of the patient, a systematic

and thorough evaluation of the cause of respiratory failure can safely be carried out.

Clinical Evaluation of Respiratory Failure Based on Physiologic Principles
Simple bedside techniques can be used to assess which of the five components of the respiratory system are no longer functioning normally in a patient with respiratory failure (Table 250-1). This assessment can provide great insight into the clinical cause of respiratory failure and assist with management planning.

CONTROLLER DYSFUNCTION This is perhaps the least common primary cause of respiratory failure, and it can be difficult to assess in the intubated ICU patient because many medications used to ensure comfort also affect the level of consciousness and limit respiratory drive. Nevertheless, useful information can frequently be obtained about respiratory drive by simple observation and history. The most frequent cause of controller dysfunction is the presence of medications that impair respiratory drive, many of which also impair the level of consciousness. A history of the use of respiratory depressants or an impaired level of consciousness prior to the administration of medications to facilitate intubation suggests the possibility of controller dysfunction. The awake, minimally sedated patient with either significant hypercarbia or hypoxemia who demonstrates no elevation in respiratory rate (i.e., <12 breaths/min) and no use of accessory muscles is likely to have a defect in regulating respiratory drive. In respiratory failure due solely to controller dysfunction, such as an opiate overdose, the degree of hypoxemia is in direct proportion to the degree of hypercarbia, i.e., the patient will have a normal alveolar-arterial gradient (Chap. 234). This can be calculated with the information obtained from an arterial blood-gas measurement. More formal tests of respiratory drive, including determining if the respiratory rate increases to at least 25 breaths/min when the patient inhales a mixture of 5% CO_2 and 15% O_2 (the CO_2 challenge test) and measuring the pressure generated 0.1 s after the start of inhalation (the $P_{0.1}$ test), have been described for outpatient investigation of respiratory controller problems, but they are not used in the ICU setting.

PUMP DYSFUNCTION This is a common cause of respiratory failure in ICU patients with respiratory failure and is usually multifactorial. Various medications, prolonged periods of mechanical ventilator support, and polyradiculopathy associated with critical illness can all adversely affect the respiratory muscles. In the patient who is not intubated, one must assess degree of respiratory distress as described above. In addition, abdominal paradoxus indicates diaphragmatic fatigue, a hallmark of pump failure. For patients who are mechanically ventilated, a

TABLE 250-1 *Methods for Assessing Controller, Pump, Airway, Alveolar Compartment, and Pulmonary Vascular Dysfunction at the Bedside*

Type of Dysfunction	Test	Method of Determination	Findings Consistent with Dysfunction
Controller	Respiratory rate	Clinical observation in spontaneously breathing patient	< 12/min in presence of hypoxia or hypercarbia and acidemia
Pump	Vital capacity, inspiratory force	Bedside measurement in awake patient	Presence of paradoxical respiratory motions. VC < 10 mL/kg IF < −20 cmH$_2$O RSBI > 105
Airway	Wheezing or ronchi on auscultation	Physical examination	Presence of wheezing
	Airway resistance measurement	Bedside measurement in cooperative or sedated patient	Raw > 10 cmH$_2$O/L per second
	Clinical evidence of auto-PEEP	Auscultation or bedside measurement in sedated patient	Presence of autoPEEP
Alveolar	Arterial blood gas	Arterial blood sample	Exam suggestive of consolidation
	Respiratory system compliance	Bedside measurement in sedated patient	Abnormal Pa$_{O_2}$/Fi$_{O_2}$ ratio or elevated Pa$_{CO_2}$; Crs > 30 mL/cmH$_2$O
	Chest radiograph	Bedside x-ray	Alveolar infiltrates
Pulmonary vascular	Assessment of right heart function	JVP–central venous pressure	Elevation
	ECG		Right heart strain or RBBB

Note: VC, vital capacity; IF, inspiratory force; RSBI, rapid-shallow-breathing index; raw, raw airway resistance; auto-PEEP, intrinsic positive end-expiratory pressure; Crs, respiratory system compliance; JVP, jugular venous pressure; ECG, electrocardiogram; RBBB, right bundle branch block.

variety of simple bedside tests have been used to assess respiratory muscle function. Measurement of vital capacity and inspiratory force are the most frequently used; they provide an assessment of both the volume the respiratory muscles can generate against the impedance of the respiratory system and the isovolumetric pressure the respiratory muscles can generate during a maximal effort. Vital capacity < 10 mL/kg and inspiratory force measurements that fail to achieve a negative pressure of at least −20 cmH₂0 indicate a component of respiratory muscle insufficiency. The rapid-shallow-breathing index (respiratory rate/tidal volume) is an integrative index of respiratory performance that predicts success of liberation from mechanical ventilation when it is <105. More sophisticated measurements of respiratory muscle function, including transdiaphragmatic pressure measurements using esophageal balloons and bedside electromyography and nerve conduction studies, can be used in special circumstances to obtain detailed information about respiratory muscle dysfunction when warranted.

AIRWAY DYSFUNCTION   This can also be readily assessed at the bedside in the patient with respiratory failure using simple bedside measurements and clinical assessment. Stridor suggests the presence of large airway or laryngeal obstruction. Bronchospasm can be diagnosed by auscultation and detection of wheezing and/or rhonchi. Coarse breath sounds or rhonchi present during the inspiratory phase of respiration usually indicate obstruction of the large airways, frequently from retained secretions. High-pitched wheezing during expiration indicates obstruction of the small airways and is commonly associated with bronchospasm. In cases of severe airflow obstruction, wheezing may be reduced because airflow is minimal. In these cases, the obstruction may be manifest as dynamic hyperinflation or intrinsic positive end-expiratory pressure (autoPEEP), and detected by persistent, faint wheezing that continues throughout expiration to the point of initiation of the subsequent inspiration.

Simple bedside measurements can also be used to detect airflow obstruction, although they require that the patient be synchronous with the ventilator and not tachypneic. Therefore these tests are best performed in the sedated patient. By programming the ventilator to impose a brief pause (0.5 to 1 s in duration) at the end of inspiration, the driving pressure to overcome airway resistance during inspiration, equal to the peak inspiratory pressure minus the airway pressure measured at the end of the pause (i.e., plateau pressure), can be determined. Dividing this pressure difference by the end-inspiratory flow rate gives an estimate of airway resistance. Normal values in the intubated patient range from 3 to 8 cmH₂O/L per second, depending upon the size of the endotracheal tube. Values significantly greater than this indicate airflow obstruction. More detailed information about lung impedance, including airway resistance and dynamic compliance, can be obtained by measuring transpulmonary pressures, volumes, and flows using an esophageal balloon and bedside pneumotachograph system. However, such detailed measurements are usually made only for research purposes.

ALVEOLAR COMPARTMENT DYSFUNCTION   This can be assessed using several distinct and complementary bedside techniques, in addition to simple gas exchange measurements. Findings on physical examination that are suggestive of consolidation, such as tubular breath sounds, dullness to percussion, and egophony, establish alveolar compartment dysfunction. Lung stiffness, as reflected in static respiratory system compliance, can be assessed by measuring the distending pressure required to inflate the lung once inspiratory flow has ceased. This is calculated by measuring the end-inspiratory plateau pressure and dividing the inspiratory volume by end-inspiratory plateau pressure minus whatever level of PEEP is being applied. A normal value of static respiratory system compliance measured using this approach is 35 to 50 mL/cmH₂O. Values <30 during conventional tidal volume inflation (7 to 12 mL/kg tidal volumes) indicate increased stiffness of the lung, chest wall, or both.

The chest radiograph is also a useful tool for assessing the pathology of the alveolar compartment. Radiographic densities consistent with air-space disease point to alveolar infection, injury, or flooding and, together with a reduced lung compliance and reduced arterial oxygen level, favor a diagnosis of alveolar compartment dysfunction.

PULMONARY VASCULAR DYSFUNCTION   This cannot be directly assessed at the bedside but may be reflected by signs of right heart dysfunction, such as elevated jugular venous pressures, a pronounced or delayed pulmonic component of the second heart sound, a right-sided heave, a right-sided third heart sound, or a murmur of tricuspid regurgitation. In the absence of these signs it can be suggested by exclusion in cases where abnormal gas exchange exists in the apparent absence of controller, pump, airway, or alveolar compartment dysfunction. Pulmonary vascular disease can cause abnormalities in routine clinical tests including the electrocardiogram (ECG) and chest radiograph. It can cause right heart strain or right bundle branch block which will show on the electrocardiogram, and pulmonary artery enlargement can be seen on radiographic studies. More definitive testing including echocardiography, right heart catheterization, or contrast-enhanced computed tomography of the chest is often required to identify the presence of pulmonary vascular disease.

Making a Definitive Diagnosis   Approaching respiratory failure from a physiologic perspective can provide important clues about its specific etiology, which in turn can lead to the formulation of a more effective diagnostic approach and a definitive therapeutic plan. Once a patient has been stabilized by establishing a stable airway and providing mechanical ventilatory support (if indicated), a thorough evaluation of the cause of respiratory failure can be safely undertaken. Table 250-2 summarizes common disease states representative of each type of respiratory system dysfunction listed above. The associated blood-gas findings and additional confirmatory tests that may be useful in further evaluating each of these conditions are also presented.

INITIAL MANAGEMENT   Treatment for many of the specific disorders identified in Table 250-2 is addressed in subsequent chapters; in this chapter the focus is on the initial management that is common to all patients with respiratory failure. As discussed above, one must first focus on physiologic stabilization. The first priority is to establish adequate oxygenation through the administration of supplemental oxygen in patients with hypoxemia. For patients with hypercarbic respiratory failure leading to significant acidemia or hypoxemia inadequately corrected by supplemental oxygen, the mainstay of supportive care for respiratory failure is mechanical ventilation (Chap. 252). Although mechanical ventilation can sometimes be provided without placement of an artificial airway (i.e., mask ventilation), in the majority of cases the first step in stabilizing the patient with respiratory failure involves placement of an endotracheal tube. This can be achieved via either the orotracheal or nasotracheal route, usually using a combination of parenteral and local anesthesia to ensure patient comfort. Following placement, the tube must be secured and its position verified so as to provide 100% O₂ and adequate ventilation immediately.

Obstruction of the upper airway is a medical emergency. In an unconscious patient this is often due to occlusion by the tongue or soft tissues of the pharynx. The airway is immediately opened with the head tilt−chin lift maneuver and the patient assessed for spontaneous respirations. When a spontaneously breathing patient is unable to dislodge a foreign object, a forceful subdiaphragmatic thrust can facilitate removal of the object. Removal may require laryngoscopy and removal with forceps. Liquids such as vomitus or blood are removed by suctioning under direct vision. In some cases of respiratory failure the airway is secure without instrumentation, but in most a stable airway is achieved by passing an endotracheal tube. When the airway cannot be secured using these techniques a tracheostomy or cricothyrotomy should be performed.

One of the most effective ways to improve the O₂ content of blood is to increase its concentration in alveolar gas by administering O₂, initally with an FI$_{O_2}$ of 100%. Oxygen delivery to the alveoli can also

TABLE 250-2 *Clinical Syndromes Associated with Dysfunction of the Components of the Respiratory System*

Type of Dysfunction	Specific Representative Conditions	Predominant Gas Exchange Abnormality	Additional Testing/Evaluation
Controller	Sedative medications	Hypercarbia	Review of medications
	Chronic obstructive or interstitial lung disease	Hypoxemia + hypercarbia	History of daytime somnulence, lung function
	Toxic overdoses	Hypoxemia + hypercarbia	Toxicology screen
	Hypothermia post operatively	Hypercarbia	Measurement of core body temperature
	Brainstem stroke	Hypercarbia	Head CT/MRI scans

Pump	Medications/toxins
	  Paralytics
	  Aminoglycosides
	  Steroids
	  Botulism
		Hypercarbia	Review of medical history

	Myopathy	Hypercarbia	Strength testing, EMG/NCV studies
	Myositis	Hypercarbia	Clinical exam, serum CK and aldolase

	Metabolic abnormalities
	  Hypothyroidism
	  Hypophosphatemia
		Hypercarbia	TSH, serum phosphate

	Myasthenia gravis	Hypercarbia	EMG/NVC studies, Tensilon test
	Guillain-Barré syndrome	Hypercarbia	Clinical evaluation, EMG/NCV studies
	Paraneoplastic syndromes	Hypercarbia	Clinical evaluation, EMG/NCV studies
	Polyradiculopathy of critical illness	Hypercarbia	Clinical evaluation, EMG/NCV studies
	Postoperative or postradiation therapy phrenic nerve dysfunction	Hypercarbia	Diaphragmatic ultrasound, fluoroscopy of diaphragm
	Postoperative pain/splitting	Hypoxemia + hypercarbia	Clinical assessment
Airway	Asthma	Mild: hypoxemia + hypocarbia Severe: hypoxemia + hypercarbia	Pulmonary function testing Functional response to bronchodilators
	Emphysema/chronic bronchitis	Hypoxemia + hypercarbia	Pulmonary function testing, chest x-ray
	Bronchiolitis	Hypoxemia + hypercarbia	Pulmonary function testing, chest CT, lung biopsy
	Endobronchial tumor, mass, or stricture	Variable	Pulmonary function testing, CT imaging, bronchoscopy
Alveolar	Pneumonia	Hypoxemia + hypercarbia	Smear and culture of secretions
	Pulmonary edema	Hypoxemia + hypercarbia	Examination of the heart Chest x-ray
	Pulmonary hemorrhage	Hypoxemia + hypercarbia	Chest x-ray, bronchoscopy
	ARDS	Hypoxemia + hypercarbia	Chest x-ray, arterial blood gas
	Drug reaction	Hypoxemia + hypercarbia	Drug exposure, toxicology screen, lung biopsy
	Pulmonary contusion	Hypoxemia + hypercarbia	Chest wall pain, chest x-ray
Pulmonary vascular	Acute pulmonary embolus	New-onset hypoxemia with or without hypercarbia	Ventilation-perfusion scanning, CT pulmonary embolism study
	Pulmonary hypertension	Exertional hypoxemia	Echocardiogram, right heart catheterization
	AVM or intracardiac shunt	Hypoxemia that is refractory to oxygen therapy	Echocardiogram with bubble study, high-resolution CT scan

Note: CT, computed tomography; MRI, magnetic resonance imaging; CK, creatine kinase; TSH, thyroid stimulating hormone; EMG, electromyography; NCV, nerve conduction velocity study; ARDS, adult respiratory distress syndrome; AVM, arteriovenous malformation.

be improved by applying PEEP in patients receiving mechanical ventilatory support. Increasing alveolar ventilation with a mechanical ventilator eliminates CO_2 and corrects acidemia. In the setting of acute respiratory failure, it is important to document that adequate oxygenation and elimination of CO_2 have been achieved before adjustment of the O_2 content and other ventilator settings.

The effective management of respiratory failure depends on identifying and optimally managing all of the treatable factors that impair the respiratory system. This includes removing excess secretion by suctioning, treating infections with effective antimicrobials, suppressing inflammation with anti-inflammatory or immunosuppressive drugs, treating obstruction with bronchodilators, avoiding the harmful effects of excess oxygen or mechanical forces from the mechanical ventilator, dissolving blood clots with anticoagulants or thrombolytics, providing pulmonary vasodilatation, and removing transudated fluid with diuretics. Some forms of chronic respiratory system failure, such as sleep apnea syndrome and post-polio syndrome, are ultimately responsive to nocturnal mechanical ventilation or continuous positive airway pressure (Chap. 252). Finally, selected patients with isolated severe chronic respiratory failure may have the quality of their lives improved by lung transplantation.

FURTHER READING

BEHRENDT CF: Acute respiratory failure in the United States: Incidence and 31-day survival. Chest 118:1100, 2000

HERTZ MI et al: The registry of the international society for heart and lung transplantation: Nineteenth official report: 2002. J Heart Lung Transplant 21:950, 2002

TOBIN MJ: *Principles and Practice of Mechanical Ventilation.* New York, McGraw-Hill, 1994

———: Advances in mechanical ventilation. N Engl J Med 344:1986, 2001

VINCENT JL et al: The epidemiology of acute respiratory failure in critically ill patients. Chest 121:1602, 2002

YANG KI, TOBIN MJ: A prospective study of indexes predicting the outcome of trials of weaning from mechanical ventilation. N Engl J Med 324:1445, 1991

Acute respiratory distress syndrome (ARDS) is a clinical syndrome of severe dyspnea of rapid onset, hypoxemia, and diffuse pulmonary infiltrates leading to respiratory failure. ARDS is caused by diffuse lung injury from many underlying medical and surgical disorders. The lung injury may be direct, as occurs in toxic inhalation, or indirect, as occurs in sepsis (Table 251-1). The clinical features of ARDS are listed in Table 251-2. Acute lung injury (ALI) is a less severe disorder but has the potential to evolve into ARDS (Table 251-2). The arterial (a) P_{O_2} (in mmHg)/ FI_{O_2} (inspiratory O_2 fraction) <200 mmHg is characteristic of ARDS, while a Pa_{O_2}/FI_{O_2} between 200 and 300 identifies patients with ALI who are likely to benefit from aggressive therapy.

The annual incidences of ALI and ARDS are estimated to be 30/100,000 and 10/100,000, respectively. Approximately 10% of all intensive care unit (ICU) admissions suffer from acute respiratory failure (Chap. 250), with ~20% of these patients meeting criteria for ALI or ARDS.

ETIOLOGY While many medical and surgical illnesses have been associated with the development of ALI and ARDS, most cases (>80%) are caused by a relatively small number of clinical disorders, namely, severe sepsis syndrome and/or bacterial pneumonia (~40 to 50%), trauma, multiple transfusions, aspiration of gastric contents, and drug overdose. Among patients with trauma, pulmonary contusion, multiple bone fractures, and chest wall trauma/flail chest are the most frequently reported surgical conditions in ARDS, whereas head trauma, near-drowning, toxic inhalation, and burns are rare causes. The risks of developing ARDS are increased in patients suffering from more than one predisposing medical or surgical condition; e.g., the risk for ARDS increases from 25% in patients with severe trauma to 56% in patients with trauma and sepsis.

Several other clinical variables have been associated with the development of ARDS. These include older age, chronic alcohol abuse, metabolic acidosis, and severity of critical illness. Trauma patients with an acute physiology and chronic health evaluation (APACHE) II score ≥ 16 (Chap. 249) have a 2.5-fold increase in the risk of developing ARDS, and those with a score > 20 have an incidence of ARDS that is more threefold greater than those with APACHE II scores ≤ 9.

CLINICAL COURSE AND PATHOPHYSIOLOGY The natural history of ARDS is marked by three phases—exudative, proliferative, and fibrotic—each with characteristic clinical and pathologic features (Fig. 251-1).

Exudative Phase In this phase, alveolar capillary endothelial cells and type I pneumocytes (alveolar epithelial cells) are injured, leading to the loss of the normally tight alveolar barrier to fluid and macromolecules. Edema fluid that is rich in protein accumulates in the interstitial and alveolar spaces. Significant concentrations of cytokines (e.g., interleukin 1, interleukin 8, and tumor necrosis factor α) and lipid mediators (e.g., leukotriene B_4) are present in the lung in this early phase. In response to proinflammatory mediators, leukocytes (especially neutrophils) traffick into the pulmonary interstitium and alveoli. In addi-

tion, condensed plasma proteins aggregate in the air spaces with cellular debris and dysfunctional pulmonary surfactant to form hyaline membrane whorls. Pulmonary vascular injury also occurs early in ARDS, with vascular obliteration by microthrombi and fibrocellular proliferation.

Alveolar edema predominantly involves *dependent* portions of the lung, leading to diminished aeration and atelectasis. Collapse of large sections of dependent lung markedly decreases lung compliance. Consequently, intrapulmonary shunting and hypoxemia develop and the work of breathing rises, leading to dyspnea. The pathophysiologic alterations in alveolar spaces are exacerbated by microvascular occlusion, which leads to reductions in pulmonary arterial blood flow to ventilated portions of the lung, increasing the dead space, and pulmonary hypertension. Thus, in addition to severe hypoxemia, hypercapnia secondary to an increase in pulmonary dead space is also prominent in early ARDS.

The exudative phase encompasses the first 7 days of illness after exposure to a precipitating ARDS risk factor, with the patient experiencing the onset of respiratory symptoms. Although usually present within 12 to 36 h after the initial insult, symptoms can be delayed by 5 to 7 days. Dyspnea develops with a sensation of rapid shallow breathing and an inability to get enough air. Tachypnea and increased work of breathing frequently result in respiratory fatigue and ultimately in respiratory failure. Laboratory values are generally nonspecific and primarily indicative of underlying clinical disorders. The chest radiograph usually reveals alveolar and interstitial opacities involving at least three-quarters of the lung fields (Fig. 251-2). While characteristic for ARDS or ALI, these radiographic findings are not specific and can be indistinguishable from cardiogenic pulmonary edema (Chaps. 29 and 255). Unlike the latter, however, the chest x-ray in ARDS rarely shows cardiomegaly, pleural effusions or pulmonary vascular redistribution. Chest computed tomography (CT) scanning in ARDS reveals extensive heterogeneity of lung involvement (Fig. 251-3).

Because the early features of ARDS and ALI are nonspecific, alternative diagnoses must be considered. In the differential diagnosis of ARDS, the most common disorders are cardiogenic pulmonary edema, diffuse pneumonia, and alveolar hemorrhage. Less frequent diagnoses to consider include acute interstitial lung diseases [e.g., acute interstitial pneumonitis (Chap. 243)], acute immunologic injury [e.g, hypersensitivity pneumonitis (Chap. 237)], toxin injury (e.g., radiation pneumonitis), and neurogenic pulmonary edema (Chap. 29).

Proliferative Phase This phase of ARDS usually lasts from day 7 to day 21. Most patients recover rapidly and are liberated from mechanical ventilation during this phase. Despite this improvement, many still experience dyspnea, tachypnea, and hypoxemia. Some patients develop progressive lung injury and early changes of pulmonary fibrosis during the proliferative phase. Histologically, the first signs of resolution are often evident in this phase with the initiation of lung repair,

TABLE 251-1 *Clinical Disorders Commonly Associated with ARDS*

Direct Lung Injury	Indirect Lung Injury
Pneumonia	Sepsis
Aspiration of gastric contents	Severe trauma
Pulmonary contusion	Multiple bone fractures
Near-drowning	Flail chest
Toxic inhalation injury	Head trauma
	Burns
	Multiple transfusions
	Drug overdose
	Pancreatitis
	Post-cardiopulmonary bypass

TABLE 251-2 *Diagnostic Criteria for ALI and ARDS*

Oxygenation	Onset	Chest Radiograph	Absence of Left Atrial Hypertension

ALI:
  $Pa_{O_2}/FI_{O_2} \leq$ 300 mmHg
ARDS:
  $Pa_{O_2}/FI_{O_2} \leq$ 200 mmHg
	Acute	Bilateral alveolar or interstitial infiltrates	PCWP ≤ 18 mmHg *or* no clinical evidence of increased left atrial pressure

Note: ALI, acute lung injury; ARDS, acute respiratory distress syndrome; Pa_{O_2} = arterial partial pressure of O_2; FI_{O_2}, inspired O_2 percentage; PCWP, pulmonary capillary wedge pressure.

Exudative   Proliferative   Fibrotic

Hyaline   Interstitial Inflammation   Fibrosis
Membranes   Interstitial Fibrosis
Edema

Day: 0 2   7   14   21...

FIGURE 251-1 Diagram illustrating the time course for the development and resolution of ARDS. The exudative phase is notable for early alveolar edema and neutrophil-rich leukocytic infiltration of the lungs with subsequent formation of hyaline membranes from diffuse alveolar damage. Within 7 days, a proliferative phase ensues with prominent interstitial inflammation and early fibrotic changes. Approximately 3 weeks after the initial pulmonary injury, some patients enter the fibrotic phase, with substantial fibrosis and bullae formation.

organization of alveolar exudates, and a shift from a neutrophil to a lymphocyte-predominant pulmonary infiltrate. As part of the reparative process, there is a proliferation of type II pneumocytes along alveolar basement membranes. These specialized epithelial cells synthesize new pulmonary surfactant and differentiate into type I pneumocytes. The presence of alveolar type III procollagen peptide, a marker of pulmonary fibrosis, is associated with a protracted clinical course and increased mortality from ARDS.

Fibrotic Phase While many patients with ARDS recover lung function 3 to 4 weeks after the initial pulmonary injury, some will enter a fibrotic phase that may require long-term support on mechanical ventilators and/or supplemental oxygen. Histologically, the alveolar edema and inflammatory exudates of earlier phases are now converted to extensive ductal and interstitial fibrosis. Acinar architecture is markedly disrupted, leading to emphysema-like changes with large bullae. Intimal fibroproliferation in the pulmonary microcirculation leads to progressive vascular occlusion and pulmonary hypertension. The physiologic consequences include an increased risk of pneumothorax, reductions in lung compliance, and increased pulmonary dead space. Patients in this late phase experience a substantial burden of excess morbidity. Lung biopsy evidence for pulmonary fibrosis in any phase of ARDS is associated with increased mortality.

℞ TREATMENT

General Principles Recent reductions in ARDS/ALI mortality are largely the result of general advances in the care of critically ill patients (Chap. 249). Thus, caring for these patients requires close attention to: (1) the recognition and treatment of the underlying medical and surgical disorders (e.g., sepsis, aspiration, trauma); (2) minimizing

procedures and their complications; (3) prophylaxis against venous thromboembolism, gastrointestinal bleeding, and central venous catheter infections; (4) the prompt recognition of nosocomial infections; and (5) provision of adequate nutrition.

Management of Mechanical Ventilation (See also Chap. 252) ■ *VENTILATOR-INDUCED LUNG INJURY* Despite its life-saving potential, mechanical ventilation can aggravate lung injury. Experimental models have demonstrated that ventilator-induced lung injury appears to require two processes: repeated alveolar overdistention and recurrent alveolar collapse. Clearly evident by chest CT (Fig. 251-3), ARDS is a heterogeneous disorder, principally involving dependent portions of the lung with relative sparing of other regions. Because of their differing compliance, attempts to fully inflate the consolidated lung may lead to overdistention and injury to the more "normal" areas of lung. Ventilator-induced injury can be demonstrated in experimental models of ALI, with high tidal volume ventilation resulting in additional, synergistic alveolar damage. These findings led to the hypothesis that ventilating patients suffering from ALI or ARDS with lower tidal volumes would protect against ventilator-induced lung injury and improve clinical outcomes.

A large-scale, randomized controlled trial sponsored by the National Institutes of Health and conducted by the ARDS Network compared low tidal volume (6 mL/kg predicted body weight) ventilation to conventional tidal volume (12 mL/kg predicted body weight) ventilation. Mortality was significantly lower in the low tidal volume patients (31%) compared to the conventional tidal volume patients (40%). This improvement in survival represents the most substantial benefit in ARDS mortality demonstrated for *any* therapeutic intervention in ARDS to date.

PREVENTION OF ALVEOLAR COLLAPSE In ARDS, the presence of alveolar and interstitial fluid and the loss of surfactant can lead to a marked reduction of lung compliance. Without an increase in end-expiratory pressure, significant alveolar collapse can occur at end-expiration, impairing oxygenation. In most clinical settings, positive end-expiratory pressure (PEEP) is empirically set to minimize F_{IO_2} and maximize Pa_{O_2}. On most modern mechanical ventilators, it is possible to construct a static pressure–volume curve for the respiratory system. The lower inflection point on the curve represents alveolar opening (or "recruitment"). The pressure at this point, usually 12 to 15 mmHg in ARDS, is a theoretical "optimal PEEP" for alveolar recruitment. Titration of the PEEP to the lower inflection point on the static pressure–volume curve has been hypothesized to keep the lung open, improving oxygenation and protecting against lung injury. The ARDS Network investigators are currently studying the effect of PEEP on clinical out-

FIGURE 251-2 A representative anteroposterior (AP) chest x-ray in the exudative phase of ARDS that shows diffuse interstitial and alveolar infiltrates, which can be difficult to distinguish from left ventricular failure.

FIGURE 251-3 A representative computed tomographic scan of the chest during the exudative phase of ARDS in which *dependent* alveolar edema and atelectasis predominate.

TABLE 251-3 A Stepwise Approach to Mechanical Ventilation in ARDS

1. Calculate predicted body weight (PBW) in kilogram	Men = 50 + 5.42[height (cm) − 60] Women = 45.5 + 5.42[height (cm) − 60]
2. Ventilator mode	Volume cycle, assist control
3. Tidal volume (V_T)	Initial V_T 8 mL/kg PBW Reduce to 6 mL/kg over 2–4 h if ventilation adequate Goal inspiratory plateau pressures < 30 cmH$_2$O; reduce V_T to as low as 4 mL/kg as needed (and permitted by ventilation) to achieve this goal
4. Oxygenation	Pa$_{O_2}$ goal = 55 – 80 mmHg or pulse oximetry oxygen saturation 88–95% Use the minimal amount of PEEP to keep Fi$_{O_2}$ ≤ 0.6 and meet Pa$_{O_2}$ goal
5. Respiratory rate and acidosis management	Goal arterial pH = 7.30–7.40 If pH < 7.30, increase respiratory rate up to 35 breaths/min If pH < 7.30 and respiratory rate = 35, consider starting intravenous bicarbonate (or equivalent buffer)

If the above strategy fails and the patient is suffering from persistent hypoxemic respiratory failure, *consider* the following:
1. Neuromuscular blocking agents (if not already in use)
2. Prone position ventilation
3. Recruitment maneuvers
4. Inverse ratio ventilation, nitric oxide, high-frequency ventilation, extracorporeal membrane oxygenation, or partial liquid ventilation as part of a clinical research trial.

Note: PEEP, positive end-expiratory pressure.

comes in ARDS; until the results of these studies are available, it is advisable to set PEEP to minimize Fi$_{O_2}$ and optimize Pa$_{O_2}$ using parameters similar to those used by the ARDS Network (Table 251-3).

Oxygenation can also be improved by increasing mean airway pressure with "inverse ratio ventilation." In this technique, the inspiratory (*I*) time is lengthened so that it is longer than the expiratory (*E*) time (*I:E* >1:1). With diminished time to exhale, dynamic hyperinflation leads to increased end-expiratory pressure, similar to ventilator-prescribed PEEP. This mode of ventilation has the advantage of improving oxygenation with lower peak pressures than conventional ventilation. Although inverse ratio ventilation can improve oxygenation and help reduce Fi$_{O_2}$ to ≤ 0.60 to avoid possible oxygen toxicity, no mortality benefit in ARDS has been demonstrated.

Mechanical ventilation in the prone position improves arterial oxygenation, but its effect on important clinical outcomes remains uncertain. Moreover, unless the critical care team is experienced in "proning," repositioning critically ill patients can be hazardous, leading to accidental endotracheal extubation, loss of central venous catheters, and orthopedic injury. Until further studies validate its efficacy, prone position ventilation should be reserved for only the most critically ill ARDS patients.

OTHER STRATEGIES IN MECHANICAL VENTILATION Several additional mechanical ventilation strategies that utilize specialized equipment have been tested in ARDS patients, most with mixed or disappointing results in adults. These include high-frequency ventilation (HFV), i.e., ventilating at extremely high respiratory rates (5 to 20 cycles per second) and low tidal volumes (1 to 2 mL/kg). Also, lung replacement therapy with extracorporeal membrane oxygenation (ECMO), which provides a clear survival benefit in neonatal respiratory distress syndrome, has yet to have proven survival benefit in adults with ARDS. Ongoing research on partial liquid ventilation (PLV) with perfluorocarbon, an inert, high-density liquid that easily solubilizes oxygen and carbon dioxide, has revealed promising preliminary data on pulmonary function in patients with ARDS, but also without survival benefit.

RECOMMENDATIONS Based on current evidence, the approach to mechanical ventilation in Table 251-3 is recommended. Data in support of the efficacy of "adjunctive" ventilator therapies (e.g., high PEEP, inverse ratio ventilation, prone positioning, HFV, ECMO, and PLV) remain incomplete, so these modalities are not routinely used.

Fluid Management Increased pulmonary vascular permeability leading to interstitial and alveolar edema rich in protein is a central feature of ARDS. In addition, impaired vascular integrity augments the normal increase in extravascular lung water that occurs with increasing left atrial pressure. Maintaining a normal or low left atrial filling pressure minimizes pulmonary edema and prevents further decrements in arterial oxygenation and lung compliance, improves pulmonary mechanics, shortens ICU stay and the duration of mechanical ventilation, and is associated with a lower mortality. Thus, aggressive attempts to reduce left atrial filling pressures with fluid restriction and diuretics should be an important aspect of ARDS management, limited only by hypotension and hypoperfusion of critical organs, such as the kidneys.

Glucocorticoids Inflammatory mediators and leukocytes are abundant in the lungs of patients with ARDS. Many attempts have been made to treat both early and late ARDS with glucocorticoids to reduce this potentially deleterious pulmonary inflammation. Few studies have shown any benefit. The ARDS Network is currently conducting a large-scale study of glucocorticoids in ALI and ARDS. Current evidence does *not* support their use in the care of early ARDS patients. On the other hand, if patients fail to improve after 1 week of supportive therapy and have no contraindications to glucocorticoid therapy, providers may wish to consider an *empirical* trial of them in an attempt to speed ARDS resolution.

Other Therapies Clinical trials of surfactant replacement therapy have proven disappointing. Similarly, although several randomized clinical trials of inhaled nitric oxide (NO) in ARDS have demonstrated improved oxygenation, no significant improvement in survival or decrements in time on mechanical ventilation has been observed. Therefore, the use of NO is *not* currently recommended in ARDS.

Recommendations Many clinical trials have been undertaken to improve the outcome of patients with ARDS; most have been unsuccessful in modifying the natural history. The large number and uncertain clinical efficacy of ARDS therapies can make it difficult for clinicians to select a rational treatment plan, and these patients' critical illness can tempt physicians to try unproven and potentially harmful therapies. While results of large clinical trials must be judiciously administered to *individual* patients, an evidenced-based recommendation for ARDS management is summarized in Table 251-4.

PROGNOSIS ■ Mortality Recent mortality estimates for ARDS range from 41 to 65%. There is substantial variability, but a trend towards improved ARDS outcomes appears evident. Of interest, mortality in ARDS

TABLE 251-4 Evidence-Based Recommendations for ARDS Therapies

Treatment	Recommendation[a]
Mechanical ventilation:	
Low tidal volume	A
High-PEEP or "open-lung"	C
Prone position	C
High-frequency ventilation and ECMO	D
Minimize left atrial filling pressures	B
Glucocorticoids	C
Surfactant replacement, inhaled nitric oxide, and other anti-inflammatory therapy (e.g., ketoconazole, PGE$_1$, NSAIDs)	D

[a] **A**, recommended therapy based on strong clinical evidence from randomized clinical trials; **B**, recommended therapy based on supportive but limited clinical data; **C**, indeterminate evidence: recommended only as alternative therapy; **D**, not recommended based on clinical evidence against efficacy of therapy.
Note: PEEP, positive end-expiratory pressure; ECMO, extracorporeal membrane oxygenation; PGE$_1$, prostaglandin E$_1$; NSAIDs, nonsteroidal anti-inflammatory drugs.

is largely attributable to nonpulmonary causes, with sepsis and nonpulmonary organ failure accounting for >80% of deaths. Thus, improvement in survival is likely secondary to advances in the care of septic/infected patients and those with multiple organ failure (Chap. 249).

Several risk factors for mortality to help estimate prognosis have been identified. Similar to the risk factors for developing ARDS, the major risk factors for ARDS mortality are also nonpulmonary. Advanced age is an important risk factor. Patients >75 years have a substantially increased mortality (~60%) compared to those <45 (~20%). Also, patients >60 years with ARDS and sepsis have a threefold higher mortality compared to those <60. Preexisting organ dysfunction from chronic medical illness is an important additional risk factor. In particular, chronic liver disease, cirrhosis, chronic alcohol abuse, chronic immunosuppression, sepsis, chronic renal disease, any nonpulmonary organ failure, and increased APACHE II scores (Chap. 249) have also been linked to increased ARDS mortality. Several factors related to the presenting clinical disorders also increase risk for ARDS mortality. Patients with ARDS from direct lung injury (including pneumonia, pulmonary contusion, and aspiration; Table 251-1) have nearly twice the mortality of those with indirect causes of lung injury, while surgical and trauma patients with ARDS, especially those without direct lung injury, have a better survival rate than other ARDS patients.

Surprisingly, there is little value in predicting ARDS mortality from the extent of hypoxemia and any of the following measures of the severity of lung injury: the level of PEEP used in mechanical ventilation, the respiratory compliance, the extent of alveolar infiltrates on chest radiography, and the lung injury score (a composite of all these variables). However, recent data indicate that an early (within 24 h of presentation) elevation in dead space may predict increased mortality from ARDS.

Functional Recovery in ARDS Survivors While it is common for patients with ARDS to experience prolonged respiratory failure and remain dependent on mechanical ventilation for survival, it is a testament to the resolving powers of the lung that the majority of patients recover nearly normal lung function. Patients usually recover their maximum lung function within 6 months. One year after endotracheal extubation, over a third of ARDS survivors have normal spirometry values and diffusion capacity. Most of the remaining patients have only mild abnormalities in their pulmonary function. Unlike the risk for mortality, recovery of lung function is strongly associated with the extent of lung injury in early ARDS. Low static respiratory compliance, high levels of required PEEP, longer durations of mechanical ventilation, and high lung injury scores are all associated with worse recovery of pulmonary function. When caring for ARDS survivors it is important to be aware of the potential for a substantial burden of emotional and respiratory symptoms. There are significant rates of depression and posttraumatic stress disorder in ARDS survivors.

FURTHER READING

BERNSTEN AD et al: Incidence and mortality of acute lung injury and the acute respiratory distress syndrome in three Australian states. Am J Respir Crit Care Med 165:443, 2002

GATTINONI L et al: Lung structure and function in different stages of severe adult respiratory distress syndrome. JAMA, 271:1772, 1994

HERRIDGE MS et al: One-year outcomes in survivors of the acute respiratory distress syndrome. N Engl J Med 348:683, 2003

MILBERG JA et al: Improved survival of patients with acute respiratory distress syndrome (ARDS): 1983–1993. JAMA 273:306, 1995

THE ACUTE RESPIRATORY DISTRESS SYNDROME NETWORK: Ventilation with lower tidal volumes as compared with traditional tidal volumes for acute lung injury and the acute respiratory distress syndrome. N Engl J Med 342:1301, 2000

WARE LB and MATTHAY MA, The acute respiratory distress syndrome. N Engl J Med 342:1334, 2000

252 MECHANICAL VENTILATORY SUPPORT
Edward P. Ingenito, Jeffrey M. Drazen

Ventilators are specially designed pumps that can support the ventilatory function of the respiratory system and improve oxygenation through application of high oxygen content gas and positive pressure. They are a mainstay of physiologic supportive care (see also Chap. 249).

INDICATIONS FOR MECHANICAL VENTILATION

There are two basic types of respiratory failure, the primary indication for initiation of mechanical ventilation (see also Chap. 250).

1. *Hypoxemic respiratory failure* most commonly results from pulmonary conditions such as severe pneumonia, pulmonary edema, pulmonary hemorrhage, and respiratory distress syndrome causing ventilation-perfusion ($\dot{V}/\dot{Q}$) mismatch and shunt. Hypoxemic respiratory failure is present when arterial O_2 saturation (Sa_{O_2}) < 90% is observed despite an inspired O_2 fraction (FI_{O_2}) > 0.6. The goal of ventilator treatment in this setting is to provide adequate Sa_{O_2} through a combination of supplemental O_2 and specific patterns of ventilation that enhance oxygenation by improving $\dot{V}/\dot{Q}$ matching and reducing intrapulmonary shunt.

2. *Hypercarbic respiratory failure* results from disease states causing either a decrease in minute ventilation or an increase in physiologic dead space such that, despite adequate total minute ventilation, alveolar ventilation is inadequate to meet metabolic demands. Common clinical conditions associated with hypercarbic respiratory failure include neuromuscular diseases, such as myasthenia gravis, ascending polyradiculopathy, and myopathies, and diseases that cause respiratory muscle fatigue due to increased workload, such as asthma, chronic obstructive pulmonary disease, and restrictive lung disease. *Acute* hypercarbic respiratory failure is characterized by arterial P_{CO_2} values >50 mmHg and an arterial pH <7.30.

Mechanical ventilation generally should be instituted in acute hypercarbic respiratory failure. In contrast, the decision to institute ventilator support when components of both acute and chronic hypercarbic respiratory failure are present depends on blood gas parameters and clinical evaluation. In particular, if a patient is not in respiratory distress and is not mentally impaired by CO_2 accumulation, it is not mandatory to initiate mechanical ventilation while other forms of treatment are being administered. The goal of ventilator treatment in hypercarbic respiratory failure is to normalize arterial pH through changes in CO_2 tensions. In patients with severe obstructive or restrictive lung disease, potentially injurious elevation in airway pressures may limit tidal volumes to the extent that normalization of pH is not possible, a situation known as *permissive hypercapnia*.

Accepted therapeutic applications of mechanical ventilation include controlled hyperventilation to reduce cerebral blood flow in patients with increased intracranial pressure (ICP) or to improve pulmonary hemodynamics in patients with postoperative pulmonary hypertension. Mechanical ventilation has also been used to reduce the work of breathing in patients with congestive heart failure, especially in the presence of myocardial ischemia. Ventilator support is also frequently used in conjunction with endotracheal intubation to prevent aspiration of gastric contents in otherwise unstable patients during gastric lavage for suspected drug overdose or during upper gastrointestinal endoscopy. In the critically ill patient, intubation and mechanical ventilation are indicated before essential diagnostic or therapeutic studies if it appears that respiratory failure may occur during these maneuvers.

PHYSIOLOGIC ASPECTS OF MECHANICAL VENTILATION

Mechanical ventilators provide warmed and humidified gas to the airway opening in conformance with various specific volume, pressure, and time patterns. The ventilator serves as the energy source for inspiration, replacing the muscles of the diaphragm and chest wall. Expiration is passive, driven by the recoil of the lungs and chest wall; at the completion of inspiration, internal ventilator circuitry vents the airway to atmospheric pressure or a specified level of positive end-expiratory pressure (PEEP).

PEEP helps maintain patency of alveoli and small airways in the presence of destabilizing factors and therefore reverses hypoxemia and atelectasis by improving matching of ventilation and perfusion. PEEP levels between 0 and 10 cmH$_2$O are generally safe and effective; higher levels are recommended only in the management of significant refractory hypoxemia unresponsive to increments in FI$_{O_2}$ up to 0.6.

ESTABLISHING AND MAINTAINING AN AIRWAY   A cuffed endotracheal tube is often inserted to allow positive-pressure ventilators to deliver conditioned gas, at pressures above atmospheric pressure, to the lungs in a controlled fashion. If neuromuscular paralysis is to be induced during intubation, the use of agents whose mechanism of action includes depolarization at the neuromuscular junction, such as succinylcholine chloride, should be avoided in patients with renal failure, tumor lysis syndrome, crush injuries, medical conditions associated with elevated serum potassium levels, and muscular dystrophy syndromes. Opiates and benzodiazepines can have a deleterious effect on hemodynamics in patients with depressed cardiac function or low systemic vascular resistance and should be used cautiously in this setting. Morphine can promote histamine release from tissue mast cells and may worsen

bronchospasm in patients with asthma; fentanyl, sufentanil, and alfentanil are acceptable alternatives to morphine. Ketamine may increase systemic arterial pressure as well as ICP and has been associated with dramatic hallucinatory responses; it should be used with caution in patients with hypertensive crisis, increased ICP, or a history of psychiatric disorders. Newer agents such as etomidate and propofol have also been used for both induction and maintenance of anesthesia in patients receiving mechanical ventilator support. They are shorter acting and have fewer adverse hemodynamic effects, but are significantly more expensive than older agents.

Patients who require ventilator support for extended periods of time may be candidates for tracheostomy. Although definitive guidelines for performing a tracheostomy in the ventilated patient have not been established, in current clinical practice patients who are anticipated to require ventilator therapy for more than 3 weeks should be considered for this procedure. While it does not clearly reduce the incidence of laryngeal injury or tracheal stenosis, tracheostomy has been associated with improved patient comfort and enhanced ability to partake in rehabilitation-oriented activities.

VENTILATOR MODES   *Mode* refers to the manner in which ventilator breaths are triggered, cycled, and limited; commonly used modes of mechanical ventilation are given in Table 252-1. The *trigger*, either an inspiratory effort or a time-based signal, defines what the ventilator senses to initiate an assisted breath. *Cycle* refers to the factors that determine the end of inspiration. For example, in volume-cycled ventilation, inspiration ends when a specific tidal volume is delivered to the patient. Other types of cycling include pressure cycling, time cycling, and flow cycling. *Limiting factors* are operator-specified values, such as airway pressure, that are monitored by transducers internal to the ventilator circuit throughout the respiratory cycle; if the specified

TABLE 252-1	*Clinical Characteristics of Commonly Used Modes of Mechanical Ventilation*					
Ventilator Mode	Independent Variables (Set by User)	Dependent Variables (Monitored by User)	Trigger/Cycle Limit	Advantages	Disadvantages	Initial Settings
ACMV[a]	FI$_{O_2}$ Tidal volume Ventilator rate Level of PEEP Inspiratory flow pattern Peak inspiratory flow Pressure limit	Peak airway pressure, Pa$_{O_2}$, Pa$_{CO_2}$ Mean airway pressure I/E ratio	Patient/timer Pressure limit	Timer backup Patient-vent synchrony Patient controls minute ventilation	Not useful for weaning Potential for dangerous respiratory alkalosis	FI$_{O_2}$ = 1.0[b] V$_t$ = 10–15 mL/kg[a] f = 12–15/min PEEP = 0–5 cmH$_2$O Inspiratory flow = 60 L/min
SIMV[a]	Same as for ACMV	Same as for ACMV	Same as for ACMV	Timer backup useful for weaning	Potential dysynchrony	Same as for ACMV[a]
CPAP	FI$_{O_2}$ Level of CPAP	Tidal volume Rate, flow pattern Airway pressure Pa$_{O_2}$, Pa$_{CO_2}$, I/E ratio	No trigger Pressure limit	Allows assessment of spontaneous function Helps prevent atelectasis	No backup	FI$_{O_2}$ = 0.5–1.0[b] CPAP = 5–15 cmH$_2$O
PCV[a]	FI$_{O_2}$ Inspiratory pressure level Ventilator rate Level of PEEP Pressure limit I/E ratio	Tidal volume Flow rate, pattern Minute ventilation Pa$_{O_2}$, Pa$_{CO_2}$	Timer/patient Timer/pressure limit	System pressures regulated Useful for barotrauma treatment Timer backup	Requires heavy sedation Not useful for weaning	FI$_{O_2}$ = 1.0[b] PC = 20–40 cmH$_2$O[a] PEEP = 5–10 cmH$_2$O f = 12–15/min I/E = 0.7/1–4/1
PSV	FI$_{O_2}$ Inspiratory pressure level PEEP Pressure limit	Same as for PCV + I/E ratio	Inspiratory flow Pressure limit	Assures synchrony Good for weaning	No timer backup	FI$_{O_2}$ = 0.5–1.0[b] PS = 10–30 cmH$_2$O 5 cmH$_2$O usually the level used PEEP = 0–5 cmH$_2$O

[a] Open lung ventilation (OLV) involves the use of any of these specific modes with tidal volumes (or applied pressures) to achieve 5–6 mL/kg, and positive end expiratory pressures achieve maximal alveolar recruitment.

[b] FI$_{O_2}$ is usually set to 1.0 initially, unless there is a specific clinical indication to minimize FI$_{O_2}$, such as history of chemotherapy with bleomycin. Once adequate oxygenation is documented by blood gas analysis, FI$_{O_2}$ should be decreased in decrements of 0.1–0.2 as tolerated, until the lowest FI$_{O_2}$ required for an Sa$_{O_2}$ >90% is achieved.

Abbreviations: f, frequency; I/E, inspiration/expiration; FI$_{O_2}$, inspired O$_2$; PEEP, positive end-expiratory pressure; for ventilator modes, see text; V$_t$, tidal ventilation.

values are exceeded, inspiratory flow is immediately stopped, and the ventilator circuit is vented to atmospheric pressure or the specified PEEP.

Assist Control Mode Ventilation (ACMV)   An inspiratory cycle is initiated either by the patient's inspiratory effort or, if no patient effort is detected within a specified time window, by a timer signal within the ventilator. Every breath delivered, whether patient or timer triggered, consists of the operator-specified tidal volume. Ventilatory rate is determined either by the patient or by the operator-specified backup rate, whichever is of higher frequency (Fig. 252-1A). ACMV is commonly used for initiation of mechanical ventilation because it ensures a backup minute ventilation in the absence of an intact respiratory drive

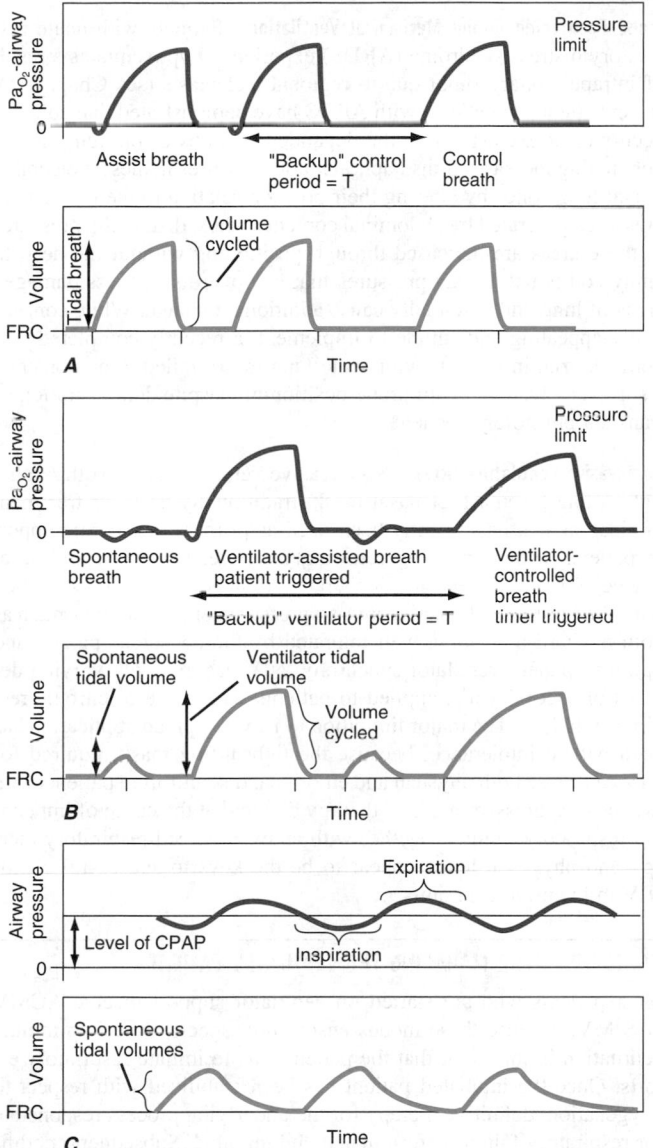

A. Airway pressure and lung volume versus time profile during assist control mode ventilation (ACMV). Assisted breaths are triggered by the patient's effort. Controlled breaths are triggered by the ventilator timer. Every breath, whether triggered by the patient or by the timer, is a complete volume-cycled breath, with airway pressure as a dependent variable. The pressure limit is set above the peak inspiratory pressure. **B.** Airway pressure and lung volume versus time profiles during synchronized intermittent mandatory ventilation (SIMV). Spontaneous breaths occur between patient-triggered assisted breaths and timer-triggered breaths. The tidal volume of the spontaneous breaths is determined by the patient's effort and lung impedance. Assisted and controlled breaths are volume cycled. **C.** Airway pressure and lung volume versus time profiles during continuous positive airway pressure (CPAP). Breathing is spontaneous, and no ventilator assist is provided. The spontaneous profile is superimposed on an elevated mean airway pressure that the user specifies. FRC, functional residual capacity.

and allows for synchronization of the ventilator cycle with the patient's inspiratory effort.

Problems can arise when ACMV is used in patients with tachypnea due to nonrespiratory or nonmetabolic factors such as anxiety, pain, or airway irritation. Respiratory alkalemia may develop and trigger myoclonus or seizures. Dynamic hyperinflation (so-called auto-PEEP) may occur if the patient's respiratory mechanics are such that inadequate time is available for complete exhalation between inspiratory cycles. Auto-PEEP can limit venous return, decrease cardiac output, and increase airway pressures, predisposing to barotrauma. ACMV is not effective for weaning patients from mechanical ventilation because it provides full ventilator assistance on each patient-initiated breath.

Synchronized Intermittent Mandatory Ventilation (SIMV)   The major difference between SIMV and ACMV is that in the former the patient is allowed to breathe spontaneously, i.e., without ventilator assist, between delivered ventilator breaths. However, mandatory breaths are delivered in synchrony with the patient's inspiratory efforts at a frequency determined by the operator. If the patient fails to initiate a breath, the ventilator delivers a fixed-tidal-volume breath and resets the internal timer for the next inspiratory cycle (Fig. 252-1B). SIMV differs from ACMV in that only the preset number of breaths is ventilator-assisted.

SIMV allows patients with an intact respiratory drive to exercise inspiratory muscles between assisted breaths, making it useful for both supporting and weaning intubated patients. SIMV may be difficult to use in patients with tachypnea because they may attempt to exhale during the ventilator-programmed inspiratory cycle. When this occurs, the airway pressure may exceed the inspiratory pressure limit, the ventilator-assisted breath will be aborted, and minute volume may drop below that programmed by the operator. In this setting, if the tachypnea is in response to respiratory or metabolic acidosis, a change to ACMV will increase minute ventilation and help normalize the pH while the underlying process is further evaluated.

Continuous Positive Airway Pressure (CPAP)   This is not a true support-mode of ventilation, inasmuch as all ventilation occurs through the patient's spontaneous efforts. The ventilator provides fresh gas to the breathing circuit with each inspiration and charges the circuit to a constant, operator-specified pressure that can range from 0 to 20 cmH₂O (Fig. 252-1C). CPAP is used to assess extubation potential in patients who have been effectively weaned and are requiring little ventilator support and in patients with intact respiratory system function who require an endotracheal tube for airway protection.

Pressure-Control Ventilation (PCV)   This form of ventilation is time triggered, time cycled, and pressure limited. During the inspiratory phase, a given pressure is imposed at the airway opening, and the pressure remains at this user-specified level throughout inspiration (Fig. 252-2A). Since inspiratory airway pressure is specified by the operator, tidal volume and inspiratory flow rate are *dependent* rather than *independent* variables and are not user specified. PCV is the preferred mode of ventilation for patients with documented barotrauma, because airway pressures can be limited, and for postoperative thoracic surgical patients, in whom the shear forces across a fresh suture line should be limited. When PCV is used, minute ventilation and tidal volume must be monitored; minute ventilation is altered through changes in rate or in the pressure-control value.

PCV with the use of a prolonged inspiratory time is frequently applied to patients with severe hypoxemic respiratory failure. This approach, called inverse inspiratory-to-expiratory ratio ventilation (IRV), increases mean distending pressures without increasing peak airway pressures. It is thought to work in conjunction with PEEP to open collapsed alveoli and improve oxygenation. IRV may be associated with fewer deleterious effects than conventional volume-cycled ventilation, which requires higher peak airway pressures to achieve an equivalent reduction in shunt fraction, but there are no convincing data to show that IRV improves outcomes.

FIGURE 252-1

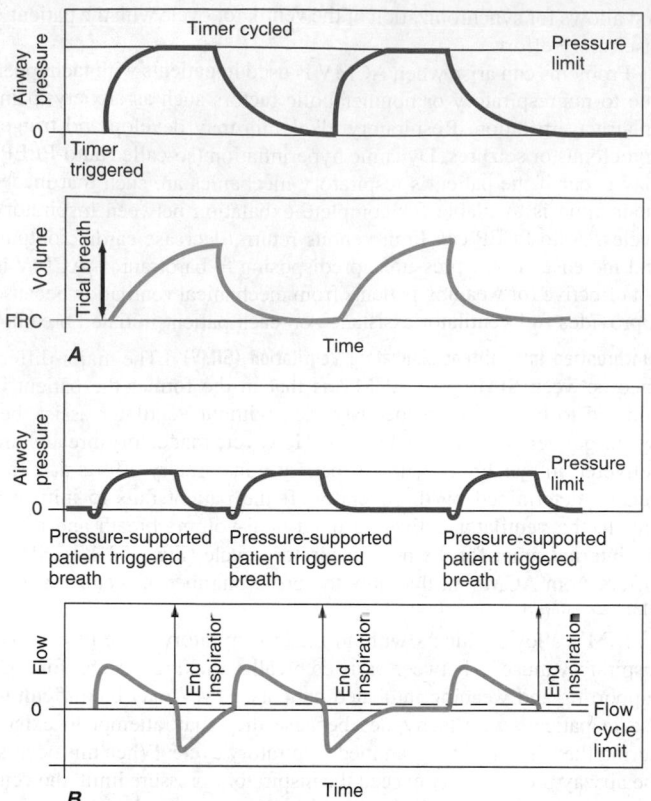

FIGURE 252-2 *A.* Airway pressure and lung volume versus time profiles during pressure-control ventilation (PCV). All breaths are timer triggered, timer cycled, and pressure limited. Peak airway pressure is set by the operator, and tidal volume is a dependent variable. The profiles shown here display the pressure limit as slightly higher than pressure-control level. This need not be the case, but it is appropriate to set the pressure limit only slightly above the pressure-control level when using this mode of ventilation for management of the patient with barotrauma. *B.* Airway pressure and airway flow versus time profiles during pressure-support ventilation (PSV). All breaths are patient triggered and flow cycled. Inspiration is cycled off when the inspiratory flow drops below a predetermined threshold internally set in the ventilator circuit. In the example shown, the pressure limit is slightly greater than the pressure-support level. Since each can be set independently, this need not be the case. FRC, functional residual capacity.

Pressure-Support Ventilation (PSV)   This form of ventilation is patient triggered, flow cycled, and pressure limited; it is specifically designed for use in the weaning process. During PSV, the inspiratory phase is terminated when inspiratory airflow falls below a certain level; in most ventilators this flow rate cannot be adjusted by the operator. When PSV is used, patients receive ventilator assist only when the ventilator detects an inspiratory effort (Fig. 252-2*B*). PSV can also be used in combination with SIMV to ensure volume-cycled backup for patients whose respiratory drive is depressed.

PSV is well tolerated by most patients who are being weaned; PSV parameters can be set to provide fully or nearly fully ventilatory support and can be withdrawn slowly over a period of days in a systematic fashion to gradually load the respiratory muscles.

Open Lung Ventilation (OLV)   OLV is not a distinct mode of ventilation, but rather a strategy for applying either volume-cycled or pressure-control ventilation to patients with severe respiratory failure. In OLV, the primary objectives of ventilator support are maintenance of adequate oxygenation and avoidance of cyclic opening and closing of alveolar units by selecting a level of PEEP that allows the majority of units to remain inflated during tidal ventilation. Achievement of eucapnia and normal blood pH through adjustments in ventilator tidal volume and breathing frequency are of lower priority. Clinical and experimental observations indicate that high airway pressures and repeated opening and closing of alveoli can cause microstructural lung

damage, propagation of lung injury through generation of inflammatory cytokines, and direct barotrauma. Current data suggest that a small tidal volume (i.e., 6 mL/kg) provides adequate ventilatory support with a lower incidence of adverse effects than more conventional tidal volumes of 10 to 15 mL/kg. Hypercapnia and consequent respiratory acidosis tend to be well tolerated physiologically, except in patients with significant hemodynamic compromise, ventricular dysfunction, cardiac dysrrhythmias, or increased ICP. Furthermore, there are recent data to suggest that hypercapnia may have direct beneficial anti-inflammatory effects. OLV has been used most extensively in the management of patients with hypoxemic respiratory failure due to acute lung injury. Although few randomized clinical trials of OLV have been performed, available data suggest that this strategy reduces the mortality rate and improves gas exhange in patients with acute lung injury.

Prone Positioning during Mechanical Ventilation   Patients with acute respiratory distress syndrome (ARDS) experience hypoxemia as a result of intrapulmonary shunt due to regional atelectasis (see Chap. 251). Recent studies in patients with ARDS have demonstrated that collapse occurs most extensively in the dependent regions of the lung. Prone positioning increases transdiaphragmatic pressures in these atelectatic, dorsal lung zones by altering their position relative to the hydrostatic pressures generated by abdominal contents. Thus, distending pressures in these areas are increased through positioning without the need to apply additional airway pressures that can overdistend less damaged areas of lung and potentially cause additional damage. While conceptually appealing and simple to implement, a recently completed randomized trial in patients with acute lung injury failed to demonstrate a survival advantage with prone positioning despite demonstration of transient physiologic benefit.

Noninvasive Ventilation (NIV)   Noninvasive ventilator support through a tight-fitting facemask or nasal mask, traditionally used for treatment of sleep apnea, has recently been used as primary ventilator support in patients with impending respiratory failure. Facemask and nasal devices for administering NIV therapy are most frequently combined with PSV or bi-level positive airway pressure ventilation, inasmuch as both of these modes are well tolerated by the conscious patient and optimize patient-ventilator synchrony. NIV has met with varying degrees of success when applied to patients with acute or chronic respiratory failure. The major limitation to its widespread application has been patient intolerance, because the tight-fitting mask required for NIV can cause both physical and emotional discomfort in patients with dyspnea. Aggressive medical therapy directed at the cause of impending respiratory failure, together with an experienced respiratory therapy and physician team, appear to be the keys to successful use of NIV in intensive care units.

GUIDELINES FOR MANAGING THE VENTILATED PATIENT

Most patients who are started on ventilator support receive ACMV or SIMV, because these modes ensure user-specified backup minute ventilation in the event that the patient fails to initiate respiratory efforts. Once the intubated patient has been stabilized with respect to oxygenation, definitive therapy for the underlying process responsible for respiratory failure is formulated and initiated. Subsequent modifications in ventilator therapy must be provided in parallel with changes in the patient's clinical status. As improvement in respiratory function is noted, the first priorities are to reduce PEEP and supplemental O_2. Once a patient can achieve adequate arterial saturation with an $FI_{O_2} \leq 0.5$ and 5 cmH$_2$O PEEP, attempts should be made to reduce the level of mechanical ventilatory support. Patients previously on full ventilator support should be switched to a ventilator mode that allows for weaning, such as SIMV, PSV, or SIMV combined with PSV. Ventilator therapy can then be gradually removed, as outlined in the section on weaning. Patients whose condition continues to deteriorate after ventilator support is initiated may require increased O_2, PEEP, and alternative modes of ventilation such as IRV or OLV.

GENERAL SUPPORT IN THE VENTILATED PATIENT

Patients who are started on mechanical ventilation usually require some form of sedation and analgesia to maintain an acceptable level of comfort. Often, this regimen consists of a combination of a benzodiazepine and opiate administered intravenously. Medications commonly used for this purpose include lorazepam, midazolam, diazepam, morphine, and fentanyl.

Immobilized patients in the intensive care unit on mechanical ventilator support are at increased risk for deep venous thrombosis; accepted practice consists of administering prophylaxis in the form of subcutaneous heparin and/or pneumatic compression boots. Fractionated low-molecular-weight heparin has also been used for this purpose; it appears to be equally effective and is associated with a decreased incidence of heparin-associated thrombocytopenia.

Prophylaxis against diffuse gastrointestinal mucosal injury is indicated for patients who have suffered a neurologic insult or those with severe respiratory failure in association with ARDS. Histamine receptor antagonists (H_2-receptor antagonists), antacids, and cytoprotective agents such as carafate have all been used for this purpose and appear to be effective. Recent data suggest that carafate use is associated with a reduction in the incidence of nosocomial pneumonias, since it does not cause changes in stomach pH and is less likely to permit colonization of the gastrointestinal tract by nosocomial organisms at neutral pH.

Nutrition support by enteral feeding through either a nasogastric or an orogastric tube should be maintained in all intubated patients whenever possible. In those patients with a normal baseline nutritional state, support should be initiated within 7 days. In malnourished patients, nutrition support should be initiated within 72 h. Delayed gastric emptying is common in critically ill patients on sedative medications but often responds to promotility agents such as metoclopramide. Parenteral nutrition is an alternative to enteral nutrition in patients with severe gastrointestinal pathology.

COMPLICATIONS OF MECHANICAL VENTILATION

Endotracheal intubation and positive-pressure mechanical ventilation have direct and indirect effects on several organ systems, including the lung and upper airways, the cardiovascular system, and the gastrointestinal system. Pulmonary complications include barotrauma, nosocomial pneumonia, oxygen toxicity, tracheal stenosis, and deconditioning of respiratory muscles. *Barotrauma*, which occurs when high pressures (i.e., > 50 cmH_2O) overdistend and disrupt lung tissue, is clinically manifest by interstitial emphysema, pneumomediastinum, subcutaneous emphysema, or pneumothorax. Although the first three conditions may resolve simply through the reduction of airway pressures, clinically significant pneumothorax, as indicated by hypoxemia, decreased lung compliance, and hemodynamic compromise, requires tube thoracostomy.

Patients intubated for longer than 72 h are at high risk for ventilator associated pneumonia as a result of aspiration from the upper airways through small leaks around the endotracheal tube cuff; the most common organisms responsible for this condition are enteric gram-negative rods, *Staphylococcus aureus*, and anaerobic bacteria. Because the endotracheal tube and upper airways of patients on mechanical ventilation are commonly colonized with bacteria, the diagnosis of nosocomial pneumonia requires "protected brush" bronchoscopic sampling of airway secretions coupled with quantitative microbiologic techniques to differentiate colonization from infection.

Hypotension resulting from elevated intrathoracic pressures with decreased venous return is almost always responsive to intravascular volume repletion. In patients judged to have hypotension or respiratory failure on the basis of alveolar edema, hemodynamic monitoring with a pulmonary arterial catheter may be of value in optimizing O_2 delivery via manipulation of intravascular volume and FI_{O_2} and PEEP levels.

Gastrointestinal effects of positive-pressure ventilation include *stress ulceration* and *mild to moderate cholestasis*. It is common practice to provide prophylaxis with H_2-receptor antagonists or sucralfate for stress-related ulcers. Mild cholestasis [i.e., total bilirubin values ≤ 68 $\mu mol/L$ (≤ 4.0 mg/dL)] attributable to the effects of increased intrathoracic pressures on portal vein pressures is common and generally self-limited. Cholestasis of a more severe degree should not be attributed to a positive-pressure ventilation response and is more likely due to a primary hepatic process.

WEANING FROM MECHANICAL VENTILATION

Removal of mechanical ventilator support requires that a number of criteria be met. Upper airway function must be intact for a patient to remain extubated but is difficult to assess in the intubated patient. Therefore, if a patient can breathe on his or her own through an endotracheal tube but develops stridor or recurrent aspiration once the tube is removed, upper airway dysfunction or an abnormal swallowing mechanism should be suspected and plans for achieving a stable airway developed. An intact cough during suctioning is a good indicator of a patient's ability to mobilize secretions. Respiratory drive and chest wall function are assessed by observation of respiratory rate, tidal volume, inspiratory pressure, and vital capacity. The weaning index, defined as the ratio of breathing frequency to tidal volume (breaths per minute per liter), is both sensitive and specific for predicting the likelihood of successful extubation. When this ratio is less than 105 with the patient breathing without mechanical assistance through an endotracheal tube, successful extubation is likely. An inspiratory pressure of more than -30 cmH_2O and a vital capacity of greater than 10 mL/kg are considered indicators of acceptable chest wall and diaphragm function. Alveolar ventilation is generally adequate when elimination of CO_2 is sufficient to maintain arterial pH in the range of 7.35 to 7.40, and an $Sa_{O_2} > 90\%$ can be achieved with an $FI_{O_2} < 0.5$ and a PEEP ≤ 5 cmH_2O. Although many patients may not meet all criteria for weaning, the likelihood that a patient will tolerate extubation without difficulty increases as more criteria are met.

Many approaches to weaning patients from ventilator support have been advocated. T-piece and CPAP weaning are best tolerated by patients who have undergone mechanical ventilation for brief periods and require little respiratory muscle reconditioning, whereas SIMV and PSV are best for patients who have been intubated for extended periods and require gradual respiratory-muscle reconditioning.

T-piece weaning involves brief spontaneous breathing trials with supplemental O_2. These trials are usually initiated for 5 min/h followed by a 1-h interval of rest. T-piece trials are increased in 5- to 10-min increments until the patient can remain ventilator independent for periods of several hours. Extubation can then be attempted. CPAP weaning is similar to T-piece weaning except that trials of spontaneous breathing are conducted on the ventilator in CPAP mode.

Weaning by means of SIMV involves gradually tapering the mandatory backup rate in increments of 2 to 4 breaths per minute while monitoring blood gas parameters and respiratory rates. Rates of greater than 25 breaths per minute on withdrawal of mandatory ventilator breaths generally indicate respiratory muscle fatigue and the need to combine periods of exercise with periods of rest. Exercise periods are gradually increased until a patient remains stable on SIMV at 4 breaths per minute or less without needing rest at higher SIMV rates. A CPAP or T-piece trial can then be attempted before planned extubation.

PSV, as described in detail above, is used primarily for weaning from mechanical ventilation. PSV is usually initiated at a level adequate for full ventilator support (PSV_{max}); i.e., PSV is set slightly below the peak inspiratory pressures required by the patient during volume-cycled ventilation. The level of pressure support is then gradually withdrawn in increments of 5 cmH_2O until a level is reached at which the respiratory rate increases to 25 breaths per minute. At this point, intermittent periods of higher-pressure support are alternated with periods of lower-pressure support to provide muscle reconditioning without causing diaphragmatic fatigue. Gradual withdrawal of PSV continues until the level of support is just adequate to overcome the resistance of the endotracheal tube (approximately 5 to 10 cmH_2O). Support can be discontinued and the patient extubated.

FURTHER READING

AMATO MBP et al: Effect of a protective-ventilation strategy on mortality in the acute respiratory distress syndrome. N Engl J Med 338:347, 1998

BOZEMAN YP et al: Etomidate as a sole agent for endotracheal intubation in the prehospital air medical setting. Air Med J 21:32, 2002

ESTEBAN A et al: A comparison of four methods of weaning patients from mechanical ventilation. N Engl J Med 332:345, 1995

GATTINONI L et al: Effect of prone positioning on the survival of patients with acute respiratory failure. N Engl J Med 345:568, 2001

INGENITO EP, DRAZEN JM: Mechanical ventilators, in *Principles of Critical Care*, 2d ed, JB Hall, GA Schmidt, LDH Wood (eds). New York, McGraw-Hill, 1997, pp 142–154

TOBIN MJ: Advances in mechanical ventilation. N Engl J Med 344:1986, 2001

Section 2   Shock and Cardiac Arrest

253   APPROACH TO THE PATIENT WITH SHOCK
Ronald V. Maier

Shock is the clinical syndrome that results from inadequate tissue perfusion. Irrespective of cause, the hypoperfusion-induced imbalance between the delivery of and requirements for oxygen and substrate leads to cellular dysfunction. The cellular injury created by the inadequate delivery of oxygen and substrates also induces the production and release of inflammatory mediators that further compromise perfusion through functional and structural changes within the microvasculature. This leads to a vicious cycle in which impaired perfusion is responsible for cellular injury which causes maldistribution of blood flow, further compromising cellular perfusion; the latter causes multiple organ failure and, if the process is not interrupted, leads to the death of the patient. The clinical manifestations of shock are the result, in part, of sympathetic neuroendocrine responses to hypoperfusion as well as the breakdown in organ function induced by severe cellular dysfunction.

When very severe and/or persistent, inadequate oxygen delivery leads to irreversible cell injury; thus, only rapid restoration of oxygen delivery can reverse the progression of the shock state. The fundamental approach to management, therefore, is to recognize overt and impending shock in a timely fashion and to intervene emergently to restore perfusion. This requires the expansion or reexpansion of blood volume. Control of any inciting pathologic process, e.g., continued hemorrhage, impairment of cardiac function, or infection, must occur simultaneously.

Clinical shock is usually accompanied by hypotension, i.e., a mean arterial pressure <60 mmHg in previously normotensive persons. Multiple classification schemes have been developed in an attempt to synthesize the seemingly dissimilar processes leading to shock. Strict adherence to a classification scheme may be difficult from a clinical standpoint because of the frequent combination of two or more causes of shock in any individual patient, but the classification shown in Table 253-1 provides a useful reference point from which to discuss and further delineate the underlying processes.

PATHOGENESIS AND ORGAN RESPONSE

MICROCIRCULATION Normally when cardiac output falls, systemic vascular resistance rises to maintain a level of systemic pressure that is adequate for perfusion of the heart and brain at the expense of other tissues such as muscle, skin, and especially the gastrointestinal tract. Systemic vascular resistance is determined primarily by the luminal diameter of arterioles. The metabolic rates of the heart and brain are high, and their stores of energy substrate are low. These organs are critically dependent on a continuous supply of oxygen and nutrients, and neither tolerates severe ischemia for more than brief periods. Autoregulation, i.e., the maintenance of blood flow over a wide range of perfusion pressures, is critical in sustaining cerebral and coronary perfusion despite significant hypotension. However, when mean arterial pressure drops to ≤60 mmHg, flow to these organs falls and their function deteriorates.

Arteriolar vascular smooth muscle has both α- and β-adrenergic receptors. The α_1 receptors mediate vasoconstriction, while the β_2 receptors mediate vasodilation. Efferent sympathetic fibers release norepinephrine, which acts primarily on α_1 receptors in one of the most fundamental compensatory responses to reduced perfusion pressure. Other constrictor substances that are increased in most forms of shock include angiotensin II, vasopressin, endothelin-1, and thromboxane A_2. Both norepinephrine and epinephrine are released by the adrenal medulla, and the concentrations of these catecholamines in the bloodstream rise. Circulating vasodilators in shock include prostacyclin [prostaglandin (PG)I_2], nitric oxide (NO), and, importantly, products of local metabolism such as adenosine that match flow to the metabolic needs of the tissue. The balance between these various vasoconstrictor and vasodilator influences acting upon the microcirculation determines local perfusion.

Transport to cells depends on microcirculatory flow; capillary permeability; the diffusion of oxygen, carbon dioxide, nutrients, and products of metabolism through the interstitium; and the exchange of these products across cell membranes. Impairment of the microcirculation, which is central to the pathophysiologic responses in the late stages of all forms of shock, results in the derangement of cellular metabolism, which is ultimately responsible for organ failure.

The endogenous response to mild or moderate hypovolemia is an attempt at restitution of intravascular volume through alterations in hydrostatic pressure and osmolarity. Constriction of arterioles leads to reductions in both the capillary hydrostatic pressure and the number of capillary beds perfused, thereby limiting the capillary surface area across which filtration occurs. When filtration is reduced while intravascular oncotic pressure remains constant or rises, there is net reabsorption of fluid into the vascular bed, in accord with Starling's law of capillary-interstitial liquid exchange (Chap. 29). Metabolic changes (including hyperglycemia and elevations in the products of glycolysis, lipolysis, and proteolysis) raise extracellular osmolarity, leading to an osmotic gradient between cells and interstitium that increases interstitial and intravascular volume at the expense of intracellular volume.

CELLULAR RESPONSES Interstitial transport of nutrients is impaired, leading to a decline of intracellular high-energy phosphate stores. Mitochondrial dysfunction and uncoupling of oxidative phosphorylation are the most likely causes for decreased amounts of ATP. As a consequence, there is an accumulation of hydrogen ions, lactate, and other products of anaerobic metabolism. As shock progresses, these vasodilator metabolites override vasomotor tone, causing further hypotension and hypoperfusion. Dysfunction of cell membranes is thought to represent a common end-stage pathophysiologic pathway in the various forms of shock. Normal cellular transmembrane potential falls,

TABLE 253-1   *Classification of Shock*

Hypovolemic	Septic
Traumatic	Hyperdynamic
Cardiogenic	Hypodynamic
Intrinsic	Neurogenic
Compressive	Hypoadrenal

and there is an associated increase in intracellular sodium and water, leading to cell swelling, which interferes further with microvascular perfusion.

NEUROENDOCRINE RESPONSE Hypovolemia, hypotension, and hypoxia are sensed by baroreceptors and chemoreceptors, which contribute to an autonomic response that attempts to restore blood volume, maintain central perfusion, and mobilize metabolic substrates. Hypotension disinhibits the vasomotor center, resulting in increased adrenergic output and reduced vagal activity. Release of norepinephrine induces peripheral and splanchnic vasoconstriction, a major contributor to the maintenance of central organ perfusion, while reduced vagal activity increases the heart rate and cardiac output. The effects of circulating epinephrine released by the adrenal medulla in shock are largely metabolic, causing increased glycogenolysis and gluconeogenesis and reduced pancreatic insulin release. Epinephrine also inhibits production and release of inflammatory mediators through stimulation of β-adrenergic receptors on innate immune cells.

Severe pain and other severe stress cause the hypothalamic release of adrenocorticotropic hormone (ACTH). This stimulates cortisol secretion, which contributes to decreased peripheral uptake of glucose and amino acids, enhances lipolysis, and increases gluconeogenesis. Increased pancreatic secretion of glucagon during stress accelerates hepatic gluconeogenesis and further elevates blood glucose concentration. These hormonal actions act synergistically in the maintenance of blood volume. Many critically ill patients exhibit low plasma cortisol levels and an impaired response to ACTH stimulation. The importance of the cortisol response to stress is illustrated by the profound circulatory collapse that occurs in hypoadrenal patients (see below).

Renin release is increased in response to adrenergic discharge and reduced perfusion of the juxtaglomerular apparatus in the kidney. Renin induces the formation of angiotensin I, which is then converted to angiotensin II, an extremely potent vasoconstrictor and stimulator of aldosterone release by the adrenal cortex and of vasopressin by the posterior pituitary. Aldosterone contributes to the maintainance of intravascular volume by enhancing renal tubular reabsorption of sodium, resulting in the excretion of a low-volume, concentrated, sodium-free urine. Vasopressin has a direct action on vascular smooth muscle, contributing to vasoconstriction, and acts on the distal renal tubules to enhance water reabsorption.

CARDIOVASCULAR RESPONSE Three variables—ventricular filling (preload), the resistance to ventricular ejection (afterload), and myocardial contractility—are paramount in controlling stroke volume (Chap. 215). Cardiac output, the major determinant of tissue perfusion, is the product of stroke volume and heart rate. Hypovolemia leads to decreased ventricular preload, which in turn reduces the stroke volume. An increase in heart rate is a useful but limited compensatory mechanism to maintain cardiac output. A shock-induced reduction in myocardial compliance is frequent, reducing ventricular end-diastolic volume and hence stroke volume at any given ventricular filling pressure. Restoration of intravascular volume returns stroke volume to normal but only at elevated filling pressures. In addition, sepsis, ischemia, myocardial infarction, severe tissue trauma, hypothermia, general anesthesia, prolonged hypotension, and acidemia may all impair myocardial contractility and also reduce the stroke volume at any given ventricular end-diastolic volume. The resistance to ventricular ejection is significantly influenced by the systemic vascular resistance, which is elevated in most forms of shock. However, resistance is depressed in the early hyperdynamic stage of septic shock (see below), thereby allowing the cardiac output to be maintained or elevated.

The venous system contains nearly two-thirds of the total circulating blood volume, most in the small veins, and serves as a dynamic reservoir for autoinfusion of blood. Active venoconstriction as a consequence of α-adrenergic activity is an important compensatory mechanism for the maintenance of venous return and therefore of ventricular filling during shock. On the other hand, venous dilatation, as occurs in neurogenic shock, reduces ventricular filling and hence stroke volume and cardiac output (see below).

PULMONARY RESPONSE The response of the pulmonary vascular bed to shock parallels that of the systemic vascular bed, and the relative increase in pulmonary vascular resistance, particularly in septic shock, may exceed that of the systemic vascular resistance. Shock-induced tachypnea reduces tidal volume and increases both dead space and minute ventilation. Relative hypoxia and the subsequent tachypnea induce a respiratory alkalosis. Recumbency and involuntary restriction of ventilation secondary to pain reduce functional residual capacity and may lead to atelectasis. Shock is recognized as a major cause of acute lung injury and subsequent acute respiratory distress syndrome (ARDS; Chap. 251). These disorders are characterized by noncardiogenic pulmonary edema secondary to diffuse pulmonary capillary endothelial and alveolar epithelial injury, hypoxemia, and bilateral diffuse pulmonary infiltrates. Hypoxemia results from perfusion of underventilated and nonventilated alveoli. Loss of surfactant and lung volume in combination with increased interstitial and alveolar edema reduce lung compliance. The work of breathing and the oxygen requirements of respiratory muscles increase.

RENAL RESPONSE Acute renal failure (Chap. 260), a serious complication of shock and hypoperfusion, occurs less frequently than heretofore because of early aggressive volume repletion. Acute tubular necrosis is now more frequently seen as a result of the interactions of shock, sepsis, the administration of nephrotoxic agents (such as aminoglycosides and angiographic contrast media), and rhabdomyolysis; the latter may be particularly severe in skeletal muscle trauma. The physiologic response of the kidney to hypoperfusion is to conserve salt and water. In addition to decreased renal blood flow, increased afferent arteriolar resistance accounts for diminished glomerular filtration rate, which together with increased aldosterone and vasopressin is responsible for reduced urine formation. Toxic injury causes necrosis of tubular epithelium and tubular obstruction by cellular debris with back-leak of filtrate. The depletion of renal ATP stores that occurs with prolonged renal hypoperfusion contributes to subsequent impairment of renal function. There is no convincing evidence that low-dose dopamine protects against acute renal failure.

METABOLIC DERANGEMENTS During shock, there is disruption of the normal cycles of carbohydrate, lipid, and protein metabolism. Through the citric acid cycle, alanine in conjunction with lactate (which is converted from pyruvate in the periphery in the presence of oxygen deprivation) enhances the hepatic production of glucose. With reduced availability of oxygen, the breakdown of glucose to pyruvate and ultimately lactate represents an inefficient cycling of substrate with minimal net energy production. An elevated plasma lactate/pyruvate ratio is consistent with anaerobic metabolism and reflects inadequate tissue perfusion. Decreased clearance of exogenous triglycerides coupled with increased hepatic lipogenesis causes a significant rise in serum triglyceride concentrations. There is increased protein catabolism, a negative nitrogen balance, and, if the process is prolonged, severe muscle wasting.

INFLAMMATORY RESPONSES Activation of an extensive network of proinflammatory mediator systems plays a significant role in the progression of shock and contributes importantly to the development of organ injury and failure.

Multiple humoral mediators are activated during shock and tissue injury. The complement cascade, activated through both the classic and alternate pathways, generates the anaphylatoxins C3a and C5a. Direct complement fixation to injured tissues can progress to the C5-C9 attack complex, causing further cell damage. Activation of the coagulation cascade causes microvascular thrombosis, with subsequent lysis leading to repeated episodes of ischemia and reperfusion. Components of the coagulation system, such as thrombin, are potent proinflammatory mediators that cause expression of adhesion molecules on endothelial cells and activation of neutrophils, leading to microvascular injury. Coagulation also activates the kallekrein-kininogen cascade, contributing to hypotension.

TABLE 253-2 *Normal Hemodynamic Parameters*

Parameter	Calculation	Normal Values
Cardiac output (CO)	SV × HR	4–8 L/min
Cardiac index (CI)	CO/BSA	2.6–4.2 (L/min)/m²
Stroke volume (SV)	CO/HR	50–100 mL/beat
Systemic vascular resistance (SVR)	[(MAP − RAP)/CO] × 80	700–1600 dynes · s/cm⁵
Pulmonary vascular resistance (PVR)	[(PAP$_m$ − PCWP)/CO] × 80	20–130 dynes · s/cm⁵
Left ventricular stroke work (LVSW)	SV(MAP − PCWP) × 0.0136	60–80 g-m/beat
Right ventricular stroke work (RVSW)	SV(PAP$_m$ − RAP)	10–15 g-m/beat

Note: HR, heart rate; BSA, body surface area; MAP, mean arterial pressure; RAP, right atrial pressure; PAP$_m$, pulmonary artery pressure—mean; PCWP, pulmonary capillary wedge pressure.

Eicosanoids are vasoactive and immunomodulatory products of arachidonic acid metabolism that include cyclooxygenase-derived prostaglandins and thromboxane A_2 as well as lipoxygenase-derived leukotrienes and lipoxins. Thromboxane A_2 is a potent vasoconstrictor that contributes to the pulmonary hypertension and acute tubular necrosis of shock. PGI_2 and PGE_2 are potent vasodilators that enhance capillary permeability and edema formation. The cysteinyl leukotrienes LTC_4 and LTD_4 are pivotal mediators of the vascular sequelae of anaphylaxis, as well as of shock states resulting from sepsis or tissue injury. LTB_4 is a potent neutrophil chemoattractant and secretagogue that stimulates the formation of reactive oxygen species. Platelet-activating factor, an ether-linked, arachidonyl-containing phospholipid mediator, causes pulmonary vasoconstriction, bronchoconstriction, systemic vasodilation, increased capillary permeability, and the priming of macrophages and neutrophils to produce enhanced levels of inflammatory mediators.

Tumor necrosis factor (TNF) α, produced by activated macrophages, reproduces many components of the shock state including hypotension, lactic acidosis, and respiratory failure. Interleukin (IL) 1, produced by tissue-fixed macrophages, is critical to the inflammatory response. Chemokines such as IL-8 are potent neutrophil chemoattractants and activators that upregulate adhesion molecules on the neutrophil to enhance aggregation, adherence, and damage to the vascular endothelium. While the endothelium normally produces nitric oxide (NO), the inflammatory response stimulates the inducible isoform of NO synthase (iNOS), which is overexpressed and produces toxic NO and oxygen-derived free radicals which contribute to the hyperdynamic cardiovascular response in sepsis.

Multiple inflammatory cells, including neutrophils, macrophages, and platelets, are a major contributor to inflammation-induced injury. Margination of activated neutrophils in the microcirculation is a common pathologic finding in shock, causing secondary injury due to the release of toxic oxygen radicals and proteases. Tissue-fixed macrophages produce virtually all major components of the inflammatory response and orchestrate the progression and duration of the inflammatory response.

Monitoring Patients in shock require care in an intensive care unit. Careful and continuous assessment of the physiologic status is necessary. Arterial pressure through an indwelling line, pulse, and respiratory rate should be monitored continuously; a Foley catheter should be inserted to follow urine flow; and mental status assessed frequently.

Although there is ongoing debate as to the indications for using the flow-directed pulmonary artery catheter (PAC, Swan-Ganz catheter), most intensivists believe that the ability to predict the hemodynamic profiles of patients in shock accurately without a PAC is poor. The PAC is placed percutaneously via the subclavian or jugular vein through the central venous circulation and right heart into the pulmonary artery. There are ports both proximal in the right atrium and distal in the pulmonary artery to provide access for infusions and for cardiac output measurements. Right atrial and pulmonary artery pressures are measured, and the pulmonary capillary wedge pressure (PCWP) serves as an approximation of the left atrial pressure. Normal hemodynamic parameters are shown in Table 212-3 and Table 253-2.

Cardiac output is determined by the thermodilution technique, and high-resolution thermistors can also be used to determine right ventricular end-diastolic volume to monitor further the response of the right heart to fluid resuscitation. A PAC with an oximeter port offers the additional advantage of on-line monitoring of the mixed venous oxygen saturation, an important index of tissue perfusion. Systemic and pulmonary vascular resistances are calculated as the ratio of the pressure drop across these vascular beds to the cardiac output (Chap. 212). Determinations of oxygen content in arterial and venous blood, together with cardiac output and hemoglobin concentration, allow calculation of oxygen delivery, oxygen consumption, and oxygen-extraction ratio (Table 253-3). The hemodynamic patterns associated with the various forms of shock are shown in Table 253-4.

In resuscitation from shock, it is critical to restore tissue perfusion and optimize oxygen delivery, hemodynamics, and cardiac function rapidly. A reasonable goal of therapy is to achieve normal mixed venous oxygen saturation and arteriovenous oxygen-extraction ratio. To enhance oxygen delivery, red cell mass, arterial oxygen saturation, and cardiac output may be augmented singly or simultaneously. An increase in oxygen delivery not accompanied by an increase in oxygen consumption implies that oxygen availability is adequate and that oxygen consumption is not flow-dependent. Conversely, an elevation of oxygen consumption with increased cardiac output implies that the oxygen supply was inadequate. A reduction in systemic vascular resistance accompanying an increase in cardiac output indicates that compensatory vasoconstriction is reversing due to improved tissue perfusion. The determination of stepwise expansion of blood volume on cardiac performance allows identification of the optimum preload (Starling's law). An algorithm for the resuscitation of the patient in shock is shown in Fig. 253-1.

TABLE 253-3 *Oxygen Transport Calculations*

Parameter	Calculation	Normal Values
Oxygen-carrying capacity of hemoglobin		1.39 mL/g
Plasma O_2 concentration		P_{O_2} × 0.0031
Arterial O_2 concentration (Ca$_{O_2}$)	1.39 Sa$_{O_2}$ + 0.0031 Pa$_{O_2}$	20 vol%
Venous O_2 concentration (Cv$_{O_2}$)	1.39 Sv$_{O_2}$ + 0.0031 Pv$_{O_2}$	15.5 vol%
Arteriovenous O_2 difference (Ca$_{O_2}$ − Cv$_{O_2}$)	1.39 (Sa$_{O_2}$ − Sv$_{O_2}$) + 0.0031 (Pa$_{O_2}$ − Pv$_{O_2}$)	3.5 vol%
Oxygen delivery (D$_{O_2}$)	Ca$_{O_2}$ × CO (L/min) × 10 (dL/L) 1.39 Sa$_{O_2}$ × CO × 10	800–1600 mL/min
Oxygen uptake (V$_{O_2}$)	(Ca$_{O_2}$ − Cv$_{O_2}$) × CO × 10 1.39 (Sa$_{O_2}$ − Sv$_{O_2}$) × CO × 10	150–400 mL/min
Oxygen delivery index (D$_{O_2}$I)	D$_{O_2}$/BSA	520–720 (mL/min)/m²
Oxygen uptake index (V$_{O_2}$I)	V$_{O_2}$/BSA	115–165 (mL/min)/m²
Oxygen extraction ratio (O$_2$ER)	[1 − (V̇$_{O_2}$/Ḋ$_{O_2}$)] × 100	22–32%

Note: P_{O_2}, partial pressure of oxygen; Sa$_{O_2}$, saturation of hemoglobin with O_2 in arterial blood; Pa$_{O_2}$, partial pressure of O_2 in arterial blood; Sv$_{O_2}$, saturation of hemoglobin with O_2 in venous blood; Pv$_{O_2}$, partial pressure of O_2 in venous blood; CO, cardiac output; BSA, body surface area.

SPECIFIC FORMS OF SHOCK

HYPOVOLEMIC SHOCK This most common form of shock results either from the loss of red blood cell mass and plasma from hemorrhage or from the loss of plasma volume alone arising

Type of Shock	CVP and PCWP	Cardiac Output	Systemic Vascular Resistance	Venous O_2 Saturation
Hypovolemic	↓	↓	↑	↓
Cardiogenic	↑	↓	↑	↓
Septic				
Hyperdynamic	↓↑	↑	↓	↑
Hypodynamic	↓↑	↓	↑	↑↓
Traumatic	↓	↓↑	↑↓	↓
Neurogenic	↓	↓	↓	↓
Hypoadrenal	↓↑	↓	=↓	↓

Note: CVP, central venous pressure; PCWP, pulmonary capillary wedge pressure.

from extravascular fluid sequestration or gastrointestinal, urinary, and insensible losses. The signs and symptoms of nonhemorrhagic hypovolemic shock are the same as those of hemorrhagic shock, although they may have a more insidious onset. The normal physiologic response to hypovolemia is to maintain perfusion of the brain and heart while restoring an effective circulating blood volume. There is an increase in sympathetic activity, hyperventilation, collapse of venous capacitance vessels, release of stress hormones, and expansion of intravascular volume through the recruitment of interstitial and intracellular fluid and reduction of urine output.

Mild hypovolemia (≤20% of the blood volume) generates mild tachycardia but relatively few external signs, especially in a supine resting young patient (Table 253-5). With moderate hypovolemia (~20 to 40% of the blood volume) the patient becomes increasingly anxious and tachycardic; although normal blood pressure may be maintained in the supine position, there may be significant postural hypotension and tachycardia. If hypovolemia is severe (≥~40% of the blood volume), the classic signs of shock appear; the blood pressure declines and becomes unstable even in the supine position, and the patient develops marked tachycardia, oliguria, and agitation or confusion. Perfusion of the central nervous system is well maintained until shock becomes severe. Hence, mental obtundation is an ominous clinical sign. The transition from mild to severe hypovolemic shock can be insidious or extremely rapid. If severe shock is not reversed rapidly, especially in elderly patients and those with comorbid illnesses, death is imminent. A very narrow time frame separates the derangements found in severe shock that can be reversed with aggressive resuscitation from those of progressive decompensation and irreversible cell injury.

Diagnosis Hypovolemic shock is readily diagnosed when there are signs of hemodynamic instability and the source of volume loss is obvious. The diagnosis is more difficult when the source of blood loss is occult, as into the gastrointestinal tract, or when plasma volume alone is depleted. After acute hemorrhage, hemoglobin and hematocrit values do not change until compensatory fluid shifts have occurred or exogenous fluid is administered. Thus, an initial normal hematocrit does not disprove

the presence of significant blood loss. Plasma losses cause hemoconcentration, and free water loss leads to hypernatremia. These findings should suggest the presence of hypovolemia.

It is essential to distinguish between hypovolemic and cardiogenic shock (see below) because definitive therapy differs significantly. Both forms are associated with a reduced cardiac output and a compensatory sympathetic mediated response characterized by tachycardia and elevated systemic vascular resistance. However, the findings in cardiogenic shock of jugular venous distention, rales, and an S_3 gallop distinguish it from hypovolemic shock and signify that ongoing volume expansion is undesirable.

℞ TREATMENT

Initial resuscitation requires rapid reexpansion of the circulating blood volume along with interventions to control ongoing losses. In accordance with Starling's law (Chap. 215), stroke volume and cardiac output rise with the increase in preload. After resuscitation, the compliance of the ventricles may remain reduced due to increased interstitial fluid in the myocardium. Therefore, elevated filling pressures are required to maintain adequate ventricular performance.

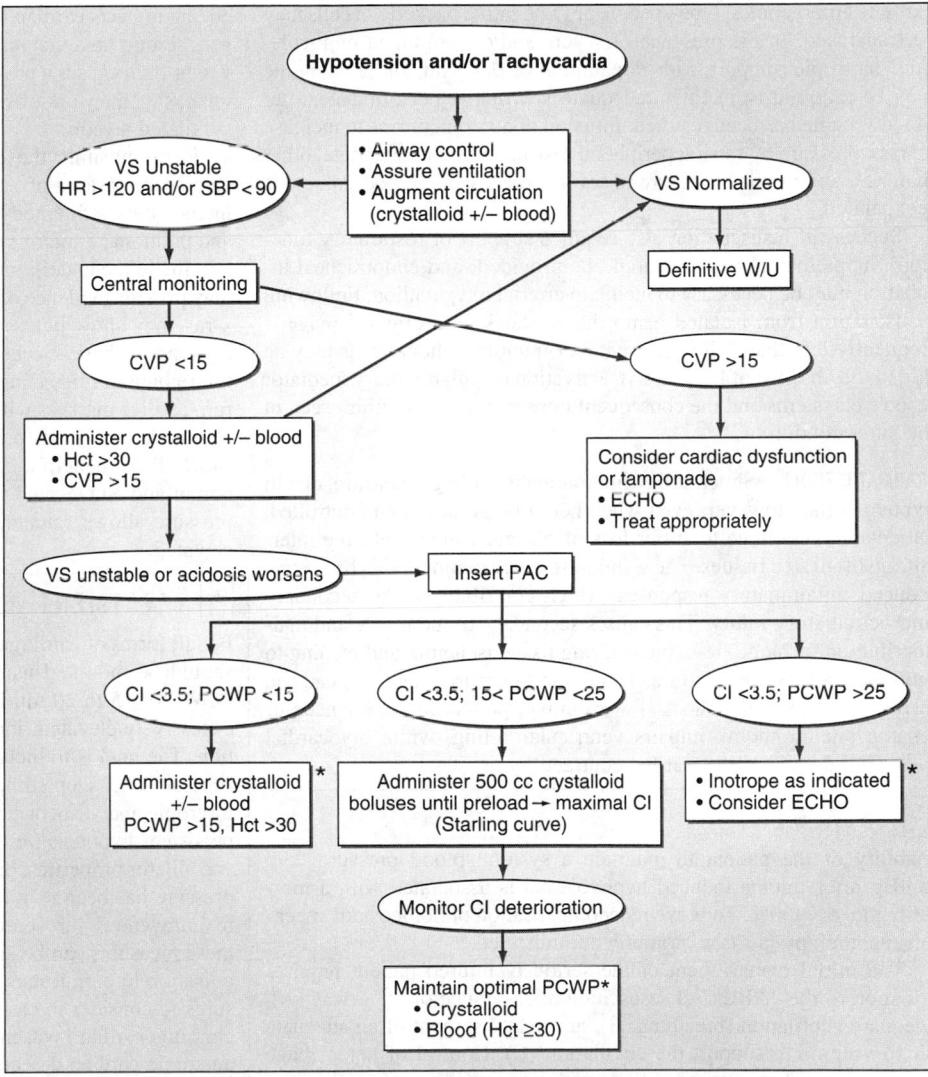

FIGURE 253-1   An algorithm for the resuscitation of the patient in shock. VS, vital signs; HR, heart rate; SBP, systolic blood pressure; W/U, work up; CVP, central venous pressure; Hct, hematocrit; ECHO, echocardiogram; PAC, pulmonary artery catheter; CI, cardiac index in (L/min)/m²; PCWP, pulmonary capillary wedge pressure in mmHg.

*Monitor SV_{O_2}, SVRI, and RVEDVI as additional markers of correction for perfusion and hypovolemia. Consider age-adjusted CI. SV_{O_2}, saturation of hemoglobin with O_2 in venous blood; SVRI, systemic vascular resistance index; RVEDVI, right-ventricular end-diastolic volume index.

TABLE 253-5 *Hypovolemic Shock*

Mild (<20% Blood Volume)	Moderate (20–40% Blood Volume)	Severe (>40% Blood Volume)
Cool extremities	Same, plus:	Same, plus:
Increased capillary refill time	Tachycardia	Hemodynamic instability
	Tachypnea	Marked tachycardia
Diaphoresis	Oliguria	Hypotension
Collapsed veins	Postural changes	Mental status
Anxiety		deterioration (coma)

Volume resuscitation is initiated with the rapid infusion of isotonic saline (although care must be taken to avoid hyperchloremic acidosis) or a balanced salt solution such as Ringer's lactate through large-bore intravenous lines. No distinct benefit from the use of colloid has been demonstrated and, in trauma patients, it is associated with a higher mortality. The infusion of 2 to 3 L over 20 to 30 min should restore normal hemodynamic parameters. Continued hemodynamic instability implies that shock has not been reversed and/or that there are significant ongoing blood or volume losses. Continuing blood loss, with hemoglobin concentrations declining to ≤100 g/L (10 g/dL), should initiate blood transfusion, preferably as fully cross-matched blood. In extreme emergencies, type-specific or O-negative packed red cells may be transfused. In the presence of severe and/or prolonged hypovolemia, inotropic support with dopamine, vasopressin, or dobutamine may be required to maintain adequate ventricular performance, after blood volume has been restored. Infusion of norepinephrine to increase arterial pressure by raising peripheral resistance is inappropriate, other than as a temporizing measure in severe shock while blood volume is reexpanded.

Successful resuscitation also requires support of respiratory function. Supplemental oxygen should be provided, and endotracheal intubation may be necessary to maintain arterial oxygenation. Following resuscitation from isolated hemorrhagic shock, end-organ damage is frequently less than following septic or traumatic shock. This may be due to the absence of the massive activation of inflammatory mediator response systems and the consequent nonspecific organ injury seen in the latter conditions.

TRAUMATIC SHOCK   Shock following trauma is, in large measure, due to hypovolemia. However, even when hemorrhage has been controlled, patients can continue to suffer loss of plasma volume into the interstitium of injured tissues. These fluid losses are compounded by injury-induced inflammatory responses, which contribute to the secondary microcirculatory injury. This causes secondary tissue injury and maldistribution of blood flow, intensifying tissue ischemia and leading to multiple organ system failure. Trauma to the heart, chest, or head can also contribute to the shock. For example, pericardial tamponade or tension pneumothorax impairs ventricular filling, while myocardial contusion depresses myocardial contractility.

℞ TREATMENT

Inability of the patient to maintain a systolic blood pressure ≥90 mmHg after trauma-induced hypovolemia is associated with a mortality rate of ~50%. To prevent decompensation of homeostatic mechanisms, therapy must be promptly administered.

The initial management of the seriously injured patient requires attention to the "ABCs" of resuscitation: assurance of an airway (A), adequate ventilation (breathing, B), and establishment of an adequate blood volume to support the circulation (C). Control of hemorrhage requires immediate attention. Early stabilization of fractures, debridement of devitalized or contaminated tissues, and evacuation of hematomata all reduce the subsequent inflammatory response to the initial insult and minimize subsequent organ injury. Supplementation of depleted endogenous antioxidants also reduces subsequent organ failure and mortality.

INTRINSIC CARDIOGENIC SHOCK   This form of shock is caused by failure, often sudden, of the heart as an effective pump. It occurs most commonly as a complication of acute myocardial infarction (AMI; Chaps. 228 and 255), but it may also be seen in patients with severe brady- or tachyarrhythmias, valvular heart disease, significant cardiac contusion, or in the terminal stage of chronic heart failure of any cause, including ischemic heart disease and dilated cardiomyopathy. Cardiogenic shock is characterized by a low cardiac output, diminished peripheral perfusion, pulmonary congestion, and elevation of systemic vascular resistance and pulmonary vascular pressures. Acute right heart failure can arise as the result of right ventricular infarction or may complicate ARDS and severe pulmonary hypertension of any etiology. As a consequence of right ventricular failure, left ventricular preload falls, and this, in turn, reduces systemic perfusion. In contrast to other forms of shock, absolute or relative hypovolemia is usually not present in cardiogenic shock.

The ineffective contractile activity of either the right or left side of the heart leads to the accumulation of blood in the venous circulation upstream to the failing ventricle. Cardiogenic shock with left-sided heart failure increases fluid in the lungs that can overwhelm the capacity of the pulmonary lymphatics and causes interstitial and eventually alveolar edema. Interstitial lung edema usually occurs at pulmonary capillary pressures >18 mmHg, and overt pulmonary alveolar edema develops at pressures >24 mmHg (Chap. 29). Pulmonary edema impacts cardiac function further by impairing diffusion of oxygen, setting up a vicious cycle. The increase in interstitial and intraalveolar fluid causes a progressive reduction in lung compliance, thereby increasing the work of ventilation while increasing perfusion of poorly ventilated alveoli.

In establishing the diagnosis of cardiogenic shock, a history of cardiac disease or of AMI is of value. Associated physical findings include those of hemodynamic instability, peripheral vasoconstriction, and pulmonary and/or systemic venous congestion, as well as findings specific to the underlying cardiac abnormalities. An electrocardiogram may provide evidence of AMI or preexisting cardiac disease. The chest x-ray may show pulmonary edema and cardiomegaly. Transthoracic or transesophageal echocardiograms assist in the diagnosis of structural abnormalities and/or functional impairment of contractility. Serum cardiac markers will support the diagnosis of acute cardiac injury. Hemodynamic monitoring is usually necessary in the presence of shock. Placement of a PAC is helpful and will show a reduced cardiac output and an elevated PCWP, and direct measurement of right atrial pressure allows calculation of systemic vascular resistance which is elevated.

℞ TREATMENT

For all forms of cardiogenic shock, preload, afterload, and contractility should be modified using the information provided by the PAC. A PCWP of 15 to 20 mmHg should be the initial goal. If the PCWP is excessively elevated, inotropic agents may provide significant reduction. The goal is to increase contractility without significant increases in heart rate. Dopamine, norepinephrine, or vasopressin exert both inotropic and vasoconstrictor actions that are useful in the presence of persistent hypotension. Dobutamine, a positive inotropic agent with vasodilator properties, or vasodilators may be substituted when arterial pressure has been restored. Pulmonary congestion may be responsive to intravenous furosemide. Patients with an inadequate response to these measures can be supported by using intraaortic balloon counterpulsation to permit recovery of myocardial function. Additional measures to consider in cases of refractory cardiogenic shock include urgent myocardial revascularization in patients with AMI, correction of anatomic cardiac defects such as rupture of the papillary muscles of the interventricular septum, the placement of ventricular assist devices, and even urgent cardiac transplantation.

COMPRESSIVE CARDIOGENIC SHOCK   With compression, the heart and surrounding structures are less compliant and, thus, normal filling pressures generate inadequate diastolic filling. Blood or fluid within the poorly distensible pericardial sac may cause tamponade (Chap. 222). Any cause of increased intrathoracic pressure, such as tension pneumothorax, herniation of abdominal viscera through a diaphragmatic hernia, or excessive positive pressure ventilation to support pulmonary function, can also cause compressive cardiogenic shock while simultaneously impeding venous return. Acute right heart failure with a sudden decline in cardiac output can be caused by pulmonary embolism obstructing right ventricular outflow and impairing left ventricular filling. Although initially responsive to increased filling pressures produced by volume expansion, as compression increases, cardiogenic shock recurs.

The diagnosis of compressive cardiogenic shock is most frequently based on clinical findings, the chest radiograph, and an echocardiogram. The diagnosis of compressive cardiac shock may be more difficult to establish in the setting of trauma when hypovolemia and cardiac compression are present simultaneously. The classic findings of pericardial tamponade include the triad of hypotension, neck vein distention, and muffled heart sounds (Chap. 222). Pulsus paradoxus, i.e., an inspiratory reduction in systolic pressure >10 mmHg, may also be noted. The diagnosis is confirmed by echocardiography, and treatment consists of immediate pericardiocentesis. A tension pneumothorax produces ipsilateral decreased breath sounds, tracheal deviation away from the affected thorax, and jugular venous distention. Radiographic findings include increased intrathoracic volume, depression of the diaphragm of the affected hemithorax, and shifting of the mediastinum to the contralateral side. Chest decompression must be carried out immediately. Release of air and restoration of normal cardiovascular dynamics are both diagnostic and therapeutic.

SEPTIC SHOCK (See also Chap. 254) This form of shock is caused by the systemic response to a severe infection. It occurs most frequently in elderly or immunocompromised patients and in those who have undergone an invasive procedure in which bacterial contamination has occurred. Infections of the lung, abdomen, or urinary tract are most common, and approximately half of the patients have bacteremia. Gram-positive and -negative bacteria, viruses, fungi, rickettsiae, and protozoa have all been reported to produce the clinical picture of septic shock, and the overall response is generally independent of the specific type of invading organism. The clinical findings in septic shock are a consequence of the combination of metabolic and circulatory derangements driven by the systemic infection and the release of toxic components of the infectious organisms, e.g., the endotoxin of gram-negative bacteria or the exotoxins and enterotoxins of gram-positive bacteria. Organism toxins lead to the release of cytokines, including IL-1 and TNF-α, from tissue macrophages. Tissue factor expression and fibrin deposition are increased, and disseminated intravascular coagulation may develop. The inducible form of NO synthase is stimulated, and NO, a powerful vasodilator, is released. Hemodynamic changes in septic shock occur in two characteristic patterns: early, or hyperdynamic, and late, or hypodynamic, septic shock.

Hyperdynamic Response In hyperdynamic septic shock, tachycardia is present, the cardiac output is normal or elevated, and the systemic vascular resistance is reduced while the pulmonary vascular resistance is elevated. The extremities are usually warm. However, splanchnic vasoconstriction with decreased visceral flow is present. The venous capacitance is increased, which decreases venous return. With volume expansion cardiac output becomes supranormal. Myocardial contractility is depressed in septic shock by mediators including NO, IL-1, and/or TNF-α. Inflammatory mediator–induced processes include increased capillary permeability and continued loss of intravascular volume.

In septic shock, in contrast to other types of shock, total oxygen delivery may be increased while oxygen extraction is reduced due to maldistribution of microcirculatory perfusion and impaired mitochondrial utilization. In this setting the presence of a normal mixed venous oxygen saturation is not indicative of adequate peripheral perfusion, and even though the cardiac output may be elevated, it is still inadequate to meet the total metabolic needs. The toxicity of the infectious agents and their byproducts and the subsequent metabolic dysfunction drive the progressive deterioration of cellular and organ function. ARDS, thrombocytopenia, and neutropenia are common complications.

Hypodynamic Response As sepsis progresses, vasoconstriction occurs and the cardiac output declines. The patient usually becomes markedly tachypneic, febrile, diaphoretic, and obtunded, with cool, mottled, and often cyanotic extremities. Oliguria, renal failure, and hypothermia develop; there may be striking increases in serum lactate.

Rx TREATMENT

Aggressive volume expansion with a crystalloid solution to a PCWP of ~15 mmHg and the restoration of arterial oxygenation with inspired oxygen and frequently with mechanical ventilation are the highest priorities. In the presence of sepsis, augmentation of cardiac output may require inotropic support with dopamine, norepinephrine, or vasopressin in the presence of hypotension or with dobutamine if arterial pressure is normal. High-dose, *a*ctivated *p*rotein *C* (APC) provides a survival benefit in patients with severe sepsis and septic shock. Antibiotics should be administered, either appropriate for the results of cultures or empirical therapy based on the likely source of infection. Surgical debridement or drainage may also be necessary to control the infection.

NEUROGENIC SHOCK Interruption of sympathetic vasomotor input after a high cervical spinal cord injury, inadvertent cephalad migration of spinal anesthesia, or severe head injury may result in neurogenic shock. In addition to arteriolar dilatation, venodilation causes pooling in the venous system, which decreases venous return and cardiac output. The extremities are often warm, in contrast to the usual vasoconstriction-induced coolness in hypovolemic or cardiogenic shock. Treatment involves a simultaneous approach to the relative hypovolemia and to the loss of vasomotor tone. Excessive volumes of fluid may be required to restore normal hemodynamics. Once hemorrhage has been ruled out, norepinephrine may be necessary to augment vascular resistance.

HYPOADRENAL SHOCK (See also Chap. 321) The normal host response to the stress of illness, operation, or trauma requires that the adrenal glands hypersecrete cortisol in excess of that normally required. Hypoadrenal shock occurs in settings in which unrecognized adrenal insufficiency complicates the host response to the stress induced by acute illness or major surgery. Adrenocortical insufficiency may occur as a consequence of the chronic administration of high doses of exogenous glucocorticoids. Recent studies have shown that critical illness, including trauma and sepsis, may also induce a relative hypoadrenal state. Other, less common causes include adrenal insufficiency secondary to idiopathic atrophy, tuberculosis, metastatic disease, bilateral hemorrhage, and amyloidosis. The shock produced by adrenal insufficiency is characterized by reductions in systemic vascular resistance, hypovolemia, and reduced cardiac output. The diagnosis of adrenal insufficiency may be established by means of an ACTH stimulation test.

Rx TREATMENT

In the hemodynamically unstable patient, dexamethasone sodium phosphate, 4 mg, should be given intravenously. This agent is preferred because unlike hydrocortisone it does not interfere with the ACTH stimulation test. If the diagnosis of absolute or relative adrenal insufficiency has been established as shown by non-response to corticotropin stimulation, the patient has a reduced risk of death if treated with hydrocortisone, 100 mg every 6 to 8 h, and tapered as the patient achieves hemodynamic stability. Simultaneous volume resuscitation and pressor support are required.

ADJUNCTIVE THERAPIES

As described above, the sympathomimetic amines dobutamine, dopamine, and norepinephrine are widely used in the treatment of all forms of shock. Arginine-vasopressin (antidiuretic hormone) is also being used increasingly and may better protect vital organ blood flow and prevent pathologic vasodilation.

POSITIONING   Positioning of the patient may be a valuable adjunct in the initial treatment of hypovolemic shock. Elevating the foot of the bed (i.e., placing it on "shock blocks") and assumption of the Trendelenburg position without flexion at the knees are effective but may increase work of breathing and risk for aspiration. Simply elevating both legs may be the optimal approach.

PNEUMATIC ANTISHOCK GARMENT (PASG)   The PASG and the military antishock trousers (MAST) are inflatable external compression devices that can be wrapped around the legs and abdomen and have been widely used in the prehospital setting as a means of providing temporary support of central hemodynamics in shock. They cause an increase in systemic vascular resistance and blood pressure by arterial compression, without causing a significant change in cardiac output. The most appropriate use appears to be as a means to tamponade bleeding and augment hemostasis. Inflation of the suit provides splinting of fractures of the pelvis and lower extremities and arrests hemorrhage.

REWARMING   Hypothermia is a potential adverse consequence of massive volume resuscitation. The infusion of large volumes of refrigerated blood products and room-temperature crystalloid solutions can rapidly drop core temperatures if fluid is not run through warming devices. Hypothermia may depress cardiac contractility and thereby further impair cardiac output and oxygen delivery. Hypothermia, particularly temperatures <35° C, directly impairs the coagulation pathway, sometimes causing a significant coagulopathy. Rapid rewarming to >35° C significantly decreases the requirement for blood products and produces an improvement in cardiac function. The most effective method for rewarming is extracorporeal countercurrent warmers through femoral artery and vein cannulation. This process does not require a pump and can rewarm from 30° to 35°C in <30 min.

FURTHER READING

ANNANE D et al: Effect of treatment with low doses of hydrocortisone and fludrocortisone on mortality in patients with septic shock. JAMA 288:862, 2002

BERNARD GR et al: Pulmonary artery catheterization and clinical outcomes: National Heart, Lung, and Blood Institute and Food and Drug Administration Workshop Report Consensus Statement. JAMA 283:2568, 2000

CHEN P: Vasopressin: New uses in critical care. Am J Med Sci 324:146, 2002

CHOI PT et al: Crystalloids vs. colloids in fluid resuscitation: A systematic review. Crit Care Med 27:200, 1999

MCGEE S et al: The rational clinical examination. Is this patient hypovolemic? JAMA 281:1022, 1999

RIVERS E et al: Early goal-directed therapy in the treatment of severe sepsis and septic shock. N Engl J Med 345:1368, 2001

254   SEVERE SEPSIS AND SEPTIC SHOCK
Robert S. Munford

DEFINITIONS (See Table 254-1)   Animals mount both local and systemic responses to microbes that traverse epithelial barriers and invade underlying tissues. Fever or hypothermia, leukocytosis or leukopenia, tachypnea, and tachycardia are the cardinal signs of the systemic response often called the *systemic inflammatory response syndrome* (SIRS). SIRS may have an infectious or a noninfectious etiology. If infection is suspected or proven, a patient with SIRS is said to have *sepsis*. When sepsis is associated with dysfunction of organs distant from the site of infection, the patient has *severe sepsis*. Severe sepsis may be accompanied by hypotension or evidence of hypoperfusion. When hypotension cannot be corrected by infusing fluids, the diagnosis is *septic shock*. These definitions were proposed by a consensus conference committee in 1992 and are now widely used; there is evidence that the different stages form a continuum. As sepsis progresses to septic shock, the risk of dying increases substantially. Sepsis is usually reversible, whereas patients with septic shock often succumb despite aggressive therapy.

ETIOLOGY   Severe sepsis can be a response to any class of microorganism. Microbial invasion of the bloodstream is not essential for the development of severe sepsis, since local inflammation can also elicit distant organ dysfunction and hypotension. In fact, blood cultures yield bacteria or fungi in only ~20 to 40% of cases of severe sepsis and 40 to 70% of cases of septic shock. Individual gram-negative or gram-positive bacteria account for ~70% of these isolates; the remainder are fungi or a mixture of microorganisms (Table 254-2). In patients whose blood cultures are negative, the etiologic agent is often established by culture or microscopic examination of infected material from a local site. In some case series, a majority of patients with a clinical picture of severe sepsis or septic shock have had negative microbiologic data. Factors that predispose to infections with positive blood cultures are listed in (Table 254-3). Among patients who have positive blood cultures, the risk of developing severe sepsis is greater in persons >50 years old and in those with a primary pulmonary, abdominal, or neuromeningeal site of infection.

EPIDEMIOLOGY   The septic response is a contributing factor in >200,000 deaths per year in the United States. The incidence of severe sepsis and septic shock has increased over the past 20 years, and the annual number of cases is now >300,000. Approximately two-thirds of cases occur in patients hospitalized for other illnesses. The increasing incidence of severe sepsis in the United States is attributable to the aging of the population, the increasing longevity of patients with chronic diseases, and the relatively high frequency with which sepsis develops in patients with AIDS. The widespread use of antimicrobial agents, glucocorticoids, indwelling catheters and mechanical devices, and mechanical ventilation also plays a role.

PATHOPHYSIOLOGY   Most cases of severe sepsis are triggered by bacteria or fungi that do not ordinarily cause systemic disease in immunocompetent hosts (Table 254-2). These microbes probably exploit deficiencies in innate host defenses (e.g., phagocytes, complement, and natural antibodies) to survive within the body. Microbial pathogens, in contrast, are able to circumvent innate defenses by elaborating toxins or other virulence factors. In both cases, the body can fail to kill the invaders despite mounting a vigorous inflammatory reaction that can progress to severe sepsis. The septic response may also be induced by microbial exotoxins that act as superantigens (e.g., toxic shock syndrome toxin 1; Chap. 120).

Host Mechanisms for Sensing Microbes   Animals have exquisitely sensitive mechanisms for recognizing and responding to conserved microbial molecules. The lipid A moiety of lipopolysaccharide (LPS, also called *endotoxin*; Chap. 105) is the best-studied example. Lipid A is the bioactive center of the LPS of all gram-negative bacteria found in nature. A host protein (LPS-binding protein, or LBP) binds lipid A and transfers LPS to CD14 on the surfaces of monocytes, macrophages, and neutrophils. LPS and CD14 then interact with toll-like receptor (TLR) 4 and MD-2 to form a molecular complex that transduces the LPS signal to the interior of the cell. This signal rapidly triggers the production and release of mediators, such as tumor necrosis factor (TNF) α (see below), that amplify the LPS signal and transmit it to other cells and tissues. Bacterial peptidoglycan, lipoteichoic acids, DNA, certain polysaccharides, and fimbriae elicit responses in animals that are similar to those induced by LPS; whereas some of

TABLE 254-1 *Definitions Used to Describe the Condition of Septic Patients*

Bacteremia	Presence of bacteria in blood, as evidenced by positive blood cultures
Septicemia	Presence of microbes or their toxins in blood
Systemic inflammatory response syndrome (SIRS)	Two or more of the following conditions: (1) fever (oral temperature >38°C) or hypothermia (<36°C); (2) tachypnea (>24 breaths/min); (3) tachycardia (heart rate > 90 beats/min); (4) leukocytosis (>12,000/μL), leukopenia (<4,000/μL), or >10% bands; may have a noninfectious etiology
Sepsis	SIRS that has a proven or suspected microbial etiology
Severe sepsis (similar to "sepsis syndrome")	Sepsis with one or more signs of organ dysfunction—for example: 1. *Cardiovascular:* Arterial systolic blood pressure ≤90 mmHg or mean arterial pressure ≤ 70 mmHg that responds to administration of intravenous fluid 2. *Renal:* Urine output < 0.5 mL/kg per hour for 1 h despite adequate fluid resuscitation 3. *Respiratory:* $Pa_{O_2}/FI_{O_2} \leq 250$ or, if the lung is the only dysfunctional organ, ≤200 4. *Hematologic:* Platelet count < 80,000/μL or 50% decrease in platelet count from highest value recorded over previous 3 days 5. *Unexplained metabolic acidosis:* A pH ≤ 7.30 or a base deficit ≥ 5.0 mEq/L and a plasma lactate level > 1.5 times upper limit of normal for reporting lab 6. *Adequate fluid resuscitation:* Pulmonary artery wedge pressure ≥ 12 mmHg or central venous pressure ≥ 8 mmHg
Septic shock	Sepsis with hypotension (arterial blood pressure <90 mmHg systolic, or 40 mmHg less than patient's normal blood pressure) for at least 1 h despite adequate fluid resuscitation; *or* Need for vasopressors to maintain systolic blood pressure ≥ 90 mmHg *or* mean arterial pressure ≥ 70 mmHg
Refractory septic shock	Septic shock that lasts for >1 h and does not respond to fluid or pressor administration
Multiple-organ dysfunction syndrome (MODS)	Dysfunction of more than one organ, requiring intervention to maintain homeostasis

Source: Adapted from the American College of Chest Physicians/Society of Critical Care Medicine Consensus Conference Committee and Bernard et al.

these molecules also bind CD14, they interact with several different TLRs. CD14 thus attracts numerous non-self molecules to the surfaces of cells, greatly increasing the sensitivity with which these molecules can be recognized by the host. Having numerous TLR-based receptor complexes (10 different TLRs have been identified so far) allows cells to recognize many conserved microbial molecules. The ability of some

TABLE 254-2 *Microorganisms Involved in Episodes of Severe Sepsis at Eight Academic Medical Centers*

Microorganisms	Episodes with Blood-stream Infection, % (n = 436)	Episodes with Documented Infection but No Bloodstream Infection, % (n = 430)	Total Episodes, % (n = 866)
Gram-negative bacteria[a]	35	44	40
Gram-positive bacteria[b]	40	24	31
Fungi	7	5	6
Polymicrobial	11	21	16
Classic pathogens[c]	<5	<5	<5

[a] Enterobacteriaceae, pseudomonads, *Haemophilus* spp., other gram-negative bacteria.
[b] *Staphylococcus aureus*, coagulase-negative staphylococci, enterococci, *Streptococcus pneumoniae*, other streptococci, other gram-positive bacteria.
[c] Such as *Neisseria meningitidis*, *S. pneumoniae*, *H. influenzae*, and *Streptococcus pyogenes*.
Source: Adapted from Sands et al.

TABLE 254-3 *Conditions That May Predispose to Infections with Positive Blood Cultures*

Microbial Isolate	Condition
Gram-negative bacilli	Diabetes mellitus Lymphoproliferative diseases Cirrhosis of the liver Burns Invasive procedures or devices Neutropenia Indwelling urinary catheter Diverticulitis, perforated viscus
Gram-positive bacteria	Intravascular catheters Indwelling mechanical devices Burns Neutropenia Intravenous drug use Infection with superantigen-producing *Streptococcus pyogenes*
Fungi	Neutropenia Broad-spectrum antimicrobial therapy

of the TLRs to serve as receptors for host ligands (e.g., hyaluronans) raises the possibility that they play a role in producing noninfectious sepsis-like states. Other molecular pattern-recognition proteins that are important for sensing microbial invasion include complement (principally the alternative pathway), mannose-binding lectin, bactericidal permeability-increasing protein, and C-reactive protein.

Local and Systemic Host Responses to Invading Microbes Recognition of microbial molecules by tissue phagocytes triggers the production and/or release of numerous host molecules (cytokines, chemokines, prostanoids, leukotrienes, and others) that increase blood flow to the infected tissue, enhance the permeability of local blood vessels, recruit neutrophils to the site of infection, and elicit pain. These phenomena are familiar elements of local inflammation, the body's major innate immune mechanism for eliminating microbial invaders. Systemic responses may be activated by neural and/or humoral communication with the hypothalamus and brainstem; these responses may enhance local defenses by increasing blood flow to the infected area, augmenting the number of circulating neutrophils, and elevating blood levels of numerous molecules (such as the microbial recognition proteins discussed above) that have anti-infective functions.

CYTOKINES AND OTHER MEDIATORS Cytokines can exert endocrine, paracrine, and autocrine effects (Chap. 295). TNF-α stimulates leukocytes and vascular endothelial cells to release other cytokines (as well as additional TNF-α), to express cell-surface molecules that enhance neutrophil-endothelial adhesion at sites of infection, and to increase prostaglandin and leukotriene production. Animals that are unable to produce or respond to TNF-α are abnormally susceptible to infection. Whereas blood levels of TNF-α are not elevated in individuals with localized infections, they increase in most patients with severe sepsis or septic shock. Moreover, intravenous infusion of TNF-α can elicit many of the characteristic abnormalities of sepsis, including fever, tachycardia, tachypnea, leukocytosis, myalgias, and somnolence. In animals, larger doses of TNF-α induce shock, disseminated intravascular coagulation (DIC), and death.

Although TNF-α is a central mediator, it is only one of many proinflammatory molecules that contribute to innate host defense. Chemokines, most prominently interleukin (IL) 8, attract circulating neutrophils to the infection site. IL-1β exhibits many of the same activities as TNF-α. TNF-α, IL-1β, interferon γ, IL-12, and other cytokines probably interact synergistically with one another and with additional mediators. Recent evidence suggests that proinflammatory cytokines that circulate in blood often originate in an inflamed local site.

COAGULATION FACTORS Intravascular thrombosis, a hallmark of the local inflammatory response, may help wall off invading microbes and prevent infection and inflammation from spreading to other tissues. Intravascular fibrin deposition, thrombosis, and DIC can also be important features of the systemic response. IL-6 and other mediators promote intravascular coagulation initially by inducing blood monocytes and vascular endothelial cells to express tissue factor (Chap. 53). When tissue factor is expressed on cell surfaces, it binds to factor VIIa to form an active complex that can convert factors X and IX to enzymatically active forms. The result is activation of both extrinsic and intrinsic clotting pathways, culminating in the generation of fibrin. Clotting is also favored by impaired function of the protein C–protein S inhibitory pathway and depletion of antithrombin and protein C, while fibrinolysis is prevented by increased plasma levels of plasminogen activator inhibitor 1. Thus, there may be a striking propensity to intravascular fibrin deposition, thrombosis, and bleeding (Chap. 127). Contact-system activation occurs during sepsis but contributes more to the development of hypotension than to DIC.

CONTROL MECHANISMS   Elaborate control mechanisms operate within both local sites of inflammation and the systemic circulation. The available evidence suggests that the body's systemic responses to injury and infection normally prevent inflammation within organs distant from a site of infection.

The signaling apparatus that links microbial recognition to cellular responses is greatly diminished in the blood. Whereas LBP plays a role in recognizing the presence of LPS, for example, in plasma it also prevents LPS signaling by transferring LPS molecules into plasma lipoprotein particles, which sequester the lipid A moiety so that it cannot interact with cells. At concentrations found in blood, LBP also inhibits monocyte responses to LPS, and the soluble (circulating) form of CD14 strips off LPS that has bound to monocyte cell surfaces. The blood concentrations of both LBP and soluble CD14 increase during the response to infection, enhancing the body's ability to prevent activation of blood cells by LPS.

Systemic responses to infection also diminish cellular responses to microbial molecules. Circulating levels of anti-inflammatory cytokines (e.g., IL-6 and IL-10) increase even in patients with mild infections. Glucocorticoids inhibit cytokine synthesis by monocytes in vitro; the increase in blood cortisol levels early in the systemic response presumably plays a similar inhibitory role. Epinephrine inhibits the TNF-α response to endotoxin infusion in humans while augmenting and accelerating the release of IL-10; prostaglandin E_2 has a similar "reprogramming" effect on the responses of circulating monocytes to LPS and other bacterial agonists. Cortisol, epinephrine, IL-10, and C reactive protein reduce the ability of neutrophils to attach to vascular endothelium, favoring their demargination and thus contributing to leukocytosis while preventing neutrophil-endothelial adhesion in uninflamed organs.

The acute-phase response increases the blood concentrations of numerous molecules that have anti-inflammatory actions. Blood levels of IL-1 receptor antagonist (IL-1Ra) often greatly exceed those of circulating IL-1β, for example, and this excess may result in inhibition of the binding of IL-1β to its receptors. High levels of soluble TNF receptors neutralize TNF-α that enters the circulation. Other acute-phase proteins are protease inhibitors; these may neutralize proteases released from neutrophils and other inflammatory cells.

Organ Dysfunction and Shock   As the body's responses to infection intensify, the mixture of circulating cytokines and other molecules becomes very complex: elevated blood levels of more than 50 molecules have been found in patients with septic shock. Although high concentrations of both pro- and anti-inflammatory molecules are found, the net mediator balance in the plasma of these extremely sick patients may actually be anti-inflammatory. In addition, blood leukocytes from patients with severe sepsis are often hyporesponsive to agonists such as LPS. In patients with severe sepsis, persistence of leukocyte hyporesponsiveness has been associated with an increased risk of dying. How the body's pro- and anti-inflammatory forces contribute to hy-

potension and the dysfunction of organs distant from a site of infection is not known.

ENDOTHELIAL INJURY   Most investigators have favored widespread vascular endothelial injury as the major mechanism for multiorgan dysfunction. In keeping with this idea, one study found high numbers of vascular endothelial cells in the peripheral blood of septic patients. Leukocyte-derived mediators and platelet-leukocyte-fibrin thrombi may contribute to vascular injury, but the vascular endothelium also seems to play an active role. Stimuli such as TNF-α induce vascular endothelial cells to produce and release cytokines, procoagulant molecules, platelet-activating factor (PAF), nitric oxide, and other mediators. In addition, regulated cell-adhesion molecules promote the adherence of neutrophils to endothelial cells. While these responses can attract phagocytes to infected sites and activate their antimicrobial arsenals, endothelial cell activation can also promote increased vascular permeability, microvascular thrombosis, DIC, and hypotension.

Tissue oxygenation may be diminished as the number of functional capillaries is reduced by luminal obstruction due to swollen endothelial cells, decreased deformability of circulating erythrocytes, leukocyte-platelet-fibrin thrombi, or compression by edema fluid. One study using orthogonal polarization spectral imaging of the microcirculation in the tongue found that sepsis-associated derangements in capillary flow could be reversed by applying acetylcholine to the surface of the tongue; this observation suggested a neuroendocrine basis for the loss of capillary filling. Cellular ATP and antioxidant stores may become depleted as the production of lactate increases. Programmed cell death may ensue.

SEPTIC SHOCK   The hallmark of septic shock is a decrease in peripheral vascular resistance that occurs despite increased levels of vasopressor catecholamines. Cardiac output increases, as does blood flow to peripheral tissues. Oxygen utilization by these tissues may be greatly impaired by maldistribution of blood flow as well as by microcirculatory dysfunction (see above).

Prominent hypotensive molecules include nitric oxide, β-endorphin, bradykinin, PAF, and prostacyclin. Agents that inhibit the synthesis or action of each of these mediators can prevent or reverse endotoxic shock in animals. However, in clinical trials, neither a PAF receptor antagonist nor a bradykinin antagonist improved the survival rate of patients with septic shock, and a nitric oxide synthetase inhibitor, L-N^G-methylarginine HCl, actually increased the mortality rate.

Patients with septic shock often show diminished vasoconstrictor responses to catecholamines. This loss of sensitivity has been attributed to downregulation of adrenergic receptors and to elevated levels of nitric oxide. In patients with septic shock, plasma vasopressin levels do not increase to augment vasoconstriction; in several small series of patients with septic shock, infusion of vasopressin has increased blood pressure and reduced the requirement for catecholamine infusion. Administering hydrocortisone may also improve vascular sensitivity to catecholamines in many patients with septic shock.

Severe Sepsis: A Single Pathogenesis?   In some cases, circulating bacteria and their products almost certainly elicit multiorgan dysfunction and hypotension by directly stimulating inflammatory responses within the vasculature. In patients with fulminant meningococcemia, for example, mortality has correlated well with blood endotoxin levels and with the occurrence of DIC (Chap. 127). In most patients with nosocomial infections, in contrast, circulating bacteria or bacterial molecules may reflect uncontrolled infection at a local tissue site and have little or no direct impact on distant organs; in these patients, inflammatory mediators arising from the local site seem to be the key triggers for severe sepsis and septic shock. Support for this concept comes from a study in which *Pseudomonas aeruginosa* bacteremia was induced in rabbits either by constant intravenous infusion of bacteria or by intratracheal inoculation to produce pneumonia. Only the animals with pneumonia developed septic shock. Hypotension occurred only when TNF could move from the lungs into the blood. Shock could be prevented by use of a *P. aeruginosa* strain that did not disrupt alveolar epithelial permeability or by administration of an anti-TNF antibody prior to the onset of pneumonia. Clinical observations also suggest that uncontrolled local inflammation may drive the septic reaction. In a large series of patients with positive blood cultures, the risk of developing severe sepsis was strongly related to the site of primary infection: bacteremia arising from a pulmonary or abdominal source was eightfold more likely to be associated with severe sepsis than was bacteremic urinary tract infection, even after controlling for age, the kind of bacteria isolated from the blood, and other factors. A third pathogenesis may be represented by severe sepsis due to superantigen-producing *Staphylococcus aureus* or *Streptococcus pyogenes*, since the T cell activation induced by these toxins produces a cytokine profile that differs substantially from that elicited by gram-negative bacterial infection.

In summary, the pathogenesis of severe sepsis may differ according to the infecting microbe, the site of the primary infection, the presence or absence of immune defects, and the prior physiologic status of the host. Genetic factors may also be important. In patients who have sustained major trauma, for example, studies in different ethnic groups have identified associations between allelic polymorphisms in TNF-α and interferon-γ genes and risk of developing severe sepsis. Further studies in this area are needed.

CLINICAL MANIFESTATIONS

The manifestations of the septic response are usually superimposed on the symptoms and signs of the patient's underlying illness and primary infection. The rate at which signs and symptoms develop may differ from patient to patient, and there are striking individual variations in presentation. For example, some patients with sepsis are normo- or hypothermic; the absence of fever is most common in neonates, in elderly patients, and in persons with uremia or alcoholism.

Hyperventilation is often an early sign. Disorientation, confusion, and other manifestations of encephalopathy may also develop early in the septic response, particularly in the elderly and in individuals with preexisting neurologic impairment. Focal neurologic signs are uncommon, although preexisting focal deficits may become more prominent.

Hypotension and DIC predispose to acrocyanosis and ischemic necrosis of peripheral tissues, most commonly the digits. Cellulitis, pustules, bullae, or hemorrhagic lesions may develop when hematogenous bacteria or fungi seed the skin or underlying soft tissue. Bacterial toxins may also be distributed hematogenously and elicit diffuse cutaneous reactions. On occasion, skin lesions may suggest specific pathogens. When sepsis is accompanied by cutaneous petechiae or purpura, infection with *Neisseria meningitidis* (or, less commonly, *Haemophilus influenzae*) should be suspected (Fig. 127-1); in a patient who has been bitten by a tick while in an endemic area, petechial lesions also suggest Rocky Mountain spotted fever (Fig. 158-1). A cutaneous lesion seen almost exclusively in neutropenic patients is ecthyma gangrenosum, usually caused by *P. aeruginosa*. It is a bullous lesion, surrounded by edema, that undergoes central hemorrhage and necrosis (see Fig. 136-1). Histopathologic examination shows bacteria in and around the wall of a small vessel, with little or no neutrophilic response. Hemorrhagic or bullous lesions in a septic patient who has recently eaten raw oysters suggest *Vibrio vulnificus* bacteremia, while such lesions in a patient who has recently suffered a dog bite may indicate bloodstream infection due to *Capnocytophaga canimorsus* or *C. cynodegmi*. Generalized erythroderma in a septic patient suggests the toxic shock syndrome due to *S. aureus* or *S. pyogenes*.

Gastrointestinal manifestations such as nausea, vomiting, diarrhea, and ileus may suggest acute gastroenteritis. Stress ulceration can lead to upper gastrointestinal bleeding. Cholestatic jaundice, with elevated levels of serum bilirubin (mostly conjugated) and alkaline phosphatase, may precede other signs of sepsis. Hepatocellular or canalicular dysfunction appears to underlie most cases, and the results of hepatic function tests return to normal with resolution of the infection. Prolonged or severe hypotension may induce acute hepatic injury or ischemic bowel necrosis.

Many tissues may be unable to extract oxygen normally from the blood, so that anaerobic metabolism occurs despite near-normal mixed

venous oxygen saturation. Blood lactate levels rise early, in part because of increased glycolysis with impaired clearance of the resulting lactate and pyruvate by the liver and kidneys. As hypoperfusion develops, tissue hypoxia generates more lactic acid, contributing to metabolic acidosis. The blood glucose concentration often increases, particularly in patients with diabetes, although impaired gluconeogenesis and excessive insulin release on occasion produce hypoglycemia. The cytokine-driven acute-phase response inhibits the synthesis of transthyretin while enhancing the production of C-reactive protein, fibrinogen, and complement components. Protein catabolism is often markedly accelerated.

MAJOR COMPLICATIONS ■ Cardiopulmonary Complications

Ventilation-perfusion mismatching produces a fall in arterial P_{O_2} early in the course. Increasing alveolar capillary permeability results in an increased pulmonary water content, which decreases pulmonary compliance and interferes with oxygen exchange. Progressive diffuse pulmonary infiltrates and arterial hypoxemia (Pa_{O_2}/Fi_{O_2}, < 200) indicate the development of the acute respiratory distress syndrome (ARDS). ARDS develops in ~50% of patients with severe sepsis or septic shock. The failure of the respiratory muscles can exacerbate hypoxemia and hypercapnia. An elevated pulmonary capillary wedge pressure (>18 mmHg) suggests fluid volume overload or cardiac failure rather than ARDS. Pneumonia caused by viruses or by *Pneumocystis* may be clinically indistinguishable from ARDS.

Sepsis-induced hypotension (see "Septic Shock," above) usually results from a generalized maldistribution of blood flow and blood volume and from hypovolemia that is due, at least in part, to diffuse capillary leakage of intravascular fluid. Other factors that may decrease effective intravascular volume include dehydration from antecedent disease or insensible fluid losses, vomiting or diarrhea, and polyuria. During early septic shock, systemic vascular resistance is usually elevated and cardiac output may be low. After fluid repletion, in contrast, cardiac output typically increases and systemic vascular resistance falls. Indeed, normal or increased cardiac output and decreased systemic vascular resistance distinguish septic shock from cardiogenic, extracardiac obstructive, and hypovolemic shock; other processes that can produce this combination include anaphylaxis, beriberi, cirrhosis, and overdoses of nitroprusside or narcotics.

Depression of myocardial function, manifested as increased end-diastolic and systolic ventricular volumes with a decreased ejection fraction, develops within 24 h in most patients with severe sepsis. Cardiac output is maintained despite the low ejection fraction because ventricular dilatation permits a normal stroke volume. In survivors, myocardial function returns to normal over several days. Although myocardial dysfunction may contribute to hypotension, refractory hypotension is usually due to a low systemic vascular resistance, and death results from refractory shock or the failure of multiple organs rather than from cardiac dysfunction per se.

Renal Complications

Oliguria, azotemia, proteinuria, and nonspecific urinary casts are frequently found. Many patients are inappropriately polyuric; hyperglycemia may exacerbate this tendency. Most renal failure is due to acute tubular necrosis induced by hypotension or capillary injury, although some patients also have glomerulonephritis, renal cortical necrosis, or interstitial nephritis. Drug-induced renal damage may complicate therapy, particularly when hypotensive patients are given aminoglycoside antibiotics.

Coagulation

Although thrombocytopenia occurs in 10 to 30% of patients, the underlying mechanisms are not understood. Platelet counts are usually very low (<50,000/μL) in patients with DIC; these low counts may reflect diffuse endothelial injury or microvascular thrombosis.

Neurologic Complications

When the septic illness lasts for weeks to months, "critical-illness" polyneuropathy may prevent weaning from ventilatory support and produce distal motor weakness. Electrophysiologic studies are diagnostic. Guillain-Barré syndrome, metabolic disturbances, and toxin activity must be ruled out.

LABORATORY FINDINGS Abnormalities that occur early in the septic response may include leukocytosis with a left shift, thrombocytopenia, hyperbilirubinemia, and proteinuria. Leukopenia may develop. The neutrophils may contain toxic granulations, Döhle bodies, or cytoplasmic vacuoles. As the septic response becomes more severe, thrombocytopenia worsens (often with prolongation of the thrombin time, decreased fibrinogen, and the presence of D-dimers, suggesting DIC), azotemia and hyperbilirubinemia become more prominent, and levels of aminotransferases rise. Active hemolysis suggests clostridial bacteremia, malaria, a drug reaction, or DIC; in the case of DIC, microangiopathic changes may be seen on a blood smear.

During early sepsis, hyperventilation induces respiratory alkalosis. With respiratory muscle fatigue and the accumulation of lactate, metabolic acidosis (with increased anion gap) typically supervenes. Evaluation of arterial blood gases reveals hypoxemia, which is initially correctable with supplemental oxygen but whose later refractoriness to 100% oxygen inhalation indicates right-to-left shunting. The chest radiograph may be normal or may show evidence of underlying pneumonia, volume overload, or the diffuse infiltrates of ARDS. The electrocardiogram may show only sinus tachycardia or nonspecific ST–T–wave abnormalities.

Most diabetic patients with sepsis develop hyperglycemia. Severe infection may precipitate diabetic ketoacidosis, which may exacerbate hypotension (Chap. 323). Hypoglycemia occurs rarely. The serum albumin level, initially within the normal range, declines as sepsis continues. Serum lipid concentrations are often elevated. Hypocalcemia is rare.

DIAGNOSIS There is no specific diagnostic test for the septic response. Diagnostically sensitive findings in a patient with suspected or proven infection include fever or hypothermia, tachypnea, tachycardia, and leukocytosis or leukopenia (Table 254-1); acutely altered mental status, thrombocytopenia, or hypotension also suggests the diagnosis. The septic response can be quite variable, however. In one study, 36% of patients with severe sepsis had a normal temperature, 40% had a normal respiratory rate, 10% had a normal pulse rate, and 33% had normal white blood cell counts. Moreover, the systemic responses of uninfected patients with other conditions may be similar to those characteristic of sepsis. Noninfectious etiologies of SIRS (Table 254-1) include pancreatitis, burns, trauma, adrenal insufficiency, pulmonary embolism, dissecting or ruptured aortic aneurysm, myocardial infarction, occult hemorrhage, cardiac tamponade, post-cardiopulmonary bypass syndrome, anaphylaxis, and drug overdose.

Definitive etiologic diagnosis requires isolation of the microorganism from blood or a local site of infection. At least two blood samples (10 mL each) should be obtained (from different venipuncture sites) for culture. Because gram-negative bacteremia is typically low-grade (<10 organisms per milliliter of blood), multiple blood cultures or prolonged incubation of cultures may be necessary; *S. aureus* grows more readily and is detectable in blood cultures within 48 h in most instances. In many cases, blood cultures are negative; this result can reflect prior antibiotic administration, the presence of slow-growing or fastidious organisms, or the absence of microbial invasion of the bloodstream. In these cases, Gram's staining and culture of material from the primary site of infection or of infected cutaneous lesions may help establish the microbial etiology. The skin and mucosae should be examined carefully and repeatedly for lesions that might yield diagnostic information. With overwhelming bacteremia (e.g., pneumococcal sepsis in splenectomized individuals or fulminant meningococcemia), microorganisms are sometimes visible on buffy coat smears of peripheral blood.

Detection of endotoxin in blood by the limulus lysate test may portend a poor outcome, but this assay is not useful for diagnosing gram-negative bacterial infections, including gram-negative bacteremia. Although blood levels of IL-6 may also correlate with prognosis, cytokine assays are poorly standardized and currently have limited clinical value.

℞ TREATMENT

Patients in whom sepsis is suspected must be managed expeditiously. This task is best accomplished by personnel who are experienced in the care of the critically ill. Successful management requires urgent measures to treat the local site of infection, to provide hemodynamic and respiratory support, and to eliminate the offending microorganism. The outcome is also influenced by the patient's underlying disease, which should be managed aggressively.

ANTIMICROBIAL AGENTS Antimicrobial chemotherapy should be initiated as soon as samples of blood and other relevant sites have been cultured. The choice of initial therapy is based on knowledge of the likely pathogens at specific sites of local infection. Available information about patterns of antimicrobial susceptibility among bacterial isolates from the community, the hospital, and the patient also should be taken into account. It is important, pending culture results, to initiate empirical antimicrobial therapy that is effective against both gram-positive and gram-negative bacteria (Table 254-4). Maximal recommended doses of antimicrobial drugs should be given intravenously, with adjustment for impaired renal function when necessary. When culture results become available, the regimen can often be simplified, as a single antimicrobial agent is frequently adequate for the treatment of a known pathogen. Most patients require antimicrobial therapy for at least 1 week; the duration of treatment is typically influenced by factors such as the site of tissue infection, the adequacy of surgical drainage, the patient's underlying disease, and the antimicrobial susceptibility of the bacterial isolate(s).

REMOVAL OF THE SOURCE OF INFECTION Removal or drainage of a focal source of infection is essential. Sites of occult infection should be sought carefully. Indwelling intravenous catheters should be removed, the tip rolled over a blood agar plate for quantitative culture, and a new catheter inserted at a different site. Foley and drainage catheters should be replaced. The possibility of paranasal sinusitis (often caused by gram-negative bacteria) should be considered if the patient has undergone nasal intubation. In patients with extensive abnormalities on chest radiographs, computed tomography (CT) of the chest may identify unsuspected parenchymal, mediastinal, or pleural disease. In the neutropenic patient, cutaneous sites of tenderness and erythema, particularly in the perianal region, must be carefully sought. In patients with sacral or ischial decubitus ulcers, it is important to exclude pelvic or other soft tissue pus collections (by CT or magnetic resonance imaging, if necessary). In patients with severe sepsis arising from the urinary tract, sonography or CT should be used to rule out ureteral obstruction, perinephric abscess, and renal abscess. These studies are not so urgent in patients with less severe urosepsis, provided that a clinical response is evident within 48 to 72 h.

HEMODYNAMIC, RESPIRATORY, AND METABOLIC SUPPORT The primary goal is to restore adequate oxygen and substrate delivery to the tissues. Adequate organ perfusion is essential. Effective intravascular volume depletion is common in patients with sepsis, and initial management of hypotension should include the administration of intravenous fluids, typically 1 to 2 L of normal saline over 1 to 2 h. To avoid pulmonary edema, the pulmonary capillary wedge pressure should be maintained between 12 and 16 mmHg or the central venous pressure between 8 and 12 cmH$_2$O. The urine output rate should be kept at >0.5 mL/kg per hour by continuing fluid administration; a diuretic such as furosemide may be used if needed. In about one-third of patients, hypotension and organ hypoperfusion respond to fluid resuscitation; a reasonable goal is to maintain a mean arterial blood pressure of >65 mmHg (systolic pressure, >90 mmHg) and a cardiac index of ≥4 L/min per m². If these guidelines cannot be met by volume infusion, inotropic and vasopressor therapy is indicated. Circulatory adequacy is also assessed by clinical parameters (mentation, urine output, skin perfusion) and, when possible, by measurements of oxygen delivery and consumption. A recent study found that prompt resuscitative measures, including maintenance of central venous oxygen saturation at >70% (by administration of dobutamine, if needed), were associated with significantly improved survival in patients who were admitted to the emergency department with severe sepsis.

Adrenal insufficiency should be considered in septic patients with refractory hypotension, fulminant *N. meningitidis* bacteremia, prior glucocorticoid use, disseminated tuberculosis, or AIDS. The cosyntropin (α^{1-24}-ACTH) stimulation test (Chap. 321) may suggest absolute or partial adrenal insufficiency. Supplemental hydrocortisone (50 mg intravenously every 6 h) may be given while the results of the cosyntropin test are awaited (see "Antimediator Agents," below).

Plasma vasopressin levels do not increase in patients with septic shock. Recent studies have found that vasopressin infusion can reverse septic shock in some patients, reducing or eliminating the need for catecholamine pressors. An adequately powered and randomized trial of vasopressin infusion has not been performed, however, and its impact on end-organ function and survival is not known.

Ventilator therapy is indicated for progressive hypoxemia, hypercapnia, neurologic deterioration, or respiratory muscle failure. Sustained tachypnea (respiratory rate, >30 breaths/min) is frequently a harbinger of impending respiratory collapse; mechanical ventilation is often initiated to ensure adequate oxygenation, divert blood from the muscles of respiration, prevent aspiration of oropharyngeal contents, and reduce the cardiac afterload. Erythrocyte transfusion is indicated if oxygen delivery is compromised by a low hemoglobin concentration (<7 g/dL).

Bicarbonate is sometimes administered for severe metabolic acidosis (arterial pH <7.2). DIC, if complicated by major bleeding, should be treated with transfusion of fresh-frozen plasma and platelets. Successful treatment of the underlying infection is essential to reverse both acidosis and DIC.

GENERAL SUPPORT In patients with prolonged severe sepsis (i.e., that lasting more than 2 or 3 days), nutritional supplementation may reduce the impact of protein hypercatabolism; available evidence favors the enteral delivery route. Recovery is also assisted by preventing skin breakdown, deep venous thrombosis, nosocomial infections, and stress ulcers.

OTHER MEASURES Despite aggressive management, many patients with severe sepsis or septic shock die. Three kinds of agents that may help prevent these deaths are being investigated: (1) drugs that neutralize bacterial endotoxin, thereby potentially benefiting the fraction (approximately half) of septic patients who have gram-negative bacterial infection; (2) anti-inflammatory drugs that interfere with one or more mediators of the inflammatory response; and (3) anticoagulant drugs intended to prevent or reverse microthrombosis.

Antiendotoxin Agents Despite much effort to develop drugs that neutralize endotoxin in vivo, the potential of endotoxin as a target for therapeutic intervention remains controversial. In placebo-controlled clinical trials, two monoclonal antibodies to endotoxin did not prevent the

TABLE 254-4 *Initial Antimicrobial Therapy for Severe Sepsis with No Obvious Source in Adults with Normal Renal Function*

Clinical Condition	Antimicrobial Regimens (Intravenous Therapy)
Immunocompetent adult	The many acceptable regimens include (1) ceftriaxone (2 g q24h) *or* ticarcillin-clavulanate (3.1 g q4–6h) *or* piperacillin-tazobactam (3.375 g q4–6h); (2) imipenem-cilastatin (0.5 g q6h) *or* meropenem (1 g q8h) *or* cefepime (2 g q12h). Gentamicin *or* tobramycin (5–7 mg/kg q24h) may be *added* to either regimen. If the patient is allergic to β-lactam agents, use ciprofloxacin (400 mg q12h) *or* levofloxacin (500–750 mg q12h) *plus* clindamycin (600 mg q8h). If the institution has a high incidence of MRSA infections, add vancomycin (15 mg/kg q12h) to each of the above regimens.
Neutropenia[a] (<500 neutrophils/μL)	Regimens include (1) imipenem-cilastatin (0.5 g q6h) *or* meropenem (1 g q8h) *or* cefepime (2 g q8h); (2) ticarcillin-clavulanate (3.1 g q4h) *or* piperacillin-tazobactam (3.375 g q4h) *plus* tobramycin (5–7 mg/kg q24h). Vancomycin (15 mg/kg q12h) and cefepime should be used if the patient has an infected vascular catheter, if staphylococci are suspected, if the patient has received quinolone prophylaxis, if the patient has received intensive chemotherapy that produces mucosal damage, or if the institution has a high incidence of MRSA infections.
Splenectomy	Cefotaxime (2 g q6–8h) *or* ceftriaxone (2 g q12h) should be used. If the local prevalence of cephalosporin-resistant pneumococci is high, *add* vancomycin. If the patient is allergic to β-lactam drugs, vancomycin (15 mg/kg q12h) *plus* ciprofloxacin (400 mg q12h) *or* levofloxacin (750 mg q12h) *or* aztreonam (2 g q8h) should be used.
IV drug user	Nafcillin or oxacillin (2 g q8h) plus gentamicin (5–7 mg/kg q24h). If the local prevalence of MRSA is high or if the patient is allergic to β-lactam drugs, vancomycin (15 mg/kg q12h) with gentamicin should be used.
AIDS	Cefepime (2 g q8h), ticarcillin-clavulanate (3.1 g q4h), *or* piperacillin-tazobactam (3.375 g q4h) *plus* tobramycin (5–7 mg/kg q24h) should be used. If the patient is allergic to β-lactam drugs, ciprofloxacin (400 mg q12h) *or* levofloxacin (750 mg q12h) *plus* vancomycin (15 mg/kg q12h) *plus* tobramycin should be used.

[a] Adapted in part from WT Hughes et al: Clin Infect Dis 25:551, 1997.
Note: MRSA, methicillin-resistant *Staphylococcus aureus*.

death of patients with severe gram-negative bacterial sepsis. These antibodies did not bind to LPS with high affinity, and one was later reported to be a polyreactive autoantibody. A theoretically more promising agent is bactericidal permeability-increasing (BPI) protein, a human neutrophil protein that neutralizes lipid A and may be lethal for many gram-negative bacteria. In one clinical trial, infusion of BPI protein decreased the incidence of severe thrombotic events among children with fulminant meningococcemia. Other investigational drugs include nontoxic lipid A analogues that reduce host responses to endotoxins by competing with lipid A for interaction with the TLR4 signaling complex.

Antimediator Agents Other adjunctive therapies are intended to control the inflammatory response, regardless of the microbial stimulus. However, numerous agents that directly or indirectly interfere with the actions of inflammatory mediators have not prevented the death of patients with severe sepsis or septic shock. Many factors have probably contributed to the unsuccessful outcomes of these trials, including problems with study design (inappropriate end points, inadequate sample size, population heterogeneity, multiple covariates) and drug administration (wrong dose, time, or duration of administration). Anti-inflammatory drugs tested in clinical trials include methylprednisolone, dexamethasone, ibuprofen, PAF antagonists, recombinant IL-1Ra, genetically engineered soluble receptors for TNF-α, and monoclonal antibodies to TNF-α.

Whereas large doses of glucocorticoids have not improved survival, recent evidence suggests that many septic patients have inadequate adrenal reserve and that these individuals may benefit from low doses of glucocorticoid and mineralocorticoid. A recent study measured each patient's plasma cortisol response to a bolus infusion of 250 μg of synthetic ACTH. In the study population of severely septic patients, an increment of ≤9 μg/dL correlated with partial adrenal insufficiency and identified a group of patients who benefited from the administration of hydrocortisone (50 mg intravenously every 6 h) and 9-α-fludrocortisone (50 μg/d via nasogastric tube) for 7 days. The 28-day mortality was 53% among adrenal-deficient (nonresponder) patients who received combined steroid therapy and 63% in the placebo group (*p* < .02). Patients who had normal adrenal reserve did not benefit from steroid administration. Although these results have not been confirmed in a second clinical trial, the strategy has a strong physiologic rationale.

Anticoagulant Agents   Recombinant activated protein C (aPC) recently became the first drug to be approved by the U.S. Food and Drug Administration (FDA) for the treatment of patients with severe sepsis or septic shock. In a randomized controlled trial in which drug or placebo was given within 24 h of the patient's first sepsis-related organ dysfunction, 28-day mortality was significantly lower among recipients of aPC than among patients who received placebo (24.7% vs. 30.8%; *p* < .005). In addition, aPC recipients were more likely than placebo recipients to have severe bleeding (3% vs. 2%). Survival improved only for patients who had an APACHE II score of ≥25 during the 24 h before initiation of aPC infusion. Specifically, the FDA has approved aPC for use in adults (>18 years of age) who meet the APACHE II criterion and have a low risk of hemorrhage-related side effects. The drug is administered as a constant intravenous infusion of 24 μg/kg per hour for 96 h. Each patient's clotting parameters must be monitored carefully. Intracranial hemorrhage, the most serious complication noted to date, has occurred infrequently but seems to be more common among patients with platelet counts of <30,000/μL or meningitis at the time of infusion.

The long-term impact of aPC treatment is uncertain. In the pivotal clinical trial, the treatment and placebo groups did not differ significantly in the percentage of patients who had been discharged from the hospital by treatment day 28. Long-term survival data have not been released by the sponsor. Although the theoretical rationale for treating septic patients with anticoagulants is strong, two other human anticoagulant proteins (antithrombin III and tissue factor pathway inhibitor) did not improve patient survival in recent clinical trials, and the apparent efficacy of aPC did not correlate with preinfusion blood levels of protein C or other clotting parameters. In vitro studies suggest that aPC has anti-inflammatory activities that could contribute to its therapeutic effect.

Studies are needed to determine the relative benefits of hydrocortisone and mineralocorticoid treatment (in patients with adrenal insufficiency), vasopressin, and aPC and to learn how these agents should best be used—singly, together, or in combination with other agents.

PROGNOSIS   Approximately 20 to 35% of patients with severe sepsis and 40 to 60% of patients with septic shock die within 30 days. Others die within the ensuing 6 months. Late deaths often result from poorly controlled infection, complications of intensive care, failure of multiple organs, or the patient's underlying disease.

Prognostic stratification systems such as APACHE II indicate that factoring in the patient's age, underlying condition, and various physiologic variables can yield estimates of the risk of dying of severe sepsis. Of the individual covariates, the severity of underlying disease most strongly influences the risk of dying. Septic shock is also a strong predictor of short- and long-term mortality. Case-fatality rates are similar for culture-positive and culture-negative severe sepsis.

PREVENTION   Prevention offers the best opportunity to reduce morbidity and mortality. In developed countries, most episodes of severe sepsis and septic shock are complications of nosocomial infections. These cases might be prevented by reducing the number of invasive procedures undertaken, by limiting the use (and duration of use) of indwelling vascular and bladder catheters, by reducing the incidence and duration of profound neutropenia (<500 neutrophils/μL), and by more aggressively treating localized nosocomial infections. Indiscriminate use of antimicrobial agents and glucocorticoids should be avoided, and optimal infection-control measures (Chap. 116) should be used. Several studies point to associations between allelic polymorphisms in cytokine genes and risk of developing severe sepsis; if these associations prove to be broadly applicable, such polymorphisms can be used prospectively to identify high-risk patients and to target preventive and/or therapeutic measures to them. Studies indicate that 50 to 70% of patients who develop nosocomial severe sepsis or septic shock have experienced a less severe stage of the septic response (e.g., SIRS, sepsis) on at least one previous day in the hospital. Research is needed to develop adjunctive agents that can damp the septic response before organ dysfunction or hypotension occurs.

FURTHER READING

ANNANE D et al: Effect of treatment with low doses of hydrocortisone and fludrocortisone on mortality in patients with septic shock. JAMA 288:862, 2002

BERNARD GR et al: Efficacy and safety of recombinant human activated protein C for severe sepsis. N Engl J Med 344:699, 2001

DE BACKER D et al: Microvascular blood flow is altered in patients with sepsis. Am J Respir Crit Care Med 166:98, 2002

HOLMES CL et al: Physiology of vasopressin relevant to management of septic shock. Chest 120:989, 2001

HOTCHKISS RS, KARL IE: The pathophysiology and treatment of sepsis. N Engl J Med 348:138, 2003

MUNFORD RS, PUGIN J: Normal responses to injury prevent systemic inflammation and can be immunosuppressive. Am J Respir Crit Care Med 163:316, 2001

RIVERS E et al: Early goal-directed therapy in the treatment of severe sepsis and septic shock. N Engl J Med 345:1368, 2001

SANDS KE et al: Epidemiology of sepsis syndrome in 8 academic medical centers. JAMA 278:234, 1997

255   CARDIOGENIC SHOCK AND PULMONARY EDEMA
Judith S. Hochman, David Ingbar

Cardiogenic shock and pulmonary edema are life-threatening conditions that should be treated as medical emergencies. The most common etiology for both is severe left ventricular (LV) dysfunction, leading to pulmonary congestion and/or systemic hypoperfusion (Fig. 255-1). →*The pathophysiology of pulmonary edema and shock are discussed in Chaps. 29 and 253, respectively.*

CARDIOGENIC SHOCK

Cardiogenic shock (CS) is characterized by systemic hypoperfusion due to severe depression of the cardiac index [<2.2 (L/min)/m²] and sustained systolic arterial hypotension (<90 mmHg), despite an elevated filling pressure [pulmonary capillary wedge pressure (PCWP) > 18 mmHg]. It is associated with in-hospital mortality rates >50%. The major causes of CS are listed in Table 255-1. Circulatory failure based on cardiac dysfunction may be caused by primary myocardial failure, most commonly secondary to acute myocardial infarction (MI) (Chap. 228), and less frequently by cardiomyopathy or myocarditis (Chap. 221) or cardiac tamponade (Chap. 222).

INCIDENCE   CS is the leading cause of death of patients hospitalized with MI. Early reperfusion therapy for acute MI decreases the incidence of CS. The rate of CS complicating acute MI fell from 20% in the 1960s but has plateaued at ~8% for over 20 years. Shock is typically associated with ST elevation MI and is less common with non-ST elevation MI (Chap. 228).

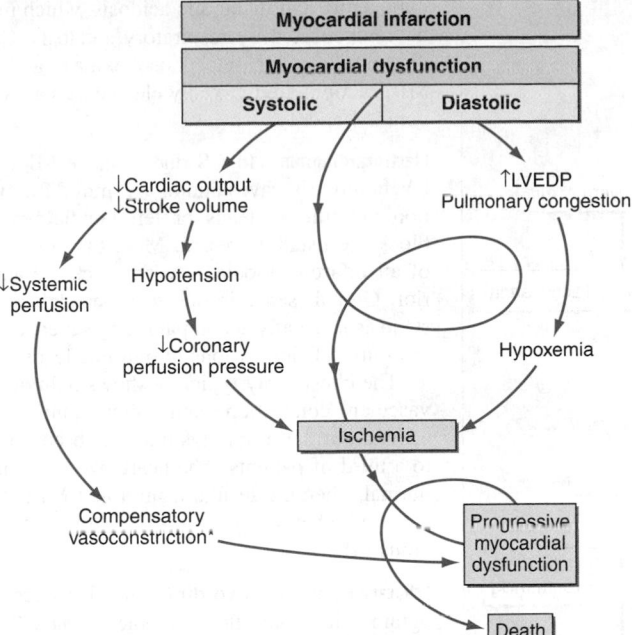

FIGURE 255-1 Pathophysiology of cardiogenic shock. Systolic and diastolic myocardial dysfunction result in a reduction in cardiac output and often pulmonary congestion. Systemic and coronary hypoperfusion occur, resulting in progressive ischemia. Although a number of compensatory mechanisms are activated in an attempt to support the circulation, these compensatory mechanisms may become maladaptive and produce a worsening of hemodynamics. *Release of inflammatory cytokines after myocardial infarction may lead to inducible nitrous oxide expression, excess NO, and inappropriate vasodilation. This causes further reduction in systemic and coronary perfusion. A vicious spiral of progressive myocardial dysfunction occurs that ultimately results in death if it is not interrupted. LVEDP, left ventricular end-diastolic pressure. *(From SM Hollenberg et al: Ann Intern Med 131:47, 1999.)*

LV failure accounts for ~80% of the cases of CS complicating acute MI. Acute severe mitral regurgitation (MR), ventricular septal rupture (VSR), predominant right ventricular (RV) failure, and free wall rupture or tamponade account for the remainder.

PATHOPHYSIOLOGY CS is characterized by a vicious circle in which depression of myocardial contractility, usually due to ischemia, results in reduced cardiac output and arterial pressure, which result in hypoperfusion of the myocardium and further ischemia and depression of the cardiac output (Fig. 255-1). Systolic myocardial dysfunction reduces stroke volume and, together with diastolic dysfunction, leads to elevated LV end-diastolic pressure and PCWP as well as to pulmonary congestion. Reduced coronary perfusion leads to worsening ischemia and progressive myocardial dysfunction and a rapid downward spiral, which, if uninterrupted, is often fatal. A systemic inflammatory response syndrome may accompany large infarctions and shock. Inflammatory cytokines, inducible nitric oxide synthase, and excess nitric oxide and peroxynitrite may contribute to the genesis of CS as they do to other forms of shock (Chap. 253). Hypoxemia and lactic acidosis develop as a result of pump failure and then contribute to the vicious circle by worsening myocardial ischemia and hypotension. Severe acidosis (pH <7.25) reduces the efficacy of endogenous and exogenously administered catecholamines. Refractory sustained ventricular or atrial tachyarrhythmias can cause or exacerbate CS.

Autopsy specimens often reflect the stuttering course and piecemeal necrosis of the left ventricle, often showing varying stages of infarction. Reinfarction is apparent as new areas of necrosis contiguous with or remote from a slightly older infarct. Typically, at least 40% of the LV myocardium is damaged by a combination of old scar and new infarcts. Infarctions that extend through the full myocardial thickness and result in rupture of the interventricular septum, papillary muscle, or ventricular free wall may result in shock (Chap. 228 and p. 1616).

PATIENT PROFILE In patients with acute MI, older age, female sex, prior MI, diabetes, and anterior MI location are all associated with increased risk of CS. Shock associated with a first inferior MI should prompt a search for a mechanical cause. In patients with non-ST elevation acute coronary syndrome (ACS), prior heart failure (HF), coronary artery bypass graft (CABG) surgery, and peripheral vascular disease are additional important risk factors. Reinfarction soon after MI increases the risk of CS. Severe and extensive coronary artery atherosclerotic lesions are typically present in MI patients who develop shock. Two-thirds of patients with CS have flow-limiting stenoses in all three major coronary arteries, and 20% have left main coronary artery stenosis.

TIMING Shock is present on admission in only 10 to 15% of patients who develop CS complicating MI; one-half develop it rapidly thereafter, within 6 h of MI onset. Another quarter develop shock later on the first day. Subsequent onset of CS may be due to reinfarction, marked infarct expansion, or a mechanical complication.

DIAGNOSIS Due to the unstable condition of these patients, supportive therapy must be initiated simultaneously with diagnostic evaluation (Fig. 255-2). A focused history and physical examination should be performed, blood specimens sent to the laboratory, and an electrocardiogram and chest x-ray obtained. A two-dimensional echocardiogram with color flow Doppler is an invaluable diagnostic tool in patients suspected of CS.

Clinical Findings Most patients have continuing chest pain and dyspnea and appear pale, apprehensive, cyanotic, and diaphoretic. Mentation may be altered, with varying degrees of somnolence, confusion, and

TABLE 255-1 *Etiologies of Cardiogenic Shock (CS)[a] and Cardiogenic Pulmonary Edema[b]*

ETIOLOGIES OF CARDIOGENIC SHOCK OR PULMONARY EDEMA

Acute myocardial infarction/ischemia
  LV failure
  VSR
  Papillary muscle/chordal rupture—severe MR
  Ventricular free wall rupture with subacute tamponade
  Other conditions complicating large MIs
    Hemorrhage
    Infection
    Excess negative inotropic or vasodilator medications
    Prior valvular heart disease
    Hyperglycemia/ketoacidosis
Post-cardiac arrest
Post-cardiotomy
Refractory sustained tachyarrhythmias
Acute fulminant myocarditis
End-stage cardiomyopathy
Hypertrophic cardiomyopathy with severe outflow obstruction
Aortic dissection with aortic insufficiency or tamponade
Pulmonary embolus
Severe valvular heart disease
  Critical aortic or mitral stenosis
  Acute severe aortic or MR
Toxic-metabolic
  Beta-blocker or calcium channel antagonist overdose

OTHER ETIOLOGIES OF CARDIOGENIC SHOCK[c]

RV failure due to:
  Acute myocardial infarction
  Acute coronary pulmonale
Refractory sustained bradyarrhythmias
Pericardial tamponade
Toxic/metabolic
  Severe acidosis, severe hypoxemia

[a] The etiologies of CS are listed. Most of these can cause pulmonary edema instead of shock or pulmonary edema with CS.
[b] Etiologies of noncardiogenic pulmonary edema are in Chap. 29.
[c] These cause CS but not pulmonary edema.
Note: LV, left ventricular; VSR, ventricular septal rupture; MR, mitral regurgitation; RV, right ventricular.

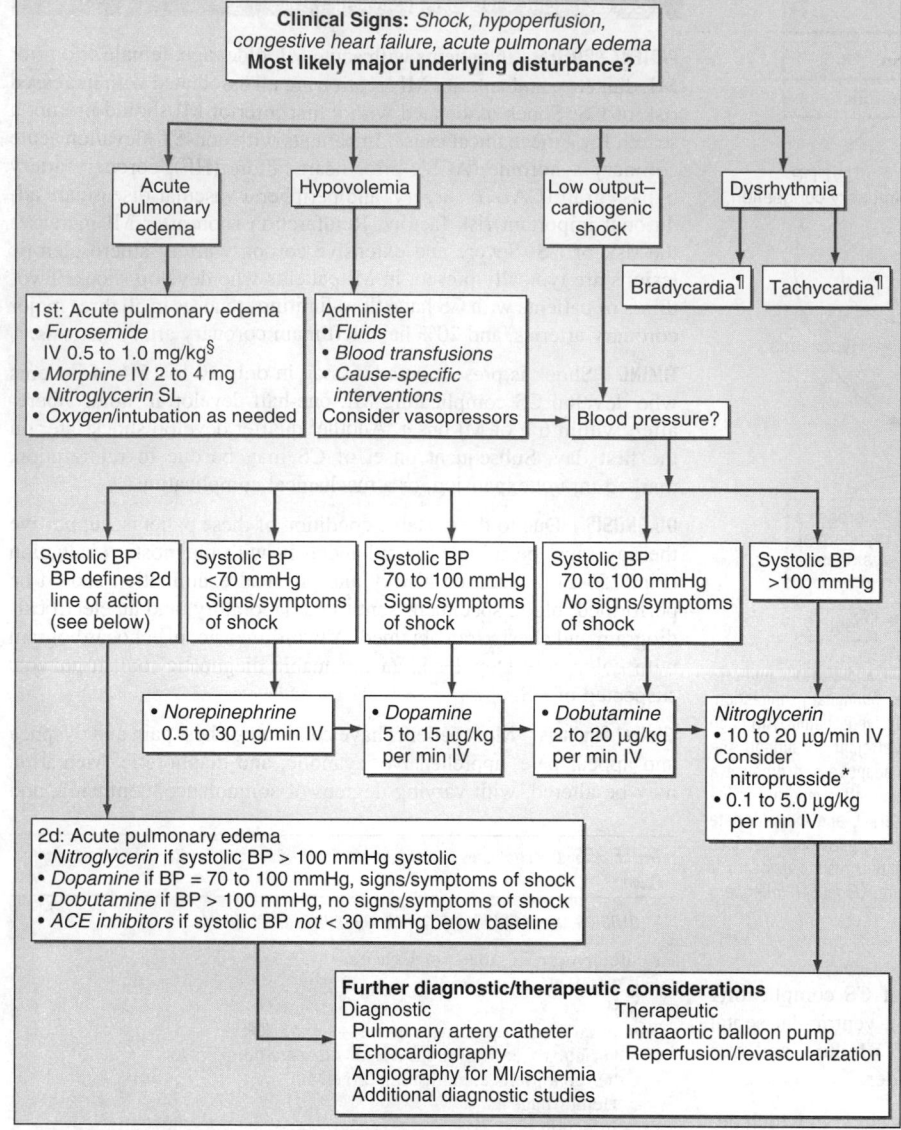

Clinical Signs: *Shock, hypoperfusion, congestive heart failure, acute pulmonary edema*
Most likely major underlying disturbance?

- Acute pulmonary edema
- Hypovolemia
- Low output–cardiogenic shock
- Dysrhythmia
  - Bradycardia¶
  - Tachycardia¶

1st: Acute pulmonary edema
- *Furosemide* IV 0.5 to 1.0 mg/kg§
- *Morphine* IV 2 to 4 mg
- *Nitroglycerin* SL
- *Oxygen*/intubation as needed

Administer
- *Fluids*
- *Blood transfusions*
- *Cause-specific interventions*
Consider vasopressors

Blood pressure?

| Systolic BP BP defines 2d line of action (see below) | Systolic BP <70 mmHg Signs/symptoms of shock | Systolic BP 70 to 100 mmHg Signs/symptoms of shock | Systolic BP 70 to 100 mmHg *No* signs/symptoms of shock | Systolic BP >100 mmHg |

- *Norepinephrine* 0.5 to 30 µg/min IV
- *Dopamine* 5 to 15 µg/kg per min IV
- *Dobutamine* 2 to 20 µg/kg per min IV
- Nitroglycerin
  - 10 to 20 µg/min IV
  - Consider nitroprusside*
  - 0.1 to 5.0 µg/kg per min IV

2d: Acute pulmonary edema
- *Nitroglycerin* if systolic BP > 100 mmHg systolic
- *Dopamine* if BP = 70 to 100 mmHg, signs/symptoms of shock
- *Dobutamine* if BP > 100 mmHg, no signs/symptoms of shock
- *ACE inhibitors* if systolic BP *not* < 30 mmHg below baseline

Further diagnostic/therapeutic considerations

Diagnostic
- Pulmonary artery catheter
- Echocardiography
- Angiography for MI/ischemia
- Additional diagnostic studies

Therapeutic
- Intraaortic balloon pump
- Reperfusion/revascularization

FIGURE 255-2 The emergency management of patients with cardiogenic shock, acute pulmonary edema, or both is outlined. *Nitroprusside is contraindicated in states of reduced coronary artery perfusion. §Furosemide: <0.5 mg/kg for new-onset acute pulmonary edema without hypervolemia; 1 mg/kg for acute on chronic volume overload, renal insufficiency. ¶For management of bradycardia and tachycardia, see Chaps. 213 and 214. ACE, angiotensin-converting enzyme; BP, blood pressure; MI, myocardial infarction. [*Modified from Guidelines 2000 for Cardiopulmonary Resuscitation and Emergency Cardiovascular Care Part 7: The Era of Reperfusion. Section 1: Acute Coronary Syndromes (Acute Myocardial Infarction). Circulation 102 (suppl): I-172, 2000. Reprinted with permission from Circulation*].

agitation. The pulse is typically weak and rapid, often in the range of 90 to 110 beats/min, or severe bradycardia due to high-grade heart block may be present. Systolic arterial pressure is reduced (<90 mmHg) with a narrow pulse pressure (<30 mmHg), but occasionally arterial pressure may be maintained by very high systemic vascular resistance. Tachypnea, Cheyne-Stokes respirations, and jugular venous distention may be present. The precordium is typically quiet, with a weak apical pulse. S1 is usually soft, and an S3 gallop may be audible. Acute, severe MR and VSR are usually associated with characteristic systolic murmurs (Chap. 228). Rales are audible in most patients with LV failure causing CS. Oliguria (urine output < 30 mL/h) is common.

Laboratory Findings The white blood cell count is typically elevated with a left shift. In the absence of prior renal insufficiency, renal function is initially normal, but blood urea nitrogen and creatinine rise progressively. Hepatic transaminases may be markedly elevated due to liver hypoperfusion. Lactic acid levels are elevated in severe shock, and electrolytes may reflect anion-gap acidosis. Prior to ventilatory support with supplemental O_2, arterial blood gases usually demonstrate

hypoxemia and metabolic acidosis, which may be compensated by respiratory alkalosis. Cardiac markers, creatine phosphokinase and its MB fraction, are markedly elevated, as are troponins I and T.

Electrocardiogram In CS due to acute MI with LV failure, Q waves and/or >2-mm ST elevation in multiple leads or left bundle branch block are usually present. More than one-half of all infarcts associated with shock are anterior. Global ischemia due to severe left main stenosis is usually accompanied by severe (e.g., >3 mm) ST depressions in multiple leads.

The chest x-ray typically shows pulmonary vascular congestion and often pulmonary edema, but these findings may be absent in up to a third of patients. The heart size is usually normal when CS results from a first MI but is enlarged when it occurs in a patient with a previous MI.

Echocardiogram A two-dimensional echocardiogram with color flow Doppler (Chap. 211) should be obtained promptly in patients with suspected CS to help define its etiology. Doppler mapping demonstrates a left-to-right shunt in patients with VSR and the severity of MR when the latter is present. Proximal aortic dissection with aortic regurgitation or tamponade may be visualized or evidence for pulmonary embolism obtained (Chap. 244).

Pulmonary Artery Catheterization There is controversy regarding the use of pulmonary artery balloon flotation (Swan-Ganz) catheters in patients with established or suspected CS (Chaps. 212 and 249). However, given the ominous prognosis, their use is generally recommended for measurement of filling pressures and cardiac output to confirm the diagnosis and help optimize use of intravenous fluids, inotropic agents, and vasopressors (Table 255-2). Blood samples for O_2 saturation measurement should be obtained from the right atrium, right ventricle, and pulmonary artery to rule out a left-to-right shunt. Mixed venous O_2 saturations are low and arterial-venous O_2 differences are elevated, reflecting increased O_2 extraction and low cardiac index, and the PCWP is elevated. However, these measurements, as well as systemic arterial pressure, may have returned toward normal in the presence of sympathomimetic amines. Systemic vascular resistance may be normal or elevated in CS. Equalization of right- and left-sided filling pressures (right atrial and PCWP) suggests cardiac tamponade as the cause of CS (Chap. 222).

Left Heart Catheterization and Coronary Angiography Measurement of LV pressure, definition of the coronary anatomy, and left ventriculography provide useful information and are indicated in most patients with CS complicating MI. Because of the procedural risk in this critically ill population, cardiac catheterization should be performed when there is a plan and capability for immediate coronary intervention (see below) or when a definitive diagnosis has not been made by other tests.

℞ TREATMENT (Fig. 255-2)

General Measures In addition to the usual treatment of acute MI (Chap. 228), initial therapy is aimed at maintaining systemic and coronary perfusion by raising systolic blood pressure to ~90 mmHg with vaso-

TABLE 255-2 Hemodynamic Patterns[a]

	RA, mmHg	RVS, mmHg	RVD, mmHg	PAS, mmHg	PAD, mmHg	PCW, mmHg	CI, (L/min)/m²	SVR, (dyn · s)/cm⁵
Normal values	< 6	< 25	0–12	< 25	0–12	< 6–12	≥2.5	(800–1600)
MI without pulmonary edema[b]	—	—	—	—	—	~13 (5–18)	~2.7 (2.2–4.3)	—
Pulmonary edema	↔↑	↔↑	↔↑	↑	↑	↑	↔↓	↑
Cardiogenic shock								
LV failure[c]	↔↑	↔↑	↔↑	↑	↑	↑	↓	↔↑
RV failure[c]	↑	↓↔↑ᵈ	↑	↓↔↑ᵈ	↔↓↑ᵈ	↓↔↑ᵈ	↓	↔↑
Cardiac tamponade	↑	↔↑	↑	↑	↑	↔↑	↓	↔↑
Acute mitral regurgitation	↔↑	↑	↔↑	↑	↑	↑	↔↓	↔↑
Ventricular septal rupture	↑	↔↑	↑	↔↑	↔↑	↔↑	↑ PBF ↓ SBF	↔↑
Hypovolemic shock	↓	↔↓	↔↓	↓	↓	↓	↓	↑
Septic shock	↓	↔↓	↔↓	↓	↓	↓	↓	↑

[a] There is significant patient-to-patient variation. Pressure may be normalized if cardiac output is low.

[b] Forrester et al classified non-reperfused MI patients into four hemodynamic subsets. (From Forrester JS et al: N Engl J Med 295:1356, 1976.) PCWP and CI in clinically stable subset 1 patients are shown. Values in parentheses represent range.

[c] "Isolated" or predominant RV failure.

[d] PCW and PA pressures may rise in RV failure after volume loading due to RV dilation, right to left shift of the interventricular septum, resulting in impaired LV filling. When biventricular failure is present, the patterns are similar to those shown for LV failure.

Note: RA, right atrium; RVS/D, right ventricular systolic/diastolic; PAS/D, pulmonary artery systolic/diastolic; PCW, pulmonary capillary wedge; CI, cardiac index; SVR, systemic vascular resistance; MI, myocardial infarction; P/SBF, pulmonary/systemic blood flow.

Source: Table prepared with the assistance of Krishnan Ramanathan, MD.

pressors and adjusting volume status to a level that ensures optimum LV filling pressure (PCWP ~ 20 mmHg). Hypoxemia and acidosis must be corrected; most patients require endotracheal intubation to correct these abnormalities and reduce the work of breathing (see "Pulmonary Edema," below). Negative inotropic agents should be discontinued and the doses of renally cleared medications adjusted. Hyperglycemia should be corrected with continuous infusion of insulin. Bradyarrhythmias may require transvenous pacing. Recurrent ventricular tachycardia or rapid atrial fibrillation may require immediate treatment (Chap. 214).

Vasopressors Various intravenous drugs may be used to augment blood pressure and cardiac output in patients with CS. All have important disadvantages, and none has been shown to change the outcome in patients with established shock. *Norepinephrine* is a potent vasoconstrictor and inotropic stimulant that increases myocardial O₂ consumption; it should be reserved for patients with CS and refractory hypotension without elevated systemic vascular resistance. It should be started at a dosage of 2 to 4 μg/min and titrated upward as necessary. If systolic pressure cannot be maintained at 90 mmHg with a dosage of 15 μg/min, it is unlikely that a further increase will be beneficial.

Dopamine is useful in many patients; at low doses (≤2 μg/kg per min), it dilates the renal vascular bed; at moderate doses (2 to 10 μg/kg per min), it has positive chronotropic and inotropic effects as a consequence of β-receptor stimulation. At higher doses, a vasoconstrictor effect results from α-receptor stimulation. It is started at an infusion rate of 2 to 5 μg/kg per min, and the dosage is increased every 2 to 5 min to a maximum of 20 to 50 μg/kg per min. Systolic blood pressure should be maintained at ~90 mmHg. *Dobutamine* is a synthetic sympathomimetic amine with positive inotropic action and minimal positive chronotropic activity at low doses (2.5 μg/kg per min) but moderate chronotropic activity at higher doses. Although the usual dosage is up to 10 μg/kg per min, its vasodilating activity precludes its use when a vasoconstrictor effect is required.

Aortic Counterpulsation In CS, mechanical assistance with an intraaortic balloon pumping (IABP) system capable of augmenting both arterial diastolic pressure and cardiac output is helpful in rapidly stabilizing patients. A sausage-shaped balloon at the end of a catheter is introduced into the aorta percutaneously via the femoral artery, and the balloon is automatically inflated during early diastole, augmenting coronary blood flow. The balloon collapses in early systole, reducing the afterload against which the left ventricle ejects. IABP improves hemodynamic status at least temporarily in the majority of patients. In contrast to vasopressors and inotropic agents, myocardial O₂ consumption is reduced, leading to amelioration of ischemia. In the ab-

sence of early revascularization, however, long-term survival after this mode of therapy in patients with CS is disappointing. IABP is useful as a stabilizing measure in patients with CS prior to and during cardiac catheterization and percutaneous coronary intervention (PCI) or prior to urgent surgery. IABP is contraindicated if aortic regurgitation is present or aortic dissection is suspected. Ventricular assist devices may be considered for eligible young patients with refractory shock as a bridge to cardiac transplantation.

Reperfusion-Revascularization The rapid establishment of blood flow in the infarct-related artery is essential in the management of CS and forms the centerpiece of management. The randomized SHOCK Trial demonstrated 132 lives saved per 1000 patients treated with early revascularization with PCI or CABG compared to initial medical therapy including IABP with fibrinolytics followed by delayed revascularization (Fig. 255-3). The greatest benefit was in patients <75 years. Early revascularization with PCI or CABG is a class I recommendation for such patients with ST elevation or left bundle branch block MI who develop CS within 36 h of MI and who can be revascularized within 18 h of development of shock. When mechanical revascularization is not possible, IABP and fibrinolytic therapy are recommended. Older patients should be managed on an individual basis.

No. at risk

ERV	152	76	72	70
IMS	149	58	53	49

FIGURE 255-3 Early revascularization (ERV) (percutaneous coronary intervention or coronary artery bypass graft) for cardiogenic shock complicating acute myocardial infarction resulted in substantially improved 1-year survival compared to initial mechanical stabilization (IMS), including intraaortic balloon pumping and fibrinolytic agents, followed by selective delayed revascularization in the SHOCK Trial (SHould we emergently revascularize Occluded coronaries for Cardiogenic shocK?) *(Reprinted with permission from JAMA.)*

PROGNOSIS Within this high-risk condition, there is a wide range of expected death rates based on age, severity of hemodynamic abnormalities, severity of the clinical manifestations of hypoperfusion, and the performance of early revascularization. Independent risk factors are advanced age; depressed cardiac index, ejection fraction, and arterial pressure; elevated PCWP; more extensive coronary artery disease; and renal insufficiency.

SHOCK SECONDARY TO RIGHT VENTRICULAR INFARCTION Although transient hypotension is common in patients with RV infarction and inferior MI (Chap. 228), persistent CS due to RV failure accounts for only 3% of CS complicating MI. The salient features of RV shock are absence of pulmonary congestion, high right atrial pressure (which may be seen only after volume loading), RV dilatation and dysfunction, only mildly or moderately depressed LV function, and predominance of single-vessel proximal right coronary artery occlusion. Management includes intravenous fluid administration to optimize right atrial pressure (10 to 15 mmHg); avoidance of excess fluids, which cause a shift of the interventricular septum into the LV; sympathomimetic amines; IABP; and the early reestablishment of infarct-artery flow.

MITRAL REGURGITATION (See also Chap 228) Acute severe MR may complicate MI and result in CS and/or pulmonary edema. This complication most often occurs on the first day, with a second peak several days later. The diagnosis is confirmed by echo-Doppler. Rapid stabilization with IABP is recommended, with administration of dobutamine as needed to raise cardiac output. Reducing the load against which the left ventricle pumps (afterload) reduces the volume of regurgitant flow of blood into the left atrium. Mitral valve surgery is the definitive therapy and should be performed early in the course in suitable candidates.

VENTRICULAR SEPTAL RUPTURE (See also Chap 228) Echo-Doppler demonstrates shunting of blood from the left to the right ventricle and may visualize the opening in the interventricular septum. Timing and management are similar to that for MR with IABP support and surgical correction for suitable candidates.

FREE WALL RUPTURE Myocardial rupture is a dramatic complication of STEMI that is most likely to occur during the first week after the onset of symptoms; its frequency increases with the age of the patient. First infarction, a history of hypertension, no history of angina pectoris, and a relatively large Q-wave infarct are associated with a higher incidence of cardiac rupture. The clinical presentation typically is a sudden loss of pulse, blood pressure, and consciousness while the ECG continues to show sinus rhythm (apparent electromechanical dissociation or pulseless electrical activity). The myocardium continues to contract, but forward flow is not maintained as blood escapes into the pericardium. Cardiac tamponade (Chap. 222) ensues, and closed-chest massage is ineffective. This condition is almost universally fatal, although dramatic cases of urgent pericardiotensis followed by successful surgical repair have been reported.

ACUTE FULMINANT MYOCARDITIS (See also Chap 221) Myocarditis can mimic acute MI with ST deviation or bundle branch block on the electrocardiogram and marked elevation of cardiac markers. Acute myocarditis causes CS in ~15% of cases. These patients are typically younger than those with CS due to acute MI and often do not have typical ischemic chest pain. Echocardiography typically shows global LV dysfunction. Initial management is the same as for CS complicating acute MI (Fig. 255-2) but of course does not involve coronary revascularization.

PULMONARY EDEMA

→*The etiologies and pathophysiology of pulmonary edema are discussed in Chap. 29.*

DIAGNOSIS

Acute pulmonary edema usually presents with the rapid onset or aggravation of dyspnea at rest, tachypnea, tachycardia, and severe hypoxemia. In addition to rales, wheezing due to airway compression from peribronchial cuffing may be audible. Hypertension is usually present due to endogenous release of catecholamines.

It is often difficult to distinguish cardiogenic and noncardiogenic causes of acute pulmonary edema. *Echocardiography* with color flow Doppler may identify systolic and diastolic ventricular dysfunction and valvular lesions and aid in the differentiation of these two causes. Pulmonary edema associated with electrocardiographic ST elevation and evolving Q waves is usually diagnostic of acute MI and should prompt immediate institution of MI protocols and coronary artery reperfusion therapy (Chap. 228). Brain natriuretic peptide levels, when elevated, support heart failure as the etiology of acute dyspnea with pulmonary edema (Chap. 216).

The use of a *balloon flotation catheter* permits measurement of PCWP and helps to differentiate high pressure (cardiogenic) and normal pressure (noncardiogenic) causes of pulmonary edema. Pulmonary artery catheterization (see p. 1614) is indicated when the etiology of the pulmonary edema is uncertain, when it is refractory to therapy, or when it is accompanied by hypotension.

℞ TREATMENT

The treatment of pulmonary edema depends upon the specific etiology. Given the acute, life-threatening nature of the condition, a number of measures must be applied immediately to support the circulation, gas exchange, and lung mechanics as outlined in Fig. 255-2. In addition, conditions that frequently complicate pulmonary edema, such as infection, acidemia, anemia, and renal failure, must be corrected.

Support of Oxygenation and Ventilation Patients with acute cardiogenic pulmonary edema often have an identifiable cause of acute LV failure such as arrhythmia, ischemia, or myocardial decompensation (Chap. 216) that can be rapidly treated, with improvement in gas exchange. In contrast, noncardiogenic edema usually resolves much less quickly, and most patients require mechanical ventilation.

OXYGEN THERAPY Support of oxygenation is essential to ensure adequate O_2 delivery to peripheral tissues, including the heart.

POSITIVE PRESSURE VENTILATION The work of breathing and the O_2 requirements of this work are increased and may pose a significant physiologic stress on the heart. For patients with inadequate oxygenation or ventilation in spite of supplemental O_2, assisted ventilation should be initiated. This can be accomplished either by noninvasive ventilation using a face or nasal mask or by endotracheal intubation and ventilation. Continuous or bilevel positive airway pressure (Chap. 252) can rest the respiratory muscles, improve oxygenation and cardiac function, and reduce the need for intubation. In refractory cases, mechanical ventilation can relieve the work of breathing more completely than noninvasive ventilation. Mechanical ventilation with positive end-expiratory pressure can have multiple beneficial effects on pulmonary edema: (1) it can decrease both preload and afterload, thereby improving cardiac function; (2) it can redistribute lung water from the intraalveolar to the extraalveolar space where it does not interfere as much with gas exchange; and (3) it can increase lung volume to avoid atelectasis.

Reduction of Preload In most forms of pulmonary edema, the quantity of extravascular lung water is related to both the PCWP and the intravascular volume status.

DIURETICS The "loop diuretics" furosemide, bumetanide, and torsemide are effective in most forms of pulmonary edema, even in the presence of hypoalbuminemia, hyponatremia, or hypochloremia. Furosemide is also a venodilator that can reduce preload rapidly, prior to any diuresis, and is the diuretic of choice. The initial dose of furosemide should be ≤0.5 mg/kg, but a higher dose (1 mg/kg) is required in patients with renal insufficiency, chronic diuretic use, or hypervolemia or after failure of a lower dose.

NITRATES Nitroglycerin and isosorbide dinitrate act predominantly as venodilators, with coronary vasodilating properties as well. They are rapid in onset and effective when administered by a variety of routes. Sublingual nitroglycerin (0.4 mg × 3 every 5 min) is first-line therapy for acute cardiogenic pulmonary edema. If pulmonary edema persists and in the absence of hypotension, sublingual may be followed by intravenous nitroglycerin, commencing at 5 to 10 μg/min. Intravenous nitroprusside (0.1 to 5 μg/kg per min) is a potent and predominantly arterial vasodilator that is useful for patients with pulmonary edema and hypertension and for cautious afterload and preload reduction if systolic pressure >100 mmHg. It requires close monitoring and titration, including the use of an arterial catheter for continuous blood pressure measurement in the intensive care unit.

MORPHINE Given in 2- to 4-mg intravenous boluses, morphine is a transient venodilator that reduces preload while relieving dyspnea and anxiety. These effects can diminish stress, catecholamine levels, tachycardia, and ventricular afterload in patients with pulmonary edema and systemic hypertension.

ANGIOTENSIN-CONVERTING ENZYME (ACE) INHIBITORS ACE inhibitors reduce both afterload and preload and are recommended in hypertensive patients. A low dose of a short-acting agent may be initiated and followed by increasing oral doses. In acute MI with heart failure, ACE inhibitors reduce short- and long-term mortality.

OTHER PRELOAD-REDUCING AGENTS Intravenous recombinant brain natriuretic peptide (nesiritide) is a potent vasodilator with diuretic properties and is effective in the treatment of pulmonary edema. The starting dose is a 2-μg/kg intravenous bolus, followed by a 0.01-μg/kg per min infusion.

PHYSICAL METHODS Reduction of venous return reduces preload. Patients without hypotension should be maintained in the sitting position with the legs dangling along the side of the bed.

INOTROPIC AND INODILATOR DRUGS The sympathomimetic amines dopamine and dobutamine (see above) are potent inotropic agents. The bipyridine phosphodiesterase-3 inhibitors (inodilators), such as amrinone (0.75-mg/kg loading dose followed by 5 to 20 μg/kg per min) or milrinone (50 μg/kg followed by 0.25 to 0.75 μg/kg per min) stimulate myocardial contractility while promoting peripheral and pulmonary vasodilation. Such agents are indicated in patients with cardiogenic pulmonary edema and severe LV dysfunction.

DIGITALIS GLYCOSIDES Once a mainstay of treatment because of their positive inotropic action (Chap. 216), digitalis glycosides are rarely used at present. However, they may be useful for control of ventricular rate in patients with rapid atrial fibrillation or flutter and LV dysfunction, since they do not have the negative inotropic effects of other drugs that inhibit atrioventricular nodal conduction.

INTRAAORTIC COUNTERPULSATION IABP may help to relieve cardiogenic pulmonary edema. It is indicated as a stabilizing measure when acute severe mitral regurgitation or ventricular septal rupture cause refractory pulmonary edema, especially in preparation for surgical repair. IABP or LV-assist devices (Chap. 217) are useful as bridging therapy to cardiac transplantation in patients with refractory pulmonary edema secondary to myocarditis or cardiomyopathy.

TREATMENT OF TACHYARRHYTHMIAS AND ATRIAL-VENTRICULAR RESYNCHRONIZATION (See also Chap. 214) Sinus tachycardia or atrial fibrillation results from elevated left atrial pressure and sympathetic stimulation. Tachycardia itself can also limit LV filling time and raise left atrial pressure further. While relief of pulmonary congestion will slow the sinus rate or ventricular response in atrial fibrillation, a primary tachyarrhythmia may require cardioversion. In patients with reduced LV function and without atrial contraction or with lack of synchronized atrioventricular

contraction, placement of an atrioventricular sequential pacemaker should be considered (Chap. 213).

Special Considerations ■ *THE RISK OF IATROGENIC CARDIOGENIC SHOCK* In the treatment of pulmonary edema vasodilators lower blood pressure, and, particularly when used in combination, their use may lead to hypotension, coronary artery hypoperfusion, and shock (Fig. 255-1). In general, patients with a *hypertensive* response to pulmonary edema tolerate and are benefited by these medications. In normotensive patients, low doses of single agents should be instituted sequentially, as needed.

ACUTE CORONARY SYNDROMES Acute ST-segment elevation MI complicated by pulmonary edema is associated with in-hospital mortality rates of 20 to 40%. After immediate stabilization, coronary artery blood flow must be rapidly reestablished. When available, primary PCI is preferable; alternatively, a fibrinolytic agent should be administered. Early coronary angiography and revascularization by PCI or CABG are also indicated for patients with non-ST elevation acute coronary syndrome. IABP use may be required to stabilize patients for coronary angiography if hypotension develops or for refractory pulmonary edema in patients with LV failure who are candidates for revascularization (Chap. 228).

UNUSUAL TYPES OF EDEMA Specific etiologies of pulmonary edema may require particular therapy. One type is reexpansion pulmonary edema that develops after removal of air or fluid that has been in the pleural space for some time. These patients may develop hypotension or oliguria resulting from rapid fluid shifts into the lung. Diuretics and preload reduction are contraindicated, and intravascular volume repletion is often needed while supporting oxygenation and gas exchange.

The risk of development of high-altitude pulmonary edema can be prevented by use of dexamethasone, calcium channel-blocking drugs, or long-acting inhaled β_2-adrenergic agonists. Treatment includes descent from altitude, bed rest, oxygen, and, if feasible, inhaled nitric oxide; nifedipine may also be effective.

For pulmonary edema resulting from upper airway obstruction, recognition of the obstructing cause is key, since treatment then is to relieve or bypass the obstruction.

FURTHER READING

ANTMAN EM: Treatment of ST elevation myocardial infarction, in *Braunwald's Heart Disease*, 7th ed, D Zipes et al (eds). Philadelphia, Saunders, 2005

ANTMAN EM et al: ACC/AHA guidelines for the management of patients with ST-segment elevation myocardial infarction. J Am Coll Cardiol (In press)

COTTER G et al: Randomised trial of high-dose isosorbide dinitrate plus low-dose furosemide versus high-dose furosemide plus low-dose isosorbide dinitrate in severe pulmonary oedema. Lancet 351:389, 1998

——— et al: The role of cardiac power and systemic vascular resistance in the pathophysiology and diagnosis of patients with acute congestive heart failure. Eur J Heart Fail (In press)

GOLDBERG RJ et al: Temporal trends in cardiogenic shock complicating acute myocardial infarction. N Engl J Med 340:1162, 1999

HOCHMAN JS: Cardiogenic shock complicating acute myocardial infarction: Expanding the paradigm. Circulation 107:2998, 2003

——— et al: Early revascularization in acute myocardial infarction complicated by cardiogenic shock. N Engl J Med 341:625, 1999

——— et al: One-year survival following early revascularization for cardiogenic shock. JAMA 285:190, 2001

JACOBS AK et al: Cardiogenic shock caused by right ventricular infarction: A report from the SHOCK Registry. J Am Coll Cardiol 41:159, 2003

MAISEL AS et al: Rapid measurement of B-type natriuretic peptide in the emergency diagnosis of heart failure. N Engl J Med 347:161, 2002

MASIP J et al: Non-invasive pressure support ventilation versus conventional oxygen therapy in acute cardiogenic pulmonary oedema. Lancet 356:2126, 2000

MENON V et al: Acute myocardial infarction complicated by systemic hypoperfusion without hypotension: Report of the SHOCK Trial Registry. Am J Med 108:374, 2000

OVERVIEW AND DEFINITIONS

The vast majority of naturally occurring sudden deaths are caused by cardiac disorders. The magnitude of sudden *cardiac* death (SCD) as a public health problem is highlighted by estimates that more than 400,000 deaths occur each year in the United States by this mechanism, accounting for 50% of all cardiac deaths. SCD is a direct consequence of cardiac arrest, which is potentially reversible if responded to promptly. Since resuscitation techniques and emergency rescue systems are available to respond to and save victims of out-of-hospital cardiac arrest, which was uniformly fatal in the past, understanding the SCD problem has practical importance.

SCD must be defined carefully. In the context of time, "sudden" is defined, for most clinical and epidemiologic purposes, as 1 h or less between a change in clinical status heralding the onset of the terminal clinical event, and the cardiac arrest itself. An exception is unwitnessed deaths in which pathologists may expand the definition of time to 24 h after the victim was last seen to be alive and stable.

Because of community-based interventions, victims may remain biologically alive for days or even weeks after a cardiac arrest that has resulted in irreversible central nervous system damage. Confusion in terms can be avoided by adhering strictly to definitions of cardiovascular collapse, cardiac arrest, and death (Table 256-1). Death is biologically, legally, and literally an absolute and irreversible event. Death may be delayed in a survivor of cardiac arrest, but "survival after sudden death" is an irrational term. A generally accepted definition of SCD is *natural death due to cardiac causes*, heralded by abrupt loss of consciousness within *1 h* of the onset of acute symptoms, in an individual who may have known *preexisting* heart disease but in whom the *time* and *mode* of death are *unexpected*. When biologic death of the cardiac arrest victim is delayed because of interventions, the relevant pathophysiologic event remains the sudden and unexpected cardiac arrest that leads ultimately to death, even though delayed by artificial methods. The language used should reflect the fact that the index event was a cardiac arrest and that death was due to its delayed consequences.

TABLE 256-1 *Distinction Between Cardiovascular Collapse, Cardiac Arrest, and Death*

Term	Definition	Qualifiers or Exceptions
Cardiovascular collapse	A sudden loss of effective blood flow due to cardiac and/or peripheral vascular factors which may reverse spontaneously (e.g., neurocardiogenic syncope; vasovagal syncope) or only with interventions (e.g., cardiac arrest)	Nonspecific term that includes cardiac arrest and its consequences and also events that characteristically revert spontaneously
Cardiac arrest	Abrupt cessation of cardiac pump function which may be reversible by a prompt intervention but will lead to death in its absence	Rare spontaneous reversions; likelihood of successful interventions relates to mechanism of arrest, clinical setting, and prompt return of circulation
Death	Irreversible cessation of all biologic functions	None

CLINICAL DEFINITION OF FORMS OF CARDIOVASCULAR COLLAPSE

Cardiovascular collapse is a general term connoting loss of effective blood flow due to acute dysfunction of the heart and/or peripheral vasculature. Cardiovascular collapse may be caused by vasodepressor syncope (vasovagal syncope, postural hypotension with syncope, neurocardiogenic syncope; Chap. 20), a transient severe bradycardia, or cardiac arrest. The latter is distinguished from the transient forms of cardiovascular collapse in that it usually requires an intervention to achieve resuscitation. In contrast, vasodepressor syncope and many primary bradyarrhythmic syncopal events are transient and non-life-threatening, with spontaneous return of consciousness.

The most common electrical mechanism for true cardiac arrest is ventricular fibrillation (VF), which is responsible for 65 to 80% of cardiac arrests. Severe persistent bradyarrhythmias, asystole, and pulseless electrical activity (PEA; an organized electrical activity without mechanical response, formerly called electromechanical dissociation) cause another 20 to 30%. Sustained ventricular tachycardia (VT) with hypotension is a less common cause. Acute low cardiac output states, having precipitous onset, may also present clinically as a cardiac arrest. These hemodynamic causes include massive acute pulmonary emboli, internal blood loss from ruptured aortic aneurysm, intense anaphylaxis, and cardiac rupture after myocardial infarction (MI).

ETIOLOGY, INITIATING EVENTS, AND CLINICAL EPIDEMIOLOGY

Clinical and epidemiologic studies have identified population subgroups at high risk for SCD. In addition, a large body of pathologic data provides information on the underlying *structural abnormalities* in victims of SCD, and studies of clinical physiology have begun to identify a group of *transient functional factors* that may convert a long-standing underlying structural abnormality from a stable to an unstable state (Table 256-2). This information has developed into an understanding of the causes and mechanisms of SCD.

Cardiac disorders constitute the most common causes of sudden *natural* death. After an initial peak incidence of sudden death between birth and 6 months of age (the sudden infant death syndrome), the incidence of sudden death declines sharply and remains low through childhood and adolescence. Among adolescents and young adults, the incidence of SCD is approximately 1 per 100,000 population per year. The incidence begins to increase in adults over the age of 30 years, reaching a second peak in the age range of 45 to 75 years, when the incidence approximates 1 to 2 per 1000 per year among the unselected adult population. Increasing age within this range is associated with increasing risk for sudden *cardiac* death, and the proportion of cardiac causes among all sudden natural deaths increases dramatically with advancing years. From 1 to 13 years of age, only one of five sudden *natural* deaths is due to cardiac causes. Between 14 and 21 years of age, the proportion increases to 30%, and then to 88% in the middle-aged and elderly.

Young and middle-aged men and women have very different susceptibilities to SCD, but the gender differences decrease with advancing age. In the 45- to 64-year-old age group, the male SCD excess is nearly 7:1. It falls to less than 2:1 in the 65- to 74-year-old age group. The difference in risk for SCD parallels the differences in age-related risks for other manifestations of coronary heart disease (CHD) between men and women. As the gender gap for manifestations of CHD closes in the seventh and eighth decades of life, the excess risk of SCD in males also narrows. Despite the lower incidence among younger women, coronary risk factors such as cigarette smoking, diabetes, hyperlipidemia, and hypertension are highly influential, and SCD remains an important clinical and epidemiologic problem. The inci-

TABLE 256-2 *Cardiac Arrest and Sudden Cardiac Death*

STRUCTURAL CAUSES

I. Coronary heart disease
  A. Coronary artery abnormalities
    1. Chronic atherosclerotic lesions
    2. Acute (active) lesions (plaque fissuring, platelet aggregation, acute thrombosis)
    3. Anomalous coronary artery anatomy
  B. Myocardial infarction
    1. Healed
    2. Acute
II. Myocardial hypertrophy
  A. Secondary
  B. Hypertrophic cardiomyopathy
    1. Obstructive
    2. Nonobstructive
III. Dilated cardiomyopathy—primary muscle disease
IV. Inflammatory and infiltrative disorders
  A. Myocarditis
  B. Noninfectious inflammatory diseases
  C. Infiltrative diseases
  D. Right ventricular dysplasia
V. Valvular heart disease
VI. Electrophysiologic abnormalities, structural
  A. Anomalous pathways in Wolff-Parkinson-White syndrome
  B. Conducting system disease
VII. Inherited disorders of molecular structure associated with electrophysiologic abnormalities (e.g., congenital long QT syndromes, Brugada syndrome)

FUNCTIONAL CONTRIBUTING FACTORS

I. Alterations of coronary blood flow
  A. Transient ischemia
  B. Reperfusion after ischemia
II. Low cardiac output states
  A. Heart failure
    1. Chronic
    2. Acute decompensation
  B. Shock
III. Systemic metabolic abnormalities
  A. Electrolyte imbalance (e.g., hypokalemia)
  B. Hypoxemia, acidosis
IV. Neurophysiologic disturbances
  A. Autonomic fluctuations: central, neural, humoral
  B. Receptor function
V. Toxic responses
  A. Proarrhythmic drug effects
  B. Cardiac toxins (e.g., cocaine, digitalis intoxication)
  C. Drug interactions

dence of SCD among the African-American population appears to be higher than among the white population, but the reasons remain uncertain.

Hereditary factors contribute to the risk of SCD. In a nonspecific sense, they represent expressions of the hereditary predisposition to CHD. In addition, however, there are recent data suggesting a familial predisposition to SCD as a specific form of expression of CHD. In a few syndromes, such as hypertrophic cardiomyopathy, congenital long QT interval syndromes, right ventricular dysplasia, and the syndrome of right bundle branch block and non-ischemic ST-segment elevations (Brugada syndrome), there is a specific inherited risk of SCD (Chap. 214).

The structural causes of and functional factors contributing to the SCD syndrome are listed in Table 256-2. Worldwide, and especially in western cultures, coronary atherosclerotic heart disease is the most common structural abnormality associated with SCD in middle-aged and older adults. Up to 80% of all SCDs in the United States are due to the consequences of coronary atherosclerosis. The cardiomyopathies (dilated and hypertrophic, collectively; Chap. 221) account for another 10 to 15% of SCDs, and all the remaining diverse etiologies cause only 5 to 10% of all SCDs. The inherited arrhythmia syndromes

(see above and Table 256-2) are more common causes in adolescents and young adults.

Transient ischemia in the previously scarred or hypertrophied heart, hemodynamic and fluid and electrolyte disturbances, fluctuations in autonomic nervous system activity, and transient electrophysiologic changes caused by drugs or other chemicals (e.g., proarrhythmia) have all been implicated as mechanisms responsible for transition from electrophysiologic stability to instability. In addition, reperfusion of ischemic myocardium may cause transient electrophysiologic instability and arrhythmias.

PATHOLOGY

Data from postmortem examinations of SCD victims parallel the clinical observations on the prevalence of CHD as the major structural etiologic factor. More than 80% of SCD victims have pathologic findings of CHD. The pathologic description often includes a combination of long-standing, extensive atherosclerosis of the epicardial coronary arteries and unstable coronary artery lesions, which include a combination of fissured or ruptured plaques, platelet aggregates, hemorrhage, and thombosis. In one study, chronic coronary atherosclerosis involving two or more major vessels with ≥75% stenosis was observed in 75% of the victims. In another study, atherosclerotic plaque fissuring, platelet aggregates, and/or acute thrombosis were observed in 95 of 100 individuals who had pathologic studies after SCD.

As many as 70 to 75% of males who die suddenly have preexisting healed MIs, while only 20 to 30% have recent acute MIs, despite the prevalence of unstable plaques and thrombi. Regional or global left ventricular (LV) hypertrophy coexists with prior MIs.

PREDICTION AND PREVENTION OF CARDIAC ARREST AND SUDDEN CARDIAC DEATH

SCD accounts for approximately one-half the total cardiovascular mortality rate. As shown in Fig. 256-1A, the very high risk subgroups provide more focused populations ("percent per year") for predicting cardiac arrest or SCD; but the impact of such subgroups on the overall problem of SCD, indicated by the absolute number of preventable events ("events per year"), is relatively small. The requirements for achieving a major population impact are effective prevention of underlying diseases and/or new epidemiologic probes that will allow better resolution of subgroups at specific risk within the large general populations.

Strategies for predicting and preventing SCD are categorized as primary and secondary, in addition to responses intended to abort cardiac arrests. *Primary prevention* refers to the attempt to identify individual patients at specific risk for SCD and institute preventive strategies. *Secondary prevention* refers to measures taken to prevent recurrent cardiac arrest or death in individuals who have survived a previous cardiac arrest. The primary prevention strategies currently used depend upon magnitude of risk among the various population subgroups. Because the annual incidence of SCD among the unselected adult population is limited to 1 to 2 per 1000 population per year (Fig. 256-1A), and more than 30% of all SCDs due to coronary artery disease occur as the first clinical manifestation of the disease (Fig. 256-2A), the only practical strategies are profiling for risk of developing CHD and risk factor control (Fig. 256-2B). The most powerful long-term risk factors include age, cigarette smoking, elevated serum cholesterol, diabetes mellitus, elevated blood pressure, LV hypertrophy, and nonspecific electrocardiographic abnormalities. Markers of inflammation (e.g., C-reactive protein levels) that may predict plaque destabilization, have recently been added to risk classifications. The presence of multiple risk factors progressively increases incidence, but not sufficiently or specifically enough to warrant therapies targeted to potentially fatal arrhythmias (Fig. 256-1A). However, recent studies offer the hope that genetic markers for specific risk may

A

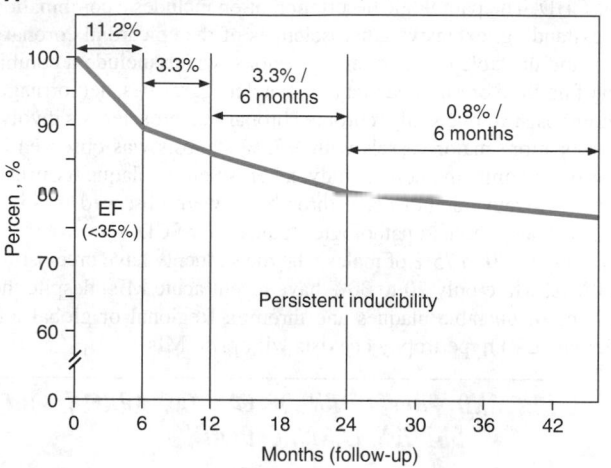

B

FIGURE 256-1 *A.* Incidence of sudden and nonsudden cardiac deaths in population subgroups, and the relation of total number of events per year to incidence figures. Approximations of subgroup incidence figures, and the related population pool from which they are derived, are presented. Approximately 50% of all cardiac deaths are sudden and unexpected. The incidence triangle on the left ("Percent/Year") indicates the approximate percentage of sudden and nonsudden deaths in each of the population subgroups indicated, ranging from the lowest percentage in unselected adult populations (0.1 to 2% per year) to the highest percentage in patients with VT or VF during convalescence after an MI (approximately 50% per year). The triangle on the right indicates the total number of events per year in each of these groups, to reflect incidence in context with the size of the population subgroups. The highest risk categories identify the smallest number of total annual events, and the lowest incidence category accounts for the largest number of events per year. (EF, ejection fraction; VT, ventricular tachycardia; VF, ventricular fibrillation; MI, myocardial infarction.) *B.* Time dependence of risk among survivors of out-of-hospital cardiac arrest. Recurrence risk is highest in the first 6 months of the index event. Survival is expressed as a percentage. High risk is best predicted initially by an ejection fraction ≤ 35% during the first 6 months, and subsequently persistent inducibility of VT during electrophysiologic testing becomes an added major risk. *n* = 101 at *t* = 0. [*After T Furukawa et al, in RJ Myerburg et al, Circulation 85(Suppl 1):2, 1992. Reproduced with permission of the American Heart Association.*]

be available in the future. These studies suggest that a family history of SCD associated with acute coronary syndromes predicts a higher likelihood of cardiac arrest as the initial manifestation of coronary artery disease in first-degree family members.

After coronary artery disease has been identified in a patient, additional strategies for risk profiling become available (Fig. 256-2*B*), but the majority of SCDs occur among the large unselected groups rather than in the specific high-risk subgroups that become evident among populations with established disease (compare events per year with percent per year in Fig. 256-1*A*). Under most conditions of higher level of risk, particularly those indexed to a major recent cardiovascular event (e.g., MI, recent onset of heart failure, survival after out-of-hospital cardiac arrest), the highest risk of SCD occurs during the

initial 6 to 18 months and then plateaus towards the baseline risk of the underlying disease (Fig. 256-1*B*). Accordingly, preventive interventions are more likely to be effective when initiated early.

Among patients in the acute, convalescent, and chronic phases of myocardial infarction (Chap. 228), subgroups at high absolute risk of SCD can be identified. During the acute phase, the potential risk of cardiac arrest from onset through the first 48 hours may be as high as 15 to 20%, emphasizing the importance for patients to respond promptly to the onset of symptoms. Those who survive acute-phase VF, however, are not at continuing risk for recurrent cardiac arrest indexed to that event. During the convalescent phase after MI (3 days to ~6 weeks), an episode of sustained VT or VF predicts a mortality risk of up to 50% at 12 months. At least 50% of the deaths are sudden. Aggressive intervention techniques may reduce this incidence.

After passage into the chronic phase of MI, the longer-term risk for total and SCD mortality is predicted by a number of factors (Fig. 256-2*B*). The most important for both SCD and non-sudden death is the extent of myocardial damage sustained as a result of the acute MI. This is measured by the magnitude of reduction of the ejection fraction (EF), functional capacity, and/or the occurrence of heart failure. Various studies have demonstrated that an EF < 40% contributes significantly to this risk. In addition, inducibility of VT or VF during electrophysiologic testing of patients who have ambient ventricular arrhythmias [premature ventricular contractions (PVCs) and nonsustained VT] and an EF < 35 or 40% is a strong predictor of SCD risk. Patients in this subgroup are now considered candidates for implantable cardioverter defibrillators (ICDs) (see below). Risk falls off sharply with EFs > 40% after MI and the absence of ambient arrhythmias, and conversely continues to rise with EFs < 30% even without the ambient arrhythmia markers.

The cardiomyopathies (dilated and hypertrophic) are the second most common category of diseases associated with risk of SCD, following CHD (Table 256-2). Some risk factors have been identified, largely related to extent of disease, documented ventricular arrhythmias, and symptoms of arrhythmias (e.g., unexplained syncope). The rare diseases associated with SCD in younger populations (adolescents, young adults, competitive athletes), such as the long QT interval syndromes, right ventricular dysplasia, hypertrophic cardiomyopathy, and Brugada syndrome, may be recognized or suspected based on symptoms, family history of premature sudden death or known presence of the specific entity, or incidental clinical data. Despite the low absolute incidence of SCD among the younger population (<1/100,000 per year), routine electrocardiographic (ECG) screening has been suggested for identifying individuals at risk.

Secondary prevention strategies are applied to surviving victims of a cardiac arrest that was not associated with an acute MI or a transient risk of SCD (e.g., drug exposures, correctable electrolyte imbalances). The extent of underlying disease (CHD, dilated cardiomyopathy), or merely its presences in association with life-threatening arrhythmias (e.g., long QT syndromes, right ventricular dysplasia) predicts a 1- to 2-year SCD or cardiac arrest recurrence risk of up to 30% in the absence of specific interventions (see below).

CLINICAL CHARACTERISTICS OF CARDIAC ARREST

PRODROME, ONSET, ARREST, DEATH

SCD may be presaged by days, weeks, or months of increasing angina, dyspnea, palpitations, easy fatigability, and other nonspecific complaints. However, these *prodromal complaints* are generally predictive of any major cardiac event; they are not specific for predicting SCD.

The *onset of the terminal event*, leading to cardiac arrest, is defined as an acute change in cardiovascular status preceding cardiac arrest by up to 1 h. When the onset is instantaneous or abrupt, the probability that the arrest is cardiac in origin is >95%. Continuous ECG recordings, fortuitously obtained at the onset of a cardiac arrest, commonly demonstrate changes in cardiac electrical activity during the minutes or hours before the event. There is a tendency for the heart rate to increase and for advanced grades of PVCs to evolve. Most cardiac arrests that are caused by VF begin with a run of sustained or nonsustained VT, which then degenerates into VF.

Sudden unexpected loss of effective circulation may be separated into "arrhythmic events" and "circulatory failure." Arrhythmic events are characterized by a high likelihood of patients being awake and active immediately prior to the event, are dominated by VF as the electrical mechanism, and have a short duration of terminal illness (<1 h). In contrast, circulatory failure deaths occur in patients who are inactive or comatose, have a higher incidence of asystole than VF, have a tendency to a longer duration of terminal illness, and are dominated by noncardiac events preceding the terminal illness.

The onset of cardiac arrest may be characterized by typical symptoms of an acute cardiac event, such as prolonged angina or the pain of onset of MI; acute dyspnea or orthopnea; or the sudden onset of palpitations, sustained tachycardia, or light-headedness. However, in many patients, the onset is precipitous, with minimal forewarning.

Cardiac arrest is, by definition, abrupt. Mentation may be impaired in patients with sustained VT during the onset of the terminal event. However, complete loss of consciousness is *a sine qua non* in cardiac arrest. Although rare spontaneous reversions occur, it is usual that cardiac arrest progresses to death within minutes (i.e., SCD has occurred) if active interventions are not undertaken promptly.

The probability of achieving successful resuscitation from cardiac arrest is related to the interval from onset to institution of resuscitative efforts, the

FIGURE 256-2 Population subsets, risk predictors, and distribution of sudden cardiac deaths (SCDs) according to clinical circumstances. *A.* The population subset with high-risk arrhythmia markers in conjunction with low ejection fraction is a group at high risk of SCD, but accounts for <10% of the total SCD burden attributable to coronary artery disease. In contrast, nearly two-thirds of all SCD victims present with SCD as the first and only manifestation of underlying disease or have known disease but are considered relatively low-risk, because of the absence of high-risk markers. *B.* Risk profile for prediction and prevention of SCD is difficult. The highest absolute numbers of events occur among the general population who may have risk factors for coronary heart disease or expressions of disease that do not predict high risk. This results in a low sensitivity for predicting and preventing SCD. New approaches that include epidemiologic modeling of transient risk factors and methods of predicting individual patient risk offer hope for greater sensitivity in the future. AP, anginapectoris; ASHD, arteriosclerotic heart disease; CAD, coronary artery disease; EPS, electrophysiologic study; HRV, heart rate variability. *(From Myerburg, reproduced with permission of the publisher).*

setting in which the event occurs, the mechanism (VF, VT, pulseless electrical activity, asystole), and the clinical status of the patient prior to the cardiac arrest. Return of circulation and survival rates as a result of defibrillation decrease linearly from the first minute to 10 minutes. By 5 minutes, survival rates are no better than 25 to 30% in out-of-hospital settings. Those settings in which it is possible to institute prompt cardiopulmonary resuscitation (CPR) with rapid defibrillation of VF provide a better chance of a successful outcome. However, the outcome in intensive care units and other in-hospital environments is heavily influenced by the patient's preceding clinical status. The immediate outcome is good for cardiac arrest occurring in the intensive care unit in the presence of an acute cardiac event or transient metabolic disturbance, but survival among patients with far-advanced chronic cardiac disease or advanced noncardiac diseases (e.g., renal failure, pneumonia, sepsis, diabetes, cancer) is low, and not much more successful in the in-hospital than in the out-of-hospital setting.

The success rate for initial resuscitation and survival to hospital discharge after an out-of-hospital cardiac arrest depends heavily on the mechanism of the event. When the mechanism is VT, the outcome is best; VF is the next most successful; and asystole and PEA generate dismal outcome statistics. Advanced age also influences adversely the chances of successful resuscitation.

Progression to biologic death is a function of the mechanism of cardiac arrest and the length of the delay before interventions. VF or

asystole without CPR within the first 4 to 6 min has a poor outcome even if defibrillation is successful, because of superimposed brain damage; and there are few survivors among patients who had no life support activities for the first 8 min after onset. Outcome statistics are improved by lay bystander intervention (basic life support—see below) prior to definitive interventions (advanced life support), and even more by early defibrillation. In regard to the latter, evaluations of deployment of automatic external defibrillators (AEDs) in communities (e.g., police vehicles, large buildings, stadiums) are beginning to generate encouraging data.

Death during the hospitalization after a successfully resuscitated cardiac arrest relates closely to the severity of central nervous system injury. Anoxic encephalopathy and infections subsequent to prolonged respirator dependence account for 60% of the deaths. Another 30% occur as a consequence of low cardiac output states that fail to respond to interventions. Recurrent arrhythmias are the least common cause of death, accounting for only 10% of in-hospital deaths.

In the setting of acute MI, it is important to distinguish between primary and secondary cardiac arrests. *Primary cardiac arrests* refer to those that occur in the absence of hemodynamic instability, and *secondary cardiac arrests* are those that occur in patients in whom abnormal hemodynamics dominate the clinical picture before cardiac arrest. The success rate for immediate resuscitation in primary cardiac arrest during acute MI in a monitored setting should approach 100%.

In contrast, as many as 70% of patients with secondary cardiac arrest succumb immediately or during the same hospitalization.

℞ TREATMENT

The individual who collapses suddenly is managed in four stages: (1) the initial response and basic life support, (2) advanced life support, (3) postresuscitation care, and (4) long-term management. The initial response and basic life support can be carried out by physicians, nurses, paramedical personnel, and trained lay persons. There is a requirement for increasingly specialized skills as the patient moves through the stages of advanced life support, postresuscitation care, and long-term management.

Initial Response and Basic Life Support   The initial evaluation will confirm whether a sudden collapse is indeed due to a cardiac arrest. Observations of the state of consciousness, respiratory movements, skin color, and the presence or absence of pulses in the carotid or femoral arteries will promptly determine whether a life-threatening cardiac arrest has occurred. For lay responders, the pulse check is no longer recommended. As soon as a cardiac arrest is suspected, confirmed, or even considered to be impending, calling an emergency rescue system (e.g., 911) is the immediate priority. With the development of AEDs that are easily used by nonconventional emergency responders, an additional layer for response has evolved. Immediate defibrillation by emergency medical rescue personnel on fire rescue vehicles, police, public conveyance personnel, security officers in various locations with large numbers of people, and trained lay persons is becoming available to save more cardiac arrest victims.

Agonal respiratory movements may persist for a short time after the onset of cardiac arrest, but it is important to observe for severe stridor with a persistent pulse as a clue to aspiration of a foreign body or food. If this is suspected, a Heimlich maneuver (see below) may dislodge the obstructing body. A precordial blow, or "thump," delivered firmly by the clenched fist to the junction of the middle and lower third of the sternum may occasionally revert VT or VF, but there is concern about converting VT to VF. Therefore, it has been recommended to use precordial thumps as an advanced life support technique when monitoring and defibrillation are available. This conservative application of the technique remains controversial.

The third action during the initial response is to clear the airway. The head is tilted back and chin lifted so that the oropharynx can be explored to clear the airway. Dentures or foreign bodies are removed, and the Heimlich maneuver is performed if there is reason to suspect that a foreign body is lodged in the oropharynx. If respiratory arrest precipitating cardiac arrest is suspected, a second precordial thump is delivered after the airway is cleared.

Basic life support, more popularly known as CPR, is intended to maintain organ perfusion until definitive interventions can be instituted. The elements of CPR are the maintenance of ventilation of the lungs and compression of the chest. Mouth-to-mouth respiration may be used if no specific rescue equipment is immediately available (e.g., plastic oropharyngeal airways, esophageal obturators, masked Ambu bag). Conventional ventilation techniques during CPR require the lungs to be inflated twice in succession every 15 chest compressions.

Chest compression is based on the assumption that cardiac compression allows the heart to maintain a pump function by sequential filling and emptying of its chambers, with competent valves maintaining forward direction of flow. The palm of one hand is placed over the lower sternum, with the heel of the other resting on the dorsum of the lower hand. The sternum is depressed, with the arms remaining straight, at a rate of approximately 100 per minute. Sufficient force is applied to depress the sternum 4 to 5 cm, and relaxation is abrupt.

Advanced Life Support   Advanced life support is intended to achieve adequate ventilation, control cardiac arrhythmias, stabilize blood pressure and cardiac output, and restore organ perfusion. The activities carried out to achieve these goals include (1) defibrillation/cardiover-

sion and/or pacing, (2) intubation with an endotracheal tube, and (3) insertion of an intravenous line. The speed with which defibrillation/ cardioversion is carried out is an important element for successful resuscitation, both for restoration of spontaneous circulation and protection of the central nervous system. Immediate defibrillation should precede intubation and insertion of an intravenous line; CPR should be carried out while the defibrillator is being charged. As soon as a diagnosis of VF or VT is established, a shock of at least 200 J should be delivered. Additional shocks at higher energies, up to a maximum of 360 J, are tried if the initial shock does not successfully abolish VT or VF. Epinephrine, 1 mg intravenously, is given after failed defibrillation, and attempts to defibrillate are repeated. The dose of epinephrine may be repeated after intervals of 3 to 5 min (Fig. 256-3A). Vasopressin (a single 40 Unit dose given IV) has been suggested as an alternative to epinephrine.

If the patient is less than fully conscious upon reversion, or if two or three attempts fail, prompt intubation, ventilation, and arterial blood gas analysis should be carried out. Ventilation with O_2 (room air if O_2 is not immediately available) may promptly reverse hypoxemia and acidosis. The patient who is persistently acidotic after successful defibrillation and intubation should be given 1 meq/kg $NaHCO_3$ initially and an additional 50% of the dose repeated every 10 to 15 min. However, it should not be used routinely.

After initial unsuccessful defibrillation attempts, or with persistent/ recurrent electrical instability, antiarrhythmic therapy should be instituted. Intravenous amiodarone has emerged as the initial treatment of choice (150 mg over 10 min, followed by 1 mg/min for up to 6 h and 0.5 mg/min thereafter) (Fig. 256-3A). A bolus of 1 mg/kg of lidocaine may be given intravenously (Chap. 228), and the dose repeated in 2 min, in those patients in whom amiodarone is unsuccessful, and possibly in those who clearly have an acute MI as the triggering mechanism for the cardiac arrest. Intravenous procainamide (loading infusion of 100 mg/5 min to a total dose of 500 to 800 mg, followed by continuous infusion at 2 to 5 mg/min) is rarely used in this setting any longer but may be tried for persisting, hemodynamically stable arrhythmias. Intravenous calcium gluconate is no longer considered safe or necessary for routine administration. It is used only in patients in whom acute hyperkalemia is known to be the triggering event for resistant VF, in the presence of known hypocalcemia, or in patients who have received toxic doses of calcium channel antagonists.

Cardiac arrest secondary to bradyarrhythmias or asystole is managed differently (Fig. 256-3B). The patient is promptly intubated, CPR is continued, and an attempt is made to control hypoxemia and acidosis. Epinephrine and/or atropine are given intravenously or by an intracardiac route. External pacing devices are now available to attempt to establish a regular rhythm, but the prognosis is generally very poor in this form of cardiac arrest, even with successful electrical pacing. PEA is treated similarly to bradyarrhythmias, but its outcome is also dismal. The one exception is bradyarrhythmic/asystolic cardiac arrest secondary to airway obstruction. This form of cardiac arrest may respond promptly to removal of foreign bodies by the Heimlich maneuver or, in hospitalized patients, by intubation and suctioning of obstructing secretions in the airway.

Postresuscitation Care   This phase of management is determined by the clinical setting of the cardiac arrest. Primary VF in acute MI (Chap. 228) is generally very responsive to life-support techniques and easily controlled after the initial event. In the in-hospital setting, respirator support is usually not necessary or is needed for only a short time, and hemodynamics stabilize promptly after defibrillation or cardioversion. In secondary VF in acute MI (those events in which hemodynamic abnormalities predispose to the potentially fatal arrhythmia), resuscitative efforts are less often successful; and in those patients who are successfully resuscitated, the recurrence rate is high. The clinical picture and outcome are dominated by hemodynamic instability and the ability to control hemodynamic dysfunction. Bradyarrhythmias, asystole, and PEA are commonly secondary events in hemodynamically unstable patients. The in-hospital phase of care of the out-of-hospital

FIGURE 256-3 Management of cardiac arrest. *A.* The algorithm of ventricular fibrillation or hypotensive ventricular tachycardia begins with defibrillation attempts. If that fails, it is followed by epinephrine and then antiarrhythmic drugs. See text for details. *B.* The algorithms for bradyarrhythmia/asystole (left) or pulseless electrical activity (right) is dominated first by continued life support and a search for reversible causes. Subsequent therapy is nonspecific and accompanied by a low success rate. See text for details. CPR, cardiopulmonary resuscitation; MI, myocardial infarction.

cardiac arrest survivor is dictated by specific clinical circumstances. The most difficult is the presence of anoxic encephalopathy which is a strong predictor of in-hospital death. A recent addition to the management of this condition is induced hypothermia to reduce metabolic demands and cerebral edema.

The outcome after in-hospital cardiac arrest associated with non-cardiac diseases is poor, and in the few successfully resuscitated patients, the postresuscitation course is dominated by the nature of the underlying disease. Patients with cancer, renal failure, acute central nervous system disease, and uncontrolled infections, as a group, have a survival rate of less than 10% after in-hospital cardiac arrest. Some major exceptions are patients with transient airway obstruction, electrolyte disturbances, proarrhythmic effects of drugs, and severe metabolic abnormalities, most of whom may have an excellent chance of survival if they can be resuscitated promptly and maintained while the transient abnormalities are being corrected.

Long-Term Management after Survival of Out-of-Hospital Cardiac Arrest Patients who survive cardiac arrest without irreversible damage to the central nervous system, and who achieve hemodynamic stability, should have extensive diagnostic testing and appropriate therapeutic interventions for their long-term management. This aggressive approach is driven by the fact that survival after out-of-hospital cardiac arrest was followed by a 25 to 30% mortality rate during the first 2 years after the event, and there are data suggesting that significant reductions in risk can be achieved by appropriate therapy.

Among patients in whom an acute transmural MI is identified as the specific mechanism triggering an out-of-hospital cardiac arrest, the management is dictated in part by the known transient nature of life-threatening arrhythmia risk in the acute phase of MI, and in part by the extent of permanent myocardial damage that results. Several clinical trials have now documented an improved mortality among cardiac arrest survivors who have EFs < 40% and receive ICDs. It is not clear whether ICDs provide a benefit over aminodarone therapy when the EF is between 35 and 40% or >40%, but the data support the use of ICDs when the EF < 35%. Since is is usually not possible to determine whether the EF reduction was preexisting or a consequence of the MI, the cut-offs described are those generally used as ICD indications. Earlier studies had suggested that inducibility of ventricular arrhythmias during programmed electrical stimulation (E-P) studies in the electrophysiology laboratory could stratify risk prediction, but this is not universally used any longer for patients with low EFs, since even without inducible arrhythmias, the risk remains high enough to warrant ICDs in these cardiac arrest survivors.

For patients with cardiac arrest thought to be due to a transient ischemic mechanism, particularly with higher EFs, anti-ischemic therapy by pharmacologic or interventional methods is generally accepted as appropriate management. However, despite the absence of supportive clinical trial evidence, some adopt a more aggressive attitude about the use of ICDs in this group of cardiac arrest survivors as well, given the unpredictability of recurrent ischemia as a triggering mechanism.

The principles guiding therapy for patients with coronary artery disease who survive a cardiac arrest generally apply to the other cardiac disorders as well, with the exception that there is less focus on the extent of disease in certain disorders. Generally, cardiac arrest survivors from other categories of disease, such as the hypertrophic or dilated cardiomyopathies and various rare inherited disorders (e.g., RV dysplasia, long QT syndrome, Brugada syndrome, arrhythmic VF) are all considered ICD candidates.

PREVENTION OF SCD IN HIGH-RISK INDIVIDUALS WITHOUT PRIOR CARDIAC ARREST

Post-MI patients have been the subject of clinical trials for ICD benefit. It is now established that for post-MI patients with EFs < 40%, ambient ventricular arrhythmias, and inducible ventricular tachyarrhythmias in the electrophysiology laboratory, ICDs provide a significant reduction in relative risk of SCD and total mortality. Total mortality benefits in the range of a 20 to 30% reduction over 2 to 3 years have been observed, and ICD has emerged as preferred therapy for such patients. One study suggests that when the EF < 30%, electrophysiologic testing is not necessary to identify ICD benefit (see Chaps. 214 and 216).

Decision-making for primary prevention in disorders other than coronary artery disease is generally driven by observational data and judgment based on clinical observations. Controlled clinical trials providing evidence-based indicators for ICDs are lacking for these smaller population subgroups. In general, for both the cardiomyopathies and the rare disorders listed above, indicators of arrhythmic risk such as syncope, documented ventricular tachyarrhythmias, aborted cardiac arrest or perhaps a family history of SCD, and a number of other clinical or ECG markers, may be used as indicators for ICDs.

FURTHER READING

AMERICAN HEART ASSOCIATION: International Guidelines 2000 for CPR and ECC. Circulation 102(Suppl I):I-1, 2000

EWY GA, ORNATO JP: Emergency Cardiac Care Task Force 1: Cardiac arrest. J Am Coll Cardiol 35:832, 2000

HUIKURI H et al: Sudden death due to cardiac arrhythmias. N Engl J Med 345: 1473, 2001

MARENCO JP et al: Improving survival from sudden cardiac arrest: The role of the automated external defibrillator. JAMA 285:1193, 2001

MYERBURG RJ: Sudden cardiac death: Exploring the limits of our knowledge. J Cardiovasc Electrophysiol 12:369, 2001

——, CASTELLANOS A: Cardiac arrest and sudden cardiac death, in *Braunwald's Heart Disease*, 7th ed, D Zipes et al (eds). Philadelphia, Saunders, 2005

ORNATO JP: Use of adrenergic agonists during CPR in adults. Ann Emerg Med 22:411, 1993

ZHENG ZJ et al: Sudden cardiac death in the United States, 1989 to 1998. Circulation 104:2158, 2001

Section 3 Neurologic Critical Care

257 ACUTE CONFUSIONAL STATES AND COMA
Allan H. Ropper

Confusional states and coma are among the most common problems in general medicine. They account for a substantial portion of admissions to emergency wards and occur frequently on all hospital services. Because confusion and a diminished level of consciousness frequently coexist and are caused by many of the same diseases, they are presented together here, but from a medical perspective they have different clinical characteristics and physiologic explanations.

Almost all instances of diminished alertness can be traced to widespread abnormalities of the cerebral hemispheres or to reduced activity of a special thalamocortical alerting system termed the *reticular activating system* (RAS). The proper functioning of this system, its ascending projections to the cortex, and the cortex itself are required to maintain alertness and coherence of thought.

THE CONFUSIONAL STATE

Confusion is a mental and behavioral state of reduced comprehension, coherence, and capacity to reason. Inattention, as defined by the inability to sustain uninterrupted thought and actions, and disorientation are its earliest outward signs. As the state of confusion worsens, there are more global mental failings, including impairments of memory, perception, comprehension, problem solving, language, praxis, visuospatial function, and various aspects of emotional behavior that are attributable to particular regions of the brain. In some instances an apparent confusional state may be due to an isolated deficit in mental function such as an impairment of language (*aphasia*), loss of memory (*amnesia*), or lack of appreciation of spatial relations of self or the external environment (*agnosia*) (Chap. 23). Confusion is also a feature of dementia (Chap. 350), in which case the chronicity of the process distinguishes it from an acute encephalopathy.

The confused patient is usually subdued, not inclined to speak, and is physically inactive. A state of confusion that is accompanied by agitation, hallucinations, tremor, and illusions (misperceptions of environmental sight, sound, or touch) is termed *delirium*, as typified by delirium tremens from alcohol or drug withdrawal.

APPROACH TO THE PATIENT

Confusion and delirium always signify a disorder of the nervous system. They may be the major manifestations of a head injury; a seizure; drug toxicity (or drug withdrawal); a metabolic disorder resulting from hepatic, renal, pulmonary or cardiac failure; a systemic infection; meningitis or encephalitis; or a chronic dementing disease.

Evaluation begins with a careful history emphasizing the patient's condition before the onset of confusion. The clinical examination should focus on signs of diminished attentiveness, disorientation, and drowsiness and on the presence of localizing neurologic signs. From the clinical data the clinician is directed to the appropriate laboratory tests (see below.). Often, even after all diagnostic tests are completed, one may still not know the cause of a confusional state. The patient should then be observed in the hospital for a number of days under stable conditions. New clues may appear or confusion caused by a medication may resolve.

Orientation and memory are tested by asking the patient the date, inclusive of month, day, year, and day of week; the precise place; and some items of universally known information (the names of the President and Vice President, a recent national event, the state capital). Further probing may be necessary to reveal a defect in clarity—why is the patient in the hospital; what is his or her address, zip code, telephone number, social security number? Problems of increasing complexity may be pursued, but they usually provide little additional information. Attention and coherence of thought can be gauged by the accuracy and speed of responses but are examined more explicitly by having the patient repeat strings of numbers (most adults easily retain seven digits forward and four backward), spell a word such as "world" backwards, and perform serial calculations—tests of serial subtraction of 3 from 30 or 7 from 100 are useful. It is the inability to sustain coherent mental activity in performing tasks such as these that exposes the most subtle confusional states.

Other salient findings are the level of alertness, which fluctuates if there is drowsiness; indications of focal damage of the cerebrum such as hemiparesis, hemianopia, and aphasia; or adventitious movements of myoclonus or partial convulsions. The language of the confused patient may be disorganized and rambling, even to the extent of incorporating paraphasic words. These features, along with impaired comprehension that is due mainly to inattention, may be mistaken for aphasia.

One of the most specific signs of a metabolic encephalopathy is *asterixis*, which is an arrhythmic flapping tremor that is typically elicited by asking the patient to hold the arms outstretched with the wrists and hands fully extended. After a few seconds, there is a large jerking lapse in the posture of the hand and then a rapid return to the original position. The same movements can be found in any tonically held posture, even of the protruded tongue. Bilateral asterixis always signifies a metabolic encephalopathy, e.g., from hepatic failure, hypercapnia, or drug intoxication, especially with anticonvulsant medications. Myoclonic jerking and tremor are typical of uremic encephalopathy or exposure to antipsychotic drugs such as lithium, phenothiazines, or butyrophenones; myoclonus is also common with severe anoxic cerebral damage.

Confusion in the postoperative period, particularly after cardiac and extensive orthopedic procedures, is common but at times so subtle as to escape attention. Often a careful history will reveal that a mild but compensated dementia existed prior to the operation. Medications, particularly those with anticholinergic activity (including meperidine), inadvertent withdrawal from sleeping pills or alcohol, fever, and any of the endogenous metabolic derangements listed above may be responsible, or a stroke may have occurred. In many cases, particularly in the elderly, transient confusion and drowsiness arise with a febrile infection of the urinary tract, lungs, blood, or peritoneum. The term *septic encephalopathy* is used to describe this association, but the mechanism by which systemic infection leads to cerebral dysfunction is unknown.

Distinguishing dementia from an acute confusional state is a problem in the elderly. The two may coexist if an acute medical problem or a poorly tolerated medication supervenes in a mildly demented patient, producing a so-called beclouded dementia. The memory loss of dementia brings about a confusional state that varies little in severity from day to day. Poor mental performance in dementia is manifested primarily as incomplete recollection; inadequate access to names and words, and ideas; and the inability to retain new information, thus affecting orientation and factual knowledge. In contrast to the acute confusional states, attention, alertness, and coherence are preserved until the most advanced stages. Dementia in its advanced stages produces a chronic confusion with breakdown of all types of mental performance; the distinction from an acute encephalopathy then depends mainly on the longstanding nature of the condition.

Treatment of the confused patient requires that all unnecessary medication be stopped, metabolic alterations be rectified, and infection be treated. Skilled nursing and a quiet room with a window are important. Careful explanations should be given at regular intervals to the family. In the elderly, regular reorientation and active measures to lessen risk factors (sleep deprivation, immobility, and vision and hearing impairments) have been shown to reduce the number and severity of episodes of delirium in hospitalized patients.

COMA AND RELATED DISORDERS OF CONSCIOUSNESS

States of reduced alertness and responsiveness represent a continuum that in its severest form is called *coma*, a deep sleeplike state from which the patient cannot be aroused. *Stupor* refers to lesser degrees of unarousability in which the patient can be awakened only by vigorous stimuli, accompanied by motor behavior that leads to avoidance of uncomfortable or aggravating stimuli. *Drowsiness*, which is familiar to all persons, simulates light sleep and is characterized by easy arousal and the persistence of alertness for brief periods. Drowsiness and stupor are usually attended by some degree of confusion. A narrative description of the level of arousal and of the type of responses evoked by various stimuli precisely as observed at the bedside is preferable to ambiguous terms such as semicoma or obtundation.

Several other neurologic conditions render patients apparently unresponsive and simulate coma, and certain subsyndromes of coma must be considered separately because of their special significance. Among the latter, the *vegetative state* signifies an awake but unresponsive state. These patients have emerged from coma after a period of days or weeks to an unresponsive state in which the eyelids are open, giving the appearance of wakefulness. Yawning, coughing, swallowing, as well as limb and head movements persist, but there are few, if any, meaningful responses to the external and internal environment—in essence, an "awake coma." Respiratory and autonomic functions are retained. The term "vegetative" is unfortunate as it is subject to misinterpretation by lay persons. There are always accompanying signs that indicate extensive damage in both cerebral hemispheres, e.g., decerebrate or decorticate limb posturing and absent responses to visual stimuli (see below). In the closely related *minimally conscious state* the patient may make intermittent rudimentary vocal or motor responses. Cardiac arrest and head injuries are the most common causes of the vegetative state (Chaps. 258 and 357). The prognosis for regaining mental faculties once the vegetative state has supervened for several months is almost nil, hence the term *persistent vegetative state*. Most reports of dramatic recovery, when investigated carefully, are found to yield to the usual rules for prognosis, but there have been rare instances of awakening to a demented condition.

Certain clinical states are prone to be misinterpreted as stupor or coma. *Akinetic mutism* refers to a partially or fully awake patient who is able to form impressions and think but remains immobile and mute, particularly when unstimulated. The condition results from damage in the regions of the medial thalamic nuclei, the frontal lobes (particularly situated deeply or on the orbitofrontal surfaces), or from hydrocephalus. The term *abulia* is used to describe a mental and physical slowness and diminished ability to initiate activity that is in essence a mild form of akinetic mutism, with the same anatomic origins. *Catatonia* is a curious hypomobile and mute syndrome associated with a major psychosis. In the typical form patients appear awake with eyes open but make no voluntary or responsive movements, although they blink spontaneously, swallow, and may not appear distressed. Often, the eyes are half-open as if the patient is in a fog or light sleep. There are signs that indicate the patient is responsive, though it may take some ingenuity on the part of the examiner to demonstrate these. For example, eyelid elevation is actively resisted, blinking occurs in response to a visual threat, and the eyes move concomitantly with head rotation, all of which are inconsistent with a brain lesion. It is characteristic but not invariable in catatonia for the limbs to retain the posture, no matter how bizarre, in which they have been placed by the examiner ("waxy flexibility," or catalepsy.) Upon recovery, such patients have some memory of events that occurred during their catatonic stupor. The appearance is superficially similar to akinetic mutism, but clinical evidence of cerebral damage is lacking.

The *locked-in state* describes a pseudocoma in which an awake patient has no means of producing speech or volitional movement in order to indicate that he is awake, but vertical eye movements and lid elevation remain unimpaired, thus allowing the patient to signal. Such individuals have written entire treatises using Morse code. Infarction or hemorrhage of the ventral pons, which transects all descending corticospinal and corticobulbar pathways, is the usual cause. A similar awake but de-efferented state occurs as a result of total paralysis of the musculature in severe cases of Guillain-Barré syndrome (Chap. 365), critical illness neuropathy (Chap. 258), and pharmacologic neuromuscular blockade.

THE ANATOMY AND PHYSIOLOGY OF UNCONSCIOUSNESS To the extent that all complex waking behaviors require the widespread participation of the cerebral cortex, consciousness cannot exist without the activity of this structure. The RAS, a loosely grouped aggregation of neurons located in the upper brainstem and medial thalamus, maintains the cerebral cortex in a state of wakeful consciousness. It follows that the principal causes of coma are (1) lesions that damage the RAS or its projections; (2) destruction of large portions of both cerebral hemispheres; and (3) suppression of reticulo-cerebral function by drugs, toxins, or metabolic derangements such as hypoglycemia, anoxia, azotemia, or hepatic failure.

The regions of the reticular formation that are critical to the maintenance of wakefulness extend from the caudal midbrain to the lower thalamus. The neurons of the RAS project rostrally to the cortex primarily via thalamic relay nuclei that in turn exert a tonic influence on the activity of the entire cerebral cortex. The behavioral arousal ef-

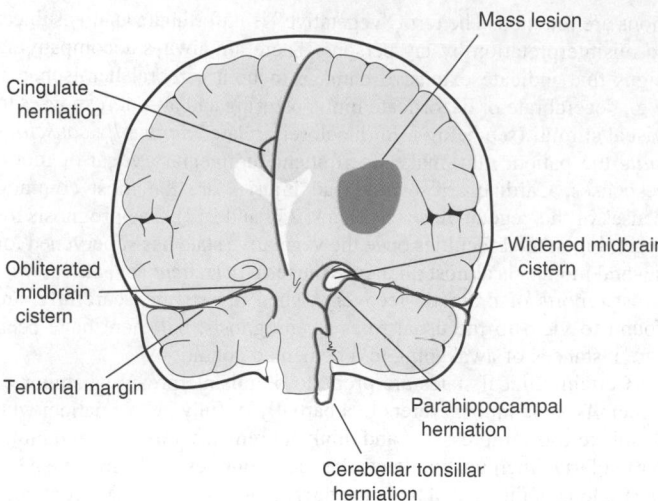

FIGURE 257-1   Types of cerebral herniation.

fected by somesthetic, auditory, and visual stimuli depends upon the rich reciprocal innervation that the RAS receives from these sensory systems. A most important practical consideration derives from the anatomic proximity of the RAS to structures that control pupillary function and eye movements. Pupillary enlargement and loss of vertical and adduction movements of the globes suggest that upper brainstem damage may be the source of coma.

Coma due to Cerebral Mass Lesions and Herniations   The cranial cavity is separated into compartments by infoldings of the dura—the two cerebral hemispheres are separated by the falx, and the anterior and posterior fossae by the tentorium. *Herniation* refers to displacement of brain tissue into a compartment that it normally does not occupy. Many of the signs associated with coma, and indeed coma itself, can be attributed to these tissue shifts (Fig. 257-1).

Uncal transtentorial herniation refers to impaction of the anterior medial temporal gyrus (the uncus) into the anterior portion of the tentorial opening. The displaced tissue compresses the third nerve as it traverses the subarachnoid space and results in enlargement of the ipsilateral pupil (putatively because the fibers subserving parasympathetic pupillary function are located peripherally in the nerve). The coma that follows may be due to lateral compression of the midbrain

against the opposite tentorial edge by the displaced parahippocampal gyrus (Fig. 257-2). In some cases the lateral displacement causes compression of the opposite cerebral peduncle, producing a Babinski response and hemiparesis contralateral to the original hemiparesis (the Kernohan-Woltman sign). In addition to compressing the upper brainstem, tissue shifts, including herniations, may compress major blood vessels, particularly the anterior and posterior cerebral arteries as they pass over the tentorial reflections, thus producing brain infarctions. The distortions may also entrap portions of the ventricular system, resulting in regional hydrocephalus.

Central transtentorial herniation denotes a symmetric downward movement of the upper thalamic region through the tentorial opening. Miotic pupils and drowsiness are the heralding signs. Both temporal and central herniations are thought to cause progressive compression of the brainstem from above: first the midbrain, then the pons, and finally the medulla. The result is a sequential appearance of neurologic signs that correspond to the affected level. Other forms of herniation are *transfalcial herniation* (displacement of the cingulate gyrus under the falx and across the midline), and *foraminal herniation* (downward forcing of the cerebellar tonsils into the foramen magnum).

A direct relationship between the various configurations of transtentorial herniations and coma is not always found. Displacement of deep brain structures by a mass in any direction, with or without herniation, is adequate to compress the region of the RAS and result in coma. Furthermore, drowsiness and stupor typically occur with moderate horizontal shifts at the level of the diencephalon (thalami) well before transtentorial or other herniations are evident. Lateral shift is easily quantified on axial images of computed tomography (CT) and magnetic resonance imaging (MRI) scans (Fig. 257-2). In cases of *acutely appearing masses*, a fairly consistent relationship exists between the degree of horizontal displacement of midline structures and the level of consciousness. Specifically, horizontal displacement of the pineal calcification of 3 to 5 mm is generally associated with drowsiness, 6 to 8 mm with stupor, and >9 mm with coma. At the same time, intrusion of the medial temporal lobe into the tentorial opening may be apparent on MRI and CT scan by an obliteration of the cisterns that surround the upper brainstem.

Coma and Confusional States due to Metabolic Disorders   Many systemic metabolic abnormalities cause coma by interrupting the delivery of energy substrates (hypoxia, ischemia, hypoglycemia) or by altering neuronal excitability (drug and alcohol intoxication, anesthesia, and epilepsy). The same metabolic abnormalities that produce coma may in milder form induce widespread cortical dysfunction and an acute confusional state. Thus, in metabolic encephalopathies, clouded consciousness and coma are in a continuum. Neuropathologic changes are variable—prominent in hypoxia-ischemia, evident as astrocytic changes in hepatic coma, and negligible in renal and other metabolic encephalopathies.

Cerebral neurons are fully dependent on cerebral blood flow (CBF) and the related delivery of oxygen and glucose. CBF approximates 75 mL per 100 g/min in gray matter and 30 mL per 100 g/min in white matter (mean = 55 mL per 100 g/min); oxygen consumption is 3.5 mL per 100 g/min, and glucose utilization is 5 mg per 100 g/min. Brain stores of glucose provide energy for approximately 2 min after blood flow is interrupted, and oxygen stores last 8 to 10 s after the cessation of blood flow. Simultaneous hypoxia and ischemia exhaust glucose more rapidly. The electroencephalogram (EEG) rhythm in these circumstances becomes diffusely slowed, typical of metabolic encephalopathies, and as conditions of substrate delivery worsen, eventually all recordable brain electrical activity ceases. In almost all instances of metabolic encephalopathy, the global metabolic activity of the brain is reduced in proportion to the degree of unconsciousness.

Conditions such as hypoglycemia, hyponatremia, hyperosmolarity, hypercapnia, hypercalcemia, and hepatic and renal failure are associated with a variety of alterations in neurons and

FIGURE 257-2   Coronal (*A*) and axial (*B*) magnetic resonance images from a stuporous patient with a left third nerve palsy as a result of a large left-sided subdural hematoma (seen as a gray-white rim). The upper midbrain and lower thalamic regions are compressed and displaced horizontally away from the mass, and there is transtentorial herniation of the medial temporal lobe structures, including the uncus anteriorly. The lateral ventricle opposite to the hematoma has become enlarged as a result of compression of the third ventricle.

astrocytes. The reversible effects of these conditions on the brain are not understood, but may result from impaired energy supplies, changes in ion fluxes across neuronal membranes, and neurotransmitter abnormalities. For example, the high brain ammonia concentration of hepatic coma interferes with cerebral energy metabolism and with the Na$^+$, K$^+$-ATPase pump, increases the number and size of astrocytes, alters nerve cell function, and causes increased concentrations of potentially toxic products of ammonia metabolism; it may also result in abnormalities of neurotransmitters, including putative "false" neurotransmitters that are active at receptor sites. Apart from hyperammonemia, which of these mechanisms is of critical importance is not clear. The mechanism of the encephalopathy of renal failure is also not known. Unlike ammonia, urea itself does not produce central nervous system (CNS) toxicity. A multifactorial causation has been proposed, including increased permeability of the blood-brain barrier to toxic substances such as organic acids and an increase in brain calcium or cerebrospinal fluid (CSF) phosphate content.

Coma and seizures are a common accompaniment of any large shifts in sodium and water balance. These changes in osmolarity arise from systemic medical disorders including diabetic ketoacidosis, the nonketotic hyperosmolar state, and hyponatremia from any cause (e.g., water intoxication, excessive secretion of antidiuretic hormone or atrial natriuretic peptides). The volume of brain water correlates with the level of consciousness in these states, but other factors also play a role. Sodium levels below 125 mmol/L induce confusion, and below 115 mmol/L are associated with coma and convulsions. In hyperosmolar coma the serum osmolarity generally exceeds 350 mosmol/L. *As in most other metabolic encephalopathies, the severity of neurologic change depends to a large degree on the rapidity with which the serum changes occur.* Hypercapnia depresses the level of consciousness in proportion to the rise in CO$_2$ tension in the blood; the level of consciousness also depends on the rapidity of change. The pathophysiology of other metabolic encephalopathies such as hypercalcemia, hypothyroidism, vitamin B$_{12}$ deficiency, and hypothermia are incompletely understood but must also reflect derangements of CNS biochemistry and membrane function.

Epileptic Coma Continuous, generalized electrical discharges of the cortex (*seizures*) are associated with coma even in the absence of epileptic motor activity (*convulsions*). The self-limited coma that follows seizures, termed the *postictal state*, may be due to exhaustion of energy reserves or effects of locally toxic molecules that are the byproduct of seizures. The postictal state produces a pattern of continuous, generalized slowing of the background EEG activity similar to that of other metabolic encephalopathies.

Pharmacologic Coma This class of encephalopathy is in large measure reversible and leaves no residual damage providing hypoxia does not supervene. Many drugs and toxins are capable of depressing nervous system function. Some produce coma by affecting both the brainstem nuclei, including the RAS, and the cerebral cortex. The combination of cortical and brainstem signs, which occurs in certain drug overdoses, may lead to an incorrect diagnosis of structural brainstem disease.

APPROACH TO THE PATIENT

Acute respiratory and cardiovascular problems should be attended to prior to neurologic assessment. In most instances, a complete medical evaluation, except for vital signs, funduscopy, and examination for nuchal rigidity, may be deferred until the neurologic evaluation has established the severity and nature of coma. →*The approach to the patient with trauma is discussed in Chap. 357.*

History In many cases, the cause of coma is immediately evident (e.g., trauma, cardiac arrest, or known drug ingestion). In the remainder, certain points are especially useful: (1) the circumstances and rapidity with which neurologic symptoms developed; (2) the antecedent symptoms (confusion, weakness, headache, fever, seizures, dizziness, double vision, or vomiting); (3) the use of medi-

cations, illicit drugs, or alcohol; and (4) chronic liver, kidney, lung, heart, or other medical disease. Direct interrogation or telephone calls to family and observers on the scene are an important part of the initial evaluation. Ambulance technicians often provide the most useful information.

General Physical Examination The temperature, pulse, respiratory rate and pattern, and blood pressure should be measured quickly. Fever suggests a systemic infection, bacterial meningitis, or encephalitis; only rarely is it attributable to a brain lesion that has disturbed temperature-regulating centers. A slight elevation in temperature may follow vigorous convulsions. High body temperature, 42 to 44°C, associated with dry skin should arouse the suspicion of heat stroke or anticholinergic drug intoxication. Hypothermia is observed with alcoholic, barbiturate, sedative, or phenothiazine intoxication; hypoglycemia; peripheral circulatory failure; or hypothyroidism. Hypothermia itself causes coma only when the temperature is <31°C. Tachypnea may indicate acidosis or pneumonia. Aberrant respiratory patterns that reflect brainstem disorders are discussed below. Marked hypertension indicates hypertensive encephalopathy or a rapid rise in intracranial pressure (ICP) and may occur acutely after head injury. Hypotension is characteristic of coma from alcohol or barbiturate intoxication, internal hemorrhage, myocardial infarction, sepsis, profound hypothyroidism, or Addisonian crisis. The funduscopic examination can detect subarachnoid hemorrhage (subhyaloid hemorrhages), hypertensive encephalopathy (exudates, hemorrhages, vessel-crossing changes, papilledema), and increased ICP (papilledema). Petechiae suggest thrombotic thrombocytopenic purpura, meningococcemia, or a bleeding diathesis from which an intracerebral hemorrhage arises.

Neurologic Assessment First, the patient should be observed without intervention by the examiner. Patients who toss about, reach up toward the face, cross their legs, yawn, swallow, cough, or moan are close to being awake. Lack of restless movements on one side or an outturned leg suggests a hemiplegia. Intermittent twitching movements of a foot, finger, or facial muscle may be the only sign of seizures. Multifocal myoclonus almost always indicates a metabolic disorder, particularly uremia, anoxia, or drug intoxication (lithium and haloperidol are particularly likely to cause this sign), or the rarer conditions of spongiform encephalopathy and Hashimoto disease. In a drowsy and confused patient bilateral asterixis is a certain sign of metabolic encephalopathy or drug intoxication.

The terms *decorticate rigidity* and *decerebrate rigidity*, or "posturing," describe stereotyped arm and leg movements occurring spontaneously or elicited by sensory stimulation. Flexion of the elbows and wrists and supination of the arm (decortication) suggests bilateral damage rostral to the midbrain, whereas extension of the elbows and wrists with pronation (decerebration) indicates damage to motor tracts in the midbrain or caudal diencephalon. The less frequent combination of arm extension with leg flexion or flaccid legs is associated with lesions in the pons. These concepts have been adapted from animal work and cannot be applied with the same precision to coma in humans. In fact, acute and widespread cerebral disorders of any type, regardless of location, frequently cause limb extension, and almost all such extensor posturing becomes predominantly flexor as time passes. Posturing may also be unilateral and may coexist with purposeful limb movements, usually reflecting incomplete damage to the motor system.

Level of Arousal and Elicited Movements If the patient is not aroused by a conversational volume of voice, a sequence of increasingly intense stimuli is used to determine the threshold for arousal and the optimal motor response of each side of the body. The results of testing may vary from minute to minute and serial examinations are most useful. Tickling the nostrils with a cotton wisp is a moderate stimulus to arousal—all but deeply stuporous and comatose patients will move the head away and rouse to some degree. Using the hand to remove the offending stimulus represents an even greater degree of responsiveness.

Responses to noxious stimuli should be appraised critically. Stereotyped posturing indicates severe dysfunction of the corticospinal system. Abduction-avoidance movement of a limb is usually purposeful and denotes an intact corticospinal system. Pressure on the knuckles or bony prominences and pinprick are humane forms of noxious stimuli; pinching the skin causes unsightly ecchymoses and is generally not necessary but may be useful in eliciting abduction withdrawal movements of the limbs.

Brainstem Reflexes   Assessment of brainstem function is essential to localization of the lesion in coma (Fig. 257-3). The brainstem reflexes that are conveniently examined are pupillary responses to light, spontaneous and elicited eye movements, corneal responses, and the respiratory pattern. As a rule, when these brainstem activities are preserved, particularly the pupil reactions and eye movements, coma must be ascribed to bilateral hemispheral disease. The converse, however, is not always true as a mass in the hemispheres may be the underlying cause of coma but nonetheless produce brainstem signs.

PUPILS   Pupillary reactions are examined with a bright, diffuse light (not an ophthalmoscope); if the response is absent, this should be confirmed by observation through a magnifying lens. Normally reactive and round pupils of midsize (2.5 to 5 mm) essentially exclude midbrain damage, either primary or secondary to compression. Reaction to light is often difficult to appreciate in pupils <2 mm in diameter, and bright room lighting mutes pupillary reactivity. One unreactive and enlarged pupil (>6 mm) or one that is poorly reactive signifies a compression or stretching of the third nerve from the effects of a mass above. Enlargement of the pupil contralateral to a mass may occur first but is infrequent. An oval and slightly eccentric pupil is a transitional sign that accompanies early midbrain–third nerve compression. The most extreme pupillary sign, bilaterally dilated and unreactive pupils, indicates severe midbrain damage, usually from compression by a mass. Ingestion of drugs with anticholinergic activity, the use of mydriatic eye drops, and direct ocular trauma are among the causes of misleading pupillary enlargement.

Unilateral miosis in coma has been attributed to dysfunction of sympathetic efferents originating in the posterior hypothalamus and descending in the tegmentum of the brainstem to the cervical cord. It is an occasional finding with a large cerebral hemorrhage that affects the thalamus. Reactive and bilaterally small (1 to 2.5 mm) but not pinpoint pupils are seen in metabolic encephalopathies or in deep bilateral hemispheral lesions such as hydrocephalus or thalamic hemorrhage. Very small but reactive pupils (<1 mm) characterize narcotic or barbiturate overdoses but also occur with extensive pontine hemorrhage. The response to naloxone and the presence of reflex eye movements (see below) distinguish these.

OCULAR MOVEMENTS   The eyes are first observed by elevating the lids and noting the resting position and spontaneous movements of the globes. Lid tone, tested by lifting the eyelids and noting their resistance to opening and the speed of closure, is reduced progressively as coma deepens. Horizontal divergence of the eyes at rest is normal in drowsiness. As coma deepens, the ocular axes may become parallel again.

Spontaneous eye movements in coma often take the form of conjugate horizontal roving. This finding alone exonerates the midbrain and pons and has the same significance as normal reflex eye movements (see below). Conjugate horizontal ocular deviation to one side indicates damage to the pons on the opposite side or a lesion in the frontal lobe on the same side. This phenomenon may

FIGURE 257-3   Examination of brainstem reflexes in coma. Midbrain and third nerve function are tested by pupillary reaction to light, pontine function by spontaneous and reflex eye movements and corneal responses, and medullary function by respiratory and pharyngeal responses. Reflex conjugate, horizontal eye movements are dependent on the medial longitudinal fasciculus (MLF) interconnecting the sixth and contralateral third nerve nuclei. Head rotation (oculocephalic reflex) or caloric stimulation of the labyrinths (oculovestibular reflex) elicits contraversive eye movements (for details see text).

be summarized by the following maxim: *The eyes look toward a hemispheral lesion and away from a brainstem lesion.* Seizures also drive the eyes to one side. On rare occasions, the eyes may turn paradoxically away from the side of a deep hemispheral lesion ("wrong-way eyes"). The eyes turn down and inward as a result of thalamic and upper midbrain lesions, typically with thalamic hemorrhage. "Ocular bobbing" describes a brisk downward and slow upward movement of the eyes associated with loss of horizontal eye movements and is diagnostic of bilateral pontine damage, usually from thrombosis of the basilar artery. "Ocular dipping" is a slower, arrhythmic downward movement followed by a faster upward movement in patients with normal reflex horizontal gaze; it indicates diffuse cortical anoxic damage. Many other complex eye movements are known but do not have the same significance as the ones already mentioned.

The oculocephalic reflexes depend on the integrity of the ocular motor nuclei and their interconnecting tracts that extend from the midbrain to the pons and medulla. These reflexes are elicited by moving the head from side to side or vertically and observing evoked eye movements in the direction opposite to the head movement (Fig. 257-3). These movements, called somewhat inappropriately "doll's eyes" (which refers more accurately to the reflex elevation of the eyelids with flexion of the neck), are normally suppressed in the awake patient by visual fixation. Their presence therefore indicates a reduced cortical influence on the brainstem. Furthermore, preservation of evoked reflex eye movements signifies the integrity of the brainstem and, by implication, that the origin of unconsciousness lies in the cerebral hemispheres. The opposite—the absence of reflex eye movements—signifies damage within the brainstem but can be produced infrequently by profound overdoses of certain drugs. Normal pupillary size and light reaction distinguishes most drug-induced comas from structural brainstem damage.

Thermal, or "caloric," stimulation of the vestibular apparatus (oculovestibular response) provides a more intense stimulus for the oculocephalic reflex but gives fundamentally the same information. The test is performed by irrigating the external auditory canal with cool water in order to induce convection currents in the labyrinths. After a brief latency, the result is tonic deviation of both eyes to the side of cool-water irrigation and nystagmus in the opposite direction. (The acronym "COWS" has been used to remind generations of medical students of the direction of nystagmus—"cold water opposite, warm water same"). The absence of nystagmus despite conjugate deviation of the globes signifies that the cerebral hemispheres are damaged or suppressed. The loss of conjugate ocular movements indicates brainstem damage.

By touching the cornea with a wisp of cotton, a response consisting of brief bilateral lid closure is normally observed. The corneal reflexes depend on the integrity of pontine pathways between the fifth (afferent) and both seventh (efferent) cranial nerves; although rarely useful alone, in conjunction with reflex eye movements they are important clinical tests of pontine function. CNS depressant drugs diminish or eliminate the corneal responses soon after reflex eye movements are paralyzed but before the pupils become unreactive to light. The corneal (and pharyngeal) response may be lost for a time on the side of an acute hemiplegia.

RESPIRATION Respiratory patterns are of less localizing value in comparison to other brainstem signs. Shallow, slow, but regular breathing suggests metabolic or drug depression. Cheyne-Stokes respiration in its classic cyclic form, ending with a brief apneic period, signifies bihemispheral damage or metabolic suppression and commonly accompanies light coma. Rapid, deep (Kussmaul) breathing usually implies metabolic acidosis but may also occur with pontomesencephalic lesions. Agonal gasps reflect bilateral lower brainstem damage and are well known as the terminal respiratory pattern of severe brain damage. A number of other cyclic breathing variations are of lesser significance.

LABORATORY STUDIES AND IMAGING The studies that are most useful in the diagnosis of confusional states and coma are: chemical-toxicologic analysis of blood and urine, cranial CT or MRI, EEG, and CSF examination. Arterial blood-gas analysis is helpful in patients with lung disease and acid-base disorders. The metabolic aberrations commonly encountered in clinical practice require measurements of electrolytes, glucose, calcium, osmolarity, and renal (blood urea nitrogen) and hepatic (NH_3) function. Toxicologic analysis is necessary in any case of coma where the diagnosis is not immediately clear. However, the presence of exogenous drugs or toxins, especially alcohol, does not exclude the possibility that other factors, particularly head trauma, are also contributing to the clinical state. An ethanol level of 43 mmol/L (200 mg/dL) in nonhabituated patients generally causes impaired mental activity and of >65 mmol/L (300 mg/dL) is associated with stupor. The development of tolerance may allow the chronic alcoholic to remain awake at levels >87 mmol/L (400 mg/dL).

The availability of CT and MRI has focused attention on causes of coma that are radiologically detectable (e.g., hemorrhages, tumors, or hydrocephalus). Resorting primarily to this approach, although at times expedient, is imprudent because most cases of coma (and confusion) are metabolic or toxic in origin. The notion that a normal CT scan excludes anatomic lesions as the cause of coma is also erroneous. Bilateral hemisphere infarction, small brainstem lesions, encephalitis, meningitis, mechanical shearing of axons as a result of closed head trauma, sagittal sinus thrombosis, and subdural hematomas that are isodense to adjacent brain are some of the disorders that may not be detected. Nevertheless, if the source of coma remains unknown, a scan should be obtained.

The EEG is useful in metabolic or drug-induced confusional states but is rarely diagnostic, except when coma is due to clinically unrecognized seizures, to herpesvirus encephalitis, or to Creutzfeldt-Jakob disease. The amount of background slowing of the EEG is a reflection of the severity of any diffuse encephalopathy. Predominant high-voltage slowing (δ or triphasic waves) in the frontal regions is typical of metabolic coma, as from hepatic failure, and widespread fast (β) activity implicates sedative drugs (e.g., diazepines, barbiturates). A special pattern of "α coma," defined by widespread, variable 8- to 12-Hz activity, superficially resembles the normal α rhythm of waking but is unresponsive to environmental stimuli. It results from pontine or diffuse cortical damage and is associated with a poor prognosis. Most importantly, EEG recordings may reveal clinically inapparent epileptic discharges in a patient with coma. Normal α activity on the EEG also alerts the clinician to the locked-in syndrome or to hysteria or catatonia.

Lumbar puncture is performed less frequently than in the past because neuroimaging scans effectively exclude intracerebral and subarachnoid hemorrhages that are severe enough to cause coma. However, examination of the CSF is indispensable in the diagnosis of meningitis and encephalitis. Lumbar puncture should therefore not be deferred if meningitis is a possibility.

DIFFERENTIAL DIAGNOSIS OF COMA (Table 257-1) The causes of coma can be conceptualized in three broad categories: those without focal neurologic signs (e.g., metabolic encephalopathies); meningitis syndromes, characterized by fever or stiff neck and an excess of cells in the spinal fluid (e.g., bacterial meningitis, subarachnoid hemorrhage);

TABLE 257-1 *Differential Diagnosis of Coma*

1. Diseases that cause no focal or lateralizing neurologic signs, usually with normal brainstem functions; CT scan and cellular content of the CSF are normal
   a. Intoxications: alcohol, sedative drugs, opiates, etc.
   b. Metabolic disturbances: anoxia, hyponatremia, hypernatremia, hypercalcemia, diabetic acidosis, nonketotic hyperosmolar hyperglycemia, hypoglycemia, uremia, hepatic coma, hypercarbia, addisonian crisis, hypo- and hyperthyroid states, profound nutritional deficiency
   c. Severe systemic infections: pneumonia, septicemia, typhoid fever, malaria, Waterhouse-Friderichsen syndrome
   d. Shock from any cause
   e. Postseizure states, status epilepticus, subclinical epilepsy
   f. Hypertensive encephalopathy, eclampsia
   g. Severe hyperthermia, hypothermia
   h. Concussion
   i. Acute hydrocephalus
2. Diseases that cause meningeal irritation with or without fever, and with an excess of WBCs or RBCs in the CSF, usually without focal or lateralizing cerebral or brainstem signs; CT or MRI shows no mass lesion
   a. Subarachnoid hemorrhage from ruptured aneurysm, arteriovenous malformation, trauma
   b. Acute bacterial meningitis
   c. Viral encephalitis
   d. Miscellaneous: Fat embolism, cholesterol embolism, carcinomatous and lymphomatous meningitis, etc.
3. Diseases that cause focal brainstem or lateralizing cerebral signs, with or without changes in the CSF; CT and MRI are abnormal
   a. Hemispheral hemorrhage (basal ganglionic, thalamic) or infarction (large middle cerebral artery territory) with secondary brainstem compression
   b. Brainstem infarction due to basilar artery thrombosis or embolism
   c. Brain abscess, subdural empyema
   d. Epidural and subdural hemorrhage, brain contusion
   e. Brain tumor with surrounding edema
   f. Cerebellar and pontine hemorrhage and infarction
   g. Widespread traumatic brain injury
   h. Metabolic coma (see above) with preexisting focal damage
   i. Miscellaneous: cortical vein thrombosis, herpes simplex encephalitis, multiple cerebral emboli due to bacterial endocarditis, acute hemorrhagic leukoencephalitis, acute disseminated (postinfectious) encephalomyelitis, thrombotic thrombocytopenic purpura, cerebral vasculitis, gliomatosis cerebri, pituitary apoplexy, intravascular lymphoma, etc.

Note: CT, computed tomography; CSF, cerebrospinal fluid; WBCs, white blood cells; RBCs, red blood cells; MRI, magnetic resonance imaging.

and those with prominent focal signs (e.g., stroke, cerebral hemorrhage). In most instances confusion and coma are part of an obvious medical problem such as drug ingestion, hypoxia, stroke, trauma, or liver or kidney failure. Conditions that cause sudden coma include drug ingestion, cerebral hemorrhage, trauma, cardiac arrest, epilepsy, or basilar artery embolism. Coma that appears subacutely is usually related to a preceding medical or neurologic problem, including the secondary brain swelling of a mass lesion such as tumor or cerebral infarction.

Cerebrovascular diseases cause the greatest difficulty in coma diagnosis (Chap. 349). These may be summarized as follows: (1) basal ganglia and thalamic hemorrhage (acute but not instantaneous onset, vomiting, headache, hemiplegia, and characteristic eye signs); (2) pontine hemorrhage (sudden onset, pinpoint pupils, loss of reflex eye movements and corneal responses, ocular bobbing, posturing, hyperventilation, and excessive sweating); (3) cerebellar hemorrhage (occipital headache, vomiting, gaze paresis, and inability to stand); (4) basilar artery thrombosis (neurologic prodrome or warning spells, diplopia, dysarthria, vomiting, eye movement and corneal response abnormalities, and asymmetric limb paresis); and (5) subarachnoid hemorrhage (precipitous coma after headache and vomiting). The most common stroke, infarction in the territory of the middle cerebral artery, does not cause coma, but edema surrounding large infarcts may expand during the first few days and act as a mass. The syndrome of acute hydrocephalus accompanies many intracranial diseases, particularly subarachnoid hemorrhage. It is characterized by headache and sometimes vomiting that may progress quickly to coma, with extensor posturing of the limbs, bilateral Babinski signs, small nonreactive pupils, and impaired oculocephalic movements in the vertical direction.

If the history and examination do not indicate the cause of coma, then information obtained from CT or MRI may be needed. As mentioned earlier, the majority of medical causes of coma can be established without a neuroimaging study.

BRAIN DEATH   This is a state in which there has been cessation of cerebral blood flow; as a result there is global loss of brain function while respiration is maintained by artificial means and the heart continues to pump. It is the only type of brain damage that is recognized as equivalent to death. Many roughly equivalent criteria have been advanced for the diagnosis of brain death, and it is essential to adhere to those standards endorsed by the local medical community. Ideal criteria are simple, can be conducted at the bedside, and allow no chance of diagnostic error. They contain three essential elements: (1) widespread cortical destruction shown by deep coma—unresponsiveness to all forms of stimulation; (2) global brainstem damage demonstrated by absent pupillary light reaction and the loss of oculovestibular and corneal reflexes; and (3) destruction of the medulla manifested by complete apnea. The pulse rate is invariant and unresponsive to atropine. Diabetes insipidus is often present, but may develop hours or days after the other clinical signs of brain death. The pupils are often enlarged but may be mid-sized; they should not be constricted. The absence of deep tendon reflexes is not required because the spinal cord remains functional.

Demonstration that apnea is due to irreversible medullary damage requires that the P_{CO_2} be high enough to stimulate respiration during a test of spontaneous breathing (apnea test). This can be done safely by the use, prior to removing the ventilator, of diffusion oxygenation. This is accomplished by preoxygenation with 100% oxygen, which is then sustained during the test by oxygen administered through a tracheal cannula. CO_2 tension increases approximately 0.3 to 0.4 kPa/min (2 to 3 mmHg/min) during apnea. At the end of the period of observation, typically several minutes in duration, arterial P_{CO_2} should be at least >6.6 to 8.0 kPa (50 to 60 mmHg) for the test to be valid. Complete apnea is considered to be present if no respiratory effort is observed in the presence of a sufficiently elevated P_{CO_2}.

The possibility of profound drug-induced or hypothermic depression of the nervous system should be excluded, and some period of observation, usually 6 to 24 h, is desirable during which this state is shown to be sustained. It is particularly advisable to delay clinical testing for at least 24 h if a cardiac arrest has caused brain death or if the inciting disease is not known. An isoelectric EEG may be used as a confirmatory test for total cerebral damage but is not absolutely necessary. Radionuclide brain scanning, cerebral angiography, or transcranial Doppler measurements may also be used to demonstrate the absence of cerebral blood flow but they have not been extensively correlated with pathologic changes.

There is no compelling reason to embark on the demonstration of brain death except when organ transplantation is involved. Although it is largely accepted in western society that the respirator can be disconnected from a brain-dead patient, problems frequently arise because of poor communication and inadequate preparation of the family by the physician. Reasonable medical practice allows the removal of support or transfer out of an intensive care unit of patients who are not brain dead but whose condition is nonetheless hopeless and are likely to live for only a brief time.

℞ TREATMENT

The immediate goal is prevention of further nervous system damage. Hypotension, hypoglycemia, hypercalcemia, hypoxia, hypercapnia, and hyperthermia should be corrected rapidly. An oropharyngeal airway is adequate to keep the pharynx open in drowsy patients who are breathing normally. Tracheal intubation is indicated if there is apnea, upper airway obstruction, hypoventilation, or emesis, or if the patient is liable to aspirate because of coma. Mechanical ventilation is required if there is hypoventilation or a need to induce hypocapnia in order to lower ICP as described below. Intravenous access is established, and naloxone and dextrose are administered if narcotic overdose or hypoglycemia are even remote possibilities; thiamine is given along with glucose to avoid provoking Wernicke disease in malnourished patients. In cases of suspected basilar thrombosis with brainstem ischemia, intravenous heparin or a thrombolytic agent is often utilized, after cerebral hemorrhage is excluded by a neuroimaging study. Physostigmine may awaken patients with anticholinergic-type drug overdose, but must be used only by experienced physicians and with careful monitoring; many physicians believe that it should only be used to treat anticholinergic overdose–associated cardiac arrhythmias. The use of benzodiazepine antagonists offers some prospect of improvement after overdoses of soporific drugs and has transient benefit in hepatic encephalopathy. Intravenous administration of hypotonic solutions should be monitored carefully in any serious acute brain illness because of the potential for exacerbating brain swelling. Cervical spine injuries must not be overlooked, particularly prior to attempting intubation or evaluating of oculocephalic responses. Headache accompanied by fever and meningismus indicates an urgent need for examination of the CSF to diagnose meningitis. If the lumbar puncture in a case of suspected meningitis is delayed for any reason, an antibiotic such as a third-generation cephalosporin should be administered as soon as possible, preferably after obtaining blood cultures. The management of raised ICP is discussed in Chap. 258.

PROGNOSIS   The prediction of the outcome of coma must be considered in reference to long-term care and medical resources. One hopes to avoid the emotionally painful, hopeless outcome of a patient who is left severely disabled or vegetative. The uniformly pessimistic outcome of the persistent vegetative state has already been mentioned. Children and young adults may have ominous early clinical findings such as abnormal brainstem reflexes and yet recover, so that temporization in offering a prognosis in this group of patients is wise. Metabolic comas have a far better prognosis than traumatic comas. All schemes for prognosis in adults should be taken as approximations, and medical judgments must be tempered by factors such as age, underlying systemic disease, and general medical condition. In an attempt to collect prognostic information from large numbers of patients with head injury, the Glasgow Coma Scale was devised; empirically it has predictive value in cases of brain trauma (Chap. 357). For anoxic and metabolic coma, clinical signs such as the pupillary and motor responses after 1 day, 3 days, and 1 week have been shown to have predictive value (Chap. 258). The absence of the cortical waves of the somatosensory evoked potentials has also proved a strong indicator of poor outcome in coma from any cause.

FURTHER READING

PARVIZI J, DAMASIO AR: Neuroanatomical correlates of brainstem coma. Brain 126:1524, 2003

ROPPER AH: *Neurological and Neurosurgical Intensive Care*, 4th ed. New York, Lippincott, Williams & Wilkins, 2004

---

258 CRITICAL CARE NEUROLOGY
J. Claude Hemphill

Life-threatening neurologic illness may be caused by a primary disorder affecting any region of the neuroaxis or may occur as a consequence of a systemic disorder such as hepatic failure, multisystem organ failure, or cardiac arrest (Table 258-1). Neurologic critical care focuses on preservation of neurologic tissue and prevention of secondary brain injury caused by ischemia, edema, and elevated intracranial pressure (ICP).

PATHOPHYSIOLOGY ■ Brain Edema
Swelling, or edema, of brain tissue occurs with many types of brain injury. The two principal types of edema are vasogenic and cytotoxic. *Vasogenic edema* refers to the influx of fluid and solutes into the brain through an incompetent blood-brain barrier (BBB). In the normal cerebral vasculature, endothelial tight junctions associated with astrocytes create an impermeable barrier (the BBB), through which access into the brain interstitium is dependent upon specific transport mechanisms (Chap. 345). The BBB may be compromised in ischemia, trauma, infection, and metabolic derangements. Typically, vasogenic edema develops rapidly following injury. *Cytotoxic edema* refers to cellular swelling and occurs in a variety of settings including brain ischemia and trauma. Early astrocytic swelling is a hallmark of ischemia. Brain edema that is clinically significant usually represents a combination of vasogenic and cellular components. Edema can lead to increased ICP as well as tissue shifts and brain displacement from focal processes. These tissue shifts can cause injury by mechanical distraction and compression in addition to the ischemia of impaired perfusion consequent to the elevated ICP.

Ischemic Cascade and Cellular Injury
When delivery of substrates, principally oxygen and glucose, is inadequate to sustain cellular function, a series of interrelated biochemical reactions known as the *ischemic cascade* is initiated. The release of excitatory amino acids, especially glutamate, leads to influx of calcium and sodium ions, which disrupt cellular homeostasis. An increased intracellular calcium concentration may activate proteases and lipases, which then lead to lipid peroxidation and free radical–mediated cell membrane injury. Cytoxic edema ensues, and ultimately necrotic cell death and tissue infarction occur. This pathway to irreversible cell death is common to ischemic stroke, global cerebral ischemia, and traumatic brain injury. *Penumbra* refers to ischemic brain tissue that has not yet undergone irreversible infarction, implying that the region is potentially salvageable if ischemia can be reversed. Factors that may exacerbate ischemic

TABLE 258-1 *Neurologic Disorders in Critical Illness*

Localization Along Neuroaxis	Syndrome
CENTRAL NERVOUS SYSTEM	
Brain: Cerebral hemispheres	Global encephalopathy
	Sepsis
	Organ failure—hepatic, renal
	Medication related
	Sedatives/hypnotics/analgesics
	H$_2$ blockers, antihypertensives
	Drug overdose
	Electrolyte disturbance—hyponatremia; hypoglycemia
	Hypotension/hypoperfusion
	Hypoxia
	Meningitis
	Subarachnoid hemorrhage
	Wernicke's disease
	Seizure—postictal or nonconvulsive status
	Hypertensive encephalopathy
	Hypothyroidism—myxedema
	Focal deficits
	Ischemic stroke
	Tumor
	Abscess, subdural empyema
	Subdural/epidural hematoma
Brainstem	Mass effect and compression
	Ischemic stroke, intraparenchymal hemorrhage
	Hypoxia
Spinal cord	Mass effect and compression
	Disc herniation
	Epidural hematoma
	Ischemia—hypotension/embolic
	Subdural empyema
	Trauma, central cord syndrome
PERIPHERAL NERVOUS SYSTEM	
Peripheral nerve	
Axonal	Critical illness polyneuropathy
	Possible neuromuscular blocking agent complication
	Metabolic disturbances, uremia—hyperglycemia
	Medication effects—chemotherapeutic, antiretroviral
Demyelinating	Guillian-Barré syndrome
	Chronic inflammatory demyelinating polyneuropathy
Neuromuscular junction	Prolonged effect of neuromuscular blockade
	Medication effects—aminoglycosides
	Myasthenia-gravis, Lambert-Eaton syndrome
Muscle	Septic myopathy
	Cachectic myopathy—with or without disuse atrophy
	Electrolyte disturbances—hypokalemia/hyperkalemia; hypophosphatemia
	Acute quadriplegic myopathy

brain injury include systemic hypotension and hypoxia, which further reduce substrate delivery to vulnerable brain tissue, and fever, seizures, and hyperglycemia, which can increase cellular metabolism outstripping compensatory processes. Clinically, these events are known as *secondary brain insults* because they lead to exacerbation of the primary brain injury. Prevention, identification, and treatment of secondary brain insults are fundamental goals of management.

An alternative pathway of cellular injury is *apoptosis*. This process implies programmed cell death, which may occur in the setting of ischemic stroke, global cerebral ischemia, traumatic brain injury, and possibly intracerebral hemorrhage. Apoptotic cell death can be distinguished histologically from the necrotic cell death of ischemia and is mediated through a different set of biochemical pathways. At present, interventions for prevention and treatment of apoptotic cell death remain less well defined than those for ischemia. →*Excitotoxicity and mechanisms of cell death are discussed in more detail in Chap. 345.*

Cerebral Perfusion and Autoregulation   Brain tissue requires constant perfusion in order to ensure adequate delivery of substrate. The hemodynamic response of the brain has the capacity to preserve perfusion across a wide range of systemic blood pressures. Cerebral perfusion pressure (CPP), defined as the mean systemic arterial pressure (MAP) minus the ICP, provides the driving force for circulation across the capillary beds of the brain. *Autoregulation* refers to the physiologic response whereby cerebral blood flow (CBF) remains relatively constant over a wide range of blood pressures as a consequence of alterations of cerebrovascular resistance (Fig. 258-1). If systemic blood pressure drops, cerebral perfusion is preserved through vasodilation of arterioles in the brain; likewise, arteriolar vasoconstriction occurs at high systemic pressures to prevent hyperperfusion. At the extreme limits of MAP or CPP (high or low), flow becomes directly related to perfusion pressure. These autoregulatory changes occur in the microcirculation and are mediated by vessels below the resolution of those seen on angiography. CBF is also strongly influenced by pH and P_{CO_2}. CBF increases with hypercapnia and acidosis and decreases with hypocapnia and alkalosis. This forms the basis for the use of hyperventilation to lower ICP, and this effect on ICP is mediated through a decrease in intracranial blood volume. Cerebral autoregulation is critical to the normal homeostatic functioning of the brain, and this process may be disordered focally and unpredictably in disease states such as traumatic brain injury and severe focal cerebral ischemia.

Cerebrospinal Fluid and Intracranial Pressure   The cranial contents consist essentially of brain, cerebrospinal fluid (CSF), and blood. CSF is pro-

duced principally in the choroid plexus of each lateral ventricle, exits the brain via the foramina of Luschka and Magendi, and flows over the cortex to be absorbed into the venous system along the superior sagittal sinus. Approximately 150 mL of CSF are contained within the ventricles and surrounding the brain and spinal cord; the cerebral blood volume is also ~150 mL. The bony skull offers excellent protection for the brain but allows little tolerance for additional volume. Significant increases in volume eventually result in increased ICP. Obstruction of CSF outflow, edema of cerebral tissue, or increases in volume from tumor or hematoma may increase ICP. Elevated ICP diminishes cerebral perfusion and can lead to tissue ischemia. Ischemia in turn may lead to vasodilatation via autoregulatory mechanisms designed to restore cerebral perfusion. However, vasodilatation also increases cerebral blood volume, which in turn then increases ICP, lowers CPP, and provokes further ischemia (Fig. 258-2). This vicious cycle is commonly seen in traumatic brain injury, massive intracerebral hemorrhage, and large hemispheric infarcts with significant tissue shift.

APPROACH TO THE PATIENT

Critically ill patients with severe central nervous system dysfunction require rapid evaluation and intervention in order to limit primary and secondary brain injury. Initial neurologic evaluation should be performed concurrent with stabilization of basic respiratory, cardiac, and hemodynamic parameters. Significant barriers may exist to neurologic assessment in the critical care unit. Endotracheal intubation and the use of sedative or paralytic agents to facilitate critical care procedures can make clinical assessment challenging.

An impaired level of consciousness is frequent in critically ill patients. The essential first task in assessment is to determine whether the cause of dysfunction is related to a diffuse, usually metabolic, process or whether a focal, usually structural, process is implicated. Examples of diffuse processes include metabolic encephalopathies related to organ failure, drug overdose, or hypoxia-ischemia. Focal processes include ischemic and hemorrhagic stroke and traumatic brain injury, especially with intracranial hematomas. Since these two categories of disorders have fundamentally different causes, treatments, and prognoses, the initial focus is on making this distinction rapidly and accurately. →*The approach to the confused or comatose patient is discussed in Chap. 257; etiologies are listed in Table 257-1.*

Minor focal deficits may be present on the neurologic examination in patients with metabolic encephalopathies. However, the finding of prominent focal signs such as pupillary asymmetry, hemiparesis, gaze palsy, or paraplegia should alert the examiner to the possibility of a structural lesion. All patients with a decreased level of consciousness associated with focal findings should undergo an urgent neuroimaging procedure, as should all patients

FIGURE 258-1   Autoregulation of cerebral blood flow (solid line). Cerebral perfusion is constant over a wide range of systemic blood pressure. Perfusion is increased in the setting of hypoxia or hypercarbia. BP, blood pressure; CBF, cerebral blood flow. (*Reprinted with permission from Anesthesiology 43:447, 1975. Copyright 1975, Lippincott Company.*)

FIGURE 258-2   Ischemia and vasodilatation. Reduced cerebral perfusion pressure (CPP) leads to increased ischemia, vasodilatation, increased intracranial pressure (ICP), and further reductions in CPP, a cycle leading to further neurologic injury. CBV, cerebral blood volume; CMR, cerebral metabolic rate; CSF, cerebrospinal fluid; SABP, systolic arterial blood pressure. (*From MJ Rosner et al: J Neurosurg 83:949, 1995; with permission.*)

with coma of unknown etiology. Computed tomographic (CT) scanning is usually the most appropriate initial study because it can be performed quickly in critically ill patients and demonstrates hemorrhage, hydrocephalus, and intracranial tissue shifts well. Magnetic resonance imaging (MRI) may provide more specific information in some situations, such as acute ischemic stroke (diffusion-weighted imaging, DWI) and cerebral venous sinus thrombosis (magnetic resonance venography, MRV). Any suggestion of trauma from the history or examination should alert the examiner to the possibility of cervical spine injury and prompt an imaging evaluation using plain x-rays, MRI, or CT.

Other diagnostic studies are best utilized in specific circumstances, usually when neuroimaging studies fail to reveal a structural lesion and the etiology of the altered mental state remains uncertain. Electroencephalography (EEG) can be important in the evaluation of critically ill patients with severe brain dysfunction. The EEG of metabolic encephalopathy typically reveals generalized slowing. One of the most important uses of EEG is to help exclude inapparent seizures, especially nonconvulsive status epilepticus. Untreated continuous or frequently recurrent seizures may cause neuronal injury, making the diagnosis and treatment of seizure crucial in this patient group. Lumbar puncture (LP) may be necessary to exclude infectious processes, and an elevated opening pressure may be an important clue to cerebral venous sinus thrombosis. In patients with coma or profound encephalopathy, it is preferable to perform a neuroimaging study prior to LP. If bacterial meningitis is suspected, an LP may be performed first or antibiotics may be empirically administered before the diagnostic studies are completed. Standard laboratory evaluation of critically ill patients should include assessment of serum electrolytes (especially sodium and calcium), glucose, renal and hepatic function, complete blood counts, and coagulation. Serum or urine toxicology screens should be performed in patients with encephalopathy of unknown cause. EEG, LP, and other specific laboratory tests are most useful when the mechanism of the altered level of consciousness is uncertain; they are not routinely performed in clear-cut cases of stroke or traumatic brain injury.

Monitoring of ICP can be an important tool in selected patients. Indications for ICP monitoring, as well as specific types of monitors, vary. In general, patients who should be considered for ICP monitoring are those with primary neurologic disorders, such as stroke or traumatic brain injury, who are at significant risk for secondary brain injury due to elevated ICP and decreased CPP. Such patients include those with severe traumatic brain injury resulting in coma [Glasgow Coma Scale (GCS) score of ≤8 (Table 357-1)]; those with large tissue shifts from supratentorial ischemic or hemorrhagic stroke resulting in decreased consciousness; and those with (or at risk for) hydrocephalus from subarachnoid hemorrhage, intraventricular hemorrhage, or posterior fossa stroke. An additional disorder in which ICP monitoring can add important information is fulminant hepatic failure, in which elevated ICP may be treated with barbiturates or, eventually, liver transplantation. In general, ventriculostomy is preferable to ICP monitoring devices that are placed in brain parenchyma, because ventriculostomy allows CSF drainage as a method of treating elevated ICP. However, parenchymal ICP monitoring is most appropriate for patients with diffuse edema and small ventricles (which may make ventriculostomy placement more difficult) or any degree of coagulopathy (in which ventriculostomy carries a higher risk of hemorrhagic complications).

Treatment of Elevated ICP   Elevated ICP may occur in a wide range of disorders including head trauma, intracerebral hemorrhage, subarachnoid hemorrhage with hydrocephalus, and fulminant hepatic failure. Because CSF and blood volume can be redistributed initially, by the time elevated ICP occurs intracranial compliance is severely impaired. At this point, small changes in the volume of CSF, intravascular blood, edema, or a mass lesion may result in significant changes in ICP. Elevated ICP then diminishes cerebral

perfusion. This is a fundamental mechanism of secondary ischemic brain injury and constitutes an emergency that requires immediate attention. Specific thresholds of ICP vary, but in general, ICP should be maintained at <20 mmHg and CPP should be maintained at ≥70 mmHg.

A number of different interventions may lower ICP, and ideally the selection of treatment will be based on the underlying mechanism responsible for the elevated ICP (Table 258-2). For example, in hydrocephalus from subarachnoid hemorrhage, the principal cause of elevated ICP is impairment of CSF drainage. In this setting, ventricular drainage of CSF is likely to be sufficient and most appropriate. In head trauma and stroke, cytotoxic edema may be most responsible, and the use of osmotic diuretics such as mannitol becomes an appropriate early step. As described above, elevated ICP may cause tissue ischemia, and, if cerebral autoregulation is intact, the resulting vasodilatation can lead to a cycle of worsening ischemia. Paradoxically, administration of vasopressor agents to increase mean arterial pressure may actually lower ICP by improving perfusion, thereby allowing autoregulatory vasoconstriction as ischemia is relieved and ultimately decreasing intracranial blood volume.

Early signs of elevated ICP include drowsiness and a diminished level of consciousness. Neuroimaging studies may reveal evidence of edema and mass effect. Hypotonic intravenous fluids should be avoided, and elevation of the head of the bed is recommended. Patients must be carefully observed for risk of aspiration and compromise of the airway as the level of alertness declines. Coma and unilateral pupillary changes are late signs and require immediate intervention. Emergent treatment of elevated ICP is most quickly achieved by intubation and hyperventilation, which causes vasoconstriction and reduces cerebral blood volume. Because of the concern of provoking or worsening cerebral ischemia, hyperventilation is best used for short periods of time until a more definitive treatment can be instituted. Furthermore, the effects of continued hyperventilation on ICP are short-lived, often only for several hours because of the buffering capacity of the cerebral interstitium, and rebound elevated ICP may accompany abrupt discontinuation of hyperventilation. As the level of consciousness declines to coma, the ability to follow the neurologic status of the patient by examination deteriorates and measurement of ICP must be considered. If a ventriculostomy device is in place, direct drain-

TABLE 258-2   *Stepwise Approach to Treatment of Elevated Intracranial Pressure*[a]

Insert ICP monitor—ventriculostomy versus parenchymal device
General goals: maintain ICP < 20 mmHg and CPP > 70 mmHg

For ICP > 20–25 mmHg for >5 min:
1. Drain CSF via ventriculostomy (if in place)
2. Elevate head of the bed
3. Osmotherapy—mannitol 25–100 g q4h as needed
   (maintain serum osmolality <320 mosmol)
4. Glucocorticoids—dexamethasone 4 mg q6h for vasogenic edema from tumor, abscess (avoid glucocorticoids in head trauma, ischemic and hemorrhagic stroke)
5. Sedation (e.g., morphine, propofol, or midazolam); add neuromuscular paralysis if necessary (patient will require endotracheal intubation and mechanical ventilation at this point, if not before)
6. Hyperventilation—to Pa_{CO_2} 30–35 mmHg
7. Pressor therapy—phenylephrine, dopamine, or norepinephrine to maintain adequate MAP to ensure CPP > 70 mmHg (maintain euvolemia to minimize deleterious systemic effects of pressors)
8. Consider second-tier therapies for refractory elevated ICP
   a. High-dose barbiturate therapy ("pentobarb coma")
   b. Aggressive hyperventilation to Pa_{CO_2} < 30 mmHg
   c. Hemicraniectomy

[a] Throughout ICP treatment algorithm, consider repeat head CT to identify mass lesions amenable to surgical evacuation.
Note: CPP, cerebral perfusion pressure; MAP, mean arterial pressure; Pa_{CO_2}, arterial partial pressure of carbon dioxide.

age of CSF to reduce ICP is possible. Finally, high-dose barbiturates or hypothermia are sometimes used for refractory elevated ICP, although these have significant side effects and have not been shown to improve outcome.

Secondary Brain Insults   Patients with primary brain injuries, whether trauma or stroke, are at significant risk for ongoing secondary ischemic brain injury. Because secondary brain injury can be a major determinant of a poor outcome, strategies for minimizing secondary brain insults are an integral part of the critical care of all patients. While elevated ICP may lead to secondary ischemia, most secondary brain injury is mediated through other clinical events that exacerbate the ischemic cascade already initiated by the primary brain injury. Episodes of secondary brain insults are usually not associated with apparent neurologic worsening. Rather, they lead to cumulative injury, which manifests as higher mortality or worsened long-term functional outcome. Thus, clinical strategies involve close monitoring of vital signs and early intervention to prevent secondary ischemia. Avoiding hypotension and hypoxia is critical, as significant hypotensive events (systolic blood pressure < 90 mmHg) as short as 10 min in duration have been shown to adversely influence outcome after traumatic brain injury. Even in patients with stroke or head trauma who do not require ICP monitoring, close attention to adequate cerebral perfusion is warranted. Hypoxia (percutaneous oxygen saturation < 90%), alone or in combination with hypotension, also leads to secondary brain injury. Likewise, fever and hyperglycemia both worsen experimental ischemia and have been associated with worsened clinical outcome after stroke and head trauma. Aggressive control of fever with a goal of normothermia is warranted and can usually be achieved with antipyretic medications and cooling blankets. The use of intravenous insulin infusion is encouraged for control of hyperglycemia as this allows better regulation of serum glucose levels than subcutaneous insulin. A reasonable goal is to maintain the serum glucose level at <160 mg/dL, although some experts believe that even tighter control is appropriate. New cerebral monitoring tools that allow continuous evaluation of brain tissue oxygen tension, CBF, and metabolism (via microdialysis) may further improve the management of secondary brain injury.

CRITICAL CARE DISORDERS OF THE CENTRAL NERVOUS SYSTEM ASSOCIATED WITH SYSTEMIC DISEASE

HYPOXIC-ISCHEMIC ENCEPHALOPATHY   This occurs from lack of delivery of oxygen to the brain because of hypotension or respiratory failure. The most common causes are myocardial infarction, cardiac arrest, shock, asphyxiation, paralysis of respiration, and carbon monoxide or cyanide poisoning. In some circumstances, hypoxia may predominate. Carbon monoxide and cyanide poisoning are termed *histotoxic hypoxia* since they cause a direct impairment of the respiratory chain.

Clinical Manifestations   Mild degrees of pure hypoxia, such as occur at high altitudes, cause impaired judgment, inattentiveness, motor incoordination, and, at times, euphoria. However, with hypoxia-ischemia, such as occurs with circulatory arrest, consciousness is lost within seconds. If circulation is restored within 3 to 5 min, full recovery may occur, but if hypoxia-ischemia lasts beyond 3 to 5 min, some degree of permanent cerebral damage is the rule. Except in extreme cases, it may be difficult to judge the precise degree of hypoxia-ischemia, and some patients make a relatively full recovery after even 8 to 10 min of global cerebral ischemia. The distinction between pure hypoxia and hypoxia-ischemia is important, since a Pa_{O_2} as low as 20 mmHg (2.7 kPa) can be well tolerated if it develops gradually and normal blood pressure is maintained, but short durations of very low or absent cerebral circulation may result in permanent impairment.

Clinical examination at different time points after a hypoxic-ischemic insult (especially cardiac arrest) is useful in assessing prognosis

for long-term neurologic outcome. The prognosis is better for patients with intact brainstem function, as indicated by normal pupillary light responses and intact oculocephalic (doll's-eyes), oculovestibular (caloric), and corneal reflexes (Fig. 258-3). Absence of these reflexes and the presence of persistently dilated pupils that do not react to light are grave prognostic signs. A uniformly dismal prognosis from hypoxic-ischemic coma is conveyed by the clinical findings of absence of pupillary light reflex or absence of a motor response to pain on day 3 following the injury. Electrophysiologically, the finding of bilateral absence of the early cortical somatosensory evoked response (SSEPs) in the first week also conveys a poor prognosis. Whether administration of mild hypothermia after cardiac arrest (see "Treatment") will alter the usefulness of these clinical and electrophysiologic predictors is unknown. Long-term consequences of hypoxic-ischemic encepha-

FIGURE 258-3   Clinical examination at day 1 provides useful prognostic information in hypoxic-ischemic encephalopathy. Numbers in parentheses represent 95% confidence intervals. Recov, recovery; veg, vegetative; sev, severe; mod, moderate; spont eye movt, spontaneous eye movement; rov conj, roving conjugate. (*From DE Levy et al: JAMA 253:1420, 1985; with permission.*)

lopathy include persistent coma or vegetative state (Chap. 257), dementia, visual agnosia (Chap. 23), parkinsonism, choreoathetosis, cerebellar ataxia, myoclonus, seizures, and an amnestic state, which may be a consequence of selective damage to the hippocampus.

Pathologic Findings Principal histologic findings are extensive multifocal or diffuse laminar cortical necrosis (Fig. 258-4), with almost invariable involvement of the hippocampus. The hippocampal CA1 neurons (Fig. 350-1) are vulnerable to even brief episodes of hypoxia-ischemia, perhaps explaining why selective persistent memory deficits may occur after brief cardiac arrest. Scattered small areas of infarction or neuronal loss may be present in the basal ganglia, hypothalamus, or brainstem. In some cases, extensive bilateral thalamic scarring may affect pathways that mediate arousal, and this pathology may be responsible for the persistent vegetative state. A specific form of hypoxic-ischemic encephalopathy, so-called watershed infarcts, occurs at the distal territories between the major cerebral arteries and can cause cognitive deficits, including visual agnosia, and weakness that is greater in proximal than in distal muscle groups.

Diagnosis Diagnosis is based upon the history of a hypoxic-ischemic event such as cardiac arrest. Blood pressure <70 mmHg systolic or Pa_{O_2} < 40 mmHg is usually necessary, although both absolute levels as well as duration of exposure are important determinants of cellular injury. Occasionally the clinical and radiographic features of a hypoxic-ischemic syndrome are seen without documented profound hypotension or hypoxia. Carbon monoxide intoxication can be confirmed by measurement of carboxyhemoglobin and is suggested by a cherry red color of the skin, although the latter is an inconsistent clinical finding.

℞ TREATMENT

Treatment should be directed at restoration of normal cardiorespiratory function. This includes securing a clear airway, ensuring adequate oxygenation and ventilation, and restoring cerebral perfusion, whether by cardiopulmonary resuscitation, fluid, pressors, or cardiac pacing. Hypothermia may target the neuronal cell injury cascade and has substantial neuroprotective properties in experimental models of brain injury. In two recently reported clinical trials, mild hypothermia (33°C) improved functional outcome in patients who remained comatose after resuscitation from a cardiac arrest. Treatment was initiated within minutes of cardiac resuscitation and continued for 12 h in one study and 24 h in the other. Potential complications of hypothermia treatment include coagulopathy and an increased risk of infection.

Severe carbon monoxide intoxication may be treated with hyper-

FIGURE 258-4 Cortical laminar necrosis in hypoxic-ischemic encephalopathy. T1-weighted postcontrast magnetic resonance image shows cortical enhancement in a watershed distribution consistent with laminar necrosis.

baric oxygen. Anticonvulsants may be needed to control seizures, although these are not usually given prophylactically. Posthypoxic myoclonus may respond to oral administration of clonazepam at doses of 1.5 to 10 mg daily or valproate at doses of 300 mg to 1200 mg daily in divided doses. Myoclonic status epilepticus after a severe hypoxic-ischemic insult portends a universally poor prognosis, even if seizures are controlled.

DELAYED POSTANOXIC ENCEPHALOPATHY Delayed postanoxic encephalopathy is an uncommon phenomenon in which patients appear to make an initial recovery from hypoxic-ischemic insult but then develop a relapse characterized by apathy, confusion, and agitation. Progressive neurologic deficits may include shuffling gait, diffuse rigidity and spasticity, persistent parkinsonism or myoclonus, and, on occasion, coma and death after 1 to 2 weeks. Widespread cerebral demyelination may be present.

Carbon monoxide and cyanide intoxication can also cause a delayed encephalopathy. Little clinical impairment is evident when the patient first regains consciousness, but a parkinsonian syndrome characterized by akinesia and rigidity without tremor may develop. Symptoms can worsen over months, accompanied by increasing evidence of damage in the basal ganglia as seen on both CT and MRI.

METABOLIC ENCEPHALOPATHIES Altered mental states, variously described as confusion, delirium, disorientation, and encephalopathy, are present in many patients with severe illness in an intensive care unit (ICU). Older patients are particularly vulnerable to delirium, a confusional state characterized by disordered perception, frequent hallucinations, delusions, and sleep disturbance. This is often attributed to medication effects, sleep deprivation, pain, and anxiety. The term *ICU psychosis* has been used to describe a mental state with profound agitation occurring in this setting. The presence of family members in the ICU may help to calm and orient agitated patients, and in severe cases, low doses of neuroleptics (e.g., haloperidol 0.5 to 1 mg) can be useful. Ultimately, the psychosis resolves with improvement in the underlying illness and a return to familiar surroundings.

In the ICU setting, several metabolic causes of an altered level of consciousness predominate. Hypercarbic encephalopathy can present with headache, confusion, stupor, or coma. Hypoventilation syndrome occurs most frequently in patients with a history of chronic CO_2 retention who are receiving oxygen therapy for emphysema or chronic pulmonary disease (Chap. 246). The elevated Pa_{CO_2} leading to CO_2 narcosis may have a direct anesthetic effect, and cerebral vasodilation from increased Pa_{CO_2} can lead to increased ICP. Hepatic encephalopathy is suggested by asterixis and can occur in chronic liver failure or acute fulminant hepatic failure. Both hyperglycemia and hypoglycemia can cause encephalopathy, as can hypernatremia and hyponatremia. Confusion, impairment of eye movements, and gait ataxia are the hallmarks of acute Wernicke's disease (see below).

SEPTIC ENCEPHALOPATHY ■ Pathogenesis In patients with sepsis, the systemic response to infectious agents leads to the release of circulating inflammatory mediators that appear to contribute to encephalopathy. Critical illness, in association with the systemic inflammatory response syndrome (SIRS), can lead to multisystem organ failure. This syndrome can occur in the setting of apparent sepsis, severe burns, or trauma, even without clear identification of an infectious agent. Many patients with critical illness, sepsis, or SIRS develop encephalopathy without obvious explanation. This condition is broadly termed *septic encephalopathy*. While the specific mediators leading to neurologic dysfunction remain uncertain, it is clear that the encephalopathy is not simply the result of metabolic derangements of multiorgan failure. The cytokines tumor necrosis factor α, interleukin (IL) 1, IL-2, and IL-6 are thought to play a role in this syndrome.

Diagnosis Septic encephalopathy presents clinically as a diffuse dysfunction of the brain without prominent focal findings. Confusion, disorientation, agitation, and fluctuations in level of alertness are typical. In more profound cases, especially with hemodynamic compromise, the decrease in level of alertness can be more prominent, at times resulting in coma. Hyperreflexia and frontal release signs such as a grasp or snout reflex (Chap. 23) can be seen. Abnormal movements such as myoclonus, tremor, or asterixis can occur. Septic encephalopathy is quite common, occurring in the majority of patients with sepsis and multisystem organ failure. Diagnosis is often difficult because of the multiple potential causes of neurologic dysfunction in critically ill patients, and requires exclusion of structural, metabolic, toxic, and infectious (e.g., meningitis or encephalitis) causes. Although the mortality of patients with septic encephalopathy severe enough to produce coma approaches 50%, this reflects the severity of the underlying critical illness and is not a direct result of the septic encephalopathy. Neurologically, successful treatment of the underlying critical illness almost always results in complete resolution of the encephalopathy, without significant residua.

CENTRAL PONTINE MYELINOLYSIS This disorder typically presents in a devastating fashion as quadriplegia and pseudobulbar palsy. Predisposing factors include severe underlying medical illness or nutritional deficiency; most cases are associated with rapid correction of hyponatremia or with hyperosmolar states. The pathology consists of demyelination without inflammation in the base of the pons, with relative sparing of axons and nerve cells. MRI is useful in establishing the diagnosis (Fig. 258-5) and may also identify partial forms that present as confusion, dysarthria, and/or disturbances of conjugate gaze without quadriplegia. Therapeutic guidelines for the restoration of severe hyponatremia should aim for gradual correction, i.e., by ≤10 mmol/L (10 meq/L) within 24 h and 20 mmol/L (20 meq/L) within 48 h.

WERNICKE'S DISEASE Wernicke's disease is a common and preventable disorder due to a deficiency of thiamine (Chap. 61). In the United States, alcoholics account for most cases, but patients with malnutrition due to hyperemesis, starvation, renal dialysis, cancer, or AIDS are also at risk. The characteristic clinical triad is that of ophthalmoplegia, ataxia, and global confusion. However, only one-third of patients with acute Wernicke's disease present with the classic clinical triad. Most patients are profoundly disoriented, indifferent, and inattentive, although rarely they have an agitated delirium related to ethanol withdrawal. If the disease is not treated, stupor, coma, and death may ensue. Ocular motor abnormalities include horizontal nystagmus on lateral gaze, lateral rectus palsy (usually bilateral), conjugate gaze palsies, and rarely ptosis. Gait ataxia probably results from a combination of polyneuropathy, cerebellar involvement, and vestibular paresis. The pupils are usually spared, but they may become miotic with advanced disease.

Wernicke's disease is usually associated with other manifestations of nutritional disease, such as polyneuropathy. Rarely, amblyopia or myelopathy occurs. Tachycardia and postural hypotension may be related to impaired function of the autonomic nervous system or to the coexistence of cardiovascular beriberi. Patients who recover show improvement in ocular palsies within hours after the administration of thiamine, but horizontal nystagmus may persist. Ataxia improves more slowly than the ocular motor abnormalities. Approximately half recover incompletely and are left with a slow, shuffling, wide-based gait and an inability to tandem walk. Apathy, drowsiness, and confusion improve more gradually. As these symptoms recede, an amnestic state with impairment in recent memory and learning may become more apparent (*Korsakoff's psychosis*). Korsakoff's psychosis is frequently persistent; the residual mental state is characterized by gaps in memory, confabulation, and disordered temporal sequencing.

Pathology Lesions in the periventricular regions of the diencephalon, midbrain, and brainstem as well as the superior vermis of the cerebellum consist of symmetric discoloration of structures surrounding the third ventricle, aqueduct, and fourth ventricle, with petechial hemorrhages in occasional acute cases and atrophy of the mamillary bodies in most chronic cases. There is frequently endothelial proliferation,

FIGURE 258-5 Central pontine myelinolysis. Axial T2-weighted magnetic resonance scan through the pons reveals a symmetric area of abnormal high signal intensity within the basis pontis (*arrows*).

demyelination, and some neuronal loss. These changes may be detected by MRI scanning (Fig. 258-6). The amnestic defect is related to lesions in the dorsal medial nuclei of the thalamus.

Pathogenesis Thiamine is a cofactor of several enzymes, including transketolase, pyruvate dehydrogenase, and α-ketoglutarate dehydrogenase. Thiamine deficiency produces a diffuse decrease in cerebral glucose utilization and results in mitochondrial damage. Glutamate accumulates owing to impairment of α-ketoglutarate dehydrogenase activity and, in combination with the energy deficiency, may result in excitotoxic cell damage.

℞ **TREATMENT**

Wernicke's disease is a medical emergency and requires immediate administration of thiamine, in a dose of 100 mg either intravenously or intramuscularly. The dose should be given daily until the patient resumes a normal diet and should be begun prior to treatment with intravenous glucose solutions. Glucose infusions may precipitate Wernicke's disease in a previously unaffected patient or cause a rapid worsening of an early form of the disease. For this reason, thiamine should be administered to all alcoholic patients requiring parenteral glucose.

CRITICAL CARE DISORDERS OF THE PERIPHERAL NERVOUS SYSTEM ASSOCIATED WITH SYSTEMIC DISEASE

Critical illness with disorders of the peripheral nervous system (PNS) arises in two contexts: (1) primary neurologic diseases that require critical care interventions such as intubation and mechanical ventilation, and (2) secondary PNS manifestations of systemic critical illness, often involving multisystem organ failure. The former include acute polyneuropathies such as Guillain-Barré syndrome (Chap. 365), neuromuscular junction disorders including myasthenia gravis (Chap.

FIGURE 258-6 Wernicke's disease. Coronal T1-weighted postcontrast magnetic resonance image reveals abnormal enhancement of the mammillary bodies (*arrows*), typical of acute Wernicke's encephalopathy.

366) and botulism (Chap. 125), and primary muscle disorders such as polymyositis (Chap. 369). The latter result either from the systemic disease itself or as a consequence of interventions.

General principles of respiratory evaluation in patients with PNS involvement, regardless of cause, include assessment of pulmonary mechanics, such as maximal inspiratory force (MIF) and vital capacity (VC), and evaluation of strength of bulbar muscles. Regardless of the cause of weakness, endotracheal intubation should be considered when the MIF falls to < -25 cmH$_2$O or the VC is <1 L. Also, patients with severe palatal weakness may require endotracheal intubation in order to prevent acute upper airway obstruction or recurrent aspiration. Arterial blood gases and percutaneous oxygen saturation are used to follow patients with potential respiratory compromise from PNS dysfunction. However, intubation and mechanical ventilation should be undertaken based on clinical assessment rather than waiting until oxygen saturation drops or CO$_2$ retention develops from hypoventilation. →*Principles of mechanical ventilation are discussed in Chap. 252.*

NEUROPATHY   While encephalopathy may be the most obvious neurologic dysfunction in critically ill patients, dysfunction of the PNS is also quite common. It is typically present in patients with prolonged critical illnesses lasting several weeks and involving sepsis; clinical suspicion is aroused when there is failure to wean from mechanical ventilation despite improvement of the underlying sepsis and critical illness. *Critical illness polyneuropathy* refers to the most common PNS complication related to critical illness; it is seen in the setting of prolonged critical illness, sepsis, and multisystem organ failure. Neurologic findings include diffuse weakness, decreased reflexes, and distal sensory loss. Electrophysiologic studies demonstrate a diffuse, symmetric, distal axonal sensorimotor neuropathy, and pathologic studies have confirmed axonal degeneration. The precise mechanism of critical illness polyneuropathy remains unclear, but circulating factors such as cytokines, which are associated with sepsis and SIRS, are thought to play a role. It has been reported that up to 70% of patients with the sepsis syndrome have some degree of neuropathy, although far fewer have a clinical syndrome profound enough to cause severe respiratory muscle weakness requiring prolonged mechanical ventilation or resulting in failure to wean. Treatment is supportive, with specific intervention directed at treating the underlying illness. While spontaneous recovery is usually seen, the time course may extend over weeks to months and necessitate long-term ventilatory support and care even after the underlying critical illness has resolved.

DISORDERS OF NEUROMUSCULAR TRANSMISSION   A defect in neuromuscular transmission may be a source of weakness in critically ill patients. Myasthenia gravis may be a consideration; however, persistent weakness secondary to impaired neuromuscular junction transmission is almost always due to administration of drugs. A number of medications impair neuromuscular transmission; these include antibiotics, especially aminoglycosides, and beta-blocking agents. In the ICU, the nondepolarizing neuromuscular blocking agents (nd-NMBAs), also known as muscle relaxants, are most commonly responsible. Included in this group of drugs are such agents as pancuronium, vecuronium, rocuronium, and atracurium. They are often used to facilitate mechanical ventilation or other critical care procedures, but with prolonged use persistent neuromuscular blockade may result in weakness even after discontinuation of these agents hours or days earlier. Risk factors for this prolonged action of neuromuscular blocking agents include female sex, metabolic acidosis, and renal failure.

Prolonged neuromuscular blockade does not appear to produce permanent damage to the PNS. Once the offending medications are discontinued, full strength is restored, although this may take days. In general, the lowest dose of neuromuscular blocking agent should be used to achieve the desired result, and, when these agents are used in the ICU, a peripheral nerve stimulator should be used to monitor neuromuscular junction function.

MYOPATHY   Critically ill patients, especially those with sepsis, frequently develop muscle wasting, often in the face of seemingly adequate nutritional support. The assumption has been that this represents a catabolic myopathy brought about as a result of multiple factors, including elevated cortisol and catecholamine release and other circulating factors induced by the SIRS. In this syndrome, known as *cachectic myopathy*, serum creatine kinase levels and electromyography (EMG) are normal. Muscle biopsy shows type II fiber atrophy. Panfascicular muscle fiber necrosis may also occur in the setting of profound sepsis. This so-called *septic myopathy* is characterized clinically by weakness progressing to a profound level over just a few days. There may be associated elevations in serum creatine kinase and urine myoglobin. Both EMG and muscle biopsy may be normal initially but eventually show abnormal spontaneous activity and panfascicular necrosis with an accompanying inflammatory reaction.

Acute quadriplegic myopathy describes a clinical syndrome of severe weakness seen in the setting of glucocorticoid and nd-NMBA use. The most frequent scenario in which this is encountered is the asthmatic patient who requires high-dose glucocorticoids and nd-NMBA to facilitate mechanical ventilation. This muscle disorder is not due to prolonged action of nd-NMBAs at the neuromuscular junction but, rather, is an actual myopathy with muscle damage; it has occasionally been described with high-dose glucocorticoid use alone. Clinically this syndrome is most often recognized when a patient fails to wean from mechanical ventilation despite resolution of the primary pulmonary process. Pathologically, there may be vacuolar changes in both type I and type II muscle fibers with evidence of regeneration. Acute quadriplegic myopathy has a good prognosis. If patients survive their underlying critical illness, the myopathy invariably improves and patients usually return to normal. However, because this syndrome is a result of true muscle damage, not just prolonged blockade at the neuromuscular junction, this process may take weeks or months, and tracheostomy with prolonged ventilatory support may be necessary. At present, it is unclear how to prevent this myopathic complication, except by avoiding use of nd-NMBAs, a strategy not always possible. Monitoring with a peripheral nerve stimulator can help to avoid the overuse of these agents. However, this is more likely to prevent the complication of prolonged neuromuscular junction blockade than it is to prevent this myopathy.

FURTHER READING

THE HYPOTHERMIA AFTER CARDIAC ARREST STUDY GROUP: Mild therapeutic hypothermia to improve the neurologic outcome after cardiac arrest. N Engl J Med 346:549, 2002

LIOU AK et al: To die or not to die for neurons in ischemia, traumatic brain injury and epilepsy: A review on the stress-activated signaling pathways and apoptotic pathways. Prog Neurobiol 69:103, 2003

VAN MOOK WN and HULSEWE-EVERS RP: Critical illness polyneuropathy. Curr Opin Crit Care 8:302, 2002

259 | ADAPTATION TO RENAL INJURY
Robert M. Brenner, Barry M. Brenner

Near constancy of the internal environment, including the volume, composition, and compartmental distribution of the body fluids, is essential to survival. With normal day-to-day variations in the intake of food and water, preservation of the internal environment requires the excretion in amounts that balance the quantities ingested. While losses from intestines, lungs, and skin contribute, the greatest responsibility for solute and water excretion is borne by the kidneys. This chapter reviews the excretory functions of the kidney and examines how these functions are affected by chronic renal disease.

EFFECTS OF NEPHRON LOSS ON RENAL EXCRETORY MECHANISMS

GLOMERULAR ULTRAFILTRATION Urine production begins at the glomerulus where an ultrafiltrate of plasma is formed. The rate of glomerular ultrafiltration (glomerular filtration rate, GFR) is governed chiefly by forces favoring filtration on the one hand (hydraulic pressure in the glomerular capillaries) and forces opposing filtration on the other (the sum of hydraulic pressure in Bowman's space and colloid osmotic pressure of blood in the glomerular capillaries). The rate of glomerular plasma flow and the total surface area of the glomerular capillaries are also determinants of GFR. Decreased GFR can therefore be expected when (1) glomerular hydraulic pressure is reduced (as in circulatory shock); (2) tubule (hence Bowman's space) hydraulic pressure is elevated, as in urinary tract obstruction; (3) plasma colloid osmotic pressure rises to high levels (hemoconcentration due to severe volume depletion, or myeloma, other dysproteinemias); (4) renal, and hence glomerular, blood flow is reduced (severe hypovolemia, cardiac failure); (5) permeability is reduced (diffuse glomerular disease); or (6) filtration surface area is diminished, through nephron loss in progressive renal failure.

The glomerular capillary wall is specially adapted to allow passage of extremely large volumes of water while retaining all but the smallest solute molecules. Molecules the size of inulin (approximately 5200 mol wt) pass freely across the glomerular filtration barrier, appearing at approximately the same concentration in Bowman's space as in plasma. The passage of solutes across the glomerular barrier decreases progressively with increasing molecular size such that, as the molecular weight of albumin is approached, most of the solute is retained in the plasma. Albumin, a polyanionic molecule in plasma, is further retarded at the glomerular filtration barrier by *electrostatic forces* imparted by negatively charged cell-surface molecules on the epithelial foot processes that form the *filtration slits* and the *slit diaphragms*. With disruption of these structural and electrostatic barriers, as in many forms of glomerular injury (Chap. 264), large quantities of plasma proteins gain access to the glomerular filtrate.

GLOMERULAR ADAPTATIONS TO NEPHRON LOSS With loss of nephron mass, the remaining functional (or least injured) nephrons tend to hypertrophy and take on an increased workload so that the overall loss of function is minimized. For example, a patient with a unilateral nephrectomy loses one-half of the nephron mass, resulting in a 50% reduction in GFR at the time of surgery. However, within several months total GFR may rise to 80% of the preoperative value. This indicates that the GFR of the individual remaining nephrons has increased above normal, a state known as *hyperfiltration*. Increases in single-nephron GFR may be achieved by renal hemodynamic adjustments (increased glomerular plasma flow and increased glomerular capillary hydraulic pressure), which augment the forces driving ultra-

filtration, and by glomerular hypertrophy, which increases the maximum surface area available for filtration. These structural adaptations are evident from the enlargement of glomeruli (and tubules) seen on histologic sections from persons with single kidneys. Similar structural changes are observed in kidneys damaged by chronic disease processes; foci of hypertrophied glomeruli and tubules are interspersed with areas of atrophic or scarred parenchyma. Although direct measurements of single-nephron GFR cannot be made in humans, it is reasonable to conclude that focal nephron enlargement as occurs in chronically diseased kidneys generally signifies focally increased single-nephron GFR, and that these dynamic adaptations represent compensatory adjustments for the effects of nephron loss through disease.

GLOMERULOTUBULAR BALANCE The close integration of glomerular and tubular functions (*glomerulotubular balance*) seen in chronic renal failure (CRF) supports the notion that progressive nephron obliteration is the usual mode of GFR reduction in CRF. Preservation of glomerulotubular balance until the terminal stages of CRF is fundamental to the *intact-nephron hypothesis*, which states that as CRF advances, kidney function is supported by a diminishing pool of functioning (or hyperfunctioning) nephrons, rather than relatively constant numbers of nephrons, each with diminishing function. This hypothesis has important implications for the mechanisms of disease progression in CRF. A considerable amount of evidence suggests that nephrons subjected to increased excretory burdens for prolonged periods actually sustain injury as a result of these adaptations: thus the cost of these compensatory adaptations to nephron loss may ultimately be relentless destruction of the remaining nephron pool.

The magnitude of the single-nephron hyperfiltration induced by loss of 50% of the total nephron mass usually has no serious adverse clinical consequences, even when sustained over two to three decades. When more than 50% of the total nephron mass is lost, however, as in renal-sparing surgery for bilateral trauma or neoplasm or from a renal disease whose activity has abated, the remaining nephrons are forced to the limits of their compensatory capacity. While these adaptations achieve remarkable short-term success at offsetting the tendency for GFR to fall, over time, proteinuria and focal and segmental glomerulosclerosis develop, the more so where greater amounts of nephrons are lost or removed. As a result, a progressive decline in GFR ensues. Experimental study of the processes that advance glomerular injury show that the adverse long-term consequences of severe nephron deficits are invariably preceded by increases in glomerular capillary hydraulic pressure (glomerular capillary hypertension), glomerular hyperperfusion, and hypertrophy. Interventions directed against these compensatory and maladaptive responses can greatly ameliorate the subsequent development of renal failure. In particular, drugs (e.g., angiotensin-converting enzyme inhibitors and angiotensin II receptor blockers) and other interventions (such as dietary protein restriction) that lower glomerular pressure can slow the rate of progression of experimental and human renal disease. In the absence of such interventions, more and more glomeruli cease to function through advancing glomerulosclerosis and disruption of tubule structure and function, leading eventually to marked or even total loss of GFR (i.e., end-stage renal disease). This *final common pathway* for chronic renal injury helps to explain the observed progressive nature of chronic renal failure resulting from many different kidney diseases.

BIOLOGIC CONSEQUENCES OF SUSTAINED REDUCTIONS IN GFR

Figure 259-1 depicts the major types of response to impaired GFR. The degree of reduction in total GFR is plotted on the abscissa, expressed as a percentage of normal (100%). The renal handling of most solutes normally present in glomerular filtrate conforms to one of three

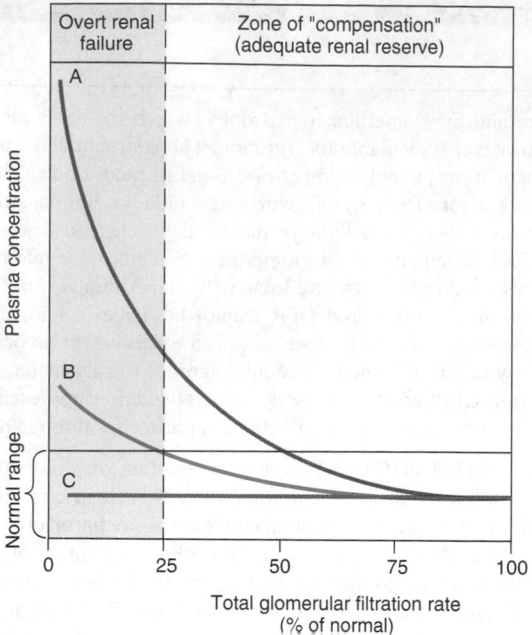

FIGURE 259-1   Representative patterns of adaptation for different types of solutes in body fluids in chronic renal failure. [*After NS Bricker et al, in BM Brenner (ed): Brenner and Rector's The Kidney, 6th ed. Philadelphia, Saunders, 2000.*]

patterns. Curve *A* describes the pattern with substances such as creatinine and urea that normally depend largely on glomerular filtration for urinary excretion, i.e., secretion contributes little to overall excretion. Therefore, as illustrated, gradual reductions in GFR are accompanied by progressive increases in plasma levels of creatinine, urea, and other substances normally excreted primarily by filtration.

The clinical course of CRF usually also approximates the pattern described by curve *A*. Patients with CRF usually pass from a long asymptomatic period of "compensation" to a more accelerated and clinically overt terminal phase. In other words, despite chronic injury leading to destruction of more than 50% of nephrons, plasma elevations of creatinine and urea may still lie within the normal limits for these substances. With further nephron loss and reduction in GFR, however, the limits of renal reserve are exceeded and continued accumulations of curve *A*–type solutes lead to abnormally elevated plasma concentrations (Fig. 259-1). Because some of these retained solutes are thought to exert "toxic" effects on all organ systems, clinical manifestations of CRF may now become apparent.

The accumulation of curve *A*–type solutes with chronic loss of renal function proceeds until external balance is restored, i.e., intake and/or production rates exactly match excretion rates. In the case of creatinine, for example, assuming a constant rate of creatinine production, a 50% reduction in GFR results in an approximate doubling of the plasma creatinine concentration. The latter restores the filtered load of creatinine (i.e., the product of GFR and plasma creatinine concentration) to normal, and the urinary excretion rate once again is equivalent to creatinine production. *In practice, so long as the net rates of acquisition and production (i.e., liver function and muscle mass) remain reasonably constant, the inverse relationship between plasma concentrations of solutes such as creatinine and urea and GFR is sufficiently reliable to serve as clinical indices of GFR.* However, where muscle mass is low, as with severe weight loss, even normal plasma levels of creatinine may belie substantial reductions in GFR.

In contrast to solutes of the curve *A* type, plasma levels of phosphate (PO_4^{3-}), urate, and potassium (K^+) and hydrogen (H^+) ions usually do not rise until the GFR falls to a small percentage of normal. With progressive renal failure this pattern of response (curve *B* in Fig. 259-1) reflects the participation of tubule transport mechanisms in the excretion of these substances. In other words, *as GFR declines, the*

tubules facilitate greater elimination of these substances, by enhancing secretion and/or by diminishing reabsorption, so that a greater fraction of the filtered load is excreted. Plasma levels of curve *B*–type solutes, therefore, rise less than those of curve *A* because, with progressive reductions in GFR, *excretion rate per nephron* and therefore *fractional excretion* both increase. Eventually, however, with further loss of GFR, enhanced fractional excretion can no longer mitigate the reduction in net filtered load of these solutes and plasma levels rise (Fig. 259-1). For urate, PO_4^{3-}, and K^+, at least, increased fractional excretion serves to maintain normal plasma levels until GFR falls to less than one-fourth of normal.

Finally, for certain solutes, such as sodium chloride (NaCl), plasma concentrations remain normal throughout the course of CRF, despite unrestricted intake of these substances (curve *C* in Fig. 259-1). The compensatory mechanism required to achieve this represents a fundamental adaptation to chronic renal injury. To illustrate the magnitude of this adaptation, it is useful to compare the excretion of sodium (Na^+) in a normal individual (GFR of 125 mL/min) with that of a patient with advanced renal failure (GFR of 2 mL/min). Both individuals consume a conventional diet containing 7 g/d of salt (120 mmol Na^+). With a serum Na^+ concentration of 140 mmol/L, external Na^+ balance is achieved in the normal subject by excreting approximately 0.5% of the filtered load. By contrast, for external balance to be maintained in the patient with CRF, fractional excretion of Na^+ must rise to 30%. In other words, *to maintain external Na^+ balance*, the same amount of Na^+ must be excreted into the urine each day in the patient with CRF as in the normal individual. Given the drastic reduction in GFR in CRF, external balance can only be maintained by marked adaptations in the reabsorptive processes in surviving tubules. In this manner, a progressively larger fraction of the filtered load escapes reabsorption and appears in the final urine.

ADAPTATIONS IN TUBULE TRANSPORT MECHANISMS IN RESPONSE TO NEPHRON LOSS

Despite progressive nephron loss, many mechanisms that regulate renal solute and water balance differ only quantitatively, and not qualitatively, from those that operate normally. Thus, glomerulotubular balance is maintained. The most important of these mechanisms are considered below.

TUBULAR TRANSPORT OF SODIUM CHLORIDE AND WATER   Most of the filtered water and sodium salts are reabsorbed by the tubules, leaving small and variable amounts, equivalent on average to the quantities ingested, to reach the final urine. About two-thirds of the glomerular ultrafiltrate is reabsorbed in the *proximal tubule* with little change in the osmolality or Na^+ concentration of the unreabsorbed fraction (Fig. 259-2). In other words, fluid reabsorption in the proximal tubule is nearly *isosmotic* and is coupled to the active transport of Na^+. Since chloride (Cl^-) and bicarbonate (HCO_3^-) are the primary anions in the extracellular fluid, they constitute the main solutes that accompany Na^+ reabsorption in the renal tubules. In the earliest portion of the proximal tubule, bicarbonate is the principal anion that accompanies the reabsorption of Na^+. This process occurs via a Na^+/H^+ exchanger at the luminal brush border and is dependent on the activity of carbonic anhydrase. Glucose, amino acids, and other organic solutes (e.g., lactate) are also extensively reabsorbed in the proximal tubule by cotransport mechanisms that link the cellular entry of these organic molecules with Na^+.

The coupling of water absorption (i.e., volume) with solute absorption appears to be dependent upon three processes. First, given the remarkably high water permeability of this segment, very small transepithelial osmolality differences, i.e., *luminal hypotonicity* of the order of 2 to 3 mosmol/L produced by solute absorption, could drive water absorption. Second, due to preferential absorption of HCO_3^- and organic solutes in the early portions of the proximal tubule, the concentrations of these substances decrease along the proximal tubule while that of chloride increases. Volume reabsorption would then occur if the diffusion of Na^+ and Cl^- down their respective electrochemical gradients across the proximal tubule epithelium occurred more easily than the back-diffusion of sodium bicarbonate into the lumen, creating an *effective osmotic pressure gradient*. Finally, *lateral interstitial space hypertonicity* produced by differences in the rates at which solutes are transported into the spaces or exit them by diffusion may also contribute to the coupling of water and solute reabsorption.

Reabsorption of Fluid from Proximal Convoluted Tubules This is sensitive to *Starling forces*, i.e., the hydraulic and colloid osmotic (or oncotic) pressures acting across the walls of the peritubular capillaries. Because the plasma proteins in glomerular capillaries are concentrated by ultrafiltration, oncotic pressure rises along the glomerular capillary network. This step-up in oncotic pressure is transmitted largely unchanged to the first branches of the peritubular capillaries via the efferent arterioles. These resistance vessels cause a substantial drop in hydraulic pressure, however, so that when the plasma reaches the peritubular capillaries, oncotic pressure greatly exceeds hydraulic pressure. The Starling forces are therefore oriented in an *uptake* mode, in contrast to their configuration at the glomerulus where hydraulic pressure exceeds oncotic pressure, favoring *filtration*. The extent to which oncotic pressure exceeds hydraulic pressure in the peritubular capillary network modulates the overall rate of fluid absorption by the peritubular capillaries. Therefore, when peritubular capillary oncotic pressure falls, or hydraulic pressure rises, uptake of fluid by these capillaries is reduced. As a result, fluid is retained in the interstitial space, tending to increase hydraulic pressure, ultimately retarding the egress of fluid from the lateral intercellular channels.

Without an adequate route of drainage, fluid in the intercellular channels leaks back into the tubule lumen, thereby *diminishing net fluid reabsorption* from this tubule segment. The opposite occurs in states where peritubular oncotic pressure is increased (increased filtration fraction) or hydraulic pressure is decreased (enhanced efferent arteriolar tone). Under these circumstances, peritubular capillary uptake of reabsorbate is augmented, leading ultimately to *enhanced net fluid reabsorption* by the proximal tubule. Although physical factors appear to be the major determinants of fluid reabsorption in the proximal tubule, hormones (e.g., angiotensin II) may also modulate fluid reabsorption directly, by enhancing luminal Na^+ entry into proximal tubule cells via an apical Na^+/H^+ exchanger.

The Limbs of Henle's Loop In contrast to the proximal tubule, active outward transport of Na^+ has not been established for the *thin descending or ascending limbs of Henle's loop*. However, passive outward salt transport does occur, as indicated in Fig. 259-2. In the next nephron segment, the *medullary thick ascending limb of Henle*, the concentration of NaCl is reduced as fluid traverses this segment. Here Cl^- absorption occurs by an active process involving a $Na^+:K^+:2Cl^-$ cotransport mechanism in the luminal membrane, with one-half of Na^+ absorption pro-

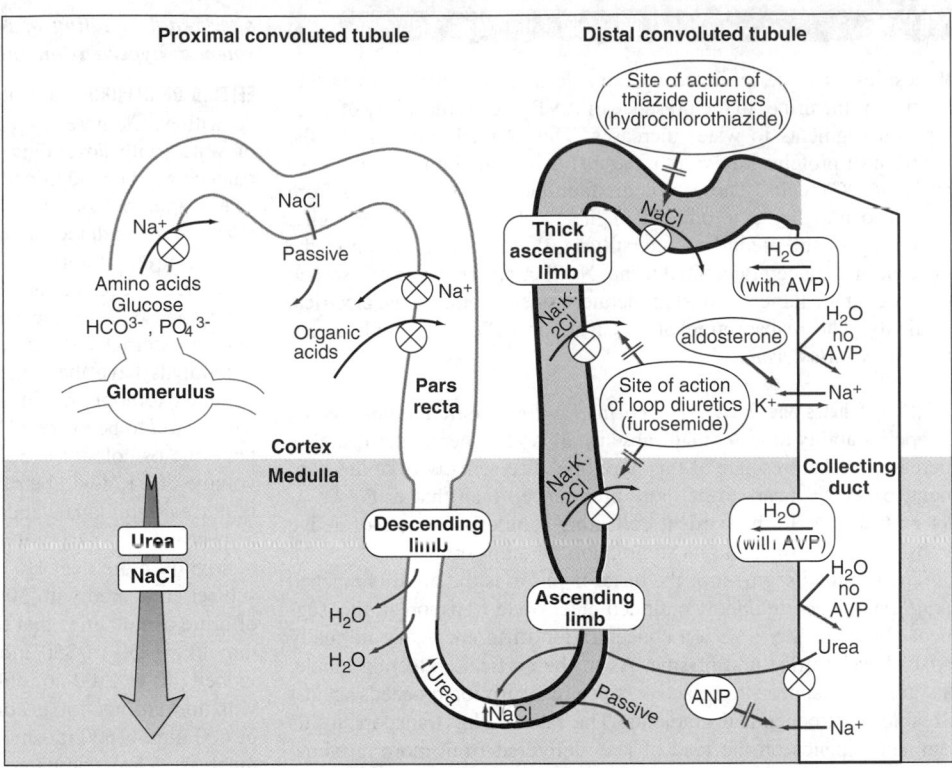

FIGURE 259-2 Transport functions of the various anatomic segments of the mammalian nephron. Fluid reabsorption across the proximal tubule is isosmotic and accounts for reabsorption of approximately two-thirds of the filtered Na^+ and H_2O. The major portions of the filtered HCO_3^-, amino acids, glucose, and phosphate are reabsorbed in the early proximal convoluted tubule. Reabsorption of glucose and amino acids is coupled to Na^+ transport and thereby generates a negative potential difference within the tubule lumen. At the same time, HCO_3^- is reabsorbed by a nonelectrogenic mechanism, via H^+ secretion. The active transport of these solutes results in transepithelial concentration and effective osmotic pressure gradients promoting H_2O flow across the proximal tubule, into the peritubular capillaries. The rise in tubule fluid Cl^- concentration is a necessary reciprocal consequence of the decreased luminal HCO_3^- concentration. The resultant high concentration of Cl^- becomes an important force for the outward passive transport of Cl^- down its concentration gradient, resulting in a lumen-positive potential difference in the late proximal convoluted tubule.

The pars recta of the proximal tubule is capable of active electrogenic transport of Na^+ independent of organic solute transport. Under normal conditions, approximately one-third of the glomerular filtrate enters the descending limb of Henle's loop. This segment is incapable of active outward NaCl transport and is characterized by low permeability to Na^+ but high H_2O permeability. H_2O is abstracted passively as the fluid approaches the bend of Henle's loop. Hypertonic fluid with a greater NaCl concentration but lower urea concentration than the surrounding medullary interstitium thus enters the thin ascending limb of Henle, which is largely impermeable to H_2O and urea but highly permeable to NaCl. This permits passive outward diffusion of NaCl. Active $Na:K:2Cl$ transport across the water-impermeable thick ascending limb of Henle enables tubule fluid to become dilute and the medullary interstitium hypertonic.

Irrespective of the final osmolality of the urine, the fluid that enters the distal convoluted tubule (DCT) is always hypoosmotic. This segment exhibits active Na^+ reabsorption. All but the terminal portion of the DCT is water-impermeable, even in the presence of arginine vasopressin (AVP). Aldosterone exerts its effect in this segment by enhancing Na^+ reabsorption, which is variably coupled to K^+ and H^+ secretion. The cortical and papillary portions of the collecting duct are sites where AVP exerts its principal effect. The permeability of these segments to H_2O in the absence of AVP is very low but can be greatly enhanced in the presence of AVP. These segments are also characterized by active Na^+ reabsorption, which appears to depend on the presence of mineralocorticoid. In the absence of AVP, the collecting tubule is water-impermeable so that hypotonic tubule fluid courses through it. However, in the presence of AVP, water is avidly reabsorbed here, resulting in hypertonic final urine. Sites of action of furosemide and thiazide diuretics and of aldosterone and atrial natriuretic peptide (ANP) are shown.

ceeding passively, driven by the lumen positive transepithelial voltage difference. This cotransporter is the site of action of the powerful loop diuretics, and mutations give rise to Bartter's syndrome. Since the ascending limb of Henle is impermeable to water, net NaCl reabsorption generates a hypotonic tubule fluid and gives rise to the high NaCl concentration of the outer medullary interstitium (Fig. 259-2).

Distal Tubule The fluid leaving the thick ascending limb of Henle is normally of low NaCl concentration, a characteristic independent of the organism's hydration status. In the *distal tubule*, water reabsorption is variable, depending on the state of hydration or, specifically, on the presence or absence of arginine vasopressin (AVP) in plasma. In the absence of AVP, this and more distal nephron segments are impermeable to water, so that hypotonic fluid entering this segment is excreted as *dilute urine*. Indeed, continued salt reabsorption along the distal convoluted tubule (DCT) and connecting tubule segments, a process that can be inhibited by thiazide diuretics, results in further dilution of the urine. In the presence of AVP, the permeability of these nephron segments to water increases. This is made possible by the insertion of proteins known as *aquaporins* into the luminal cell membrane of DCT cells. These proteins facilitate water movement from the low-osmolality environment of the DCT lumen into the higher osmolality of the medullary interstitium, thereby contributing to the creation of a concentrated final urine. NaCl continues to be reabsorbed from the tubule lumen against moderately steep chemical and electrical gradients. The reabsorption of NaCl at the collecting tubule is enhanced by *aldosterone.*

Collecting Tubules and Ducts The *cortical collecting tubule* possesses a low permeability to water in the absence of AVP, whereas permeability increases in the presence of this hormone. The sensitivity of this segment to AVP appears to be more pronounced than that of the DCT. As with the DCT, the cortical collecting tubule is capable of active reabsorption of NaCl and its stimulation by aldosterone.

The terminal segment of the distal nephron is the highly branched *papillary collecting duct.* Continued electrolyte transport in this segment results in the large ion concentration differences that normally exist between urine and plasma. As in the cortical collecting tubule, Na^+ transport appears to be active, since reabsorption proceeds against sizeable electrochemical gradients. The rate of Na^+ transport in this segment depends on the load of Na^+ delivered from more proximal segments and is also affected by aldosterone. The permeability to water is also increased markedly in the presence of AVP.

EFFECTS OF NEPHRON LOSS ON SODIUM CHLORIDE TRANSPORT IN SURVIVING NEPHRONS With progressive nephron loss, *maintenance of external balance for NaCl requires that fractional salt excretion increases in concert with the decline in GFR.* Several mechanisms contribute to this adaptive increase in fractional Na^+ excretion. With loss of functioning nephrons, peritubular capillary Starling forces are altered in directions that serve to reduce proximal tubule reabsorption of NaCl and water. For example, a rise in peritubular capillary hydraulic pressure, which tends to inhibit net proximal fluid reabsorption, might be anticipated with systemic hypertension, a common feature of CRF. Similarly, reductions in peritubular capillary oncotic pressures may be anticipated due to reductions in both filtration fraction and hypoalbuminemia.

Several factors that regulate NaCl transport across tubules under normal conditions are also likely to contribute to the enhanced fractional excretion of NaCl in renal insufficiency. Atrial natriuretic peptides are released from the heart in response to elevated cardiac (atrial) filling pressures as seen with increased plasma volume or atrial tachyarrhythmias. These peptides affect natriuresis by reducing net Na^+ reabsorption through complementary actions on Na^+ transport in the collecting duct and by altering Starling forces in the adjacent vasa recta. Other modulators of tubule transport processes may also contribute to increased single-nephron natriuresis in the setting of nephron loss. Vasodilator prostaglandins are present at increased plasma levels in CRF, as are other inhibitors of transport, including inhibitor(s) of the Na^+,K^+-ATPase. Serum and urine from patients with uremia contain retained toxins capable of inhibiting this enzyme.

The obligatory high rate of solute excretion per surviving nephron (so-called osmotic diuresis due to urea and other retained solutes) also contributes to enhancing fractional NaCl excretion, much as occurs in normal individuals after the administration of mannitol or other nonreabsorbable solutes. Finally, certain forms of CRF are associated with unusually large losses of salt in the urine. These *salt-wasting nephropathies* include chronic pyelonephritis and other tubulointerstitial diseases (Chap. 266) as well as polycystic and medullary cystic diseases. These disorders have in common greater destruction of medullary and tubulointerstitial, rather than cortical and glomerular, portions of the renal parenchyma. →*For discussion of clinical derangements that alter renal handling of NaCl in CRF (including hypo- and hypervolemia, hypertension, etc.), see Chap. 261.*

EFFECTS OF NEPHRON LOSS ON WATER REABSORPTION IN SURVIVING NEPHRONS As with NaCl, there is a progressive increase in the fractional excretion of water with advancing renal insufficiency, so that external water balance can be maintained even with a total GFR of 5 mL/min or less. The adaptations of water handling by the diseased kidney are of importance in the defects in urinary concentration and dilution and hence the polyuria, nocturia, and tendency to develop water retention encountered in CRF (Chap. 40). To appreciate the mechanisms involved, the responses of a normal individual and a patient with CRF maintaining external water balance need to be considered. Assuming both individuals have the same dietary and fluid intakes, total solute and volume excretion in both should be identical as well. If the *obligatory solute load* to be excreted by each is 600 mmol/d (600 mosmol/d) and the urine osmolality is 300 mmol/kg water (300 mosmol/kg), a urine volume of 2 L/d will be required to excrete the total solute. If the GFR in normal individuals and the patient with CRF totals 180 and 4 L/d, respectively, urinary volume excretion of 2 L/d represents excretion of slightly more than 1% of the total glomerular filtrate in the normal subject compared with 50% in the patient with CRF. Since the range of urine osmolalities that the diseased kidney can achieve [250 to 350 mmol/kg (250 to 350 mosmol/kg)] is narrower than in the normal kidney [40 to 1200 mmol/kg (40 to 1200 mosmol/kg)], the individual with normal function is able to excrete the obligatory daily solute load of 600 mmol (600 mosmol) in as little as 500 mL urine per day or as much as 15 L/d, compared with the narrower range in CRF, from about 1.7 to 2.4 L/d.

In CRF, the limited capacity to concentrate the urine often correlates with other measures of impaired renal function. Isosthenuria (urine of similar osmolality to plasma) is therefore an almost universal finding when the GFR falls below 25 mL/min. At this level of GFR and below, urine osmolality does not rise even when supraphysiologic doses of AVP are administered, suggesting that the concentrating defect relates to impaired concentrating capacity in surviving nephrons. The associated increased fractional excretion per nephron of a variety of solutes produces an obligatory water loss (solute diuresis) at roughly isotonic proportions. Consequently, formation of a concentrated urine is prevented. Disease-induced abnormalities of the architecture of the renal medulla (loops of Henle, vasa recta), aberrations in medullary blood flow, and defective transport of NaCl in the ascending limb of Henle also contribute to this defect in urine concentration.

Since patients with CRF are unable to excrete concentrated or dilute urine, they must have access to adequate, and to some extent, relatively constant amounts of water per day to ensure that they have adequate water to eliminate total daily solute loads. For this reason, restriction of fluid intake may be hazardous in patients with CRF. Likewise, impairment of diluting capacity may prevent many patients from excreting excess ingested fluid. →*For discussion of the consequences of the abnormal patterns of water excretion, and the attendant susceptibilities to develop hypo- and hypernatremia, see Chaps. 41 and 261.*

TUBULE TRANSPORT OF PHOSPHATE WITH NORMAL AND REDUCED NEPHRON MASS Under normal physiologic conditions, about 80 to 90% of phosphate is reabsorbed, mainly in the proximal tubule. *Parathyroid hormone* (PTH), by augmenting phosphate excretion via inhibition of this proximal reabsorptive process (Chap. 331), plays a central role in phosphate homeostasis. When dietary phosphate intake increases, a *transient* rise in plasma phosphate concentration is usually observed. This results in a similarly transient reduction in the plasma ionized calcium level (due largely to deposition of calcium phosphate in bone), which is sensed by a specific receptor on parathyroid cells, stimulating PTH secretion. By enhancing fractional phosphate excretion, PTH restores external phosphate balance and normophosphatemia. This enables plasma ionized calcium and hence phosphate levels to return to normal, thereby removing the stimulus to PTH release.

With advancing renal failure and constant dietary intake of phosphate, external phosphate balance is achieved by progressive reduction in fractional phosphate reabsorption. Enhanced PTH secretion is an important determinant of this phosphaturic response. With succeeding decrements in total GFR, the amount of phosphate filtered by surviving glomeruli is reduced, leading to transient phosphate retention and, therefore, a rise (albeit small) in plasma phosphate concentration. This leads to a small, reciprocal decline in plasma levels of ionized calcium and a corresponding increase in PTH secretion. Although the phosphaturic response of surviving tubules to this elevation in circulating PTH restores plasma phosphate and calcium to normal levels (at least in the "compensated" stage of CRF described by curve *B* in Fig. 259-1), the new steady-state conditions are only achieved at the cost of *persistently elevated plasma PTH levels*. With progressive reductions in GFR, the process is repeated, resulting in substantially elevated PTH levels.

Alterations in Vitamin D Metabolism The kidney is normally the major site of *conversion of vitamin D to its active metabolites*. As discussed in Chap. 331, vitamin D, synthesized in skin or acquired in the diet, undergoes initial hydroxylation in the liver to form 25-hydroxyvitamin D [25(OH)D]. The kidney is the site of a second important conversion to 1,25-dihydroxyvitamin D [1,25(OH)$_2$D]. This active form of vitamin D acts directly on the parathyroid gland to suppress PTH secretion as well as to enhance intestinal absorption of calcium and promote its resorption from bone. With advancing renal disease, nephron loss reduces the renal capacity for vitamin D hydroxylation; phosphate retention also impairs this reaction. Not only are the circulating levels of 1,25(OH)$_2$D diminished in CRF, but the receptors that mediate its action at the parathyroid gland are also diminished. These two effects remove inhibitory influences on PTH secretion, leading again to increased plasma PTH levels. Reduction in circulating 1,25(OH)$_2$D levels, by suppressing intestinal calcium absorption, contributes to the development of the hypocalcemia and hyperparathyroidism of CRF (Chap. 261). →*For a discussion of hyperparathyroidism in chronic renal failure, see Chap. 261.*

HYDROGEN AND BICARBONATE TRANSPORT WITH NORMAL AND REDUCED RENAL MASS As discussed in Chap. 42, the pH of extracellular fluid is normally maintained within a narrow range (7.36 to 7.44) despite day-to-day fluctuations in the quantity of acids added to the extracellular fluid from dietary and metabolic sources (approximately 1 mmol H$^+$ per kilogram of body weight per day). These acids consume buffers from both extracellular and intracellular fluid, of which HCO$_3^-$ is the most important in the intracellular compartment. Such buffering minimizes changes in pH. Long-term effectiveness of the HCO$_3^-$ buffer system, however, requires mechanisms for replenishment, otherwise unrelenting acquisition of nonvolatile acids from dietary and metabolic sources would ultimately exhaust buffering capacity, culminating in fatal acidosis. The kidneys normally function to prevent this eventuality by *regenerating* bicarbonate, thereby maintaining plasma concentrations of HCO$_3^-$. In addition, the kidneys also *reclaim* HCO$_3^-$ in the glomerular ultrafiltrate.

The *reabsorption* of filtered HCO$_3^-$ occurs by the following mechanism. Filtered bicarbonate combines with H$^+$ secreted from proximal tubule cells via the Na$^+$/H$^+$ exchange, to form carbonic acid (H$_2$CO$_3$). Dehydration of carbonic acid under the influence of *luminal* carbonic anhydrase yields H$_2$O and CO$_2$, which is free to diffuse from lumen to peritubular blood. In the proximal tubule cell, the OH$^-$ left behind by the H$^+$ secretion reacts with CO$_2$, under the influence of *intracellular* carbonic anhydrase, forming HCO$_3^-$. This ion is transported across the contraluminal proximal tubule cell membrane, via an electrogenic Na/HCO$_3^-$ cotransporter, to reenter the extracellular HCO$_3^-$ pool. The net result is *reclamation of a filtered bicarbonate ion*. Hydrogen ions in the urine are bound to filtered buffers (e.g., phosphate) in amounts equivalent to the amounts of alkali required to titrate the pH of the urine up to the pH of the blood (the so-called titratable acid). It is not usually possible to excrete all the daily acid load in the form of titratable acid due to limits of urinary pH. Metabolism of glutamine by proximal tubule cells to yield ammonium (ammoniagenesis) serves as an additional mechanism for H$^+$ elimination and bicarbonate re-

generation. Glutamine metabolism forms not only NH$_4^+$ (i.e., NH$_3$ plus H$^+$) but also HCO$_3^-$, which is transported across the proximal tubule (HCO$_3^-$ regeneration). The NH$_4^+$ must be excreted in the urine for this process to be effective in bicarbonate regeneration. *Ammoniagenesis* is responsive to the acid-base needs of the individual. When faced with an acute acid burden and an increased need for HCO$_3^-$ regeneration, the rate of renal ammonia synthesis increases sharply.

The quantity of hydrogen ions excreted as titratable acid and NH$_4^+$ is equal to the quantity of HCO$_3^-$ regenerated in tubule cells and added to plasma. Under steady-state conditions, the net quantity of acid excreted into the urine (the sum of titratable acid and NH$_4^+$ less HCO$_3^-$) must equal the quantity of acid gained by the extracellular fluid from all sources. Metabolic acidosis and alkalosis result when this delicate balance is perturbed, the former the result of insufficient net acid excretion, and the latter due to excessive acid excretion (Chap. 42).

Progressive loss of renal function usually causes little or no change in arterial pH, plasma bicarbonate concentration, or arterial carbon dioxide tension (P$_{CO_2}$) until GFR falls below 25% of normal. Thereafter, all three tend to decline as *metabolic acidosis* ensues. In general, the metabolic acidosis of CRF is not due to overproduction of acids but is rather a reflection of nephron loss, which limits the amount of NH$_3$ (and therefore also HCO$_3^-$) that can be generated. Although surviving nephrons appear to be capable of generating supranormal amounts of NH$_3$ *per nephron*, the diminished nephron population causes overall production to be reduced to an extent that is insufficient to permit adequate buffering of H$^+$ in urine. As a result, although patients with CRF may be able to acidify their urine normally (i.e., urine pH as low as 4.5), the defect in NH$_3$ production limits daily net acid excretion to 30 to 40 mmol, or one-half to two-thirds the quantity of nonvolatile acid added to the extracellular fluid in the same time period. Metabolic acidosis resulting from this daily positive balance of H$^+$ is seldom florid in CRF of mild to moderate severity. Relative stability of plasma bicarbonate (albeit at reduced levels of 14 to 18 mmol/L) is maintained at the expense of buffering by bone. Because it contains large reserves of alkaline salts (calcium phosphate and calcium bicarbonate), bone constitutes a major reserve of buffering capacity. Dissolution of these buffers contributes to the osteodystrophy of CRF (see Fig. 261-1).

Although the acidosis of CRF is due to loss of tubule mass, it nevertheless depends to a large part on the level of GFR. When GFR is reduced to only a moderate extent (i.e., to about 50% of normal), retention of anions, principally sulfates and phosphates, is not pronounced. Therefore, as the plasma HCO$_3^-$ falls owing to dysfunction or loss of tubules, retention of Cl$^-$ by the kidneys leads to a *hyperchloremic acidosis*. At this stage *the anion gap is normal*. With further reductions in GFR and progressive azotemia, however, the retention of phosphates, sulfates, and other *unmeasured* anions ensues and plasma Cl$^-$ falls to normal levels despite the reduction in plasma HCO$_3^-$ concentration. *An elevated anion gap therefore develops.*

TUBULE POTASSIUM TRANSPORT WITH NORMAL AND REDUCED NEPHRON MASS As with H$^+$, the concentration of K$^+$ in extracellular fluid is normally maintained within a relatively narrow range, 4 to 5 mmol/L. At least 95% of total-body K$^+$ is in the intracellular compartment, where the intracellular concentration is approximately 160 mmol/L. Normal individuals maintain external K$^+$ balance by excreting amounts into the urine that equal the intake, less the relatively small losses in stool and sweat. K$^+$ is freely filtered at the glomerulus, although the amount excreted usually represents no more than about 20% of the quantity filtered. The great bulk of the K$^+$ filtered is reabsorbed in the early portions of the nephron, about two-thirds in the proximal tubule, and an additional 20 to 25% in the loop of Henle. A *K$^+$* secretory process operates in the distal tubule and terminal nephron segments. This process is largely dependent on Na$^+$ reabsorption and the accompanying lumen-negative voltage creating an electrical gradient across the tubule wall, favoring K$^+$ secretion into the lumen of the distal tubule and collecting duct.

The ability to maintain external K^+ balance and normal plasma K^+ concentration until relatively late in the course of CRF is a consequence primarily of a progressive increase in fractional excretion of K^+. Greatly enhanced rates of K^+ secretion occur in distal portions of surviving tubules. The augmented secretion rate of aldosterone contributes to enhanced tubule secretion of K^+. In addition, both the increased distal tubule flow rates in surviving nephrons, due to the osmotic diuresis, and enhanced luminal electronegativity, created by the increased presence of highly impermeable anions such as phosphate and sulfate, enhance K^+ secretion. Aldosterone also stimulates net entry of K^+ into the lumen of the colon, a mechanism known to be enhanced in CRF. →*For more detailed discussions of abnormal K^+ homeostasis in acute and chronic forms of renal failure, see Chaps. 260 and 261.*

FURTHER READING

BRENNER BM et al: Diverse biological actions of atrial natriuretic peptides. Physiol Rev 70:665, 1990

O'CALLAGHAN CA, BRENNER BM: *The Kidney at a Glance.* Oxford, Blackwell Science Ltd., 2000

TAAL MW et al: Adaptation to nephron loss, in *Brenner and Rector's The Kidney,* 7th ed, BM Brenner, (ed). Philadelphia, Saunders, 2004

TAAL MW, BRENNER BM: Renoprotective benefits of RAS inhibition: From ACEI to angiotensin II antagonists. Kidney Int 57:1803, 2000

260 ACUTE RENAL FAILURE
Hugh R. Brady, Barry M. Brenner

Acute renal failure (ARF) is a syndrome characterized by rapid decline in glomerular filtration rate (hours to days), retention of nitrogenous waste products, and perturbation of extracellular fluid volume and electrolyte and acid-base homeostasis. ARF complicates approximately 5% of hospital admissions and up to 30% of admissions to intensive care units. Oliguria (urine output < 400 mL/d) is a frequent but not invariable clinical feature (~50%). ARF is usually asymptomatic and diagnosed when biochemical monitoring of hospitalized patients reveals a recent increase in blood urea and creatinine concentrations. It may complicate a wide range of diseases, which for purposes of diagnosis and management are conveniently divided into three categories: (1) diseases that cause renal hypoperfusion without compromising the integrity of renal parenchyma (*prerenal ARF,* prerenal azotemia) (~55%); (2) diseases that directly involve renal parenchyma (*intrinsic renal ARF,* renal azotemia) (~40%); and (3) diseases associated with urinary tract obstruction (*postrenal ARF,* postrenal azotemia) (~5%). Most ARF is reversible, the kidney being relatively unique among major organs in its ability to recover from almost complete loss of function. Nevertheless, ARF is associated with major in-hospital morbidity and mortality, in large part due to the serious nature of the illnesses that precipitate the ARF.

ETIOLOGY AND PATHOPHYSIOLOGY

PRERENAL ARF (PRERENAL AZOTEMIA)   Prerenal ARF is the most common form of ARF and represents a physiologic response to mild to moderate renal hypoperfusion. Prerenal ARF is by definition rapidly reversible upon restoration of renal blood flow and glomerular ultrafiltration pressure. Renal parenchymal tissue is not damaged; indeed, kidneys from individuals with prerenal ARF function well when transplanted into recipients with normal cardiovascular function. More severe hypoperfusion may lead to ischemic injury of renal parenchyma and intrinsic renal ARF (see below). Thus, prerenal ARF and intrinsic renal ARF due to ischemia are part of a spectrum of manifestations of renal hypoperfusion. As shown in Table 260-1, prerenal ARF can complicate any disease that induces hypovolemia, low cardiac output, systemic vasodilatation, or selective intrarenal vasoconstriction.

Hypovolemia leads to a fall in mean systemic arterial pressure, which is detected as reduced stretch by arterial (e.g., carotid sinus) and cardiac baroreceptors. Activated baroreceptors trigger a coordinated series of neural and humoral responses designed to restore blood volume and arterial pressure. These include activation of the sympathetic nervous system and renin-angiotensin-aldosterone system and release of arginine vasopressin (AVP; formerly called antidiuretic hormone). Norepinephrine, angiotensin II, and AVP act in concert in an attempt to preserve cardiac and cerebral perfusion by stimulating vasoconstriction in relatively "nonessential" vascular beds, such as the musculocutaneous and splanchnic circulations, by inhibiting salt loss through sweat glands, by stimulating thirst and salt appetite, and by promoting renal salt and water retention. Glomerular perfusion, ultrafiltration pressure, and filtration rate are preserved during mild hypoperfusion through several compensatory mechanisms. Stretch receptors in afferent arterioles, in response to a reduction in perfusion pressure, trigger afferent arteriolar vasodilatation through a local myogenic reflex (autoregulation). Biosynthesis of vasodilator prostaglandins (e.g., prostaglandin E_2 and prostacyclin) is also enhanced, and these compounds preferentially dilate afferent arterioles. In addition, angiotensin II induces preferential constriction of efferent arterioles. As a result, intraglomerular pressure is maintained, the fraction of plasma flowing through glomerular capillaries that is filtered is increased (filtration fraction), and glomerular filtration rate (GFR) is preserved. During states of more severe hypoperfusion, these compensatory responses are overwhelmed and GFR falls, leading to prerenal ARF.

Autoregulatory dilatation of afferent arterioles is maximal at mean systemic arterial blood pressures of ~80 mmHg, and hypotension below this level is associated with a precipitous decline in GFR. Lesser degrees of hypotension may provoke prerenal ARF in the elderly and in patients with diseases affecting the integrity of afferent arterioles (e.g., hypertensive nephrosclerosis, diabetic vasculopathy). In addition, drugs that interfere with adaptive responses in the renal microcirculation may convert compensated renal hypoperfusion into overt prerenal ARF or trigger progression of prerenal ARF to ischemic intrinsic renal ARF (see below). Pharmacologic inhibitors of either renal prostaglandin biosynthesis [*cyclooxygenase inhibitors*; nonsteroidal anti-inflammatory drugs (NSAIDs)] or angiotensin-converting enzyme (ACE) activity (ACE inhibitors) and angiotensin II receptor blockers are the major culprits and should be used judiciously in the setting of suspected renal hypoperfusion. NSAIDs do not compromise GFR in healthy individuals but may precipitate prerenal ARF in patients with volume depletion or in those with chronic renal insufficiency in whom GFR is maintained, in part, through prostaglandin-mediated hyperfiltration by the remaining functional nephrons. ACE inhibitors should be used with special care in patients with bilateral renal artery stenosis or unilateral stenosis in a solitary functioning kidney. In these settings glomerular perfusion and filtration may be exquisitely dependent on the actions of angiotensin II. Angiotensin II preserves glomerular filtration pressure distal to stenoses by elevating systemic arterial pressure and by triggering selective constriction of efferent arterioles. ACE inhibitors blunt these responses and precipitate ARF, usually reversible, in ~30% of these patients.

Hepatorenal Syndrome   This is a particularly aggressive form of ARF, with many of the features of prerenal ARF, that frequently complicates hepatic failure due to advanced cirrhosis or other liver diseases, including malignancy, hepatic resection, and biliary obstruction. In full-blown hepatorenal syndrome, ARF progresses even after optimization

TABLE 260-1 Classification and Major Causes of Acute Renal Failure (ARF)

PRERENAL ARF

I. Hypovolemia
   A. Hemorrhage, burns, dehydration
   B. Gastrointestinal fluid loss: vomiting, surgical drainage, diarrhea
   C. Renal fluid loss: diuretics, osmotic diuresis (e.g., diabetes mellitus), hypoadrenalism
   D. Sequestration in extravascular space: pancreatitis, peritonitis, trauma, burns, severe hypoalbuminemia

II. Low cardiac output
   A. Diseases of myocardium, valves, and pericardium; arrhythmias; tamponade
   B. Other: pulmonary hypertension, massive pulmonary embolus, positive pressure mechanical ventilation

III. Altered renal systemic vascular resistance ratio
   A. Systemic vasodilatation: sepsis, antihypertensives, afterload reducers, anesthesia, anaphylaxis
   B. Renal vasoconstriction: hypercalcemia, norepinephrine, epinephrine, cyclosporine, tacrolimus, amphotericin B
   C. Cirrhosis with ascites (hepatorenal syndrome)

IV. Renal hypoperfusion with impairment of renal autoregulatory responses
   Cyclooxygenase inhibitors, angiotensin-converting enzyme inhibitors

V. Hyperviscosity syndrome (rare)
   Multiple myeloma, macroglobulinemia, polycythemia

INTRINSIC RENAL ARF

I. Renovascular obstruction (bilateral or unilateral in the setting of one functioning kidney)
   A. Renal artery obstruction: atherosclerotic plaque, thrombosis, embolism, dissecting aneurysm, vasculitis
   B. Renal vein obstruction: thrombosis, compression

II. Disease of glomeruli or renal microvasculature
   A. Glomerulonephritis and vasculitis
   B. Hemolytic uremic syndrome, thrombotic thrombocytopenic purpura, disseminated intravascular coagulation, toxemia of pregnancy, accelerated hypertension, radiation nephritis, systemic lupus erythematosus, scleroderma

III. Acute tubular necrosis
   A. Ischemia: as for prerenal ARF (hypovolemia, low cardiac output, renal vasoconstriction, systemic vasodilatation), obstetric complications (abruptio placentae, postpartum hemorrhage)
   B. Toxins
      1. Exogenous: radiocontrast, cyclosporine, antibiotics (e.g., aminoglycosides), chemotherapy (e.g., cisplatin), organic solvents (e.g., ethylene glycol), acetaminophen, illegal abortifacients
      2. Endogenous: rhabdomyolysis, hemolysis, uric acid, oxalate, plasma cell dyscrasia (e.g., myeloma)

IV. Interstitial nephritis
   A. Allergic: antibiotics (e.g., β-lactams, sulfonamides, trimethoprim, rifampicin), nonsteroidal anti-inflammatory agents, diuretics, captopril
   B. Infection: bacterial (e.g., acute pyelonephritis, leptospirosis), viral (e.g., cytomegalovirus), fungal (e.g., candidiasis)
   C. Infiltration: lymphoma, leukemia, sarcoidosis
   D. Idiopathic

V. Intratubular deposition and obstruction
   Myeloma proteins, uric acid, oxalate, acyclovir, methotrexate, sulphonamides

VI. Renal allograft rejection

POSTRENAL ARF (OBSTRUCTION)

I. Ureteric
   Calculi, blood clot, sloughed papillae, cancer, external compression (e.g., retroperitoneal fibrosis)

II. Bladder neck
   Neurogenic bladder, prostatic hypertrophy, calculi, cancer, blood clot

III. Urethra
   Stricture, congenital valve, phimosis

of systemic hemodynamics and carries a mortality rate of >90%. →*The diagnosis and management of this condition are discussed in Chaps. 289 and 291.*

INTRINSIC RENAL ARF (INTRINSIC RENAL AZOTEMIA) Intrinsic renal ARF can complicate many diverse diseases of the renal parenchyma. From a clinicopathologic viewpoint, it is useful to divide the causes of intrinsic

renal ARF into (1) diseases of larger renal vessels, (2) diseases of the renal microcirculation and glomeruli, (3) ischemic and nephrotoxic ARF, and (4) tubulointerstitial inflammation (Table 260-1). Most intrinsic renal ARF is triggered by ischemia (ischemic ARF) or nephrotoxins (nephrotoxic ARF), insults that classically induce acute tubular necrosis (ATN). Accordingly, the terms ARF and ATN are usually used interchangeably in these settings. However, as many as 20 to 30% of patients with ischemic or nephrotoxic ARF do not have clinical (granular or tubular cell urinary casts) or morphologic evidence of tubular necrosis, underscoring the role of sublethal injury to tubular epithelium and injury to other renal cells (e.g., endothelial cells) in the pathophysiology of this syndrome.

Etiology and Pathophysiology of Ischemic ARF Prerenal ARF and ischemic ARF are part of a spectrum of manifestations of renal hypoperfusion. Ischemic ARF differs from prerenal ARF in that the hypoperfusion induces ischemic injury to renal parenchymal cells, particularly tubular epithelium, and recovery typically takes 1 to 2 weeks after normalization of renal perfusion as it requires repair and regeneration of renal cells. In its most extreme form, ischemia leads to bilateral renal cortical necrosis and irreversible renal failure. Ischemic ARF occurs most frequently in patients undergoing major cardiovascular surgery or suffering severe trauma, hemorrhage, sepsis, and/or volume depletion (Table 260-1). Ischemic ARF can also complicate milder forms of true hypovolemia or reduced "effective" arterial blood volume if they occur in the presence of other insults (e.g., nephrotoxins or sepsis) or in patients with compromised autoregulatory defense mechanisms or preexisting renal disease.

The course of ischemic ARF is typically characterized by three phases: the initiation, maintenance, and recovery phases. The *initiation phase* (hours to days) is the initial period of renal hypoperfusion during which ischemic injury is evolving. GFR declines because (1) glomerular ultrafiltration pressure is reduced as a consequence of the fall in renal blood flow, (2) the flow of glomerular filtrate within tubules is obstructed by casts comprised of epithelial cells and necrotic debris derived from ischemic tubule epithelium, and (3) there is backleak of glomerular filtrate through injured tubular epithelium (Fig. 260-1). Ischemic injury is most prominent in the terminal medullary portion of the proximal tubule (S_3 segment, pars recta) and the medullary portion of the thick ascending limb of the loop of Henle. Both segments have high rates of active (ATP-dependent) solute transport and oxygen consumption and are located in a zone of the kidney (the outer medulla) that is relatively ischemic, even under basal conditions, by virtue of the unique countercurrent arrangement of the medullary vasculature. Cellular ischemia results in a series of alterations in energetics, ion transport, and membrane integrity that ultimately lead to cell injury and, if severe, cell apoptosis or necrosis. These alterations include depletion of ATP, inhibition of active sodium transport and transport of other solutes, impairment of cell volume regulation and cell swelling, cytoskeletal disruption and loss of cell polarity, cell-cell and cell-matrix attachment, accumulation of intracellular calcium, altered phospholipid metabolism, oxygen free radical formation, and peroxidation of membrane lipids. Importantly, renal injury can be limited by restoration of renal blood flow during this period.

The initiation phase is followed by a *maintenance phase* (typically 1 to 2 weeks) during which renal cell injury is established, GFR stabilizes at its nadir (typically 5 to 10 mL/min), urine output is lowest, and uremic complications arise (see below). The reasons why the GFR remains low during this phase, despite correction of systemic hemodynamics, are still being defined. Putative mechanisms include persistent intrarenal vasoconstriction and medullary ischemia triggered by dysregulated release of vasoactive mediators from injured endothelial cells (e.g., decreased nitric oxide, increased endothelin-1, adenosine, and platelet-activating factor), congestion of medullary blood vessels, and reperfusion injury induced by reactive oxygen species and other mediators derived from leukocytes or renal parenchymal cells

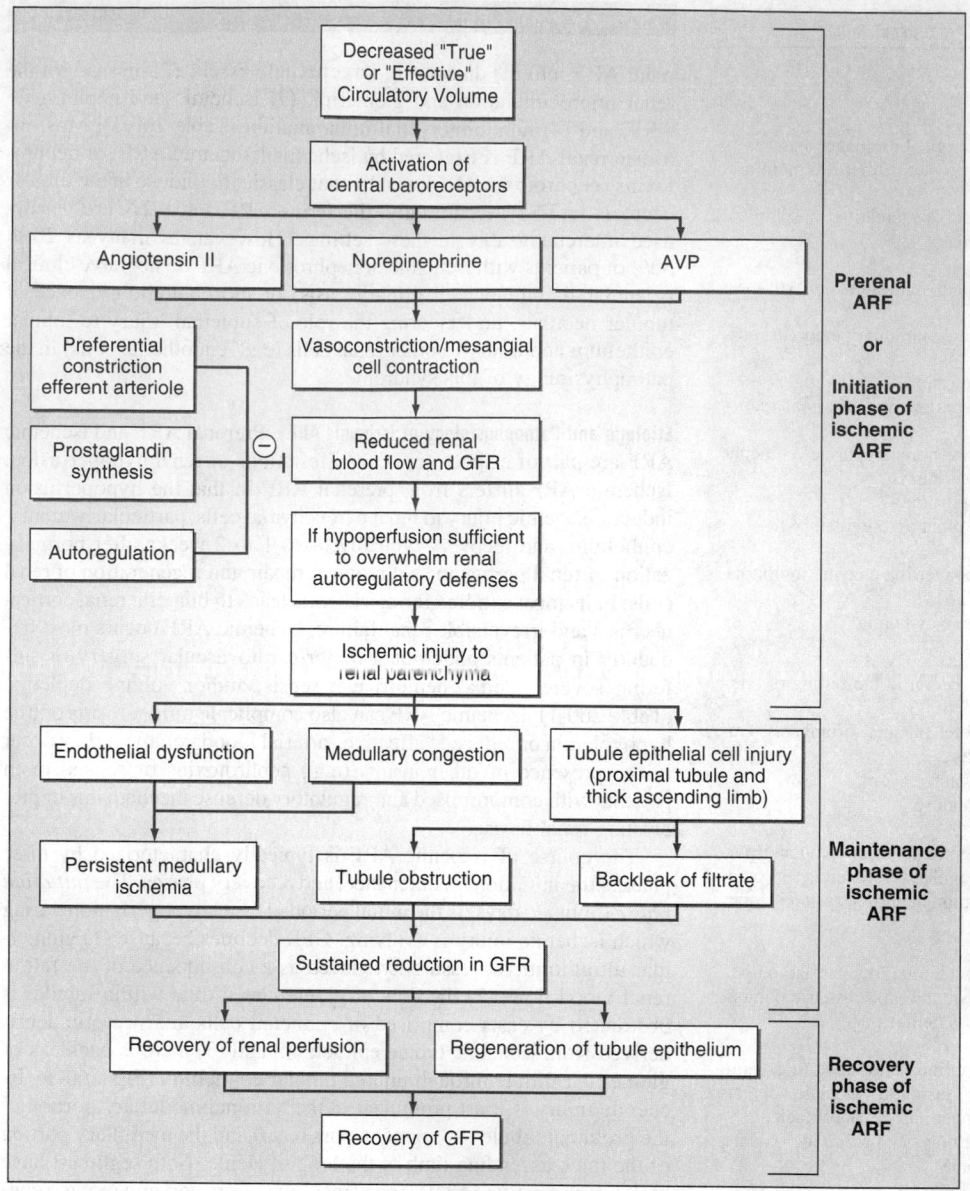

FIGURE 260-1 Overview of the pathophysiology of prerenal ARF and ischemic intrinsic renal ARF: A spectrum of manifestations of renal hypoperfusion. ARF, acute renal failure; AVP, arginine vasopressin; GFR, glomerular filtration rate.

Intrarenal vasoconstriction is a pivotal event in ARF that is triggered by *radiocontrast agents* (contrast nephropathy), *cyclosporine*, and *tacrolimus (FK506)*. In keeping with this pathophysiology, both agents induce ARF that shares features with prerenal ARF: namely, an acute fall in renal blood flow and GFR, a relatively benign urine sediment, and a low fractional excretion of sodium (see below). Severe cases may show clinical or pathologic evidence of ATN. Contrast nephropathy classically presents as an acute (onset within 24 to 48 h) but reversible (peak 3 to 5 days, resolution within 1 week) rise in blood urea nitrogen and creatinine and is most common in individuals with preexisting chronic renal insufficiency, diabetes mellitus, congestive heart failure, hypovolemia, or multiple myeloma. The syndrome appears to be dose-related, and its incidence is only slightly reduced in high-risk individuals by use of more expensive low osmolality, nonionic contrast agents.

Direct toxicity to tubule epithelial cells and/or intratubular obstruction are major pathophysiologic events in ARF induced by many antibiotics and anticancer drugs. Frequent offenders are the antimicrobial agents, such as acyclovir, foscarnet, aminoglycosides, amphotericin B, and pentamidine, and chemotherapeutic agents, such as cisplatin, carboplatin, and ifosfamide. ARF complicates 10 to 30% of courses of *aminoglycoside antibiotics*, even in the presence of therapeutic levels. *Amphotericin B* causes dose-related ARF through intrarenal vasoconstriction and direct toxicity to proximal tubule epithelium. Cisplatin and carboplatin, like the aminoglycosides, are accumulated by proximal tubule cells and typically provoke ARF after 7 to 10 days of exposure by inducing mitochondrial injury, inhibition of ATPase activity and solute transport, free radical–mediated injury to cell membranes, apoptosis, and/or necrosis.

The most common endogenous nephrotoxins are calcium, myoglobin, hemoglobin, urate, oxalate, and myeloma light chains. Hypercalcemia can compromise GFR, predominantly by inducing intrarenal vasoconstriction. Calcium phosphate deposition within the kidney may also contribute. Both *rhabdomyolysis* and *hemolysis* can induce ARF, particularly in hypovolemic or acidotic individuals. Myoglobinuric ARF complicates approximately 30% of cases of rhabdomyolysis. Common causes of the latter include traumatic crush injury, acute muscle ischemia, seizures, excessive exercise, heat stroke or malignant hyperthermia, intoxications (e.g., alcohol, cocaine), and infectious or metabolic disorders. ARF due to hemolysis is relatively rare and is observed following massive blood transfusion reactions. It has been postulated that myoglobin and hemoglobin or other compounds released from muscle or red blood cells cause ARF via toxic effects on tubule epithelial cells, by promoting intrarenal oxidative stress and by inducing intratubular cast formation. Hypovolemia or acidosis may contribute to the pathogenesis of ARF in this setting by promoting intratubular cast formation. In addition, both hemoglobin and myoglobin are potent inhibitors of nitric oxide bioactivity and may trigger

(Fig. 260-1). In addition, epithelial cell injury per se may contribute to persistent intrarenal vasoconstriction by a process termed *tubuloglomerular feedback*. Specialized epithelial cells in the macula densa region of distal tubules detect increases in distal salt (probably chloride) delivery that occur as a consequence of impaired reabsorption by more proximal nephron segments. Macula densa cells in turn stimulate constriction of adjacent afferent arterioles by a poorly defined mechanism and further compromise glomerular perfusion and filtration, thereby contributing to a vicious cycle. A *recovery phase* is characterized by renal parenchymal cell, particularly tubule epithelial cell, repair and regeneration and a gradual return of GFR to or towards premorbid levels. The recovery phase may be complicated by a marked diuretic phase due to excretion of retained salt and water and other solutes, continued use of diuretics, and/or delayed recovery of epithelial cell function (solute and water reabsorption) relative to glomerular filtration (see below).

Etiology and Pathophysiology of Nephrotoxic ARF Acute intrinsic renal ARF can complicate exposure to many structurally diverse pharmacologic agents (Table 260-1). With most nephrotoxins, the incidence of ARF is increased in the elderly and in patients with preexisting chronic renal insufficiency, true or "effective" hypovolemia, or concomitant exposure to other toxins.

intrarenal vasoconstriction and ischemia in patients with borderline renal hypoperfusion. The formation of intratubular casts containing filtered immunoglobulin light chains and other proteins, including Tamm-Horsfall protein produced by thick ascending limb cells, is the major trigger for ARF in patients with *multiple myeloma* (myeloma cast nephropathy). In addition, light chains are directly toxic to tubule epithelial cells. Intratubular obstruction is also an important cause of ARF in patients with severe *hyperuricosuria* or *hyperoxaluria*. Acute uric acid nephropathy typically complicates treatment of lymphoproliferative or myeloproliferative disorders but occasionally occurs in other forms of primary or secondary hyperuricemia if the urine is concentrated.

Pathology of Ischemic and Nephrotoxic ARF The classic pathologic features of ischemic ARF are patchy and focal necrosis of tubule epithelium with detachment from its basement membrane and occlusion of tubule lumens with casts composed of intact or degenerating epithelial cells, cellular debris, Tamm-Horsfall mucoprotein, and pigments. Leukocyte accumulation is frequently observed in vasa recta; however, the morphology of the glomeruli and renal vasculature is characteristically normal. Necrosis is most severe in the straight portion (pars recta) of proximal tubules but may also affect the medullary thick ascending limb of the loop of Henle.

In nephrotoxic ARF, morphologic changes tend to be most prominent in both the convoluted and straight portions of proximal tubules. Tubule cell necrosis is less pronounced than in ischemic ARF.

Other Causes of Intrinsic Renal ARF Patients with advanced atherosclerosis can develop ARF after manipulation of the aorta or renal arteries at surgery or angiography, following trauma, or, rarely, spontaneously due to embolization of cholesterol crystals to the renal vasculature (atheroembolic ARF). Cholesterol crystals lodge in small- and medium-sized arteries and incite a giant cell and fibrotic reaction in the vessel wall with narrowing or obstruction of the vessel lumen. Atheroembolic ARF is frequently irreversible. A myriad of structurally diverse pharmacologic agents induce ARF by triggering allergic interstitial nephritis, a disease characterized by infiltration of the tubulointerstitium by granulocytes (typically but not invariably eosinophils), macrophages, and/or lymphocytes and by interstitial edema. The most common offenders are antibiotics (e.g., penicillins, cephalosporins, trimethoprim, sulfonamides, rifampicin) and NSAIDs (Table 260-1).

POSTRENAL ARF (See also Chap. 270) Urinary tract obstruction accounts for fewer than 5% of cases of ARF. Because one kidney has sufficient clearance capacity to excrete the nitrogenous waste products generated daily, ARF from obstruction requires obstruction to urine flow between the external urethral meatus and bladder neck, bilateral ureteric obstruction, or unilateral ureteric obstruction in a patient with one functioning kidney or with preexisting chronic renal insufficiency. Bladder neck obstruction represents the most common cause of postrenal ARF and is usually due to prostatic disease (e.g., hypertrophy, neoplasia, or infection), neurogenic bladder, or therapy with anticholinergic drugs. Less common causes of acute lower urinary tract obstruction include blood clots, calculi, and urethritis with spasm. Ureteric obstruction may result from intraluminal obstruction (e.g., calculi, blood clots, sloughed renal papillae), infiltration of the ureteric wall (e.g., neoplasia), or external compression (e.g., retroperitoneal fibrosis, neoplasia or abscess, inadvertent surgical ligature). During the early stages of obstruction (hours to days), continued glomerular filtration leads to increased intraluminal pressure upstream to the site of obstruction. As a result there is gradual distention of the proximal ureter, renal pelvis, and calyces and a fall in GFR. Acute obstruction is initially associated with modest increase in renal blood flow, but arteriolar vasoconstriction soon supervenes, leading to a further decline in glomerular filtration.

CLINICAL FEATURES AND DIFFERENTIAL DIAGNOSIS

Patients presenting with renal failure should be assessed initially to determine if the decline in GFR is acute or chronic. An acute process is easily established if a review of laboratory records reveals a recent rise in blood urea and creatinine levels, but previous measurements are not always available. Findings that suggest chronic renal failure (Chap. 261) include anemia, neuropathy, and radiologic evidence of renal osteodystrophy or small scarred kidneys. However, it should be noted that anemia may also complicate ARF (see below), and renal size may be normal or increased in several chronic renal diseases (e.g., diabetic nephropathy, amyloidosis, polycystic kidney disease). Once a diagnosis of ARF has been established, several issues should be addressed promptly: (1) the identification of the cause of ARF, (2) the elimination of the triggering insult (e.g., nephrotoxin) and/or institution of disease-specific therapies, and (3) the prevention and management of uremic complications.

CLINICAL ASSESSMENT Clinical clues to *prerenal* ARF are symptoms of thirst and orthostatic dizziness and physical evidence of orthostatic hypotension and tachycardia, reduced jugular venous pressure, decreased skin turgor, dry mucous membranes, and reduced axillary sweating. Case records should be reviewed for documentation of a progressive fall in urine output and body weight and recent initiation of treatment with NSAIDs, ACE inhibitors, or angiotensin II receptor blockers. Careful clinical examination may reveal stigmata of chronic liver disease and portal hypertension, advanced cardiac failure, sepsis, or other causes of reduced "effective" arterial blood volume (Table 260-1).

Intrinsic renal ARF due to ischemia is likely following severe renal hypoperfusion complicating hypovolemic or septic shock or following major surgery. The likelihood of ischemic ARF is increased further if ARF persists despite normalization of systemic hemodynamics. Diagnosis of nephrotoxic ARF requires careful review of the clinical data and pharmacy, nursing, and radiology records for evidence of recent exposure to nephrotoxic medications or radiocontrast agents or to endogenous toxins (e.g., myoglobin, hemoglobin, uric acid, myeloma protein, or elevated levels of serum calcium).

Although ischemic and nephrotoxic ARF account for more than 90% of cases of intrinsic renal ARF, other renal parenchymal diseases must be considered (Table 260-2). Flank pain may be a prominent symptom following occlusion of a renal artery or vein and with other parenchymal diseases distending the renal capsule (e.g., severe glomerulonephritis or pyelonephritis). Subcutaneous nodules, livedo reticularis, bright orange retinal arteriolar plaques, and digital ischemia, despite palpable pedal pulses, are clues to atheroembolization. ARF in association with oliguria, edema, hypertension, and an "active" urine sediment (nephritic syndrome) suggests acute glomerulonephritis or vasculitis. Malignant hypertension is a likely cause of ARF in patients with severe hypertension and evidence of hypertensive injury to other organs (e.g., left ventricular hypertrophy and failure, hypertensive retinopathy and papilledema, neurologic dysfunction). Fever, arthralgias, and a pruritic erythematous rash following exposure to a new drug suggest allergic interstitial nephritis, although systemic features of hypersensitivity are frequently absent.

Postrenal ARF presents with suprapubic and flank pain due to distention of the bladder and of the renal collecting system and capsule, respectively. Colicky flank pain radiating to the groin suggests acute ureteric obstruction. Prostatic disease is likely if there is a history of nocturia, frequency, and hesitancy and enlargement or induration of the prostate on rectal examination. Neurogenic bladder should be suspected in patients receiving anticholinergic medications or with physical evidence of autonomic dysfunction. Definitive diagnosis of postrenal ARF hinges on judicious use of radiologic investigations and rapid improvement in renal function following relief of obstruction.

URINALYSIS Anuria suggests complete urinary tract obstruction but may complicate severe cases of prerenal or intrinsic renal ARF. Wide fluctuations in urine output raise the possibility of intermittent obstruction, whereas patients with partial urinary tract obstruction can present with polyuria due to impairment of urine concentrating mechanisms.

Cause of Acute Renal Failure	Suggestive Clinical Features	Typical Urinalysis	Some Confirmatory Tests
I. Prerenal ARF	Evidence of true volume depletion (thirst, postural or absolute hypotension and tachycardia, low jugular venous pressure, dry mucous membranes/axillae, weight loss, fluid output > input) or decreased "effective" circulatory volume (e.g., heart failure, liver failure), treatment with NSAIDs or ACE inhibitors	Hyaline casts FE_{Na} <1% U_{Na} <10 mmol/L SG >1.018	Occasionally requires invasive hemodynamic monitoring; rapid resolution of ARF upon restoration of renal perfusion
II. Intrinsic renal ARF			
A. Diseases involving large renal vessels			
1. Renal artery thrombosis	History of atrial fibrillation or recent myocardial infarct; flank or abdominal pain	Mild proteinuria Occasionally red cells	Elevated LDH with normal transaminases, renal arteriogram
2. Atheroembolism	Age usually > 50 years, recent manipulation of aorta, retinal plaques, subcutaneous nodules, palpable purpura, livedo reticularis, vasculopathy, hypertension, anticoagulation	Often normal, eosinophiluria, rarely casts	Eosinophilia, hypocomplementemia, skin biopsy, renal biopsy
3. Renal vein thrombosis	Evidence of nephrotic syndrome or pulmonary embolism, flank pain	Proteinuria, hematuria	Inferior vena cavagram and selective renal venogram
B. Diseases of small vessels and glomeruli			
1. Glomerulonephritis/vasculitis	Compatible clinical history (e.g., recent infection), sinusitis, lung hemorrhage, skin rash or ulcers, arthralgias, new cardiac murmur, history of hepatitis B or C infection	Red cell or granular casts, red cells, white cells, mild proteinuria	Low C3, ANCA, anti-GBM Ab, ANA, ASO, anti-DNase, cryoglobulins, blood cultures, renal biopsy
2. Hemolytic-uremic syndrome/thrombotic thrombocytopenic purpura	Compatible clinical history (e.g., recent gastrointestinal infection, cyclosporine, anovulants), fever, pallor, ecchymoses, neurologic abnormalities	May be normal, red cells, mild proteinuria, rarely red cell/granular casts	Anemia, thrombocytopenia, schistocytes on blood smear, increased LDH, renal biopsy
3. Malignant hypertension	Severe hypertension with headaches, cardiac failure, retinopathy, neurologic dysfunction, papilledema	Red cells, red cell casts, proteinuria	LVH by echocardiography/ECG, resolution of ARF with control of blood pressure
C. ARF mediated by ischemia or toxins (ATN)			
1. Ischemia	Recent hemorrhage, hypotension (e.g., cardiac arrest), surgery	Muddy brown granular or tubular epithelial cell casts FE_{Na} >1% U_{Na} >20 mmol/L SG <1.015	Clinical assessment and urinalysis usually sufficient for diagnosis
2. Exogenous toxins	Recent radiocontrast study, nephrotoxic antibiotics or anticancer agents often coexistent with volume depletion, sepsis, or chronic renal insufficiency	Muddy brown granular or tubular epithelial cell casts FE_{Na} >1% U_{Na} >20 mmol/L SG <1.015	Clinical assessment and urinalysis usually sufficient for diagnosis
3. Endogenous toxins	History suggestive of rhabdomyolysis (seizures, coma, ethanol abuse, trauma)	Urine supernatant positive for heme	Hyperkalemia, hyperphosphatemia, hypocalcemia, increased circulating myoglobin, CPK (MM), and uric acid
	History suggestive of hemolysis (blood transfusion)	Urine supernatant pink and positive for heme	Hyperkalemia, hyperphosphatemia, hypocalcemia, hyperuricemia, pink plasma positive for hemoglobin
	History suggestive of tumor lysis (recent chemotherapy), myeloma (bone pain), or ethylene glycol ingestion	Urate crystals, dipstick-negative proteinuria, oxalate crystals, respectively	Hyperuricemia, hyperkalemia, hyperphosphatemia (for tumor lysis); circulating or urinary monoclonal spike (for myeloma); toxicology screen, acidosis, osmolal gap (for ethylene glycol)
D. Acute diseases of the tubulointerstitium			
1. Allergic interstitial nephritis	Recent ingestion of drug, and fever, rash, or arthralgias	White cell casts, white cells (frequently eosinophiluria), red cells, rarely red cell casts, proteinuria (occasionally nephrotic)	Systemic eosinophilia, skin biopsy of rash (leukocytoclastic vasculitis), renal biopsy
2. Acute bilateral pyelonephritis	Flank pain and tenderness, toxic, febrile	Leukocytes, proteinuria, red cells, bacteria	Urine and blood cultures
III. Postrenal ARF	Abdominal or flank pain, palpable bladder	Frequently normal, hematuria if stones, hemorrhage, malignancy, or prostatic hypertrophy	Plain film, renal ultrasound, IVP, retrograde or anterograde pyelography, CT scan

Note: U_{Na}, urine sodium concentration; SG, specific gravity; LDH, lactate dehydrogenase; C3, complement component; ANCA, antineutrophil cytoplasmic autoantibody; anti-GBM Ab, anti-glomerular basement membrane antibody; ANA, antinuclear antibody; ASO, antistreptolysin O; LVH, left ventricular hypertrophy; ECG, electrocardiogram; CK, creatine kinase; IVP, intravenous pyelogram; CT, computed tomography.
Source: Adapted with permission from Brady et al.

In prerenal ARF, the sediment is characteristically acellular and contains transparent hyaline casts ("bland," "benign," "inactive" urine sediment). Hyaline casts are formed in concentrated urine from normal constituents of urine—principally Tamm-Horsfall protein, which is secreted by epithelial cells of the loop of Henle. Postrenal ARF may also present with an inactive sediment, although hematuria and pyuria are common in patients with intraluminal obstruction or prostatic disease. Pigmented "muddy brown" granular casts and casts containing tubule epithelial cells are characteristic of ATN and suggest ischemic or nephrotoxic ARF. They are usually found in association with microscopic hematuria and mild "tubular" proteinuria (<1 g/d); the latter reflects impaired reabsorption and processing of filtered proteins by injured proximal tubules. Casts are absent, however, in 20 to 30% of patients with ischemic or nephrotoxic ARF and are not a requisite for diagnosis. In general, red blood cell casts indicate glomerular injury or, less often, acute tubulointerstitial nephritis. White cell casts and nonpigmented granular casts suggest interstitial nephritis, whereas broad granular casts are characteristic of chronic renal disease and probably reflect interstitial fibrosis and dilatation of tubules. Eosinophiluria (>5% of urine leukocytes) is a common finding (~90%) in antibiotic-induced allergic interstitial nephritis when studied using Hansel's stain; however, lymphocytes may predominate in allergic interstitial nephritis induced by NSAIDs. Eosinophiluria is also a feature of atheroembolic ARF. Occasional uric acid crystals (pleomorphic in shape) are common in the concentrated urine of prerenal ARF but suggest acute urate nephropathy if seen in abundance. Oxalate (envelope-shaped) and hippurate (needle-shaped) crystals raise the possibility of ethylene glycol ingestion and toxicity.

Proteinuria of >1 g/d suggests injury to the glomerular ultrafiltration barrier ("glomerular proteinuria") or excretion of myeloma light chains. The latter are not detected by conventional dipsticks (which detect albumin) and must be sought by other means (e.g., sulfosalicylic acid test, immunoelectrophoresis). Heavy proteinuria is also a frequent finding (~80%) in patients who develop combined allergic interstitial nephritis and minimal change glomerulopathy when treated with NSAIDs. A similar syndrome can be triggered by ampicillin, rifampicin, or interferon α. Hemoglobinuria or myoglobinuria should be suspected if urine is strongly positive for heme by dipstick, but contains few red cells, and if the supernatant of centrifuged urine is positive for free heme. Bilirubinuria may provide a clue to the presence of hepatorenal syndrome.

RENAL FAILURE INDICES Analysis of urine and blood biochemistry is particularly useful for distinguishing prerenal ARF from ischemic or nephrotoxic intrinsic renal ARF (Table 260-3). The fractional excretion of sodium (FE_{Na}) is most useful in this regard. The FE_{Na} relates sodium clearance to creatinine clearance. Sodium is reabsorbed avidly from glomerular filtrate in patients with prerenal ARF, in an attempt to restore intravascular volume, but not in patients with ischemic or nephrotoxic intrinsic ARF, as a result of tubular epithelial cell injury. In contrast, creatinine is not reabsorbed in either setting. Consequently, patients with prerenal ARF typically have a FE_{Na} of <1.0% (frequently <0.1%), whereas the FE_{Na} in patients with ischemic or nephrotoxic ARF is usually >1.0%. The *renal failure index* (Table 260-3) provides comparable information, since clinical variations in serum sodium concentration are relatively small. *Urine sodium concentration* is a less sensitive index for distinguishing prerenal ARF from ischemic and nephrotoxic ARF as values overlap between groups. Similarly, indices of urinary concentrating ability such as urine specific gravity, urine osmolality, urine-to-plasma urea ratio, and blood urea-to-creatinine ratio are of limited value in differential diagnosis.

Many caveats apply when interpreting biochemical renal failure indices. FE_{Na} may be >1.0% in prerenal ARF if patients are receiving diuretics or have bicarbonaturia (accompanied by sodium to maintain electroneutrality), preexisting chronic renal failure complicated by salt wasting, or adrenal insufficiency. In contrast, the FE_{Na} is <1.0% in approximately 15% of patients with nonoliguric ischemic or nephrotoxic ARF, probably reflecting patchy injury to tubular epithelium with

TABLE 260-3 *Urine Diagnostic Indices in Differentiation of Prerenal versus Intrinsic Renal ARF*

Diagnostic Index	Typical Findings in ARF	
	Prerenal	Intrinsic Renal
Fractional excretion of sodium (%)[a] $$\frac{U_{Na} \times P_{Cr}}{P_{Na} \times U_{Cr}} \times 100$$	<1	>1
Urine sodium concentration (mmol/L)	<10	>20
Urine creatinine to plasma creatinine ratio	>40	<20
Urine urea nitrogen to plasma urea nitrogen ratio	>8	<3
Urine specific gravity	>1.020	~1.010
Urine osmolality (mosmol/kg H_2O)	>500	~300
Plasma BUN/creatinine ratio	>20	<10–15
Renal failure index[a] $$\frac{U_{Na}}{U_{Cr}/P_{Cr}}$$	<1	>1
Urinary sediment	Hyaline casts	Muddy brown granular casts

[a] Most sensitive indices.

Note: U_{Na}, urine sodium concentration; P_{Cr}, plasma creatinine concentration; P_{Na}, plasma sodium concentration; U_{Cr}, urine creatinine concentration; BUN, blood urea nitrogen.

preservation of reabsorptive function in some areas. The FE_{Na} is also often <1.0% in ARF due to urinary tract obstruction, glomerulonephritis, and vascular diseases.

LABORATORY FINDINGS Serial measurements of serum creatinine can provide useful pointers to the cause of ARF. Prerenal ARF is typified by fluctuating levels that parallel changes in hemodynamic function. Creatinine rises rapidly (within 24 to 48 h) in patients with ARF following renal ischemia, atheroembolization, and radiocontrast exposure. Peak creatinine levels are observed after 3 to 5 days with contrast nephropathy and return to baseline after 5 to 7 days. In contrast, creatinine levels typically peak later (7 to 10 days) in ischemic ARF and atheroembolic disease. The initial rise in serum creatinine is characteristically delayed until the second week of therapy with many tubule epithelial cell toxins (e.g., aminoglycosides, cisplatin) and probably reflects the need for accumulation of these agents within cells before GFR falls.

Hyperkalemia, hyperphosphatemia, hypocalcemia, and elevations in serum uric acid and creatine kinase (MM isoenzyme) levels at presentation suggest a diagnosis of rhabdomyolysis. Hyperuricemia [>890 μmol/L (>15 mg/dL)] in association with hyperkalemia, hyperphosphatemia, and increased circulating levels of intracellular enzymes such as lactate dehydrogenase may indicate acute urate nephropathy and tumor lysis syndrome following cancer chemotherapy. A wide serum anion and osmolal gap (measured serum osmolality minus the serum osmolality calculated from serum sodium, glucose, and urea concentrations) indicate the presence of an unusual anion or osmole in the circulation and are clues to diagnosis of ethylene glycol or methanol ingestion. Severe anemia in the absence of hemorrhage raises the possibility of hemolysis, multiple myeloma, or thrombotic microangiopathy. Systemic eosinophilia suggests allergic interstitial nephritis but is also a feature of atheroembolic disease and polyangiitis nodosa.

RADIOLOGIC FINDINGS Imaging of the urinary tract by ultrasonography is useful to exclude postrenal ARF. Computed tomography and magnetic resonance imaging are alternative imaging modalities. Whereas pelvicalyceal dilatation is usual with urinary tract obstruction (98% sensitivity), dilatation may be absent immediately following obstruction or in patients with ureteric encasement (e.g., retroperitoneal fibrosis, neoplasia). Retrograde or anterograde pyelography are more definitive investigations in complex cases and provide precise localization of the site of obstruction. A plain film of the abdomen, with tomography if necessary, is a valuable initial screening technique in patients with suspected nephrolithiasis. Doppler ultrasonography and magnetic resonance angiography are useful for assessment of patency of renal arteries and veins in patients with suspected vascular obstruction; however, contrast angiography is usually required for definitive diagnosis.

RENAL BIOPSY Biopsy is reserved for patients in whom prerenal and postrenal ARF have been excluded and the cause of intrinsic renal ARF is unclear. Renal biopsy is particularly useful when clinical assessment and laboratory investigations suggest diagnoses other than ischemic or nephrotoxic injury that may respond to disease-specific therapy. Examples include glomerulonephritis, vasculitis, hemolytic-uremic syndrome, thrombotic thrombocytopenic purpura, and allergic interstitial nephritis.

COMPLICATIONS

ARF impairs renal excretion of sodium, potassium, and water and perturbs divalent cation homeostasis and urinary acidification mechanisms. As a result, ARF is frequently complicated by intravascular volume overload, hyponatremia, hyperkalemia, hyperphosphatemia, hypocalcemia, hypermagnesemia, and metabolic acidosis. In addition, patients are unable to excrete nitrogenous waste products and are prone to develop the uremic syndrome (Chap. 261). The speed of development and the severity of these complications reflect the degree of renal impairment and catabolic state of the patient.

Expansion of extracellular fluid volume is an inevitable consequence of diminished salt and water excretion in oliguric or anuric individuals. Whereas milder forms are characterized by weight gain, bibasilar lung rales, raised jugular venous pressure, and dependent edema, continued volume expansion may precipitate life-threatening pulmonary edema. Hypervolemia may be particularly problematic in patients receiving multiple intravenous medications and enteral or parenteral nutrition. Excessive administration of free water either through ingestion and nasogastric administration or as hypotonic saline or isotonic dextrose solutions (dextrose being metabolized) can induce *hypoosmolality* and *hyponatremia*, which, if severe, lead to cerebral edema and neurologic abnormalities, including seizures.

Hyperkalemia is a frequent complication of ARF. Serum potassium typically rises by 0.5 mmol/L per day in oliguric and anuric patients due to impaired excretion of ingested or infused potassium and potassium released from injured tissue. Coexistent metabolic acidosis may exacerbate hyperkalemia by promoting potassium efflux from cells. Hyperkalemia may be particularly severe, even at the time of diagnosis, in patients with rhabdomyolysis, hemolysis, and tumor lysis syndrome. Mild hyperkalemia (<6.0 mmol/L) is usually asymptomatic. Higher levels may trigger electrocardiographic abnormalities and/or arrythmias (Chap. 210).

Metabolism of dietary protein yields between 50 and 100 mmol/d of fixed nonvolatile acids that are normally excreted by the kidneys. Consequently, ARF is typically complicated by *metabolic acidosis*, often with an increased serum anion gap (Chap. 42). Acidosis can be particularly severe when endogenous production of hydrogen ions is increased by other mechanisms (e.g., diabetic or fasting ketoacidosis; lactic acidosis complicating generalized tissue hypoperfusion, liver disease, or sepsis; metabolism of ethylene glycol or methanol).

Mild *hyperphosphatemia* is an almost invariable complication of ARF. Severe hyperphosphatemia may develop in highly catabolic patients or following rhabdomyolysis, hemolysis, or tumor lysis. Metastatic deposition of calcium phosphate can lead to *hypocalcemia*, particularly when the product of serum calcium (mg/dL) and phosphate (mg/dL) concentrations exceeds 70. Other factors that contribute

to hypocalcemia include tissue resistance to the actions of parathyroid hormone and reduced levels of 1,25-dihydroxyvitamin D. Hypocalcemia is often asymptomatic but can cause perioral paresthesia, muscle cramps, seizures, hallucinations and confusion, and prolongation of the QT interval and nonspecific T-wave changes on electrocardiography (Chap. 332).

Anemia develops rapidly in ARF and is usually mild and multifactorial in origin. Contributing factors include impaired erythropoiesis, hemolysis, bleeding, hemodilution, and reduced red cell survival time. Prolongation of the *bleeding time* and *leukocytosis* are also common. Common contributors to the bleeding diathesis include mild thrombocytopenia, platelet dysfunction, and/or clotting factor abnormalities (e.g., factor VIII dysfunction), whereas leukocytosis usually reflects sepsis, a stress response, or other concurrent illness. *Infection* is a common and serious complication of ARF, occurring in 50 to 90% of cases and accounting for up to 75% of deaths. It is unclear whether patients with ARF have a clinically significant defect in host immune responses or whether the high incidence of infection reflects repeated breaches of mucocutaneous barriers (e.g., intravenous cannulae, mechanical ventilation, bladder catheterization). *Cardiopulmonary complications* of ARF include arrhythmias, myocardial infarction, pericarditis and pericardial effusion, pulmonary edema, and pulmonary embolism. Mild *gastrointestinal bleeding* is common (10 to 30%) and is usually due to stress ulceration of gastric or small intestinal mucosa.

Protracted periods of severe ARF are invariably associated with the development of the *uremic syndrome* (Chap. 261).

A *vigorous diuresis* can occur during the recovery phase of ARF (see above), which may on occasions be inappropriate and lead to intravascular volume depletion and delayed recovery of GFR by causing secondary prerenal ARF. *Hypernatremia* can also complicate recovery if water losses via hypotonic urine are not replaced or if losses are inappropriately replaced by relatively hypertonic saline solutions. *Hypokalemia, hypomagnesemia, hypophosphatemia,* and *hypocalcemia* are less common metabolic complications during this period.

$\boxed{R_x}$ TREATMENT

Prevention Because there are no specific therapies for ischemic or nephrotoxic ARF, prevention is of paramount importance. Many cases of ischemic ARF can be avoided by close attention to cardiovascular function and intravascular volume in high-risk patients, such as the elderly and those with preexisting renal insufficiency. Indeed, aggressive restoration of intravascular volume has been shown to reduce dramatically the incidence of ischemic ARF after major surgery or trauma, burns, or cholera. The incidence of nephrotoxic ARF can be reduced by tailoring the dosage of nephrotoxic drugs to body size and GFR; for example, reducing the dose or frequency of administration of drugs in patients with preexisting renal impairment. In this regard, it should be noted that serum creatinine is a relatively insensitive index of GFR and may overestimate GFR considerably in small or elderly patients. For purposes of drug dosing, it is advisable to estimate the GFR using the Cockcroft-Gault formula, which factors in the variables of age and weight (Chap. 40). Adjusting drug dosage according to circulating drug levels also appears to limit renal injury in patients receiving aminoglycoside antibiotics, cyclosporine, or tacrolimus. Diuretics, cyclooxygenase inhibitors, ACE inhibitors, angiotensin II receptor blockers, and other vasodilators should be used with caution in patients with suspected true or "effective" hypovolemia or renovascular disease as they may precipitate prerenal ARF or convert the latter to ischemic ARF. Allopurinol and forced alkaline diuresis are useful prophylactic measures in patients at high risk for acute urate nephropathy (e.g., cancer chemotherapy in hematologic malignancies) to limit uric acid generation and prevent precipitation of urate crystals in renal tubules. Forced alkaline diuresis may also prevent or attenuate ARF in patients receiving high-dose methotrexate or suffering from rhabdomyolysis. *N*-acetylcysteine limits acetaminophen-induced renal injury if given within 24 h of ingestion. Dimercaprol, a chelating agent, may prevent heavy metal nephrotoxicity. Ethanol inhibits ethylene glycol metabolism to oxalic acid and other toxic metabolites and is an important adjunct to hemodialysis in the emergency management of ethylene glycol intoxication.

Specific Therapies By definition, prerenal ARF is rapidly reversible upon correction of the primary hemodynamic abnormality, and postrenal ARF resolves upon relief of obstruction. To date, there are no specific therapies for established intrinsic renal ARF due to ischemia or nephrotoxicity. Management of these disorders should focus on elimination of the causative hemodynamic abnormality or toxin, avoidance of additional insults, and prevention and treatment of complications. Specific treatment of other causes of intrinsic renal ARF depends on the underlying pathology.

PRERENAL ARF The composition of replacement fluids for treatment of prerenal ARF due to hypovolemia must be tailored according to the composition of the lost fluid. Severe hypovolemia due to hemorrhage should be corrected with packed red cells, whereas isotonic saline is usually appropriate replacement for mild to moderate hemorrhage or plasma loss (e.g., burns, pancreatitis). Urinary and gastrointestinal fluids can vary greatly in composition but are usually hypotonic. Hypotonic solutions (e.g., 0.45% saline) are usually recommended as initial replacement in patients with prerenal ARF due to increased urinary or gastrointestinal fluid losses, although isotonic saline may be more appropriate in severe cases. Subsequent therapy should be based on measurements of the volume and ionic content of excreted or drained fluids. Serum potassium and acid-base status should be monitored carefully, and potassium and bicarbonate supplemented as appropriate. Cardiac failure may require aggressive management with positive inotropes, preload and afterload reducing agents, antiarrhythmic drugs, and mechanical aids such as intraaortic balloon pumps. Invasive hemodynamic monitoring may be required to guide therapy for complications in patients in whom clinical assessment of cardiovascular function and intravascular volume is difficult.

Fluid management may be particularly challenging in patients with cirrhosis complicated by ascites. In this setting, it is important to distinguish between full-blown hepatorenal syndrome (Chap. 289), which carries a grave prognosis, and reversible ARF due to true or "effective" hypovolemia induced by overzealous use of diuretics or sepsis (e.g., spontaneous bacterial peritonitis). The contribution of hypovolemia to ARF can be definitively assessed only by administration of a fluid challenge. Fluids should be administered slowly and titrated against jugular venous pressure and, if necessary, central venous and pulmonary capillary wedge pressure, abdominal girth, and urine output. Patients with a reversible prerenal component typically have an increase in urine output and fall in serum creatinine, whereas patients with hepatorenal syndrome do not and may suffer increased ascites formation and pulmonary compromise if not monitored closely. Large volumes of ascitic fluid can usually be drained by paracentesis without deterioration in renal function if intravenous albumin is administered simultaneously. Indeed, "large-volume paracentesis" may afford an increase in GFR, possibly by lowering intraabdominal pressure and improving flow in renal veins. Shunting of ascitic fluid from the peritoneum to a central vein (peritoneojugular shunt, LeVeen or Denver shunts) is an alternative approach in refractory cases but has not been shown to improve survival in controlled trials. The efficacy of the newer technique of transjugular intrahepatic portosystemic shunting (TIPS procedure) is currently undergoing rigorous clinical assessment. Shunting can also improve GFR and sodium excretion transiently, probably because the increase in central blood volume stimulates release of atrial natriuretic peptides (ANPs) and inhibits secretion of aldosterone and norepinephrine.

INTRINSIC RENAL ARF Many different approaches have been tested for their ability to attenuate injury or hasten recovery in ischemic and nephrotoxic ARF. These include ANP, low-dose dopamine, endothelin antagonists, loop-blocking diuretics, calcium channel blockers, α-adrenoreceptor blockers, prostaglandin analogues, antioxidants, antibodies against leukocyte adhesion molecules, and insulin-like growth factor type I. Whereas many of these are beneficial in experimental models of ischemic or nephrotoxic ARF, they have either failed to confer consistent benefit or proved ineffective in humans.

ARF due to other intrinsic renal diseases such as acute glomerulonephritis or vasculitis may respond to glucocorticoids, alkylating agents, and/or plasmapheresis, depending on the primary pathology. Glucocorticoids also hasten remission in some cases of allergic interstitial nephritis. Aggressive control of systemic arterial pressure is of paramount importance in limiting renal injury in malignant hypertensive nephrosclerosis, toxemia of pregnancy, and other vascular diseases. Hypertension and ARF due to scleroderma may be exquisitely sensitive to treatment with ACE inhibitors.

POSTRENAL ARF Management of postrenal ARF requires close collaboration between nephrologist, urologist, and radiologist. Obstruction of the urethra or bladder neck is usually managed initially by transurethral or suprapubic placement of a bladder catheter, which provides temporary relief while the obstructing lesion is identified and treated definitively. Similarly, ureteric obstruction may be treated initially by percutaneous catheterization of the dilated renal pelvis or ureter. Indeed, obstructing lesions can often be removed percutaneously (e.g., calculus, sloughed papilla) or bypassed by insertion of a ureteric stent (e.g., carcinoma). Most patients experience an appropriate diuresis for several days following relief of obstruction. Approximately 5% of patients develop a transient salt-wasting syndrome that may require administration of intravenous saline to maintain blood pressure.

Supportive Measures (Table 260-4) Following correction of hypovolemia, salt and water intake are tailored to match losses. Hypervolemia can usually be managed by restriction of salt and water intake and diuretics. Indeed, there is, as yet, no proven rationale for administration of diuretics in ARF except to treat this complication. High doses of loop-blocking diuretics such as furosemide (up to 200 to 400 mg intravenously) or bumetanide (up to 10 mg intravenously administered as a bolus or by continuous infusion) may promote diuresis in patients who fail to respond to conventional doses. Despite the fact that subpressor doses of dopamine may transiently promote salt and water excretion by increasing renal blood flow and GFR and by inhibiting tubule sodium reabsorption, subpressor ("low-dose," "renal-dose,") dopamine has proved ineffective in clinical trials, may trigger arrythmias and sudden cardiac death in critically ill patients, and should not be used as a renoprotective agent in this setting. Ultrafiltration or dialysis is used to treat severe hypervolemia when conservative measures fail. Hyponatremia and hypoosmolality can usually be controlled by restriction of free water intake. Conversely, hypernatremia is treated by administration of water or intravenous hypotonic saline or isotonic dextrose-containing solutions. →*The management of hyperkalemia is described in Chap. 41.*

Metabolic acidosis is not usually treated unless serum bicarbonate concentration falls below 15 mmol/L or arterial pH falls below 7.2. More severe acidosis is corrected by oral or intravenous sodium bicarbonate. Initial rates of replacement are guided by estimates of bicarbonate deficit and adjusted thereafter according to serum levels (Chap. 42). Patients are monitored for complications of sodium bicarbonate administration such as hypervolemia, metabolic alkalosis, hypocalcemia, and hypokalemia. From a practical point of view, most patients requiring sodium bicarbonate need emergency dialysis within days. Hyperphosphatemia is usually controlled by restriction of dietary phosphate and by oral aluminum hydroxide or calcium carbonate, which reduce gastrointestinal absorption of phosphate. Hypocalcemia does not usually require treatment unless severe, as may occur with rhabdomyolysis or pancreatitis or following admininstration of bicarbonate. Hyperuricemia is typically mild [<890 μmol/L (< 15 mg/dL)] and does not require intervention.

The objective of *nutritional management* during the maintenance phase of ARF is to provide sufficient calories to avoid catabolism and starvation ketoacidosis, while minimizing production of nitrogenous

TABLE 260-4 *Management of Ischemic and Nephrotoxic Acute Renal Failure[a]*

Management Issue	Therapy
REVERSE CAUSATIVE RENAL INSULT	
Ischemic ARF	Restore systemic hemodynamics and renal perfusion
Nephrotoxic ARF	Eliminate nephrotoxins
	Consider specific measures (e.g., forced alkaline diuresis, chelators: see text)
PREVENTION AND TREATMENT OF COMPLICATIONS	
Intravascular volume overload	Salt (1–2 g/d) and water (usually <1 L/d) restriction
	Diuretics (usually loop blockers ± thiazide)
	Ultrafiltration or dialysis
Hyponatremia	Restriction of enteral free water intake (<1 L/d)
	Avoid hypotonic intravenous solutions (including dextrose solutions)
Hyperkalemia	Restriction of dietary K^+ intake (usually <40 mmol/d)
	Eliminate K^+ supplements and K^+-sparing diuretics
	Potassium-binding ion-exchange resins (e.g., sodium polystyrene sulphonate)
	Glucose (50 mL of 50% dextrose) and insulin (10 units regular)
	Sodium bicarbonate (usually 50–100 mmol)
	Calcium gluconate (10 mL of 10% solution over 5 min)
	Dialysis (with low K^+ dialysate)
Metabolic acidosis	Restriction of dietary protein (usually 0.6 g/kg per day of high biologic value)
	Sodium bicarbonate (maintain serum bicarbonate >15 mmol/L or arterial pH >7.2)
	Dialysis
Hyperphosphatemia	Restriction of dietary phosphate intake (usually <800 mg/d)
	Phosphate binding agents (calcium carbonate, aluminum hydroxide)
Hypocalcemia	Calcium carbonate (if symptomatic or if sodium bicarbonate to be administered)
	Calcium gluconate (10–20 mL of 10% solution)
Hypermagnesemia	Discontinue Mg^{2+}-containing antacids
Hyperuricemia	Treatment usually not necessary [if <890 μmol/L (<15 mg/dL)]
Nutrition	Restriction of dietary protein (~0.6 g/kg per day)
	Carbohydrate (~100 g/d)
	Enteral or parenteral nutrition (if recovery prolonged or patient very catabolic)
Indications for dialysis	Clinical evidence (symptoms or signs) of uremia
	Intractable intravascular volume overload
	Hyperkalemia or severe acidosis resistant to conservative measures
	?Prophylactic dialysis when urea >100–150 mg/dL or creatinine >8–10 mg/dL
PRESCRIBING OF MEDICATIONS	
Choice of agents	Avoid other nephrotoxins, ACE inhibitors, cyclooxygenase inhibitors, and radiocontrast unless absolute indication and no alternative agent
Drug dosing	Adjust doses and frequency of administration for degree of renal impairment

[a] These are general recommendations and must be tailored to needs of individual patients.

waste. This is best achieved by restricting dietary protein to approximately 0.6 g/kg per day of protein of high biologic value (i.e., rich in essential amino acids) and to provide most calories as carbohydrate (approximately 100 g daily). Nutritional management is easier in nonoliguric patients and following institution of dialysis. Vigorous parenteral hyperalimentation is claimed to improve prognosis; however, convincing benefit has yet to be demonstrated in controlled trials.

Anemia may necessitate blood transfusion if severe or if recovery is delayed. In contrast to chronic renal failure, recombinant human erythropoietin is rarely used in ARF because bone marrow resistance to erythropoietin is common, more immediate treatment of anemia (if any) is required, and renal failure is usually self-limiting. Uremic bleeding usually responds to correction of anemia, administration of desmopressin or estrogens, or dialysis. Regular doses of antacids appear to reduce the incidence of gastrointestinal hemorrhage significantly and may be more effective in this regard than H_2 antagonists or proton pump inhibitors. Meticulous care of intravenous cannulae, bladder catheters, and other invasive devices is mandatory to avoid infections. Unfortunately, prophylactic antibiotics have not been shown to reduce the incidence of infection in these high-risk patients.

INDICATIONS AND MODALITIES OF DIALYSIS (See also Chap. 262) Dialysis replaces renal function until regeneration and repair restore renal function. Hemodialysis and peritoneal dialysis appear equally effective for management of ARF. Thus, the dialysis modality is chosen according to the needs of individual patients (e.g., peritoneal dialysis may be preferable if the patient is hemodynamically unstable, and hemodialysis after abdominal surgery involving the peritoneum), the expertise of the nephrologist, and the facilities of the institution. Vascular access for conventional intermittent hemodialysis is best achieved by insertion of a temporary double-lumen hemodialysis catheter into the internal jugular vein. The subclavian and femoral veins are alternative access sites. Peritoneal dialysis is achieved by insertion of a cuffed catheter into the peritoneal cavity. Absolute indications for dialysis include symptoms or signs of the uremic syndrome and management of refractory hypervolemia, hyperkalemia, or acidosis. Most nephrologists also initiate dialysis empirically for blood urea levels of >100 mg/dL, even in the absence of clinical uremia; however, this approach has yet to be validated in controlled clinical trials. Recent evidence suggests that more intensive hemodialysis (e.g., daily rather than alternate-day intermittent dialysis) is clinically superior and confers improved survival in ARF once dialysis is required. This conclusion may not be as intuitive as it first appears as dialysis itself has been postulated to prolong the period of oliguria in some cases by inducing hypotension and further renal ischemia and through activation of leukocytes on the dialysis membrane, which may then proceed to aggravate renal injury.

Continuous renal replacement therapies (CRRTs) are alternatives to conventional intermittent hemodialysis techniques for treatment of ARF. They are particularly valuable techniques in patients in whom intermittent hemodialysis fails to control hypervolemia or uremia and for those who do not tolerate intermittent hemodialysis and in whom peritoneal dialysis is not possible. Continuous arteriovenous hemodiafiltration (CAVHD) requires both arterial and venous access. The patient's own blood pressure generates an ultrafiltrate of plasma across a porous biocompatible dialysis membrane. A physiologic crystalloid solution is passed along the other side of the membrane to achieve diffusive clearance. Continuous venovenous hemodiafiltration (CVVHD), in contrast, requires only a double-lumen venous catheter as a blood pump generates ultrafiltration pressure across the dialysis membrane. In the more simple techniques of continuous arteriovenous hemofiltration (CAVH) and continuous venovenous hemofiltration (CVVH) the dialysis step is eliminated and an ultrafiltrate of plasma is removed across the dialysis membrane and replaced by a physiologic crystalloid solution. The bulk of evidence to date suggests that intermittent and continuous dialytic therapies are equally effective in the context of ARF. The choice of technique is currently tailored to the specific needs of the patient, the resources of the institution, and the expertise of the physician. Potential disadvantages of continuous hemodialysis techniques are the need for prolonged immobilization in bed, systemic anticoagulation, arterial cannulation (in CAVH), and prolonged exposure of blood to synthetic, albeit relatively biocompatible, dialysis membranes.

The mortality rate among patients with ARF approximates 50% and has changed little over the past 30 years. It should be stressed, however, that patients usually die from sequelae of the primary illness that induced ARF and not from ARF itself. Indeed, the kidney is one of the few organs whose function can be replaced artificially (i.e., by dialysis) for protracted periods of time. In agreement with this interpretation, mortality rates vary greatly depending on the cause of ARF: ~15% in obstetric patients, ~30% in toxin-related ARF, and ~60% following trauma or major surgery. Oliguria (<400 mL/d) at time of presentation and a rise in serum creatinine of >265 μmol/L (>3 mg/dL) are associated with a poor prognosis and probably reflect the severity of renal injury and of the primary illness. Mortality rates are higher in older debilitated patients and in those with multiple organ failure. Most patients who survive an episode of ARF recover sufficient renal function to live normal lives. However, 50% have subclinical impairment of renal function or residual scarring on renal biopsy. Approximately 5% of patients never recover function and require long-

term renal replacement with dialysis or transplantation. An additional 5% suffer progressive decline in GFR, following an initial recovery phase, probably due to hemodynamic stress and sclerosis of remnant glomeruli (Chap. 264).

FURTHER READING

BRADY HR et al: Acute renal failure, in *Brenner and Rector's The Kidney*, 7th ed., BM Brenner (ed). Philadelphia, Saunders, 2004

DAUGIRDAS JT et al: (eds): *Handbook of Dialysis*. New York, Little, Brown, 2001

DENTON MD et al: "Renal-dose" dopamine for the treatment of acute renal failure: Scientific rationale, experimental studies and clinical trials. Kidney Int 49:4, 1996

RONCO C et al: Effect of different doses of continuous veno-venous haemofiltration on outcomes of acute renal failure: A prospective randomised trial. Lancet 355:26, 2000

SCHIFFL H et al: Daily hemodialysis and the outcome of acute renal failure. N Engl J Med 346:305; 2002

261 CHRONIC RENAL FAILURE
Karl Skorecki, Jacob Green,[†] Barry M. Brenner

MECHANISMS OF CHRONIC RENAL FAILURE

DEFINITIONS *Chronic renal disease* (CRD) is a pathophysiologic process with multiple etiologies, resulting in the inexorable attrition of nephron number and function and frequently leading to *end-stage renal disease* (ESRD). In turn, ESRD represents a clinical state or condition in which there has been an irreversible loss of endogenous renal function, of a degree sufficient to render the patient permanently dependent upon renal replacement therapy (dialysis or transplantation) in order to avoid life-threatening *uremia*. Uremia is the clinical and laboratory syndrome, reflecting dysfunction of all organ systems as a result of untreated or undertreated acute or chronic renal failure. Given the capacity of the kidneys to regain function following acute injury (Chap. 260), the vast majority (>90%) of patients with ESRD have reached this state as a result of CRD.

PATHOPHYSIOLOGY OF CRD (See also Chap. 259) The pathophysiology of CRD involves initiating mechanisms specific to the underlying etiology as well as a set of progressive mechanisms that are a common consequence following long-term reduction of renal mass, irrespective of etiology. Such reduction of renal mass causes structural and functional hypertrophy of surviving nephrons. This compensatory hypertrophy is mediated by vasoactive molecules, cytokines, and growth factors and is due initially to adaptive hyperfiltration, in turn mediated by increases in glomerular capillary pressure and flow. Eventually, these short-term adaptations prove maladaptive, in that they predispose to sclerosis of the remaining viable nephron population. Increased intrarenal activity of the renin-angiotensin axis appears to contribute both to the initial adaptive hyperfiltration and to the subsequent maladaptive hypertrophy and sclerosis.

The definition of CRD requires that the pathophysiologic process described above last more than 3 months. A recently widely accepted international classification divides CRD into a number of stages (Table 261-1) defined by clinical estimation of the glomerular filtration rate (GFR). These stages help guide clinical diagnostic and management approaches. First, it is important to identify factors that increase the risk for CRD, even in individuals with normal GFR. Such factors include family history of heritable renal disease, hypertension, diabetes, autoimmune disease, older age, past episode of acute renal failure, and current evidence of kidney damage with normal or even

increased GFR. Such evidence of kidney damage in the face of normal or increased GFR places affected individuals into stage 1 CRD and includes proteinuria, abnormal urinary sediment, or urinary tract structural abnormalities (e.g., vesicoureteric reflux) evident on imaging studies. Even at this stage, when baseline GFR is normal, there is often a characteristic loss of renal reserve. This early stage is particularly well documented in diabetic nephropathy. Further stages in the pathogenesis of CRD are characterized by a progressive decline in estimated GFR with mild, moderate, and severe stages defined at GFR levels (mL/min per 1.73 m²) of 60 to 89, 30 to 59, and 15 to 29, respectively. At a GFR < 15 mL/min per 1.73 m², renal replacement therapy may be indicated if uremia is present. For purposes of staging CRD, current guidelines recommend estimating GFR using one of the two equations shown in Table 261-2, based on measured plasma creatinine concentration, age, gender, and ethnic origin. The normal annual mean decline in GFR with age beginning at age 20 to 30 years is 1 mL/min per 1.73 m², reaching a mean value in males of 70 at age 70. GFR is slightly lower in women than men. By the time plasma creatinine concentration is even mildly elevated, substantial chronic nephron injury has already occurred.

Albuminuria serves as a key adjunctive tool for monitoring nephron injury and response to therapy in many forms of CRD. Current guidelines recommend use of albumin-specific dipstick measurement or quantitation by measurement of albumin-to-creatinine ratio in a spot first morning urine sample. Persistence of >17 mg albumin per gram of creatinine in adult males and 25 mg albumin per gram of creatinine in adult females usually signifies chronic renal damage, irrespective of GFR, and can be followed in monitoring natural history and response to therapy, especially in CRD consequent to diabetes, hypertension, or glomerulonephritis. →*Further considerations in the overall clinical approach to proteinuria are provided in Chap. 40.*

During stages 1 and 2 CRD, patients often remain free of symp-

TABLE 261-1 *Stages of Chronic Renal Disease CRD*

Stage	Description	GFR, mL/min per 1.73 m²
	At increased risk	90 (with CRD risk factors)
1	Kidney damage with normal or increased GFR	90
2	Kidney damage with mildly decreased GFR	60–89
3	Moderately decreased GFR	30–59
4	Severely decreased GFR	15–29
5	Renal failure	<15 (or dialysis)

Note: GFR, glomerular filtration rate.
Source: Adapted from Levey, with permission.

†Deceased

TABLE 261-2 *Recommended Equations for Estimation of Glomerular Filtration Rate (GFR) from Laboratory-Validated Plasma Creatinine Concentration (P_{Cr})*

1. Equation from the Modification of Diet in Renal Disease study[a]
   Estimated GFR (mL/min per 1.73 m²) = $1.86 \times (P_{Cr})^{-1.154} \times (age)^{-0.203}$
      Multiply by 0.742 for women
      Multiply by 1.21 for African Americans
2. Cockcroft-Gault equation
   Estimated creatinine clearance (mL/min) =
   $$\frac{(140 - age) \times body\ weight\ (kg)}{72 \times P_{Cr}\ (mg/dL)}$$
      Multiply by 0.85 for women

[a] Equation is *available* in hand-held calculators and in tabular form.
Source: Adapted from Levey, with permission.

TABLE 261-3 *Summary of Clinical Presentations That may Suggest Given Major Categories of Causes of Chronic Renal Disease*

Cause	Clinical Presentation
Diabetic kidney disease	History of diabetes, proteinuria, retinopathy
Hypertension	Elevated blood pressure, normal urinalysis, family history.
Nondiabetic glomerular disease	Nephritic or nephrotic presentations (Chap. 264)
Cystic kidney disease	Urinary tract symptoms, abnormal urinary sediment, radiologic imaging abnormalities
Tubulointerstitial disease	History of urinary tract infections and reflux, chronic medication and drug exposure, abnormalities in urinary tract imaging, tubular syndromes including urine-concentrating defect, abnormal urinalysis

Source: Adapted from Levey, with permission.

toms, other than those that might accompany the underlying etiologic process causing renal disease. As the decline in GFR progresses to stages 3 and 4 (GFR < 60 mL/min per 1.73 m²), clinical and laboratory complications of CRD become progressively more prominent. Virtually all organ systems are affected, but the most evident complications include anemia and loss of energy; decreasing appetite and disturbances in nutritional status; abnormalities in calcium and phosphorus metabolism accompanied by metabolic bone disease; and abnormalities in sodium, water, potassium, and acid-base homeostasis. When GFR falls to <15 mL/min per 1.73 m², patients usually experience a severe disturbance in their activities of daily living, sense of well-being, nutritional status, and water and electrolyte homeostasis, eventuating in an overtly uremic state wherein continued survival without renal replacement therapy becomes impossible.

ETIOLOGY AND EPIDEMIOLOGY It has been estimated that at least 6% of the adult U.S. population have chronic renal damage with a GFR > 60 mL/min per 1.73 m² (stages 1 and 2 CRD) and hence are at imminent risk of a progressive further decline in GFR. An additional ~4.5% of the U.S. population are in stages 3 and 4 CRD. Diabetic and hypertensive nephropathy are the leading underlying etiologies of both CRD and ESRD. Hypertension is a particularly common cause and consequence of CRD in the elderly, in whom chronic renal ischemia due to renovascular disease may be an underrecognized additional contribution to the pathophysiologic process. It should be noted that cardiovascular mortality precludes most patients with CRD from reaching the stage of ESRD. Identification of CRD as a major risk factor for cardiovascular morbidity and mortality, and the expectation of effective interventions to diminish premature cardiovascular mortality, and increasing longevity overall, will increase the cohort of patients reaching ESRD.

Although the clinical manifestations of the declining GFR per se dominate the clinical presentation in all forms of CRD, in many cases the underlying etiology can be presumed from associated additional clinical information (Table 261-3).

GENETIC CONSIDERATIONS Disorders with clear-cut monogenic inheritance comprise a small but important component among the etiologies of CRD. Among these, autosomal dominant polycystic kidney disease is the most common on a world-wide basis (Chap. 265). Alport's hereditary nephritis (Chap. 264) is a less common cause of both benign hematuria without progression to CRD and more severe nephron injury with progression to ESRD, and it most often displays an X-linked pattern of inheritance. Several genetic loci have been identified that encode important components of the glomerular podocyte-associated filtration barrier, and mutations in these genes cause inherited forms of focal segmental glomerular sclerosis with glucocorticoid nonresponsive nephrotic syndrome and progression to ESRD. Nephronopthisis, medullary cystic kidney disease, and Fabry's disease are among other rare causes of progressive CRD with monogenic inheritance based on well-characterized genetic loci. In contrast, the two most common etiologies of CRD, diabetes mellitus (both types

1 and 2) and essential hypertension, display complex polygenic patterns of inheritance.

The striking interindividual variability in the rate of progression to ESRD has an important heritable component, and a number of genetic loci that contribute to the progression of CRD have been identified. Most extensively studied has been an insertion/deletion polymorphism of the angiotensin-converting enzyme (ACE) gene. The homozygous deletion (D/D) variant is associated with the highest expression of endogenous ACE activity and a greater risk of CRD progression. This finding leads to the prediction that ACE inhibitor therapy might be most effective in patients who are homozygous for the "at-risk" allele. Similar conclusions have been reached with respect to genes encoding other components of the renin-angiotensin axis. More recent studies of genetic association with renal failure progression have focused on a region of human chromosome 10, homologous to a well-characterized rodent renal failure susceptibility gene (Rf1).

PATHOPHYSIOLOGY AND BIOCHEMISTRY OF UREMIA *Azotemia* refers to the retention of nitrogenous waste products as renal insufficiency develops. *Uremia* refers to the more advanced stages of progressive renal insufficiency when the complex, multiorgan system derangements become clinically manifest.

Although not the major cause of overt uremic toxicity, urea may contribute to some of the clinical abnormalities, including anorexia, malaise, vomiting, and headache. Additional categories of nitrogenous excretory products include guanido compounds, urates and hippurates, end products of nucleic acid metabolism, polyamines, myoinositol, phenols, benzoates, and indoles, among others. Nitrogenous compounds with a molecular mass of 500 to 12,000 Da (so-called middle molecules) are also retained in CRD and similarly are believed to contribute to morbidity and mortality in uremic subjects. However, uremia involves more than renal excretory failure alone. A host of metabolic and endocrine functions normally subserved by the kidney are also impaired, resulting in anemia; malnutrition; impaired metabolism of carbohydrates, fats, and proteins; defective utilization of energy; and metabolic bone disease. Furthermore, plasma levels of many polypeptide hormones, including parathyroid hormone (PTH), insulin, glucagon, luteinizing hormone, and prolactin, rise with renal failure, not only because of impaired renal catabolism but also because of enhanced endocrine secretion, occurring as a secondary consequence of primary excretory or synthetic renal dysfynction. On the other hand, the renal production of erythropoietin (EPO) and 1,25-dihydroxycholecalciferol is impaired. Thus, the pathophysiology of the uremic syndrome can be divided into two sets of abnormalities: (1) those consequent to the accumulation of products of protein metabolism; and (2) those consequent to the loss of other renal functions, such as fluid and electrolyte homeostasis and hormonal abnormalities.

Uremia leads to disturbances in the function of every organ system. Chronic dialysis (Chap. 262) reduces the incidence and severity of these disturbances, so that, where modern medicine is practiced, the overt and florid manifestations of uremia have largely disappeared. Unfortunately, as indicated in Table 261-4, even optimal dialysis therapy is not a panacea, because some disturbances resulting from impaired renal function fail to respond fully, while others continue to progress.

FLUID, ELECTROLYTE, AND ACID-BASE DISORDERS (See also Chaps. 41, 42, and 259) ■ Sodium and Water Homeostasis

In most patients with stable CRD, the total body contents of Na^+ and H_2O are increased modestly, although this may not be clinically apparent. The underlying etiologic disease process may itself disrupt glomerulotubular balance and promote Na^+ retention (e.g., glomerulonephritis), or excessive Na^+ ingestion may lead to cumulative positive Na^+ balance and attendant extracellular fluid volume (ECFV) expansion. Such ECFV expansion contributes to hypertension, which in turn accelerates further the progression of nephron injury. As long as water intake does not exceed the capacity for free water clearance, the ECFV expansion will be isotonic and the patient will remain normonatremic. Hyponatremia is an uncommon complication in predialysis patients, and water restriction is only necessary when hyponatremia is documented. Weight gain usually associated with volume expansion may be offset in patients with CRD by concomitant loss of lean body mass. In the CRD patient who is not yet on dialysis but has clear evidence of ECFV expansion, administration of loop diuretics coupled with restriction of salt intake are the mainstays of therapy. It should be noted that resistance to loop diuretics in renal failure often mandates use of higher doses than those usually used when GFR is well preserved. The combination of loop diuretics with metalozone, which inhibits the Na^+Cl^- cotransporter of the distal convoluted tubule, can sometimes overcome diuretic resistance. When the GFR falls to <5 to 10 mL/min per 1.73 m^2, even high doses of combination diuretics are ineffective. ECFV expansion under these circumstances usually means that dialysis is indicated.

Patients with CRD also have impaired renal mechanisms for conserving Na^+ and H_2O (Chap. 259). When an *extrarenal* cause for fluid loss is present (e.g., vomiting, diarrhea, sweating, fever), these patients are prone to volume depletion. Depletion of ECFV may compromise residual renal function with resulting signs and symptoms of overt uremia. Because of impaired renal Na^+ and H_2O conservation, the usual indices of prerenal azotemia (oliguria, high urine osmolality, low urinary Na^+ concentration, and low fractional excretion of Na^+) are not useful. Cautious volume repletion, usually with normal saline, returns ECFV to normal and usually restores renal function to prior levels.

Potassium Homeostasis (See also Chap. 41)

In CRD, the decline in GFR is not necessarily accompanied by a concomitant and proportionate decline in urinary K^+ excretion. In addition, K^+ excretion in the gastrointestinal tract is augmented in patients with CRD. However, hyperkalemia may be precipitated in a number of clinical situations, including constipation, augmented dietary intake, protein catabolism, hemolysis, hemorrhage, transfusion of stored red blood cells, metabolic acidosis, and following the exposure to a variety of medications that inhibit K^+ entry into cells or K^+ secretion in the distal nephron. Most commonly encountered medications in this regard are beta blockers, ACE inhibitors and angiotensin receptor blockers, K^+-sparing diuretics (amiloride, triamterene, spironolactone), and nonsteroidal anti-inflammatory drugs (NSAIDs). In addition, certain etiologies of CRD may be associated with earlier and more severe disruption of K^+ secretory mechanisms in the distal nephron, relative to the reduction in GFR. Most important are conditions associated with hyporeninemic hypoaldosteronism (e.g., diabetic nephropathy and certain forms of distal renal tubular acidosis; Chaps. 264 and 265).

Hypokalemia is uncommon in CRD and usually reflects markedly reduced dietary K^+ intake, in association with excessive diuretic therapy or gastrointestinal losses. Hypokalemia occurs as a result of primary renal K^+ wasting in association with other solute transport abnormalities, as in Fanconi's syndrome, renal tubular acidosis, or other forms of hereditary or acquired tubulointerstitial diseases. However, even under these circumstances, as GFR declines, the tendency

---

TABLE 261-4   Clinical Abnormalities in Uremia[a]

Fluid and electrolyte disturbances	Neuromuscular disturbances	Dermatologic disturbances
Volume expansion and contraction (I)	Fatigue (I)[b]	Pallor (I)[b]
Hypernatremia and hyponatremia (I)	Sleep disorders (P)	Hyperpigmentation (I, P, or D)
Hyperkalemia and hypokalemia (I)	Headache (I or P)	Pruritus (P)
Metabolic acidosis (I)	Impaired mentation (I)[b]	Ecchymoses (I)
Hyperphosphatemia (I)	Lethargy (I)[b]	Uremic frost (I)
Hypocalcemia (I)	Asterixis (I)	
	Muscular irritability (I)	**Gastrointestinal disturbances**
Endocrine-metabolic disturbances	Peripheral neuropathy (I or P)	Anorexia (I)
Secondary hyperparathyroidism (I or P)	Restless legs syndrome (I or P)	Nausea and vomiting (I)
Adynamic osteomalacia (D)	Paralysis (I or P)	Uremic fetor (I)
Vitamin D–deficient osteomalacia (I)	Myoclonus (I)	Gastroenteritis (I)
Carbohydrate intolerance (I)	Seizures (I or P)	Peptic ulcer (I or P)
Hyperuricemia (I or P)	Coma (I)	Gastrointestinal bleeding (I, P, or D)
Hypertriglyceridemia (I or P)	Muscle cramps (P or D)	Hepatitis (D)
Increased Lp(a) level (P)	Dialysis disequilibrium syndrome (D)	Idiopathic ascites (D)
Decreased high-density lipoprotein level (P)	Myopathy (P or D)	Peritonitis (D)
Protein-energy malnutrition (I or P)		
Impaired growth and development (P)	**Cardiovascular and pulmonary disturbances**	**Hematologic and immunologic disturbances**
Infertility and sexual dysfunction (P)	Arterial hypertension (I or P)	Anemia (I)[b]
Amenorrhea (P)	Congestive heart failure or pulmonary edema (I)	Lymphocytopenia (P)
Hypothermia (I)	Pericarditis (I)	Bleeding diathesis (I or D)[b]
β_2-Microglobulin deposition (P or D)	Cardiomyopathy (I or P)	Increased susceptibility to infection (I or P)
Associated amyloidosis (P)	Uremic lung (I)	Splenomegaly and hypersplenism (P)
	Accelerated atherosclerosis (P or D)	Leukopenia (D)
	Hypotension and arrhythmias (D)	Hypocomplementemia (D)
	Vascular calcification (P or D)	

[a] Virtually all abnormalities in this table are completely reversed in time by successful renal transplantation. The response of these abnormalities to hemodialysis or peritoneal dialysis therapy is more variable. (I) denotes an abnormality that usually improves with an optimal program of dialysis and related therapy; (P) denotes an abnormality that tends to persist or even progress, despite an optimal program; (D) denotes an abnormality that develops only after initiation of dialysis therapy.
[b] Improves with dialysis and erythropoietin therapy.
Note: Lp(a), lipoprotein A.

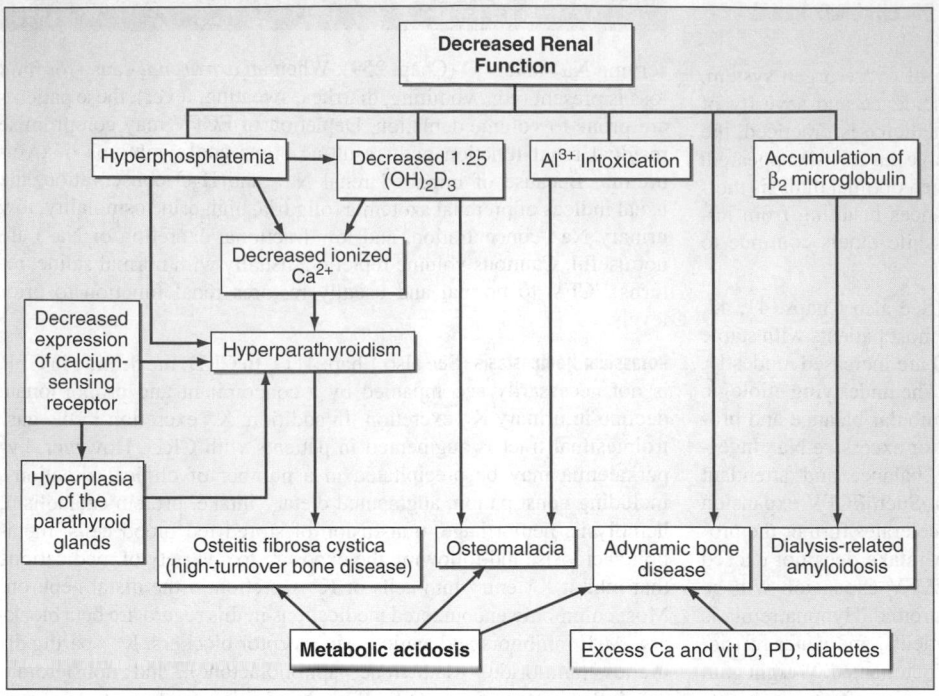

FIGURE 261-1   Flowchart for the development of bone, phosphate, and calcium abnormalities in chronic renal disease. (PD, peritoneal dialysis).

to hypokalemia diminishes and hyperkalemia may supervene. Accordingly, K^+ supplementation and K^+-sparing diuretics should generally be avoided as GFR declines.

Metabolic Acidosis (See also Chap. 42)   Acidosis is a common disturbance during the advanced stages of CRD. Although in a majority of patients with CRD the urine can be acidified normally, these patients have a reduced ability to produce ammonia. Hyperkalemia further depresses urinary ammonium excretion. The combination of hyperkalemia and hyperchloremic metabolic acidosis (known as type IV renal tubular acidosis, or hyporeninemic hypoaldosteronism) is most characteristically seen in patients with diabetes or in those with predominantly tubulointerstitial disease. Treatment of the hyperkalemia frequently improves the acidosis as well.

With advancing renal failure, total urinary net daily acid excretion is usually limited to 30 to 40 mmol, and an anion gap of ~20 mmol/L with a reciprocal fall in plasma $[HCO_3^-]$ may develop. In most patients, the metabolic acidosis is mild; the pH is rarely <7.35 and can usually be corrected by treating the patient with 20 to 30 mmol of $NaHCO_3$ or sodium citrate daily. However, the concomitant Na^+ load mandates careful attention to volume status and the potential need for diuretic agents. Also, citrate enhances aluminum absorption in the large bowel, and citrate-containing agents should be avoided if aluminum-containing drugs are also administered. Severe symptomatic manifestations of acid-base imbalance may occur when the patient is challenged with an excessive endogenous or exogenous acid load or loses excessive alkali (e.g., with diarrhea).

℞ TREATMENT

Adjustments in dietary intake and use of loop diuretics, occasionally in combination with metalozone, may be needed to maintain salt and hence extracellular fluid volume balance. In contrast, overzealous salt restriction and diuretic use may cause hypovolemia and precipitate a further decline in GFR. Occasional patients with salt-wasting states need to be given sodium-rich diets or sodium supplements. Water restriction is indicated only if there is a demonstrated propensity to hyponatremia. Intractable ECFV expansion, despite dietary restriction and diuretic use, indicates the need to initiate renal replacement therapy. Hyperkalemia often responds to dietary restriction of potassium, avoidance of potassium-containing or -retaining medications, and to

the use of diuretics if they are also indicated for management of sodium balance. Many salt substitutes contain potassium instead of sodium, and patients with CRD seeking to avoid sodium should be cautioned accordingly as part of their dietary counseling. Potassium-binding resins taken with cathartics can promote gastrointestinal potassium losses and thus are useful as temporizing measures in the treatment or avoidance of hyperkalemia in CRD patients. However, the need for such treatment over a prolonged period, in the absence of other reversible causes of hyperkalemia, usually signifies the need to initiate renal replacement therapy.

BONE DISEASE AND DISORDERS OF CALCIUM AND PHOSPHATE METABOLISM (Fig. 261-1; see also Chaps. 331 and 332)   The major disorders of bone disease in CRD can be classified into those associated with high bone turnover and high PTH levels (including osteitis fibrosa, the hallmark lesion of secondary hyperparathyroidism) and low bone turnover with low or normal PTH levels (osteomalacia and adynamic bone disease).

The pathophysiology of bone disease due to secondary hyperparathyroidism is related to abnormal mineral metabolism. (1) Decreased GFR leads to reduced inorganic phosphate (PO_4^{3-}) excretion and consequent PO_4^{3-} retention, (2) retained PO_4^{3-} has a direct stimulatory effect on PTH synthesis and on cellular mass of the parathyroid glands, (3) retained PO_4^{3-} also indirectly causes excessive production and secretion of PTH through lowering of ionized Ca^{2+} and by suppression of calcitriol (1,25-dihydroxycholecalciferol) production, and (4) reduced calcitriol production in CRD results both from decreased synthesis due to reduced kidney mass and from hyperphosphatemia. Low calcitriol levels, in turn, lead to hyperparathyroidism via both direct and indirect mechanisms. Calcitriol is known to have a direct suppressive effect on PTH transcription (i.e., a genomic effect), and therefore reduced calcitriol in CRD causes elevated levels of PTH. In addition, reduced calcitriol leads to impaired Ca^{2+} absorption from the gastrointestinal tract, thereby leading to hypocalcemia, which then increases PTH secretion and production. Taken together, hyperphosphatemia, hypocalcemia, and reduced calcitriol synthesis all promote the production of PTH and the proliferation of parathyroid cells, resulting in secondary hyperparathyroidism.

In addition to excessive release of PTH from individual parathyroid cells, the mass of parathyroid cells increases progressively with CRD. Excessive parathyroid gland cellular mass may assume one of the following patterns: (1) diffuse hyperplasia (polyclonal), (2) nodular growth (monoclonal) within diffuse hyperplastic tissue, or (3) diffuse monoclonal hyperplasia ("adenoma" or tertiary autonomous hyperparathyroidism). Patients with monoclonal ("autonomous") hyperplasia are especially prone to develop hypercalcemia following successful kidney transplantation, often necessitating parathyroidectomy. High PTH levels stimulate osteoblasts and result in high bone turnover, which leads to *osteitis fibrosa cystica*. The latter is characterized by irregularly woven abnormal osteoid, fibrosis, and cyst formation, which result in decreased cortical bone and bone strength and an increased risk of fracture.

Low-turnover bone disease can be classified into two categories—osteomalalcia and adynamic bone disease. Both lesions are characterized by a reduced number of osteoclasts and osteoblasts and decreased activity of the latter. In *osteomalacia* there is an accumulation of unmineralized bone matrix, or increased osteoid volume, which may be caused by vitamin D deficiency, excess aluminum deposition, or metabolic acidosis. Adynamic bone disease is now recognized to be as prevalent as the hyperparathyroid bone lesion in patients with CRD and ESRD, and is especially common among diabetic patients. *Adynamic bone disease* is characterized by reduced bone volume and mineralization and may result in part from excessive suppression of PTH production with calcitriol treatment or, currently less common, from aluminium exposure.

Irrespective of the cause for skeletal abnormalities in CRD, bone disease can lead to pain, increased incidence of fractures, and severe incapacity. Bone fractures complicate both the high- and low-turnover types of bone disease, and it is now appreciated that patients with adynamic bone may be more predisposed to fractures than those with osteitis fibrosa cystica. In the latter disorder, however, a PTH-associated proximal myopathy often coexists, giving rise to gait abnormalities and impaired ambulation.

Other Complications of Abnormal Calcium-Phosphate Product Metabolism

In addition to abnormalities in bone metabolism, abnormal calcium-phosphate product metabolism may lead to *calciphylaxis*, i.e., extraosseous ("metastatic") calcification of soft tissue and blood vessels. Electron beam computed tomography in patients with CRD has revealed highly elevated coronary calcification scores, which likely represent a major factor in the predisposition to occlusive coronary vascular disease in the CRD and ESRD populations. The pathogenesis remains unclear, but hyperphosphatemia, hypercalcemia, elevated calcium-phosphate product, and increased PTH levels are all thought to contribute to this process. Calciphylaxis represents a severe and systemic form of vascular and soft tissue calcium-phosphate product deposition associated with skin and soft tissue necrosis, which can lead to extremity loss.

℞ TREATMENT

Secondary hyperparathyroidism and osteitis fibrosa are best prevented and treated by reducing the plasma PO_4^{3-} concentration through the use of a phosphate-restricted diet as well as oral phosphate-binding agents. Calcium carbonate and calcium acetate are useful phosphate-binding agents. Sevelamer, a nonabsorbable, non-calcium-containing polymer has been recently added to the phosphate-lowering armamentarium. It has an advantage over the calcium-based phosphate chelating agents in that it does not predispose CRD patients to hypercalcemia and attenuates calcium deposition in the coronary arteries and aorta.

Daily oral calcitriol, or intermittent oral or intravenous pulses, appears to exert a direct suppressive effect on PTH secretion, in addition to the indirect effect mediated through raising plasma Ca^{2+} concentration. The use of calcitriol and calcium preparations in the predialysis population must take into account potential effects of increased PO_4^{3-} and Ca^{2+} on the rate of progression of CRD. The recommended target plasma PO_4^{3-} concentration is approximately 1.4 mmol/L (4.5 mg/dL), with a corresponding plasma Ca^{2+} concentration of approximately 2.5 mmol/L (10 mg/dL) in an attempt to suppress parathyroid hyperplasia, thus avoiding or reversing osteitis fibrosa cystica, osteomalacia, and myopathy. It is particularly important to maintain the calcium-phosphate product in the normal range to avoid metastatic calcification. Recognition of the role of the extracellular calcium–sensing receptor has led to the development of calcimimetic agents that enhance the sensitivity to Ca^{2+}-suppressive effects on PTH secretion. The first-generation calcimimetic agent tested produced a dose-dependent reduction in PTH and plasma Ca^{2+} concentration, and subsequent formulations with improved pharmacokinetic profiles show great promise as effective and safe treatments for secondary hyperparathyroidism. However, since adynamic bone disease is often a consequence of overzealous treatment of secondary hyperparathyroidism, suppression of PTH levels to <120 pg/mL in CRD patients may not be desirable.

The incidence of aluminum-induced osteomalacia has been greatly reduced with the recognition of aluminum as the principal culprit. Therapy for this disorder is based on the complete cessation of the use of aluminum combined with the use of a chelating agent such as deferoxamine.

Management of metabolic acidosis should aim to maintain a nearly normal level of plasma bicarbonate with the administration of calcium acetate or calcium carbonate, with the addition of sodium bicarbonate (limited by considerations of sodium load) if necessary. Excessive administration of alkali should be avoided to minimize risk of urinary precipitation of Ca^{2+} phosphate.

CARDIOVASCULAR ABNORMALITIES

Cardiovascular disease is the leading cause of morbidity and mortality in patients with CRD at all stages. Estimates of the increase in cardiovascular disease risk attributable to CRD range from 10- to 200-fold, depending on the stage of CRD, other risk factors, and comorbid conditions. Between 30 and 45% of patients reaching ESRD already have advanced cardiovascular complications. Thus the management of patients with CRD should emphasize prevention of cardiovascular complications as well as measures aimed at alleviating the progression and complications of CRD itself.

Ischemic Cardiovascular Disease

CRD at all stages constitutes a major risk factor for ischemic cardiovascular disease, including occlusive coronary heart, cerebrovascular, and peripheral vascular diseases. Increased prevalence of coronary heart disease in CRD derives from both traditional ("classic") and CRD-related ("nontraditional") risk factors. The former include hypertension (see below), hypervolemia, dyslipidemia, sympathetic overactivity, and hyperhomocysteinemia. The CRD-related risks include anemia, hyperphosphatemia, hyperparathyroidism, and a state of "microinflammation" that can be found at all stages of CRD but is undoubtedly aggravated by dialysis. The inflammatory state elicits a rise in acute-phase reactants such as interleukin 6 and C-reactive protein, which contribute to the coronary occlusive process and are predictors of cardiovascular disease risk. Other abnormalities augment myocardial ischemia. These include reduced myocardial tolerance to ischemia due to left ventricular hypertrophy (see below) and microvascular disease. Also, coronary reserve, defined as the increase in coronary blood flow in response to greater demand, is attenuated. Nitric oxide is an important mediator for vascular dilatation. Its availability in CRD is decreased because of increased concentrations of asymmetric dimethyl-l-arginine, even at early stages of CRD, and also because nitric oxide is scavenged by reactive oxygen species. In addition, coronary arteriolar hypertrophy/hyperplasia limits vasodilatory capacity.

Congestive Heart Failure (See also Chap. 216)

Abnormal cardiac function secondary to myocardial ischemic disease and/or left ventricular hypertrophy, together with salt and water retention in uremia, often result in congestive heart failure and/or pulmonary edema. A unique form of pulmonary congestion and edema may occur even in the absence of volume overload and is associated with normal or mildly elevated intracardiac and pulmonary capillary wedge pressures. This entity, characterized radiologically by peripheral vascular congestion giving rise to a "butterfly wing" distribution, is due to increased permeability of alveolar capillary membranes. This "low-pressure" pulmonary edema as well as cardiopulmonary abnormalities associated with circulatory overload usually respond promptly to vigorous dialysis.

Hypertension and Left Ventricular Hypertrophy (See also Chap. 230)

Hypertension is the most common complication of CRD and ESRD. It may develop early during the course of CRD and is associated with adverse outcomes—in particular, more rapid loss of renal function and development of cardiovascular disease. Numerous epidemiologic studies and clinical trials have shown a relationship between the level of blood pressure and rate of progression of diabetic and non-diabetic kidney disease (see below).

Administration of EPO (p. 1658) may raise blood pressure and increase the requirement for antihypertensive drugs in CRD patients. Left ventricular hypertrophy and dilated cardiomyopathy are among the most ominous risk factors for excess cardiovascular morbidity and mortality in patients with CRD and ESRD and are thought to be related primarily to prolonged hypertension and ECFV overload. In addition, anemia and the surgical placement of an arteriovenous anastomosis for future or ongoing dialysis access may generate a high cardiac output state and pulmonary hypertension, which also intensify the burden placed on the left ventricle. *Absence* of hypertension may signify the presence of a salt-wasting form of renal disease (e.g., medullary cystic disease, chronic tubulointerstitial disease, or papillary necrosis), ongoing antihypertensive therapy, volume-depletion due to gastrointestinal causes or diuretic therapy, or reduced cardiac index.

Since volume overload is the major cause of hypertension in uremia, the normotensive state can often be restored by appropriate (not overzealous) use of salt restriction and natriuretic drugs or ultrafiltration in the dialysis setting. Nevertheless, because of hyperreninemia and other disturbances in renal vasoconstrictors and vasodilators, some patients remain hypertensive despite rigorous salt and water restriction and ultrafiltration. Rarely, such patients may develop accelerated or malignant hypertension. Intravenous labetolol, or more recently approved agents such as fenoldopam or urapidil, together with control of ECFV generally control such hypertension. Enalaprilat or other ACE inhibitors may also be considered, but in the face of bilateral renovascular disease they have the potential to further reduce GFR abruptly.

℞ TREATMENT

Management of Hypertension (See also Chap. 230)   There are two overall goals: to slow the progression of CRD itself and to prevent the extrarenal complications of hypertension, such as cardiovascular disease and stroke. In all patients with CRD, blood pressure should be controlled to at least the level established in the guidelines of the Sixth Joint National Commission on Hypertension Detection Education and Follow-up Program (130/80 to 85 mmHg). In CRD patients with diabetes or proteinuria >1 g per 24 h, blood pressure should be further reduced to 125/75 mmHg. Volume control with salt restriction and diuretics is the mainstay of therapy. When volume management is not sufficient, the choice of antihypertensive agent is similar to that in the general population, with the added consideration of cardioprotective benefit provided by ACE inhibition, or angiotensin receptor blockade. The choice of antihypertensive agents may come from all the major classes, with careful consideration of comorbid conditions. However, powerful direct-acting vasodilators, such as hydralazine or minoxidil, may perpetuate the tendency to cardiac hypertrophy, despite the lowering of blood pressure. Therefore, prolonged use of such agents should be reserved for those very rare patients in whom severe refractory hypertension persists, despite adequate volume reduction and compliance with all other classes of antihypertensives.

Management of Cardiovascular Disease   Hypertension, hyperhomocysteinemia, and lipid abnormalities promote atherosclerosis but are potentially treatable complications of CRD. Ongoing or prior nephrotic syndrome is also associated with hyperlipidemia and hypercoagulability, which increase the risk of occlusive vascular disease. Since diabetes mellitus and hypertension are themselves the two most frequent etiologies of CRD, it is not surprising that cardiovascular disease is the most frequent cause of death in ESRD patients. Therefore, accepted life-style changes and therapeutic measures for cardiac risk reduction (Chap. 225) are especially important in this group of patients. Hyperhomocysteinemia may respond to vitamin therapy, which includes folate supplementation to between 1 and 5 mg/d. Hyperlipidemia in patients with CRD and ESRD should be managed aggressively according to the guidelines of the National Cholesterol Education Program (Chap. 335). If dietary measures are inadequate, the preferred lipid-lowering medications are gemfibrozil and an HMG-CoA reductase inhibitor. However, caution should be exercised in combining these two classes of agents because of an increased risk of myositis and rhabdomyolysis in CRD and ESRD patients.

Pericarditis (See also Chap. 222)   With the advent of early initiation of renal replacement therapy, pericarditis is now observed more often in underdialyzed patients than in predialysis CRD patients. Pericardial pain with respiratory accentuation, accompanied by a friction rub, are the hallmarks of uremic pericarditis. The finding of a multicomponent friction rub strongly supports the diagnosis. Classic electrocardiographic abnormalities include PR-interval depression and diffuse ST-segment elevation. Pericarditis may be accompanied by the accumulation of pericardial fluid that is readily detected by echocardiography and that sometimes leads to cardiac tamponade. Pericardial fluid in uremic pericarditis is more often hemorrhagic than in viral pericarditis.

℞ TREATMENT

Uremic pericarditis is an absolute indication for initiation of dialysis or for intensification of the dialysis prescription in those already on dialysis. Because of the propensity to hemorrhagic pericardial fluid, heparin-free dialysis is indicated. Pericardiectomy should be considered only if more conservative measures fail. Nonuremic causes of pericarditis and pericardial effusion include viral, malignant, and tuberculous pericarditis and pericarditis associated with myocardial infarction; these are also more frequent in patients with ESRD and should be managed according to the dictates of the underlying disease process.

HEMATOLOGIC ABNORMALITIES ■ Anemia   A normocytic, normochromic anemia attributable to CRD is observed beginning at stage 3 CRD and is almost universal at stage 4. If untreated, the anemia of CRD is associated with a number of physiologic abnormalities, including decreased tissue oxygen delivery and utilization, increased cardiac output, cardiac enlargement, ventricular hypertrophy, angina, congestive heart failure, decreased cognition and mental acuity, altered menstrual cycles, and impaired host defense against infection. In addition, anemia may play a role in growth retardation in children with CRD. The primary cause of anemia in patients with CRD is insufficient production of EPO by the diseased kidneys. Additional factors include iron and folate deficiency, severe hyperparathyroidism, acute and chronic inflammation, aluminum toxicity, shortened red cell survival, and associated comorbid conditions such as hemoglobinopathies. These potential contributing factors should be considered and addressed, especially in EPO-resistant patients.

℞ TREATMENT

The anemia of CRD is due to several factors including chronic blood loss, hemolysis, marrow suppression by retained uremic factors and reduced renal production of EPO. The availability of recombinant human EPO, epoetin alfa, has made possible one of the most significant advances in the care of renal patients since the introduction of dialysis and transplantation. More recently, a novel erythropoiesis-stimulating protein has been introduced for the treatment of anemia in CRD patients. This protein, darbopoetin alfa, is a hyperglycosylated analogue of recombinant human EPO that possesses greater biologic activity and prolonged half-life. Thus, dose intervals can be extended and still effectively correct renal anemia in both predialysis and dialysis patients. Guidelines for using epoetin and darbopoetin alfa for the management of anemia of CRD are provided in Table 261-5.

The iron status of the patient with CRD must be assessed, and adequate iron stores should be available before treatment with EPO is initiated. Iron supplementation is usually essential to ensure an adequate response to EPO in patients with CRD, because the demands for iron by the erythroid marrow frequently exceed the amount of iron that is immediately available for erythropoiesis (as measured by percent transferrin saturation) as well as iron stores (as measured by serum ferritin). In most cases, intravenous iron is required to achieve and/or maintain adequate iron. However, excessive iron therapy may be associated with a number of complications, including hemosiderosis, accelerated atherosclerosis, increased susceptibility to infection, and possibly an increased propensity to the emergence of malignancies. In addition to iron, an adequate supply of the other major substrates and cofactors for erythrocyte production must be assured, especially vitamin B_{12} and folate. Anemia resistant to recommended doses of EPO in the face of adequate availability of iron and vitamin factors often suggests inadequate dialysis; uncontrolled hyperparathyroidism; aluminum toxicity; chronic blood loss or hemolysis; associated hemoglobinopathy, malnutrition, chronic infection, multiple myeloma, or another malignancy. Blood transfusions may contribute to suppression of erythropoiesis in CRD; because they increase the risk of hepatitis, hemosiderosis, and transplant sensitization, they should be avoided unless the anemia fails to respond to erythropoietin and the patient is symptomatic.

TABLE 261-5 *Management Guidelines for Correction of Anemia of Chronic Renal Disease*

Erythropoietin

Starting dosage:	50–150 units/kg per week IV or SC (once, twice, or three times per week)
Target hemoglobin (Hb):	11–12 g/dL
Optimal rate of correction[a]	Increase Hb by 1–2 g/dL over 4-week period

Darbepoetin alfa

Starting dosage:	0.45 μg/kg administered as a single IV or SC injection once weekly
	0.75 μg/kg administered as a single IV or SC injection once every 2 weeks
Target Hb:	$\leq$12 g/dL
Optimal rate of correction	Increase Hb by 1–2 g/dL over 4-week period

Iron

1. Monitor iron stores by percent transferrin saturation (TSat) and serum ferritin.
2. If patient is iron-deficient (TSat <20%; serum ferritin <100 μg/L), administer iron, 50–100 mg IV twice per week for 5 weeks; if iron indices are still low, repeat the same course.
3. If iron indices are normal yet Hb is still inadequate, administer IV iron as outlined above; monitor Hb, TSat, and ferritin.
4. Withhold iron therapy when TSat > 50% and/or ferritin > 800 ng/mL (>800 g/L).

[a] If correction of anemia is inadequate, consider causes for refractoriness as outlined in text. Recent reports of pure red blood cell aplasia, may lead to preferences for IV route for some EPO formulations.

Abnormal Hemostasis This is common in CRD and is associated with prolongation of bleeding time, decreased activity of platelet factor III, abnormal platelet aggregation and adhesiveness, and impaired prothrombin consumption. Clinical manifestations include an increased tendency to abnormal bleeding and bruising; bleeding from surgical wounds; and spontaneous bleeding into the gastrointestinal tract, pericardial sac, or intracranial vault (in the form of subdural hematoma or intracerebral hemorrhage). Notwithstanding these abnormalities in hemostasis, CRD patients have a greater susceptibility to thromboembolic complications, particularly if their underlying disease was characterized by a nephrotic presentation.

Rx TREATMENT

Abnormal bleeding times and coagulopathy in patients with renal failure may be reversed with desmopressin, cryoprecipitate, conjugated estrogens, and blood transfusions, as well as EPO. On the other hand, patients with CRD should also be viewed as being at greater risk for thromboembolic complications and receive appropriate anticoagulant prophylaxis when indicated. Avoidance or dose adjustment of certain anticoagulants, such as fractionated low-molecular-weight heparin, is necessary in CRD patients.

NEUROMUSCULAR ABNORMALITIES Central, peripheral, and autonomic neuropathy, as well as abnormalities in muscle composition and function, are all common complications in CRD. Retained nitrogenous metabolites and middle molecules as well as PTH all contribute to the pathophysiology of neuromuscular abnormalities. Subtle clinical manifestations of uremic neuromuscular disease usually become evident beginning at stage 3 CRD. Early manifestations of central nervous system complications include mild disturbances in memory and concentration and sleep disturbance. Neuromuscular irritability, including hiccups, cramps, and fasciculations/twitching of muscles, becomes evident at later stages. Asterixis, myoclonus, and chorea are common in terminal uremia, which may also be associated with seizures and coma.

Peripheral neuropathy usually becomes clinically evident when the patient has been at stage 4 CRD for >6 months, although electrophysiologic and histologic evidence of peripheral neuropathy occurs earlier. Initially, sensory nerves are involved more than motor nerves, lower extremities more than upper, and distal portions of the extremities more than proximal. The "restless legs syndrome" is characterized by ill-defined sensations of discomfort in the legs and feet requiring frequent leg movement. If dialysis is not instituted soon after onset of sensory abnormalities, motor involvement follows, including muscle weakness and loss of deep tendon reflexes. Accordingly, evidence of peripheral neuropathy is a firm indication for renal replacement therapy. Some of the central nervous system and neuromuscular complications of advanced uremia resolve with dialysis, although nonspecific electroencephalographic abnormalities may persist. Successful transplantation may reverse residual peripheral neuropathy.

GASTROINTESTINAL AND NUTRITIONAL ABNORMALITIES *Uremic fetor*, a uriniferous odor to the breath, derives from the breakdown of urea to ammonia in saliva and is often associated with an unpleasant metallic taste sensation. Gastritis, peptic disease, and mucosal ulcerations at any level of the gastrointestinal tract occur in uremic patients and can lead to abdominal pain, nausea, vomiting, and blood loss. Other gastrointestinal complications of CRD include an increased incidence of diverticulosis, particularly in patients with polycystic kidney disease, and an increased incidence of pancreatitis. In addition, central nervous system effects of uremia contribute to anorexia, hiccups, nausea, and vomiting. Protein restriction is useful in diminishing nausea and vomiting late in the course of renal failure. However, protein restriction should not be implemented in patients with signs of protein-energy malnutrition, which is a consequence of low protein and caloric intake, resistance to anabolic actions of insulin and other hormones and growth factors, disturbed dietary protein utilization, proinflammatory cytokine activation, and metabolic acidosis. Assessment for protein-energy malnutrition should begin at stage 3 CRD (GFR < 60 mL/min per 1.73 m^2). A number of indices are useful in this assessment and include dietary history, edema-free body weight, measurement of urinary protein nitrogen appearance, and plasma markers, of which albumin is the most useful. Guidelines for calorie and protein intake in patients with CRD are provided below (p. 1661).

ENDOCRINE-METABOLIC DISTURBANCES Disturbances in parathyroid function have already been considered (p. 1656).

Glucose metabolism is impaired in CRD, as evidenced by a slowing of the rate at which blood glucose levels decline after a glucose load. Fasting blood glucose is usually normal or only slightly elevated, and the mild glucose intolerance related to uremia per se, when present, does not require specific therapy. Because the kidney contributes significantly to insulin removal from the circulation, plasma levels of insulin are slightly to moderately elevated in most uremic subjects, both in the fasting and postprandial states. However, the response to insulin and glucose utilization is impaired in CRD. Many hypoglycemic drugs require dose reduction in renal failure, and some, such as metformin, are contraindicated when the GFR has diminished by more than approximately 25 to 50%.

In women, *estrogen levels* are low, and amenorrhea and inability to carry pregnancies to term are common manifestations of uremia. When the GFR has declined by ~30%, pregnancy may hasten the progression of CRD. In men with CRD, including those receiving chronic dialysis, impotence, oligospermia, and germinal cell dysplasia are common, as are reduced plasma testosterone levels. Like growth, sexual maturation is often impaired in adolescent children with CRD, even among those treated with chronic dialysis. Many of these abnormalities improve or reverse with successful renal transplantation.

DERMATOLOGIC ABNORMALITIES The skin may show evidence of anemia (pallor), defective hemostasis (ecchymoses and hematomas), calcium-phosphate deposition and secondary hyperparathyroidism (pruritus, excoriations), and deposition of pigmented metabolites or *urochromes* (yellow discoloration) or urea itself (uremic frost). Although many of these cutaneous abnormalities improve with dialysis, *uremic pruritus* often remains a problem. The first lines of management are to rule out unrelated skin disorders and to control PO_4^{3-} concentration with avoidance of an elevated calcium-phosphate product. Occasionally, pruritus remains refractory to these measures and to other nonspecific systemic and topical therapies. Skin necrosis can occur as part of the calciphylaxis syndrome, which also includes subcutaneous, vascular, joint, and visceral calcification in patients with poorly controlled calcium-phosphate product.

EVALUATION AND MANAGEMENT OF PATIENTS WITH CRD

INITIAL APPROACH ■ History and Physical Examination Complaints referred to the kidneys themselves are often conspicuously absent in CRD, and this often surprises patients and is a cause of skepticism and denial. Of special importance in establishing the etiology of CRD are a history of hypertension; diabetes; systemic infectious, inflammatory, or metabolic diseases; exposure to drugs and toxins; and a family history of renal and urologic disease. Drugs of particular importance include analgesics (usage frequently underestimated or denied by the patient), NSAIDs, gold, penicillamine, antimicrobials, lithium, and ACE inhibitors. In evaluating the uremic syndrome, questions about appetite, diet, nausea, vomiting, hiccupping, shortness of breath, edema, weight change, muscle cramps, pruritus, mental acuity, and activities of daily living are especially helpful.

On physical examination, particular attention should be paid to blood pressure, fundoscopy, precordial examination, examination of the abdomen for bruits and palpable renal masses, examination for edema, and neurologic examination for the presence of asterixis, muscle weakness, and neuropathy. In addition the evaluation of prostate size in men, and potential pelvic masses in women should be undertaken.

Laboratory Investigations These should also focus on a search for clues to an underlying disease process and its continued activity. Therefore, if the history and physical examination warrant, immunologic tests for systemic lupus erythematosus and vasculitis might be considered. Serum and urinary protein electrophoresis should be undertaken in all patients >40 years with unexplained CRD and anemia, to rule out paraproteinemia. Other tests to determine the stage and chronicity of the disease, including complications of the uremic syndrome, include serial measurements of plasma creatinine and estimation of GFR, urea, electrolytes (including HCO_3^-, Ca^{2+}, and PO_4^{3-}), and alkaline phosphatase to assess metabolic bone disease as well as hemoglobin. Urinalysis may be helpful in assessing the presence of ongoing activity of the underlying inflammatory or proteinuric disease process and, when indicated, should be supplemented by a 24-h urine collection for protein excretion. The latter is particularly helpful in guiding management strategies aimed at ameliorating the progression of CRD. The presence of broad casts on examination of the urinary sediment is a nonspecific finding seen with all underlying etiologies and reflects chronic tubulointerstitial scarring and tubular atrophy with widened tubule diameter, usually signifying an advanced stage of CRD.

Imaging Studies The most useful imaging study is renal ultrasonography. An ultrasound examination of the kidneys can verify the presence of two symmetric kidneys, provide an estimate of kidney size, and rule out renal masses and obstructive uropathy. The documentation

of symmetric small kidneys supports the diagnosis of progressive CRD with an irreversible component of scarring. Normal kidney size suggests the possibility of an acute rather than chronic process. However, polycystic kidney disease, amyloidosis, diabetes, and HIV-associated renal disease (Chap. 173) may lead to CRD with normal kidney size. Documentation of asymmetric kidney size suggests either a unilateral developmental abnormality or chronic renovascular disease. In the latter case, a vascular imaging procedure, such as duplex doppler sonography of the renal arteries, radionuclide scintigraphy, or magnetic resonance angiography should be strongly considered if the possibility of revascularization is feasible. A spiral computed tomographic scan without contrast may be useful in assessing kidney stone activity. Voiding cystourethrography to rule out reflux may be indicated in some patients with a history of enuresis or with a family history of reflux. However, in most cases by the time CRD is established, reflux has resolved, and even if present, its repair does not stabilize renal function. In any case, imaging studies should avoid exposure to intravenous radiocontrast dye where possible because of its nephrotoxicity.

Renal Biopsy This procedure should be reserved for patients with near-normal kidney size, in whom a clear-cut diagnosis cannot be made by less invasive means and when the possibility of a reversible underlying disease process remains tenable, such that clarification of the underlying etiology may alter management. The extent of tubulointerstitial scarring on kidney biopsy generally provides the most reliable pathologic correlate indicating prognosis for continued deterioration toward ESRD. Contraindications to renal biopsy include bilateral small kidneys, polycystic kidney disease, uncontrolled hypertension, urinary tract or perinephric infection, bleeding diathesis, respiratory distress, and morbid obesity. Ultrasound-guided percutaneous biopsy is the favored approach, but surgical approaches, including laparoscopic biopsy, may be considered in special circumstances such as biopsy of a solitary kidney.

ESTABLISHING THE DIAGNOSIS AND ETIOLOGY OF CRD The most important initial step in the evaluation of a patient presenting de novo with biochemical or clinical evidence of renal failure is to distinguish newly diagnosed CRD from acute renal failure. Availability of past medical records documenting serial measurements of the plasma urea and/or creatinine concentrations can be of great help in this regard. In the absence of such information, some of the laboratory tests and imaging studies outlined above can be useful. In particular, a urinary sediment that is inactive or reveals proteinuria and broad casts; the demonstration of evidence of chronic metabolic bone disease with hyperphosphatemia, hypocalcemia, elevated PTH levels, and radiologic bone disease; normocytic and normochromic anemia; and the finding of bilaterally reduced kidney size (< 8.5 cm) by imaging studies, strongly favor a long-standing process consistent with CRD. However, these findings do not rule out the superimposition of an acute and reversible exacerbating factor that may have accelerated the decline in GFR (see below).

In the early stages of CRD it is often possible to establish the underlying etiology. Integration of a particular constellation of clinical, laboratory, and imaging findings based on the approach noted above strongly supports a particular presumed underlying etiologic disease process. For example, in a patient with insulin-dependent type 1 diabetes mellitus of 15 to 20 years duration, diabetic retinopathy, and nephrotic-range albuminuria without hematuria, the diagnosis of *diabetic nephropathy* is likely. The diagnosis of *chronic hypertensive nephrosclerosis* requires a history of long-standing hypertension, in the absence of evidence for another renal disease process, and hence it is usually a diagnosis of exclusion. Usually proteinura is mild to moderate (< 3 g/d) and the urine sediment inactive. It should be noted that in many cases of presumed hypertensive nephrosclerosis, renovascular disease not only may be the cause of hypertension but also may cause ischemic renal damage. In this regard, bilateral renovascular ischemic disease may be a greatly underdiagnosed cause of CRD. This is of therapeutic significance from two points of view: (1) documentation of ischemic renal disease secondary to occlusive vascular disease may prompt revascularization therapy in some subgroups of patients, with occasional stabilization and improvement in renal function; (2) renovascular ischemic disease is a contraindication to ACE inhibitor therapy in most cases. *Analgesic-associated chronic tubulointerstitial nephropathy* is also an underdiagnosed cause of CRD. Imaging studies, including computed tomography, often reveal pathognomonic features such as papillary calcification and necrosis. Under such circumstances, cessation of analgesic exposure may dramatically stabilize renal function.

In the absence of an etiologically suggestive clinical constellation, renal biopsy may be the only recourse to establish etiology in early CRD. However, in advanced stages of CRD, definitively establishing an underlying etiology becomes less feasible and is also of less therapeutic significance.

℞ TREATMENT

Specific treatments aimed at selected underlying etiologies of CRD are provided in the respective chapters describing these disease states. The optimal time for such therapy is usually well before there has been a measurable decline in baseline GFR and usually well before CRD is established. It is of benefit to follow and plot the rate of decline in GFR in all patients. Any acceleration in the rate of decline should prompt a search for superimposed acute processes that may lead to an acute and reversible decline in GFR in patients with CRD. These include superimposed volume depletion, accelerated and uncontrolled hypertension, urinary tract infection, superimposed obstructive uropathy (e.g., due to stone disease, papillary necrosis), nephrotoxic effect of medications (e.g., NSAIDs) and radiocontrast agents, and reactivation or flare of the original underlying etiologic disease process.

SLOWING THE PROGRESSION OF CRD While there is great interindividual variation in the rate of decline of GFR in patients with CRD, a series of therapeutic interventions should be pursued that aim to stabilize the GFR or reduce the annual rate of decline.

Protein Restriction (Table 261-6) A major goal of protein restriction in CRD, beyond ameliorating the complications of uremia, is to slow the rate of nephron injury. This concept is based on clinical and experimental evidence demonstrating the role of protein-mediated hyperfiltration in progressive nephron injury. The effectiveness of protein restriction in slowing the progression of CRD has been shown in controlled clinical trials in patients with both diabetic and nondiabetic renal disease.

Protein restriction should be carried out in the context of an overall dietary program that optimizes nutritional status and avoids malnutrition, especially as patients near dialysis or transplantation. Metabolic and nutritional studies indicate that protein requirements for patients with CRD are similar to those for normal adults and are in the range

of 0.6 g/kg per day. However, there is a particular requirement in patients with CRD that the composition of dietary protein be higher in essential amino acids, and that this be combined with an overall energy supply sufficient to mitigate a catabolic state. Energy requirements in the range of 35 kcal/kg per day are recommended. Fortunately, even patients with advanced CRD (GFR ~ 10 to 15 mL/min per 1.73 m²) are able to activate the same adaptive responses to dietary protein restriction as healthy individuals, i.e., a postprandial suppression of whole-body protein degradation and a marked inhibition of amino acid oxidation. These compensatory responses to dietary protein restriction and nutritional indices are sustained during long-term therapy.

Reducing Intraglomerular Hypertension and Proteinuria (See also p. 1657) In addition to reduction of cardiovascular disease risk, antihypertensive therapy in patients with CRD also aims to slow the progression of nephron injury, by ameliorating intraglomerular hypertension and hypertrophy. Progressive renal injury in CRD appears to be most closely related to the height of intraglomerular pressure and/or the extent of glomerular hypertrophy. Control of hypertension is as at least as important as dietary protein restriction in slowing the progression of CRD. Furthermore, the target for pharmacologic therapy is highly dependent on the level of proteinuria. Indeed, proteinuria is now considered a risk factor for both progressive nephron injury as well cardiovascular disease. Elevated blood pressure increases proteinuria due to the transmission to the glomeruli of the elevated systemic pressure. Conversely, the renoprotective effect of antihypertensive medications is evident through the curtailment of proteinuria. Thus, the more effective a given treatment is in lowering proteinuria, the greater the subsequent impact on protection from GFR decline. This is the basis for the treatment guideline establishing 125/75 mmHg as the target blood pressure value in proteinuric CRD patients.

Owing to their unique effect on the glomerular microcirculation (i.e., dilatation of the efferent arteriole), which is related to inhibition of the renin-angiotensin system, ACE inhibitors and angiotensin receptor blockers are now clearly established as effective, antiproteinuric agents. Several multicenter studies have shown that these drugs are effective in slowing the progression of renal failure in patients with both diabetic and nondiabetic renal failure. The slowing in the progression of renal failure by these drugs is strongly related to their proteinuria-lowering effect. In the absence of a significant antiproteinuric response, combined treatment with both an ACE inhibitor and angiotensin receptor blocker can be tried. Contraindications to or adverse effects of the use of these classes of agents (e.g., intractable cough, anaphylaxis, hyperkalemia not controlled by dietary restriction) may prompt the choice of calcium channel blockers as a second-line therapeutic approach. Among the calcium channel blockers, diltiazem and verapamil may exhibit superior antiproteinuric and renal protective effects. Available clinical studies have indicated that calcium antagonists as a group do not adversely affect renal function in patients with nondiabetic renal insufficiency, and also indicate that they may be more effective in preventing or ameliorating progressive renal injury than some other classes of antihypertensive drugs in this group of patients. Thus, it appears that at least two different categories of responses may exist: one in which progression is strongly associated with systemic and intraglomerular hypertension and with proteinuria (e.g., diabetic nephropathy, glomerular diseases) and in which ACE inhibitors and angiotensin receptor blockers are likely to be the first choice; and the second in which proteinuria is mild or absent (e.g., adult polycystic kidney disease), probably with a less prominent role for intraglomerular hypertension, and which might respond as well to calcium entry blockers.

SLOWING DIABETIC RENAL DISEASE (See also Chap. 323) Diabetic nephropathy is now the leading cause of CRD eventuating in ESRD in many parts of the world. Furthermore, the prognosis of diabetic patients on chronic renal replacement therapy is very poor, owing to

TABLE 261-6 *Management Guidelines for Dietary Protein Restriction in CRD*

CRD Stage	Protein, g/kg per d	Phosphorus, g/kg per d
Stages 1 and 2	Protein restriction not usually recommended	No restriction
Stage 3	0.6 g/kg per d including ≥0.35 g/kg per d of HBV	≤10
Stages 4 and 5	0.6 g/kg per d including ≥0.35 g/kg per d of HBV *or*	≤10
	0.3 g/kg per d supplemented with EAA or KA	≤9
GFR <60 mL/min per 1.73 m² (nephrotic syndrome)	0.8 g/kg per d (plus 1 g protein/g proteinuria) *or*	≤12
	0.3 g/kg per d supplemented with EAA or KA (plus 1 g protein/g proteinuria)	≤9

Note: CRD, chronic renal disease; GFR, glomerular filtration rate; HBV, high biologic value protein; EAA, essential amino acid supplement; KA, ketoanalogue supplement.

accelerated cardiovascular disease. Therefore, it is particularly compelling to search for strategies whose aim is to prevent or slow the progression of this complication of diabetes mellitus.

Glucose Control   Although tight glycemic control reduces the risk of kidney disease in patients with type 1 diabetes, there has been prolonged controversy over whether the same is true in patients with type 2 diabetes. The results of recent controlled prospective studies provide incontrovertible evidence that in type 2 diabetes mellitus the risk of the development and progression of albuminuria and CRD can also be substantially reduced by improving glycemic control. The United Kingdom Prospective Diabetes Study showed that the way in which glycemic control was achieved, whether by insulin or oral antihyperglycemic agents such as sulfonylureas or metformin, was far less important than success in achieving control. Achieving a target hemoglobin A_{1C} level of $<7.2\%$, as compared to $>9\%$, is associated with an approximately 50% reduction in the occurrence of indices of progressive nephropathy. As a result of these findings, recommendations for glucose control aim to achieve plasma values for preprandial glucose in the range of 90 to 130 mg/dL, and for average bedtime glucose of 110 to 150 mg/dL and hemoglobin $A_{1C} < 7\%$. Reduction in GFR mandates dose adjustment of many antihyperglycemic agents, and in particular the discontinuation of metformin when the plasma creatinine is >133 μmol/L (1.5 mg/dL).

Control of Blood Pressure and Proteinuria   Hypertension or an abnormal circadian blood pressure profile is found in 80% of type 2 diabetic patients at the time of diagnosis. Both of these findings correlate with the presence of albuminuria and are powerful predictors of cardiovascular and renal events. The onset of microalbuminuria precedes the decline in GFR in diabetic patients and heralds renal as well as cardiovascular complications. Therefore, microalbuminuria testing is recommended in all diabetic patients at least annually, and more frequently to follow therapeutic interventions. Antihypertensive treatment reduces albuminuria and diminishes the risk of progression of albuminuria even in normotensive patients with diabetes. There is now compelling evidence that ACE inhibitors and angiotensin receptor blockers have specific renoprotective properties in diabetic patients with microalbuminuria or overt proteinuria. These salutary effects are almost certainly mediated by reducing intraglomerular pressure and inhibition of transforming growth factor β–mediated sclerosing pathways.

MANAGING OTHER COMPLICATIONS OF CHRONIC RENAL FAILURE ■ **Impending Uremic Symptomatology**   Temporary relief of symptoms and signs of impending uremia, such as anorexia, nausea, vomiting, asterixis, lassitude, and other central nervous system manifestations, may be achieved with protein restriction. However, this must be associated with careful monitoring of nutritional status, so as to avoid protein-energy malnutrition, evidence of which serves as a clear-cut indication for initiation of renal replacement therapy.

Medication Dose Adjustment (See also Chap. 3)   Although the loading dose of most drugs is not affected by CRD, maintenance doses of many drugs need to be adjusted. For those drugs in which >70% excretion is by a nonrenal (e.g., hepatic or intestinal) route, dosage adjustment may not be needed. Some drugs that should be entirely avoided include meperidine, metformin, and other oral hypoglycemics with a renal route of elimination. Commonly used medications that require either a reduction in dosage or changes in interval include allopurinol, many antibiotics, several antihypertensives, and antiarrhythmics. For a comprehensive detailed and authoritative listing of the recommended dose adjustment for most of the commonly used medications, the reader is referred to the American College of Physicians' handbook *Drug Prescribing in Renal Failure* (see *www.acponline.org*). In addition to dose adjustment requirements, many drugs have nephrotoxicity as a prominent side effect, to which patients with CRD are more susceptible. Of particular notoriety in this regard are NSAIDs, because of

their widespread availability and usage. These drugs aggravate the tendency to sodium retention, hypertension, hyperkalemia, and hyponatremia and further reduce GFR in patients with CRD. In this regard, there is no advantage to more selective inhibitors of cyclooxygenase-2.

Preparation for Renal Replacement Therapy (See also Chaps. 262 and 263)   Over the past 40 years, renal replacement therapy using dialysis and transplantation has prolonged the lives of hundreds of thousands of patients with ESRD. Renal replacement therapy should *not* be initiated when the patient is totally asymptomatic; however, dialysis and/or transplantation should be started sufficiently early to prevent serious complications of the uremic state. Clear indications for initiation of renal replacement therapy include pericarditis, progressive neuropathy attributable to uremia, encephalopathy, muscle irritability, anorexia and nausea that are not ameliorated by reasonable protein restriction, evidence of protein-energy malnutrition, and fluid and electrolyte abnormalities that are refractory to conservative measures. The latter include volume overload unresponsive to diuretic therapy, hyperkalemia unresponsive to dietary potassium restriction, and progressive metabolic acidosis that cannot be managed with alkali therapy. Clinical clues indicating the imminent development of uremic complications are a history of hiccupping, intractable pruritus, morning nausea and vomiting, muscle twitching and cramps, and the presence of asterixis on physical examination. In addition, the patient whose follow-up and compliance with conservative management are questionable should be considered for earlier initiation of renal replacement therapy, lest potentially life-threatening uremic complications or electrolyte disturbances supervene.

Since there is considerable interindividual variability in the severity of uremic symptoms and renal function, it is ill-advised to assign a certain "usual" level of blood urea nitrogen, serum creatinine, or GFR to the need to start dialysis. Nevertheless, in the United States, the Health Care Financing Administration has assigned levels of serum creatinine and creatinine clearance to qualify for reimbursement from Medicare for patients receiving dialysis. Serum creatinine must be ≥ 700 μmol/L (≥ 8.0 mg/dL) and the creatinine clearance must be ≤ 10 mL/min. Recent controlled studies have failed to show a survival advantage for early initiation of renal replacement therapy prior to onset of clinical indications.

Patient Education and Adjustment   Social, psychological, and physical preparation for the transition to renal replacement therapy and choice of the optimal initial modality is best accomplished with a gradual approach involving a multidisciplinary team. While conservative measures are being carried out in patients with CRD, it is important to prepare them with an intensive educational program, explaining the likelihood and timing of initiation of renal replacement therapy and the various forms of therapy available. The more knowledgable patients are concerning hemodialysis, peritoneal dialysis, and transplantation, the easier and more appropriate will be their decisions at a later time. Exploration of social service support resources is of great importance. In those who may perform home dialysis or undergo transplantation, early education of family members for selection and preparation as a home dialysis helper or a related donor for transplantation should occur long before the onset of symptomatic renal failure.

Selection of patients to be treated with various modalities of dialysis or transplantation is a matter of some debate, with considerable variation in different parts of the world. In general, in the United States and some other countries, nearly all patients who have reached ESRD are accepted for dialysis if they or their families desire prolongation of life, irrespective of age.

Only kidney transplantation (Chap. 263) offers the potential for nearly complete rehabilitation. This is because dialysis techniques replace only 10 to 15% of normal kidney function at the level of small-solute removal and are even less efficient at the removal of larger solutes. Generally, kidney transplantation follows a prior period of dialysis treatment. All patients in whom an acute reversible component of renal failure has not been completely excluded should be supported with dialysis first, at least for some period of time, to allow for possible return of renal function before consideration of transplantation. Recovery of endogenous renal function in patients treated with dialysis for >6 months is a rare occurrence. For patients approaching ESRD in whom a reversible component has been excluded, and who have a good antigenic match with a willing donor, consideration should be given to preemptive or primary transplantation without intervening dialysis.

FURTHER READING

ALJAMA P et al: New insights in ESRD. Kidney Int (Suppl) No. 80, 2002

BRENNER BM et al: For the RENAAL Study Investigators: Effects of Losartan on renal and cardiovascular outcomes in patients with type 2 diabetes and nephropathy. N Engl J Med 345:861, 2001

COZZOLINO M et al: Role of calcium-phosphate product and bone-associated proteins on vascular calcification in renal failure. J Am Soc Nephrol 12: 2511, 2001

GOODMAN WG: Recent developments in the management of secondary hyperparathyroidism. Kidney Int 59:1187, 2001

LEVEY AS et al: National Kidney Foundation K/DOQI *Clinical Practice Guidelines for Chronic Kidney Disease: Evaluation, Classification and Stratification.* Am J Kidney Dis 39(Suppl 1):S1, 2002

LIM VS et al: Protein metabolism in patients with chronic renal failure: Role of uremia and dialysis. Kidney Int 58:1, 2000

MAXWELL AP: Novel erythropoiesis-stimulating protein in the management of the anemia of chronic renal failure. Kidney Int 62:720, 2002

262 DIALYSIS IN THE TREATMENT OF RENAL FAILURE
Ajay K. Singh, Barry M. Brenner

With the widespread availability of dialysis, the lives of hundreds of thousands of patients with end-stage renal disease (ESRD) have been prolonged. In the United States alone, there are now approximately 400,000 patients with ESRD. The overall incidence of ESRD is 260 cases per million population per year. The incident population of patients with ESRD is increasing at approximately 6% each year. The incidence of ESRD is disproportionately higher in African Americans (843 per million population per year) as compared with white Americans (189 per million population per year). In the United States, the leading cause of ESRD is diabetes mellitus, currently accounting for nearly 45% of newly diagnosed cases of ESRD. The second most common cause is hypertension, which is estimated to cause 28% of ESRD cases. Other causes of ESRD include glomerulonephritis, polycystic kidney disease, and obstructive uropathy. The mortality of patients with ESRD is lowest in Europe and Japan but is very high in the developing world because of the limited availability of dialysis. In the United States, the mortality rate of patients on dialysis is approximately 18% per year. Deaths are due mainly to cardiovascular diseases and infections (approximately 50% and 15% of deaths, respectively).

TREATMENT OPTIONS FOR ESRD PATIENTS

Commonly accepted criteria for placing patients on dialysis include the presence of the uremic syndrome; the presence of hyperkalemia unresponsive to conservative measures; extracellular volume expansion; acidosis refractory to medical therapy; a bleeding diathesis; and a creatinine clearance of 10 mL/min per 1.73 m². Early referral to a nephrologist for advanced planning and creation of a dialysis access, education about ESRD treatment options, and the aggressive management of the complications of chronic renal failure, including acidosis, anemia, and hyperparathyroidism, are important. In addition to care fully evaluating patients for the onset of uremia (Chap. 261), regular measurement of renal function is important.

Renal function can be assessed indirectly by measurement of serum creatinine and blood urea nitrogen or of creatinine and urea clearance, or directly by measurement of glomerular filtration rate (GFR) using a radioisotope such as iothalamate. Creatinine clearance usually overestimates GFR because a substantial fraction of creatinine excretion in advanced renal failure occurs as a consequence of proximal tubular secretion. On the other hand, urea clearance invariably underestimates GFR because urea is reabsorbed in the distal nephron. Thus, when measurement of GFR by a direct test is not available, the average of the sum of the creatinine and urea clearance, or a cimetidine-blocked creatinine clearance (cimetidine blocks proximal tubular secretion), is recommended. Alternatively, the GFR can be estimated using a prediction equation that computes a calculated value for GFR. Examples of such equations include the Cockcroft-Gault equation and the Modification of Diet in Renal Disease (MDRD) equation.

The treatment options available for patients with renal failure depend on whether it is acute or chronic (Fig. 262-1). In acute renal failure, treatments include hemodialysis, continuous renal replacement therapies (Chap. 260), and peritoneal dialysis. In chronic renal failure (ESRD) the options include hemodialysis (in center or at home); peritoneal dialysis, as either continuous ambulatory peritoneal dialysis (CAPD) or continuous cyclic peritoneal dialysis (CCPD); or transplantation (Chap. 263). Although there are geographic variations, hemodialysis remains the most common therapeutic modality for ESRD (>80% of patients in the United States). The choice between hemodialysis and peritoneal dialysis involves the interplay of various factors that include the patient's age, the presence of comorbid conditions, the ability to perform the procedure, and the patient's own conceptions about the therapy. Peritoneal dialysis is favored in younger patients because of their better manual dexterity and greater visual acuity, and because younger patients prefer the independence and flexibility of home-based peritoneal dialysis treatment. In contrast, larger patients (>80 kg), patients with no residual renal function, and patients who have truncal obesity with or without prior abdominal surgery may be more suited to hemodialysis. Larger patients with no residual renal function are more appropriate for hemodialysis because these patients have a large volume of distribution of urea and require significantly higher amounts of peritoneal dialysis, which may be difficult to achieve because of the limited willingness of patients to perform more than four exchanges each day. In some patients, the inability to obtain vascular access necessitates a switch from hemodialysis to peritoneal dialysis.

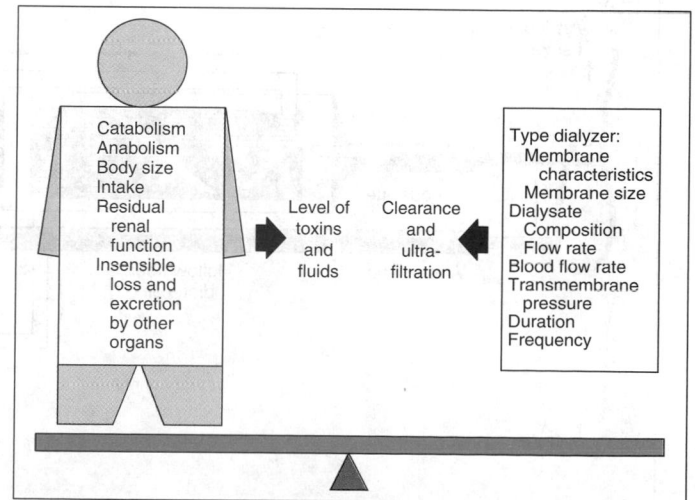

FIGURE 262-1 Factors in the development of the uremic syndrome and considerations in its treatment.

HEMODIALYSIS

Hemodialysis relies on the principles of solute diffusion across a semipermeable membrane. Movement of metabolic waste products takes place down a concentration gradient from the circulation into the dialysate. The rate of diffusive transport increases in response to several factors, including the magnitude of the concentration gradient, the membrane surface area, and the mass transfer coefficient of the membrane. The latter is a function of the porosity and thickness of the membrane, the size of the solute molecule, and the conditions of flow on the two sides of the membrane. According to the laws of diffusion, the larger the molecule, the slower its rate of transfer across the membrane. A small molecule such as urea (60 Da) undergoes substantial clearance, whereas a larger molecule such as creatinine (113 Da) is cleared less efficiently. In addition to diffusive clearance, movement of toxic materials such as urea from the circulation into the dialysate may occur as a result of ultrafiltration. Convective clearance occurs because of solvent drag with solutes getting swept along with water across the semipermeable dialysis membrane.

THE DIALYZER There are three essential components to dialysis: the dialyzer, the composition and delivery of the dialysate, and the blood delivery system (Fig. 262-2). The dialyzer consists of a plastic device with the facility to perfuse blood and dialysate compartments at very high flow rates. The surface area of dialysis membranes in adult patients is usually in the range of 0.8 to 1.2 m².

There are currently two geometric configurations for dialyzers: hollow fiber and flat plate. The hollow fiber dialyzer is the most common in use in the United States. These dialyzers are composed of bundles of capillary tubes through which blood circulates while dialysate travels on the outside of the fiber bundle. In contrast, the less frequently utilized flat plate dialyzers are composed of sandwiched sheets of membrane in a parallel plate configuration. The advantage of the hollow fiber construction is the lower priming volume (60 to 90 mL vs 100 to 120 mL for the flat plate) and easier reprocessing of the filter for reuse in future dialysis treatments.

Recent advances have led to the development of many different types of membrane material. Broadly, there are four categories of dialysis membranes: cellulose, substituted cellulose, cellulosynthetic, and synthetic. Over the past two decades, there has been a gradual switch from cellulose-derived to synthetic membranes, because the latter are more biocompatible. Bioincompatibility may be defined as the ability of the membrane to activate the complement cascade. Cellulosic membranes are bioincompatible because of the presence of free hydroxyl groups on the membrane surface. In contrast, with the substituted cellulose membranes (e.g., cellulose acetate) or the cellulosynthetic membranes, the hydroxyl groups are chemically bonded to either acetate or tertiary amino groups, resulting in limited complement activation. Synthetic membranes, such as polysulfone, polymethylmethacrylate, and polyacrylonitrile membranes, are more biocompatible because of the absence of these hydroxyl groups. Polysulfone membranes are now used in over 60% of the dialysis treatments in the United States.

Reprocessing and reuse of hemodialyzers are employed for patients on chronic hemodialysis in nearly 80% of dialysis centers in the United States, in large part because of the expense of individual dialyzers. Evidence also suggests that reuse reduces complement activation, the incidence of anaphylactoid reactions to the membrane (first-use syndrome), and, in some studies, mortality rates among dialysis patients. In most centers, only the dialyzer unit is reprocessed and reused, whereas in the developing world blood lines are also frequently reused. The reprocessing procedure can be either manual or automated. It consists of the sequential rinsing of the blood and dialysate compartments with water, a chemical cleansing step with reverse ultrafiltration from the dialysate to the blood compartment, the testing of the patency of the dialyzer, and, finally, disinfection of the dialyzer. Formaldehyde, peracetic acid–hydrogen peroxide, and glutaraldehyde are the most frequently used reprocessing agents, with peracetic acid–hydrogen peroxide being the most common.

DIALYSATE The composition of dialysate is listed in Table 262-1. Bicarbonate has replaced acetate as the preferred buffer in the United States. This change has resulted in fewer episodes of hypotension dur-

FIGURE 262-2 Schema for hemodialysis.

TABLE 262-1 *Composition of Commercial Dialysate for Hemodialysate*

Solute	Bicarbonate Dialysate
Sodium (meq/L)	137–143
Potassium (meq/L)	0–4.0
Chloride (meq/L)	100–111
Calcium (meq/L)	0–3.5
Magnesium (meq/L)	0.75–1.5
Acetate (meq/L)	2.0–4.5
Bicarbonate (meq/L)	30–35
Glucose (mg/dL)	0–0.25

ing dialysis. The potassium concentration of dialysate may be varied from 0 to 4 mmol/L depending on the predialysis plasma potassium concentration. The usual dialysate calcium concentration is 1.25 mmol/L (2.5 meq/L). The usual dialysate sodium concentration is 140 mmol/L. Lower dialysate sodium concentrations are associated with a higher frequency of hypotension, cramping, nausea, vomiting, fatigue, and dizziness. In patients who frequently develop hypotension during their dialysis run, sodium modeling to counterbalance urea-related osmolar gradients is now widely used. In this technique, the dialysate sodium concentration is gradually lowered from the range of 148 to 160 meq/L to isotonic levels (140 meq/L) near the end of the dialysis treatment. A dialysate glucose concentration of 200 mg/dL (11 mmol/L) is used to optimize blood glucose concentrations. Because patients are exposed to approximately 120 L of water during each dialysis treatment, untreated water could expose them to a variety of environmental contaminants. Therefore, in 98% of U.S. dialysis centers, water used for the dialysate is subjected to filtration, softening, deionization, and, ultimately, reverse osmosis. During the reverse osmosis process, water is forced through a semipermeable membrane at very high pressure to remove microbiologic contaminants and more than 90% of dissolved ions.

BLOOD DELIVERY SYSTEM   The blood delivery system is composed of the extracorporeal circuit in the dialysis machine and the dialysis access. The dialysis machine consists of a blood pump, dialysis solution delivery system, and various safety monitors. The blood pump, using a roller mechanism, moves blood from the access site, through the dialyzer, and back to the patient. The blood flow rate may range from 250 to 500 mL/min. Negative hydrostatic pressure on the dialysate side can be manipulated to achieve desirable fluid removal: so-called *ultrafiltration*. Dialysis membranes have different ultrafiltration coefficients (i.e., mL removed/min per mmHg) so that along with hydrostatic changes, fluid removal can be varied. The dialysis solution delivery system dilutes the dialysate concentrate with water and monitors the temperature, conductivity, and flow of dialysate. The dialysate may be delivered to the dialyzer from a storage tank or a proportioning system that manufactures dialysate online.

Dialysis Access   The fistula, graft, or catheter through which blood is obtained for hemodialysis is often referred to as a *dialysis access*. A native fistula created by the anastomosis of an artery to a vein (e.g., the Cimino-Breschia fistula, in which the cephalic vein is anastomosed to the radial artery) results in arterialization of the vein. This facilitates its subsequent use in the placement of large needles (typically 15 gauge) to access the circulation. Although fistulas have a high patency rate (approximately 60% are patent at 3 years following creation), fistulas are created in only approximately 30% of patients in the United States. In the majority of U.S. dialysis patients, the dialysis access consists of an arteriovenous graft that interposes prosthetic material, such as polytetrafluoroethylene, between an artery and a vein. Reasons for the higher rates of graft placement include the late referral of patients to vascular access surgeons so that by the time surgery is planned, the patient's arm veins have already been obliterated through multiple blood draws; the high prevalence of patients with diabetes mellitus and its associated microvascular disease; and the greater surgical skill required in creating a fistula. However, by 3 years most grafts fail because of thrombosis or infection. Fortunately, grafts may

be inserted in one of several locations: the arm (brachial artery to basilic vein), the chest wall (axillary artery to axillary vein), or the leg (femoral artery to femoral vein). The most common access-related complication is thrombosis due to intimal hyperplasia, which results in stenosis 2 to 3 cm proximal to the venous anastomosis.

A double-lumen cuffed catheter is used in approximately 20% of patients on chronic hemodialysis in the United States. These catheters are used as an alternative to either a native arteriovenous fistula or a graft in selected patients in whom dialysis is required relatively urgently, such as patients who manifest delayed recovery from acute renal failure, or where a further permanent access procedure (e.g., arteriovenous fistula or arteriovenous graft) is not feasible for anatomical reasons. Although double-lumen catheters may permit blood flows comparable to a permanent arteriovenous access, these catheters are prone to infection and to occlusion because of thrombosis. Temporary double-lumen catheters in either the femoral vein or the internal jugular or subclavian vein are usually employed in patients with acute renal failure. The jugular is preferred to the subclavian vein because, for unclear reasons, a catheter placed in a subclavian vein appears to be associated with a higher rate of venous stenosis. Temporary access can be used for 2 to 3 weeks. Thrombosis, low blood flow, and infection limit the life of the catheter.

GOALS OF DIALYSIS   The hemodialysis procedure is targeted at removing both low- and high-molecular-weight solutes. The procedure consists of pumping heparinized blood through the dialyzer at a flow rate of 300 to 500 mL/min, while dialysate flows in an opposite *countercurrent* direction at 500 to 800 mL/min. The clearance of urea ranges from 200 to 350 mL/min, while the clearance of α_2 microglobulin is more modest and ranges from 20 to 25 mL/min. The efficiency of dialysis is determined by blood and dialysate flow through the dialyzer, as well as dialyzer characteristics (i.e., its efficiency in removing solute). The *dose* of dialysis, which is defined as the magnitude of urea clearance during a single dialysis treatment, is further governed by patient size, residual renal function, dietary protein intake, the degree of anabolism or catabolism, and the presence of comorbid conditions.

Since the landmark studies of Sargent and Gatch relating the measurement of the dose of dialysis using urea concentration with patient outcome, the *delivered* dose of dialysis has been correlated with morbidity and mortality. This has led to the development of two major models for assessing the adequacy of the dialysis dose. Fundamentally, these two widely used measures of the adequacy of dialysis are calculated from the decrease in the blood urea nitrogen concentration during the dialysis treatment—that is, the urea reduction ratio (URR), and KT/V, an index based on the urea clearance rate, K, and the size of the urea pool, represented as the urea distribution volume, V. K, which is the sum of clearance by the dialyzer plus renal clearance, is multiplied by the time spent on dialysis, T. Increasingly, KT/V has become the preferred marker for dialysis adequacy. Currently, a URR of 65% and a KT/V of 1.2 per treatment are minimal standards for adequacy among ESRD patients; lower levels of dialysis treatment are associated with increased morbidity and mortality. The HEMO study examined the effect of dialysis dose and the level of flux of the dialyzer membrane on mortality and morbidity and found that a higher dialysis dose (single pool KT/V of 1.71 ± 0.11) did not confer a benefit over a standard dialysis dose (single pool KT/V of 1.32 ± 0.09). Thus, the study supported the continued use of current US Practice Guidelines, which recommend a KT/V of at least 1.2. Furthermore, since no benefit of a high flux dialyzer was demonstrated in the study, the use of a high flux dialyzer was also not supported.

For the majority of patients with chronic renal failure, between 9 and 12 h of dialysis is required each week, usually divided into three equal sessions. However, the dialysis dose must be individualized. Recently there has been much interest in the possibility that more frequent dialysis may be associated with improved outcomes in paticnts with acute or chronic renal failure. Indeed, it has been suggested that among patients with acute renal failure, daily dialysis may better control uremia, reduce hypotensive episodes, more rapidly resolve acute renal failure, and significantly lower mortality. Therefore, the measurement of dialysis adequacy using KT/V or the URR should serve only as a guide; body size, residual renal function, dietary intake, complicating illness, degree of anabolism or catabolism, and the presence of large interdialytic fluid gains should be important factors that are taken into consideration in the dialysis prescription.

COMPLICATIONS DURING HEMODIALYSIS   Hypotension is the most common acute complication of hemodialysis, particularly among diabetics. Numerous factors appear to increase the risk of hypotension, including excessive ultrafiltration with inadequate compensatory vascular filling, impaired vasoactive or autonomic responses, osmolar shifts, food ingestion, impaired cardiac reserve, diastolic dysfunction, the use of antihypertensive drugs, anemia, and vasodilation due to the use of warm dialysate. Because of the vasodilatory and cardiodepressive effects of acetate, the use of acetate as the buffer in dialysate was once a common cause of hypotension. Since the introduction of bicarbonate-containing dialysate, dialysis-associated hypotension has become less common. The management of hypotension during dialysis consists of discontinuing ultrafiltration, the administration of 100 to 250 mL of isotonic saline or 10 mL of 23% saturated hypertonic saline, and administration of salt-poor albumin. Hypotension during dialysis can frequently be prevented by careful evaluation of the dry weight, withholding of antihypertensive medications on the day prior to and on the day of dialysis, and avoiding heavy meals during dialysis. Additional maneuvers include ultrafiltration modeling, such that more fluid is ultrafiltered at the beginning rather than the end of the dialysis procedure; the performance of sequential ultrafiltration followed by dialysis; the use of midodrine, a selective α_1-adrenergic pressor agent; and cooling of the dialysate during dialysis treatment.

Muscle cramps during dialysis are also a common complication of the procedure. However, since the introduction of volumetric controls on dialysis machines and sodium modeling, the incidence of cramps has fallen. The etiology of dialysis-associated cramps remains obscure. Changes in muscle perfusion because of excessively aggressive volume removal, particularly below the estimated dry weight, and the use of low-sodium-containing dialysate, have been proposed as precipitants of dialysis-associated cramps. Strategies that may be used to prevent cramps include reducing volume removal during dialysis, the use of higher concentrations of sodium in the dialysate, and the use of quinine sulfate (260 mg 2 h before treatment).

Anaphylactoid reactions to the dialyzer, particularly on its first use, have been reported most frequently with the bioincompatible cellulosic-containing membranes. With the gradual phasing out of cuprophane membranes in the United States, the first-use syndrome has become relatively uncommon. The first-use syndrome consists of either an intermediate hypersensitivity reaction due to an IgE-mediated reaction to ethylene oxide used in the sterilization of new dialyzers, or a symptom complex of nonspecific chest and back pain, which appears to result from complement activation and cytokine release.

The major cause of death in patients with ESRD receiving chronic dialysis is cardiovascular disease. The rate of death from cardiac disease is higher in patients on hemodialysis as compared to patients on peritoneal dialysis and renal transplantation. The underlying cause of cardiovascular disease is unclear but may be related to the inadequate treatment of hypertension; the presence of hyperlipidemia, homocystinemia and anemia; the calcification of coronary arteries in patients with an elevated calcium-phosphorus product; and perhaps alterations in cardiovascular dynamics during the dialysis treatment. Intensive investigation of the mechanisms and potential interventions that could impact on reducing the mortality from cardiovascular causes is currently underway.

CONTINUOUS RENAL REPLACEMENT THERAPY   Continuous renal replacement therapies (CRRT) have become increasingly prevalent in the intensive care unit (ICU) setting for management of acute renal failure. The advantages of CRRT over intermittent hemodialysis are that it is usually better tolerated hemodynamically; it facilitates gradual correction of biochemical abnormalities; it is highly effective in removing fluid; and it is technically simple to perform. Clearance of toxic materials (using urea as the marker) can occur with CRRT from convective clearance alone if the ultrafiltration rate is high and with diffusive clearance if dialysis accompanies ultrafiltration. CRRT techniques include continuous arteriovenous hemodiafiltration (CAVH/D) with or without dialysis, and continuous veno-venous hemodiafiltration (CVVH/D) with or without dialysis.

Veno-venous therapies differ fundamentally from arteriovenous therapies in that veno-venous therapies do not require arterial access. This allows obtaining less risky and easier vascular access. However, because there is no systemic arterial pressure to drive hemofiltration, veno-venous therapies require a blood pump in the extracorporeal circuit. Veno-venous therapies such as CVVH provide substantial flexibility because changing the blood flow rate in the pump can change the ultrafiltration and clearance rates. In contrast, arteriovenous therapies such as CAVH are associated with variable efficiency because the systemic blood pressure is frequently low or unstable in patients with acute renal failure. Furthermore, low blood flow with CAVH may also result in clotting of the extracorporeal circuit. CAVH often results in clearance rates as low as 10 to 15 mL/min, whereas CVVH may generate clearances in the range of 30 to 40 mL/min. Thus, in light of these advantages of CVVH, many centers have completely switched from arteriovenous to veno-venous therapies in patients with acute renal failure in the ICU setting.

Vascular access in patients on CVVH is usually achieved by the insertion of a double-lumen catheter into the femoral vein. The blood pump is typically set to deliver approximately 150 to 180 mL/min. In automated systems, (e.g., the Cobe Prisma system), the treatment is volumetrically governed by continuously weighing the effluent and replacement solutions and using a servomechanism to drive the replacement fluid pump at a rate computed either to balance the inflow and loss of fluid or to maintain a predetermined rate of fluid loss. Anticoagulation of the extracorporeal circuit is via a heparin infusion (200 to 1600 U/h) through the inflow side of the circuit. Alternatively, citrate can be used to chelate calcium in the extracorporeal circuit to provide regional anticoagulation in selected patients who cannot undergo systemic heparinization. The replacement solution in continuous therapies is designed specifically to replace calcium, magnesium, and bicarbonate. In place of bicarbonate, lactate or citrate is the buffer in the replacement solution. However, bicarbonate-based replacement fluid is the preferred option in patients with liver failure because of the impaired ability of the liver to metabolize either lactate or acetate into bicarbonate.

PERITONEAL DIALYSIS

Peritoneal dialysis consists of infusing 1 to 3 L of a dextrose-containing solution into the peritoneal cavity and allowing the fluid to dwell for 2 to 4 h. As with hemodialysis, toxic materials are removed through a combination of convective clearance generated through ultrafiltration, and diffusive clearance down a concentration gradient. The clearance of solute and water during a peritoneal dialysis exchange depends on the balance between the movement of solute and water into the peritoneal cavity versus absorption from the peritoneal cavity. The rate of diffusion diminishes with time and eventually stops when equilibration between plasma and dialysate is reached. Absorption of solutes and water from the peritoneal cavity occurs across the peritoneal membrane into the peritoneal capillary circulation and via peritoneal lymphatics into the lymphatic circulation. The rate of peritoneal solute transport varies from patient to patient and may be altered by the presence of infection (peritonitis), drugs such as beta blockers and calcium channel blockers, and physical factors such as position and exercise.

FORMS OF PERITONEAL DIALYSIS Peritoneal dialysis may be carried out as continuous ambulatory peritoneal dialysis (CAPD), continuous cyclic peritoneal dialysis (CCPD), or nocturnal intermittent peritoneal dialysis (NIPD). In CAPD, dialysis solution is manually infused into the peritoneal cavity during the day and exchanged three to four times daily. A nighttime dwell is frequently instilled at bedtime and remains in the peritoneal cavity through the night. The drainage of spent dialysate (effluence) is performed manually with the assistance of gravity to move fluid out of the abdomen. In CCPD, exchanges are performed in an automated fashion, usually at night; the patient is connected to the automated cycler, which then performs four to five exchange cycles while the patient sleeps. Peritoneal dialysis cyclers automatically cycle dialysate in and out of the abdominal cavity. In the morning the patient, with the last exchange remaining in the abdomen, is disconnected from the cycler and goes about his regular daily activities. In NIPD, the patient is given approximately 10 h of cycling each night, with the abdomen left dry during the day.

Peritoneal dialysis solutions are available in various volumes ranging from 0.5 to 3.0 L. The electrolyte composition is shown in Table 262-2. Lactate is the preferred buffer in peritoneal dialysis solutions. Acetate in peritoneal dialysis solutions appears to accelerate peritoneal sclerosis, whereas use of bicarbonate results in precipitation of calcium and caramelization of glucose. The most common additives to peritoneal dialysis solutions are heparin and antibiotics during an episode of acute peritonitis. Insulin may also be added in patients with diabetes mellitus.

ACCESS TO THE PERITONEAL CAVITY This is obtained through a peritoneal catheter. These are either *acute* catheters, used to perform acute continuous peritoneal dialysis, usually in an emergency setting, or *chronic* catheters, which have either one or two Dacron cuffs and are tunneled under the skin into the peritoneal cavity. An acute catheter consists of a straight or slightly curved rigid tube with several holes at its distal end. Catheters can be inserted at the bedside by making a small incision in the anterior abdominal wall; the catheter is inserted with the assistance of a guidewire or stylet. Acute catheters are anchored externally with adhesives or sutures and are usually reserved for temporary use because of the risk of infection, which increases after 72 h of use. In contrast, chronic catheters are flexible and made of silicon rubber with numerous side holes at the distal end. These chronic catheters usually have two Dacron cuffs to promote fibroblast proliferation, granulation, and invasion of the cuff. The scarring that occurs around the cuffs anchors the catheter and seals it from bacteria tracking from the skin surface into the peritoneal cavity; it also prevents the external leakage of fluid from the peritoneal cavity. The cuffs are placed in the preperitoneal plane and approximately 2 cm from the skin surface. The most common chronic peritoneal dialysis catheter in use is the Tenckhoff catheter, which contains two cuffs.

The initial CAPD prescription consists of the infusion of a 2-L volume of a 1.5% dextrose concentration peritoneal dialysis solution into the peritoneal cavity over 10 min and allowing it to dwell for 2.5 h. The effluent solution is then drained over 20 min before the next exchange. Three daytime exchanges are accompanied by a 2-L nighttime dwell as the standard prescription. Because peritoneal membrane characteristics vary from one individual to another, the peritoneal equilibrium test should be employed within 2 months of a patient initiating peritoneal dialysis. This test measures the peritoneal membrane transfer rate for solutes (usually urea and creatinine) based on the ratio of their concentration in dialysate and plasma at specific times during the dialysate dwell. It allows patients to be classified as low, low–average, high–average, and high transporters. Approximately 10 to 17% of patients are high transporters, 50% high–average transporters, 25 to 30% low–average transporters, and 1 to 5% low transporters. Identifying the high transporters early is important, since these patients not only demonstrate excellent solute removal, they also absorb glucose rapidly; maximum ultrafiltration occurs early in the dwell, followed by reabsorption of water back into the circulation over the course of the dwell. Such patients benefit from either NIPD or CAPD without a nighttime dwell.

The dose of peritoneal dialysis required to provide adequate or optimal dialysis as measured by patient outcomes is not known. However, there is emerging consensus that the weekly KT/V should be >2.0 and the creatinine clearance >65 L/week per 1.73 m². The most frequently utilized approach to calculating a weekly KT/V and creatinine clearance is to collect the spent dialysate and urine over a 24-h period. The peritoneal dialysis prescription can be tailored to improve suboptimal clearance values by increasing the volume of individual exchanges, increasing the number of exchanges, or combining the CAPD and CCPD techniques. In combining these techniques, the CAPD patient hooks up to a cycler at night and the machine automatically performs one or two nocturnal exchanges, whereas the CCPD patient makes an additional manual daytime exchange.

FURTHER READING

BURKART JM et al: Peritoneal dialysis, in *Brenner and Rector's The Kidney*, 7th ed, BM Brenner (ed). Philadelphia, Saunders, 2004

DIAZ-BUXO JA: Early referral and selection of peritoneal dialysis as a treatment modality. Nephrol Dial Transplant 15:147, 2000

EKNOYAN G et al: Effect of dialysis dose and membrane flux in maintenance hemodialysis. N Engl J Med 346:2010, 2002

EKNOYAN G, LEVIN N: NKF-DOQ1 clinical practice guidelines: Update 2000. Am J Kidney Dis 37(Suppl 1):55, 2001

FORNI LG, HILTON PJ: Current concepts: Continuous hemofiltration in the treatment of acute renal failure. N Engl J Med 336:1303, 1997

IFUDU O: Care of patients undergoing hemodialysis. N Engl J Med 339:1054, 1998

MEYER MM: Renal replacement therapies. Crit Care Clin 16:29, 2000

SCHIFFL H et al: Daily hemodialysis and the outcome of acute renal failure. N Engl J Med 346:305, 2002

U.S. RENAL DATA SYSTEM: USRDS 2001 Annual Report: Atlas of End-Stage Renal Disease in the United States. Bethesda, National Institutes of Health, National Institute of Diabetes and Digestive and Kidney Disease, 2001

TABLE 262-2 *Composition of Peritoneal Dialysate*

Solute	Dianeal (PD-2)
Sodium (meq/L)	132
Potassium (meq/L)	0
Chloride (meq/L)	96
Calcium (meq/L)	3.5
Magnesium (meq/L)	0.5
D,L-Lactate (meq/L)	40
Glucose (g%)	
1.5	
2.5	
4.25	
pH	5.2

Transplantation of the human kidney is frequently the most effective treatment of advanced chronic renal failure. Worldwide, tens of thousands of such procedures have been performed. When azathioprine and prednisone were initially used as immunosuppressive drugs in the 1960s, the results with properly matched familial donors were superior to those with organs from cadaveric donors, namely, 75 to 90% compared with 50 to 60% graft survival rates at 1 year. During the 1970s and 1980s, the success rate at the 1-year mark for cadaveric transplants rose progressively. By the time cyclosporine was introduced in the early 1980s, cadaveric donor grafts had a 70% 1-year survival and reached the 82% level in the mid-1990s and 88% by 1998 (Fig. 263-1). After the first year, graft survival curves show an exponential decline in numbers of functioning grafts from which a half-life ($t_{1/2}$) in years is calculated; this has increased by 2 years since the 1980s (Fig. 263-1).

Mortality rates after transplantation are highest in the first year and are age-related: 2% for ages 18 to 34 years, 3% for ages 35 to 49 years, and 6.8% for ages over 50 to 60 years. These rates compare favorably to those in the chronic dialysis population, even after risk adjustments for age, diabetes, and cardiovascular status. Occasionally, acute irreversible rejection may occur after many months of good function, especially if the patient neglects to take the immunosuppressive drugs. Most grafts, however, succumb at varying rates to a chronic vascular and interstitial obliterative process termed *chronic rejection*, although its pathogenesis is incompletely understood. Overall, transplantation returns the majority of patients to an improved lifestyle and an improved life expectancy, as compared to patients on dialysis; however, careful prospective cohort studies have yet to be reported.

RECIPIENT SELECTION There are few absolute contraindications to renal transplantation. The transplant procedure is relatively noninvasive, as the organ is placed in the inguinal fossa without entering the peritoneal cavity. Recipients without perioperative complications can often be discharged from the hospital in excellent condition within 5 days of the operation.

Virtually all end-stage renal disease (ESRD) patients who receive a transplant have a higher life expectancy than risk-matched patients who remain on dialysis. Even though diabetics or older candidates have a higher mortality rate than other transplant recipients, their survival is improved with transplantation compared to remaining on dialysis. This global benefit of transplantation as a treatment modality poses substantial ethical issues for policy makers, as the number of cadaveric kidneys available is far from sufficient to meet the current needs of the candidates. Waiting lists continue to grow, and the average wait time for a cadaver kidney is now >4 years in many locales. The current standard of care is that the candidate should have a life expectancy of >5 years to be put on a cadaver organ wait list. Even for living donation, the candidate should have >5 years of life expectancy. This is because the benefits of kidney transplantation over dialysis are only realized after a perioperative period in which the mortality is higher in transplanted patients than in dialysis patients with comparable risk profile.

All candidates must have a thorough risk/benefit evaluation prior to being approved for transplantation. In particular, an aggressive approach to diagnosis of correctable coronary artery disease, presence of latent or indolent infection (HIV, hepatitis B or C, tuberculosis), and neoplasm should be a routine part of the candidate workup. Most transplant centers consider overt AIDS and active hepatitis to be an absolute contraindication to transplantation because of the high risk of opportunistic infection. Some centers are now transplanting individuals with hepatitis and even HIV infection under strict protocols to determine whether the risks and benefits favor transplantation over dialysis.

Among the few absolute contraindications to transplantation is the presence of potentially harmful antibody against the donor kidney at the time of the anticipated transplant. Harmful antibodies that can cause very early graft loss include natural antibodies against the ABO blood group antigens and antibodies against HLA-class I (A, B, C) or class II (DR) antigens. These antibodies are routinely excluded by proper pretransplant screening of the candidates, ABO and HLA typing of donor and recipient, and cross-matching of candidate serum with that of the donor.

DONOR SELECTION Donors can be cadavers or volunteer living donors. The latter are usually family members selected to have at least partial compatibility for HLA antigens. Living volunteer donors should be normal on physical examination and of the same major ABO blood group, because crossing major blood group barriers prejudices survival of the allograft. It is possible, however, to transplant a kidney of a type O donor into an A, B, or AB recipient. Selective renal arteriography should be performed on donors to rule out the presence of multiple or abnormal renal arteries, because the surgical procedure is difficult and the ischemic time of the transplanted kidney long when vascular abnormalities exist. Transplant surgeons are now using a laparoscopic method to isolate and remove the living donor kidney. This operation has the advantage of less evident surgical scars, and, because there is less tissue trauma, the laparoscopic donors have a substantially shorter hospital stay and less discomfort than those who have the traditional surgery. Cadaveric donors should be free of malignant neoplastic disease, hepatitis, and HIV because of possible transmission to the recipient. Increased risk of graft failure exists when the donor is elderly or has renal failure and when the kidney has a prolonged period of ischemia and storage.

In the United States, there is a coordinated national system of regulations, allocation support, and outcomes analysis for kidney transplantation called the Organ Procurement Transplant Network. It is now possible to remove cadaver kidneys and to maintain them for up to 48 h on cold pulsatile perfusion or simple flushing and cooling. This permits adequate time for typing, cross-matching, transportation, and selection problems to be solved.

TISSUE TYPING AND CLINICAL IMMUNOGENETICS Matching for antigens of the HLA major histocompatibility gene complex (Chap. 296) is an

FIGURE 263-1 One-year actuarial graft survival of cohorts of first cadaver kidney transplants performed from 1975 through 1998 is displayed (in purple) along with $t_{1/2}$ or post-year-one half-life of the same cohorts (green). These registry data are derived from the U.S. Renal Data System 2002 Annual Report. The upper curve represents the 1-year actual graft survival, which approaches 90% by 1998. From 1982 to 1985 there was an impressive rise in the 1-year survival, partially attributable to the introduction of cyclosporine. Since 1985, there has been a consistent, slow increase in 1-year survival. The lower curve represents long-term graft survival, expressed as the half-life ($t_{1/2}$), which has been relatively stable over the past decade.

important criterion for selection of donors for renal allografts. Each mammalian species has a single chromosomal region that encodes the strong, or major, transplantation antigens, and this region on the human sixth chromosome is called *HLA*. HLA antigens have been classically defined by serologic techniques, but methods to define specific nucleotide sequences in genomic DNA are increasingly being used. Other antigens, called "minor," may nevertheless play crucial roles, in addition to the ABH(O) blood groups and endothelial antigens that are not shared with lymphocytes. The Rh system is not expressed on graft tissue. Evidence for designation of HLA as the genetic region encoding major transplantation antigens comes from the success rate in living related donor renal and bone marrow transplantation, with superior results in HLA-identical sibling pairs. Nevertheless, 5% of HLA-identical renal allografts are rejected, often within the first weeks after transplantation. These failures represent states of prior sensitization to non-HLA antigens. Non-HLA minor antigens are relatively weak when initially encountered and are therefore suppressible by conventional immunosuppressive therapy. Once priming has occurred, however, secondary responses are much more refractory to treatment. ABO incompatibilities are hazardous because of the presence of natural anti-A and anti-B antibodies in recipients and the normal expression of A and B blood group substances on endothelium, resulting in immediate vascular injury.

Living Donors When first-degree relatives are donors, graft survival rates at 1 year are 5 to 7% greater than those for cadaver grafts. The 5-year survival rates still favor the partially matched (3/6 HLA mismatched) family donor over a randomly selected cadaver donor (Table 263-1). In addition, living donors provide the advantage of immediate availability. For both living and cadaveric donors, the 5-year outcomes are poor if there is a complete (6/6) HLA mismatch. Waiting lists for cadaveric kidneys have grown faster than the available organ supply, to the point where most new patients with ESRD wait for >4 years. In response to this increasing disparity between cadaver donor supply and patient demand, living unrelated volunteers, usually spouses or close friends, are being accepted as donors in increasing numbers. The survival rate of living unrelated renal allografts is as good or better than that of perfectly HLA matched cadaver renal transplants and comparable to that of kidneys from living relatives. This is likely to be a consequence both of short cold ischemia time and the extra care taken to document that the condition and renal function of the donor are optimal before proceeding with a living unrelated donation (Table 263-1). It is illegal in the United States to purchase organs for transplantation.

Concern has been expressed regarding the potential risk to a volunteer kidney donor of premature renal failure after several years of increased blood flow and hyperfiltration per nephron in the remaining kidney. There are a few reports of the development of hypertension, proteinuria, and even lesions of focal segmental sclerosis in donors under long-term follow-up. Difficulties in donors followed for ≥20 years are unusual, however, and it may be that having a single kidney becomes significant only when another condition, such as hyperten-

sion, is superimposed. It is also desirable to consider the risk of development of type 1 diabetes mellitus in a family member who is a potential donor to a diabetic renal failure patient. Anti-insulin and anti-islet antibodies should be measured, and glucose tolerance tests should be performed in such donors to rule out a prediabetic state.

HLA Matching and Cadaveric Donors The question of whether matching of HLA antigens in unrelated donor-recipient pairs would approximate the high initial success rates and slow rates of subsequent graft loss with HLA-identical sib pairs could not be answered until the late 1980s when reliable class II histocompatibility (DR) typing became widely available. Now that pooled data on tens of thousands of cadaveric renal transplants from all over the world are available, the HLA-matching effect can be clearly seen, especially in the long-term survival figures. It is shown in Table 263-1 that there is an overall beneficial effect of HLA matching in cadaveric grafts. With increasing numbers of mismatches for cadaveric donors, the 5-year survival drops from 68.2% to 55.3%. The survival rates at the 10-year mark are projected to range from 65 (zero mismatches) to 34% (six mismatches). There is controversy regarding the value of cadaveric organ-sharing rules that are based entirely upon the numbers of HLA mismatches. Giving preference to HLA zero-mismatched candidates (Table 263-1) is a top priority in the United States, however, and 20% of kidneys are transplanted on this basis. Table 263-1 also shows the interaction of HLA matching and graft ischemia on results; namely, kidneys from HLA-incompatible unrelated or spousal donors do better than those from similarly mismatched cadaver donors, suggesting that the additional ischemic injury of organ storage is important. Nevertheless, when such a cadaveric donor is HLA-compatible, the benefit of matching can still be seen.

Presensitization A positive cross match of recipient serum with donor T lymphocytes representing anti-HLA class I is usually predictive of an acute vasculitic event termed *hyperacute rejection*. Patients with anti-HLA antibodies can be safely transplanted if careful cross-matching of donor blood lymphocytes with recipient serum is performed. Patients sustained by dialysis often show fluctuating antibody titers and specificity patterns. At the time of assignment of a cadaveric kidney, cross matches are performed with at least a current serum. Previously analyzed antibody specificities and additional cross matches are performed accordingly. Techniques for cross-matching are not universally standardized; however, at least two techniques are employed in most laboratories. The minimal purpose for the cross match is avoidance of hyperacute rejection mediated by recipient antibodies to donor HLA class I antigens. Sensitive tests, such as the use of flow cytometry, can be useful for avoidance of accelerated, and often untreatable, early graft rejection in patients receiving second or third transplants. Donor T lymphocytes, which express only class I antigens, are used as targets for detection of anti-class I (HLA-A and -B) antibodies. Preformed anti-class II (HLA-DR) antibodies against the donor carry a higher risk of graft loss as well, particularly in recipients who have suffered early loss of a prior kidney transplant. B lymphocytes expressing both class I and class II antigens are used in these assays. Non-HLA antigens restricted in expression to endothelium and sometimes monocytes have been described, but clinical relevance is not well established. A series of minor histocompatibility antigens do not elicit antibodies, and sensitization to these is detectable only by cytotoxic T cells, an assay too cumbersome for routine use.

Blood Transfusions Exposure to leukocyte HLA antigens during transfusions is a major cause of sensitization that limits transplantation access and increases the risk of early graft rejection. In the 1970s, attempts to avoid all blood exposure in dialysed patients paradoxically increased the risk of graft rejection. The beneficial "transfusion effect" was never fully explained, and it almost disappeared in the 1980s as overall management of patients improved with the use of cyclosporine and more effective means of rejection treatment. Currently, with the use of erythropoietin the need for transfusion is much reduced. It has

TABLE 263-1 *Effect of HLA-A, -B, -DR Mismatching on Kidney Graft Survival*[a]

Degree of Donor Mismatch	1-Year Survival, %	5-Year Survival, %
Cadaver donor (all)	89.2	61.3
0/6-HLA mismatch	91.3	68.2
3/6-HLA mismatch	90.1	60.8
6/6-HLA mismatch	85.2	55.3
Living related donor (all)	94.7	76.0
0/6-HLA mismatch	96.7	87.0
3/6-HLA mismatch	94.3	73.2
6/6-HLA mismatch	92.7	57.7
Living unrelated donor	95.3	77.4

Note: 0-mismatched related donor transplants are virtually all from HLA-identical siblings, while 3/6-mismatched transplants can be one haplotype mismatched (1-A, 1-B, and 1-DR antigen) from parent, child or sibling; 6/6-HLA-mismatched living related kidneys are derived from siblings or relatives outside of the nuclear family.

been noted, however, that nontransfused patients do have more rejection activity.

IMMUNOLOGY OF REJECTION Both cellular and humoral (antibody-mediated) effector mechanisms can play roles in kidney transplant rejection. Antibodies directed against ABO blood group antigens and HLA class I or class II antigens can cause hyperacute rejection within minutes to hours of engraftment if they are present in the recipient at the time of engraftment. Such antibodies bind to vascular endothelium, cause activation of the complement cascade, and direct endothelial damage, platelet aggregation, microvascular thrombi, and in the most severe cases ischemic necrosis of the organ. Antibodies against ABO are naturally found in humans. Anti-HLA antibodies are produced as a consequence of prior blood transfusions, multiple pregnancies, or rejection of a prior HLA-incompatible transplant. Antibodies that bind to cells within the transplant can also initiate a form of antibody-dependent cell death mediated by recipient cells that bear receptors for the Fc portion of immunoglobulin.

Cellular rejection is mediated by lymphocytes that respond to HLA antigens expressed within the organ. The CD4+ lymphocyte responds to class II (HLA-DR) incompatibility by proliferating and releasing proinflammatory cytokines that augment the proliferative response of both CD4+ and CD8+ cells. CD8+ cytotoxic lymphocyte precursors respond primarily to class I (HLA-A, -B) antigens and mature into cytotoxic effector cells. The cytotoxic effector, or "killer" T, cells cause organ damage through direct contact and lysis of donor target cells. The natural role of HLA antigens is to present processed peptide fragments of antigen to T lymphocytes, the fragments residing in a "groove" of the HLA molecule distal to the cell surface. T cells can be directly stimulated by non-self HLA antigen expressed on donor parenchymal cells and residual donor leukocytes residing in the kidney interstitium. In addition, donor HLA molecules can be processed by a variety of donor or recipient cells capable of antigen presentation and then presented to T cells in the same manner as most other antigens. The former mode of stimulation is sometimes called *direct presentation* and the latter mode called *indirect presentation* (Fig. 263-2). There is evidence that non-HLA antigens can also play a role in renal transplant rejection episodes. Recipients who receive a kidney from an HLA-identical sibling can have rejection episodes and require maintenance immunosuppression, while identical twin transplants require no immunosuppression. There are documented non-HLA antigens, such as an endothelial-specific antigen system with limited polymorphism and a tubular antigen, which can be targets of humoral or cellular rejection responses, respectively.

IMMUNOSUPPRESSIVE TREATMENT Immunosuppressive therapy, as presently available, generally suppresses all immune responses, including those to bacteria, fungi, and even malignant tumors. In the 1950s when clinical renal transplantation began, sublethal total-body irradiation was employed. We have now reached the point where sophisticated pharmacologic immunosuppression is available, but it still has the hazard of promoting infection and malignancy. In general, all clinically useful drugs are more selective to primary than to memory immune responses. Agents to suppress the immune response are discussed in the following paragraphs, and those currently in clinical use are listed in Table 263-2.

Drugs *Azathioprine*, an analogue of mercaptopurine, was for two decades the keystone to immunosuppressive therapy in humans. This agent can inhibit synthesis of DNA, RNA, or both. Because cell division and proliferation are a necessary part of the immune response to antigenic stimulation, suppression by this agent may be mediated by the inhibition of mitosis of immunologically competent lymphoid cells, interfering with synthesis of DNA. Alternatively, immunosuppression may be brought about by blocking the synthesis of RNA (possibly messenger RNA), inhibiting processing of antigens prior to lymphocyte stimulation. Therapy with azathioprine in doses of 1.5 to

FIGURE 263-2 Recognition pathways for major histocompatibility complex (MHC) antigens. Graft rejection is initiated by CD4 helper T lymphocytes (T_H) having antigen receptors that bind to specific complexes of peptides and MHC class II molecules on antigen-presenting cells (APC). In transplantation, in contrast to other immunologic responses, there are two sets of T cell clones involved in rejection. In the direct pathway the class II MHC of donor allogeneic APCs is recognized by CD4 T_H cells that bind to the intact MHC molecule, and class I MHC allogeneic cells are recognized by CD8 T cells. The latter generally proliferate into cytotoxic cells (T_C). In the indirect pathway, the incompatible MHC molecules are processed into peptides that are presented by the self-APCs of the recipient. The indirect, but not the direct, pathway is the normal physiologic process in T cell recognition of foreign antigens. Once T_H cells are activated, they proliferate, and by secretion of cytokines and direct contact exert strong helper effects on macrophages, T_C, and B cells. (*From Sayegh and Turka, Copyright 1998, Massachusetts Medical Society. All rights reserved.*)

2.0 mg/kg per day is generally added to cyclosporine as a means of decreasing the requirements for the latter. Because azathioprine is rapidly metabolized by the liver, its dosage need not be varied directly in relation to renal function, even though renal failure results in retention of the metabolites of azathioprine. Reduction in dosage is required because of leukopenia and occasionally thrombocytopenia. Excessive amounts of azathioprine may also cause jaundice, anemia, and alopecia. If it is essential to administer allopurinol concurrently, the azathioprine dose must be reduced, since inhibition of xanthine oxidase delays degradation. This combination is best avoided.

Mycophenolate mofetil is now used in place of azathioprine in many centers. It has a similar mode of action and a mild degree of gastrointestinal toxicity but produces minimal bone marrow suppression. Its advantage is its increased potency in preventing or reversing rejection. Patients with hyperuricemia can be given allopurinol without adjustment of the mycophenylate dose.

Glucocorticoids are important adjuncts to immunosuppressive therapy. Of all the agents employed, prednisone has effects that are easiest to assess, and in large doses it is usually effective for the reversal of rejection. In general, 200 to 300 mg prednisone is given immediately prior to or at the time of transplantation, and the dosage is reduced to 30 mg within a week. The side effects of the glucocorticoids, particularly impairment of wound healing and predisposition to infection, make it desirable to taper the dose as rapidly as possible in the immediate postoperative period. Customarily, methylprednisolone, 0.5 to 1.0 g intravenously, is administered immediately upon diagnosis of beginning rejection and continued once daily for 3 days. When the drug is effective, the results are usually apparent within 96 h. Such "pulse" doses are not effective in chronic rejection. Most patients whose renal function is stable after 6 months or a year do not require large doses of prednisone; maintenance doses of 10 to 15 mg/d are the rule. Many patients tolerate an alternate-day course of steroids without an increased risk of rejection.

A major effect of steroids is on the monocyte-macrophage system, preventing the release of interleukin (IL) 6 and IL-1. Lymphopenia after large doses of glucocorticoids is primarily due to sequestration of recirculating blood lymphocytes to lymphoid tissue.

Cyclosporine is a fungal peptide with potent immunosuppressive activity. It acts on the calcineurin pathway to block transcription of mRNA for IL-2 and other proinflammatory cytokines, thereby inhibiting T cell proliferation. Although it works alone, cyclosporine is more effective in conjunction with glucocorticoids. Since cyclosporine blocks production of IL-2 by T cells, its combination with steroids is expected to produce a double block in the macrophage → IL-6/IL-1 → T cell → IL-2 sequence. Clinical results with tens of thousands of renal transplants have been impressive. Of its toxic effects (nephrotoxicity, hepatotoxicity, hirsutism, tremor, gingival hyperplasia, diabetes), only nephrotoxicity presents a serious management problem and is further discussed below.

TABLE 263-2	*Maintenance Immunosuppressive Drugs*		
Agent	Pharmacology	Mechanisms	Side Effects
Glucocorticoids	Increased bioavailability with hypoalbuminemia and liver disease; prednisone/prednisolone generally used	Binds cytosolic receptors and heat shock proteins. Blocks transcription of IL-1,-2,-3,-6, TNF-α, and IFN-γ	Hypertension, glucose intolerance, dyslipidemia, osteoporosis
Cyclosporine (CsA)	Lipid-soluble polypeptide, variable absorption, microemulsion more predictable	Trimolecular complex with cyclophilin and calcineurin → block in cytokine (e.g., IL-2) production; however, stimulates TGF-β production	Nephrotoxicity, hypertension, dyslipidemia, glucose intolerance, hirsutism/ hyperplasia of gums
Tacrolimus (FK506)	Macrolide, well absorbed	Trimolecular complex with FKBP-12 and calcineurin → block in cytokine (e.g., IL-2) production; may stimulate TGF-β production	Similar to CsA, but hirsutism/hyperplasia of gums unusual, and diabetes more likely
Azathioprine	Mercaptopurine analogue	Hepatic metabolites inhibit purine synthesis	Marrow suppression (WBC > RBC > platelets)
Mycophenolate mofetil (MMF)	Metabolized to mycophenolic acid	Inhibits purine synthesis via inosine monophosphate dehydrogenase	Diarrhea/cramps; dose-related liver and marrow suppression is uncommon
Sirolimus	Macrolide, poor oral bioavailability	Complexes with FKBP-12 and then blocks p70 S6 kinase in the IL-2 receptor pathway for proliferation	Hyperlipidemia, thrombocytopenia

Note: IL, interleukin; TNF, tumor necrosis factor; IFN, interferon; TGF, transforming growth factor; FKBP-12, FK506 binding protein 12; WBC, white blood cells; RBC, red blood cells.

Tacrolimus (FK-506) is a fungal macrolide that has the same mode of action, and a similar side effect profile, as cyclosporine. It does not produce hirsutism or gingival hyperplasia, however. De novo induction of diabetes mellitus is more common with tacrolimus. The drug was first used in liver transplantation and may substitute for cyclosporine entirely or be tried as an alternative in renal patients whose rejections are poorly controlled by cyclosporine.

Sirolimus (previously called rapamycin) is another fungal macrolide but has a different mode of action, i.e., it inhibits T cell growth factor pathways, preventing the response to IL-2 and other cytokines. Sirolimus can be used in conjunction with cyclosporine or tacrolimus as an alternative immunosuppressive regimen. Its use with tacrolimus alone shows promise as a steroid-sparing regimen, especially in patients who would benefit from pancreatic islet transplantation, where steroids have an adverse effect on islet survival.

Antibodies to Lymphocytes When serum from animals made immune to host lymphocytes is injected into the recipient, a marked suppression of cellular immunity to the tissue graft results. The action on cell-mediated immunity is greater than on humoral immunity. A globulin fraction of serum [antilymphocyte globulin (ALG)] is the agent generally employed. For use in humans, peripheral human lymphocytes, thymocytes, or lymphocytes from spleens or thoracic duct fistulas have been injected into horses, rabbits, or goats to produce antilymphocyte serum, from which the globulin fraction is then separated. Monoclonal antibodies against defined lymphocyte subsets offer a more precise and standardized form of therapy. OKT3 is directed to the CD3 molecules that form a portion of the T cell antigen-receptor complex; hence CD3 is expressed on all mature T cells. CD4 or CD8 molecules also form part of the fully activated cluster of molecules, and monoclonal antibodies to these offer the potential for more selective targeting of T cell subsets.

Another approach to more selective therapy is to target the 55-kDa alpha chain of the IL-2 receptor, expressed only on T cells that have been recently activated. The problem with such mouse antibodies is the potential for developing human antimouse antibodies (HAMA), an event that limits the effective period of use. Genetically engineered monoclonal antibodies can solve this problem. Two such antibodies to the IL-2 receptor, in which either a chimeric protein has been made between mouse Fab with human Fc (basiliximab) or "humanized" by splicing the combining sites of the mouse into a molecule that is 90% human IgG (daclizumab), have been approved for prophylaxis of acute rejection in the immediate posttransplant period. They are effective at decreasing the acute rejection rate and have few adverse side effects.

CLINICAL COURSE AND MANAGEMENT OF THE RECIPIENT Adequate hemodialysis should be performed within 48 h of surgery, and care should be taken that the serum potassium level is not markedly elevated so that intraoperative cardiac arrhythmias can be averted. The diuresis that commonly occurs postoperatively must be carefully monitored; in some instances it may be massive, reflecting the inability of ischemic tubules to regulate sodium and water excretion; with large diureses, massive potassium losses may occur. Most chronically uremic patients have some excess of extracellular fluid, and it is useful to maintain an expanded fluid volume in the immediate postoperative period. Acute tubular necrosis (ATN) may cause immediate oliguria or may follow an initial short period of graft function. ATN is most likely when cadaveric donors have been hypotensive or if the interval between cessation of blood flow and organ harvest (warm ischemic time) is more than a few minutes. Recovery usually occurs within 3 weeks, although periods as long as 6 weeks have been reported. Superimposition of rejection on ATN is common, and the differential diagnosis may be difficult without a graft biopsy. Cyclosporine therapy prolongs ATN, and some patients do not diurese until the dose is drastically reduced. Many centers avoid starting cyclosporine for the first several days, using ALG or a monoclonal antibody along with mycophenolate mofetil and prednisone until renal function is established. Fig. 263-3 illustrates an algorithm followed by many transplant centers for early

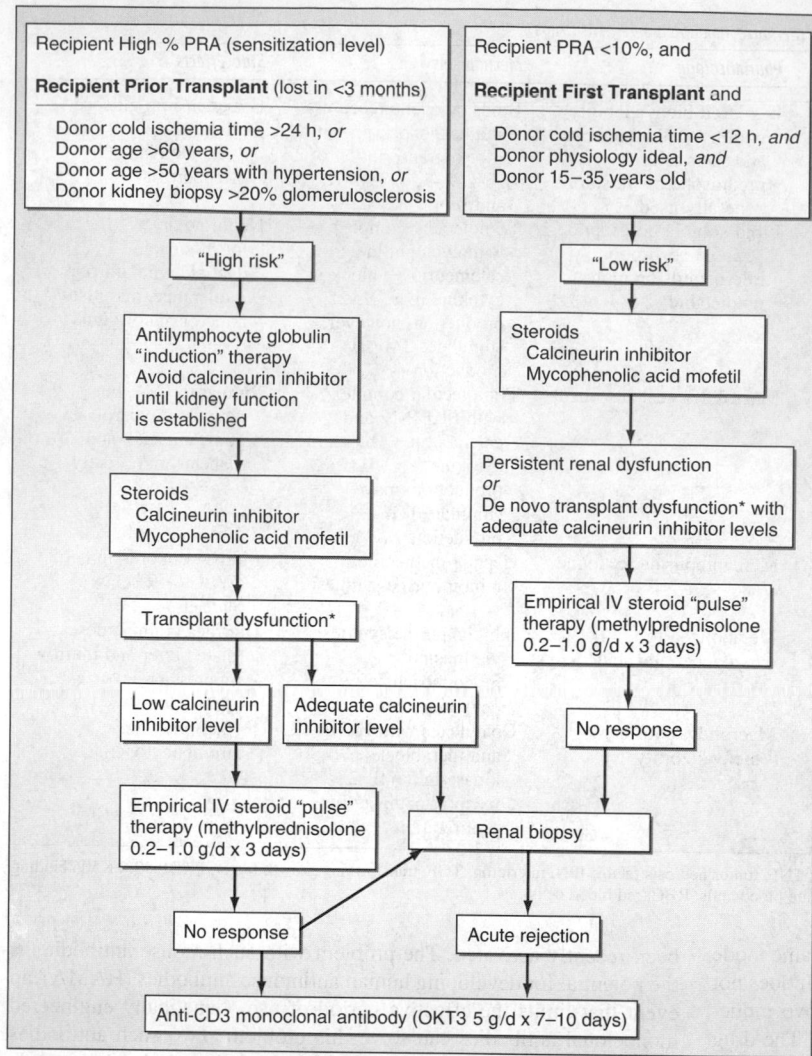

FIGURE 263-3 A typical algorithm for early posttransplant care of the kidney recipient. If any of the recipient or donor "high-risk" factors exist, more aggressive management is called for. Low-risk patients can be treated with a standard immunosuppressive regimen. Patients at higher risk of rejection or early ischemic and nephrotoxic transplant dysfunction are often induced with an antilymphocyte globulin to provide more potent early immunosuppression or to spare calcineurin nephrotoxicity. *When there is early transplant dysfunction, prerenal, obstructive, and vascular causes must be ruled out by ultrasonographic examination. The panel reactive antibody (PRA) is a quantitation of how much antibody is present in a candidate against a panel of cells representing the distribution of antigens in the donor pool.

posttransplant management of recipients at high or low risk of early renal dysfunction.

The Rejection Episode Early diagnosis of rejection allows prompt institution of therapy to preserve renal function and prevent irreversible damage. Clinical evidence of rejection is rarely characterized by fever, swelling, and tenderness over the allograft. Rejection may present only with a rise in serum creatinine, with or without a reduction in urine volume. The focus should be on ruling out other causes of functional deterioration.

Arteriography and radioactive iodohippurate sodium renograms of the transplanted kidney may be useful in ascertaining changes in the renal vasculature and in renal blood flow, even in the absence of urinary flow. Thrombosis of the renal vein occurs rarely; it may be reversible if caused by technical factors and intervention is prompt. Diagnostic ultrasound is the procedure of choice to rule out urinary obstruction or to confirm the presence of perirenal collections of urine, blood, or lymph. When renal function has been good initially, a rise in the serum creatinine level is the most sensitive and reliable indicator of possible rejection and may be the only sign.

Calcineurin inhibitors (cyclosporine or tacrolimus) may cause de-

terioration in renal function in a manner similar to a rejection episode. In fact, rejection processes tend to be more indolent with these inhibitors, and the only way to make a diagnosis may be by renal biopsy. Calcineurin inhibitors have an afferent arteriolar constrictor effect on the kidney and may produce permanent vascular and interstitial injury after sustained high-dose therapy. Addition of angiotensin-converting enzyme (ACE) inhibitors or nonsteroidal anti-inflammatory drugs are likely to raise serum creatinine levels. The former are generally safe to use after the early months, while the latter are best avoided in all renal transplant patients. There is no universally accepted lesion(s) that makes a diagnosis of calcineurin inhibitor toxicity, although interstitial fibrosis, isometric tubular vacuolization, and thickening of arteriolar walls have been noted by some. Basically, if the biopsy does not reveal moderate and active cellular rejection activity, the serum creatinine will most likely respond to a reduction in dose. Blood levels of drug can be useful if very high or very low but do not correlate precisely with renal function, although serial changes in a patient can be useful. If rejection activity is present in the biopsy, appropriate therapy is indicated. The first rejection episode is usually treated with intravenous administration of methylprednisolone, 500 to 1000 mg daily for 3 days. Failure to respond is indication for antibody therapy, usually with OKT3.

OKT3 monoclonal antibody, given intravenously for 10 to 14 days, is effective in >90% of first rejections but less so if methylprednisolone pulses have failed and in cases of severe recurrent rejection activity. A major problem with OKT3 is that severe systemic reactions may be produced during the first day or two of therapy. Chills, fever, hypotension, and headache are the direct result of the antibody effects on the targeted T cells, most likely related to the known potential of OKT3 to activate T cells nonspecifically with release of cytokines, especially tumor necrosis factor α. If the antibody is administered to overhydrated oliguric patients, pulmonary edema may be induced. These reactions are not characteristic of other monoclonal antibodies, such as those to the IL-2 receptor. Recurrent or rebound rejection activity may require additional therapy. In such circumstances, methylprednisolone may be effective even though it failed initially. Second courses of OKT3 may be given in spite of HAMA generated in response to the first course if the titers are low and the human antibodies are not directed to the combining-site region (idiotype) of the OKT3.

Management Problems The usual clinical manifestations of infection in the posttransplant period are blunted by immunosuppressive therapy. The major toxic effect of azathioprine is bone marrow suppression, which is less likely with mycophenolate mofetil, while calcineurin inhibitors have no marrow effects. All drugs predispose to unusual opportunistic infections, however. The typical times posttransplant when the most common opportunistic infections occur are tabulated in Table 263-3. The signs and symptoms of infection may be masked or distorted. Fever without obvious cause is common and only after days or weeks may it become apparent that it has a viral or fungal origin. Bacterial infections are most common during the first month after transplantation. The importance of blood cultures in such patients cannot be overemphasized, because systemic infection without obvious foci is frequent, although wound infections with or without urinary fistulas are most common. Particularly ominous are rapidly occurring pulmonary lesions, which may result in death within 5 days of onset. When these become apparent, immunosuppressive agents should be discontinued, except for maintenance doses of prednisone.

TABLE 263-3 *The Most Common Opportunistic Infections in the Renal Transplant Recipient*

Peritransplant (<1 month)	Late (>6 months)
Wound infections	*Aspergillus*
Herpesvirus	*Nocardia*
Oral candidiasis	BK virus (polyoma)
Urinary tract infection	Herpes zoster
Early (1–6 months)	Hepatitis B
Pneumocystis carinii	Hepatitis C
Cytomegalovirus	
Legionella	
Listeria	
Hepatitis B	
Hepatitis C	

Aggressive diagnostic procedures, including transbronchial and open lung biopsy, are frequently indicated. In the case of *Pneumocystis carinii* (Chap. 191) infection, trimethoprim-sulfamethoxazole is the treatment of choice; amphotericin B has been used effectively in systemic fungal infections. Prophylaxis against *P. carinii* with daily or alternate day low-dose trimethoprim-sulfamethoxazole is very effective. Involvement of the oropharynx with *Candida* (Chap. 187) may be treated with local nystatin. Tissue-invasive fungal infections require treatment with systemic agents such as fluconazole. Small doses (a total of 300 mg) of amphotericin given over a period of 2 weeks may be effective in fungal infections refractory to fluconazole. Macrolide antibiotics, especially ketoconazole and erythromycin, and some calcium channel blockers (diltiazem, verapamil) compete with calcineurin inhibitors for P450 catabolism and cause elevated levels of these immunosuppressive drugs. Analeptics, such as phenytoin and carbamazepine, will increase catabolism to result in low levels. *Aspergillus* (Chap. 188), *Nocardia* (Chap. 146), and cytomegalovirus (CMV) (Chap. 166) infections also occur.

CMV is a common and dangerous infection in transplant recipients. It does not generally appear until the end of the first posttransplant month. Active CMV infection is sometimes associated, or occasionally confused, with rejection episodes. Patients at highest risk for severe CMV disease are those without anti-CMV antibodies who receive a graft from a CMV antibody–positive donor (15% mortality). Serial intravenous administration of high-titer CMV immune globulin is effective in reducing this risk. Prophylactic use of ganciclovir is an effective alternative. Valganciclovir is a cost-effective and bioavailable oral form of ganciclovir that has proven effective in both prophylaxis and treatment of CMV disease. Early diagnosis in a febrile patient can be made by detecting CMV antigens in the blood. A rise in IgM antibodies to CMV is also diagnostic. Culture of CMV from blood may be less sensitive. Tissue invasion of CMV is common in the gastrointestinal tract and lungs. CMV retinopathy occurs late in the course, if untreated. Treatment of active CMV disease with valganciclovir is always indicated. Many patients immune to CMV can activate the virus after heavy immunosuppression, such as with OKT3. Concurrent treatment with ganciclovir during OKT3 administration appears to be effective for prophylaxis of CMV activation. The complications of glucocorticoid therapy are well known and include gastrointestinal bleeding, impairment of wound healing, osteoporosis, diabetes mellitus, cataract formation, and hemorrhagic pancreatitis. The treatment of unexplained jaundice in transplant patients should include cessation or reduction of immunosuppressive drugs if hepatitis or drug toxicity is suspected. It is surprising that cessation of azathioprine or calcineurin inhibitor therapy in such circumstances often does not result in rejection of a graft, at least for several weeks. Acyclovir is effective in therapy of herpes simplex virus infections.

Chronic Lesions of the Transplanted Kidney While 1-year transplant survival is excellent, most recipients experience progressive decline in kidney function over time thereafter. The chronic renal transplant dysfunction can be caused by recurrent disease, hypertension, cyclosporine or tacrolimus nephrotoxicity, chronic immunologic rejection,

secondary focal glomerulosclerosis, or a combination of these pathophysiologies. Chronic vascular changes with intimal proliferation and medial hypertrophy are commonly found. Control of systemic and intrarenal hypertension with ACE inhibitors is thought to have a beneficial influence on the rate of progression of chronic renal transplant dysfunction. Renal biopsy can distinguish subacute cellular rejection from recurrent disease or secondary focal sclerosis.

Malignancy The incidence of tumors in patients on immunosuppressive therapy is 5 to 6%, or approximately 100 times greater than that in the general population of the same age range. The most common lesions are cancer of the skin and lips and carcinoma in situ of the cervix, as well as lymphomas, such as non-Hodgkin's lymphomas. The risks are increased in proportion to the total immunosuppressive load administered and time elapsed since transplantation. Surveillance for skin and cervical cancers is necessary.

Other Complications *Hypercalcemia* after transplantation may indicate failure of hyperplastic parathyroid glands to regress. Aseptic necrosis of the head of the femur is probably due to preexisting hyperparathyroidism, with aggravation by glucocorticoid treatment. With improved management of calcium and phosphorus metabolism during chronic dialysis, the incidence of parathyroid-related complications has fallen dramatically. Persistent hyperparathyroid activity may require subtotal parathyroidectomy.

Hypertension may be caused by (1) native kidneys; (2) rejection activity in the transplant; (3) renal artery stenosis, if an end-to-end anastomosis was constructed with an iliac artery branch; and (4) renal calcineurin inhibitor toxicity. The latter may improve with reduction in dose. Whereas ACE inhibitors may be useful, calcium channel blockers are more frequently used initially. Amelioration of hypertension to the 120 to 130/70 to 80 mmHg range should be the goal in all patients.

While most transplant patients have a robust production of erythropoietin and normalization of the hemoglobin without exogenous erythropoietin administration, *anemia* is commonly seen in the posttransplant period. Often the anemia is attributable to bone marrow–suppressant immunosuppressive medications such as azathioprine, mycophenolate mofetil, or sirolimus. Gastrointestinal bleeding is a common side effect of high-dose and long-term steroid administration. Many transplant patients have creatinine clearances of 30 to 50 mL/min and can be considered in the same way as other patients with chronic renal insufficiency for anemia management, including supplemental erythropoietin.

Chronic hepatitis, particularly when due to hepatitis B virus, can be a progressive, fatal disease over a decade or so. Patients who are persistently hepatitis B surface antigen–positive are at higher risk, according to some studies, but the presence of hepatitis C virus is also a concern when one embarks on a course of immunosuppression in a transplant recipient.

Both chronic dialysis and renal transplant patients have a higher incidence of death from myocardial infarction and stroke than in the population at large, and this is particularly true in diabetic patients. Contributing factors are the use of glucocorticoids, hypertension, and hypertriglyceridemia. Increased low-density lipoprotein cholesterol and depressed high-density lipoprotein cholesterol concentrations may be exaggerated after transplantation and require treatment, particularly in patients receiving sirolimus. Recipients of renal transplants have a high prevalence of coronary artery and peripheral vascular diseases. The percentage of deaths from these causes has been slowly rising as the numbers of transplanted diabetic patients and the average age of all recipients increase. More than 50% of renal recipient mortality is attributable to cardiovascular disease. In addition to strict control of blood pressure and blood lipid levels, close monitoring of patients for indications of further medical or surgical intervention is an important part of management.

FURTHER READING

CHANDRAKER A et al: Transplantation immunobiology, in *Brenner and Rector's The Kidney*, 7th ed, B Brenner (ed). Philadelphia, Saunders, 2004, pp 2759–84

LIMAYE AP et al: Quantitation of BK virus load in serum for the diagnosis of BK virus–associated nephropathy in renal transplant recipients. J Infect Dis 183:1669, 2001

MACDONALD AS: A worldwide, phase III, randomized, controlled, safety and efficacy study of a sirolimus/cyclosporine regimen for prevention of acute rejection in recipients of primary mismatched renal allografts. Transplantation 71:271, 2001

MAHONEY RJ et al: B-Cell crossmatching and kidney allograft outcome in 9031 United States transplant recipients. Hum Immunol 63:324, 2002

PESCOVITZ MD, GOVANI M: Sirolimus and mycophenolate mofetil for calcineurin-free immunosuppression in renal transplant recipients. Am J Kidney Dis 38:S16, 2001

SAYEGH MH, TURKA LA: The role of T-cell costimulatory activation pathways in transplant rejection. N Engl J Med 338:1813, 1998

VELIDEDEOGLU E et al: Comparison of open, laparoscopic, and hand-assisted approaches to live-donor nephrectomy. Transplantation 74:169, 2002

264 GLOMERULAR DISEASES
Hugh R. Brady, Yvonne M. O'Meara, Barry M. Brenner

PATHOGENESIS

The glomerulus is a modified capillary network that delivers an ultrafiltrate of plasma to Bowman's space, the most proximal portion of the renal tubule. Approximately 1.6 million glomeruli are present in two mature kidneys (range 0.5 to 2.4 million) and collectively they produce 120 to 180 L of ultrafiltrate daily. Glomerular filtration rate (GFR) is dependent on glomerular blood flow, ultrafiltration pressure, and the area and composition of the filtration barrier. These parameters are tightly regulated through changes in afferent and efferent arteriolar tone (for blood flow and ultrafiltration pressure) and mesangial cell contractility (for filtration surface area). Arteriolar tone and mesangial cell contractility are, in turn, modulated by neurohumoral factors, local myenteric reflexes, and endothelium-derived vasoactive substances, such as nitric oxide, prostanoids, and endothelins. In health, glomerular endothelium is also antithrombotic and antiadhesive for leukocytes and platelets, thereby preventing inappropriate vascular thrombosis and inflammation during the filtration process. Filtration of most plasma proteins and all blood cells is normally prevented as a consequence of the physiochemical and electrostatic charge characteristics of the glomerular filtration barrier, the latter being composed of fenestrated glomerular endothelium, basement membrane, and the foot processes and slit diaphragms of visceral epithelial cells (podocytes). Parietal epithelium facilitates glomerular filtration by maintaining the integrity of Bowman's space. In keeping with the physiologic functions of the glomerulus outlined above, virtually all glomerular injury results in impairment of glomerular filtration and/or the inappropriate appearance of plasma proteins and blood cells in the urine.

CLINICOPATHOLOGIC CORRELATES IN GLOMERULAR DISEASE The major morphologic patterns of glomerular disease and their clinical features are summarized in Table 264-1. These clinicopathologic entities can be induced by a variety of mechanisms. Prompt diagnosis, optimal management, and accurate prognostication is a multistep process that requires (1) recognition of the presenting clinical syndrome, (2) delineation of the underlying morphologic pattern of glomerular injury, and (3) elucidation of the specific renal-limited or systemic disease that triggered glomerular dysfunction.

Nomenclature The terms *glomerulonephritis* and *glomerulopathy* are usually used interchangeably to denote glomerular injury, although some authorities reserve the former term for injury with evidence of inflammation such as leukocyte infiltration, antibody deposition, and complement activation. Glomerular diseases are classified as *primary* when the pathology is confined to the kidney and any systemic features are a direct consequence of glomerular dysfunction (e.g., pulmonary edema, hypertension, the uremic syndrome). Usually, but not always, the term primary is synonymous with *idiopathic*. Glomerular diseases are classified as *secondary* when part of a multisystem disorder. In general, *acute* refers to glomerular injury occurring over days or weeks, *subacute* or *rapidly progressive* over weeks or a few months, and *chronic* over many months or years. Lesions are classified as *focal* or *diffuse* when they involve the minority (<50%) or majority (≥50%) of glomeruli, respectively. Lesions are termed *segmental* or *global* when they involve part of or almost all of the glomerular tuft, respectively. *Proliferative* is used to describe an increase in glomerular cell number, which can be either true proliferation of resident glomerular cells or glomerular hypercellularity caused by infiltration by leukocytes.

Proliferation of resident glomerular cells is classified as *intracapillary* or *endocapillary* when referring to endothelial or mesangial cells and *extracapillary* when referring to cells in Bowman's space. A *crescent* is a half-moon-shaped collection of cells in Bowman's space, usually composed of proliferating parietal epithelial cells and infiltrating macrophages. Because crescentic glomerulonephritis is often associated with renal failure that progresses rapidly over weeks to months, the clinical term *rapidly progressive glomerulonephritis* and pathologic term *crescentic glomerulonephritis* are often used interchangeably. The description *membranous* is applied to glomerulonephritis dominated by expansion of the glomerular basement membrane (GBM) by immune deposits. *Sclerosis* refers to an increase in the amount of homogeneous nonfibrillar extracellular material of similar composition to GBM and mesangial matrix. This process is distinct from *fibrosis*, which involves deposition of collagens type I and III and is more commonly a consequence of healing of crescents or tubulointerstitial inflammation.

Major Clinicopathologic Entities In the absence of comprehensive knowledge of disease etiology, most glomerulopathies are still classified and named according to their morphologic features (Table 264-1). The major inflammatory glomerulopathies are *focal proliferative glomerulonephritis* (termed *mesangial proliferative glomerulonephritis* if the proliferating cells are predominantly mesangial cells), *diffuse proliferative glomerulonephritis*, and *crescentic glomerulonephritis*. These diseases typically present with a *nephritic-type* "active" urine sediment characterized by the presence of red blood cells, red blood cell casts, leukocytes, and *subnephrotic* proteinuria of <3 g/24 h. The severity of renal insufficiency varies in proportion to the degree of glomerular inflammation.

The major morphologic patterns affecting the glomerular filtration barrier for proteins, namely the GBM and visceral epithelial cells, are *membranous glomerulopathy, minimal change disease* (MCD), and *focal and segmental glomerulosclerosis* (FSGS). These entities typically present with *nephrotic-range* proteinuria of ≥3 g/24 h and the presence of relatively few red blood cells, leukocytes, or cellular casts. As a consequence of the heavy proteinuria, nephrotic syndrome is associated with hypoalbuminemia, edema, hyperlipidemia, and lipiduria, and a prothrombotic state. *Membranoproliferative glomerulonephritis*, as the name suggests, is a hybrid lesion that presents with a combination of nephritic and nephrotic features.

The *glomerular deposition diseases* are a group of disorders characterized by prominent extravascular deposition of a paraprotein or fibrillar material. These diseases can trigger either nephritic-type or nephrotic-type responses (or a combination of both) and thus show marked clinical and morphologic overlap with the entities described above.

TABLE 264-1 Major Clinicopathologic Presentation of Glomerular Disease

Structural Pattern	Typical Clinical Presentation	Typical Pathology Findings	Most Common Etiologies
Diffuse proliferative GN	Acute nephritic syndrome: Acute renal failure over days to weeks, hypertension, edema, oliguria, active urine sediment, subnephrotic proteinuria	Diffuse increase in cellularity of tufts of most glomeruli due to infiltration by neutrophils and monocytes, and proliferation of glomerular endothelial and mesangial cells	Immune complex GN: idiopathic, postinfectious, SLE, SBE, cryoglobulinemia, HSP Pauci-immune GN and anti-GBM disease (crescentic GN common—see below)
Crescentic GN	Rapidly progressive glomerulonephritis (RPGN): Subacute renal failure over weeks to months, active urine sediment, variable amount of hypertension, edema, oliguria, and proteinuria	Majority of glomeruli contain areas of fibrinoid necrosis and crescents in Bowman's space, composed of proliferating parietal epithelial cells, infiltrating macrophages, and fibrin	Immune complex GN (as above) Pauci-immune GN: Wegener's granulomatosis, microscopic polyarteritis nodosa, renal-limited crescentic GN Anti-GBM disease (Goodpasture's syndrome if lung hemorrhage)
Focal proliferative GN	Mild to moderate glomerular inflammation: Active urine sediment and mild to moderate decline in GFR	Segmental areas of proliferation and necrosis in less than 50% of glomeruli, occasionally with crescent formation	Early and milder forms, or recovery phase of most diseases causing diffuse proliferative and crescentic GN IgA nephropathy/HSP
Mesangial proliferative GN	Chronic glomerular inflammation: Proteinuria, hematuria, hypertension, variable effect on GFR	Proliferation of mesangial cells and matrix	IgA nephropathy/HSP Early and milder forms, or recovery phases of most diseases that cause diffuse proliferative and crescentic GN (see above) In association with minimal change glomerulopathy and FSGS
Membranoproliferative GN	Variable combination of nephritic and nephrotic features: Acute or subacute decline in GFR, active urine sediment, proteinuria often in nephrotic range	Diffuse proliferation of mesangial cells and infiltration of glomeruli by macrophages; increased mesangial matrix and thickening and reduplication of glomerular basement membrane	Immune complex GN (as for diffuse proliferative GN) In association with thrombotic microangiopathies (see below) In association with deposition diseases (see below) Postrenal or -marrow transplantation
Minimal change GN	Nephrotic syndrome: Proteinuria of >3–3.5 g/d, hypoalbuminemia, edema, hyperlipidemia, lipiduria, thrombotic diathesis, slow decline in GFR in 10–30%.	Light microscopy normal, but electron microscopy (EM) shows foot process effacement	Idiopathic In association with drug-induced interstitial nephritis, HIV infection, heroin, Hodgkin's and other lymphomas
Focal segmental glomerulosclerosis	Nephrotic syndrome: Proteinuria of >3–3.5 g/d, hypoalbuminemia, edema, hyperlipidemia, lipiduria, thrombotic diathesis, slow decline in GFR in 10–30%.	Segmental capillary collapse affecting <50% of glomeruli with entrapment of amorphous hyaline material. EM shows foot process effacement	Primary FSGS: idiopathic, HIV, heroin, lysosomal diseases, Charcot-Marie-Tooth Secondary response to reduction in nephron number from any cause (hyperfiltration injury)
Nodular or global sclerosis	Proteinuria and chronic renal failure	Sclerosis of most glomeruli with interstitial fibrosis	Diabetic nephropathy Potential long-term consequence of most glomerulopathies listed above
Membranous GN	Nephrotic syndrome: Proteinuria of >3–3.5 g/d, hypoalbuminemia, edema, hyperlipidemia, lipiduria, thrombotic diathesis, slow decline in GFR in 10–30%	Diffuse thickening of the glomerular basement membrane with subepithelial projections ("spikes") around immune deposits	Idiopathic Infections (e.g., hepatitis B & C, syphilis, schistasomiasis, malaria, leprosy) Drugs (e.g., gold, penicillamine, captopril) Autoimmune diseases (SLE, rheumatoid arthritis) Paraneoplastic
Deposition diseases	Combination of nephritic and nephrotic features: Renal failure over months to years, proteinuria, hematuria, and hypertension.	Mesangial expansion and thickening of glomerular capillary wall; variable cellular proliferation and crescent formation	Amyloid Cryoglobulinemia Light chain deposition disease Fibrillary/immunotactoid GN
Thrombotic microangiopathy	Acute or subacute renal failure: Variable degree of hypertension, edema and proteinuria, urine sediment usually contains red blood cells, but less activity than patients with nephrotic syndrome or RPGN	Microthrombi in glomerular capillaries ± endothelial injury	Idiopathic In association with gastrointestinal infections, or drugs such as anovulants, mitomycin C, cyclosporine Other diseases: SLE, scleroderma, toxemia, malignant hypertension
Nonimmune basement membrane abnormalities	Asymptomatic hematuria and variable renal failure	Alport's syndrome—mesangial hypercellularity with focal sclerosis and interstitial fibrosis; splintering of GBM on EM.	Alport's syndrome, Thin basement membrane disease. Nail-patella syndrome, Lecithin–cholesterol acyltransferase deficiency

Note: Diffuse, affecting ≥50% of glomeruli; focal, affecting <50% of glomeruli; global, affecting ≥50% of glomerular tuft; segmental, affecting <50% of glomerular tuft; GN, glomerulonephritis; FSGS, focal segmental glomerulosclerosis; HSP, Henoch-Schönlein purpura; SLE, systemic lupus erythematosus; SBE, subacute bacterial endocarditis; GBM, glomerular basement membrane; GFR, glomerular filtration rate.

TABLE 264-2 *Primary Mechanisms of Glomerular Injury*

Mechanism of Injury	Some Renal Insults/Defects	Glomerular Disease
Immunologic[a]	Immunoglobulin[b]	Immune complex–mediated glomerulonephritis
	Cell-mediated injury[b]	Pauci-immune glomerulonephritis
	Cytokine (or other soluble factor)	Primary focal segmental glomerulosclerosis
	Persistent complement activation	Membranoproliferative glomerulonephritis (type II)
Metabolic[a]	Hyperglycemia[b]	Diabetic nephropathy
	Fabry's disease and sialidosis	Focal segmental glomerulosclerosis
Hemodynamic[a]	Systemic hypertension[b]	Hypertensive nephrosclerosis
	Intraglomerular hypertension[b]	Secondary focal segmental glomerulosclerosis
Toxic	E. coli–derived verotoxin	Thrombotic microangiopathy
	Therapeutic drugs (e.g., NSAIDs)	Minimal change disease
	Recreational drugs (heroin)	Focal segmental glomerulosclerosis
Deposition	Amyloid fibrils	Amyloid nephropathy
Infectious	HIV	HIV nephropathy
	Subacute bacterial endocarditis	Immune complex glomerulonephritis
Inherited	Defect in gene for α5 chain of type IV collagen	Alport's syndrome
	Abnormally thin basement membrane	Thin basement membrane disease

[a] Most common categories.
[b] Most common insults within these categories.

Note: NSAIDs, nonsteroidal anti-inflammatory drugs.

The *thrombotic microangiopathies* are a family of diseases in which the pathologic presentation is dominated by coagulation disturbances or endothelial cell injury that result in the formation of thrombi within the renal microvasculature, often leading to renal insufficiency. →*For further discussion of this category of glomerular diseases see Chap. 267.*

MAJOR DETERMINANTS OF GLOMERULAR INJURY The important determinants of the extent and severity of glomerular injury, and accordingly of the clinical presentation, include (1) the nature of the primary insult and the secondary mediator systems that it invokes; (2) the site of injury within the glomerulus; and (3) the speed of onset, the extent, and intensity of disease.

Primary Insult Glomeruli are susceptible to a variety of inflammatory, metabolic, hemodynamic, toxic, and infectious insults (Table 264-2). Most human glomerular disease is triggered by either immune attack (e.g., most forms of inflammatory glomerulonephritis), metabolic stress (e.g., diabetic nephropathy), or mechanical stress (e.g., hypertension). Diverse insults can induce similar clinicopathologic presentations, suggesting marked overlap among downstream molecular and cellular responses. For example, immune complex deposition triggered by streptococcal pharyngitis and antibody-independent glomerular injury in microscopic polyarteritis can each induce proliferative glomerulonephritis. Similarly, metabolic (e.g., diabetes mellitus) and deposition diseases (e.g., amyloid) can each induce glomerulosclerosis with nephrotic syndrome.

Site of Injury The consequences of injury at different sites within the glomerulus can be predicted from the physiologic functions of the cells within the local milieu. In health the renal endothelium is antiadhesive for leukocytes and antithrombotic and maintains the diameter of the vascular lumen through release of nitric oxide and prostacyclin. The major sequelae of injury to the endothelium and subendothelial aspect of the GBM are (1) recruitment of leukocytes leading to inflammatory glomerulonephritis, or (2) perturbed hemostasis leading to thrombotic microangiopathy. It is usual for one of these phenotypes to dominate; however, hybrid lesions may occur (e.g., in lupus nephritis; see below). Intrarenal vasoconstriction and mesangial cell contraction can complicate each phenotype and thereby contribute to renal failure. Injury localized to the mesangial area typically presents as asymptomatic abnormalities of the urinary sediment and mild renal insufficiency. Proteinuria dominates the clinical presentation of injury to the subepithelial aspect of the GBM and visceral epithelial cells. As with mesangial injury, GFR is often only mildly compromised in this set-

ting unless there is concomitant tubulointerstitial injury. The classic pathologic manifestation of parietal epithelial cell injury is crescent formation, which typically presents with acute or subacute renal failure. Crescents can be the dominant morphologic presentation of glomerular disease or complicate proliferative or membranous lesions.

Speed of Onset, Intensity, and Extent of Injury To illustrate the importance of the speed of onset, extent, and intensity of glomerular injury, it is instructive to compare two forms of immune complex glomerulonephritis, i.e., acute postinfectious glomerulonephritis and IgA nephropathy. Poststreptococcal glomerulonephritis is characterized by rapid deposition of immune complexes throughout the glomerular capillary wall, which often provokes acute diffuse proliferative glomerulonephritis with the classic hallmarks of acute inflammation (i.e., complement activation, leukocyte recruitment, lysosomal enzyme release, free radical generation, and perturbation of vascular tone and permeability) with resultant acute renal failure. In contrast, IgA nephropathy is characterized by slow, but sustained, formation of IgA-containing immune complexes, largely confined to the mesangium; less dramatic activation of complement and other mediator systems; and either stability of GFR or progressive renal insufficiency over decades.

MAJOR MECHANISMS OF GLOMERULAR INJURY

Hereditary defects accounts for a minority of glomerular disease. Most acquired glomerular disease is triggered by immune-mediated injury, metabolic stress, or mechanical stress.

INHERITED GLOMERULAR DISEASES *Alport's syndrome* (hereditary nephritis; p. 1691 and Chap. 342), the prototypical inherited glomerular disease, is usually transmitted as an X-linked dominant trait, although autosomal dominant and recessive forms have been reported. Patients afflicted with the classic X-linked form have a mutation in the COL4A5 gene that encodes the α5 chain of type IV collagen located on the X chromosome. As a result, the GBM is irregular with longitudinal layering, splitting, or thickening, and patients develop hematuria, progressive glomerulosclerosis, and renal failure. Other inherited glomerular diseases include *thin basement membrane disease* (p. 1690), *nail-patella syndrome* (osteoonychodysplasia), *partial lipodystrophy*, and *familial lecithin–cholesterol acyltransferase deficiency*. These will be discussed later in this chapter.

IMMUNOLOGIC GLOMERULAR INJURY Immune-mediated glomerulonephritis accounts for a large fraction of acquired renal disease (Fig. 264-1). The majority of cases are associated with the deposition of antibodies, often autoantibodies, within the glomerular tuft, indicating dysregulation of humoral immunity. Cellular immune mechanisms contribute to the pathogenesis of antibody-mediated glomerulonephritis by modulating antibody production and through antibody-dependent cell cytotoxicity (see below). Cellular immune mechanisms also play a dominant role in the pathophysiology of "pauci-immune" glomerulonephritis, notable for robust glomerular inflammation without immunoglobulin deposition.

Humoral Antibody-Mediated Injury Most antibody-mediated glomerulonephritis in humans is initiated by reactivity of circulating antibodies with glomerular antigens. The major mechanisms of antibody deposition within the glomerulus are (1) reactivity of circulating autoantibodies with intrinsic autoantigens that are components of normal glomerular parenchyma, as occurs in anti-GBM disease (Goodpasture's syndrome); (2) in situ formation of immune complexes within glomeruli through interaction of circulating antibodies with extrinsic antigens that have been trapped, or "planted," within the glomerulus, as occurs in postinfectious glomerulonephritis; and (3) intraglomerular trapping of immune complexes that have formed in the systemic circulation, as occurs in cryoglobulinemia-associated glomerulonephritis. Circulating autoantibodies against neutrophil cytoplasmic antigens (antineutrophil cytoplasmic antibodies, ANCA) and endothelial antigens (antiendothelial cell antibodies, AECA) may represent additional mechanisms of antibody-mediated glomerular injury in patients without discernible immune complexes in the glomerular parenchyma.

GENERATION OF NEPHRITOGENIC ANTIBODIES Exposure of the host to a foreign antigen (e.g., a prodromal infection) has been implicated as the trigger for the generation of nephritogenic autoantibodies in several forms of glomerulonephritis. Foreign antigens can provoke autoantibody formation through several mechanisms. First, a foreign antigen, whose structure resembles that of a host glomerular antigen, may stimulate the production of autoantibodies that cross-react with the intrinsic glomerular antigen (*molecular mimicry*). Second, the foreign antigen may trigger aberrant expression of major histocompatibility complex (MHC) class II molecules on glomerular cells, which present previously "invisible" autoantigens to T lymphocytes and thereby generate an autoimmune response. Third, the foreign antigen can trigger polyclonal activation of B lymphocytes, some of which generate nephritogenic antibodies. Alternatively, individuals may suffer a breakdown of immune tolerance through other mechanisms (e.g., genetically programmed).

Autoreactive B cells are usually deleted in the thymus during development (*clonal deletion*) or rendered anergic in peripheral lymphoid tissue (*clonal anergy*). Similar tolerogenic mechanisms exist for deleting or anergizing autoreactive T helper cells that modulate immunoglobulin production by autoreactive B cells. Perturbation of these tolerogenic mechanisms could drive immunoglobulin production in some forms of autoimmune glomerulonephritis. Indeed, defective clonal deletion of autoreactive T cells has been demonstrated in experimental lupus nephritis due to defective synthesis of Fas, a cell-surface receptor that modulates T cell deletion through *apoptosis* (programmed cell death) within the thymus.

DEPOSITION OF NEPHRITOGENIC ANTIBODIES WITHIN THE GLOMERULUS (Fig. 264-1) The site of antibody deposition within the glomerulus is a critical determinant of the clinicopathologic presentation and is determined by the avidity, affinity, and quantity of the antibody; the size, charge, and site of the antigen; the size of the immune complexes; the efficiency of the clearance mechanisms for immune complexes; and local hemodynamic factors. Relatively anionic antigens are repelled by the GBM, which is negatively charged, and tend to be trapped in the subendothelial cell space and mesangium. In contrast, relatively cationic antigens tend to permeate the GBM and deposit within the GBM or in the subepithelial space.

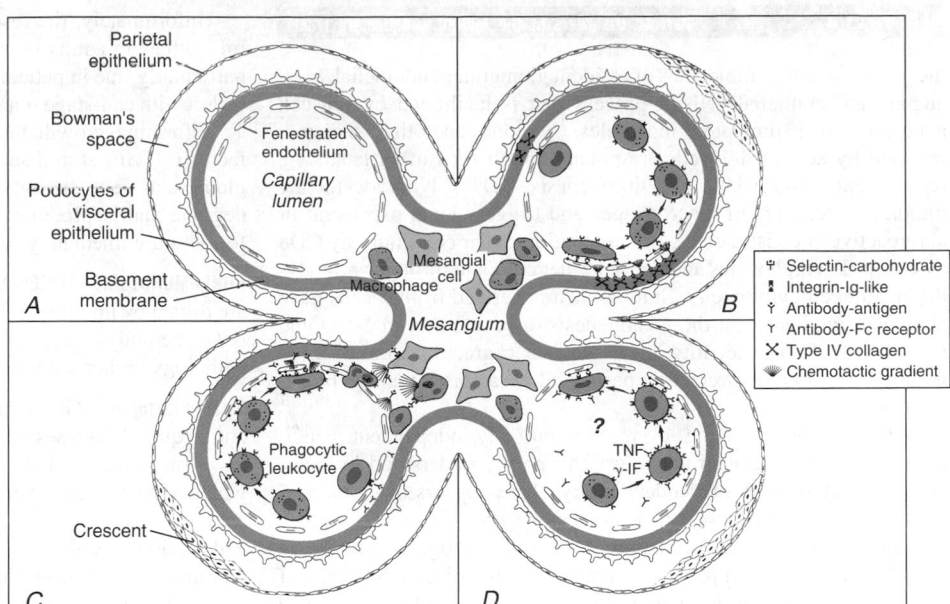

FIGURE 264-1 Major mechanisms of antibody-mediated injury in glomerulonephritis. *A.* Normal glomerulus. Key components of "healthy" glomerular capillary loop. *B.* Antiglomerular basement membrane antibody-mediated glomerulonephritis. Linear deposition of IgG against the Goodpasture antigen. The latter autoantigen is a normal constituent of the noncollagenous domain of $\alpha 3$ chain of type IV collagen, whose "chicken wire"–like structure is essential for maintenance of normal glomerular basement membrane architecture and function. *C.* Immune complex–mediated glomerulonephritis. Immune complexes scattered throughout the glomerular capillary wall, e.g., as can occur in lupus nephritis or postinfectious glomerulonephritis. In mechanisms *B* and *C*, leukocyte chemotaxis is triggered by complement components, chemokines, and other inflammatory mediators. Leukocyte–endothelial cell adhesion is supported by four major classes of adhesion molecules: the selectins and their diverse carbohydrate-bearing ligands, the leukocyte integrins, and immunoglobulin-like molecules such as intercellular adhesion molecule-1. Leukocytes also adhere through binding of their Fc receptors to the Fc domains of immunoglobulin. *D.* Antineutrophil cytoplasmic antibody (ANCA)-associated glomerulonephritis. In diseases such as Wegener's granulomatosis, ANCA are postulated to induce glomerular injury by interacting with neutrophil granule components that have migrated to the cell surface following priming of neutrophils by cytokines, as may occur during a prodromal viral illness. Reactivity of ANCA with neutrophil granule components in vitro triggers neutrophil activation and endothelial cell injury. This mechanism of glomerular injury remains to be established definitively in vivo, however, hence the symbol "?" in the cartoon. Crescents are formed by proliferation of parietal epithelial cells and migration of monocyte-macrophages into the glomerulus from the glomerular capillary lumen and tubulointerstitial space. As they expand, crescents compress the glomerular capillary tuft and are a rich source of mediators that further amplify the inflammatory response. TNF, tumor necrosis factor; γ-IF, interferon γ.

Acute deposition of antibody in the subendothelial cell space (e.g., poststreptococcal glomerulonephritis) or mesangium (e.g., Henoch-Schönlein purpura) typically triggers a nephritic-type response characterized by rapid recruitment of leukocytes and platelets, probably because inflammatory mediators generated at these sites are strategically positioned to activate endothelial and hematogenous cells. Leukocyte-derived products, such as reactive oxygen species, lysosomal enzymes and cytokines, complement components, and other toxic moieties generated in the local inflammatory milieu are both injurious to the glomerular vascular wall and filtration barrier and attract subsequent waves of leukocytes from the circulation. Antibody deposition in the subepithelial cell space (e.g., membranous nephropathy) typically induces a nephrotic-type response characterized by proteinuria without a pronounced inflammatory cell infiltrate, probably because the immune complexes are shielded from circulating inflammatory cells by the GBM and because the large fluid flux from blood to Bowman's space minimizes back-diffusion of inflammatory mediators towards the endothelium and vascular lumen. In this setting, complement components such as the membrane attack complex (C5b-9) appear to be the major effectors of glomerular injury.

Cellular Antibody-Independent Glomerular Injury Although cell-mediated injury is, as yet, less well defined than antibody-mediated glomerular injury, T cells have also been implicated as independent mediators of glomerular injury and as modulators of the production of nephritogenic antibodies. T cells may be particularly important as initiators of injury in pauci-immune glomerulonephritis. T cells interact, through their cell-surface T cell receptor/CD3 complex, with antigens presented in the groove of MHC molecules of resident glomerular endothelial, mesangial, and epithelial cells, a process that is facilitated by cell-cell adhesion and costimulatory molecules. Cytokines and other mediators released by activated T cells are potent stimuli for further leukocyte recruitment, cytotoxicity, and fibrogenesis. CD4 T lymphocytes are important recruiters of macrophages and trigger clonal expansion of autoreactive B cells; they also promote glomerular cell injury by CD8 cytotoxic T lymphocytes and natural killer cells and through antibody-dependent cell cytotoxicity. Soluble factors derived from T cells have also been implicated in the pathogenesis of proteinuria in MCD and primary FSGS. The identity and molecular characterization of these nonimmunoglobulin circulating permeability factors remain to be determined.

Whereas the initiating events in antibody-independent pauci-immune forms of glomerular injury are poorly understood by comparison with antibody-dependent injury, there appears to be marked overlap between the downstream mediator systems that perturb glomerular morphology and function. Thus key pathogenic roles have already been defined in pauci-immune glomerular disease for many of the mediator systems discussed above including leukocyte-derived toxic moieties, such as reactive oxygen species, proteases, cytokines, chemokines, and other inflammatory mediators derived from recruited and resident renal cells.

Cell Proliferation and Accumulation of Extracellular Matrix A hallmark of the nephritic-type proliferative glomerulopathies is an increase in glomerular cell number. Initially, this hypercellularity is due predominantly to infiltration of the glomerular tuft by leukocytes. Subsequently, resident glomerular cells proliferate in response to growth factors [e.g., epidermal growth factor (EGF), platelet-derived growth factor (PDGF)] released into the local inflammatory milieu. The proliferating cells are typically mesangial in mesangioproliferative glomerulonephritis and both endothelial and mesangial cells in diffuse proliferative glomerulonephritis. The visceral epithelial cell is, for the most part, a terminally differentiated cell that does not proliferate rapidly, even when injured.

Whereas acute antibody-mediated glomerulonephritis typically induces acute diffuse proliferative glomerulonephritis and acute renal failure over days to weeks (nephritic syndrome), subacute immune injury often induces the formation of glomerular crescents and renal failure over weeks to months (termed *rapidly progressive glomerulonephritis* (RPGN). As discussed above, crescents are extracapillary proliferations of cells in Bowman's space, composed of infiltrating monocytes, proliferating parietal epithelial cells, and fibrin.

Sustained low-level immune complex deposition over months to years can provoke a marked increase in basement membrane or mesangial matrix production. Mild to moderate accumulation of matrix usually manifests as proteinuria due to disruption of the glomerular filtration barrier; however, in its most severe form, matrix accumulation causes glomerulosclerosis and chronic renal insufficiency.

Determinants of Resolution, Repair, and Scarring Glomerular inflammation can resolve with complete recovery of renal function or with a variable amount of scarring and chronic renal insufficiency. Acute poststreptococcal glomerulonephritis, for example, usually resolves spontaneously and fully in children, whereas adults may be left with residual renal impairment. The resolution process requires cessation of further antibody production and immune complex formation, removal of deposited and circulating immune complexes, inhibition of further recruitment of inflammatory cells, dissipation of the gradients of inflammatory mediators, restoration of normal endothelial adhesiveness and permeability, normalization of vascular tone, and clearance of infiltrating inflammatory cells and proliferating resident glomerular cells. Putative pro-resolution signals in spontaneously resolving glomerular inflammation include the lipoxygenase-derived eicosanoids, the lipoxins, and cytokines such as interleukin (IL)-4, -10, and -13.

Unfortunately, the resolution phase of most inflammatory glomerulopathies in adults terminates in some glomerular scarring. This is particularly true in patients with crescentic glomerulopathies who may be left with end-stage renal failure requiring dialysis or transplantation. Transforming growth factor (TGF) β and connective tissue growth factor (CTGF) stimulate production of extracellular matrix by most glomerular cells, inhibits synthesis of tissue proteases that normally degrade matrix proteins, and appear to be important stimuli for scar formation immediately following glomerular injury.

NONIMMUNOLOGIC GLOMERULAR INJURY While many glomerular diseases are driven by immunologic events, a variety of nonimmunologic metabolic, hemodynamic, and toxic stresses can each induce glomerular pathology, either alone or in concert with immunologic processes.

Metabolic Injury Glomerulopathy complicates a variety of inherited and acquired diseases of carbohydrate and lipid metabolism. Hyperglycemia is a central event in the injury process. The mechanisms by which hyperglycemia perturbs renal function in diabetes are still being appreciated and include (1) the interactions of advanced glycosylation end-products (AGEs) with renal cells; (2) direct effects of high glucose on renal cells mediated through the generation of reactive oxygen species, cell sorbitol accumulation, activation of protein kinase C, and mitogen-activated protein kinases; and (3) high glucose–triggered glomerular hypertension. Important functional consequences of these high glucose–triggered events include mesangial cell hypertrophy, increased mesangial cell matrix production, reduced matrix catabolism, and glomerulosclerosis.

Several rare inherited lysosomal enzyme defects induce focal segmental glomerulosclerosis, probably by allowing accumulation of toxic metabolites in renal cells. *Fabry's disease* (α-galactosidase deficiency) and *sialidosis* (N-acetylneuraminic acid hydrolase deficiency) are the major culprits in this regard.

Hemodynamic Glomerular Injury High intraglomerular pressure is a major cause of glomerular injury and can result from systemic hypertension or from local change in glomerular hemodynamics leading to glomerular hypertension.

Systemic Hypertension (See also Chap. 230) Although the kidneys have evolved sophisticated mechanisms for autoregulating glomerular blood flow and pressure, marked or sustained increments in systemic blood pressure can overwhelm these compensatory systems and perturb glomerular morphology and function. In its most dramatic form, namely malignant hypertension, hemodynamic stress causes massive fibrinoid necrosis of afferent arterioles and glomeruli, thrombotic microangiopathy, a nephritic urinary sediment, and acute renal failure. Chronic sustained hypertension typically leads to arteriolar vasoconstriction and sclerosis, which, in turn, cause secondary atrophy and sclerosis of glomeruli and the tubulointerstitium. A variety of molecular signals appear to couple elevations in intravascular pressure to myointimal proliferation and eventually sclerosis of the vessel wall. These include growth factors such as angiotensin II, EGF, PDGF, and CTGF; cytokines such as TGF-β; and activation of stretch-activated ion channels and early response genes.

Glomerular Hypertension As discussed below, glomerular hypertension is also a key factor in the pathogenesis of the progressive glomerulosclerosis and renal failure. Glomerular hypertension is an adaptive response to increased workload in the remaining functioning nephrons following loss of other nephrons from any cause, including chronic allograft failure. While appropriate in the short term, sustained glomerular hypertension is a stimulus for increased mesangial matrix production and glomerulosclerosis. Importantly, glomerular hypertension appears to precede the development of systemic hypertension in many forms of glomerular disease where it is an independent risk factor for glomerular injury.

Miscellaneous Mechanisms of Nonimmunologic Glomerular Injury In addition to the major immune, metabolic, and mechanical mechanisms of glomeruli injury described above, glomerulopathy can be precipitated by a variety of infectious and toxic agents; the latter include both exogenous (e.g., drugs) and endogenous (e.g., fibril deposition) toxins.

FINAL COMMON PATHWAYS OF INJURY IN GLOMERULAR DISEASE Two pathologic features dominate most cases of chronic progressive glomerular disease, i.e., focal segmental glomerulosclerosis and tubulointerstitial fibrosis. By elucidating the molecular events that contribute to these final common pathways of injury, it should be possible to design new renoprotective therapies. Indeed, the identification of glomerular hypertension as a major stimulus for secondary focal segmental glomerulosclerosis has already led to the use of angiotensin-converting enzyme (ACE) inhibitors and angiotensin II receptor blockers (ARBs) as specific renoprotective agents in clinical practice.

Secondary Focal Segmental Glomerulosclerosis Nephron loss, from any cause, is followed by compensatory vasodilation of afferent arterioles, increased glomerular pressure (*glomerular hypertension*), and increased filtration (*glomerular hyperfiltration*) in the remaining functional glomeruli. This adaptive response is appropriate in the short term and maintains GFR. Over years, however, sustained glomerular hypertension and hyperfiltration induce focal and segmental glomerulosclerosis and eventually global sclerosis, which manifests clinically as proteinuria, hypertension, and progressive renal insufficiency. Glomerular hypertension, in particular, has been implicated as a major stimulus for glomerulosclerosis in this setting. Increased glomerular blood flow and ultrafiltration pressure are early findings in remnant nephrons in most experimental models in which the function of >50% of nephron mass has been lost through surgical ablation, immunologic or toxic injury, or other mechanisms.

Sustained glomerular hypertension is thought to stimulate the accumulation of extracellular matrix by perturbing the function of visceral epithelial and mesangial cells, either directly or by increasing the flux of circulating macromolecules through the glomerular capillary wall. As with most forms of glomerulosclerosis, TGF-β may be an important regulator of matrix accumulation in remnant nephrons. Angiotensin II, PDGF, CTGF, and endothelins are other potential modulators of this process. Maneuvers that lower intraglomerular pressure, such as a low-protein diet or treatment with ACE inhibitors or ARBs, slow the development of glomerulosclerosis and renal failure. Glomerular hypertrophy, intracapillary microthrombi, recruited macrophages, and hyperlipidemia are other potential stimuli for glomerulosclerosis. Indeed, glomerular capillary hypertension and hypertrophy appear to be independent risk factors that could act synergistically to cause progressive renal insufficiency. Intriguingly, angiotensin II may trigger TGF-β production, and engagement of angiotensin II receptors may trigger activation of growth factor receptor signaling pathways (so-called *receptor transactivation*) in remnant nephrons, suggesting that ACE inhibitors and ARBs may be renoprotective through complementary effects on glomerular hemodynamics and matrix production.

Tubulointerstitial Inflammation and Fibrosis Downstream from Glomerular Injury Moderate-to-severe glomerulonephritis is usually associated with a variable degree of tubulointerstitial inflammation and scarring in addition to glomerular injury. Indeed, the severity of tubulointerstitial injury usually correlates closely with long-term impairment of renal function. The pathogenesis of tubulointerstitial inflammation in this setting is unclear. Potential mechanisms include: (1) primary involvement of both the glomeruli and the tubulointerstitium in autoimmune disease; (2) induction of tubulointerstitial inflammation by mediators generated by diseased glomeruli, which then diffuse into the tubulointerstitium via blood, tubular fluid, or the interstitial space; (3) injury to tubule epithelial cells by excessive filtered proteins ("protein overload" hypothesis); and (4) ischemia to areas of the tubulointerstitium downstream to areas of vigorous glomerular inflammation or severe glomerulosclerosis.

CLINICAL PRESENTATIONS

ACUTE NEPHRITIC SYNDROME AND RAPIDLY PROGRESSIVE GLOMERULONEPHRITIS

CLINICAL FEATURES AND CLINICOPATHOLOGIC CORRELATES The *acute nephritic syndrome* is the clinical correlate of acute glomerular inflammation. In its most dramatic form, the acute nephritic syndrome is characterized by sudden onset (i.e., over days to weeks) of acute renal failure and oliguria (400 mL/day of urine). Renal blood flow and GFR fall as a result of obstruction of the glomerular capillary lumen by infiltrating inflammatory cells and proliferating resident glomerular cells. Renal blood flow and GFR are further compromised by intrarenal vasoconstriction and mesangial cell contraction that result from local imbalances of vasoconstrictor (e.g., leukotrienes, platelet-activating factor, thromboxanes, endothelins) and vasodilator substances (e.g., nitric oxide, prostacyclin) within the renal microcirculation. Extracellular fluid volume expansion, edema, and hypertension develop because of impaired GFR and enhanced tubular reabsorption of salt and water. As a result of injury to the glomerular capillary wall, urinalysis typically reveals red blood cell casts, dysmorphic red blood cells, leukocytes, and subnephrotic proteinuria of <3.0 g per 24 h ("nephritic urinary sediment"). Hematuria is often macroscopic.

The classic pathologic correlate of the nephritic syndrome is *proliferative glomerulonephritis*. The proliferation of glomerular cells is due initially to infiltration of the glomerular tuft by neutrophils and monocytes and subsequently to true proliferation of resident glomerular endothelial and mesangial cells (endocapillary proliferation). In its most severe form, the nephritic syndrome is associated with acute inflammation of most glomeruli, i.e., *acute diffuse proliferative glomerulonephritis*. When less vigorous, <50% of glomeruli may be involved, i.e., *focal proliferative glomerulonephritis*. In milder forms of nephritic injury, cellular proliferation may be confined to the mesangium, i.e., *mesangioproliferative glomerulonephritis*.

RPGN is the clinical correlate of more subacute glomerular inflammation. Patients develop renal failure over weeks to months in association with a nephritic urinary sediment, subnephrotic proteinuria and variable oliguria, hypervolemia, edema, and hypertension. The classic pathologic correlate of RPGN is crescent formation involving most glomeruli (*crescentic glomerulonephritis*). In practice, the clinical term *rapidly progressive glomerulonephritis* and the pathologic term *crescentic glomerulonephritis* are often used interchangeably. In addition to classic crescentic glomerulonephritis, in which crescents dominate the glomerular pathology, crescents can also develop concomitantly with proliferative glomerulonephritis or as a complication of membranous glomerulopathy and other more indolent forms of glomerular inflammation.

The acute nephritic syndrome and RPGN are part of a spectrum of presentations of immunologically mediated proliferative glomerulonephritis. Studies of experimental models suggest that nephritic syndrome and diffuse proliferative glomerulonephritis represent an acute immune response to a sudden large antigen load, whereas RPGN and crescentic glomerulonephritis represent a more subacute immune response to a smaller antigen load in presensitized individuals. At the other end of the spectrum, chronic low-grade immune injury presents with slowly progressive renal insufficiency or asymptomatic hematuria in association with focal proliferative or mesangioproliferative glomerulonephritis. These more indolent forms of immune-mediated glomerulonephritis are discussed later in this chapter.

ETIOLOGY AND DIFFERENTIAL DIAGNOSIS Acute nephritic syndrome and RPGN can result from renal-limited *primary* glomerulopathy or from *secondary* glomerulopathy complicating systemic disease. Figure 264-2 highlights the histopathologic and serologic features that help distinguish among the major causes of nephritic syndrome and RPGN. In general, rapid diagnosis and prompt treatment are critical to avoid

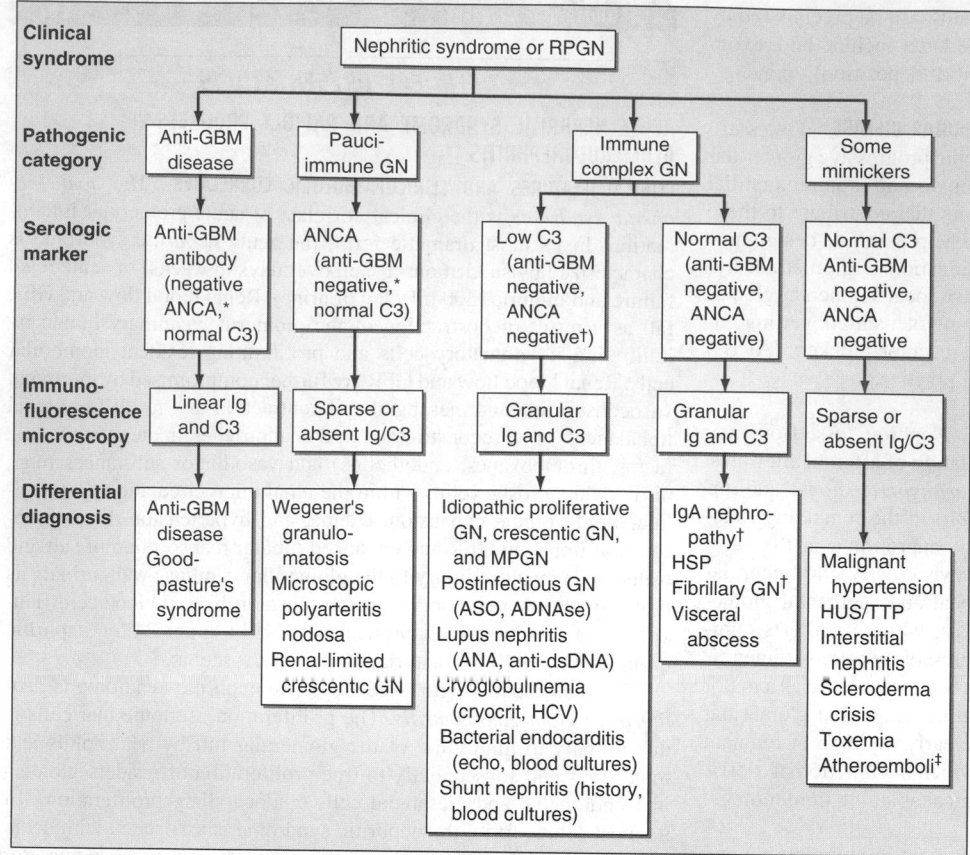

FIGURE 264-2 Differential diagnosis of nephritic syndrome and rapidly progressive glomerulonephritis. Abbreviations: GN, glomerulonephritis; RPGN, rapidly progressive glomerulonephritis; MPGN, membranoproliferative glomerulonephritis; GBM, glomerular basement membrane; ANCA, antineutrophil cytoplasmic antibodies; Ig, immunoglobulin; C3, third component of complement; ASO, antistreptolysin O antibody titer; ADNAse, anti-deoxyribonuclease antibody titer; ANA, antinuclear antibody; anti-dsDNA, anti-double-stranded DNA antibody; HCV, hepatitis C virus; echo, echocardiogram; HSP, Henoch-Schönlein purpura; HUS, hemolytic-uremic syndrome; TTP, thrombotic thrombocytopenic purpura. *Approximately 20% of patients with anti-GBM disease have ANCA, which may portend a better prognosis. †Nephritic syndrome and RPGN are unusual presentations of IgA nephropathy and fibrillary GN. ‡Atheroembolic renal disease may cause transient hypocomplementemia.

the development of irreversible renal failure. Renal biopsy remains the "gold standard" for diagnosis. *Immunofluorescence microscopy* is particularly helpful and identifies three major patterns of deposition of immunoglobulin that define three broad diagnostic categories: (1) scattered *granular* deposits of immunoglobulin, a hallmark of *immune-complex glomerulonephritis*; (2) more discrete *linear* deposition of immunoglobulin along the GBM, characteristic of *anti-GBM disease*; and (3) paucity or absence of immunoglobulin—*pauci-immune glomerulonephritis* (Figs. 264-1 and 264-3). Most patients (≥70%) with full-blown acute nephritic syndrome have immune-complex glomerulonephritis. Pauci-immune glomerulonephritis is less common in this setting (<30%), and anti-GBM disease is rare (<1%). Among patients with RPGN, immune-complex glomerulonephritis and pauci-immune glomerulonephritis are equally prevalent (~45% each), whereas anti-GBM disease again accounts for a minority of cases (<10%).

Three *serologic markers* often predict the immunofluorescence microscopy findings in nephritic syndrome and RPGN and may obviate the need for renal biopsy in classic cases. They are the serum C3 level and titers of anti-GBM antibody and ANCA. As discussed in previous sections, the kidney is host to immune attack in immune-complex glomerulonephritis, most cases being initiated either by in situ formation of immune complexes or less commonly by glomerular trapping of circulating immune complexes. These patients typically have hypocomplementemia (low C3 in 90%) and negative anti-GBM and ANCA serology, the major exception being IgA nephropathy/Henoch Schönlein purpura where complement levels are typically normal. The glomerulus is the direct target of immune attack in anti-GBM disease, glomerular inflammation being initiated by an autoantibody directed at a 28-kDa autoantigen on the α3 chain of type IV collagen. Approx-

imately 90 to 95% of patients with anti-GBM disease have circulating anti-GBM autoantibodies detectable by immunoassay; serum complement levels are typically normal, and ANCA are usually not detected. The pathogenesis of pauci-immune glomerulonephritis is still being defined; however, most patients have circulating ANCA. Serum complement levels are typically normal, and anti-GBM titers are usually negative in ANCA-associated renal disease. It should be noted, however, that there may be some serologic overlap, with as many as 20% of patients with immune complex or anti-GBM glomerulonephritis also having at least low levels of circulating ANCA.

NEPHRITIC SYNDROME AND RPGN DUE TO IMMUNE-COMPLEX GLOMERULONEPHRITIS

Nephritic syndrome induced by immune-complex glomerulonephritis may be (1) be idiopathic, (2) represent a response to a known antigenic stimulus (e.g., glomerulonephritis triggered by bacterial endocarditis or streptococcal infection, or hepatitis B or C infection in cryoglobulinemic glomerulonephritis), or (3) form part of a multisystem immune-complex disorder (e.g., lupus nephritis, Henoch-Schönlein purpura; Table 264-1, Figs. 264-1 to 264-3).

INFECTION-ASSOCIATED GLOMERULONEPHRITIS INCLUDING GLOMERULONEPHRITIS ASSOCIATED WITH STREPTOCOCCAL INFECTION AND INFECTIVE ENDOCARDITIS   A variety of infections can precipitate immune-complex glomerulonephritis. The most common clinicopathologic lesion in this setting is acute diffuse proliferative glomerulonephritis presenting as the acute nephritic syndrome; however, depending on the speed of onset and site and extent of immune complex formation, infection-associated immune complex formation can trigger mesangioproliferative, focal proliferative, membranoproliferative, or membranous glomerulopathy.

Poststreptococcal glomerulonephritis is the prototypical *postinfectious glomerulonephritis* and a leading cause of acute nephritic syndrome. Most cases are sporadic, though the disease can occur as an epidemic. Glomerulonephritis develops, on average, 10 days after pharyngitis or 2 weeks after a skin infection (impetigo) with a nephritogenic strain of group A β-hemolytic streptococcus. The known nephritic strains include M types 1, 2, 4, 12, 18, 25, 49, 55, 57, and 60. Immunity to these strains is type-specific and long-lasting, and repeated infection and nephritis are rare. Epidemic poststreptococcal glomerulonephritis is most commonly encountered in children of 2 to 6 years of age with pharyngitis during the winter months. This entity appears to be decreasing in frequency, possibly due to more widespread and prompt use of antibiotics. Poststreptococcal glomerulonephritis in association with cutaneous infections usually occurs in a setting of poor personal hygiene or streptococcal superinfection of another skin disease.

The classic clinical presentation of poststreptococcal glomerulonephritis is full-blown nephritic syndrome with oliguric acute renal failure; however, most patients have milder disease. Indeed, subclinical cases outnumber overt cases by four- to tenfold during epidemics. Patients with overt disease present with gross hematuria (red or

FIGURE 264-3 Typical findings on immunofluorescence microscopy of renal biopsy specimens from patients with anti-glomerular basement membrane antibody disease, immune complex–mediated glomerulonephritis, and pauci-immune glomerulonephritis. Specimens in the upper and middle panels were stained for immunoglobulin and show the classic linear "ribbon-like" pattern of anti-GBM disease (*A*) and granular pattern of immune complex–mediated glomerulonephritis (*B*). Immunoglobulin is sparse or absent in patients with pauci-immune glomerulonephritis (not shown); however, abundant fibrin is detected in crescents (*C*). *(Micrographs courtesy of Dr. Helmut Rennke.)*

"smoky" urine), headache, and generalized symptoms such as anorexia, nausea, vomiting, and malaise. Swelling of the renal capsule can cause flank or back pain. Physical examination reveals hypervolemia, edema, and hypertension. The urinary sediment is nephritic, with dys-

morphic red blood cells, red cell casts, leukocytes, occasionally leukocyte casts, and subnephrotic proteinuria. Fewer than 5% of patients develop nephrotic-range proteinuria. The latter may only manifest as acute nephritis resolves and renal blood flow and GFR recover. Coexistent rheumatic fever is extremely rare.

The serum creatinine is often mildly elevated at presentation. Serum C3 levels and CH_{50} are depressed within 2 weeks in ~90% of cases. C4 levels are characteristically normal, indicating activation of the alternate pathway of complement. Complement levels usually return to normal within 6 to 8 weeks. Persistently depressed levels after this period should suggest another cause, such as the presence of a C3 nephritic factor (see "Membranoproliferative Glomerulonephritis," p. 1687). The majority of patients (>75%) have transient hypergammaglobulinemia and mixed cryoglobulinemia. The antecedent streptococcal infection may still be evident or may have resolved either spontaneously or in response to antibiotic therapy. Most patients (>90%) have circulating antibodies against streptococcal exoenzymes such as antistreptolysin O (ASO), anti-deoxyribonuclease B (anti-DNAse B), antistreptokinase (ASKase), anti-nicotinyl adenine dinucleotidase (anti-NADasc), and antihyaluronidase (AHase).

Acute poststreptococcal glomerulonephritis is usually diagnosed on clinical and serologic grounds, without resort to renal biopsy, especially in children with a typical antecedent history. The characteristic lesion on light microscopy is diffuse proliferative glomerulonephritis. Crescents are uncommon, and extraglomerular involvement is usually mild. Immunofluorescence microscopy reveals diffuse granular deposition of IgG and C3, giving rise to a "starry sky" appearance (Figs. 264-1 and 264-3). The characteristic finding on electron microscopy is the presence of large electron-dense immune deposits in the subendothelial, subepithelial, and mesangial areas.

In addition to poststreptococcal glomerulonephritis, the nephritic syndrome and RPGN can complicate acute immune-complex glomerulonephritis due to other viral, bacterial, fungal, and parasitic infections. Diffuse proliferative immune-complex glomerulonephritis is a well-described complication of acute and *subacute infective endocarditis* and is usually associated with hypocomplementemia. The glomerular lesion typically resolves following eradication of the cardiac infection.

℞ **TREATMENT**

Treatment of poststreptococcal glomerulonephritis focuses on eliminating the streptococcal infection with antibiotics and providing supportive therapy until spontaneous resolution of glomerular inflammation occurs. Patients are usually confined to bed during the acute inflammatory phase. Diuretics and antihypertensive agents are employed to control extracellular fluid volume and blood pressure. Dialysis is rarely needed to control hypervolemia or the uremic syndrome. Poststreptococcal glomerulonephritis carries an excellent prognosis and rarely causes end-stage renal disease (ESRD). Whereas spontaneous resolution of the glomerular lesion and nephritic syndrome is the norm in children within 6 to 8 weeks, >20% of adults may have some degree of persistent proteinuria and/or compromise of GFR 1 year after presentation. As with poststreptoccal glomerulonephritis, treatment of immune complex glomerulonephritis in association with bacterial endocarditis and other forms of infection is supportive until the causative infection is eliminated.

SYSTEMIC LUPUS ERYTHEMATOSUS (SLE) (LUPUS NEPHRITIS) (See also Chap. 300) Renal involvement is clinically evident in 40 to 85% of patients with SLE; it varies from isolated abnormalities of the urinary sediment to full-blown nephritic or nephrotic syndrome or chronic renal failure. Most glomerular injury is triggered by the formation of immune complexes within the glomerular capillary wall; however, thrombotic microangiopathy may be the dominant reason for renal dysfunction in a small subset of patients with the antiphospholipid antibody syndrome. Renal biopsy has proven very useful for identifying the different patterns of immune-complex glomerulonephritis in SLE, which are diverse, portend different prognoses, and do not necessarily correlate with the clinical findings. Indeed, clinically silent lupus nephritis is well described as having a urinalysis virtually normal but renal biopsy demonstrating varying degrees of injury.

Patients with active lupus nephritis have a range of serologic abnormalities. Hypocomplementemia is present in 75 to 90% of patients and is most striking with diffuse proliferative glomerulonephritis. Antinuclear antibodies (ANA) are usually detected (95 to 99%), although not specific for SLE. ANA titers tend to fall with treatment, and ANA may not be detected during remissions. Anti-double-stranded DNA (dsDNA) antibodies are highly specific for SLE, and changes in their titers correlate with the activity of lupus nephritis.

Patients with the lupus-related antiphospholipid antibody syndrome can develop a variable degree of renal impairment due to thrombotic microangiopathy. The latter typically affects the interlobular arteries, arterioles, and glomerular capillaries and is characterized by intravascular microthrombi and swelling of endothelial cells. Decreased levels of tissue plasminogen activator and increased levels of α_2-antiplasmin, both of which would tend to promote thrombosis, have been described in this syndrome.

R_x TREATMENT

The treatment of lupus nephritis is controversial and based largely on the class of injury and disease activity. Because there is relatively poor correlation between clinical features (urinalysis findings, serum creatinine) and histologic class, the renal biopsy findings are an important guide to therapy. Treatment is not indicated for those with a normal biopsy or only mesangial deposits of immunoglobulins, as these histologic patterns portend an excellent prognosis (100% and 90% 5-year survival rates, respectively). Extrarenal manifestations may warrant treatment with glucocorticoids, salicylates, or antimalarials. Glucocorticoids and cyclophosphamide are the mainstays of therapy for patients with proliferative nephritis. High-dose steroids given as intravenous boluses (pulse therapy) are usually effective at rapidly controlling acute glomerular inflammation. Cyclophosphamide and azathioprine are important adjuncts to steroid therapy and appear to afford better long-term preservation of renal function than steroids alone. Intravenous pulse cyclophosphamide is as efficacious as oral therapy and appears to be less toxic. An initial regimen of monthly intravenous boluses of cyclophosphamide for 6 months should be administered. Subsequent therapy is tailored to disease activity and typically involves dosing every 3 to 6 months for a total treatment period of 12 to 24 months.

The initial dose of cyclophosphamide is 0.5 g/m², and the dose is increased gradually to a maximum of 1 g/m² unless patients develop leukopenia or other side effects. Steroids are usually started simultaneously at 1 mg/kg per day and are tapered over the first 6 months to a maintenance dose of 5 to 10 mg/d for the duration of cyclophosphamide therapy. Cyclophosphamide may be stopped after 6 months and replaced with either azathioprine or mycophenolate provided that partial or complete remission has been achieved. Five-year renal survival rates of 60 to 90% have been obtained with these regimens. Mycophenolate mofetil has also been used as a therapeutic option in patients resistant to cyclophosphamide. A large randomized, prospective trial indicated that plasmapheresis does not offer additional benefit in patients with severe proliferative lupus nephritis.

The management of membranous lupus nephritis (see "Nephrotic Syndrome," below) is less well defined. As with idiopathic membranous glomerulopathy, the incidence of spontaneous remission approaches 50% in membranous lupus nephritis, and the course of the disease is generally indolent, with a 70 to 90% renal survival rate at 5 years. Some authorities advocate steroids at the time of diagnosis, whereas others reserve them for patients with progressive renal insufficiency or severe nephrotic syndrome. Useful parameters for monitoring the response to therapy and predicting relapse include the activity of the urine sediment, proteinuria, GFR, serum complement levels, and anti-dsDNA titers. As in other proteinuric renal diseases, ACE inhibitors or ARBs are usually prescribed as adjunctive treatment. Despite maximal immunosuppressive therapy, about 20% of patients with aggressive lupus nephritis develop ESRD requiring dialysis. SLE tends to become quiescent with advanced uremia, and patients rarely develop systemic flares once they commence dialysis. Recurrence of nephritis and systemic flares are also very uncommon after renal transplantation, and allograft survival rates are comparable to those in patients with other causes of ESRD.

In patients with thrombotic microangiopathy due to lupus-related antiphospholipid antibody syndrome, anticoagulation to maintain the Internalized Normal Ratio (INR) at 3.0 may be beneficial in reducing the incidence of recurrent thromboses. There are uncontrolled reports of a benefit of plasmapheresis in the setting of acute renal failure secondary to thrombotic microangiopathy.

CRYOGLOBULINEMIA GLOMERULOPATHY (See also Chap. 306) Renal involvement is most common with the mixed cryoglobulinemias (types II and III), which are more common in females and usually begin in the sixth decade. Most patients present with a variable combination of leukocytoclastic vasculitis, skin ulcerations, arthralgias, fatigue, and Raynaud's phenomenon. Renal disease is a complication in 50% of patients and usually develops after 12 to 24 months. The typical clinical renal manifestations are nephrotic-range proteinuria, microscopic hematuria, and hypertension. Acute nephritic syndrome occurs in 20 to 30%, and oliguric acute renal failure in about 5% of patients with renal disease.

Circulating levels of C3, C4, and CH50 are depressed in about 80% of patients with renal involvement, and a transient ANA (speckled pattern) is sometimes detected. Hepatitis C virus (HCV) RNA has been isolated from the serum of patients with essential mixed cryoglobulinemia (EMC).

R_x TREATMENT

Traditionally, glucocorticoids, with or without cyclophosphamide, and plasmapheresis were the standard treatment for EMC, with poor results. With the recognition that many cases are triggered by HCV infection, interferon α has been employed to successfully control viral replication and stabilize renal function in most HCV-positive patients. Unfortunately, relapse is common when interferon α is discontinued, a major problem given the cost of this agent. In general, patient and renal survival are good in EMC, with 75% of patients being alive at 10 years.

IGA NEPHROPATHY AND HENOCH-SCHÖNLEIN PURPURA IgA nephropathy (Berger's disease) is a renal-limited form of glomerulonephritis characterized by deposition of IgA-containing immune deposits in the glomerular mesangium (p. 1690). Henoch-Schönlein purpura (Chap. 306) is a systemic disease characterized by a petechial rash on the extremities, arthropathy, abdominal pain, and glomerulonephritis. Because the glomerular lesion is identical to that found in IgA nephropathy, Henoch-Schönlein nephritis and IgA nephropathy may be part of a spectrum of manifestations of a single disease. Nephritis is present in 80% of patients and manifests as a nephritic urine sediment and moderate proteinuria. Macroscopic hematuria and nephrotic-range proteinuria are uncommon. Light-microscopic appears can vary from mild mesangial proliferation and expansion to diffuse proliferation with glomerular crescents. The sine qua non for diagnosis is the presence of mesangial IgA deposition on immunofluorescence microscopy. IgG and C3 are also detected. Electron microscopy reveals mesangial immune deposits. Immune complexes may also be present in the peripheral glomerular capillary wall and paramesangial areas. Biopsy of involved skin reveals dermal IgA deposition and leukocytoclastic vasculitis. IgA deposition is also seen in areas of uninvolved skin.

℞ TREATMENT

Since there is no proven therapy for Henoch-Schönlein nephritis, treatment is supportive. Steroids and/or cytotoxic agents are often tried in patients with severe disease, but without compelling scientific evidence to support their use. The disease typically undergoes clinical exacerbations and remissions in the first year and then enters long-term remission. The prognosis is generally excellent; chronic renal failure and persistent hypertension occur in <10% of patients. The treatment of IgA nephropathy will be discussed later.

NEPHRITIC SYNDROME AND RPGN DUE TO ANTI-GLOMERULAR BASEMENT MEMBRANE DISEASE (GOODPASTURE'S SYNDROME)

Anti-GBM disease is an autoimmune disease in which autoantibodies directed against type IV collagen induce RPGN and crescentic glomerulonephritis (Figs. 264-1 to 264-3). Acute nephritic syndrome is rare. Between 50 and 70% of patients have lung hemorrhage; the clinical complex of anti-GBM nephritis and lung hemorrhage is referred to as *Goodpasture's syndrome*. Patients with this syndrome are typically young males (5 to 40 years; male-female ratio of 6:1). In contrast, patients presenting during the second peak in the sixth decade rarely suffer lung hemorrhage and have an almost equal sex distribution. The target antigen is a component of the noncollagenous (NCI) domain of the $\alpha3$ chain of type IV collagen, the $\alpha3$ chain being preferentially expressed in glomerular and pulmonary alveolar basement membrane.

Anti-GBM disease commonly presents with hematuria, nephritic urinary sediment, subnephrotic proteinuria, and rapidly progressive renal failure over weeks, with or without pulmonary hemorrhage. When pulmonary hemorrhage occurs, it usually predates nephritis by weeks or months. Hemoptysis can vary from fluffy pulmonary infiltrates on chest x-ray and mild dyspnea on exertion to life-threatening pulmonary hemorrhage; hypertension is unusual.

The diagnostic serologic marker is circulating anti-GBM antibodies with a specificity for the NCI domain of the $\alpha3$ chain of type IV collagen. Anti-GBM antibodies are detected in the serum of >90% of patients with anti-GBM nephritis by specific immunoassay. Renal biopsy is the gold standard for diagnosis of anti-GBM nephritis. The typical morphologic pattern on light microscopy is diffuse proliferative glomerulonephritis, with focal necrotizing lesions and crescents in >50% of glomeruli (crescentic glomerulonephritis). Immunofluorescence microscopy reveals linear ribbon-like deposition of IgG along the GBM (Fig. 264-3).

℞ TREATMENT

Prior to the introduction of immunosuppressive therapy, >80% of patients with anti-GBM nephritis developed ESRD within 1 year, and many patients died from pulmonary hemorrhage or complications of uremia. With early and aggressive use of plasmapheresis, glucocorticoids, cyclophosphamide, and azathioprine, renal and patient survival have improved dramatically. In general, emergency plasmapheresis is performed daily or on alternate days until anti-GBM antibodies are not detected in the circulation (usually 1 to 2 weeks). Prednisone (1 mg/kg per day) is started simultaneously, in combination with either cyclophosphamide (2 to 3 mg/kg per day) or azathioprine (1 to 2 mg/kg per day) to suppress new synthesis of anti-GBM antibodies. The speed of initiation of therapy is a critical determinant of outcome. One-year renal survival approaches 90% if treatment is started before serum creatinine exceeds 442 μmol/L (5 mg/dL) and falls to about 10% if renal failure is more advanced. Patients who require dialysis at presentation rarely recover renal function. Serial anti-GBM titers are monitored to gauge response to therapy. Relapses are not unusual and are often heralded by rising antibody titers. In patients with ESRD, renal transplantation is a viable treatment option. Recurrence of anti-GBM nephritis in the allograft is extremely unusual provided that anti-GBM antibody titers have been consistently negative for 6 to 12 months prior to transplantation. However, in occasional patients with Alport's syndrome, when the allograft presents normal GBM components to the immune system of the recipient for the first time, anti-GBM nephritis can occur de novo in renal allografts.

NEPHRITIC SYNDROME AND RPGN DUE TO PAUCI-IMMUNE GLOMERULONEPHRITIS

The major pauci-immune glomerulonephritides are *idiopathic renal-limited crescentic glomerulonephritis, microscopic polyangiitis nodosa* (PAN), and *Wegener's granulomatosis* (Figs. 264-1 to 264-3). Significant glomerular disease may also complicate the Churg-Strauss syndrome and classic forms of PAN, albeit less frequently than the aforementioned three conditions. RPGN is a more common clinical presentation than acute nephritic syndrome, and the usual pathology is necrotizing glomerulonephritis with crescents affecting 50% of glomeruli (crescentic glomerulonephritis). The marked overlap of clinical features and glomerular histopathology, and the presence of circulating ANCA in most patients, suggest that these entities are a spectrum of a single disease. Indeed this group of diseases is frequently categorized under the all-encompassing term *ANCA-associated small vessel vasculitis*. They are more common in whites and older patients (mean age 57 years) and typically present with nonspecific constitutional symptoms and signs such as lethargy, malaise, anorexia, weight loss, fever, arthralgias, and myalgias. Nonspecific laboratory abnormalities include a rapid sedimentation rate, elevated C-reactive protein, leukocytosis, thrombocytosis, and normochromic, normocytic anemia. Serum complement levels are typically normal.

ANCA-Associated Renal Disease Patients with ANCA-associated renal disease usually present with a nephritic urine sediment and subnephrotic proteinuria. Renal dysfunction can vary from a mild decrement in GFR to RPGN. Renal biopsy typically reveals focal, segmental, necrotizing glomerulonephritis with crescent formation. Immunofluorescence and electron microscopy are remarkable for the paucity or absence of immunoglobulin, complement, and immune deposits: hence the term *pauci-immune glomerulonephritis*.

Idiopathic Renal-Limited Crescentic Glomerulonephritis This is more common in middle-aged and older patients and shows a slight male preponderance. Patients typically present with RPGN, nephritic syndrome being rare. ANCA, usually a perinuclear ANCA IgG with specificity for myeloperoxidase, are detected in 70 to 90% of patients. The erythrocyte sedimentation rate and C-reactive protein levels may be elevated; however, C3 levels are typically normal, and circulating immune complexes, cryoglobulins, and anti-GBM antibodies are not detected. Most patients have crescents on light microscopy, often associated with necrotizing glomerulonephritis. Immune deposits are scanty or absent. Immunofluorescence microscopy reveals abundant fibrin deposits within crescents (Fig. 264-3).

Wegener's Granulomatosis (See also Chap. 306) Renal injury occurs in 80% of patients with Wegener's granulomatosis and varies from indolent smoldering inflammation to rapidly progressive renal failure. Cytoplasmic ANCA are detected at presentation in 80% of patients with renal disease and in 10% more on follow-up. Renal biopsy typically reveals focal, segmental, necrotizing pauci-immune glomerulonephritis with crescent formation. In contrast to the lung, granulomas are rarely seen in the kidney.

Microscopic Polyangiitis Nodosa (See also Chap. 306) Microscopic PAN is a systemic disease characterized by leukocytoclastic vasculitis involving multiple organ systems including the lungs, skin, joints, and kidneys. Clinical renal disease ranges from a nephritic urinary sediment with mild impairment of GFR to RPGN. The usual histopathologic lesion is pauci-immune focal segmental necrotizing and crescentic glomerulonephritis. Circulating ANCA are detected in 70 to 80% of patients at presentation, with cANCA or pANCA being equally prevalent.

Churg-Strauss Syndrome (See also Chap. 306) Clinical renal involvement in Churg-Strauss syndrome is relatively infrequent and usually limited to mild proteinuria and hematuria. Evolution to chronic renal failure is rare. Renal biopsy most frequently reveals extraglomerular pathology, with involvement of the renal vasculature and tubulointerstitium by granulomatous vasculitis. Focal segmental glomerulonephritis with crescents is also seen. A minority of patients have focal segmental necrotizing glomerulonephritis.

CLASSIC POLYANGIITIS NODOSA AND LARGE VESSEL VASCULITIDES

(See also Chap. 306) In contrast to the small vessel vasculitides discussed above, it is unusual to detect ANCA in classic PAN and the major large-vessel vasculitides. The typical glomerular lesion in classic PAN is ischemic collapse and obsolescence. Characteristic clinical and serologic features are hypertension, a bland urine sediment with subnephrotic proteinuria, slowly progressive renal insufficiency, normal serum complement levels, and absence of ANCA. Glomerular involvement is exceedingly rare in the major large vessel vasculitides such as Takayasu's disease and giant cell arteritis.

℞ TREATMENT

Glucocorticoids and cyclophosphamide are the mainstays of treatment and dramatically ameliorate glomerular injury in pauci-immune glomerulonephritis. Steroids are usually administered initially by pulse intravenous therapy on three consecutive days, followed by a daily oral dose of about 1 mg/kg body weight tapered to a maintenance doses of 5 to 10 mg every day or alternate day over 3 to 6 months. Cyclophosphamide is typically administered orally at a daily dose of 1 to 2 mg/kg or as six monthly intravenous pulses of 1 g/m² of body surface area followed by pulses every 3 months for a maximum of 1 to 2 years. Alternatively, patients are switched from cyclophosphamide to either azathioprine or mycophenolate after 6 months in an effort to avoid cyclophosphamide toxicity and treatment is continued for a total duration of at least 1 year. Plasmapheresis may be a useful adjunct in patients with severe nephritis requiring dialysis. As many as 30% of patients relapse after treatment-induced remission. As with all patients receiving potent immunosuppressive therapy, the benefits of immunosuppression must be balanced against the risk of toxicity, and factors such as patient age co-morbidity, and the intensity of the vasculitic process must be taken into account. A persistently elevated or rising ANCA titer may predict relapse in individual patients; however, this relationship is not strong enough to justify treatment based on titers alone. Recent studies demonstrate that administration of trimethoprim-sulfamethoxazole reduces the relapse rate, possibly by eradicating nasal carriage of *Staphylococcus aureus*. Dialysis and renal transplantation afford excellent survival in patients with ESRD. Recurrence of Wegener's granulomatosis in the allograft is rare. ACE inhibitors may help to slow the progression to end-stage renal failure.

NEPHROTIC SYNDROME

Proteinuria >150 mg per 24 h is abnormal and can result from a number of mechanisms. *Glomerular proteinuria* results from leakage of plasma proteins through a perturbed glomerular filtration barrier; *tubular proteinuria* results from failure of tubular reabsorption of low-molecular-weight plasma proteins that are normally filtered and then reabsorbed and metabolized by tubular epithelium; *overflow proteinuria* results from filtration of proteins, usually immunoglobulin light chains, that are present in excess in the circulation. Tubular proteinuria virtually never exceeds 2 g per 24 h and thus, by definition, never causes nephrotic syndrome. Overflow proteinuria should be suspected in patients with clinical or laboratory evidence of multiple myeloma or other lymphoproliferative malignancy. Suspicion is heightened when there is a discrepancy between proteinuria detected by dipstick, the latter being sensitive to albumin but not light chains, and the sulfosalicylic acid precipitation method, which detects both.

DEFINITION The *nephrotic syndrome* is a clinical complex characterized by a number of renal and extrarenal features, the most prominent of which are proteinuria of >3.5 g per 1.73 m² per 24 h (in practice, >3.0 to 3.5 g per 24 h), hypoalbuminemia, edema, hyperlipidemia,

lipiduria, and hypercoagulability. Nephrotic syndrome can complicate any disease that perturbs the negative electrostatic charge or architecture of the GBM and the podocytes and their slit diaphragms. Recent attention has focused on several key molecules that mediate GBM-podocyte-slit diaphragm interactions such as nephrin, podocin, and alpha-actinin-4. Six entities account for >90% of cases of nephrotic syndrome in adults: minimal change disease (MCD), focal and segmental glomerulosclerosis (FSGS), membranous glomerulopathy, membranoproliferative glomerulonephritis (MPGN), diabetic nephropathy, and amyloidosis. *Renal biopsy* is a valuable tool in adults with nephrotic syndrome for establishing a definitive diagnosis, guiding therapy, and assessing prognosis. Renal biopsy is not required in the majority of children with nephrotic syndrome as most cases are due to MCD and respond to empirical treatment with glucocorticoids.

It should be stressed that the key component of nephrotic syndrome is *proteinuria*, which results from altered permeability of the glomerular filtration barrier for protein, namely the GBM and the podocytes and their slit diaphragms. The other components of the nephrotic syndrome and the ensuing metabolic complications are all secondary to urine protein loss and can occur with lesser degrees of proteinuria or may be absent even in patients with massive proteinuria.

PATHOPHYSIOLOGY In general, the greater the proteinuria, the lower the serum albumin level. *Hypoalbuminemia* is compounded further by increased renal catabolism and inadequate, albeit usually increased, hepatic synthesis of albumin. The pathophysiology of *edema* formation in nephrotic syndrome is poorly understood. The *underfilling hypothesis* postulates that hypoalbuminemia results in decreased intravascular oncotic pressure, leading to leakage of extracellular fluid from blood to the interstitium. Intravascular volume falls, thereby stimulating activation of the renin-angiotensin-aldosterone axis and the sympathetic nervous system and release of vasopressin (antidiuretic hormone), and suppressing atrial natriuretic peptide release. These neural and hormonal responses promote renal salt and water retention, thereby restoring intravascular volume and triggering further leakage of fluid to the interstitium. This hypothesis does not, however, explain the occurrence of edema in many patients in whom plasma volume is expanded and the renin-angiotensin-aldosterone axis is suppressed. The latter finding suggests that *primary renal salt and water retention* may also contribute to edema formation in some cases.

Hyperlipidemia is believed to be a consequence of increased hepatic lipoprotein synthesis that is triggered by reduced oncotic pressure and may be compounded by increased urinary loss of proteins that regulate lipid homeostasis. Defective lipid catabolism is also thought to play an important role. Low-density lipoproteins and cholesterol are increased in the majority of patients, whereas very low density lipoproteins and triglycerides tend to rise in patients with severe disease. Although not proven conclusively, hyperlipidemia may accelerate atherosclerosis and progression of renal disease.

Hypercoagulability is probably multifactorial in origin and is caused, at least in part, by increased urinary loss of antithrombin III, altered levels and/or activity of proteins C and S, hyperfibrinogenemia due to increased hepatic synthesis, impaired fibrinolysis, and increased platelet aggregability. As a consequence of these perturbations, patients can develop spontaneous *peripheral arterial or venous thrombosis, renal vein thrombosis,* and *pulmonary embolism.* Clinical features that suggest acute renal vein thrombosis include sudden onset of flank or abdominal pain, gross hematuria, a left-sided varicocele (the left testicular vein drains into the renal vein), increased proteinuria, and an acute decline in GFR. Chronic renal vein thrombosis is usually asymptomatic. Renal vein thrombosis is particularly common (up to 40%) in patients with nephrotic syndrome due to membranous glomerulopathy, membranoproliferative glomerulonephritis, and amyloidosis.

Other metabolic complications of nephrotic syndrome include *protein malnutrition* and iron-resistant *microcytic hypochromic anemia* due to transferrin loss. *Hypocalcemia* and secondary hyperparathyroidism can occur as a consequence of vitamin D deficiency due to enhanced urinary excretion of cholecalciferol-binding protein, whereas loss of thyroxine-binding globulin can result in *depressed thyroxine levels*. An increased *susceptibility to infection* may reflect low levels of IgG that result from urinary loss and increased catabolism. In addition, patients are prone to unpredictable changes in the *pharmacokinetics* of therapeutic agents that are normally bound to plasma proteins.

Ⓡ TREATMENT

GENERAL MANAGEMENT OF NEPHROTIC SYNDROME AND COMPLICATIONS The treatment of nephrotic syndrome involves (1) specific treatment of the underlying morphologic entity and, when possible, causative disease (see above); (2) general measures to control proteinuria if remission is not achieved through immunosuppressive therapy and other specific measures; and (3) general measures to control nephrotic complications.

General measures may be warranted to control proteinuria in nephrotic syndrome if patients do not respond to immunosuppressive therapy and other specific measures and suffer progressive renal failure or severe nephrotic complications. Nonspecific measures that may reduce proteinuria include ACE inhibitors, ARBs, and nonsteroidal anti-inflammatory drugs (NSAIDs). ACE inhibitors and ARBs reduce proteinuria and slow the rate of progression of renal failure by lowering intraglomerular pressure and preventing the development of hemodynamically mediated focal segmental glomerulosclerosis. There is conclusive evidence that these drugs are renoprotective in human diabetic nephropathy and many other proteinuric glomerulopathies, including secondary FSGS. NSAIDs also reduce proteinuria in some patients with nephrotic syndrome, probably by altering glomerular hemodynamics and GBM permeability characteristics. This potential benefit must be balanced against the risk of inducing acute renal failure, hyperkalemia, salt and water retention, and other side effects.

Complications of nephrotic syndrome that may require treatment include edema, hyperlipidemia, thromboembolism, malnutrition, and vitamin D deficiency. Edema should be managed cautiously by moderate *salt restriction*, usually 1 to 2 g per day, and the judicious use of *loop diuretics*. It is unwise to remove >1.0 kg of edema per day without close monitoring as more aggressive diuresis may precipitate intravascular volume depletion and prerenal azotemia. Administration of salt-poor albumin is not recommended as most is excreted within 24 to 48 h. Whereas many nephrologists advocate lowering low-density lipoproteins and cholesterol levels with *lipid-lowering drugs*, specifically HMG CoA reductase inhibitors to prevent accelerated atherosclerosis and possibly slow the rate of decline of GFR, the value of such interventions in this setting has not been conclusively shown.

Anticoagulation is indicated for patients with deep venous thrombosis, arterial thrombosis, and pulmonary embolism. Patients may be relatively resistant to heparin as a consequence of antithrombin III deficiency. Renal vein and vena caval angiography are probably indicated only when embolization occurs on anticoagulation and insertion of a caval filter is contemplated. There is no consensus regarding the optimal *diet* for patients with nephrotic syndrome. High-protein diets to prevent protein malnutrition are now in disfavor, since protein supplements have little, if any, effect on serum albumin levels and may hasten the progression of renal disease by increasing urinary protein excretion. The potential value of dietary protein restriction for reducing proteinuria must be balanced against the risk of contributing to malnutrition. *Vitamin D* supplementation is advisable in patients with clinical or biochemical evidence of vitamin D deficiency.

MINIMAL CHANGE DISEASE (MINIMAL CHANGE GLOMERULOPATHY) MCD accounts for about 80% of nephrotic syndrome in children younger than 16 years and 20% in adults (Table 264-3). The peak incidence is between 6 and 8 years. Patients typically present with nephrotic syndrome and benign urinary sediment. Microscopic hematuria is present in 20 to 30%. Hypertension and renal insufficiency are very rare.

MCD (also called nil disease, lipoid nephrosis, or foot process disease) is so named because glomerular size and architecture are normal by light microscopy. Immunofluorescence studies are typically nega-

TABLE 264-3 Major Causes of Minimal Change Disease (Nil Disease, Lipoid Nephrosis)

Idiopathic (majority)
In association with systemic diseases or drugs
  Drug-induced interstitial nephritis induced by NSAIDs, rifampin, interferon α
  Hodgkin's disease and other lymphoproliferative malignancy
  HIV infection

Note: NSAIDs, nonsteroidal anti-inflammatory drugs.

tive for immunoglobulin and C3. The findings of mesangial hypercellularity and sparse deposits of C3 and IgM portend a worse prognosis. Electron microscopy reveals characteristic *diffuse effacement of the foot processes of visceral epithelial cells* (Fig. 264-4). This morphologic finding is referred to as foot process fusion in the older literature.

The etiology of MCD is unknown, and the vast majority of cases are idiopathic (Table 264-3). MCD occasionally develops after upper respiratory tract infection, immunizations, and atopic attacks. Patients with atopy and MCD have an increased incidence of HLA-B12, suggesting a genetic predisposition. MCD, often in association with interstitial nephritis, is a rare side effect of NSAIDs, rifampin, and interferon α. The occasional association with lymphoproliferative malignancies (such as Hodgkin's lymphoma), the tendency for idiopathic MCD to remit during intercurrent viral infection such as measles, and the good response of idiopathic forms to immunosuppressive agents (see below) suggest an immune etiology. In children, the urine contains albumin principally and minimal amounts of higher molecular weight proteins such as IgG and α_2-macroglobulin. This *selective proteinuria* in conjunction with foot process effacement suggests injury to podocytes and loss of the fixed *negative charge* in the glomerular filtration barrier for protein. Proteinuria is typically nonselective in adults, suggesting more extensive perturbation of membrane permeability. Mutations in nephrin, α-actinin-4, and podocin, molecules that pay central roles in the anchoring of podocytes together through their slit diaphragms and to the GBM, cause proteinuria and glomerular morphologic changes that are virtually identical to those observed with acquired MCD and FSGS. There is increasing evidence that the expression and/or function of these and related molecules is also perturbed in acquired MCD and FSGS.

Ⓡ TREATMENT

MCD is highly steroid-responsive and carries an excellent prognosis. Spontaneous remission occurs in 30 to 40% of childhood cases but is less common in adults. Approximately 90% of children and 50% of adults enter remission following 8 weeks of high-dose oral glucocorticoids. In a typical regimen using prednisone, children receive 60 mg/m² of body surface area daily for 4 weeks, followed by 40 mg/m² on alternate days for an additional 4 weeks; adults receive 1 to 1.5 mg/kg body weight per day for 4 weeks, followed by 1 mg/kg per day on alternate days for 4 weeks. Up to 90% of adults enter remission if therapy is extended for 20 to 24 weeks. Nephrotic syndrome relapses in over >50% of cases following withdrawal of glucocorticoids. Alkylating agents are reserved for the small number of patients who fail to achieve lasting remission. These include patients who relapse during or shortly after withdrawal of steroids (steroid-dependent) and those who relapse more than three times per year (frequently relapsing). In these settings, cyclophosphamide (2 to 3 mg/kg per day) or chlorambucil (0.1 to 0.2 mg/kg per day) is started after steroid-induced remission and continued for 8 to 12 weeks. Cytotoxic agents may also induce remission in occasional steroid-resistant cases. These benefits must be balanced against the risk of infertility, cystitis, alopecia, infection, and secondary malignancies, particularly in children and young adults. Azathioprine has not been proven to be a useful adjunct to steroid therapy. Cyclosporine induces remission in 60 to 80% of patients; it is an alternative to cytotoxic agents and an option in patients who are resistant to cytotoxic agents. Unfortunately, relapse is usual

A

B

C

FIGURE 264-4 Typical findings on electron microscopy of renal biopsy specimens from patients with minimal change glomerulopathy, membranous glomerulopathy, and membranoproliferative glomerulonephritis. The pathognomonic feature of minimal change glomerulopathy (*A*) is effacement of foot processes of visceral epithelial cells (podocytes), giving the impression of foot process fusion. Foot process effacement is also evident in focal and segmental glomerulosclerosis (not shown here); in addition, there is typically detachment of podocytes from basement membrane, areas of glomerular capillary collapse, deposits of hyaline material, and sclerosis. Membranous nephropathy (*B*) is characterized by immune complexes in the subepithelial space. These electron-dense immune deposits stimulate production of new GBM, which eventually surrounds and incorporates the immune deposits into the GBM. The hallmarks of type I membranoproliferative glomerulonephritis (*C*) are increased mesangial cellularity and matrix and thickening and reduplication of the GBM. The latter is initiated by formation of electron-dense immune complexes on the subendothelial aspect of the GBM, which are subsequently covered by a new layer of GBM, probably produced by regenerating endothelial cells. (*Micrographs courtesy of Dr. Helmut Rennke.*)

when cyclosporine is withdrawn, and long-term therapy carries the risk of nephrotoxicity and other side effects. Long-term renal and patient survival is excellent in MCD.

FOCAL AND SEGMENTAL GLOMERULOSCLEROSIS The pathognomonic morphologic lesion in FSGS is sclerosis with hyalinosis involving portions (segmental) of fewer than 50% (focal) of glomeruli on a tissue section. The incidence of idiopathic (primary) FSGS has increased over the past two decades so that it now accounts for about one-third of cases of nephrotic syndrome in adults and as many as one-half of cases of nephrotic syndrome in blacks. Secondary FSGS can complicate a number of systemic diseases and sustained glomerular capillary hypertension following nephron loss from any cause (Table 264-4).

Idiopathic FSGS typically presents as nephrotic syndrome (~66%) or subnephrotic proteinuria (~33%) in association with hypertension, mild renal insufficiency, and an abnormal urine sediment that contains red blood cells and leukocytes. Proteinuria is nonselective in most cases.

Light microscopy of renal biopsy tissue reveals FSGS with entrapment of amorphous hyaline material, a process that shows a predilection for juxtamedullary glomeruli. Electron microscopy reveals evidence of damage to visceral epithelial cell.

The etiology of primary FSGS is unclear, but appears to be, at least in part, immunologic. There is evidence that a circulating nonimmunoglobulin permeability factor, possibly a lymphokine, triggers FSGS in at least a subgroup of patients. Plasmapharesis has been employed with variable success to control the nephrotic syndrome in this group. Secondary FSGS is a potential long-term consequence of nephron loss from any cause. It can complicate congenital renal diseases such as congenital oligomeganephronia, in which both kidneys have a reduced

complement of nephrons, and congenital unilateral agenesis. In addition, FSGS may develop following acquired loss of nephrons from extensive surgical ablation of renal mass; reflux nephropathy; glomerulonephritis; interstitial nephritis; sickle cell disease; and the combined effects of ischemia, cyclosporine nephrotoxicity, and rejection on renal allograft function (Table 264-4). It appears that >50% of nephrons must be lost for development of secondary FSGS.

TABLE 264-4 *Etiology of Focal and Segmental Glomerulosclerosis*

Idiopathic (majority)
In association with systemic diseases or drugs
  HIV infection
  Diabetes mellitus
  Fabry's disease
  Sialidosis
  Charcot-Marie-Tooth disease
As consequence of sustained glomerular capillary hypertension
  Congenital oligonephropathies
    Unilateral renal agenesis
    Oligomeganephronia
  Acquired nephron loss
    Surgical resection
    Reflux nephropathy
    Glomerulonephritis or tubulointerstitial nephritis
  Other adaptive responses
    Sickle cell nephropathy
    Obesity with sleep apnea syndrome
    Familial dysautonomia
Miscellaneous
  Heroin use

℞ TREATMENT

Spontaneous remission of primary FSGS is rare and renal prognosis is relatively poor. Proteinuria remits in only 20 to 40% of patients treated with glucocorticoids for 8 weeks. Uncontrolled studies suggest that up to 70% respond when steroid therapy is prolonged for 16 to 24 weeks. Cyclophosphamide and cyclosporine, when used at doses described above for MCD, induce partial or complete remission in 50 to 60% of steroid-responsive patients but are generally ineffective in steroid-resistant cases. Mycophenolate mofetil is another option in resistant cases. Poor prognostic factors at presentation include hypertension, abnormal renal function, black race, and persistent heavy proteinuria. Renal transplantation is complicated by recurrence of FSGS in the allograft in about 50% of cases and graft loss in about 10%. Factors associated with an increased risk of recurrence include a short time interval between the onset of the FSGS and ESRD, young age at onset, and possibly the presence of mesangial hypercellularity on renal biopsy.

MEMBRANOUS GLOMERULOPATHY (MEMBRANOUS NEPHROPATHY) This morphologic lesion is a leading cause of idiopathic nephrotic syndrome in adults (30 to 40%) and a rare cause in children (<5%). It has a peak incidence between the ages of 30 to 50 years and a male-female ratio of 2:1 (Fig. 264-4 and Table 264-5). Membranous glomerulopathy derives its name from the characteristic light-microscopic appearance on renal biopsy, namely diffuse thickening of the GBM, which is most apparent upon staining with periodic acid–Schiff (PAS). Most patients (>80%) present with nephrotic syndrome, proteinuria usually being nonselective. Microscopic hematuria is present in up to 50% of cases. Hypertension is documented in only 10 to 30% of patients at the outset but is common later in patients with progressive renal failure. Serologic tests such as antinuclear antibody, ANCA, anti-GBM antibody, cryoglobulin titers, and complement levels are normal in the idiopathic form.

Light microscopy of renal biopsy sections reveals diffuse thickening of the GBM without evidence of inflammation or cellular proliferation. Immunofluorescence reveals granular deposition of IgG, C3, and the terminal components of complement (C5b–9) along the glomerular capillary wall.

The pathogenesis of idiopathic human membranous glomerulopathy is incompletely understood. The presence of electron-dense immune deposits that contain IgG and C3 suggest an immune process. About one-third of adult membranous nephropathy occurs in association with systemic diseases such as SLE, infections such as hepatitis B, malignancy, and drug therapy with gold and penicillamine (Table 264-5).

Nephrotic syndrome remits spontaneously and completely in up to 40% of patients. The natural history of another 30 to 40% is characterized by repeated relapses and remissions. The final 10 to 20% suffer a slow progressive decline in GFR that typically culminates in ESRD after 10 to 15 years. Presenting features that predict a poor prognosis include male gender, older age, hypertension, severe proteinuria and hyperlipidemia, and impaired renal function. Controlled trials of glucocorticoids have failed to show consistent improvement in proteinuria or renal protection. Cyclophosphamide, chlorambucil, and cyclosporine have each been shown to reduce proteinuria and/or slow the decline in GFR in patients with progressive disease in small or uncontrolled studies. These observations need to be confirmed in controlled prospective studies. Transplantation is a successful treatment option for patients who reach ESRD.

MEMBRANOPROLIFERATIVE GLOMERULONEPHRITIS This morphologic entity, also known as mesangiocapillary glomerulonephritis, is characterized by thickening of the GBM and proliferative changes on light microscopy (Fig. 264-4 and Table 264-6). Two major types are identified; both are characterized by a diffuse increase in mesangial cellularity and matrix, and by thickening and reduplication of the GBM such that the lobular pattern of the glomerular tuft is exaggerated. The hallmark of type I MPGN is the presence of subendothelial and mesangial deposits on electron microscopy that contain C3 and IgG or IgM; rarely, IgA deposits are demonstrated by immunofluorescence microscopy. The hallmark of type II MPGN (dense deposit disease) is the presence of electron-dense deposits within the GBM and other renal basement membranes (shown by electron microscopy) that stain for C3, but little or no immunoglobulin.

Most patients with type I MPGN present with heavy proteinuria or nephrotic syndrome, active urinary sediment, and normal or mildly impaired GFR. C3 levels are usually depressed, and C1q and C4 levels are borderline or low. Type I MPGN is an immune-complex glomerulonephritis and can be associated with a variety of chronic infections (e.g., bacterial endocarditis, HIV, hepatitis B and C), systemic immune-complex diseases (e.g., SLE, cryoglobulinemia), and malignancies (e.g., leukemias, lymphomas). Type I MPGN usually has a protracted course, and as many as 50% of patients reach ESRD by 10 years. There is no proven therapy for patients with progressive disease beyond eradicating the underlying infection, malignancy, or systemic disease, when possible. The incidence of type I MPGN appears to be falling, possibly because the overall incidence of HCV infection has fallen dramatically in western society over the past decade.

TABLE 264-5 *Conditions Associated with Membranous Glomerulopathy*

Idiopathic (majority)
In association with systemic diseases or drugs
  Infection
    Hepatitis B and C, secondary and congenital syphilis, malaria, schistosomiasis, leprosy, hydatid disease, filariasis, enterococcal endocarditis
  Systemic autoimmune diseases
    SLE, rheumatoid disease, Sjögren's syndrome, Hashimoto's disease, Graves' disease, mixed connective tissue disease, primary biliary cirrhosis, ankylosing spondylitis, dermatitis herpetiformis, bullous pemphigoid, myasthenia gravis
  Neoplasia
    Carcinoma of the breast, lung, colon, stomach, and esophagus; melanoma; renal cell carcinoma; neuroblastoma; carotid body tumor
  Drugs
    Gold, penicillamine, captopril, NSAIDs, probenecid, trimethadione, chlormethiazole, mercury
  Miscellaneous
    Sarcoidosis, diabetes mellitus, sickle cell disease, Crohn's disease, Guillain-Barré syndrome, Weber-Christian disease, Fanconi's syndrome, α_1 antitrypsin deficiency, angiofollicular lymph node hyperplasia

Note: SLE, systemic lupus erythematosus; NSAIDs, nonsteroidal anti-inflammatory drugs.

TABLE 264-6 *Causes of Membranoproliferative (Mesangiocapillary) Glomerulonephritis (MPGN)*

Idiopathic	
Type I	With subendothelial and mesangial immune deposits
Type II	With intramembranous dense deposits containing sparse or no Ig; associated with C3 nephritic factor
Type III	Features of type I MPGN and membranous nephropathy
In association with systemic diseases or drugs[a]	
Systemic immune-complex disease	SLE, mixed cryoglobulinemia, Sjögren's syndrome
Chronic infections	Hepatitis B and C, HIV, bacterial endocarditis, ventriculoatrial shunts, visceral abscess
Malignancy	Leukemias, lymphomas
Liver disease	Chronic active hepatitis and cirrhosis (usually associated with hepatitis B or C)
Miscellaneous	Partial lipodystrophy, heroin use, sarcoidosis, inherited C2 deficiency, thrombotic microangiopathies

[a] Usual with morphologic features of idiopathic type I MPGN (see above).
Note: SLE, systemic lupus erythematosus.

Type II MPGN can also present with proteinuria and nephrotic syndrome; however, some patients present with nephritic syndrome, RPGN, or recurrent macroscopic hematuria. Type II MPGN is an autoimmune disease in which patients have an IgG autoantibody, termed *C3 nephritic factor*, that binds to C3 convertase, the enzyme that metabolizes C3, and renders it resistant to inactivation. Type II MPGN runs a variable course; the GFR remains stable in some patients and declines gradually to ESRD over 5 to 10 years in others. There is no effective therapy for this disease, which may be associated with partial lipodystrophy, although corticosteroids are sometimes used.

A third, rarer form of MPGN is associated with subepithelial immune deposits. It should be noted that a membranoproliferative pattern of glomerular injury may also complicate thrombotic microangiopathies (e.g., antiphospholipid antibody syndrome, chronic allograft rejection, healing phase of hemolytic-uremic syndrome, or thrombotic thrombocytopenic purpura) and glomerular deposition disease (e.g., fibrillary glomerulopathy—see below).

MESANGIOPROLIFERATIVE GLOMERULONEPHRITIS In 5 to 10% of patients with idiopathic nephrotic syndrome, renal biopsy reveals a diffuse increase in glomerular cellularity, predominantly due to proliferation of mesangial and endothelial cells, and infiltration by monocytes. Findings on immunofluorescence microscopy vary and include deposits of IgA, IgG, IgM, and/or complement, or absence of immune reactants. It is likely that this morphologic entity is, in fact, a heterogeneous group of diseases that includes atypical forms of MCD and FSGS and milder or resolving forms of the immune-complex and pauci-immune glomerulopathies described above under nephritic syndrome and RPGN. In keeping with the heterogeneity of this diagnosis, the prognosis is variable. In general, persistent nephrotic-range proteinuria signals a poor prognosis, with many patients progressing to ESRD over 10 to 20 years despite immunosuppressive therapy.

DIABETIC NEPHROPATHY (See also Chap. 323)   Diabetic nephropathy is the leading cause of ESRD in western societies and accounts for 30 to 35% of patients on renal replacement therapy in North America. Type 1 diabetes mellitus (DM; formerly, insulin-dependent diabetes mellitus) and type 2 DM (formerly, non-insulin-dependent diabetes mellitus) affect approximately 0.5 and 4% of the population, respectively. Nephropathy complicates 30% of cases of type 1 DM and approximately 20% of cases of type 2 DM. However, most diabetic patients with ESRD have type 2 DM because of the greater prevalence of type 2 DM worldwide (90% of all individuals with diabetes). Risk factors for the development of diabetic nephropathy include hyperglycemia, systemic hypertension, glomerular hypertension and hyperfiltration, proteinuria, and possibly cigarette smoking, hyperlipidemia, and gene polymorphisms affecting the activity of the renin-angiotensin-aldosterone axis. For reasons that are unclear, ESRD from diabetic nephropathy is more common in blacks with type 2 DM than in whites (4:1 ratio), whereas the reverse is true for type 1 DM.

Pathophysiology   The pathophysiology, clinical features, and morphology of diabetic nephropathy appears similar in type 1 and type 2 DM, although the true incidence and precise time course of nephropathy in type 2 DM is still debated. Glomerular hypertension and hyperfiltration are the earliest renal abnormalities in experimental and human diabetes and are observed within days to weeks of diagnosis. Microalbuminuria, so named because the abnormal albumin excretion of 30 to 300 mg/24 h is below the limits of detection of standard dipsticks, develops after approximately 5 years of sustained glomerular hypertension and hyperfiltration in type 1 DM.

Microalbuminuria is the first manifestation of injury to the glomerular filtration barrier and predicts the development of overt nephropathy. Dipstick-positive proteinuria, ultimately reaching nephrotic levels, typically develops 5 to 10 years after the onset of microalbuminuria (i.e., 10 to 15 years after the onset of diabetes) and is associated with hypertension and progressive loss of renal function.

In addition, patients can display features of tubulointerstitial disease such as hyperkalemia and type IV renal tubular acidosis. ESRD typically develops 5 to 10 years after the development of overt nephropathy. As noted above, the course of diabetic nephropathy may be shorter in type 2 DM, and many patients present with established nephropathy and hypertension. Diabetic nephropathy is usually diagnosed on clinical grounds without a renal biopsy. Supportive clues are the presence of normal sized or enlarged kidneys, evidence of proliferative diabetic retinopathy, and a bland urinary sediment. Retinopathy is found in 90% and 60% of patients with type 1 and type 2 DM, respectively, who develop nephropathy.

Pathologic Changes   The earliest morphologic abnormalities in diabetic nephropathy are thickening of the GBM and expansion of the mesangium due to accumulation of extracellular matrix. With time, matrix accumulation becomes diffuse and is evident as eosinophilic, PAS-positive glomerulosclerosis on renal biopsy. Prominent areas of nodular matrix expansion (nodular glomerulosclerosis, the classic Kimmelsteil-Wilson lesion) are often superimposed on this background. The glomeruli and kidneys are typically normal or increased in size, distinguishing diabetic nephropathy from most other forms of chronic renal insufficiency (renal amyloidosis and polycystic kidney disease being other important exceptions). Immunofluorescence microscopy may reveal deposition of IgG along the GBM in a linear pattern, but this does not appear to be immunopathogenetic as in anti-GBM disease. Immune deposits are not seen. The renal vasculature typically displays evidence of atherosclerosis, as a consequence of hyperlipidemia, and hypertensive arteriosclerosis.

Factors implicated as triggers for increased matrix production in DM include glomerular hypertension; the direct effects of hyperglycemia on mesangial cells; advanced glycosylation end-products; growth factors such as growth hormone, insulin-like growth factor 1, angiotensin II, CTGF; cytokines such as TGF-β; hyperlipidemia; and cell sorbitol accumulation. Complementary clinical and laboratory approaches suggest an important role for hemodynamic factors. Glomerular hydrostatic pressure and GFR increase within months of the development of hyperglycemia. The mechanism by which DM induces glomerular hypertension is still being defined and appears to involve circulating factors such as atrial natriuretic peptide acting in concert with the direct effects of high glucose on the actin cytoskeleton of renal mesangial and vascular smooth-muscle cells.

In this framework, glycosuria triggers increased reabsorption of glucose coupled to sodium in the proximal tubule, thereby increasing total-body sodium and extracellular fluid volume. As a compensatory response, atrial natriuretic peptide is released from cardiac myocytes and induces natriuresis in part by triggering afferent arteriolar dilatation and thereby increasing intraglomerular pressure and GFR. Whereas this compensatory response is appropriate in the short term, sustained glomerular hypertension provokes thickening of the GBM, increased mesangial matrix production, and glomerulosclerosis and disruption of barrier function. Exposure of mesangial cells and vascular smooth-muscle cells to high glucose in vitro and in vivo results in disruption of the actin cytoskeleton, possibly through the action of reactive oxygen species, rendering the cells relatively unresponsive to vasoconstrictors and further contributing to afferent arteriolar vasodilatation and glomerular hypertension. In keeping with a central role for intraglomerular pressure in the pathogenesis of diabetic nephropathy, ACE inhibitors and ARBs, which lower intraglomerular pressure, slow the progression of diabetic nephropathy, even in normotensive patients.

It remains to be determined why DM and glomerular hypertension induce glomerulosclerosis in some but not all individuals. Epidemiologic studies and studies of disease concordance in identical twins suggest that important, but as yet unidentified, genetic factors may play a role. It is likely that hemodynamic and metabolic factors act in concert to generate the final glomerulosclerotic phenotype in genetically predisposed patients.

TREATMENT

Therapy is aimed at retarding the progression of nephropathy through control of blood sugar, systemic blood pressure, and glomerular capillary pressure. Glycemic control is achieved through regulation of diet and administration of oral hypoglycemic agents and insulin. ACE inhibitors and ARBs are the drugs of choice as they control both systemic hypertension and intraglomerular hypertension by inhibiting the actions of angiotensin II on the systemic vasculature and renal efferent arterioles. In addition, these agents also attenuate the stimulatory effect of angiotensin II on glomerular cell growth and matrix production. Because ACE inhibitors conclusively delayed the time to ESRD by 50% in patients with type 1 DM in several randomized controlled trials and probably delay progression in type 2 DM, it is recommended that all patients with diabetes over the age of 12 should be screened annually for microalbuminuria and should receive an ACE inhibitor on the development of microalbuminuria, even in the absence of systemic hypertension. ARBs slowed the rate of progression of diabetic nephropathy in patients with type 2 DM in two recent randomized controlled trials and are an alternative to ACE inhibitors for renoprotection. Approximately 80% of patients with DM require more than one drug to control systemic hypertension, and aggressive lowering of blood pressure in these patients retards the rate of progression of nephropathy and other diabetic complications.

Diabetic nephropathy is the most common cause of ESRD requiring renal replacement therapy, and patients with DM have the highest annual mortality rate (20 to 30%) of any group on dialysis, in large part as a result of accelerated atherosclerosis. The survival rates of younger patients undergoing either peritoneal dialysis or hemodialysis are comparable; however, older patients with DM appear to have a higher mortality rate on peritoneal dialysis. Renal transplantation, with or without pancreas transplantation, is the preferred mode of renal replacement therapy in patients who are otherwise medically suitable.

GLOMERULAR DEPOSITION DISEASES The glomerular deposition diseases are characterized by deposition of abnormal proteins, usually immunoglobulins or fragments thereof, within the glomerulus. They include amyloidosis, light and heavy chain deposition disease, cryoglobulinemia, and fibrillary/immunotactoid glomerulonephritis below.

Renal Amyloidosis Amyloidosis is classified according to the major component of its fibrils (Chap. 310). There is substantial overlap in the renal clinicopathologic presentations of amyloid (AL) and amyloid A (AA) disease. Glomeruli are involved in 75 to 90% of patients, usually in association with involvement of other organs. The clinical correlate of glomerular amyloid deposition is nephrotic-range proteinuria. In addition, >50% of patients have impaired glomerular filtration at diagnosis. Hypertension is present in about 20 to 25%. Renal size is usually normal or slightly enlarged. A minority of patients present with renal failure due to amyloid deposition in the renal vasculature or with Fanconi's syndrome, nephrogenic diabetes insipidus, or renal tubular acidosis due to involvement of the tubulointerstitium. Rectal biopsy and abdominal fat pad biopsy reveal amyloid deposits in about 70% of patients and may obviate the need for renal biopsy.

Renal biopsy gives a very high yield if there is clinical evidence of renal involvement. The earliest pathologic changes are mesangial expansion by amorphous hyaline material and thickening of the GBM. Further amyloid deposition results in the development of large nodular eosinophilic masses. When stained with Congo red, these deposits show apple-green birefringence under polarized light. Electron microscopy reveals the characteristic nonbranching extracellular amyloid fibrils of 7.5 to 10 nm in diameter. Tubulointerstitial and vascular deposits of amyloid are also seen and may occasionally be more prominent than glomerular deposits.

TREATMENT

Most patients with renal involvement by AL amyloidosis develop ESRD within 2 to 5 years. No treatment has been shown consistently to improve this prognosis; however, some success has been reported with a combination of melphalan and prednisone. Preliminary studies have reported a benefit of high-dose melphalan with autologous stem cell transplantation. Colchicine delays the onset of nephropathy in patients with familial Mediterranean fever but has not proved useful in patients with established disease or with other forms of amyloid. Remissions may be achieved in AA amyloidosis by eradication of the underlying cause. Renal replacement therapy is offered to patients who reach ESRD; however, the 1-year survival rate on dialysis is low (~66%) by comparison with other causes of ESRD. Most patients die from extrarenal complications, particularly cardiovascular disease. Renal transplantation is a viable option in patients with AA amyloidosis whose primary disease has been eradicated. Transplantation is also an option for patients with AL amyloidosis, although a poor prognosis because of extrarenal organ involvement may preclude them as candidates. Here again, the survival rate is lower by comparison with other causes of ESRD; most of the excess mortality is due to infectious and cardiovascular complications. Recurrence of amyloidosis in the allograft is common but rarely leads to graft loss.

LIGHT CHAIN DEPOSITION DISEASE (LCDD) (See also Chap. 98) Renal involvement is a complication in 90% of patients with LCDD and is often the dominant feature. Nephrotic syndrome and renal impairment are the usual presenting features. Microscopic hematuria occurs in about 20% of patients. Defective hydrogen ion and potassium excretion and urinary concentration may be evident if light chains are deposited predominantly in the tubules. The most common pathologic lesion on renal biopsy is ribbon-like thickening of the tubular basement membrane due to light chain deposition. Mesangial expansion and nodular glomerulosclerosis are found in about 33% of patients. This light-microscopic appearance resembles that of idiopathic membranoproliferative glomerulonephritis and diabetic nephropathy. Superimposed crescentic change is occasionally seen. Immunofluorescence studies are strongly positive for monoclonal light chains, in contrast to AL amyloid, because the constant region of the immunoglobulin is typically deposited. The tissue deposits in LCDD are granular rather than fibrillar on electron microscopy, appear more amorphous in character, do not stain with Congo red, and seem to have a greater affinity for basement membranes.

The prognosis of LCDD is poor when it is associated with multiple myeloma, and most patients progress rapidly to ESRD. Treatment with melphalan and prednisone has been reported to reduce proteinuria and stabilize renal function in uncontrolled studies. In the absence of myeloma, the prognosis is somewhat more variable, and several patients have undergone successful renal transplantation.

WALDENSTRÖM'S MACROGLOBULINEMIA (See also Chap. 98) This disorder is characterized by monoclonal proliferation of an IgM-secreting clone of plasma cells. The circulating IgM paraprotein frequently gives rise to the hyperviscosity syndrome, which may compromise renal blood flow and GFR. Direct renal involvement is rare and, when present, involves deposition of large amorphous deposits of eosinophilic material in the glomerular capillaries. Renal amyloidosis can also occur.

FIBRILLARY-IMMUNOTACTOID GLOMERULOPATHY This emerging clinicopathologic entity accounts for 1% of diagnoses in most large renal biopsy series. Virtually all patients present with proteinuria, and ~50% have nephrotic syndrome. The majority of patients also have hematuria, hypertension, and renal insufficiency. The light-microscopic appearances vary from mesangial expansion and basement membrane thickening with PAS-positive material to proliferative and crescentic glomerulonephritis. On electron microscopy, this PAS-positive material is observed to be composed of randomly arranged (fibrillary glomerulopathy) or organized bundles (immunotactoid glomerulopathy) of microfibrils and microtubules, the composition of which has yet to be defined. The etiology of fibrillary-immunotactoid glomerulopathy remains to be determined. Patients with the immunotactoid variant have an increased incidence of lymphoproliferative malignancy. There is no proven therapy for fibrillary-immunotactoid glomerulopathy, and many patients progress to ESRD over 1 to 10 years. Transplantation appears to be a viable option in the latter setting.

ASYMPTOMATIC ABNORMALITIES OF THE URINARY SEDIMENT

Many cases of glomerular disease are diagnosed when asymptomatic hematuria or proteinuria are detected on routine examination of the urinary sediment as part of preemployment or insurance-related medical assessments.

HEMATURIA Most asymptomatic glomerular hematuria is due to IgA nephropathy (Berger's disease) or thin basement membrane (TBM) disease (benign hematuria). A rarer but more ominous cause of isolated hematuria is Alport's syndrome (p. 1691). The latter is the most common form of hereditary nephritis, is usually transmitted as an X-linked dominant trait, and is associated with sensorineural deafness, ophthalmologic abnormalities, and progressive renal insufficiency. TBM disease is sometimes familial but, in contrast to Alport's syndrome, is usually a benign disorder. Asymptomatic hematuria may also be the presenting feature of indolent forms of most other primary and secondary proliferative glomerulopathies. Glomerular hematuria must be distinguished from a variety of renal parenchymal and extrarenal causes of hematuria. It is particularly important to exclude malignancy of the kidney or urinary tract, particularly in older male patients. Other potential diagnoses include vascular, cystic, and tubulointerstitial diseases; papillary necrosis; hypercalciuria and hyperuricosuria; benign prostatic hypertrophy; and renal calculi. Important clues to the presence of glomerular hematuria are the presence of urinary red blood cell casts; dysmorphic urinary red blood cells; proteinuria >2.0 g per 24 h; and clinical or serologic evidence of nephritic syndrome, RPGN, or a compatible systemic disease.

IGA NEPHROPATHY (BERGER'S DISEASE) IgA nephropathy is the most common glomerulopathy worldwide and accounts for 10 to 40% of glomerulonephritis in most series (Table 264-7). The disease is particularly common in southern Europe and Asia and appears to be more common in blacks than whites. Familial clustering has been reported but is rare. Most cases are idiopathic. The renal and serologic abnormalities in IgA nephropathy and Henoch-Schönlein purpura are indistinguishable, and most authorities consider these to be a spectrum of a single disease. Less commonly, IgA nephropathy is found in association with systemic diseases, including chronic liver disease, Crohn's

TABLE 264-7 *Diseases Associated with IgA Nephropathy*

Idiopathic (majority)
  Renal-limited or as component of Henoch-Schönlein purpura
In association with systemic diseases or drugs[a]

Liver	Chronic liver disease with involvement of biliary tree
Gastrointestinal	Celiac disease, Crohn's disease, adenocarcinoma
Respiratory	Idiopathic interstitial pneumonitis, obstructive bronchiolitis, adenocarcinoma
Skin	Dermatitis herpetiformis, mycosis fungoides, leprosy
Eyes	Episcleritis, anterior uveitis
Miscellaneous	Ankylosing spondylitis, relapsing polychondritis, Sjögren's syndrome, monoclonal IgA gammopathy, schistosomiasis

[a] Although prominent deposition of IgA has been reported with each of these conditions, significant glomerular inflammation and dysfunction are rare.

disease, gastrointestinal adenocarcinoma, chronic obstructive bronchiolitis, idiopathic interstitial pneumonia, dermatitis herpetiformis, mycosis fungoides, leprosy, ankylosing spondylitis, relapsing polychondritis, and Sjögren's syndrome. In many of these conditions, IgA is deposited in the glomerulus without inducing inflammation, and this may be a clinically insignificant consequence of perturbed IgA homeostasis.

Patients with IgA nephropathy typically present with gross hematuria, often 24 to 48 h after a pharyngeal or gastrointestinal infection, vaccination, or strenuous exercise. Other cases are diagnosed upon detection of microscopic hematuria during routine physical examinations. Hypertension (20 to 30%) and nephrotic syndrome (~10%) are unusual at presentation. Light microscopy of renal biopsy specimens typically shows mesangial expansion by increased matrix and cells. Diffuse proliferation, cellular crescents, interstitial inflammation, and areas of glomerulosclerosis may be evident in severe cases. The diagnostic finding, for which the disease is named, is mesangial deposition of IgA, detected by immunofluorescence microscopy. C3 is usually detected in the area of immune deposits, and IgG is observed in 50% of cases. Electron microscopy reveals electron-dense deposits in the mesangium and, in severe cases, these extend into the paramesangial subendothelial space. The pathogenesis of IgA nephropathy is incompletely understood. Among the major abnormalities in IgA metabolism described in this setting are increased IgA production, abnormal IgA glycosylation, and impaired IgA clearance. Although IgA nephropathy is associated with altered mucosal immunity, most IgA deposited in the kidney appears to be derived from bone marrow cells.

℞ TREATMENT

The optimal treatment of IgA nephropathy is a subject of ongoing debate and controversy. Most authorities advise observation only in patients whose GFR is not compromised and whose proteinuria is <1 g/day. ACE inhibitors are usually prescribed for their renoprotective effect in patients with more severe disease. One trial has suggested a role for prolonged (6 months) high-dose glucocorticoids in patients presenting with impaired GFR and >1 g of proteinuria. Randomized controlled trials evaluating the efficacy of daily fish oils have yielded conflicting results. The case for other immunosuppressive agents such as cyclophosphamide and mycophenolate mofetil is unproven, and such agents are usually reserved for the minority of patients presenting with nephritic syndrome or RPGN, and with aggressive crescent formation and marked glomerular inflammation on renal biopsy.

IgA nephropathy typically smolders for decades, with patients often suffering exacerbations of hematuria and renal impairment during intercurrent infections. As many as 20 to 50% of patients develop ESRD within 20 years. Clinical predictors of a poor prognosis include older age, male sex, hypertension, nephrotic-range proteinuria, and renal insufficiency at presentation. Histologic features that predict an aggressive course include diffuse severe disease, extracapillary proliferation (crescents), extension of immune attack into the paramesangial subendothelial space, glomerulosclerosis, interstitial fibrosis, and arteriolar hyalinosis.

THIN BASEMENT MEMBRANE DISEASE (BENIGN HEMATURIA) This disorder can be heredofamilial or sporadic and is as common as IgA nephropathy in some series of asymptomatic hematuria. When familial, it is usually inherited as an autosomal dominant trait and is due to a defect in the gene encoding the $\alpha 4$ chain of type IV collagen. The molecular basis for the sporadic form of TBM disease has not been determined. TBM disease typically manifests in childhood as persistent hematuria. Intermittent hematuria and exacerbation of hematuria during upper respiratory tract infections have also been reported. The kidney is normal on light and immunofluorescence microscopy. The GBM is thin by comparison with normal subjects. TBM disease is usually a benign condition, and progressive renal impairment or proteinuria should prompt a search for an alternative diagnosis. A small proportion of patients do, however, appear to develop hypertension and focal glomerulosclerosis upon long-term follow-up, and ACE inhibitors are usually prescribed in this group in an effort to attenuate renal injury.

ALPORT'S SYNDROME (HEREDITARY NEPHRITIS) Alport's syndrome is the most common hereditary nephritis and is usually transmitted as an X-linked dominant trait. The genetic defect resides in the gene for the $\alpha 5$ chain of type IV collagen located on the long arm of the X chromosome; type IV collagen is a major structural component of the GBM. Numerous genetic mutations have been detected (Chap. 342).

Typical light-microscopic features on renal biopsy include mesangial hypercellularity, focal and segmental glomerulosclerosis, chronic tubulointerstitial fibrosis, atrophy, and accumulation of foam cells. Electron microscopy reveals thickening, fragmentation, and lamellation of the lamina densa of the GBM.

Males with the disease tend to progress to ESRD and are suitable candidates for dialysis and transplantation. ACE inhibitors are typically prescribed in the predialysis phase in an effort to slow the decline in GFR. About 5% of transplant recipients develop anti-GBM disease in the renal allograft; their immune system recognizes normal GBM of the transplanted kidney as a foreign antigen. These patients can have antibodies against the $\alpha 3$ (Goodpasture antigen) or $\alpha 5$ chains of type IV collagen, probably because defective synthesis of the $\alpha 5$ chain results in defective incorporation or orientation of the $\alpha 3$ chain in the GBM. In the majority of patients this posttransplant anti-GBM disease does not significantly compromise GFR.

PROTEINURIA Between 0.5 and 10% of the population have isolated proteinuria, defined as proteinuria in the presence of an otherwise normal urinary sediment, a radiologically normal urinary tract, and the absence of known renal disease. The majority of these patients excrete <2 g of protein per day, and more than 80% have an excellent prognosis (*benign isolated proteinuria*). A minority (10 to 25%) are found to have persistent proteinuria (*persistent isolated proteinuria*), some of whom develop progressive renal insufficiency over 10 to 20 years.

Benign Isolated Proteinuria The major categories of benign isolated proteinuria are idiopathic transient proteinuria, functional proteinuria, intermittent proteinuria, and postural proteinuria. *Idiopathic transient proteinuria* is usually observed in young adults and refers to dipstick-positive proteinuria in an otherwise healthy individual that disappears spontaneously by the next clinic visit. *Functional proteinuria* refers to transient proteinuria during fever, exposure to cold, emotional stress, congestive cardiac failure, or obstructive sleep apnea. This phenomenon is presumed to be mediated through changes in glomerular ultrafiltration pressure and/or membrane permeability. Patients with *intermittent proteinuria* have proteinuria in approximately half of their urine samples in the absence of other renal or systemic abnormalities. *Postural proteinuria* is proteinuria (usually <2.0 g per 24 h) that is evident only in the upright position. This disorder affects 2 to 5% of adolescents and may be transient (~80%) or fixed (~20%). Fixed postural proteinuria resolves within 10 to 20 years in most cases. In each of these conditions, renal biopsy reveals either normal renal parenchyma or mild and nonspecific changes involving podocytes or the mesangium. All carry an excellent prognosis.

Persistent Isolated Proteinuria Isolated proteinuria detected on multiple ambulatory clinic visits in both the recumbent and upright position usually signals a structural renal lesion. Virtually all glomerulopathies that induce nephrotic syndrome (see above) can cause persistent isolated proteinuria. The most common lesion on renal biopsy is mild mesangial proliferative glomerulonephritis with or without focal and segmental glomerulosclerosis (30 to 70%), followed by focal or diffuse proliferative glomerulonephritis (~15%) and interstitial nephritis (~5%). Although this clinical entity carries a worse prognosis than benign isolated proteinuria, the prognosis is still relatively good, with only 20 to 40% of patients developing renal insufficiency after 20 years. Furthermore, progression to ESRD is extremely rare. It is wise to exclude monoclonal gammopathy by urinary electrophoresis in older patients.

CHRONIC GLOMERULONEPHRITIS AND OTHER GLOMERULAR ABNORMALITIES

This syndrome is characterized by persistent proteinuria and/or hematuria and renal insufficiency that progresses slowly over years. Chronic glomerulonephritis usually comes to light either (1) upon routine urinalysis, (2) when routine blood tests reveal unexplained anemia or elevated blood urea nitrogen and creatinine, (3) following discovery of bilateral small kidneys on abdominal imaging, (4) during evaluation for secondary causes of hypertension, or (5) during a clinical exacerbation of glomerulonephritis triggered by pharyngitis (synpharyngitic) or other infections. Chronic glomerulonephritis can be a manifestation of virtually all of the major glomerulopathies. While renal biopsy may reveal the causative glomerular lesion, glomerular scarring and sclerosis are frequently so advanced by the time patients present that it may be impossible to define the primary diagnosis. Tubulointerstitial inflammation and scarring are frequent additional findings and portend a poor prognosis. Glomerular hypertension and hyperfiltration through remnant functioning nephrons can hasten progression to ESRD. Treatment is directed at lowering systemic and glomerular hypertension, usually with an ACE inhibitor or ARB, and controlling extracellular fluid volume, anemia, metabolic abnormalities, and the uremic syndrome through judicious use of diuretics, erythropoietin, and dietary modification. Some patients develop ESRD and require renal replacement therapy with dialysis or transplantation.

GLOMERULAR DISEASES IN SPECIFIC CLINICAL SITUATIONS

When considering the clinical approach to patients presenting with abnormalities of the urinary sediment, it is worth considering several specific clinical scenarios: (1) patients whose presentation or family history suggests a hereditary disease, (2) patients on therapeutic or recreational drugs, (3) glomerular disease in the setting of a systemic infection, (4) glomerular disease in a patient with neoplasia, and (5) glomerular disease in patients with arthritis and connective tissue diseases.

HEREDITARY DISEASE WITH GLOMERULAR INVOLVEMENT Although relatively rare, hereditary glomerular diseases are an important category of glomerular disease because of their propensity to cause progressive loss of renal function and for transmission down the generations. Furthermore, studies into the pathogenesis of these disorders have shed important new insights on renal physiology and pathophysiology that are relevant to a wider group of glomerulopathies.

Alport's Syndrome Alport's syndrome is the most common form of hereditary glomerular disease (Chap. 342).

Sickle Cell Disease (See also Chap. 91) Glomerular disease is common (15 to 30%) in homozygotes for sickle cell disease. Glomerular hyperfiltration and hypertrophy occur within the first 5 years of life. Approximately 15 to 30% of patients develop proteinuria in the first three decades, and 5% develop ESRD. The glomerular pathology is usually focal segmental glomerulosclerosis, probably due to sustained glomerular capillary hypertension. MPGN is also seen on occasion. Predictors of chronic renal failure are worsening anemia, proteinuria, nephrotic syndrome, and hypertension. ACE inhibitors and ARBs may slow the progression of renal disease by lowering systemic and glomerular capillary hypertension.

Fabry's Disease (See also Chap. 340) In patients with Fabry's disease, renal biopsy reveals accumulation of neutral glycosphingolipids with terminal α-galactosyl moieties in lysosomes of glomerular, tubular, vascular, and interstitial cells. Focal and global glomerulosclerosis are later features. Electron microscopy reveals stacked, concentric lamellar profiles known as "myeloid" bodies, which are characteristic. Renal disease manifests in the late teens to early twenties with lipiduria, proteinuria with minimal hematuria, nephrotic syndrome, hypertension, and progressive renal insufficiency. The renal lesion is progressive, and these patients often tolerate hemodynamic changes during dialysis poorly because of progressive vascular disease. Significant slowing of disease progression has been demonstrated in early trials of enzyme replacement with recombinant human α-galactosidase A. Successful renal transplantation has been reported despite recurrence in the allograft.

Nail-Patella Syndrome The nail-patella syndrome is a rare hereditary disorder transmitted as an autosomal dominant trait. The abnormal gene is located on the long arm of chromosome 9 and encodes transcription factor of the LIM-homeodomain type, namely LMX1B. The phenotype is characterized by multiple osseous abnormalities, primarily affecting the elbows and knees, and nail dysplasia. About 50% of patients have clinically evident nephropathy. The light-microscopic features on renal biopsy include local GBM thickening, tubular atrophy, interstitial fibrosis, and varying degrees of glomerular sclerosis. The disease usually manifests clinically as asymptomatic hematuria and proteinuria, occasionally in the nephrotic range, but it may be silent. The renal lesion is relatively benign, and progression to ESRD occurs in 10 to 30% of patients.

Lipodystrophy MPGN type II (dense deposit disease) is the most frequent glomerular lesion in patients with lipodystrophy (80%), whereas MPGN type I affects the remainder (20%). The disease occurs mostly in females between the ages of 5 and 15 years, and the clinical presentation and course are similar to those of idiopathic MPGN, namely nephrotic-range proteinuria and progressive renal insufficiency. Low C3 levels are common in association with C3 nephritic factor (p. 1680).

Lecithin-Cholesterol Acyltransferase Deficiency (See also Chap. 335) Renal manifestations of this disease include proteinuria, microscopic hematuria, and progressive renal insufficiency. Renal biopsy typically reveals focal and segmental glomerulosclerosis. Endothelial cell detachment is also evident, and capillary lumens may be occluded by vacuolated foam cells. Recurrence of the disease has been documented in the renal allograft but without marked impairment of graft function.

DRUG-INDUCED GLOMERULAR DISEASE A variety of drugs damage the glomerular filtration barrier and induce proteinuria and nephrotic syndrome (Table 264-8). In contrast, drug-induced proliferative glomerulonephritis is rare. The more common drug-induced glomerulopathies are discussed here.

NSAIDs have a variety of renal side effects, including hemodynamically mediated acute renal failure, salt and water retention, hyponatremia, hyperkalemia, papillary necrosis, acute interstitial nephritis, nephrotic syndrome, and ESRD. Nephrotic syndrome and acute renal failure frequently coexist due to a combination of acute interstitial nephritis and a glomerular lesion that is identical to that of MCD. This entity occurs most commonly in patients on propionic acid derivatives such as fenoprofen, ibuprofen, and naproxen but can occur with other NSAIDs, ampicillin, rifampin, and interferon α. Withdrawal of the drug usually results in resolution of renal disease. Membranous nephropathy is also described as an idiosyncratic reaction to NSAIDs. While the more selective inhibitors of cyclooxygenase (COX)-2 appear to have less renal toxicity, many of the renal syndromes described for NSAIDs have also been reported with COX-2 inhibitors.

Gold therapy, administered by injection or orally, induces proteinuria in 5 to 25% of patients with rheumatoid arthritis. Proteinuria develops after 4 to 6 months of therapy, and up to 33% of patients develop full-blown nephrotic syndrome. Renal biopsy typically reveals membranous glomerulopathy, though MCD or mesangial proliferative lesions have also been described. Progressive renal impairment is rare. Nephrotic syndrome is more common in patients who are HLA-B8/DR3 positive, suggesting a genetic susceptibility. Withdrawal of the drug leads to gradual resolution of the proteinuria.

Penicillamine also induces proteinuria in 5 to 30% of patients. As with gold, the underlying glomerular lesion is usually membranous glomerulopathy, and proteinuria gradually resolves after withdrawal

TABLE 264-8 *Drug-Induced Glomerular Disease*

Morphologic Lesion	Causative Agent
Minimal change diseases (usually with interstitial nephritis)	Nonsteroidal anti-inflammatory agents Recombinant interferon α Rifampin Ampicillin
Membranous nephropathy	Penicillamine Gold Mercury Trimethadione Captopril Chlormethiazole
Focal segmental glomerulosclerosis	Heroin
Pauci-immune necrotizing GN	Ciprofloxacin Hydralazine
Proliferative GN with vasculitis	Allopurinol Penicillin Sulfonamides Thiazides Intravenous amphetamines
RPGN	Rifampin Warfarin Carbimazole Amoxicillin Penicillamine

Note: GN, glomerulonephritis; RPGN, rapidly progressive glomerulonephritis.

of the drug. Acute renal failure secondary to crescentic glomerulonephritis with immune deposits has also been described.

Intravenous heroin use is associated with an increased incidence of focal and segmental glomerulosclerosis (heroin-associated nephropathy). It is not clear whether the nephrotoxin in this setting is heroin itself or a contaminant. Heroin-associated nephropathy occurs predominantly in blacks and is characterized by nephrotic syndrome, hypertension, and a gradual progression to ESRD over a period of 3 to 5 years. The pathologic features are similar to those of idiopathic FSGS, although mesangial deposition of IgM and C3 may be more prominent. The incidence of this disease appears to be declining steadily. Potential reasons for the decline include increased purity of street heroin and a bias to attribute FSGS to HIV infection when both risk factors coexist. Intravenous *amphetamine* abuse is a rare cause of systemic necrotizing vasculitis.

GLOMERULAR LESIONS ASSOCIATED WITH INFECTIOUS DISEASES Infectious organisms can induce glomerular disease through several different mechanisms: (1) by direct infection of renal cells, (2) by elaborating nephrotoxins such as *Escherichia coli*-derived verotoxin, (3) by inciting intraglomerular deposition of immune complexes (e.g., postinfectious glomerulonephritis) or cryoglobulins (e.g., hepatitis B or C), and (4) by providing a chronic stimulus for amyloid fibril formation, as in AA amyloidosis. Direct infection of glomerular cells is a relatively rare mechanism of injury but has been implicated in the pathogenesis of nephropathy associated with HIV (Chap. 173 and below).

Viral Infections ■ *HEPATITIS B VIRUS (HBV) INFECTION* (See also Chap. 285) Infectious HBV, HCV, and HIV are strongly associated with glomerular disease. Glomerular lesions associated with HBV infection include membranous glomerulopathy, MPGN, IgA nephropathy, essential mixed cryoglobulinemia, and polyarteritis nodosa. Membranous glomerulopathy is most common. In endemic areas, such as Asia and Africa, 80 to 100% of children and 30 to 45% of adults with membranous glomerulopathy have HBV surface antigenemia. HBV antigens have been identified in renal immune deposits, suggesting in situ immune-complex formation after planting of HBV antigens or trapping of circulating immune complexes containing HBV antigens. Patients typically present with nephrotic syndrome and microscopic hematuria. Hypertension and renal impairment are rare. The most common associated hepatic lesion is chronic persistent or chronic active hepatitis. In nonendemic areas there is a male preponderance, and many patients are intravenous drug users or have other risk factor for acquisition of HBV. The asymptomatic carrier state of HBV is frequently associated with MPGN in endemic areas. Hypertension and azotemia are more common with this morphologic pattern than with membranous glomerulopathy. Children with HBV-associated membranous glomerulonephritis have a good prognosis, and almost two-thirds enter spontaneous remission within 3 years. ESRD is rare. In contrast, 30% of adults develop progressive renal failure within 5 years, with 10% reaching ESRD. Steroids and cytotoxic agents are contraindicated as they may lead to increased viral replication and worsening of liver disease. Interferon α may reduce proteinuria and stabilize renal function in patients with progressive disease.

HEPATITIS C VIRUS INFECTION (See also Chap. 285)   This should be considered in all patients with cryoglobulinemic proliferative glomerulonephritis, MPGN, and membranous glomerulopathy. These three clinicopathologic entities may represent a spectrum of morphologic manifestations of the same pathogenetic process, namely HCV-induced immune-complex disease. Up to 30% of patients with chronic HCV infection have an abnormal urinary sediment. HCV infection accounts for 10 to 20% of type I MPGN and is a major cause of essential mixed cryoglobulinemia. Renal biopsy reveals typical features of type I MPGN and IgG, IgM, C3, and/or cryoglobulin deposits. Most patients present with nephrotic syndrome and microscopic hematuria and may have red blood cell casts. Liver function tests are usually abnormal, and C3 levels are typically depressed. Anti-HCV antibodies are detected in most patients, and viral RNA has been documented in blood and cryoglobulins. Various treatments have been reported to be useful in HCV-induced renal disease including steroids, cytotoxic agents, and plasmapheresis; however, controlled trials to support their use are lacking. Interferon α has been demonstrated to clear antigenemia, lower cryoglobulin levels, and stabilize renal disease. Unfortunately, relapse is usual once the drug is discontinued.

HIV INFECTION (See also Chap. 173)   This condition has been associated with focal segmental glomerulosclerosis, acute diffuse proliferative glomerulonephritis, and mesangioproliferative glomerulonephritis, including IgA nephropathy, MPGN, and membranous glomerulopathy. The classic and most common HIV-associated glomerulopathy is an aggressive form of focal segmental glomerulosclerosis, an entity that is termed *HIV-associated nephropathy* (HIVAN). This disease may be the first manifestation of infection in otherwise asymptomatic patients. HIVAN is more common in blacks than in other ethnic groups and is more frequent in intravenous drug abusers with HIV infection than in homosexuals. The disease has been described in all high-risk groups, however, including infants of HIV-positive mothers. Renal biopsy typically reveals visceral epithelial cell swelling, collapse of the glomerular capillary tuft, severe tubulointerstitial inflammation, and microcystic dilatation of renal tubules. The presence of tubuloreticular inclusions and the aggressive clinical course distinguish HIVAN from idiopathic focal segmental glomerulosclerosis. The mechanisms of renal cell injury are still being defined. Viral DNA has been demonstrated in the renal epithelia of HIV-infected patients with and without nephropathy, suggesting that pathogenetic factors, other than infection of cells, are required for induction of disease. The typical clinical correlates of HIVAN are severe nephrotic syndrome and rapid progression to ESRD, occurring in weeks to months. Despite early reports of poor survival of patients on dialysis, more recent studies indicate improved survival for both asymptomatic patients with HIV and patients with full-blown AIDS.

There is no proven therapy for HIVAN. The initial experience with combined highly active antiretroviral therapy (triple therapy) suggests that these regimens have reduced the incidence of nephropathy in HIV-infected patients and improved prognosis in patients with established nephropathy. A number of retrospective studies of glucocorticoids alone or in combination with triple therapy have demonstrated a reduction in proteinuria and slowing of renal progression in some patients with established nephropathy. The precise role of steroids requires further study. ACE inhibitors may confer renoprotection as in other proteinuric renal diseases.

Bacterial Infections   Immune-complex glomerulonephritis is a relatively frequent complication of *infective endocarditis* (Chap. 109). Other mechanisms of renal injury in bacterial endocarditis include embolic renal infarction, septic abscesses, acute tubular necrosis secondary to septicemia and drug therapy, disseminated intravascular coagulation, and antibiotic-induced acute interstitial nephritis. Patients typically present with microscopic hematuria, urinary red blood cell casts, pyuria and modest proteinuria (nephrotic range in 25% of patients), and variable degrees of renal failure. Rheumatoid factor is present in 10 to 70%, and circulating immune complexes in 90%. Serum complement levels are usually depressed. Renal biopsy reveals mild focal proliferative glomerulonephritis with mesangial and capillary wall deposition of IgG and C3 by immunofluorescence microscopy and subendothelial, mesangial, and subepithelial electron-dense deposits by electron microscopy. Occasional patients develop diffuse necrotizing glomerulonephritis with crescent formation and present with nephritic syndrome or RPGN. Endocarditis-associated glomerulonephritis typically has a good prognosis and resolves with eradication of the underlying infection.

Suppurative infections such as intrathoracic and intraabdominal abscesses, osteomyelitis, and dental abscesses have been associated with glomerulonephritis. The usual presentation is hematuria, urinary red blood cell casts, proteinuria, and acute renal failure. Oliguria and hypertension are common. Pathologic renal lesions include mesangial proliferative, membranoproliferative, and diffuse proliferative glomerulonephritis with crescents. Immunofluorescence reveals mesangial and capillary wall deposition predominantly of C3, although IgG and IgM may also be seen.

Nephrotic syndrome is a complication in 0.3% of patients with secondary *syphilis* and 8% of patients with congenital syphilis. The usual pathology is membranous glomerulopathy.

Leprosy most commonly causes AA amyloidosis; however, a syndrome resembling acute poststreptococcal glomerulonephritis has also been described.

Protozoan and Parasitic Infections   Transient proteinuria (50% of patients) and nephrotic syndrome (<1% of patients) are complications of infection with *Plasmodium falciparum*. Membranoproliferative glomerulonephritis is the usual pathologic lesion and may respond to eradication of infection. *P. malariae* has been associated with diffuse or focal proliferative glomerulonephritis, membranous glomerulopathy, and minimal change disease. Eradication of the malarial infection does not consistently induce remission of the nephrotic syndrome. *Schistosoma mansoni* causes nephrotic syndrome in 5 to 10% of patients, and progression to ESRD is common. The usual pathology is MPGN or mesangial proliferative glomerulonephritis, although membranous glomerulonephritis and amyloidosis are occasionally seen. *Filariasis* can trigger membranous glomerulonephritis (*Loa loa*) and occasionally induces proliferative glomerulonephritis (*Onchocerca volvulus*). *Congenital toxoplasmosis* infection occasionally induces immune-complex glomerulonephritis characterized by mesangial and subendothelial immune deposits that contain *Toxoplasma* antigens. Membranous glomerulopathy and proliferative glomerulonephritis are occasional complications of *hydatid disease* and *trichinosis*, respectively.

GLOMERULAR LESIONS ASSOCIATED WITH NEOPLASIA   Infectious glomerulopathies associated with neoplasia include membranous glomerulopathy, MCD, FSGS, immune-complex glomerulonephritis, fibrillary/immunotactoid glomerulonephritis, LCDD, and amyloidosis. Mild proteinuria is common in patients with *solid tumors*, but overt glomerulonephritis is rare. Occasional patients with solid tumors of the lung, gastrointestinal tract, breast, kidney, and ovary develop full-blown nephrotic syndrome, usually due to a membranous glomerulopathy. Estimates of the incidence of occult malignancy in patients presenting with membranous glomerulopathy range from 0.1 to 10%. Most authorities agree that an extensive search for malignancy is not indicated, unless there are other suggestive clinical features. As many as 35% of patients with renal cell carcinoma have mesangial deposition of IgG and C3 visible on immunofluorescence; however, morphologic abnormalities are detected in only 50% of these patients, and clinically significant glomerulopathy is rare. Glomerular amyloidosis has also been described in association with this tumor.

An array of glomerular disease has been reported in patients with lymphoproliferative malignancy. Nephrotic syndrome is a recognized complication of *Hodgkin's lymphoma*, with 70% of cases due to MCD. The latter may occur concurrently with (40 to 45%), precede (10 to 15%), or follow (40 to 50%) diagnosis of the malignancy. It is postulated that a lymphokine or other mediator released by malignant T lymphocytes perturbs podocyte function and alters glomerular permeability in this setting. Nephrotic syndrome typically resolves with successful treatment and relapses with recurrence of disease. Less frequent associations with Hodgkin's lymphoma include FSGS, membranous glomerulopathy, MPGN, proliferative glomerulonephritis, and crescentic glomerulonephritis. MCD, membranous glomerulopathy, MPGN, and crescentic glomerulonephritis have also been reported in patients with *non-Hodgkin's lymphoma*. Glomerulopathy in the context of leukemia is rare. MPGN can complicate *chronic lymphatic leukemia* and related *B cell lymphomas*, particularly when associated with cryoglobulinemia. Other glomerular lesions associated with *paraproteinemia* include primary amyloid, LCDD, proliferative glomerulonephritis induced by cryoglobulinemia, and fibrillary/immunotactoid glomerulopathy. Here again, the renal lesion frequently improves or resolves with successful treatment of the underlying malignancy.

GLOMERULAR LESIONS ASSOCIATED WITH ARTHRITIS AND OTHER FORMS OF CONNECTIVE TISSUE DISEASE Although extraarticular manifestations are present in 35% of patients with rheumatoid arthritis, direct involvement of the kidney by rheumatoid disease is rare, and glomerular injury is usually secondary to AA amyloidosis or a side effect of drug therapy. AA amyloidosis is a complication experienced by 10 to 20% of patients with rheumatoid arthritis, and renal involvement is evident clinically in 3 to 10% of these patients (nephrotic syndrome, renal insufficiency). Amyloidosis is more frequent in patients with rheumatoid arthritis of long duration (>10 years), with circulating rheumatoid factor, and with destructive arthropathy. Less frequent glomerular lesions include mesangial proliferative glomerulonephritis and basement membrane thickening by subepithelial immune deposits. Gold and penicillamine may cause nephrotic syndrome by inducing membranous glomerulopathy, whereas NSAIDs can trigger the nephrotic syndrome by inducing minimal change nephropathy, usually in association with acute interstitial nephritis (see above). Tubulointerstitial injury is the most common form of renal involvement in Sjögren's syndrome and usually presents as either Fanconi's syndrome, distal renal tubular acidosis, or impairment of renal concentrating ability. Glomerulonephritis is relatively rare and should prompt a search for other causes. Membranous glomerulopathy and MPGN are the most common lesions. Anecdotal reports describe successful therapy with glucocorticoids and cytotoxic agents. Occasional cases of focal mesangial proliferative glomerulonephritis with mesangial deposition of IgG and complement have been described in polymyositis/dermatomyositis. Membranous glomerulopathy has also been reported, particularly when polymyositis/dermatomyositis is associated with malignancy. Mixed connective tissue disease is a syndrome that includes features of SLE, scleroderma, and polymyositis and is associated with high titers of anti-ribonucleoprotein antibodies and negative anti-smooth-muscle antibodies. Renal involvement occurs in fewer than 15% of patients and manifests as hematuria and subnephrotic proteinuria. The usual pathologic lesion is membranous glomerulopathy or MPGN. The prognosis is usually excellent, and steroid therapy may be useful in rare patients with progressive renal disease.

FURTHER READING

APPEL G et al: Secondary glomerular diseases, in *Brenner & Rector's The Kidney*, 7th ed, BM Brenner (ed). Philadelphia, Saunders, 2004, p 1381

BRENNER BM et al: Effects of losartan on renal and cardiovascular outcomes in patients with type 2 diabetes and nephropathy. N Engl J Med 345:861, 2001

DAGHESTANI L et al: Renal manifestations of hepatitis C infection. Am J Med 106:347, 1999

FALK R et al: Primary glomerular diseases, in *Brenner & Rector's The Kidney*, 7th ed, BM Brenner (ed). Philadelphia, Saunders, 2004, pp 1293–1380

LEWIS EJ et al: Renoprotective effect of the angiotensin receptor antagonist irbesartan in patients with nephropathy due to type 2 diabetes. N Engl J Med 345:851, 2001

ORTH SR, RITZ E: The nephrotic syndrome. N Engl J Med 338:1202, 1998

PARVING HH et al: Diabetic nephropathy, in *Brenner & Rector's The Kidney*, 7th ed, BM Brenner (ed). Philadelphia, Saunders, 2004, pp 1777–1818

STEHMAN-BREEN C, JOHNSON RJ: Hepatitis C virus–associated glomerulonephritis. Adv Intern Med 43:79, 1998

TAAL MW, BRENNER BM: Renoprotective effects of RAS inhibition: From ACEI to angiotensin II antagonists. Kidney Int 57:1803, 2000

---

265 TUBULAR DISORDERS
John R. Asplin, Fredric L. Coe

The renal tubular disorders and their morphologic and functional abnormalities, mode of inheritance, and associated abnormalities are summarized in Table 265-1. The individual disorders are discussed in detail below.

AUTOSOMAL DOMINANT POLYCYSTIC KIDNEY DISEASE

Etiology and Pathology Autosomal dominant polycystic kidney disease (ADPKD) has a prevalence of 1:300 to 1:1000 and accounts for ~4% of end-stage renal disease (ESRD) in the United States. Some 90% of cases are inherited as an autosomal dominant trait, and ~10% are spontaneous mutations.

GENETIC CONSIDERATIONS Three forms of ADPKD have been identified. ADPKD-1 accounts for 85% of cases, and the gene has been mapped to chromosome 16p13.3. The gene for ADPKD-2 has been mapped to chromosome 4q21-23. The protein products of the two genes form the polycystin complex, which may regulate cell-cell or cell-matrix interactions. A defect in either of these proteins interrupts the normal function of the polycystin complex, resulting in the same phenotype for two distinct genetic abnormalities. ADPKD-2 appears to have a later age of onset of symptoms and renal failure than ADPKD-1. A rare third form has been described but has not been mapped to a gene at this point.

The kidneys are grossly enlarged, with multiple cysts studding the surface of the kidney. The cysts contain straw-colored fluid that may become hemorrhagic. The cysts are spherical, vary in size from a few millimeters to centimeters, and are distributed evenly throughout the cortex and medulla. Only 1 to 5% of nephrons will develop cysts. Cysts form when a "second hit" causes a somatic mutation in the normal allele of a tubule cell, leading to monoclonal proliferation of the tubular epithelium. The remaining renal parenchyma reveals varying degrees of tubular atrophy, interstitial fibrosis, and nephrosclerosis.

TABLE 265-1 *Renal Tubule Defects*

Disease	Renal Morphologic Abnormalities	Renal Functional Abnormalities	Mode of Inheritance	Associated Abnormalities
Autosomal dominant polycystic disease	Cortical and medullary cysts	Chronic renal failure, >20 yr	AD	Hepatic cysts, intracranial aneurysms, colonic diverticula
Autosomal recessive polycystic disease	Distal tubule and collecting duct cysts	Chronic renal failure, <20 yr	AR	Congenital hepatic fibrosis
Tuberous sclerosis	Renal cysts and angiomyolipomas	None	AD, S	Skin lesions, hamartomas of the central nervous system
Von Hippel–Lindau disease	Renal cysts, increased risk of renal cell cancer	None	AD	Hemangioblastoma of the retina and central nervous system
Medullary sponge kidney	Dilated collecting ducts	Nephrocalcinosis, hematuria	AD, S	None
Nephronophthisis	Medullary cysts, small kidneys	Chronic renal failure, <20 yr polyuria, salt wasting	AR	Hepatic fibrosis, retinal abnormalities
Medullary cystic disease	Medullary cysts, small kidneys	Chronic renal failure, >20 yr polyuria, salt wasting	AD	None
Liddle's syndrome	None	Hypokalemia, alkalosis, low aldosterone levels	AD	Hypertension
Bartter's syndrome	Juxtaglomerular apparatus hyperplasia	Hypokalemia, alkalosis, high aldosterone levels	AR	None
Gitelman's syndrome	Juxtaglomerular apparatus hypertrophy	Hypokalemia, alkalosis, hypocalciuria	AR	None
Congenital nephrogenic diabetes insipidus	None	Vasopressin renal concentrating defect	XL, AR	None
Renal tubular acidosis, type 1	Nephrocalcinosis	Impaired proton secretion in distal tubule, non-anion-gap metabolic acidosis	AD, AR, S, ACQ	Rickets, osteomalacia, nephrolithiasis
Renal tubular acidosis, type 2	None	Reduced bicarbonate reabsorption, non-anion-gap metabolic acidosis	AR, AD, ACQ	Fanconi syndrome, rickets
Renal tubular acidosis, type 4	Chronic renal insufficiency	Reduced proton and potassium secretion	ACQ	Renal insufficiency
X-linked hypophosphatemia	None	Reduced phosphate reabsorption	XL	Rickets, osteomalacia, normal serum 1,25(OH)$_2$D$_3$
Autosomal dominant hypophosphatemic rickets	None	Reduced phosphate reabsorption	AD	Rickets, osteomalacia
Vitamin D–dependent rickets, type 1	None	Defective renal 1,25(OH)$_2$D$_3$ production	AR	Rickets, osteomalacia, low serum 1,25(OH)$_2$D$_3$
Vitamin D–dependent rickets, type 2	None	Renal resistance to 1,25(OH)$_2$D$_3$	AR, S	Rickets, osteomalacia, high serum 1,25(OH)$_2$D$_3$
Oncogenic osteomalacia	None	Reduced phosphate reabsorption	ACQ	Osteomalacia, mesenchymal tumors
Dent's disease	Interstitial fibrosis, medullary calcifications	Hypercalciuria, low-molecular-weight proteinuria	XL	Renal failure
Isolated hyperuricemia	None	Reduced urate reabsorption	AR	Variable hypercalciuria
Hartnup disorder	None	Reduced reabsorption of neutral amino acids	AR	Dermatitis, diarrhea, dementia
Cystinuria	Cystine stones	Reduced reabsorption of dibasic amino acids	AR	Short stature
Iminoglycinuria	None	Reduced reabsorption of proline, hydroxyproline, and glycine	AR	None
Fanconi syndrome	Swan neck deformity of proximal tubule	Reduced reabsorption of bicarbonate, glucose, phosphate, uric acid, and amino acids	AR	Rickets, osteomalacia, hypokalemia, metabolic acidosis

Note: AD, autosomal dominant; AR, autosomal recessive; S, sporadic; XL, X-linked; ACQ, acquired

Clinical Features The disease may present at any age but most frequently causes symptoms in the third or fourth decade. Patients may develop chronic flank pain from the mass effect of the enlarged kidneys. Acute pain indicates infection, urinary tract obstruction by clot or stone, or sudden hemorrhage into a cyst. Gross and microscopic hematuria are common, and impaired renal concentrating ability frequently leads to nocturia. Nephrolithiasis occurs in 15 to 20% of patients, calcium oxalate and uric acid stones being most common. Low urine pH, low urine citrate, and urinary stasis from distortion of the collecting system by cysts all play a role in stone formation. Hypertension is found in 20 to 30% of children and up to 75% of adults. It is secondary to intrarenal ischemia from distortion of the renal architecture, leading to activation of the renin-angiotensin system. Patients with hypertension have a much more rapid progression to ESRD. Urinary tract infection is common and may involve the bladder or renal interstitium (pyelonephritis) or infect a cyst (pyocyst). Pyocysts can be difficult to diagnose but are more likely to be present if the patient has positive blood cultures, new renal pain, or failed to improve clinically after a standard course of antibiotic therapy.

Progressive decline in renal function is common, with ~50% of patients developing ESRD by age 60. However, there is considerable variation in age of onset of renal failure, even within the same family. Hypertension, recurrent infections, male sex, and early age of diagnosis are related to early onset renal failure. Renal failure usually progresses slowly; if a sudden decrement in kidney function occurs, ureteral obstruction from stone, clot, or compression by a cyst are likely causes. Patients usually have high hematocrits for their level of renal function, as erythropoietin production is high. Fluid overload is uncommon because of a tendency for renal salt wasting.

Extrarenal manifestations of this disease are frequent and underscore the systemic nature of the defect. Hepatic cysts occur in 50 to 70% of patients. Cysts are generally asymptomatic, and liver function is normal, though women may develop massive hepatic cystic disease on occasion. Cyst formation has also been observed in the spleen, pancreas, and ovaries. Intracranial aneurysms are present in 5 to 10% of asymptomatic patients, with potential for permanent neurologic injury or death from subarachnoid hemorrhage. Screening of all ADPKD patients for aneurysms is not recommended, but patients with a family history of subarachnoid hemorrhage should be studied noninvasively with magnetic resonance imaging angiography. Colonic diverticular disease is common, and patients are more likely to develop perforation than the general population with colonic diverticula. Mitral valve prolapse is found in 25% of patients, and the prevalence of aortic and tricuspid valve insufficiency is increased.

Diagnosis Ultrasound is the preferred technique for diagnosis of symptomatic patients and for screening asymptomatic family members. The ability to detect cysts increases with the subject's age: 80 to 90% of ADPKD patients over the age of 20 will have detectable cysts, and almost 100% over the age of 30 will have cysts. At least three to five cysts in each kidney is the standard diagnostic criteria for ADPKD. Computed tomography (CT) scan may be more sensitive than ultrasound in detection of small cysts. Genetic linkage analysis is now available for diagnosis of ADPKD but is reserved for cases where radiographic imaging is negative and the need for definitive diagnosis critical, such as screening family members for potential kidney donation.

℞ TREATMENT

The goals of treatment are to slow the rate of progression of renal disease and minimize symptoms. Hypertension and renal infection should be treated aggressively to maintain renal function. Converting enzyme inhibitors are effective antihypertensive agents, though patients should be closely monitored as some develop renal insufficiency and hyperkalemia. Urinary infection is treated in a standard manner unless a pyocyst is suspected, in which case antibiotics that penetrate cysts should be used, such as trimethoprim-sulfamethoxazole, ciprofloxacin, and chloramphenicol. Chronic pain from cysts can be managed by cyst puncture and sclerosis with ethanol.

AUTOSOMAL RECESSIVE POLYCYSTIC KIDNEY DISEASE

GENETIC CONSIDERATIONS Autosomal recessive polycystic kidney disease (ARPKD) is a rare genetic disease with an incidence of 1:20,000 births. The gene for ARPKD has been localized to chromosome 6p21 and encodes a large novel protein whose function has not yet been determined. In the past, ARPKD was categorized as being of neonatal, infantile, or juvenile form depending on the age of onset and the relative degree of involvement of the kidneys and liver. However, variable clinical presentations within siblings in the same family, as well as the localization of the disease to chromosome 6 in multiple families, support the premise that this is a single genetic disease with variable phenotypic presentation.

At birth the kidneys are enlarged with a smooth external surface. The distal tubules and collecting ducts are dilated into elongated cysts that are arranged in a radial fashion. As the patient ages, the cysts may become more spherical and the disease can be confused with ADPKD. Interstitial fibrosis is also seen as renal function deteriorates. Liver involvement includes proliferation and dilation of intrahepatic bile ducts as well as periportal fibrosis.

Clinical Features The majority of cases are diagnosed in the first year of life, presenting as bilateral abdominal masses. Death in the neonatal period is most commonly due to pulmonary hypoplasia. Hypertension and impaired urinary concentrating ability are common. The time course to ESRD is variable, though many children maintain adequate kidney function for years. Older children present with complications secondary to congenital hepatic fibrosis and generally have less severe kidney disease. Hepatosplenomegaly, portal hypertension, and esophageal varices are frequent complications of ARPKD.

Diagnosis Ultrasound is the most common technique used to diagnose ARPKD, prenatally and in childhood. Ultrasound examination reveals enlarged kidneys with increased echogenicity. At times spherical cysts may be seen, potentially leading to an incorrect diagnosis of ADPKD. A thorough family history and imaging the kidneys of the parents aids in differentiation from other cystic diseases. Hepatic fibrosis seen on imaging studies in association with cystic kidneys supports the diagnosis of ARPKD.

℞ TREATMENT

Aggressive treatment of hypertension and urinary tract infection are the major goals of therapy in order to maintain native renal function as long as possible. Dialysis and transplant are appropriate when kidney failure occurs. Hepatic fibrosis may lead to life-threatening variceal hemorrhage, requiring sclerotherapy or portosystemic shunts.

TUBEROUS SCLEROSIS

Patients with this multisystem disease most commonly present with skin lesions and benign tumors of the central nervous system (Chap. 358). Renal involvement is common; angiomyolipomas are the most frequent abnormality and are usually bilateral. Renal cysts may be present as well and can give an appearance similar to that of ADPKD. Histologically, the cysts are unique—the cyst lining cells are large with an eosinophilic staining cytoplasm and may form hyperplastic nodules that can fill the cyst space.

GENETIC CONSIDERATIONS One-third of cases are inherited as an autosomal dominant trait, the rest are due to sporadic mutations. Mutations of tumor-suppression genes have been identified on chromosomes 9q34 (*TSC1*) and 16p13 (*TSC2*). Mutations of *TSC2* account for the majority of cases and are more likely to be associated with mental retardation and polycystic kidneys. Tuberous sclerosis may be confused with ADPKD if extrarenal manifestations are minimal.

VON HIPPEL–LINDAU DISEASE

This autosomal dominant disease is characterized by hemangioblastomas of the retina and the central nervous system (Chap. 358). Renal cysts occur in the majority of cases and are usually bilateral. The *VHL* gene, located on chromosome 3p25, is a tumor-suppressor gene that regulates hypoxia-induced transcription factors. It is the same gene that is mutated in sporadic renal cell carcinoma. Renal cell carcinoma may be found in 40 to 70% of patients with von Hippel–Lindau disease and is frequently multifocal. Yearly screening of adults using CT scans has been recommended in an attempt to diagnose renal cell cancers at an early stage.

MEDULLARY SPONGE KIDNEY

Etiology and Pathology Medullary sponge kidney (MSK) is a congenital disorder. Although some cases have apparent autosomal dominant inheritance, most are sporadic. It is found in 0.5 to 1% of all intravenous pyelograms. Males and females are affected equally. The pathologic lesion is cystic dilation of the inner medullary and papillary collecting ducts. Bilateral renal involvement is present in 70% of cases, but not all papillae are equally affected. The dilated ducts are lined by cuboidal epithelium with areas of pseudostratified and stratified squamous epithelium. Calculi are frequently found in the dilated collecting ducts.

FIGURE 265 1 *A. Radiographic appearance of medullary sponge kidney. Abdominal flat plate reveals multiple bilateral calcifications. B. Radiographic contrast material* accumulates in the dilated and cystic terminal collecting ducts and obscures the calcifications.

Clinical Features Patients generally present in the third or fourth decade with kidney stones, infection, or recurrent hematuria. The disease is most commonly diagnosed by intravenous pyelogram, which shows linear striations radiating into the renal papillae or small cystic collections of contrast in the dilated ducts (Fig. 265-1). Approximately 60% of patients with MSK have stones, and 12% of all stone formers will have MSK. Hypercalciuria occurs with the same frequency in MSK as it does in random stone formers. Papillary nephrocalcinosis occurs more frequently in patients with MSK than in the random stone former. Proteinuria is minimal, if present at all, and renal function is normally preserved unless there is renal damage from recurrent infection or severe stone disease.

℞ TREATMENT

Asymptomatic patients require no specific therapy except to maintain high fluid intake to reduce the risk of nephrolithiasis. If stones are present, standard laboratory evaluation should be done and metabolic abnormalities treated as in any stone former (Chap. 268). Infection should be treated aggressively, and instrumentation of the urinary tract should be minimized to avoid introducing infection.

NEPHRONOPHTHISIS/MEDULLARY CYSTIC DISEASE

GENETIC CONSIDERATIONS Nephronophthisis (NPH) and medullary cystic disease (MCD) have similar pathologic findings but differ in inheritance pattern and age of onset. NPH is inherited as an autosomal recessive disease. Three forms have been identified, the most common is juvenile (NPH1), which maps to a gene on chromosome 2q13. The infantile form (NPH2) maps to chromosome 9, and the adolescent form (NPH3) maps to chromosome 3. MCD is an autosomal dominant disease. Two loci have been associated with MCD, one on chromosome 1q21 and the other on 16p12. In both NPH and MCD the kidneys tend to be small, with cysts throughout the medulla; the cortex and papilla rarely have cysts. The cysts originate in the collecting ducts, distal convoluted tubules, and loops of Henle and range in size from 1 to 10 mm. Sclerotic glomeruli, tubule atrophy, and interstitial fibrosis are frequent findings on biopsy.

Clinical Features Patients with NPH present during childhood with symptoms of polyuria, growth retardation, anemia, and progressive renal insufficiency. ESRD develops at an average age of 2 years in NPH2, 13 years in NPH1, and 19 years in NPH3. NPH accounts for 2 to 10% of renal failure in children. Hepatic fibrosis and cerebellar ataxia have been reported in association with NPH. MCD presents in the third or fourth decade, though some cases may be diagnosed in the

elderly population. Presenting symptoms in MCD are the same as in NPH except for growth retardation. In addition, MCD does not have extrarenal abnormalities. Severe salt wasting can be seen, though this is usually a transient phase that resolves as the disease progresses to ESRD. Other features of tubule damage are often found, including hyperkalemia and hyperchloremic metabolic acidosis. Proteinuria is mild, and hematuria is rare.

Diagnosis The diagnosis is suggested by a family history of renal disease. The pattern of inheritance and age of onset aid in distinguishing NPH/MCD from other inherited diseases. Radiographic studies show small kidneys, loss of the corticomedullary junction, and multiple cysts in the medulla. CT scan is more sensitive than ultrasound in making the diagnosis. The majority of cases of NPH can be diagnosed using molecular genetics techniques. Open renal biopsy, including medullary tissue, may be required for diagnosis in some cases.

℞ TREATMENT

Treatment is mainly supportive, as there is no specific therapy to prevent loss of renal function. Patients with salt wasting require a large oral intake of salt and water to maintain adequate extracellular volume. Alkali replacement and erythropoietin are required for acidosis and anemia, respectively. Renal transplantation has been performed in numerous patients, and the disease does not recur.

LIDDLE'S SYNDROME

Liddle's syndrome is a rare autosomal dominant disorder with a clinical presentation of hyperaldosteronism, consisting of hypertension, hypokalemia, and metabolic alkalosis. However, aldosterone levels are undetectable and renin levels are suppressed. The syndrome is caused by activating mutations in the amiloride-sensitive sodium channel, which leads to increased distal tubule sodium reabsorption and potassium wasting. Potassium-sparing diuretics that block the sodium channel, such as amiloride and triamterene, used in conjunction with a low-sodium diet, are effective in treating the hypertension and electrolyte abnormalities. Spironolactone is ineffective, since the disease is not mediated via the aldosterone receptor.

BARTTER'S SYNDROME

Clinical Features Hypokalemia secondary to renal potassium wasting, metabolic alkalosis, and normal to low blood pressure are the clinical features of Bartter's syndrome. Two variants of Bartter's syndrome have been described. *Antenatal Bartter's syndrome* (also known as *hyperprostaglandin E syndrome*) is characterized by polyhydramnios and premature delivery. During infancy, episodes of fever and dehydration are common and can lead to growth retardation. Nephrocalcinosis secondary to hypercalciuria is frequent. Prostaglandin E production is very high. Most cases of *classic Bartter's syndrome* present during childhood. Symptoms such as weakness and cramps are secondary to the hypokalemia. Polyuria and nocturia are common due to the hypokalemia-induced nephrogenic diabetes insipidus. Nephrocalcinosis is less common than in the antenatal form. Both forms are inherited as autosomal recessive traits. Although rarely required for diagnosis, renal biopsy reveals hyperplasia of the juxtaglomerular apparatus and prominence of medullary interstitial cells, with variable degrees of interstitial fibrosis, though these are not pathognomonic for the syndrome.

GENETIC CONSIDERATIONS Abnormalities in three renal tubule transport proteins have been shown to cause Bartter's syndrome. Mutations in either the bumetanide-sensitive Na-K-2Cl cotransporter or the apical K^+ channel (ROMK) have been described in antenatal Bartter's. Mutations of a basolateral chloride channel (CLC-Kb) are found in patients with classic Bartter's syndrome. All of these mutations lead to a loss of Na^+ and Cl^- reabsorption in the loop of Henle. The resultant volume depletion activates the renin-angiotensin system. Distal delivery of NaCl and water are high in the presence of high aldosterone, promoting secretion of K^+ and H^+ ions. Prostaglandin overproduction is mediated by volume depletion, hypokalemia, and high angiotensin II and kallikrein levels. Increased prostaglandin production contributes to the severity of disease by inducing resistance to the pressor effects of angiotensin II and reducing reabsorption in the thick ascending limb of the loop of Henle.

Diagnosis Hypokalemia, metabolic alkalosis, and normal to low blood pressure are the clinical findings characteristic of Bartter's syndrome. The differential diagnosis includes vomiting, surreptitious diuretic abuse, and magnesium deficiency. Chronic vomiting can be diagnosed by a low urine Cl^- concentration. Magnesium deficiency causes kaluresis and alkalosis, simulating Bartter's syndrome. Serum and urine magnesium will be low in such cases. Diuretic abuse produces metabolic abnormalities indistinguishable from Bartter's syndrome. Urine should be screened for diuretics multiple times before the diagnosis of Bartter's is made in a patient without a family history of the disorder.

TREATMENT

Dietary intake of sodium and potassium should be liberal. Potassium supplements are usually required. Spironolactone will reduce potassium wasting. Nonsteroidal antiinflammatory drugs (NSAIDs) are useful, particularly in patients with antenatal Bartter's syndrome, since they reduce prostaglandin production. Angiotensin-converting enzyme (ACE) inhibitors may be beneficial in some patients.

GITELMAN'S SYNDROME

Gitelman's syndrome shares many features with Bartter's syndrome including hypokalemia, metabolic alkalosis, salt wasting, elevated renin and aldosterone levels, and normal blood pressure. Clinically it is distinguished from Bartter's by hypomagnesemia and hypocalciuria. Gitelman's syndrome is usually diagnosed during adolescence or adulthood, with weakness, fatigue, muscle cramps, and nocturia being the most common symptoms. The syndrome is inherited as an autosomal recessive trait and is due to mutations in the thiazide-sensitive Na-Cl transporter. The reduced Na^+ reabsorption in the distal convoluted tubule leads to volume depletion and hypokalemia. Loss of activity of the thiazide-sensitive transporter increases tubule calcium reabsorption, leading to the classic finding of hypocalciuria in Gitelman's syndrome. Treatment consists of liberal dietary sodium intake, potassium and magnesium supplements, and potassium sparing diuretics. Unlike in Bartter's syndrome, NSAIDs and ACE inhibitors are not effective.

CONGENITAL NEPHROGENIC DIABETES INSIPIDUS

GENETIC CONSIDERATIONS This rare genetic disorder is most commonly inherited as an X-linked disease, with full expression in males and variable penetrance in females. Vasopressin acts through two receptors; type 1 receptors are located in the vasculature, while type 2 receptors are found in the collecting ducts of the kidney. In X-linked nephrogenic diabetes insipidus (NDI), only the actions requiring type 2 receptors are abnormal. Mutations of the type 2 vasopressin receptor lead to misfolding and trapping of the receptor in the endoplasmic reticulum, with no receptor present on the cell surface. Less frequently, NDI may be inherited as an autosomal trait, either recessive or dominant, in which mutations in the gene for the water channels in collecting duct cells (aquaporin 2) lead to abnormal cell routing of aquaporin 2.

Clinical Features The clinical presentation is that of persistent polyuria, dehydration, and hypotonic urine in the presence of hypernatremia. Vasopressin levels are appropriately elevated in the hypertonic state, but renal response is lacking. About 90% of cases are diagnosed in the first 2.5 years of life. Recurrent hypernatremia may lead to seizures or mental retardation. Once old enough to satisfy their thirst, children will be clinically stable though in a chronic state of polyuria and polydypsia. Renal function is normal, and radiographic studies of the urinary system reveal dilated ureters and bladder secondary to the chronically high urine flow. Since the most common form of the disease is X-linked, most patients are male. Heterozygous females generally have mild concentrating defects, though a few have phenotypic expression similar to males due to skewed X-chromosome inactivation.

TREATMENT

Treatment is aimed at maintaining adequate hydration. In the infant, low-solute feedings and high water intake are generally adequate. Addition of a thiazide diuretic reduces urine flow by inhibiting sodium reabsorption in the distal convoluted tubule. This lowers free water production and, by causing extracellular volume contraction, increases proximal salt and water reabsorption, reducing delivery to the distal nephron. Amiloride or indomethacin are frequently used to potentiate the effects of thiazide diuretics. Administration of vasopressin and its analogues has no role in the management of this disorder.

RENAL TUBULAR ACIDOSIS

Renal tubular acidosis (RTA) is a disorder of renal acidification out of proportion to the reduction in glomerular filtration rate. RTA is characterized by hyperchloremic metabolic acidosis with a normal serum anion gap $[Na^+ - (Cl^- + HCO_3^-)]$. There are multiple forms of RTA, depending on which aspects of renal acid handling have been affected. Defective bicarbonate reabsorption in the proximal tubule, suppressed renal ammoniagenesis, and inadequate distal tubule proton secretion are the abnormalities that produce RTA. Three major forms of RTA exist (Table 265-2). Types 1 and 2 may be inherited or acquired. Type 4 is usually acquired and is associated with either hypoaldosteronism or tubular hyporesponsiveness to mineralocorticoids. *Type 3 is a very rare form of RTA with features of both type 1 and type 2 RTA. It is due to deficiency carbonic anhydrase II, an enzyme present in both the proximal and distal tubules. It is an autosomal recessive disease associated with osteopetrosis and mental retardation.*

TYPE 1 (DISTAL) RTA In this disorder the distal nephron does not lower urine pH normally, either because the collecting ducts permit excessive back-diffusion of hydrogen ions from lumen to blood or because there is inadequate transport of hydrogen ions. Excretion of titratable acid is low, as inadequate proton secretion prevents titration of urinary buffers such as phosphate. Urine ammonium excretion is inappropriately low for the level of acidosis, as the defect in acidification reduces the ion trapping required for ammonium excretion. Urinary concentration and potassium conservation also tend to be impaired.

Chronic acidosis lowers tubule reabsorption of calcium, causing renal hypercalciuria and mild secondary hyperparathyroidism. Buffering of bone by the daily metabolic acid load contributes to hypercalciuria. Urine citrate excretion is low, as acidosis and hypokalemia stimulate proximal tubule reabsorption of citrate. The hypercalciuria, alkaline urine, and low levels of urine citrate cause calcium phosphate stones and nephrocalcinosis. Growth retardation is common and improves with correction of the acidosis by alkali. In both children and adults, bone diseases may result, in part, from acidosis-induced loss of bone material and inadequate production of 1,25-dihydroxyvitamin D_3 [1,25(OH)$_2$D$_3$]. Since the kidney does not conserve potassium or concentrate the urine normally, polyuria and hypokalemia occur. With the stress of an intercurrent illness, acidosis and hypokalemia can be life-threatening.

TABLE 265-2 *Comparison of Normal Anion-Gap Acidoses*

Finding	Type 1 RTA	Type 2 RTA	Type 4 RTA	GI Bicarbonate Loss
Normal anion-gap acidosis	Yes	Yes	Yes	Yes
Minimum urine pH	>5.5	<5.5	<5.5	5 to 6
% Filtered bicarbonate excreted	<10	>15	<10	<10
Serum potassium	Low	Low	High	Low
Fanconi syndrome	No	Yes	No	No
Stones/nephrocalcinosis	Yes	No	No	No
Daily acid excretion	Low	Normal	Low	High
Urine anion gap	Positive	Positive	Positive	Negative
Daily bicarbonate replacement needs	<4 mmol/kg	>4 mmol/kg	<4 mmol/kg	Variable

Note: RTA, renal tubular acidosis.

GENETIC CONSIDERATIONS Type 1 RTA can be familial, with autosomal dominant as the most common mode of inheritance. Autosomal recessive and sporadic cases have been reported. Mutations in the basolateral chloride-bicarbonate exchanger (*AE1*) of intercalated cells have been identified in the autosomal dominant form. The autosomal recessive form has been associated with mutations in the H$^+$-ATPase in some families. Sensorineural deafness frequently accompanies the H$^+$-ATPase mutation. Other hereditary diseases that cause type 1 RTA include galactosemia, Ehler-Danlos syndrome, Fabry's disease, MSK, Wilson's disease, and hereditary elliptocytosis. The majority of cases of type 1 RTA are secondary to a systemic disorder such as Sjögren's syndrome, hypergammaglobulinemia, chronic active hepatitis, or lupus.

Diagnosis The diagnosis of type 1 RTA is suggested by a normal anion gap metabolic acidosis with a simultaneous urine pH > 5.5. Calcium phosphate stones or nephrocalcinosis support the diagnosis, though they are not present in all cases. Bicarbonaturia is not present, which distinguishes this disorder from type 2 RTA. If acidosis is not severe and urine pH is equivocal, an oral ammonium chloride loading test may confirm the diagnosis. As systemic acidosis worsens with ammonium chloride, urine pH does not fall below 5.5 in patients with type I RTA.

Chronic diarrheal states cause normal anion gap acidosis and hypokalemia; urine pH may be >5.5 if ammonium production is very high. The urine anion gap (Na$^+$ + K$^+$ − Cl$^-$) can be used to estimate renal ammonium production and distinguish RTA from gastrointestinal bicarbonate loss. Normally the urine anion gap is positive, as unmeasured anions exceed unmeasured cations. If urine ammonium levels are high, urine chloride concentration increases to balance the charge. Unmeasured cation (predominantly ammonium) now exceeds unmeasured anion, and the urine anion gap is negative. During metabolic acidosis, a negative urine anion gap suggests an extrarenal cause of acidosis, whereas a positive urine anion gap suggests RTA. The urine anion gap cannot be used if there are large amounts of unmeasured anions, such as bicarbonate or ketones, in the urine.

TREATMENT

Alkali supplements are the standard therapy. Enough alkali is prescribed to titrate the daily metabolic acid production, usually in the range of 0.5 to 2.0 mmol/kg body weight in four to six divided doses per day. Sodium bicarbonate and Shohl's solution are common treatments. Potassium alkali salts can be used if hypokalemia is a persistent problem. Citrate requires less frequent dosing than bicarbonate salts as it is metabolized to bicarbonate after absorption. The dose of alkali should be raised until acidosis and hypercalciuria are both eliminated.

Requirements for alkali may rise during intercurrent illnesses but are <4 mmol/kg body weight per day. The relatives of patients with idiopathic type 1 RTA should be screened for this disorder, as timely treatment can prevent growth retardation in children. Incomplete RTA secondary to idiopathic hypercalciuria is best treated using thiazide diuretics in conjunction with potassium citrate (Chap. 268).

TYPE 2 (PROXIMAL) RTA Type 2 RTA usually occurs as part of a generalized disorder of proximal tubule function, presenting as hyperchloremic acidosis with other features of Fanconi syndrome. Bicarbonate reabsorption in the proximal tubule is defective. At normal concentrations of plasma bicarbonate, large amounts of bicarbonate are delivered to the distal tubule, overwhelming the absorptive capacity of the distal tubule and resulting in bicarbonaturia. As plasma bicarbonate levels fall, the lower filtered load of bicarbonate can be reabsorbed by the proximal tubule, resulting in normal distal delivery of bicarbonate. At this point the distal nephron can acidify the urine normally, resulting in normal excretion of daily metabolic acid production, albeit at a low serum bicarbonate level. Hypophosphatemia and low calcitriol levels are common and may lead to rickets or osteomalacia. Hypercalciuria occurs, but stone formation is unusual since urine citrate levels are normal or high because of reduced proximal tubule citrate reabsorption. Type 2 RTA without Fanconi syndrome may be inherited as an autosomal dominant or recessive disorder. Mutations in the Na$^+$-HCO$_3^-$ cotransporter (NBC-1) have been reported in some families with the autosomal recessive form. Type 2 RTA may be acquired in association with other diseases (see "Fanconi Syndrome," below) or be secondary to drugs that inhibit carbonic anhydrase activity, such as acetazolamide.

Type 2 RTA may be distinguished from type 1 RTA by the ability to normally acidify urine during spontaneous or ammonium chloride–induced acidosis. Correction of acidosis with bicarbonate will result in bicarbonaturia in type 2 RTA but not in type 1 RTA. Fractional excretion of bicarbonate is >15% at normal or near-normal serum bicarbonate levels. In distal RTA it is <10%. It is unusual for serum bicarbonate levels to fall below 15 mmol/L in proximal RTA. The urine anion gap will be positive, as ammonium excretion is normal to handle daily acid production but is not elevated as in nonrenal causes of acidosis.

TREATMENT

Children should be treated to prevent growth retardation. Alkali must be given in large amounts daily, 5 to 15 mmol/kg body weight per day, because bicarbonate is rapidly excreted in the urine. A thiazide diuretic can be used in conjunction with a low-salt diet to reduce the amount of bicarbonate required. Potassium requirements increase during alkali therapy due to increased renal loss of potassium from bicarbonaturia.

TYPE 4 RTA In type 4 RTA, also called *hyperkalemic distal RTA*, distal tubule secretion of both potassium and hydrogen ions is abnormal, resulting in hyperchloremic acidosis with hyperkalemia. Type 4 RTA is an acquired disorder; a moderate degree of renal insufficiency is present in the majority of patients. Patients with type 4 RTA can be differentiated from patients with type 1 since they have an acid urine (pH < 5.5) during periods of acidosis (Table 265-2) and hyperkalemia. They differ from type 2 patients by having a fractional excretion of bicarbonate <10% and a daily bicarbonate requirement of 1 to 3 mmol/kg body weight per day. Because potassium and hydrogen ion excretion are abnormal, such patients are considered to have generalized distal nephron dysfunction due to either insufficient aldosterone production or intrinsic renal disease causing aldosterone resistance. The resulting hyperkalemia reduces proximal tubule ammonia production, in addition to the inadequate proton secretion, leading to inadequate excretion of the daily metabolic proton load. These patients have an acid urine despite reduced proton secretion because there is inadequate ammonia to buffer protons in the distal tubule. If buffer delivery to the distal nephron is increased, urine pH will rise despite persistent acidosis.

Type 4 RTA due to inadequate aldosterone production has multiple etiologies. Hyporeninemic hypoaldosteronism is the most common cause of type 4 RTA and is usually associated with diabetic nephropathy. Plasma levels of renin and aldosterone are subnormal, even during extracellular volume depletion. NSAIDs, ACE inhibitors, trimethoprim, and heparin can reduce aldosterone production and produce a type 4 RTA. Drug-induced type 4 RTA is usually seen in patients with preexisting renal insufficiency. Reduced aldosterone production may be due to adrenal disease, occurring as either an isolated defect or as part of a more generalized adrenal disorder (Chap. 321). Renin levels are normal to high in adrenal disorders.

Patients with tubular resistance to aldosterone present with the same clinical features as those with hyporeninemic hypoaldosteronism. A tubulointerstitial process damages the distal tubule, restricting potassium and hydrogen ion excretion, despite adequate aldosterone levels. Obstructive uropathy and sickle cell disease are the most common causes of acquired tubular resistance to aldosterone. Hyporeninemic hypoaldosteronism can be found in addition to tubular aldosterone resistance in many patients. Potassium-sparing diuretics can cause a type 4 RTA by producing an aldosterone resistant state.

℞ TREATMENT

The main goal of therapy is to reduce serum potassium, as acidosis will usually improve once the hyperkalemic block of ammonium production is removed. All patients should be placed on a low-potassium diet. Any drug that suppresses aldosterone production or blocks aldosterone effect should be discontinued. Mineralocorticoid supplementation with fludrocortisone, 0.1 to 0.2 mg/d, will improve hyperkalemia and acidosis; however, the patients who also have a partial tubule resistance to mineralocorticoid will require a higher dose. Mineralocorticoid replacement may not be appropriate for patients with hypertension or a history of heart failure. In such situations, a loop diuretic with a liberal sodium intake can usually promote adequate potassium excretion. Exchange resins will reduce potassium levels but are usually not tolerated well enough to be used for long-term treatment.

PSEUDOHYPOALDOSTERONISM

GENETIC CONSIDERATIONS Type I pseudohyperaldosteronism is transmitted as either an autosomal dominant or recessive trait. The autosomal dominant form is caused by mutations in the mineralocorticoid receptor gene; the autosomal recessive disease is caused by inactivating mutations in the amiloride-sensitive epithelial sodium channel. The aldosterone resistance leads to hyperkalemia, metabolic acidosis, salt wasting, and volume depletion, which present during childhood. Plasma renin and aldosterone levels are elevated. Treatment includes salt supplements, alkali, and potassium restriction.

Type II pseudohypoaldosteronism (also known as *Gordon syn-*

drome) presents as hypertension, hyperkalemia, and metabolic acidosis with normal renal function. The disease is inherited as an autosomal dominant trait and appears to be secondary to overactivity of the thiazide sensitive Na-Cl cotransporter. Two genes have been linked to the disease and both encode WNK kinases that are expressed in the distal tubule. Thiazide diuretics control the hypertension and correct the electrolyte disorders.

VITAMIN D DISORDERS

X-LINKED HYPOPHOSPHATEMIC RICKETS (See also Chap. 331) This disorder is an X-linked dominant disorder characterized by hypophosphatemia with renal phosphate wasting, rickets, and short stature. Hypophosphatemia is present soon after birth; rachitic bowing of the legs develops when the child begins to walk. Children have growth retardation, which is limited almost entirely to the lower extremities. Dentition is delayed, and skull abnormalities are common. Presentation in adults ranges from disabling bone pain to no active symptoms, but generally some physical sign of childhood disease, such as short stature or bowed legs, is present. Overgrowth of bone at joints or sites of muscle attachment may reduce the mobility of the joint or cause nerve entrapment.

Hypophosphatemia secondary to reduced renal phosphate reabsorption is the hallmark of the disease. Serum calcium levels are usually normal, with low intestinal absorption and renal excretion of calcium. Serum alkaline phosphatase and osteocalcin levels are elevated. Parathyroid hormone levels are normal, as would be expected with normal serum calcium. $1,25(OH)_2D_3$ levels are usually normal, though in the setting of hypophosphatemia $1,25(OH)_2D_3$ levels should be elevated. The disease is caused by inactivating mutations in the PHEX gene, located on chromosome Xp22.1, which codes for a membrane-bound endopeptidase. Circulating humoral factors, phosphatonins, that are normally inactivated by the PHEX endopeptidase accumulate in the serum and reduce proximal tubule phosphate reabsorption and $1,25(OH)_2D_3$ production.

℞ TREATMENT

The goal of therapy is to raise serum phosphorous to normal or near-normal levels to improve bone mineralization. Oral neutral phosphate, 1 to 4 g/d in four to six doses, combined with calcitriol is an effective therapy that improves growth rate, reduces bone pain, and leads to radiographically evident improvement of the bone disease. Patients should be closely monitored during therapy as they may develop nephrocalcinosis and renal insufficiency.

AUTOSOMAL DOMINANT HYPOPHOSPHATEMIC RICKETS This disorder usually presents during childhood with low serum phosphate from renal phosphate wasting, rickets, and dental abnormalities. There is significant phenotypic variability with some subjects not presenting until adulthood and other cases spontaneously correcting metabolic abnormalities after puberty. The disorder has been linked to a locus on chromosome 12p13, and mutations have been identified in the gene product, fibroblast growth factor (FGF-23). FGF-23 may act as a phosphatonin and promote renal phosphate wasting.

VITAMIN D–DEPENDENT RICKETS TYPE I

GENETIC CONSIDERATIONS This is an autosomal recessive disorder in which $1,25(OH)_2D_3$ levels are very low but 25-hydroxyvitamin D levels are normal. The disease is caused by inactivating mutations in the gene encoding the 1α-hydroxylase enzyme, leading to a clinical syndrome of vitamin D deficiency.

Symptoms usually appear before the age of 2, including rickets and growth retardation. Levels of serum calcium and phosphorous are low, but that of alkaline phosphatase is elevated. Intestinal calcium absorption and urinary calcium excretion are low. Parathyroid hormone is elevated in response to the hypocalcemia, resulting in increased urinary phosphate losses.

℞ TREATMENT

Calcitriol (0.5 to 1 $\mu g/d$) leads to rapid correction of the biochemical abnormalities and resolution of the bone disease. Calcium and phosphorous supplementation are usually not required.

VITAMIN D–DEPENDENT RICKETS TYPE II (See also Chap. 331)   End-organ resistance to $1,25(OH)_2D_3$ is the pathogenesis of this disorder. Serum calcium and phosphate levels are low, secondary hyperparathyroidism is present, and $1,25(OH)_2D_3$ levels are elevated. Inheritance is usually autosomal recessive, though sporadic cases have been reported. Most patients present during childhood with rickets, though some have a milder form of disease not recognized until adulthood. Alopecia is common and tends to be associated with the more severe childhood form of the disease. Mutations in the vitamin D receptor reduce tissue response to $1,25(OH)_2D_3$. Pharmacologic doses of calcitriol (5 to 30 $\mu g/d$) along with mineral supplementation will improve the biochemical disorders and bone disease, though some patients have no response to massive doses of calcitriol.

ONCOGENIC OSTEOMALACIA   This syndrome generally occurs in adults with highly vascular mesenchymal tumors. Patients present with bone pain and muscle weakness. Symptoms may be present for years before the correct diagnosis is made. Over 90% of the tumors are benign, and most are found in the extremities or maxillofacial region. Hypophosphatemia secondary to renal phosphate wasting and low levels of $1,25(OH)_2D_3$ are the major biochemical abnormalities. Serum calcium and parathyroid hormone levels are normal. The tumors produce humoral agents, phosphatonins, that reduce proximal tubule phosphate reabsorption and 1α-hydroxylase activity. FGF-23 is a fibroblast growth factor that has been identified as a potential phosphatonin. Removal of the tumor leads to rapid resolution of the disease. Octreotide therapy reduces secretion of phosphatonins and improves serum phosphorus in some patients with oncogenic osteomalacia.

DENT'S DISEASE

This disorder presents as hypercalciuria, low-molecular-weight proteinuria, calcium nephrolithiasis, and nephrocalcinosis in male children. Progression to renal failure is common. Phosphaturia, glycosuria, aminoaciduria, and other features of Fanconi's syndrome may be present. Females carrying the gene are asymptomatic except for low-molecular-weight proteinuria. Kidney biopsy reveals tubular atrophy, interstitial fibrosis, and medullary calcifications. The gene has been mapped to the short arm of the X chromosome and encodes a voltage-gated chloride channel (CLC-5). Treatment with thiazide diuretics improves the hypercalciuria, but whether thiazides help preserve renal function is not known.

ISOLATED HYPOURICEMIA (See also Chap. 338)

This disorder is generally inherited as an autosomal recessive trait. Most commonly there is deficient urate reabsorption in the proximal tubule, though some patients have been demonstrated to oversecrete urate. Serum uric acid is usually $<120\ \mu mol/L$ (2 mg/dL) and hyperuricosuria is common, possibly due to decreased intestinal urate excretion. Hypouricemia is usually an incidental finding, as patients with this disorder are asymptomatic except for an increased risk of nephrolithiasis. Other disorders associated with hypouricemia include Fanconi syndrome, Wilson's disease, Hodgkin's disease, and Hartnup disease. No treatment is required except for high fluid intake to prevent kidney stones. Alkali and allopurinol may be used to prevent stones if fluids alone are not sufficient.

SELECTED DISORDERS OF AMINO ACID TRANSPORT

HARTNUP DISEASE   This disorder is characterized by reduced intestinal absorption and renal reabsorption of neutral amino acids. The defect involves an amino acid transporter on the brush border of the jejunum and the proximal tubule. Intestinal absorption of free amino acids is reduced, though the neutral amino acids can be absorbed when present

in di- and tripeptides. Degradation of unabsorbed tryptophan by intestinal bacteria produces indolic acids that are absorbed and subsequently excreted at high levels in the urine of these patients. The disorder is inherited as an autosomal recessive trait with an estimated incidence of 1 in 24,000 live births. Linkage analysis suggests a locus on chromosome 5.

The majority of individuals with this disorder are asymptomatic. Approximately 10 to 20% present with clinical symptoms similar to those seen in pellagra, including a photosensitive erythematous scaly rash, intermittent cerebral ataxia, delirium, and diarrhea. Short stature is noted in some patients. The symptoms are thought to be due to deficiency in the essential amino acid tryptophan and resultant inadequate synthesis of nicotinamide. Though the inheritance of the disorder is autosomal recessive, the development of symptomatic disease appears to be multifactorial. Diet, environment, and polygenic traits controlling plasma amino acid levels all contribute to development of symptoms.

Clinically affected patients can be differentiated from patients with pellagra by dietary history and the presence of aminoaciduria. Diagnosis is made by the characteristic finding of large amounts of neutral amino acids in the urine. It can easily be distinguished from generalized aminoaciduria by the normal excretion of proline. There are no other renal tubule defects as in Fanconi syndrome. Heterozygotes have normal urinary amino acid excretion.

℞ TREATMENT

Symptomatic individuals should receive oral nicotinamide, 40 to 200 mg/d, and a high-protein diet to compensate for the poor amino acid absorption. Some patients who do not respond to nicotinamide may improve with tryptophan ethyl ester, which is lipid soluble and can be absorbed without an active transport system.

FANCONI SYNDROME

⟨S⟩ GENETIC CONSIDERATIONS   Fanconi syndrome is a generalized defect in proximal tubule transport involving amino acids, glucose, phosphate, uric acid, sodium, potassium, bicarbonate, and proteins. Idiopathic Fanconi syndrome may be inherited as an autosomal dominant, autosomal recessive, or X-linked trait. The autosomal dominant form has been mapped to chromosome 15. Sporadic cases are also seen. A variety of inherited systemic disorders are also associated with Fanconi syndrome including Wilson's disease, galactosemia, tyrosinemia, cystinosis, fructose intolerance, and Lowe's oculocerebral syndrome. The syndrome may be acquired in multiple myeloma, amyloid, heavy metal toxicity, and from chemotherapeutic drugs.

The patients may present with a wide array of laboratory abnormalities including proximal renal tubular acidosis, glucosuria with a normal serum glucose, hypophosphatemia, hypouricemia, hypokalemia, generalized aminoaciduria, and low-molecular-weight proteinuria. Some patients do not have abnormalities in all proximal tubule transporters and may present with only a few of the laboratory findings. Rickets and osteomalacia are common findings secondary to the hypophosphatemia; production of calcitriol may also be abnormal. Metabolic acidosis also contributes to the bone disease. Polyuria, salt wasting, and hypokalemia may be quite severe.

℞ TREATMENT

Treatment includes phosphate supplements and calcitriol to heal the bone lesions, alkali for the acidosis, and liberal intake of salt and water. Alkali in the form of potassium salts may be particularly useful in the patient with RTA and hypokalemia. Aminoaciduria, glucosuria, hypouricemia, and low-molecular-weight proteinuria do not require treatment.

FURTHER READING

CRUZ DN et al: Gitelman's syndrome revisited: An evaluation of symptoms and health-related quality of life. Kidney Int 59:710, 2001

HILDEBRANDT F, OTTO E: Molecular genetics of nephronophthisis and medullary cystic kidney disease. J Am Soc Nephrol 11:1753, 2000

IGARISH P, SOMLO S: Genetics and pathogenesis of polycystic kidney disease. J Am Soc Nephrol 13:2384, 2002

JAN SM, LEVINE MA: Molecular pathogenesis of hypophosphatemic rickets. J Clin Endocrinol Metab 87:2467, 2002

PIRSON Y et al: Management of cerebral aneurysms in autosomal dominant polycystic kidney disease. J Am Soc Nephrol 13:269, 2002

SEUFERT J et al: Octreotide therapy for tumor-induced osteomalacia. N Engl J Med 345:1883, 2001

SORIANO JR: Renal tubular acidosis: The clinical entity. J Am Soc Nephrol 13:2160, 2002

WARD CJ et al: The gene mutated in autosomal recessive polycystic kidney disease encodes a large, receptor-like protein. Nat Genet 30:259, 2002

WILSON FH et al: Human hypertension caused by mutations in WNK kinases. Science 293:1107, 2001

266   TUBULOINTERSTITIAL DISEASES OF THE KIDNEY
Alan S. L. Yu, Barry M. Brenner

Primary tubulointerstitial diseases of the kidney, as distinct from the disorders considered in Chaps. 264 and 267, are characterized by histologic and functional abnormalities that involve the tubules and interstitium to a greater degree than the glomeruli and renal vasculature (Table 266-1). Secondary tubulointerstitial disease occurs as a consequence of progressive glomerular or vascular injury. Morphologically, acute forms of these disorders are characterized by interstitial edema, often associated with cortical and medullary infiltration by both mononuclear cells and polymorphonuclear leukocytes, and patchy areas of tubule cell necrosis. In more chronic forms, interstitial fibrosis predominates, inflammatory cells are typically mononuclear, and abnormalities of the tubules tend to be more widespread, as evidenced by atrophy, luminal dilatation, and thickening of tubule basement membranes. Because of the nonspecific nature of the histology, particularly in chronic tubulointerstitial diseases, biopsy specimens rarely provide a specific diagnosis. The urine sediment is also unlikely to be diagnostic, except in allergic forms of acute tubulointerstitial disease, in which eosinophils may predominate in the urinary sediment.

Defects in renal function often accompany these alterations of tubule and interstitial structure (Table 266-2). Proximal tubule dysfunction may be manifested as selective reabsorptive defects leading to hypokalemia, aminoaciduria, glycosuria, phosphaturia, uricosuria, or bicarbonaturia [proximal or type II renal tubular acidosis (RTA); Chap. 265]. In combination, these defects constitute the *Fanconi syndrome*. Proteinuria, predominantly of low-molecular-weight proteins, is usually modest, rarely exceeding 2 g/d.

Defects in urinary acidification and concentrating ability often represent the most troublesome of the tubule dysfunctions encountered in patients with tubulointerstitial disease. Hyperchloremic metabolic acidosis often develops at a relatively early stage in the course. Patients with this finding generally elaborate urine of maximal acidity (pH ≤ 5.3). In such patients the defect in acid excretion is usually caused by a reduced capacity to generate and excrete ammonia due to the reduction in renal mass. Preferential damage to the collecting ducts, as in amyloidosis or chronic obstructive uropathy, may also predispose to distal or type I RTA, characterized by high urine pH (≥5.5) during spontaneous or NH_4Cl-induced metabolic acidosis. Patients with tubulointerstitial diseases affecting predominantly medullary and papillary structures may also exhibit concentrating defects, with resultant nocturia and polyuria. Analgesic nephropathy and sickle cell disease are prototypes of this form of injury.

TOXINS

Although the kidney is vulnerable to toxic injury, renal damage by a variety of nephrotoxins often goes unrecognized because the manifestations of such injury are usually nonspecific in nature and insidious in onset. Diagnosis largely depends on a history of exposure to a certain toxin. Particular attention should be paid to the occupational history, as well as to an assessment of exposure—current and remote—to drugs, especially antibiotics and analgesics, and to dietary supplements or herbal remedies. The recognition of a potential association between a patient's renal disease and exposure to a nephrotoxin is crucial, because, unlike many other forms of renal disease, progression of the functional and morphologic abnormalities associated with toxin-induced nephropathies may be prevented, and even reversed, by eliminating additional exposure.

TABLE 266-1   *Principal Causes of Tubulointerstitial Disease of the Kidney*

ACUTE INTERSTITIAL NEPHRITIS

Drugs[a]
  Antibiotics (β-lactams, sulfonamides, quinolones, vancomycin, erythromycin, minocycline, rifampin, ethambutol, acyclovir)
  Nonsteroidal anti-inflammatory drugs
  Diuretics (thiazides, furosemide, triamterene)
  Anticonvulsants (phenytoin, phenobarbital, carbamazepine, valproic acid)
  Miscellaneous (captopril, H_2 receptor blockers, omeprazole, mesalazine, indinavir, allopurinol)
Infection
  Bacteria (*Streptococcus, Staphylococcus, Legionella, Salmonella, Brucella, Yersinia, Corynebacterium diphtheriae*)
  Viruses (Epstein-Barr virus, cytomegalovirus, Hantavirus, HIV)
  Miscellaneous (*Leptospira, Rickettsia, Mycoplasma*)
Idiopathic
  Tubulointerstitial nephritis–uveitis syndrome
  Anti-tubule basement membrane disease
  Sarcoidosis

CHRONIC TUBULOINTERSTITIAL DISEASES

Hereditary renal diseases
  Polycystic kidney disease[a] (Chap. 276)
  Medullary cystic disease (Chap. 276)
  Medullary sponge kidney (Chap. 276)
Exogenous toxins
  Analgesic nephropathy[a]
  Lead nephropathy
  Miscellaneous nephrotoxins (e.g. lithium[a], cyclosporine[a], heavy metals, slimming regimens with Chinese herbs)
Metabolic toxins
  Hyperuricemia[a]
  Hypercalcemia
  Miscellaneous metabolic toxins (e.g., hypokalemia, hyperoxaluria, cystinosis, Fabry's disease)
Autoimmune disorders
  Sjögren's syndrome
Neoplastic disorders
  Leukemia
  Lymphoma
  Multiple myeloma[a]
Miscellaneous disorders
  Sickle cell nephropathy
  Chronic pyelonephritis
  Chronic urinary tract obstruction
  Vesicoureteral reflux[a]
  Radiation nephritis
  Balkan nephropathy
  Tubulointerstitial disease secondary to glomerular and vascular disease

[a] Common

TABLE 266-2 *Functional Consequences of Tubulointerstitial Disease*

Defect	Cause(s)
Reduced glomerular filtration rate[a]	Obliteration of microvasculature and obstruction of tubules
Fanconi syndrome	Damage to proximal tubular reabsorption of glucose, amino acids, phosphate, and bicarbonate
Hyperchloremic acidosis[a]	1. Reduced ammonia production 2. Inability to acidify the collecting duct fluid (distal renal tubular acidosis) 3. Proximal bicarbonate wasting
Tubular or small-molecular-weight proteinuria[a]	Failure of proximal tubule protein reabsorption
Polyuria, isothenuria[a]	Damage to medullary tubules and vasculature
Hyperkalemia[a]	Potassium secretory defects including aldosterone resistance
Salt wasting	Distal tubular damage with impaired sodium reabsorption

[a] Common

EXOGENOUS TOXINS ■ **Analgesic Nephropathy** A distinct clinicopathologic syndrome has been described in heavy users of analgesic mixtures containing phenacetin in combination with aspirin, acetaminophen, or caffeine. Morphologically, analgesic nephropathy is characterized by papillary necrosis and tubulointerstitial inflammation. At an early stage, damage to the vascular supply of the inner medulla (vasa recta) leads to a local interstitial inflammatory reaction and, eventually, to papillary ischemia, necrosis, fibrosis, and calcification. The susceptibility of the renal papillae to damage by phenacetin is believed to be related to the establishment of a renal gradient for its acetaminophen metabolite, resulting in papillary tip concentrations tenfold higher than those in renal cortex. Aspirin in these analgesic compounds contributes to renal injury by uncoupling oxidative phosphorylation in renal mitochondria and by inhibiting the synthesis of renal prostaglandins, which are potent endogenous renal vasodilator hormones.

In analgesic nephropathy, renal function usually declines gradually. Occasionally, papillary necrosis may be associated with hematuria and even renal colic owing to obstruction of a ureter by necrotic tissue. More than half of patients with analgesic nephropathy have pyuria, which, if persistently associated with sterile urine, provides an important clue to the diagnosis. Nonetheless, active pyelonephritis may coexist in patients with analgesic nephropathy. Proteinuria, if present, is typically mild (< 1 g/d). Patients with analgesic nephropathy are usually unable to generate maximally concentrated urine, reflecting the underlying medullary and papillary damage. An acquired form of distal RTA (Chap. 265) may contribute to the development of *nephrocalcinosis*. The occurrence of anemia out of proportion to the degree of azotemia may also provide a clue to the diagnosis of analgesic nephropathy. When analgesic nephropathy has progressed to renal insufficiency, the kidneys usually appear bilaterally shrunken on intravenous pyelography, and the calyces are deformed. A "ring sign" on the pyelogram is pathognomonic of papillary necrosis and represents the radiolucent sloughed papilla surrounded by the radiodense contrast material in the calyx. Computed tomography may reveal papillary calcifications surrounding the central sinus complex in a "garland" pattern. Transitional cell carcinoma may develop in the urinary pelvis or ureters as a late complication of analgesic abuse.

Whether non-phenacetin analgesics, alone or in combination, cause renal disease is controversial. A recent cohort study of men with normal baseline renal function found no association between moderate analgesic use and subsequent renal dysfunction, suggesting that the risk, if any, is low. Until conclusive evidence is available, however, physicians should consider screening heavy users of acetaminophen and nonsteroidal anti-inflammatory drugs (NSAIDs) for evidence of renal disease, and discouraging their use of these drugs.

Lead Nephropathy (See also Chap. 376) Lead intoxication may produce a chronic tubulointerstitial renal disease. Children who repeatedly ingest lead-based paints (pica) may develop kidney disease as adults. Significant occupational exposure may occur in workplaces where lead-containing metals or paints are heated to high temperatures, such as battery factories, smelters, salvage yards, and weapon firing ranges. Alcohol, illegally distilled in an apparatus constructed from automobile radiators (so-called moonshine), is another cause of lead poisoning. Environmental lead exposure, particularly in industrial regions, may be great enough to produce changes in renal function.

Tubule transport processes enhance the accumulation of lead within renal cells, particularly in the proximal convoluted tubule, leading to cell degeneration, mitochondrial swelling, and eosinophilic intranuclear inclusion bodies rich in lead. In addition, lead nephropathy is associated with ischemic changes in the glomeruli, fibrosis of the adventitia of small renal arterioles, and focal areas of cortical scarring. Eventually, the kidneys become atrophic. Urinary excretion of lead, porphyrin precursors such as δ-aminolevulinic acid and coproporphyrin, and urobilinogen may be increased. Patients with chronic lead nephropathy are characteristically *hyperuricemic*, a consequence of enhanced reabsorption of filtered urate. Acute gouty arthritis (so-called saturnine gout) develops in about 50% of patients with lead nephropathy, in striking contrast to other forms of chronic renal failure in which de novo gout is rare (Chap. 338). Hypertension is also a complication. Therefore, in any patient with slowly progressive renal failure, atrophic kidneys, gout, and hypertension, the diagnosis of lead intoxication should be considered. Features of acute lead intoxication (abdominal colic, anemia, peripheral neuropathy, and encephalopathy) are usually absent.

The diagnosis may be suspected by finding elevated serum levels of lead. However, because blood levels may not be elevated even in the presence of a toxic total-body burden of lead, the quantitation of lead excretion following infusion of the chelating agent calcium disodium edetate is a more reliable indicator of serious lead exposure. While urinary excretion of more than 0.6 mg/d of lead is generally considered to be indicative of overt or potential toxicity, recent evidence suggests that even lead burdens of 0.15 to 0.6 mg/d may cause progressive loss of renal function.

℞ **TREATMENT**

Treatment includes removing the patient from the source of exposure and augmenting lead excretion with a chelating agent such as calcium disodium edetate.

Lithium Use of lithium salts for bipolar disorder (Chap. 371) is associated with chronic tubulointerstitial nephropathy, generally manifest as the insidious development of chronic renal insufficiency. Nephrogenic diabetes insipidus, which may occur alone or in association with the renal insufficiency, is common. It manifests as polyuria and polydipsia, and is due to lithium-induced downregulation of the vasopressin-regulated water channels in the collecting duct. Mild proteinuria can occur. The predominant finding on renal biopsy is tubular atrophy and interstitial fibrosis out of proportion to the extent of glomerular or vascular disease. Tubular cysts are common, and concomitant focal segmental glomerulosclerosis can be observed.

Renal function should be followed in patients taking this drug, and caution should be exercised if lithium is employed in patients with underlying renal disease. Once renal impairment occurs, lithium therapy should be stopped and an alternative agent substituted. Despite discontinuation of lithium, chronic renal disease in such patients is often irreversible and can progress to end-stage renal failure.

Miscellaneous Nephrotoxins The immunosuppressant *cyclosporine* causes both acute and chronic renal injury. The acute injury and the use of cyclosporine in transplantation are discussed in Chap. 263. The chronic injury results in an irreversible reduction in glomerular filtration rate (GFR), with mild proteinuria and arterial hypertension. Hyperkalemia is a relatively common complication and results in part from tubule resistance to aldosterone. The histologic changes in renal tissue include patchy interstitial fibrosis and tubular atrophy. In addition, the intrarenal vasculature often demonstrates hyalinosis, and focal segmental glomerular sclerosis can be present as well. Fibrosis may be the result of a cyclosporine-induced increase in renal collagen production. Vasoconstrictive mediators, such as angiotensin II, may also play a role in chronic cyclosporine toxicity. In patients receiving this drug for renal transplantation (Chap. 263), chronic graft dysfunction and recurrence of the primary disease may coincide with chronic cyclosporine injury, and on clinical grounds, distinction among these may be difficult. Cyclosporine nephrotoxicity is also seen in patients undergoing heart or lung transplantation, as well as in patients receiving cyclosporine as an immunosuppressant in a variety of inflammatory and autoimmune disorders. Dose reduction appears to mitigate cyclosporine-associated renal fibrosis but may increase the risk of rejection and graft loss. Treatment of any associated arterial hypertension may lessen renal injury.

Chinese herbs nephropathy is characterized by rapidly progressive interstitial renal fibrosis in young women due to ingestion of slimming pills containing Chinese herbs. At least one of the culprit ingredients is aristolochic acid. Clinically, patients present with progressive chronic renal insufficiency with sterile pyuria and anemia that is disproportionately severe relative to the level of renal function. The pathologic findings are interstitial fibrosis and tubular atrophy that affects the cortex in preference to the medulla, fibrous intimal thickening of the interlobular arteries, and a relative paucity of cellular infiltrates.

Many agents that commonly lead to acute renal failure are also capable of producing tubulointerstitial injury (Chap. 260). These include antibiotics (e.g., aminoglycosides, amphotericin B), radiographic contrast agents, various hydrocarbons (e.g., carbon tetrachloride), and heavy metals (e.g., mercury, cadmium, and bismuth).

METABOLIC TOXINS ■ Acute Uric Acid Nephropathy (See also Chap. 313) Acute overproduction of uric acid and extreme hyperuricemia often lead to a rapidly progressive renal insufficiency, so-called acute uric acid nephropathy. This tubulointerstitial disease is usually seen as part of the tumor lysis syndrome in patients given cytotoxic drugs for the treatment of lymphoproliferative or myeloproliferative disorders but may also occur in these patients before such treatment is begun. The pathologic changes are largely the result of deposition of uric acid crystals in the kidneys and their collecting systems, leading to partial or complete obstruction of collecting ducts, renal pelvis, or ureter. Since obstruction is often bilateral, patients typically follow the clinical course of acute renal failure, characterized by oliguria and rapidly rising serum creatinine concentration. In the early phase uric acid crystals can be found in urine, usually in association with microscopic or gross hematuria. Hyperuricemia can also be a consequence of renal failure of any etiology. The finding of a urine/uric acid creatinine ratio greater than 1 mg/mg (0.7 mol/mol) distinguishes acute uric acid nephropathy from other causes of renal failure.

Prevention of hyperuricemia in patients at risk by treatment with allopurinol in doses of 200 to 800 mg/d prior to cytotoxic therapy reduces the danger of acute uric acid nephropathy. Once hyperuricemia develops, however, efforts should be directed to preventing deposition of uric acid within the urinary tract. Increasing urine volume with potent diuretics (furosemide or mannitol) effectively lowers intratubular uric acid concentrations, and alkalinization of the urine to pH 7 or greater with sodium bicarbonate and/or a carbonic anhydrase inhibitor (acetazolamide) enhances uric acid solubility. If these efforts, together with allopurinol therapy, are ineffective in preventing acute renal failure, dialysis should be instituted to lower the serum uric acid concentration as well as to treat the acute manifestations of uremia.

Gouty Nephropathy (See also Chap. 313) Patients with less severe but prolonged forms of hyperuricemia are predisposed to a more chronic tubulointerstitial disorder, often referred to as *gouty nephropathy*. The severity of renal involvement correlates with the duration and magnitude of the elevation of the serum uric acid concentration. Histologically, the distinctive feature of gouty nephropathy is the presence of crystalline deposits of uric acid and monosodium urate salts in kidney parenchyma. These deposits not only cause intrarenal obstruction but also incite an inflammatory response, leading to lymphocytic infiltration, foreign-body giant cell reaction, and eventual fibrosis, especially of medullary and papillary regions of the kidney. Bacteriuria and pyelonephritis occur in about one-fourth of cases, presumably as complications of intrarenal urinary stasis. Since patients with gout frequently suffer from hypertension and hyperlipidemia, degenerative changes of the renal arterioles may constitute a striking feature of the histologic abnormality, often out of proportion to other morphologic defects. Clinically, gouty nephropathy is an insidious cause of renal insufficiency. Early in its course, GFR may be near normal, often despite focal morphologic changes in medullary and cortical interstitium, proteinuria, and diminished urinary concentrating ability. Whether reducing serum uric acid levels with allopurinol exerts a beneficial effect on the kidney remains to be demonstrated. Although such undesirable consequences of hyperuricemia as gout and uric acid stones respond well to allopurinol, use of this drug in asymptomatic hyperuricemia has not been shown to improve renal function consistently. On the other hand, uricosuric agents such as probenecid, which may increase uric acid stone production, clearly have no role in the treatment of renal disease associated with hyperuricemia.

Hypercalcemic Nephropathy (See also Chap. 332) Chronic hypercalcemia, as occurs in primary hyperparathyroidism, sarcoidosis, multiple myeloma, vitamin D intoxication, or metastatic bone disease, can cause tubulointerstitial damage and progressive renal insufficiency. The earliest lesion is a focal degenerative change in renal epithelia, primarily in collecting ducts, distal convoluted tubules, and loops of Henle. Tubule cell necrosis leads to nephron obstruction and stasis of intrarenal urine, favoring local precipitation of calcium salts and infection. Dilatation and atrophy of tubules eventually occur, as do interstitial fibrosis, mononuclear leukocyte infiltration, and interstitial calcium deposition (nephrocalcinosis). Calcium deposition may also occur in glomeruli and the walls of renal arterioles.

Clinically, the most striking defect is an inability to concentrate the urine maximally, resulting in polyuria and nocturia. Reduced collecting duct responsiveness to vasopressin and defective transport of NaCl in the ascending limb of Henle's loop are responsible for this concentrating defect. Reductions in GFR and renal blood flow also occur, both in acute severe hypercalcemia and with prolonged hypercalcemia of lesser severity. Distal RTA and sodium and potassium wasting have also been described in these chronic states. Eventually, uncontrolled hypercalcemia leads to severe tubulointerstitial damage and overt renal failure. Abdominal x-rays may demonstrate nephrocalcinosis as well as nephrolithiasis, the latter due to the hypercalciuria that often accompanies hypercalcemia.

℞ **TREATMENT**

This consists of reducing the serum calcium concentration toward normal and correcting the primary abnormality of calcium metabolism. The management of hypercalcemia is discussed in Chap. 332. Prognosis for recovery of renal function depends on the severity of the renal lesion at the time hypercalcemia is corrected. Renal dysfunction of acute hypercalcemia may be completely reversible. Gradual, progressive renal insufficiency related to chronic hypercalcemia, however, may not improve with correction of the calcium disorder. Nonetheless, every effort should be made to return serum calcium concentration to normal to minimize further loss of renal function.

RENAL PARENCHYMAL DISEASE ASSOCIATED WITH EXTRARENAL NEOPLASM

Except for the glomerulopathies associated with lymphomas and several solid tumors (Chap. 264), the renal manifestations of primary extrarenal neoplastic processes are confined mainly to the interstitium and tubules. Although metastatic renal involvement by solid tumors is unusual, the kidneys are often invaded by neoplastic cells in hematologic malignancies. In postmortem studies of patients with *lymphoma* and *leukemia*, renal involvement is found in approximately half. Diffuse infiltration of the renal parenchyma with malignant cells is seen most commonly. There may be flank pain, and x-rays may show enlargement of one or both kidneys. Renal insufficiency occurs in a minority of cases, and overt uremia is rare. Treatment of the primary disease may improve renal function in these cases.

PLASMA CELL DYSCRASIAS Several glomerular and tubulointerstitial disorders may occur in association with plasma cell dyscrasias (Chap. 98). Infiltration of the kidneys with myeloma cells is infrequent. When it occurs, the process is usually focal, so renal insufficiency from this cause is also uncommon. The more usual lesion is *myeloma kidney*, characterized histologically by atrophic tubules, many with eosinophilic intraluminal casts, and numerous multinucleated giant cells within tubule walls and in the interstitium. The frequent occurrence of myeloma kidney in patients with Bence Jones proteinuria has suggested a causal relation. Bence Jones proteins are thought to cause myeloma kidney through direct toxicity to renal tubule cells. In addition, Bence Jones proteins may precipitate within the distal nephron where the high concentrations of these proteins and the acid composition of the tubule fluid favor intraluminal cast formation and intrarenal obstruction. Occasionally, acute renal failure occurs after intravenous pyelography in patients with multiple myeloma and is believed to result from the further precipitation of Bence Jones proteins induced by dehydration prior to radiographic study. Dehydration of the patient with myeloma in preparation for intravenous pyelography should therefore be avoided. Multiple myeloma may also affect the kidneys indirectly. Hypercalcemia or hyperuricemia may lead to the nephropathies described above. Proximal tubule disorders are also seen occasionally, including type II proximal RTA and the Fanconi syndrome.

AMYLOIDOSIS (See also Chaps. 264 and 310) Glomerular pathology usually predominates and leads to heavy proteinuria and azotemia. However, tubule function may also be deranged, giving rise to a nephrogenic diabetes insipidus and to distal (type I) RTA. In several cases these functional abnormalities correlated with peritubular deposition of amyloid, particularly in areas surrounding vasa rectae, loops of Henle, and collecting ducts. Bilateral enlargement of the kidneys, especially in a patient with massive proteinuria and tubule dysfunction, should raise the possibility of amyloid renal disease.

IMMUNE DISORDERS

ALLERGIC INTERSTITIAL NEPHRITIS An acute diffuse tubulointerstitial reaction may result from hypersensitivity to a number of drugs, including sulfonamides, many penicillins and cephalosporins, the fluoroquinolone antibiotics ciprofloxacin and norfloxacin, and the antituberculous drugs isoniazid and rifampin. Acute tubulointerstitial damage has also occurred after use of thiazide and loop diuretics, antiulcer medications (cimetidine, ranitidine, and omeprazole), allopurinol, and NSAIDs. Of note, the tubulointerstitial nephropathy that develops in some patients taking NSAIDs may be associated with nephrotic-range proteinuria and histologic evidence of either minimal change or membranous glomerulopathy. The use of mesalazine for the treatment of inflammatory bowel disease is associated with a more subacute disorder in which a severe indolent interstitial nephritis occurs several months after the initiation of the drug. Grossly, the kidneys are usually enlarged. Histologically, the glomeruli appear normal. The principal pathologic abnormalities are in the interstitium of the kidney, which reveals pronounced edema and infiltration with polymorphonuclear leukocytes, lymphocytes, plasma cells, and, in some cases, large numbers of eosinophils. If the process is severe, tubule cell necrosis and regeneration may also be apparent. Immunofluorescence studies have either been unrevealing or demonstrated a linear pattern of immunoglobulin and complement deposition along tubule basement membranes.

Most patients require several weeks of drug exposure before developing evidence of renal injury. Rare cases have occurred after only a few doses or after a year or more of use. Azotemia is usually present; a diagnostic triad of fever, skin rash, and peripheral blood eosinophilia is highly suggestive of acute tubulointerstitial nephritis but is often absent. Examination of the urine sediment reveals hematuria and often pyuria; occasionally, eosinophils may be present. Proteinuria is usually mild to moderate, except in cases of NSAID-induced tubulointerstitial nephritis with minimal change glomerulopathy. The clinical picture may be confused with acute glomerulonephritis, but when acute azotemia and hematuria are accompanied by eosinophilia, skin rash, and a history of drug exposure, a hypersensitivity reaction leading to acute tubulointerstitial nephritis should be regarded as the leading diagnostic possibility. Discontinuation of the drug usually results in complete reversal of the renal injury; rarely, renal damage may be irreversible. Glucocorticoids may accelerate renal recovery, but their value has not been definitively established.

SJÖGREN'S SYNDROME (See also Chap. 304) When the kidneys are involved in this disorder, the predominant histologic findings are those of chronic tubulointerstitial disease. Interstitial infiltrates are composed primarily of lymphocytes, causing the histology of the renal parenchyma in these patients to resemble that of the salivary and lacrimal glands. Renal functional defects include diminished urinary concentrating ability and distal (type I) RTA. Urinalysis may show pyuria (predominantly lymphocyturia) and mild proteinuria.

TUBULOINTERSTITIAL ABNORMALITIES ASSOCIATED WITH GLOMERULONEPHRITIS Primary glomerulopathies are often associated with damage to tubules and the interstitium. Occasionally, the primary disorder may affect glomeruli and tubules directly. For example, in more than half of patients with the nephropathy of systemic lupus erythematosus, deposits of immune complexes can be identified in tubule basement membranes, usually accompanied by an interstitial mononuclear inflammatory reaction. Similarly, in many patients with glomerulonephritis associated with anti-glomerular basement membrane antibody, the same antibody is reactive against tubule basement membranes as well. More frequently, tubulointerstitial damage is a secondary consequence of glomerular dysfunction. The extent of tubulointerstitial fibrosis correlates closely with the degree of renal impairment. Potential mechanisms by which glomerular disease might cause tubulointerstitial injury include glomerular leak of plasma proteins toxic to epithelial cells, activation of tubule epithelial cells by glomerulus-derived cytokines, reduced peritubular blood flow leading to downstream tubulointerstitial ischemia, and hyperfunction of remnant tubules.

MISCELLANEOUS DISORDERS

VESICOURETERAL REFLUX (See also Chap. 270) When the function of the ureterovesical junction is impaired, urine may reflux into the ureters due to the high intravesical pressure that develops during voiding. Clinically, reflux is often detected on the voiding and postvoiding films obtained during intravenous pyelography, although voiding cystourethrography may be required for definitive diagnosis. Bladder infection may ascend the urinary tract to the kidneys through incompetent ureterovesical sphincters. Not surprisingly, therefore, reflux is often discovered in patients with acute and/or chronic urinary tract infections. With more severe degrees of reflux, characterized by dilatation of ureters and renal pelves, progressive renal damage often appears, and although active infection may also be present, uncertainty exists as to the necessity of infection in producing the scarred kidney of reflux nephropathy. Substantial proteinuria is often present, and glomerular lesions similar to those of idiopathic focal glomerulosclerosis (Chap. 264) are often found in addition to the changes of chronic tubulointerstitial disease. Surgical correction of reflux is usually necessary only with the more severe degrees of reflux since renal damage correlates with the extent of reflux. Obviously, if extensive glomerulosclerosis already exists, urologic repair may no longer be warranted.

RADIATION NEPHRITIS Renal dysfunction can be expected to occur if 23 Gy (2300 rad) or more of x-ray irradiation is administered to both kidneys during a period of 5 weeks or less. Histologic examination of the kidneys reveals hyalinized glomeruli, atrophic tubules, extensive interstitial fibrosis, and hyalinization of the media of renal arterioles. Radiation-induced renal ischemia is believed to be the main pathogenic factor responsible for the tubulointerstitial damage, which may not become evident clinically for months after completion of radiation. The presentation of acute radiation nephritis includes rapidly progressive azotemia, moderate to malignant hypertension, anemia, and proteinuria that may reach the nephrotic range. More than 50% progress to chronic renal failure. A more insidious form is characterized by slower development of azotemia, anemia, and nephrotic syndrome. Malignant hypertension may follow unilateral renal irradiation and resolve with ipsilateral nephrectomy. Radiation nephritis has all but vanished because of heightened awareness of its pathogenesis by radiotherapists.

FURTHER READING

GOBEL U et al: The protean face of renal sarcoidosis. J Am Soc Nephrol 12: 616, 2001

HARRIS DC: Tubulointerstitial renal disease. Curr Opin Nephrol Hypertens 10: 303, 2001

KELLY CJ, NEILSON EG: Tubulointerstitial diseases, in BM Brenner (ed): *Brenner and Rector's The Kidney*, 7th ed. Philadelphia, Saunders, 2004, pp 1483–1512

MARKOWITZ GS et al: Lithium nephrotoxicity: A progressive combined glomerular and tubulointerstitial nephropathy. J Am Soc Nephrol 11:1439, 2000

REXRODE KM et al: Analgesic use and renal function in men. JAMA 286:315, 2001

SKOPOULI FN: Kidney injury in Sjogren's syndrome. Nephrol Dial Transplant 16:63, 2001

267 VASCULAR INJURY TO THE KIDNEY
Kamal F. Badr, Barry M. Brenner

Adequate delivery of blood to the glomerular capillary network is crucial for glomerular filtration and overall salt and water balance. Thus, in addition to the threat to the viability of renal tissue, vascular injury to the kidney may compromise the maintenance of body fluid volume and composition. Involvement of the renal vessels by atherosclerotic, hypertensive, embolic, inflammatory, and hematologic disorders is usually a manifestation of generalized vascular pathology. The morphologic and clinical responses to these insults are considered in this chapter.

THROMBOEMBOLIC DISEASES OF THE RENAL ARTERIES

Thrombosis of the major renal arteries or their branches is an important cause of deterioration of renal function, especially in the elderly. It is often difficult to diagnose and therefore requires a high index of suspicion. Thrombosis may occur as a result of intrinsic pathology in the renal vessels (posttraumatic, atherosclerotic, or inflammatory) or as a result of emboli originating in distant vessels, most commonly fat emboli, emboli originating in the left heart (mural thrombi following myocardial infarction, bacterial endocarditis, or aseptic vegetations), or "paradoxical" emboli passing from the right side of the circulation via a patent foramen ovale or atrial septal defect. Renal emboli are bilateral in 15 to 30% of cases.

The clinical presentation is variable, depending on the time course and the extent of the occlusive event. Acute thrombosis and infarction, such as follows embolization, may result in sudden onset of flank pain and tenderness, fever, hematuria, leukocytosis, nausea, and vomiting. If infarction occurs, renal enzymes may be elevated, namely aspartate aminotransferase (AST), lactate dehydrogenase (LDH), and alkaline phosphatase, which rise and fall in the order listed. Urinary LDH and alkaline phosphatase may also increase after infarction. Renal function deteriorates acutely, leading in bilateral thrombosis to acute oliguric renal failure. More gradual (i.e., atherosclerotic) occlusion of a single renal artery may go undetected. A spectrum of clinical presentations lies between these two extremes. Hypertension usually follows renal infarction and results from renin release in the peri-infarction zone. Hypertension is usually transient but may be persistent. Diagnosis is established by renal arteriography.

℞ TREATMENT

Management of *acute* renal arterial thrombosis includes surgical intervention, anticoagulant therapy, conservative and supportive therapy, and control of hypertension. The choice of treatment depends mainly on (1) the condition of the patient, in particular the patient's ability to withstand major surgery, and (2) the extent of renovascular occlusion and amount of renal mass at risk of infarction. In general, supportive care and anticoagulant therapy are indicated in unilateral disease. In *acute* bilateral thrombosis, medical and surgical therapies yield comparable results. Twenty-five percent of patients die during the acute episode, usually from extrarenal complications. In *chronic* ischemic renal disease, surgical revascularization is more likely to preserve and improve renal function (see below).

ATHEROEMBOLIC DISEASE OF THE RENAL ARTERIES

Atheroembolic renal disease is part of a systemic syndrome characterized by cholesterol crystal embolization. Renal damage results from embolization of cholesterol crystals from atherosclerotic plaques present in large arteries, such as the aorta, to small arteries in the renal vasculature. Atheroembolic renal disease is an increasingly common and often underdiagnosed cause of renal insufficiency in the elderly. A review of 372 autopsies identified cholesterol emboli in 2.4% of renal tissue samples. Male gender, older age, hypertension, and diabetes mellitus are important predisposing factors, present in 85% of cases. Patients with cholesterol embolization syndrome also often have a history of ischemic cardiovascular disease, aortic aneurysm, cerebrovascular disease, congestive heart failure, or renal insufficiency. A significant association is present between renal artery stenosis and atheroembolic renal disease. Inciting events, which include vascular surgery, arteriography, angioplasty, anticoagulation with heparin, and thrombolytic therapy, can be identified in about 50% of cases. Arteriographic procedures constitute the most common cause of cholesterol embolization.

Clinical manifestations usually appear 1 to 14 days after an inciting event, but their onset can be more insidious. Systemic manifestations occur in fewer than half of the patients and include fever, myalgias, headaches, and weight loss. Cutaneous manifestations such as livedo reticularis, "purple" toes, and toe gangrene occur in 50 to 90% of patients and constitute the most common extrarenal findings. Other targets of cholesterol embolization include the retina, musculoskeletal system, nervous system, and gut. Accelerated or labile hypertension is present in one-half of patients. Malignant hypertension has been described. Renal insufficiency is usually subacute and advances in a stepwise fashion over a period of several weeks. Renal failure, however, can be acute and oliguric. Uremic signs and symptoms requiring dialytic therapy develop in 40% of patients, only half of whom recover sufficient renal function to stop dialysis after 1 year. More recent data suggest less inexorable deterioration with a possibility of recovery of renal function in about one-third of patients after variable periods of dialytic support. Renal infarction secondary to cholesterol embolization is rare. Cholesterol embolic disease in renal allografts has been reported and can be of donor or of recipient origin.

Antemortem diagnosis of atherosclerotic renal emboli is difficult. The demonstration of cholesterol emboli in the retina is helpful, but a firm diagnosis is established only by demonstration of cholesterol crystals in the smaller arteries and arterioles on renal biopsy. These may also be seen in asymptomatic skeletal muscle or skin. Atheroembolic renal disease is associated with a 64 to 81% mortality rate.

TREATMENT

No effective therapy for atheroembolic renal disease is available. Withdrawal of anticoagulation may be beneficial. In some patients, kidney function improved even after a prolonged period of renal insufficiency. Cholesterol-lowering agents may also improve outcome. An aggressive therapeutic approach with patient-tailored supportive measures may be associated with more favorable clinical outcome.

RENAL VEIN THROMBOSIS (RVT)

Thrombosis of one or both main renal veins occurs in a variety of settings (Table 267-1). Nephrotic syndrome accompanying membranous glomerulopathy and certain carcinomas seems to predispose to the development of RVT, which occurs in 10 to 50% of patients with these disorders. RVT may exacerbate preexisting proteinuria but is infrequently the cause of the nephrotic syndrome.

The clinical manifestations depend on the severity and abruptness of its occurrence. Acute cases occur typically in children and are characterized by sudden loss of renal function, often accompanied by fever, chills, lumbar tenderness (with kidney enlargement), leukocytosis, and hematuria. Hemorrhagic infarction and renal rupture may lead to hypovolemic shock. In young adults RVT is usually suspected from an unexpected and relatively acute or subacute deterioration of renal function and/or exacerbation of proteinuria and hematuria in the appropriate clinical setting. In cases of gradual thrombosis, usually occurring in the elderly, the only manifestation may be recurrent pulmonary emboli or development of hypertension. A Fanconi-like syndrome and proximal renal tubular acidosis have been described.

The definitive diagnosis can only be established through selective renal venography with visualization of the occluding thrombus. Short of angiography, Doppler ultrasound, contrast-enhanced computed tomography (CT), and magnetic resonance imaging (MRI) often provides definitive evidence of thrombus.

TREATMENT

Treatment consists of anticoagulation, the main purpose of which is prevention of pulmonary embolization, although some authors have also claimed improvement in renal function and proteinuria. Encouraging reports have appeared concerning the use of streptokinase. Spontaneous recanalization with clinical improvement has also been observed. Anticoagulant therapy is more rewarding in the acute thrombosis seen in younger individuals. Nephrectomy is advocated in infants with life-threatening renal infarction. Thrombectomy is effective in some cases.

RENAL ARTERY STENOSIS (RAS)/ISCHEMIC RENAL DISEASE

Ischemic renal disease underlies end-stage renal disease in 15 to 20% of uremic patients over 50 years of age. Stenosis of the main renal artery and/or its major branches is causative in 2 to 5% of patients with hypertension (Chap. 230). The common cause in the middle-aged and elderly is an atheromatous plaque at the origin of the renal artery. In a large unselected autopsy series, stenosis producing >50% renal artery diameter reduction was found in 18% of those between 65 and 74 years of age and in 42% of those older than 75 years. Bilateral

involvement is present in half of the affected cases in both age groups. It should be considered seriously in elderly individuals, particularly in those with evidence of hypertension, diabetes, and atherosclerotic arterial disease elsewhere. In this population, the incidence of renal arterial stenosis can be as high as 40%. Established plaques progress in >50% of cases over 5 years (15% to total occlusion). Renal hypertrophy is detectable in 20% of affected kidneys. In younger women, stenosis is due to intrinsic structural abnormalities of the arterial wall caused by a heterogeneous group of lesions termed *fibromuscular dysplasia*. Clinical settings in which RAS should be considered are listed in Table 267-2.

DIAGNOSIS Diagnostic evaluation for significant RAS should begin with noninvasive approaches. An initial screening test is Doppler ultrasonography, which provides information on blood-flow velocity and pressure waveforms in the renal arteries and, when positive, is helpful. Its limitations, however, include significant operator dependence, technical difficulty in obese patients, and poor sensitivity in the presence of multiple renal arteries, distal stenoses, and total occlusion. Measurement of the intrarenal resistance index (RI) by Doppler ultrasonography provides valuable information on the extent of parenchymal tissue loss in stenosed and nonstenosed kidneys and hence on the prognosis for functional recovery following revascularization procedures.

Absence of compensatory hypertrophy in the contralateral kidney should raise the suspicion of bilateral stenosis or superimposed parenchymal renal disease, most commonly hypertensive or diabetic nephropathy. Because angiotensin-converting enzyme (ACE) inhibitors magnify the impairment in renal blood flow and glomerular filtration rate (GFR) caused by functionally significant renal artery stenosis, use of these drugs in association with ^{99m}Tc-labeled pentetic acid (DTPA) or ^{99m}Tc-labeled mertiatide (MAG$_3$) renography enhances diagnostic precision and is of additional predictive value. Gadolinium-enhanced three-dimensional magnetic resonance angiography (MRA) has replaced previous modalities as the most sensitive (>90%) and specific (95%) test for the diagnosis of RAS. The most definitive diagnostic procedure is contrast-enhanced arteriography. Intraarterial digital subtraction techniques minimize the requirements for contrast, reducing the risk of renal toxicity.

TREATMENT

Interventional therapy RAS (i.e., surgery or angioplasty) is superior to medical therapy. Success rates with conventional percutaneous transluminal angioplasty in young patients with fibromuscular dysplasia are 50% cure and improvement in blood pressure control in another

---

TABLE 267-1 Conditions Associated with Renal Vein Thrombosis

Trauma
Extrinsic compression (lymph nodes, aortic aneurysm, tumor)
Invasion by renal cell carcinoma
Dehydration (infants)
Nephrotic syndrome
Pregnancy or oral contraceptives

TABLE 267-2 Clinical Findings Associated with Renal Artery Stenosis

Hypertension
  Abrupt onset of hypertension before the age of 50 years (suggestive of fibromuscular dysplasia)
  Abrupt onset of hypertension at or after the age of 50 years (suggestive of atherosclerotic renal artery stenosis)
  Accelerated or malignant hypertension
  Refractory hypertension (not responsive to therapy with ≥3 drugs)
Renal abnormalities
  Unexplained azotemia (suggestive of atherosclerotic renal artery stenosis)
  Azotemia induced by treatment with an angiotensin-converting enzyme inhibitor
  Unilateral small kidney
  Unexplained hypokalemia
Other findings
  Abdominal bruit, flank bruit, or both
  Severe retinopathy
  Carotid, coronary, or peripheral vascular disease
  Unexplained congestive heart failure or acute pulmonary edema

Source: From Safian and Textor, reprinted with permission.

30%. For atherosclerotic lesions, conventional balloon angioplasty is associated with high restenosis rates (up to 47%) and either stent placement or surgery is recommended. About half of those with reduced renal function as a result of RAS improve following angioplasty or surgery, even when preintervention arteriography shows little evidence of cortical perfusion. In the presence of unilateral RAS and normal overall GFR, the decision for angiographic or surgical revascularization may depend on the results of fractional flow and filtration rate studies to each kidney with ^{99m}TC-DTPA or ^{99m}Tc-MAG$_3$. These techniques can also be used to assess the response to revascularization. Three-year survival is influenced by baseline renal function, being 94% in the presence of normal baseline renal function and falling to 52% in patients with serum creatinine >177 μmol/L (>2.0 mg/dL). Renal parenchymal damage, as reflected in noninvasive imaging and degree of proteinuria, is the major predictor of functional outcome and should be used for risk stratification. Rapid decline in renal function is associated with a favorable response to intervention.

Despite the risks associated with surgery, long-term follow-up studies demonstrate an advantage of surgery over angioplasty both with regard to the incidence of restenosis and to the preservation or improvement in GFR. Surgery, however, is restricted to those patients in whom angioplasty and stenting are not feasible. As with coronary angioplasty, stenting of renal arteries following balloon angioplasty is being used increasingly. Results are highly encouraging, with resten-

nosis rates <15% at 1 year. Renal functional recovery or stabilization of renal function is seen in approximately 70% of patients. An illustrative example of renal artery stenting is shown in Fig. 267-1.

HEMOLYTIC UREMIC SYNDROME (HUS) AND THROMBOTIC THROMBOCYTOPENIC PURPURA (TTP) (See also Chap. 101)

HUS and TTP, consumptive coagulopathies characterized by microangiopathic hemolytic anemia and thrombocytopenia, have a particular predilection for the kidney and the central nervous system, the latter especially in TTP. The kidneys of patients with HUS or TTP often exhibit a "flea-bitten" appearance, the result of multiple cortical hemorrhagic infarcts. The major sites of pathology are the small renal arteries and afferent arterioles, which are nearly occluded as a result of marked intimal hyperplasia (particularly in TTP) and fibrin deposits in the subintimal regions. When the vasoocclusive process is extensive, bilateral cortical necrosis may occur. In addition, arteriolar microaneurysms, glomerular infarction, or nonspecific focal changes may be seen. In keeping with the focal nature of the vascular lesions, patchy areas of interstitial edema, tubular necrosis, and, eventually, fibrosis occur. By immunofluorescence staining, complement components and immunoglobulins may be demonstrated in the arterioles, and fibrinogen deposits are present in arteries, arterioles, and glomerular capillary loops.

Endothelial cell injury appears to be the initiating pathophysiologic event in HUS/TTP. Injurious agents include bacterial toxins (Shiga toxin–like) mostly from specific *Escherichia coli* genotypes, endotoxin (lipopolysaccharides, LPS), bacterial neuraminidases, immune complexes, and drugs. Among the latter, most commonly associated with HUS/TTP are chemotherapeutic agents, cyclosporine, clopidogrel, and quinine. Also implicated in endothelial cell injury are intrinsic abnormalities of the complement sytem and the von Willebrand factor pathways, which may account for the genetic predisposition observed in familial forms of the disease.

Renal failure is common in both HUS and TTP, usually manifested by azotemia, mild proteinuria, and microscopic and/or gross hematuria. Patients with HUS have more severe renal failure, often marked by oligoanuria and hypertension and commonly progressing to chronic renal failure. The prognosis in HUS is better in children than in adults. In TTP, the course of which may span days to months, renal failure is usually less severe.

$\boxed{\text{R}_\text{X}}$ TREATMENT

In TTP, high-dose glucocorticoids and plasma exchange often provide complete remission or cure. Plasma exchange should be initiated as early as possible, and the treatment cycles can be repeated if thrombocytopenia recurs. Splenectomy and antiplatelet therapy have also been used with varying degrees of success. The success of plasma exchange in adult HUS is less well established than in TTP.

ARTERIOLAR NEPHROSCLEROSIS (See also Chaps. 224 and 230)

Whether hypertension is "essential" or of known etiology, persistent exposure of the renal circulation to elevated intraluminal pressures results in development of intrinsic lesions of the renal arterioles (hyaline arteriolosclerosis) that eventually lead to loss of function (nephrosclerosis). Nephrosclerosis is divided into two distinct entities: "benign" and "malignant" (or accelerated).

BENIGN ARTERIOLAR NEPHROSCLEROSIS   Benign arteriolar nephrosclerosis is seen in patients who are hypertensive for an extended period of time (blood pressure >150/90 mmHg) but whose hypertension has not progressed to a malignant form (described below). Such patients, usually in the older age group, are often discovered to be hypertensive on routine physical examination or as a result of nonspecific symptomatology (e.g., headaches, weakness, palpitations).

Kidney size is normal to reduced, with loss of cortical mass leading to a fine granularity. Although the larger arteries may show atherosclerotic changes, the characteristic pathology is in the afferent arterioles, which have thickened walls due to deposition of homogeneous

FIGURE 267-1   Bilateral severe ostial renal artery stenosis prior to and following balloon dilatation and stent placement in a patient with severe hypertension and renal insufficiency.

PRE STENT

eosinophilic material (hyaline arteriolosclerosis). Narrowing of vascular lumina results, with consequent ischemic injury to glomeruli and tubules.

Nephrosclerosis accompanying long-standing systemic arterial hypertension is only one manifestation of a generalized process affecting the cardiovascular system. Physical examination, therefore, may reveal changes in retinal vessels (arteriolar narrowing and/or flame-shaped hemorrhages), cardiac hypertrophy, and possibly signs of congestive heart failure. Renal disease may manifest as a mild to moderate elevation of serum creatinine concentration and/or mild proteinuria. In general, clinical evaluation does not reveal significant renal abnormalities. More specialized examination may disclose elevated urinary albumin excretion, tapering and loss of caliber of intrarenal vessels on arteriography, and an exaggerated natriuresis in response to a fluid challenge. Patients with benign nephrosclerosis generally maintain a near-normal GFR despite a reduction in renal blood flow.

MALIGNANT ARTERIOLAR NEPHROSCLEROSIS Patients with long-standing benign hypertension or patients not previously known to be hypertensive may develop malignant hypertension characterized by a sudden (accelerated) elevation of blood pressure (diastolic often >130 mmHg) accompanied by papilledema, central nervous system manifestations, cardiac decompensation, and acute progressive deterioration of renal function. The absence of papilledema does not rule out the diagnosis in a patient with markedly elevated blood pressure and rapidly declining renal function. The kidneys are characterized by a flea-bitten appearance resulting from hemorrhages in surface capillaries. Histologically, two distinct vascular lesions can be seen. The first, affecting arterioles, is fibrinoid necrosis, i.e., infiltration of arteriolar walls with eosinophilic material including fibrin, thickening of vessel walls and, occasionally, an inflammatory infiltrate (necrotizing arteriolitis). The second lesion, involving the interlobular arteries, is a concentric hyperplastic proliferation of the cellular elements of the vascular wall with deposition of collagen to form a hyperplastic arteriolitis (onion-skin lesion). Fibrinoid necrosis occasionally extends into the glomeruli, which may also undergo proliferative changes or total necrosis. Most glomerular and tubular changes are secondary to ischemia and infarction. The sequence of events leading to the development of malignant hypertension is poorly defined. Two pathophysiologic alterations appear central in its initiation and/or perpetuation: (1) increased permeability of vessel walls to invasion by plasma components, particularly fibrin, which activates clotting mechanisms leading to a microangiopathic hemolytic anemia, thus perpetuating the vascular pathology; and (2) activation of the renin-angiotensin-aldosterone system at some point in the disease process, which contributes to the acceleration and maintenance of blood pressure elevation and, in turn, to vascular injury.

Malignant hypertension is most likely to develop in a previously hypertensive individual, usually in the third or fourth decade of life. There is a higher incidence among men, particularly black men. The presenting symptoms are usually neurologic (dizziness, headache, blurring of vision, altered states of consciousness, and focal or generalized seizures). Cardiac decompensation and renal failure appear thereafter. Renal abnormalities include a rapid rise in serum creatinine, hematuria (at times macroscopic), proteinuria, and red and white blood cell casts in the sediment. Nephrotic syndrome may be present. Elevated plasma aldosterone levels cause hypokalemic metabolic alkalosis in the early phase. Uremic acidosis and hyperkalemia eventually obscure these early findings. Hematologic indices of microangiopathic hemolytic anemia (i.e., schistocytes) are often seen.

℞ TREATMENT

Control of hypertension is the principal goal of therapy for both benign and malignant forms. The time of initiation of therapy, its effectiveness, and patient compliance are crucial factors in arresting the progression of benign nephrosclerosis. Untreated, most of these patients succumb to the extrarenal complications of hypertension. In contrast, malignant hypertension is a medical emergency; its natural course includes a death rate of 80 to 90% within 1 year of onset, almost always due to uremia. Supportive measures should be instituted to control the neurologic, cardiac, and other complications of acute renal failure, but the mainstay of therapy is prompt and aggressive reduction of blood pressure, which, if successful, can reverse all complications in the majority of patients. Presently, 5-year survival is 50%, and some patients have evidence of partial reversal of the vascular lesions and a return of renal function to near-normal levels.

SCLERODERMA (PROGRESSIVE SYSTEMIC SCLEROSIS)
(See also Chap. 303)

Renal involvement can present in one of two ways, depending on whether malignant hypertension is superimposed on the renal pathology: (1) *Persistent urinary abnormalities* with or without hypertension tend to follow an indolent course with mild proteinuria, occasional casts, cellular elements in the urinary sediment, and a propensity for development of hypertension. Azotemia is absent initially, but when it develops, dialysis is required within 1 year. (2) *Scleroderma renal crisis* (SRC) is a rapid deterioration in renal function, usually accompanied by malignant hypertension, oliguria, fluid retention, microangiopathic hemolytic anemia, and central nervous system involvement. It occurs in 5 to 15% of patients, most commonly in the first 5 years following diagnosis, particularly in patients with diffuse cutaneous involvement. SRC may occur in patients with previously undemonstrable or slowly progressive renal disease. Untreated, it leads to chronic renal failure within days to months.

℞ TREATMENT

The prognosis of scleroderma renal disease is generally poor, particularly following the onset of azotemia. Aggressive antihypertensive therapy may be effective in delaying the progression of renal failure. In SRC, prompt treatment with ACE inhibitors may reverse acute renal failure. Recently, a prospective study on short- and long-term outcomes of SRC in patients who received ACE inhibitors showed that 61% of patients had favorable outcomes (no dialysis or temporary dialysis) with a survival rate at 8 years of 80 to 85%, similar to that of patients with diffuse scleroderma who did not have renal crisis. Moreover, more than half of patients with SRC who initially required dialysis and were treated aggressively with ACE inhibitors were able to discontinue dialysis 3 to 18 months later, suggesting that patients should continue to take ACE inhibitors even after beginning dialysis, in hope of discontinuing it. A significant association exists between antecedent high-dose glucocorticoid therapy and the development of SRC.

SICKLE CELL NEPHROPATHY (See also Chap. 91)

Sickle cell disease causes renal complications that arise mainly as a result of sickling of red blood cells in the microvasculature. The hypertonic and relatively hypoxic environment of the renal medulla, coupled with the slow blood flow in the vasa recta, favors the sickling of red blood cells, with resultant local infarction (papillary necrosis). Functional tubule defects in patients with sickle cell disease are likely the result of partial ischemic injury to the renal tubules.

In addition to the intrarenal microvascular pathology described above, young patients with sickle cell disease are characterized by renal hyperperfusion, glomerular hypertrophy, and hyperfiltration. Many of these individuals eventually develop a glomerulopathy leading to glomerular proteinuria (present in as many as 30%) and, in some, the nephrotic syndrome. Co-inheritance of microdeletions in the α-globin gene (α thalassemia) appear to protect against the development of nephropathy, associated with lower mean arterial pressure and less proteinuria.

Mild azotemia and hyperuricemia can also develop. Advanced renal failure and uremia occur in 4 to 18% of cases. Pathologic examination reveals the typical lesion of "hyperfiltration nephropathy," namely, focal segmental glomerular sclerosis. This finding has led to the suggestion that anemia-induced hyperfiltration in childhood is the principal cause of the adult glomerulopathy. Nephron loss secondary to ischemic injury also contributes to the development of azotemia in these patients.

In addition to the glomerulopathy described above, renal complications of sickle cell disease include the following: *Cortical infarcts* can cause loss of function, persistent hematuria, and perinephric hematomas. *Papillary infarcts*, demonstrated radiographically in 50% of patients with sickle trait, lead to an increased risk of bacterial infection in the scarred renal tissues and functional tubule abnormalities. Painless gross hematuria occurs with a higher frequency in sickle trait than in sickle cell disease and likely results from infarctive episodes in the renal medulla. *Functional tubule abnormalities* such as nephrogenic diabetes insipidus result from marked reduction in vasa recta blood flow, combined with ischemic tubule injury. This concentrating defect places these patients at increased risk of dehydration and, hence, sickling crises. The concentrating defect also occurs in individuals with sickle trait. Other tubule defects involve potassium and hydrogen ion excretion, occasionally leading to hyperkalemic metabolic acidosis and a defect in uric acid excretion which, combined with increased purine synthesis in the bone marrow, results in hyperuricemia.

Management of sickle nephropathy is not separate from that of overall patient management (Chap. 91). In addition, however, the use of ACE inhibitors has been associated with improvement of the hyperfiltration glomerulopathy. Three-year graft and patient survival in renal transplant recipients with sickle nephropathy is diminished as compared to those with other causes of end-stage renal disease.

TOXEMIAS OF PREGNANCY See also Chap. 6

BILATERAL CORTICAL NECROSIS

Acute bilateral cortical necrosis is associated with septic abortions, abruptio placentae, and preeclampsia. Coagulation in cortical vessels and arterioles leads to renal tissue necrosis. Anuria and renal failure ensue and may be irreversible. In other cases, renal function returns partially, but on long-term follow-up most patients slowly progress to uremia.

FURTHER READING

BOUDEWIJN G et al: Diagnostic tests for renal artery stenosis in patients suspected of having renovascular hypertension: A meta-analysis. Ann Intern Med 135:401, 2001

CAREY RM et al: Role of the angiotensin type 2 receptor in the regulation of blood pressure and renal function. Hypertension 35:155, 2000

CHATZIANTONIOU C, DUSSAULE JC: Endothelin and renal vascular fibrosis: Of mice and men. Curr Opin Nephrol Hypertens 9:31, 2000

GHANIOUS VE et al: Evaluating patients with renal failure for renal artery stenosis with gadolinium-enhanced magnetic resonance angiography. Am J Kidney Dis 33:36, 1999

GREENBERG A et al: Focal segmental glomerulosclerosis associated with nephrotic syndrome in cholesterol atheroembolism. Clinicopathologic correlations. Am J Kidney Dis 29:344, 1997

MODI KS et al: Atheroembolic renal disease. J Am Soc Nephrol 12:1781, 2001

MURAY S et al: Rapid decline in renal function reflects reversibility and predicts the outcome after angioplasty in renal artery stenosis. Am J Kidney Dis 39:60, 2002

PHUONG-THU T. PHAM et al: Renal abnormalities in sickle cell disease. Kidney Intl 157:1, 2000

RADERMACHER J et al: Techniques for predicting a favourable response to renal angioplasty in patients with renovascular disease. Curr Opin Nephrol Hypertens 10:799, 2001

RUGGENENTI P et al: Thrombotic microangiopathy, hemolytic uremic syndrome, and thrombotic thrombocytopenic purpura. Kidney Intl 60:831, 2001

SABORIO P et al: Sickle cell nephropathy. J Am Soc Nephrol 10:187, 1999

SAFIAN RD, TEXTOR SC: Renal-artery stenosis. N Engl J Med 344:431, 2001

SCOLARI F et al: Cholesterol crystal embolism: A recognizable cause of renal disease. Am J Kidney Dis 36:1089, 2000

TUTTLE KR, RAABE RD: Endovascular stents for renal artery revascularization. Curr Opin Nephrol Hypertens 7:695, 1998

WRIGHT JR et al: A prospective study of the determinants of renal functional outcome and mortality in atherosclerotic renovascular disease. Am J Kidney Dis 39:1153, 2002

YUDD M, LLACH F: Disorders of the renal arteries and veins in BM Brenner (ed): *The Kidney*, 7th ed. Philadelphia, Saunders, 2004, pp 1571–1600

268 | NEPHROLITHIASIS
John R. Asplin, Fredric L. Coe, Murray J. Favus

TYPES OF STONES

Calcium salts, uric acid, cystine, and struvite ($MgNH_4PO_4$) are the basic constituents of most kidney stones in the western hemisphere. Calcium oxalate and calcium phosphate stones make up 75 to 85% of the total (Table 268-1) and may be admixed in the same stone. Calcium phosphate in stones is usually hydroxyapatite [$Ca_5(PO_4)_3OH$] or, less commonly, brushite ($CaHPO_4H_2O$).

Calcium stones are more common in men; the average age of onset is the third to fourth decade. Approximately 50% of people who form a single calcium stone eventually form another within the next 10 years. The average rate of new stone formation in recurrent stone formers is about one stone every 2 or 3 years. Calcium stone disease is frequently familial. *Uric acid stones* are radiolucent and are also more common in men. Half of patients with uric acid stones have gout; uric acid lithiasis is usually familial whether or not gout is present. *Cystine stones* are uncommon; their radiopacity is due to the sulfur content. Cystine crystals appear in the urine as flat, hexagonal plates. *Struvite stones* are common and potentially dangerous. These stones occur mainly in women or patients who require chronic bladder catheterization and result from urinary tract infection with urease-producing bacteria, usually *Proteus* species. The stones can grow to a large size and fill the renal pelvis and calyces to produce a "staghorn" appearance. They are radiopaque and have a variable internal density. In urine, struvite crystals are rectangular prisms said to resemble coffin lids.

MANIFESTATIONS OF STONES

As stones grow on the surfaces of the renal papillae or within the collecting system, they need not produce symptoms. Asymptomatic stones may be discovered during the course of radiographic studies undertaken for unrelated reasons. Stones rank, along with benign and malignant neoplasms, and renal cysts, among the common causes of isolated hematuria. Much of the time, however, stones break loose and enter the ureter or occlude the ureteropelvic junction, causing pain and obstruction.

STONE PASSAGE   A stone can traverse the ureter without symptoms, but passage usually produces pain and bleeding. The pain begins gradually, usually in the flank, but increases over the next 20 to 60 min to become so severe that narcotic drugs may be needed for its control. The pain may remain in the flank or spread downward and anteriorly toward the ipsilateral loin, testis, or vulva. Pain that migrates downward indicates that the stone has passed to the lower third of the ureter, but if the pain does not migrate, the position of the stone cannot be predicted. A stone in the portion of the ureter within the bladder wall causes frequency, urgency, and dysuria that may be confused with urinary tract infection. The vast majority of ureteral stones less than 0.5 cm in diameter will pass spontaneously.

It has been standard practice to diagnose acute renal colic by intravenous pyelography; however, helical computed tomography (CT) scan without radiocontrast enhancement is now the preferred proce-

TABLE 268-1 Major Causes of Renal Stones

Stone Type and Causes	Percent of all Stones[a]	Percent Occurrence of Specific Causes[a]	Ratio of Males to Females	Etiology	Diagnosis	Treatment
Calcium stones	75–85		2:1 to 3:1			
Idiopathic hypercalciuria		50–55	2:1	Hereditary (?)	Normocalcemia, unexplained hypercalciuria[b]	Thiazide diuretic agents
Hyperuricosuria		20	4:1	Diet	Urine uric acid >750 mg per 24 h (women), >800 mg per 24 h (men)	Allopurinol or diet
Primary hyperparathyroidism		5	3:10	Neoplasia	Unexplained hypercalcemia	Surgery
Distal renal tubular acidosis		Rare	1:1	Hereditary	Hyperchloremic acidosis, minimum urine pH >5.5	Alkali replacement
Dietary hyperoxaluria		10–30	1:1	High oxalate diet or low calcium diet	Urine oxalate >50 mg per 24 h	Low oxalate diet
Enteric hyperoxaluria		~1–2	1:1	Bowel surgery	Urine oxalate >75 mg per 24 h	Cholestyramine or oral calcium loading
Hereditary hyperoxaluria		Rare	1:1	Hereditary	Urine oxalate and glycolic or l-glyceric acid increased	Fluids and pyridoxine
Hypocitraturia		15–60	2:1 to 5:1	Hereditary (?), diet	Urine citrate <320 mg per 24 h	Alkali supplements
Idiopathic stone disease		20	2:1	Unknown	None of the above present	Oral phosphate, fluids
Uric acid stones	5–8					
Gout		~50	3:1 to 4:1	Hereditary	Clinical diagnosis	Alkali and allopurinol
Idiopathic		~50	1:1	Hereditary (?)	Uric acid stones, no gout	Alkali and allopurinol if daily urine uric acid above 1000 mg
Dehydration		?	1:1	Intestinal, habit	History, intestinal fluid loss	Alkali, fluids, reversal of cause
Lesch-Nyhan syndrome		Rare	Males only	Hereditary	Reduced hypoxanthine-guanine phosphoribosyltransferase level	Allopurinol
Malignant tumors		Rare	1:1	Neoplasia	Clinical diagnosis	Allopurinol
Cystine stones	1		1:1	Hereditary	Stone type; elevated cystine excretion	Massive fluids, alkali, D-penicillamine if needed
Struvite stones	10–15		2:10	Infection	Stone type	Antimicrobial agents and judicious surgery

[a] Values are percent of patients who form a particular type of stone and who display each specific cause of stones.

[b] Urine calcium above 300 mg/24 h (men), 250 mg/24 h (women), or 4 mg/kg per 24 h either sex. Hyperthyroidism, Cushing syndrome, sarcoidosis, malignant tumors, immobilization, vitamin D intoxication, rapidly progressive bone disease, and Paget's disease all cause hypercalciuria and must be excluded in diagnosis of idiopathic hypercalciuria.

dure. The advantages of CT include detection of uric acid stones in addition to the traditional radiopaque stones, no exposure to the risk of radiocontrast agents, and possible diagnosis of other causes of abdominal pain in a patient suspected of having renal colic from stones. Ultrasound is not as sensitive as CT in detecting renal or ureteral stones.

OTHER SYNDROMES ▪ Staghorn Calculi Struvite, cystine, and uric acid stones often grow too large to enter the ureter. They gradually fill the renal pelvis and may extend outward through the infundibula to the calyces themselves.

Nephrocalcinosis Calcium stones grow on the papillae. Most break loose and cause colic, but they may remain in place so that multiple papillary calcifications are found by x-ray, a condition termed *nephrocalcinosis*. Papillary nephrocalcinosis is common in hereditary distal renal tubular acidosis (RTA) and in other types of severe hypercalciuria. In medullary sponge kidney disease (Chap. 265), calcification may occur in dilated distal collecting ducts.

Sludge Sufficient uric acid or cystine in the urine may plug both ureters with precipitate. Calcium oxalate crystals do not do this because less than 100 mg oxalate usually is excreted daily in the urine even in severe hyperoxaluric states, compared with 1000 mg uric acid in patients with hyperuricosuria and 400 to 800 mg cystine in patients with cystinuria. Calcium phosphate crystals can render the urine milky but do not plug the urinary tract.

INFECTION Although urinary tract infection is not a direct consequence of stone disease, it can occur after instrumentation and surgery of the urinary tract, which are frequent in the treatment of stone disease. Stone disease and urinary tract infection can enhance their respective seriousness and interfere with treatment. Obstruction of an infected kidney by a stone may lead to sepsis and extensive damage of renal tissue, since it converts the urinary tract proximal to the obstruction into a closed, or partially closed, space that can become an abscess. Stones may harbor bacteria in the stone matrix, leading to recurrent urinary tract infection. On the other hand, infection due to bacteria that possess the enzyme urease can cause stones composed of struvite.

ACTIVITY OF STONE DISEASE Active disease means that new stones are forming or that preformed stones are growing. Sequential radiographs of the renal areas are needed to document the growth or appearance of new stones and to ensure that passed stones are actually newly formed, not preexistent ones.

PATHOGENESIS OF STONES

Urinary stones usually arise because of the breakdown of a delicate balance. The kidneys must conserve water, but they must excrete materials that have a low solubility. These two opposing requirements must be balanced during adaptation to diet, climate, and activity. The problem is mitigated to some extent by the fact that urine contains substances that inhibit crystallization of calcium salts and others that bind calcium in soluble complexes. These protective mechanisms are less than perfect. When the urine becomes supersaturated with insoluble materials, because excretion rates are excessive and/or because water conservation is extreme, crystals form and may grow and aggregate to form a stone.

SUPERSATURATION   In a solution in equilibrium with crystals of calcium oxalate, the product of the chemical activities of the calcium and oxalate ions in the solution is termed the *equilibrium solubility product*. If crystals are removed, and if either calcium or oxalate ions are added to the solution, the activity product increases, but no new crystals form. Such a solution is *metastably supersaturated*. If new calcium oxalate seed crystals are now added, they will grow in size. Ultimately, as calcium or oxalate are added to the solution, the activity product reaches a critical value at which a solid phase begins to develop spontaneously. This value is called the *upper limit of metastability*. Stone growth in the urinary tract requires a urine that, on average, is above the equilibrium solubility product. Excessive supersaturation is common in stone formation.

Calcium, oxalate, and phosphate form many stable soluble complexes among themselves and with other substances in urine, such as citrate. As a result, their free ion activities are below their chemical concentrations and can be measured only by indirect techniques. Reduction in ligands such as citrate can increase ion activity, and therefore supersaturation, without changing total urinary calcium. Urine supersaturation can be increased by dehydration or by overexcretion of calcium, oxalate, phosphate, cystine, or uric acid. Urine pH is also important; phosphate and uric acid are weak acids that dissociate readily over the physiologic range of urine pH. Alkaline urine contains more dibasic phosphate, favoring deposits of brushite and apatite. Below a urine pH of 5.5, uric acid crystals (pK 5.47) predominate, whereas phosphate crystals are rare. The solubility of calcium oxalate, on the other hand, is not influenced by changes in urine pH. Measurements of supersaturation in a pooled 24-h urine sample probably underestimate the risk of precipitation. Transient dehydration, variation of urine pH, and postprandial bursts of overexcretion may cause values considerably above average.

NUCLEATION   In urine that is supersaturated with respect to calcium oxalate, these two ions form clusters. Most small clusters eventually disperse because the internal forces that hold them together are too weak to overcome the random tendency of ions to move away. Large ion clusters can remain stable because attractive forces balance surface losses. Once they are stable, nuclei can grow at levels of supersaturation below that needed for their creation. Cell debris, calcifications on the renal papillae, and other urinary crystals can serve as templates for crystal formation, a process known as *heterogeneous nucleation*. Heterogeneous nucleation lowers the level of supersaturation required for crystal formation and is likely the mechanism by which stones form in human urine.

INHIBITORS OF CRYSTAL FORMATION   Stable nuclei must grow and aggregate to produce a stone of clinical significance. Urine contains potent inhibitors of nucleation, growth, and aggregation for calcium oxalate and calcium phosphate but not for uric acid, cystine, or struvite. Inorganic pyrophosphate is a potent inhibitor that appears to affect calcium phosphate more than calcium oxalate crystals. Citrate inhibits crystal growth and nucleation, though most of the stone inhibitory activity of citrate is due to lowering urine supersaturation via complexation of calcium. Other urine components such as glycoproteins inhibit all three processes of calcium oxalate stone formation. As a consequence of the presence of these inhibitors, crystal growth in urine is slow compared with growth in simple salt solutions, and the upper limit of metastability is higher.

EVALUATION AND TREATMENT OF PATIENTS WITH NEPHROLITHIASIS

Most patients with nephrolithiasis have remediable metabolic disorders that cause stones and can be detected by chemical analyses of serum and urine. Adults with recurrent kidney stones and children with

even a single kidney stone should be evaluated. A practical outpatient evaluation consists of two or three 24-h urine collections, with a corresponding blood sample; measurements of serum and urine calcium, uric acid, electrolytes, and creatinine, and urine pH, volume, oxalate, and citrate should be made. Since stone risks vary with diet, activity, and environment, at least one urine collection should be made on a weekend when the patient is at home and another on a work day. When possible, the composition of kidney stones should be determined because treatment depends on stone type (Table 268-1). No matter what disorders are found, every patient should be counseled to avoid dehydration and to drink copious amounts of water. The efficacy of high fluid intake was confirmed in a prospective study of first-time stone formers. Increasing urine volume to 2.5 L per day resulted in a 50% reduction of stone recurrence compared to the control group. Because treatment is prolonged, the use of medications must be justified by the activity and severity of stone disease and the importance of protection against new stones.

℞ TREATMENT

The management of stones already present in the kidneys or urinary tract requires a combined medical and surgical approach. The specific treatment depends on the location of the stone, the extent of obstruction, the function of the affected and unaffected kidney, the presence or absence of urinary tract infection, the progress of stone passage, and the risks of operation or anesthesia given the clinical state of the patient. In general, severe obstruction, infection, intractable pain, and serious bleeding are indications for removal of a stone.

In the past, stones were removed by operation or by passing a flexible basket retrograde up the ureter from the bladder during cystoscopy. There are now three alternatives. *Extracorporeal lithotripsy* causes the in situ fragmentation of stones in the kidney, renal pelvis, or ureter by exposing them to shock waves. The kidney stone is centered at a focal point of parabolic reflectors, and high-intensity shock waves are created by high-voltage discharge. The waves are transmitted to the patient using water as a conduction medium, either by placing the patient in a water tank or by placing water-filled cushions between the patient and the shock wave generators. After multiple discharges, most stones are reduced to powder that moves through the ureter into the bladder. *Percutaneous nephrolithotomy* requires the passage of a cystoscope-like instrument into the renal pelvis through a small incision in the flank. Stones are then disrupted by a small ultrasound transducer or holmium laser. The last method is *lithotripsy via a ureteroscope* for removal of ureteral stones. These various forms of lithotripsy have largely replaced pyelolithotomy and ureterolithotomy.

CALCIUM STONES ■ **Idiopathic Hypercalciuria** (See also Chap. 332) This condition appears to be hereditary, and its diagnosis is straightforward (Table 268-1). In some patients, primary intestinal hyperabsorption of calcium causes transient postprandial hypercalcemia that suppresses secretion of parathyroid hormone. The renal tubules are deprived of the normal stimulus to reabsorb calcium at the same time that the filtered load of calcium is increased. In other patients, reabsorption of calcium by the renal tubules appears to be defective, and secondary hyperparathyroidism is evoked by urinary losses of calcium. Renal synthesis of 1,25-dihydroxyvitamin D is increased, enhancing intestinal absorption of calcium. In the past, the separation of "absorptive" and "renal" forms of hypercalciuria was used to guide treatment. However, these may not be distinct entities but the extremes of a continuum of behavior. Vitamin D overactivity, either through high calcitriol levels or excess vitamin D receptor, is a likely explanation for the hypercalciuria in many of these patients. Hypercalciuria contributes to stone formation by raising urine saturation with respect to calcium oxalate and calcium phosphate.

℞ TREATMENT

For many years the standard therapy for hypercalciuria was dietary calcium restriction. However, recent studies have shown that low-calcium diets increase the risk of incident stone formation. In addition, hypercalciuric stone formers have reduced bone mineral density and an increased risk of fracture compared to the non-stone-forming population. Low calcium intake likely contributes to the low bone mineral density. A recent prospective trial compared the efficacy of a low-calcium diet to a low-protein, low-sodium, normal-calcium diet in preventing stone recurrence in male calcium stone formers. The group on the low-calcium diet had a significantly greater rate of stone relapse. As a whole, low-calcium diets do not appear to be efficacious and carry a long-term risk of bone disease in the stone-forming population. Low-sodium and low-protein diets are a superior option in stone formers. If diet therapy is not sufficient to prevent stones, then thiazide diuretics may be used. Thiazide diuretics lower urine calcium and are effective in preventing the formation of stones. Three 3-year randomized trials have shown a 50% decrease in stone formation in the thiazide-treated groups as compared to the placebo-treated controls. The drug effect requires slight contraction of the extracellular fluid volume, and massive use of NaCl reduces its therapeutic effect. Thiazide-induced hypokalemia should be aggressively treated since hypokalemia will reduce urine citrate, increasing urine calcium ion levels.

Hyperuricosuria   About 20% of calcium oxalate stone formers are hyperuricosuric, primarily because of an excessive intake of purine from meat, fish, and poultry. The mechanism of stone formation is probably due to salting out calcium oxalate by urate. A low-purine diet is desirable but difficult for many patients to achieve. The alternative is allopurinol, which has been shown to be effective in a randomized, controlled trial. A dose of 100 mg bid is usually sufficient.

Primary Hyperparathyroidism (See also Chap. 332)   The diagnosis of this condition is established by documenting that hypercalcemia that cannot be otherwise explained is accompanied by inappropriately elevated serum concentrations of parathyroid hormone. Hypercalciuria, usually present, raises the urine supersaturation of calcium phosphate and/or calcium oxalate (Table 268-1). Prompt diagnosis is important because parathyroidectomy should be carried out before renal damage or bone disease occurs.

Distal Renal Tubular Acidosis (See also Chap. 265)   The defect in this condition seems to reside in the distal nephron, which cannot establish a normal pH gradient between urine and blood, leading to hyperchloremic acidosis. The diagnosis is suggested by a minimum urine pH above 5.5 in the presence of systemic acidosis. If the diagnosis is in doubt because metabolic abnormalities are mild, oral challenge with NH_4Cl, 1.9 mmol/kg of body weight, will not lower urine pH below 5.5 in patients with distal RTA. Hypercalciuria, an alkaline urine, and a low urine citrate level cause supersaturation with respect to calcium phosphate. Calcium phosphate stones form, nephrocalcinosis is common, and osteomalacia or rickets may occur. Renal damage is frequent, and glomerular filtration rate falls gradually.

Treatment with supplemental alkali reverses hypercalciuria and limits the production of new stones. The usual dose of sodium bicarbonate is 0.5 to 2.0 mmol/kg of body weight per day in four to six divided doses. An alternative is potassium citrate supplementation, given at the same dose per day but needing to be given only three to four times per day. In incomplete distal RTA, systemic acidosis is absent, but urine pH cannot be lowered below 5.5 after an exogenous acid load such as ammonium chloride. Incomplete RTA may develop in some patients who form calcium oxalate stones because of idiopathic hypercalciuria; the importance of RTA in producing stones in this situation is uncertain, and thiazide treatment is a reasonable alternative. Some patients with incomplete RTA form calcium phosphate stones because of low urine citrate and an alkaline urine and are best treated with alkali as if RTA were complete. When treating patients with alkali it is prudent to monitor changes in urine citrate and pH. If urine pH increases without an increase in citrate then calcium phosphate supersaturation will increase and stone disease may worsen.

Hyperoxaluria   Oxalate is a metabolic end product in humans. Urine oxalate comes from diet and endogenous metabolic production, with

approximately 40 to 50% originating from dietary sources. The upper limit of normal for oxalate excretion is generally considered to be 40 to 50 mg per day. Mild hyperoxaluria (50 to 80 mg/d) is usually caused by excessive intake of high-oxalate foods such as spinach, nuts, and chocolate. In addition, low-calcium diets may promote hyperoxaluria as there is less calcium binding oxalate in the intestine, increasing the amount of oxalate available for absorption. Enteric hyperoxaluria is a consequence of small bowel disease resulting in fat malabsorption. Oxalate excretion is often over 100 mg per day. Enteric hyperoxaluria may be caused by jejunoileal bypass for obesity, bacterial overgrowth syndromes, pancreatic insufficiency, or extensive small intestine involvement from Crohn's disease. With fat malabsorption, calcium in the bowel lumen is bound by fatty acids instead of oxalate, which is left free for absorption in the colon. Delivery of unabsorbed fatty acids and bile salts to the colon may injure the colonic mucosa and enhance oxalate absorption. Hereditary hyperoxaluria states are rare causes of severe hyperoxaluria, often greater than 150 mg per day. Patients usually present with recurrent calcium oxalate stones during childhood. Type I hereditary hyperoxaluria is inherited as an autosomal recessive trait and is due to a deficiency in the peroxisomal enzyme alanine: glyoxylate aminotransferase. Type II is due to a deficiency of D-glyceric dehydrogenase. Severe hyperoxaluria from any cause can produce tubulointerstitial nephropathy (Chap. 266) and lead to stone formation.

℞ TREATMENT

Patients with mild to moderate hyperoxaluria should be treated with a diet low in oxalate and with a normal intake of calcium and magnesium to reduce oxalate absorption. Enteric hyperoxaluria can be treated with the oxalate-binding resin cholestyramine at a dose of 8 to 16 g/d, correction of fat malabsorption, and a low-fat, low-oxalate diet. Calcium supplements, given with meals, precipitate oxalate in the gut lumen, providing an additional form of therapy. Treatment for hereditary hyperoxaluria includes a high fluid intake, neutral phosphate, and pyridoxine (25 to 200 mg/d). Citrate supplementation may also have some benefit. Even with aggressive therapy, irreversible renal failure secondary to recurrent stone formation often occurs. Segmental liver transplant, to correct the enzyme defect, combined with a kidney transplant has been successfully utilized in patients with hereditary hyperoxaluria.

Hypocitraturia   Urine citrate prevents calcium stone formation by creating a soluble complex with calcium, effectively reducing free urine calcium. Hypocitraturia is found in 15 to 60% of stone formers, either as a single disorder or in combination with other metabolic abnormalities. It can be secondary to systemic disorders, such as RTA, chronic diarrheal illness, or hypokalemia, or it may be a primary disorder, in which case it is called *idiopathic hypocitraturia*.

℞ TREATMENT

Treatment is with alkali, which increases urine citrate excretion; generally bicarbonate or citrate salts are used. Potassium salts are preferred as sodium loading increases urinary excretion of calcium, reducing the effectiveness of treatment. Two randomized, placebo-controlled trials have demonstrated the effectiveness of citrate supplements in calcium oxalate stone formers.

Idiopathic Calcium Lithiasis   Some patients have no metabolic cause for stones despite a thorough metabolic evaluation (Table 268-1). The best treatment appears to be high fluid intake so that the urine specific gravity remains at 1.005 or below throughout the day and night. Thiazide diuretics, allopurinol, and citrate therapy may help reduce crystallization of calcium salts, but there are no prospective trials in this patient population. Oral phosphate at a dose of 2 g phosphorus daily may lower urine calcium and increase urine pyrophosphate and thereby reduce the rate of recurrence. Orthophosphate causes mild nausea and diarrhea, but tolerance may improve with continued intake.

URIC ACID STONES These stones form because the urine becomes supersaturated with undissociated uric acid that is protonated at its N-9 position. In gout, idiopathic uric acid lithiasis, and dehydration, the average pH is usually below 5.4 and often below 5.0. Undissociated uric acid therefore predominates and is soluble in urine only in concentrations of 100 mg/L. Concentrations above this level represent supersaturation that causes crystals and stones to form. Hyperuricosuria, when present, increases supersaturation, but urine of low pH can be supersaturated with undissociated uric acid even though the daily excretion rate is normal. Myeloproliferative syndromes, chemotherapy of malignant tumors, and Lesch-Nyhan syndrome cause such massive production of uric acid and consequent hyperuricosuria that stones and uric acid sludge form even at a normal urine pH. Plugging of the renal collecting tubules by uric acid crystals can cause acute renal failure.

℞ TREATMENT

The two goals of treatment are to raise urine pH and to lower excessive urine uric acid excretion to less than 1 g/d. Supplemental alkali, 1 to 3 mmol/kg of body weight per day, should be given in three or four evenly spaced, divided doses, one of which should be given at bedtime. The form of the alkali may be important. Potassium citrate may reduce the risk of calcium salts crystallizing when urine pH is increased, whereas sodium citrate or sodium bicarbonate may increase the risk. If the overnight urine pH is below 5.5, the evening dose of alkali may be raised or 250 mg acetazolamide added at bedtime. A low-purine diet should be instituted in those uric acid stone formers with hyperuricosuria. Patients who continue to form uric acid stones despite treatment with fluids, alkali, and a low-purine diet should have allopurinol added to their regimen. If hypercalciuria is also present, it should be specifically treated, as alkali alone could lead to calcium phosphate stone formation.

CYSTINURIA AND CYSTINE STONES (See also Chap. 343) In this autosomal recessive disorder, proximal tubular and jejunal transport of the dibasic amino acids cystine, lysine, arginine, and ornithine are defective, and excessive amounts are lost in the urine. Clinical disease is due solely to the insolubility of cystine, which forms stones.

Pathogenesis Cystinuria occurs because of defective transport of dibasic amino acids by the brush borders of renal tubule and intestinal epithelial cells. The disease classically has been broken into three types based on differences in intestinal and renal amino acid handling in families. However, genomic studies suggest type II and type III cystinuria are due to defects in the same protein. Disease-causing mutations have been identified in both the heavy and light chain of a heteromeric amino acid transporter found in the proximal tubule of the kidney. A gene located on chromosome 2 and designated *SLC3A1* encodes the heavy chain of the transporter and has been found to be abnormal in type I cystinuria. Non-type-I cystinuria is due to mutations in the *SLC7A9* gene on chromosome 19, which encodes the light chain of the heteromeric transporter.

Diagnosis Cystine stones are formed only by patients with cystinuria, but 10% of stones in cystinuric patients do not contain cystine; therefore, every stone former should be screened for the disease. The sediment from a first morning urine specimen in many patients with homozygous cystinuria reveals typical flat, hexagonal, platelike cystine crystals. Cystinuria also can be detected using the urine sodium nitroprusside test. Because the test is sensitive, it is positive in many asymptomatic heterozygotes for cystinuria. A positive nitroprusside

test or the finding of cystine crystals in the urine sediment should be evaluated by measurement of daily cystine excretion. Normal adults excrete 40 to 60 mg cystine per gram of creatinine, heterozygotes usually excrete less than 300 mg/g, and homozygotes almost always excrete greater than 250 mg/g.

℞ TREATMENT

High fluid intake, even at night, is the cornerstone of therapy. Daily urine volume should exceed 3 L. Raising urine pH with alkali is helpful, provided the urine pH exceeds 7.5. A low-salt diet (100 mmol/d) can reduce cystine excretion up to 40%. Because side effects are frequent, drugs such as penicillamine and tiopronin, which form the soluble disulfide cysteine-drug complexes, should be used only when fluid loading, salt reduction, and alkali therapy are ineffective. Captopril, which has a free sulfhydryl group to bind cysteine, has been used in a limited number of patients with some success. Low-methionine diets have not proved to be practical for clinical use, but patients should avoid protein gluttony.

STRUVITE STONES These stones are a result of urinary infection with bacteria, usually *Proteus* species, which possess urease, an enzyme that degrades urea to NH_3 and CO_2. The NH_3 hydrolyzes to NH_4^+ and raises urine pH to 8 or 9. The CO_2 hydrates to H_2CO_3 and then dissociates to CO_3^{2-} that precipitates with calcium as $CaCO_3$. The NH_4^+ precipitates PO_4^{3-} and Mg^{2+} to form $MgNH_4PO_4$ (struvite). The result is a stone of calcium carbonate admixed with struvite. Struvite does not form in urine in the absence of infection, because NH_4^+ concentration is low in urine that is alkaline in response to physiologic stimuli. Chronic *Proteus* infection can occur because of impaired urinary drainage, urologic instrumentation or surgery, and especially with chronic antibiotic treatment, which can favor the dominance of *Proteus* in the urinary tract.

℞ TREATMENT

Complete removal of the stone with subsequent sterilization of the urinary tract is the treatment of choice for patients who can tolerate the procedures. Open surgery is successful in debulking the stone and improving renal function if obstruction is present; however, there is recurrence of stone in 25% of the patients. Irrigation of the renal pelvis and calyces with hemiacidrin, a solution that dissolves struvite, can reduce recurrence after surgery. Newer procedures such as lithotripsy and percutaneous nephrolithotomy, alone or in combination, have largely replaced open surgery. Stone-free rates of 50 to 90% have been reported after these procedures. Antimicrobial treatment is best reserved for dealing with acute infection and for maintenance of a sterile urine after surgery. Urine cultures and culture of stone fragments removed at surgery should guide the choice of antibiotic. For patients who are not candidates for surgical removal of stone, acetohydroxamic acid, an inhibitor of urease, can be used. Though effective in treating the stones, acetohydroxamic acid has many side effects, such as headache, tremor, and thrombophlebitis, that limit its use.

FURTHER READING

BUSHINSKY DA: Kidney stones. Adv Intern Med 47:219, 2001

CHILLARON J et al: Heteromeric amino acid transporters: Biochemistry, genetics, and physiology. Am J Physiol Renal Physiol 281:F995, 2001

FOWLER KA et al: Ultrasound for detecting renal calculi with nonenhanced CT as a reference standard. Radiology 222:09, 2002

HOLMES RP et al: Contribution of dietary oxalate to urinary oxalate excretion. Kidney Int 59:270, 2001

LAUDERDALE DS et al: Bone mineral density and fracture among prevalent kidney stone cases in the Third National Health and Nutrition Examination Survey. J Bone Miner Res 16:1893, 2001

PARKS JH et al: A single 24-hour urine collection is inadequate for the medical evaluation of nephrolithiasis. J Urol 167:1607, 2002

DEFINITIONS Acute infections of the urinary tract can be subdivided into two general anatomic categories: lower tract infection (urethritis and cystitis) and upper tract infection (acute pyelonephritis, prostatitis, and intrarenal and perinephric abscesses). Infections at these various sites may occur together or independently and may either be asymptomatic or present as one of the clinical syndromes described below. Infections of the urethra and bladder are often considered superficial (or mucosal) infections, while prostatitis, pyelonephritis, and renal suppuration signify tissue invasion.

From a microbiologic perspective, urinary tract infection (UTI) exists when pathogenic microorganisms are detected in the urine, urethra, bladder, kidney, or prostate. In most instances, growth of $>10^5$ organisms per milliliter from a properly collected midstream "clean-catch" urine sample indicates infection. However, significant bacteriuria is lacking in some cases of true UTI. Especially in symptomatic patients, a smaller number of bacteria (10^2 to 10^4/mL) may signify infection. In urine specimens obtained by suprapubic aspiration or "in-and-out" catheterization and in samples from a patient with an indwelling catheter, colony counts of 10^2 to 10^4/mL generally indicate infection. Conversely, colony counts of $>10^5$/mL of midstream urine are occasionally due to specimen contamination, which is especially likely when multiple bacterial species are found.

Infections that recur after antibiotic therapy can be due to the persistence of the originally infecting strain (as judged by species, antibiogram, serotype, and molecular type) or to reinfection with a new strain. "Same-strain" recurrent infections that become evident within 2 weeks of cessation of therapy can be the result of unresolved renal or prostatic infection (termed *relapse*) or of persistent vaginal or intestinal colonization leading to rapid reinfection of the bladder.

Symptoms of dysuria, urgency, and frequency that are unaccompanied by significant bacteriuria have been termed the *acute urethral syndrome*. Although widely used, this term lacks anatomic precision because many cases so designated are actually bladder infections. Moreover, since the causative agent can usually be identified in these patients, the term *syndrome*—implying unknown causation—is inappropriate.

Chronic pyelonephritis refers to chronic interstitial nephritis believed to result from bacterial infection of the kidney (Chap. 266). Many noninfectious diseases also cause an interstitial nephritis that is indistinguishable pathologically from chronic pyelonephritis.

ACUTE UTIs: URETHRITIS, CYSTITIS, AND PYELONEPHRITIS

EPIDEMIOLOGY Epidemiologically, UTIs are subdivided into catheter-associated (or nosocomial) infections and non-catheter-associated (or community-acquired) infections. Infections in either category may be symptomatic or asymptomatic. Acute community-acquired infections are very common and account for more than 7 million office visits annually in the United States. These infections occur in 1 to 3% of schoolgirls and then increase markedly in incidence with the onset of sexual activity in adolescence. The vast majority of acute symptomatic infections involve young women; a prospective study demonstrated an annual incidence of 0.5 to 0.7 infections per patient-year in this group. Acute symptomatic UTIs are unusual in men under the age of 50. The development of asymptomatic bacteriuria parallels that of symptomatic infection and is rare among men under 50 but common among women between 20 and 50. Asymptomatic bacteriuria is more common among elderly men and women, with rates as high as 40 to 50% in some studies.

ETIOLOGY Many different microorganisms can infect the urinary tract, but by far the most common agents are the gram-negative bacilli. *Escherichia coli* causes ~80% of acute infections in patients without catheters, urologic abnormalities, or calculi. Other gram-negative rods, especially *Proteus* and *Klebsiella* and occasionally *Enterobacter*, account for a smaller proportion of uncomplicated infections. These organisms, plus *Serratia* and *Pseudomonas*, assume increasing importance in recurrent infections and in infections associated with urologic manipulation, calculi, or obstruction. They play a major role in nosocomial, catheter-associated infections (see below). *Proteus* spp., by virtue of urease production, and *Klebsiella* spp., through the production of extracellular slime and polysaccharides, predispose to stone formation and are isolated more frequently from patients with calculi.

Gram-positive cocci play a lesser role in UTIs. However, *Staphylococcus saprophyticus*—a novobiocin-resistant, coagulase-negative species—accounts for 10 to 15% of acute symptomatic UTIs in young females. Enterococci occasionally cause acute uncomplicated cystitis in women. More commonly, enterococci and *Staphylococcus aureus* cause infections in patients with renal stones or previous instrumentation or surgery. Isolation of *S. aureus* from the urine should arouse suspicion of bacteremic infection of the kidney.

About one-third of women with dysuria and frequency have either an insignificant number of bacteria in midstream urine cultures or completely sterile cultures and have been previously defined as having the urethral syndrome. About three-quarters of these women have pyuria, while one-quarter have no pyuria and little objective evidence of infection. In the women with pyuria, two groups of pathogens account for most infections. Low counts (10^2 to 10^4/mL) of typical bacterial uropathogens such as *E. coli*, *S. saprophyticus*, *Klebsiella*, or *Proteus* are found in midstream urine specimens from most of these women. These bacteria are probably the causative agents in these infections because they can usually be isolated from a suprapubic aspirate, are associated with pyuria, and respond to appropriate antimicrobial therapy. In other women with acute urinary symptoms, pyuria, and urine that is sterile (even when obtained by suprapubic aspiration), sexually transmitted urethritis-producing agents such as *Chlamydia trachomatis*, *Neisseria gonorrhoeae*, and herpes simplex virus are etiologically important. These agents are found most frequently in young, sexually active women with new sexual partners.

The causative role of several more unusual bacterial and nonbacterial pathogens in UTIs remains poorly defined. *Ureaplasma urealyticum* has frequently been isolated from the urethra and urine of patients with acute dysuria and frequency but is also found in specimens from many patients without urinary symptoms. Ureaplasmas probably account for some cases of urethritis and cystitis. *U. urealyticum* and *Mycoplasma hominis* have been isolated from prostatic and renal tissues of patients with acute prostatitis and pyelonephritis, respectively, and are probably responsible for some of these infections as well. Adenoviruses cause acute hemorrhagic cystitis in children and in some young adults, often in epidemics. Although other viruses can be isolated from urine (e.g., cytomegalovirus), they are thought not to cause acute UTI. Colonization of the urine of catheterized or diabetic patients by *Candida* and other fungal species is common and sometimes progresses to symptomatic invasive infection (Chap. 187). →*Mycobacterial infection of the genitourinary tract is discussed in Chap. 150.*

PATHOGENESIS AND SOURCES OF INFECTION The urinary tract should be viewed as a single anatomic unit that is united by a continuous column of urine extending from the urethra to the kidney. In the vast majority of UTIs, bacteria gain access to the bladder via the urethra. Ascent of bacteria from the bladder may follow and is probably the pathway for most renal parenchymal infections.

The vaginal introitus and distal urethra are normally colonized by diphtheroids, streptococcal species, lactobacilli, and staphylococcal species but not by the enteric gram-negative bacilli that commonly cause UTIs. In females prone to the development of cystitis, however, enteric gram-negative organisms residing in the bowel colonize the introitus, the periurethral skin, and the distal urethra before and during episodes of bacteriuria. The factors that predispose to periurethral colonization with gram-negative bacilli remain poorly understood, but alteration of the normal vaginal flora by antibiotics, other genital infections, or contraceptives (especially spermicide) appears to play an important role. Loss of the normally dominant H_2O_2-producing lactobacilli in the vaginal flora appears to facilitate colonization by *E. coli*. Small numbers of periurethral bacteria probably gain entry to the bladder frequently, a process that is facilitated in some cases by urethral massage during intercourse. Whether bladder infection ensues depends on interacting effects of the pathogenicity of the strain, the inoculum size, and the local and systemic host defense mechanisms.

Under normal circumstances, bacteria placed in the bladder are rapidly cleared, partly through the flushing and dilutional effects of voiding but also as a result of the antibacterial properties of urine and the bladder mucosa. Owing mostly to a high urea concentration and high osmolarity, the bladder urine of many normal persons inhibits or kills bacteria. Prostatic secretions possess antibacterial properties as well. Polymorphonuclear leukocytes enter the bladder epithelium and the urine soon after infection arises and play a role in clearing bacteriuria. The role of locally produced antibody remains unclear.

Hematogenous pyelonephritis occurs most often in debilitated patients who are either chronically ill or receiving immunosuppressive therapy. Metastatic staphylococcal or candidal infections of the kidney may follow bacteremia or fungemia, spreading from distant foci of infection in the bone, skin, vasculature, or elsewhere.

CONDITIONS AFFECTING PATHOGENESIS ■ **Gender and Sexual Activity** The female urethra appears to be particularly prone to colonization with colonic gram-negative bacilli because of its proximity to the anus, its short length (~4 cm), and its termination beneath the labia. Sexual intercourse causes the introduction of bacteria into the bladder and is temporally associated with the onset of cystitis; it thus appears to be important in the pathogenesis of UTIs in younger women. Voiding after intercourse reduces the risk of cystitis, probably because it promotes the clearance of bacteria introduced during intercourse. Use of spermicidal compounds with a diaphragm or cervical cap or use of spermicide-coated condoms dramatically alters the normal introital bacterial flora and has been associated with marked increases in vaginal colonization with *E. coli* and in the risk of UTI.

In males who are <50 years old and who have no history of heterosexual or homosexual rectal intercourse, UTI is exceedingly uncommon, and this diagnosis should be questioned in the absence of clear documentation. An important factor predisposing to bacteriuria in men is urethral obstruction due to prostatic hypertrophy. Insertive rectal intercourse is also associated with an increased risk of cystitis in men. Men (and women) who are infected with HIV and who have CD4+ T cell counts of <200/μL are at increased risk of both bacteriuria and symptomatic UTI. Finally, lack of circumcision has been identified as a risk factor for UTI in both neonates and young men.

Pregnancy UTIs are detected in 2 to 8% of pregnant women. Symptomatic upper tract infections, in particular, are unusually common during pregnancy; fully 20 to 30% of pregnant women with asymptomatic bacteriuria subsequently develop pyelonephritis. This predisposition to upper tract infection during pregnancy results from decreased ureteral tone, decreased ureteral peristalsis, and temporary incompetence of the vesicoureteral valves. Bladder catheterization during or after delivery causes additional infections. Increased incidences of low-birth-weight infants, premature delivery, and newborn mortality result from UTIs during pregnancy, particularly those infections involving the upper tract.

Obstruction Any impediment to the free flow of urine—tumor, stricture, stone, or prostatic hypertrophy—results in hydronephrosis and a greatly increased frequency of UTI. Infection superimposed on urinary tract obstruction may lead to rapid destruction of renal tissue. It is of utmost importance, therefore, when infection is present, to identify and repair obstructive lesions. On the other hand, when an obstruction is minor and is not progressive or associated with infection, great caution should be exercised in attempting surgical correction. The introduction of infection in such cases may be more damaging than an uncorrected minor obstruction that does not significantly impair renal function.

Neurogenic Bladder Dysfunction Interference with bladder enervation, as in spinal cord injury, tabes dorsalis, multiple sclerosis, diabetes, and other diseases, may be associated with UTI. The infection may be initiated by the use of catheters for bladder drainage and is favored by the prolonged stasis of urine in the bladder. An additional factor often operative in these cases is bone demineralization due to immobilization, which causes hypercalciuria, calculus formation, and obstructive uropathy.

Vesicoureteral Reflux Defined as reflux of urine from the bladder cavity up into the ureters and sometimes into the renal pelvis, vesicoureteral reflux occurs during voiding or with elevation of pressure in the bladder. In practice, this condition is demonstrated by the finding of retrograde movement of radiopaque or radioactive material during a voiding cystourethrogram. An anatomically impaired vesicoureteral junction facilitates reflux of bacteria and thus upper tract infection. However, since a fluid connection between the bladder and the kidney always exists, even in the normal urinary system, some retrograde movement of bacteria probably takes place during infection but is not detected by radiologic techniques.

Vesicoureteral reflux is common among children with anatomic abnormalities of the urinary tract as well as among children with anatomically normal but infected urinary tracts. In the latter group, reflux disappears with advancing age and is probably attributable to factors other than UTI. Long-term follow-up of children with UTI who have reflux has established that renal damage correlates with marked reflux, not with infection.

The routine search for reflux would be aided by the development of noninvasive tests applicable to young children, in whom the need for an effective technique is greatest. In the meantime, it appears reasonable to search for reflux in anyone with unexplained failure of renal growth or with renal scarring, because UTI per se is an insufficient explanation for these abnormalities. On the other hand, it is doubtful that all children who have recurrent UTIs but whose urinary tract appears normal on pyelography should be subjected to voiding cystoureterography merely for the detection of the rare patient with marked reflux not revealed by the intravenous pyelogram.

Bacterial Virulence Factors Not all strains of *E. coli* are equally capable of infecting the intact urinary tract. Bacterial virulence factors markedly influence the likelihood that a given strain, once introduced into the bladder, will cause UTI. Most *E. coli* strains that cause symptomatic UTIs in noncatheterized patients belong to a small number of specific O, K, and H serogroups. These uropathogenic clones have accumulated a number of virulence genes that are often closely linked on the bacterial chromosome in "virulence islands." Adherence of bacteria to uroepithelial cells is a critical first step in the initiation of infection. For both *E. coli* and *Proteus*, fimbriae (hairlike proteinaceous surface appendages) mediate the attachment of bacteria to specific receptors on epithelial cells. The attachment of bacteria to uroepithelial cells initiates a number of important events in the mucosal epithelial cell, including secretion of interleukin (IL) 6 and IL-8 (with subsequent chemotaxis of leukocytes to the bladder mucosa) and induction of apoptosis and epithelial cell desquamation. Besides fimbriae, uropathogenic *E. coli* strains usually produce hemolysin and aerobactin (a siderophore for scavenging iron) and are resistant to the bactericidal action of human serum. Nearly all *E. coli* strains causing acute pyelonephritis and most of those causing acute cystitis are uropathogenic. In contrast, infections in patients with structural or functional abnormalities of the urinary tract are generally caused by bacterial strains that lack these uropathogenic properties; the implication is that these properties are not needed for infection of the compromised urinary tract.

Genetic Factors Increasing evidence suggests that host genetic factors influence susceptibility to UTI. A maternal history of UTI is more often found among women who have experienced recurrent UTIs than among controls. The number and type of receptors on uroepithelial cells to which bacteria may attach are at least in part genetically determined. Many of these structures are components of blood group antigens and are present on both erythrocytes and uroepithelial cells. For example, P fimbriae mediate attachment of *E. coli* to P-positive erythrocytes and are found on nearly all strains causing acute uncomplicated pyelonephritis. Conversely, P blood group–negative individuals, who lack these receptors, have a decreased likelihood of pyelonephritis. It has also been demonstrated that nonsecretors of blood group antigens are at increased risk of recurrent UTI; this predisposition may relate to a different profile of genetically determined glycolipids on uroepithelial cells. Mutations in host genes integral to the immune response (interferon γ receptors and others) may also affect susceptibility to UTI.

LOCALIZATION OF INFECTION Unfortunately, currently available methods of distinguishing renal parenchymal infection from cystitis are neither reliable nor convenient enough for routine clinical use. Fever or an elevated level of C-reactive protein often accompanies acute pyelonephritis and is found in rare cases of cystitis but also occurs in infections other than pyelonephritis.

CLINICAL PRESENTATION ■ **Cystitis** Patients with cystitis usually report dysuria, frequency, urgency, and suprapubic pain. The urine often becomes grossly cloudy and malodorous, and it is bloody in ~30% of cases. White cells and bacteria can be detected by examination of unspun urine in most cases. However, some women with cystitis have only 10^2 to 10^4 bacteria per milliliter of urine, and in these instances bacteria cannot be seen in a Gram-stained preparation of unspun urine. Physical examination generally reveals only tenderness of the urethra or the suprapubic area. If a genital lesion or a vaginal discharge is evident, especially in conjunction with $<10^5$ bacteria per milliliter on urine culture, then pathogens that may cause urethritis, vaginitis, or cervicitis, such as *C. trachomatis, N. gonorrhoeae, Trichomonas, Candida*, and herpes simplex virus, should be considered. Prominent systemic manifestations, such as a temperature of $>38.3°C$ ($>101°F$), nausea, and vomiting, usually indicate concomitant renal infection, as does costovertebral angle tenderness. However, the absence of these findings does not ensure that infection is limited to the bladder and urethra.

Acute Pyelonephritis Symptoms of acute pyelonephritis generally develop rapidly over a few hours or a day and include a fever, shaking chills, nausea, vomiting, and diarrhea. Symptoms of cystitis may or may not be present. Besides fever, tachycardia, and generalized muscle tenderness, physical examination reveals marked tenderness on deep pressure in one or both costovertebral angles or on deep abdominal palpation. In some patients, signs and symptoms of gram-negative sepsis predominate. Most patients have significant leukocytosis and bacteria detectable in Gram-stained unspun urine. Leukocyte casts are present in the urine of some patients, and the detection of these casts is pathognomonic. Hematuria may be demonstrated during the acute phase of the disease; if it persists after acute manifestations of infection have subsided, a stone, a tumor, or tuberculosis should be considered.

Except in individuals with papillary necrosis, abscess formation, or urinary obstruction, the manifestations of acute pyelonephritis usually respond to therapy within 48 to 72 h. However, despite the absence of symptoms, bacteriuria or pyuria may persist. In severe pyelonephritis, fever subsides more slowly and may not disappear for several days, even after appropriate antibiotic treatment has been instituted.

Urethritis Approximately 30% of women with acute dysuria, frequency, and pyuria have midstream urine cultures that show either no growth or insignificant bacterial growth. Clinically, these women cannot always be readily distinguished from those with cystitis. In this situation, a distinction should be made between women infected with sexually transmitted pathogens, such as *C. trachomatis, N. gonorrhoeae*, or herpes simplex virus, and those with low-count *E. coli* or staphylococcal infection of the urethra and bladder. Chlamydial or gonococcal infection should be suspected in women with a gradual onset of illness, no hematuria, no suprapubic pain, and >7 days of symptoms. The additional history of a recent sex-partner change, especially if the patient's partner has recently had chlamydial or gonococcal urethritis, should heighten the suspicion of a sexually transmitted infection, as should the finding of mucopurulent cervicitis (Chap. 115). Gross hematuria, suprapubic pain, an abrupt onset of illness, a duration of illness of <3 days, and a history of UTIs favor the diagnosis of *E. coli* UTI.

Catheter-Associated UTIs (See also Chap. 116) Bacteriuria develops in at least 10 to 15% of hospitalized patients with indwelling urethral catheters. The risk of infection is ~3 to 5% per day of catheterization. *E. coli, Proteus, Pseudomonas, Klebsiella, Serratia*, staphylococci, enterococci, and *Candida* usually cause these infections. Many infecting strains display markedly greater antimicrobial resistance than organisms that cause community-acquired UTIs. Factors associated with an increased risk of catheter-associated UTI include female sex, prolonged catheterization, severe underlying illness, disconnection of the catheter and drainage tube, other types of faulty catheter care, and lack of systemic antimicrobial therapy.

Infection occurs when bacteria reach the bladder by one of two routes: by migrating through the column of urine in the catheter lumen (intraluminal route) or by moving up the mucous sheath outside the catheter (periurethral route). Hospital-acquired pathogens reach the patient's catheter or urine-collecting system on the hands of hospital personnel, in contaminated solutions or irrigants, and via contaminated instruments or disinfectants. Bacteria usually enter the catheter system at the catheter–collecting tube junction or at the drainage bag portal. The organisms then ascend intraluminally into the bladder within 24 to 72 h. Alternatively, the patient's own bowel flora may colonize the perineal skin and periurethral area and reach the bladder via the external surface of the catheter. This route is particularly common in women. Studies have demonstrated the importance of the attachment and growth of bacteria on the surfaces of the catheter in the pathogenesis of catheter-associated UTI. Such bacteria growing in biofilms on the catheter eventually produce encrustations consisting of bacteria, bacterial glycocalyces, host urinary proteins, and urinary salts. These encrustations provide a refuge for bacteria and may protect them from antimicrobial agents and phagocytes.

Clinically, most catheter-associated infections cause minimal symptoms and no fever and often resolve after withdrawal of the catheter. The frequency of upper tract infection associated with catheter-induced bacteriuria is unknown. Gram-negative bacteremia, which follows catheter-associated bacteriuria in 1 to 2% of cases, is the most significant recognized complication of catheter-induced UTIs. The catheterized urinary tract has repeatedly been demonstrated to be the most common source of gram-negative bacteremia in hospitalized patients, generally accounting for ~30% of cases.

Catheter-associated UTIs can sometimes be prevented in patients catheterized for <2 weeks by use of a sterile closed collecting system, by attention to aseptic technique during insertion and care of the catheter, and by measures to minimize cross-infection. Other preventive approaches, including short courses of systemic antimicrobial therapy, topical application of periurethral antimicrobial ointments, use of preconnected catheter–drainage tube units, use of catheters impregnated with antimicrobial agents, and addition of antimicrobial drugs to the drainage bag, have all been protective in at least one controlled trial but are not recommended for general use. Despite precautions, the majority of patients catheterized for >2 weeks eventually develop bacteriuria. For example, because of spinal cord injury, incontinence, or other factors, some patients in hospitals or nursing homes require long-term or semipermanent bladder catheterization. Measures intended to prevent infection have been largely unsuccessful, and essentially all such chronically catheterized patients develop bacteriuria. If feasible, intermittent catheterization by a nurse or by the patient appears to reduce the incidence of bacteriuria and associated complications in such patients. Treatment should be provided when symptomatic infections arise, but treatment of asymptomatic bacteriuria in such patients has no apparent benefit.

DIAGNOSTIC TESTING   Determination of the number and type of bacteria in the urine is an extremely important diagnostic procedure. In symptomatic patients, bacteria are usually present in the urine in large numbers ($\geq 10^5$/mL). In asymptomatic patients, two consecutive urine specimens should be examined bacteriologically before therapy is instituted, and $\geq 10^5$ bacteria of a single species per milliliter should be demonstrable in both specimens. Since the large number of bacteria in the bladder urine is due in part to bacterial multiplication during residence in the bladder cavity, samples of urine from the ureters or renal pelvis may contain $<10^5$ bacteria per milliliter and yet indicate infection. Similarly, the presence of bacteriuria of any degree in suprapubic aspirates or of $\geq 10^2$ bacteria per milliliter of urine obtained by catheterization usually indicates infection. In some circumstances (antibiotic treatment, high urea concentration, high osmolarity, low pH), urine inhibits bacterial multiplication, resulting in relatively low bacterial colony counts despite infection. For this reason, antiseptic solutions should not be used in washing the periurethral area before collection of the urine specimen. Water diuresis or recent voiding also reduces bacterial counts in urine.

Microscopy of urine from symptomatic patients can be of great diagnostic value. Microscopic bacteriuria, which is best assessed with Gram-stained uncentrifuged urine, is found in $>90\%$ of specimens from patients whose infections are associated with colony counts of at least 10^5/mL, and this finding is very specific. However, bacteria cannot usually be detected microscopically in infections with lower colony counts (10^2 to 10^4/mL). The detection of bacteria by urinary microscopy thus constitutes firm evidence of infection, but the absence of microscopically detectable bacteria does not exclude the diagnosis. When carefully sought by means of chamber-count microscopy, pyuria is a highly sensitive indicator of UTI in symptomatic patients. Pyuria is demonstrated in nearly all acute bacterial UTIs, and its absence calls the diagnosis into question. The leukocyte esterase "dipstick" method is less sensitive than microscopy in identifying pyuria but is a useful alternative where microscopy is not feasible. Pyuria in the absence of bacteriuria (sterile pyuria) may indicate infection with unusual bacterial agents such as *C. trachomatis*, *U. urealyticum*, and *Mycobacterium tuberculosis* or with fungi. Alternatively, sterile pyuria may be demonstrated in noninfectious urologic conditions such as calculi, anatomic abnormality, nephrocalcinosis, vesicoureteral reflux, interstitial nephritis, or polycystic disease.

Although many authorities have recommended that urine culture and antimicrobial susceptibility testing be performed for any patient with a suspected UTI, it may be more practical and cost-effective to manage women who have symptoms characteristic of acute uncomplicated cystitis without an initial urine culture. Two approaches to presumptive therapy have generally been used. In the first, treatment is initiated solely on the basis of a typical history and/or typical findings on physical examination. In the second, women with symptoms and signs of acute cystitis and without complicating factors are managed with urinary microscopy (or, alternatively, with a leukocyte esterase test). A positive result for pyuria and/or bacteriuria provides enough evidence of infection to indicate that urine culture and susceptibility testing can be omitted and the patient treated empirically. Urine should be cultured, however, when a woman's symptoms and urine-examination findings leave the diagnosis of cystitis in question. Pretherapy cultures and susceptibility testing are also essential in the management of all patients with suspected upper tract infections and of those with complicating factors, as in these situations any of a variety

of pathogens may be involved and antibiotic therapy is best tailored to the individual organism.

℞ TREATMENT

The following principles underlie the treatment of UTIs:

1. Except in acute uncomplicated cystitis in women, a quantitative urine culture or a comparable alternative diagnostic test should be performed to confirm infection before empirical treatment is begun. When culture results become available, antimicrobial sensitivity testing should be used to further direct therapy.

2. Factors predisposing to infection, such as obstruction and calculi, should be identified and corrected if possible.

3. Relief of clinical symptoms does not always indicate bacteriologic cure.

4. Each course of treatment should be classified after its completion as a failure (symptoms and/or bacteriuria not eradicated during therapy or in the immediate posttreatment culture) or a cure (resolution of symptoms and elimination of bacteriuria). Recurrent infections should be classified as same-strain or different-strain and as early (occurring within 2 weeks of the end of therapy) or late.

5. In general, uncomplicated infections confined to the lower urinary tract respond to short courses of therapy, while upper tract infections require longer treatment. After therapy, early recurrences due to the same strain may result from an unresolved upper tract focus of infection but often (especially after short-course therapy for cystitis) result from persistent vaginal colonization. Recurrences >2 weeks after the cessation of therapy nearly always represent reinfection with a new strain or with the previously infecting strain that has persisted in the vaginal and rectal flora.

6. Despite increasing resistance, community-acquired infections, especially initial infections, are usually due to more antibiotic-sensitive strains.

7. In patients with repeated infections, instrumentation, or recent hospitalization, the presence of antibiotic-resistant strains should be suspected. Although many antimicrobial agents reach high concentrations in urine, in vitro resistance usually predicts a substantially higher failure rate.

The anatomic location of a UTI greatly influences the success or failure of a therapeutic regimen. Bladder bacteriuria (cystitis) can usually be eliminated with nearly any antimicrobial agent to which the infecting strain is sensitive; in the past, it was demonstrated that as little as a single dose of 500 mg of intramuscular kanamycin eliminated bladder bacteriuria in most cases. With upper tract infections, however, single-dose therapy fails in the majority of cases, and even a 7-day course is unsuccessful in many instances. Longer periods of treatment (2 to 6 weeks) aimed at eradicating a persistent focus of infection may be necessary in some cases.

In *acute uncomplicated cystitis*, more than 90 to 95% of infections are due to one of two organisms: *E. coli* or *S. saprophyticus*. Although resistance patterns vary geographically and resistance has increased in many areas, most strains are sensitive to many antibiotics. In most parts of the United States, more than one-quarter of *E. coli* strains causing acute cystitis are resistant to amoxicillin, sulfa drugs, and cephalexin; resistance to trimethoprim (TMP) and trimethoprim-sulfamethoxazole (TMP-SMX) is now approaching these levels as well in many areas. Substantially higher rates of resistance to TMP-SMX have been documented in some other countries, as has resistance to fluoroquinolones.

Many have advocated single-dose treatment for acute cystitis. The advantages of single-dose therapy include less expense, ensured compliance, fewer side effects, and perhaps less intense pressure favoring the selection of resistant organisms in the intestinal, vaginal, or perineal flora. However, more frequent recurrences develop shortly after single-dose therapy than after 3-day treatment, and single-dose therapy does not eradicate vaginal colonization with *E. coli* as effectively as do longer regimens. A 3-day course of therapy with TMP-SMX, TMP, norfloxacin, ciprofloxacin, or ofloxacin appears to preserve the low rate of side effects of single-dose therapy while improving efficacy (Table 269-1); thus 3-day regimens are currently preferred for acute cystitis. In areas where TMP-SMX resistance exceeds 20%, either a fluoroquinolone or nitrofurantoin can be used (Table 269-1). Neither single-dose nor 3-day therapy should be used for women with symptoms or signs of pyelonephritis, urologic abnormalities or stones, or previous infections due to antibiotic-resistant organisms. Males with UTI often have urologic abnormalities or prostatic involvement and hence are not candidates for single-dose or 3-day therapy. For empirical therapy, they should generally receive a 7- to 14-day course of a fluoroquinolone (Table 269-1).

The choice of treatment for women with acute urethritis depends on the etiologic agent involved. In chlamydial infection, azithromycin (1 g in a single oral dose) or doxycycline (100 mg twice daily by mouth for 7 days) should be used. Women with acute dysuria and frequency, negative urine cultures, and no pyuria usually do not respond to antimicrobial agents.

In women, *acute uncomplicated pyelonephritis* without accompanying clinical evidence of calculi or urologic disease is due to *E. coli* in most cases. Although the optimal route and duration of therapy have not been established, a 7- to 14-day course of a fluoroquinolone, an aminoglycoside, or a third-generation cephalosporin is usually adequate. Neither ampicillin nor TMP-SMX should be used as initial therapy because >25% of strains of *E. coli* causing pyelonephritis are now resistant to these drugs in vitro. For at least the first few days of treatment, antibiotics should probably be given intravenously to most patients, but patients with mild symptoms can be treated for 7 to 14 days with an oral antibiotic (usually ciprofloxacin or ofloxacin), with or without an initial single parenteral dose (Table 269-1). Patients who fail to respond to treatment within 72 h or who relapse after therapy should be evaluated for unrecognized suppurative foci, calculi, or urologic disease.

Complicated UTIs (those arising in a setting of catheterization, instrumentation, urologic anatomic or functional abnormalities, stones, obstruction, immunosuppression, renal disease, or diabetes) are typically due to hospital-acquired bacteria, including *E. coli*, *Klebsiella*, *Proteus*, *Serratia*, *Pseudomonas*, enterococci, and staphylococci. Many of the infecting strains are antibiotic-resistant. Empirical antibiotic therapy ideally provides broad-spectrum coverage against these pathogens. In patients with minimal or mild symptoms, oral therapy with a fluoroquinolone, such as ciprofloxacin or ofloxacin, can be administered until culture results and antibiotic sensitivities are known. In patients with more severe illness, including acute pyelonephritis or suspected urosepsis, hospitalization and parenteral therapy should be undertaken. Commonly used empirical regimens include imipenem alone, a penicillin or cephalosporin plus an aminoglycoside, and (when the involvement of enterococci is unlikely) ceftriaxone or ceftazidime. When information on the antimicrobial sensitivity pattern of the infecting strain becomes available, a more specific antimicrobial regimen can be selected. Therapy should generally be administered for 10 to 21 days, with the exact duration depending on the severity of the infection and the susceptibility of the infecting strain. Follow-up cultures 2 to 4 weeks after cessation of therapy should be performed to demonstrate cure.

The need for treatment as well as the optimal type and duration of treatment for *catheterized patients with asymptomatic bacteriuria* have not been established. Removal of the catheter in conjunction with a

---

TABLE 269-1 *Treatment Regimens for Bacterial Urinary Tract Infections*

Condition	Characteristic Pathogens	Mitigating Circumstances	Recommended Empirical Treatment[a]
Acute uncomplicated cystitis in women	*Escherichia coli*, *Staphylococcus saprophyticus*, *Proteus mirabilis*, *Klebsiella pneumoniae*	None	3-Day regimens: oral TMP-SMX, TMP, quinolone; 7-day regimen: macrocrystalline nitrofurantoin[b]
		Diabetes, symptoms for >7 d, recent UTI, use of diaphragm, age >65 years	Consider 7-day regimen: oral TMP-SMX, TMP, quinolone[b]
		Pregnancy	Consider 7-day regimen: oral amoxicillin, macrocrystalline nitrofurantoin, cefpodoxime proxetil, or TMP-SMX[b]
Acute uncomplicated pyelonephritis in women	*E. coli*, *P. mirabilis*, *S. saprophyticus*	Mild to moderate illness, no nausea or vomiting; outpatient therapy	Oral[c] quinolone for 7–14 d (initial dose given IV if desired); or single-dose ceftriaxone (1 g) or gentamicin (3–5 mg/kg) IV followed by oral TMP-SMX[b] for 14 d
		Severe illness or possible urosepsis: hospitalization required	Parenteral[d] quinolone, gentamicin (± ampicillin), ceftriaxone, or aztreonam until defervescence; then oral[c] quinolone, cephalosporin, or TMP-SMX for 14 d
Complicated UTI in men and women	*E. coli*, *Proteus*, *Klebsiella*, *Pseudomonas*, *Serratia*, enterococci, staphylococci	Mild to moderate illness, no nausea or vomiting: outpatient therapy	Oral[c] quinolone for 10–14 d
		Severe illness or possible urosepsis: hospitalization required	Parenteral[d] ampicillin and gentamicin, quinolone, ceftriaxone, aztreonam, ticarcillin/clavulanate, or imipenem-cilastatin until defervescence; then oral[c] quinolone or TMP-SMX for 10–21 d

[a] Treatments listed are those to be prescribed before the etiologic agent is known; Gram's staining can be helpful in the selection of empirical therapy. Such therapy can be modified once the infecting agent has been identified. Fluoroquinolones should not be used in pregnancy. TMP-SMX, although not approved for use in pregnancy, has been widely used. Gentamicin should be used with caution in pregnancy because of its possible toxicity to eighth-nerve development in the fetus.
[b] Multiday oral regimens for cystitis are as follows: TMP-SMX, 160/800 mg q12h; TMP, 100 mg q12h; norfloxacin, 400 mg q12h; ciprofloxacin, 250 mg q12h; ofloxacin, 200 mg q12h; levofloxacin, 250 mg q12h; gatifloxacin, 200 or 400 mg/d; moxifloxacin, 400 mg/d; lomefloxacin, 400 mg/d; enoxacin, 400 mg/d; macrocrystalline nitrofurantoin, 100 mg qid; amoxicillin, 250 mg q8h; cefpodoxime proxetil, 100 mg q12h.
[c] Oral regimens for pyelonephritis and complicated UTI are as follows: TMP-SMX, 160/800 mg q12h; ciprofloxacin, 500 mg q12h; ofloxacin, 200–300 mg q12h; lomefloxacin, 400 mg/d; enoxacin, 400 mg q12h; gatifloxacin, 400 mg/d; levofloxacin, 200 mg q12h; moxifloxacin, 400 mg/d; amoxicillin, 500 mg q8h; cefpodoxime proxetil, 200 mg q12h.
[d] Parenteral regimens are as follows: ciprofloxacin, 400 mg q12h; ofloxacin, 400 mg q12h; gatifloxacin, 400 mg/d; levofloxacin, 500 mg/d; gentamicin, 1 mg/kg q8h; ceftriaxone, 1–2 g/d; ampicillin, 1 g q6h; imipenem-cilastatin, 250–500 mg q6–8h; ticarcillin/clavulanate, 3.2 g q8h; aztreonam, 1 g q8–12h.
Note: UTI, urinary tract infection; TMP, trimethoprim; TMP-SMX, trimethoprim-sulfamethoxazole.

short course of antibiotics to which the organism is susceptible probably constitutes the best course of action and nearly always eradicates bacteriuria. Treatment of asymptomatic catheter-associated bacteriuria may be of greatest benefit to elderly women, who most often develop symptoms if left untreated. If the catheter cannot be removed, antibiotic therapy usually proves to be unsuccessful and may in fact result in infection with a more resistant strain. In this situation, the bacteriuria should be ignored unless the patient develops symptoms or is at high risk of developing bacteremia. In these cases, use of systemic antibiotics or urinary bladder antiseptics may reduce the degree of bacteriuria and the likelihood of bacteremia.

In *pregnancy*, acute cystitis can be managed with 7 days of treatment with amoxicillin, nitrofurantoin, or a cephalosporin. All pregnant women should be screened for asymptomatic bacteriuria during the first trimester and, if bacteriuric, should be treated with one of the regimens listed in Table 269-1. After treatment, a culture should be performed to ensure cure, and cultures should be repeated monthly thereafter until delivery. Acute pyelonephritis in pregnancy should be managed with hospitalization and parenteral antibiotic therapy, generally with a cephalosporin or an extended-spectrum penicillin. Continuous low-dose prophylaxis with nitrofurantoin should be given to women who have recurrent infections during pregnancy.

Asymptomatic bacteriuria in noncatheterized patients is common, especially among elderly patients, but has not been linked to adverse outcomes in most circumstances other than pregnancy. Thus antimicrobial therapy is unnecessary and may in fact promote the emergence of resistant strains in most patients with asymptomatic bacteriuria. High-risk patients with neutropenia, renal transplants, obstruction, or other complicating conditions may require treatment when asymptomatic bacteriuria occurs. Seven days of therapy with an oral agent to which the organism is sensitive should be given initially. If bacteriuria persists, it can be monitored without further treatment in most patients. Longer-term therapy (4 to 6 weeks) may be necessary in high-risk patients with persistent asymptomatic bacteriuria.

UROLOGIC EVALUATION   Very few women with recurrent UTIs have correctable lesions discovered at cystoscopy or upon intravenous pyelography, and these procedures should not be undertaken routinely in such cases. Urologic evaluation should be performed in selected instances—namely, in women with relapsing infection, a history of childhood infections, stones or painless hematuria, or recurrent pyelonephritis. Most males with UTI should be considered to have complicated infection and thus should be evaluated urologically. Possible exceptions include young men who have cystitis associated with sexual activity, who are uncircumcised, or who have AIDS. Men or women presenting with acute infection and signs or symptoms suggestive of an obstruction or stones should undergo prompt urologic evaluation, generally by means of ultrasound.

PROGNOSIS   In patients with uncomplicated cystitis or pyelonephritis, treatment ordinarily results in complete resolution of symptoms. Lower tract infections in women are of concern mainly because they cause discomfort, morbidity, loss of time from work, and substantial health care costs. Cystitis may also result in upper tract infection or in bacteremia (especially during instrumentation), but little evidence suggests that renal impairment follows. When repeated episodes of cystitis occur, they are more commonly reinfections rather than relapses.

Acute uncomplicated pyelonephritis in adults rarely progresses to renal functional impairment and chronic renal disease. Repeated upper tract infections often represent relapse rather than reinfection, and a vigorous search for renal calculi or an underlying urologic abnormality should be undertaken. If neither is found, 6 weeks of chemotherapy may be useful in eradicating an unresolved focus of infection.

Repeated symptomatic UTIs in children and in adults with obstructive uropathy, neurogenic bladder, structural renal disease, or diabetes progress to chronic renal disease with unusual frequency. Asymptomatic bacteriuria in these groups as well as in adults without urologic disease or obstruction predisposes to increased numbers of episodes of symptomatic infection but does not result in renal impairment in most instances.

PREVENTION   Women who experience frequent symptomatic UTIs (≥ 3 per year on average) are candidates for long-term administration of low-dose antibiotics directed at preventing recurrences. Such women should be advised to avoid spermicide use and to void soon after intercourse. Daily or thrice-weekly administration of a single dose of TMP-SMX (80/400 mg), TMP alone (100 mg), or nitrofurantoin (50 mg) has been particularly effective. Norfloxacin and other fluoroquinolones have also been used for prophylaxis. Prophylaxis should be initiated only after bacteriuria has been eradicated with a full-dose treatment regimen. The same prophylactic regimens can be used after sexual intercourse to prevent episodes of symptomatic infection in women in whom UTIs are temporally related to intercourse. Other patients for whom prophylaxis appears to have some merit include men with chronic prostatitis; patients undergoing prostatectomy, both during the operation and in the postoperative period; and pregnant women with asymptomatic bacteriuria. All pregnant women should be screened for bacteriuria in the first trimester and should be treated if bacteriuria is demonstrated.

PAPILLARY NECROSIS

When infection of the renal pyramids develops in association with vascular diseases of the kidney or with urinary tract obstruction, renal papillary necrosis is likely to result. Patients with diabetes, sickle cell disease, chronic alcoholism, and vascular disease seem peculiarly susceptible to this complication. Hematuria, pain in the flank or abdomen, and chills and fever are the most common presenting symptoms. Acute renal failure with oliguria or anuria sometimes develops. Rarely, sloughing of a pyramid may take place without symptoms in a patient with chronic UTI, and the diagnosis is made when the necrotic tissue is passed in the urine or identified as a "ring shadow" on pyelography. If renal function deteriorates suddenly in a diabetic individual or a patient with chronic obstruction, the diagnosis of renal papillary necrosis should be entertained, even in the absence of fever or pain. Renal papillary necrosis is often bilateral; when it is unilateral, however, nephrectomy may be a life-saving approach to the management of overwhelming infection.

EMPHYSEMATOUS PYELONEPHRITIS AND CYSTITIS

These unusual clinical entities almost always occur in diabetic patients, often in concert with urinary obstruction and chronic infection. Emphysematous pyelonephritis is usually characterized by a rapidly progressive clinical course, with high fever, leukocytosis, renal parenchymal necrosis, and accumulation of fermentative gases in the kidney and perinephric tissues. Most patients also have pyuria and glucosuria. *E. coli* causes most cases, but occasionally other Enterobacteriaceae are isolated. Gas in tissues can often be seen on plain films and can best be confirmed and localized by computed tomography. Surgical resection of the involved tissue in addition to systemic antimicrobial therapy is usually needed to prevent a fatal outcome in emphysematous pyelonephritis.

Emphysematous cystitis also occurs primarily in diabetic patients, usually in association with *E. coli* or other facultative gram-negative rods and often in relation to bladder outlet obstruction. Patients with this condition are generally less severely ill and have less rapidly progressive disease than those with emphysematous pyelonephritis. The patient typically reports abdominal pain, dysuria, frequency, and (in some cases) pneumaturia. Computed tomography shows gas within both the bladder lumen and the bladder wall. Generally, conservative therapy with systemic antimicrobial agents and relief of outlet obstruction are effective, but some patients do not respond to these measures and require cystectomy.

RENAL AND PERINEPHRIC ABSCESS

See Chap. 112.

PROSTATITIS

The term *prostatitis* has been used for various inflammatory conditions affecting the prostate, including acute and chronic infections with specific bacteria and, more commonly, instances in which signs and symptoms of prostatic inflammation are present but no specific organisms can be detected. Patients with acute bacterial prostatitis can usually be readily identified on the basis of typical symptoms and signs, pyuria, and bacteriuria. To classify a patient with suspected chronic prostatitis correctly, first-void and midstream urine specimens, a prostatic expressate, and a postmassage urine specimen should be quantitatively cultured and evaluated for numbers of leukocytes. On the basis of the results of these studies and other considerations, a panel of the National Institutes of Health has recommended that patients with suspected chronic prostatitis be categorized as having chronic bacterial prostatitis, chronic pelvic pain syndrome, or asymptomatic inflammatory prostatitis. Each of these groups is discussed below.

ACUTE BACTERIAL PROSTATITIS When it occurs spontaneously, this disease generally affects young men; however, it may also be associated with an indwelling urethral catheter in older men. It is characterized by fever, chills, dysuria, and a tense or boggy, extremely tender prostate. Although prostatic massage usually produces purulent secretions with a large number of bacteria on culture, bacteremia may result from manipulation of the inflamed gland. For this reason and because the etiologic agent can usually be identified by Gram's staining and culture of urine, vigorous prostatic massage should be avoided. In non-catheter-associated cases, the infection is generally due to common gram-negative urinary tract pathogens (*E. coli* or *Klebsiella*). Initially, an intravenous fluoroquinolone, third-generation cephalosporin, or aminoglycoside can be administered. The response to antibiotics in acute bacterial prostatitis is usually prompt, perhaps because drugs penetrate more readily into the acutely inflamed prostate. In catheter-associated cases, the spectrum of etiologic agents is broader, including hospital-acquired gram-negative rods and enterococci. The urinary Gram stain may be particularly helpful in such cases. Imipenem, an aminoglycoside, a fluoroquinolone, or a third-generation cephalosporin should be used for initial therapy until the organism has been isolated and its susceptibilities have been determined. The long-term prognosis is good, although in some instances acute infection may result in abscess formation, epididymoorchitis, seminal vesiculitis, septicemia, and residual chronic bacterial prostatitis. Since the advent of antibiotics, the frequency of acute bacterial prostatitis has diminished markedly.

CHRONIC BACTERIAL PROSTATITIS This entity is now infrequent but should be considered in men with a history of recurrent bacteriuria. Symptoms are often lacking between episodes, and the prostate usually feels normal on palpation. Obstructive symptoms or perineal pain develops in some patients. Intermittently, infection spreads to the bladder, producing frequency, urgency, and dysuria. A pattern of relapsing infection in a middle-aged man strongly suggests chronic bacterial prostatitis. Classically, the diagnosis is established by culture of *E. coli*, *Klebsiella*, *Proteus*, or other uropathogenic bacteria from the expressed prostatic secretion or postmassage urine in higher quantities than are found in first-void or midstream urine. Antibiotics promptly relieve the symptoms associated with acute exacerbations but have been less effective in eradicating the focus of chronic infection in the prostate. The relative ineffectiveness of antimicrobial agents in achieving long-term cure has in part been due to the poor penetration into the prostate by most of these drugs. Fluoroquinolones have been considerably more successful than other antimicrobials, but even they must gener-

ally be given for at least 12 weeks to be effective. Patients with frequent episodes of acute cystitis in whom attempts at curative therapy fail can be managed with prolonged courses of low-dose antimicrobial agents (usually a sulfonamide, TMP, or nitrofurantoin), with a view toward suppressing symptoms and keeping the bladder urine sterile. Total prostatectomy obviously results in the cure of chronic prostatitis but is associated with considerable morbidity. Transurethral prostatectomy is safer but cures only one-third of patients.

CHRONIC PELVIC PAIN SYNDROME (FORMERLY NONBACTERIAL PROSTATITIS)
Patients who present with symptoms of prostatitis (intermittent perineal and low-back pain, obstructive voiding symptoms), few signs on examination, no bacterial growth in cultures, and no history of recurrent episodes of bacterial prostatitis are classified as having chronic pelvic pain syndrome (CPPS). Patients with CPPS are divided into inflammatory and noninflammatory subgroups based on the presence or absence of prostatic inflammation. Prostatic inflammation can be considered present when the expressed prostatic secretion and postmassage urine contain at least tenfold more leukocytes than the first-void and midstream urine specimens or when the expressed prostatic secretion contains ≥ 1000 leukocytes per microliter.

The likely etiology of CPPS associated with inflammation would be an infectious agent, but the agent has not yet been identified. Evidence for a causative role of both *U. urealyticum* and *C. trachomatis* has been presented but is not conclusive. Since most cases of inflammatory CPPS occur in young, sexually active men and since many cases follow an episode of nonspecific urethritis, the causative agent may well be sexually transmitted. The effectiveness of antimicrobial agents in this condition remains uncertain. Some patients benefit from a 4- to 6-week course of treatment with erythromycin, doxycycline, TMP-SMX, or a fluoroquinolone, but controlled trials are lacking. Patients who have symptoms and signs of prostatitis but who have no evidence of prostatic inflammation (normal leukocyte counts) and negative urine cultures are classified as having noninflammatory CPPS. Despite their symptoms, these patients most likely do not have prostatic infection and should not be given antimicrobial agents.

FURTHER READING
FIHN SD et al: Clinical practice: Acute uncomplicated urinary tract infection in women. N Engl J Med 349:259, 2003

GUPTA K et al: Increasing antimicrobial resistance and the management of uncomplicated community-acquired urinary tract infections. Ann Intern Med 135:41, 2001

HOOTON TM, STAMM WE: Diagnosis and treatment of uncomplicated urinary tract infection. Infect Dis Clin North Am 11:551, 1997

———— et al: Randomized comparative trial and cost analysis of 3-day antimicrobial regimens for treatment of acute cystitis in women. JAMA 273: 41, 1995

———— et al: A prospective study of risk factors for symptomatic urinary tract infection in young women. N Engl J Med 335:468, 1996

SAINT S et al: Enhancing the safety of critically ill patients by reducing urinary and central venous catheter–related infections. Am J Respir Crit Care Med 165:1475, 2002

STAMM WE, SCHAEFFER AJ (eds): *The State of the Art in the Management of Urinary Tract Infections.* Am J Med 113(Suppl 1A):1S–84S, 2002

TALAN DA et al: Comparison of ciprofloxacin (7 days) and trimethoprim-sulfamethoxazole (14 days) for acute uncomplicated pyelonephritis in women. JAMA 283:1583, 2000

WARREN JW et al: Guidelines for antimicrobial therapy of uncomplicated acute bacterial cystitis and acute pyelonephritis in women. Clin Infect Dis 29:745, 1999

Obstruction to the flow of urine, with attendant stasis and elevation in urinary tract pressure, impairs renal and urinary conduit functions and is a common cause of acute and chronic renal failure. With early relief of obstruction, the defects in function usually disappear completely. However, chronic obstruction may produce permanent loss of renal mass (renal atrophy) and excretory capability, as well as enhanced susceptibility to local infection and stone formation. Early diagnosis and prompt therapy are therefore essential to minimize the otherwise devastating effects of obstruction on kidney structure and function.

ETIOLOGY Obstruction to urine flow can result from *intrinsic* or *extrinsic mechanical blockade* as well as from *functional defects* not associated with fixed occlusion of the urinary drainage system. Mechanical obstruction can occur at any level of the urinary tract, from the renal calyces to the external urethral meatus. Normal points of narrowing, such as the ureteropelvic and ureterovesical junctions, bladder neck, and urethral meatus, are common sites of obstruction. When blockage is above the level of the bladder, unilateral dilatation of the ureter (*hydroureter*) and renal pyelocalyceal system (*hydronephrosis*) occur; lesions at or below the level of the bladder cause bilateral involvement.

Common forms of obstruction are listed in Table 270-1. Childhood causes include *congenital malformations* such as narrowing of the ureteropelvic junction and anomalous (retrocaval) location of the ureter. Posterior urethral valves are the most common cause of bilateral hydronephrosis in boys. Bladder dysfunction may be secondary to congenital urethral stricture, urethral meatal stenosis, or bladder neck obstruction. In adults, urinary tract obstruction is due mainly to *acquired defects*. Pelvic tumors, calculi, and urethral stricture predominate. Ligation of, or injury to, the ureter during pelvic or colonic surgery can lead to hydronephrosis which, if unilateral, may remain relatively silent and undetected. *Schistosoma haematobium* and genitourinary tuberculosis are infectious causes of ureteral obstruction. Obstructive uropathy may also result from extrinsic neoplastic (carcinoma of cervix or colon) or inflammatory disorders. Retroperitoneal fibrosis, an inflammatory condition in middle-aged men, must be distinguished from other retroperitoneal causes of ureteral obstruction, particularly lymphomas and pelvic neoplasms.

Functional impairment of urine flow usually results from disorders that involve both the ureter and bladder. Causes include neurogenic bladder, often with adynamic ureter, and vesicoureteral reflux. Reflux of urine from bladder to ureter(s) is more common in children, may result in severe unilateral or bilateral hydroureter and hydronephrosis. Abnormal insertion of the ureter into the bladder is the most common cause. Vesicoureteral reflux in the absence of urinary tract infection or bladder neck obstruction usually does not lead to renal parenchymal damage and often resolves with age. Reinsertion of the ureter into the bladder is indicated if reflux is severe and unlikely to improve spontaneously, if renal function deteriorates, or if urinary tract infections recur despite chronic antimicrobial therapy. Hydronephrosis is common in pregnancy, due both to ureteral compression by the enlarged uterus and to functional effects of progesterone.

CLINICAL FEATURES The pathophysiology and clinical features of urinary tract obstruction are summarized in Table 270-2. *Pain*, the symptom that most commonly leads to medical attention, is due to distention of the collecting system or renal capsule. Pain severity is influenced more by the rate at which distention develops than by the degree of distention. Acute supravesical obstruction, as from a stone lodged in a ureter (Chap. 268), is associated with excruciatingly severe pain, usually called *renal colic*. This pain is relatively steady and continuous, with little fluctuation in intensity, and often radiates to the lower abdomen, testes, or labia. By contrast, more insidious causes of obstruction, such as chronic narrowing of the ureteropelvic junction, may produce little or no pain yet result in total destruction of the affected kidney. Flank pain that occurs only with micturition is pathognomonic of vesicoureteral reflux.

Azotemia develops when overall excretory function is impaired, often in the setting of bladder outlet obstruction, bilateral renal pelvic or ureteric obstruction, or unilateral disease in a patient with a solitary functioning kidney. Complete bilateral obstruction should be suspected when acute renal failure is accompanied by anuria. Any patient with renal failure otherwise unexplained, or with a history of nephrolithiasis, hematuria, diabetes mellitus, prostatic enlargement, pelvic surgery, trauma, or tumor should be evaluated for urinary tract obstruction.

In the acute setting, bilateral obstruction may mimic prerenal azotemia. However, with more prolonged obstruction, symptoms of *polyuria* and *nocturia* commonly accompany partial urinary tract obstruction and result from impaired renal concentrating ability. This defect usually does not improve with administration of vasopressin and is therefore a form of acquired nephrogenic diabetes insipidus. Disturbances in sodium chloride transport in the ascending limb of Henle and, in azotemic patients, the osmotic (urea) diuresis per nephron lead to decreased medullary hypertonicity and hence a concentrating defect. Partial obstruction, therefore, may be associated with increased rather than decreased urine output. Indeed, wide fluctuations in urine output in a patient with azotemia should always raise the possibility of intermittent or partial urinary tract obstruction. If fluid intake is inadequate, severe dehydration and hypernatremia may develop. Hesitancy and straining to initiate the urinary

TABLE 270-1 *Common Mechanical Causes of Urinary Tract Obstruction*

Ureter	Bladder Outlet	Urethra
CONGENITAL		
Ureteropelvic junction narrowing or obstruction	Bladder neck obstruction	Posterior urethral valves
Ureterovesical junction narrowing or obstruction	Ureterocele	Anterior urethral valves
Ureterocele		Stricture
Retrocaval ureter		Meatal stenosis
		Phimosis
ACQUIRED INTRINSIC DEFECTS		
Calculi	Benign prostatic hyperplasia	Stricture
Inflammation	Cancer of prostate	Tumor
Trauma	Cancer of bladder	Calculi
Sloughed papillae	Calculi	Trauma
Tumor	Diabetic neuropathy	Phimosis
Blood clots	Spinal cord disease	
Uric acid crystals	Anticholinergic drugs and α-adrenergic antagonists	
ACQUIRED EXTRINSIC DEFECTS		
Pregnant uterus	Carcinoma of cervix, colon	Trauma
Retroperitoneal fibrosis	Trauma	
Aortic aneurysm		
Uterine leiomyomata		
Carcinoma of uterus, prostate, bladder, colon, rectum		
Lymphoma, pelvic inflammatory disease		
Accidental surgical ligation		

stream, postvoid dribbling, urinary frequency, and incontinence are common with obstruction at or below the level of the bladder.

Partial bilateral urinary tract obstruction often results in *acquired distal renal tubular acidosis, hyperkalemia,* and *renal salt wasting.* These defects in tubule function are often accompanied by renal tubulointerstitial damage. Initially the interstitium becomes edematous and infiltrated with mononuclear inflammatory cells. Later, interstitial fibrosis and atrophy of the papillae and medulla occur and precede these processes in the cortex.

Urinary tract obstruction must always be considered in patients with urinary tract infections or urolithiasis. Urinary stasis encourages the growth of organisms. Urea-splitting bacteria are associated with magnesium ammonium phosphate (struvite) calculi. *Hypertension* is frequent in acute and subacute unilateral obstruction and is usually a consequence of increased release of renin by the involved kidney. Chronic hydronephrosis, in the presence of extracellular volume expansion, may result in significant hypertension. *Erythrocytosis,* an infrequent complication of obstructive uropathy, is probably secondary to increased erythropoietin production.

DIAGNOSIS A history of difficulty in voiding, pain, infection, or changes in urinary volume is common. Evidence for distention of the kidney or urinary bladder can often be obtained by palpation and percussion of the abdomen. A careful rectal examination may reveal enlargement or nodularity of the prostate, abnormal rectal sphincter tone, or a rectal or pelvic mass. The penis should be inspected for evidence of meatal stenosis or phimosis. In the female, vaginal, uterine, and rectal lesions responsible for urinary tract obstruction are usually revealed by inspection and palpation.

Urinalysis may reveal hematuria, pyuria, and bacteriuria. The urine sediment is often normal, even when obstruction leads to marked azotemia and extensive structural damage. An abdominal scout film may detect nephrocalcinosis or a radiopaque stone. As indicated in Fig. 270-1, if urinary tract obstruction is suspected, a bladder catheter should be inserted. If diuresis does not follow, then abdominal ultrasonography should be performed to evaluate renal and bladder size, as well as pyelocalyceal contour. Ultrasonography is approximately 90% specific and sensitive for detection of hydronephrosis. False-positive results are associated with diuresis, renal cysts, or presence of an extrarenal pelvis, a normal congenital variant. Hydronephrosis may be absent on ultrasound when obstruction is associated with volume contraction, staghorn calculi, retroperitoneal fibrosis, or infiltrative renal disease.

In some cases, the intravenous urogram may define the site of obstruction. In the presence of obstruction, the appearance time of the nephrogram is delayed. Eventually the renal image becomes more dense than normal because of slow tubular fluid flow rate, which results in greater concentration of contrast medium. The kidney involved by an acute obstructive process is usually slightly enlarged, and there is dilatation of the calyces, renal pelvis, and ureter above the obstruction. The ureter is not tortuous as in chronic obstruction. In comparison with the nephrogram, the urogram may be faint, especially if the dilated renal pelvis is voluminous, causing dilution of the contrast medium. The radiographic study should be continued until the site of obstruction is determined or the contrast medium is excreted. Radionuclide scans, though sensitive for the detection of obstruction, define less anatomic detail than intravenous urography and, like the urogram, are of limited value when renal function is poor. They have a role in

patients at high risk for reaction to intravenous contrast. Patients suspected of having intermittent ureteropelvic obstruction should have radiologic evaluation while in pain, since a normal urogram is commonly seen during asymptomatic periods. Hydration often helps to provoke a symptomatic attack.

To facilitate visualization of a suspected lesion in a ureter or renal pelvis, *retrograde* or *antegrade urography* should be attempted. These diagnostic studies may be preferable to the intravenous urogram in the azotemic patient, in whom poor excretory function precludes adequate visualization of the collecting system. Furthermore, intravenous urography carries the risk of contrast-induced acute renal failure in patients with proteinuria, renal insufficiency, diabetes mellitus, or mul-

TABLE 270-2 *Pathophysiology of Bilateral Ureteral Obstruction*

Hemodynamic Effects	Tubule Effects	Clinical Features
ACUTE		
↑Renal blood flow ↓GFR ↓Medullary blood flow ↑Vasodilator prostaglandins	↑Ureteral and tubule pressures ↑Reabsorption of Na⁺, urea, water	Pain (capsule distention) Azotemia Oliguria or anuria
CHRONIC		
↓Renal blood flow ↓↓GFR ↑Vasoconstrictor prostaglandins ↑Renin-angiotensin production	↓Medullary osmolarity ↓Concentrating ability Structural damage; parenchymal atrophy ↓Transport functions for Na⁺, K⁺, H⁺	Azotemia Hypertension ADH-insensitive polyuria Natriuresis Hyperkalemic, hyperchloremic acidosis
RELEASE OF OBSTRUCTION		
Slow ↑ in GFR (variable)	↓Tubule pressure ↑Solute load per nephron (urea, NaCl) Natriuretic factors present	Postobstructive diuresis Potential for volume depletion and electrolyte imbalance due to losses of Na⁺, K⁺, PO₄³⁻, Mg²⁺, and water

Note: GFR, glomerular filtration rate.

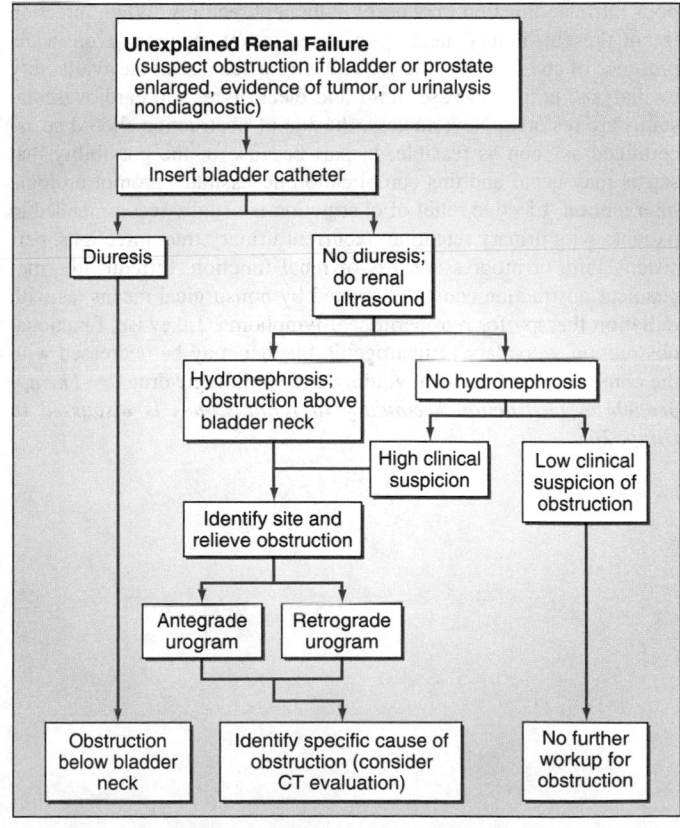

FIGURE 270-1 Diagnostic approach for urinary tract obstruction in unexplained renal failure. CT, computed tomography.

tiple myeloma, particularly if they are dehydrated. The retrograde approach involves catheterization of the involved ureter under cystoscopic control, while the antegrade technique necessitates placement of a catheter into the renal pelvis via a needle inserted percutaneously under ultrasonic or fluoroscopic guidance. While the antegrade approach may provide immediate decompression of a unilateral obstructing lesion, many urologists initially attempt the retrograde approach unless the catheterization is unsuccessful or general anesthesia is contraindicated.

Voiding cystourethrography is of value in the diagnosis of vesicoureteral reflux and bladder neck and urethral obstructions. Patients with obstruction at or below the level of the bladder exhibit thickening, trabeculation, and diverticula of the bladder wall. Postvoiding films reveal residual urine. If these radiographic studies fail to provide adequate information for diagnosis, endoscopic visualization by the urologist often permits precise identification of lesions involving the urethra, prostate, bladder, and ureteral orifices.

Computed tomography (CT) is useful in the diagnosis of specific intraabdominal and retroperitoneal causes of obstruction. The spiral CT is the preferred study to image urinary calculi. Magnetic resonance imaging may also be useful in the identification of specific obstructive causes.

R͙x TREATMENT

Urinary tract obstruction complicated by infection requires relief of obstruction as soon as possible to prevent development of generalized sepsis and progressive renal damage. On a temporary basis, drainage is often satisfactorily achieved by nephrostomy, ureterostomy, or ureteral, urethral, or suprapubic catheterization. The patient with acute urinary tract infection and obstruction should be given appropriate antibiotics based on in vitro bacterial sensitivity and the ability of the drug to concentrate in the urine. Treatment may be required for 3 to 4 weeks. Chronic or recurrent infections in an obstructed kidney with poor intrinsic function may necessitate nephrectomy. When infection is not present, immediate surgery often is not required, even in the presence of complete obstruction and anuria because of the availability of dialysis, until acid-base, fluid and electrolyte, and cardiovascular status are restored. Nevertheless, the site of obstruction should be ascertained as soon as feasible, in part because of the possibility that sepsis may occur and this complication necessitates prompt urologic intervention. Elective relief of obstruction is usually recommended in patients with urinary retention, recurrent urinary tract infections, persistent pain, or progressive loss of renal function. Infrequently, mechanical obstruction can be alleviated by nonsurgical means, as with radiation therapy for retroperitoneal lymphoma. Likewise, functional obstruction secondary to neurogenic bladder may be decreased with the combination of frequent voiding and cholinergic drugs. →*The approach to obstruction secondary to renal stones is discussed in Chap. 268.*

PROGNOSIS   With relief of obstruction, the prognosis regarding return of renal function depends largely on whether irreversible renal damage has occurred. When obstruction is not relieved, the course will depend mainly on whether the obstruction is complete or incomplete, bilateral or unilateral, and whether urinary tract infection is also present. Complete obstruction with infection can lead to total destruction of the kidney within days. Partial return of glomerular filtration rate may follow relief of complete obstruction of 1 and 2 weeks' duration but after 8 weeks of obstruction, recovery is unlikely. In the absence of definitive evidence of irreversibility, every effort should be made to decompress the obstruction in the hope of restoring renal function at least partially. A renal radionuclide scan, performed after a prolonged period of decompression, may be used to predict reversible renal function.

POSTOBSTRUCTIVE DIURESIS   Relief of bilateral, but not unilateral, complete obstruction commonly results in polyuria, which may be massive. The urine is usually hypotonic and may contain large amounts of sodium chloride, potassium, and magnesium. The natriuresis is due in part to the excretion of retained urea (osmotic diuresis). The increase in intratubular pressure very likely also contributes to the impairment in net sodium chloride reabsorption, especially in the terminal nephron segments. Natriuretic factors may also accumulate during uremia and depress salt and water reabsorption when urine flow is reestablished. In the majority of patients this diuresis results in the *appropriate* excretion of the excesses of retained salt and water. When extracellular volume and composition return to normal, the diuresis usually abates spontaneously. Therefore, replacement of urinary losses should only be done in the setting of hypovolemia, hypotension, or disturbances in serum electrolyte concentrations. Occasionally, iatrogenic expansion of extracellular volume is responsible for, or sustains, the diuresis observed in the postobstructive period. Replacement of no more than two-thirds of urinary volume losses per day is usually effective in avoiding this complication. The loss of electrolyte-free water with urea may result in hypernatremia. Serum and urine sodium and osmolal concentrations should guide the use of appropriate intravenous replacement. Often replacement with 0.45% saline is required. In a rare patient, relief of obstruction may be followed by urinary salt and water losses severe enough to provoke profound dehydration and vascular collapse. In these patients, an intrinsic defect in tubule reabsorptive function is probably responsible for the marked diuresis. Appropriate therapy in such patients includes intravenous administration of salt-containing solutions to replace sodium and volume deficits.

FURTHER READING

GULMI FA et al: Pathophysiology of urinary tract obstruction, in PC Walsh et al (eds): *Campbell's Urology*, 8th ed. Philadelphia, Saunders, 2002, pp 411–463

KLAHR S: Urinary tract obstruction, in RW Schrier, CW Gottschalk (eds): *Diseases of the Kidney*, 7th ed. Boston, Little, Brown, 2001, pp 751–787

WILSON DR: Renal function during and following obstruction. Ann Rev Med 28:329, 1977

ZEIDEL ML, PIRTSKHALAISHVILI G: Urinary tract obstruction, in BM Brenner (ed): *Brenner and Rector's The Kidney*, 7th ed. Philadelphia, Saunders, 2004, pp 1867–1894

271 | APPROACH TO THE PATIENT WITH GASTROINTESTINAL DISEASE
William L. Hasler, Chung Owyang

ANATOMIC CONSIDERATIONS

The gastrointestinal (GI) tract extends from the mouth to the anus and comprises several organs with distinct functions. The organs are separated by specialized independently controlled thickened sphincters that assist in gut compartmentalization. The gut wall is organized into well-defined layers that contribute to the functional activities in each region. The mucosa serves as a barrier to luminal contents or as a site for transfer of fluids or nutrients. Gut smooth muscle mediates propulsion from one region to the next. Many GI organs possess a serosal layer that not only provides a supportive foundation but also permits external input.

Interactions with other organ systems serve the needs both of the gut and the body. Pancreaticobiliary conduits deliver bile and enzymes into the duodenum. A rich vascular supply is modulated by GI tract activity. Lymphatic channels assist in gut immune activities. Intrinsic gut wall nerves provide the basic controls for propulsion and fluid regulation. Extrinsic neural input provides volitional or involuntary control to degrees that are specific for each gut region.

FUNCTIONS OF THE GASTROINTESTINAL TRACT

The GI tract serves two main functions—assimilation of nutrients and elimination of waste. The gut anatomy is organized to serve these functions. In the mouth, food is processed, mixed with salivary amylase, and delivered to the luminal GI tract. The esophagus propels the bolus into the stomach, and the lower esophageal sphincter prevents oral reflux of gastric contents. The esophageal mucosa has a protective squamous histology that does not permit significant diffusion or absorption. The propulsive activities of the esophagus are exclusively aboral and are coordinated with relaxation of the upper and lower esophageal sphincters upon swallowing.

The stomach furthers food preparation by triturating and mixing the bolus with pepsin and acid. Gastric acid also sterilizes the upper gut. Gastric motor activities exhibit regional variability: (1) the proximal stomach serves a storage function by relaxing to accommodate the meal; (2) the distal stomach exhibits phasic contractions that propel solid food residue against the pylorus, where it is repeatedly propelled proximally for further mixing before it is emptied into the duodenum; and (3) finally, the stomach secretes intrinsic factor for vitamin B_{12} absorption.

The small intestine serves most of the nutrient absorptive function of the gut. The intestinal mucosa exhibits villous architecture to provide maximal surface area for absorption and is endowed with specialized enzymes and transporters. Triturated food from the stomach is mixed with pancreatic juice and bile in the proximal duodenum to facilitate digestion. Pancreatic juice contains the main enzymes for carbohydrate, protein, and fat digestion as well as bicarbonate to optimize the pH for activation of these enzymes. Bile secreted by the liver and stored in the gallbladder is essential for intestinal lipid digestion. The proximal intestine is optimized for rapid absorption of nutrient breakdown products and most minerals, while the ileum is better suited for absorption of vitamin B_{12} and bile acids. The small intestine also aids in waste elimination. Bile contains byproducts of erythrocyte degradation, toxins, metabolized and unmetabolized medications, and cholesterol. Motor function of the small intestine delivers indigestible food residue and sloughed enterocytes into the colon for further processing. The small intestine terminates in the ileocecal junc-

tion, a sphincteric structure that prevents coloileal reflux and maintains small-intestinal sterility.

The colon prepares the waste material for controlled evacuation. The colonic mucosa dehydrates the stool, decreasing daily fecal volumes from the 1000 to 1500 mL delivered from the ileum to the 100 to 200 mL expelled from the rectum. The colonic lumen possesses a dense bacterial colonization that ferments undigested carbohydrates and short-chain fatty acids. Whereas transit times in the esophagus are on the order of seconds and times in the stomach and small intestine range from minutes to a few hours, propagation through the colon takes >1 day in most individuals. Colonic motor patterns exhibit a to-and-fro character that facilitates slow fecal desiccation. The proximal colon serves to mix and absorb fluid, while the distal colon exhibits peristaltic contractions and mass actions that function to expel the stool. The colon terminates in the anus, a structure with volitional and involuntary controls to permit retention of the fecal bolus until it can be released in a socially convenient setting.

EXTRINSIC MODULATION OF GUT FUNCTION

GI function is modified by influences outside of the gut. Unlike other organ systems, the gut is in physical continuity with the outside environment. Thus, protective mechanisms are vigilant against the deleterious effects of consumed foods, medications, toxins, and infectious organisms. Mucosal immune mechanisms include a lymphocyte and plasma cell population that resides in the epithelial layer and lamina propria backed up by lymph node chains to prevent noxious agents from entering the circulation. All substances absorbed into the bloodstream are filtered through the liver via the portal venous circulation. In the liver, many drugs and toxins are detoxified by a variety of mechanisms. Although intrinsic nerves control most basic gut activities, extrinsic neural input modulates a number of functions. The two activities under voluntary control are swallowing and defecation. Many normal GI reflexes involve extrinsic vagus or splanchnic nerve pathways. An active brain-gut axis further alters function in regions not under volitional regulation. As an example, stress alters GI transit as well as gut immune function.

OVERVIEW OF GASTROINTESTINAL DISEASES

GI diseases develop as a consequence of abnormalities within or outside of the gut and range in severity from those that produce mild symptoms and no long-term morbidity to those with intractable symptoms or an adverse outcome. Diseases may be localized to a single organ or exhibit diffuse involvement at a number of sites.

CLASSIFICATION OF GI DISEASES GI diseases are manifestations of alterations in nutrient assimilation or waste evacuation or in the activities supporting these main functions.

Impaired Digestion and Absorption Diseases of the stomach, intestine, biliary tree, and pancreas can disrupt nutrient digestion and absorption. Gastric hypersecretory conditions such as Zollinger-Ellison syndrome damage the intestinal mucosa and accelerate transit due to excess gastric acid. The most common intestinal maldigestion syndrome, lactase deficiency, produces flatus and diarrhea after dairy product ingestion and has no other adverse outcomes. Other intestinal enzyme deficiencies produce similar symptoms with ingestion of other simple sugars. Conversely, celiac disease, bacterial overgrowth, infectious enteritis, Crohn's ileitis, and radiation damage produce anemia, dehydration, electrolyte disorders, or malnutrition. Biliary obstruction from stricture or neoplasm may impair fat digestion. Impaired release of pancreatic enzymes in chronic pancreatitis or pancreatic cancer decreases intraluminal digestion and can lead to profound malnutrition.

Altered Secretion   Selected GI diseases result from dysregulation of gut secretion. Gastric acid hypersecretion occurs in Zollinger-Ellison syndrome, G-cell hyperplasia, retained antrum syndrome, and in some individuals with duodenal ulcer disease. Conversely, patients with atrophic gastritis or pernicious anemia release little or no gastric acid. Inflammatory and infectious small-intestinal and colonic diseases produce fluid loss through impaired absorption or enhanced secretion but do not usually cause malnutrition. Common intestinal and colonic hypersecretory conditions include acute viral infection, chronic *Giardia* or cryptosporidia infections, small-intestinal bacterial overgrowth, microscopic colitis, diabetic diarrhea, and abuse of certain laxatives. Less common causes include large colonic villous adenomas and endocrine neoplasias with tumor overproduction of secretagogue transmitters such as vasoactive intestinal polypeptide.

Altered Gut Transit   Alterations in gut transit are commonly secondary to mechanical obstruction. Esophageal occlusion often results from acid-induced stricture or neoplasm. Gastric outlet obstruction develops from peptic ulcer disease or gastric cancer. Small-intestinal obstruction most commonly results from adhesions but may also occur with Crohn's disease, radiation- or drug-induced strictures, and, less likely, malignancy. The most common cause of colonic obstruction is colon cancer, although inflammatory strictures develop in patients with inflammatory bowel disease, after certain infections, or with some drugs.

Retardation of propulsion also develops from disordered gut motor function. *Achalasia* is characterized by impaired esophageal body peristalsis and incomplete lower esophageal sphincter relaxation. *Gastroparesis* is the symptomatic delay in gastric emptying of solid or liquid meals. Intestinal pseudoobstruction causes marked delays in small-bowel transit due to injury to enteric nerves or intestinal smooth muscle. Slow transit constipation is produced by diffusely impaired colonic propulsion. Constipation is also produced by outlet abnormalities such as rectal prolapse, intussusception, or failure of anal relaxation upon attempted defecation.

Disorders of rapid propulsion are less common than those with delayed transit. Rapid gastric emptying occurs in postvagotomy dumping syndrome and with gastric hypersecretion. Exaggerated intestinal or colonic motor patterns are minor factors in symptoms with selected diarrheal conditions. Accelerated transit with hyperdefecation is noted in hyperthyroidism.

Immune Dysregulation   Many inflammatory GI conditions are consequences of altered gut immune function. The mucosal inflammation of *celiac disease* results from dietary ingestion of gluten-containing grains. Some patients with food allergy also exhibit altered immune populations. *Eosinophilic gastroenteritis* is an inflammatory condition with prominent mucosal eosinophils. *Ulcerative colitis* and *Crohn's disease* are disorders of uncertain etiology that produce mucosal injury primarily in the lower gut. The microscopic colitides, lymphocytic and collagenous colitis, exhibit colonic subepithelial infiltrates without visible mucosal damage. Bacterial, viral, and protozoal organisms may produce ileitis or colitis in selected patient populations.

Impaired Gut Blood Flow   Different GI regions are at variable risk for ischemic damage from impaired blood flow. Rare cases of gastroparesis result from blockage of the celiac and superior mesenteric arteries. More commonly encountered are intestinal and colonic ischemia, which are consequences of arterial embolus; arterial thrombosis; venous thrombosis; or hypoperfusion from dehydration, sepsis, hemorrhage, or reduced cardiac output. These may produce mucosal injury, hemorrhage, or even perforation. Some cases of radiation enterocolitis exhibit reduced mucosal blood flow.

Neoplastic Degeneration   All GI regions are susceptible to malignant degeneration to varying degrees. In the United States, colorectal cancer is most common and typically presents after age 50. Worldwide, gastric cancer is especially prevalent in certain Asian regions. Esophageal cancer develops with chronic acid reflux or in those with an extensive alcohol or tobacco use history. Small-intestinal neoplasms are rare and occur with underlying inflammatory disease. Anal cancers may arise with prior anal infection or inflammation. Pancreatic and biliary cancers elicit severe pain, weight loss, and jaundice and have poor prognoses. Hepatocellular carcinoma usually arises in the setting of chronic viral hepatitis or cirrhosis secondary to other causes. Most GI cancers are epithelial-derived; however, lymphomas and other cell types are also observed.

Disorders without Obvious Organic Abnormalities   The most common GI disorders show no abnormalities on biochemical or structural testing and include irritable bowel syndrome (IBS), functional dyspepsia, noncardiac chest pain, and functional heartburn. These functional bowel disorders exhibit altered gut motor function; however, the pathogenic relevance of these abnormalities is uncertain. Exaggerated visceral sensory responses to noxious stimulation may cause discomfort in these disorders. Symptoms in some patients result from altered processing of visceral pain sensations in the central nervous system. Patients with functional bowel abnormalities with severe symptoms may exhibit significant emotional disturbances on psychometric testing.

Genetic Influences   Although many GI diseases result from environmental factors, others exhibit hereditary components. Family members of inflammatory bowel disease (IBD) patients show a genetic predisposition to disease development themselves. Colonic and esophageal malignancies arise in certain inherited disorders. Hereditary pancreatitis is caused by mutation in the cationic trypsinogen gene. Rare genetic dysmotility syndromes are described. Familial clustering is even observed in the functional bowel disorders, although this may be secondary to learned familial illness behavior rather than a true hereditary factor.

SYMPTOMS OF GASTROINTESTINAL DISEASE   The most common GI symptoms are abdominal pain, heartburn, nausea and vomiting, altered bowel habits, GI bleeding, and jaundice (Table 271-1). Others are dysphagia, anorexia, weight loss, fatigue, and extraintestinal symptoms.

Abdominal Pain   Abdominal pain results from GI disease and extraintestinal conditions involving the genitourinary tract, abdominal wall, thorax, or spine. Visceral pain is generally midline in location and vague in character, while parietal pain is localized and precisely described. Common inflammatory diseases with pain include peptic ulcer, appendicitis, diverticulitis, IBD, and infectious enterocolitis. Other intraabdominal causes of pain include gallstone disease and pancreatitis. Noninflammatory visceral sources include mesenteric ischemia and neoplasia. The most common causes of abdominal pain are IBS and functional dyspepsia.

Heartburn   Heartburn, a burning substernal sensation, is reported intermittently by at least 40% of the population. Classically, heartburn is felt to result from excess gastroesophageal reflux of acid. However, some cases exhibit normal esophageal acid exposure and may result from heightened sensitivity of esophageal mucosal nerves.

Nausea and Vomiting   Nausea and vomiting are caused by GI diseases, medications, toxins, acute and chronic infection, endocrine disorders, labyrinthine conditions, and central nervous system disease. The best-characterized GI etiologies relate to mechanical obstruction of the upper gut; however, disorders of propulsion including gastroparesis and intestinal pseudoobstruction also elicit prominent symptoms. As with abdominal pain, IBS and functional dyspepsia commonly present with nausea and vomiting.

Altered Bowel Habits   Altered bowel habits are common complaints of patients with GI disease. Constipation is reported as infrequent defecation, straining with defecation, passage of hard stools, or a sense of

TABLE 271-1   *Common Causes of Common GI Symptoms*

Abdominal Pain	Nausea and Vomiting	Diarrhea	GI Bleeding	Obstructive Jaundice
Appendicitis	Medications	Infection	Ulcer disease	Bile duct stones
Gallstone disease	GI obstruction	Poorly absorbed sugars	Esophagitis	Cholangiocarcinoma
Pancreatitis	Motor disorders	Inflammatory bowel disease	Varices	Cholangitis
Diverticulitis	Functional bowel disorder	Microscopic colitis	Vascular lesions	Sclerosing cholangitis
Ulcer disease	Enteric infection	Functional bowel disorder	Neoplasm	Ampullary stenosis
Esophagitis	Pregnancy	Celiac disease	Diverticula	Ampullary carcinoma
GI obstruction	Endocrine disease	Pancreatic insufficiency	Hemorrhoids	Pancreatitis
Inflammatory bowel disease	Motion sickness	Hyperthyroidism	Fissures	Pancreatic tumor
Functional bowel disorder	Central nervous system disease	Ischemia	Inflammatory bowel disease	
Vascular disease		Endocrine tumor	Infectious colitis	
Gynecologic causes				
Renal stone				

incomplete fecal evacuation. Causes of constipation include obstruction, motor disorders of the colon, medications, and endocrine diseases such as hypothyroidism and hyperparathyroidism. Diarrhea is reported as frequent defecation, passage of loose or watery stools, fecal urgency, or a similar sense of incomplete evacuation. The differential diagnosis of diarrhea is broad and includes infections, inflammatory causes, malabsorption, and medications. IBS produces constipation, diarrhea, or an alternating bowel pattern. Fecal mucus is common in IBS, while pus characterizes inflammatory disease. Steatorrhea develops with malabsorption.

GI Bleeding Hemorrhage may develop from any gut organ. Most commonly, upper GI bleeding presents with melena or hematemesis, whereas lower GI bleeding produces passage of bright red or maroon stools. However, briskly bleeding upper sites can elicit voluminous red rectal bleeding, while slowly bleeding ascending colon sites may produce melena. Chronic slow GI bleeding may present with iron-deficiency anemia. The most common upper GI causes of bleeding are ulcer disease, gastroduodenitis, and esophagitis. Other etiologies include portal hypertensive causes, malignancy, tears across the gastroesophageal junction, and vascular lesions. The most prevalent lower GI sources of hemorrhage include hemorrhoids, anal fissures, diverticula, and arteriovenous malformations. Other causes include neoplasm, IBD, ischemia, infectious colitis, and other vascular lesions.

Jaundice Jaundice results from prehepatic, intrahepatic, or posthepatic disease. Posthepatic causes of jaundice include biliary diseases such as choledocholithiasis, cholangitis, stricture, and neoplasm and pancreatic disorders such as acute and chronic pancreatitis, stricture, and malignancy.

Other Symptoms Other symptoms are manifestations of GI disease. Dysphagia, odynophagia, and unexplained chest pain suggest esophageal disease. A globus sensation is reported with esophagopharyngeal conditions but also occurs with functional GI disorders. Weight loss, anorexia, and fatigue are nonspecific symptoms of neoplastic, inflammatory, gut motor, pancreatic, small bowel mucosal, and psychiatric conditions. Fever is reported with inflammatory illness, but malignancies also evoke febrile responses. GI disorders also produce extraintestinal symptoms. IBD is associated with hepatobiliary dysfunction, skin and eye lesions, and arthritis. Celiac disease may present with dermatitis herpetiformis. Jaundice can produce pruritus. Conversely, systemic diseases can have GI consequences. Systemic lupus may cause gut ischemia, presenting with pain or bleeding. Overwhelming stress or severe burns may lead to gastric ulcer formation.

EVALUATION OF THE PATIENT WITH GASTROINTESTINAL DISEASE

Evaluation of the patient with GI disease begins with a careful history and physical examination. Subsequent investigation with a variety of tools designed to test the structure or function of the gut are indicated in selected cases. Some patients exhibit normal findings on diagnostic testing. In these individuals, validated symptom profiles are employed for confident diagnosis of a functional bowel disorder.

HISTORY The history of the patient with suspected GI disease has several components. Symptom timing can suggest specific etiologies. Symptoms of short duration commonly result from acute infection, toxin exposure, or abrupt inflammation or ischemia. Long-standing symptoms point to an underlying chronic inflammatory or neoplastic condition or a functional bowel disorder. Symptoms from mechanical obstruction, ischemia, IBD, and functional bowel disorders are worsened by meal ingestion. Conversely, ulcer symptoms may be relieved by eating or antacids. The symptom pattern and duration may suggest underlying etiologies. Ulcer pain occurs at intermittent intervals lasting weeks to months, whereas biliary colic has a sudden onset and lasts up to several hours. Pain from acute inflammation, as with acute pancreatitis, is severe and persists for days to weeks. Meals elicit diarrhea in some cases of IBD and IBS, while defecation relieves discomfort in these conditions. Functional bowel disorders are exacerbated by stress. Sudden awakening from sleep suggests organic disease rather than a functional bowel disorder. Diarrhea from malabsorption usually improves with fasting, while secretory diarrhea persists without oral intake.

Symptom relation to other factors narrows the list of diagnostic possibilities. Obstructive symptoms with prior abdominal surgery raise concern for adhesions, whereas loose stools after gastrectomy or gallbladder excision suggest dumping syndrome or post-cholecystectomy diarrhea. Symptom onset after travel prompts a search for enteric infection. Medications produce pain, altered bowel habits, or GI bleeding. Lower GI bleeding likely results from neoplasm, diverticula, or vascular lesions in an older person and anorectal abnormalities or IBD in a younger individual. Celiac disease is prevalent in people of Irish descent, whereas IBD is more common in certain Jewish populations. A sexual history may raise concern for sexually transmitted diseases or immunodeficiency.

Over the past two decades, working groups have been convened to devise symptom criteria to improve the confident diagnosis of the functional bowel disorders and to minimize the number of unnecessary diagnostic tests performed. The most widely accepted symptom-based criteria are the *Rome criteria*. When tested against findings of structural investigations, the Rome criteria exhibit diagnostic specificities >90% for many of the functional bowel disorders.

PHYSICAL EXAMINATION The physical examination complements information from the history. Abnormal vital signs provide diagnostic clues and determine the need for acute intervention. Fever suggests inflammation or neoplasm. Orthostasis is found with significant blood loss, dehydration, sepsis, or autonomic neuropathy. Skin, eye, or joint findings may point to specific diagnoses. Neck examination with swallowing assessment evaluates dysphagia. Cardiopulmonary disease may present with abdominal pain or nausea; thus lung and cardiac examinations are important. Pelvic examination tests for a gynecologic source of abdominal pain. Rectal examination may detect blood, indicating gut mucosal injury or neoplasm, or a palpable inflammatory mass in appendicitis. Metabolic conditions and gut motor disorders have associated peripheral neuropathy.

Inspection of the abdomen may reveal distention from obstruction, tumor, or ascites or vascular abnormalities with liver disease. Ecchymoses develop with severe pancreatitis. Auscultation can detect bruits or friction rubs from vascular disease or hepatic tumors. Loss of bowel sounds signifies ileus, while high-pitched, hyperactive sounds characterize intestinal obstruction. Percussion assesses liver size and can detect shifting dullness from ascites. Palpation assesses for hepatosplenomegaly as well as neoplastic or inflammatory masses. Abdominal examination is helpful in evaluating unexplained pain. Intestinal ischemia elicits severe pain but little tenderness. Patients with visceral pain may exhibit generalized discomfort, while those with parietal pain or peritonitis have directed pain often with involuntary guarding, rigidity, or rebound. Patients with musculoskeletal abdominal wall pain may note tenderness exacerbated by Valsalva or straight leg lift maneuvers.

TOOLS FOR PATIENT EVALUATION Laboratory, radiographic, and scintigraphic tests can assist in diagnosis of suspected GI disease. The GI tract is also amenable to internal evaluation with upper and lower endoscopy and to examination of luminal contents. Histopathologic examinations of gastrointestinal tissues complement these tests.

Laboratory Selected laboratory tests facilitate the diagnosis of GI disease. Iron-deficiency anemia suggests mucosal blood loss, whereas vitamin B_{12} deficiency results from small-intestinal, gastric, or pancreatic disease. Either can also result from inadequate oral intake. Leukocytosis and increased erythrocyte sedimentation rates are found in inflammatory conditions, while leukopenia is seen in viremic illness. Severe vomiting or diarrhea elicits electrolyte disturbances, acid-base abnormalities, and elevated blood urea nitrogen. Pancreaticobiliary or liver disease is suggested by elevated pancreatic or liver chemistries. Thyroid chemistries, cortisol, and calcium levels are obtained to exclude endocrinologic causes of GI symptoms. Pregnancy testing is considered for young women with unexplained nausea. Serologic tests are available for rheumatologic diseases such as systemic lupus erythematosus or scleroderma. Hormone levels are obtained for suspected endocrine neoplasia. Intraabdominal malignancies produce tumor markers including carcinoembryonic antigen, while paraneoplastic dysmotility is associated with antineuronal antibodies. Other body fluids are sampled under certain circumstances. Ascitic fluid is analyzed for infection, malignancy, or findings of portal hypertension. Cerebrospinal fluid is obtained for suspected central nervous system causes of vomiting. Urine samples screen for carcinoid, porphyria, and heavy metal intoxication.

Luminal Contents Luminal contents can be examined for diagnostic clues. Stool samples are cultured for bacterial pathogens or examined for leukocytes or parasites. Duodenal aspirates can be examined for parasites or cultured for bacterial overgrowth. Fecal fat is quantified in possible malabsorption. Stool electrolytes and osmolarity can be measured in diarrheal conditions. A stool osmotic gap >100 mosmol/L indicates osmotic diarrhea. Laxative screens are done when laxative abuse is suspected. Gastric acid is quantified to rule out Zollinger-Ellison syndrome. Esophageal pH testing is done for refractory symptoms of acid reflux. Pancreatic juice is analyzed for enzyme or bicarbonate content to exclude pancreatic exocrine insufficiency.

Endoscopy The gut is accessible by means of endoscopy, which can provide the diagnosis of the causes of bleeding, pain, nausea and vomiting, weight loss, altered bowel function, and fever. Table 271-2 lists the most common indications for the major endoscopic procedures. Upper endoscopy evaluates the esophagus, stomach, and duodenum, while colonoscopy assesses the colon and distal ileum. Upper endoscopy is advocated as the initial structural test performed in patients with upper GI bleeding, suspected ulcer disease, esophagitis, neoplasm, malabsorption, and Barrett's metaplasia because of its ability both to visualize the abnormality directly and to biopsy it. Colonoscopy is the procedure of choice for colon cancer screening and surveillance; diagnosis of colitis secondary to infection, ischemia, radiation, and IBD; and characterization of causes of lower GI bleeding. Sigmoidoscopy examines the colon up to the splenic flexure and is currently used to exclude distal colonic inflammation or obstruction in young patients not at significant risk for colon cancer. For elusive GI bleeding secondary to arteriovenous malformations or superficial ulcers, small-intestinal examination is performed with push enteroscopy or capsule endoscopy. Endoscopic retrograde cholangiopancreaticography (ERCP) provides diagnoses of pancreatic and biliary disease. Endoscopic ultrasound is useful for evaluating the extent of disease in GI malignancy as well as exclusion of choledocholithiasis, evaluation of pancreatitis, drainage of pancreatic pseudocysts, and assessment of anal continuity.

Radiography/Nuclear Medicine Radiographic tests evaluate diseases of the gut and extraluminal structures. Oral or rectal contrast agents such as barium provide mucosal definition from the esophagus to the rectum. Contrast radiography also assesses gut transit and pelvic floor dysfunction. Barium swallow is the initial procedure for evaluation of dysphagia to exclude subtle rings or strictures and assess for achalasia, whereas small-bowel contrast radiology reliably diagnoses intestinal tumors and Crohn's ileitis. Contrast enemas are performed when colonoscopy is unsuccessful or contraindicated. Ultrasound and computed tomography (CT) evaluate regions not accessible by endoscopy or contrast studies, including the liver, pancreas, gallbladder, kidneys, and retroperitoneum. These tests are useful for diagnosis of mass lesions, fluid collections, and organ enlargement. Ultrasound is the initial test to evaluate for gallstone disease. Virtual CT colonoscopy is being evaluated as a method of colon cancer screening. Magnetic res-

TABLE 271-2 *Common Indications for Endoscopy*

Upper Endoscopy	Colonoscopy	Endoscopic Retrograde Cholangiopancreatography	Endoscopic Ultrasound
Dyspepsia despite treatment	Cancer screening	Jaundice	Staging of malignancy
Dyspepsia with signs of organic disease	Lower bleeding	Postbiliary surgery complaints	Characterize and biopsy submucosal mass
Refractory vomiting	Anemia	Cholangitis	Bile duct stones
Dysphagia	Diarrhea	Gallstone pancreatitis	Chronic pancreatitis
Upper bleeding	Polypectomy	Pancreatic/biliary/ampullary tumor	Drain pseudocyst
Anemia	Obstruction	Unexplained pancreatitis	Large gastric folds
Weight loss	Biopsy radiologic abnormality	Pancreatitis with unrelenting pain	Anal continuity
Malabsorption	Cancer surveillance:	Fistulas	
Biopsy radiologic abnormality	Family history, prior polyp/cancer, colitis	Biopsy radiologic abnormality	
Polypectomy	Palliate neoplasm	Pancreaticobiliary drainage	
Place gastrostomy	Remove foreign body	Sample bile	
Barrett's metaplasia surveillance		Sphincter of Oddi manometry	
Palliate neoplasm			
Sample duodenal tissue/fluid			
Remove foreign body			

onance imaging assesses the mesenteric circulation to screen for arterial exclusion; the pancreaticobiliary ducts to exclude neoplasm, stones, and sclerosing cholangitis; and the liver to characterize benign and malignant tumors. Angiography excludes mesenteric ischemia and determines spread of malignancy. Angiographic techniques also access the biliary tree in obstructive jaundice. Positron emission tomography may become useful in distinguishing malignant from benign pancreatic disease.

Scintigraphy both evaluates structural abnormalities and quantifies luminal transit. Radionuclide bleeding scans localize bleeding sites in patients with brisk hemorrhage so that therapy with endoscopy, angiography, or surgery may be directed. Radiolabeled leukocyte scans can search for intraabdominal abscesses not visualized on CT. Biliary scintigraphy is complementary to ultrasound in the assessment of cholecystitis. Scintigraphy to quantify esophageal and gastric emptying are well established, while techniques to measure small-intestinal or colonic transit are less widely used.

Histopathology Gut mucosal biopsies obtained at endoscopy evaluate for inflammatory, infectious, and neoplastic disease. Deep rectal biopsies assist with diagnosis of Hirschsprung's disease or amyloid. Liver biopsy is indicated in cases with abnormal liver chemistries, unexplained jaundice, following liver transplant to exclude rejection, and to characterize the degree of inflammation in patients with chronic viral hepatitis prior to initiating antiviral therapy. Biopsies obtained during CT or ultrasound can evaluate for other intraabdominal conditions not accessible by endoscopy.

Functional Testing Tests of gut function provide important data when structural testing is nondiagnostic. In addition to gastric acid and pancreatic function testing, functional testing of motor activity is provided by regional manometric techniques. Esophageal manometry is useful for suspected achalasia, whereas small-intestinal manometry tests for pseudoobstruction. Anorectal manometry is employed for unexplained incontinence or constipation from outlet dysfunction. Biliary manometry tests for sphincter of Oddi dysfunction with unexplained biliary pain. Electrogastrography measures gastric electrical activity in individuals with nausea and vomiting, whereas electromyography assesses anal function in fecal incontinence.

℞ TREATMENT

Management options for the patient with GI disease depend on the cause of symptoms. Available treatments include modifications in dietary intake, medications, interventional endoscopy or radiology techniques, surgery, and therapies directed to external influences.

Nutritional Manipulation Dietary modifications for GI disease include treatments that only reduce symptoms, therapies that correct pathologic defects, and measures that replace normal food intake with enteral or parenteral formulations. Changes that improve symptoms but do not reverse an organic abnormality include lactose restriction for lactase deficiency, liquid meals in gastroparesis, carbohydrate restrictions in dumping syndrome, and high-fiber diets in IBS. The gluten-free diet for celiac disease exemplifies a modification that serves as primary therapy to reduce mucosal inflammation. Enteral medium-chain triglycerides replace normal fats in patients with short-gut syndrome or severe ileal disease. Perfusion of liquid meals through a gastrostomy is performed in those who cannot swallow safely. Enteral feeding through a jejunostomy is considered for gastric dysmotility syndromes that preclude feeding into the stomach. Intravenous hyperalimentation is employed for individuals with generalized gut malfunction who cannot tolerate or who cannot be sustained with enteral nutrition.

Pharmacotherapy Several medications are available to treat GI diseases. Considerable health care resources are expended on over-the-counter (OTC) remedies. Many prescription drug classes are offered as short-term or continuous therapy of GI illness. A plethora of alternative treatments have gained popularity in GI conditions for which traditional therapies provide incomplete relief.

OVER-THE-COUNTER AGENTS OTC agents are reserved for mild GI symptoms. Antacids and histamine H_2 antagonists decrease symptoms in gastroesophageal reflux and dyspepsia, whereas antiflatulents and adsorbents reduce gaseous symptoms. Fiber supplements, stool softeners, enemas, and laxatives are used for constipation. Laxatives are categorized as stimulants, saline cathartics, and poorly absorbed sugars. Nonprescription antidiarrheal agents include kaolin-pectin combinations and loperamide. Supplemental enzymes include lactase pills for lactose intolerance and bacterial α-galactosidase to treat excess gas. In general, use of a nonprescription drug for more than a short time should be supervised by a health care provider.

PRESCRIPTION DRUGS Prescription drugs for GI diseases are a major focus of attention from pharmaceutical companies. Potent acid suppressants, including drugs that inhibit the proton pump, are advocated for acid reflux when OTC preparations are inadequate. Cytoprotective agents are sometimes used for upper gut ulcers. Prokinetic drugs stimulate GI propulsion in gastroparesis, pseudoobstruction, and constipation as well as the functional bowel disorders. Isotonic solutions containing polyethylene glycol are prescribed for constipation refractory to other agents. Prescription antidiarrheals include opiate drugs, anticholinergic antispasmodics, tricyclics, bile acid binders, and serotonin antagonists. Antispasmodics, tricyclic antidepressants, and selective serotonin reuptake inhibitors are also useful for functional abdominal pain and IBS, whereas narcotics are used for organic conditions such as disseminated malignancy and chronic pancreatitis. Antiemetics in several classes reduce nausea and vomiting. Potent pancreatic enzymes decrease malabsorption and pain from pancreatic disease. Antisecretory drugs such as somatostatin analogue, octreotide, treat hypersecretory states. Antibiotics treat ulcer disease secondary to *Helicobacter pylori*, infectious diarrhea, diverticulitis, intestinal bacterial overgrowth, and Crohn's disease. Anti-inflammatory and immunosuppressive drugs are used in ulcerative colitis, Crohn's disease, microscopic colitis, and refractory celiac disease. Chemotherapy with or without radiotherapy is offered for GI malignancies. Most GI carcinomas respond poorly to therapy, whereas lymphomas may be cured with appropriate intervention.

ALTERNATIVE THERAPIES Alternative treatments are marketed to treat selected GI symptoms. Ginger, acupressure, and acustimulation have been advocated for nausea, while pyridoxine has been investigated for nausea of first trimester pregnancy. Probiotics containing active bacterial cultures are used as adjuncts in some cases of refractory infectious diarrhea and have been used as primary therapy of IBS. Low-potency pancreatic enzyme preparations are sold as general digestive aids but have little evidence to support their efficacy.

Enteric Therapies/Interventional Endoscopy and Radiology Simple luminal interventions are commonly performed for GI diseases. Nasogastric tube suction decompresses the upper gut in ileus or mechanical obstruction. Nasogastric lavage using saline or water in the patient with upper GI hemorrhage determines the rate of bleeding and helps evacuate blood prior to endoscopy. Enteral feedings can be initiated through a nasogastric or nasoenteric tube. Enemas relieve fecal impaction or assist in gas evacuation in acute colonic pseudoobstruction. A rectal tube can be left in place to vent the distal colon.

In addition to its diagnostic role, endoscopy has therapeutic capabilities in certain settings. Cautery techniques can stop hemorrhage from ulcers, vascular malformations, and tumors. Injection with vasoconstrictor substances or sclerosants is used for bleeding ulcers, vascular malformations, varices, and hemorrhoids. Endoscopic encirclement of varices and hemorrhoids with constricting bands stops hemorrhage from these sites. Endoscopy can remove polyps or debulk lumen-narrowing malignancies. Endoscopic sphincterotomy of the ampulla of Vater relieves symptoms of choledocholithiasis. Obstructions of the gut lumen and pancreaticobiliary tree are relieved by endoscopic dilation or placement of plastic or expandable metal stents. In cases of acute colonic pseudoobstruction, colonoscopy is employed to withdraw luminal gas. Finally, endoscopy is commonly used to insert feeding tubes.

Radiologic measures are also useful in GI disease. Angiographic embolization or vasoconstriction decreases bleeding from sites not amenable to endoscopic intervention. Dilation or stenting with fluoroscopic guidance relieves luminal strictures. Contrast enemas can reduce volvulus and evacuate air in acute colonic pseudoobstruction. CT and ultrasound help drain abdominal fluid collections, in many cases obviating the need for surgery. Percutaneous transhepatic cholangiography relieves biliary obstruction when ERCP is contraindicated. Lithotripsy can fragment gallstones in patients who are not candidates for surgery. In some instances, radiologic approaches offer advantages over endoscopy for gastrostomy placement. Finally, central venous catheters for parenteral nutrition may be placed using radiographic techniques.

Surgery   Surgery is performed to cure GI disease, control symptoms without cure, maintain nutrition, or palliate unresectable neoplasm. Medication-unresponsive ulcerative colitis, diverticulitis, cholecystitis, appendicitis, and intraabdominal abscess are curable with surgery, whereas only symptom control without cure is possible with Crohn's disease. Surgery is mandated for ulcer complications such as bleeding, obstruction, or perforation and intestinal obstructions that do not resolve with conservative care. Fundoplication of the gastroesophageal junction is performed for presentations ranging from ulcerative esophagitis to drug-refractory symptoms of acid reflux. Achalasia responds to operations to relieve lower esophageal sphincter pressure. Surgery may be needed to place a jejunostomy for long-term enteral feedings. The threshold for performing surgery depends on the clinical setting. In all cases, the benefits of operation must be weighed against the potential for post-operative complications.

Therapy Directed to External Influences   In some conditions, GI symptoms respond to treatments directed outside the gut. Systemic anti-inflammatory or immunosuppressive drugs decrease GI manifestations of gut vasculitis. Plasma expanders may improve gut perfusion in bowel ischemia secondary to hypoperfusion. Finally, psychological therapies including psychotherapy, behavior modification, hypnosis, and biofeedback have shown efficacy in functional bowel disorders. Patients with significant psychological dysfunction and those with little response to treatments targeting the gut are likely to benefit from this form of therapy.

FURTHER READING

AMERICAN SOCIETY FOR GASTROINTESTINAL ENDOSCOPY: *Appropriate Use of Gastrointestinal Endoscopy Consensus Statement.* Manchester, MA, ASGE, 1992

FELMAN M et al: *Sleisenger and Fordtran's Gastrointestinal and Liver Disease,* 7th ed. Philadelphia, Saunders, 2002

YAMADA T (ed): *Textbook of Gastroenterology and Hepatology,* 4th ed. Philadelphia, Lippincott Williams & Wilkins, 2003

272   GASTROINTESTINAL ENDOSCOPY
Mark Topazian

Gastrointestinal endoscopy has been attempted for over 200 years, but the introduction of semi-rigid gastroscopes in the middle of the twentieth century marked the dawn of the modern endoscopic era. Since then, rapid advances in endoscopic technology have led to dramatic changes in the diagnosis and treatment of many digestive diseases. Innovative endoscopic devices and new endoscopic treatment modalities continue to expand the use of endoscopy in patient care.

Flexible endoscopes provide either an optical image (transmitted over fiberoptic bundles) or an electronic video image (generated by a charge-coupled device in the tip of the endoscope). Operator controls permit deflection of the endoscope tip; fiberoptic bundles bring light to the tip of the endoscope; and working channels allow washing, suctioning, and the passage of instruments. Progressive changes in the diameter and stiffness of endoscopes have improved the ease and patient tolerance of endoscopy.

ENDOSCOPIC PROCEDURES

Upper Endoscopy   Upper endoscopy, also referred to as esophagogastroduodenoscopy (EGD), is performed by passing a flexible endoscope through the mouth into the esophagus (Figs. 272-1 to 272-5), stomach (Figs. 272-6 to 272-10), bulb (Figs. 272-11, -12), and second duodenum. The procedure is the best method of examining the upper gastrointestinal mucosa. While the upper gastrointestinal radiographic series has similar accuracy for diagnosis of duodenal ulcer, EGD is superior for detection of gastric ulcers, detects flat mucosal lesions such as those of Barrett's esophagus, and permits directed biopsy and endoscopic therapy, if needed. Topical pharyngeal anesthesia is used, and intravenous conscious sedation is given to most patients in the United States to ease the anxiety and discomfort of the procedure, although in many countries EGD is routinely performed without sedation. Patient tolerance of unsedated EGD is improved by the use of an ultrathin, 5-mm diameter endoscope.

Colonoscopy   Colonoscopy is performed by passing a flexible colonoscope through the anal canal into the rectum and colon. The cecum is reached in >95% of cases, and the terminal ileum can often be examined. Colonoscopy is the "gold standard" for diagnosis of colonic mucosal disease (Figs. 272-13 to 272-21). Barium enema is more accurate for evaluation of diverticula and for accurate measurement of colonic strictures, but colonoscopy has greater sensitivity for colitis, polyps, and cancers. Conscious sedation is usually given before colonoscopy in the United States, although a willing patient and a skilled examiner can complete the procedure without sedation in many cases.

Flexible Sigmoidoscopy   Flexible sigmoidoscopy is similar to colonoscopy but visualizes only the rectum and a variable portion of the left colon, typically to 60 cm from the anal verge. This procedure causes abdominal cramping, but it is brief and is almost always performed without sedation. Flexible sigmoidoscopy is used for colorectal cancer screening and for evaluation of diarrhea and hematochezia.

Small-Bowel Enteroscopy   Two techniques are currently used to evaluate the small intestine, most often in patients with unexplained small-bowel bleeding. *Push enteroscopy* is performed with a long endoscope similar in design to an upper endoscope. The enteroscope is pushed down the small bowel with the help of a stiffening overtube that extends from the mouth to the duodenum. The mid-jejunum is usually reached, and the endoscope's instrument channel allows for biopsies or endoscopic therapy.

Capsule endoscopy involves the patient swallowing a disposable capsule containing a charge-coupled device chip. Color still images (Fig. 272-22) are transmitted wirelessly to an external receiver at fixed intervals until the capsule's battery is exhausted or it is passed into the toilet. Much of the jejunal and ileal mucosa is usually visualized.

Endoscopic Retrograde Cholangiopancreatography (ERCP)   During ERCP, a side-viewing endoscope is passed through the mouth to the duodenum, the ampulla of Vater is identified and cannulated with a thin plastic catheter, and radiographic contrast material is injected into the bile duct and pancreatic duct under fluoroscopic guidance (Fig. 272-23 to 272-25). When indicated, the sphincter of Oddi can be opened using the technique of endoscopic sphincterotomy (Fig. 272-26). Stones can be retrieved from the ducts, and strictures of the ducts can be biopsied, dilated, and stented. ERCP is often performed for therapy but remains important in diagnosis, especially for bile duct stones.

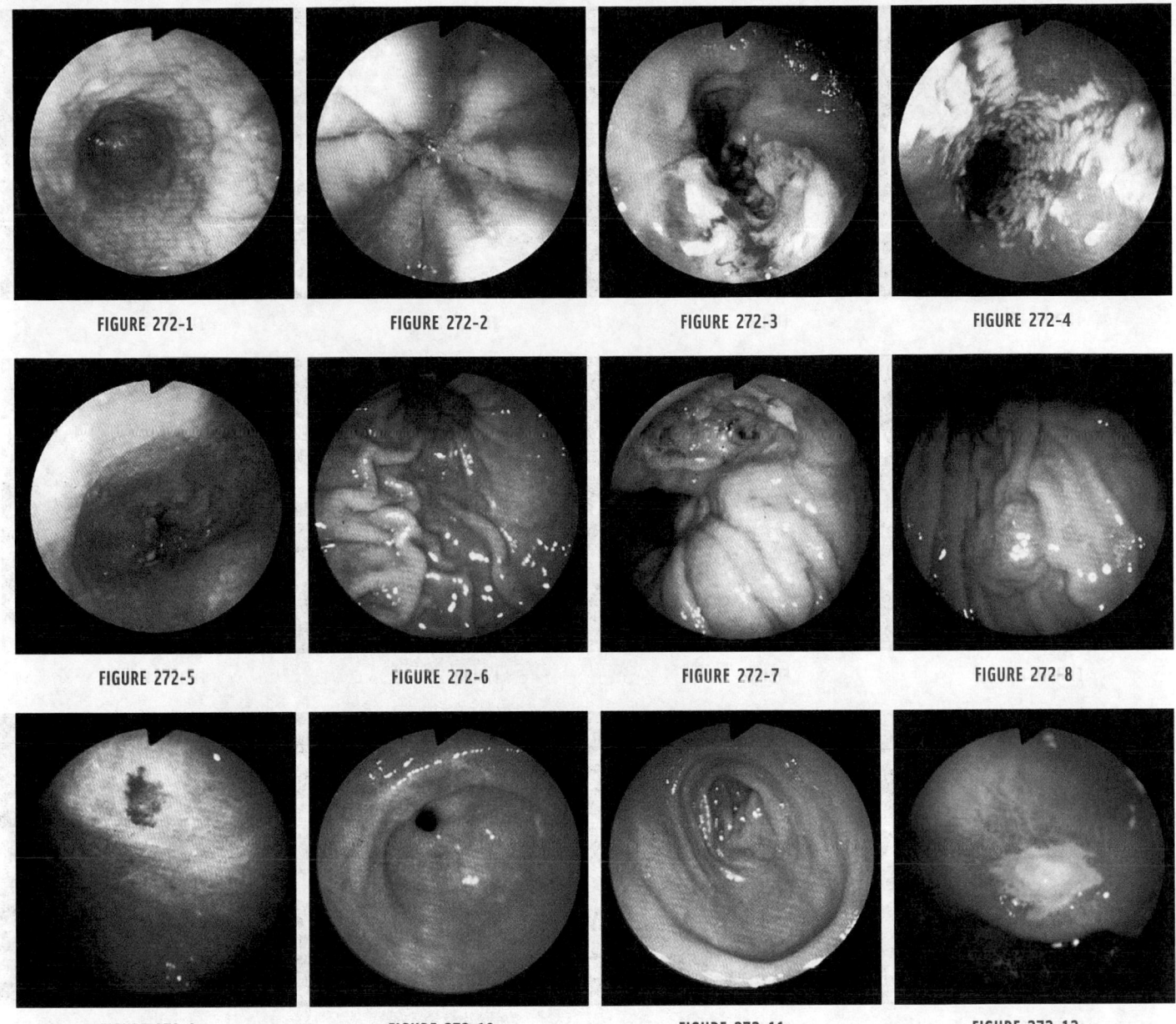

FIGURE 272-1 **FIGURE 272-2** **FIGURE 272-3** **FIGURE 272-4**

FIGURE 272-5 **FIGURE 272-6** **FIGURE 272-7** **FIGURE 272-8**

FIGURE 272-9 **FIGURE 272-10** **FIGURE 272-11** **FIGURE 272-12**

FIGURES 272-1 Normal esophagus where fine vasculature can be seen. **272-2** Linear red streaks with a central white streak extend up the esophagus in a peptic regurgitant esophagitis. **272-3** Ulcerated squamous cell carcinoma, with a depressed center, involving one wall of the esophagus. **272-4** Moniliasis of the esophagus—a white exudate is seen with underlying erythematous mucosa. **272-5** Barrett's metaplasia of the esophagus with an adenocarcinoma. The squamocolumnar junction is noted in the proximal esophagus. A mucosal irregularity in the center of the photograph was an adenocarcinoma. **272-6** Normal body of the stomach with rugal folds. **272-7** Large, benign, lesser curve gastric ulcer—the folds end at the ulcer margin. **272-8** The histologic type of this gastric polyp must be determined by excision and pathologic examination. **272-9** An arteriovenus malformation of the gastric mucosa. **272-10** A normal pylorus. Note the absence of gastric rugal folds in the antrum proximal to the pylorus. **272-11** A normal duodenal bulb. **272-12** A typical duodenal ulcer with a clean base is seen on the anterior surface of the duodenal bulb.

Endoscopic Ultrasound (EUS) EUS utilizes high-frequency ultrasound transducers incorporated into the tip of a flexible endoscope. Ultrasound images are obtained of the gut wall and adjacent organs, vessels, and lymph nodes. By sacrificing depth of ultrasound penetration and bringing the ultrasound transducer close to the area of interest via endoscopy, very high resolution images are obtained. EUS provides the most accurate preoperative local staging of esophageal, pancreatic, and rectal malignancies, although it does not detect most distant metastases. Examples of EUS tumor staging are shown in Fig. 272-27. EUS is also highly sensitive for diagnosis of bile duct stones, gallbladder disease, submucosal gastrointestinal lesions, and chronic pancreatitis. Fine-needle aspiration of masses and lymph nodes in the posterior mediastinum, abdomen, and pelvis can be performed under EUS guidance (Fig. 272-28).

RISKS OF ENDOSCOPY

All endoscopic procedures carry some risk of bleeding and gastrointestinal perforation. These risks are quite low with diagnostic upper endoscopy and colonoscopy (<1:1000 procedures), although the risk is as high as 2:100 when therapeutic procedures such as polypectomy, control of hemorrhage, or stricture dilation are performed. Bleeding and perforation are rare with flexible sigmoidoscopy. The risks for diagnostic EUS (without needle aspiration) are similar to the risks for diagnostic upper endoscopy.

Infectious complications are unusual with most endoscopic procedures. Some procedures carry a higher incidence of postprocedure bacteremia, and prophylactic antibiotics may be indicated for these procedures in some patients (Table 272-1).

FIGURE 272-13   **FIGURE 272-14**   **FIGURE 272-15**   **FIGURE 272-16**

FIGURE 272-17   **FIGURE 272-18**   **FIGURE 272-19**   **FIGURE 272-20**

FIGURE 272-21   **FIGURE 272-22**   **FIGURE 272-23**   **FIGURE 272-24**

FIGURES 272-13   Typical folds and vascular pattern can be seen in a normal colon.   **272-14**   This colonic adenomatous polyp is erythematous; a stalk is seen covered with normal mucosa.   **272-15**   Multiple, small, colonic adenomatous polyps in a case of familial polyposis coli. This colon was removed to prevent the development of cancer.   **272-16**   Colon adenocarcinoma—the cancer is multilobed and growing into the lumen.   **272-17**   Crohn's colitis with linear, serpiginous, white-based ulcers surrounded by colonic mucosa which is relatively normal.   **272-18**   Severe ulcerative colitis with diffuse ulceration, bleeding, and exudation.   **272-19**   Kaposi's sarcoma involving the colon in a patient with AIDS. The erythematous lesions involve most of the colonic mucosa in the photograph.   **272-20**   In this case of colonic varices, multiple, serpiginous, subephithelial structures impinge on the colonic lumen.   **272-21**   The mucosa appears normal in this pouch reconstructed from ileum to provide a reservoir after total proctocolectomy and ileoanal anastomosis.   **272-22**   Capsule endoscopy image of a jejunal vascular ectasia. (*Courtesy of Dr. Blair Lewis.*)   **272-23**   Normal papilla of Vater—bile is seen adjacent to the papilla.   **272-24**   Periampullary carcinoma—the mass at the papilla of Vater has been catheterized during ERCP.

ERCP carries additional risks. Pancreatitis occurs in about 5% of patients undergoing ERCP and is seen in up to 25% of patients with sphincter of Oddi dysfunction. Young anicteric patients with normal ducts are at increased risk. Post-ERCP pancreatitis is usually mild and self-limited but may infrequently result in prolonged hospitalization, surgery, diabetes, or death. Bleeding occurs after 1% of endoscopic sphincterotomies. Ascending cholangitis, pseudocyst infection, and retroperitoneal perforation and abscess may all occur as a result of ERCP.

The conscious sedation administered during endoscopy may cause respiratory depression or allergic reactions. Percutaneous gastrostomy tube placement during EGD is associated with a 10 to 15% incidence of complications, most often wound infections. Fasciitis, pneumonia, bleeding, and colonic injury may result from gastrostomy placement.

URGENT ENDOSCOPY

ACUTE GASTROINTESTINAL HEMORRHAGE   Endoscopy is an important diagnostic and therapeutic technique for patients with acute gastrointestinal hemorrhage. Although most gastrointestinal bleeding stops spontaneously, a minority of patients will have persistent or recurrent hemorrhage that may be life-threatening. Clinical predictors of rebleeding help identify patients most likely to benefit from urgent endoscopy and endoscopic, angiographic, or surgical hemostasis.

Initial Evaluation   The initial evaluation of the bleeding patient focuses on the magnitude of hemorrhage as reflected by the postural vital signs, the frequency of hematemesis or melena, and (in some cases) findings on nasogastric lavage. Decreases in hematocrit and hemoglobin lag the clinical course and are not reliable gauges of the magnitude of acute bleeding. This initial evaluation, completed well before the bleeding source is confidently identified, guides immediate supportive care of the patient and helps determine the timing of endoscopy. The magnitude of the initial hemorrhage is probably the most important indication for urgent endoscopy, since a large initial bleed increases the likelihood of ongoing or recurrent bleeding. Patients with resting hypotension, repeated hematemesis, nasogastric aspirate that does not clear with large volume lavage, orthostatic change in vital signs, or those requiring blood transfusions should be considered for urgent endoscopy. In addition, patients with cirrhosis, coagulopathy, or respiratory or renal failure and those over 70 years are more likely to have significant rebleeding.

Bedside evaluation also suggests an upper or lower gastrointestinal source of bleeding in most patients. Over 95% of patients with melena are bleeding proximal to the ligament of Treitz, and about 90% of patients with hematochezia are bleeding from the colon. Melena can result from bleeding in the small bowel or right colon, especially in older patients with slow colonic transit. Conversely, some patients with massive hematochezia are bleeding from a duodenal ulcer, with rapid intestinal transit. Early upper endoscopy should be considered in such patients.

Endoscopy should be performed after the patient has been resuscitated with intravenous fluids and transfusions as necessary. Marked coagulopathy or thrombocytopenia is usually treated before endoscopy, since correction of these abnormalities may lead to resolution of bleeding, and techniques for endoscopic hemostasis are limited in such patients. Metabolic derangements should also be addressed. Tracheal intubation for airway protection should be considered before upper endoscopy in patients with repeated hematemesis and suspected variceal hemorrhage.

Most patients with impressive hematochezia can undergo colonoscopy after a rapid colonic purge with a polyethylene glycol solution; the preparation fluid is often administered via a nasogastric tube. Colonoscopy has a higher diagnostic yield than angiography in lower gastrointestinal bleeding, and endoscopic therapy is appropriate in some cases. In a small minority of cases, persistent bleeding and recurrent hemodynamic instability prevent endoscopic visualization of the colonic mucosa, and other techniques (such as bleeding scans, angiography, or emergency subtotal colectomy) must be employed. Even in these cases, the anal and rectal mucosa should be visualized endoscopically early in the course, since bleeding lesions in or close to the anal canal are often amenable to surgical transanal hemostatic techniques.

Peptic Ulcer The endoscopic appearance of peptic ulcers provides useful prognostic information in patients with acute hemorrhage. When a platelet plug is seen protruding from a vessel wall in the base of an ulcer (a so-called sentinel clot or visible vessel), risk of major rebleeding from the ulcer is 40%. This finding often leads to local endoscopic therapy to decrease the rebleeding rate. A clean-based ulcer is associated with low (3 to 5%) risk of rebleeding; patients with melena and a clean-based duodenal ulcer are often discharged home from the emergency room or endoscopy suite if they are young, reliable, and otherwise healthy. Other findings have an intermediate risk of rebleeding: flat red or purple spots in the ulcer base have a 10% risk, and large adherent clots covering the ulcer base have a 20% risk. Occasionally, active spurting from an ulcer is seen (with >90% risk of ongoing bleeding). Examples of endoscopic stigmata of recent hemorrhage are shown in Fig. 272-29.

FIGURE 272-25 Endoscopic retrograde cholangiopancreatography (ERCP) for bile duct stones with cholangitis. *A.* Faceted bile duct stones are demonstrated in the common bile duct. *B.* After endoscopic sphincterotomy, the stones are extracted with a Dormia basket. A small abscess communicates with the left intrahepatic duct.

Patients with a visible vessel or active bleeding are usually treated endoscopically, decreasing rebleeding rates by about half. Hemostatic techniques include "coaptive coagulation" of the vessel in the base of the ulcer, using a thermal probe that is pressed against the site of bleeding, or injection of epinephrine or sclerosant into and around the vessel.

Varices Two complementary strategies guide therapy of bleeding varices: local treatment of the bleeding vessel and treatment of underlying portal hypertension. Local therapies (including endoscopic sclerotherapy, endoscopic band ligation, and balloon tamponade with a Sengstaken-Blakemore tube) effectively control acute hemorrhage in most patients and are the mainstay of acute treatment, although therapies that decrease portal pressures (pharmacologic treatment, surgical

FIGURE 272-26 Endoscopic sphincterotomy. *A.* A normal-appearing ampulla of Vater. *B.* Sphincterotomy is performed with electrocautery. *C.* Bile duct stones are extracted with a balloon catheter. *D.* Final appearance of the sphincterotomy.

FIGURE 272-27 Local staging of gastrointestinal cancers with endoscopic ultrasound. In each example the white arrowhead marks the primary tumor and the black arrow indicates the muscularis propria (mp) of the intestinal wall. "AO" indicates aorta.

A. T1 gastric cancer. The tumor does not invade the mp. *B.* T2 esophageal cancer. The tumor invades the mp. *C.* T3 esophageal cancer. The tumor extends through the mp into the surrounding tissue, and focally abuts the aorta.

shunts, or radiologically placed intrahepatic shunts) also play an important role.

Endoscopic band ligation is the preferred local therapy for bleeding esophageal varices. In this technique a varix is suctioned into a cap fitted on the end of the endoscope, and a rubber band is then released from the cap, ligating the varix. Acute hemorrhage can be controlled in up to 90% of patients, and complications (such as sepsis, symptomatic esophageal ulceration, or esophageal stenosis) are uncommon. Endoscopic sclerotherapy is another technique in which a sclerosing, thrombogenic solution is injected into or next to esophageal varices. Sclerotherapy also controls acute hemorrhage in most patients but has higher complication rates. These techniques are used when varices are actively bleeding during endoscopy or (more commonly) when varices are the only identifiable cause of acute hemorrhage.

After treatment of the acute hemorrhage, an elective course of endoscopic therapy can be undertaken with the goal of eradicating esophageal varices and preventing rebleeding months to years later. This chronic therapy is less successful, preventing long-term rebleeding in ~50% of patients. Pharmacologic therapies that decrease portal pressure have similar efficacy, and the two modalities may be combined.

Gastric varices are less amenable to endoscopic therapy and are best treated with a portal decompressive procedure (surgical portosystemic shunt or radiologic transjugular portosystemic shunt). Endoscopic therapy of gastric varices is usually reserved for actively bleeding varices or for patients with thrombosis of the portal venous system.

Dieulafoy's Lesion This lesion, also called *persistent caliber artery*, is a large-caliber arteriole that runs immediately beneath the gastrointestinal mucosa and bleeds through a pinpoint mucosal erosion. Dieulafoy's lesion is seen most commonly on the lesser curvature of the proximal stomach, causes impressive arterial hemorrhage, and is difficult to diagnose; it is often recognized only after repeated endoscopy for recurrent bleeding. Endoscopic therapy with a thermal probe usually controls acute bleeding and successfully ablates the underlying vessel once the bleeding site has been identified. Embolization or surgical oversewing are sometimes required.

Mallory-Weiss Tear A Mallory Weiss tear is a linear mucosal rent near or across the gastroesophageal junction that is often associated with retching or vomiting. When the tear disrupts a submucosal arteriole, brisk hemorrhage may result. Endoscopy is the best method of diagnosis, and an actively bleeding tear can be treated endoscopically with coaptive coagulation using a thermal probe or by injection of dilute epinephrine. Since Mallory-Weiss tears only rarely rebleed, a sentinel clot in the base of the tear is usually not treated endoscopically.

Vascular Ectasias Vascular ectasias are flat mucosal vascular anomalies best diagnosed by endoscopy. They usually cause slow intestinal blood loss and have several characteristic distributions in the gastrointestinal tract. When limited to the cecum, where they occur as senile lesions, or the gastric antrum (gastric antral vascular ectasias, or "watermelon stomach"), ectasias are often responsive to local endoscopic ablative therapy. Patients with diffuse small-bowel vascular ectasias (associated with chronic renal failure and with hereditary hemorrhagic telangiectasia) often continue to bleed despite endoscopic treatment of accessible lesions and may benefit from octreotide or estrogen/progesterone therapy.

Colonic Diverticula Diverticula form where nutrient arteries penetrate the muscular wall of the colon en route to the colonic mucosa. The artery found in the base of a diverticulum may bleed, causing painless and impressive hematochezia. Colonoscopy is indicated in patients with hematochezia and suspected diverticular hemorrhage, since other causes of bleeding (such as vascular ectasias, colitis, and colonic cancer) must be excluded. In addition, an actively bleeding diverticulum is occasionally seen and treated during colonoscopy.

GASTROINTESTINAL OBSTRUCTION AND PSEUDO-OBSTRUCTION Endoscopy is useful for evaluation and treatment of some forms of gastrointestinal obstruction. An important exception is small-bowel obstruction, which is generally not diagnosed by endoscopy or amenable to endoscopic therapy. Esophageal, gastroduodenal, and colonic obstruction or pseudoobstruction can all be diagnosed and often managed endoscopically.

Acute Esophageal Obstruction Esophageal obstruction by impacted food or an ingested foreign body is a potentially life-threatening

FIGURE 272-28 Endoscopic ultrasound (EUS)–guided needle aspiration. *A.* Ultrasound image of a 22-gauge needle passed through the duodenal wall and positioned in a hypoechoic pancreatic head mass. *B.* Micrograph of aspirated malignant cells. (*Image B courtesy of Dr. Mary Chacho.*)

TABLE 272-1 *Antibiotic Prophylaxis for Selected Endoscopic Procedures*

Patient Condition	Procedure Contemplated	Antibiotic Prophylaxis[a]
Prosthetic valve, history of endocarditis, systemic-pulmonary shunt, synthetic vascular graft (<1 year old)	High risk[b]	Recommended
	Low risk[c]	Optional[d] (insufficient data)
Rheumatic valvular disease, mitral valve prolapse with insufficiency, congenital cardiac malformations, hypertrophic cardiomyopathy	High risk	Optional[d] (insufficient data)
	Low risk	Not recommended[d]
Pacemakers, implantable defibrillators, prior coronary artery bypass grafts; prosthetic joints	High or low risk	Not recommended

[a] Acceptable antibiotic regimens for esophageal procedures include amoxicillin, 2 g PO, 1 h before, or ampicillin, 2 g IV, 30 min before upper endoscopy; clindamycin, 600 mg PO, may be substituted in penicillin-allergic patients. Acceptable regimens for colonic procedures in high-risk patients include gentamicin, 1.5 mg/kg (not to exceed 120 mg), and ampicillin, 2 g IV, within 30 min of colonoscopy, with or without amoxicillin, 1 g orally, 6 h later; vancomycin, 1 g IV, may be substituted for penicillins in penicillin-allergic patients. For colonic procedures in moderate-risk patients, amoxicillin, 2 g PO, 1 h before the procedure or vancomycin, 1 g IV, are sufficient.

[b] High-risk endoscopic procedures: stricture dilation, variceal sclerosis, endoscopic ultrasound with fine-needle aspiration, endoscopic retrograde cholangiopancreatography with an obstructed biliary tree.

[c] Low-risk endoscopic procedures: esophagogastroduodenoscopy and colonoscopy with or without biopsy and polyp removal, variceal ligation.

[d] Controversy exists and recommendations vary. For more detailed discussion, see Dajani AS et al: Clin Infect Dis 25:1448, 1997.

Source: Adapted from *Antibiotic Prophylaxis for Endoscopic Procedures*, American Society for Gastrointestinal Endoscopy, 1998.

event. Left untreated, the patient may develop esophageal ulceration, ischemia, and perforation. Patients with persistent esophageal obstruction often have hypersalivation and are usually unable to swallow water; endoscopy is generally the best initial test in such patients, since endoscopic removal of the obstructing material is usually possible, and the presence of an underlying esophageal stricture can often be determined. Radiographs of the chest and neck should be considered before endoscopy in patients with fever, obstruction for ≥24 h, or ingestion of a sharp object such as a fishbone. Radiographic contrast studies interfere with subsequent endoscopy and are not advisable in most patients with a clinical picture of esophageal obstruction. Occasionally, sublingual nifedipine or nitrates, or intravenous glucagon, may resolve an esophageal food impaction, but in most patients an underlying web, ring, or stricture is present and endoscopic removal of the obstructing food bolus is necessary.

Gastric Outlet Obstruction Obstruction of the gastric outlet is commonly caused by malignancy of the prepyloric gastric antrum or chronic peptic ulceration with stenosis of the pylorus. Patients vomit partially digested food many hours after eating. Gastric decompression with a nasogastric tube and subsequent lavage for removal of retained ma-

terial is the first step in treatment. The diagnosis can then be confirmed with a saline load test, if desired. Endoscopy is useful for diagnosis and treatment. Patients with pyloric stenosis may be treated with endoscopic balloon dilation of the pylorus, and a course of endoscopic dilation results in long-term relief of symptoms in about 50% of patients. Malignant pyloric obstruction can be treated with endoscopically placed expandable stents if the patient is deemed a poor surgical candidate.

Colonic Obstruction and Pseudoobstruction These both present with abdominal distention and discomfort; tympany; and a dilated, air-filled colon on plain abdominal radiography. Both conditions may lead to colonic perforation if untreated. Acute colonic pseudoobstruction is a form of colonic ileus that is usually attributable to electrolyte disorders, narcotic and anticholinergic medications, immobility (as after surgery), and retroperitoneal hemorrhage or mass. Multiple causative factors are often present. Either colonoscopy or a water-soluble contrast enema may be used to look for an obstructing lesion and differentiate obstruction from pseudoobstruction. One of these diagnostic studies should be strongly considered if the patient does not have clear risk factors for pseudoobstruction, if radiographs do not show air in the rectum, or if the patient fails to improve when the underlying causes of pseudoobstruction have been addressed. The risk of cecal perforation in pseudoobstruction rises when the cecal diameter exceeds 12 cm, and in such patients decompression of the colon may be achieved using intravenous neostigmine, colonoscopic decompression, or placement of a cecostomy tube. Most patients should receive a trial of conservative therapy (with correction of electrolyte disorders, removal of offending medications, and increased mobilization) before undergoing an invasive decompressive procedure.

Colonic obstruction is an indication for urgent intervention. Emergency diverting colostomy is often performed with a subsequent operation after bowel preparation to address the underlying cause. Colonscopic placement of an expandable stent is an alternative that can relieve malignant obstruction without emergency surgery and permit bowel preparation for elective surgery.

ACUTE BILIARY OBSTRUCTION The steady, severe pain that occurs when a gallstone acutely obstructs the common bile duct often brings patients to a hospital. The diagnosis of a ductal stone is suspected when the patient is jaundiced or when serum liver tests or pancreatic enzyme levels are elevated, and confirmed by direct cholangiography (performed endoscopically, percutaneously, or during surgery). ERCP is currently the primary means of diagnosing and treating common bile duct stones in most hospitals in the United States.

Bile Duct Imaging While transabdominal ultrasound and biliary scintigraphy are not sufficiently accurate for reliable diagnosis of bile duct stones, newer imaging modalities such as spiral computed tomography (CT), magnetic resonance cholangiopancreatography (MRCP), and EUS are more accurate and have an emerging role in diagnosis. Ex-

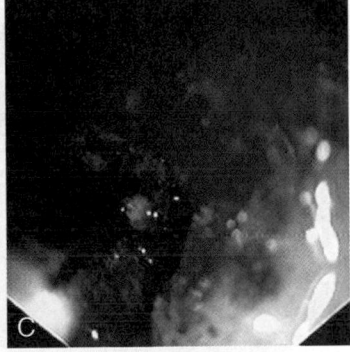

FIGURE 272-29 Endoscopic stigmata of recent bleeding in peptic ulcers. *A.* A flat red spot in an ulcer base. *B.* A sentinel clot protruding from an ulcer base. *C.* Coagulation of the sentinel clot shown in (*B*) with a thermal probe. (*Courtesy of American Society for Gastrointestinal Endoscopy.*)

amples of these modalities are shown in Fig. 272-30. During MRCP, images are obtained that demonstrate stagnant or slowly flowing fluid and subtract all other tissue. The resulting images of the right upper quadrant are strikingly similar to a direct cholangiogram, although with less resolution. MRCP can be performed rapidly without sedation and does not require any radiographic contrast. When an echo-endoscope is passed into the duodenum, detailed EUS views of the adjacent bile duct are readily obtained. While this procedure requires intravenous sedation, it has a very low incidence of complications, in contradistinction to ERCP. Spiral CT has a sensitivity of 85% for diagnosis of bile duct stones, MRCP has a sensitivity of 85 to 95%, and EUS has a sensitivity of 88 to 98%. EUS is more accurate than ERCP in some hands.

When a bile duct stone is highly likely and urgent treatment is required (as in a patient with jaundice and biliary sepsis), ERCP is the procedure of choice, since it remains the gold standard for diagnosis and provides immediate treatment. When a persistent bile duct stone is relatively unlikely (as in a patient with gallstone pancreatitis), less-invasive imaging techniques may supplant ERCP or intraoperative cholangiography.

Ascending Cholangitis Charcot's triad of jaundice, abdominal pain, and fever is present in about 70% of patients with ascending cholangitis and biliary sepsis. Initially, such patients are managed with fluid resuscitation and intravenous antibiotics. Abdominal ultrasound is often done to look for gallbladder stones and bile duct dilation. The bile duct may not be dilated early in the course of acute biliary obstruction, however. Medical management usually improves the patient's clinical status, providing a window of approximately 24 h during which biliary drainage should be established, typically by ERCP. Undue delay can result in recrudesence of overt sepsis and increased morbidity. If, in addition to Charcot's triad, shock and confusion are present (Reynolds's pentad), urgent attempts to restore biliary drainage are usually indicated.

Gallstone Pancreatitis Gallstones may cause acute pancreatitis as they pass through the ampulla of Vater. The occurrence of gallstone pancreatitis usually implies passage of a stone into the duodenum, and only about 20% of patients harbor a persistent stone in the ampulla or the common bile duct. Retained stones are more common in patients with jaundice, severe pancreatitis, or superimposed ascending cholangitis.

Urgent ERCP decreases the morbidity of gallstone pancreatitis in some subsets of patients. It remains unclear whether the benefit of ERCP is mainly attributable to treatment and prevention of ascending cholangitis or to relief of pancreatic duct obstruction. ERCP is warranted early in the course of gallstone pancreatitis if ascending cho-

langitis is also suspected, especially in a jaundiced patient. Urgent ERCP appears to benefit patients predicted to have severe pancreatitis using a clinical index of severity (such as the Glasgow or Ranson score).

ELECTIVE ENDOSCOPY

Dyspepsia and Reflux Dyspepsia is a chronic or recurrent burning discomfort or pain in the upper abdomen that may be caused by diverse processes such as gastroesophageal reflux, peptic ulcer disease, and "nonulcer dyspepsia," a heterogeneous category that includes disorders of motility, sensation, and somatization. Gastric and esophageal malignancies are less common causes of dyspepsia. Careful history-taking allows accurate differential diagnosis of dyspepsia in only about half of patients. In the remainder, endoscopy can be a useful diagnostic tool, especially in those patients whose symptoms are not resolved by an empirical trial of symptomatic treatment.

Gastroesophageal Reflux Disease (GERD) When classic symptoms of gastroesophageal reflux are present, such as water brash and substernal heartburn, presumptive diagnosis and empirical treatment are often sufficient. Although endoscopy is sensitive for diagnosis of esophagitis, it can miss cases of reflux, since some patients have symptomatic reflux without esophagitis. The most sensitive test for diagnosis of GERD is 24-h ambulatory pH monitoring. Endoscopy is indicated in patients with resistant reflux symptoms and in those with recurrent dyspepsia after treatment that is not clearly due to reflux on clinical grounds alone, to assess the esophagus and exclude other diseases. Endoscopy is also advised in a patient with reflux and dysphagia, to look for a stricture or malignancy. Endoscopy may be indicated in patients with long-standing ($\geq$10 years) frequent heartburn, who are at sixfold increased risk of Barrett's esophagus compared to a patient with <1 year of reflux symptoms. Patients with Barrett's esophagus usually enter a program of periodic endoscopy with biopsies, to detect dysplasia or early carcinoma.

Peptic Ulcer Peptic ulcer classically causes epigastric gnawing or burning, often occurring nocturnally and promptly relieved by food or antacids. Although endoscopy is the most sensitive diagnostic test for peptic ulcer, immediate endoscopy is not a cost-effective strategy in young patients with ulcer-like dyspeptic symptoms unless endoscopy is available at low cost. Patients with suspected peptic ulcer should be evaluated for *Helicobacter pylori* infection. Serology (past or present infection), urea breath testing (current infection), and stool tests are less invasive and costly than endoscopy with biopsy. Patients with ulcer-like symptoms despite treatment should undergo endoscopy to exclude gastric malignancy, and patients with "alarm symptoms" (weight loss, anemia, bleeding) should also undergo endoscopy.

Nonulcer Dyspepsia This may be associated with bloating and, unlike peptic ulcer, tends not to remit and recur. Most patients do not respond

FIGURE 272-30 Methods of bile duct imaging. Arrows mark bile duct stones. Arrowheads indicate the common bile duct, and the asterisk marks the portal vein. *A.* Endoscopic ultrasonography (EUS). *B.* Magnetic resonance cholangiography (MRCP). *C.* Helical computed tomography.

to acid-reducing, prokinetic, or anti-*Helicobacter* therapy and are referred for endoscopy to exclude a refractory ulcer. While endoscopy usefully excludes other diagnoses, it generally does little to improve the treatment of patients with nonulcer dyspepsia.

Dysphagia About 50% of patients with difficulty swallowing have a mechanical obstruction; the remainder have a motor disorder. Careful history-taking often suggests a diagnosis and leads to the appropriate use of diagnostic tests. Esophageal strictures typically cause progressive dysphagia, first for solids, then liquids; motor disorders often cause intermittent dysphagia for both solids and liquids. Some underlying disorders have characteristic historic features: Schatzki's ring causes episodic dysphagia for solids, typically at the beginning of a meal; pharyngeal motor disorders are associated with difficulty initiating deglutition ("transfer dysphagia") and nasal reflux with swallowing; and achalasia may cause nocturnal regurgitation of undigested food.

When mechanical obstruction is suspected, endoscopy is a useful initial diagnostic test, since it permits immediate biopsy and dilation of strictures, masses, or rings. Blind or forceful passage of an endoscope may lead to perforation in a patient with stenosis of the cervical esophagus or a Zencker's diverticulum, but gentle passage of an endoscope under direct visual guidance is reasonably safe. Endoscopy can miss a subtle stricture or ring in some patients.

When a motor disorder is suspected, esophageal radiography is the best initial diagnostic test. The pharyngeal swallowing mechanism, esophageal peristalsis, and the lower esophageal sphincter can all be assessed. In some disorders, subsequent esophageal manometry may also be important for diagnosis.

Anemia and Occult Blood in the Stool Iron-deficiency anemia may be attributed to poor iron absorption (as in celiac sprue) or, more commonly, chronic blood loss. Intestinal bleeding should be strongly suspected in men and postmenopausal women with iron-deficiency anemia, and colonoscopy is indicated in such patients, even in the absence of detectable occult blood in the stool. Some 30% will have large colonic polyps, 10% will have colorectal cancer, and additional patients will have colonic vascular lesions. When a convincing source of blood loss is not found in the colon, upper gastrointestinal endoscopy should also be performed; if no lesion is found, duodenal biopsies should be obtained to exclude sprue. Small-bowel evaluation may be appropriate if both EGD and colonoscopy are unrevealing.

Tests for occult blood in the stool detect hemoglobin or the heme moiety and are most sensitive for colonic blood loss, although they will also detect larger amounts of upper gastrointestinal bleeding. Patients over 50 with occult blood in normal-appearing stool should undergo colonoscopy to diagnose or exclude colorectal neoplasia. The diagnostic yield is lower than in iron-deficiency anemia. Whether upper endoscopy is also indicated largely depends on the patient's symptoms.

The small intestine may be the source of chronic intestinal bleeding, especially if colonoscopy and upper endoscopy are not diagnostic. The utility of small-bowel evaluation varies with the clinical setting and is most important in patients whose bleeding causes chronic or recurrent anemia. While small-bowel radiography is usually normal, capsule endoscopy yields a specific diagnosis in about 50% of such patients. The most common finding is mucosal vascular ectasias.

Colorectal Cancer Screening Most colon cancers develop from preexisting colonic adenomas, and colorectal cancer can be largely prevented by the detection and removal of adenomatous polyps. Screening for polyps and early, asymptomatic cancers can be accomplished both by testing stool specimens for occult blood and by directly examining the colonic mucosa. Since tests for occult blood are insensitive, detecting only about one-fourth of colon cancers and large polyps, visualization of at least a part of the colon is an important component of colorectal cancer screening.

The choice of screening strategy for an asymptomatic patient depends in part on their personal and family history. Patients at increased risk for colon cancer include those with a past history of inflammatory

bowel disease, colorectal polyps, a family history of first-degree family members with adenomatous polyps or cancer, or certain familial cancer syndromes. These considerations alter screening recommendations. An individual without these factors is generally considered at average risk.

Screening strategies are summarized in Table 272-2. Either sigmoidoscopy or colonoscopy may be used for cancer screening in asymptomatic average-risk patients. Use of sigmoidoscopy was based on the historic finding that the majority of colorectal cancers occurred in the rectum and left colon, and that patients with right-sided colon cancers had left-sided polyps. Over the past several decades, however, the distribution of colon cancers has changed, with proportionally fewer rectal and left-sided cancers than in the past. Large studies of colonoscopy for screening of average-risk individuals show that cancers are roughly equally distributed between left and right colon and half of patients with right-sided lesions have no polyps in the left colon. In addition, the new imaging technique of "virtual colonoscopy" holds considerable promise. This modality uses data from helical CT to generate a graphic display of a "flight" down the colonic lumen.

TABLE 272-2 *Colorectal Cancer Screening Strategies*

	Recommendation
AVERAGE-RISK PATIENTS	
Asymptomatic individuals ≥ 50 years of age	Colonscopy every 10 years, *or* Annual fecal occult blood test and flexible sigmoidoscopy every 5 years, or Double-contrast barium enema every 5 to 10 years
HIGH-RISK PATIENTS[a]	
Personal history	
History of colon cancer	Evaluate entire colon around the time of resection, then colonoscopy every 3 to 5 years
History of colonic adenomas	Colonoscopy every 3 to 5 years
Ulcerative pancolitis of 8 years' duration, left-sided colitis >15 years' duration	Colonoscopy with biopsies every 1 to 3 years
Family history	
Familial adenomatous polyposis	Consider genetic testing Annual sigmoidoscopy beginning at age 10 to 12; consider colectomy when polyps develop; if no polyps, annual sigmoidoscopy until age 40, then every 3 to 5 years
Hereditary nonpolyposis colorectal cancer (HNPCC)	Consider genetic testing Colonoscopy every 2 years beginning at 25 or when 5 years younger than the youngest affected relative; annual colonoscopy after age 40
Two first-degree relatives with colorectal cancer or adenomas	Colonoscopy every 3 to 5 years, beginning when 10 years younger than the youngest affected relative
One first-degree relative with sporadic colorectal cancer or adenoma before age 60	Same as above

[a] High-risk patients: Past history of inflammatory bowel disease, colorectal adenomatous polyps, or colorectal cancer; family history of colorectal adenomatous polyps, colorectal cancer, or certain familial cancer syndromes.

Source: Adapted from *Recommendations for Colorectal Cancer Screening and Surveillance in People at Average and at Increased Risk*, American Medical Association Council on Scientific Affairs, 2001; and *Screening and Surveillance Colonoscopy in Individuals at Increased Risk for Colorectal Cancer*, American Society for Gastrointestinal Endoscopy, 1998.

This technique is not yet sufficiently sensitive for routine clinical use, but further refinement may result in a useful noninvasive screening method.

Diarrhea Most cases of diarrhea are acute, self-limited, and due to infections or medication. Chronic diarrhea (lasting >6 weeks) is more often due to a primary inflammatory or malabsorptive disorder, is less likely to resolve spontaneously, and generally requires diagnostic evaluation. Patients with chronic diarrhea or severe, unexplained acute diarrhea often undergo endoscopy if stool tests for pathogens are unrevealing. The choice of endoscopic test depends on the clinical setting.

Patients with colonic symptoms and findings such as bloody diarrhea, tenesmus, fever, or leukocytes in stool generally undergo sigmoidoscopy or colonoscopy to look for colitis. Sigmoidoscopy is often adequate and is the best initial test in most such patients. On the other hand, patients with symptoms and findings suggesting small-bowel disease such as large-volume watery stools, substantial weight loss, and malabsorption of iron, calcium, or fat may undergo upper endoscopy with duodenal biopsies.

Many patients with chronic diarrhea do not fit either of these patterns. When there is a long-standing history of alternating constipation and diarrhea dating to early adulthood, without findings such as blood in the stool or anemia, a diagnosis of irritable bowel syndrome may be made without direct visualization of the bowel. Steatorrhea and upper abdominal pain may prompt evaluation of the pancreas rather than the gut. Patients whose chronic diarrhea is not easily categorized often undergo initial colonoscopy to examine the entire colon (and terminal ileum) for inflammatory or neoplastic disease.

Minor Hematochezia Bright red blood passed with or on formed brown stool usually has a rectal, anal, or distal sigmoid source. Patients with even trivial amounts of hematochezia should be investigated with flexible sigmoidoscopy to exclude large polyps or cancers in the distal bowel. Patients who report red blood on the toilet tissue only, without blood in the toilet or on the stool, are bleeding from a lesion in the anal canal, and careful external and digital examinations and anoscopy are sufficient for diagnosis in most cases.

Unexplained Pancreatitis About 20% of patients with pancreatitis have no identified cause after routine clinical investigation (including a review of medication and alcohol use, measurement of serum triglyceride and calcium levels, abdominal ultrasonography, and CT). Endoscopic techniques lead to a specific diagnosis in the majority of such patients, often altering clinical management. Endoscopic investigation is particularly appropriate if the patient has had more than one episode of pancreatitis.

Microlithiasis, or the presence of microscopic crystals in bile, is a leading cause of previously unexplained acute pancreatitis and is sometimes seen during abdominal ultrasonography as layering sludge or flecks of floating, echogenic material in the gallbladder. Gallbladder bile can be obtained for microscopic analysis by administering a cholecystokinin analogue during endoscopy, causing contraction of the gallbladder. Bile is suctioned from the duodenum as it drains from the papilla, and the darkest fraction is examined for cholesterol crystals or bilirubinate granules. Combined EUS of the gallbladder and bile microscopy is probably the most sensitive means of diagnosing microlithiasis.

Previously undetected chronic pancreatitis, pancreatic malignancy, or pancreas divisum may be diagnosed by either ERCP or EUS. Sphincter of Oddi dysfunction probably causes some cases of pancreatitis and can be diagnosed by manometric studies performed during ERCP.

Cancer Staging Local staging of esophageal, gastric, pancreatic, bile duct, and rectal cancers can be obtained with EUS. EUS with fine-needle aspiration (Fig. 272-28) currently provides the most accurate preoperative assessment of local tumor and nodal staging, but it does not detect distant metastases. Details of the local tumor stage can guide treatment decisions including resectability and need for neoadjuvant therapy. EUS with transesophageal needle biopsy may also be used to assess the presence of non-small cell lung cancer in mediastinal nodes.

OPEN-ACCESS ENDOSCOPY

While gastroenterologists have traditionally seen patients in consultation before arranging an endoscopic procedure, direct scheduling of endoscopic procedures by primary care physicians, or *open-access endoscopy*, is an increasingly common practice. When the indications for endoscopy are clear cut and appropriate, the procedural risks are low, and the patient understands what to expect, open-access endoscopy streamlines patient care and decreases costs.

Patients referred for open-access endoscopy should have a recent history, physical examination, and medication review. A copy of such an evaluation should be available when the patient comes to the endoscopy suite. Patients with unstable cardiovascular or respiratory conditions should not be referred directly for open-access endoscopy. Patients with selected cardiac conditions undergoing certain procedures should be prescribed prophylactic antibiotics prior to endoscopy, as described in Table 272-1. In addition, patients taking anticoagulants may need changes in treatment before endoscopy, as detailed in Table 272-3. While many endoscopists recommend discontinuing aspirin for 5 days before elective endoscopic procedures, most evidence suggests that in the absence of a preexisting bleeding disorder it is safe to perform endoscopic procedures in patients taking aspirin and nonsteroidal anti-inflammatory drugs.

Common indications for open-access EGD include dyspepsia resistant to a trial of appropriate therapy; gastrointestinal bleeding; and persistent anorexia, or early satiety. Open-access colonoscopy is often requested in men or postmenopausal women with iron-deficiency anemia, patients over age 50 with occult blood in the stool, patients with a previous history of colorectal adenomatous polyps or cancer, and for colorectal cancer screening. Flexible sigmoidoscopy is commonly performed as an open-access procedure.

When patients are referred for open-access colonoscopy, the primary care provider may need to choose a colonic preparation. Commonly used oral preparations include polyethelene glycol lavage solution and sodium phosphate. Sodium phosphate may cause fluid and electrolyte abnormalities, especially in patients with renal failure, congestive heart failure, and patients over 70 years of age.

TABLE 272-3 *Management of Anticoagulation before Endoscopic Procedures*

	High Patient Risk of Thromboembolism[a]	Low Patient Risk of Thromboembolism[b]
High-risk procedure[c]	Stop warfarin 3–5 days before the procedure; consider heparin when INR is below the therapeutic range	Stop warfarin 3–5 days before the procedure; restart warfarin after the procedure
Low-risk procedure[d]	No change in anticoagulation; elective procedures should be delayed while INR is above the therapeutic range	No change in anticoagulation; elective procedures should be delayed while INR is above the therapeutic range

[a] High-risk conditions: atrial fibrillation associated with valvular heart disease, mechanical valve in the mitral position, mechanical valve and prior thromboembolic event.

[b] Low-risk conditions: Uncomplicated or paroxysmal nonvalvular atrial fibrillation, mechanical valve in the aortic position, bioprosthetic valve, deep vein thrombosis.

[c] High-risk procedures: Polypectomy, stricture dilation, treatment of varices, gastrostomy placement, biliary sphincterotomy, endoscopic ultrasound with needle aspiration.

[d] Low-risk procedures: Diagnostic upper endoscopy, colonoscopy, sigmoidoscopy with or without biopsy, diagnostic endoscopic retrograde cholangiopancreatography, endoscopic ultrasound without needle aspiration.

Note: INR, international normalized ratio.

Source: Adapted from *The Management of Anticoagulants and Anti-Inflammatory Medications in Patients Undergoing Endoscopic Procedures*, American Society for Gastrointestinal Endoscopy, 1998.

FURTHER READING

BARON TH: Expandable metal stents for the treatment of cancerous obstruction of the gastrointestinal tract. N Engl J Med 344:1681, 2001

DAJANI AS et al: Prevention of bacterial endocarditis: Recommendations by the American Heart Association. Clin Infect Dis 25:1448, 1997

IMPERIALE TF et al: Risk of advanced proximal neoplasms in asymptomatic adults according to the distal colorectal findings. N Engl J Med 343:169, 2000

JENSEN DM et al: Urgent colonoscopy for the diagnosis and treatment of severe diverticular hemorrhage. N Engl J Med 342:78, 2000

LIEBERMAN DA et al: Use of colonoscopy to screen asymptomatic adults for colorectal cancer. N Engl J Med 343:162, 2000

OFMAN JJ, RABENECK L: The effectiveness of endoscopy in the management of dyspepsia: A qualitative systematic review. Am J Med 106:335, 1999

273 DISEASES OF THE ESOPHAGUS
Raj K. Goyal

The two major functions of the esophagus are the transport of the food bolus from the mouth to the stomach and the prevention of retrograde flow of gastrointestinal contents. The transport function is achieved by peristaltic contractions in the pharynx and esophagus associated with relaxation of upper and lower esophageal sphincters (Chap. 33). Retrograde flow is prevented by the two esophageal sphincters, which remain closed between swallows. The upper esophageal sphincter (UES) consists of the cricopharyngeus and inferior pharyngeal constrictor muscles, both of which are striated muscles innervated by excitatory somatic lower motor neurons. These muscles exhibit no myogenic tone and receive no inhibitory innervation. The UES remains closed owing to the elastic properties of its wall and to neurogenic tonic contraction of the sphincter muscles. Inhibition in the central nervous system opens the sphincter muscles in concert with forward displacement of the larynx by the suprahyoid muscles. In contrast, the lower esophageal sphincter (LES) is composed of smooth muscle and is innervated by parallel sets of parasympathetic excitatory and inhibitory pathways. It remains closed because of its intrinsic myogenic tone, which is modulated by the excitatory and inhibitory nerves. It opens in response to the activity of the inhibitory nerves. The neurotransmitters of the excitatory nerves are acetylcholine and substance P, and those of the inhibitory nerves are vasoactive intestinal peptide (VIP) and nitric oxide. The function of the LES is supplemented by the striated muscle of the diaphragmatic crura, which surrounds the LES and acts as an external LES. Relaxation of the LES without esophageal contraction occurs during belching and gastric distention. Gastric distention–evoked transient lower esophageal sphincter relaxation (tLESR) is a vasovagal reflex. Fatty meals, smoking, and beverages with a high xanthine content (tea, coffee, cola) also cause a reduction in sphincter pressure. Many hormones and neurotransmitters can modify LES pressure. Muscarinic M_2 and M_3 receptor agonists, α-adrenergic agonists, gastrin, substance P, and prostaglandin $F_{2\alpha}$ cause contraction. Nicotine, β-adrenergic agonists, dopamine, cholecystokinin, secretin, VIP, calcitonin gene–related peptide (CGRP), adenosine, prostaglandin E, and nitric oxide donors such as nitrates reduce sphincter pressure.

SYMPTOMS

DYSPHAGIA See Chap. 33

ESOPHAGEAL PAIN *Heartburn*, or pyrosis, is characterized by burning retrosternal discomfort that may move up and down the chest like a wave. When severe, it may radiate to the sides of the chest, the neck, and the angles of the jaw. Heartburn is a characteristic symptom of reflux esophagitis and may be associated with regurgitation or a feeling of warm fluid climbing up the throat. It is aggravated by bending forward, straining, or lying recumbent and is worse after meals. It is relieved by an upright posture, by the swallowing of saliva or water, and, more reliably, by antacids. Heartburn is produced by heightened mucosal sensitivity and can be reproduced by infusion of dilute (0.1 *N*) hydrochloric acid (Bernstein test) or neutral hyperosmolar solutions into the esophagus.

Odynophagia, or painful swallowing, is characteristic of nonreflux esophagitis, particularly monilial and herpes esophagitis. Odynophagia may occur with peptic ulcer of the esophagus (Barrett's ulcer), carcinoma with periesophageal involvement, caustic damage of the esophagus, and esophageal perforation. Odynophagia is unusual in uncomplicated reflux esophagitis. Crampy chest pain associated with impaction of a food bolus should be distinguished from odynophagia.

Atypical chest pain other than heartburn and odynophagia occurs in reflux esophagitis or esophageal motility disorders such as diffuse esophageal spasm. Spasm may occur spontaneously or during a meal. Chest pain due to periesophageal involvement with carcinoma or peptic ulcer may be constant and agonizing. Sometimes different types of esophageal pains exist together in the same patient, and frequently patients are not able to describe the pain accurately enough to allow its classification. Coronary artery disease should always be excluded before the esophagus is considered as the cause of atypical chest pain. The most frequent esophageal cause of chest pain is reflux esophagitis. Some patients with atypical chest pain have nonspecific esophageal motor abnormalities of uncertain significance. Many of these patients have behavioral abnormalities, psychosomatic disorders, depression, anxiety, panic reactions, and other psychological disorders.

REGURGITATION *Regurgitation* is the effortless appearance of gastric or esophageal contents in the mouth. In distal esophageal obstruction and stasis, as in achalasia or the presence of a large diverticulum, the regurgitated material consists of tasteless mucoid fluid or undigested food. Regurgitation of sour or bitter-tasting material occurs in severe gastroesophageal reflux and is associated with incompetence of both the UES and the LES. Regurgitation may result in laryngeal aspiration, with spells of coughing and choking that awaken the patient from sleep, and in aspiration pneumonia. Water brash is reflex salivary hypersecretion that occurs in response to peptic esophagitis and should not be confused with regurgitation.

DIAGNOSTIC TESTS

RADIOLOGIC STUDIES Barium swallow with fluoroscopy and an esophagogram is a widely used test for the diagnosis of esophageal disease and can be used to evaluate both structural and motor disorders. Spontaneous reflux of barium from the stomach into the esophagus suggests gastroesophageal reflux. Esophageal peristalsis is best studied in the recumbent position, because in the upright position barium passage occurs largely by gravity alone. A double-contrast esophagogram, obtained by coating the esophageal mucosa with barium and distending the esophageal lumen with air using effervescent granules, is particularly useful in demonstrating mucosal ulcers and early cancers. A barium-soaked piece of bread or a 13-mm barium tablet is sometimes used to demonstrate an obstructive lesion. Figures 273-1 and 273-2 illustrate the radiographic appearance of some esophageal disorders. Since the oropharyngeal phase of swallowing lasts no more than a second, videofluoroscopy is necessary to permit detection and analysis of abnormalities of oral and pharyngeal function. The pharynx is examined to detect stasis of barium in the valleculae and piriform sinuses and regurgitation of barium into the nose and tracheobronchial tree.

ESOPHAGOSCOPY Esophagoscopy is the direct method of establishing the cause of mechanical dysphagia and of identifying mucosal lesions that may not be identified by the usual barium swallow. If the lumen is markedly narrowed, use of a smaller-caliber endoscope may be needed; on occasion a stricture must be dilated before the examination can be completed. Endoscopic biopsies are useful in diagnosing car-

FIGURE 273-1 Radiographic appearance of some motor disorders of the pharynx and esophagus. (1) Pharyngeal paralysis with tracheal aspiration (*arrow*). (2) Cricopharyngeal achalasia. Note the prominent cricopharyngeus, which is recognized by its smoothness and location in the posterior wall. (3) Diffuse esophageal spasm. Note the typical corkscrew appearance of the lower part of the esophagus. (4) Achalasia, showing a dilated esophageal body with an air-fluid level and a closed lower esophageal sphincter. (5) Muscular (contractile) lower esophageal ring. The asymmetric contraction visible in (5A) has disappeared in (5B), obtained during the same examination. (6) Scleroderma esophagus showing dilated esophagus with a stricture (6A) and reflux of barium from the stomach into the esophagus (6B). (Courtesy of Dr. Harvey Goldstein.)

cinoma, reflux esophagitis, and other mucosal diseases. Cells obtained by a cytology balloon or brushing the mucosa can be evaluated for carcinoma. Endoscopic ultrasonography permits evaluation of intramural masses and staging of esophageal cancer.

ESOPHAGEAL MOTILITY The study of esophageal motility entails simultaneous recording of pressures from different sites in the esophageal lumen with an assembly of pressure sensors positioned 5 cm apart. The UES and LES appear as zones of high pressure that relax on swallowing. The pharynx and esophagus normally show peristaltic waves with each swallow.

Esophageal motility studies are helpful in the diagnosis of esophageal motor disorders (achalasia, spasm, scleroderma) (Fig. 273-3) but

are of little value in the diagnosis of mechanical dysphagia. In patients with reflux esophagitis, esophageal manometry is useful in quantitating lower esophageal competence and providing information on the status of the esophageal body motor activity. Manometry provides quantitative data that cannot be obtained by barium swallow or endoscopy. Tests for reflux esophagitis are described later.

MOTOR DISORDERS

STRIATED MUSCLE ■ Oropharyngeal Paralysis Paralysis of oral muscles leads to difficulty initiating swallowing and drooling of food out of the mouth. Pharyngeal paralysis, characterized by dysphagia, nasal regurgitation, and aspiration during swallowing, occurs in a variety of

FIGURE 273-2 Selected structural lesions of the esophagus. (1) Carcinoma of the esophagus, with typical annular narrowing with overhanging margins and destruction of the mucosa. (2) Leiomyoma of the esophagus, with a smooth filling defect and right angles of origin from the esophageal wall. (3) Esophageal ulcer in columnar cell–lined esophagus (Barrett's esophagus). (4) Monilial esophagitis, with irregular plaquelike filling defects. (5) Long stricture secondary to lye ingestion. (6) Peptic stricture, short and tubular, with associated hiatal hernia. (7) Lower esophageal mucosal (Schatzki) ring. A thin, weblike annular constriction at the esophagogastric junction is associated with a small hiatal hernia. (Courtesy of Dr. Harvey Goldstein.)

neuromuscular disorders (see Table 33-1). Some of these disorders also involve laryngeal muscles, causing hoarseness. When the suprahyoid muscles are paralyzed, the UES does not open with swallowing, leading to paralytic achalasia of the UES and severe dysphagia.

Videofluoroscopy with barium of various consistencies may reveal difficulties in the oral phase of swallowing. The test may show stasis of barium in the valleculae and piriform sinuses, nasal and tracheal aspiration, failure of the upper sphincter to open, and/or abnormal movement of the hyoid bone and the larynx with a swallow (Fig. 273-1 panel 1). Motility studies demonstrate a reduced amplitude of pharyngeal and upper esophageal contractions and reduced basal upper esophageal sphincter pressure without further relaxation on swallowing (Fig. 273-3). Patients with myasthenia gravis (Chap. 366) and polymyositis (Chap. 369) respond to treatment. Dysphagia resulting from a cerebrovascular accident improves with time, although often not completely. Treatment consists of maneuvers to reduce pharyngeal stasis and enhance airway protection under the direction of a trained swallow therapist. Feeding by a nasogastric tube or an endoscopically placed gastrostomy tube may be necessary for nutritional support; however, these maneuvers do not provide protection against aspiration of salivary secretions. Cricopharyngeal myotomy is sometimes performed, but its usefulness is unproven. Extensive operative procedures to prevent aspiration are rarely needed. Death is often due to pulmonary complications.

Cricopharyngeal Bar Failure of the cricopharyngeus to relax on swallowing appears as a prominent bar on the posterior wall of the pharynx on barium swallow (Fig. 273-1 panel 2). A transient cricopharyngeal bar is seen in up to 5% of individuals without dysphagia undergoing upper gastrointestinal studies; it can be produced in normal individuals during a Valsalva maneuver. A persistent cricopharyngeal bar may be caused by fibrosis in the cricopharyngeus. Some of these patients complain of food sticking in their throats. Cricopharyngeal myotomy may be helpful but is contraindicated in the presence of gastroesophageal reflux because it may lead to pharyngeal and pulmonary aspiration.

Globus Pharyngeus A sensation of a constant lump in the throat, but no difficulty in swallowing, occurs especially in individuals with emotional disorders, particularly women. Results of barium studies and manometry are normal. Treatment consists primarily of reassurance. Some patients with globus pharyngeus have associated reflux esophagitis, and they may respond to treatment of the esophagitis.

SMOOTH MUSCLE ■ Achalasia Achalasia is a motor disorder of the esophageal smooth muscle in which the LES does not relax normally with swallowing, and the esophageal body undergoes nonperistaltic contractions.

PATHOPHYSIOLOGY The underlying abnormality is the loss of intramural neurons. Inhibitory neurons containing VIP and nitric oxide synthase are predominantly involved, but cholinergic neurons are also affected in advanced disease. Primary idiopathic achalasia accounts for most of the patients seen in the United States. Secondary achalasia may be caused by gastric carcinoma that infiltrates the esophagus, lymphoma, Chagas' disease, certain viral infections, eosinophilic gastroenteritis, and neurodegenerative disorders.

CLINICAL FEATURES Achalasia affects patients of all ages and both sexes. Dysphagia, chest pain, and regurgitation are the main symptoms. Dysphagia appears early, occurs with both liquids and solids, and is worsened by emotional stress and hurried eating. Various maneuvers designed to increase intraesophageal pressure, including the Valsalva

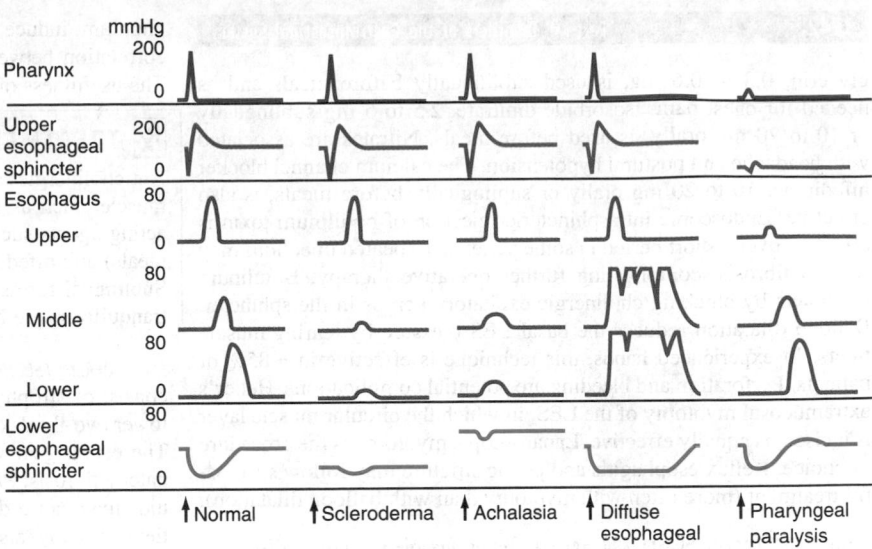

FIGURE 273-3 Motility patterns in selected esophageal and pharyngeal disorders. In normal individuals, the upper and lower esophageal sphincters (UES and LES) appear as zones of high pressure. With a swallow (indicated by ↑), pressure in the sphincters falls and a contraction wave starts in the pharynx and progresses down the esophagus. In scleroderma, the lower part of the esophagus (smooth muscle) shows a reduced amplitude of contractions, which may be peristaltic or simultaneous in onset, and hypotension of the LES. In achalasia, the lower part of the esophagus shows contractions that are reduced in amplitude and simultaneous in onset. In contrast to scleroderma, the LES in achalasia is hypertensive and fails to relax in response to a swallow. In diffuse esophageal spasm, the lower part of the esophagus shows simultaneous-onset, large-amplitude, prolonged, repetitive contractions. In pharyngeal paralysis, the smooth-muscle part of the esophagus is normal. The skeletal muscle part shows a reduced amplitude of contractions. The UES is hypotensive and may not relax normally on swallowing due to associated weakness of the suprahyoid muscles.

maneuver, may aid the passage of the bolus into the stomach. Regurgitation and pulmonary aspiration occur because of retention of large volumes of saliva and ingested food in the esophagus. Patients may complain of difficulty belching. The presence of gastroesophageal reflux argues against achalasia; in patients with long-standing heartburn, cessation of heartburn and appearance of dysphagia suggest development of achalasia on top of reflux esophagitis. The course is usually chronic, with progressive dysphagia and weight loss over months to years. Achalasia associated with carcinoma is characterized by severe weight loss and a rapid downhill course if untreated.

DIAGNOSIS A chest x-ray shows absence of the gastric air bubble and sometimes a tubular mediastinal mass beside the aorta. An air-fluid level in the mediastinum in the upright position represents retained food in the esophagus. Barium swallow shows esophageal dilation, and in advanced cases the esophagus may become sigmoid. On fluoroscopy, normal peristalsis is lost in the lower two-thirds of the esophagus. The terminal part of the esophagus shows a persistent beaklike narrowing representing the nonrelaxing LES (Fig. 273-1 panel 4).

Manometry shows the basal LES pressure to be normal or elevated, and swallow-induced relaxation either does not occur or is reduced in degree, duration, and consistency. The esophageal body shows an elevated resting pressure. In response to swallows, primary peristaltic waves are replaced by simultaneous-onset contractions (Fig. 273-3). These contractions may be of poor amplitude (classic achalasia) or of large amplitude and long duration (vigorous achalasia). Cholecystokinin (CCK), which normally causes a fall in the sphincter pressure, paradoxically causes contraction of the LES (the CCK test). This paradoxical response occurs because, in achalasia, the neurally transmitted inhibitory effect of CCK is absent owing to the loss of inhibitory neurons. Endoscopy is helpful in excluding the secondary causes of achalasia, particularly gastric carcinoma.

℞ TREATMENT

Treatment with soft foods, sedatives, and anticholinergic drugs is usually unsatisfactory. Nitrates and calcium channel blockers provide short-term benefit, but their use may be limited by side effects. Nitroglycerin, 0.3 to 0.6 mg, is used sublingually before meals and as needed for chest pain. Isosorbide dinitrate, 2.5 to 5 mg sublingually or 10 to 20 mg orally, is used before meals. Nitrates are associated with headache and postural hypotension. The calcium channel blocker nifedipine, 10 to 20 mg orally or sublingually before meals, is also effective. Endoscopic intrasphincteric injection of botulinum toxin is effective over a short period in some patients. Repeated injections may lead to fibrosis, complicating further operative therapy. Botulinum toxin acts by blocking cholinergic excitatory nerves in the sphincter. Balloon dilatation reduces the basal LES pressure by tearing muscle fibers. In experienced hands, this technique is effective in ~85% of patients. Perforation and bleeding are potential complications. Heller's extramucosal myotomy of the LES, in which the circular muscle layer is incised, is equally effective. Laparoscopic myotomy is the procedure of choice. Reflux esophagitis and peptic stricture may follow successful treatment (more often with myotomy than with balloon dilatation).

Diffuse Esophageal Spasm and Related Motor Disorders These disorders present with clinical symptoms of chest pain and dysphagia and are recognized by their manometric features. In pure form, they all show normal relaxation to swallows. Diffuse esophageal spasm is characterized by nonperistaltic contractions, usually of large amplitude and long duration. An esophageal motility pattern showing hypertensive but peristaltic contractions has been called "nutcracker esophagus."

PATHOPHYSIOLOGY Nonperistaltic contractions are due to dysfunction of inhibitory nerves. Histopathologic studies show patchy neural degeneration localized to nerve processes, rather than the prominent degeneration of nerve cell bodies seen in achalasia. Diffuse esophageal spasm may progress to achalasia. Hypertensive peristaltic contractions and hypertensive or hypercontracting LES may represent cholinergic or myogenic hyperactivity.

CLINICAL FEATURES Diffuse spasm and related motor disorders (hypertensive peristaltic contraction, hypertensive LES, and hypercontracting LES) cannot be distinguished clinically. They all present with chest pain, dysphagia, or both. Chest pain is particularly marked in patients with esophageal contractions of large amplitude and long duration. Chest pain usually occurs at rest but may be brought on by swallowing or by emotional stress. The pain is retrosternal; it may radiate to the back, the sides of the chest, both arms, or the sides of the jaw and may last from a few seconds to several minutes. Pain may be acute and severe, mimicking the pain of myocardial ischemia. Dysphagia for solids and liquids may occur with or without chest pain and is correlated with simultaneous-onset contractions.

Diffuse esophageal spasm and related esophageal motor disorders must be differentiated from other causes of chest pain, particularly ischemic heart disease with atypical angina. A complete cardiac workup should be done before a noncardiac etiology is considered seriously. The presence of dysphagia in association with pain should point to the esophagus as the site of disease. Esophageal motility disorders are an uncommon cause of noncardiac chest pain, which is more commonly due to reflux esophagitis or visceral hypersensitivity.

DIAGNOSIS In diffuse esophageal spasm, barium swallow shows that normal sequential peristalsis below the aortic arch is replaced by uncoordinated simultaneous contractions that produce the appearance of curling or multiple ripples in the wall, sacculations, and pseudodiverticula—the "corkscrew" esophagus (Fig. 273-1 panel 3). Sometimes an esophageal contraction obliterates the lumen, and barium is pushed away in both directions. The barium swallow is frequently normal in diffuse esophageal spasm and mostly normal in the related disorders.

Diffuse esophageal spasm (Fig. 273-3) and related motor disorders are manometric diagnoses. Because these abnormalities may be episodic, the results of manometry may be normal at the time of the study. Several techniques are used to provoke esophageal spasm. Cold swallows produce chest pain but do not produce spasm on manometric studies. Solid boluses and pharmacologic agents, particularly edro-

phonium, induce both chest pain and motor abnormalities. However, correlation between induction of pain and motility changes is poor. The usefulness of pharmacologic provocative tests is limited.

Anticholinergics are usually of limited value. Agents that relax smooth muscle, such as sublingual nitroglycerin (0.3 to 0.6 mg) or longer-acting agents such as isosorbide dinitrate (10 to 30 mg orally before meals) and nifedipine (10 to 20 mg orally before meals), are helpful. Sublingual forms of these agents can also be used. Reassurance and tranquilizers are helpful in allaying apprehension.

SCLERODERMA ESOPHAGUS The esophageal lesions in systemic sclerosis consist of atrophy of smooth muscle, manifested by weakness in the lower two-thirds of the esophageal body and incompetence of the LES. The esophageal wall is thin and atrophic and may exhibit areas of patchy fibrosis. Patients usually present with dysphagia to solids. Liquids may cause dysphagia when the patient is recumbent. These patients usually also complain of heartburn, regurgitation, and other symptoms of gastroesophageal reflux disease (GERD). Barium swallow shows dilation and loss of peristaltic contractions in the middle and distal portions of the esophagus. The LES is patulous, and gastroesophageal reflux may occur freely (Fig. 273-1 panel 6). Mucosal changes due to esophageal ulceration and esophageal stricture may be present. Motility studies show a marked reduction in the amplitude of smooth-muscle contractions, which may be peristaltic or nonperistaltic. The resting pressure of the LES is subnormal, but sphincter relaxation is normal (Fig. 273-3). Similar esophageal motor abnormalities are found in other collagen vascular diseases and in Raynaud's syndrome alone. Dietary adjustments with the use of soft foods are helpful in management. GERD and its complications should be treated aggressively.

GASTROESOPHAGEAL REFLUX DISEASE

GERD is one of the most prevalent gastrointestinal disorders. Population-based studies show that up to 15% of individuals have heartburn and/or regurgitation at least once a week and 7% have symptoms daily. Symptoms are caused by backflow of gastric acid and other gastric contents into the esophagus due to incompetent barriers at the gastroesophageal junction.

Pathophysiology The normal antireflux mechanisms consist of the LES, the crural diaphragm, and the anatomical location of the gastroesophageal junction below the diaphragmatic hiatus. Reflux occurs only when the gradient of pressure between the LES and the stomach is lost. It can be caused by a sustained or transient decrease in LES tone. A sustained hypotension of the LES may be due to muscle weakness that is often without apparent cause. Secondary causes of sustained LES incompetence include scleroderma-like diseases, myopathy associated with chronic intestinal pseudo-obstruction, pregnancy, smoking, anticholinergic drugs, smooth-muscle relaxants [β-adrenergic agents, aminophylline, nitrates, calcium channel blockers, phosphodiesterase inhibitors that increase cyclic AMP or cyclic GMP (including sildenafil)], surgical damage to the LES, and esophagitis. tLESR without associated esophageal contraction is due to a vagal reflex in which LES relaxation is elicited by gastric distention. Increased episodes of tLESR are associated with GERD. A similar reflex operates during belching. Apart from incompetent barriers, gastric contents are most likely to reflux (1) when gastric volume is increased (after meals, in pyloric obstruction, in gastric stasis, during acid hypersecretion states), (2) when gastric contents are near the gastroesophageal junction (in recumbency, bending down, hiatal hernia), and (3) when gastric pressure is increased (obesity, pregnancy, ascites, tight clothes). Incompetence of the diaphragmatic crural muscle, which surrounds the esophageal hiatus in the diaphragm and functions as an external LES, also predisposes to GERD.

Exposure of the esophagus to refluxed acid correlates with potential for mucosal damage. Exposure depends on the amount of refluxed material per episode, frequency of episodes, and rate of clearing the esophagus by gravity and peristaltic contractions. When peristaltic contractions are impaired, esophageal clearance is impaired. Acid refluxed into the esophagus is neutralized by saliva. Thus, impaired salivary secretion also increases esophageal exposure time. If the refluxed material extends to the cervical esophagus and breaches the upper sphincter, it can enter the pharynx, larynx, and trachea.

Reflux esophagitis is a complication of reflux and develops when mucosal defenses are unable to counteract the damage done by acid, pepsin, and bile. *Mild esophagitis* involves microscopic changes of mucosal infiltration with granulocytes or eosinophils, hyperplasia of basal cells, and elongation of dermal pegs. In nonerosive reflux disease, endoscopic appearance may be normal or show mild erythema. *Erosive esophagitis* shows endoscopically apparent mucosal damage, redness, friability, bleeding, superficial linear ulcers, and exudates. Histology shows polymorphic infiltrates and granulation tissue. *Peptic stricture* results from fibrosis that causes luminal constriction. These strictures occur in ~10% of patients with untreated GERD. Short strictures caused by spontaneous reflux are usually 1 to 3 cm long and are present in the distal esophagus near the squamocolumnar junction (Fig. 273-2 panel 6). Long, tubular peptic strictures can result from persistent vomiting or prolonged nasogastric intubation. Erosive esophagitis may heal by intestinal metaplasia (*Barrett's esophagus*), which is a risk factor for adenocarcinoma.

Clinical Features   Regurgitation of sour material in the mouth and heartburn are the characteristic symptoms of GERD. Reflux into the pharynx, larynx, and tracheobronchial tree can cause chronic cough, bronchoconstriction, pharyngitis, laryngitis, bronchitis, or pneumonia. Morning hoarseness may be noted. Recurrent pulmonary aspiration can cause aspiration pneumonia, pulmonary fibrosis, or chronic asthma. Heartburn is produced by the contact of refluxed material with the sensitized or ulcerated esophageal mucosa. Angina-like or atypical chest pain occurs in some patients, while others experience no heartburn or chest pain. Persistent dysphagia suggests development of a peptic stricture. Most patients with peptic stricture have a history of several years of heartburn preceding dysphagia. However, in one-third of patients, dysphagia is the presenting symptom. Rapidly progressive dysphagia and weight loss may indicate the development of adenocarcinoma in Barrett's esophagus. Bleeding occurs due to mucosal erosions or Barrett's ulcer. Many patients with GERD remain asymptomatic or self-treated and do not seek attention until severe complications occur.

Diagnosis   The diagnosis is easily made by history alone. Diagnostic studies are indicated in patients with persistent symptoms or complications or those who do not respond to therapy. The diagnostic approach to GERD can be divided into three categories:

1. documentation of mucosal injury,
2. documentation and quantitation of reflux, and
3. definition of the pathophysiology.

Mucosal damage is documented by the use of barium swallow, esophagoscopy, and mucosal biopsy. The results of barium swallow are usually normal in uncomplicated esophagitis but may reveal a stricture or ulcer. A high esophageal peptic stricture, a deep ulcer, or adenocarcinoma suggest Barrett's esophagus. Esophagoscopy may reveal the presence of erosive esophagitis, distal peptic stricture, or columnar cell–lined lower esophagus with or without a proximally located peptic stricture, ulcer, or adenocarcinoma. Results of esophagoscopy are normal in patients with nonerosive esophagitis; in such patients, mucosal biopsies and the Bernstein test are helpful. The mucosal biopsies should be performed at least 5 cm above the LES, as the esophageal mucosal changes of chronic esophagitis are quite frequent in the most distal esophagus in otherwise normal individuals. The Bernstein test involves the infusion of solutions of 0.1 N HCl or normal saline into the esophagus. In patients with symptomatic esophagitis, infusion of acid, but not of saline, reproduces the symptoms of heartburn. Infusion of acid in normal individuals usually produces no

symptoms. Supraesophageal manifestations are diagnosed by careful otolaryngologic exam.

A therapeutic trial with a proton pump inhibitor (PPI) (such as omeprazole, 40 mg bid) for 1 week provides strong support for the diagnosis of GERD.

Documentation and quantitation of reflux, when necessary, can be done by ambulatory long-term (24-h) esophageal pH recording. For evaluation of pharyngeal reflux, a system of recording simultaneously from pharyngeal and esophageal sites may be useful. The pH recordings are helpful only in the evaluation of acid reflux. Documentation of reflux is necessary only when the role of reflux in the symptom complex is unclear, particularly in evaluation of supraesophageal symptoms and chest pain without endoscopic evidence of esophagitis.

Definition of pathophysiologic factors in GERD is sometimes indicated for management decisions such as antireflux surgery. Esophageal motility studies may provide useful quantitative information on the competence of the LES and on esophageal motor function.

℞ TREATMENT

The goals of treatment are to provide symptom relief, heal erosive esophagitis, and prevent complications. The management of mild cases includes weight reduction, sleeping with the head of the bed elevated by about 4 to 6 in. with blocks, and elimination of factors that increase abdominal pressure. Patients should not smoke and should avoid consuming fatty foods, coffee, chocolate, alcohol, mint, orange juice, and certain medications (such as anticholinergic drugs, calcium channel blockers, and other smooth-muscle relaxants). They should also avoid ingesting large quantities of fluids with meals. In mild cases, lifestyle changes and over-the-counter antisecretory agents may be adequate. H_2 receptor blocking agents (cimetidine, 300 mg; ranitidine, 150 mg bid; famotidine, 20 mg bid; nizatidine, 150 mg bid) are effective in symptom relief. PPIs are more effective in symptom relief and more commonly used.

The PPIs are comparably effective: omeprazole (20 mg/d), lansoprazole (30 mg/d), pantoprazole (40 mg/d), esomeprazole (40 mg/d), or rabeprazole (20 mg/d) for 8 weeks can heal erosive esophagitis in up to 90% of patients. The drug is taken 15 to 30 min before breakfast and can be maintained indefinitely. Refractory patients can double the dose and administer it twice a day before meals. Side effects are minimal. Aggressive acid suppression causes hypergastrinemia but does not increase the risk for carcinoid tumors or gastrinomas. Vitamin B_{12} absorption is compromised by the treatment. Patients who have Barrett's esophagus with concomitant esophagitis should be similarly treated; however, acid suppression does not lead to resolution of the Barrett's metaplasia or cancer prevention. Patients who have an associated peptic stricture are treated with dilators to relieve dysphagia, and such patients are provided with vigorous treatment for reflux. Esophagoscopy should be performed in patients suspected of complications such as bleeding, stricture, or development of cancer.

Antireflux surgery, in which the gastric fundus is wrapped around the esophagus (fundoplication), increases the LES pressure and should be considered as an alternative for patients who require long-term, high-dose PPIs. Laparoscopic fundoplication is the surgery of choice. Ideal candidates for fundoplication are those in whom motility studies show persistently inadequate LES pressure but normal peristaltic contractions in the esophageal body.

Patients with alkaline esophagitis are treated with general antireflux measures and neutralization of bile salts with cholestyramine, aluminum hydroxide, or sucralfate. Sucralfate is particularly useful in these cases, as it also serves as a mucosal protector.

BARRETT'S ESOPHAGUS   The metaplasia of esophageal squamous epithelium to columnar epithelium (Barrett's esophagus) is a complication of severe reflux esophagitis, and it is a risk factor for esophageal adenocarcinoma (Chap. 77). Metaplastic columnar epithelium develops during healing of erosive esophagitis with continued acid reflux because columnar epithelium is more resistant to acid-pepsin damage than is squamous epithelium. The metaplastic epithelium is a mosaic of different epithelial types including goblet cells and columnar cells that have features of both secretory and absorptive cells (incomplete or type III metaplasia). Barrett's esophagus is arbitrarily divided into long-segment (>2–3 cm) or short-segment (<2–3 cm) groups; long-segment disease is present in 0.5% of the population and short-segment disease may occur in up to 15%.

Barrett's epithelium progresses through a dysplastic stage before developing into adenocarcinoma. The rate of cancer development is 0.5% per year; those with long-segment disease have a risk of developing esophageal cancer that is 30 to 125 times the risk of the general population. Barrett's esophagus can also lead to chronic peptic ulcer of the esophagus with high (midesophageal) and long strictures.

Given the natural history, erosive esophagitis should be aggressively treated. The prevalence of intestinal metaplasia is estimated at 4 to 10% of patients with significant heartburn. Barrett's esophagus is more common in men, particularly white men, and prevalence increases with age. A one-time esophagoscopy is recommended in patients with persistent GERD symptoms at age 50 to identify patients with Barrett's esophagus. Established metaplasia does not regress with treatment; thus, acid suppression and fundoplication are indicated only when active esophagitis is also present.

The need and frequency of surveillance endoscopies in patients with established Barrett's esophagus are debated. The risk of developing esophageal adenocarcinoma is related to the length of involved esophageal mucosa. People with short segments of Barrett's esophagus (distal 2 to 3 cm) account for up to 25% of unselected patients undergoing endoscopy with or without GERD symptoms and appear to be at low risk. They are not routinely surveyed. However, those with long-segment Barrett's esophagus are advised to have endoscopic surveillance at 1-year intervals for 2 years and then every 2 to 3 years. The frequency is increased if dysplasia is detected independent of the length of the metaplasia. Optical methods of recognizing dysplasia during the endoscopy (laser-induced fluorescence spectroscopy, optical coherence tomography) are being developed. Once high-grade dysplasia is detected, treatment of choice is esophagectomy of the Barrett's segment. Photodynamic laser or thermocoagulative mucosal ablation and endoscopic mucosal resection are being evaluated as alternatives.

INFLAMMATORY DISORDERS

INFECTIOUS ESOPHAGITIS Infectious esophagitis can be due to viral, bacterial, fungal, or parasitic organisms. In severely immunocompromised patients, multiple organisms may coexist.

Viral Esophagitis *Herpes simplex virus* (HSV) type 1 occasionally causes esophagitis in immunocompetent individuals, but either HSV type 1 or HSV type 2 may afflict patients who are immunosuppressed (Chap. 163). Patients complain of an acute onset of chest pain, odynophagia, and dysphagia. Bleeding may occur in severe cases; tracheoesophageal fistula and food impaction have been noted. Systemic manifestations such as nausea, vomiting, fever, chills, and mild leukocytosis may be present. Herpetic vesicles on the nose and lips may provide a clue to the diagnosis. Barium swallow is inadequate to detect early lesions and cannot reliably distinguish HSV infection from other types of infections. Endoscopy shows vesicles and small, discrete, punched-out ("volcano-like") superficial ulcerations with or without a fibrinous exudate. In later stages, a diffuse erosive esophagitis develops from enlargement and coalescence of the ulcers. Mucosal cells from a biopsy sample taken at the edge of an ulcer or from a cytologic smear show ballooning degeneration, ground-glass changes in the nuclei with eosinophilic intranuclear inclusions (Cowdry type A), and giant cell formation on routine stains. Culture for HSV becomes positive within days and is helpful in diagnosis and to identify acyclovir-resistant virus. Acyclovir (400 mg 5 times a day for 14 to 21 days) is

effective. In patients with severe odynophagia, intravenous acyclovir, 5 mg/kg every 8 h for 7 to 14 days is used. Symptoms usually resolve in 1 week, but large ulcerations may take longer to heal. Foscarnet (90 mg/kg intravenously bid for 2 to 4 weeks) is used if resistance to acyclovir occurs.

Varicella-zoster virus (VZV) (Chap. 164) sometimes produces esophagitis in children with chickenpox and adults with herpes zoster. Esophageal VZV also can be the source of disseminated VZV infection without skin involvement. In an immunocompromised host, VZV esophagitis causes vesicles and confluent ulcers and usually resolves spontaneously, but it may cause necrotizing esophagitis in a severely compromised host. On routine histologic examination of mucosal biopsy samples or cytology specimens, VZV is difficult to distinguish from HSV, but the distinction can be made immunohistologically or by culture. Acyclovir reduces the duration of symptoms in VZV esophagitis.

Cytomegalovirus (CMV) infections (Chap. 166) occur only in immunocompromised patients. CMV is usually activated from a latent stage or may be acquired from blood product transfusions. CMV lesions initially appear as serpiginous ulcers in an otherwise normal mucosa. These may coalesce to form giant ulcers, particularly in the distal esophagus.

Patients present with odynophagia, persistent and focal chest pain, hematemesis, nausea, and vomiting. Diagnosis requires endoscopy and biopsies of the ulcer. Mucosal brushings are not useful. Routine histologic examination shows intranuclear and small intracytoplasmic inclusions in large fibroblasts and endothelial cells. Immunohistology with monoclonal antibodies to CMV and in situ hybridization of CMV DNA on centrifugation culture and are useful for early diagnosis. Ganciclovir, 5 mg/kg every 12 h intravenously, is the treatment of choice. Valganciclovir (900 mg bid) is an oral formulation of ganciclovir. Foscarnet (90 mg/kg every 12 h intravenously) is used in resistant cases. Therapy is continued until healing occurs, which may take 2 to 4 weeks.

HIV (Chap. 173) may be associated with a self-limited syndrome of acute esophageal ulceration associated with oral ulcers and a maculopapular skin rash, which occurs at the time of HIV seroconversion. Some patients with advanced disease have deep, persistent esophageal ulcers requiring treatment with oral glucocorticoids or thalidomide. Some ulcers respond to local steroid injection.

Bacterial and Fungal Esophagitis *Bacterial esophagitis* is unusual, but esophagitis caused by *Lactobacillus* and β-hemolytic streptococci can occur in the immunocompromised host. In patients with profound granulocytopenia and patients with cancer, bacterial esophagitis is often overlooked because it is commonly present with other organisms, including viruses and fungi. In patients with AIDS, infection with *Cryptosporidium* or *Pneumocystis carinii* may cause nonspecific inflammation, and *Mycobacterium tuberculosis* infection may cause deep ulcerations of the distal esophagus. Very rarely, other types of fungi may cause esophagitis.

CANDIDA ESOPHAGITIS

Candida species are normal commensals in the throat but become pathogenic and produce esophagitis in immunodeficiency states. Candida esophagitis can occur without any predisposing factors. Patients may be asymptomatic or complain of odynophagia and dysphagia. Oral thrush or other evidence of mucocutaneous candidiasis may be absent. Rarely, Candida esophagitis is complicated by esophageal bleeding, perforation, and stricture or by systemic invasion. Barium swallow may be normal or show multiple nodular filling defects of various sizes (Fig. 273-2 panel 4). Large nodular defects may resemble grape clusters. Endoscopy shows small, yellow-white raised plaques with surrounding erythema in mild disease. Confluent linear and nodular plaques reflect extensive disease. Diagnosis is made by demonstration of yeast or hyphal forms in plaque smears and exudate stained with periodic acid–Schiff or Gomori silver stains. Histologic examination is often negative. Culture is not useful in diagnosis but may define the species and the drug sensitivities of the yeast; *Candida albicans* is most common (Chap. 187). Empirical therapy with fluconazole for 7 days is appropriate for suspected cases. Oral fluconazole (200 mg on the first day, followed by 100 mg daily) is the preferred treatment. Patients refractory to fluconazole often respond to itraconazole. Patients who respond poorly or cannot swallow oral medications are treated with amphotericin B (10 to 15 mg as an intravenous infusion for 6 h daily to a total dose of 300 to 500 mg) or intravenous fluconazole. Nystatin oral suspension (100,000 units per mL) in doses of 10 to 20 mL every 6 h is effective for oral thrush. In resistant cases, amphotericin lozenges are used for 7 to 10 days followed by nystatin or fluconazole for as long as the host resistance remains low.

OTHER TYPES OF ESOPHAGITIS *Radiation esophagitis* is a common occurrence during radiation treatment for thoracic cancers. The frequency and severity of esophagitis increase with the amount of radiation delivered and may be enhanced by radiosensitizing drugs like doxorubicin, bleomycin, cyclophosphamide, and cisplatin. Dysphagia and odynophagia may last several weeks to several months after therapy. The esophageal mucosa becomes erythematous, edematous, and friable. Superficial erosions coalesce to form larger superficial ulcers. Submucosal fibrosis and degenerative changes in the blood vessels, muscles, and myenteric neurons may occur. The treatment is relief of pain with viscous lidocaine during the acute phase; indomethacin treatment may reduce radiation damage. Esophageal stricture may develop.

Corrosive esophagitis is caused by the ingestion of caustic agents, such as strong alkali or acid. Severe corrosive injury may lead to esophageal perforation, bleeding, and death. Glucocorticoids are not useful in acute corrosive esophagitis. Healing is usually associated with stricture formation. Caustic strictures are usually long and rigid (Fig. 273-2 panel 5) and generally require dilatation with dilators passed over a guidewire through the stricture. *Pill-induced esophagitis* is associated with the ingestion of certain types of pills and occurs most often in bedridden patients. Antibiotics such as doxycycline, tetracycline, oxytetracycline, minocycline, penicillin, and clindamycin account for more than half the cases. Nonsteroidal anti-inflammatory agents such as aspirin, indomethacin, and ibuprofen may cause injury. Other commonly prescribed pills that cause esophageal injury include potassium chloride, ferrous sulfate or succinate, quinidine, alprenolol, theophylline, ascorbic acid, and pinaverium bromide. Bisphosphonates, particularly alendronate and pamidronate, are more common offenders. Pill esophagitis can be prevented by avoiding the offending agents or by having patients take pills in the upright position and wash them down with copious amounts of fluids.

Sclerotherapy for bleeding esophageal varices usually produces transient retrosternal chest pain and dysphagia; esophageal ulcer, stricture, hematoma, or perforation may occur. Variceal banding causes similar complications but less frequently. *Esophagitis* associated with mucocutaneous and systemic diseases is usually associated with blister and bulla formation, epithelial desquamation, and thin, weblike, or dense esophageal strictures. Pemphigus vulgaris and bullous pemphigoid form intraepithelial and subepithelial bullae, respectively, and can be distinguished by specific immunohistology; both are characterized by sloughing of epithelium or the presence of esophageal casts. Glucocorticoid treatment is usually effective. Cicatricial pemphigoid, Stevens-Johnson syndrome, and toxic epidermolysis bullosa can produce esophageal bullous lesions and strictures requiring gentle dilatation. Graft-versus-host disease occurs in patients who have received allogeneic bone marrow transplants and is associated with generalized desquamation and esophageal strictures. Behçet's disease and eosinophilic gastroenteritis may involve the esophagus and may respond to glucocorticoid therapy. An erosive lichen planus also can involve the esophagus. Crohn's disease may cause inflammatory strictures, sinus tracts, filiform polyps, and fistulas in the esophagus.

OTHER ESOPHAGEAL DISORDERS

DIVERTICULA Diverticula are outpouchings of the wall of the esophagus. A *Zenker's diverticulum* appears in the natural zone of weakness in the posterior hypopharyngeal wall (Killian's triangle) and causes halitosis and regurgitation of saliva and food particles consumed several days previously. When it becomes large and filled with food, such a diverticulum can compress the esophagus and cause dysphagia or complete obstruction. Nasogastric intubation and endoscopy should be performed with utmost care in these patients, since they may cause perforation of the diverticulum. A *midesophageal diverticulum* may be caused by traction from old adhesions or by propulsion associated with esophageal motor abnormalities. An *epiphrenic diverticulum* may be associated with achalasia. Small or medium-sized diverticula and midesophageal and epiphrenic diverticula are usually asymptomatic. *Diffuse intramural diverticulosis* of the esophagus is due to dilation of the deep esophageal glands and may lead to chronic candidiasis or to the development of a stricture high up in the esophagus. These patients may present with dysphagia. Symptomatic Zenker's diverticula are treated by cricopharyngeal myotomy with or without diverticulectomy. Large symptomatic esophageal diverticula are removed surgically. When they are associated with motor abnormalities, distal myotomy is performed. Strictures associated with diffuse intramural diverticulosis are treated with rubber dilators.

WEBS AND RINGS Weblike constrictions of the esophagus are usually congenital or inflammatory in origin. Asymptomatic hypopharyngeal webs are demonstrated in <10% of normal individuals. When concentric, they cause intermittent dysphagia to solids. The combination of symptomatic hypopharyngeal webs and iron-deficiency anemia in middle aged women constitutes *Plummer-Vinson syndrome*. The clinical importance of this syndrome is uncertain. Midesophageal webs are rare. A *lower esophageal mucosal ring* (Schatzki ring) is a thin, weblike constriction located at the squamocolumnar mucosal junction at or near the border of the LES (Fig. 273-2 panel 7). It invariably produces dysphagia when the lumen diameter is <1.3 cm. Dysphagia to solids is the only symptom, and it is usually episodic. Asymptomatic rings may be present in ~10% of normal individuals. A lower esophageal ring is one of the common causes of dysphagia. Symptomatic webs and mucosal lower esophageal rings are easily treated by dilatation. A *lower esophageal muscular ring* (contractile ring) is located proximal to the site of mucosal rings and may represent an abnormal uppermost segment of the LES. These rings can be recognized by the fact that they are not constant in size and shape. They also may cause dysphagia and should be differentiated from peptic strictures, achalasia, and lower esophageal mucosal rings. Muscular rings do not respond well to dilatation.

HIATAL HERNIA A *hiatal hernia* is a herniation of part of the stomach into the thoracic cavity through the esophageal hiatus in the diaphragm. A *sliding hiatal hernia* is one in which the gastroesophageal junction and fundus of the stomach slide upward. A sliding hernia may result from weakening of the anchors of the gastroesophageal junction to the diaphragm, from longitudinal contraction of the esophagus, or from increased intra-abdominal pressure. Small sliding hernias can be demonstrated commonly during barium studies if intra-abdominal pressure is increased. Incidence increases with age; in individuals in the sixth decade of life, the prevalence of such hernias is ~60%. Small sliding hiatal hernias alone probably produce no symptoms but can contribute to reflux esophagitis. A *paraesophageal hernia* is one in which the esophagogastric junction remains fixed in its normal location and a pouch of stomach is herniated beside the gastroesophageal junction through the esophageal hiatus. A paraesophageal or mixed paraesophageal and sliding hernia may become incarcerated and strangulate, leading to acute chest pain, dysphagia, and a mediastinal mass and requiring surgery. A herniated gastric pouch may cause dysphagia, develop gastritis, or ulcerate, causing chronic blood loss. Large paraesophageal hernias should be surgically repaired.

MECHANICAL TRAUMA *Esophageal rupture* may be caused by (1) iatrogenic damage from instrumentation of the esophagus or external trauma, (2) increased intraesophageal pressure associated with forceful vomiting or retching (*spontaneous rupture* or *Boerhaave's syndrome*), or (3) diseases of the esophagus such as corrosive esophagitis, esophageal ulcer, and neoplasm. The site of perforation depends on the cause. Instrumental perforation usually occurs in the pharynx or lower esophagus, just above the diaphragm in the posterolateral wall. Esophageal perforation causes severe retrosternal chest pain, which may be worsened by swallowing and breathing. Free air enters the mediastinum and spreads to neighboring structures, causing palpable subcutaneous emphysema in the neck, mediastinal crackling sounds on auscultation, and pneumothorax. With time, secondary infection supervenes, and mediastinal abscess may develop. Esophageal perforation associated with vomiting usually deposits gastric contents in the mediastinum and causes severe mediastinal complications. By contrast, instrumental perforation may be clinically mild and free of severe complications. Spontaneous rupture of the esophagus may mimic myocardial infarction, pancreatitis, or rupture of an abdominal viscus. Symptoms of chest pain may be mild, particularly in the elderly. Mediastinal emphysema may develop late. An x-ray of the chest shows abnormalities in most patients, but computed tomography (CT) of the chest is more sensitive in detecting mediastinal air. Fluid from pleural effusions may have a high content of (salivary) amylase. The diagnosis is confirmed by swallow of radiopaque contrast material. Gastrograffin is used initially, and if no leak is found, a small amount of thin barium is used to confirm the diagnosis. Treatment includes esophageal and gastric suction and parenteral broad-spectrum antibiotics. Surgical drainage and repair of the laceration should be performed as soon as possible. In patients with terminal carcinoma, surgical repair may not be feasible, and patients with minor instrumental perforation can be treated conservatively. Extensive corrosive damage may require esophageal diversion and excision of the damaged portion.

Mucosal Tear (Mallory-Weiss Syndrome)

This tear is usually caused by vomiting, retching, or vigorous coughing. The tear usually involves the gastric mucosa near the squamocolumnar mucosal junction. Patients present with upper gastrointestinal bleeding, which may be severe. In most patients bleeding ceases spontaneously; continued bleeding may respond to vasopressin therapy or angiographic embolization. Surgery is rarely needed.

Intramural Hematoma   Emetogenic injury, particularly in patients with bleeding abnormalities, can cause bleeding between the mucosal and muscle layers of the esophagus. The patients develop sudden dysphagia. The diagnosis is made by barium swallow and CT. Resolution is usually spontaneous.

FOREIGN BODIES   Foreign bodies may lodge in the cervical esophagus just beyond the UES, near the aortic arch, or above the LES. Impaction of a bolus of food, particularly a piece of meat or bread, may occur when the esophageal lumen is narrowed due to stricture, carcinoma, or a lower esophageal ring. Acute impaction causes a complete inability to swallow and severe chest pain. Both foreign bodies and food boluses may be removed endoscopically. Use of a meat tenderizer to facilitate passage of a meat bolus is discouraged because of potential esophageal perforation and aspiration pneumonia.

FURTHER READING

DEMEESTER SR et al: Barrett's esophagus. Curr Probl Surg 38:558, 2001

HIRANO I: Pathophysiology of achalasia. Curr Gastroenterol Rep 1:198, 1999

ONLANDO RC: Pathogenesis of gastroesophageal reflux disease. Gastroenterol Clin North Am 31:S35, 2002

PATERSON WG: Extraesophageal manifestations of reflux disease: Myths and reality. Chest Surg Clin N Am 11:523, 2001

RAMAKRISHNAN A, KATZ PO: Pharmacologic management of gastroesophageal reflux disease. Curr Gastroenterol Rep 4:218, 2002

SPECHLER SJ: Barrett's esophagus and esophageal adenocarcinoma: Pathogenesis, diagnosis and therapy. Med Clin North Am 86:1423, 2002

———: AGA technical review on treatment of patients with dysphagia caused by benign disorders of the distal esophagus. Gastroenterology 117:233, 1999

WARING JP: Surgical and endoscopic treatment of gastroesophageal reflux disease. Gastroenterol Clin North Am 31:S89, 2002

274   PEPTIC ULCER DISEASE AND RELATED DISORDERS
John Del Valle

PEPTIC ULCER DISEASE

Burning epigastric pain exacerbated by fasting and improved with meals is a symptom complex associated with peptic ulcer disease (PUD). An *ulcer* is defined as disruption of the mucosal integrity of the stomach and/or duodenum leading to a local defect or excavation due to active inflammation. Ulcers occur within the stomach and/or duodenum and are often chronic in nature. Acid peptic disorders are very common in the United States, with 4 million individuals (new cases and recurrences) affected per year. Lifetime prevalence of PUD in the United States is ~12% in men and 10% in women. Moreover, an estimated 15,000 deaths per year occur as a consequence of complicated PUD. The financial impact of these common disorders has been substantial, with an estimated burden on direct and indirect health care costs of ~$10 billion per year in the United States.

GASTRIC PHYSIOLOGY   Despite the constant attack on the gastroduodenal mucosa by a host of noxious agents (acid, pepsin, bile acids, pancreatic enzymes, drugs, and bacteria), integrity is maintained by an intricate system that provides mucosal defense and repair.

Gastric Anatomy   The gastric epithelial lining consists of rugae that contain microscopic gastric pits, each branching into four or five gastric glands made up of highly specialized epithelial cells. The makeup of gastric glands varies with their anatomic location. Glands within the gastric cardia comprise <5% of the gastric gland area and contain mucous and endocrine cells. The majority of gastric glands (75%) are found within the oxyntic mucosa and contain mucous neck, parietal, chief, endocrine, and enterochromaffin cells (Fig. 274-1). Pyloric glands contain mucous and endocrine cells (including gastrin cells) and are found in the antrum.

The parietal cell, also known as the oxyntic cell, is usually found in the neck, or isthmus, or the oxyntic gland. The resting, or unstimulated, parietal cell has prominent cytoplasmic tubulovesicles and intracellular canaliculi containing short microvilli along its apical surface (Fig. 274-2). H+, K+-ATPase is expressed in the tubulovesicle membrane; upon cell stimulation, this membrane, along with apical membranes, transforms into a dense network of apical intracellular canaliculi containing long microvilli. Acid secretion, a process requiring high energy, occurs at the apical canalicular surface. Numerous mitochondria (30 to 40% of total cell volume) generate the energy required for secretion.

Gastroduodenal Mucosal Defense   The gastric epithelium is under a constant assault by a series of endogenous noxious factors including HCl, pepsinogen/pepsin, and bile salts. In addition, a steady flow of exogenous substances such as medications, alcohol, and bacteria encounter the gastric mucosa. A highly intricate biologic system is in place to provide defense from mucosal injury and to repair any injury that may occur.

The mucosal defense system can be envisioned as a three-level barrier, composed of preepithelial, epithelial, and subepithelial elements (Fig. 274-3). The first line of defense is a mucus-bicarbonate

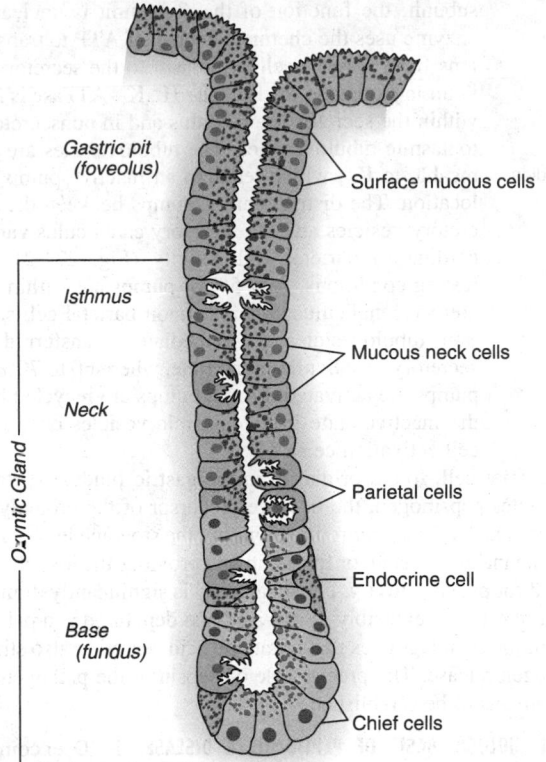

FIGURE 274-1 Diagramatic representation of the oxyntic gastric gland. *(Adapted from S Ito, RJ Winchester. Cell Biol 16:541, 1963.)*

layer, which serves as a physicochemical barrier to multiple molecules including hydrogen ions. Mucus is secreted in a regulated fashion by gastroduodenal surface epithelial cells. It consists primarily of water (95%) and a mixture of lipids and glycoproteins. Mucin is the constituent glycoprotein that, in combination with phospholipids (also secreted by gastric mucous cells), forms a hydrophobic surface with fatty acids that extend into the lumen from the cell membrane. The mucous gel functions as a nonstirred water layer impeding diffusion of ions and molecules such as pepsin. Bicarbonate, secreted by surface epithelial cells of the gastroduodenal mucosa into the mucous gel, forms a pH gradient ranging from 1 to 2 at the gastric luminal surface and reaching 6 to 7 along the epithelial cell surface. Bicarbonate secretion is stimulated by calcium, prostaglandins, cholinergic input, and luminal acidification.

Surface epithelial cells provide the next line of defense through several factors, including mucus production, epithelial cell ionic transporters that maintain intracellular pH and bicarbonate production, and intracellular tight junctions. If the preepithelial barrier were breached,

FIGURE 274-2 Gastric parietal cell undergoing transformation after secretagogue-mediated stimulation. *(Adapted from SJ Hersey, G Sachs: Physiol Rev 75:155, 1995.)*

gastric epithelial cells bordering a site of injury can migrate to restore a damaged region (*restitution*). This process occurs independent of cell division and requires uninterrupted blood flow and an alkaline pH in the surrounding environment. Several growth factors including epidermal growth factor (EGF), transforming growth factor (TGF) α, and basic fibroblast growth factor (FGF) modulate the process of restitution. Larger defects that are not effectively repaired by restitution require cell proliferation. Epithelial cell regeneration is regulated by prostaglandins and growth factors such as EGF and TGF-α. In tandem with epithelial cell renewal, formation of new vessels (*angiogenesis*) within the injured microvascular bed occurs. Both FGF and vascular endothelial growth factor (VEGF) are important in regulating angiogenesis in the gastric mucosa.

An elaborate microvascular system within the gastric submucosal layer is the key component of the subepithelial defense/repair system. A rich submucosal circulatory bed provides HCO_3^-, which neutralizes the acid generated by parietal cell secretion of HCl. Moreover, this microcirculatory bed provides an adequate supply of micronutrients and oxygen while removing toxic metabolic by-products.

Prostaglandins play a central role in gastric epithelial defense/repair (Fig. 274-4). The gastric mucosa contains abundant levels of prostaglandins. These metabolites of arachidonic acid regulate the release of mucosal bicarbonate and mucus, inhibit parietal cell secretion, and are important in maintaining mucosal blood flow and epithelial cell restitution. Prostaglandins are derived from esterified arachidonic acid, which is formed from phospholipids (cell membrane) by the action of phospholipase A_2. A key enzyme that controls the rate-limiting step in prostaglandin synthesis is cyclooxygenase (COX), which is present in two isoforms (COX-1, COX-2), each having distinct characteristics regarding structure, tissue distribution, and expression. COX-1 is expressed in a host of tissues including the stomach, platelets, kidneys, and endothelial cells. This isoform is expressed in a constitutive manner and plays an important role in maintaining the integrity of renal function, platelet aggregation, and gastrointestinal mucosal integrity. In contrast, the expression of COX-2 is inducible by inflammatory stimuli, and it is expressed in macrophages, leukocytes, fibroblasts, and synovial cells. The beneficial effects of nonsteroidal anti-inflammatory drugs (NSAIDs) on tissue inflammation are due to inhibition of COX-2; the toxicity of these drugs (e.g., gastrointestinal mucosal ulceration and renal dysfunction) is related to inhibition of the COX-1 isoform. The highly COX-2-selective NSAIDs have the potential to provide the beneficial effect of decreasing tissue inflammation while minimizing toxicity in the gastrointestinal tract.

Physiology of Gastric Secretion Hydrochloric acid and pepsinogen are the two principal gastric secretory products capable of inducing mucosal injury. Acid secretion should be viewed as occurring under basal and stimulated conditions. Basal acid production occurs in a circadian pattern, with highest levels occurring during the night and lowest levels during the morning hours. Cholinergic input via the vagus nerve and histaminergic input from local gastric sources are the principal contributors to basal acid secretion. Stimulated gastric acid secretion occurs primarily in three phases based on the site where the signal originates (cephalic, gastric, and intestinal). Sight, smell, and taste of food are the components of the cephalic phase, which stimulates gastric secretion via the vagus nerve. The gastric phase is activated once food enters the stomach. This component of secretion is driven by nutrients (amino acids and amines) that directly stimulate the G cell to release gastrin, which in turn activates the parietal cell via direct and indirect mechanisms. Distention of the stomach wall also leads to gastrin release and acid production. The last phase of gastric acid secretion is initiated as food enters the intestine and is mediated by luminal distention and nutrient assimilation. A series of pathways that inhibit gastric acid production are also set into motion during these phases. The gastrointestinal hormone somatostatin is released from endocrine cells found in the gastric mucosa (D cells) in response to HCl. Somatostatin can inhibit acid production by both direct (parietal

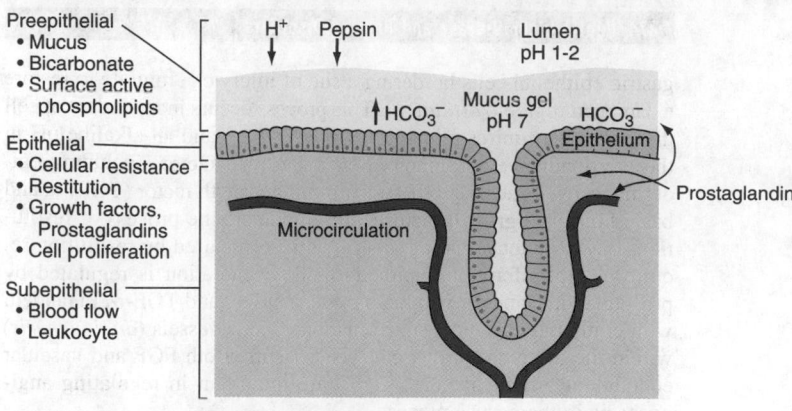

Preepithelial
• Mucus
• Bicarbonate
• Surface active phospholipids

Epithelial
• Cellular resistance
• Restitution
• Growth factors, Prostaglandins
• Cell proliferation

Subepithelial
• Blood flow
• Leukocyte

FIGURE 274-3 Components involved in providing gastroduodenal mucosal defense and repair.

cell) and indirect mechanisms [decreased histamine release from enterochromaffin-like (ECL) cells and gastrin release from G cells. Additional neural (central and peripheral) and hormonal (secretin, cholecystokinin) factors play a role in counterbalancing acid secretion. Under physiologic circumstances, these phases are occurring simultaneously.

The acid-secreting parietal cell is located in the oxyntic gland, adjacent to other cellular elements (ECL cell, D cell) important in the gastric secretory process (Fig. 274-5). This unique cell also secretes intrinsic factor (IF). The parietal cell expresses receptors for several stimulants of acid secretion including histamine (H_2), gastrin (cholecystokinin B/gastrin receptor), and acetylcholine (muscarinic, M_3). Each of these are G protein–linked, seven transmembrane–spanning receptors. Binding of histamine to the H_2 receptor leads to activation of adenylate cyclase and an increase in cyclic AMP. Activation of the gastrin and muscarinic receptors results in activation of the protein kinase C/phosphoinositide signaling pathway. Each of these signaling pathways in turn regulates a series of downstream kinase cascades, which control the acid-secreting pump, H^+, K^+-ATPase. The discovery that different ligands and their corresponding receptors lead to activation of different signaling pathways explains the potentiation of acid secretion that occurs when histamine and gastrin or acetylcholine are combined. More importantly, this observation explains why blocking one receptor type (H_2) decreases acid secretion stimulated by agents that activate a different pathway (gastrin, acetylcholine). Parietal cells also express receptors for ligands that inhibit acid production (prostaglandins, somatostatin, and EGF).

The enzyme H^+, K^+-ATPase is responsible for generating the large concentration of H^+. It is a membrane-bound protein that consists of two subunits, α and β. The active catalytic site is found within the α subunit; the function of the β subunit is unclear. This enzyme uses the chemical energy of ATP to transfer H^+ ions from parietal cell cytoplasm to the secretory canaliculi in exchange for K^+. The H^+,K^+-ATPase is located within the secretory canaliculus and in nonsecretory cytoplasmic tubulovesicles. The tubulovesicles are impermeable to K^+, which leads to an inactive pump in this location. The distribution of pumps between the nonsecretory vesicles and the secretory canaliculus varies according to parietal cell activity (Fig. 274-2). Under resting conditions, only 5% of pumps are within the secretory canaliculus, whereas upon parietal cell stimulation, tubulovesicles are immediately transferred to the secretory canalicular membrane, where 60 to 70% of the pumps are activated. Proton pumps are recycled back to the inactive state in cytoplasmic vesicles once parietal cell activation ceases.

The chief cell, found primarily in the gastric fundus, synthesizes and secretes pepsinogen, the inactive precursor of the proteolytic enzyme pepsin. The acid environment within the stomach leads to cleavage of the inactive precursor to pepsin and provides the low pH (<2.0) required for pepsin activity. Pepsin activity is significantly diminished at a pH of 4 and irreversibly inactivated and denatured at a pH of ≥7. Many of the secretagogues that stimulate acid secretion also stimulate pepsinogen release. The precise role of pepsin in the pathogenesis of PUD remains to be established.

PATHOPHYSIOLOGIC BASIS OF PEPTIC ULCER DISEASE PUD encompasses both gastric and duodenal ulcers. Ulcers are defined as a break in the mucosal surface >5 mm in size, with depth to the submucosa. Duodenal ulcers (DUs) and gastric ulcers (GUs); share many common features in terms of pathogenesis, diagnosis, and treatment, but several factors distinguish them from one another.

Epidemiology ■ *DUODENAL ULCERS* DUs are estimated to occur in 6 to 15% of the western population. The incidence of DUs declined steadily from 1960 to 1980 and has remained stable since then. The death rates, need for surgery, and physician visits have decreased by >50% over the past 30 years. The reason for the reduction in the frequency of DUs is likely related to the decreasing frequency of *Helicobacter pylori*. Before the discovery of *H. pylori*, the natural history of DUs was typified by frequent recurrences after initial therapy. Eradication of *H. pylori* has greatly reduced these recurrence rates.

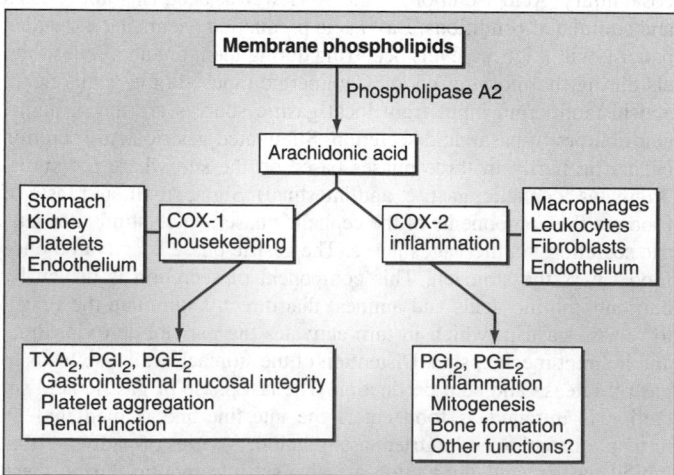

FIGURE 274-4 Schematic representation of the steps involved in synthesis of prostaglandin E_2 (PGE$_2$) and prostacyclin (PGI$_2$). Characteristics and distribution of the cyclooxgenase (COX) enzymes 1 and 2 are also shown. TXA$_2$, thromboxane A$_2$.

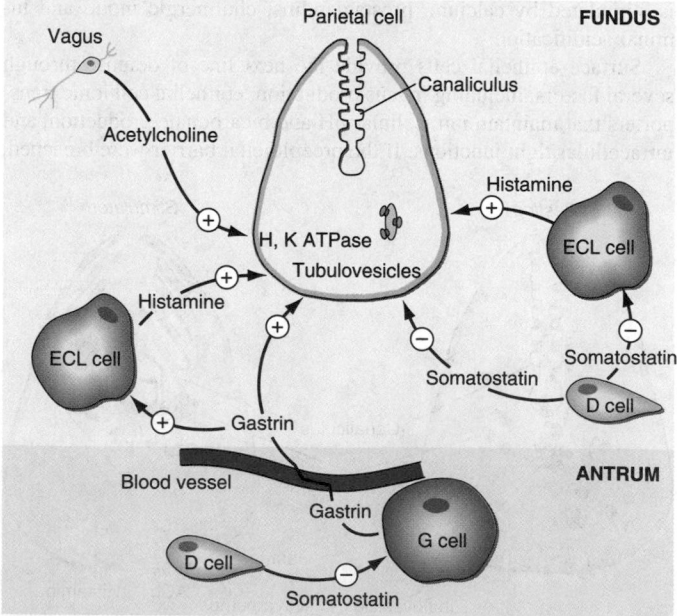

FIGURE 274-5 Regulation of gastric acid secretion at the cellular level. ECL cell, enterochromaffin-like cell.

GASTRIC ULCERS GUs tend to occur later in life than duodenal lesions, with a peak incidence reported in the sixth decade. More than half of GUs occur in males and are less common than DUs, perhaps due to the higher likelihood of GUs being silent and presenting only after a complication develops. Autopsy studies suggest a similar incidence of DUs and GUs.

Pathology ■ *DUODENAL ULCERS* DUs occur most often in the first portion of duodenum (>95%), with ~90% located within 3 cm of the pylorus. They are usually ≤1 cm in diameter but can occasionally reach 3 to 6 cm (giant ulcer). Ulcers are sharply demarcated, with depth at times reaching the muscularis propria. The base of the ulcer often consists of a zone of eosinophilic necrosis with surrounding fibrosis. Malignant duodenal ulcers are extremely rare.

GASTRIC ULCERS In contrast to DUs, GUs can represent a malignancy. Benign GUs are most often found distal to the junction between the antrum and the acid secretory mucosa. This junction is variable, but in general the antral mucosa extends about two-thirds of the distance of the lesser curvature and one-third the way up the greater curvature. Benign GUs are quite rare in the gastric fundus and are histologically similar to DUs. Benign GUs associated with *H. pylori* are associated with antral gastritis. In contrast, NSAID-related GUs are not accompanied by chronic active gastritis but may instead have evidence of a chemical gastropathy.

Pathophysiology It is now clear that *H. pylori* and NSAID-induced injury account for the majority of DUs. Gastric acid contributes to mucosal injury but does not play a primary role.

DUODENAL ULCERS Many acid secretory abnormalities have been described in DU patients. Of these, average basal and nocturnal gastric acid secretion appear to be increased in DU patients as compared to control; however, the level of overlap between DU patients and control subjects is substantial. The reason for this altered secretory process is unclear, but *H. pylori* infection may contribute to this finding. Accelerated gastric emptying of liquids has been noted in some DU patients but is not consistently observed; its role in DU formation, if any, is unclear. Bicarbonate secretion is significantly decreased in the duodenal bulb of patients with an active DU as compared to control subjects. *H. pylori* infection may also play a role in this process.

GASTRIC ULCERS As in DUs, the majority of GUs can be attributed to either *H. pylori* or NSAID-induced mucosal damage. GUs that occur in the prepyloric area or those in the body associated with a DU or a duodenal scar are similar in pathogenesis to DUs. Gastric acid output (basal and stimulated) tends to be normal or decreased in GU patients. When GUs develop in the presence of minimal acid levels, impairment of mucosal defense factors may be present.

Abnormalities in resting and stimulated pyloric sphincter pressure with a concomitant increase in duodenal gastric reflux have been implicated in some GU patients. Although bile acids, lysolecithin, and pancreatic enzymes may injure gastric mucosa, a definite role for these in GU pathogenesis has not been established. Delayed gastric emptying of solids has been described in GU patients but has not been reported consistently. The observation that patients who have undergone disruption of the normal pyloric barrier (pyloroplasty, gastroenterostomy) often have superficial gastritis without frank ulceration decreases enthusiasm for duodenal gastric reflux as an explanation for GU pathogenesis.

H. PYLORI AND ACID PEPTIC DISORDERS Gastric infection with the bacterium *H. pylori* accounts for the majority of PUD. This organism also plays a role in the development of gastric mucosal-associated lymphoid tissue (MALT) lymphoma and gastric adenocarcinoma. Although the entire genome of *H. pylori* has been sequenced, it is still not clear how this organism, which is in the stomach, causes ulceration in the duodenum, or whether its eradication will lead to a decrease in gastric cancer.

The Bacterium The bacterium, initially named *Campylobacter pyloridis*, is a gram-negative microaerophilic rod found most commonly in the deeper portions of the mucous gel coating the gastric mucosa or between the mucous layer and the gastric epithelium. It may attach to gastric epithelium but under normal circumstances does not appear to invade cells. It is strategically designed to live within the aggressive environment of the stomach. It is S-shaped (~0.5 × 3 μm in size) and contains multiple sheathed flagella. Initially, *H. pylori* resides in the antrum but, over time, migrates toward the more proximal segments of the stomach. The organism is capable of transforming into a coccoid form, which represents a dormant state that may facilitate survival in adverse conditions. The genome of *H. pylori* has been sequenced (1.65 million base pairs) and encodes ~1500 proteins. Amongst this multitude of proteins there are factors that are essential determinants of *H. pylori*–mediated pathogenesis and colonization such as the outer membrane protein (Hop proteins), urease, and the vacuolating cytotoxin (Vac A). Moreover, the majority of *H. pylori* strains contain a genomic fragment, which encodes the cag pathogenicity island (cag-PAI). Several of the genes that make up cag-PAI encode components of a type IV secretion island that translocates Cag A into host cells. Once in the cell, Cag A activates a series of cellular events important in cell growth and cytokine production. The first step in infection by *H. pylori* is dependent on the bacteria's motility and its ability to produce urease. Urease produces ammonia from urea, an essential step in alkalinizing the surrounding pH. Additional bacterial factors include catalase, lipase, adhesins, platelet-activating factor, and pic B (induces cytokines). Multiple strains of *H. pylori* exist and are characterized by their ability to express several of these factors (Cag A, Vac A, etc.). It is possible that the different diseases related to *H. pylori* infection can be attributed to different strains of the organism with distinct pathogenic features.

Epidemiology The prevalence of *H. pylori* varies throughout the world and depends to a great extent on the overall standard of living in the region. In developing parts of the world, 80% of the population may be infected by the age of 20, whereas the prevalence is 20 to 50% in industrialized countries. In contrast, in the United States, this organism is rare in childhood. The overall prevalence of *H. pylori* in the United States is ~30%, with individuals born before 1950 having a higher rate of infection than those born later. About 10% of Americans <30 are colonized with the bacteria. The rate of infection with *H. pylori* in industrialized countries has decreased substantially in recent decades. The steady increase in the prevalence of *H. pylori* noted with increasing age is due primarily to a cohort effect, reflecting higher transmission during a period in which the earlier cohorts were children. It has been calculated, through mathematical models, that improved sanitation during the latter half of the nineteenth century dramatically decreased transmission of *H. pylori*. Moreover, with the present rate of intervention, it is predicted that the organism will be ultimately eliminated from the United States. Two factors that predispose to higher colonization rates include poor socioeconomic status and less education. These factors, not race, are responsible for the rate of *H. pylori* infection in blacks and Hispanic Americans being double the rate seen in whites of comparable age. Other risk factors for *H. pylori* infection are (1) birth or residence in a developing country, (2) domestic crowding, (3) unsanitary living conditions, (4) unclean food or water, and (5) exposure to gastric contents of an infected individual.

Transmission of *H. pylori* occurs from person to person, following an oral-oral or fecal-oral route. The risk of *H. pylori* infection is declining in developing countries. The rate of infection in the United States has fallen by >50% when compared to 30 years ago.

Pathophysiology *H. pylori* infection is virtually always associated with a chronic active gastritis, but only 10 to 15% of infected individuals develop frank peptic ulceration. The basis for this difference is unknown. Initial studies suggested that >90% of all DUs were associated with *H. pylori*, but *H. pylori* is present in only 30 to 60% of individuals with GUs and 70% of patients with DUs. The pathophysiology of ulcers not associated with *H. pylori* or NSAID ingestion [or the rare Zollinger-Ellison syndrome (ZES)] is unclear.

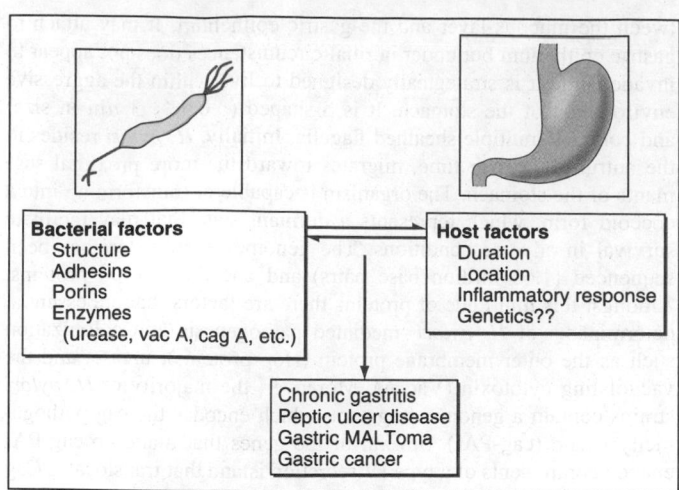

FIGURE 274-6 Outline of the bacterial and host factors important in determining *H. pylori*–induced gastrointestinal disease. MALT, mucosal-associated lymphoid tissue.

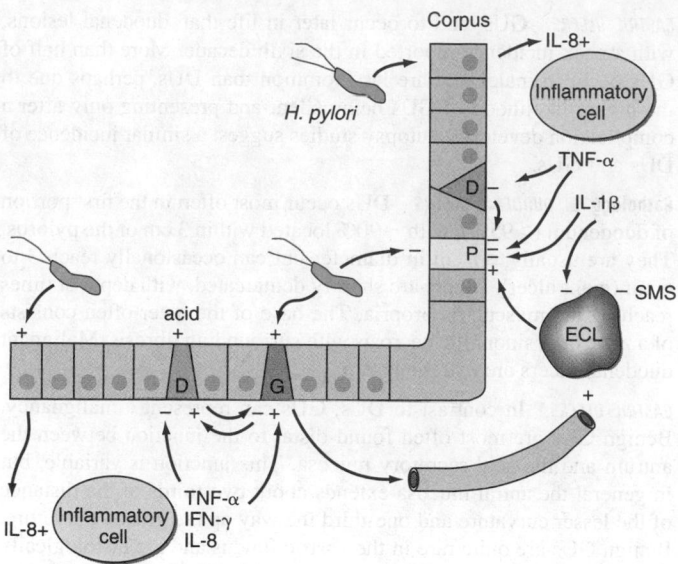

FIGURE 274-7 Summary of potential mechanisms by which *H. pylori* may lead to gastric secretory abnormalities. D, somatostatin cell; ECL, enterochromaffin-like; G, G cell; IFN, interferon; IL, interleukin; P, parietal cell; SMS, somatostatin; TNF, tumor necrosis factor. *(Adapted from J Calam et al: Gastroenterology 113:543, 1997.)*

The particular end result of *H. pylori* infection (gastritis, PUD, gastric MALT lymphoma, gastric cancer) is determined by a complex interplay between bacterial and host factors (Fig. 274-6).

1. *Bacterial factors*: *H. pylori* is able to facilitate gastric residence, induce mucosal injury, and avoid host defense. Different strains of *H. pylori* produce different virulence factors. A specific region of the bacterial genome, the pathogenicity island, encodes the virulence factors Cag A and pic B. Vac A also contributes to pathogenicity, though it is not encoded within the pathogenicity island. These virulence factors, in conjunction with additional bacterial constituents, can cause mucosal damage. Urease, which allows the bacteria to reside in the acidic stomach, generates NH_3, which can damage epithelial cells. The bacteria produce surface factors that are chemotactic for neutrophils and monocytes, which in turn contribute to epithelial cell injury (see below). *H. pylori* makes proteases and phospholipases that break down the glycoprotein lipid complex of the mucous gel, thus reducing the efficacy of this first line of mucosal defense. *H. pylori* expresses adhesins, which facilitate attachment of the bacteria to gastric epithelial cells. Although lipopolysaccharide (LPS) of gram-negative bacteria often plays an important role in the infection, *H. pylori* LPS has low immunologic activity compared to that of other organisms. It may promote a smoldering chronic inflammation.

2. *Host factors*: The inflammatory response to *H. pylori* includes recruitment of neutrophils, lymphocytes (T and B), macrophages, and plasma cells. The pathogen leads to local injury by binding to class II MHC molecules expressed on gastric epithelial cells leading to cell death (*apoptosis*). Moreover, bacterial strains that encode cag-PAI can introduce Cag A into the host cells, leading to further cell injury and activation of cellular pathways involved in cytokine production. Elevated concentrations of multiple cytokines are found in the gastric epithelium of *H. pylori*–infected individuals, including interleukin (IL) $1\alpha/\beta$, IL-2, IL-6, IL-8, tumor necrosis factor (TNF) α and interferon (IFN) γ. *H. pylori* infection also leads to both a mucosal and systemic humoral response, which does not lead to eradication of the bacteria but further compounds epithelial cell injury. Additional mechanisms by which *H. pylori* may cause epithelial cell injury include: activated neutrophil-mediated production of reactive oxygen or nitrogen species and enhanced epithelial cell turnover and apoptosis related to interaction with T cells (T helper 1, or T_H1, cells) and interferon-γ.

The reason for *H. pylori*–mediated duodenal ulceration remains unclear. One potential explanation is that gastric metaplasia in the duodenum of DU patients permits *H. pylori* to bind to it and produce local injury secondary to the host response. Another hypothesis is that *H. pylori* antral infection could lead to increased acid production, in-

creased duodenal acid, and mucosal injury. Basal and stimulated [meal, gastrin-releasing peptide (GRP)] gastrin release are increased in *H. pylori*–infected individuals, and somatostatin-secreting D cells may be decreased. *H. pylori* infection might induce increased acid secretion through both direct and indirect actions of *H. pylori* and proinflammatory cytokines (IL-8, TNF, and IL-1) on G, D, and parietal cells (Fig. 274-7). *H. pylori* infection has also been associated with decreased duodenal mucosal bicarbonate production. Data supporting and contradicting each of these interesting theories have been demonstrated. Thus, the mechanism by which *H. pylori* infection of the stomach leads to duodenal ulceration remains to be established.

In summary, the final effect of *H. pylori* on the gastrointestinal tract is variable and determined by microbial and host factors. The type and distribution of gastritis correlate with the ultimate gastric and duodenal pathology observed. Specifically, the presence of antral-predominant gastritis is associated with DU formation; gastritis involving primarily the corpus predisposes to the development of GUs, gastric atrophy, and ultimately gastric carcinoma (Figure 274-8).

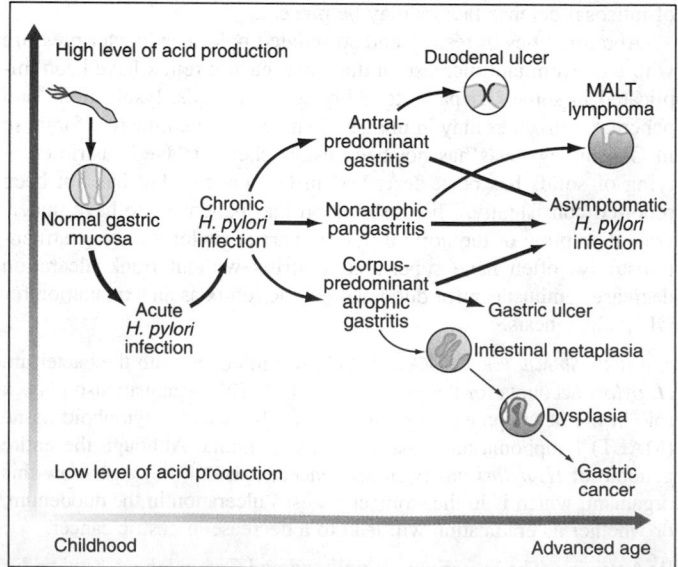

FIGURE 274-8 Natural history of *H. pylori* infection. *(Used with permission from Suerbaum and Michetti.)*

NSAIDS-INDUCED DISEASE ■ *Epidemiology* NSAIDs represent one of the most commonly used medications in the United States. More than 30 billion over-the-counter tablets and 70 million prescriptions are sold yearly in the United States alone. In fact, after the introduction of COX-2 inhibitors in the year 2000, the number of prescriptions written for NSAIDs was >111 million at a cost of $4.8 billion. The spectrum of NSAID-induced morbidity ranges from nausea and dyspepsia (prevalence reported as high as 50 to 60%) to a serious gastrointestinal complication such as frank peptic ulceration (3 to 4%) complicated by bleeding or perforation in as many as 1.5% of users per year. About 20,000 patients die each year from serious gastrointestinal complications from NSAIDs. Unfortunately, dyspeptic symptoms do not correlate with NSAID-induced pathology. Over 80% of patients with serious NSAID-related complications did not have preceding dyspepsia. In view of the lack of warning signs, it is important to identify patients who are at increased risk for morbidity and mortality related to NSAID usage. Even 75 mg/d of aspirin may lead to serious gastrointestinal ulceration, thus no dose of NSAID is completely safe. Established risk factors include advanced age, history of ulcer, concomitant use of glucocorticoids, high dose NSAIDs, multiple NSAIDs, concomitant use of anticoagulants, and serious or multisystem disease. Possible risk factors include concomitant infection with *H. pylori*, cigarette smoking, and alcohol consumption.

Pathophysiology Prostaglandins play a critical role in maintaining gastroduodenal mucosal integrity and repair. It therefore follows that interruption of prostaglandin synthesis can impair mucosal defense and repair, thus facilitating mucosal injury via a systemic mechanism. A summary of the pathogenetic pathways by which systemically administered NSAIDs may lead to mucosal injury is shown in Fig. 274-9.

Injury to the mucosa also occurs as a result of the topical encounter with NSAIDs. Aspirin and many NSAIDs are weak acids that remain in a nonionized lipophilic form when found within the acid environment of the stomach. Under these conditions, NSAIDs migrate across lipid membranes of epithelial cells, leading to cell injury once trapped intracellularly in an ionized form. Topical NSAIDs can also alter the surface mucous layer, permitting back diffusion of H+ and pepsin, leading to further epithelial cell damage. Moreover, enteric-coated or buffered preparations are also associated with risk of peptic ulceration.

MISCELLANEOUS PATHOGENETIC FACTORS IN ACID PEPTIC DISEASE Cigarette smoking has been implicated in the pathogenesis of PUD. Not only have smokers been found to have ulcers more frequently than do nonsmokers, but smoking appears to decrease healing rates, impair response to therapy, and increase ulcer-related complications such as perforation. The mechanism responsible for increased ulcer diathesis in smokers is unknown. Theories have included altered gastric emptying, decreased proximal duodenal bicarbonate production, increased risk for

H. pylori infection, and cigarette-induced generation of noxious mucosal free radicals. Acid secretion is not abnormal in smokers. Despite these interesting theories, a unifying mechanism for cigarette-induced peptic ulcer diathesis has not been established.

Genetic predisposition has also been considered to play a role in ulcer development. First-degree relatives of DU patients are three times as likely to develop an ulcer; however, the potential role of *H. pylori* infection in contacts is a major consideration. Increased frequency of blood group O and of the nonsecretor status have also been implicated as genetic risk factors for peptic diathesis. However, *H. pylori* preferentially binds to group O antigens. Therefore, the role of genetic predisposition in common PUD has not been established.

Psychological stress has been thought to contribute to PUD, but studies examining the role of psychological factors in its pathogenesis have generated conflicting results. Although PUD is associated with certain personality traits (neuroticism), these same traits are also present in individuals with nonulcer dyspepsia (NUD) and other functional and organic disorders. Although more work in this area is needed, no typical PUD personality has been found.

Diet has also been thought to play a role in peptic diseases. Certain foods can cause dyspepsia, but no convincing studies indicate an association between ulcer formation and a specific diet. This is also true for beverages containing alcohol and caffeine. Specific chronic disorders have been associated with PUD. Those with a strong association are (1) systemic mastocytosis, (2) chronic pulmonary disease, (3) chronic renal failure, (4) cirrhosis, (5) nephrolithiasis, and (6) α_1-antitrypsin deficiency. Those with a possible association are (1) hyperparathyroidism, (2) coronary artery disease, (3) polycythemia vera, and (4) chronic pancreatitis.

Multiple factors play a role in the pathogenesis of PUD. The two predominant causes are *H. pylori* infection and NSAID ingestion. PUD not related to *H. pylori* or NSAIDs may be increasing. Independent of the inciting or injurious agent, peptic ulcers develop as a result of an imbalance between mucosal protection/repair and aggressive factors. Gastric acid plays an essential role in mucosal injury.

CLINICAL FEATURES ■ **History** Abdominal pain is common to many gastrointestinal disorders, including DU and GU, but has a poor predictive value for the presence of either DU or GU. Up to 10% of patients with NSAID-induced mucosal disease can present with a complication (bleeding, perforation, and obstruction) without antecedent symptoms. Despite this poor correlation, a careful history and physical examination are essential components of the approach to a patient suspected of having peptic ulcers.

Epigastric pain described as a burning or gnawing discomfort can be present in both DU and GU. The discomfort is also described as an ill-defined, aching sensation or as hunger pain. The typical pain pattern in DU occurs 90 min to 3 h after a meal and is frequently relieved by antacids or food. Pain that awakes the patient from sleep (between midnight and 3 A.M.) is the most discriminating symptom, with two-thirds of DU patients describing this complaint. Unfortunately, this symptom is also present in one-third of patients with NUD. The pain pattern in GU patients may be different from that in DU patients, where discomfort may actually be precipitated by food. Nausea and weight loss occur more commonly in GU patients. In the United States, endoscopy detects ulcers in <30% of patients who have dyspepsia. Despite this, 40% of these individuals with typical ulcer symptoms had an ulcer crater, and 40% had gastroduodenitis on endoscopic examination.

The mechanism for development of abdominal pain in ulcer patients is unknown. Several possible explanations include acid-induced activation of chemical receptors in the duodenum, enhanced duodenal sensitivity to bile acids and pepsin, or altered gastroduodenal motility.

Variation in the intensity or distribution of the abdominal pain, as well as the onset of associated symptoms such as nausea and/or vomiting, may be indicative of an ulcer complication. Dyspepsia that be-

FIGURE 274-9 Mechanisms by which NSAIDs may induce mucosal injury. *(Adapted from J Scheiman et al: J Clin Outcomes Management 3:23, 1996.)*

comes constant, is no longer relieved by food or antacids, or radiates to the back may indicate a penetrating ulcer (pancreas). Sudden onset of severe, generalized abdominal pain may indicate perforation. Pain worsening with meals, nausea, and vomiting of undigested food suggest gastric outlet obstruction. Tarry stools or coffee ground emesis indicate bleeding.

Physical Examination   Epigastric tenderness is the most frequent finding in patients with GU or DU. Pain may be found to the right of the midline in 20% of patients. Unfortunately, the predictive value of this finding is rather low. Physical examination is critically important for discovering evidence of ulcer complication. Tachycardia and orthostasis suggest dehydration secondary to vomiting or active gastrointestinal blood loss. A severely tender, boardlike abdomen suggests a perforation. Presence of a succussion splash indicates retained fluid in the stomach, suggesting gastric outlet obstruction.

PUD-Related Complications ■ *GASTROINTESTINAL BLEEDING*   Gastrointestinal bleeding is the most common complication observed in PUD. It occurs in ~15% of patients and more often in individuals >60 years old. The higher incidence in the elderly is likely due to the increased use of NSAIDs in this group. As many as 20% of patients with ulcer-related hemorrhage bleed without any preceding warning signs or symptoms.

PERFORATION   The second most common ulcer-related complication is perforation, being reported in as many as 6 to 7% of PUD patients. As in the case of bleeding, the incidence of perforation in the elderly appears to be increasing secondary to increased use of NSAIDs. Penetration is a form of perforation in which the ulcer bed tunnels into an adjacent organ. DUs tend to penetrate posteriorly into the pancreas, leading to pancreatitis, whereas GUs tend to penetrate into the left hepatic lobe. Gastrocolic fistulas associated with GUs have also been described.

GASTRIC OUTLET OBSTRUCTION   Gastric outlet obstruction is the least common ulcer-related complication, occurring in 1 to 2% of patients. A patient may have relative obstruction secondary to ulcer-related inflammation and edema in the peripyloric region. This process often resolves with ulcer healing. A fixed, mechanical obstruction secondary to scar formation in the peripyloric areas is also possible. The latter requires endoscopic (balloon dilation) or surgical intervention. Signs and symptoms relative to mechanical obstruction may develop insidiously. New onset of early satiety, nausea, vomiting, increase of postprandial abdominal pain, and weight loss should make gastric outlet obstruction a possible diagnosis.

Differential Diagnosis   The list of gastrointestinal and nongastrointestinal disorders that can mimic ulceration of the stomach or duodenum is quite extensive. The most commonly encountered diagnosis among patients seen for upper abdominal discomfort is NUD. NUD, also known as *functional dyspepsia* or *essential dyspepsia*, refers to a group of heterogeneous disorders typified by upper abdominal pain without the presence of an ulcer. Dyspepsia has been reported to occur in up to 30% of the U.S. population. Up to 60% of patients seeking medical care for dyspepsia have a negative diagnostic evaluation. The etiology of NUD is not established, and the potential role of *H. pylori* in NUD remains controversial.

Several additional disease processes that may present with "ulcer-like" symptoms include proximal gastrointestinal tumors, gastroesophageal reflux, vascular disease, pancreaticobiliary disease (biliary colic, chronic pancreatitis), and gastroduodenal Crohn's disease.

Diagnostic Evaluation   In view of the poor predictive value of abdominal pain for the presence of a gastroduodenal ulcer and the multiple disease processes that can mimic this disease, the clinician is often confronted with having to establish the presence of an ulcer. Documentation of an ulcer requires either a radiographic (barium study) or an endoscopic procedure. However, a large percentage of patients with symptoms suggestive of an ulcer have NUD; empirical therapy is appropriate for

individuals who are otherwise healthy and <45, before embarking on a diagnostic evaluation (Chap. 34).

Barium studies of the proximal gastrointestinal tract are still commonly used as a first test for documenting an ulcer. The sensitivity of older single-contrast barium meals for detecting a DU is as high as 80%, with a double-contrast study providing detection rates as high as 90%. Sensitivity for detection is decreased in small ulcers (<0.5 cm), presence of previous scarring, or in postoperative patients. A DU appears as a well-demarcated crater, most often seen in the bulb. A GU may represent benign or malignant disease. Typically, a benign GU also appears as a discrete crater with radiating mucosal folds originating from the ulcer margin. Ulcers >3 cm in size or those associated with a mass are more often malignant. Unfortunately, up to 8% of GUs that appear to be benign by radiographic appearance are malignant by endoscopy or surgery. Radiographic studies that show a GU must be followed by endoscopy and biopsy.

Endoscopy provides the most sensitive and specific approach for examining the upper gastrointestinal tract. In addition to permitting direct visualization of the mucosa, endoscopy facilitates photographic documentation of a mucosal defect and tissue biopsy to rule out malignancy (GU) or *H. pylori*. Endoscopic examination is particularly helpful in identifying lesions too small to detect by radiographic examination, for evaluation of atypical radiographic abnormalities, or to determine if an ulcer is a source of blood loss.

Although the methods for diagnosing *H. pylori* are outlined in Chap. 135, a brief summary will be included here (Table 274-1). Several biopsy urease tests have been developed (PyloriTek, Clotest, Hpfast, Pronto Dry) and have a sensitivity and specificity of >90 to 95%. Several noninvasive methods for detecting this organism have been developed. Three types of studies routinely used include serologic testing, the ^{13}C- or ^{14}C-urea breath test (UBT), and the fecal *H. pylori* antigen test.

Occasionally, specialized testing such as serum gastrin and gastric acid analysis or sham feeding may be needed in individuals with complicated or refractory PUD (see "Zollinger-Ellison Syndrome," below). Screening for aspirin or NSAIDS (blood or urine) may also be necessary in refractory *H. pylori*–negative PUD patients.

℞ **TREATMENT**

Before the discovery of *H. pylori*, the therapy of PUD disease was centered on the old dictum by Schwartz of "no acid, no ulcer." Al-

TABLE 274-1   *Tests for Detection of H. pylori*

Test	Sensitivity/ Specificity, %	Comments
INVASIVE (ENDOSCOPY/BIOPSY REQUIRED)		
Rapid urease	80–95/95–100	Simple, false negative with recent use of PPIs, antibiotics, or bismuth compounds
Histology	80–90/>95	Requires pathology processing and staining; provides histologic information
Culture	—/—	Time-consuming, expensive, dependent on experience; allows determination of antibiotic susceptibility
NON-INVASIVE		
Serology	>80/>90	Inexpensive, convenient; not useful for early follow-up
Urea breath test	>90/>90	Simple, rapid; useful for early follow-up; false negatives with recent therapy (see rapid urease test); exposure to low-dose radiation with ^{14}C test
Stool antigen	>90/>90	Inexpensive, convenient; not established for eradication but promising

Note: PPIs, proton pump inhibitors.

though acid secretion is still important in the pathogenesis of PUD, eradication of *H. pylori* and therapy/prevention of NSAID-induced disease is the mainstay. A summary of commonly used drugs for treatment of acid peptic disorders is shown in Table 274-2.

Acid Neutralizing/Inhibitory Drugs ■ *ANTACIDS* Before we understood the important role of histamine in stimulating parietal cell activity, neutralization of secreted acid with antacids constituted the main form of therapy for peptic ulcers. They are now rarely, if ever, used as the primary therapeutic agent but instead are often used by patients for symptomatic relief of dyspepsia. The most commonly used agents are mixtures of aluminum hydroxide and magnesium hydroxide. Aluminum hydroxide can produce constipation and phosphate depletion; magnesium hydroxide may cause loose stools. Many of the commonly used antacids (e.g., Maalox, Mylanta) have a combination of both aluminum and magnesium hydroxide in order to avoid these side effects. The magnesium-containing preparation should not be used in chronic renal failure patients because of possible hypermagnesemia, and aluminum may cause chronic neurotoxicity in these patients.

Calcium carbonate and sodium bicarbonate are potent antacids with varying levels of potential problems. The long-term use of calcium carbonate (converts to calcium chloride in the stomach) can lead to milk-alkali syndrome (hypercalcemia, hyperphosphatemia with possible renal calcinosis and progression to renal insufficiency). Sodium bicarbonate may induce systemic alkalosis.

H₂ RECEPTOR ANTAGONISTS Four of these agents are presently available (cimetidine, ranitidine, famotidine, and nizatidine), and their structures share homology with histamine. Although each has different potency, all will significantly inhibit basal and stimulated acid secretion to comparable levels when used at therapeutic doses. Moreover, similar ulcer-healing rates are achieved with each drug when used at the correct dosage. Presently, this class of drug is often used for treatment of active ulcers (4 to 6 weeks) in combination with antibiotics directed at eradicating *H. pylori* (see below).

Cimetidine was the first H_2 receptor antagonist used for the treatment of acid peptic disorders. The initial recommended dosing profile for cimetidine was 300 mg four times per day. Subsequent studies have documented the efficacy of using 800 mg at bedtime for treatment of active ulcer, with healing rates approaching 80% at 4 weeks. Cimetidine may have weak antiandrogenic side effects resulting in reversible gynecomastia and impotence, primarily in patients receiving high doses for prolonged periods of time (months to years, as in ZES). In view of cimetidine's ability to inhibit cytochrome P450, careful monitoring of drugs such as warfarin, phenytoin, and theophylline is indicated with long-term usage. Other rare reversible adverse effects reported with cimetidine include confusion and elevated levels of serum aminotransferases, creatinine, and serum prolactin. Ranitidine, famotidine, and nizatidine are more potent H_2 receptor antagonists than cimetidine. Each can be used once a day at bedtime. Comparable nighttime dosing regimens are ranitidine, 300 mg, famotidine, 40 mg, and nizatidine, 300 mg.

Additional rare, reversible systemic toxicities reported with H_2 receptor antagonists include pancytopenia, neutropenia, anemia, and thrombocytopenia, with a prevalence rate varying from 0.01 to 0.2%. Cimetidine and rantidine (to a lesser extent) can bind to hepatic cytochrome P450; famotidine and nizatidine do not.

PROTON PUMP (H⁺,K⁺-ATPASE) INHIBITORS Omeprazole, esomeprazole, lansoprazole, rabeprazole, and pantoprazole are substituted benzimidazole derivatives that covalently bind and irreversibly inhibit H⁺,K⁺-ATPase. Esomeprazole, the newest member of this drug class, is the S-enantiomer of omeprazole, which is a racemic mixture of both S- and R-optical isomers. These are the most potent acid inhibitory agents available. Omeprazole and lansoprazole are the proton pump inhibitors (PPIs) that have been used for the longest time. Both are acid labile and are administered as enteric-coated granules in a sustained-release capsule that dissolves within the small intestine at a pH of 6. Pantoprazole and rabeprazole are available as enteric-coated tablets. Pantoprazole is also available as a parenteral formulation for intravenous use. These agents are lipophilic compounds; upon entering the parietal cell, they are protonated and trapped within the acid environment of the tubulovesicular and canalicular system. These agents potently inhibit all phases of gastric acid secretion. Onset of action is rapid, with a maximum acid inhibitory effect between 2 and 6 h after administration and duration of inhibition lasting up to 72 to 96 h. With repeated daily dosing, progressive acid inhibitory effects are observed, with basal and secretagogue-stimulated acid production being inhibited by >95% after 1 week of therapy. The half-life of PPIs is ~18 h; thus it can take between 2 and 5 days for gastric acid secretion to return to normal levels once these drugs have been discontinued. Because the pumps need to be activated for these agents to be effective, their efficacy is maximized if they are administered before a meal (e.g., in the morning before breakfast). Standard dosing for omeprazole and lansoprazole is 20 mg and 30 mg once per day, respectively. Mild to moderate hypergastrinemia has been observed in patients taking these drugs. Carcinoid tumors developed in some animals given the drugs preclinically; however, extensive experience has failed to demonstrate gastric carcinoid tumor development in humans. Serum gastrin levels return to normal levels within 1 to 2 weeks after drug cessation. As with any agent that leads to significant hypochlorhydria, PPIs may interfere with absorption of drugs such as ketoconazole, ampicillin, iron, and digoxin. Hepatic cytochrome P450 can be inhibited by the earlier PPIs (omeprazole, lansoprazole). Rabeprazole, pantoprazole, and esomeprazole do not appear to interact significantly with drugs metabolized by the cytochrome P450 system. The overall clinical significance of this observation is not definitely established. Caution should be taken when using warfarin, diazepam, and phenytoin concomitantly with PPIs.

Cytoprotective Agents ■ *SUCRALFATE* Sucralfate is a complex sucrose salt in which the hydroxyl groups have been substituted by aluminum hydroxide and sulfate. This compound is insoluble in water and becomes a viscous paste within the stomach and duodenum, binding primarily to sites of active ulceration. Sucralfate may act by several mechanisms. In the gastric environment, aluminum hydroxide dissociates, leaving the polar sulfate anion, which can bind to positively charged tissue proteins found within the ulcer bed, and providing a physicochemical barrier impeding further tissue injury by acid and pepsin. Sucralfate may also induce a trophic effect by binding growth factors such as EGF, enhance prostaglandin synthesis, stimulate mucous and bicarbonate secretion, and enhance mucosal defense and repair. Toxicity from this drug is rare, with constipation being the most common one reported (2 to 3%). It should be avoided in patients with chronic renal

TABLE 274-2 Drugs Used in the Treatment of Peptic Ulcer Disease		
Drug Type/Mechanism	**Examples**	**Dose**
Acid-suppressing drugs		
Antacids	Mylanta, Maalox, Tums, Gaviscon	100–140 meq/L 1 and 3 h after meals and hs
H₂ receptor antagonists	Cimetidine	400 mg bid
	Ranitidine	300 mg hs
	Famotidine	40 mg hs
	Nizatidine	300 mg hs
Proton pump inhibitors	Omeprazole	20 mg/d
	Lansoprazole	30 mg/d
	Rabeprazole	20 mg/d
	Pantoprazole	40 mg/d
	Esomeprazole	20 mg/d
Mucosal protective agents		
Sucralfate	Sucralfate	1 g qid
Prostaglandin analogue	Misoprostol	200 μg qid
Bismuth-containing compounds	Bismuth subsalicylate (BSS)	See anti-*H. pylori* regimens (Table 274-3)

insufficiency to prevent aluminum-induced neurotoxicity. Hypophosphatemia and gastric bezoar formation have also been rarely reported. Standard dosing of sucralfate is 1 g four times per day.

BISMUTH-CONTAINING PREPARATIONS Sir William Osler considered bismuth-containing compounds the drug of choice for treating PUD. The resurgence in the use of these agents is due to their effect against *H. pylori*. Colloidal bismuth subcitrate (CBS) and bismuth subsalicylate (BSS, Pepto-Bismol) are the most widely used preparations. The mechanism by which these agents induce ulcer healing is unclear. Potential mechanisms include ulcer coating; prevention of further pepsin/HCl-induced damage; binding of pepsin; and stimulation of prostaglandins, bicarbonate, and mucous secretion. Adverse effects with short-term usage are rare with bismuth compounds. Long-term usage with high doses, especially with the avidly absorbed CBS, may lead to neurotoxicity. These compounds are commonly used as one of the agents in an anti-*H. pylori* regimen (see below).

PROSTAGLANDIN ANALOGUES In view of their central role in maintaining mucosal integrity and repair, stable prostaglandin analogues were developed for the treatment of PUD. The prostaglandin E_1 derivative misoprostal is the only agent of this class approved by the U.S. Food and Drug Administration for clinical use in the prevention of NSAID-induced gastroduodenal mucosal injury (see below). The mechanism by which this rapidly absorbed drug provides its therapeutic effect is through enhancement of mucosal defense and repair. Prostaglandin analogues enhance mucous bicarbonate secretion, stimulate mucosal blood flow, and decrease mucosal cell turnover. The most common toxicity noted with this drug is diarrhea (10 to 30% incidence). Other major toxicities include uterine bleeding and contractions; misoprostal is contraindicated in women who may be pregnant, and women of childbearing age must be made clearly aware of this potential drug toxicity. The standard therapeutic dose is 200 μg four times per day.

MISCELLANEOUS DRUGS A number of drugs aimed at treating acid peptic disorders have been developed over the years. In view of their limited utilization in the United States, if any, they will only be listed briefly. Anticholinergics, designed to inhibit activation of the muscarinic receptor in parietal cells, met with limited success due to their relatively weak acid-inhibiting effect and significant side effects (dry eyes, dry mouth, urinary retention). Tricyclic antidepressants have been suggested by some, but again the toxicity of these agents in comparison to the safe, effective drugs already described precludes their utility. Finally, the licorice extract carbenoxolone has aldosterone-like side effects with fluid retention and hypokalemia, making it an undesirable therapeutic option.

Therapy of *H. pylori* Extensive effort has been placed into determining who of the many individuals with *H. pylori* infection should be treated. The common conclusion arrived at by multiple consensus conferences (National Institutes of Health Consensus Development, American Digestive Health Foundation International Update Conference, European Maastricht Consensus, and Asia Pacific Consensus Conference) is that *H. pylori* should be eradicated in patients with documented PUD. This holds true independent of time of presentation (first episode or not), severity of symptoms, presence of confounding factors such as ingestion of NSAIDs, or whether the ulcer is in remission. Some have advocated treating patients with a history of documented PUD who are found to be *H. pylori*–positive by serology or breath testing. Over half of patients with gastric MALT lymphoma experience complete remission of the tumor in response to *H. pylori* eradication. Treating patients with NUD to prevent gastric cancer or patients with gastroesophageal reflux disease requiring long-term acid suppression remains controversial.

Multiple drugs have been evaluated in the therapy of *H. pylori*. No single agent is effective in eradicating the organism. Combination therapy for 14 days provides the greatest efficacy. A short-time course administration (7 to 10 days), although attractive, has not proved as successful as the 14-day regimens. The agents used with the greatest frequency include amoxicillin, metronidazole, tetracycline, clarithromycin, and bismuth compounds.

The physician's goal in treating PUD is to provide relief of symptoms (pain or dyspepsia), promote ulcer healing, and ultimately prevent ulcer recurrence and complications. The greatest impact of understanding the role of *H. pylori* in peptic disease has been the ability to prevent recurrence of what was often a recurring disease. Documented eradication of *H. pylori* in patients with PUD is associated with a dramatic decrease in ulcer recurrence to 4% (as compared to 59%) in GU patients and 6% (compared to 67%) in DU patients. Eradication of the organism may lead to diminished recurrent ulcer bleeding. The impact of its eradication on ulcer perforation is unclear.

Suggested treatment regimens for *H. pylori* are outlined in Table 274-3. Choice of a particular regimen will be influenced by several factors including efficacy, patient tolerance, existing antibiotic resistance, and cost of the drugs. The aim for initial eradication rates should be 85 to 90%. Dual therapy [PPI plus amoxicillin, PPI plus clarithromycin, ranitidine bismuth citrate (Tritec) plus clarithromycin] are not recommended in view of studies demonstrating eradication rates of <80 to 85%. The combination of bismuth, metronidazole, and tetracycline was the first triple regimen found effective against *H. pylori*. The combination of two antibiotics plus either a PPI, H_2 blocker, or bismuth compound has comparable success rates. Addition of acid suppression assists in providing early symptom relief and may enhance bacterial eradication.

Triple therapy, although effective, has several drawbacks, including the potential for poor patient compliance and drug-induced side effects. Compliance is being addressed somewhat by simplifying the regimens so that patients can take the medications twice a day. Simpler (dual therapy) and shorter regimens (7 and 10 days) are not as effective as triple therapy for 14 days. Two anti-*H. pylori* regimens are available in prepackaged formulation: Prevpac (lansoprazole, clarithromycin, and amoxicillin) and Helidac (bismuth subsalicylate, tetracycline, and metronidazole). The contents of the Prevpac are to be taken twice per day for 14 days, whereas Helidac constituents are taken four times per day with an antisecretory agent (PPI or H_2 blocker), also taken for at least 14 days.

Side effects have been reported in up to 20 to 30% of patients on triple therapy. Bismuth may cause black stools, constipation, or darkening of the tongue. The most feared complication with amoxicillin is pseudomembranous colitis, but this occurs in <1 to 2% of patients. Amoxicillin can also lead to antibiotic-associated diarrhea, nausea, vomiting, skin rash, and allergic reaction. Tetracycline has been reported to cause rashes and very rarely hepatotoxicity and anaphylaxis.

TABLE 274-3 Regimens Recommended for Eradication of *H. pylori* Infection	
Drug	Dose
TRIPLE THERAPY	
1. Bismuth subsalicylate *plus*	2 tablets qid
Metronidazole *plus*	250 mg qid
Tetracycline[a]	500 mg qid
2. Ranitidine bismuth citrate *plus*	400 mg bid
Tetracycline *plus*	500 mg bid
Clarithromycin or metronidazole	500 mg bid
3. Omeprazole (lansoprazole) *plus*	20 mg bid (30 mg bid)
Clarithromycin *plus*	250 or 500 mg bid
Metronidazole[b] *or*	500 mg bid
Amoxicillin[c]	1 gr bid
QUADRUPLE THERAPY	
Omeprazole (lansoprazole)	20 mg (30 mg) daily
Bismuth subsalicylate	2 tablets qid
Metronidazole	250 mg qid
Tetracycline	500 mg qid

[a] Alternative: use prepacked Helidac (see text).
[b] Alternative: use prepacked Prevpac (see text).
[c] Use either metronidazole or amoxicillin, not both.

One important concern with treating patients who may not need treatment is the potential for development of antibiotic-resistant strains. The incidence and type of antibiotic-resistant *H. pylori* strains vary worldwide. Strains resistant to metronidazole, clarithromycin, amoxicillin, and tetracycline have been described, with the latter two being uncommon. Antibiotic-resistant strains are the most common cause for treatment failure in compliant patients. Unfortunately, in vitro resistance does not predict outcome in patients. Culture and sensitivity testing of *H. pylori* is not performed routinely. Although resistance to metronidazole has been found in as many as 30% and 95% of isolates in North America and Asia, respectively, triple therapy is effective in eradicating the organism in >50% of patients infected with a resistant strain. Clarithromycin resistance is seen in about 10% of persons in the United States.

Failure of *H. pylori* eradication with triple therapy is usually due to infection with a resistant organism. Quadruple therapy (Table 274-3), where clarithromycin is substituted for metronidazole (or vice versa), should be the next step. The combination of pantoprazole, amoxicillin, and rifabutin for 10 days has also been used successfully (86% cure rate) in patients infected with resistant strains. If eradication is still not achieved in a compliant patient, then culture and sensitivity of the organism should be considered.

Reinfection after successful eradication of *H. pylori* is rare in the United States (<1%/year). If recurrent infection occurs within the first 6 months after completing therapy, the most likely explanation is recrudescence as opposed to reinfection, which occurs later in time.

Therapy of NSAID-Related Gastric or Duodenal Injury Medical intervention for NSAID-related mucosal injury includes treatment of an active ulcer and prevention of future injury. Recommendations for the treatment and prevention of NSAID-related mucosal injury are in Table 274-4. Ideally the injurious agent should be stopped as the first step in the therapy of an active NSAID-induced ulcer. If that is possible, then treatment with one of the acid inhibitory agents (H_2 blockers, PPIs) is indicated. Cessation of NSAIDs is not always possible because of the patient's severe underlying disease. Only PPIs can heal GUs or DUs, independent of whether NSAIDs are discontinued.

Prevention of NSAID-induced ulceration can be accomplished by misoprostol (200 μg qid) or a PPI. High-dose H_2 blockers (famotidine, 40 mg bid) have also shown some promise, although PPIs are superior. The use of COX-2-selective NSAIDs may also reduce injury to gastric mucosa. Two highly selective COX-2 inhibitors, celecoxib and rofecoxib, are 100 times more selective inhibitors of COX-2 than standard NSAIDs, leading to gastric or duodenal mucosal injury that is comparable to placebo. However, several issues regarding the safety of these selective COX-2 inhibitors require clarification. Specifically, the CLASS study demonstrates that the advantage of celecoxib in preventing gastrointestinal complications was offset when low-dose aspirin was used simultaneously. Therefore, gastric protection therapy is required in individuals taking COX-2 inhibitors and aspirin prophylaxis. In addition, COX-2 inhibitors delay experimental ulcer healing in animal models and may promote cardiovascular thrombosis. Finally, much of the work performed demonstrating the benefit of COX-2 inhibitors and PPIs on gastrointestinal injury has been performed in individuals of average risk; it is unclear if the same level of benefit will be achieved in high-risk patients.

Approach and Therapy: Summary Controversy continues regarding the best approach to the patient who presents with dyspepsia (Chap. 34). The discovery of *H. pylori* and its role in pathogenesis of ulcers has added a new variable to the equation. Previously, if a patient <50 presented with dyspepsia and without alarming signs or symptoms suggestive of an ulcer complication or malignancy, an empirical therapeutic trial with acid suppression was commonly recommended. Although this approach is practiced by some today, an approach presently gaining approval for the treatment of patients with dyspepsia is outlined in Fig. 274-10. The referral to a gastroenterologist is for the potential need of endoscopy and subsequent evaluation and treatment if the endoscopy is negative.

TABLE 274-4	*Recommendations for Treatment of NSAID-Related Mucosal Injury*
Clinical Setting	**Recommendation**
Active ulcer	
NSAID discontinued	H_2 receptor antagonist or PPI
NSAID continued	PPI
Prophylactic therapy	Misoprostol
	PPI
	Selective COX-2 inhibitor
H. pylori infection	Eradication if active ulcer present or there is a past history of peptic ulcer disease

Note: PPI, proton pump inhibitor; COX-2, isoenzyme of cyclooxygenase.

Once an ulcer (GU or DU) is documented, then the main issue at stake is whether *H. pylori* or an NSAID is involved. With *H. pylori* present, independent of the NSAID status, triple therapy is recommended for 14 days, followed by continued acid-suppressing drugs (H_2 receptor antagonist or PPIs) for a total of 4 to 6 weeks. Selection of patients for documentation of *H. pylori* eradication (organisms gone at least 4 weeks after completing antibiotics) is an area of some debate. The test of choice for documenting eradication is the UBT. The stool antigen study may also hold promise for this purpose, but the data have not been as clear cut as in the case of using the stool antigen test for primary diagnosis. Further studies are warranted, but if the UBT is not available, a stool antigen should be considered to document eradication. Serologic testing is not useful for the purpose of documenting eradication since antibody titers fall slowly and often do not become undetectable. Two approaches toward documentation of eradication exist: (1) test for eradication only in individuals with a complicated course or in individuals who are frail or with multisystem disease who would do poorly with an ulcer recurrence, and (2) test all patients for successful eradication. Some recommend that patients with complicated ulcer disease or who are frail should be treated with long-term acid suppression, thus making documentation of *H. pylori* eradication a moot point. In view of this discrepancy in practice, it would be best to discuss with the patient the different options available.

Several issues differentiate the approach to a GU versus a DU. GUs,

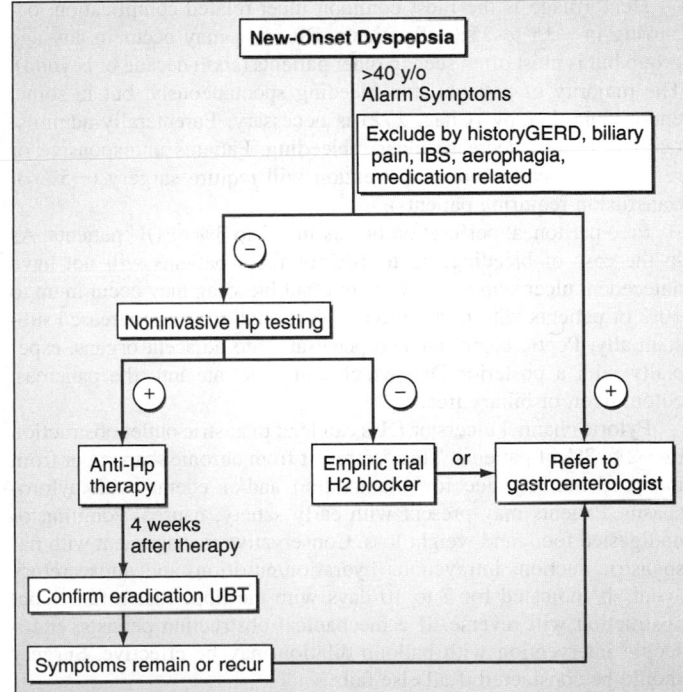

FIGURE 274-10 Overview of new-onset dyspepsia. Hp, *H. pylori*; UBT, urea breath test; IBS, irritable bowel syndrome. (*Adapted from BS Anand and DY Graham: Endoscopy 31:215, 1999.*)

especially of the body and fundus, have the potential of being malignant. Multiple biopsies of a GU should be taken initially; even if these are negative for neoplasm, repeat endoscopy to document healing at 8 to 12 weeks should be performed, with biopsy if the ulcer is still present. About 70% of GUs eventually found to be malignant undergo significant (usually incomplete) healing.

The majority (>90%) of GUs and DUs heal with the conventional therapy outlined above. A GU that fails to heal after 12 weeks and a DU that does not heal after 8 weeks of therapy should be considered refractory. Once poor compliance and persistent *H. pylori* infection have been excluded, NSAID use, either inadvertent or surreptitious, must be excluded. In addition, cigarette smoking must be eliminated. For a GU, malignancy must be meticulously excluded. Next, consideration should be given to a gastric hypersecretory state, which can be excluded with gastric acid analysis. Although a subset of patients have gastric acid hypersecretion of unclear etiology as a contributing factor to refractory ulcers, ZES should be excluded with a fasting gastrin or secretin stimulation test (see below). More than 90% of refractory ulcers (either DUs or GUs) heal after 8 weeks of treatment with higher doses of PPI (omeprazole, 40 mg/d; lansoprazole 30 to 60 mg/d). This higher dose is also effective in maintaining remission. Surgical intervention may be a consideration at this point; however, other rare causes of refractory ulcers must be excluded before recommending surgery. Rare etiologies of refractory ulcers that may be diagnosed by gastric or duodenal biopsies include: ischemia, Crohn's disease, amyloidosis, sarcoidosis, lymphoma, eosinophilic gastroenteritis, or infection [cytomegalovirus (CMV), tuberculosis, or syphilis].

Surgical Therapy   Surgical intervention in PUD can be viewed as being either elective, for treatment of medically refractory disease, or as urgent/emergent, for the treatment of an ulcer-related complication. The development of pharmacologic and endoscopic approaches for the treatment of peptic disease has led to a substantial decrease in the number operations needed for this disorder. Refractory ulcers are an exceedingly rare occurrence. Surgery is more often required for treatment of an ulcer-related complication. Gastrointestinal bleeding (Chap. 37), perforation, and gastric outlet obstruction are the three complications that may require surgical intervention.

Hemorrhage is the most common ulcer-related complication, occurring in ~15 to 25% of patients. Bleeding may occur in any age group but is most often seen in older patients (sixth decade or beyond). The majority of patients stop bleeding spontaneously, but in some, endoscopic therapy (Chap. 272) is necessary. Parenterally administered PPIs also decrease ulcer rebleeding. Patients unresponsive or refractory to endoscopic intervention will require surgery (~5% of transfusion-requiring patients).

Free peritoneal perforation occurs in ~2 to 3% of DU patients. As in the case of bleeding, up to 10% of these patients will not have antecedent ulcer symptoms. Concomitant bleeding may occur in up to 10% of patients with perforation, with mortality being increased substantially. Peptic ulcer can also penetrate into adjacent organs, especially with a posterior DU, which can penetrate into the pancreas, colon, liver, or biliary tree.

Pyloric channel ulcers or DUs can lead to gastric outlet obstruction in ~2 to 3% of patients. This can result from chronic scarring or from impaired motility due to inflammation and/or edema with pylorospasm. Patients may present with early satiety, nausea, vomiting of undigested food, and weight loss. Conservative management with nasogastric suction, intravenous hydration/nutrition, and antisecretory agents is indicated for 7 to 10 days with the hope that a functional obstruction will reverse. If a mechanical obstruction persists, endoscopic intervention with balloon dilation may be effective. Surgery should be considered if all else fails.

Specific Operations for Duodenal Ulcers   Surgical treatment is designed to decrease gastric acid secretion. Operations most commonly performed include (1) vagotomy and drainage (by pyloroplasty, gastroduodenostomy, or gastrojejunostomy), (2) highly selective vagotomy (which does not require a drainage procedure), and (3) vagotomy with antrectomy. The specific procedure performed is dictated by the underlying circumstances: elective vs. emergency, the degree and extent of duodenal ulceration, and the expertise of the surgeon.

Vagotomy is a component of each of these procedures and is aimed at decreasing acid secretion through ablating cholinergic input to the stomach. Unfortunately, both truncal and selective vagotomy (preserves the celiac and hepatic branches) result in gastric atony despite successful reduction of both basal acid output (BAO, decreased by 85%) and maximal acid output (MAO, decreased by 50%). Drainage through pyloroplasty or gastroduodenostomy is required in an effort to compensate for the vagotomy-induced gastric motility disorder. This procedure has an intermediate complication rate and a 10% ulcer recurrence rate. To minimize gastric dysmotility, highly selective vagotomy (also known as parietal cell, super selective, and proximal vagotomy) was developed. Only the vagal fibers innervating the portion of the stomach that contains parietal cells is transected, thus leaving fibers important for regulating gastric motility intact. Although this procedure leads to an immediate decrease in both BAO and stimulated acid output, acid secretion recovers over time. By the end of the first postoperative year, basal and stimulated acid output are ~30 and 50%, respectively, of preoperative levels. Ulcer recurrence rates are higher with highly selective vagotomy (≥10%), although the overall complication rates are the lowest of the three procedures.

The procedure that provides the lowest rates of ulcer recurrence (1%) but has the highest complication rate is vagotomy (truncal or selective) in combination with antrectomy. Antrectomy is aimed at eliminating an additional stimulant of gastric acid secretion, gastrin. Gastrin originates from G cells found in the antrum. Two principal types of reanastomoses are used after antrectomy, gastroduodenostomy (Billroth I) or gastrojejunostomy (Billroth II) (Fig. 274-11). Although Billroth I is often preferred over II, severe duodenal inflammation or scarring may preclude its performance.

Of these procedures, highly selective vagotomy may be the one of choice in the elective setting, except in situations where ulcer recurrence rates are high (prepyloric ulcers and those refractory to H₂ therapy). Selection of vagotomy and antrectomy may be more appropriate in these circumstances.

These procedures have been traditionally performed by standard laparotomy. The advent of laparoscopic surgery has led several surgical teams to successfully perform highly selective vagotomy, truncal vagotomy/pyloroplasty, and truncal vagotomy/antrectomy through

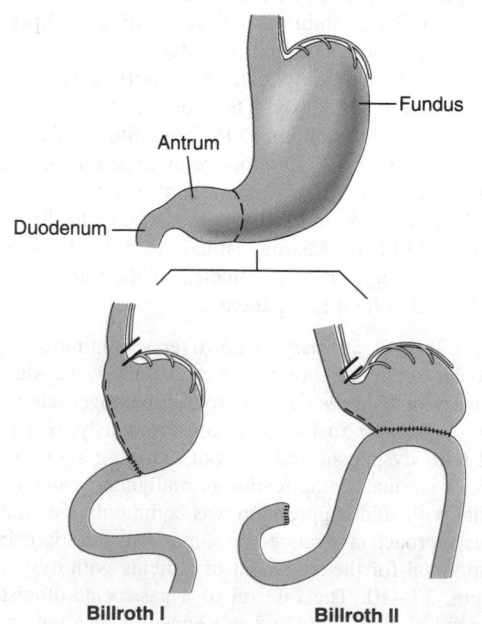

FIGURE 274-11   Schematic representation of Billroth I and II procedures.

this approach. An increase in the number of laparoscopic procedures for treatment of PUD is expected.

Specific Operations for Gastric Ulcers The location and the presence of a concomitant DU dictate the operative procedure performed for a GU. Antrectomy (including the ulcer) with a Billroth I anastomosis is the treatment of choice for an antral ulcer. Vagotomy is performed only if a DU is present. Although ulcer excision with vagotomy and drainage procedure has been proposed, the higher incidence of ulcer recurrence makes this a less desirable approach. Ulcers located near the esophagogastric junction may require a more radical approach, a subtotal gastrectomy with a Roux-en-Y esophagogastrojejunostomy (Csende's procedure). A less aggressive approach including antrectomy, intraoperative ulcer biopsy, and vagotomy (Kelling-Madlener procedure) may be indicated in fragile patients with a high GU. Ulcer recurrence approaches 30% with this procedure.

Surgery-Related Complications Complications seen after surgery for PUD are related primarily to the extent of the anatomical modification performed. Minimal alteration (highly selective vagotomy) is associated with higher rates of ulcer recurrence and less gastrointestinal disturbance. More aggressive surgical procedures have a lower rate of ulcer recurrence but a greater incidence of gastrointestinal dysfunction. Overall, morbidity and mortality related to these procedures are quite low. Morbidity associated with vagotomy and antrectomy or pyloroplasty is ≤5%, with mortality ~1%. Highly selective vagotomy has lower morbidity and mortality rates of 1 and 0.3%, respectively.

In addition to the potential early consequences of any intraabdominal procedure (bleeding, infection, thromboembolism), gastroparesis, duodenal stump leak, and efferent loop obstruction can be observed.

RECURRENT ULCERATION The risk of ulcer recurrence is directly related to the procedure performed. Ulcers that recur after partial gastric resection tend to develop at the anastomosis (stomal or marginal ulcer). Epigastric abdominal pain is the most frequent presenting complaint. Severity and duration of pain tend to be more progressive than observed with DUs before surgery.

Ulcers may recur for several reasons including incomplete vagotomy, retained antrum, and, less likely, persistent or recurrent *H. pylori* infection. ZES should have been excluded preoperatively. More recently, surreptitious use of NSAIDs has been found to be a reason for recurrent ulcers after surgery, especially if the initial procedure was done for an NSAID-induced ulcer. Once *H. pylori* and NSAIDs have been excluded as etiologic factors, the question of incomplete vagotomy or retained gastric antrum should be explored. For the latter, fasting plasma gastrin levels should be determined. If elevated, retained antrum or ZES (see below) should be considered. A combination of acid secretory analysis and secretin stimulation (see below) can assist in this differential diagnosis. Incomplete vagotomy can be ruled out by gastric acid analysis coupled with sham feeding. In this test, gastric acid output is measured while the patient sees, smells, and chews a meal (without swallowing). The cephalic phase of gastric secretion, which is mediated by the vagus, is being assessed with this study. An increase in gastric acid output in response to sham feeding is evidence that the vagus nerve is intact.

Medical therapy with H$_2$ blockers will heal postoperative ulceration in 70 to 90% of patients. The efficacy of PPIs has not been fully assessed in this group, but one may anticipate greater rates of ulcer healing compared to those obtained with H$_2$ blockers. Repeat operation (complete vagotomy, partial gastrectomy) may be required in a small subgroup of patients who have not responded to aggressive medical management.

AFFERENT LOOP SYNDROMES Two types of afferent loop syndrome can occur in patients who have undergone partial gastric resection with Billroth II anastomosis. The most common of the two is bacterial overgrowth in the afferent limb secondary to stasis. Patients may experience postprandial abdominal pain, bloating, and diarrhea with concomitant malabsorption of fats and vitamin B$_{12}$. Cases refractory to antibiotics may require surgical revision of the loop. The less common

afferent loop syndrome can present with severe abdominal pain and bloating that occur 20 to 60 min after meals. Pain is often followed by nausea and vomiting of bile-containing material. The pain and bloating may improve after emesis. The cause of this clinical picture is theorized to be incomplete drainage of bile and pancreatic secretions from an afferent loop that is partially obstructed. Cases refractory to dietary measures may need surgical revision.

DUMPING SYNDROME Dumping syndrome consists of a series of vasomotor and gastrointestinal signs and symptoms and occurs in patients who have undergone vagotomy and drainage (especially Billroth procedures). Two phases of dumping, early and late, can occur. Early dumping takes place 15 to 30 min after meals and consists of crampy abdominal discomfort, nausea, diarrhea, belching, tachycardia, palpitations, diaphoresis, light-headedness, and, rarely, syncope. These signs and symptoms arise from the rapid emptying of hyperosmolar gastric contents into the small intestine, resulting in a fluid shift into the gut lumen with plasma volume contraction and acute intestinal distention. Release of vasoactive gastrointestinal hormones (vasoactive intestinal polypeptide, neurotensin, motilin) is also theorized to play a role in early dumping.

The late phase of dumping typically occurs 90 min to 3 h after meals. Vasomotor symptoms (light-headedness, diaphoresis, palpitations, tachycardia, and syncope) predominate during this phase. This component of dumping is thought to be secondary to hypoglycemia from excessive insulin release.

Dumping syndrome is most noticeable after meals rich in simple carbohydrates (especially sucrose) and high osmolarity. Ingestion of large amounts of fluids may also contribute. Up to 50% of postvagotomy and drainage patients will experience dumping syndrome to some degree. Signs and symptoms often improve with time, but a severe protracted picture can occur in up to 1% of patients.

Dietary modification is the cornerstone of therapy for patients with dumping syndrome. Small, multiple (six) meals devoid of simple carbohydrates coupled with elimination of liquids during meals is important. Antidiarrheals and anticholinergic agents are complementary to diet. Guar and pectin, which increase the viscosity of intraluminal contents, may be beneficial in more symptomatic individuals. Acarbose, an α-glucosidase inhibitor that delays digestion of ingested carbohydrates, has also been shown to be beneficial in the treatment of the late phases of dumping. The somatostatin analogue octreotide has been successful in diet-refractory cases. This drug is administered subcutaneously (50 μg tid), titrated according to clinical response. Recently a long-acting formulation has become available, but its use in dumping syndrome has not been examined.

POSTVAGOTOMY DIARRHEA Up to 10% of patients may seek medical attention for the treatment of postvagotomy diarrhea. This complication is most commonly observed after truncal vagotomy. Patients may complain of intermittent diarrhea that occurs typically 1 to 2 h after meals. Occasionally the symptoms may be severe and relentless. This is due to a motility disorder from interruption of the vagal fibers supplying the luminal gut. Other contributing factors may include decreased absorption of nutrients (see below), increased excretion of bile acids, and release of luminal factors that promote secretion. Diphenoxylate or loperamide is often useful in symptom control. The bile salt–binding agent cholestyramine may be helpful in severe cases. Surgical reversal of a 10-cm segment of jejunum may yield a substantial improvement in bowel frequency in a subset of patients.

BILE REFLUX GASTROPATHY A subset of post-partial gastrectomy patients will present with abdominal pain, early satiety, nausea, and vomiting, who have as the only finding mucosal erythema of the gastric remnant. Histologic examination of the gastric mucosa reveals minimal inflammation but the presence of epithelial cell injury. This clinical picture is categorized as bile or alkaline reflux gastropathy/gastritis. Although reflux of bile is implicated as the reason for this disorder, the mechanism is unknown. Prokinetic agents (cisapride, 10 to 20 mg before meals and at bedtime) and cholestyramine have been effective treatments. Cisapride is no longer available because it induces cardiac arrhythmias. Severe refractory symptoms may require using either nuclear scanning with ^{99m}Tc-HIDA, to document reflux, or an alkaline challenge test, where 0.1 N NaOH is infused into the stomach in an effort to reproduce the patient's symptoms. Surgical diversion of pancreaticobiliary secretions away from the gastric remnant with a Roux-en-Y gastrojejunostomy consisting of a long (50 to 60 cm) Roux limb has been used in severe cases. Bilious vomiting improves, but early satiety and bloating may persist in up to 50% of patients.

MALDIGESTION AND MALABSORPTION Weight loss can be observed in up to 60% of patients after partial gastric resection. A significant component of this weight reduction is due to decreased oral intake. However, mild steatorrhea can also develop. Reasons for maldigestion/malabsorption include decreased gastric acid production, rapid gastric emptying, decreased food dispersion in the stomach, reduced luminal bile concentration, reduced pancreatic secretory response to feeding, and rapid intestinal transit.

Decreased serum vitamin B$_{12}$ levels can be observed after partial gastrectomy. This is usually not due to deficiency of IF, since a minimal amount of parietal cells (source of IF) are removed during antrectomy. Reduced vitamin B$_{12}$ may be due to competition for the vitamin by bacterial overgrowth or inability to split the vitamin from its protein-bound source due to hypochlorhydria.

Iron-deficiency anemia may be a consequence of impaired absorption of dietary iron in patients with a Billroth II gastrojejunostomy. Absorption of iron salts is normal in these individuals; thus a favorable response to oral iron supplementation can be anticipated. Folate deficiency with concomitant anemia can also develop in these patients. This deficiency may be secondary to decreased absorption or diminished oral intake.

Malabsorption of vitamin D and calcium resulting in osteoporosis and osteomalacia is common after partial gastrectomy and gastrojejunostomy (Billroth II). Osteomalacia can occur as a late complication in up to 25% of post-partial gastrectomy patients. Bone fractures occur twice as commonly in men after gastric surgery as in a control population. It may take years before x-ray findings demonstrate diminished bone density. Elevated alkaline phosphatase, reduced serum calcium, bone pain, and pathologic fractures may be seen in patients with osteomalacia. The high incidence of these abnormalities in this subgroup of patients justifies treating them with vitamin D and calcium supplementation indefinitely. Therapy is especially important in females.

GASTRIC ADENOCARCINOMA The incidence of adenocarcinoma in the gastric stump is increased 15 years after resection. Some have reported a four- to fivefold increase in gastric cancer 20 to 25 years after resection. The pathogenesis is unclear but may involve alkaline reflux, bacterial proliferation, or hypochlorhydria. Endoscopic screening every other year may detect surgically treatable disease.

RELATED CONDITIONS

ZOLLINGER-ELLISON SYNDROME Severe peptic ulcer diathesis secondary to gastric acid hypersecretion due to unregulated gastrin release from a non-β cell endocrine tumor (gastrinoma) defines the components of the ZES. Initially, ZES was typified by aggressive and refractory ulceration in which total gastrectomy provided the only chance for enhancing survival. Today ZES can be cured by surgical resection in up to 30% of patients.

Epidemiology The incidence of ZES varies from 0.1 to 1% of individuals presenting with PUD. Males are more commonly affected than females, and the majority of patients are diagnosed between ages 30 and 50. Gastrinomas are classified into sporadic tumors (more common) and those associated with multiple endocrine neoplasia (MEN) type I (see below).

Pathophysiology Hypergastremia originating from an autonomous neoplasm is the driving force responsible for the clinical manifestations in ZES. Gastrin stimulates acid secretion through gastrin receptors on parietal cells and by inducing histamine release from ECL cells. Gastrin also has a trophic action on gastric epithelial cells. Long-standing hypergastrinemia leads to markedly increased gastric acid secretion through both parietal cell stimulation and increased parietal cell mass. The increased gastric acid output leads to the peptic ulcer diathesis, erosive esophagitis, and diarrhea.

Tumor Distribution Although early studies suggested that the vast majority of gastrinomas occurred within the pancreas, a significant number of these lesions are extrapancreatic. Over 80% of these tumors are found within the hypothetical gastrinoma triangle (confluence of the cystic and common bile ducts superiorly, junction of the second and third portions of the duodenum inferiorly, and junction of the neck and body of the pancreas medially). Duodenal tumors constitute the most common nonpancreatic lesion; up to 50% of gastrinomas are found here. Less common extrapancreatic sites include stomach, bones, ovaries, heart, liver, and lymph nodes. More than 60% of tumors are considered malignant, with up to 30 to 50% of patients having multiple lesions or metastatic disease at presentation. Histologically, gastrin-producing cells appear well differentiated, expressing markers typically found in endocrine neoplasms (chromogranin, neuron-specific enolase).

Clinical Manifestations Gastric acid hypersecretion is responsible for the signs and symptoms observed in patients with ZES. Peptic ulcer is the most common clinical manifestation, occurring in >90% of gastrinoma patients. Initial presentation and ulcer location (duodenal bulb) may be indistinguishable from common PUD. Clinical situations that should create suspicion of gastrinoma are ulcers in unusual locations (second part of the duodenum and beyond), ulcers refractory to standard medical therapy, ulcer recurrence after acid-reducing surgery, ulcers presenting with frank complications (bleeding, obstruction, and perforation), or ulcers in the absence of *H. pylori* or NSAID ingestion. Symptoms of esophageal origin are present in up to two-thirds of patients with ZES, with a spectrum ranging from mild esophagitis to frank ulceration with stricture and Barrett's mucosa.

Diarrhea is the next most common clinical manifestation, in up to 50% of patients. Although diarrhea often occurs concomitantly with acid peptic disease, it may also occur independent of an ulcer. Etiology of the diarrhea is multifactorial, resulting from marked volume overload to the small bowel, pancreatic enzyme inactivation by acid, and damage of the intestinal epithelial surface by acid. The epithelial damage can lead to a mild degree of maldigestion and malabsorption of nutrients. The diarrhea may also have a secretory component due to the direct stimulatory effect of gastrin on enterocytes or the cosecretion of additional hormones from the tumor, such as vasoactive intestinal peptide.

Gastrinomas can develop in the presence of MEN I syndrome (Chap. 329) in ~25% of patients. This autosomal dominant disorder involves primarily three organ sites: the parathyroid glands (80 to 90%), pancreas (40 to 80%), and pituitary gland (30 to 60%). The genetic defect in MEN I is in the long arm of chromosome 11 (11q11-q13). In view of the stimulatory effect of calcium on gastric secretion, the hyperparathyroidism and hypercalcemia seen in MEN I patients may have a direct effect on ulcer disease. Resolution of hypercalcemia by parathyroidectomy reduces gastrin and gastric acid output in gastrinoma patients. An additional distinguishing feature in ZES patients with MEN I is the higher incidence of gastric carcinoid tumor development (as compared to patients with sporadic gastrinomas). Gastrinomas tend to be smaller, multiple, and located in the duodenal wall more often than is seen in patients with sporadic ZES. Establishing the diagnosis of MEN I is critical not only from the standpoint of providing genetic counseling to the patient and his or her family but also from the surgical approach recommended.

TABLE 274-5 *When to Obtain a Fasting Serum Gastrin Level*

Multiple ulcers
Ulcers in unusual locations; associated with severe esophagitis; resistant to therapy with frequent recurrences; in the absence of NSAID ingestion or *H. pylori* infection
Ulcer patients awaiting surgery
Extensive family history for peptic ulcer disease
Postoperative ulcer recurrence
Basal hyperchlorhydria
Unexplained diarrhea or steatorrhea
Hypercalcemia
Family history of pancreatic islet, pituitary, or parathyroid tumor
Prominent gastric or duodenal folds

Diagnosis The first step in the evaluation of a patient suspected of having ZES is to obtain a fasting gastrin level. A list of clinical scenarios that should arouse suspicion regarding this diagnosis is shown in Table 274-5. Fasting gastrin levels are usually <150 pg/mL. Virtually all gastrinoma patients will have a gastrin level >150 to 200 pg/mL. Measurement of fasting gastrin should be repeated to confirm the clinical suspicion.

Multiple processes can lead to an elevated fasting gastrin level: gastric hypochlorhydria or achlorhydria (the most frequent), with or without pernicious anemia; retained gastric antrum; G cell hyperplasia; gastric outlet obstruction; renal insufficiency; massive small-bowel obstruction; and conditions such as rheumatoid arthritis, vitiligo, diabetes mellitus, and pheochromocytoma. Gastric acid induces feedback inhibition of gastrin release. A decrease in acid production will subsequently lead to failure of the feedback inhibitory pathway, resulting in net hypergastrinemia. Gastrin levels will thus be high in patients using antisecretory agents for the treatment of acid peptic disorders and dyspepsia. *H. pylori* infection can also cause hypergastrinemia.

The next step in establishing a biochemical diagnosis of gastrinoma is to assess acid secretion. Nothing further needs to be done if decreased acid output is observed. In contrast, normal or elevated gastric acid output suggests a need for additional tests. Gastric acid analysis is performed by placing a nasogastric tube in the stomach and drawing samples at 15-min intervals for 1 h during unstimulated or basal state (BAO), followed by continued sampling after administration of intravenous pentagastrin (MAO). Up to 90% of gastrinoma patients may have a BAO of ≥15 meq/h (normal, <4 meq/h). Up to 12% of patients with common PUD may have comparable levels of acid secretion. A BAO/MAO ratio >0.6 is highly suggestive of ZES, but a ratio <0.6 does not exclude the diagnosis. Pentagastrin is no longer available in the United States, making measurement of MAO virtually impossible. If the technology for measuring gastric acid secretion is not available, a basal gastric pH ≥3 virtually excludes a gastrinoma.

Gastrin provocative tests have been developed in an effort to differentiate between the causes of hypergastrinemia and are especially helpful in patients with indeterminant acid secretory studies. The tests are the secretin stimulation test, the calcium infusion study, and a standard meal test. In each of these, a fasted patient has an indwelling intravenous catheter in place for serial blood sampling and an intravenous line in place for secretin or calcium infusion. The patient receives either secretin (intravenous bolus of 2 μg/kg) or calcium (calcium gluconate, 5 mg/kg body weight over 3 h) or is fed a meal. Blood is then drawn at predetermined intervals (10 min and 1 min before and at 2, 5, 10, 15, 20, and 30 min after injection for secretin stimulation and at 30-min intervals during the calcium infusion). The most sensitive and specific gastrin provocative test for the diagnosis of gastrinoma is the secretin study. An increase in gastrin of ≥200 pg within 15 min of secretin injection has a sensitivity and specificity of >90% for ZES. The calcium infusion study is less sensitive and specific than the secretin test, with a rise of >400 pg/mL observed in ~80% of gastrinoma patients. The lower accuracy, coupled with it being a more cumbersome study with greater potential for adverse effects, makes calcium infusion less useful and therefore rarely, if ever,

utilized. Rarely, one may observe increased BAO and hypergastrinemia in a patient who in the past has been categorized as having G cell hyperplasia or hyperfunction. This set of findings may have been due to *H. pylori*. The standard meal test was devised to assist in making the diagnosis of G cell–related hyperactivity, by observing a dramatic increase in gastrin after a meal (>200%). This test is not useful in differentiating between G cell hyperfunction and ZES.

Tumor Localization Once the biochemical diagnosis of gastrinoma has been confirmed, the tumor must be located. Multiple imaging studies have been utilized in an effort to enhance tumor localization (Table 274-6). The broad range of sensitivity is due to the variable success rates achieved by the different investigative groups. Endoscopic ultrasound (EUS) permits imaging of the pancreas with a high degree of resolution (<5 mm). This modality is particularly helpful in excluding small neoplasms within the pancreas and in assessing the presence of surrounding lymph nodes and vascular involvement. Several types of endocrine tumors express cell-surface receptors for somatostatin. This permits the localization of gastrinomas by measuring the uptake of the stable somatostatin analogue ^{111}In-pentreotide (octreoscan) with sensitivity and specificity rates of >75%.

Up to 50% of patients have metastatic disease at diagnosis. Success in controlling gastric acid hypersecretion has shifted the emphasis of therapy towards providing a surgical cure. Detecting the primary tumor and excluding metastatic disease are critical in view of this paradigm shift. Once a biochemical diagnosis has been confirmed, the patient should first undergo an abdominal computed tomographic scan, magnetic resonance imaging, or octreoscan (depending on availability) to exclude metastatic disease. Once metastatic disease has been excluded, an experienced endocrine surgeon may opt for exploratory laparotomy with intraoperative ultrasound or transillumination. In other centers, careful examination of the peripancreatic area with EUS, accompanied by endoscopic exploration of the duodenum for primary tumors, will be performed before surgery. Selective arterial secretin injection may be a useful adjuvant for localizing tumors in a subset of patients.

℞ TREATMENT

Treatment of functional endocrine tumors is directed at ameliorating the signs and symptoms related to hormone overproduction, curative resection of the neoplasm, and attempts to control tumor growth in metastatic disease.

PPIs are the treatment of choice and have decreased the need for total gastrectomy. Initial doses of omeprazole or lansoprazole should be in the range of 60 mg/d. Dosing can be adjusted to achieve a BAO <10 meq/h (at the drug trough) in surgery-naive patients and to <5 meq/h in individuals who have previously undergone an acid-reducing operation. Although the somatostatin analogue has inhibitory effects on gastrin release from receptor-bearing tumors and inhibits gastric

TABLE 274-6 *Sensitivity of Imaging Studies in Zollinger Ellison Syndrome*

	Sensitivity, %	
Study	Primary Gastrinoma	Metastatic Gastrinoma
Ultrasound	21–28	14
CT scan	35–59	35–72
Selective angiography	35–68	33–86
Portal venous sampling	70–90	N/A
SASI	55–78	41
MRI	30–60	71
Octreoscan	67–86	80–100
EUS	80–100	N/A

Note: CT, computed tomography; SASI, selective arterial secretin injection; MRI, magnetic resonance imaging; octreoscan, imaging with ^{111}In-pentreotide; EUS, endoscopic ultrasonography.

acid secretion to some extent, PPIs have the advantage of reducing parietal cell activity to a greater degree.

The ultimate goal of surgery would be to provide a definitive cure. Improved understanding of tumor distribution has led to 10-year disease-free intervals as high as 34% in sporadic gastrinoma patients undergoing surgery. A positive outcome is highly dependent on the experience of the surgical team treating these rare tumors. Surgical therapy of gastrinoma patients with MEN I remains controversial because of the difficulty in rendering these patients disease free with surgery. In contrast to the encouraging postoperative results observed in patients with sporadic disease, only 6% of MEN I patients are disease free 5 years after an operation. Some groups suggest surgery only if a clearly identifiable, nonmetastatic lesion is documented by structural studies. Others advocate a more aggressive approach, where all patients free of hepatic metastasis are explored and all detected tumors in the duodenum are resected; this is followed by enucleation of lesions in the pancreatic head, with a distal pancreatectomy to follow. The outcome of the two approaches has not been clearly defined.

Therapy of metastatic endocrine tumors in general remains suboptimal; gastrinomas are no exception. A host of medical therapeutic approaches including chemotherapy (streptozotocin, 5-fluorouracil, and doxorubicin), IFN-α, and hepatic artery embolization lead to significant toxicity without a substantial improvement in overall survival. ^{111}In-pentetreotide has been utilized in the therapy of metastatic neuroendocrine tumors; further studies are needed. Surgical approaches including debulking surgery and liver transplantation for hepatic metastasis have also produced limited benefit. Therefore, early recognition and surgery are the only chances for curing this disease.

The 5- and 10-year survival rates for gastrinoma patients are 62 to 75% and 47 to 53%, respectively. Individuals with the entire tumor resected or those with a negative laparotomy have 5- and 10-year survival rates >90%. Patients with incompletely resected tumors have 5- and 10-year survival of 43% and 25%, respectively. Patients with hepatic metastasis have <20% survival at 5 years. Favorable prognostic indicators include primary duodenal wall tumors, isolated lymph node tumor, and undetectable tumor upon surgical exploration. Poor outcome is seen in patients with shorter disease duration, higher gastrin levels (>10,000 pg/mL); large pancreatic primary tumors (>3 cm), metastatic disease to lymph nodes, liver, and bone; and Cushing's syndrome. Rapid growth of hepatic metastases is also predictive of poor outcome.

STRESS-RELATED MUCOSAL INJURY

Patients suffering from shock, sepsis, massive burns, severe trauma, or head injury can develop acute erosive gastric mucosal changes or frank ulceration with bleeding. Classified as stress-induced gastritis or ulcers, injury is most commonly observed in the acid-producing (fundus and body) portions of the stomach. The most common presentation is gastrointestinal bleeding, which is usually minimal but can occasionally be life-threatening. Respiratory failure requiring mechanical ventilation and underlying coagulopathy are risk factors for bleeding, which tends to occur 48 to 72 h after the acute injury or insult.

Histologically, stress injury does not contain inflammation or *H. pylori*; thus "gastritis" is a misnomer. Although elevated gastric acid secretion may be noted in patients with stress ulceration after head trauma (Cushing's ulcer) and severe burns (Curling's ulcer), mucosal ischemia and breakdown of the normal protective barriers of the stomach also play an important role in the pathogenesis. Acid must contribute to injury in view of the significant drop in bleeding noted when acid inhibitors are used as a prophylactic measure for stress gastritis.

Improvement in the general management of intensive care unit patients has led to a significant decrease in the incidence of gastrointestinal bleeding due to stress ulceration. The estimated decrease in bleeding is from 20 to 30% to <5%. This improvement has led to some debate regarding the need for prophylactic therapy. The limited benefit of medical (endoscopic, angiographic) and surgical therapy in

a patient with hemodynamically compromising bleeding associated with stress ulcer/gastritis supports the use of preventive measures in high-risk patients (mechanically ventilated, coagulopathy, multiorgan failure, or severe burns). Maintenance of gastric pH > 3.5 with continuous infusion of H_2 blockers or liquid antacids administered every 2 to 3 h are viable options. Sucralfate slurry (1 g every 4 to 6 h) has also been successful. If bleeding occurs despite these measures, endoscopy, intraarterial vasopressin, or embolization are options. If all else fails, then surgery should be considered. Although vagotomy and antrectomy may be used, the better approach would be a total gastrectomy, which has an exceedingly high mortality rate in this setting.

GASTRITIS The term *gastritis* should be reserved for histologically documented inflammation of the gastric mucosa. Gastritis is not the mucosal erythema seen during endoscopy and is not interchangeable with "dyspepsia." The etiologic factors leading to gastritis are broad and heterogeneous. Gastritis has been classified based on time course (acute vs. chronic), histologic features, and anatomical distribution or proposed pathogenic mechanism (Table 274-7).

The correlation between the histologic findings of gastritis, the clinical picture of abdominal pain or dyspepsia, and endoscopic findings noted on gross inspection of the gastric mucosa is poor. Therefore, there is no typical clinical manifestation of gastritis.

Acute Gastritis The most common causes of acute gastritis are infectious. Acute infection with *H. pylori* induces gastritis. However, *H. pylori* acute gastritis has not been extensively studied. Reported as presenting with sudden onset of epigastric pain, nausea, and vomiting, limited mucosal histologic studies demonstrate a marked infiltrate of neutrophils with edema and hyperemia. If not treated, this picture will evolve into one of chronic gastritis. Hypochlorhydria lasting for up to 1 year may follow acute *H. pylori* infection.

The highly acidic gastric environment may be one reason why infectious processes of the stomach are rare. Bacterial infection of the stomach or phlegmonous gastritis is a rare potentially life-threatening disorder, characterized by marked and diffuse acute inflammatory infiltrates of the entire gastric wall, at times accompanied by necrosis. Elderly individuals, alcoholics, and AIDS patients may be affected. Potential iatrogenic causes include polypectomy and mucosal injection with India ink. Organisms associated with this entity include streptococci, staphylococci, *Escherichia coli*, *Proteus*, and *Haemophilus* sp. Failure of supportive measures and antibiotics may result in gastrectomy.

Other types of infectious gastritis may occur in immunocompromised individuals such as AIDS patients. Examples include herpetic (herpes simplex) or CMV gastritis. The histologic finding of intranuclear inclusions would be observed in the latter.

Chronic Gastritis Chronic gastritis is identified histologically by an inflammatory cell infiltrate consisting primarily of lymphocytes and plasma cells, with very scant neutrophil involvement. Distribution of the inflammation may be patchy, initially involving superficial and glandular portions of the gastric mucosa. This picture may progress to more severe glandular destruction, with atrophy and metaplasia.

TABLE 274-7 *Classification of Gastritis*

I. Acute gastritis	II. Chronic atrophic gastritis
A. Acute *H. pylori* infection	A. Type A: Autoimmune, body-predominant
B. Other acute infectious gastritides	B. Type B: *H. pylori*–related, antral-predominant
1. Bacterial (other than *H. pylori*)	C. Indeterminant
2. *Helicobacter helmanni*	III. Uncommon Forms of Gastritis
3. Phlegmonous	A. Lymphocytic
4. Mycobacterial	B. Eosinophilic
5. Syphilitic	C. Crohn's disease
6. Viral	D. Sarcoidosis
7. Parasitic	E. Isolated granulomatous gastritis
8. Fungal	

Chronic gastritis has been classified according to histologic characteristics. These include superficial atrophic changes and gastric atrophy.

The early phase of chronic gastritis is *superficial gastritis*. The inflammatory changes are limited to the lamina propria of the surface mucosa, with edema and cellular infiltrates separating intact gastric glands. Additional findings may include decreased mucus in the mucous cells and decreased mitotic figures in the glandular cells. The next stage is *atrophic gastritis*. The inflammatory infiltrate extends deeper into the mucosa, with progressive distortion and destruction of the glands. The final stage of chronic gastritis is *gastric atrophy*. Glandular structures are lost; there is a paucity of inflammatory infiltrates. Endoscopically the mucosa may be substantially thin, permitting clear visualization of the underlying blood vessels.

Gastric glands may undergo morphologic transformation in chronic gastritis. Intestinal metaplasia denotes the conversion of gastric glands to a small intestinal phenotype with small-bowel mucosal glands containing goblet cells. The metaplastic changes may vary in distribution from patchy to fairly extensive gastric involvement. Intestinal metaplasia is an important predisposing factor for gastric cancer (Chap. 77).

Chronic gastritis is also classified according to the predominant site of involvement. Type A refers to the body-predominant form (autoimmune) and type B is the central-predominant form (*H. pylori*–related). This classification is artificial in view of the difficulty in distinguishing these two entities. The term *AB gastritis* has been used to refer to a mixed antral/body picture.

TYPE A GASTRITIS   The less common of the two forms involves primarily the fundus and body, with antral sparing. Traditionally, this form of gastritis has been associated with pernicious anemia (Chap. 92) in the presence of circulating antibodies against parietal cells and IF; thus it is also called *autoimmune gastritis. H. pylori* infection can lead to a similar distribution of gastritis. The characteristics of an autoimmune picture are not always present.

Antibodies to parietal cells have been detected in >90% of patients with pernicious anemia and in up to 50% of patients with type A gastritis. The parietal cell antibody is directed against H^+,K^+-ATPase. T cells are also implicated in the injury pattern of this form of gastritis.

Parietal cell antibodies and atrophic gastritis are observed in family members of patients with pernicious anemia. These antibodies are observed in up to 20% of individuals over age 60 and in ~20% of patients with vitiligo and Addison's disease. About half of patients with pernicious anemia have antibodies to thyroid antigens, and about 30% of patients with thyroid disease have circulating anti-parietal cell antibodies. Anti-IF antibodies are more specific than parietal cell antibodies for type A gastritis, being present in ~40% of patients with pernicious anemia. Another parameter consistent with this form of gastritis being autoimmune in origin is the higher incidence of specific familial histocompatibility haplotypes such as HLA-B8 and -DR3.

The parietal cell–containing gastric gland is preferentially targeted in this form of gastritis, and achlorhydria results. Parietal cells are the source of IF, lack of which will lead to vitamin B_{12} deficiency and its sequelae (megaloblastic anemia, neurologic dysfunction).

Gastric acid plays an important role in feedback inhibition of gastrin release from G cells. Achlorhydria, coupled with relative sparing of the antral mucosa (site of G cells), leads to hypergastrinemia. Gastrin levels can be markedly elevated (>500 pg/mL) in patients with pernicious anemia. ECL cell hyperplasia with frank development of gastric carcinoid tumors may result from gastrin trophic effects. The role of gastrin in carcinoid development is confirmed by the observation that antrectomy leads to regression of these lesions. Hypergastrinemia and achlorhydria may also be seen in non-pernicious anemia–associated type A gastritis.

TYPE B GASTRITIS   Type B, or antral-predominant, gastritis is the more common form of chronic gastritis. *H. pylori* infection is the cause of this entity. Although described as "antral-predominant," this is likely a misnomer in view of studies documenting the progression of the inflammatory process towards the body and fundus of infected individuals. The conversion to a pan-gastritis is time-dependent—estimated to require 15 to 20 years. This form of gastritis increases with age, being present in up to 100% of persons over age 70. Histology improves after *H. pylori* eradication. The number of *H. pylori* organisms decreases dramatically with progression to gastric atrophy, and the degree of inflammation correlates with the level of these organisms. Early on, with antral-predominant findings, the quantity of *H. pylori* is highest and a dense chronic inflammatory infiltrate of the lamina propria is noted accompanied by epithelial cell infiltration with polymorphonuclear leukocytes (Fig. 274-12).

Multifocal atrophic gastritis, gastric atrophy with subsequent metaplasia, has been observed in chronic *H. pylori*–induced gastritis. This may ultimately lead to development of gastric adenocarcinoma (Fig. 274-8; Chap. 77). *H. pylori* infection is now considered an independent risk factor for gastric cancer. Worldwide epidemiologic studies have documented a higher incidence of *H. pylori* infection in patients with adenocarcinoma of the stomach as compared to control subjects. Seropositivity for *H. pylori* is associated with a three- to sixfold increased risk of gastric cancer. This risk may be as high as ninefold after adjusting for the inaccuracy of serologic testing in the elderly. The mechanism by which *H. pylori* infection leads to cancer is unknown. However, eradication of *H. pylori* as a general preventative measure for gastric cancer is not recommended.

Infection with *H. pylori* is also associated with development of a low-grade B cell lymphoma, gastric MALT lymphoma (Chap. 97).

FIGURE 274-12   Chronic gastritis and *Helicobacter pylori* organisms. *A.* H&E stain of gastric mucosa showing surface foveolar cells, adherent mucus, and scattered bacillary forms within the mucus. *B.* Steiner silver stain of superficial gastric mucosa, showing abundant darkly staining microorganisms layered over the apical portion of the surface epithelium. Note that there is no tissue invasion. *[Courtesy of James M. Crawford, M.D., Ph.D. Reprinted with permission from JM Crawford, in V Kumar et al (eds): Basic Pathology. Philadelphia, Saunders, 1997.]*

The chronic T cell stimulation caused by the infection leads to production of cytokines that promote the B cell tumor. Tumor growth remains dependent upon the presence of *H. pylori* in that its eradication is often associated with complete regression of the tumor. The tumor may take more than a year to regress after treating the infection. Such patients should be followed by EUS every 2 to 3 months. If the tumor is stable or decreasing in size, no other therapy is necessary. If the tumor grows, it may have become a high-grade B cell lymphoma. When the tumor becomes a high-grade aggressive lymphoma histologically, it loses responsiveness to *H. pylori* eradication.

℞ TREATMENT

Treatment in chronic gastritis is aimed at the sequelae and not the underlying inflammation. Patients with pernicious anemia will require parenteral vitamin B_{12} supplementation on a long-term basis. Eradication of *H. pylori* is not routinely recommended unless PUD or a low-grade MALT lymphoma is present.

Miscellaneous Forms of Gastritis Lymphocytic gastritis is characterized histologically by intense infiltration of the surface epithelium with lymphocytes. The infiltrative process is primarily in the body of the stomach and consists of mature T cells and plasmacytes. The etiology of this form of chronic gastritis is unknown. It has been described in patients with celiac sprue, but whether there is a common factor associating these two entities is unknown. No specific symptoms suggest lymphocytic gastritis. A subgroup of patients have thickened folds noted on endoscopy. These folds are often capped by small nodules that contain a central depression or erosion; this form of the disease is called *varioliform gastritis*. *H. pylori* probably plays no significant role in lymphocytic gastritis. Therapy with glucocorticoids or sodium cromoglycate has obtained unclear results.

Marked eosinophilic infiltration involving any layer of the stomach (mucosa, muscularis propria, and serosa) is characteristic of *eosinophilic gastritis*. Affected individuals will often have circulating eosinophilia with clinical manifestation of systemic allergy. Involvement may range from isolated gastric disease to diffuse eosinophilic gastroenteritis. Antral involvement predominates, with prominent edematous folds being observed on endoscopy. These prominent antral folds can lead to outlet obstruction. Patients can present with epigastric discomfort, nausea, and vomiting. Treatment with glucocorticoids has been successful.

Several systemic disorders may be associated with *granulomatous gastritis*. Gastric involvement has been observed in Crohn's disease. Involvement may range from granulomatous infiltrates noted only on gastric biopsies to frank ulceration and stricture formation. Gastric Crohn's disease usually occurs in the presence of small-intestinal disease. Several rare infectious processes can lead to granulomatous gastritis, including histoplasmosis, candidiasis, syphilis, and tuberculosis. Other unusual causes of this form of gastritis include sarcoidosis, idiopathic granulomatous gastritis, and eosinophilic granulomas involving the stomach. Establishing the specific etiologic agent in this form of gastritis can be difficult, at times requiring repeat endoscopy with biopsy and cytology. Occasionally, a surgically obtained full-thickness biopsy of the stomach may be required to exclude malignancy.

MÉNÉTRIER'S DISEASE Ménétrier's disease is a rare entity characterized by large, tortuous gastric mucosal folds. The differential diagnosis of large gastric folds includes ZES, malignancy, infectious etiologies (CMV, histoplasmosis, syphilis), and infiltrative disorders such as sarcoidosis. The mucosal folds in Ménétrier's disease are often most prominent in the body and fundus. Histologically, massive foveolar hyperplasia (hyperplasia of surface and glandular mucous cells) is noted, which replaces most of the chief and parietal cells. This hyperplasia produces the prominent folds observed. The pits of the gastric glands elongate and may become extremely tortuous. Although the lamina propria may contain a mild chronic inflammatory infiltrate, Ménétrier's disease is not considered a form of gastritis. The etiology of this unusual clinical picture is unknown. Overexpression of growth factors such as TGF-α may be involved in the process.

Epigastric pain at times accompanied by nausea, vomiting, anorexia, and weight loss are signs and symptoms in patients with Ménétrier's disease. Occult gastrointestinal bleeding may occur, but overt bleeding is unusual and, when present, is due to superficial mucosal erosions. Twenty to 100% of patients (depending on time of presentation) develop a protein-losing gastropathy accompanied by hypoalbuminemia and edema. Gastric acid secretion is usually reduced or absent because of the replacement of parietal cells. Large gastric folds are readily detectable by either radiographic (barium meal) or endoscopic methods. Endoscopy with deep mucosal biopsy (and cytology) is required to establish the diagnosis and exclude other entities that may present similarly. A nondiagnostic biopsy may lead to a surgically obtained full-thickness biopsy to exclude malignancy.

℞ TREATMENT

Medical therapy with anticholinergic agents, prostaglandins, PPIs, prednisone, and H_2 receptor antagonists has obtained varying results. Anticholinergics decrease protein loss. A high-protein diet should be recommended to replace protein loss in patients with hypoalbuminemia. Ulcers should be treated with a standard approach. Severe disease with persistent and substantial protein loss may require total gastrectomy. Subtotal gastrectomy is performed by some; it may be associated with higher morbidity and mortality secondary to the difficulty in obtaining a patent and long-lasting anastomosis between normal and hyperplastic tissues.

ACKNOWLEDGMENT
The author acknowledges the contribution of material to this chapter by Dr. Lawrence Friedman and Dr. Walter Peterson from their chapter on this subject in the 14th edition of Harrison's.

FURTHER READING

CHAN FK et al: Preventing recurrent upper gastrointestinal bleeding in patients with *Helicobacter pylori* infection who are taking low-dose aspirin or naproxen. N Engl J Med 344:967, 2001

CHAN FKL, LEUNG WK: Peptic-ulcer disease. Lancet 360:933, 2002

———— et al: Celecoxib versus diclofenac and omeprazole in reducing the risk of recurrent ulcer bleeding in patients with arthritis. N Engl J Med 347:2104, 2002

LAI KC et al: Lansoprazole for the prevention of recurrences of ulcer complications from long-term low-dose aspirin use. N Engl J Med 346:2033, 2002

LAINE L: Approaches to nonsteroidal anti-inflammatory drug use in the high-risk patient. Gastroenterology 120:594, 2001

————: Gastrointestinal effects of NSAIDs and coxibs. J Pain Symptom Manage 25 (suppl 2):532, 2003

MOAYYEDI P et al: An update of the Cochrane systematic review of *Helicobacter pylori* eradication therapy in nonulcer dyspepsia: Resolving the discrepancy between systematic reviews. Am J Gastroenterol 98:2621, 2003

ROY PK et al: Gastric secretion in Zollinger-Ellison syndrome. Correlation with clinical expression, tumor extent and role in diagnosis—a prospective NIH study of 235 patients and a review of 984 cases in the literature. Medicine (Baltimore) 80:189, 2001

SUERBAUM S, MICHETTI P: *Helicobacter pylori* infection. N Engl J Med 347:1175, 2002

UEMURA N et al: *Helicobacter pylori* infection and the development of gastric cancer. N Engl J Med 345:784, 2001

Disorders of absorption constitute a broad spectrum of conditions with multiple etiologies and varied clinical manifestations. Almost all of these clinical problems are associated with *diminished* intestinal absorption of one or more dietary nutrients and are often referred to as the *malabsorption syndrome*. This latter term is not ideal as it represents a pathophysiologic state, does *not* provide an etiologic explanation for the underlying problem, and should not be considered an adequate final diagnosis. The only clinical situations in which absorption is *increased* are hemochromatosis and Wilson's disease, in which there is increased absorption of iron and copper, respectively.

Most, but not all, of these clinical conditions are associated with *steatorrhea*, an increase in stool fat excretion of >6% of dietary fat intake. Some disorders of absorption are not associated with steatorrhea: Primary lactase deficiency, which represents a congenital absence of the small intestinal brush border disaccharidase enzyme lactase, is associated with lactose "malabsorption," and pernicious anemia is associated with a marked decrease in intestinal absorption of cobalamin (vitamin B_{12}) due to an absence of gastric parietal cell intrinsic factor required for cobalamin absorption.

Disorders of absorption must be included in the differential diagnosis of diarrhea (Chap. 35). First, diarrhea is frequently associated with and/or is a consequence of the diminished absorption of one or more dietary nutrients. The diarrhea may be secondary either to the intestinal process that is responsible for the steatorrhea or to steatorrhea per se. Thus, celiac sprue (see below) is associated with both extensive morphologic changes in the small intestinal mucosa and reduced absorption of several dietary nutrients; in contrast, the diarrhea of steatorrhea is the result of the effect of nonabsorbed dietary fatty acids on intestinal, usually colonic, ion transport. For example, oleic acid and ricinoleic acid (a bacterially hydroxylated fatty acid that is also the active ingredient in castor oil, a widely used laxative) induce active colonic Cl ion secretion, most likely secondary to increasing intracellular Ca. In addition, diarrhea per se may result in mild steatorrhea (<11 g fat excretion while on a 100-g fat diet). Second, as diarrhea is both a symptom and a sign, most patients will indicate that they have diarrhea, not that they have fat malabsorption. Third, many intestinal disorders that have diarrhea as a prominent symptom (e.g., ulcerative colitis, traveler's diarrhea secondary to an enterotoxin produced by *Escherichia coli*) do not necessarily have diminished absorption of any dietary nutrient.

Diarrhea as a *symptom* (i.e., when used by patients to describe their bowel movement pattern) may be either a decrease in stool consistency, an increase in stool volume, an increase in number of bowel movements, or any combination of these three changes. In contrast, diarrhea as a *sign* is a quantitative increase in stool water or weight of >200 to 225 mL, or gram per 24 h, when a western-type diet is consumed. Individuals consuming a diet with a higher fiber content may normally have a stool weight of up to 400 g per 24 h. Thus, the clinician must clarify what an individual patient means by diarrhea. Some 10% of patients referred to gastroenterologists for further evaluation of unexplained diarrhea do not have an increase in stool water when it is determined quantitatively. Such patients may have small, frequent, somewhat loose bowel movements with stool urgency that is indicative of proctitis but do not have an increase in stool weight or volume.

It is also critical to establish whether a patient's diarrhea is secondary to diminished absorption of one or more dietary nutrients, in contrast to diarrhea that is due to small- and/or large-intestinal fluid and electrolyte secretion. The former has often been termed *osmotic diarrhea*, while the latter has been referred to as *secretory diarrhea*. Unfortunately, both secretory and osmotic elements can be present simultaneously in the same disorder; thus, this separation is not always precise. Nonetheless, two studies—determination of stool electrolytes and observation of the effect of a fast on stool output—can help make this distinction.

The demonstration of the effect of prolonged (>24 h) fasting on stool output can be very effective in suggesting that a *dietary nutrient* is responsible for the individual's diarrhea. A secretory diarrhea associated with enterotoxin-induced traveler's diarrhea would not be affected by prolonged fasting, as enterotoxin-induced stimulation of intestinal fluid and electrolyte secretion is not altered by eating. In contrast, diarrhea secondary to lactose malabsorption in primary lactase deficiency would undoubtedly cease during a prolonged fast. Thus, a substantial decrease in stool output while fasting during a quantitative stool collection of at least 24 h is presumptive evidence that the diarrhea is related to malabsorption of a dietary nutrient. The persistence of stool output while fasting indicates that the diarrhea is likely secretory and that the cause of diarrhea is *not* due to a dietary nutrient. Either a luminal (e.g., *E. coli* enterotoxin) or circulating (e.g., vasoactive intestinal peptide) secretagogue could be responsible for the patient's diarrhea persisting unaltered during a prolonged fast. The observed effects of fasting can be compared and correlated with stool electrolyte and osmolality determinations.

Measurement of stool electrolytes and osmolality requires the comparison of stool Na^+ and K^+ concentrations determined in liquid stool to the stool osmolality to determine the presence or absence of a so-called stool osmotic gap. The following formula is used:

$$2 \times (\text{stool } [Na^+] + \text{stool } [K^+]) \leq \text{stool osmolality}$$

The cation concentrations are doubled to estimate stool anion concentrations. The presence of a significant osmotic gap suggests the presence in stool water of a substance (or substances) other than Na/K/anions that presumably is responsible for the patient's diarrhea. Originally, stool osmolality was measured, but it is almost invariably greater than the required 290 to 300 mosmol/kg H_2O, reflecting bacterial degradation of nonabsorbed carbohydrate either immediately before defecation or in the stool jar while awaiting chemical analysis, even when the stool is refrigerated. As a result, the stool osmolality should be assumed to be 300 mosmol/kg H_2O. When the calculated difference is >50, an osmotic gap is present, suggesting that the diarrhea is due to a nonabsorbed dietary nutrient, e.g., a fatty acid and/or carbohydrate. When this difference is <25, it is presumed that a dietary nutrient is not responsible for the diarrhea. Since elements of both osmotic (i.e., malabsorption of a dietary nutrient) and secretory diarrhea may be present, this separation at times is less clear-cut at the bedside than when used as a teaching example. Ideally, the presence of an osmotic gap will be associated with a marked decrease in stool output during a prolonged fast, while the absence of an osmotic gap will likely be present in an individual whose stool output had not been reduced substantially during a period of fasting.

NUTRIENT DIGESTION AND ABSORPTION

The lengths of the small intestine and colon are ~300 cm and ~80 cm, respectively. However, the effective functional surface area is approximately 600-fold greater than that of a hollow tube as a result of the presence of folds, villi (in the small intestine), and microvilli. The functional surface area of the small intestine is somewhat greater than that of a doubles tennis court. In addition to nutrient digestion and absorption, the intestinal epithelia have several other functions:

1. *Barrier and immune defense.* The intestine is exposed to a large number of potential antigens and enteric and invasive microorganisms, and it is extremely effective preventing the entry of almost all these agents. The intestinal mucosa also synthesizes and secretes secretory IgA.

2. *Fluid and electrolyte absorption and secretion.* The intestine absorbs ~7 to 8 L of fluid daily, comprising dietary fluid intake (1 to 2 L/d) and salivary, gastric, pancreatic, biliary, and intestinal fluid (6 to 7 L/d). The intestine also responds to several stimuli, especially bacteria and bacterial enterotoxins, that induce fluid and electrolyte secretion, often leading to diarrhea (Chap. 113).

3. *Synthesis and secretion of several proteins.* The intestinal mucosa

is a major site for the production of proteins, including apolipo-proteins.

4. *Production of several bioactive amines and peptides.* The intestine is one of the largest endocrine organs in the body and produces several amines and peptides that serve as paracrine and hormonal mediators of intestinal function.

The small and large intestine are anatomically distinct in that villi are present in the small intestine but are absent in the colon and functionally distinct in that nutrient digestion and absorption take place in the small intestine but not in the colon. No precise anatomical characteristics separate duodenum, jejunum, and ileum, although certain nutrients are absorbed exclusively in specific areas of the small intestine. However, villus cells in the small intestine (and surface epithelial cells in the colon) and crypt cells have distinct anatomical and functional characteristics. Intestinal epithelial cells are continuously renewed, with new proliferating epithelial cells at the base of the crypt migrating over 48 to 72 h to the tip of the villus (or surface of the colon), where they are well-developed epithelial cells with digestive and absorptive function. This high rate of cell turnover explains the relatively rapid resolution of diarrhea and other digestive tract side effects during chemotherapy as new cells not exposed to these toxic agents are produced. Equally important is the paradigm of separation of villus/surface cell and crypt cell function: digestive hydrolytic enzymes are present primarily in the brush border of villus epithelial cells. Absorptive and secretory functions are also separated, with villus/surface cells primarily, but not exclusively, being the site for absorptive function, while secretory function is present in crypts of both the small and large intestine.

Nutrients, minerals, and vitamins are absorbed by one or more active transport mechanisms. (The mechanisms of intestinal fluid and electrolyte absorption and secretion are discussed in Chap. 35.) Active transport mechanisms are energy-dependent and mediated by membrane transport proteins. These transport processes will result in the *net* movement of a substance against or in the absence of an electrochemical concentration gradient. Intestinal absorption of amino acids and monosaccharides, e.g., glucose, is also a specialized form of active transport—*secondary active transport*. The movement of these actively transported nutrients against a concentration gradient is Na^+-dependent and is due to a Na^+ gradient across the apical membrane. The Na^+ gradient is maintained by Na^+,K^+-ATPase, the so-called Na^+ pump located on the basolateral membrane, which extrudes Na^+ and maintains a low intracellular [Na] as well as the Na^+ gradient across the apical membrane. As a result, active glucose absorption and glucose-stimulated Na^+ absorption require both the apical membrane transport protein, SGLT, and the basolateral Na^+,K^+-ATPase. In addition to glucose absorption being Na^+-dependent, glucose also stimulates Na^+ and fluid absorption, which is the physiologic basis of oral rehydration therapy for the treatment of diarrhea (Chap. 35).

Although the intestinal epithelial cells are crucial mediators of absorption and ion and water flow, the several cell types in the lamina propria (e.g., mast cells, macrophages, myofibroblasts) and the enteric nervous system interact with the epithelium to regulate mucosal cell function. The function of the intestine is the result of the integrated responses of and interactions between both intestinal epithelial cells and intestinal muscle.

ENTEROHEPATIC CIRCULATION OF BILE ACIDS   Bile acids are not present in the diet but are synthesized in the liver by a series of enzymatic steps that also include cholesterol catabolism. Indeed, interruption of the enterohepatic circulation of bile acids can reduce serum cholesterol levels by 10% before a new steady state is established. Bile acids are either primary or secondary: primary bile acids are synthesized in the liver from cholesterol, and secondary bile acids are synthesized from primary bile acids in the intestine by colonic bacterial enzymes. The two primary bile acids in humans are cholic acid and chenodeoxycholic acid; the two most abundant secondary bile acids are deoxycholic

acid and lithocholic acid. Approximately 500 mg bile acids are synthesized in the liver daily, conjugated to either taurine or glycine to form tauro-conjugated or glyco-conjugated bile acids, respectively, and are secreted into the duodenum in bile. The primary functions of bile acids are (1) to promote bile flow, (2) to solubilize cholesterol and phospholipid in the gallbladder by mixed micelle formation, and (3) to enhance dietary lipid digestion and absorption by forming mixed micelles in the proximal small intestine.

Bile acids are primarily absorbed by an active, Na^+-dependent process that is located exclusively in the ileum, though bile acids can also be absorbed to a lesser extent by non-carrier-mediated transport processes in the jejunum, ileum, and colon. Conjugated bile acids that enter the colon are deconjugated by colonic bacterial enzymes to unconjugated bile acids and are rapidly absorbed. Colonic bacterial enzymes also dehydroxylate bile acids to secondary bile acids.

Bile acids absorbed from the intestine return to the liver via the portal vein where they are resecreted (Fig. 275-1). Bile acid synthesis is largely autoregulated by 7α-hydroxylase, the initial enzyme in cholesterol degradation. A decrease in the amount of bile acids returning to the liver from the intestine is associated with an increase in bile acid synthesis/cholesterol catabolism, which helps keep the bile acid pool size relatively constant. However, there is a relatively limited capacity for an increase in bile acid synthesis—about two to two and one-half times (see below). The bile acid pool size is approximately 1 g and is circulated via the enterohepatic circulation about twice during each meal, or six to eight times during a 24-h period. A relatively small quantity of bile acids is not absorbed and is excreted in stool daily; this fecal loss is matched by hepatic bile acid synthesis.

Defects in any of the steps of the enterohepatic circulation of bile acids can result in a decrease in duodenal concentration of conjugated bile acids and, as a result, steatorrhea. Thus, steatorrhea can be caused by abnormalities in bile acid synthesis and excretion, their physical state in the intestinal lumen, and reabsorption (Table 275-1).

Synthesis   Decreased bile acid synthesis and steatorrhea have been demonstrated in chronic liver disease, but steatorrhea is often not a major component of the illness of these patients.

Secretion   Although bile acid secretion may be reduced or absent in biliary obstruction, steatorrhea is rarely a significant medical problem in these patients. In contrast, primary biliary cirrhosis represents a

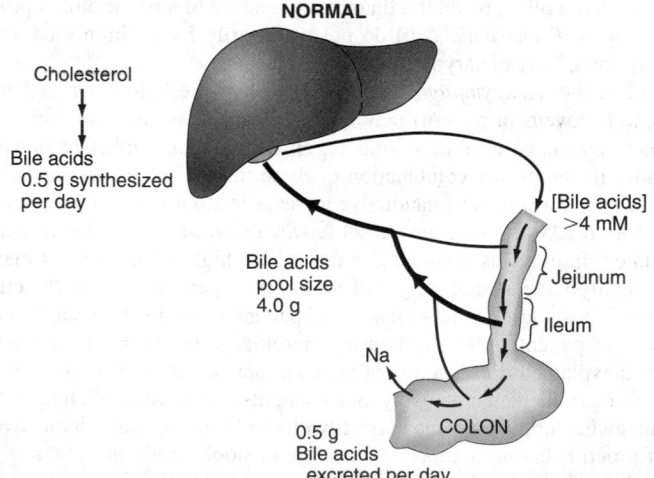

FIGURE 275-1   Schematic representation of the enterohepatic circulation of bile acids. Bile acid synthesis is cholesterol catabolism and occurs in the liver. Bile acids are secreted in bile and are stored in the gallbladder between meals and at night. Food in the duodenum induces the release of cholecystokinin, which is a potent stimulus for gallbladder contraction resulting in bile acid entry into the duodenum. Bile acids are primarily absorbed via a Na-dependent transport process that is located only in the ileum. A relatively small quantity of bile acids (~500 mg) is not absorbed in a 24-h period and is lost in stool. Fecal bile acid losses are matched by bile acid synthesis. The bile acid pool, i.e., the total amount of bile acids in the body at any time, is ~4 g and is circulated twice during each meal or six to eight times in a 24-h period.

TABLE 275-1 *Defects in Enterohepatic Circulation of Bile Acids*

Process	Pathophysiologic Defect	Disease Example
Synthesis	Decreased hepatic function	Cirrhosis
Biliary secretion	Altered canalicular function	Primary biliary cirrhosis
Maintenance of conjugated bile acids	Bacterial overgrowth	Jejunal diverticulosis
Reabsorption	Abnormal ileal function	Crohn's disease

defect in canalicular excretion of organic anions, including bile acids, and not infrequently is associated with steatorrhea and its consequences, e.g., chronic bone disease. Thus, the osteomalacia and other chronic bone abnormalities often present in patients with primary biliary cirrhosis and other cholestatic syndromes are secondary to steatorrhea that then leads to calcium and vitamin D malabsorption.

Maintenance of Conjugated Bile Acids In bacterial overgrowth syndromes associated with diarrhea, steatorrhea, and macrocytic anemia, there is an increase in a colonic type of bacterial flora in the small intestine. The steatorrhea is primarily a result of the decrease in conjugated bile acids secondary to their deconjugation by colonic-type bacteria. Two complementary explanations account for the resulting impairment of micelle formation: (1) unconjugated bile acids are rapidly absorbed in the jejunum by nonionic diffusion, resulting in a reduced concentration of duodenal bile acids; and (2) the critical micellar concentration (CMC) of unconjugated bile acids is higher than that of conjugated bile acids, and therefore unconjugated bile acids are less effective than conjugated bile acids in micelle formation.

Reabsorption Ileal dysfunction caused by either Crohn's disease or surgical resection results in a decrease in bile acid reabsorption in the ileum and an *increase* in the delivery of bile acids to the large intestine. The resulting clinical consequences—diarrhea with or without steatorrhea—are determined by the *degree* of ileal dysfunction and the *response* of the enterohepatic circulation to bile acid losses (Table 275-2). Patients with limited ileal disease or resection will often have diarrhea, but not steatorrhea. The diarrhea, a result of bile acids in the colon stimulating active Cl secretion, has been called *bile acid diarrhea*, or cholorrheic enteropathy, and responds promptly to cholestyramine, an anion-binding resin. Such patients do not develop steatorrhea because hepatic synthesis of bile acids increases to compensate for the rate of fecal bile acid losses, resulting in maintenance of both the bile acid pool size and the intraduodenal concentrations of bile acids. In contrast, patients with greater degrees of ileal disease and/or resection will often have diarrhea and steatorrhea that do not respond to cholestyramine. In this situation, ileal disease is also associated with increased amounts of bile acids entering the colon; however, hepatic synthesis can no longer increase sufficiently to maintain the bile acid pool size. As a consequence, the intraduodenal concentration of bile acids is also reduced to less than the CMC, resulting in impaired micelle formation and steatorrhea. This second situation is often called *fatty acid diarrhea*. Although cholestyramine may not be effective (and may even increase the diarrhea by further depleting the intraduodenal bile acid concentration), a low-fat diet to reduce fatty acids entering the colon can be effective. Two clinical features, the length

TABLE 275-2 *Comparison of Bile Acid and Fatty Acid Diarrhea*

	Bile Acid Diarrhea	Fatty Acid Diarrhea
Extent of ileal disease	Limited	Extensive
Ileal bile acid absorption	Reduced	Reduced
Fecal bile acid excretion	Increased	Increased
Fecal bile acid loss compensated by hepatic synthesis	Yes	No
Bile acid pool size	Normal	Reduced
Intraduodenal [bile acid]	Normal	Reduced
Steatorrhea	None or mild	>20 g
Response to cholestyramine	Yes	No
Response to low-fat diet	No	Yes

TABLE 275-3 *Comparison of Different Types of Fatty Acids*

	Long-Chain	Medium-Chain	Short-Chain
Carbon chain length	>12	8–12	<8
Present in diet	In large amounts	In small amounts	No
Origin	In diet as triglycerides	Only in small amounts in diet as triglycerides	Bacterial degradation in colon of nonabsorbed carbohydrate to fatty acids
Primary site of absorption	Small intestine	Small intestine	Colon
Requires pancreatic lipolysis	Yes	No	No
Requires micelle formation	Yes	No	No
Presence in stool	Minimal	No	Substantial

of ileum removed and the degree of steatorrhea, can predict whether an individual patient will respond to cholestyramine. Unfortunately, these predictors are imperfect, and a therapeutic trial of cholestyramine is often necessary to establish whether an individual patient will benefit from cholestyramine. Table 275-2 contrasts the characteristics of bile acid diarrhea (small ileal dysfunction) and fatty acid diarrhea (large ileal dysfunction).

LIPIDS Steatorrhea is caused by one or more defects in the digestion and absorption of dietary fat. Average intake of dietary fat in the United States is approximately 120 to 150 g/d, and fat absorption is linear to dietary fat intake. The total load of fat presented to the small intestine is considerably greater, as substantial amounts of lipid are secreted in bile each day. (See above for discussion of enterohepatic circulation of bile acids.) Three types of fatty acids compose fats: long-chain fatty acids (LCFAs), medium-chain fatty acids (MCFAs), and short-chain fatty acids (SCFAs) (Table 275-3). Dietary fat is exclusively composed of long-chain triglycerides (LCTs), i.e., glycerol that is bound via ester-linkages to three LCFAs. While the majority of dietary LCFAs have carbon chain lengths of 16 or 18, fatty acids of carbon chain length >12 are metabolized in the same manner; saturated and unsaturated fatty acids are handled identically.

Assimilation of dietary lipid requires several integrated processes that can be divided into (1) an intraluminal, or digestive, phase; (2) a mucosal, or absorptive, phase; and (3) a delivery, or postabsorptive, phase. An abnormality at any site of this process can cause steatorrhea (Table 275-4). Therefore, it is essential that any patient with steatorrhea be evaluated to identify the specific physiologic defect in overall

TABLE 275-4 *Defects in Lipid Digestion and Absorption in Steatorrhea*

Phase: Process	Pathophysiologic Defect	Disease Example
Digestive		
Lipolysis formation	Decrease lipase secretion	Chronic pancreatitis
Micelle formation	Decreased intraduodenal [bile acids]	See Table 275-1
Absorptive		
Mucosal uptake and resterification	Mucosal dysfunction	Celiac sprue
Post-absorptive		
Chylomicron formation	Absent betalipoproteins	Abetalipoproteinemia
Delivery from intestine	Abnormal lymphatics	Intestinal lymphangiectasia

FIGURE 275-2   Schematic representation of lipid digestion and absorption. Dietary lipid is in the form of long-chain triglycerides (LCTs). The overall process can be divided into (1) a digestive phase that includes both lipolysis and micelle formation requiring pancreatic lipase and conjugated bile acids, respectively, in the duodenum; (2) an absorptive phase for mucosal uptake and reesterification; and (3) a postabsorptive phase that includes chylomicron formation and exit from the intestinal epithelial cell via lymphatics. (*Courtesy of John M. Dietschy, MD.*)

lipid digestion-absorption as therapy will be determined by the specific cause responsible for the steatorrhea.

The digestive phase has two components, *lipolysis* and *micellar formation*. Although dietary lipid is in the form of LCTs, the intestinal mucosa does not absorb triglycerides; they must first be hydrolyzed (Fig. 275-2). The initial step in lipid digestion is the formation of emulsions of finely dispersed lipid, which is accomplished by mastication and gastric contractions. Lipolysis, the hydrolysis of triglycerides to free fatty acids, monoglycerides, and glycerol by lipase, is initiated in the stomach by a gastric lipase that has a pH optimum of 4.5 to 6.0. About 20 to 30% of total lipolysis occurs in the stomach. Lipolysis is completed in the duodenum and jejunum by pancreatic lipase, which is inactivated by pH <7.0. Pancreatic lipolysis is greatly enhanced by the presence of a second pancreatic enzyme, colipase, which facilitates the movement of lipase to the triglyceride.

Impaired lipolysis can lead to steatorrhea and can occur in the presence of pancreatic insufficiency due to chronic pancreatitis in adults or cystic fibrosis in children and adolescents. Normal lipolysis can be maintained by approximately 5% of maximal pancreatic lipase secretion; thus, steatorrhea is a late manifestation of these disorders. A reduction in intraduodenal pH can also result in altered lipolysis as pancreatic lipase is inactivated at pH <7. Thus, ~15% of patients with gastrinoma (Chap. 274) with substantial increases in gastric acid secretion from ectopic production of gastrin (usually from an islet cell adenoma) have diarrhea, and some will have steatorrhea believed secondary to acid-inactivation of pancreatic lipase. Similarly, patients with chronic pancreatitis (who have reduced lipase secretion) often have a decrease in pancreatic bicarbonate secretion, which will also result in a decrease in intraduodenal pH and inactivation of endogenous pancreatic lipase or of therapeutically administered lipase.

Overlying the microvillus membrane of the small intestine is the so-called unstirred water layer, a relatively stagnant aqueous phase that must be traversed by the products of lipolysis that are primarily water-insoluble. Water-soluble mixed micelles provide a mechanism for the water-insoluble products of lipolysis to reach the luminal plasma membrane of villus epithelial cells, the site for lipid absorption. Mixed micelles are molecular aggregates composed of fatty acids, monoglycerides, phospholipids, cholesterol, and conjugated bile acids. Mixed micelles are formed when the concentration of conjugated bile acids is greater than its CMC, which differs among the several bile acids present in the small intestinal lumen. Conjugated bile acids, synthesized in the liver and excreted into the duodenum in bile, are regulated by the enterohepatic circulation (see above). Steatorrhea can result from impaired movement of fatty acids across the unstirred aqueous fluid layer in two situations: (1) an increase in the relative thickness of the unstirred water layer that occurs in bacterial overgrowth syndromes (see below) secondary to functional stasis (e.g., scleroderma), and (2) a decrease in the *duodenal* concentration of con-

jugated bile acids below its CMC, resulting in impaired micelle formation. Thus, steatorrhea can be caused by one or more defects in the enterohepatic circulation of bile acids.

Uptake and reesterification constitute the *absorptive phase* of lipid digestion-absorption. Although passive diffusion has been thought responsible, a carrier-mediated process may mediate fatty acid and monoglyceride uptake. Regardless of the uptake process, fatty acids and monoglycerides are reesterified by a series of enzymatic steps in the endoplasmic reticulum and Golgi to form triglycerides, the form in which lipid exits from the intestinal epithelial cell. Impaired lipid absorption as a result of either mucosal inflammation (e.g., celiac sprue) and/or intestinal resection can also lead to steatorrhea.

The reesterified triglycerides require the formation of *chylomicrons* to permit their exit from the small-intestinal epithelial cell and their delivery to the liver via the *lymphatics*. Chylomicrons are composed of β-lipoprotein and contain triglycerides, cholesterol, cholesterol esters, and phospholipids and enter the lymphatics, not the portal vein. Defects in the *postabsorptive phase* of lipid digestion-absorption can also result in steatorrhea, but these disorders are uncommon. Abetalipoproteinemia, or acanthocytosis, is a rare disorder of impaired synthesis of β-lipoprotein associated with abnormal erythrocytes (acanthocytes), neurologic problems, and steatorrhea. Lipolysis, micelle formation, and lipid uptake are all normal in patients with abetalipoproteinemia, but the reesterified triglyceride cannot exit from the epithelial cell because of the failure to produce chylomicrons. Small-intestinal biopsies of these rare patients in the postprandial state reveal lipid-laden small-intestinal epithelial cells that become perfectly normal in appearance following a 72- to 96-h fast. Similarly, abnormalities of intestinal lymphatics (e.g., intestinal lymphangiectasia) may also be associated with steatorrhea as well as protein loss (see below). Steatorrhea can result from defects at any of the several steps in lipid digestion-absorption. The mechanism of lipid digestion-absorption outlined above is limited to *dietary* lipid that is almost exclusively in the form of LCTs (Table 275-3). Medium-chain triglycerides (MCTs), composed of fatty acids with carbon chain lengths of 8 to 10, are present in large amounts in coconut oil and are used as a nutritional supplement. MCTs can be digested and absorbed by a different pathway from LCTs and at one time held promise as an important treatment of steatorrhea of almost all etiologies. Unfortunately, their therapeutic effects have been less than expected because their use is often not associated with an increase in body weight for reasons that are not completely understood.

MCTs, in contrast to LCTs, do not require pancreatic lipolysis as the triglyceride can be absorbed intact by the intestinal epithelial cell. Further, micelle formation is not necessary for the absorption of MCTs or medium-chain fatty acids, if hydrolyzed by pancreatic lipase. MCTs are absorbed more efficiently than LCTs for the following reasons: (1) the rate of MCT absorption is greater than that of long-chain fatty acids; (2) medium-chain fatty acids following absorption are not reesterified; (3) following absorption, MCTs are hydrolyzed to medium-chain fatty acids; (4) MCTs do not require chylomicron formation for their exit from the intestinal epithelial cells; and (5) their route of exit is via the portal vein and not via lymphatics. Thus, the absorption of MCTs is greater than that of LCTs in pancreatic insufficiency, conditions with reduced intraduodenal bile acid concentrations, small-intestinal mucosal disease, abetalipoproteinemia, and intestinal lymphangiectasia.

SCFAs are not dietary lipids but are synthesized by colonic bacterial enzymes from nonabsorbed carbohydrate and are the anions in highest concentration in stool (between 80 and 130 mM). The SCFAs present in stool are primarily acetate, propionate, and butyrate, whose carbon chain lengths are 2, 3, and 4, respectively. Butyrate is the primary nutrient for colonic epithelial cells, and its deficiency may be associated with one or more colitides. SCFAs conserve calories and carbohydrate, because carbohydrates not completely absorbed in the small intestine will not be absorbed in the large intestine due to the absence of both disaccharidases and SGLT, the transport protein that mediates monosaccharide absorption. In contrast, SCFAs are rapidly absorbed and stimulate colonic Na-Cl and fluid absorption. Most non–*Clostridium difficile* antibiotic-associated diarrhea is due to antibiotic suppression of colonic microflora, with a resulting decrease in SCFA production. As *C. difficile* accounts for about 10 to 15% of all antibiotic-associated diarrhea, a relative decrease in colonic production of SCFAs is likely the cause of most antibiotic-associated diarrhea.

The clinical manifestations of steatorrhea are a consequence of both the underlying disorder responsible for the development of steatorrhea and steatorrhea per se. Depending on the degree of steatorrhea and the level of dietary intake, significant fat malabsorption may lead to weight loss. Steatorrhea per se can be responsible for diarrhea; if the primary cause of the steatorrhea has not been identified, a low-fat diet can often ameliorate the diarrhea by decreasing fecal fat excretion. Steatorrhea is often associated with fat-soluble vitamin deficiency, which will require replacement with water-soluble preparations of these vitamins.

Disorders of absorption may also be associated with malabsorption of other dietary nutrients, most often carbohydrates, with or without a decrease in dietary lipid digestion and absorption. Therefore, knowledge of the mechanism of the digestion and absorption of carbohydrates, proteins, and other minerals and vitamins is useful in the evaluation of patients with altered intestinal nutrient absorption.

CARBOHYDRATES Carbohydrates in the diet are present in the form of starch, disaccharides (sucrose and lactose), and glucose. Carbohydrates are absorbed only in the small intestine and only in the form of monosaccharides. Therefore, before their absorption, starch and disaccharides must first be digested by pancreatic amylase and intestinal brush border disaccharidases to monosaccharides. Monosaccharide absorption occurs by a Na-dependent process mediated by the brush border transport protein SGLT.

Lactose malabsorption is the only clinically important disorder of carbohydrate absorption. Lactose, the disaccharide present in milk, requires digestion by brush border lactase to its two constituent monosaccharides, glucose and galactose. Lactase is present in almost all species in the postnatal period but then disappears throughout the animal kingdom, except in humans. Lactase activity persists in many individuals throughout life. Two different types of lactase deficiency exist—primary and secondary. In *primary lactase deficiency*, a genetically determined decrease or absence of lactase is noted, while all other aspects of both intestinal absorption and brush border enzymes are normal. In a number of non-Caucasian groups, primary lactase deficiency is common in adulthood. Table 275-5 presents the incidence of primary lactase deficiency in several different ethnic groups. Northern European and North American Caucasians are the only population group to maintain small-intestinal lactase activity throughout adult life. The persistence of lactase is the abnormality due to a defect in the regulation of its maturation. In contrast, *secondary lactase deficiency* occurs in association with small-intestinal mucosal disease with abnormalities in both structure and function of other brush border

enzymes and transport processes. Secondary lactase deficiency is often seen in celiac sprue.

As lactose digestion is rate-limiting compared to glucose/galactose absorption, lactase deficiency is associated with significant lactose malabsorption. Some individuals with lactose malabsorption develop symptoms such as diarrhea, abdominal pain, cramps, and/or flatus. Most individuals with primary lactase deficiency do not have symptoms. Since lactose intolerance may be associated with symptoms suggestive of an irritable bowel syndrome, persistence of such symptoms in an individual with lactose intolerance while on a strict lactose-free diet would suggest that the individual's symptoms were related to irritable bowel syndrome.

Development of symptoms of lactose intolerance is related to several factors:

1. *Amount of lactose in the diet.*
2. *Rate of gastric emptying.* Symptoms are more likely when gastric emptying is rapid than when gastric emptying is slower. Therefore, it is more likely that skim milk will be associated with symptoms of lactose intolerance than will whole milk, as the rate of gastric emptying following skim milk intake is more rapid. Similarly, the diarrhea observed following subtotal gastrectomy is often a result of lactose intolerance, as gastric emptying is accelerated in patients with a gastrojejunostomy.
3. *Small-intestinal transit time.* Although the small and large intestine contribute to the development of symptoms, many of the symptoms of lactase deficiency are related to the interaction of colonic bacteria and nonabsorbed lactose. More rapid small-intestinal transit makes symptoms more likely.
4. *Colonic compensation by production of SCFAs* from nonabsorbed lactose. Reduced levels of colonic microflora, which can occur following antibiotic use, will also be associated with increased symptoms following lactose ingestion, especially in a lactase-deficient individual.

Glucose-galactose or monosaccharide malabsorption may also be associated with diarrhea and is due to a congenital absence of SGLT. Diarrhea is present when individuals with this disorder ingest carbohydrates that contain actively transported monosaccharides (e.g., glucose, galactose) but not monosaccharides that are not actively transported (e.g., fructose). Fructose is absorbed by the brush border transport protein GLUT 5, a facilitated diffusion process that is not Na-dependent and is distinct from SGLT. In contrast, some individuals develop diarrhea as a result of consuming large quantities of sorbitol, a sugar used in diabetic candy; sorbitol is only minimally absorbed due to the absence of an intestinal absorptive transport mechanism for sorbitol.

PROTEINS Protein is present in food almost exclusively as polypeptides and requires extensive hydrolysis to di- and tripeptides and amino acids before absorption. Proteolysis occurs in both the stomach and small intestine; it is mediated by pepsin secreted as pepsinogen by gastric chief cells and trypsinogen and other peptidases from pancreatic acinar cells. These proenzymes, pepsinogen and trypsinogen, must be activated to pepsin (by pepsin in the presence of a pH <5) and trypsin (by the intestinal brush border enzyme enterokinase, and subsequently by trypsin). Proteins are absorbed by separate transport systems for di- and tripeptides and for different types of amino acids, e.g., neutral and dibasic. Alterations in either protein or amino acid digestion and absorption are rarely observed clinically, even in the presence of extensive small-intestinal mucosal inflammation. However, three rare genetic disorders involve protein digestion-absorption: (1) *enterokinase deficiency* is due to an absence of the brush border enzyme that converts the proenzyme trypsinogen to trypsin and is associated with diarrhea, growth retardation, and hypoproteinemia; (2) *Hartnup syndrome*, a defect in neutral amino acid transport, is characterized by a pellagra-like rash and neuropsychiatric symptoms; and (3) *cystinu-*

TABLE 275-5 *Primary Lactase Deficiency in Different Adult Ethnic Groups*

Ethnic Group	Prevalence of Lactase Deficiency, %
Northern European	5–15
Mediterranean	60–85
African black	85–100
American black	45–80
American Caucasian	10–25
Native American	50–95
Mexican American	40–75
Asian	90–100

Source: From FJ Simons: Am J Dig Dis 23:963, 1978.

ria, a defect in dibasic amino acid transport, is associated with renal calculi and chronic pancreatitis.

EVALUATION OF MALABSORPTION

The clues provided by the history, symptoms, and initial preliminary observations will serve to limit extensive, ill-focused, and expensive laboratory and imaging studies. For example, a clinician evaluating a patient with symptoms suggestive of malabsorption who recently had extensive small-intestinal resection for mesenteric ischemia should direct the initial assessment almost exclusively to define whether a short bowel syndrome might explain the entire clinical picture. Similarly, the development of a pattern of bowel movements suggestive of steatorrhea in a patient with long-standing alcohol abuse and chronic pancreatitis should lead toward assessing pancreatic exocrine function.

The classic picture of malabsorption described in textbooks >30 years ago is rarely seen today in most parts of the United States. As a consequence, diseases with malabsorption must be suspected in individuals with less severe symptoms and signs and with subtle evidence of the altered absorption of only a *single* nutrient rather than obvious evidence of the malabsorption of multiple nutrients.

Although diarrhea can be caused by changes in fluid and electrolyte movement in either the small or the large intestine, dietary nutrients are absorbed almost exclusively in the small intestine. Therefore, the demonstration of diminished absorption of a dietary nutrient provides unequivocal evidence of small-intestinal disease, although colonic dysfunction may also be present (e.g., Crohn's disease may involve both small and large intestine). Dietary nutrient absorption may be segmental or diffuse along the small intestine and is site-specific. Thus, for example, calcium, iron, and folic acid are exclusively absorbed by active transport processes in the proximal small intestine, especially the duodenum; in contrast, the active transport mechanisms for both cobalamin and bile acids are present only in the ileum. Therefore, in an individual who years previously had had an intestinal resection, the details of which are not presently available, a presentation with evidence of calcium, folic acid, and iron malabsorption but without cobalamin deficiency would make it likely that the duodenum and jejunum, but not ileum, had been resected.

Some nutrients, e.g., glucose, amino acids, and lipids, are absorbed throughout the small intestine, though there is evidence that their rate of absorption is greater in the proximal than in the distal segments. However, following segmental resection of the small intestine, the remaining segments will undergo both morphologic and functional "adaptation" to enhance absorption. Such adaptation is secondary to the presence of luminal nutrients and hormonal stimuli and may not be complete in humans for several months following the resection. Adaptation is critical for individuals who have undergone massive resection of the small intestine and/or colon to help ensure survival.

Establishing the presence of steatorrhea and identifying its specific cause are often quite difficult for several reasons. Despite attempts to develop tests that do *not* require the collection of stool to document the presence of steatorrhea, the "gold standard" still remains a timed, quantitative stool fat determination. On a practical basis, stool collections are invariably difficult and often incomplete as nobody wants to handle stool. A qualitative test—Sudan III stain—has long been available to establish the presence of an increase in stool fat. This test is rapid and inexpensive but, as a qualitative test, does not establish the degree of fat malabsorption and is best used as a preliminary screening study. Many of the blood, breath, and isotopic tests that have been developed either (1) do not directly measure fat absorption, (2) have excellent sensitivity when steatorrhea is obvious and severe but have poor sensitivity when steatorrhea is mild, or (3) have not survived the transition from their development in a laboratory to commercial utilization and dissemination.

Despite this situation, the use of routine laboratory studies (i.e., complete blood count, prothrombin time, serum protein determination, alkaline phosphatase) may suggest the presence of dietary nutrient

depletion, especially iron, folate, cobalamin, and vitamins D and K. Additional studies include measurement of serum carotene, cholesterol, albumin, iron, folate, and cobalamin levels. The serum carotene level can also be reduced if the patient has poor dietary intake of leafy vegetables.

If steatorrhea and/or altered absorption of other nutrients are suspected, the history, clinical observations, and laboratory testing can help detect deficiency of a dietary nutrient, especially the fat-soluble vitamins A, D, E, or K. Thus, evidence of metabolic bone disease with elevated alkaline phosphatase and/or reduced serum calcium levels would suggest vitamin D malabsorption. A deficiency of vitamin K would be suggested by an elevated prothrombin time in an individual without liver disease who was not taking anticoagulants. Macrocytic anemia would lead to evaluation of whether cobalamin or folic acid malabsorption was present. The presence of iron-deficiency anemia in the absence of occult bleeding from the gastrointestinal tract in either a male or a nonmenstruating female would require evaluation of iron malabsorption and the exclusion of celiac sprue, as iron is absorbed exclusively in the proximal small intestine.

At times, however, a timed (72-h) quantitative stool collection, preferably on a defined diet, must be obtained to determine stool fat content and establish the presence of steatorrhea. The presence of steatorrhea then requires further assessment to establish the pathophysiologic process(es) responsible for the defect in dietary lipid digestion-absorption (Table 275-4). Some of the other studies include the Schilling test, D-xylose test, duodenal mucosal biopsy, small-intestinal radiologic examination, and tests of pancreatic exocrine function.

THE SCHILLING TEST   This test is performed to determine the cause for cobalamin malabsorption. Since cobalamin absorption requires multiple steps, including gastric, pancreatic, and ileal processes, the Schilling test can also be used to assess the integrity of these other organs (Chap. 92). Cobalamin is present primarily in meat. Except in strict vegans, *dietary* cobalamin deficiency is exceedingly uncommon. Dietary cobalamin is bound in the stomach to a glycoprotein called *R-binder protein*, which is synthesized in both the stomach and salivary glands. This cobalamin–R binder complex is formed in the acid milieu of the stomach. Cobalamin absorption has an absolute requirement for intrinsic factor, another glycoprotein synthesized and released by gastric parietal cells, to promote its uptake by specific cobalamin receptors on the brush border of ileal enterocytes. Pancreatic protease enzymes split the cobalamin–R binder complex to release cobalamin in the proximal small intestine, where cobalamin is then bound by intrinsic factor.

As a consequence, cobalamin absorption may be abnormal in the following:

1. Pernicious anemia, a disease in which immunologically mediated atrophy of gastric parietal cells leads to an absence of both gastric acid and intrinsic factor secretion.
2. Chronic pancreatitis as a result of deficiency of pancreatic proteases to split the cobalamin–R binder complex. Although 50% of patients with chronic pancreatitis have been reported to have an abnormal Schilling test that was corrected by pancreatic enzyme replacement, the presence of a cobalamin-responsive macrocytic anemia in chronic pancreatitis is extremely rare. Although this probably reflects a difference in the digestion/absorption of cobalamin in food versus that in a crystalline form, the Schilling test can still be used to assess pancreatic exocrine function.
3. Achlorhydria or absence of another factor secreted with acid that is responsible for splitting cobalamin away from the proteins in food to which it is bound. Up to one-third of individuals >60 years of age have marginal vitamin B_{12} absorption because of the inability to release cobalamin from food; these people have no defects in absorbing crystalline vitamin B_{12}.
4. Bacterial overgrowth syndromes, which are most often secondary to stasis in the small intestine, leading to bacterial utilization of cobalamin (often referred to as *stagnant bowel syndrome*) (see below).

5. Ileal dysfunction (as a result of either inflammation or prior intestinal resection) due to impaired function of the mechanism of cobalamin–intrinsic factor uptake by ileal intestinal epithelial cells.

The Schilling test is performed by administering ⁵⁸Co-labeled cobalamin and collecting urine for 24 h and is dependent on normal renal and bladder function. Urinary excretion of cobalamin will reflect cobalamin absorption provided that intrahepatic binding sites for cobalamin are fully occupied. To ensure saturation of hepatic cobalamin binding sites so that all absorbed radiolabeled cobalamin will be excreted in urine, 1 mg cobalamin is administered intramuscularly 1 h following ingestion of the radiolabeled cobalamin. The Schilling test may be abnormal (usually defined as <10% excretion in 24 h) in pernicious anemia, chronic pancreatitis, blind loop syndrome, and ileal disease (Table 275-6). Therefore, whenever an abnormal Schilling test is found, ⁵⁸Co-labeled cobalamin should be administered on another occasion either bound to intrinsic factor, with pancreatic enzymes, or following a 5-day course of antibiotics (often tetracycline). A variation of the Schilling test can detect failure to split cobalamin from food proteins. The labeled cobalamin is cooked together with a scrambled egg and administered orally. People with achlorydria will excrete <10% of the labeled cobalamin in the urine. In addition to establishing the etiology for cobalamin deficiency, the Schilling test can be used to help delineate the pathologic process responsible for steatorrhea by assessing ileal, pancreatic, and small-intestinal luminal function. Unfortunately, in recent years the Schilling test has been infrequently performed because radiolabeled cobalamin is often not available.

FIGURE 275-3 Barium contrast small-intestinal radiologic examinations. *A.* Normal individual. *B.* Celiac sprue. *C.* Jejunal diverticulosis. *D.* Crohn's disease. *(Courtesy of Morton Burrell, MD, Yale University.)*

URINARY D-XYLOSE TEST The urinary D-xylose test for carbohydrate absorption provides an assessment of proximal small-intestinal mucosal function. D-Xylose, a pentose, is absorbed almost exclusively in the proximal small intestine. The D-xylose test is usually performed by giving 25 g D-xylose and collecting urine for 5 h. An abnormal test (<4.5 g excretion) primarily reflects the presence of duodenal/jejunal mucosal disease. The D-xylose test can also be abnormal in patients with blind loop syndrome (as a consequence primarily of abnormal intestinal mucosa) and, as a false-positive study, in patients with large collections of fluid in a third space (i.e., ascites, pleural fluid). The ease of obtaining a mucosal biopsy of the small intestine by endoscopy and the false-negative rate of the D-xylose test have led to its diminished use. When small-intestinal mucosal disease is suspected, a small-intestinal mucosal biopsy should be performed.

RADIOLOGIC EXAMINATION Radiologic examination of the small intestine using barium contrast (small-bowel series or study) can provide important information in the evaluation of the patient with presumed or suspected malabsorption. These studies are most often performed in conjunction with the examination of the esophagus, stomach, and duodenal bulb, and insufficient barium is given to the patient to permit an adequate examination of the small-intestinal mucosa, especially the ileum. As a result, many gastrointestinal radiologists alter the procedure of a barium contrast examination of the small intestine by performing either a small-bowel series in which a large amount of barium is given by mouth without concurrent examination of the esophagus and stomach or an enteroclysis study in which a large amount of barium is introduced into the duodenum via a fluoroscopically placed tube. In addition, many of the diagnostic features initially described by radiologists to denote the presence of small-intestinal disease (e.g., flocculation, segmentation) are rarely seen with current barium suspensions. Nonetheless, in skilled hands barium contrast examination of the small intestine can yield important information. For example, with extensive mucosal disease, dilation of intestine can be seen, as candilution of barium from increased intestinal fluid secretion (Fig. 275-3). A normal barium contrast study does *not* exclude the possibility of small-intestinal disease. However, a small-bowel series remains a very useful examination to assess for the presence of anatomical abnormalities, such as strictures and fistulas (as in Crohn's disease) or blind loop syndrome (e.g., multiple jejunal diverticula), and to define the extent of a previous surgical resection.

TABLE 275-6 *Differential Results of Schilling Test in Several Diseases Associated with Cobalamin (Cbl) Malabsorption*

	⁵⁸Co-Cbl	With Intrinsic Factor	With Pancreatic Enzymes	After 5 Days of Antibiotics
Pernicious anemia	Reduced	Normal	Reduced	Reduced
Chronic pancreatitis	Reduced	Reduced	Normal	Reduced
Bacterial overgrowth	Reduced	Reduced	Reduced	Normal
Ileal disease	Reduced	Reduced	Reduced	Reduced

BIOPSY OF SMALL-INTESTINAL MUCOSA A small-intestinal mucosal biopsy is essential in the evaluation of a patient with documented steatorrhea or chronic diarrhea (lasting >3 weeks) (Chap. 35). The ready availability of endoscopic equipment to examine the stomach and duodenum has led to its almost uniform use as the preferred method to obtain histologic material of proximal small-intestinal mucosa. The primary indications for a small-intestinal biopsy are (1) evaluation of a patient either with documented or suspected steatorrhea or with chronic diarrhea, and (2) diffuse or focal abnormalities of the small intestine defined on a small-intestinal series. Lesions seen on small-bowel biopsy can be classified into three different categories (Table 275-7): (1) diffuse, specific; (2) patchy, specific; and (3) diffuse, nonspecific.

1. *Diffuse, specific lesions.* Relatively few diseases associated with altered nutrient absorption have specific histopathologic abnormalities on small-intestinal mucosal biopsy, and they are uncommon. Whipple's disease is characterized by the presence of periodic acid–Schiff (PAS)-positive macrophages in the lamina propria, while the bacilli that are also present may require electron-microscopic examination for identification (Fig. 275-4). *Abetalipoproteinemia* is characterized by a normal mucosal appearance except for the presence of mucosal absorptive cells that contain lipid postprandially and disappear following a prolonged period of either fat-free intake or fasting. *Immune globulin deficiency* is associated with a variety of histopathologic findings on small-intestinal mucosal biopsy. The characteristic feature is the absence of or substantial reduction in the number of plasma cells in the lamina propria; the mucosal architecture may be either per-

fectly normal or flat, i.e., villus atrophy. As patients with immune globulin deficiency are often infected with *Giardia lamblia*, *Giardia* trophozoites may also be seen in the biopsy.

2. *Patchy, specific lesions.* Several diseases are associated with abnormal small-intestinal mucosal biopsies, but the characteristic features that are present have a patchy distribution. As a result, biopsies obtained randomly or in the absence of abnormalities visualized endoscopically may not reveal these diagnostic features. Intestinal *lymphoma* can at times be diagnosed on mucosal biopsy by the identification of malignant lymphoma cells in the lamina propria and submucosa (Chap. 97). The presence of dilated lymphatics in the submucosa and sometimes in the lamina propria indicates the presence of *lymphangiectasia* associated with hypoproteinemia secondary to protein loss into the intestine. *Eosinophilic gastroenteritis* comprises a heterogeneous group of disorders with a spectrum of presentations and symptoms with an eosinophilic infiltrate of the lamina propria, with or without peripheral eosinophilia. The patchy nature of the infiltrate as well as its presence in the submucosa often leads to an absence of histopathologic findings on mucosal biopsy. As the involvement of the duodenum in *Crohn's disease* is also submucosal and not necessarily continuous, mucosal biopsies are not the most direct approach to the diagnosis of duodenal Crohn's disease (Chap. 276). Amyloid deposition can be identified by Congo Red stain in some patients with *amyloidosis* involving the duodenum (Chap. 310).

Several microorganisms can be identified on small-intestinal biopsies, establishing a correct diagnosis. Many of these microorganisms are associated with diarrhea that occurs in immunodeficient individuals, especially those with HIV infection, and include *Cryptosporidium*, *Isospora belli*, cytomegalovirus, *Mycobacterium avium-intracellulare*, and *G. lamblia*.

3. *Diffuse, nonspecific lesions.* Celiac sprue presents with a characteristic mucosal appearance on duodenal/proximal jejunal mucosal biopsy that is not diagnostic of the disease. The diagnosis of celiac sprue is established by clinical, histologic, and immunologic response to a gluten-free diet. *Tropical sprue* is associated with histopathologic findings similar to those of celiac sprue after a tropical or subtropical exposure but does not respond to gluten restriction; most often symptoms improve with antibiotics and folate administration.

Patients with steatorrhea require assessment of *pancreatic exocrine function*, which is often abnormal in chronic pancreatitis. No test assesses pancreatic exocrine function well. Endoscopic approaches provide excellent assessment of pancreatic duct anatomy but do **not** assess exocrine function (Chap. 293). One noninvasive study (bentiromide test) of pancreatic exocrine function is based on the feeding of a tripeptide containing *p*-aminobenzoic acid (PABA). Following splitting of PABA by pancreatic proteases, PABA is liberated, absorbed, and excreted in urine. Reduced proteolysis results in reduced urinary excretion of PABA. This test is neither sensitive nor specific.

Table 275-8 summarizes the results of the D-xylose test, Schilling test, and small-intestinal mucosal biopsy in patients with five different causes of steatorrhea.

SPECIFIC DISEASE ENTITIES

CELIAC SPRUE Celiac sprue is a common cause of malabsorption of one or more nutrients in Caucasians, especially those of European descent. Estimated incidence in the United States may be as high as 1:13 people. Celiac sprue has had several other names including nontropical sprue, celiac disease (in children), adult celiac disease, and gluten-sensitive enteropathy. The etiology of celiac sprue is not known, but environmental, immunologic, and genetic factors are important. Celiac sprue has protean manifestations, almost all of which are secondary to nutrient malabsorption, and a varied natural history, with the onset of symptoms occurring at ages ranging from the first year of life through the eighth decade.

The hallmark of celiac sprue is the presence of an abnormal small-intestinal biopsy (Fig. 275-4) and the response of both symptoms—

TABLE 275-7 *Disease that Can be Diagnosed by Small-Intestinal Mucosal Biopsies*

Lesions	Pathologic Findings
Diffuse, specific	
Whipple's disease	Lamina propria contains macrophages containing PAS+ material
Agammaglobulinemia	No plasma cells; either normal or absent villi ("flat mucosa");
Abetalipoproteinemia	Normal villi; epithelial cells vacuolated with fat postprandially
Patchy, specific	
Intestinal lymphoma	Malignant cells in lamina propria and submucosa
Intestinal lymphangiectasia	Dilated lymphatics; clubbed villi
Eosinophilic gastroenteritis	Eosinophil infiltration of lamina propria and mucosa
Amyloidosis	Amyloid deposits
Crohn's disease	Noncaseating granulomas
Infection by one or more microorganisms (see text)	Specific organisms
Mastocytosis	Mast cell infiltration of lamina propria
Diffuse, nonspecific	
Celiac sprue	Short or absent villi; mononuclear infiltrate; epithelial cell damage; hypertrophy of crypts
Tropical sprue	Similar to celiac sprue
Bacterial overgrowth	Patchy damage to villi; lymphocyte infiltration
Folate deficiency	Short villi; decreased mitosis in crypts; megalocytosis
Vitamin B_{12} deficiency	Similar to folate deficiency
Radiation enteritis	Similar to folate deficiency
Zollinger-Ellison syndrome	Mucosal ulceration and erosion from acid
Protein-calorie malnutrition	Villous atrophy; secondary bacterial overgrowth
Drug-induced enteritis	Variable histology

Note: PAS+, periodic acid–Schiff positive.

evidence of malabsorption and the histopathologic changes on the small-intestinal biopsy—to the elimination of gluten from the diet. The histopathologic changes have a proximal to distal intestinal distribution of severity, which probably reflects the exposure of the intestinal mucosa to varied amounts of dietary gluten; the degree of symptoms is often related to the extent of these histopathologic changes.

The symptoms of celiac sprue may appear with the introduction of cereals in an infant's diet, although there is frequently a spontaneous remission during the second decade of life that may be either permanent or followed by the reappearance of symptoms over several years. Alternatively, the symptoms of celiac sprue may first become evident at almost any age throughout adulthood. In many patients, frequent spontaneous remissions and exacerbations occur. The symptoms range from significant malabsorption of multiple nutrients with diarrhea, steatorrhea, weight loss, and the consequences of nutrient depletion (i.e., anemia and metabolic bone disease) to the absence of any gastrointestinal symptoms but with evidence of the depletion of a single nutrient (e.g., iron or folate deficiency, osteomalacia, edema from protein loss). Asymptomatic relatives of patients with celiac sprue have been identified as having this disease either by small-intestinal biopsy or by serologic studies (e.g., antiendomysial antibodies).

Etiology   The etiology of celiac sprue is not known, but environmental, immunologic, and genetic factors all appear to contribute to the disease.

One *environmental* factor is the clear association of the disease with gliadin, a component of gluten that is present in wheat, barley, rye, and, in smaller amounts, oats. In addition to the role of gluten restriction in treatment, the instillation of gluten into both normal-appearing rectum and distal ileum of patients with celiac sprue results within hours in morphologic changes.

An *immunologic* component to etiology is suspected for three reasons. First, serum antibodies—IgA antigliadin, IgA antiendomysial, and IgA anti-tissue transglutaminase (tTG) antibodies—are present, but it is also not known whether such antibodies are primary or secondary to the tissue damage. The antiendomysial antibody has 90 to 95% sensitivity and 90 to 95% specificity, and the antigen recognized by the antiendomysial antibody test is tissue transglutaminase. Antibody studies are frequently used to identify patients with celiac sprue; patients with these antibodies should undergo duodenal biopsy. The relationship of this autoantibody to a pathogenetic mechanism (or mechanisms) responsible for celiac sprue remains to be established. Nonetheless, this antibody will undoubtedly prove extremely useful in establishing the true prevalence of celiac sprue in the general population and may provide important clues to its etiology. Second, treatment with prednisolone for 4 weeks of a patient with celiac sprue who continues to eat gluten will induce a remission and convert the "flat" abnormal duodenal biopsy to a more normal-appearing one. Third, gliadin peptides may interact with gliadin-specific T cells that may either mediate tissue injury or induce the release of one or more cytokines that are responsible for the tissue injury.

Genetic factor(s) also appear to be involved in celiac sprue. The incidence of celiac sprue varies widely in different population groups (high in Caucasians, low in blacks and Asians) and is 10% in first-

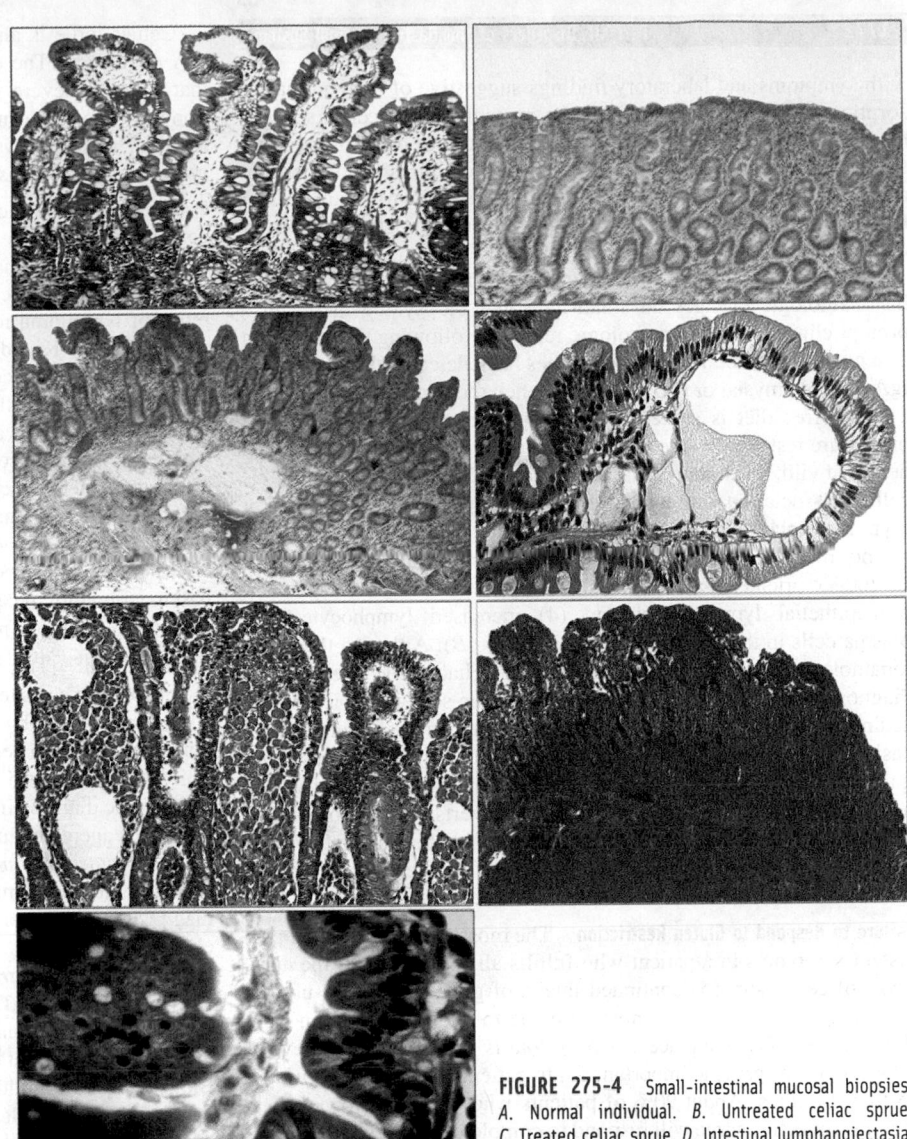

FIGURE 275-4   Small-intestinal mucosal biopsies. *A.* Normal individual. *B.* Untreated celiac sprue. *C.* Treated celiac sprue. *D.* Intestinal lymphangiectasia. *E.* Whipple's disease. *F.* Lymphoma. *G.* Giardiasis. *(Courtesy of Marie Robert, MD, Yale University.)*

degree relatives of celiac sprue patients. Furthermore, about 95% of patients with celiac sprue express the HLA-DQ2 allele, though only a minority of all persons expressing DQ2 have celiac sprue.

Diagnosis   A small-intestinal biopsy is required to establish a diagnosis of celiac sprue (Fig. 275-4). A biopsy should be performed in patients

TABLE 275-8   *Results of Diagnostic Studies in Different Causes of Steatorrhea*

	D-Xylose Test	Schilling Test	Duodenal Mucosal Biopsy
Chronic pancreatitis	Normal	50% abnormal; if abnormal, normal with pancreatic enzymes	Normal
Bacterial overgrowth syndrome	Normal or only modestly abnormal	Often abnormal; if abnormal, normal after antibiotics	Usually normal
Ileal disease	Normal	Abnormal	Normal
Celiac sprue	Decreased	Normal	Abnormal: probably "flat"
Intestinal lymph-angiectasia	Normal	Normal	Abnormal: "dilated lymphatics"

with symptoms and laboratory findings suggestive of nutrient malabsorption and/or deficiency. Since the presentation of celiac sprue is often subtle, without overt evidence of malabsorption or nutrient deficiency, it is important to have a relatively low threshold to perform a biopsy. It is more prudent to perform a biopsy than to obtain another test of intestinal absorption, which can never completely exclude or establish this diagnosis.

The diagnosis of celiac sprue requires the presence of characteristic histopathologic changes on small-intestinal biopsy together with a prompt clinical and histopathologic response following the institution of a gluten-free diet. If serologic studies have detected the presence of IgA antiendomysial or tTG antibodies, they too should disappear after a gluten-free diet is started. The changes seen on duodenal/jejunal biopsy are restricted to the mucosa and include (1) absence or reduced height of villi, resulting in a flat appearance; (2) increased loss of villus cells in association with increased crypt cell proliferation resulting in crypt hyperplasia and loss of villus structure, with consequent villus, but not mucosal, atrophy; (3) cuboidal appearance and nuclei that are no longer oriented basally in surface epithelial cells and increased intraepithelial lymphocytes; and (4) increased lymphocytes and plasma cells in the lamina propria (Fig. 275-4*B*). Although these histopathologic features are characteristic of celiac sprue, they are *not* diagnostic because a similar appearance can be seen in tropical sprue, eosinophilic enteritis, and milk-protein intolerance in children and occasionally in lymphoma, bacterial overgrowth, Crohn's disease, and gastrinoma with acid hypersecretion. However, the presence of a characteristic histopathologic appearance that reverts toward normal following the initiation of a gluten-free diet establishes the diagnosis of celiac sprue (Fig. 275-4*C*). Readministration of gluten with or without an additional small-intestinal biopsy is not necessary.

Failure to Respond to Gluten Restriction The most common cause of persistent symptoms in a patient who fulfills all the criteria of the diagnosis of celiac sprue is continued intake of gluten. Gluten is ubiquitous, and significant effort must be made to exclude all gluten from the diet. Use of rice in place of wheat flour is very helpful, and several support groups provide important aid to patients with celiac sprue and to their families. About 90% of patients who have the characteristic findings of celiac sprue will respond to complete dietary gluten restriction. The remainder constitute a heterogeneous group (whose condition is often called *refractory sprue*) that includes some patients who (1) respond to restriction of other dietary protein, e.g., soy; (2) respond to glucocorticoids; (3) are "temporary," i.e., the clinical and morphologic findings disappear after several months or years; or (4) fail to respond to all measures and have a fatal outcome, with or without documented complications of celiac sprue, such as development of intestinal T cell lymphoma.

Mechanism of Diarrhea The diarrhea in celiac sprue has several pathogenetic mechanisms. Diarrhea may be secondary to (1) steatorrhea, which is primarily a result of the changes in jejunal mucosal function; (2) secondary lactase deficiency, a consequence of changes in jejunal brush border enzymatic function; (3) bile acid malabsorption resulting in bile acid–induced fluid secretion in the colon, in cases with more extensive disease involving the ileum; and (4) endogenous fluid secretion resulting from the crypt hyperplasia. Patients with more severe involvement with celiac sprue may obtain temporary improvement with *dietary lactose and fat restriction* while awaiting the full effects of total gluten restriction, which is primary therapy.

Associated Diseases Celiac sprue is associated with dermatitis herpetiformis (DH), though the association has not been explained. Patients with DH have characteristic papulovesicular lesions that respond to dapsone. Almost all patients with DH have histopathologic changes in the small intestine consistent with celiac sprue, although usually much milder and less diffuse in distribution. Most patients with DH have mild, or no, gastrointestinal symptoms. In contrast, relatively few patients with celiac sprue have DH.

Celiac sprue is also associated with diabetes mellitus type 1 and IgA deficiency. The clinical importance of the former association is that although severe watery diarrhea without evidence of malabsorption is most often seen in patients with "diabetic diarrhea" (Chap. 323), assay of antiendomysial antibodies and/or a small-intestinal biopsy must at times be considered to exclude this association.

Complications The most important complication of celiac sprue is the development of cancer. An increased incidence of both gastrointestinal and nongastrointestinal neoplasms as well as intestinal lymphoma exists in patients with celiac sprue. For unexplained reasons the occurrence of lymphoma in patients with celiac sprue is higher in Ireland and the United Kingdom than in the United States. The possibility of lymphoma must be considered whenever a patient with celiac sprue previously doing well on a gluten-free diet is no longer responsive to gluten restriction or a patient who presents with clinical and histopathologic features consistent with celiac sprue does not respond to a gluten-free diet. Other complications of celiac sprue include the development of intestinal ulceration independent of lymphoma and socalled refractory sprue (see above) and collagenous sprue. In *collagenous sprue*, a layer of collagen-like material is present beneath the basement membrane; patients with collagenous sprue generally do not respond to a gluten-free diet and often have a poor prognosis.

TROPICAL SPRUE Tropical sprue is a poorly understood syndrome that affects both expatriates and natives in certain but not all tropical areas and is manifested by chronic diarrhea, steatorrhea, weight loss, and nutritional deficiencies, including those of both folate and cobalamin. This disease affects 5 to 10% of the population in some tropical areas.

Chronic diarrhea in a tropical environment is most often caused by infectious agents including *G. lamblia*, *Yersinia enterocolitica*, *C. difficile*, *Cryptosporidium parvum*, and *Cyclospora cayetanensis*, among other organisms. Tropical sprue should not be entertained as a possible diagnosis until the presence of cysts and trophozoites has been excluded in three stool samples. →*Chronic infections of the gastrointestinal tract and diarrhea in patients with or without AIDS are discussed in Chaps. 113 and 173.*

The small-intestinal mucosa in individuals living in tropical areas is not identical to that of individuals who reside in temperate climates. Biopsies reveal a mild alteration of villus architecture with a modest increase in mononuclear cells in the lamina propria, which on occasion can be as severe as that seen in celiac sprue. These changes are observed both in native residents and in expatriates living in tropical regions and are usually associated with mild decreases in absorptive function, but revert to "normal" when an individual moves or returns to a temperate area. Some have suggested that the changes seen in tropical enteropathy and in tropical sprue represent different ends of the spectrum of a single entity, but convincing evidence to support this concept is lacking.

Etiology The etiology of tropical sprue is not known, though because tropical sprue responds to antibiotics, the consensus is that tropical sprue may be caused by one or more infectious agents. Nonetheless, there are multiple uncertainties regarding the etiology and pathogenesis of tropical sprue. First, its occurrence is not evenly distributed in all tropical areas; rather, it is found in specific locations including South India, the Philippines, and several Caribbean islands (e.g., Puerto Rico, Haiti) but is rarely observed in Africa, Jamaica, or Southeast Asia. Second, an occasional individual will not develop symptoms of tropical sprue until long after having left an endemic area. This is the reason why the original term for celiac sprue was *nontropical sprue* to distinguish it from tropical sprue. Third, multiple microorganisms have been identified on jejunal aspirate with relatively little consistency among studies. *Klebsiella pneumoniae*, *Enterobacter cloacae*, or *E. coli* have been implicated in some studies of tropical sprue, while other investigations have favored a role for a toxin produced by one or more of these bacteria. Fourth, the incidence of tropical sprue appears to have decreased substantially during the past decade. One speculation for this reduced occurrence of tropical sprue is the wider use of antibiotics in acute diarrhea, especially in travelers to tropical areas from temperate countries. Fifth, the role of folic acid deficiency in the pathogenesis of tropical sprue requires clarification. Folic acid is absorbed exclusively in the duodenum and proximal jejunum, and most patients with tropical sprue have evidence of folate malabsorption and depletion. Although folate deficiency can cause changes in small-intestinal mucosa that are corrected by folate replacement, the several earlier studies reporting that tropical sprue could be cured by folic acid did not provide an explanation for the "insult" that was initially responsible for folate malabsorption.

The clinical pattern of tropical sprue varies in different areas of the world (e.g., India vs Puerto Rico). Not infrequently, individuals in South India initially will report the occurrence of an acute enteritis before the development of steatorrhea and malabsorption. In contrast, in Puerto Rico, a most insidious onset of symptoms and a more dramatic response to antibiotics is seen when compared to some other locations. Tropical sprue in different areas of the world may not be the same disease; similar clinical entities may have different etiologies.

Diagnosis The diagnosis of tropical sprue is best made by the presence of an abnormal small-intestinal mucosal biopsy in an individual with chronic diarrhea and evidence of malabsorption who is either residing or has recently lived in a tropic country. The small-intestinal biopsy in tropical sprue does not have pathognomonic features but resembles, and can often be indistinguishable from, that seen in celiac sprue (Fig. 275-4). The biopsy in tropical sprue will have less villus architectural alteration and more mononuclear cell infiltrate in the lamina propria. In contrast to celiac sprue, the histopathologic features of tropical sprue are present with a similar degree of severity throughout the small intestine, and a gluten-free diet does not result in either clinical or histopathologic improvement in tropical sprue.

℞ TREATMENT

Broad-spectrum antibiotics and folic acid are most often curative, especially if the patient leaves the tropical area and does not return. Tetracycline should be used for up to 6 months and may be associated with improvement within 1 to 2 weeks. Folic acid alone will induce a hematologic remission as well as improvement in appetite, weight gain, and some morphologic changes in small intestinal biopsy. Because of the presence of marked folate deficiency, folic acid is most often given together with antibiotics.

SHORT BOWEL SYNDROME This is a descriptive term for the myriad clinical problems that often occur following resection of varying lengths of small intestine. The factors that determine both the type and degree of symptoms include (1) the specific segment (jejunum vs ileum) resected, (2) the length of the resected segment, (3) the integrity of the ileocecal valve, (4) whether any large intestine has also been removed, (5) residual disease in the remaining small and/or large intestine (e.g., Crohn's disease, mesenteric artery disease), and (6) the degree of adaptation in the remaining intestine. Short bowel syndrome can occur at any age from neonates through the elderly.

Three different situations in adults demand intestinal resections: (1) mesenteric vascular disease including atherosclerosis, thrombotic phenomena, and vasculitides; (2) primary mucosal and submucosal disease, e.g., Crohn's disease; and (3) operations without preexisting small intestinal disease, such as trauma and jejunoileal bypass for obesity.

Following resection of the small intestine, the residual intestine undergoes adaptation of both structure and function that may last for up to 6 to 12 months. Continued intake of dietary nutrients and calories is required to stimulate adaptation via direct contact with intestinal mucosa, the release of one or more intestinal hormones, and pancreatic and biliary secretions. Thus, enteral nutrition and calorie administration must be maintained, especially in the early postoperative period, even if an extensive intestinal resection requiring total parenteral nutrition (TPN) was performed. The subsequent ability of such patients to absorb nutrients will not be known for several months, until adaptation is completed.

Multiple factors besides the absence of intestinal mucosa (required

for lipid, fluid, and electrolyte absorption) contribute to the diarrhea and steatorrhea in these patients. Removal of the ileum and especially the ileocecal valve is often associated with more severe diarrhea than jejunal resection. Without part or all of the ileum, diarrhea can be caused by an increase in bile acids entering the colon, leading to their stimulation of colonic fluid and electrolyte secretion. Absence of the ileocecal valve is also associated with a decrease in intestinal transit time and bacterial overgrowth from the colon. Lactose intolerance as a result of the removal of lactase-containing mucosa as well as gastric hypersecretion will also contribute to the diarrhea.

In addition to diarrhea and/or steatorrhea, a range of nonintestinal symptoms is also observed in some patients. A significant increase in renal calcium oxalate calculi is observed in patients with a small-intestinal resection with an intact colon and is due to an increase in oxalate absorption by the large intestine, with subsequent hyperoxaluria (called *enteric hyperoxaluria*). Since oxalate is high in relatively few foods (e.g., spinach, rhubarb, tea), dietary restrictions alone are not adequate treatment. Cholestyramine, an anion-binding resin, and calcium have proved useful in reducing the hyperoxaluria. Similarly, an increase in cholesterol gallstones is related to a decrease in the bile acid pool size, which results in the generation of cholesterol supersaturation in gallbladder bile. Gastric hypersecretion of acid occurs in many patients following large resections of the small intestine. The etiology is unclear but may be related to either reduced hormonal inhibition of acid secretion or increased gastrin levels due to reduced small-intestinal catabolism of circulating gastrin. The resulting gastric acid secretion may be an important factor contributing to the diarrhea and steatorrhea. A reduced pH in the duodenum can inactivate pancreatic lipase and/or precipitate duodenal bile acids, thereby increasing steatorrhea, and an increase in gastric secretion can create a volume overload relative to the reduced small-intestinal absorptive capacity. Inhibition of gastric acid secretion with either proton pump inhibitors or H_2 receptor antagonists can help in reducing the diarrhea and steatorrhea.

℞ TREATMENT

Treatment of short bowel syndrome depends on the severity of symptoms and whether the individual is able to maintain caloric and electrolyte balance with oral intake alone. Initial treatment includes judicious use of opiates (including codeine) to reduce stool output and to establish an effective diet. An initial diet should be low-fat and high-carbohydrate to minimize the diarrhea from fatty acid stimulation of colonic fluid secretion. MCTs (see above), a low-lactose diet, and various fiber-containing diets should also be tried. In the absence of an ileocecal valve, the possibility of bacterial overgrowth must be considered and treated. If gastric acid hypersecretion is contributing to the diarrhea and steatorrhea, a proton pump inhibitor may be helpful. Usually none of these therapeutic approaches will provide an instant solution but they can reduce disabling diarrhea.

The patient's vitamin and mineral status must also be monitored; replacement therapy should be initiated if indicated. Fat-soluble vitamins, folate, cobalamin, calcium, iron, magnesium, and zinc are the most critical factors to monitor on a regular basis. If these approaches are not successful, home TPN is an established therapy that can be maintained for many years. Intestinal transplantation is becoming established as a possible approach for individuals with extensive intestinal resection who cannot be maintained without TPN.

BACTERIAL OVERGROWTH SYNDROME Bacterial overgrowth syndrome comprises a group of disorders with diarrhea, steatorrhea, and macrocytic anemia whose common feature is the proliferation of colon-type bacteria within the small intestine. This bacterial proliferation is due to stasis caused by impaired peristalsis (i.e., *functional stasis*), changes in intestinal anatomy (i.e., *anatomic stasis*), or direct communication between the small and large intestine. These conditions have also been referred to as *stagnant bowel syndrome* or *blind loop syndrome*.

Pathogenesis   The manifestations of bacterial overgrowth syndromes are a direct consequence of the presence of increased amounts of a colonic-type bacterial flora, such as *E. coli* or *Bacteroides*, in the small intestine. *Macrocytic anemia* is due to cobalamin, not folate, deficiency. Most bacteria require cobalamin for growth, and increasing concentrations of bacteria use up the relatively small amounts of dietary cobalamin. *Steatorrhea* is due to impaired micelle formation as a consequence of a reduced intraduodenal concentration of conjugated bile acids and the presence of unconjugated bile acids. Certain bacteria, e.g., *Bacteroides*, deconjugate conjugated bile acids to unconjugated bile acids. In the presence of bacterial overgrowth, unconjugated bile acids will be absorbed more rapidly than conjugated bile acids, and, as a result, the intraduodenal concentration of bile acids will be reduced. In addition, the CMC of unconjugated bile acids is higher than that of conjugated bile acids, resulting in a decrease in micelle formation. *Diarrhea* is due, at least in part, to the steatorrhea, when it is present. However, some patients manifest diarrhea *without* steatorrhea, and it is assumed that the colonic-type bacteria in these patients are producing one or more bacterial enterotoxins that are responsible for fluid secretion and diarrhea.

Etiology   The etiology of these different disorders is bacterial proliferation in the small intestinal lumen secondary to either anatomical or functional stasis or to a communication between the relatively sterile small intestine and the colon with its high levels of aerobic and anaerobic bacteria. Several examples of anatomical stasis have been identified: (1) one or more diverticula (both duodenal and jejunal) (Fig. 275-3*C*); (2) fistulas and strictures related to Crohn's disease (Fig. 275-3*D*); (3) a proximal duodenal afferent loop following a subtotal gastrectomy and gastrojejunostomy; (4) a bypass of the intestine, e.g., jejunoileal bypass for obesity; and (5) dilation at the site of a previous intestinal anastomosis. These anatomical derangements are often associated with the presence of a segment (or segments) of intestine out of continuity of propagated peristalsis, resulting in stasis and bacterial proliferation. Bacterial overgrowth syndromes can also occur in the absence of an anatomical blind loop when functional stasis is present. Impaired peristalsis and bacterial overgrowth in the absence of a blind loop occur in scleroderma, where motility abnormalities exist in both the esophagus and small intestine (Chap. 303), and in small-intestinal stricture associated with either Crohn's disease or an intestinal anastomosis. Functional stasis and bacterial overgrowth can also occur in association with diabetes mellitus and in the small intestine when a direct connection exists between the small and large intestine, including an ileocolonic resection, or occasionally following an enterocolic anastomosis that permits entry of bacteria into the small intestine as a result of bypassing the ileocecal valve.

Diagnosis   The diagnosis may be suspected from the combination of a low serum cobalamin level and an elevated serum folate level as enteric bacteria frequently produce folate compounds that will be absorbed in the duodenum. Ideally, the diagnosis of the bacterial overgrowth syndrome is the demonstration of increased levels of aerobic and/or anaerobic colonic-type bacteria in a jejunal aspirate obtained by intubation. This specialized test is rarely available, and bacterial overgrowth is best established by a Schilling test (Table 275-6), which should be abnormal following the administration of ^{58}Co-labeled cobalamin, with or without the administration of intrinsic factor. Following the administration of tetracycline for 5 days, the Schilling test will become normal, confirming the diagnosis of bacterial overgrowth. Breath hydrogen testing following lactose administration has also been used to detect bacterial overgrowth.

℞ TREATMENT

Primary treatment should be directed, if at all possible, to the surgical correction of an anatomical blind loop. In the absence of functional stasis, it is important to define the anatomical relationships responsible for stasis and bacterial overgrowth. For example, bacterial overgrowth

secondary to strictures, one or more diverticula, or a proximal afferent loop can potentially be cured by surgical correction of the anatomical state. In contrast, the functional stasis of scleroderma or certain anatomical stasis states (e.g., multiple jejunal diverticula), cannot be corrected surgically, and these conditions should be treated with broad-spectrum antibiotics. Tetracycline used to be the initial treatment of choice but, due to increasing resistance, other antibiotics such as metronidazole, amoxicillin/clavulanic acid, and cephalosporins have been employed. The antibiotic should be given for approximately 3 weeks or until symptoms remit. Since the natural history of these conditions is chronic, antibiotics should not be given continuously, and symptoms usually remit within 2 to 3 weeks of initial antibiotic therapy. Therapy need not be repeated until symptoms recur. In the presence of frequent recurrences several treatment strategies exist, but the use of antibiotics for 1 week per month whether or not symptoms are present is often most effective.

Unfortunately, therapy for bacterial overgrowth syndrome is largely empirical, with an absence of clinical trials on which to base decisions regarding the antibiotic to be used, the duration of treatment, and/or the best approach for treating recurrences. Bacterial overgrowth may also occur as a component of another chronic disease, e.g., Crohn's disease, radiation enteritis, or short bowel syndrome. Treatment of the bacterial overgrowth in these settings will not cure the underlying problem but may be very important in ameliorating a subset of clinical problems that are related to bacterial overgrowth.

WHIPPLE'S DISEASE   Whipple's disease is a chronic multisystem disease associated with diarrhea, steatorrhea, weight loss, arthralgia, and central nervous system and cardiac problems; it is caused by the bacteria *Tropheryma whipplei*. Until the identification of *T. whipplei* by polymerase chain reaction, the hallmark of Whipple's disease had been the presence of PAS-positive macrophages in the small intestine (Fig. 275-4*E*) and other organs with evidence of disease.

Long before the establishment of *T. whipplei* as the causative agent of Whipple's disease, gram-positive bacilli had been identified both within and outside of macrophages.

Etiology   Whipple's disease is caused by a small gram-positive bacillus, *T. whipplei*. The bacillus, an actinobacterium, has low virulence but high infectivity, and relatively minimal symptoms are observed compared to the extent of the bacilli in multiple tissues.

Clinical Presentation   The onset of Whipple's disease is insidious and is characterized by diarrhea, steatorrhea, abdominal pain, weight loss, migratory large-joint arthropathy, and fever as well as ophthalmologic and central nervous system symptoms. The development of dementia is a relatively late symptom and is an extremely poor prognostic sign, especially in patients who relapse following the induction of a remission with antibiotics. For unexplained reasons, the disease occurs primarily in middle-aged Caucasian men. The steatorrhea in these patients is generally believed secondary to both small-intestinal mucosal injury and lymphatic obstruction secondary to the increased number of PAS-positive macrophages in the lamina propria of the small intestine.

Diagnosis   The diagnosis of Whipple's disease is suggested by a multisystem disease in a man with diarrhea and steatorrhea. Obtaining tissue biopsies from the small intestine and/or other organs that may be involved (e.g., liver, lymph nodes, heart, eyes, central nervous system, or synovial membranes), based on the patient's symptoms, is the primary approach to establish the diagnosis of Whipple's disease. The presence of PAS-positive macrophages containing the characteristic small (0.25 × 1 to 2 mm) bacilli is suggestive of this diagnosis. However, Whipple's disease can be confused with the PAS-positive macrophages containing *M. avium* complex, which may be a cause of diarrhea in AIDS. The presence of the *T. whipplei* bacillus outside of macrophages is a more important indicator of active disease than is their presence within the macrophages. *T. whipplei* has now been successfully grown in culture.

TABLE 275-9 *Classification of Malabsorption Syndromes*

Inadequate digestion
  Postgastrectomy[a]
  Deficiency or inactivation of pancreatic lipase
    Exocrine pancreatic insufficiency
      Chronic pancreatitis
      Pancreatic carcinoma
      Cystic fibrosis
      Pancreatic insufficiency—congenital or acquired
    Gastrinoma—acid inactivation of lipase[a]
    Drugs—orlistat
Reduced intraduodenal bile acid concentration/impaired micelle
  formation
  Liver disease
    Parenchymal liver disease
    Cholestatic liver disease
  Bacterial overgrowth in small intestine:

Anatomic stasis	Functional stasis
Afferent loop stasis/blind	Diabetes[a]
loop/strictures/fistulae	Scleroderma[a]
	Intestinal pseudoobstruction

  Interrupted enterohepatic circulation of bile salts
    Ileal resection
    Crohn's disease[a]
  Drugs (bind or precipitate bile salts)—neomycin, cholestyramine,
    calcium carbonate
Impaired mucosal absorption/mucosal loss or defect
  Intestinal resection or bypass[a]
  Inflammation, infiltration, or infection:

Crohn's disease[a]	Celiac sprue
Amyloidosis	Collagenous sprue
Scleroderma[a]	Whipple's disease[a]
Lymphoma[a]	Radiation enteritis[a]
Eosinophilic enteritis	Folate and vitamin B_{12} deficiency
Mastocytosis	Infections—giardiasis
Tropical sprue	Graft-vs.-host disease

  Genetic disorders
    Disaccharidase deficiency
    Agammaglobulinemia
    Abetalipoproteinemia
    Hartnup disease
    Cystinuria
Impaired nutrient delivery to and/or from intestine:

Lymphatic obstruction	Circulatory disorders
Lymphoma[a]	Congestive heart failure
Lymphangiectasia	Constrictive pericarditis
	Mesenteric artery atherosclerosis
	Vasculitis

Endocrine and metabolic disorders
  Diabetes[a]
  Hypoparathyroidism
  Adrenal insufficiency
  Hyperthyroidism
  Carcinoid syndrome

[a] Malabsorption caused by more than one mechanism.

℞ TREATMENT

The treatment for Whipple's disease is prolonged use of antibiotics. The current drug of choice is double-strength trimethoprim/sulfamethoxazole for approximately 1 year. PAS-positive macrophages can persist following successful treatment, and the presence of bacilli outside of macrophages is indicative of persistent infection or an early sign of recurrence. Recurrence of disease activity, especially with dementia, is an extremely poor prognostic sign and requires an antibiotic that crosses the blood-brain barrier. If trimethoprim/sulfamethoxazole is not tolerated, chloramphenicol is an appropriate second choice.

PROTEIN-LOSING ENTEROPATHY Protein-losing enteropathy is not a specific disease but rather describes a group of gastrointestinal and nongastrointestinal disorders with hypoproteinemia and edema in the absence of either proteinuria or defects in protein synthesis, e.g., chronic liver disease. These diseases are characterized by excess protein loss into the gastrointestinal tract. Normally, about 10% of the total protein catabolism occurs via the gastrointestinal tract. Evidence of increased protein loss into the gastrointestinal tract has been established in more than 65 different diseases, which can be classified into three primary groups: (1) mucosal ulceration such that the protein loss primarily represents exudation across damaged mucosa, e.g., ulcerative colitis, gastrointestinal carcinomas, and peptic ulcer; (2) nonulcerated mucosa but with evidence of mucosal damage so that the protein loss represents loss across epithelia with altered permeability, e.g., celiac sprue and Ménétrier's disease in the small intestine and stomach, respectively; and (3) lymphatic dysfunction, either representing primary lymphatic disease or secondary to partial lymphatic obstruction that may occur as a result of enlarged lymph nodes or cardiac disease.

Diagnosis The diagnosis of protein-losing enteropathy is suggested by the presence of peripheral edema and low serum albumin and globulin levels in the absence of renal and hepatic disease. It is extremely rare for an individual with protein-losing enteropathy to have selective loss of *only* albumin or *only* globulins. Therefore, marked reduction of serum albumin with normal serum globulins should not initiate an evaluation for protein-losing enteropathy but should suggest the presence of renal and/or hepatic disease. Likewise, reduced serum globulins with normal serum albumin levels are more likely a result of reduced globulin synthesis rather than enhanced globulin loss into the intestine. Documentation of an increase in protein loss into the gastrointestinal tract has been established by the administration of one of several radiolabeled proteins and its quantitation in stool during a 24- or 48-h period. Unfortunately, none of these radiolabeled proteins is available for routine clinical use. α_1 Antitrypsin, a protein that amounts to approximately 4% of total serum proteins and is resistant to proteolysis, can be used to document enhanced rates of serum protein loss into the intestinal tract but cannot be used to assess gastric protein loss due to its degradation in an acid milieu. α_1 Antitrypsin clearance is measured by determining stool volume and both stool and plasma α_1 antitrypsin concentrations. In addition to the loss of protein via abnormal and distended lymphatics, peripheral lymphocytes may also be lost via lymphatics, resulting in a relative lymphopenia. Thus, the pres-

TABLE 275-10 *Pathophysiology of Clinical Manifestations of Malabsorption Disorders*

Symptom or Sign	Mechanism
Weight loss/malnutrition	Anorexia, malabsorption of nutrients
Diarrhea	Impaired absorption or secretion of water and electrolytes; colonic fluid secretion secondary to unabsorbed dihydroxy bile acids and fatty acids
Flatus	Bacterial fermentation of unabsorbed carbohydrate
Glossitis, cheilosis, stomatitis	Deficiency of iron, vitamin B_{12}, folate, and vitamin A
Abdominal pain	Bowel distention or inflammation, pancreatitis
Bone pain	Calcium, vitamin D malabsorption, protein deficiency, osteoporosis
Tetany, paresthesia	Calcium and magnesium malabsorption
Weakness	Anemia, electrolyte depletion (particularly K^+)
Azotemia, hypotension	Fluid and electrolyte depletion
Amenorrhea, decreased libido	Protein depletion, decreased calories, secondary hypopituitarism
Anemia	Impaired absorption of iron, folate, vitamin B_{12}
Bleeding	Vitamin K malabsorption, hypoprothrombinemia
Night blindness/ xerophthalmia	Vitamin A malabsorption
Peripheral neuropathy	Vitamin B_{12} and thiamine deficiency
Dermatitis	Deficiency of vitamin A, zinc, and essential fatty acid

ence of lymphopenia in a patient with hypoproteinemia supports the presence of increased loss of protein into the gastrointestinal tract.

Patients with increased protein loss into the gastrointestinal tract from lymphatic obstruction often have steatorrhea and diarrhea. The steatorrhea is a result of altered lymphatic flow as lipid-containing chylomicrons exit from intestinal epithelial cells via intestinal lymphatics (Table 275-4; Fig. 275-4). In the absence of mechanical or anatomical lymphatic obstruction, intrinsic intestinal lymphatic dysfunction, with or without lymphatic dysfunction in the peripheral extremities, has been named *intestinal lymphangiectasia*. Similarly, about 50% of individuals with intrinsic peripheral lymphatic disease (Milroy disease) will also have intestinal lymphangiectasia and hypoproteinemia. Other than steatorrhea and enhanced protein loss into the gastrointestinal tract, all other aspects of intestinal absorptive function are normal in intestinal lymphangiectasia.

Other Causes Patients who appear to have idiopathic protein-losing enteropathy without any evidence of gastrointestinal disease should be examined for cardiac disease—especially right-sided valvular disease and chronic pericarditis (Chaps. 219 and 222). On occasion, hypoproteinemia can be the only presentation for these two types of heart disease. Ménétrier's disease (also called *hypertrophic gastropathy*) is an uncommon entity that involves the body and fundus of the stomach and is characterized by large gastric folds, reduced gastric acid secretion, and, at times, enhanced protein loss into the stomach.

℞ TREATMENT

As excess protein loss into the gastrointestinal tract is most often secondary to a specific disease, treatment should be directed primarily to the underlying disease process and not to the hypoproteinemia. For example, if significant hypoproteinemia with resulting peripheral edema is present secondary to either celiac sprue or ulcerative colitis, a gluten-free diet or mesalamine, respectively, would be the initial

therapy. When enhanced protein loss is secondary to lymphatic obstruction, it is critical to establish the nature of this obstruction. Identification of mesenteric nodes or lymphoma may be possible by imaging studies. Similarly, it is important to exclude cardiac disease as a cause of protein-losing enteropathy either by echosonography or, on occasion, by a right-heart catheterization.

The increased protein loss that occurs in intestinal lymphangiectasia is a result of distended lymphatics associated with lipid malabsorption. Treatment of the hypoproteinemia is accomplished by a low-fat diet and the administration of MCTs (Table 275-3), which do not exit from the intestinal epithelial cells via lymphatics but are delivered to the body via the portal vein.

SUMMARY

A pathophysiologic classification of the many conditions that can produce malabsorption is given in Table 275-9. A summary of the pathophysiology of the various clinical manifestations of malabsorption is given in Table 275-10.

FURTHER READING

AMERICAN GASTROENTEROLOGICAL ASSOCIATION: AGA technical review on the evaluation and management of chronic diarrhea. Gastroenterology 116:1464, 1999

COOK SI, SELLIN JH: Short chain fatty acids in health and disease. Aliment Pharmacol Ther 12:499, 1998

CRAIG RM, EHRENPREIS ED: D-Xylose testing. J Clin Gastroenterol 29:143, 1999

FENOLLAR F, RAOULT D: Whipple's disease. Curr Gastroenterol Rep 5:379, 2003

GREEN PH, JABRI B: Coeliac disease. Lancet 362:383, 2003

GREENBERGER NJ: Enzymatic therapy in patients with chronic pancreatitis. Gastroenterol Clin North Am 28:687, 1999

HAREWOOD GC, MURRAY JA: Approaching the patient with chronic malabsorption syndrome. Semin Gastrointest Dis 10:138, 1999

SHAW AD, DAVIES GJ: Lactose intolerance: Problems in diagnosis and treatment. J Clin Gastroenterol 28:208, 1999

276 INFLAMMATORY BOWEL DISEASE
Sonia Friedman, Richard S. Blumberg

Inflammatory bowel disease (IBD) is an idiopathic and chronic intestinal inflammation. Ulcerative colitis (UC) and Crohn's disease (CD) are the two major types of IBD.

EPIDEMIOLOGY

The incidence of IBD varies within different geographic areas. Northern countries, such as the United States, United Kingdom, Norway, and Sweden, have the highest rates. The incidence rates of UC and CD in the United States are about 11 per 100,000 and 7 per 100,000, respectively (Table 276-1). Countries in southern Europe, South Africa, and Australia have lower incidence rates: 2 to 6.3 per 100,000 for UC, and 0.9 to 3.1 per 100,000 for CD. In Asia and South America, IBD is rare; incidence rates of UC and CD are 0.5 and 0.08 per 100,000, respectively. The highest mortality in IBD patients is during the first years of disease and in long-duration disease due to the risk of colon cancer. In a Swedish population study, the standardized mortality ratios for CD and UC were 1.51 and 1.37, respectively.

The peak age of onset of UC and CD is between 15 and 30 years. A second peak occurs between the ages of 60 and 80. The male to female ratio for UC is 1:1 and for CD is 1.1 to 1.8:1. A two- to fourfold increased frequency of UC and CD in Jewish populations has been described in the United States, Europe, and South Africa. Furthermore, disease frequency differs within the Jewish populations. The prevalence of IBD in Ashkenazi Jews is about twice that of Israeli-born, Sephardic, or Oriental Jews. The prevalence decreases progressively

TABLE 276-1 *Epidemiology of IBD*

	Ulcerative Colitis	Crohn's Disease
Incidence (U.S.)	11/100,000	7/100,000
Age of onset	15–30 & 60–80	15–30 & 60–80
Ethnicity	Jewish > Non-Jewish Caucasian > African American > Hispanic > Asian	
Male:female ratio	1:1	1.1–1.8:1
Smoking	May prevent disease	May cause disease
Oral contraceptives	No increased risk	Relative risk 1.9
Appendectomy	Protective	Not protective
Monozygotic twins	20% concordance	67% concordance
Dizygotic twins	0% concordance	8% concordance

in non-Jewish Caucasian, African-American, Hispanic, and Asian populations. Urban areas have a higher prevalence of IBD than rural areas, and high socioeconomic classes have a higher prevalence than lower socioeconomic classes.

The effects of cigarette smoking are different in UC and CD. The risk of UC in smokers is 40% that of nonsmokers. Additionally, former smokers have a 1.7-fold increased risk for UC than people who have never smoked. In contrast, smoking is associated with a twofold increased risk of CD. Oral contraceptives are also linked to CD; the relative risk of CD for oral contraceptive users is about 1.9. Appendectomy appears to be protective against UC, but no studies have applied this as a preventive intervention.

IBD runs in families. If a patient has IBD, the lifetime risk that a first-degree relative will be affected is ~10%. If two parents have IBD, each child has a 36% chance of being affected. In twin studies, 67% of monozygotic twins are concordant for CD and 20% are concordant for UC, whereas 8% of dizygotic twins are concordant for CD and none are concordant for UC. Anatomic site and clinical type of CD is also concordant within families.

Additional evidence for genetic predisposition to IBD comes from its association with certain genetic syndromes. UC and CD are both associated with Turner's syndrome, and Hermansky-Pudlak syndrome is associated with a granulomatous colitis. Glycogen storage disease type 1b can present with Crohn's-like lesions of the large and small bowel. Other immunodeficiency disorders, such as hypogammaglobulinemia, selective IgA deficiency, and hereditary angioedema, also exhibit an increased association with IBD.

ETIOLOGY AND PATHOGENESIS

Although IBD has been described as a clinical entity for over 100 years, its etiology and pathogenesis have not been defined. A consensus hypothesis is that in genetically predisposed individuals, both exogenous factors (e.g., infectious agents, normal lumenal flora) and host factors (e.g., intestinal epithelial cell barrier function, vascular supply, neuronal activity) cause a chronic state of dysregulated mucosal immune function that is further modified by specific environmental factors (e.g., smoking). Although it is possible that the chronic activation of the mucosal immune system may represent an appropriate response to an unidentified infectious agent, a search for such an agent has thus far been unrewarding. As such, IBD is currently considered an inappropriate response to either the endogenous microbial flora within the intestine, with or without some component of autoimmunity. Importantly, the normal intestine contains a large number of immune cells in a chronic state of so-called physiologic inflammation, in which the gut is poised for, but actively restrained from, full immunologic responses. During the course of infections in the normal host, full activation of the gut-associated lymphoid tissue occurs but is rapidly superceded by dampening the immune response and tissue repair. In IBD this process is not regulated normally.

GENETIC CONSIDERATIONS IBD is a polygenic disorder that gives rise to multiple clinical subgroups within UC and CD. Genome-wide searches have shown potential disease-associated loci on chromosomes 16, 12, 7, 5, 3, and 1, although the specific gene associations are mostly undefined. The disease-related gene on chromosome 16 is *NOD-2*, an intracellular molecule that senses bacterial peptidoglycan and regulates NF-κB signaling. Homozygosity for mutant alleles confers up to a 40-fold increased risk for fibrostenosing CD, especially in the ileum. HLA alleles may also play a role. UC patients disproportionately express DR2-related alleles, whereas in CD an increased use of the DR5 DQ1 haplotype or the DRB*0301 allele has been described. In UC patients with pancolitis undergoing total proctocolectomy, 14.3% versus 3.2% of non-IBD controls express the HLA DRB1*0103 allele. This allele is associated with extensive disease and extraintestinal manifestations such as mouth ulcers, arthritis, and uveitis. Other associations with immunoregulatory genes include the intercellular adhesion molecule R241 allele in UC and CD and the interleukin (IL) 1 receptor antagonist allele 2 in UC patients that is associated with total colonic inflammation. Patients with IBD and their first-degree relatives may also exhibit diminished intestinal epithelial cell barrier function.

DEFECTIVE IMMUNE REGULATION IN IBD The normal state of the mucosal immune system is one of inhibited immune responses to lumenal contents due to oral tolerance that occurs in the normal individual. When soluble antigens are administered orally rather than subcutaneously or intramuscularly, antigen-specific non-responsiveness is induced. Multiple mechanisms are involved in the induction of oral tolerance and include deletion or anergy of antigen-reactive T cells or activation of CD4+ T cells that suppress gut inflammation through secretion of inhibitory cytokines, such as IL-10 and transforming growth factor β (TGF-β). Oral tolerance may be responsible for the lack of immune responsiveness to dietary antigens and the commensal flora in the in-

testinal lumen. In IBD this suppression of inflammation is altered, leading to uncontrolled inflammation. The mechanisms that maintain this regulated immune suppression are unknown.

Gene knockout (-/-) or transgenic (Tg) mouse models of colitis have revealed that deleting specific cytokines (e.g., IL-2, IL-10, TGF-β) or their receptors, deleting molecules associated with T cell antigen recognition (e.g., T cell antigen receptors, MHC class II), or interfering with intestinal epithelial cell barrier function (e.g., blocking N-cadherin, deleting multidrug resistance gene 1a or trefoil factor) leads to colitis. Thus, a variety of specific alterations can lead to autoimmunity directed at the colon in mice.

In both UC and CD, activated CD4+ T cells in the lamina propria and peripheral blood secrete inflammatory cytokines. Some activate other inflammatory cells (macrophages and B cells) and others act indirectly to recruit other lymphocytes, inflammatory leukocytes, and mononuclear cells from the peripheral vasculature into the gut through interactions between homing receptors on leukocytes (e.g., $\alpha 4\beta 7$ integrin) and addressins on vascular endothelium (e.g., MadCAM1). CD4+ T cells are of two major types, both of which may be associated with colitis in animal models and humans: $T_H 1$ cells [interferon (IFN) γ, tumor necrosis factor (TNF)] and $T_H 2$ cells (IL-4, IL-5, IL-13). $T_H 1$ cells appear to induce transmural granulomatous inflammation that resembles CD, and $T_H 2$ cells appear to induce superficial mucosal inflammation resembling UC. The $T_H 1$ cytokine pathway is initiated by IL-12, a key cytokine in the pathogenesis of experimental models of mucosal inflammation. Thus, use of antibodies to block proinflammatory cytokines (e.g., anti-TNF-α, anti-IL-12) or molecules associated with leukocyte recruitment (e.g., anti-$\alpha 4\beta 7$) or use of cytokines that inhibit inflammation (e.g., IL-10) or promote intestinal barrier function (e.g., IL-11) may be beneficial to humans with colitis.

THE INFLAMMATORY CASCADE IN IBD Once initiated in IBD, the immune inflammatory response is perpetuated as a consequence of T cell activation. A sequential cascade of inflammatory mediators acts to extend the response; each step is a potential target for therapy. Inflammatory cytokines, such as IL-1, IL-6, and TNF, have diverse effects on tissue. They promote fibrogenesis, collagen production, activation of tissue metalloproteinases, and the production of other inflammatory mediators; they also activate the coagulation cascade in local blood vessels (e.g., increased production of von Willebrand's factor). These cytokines are normally produced in response to infection, but are usually turned off or inhibited at the appropriate time to limit tissue damage. In IBD their activity is not regulated, resulting in an imbalance between the proinflammatory and anti-inflammatory mediators. Therapies such as the 5-ASA (5-aminosalicylic acid) compounds are potent inhibitors of these inflammatory mediators through inhibition of transcription factors such as NF-κB that regulate their expression.

EXOGENOUS FACTORS IBD may have an as yet undefined infectious etiology. Three specific agents have received the greatest attention, *Mycobacterium paratuberculosis*, Paramyxovirus, and *Helicobacter* species. The immune response to a specific organism could be expressed differently, depending upon the individual's genetic background. *M. paratuberculosis* does not have a confirmed disease association, and antimycobacterial agents are not effective in treating CD. A role for the measles virus or paramyxoviruses in the development of CD has been suggested based on an increase in the incidence of CD in England that paralleled use of the measles vaccine. However, studies in the United States have not substantiated this finding. In an animal model of IBD, *H. hepaticus* has been implicated as a trigger for the inflammatory response; evidence in humans is lacking.

Multiple pathogens (e.g., *Salmonella, Shigella* sp., *Campylobacter* sp.) may initiate IBD by triggering an inflammatory response that the mucosal immune system may fail to control. However, in an IBD patient the normal flora is likely perceived as if it were a pathogen. Anaerobic organisms, particularly *Bacteroides* species, may be responsible for the induction of inflammation. Such a notion is supported by the response in patients with CD to agents that alter the intestinal flora, such as metronidazole, ciprofloxacin, and elemental diets. CD also responds to fecal diversion, demonstrating the ability of lumenal contents to exacerbate disease. On the other hand, other bacteria, so-called probiotics (*Lactobacillus* sp.), inhibit inflammation in animal models and humans.

Psychosocial factors can contribute to worsening of symptoms. Major life events such as illness or death in the family, divorce or separation, interpersonal conflict, or other major loss are associated with an increase in IBD symptoms such as pain, bowel dysfunction, and bleeding. Acute daily stress can worsen bowel symptoms even after controlling for major life events. When the sickness-impact profile, a measurement of overall psychological and physical functioning, is used, IBD patients have functional impairment greater than that of a normal population but less than that of patients with chronic back pain or amyotrophic lateral sclerosis. IBD patients have been hypothesized to have a characteristic personality that renders them susceptible to emotional stresses. However, emotional dysfunction could also be the result of chronic illness rather than a cause.

PATHOLOGY

ULCERATIVE COLITIS: MACROSCOPIC FEATURES   UC is a mucosal disease that usually involves the rectum and extends proximally to involve all or part of the colon. About 40 to 50% of patients have disease limited to the rectum and rectosigmoid, 30 to 40% have disease extending beyond the sigmoid but not involving the whole colon, and 20% have a total colitis. Proximal spread occurs in continuity without areas of uninvolved mucosa. When the whole colon is involved, the inflammation extends 1 to 2 cm into the terminal ileum in 10 to 20% of patients. This is called *backwash ileitis* and is of little clinical significance. Although variations in macroscopic activity may suggest skip areas, biopsies from normal-appearing mucosa are usually abnormal. Thus, it is important to obtain multiple biopsies from apparently uninvolved mucosa, whether proximal or distal, during endoscopy.

With mild inflammation, the mucosa is erythematous and has a fine granular surface that looks like sandpaper. In more severe disease, the mucosa is hemorrhagic, edematous, and ulcerated (Fig. 276-1). In long-standing disease, inflammatory polyps (pseudopolyps) may be present as a result of epithelial regeneration. The mucosa may appear normal in remission, but in patients with many years of disease it appears atrophic and featureless and the entire colon becomes narrowed and shortened. Patients with fulminant disease can develop a toxic colitis or megacolon where the bowel wall thins and the mucosa is severely ulcerated; this may lead to perforation.

FIGURE 276-1   Pan-ulcerative colitis. Mucosa has a lumpy, bumpy appearance because of areas of inflamed but intact mucosa separated by ulcerated areas. (*Courtesy of Dr. EK Rosado and Dr. CA Perkos, Division of Gastrointestinal Pathology, Department of Pathology, Emory University, Atlanta, Georgia.*)

FIGURE 276-2   Characteristic findings of IBD in a case of ulcerative colitis: crypt distortion, cryptitis, and crypt abscess. (*Courtesy of Dr. EK Rosado and Dr. CA Perkos, Division of Gastrointestinal Pathology, Department of Pathology, Emory University, Atlanta, Georgia.*)

ULCERATIVE COLITIS: MICROSCOPIC FEATURES   Histologic findings correlate well with the endoscopic appearance and clinical course of UC. The process is limited to the mucosa and superficial submucosa, with deeper layers unaffected except in fulminant disease. In UC, two major histologic features are indicative of chronicity and help distinguish it from infectious or acute self-limited colitis. First, the crypt architecture of the colon is distorted; crypts may be bifid and reduced in number, often with a gap between the crypt bases and the muscularis mucosae. Second, some patients have basal plasma cells and multiple basal lymphoid aggregates. Mucosal vascular congestion with edema and focal hemorrhage, and an inflammatory cell infiltrate of neutrophils, lymphocytes, plasma cells, and macrophages may be present. The neutrophils invade the epithelium, usually in the crypts, and give rise to cryptitis and, ultimately, to crypt abscesses (Fig. 276-2).

CROHN'S DISEASE: MACROSCOPIC FEATURES   CD can affect any part of the gastrointestinal tract from the mouth to the anus. Some 30 to 40% of patients have small-bowel disease alone, 40 to 55% have disease involving both the small and large intestines, and 15 to 25% have colitis alone. In the 75% of patients with small-intestinal disease, the terminal ileum is involved in 90%. Unlike UC, which almost always involves the rectum, the rectum is often spared in CD. CD is segmental, with skip areas in the midst of diseased intestine (Fig. 276-3). Perirectal fistulas, fissures, abscesses, and anal stenosis are present in one-third

FIGURE 276-3   Portion of colon with stricture in patient with CD. (*Courtesy of Dr. EK Rosado and Dr. CA Perkos, Division of Gastrointestinal Pathology, Department of Pathology, Emory University, Atlanta, Georgia.*)

of patients with CD, particularly those with colonic involvement. CD may also involve the liver and the pancreas.

Unlike UC, CD is a transmural process. Endoscopically, aphthous or small superficial ulcerations characterize mild disease; in more active disease, stellate ulcerations fuse longitudinally and transversely to demarcate islands of mucosa that frequently are histologically normal. This "cobblestone" appearance is characteristic of CD, both endoscopically and by barium radiography. As in UC, pseudopolyps can form in CD.

Active CD is characterized by focal inflammation and formation of fistula tracts, which resolve by fibrosis and stricturing of the bowel. The bowel wall thickens and becomes narrowed and fibrotic, leading to chronic, recurrent bowel obstructions. Projections of thickened mesentery encase the bowel ("creeping fat"), and serosal and mesenteric inflammation promote adhesions and fistula formation.

CROHN'S DISEASE: MICROSCOPIC FEATURES The earliest lesions are aphthoid ulcerations and focal crypt abscesses with loose aggregations of macrophages, which form noncaseating granulomas in all layers of the bowel wall from mucosa to serosa (Fig. 276-4). Granulomas can be seen in lymph nodes, mesentery, peritoneum, liver, and pancreas. Although granulomas are a pathognomonic feature of CD, they are rarely found on mucosal biopsies. Surgical resection reveals granulomas in about half of cases. Other histologic features of CD include submucosal or subserosal lymphoid aggregates, particularly away from areas of ulceration, gross and microscopic skip areas, and transmural inflammation that is accompanied by fissures that penetrate deeply into the bowel wall and sometimes form fistulous tracts or local abscesses.

CLINICAL PRESENTATION

ULCERATIVE COLITIS ■ Signs and Symptoms The major symptoms of UC are diarrhea, rectal bleeding, tenesmus, passage of mucus, and crampy abdominal pain. The severity of symptoms correlates with the extent of disease. Although UC can present acutely, symptoms usually have been present for weeks to months. Occasionally, diarrhea and bleeding are so intermittent and mild that the patient does not seek medical attention.

Patients with proctitis usually pass fresh blood or blood-stained mucus, either mixed with stool or streaked onto the surface of a normal or hard stool. They also have tenesmus, or urgency with a feeling of incomplete evacuation. They rarely have abdominal pain. With proctitis or proctosigmoiditis, proximal transit slows, which may account

FIGURE 276-4 Granulomas (*arrow*) in bowel wall and serosa of colon, CD. (*Courtesy of Dr. EK Rosado and Dr. CA Perkos, Division of Gastrointestinal Pathology, Department of Pathology, Emory University, Atlanta, Georgia.*)

TABLE 276-2 *Ulcerative Colitis: Disease Presentation*

	Mild	Moderate	Severe
Bowel movements	<4 per day	4–6 per day	>6 per day
Blood in stool	Small	Moderate	Severe
Fever	None	<37.5°C mean	>37.5°C mean
Tachycardia	None	<90 mean pulse	>90 mean pulse
Anemia	Mild	>75%	≤75%
Sedimentation rate	<30 mm		>30 mm
Endoscopic appearance	Erythema, decreased vascular pattern, fine granularity	Marked erythema, coarse granularity, absent vascular markings, contact bleeding, no ulcerations	Spontaneous bleeding, ulcerations

for the constipation that is commonly seen in patients with distal disease.

When the disease extends beyond the rectum, blood is usually mixed with stool or grossly bloody diarrhea may be noted. Colonic motility is altered by inflammation with rapid transit through the inflamed intestine. When the disease is severe, patients pass a liquid stool containing blood, pus, and fecal matter. Diarrhea is often nocturnal and/or postprandial. Although severe pain is not a prominent symptom, some patients with active disease may experience vague lower abdominal discomfort or mild central abdominal cramping. Severe cramping and abdominal pain can occur in association with severe attacks of the disease. Other symptoms in moderate to severe disease include anorexia, nausea, vomiting, fever, and weight loss.

Physical signs of proctitis include a tender anal canal and blood on rectal examination. With more extensive disease, patients have tenderness to palpation directly over the colon. Patients with a toxic colitis have severe pain and bleeding, and those with megacolon have hepatic tympany. Both may have signs of peritonitis if a perforation has occurred. The classification of disease activity is shown in Table 276-2.

Laboratory, Endoscopic, and Radiographic Features Active disease can be associated with a rise in acute-phase reactants (C-reactive protein, orosomucoid levels), platelet count, erythrocyte sedimentation rate (ESR), and a decrease in hemoglobin. In severely ill patients, the serum albumin level will fall rather quickly. Leukocytosis may be present but is not a specific indicator of disease activity. Proctitis or proctosigmoiditis rarely causes a rise in C-reactive protein. Diagnosis relies upon the patient's history; clinical symptoms, negative stool examination for bacteria, *Clostridium difficile* toxin, and ova and parasites; sigmoidoscopic appearance (see Fig. 272-18); and histology of rectal or colonic biopsy specimens.

Sigmoidoscopy is used to assess disease activity and is often performed before treatment. If the patient is not having an acute flare, colonoscopy is used to assess disease extent and activity. Histologic features change more slowly than clinical features but can also be used to grade disease activity.

Patients with a severe attack of UC should have a plain, supine film of the abdomen. In the presence of severe disease, the margin of the colon becomes edematous and irregular. Colon thickening and toxic dilation can both be seen on a plain radiograph.

The earliest radiologic change of UC seen on single-contrast barium enema is a fine mucosal granularity (Fig. 276-5). With increasing severity, the mucosa becomes thickened and superficial ulcers are seen. Deep ulcerations can appear as "collar-button" ulcers, which indicate that the ulceration has penetrated the mucosa. Haustral folds may be normal in mild disease, but as activity progresses they become edematous and thickened. Loss of haustration can occur, especially in patients with long-standing disease. In addition, the colon becomes shortened and narrowed. Polyps in the colon may be postinflammatory polyps or pseudopolyps, adenomatous polyps, or carcinoma.

Computed tomography (CT) scanning is not as helpful as endoscopy and barium enema in making the diagnosis of UC, but typical findings include mild mural thickening (<1.5 cm), inhomogeneous

FIGURE 276-5   Barium enema in a patient with acute ulcerative colitis: inflammation of the entire colon. *(Courtesy of Dr. JM Braver, Gastrointestinal Radiology, Department of Radiology, Brigham and Women's Hospital, Boston, Massachusetts.)*

wall density, absence of small-bowel thickening, increased perirectal and presacral fat, target appearance of the rectum, and adenopathy.

Complications   Only 15% of patients with UC present initially with catastrophic illness. Massive hemorrhage occurs with severe attacks of disease in 1% of patients, and treatment for the disease usually stops the bleeding. However, if a patient requires 6 to 8 units of blood within 24 to 48 h, colectomy is indicated. Toxic megacolon is defined as a transverse colon with a diameter of >5 to 6 cm, with loss of haustration in patients with severe attacks of UC. It occurs in about 5% of attacks and can be triggered by electrolyte abnormalities and narcotics. About 50% of acute dilations will resolve with medical therapy alone, but urgent colectomy is required for those that do not improve. Perforation is the most dangerous of the local complications, and the physical signs of peritonitis may not be obvious, especially if the patient is receiving glucocorticoids. Although perforation is rare, the mortality rate for perforation complicating a toxic megacolon is about 15%. In addition, patients can develop a toxic colitis and such severe ulcerations that the bowel may perforate without first dilating.

Obstructions caused by benign stricture formation occur in 10% of patients, with one-third of the strictures occurring in the rectum. These should be surveyed endoscopically for carcinoma. UC patients occasionally develop anal fissures, perianal abscesses, or hemorrhoids, but the occurrence of extensive perianal lesions should suggest CD.

CROHN'S DISEASE ■ Signs and Symptoms   Although CD usually presents as acute or chronic bowel inflammation, the inflammatory process evolves toward one of two patterns of disease: a fibrostenotic-obstructing pattern or a penetrating-fistulous pattern, each with different treatments and prognoses. The site of disease influences the clinical manifestations.

ILEOCOLITIS   Because the most common site of inflammation is the terminal ileum, the usual presentation of ileocolitis is a chronic history of recurrent episodes of right lower quadrant pain and diarrhea. Sometimes the initial presentation mimics acute appendicitis with pronounced right lower quadrant pain, a palpable mass, fever, and

leukocytosis. Pain is usually colicky; it precedes and is relieved by defecation. A low-grade fever is usually noted. High-spiking fever suggests intraabdominal abscess formation. Weight loss is common—typically 10 to 20% of body weight—and develops as a consequence of diarrhea, anorexia, and fear of eating.

An inflammatory mass may be palpated in the right lower quadrant of the abdomen. The mass is composed of inflamed bowel, adherent and indurated mesentery, and enlarged abdominal lymph nodes. Extension of the mass can cause obstruction of the right ureter or bladder inflammation, manifested by dysuria and fever. Edema, bowel wall thickening, and fibrosis of the bowel wall within the mass account for the radiographic "string sign" of a narrowed intestinal lumen.

Bowel obstruction may take several forms. In the early stages of disease, bowel wall edema and spasm produce intermittent obstructive manifestations and increasing symptoms of postprandial pain. Over several years, persistent inflammation gradually progresses to fibrostenotic narrowing and stricture. Diarrhea will decrease and be replaced by chronic bowel obstruction. Acute episodes of obstruction occur as well, precipitated by bowel inflammation and spasm or sometimes by impaction of undigested food or medication. These episodes usually resolve with intravenous fluids and gastric decompression.

Severe inflammation of the ileocecal region may lead to localized wall thinning, with microperforation and fistula formation to the adjacent bowel, the skin, the urinary bladder, or to an abscess cavity in the mesentery. Enterovesical fistulas typically present as dysuria or recurrent bladder infections or less commonly as pneumaturia or fecaluria. Enterocutaneous fistulas follow tissue planes of least resistance, usually draining through abdominal surgical scars. Enterovaginal fistulas are rare and present as dyspareunia or as a feculent or foul-smelling, often painful vaginal discharge. They are unlikely to develop without a prior hysterectomy.

JEJUNOILEITIS   Extensive inflammatory disease is associated with a loss of digestive and absorptive surface, resulting in malabsorption and steatorrhea. Nutritional deficiencies can also result from poor intake and enteric losses of protein and other nutrients. Intestinal malabsorption can cause hypoalbuminemia, hypocalcemia, hypomagnesemia, coagulopathy, and hyperoxaluria with nephrolithiasis. Vertebral fractures are caused by a combination of vitamin D deficiency, hypocalcemia, and prolonged glucocorticoid use. Pellagra from niacin deficiency can occur in extensive small-bowel disease, and malabsorption of vitamin B_{12} can lead to a megaloblastic anemia and neurologic symptoms.

Diarrhea is characteristic of active disease; its causes include: (1) bacterial overgrowth in obstructive stasis or fistulization, (2) bile-acid malabsorption due to a diseased or resected terminal ileum, and (3) intestinal inflammation with decreased water absorption and increased secretion of electrolytes.

COLITIS AND PERIANAL DISEASE   Patients with colitis present with low-grade fevers, malaise, diarrhea, crampy abdominal pain, and sometimes hematochezia. Gross bleeding is not as common as in UC and appears in about half of patients with exclusively colonic disease. Only 1 to 2% bleed massively. Pain is caused by passage of fecal material through narrowed and inflamed segments of large bowel. Decreased rectal compliance is another cause for diarrhea in Crohn's colitis patients. Toxic megacolon is rare but may be seen with severe inflammation and short-duration disease.

Stricturing can occur in the colon and produce symptoms of bowel obstruction. Also, colonic disease may fistulize into the stomach or duodenum, causing feculent vomiting, or to the proximal or mid small bowel, causing malabsorption by "short circuiting" and bacterial overgrowth. Ten percent of women with Crohn's colitis will develop a rectovaginal fistula.

Perianal disease affects about one-third of patients with Crohn's colitis and is manifested by incontinence, large hemorrhoidal tags, anal strictures, anorectal fistulae, and perirectal abscesses. Not all patients with perianal fistula will have endoscopic evidence of colonic inflammation.

GASTRODUODENAL DISEASE   Symptoms and signs of upper gastrointestinal tract disease include nausea, vomiting, and epigastric pain. Patients usually have a *H. pylori*–negative gastritis. The second portion of the duodenum is more commonly involved than the bulb. Fistulas involving the stomach or duodenum arise from the small or large bowel and do not necessarily signify the presence of upper gastrointestinal tract involvement. Patients with advanced gastroduodenal CD may develop a chronic gastric outlet obstruction.

Laboratory, Endoscopic, and Radiographic Features   Laboratory abnormalities include elevated ESR and C-reactive protein. In more severe disease, findings include hypoalbuminemia, anemia, and leukocytosis.

Endoscopic features of CD include rectal sparing, aphthous ulcerations, fistulas, and skip lesions. Endoscopy is useful for biopsy of mass lesions or strictures, or for visualization of filling defects seen on barium enema. Colonoscopy allows examination and biopsy of the terminal ileum, and upper endoscopy is useful in diagnosing gastroduodenal involvement in patients with upper tract symptoms. Ileal or colonic strictures may be dilated with balloons introduced through the colonoscope. Endoscopic appearance correlates poorly with clinical remission; thus, repeated endoscopy is not used to monitor the inflammation.

In CD early radiographic findings in the small bowel include thickened folds and aphthous ulcerations. "Cobblestoning" from longitudinal and transverse ulcerations most frequently involves the small bowel (Fig. 276-6). In more advanced disease, strictures, fistulas (Fig. 276-7), inflammatory masses, and abscesses may be detected. The earliest macroscopic findings of colonic CD are aphthous ulcers. These small ulcers are often multiple and separated by normal intervening mucosa. As disease progresses, aphthous ulcers become enlarged, deeper, and occasionally connected to one another, forming longitudinal stellate, serpiginous, and linear ulcers (see Fig. 272-17).

The transmural inflammation of CD leads to decreased luminal diameter and limited distensibility. As ulcers progress deeper, they can lead to fistula formation. The radiographic "string sign" represents long areas of circumferential inflammation and fibrosis, resulting in long segments of luminal narrowing. The segmental nature of CD

FIGURE 276-6   Crohn's disease: small bowel series demonstrating "cobblestoning" of the terminal ileum (*arrows*). (*Courtesy of Dr. JM Braver, Gastrointestinal Radiology, Department of Radiology, Brigham and Women's Hospital, Boston, Massachusetts.*)

FIGURE 276-7   Small bowel series demonstrating distal ileal inflammation and fistulization (*arrows*) in a patient with CD. (*Courtesy of Dr. JM Braver, Gastrointestinal Radiology, Department of Radiology, Brigham and Women's Hospital, Boston, Massachusetts.*)

results in wide gaps of normal or dilated bowel between involved segments.

CT findings include mural thickening >2 cm, homogeneous wall density, mural thickening of small bowel, mesenteric fat stranding, perianal disease, and adenopathy. CT scanning can help identify abscesses, fistulas, and sinus tracts. Magnetic resonance imaging (MRI) may prove superior for demonstrating pelvic lesions such as ischiorectal abscesses.

Complications   Because CD is a transmural process, serosal adhesions develop that provide direct pathways for fistula formation and reduce the incidence of free perforation. Free perforation occurs in 1 to 2% of patients, usually in the ileum but occasionally in the jejunum or as a complication of toxic megacolon. The peritonitis of free perforation, especially colonic, may be fatal. Generalized peritonitis may also result from the rupture of an intraabdominal abscess. Other complications include intestinal obstruction in 40%, massive hemorrhage, malabsorption, and severe perianal disease.

Serologic Markers   Several serologic markers may be used to differentiate between CD and UC and help to predict the course of disease. Two antibodies that can be detected in the serum of IBD patients are perinuclear antineutrophil cytoplasmic antibodies (pANCAs) and anti-*Saccharomyces cerevisiae* antibodies (ASCAs). A distinct set of antineutrophil cytoplasmic antibodies with perinuclear staining by indirect immunofluorescence is associated with UC. The antigens to which these antibodies are directed have not been identified, but they are distinct from those associated with vasculitis and may be a marker for reactivity to enteric bacteria. pANCA positivity is found in about 60 to 70% of UC patients and 5 to 10% of CD patients; 5 to 15% of first-degree relatives of UC patients are pANCA positive, whereas only 2 to 3% of the general population is pANCA positive. pANCA may also identify specific disease phenotypes. pANCA positivity is more often associated with pancolitis, early surgery, pouchitis, or inflammation of the pouch after ileal pouch–anal anastamosis (IPAA) and primary sclerosing cholangitis. pANCA in CD is associated with colonic disease that resembles UC.

ASCA antibodies recognize mannose sequences in the cell wall mannan of *S. cerevisiae*; 60 to 70% of CD patients, 10 to 15% of UC patients, and up to 5% of non-IBD controls are ASCA positive. About 55% of CD patients are seroreactive to outer-membrane porin C (OMPC), a bacterial antigen. The combined measurement of pANCA and ASCA has been advocated as a valuable diagnostic approach to IBD. In one report, pANCA+ with ASCA− results showed a 57% sensitivity and 97% specificity for UC, whereas pANCA− with ASCA+ results showed a 49% sensitivity and 97% specificity for CD. ASCA was associated with small-bowel CD. These antibody tests may help decide whether a patient with indeterminate colitis should undergo an IPAA, because patients with predominant features of CD often have a more difficult postoperative course.

Other serologic markers in IBD patients include anti-goblet cell autoantibodies, pancreatic autoantibodies, and an autoantibody against tropomyosin isoform 5 found in colon epithelial cells. Antibodies to red cell membrane antigens that cross-react with enteropathogens such as *Campylobacter* sp. may be associated with hemolytic anemia in CD. None of these antibodies are useful in the diagnosis and management of patients with IBD.

DIFFERENTIAL DIAGNOSIS OF UC AND CD

UC and CD have similar features to many other diseases. In the absence of a key diagnostic test, a combination of clinical, laboratory, histopathologic, radiographic, and therapeutic observations is required (Table 276-3). Once a diagnosis of IBD is made, distinguishing between UC and CD is impossible in 10 to 15% of cases. These are termed *indeterminate colitis*.

INFECTIOUS DISEASE Infections of the small intestines and colon can mimic CD or UC. They may be bacterial, fungal, viral, or protozoal in origin (Table 276-4). *Campylobacter* colitis can mimic the endoscopic appearance of severe UC and can cause a relapse of established UC. *Salmonella* can cause watery or bloody diarrhea, nausea, and vomiting. Shigellosis causes watery diarrhea, abdominal pain, and fe-

TABLE 276-3 *Different Clinical, Endoscopic, and Radiographic Features*

	Ulcerative Colitis	Crohn's Disease
CLINICAL		
Gross blood in stool	Yes	Occasionally
Mucus	Yes	Occasionally
Systemic symptoms	Occasionally	Frequently
Pain	Occasionally	Frequently
Abdominal mass	Rarely	Yes
Significant perineal disease	No	Frequently
Fistulas	No	Yes
Small-intestinal obstruction	No	Frequently
Colonic obstruction	Rarely	Frequently
Response to antibiotics	No	Yes
Recurrence after surgery	No	Yes
ANCA-positive	Frequently	Rarely
ASCA-positive	Rarely	Frequently
ENDOSCOPIC		
Rectal sparing	Rarely	Frequently
Continuous disease	Yes	Occasionally
"Cobblestoning"	No	Yes
Granuloma on biopsy	No	Occasionally
RADIOGRAPHIC		
Small bowel significantly abnormal	No	Yes
Abnormal terminal ileum	Occasionally	Yes
Segmental colitis	No	Yes
Asymmetric colitis	No	Yes
Stricture	Occasionally	Frequently

Note: ANCA, antineutrophil cytoplasm antibody; ASCA, anti-Saccharomyces cerevisiae antibody.

TABLE 276-4 *Diseases that Mimic IBD*

INFECTIOUS ETIOLOGIES

Bacterial	Mycobacterial	Viral
Salmonella	Tuberculosis	Cytomegalovirus
Shigella	*Mycobacterium*	Herpes simplex
Toxigenic	*avium*	HIV
Escherichia coli	**Parasitic**	**Fungal**
Campylobacter	Amebiasis	Histoplasmosis
Yersinia	*Isospora*	*Candida*
Clostridium	*Trichuris trichura*	*Aspergillus*
difficile	Hookworm	
Gonorrhea	*Strongyloides*	
Chlamydia		
trachomatis		

NONINFECTIOUS ETIOLOGIES

Inflammatory	Neoplastic	Drugs and Chemicals
Appendicitis	Lymphoma	NSAIDs
Diverticulitis	Metastatic	Phosphasoda
Diversion colitis	carcinoma	Cathartic colon
Collagenous/	Carcinoma of the	Gold
lymphocytic	ileum	Oral contraceptives
colitis	Carcinoid	Cocaine
Ischemic colitis	Familial polyposis	Chemotherapy
Radiation colitis/		
enteritis		
Solitary rectal ulcer		
Eosinophilc		
gastroenteritis		
Neutropenic colitis		
Beçhet's syndrome		
Graft-versus-host		
disease		

Note: NSAIDs, nonsteroidal anti-inflammatory drugs.

ver followed by rectal tenesmus and by the passage of blood and mucus per rectum. All three are usually self-limited, but 1% of patients infected with *Salmonella* become asymptomatic carriers. *Yersinia enterocolitica* infection occurs mainly in the terminal ileum and causes mucosal ulceration, neutrophil invasion, and thickening of the ileal wall. Other bacterial infections that may mimic IBD include *C. difficile*, which presents with watery diarrhea, tenesmus, nausea, and vomiting; and *Escherichia coli*, three categories of which can cause colitis. These are enterohemorrhagic, enteroinvasive, and enteroadherent *E. coli*, all of which can cause bloody diarrhea and abdominal tenderness. Diagnosis of bacterial colitis is made by sending stool specimens for bacterial culture and *C. difficile* toxin analysis. Gonorrhea, *Chlamydia*, and syphilis can also cause proctitis.

Gastrointestinal involvement with mycobacterial infection occurs primarily in the immunosuppressed patient but may occur in patients with normal immunity. Distal ileal and cecal involvement predominates, and patients present with symptoms of small-bowel obstruction and a tender abdominal mass. The diagnosis is made most directly by colonoscopy with biopsy and culture. *Mycobacterium avium-intracellulare* complex infection occurs in advanced stages of HIV infection and in other immunocompromised states and usually manifests as a systemic infection with diarrhea, abdominal pain, weight loss, fever, and malabsorption. Diagnosis is established by acid-fast smear and culture of mucosal biopsies.

Although most of the patients with viral colitis are immunosuppressed, cytomegalovirus (CMV) and herpes simplex proctitis may occur in immunocompetent individuals. CMV occurs most commonly in the esophagus, colon, and rectum but may also involve the small intestine. Symptoms include abdominal pain, bloody diarrhea, fever, and weight loss. With severe disease, necrosis and perforation can occur. Diagnosis is made by identification of intranuclear inclusions in mucosal cells on biopsy. Herpes simplex infection of the gastrointestinal tract is limited to the oropharynx, anorectum, and perianal areas. Symptoms include anorectal pain, tenesmus, constipation, inguinal adenopathy, difficulty with urinary voiding, and sacral paresthesias. Diagnosis is made by rectal biopsy. HIV itself can cause diarrhea, nausea, vomiting, and anorexia. Small-intestinal biopsies show partial villus atrophy; small-bowel bacterial overgrowth and fat malabsorption may also be noted.

Protozoan parasites include *Isospora belli*, which can cause a self-limited infection in healthy hosts but causes a chronic profuse, watery diarrhea and weight loss in AIDS patients. *Entamoeba histolytica* or related species infect about 10% of the world's population; symptoms include abdominal pain, tenesmus, frequent loose stools containing blood and mucus, and abdominal tenderness. Colonoscopy reveals focal punctate ulcers with normal intervening mucosa; diagnosis is made by biopsy or serum amebic antibodies. Fulminant amebic colitis is rare but has a mortality rate of >50%.

Other parasitic infections that may mimic IBD include hookworm (*Necator americanus*), whipworm (*Trichuris trichiura*), and *Strongyloides stercoralis*. In severely immunocompromised patients *Candida* or *Aspergillus* can be identified in the submucosa. Disseminated histoplasmosis can involve the ileocecal area.

NONINFECTIOUS DISEASE Many diseases may mimic IBD (Table 276-4). Diverticulitis can be confused with CD clinically and radiographically. Both diseases cause fever, abdominal pain, tender abdominal mass, leukocytosis, elevated ESR, partial obstruction, and fistulas. Perianal disease or ileitis on small-bowel series favors the diagnosis of CD. Significant endoscopic mucosal abnormalities are more likely in CD than in diverticulitis. Endoscopic or clinical recurrence following segmental resection favors CD. Diverticular-associated colitis is similar to CD, but mucosal abnormalities are limited to the sigmoid and descending colon.

Ischemic colitis is commonly confused with IBD. The ischemic process can be chronic and diffuse as in UC, or segmental as in CD. Colonic inflammation due to ischemia may resolve quickly or may persist and result in transmural scarring and stricture formation. Ischemic bowel disease should be considered in the elderly following abdominal aortic aneurysm repair or when a patient has a hypercoagulable state or a severe cardiac or peripheral vascular disorder. Patients usually present with sudden onset of left lower quadrant pain, urgency to defecate, and the passage of bright red blood per rectum. Endoscopic examination often demonstrates a normal-appearing rectum and a sharp transition to an area of inflammation in the descending colon and splenic flexure.

The effects of radiation therapy on the gastrointestinal tract can be difficult to distinguish from IBD. Acute symptoms can occur within 1 to 2 weeks of starting radiotherapy. When the rectum and sigmoid are irradiated, patients develop bloody, mucoid diarrhea and tenesmus, as in distal UC. With small-bowel involvement, diarrhea is common. Late symptoms include malabsorption and weight loss. Stricturing with obstruction and bacterial overgrowth may occur. Fistulas can penetrate the bladder, vagina, or abdominal wall. Flexible sigmoidoscopy reveals mucosal granularity, friability, numerous telangiectasias, and occasionally discrete ulcerations. Biopsy can be diagnostic.

Solitary rectal ulcer syndrome is uncommon and can be confused with IBD. It occurs in persons of all ages and may be caused by impaired evacuation and failure of relaxation of the puborectalis muscle. Ulceration may arise from anal sphincter overactivity, higher intrarectal pressures during defecation, and digital removal of stool. Patients complain of constipation with straining and pass blood and mucus per rectum. Other symptoms include abdominal pain, diarrhea, tenesmus, and perineal pain. The ulceration, which can be as large as 5 cm in diameter, is usually seen anteriorly or anteriorlaterally 3 to 15 cm from the anal verge. Biopsies can be diagnostic.

Several types of colitis have been associated with nonsteroidal antiinflammatory drugs (NSAIDs), including de novo colitis, reactivation of IBD, and proctitis caused by use of suppositories. Most patients with NSAID-related colitis present with diarrhea and abdominal pain and complications include stricture, bleeding, obstruction, perforation,

and fistulization. Withdrawal of these agents is crucial, and in cases of reactivated IBD, standard therapies are indicated.

INDETERMINATE COLITIS Cases of IBD that cannot be categorized as UC or CD are called *indeterminate colitis*. Long-term follow-up reduces the number of cases labeled indeterminate to about 10%. The disease course of indeterminate colitis is unclear and surgical recommendations are difficult, especially since up to 20% of pouches fail, requiring ileosotomy. A multistage IPAA (the initial stage consisting of a subtotal colectomy with Hartmann pouch) with careful histologic evaluation of the resected specimen to exclude CD is advised. Medical therapy is similar to that for UC and CD; most clinicians use 5-ASA drugs, glucocorticoids, and immunomodulators as necessary.

THE ATYPICAL COLITIDIES Two atypical colitides—collagenous colitis and lymphocytic colitis—have completely normal endoscopic appearances. Collagenous colitis has two main histologic components: increased subepithelial collagen deposition and colitis with increased intraepithelial lymphocytes. Female to male ratio is 9:1, and most patients present in the sixth or seventh decades of life. The main symptom is chronic watery diarrhea. Treatments range from sulfasalazine or mesalamine and Lomotil to bismuth to glucocorticoids for refractory disease.

Lymphocytic colitis has features similar to collagenous colitis including age at onset and clinical presentation, but it has almost equal incidence in men and women and no subepithelial collagen deposition on pathologic section. However, intraepithelial lymphocytes are increased. Diarrhea stops in most patients treated with 5-ASA or prednisone.

Diversion colitis is an inflammatory process that arises in segments of the large intestine that are excluded from the fecal stream. It usually occurs in patients with ileostomy or colostomy when a mucus fistula or a Hartmann's pouch has been created. Diversion colitis is reversible by surgical reanastamosis. Clinically, patients have mucus or bloody discharge from the rectum. Erythema, granularity, friability, and, in more severe cases, ulceration can be seen on endoscopy. Histopathology shows areas of active inflammation with foci of cryptitis and crypt abscesses. Crypt architecture is normal and this differentiates it from UC. It may be impossible to distinguish it from CD. Short-chain fatty acid enemas will help in diversion colitis, but the definitive therapy is surgical reanastamosis.

EXTRAINTESTINAL MANIFESTATIONS

IBD is associated with a variety of extraintestinal manifestations; up to one-third of patients have at least one. Patients with perianal CD are at higher risk for developing extraintestinal manifestations than other IBD patients.

DERMATOLOGIC Erythema nodosum (EN) occurs in up to 15% of CD patients and 10% of UC patients. Attacks usually correlate with bowel activity; skin lesions develop after the onset of bowel symptoms, and patients frequently have concomitant active peripheral arthritis. The lesions of EN are hot, red, tender nodules measuring 1 to 5 cm in diameter and are found on the anterior surface of the lower legs, ankles, calves, thighs, and arms. Therapy is directed toward the underlying bowel disease.

Pyoderma gangrenosum (PG) is seen in 1 to 12% of UC patients and less commonly in Crohn's colitis. Although it usually presents after the diagnosis of IBD, PG may occur years before the onset of bowel symptoms, run a course independent of the bowel disease, respond poorly to colectomy, and even develop years after proctocolectomy. It is usually associated with severe disease. Lesions are commonly found on the dorsal surface of the feet and legs but may occur on the arms, chest, stoma, and even the face. PG usually begins as a pustule and then spreads concentrically to rapidly undermine healthy skin. Lesions then ulcerate, with violaceous edges surrounded by a margin of erythema. Centrally, they contain necrotic tissue with blood and exudates. Lesions may be single or multiple and grow as large as 30 cm. They are sometimes very difficult to treat and often require intravenous antibiotics, intravenous glucocorticoids, dapsone, azathioprine, thalidomide, intravenous cyclosporine, or infliximab.

Other dermatologic manifestations include pyoderma vegetans that occurs in intertriginous areas, pyostomatitis vegetans that involves the mucous membranes, Sweet's syndrome, a neutrophilic dermatosis, and metastatic CD, a rare disorder defined by cutaneous granuloma formation. Psoriasis affects 5 to 10% of patients with IBD and is unrelated to bowel activity. Perianal skin tags are found in 75 to 80% of patients with CD, especially those with colon involvement. Oral mucosal lesions are seen often in CD and rarely in UC and include aphthous stomatitis and "cobblestone" lesions of the buccal mucosa.

RHEUMATOLOGIC Peripheral arthritis develops in 15 to 20% of IBD patients, is more common in CD, and worsens with exacerbations of bowel activity. It is asymmetric, polyarticular, and migratory and most often affects large joints of the upper and lower extremities. Treatment is directed at reducing bowel inflammation. In severe UC, colectomy frequently cures the arthritis.

Ankylosing spondylitis (AS) occurs in about 10% of IBD patients and is more common in CD than UC. About two-thirds of IBD patients with AS test positive for the HLA-B27 antigen. The activity of AS is not related to bowel activity and does not remit with glucocorticoids or colectomy. It most often affects the spine and pelvis, producing symptoms of diffuse low-back pain, buttock pain, and morning stiffness. The course is continuous and progressive, leading to permanent skeletal damage and deformity.

Sacroiliitis is symmetric, occurs equally in UC and CD, is often asymptomatic, does not correlate with bowel activity, and does not always progress to AS. Other rheumatic manifestations include hypertrophic osteoarthropathy, pelvic/femoral osteomyelitis, and relapsing polychondritis.

OCULAR The incidence of ocular complications in IBD patients is 1 to 10%. The most common are conjunctivitis, anterior uveitis/iritis, and episcleritis. Uveitis is associated with both UC and Crohn's colitis, may be found during periods of remission, and may develop in patients following bowel resection. Symptoms include ocular pain, photophobia, blurred vision, and headache. Prompt intervention, sometimes with systemic glucocorticoids, is required to prevent scarring and visual impairment. Episcleritis is a benign disorder that presents with symptoms of mild ocular burning. It occurs in 3 to 4% of IBD patients, more commonly in Crohn's colitis, and is treated with topical glucocorticoids.

HEPATOBILIARY Hepatic steatosis is detectable in about half of the abnormal liver biopsies from patients with CD and UC; patients usually present with hepatomegaly. Fatty liver usually results from a combination of chronic debilitating illness, malnutrition, and glucocorticoid therapy. Cholelithiasis is more common in CD than UC and occurs in 10 to 35% of patients with ileitis or ileal resection. Gallstone formation is caused by malabsorption of bile acids resulting in depletion of the bile salt pool and the secretion of lithogenic bile.

Primary sclerosing cholangitis (PSC) is characterized by both intrahepatic and extrahepatic bile duct inflammation and fibrosis, frequently leading to biliary cirrhosis and hepatic failure; 1 to 5% of patients with IBD have PSC, but 50 to 75% of patients with PSC have IBD. Although it can be recognized after the diagnosis of IBD, PSC can be detected earlier or even years after proctocolectomy. Most patients have no symptoms at the time of diagnosis; when symptoms are present they consist of fatigue, jaundice, abdominal pain, fever, anorexia, and malaise. Diagnosis is made by endoscopic retrograde cholangiopancreatography (ERCP), which demonstrates multiple bile duct strictures alternating with relatively normal segments. The bile acid ursodeoxycholic acid (ursodiol) may reduce alkaline phosphatase and serum aminotransferase levels, but histologic improvement has been

marginal. High doses (25 to 30 mg/kg per day) may have long-term benefit. Endoscopic stenting may be palliative for cholestasis secondary to bile duct obstruction. Patients with symptomatic disease develop cirrhosis and liver failure over 5 to 10 years and eventually require liver transplantation. Ten percent of PSC patients develop cholangiocarcinoma and cannot be transplanted. Pericholangitis is a subset of PSC found in about 30% of IBD patients; it is confined to small bile ducts and is usually benign.

UROLOGIC The most frequent genitourinary complications are calculi, ureteral obstruction, and fistulas. The highest frequency of nephrolithiasis (10 to 20%) occurs in patients with CD following small-bowel resection. Calcium oxalate stones develop secondary to hyperoxaluria, which results from increased absorption of dietary oxalate. Normally, dietary calcium combines with luminal oxalate to form insoluble calcium oxalate, which is eliminated in the stool. In patients with ileal dysfunction, however, nonabsorbed fatty acids bind calcium and leave oxalate unbound. The unbound oxalate is then delivered to the colon, where it is readily absorbed, especially in the presence of colonic inflammation.

OTHER The risk of thromboembolic disease increases when IBD becomes active, and patients may present with deep vein thrombosis, pulmonary embolism, cerebrovascular accidents, and arterial emboli. Factors responsible for the hypercoagulable state include reactive thrombocytosis; increased levels of fibrinopeptide A, factor V, factor VIII, and fibrinogen; accelerated thromboplastin generation; antithrombin III deficiency secondary to increased gut losses or increased catabolism; and free protein S deficiency. A spectrum of vasculitidies involving small, medium, and large vessels has also been observed in IBD patients.

Patients with IBD have an increased prevalence of osteoporosis and osteomalacia from vitamin D deficiency, calcium malabsorption, malnutrition, glucocorticoid use, and the intestinal inflammation itself. Deficiencies of vitamin B_{12} and fat-soluble vitamins may occur after ileal resection or with ileal disease.

More common cardiopulmonary manifestations include endocarditis, myocarditis, pleuropericarditis, and interstitial lung disease. A secondary or reactive amyloidosis can occur in patients with long-standing IBD, especially in patients with CD. Amyloid material is deposited systemically and can cause diarrhea, constipation, and renal failure. The renal disease can be successfully treated with colchicine. Pancreatitis is a rare extraintestinal manifestation of IBD and results from duodenal fistulas, ampullary CD, gallstones, PSC, drugs such as 6-mercaptopurine, azathioprine, or very rarely, 5-ASA agents, autoimmune pancreatitis, and primary CD of the pancreas.

R_x TREATMENT

5-ASA AGENTS The mainstay of therapy for mild to moderate UC and Crohn's colitis is sulfasalazine and the other 5-ASA agents. These agents are effective at inducing remission in both UC and CD and in maintaining remission in UC; it remains unclear whether they have a role in remission maintenance in CD.

Sulfasalazine was originally developed to deliver both antibacterial (sulfapyridine) and anti-inflammatory (5-ASA) therapy into the connective tissues of joints and the colonic mucosa. The molecular structure provides a convenient delivery system to the colon by allowing the intact molecule to pass through the small intestine after only partial absorption, and to be broken down in the colon by bacterial azo reductases that cleave the azo bond linking the sulfa and 5-ASA moieties. Sulfasalazine is effective treatment for mild to moderate UC and Crohn's ileocolitis and colitis, but its high rate of side effects limits its use. Although sulfasalazine is more effective at higher doses, at 6 or 8 g/d up to 30% of patients experience allergic reactions or intolerable side effects such as headache, anorexia, nausea, and vomiting that are attributable to the sulfapyridine moiety. Hypersensitivity reactions, independent of sulfapyridine levels, include rash, fever, hepatitis, agranulocytosis, hypersensitivity pneumonitis, pancreatitis, worsening of colitis, and reversible sperm abnormalities. Sulfasalazine can also impair folate absorption, and patients should be given folic acid supplements.

Newer sulfa-free aminosalicylate preparations deliver increased amounts of the pharmacologically active ingredient of sulfasalazine (5-ASA, mesalamine) to the site of active bowel disease while limiting systemic toxicity. 5-ASA may function through inhibition of NF-κB activity. Sulfa-free aminosalicylate formulations include alternative azo-bonded carriers, 5-ASA dimers, pH-dependent tablets, and continuous-release preparations. Each has the same efficacy as sulfasalazine when equimolar concentrations are used. Olsalazine is composed of two 5-ASA radicals linked by an azo bond, which is split in the colon by bacterial reduction and two 5-ASA molecules are released. Olsalazine is similar in effectiveness to sulfasalazine in treating CD and UC, but up to 17% of patients experience non-bloody diarrhea caused by increased secretion of fluid in the small bowel. Balsalazide contains an azo bond binding mesalamine to the carrier molecule 4-aminobenzoyl-β-alanine; it is effective in the colon. Claversal is an enteric-coated form of 5-ASA that consists of mesalamine surrounded by an acrylic-based polymer resin and a cellulose coating that releases mesalamine at pH > 6.0, a level that is present from the mid-jejunum continuously to the distal colon.

The most commonly used drugs besides sulfasalazine in the United States are Asacol and Pentasa. Asacol is also an enteric-coated form of mesalamine, but it has a slightly different release pattern, with 5-ASA liberated at pH > 7.0. The disintegration of Asacol is variable, with complete breakup of the tablet occurring in many different parts of the gut ranging from the small intestine to the splenic flexure; it has increased gastric residence when taken with a meal. Asacol is used to induce and maintain remission in UC and to induce remission in CD ileitis, ileocolitis, and colitis. Appropriate doses of Asacol and the other 5-ASA compounds are shown in Table 276-5. Some 50 to 75% of patients with mild to moderate UC and CD improve when treated with 2 g/d of 5-ASA; the dose response continues up to at least 4.8 g/d. Doses of 1.5 to 4 g/d maintain remission in 50 to 75% of patients with UC.

Pentasa is another mesalamine formulation that uses an ethylcellulose coating to allow water absorption into small beads containing the mesalamine. Water dissolves the 5-ASA, which then diffuses out of the bead into the lumen. Disintegration of the capsule occurs in the stomach. The microspheres then disperse throughout the entire gastrointestinal tract from the small intestine through the distal colon in both fasted or fed conditions. Controlled trials of Pentasa and Asacol in active CD demonstrate a 40 to 60% clinical improvement or remission, but the data are not conclusive that these agents maintain remission in CD. 5-ASA agents may be effective in postoperative prophylaxis of CD.

Topical mesalamine enemas are effective in mild-to-moderate distal UC and CD. Clinical response occurs in up to 80% of UC patients with colitis distal to the splenic flexure. Mesalamine suppositories are effective in treating proctitis.

Glucocorticoids The majority of patients with moderate to severe UC benefit from oral or parenteral glucocorticoids. Prednisone is usually started at doses of 40 to 60 mg/d for active UC that is unresponsive to 5-ASA therapy. Parenteral glucocorticoids may be administered as intravenous hydrocortisone, 300 mg/d, or methylprednisolone, 40 to 60 mg/d. Adrenocorticotropic hormone (ACTH) is occasionally preferred for glucocorticoid-naïve patients despite a risk of adrenal hemorrhage. ACTH has equivalent efficacy to intravenous hydrocortisone in both glucocorticoid-naïve and -experienced CD patients.

Topically applied glucocorticoids are also beneficial for distal co-

Preparation	Formulation	Delivery	Dosing, g/d
AZO-BOND			
Sulfasalazine (500 mg)	Sulfapyridine-5-ASA	Colon	4–8 (acute) 2–6 (maintenance)
Olsalazine (250 mg)	5-ASA-5-ASA	Colon	1–3
Balsalazide (500–750 mg)	Aminobenzoyl-alanine-5-ASA	Colon	2.25–6.75
DELAYED-RELEASE			
Asacol (400 mg)	Eudragit S (pH 7)	Distal ileum-colon	2.4–4.8 (acute) 1.6–4.8 (maintenance)
Claversal (250–500 mg)	Eudragit L (pH 6)	Ileum-colon	1.5–3 (acute) 0.75–3 (maintenance)
SUSTAINED-RELEASE			
Pentasa (250 mg)	Ethylcellulose microgranules	Stomach-colon	2–4 (acute) 1.5–4 (maintenance)

TABLE 276-5 Oral 5-ASA Preparations

litis and may serve as an adjunct in those who have rectal involvement plus more proximal disease. Hydrocortisone enemas or foam may control active disease, although they have no proven role as maintenance therapy. These glucocorticoids are significantly absorbed from the rectum and can lead to adrenal suppression with prolonged administration.

Glucocorticoids are also effective for treatment of moderate-to-severe CD and induce a 60 to 70% remission rate compared to a 30% placebo response. The systemic effects of standard glucocorticoid formulations have led to the development of more potent formulations that are less well absorbed and have increased first-pass metabolism. Controlled ileal-release budesonide has been nearly equal to prednisone for ileocolonic CD with fewer glucocorticoid side effects. Budesonide is used for 2 to 3 months at a dose of 9 mg/d, then tapered.

Glucocorticoids play no role in maintenance therapy in either UC or CD. Once clinical remission has been induced, they should be tapered according to the clinical activity, normally at a rate of no more than 5 mg per week. They can usually be tapered to 20 mg/d within 4 to 5 weeks but often take several months to be discontinued altogether. The side effects are numerous, including fluid retention, abdominal striae, fat redistribution, hyperglycemia, subcapsular cataracts, osteonecrosis, myopathy, emotional disturbances, and withdrawal symptoms. Most of these side effects, aside from osteonecrosis, are related to the dose and duration of therapy.

ANTIBIOTICS Antibiotics have no role in the treatment of active or quiescent UC. However, pouchitis, which occurs in about a third of UC patients after colectomy and IPAA, usually responds to treatment with metronidazole or ciprofloxacin.

Metronidazole is effective in active inflammatory, fistulous, and perianal CD and may prevent recurrence after ileal resection. The most effective dose is 15 to 20 mg/kg per day in three divided doses; it is usually continued for several months. Common side effects include nausea, metallic taste, and disulfiram-like reaction. Peripheral neuropathy can occur with prolonged administration (several months) and on rare occasions is permanent despite discontinuation. Ciprofloxacin (500 mg bid) is also beneficial for inflammatory, perianal, and fistulous CD. These two antibiotics should be used as second-line drugs in active CD after 5-ASA agents and as first-line drugs in perianal and fistulous CD.

AZATHIOPRINE AND 6-MERCAPTOPURINE Azathioprine and 6-mercaptopurine (6-MP) are purine analogues commonly employed in the management of glucocorticoid-dependent IBD. Azathioprine is rapidly absorbed and converted to 6-MP, which is then metabolized to the active end product, thioinosinic acid, an inhibitor of purine ribonucleotide synthesis and cell proliferation. These agents also inhibit the immune response. Efficacy is seen at 3 to 4 weeks. Compliance can

TABLE 276-6 *Medical Management of IBD*

Ulcerative Colitis: Active Disease

	Mild	Moderate	Severe	Fulminant
Distal	5-ASA oral and/or enema	5-ASA oral and/or enema Glucocorticoid enema Oral glucocorticoid	5-ASA oral and/or enema Glucocorticoid enema Oral or IV glucocorticoid	Intravenous glucocorticoid Intravenous CSA
Extensive	5-ASA oral and/or enema	5-ASA oral and/or enema Glucocorticoid enema Oral glucocorticoid	5-ASA oral and/or enema Glucocorticoid enema Oral or IV glucocorticoid	Intravenous glucocorticoid Intravenous CSA

Ulcerative Colitis: Maintenance Therapy

Distal	5-ASA oral and/or enema 6-MP or azathioprine
Extensive	5-ASA oral and/or enema 6-MP or azathioprine

Crohn's Disease: Active Disease

Mild–Moderate	Severe	Perianal or Fistulizing Disease
5-ASA oral and/or enema Metronidazole and/or ciprofloxacin Oral glucocorticoids Infliximab Budesonide	5-ASA oral and/or enema Metronidazole and/or ciprofloxacin Oral or IV glucocorticoids Infliximab TPN or elemental diet	Metronidazole and/or ciprofloxacin Azathioprine or 6-MP Infliximab Intravenous CSA

Crohn's Disease: Maintenance Therapy

Inflammatory	Perianal or Fistulizing Disease
5-ASA oral and/or enema Azathioprine or 6-MP Infliximab	Metronidazole and/or ciprofloxacin Azathioprine or 6-MP Infliximab

Note: CSA, cyclosporine; 6-MP, 6-mercaptopurine; TPN, total parenteral nutrition.

be monitored by measuring the levels of 6-thioguanine and 6-methylmercaptopurine, end products of 6-MP metabolism. Azathioprine (2.0 to 2.5 mg/kg per day) or 6-MP (1.0 to 1.5 mg/kg per day) have been employed successfully as glucocorticoid-sparing agents in up to two-thirds of UC and CD patients previously unable to be weaned from glucocorticoids. The role of these immunomodulators as maintenance therapy in UC and CD and for treating active perianal disease and fistulas in CD appears promising. In addition, 6-MP or azathioprine may be effective for postoperative prophylaxis of CD.

Although azathioprine and 6-MP are usually well tolerated, pancreatitis occurs in 3 to 4% of patients, typically presents within the first few weeks of therapy, and is completely reversible when the drug is stopped. Other side effects include nausea, fever, rash, and hepatitis. Bone marrow suppression (particularly leukopenia) is dose-related and often delayed, necessitating regular monitoring of the complete blood count. Additionally, 1 in 300 individuals lacks thiopurine methyltransferase, the enzyme responsible for drug metabolism; an additional 11% of the population are heterozygotes with intermediate enzyme activity. Both are at increased risk of toxicity because of increased accumulation of thioguanine metabolites. No increased risk of cancer has been documented in IBD patients chronically taking these medications.

METHOTREXATE Methotrexate (MTX) inhibits dihydrofolate reductase, resulting in impaired DNA synthesis. Additional anti-inflammatory properties may be related to decreased IL-1 production. Intramuscular or subcutaneous MTX (25 mg per week) is effective in inducing remission and reducing glucocorticoid dosage, and 15 mg per week is effective in maintaining remission in active CD. Potential toxicities include leukopenia and hepatic fibrosis, necessitating periodic evaluation of complete blood counts and liver enzymes. The role of liver biopsy in patients on long-term MTX is uncertain. Hypersensitivity pneumonitis is a rare but serious complication of therapy.

CYCLOSPORINE Cyclosporine (CSA) alters the immune response by acting as a potent inhibitor of T cell–mediated responses. Although CSA acts primarily via inhibition of IL-2 production from T helper cells, it also decreases recruitment of cytotoxic T cells and blocks other cytokines, including IL-3, IL-4, IFN-γ, and TNF. It has a more rapid onset of action than 6-MP and azathioprine.

CSA is most effective given at 2 to 4 mg/kg per day intravenously in severe UC that is refractory to intravenous glucocorticoids, with 82% of patients responding. CSA can be an alternative to colectomy. The long-term success of oral CSA is not as dramatic, but if patients are started on 6-MP or azathioprine at the time of hospital discharge, remission can be maintained. Intravenous CSA is effective in 80% of patients with refractory fistulas, but 6-MP or azathioprine must be used to maintain remission. Oral CSA alone is effective only at a higher dose (7.5 mg/kg per day) in active disease but is not effective in maintaining remission without 6-MP/azathioprine. Serum levels should be monitored and kept in the range of 200 to 400 ng/mL.

CSA may cause significant toxicity; renal function should be monitored frequently. Hypertension, gingival hyperplasia, hypertrichosis, paresthesias, tremors, headaches, and electrolyte abnormalities are common side effects. Creatinine elevation calls for dose reduction or discontinuation. Seizures may also complicate therapy, especially if the patient is hypomagnesemic or if serum cholesterol levels are <3.1 mmol/L (<120 mg/dL). Opportunistic infections, most notably *Pneumocystis carinii* pneumonia, may occur with combination immunosuppressive treatment; prophylaxis should be given.

NUTRITIONAL THERAPIES Dietary antigens may stimulate the mucosal immune response. Patients with active CD respond to bowel rest, along with total enteral or total parenteral nutrition (TPN). Bowel rest and TPN are as effective as glucocorticoids at inducing remission of active CD but are not effective as maintenance therapy. Enteral nutrition in the form of elemental or peptide-based preparations are also as effective as glucocorticiods or TPN, but these diets are not palatable. Enteral diets may provide the small intestine with nutrients vital to cell growth and do not have the complications of TPN. In contrast to CD, active UC is not effectively treated with either elemental diets or TPN. Standard medical management of UC and CD is reviewed in Table 276-6.

NEWER MEDICAL THERAPIES ■ Anti-Tumor Necrosis Factor Antibody TNF is a key inflammatory cytokine and mediator of intestinal inflammation. The expression of TNF is increased in IBD. Infliximab is a chimeric mouse-human monoclonal antibody against TNF that is extremely effective in CD. It blocks TNF in the serum and at the cell surface and likely lyses TNF-producing macrophages and T cells through complement fixation and antibody-dependent cytotoxicity. Of active CD patients refractory to glucocorticoids, 6-MP, or 5-ASA, 65% will respond to intravenous infliximab (5 mg/kg); one-third will enter complete remission. Of the patients who experience an initial response, 40% will maintain remission for at least 1 year with repeated infusions of infliximab every 8 weeks.

Infliximab is also effective in CD patients with refractory perianal and enterocutaneous fistulas, with a 68% response rate (50% reduction in fistula drainage) and a 50% complete remission rate. Reinfusion, typically every 8 weeks, is necessary to continue therapeutic benefits in many patients.

The development of antibodies to infliximab (ATI) is associated with an increased risk of infusion reactions and a decreased response to treatment. Patients who receive on-demand or episodic infusions rather than periodic (every 8 weeks) infusions are more likely to develop ATI. A humanized antibody to TNF also shows some promise in early clinical testing.

Among 120,000 patients treated with infliximab, 8 developed lymphoma: 5 patients with CD and 3 with rheumatoid arthritis. As the risk of lymphoma is already increased in these conditions, it is unclear whether infliximab is the cause. Thus, infliximab is extremely effective in refractory inflammatory and fistulous CD but should be used only when necessary. Results on the efficacy of infliximab in UC are mixed.

Newer Immunosuppressive Agents Tacrolimus has a mechanism of action similar to cyclosporine. It has shown efficacy in children with refractory IBD and in adults with extensive involvement of the small bowel.

Mycophenolate mofetil is another immunomodulator that may be effective in CD patients resistant to or intolerant of 6-MP azathioprine. Patients with CD who received 15 mg/kg per day have tolerated the drug well and have experienced benefit with reduction of glucocorticoid requirements.

6-Thioguanine is the active metabolite of 6-MP and has shown activity in patients resistant to or intolerant of 6-MP/azathioprine.

Thalidomide has been shown to inhibit TNF production by monocytes and other cells. Thalidomide is effective in glucocorticoid-refractory and fistulous CD, but randomized controlled trials still need to be performed.

The $\alpha4$ integrin-specific humanized monoclonal antibody, natalizumab, prevents the migration of leukocytes into the parenchyma and blocks their activation in inflammatory sites. It seems to be effective in CD, but more trials are needed.

SURGICAL THERAPY ■ **Ulcerative Colitis** Nearly half of patients with extensive chronic UC undergo surgery within the first 10 years of their illness. The indications for surgery are listed in Table 276-7. Morbidity is about 20% in elective, 30% for urgent, and 40% for emergency proctocolectomy. The risks are primarily hemorrhage, contamination and sepsis, and neural injury. Although single-stage total proctocolec-

tomy with ileostomy has been the operation of choice, newer operations maintain continence while surgically removing the involved rectal mucosa.

The IPAA is the most frequent continence-preserving operation performed. Because UC is a mucosal disease, the rectal mucosa can be dissected out and removed down to the dentate line of the anus or about 2 cm proximal to it. The ileum is fashioned into a pouch that serves as a neorectum. This ileal pouch is then sutured circumferentially to the anus in an end-to-end fashion. If performed carefully, this operation preserves the anal sphincter and maintains continence. The overall operative morbidity is 10%, with the major complication being bowel obstruction. Pouch failure necessitating conversion to permanent ileostomy occurs in 5 to 10% of patients. Some inflamed rectal mucosa is usually left behind, and thus endoscopic surveillance is necessary. Primary dysplasia of the ileal mucosa of the pouch has occurred rarely.

Patients with IPAAs usually have about six to eight bowel movements a day. On validated quality-of-life indices, they report better performance in sports and sexual activities than ileostomy patients. The most frequent late complication of IPAA is pouchitis in about one-third of patients with UC. This syndrome consists of increased stool frequency, watery stools, cramping, urgency, nocturnal leakage of stool, arthralgias, malaise, and fever. Pouch biopsies and pANCA/ASCA/OMPC serologies can distinguish true pouchitis from underlying CD. Although it usually responds to antibiotics, in 3 to 5% of patients it is refractory and requires pouch take-down.

Crohn's Disease Most patients with CD require at least one operation in their lifetime. The need for surgery is related to duration of disease and the site of involvement. Patients with small-bowel disease have an 80% chance of requiring surgery. Those with colitis alone have a 50% chance. The indications for surgery are shown in Table 276-7.

SMALL INTESTINAL DISEASE Because CD is chronic and recurrent with no clear surgical cure, as little intestine as possible is resected. Current surgical alternatives for treatment of obstructing CD include resection of the diseased segment and strictureplasty. Surgical resection of the diseased segment is the most frequently performed operation, and in most cases primary anastomosis can be done to restore continuity. If much of the small bowel has already been resected and the strictures are short with intervening areas of normal mucosa, strictureplasties should be done to avoid a functionally insufficient length of bowel. The strictured area of intestine is incised longitudinally and the incision sutured transversely, thus widening the narrowed area. Complications of strictureplasty include prolonged ileus, hemorrhage, fistula, abscess, leak, and restricture.

COLORECTAL DISEASE A greater percentage of patients with Crohn's colitis require surgery for intractability, fulminant disease, and anorectal disease. Several alternatives are available, ranging from the use of a temporary loop ileostomy to resection of segments of diseased colon or even the entire colon and rectum. For patients with segmental involvement, segmental colon resection with primary anastomosis can be performed. In 20 to 25% of patients with extensive colitis, the rectum is spared sufficiently to consider rectal preservation. Most surgeons believe that an IPAA is contraindicated in CD due to the high incidence of pouch failure. A diverting colostomy may help heal severe perianal disease or rectovaginal fistulas, but disease almost always recurs with reanastomosis. Often, these patients require a total proctocolectomy and ileostomy.

INFLAMMATORY BOWEL DISEASE AND PREGNANCY

Patients with quiescent UC and CD have normal fertility rates; the fallopian tubes can be scarred by the inflammatory process of CD, especially on the right side because of the proximity of the terminal ileum. In addition, perirectal, perineal, and rectovaginal abscesses and fistulae can result in dyspareunia. Infertility in men can be caused by sulfasalazine but reverses when treatment is stopped.

TABLE 276-7 *Indications for Surgery*

Ulcerative Colitis	Crohn's Disease
Intractable disease	CD of Small Intestine
Fulminant disease	Stricture and obstruction
Toxic megacolon	unresponsive to medical
Colonic perforation	therapy
Massive colonic hemorrhage	Massive hemorrhage
Extracolonic disease	Refractory fistula
Colonic obstruction	Abscess
Colon cancer prophylaxis	CD of Colon and Rectum
Colon dysplasia or cancer	Intractable disease
	Fulminant disease
	Perianal disease unresponsive to
	medical therapy
	Refractory fistula
	Colonic obstruction
	Cancer prophylaxis
	Colon dysplasia or cancer

In mild or quiescent UC and CD, fetal outcome is nearly normal. Spontaneous abortions, stillbirths, and developmental defects are increased with increased disease activity, not medications. The courses of CD and UC during pregnancy mostly correlate with disease activity at the time of conception. Patients should be in remission for 6 months before conceiving. Most CD patients can deliver vaginally, but cesarean section may be the preferred route of delivery for patients with anorectal and perirectal abscesses and fistulas to reduce the likelihood of fistulas developing or extending into the episiotomy scar.

Sulfasalazine, mesalamine, and balsalazide are safe for use in pregnancy and nursing, but folate supplementation must be given with sulfasalazine. Topical 5-ASA agents are also safe during pregnancy and nursing. Glucocorticoids are generally safe for use during pregnancy and are indicated for patients with moderate to severe disease activity. The amount of glucocorticoids received by the nursing infant is minimal. The safest antibiotics to use for CD in pregnancy for short periods of time (weeks, not months) are ampicillin, cephalosporin, or flagyl. Ciprofloxacin causes cartilage lesions in immature animals and should be avoided because of the absence of data on its effects on growth and development in humans.

6-MP and azathioprine pose minimal or no risk during pregnancy, but experience is limited. If the patient cannot be weaned from the drug or has an exacerbation that requires 6-MP/azathioprine during pregnancy, she should continue the drug with informed consent. Their effects during nursing are unknown.

Little data exist on cyclosporine in pregnancy. In a small number of patients with severe IBD treated with intravenous cyclosporine during pregnancy, 80% of pregnancies were successfully completed without development of renal toxicity, congenital malformations, or developmental defects. However, because of the lack of data, cyclosporine should probably be avoided unless the patient would otherwise require surgery. Methotrexate is contraindicated in pregnancy and nursing. Based on 35 reported pregnancies, infliximab does not appear to present a risk to the mother or baby.

Surgery in UC should be performed only for emergency indications, including severe hemorrhage, perforation, and megacolon refractory to medical therapy. Total colectomy and ileostomy carry a 60% risk of postoperative spontaneous abortion. Fetal mortality is also high in CD requiring surgery. Patients with IPAAs have increased nighttime stool frequency during pregnancy that resolves post-partum. Transient small-bowel obstruction or ileus has been noted in up to 8% of patients with ileostomies.

INFLAMMATORY BOWEL DISEASE IN THE ELDERLY

The most common presenting symptoms in the elderly are diarrhea, weight loss, and abdominal pain. CD in the elderly mostly affects the colon with a distal distribution and occurs predominantly in women. Proctitis has been documented in 50% of elderly patients, and the diagnosis is often delayed. Diseases that can mimic CD in the elderly are ischemic colitis, diverticular disease, irritable bowel, infectious colitides, and malignancies, including carcinoma, lymphoma, and carcinoid. The incidence of surgery is high in elderly patients, with up to 50% of patients with ileitis, ileocolitis, or extensive colitis requiring urgent or early surgery for first-time disease. In addition, surgery has a much higher morbidity than in younger patients, although the rate of postoperative recurrence is less. Most elderly patients respond as well as younger individuals to medical management.

UC in the elderly is more common in men, presents usually with diarrhea and weight loss, and may have a more distal distribution than in younger patients. Most elderly patients have a favorable response to medical therapy, especially 5-ASA agents, and immunosuppressives used in conjunction with low doses of glucocorticoids. Cyclosporine has been used more frequently in the elderly, but the age-related decreases in renal clearance may affect dosing. Glucocorticoid complications such as osteoporosis and hyperglycemia are also increased in the elderly. 6-MP and azathioprine are well tolerated in the elderly.

Surgery also has a higher morbidity and mortality in UC, and elderly patients have a longer hospital stay than younger patients. The risk of colon cancer in UC and Crohn's colitis is no greater than that in the general population since the duration of disease is short and the extent of disease is often distal.

CANCER IN INFLAMMATORY BOWEL DISEASE

ULCERATIVE COLITIS Patients with long-standing UC are at increased risk for developing colonic epithelial dysplasia and carcinoma (Fig. 276-8). Several features distinguish sporadic colon cancer (SCC) and colitis-associated colon cancer (CAC). First, SCCs usually arise from an adenomatous polyp; CACs typically arise from either flat dysplasia or a dysplasia-associated lesion or mass (DALM). Second, multiple synchronous colon cancers occur in 3 to 5% of SCC but in 12% of CAC. Third, the mean age of individuals with SCC is in the sixties; the mean age of those with CAC is in the thirties. Fourth, SCC exhibits a left-sided predominance, whereas CAC is distributed more uniformly throughout the colon. Fifth, mucinous and anaplastic cancers are more common in CAC than SCC. At the molecular level, p53 mutations occur much earlier and *APC* gene mutations much later in CAC than in SCC.

The risk of neoplasia in chronic UC increases with duration and extent of disease. For patients with pancolitis, the risk of cancer rises 0.5 to 1% per year after 8 to 10 years of disease. This observed increase in cancer rates has led to the endorsement of surveillance colonoscopy with biopsies for patients with chronic UC as the standard of care. Annual or biennial colonoscopy with multiple biopsies has been advocated for patients with >8 to 10 years of pancolitis or 12 to 15 years of left-sided colitis and has been widely employed to screen and survey for subsequent dysplasia and carcinoma.

CROHN'S DISEASE Risk factors for developing colorectal cancer in CD are a history of colonic (or ileocolonic) involvement and long disease duration. The cancer risks in CD and UC are probably equivalent for similar extent and duration of disease. In patients with extensive

FIGURE 276-8   Low-power transition between dysplasia (D) and nondysplastic (N) mucosa in a case of ulcerative colitis. (*Courtesy of Dr. EK Rosado and Dr. CA Perkos, Division of Gastrointestinal Pathology, Department of Pathology, Emory University, Atlanta, Georgia.*)

Crohn's colitis, 22% developed dysplasia or cancer by the fourth surveillance exam after a negative screening colonoscopy. Thus, the same endoscopic surveillance strategy used for UC is recommended for patients with chronic Crohn's colitis. A pediatric colonoscope can be used to pass narrow strictures in CD patients, but surgery should be considered in symptomatic patients with impassable strictures.

MANAGEMENT OF DYSPLASIA AND CANCER Dysplasia can be flat or polypoid. If flat high-grade dysplasia (HGD) is encountered on colonoscopic surveillance, the usual treatment for UC is colectomy and for CD is either colectomy or segmental resection. If flat low-grade dysplasia (LGD) is found, most investigators recommend immediate colectomy. Adenomas may occur coincidently in UC and CD patients with chronic colitis and can be removed endoscopically provided that biopsies of the surrounding mucosa are free of dysplasia.

IBD patients are also at greater risk for other malignancies. Patients with CD may have an increased risk of developing non-Hodgkin's lymphoma and squamous cell carcinoma of the skin. Although CD patients have a twelvefold increased risk of developing small-bowel cancer, this type of carcinoma is extremely rare.

QUALITY OF LIFE IN INFLAMMATORY BOWEL DISEASE

The assessment of health-related quality of life plays an important role in the evaluation and treatment of IBD patients. Although clinical trials have generally relied upon traditional disease activity indices such as the Crohn's Disease Activity Index (CDAI) to measure therapeutic efficacy, these measures do not reflect quality of life. The Inflammatory Bowel Disease Questionnaire (IBDQ) is a validated, disease-specific instrument that has been used to measure quality of life. It is a 32-item questionnaire that measures global function, systemic and bowel symptoms, functional and social impairment, and emotional function. When compared to the general population, IBD patients have an impaired quality of life in all six categories. The most frequent concerns of UC patients are having an ostomy bag, developing cancer, effects of medication, the uncertain nature of the disease, and having surgery. The most frequent concerns of CD patients are the uncertain nature of the disease, energy level, effects of medication, having surgery, and having an ostomy bag.

FURTHER READING

CHEUNG O, REGUEIRO D: Inflammatory bowel disease emergencies. Gastroenterol Clin North Am 32:1269, 2003

FRASER AG et al: The efficacy of azathioprine for the treatment of inflammatory bowel disease: A 30-year review. Gut 50:485, 2002

FRIEDMAN S et al: Screening and surveillance colonoscopy in chronic Crohn's colitis. Gastroenterology 120:820, 2001

HANAUER SB, SANBORN W: Management of Crohn's disease in adults. Am J Gastroenterol 96:635, 2001

HUGOT JP et al: Association of NOD2 leucine-rich repeat variants with susceptibility to Crohn's disease. Nature 411:599, 2001

ITZKOWITZ SH: Cancer prevention in patients with inflammatory bowel disease. Gastroenterol Clin North Am 31:1133, 2002

KORNBLUTH A, SACHAR DB: Ulcerative colitis practice guidelines in adults. Am J Gastroenterol 92:204, 1997

NAVARRO F, HANAUER SB: Treatment of inflammatory bowel disease: Safety and tolerability issues. Am J Gastroenterol 98(Suppl 12):518, 2003

277 IRRITABLE BOWEL SYNDROME
Chung Owyang

Irritable bowel syndrome (IBS) is a gastrointestinal (GI) disorder characterized by altered bowel habits and abdominal pain in the absence of detectable structural abnormalities. No clear diagnostic markers exist for IBS, thus all definitions of the disease are based on the clinical presentation. The Rome II criteria for the diagnosis of IBS are summarized in Table 277-1. It is one of the most common conditions encountered in clinical practice but one of the least well understood. Until recently, many physicians did not consider IBS to be a disease at all; they viewed it as nothing more than a somatic manifestation of psychological stress. With the availability of better techniques to study colonic and GI motility and visceral sensory function, along with the development of newer concepts on the importance of the brain in regulating gut function, significant progress has been made toward a better understanding of the pathogenesis of IBS. This may result in improved methods of treatment.

CLINICAL FEATURES IBS is a disorder of the young, with most new patients presenting before age 45. However, some reports suggest that the elderly are troubled by IBS symptoms up to 92% as often as middle-aged persons. Indeed, many of the diagnoses of "painful diverticular disease" given to elderly patients may represent IBS. Women are diagnosed with IBS two to three times as often as men. Moreover, women make up 80% of the population with severe IBS. Patients with IBS fall into two broad clinical groups. Most commonly, patients have abdominal pain associated with altered bowel habits that consist of constipation, diarrhea, or both. In the second group, patients have painless diarrhea. This symptom in this group, who account for <20% of patients with IBS, may be caused by a separate entity. In fact, painless diarrhea does not strictly fulfill the Rome II criteria to be classified as IBS.

Abdominal Pain According to the Rome II criteria, abdominal pain or discomfort is a prerequisite clinical feature of IBS. Abdominal pain in IBS is highly variable in intensity and location; it is localized to the hypogastrium in 25%, the right side in 20%, to the left side in 20%, and the epigastrium in 10% of patients. It is frequently episodic and crampy, but it may be superimposed on a background of constant ache. Pain may be mild enough to be ignored or it may interfere with daily activities. Despite this, malnutrition due to inadequate caloric intake is exceedingly rare with IBS. Sleep deprivation is also unusual because abdominal pain is almost uniformly present only during waking hours. However, patients with severe IBS often wake repeatedly during the night, and, hence, nocturnal pain is a poor discriminating factor between organic and functional bowel disease. Pain is often exacerbated by eating or emotional stress and relieved by passage of flatus or stools. Female patients with IBS commonly report worsening symptoms during the premenstrual and menstrual phases.

Altered Bowel Habits Alteration in bowel habits is the most consistent clinical feature in IBS. It usually begins in adult life. The most common pattern is constipation alternating with diarrhea, usually with one of these symptoms predominating. At first, constipation may be episodic, but eventually it becomes continuous and increasingly intractable to treatment with laxatives. Stools are usually hard with narrowed caliber, possibly reflecting excessive dehydration caused by prolonged colonic retention and spasm. Most patients also experience a sense of incomplete evacuation, leading to repeated attempts at defecation in a short time span. Patients whose predominant symptom is constipation may have weeks or months of constipation interrupted with brief periods of diarrhea. In other patients, diarrhea may be the predominant symptom. Diarrhea resulting from IBS usually consists of small volumes of loose stools. Most patients have stool volumes of <200 mL.

TABLE 277-1 Rome II Criteria for the Diagnosis of IBS

At least 12 weeks, which need not be consecutive, in the preceding 12 months of abdominal discomfort or pain that has two of following three features:
1. Relieved by defecation
2. Onset associated with changes in stool frequency
3. Onset associated with changes in stool form

Nocturnal diarrhea does not occur in IBS. Diarrhea may be aggravated by emotional stress or eating. Stool may be accompanied by passage of large amounts of mucus; hence, the term *mucous colitis* has been used to describe IBS. This is a misnomer, since inflammation is not present. Bleeding is not a feature of IBS unless hemorrhoids are present, and malabsorption or weight loss does not occur.

Gas and Flatulence   Patients with IBS frequently complain of abdominal distention and increased belching or flatulence, all of which they attribute to increased gas. Although some patients with these symptoms actually may have a larger amount of gas, quantitative measurements reveal that most patients who complain of increased gas generate no more than a normal amount of intestinal gas. Studies have shown that most IBS patients have impaired transit and tolerance of intestinal gas loads. In addition, patients with IBS tend to reflux gas from the distal to the more proximal intestine, which may explain the belching.

Upper Gastrointestinal Symptoms   Between 25 and 50% of patients with IBS complain of dyspepsia, heartburn, nausea, and vomiting. This suggests that other areas of the gut apart from the colon may be involved. Prolonged ambulant recordings of small-bowel motility in patients with IBS show a high incidence of abnormalities in the small bowel during the diurnal (waking) period; nocturnal motor patterns are no different from those of healthy controls. A great deal of overlap is seen between dyspepsia and IBS. The prevalence of IBS is higher among individuals with dyspepsia (31.7%) than among those who report no symptoms of dyspepsia (7.9%). Conversely among those with IBS, 55.6% report symptoms of dyspepsia. In addition, the functional abdominal symptoms can change over time. Those with predominant dyspepsia or IBS can fluctuate between the two. Thus, functional dyspepsia and IBS may be two manifestations of a single, more extensive digestive system disorder. Furthermore, IBS symptoms are prevalent in noncardiac chest pain patients, suggesting overlap with other functional gut disorders.

PATHOPHYSIOLOGY   The pathogenesis of IBS is poorly understood, although roles for abnormal gut motor and sensory activity, central neural dysfunction, psychological disturbances, stress, and luminal factors have been proposed.

Studies of colonic myoelectrical and motor activity under unstimulated conditions have not shown consistent abnormalities in IBS. In contrast, colonic motor abnormalities are more prominent under stimulated conditions in IBS. IBS patients may exhibit increased rectosigmoid motor activity for up to 3 h after eating. Provocative stimuli also induce exaggerated colonic motor responses in IBS patients compared with healthy volunteers. For example, inflation of rectal balloons both in diarrhea- and constipation-predominant IBS patients leads to marked distention-evoked contractile activity, which may be prolonged. Recording from the transverse, descending, and sigmoid colon shows that the motility index and peak amplitude of high-amplitude propagating contractions in diarrhea-prone IBS patients are greatly increased compared to healthy subjects. These contractions are associated with rapid colonic transit and accompanied by abdominal pain.

As with studies of motor activity, IBS patients frequently exhibit exaggerated sensory responses to visceral stimulation. Postprandial pain has been temporally related to the entry of the food bolus into the cecum in 74% of patients. Exaggerated symptoms can be induced by visceral distention in IBS patients. Rectal balloon inflation produces nonpainful and painful sensations at lower volumes in IBS patients than in healthy controls without altering rectal tension, suggestive of visceral afferent dysfunction in IBS. The visceral hyperalgesia of IBS appears to be selective for mechanoreceptor-activated stimuli, as perception of intestinal mucosal electrical stimulation is normal in IBS. Similar studies show gastric and esophageal hypersensitivity in patients with nonulcer dyspepsia and noncardiac chest pain, raising the possibility that these conditions have a similar pathophysiologic basis. Lipids lower the thresholds for the first sensation of gas, discomfort, and pain in IBS patients. Furthermore, IBS patients have an increased

area of referred pain after lipid ingestion that is not observed in healthy subjects. Hence, postprandial symptoms in IBS patients may be explained in part by a nutrient-dependent exaggerated sensory component of the gastrocolonic response. In contrast to enhanced gut sensitivity, IBS patients do not exhibit heightened sensitivity elsewhere in the body. Thus the afferent pathway disturbances in IBS appear to be selective for visceral innervation, with sparing of somatic pathways. The mechanisms responsible for visceral hypersensitivity are still under investigation. These exaggerated responses may be due to (1) increased end-organ sensitivity with recruitment of "silent" nociceptors, (2) spinal hyperexcitability with activation of nitric oxide and possibly other neurotransmitters, (3) endogenous (cortical and brainstem) modulation of caudad nociceptive transmission, and (4) over time, the possible development of long-term hyperalgesia due to development of neuroplasticity, resulting in permanent or semipermanent changes in neural responses to chronic or recurrent visceral stimulation (Table 277-2).

The role of central nervous system (CNS) factors in the pathogenesis of IBS is strongly suggested by the clinical association of emotional disorders and stress with symptom exacerbation and the therapeutic response to therapies that act on cerebral cortical sites. Positron emission tomography has been employed to quantify regional cerebral blood flow in IBS. In healthy individuals, rectal distention increases blood flow in the anterior cingulate cortex, a region with an abundance of opiate receptors, which, when activated, may help to reduce sensory input. In contrast, IBS patients exhibit no increased blood flow in the anterior cingulate gyrus but show activation of the prefrontal cortex, either in response to rectal activation or in anticipation of rectal distention. Activation of the frontal lobes may activate a vigilance network within the brain that increases alertness. The anterior cingulate cortex and the prefrontal cortex appear to have reciprocal inhibitory associations. Thus, in patients with IBS, the preferential activation of the prefrontal lobe, without activation of the anterior cingulate cortex, may represent a form of cerebral dysfunction leading to the increased perception of visceral pain.

Abnormal psychiatric features are recorded in up to 80% of IBS patients, especially in referral centers; however, no single psychiatric diagnosis predominates. Most of these patients demonstrate exaggerated symptoms in response to visceral distention, and this abnormality persists even after exclusion of psychological factors. Psychological factors also influence pain thresholds in IBS patients; stress alters sensory thresholds. An association between prior sexual or physical abuse and development of IBS has been reported. Forms of sexual abuse associated with IBS include verbal aggression, exhibitionism, sexual harassment, sexual touching, and rape. The pathophysiologic relationship between IBS and sexual or physical abuse is unknown. Sexual abuse is not associated with a lower pain threshold in IBS patients.

Thus, patients with IBS frequently demonstrate increased motor reactivity of the colon and small bowel to a variety of stimuli and altered visceral sensation associated with lowered sensation thresholds. These may result from CNS or enteric nervous system dysregulation.

IBS may be induced by gastrointestinal infection. In an investigation of 544 patients with confirmed bacterial gastroenteritis, one-quarter subsequently developed IBS. Conversely, about a third of IBS patients experienced an acute "gastroenteritis-like" illness at the onset of their chronic IBS symptomatology. This "postinfective" IBS occurs more commonly in women and affects younger, rather than older, patients and those who have a protracted acute diarrheal illness. The

TABLE 277-2   *Proposed Mechanisms for Visceral Hypersensitivity*

End-organ sensitivity	Long-term hyperalgesia
"Silent" nociceptors	Tonic cortical regulation
CNS modulation	Neuroplasticity
Cortex	
Brainstem	

Note: CNS, central nervous system.

microbes involved in the initial infection are *Campylobacter*, *Salmonella*, and *Shigella*. Those patients infected with *Campylobacter* who are toxin-positive are more likely to develop postinfective IBS. Increased rectal mucosal enteroendocrine cells, T lymphocytes, and gut permeability are acute changes following *Campylobacter* enteritis that could persist for more than a year and may contribute to postinfective IBS.

The serotonin (5HT)-containing enterochromaffin cells in the colon are increased in diarrhea-predominant IBS patients compared to healthy subjects or to patients with ulcerative colitis. Furthermore, postprandial plasma 5HT plasma levels are significantly higher in diarrhea-predominant IBS patients compared to healthy controls. As 5HT plays an important role in the regulation of GI motility and visceral perception, the increased release of 5HT may contribute to the postprandial symptoms of these patients and provides a rationale for the use of 5HT antagonists in the treatment of this disorder.

APPROACH TO THE PATIENT

Because IBS is a disorder for which no pathognomonic abnormalities have been identified, its diagnosis relies on recognition of positive clinical features and elimination of other organic diseases. A careful history and physical examination are frequently helpful in establishing the diagnosis. Clinical features suggestive of IBS include the following: recurrence of lower abdominal pain with altered bowel habits over a period of time without progressive deterioration, onset of symptoms during periods of stress or emotional upset, absence of other systemic symptoms such as fever and weight loss, and small-volume stool without any evidence of blood.

On the other hand, the appearance of the disorder for the first time in old age, a progressive course from time of onset, persistent diarrhea after a 48-h fast, and presence of nocturnal diarrhea or steatorrheal stools argue against the diagnosis of IBS.

Because the major symptoms of IBS—abdominal pain, abdominal bloating, and alteration in bowel habits—are common complaints of many GI organic disorders, the list of differential diagnoses is long. The quality, location, and timing of pain may be helpful in suggesting specific disorders. Pain due to IBS that occurs in the epigastric or periumbilical area must be differentiated from biliary tract disease, peptic ulcer disorders, intestinal ischemia, and carcinoma of the stomach and pancreas. If pain occurs mainly in the lower abdomen, the possibility of diverticular disease of the colon, inflammatory bowel disease (including ulcerative colitis and Crohn's disease), and carcinoma of the colon must be considered. Postprandial pain accompanied by bloating, nausea, and vomiting suggests gastroparesis or partial intestinal obstruction. Intestinal infestation with *Giardia lamblia* or other parasites may cause similar symptoms. When diarrhea is the major complaint, the possibility of lactase deficiency, laxative abuse, malabsorption, hyperthyroidism, inflammatory bowel disease, or infectious diarrhea must be ruled out. On the other hand, constipation may be a side effect of many different drugs, such as anticholinergic, antihypertensive, and antidepressant medications. Endocrinopathies such as hypothyroidism and hypoparathyroidism must also be considered in the differential diagnosis of constipation, particularly if other systemic signs or symptoms of these endocrinopathies are present. In addition, acute intermittent porphyria and lead poisoning may present in a fashion similar to that of IBS, with painful constipation as the major complaint. These possibilities are suspected on the basis of their clinical presentations and are confirmed by appropriate serum and urine tests.

Because IBS is in part a diagnosis of exclusion, certain diagnostic tests should be performed routinely; others may be required depending on the specific presenting symptoms. The American Gastroenterological Association has delineated factors to be considered when determining the aggressiveness of the diagnostic evaluation. These include the duration of symptoms, the change in symptoms over time, the age and sex of the patient, the referral status of the patient, prior diagnostic studies, a family history of colorectal malignancy, and the degree of psychosocial dysfunction. Thus, a younger individual with mild symptoms requires a minimal diagnostic evaluation, while an older person or an individual with rapidly progressive symptoms should undergo a more thorough exclusion of organic disease. Most patients should have a complete blood count and sigmoidoscopic examination; in addition, stool specimens should be examined for ova and parasites. In those older than 40 years, an air-contrast barium enema or colonoscopy should also be performed. If the main symptoms are diarrhea and increased gas, the possibility of lactase deficiency should be ruled out with a hydrogen breath test or with evaluation after a 3-week lactose-free diet. In patients with concurrent symptoms of dyspepsia, upper GI radiographs or esophagogastroduodenoscopy may be advisable. In patients with postprandial right upper quadrant pain, an ultrasonogram of the gallbladder should be obtained. Laboratory features that argue against IBS include evidence of anemia, elevated sedimentation rate, presence of leukocytes or blood in stool, and stool volume >200 to 300 mL/d. These findings would necessitate other diagnostic considerations.

℞ TREATMENT

Patient Counseling and Dietary Alterations Reassurance and careful explanation of the functional nature of the disorder and of how to avoid obvious food precipitants are important first steps in patient counseling and dietary change. Occasionally, a meticulous dietary history may reveal substances (such as coffee, disaccharides, legumes, and cabbage) that aggravate symptoms. As a therapeutic trial, patients should be encouraged to eliminate any foodstuffs that appear to produce symptoms.

Stool-Bulking Agents High-fiber diets and bulking agents, such as bran or hydrophilic colloid, are frequently used in treating IBS. Dietary fiber has multiple effects on colonic physiology. The water-holding action of fiber may contribute to increased stool bulk because of the ability of fiber to increase fecal output of bacteria. Fiber also speeds up colonic transit in most persons. In diarrhea-prone patients, whole colonic transit is faster than average; however, dietary fiber can delay transit. Furthermore, because of their hydrophilic properties, stool-bulking agents bind water and thus prevent both excessive hydration or dehydration of stool. The latter observation may explain the clinical experience that a high-fiber diet relieves diarrhea in some IBS patients. More recently, fiber supplementation with psyllium has been shown to reduce perception of rectal distention, indicating that fiber may have a positive affect on visceral afferent function.

The beneficial effects of dietary fiber on colonic physiology suggest that dietary fiber should be an effective treatment for IBS patients, but controlled trials of dietary fiber have produced variable results. This is not surprising since IBS is a heterogeneous disorder, with some patients being constipated and others having predominant diarrhea. Most investigations report increases in stool weight, decreases in colonic transit times, and improvement in constipation. Others have noted benefits in patients with alternating diarrhea and constipation, pain, and bloating; however, most studies observe no responses in patients with diarrhea- or pain-predominant IBS. Different fiber preparations may have dissimilar effects on selected symptoms in IBS. A crossover comparison of different fiber preparations found that psyllium produced greater improvements in stool pattern and abdominal pain than bran. Furthermore, psyllium preparations tend to produce less bloating and distention. Despite the equivocal data regarding efficacy, most gastroenterologists consider stool-bulking agents worth trying in patients with IBS.

Antispasmodics Clinicians have observed that anticholinergic drugs may provide temporary relief for symptoms such as painful cramps related to intestinal spasm. Although controlled clinical trials have produced mixed results, evidence generally supports beneficial effects of anticholinergic drugs for pain. A meta-analysis of 26 double-blind clinical trials of antispasmodic agents in IBS reported better global improvement (62%) and abdominal pain reduction (64%) compared to placebo (35% and 45%, respectively), indicative of their symptomatic efficacy. The drugs are most effective when prescribed in anticipation of predictable pain. Physiologic studies demonstrate that anticholinergic drugs inhibit the gastrocolic reflex; hence, postprandial pain is best managed by giving antispasmodics 30 min before meals so that effective blood levels are achieved shortly before the anticipated onset of pain. Most anticholinergics contain natural belladonna alkaloids, which may cause xerostomia, urinary hesitancy and retention, blurred vision, and drowsiness. Some physicians prefer to use synthetic anticholinergics such as dicyclomine that have less effect on mucous membrane secretions and therefore produce fewer undesirable side effects.

Antidiarrheal Agents Peripherally acting opiate-based agents are the initial therapy of choice for diarrhea-predominant IBS. Physiologic studies demonstrate increases in segmenting colonic contractions, delays in fecal transit, increases in anal pressures, and reductions in rectal perception with these drugs. When diarrhea is severe, especially in the painless diarrhea variant of IBS, small doses of diphenoxylate (Lomotil), 2.5 to 5 mg every 4 to 6 h, can be prescribed. These agents are less addictive than paregoric, codeine, or tincture of opium. In general, the intestines do not become tolerant of the antidiarrheal effect of opiates, and increasing doses are not required to maintain antidiarrheal potency. These agents are most useful if taken before anticipated stressful events that are known to cause diarrhea. Treatment with antidiarrheals, however, should be considered only as temporary management; the final goal of treatment is gradual withdrawal of medication with substitution of a high-fiber diet.

Antidepressant Drugs In addition to their mood-elevating effects, antidepressant medications have several physiologic effects that may be beneficial in IBS. In diarrhea-predominant IBS patients, the tricyclic antidepressant imipramine slows jejunal migrating motor complex transit propagation and delays orocecal and whole-gut transit, indicative of a motor inhibitory effect. Tricyclic agents may also alter visceral afferent neural function.

Tricyclic antidepressants may be effective in some IBS patients. In a 2-month study of desipramine, abdominal pain improved in 86% of patients compared to 59% given a placebo. Another study of desipramine in 28 IBS patients showed improvement in stool frequency, diarrhea, pain, and depression. Improvements were observed mainly in diarrhea-predominant patients, with no improvement being noted in constipated patients. The beneficial effects of the tricyclic compounds in the treatment of IBS appear to be independent of their antidepression actions. The therapeutic benefits for the bowel symptoms occur faster and at a lower dosage. The efficacy of other classes of antidepressant agents in the management of IBS is less well evaluated. The selective serotonin reuptake inhibitor (SSRI) paroxetine accelerates orocecal transit, raising the possibility that this drug class may be useful in constipation-predominant patients. The SSRI citalopram blunts perception of rectal distention and reduces the magnitude of the gastrocolonic response in healthy volunteers. A small placebo-controlled study of citalopram in IBS patients reported reductions in pain. An

FIGURE 277-1 Therapeutic targets for irritable bowel syndrome. Patients with mild to moderate symptoms usually have intermittent symptoms that correlate with altered gut physiology. Treatments include gut-acting pharmacologic agents such as antispasmodics, antidiarrheals, fiber supplements, and gut serotonin modulators. Patients who have severe symptoms usually have constant pain and psychosocial difficulties. This group of patients are best managed with antidepressants and other psychological treatments. CNS, central nervous system; ENS, enteric nervous system.

investigation of mianserin, with serotonin $5HT_2$ and $5HT_3$ receptor antagonist and α_2-adrenoceptor antagonist effects, reported reductions in pain, distress, and functional disability compared to placebo. Despite these preliminary results, the efficacy of SSRIs in the treatment of IBS still needs further confirmation.

Antiflatulence Therapy The management of excessive gas is seldom satisfactory, except in obvious aerophagia or disaccharidase deficiency. Patients should be advised to eat slowly; avoid chewing gum or drinking carbonated beverages; and avoid consuming artificial sweeteners, legumes, and foods of the cabbage family. Simethicone, antacids, and activated charcoal have all been tried, usually with disappointing results.

Serotonin Receptor Agonists and Antagonists Serotonin receptor antagonists have been evaluated as therapies for diarrhea-predominant IBS. Serotonin acting on $5HT_3$ receptors enhances the sensitivity of afferent neurons projecting from the gut. In humans, a $5HT_3$ receptor antagonist such as alosetron reduces perception of painful visceral stimulation in IBS. It also induces rectal relaxation, increases rectal compliance, and delays colonic transit. Large, 12-week, placebo-controlled trials of alosetron reported reductions in discomfort and improvements in stool frequency, consistency, and urgency in nonconstipated IBS patients. A follow-up 48-week study confirmed the long-term efficacy of alosetron. For unclear reasons, women with IBS derived greater benefit than men. However, in postrelease surveillance, 70 cases of ischemic colitis were observed, including 10 cases requiring surgery and 3 deaths. As a consequence, the medication was voluntarily withdrawn by the manufacturer. Preliminary studies in nonconstipated IBS patients of a newer $5HT_3$ receptor antagonist, cilansetron, have shown similar improvements in abdominal pain and diarrhea as alosetron. Follow-up investigation will determine if side effects also undermine the utility of this agent.

Novel $5HT_4$ receptor agonists exhibit prokinetic activity by stimulating peristalsis. In IBS patients with constipation, tegaserod accelerated intestinal and ascending colon transit. Clinical trials involving >4000 constipation-predominant IBS patients have reported reductions in discomfort and improvements in constipation and bloating compared to placebo. Other than diarrhea, no other significant side effects were noted. Tegaserod has been approved for the treatment of constipation-predominant IBS.

Summary The treatment strategy of IBS depends on the severity of the disorder (Table 277-3). Most IBS patients have mild symptoms. They are usually cared for in primary care practices and have little or no psychosocial difficulties and do not seek health care often. Treatment usually involves education, reassurance, and dietary/lifestyle changes. A smaller proportion have moderate symptoms that are usually intermittent and correlate with altered gut physiology, such as worsening with eating or stress and relieved by defecation. Treatments include

TABLE 277-3 *Spectrum of Severity in IBS*

	Mild	Moderate	Severe
Clinical features			
Prevalence	70%	25%	5%
Correlation with gut physiology	+++	++	+
Symptoms constant	0	+	+++
Psychosocial difficulties	0	+	+++
Health care issues	+	++	+++
Practice type	Primary	Specialty	Referral

gut-acting pharmacologic agents such as antispasmodics, antidiarrheals, fiber supplements, and the newer gut serotonin modulators (Fig. 277-1). A small proportion of IBS patients have severe and refractory symptoms. They are usually seen in referral centers and frequently have constant pain and psychosocial difficulties (Fig. 277-1). This group of patients are best managed with antidepressants and other psychological treatments.

FURTHER READING

AMERICAN GASTROENTEROLOGICAL ASSOCIATION MEDICAL POSITION STATEMENT: Irritable bowel syndrome. Gastroenterology 112:2118, 1997

BUENO L et al: Mediators and pharmacology of visceral sensitivity: from basic to clinical investigations. Gastroenterology 112:1714, 1997

HASLER WL, OWYANG C: Irritable bowel syndrome, in *Textbook of Gastroenterology*, 4th ed, T Yamada (ed). Philadelphia, Lippincott Williams & Wilkins, 2003, pp 1817–1842

JACKSON JL et al: Treatment of functional gastrointestinal disorders with antidepressant medications: A meta-analysis. Am J Med 108:65, 2000

MERTZ H: Irritable bowel syndrome. N Engl J Med 349:2136, 2003

SPILLER RC et al: Increased rectal mucosal enteroendocrine cells, T lymphocytes, and increased gut permeability following acute *Campylobacter* enteritis and in post-dysenteric irritable bowel syndrome. Gut 47:804, 2000

TALLEY NJ: Evaluation of drug treatment for irritable bowel syndrome. Br J Clin Pharmacol 56:362, 2003

278 FAMILIAL MEDITERRANEAN FEVER AND OTHER HEREDITARY RECURRENT FEVERS
Daniel L. Kastner

FAMILIAL MEDITERRANEAN FEVER

Familial Mediterranean fever (FMF) is the prototype of a group of inherited diseases (Table 278-1) that are characterized by recurrent episodes of fever with serosal, synovial, or cutaneous inflammation and, in some individuals, the eventual development of systemic AA amyloidosis (Chap. 310). Because of the relative infrequency of high-titer autoantibodies or antigen-specific T cells, the term *autoinflammatory* has been proposed to describe these disorders.

BACKGROUND AND PATHOPHYSIOLOGY FMF was first recognized among Armenians, Arabs, Turks, and non-Ashkenazi (primarily North African and Iraqi) Jews. With the advent of genetic testing, FMF has been documented with increasing frequency among Ashkenazi Jews and

TABLE 278-1 *The Hereditary Periodic Fever Syndromes*

	FMF	TRAPS	HIDS	MWS	FCAS	NOMID
Ethnicity	Jewish, Arab, Turkish, Armenian, Italian	Any ethnic group	Predominantly Dutch, northern European	Any ethnic group	Any ethnic group	Any ethnic group
Inheritance	Recessive	Dominant	Recessive	Dominant	Dominant	Usually de novo mutations
Gene/chromosome	*MEFV*/16p13.3	*TNFRSF1A*/12p13	*MVK*/12q24	*CIAS1*/1q44	*CIAS1*/1q44	*CIAS1*/1q44
Protein	Pyrin	p55 TNF receptor	Mevalonate kinase	Cryopyrin	Cryopyrin	Cryopyrin
Attack length	1–3 days	Often >7 days	3–7 days	1–2 days	Minutes–3 days	Continuous, with flares
Serosa	Pleurisy, peritonitis; asymptomatic pericardial effusions	Pleurisy, peritonitis, pericarditis	Abd pain, but seldom peritonitis; pleurisy, pericarditis uncommon	Abd pain common; pleurisy, pericarditis rare	Rare	Rare
Skin	Erysipeloid erythema	Centrifugally migrating erythema	Diffuse maculopapular rash; oral, vaginal ulcers	Diffuse urticaria-like rash	Cold-induced urticaria-like rash	Diffuse urticaria-like rash
Joints	Acute monoarthritis; chronic hip arthritis (rare)	Acute monoarthritis, arthralgia	Arthralgia, oligoarthritis	Arthralgia, large-joint oligoarthritis	Polyarthralgia	Epiphyseal, patellar overgrowth, clubbing
Muscle	Exercise-induced myalgia common; protracted febrile myalgia rare	Migratory myalgia	Uncommon	Myalgia common	Sometimes myalgia	Sometimes myalgia
Eyes, ears	Uncommon	Periorbital edema, conjunctivitis, rarely uveitis	Uncommon	Conjunctivitis, episcleritis, optic disc edema; sensorineural hearing loss	Conjunctivitis	Conjunctivitis, uveitis, optic disc edema, blindness, sensorineural hearing loss
CNS	Aseptic meningitis rare	Headache	Headache	Headache	Headache	Aseptic meningitis, seizures
Amyloidosis	Most common in M694V homozygotes	~15% of cases	Not described	~25% of cases	Uncommon	Late complication
Treatment	Oral colchicine prophylaxis	Glucocorticoids, etanercept	NSAIDs for fever; etanercept investigational	NSAIDs, prednisone; anakinra investigational	NSAIDs	Anakinra investigational

Abbreviations: FMF, familial Mediterranean fever; TNF, tumor necrosis factor; TRAPS, TNF receptor-associated periodic syndrome; HIDS, hyperimmunoglobulin D with periodic fever syndrome, MWS, Muckle-Wells syndrome; FCAS, familial cold autoinflammatory syndrome; NOMID; neonatal onset multisystem inflammatory disease; Abd, abdominal; CNS, central nervous system; NSAID, nonsteroidal anti-inflammatory drug.

Italians, and occasional cases have been confirmed even in the absence of known Mediterranean ancestry. FMF is recessively inherited, but, particularly in countries where families are small, a positive family history can be elicited only in ~50% of cases. DNA testing demonstrates carrier frequencies as high as 1:3 among affected populations, suggesting a heterozygote advantage.

The FMF gene was identified by positional cloning in 1997. It encodes a 781-amino acid, ~95-kDa protein denoted *pyrin* (or *marenostrin*) that is expressed in association with the cytoskeleton in granulocytes, eosinophils, and cytokine-activated monocytes. The N-terminal 92 amino acids of pyrin define a motif, the PYRIN domain, similar in structure to death domains, death effector domains, and caspase recruitment domains. PYRIN domains mediate homotypic protein-protein interactions and have been found in several other proteins, including cryopyrin, which is mutated in three other recurrent fever syndromes. Through the interaction of this domain with an intermediary adaptor protein, pyrin regulates caspase-1 [interleukin (IL) 1β-converting enzyme], and thereby IL-1β secretion. Pyrin-deficient mice exhibit heightened sensitivity to endotoxin, excessive IL-1β production, and impaired monocyte apoptosis.

ACUTE ATTACKS Febrile episodes in FMF may begin even in early infancy; 90% of patients have had their first attack by age 20. Typical FMF episodes generally last 24 to 72 h, with arthritic attacks tending to last somewhat longer. In some patients the episodes occur with great regularity, but more often the frequency of attacks varies over time, ranging from as often as once every few days to remissions lasting several years. Attacks are often unpredictable, although some patients relate them to physical exertion, emotional stress, or menses; pregnancy may be associated with remission.

If measured, temperature elevation is nearly always present throughout FMF attacks. Severe hyperpyrexia and even febrile seizures may be seen in infants, and fever is sometimes the only manifestation of FMF in young children.

Over 90% of FMF patients experience abdominal attacks at some time. Episodes range in severity from dull, aching pain and distention with mild tenderness on direct palpation to severe generalized pain with absent bowel sounds, rigidity, rebound tenderness, and air-fluid levels on upright radiographs. Computed tomography (CT) scanning may demonstrate a small amount of fluid in the abdominal cavity. If such patients undergo exploratory laparotomy, a sterile, neutrophil-rich peritoneal exudate is present, sometimes with adhesions from previous episodes. Ascites is rare.

Pleural attacks are usually manifested by unilateral, sharp, stabbing chest pain. Radiographs may show atelectasis and sometimes an effusion; thoracentesis demonstrates an exudative fluid rich in neutrophils. After repeated attacks, pleural thickening may develop.

FMF arthritis is most frequent among individuals homozygous for the M694V mutation, which is especially common in the non-Ashkenazi Jewish population. Acute arthritis in FMF is usually monoarticular, affecting the knee, ankle, or hip, although other patterns can be seen, particularly in children. Large sterile effusions rich in neutrophils are frequent, without commensurate erythema or warmth. Even after repeated arthritic attacks, radiographic changes are rare. Before the advent of colchicine prophylaxis, chronic arthritis of the knee or hip was seen in ~5% of FMF patients with arthritis. Chronic sacroiliitis can occur in FMF irrespective of the HLA-B27 antigen, even in the face of colchicine therapy. In the United States, FMF patients are much more likely to have arthralgia than arthritis.

The most characteristic cutaneous manifestation of FMF is erysipelas-like erythema, a flat, raised erythematous rash that most commonly occurs on the dorsum of the foot, ankle, or lower leg, alone or in combination with abdominal pain, pleurisy, or arthritis. Biopsy demonstrates perivascular infiltrates of granulocytes and monocytes. This rash is seen most often in M694V homozygotes and is relatively rare in the United States.

Exercise-induced (nonfebrile) myalgia is common in FMF, and a small percentage of patients develop a protracted febrile myalgia that can last several weeks. Symptomatic pericardial disease is rare, although some patients have small pericardial effusions as an incidental echocardiographic finding. Unilateral acute scrotal inflammation may occur in prepubertal boys. Aseptic meningitis has been reported, but the causal connection is controversial. Vasculitis, including Henoch-Schönlein purpura and periarteritis nodosum (Chap. 306), may be seen at increased frequency in FMF.

Laboratory features of FMF attacks are consistent with acute inflammation and include an elevated erythrocyte sedimentation rate; leukocytosis; thrombocytosis (in children); and elevations in the C-reactive protein, fibrinogen, haptoglobin, and serum immunoglobulins. Transient albuminuria and hematuria may also be seen.

AMYLOIDOSIS Before the advent of colchicine prophylaxis, systemic amyloidosis was a common complication of FMF. It is caused by deposition of a fragment of serum amyloid A, an acute-phase reactant, in the kidneys, adrenals, intestine, spleen, lung, and testes. Amyloidosis should be suspected in patients who have proteinuria between attacks; renal or rectal biopsy is most often used to establish the diagnosis. Risk factors include the M694V homozygous genotype, positive family history (independent of FMF mutational status), the SAA 1 genotype, male gender, noncompliance with colchicine therapy, and having grown up in the Middle East.

DIAGNOSIS For typical cases, experienced physicians can often make the diagnosis on clinical grounds alone. Clinical criteria for FMF have been shown to have high sensitivity and specificity in parts of the world where the pretest probability of FMF is high. Genetic testing can provide a useful adjunct in ambiguous cases or for physicians not experienced in FMF. Most of the disease-associated FMF mutations are in exon 10 of the gene, with a smaller group of mutations in exon 2. An updated list of mutations for FMF and other hereditary periodic fevers can be found online at *http://fmf.igh.cnrs.fr/infevers/*.

Genetic testing has permitted a broadening of the clinical spectrum and geographic distribution of FMF and may be of prognostic value. Most studies indicate that M694V homozygotes have an earlier age of onset and a higher frequency of arthritis, rash, and amyloidosis. In contrast, the E148Q mutation is usually associated with milder disease. E148Q is sometimes found in *cis* with exon 10 mutations, which complicates the interpretation of genetic test results. Only ~70% of patients with clinically typical FMF have two identifiable mutations in *trans*, suggesting either that current screening methods do not detect all of the relevant mutations or that one mutation may be sufficient for disease under some circumstances. In these cases clinical judgment is very important, and sometimes a therapeutic trial of colchicine may help to confirm the diagnosis. Genetic testing of unaffected individuals is usually inadvisable because of the possibility of nonpenetrance and the potential impact of a positive test on future insurability.

If a patient is seen during their first attack, the differential diagnosis may be broad, although delimited by the specific organ involvement. After several attacks the differential diagnosis may include the other hereditary periodic fever syndromes (Table 278-1); the syndrome of periodic fever with aphthous ulcers, pharyngitis, and cervical adenopathy (PFAPA); systemic-onset juvenile rheumatoid arthritis or adult Still's disease; porphyria; hereditary angioedema; inflammatory bowel disease; and, in women, gynecologic disorders.

℞ TREATMENT

The treatment of choice for FMF is daily oral colchicine, which decreases the frequency and intensity of attacks and prevents the development of amyloidosis in compliant patients. Intermittent dosing at the onset of attacks is not as effective as daily prophylaxis and is of unproven value in preventing amyloidosis. The usual adult dose of colchicine is 1.2 to 1.8 mg/d, which causes substantial reduction in symptoms in two-thirds of patients and some improvement in >90%. Children may require lower doses, although not proportionately to body weight.

Common side effects of colchicine include bloating, abdominal cramps, lactose intolerance, and diarrhea. They can be minimized by starting at a low dose and gradually advancing as tolerated, splitting the dose, use of simethicone for flatulence, and avoidance of dairy products. If taken by either parent at the time of conception, colchicine may cause a small increase in the risk of trisomy 21 (Down syndrome). In elderly patients with renal insufficiency, colchicine can cause a myoncuropathy characterized by proximal muscle weakness and elevation of the creatine kinase. Cyclosporine inhibits hepatic excretion of colchicine by its effects on the MDR-1 transport system, sometimes leading to colchicine toxicity in patients who have undergone renal transplantation for amyloidosis. Intravenous colchicine should generally not be administered to patients already taking oral colchicine, because severe, sometimes fatal, toxicity can occur in this setting.

No alternatives have been established for the small number of patients who do not respond to colchicine or cannot tolerate therapeutic dosages, although interferon-α and tumor necrosis factor (TNF) inhibitors are investigational. Bone marrow transplantation has been suggested for refractory FMF, but the risk-benefit ratio is currently regarded as unacceptable.

OTHER HEREDITARY RECURRENT FEVERS

Within 5 years of the discovery of the FMF gene, three additional genes causing five other hereditary periodic fever syndromes were identified, catalyzing a paradigm shift in diagnosis and treatment of these disorders.

TNF RECEPTOR–ASSOCIATED PERIODIC SYNDROME (TRAPS) TRAPS is caused by dominantly inherited mutations in the extracellular domains of the 55-kDa TNF receptor (TNFRSF1A, p55). Although originally described in a large Irish family (and hence the name *familial Hibernian fever*), TRAPS has a broad ethnic distribution. TRAPS episodes often begin in childhood. The duration of attacks ranges from 1 to 2 days to as long as several weeks, and in severe cases symptoms may be nearly continuous. In addition to peritoneal, pleural, and synovial attacks similar to those in FMF, TRAPS patients frequently have ocular inflammation (most often conjunctivitis and/or periorbital edema) and a distinctive migratory myalgia with overlying painful erythema. TRAPS patients generally respond better to glucocorticoids than to prophylactic colchicine. About 15% develop amyloidosis. The diagnosis of TRAPS is based on the demonstration of *TNFRSF1A* mutations in the presence of characteristic symptoms. Leukocytes from patients with certain TRAPS mutations exhibit a defect in TNF receptor shedding, possibly impairing normal homeostasis and explaining autoinflammatory manifestations. Etanercept, a TNF inhibitor, has been shown to ameliorate TRAPS attacks, although its effect on amyloidosis is unproven.

HYPERIMMUNOGLOBULINEMIA D WITH PERIODIC FEVER SYNDROME (HIDS) HIDS is a recessively inherited recurrent fever syndrome found primarily in individuals of northern European ancestry. It is caused by mutations in mevalonate kinase (*MVK*), encoding an enzyme involved in the synthesis of cholesterol and nonsterol isoprenoids. Attacks usually begin in infancy, and last 3 to 7 days. Clinically distinctive features include painful cervical lymphadenopathy, a diffuse maculopapular rash sometimes affecting the palms and soles, and aphthous ulcers; pleurisy is rare, and amyloidosis has not yet been reported. Although originally defined by the persistent elevation of serum IgD, disease activity is not related to IgD level, and some patients with FMF or TRAPS may have modestly increased serum IgD. Moreover, occasional patients with *MVK* mutations and periodic fever have normal IgD levels. No treatment for HIDS has been established.

THE CRYOPYRINOPATHIES Three hereditary febrile syndromes, familial cold autoinflammatory syndrome (FCAS), Muckle-Wells syndrome (MWS), and neonatal onset multisystem inflammatory disease (NOMID), are all caused by mutations in *CIAS1*, the gene encoding cryopyrin, and represent a clinical spectrum of disease. FCAS patients develop chills, fever, headache, arthralgia, conjunctivitis, and an urticaria-like rash in response to generalized cold exposure. In MWS there is a similar rash, but it is not usually induced by cold. MWS patients also develop fevers, abdominal pain, limb pain, arthritis, conjunctivitis, and, over time, sensorineural hearing loss. NOMID is the most severe of the three disorders, with chronic aseptic meningitis, a characteristic arthropathy, and urticarial rash. Like the FMF protein, pyrin, cryopyrin has an N-terminal PYRIN domain and regulates IL-1β production. Initial therapeutic experience with anakinra, the IL-1 receptor antagonist, in MWS has been encouraging.

FURTHER READING

AKSENTIJEVICH I et al: De novo *CIAS1* mutations, cytokine activation, and evidence for genetic heterogeneity in patients with neonatal-onset multisystem inflammatory disease (NOMID). A new member of the expanding family of pyrin-associated autoinflammatory diseases. Arthritis Rheum 46: 3340, 2002

DRENTH JPII, VAN DER MEER JWM: Hereditary periodic fever. N Engl J Med 345:1748, 2001

HAWKINS PN et al: Interleukin-1-receptor antagonist in the Muckle-Wells syndrome. N Engl J Med 348:2583, 2003

HOFFMAN HM et al: Mutation of a new gene encoding a putative pyrin-like protein causes familial cold autoinflammatory syndrome and Muckle-Wells syndrome. Nat Genet 29:301, 2001

HULL KM et al: The TNF receptor-associated periodic syndrome (TRAPS). Emerging concepts of an autoinflammatory disorder. Medicine (Baltimore) 81:349, 2002

———: The expanding spectrum of systemic autoinflammatory disorders and their rheumatic manifestations. Curr Opin Rheumatol 15:61, 2003

LA REGINA M et al: Familial Mediterranean fever is no longer a rare disease in Italy. Eur J Hum Genet 11:50, 2003

279 COMMON DISEASES OF THE COLON AND ANORECTUM AND MESENTERIC VASCULAR INSUFFICIENCY
Susan L. Gearhart, Gregory Bulkley

COLON

DIVERTICULAR DISEASE ■ Incidence and Epidemiology Among western populations, diverticulosis affects nearly one-half of individuals over age 60. The prevalence among females and males is similar. However, males tend to present at a younger age. Fortunately, only 20% of patients with diverticulosis develop symptomatic disease. Diverticulosis is rare in underdeveloped countries, where diets include more fiber and roughage.

Anatomy and Pathophysiology Two types of diverticula occur in the intestine: true and false, or pseudodiverticula. The most common type of diverticulum affecting the colon is the pseudodiverticulum. This is a herniation or saclike projection of the mucosa through the muscularis propria. The protrusion occurs commonly at the point where the nutrient artery penetrates through the muscularis propria, resulting in a break in the integrity of the colonic wall. Diverticulosis commonly affects the sigmoid colon; only 5% of persons exhibit pancolonic diverticula. This may be a result of the relative high-pressure zone within the sigmoid colon. Thus, higher amplitude contractions combined with constipated, high-fat content stool within the sigmoid lumen results in the creation of these diverticula. *Diverticulitis*, or inflammation of a diverticulum, is related to the retention of particulate material within the diverticular sac and the formation of a fecalith. Consequently, the blood vessel is either compressed or eroded, leading to either perforation or bleeding.

Presentation, Evaluation, and Management of Diverticular Bleeding   Hemorrhage from a colonic diverticulum is the most common cause of hematochezia in patients over the age of 60, yet only 20% of patients with diverticulosis will have gastrointestinal bleeding. Patients at increased risk for bleeding tend to be hypertensive, have atherosclerosis, and regularly use nonsteroidal anti-inflammatory agents. Most bleeds are self-limited and stop spontaneously with bowel rest. The lifetime risk of rebleeding is 25%.

Localization of diverticular bleeding should include colonoscopy, which may be both diagnostic and therapeutic in the management of mild to moderate diverticular bleeding. If the patient is stable, massive bleeding is best managed by angiography. Mesenteric angiography can localize the bleeding site and occlude it successfully with a coil in 80% of cases. The patient can then be followed closely with or without repetitive endoscopy looking for evidence of colonic ischemia. With newer techniques of highly selective coil embolization, the rate of colonic ischemia is <10% and the risk of acute rebleeding is <25%. Alternatively, a selective infusion of vasopressin can be given to stop the hemorrhage. However, this has been associated with significant complications, including myocardial infarction and intestinal ischemia in >40% of patients. Furthermore, bleeding recurs in 50% of patients once the infusion is stopped. Localization studies indicate that bleeding as a result of colonic diverticulosis is more often seen from the right colon. For this reason, patients with presumed bleeding from diverticular disease requiring emergent surgery without localization should undergo a total abdominal colectomy. Current recommendations state that if the patient is unstable or has had a 6-unit bleed within 24 h, surgery should be performed. In patients without severe comorbidities, surgical resection can be performed with a primary anastomosis. A higher anastomotic leak rate has been reported in patients undergoing primary anastomosis who received >10 units of blood.

Presentation and Evaluation of Diverticulitis   Acute diverticulitis characteristically presents with fever, anorexia, left lower quadrant abdominal pain, and diarrhea. In severe cases, patients may have generalized peritonitis and obstipation. Diverticular perforation with a fistula to the bladder presents with pneumaturia or recurrent urinary tract infections. On examination, the patient may have abdominal distention and signs of localized or generalized peritonitis. Laboratory investigations will demonstrate a leukocytosis. Rarely, a patient may present with an air-fluid level in the left lower quadrant on plain abdominal film. This is a giant diverticulum of the sigmoid colon and is managed with resection to avoid impending perforation.

The diagnosis of diverticulitis is best made on computed tomography (CT) with the following findings: sigmoid diverticula; thickened colonic wall >4 mm; inflammation within the pericolic fat ± the collection of contrast material or fluid. Symptoms of irritable bowel syndrome (IBS) may mimic those of diverticulitis. Therefore, suspected diverticulitis that does not meet CT criteria or is not associated with a leukocytosis or fever is not diverticular disease. A gastrograffin enema may also be useful in the evaluation of patients with presumed diverticular disease. If the patient has diverticular disease with a contained perforation (abscess), this study will differentiate whether the abscess is communicating with the bowel lumen or not. The latter can be managed acutely with antimicrobial therapy, whereas the former has a higher rate of failure of medical management. Repeated use of CT imaging in mild disease is not recommended as the rate of perforation with abscess formation from left-sided diverticular disease is only 16%.

Barium enema or colonoscopy should not be performed in the acute setting because of the higher risk of colonic perforation associated with insufflation or insertion of barium-based contrast material under pressure. A sigmoid malignancy can masquerade as diverticular disease.

Therefore, a barium enema or colonoscopy should be performed before surgical resection.

Staging of Complicated Diverticulitis   In contrast to uncomplicated diverticulitis, *complicated diverticular disease* is defined as diverticular disease associated with a stricture, abscess, or fistula requiring surgical intervention to cure. Complicated diverticular disease is staged using the Hinchey classification system (Fig. 279-1). This staging system was developed to predict outcomes following the surgical management of complicated diverticular disease. Other preoperative risk factors influencing postoperative mortality rates include higher American Society of Anesthesia (ASA) class and preexisting organ failure.

℞ TREATMENT

Medical Management   Asymptomatic diverticular disease discovered on imaging studies or at the time of endoscopy is best managed by diet alterations. Patients should be instructed to eat a fiber-enriched diet. This diet requires that 15 to 30 g of fiber be consumed each day, best accomplished with supplementary fiber products such as Metamucil, Fibercon, or Citrucel. The patient should also be instructed to avoid nuts and popcorn.

Symptomatic diverticular disease, defined as radiographic and hematologic confirmation of inflammation and infection within the colon, should be treated initially with antibiotics and bowel rest. Nearly 75% of patients hospitalized for acute diverticulitis will respond to nonoperative treatment with a suitable antimicrobial regiment. The current recommended antimicrobial coverage is trimethoprim/sulfamethoxazole or ciprofloxacin and metronidazole targeting aerobic gram-negative rods and anaerobic bacteria. Unfortunately, this does not cover enterococci, and the addition of ampicillin to this regimen for nonresponders is recommended. Single-agent therapy with a third-generation penicillin such as piperacillin may be effective. The usual course of antibiotics is 7 to 10 days. Current recommendations concerning bowel rest suggest that patients should remain on nothing by mouth or on clear liquids until their pain resolves. A role for parenteral nutrition has not been established.

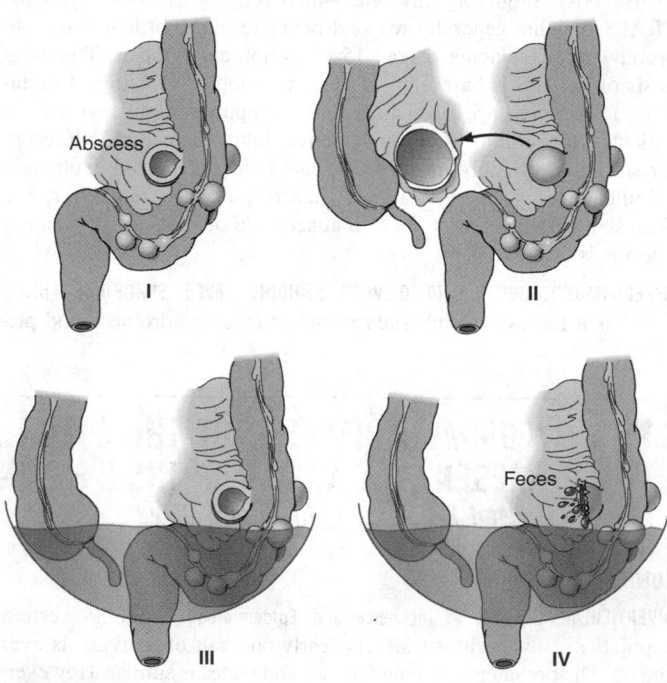

FIGURE 279-1   Hinchey classification of diverticulitis. Stage I: perforated diverticulitis with a confined paracolic abscess. Stage II: perforated diverticulitis that has closed spontaneously with distant abscess formation. Stage III: noncommunicating perforated diverticulitis with fecal peritonitis (the diverticular neck is closed off and therefore contrast will not freely expel on radiographic images). Stage IV: perforation and free communication with the peritoneum, resulting in fecal peritonitis.

Surgical Management Surgical therapy should be offered to patients who have had at least two documented attacks of diverticulitis or those who do not rapidly improve on medical therapy. Surgical therapy is indicated in all patients with complicated diverticular disease. In contrast to older patients, younger patients may experience a more aggressive form of the disease. Nearly 30% of people with diverticular disease are <40 years old. Surgical intervention is required in >70% of these patients. Patients under age 40 should undergo surgical excision following the first episode of documented diverticulitis.

The goals of surgical management of diverticular disease include controlling sepsis, eliminating complications such as fistula or obstruction, removing the diseased colonic segment, and restoring intestinal continuity. These goals must be obtained while minimizing morbidity, length of hospitalization, and cost and maximizing survival and quality of life. The options for the surgical management of diverticular disease include: (1) proximal diversion of the fecal stream with an ileostomy or colostomy and sutured omental patch with drainage, (2) resection with colostomy and mucus fistula or closure of distal bowel with formation of a Hartmann's pouch, (3) resection with anastomosis (coloproctostomy), or (4) resection with anastomosis and diversion (coloproctostomy with loop ileostomy or colostomy).

Patients with Hinchey stages I and II disease are managed with percutaneous drainage followed by resection with anastomosis about 6 weeks later. Percutaneous drainage is recommended for abscesses that are ≥5 cm with a well-defined wall that is accessible. Paracolic abscesses that are <5 cm in size will usually resolve with bowel rest and antibiotics alone. Contraindications to percutaneous drainage are pneumoperitoneum and fecal peritonitis. Urgent operative intervention is undertaken if patients develop generalized peritonitis, and most will need to be managed with a Hartmann's procedure. In selected cases, nonoperative therapy may be considered. Nonoperative management of isolated paracolic abscesses (Hinchey stage I) is associated with only a 20% recurrence rate at 2 years. Over 80% of patients with distant abscesses (Hinchey stage II) require surgical resection for recurrent symptoms.

Hinchey stage III disease is managed with a Hartman's procedure or with primary anastomosis and proximal diversion. If the patient has significant comorbidities, making operative intervention risky, a limited procedure including intraoperative peritoneal lavage (irrigation), omental patch to the oversewn perforation, and proximal diversion of the fecal stream with either an ileostomy or transverse colostomy can be performed. No anastomosis of any type should be attempted in Hinchey stage IV disease. A limited approach to these patients is associated with a decreased mortality (Table 279-1). Other important modalities in the surgical management of diverticular disease include newer minimally invasive surgical techniques. Patients undergoing successful laparoscopic resection for diverticular disease have shorter hospital stays and return to work earlier. However, conversion rates from laparoscopic to open resection are higher in patients with complicated diverticular disease.

Recurrent Symptoms Recurrent abdominal symptoms following surgical resection for diverticular disease occurs in 10% of patients. Recurrent diverticular disease develops in patients following inadequate surgical resection. A retained segment of diseased rectosigmoid colon is associated with twice the incidence of recurrence. IBS may also cause symptom recurrence. Patients undergoing surgical resection for presumed diverticulitis and symptoms of abdominal cramping and irregular loose bowel movements consistent with IBS have functionally poorer outcomes.

MESENTERIC VASCULAR INSUFFICIENCY

INTESTINAL ISCHEMIA ■ Incidence and Epidemiology Intestinal ischemia may result from either arterial occlusive and vasospastic disease or from venoocclusive disease. The most common form of intestinal ischemia is acute arterial ischemia. Risk factors for acute arterial ischemia include atrial fibrillation, recent myocardial infarction, valvular heart disease, and recent cardiac or vascular catheterization. The increased incidence of intestinal ischemia seen among western countries

TABLE 279-1 *Outcome Following Surgical Therapy for Complicated Diverticular Disease*

Hinchey Stage	Operative Procedure	Anastomotic Leak Rate, %	Overall Morbidity, %
I	Resection with primary anastomosis without diverting stoma	3.8	22
II	Resection with primary anastomosis +/− diversion	3.8	30
III	Hartmann's procedure vs. diverting colostomy and omental pedal graft	—	0 vs. 6 mortality
IV	Hartmann's procedure vs. diverting colostomy and omental pedicle graft	—	6 vs. 2 mortality

parallels atherosclerosis and the aging population. With the exception of strangulated small-bowel obstruction, ischemic colitis is the most common form of acute ischemia and the most prevalent gastrointestinal disease complicating cardiovascular surgery. The incidence of ischemic colitis following elective aortic repair is 5 to 9%, and the incidence triples in patients following emergent repair. Other less common forms of intestinal ischemia include chronic mesenteric angina associated with atherosclerotic disease and mesenteric venous thrombosis. Mesenteric venous thrombosis is associated with the presence of a hypercoaguable state including proteins C and S deficiency, antithrombin III deficiency, polycythema vera, and carcinoma.

Anatomy and Pathophysiology Intestinal ischemia occurs when insufficient perfusion to intestinal tissue produces ischemic tissue injury. The blood supply to the intestines is depicted in Fig. 279-2. To prevent ischemic injury, extensive collateralization occurs between major mesenteric trunks and branches of the mesenteric arcades (Table 279-2). Collateral vessels within the small bowel are numerous and meet

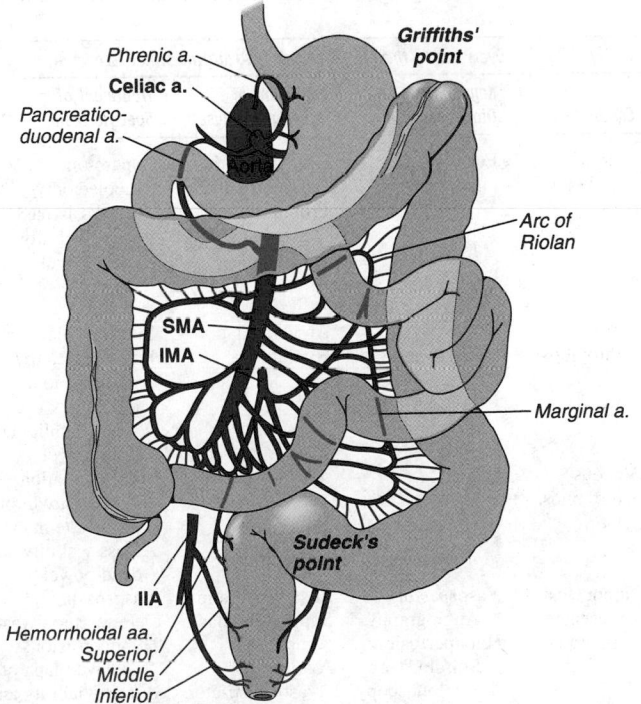

FIGURE 279-2 Blood supply to the intestines includes the celiac artery, superior mesenteric artery (SMA), inferior mesenteric artery (IMA), and branches of the internal iliac artery (IIA). Sudeck's and Griffiths' points, indicated by shaded area, are watershed areas within the colonic blood supply and common locations for ischemia.

TABLE 279-2 *Collateral Arterial Intestinal Blood Flow*

Involved Circulation	Mesenteric Artery	Adjoining Artery	Collateral Artery
Systemic	Celiac	Descending aorta	Phrenic
Systemic	IMA	Hypogastric	Middle hemorrhoidal
Mesenteric	Celiac	SMA	Superior/inferior pancreaticoduodenal
Mesenteric	SMA	IMA	Arch of Riolan
Mesenteric	SMA	Celiac/IMA	Intramesenteric
Mesenteric	SMA	IMA	Marginal

Note: IMA, inferior mesenteric artery; SMA, superior mesenteric artery.

within the duodenum and the bed of the pancreas. Collateral vessels within the colon meet at the splenic flexure and descending/sigmoid colon. These areas, which are inherently at risk for decreased blood flow, are known as *Sudek's point* and *Griffiths' point*, respectively, and are the most common locations for colonic ischemia (Fig. 279-2, shaded area). The splanchnic circulation can receive up to 30% of the cardiac output. Protective responses to prevent intestinal ischemia include abundant collateralization, autoregulation of blood flow, and the ability to increase oxygen extraction.

Intestinal ischemia may result from arterial occlusive disease, arterial nonocclusive or vasospastic disease, and venous thrombosis. Occlusive ischemia is a result of disruption of blood flow by an embolus or progressive thrombosis in a major artery supplying the intestine. Emboli originate from the heart in >75% of cases and lodge preferentially just distal to the origin of the middle colic artery from the superior mesenteric artery. Progressive thrombosis of at least two of the major vessels supplying the intestine is required for the development of chronic intestinal angina. Nonocclusive ischemia is disproportionate mesenteric vasoconstriction (arteriolar vasospasm) in response to a severe physiologic stress such as dehydration or shock. If left untreated, early mucosal stress ulceration will progress to full-thickness injury.

Presentation, Evaluation, and Management Intestinal ischemia remains one of the most challenging diagnoses. The mortality rate with intestinal ischemia is >50%. The most significant indicator of survival is the timeliness of diagnosis and treatment. An overview of diagnosis and management of each form of intestinal ischemia is given in Table 279-3.

Acute mesenteric ischemia resulting from arterial embolus or thrombosis presents with severe acute, nonremitting abdominal pain strikingly out of proportion to the physical findings. Associated symptoms may include nausea and vomiting, transient diarrhea, and bloody stools. With the exception of minimal abdominal distention and hypoactive bowel sounds, early abdominal examination is unimpressive. Later findings will demonstrate peritonitis and cardiovascular collapse. In the evaluation of acute intestinal ischemia, routine laboratory tests should be obtained, including complete blood count, serum chemistry, coagulation profile, arterial blood gas, amylase, lipase, lactic acid, blood type and cross match, and cardiac enzymes. Regardless of the need for urgent surgery, emergent admission to a monitored bed or intensive care unit is recommended for resuscitation and further evaluation. If the diagnosis of intestinal ischemia is being considered, consultation with a surgical service is necessary.

Other diagnostic modalities that may be useful in diagnosis but should not delay surgical therapy include electrocardiogram (ECG), abdominal radiographs, CT, and mesenteric angiography. The ECG may demonstrate an arrhythmia, indicating the possible source of the emboli. A plain abdominal film may show evidence of free intraperitoneal air, indicating a perforated viscus and the need for emergent exploration. Earlier features of intestinal ischemia seen on abdominal radiographs include bowel-wall edema, known as "thumbprinting." If the ischemia progresses, air can be seen within the bowel wall (*pneumatosis intestinalis*) and within the portal venous system. Other features include calcifications of the aorta and its tributaries, indicating atherosclerotic disease. With the administration of oral and intravenous contrast, dynamic CT with three-dimensional reconstruction is a highly sensitive test for intestinal ischemia. Other common causes of abdominal pain that may be identified on CT and alter the management of the patient are pancreatitis, diverticulitis, appendicitis, and small-bowel obstruction. In acute embolic disease, mesenteric angiography is best performed intraoperatively.

The "gold standard" for the diagnosis and management of acute arterial occlusive disease is laparotomy. Surgical exploration should not be delayed if suspicion of acute occlusive mesenteric ischemia is high or evidence of clinical deterioration or frank peritonitis is present. The goal of operative exploration is to resect compromised bowel and restore blood supply. Intraoperative or preoperative arteriography and systemic heparinization may assist the vascular surgeon in restoring blood supply to compromised bowel. The entire length of the small and large bowel beginning at the ligament of Treitz should be evaluated. The pattern of intestinal ischemia may indicate the level of arterial occlusion. In the case of superior mesenteric artery occlusion where the embolus usually lies just proximal to the origin of the middle colic artery, the proximal jejunum is often spared while the remainder of the small bowel to the transverse colon will be ischemic. The surgical management of acute mesenteric ischemia of the small bowel is attempted embolectomy via intra-

TABLE 279-3 *Overview of the Management of Acute Intestinal Ischemia*

Condition	Key to Early Diagnosis	Treatment of Underlying Cause	Treatment of Specific Lesion	Treatment of Systemic Consequences
Arterial embolus	Early laparotomy	Anticoagulation Cardioversion Proximal thrombectomy Aneurysmectomy	Laparotomy Embolectomy Vascular bypass Assess viability and resect dead bowel	Ensure hydration Give antibiotics Reverse acidosis Optimize oxygen delivery Support cardiac output Treat other embolic sites Avoid vasoconstrictors
Arterial thrombosis	Duplex ultrasound Angiography	Anticoagulation Hydration	Endovascular stent Endarterectomy/ thrombectomy or vascular bypass Assess viability and resect dead bowel	Give antibiotics Reverse acidosis Optimize oxygen delivery Support cardiac output Avoid vasoconstrictors
Venous thrombosis	Spiral CT	Anticoagulation Massive hydration	Anticoagulation +/− laparotomy/thrombectomy/ portasystemic shunt Assess viability and resect dead bowel	Give antibiotics Reverse acidosis Optimize oxygen delivery Support cardiac output Avoid vasoconstrictors
Nonocclusive mesenteric ischemia	Vasospasm: Angiography Hypoperfusion: Spiral CT or colonoscopy	Ensure hydration Support cardiac output Avoid vasoconstrictors Ablate renin-angiotensin axis	Vasospasm: Intraarterial vasodilators Hypoperfusion: Delayed laparotomy Assess viability and resect dead bowel	Ensure hydration Give antibiotics Reverse acidosis Optimize oxygen delivery Support cardiac output Avoid vasoconstrictors

Note: CT, computed tomography.
Source: Modified from GB Bulkley, in JL Cameron (ed): *Current Surgical Therapy*, 2d ed. Toronto, BC Decker, 1986.

operative angiography or arteriotomy. Although more commonly applied to chronic disease, acute thrombosis may be managed with angioplasty, with or without endovascular stent placement. If this is unsuccessful, a bypass from the aorta to the superior mesenteric artery is performed.

Nonocclusive or vasospastic mesenteric ischemia presents with generalized abdominal pain, anorexia, bloody stools, and abdominal distention. Often these patients are obtunded, and physical findings may not assist in the diagnosis. The presence of a leukocytosis, metabolic acidosis, elevated amylase or creatinine phosphokinase levels, and/or lactic acidosis are useful in support of the diagnosis of advanced intestinal ischemia; however, these markers may not be indicative of either reversible ischemia or frank necrosis. Newer investigational markers for intestinal ischemia that have been used include D-dimer, glutathione S-transferase, platelet-activating factor (PAF), and mucosal pH monitoring. Regardless of the need for urgent surgery, emergent admission to a monitored bed or intensive care unit is recommended for resuscitation and further evaluation. Early manifestations of intestinal ischemia include fluid sequestration within the bowel wall. This may lead to a loss of interstitial volume, and aggressive fluid resuscitation may be necessary. To optimize oxygen delivery, blood transfusions may be given. Broad-spectrum antibiotics to provide sufficient coverage for enteric pathogens, including gram-negative and anaerobic organisms, should be administered. Frequent monitoring of the patient's vital signs, urine output, blood gases, and lactate levels is paramount, as is frequent abdominal examination. All vasoconstriction agents should be avoided, allowing fluid resuscitation to maintain hemodynamics.

If ischemic colitis is a concern, colonscopy should be performed to assess the integrity of the colon mucosa (Fig. 279-3). Visualization of the rectosigmoid region may demonstrate decreased mucosal integrity, associated more commonly with nonocclusive mesenteric ischemia, or, on occasion, occlusive disease as a result of acute loss of inferior mesenteric arterial flow following aortic surgery. Ischemia of the colonic mucosa is graded as *mild* with minimal mucosal erythema or as *moderate* with pale mucosal ulcerations and evidence of exten-

sion to the muscular layer of the bowel wall. *Severe* ischemic colitis presents with severe ulcerations resulting in black or green discoloration of the mucosa, consistent with full-thickness bowel-wall necrosis. The degree of reversibility can be predicted from the mucosal findings: mild erythema is nearly 100% reversible, moderate ~50%, and frank necrosis is simply dead bowel. Follow-up colonoscopy can be performed to rule out progression of ischemic colitis.

Laparotomy for nonocclusive mesenteric ischemia is warranted for signs of peritonitis or worsening endoscopic findings and if the patient's condition does not improve with aggressive resuscitation. Ischemic colitis is optimally treated with resection of the ischemic bowel and formation of a proximal stoma. Primary anastomosis should not be performed in patients with acute intestinal ischemia.

Patients with mesenteric venous thrombosis may present with a gradual or sudden onset. Symptoms include vague abdominal pain, nausea, and vomiting. Examination findings include abdominal distention with mild to moderate tenderness and signs of dehydration. The gold standard for the diagnosis of mesenteric thrombosis is the abdominal spiral CT with oral and intravenous contrast. Findings on CT include bowel-wall thickening and ascites. Intravenous contrast will demonstrate a delayed arterial phase and clot within the superior mesenteric vein. The goal of management is to optimize hemodynamics and correct electrolyte abnormalities with massive fluid resuscitation. Intravenous antibiotics as well as anticoagulation should be initiated. If laparotomy is performed and mesenteric venous thrombosis is suspected, heparin anticoagulation is immediately initiated and clearly compromised bowel is resected.

Chronic intestinal ischemia presents with intestinal angina or abdominal pain associated with need for increased blood flow to the intestine. Patients report abdominal cramping and pain following ingestion of a meal. Weight loss and chronic diarrhea may also be noted. Abdominal pain without weight loss is not chronic mesenteric angina. Physical examination will often reveal the presence of an abdominal bruit as well as other manifestations of atherosclerosis. Duplex ultrasound evaluation of the mesenteric vessels has gained in popularity. In the absence of obesity and an increased bowel gas pattern, the radiologist may be able to identify flow disturbances within the vessels or the lack of a vasodilation response to feeding. This tool is frequently used as a screening test for patients with symptoms suggestive of chronic mesenteric ischemia. The gold standard for confirmation of mesenteric arterial occlusion is mesenteric angiography. Evaluation with mesenteric angiography allows for identification and possible intervention for the treatment of thrombus within the vessel lumen and will also evaluate the patency of remaining mesenteric vessels. The use of mesenteric angiography may be limited in the presence of renal failure or contrast allergy. Magnetic resonance angiography is an alternative if the administration of contrast dye is contraindicated.

The management of chronic intestinal ischemia includes medical management of atherosclerotic disease by lipid-lowering medications, exercise, and cessation of smoking. A full cardiac evaluation should be performed before intervention. Newer endovascular procedures may avoid an operative intervention in selective patient populations. Angioplasty with endovascular stenting in the treatment of chronic mesenteric ischemia is associated with an 80% long-term success rate. In patients requiring surgical exploration, the approach used is determined by the mesenteric angiogram. The entire length of the small and large bowel should be evaluated, beginning at the ligament of Treitz. Restoration of blood flow at the time of laparotomy is accomplished with mesenteric bypass.

Determination of intestinal viability intraoperatively in patients with suspected intestinal ischemia can be challenging. After revascularization, the bowel wall should be observed for return of a pink color and peristalsis. Palpation of major arterial vessels can be performed as well as applying a doppler flowmeter to the antimesenteric border of the bowel wall, but neither is a definitive indicator of viability. In equivocal cases, 1 g of intravenous sodium fluorescein is administered

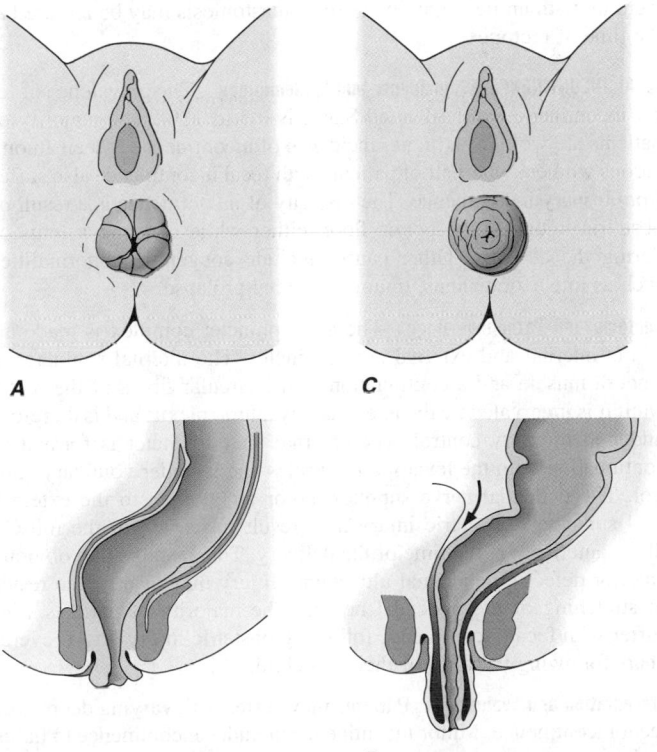

FIGURE 279-3 Degree of rectal prolapse. Mucosal prolapse only (*A, B,* sagittal view). Full-thickness prolapse associated with redundant rectosigmoid and deep pouch of Douglas (*C, D,* sagittal view).

and the pattern of bowel reperfusion is observed under ultraviolet illumination with a standard (3600 A) Wood's lamp. An area of nonfluorescence >5 mm in diameter is indicative of nonviability. If doubt still persists, reexploration should be performed 24 to 48 h following surgery. This will allow demarcation of nonviable bowel. Primary intestinal anastomosis in patients with ischemic bowel is always worrisome, and reanastomosis should be deferred to the time of second-look laparotomy.

ANORECTUM

RECTAL PROLAPSE (PROCIDENTIA) ■ Incidence and Epidemiology
The incidence of rectal prolapse peaks in women >60 years. Rectal prolapse is six times more common in women than in men. The incidence of rectal prolapse peaks in women >60 years. Women with rectal prolapse have a higher incidence of associated pelvic floor disorders including urinary incontinence, rectocele, cystocele, and enterocele. Nearly one-third of male patients with rectal prolapse suffer from a neurologic or psychiatric disorders. About 20% of children with rectal prolapse will have cystic fibrosis. All children presenting with prolapse should undergo a sweat chloride test. Less common associations include Ehlers-Danlos syndrome, solitary rectal ulcer syndrome, congenital hypothyroidism, and Hirschsprung's disease.

Anatomy and Pathophysiology
Rectal prolapse (procidentia) is a circumferential, full-thickness protrusion of the rectal wall through the anal orifice. It is often associated with a redundant sigmoid colon, pelvic laxity, and a deep pouch of Douglas. Initially, rectal prolapse was considered to be the result of early internal rectal intussusception, the first step in an inevitable progression to full-thickness external prolapse. However, only 1 of 38 patients with internal prolapse followed for >5 years developed full-thickness prolapse. Others have suggested that full-thickness prolapse is the result of damage to the pudendal nerves from repeated stretching with straining to defecate. Damage to the pudendal nerves would weaken the pelvic floor muscles, including the anal sphincters.

Presentation and Evaluation
Patients are often concerned that the symptoms they are experiencing may be a cancer. The majority of complaints include anal mass, bleeding per rectum, and a change in bowel habits. Prolapse of the rectum usually occurs following defecation. It is often associated with mild bleeding and inability to maintain good perianal hygiene. Constipation and differing degrees of fecal incontinence are common complaints associated with rectal prolapse.

To evaluate a patient's prolapse in the office, it is best to give the patient an enema in the bathroom and to have them signal when the prolapse protrudes. An important distinction should be made between full-thickness rectal prolapse and isolated mucosal prolapse associated with hemorrhoidal disease (Fig. 279-4). Mucosal prolapse is known for radial grooves rather than circumferential folds around the anus and is due to increased laxity of the connective tissue between the submucosa and underlying muscle of the anal canal. The evaluation of prolapse should also include cystoproctography and colonoscopy. These examinations evaluate for associated pelvic floor disorders and rule out a malignancy or a polyp as the lead point for prolapse. If rectal prolapse is associated with constipation, the patient should undergo a sitzmark study. For patients with fecal incontinence, endoanal ultrasound and manometric evaluation, including pudendal nerve testing of their anal sphincter muscles, should be performed before surgery for prolapse (see "Fecal Incontinence," below).

R̶x̶ TREATMENT

The medical approach to the management of rectal prolapse is limited and includes stool-bulking agents or fiber supplementation to ease the process of evacuation. Surgical correction of rectal prolapse is the mainstay of therapy. Two approaches are commonly considered, transabdominal and transperineal. Transabdominal approaches have been

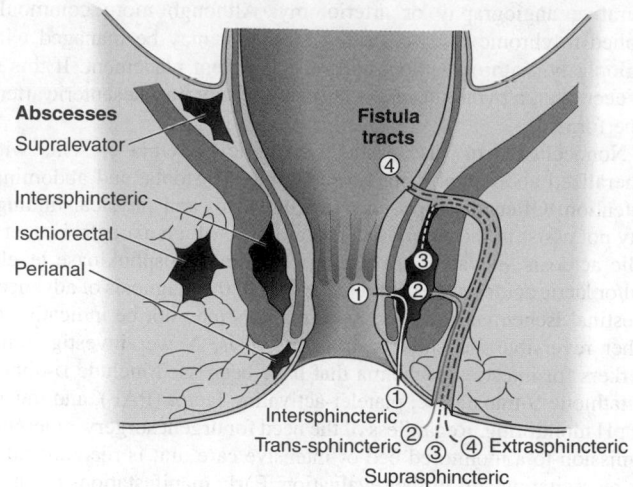

FIGURE 279-4 Common locations of anorectal abscess (*left*) and fistula in ano (*right*).

associated with lower recurrence rates, but some patients with significant comorbidities are better served by a transperineal approach.

Common transperineal approaches include a transanal proctectomy (Altmeier procedure), mucosal proctectomy (Delorme procedure), or placement of a Tirsch wire encircling the anus. The goal of the transperineal approach is to remove the redundant rectosigmoid colon. Common transabdominal approaches include presacral suture or mesh rectopexy (Ripstein) with (Frykman-Goldberg) or without resection of the redundant sigmoid. The goal of the transabdominal approach is to attempt to restore normal anatomy by removing redundant bowel and reattaching the supportive tissue of the rectum to the presacral fascia. The final alternative is abdominal proctectomy with end-sigmoid colostomy. Colon resection, in general, is reserved for patients with constipation and outlet obstruction. If total colonic inertia is present, as defined by a history of constipation and a positive sitzmark study (retention of >20% of markers 5 days after swallowing), a subtotal colectomy with an ileosigmoid or rectal anastomosis may be required at the time of rectopexy.

FECAL INCONTINENCE ■ Incidence and Epidemiology
The prevalence of fecal incontinence in the United States is 0.5 to 11%. The majority of patients are women. A higher incidence of incontinence is seen among parous women. One-half of patients with fecal incontinence also suffer from urinary incontinence. The majority of incontinence is a result of obstetric injury to the pelvic floor, either while carrying a fetus or during the delivery. Other causes include congenital abnormalities such as imperforate anus, trauma, or rectal prolapse.

Anatomy and Pathophysiology
The anal sphincter complex is made up of the internal and external anal sphincter. The internal sphincter is smooth muscle and a continuation of the circular fibers of the rectal wall. It is innervated by the intestinal myenteric plexus and is therefore under involuntary control. The external anal sphincter is formed in continuation with the levator ani muscles and is under voluntary control. The pudendal nerve supplies motor innervation to the external anal sphincter. Obstetric injury may result in tearing of the muscle fibers anteriorly at the time of the delivery. This results in an obvious anterior defect on endoanal ultrasound. Injury may also be the result of stretching of the pudendal nerves. The majority of patients who suffer with fecal incontinence following obstetric injury do so several years following the birth of their last child.

Presentation and Evaluation
Patients may suffer with varying degrees of fecal incontinence. Minor incontinence includes incontinence to flatus and occasional seepage of liquid stool. Major incontinence is frequent inability to control solid waste. As a result of fecal incontinence, patients suffer from poor perianal hygiene. Beyond the immediate problems associated with fecal incontinence, these patients are often

withdrawn and suffer from depression. For this reason, quality-of-life measures have become an important component in the evaluation of patients with fecal incontinence.

The evaluation of fecal incontinence should include a thorough history and physical examination, anal manometry, pudendal nerve terminal motor latency (PNTML), and endoanal ultrasound. Anal manometry determines the resting and squeeze pressures within the anal canal. Pudendal nerves studies evaluate the function of the nerves innervating the anal canal. Stretch injuries to these nerves will result in a delayed response of the sphincter muscle to a stimulus, indicating a prolonged latency. Finally, ultrasound will evaluate the extent of the injury to the sphincter muscles. Only PNTML has been able to predict outcome following surgical intervention.

Rarely does a pelvic floor disorder exist alone. The majority of patients with fecal incontinence will have a degree of urinary incontinence. Similarly, fecal incontinence is a part of the spectrum of pelvic organ prolapse. For this reason, patients may present with symptoms of obstructed defecation as well as fecal incontinence. Careful evaluation including cinedefography should be performed to search for other associated defects. Surgical repair of incontinence without attention to other associated defects may decrease the success of the repair.

Rx TREATMENT

The gold standard for the treatment of fecal incontinence with an isolated sphincter defect is overlapping sphincteroplasty. The external anal sphincter muscle and scar tissue as well as any identifiable internal sphincter muscle are dissected free from the surrounding adipose and connective tissue anteriorly and then an overlapping repair is performed in an attempt to rebuild the muscular ring and restore its function. Other newer approaches include radiofrequency therapy to the anal canal to aid in the development of collagen fibers and provide tensile strength to the sphincter muscles. Sacral nerve stimulation and the artificial bowel sphincter are both adaptations of procedures developed for the management of urinary incontinence. Sacral nerve stimulation is ideally suitable for patients with intact but weak anal sphincters. The artificial bowel sphincter allows the patient to manually close off the anal canal unless defecation is necessary.

Long-term results following overlapping sphincteroplasty show about a 50% failure rate over 5 years. Poorer outcome has been seen in patients with prolonged PNTML. Long-term results for sacral stimulation and the artificial bowel sphincter have not been reported. However, the artificial bowel sphincter has been associated with a 30% infection rate.

HEMORRHOIDAL DISEASE ■ **Incidence and Epidemiology** Symptomatic hemorrhoids affect >1 million individuals in western civilization per year. The prevalence of hemorrhoidal disease is not selective for age or sex. However, age is known to have a deleterious effect on the anal canal. The prevalence of hemorrhoidal disease is less in underdeveloped countries. The typical low-fiber, high-fat western diet is associated with constipation and straining, and the development of symptomatic hemorrhoids.

Anatomy and Pathophysiology Hemorrhoidal cushions are a normal part of the anal canal. The vascular structures contained within this tissue aid in continence by preventing damage to the sphincter muscle. Three main hemorrhoidal complexes traverse the anal canal—the left lateral, the right anterior, and the right posterior. Engorgement and straining results in prolapse of this tissue into the anal canal. Over time, the anatomic support system of the hemorrhoidal complex weakens, exposing this tissue to the outside of the anal canal where it is susceptible to injury. Hemorrhoids are commonly classified as internal or external. Although small external cushions do exist, the standard classification of hemorrhoidal disease is based on the progression of the disease from their normal internal location to the prolapsing external position (Table 279-4).

Presentation and Evaluation Patients commonly present to a physician for two reasons: bleeding and protrusion. Pain is less common than

TABLE 279-4 *The Staging and Treatment of Hemorrhoids*

Stage	Description of Classification	Treatment
I	Enlargement with bleeding	Fiber supplementation Cortisone suppository Sclerotherapy
II	Protrusion with spontaneous reduction	Fiber supplementation Cortisone suppository
III	Protrusion requiring manual reduction	Fiber supplementation Cortisone suppository Banding Operative hemorrhoidectomy (stapled or traditional)
IV	Irreducible protrusion	Fiber supplementation Cortisone suppository Operative hemorrhoidectomy

with fissures and, if present, is described as a dull ache from engorgement of the hemorrhoidal tissue. Severe pain may indicate a thrombosed hemorrhoid. Hemorrhoidal bleeding is described as bright red blood seen either in the toilet or upon wiping. Occasional patients can present with significant bleeding, which may be a cause of anemia; however, the presence of a colonic neoplasm must be ruled out. Patients who present with a protruding mass complain about inability to maintain perianal hygiene and are often concerned about the presence of a malignancy.

The diagnosis of hemorrhoidal disease is made on physical examination. Inspection of the perianal region for evidence of thrombosis or excoriation is performed, followed by a careful digital examination. Anoscopy is performed paying particular attention to the known position of hemorrhoidal disease. The patient is asked to strain. If this is difficult for the patient, the maneuver can be performed while sitting on a toilet. The physician is notified when the tissue prolapses. It is important to differentiate the circumferential appearance of a full-thickness rectal prolapse from the radial nature of prolapsing hemorrhoids (see "Rectal Prolapse," above). The stage and location of the hemorrhoidal complexes are defined.

Rx TREATMENT

The treatment for bleeding hemorrhoids is based upon the stage of the disease (Table 279-4). In all patients with bleeding, the possibility of other causes must be considered. In young patients without a family history of colorectal cancer, the hemorrhoidal disease may be treated first and a colonoscopic examination performed if the bleeding continues. Older patients who have not had colorectal cancer screening should undergo colonoscopy or flexible sigmoidoscopy.

With rare exceptions, the acutely thrombosed hemorrhoid should be excised with an elliptical excision. Sitz baths, fiber, and stool softeners are prescribed. Additional therapy for bleeding hemorrhoids includes banding, sclerotherapy, excisional hemorrhoidectomy, and stapled hemorrhoidectomy. Sensation begins at the dentate line; therefore, banding or sclerotherapy can be performed without discomfort in the office. Two bands (doubled) are placed around the engorged tissue, causing ischemia and fibrosis. The aids in fixing the tissue proximally in the anal canal. During sclerotherapy, 1 to 2 mL of a sclerosant (usually sodium tetradechol sulfate) is injected using a 25-gauge needle into the submucosa of the hemorrhoidal complex. Care must be taken not to inject the anal canal circumferentially or stenosis may occur. The stapled hemorrhoidectomy is associated with less discomfort. It is currently recommended that no procedures on hemorrhoids should be done in patients who are immunocompromised or who have active proctitis. Furthermore, emergent hemorrhoidectomy for bleeding hemorrhoids is associated with a higher complication rate.

Acute complications associated with the treatment of hemorrhoids include pain, infection, recurrent bleeding, and urinary retention. Care should be taken to place bands properly and to avoid overhydration in patients undergoing operative hemorrhoidectomy. Late complications include fecal incontinence as a result of injury to the sphincter during the dissection. Anal stenosis may develop from overzealous excision, with loss of mucosal skin bridges for reepithelialization. Finally, an *ectropion* (prolapse of rectal mucosa from the anal canal) may develop. Patients with an ectropion complain of a "wet" anus as a result of inability to prevent soiling once the rectal mucosa is exposed below the dentate line.

ANORECTAL ABSCESS ■ **Incidence and Epidemiology** The development of a perianal abscess is more common in men than women by a ratio of 3:1. The peak incidence is in the third to fifth decade of life. Perianal pain associated with the presence of an abscess accounts for 15% of office visits to a colorectal surgeon. The disease is more prevalent in immunocompromised patients such as diabetics, those with hematologic disorders or inflammatory bowel disease (IBD), and persons who are HIV positive. These disorders should be considered in patients with recurrent perianal infections.

Anatomy and Pathophysiology An anorectal abscess is an abnormal fluid-containing cavity in the anorectal region. Anorectal abscess results from an infection involving the glands surrounding the anal canal. Normally, these glands release mucus into the anal canal, which aids in defecation. When stool accidentally enters the anal glands, the glands become infected and an abscess develops. Anorectal abscesses are perianal in 40 to 50% of patients, ischiorectal in 20 to 25%, intersphincteric in 2 to 5%, and supralevator in 2.5% (Fig. 279-4).

Presentation and Evaluation Perianal pain and fever are the hallmarks of an abscess. Patients may have difficulty voiding and have blood in the stool. A prostatic abscess may present with similar complaints including dysuria. Patients with a prostatic abscess will often have a history of recurrent sexually transmitted diseases. On physical examination, a large fluctuant area is usually readily visible. Routine laboratory evaluation shows an elevated white blood cell count. Diagnostic procedures are rarely necessary unless evaluating a recurrent abscess. A CT scan or magnetic resonance imaging (MRI) has an accuracy of 80% in determining incomplete drainage. If there is a concern about the presence of IBD, a rigid or flexible sigmoidoscopic examination may be done at the time of drainage to evaluate for inflammation within the rectosigmoid region. A more complete evaluation for Crohn's disease would include a full colonoscopy and small-bowel series.

℞ TREATMENT

Office drainage of an uncomplicated anorectal abscess may suffice. A small incision close to the anal verge is made and a Mallenkot drain is advanced into the abscess cavity. For patients who have a complicated abscess or who are diabetic or immunocompromised, drainage should be performed in a operating room under anesthesia. These patients are at greater risk for developing necrotizing fasciitis. The course of antibiotics is controversial but should be at least 2 weeks in patients who are immunocompromised or have prosthetic heart valves, artificial joints, diabetes, or IBD.

FISTULA IN ANO ■ **Incidence and Epidemiology** The incidence and prevalence of fistulating perianal disease parallels the incidence of anorectal abscess. Some 30 to 40% of abscesses will give rise to fistula in ano. While the majority of the fistulas are cryptoglandular in origin, 10% are associated with IBD, tuberculosis, malignancy, and radiation.

Anatomy and Pathophysiology A fistula in ano is defined as a communication of an abscess cavity with an identifiable internal opening within the anal canal. This identifiable opening is most commonly located at the dentate line where the anal glands enter the anal canal. Patients experiencing continuous drainage following the treatment of a perianal abscess likely have a fistula in ano. These fistulas are classified by their relationship to the anal sphincter muscles, with 70%

being intersphincteric, 23% transsphincteric, 5% suprasphincteric, and 2% extrasphincteric (Fig. 279-4).

Presentation and Evaluation A patient with a fistula in ano will complain of constant drainage from the perianal region. The drainage may increase with defecation. Perianal hygiene is difficult to maintain. Examination under anesthesia is the best way to evaluate a fistula. At the time of the examination, anoscopy is performed to look for an internal opening. Diluted hydrogen peroxide will aid in identifying such an opening. In lieu of anesthesia, MRI with an endoanal coil will also identify tracts in 80% of the cases. After drainage of an abscess with insertion of a Mallenkot catheter, a fistulagram through the catheter can be obtained in search of an occult fistula tract. Goodsale's rule states that a posterior external fistula will enter the anal canal in the posterior midline, whereas an anterior fistula will enter at the nearest crypt. A fistula exiting >3 cm from the anal verge may have a complicated upward extension and may not obey Goodsale's rule.

℞ TREATMENT

A newly diagnosed draining fistula is best managed with placement of a seton, a vessel loop or silk tie placed through the fistula tract, which maintains the tract open and quietens the surrounding inflammation that occurs from repeated blockage of the tract (Fig. 279-4). Once the inflammation is quieted, the exact relationship of the fistula tract to the anal sphincters can be ascertained. A simple fistulotomy can be performed for intersphincteric and low (less than one-third of the muscle) transphincteric fistulas without compromising continence. For a higher transphincteric fistula, an anorectal advancement flap in combination with a drainage catheter or fibrin glue may be used. Very long (>2 cm) and narrow tracts respond better to fibrin glue than shorter tracts. Patients should be maintained on stool-bulking agents, nonnarcotic pain medication, and sitz baths. Early complications from these procedures include urinary retention and bleeding. Later complications include temporary and permanent incontinence. Recurrence following fistulotomy is 0 to 18% and following anorectal advancement flap is 20 to 30% and is related to failure to excise and close the internal opening.

ANAL FISSURE ■ **Incidence and Epidemiology** Anal fissures occur at all ages but are more common in the third through the fifth decades. A fissure is the most common cause of rectal bleeding in infancy. The prevalence is equal in males and females. It is associated with constipation, diarrhea, infectious etiologies, perianal trauma, and Crohn's disease.

Anatomy and Pathophysiology Trauma to the anal canal occurs following defecation. This injury occurs in the anterior or, more commonly, the posterior anal canal. Irritation caused by the trauma to the anal canal results in an increased resting pressure of the internal sphincter. The blood supply to the sphincter and anal mucosa enters laterally. Therefore, increased anal sphincter tone results in a relative ischemia in the region of the fissure and leads to poor healing of the anal injury. A fissure that is not in the posterior or anterior position should raise suspicion for other causes including tuberculosis, syphilis, Crohn's disease, and malignancy.

Presentation and Evaluation A fissure can be easily diagnosed on history alone. The classic complaint is pain, which is strongly associated with defecation and is relentless. The bright red bleeding that can be associated with a fissure is less extensive than that associated with hemorrhoids. On examination, most fissures are located in either the posterior or anterior position. A lateral fissure is worrisome as it may have a less benign nature, and systemic disorders should be ruled out. A chronic fissure is indicated by the presence of a hypertrophied anal papilla at the proximal end of the fissure and a sentinel pile or skin tag at the distal end. Often the circular fibers of the hypertrophied internal sphincter are visible within the base of the fissure. If anal manometry is performed, elevation in anal resting pressure and a sawtooth deformity with paradoxical contractions of the sphincter muscles are pathognomonic.

Rx TREATMENT

The management of the acute fissure is conservative. Stool softeners for those with constipation, increased dietary fiber, topical anesthetics, glucocorticoids, and sitz baths are prescribed and will heal 60 to 90% of fissures. Chronic fissures are those present for >6 weeks. These can be treated with modalities aimed at decreasing the anal canal resting pressure including nitroglycerin ointment (0.2%), applied three times a day, and botulinum toxin type A, up to 20 units, injected into the internal sphincter on each side of the fissure. Surgical management includes anal dilation and lateral internal sphincterotomy. Usually, one-third of the internal sphincter muscle is divided; it is easily identified because it is hypertrophied. Recurrence rates from medical therapy are higher, but this is offset by a risk of incontinence following sphincterotomy. Lateral internal sphincterotomy more commonly leads to incontinence in women.

ACKNOWLEDGMENT
We would like to thank Cory Sandore for providing the illustrations for this chapter.

FURTHER READING

AMBROSETTI P et al: Incidence, outcome, and proposed management of isolated abscesses complicating acute left-sided colonic diverticulitis. A prospective study of 140 patients. Dis Colon Rectum 35:1072, 1992

COLECCHIA A et al: Diverticular disease of the colon: New perspectives in symptom development and treatment. World J Gastroenterol 9:1385, 2003

JENSEN DM et al: Urgent colonoscopy for the diagnosis and treatment of severe diverticular hemorrhage. N Engl J Med 342:78, 2000

KARULF R et al: Rectal prolapse. Curr Probl Surg 38:757, 2001

LINDSEY I et al: A randomized, controlled trial of fibrin glue vs. conventional treatment for anal fistula. Dis Colon Rectum 45:1608, 2002

MATSUMOTO AH et al: Percutaneous transluminal angioplasty and stenting in the treatment of chronic mesenteric ischemia: Results and long-term follow-up. J Am Coll Surg 194 (Suppl):S22, 2002

STEIN E: Botulinum toxin and anal fissure. Curr Probl Dermatol 30:218, 2002

SUTHERLAND LM et al: A systematic review of stapled hemorrhoidectomy. Arch Surg 137:1395, 2002

WONG WD et al: Practice parameters for the treatment of sigmoid diverticulitis—supporting documentation. Dis Colon Rectum 43:290, 2000

280 ACUTE INTESTINAL OBSTRUCTION
William Silen

ETIOLOGY AND CLASSIFICATION   Intestinal obstruction may be *mechanical* or *nonmechanical* (resulting from neuromuscular disturbances that produce either adynamic or dynamic ileus). The causes of mechanical obstruction of the lumen are conveniently divided into (1) lesions *extrinsic* to the intestine, e.g., adhesive bands, internal and external hernias; (2) lesions *intrinsic* to the wall of the intestine, e.g., diverticulitis, carcinoma, regional enteritis; and (3) obturation of the lumen, e.g., gallstone obstruction, intussusception. Clinically, however, it is most useful to consider whether the obstructive mechanism involves the small or large intestine, because the causes, symptoms, and treatments are different (see below). Adhesions and external hernias are the most common causes of obstruction of the small intestine, constituting 70 to 75% of cases of this type. Adhesions, however, almost never produce obstruction of the colon, whereas carcinoma, sigmoid diverticulitis, and volvulus, in that order, are the most common causes and together account for about 90% of the cases. Primary intestinal pseudoobstruction (Chap. 279) is a chronic motility disorder that frequently mimics mechanical obstruction. Unnecessary operations in such patients should be avoided.

Adynamic ileus is probably the most common overall cause of obstruction. The development of this condition is mediated via the hormonal component of the sympathoadrenal system. Adynamic ileus may occur after any peritoneal insult, and its severity and duration will be dependent to some degree on the type of peritoneal injury. Hydrochloric acid, colonic contents, and pancreatic enzymes are among the most irritating substances, whereas blood and urine are less so. Adynamic ileus occurs to some degree after any abdominal operation. Retroperitoneal hematomas, particularly associated with vertebral fracture, commonly cause severe adynamic ileus, and the latter may occur with other retroperitoneal conditions, such as ureteral calculus or severe pyelonephritis. Thoracic diseases, including lower-lobe pneumonia, fractured ribs, and myocardial infarction, frequently produce adynamic ileus, as do electrolyte disturbances, particularly potassium depletion. Finally, intestinal ischemia, whether the result of vascular occlusion or intestinal distention itself, may perpetuate an adynamic ileus.

Spastic ileus, or *dynamic ileus*, is very uncommon and results from extreme and prolonged contraction of the intestine. It has been observed in heavy metal poisoning, uremia, porphyria, and extensive intestinal ulcerations.

PATHOPHYSIOLOGY   Distention of the intestine is caused by the accumulation of gas and fluid proximal to and within the obstructed segment. Between 70 and 80% of intestinal gas consists of swallowed air, and because this is composed mainly of nitrogen, which is poorly absorbed from the intestinal lumen, removal of air by continuous gastric suction is a useful adjunct in the treatment of intestinal distention. The accumulation of fluid proximal to the obstructing mechanism results not only from ingested fluid, swallowed saliva, gastric juice, and biliary and pancreatic secretions but also from interference with normal sodium and water transport. During the first 12 to 24 h of obstruction, there is a marked depression of flux from lumen to blood of sodium and consequently water in the distended proximal intestine. After 24 h, there is movement of sodium and water into the lumen, contributing further to the distention and fluid losses. Intraluminal pressure rises from a normal of 2 to 4 cmH$_2$O to 8 to 10 cmH$_2$O. During peristalsis, when simple obstruction or a "closed loop" is present, pressures reach 30 to 60 cmH$_2$O. Closed-loop obstruction of the small intestine results when the lumen is occluded at two points by a single mechanism such as a hernial ring or adhesive band, thus producing a closed loop whose blood supply is often obstructed at the same time. Strangulation of the loop itself is thus common in association with marked distention proximal to the involved loop. A form of closed-loop obstruction is encountered when complete obstruction of the colon exists in the presence of a competent ileocecal valve (85% of individuals). Although the blood supply of the colon is not entrapped within the obstructing mechanism, distention of the cecum is extreme because of its greater diameter (Laplace's law), and impairment of the intramural blood supply is considerable with consequent gangrene of the cecal wall, usually anteriorly. Necrosis of the small intestine may occur by the same mechanism of interference with intramural blood flow when distention is extreme, but this sequence is uncommon in the small intestine. Once impairment of blood supply occurs, bacterial invasion supervenes, and peritonitis develops. The systemic effects of extreme distention include elevation of the diaphragm with restricted ventilation and subsequent atelectasis. Venous return via the inferior vena cava may also be impaired.

The loss of fluids and electrolytes may be extreme and, unless replacement is prompt, leads to hemoconcentration, hypovolemia, renal insufficiency, shock, and death. Vomiting, accumulation of fluids within the lumen by the mechanisms described above, and the sequestration of fluid into the edematous intestinal wall and peritoneal cavity as a result of impairment of venous return from the intestine all contribute to massive loss of fluid and electrolytes, especially potassium. As soon as significant impedance to venous return is present, the intestine becomes severely congested, and blood begins to seep into the intestinal lumen. Blood loss may reach significant levels when long segments of intestine are involved.

SYMPTOMS   *Mechanical small-intestinal obstruction* is characterized by cramping midabdominal pain, which tends to be more severe the higher the obstruction. The pain occurs in paroxysms, and the patient is relatively comfortable in the intervals between the pains. Audible borborygmi are often noted by the patient simultaneously with the paroxysms of pain. The pain may become less severe as distention progresses, probably because motility is impaired in the edematous intestine. When strangulation is present, the pain is usually more localized and may be steady and severe without a colicky component, a fact that often causes delay in diagnosis of obstruction. Vomiting is almost invariable, and it is earlier and more profuse the higher the obstruction. The vomitus initially contains bile and mucus and remains as such if the obstruction is high in the intestine. With low ileal obstruction, the vomitus becomes feculent, i.e., orange-brown in color with a foul odor, which results from the overgrowth of bacteria proximal to the obstruction. Hiccups (singultus) are common. Obstipation and failure to pass gas by rectum are invariably present when the obstruction is complete, although some stool and gas may be passed spontaneously or after an enema shortly after onset of the complete obstruction. Diarrhea is occasionally observed in partial obstruction. Blood in the stool is rare but does occur in cases of intussusception. Other than some minor but inconsistent differences in pain patterns noted above, the symptoms of strangulating obstructions cannot be distinguished from those of nonstrangulating obstructions.

Mechanical colonic obstruction produces colicky abdominal pain similar in quality to that of small-intestinal obstruction but of much lower intensity. Complaints of pain are occasionally absent in stoic elderly patients. Vomiting occurs late, if at all, particularly if the ileocecal valve is competent. Paradoxically, feculent vomitus is very rare. A history of recent alterations in bowel habits and blood in the stool is common because carcinoma and diverticulitis are the most frequent causes. Constipation becomes progressive, and obstipation with failure to pass gas ensues. Acute symptoms may develop over a period of a week. Cecal volvulus more closely resembles obstruction of the small intestine clinically, whereas patients with sigmoid volvulus more typically have the picture of colonic obstruction in which marked distention predominates, with relatively less pain.

In *adynamic ileus*, colicky pain is absent, and only discomfort from distention is evident. Vomiting may be frequent but is rarely profuse. It usually consists of gastric contents and bile and is almost never feculent. Complete obstipation may or may not occur. Singultus (hiccups) is common.

PHYSICAL FINDINGS   *Abdominal distention* is the hallmark of all forms of intestinal obstruction. It is least marked in cases of obstruction high in the small intestine and most marked in colonic obstruction. Early, especially in closed-loop strangulating small-bowel obstruction, distention may be barely perceptible or absent. Tenderness and rigidity are usually minimal; the temperature is rarely >37.8°C (100°F) in nonstrangulating obstruction of the small and large intestine. Contrary to popular belief, the same is true of strangulating obstruction until very late, a fact that has often resulted in unfortunate delay in treatment. Signs and symptoms of shock also occur *very late* in strangulating obstruction. The appearance of shock, tenderness, rigidity, and fever often means that contamination of the peritoneum with infected intestinal content has occurred. Hernial orifices should always be carefully examined for the presence of a mass. The presence of a palpable abdominal mass usually signifies a closed-loop strangulating small-bowel obstruction because the tense fluid-filled loop is the palpable lesion. Auscultation may reveal loud, high-pitched borborygmi coincident with the colicky pain, but this finding is often absent late in strangulating or nonstrangulating obstruction. A quiet abdomen does

not eliminate the possibility of obstruction, nor does it necessarily establish the diagnosis of adynamic ileus.

LABORATORY AND X-RAY FINDINGS   Leukocytosis, with shift to the left, usually occurs when strangulation is present, but a normal white blood cell count does not exclude strangulation. Elevation of the serum amylase level is encountered occasionally in all forms of intestinal obstruction, especially the strangulating variety.

The x-ray is extremely valuable but under certain circumstances may also be misleading. In nonstrangulating complete small-bowel obstruction, x-rays are almost completely reliable. Distention of fluid- and gas-filled loops of small intestine usually arranged in a "stepladder" pattern with air-fluid levels and an absence or paucity of colonic gas are pathognomonic (Fig. 280-1). These findings, however, are absent in slightly over half the cases of strangulating small-bowel obstruction, especially early in the disease. A general haze due to peritoneal fluid and sometimes a "coffee bean"–shaped mass are seen in strangulating obstruction. Occasionally, the films are normal, but when symptoms are consistent with obstruction of the small intestine, a normal film should suggest strangulation. In these circumstances, computed tomography may be very useful. Roentgenographic differentiation of partial mechanical small-bowel obstruction from adynamic ileus may be impossible because gas is present in both the small and large intestines; however, colonic distention is usually more prominent in adynamic ileus. A radiopaque dye given by mouth is useful in making this distinction.

Colonic obstruction with a competent ileocecal valve is easily recognized because distention with gas is mainly confined to the colon. Barium enema, sigmoidoscopy, or colonoscopy, depending on the suspected site of obstruction, is usually advisable to determine the nature of the lesion, except when concomitant perforation is suspected, a rare occurrence. Sigmoidoscopy may be therapeutic in cases of sigmoid volvulus. When the ileocecal valve is incompetent, the films resemble those of partial small-bowel obstruction or adynamic ileus, and barium enema or colonoscopy is necessary to establish the correct diagnosis. Barium given by mouth is perfectly safe when obstruction is in the small intestine, since the barium sulfate does not become inspissated

FIGURE 280-1   Acute mechanical obstruction of small intestine (upright film). Note air-fluid levels, marked distention of bowel loops, and absence of colonic gas.

℞ TREATMENT

Small-Intestinal Obstruction The overall mortality rate for obstruction of the small intestine is about 10%, even under the most optimal conditions. While the mortality rate for nonstrangulating obstruction is as low as 5 to 8%, that for strangulating obstruction has been reported to be between 20 and 75%. Well over half the deaths from small-bowel obstruction occur in those with strangulation; however, the latter constitute only one-fourth to one-third of the cases. Careful studies indicate that the clinical, laboratory, and x-ray findings are not reliable in distinguishing strangulating from nonstrangulating obstruction when obstruction is complete. Complete obstruction is suggested when passage of gas or stool per rectum has ceased and when gas is absent in the distal intestine by x-ray. Since strangulating small-bowel obstruction is always complete, operation should always be undertaken in such patients after suitable preparation. Before operation, fluid and electrolyte balance should be restored and decompression instituted by means of a nasogastric tube. Replacement of potassium is especially important because intake is nil and losses in vomitus are large. From 6 to 8 h of preparation may be necessary. During this period, broad-spectrum antibiotics are indicated if strangulation is felt to be likely, but operation should not be delayed unless there is unequivocal clinical and roentgenographic evidence of resolution of the obstruction during the period of preparation. Attempts to pass a long tube into the small intestine usually fail while putting the patient through uncomfortable, unproductive manipulations that delay appropriate fluid replacement and decompression. *There are few, if any, indications for the use of a long intestinal tube.* Procrastination of operation because of improvement in well-being of the patient during resuscitation and gastric decompression usually leads to unnecessary and hazardous delay in proper treatment. Purely nonoperative therapy is safe only in the presence of incomplete obstruction and is best utilized in patients with (1) repeated episodes of partial obstruction, (2) recent postoperative partial obstruction, and (3) partial obstruction following a recent episode of diffuse peritonitis.

Colonic Obstruction The mortality rate for colonic obstruction is about 20%. As in small-bowel obstruction, nonoperative treatment is contraindicated unless the obstruction is incomplete. Occasionally, but not always, when the obstruction is incomplete, nonoperative therapy may result in sufficient decompression that a definitive operative procedure can be undertaken at a later date. This can usually be accomplished by discontinuation of all oral intake and perhaps by nasogastric suction, although attempts to decompress a *completely* obstructed colon by intubation are almost invariably futile. A long intestinal tube will not decompress an obstructed colon with a competent ileocecal valve. When obstruction is complete, early operation is mandatory, especially when the ileocecal valve is competent; cecal gangrene is likely if the cecal diameter is >10 cm on plain abdominal film. For obstruction on the left side of the colon, the most common site, preliminary operative decompression by cecostomy or transverse colostomy followed by definitive resection of the primary lesion has been the treatment of choice. Recently, primary resection of obstructing left-sided lesions with on-table washout of the colon has been accomplished safely. For a lesion of the right or transverse colon, primary resection and anastomosis can be performed safely because distention of the ileum with consequent discrepancy in size and hazard in suture are not present.

Adynamic Ileus This type of ileus usually responds to nonoperative continuous decompression and adequate treatment of the primary disease. The prognosis is usually good. Successful decompression of severe colonic ileus has been accomplished by colonoscopy, but this should be avoided if tenderness in the right lower quadrant suggests possible cecal gangrene. Neostigmine is effective in cases of colonic ileus that have not responded to other conservative treatment. Rarely, adynamic colonic distention may become so great that cecostomy is required if cecal gangrene is feared. Spastic ileus usually responds to treatment of the primary disease.

FURTHER READING

BULKLEY GB et al: Intraoperative determination of small intestinal viability following ischemic injury: Prospective controlled trial of two adjuvant methods (Doppler and fluorescein) compared with standard clinical judgement. Ann Surg 193:628, 1981

DUBOIS A et al: Postoperative ileus: Physiopathology, etiology and treatment. Ann Surg 178:781, 1973

ESKELINEN M et al: Contributions of history-taking, physical examination, and computer assistance to diagnosis of acute small-bowel obstruction. A prospective study of 1333 patients with acute abdominal pain. Scand J Gastroenterol 29:715, 1994

FEVANG BT et al: Complications and death after surgical treatment of small bowel obstruction: A 35-year institutional experience. Ann Surg 231:529, 2000

JACKSON BR: The diagnosis of colonic obstruction. Dis Colon Rectum 25:603, 1982

SILEN W: *Cope's Early Diagnosis of the Acute Abdomen*, 20th ed. London, Oxford, 2000

281 ACUTE APPENDICITIS AND PERITONITIS
William Silen

ACUTE APPENDICITIS

INCIDENCE AND EPIDEMIOLOGY The peak incidence of acute appendicitis is in the second and third decades of life; it is relatively rare at the extremes of age. Males and females are equally affected, except between puberty and age 25, when males predominate in a 3:2 ratio. Perforation is more common in infancy and in the aged, during which periods mortality rates are highest. The mortality rate has decreased steadily in Europe and the United States from 8.1 per 100,000 of the population in 1941 to <1 per 100,000 in 1970 and subsequently. The absolute incidence of the disease also decreased by about 40% between 1940 and 1960 but since then has remained unchanged. Although various factors such as changing dietary habits, altered intestinal flora, and better nutrition and intake of vitamins have been suggested to explain the reduced incidence, the exact reasons have not been elucidated. The overall incidence of appendicitis is much lower in underdeveloped countries, especially parts of Africa, and in lower socioeconomic groups.

PATHOGENESIS Luminal obstruction has long been considered the pathogenetic hallmark. However, obstruction can be identified in only 30 to 40% of cases; ulceration of the mucosa is the initial event in the majority. The cause of the ulceration is unknown, although a viral etiology has been postulated. Infection with *Yersinia* organisms may cause the disease, since high complement fixation antibody titers have been found in up to 30% of cases of proven appendicitis. Whether the inflammatory reaction seen with ulceration is sufficient to obstruct the tiny appendiceal lumen even transiently is not clear. Obstruction, when present, is most commonly caused by a fecalith, which results from accumulation and inspissation of fecal matter around vegetable fibers. Enlarged lymphoid follicles associated with viral infections (e.g., measles), inspissated barium, worms (e.g., pinworms, *Ascaris*, and *Tae-*

nia), and tumors (e.g., carcinoid or carcinoma) may also obstruct the lumen. Secretion of mucus distends the organ, which has a capacity of only 0.1 to 0.2 mL, and luminal pressures rise as high as 60 cmH$_2$O. Luminal bacteria multiply and invade the appendiceal wall as venous engorgement and subsequent arterial compromise result from the high intraluminal pressures. Finally, gangrene and perforation occur. If the process evolves slowly, adjacent organs such as the terminal ileum, cecum, and omentum may wall off the appendiceal area so that a localized abscess will develop, whereas rapid progression of vascular impairment may cause perforation with free access to the peritoneal cavity. Subsequent rupture of primary appendiceal abscesses may produce fistulas between the appendix and bladder, small intestine, sigmoid, or cecum. Occasionally, acute appendicitis may be the first manifestation of Crohn's disease.

While chronic infection of the appendix with tuberculosis, amebiasis, and actinomycosis may occur, a useful clinical aphorism states that *chronic appendiceal inflammation is not usually the cause of prolonged abdominal pain of weeks' or months' duration*. In contrast, recurrent acute appendicitis does occur, often with complete resolution of inflammation and symptoms between attacks. Recurrent acute appendicitis may become more frequent as antibiotics are dispensed more freely and if a long appendiceal stump is left after laparoscopic appendectomy.

CLINICAL MANIFESTATIONS The history and sequence of symptoms are important diagnostic features of appendicitis. The initial symptom is almost invariably *abdominal pain* of the visceral type, resulting from appendiceal contractions or distention of the lumen. It is usually poorly localized in the periumbilical or epigastric region with an accompanying urge to defecate or pass flatus, neither of which relieves the distress. This visceral pain is mild, often cramping, and rarely catastrophic in nature, usually lasting 4 to 6 h, but it may not be noted by stoic individuals or by some patients during sleep. As inflammation spreads to the parietal peritoneal surfaces, the pain becomes somatic, steady, and more severe, aggravated by motion or cough, and usually located in the *right lower quadrant*. Anorexia is very common; a hungry patient does not have acute appendicitis. *Nausea* and *vomiting* occur in 50 to 60% of cases, but vomiting is usually self-limited. The development of nausea and vomiting before the onset of pain is extremely rare. Change in bowel habit is of little diagnostic value, since any or no alteration may be observed, although the presence of diarrhea caused by an inflamed appendix in juxtaposition to the sigmoid may cause serious diagnostic difficulties. Urinary frequency and dysuria occur if the appendix lies adjacent to the bladder. The typical sequence of symptoms (poorly localized periumbilical pain followed by nausea and vomiting with subsequent shift of pain to the right lower quadrant) occurs in only 50 to 60% of patients.

Physical findings vary with time after onset of the illness and according to the location of the appendix, which may be situated deep in the pelvic cul-de-sac; in the right lower quadrant in any relation to the peritoneum, cecum, and small intestine; in the right upper quadrant (especially during pregnancy); or even in the left lower quadrant. *The diagnosis cannot be established unless tenderness can be elicited.* While tenderness is sometimes absent in the early visceral stage of the disease, it ultimately always develops and is found in any location corresponding to the position of the appendix. Abdominal tenderness may be completely absent if a retrocecal or pelvic appendix is present, in which case the sole physical finding may be tenderness in the flank or on rectal or pelvic examination. Percussion, rebound tenderness, and referred rebound tenderness are often, but not invariably, present; they are most likely to be absent early in the illness. Flexion of the right hip and guarded movement by the patient are due to parietal peritoneal involvement. Hyperesthesia of the skin of the right lower quadrant and a positive psoas or obturator sign are often late findings and are rarely of diagnostic value. When the inflamed appendix is in close proximity to the anterior parietal peritoneum, muscular rigidity is present yet is often minimal early.

The temperature is usually normal or slightly elevated [37.2 to 38°C (99 to 100.5°F)], but a temperature >38.3°C (101°F) should suggest perforation. Tachycardia is commensurate with the elevation of the temperature. Rigidity and tenderness become more marked as the disease progresses to perforation and localized or diffuse peritonitis. Distention is rare unless severe diffuse peritonitis has developed. The disappearance of pain and tenderness just before perforation is extremely unusual. A mass may develop if localized perforation has occurred but will not usually be detectable before 3 days after onset. Earlier presence of a mass suggests carcinoma of the cecum or Crohn's disease. Perforation is rare before 24 h after onset of symptoms, but the rate may be as high as 80% after 48 h.

Diagnosis is based primarily on clinical grounds. Although moderate leukocytosis of 10,000 to 18,000 cells/μL is frequent (with a concomitant left shift), the absence of leukocytosis does not rule out acute appendicitis. Leukocytosis of >20,000 cells/μL suggests probable perforation. Anemia and blood in the stool suggest a primary diagnosis of carcinoma of the cecum, especially in elderly individuals. The urine may contain a few white or red blood cells without bacteria if the appendix lies close to the right ureter or bladder. Urinalysis is most useful in excluding genitourinary conditions that may mimic acute appendicitis.

Radiographs are rarely of value except when an opaque fecalith (5% of patients) is observed in the right lower quadrant (especially in children). Consequently, abdominal films are not routinely obtained unless other conditions such as intestinal obstruction or ureteral calculus may be present. In some patients with recurrent or prolonged symptoms, computed tomography (CT) may reveal an extrinsic defect on the medial wall of the cecum or a calcified fecalith. The predictive value of CT scan in acute appendicitis is being evaluated. The diagnosis may also be established by the ultrasonic demonstration of an enlarged and thick-walled appendix. Ultrasound is most useful to exclude ovarian cysts, ectopic pregnancy, or tuboovarian abscess.

While the typical historic sequence and physical findings are present in 50 to 60% of cases, a wide variety of atypical patterns of disease are encountered, especially at the age extremes and during pregnancy. Infants under 2 years of age have a 70 to 80% incidence of perforation and generalized peritonitis. Any infant or child with diarrhea, vomiting, and abdominal pain is highly suspect. Fever is much more common in this age group, and abdominal distention is often the only physical finding. In the elderly, pain and tenderness are often blunted, and thus the diagnosis is frequently delayed and leads to a 30% incidence of perforation in patients over 70. Elderly patients often present initially with a slightly painful mass (a primary appendiceal abscess) or with adhesive intestinal obstruction 5 or 6 days after a previously undetected perforated appendix.

Appendicitis occurs about once in every 1000 pregnancies and is the most common extrauterine condition requiring abdominal operation. The diagnosis may be missed or delayed because of the frequent occurrence of mild abdominal discomfort and nausea and vomiting during pregnancy. During the last trimester, when the mortality rate from appendicitis is highest, uterine displacement of the appendix to the right upper quadrant and laterally leads to confusion in diagnosis because pain and tenderness are similarly displaced.

DIFFERENTIAL DIAGNOSIS Appendicitis can be confused with any condition that causes abdominal pain. Diagnostic accuracy is about 75 to 80% for experienced clinicians based solely on the clinical criteria outlined. It is probably better to err slightly in the direction of overdiagnosis, since delay is associated with perforation and increased morbidity and mortality. In unperforated appendicitis, the mortality rate is 0.1%, little more than that associated with general anesthesia; for perforated appendicitis, overall mortality is 3% (15% in the elderly). In doubtful cases, 4 to 6 h of observation is always more beneficial than harmful. The most common conditions discovered at operation when acute appendicitis is erroneously diagnosed are, in order of frequency, mesenteric lymphadenitis, no organic disease, acute pelvic inflammatory disease, ruptured graafian follicle or corpus luteum cyst, and acute gastroenteritis. In addition, acute cholecystitis, perforated ulcer, acute pancreatitis, acute diverticulitis, strangulating intestinal obstruction, ureteral calculus, and pyelonephritis may present diagnostic difficulties.

Differentiation of *pelvic inflammatory disease* from acute appendicitis on clinical grounds may be virtually impossible. Gram-negative intracellular diplococci on cervical smear are not pathognomonic unless *Neisseria gonorrhoeae* can be cultured. Pain on movement of the cervix is not specific and may occur in appendicitis if perforation has occurred or if the appendix lies adjacent to the uterus or adnexa. *Rupture of a graafian follicle* (mittelschmerz) occurs at midcycle and will spill off blood and fluid to produce pain and tenderness more diffuse and usually of a less severe degree than in appendicitis. Fever and leukocytosis are usually absent. *Rupture of a corpus luteum cyst* is identical clinically to rupture of a graafian follicle but develops about the time of menstruation. The presence of an adnexal mass, evidence of blood loss, and a positive pregnancy test help differentiate *ruptured tubal pregnancy*, but a negative pregnancy test is present when tubal abortion has occurred. *Twisted ovarian cyst* and *endometriosis* are occasionally difficult to distinguish from appendicitis. In all these female conditions, ultrasonography, laparoscopy, and occasionally CT may be of great value.

Acute mesenteric lymphadenitis is the diagnosis usually given when enlarged, slightly reddened lymph nodes at the root of the mesentery and a normal appendix are encountered at operation in a patient who usually has right lower quadrant tenderness. Whether this is a single, discrete entity is unclear, since the causative factor is not known. Some of these patients have infection with *Y. pseudotuberculosis* or *Y. enterocolitica*, in which case the diagnosis can be established by culture of the mesenteric nodes or by serologic titers (Chap. 143). The diagnosis is essentially impossible clinically, although retrospectively these patients may have a higher temperature and more diffuse pain and tenderness. Children seem to be affected more frequently than adults. *Acute gastroenteritis* usually causes profuse watery diarrhea, often with nausea and vomiting, but without localized findings. Between cramps, the abdomen is completely relaxed. In *Salmonella* gastroenteritis, the abdominal findings are similar, although the pain may be more severe and more localized, and fever and chills are common. The occurrence of similar symptoms among other members of the family may be helpful. When the diagnosis of acute pelvic appendicitis with perforation has been missed, gastroenteritis is the most common previous working diagnosis. Persistent abdominal or rectal tenderness should eliminate the diagnosis of gastroenteritis. *Regional enteritis* (Crohn's disease) is usually associated with a more prolonged history, often with previous exacerbations regarded as episodes of gastroenteritis unless the diagnosis has been established previously. *Meckel's diverticulitis* usually cannot be distinguished from acute appendicitis but is very rare.

℞ TREATMENT

Cathartics and enemas should be avoided if appendicitis is under consideration, and antibiotics should not be administered when the diagnosis is in question, since they will only mask the perforation. The treatment is early operation and appendectomy as soon as the patient can be prepared. Appendectomy is increasingly accomplished laparoscopically and may have some benefits over the open technique. Preparation for operation rarely takes more than 1 to 2 h in early appendicitis but may require 6 to 8 h in cases of severe sepsis and dehydration associated with late perforation. The *only* circumstance in which operation is *not* indicated is the presence of a palpable mass 3 to 5 days after the onset of symptoms. Should operation be undertaken at that time, a phlegmon rather than a definitive abscess will be found, and complications from its dissection are frequent. Such patients treated with broad-spectrum antibiotics, parenteral fluids, and rest usually show resolution of the mass and symptoms within 1 week. *Interval appendectomy* should be done safely 3 months later. Should the mass enlarge or the patient become more toxic, drainage of the abscess is

necessary. The complications of subphrenic, pelvic, or other intraabdominal abscesses usually follow perforation with generalized peritonitis and can be avoided by early diagnosis of the disease.

ACUTE PERITONITIS

Peritonitis is an inflammation of the peritoneum; it may be localized or diffuse in location, acute or chronic in natural history, infectious or aseptic in pathogenesis. Acute peritonitis is most often infectious and is usually related to a perforated viscus (and called secondary peritonitis). When no bacterial source is identified, infectious peritonitis is called primary or spontaneous. Acute peritonitis is associated with decreased intestinal motor activity resulting in distention of the intestinal lumen with gas and fluid. The accumulation of fluid in the bowel together with the lack of oral intake leads to rapid intravascular volume depletion with effects on cardiac, renal, and other systems.

ETIOLOGY Infectious agents gain access to the peritoneal cavity through a perforated viscus, a penetrating wound of the abdominal wall, or external introduction of a foreign object that is or becomes infected (for example, a chronic peritoneal dialysis catheter). In the absence of immune compromise, host defenses are capable of eradicating small contaminations. Large numbers of mixed aerobic and anaerobic bacteria, particularly when persistently infused, can lead to peritonitis. The conditions that most commonly result in the introduction of bacteria into the peritoneum are ruptured appendix, ruptured diverticulum, perforated peptic ulcer, incarcerated hernia, gangrenous gall bladder, volvulus, bowel infarction, cancer, inflammatory bowel disease, or intestinal obstruction. However, a wide range of mechanisms may play a role (Table 281-1). Bacterial peritonitis can also occur in the apparent absence of an intraperitoneal source of bacteria (primary or spontaneous bacterial peritonitis). This condition occurs in the setting of ascites and liver cirrhosis in 90% of the cases, usually in patients with ascites with low protein concentration (<1 g/L) (Chap. 289). →*Bacterial peritonitis is discussed in detail in Chap. 112.*

Aseptic peritonitis may be due to peritoneal irritation by abnormal presence of physiologic fluids (e.g., gastric juice, bile, pancreatic enzymes, blood, or urine) or sterile foreign bodies (e.g., surgical sponges or instruments, starch from surgical gloves) in the peritoneal cavity or as a complication of rare systemic diseases such as lupus erythematosus, porphyria, or familial Mediterranean fever (Chap. 278). Chemical irritation of the peritoneum is greatest for acidic gastric juice and pancreatic enzymes. In chemical peritonitis, a major risk of secondary bacterial infection exists.

TABLE 281-1 *Conditions Leading to Secondary Bacterial Peritonitis*

Perforations of bowel	Perforations or leaking of other organs
Trauma, blunt or penetrating	
Inflammation	Pancreas—pancreatitis
Appendicitis	Gall bladder—cholecystitis
Diverticulitis	Urinary bladder—trauma, rupture
Peptic ulcer disease	Liver—bile leak after biopsy
Inflammatory bowel disease	Fallopian tubes—salpingitis
Iatrogenic	Bleeding into the peritoneal cavity
Endoscopic perforation	**Disruption of integrity of peritoneal**
Anastomotic leaks	**cavity**
Catheter perforation	Trauma
Vascular	Continuous ambulatory peritoneal
Embolus	dialysis (indwelling catheter)
Ischemia	Intraperitoneal chemotherapy
Obstructions	Perinephric abscess
Adhesions	Iatrogenic—postoperative,
Strangulated hernias	foreign body
Volvulus	
Intussusception	
Neoplasms	
Ingested foreign body, toothpick, fish bone	

CLINICAL FEATURES The cardinal manifestations of peritonitis are acute abdominal pain and tenderness, usually with fever. The location of the pain depends on the underlying cause and whether the inflammation is localized or generalized. Localized peritonitis is most common in uncomplicated appendicitis and diverticulitis and physical findings are limited to the area of inflammation. Generalized peritonitis is associated with widespread inflammation and diffuse abdominal tenderness and rebound. Rigidity of the abdominal wall is common in both localized and generalized peritonitis. Bowel sounds are usually absent. Tachycardia, hypotension, and signs of dehydration are common. Leukocytosis and acidosis are common laboratory findings. Plain abdominal films may show dilation of large and small bowel with edema of the bowel wall. Free air under the diaphragm is associated with a perforated viscus. CT and/or ultrasonography can identify the presence of free fluid or an abscess. When ascites is present, diagnostic paracentesis with cell count (>250 neutrophils/μL is usual in peritonitis), protein and lactate dehydrogenase levels, and culture is essential. In elderly and immunosuppressed patients, signs of peritoneal irritation may be more difficult to detect.

THERAPY AND PROGNOSIS Treatment relies on rehydration, correction of electrolyte abnormalities, antibiotics, and surgical correction of the underlying defect. Mortality rates are <10% for uncomplicated peritonitis associated with a perforated ulcer or ruptured appendix or diverticulum in an otherwise healthy person. Mortality rates of ≥40% have been reported for elderly people, those with underlying illnesses, and when peritonitis has been present for >48 h.

FURTHER READING

CHEADLE WG, SPAIN DA: The continuing challenge of intraabdominal infection. Am J Surg 186(Suppl 1):15, 2003

FLUM DR et al: Has misdiagnosis of appendicitis decreased over time? A population-based analysis. JAMA 286:1748, 2001

GRONROOS JM, GRONROOS P: Leucocyte count and C-reactive protein in the diagnosis of acute appendicitis. Br J Surg 86:501, 1999

GWYNN LK: The diagnosis of acute appendicitis: Clinical assessment versus computed tomography evaluation. J Emerg Med 21:119, 2001

RAO P et al: Effect of computed tomography of the appendix on treatment of patients and use of hospital resources. N Engl J Med 338:141, 1998

WADE DS et al: Accuracy of ultrasound in the diagnosis of acute appendicitis compared with the surgeon's clinical impression. Arch Surg 128:1039, 1993

Section 2   Liver and Biliary Tract Disease

282 APPROACH TO THE PATIENT WITH LIVER DISEASE
Marc Ghany, Jay H. Hoofnagle

In most instances, a diagnosis of liver disease can be made accurately by a careful history, physical examination, and application of a few laboratory tests. In some circumstances, radiologic examinations are helpful or, indeed, diagnostic. Liver biopsy is considered the "gold standard" in evaluation of liver disease but is now needed less for diagnosis than for grading and staging disease. This chapter provides an introduction to diagnosis and management of liver disease, briefly reviewing the structure and function of the liver; the major clinical manifestations of liver disease; and the use of clinical history, physical examination, laboratory tests, imaging studies, and liver biopsy.

LIVER STRUCTURE AND FUNCTION The liver is the largest organ of the body, weighing 1 to 1.5 kg and representing 1.5 to 2.5% of the lean body mass. The size and shape of the liver vary and generally match the general body shape—long and lean or squat and square. The liver is located in the right upper quadrant of the abdomen under the right lower rib cage against the diaphragm and projects for a variable extent into the left upper quadrant. The liver is held in place by ligamentous attachments to the diaphragm, peritoneum, great vessels, and upper gastrointestinal organs. It receives a dual blood supply; approximately 20% of the blood flow is oxygen-rich blood from the hepatic artery, and 80% is nutrient-rich blood from the portal vein arising from the stomach, intestines, pancreas, and spleen.

The majority of cells in the liver are hepatocytes, which constitute two-thirds of the mass of the liver. The remaining cell types are Kupffer cells (members of the reticuloendothelial system), stellate (Ito or fat-storing) cells, endothelial cells and blood vessels, bile ductular cells, and supporting structures. Viewed by light microscopy, the liver appears to be organized in lobules, with portal areas at the periphery and central veins in the center of each lobule. However, from a functional point of view, the liver is organized into acini, with both hepatic arterial and portal venous blood entering the acinus from the portal areas (zone 1) and then flowing through the sinusoids to the terminal hepatic veins (zone 3); the intervening hepatocytes constituting zone 2. The advantage of viewing the acinus as the physiologic unit of the liver is that it helps to explain the morphologic patterns and zonality of many vascular and biliary diseases not explained by the lobular arrangement.

Portal areas of the liver consist of small veins, arteries, bile ducts, and lymphatics organized in a loose stroma of supporting matrix and small amounts of collagen. Blood flowing into the portal areas is distributed through the sinusoids, passing from zone 1 to zone 3 of the acinus and draining into the terminal hepatic veins ("central veins"). Secreted bile flows in the opposite direction, in a counter current pattern from zone 2 to zone 1. The sinusoids are lined by unique endothelial cells that have prominent fenestrae of variable size, allowing the free flow of plasma but not cellular elements. The plasma is thus in direct contact with hepatocytes in the subendothelial space of Disse.

Hepatocytes have distinct polarity. The basolateral side of the hepatocyte lines the space of Disse and is richly lined with microvilli; it demonstrates endocytotic and pinocytotic activity, with passive and active uptake of nutrients, proteins, and other molecules. The apical pole of the hepatocyte forms the cannicular membranes through which bile components are secreted. The canniculi of hepatocytes form a fine network, which fuses into the bile ductular elements near the portal areas. Kupffer cells usually lie within the sinusoidal vascular space and represent the largest group of fixed macrophages in the body. The stellate cells are located in the space of Disse but are not usually prominent unless activated, when they produce collagen and matrix. Red blood cells stay in the sinusoidal space as blood flows through the lobules, but white blood cells can migrate through or around endothelial cells into the space of Disse and from there to portal areas, where they can return to the circulation through lymphatics.

Hepatocytes perform numerous and vital roles in maintaining homeostasis and health. These functions include the synthesis of most essential serum proteins (albumin, carrier proteins, coagulation factors, many hormonal and growth factors), the production of bile and its carriers (bile acids, cholesterol, lecithin, phospholipids), the regulation of nutrients (glucose, glycogen, lipids, cholesterol, amino acids), and metabolism and conjugation of lipophilic compounds (bilirubin, anions, cations, drugs) for excretion in the bile or urine. Measurement of these activities to assess liver function is complicated by the multiplicity and variability of these functions. The most commonly used liver "function" tests are measurements of serum bilirubin, albumin, and prothrombin time. The serum bilirubin level is a measure of hepatic conjugation and excretion, and the serum albumin level and prothrombin time are measures of protein synthesis. Abnormalities of bilirubin, albumin, and prothrombin time are typical of hepatic dysfunction. Frank liver failure is incompatible with life, and the functions of the liver are too complex and diverse to be subserved by a mechanical pump; dialysis membrane; or concoction of infused hormones, proteins, and growth factors.

LIVER DISEASES While there are many causes of liver disease (Table 282-1), they generally present clinically in a few distinct patterns, usually classified as hepatocellular, cholestatic (obstructive), or mixed. In *hepatocellular diseases* (such as viral hepatitis or alcoholic liver disease), features of liver injury, inflammation, and necrosis predominate. In *cholestatic diseases* (such as gall stone or malignant obstruction, primary biliary cirrhosis, some drug-induced liver diseases), features of inhibition of bile flow predominate. In a mixed pattern, features of both hepatocellular and cholestatic injury are present (such as in cholestatic forms of viral hepatitis and many drug-induced liver diseases). The pattern of onset and prominence of symptoms can rapidly suggest a diagnosis, particularly if major risk factors are considered, such as the age and sex of the patient and a history of exposure or risk behaviors.

Typical presenting symptoms of liver disease include jaundice, fatigue, itching, right upper quadrant pain, abdominal distention, and intestinal bleeding. At present, however, many patients are diagnosed with liver disease who have no symptoms and who have been found to have abnormalities in biochemical liver tests as a part of a routine physical examination or screening for blood donation or for insurance or employment. The wide availability of batteries of liver tests makes it relatively simple to demonstrate the presence of liver injury as well as to rule it out in someone suspected of liver disease.

Evaluation of patients with liver disease should be directed at (1) establishing the etiologic diagnosis, (2) estimating the disease severity (grading), and (3) establishing the disease stage (staging). *Diagnosis* should focus on the category of disease, such as hepatocellular, cholestatic, or mixed injury, as well as on the specific etiologic diagnosis. *Grading* refers to assessing the severity or activity of disease—active or inactive, and mild, moderate, or severe. *Staging* refers to estimating the place in the course of the natural history of the disease, whether acute or chronic; early or late; precirrhotic, cirrhotic, or end-stage.

The goal of this chapter is to introduce general, salient concepts in the evaluation of patients with liver disease that help lead to the diagnoses discussed in subsequent chapters.

CLINICAL HISTORY The clinical history should focus on the symptoms of liver disease—their nature, pattern of onset, and progression—and on potential risk factors for liver disease. The symptoms of liver disease include constitutional symptoms such as fatigue, weakness, nausea, poor appetite, and malaise and the more liver-specific symptoms

TABLE 282-1 *Liver Diseases*

Inherited hyperbilirubinemia	Liver involvement in systemic diseases
Gilbert's syndrome	Sarcoidosis
Crigler-Najjar syndrome, types I and II	Amyloidosis
Dubin-Johnson syndrome	Glycogen storage diseases
Rotor syndrome	Celiac disease
Viral hepatitis	Tuberculosis
Hepatitis A	*Myobacterium avium intracellulare*
Hepatitis B	Cholestatic syndromes
Hepatitis C	Benign postoperative cholestasis
Hepatitis D	Jaundice of sepsis
Hepatitis E	Total parenteral nutrition (TPN)–induced
Others (mononucleosis, herpes, adenovirus	jaundice
hepatitis)	Cholestasis of pregnancy
Cryptogenic hepatitis	Cholangitis and cholecystitis
Immune and autoimmune liver diseases	Extrahepatic biliary obstruction (stone, stricture,
Primary biliary cirrhosis	cancer)
Autoimmune hepatitis	Biliary atresia
Sclerosing cholangitis	Caroli's disease
Overlap syndromes	Cryptosporidiosis
Graft-vs-host disease	Drug induced liver disease
Allograft rejection	Hepatocellular patterns (isoniazid, acetaminophen)
Genetic liver diseases	Cholestatic patterns (methyltestosterone)
α_1 Antitrypsin deficiency	Mixed patterns (sulfonamides, phenytoin)
Hemochromatosis	Micro- and macrovesicular steatosis
Wilson's disease	(methotrexate, fialuridine)
Benign recurrent intrahepatic cholestasis	Vascular injury
(BRIC)	Venoocclusive disease
Familial intrahepatic cholestasis (FIC),	Budd-Chiari syndrome
types I–III	Ischemic hepatitis
Others (galactosemia, tyrosinemia, cystic	Passive congestion
fibrosis, Newman-Pick disease,	Portal vein thrombosis
Gaucher's disease)	Nodular regenerative hyperplasia
Alcoholic liver disease	Mass lesions
Acute fatty liver	Hepatocellular carcinoma
Acute alcoholic hepatitis	Cholangiocarcinoma
Laennec's cirrhosis	Adenoma
Nonalcoholic fatty liver	Focal nodular hyperplasia
Steatosis	Metastatic tumors
Steatohepatitis	Abscess
Acute fatty liver of pregnancy	Cysts

of jaundice, dark urine, light stools, itching, abdominal pain, and bloating. Symptoms can also suggest the presence of cirrhosis, end-stage liver disease, or complications of cirrhosis such as portal hypertension. Generally, the constellation of symptoms and their pattern of onset rather than a specific symptom points to an etiology.

Fatigue is the most common and most characteristic symptom of liver disease. It is variously described as lethargy, weakness, listlessness, malaise, increased need for sleep, lack of stamina, and poor energy. The fatigue of liver disease typically arises after activity or exercise and is rarely present or severe in the morning after adequate rest (afternoon versus morning fatigue). Fatigue in liver disease is often intermittent and variable in severity from hour to hour and day to day. In some patients, it may not be clear whether fatigue is due to the liver disease or to other problems such as stress, anxiety, sleep disturbance, or a concurrent illness.

Nausea occurs with more severe liver disease and may accompany fatigue or be provoked by odors of food or eating fatty foods. Vomiting can occur but is rarely persistent or prominent. Poor appetite with weight loss occurs commonly in acute liver diseases but is rare in chronic disease, except when cirrhosis is present and advanced. Diarrhea is uncommon in liver disease, except with severe jaundice, where lack of bile acids reaching the intestine can lead to steatorrhea.

Right upper quadrant discomfort or ache ("liver pain") occurs in many liver diseases and is usually marked by tenderness over the liver area. The pain arises from stretching or irritation of Glisson's capsule, which surrounds the liver and is rich in nerve endings. Severe pain is most typical of gall bladder disease, liver abscess, and severe venoocclusive disease but is an occasional accompaniment of acute hepatitis.

Itching occurs with acute liver disease, appearing early in obstructive jaundice (from biliary obstruction or drug-induced cholestasis) and somewhat later in hepatocellular disease (acute hepatitis). Itching also occurs in chronic liver diseases, typically the cholestatic forms such as primary biliary cirrhosis and sclerosing cholangitis where it is often the presenting symptom, occurring before the onset of jaundice. However, itching can occur in any liver disease, particularly once cirrhosis is present.

Jaundice is the hallmark symptom of liver disease and perhaps the most reliable marker of severity. Patients usually report darkening of the urine before they notice scleral icterus. Jaundice is rarely detectable with a bilirubin level <43 μmol/L (2.5 mg/dL). With severe cholestasis there will also be lightening of the color of the stools and steatorrhea. Jaundice without dark urine usually indicates indirect (unconjugated) hyperbilirubinemia and is typical of hemolytic anemia and the genetic disorders of bilirubin conjugation, the common and benign form being Gilbert's syndrome and the rare and severe form being Crigler-Najjar syndrome. Gilbert's syndrome affects up to 5% of the population; the jaundice is more noticeable after fasting and with stress.

Major risk factors for liver disease that should be sought in the clinical history include details of alcohol use, medications (including herbal compounds, birth control pills, and over-the-counter medications), personal habits, sexual activity, travel, exposure to jaundiced or other high-risk persons, injection drug use, recent surgery, remote or recent transfusion with blood and blood products, occupation, accidental exposure to blood or needlestick, and familial history of liver disease.

For assessing the risk of viral hepatitis, a careful history of sexual activity is of particular importance and should include number of lifetime sexual partners and, for men, a history of having sex with men. Sexual exposure is a common mode of spread of hepatitis B but is rare for hepatitis C. A family history of hepatitis, liver disease, and liver cancer is also important. Maternal-infant transmission occurs with both hepatitis B and C. Vertical spread of hepatitis B can now be prevented by passive and active immunization of the infant at birth. Vertical spread of hepatitis C is uncommon, but there are no reliable means of prevention. A history of injection drug use, even in the remote past, is of great importance in assessing the risk for hepatitis B and C. Injection drug use is now the single most common risk factor for hepatitis C. Transfusion with blood or blood products is no longer an important risk factor for acute viral hepatitis. However, blood transfusions received before the introduction of sensitive enzyme immunoassays for antibody to hepatitis C virus (anti-HCV) in 1992 is an important risk factor for chronic hepatitis C. Blood transfusion before 1986, when screening for antibody to hepatitis B core antigen (anti-HBc) was introduced, is also a risk factor for hepatitis B. Travel to an underdeveloped area of the world, exposure to persons with jaundice, and exposure to young children in day-care centers are risk factors for hepatitis A. Tattooing and body piercing (for hepatitis B and C) and eating shellfish (for hepatitis A) are frequently mentioned but actually quite rare types of exposure for acquiring hepatitis.

A history of alcohol intake is important in assessing the cause of liver disease and also in planning management and recommendations. In the United States, for example, at least 70% of adults drink alcohol to some degree, but significant alcohol intake is less common; in population-based surveys, only 5% have more than two drinks per day, the average drink representing 11 to 15 g alcohol. Alcohol consumption associated with an increased rate of alcoholic liver disease is probably more than two drinks (22 to 30 g) per day in women and three drinks (33 to 45 g) in men. Most patients with alcoholic cirrhosis have a much higher daily intake and have drunk excessively for 10 years or more before onset of liver disease. In assessing alcohol intake, the history should also focus upon whether alcohol abuse or dependence is present. Alcoholism is usually defined on the behavioral patterns and consequences of alcohol intake, not on the basis of the amount of alcohol intake. *Abuse* is defined by a repetitive pattern of drinking

alcohol that has adverse effects on social, family, occupational, or health status. *Dependence* is defined by alcohol-seeking behavior, despite its adverse effects. Many alcoholics demonstrate both dependence and abuse, and dependence is considered the more serious and advanced form of alcoholism. A clinically helpful approach to diagnosis of alcohol dependence and abuse is the use of the CAGE questionnaire (Table 282-2), which is recommended in all medical history taking.

Family history can be helpful in assessing liver disease. Familial causes of liver disease include Wilson's disease; hemochromatosis and α_1 antitrypsin (α_1AT) deficiency; and the more uncommon inherited pediatric liver diseases of familial intrahepatic cholestasis, benign recurrent intrahepatic cholestasis, and Alagille's syndrome. Onset of severe liver disease in childhood or adolescence with a family history of liver disease or neuropsychiatric disturbance should lead to investigation for Wilson's disease. A family history of cirrhosis, diabetes, or endocrine failure and the appearance of liver disease in adulthood should suggest hemochromatosis and lead to investigation of iron status. Patients with abnormal iron studies warrant genotyping of the *HFE* gene for the C282Y and H63D mutations typical of genetic hemochromatosis. A family history of emphysema should provoke investigation of α_1AT levels and, if low, for Pi genotype.

PHYSICAL EXAMINATION The physical examination rarely demonstrates evidence of liver dysfunction in a patient without symptoms or laboratory findings, nor are most signs of liver disease specific to one diagnosis. Thus, the physical examination usually complements rather than replaces the need for other diagnostic approaches. In many patients, the physical examination is normal unless the disease is acute or severe and advanced. Nevertheless, the physical examination is important in that it can be the first evidence for the presence of hepatic failure, portal hypertension, and liver decompensation. In addition, the physical examination can reveal signs that point to a specific diagnosis, either in risk factors or in associated diseases or findings.

Typical physical findings in liver disease are icterus, hepatomegaly, hepatic tenderness, splenomegaly, spider angiomata, palmar erythema, and excoriations. Signs of advanced disease include muscle-wasting, ascites, edema, dilated abdominal veins, hepatic fetor, asterixis, mental confusion, stupor, and coma. In males with cirrhosis, particularly when related to alcohol, signs of hyperestrogenemia such as gynecomastia, testicular atrophy, and loss of male-pattern hair distribution may be found.

Icterus is best appreciated by inspecting the sclera under natural light. In fair-skinned individuals, a yellow color of the skin may be obvious. In dark-skinned individuals, the mucous membranes below the tongue can demonstrate jaundice. Jaundice is rarely detectable if the serum bilirubin level is <43 μmol/L (2.5 mg/dL) but may remain detectable below this level during recovery from jaundice (because of protein and tissue binding of conjugated bilirubin).

Spider angiomata and palmar erythema occur in both acute and chronic liver disease and may be especially prominent in persons with cirrhosis, but they can occur in normal individuals and are frequently present during pregnancy. Spider angiomata are superficial, tortuous arterioles and, unlike simple telangiectases, typically fill from the center outwards. Spider angiomata occur only on the arms, face, and upper torso; they can be pulsatile and may be difficult to detect in dark-skinned individuals.

TABLE 282-2 CAGE Questions[a]	
Acronym	**Question**
C	Have you ever felt you ought to *C*ut down on your drinking?
A	Have people *A*nnoyed you by criticizing your drinking?
G	Have you ever felt *G*uilty or bad about your drinking?
E	Have you ever had a drink first thing in the morning to steady your nerves or get rid of a hangover (*E*yeopener)?

[a] One "yes" response should raise suspicion of an alcohol use problem, and more than one is a strong indication that abuse or dependence exists.

Hepatomegaly is not a very reliable sign of liver disease, because of the variability of the size and shape of the liver and the physical impediments to assessing liver size by percussion and palpation. Marked hepatomegaly is typical of cirrhosis, venoocclusive disease, metastatic or primary cancers of the liver, and alcoholic hepatitis. Careful assessment of the liver edge may also demonstrate unusual firmness, irregularity of the surface, or frank nodules. Perhaps the most reliable physical finding in examining the liver is hepatic tenderness. Discomfort on touching or pressing on the liver should be carefully sought with percussive comparison of the right and left upper quadrants.

Splenomegaly occurs in many medical conditions but can be a subtle but significant physical finding in liver disease. The availability of ultrasound (US) assessment of the spleen allows for confirmation of the physical finding.

Signs of advanced liver disease include muscle-wasting and weight loss as well as hepatomegaly, bruising, ascites, and edema. Ascites is best appreciated by attempts to detect shifting dullness by careful percussion. US examination will confirm the finding of ascites in equivocal cases. Peripheral edema can occur with or without ascites. In patients with advanced liver disease, other factors frequently contribute to edema formation, including hypoalbuminemia, venous insufficiency, heart failure, and medications.

Hepatic failure is defined as the occurrence of signs or symptoms of hepatic encephalopathy in a person with severe acute or chronic liver disease. The first signs of hepatic encephalopathy can be subtle and nonspecific—change in sleep patterns, change in personality, irritability, and mental dullness. Thereafter, confusion, disorientation, stupor, and eventually coma supervene. Physical findings include asterixis and flapping tremors of the body and tongue. *Fetor hepaticus* refers to the slightly sweet, ammoniacal odor that is common in patients with liver failure, particularly if there is portal-venous shunting of blood around the liver. Other causes of coma and confusion should be excluded, mainly electrolyte imbalances, sedative use, and renal or respiratory failure. A helpful measure of hepatic encephalopathy is a careful mental status examination and use of the trail-making test, which consists of a series of 25 numbered circles that the patient is asked to connect as rapidly as possible using a pencil. The normal range for the connect-the-dot test is 15 to 30 s; it is considerably delayed in patients with early hepatic encephalopathy. Other tests include drawing abstract objects or comparison of a signature to previous examples.

Other signs of advanced liver disease include umbilical hernia from ascites, prominent veins over the abdomen, and *caput medusa*, which consists of collateral veins seen radiating from the umbilicus and resulting from the recanulation of the umbilical vein. Widened pulse pressure and signs of a hyperdynamic circulation can occur in patients with cirrhosis as a result of fluid and sodium retention, increased cardiac output, and reduced peripheral resistance. Patients with long-standing cirrhosis and portal hypertension are prone to develop the hepatopulmonary syndrome, defined by the triad of liver disease, with hypoxemia, and pulmonary arteriovenous shunting. The hepatopulmonary syndrome is characterized by platypnea and orthodeoxia, representing shortness of breath and oxygen desaturation that occur paradoxically upon assuming an upright position.

Several skin disorders and changes occur commonly in liver disease. Hyperpigmentation is typical of advanced chronic cholestatic diseases such as primary biliary cirrhosis and sclerosing cholangitis. In these same conditions, xanthelasma and tendon xanthomata occur as a result of retention and high serum levels of lipids and cholesterol. A slate-gray pigmentation to the skin also occurs with hemochromatosis if iron levels are high for a prolonged period. Mucocutaneous vasculitis with palpable purpura, especially on the lower extremities, is typical of cryoglobulinemia of chronic hepatitis C but can also occur in chronic hepatitis B.

Some physical signs point to specific liver diseases. Kayser-Fleischer rings occur in Wilson's disease and consist of a golden-brown copper pigment deposited in Disemet's membrane at the periphery of the cornea; they are best seen by slit-lamp examination. In metastatic liver disease or primary hepatocellular carcinoma, signs of cachexia and wasting may be prominent, as well as firm hepatomegaly and a hepatic bruit.

LABORATORY TESTING　Diagnosis in liver disease is greatly aided by the availability of reliable and sensitive tests of liver injury and function. Use and interpretation of liver function tests is summarized in Chap. 283. A typical battery of blood tests used for initial assessment of liver disease includes measuring levels of serum alanine and aspartate aminotransferases (ALT and AST), alkaline phosphatase, direct and total serum bilirubin, and albumin and assessing prothrombin time. The pattern of abnormalities generally points to hepatocellular versus cholestatic liver disease and will help to decide whether the disease is acute or chronic and whether cirrhosis and hepatic failure are present. Based on these results, further testing over time may be necessary. Other laboratory tests may be helpful, such as γ-glutamyl transpeptidase (GGT) to define whether alkaline phosphatase elevations are due to liver disease; hepatitis serology to define the type of viral hepatitis; and autoimmune markers to diagnose primary biliary cirrhosis (antimitochondrial antibody; AMA), sclerosing cholangitis (peripheral antineutrophil cytoplasmic antibody; P-ANCA), and autoimmune hepatitis (antinuclear, smooth-muscle, and liver-kidney microsomal antibody). A simple delineation of laboratory abnormalities and common liver diseases is given in Table 282-3.

DIAGNOSTIC IMAGING　There have been great advances made in hepatic imaging, although no method is suitably accurate in demonstrating underlying cirrhosis. There are many modalities available for imaging the liver. US, computed tomography (CT), and magnetic resonance imaging (MRI) are the most commonly employed and are complementary to each other. In general, US and CT have a high sensitivity for detecting biliary duct dilatation and are the first-line options for investigating the patient with suspected obstructive jaundice. Both US and CT can detect a fatty liver, which appears bright on both studies. Magnetic resonance cholangiopancreatography (MRCP) and endo-

TABLE 282-3　*Important Diagnostic Tests in Common Liver Diseases*

Disease	Diagnostic Test
Hepatitis A	Anti-HAV IgM
Hepatitis B	
Acute	HBsAg and anti-HBc IgM
Chronic	HBsAg and HBeAg and/or HBV DNA
Hepatitis C	Anti-HCV and HCV RNA
Hepatitis D (delta)	HBsAg and anti-HDV
Hepatitis E	Anti-HEV
Autoimmune hepatitis	ANA or SMA, elevated IgG levels, and compatible histology
Primary biliary cirrhosis	Mitochondrial antibody, elevated IgM levels, and compatible histology
Primary sclerosing cholangitis	P-ANCA, cholangiography
Drug-induced liver disease	History of drug ingestion
Alcoholic liver disease	History of excessive alcohol intake and compatible histology
Nonalcoholic steatohepatitis	Ultrasound or CT evidence of fatty liver and compatible histology
α_1 Antitrypsin disease	Reduced α_1 antitrypsin levels, phenotypes PiZZ or PiSZ
Wilson's disease	Decreased serum ceruloplasmin and increased urinary copper; increased hepatic copper level
Hemochromatosis	Elevated iron saturation and serum ferritin; genetic testing for *HFE* gene mutations
Hepatocellular cancer	Elevated α-fetoprotein level >500; ultrasound or CT image of mass

Note: HAV, HBV, HCV, HDV, HEV: hepatitis A, B, C, D, or E virus; HBsAg, hepatitis B surface antigen; anti-HBc, antibody to hepatitis B core (antigen); HBeAg, hepatitis e antigen; ANA, antinuclear antibodies; SMA, smooth-muscle antibody; P-ANCA, peripheral antineutrophil cytoplasmic antibody; CT, computed tomography.

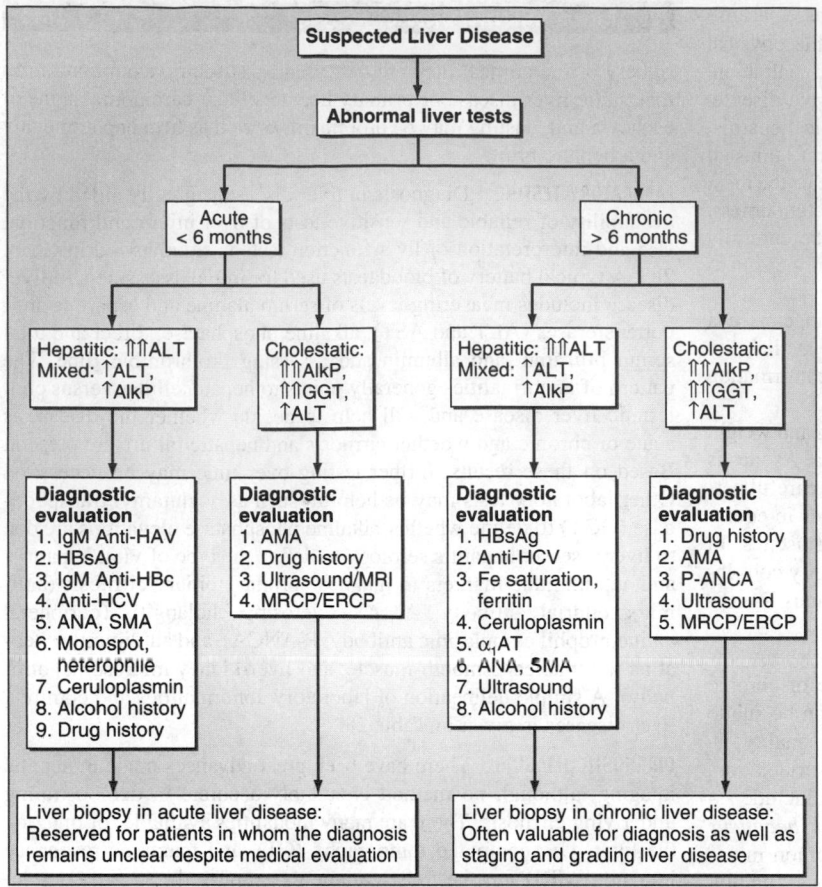

FIGURE 282-1 Algorithm for evaluation of abnormal liver tests. For patients with suspected liver disease, an appropriate approach to evaluation is initial testing for routine liver tests such as bilirubin, albumin, alanine aminotransferase (ALT), aspartate aminotransferase (AST), and alkaline phosphatase (AlkP). These results (sometimes complemented by testing of γ-glutamyl transpeptidase; GGT) will establish whether the pattern of abnormalities is hepatic, cholestatic, or mixed. In addition, the duration of symptoms or abnormalities will show whether the disease is acute or chronic. If the disease is acute and if history, laboratory tests, and imaging studies do not reveal a diagnosis, liver biopsy is appropriate to help to establish the diagnosis. If the disease is chronic, liver biopsy can be helpful not only for diagnosis, but also to grade the activity and stage the progression of disease. This approach is largely applicable to patients without immune deficiency. In patients with HIV infection or after bone marrow or solid organ transplantation, diagnostic evaluation should also include evaluation of opportunistic infections (adenovirus, cytomegalovirus, coccidioidomycosis, etc.) as well as vascular and immunologic conditions (venoocclusive disease, graft-vs-host disease). HAV, HCV: hepatitis A or C virus; HBsAg, hepatitis B surface antigen; anti-HBc, antibody to hepatitis B core (antigen); ANA, antinuclear antibodies; SMA, smooth-muscle antibody; MRI, magnetic resonance imaging; MRCP; magnetic resonance cholangiopancreatography; ERCP, endoscopic retrograde cholangiopancreatography; α_1AT, α_1 antitrypsin; AMA; antimitochondrial antibody; P-ANCA, peripheral antineutrophil cytoplasmic antibody.

scopic retrograde cholangiopancreatography (ERCP) are the procedures of choice for visualization of the biliary tree. MRCP offers several advantages over ERCP; there is no need for contrast media or ionizing radiation, images can be acquired faster, it is less operator dependent, and it carries no risk of pancreatitis. MRCP is superior to US and CT for detecting choledocholithiasis but less specific. It is useful in the diagnosis of bile duct obstruction and congenital biliary abnormalities, but ERCP is more valuable in evaluating ampullary lesions and primary sclerosing cholangitis. ERCP allows for biopsy, direct visualization of the ampulla and common bile duct, and intraductal ultrasonography. It also provides several therapeutic options in patients with obstructive jaundice, such as sphincterotomy, stone extraction, and placement of nasobiliary catheters and biliary stents. Doppler US and MRI are used to assess hepatic vasculature and hemodynamics and to monitor surgically or radiologically placed vascular shunts such as transjugular intrahepatic portosystemic shunts. CT and MRI are indicated for the identification and evaluation of hepatic masses, staging of liver tumors, and preoperative assessment. With regard to mass lesions, sensitivity of hepatic imaging continues to increase; unfortunately, specificity remains a problem, and often two

and sometimes three studies are needed before a diagnosis can be reached. Finally, interventional radiologic techniques allow the biopsy of solitary lesions, insertion of drains into hepatic abscesses, and creation of vascular shunts in patients with portal hypertension. Which modality to use depends on factors such as availability, cost, and experience of the radiologist with each technique.

LIVER BIOPSY Liver biopsy remains the gold standard in the evaluation of patients with liver disease, particularly in patients with chronic liver diseases. In selected instances, liver biopsy is necessary for diagnosis but is more often useful in assessing the severity (grade) and stage of liver damage, in predicting prognosis, and in monitoring response to treatment.

Diagnosis of Liver Disease The major causes of liver disease and key diagnostic features are outlined in Table 282-3, and an algorithm for evaluation of the patient with suspected liver disease is given in Fig. 282-1. Specifics of diagnosis are discussed in later chapters. The most common causes of acute liver disease are viral hepatitis (particularly hepatitis A, B, and C), drug-induced liver injury, cholangitis, and alcoholic liver disease. Liver biopsy is usually not needed in the diagnosis and management of acute liver disease, exceptions being situations where the diagnosis remains unclear despite thorough clinical and laboratory investigation. Liver biopsy can be helpful in the diagnosis of drug-induced liver disease and in establishing the diagnosis of acute alcoholic hepatitis.

The most common causes of chronic liver disease in general order of frequency are chronic hepatitis C, alcoholic liver disease, nonalcoholic steatohepatitis, chronic hepatitis B, autoimmune hepatitis, sclerosing cholangitis, primary biliary cirrhosis, hemochromatosis, and Wilson's disease. Strict diagnostic criteria have not been developed for most liver diseases, but liver biopsy plays an important role in the diagnosis of autoimmune hepatitis, primary biliary cirrhosis, nonalcoholic and alcoholic steatohepatitis, and Wilson's disease (with a quantitative hepatic copper level).

Grading and Staging of Liver Disease Grading refers to an assessment of the severity or activity of liver disease, whether acute or chronic; active or inactive; and mild, moderate, or severe. Liver biopsy is the most accurate means of assessing severity, particularly in chronic liver disease. Serum aminotransferase levels are used as a convenient and noninvasive means to follow disease activity, but aminotransferases are not always reliable in reflecting disease severity. Thus, normal serum aminotransferases in patients with hepatitis B surface antigen (HBsAg) in serum may indicate the inactive HBsAg carrier state or may reflect mild chronic hepatitis B or hepatitis B with fluctuating disease activity. Serum testing for hepatitis B e antigen and hepatitis B virus DNA can help resolve these different patterns, but these markers can also fluctuate and change over time. Similarly, in chronic hepatitis C, serum aminotransferases can be normal despite moderate activity of disease. Finally, in both alcoholic and nonalcoholic steatohepatitis, aminotransferases are quite unreliable in reflecting severity. In these conditions, liver biopsy is helpful in guiding management and recommending therapy, particularly if therapy is difficult, prolonged, and expensive as is often the case in chronic viral hepatitis. There are several well-verified numerical scales for grading activity in chronic liver disease, the most common being the histology activity index and the Ishak histology scale.

Liver biopsy is also the most accurate means of assessing stage of disease as early or advanced, precirrhotic, and cirrhotic. Staging of disease pertains largely to chronic liver diseases in which progression

TABLE 282-4 *Child-Pugh Classification of Cirrhosis*

Factor	Units	1	2	3
Serum bilirubin	μmol/L	<34	34–51	>51
	mg/dL	<2.0	2.0–3.0	>3.0
Serum albumin	g/L	>35	30–35	<30
	g/dL	>3.5	3.0–3.5	<3.0
Prothrombin time	second prolonged	0–4	4–6	>6
	INR	<1.7	1.7–2.3	>2.3
Ascites		None	Easily controlled	Poorly controlled
Hepatic encephalopathy		None	Minimal	Advanced

Note: The Child-Pugh score is calculated by adding the scores of the five factors and can range from 5 to 15. Child-Pugh class is either A (a score of 5 to 6), B (7 to 9), or C (10 or above). Decompensation indicates cirrhosis with a Child-Pugh score of 7 or more (Class B). This level has been the accepted criterion for listing for liver transplantation.

to cirrhosis and end-stage liver disease can occur, but which may require years or decades to develop. Clinical features, biochemical tests, and hepatic imaging studies are helpful in assessing stage but generally become abnormal only in the middle to late stages of cirrhosis. Noninvasive tests that suggest advanced fibrosis include mild elevations of bilirubin, prolongation of prothrombin time, slight decreases in serum albumin, and mild thrombocytopenia (which is often the first indication of worsening fibrosis). Early stages of cirrhosis are generally detectable only by liver biopsy. In assessing stage, the degree of fibrosis is usually used as its quantitative measure. The amount of fibrosis is generally staged on a 0 to 4+ (histology activity index) or 0 to 6+ scale (Ishak scale). The importance of staging relates primarily to prognosis and to guiding management of complications. Patients with cirrhosis are candidates for screening and surveillance for esophageal varices and hepatocellular carcinoma. Patients without advanced fibrosis need not undergo screening.

Cirrhosis can also be staged clinically. A reliable staging system is the modified Child-Pugh classification with a scoring system of 5 to 15: scores of 5 and 6 being Child-Pugh class A (consistent with "compensated cirrhosis"), scores of 7 to 9 indicating class B, and 10 to 15 class C (Table 282-4). This scoring system was initially devised to stratify patients into risk groups prior to undergoing portal decompressive surgery. The Child-Pugh score is a reasonably reliable predictor of survival in many liver diseases and predicts the likelihood of major complications of cirrhosis such as bleeding from varices and spontaneous bacterial peritonitis. It was used to assess prognosis in cirrhosis and to provide the standard criteria for listing for liver transplantation (Child-Pugh class B). Recently the Child-Pugh system has been replaced by the model for end-stage liver disease (MELD) score for assessing the need for liver transplantation. The MELD score is a prospectively derived scoring system designed to predict prognosis of patients with liver disease and portal hypertension. It is calculated using three noninvasive variables—the prothrombin time expressed as international normalized ratio (INR), serum bilirubin, and serum

creatinine (www.mayo.edu/int-med/gi/model/). MELD provides a more objective means of assessing disease severity and has less center-to-center variation than the Child-Pugh score and has a wider range of values. MELD is currently used to establish priority listing for liver transplantation in the United States.

Thus, liver biopsy is helpful not only in diagnosis but also in management of chronic liver disease and assessment of prognosis. Because liver biopsy is an invasive procedure and not without complications, it should be used only when it will contribute materially to management and therapeutic decisions.

NONSPECIFIC ISSUES IN MANAGEMENT OF PATIENTS WITH LIVER DISEASE

Specifics on management of different forms of acute or chronic liver disease are given in subsequent chapters, but certain issues are applicable to any patient with liver disease. These include advice regarding alcohol use, medications, vaccination, and surveillance for complications of liver disease. Alcohol should be used sparingly, if at all, by patients with liver disease. Abstinence from alcohol should be encouraged for all patients with alcohol-related liver disease and in patients with cirrhosis and those receiving interferon-based therapy for hepatitis B or C. Regarding vaccinations, all patients with liver disease should receive hepatitis A vaccine and those with risk factors should receive hepatitis B vaccination as well. Influenza and pneumococcal vaccination should also be encouraged. Patients with liver disease should be careful in use of any medications, other than the most necessary. Drug-induced hepatotoxicity can mimic many forms of liver disease and can cause exacerbations of chronic hepatitis and cirrhosis; drugs should be suspected in any situation where the cause of exacerbation is unknown. Finally, consideration should be given to surveillance for complications of chronic liver disease such as variceal hemorrhage and hepatocellular carcinoma. Patients with cirrhosis warrant upper endoscopy to assess the presence of varices and should be given chronic therapy with beta blockers if large varices are found. Patients with cirrhosis also warrant screening and long-term surveillance for development of hepatocellular carcinoma. While the optimal regimen for such surveillance has not been established, an appropriate approach is US of the liver at 6- to 12-month intervals.

FURTHER READING

DESMET VJ et al: Classification of chronic hepatitis: Diagnosis, grading and staging. Hepatology 19:1513, 1994

ISHAK K et al: Histological grading and staging of chronic hepatitis. J Hepatol 22:696, 1995

KAMATH PS et al: A model to predict survival in patients with end-stage liver disease. Hepatology 33:464, 2001

SCHIFF ER et al (eds): *Schiff's Diseases of the Liver,* 9th ed. Philadelphia, Lippincott Williams & Wilkins, 2002

ZAKIM D, BOYER TD (eds): *Hepatology: A Textbook of Liver Disease,* 4th ed. Philadelphia, Saunders, 2003

ZIMMERMAN HJ: *Hepatotoxicity: The Adverse Effects of Drugs and Other Chemicals on the Liver,* 2d ed. Philadelphia, Lippincott Williams & Wilkins, 1999

283 EVALUATION OF LIVER FUNCTION
Daniel S. Pratt, Marshall M. Kaplan

Several biochemical tests are useful in the evaluation and management of patients with hepatic dysfunction. These tests can be used to (1) detect the presence of liver disease, (2) distinguish among different types of liver disorders, (3) gauge the extent of known liver damage, and (4) follow the response to treatment.

Liver tests have shortcomings. They can be normal in patients with serious liver disease and abnormal in patients with diseases that do not affect the liver. Liver tests rarely suggest a specific diagnosis; rather, they suggest a general category of liver disease, such as hepatocellular or cholestatic, which then further directs the evaluation.

The liver carries out thousands of biochemical functions, most of which cannot be easily measured by blood tests. Laboratory tests measure only a limited number of these functions. In fact, many tests, such as the aminotransferases or alkaline phosphatase, do not measure liver function at all. Rather, they detect liver cell damage or interference with bile flow. Thus, no one test enables the clinician to accurately assess the liver's total functional capacity.

To increase both the sensitivity and the specificity of laboratory tests in the detection of liver disease, it is best to use them as a battery. Those tests usually employed in clinical practice include the bilirubin,

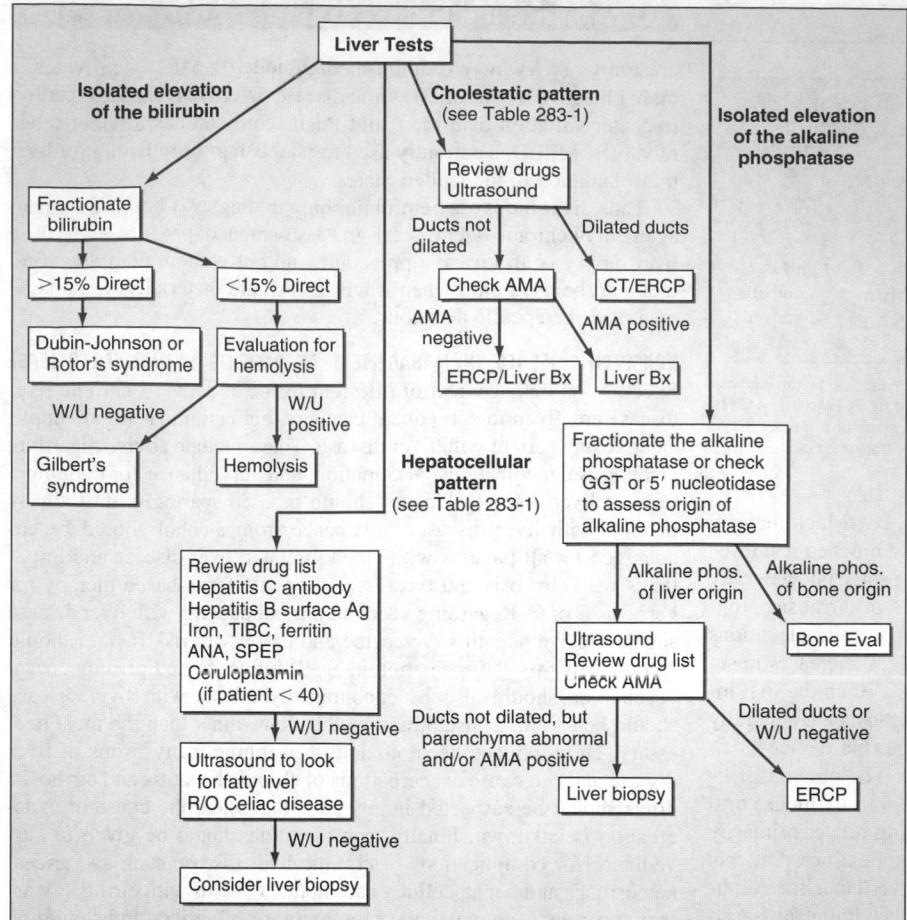

FIGURE 283-1 Algorithm for the evaluation of chronically abnormal liver tests. ERCP, endoscopic retrograde cholangiopancreatography; CT, computed tomography; AMA, antimitochondrial antibody; ANA, antinuclear antibody; SPEP, serum protein electrophoresis; TIBC, total iron-binding capacity; GGT, gamma glutamyl transpeptidase.

aminotransferases, alkaline phosphatase, albumin, and prothrombin time tests. When more than one of these tests provide abnormal findings, or the findings are persistently abnormal on serial determinations, the probability of liver disease is high. When all test results are normal, the probability of missing occult liver disease is low.

When evaluating patients with liver disorders, it is helpful to group these tests into general categories. The classification we have found most useful is given below.

TESTS BASED ON DETOXIFICATION AND EXCRETORY FUNCTIONS ■ Serum Bilirubin (See also Chap. 38)

Bilirubin, a breakdown product of the porphyrin ring of heme-containing proteins, is found in the blood in two fractions—conjugated and unconjugated. The unconjugated fraction, also termed the *indirect fraction*, is insoluble in water and is bound to albumin in the blood. The conjugated (direct) bilirubin fraction is water soluble and can therefore be excreted by the kidney. When measured by the original van den Bergh method, the normal total serum bilirubin concentration is <17 μmol/L (1 mg/dL). Up to 30%, or 5.1 μmol/L (0.3 mg/dL), of the total is direct-reacting (or conjugated) bilirubin.

Elevation of the unconjugated fraction of bilirubin is rarely due to liver disease. An isolated elevation of unconjugated bilirubin is seen primarily in hemolytic disorders and in a number of genetic conditions such as Crigler-Najjar and Gilbert's syndromes (Chap. 38). Isolated unconjugated hyperbilirubinemia (bilirubin elevated, but less than 15% direct) should prompt a workup for hemolysis (Fig. 283-1). In the absence of hemolysis, an isolated unconjugated hyperbilirubinemia in an otherwise healthy patient can be attributed to Gilbert's syndrome and no further evaluation is required.

In contrast, conjugated hyperbilirubinemia almost always implies liver or biliary tract disease. The rate-limiting step in bilirubin metab-

olism is not conjugation of bilirubin, but rather the transport of conjugated bilirubin into the bile canaliculi. Thus, elevation of the conjugated fraction may be seen in any type of liver disease. In most liver diseases, both conjugated and unconjugated fractions of the bilirubin tend to be elevated. Except in the presence of a purely unconjugated hyperbilirubinemia, fractionation of the bilirubin is rarely helpful in determining the cause of jaundice.

Urine Bilirubin Unconjugated bilirubin always binds to albumin in the serum and is not filtered by the kidney. Therefore, any bilirubin found in the urine is conjugated bilirubin; the presence of bilirubinuria implies the presence of liver disease. A urine dipstick test can theoretically give the same information as fractionation of the serum bilirubin. This test is almost 100% accurate. Phenothiazines may give a false-positive reading with the Ictotest tablet.

Blood Ammonia Ammonia is produced in the body during normal protein metabolism and by intestinal bacteria, primarily those in the colon. The liver plays a role in the detoxification of ammonia by converting it to urea, which is excreted by the kidneys. Striated muscle also plays a role in detoxification of ammonia, which is combined with glutamic acid to form glutamine. Patients with advanced liver disease typically have significant muscle wasting, which likely contributes to hyperammonemia in these patients. Some physicians use the blood ammonia for detecting encephalopathy or for monitoring hepatic synthetic function, although its use for either of these indications has problems. There is very poor correlation between either the presence or the degree of acute encephalopathy and elevation of blood ammonia; it can be occasionally useful for identifying the occult liver disease in patients with mental status changes. There is also a poor correlation of the blood serum ammonia and hepatic function. The ammonia can be elevated in patients with severe portal hypertension and portal blood shunting around the liver even in the presence of normal or near normal hepatic function.

Serum Enzymes The liver contains thousands of enzymes, some of which are also present in the serum in very low concentrations. These enzymes have no known function in the serum and behave like other serum proteins. They are distributed in the plasma and in interstitial fluid and have characteristic half-lives, usually measured in days. Very little is known about the catabolism of serum enzymes, although they are probably cleared by cells in the reticuloendothelial system. The elevation of a given enzyme activity in the serum is thought to primarily reflect its increased rate of entrance into serum from damaged liver cells.

Serum enzyme tests can be grouped into three categories: (1) enzymes whose elevation in serum reflects damage to hepatocytes, (2) enzymes whose elevation in serum reflects cholestasis, and (3) enzyme tests that do not fit precisely into either pattern.

ENZYMES THAT REFLECT DAMAGE TO HEPATOCYTES The aminotransferases (transaminases) are sensitive indicators of liver cell injury and are most helpful in recognizing acute hepatocellular diseases such as hepatitis. They include the aspartate aminotransferase (AST) and the alanine aminotransferase (ALT). AST is found in the liver, cardiac muscle, skeletal muscle, kidneys, brain, pancreas, lungs, leukocytes, and erythrocytes in decreasing order of concentration. ALT is found primarily in the liver. The aminotransferases are normally present in the serum in low concentrations. These enzymes are released into the blood in greater amounts when there is damage to the liver cell membrane resulting in increased permeability. Liver cell necrosis is not required for the release of the aminotransferases, and there is a poor correlation between the degree of liver cell damage and the level of the aminotransferases. Thus, the absolute elevation of the aminotransferases is of no prognostic significance in acute hepatocellular disorders.

Any type of liver cell injury can cause modest elevations in the serum aminotransferases. Levels of up to 300 U/L are nonspecific and may be found in any type of liver disorder. Striking elevations—i.e., aminotransferases >1000 U/L—occur almost exclusively in disorders associated with extensive hepatocellular injury such as (1) viral hepatitis, (2) ischemic liver injury (prolonged hypotension or acute heart failure), or (3) toxin or drug-induced liver injury.

The pattern of the aminotransferase elevation can be helpful diagnostically. In most acute hepatocellular disorders, the ALT is higher than or equal to the AST. An AST:ALT ratio > 2:1 is suggestive while a ratio > 3:1 is highly suggestive of alcoholic liver disease. The AST in alcoholic liver disease is rarely >300 U/L and the ALT is often normal. A low level of ALT in the serum is due to an alcohol-induced deficiency of pyridoxal phosphate.

The aminotransferases are usually not greatly elevated in obstructive jaundice. One notable exception occurs during the acute phase of biliary obstruction caused by the passage of a gallstone into the common bile duct. In this setting, the aminotransferases can briefly be in the 1000 to 2000 U/L range. However, aminotransferase levels decrease quickly, and the liver function tests rapidly evolve into one typical of cholestasis.

ENZYMES THAT REFLECT CHOLESTASIS The activities of three enzymes—alkaline phosphatase, 5′-nucleotidase, and gamma glutamyl transpeptidase (GGT)—are usually elevated in cholestasis. Alkaline phosphatase and 5′-nucleotidase are found in or near the bile canalicular membrane of hepatocytes, while GGT is located in the endoplasmic reticulum and in bile duct epithelial cells. Reflecting its more diffuse localization in the liver, GGT elevation in serum is less specific for cholestasis than are elevations of alkaline phosphatase or 5′-nucleotidase. Some have advocated the use of GGT to identify patients with occult alcohol use. Its lack of specificity makes its use in this setting questionable.

The normal serum alkaline phosphatase consists of many distinct isoenzymes found in the liver, bone, placenta, and, less commonly, small intestine. Patients over age 60 can have a mildly elevated alkaline phosphatase (1 to 1½ times normal), while individuals with blood types O and B can have an elevation of the serum alkaline phosphatase after eating a fatty meal due to the influx of intestinal alkaline phosphatase into the blood. It is also nonpathologically elevated in children and adolescents undergoing rapid bone growth because of bone alkaline phosphatase, and late in normal pregnancies due to the influx of placental alkaline phosphatase.

Elevation of liver-derived alkaline phosphatase is not totally specific for cholestasis, and a less than threefold elevation can be seen in almost any type of liver disease. Alkaline phosphatase elevations greater than four times normal occur primarily in patients with cholestatic liver disorders, infiltrative liver diseases such as cancer, and bone conditions characterized by rapid bone turnover (e.g., Paget's disease). In bone diseases, the elevation is due to increased amounts of the bone isoenzymes. In liver diseases, the elevation is almost always due to increased amounts of the liver isoenzyme.

If an elevated serum alkaline phosphatase is the only abnormal finding in an apparently healthy person, or if the degree of elevation is higher than expected in the clinical setting, identification of the source of elevated isoenzymes is helpful (Fig. 283-1). This problem can be approached in several ways. First, and most precise, is the fractionation of the alkaline phosphatase by electrophoresis. The second approach is based on the observation that alkaline phosphatases from individual tissues differ in susceptibility to inactivation by heat.

The finding of an elevated serum alkaline phosphatase level in a patient with a heat-stable fraction strongly suggests that the placenta or a tumor is the source of the elevated enzyme in serum. Susceptibility to inactivation by heat increases, respectively, for the intestinal, liver, and bone alkaline phosphatases, bone being by far the most sensitive. The third, best substantiated, and most available approach involves the measurement of serum 5′-nucleotidase or GGT. These enzymes are rarely elevated in conditions other than liver disease.

In the absence of jaundice or elevated aminotransferases, an elevated alkaline phosphatase of liver origin often, but not always, suggests early cholestasis and, less often, hepatic infiltration by tumor or granulomata. Other conditions that cause isolated elevations of the alkaline phosphatase include Hodgkin's disease, diabetes, hyperthyroidism, congestive heart failure, and inflammatory bowel disease.

The level of serum alkaline phosphatase elevation is not helpful in distinguishing between intrahepatic and extrahepatic cholestasis. There is essentially no difference among the values found in obstructive jaundice due to cancer, common duct stone, sclerosing cholangitis, or bile duct stricture. Values are similarly increased in patients with intrahepatic cholestasis due to drug-induced hepatitis, primary biliary cirrhosis, rejection of transplanted livers, and, rarely, alcohol-induced steatonecrosis. Values are also greatly elevated in hepatobiliary disorders seen in patients with AIDS (e.g., AIDS cholangiopathy due to cytomegalovirus or cryptosporidial infection and tuberculosis with hepatic involvement).

TESTS THAT MEASURE BIOSYNTHETIC FUNCTION OF THE LIVER ■ Serum Albumin

Serum albumin is synthesized exclusively by hepatocytes. Serum albumin has a long half-life: 15 to 20 days, with approximately 4% degraded per day. Because of this slow turnover, the serum albumin is not a good indicator of acute or mild hepatic dysfunction; only minimal changes in the serum albumin are seen in acute liver conditions such as viral hepatitis, drug-related hepatoxicity, and obstructive jaundice. In hepatitis, albumin levels <3 g/dL should raise the possibility of chronic liver disease. Hypoalbuminemia is more common in chronic liver disorders such as cirrhosis and usually reflects severe liver damage and decreased albumin synthesis. One exception is the patient with ascites in whom synthesis may be normal or even increased, but levels are low because of the increased volume of distribution. However, hypoalbuminemia is not specific for liver disease and may occur in protein malnutrition of any cause, as well as protein-losing enteropathies, nephrotic syndrome, and chronic infections that are associated with prolonged increases in levels of serum interleukin 1 and/or tumor necrosis factor, cytokines that inhibit albumin synthesis. Serum albumin should not be measured for screening in patients in whom there is no suspicion of liver disease. A general medical clinic study of consecutive patients in whom no indications were present for albumin measurement showed that while 12% of patients had abnormal test results, the finding was of clinical importance in only 0.4%.

Serum Globulins Serum globulins are a group of proteins made up of gamma globulins (immunoglobulins) produced by B lymphocytes and alpha and beta globulins produced primarily in hepatocytes. Gamma globulins are increased in chronic liver disease, such as chronic hepatitis and cirrhosis. In cirrhosis, the increased serum gamma globulin concentration is due to the increased synthesis of antibodies, some of which are directed against intestinal bacteria. This occurs because the cirrhotic liver fails to clear bacterial antigens that normally reach the liver through the hepatic circulation.

Increases in the concentration of specific isotypes of gamma globulins are often helpful in the recognition of certain chronic liver diseases. Diffuse polyclonal increases in IgG levels are common in autoimmune hepatitis; increases >100% should alert the clinician to this possibility. Increases in the IgM levels are common in primary biliary cirrhosis, while increases in the IgA levels occur in alcoholic liver disease.

TABLE 283-1 Liver Test Patterns in Hepatobiliary Disorders

Type of Disorder	Bilirubin	Aminotransferases	Alkaline Phosphatase	Albumin	Prothrombin Time
Hemolysis/Gilbert's syndrome	Normal to 86 μmol/L (5 mg/dl) 85% due to indirect fractions No bilirubinuria	Normal	Normal	Normal	Normal
Acute hepatocellular necrosis (viral and drug hepatitis, hepatotoxins, acute heart failure)	Both fractions may be elevated Peak usually follows aminotransferases Bilirubinuria	Elevated, often >500 IU ALT >AST	Normal to <3 times normal elevation	Normal	Usually normal. If >5X above control and not corrected by parenteral vitamin K, suggests poor prognosis
Chronic hepatocellular disorders	Both fractions may be elevated Bilirubinuria	Elevated, but usually <300 IU	Normal to <3 times normal elevation	Often decreased	Often prolonged Fails to correct with parenteral vitamin K
Alcoholic hepatitis Cirrhosis	Both fractions may be elevated Bilirubinuria	AST:ALT > 2 suggests alcoholic hepatitis or cirrhosis	Normal to <3 times normal elevation	Often decreased	Often prolonged Fails to correct with parenteral vitamin K
Intra- and extra-hepatic cholestasis (Obstructive jaundice)	Both fractions may be elevated Bilirubinuria	Normal to moderate elevation Rarely >500 IU	Elevated, often >4 times normal elevation	Normal, unless chronic	Normal If prolonged, will correct with parenteral vitamin K
Infiltrative diseases (tumor, granulomata); partial bile duct obstruction	Usually normal	Normal to slight elevation	Elevated, often >4 times normal elevation Fractionate, or confirm liver origin with 5' nucleotidase or gamma glutamyl transpeptidase	Normal	Normal

COAGULATION FACTORS   With the exception of factor VIII, the blood clotting factors are made exclusively in hepatocytes. Their serum half-lives are much shorter than albumin, ranging from 6 h for factor VII to 5 days for fibrinogen. Because of their rapid turnover, measurement of the clotting factors is the single best acute measure of hepatic synthetic function and helpful in both the diagnosis and assessing the prognosis of acute parenchymal liver disease. Useful for this purpose is the *serum prothrombin time*, which collectively measures factors II, V, VII, and X. Biosynthesis of factors II, VII, IX, and X depends on vitamin K. The prothrombin time may be elevated in hepatitis and cirrhosis as well as in disorders that lead to vitamin K deficiency such as obstructive jaundice or fat malabsorption of any kind. Marked prolongation of the prothrombin time, >5 s above control and not corrected by parenteral vitamin K administration, is a poor prognostic sign in acute viral hepatitis and other acute and chronic liver diseases.

OTHER DIAGNOSTIC TESTS   While tests may direct the physician to a category of liver disease, additional radiologic testing and procedures are often necessary to make the proper diagnosis, as shown in Fig. 283-1. The two most commonly used ancillary tests are reviewed here.

Percutaneous Liver Biopsy   Percutaneous biopsy of the liver is a safe procedure that can be easily performed at the bedside with local anesthesia. Liver biopsy is of proven value in the following situations: (1) hepatocellular disease of uncertain cause, (2) prolonged hepatitis with the possibility of chronic active hepatitis, (3) unexplained hepatomegaly, (4) unexplained splenomegaly, (5) hepatic filling defects by radiologic imaging, (6) fever of unknown origin, (7) staging of malignant lymphoma. Liver biopsy is most accurate in disorders causing diffuse changes throughout the liver and is subject to sampling error in focal infiltrative disorders such as hepatic metastases. Liver biopsy should not be the initial procedure in the diagnosis of cholestasis. The biliary tree should first be assessed for signs of obstruction.

Ultrasonography   Ultrasonography is the first diagnostic test to use in patients whose liver tests suggest cholestasis, to look for the presence of a dilated intrahepatic or extrahepatic biliary tree or to identify gallstones. In addition, it shows space-occupying lesions within the liver, enables the clinician to distinguish between cystic and solid masses, and helps direct percutaneous biopsies. Ultrasound with Doppler imaging can detect the patency of the portal vein, hepatic artery, and hepatic veins and determine the direction of blood flow. This is the first test ordered in patients suspected of having Budd-Chiari syndrome.

USE OF LIVER TESTS   As previously noted, the best way to increase the sensitivity and specificity of laboratory tests in the detection of liver disease is to employ a battery of tests that include the aminotransferases, alkaline phosphatase, bilirubin, albumin, and prothrombin time along with the judicious use of the other tests described in this chapter. Table 283-1 shows how patterns of liver tests can lead the clinician to a category of disease that will direct further evaluation. However, it is important to remember that no single set of liver tests will necessarily provide a diagnosis. It is often necessary to repeat these tests on several occasions over days to weeks for a diagnostic pattern to emerge. Figure 283-1 is an algorithm for the evaluation of chronically abnormal liver tests.

FURTHER READING

BOSMA PJ et al: The genetic basis of the reduced expression of bilirubin UDP-glucoronosyltransferase 1 in Gilbert's syndrome. N Engl J Med 333:1171, 1995

BRENSILVER HL, KAPLAN MM: Significance of elevated liver alkaline phosphatase in serum. Gastroenterology 68:1556, 1975

COHEN JA, KAPLAN MM: The SGOT/SGPT ratio: An indicator of alcoholic liver disease. Dig Dis Sci 24:835, 1979

PRATT DS, KAPLAN MM: Laboratory tests, in *Schiff's Diseases of the Liver*, 9th ed, ER Schiff et al (eds). Philadelphia, Lippincott Williams & Wilkins, 2003

WEISS JS et al: The clinical importance of a protein bound fraction of serum bilirubin in patients with hyperbilirubinemia. N Engl J Med 309:147, 1983

284 THE HYPERBILIRUBINEMIAS
Allan W. Wolkoff

BILIRUBIN METABOLISM

The details of bilirubin metabolism are presented in Chap. 38, "Jaundice." However, the hyperbilirubinemias are best understood in terms of perturbations of specific aspects of bilirubin metabolism and transport, and these will be briefly reviewed here as depicted in Fig. 284-1.

Bilirubin is the end product of heme degradation. From 70 to 90% of bilirubin is derived from degradation of the hemoglobin of senescent red blood cells. Bilirubin produced in the periphery is transported to the liver within the plasma, where, due to its insolubility in aqueous solutions, it is tightly bound to albumin. Under normal circumstances, bilirubin is removed from the circulation rapidly and efficiently by hepatocytes. Transfer of bilirubin from blood to bile involves four distinct but interrelated steps (Fig. 284-1):

1. *Hepatocellular uptake*: Uptake of bilirubin by the hepatocyte has carrier-mediated kinetics. Although a number of candidate bilirubin transporters have been proposed, the actual transporter remains elusive.

2. *Intracellular binding*: Within the hepatocyte, bilirubin is kept in solution by binding as a nonsubstrate ligand to several of the glutathione-S-transferases, formerly called ligandins.

3. *Conjugation*: Bilirubin is conjugated with one or two glucuronic acid moieties by a specific UDP-glucuronosyltransferase to form bilirubin mono- and diglucuronide, respectively. Conjugation disrupts the internal hydrogen bonding that limits aqueous solubility of bilirubin, and the resulting glucuronide conjugates are highly soluble in water. Conjugation is obligatory for excretion of bilirubin across the bile canalicular membrane into bile. The UDP-glucuronosyltransferases have been classified into gene families based on the degree of homology among the mRNAs for the various isoforms. Those that conjugate bilirubin and certain other substrates have been designated the *UGT1* family. These are expressed from a single gene complex by alternative promoter usage. This gene complex contains multiple substrate-specific first exons, designated A1, A2, etc. (Fig. 284-2), each with its own promoter and each encoding the amino-terminal half of a specific isoform. In addition, there are four common exons (exons 2 to 5) that encode the shared carboxyl-terminal half of all of the *UGT1* isoforms. The various first exons encode the specific aglycone substrate–binding sites for each isoform, while the shared exons encode the binding site for the sugar donor, UDP-glucuronic acid, and the

transmembrane domain. Exon A1 and the four common exons, collectively designated the *UGT1A1* gene (Fig. 284-2), encode the physiologically critical enzyme bilirubin-UDP-glucuronosyltransferase (UGT1A1). A functional corollary of the organization of the *UGT1* gene is that a mutation in one of the first exons will affect only a single enzyme isoform. By contrast, a mutation in exons 2 to 5 will alter all isoforms encoded by the *UGT1* gene complex.

4. *Biliary excretion*: Bilirubin mono- and diglucuronides are excreted across the canalicular plasma membrane into the bile canaliculus by an ATP-dependent transport process mediated by a canalicular membrane protein called *multidrug resistance–associated protein 2* (MRP2). Mutations of MRP2 result in the Dubin-Johnson syndrome (see below).

EXTRAHEPATIC ASPECTS OF BILIRUBIN DISPOSITION ■ Bilirubin in the Gut
Following secretion into bile, conjugated bilirubin reaches the duodenum and passes down the gastrointestinal tract without reabsorption by the intestinal mucosa. An appreciable fraction is converted by bacterial metabolism in the gut to the water-soluble colorless compound, urobilinogen. Urobilinogen undergoes enterohepatic cycling. Urobilinogen not taken up by the liver reaches the systemic circulation, from which some is cleared by the kidneys. Unconjugated bilirubin ordinarily does not reach the gut except in neonates or, by ill-defined alternative pathways, in the presence of severe unconjugated hyperbilirubinemia [e.g., Crigler-Najjar syndrome, type I (CN-I)]. Unconjugated bilirubin that reaches the gut is partly reabsorbed, amplifying any underlying hyperbilirubinemia.

Renal Excretion of Bilirubin Conjugates Unconjugated bilirubin is not excreted in urine as it is too tightly bound to albumin for effective glomerular filtration and there is no tubular mechanism for its renal secretion. In contrast, the bilirubin conjugates are readily filtered at the glomerulus and can appear in urine in disorders characterized by increased bilirubin conjugates in the circulation.

DISORDERS OF BILIRUBIN METABOLISM LEADING TO UNCONJUGATED HYPERBILIRUBINEMIA

INCREASED BILIRUBIN PRODUCTION ■ Hemolysis Increased destruction of erythrocytes leads to increased bilirubin turnover and unconjugated hyperbilirubinemia; the hyperbilirubinemia is usually modest in the presence of normal liver function. In particular, the bone marrow is only capable of a sustained eightfold increase in erythrocyte production in response to a hemolytic stress. Therefore, hemolysis alone cannot result in a sustained hyperbilirubinemia of more than approximately 68 μmol/L (4 mg/dL). Higher values imply concomitant hepatic dysfunction. When hemolysis is the only abnormality in an otherwise healthy individual, the result is a purely unconjugated hyperbilirubinemia, with the direct-reacting fraction as measured in a typical clinical laboratory being ≤15% of the total serum bilirubin. In the presence of systemic disease, which may include a degree of hepatic dysfunction, hemolysis may produce a component of conjugated hyperbilirubinemia in addition to an elevated unconjugated bilirubin concentration. Prolonged hemolysis may lead to the precipitation of bilirubin salts within the gall bladder or biliary tree, resulting in the formation of gallstones in which bilirubin, rather than cholesterol, is the major component. Such pigment stones may lead to acute or chronic cholecystitis, biliary obstruction, or any other biliary tract consequence of calculous disease.

Ineffective Erythropoiesis During erythroid maturation, small amounts of hemoglobin may be lost at the time of nuclear extrusion, and a fraction of developing erythroid cells is destroyed within the marrow. These processes normally account for a small proportion of bilirubin that is produced. In various disorders, including thalassemia major, megaloblastic anemias due to folate or vitamin B_{12} deficiency, congenital erythropoietic porphyria, lead poisoning, and various congenital and acquired dyserythropoietic anemias, the fraction of total bilirubin production derived from ineffective erythropoiesis is increased,

FIGURE 284-1 Hepatocellular bilirubin transport. Albumin-bound bilirubin in sinusoidal blood passes through endothelial cell fenestrae to reach the hepatocyte surface, entering the cell by both facilitated and simple diffusional processes. Within the cell it is bound to glutathione-S-transferases and conjugated by bilirubin-UDP-glucuronosyltransferase (UGT1A1) to mono- and diglucuronides, which are actively transported across the canalicular membrane into the bile. ALB, albumin; UCB, unconjugated bilirubin; UGT1A1, bilirubin-UDP-glucuronosyltransferase; BMG, bilirubin monoglucuronide; GST, glutathione-S-transferase; MRP2, multidrug resistance–associated protein 2; BDG, bilirubin diglucuronide; BT, proposed bilirubin transporter.

FIGURE 284-2 *Structural organization of the human UGT1 gene complex. This large complex on chromosome 2 contains at least 13 substrate-specific first exons (A1, A2, etc.). Since four of these are pseudogenes, nine UGT1 isoforms with differing substrate specificities are expressed. Each exon 1 has its own promoter and encodes the amino-terminal substrate-specific ~286 amino acids of the various UGT1-encoded isoforms, and common exons 2 to 5 that encode the 245 carboxyl-terminal amino acids common to all of the isoforms. mRNAs for specific isoforms are assembled by splicing a particular first exon such as the bilirubin-specific exon A1 to exons 2 to 5. The resulting message encodes a complete enzyme, in this particular case bilirubin-UDP-glucuronosyltransferase (UGT1A1). Mutations in a first exon affect only a single isoform. Those in exons 2 to 5 affect all enzymes encoded by the UGT1 complex.*

reaching as much as 70% of the total. This may be sufficient to produce modest degrees of unconjugated hyperbilirubinemia.

Miscellaneous   Degradation of the hemoglobin of extravascular collections of erythrocytes, such as those seen in massive tissue infarctions or large hematomas, may lead transiently to unconjugated hyperbilirubinemia.

DECREASED HEPATIC BILIRUBIN CLEARANCE ■ Decreased Hepatic Uptake   Decreased hepatic bilirubin uptake is believed to contribute to the unconjugated hyperbilirubinemia of Gilbert's syndrome (GS), although the molecular basis for this finding remains unclear (see below). Several drugs, including flavaspidic acid, novobiocin, and various cholecystographic contrast agents, have been reported to inhibit bilirubin uptake. The resulting unconjugated hyperbilirubinemia resolves with cessation of the medication.

Impaired Conjugation ■ *PHYSIOLOGIC NEONATAL JAUNDICE*   Bilirubin produced by the fetus is cleared by the placenta and eliminated by the maternal liver. Immediately after birth, the neonatal liver must assume responsibility for bilirubin clearance and excretion. However, many hepatic physiologic processes are incompletely developed at birth. Levels of UGT1A1 are low, and alternative excretory pathways allow passage of unconjugated bilirubin into the gut. Since the intestinal flora that convert bilirubin to urobilinogen are also undeveloped, an enterohepatic circulation of unconjugated bilirubin ensues. As a consequence, most neonates develop mild unconjugated hyperbilirubinemia between days 2 and 5 after birth. Peak levels are typically <85 to 170 μmol/L (5 to 10 mg/dL) and decline to normal adult concentrations within 2 weeks, as mechanisms required for bilirubin disposition mature. Prematurity, with more profound immaturity of hepatic function, or hemolysis, result in higher levels of unconjugated hyperbilirubinemia. A rapidly rising unconjugated bilirubin concentration, or absolute levels >340 μmol/L (20 mg/dL), puts the infant at risk for bilirubin encephalopathy, or kernicterus. Under these circumstances, bilirubin crosses an immature blood-brain barrier and precipitates in the basal ganglia and other areas of the brain. The consequences range from appreciable neurologic deficits to death. Treatment options include phototherapy, which converts bilirubin into water-soluble photoisomers that are excreted directly into bile, and exchange transfusion. The canalicular mechanisms responsible for bilirubin excretion are also immature at birth, and their maturation may lag behind that of UGT1A1; this can lead to transient conjugated neonatal hyperbilirubinemia, especially in infants with hemolysis.

ACQUIRED CONJUGATION DEFECTS   A modest reduction in bilirubin-conjugating capacity may be observed in advanced hepatitis or cirrhosis. However, in this setting, conjugation is better preserved than other aspects of bilirubin disposition, such as canalicular excretion. Various drugs, including pregnanediol, novobiocin, chloramphenicol, and gentami-

cin, may produce unconjugated hyperbilirubinemia by inhibiting UGT1A1 activity. Finally, bilirubin conjugation may be inhibited by certain fatty acids that are present in breast milk but not serum of mothers whose infants have excessive neonatal hyperbilirubinemia (*breast milk jaundice*). The pathogenesis of breast milk jaundice appears to differ from that of transient familial neonatal hyperbilirubinemia (Lucey-Driscoll syndrome), in which there is a UGT1A1 inhibitor in maternal serum.

HEREDITARY DEFECTS IN BILIRUBIN CONJUGATION   Three familial disorders characterized by differing degrees of unconjugated hyperbilirubinemia have long been recognized. The defining clinical features of each are described below (Table 284-1). While these disorders have been recognized for decades to reflect differing degrees of deficiency in the ability to conjugate bilirubin, recent advances in the molecular biology of the *UGT1* gene complex have elucidated their interrelationships and clarified previously puzzling features.

Crigler-Najjar Syndrome, Type I   CN-I is characterized by striking unconjugated hyperbilirubinemia of about 340 to 765 μmol/L (20 to 45 mg/dL) that appears in the neonatal period and persists for life. Other conventional hepatic biochemical tests such as serum aminotransferases and alkaline phosphatase are normal, and there is no evidence of hemolysis. Hepatic histology is also essentially normal except for the occasional presence of bile plugs within canaliculi. Bilirubin glucuronides are virtually absent from the bile, and there is no detectable constitutive expression of UGT1A1 activity in hepatic tissue. Neither UGT1A1 activity nor the serum bilirubin concentration responds to administration of phenobarbital or other enzyme inducers. In the absence of conjugation, unconjugated bilirubin accumulates in plasma, from which it is eliminated very slowly by alternative pathways that include direct passage into the bile and small intestine. These account for the small amounts of urobilinogen found in feces. No bilirubin is found in the urine. First described in 1952, the disorder is rare (estimated prevalence of 0.6 to 1.0 per million). Many patients are from geographically or socially isolated communities in which consanguinity is common, and pedigree analyses show an autosomal recessive pattern of inheritance. The majority of patients (type IA) exhibit defects in the glucuronide conjugation of a spectrum of substrates in addition to bilirubin, including various drugs and other xenobiotics. These individuals have mutations in one of the common exons (2 to 5) of the *UGT1* gene (Fig. 284-2). In a smaller subset (type IB), the defect is limited largely to bilirubin conjugation, and the causative mutation is in the bilirubin-specific exon A1. Estrogen glucuronidation is mediated by UGT1A1 and is defective in all CN-I patients. More than 30 different genetic lesions of *UGT1A1* responsible for CN-I have been identified, including deletions, insertions, alterations in intronic splice donor and acceptor sites, exon skipping, and point mutations that introduce premature stop codons or alter critical amino acids. Their common feature is that they all encode proteins with absent or, at most, traces of bilirubin-UDP-glucuronosyltransferase enzymatic activity.

Prior to the availability of phototherapy, most patients with CN-I died of bilirubin encephalopathy (*kernicterus*) in infancy or early childhood. A few lived as long as early adult life without overt neurologic damage, although more subtle testing usually indicated mild but progressive brain damage. In the absence of liver transplantation, death eventually supervened from late-onset bilirubin encephalopathy, which often followed a nonspecific febrile illness. Recent data suggest that the best hope for survival of a neurologically intact patient involves the following treatment options: (1) about 12 h/d of phototherapy-

TABLE 284-1 *Principal Differential Characteristics of Gilbert's and Crigler-Najjar Syndromes*

Feature	Crigler-Najjar Syndrome		Gilbert's Syndrome
	Type I	Type II	
Total serum bilirubin, μmol/L [mg/dL]	310–755 (usually >345) [18–45 (usually >20)]	100–430 (usually ≤345) [6–25 (usually ≤20)]	Typically ≤70 μmol/L [≤4 mg/dL] in absence of fasting or hemolysis
Routine liver tests	Normal	Normal	Normal
Response to phenobarbital	None	Decreases bilirubin by >25%	Decreases bilirubin to normal
Kernicterus	Usual	Rare	No
Hepatic histology	Normal	Normal	Usually normal; increased lipofuscin pigment in some
Bile characteristics			
Color:	Pale or colorless	Pigmented	Normal dark color
Bilirubin fractions:	>90% unconjugated	Largest fraction (mean:57%) monoconjugates	Mainly diconjugates but monoconjugates increased (mean 23%)
Bilirubin UDP-glucuronosyl-transferase activity	Typically absent; traces in some patients	Markedly reduced: 0 to 10% of normal	Reduced: typically 10–33% of normal
Inheritance (all autosomal)	Recessive	Predominantly recessive	Promoter mutation: recessive Missense mutations: 7 of 8 dominant; 1 reportedly recessive

apy from birth throughout childhood, perhaps supplemented by exchange transfusion in the immediate neonatal period; (2) use of tin-protoporphyrin, an inhibitor of heme oxygenase, to blunt transient exacerbations of hyperbilirubinemia; (3) oral administration of a combination of calcium phosphate and calcium carbonate to sequester unconjugated bilirubin in the gut; and (4) liver transplantation prior to the onset of brain damage. In a single patient, transplantation with isolated allogeneic hepatocytes produced a clinically significant reduction in serum bilirubin concentration.

Crigler-Najjar Syndrome, Type II (CN-II) This condition was recognized as a distinct entity in 1962 and is characterized by marked unconjugated hyperbilirubinemia in the absence of abnormalities of other conventional hepatic biochemical tests, hepatic histology, or hemolysis. It differs from CN-I in several specific ways (Table 284-1): (1) Although there is considerable overlap, average bilirubin concentrations are lower in CN-II; (2) accordingly, CN-II is only infrequently associated with kernicterus; (3) bile is deeply colored, and bilirubin glucuronides are present, with a striking, characteristic increase in the proportion of monoglucuronides; (4) UGT1A1 in liver is usually present at reduced levels (typically ≤10% of normal) but may be undetectable by older, less sensitive assays; (5) while typically detected in infancy, hyperbilirubinemia was not recognized in some cases until later in life and, in one instance, at age 34. As with CN-I, most CN-II cases exhibit abnormalities in the conjugation of other compounds, such as salicylamide and menthol, but in some instances the defect appears limited to bilirubin. Reduction of serum bilirubin concentrations by >25% in response to enzyme inducers such as phenobarbital distinguishes CN-II from CN-I, although this response may not be elicited in early infancy and often is not accompanied by measurable UGT1A1 induction. Bilirubin concentrations during phenobarbital administration do not return to normal but are typically in the range of 51 to 86 μmol/L (3 to 5 mg/dL). Although the incidence of kernicterus in CN-II is low, instances have occurred, not only in infants but also in adolescents and adults, often in the setting of an intercurrent illness, fasting, or another factor that temporarily raises the serum bilirubin concentration above baseline and reduces serum albumin levels. For this reason, phenobarbital therapy is widely recommended, a single bedtime dose often sufficing to maintain clinically safe plasma bilirubin concentrations.

At least 10 different mutations of *UGT1* have been identified that are associated with CN-II. Their common feature is that they encode for a bilirubin-UDP-glucuronosyltransferase with markedly reduced but detectable enzymatic activity. The spectrum of residual enzyme activity explains the spectrum of phenotypic severity of the resulting hyperbilirubinemia. Molecular analysis has established that a large majority of CN-II patients are either homozygotes or compound het-

erozygotes for CN-II mutations and that individuals carrying one mutated and one entirely normal allele have normal bilirubin concentrations. Possible inheritance of a dominant negative mutation in one case remains to be confirmed.

Gilbert's Syndrome This syndrome is characterized by mild unconjugated hyperbilirubinemia, normal values for standard hepatic biochemical tests, and normal hepatic histology other than a modest increase of lipofuscin pigment in some patients. Serum bilirubin concentrations are most often <51 μmol/L (<3 mg/dL), although both higher and lower values are frequent. The clinical spectrum of hyperbilirubinemia fades into that of CN-II at serum bilirubin concentrations of 86 to 136 μmol/L (5 to 8 mg/dL). At the other end of the scale, the distinction between mild cases of GS and a normal state is often blurred. Bilirubin concentrations may fluctuate substantially in any given individual, and at least 25% of patients will exhibit temporarily normal values during prolonged follow-up. More elevated values are associated with stress, fatigue, alcohol use, reduced caloric intake, and intercurrent illness, while increased caloric intake or administration of enzyme-inducing agents produce lower bilirubin levels. GS is most often diagnosed at or shortly after puberty or in adult life during routine examinations that include multichannel biochemical analyses. UGT1A1 activity is typically reduced to 10 to 35% of normal, and bile pigments exhibit a characteristic increase in bilirubin monoglucuronides. Studies of radiobilirubin kinetics indicate that hepatic bilirubin clearance is reduced to an average of one-third of normal. Administration of phenobarbital normalizes both the serum bilirubin concentration and hepatic bilirubin clearance; however, failure of UGT1A1 activity to improve in many such instances suggests the possible coexistence of an additional defect. Compartmental analysis of bilirubin kinetic data suggests that GS patients have a defect in bilirubin uptake as well as in conjugation. Defect(s) in the hepatic uptake of other organic anions that at least partially share an uptake mechanism with bilirubin, such as sulfobromophthalein and indocyanine green (ICG), are observed in a minority of patients. The metabolism and transport of bile acids, which do not utilize the bilirubin uptake mechanism, are normal. The magnitude of changes in the plasma bilirubin concentration induced by provocation tests such as 48 h of fasting or the intravenous administration of nicotinic acid have been reported to be of help in separating GS patients from normal individuals. Other studies dispute this assertion. Moreover, on theoretical grounds, the results of such studies should provide no more information than simple measurements of the baseline plasma bilirubin concentration. Family studies indicate that GS and hereditary hemolytic anemias such as hereditary spherocytosis, glucose-6-phosphate dehydrogenase deficiency, and β-thalassemia trait sort independently. Reports of hemolysis in up to 50% of GS patients are believed to reflect better case finding, since patients with both GS and hemolysis have higher bilirubin concentrations, and are more likely to be jaundiced, than patients with either defect alone.

GS is common, with many series placing its prevalence at ≥8%. Males predominate over females by reported ratios ranging from 1.5:1 to >7:1. However, these ratios may have a large artifactual component since normal males have higher mean bilirubin levels than normal females, but the diagnosis of GS is often based on comparison to normal ranges established in men. The high prevalence of GS in the general population may explain the reported frequency of mild unconjugated hyperbilirubinemia in liver transplant recipients. The disposition of most xenobiotics metabolized by glucuronidation appears to be normal in GS, as is oxidative drug metabolism in the majority of reported studies. The principal exception is the metabolism of the antitumor agent irinotecan (CPT-11), whose active metabolite (SN-38) is glucuronidated specifically by bilirubin-UDP-glucuronosyltransferase. Administration of CPT-11 to patients with GS has resulted in several toxicities, including intractable diarrhea and myelosuppression. Some reports also suggest abnormal disposition of menthol, estradiol benzoate, acetaminophen, tolbutamide, and rifamycin SV. Although some of these studies have been disputed, and there have been no reports of clinical complications from use of these agents in GS, prudence should be exercised in prescribing them, or any agents metabolized primarily by glucuronidation, in this condition.

Most older pedigree studies of GS were consistent with autosomal dominant inheritance with variable expressivity. However, studies of the UGT1 gene in GS have indicated a variety of molecular genetic bases for the phenotypic picture and several different patterns of inheritance. Studies in Europe and the United States found that nearly all patients had normal coding regions for UGT1A1 but were homozygous for the insertion of an extra TA (i.e., A[TA]$_7$TAA rather than A[TA]$_6$TAA) in the promoter region of the first exon. This appeared to be necessary, but not sufficient, for clinically expressed GS, since 15% of normal controls were also homozygous for this variant. While normal by standard criteria, these individuals had somewhat higher bilirubin concentrations than the rest of the controls studied. Heterozygotes for this abnormality had bilirubin concentrations identical to those homozygous for the A[TA]$_6$TAA allele. The prevalence of the A[TA]$_7$TAA allele in a general western population is 30%, in which case 9% would be homozygotes. This is slightly higher than the prevalence of GS based on purely phenotypic parameters. It was suggested that additional variables, such as mild hemolysis or a defect in bilirubin uptake, might be among the factors enhancing phenotypic expression of the defect.

Phenotypic expression of GS due solely to the A[TA]$_7$TAA promoter abnormality is inherited as an autosomal recessive trait. A number of CN-II kindreds have been identified in which there is also an allele containing a normal coding region but the A[TA]$_7$TAA promoter abnormality. CN-II heterozygotes who have the A[TA]$_6$TAA promoter are phenotypically normal, whereas those with the A[TA]$_7$TAA promoter express the phenotypic picture of GS. GS in such kindreds may also result from homozygosity for the A[TA]$_7$TAA promoter abnormality. Seven different missense mutations in the UGT1 gene that reportedly cause GS with dominant inheritance have been found in Japanese individuals. Another Japanese patient with mild unconjugated hyperbilirubinemia was homozygous for a missense mutation in exon 5. GS in her family appeared to be recessive. Missense mutations causing GS have not been reported outside of certain Asian populations.

DISORDERS OF BILIRUBIN METABOLISM LEADING TO MIXED OR PREDOMINANTLY CONJUGATED HYPERBILIRUBINEMIA

In hyperbilirubinemia due to acquired liver disease (e.g., acute hepatitis, common bile duct stone), there are usually elevations in the serum concentrations of both conjugated and unconjugated bilirubin. Although biliary tract obstruction or hepatocellular cholestatic injury may present on occasion with a predominantly conjugated hyperbilirubinemia, it is generally not possible to differentiate intrahepatic from extrahepatic causes of jaundice based upon the serum levels or relative proportions of unconjugated and conjugated bilirubin. The major reason for determining the amounts of conjugated and unconjugated bilirubin in the serum is for the initial differentiation of hepatic parenchymal and obstructive disorders (mixed conjugated and unconjugated hyperbilirubinemia) from the inheritable and hemolytic disorders discussed above that are associated with unconjugated hyperbilirubinemia.

FAMILIAL DEFECTS IN HEPATIC EXCRETORY FUNCTION ■ Dubin-Johnson Syndrome (DJS) This benign, relatively rare disorder is characterized by low-grade, predominantly conjugated hyperbilirubinemia (Table 284-2). Total bilirubin concentrations are typically between 34 and 85 μmol/L (2 and 5 mg/dL) but on occasion can be in the normal range or as high as 340 to 430 μmol/L (20 to 25 mg/dL) and can fluctuate widely in any given patient. The degree of hyperbilirubinemia may be increased by intercurrent illness, oral contraceptive use, and pregnancy. As the hyperbilirubinemia is due to a predominant rise in conjugated bilirubin, bilirubinuria is characteristically present. Aside from elevated serum bilirubin levels, other routine laboratory tests are normal. Physical examination is usually normal except for jaundice, although an occasional patient may have hepatosplenomegaly.

Patients with DJS are usually asymptomatic, although some may have vague constitutional symptoms. These latter patients have usually undergone extensive and often unnecessary diagnostic examinations for unexplained jaundice and have high levels of anxiety. In women, the condition may be subclinical until the patient becomes pregnant

TABLE 284-2 *Principal Differential Characteristics of Inheritable Disorders of Bile Canalicular Function*

	DJS	Rotor	PFIC1	BRIC	PFIC2	PFIC3
Gene	ABCCA	?	ATP8B1	ATP8B1	ABCB11	ABCB4
Protein	MRP2	?	FIC1	FIC1	BSEP	MDR3
Cholestasis	No	No	Yes	Episodic	Yes	Yes
Serum γ-GT	Normal	Normal	Normal	Normal	Normal	⇈
Serum bile acids	Normal	Normal	⇈	⇈ during episodes	⇈	⇈
Clinical features	Mild conjugated hyperbilirubinemia; otherwise normal liver function; dark pigment in liver; characteristic pattern of urinary coproporphyrins	Mild conjugated hyperbilirubinemia; otherwise normal liver function; liver without abnormal pigmentation	Severe cholestasis beginning in childhood	Recurrent episodes of cholestasis beginning at any age	Severe cholestasis beginning in childhood	Severe cholestasis beginning in childhood; decreased phospholipids in bile

Note: DJS, Dubin-Johnson syndrome; PFIC, progressive familial intrahepatic cholestasis; MRP2, multidrug resistance–associated protein 2; BSEP, bile salt excretory protein; γ-GT, γ-glutamyltransferase; ⇈, increased.

or receives oral contraceptives, at which time chemical hyperbilirubinemia becomes frank jaundice. Even in these situations, other routine liver function tests, including serum alkaline phosphatase and transaminase activities, are normal.

A cardinal feature of DJS is the accumulation in the lysosomes of centrilobular hepatocytes of dark, coarsely granular pigment. As a result, the liver may be grossly black in appearance. This pigment is thought to be derived from epinephrine metabolites that are not excreted normally. The pigment may disappear during bouts of viral hepatitis, only to reaccumulate slowly after recovery.

Biliary excretion of a number of anionic compounds is compromised in DJS. These include various cholecystographic agents, as well as sulfobromophthalein (Bromsulphalein, BSP), a synthetic dye formerly used in a test of liver function. In this test, the rate of disappearance of BSP from plasma was determined following bolus intravenous administration. BSP is conjugated with glutathione in the hepatocyte; the resulting conjugate is normally excreted rapidly into the bile canaliculus. Patients with DJS exhibit a characteristic rise in its plasma concentration at 90 min after injection, due to reflux of conjugated BSP into the circulation from the hepatocyte. Dyes such as ICG that are taken up by hepatocytes but are not further metabolized prior to biliary excretion do not show this reflux phenomenon. Continuous BSP infusion studies suggest a reduction in the t_{max} for biliary excretion. Bile acid disposition, including hepatocellular uptake and biliary excretion, is normal in DJS. These patients have normal serum and biliary bile acid concentrations and do not have pruritus.

By analogy with findings in several mutant rat strains, the selective defect in biliary excretion of bilirubin conjugates and certain other classes of organic compounds, but not of bile acids, that characterizes DJS in humans was found to reflect defective expression of MRP2, an ATP-dependent canalicular membrane transporter. Several different mutations in the *MRP2* gene produce the Dubin-Johnson phenotype, which has an autosomal recessive pattern of inheritance. Although MRP2 is undoubtedly important in the biliary excretion of conjugated bilirubin, the fact that this pigment is still excreted in the absence of MRP2 suggests that other, as yet uncharacterized, transport proteins may serve in a secondary role in this process.

Patients with DJS also have a diagnostic abnormality in urinary coproporphyrin excretion. There are two naturally occurring coproporphyrin isomers, I and III. Normally, approximately 75% of the coproporphyrin in urine is isomer III. In urine from DJS patients, total coproporphyrin content is normal, but >80% is isomer I. Heterozygotes for the syndrome show an intermediate pattern. The molecular basis for this phenomenon remains unclear.

Rotor Syndrome This benign, autosomal recessive disorder is clinically similar to DJS (Table 284-2), although it is seen even less frequently. A major phenotypic difference is that the liver in patients with Rotor syndrome has no increased pigmentation and appears totally normal. The only abnormality in routine laboratory tests is an elevation of total serum bilirubin, due to a predominant rise in conjugated bilirubin. This is accompanied by bilirubinuria. Several additional features differentiate Rotor syndrome and DJS. In Rotor syndrome, the gallbladder is usually visualized on oral cholecystography, in contrast to the nonvisualization that is typical of DJS. The pattern of urinary coproporphyrin excretion also differs. The pattern in Rotor syndrome resembles that of many acquired disorders of hepatobiliary function, in which coproporphyrin I, the major coproporphyrin isomer in bile, refluxes from the hepatocyte back into the circulation and is excreted in urine. Thus, total urinary coproporphyrin excretion is substantially increased in Rotor syndrome, in contrast to the normal levels seen in DJS. Although the fraction of coproporphyrin I in urine is elevated, it is usually <70% of the total, as compared to 80% or more in DJS. The disorders also can be distinguished by their patterns of BSP excretion. Although clearance of BSP from plasma is delayed in Rotor syndrome, there is no reflux of conjugated BSP back into the circulation as seen in DJS. Kinetic analysis of plasma BSP infusion studies suggests the presence of a defect in intrahepatocellular storage of this compound. This has never been demonstrated directly, and the molecular basis of Rotor syndrome remains unknown.

Benign Recurrent Intrahepatic Cholestasis (BRIC) This rare disorder is characterized by recurrent attacks of pruritus and jaundice. The typical episode begins with mild malaise and elevations in serum aminotransferase levels, followed rapidly by rises in alkaline phosphatase and conjugated bilirubin and onset of jaundice and itching. The first one or two episodes may be misdiagnosed as acute viral hepatitis. The cholestatic episodes, which may begin in childhood or adulthood, can vary in duration from several weeks to months, following which there is complete clinical and biochemical resolution. Intervals between attacks may vary from several months to years. Between episodes, physical examination is normal, as are serum levels of bile acids, bilirubin, transaminases, and alkaline phosphatase. The disorder is familial and has an autosomal recessive pattern of inheritance. BRIC is considered a benign disorder in that it does not lead to cirrhosis or end-stage liver disease. However, the episodes of jaundice and pruritus can be prolonged and debilitating, and some patients have undergone liver transplantation to relieve the intractable and disabling symptoms. Treatment during the cholestatic episodes is symptomatic; there is no specific treatment to prevent or shorten the occurrence of episodes.

A gene termed *FIC1* was recently identified and found to be mutated in patients with BRIC. Curiously, this gene is expressed strongly in the small intestine but only weakly in the liver. The protein encoded by *FIC1* shows little similarity to genes that have been shown to play a role in bile canalicular excretion of various compounds. Rather, it appears to be a member of a P-type ATPase family that transports aminophospholipids from the outer to the inner leaflet of a variety of cell membranes. Its relationship to the pathobiology of this disorder remains unclear.

Progressive Familial Intrahepatic Cholestasis (FIC) This name is applied to three phenotypically related syndromes (Table 284-2). Progressive FIC type 1 (Byler disease) presents in early infancy as cholestasis that may be initially episodic. However, in contrast to BRIC, Byler disease progresses to malnutrition, growth retardation, and end-stage liver disease during childhood. This disorder is also a consequence of a *FIC1* mutation. The functional relationship of the FIC1 protein to the pathogenesis of cholestasis in these disorders is unknown. Two other types of progressive FIC (types 2 and 3) have been described. Type 2 is associated with a mutation in the protein named *sister of p-glycoprotein*, which is the major bile canalicular exporter of bile acids and is also known as *bile salt excretory protein* (BSEP). Type 3 has been associated with a mutation of MDR3, a protein that is essential for normal hepatocellular excretion of phospholipids across the bile canaliculus. Although all three types of progressive FIC have similar clinical phenotypes, only type 3 is associated with high serum levels of γ-glutamyltransferase activity. In contrast, activity of this enzyme is normal or only mildly elevated in symptomatic BRIC and progressive FIC types 1 and 2.

FURTHER READING

BOSMA P et al: The genetic basis of the reduced expression of bilirubin-UDP-glucuronosyltransferase 1 in Gilbert's syndrome. N Engl J Med 333:1171, 1995

IYANAGI T et al: Biochemical and molecular aspects of genetic disorders of bilirubin metabolism. Biochim Biophys Acta 1407:173, 1998

JANSEN PL: Diagnosis and management of Crigler-Najjar syndrome. Eur J Pediatr 158:S89, 1999

ROY CHOWDHURY J et al: Hereditary jaundice and disorders of bilirubin metabolism, in *The Metabolic and Molecular Bases of Inherited Disease*, 8th ed. CR Scriver et al (eds.) New York, McGraw-Hill, 2001, pp 3063–3101

THOMPSON R et al: Genetic defects in hepatocanalicular transport. Semin Liver Dis 20:365, 2000

Acute viral hepatitis is a systemic infection affecting the liver predominantly. Almost all cases of acute viral hepatitis are caused by one of five viral agents: hepatitis A virus (HAV), hepatitis B virus (HBV), hepatitis C virus (HCV), the HBV-associated delta agent or hepatitis D virus (HDV), and hepatitis E virus (HEV). Other transfusion-transmitted agents, e.g., "hepatitis G" virus and "TT" virus, have been identified but do not cause hepatitis. All these human hepatitis viruses are RNA viruses, except for hepatitis B, which is a DNA virus. Although these agents can be distinguished by their molecular and antigenic properties, all types of viral hepatitis produce clinically similar illnesses. These range from asymptomatic and inapparent to fulminant and fatal acute infections common to all types, on the one hand, and from subclinical persistent infections to rapidly progressive chronic liver disease with cirrhosis and even hepatocellular carcinoma, common to the bloodborne types (HBV, HCV, and HDV), on the other.

VIROLOGY AND ETIOLOGY ■ Hepatitis A

Hepatitis A virus is a nonenveloped 27-nm, heat-, acid-, and ether-resistant RNA virus in the hepatovirus genus of the picornavirus family (Fig. 285-1). Its virion contains four capsid polypeptides, designated VP1 to VP4, which are cleaved posttranslationally from the polyprotein product of a 7500-nucleotide genome. Inactivation of viral activity can be achieved by boiling for 1 min, by contact with formaldehyde and chlorine, or by ultraviolet irradiation. Despite nucleotide sequence variation of up to 20% among isolates of HAV, all strains of this virus are immunologically indistinguishable and belong to one serotype. Hepatitis A has an incubation period of approximately 4 weeks. Its replication is limited to the liver, but the virus is present in the liver, bile, stools, and blood during the late incubation period and acute preicteric phase of illness. Despite persistence of virus in the liver, viral shedding in feces, viremia, and infectivity diminish rapidly once jaundice becomes apparent. HAV can be cultivated reproducibly in vitro.

Antibodies to HAV (anti-HAV) can be detected during acute illness when serum aminotransferase activity is elevated and fecal HAV shedding is still occurring. This early antibody response is predominantly of the IgM class and persists for several months, rarely for 6 to 12 months. During convalescence, however, anti-HAV of the IgG class becomes the predominant antibody (Fig. 285-2). Therefore, the diagnosis of hepatitis A is made during acute illness by demonstrating anti-HAV of the IgM class. After acute illness, anti-HAV of the IgG class remains detectable indefinitely, and patients with serum anti-HAV are immune to reinfection. Neutralizing antibody activity parallels the appearance of anti-HAV, and the IgG anti-HAV present in immune globulin accounts for the protection it affords against HAV infection.

FIGURE 285-2 Scheme of typical clinical and laboratory features of viral hepatitis A.

Hepatitis B

Hepatitis B virus is a DNA virus with a remarkably compact genomic structure; despite its small, circular, 3200-basepair size, HBV DNA codes for four sets of viral products with a complex, multiparticle structure. HBV achieves its genomic economy by relying on an efficient strategy of encoding proteins from four overlapping genes: S, C, P, and X (Fig. 285-3), as detailed below. Once thought to be unique among viruses, HBV is now recognized as one of a family of animal viruses, hepadnaviruses (hepatotropic DNA viruses), and is classified as hepadnavirus type 1. Similar viruses infect certain species of woodchucks, ground and tree squirrels, and Pekin ducks, to mention the most carefully characterized. Like HBV, all have the same distinctive three morphologic forms, have counterparts to the envelope and nucleocapsid virus antigens of HBV, replicate in the liver but exist in extrahepatic sites, contain their own endogenous DNA polymerase, have partially double-stranded and partially single-stranded genomes, are associated with acute and chronic hepatitis and hepatocellular carcinoma, and rely on a replicative strategy unique among DNA viruses but typical of retroviruses. Instead of DNA replication directly from a DNA template, hepadnaviruses rely on reverse transcription (effected by the DNA polymerase) of minus-strand DNA from a "pregenomic" RNA intermediate. Then plus-strand DNA is transcribed from the minus-strand DNA template by the DNA-dependent DNA polymerase and converted in the hepatocyte nucleus to a covalently closed circular DNA, which serves as a template for messenger RNA and pregenomic RNA. Viral proteins are translated by the messenger RNA, and the proteins and genome are packaged into virions and secreted from the hepatocyte. Although HBV is difficult to cultivate in vitro in the conventional sense from clinical material, several cell lines have been transfected with HBV DNA. Such transfected cells support in vitro replication of the intact virus and its component proteins.

VIRAL PROTEINS AND PARTICLES Of the three particulate forms of HBV (Table 285-1), the most numerous are the 22-nm particles, which appear as spherical or long filamentous forms; these are antigenically indistinguishable from the outer surface or envelope protein of HBV and are thought to represent excess viral envelope protein. Outnumbered in serum by a factor of 100 or 1000 to 1 compared with the spheres and tubules are large, 42-nm, double-shelled spherical particles, which represent the intact hepatitis B virion (Fig. 285-1) . The envelope protein expressed on the outer surface of the virion and on the smaller spherical and tubular structures is referred to as *hepatitis B surface antigen* (HBsAg). The concentration of HBsAg and virus particles in the blood may reach 500 µg/mL and 10 trillion particles per milliliter, respectively. The envelope protein, HBsAg, is the product of the S gene of HBV.

FIGURE 285-1 *Left*. Electron micrograph of 27-nm hepatitis A virus particles purified from stool of a patient with acute hepatitis A virus infection and aggregated by hepatitis A antibody. *Right*. Electron micrograph of concentrated serum from a patient with hepatitis B infection, demonstrating the 42-nm virions, tubular forms, and spherical 22-nm particles of hepatitis B surface antigen. 132,000×. (Hepatitis D resembles 42-nm virions of hepatitis B but is smaller, 35 to 37 nm; hepatitis E resembles hepatitis A virus but is slightly larger, 32 to 34 nm; hepatitis C has not been visualized definitively.)

FIGURE 285-3 Its compact genomic structure, with overlapping genes, permits HBV to code for multiple proteins. The S gene codes for the "major" envelope protein, HBsAg. Pre-S1 and pre-S2, upstream of S, combine with S to code for two larger proteins, "middle" protein, the product of pre-S2 + S, and "large" protein, the product of pre-S1 + pre-S2 + S. The largest gene, P, codes for DNA polymerase. The C gene codes for two nucleocapsid proteins, HBeAg, a soluble, secreted protein (initiation from the pre-C region of the gene) and HBcAg, the intracellular core protein (initiation after pre-C). The X gene codes for HBxAg, which can transactivate the transcription of cellular and viral genes; its clinical relevance is not known, but it may contribute to carcinogenesis by binding to p53.

A number of different HBsAg subdeterminants have been identified. There is a common group-reactive antigen, *a*, shared by all HBsAg isolates. In addition, HBsAg may contain one of several subtype-specific antigens, namely, *d* or *y*, *w* or *r*, as well as other more recently characterized specificities. Hepatitis B isolates fall into one of at least eight subtypes and seven genotypes (A–G). Geographic distribution of genotypes and subtypes varies; genotypes A (corresponding to subtype *adw* and D (*ayw*) predominate in the United States and Europe, while genotypes B (*adw*) and C (*adr*) predominate in Asia. Clinical course and outcome are independent of subtype, but preliminary reports suggest that genotype B is associated with less rapidly progressive liver disease and a lower likelihood, or delayed appearance, of hepatocellular carcinoma than genotype C. In addition, "precore" mutations are favored by certain genotypes (see below).

Upstream of the S gene are the pre-S genes (Fig. 285-3), which code for pre-S gene products, including receptors on the HBV surface for polymerized human serum albumin and for hepatocyte membrane proteins. The pre-S region actually consists of both pre-S1 and pre-S2. Depending on where translation is initiated, three potential HBsAg gene products are synthesized. The protein product of the S gene is HBsAg (*major protein*), the product of the S region plus the adjacent pre-S2 region is the *middle protein*, and the product of the pre-S1 plus pre-S2 plus S regions is the *large protein*. Compared with the smaller spherical and tubular particles of HBV, complete 42-nm virions are enriched in the large protein. Both pre-S proteins and their respective antibodies can be detected during HBV infection, and the period of pre-S antigenemia appears to coincide with other markers of virus replication, as detailed below.

The intact 42-nm virion contains a 27-nm nucleocapsid core particle. Nucleocapsid proteins are coded for by the C gene. The antigen expressed on the surface of the nucleocapsid core is referred to as *hepatitis B core antigen* (HBcAg), and its corresponding antibody is anti-HBc. A third HBV antigen is *hepatitis B e antigen* (HBeAg), a soluble, nonparticulate, nucleocapsid protein that is immunologically distinct from intact HBcAg but is a product of the same C gene. The C gene has two initiation codons, a precore and a core region (Fig. 285-3). If translation is initiated at the precore region, the protein product is HBeAg, which has a signal peptide that binds it to the smooth endoplasmic reticulum and leads to its secretion into the circulation. If translation begins with the core region, HBcAg is the protein product; it has no signal peptide, it is not secreted, but it assembles into

nucleocapsid particles, which bind to and incorporate RNA and which, ultimately, contain HBV DNA. Also packaged within the nucleocapsid core is a DNA polymerase, which directs replication and repair of HBV DNA. When packaging within viral proteins is complete, synthesis of the incomplete plus strand stops; this accounts for the single-stranded gap and for differences in the size of the gap. HBcAg particles remain in the hepatocyte, where they are readily detectable by immunohistochemical staining, and are exported after encapsidation by an envelope of HBsAg. Therefore, naked core particles do not circulate in the serum. The secreted nucleocapsid protein, HBeAg, provides a convenient, readily detectable, qualitative marker of HBV replication and relative infectivity.

HBsAg-positive serum containing HBeAg is more likely to be highly infectious and to be associated with the presence of hepatitis B virions (and detectable HBV DNA, see below) than HBeAg-negative or anti-HBe-positive serum. For example, HBsAg carrier mothers who are HBeAg-positive almost invariably (>90%) transmit hepatitis B infection to their offspring, whereas HBsAg carrier mothers with anti-HBe rarely (10 to 15%) infect their offspring.

Early during the course of acute hepatitis B, HBeAg appears transiently; its disappearance may be a harbinger of clinical improvement and resolution of infection. Persistence of HBeAg in serum beyond the first 3 months of acute infection may be predictive of the development of chronic infection, and the presence of HBeAg during chronic hepatitis B is associated with ongoing viral replication, infectivity, and inflammatory liver injury.

The third of the HBV genes is the largest, the P gene (Fig. 285-3), which codes for the DNA polymerase; as noted above, this enzyme has both DNA-dependent DNA polymerase and RNA-dependent reverse transcriptase activities. The fourth gene, X, codes for a small, nonparticulate protein, hepatitis B x antigen (HBxAg), that is capable of transactivating the transcription of both viral and cellular genes (Fig. 285-3). In the cytoplasm, HBxAg effects calcium release (possibly from mitochondria), which activates signal-transduction pathways that lead to stimulation of HBV reverse transcription and HBV DNA replication. Such transactivation may enhance the replication of HBV, leading to the clinical association observed between the expression of HBxAg and antibodies to it in patients with severe chronic hepatitis and hepatocellular carcinoma. The transactivating activity can enhance the transcription and replication of other viruses besides HBV, such as HIV. Cellular processes transactivated by X include the human interferon γ gene and class I major histocompatibility genes; potentially, these effects could contribute to enhanced susceptibility of HBV-infected hepatocytes to cytolytic T cells. The expression of X can also induce programmed cell death (apoptosis).

SEROLOGIC AND VIROLOGIC MARKERS After a person is infected with HBV, the first virologic marker detectable in serum is HBsAg (Fig. 285-4). Circulating HBsAg precedes elevations of serum aminotransferase activity and clinical symptoms and remains detectable during the entire icteric or symptomatic phase of acute hepatitis B and beyond. In typical cases, HBsAg becomes undetectable 1 to 2 months after the onset of jaundice and rarely persists beyond 6 months. After HBsAg disappears, antibody to HBsAg (anti-HBs) becomes detectable in serum and remains detectable indefinitely thereafter. Because HBcAg is sequestered within an HBsAg coat, HBcAg is not detectable routinely in the serum of patients with HBV infection. By contrast, anti-HBc is readily demonstrable in serum, beginning within the first 1 to 2 weeks after the appearance of HBsAg and preceding detectable levels of anti-HBs by weeks to months. Because variability exists in the time of appearance of anti-HBs after HBV infection, occasionally a gap of several weeks or longer may separate the disappearance of HBsAg and the appearance of anti-HBs. During this "gap" or "window" period, anti-HBc may represent serologic evidence of current or recent HBV infection, and blood containing anti-HBc in the absence of HBsAg and anti-HBs has been implicated in the development of transfusion-as-

TABLE 285-1 Nomenclature and Features of Hepatitis Viruses

Hepatitis Type	Virus Particle	Morphology	Genome[a]	Classification	Antigen(s)	Antibodies	Remarks
HAV	27 nm	Icosahedral nonenveloped	7.5-kb RNA, linear, ss, +	Hepatovirus	HAV	Anti-HAV	Early fecal shedding Diagnosis: IgM anti-HAV Previous infection: IgG anti-HAV
HBV	42 nm	Double-shelled virion (surface and core) spherical	3.2-kb DNA, circular, ss/ds	Hepadnavirus	HBsAg HBcAg HBeAg	Anti-HBs Anti-HBc Anti-HBe	Bloodborne virus; carrier state Acute diagnosis: HBsAg, IgM anti-HBc Chronic diagnosis: IgG anti-HBc, HBsAg Markers of replication: HBeAg, HBV DNA Liver, lymphocytes, other organs
	27 nm	Nucleocapsid core			HBcAg HBeAg	Anti-HBc Anti-HBe	Nucleocapsid contains DNA and DNA polymerase; present in hepatocyte nucleus; HBcAg does not circulate; HBeAg (soluble, nonparticulate) and HBV DNA circulate—correlate with infectivity and complete virions
	22 nm	Spherical and filamentous; represents excess virus coat material			HBsAg	Anti-HBs	HBsAg detectable in >95% of patients with acute hepatitis B; found in serum, body fluids, hepatocyte cytoplasm; anti-HBs appears following infection—protective antibody
HCV	Approx. 40–60 nm	Enveloped	9.4-kb RNA, linear, ss, +	Hepacivirus	HCV C100-3 C33c C22-3 NS5	Anti-HCV	Bloodborne agent, formerly labeled non-A, non-B hepatitis Acute diagnosis: anti-HCV (C33c, C22-3, NS5), HCV RNA Chronic diagnosis: anti-HCV (C100-3, C33c, C22-3, NS5) and HCV RNA; cytoplasmic location in hepatocytes
HDV	35–37 nm	Enveloped hybrid particle with HBsAg coat and HDV core	1.7-kb RNA, circular, ss, −	Resembles viroids and plant satellite viruses	HBsAg HDV antigen	Anti-HBs Anti-HDV	Defective RNA virus, requires helper function of HBV (hepadnaviruses); HDV antigen present in hepatocyte nucleus Diagnosis: anti-HDV, HDV RNA; HBV/HDV coinfection—IgM anti-HBc and anti-HDV; HDV superinfection—IgG anti-HBc and anti-HDV
HEV	32–34 nm	Nonenveloped icosahedral	7.6-kb RNA, linear, ss, +	Alphavirus-like	HEV antigen	Anti-HEV	Agent of enterically transmitted hepatitis; rare in USA; occurs in Asia, Mediterranean countries, Central America Diagnosis: IgM/IgG anti-HEV (assays being developed); virus in stool, bile, hepatocyte cytoplasm

[a] ss, single-strand; ss/ds, partially single-strand, partially double-strand; −, minus-strand; +, plus-strand.

sociated hepatitis B. In part because the sensitivity of immunoassays for HBsAg and anti-HBs has increased, however, this window period is rarely encountered. In some persons, years after HBV infection, anti-HBc may persist in the circulation longer than anti-HBs. Therefore, isolated anti-HBc does not necessarily indicate active virus replication; most instances of isolated anti-HBc represent hepatitis B infection in the remote past. Rarely, however, isolated anti-HBc represents low-

level hepatitis B viremia, with HBsAg below the detection threshold; occasionally, isolated anti-HBc represents a cross-reacting or false-positive immunologic specificity. Recent and remote HBV infections can be distinguished by determination of the immunoglobulin class of anti-HBc. Anti-HBc of the IgM class (IgM anti-HBc) predominates during the first 6 months after acute infection, whereas IgG anti-HBc is the predominant class of anti-HBc beyond 6 months. Therefore,

FIGURE 285-4 Scheme of typical clinical and laboratory features of acute viral hepatitis B.

patients with current or recent acute hepatitis B, including those in the anti-HBc window, have IgM anti-HBc in their serum. In patients who have recovered from hepatitis B in the remote past as well as those with chronic HBV infection, anti-HBc is predominantly of the IgG class. Infrequently, in no more than 1 to 5% of patients with acute HBV infection, levels of HBsAg are too low to be detected; in such cases, the presence of IgM anti-HBc establishes the diagnosis of acute hepatitis B. When isolated anti-HBc occurs in the rare patient with chronic hepatitis B whose HBsAg level is below the sensitivity threshold of contemporary immunoassays (a low-level carrier), the anti-HBc is of the IgG class. Generally, in persons who have recovered from hepatitis B, anti-HBs and anti-HBc persist indefinitely.

The temporal association between the appearance of anti-HBs and resolution of HBV infection as well as the observation that persons with anti-HBs in serum are protected against reinfection with HBV suggest that *anti-HBs is the protective antibody.* Therefore, strategies for prevention of HBV infection are based on providing susceptible persons with circulating anti-HBs (see below). Occasionally, in 10 to 20% of patients with chronic hepatitis B, low-level, low-affinity anti-HBs can be detected. This antibody is directed against a subtype determinant different from that represented by the patient's HBsAg; its presence is thought to reflect the stimulation of a related clone of antibody-forming cells, but it has no clinical relevance and does not signal imminent clearance of hepatitis B.

The other readily detectable serologic marker of HBV infection, HBeAg, appears concurrently with or shortly after HBsAg. Its appearance coincides temporally with high levels of virus replication and reflects the presence of circulating intact virions and detectable HBV DNA. Pre-S1 and pre-S2 proteins are also expressed during periods of peak replication, but assays for these gene products are not routinely available. In self-limited HBV infections, HBeAg becomes undetectable shortly after peak elevations in aminotransferase activity, before the disappearance of HBsAg, and anti-HBe then becomes detectable, coinciding with a period of relatively lower infectivity (Fig. 285-4). Because markers of HBV replication appear transiently during acute infection, testing for such markers is of little clinical utility in typical cases of acute HBV infection. In contrast, markers of HBV replication provide valuable information in patients with protracted infections.

Departing from the pattern typical of acute HBV infections, in chronic HBV infection, HBsAg remains detectable beyond 6 months, anti-HBc is primarily of the IgG class, and anti-HBs is either undetectable or detectable at low levels (see "Laboratory Features," below) (Fig. 285-5). During early chronic HBV infection, HBV DNA can be detected both in serum and in hepatocyte nuclei, where it is present in free or episomal form. This *replicative stage* of HBV infection is the time of maximal infectivity and liver injury; HBeAg is a qualitative marker and HBV DNA a quantitative marker of this replicative phase,

during which all three forms of HBV circulate, including intact virions. Over time, the replicative phase of chronic HBV infection gives way to a relatively *nonreplicative phase.* This occurs at a rate of approximately 10% per year and is accompanied by seroconversion from HBeAg-positive to anti-HBe-positive. In most cases, this seroconversion coincides with a transient, acute hepatitis-like elevation in aminotransferase activity, believed to reflect cell-mediated immune clearance of virus-infected hepatocytes. In the nonreplicative phase of chronic infection, when HBV DNA is demonstrable in hepatocyte nuclei, it tends to be integrated into the host genome. In this phase, only spherical and tubular forms of HBV, *not intact virions,* circulate, and liver injury tends to subside. Most such patients would be characterized as *inactive HBV carriers.* In reality, the designations *replicative* and *nonreplicative* are only relative; even in the so-called nonreplicative phase, HBV replication can be detected with highly sensitive amplification probes such as the polymerase chain reaction (PCR). Still, the distinctions are pathophysiologically and clinically meaningful. Occasionally, nonreplicative HBV infection converts back to replicative infection. Such spontaneous reactivations are accompanied by reexpression of HBeAg and HBV DNA, and sometimes of IgM anti-HBc, as well as by exacerbations of liver injury.

MOLECULAR VARIANTS Variation occurs throughout the HBV genome, and clinical isolates of HBV that do not express typical viral proteins have been attributed to mutations in individual or even multiple gene locations. For example, variants have been described that lack nucleocapsid proteins, envelope proteins, or both. Two categories of HBV have attracted the most attention. One of these was identified initially in Mediterranean countries among patients with an unusual serologic-clinical profile. They have severe chronic HBV infection and detectable HBV DNA but with anti-HBe instead of HBeAg. These patients were found to be infected with an HBV mutant that contained an alteration in the precore region rendering the virus incapable of encoding HBeAg. Although several potential mutation sites exist in the pre-C region, the region of the C gene necessary for the expression of HBeAg (see "Virology and Etiology," above), the most commonly encountered in such patients is a single base substitution, from G to A, which occurs in the second to last codon of the pre-C gene at nucleotide 1896. This substitution results in the replacement of the TGG tryptophan codon by a stop codon (TAG), which prevents the translation of HBeAg. Another mutation, in the core promoter region, prevents transcription of the coding region for HBeAg and yields an

FIGURE 285-5 Scheme of typical laboratory features of chronic viral hepatitis B. HBeAg and HBV DNA can be detected in serum during the *replicative phase* of chronic infection, which is associated with infectivity and liver injury. Seroconversion from the replicative phase to the *nonreplicative phase* occurs at a rate of approximately 10 to 15% per year and is heralded by an acute hepatitis–like elevation of ALT activity; during the nonreplicative phase, infectivity and liver injury are limited.

HBeAg-negative phenotype. Patients with such precore mutants that are unable to secrete HBeAg tend to have severe liver disease that progresses more rapidly to cirrhosis. Both "wild-type" HBV and precore-mutant HBV can coexist in the same patient, or mutant HBV may arise late during wild-type HBV infection. In addition, clusters of fulminant hepatitis B in Israel and Japan have been attributed to common-source infection with a precore mutant. Fulminant hepatitis B in North America and western Europe, however, occurs in patients infected with wild-type HBV, in the absence of precore mutants, and both precore mutants and other mutations throughout the HBV genome occur commonly even in patients with typical, self-limited, milder forms of HBV infection. Precore-mutant hepatitis B is now the most frequently encountered form of hepatitis B in Mediterranean countries and in Europe. In the United States, where HBV genotype A (less prone to G1896A mutation) is prevalent, precore-mutant HBV is much less common. Characteristic of such HBeAg-negative chronic hepatitis B are lower levels of HBV DNA and periodic fluctuations in hepatic necroinflammatory activity.

The second important category of HBV mutants consists of *escape mutants*, in which a single amino acid substitution, from glycine to arginine, occurs at position 145 of the immunodominant *a* determinant common to all subtypes of HBsAg. This change in HBsAg leads to a critical conformational change that results in a loss of neutralizing activity by anti-HBs. This specific HBV/*a* mutant has been observed in two situations, active and passive immunization, in which humoral immunologic pressure may favor evolutionary change ("escape") in the virus—in a small number of hepatitis B vaccine recipients who acquired HBV infection despite the prior appearance of neutralizing anti-HBs and in liver transplant recipients who underwent the procedure for hepatitis B and who were treated with a high-potency human monoclonal anti-HBs preparation. Although such mutants have not been recognized frequently, their existence raises a concern that may complicate vaccination strategies and serologic diagnosis.

EXTRAHEPATIC SITES Hepatitis B antigens and HBV DNA been identified in extrahepatic sites, including lymph nodes, bone marrow, circulating lymphocytes, spleen, and pancreas. Although the virus does not appear to be associated with tissue injury in any of these extrahepatic sites, its presence in these "remote" reservoirs has been invoked to explain the recurrence of HBV infection after orthotopic liver transplantation. A more complete understanding of the clinical relevance of extrahepatic HBV remains to be defined.

Hepatitis D The delta hepatitis agent, or HDV, is a defective RNA virus that coinfects with and requires the helper function of HBV (or other hepadnaviruses) for its replication and expression. Slightly smaller than HBV, delta is a formalin-sensitive, 35- to 37-nm virus with a hybrid structure. Its nucleocapsid expresses delta antigen, which bears no antigenic homology with any of the HBV antigens, and contains the virus genome. The delta core is "encapsidated" by an outer envelope of HBsAg, indistinguishable from that of HBV except in its relative compositions of major, middle, and large HBsAg component proteins. The genome is a small, 1700-nucleotide, circular, single-stranded RNA (minus strand) that is nonhomologous with HBV DNA (except for a small area of the polymerase gene) but that has features and the rolling circle model of replication common to genomes of plant satellite viruses or viroids. HDV RNA contains many areas of internal complementarity; therefore, it can fold on itself by internal base pairing to form an unusual, very stable, rodlike structure. HDV RNA requires host RNA polymerase II for its replication via RNA-directed RNA synthesis by transcription of genomic RNA to a complementary antigenomic (plus strand) RNA; the antigenomic RNA, in turn, serves as a template for subsequent genomic RNA synthesis. Between the genomic and antigenomic RNAs of HDV, there are coding regions for nine proteins. Delta antigen, which is a product of the antigenomic strand, exists in two forms, a small, 195-amino-acid species, which plays a role in facilitating HDV RNA replication, and a large, 214-

amino-acid species, which appears to suppress replication but is required for assembly of the antigen into virions. Delta antigens have been shown to bind directly to RNA polymerase II, resulting in stimulation of transcription. Although complete hepatitis D virions and liver injury require the cooperative helper function of HBV, intracellular replication of HDV RNA can occur without HBV. Genomic heterogeneity among HDV isolates has been described; however, pathophysiologic and clinical consequences of this genetic diversity have not been recognized.

HDV can either infect a person simultaneously with HBV (*co-infection*) or superinfect a person already infected with HBV (*super-infection*); when HDV infection is transmitted from a donor with one HBsAg subtype to an HBsAg-positive recipient with a different subtype, the HDV agent assumes the HBsAg subtype of the recipient, rather than the donor. Because HDV relies absolutely on HBV, the duration of HDV infection is determined by the duration of (and cannot outlast) HBV infection. HDV antigen is expressed primarily in hepatocyte nuclei and is occasionally detectable in serum. During acute HDV infection, anti-HDV of the IgM class predominates, and 30 to 40 days may elapse after symptoms appear before anti-HDV can be detected. In self-limited infection, anti-HDV is low titer and transient, rarely remaining detectable beyond the clearance of HBsAg and HDV antigen. In chronic HDV infection, anti-HDV circulates in high titer, and both IgM and IgG anti-HDV can be detected. HDV antigen in the liver and HDV RNA in serum and liver can be detected during HDV replication.

Hepatitis C Hepatitis C virus, which, before its identification was labeled "non-A, non-B hepatitis," is a linear, single-strand, positive-sense, 9600-nucleotide RNA virus, the genome of which is similar in organization to that of flaviviruses and pestiviruses; HCV is the only member of the genus *Hepacivirus* in the family Flaviviridae. The HCV genome contains a single large open reading frame (gene) that codes for a virus polyprotein of approximately 3000 amino acids. The 5′ end of the genome consists of an untranslated region (containing an internal ribosomal entry site) adjacent to the genes for structural proteins, the nucleocapsid core protein and two envelope glycoproteins, E1 and E2/NS1. The 5′ untranslated region and core gene are highly conserved among genotypes, but the envelope proteins are coded for by the hypervariable region, which varies from isolate to isolate and may allow the virus to evade host immunologic containment directed at accessible virus-envelope proteins. The 3′ end of the genome contains the genes for nonstructural (NS) proteins. The first reported HCV clone, 5-1-1, and the nucleotide sequence coding for C100-3, the recombinant virus protein used in the first immunoassay for antibodies to HCV, reside within the NS4 gene, and the RNA-dependent RNA polymerase, through which HCV replicates, is encoded by the NS5 region (Fig. 285-6). Because HCV does not replicate via a DNA intermediate, it does not integrate into the host genome. Because HCV tends to circulate in relatively low titer, visualization of virus particles, estimated to be 40 to 60 nm in diameter, has been difficult. Still, the replication rate of HCV is very high, 10^{12} virions per day; its half-life is 2.7 h. The chimpanzee is a helpful but cumbersome animal model. Although in vitro replication has been difficult, hepatocellular carcinoma–derived cell lines have been described (replicon systems) that support replication of genetically manipulated, truncated or full-length HCV RNA (but not intact virions). Although a robust, reproducible, small-animal model is lacking, HCV replication has been documented in an immunodeficient-mouse model containing explants of human liver.

At least six distinct genotypes, as well as subtypes within genotypes, of HCV have been identified by nucleotide sequencing. Genotypes differ one from another in sequence homology by ≥30%. Because divergence of HCV isolates within a genotype or subtype, and within the same host, may vary insufficiently to define a distinct genotype, these intragenotypic differences are referred to as *quasispecies* and differ in sequence homology by only a few percent. The genotypic and quasispecies diversity of HCV, resulting from its high mutation

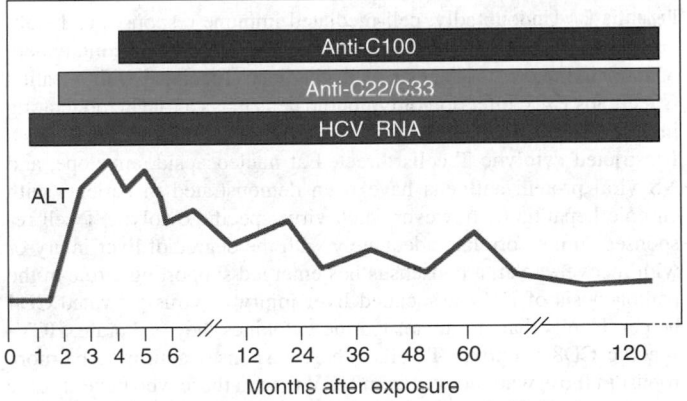

FIGURE 285-6 Organization of the hepatitis C virus genome and its associated proteins. Structural genes at the 5' end include the nucleocapsid region, C, and the envelope regions, E1 and E2. The 5' untranslated region and the C region are highly conserved among isolates, while the envelope domain E2/NS1 contains the hypervariable region. At the 3' end are five nonstructural (NS) regions. Viral proteins included in the first-generation (C100-3), second-generation (C200, a fusion protein of C100-3 and C33c, and C22-3), and third-generation (C22-3, C200, or C33c and C100-3, and NS5) immunoassays and in the recombinant immunoblot assay (5-1-1, C100-3, C33c, C22-3, NS5) are presented below their corresponding genes (AA, amino acid).

rate, interferes with effective humoral immunity. Neutralizing antibodies to HCV have been demonstrated, but they tend to be short-lived; and HCV infection does not induce lasting immunity against reinfection with different virus isolates or even the same virus isolate. Thus, neither *heterologous* nor *homologous* immunity appears to develop commonly after acute HCV infection. Some HCV genotypes are distributed worldwide, while others are more geographically confined. In addition, differences exist among genotypes in responsiveness to antiviral therapy; however, early reports of differences in pathogenicity among genotypes have not been corroborated.

As noted above, the first assay detected antibodies to C100-3, a recombinant polypeptide derived from the NS4 region of the genome. In most patients with acute hepatitis C, antibody detected with this assay appears between 1 to 3 months after the onset of acute hepatitis but sometimes not for a year or longer. Second-generation assays incorporate recombinant proteins from the nucleocapsid core region, C22-3, and the NS3 region, C33c (expressed in combination with C100-3 as C200); these assays are more sensitive (by approximately 20%) and detect anti-HCV 30 to 90 days earlier, during the period of acute hepatitis. A third-generation immunoassay, which incorporates proteins from the NS5 region and replaces some recombinant proteins with synthetic peptides, may detect anti-HCV even earlier. Because nonspecificity has been encountered in clinical samples tested for anti-HCV, a supplementary recombinant immunoblot assay was introduced. Reactivity in an immunoassay is "confirmed" by incubation with a nitrocellulose strip that contains individual bands of recombinant or synthetic HCV proteins. This approach allows the demonstration of individual antibodies to nonstructural and structural viral proteins and identifies false-positive reactivity associated with nonviral specificities. Although useful to support the validity of anti-HCV-reactive samples, especially in patients with a low prior probability of true infection (e.g., blood donors) or in patients with confounding activity in serum (such as a rheumatoid factor) that may yield false-positive antibody reactivity, immunoblotting assays have been supplanted by tests for HCV RNA. The most sensitive indicator is the presence of HCV RNA, which requires molecular amplification by (PCR) or transcription-mediated amplification (TMA) (Fig. 285-7). An alternative method for detection of HCV RNA, more easily automated but one or two orders of magnitude less sensitive, is branched-chain complementary DNA hybridization. HCV RNA can be detected within a few days of exposure to HCV, well before the appearance of anti-HCV, and tends to persist for the duration of HCV infection; however, occasionally in patients with chronic HCV infection, HCV RNA may be detectable only intermittently. Application of sensitive molecular probes for HCV RNA has revealed the presence of replicative HCV in peripheral blood lymphocytes of infected persons; however, as is

the case for HBV in lymphocytes, the clinical relevance of HCV lymphocyte infection is not known.

Hepatitis E Previously labeled *epidemic* or *enterically transmitted non-A, non-B hepatitis*, HEV is an enterically transmitted virus that occurs primarily in India, Asia, Africa, and Central America. This agent, with epidemiologic features resembling those of hepatitis A, is a 32- to 34-nm, nonenveloped, HAV-like virus with a 7600-nucleotide, single-stranded, positive-sense RNA genome. HEV has three open reading frames (genes), the largest of which encodes nonstructural proteins involved in virus replication. A middle-sized gene encodes the nucleocapsid protein, and the smallest, whose function is not known, encodes protein specificities to which antibodies appear in human serum. All HEV isolates appear to belong to a single serotype, despite genomic heterogeneity of up to 25%. There is no genomic or antigenic homology, however, between HEV and HAV or other picornaviruses; and HEV, although resembling calciviruses, appears to be sufficiently distinct from any known agent to merit a new classification of its own within the alphavirus group. The virus has been detected in stool, bile, and liver and is excreted in the stool during the late incubation period; immune responses to viral antigens occur very early during the course of acute infection. Both IgM anti-HEV and IgG anti-HEV can be detected, but both fall rapidly after acute infection, reaching low levels within 9 to 12 months. Currently, serologic testing for HEV infection is not available routinely.

PATHOGENESIS   Under ordinary circumstances, none of the hepatitis viruses is known to be directly cytopathic to hepatocytes. Evidence suggests that the clinical manifestations and outcomes after acute liver injury associated with viral hepatitis are determined by the immunologic responses of the host.

HEPATITIS B   Among the viral hepatitides, the immunopathogenesis of hepatitis B has been studied most extensively. Certainly for this agent, the existence of inactive hepatitis B carriers with normal liver histology and function suggests that the virus is not directly cytopathic. The fact that patients with defects in cellular immune competence are more likely to remain chronically infected rather than to clear the virus is cited to support the role of cellular immune responses in the pathogenesis of hepatitis B–related liver injury. The model that has the most experimental support involves cytolytic T cells sensitized specifically to recognize host and hepatitis B viral antigens on the liver cell surface. Laboratory observations suggest that nucleocapsid proteins (HBcAg and possibly HBeAg), present on the cell membrane in minute quantities, are the viral target antigens that, with host antigens, invite cytolytic T cells to destroy HBV-infected hepatocytes. Differences in the

FIGURE 285-7 Scheme of typical laboratory features during acute hepatitis C progressing to chronicity. HCV RNA is the first detectable event, preceding ALT elevation and the appearance of anti-HCV. The appearance of antibody to C100, detectable with first-generation assays, is delayed from 1 to 3 months after the appearance of antibody to C22 and C33, antibodies that are included in second-generation immunoassays. Anti-HCV detectable with second-generation assays appears during acute hepatitis C.

robustness of cytolytic T cell responsiveness and in the elaboration of antiviral cytokines by T cells have been invoked to explain differences in outcomes between those who recover after acute hepatitis and those who progress to chronic hepatitis or between those with mild and those with severe (fulminant) acute HBV infection.

Although a robust cytolytic T cell response occurs and eliminates virus-infected liver cells during acute hepatitis B, >90% of HBV DNA has been found in experimentally infected chimpanzees to disappear from the liver and blood before maximal T cell infiltration of the liver and before most of the biochemical and histologic evidence of liver injury. This observation suggests that inflammatory cytokines, independent of cytopathic antiviral mechanisms, participate in early viral clearance; this effect has been shown to represent elimination of HBV replicative intermediates from the cytoplasm and covalently closed circular viral DNA from the nucleus of infected hepatocytes.

Debate continues over the relative importance of viral and host factors in the pathogenesis of HBV-associated liver injury and its outcome. As noted above, precore genetic mutants of HBV have been associated with the more severe outcomes of HBV infection (severe chronic and fulminant hepatitis), suggesting that, under certain circumstances, relative pathogenicity is a property of the virus, not the host. The fact that concomitant HDV and HBV infections are associated with more severe liver injury than HBV infection alone and the fact that cells transfected in vitro with the gene for HDV (delta) antigen express HDV antigen and then become necrotic in the absence of any immunologic influences are also consistent with a viral effect on pathogenicity. Similarly, in patients who undergo liver transplantation for end-stage chronic hepatitis B, occasionally, rapidly progressive liver injury appears in the new liver. This clinical pattern is associated with an unusual histologic pattern in the new liver, *fibrosing cholestatic hepatitis*, which, ultrastructurally, appears to represent a choking of the cell with overwhelming quantities of HBsAg. This observation suggests that under the influence of the potent immunosuppressive agents required to prevent allograft rejection, HBV may have a direct cytopathic effect on liver cells, independent of the immune system.

Although the precise mechanism of liver injury in HBV infection remains elusive, studies of nucleocapsid proteins have shed light on the profound immunologic tolerance to HBV of babies born to mothers with highly replicative (HBeAg-positive), chronic HBV infection. In HBeAg-expressing transgenic mice, in utero exposure to HBeAg, which is sufficiently small to traverse the placenta, induces T cell tolerance to both nucleocapsid proteins. This, in turn, may explain why, when infection occurs so early in life, immunologic clearance does not occur, and protracted, lifelong infection ensues.

Hepatitis C Undoubtedly, cell-mediated immune responses and elaboration by T cells of antiviral cytokines contribute to the containment of infection and pathogenesis of liver injury associated with hepatitis C. Perhaps HCV infection of lymphoid cells plays a role in moderating immune responsiveness to the virus, as well. Intrahepatic HLA class-I-restricted cytolytic T cells directed at nucleocapsid, envelope, and NS viral protein antigens have been demonstrated in patients with chronic hepatitis C; however, such virus-specific cytolytic T cell responses do not correlate adequately with the degree of liver injury or with recovery. Yet, a consensus has emerged supporting a role in the pathogenesis of HCV-associated liver injury of virus-activated CD4 helper T cells that stimulate, via the cytokines they elaborate, HCV-specific CD8 cytotoxic T cells. These responses appear to be more robust in those who recover from HCV than in those who have chronic infection. Several HLA alleles have been linked with self-limited hepatitis C, but such associations do not apply universally. Finally, cross-reactivity between viral and host autoantigens has been invoked to explain the association between hepatitis C and a subset of patients with autoimmune hepatitis and antibodies to liver-kidney microsomal (LKM) antigen (anti-LKM) (Chap. 287).

EXTRAHEPATIC MANIFESTATIONS Immune complex–mediated tissue damage appears to play a pathogenetic role in the extrahepatic manifestations of acute hepatitis B. The occasional prodromal serum sickness–like syndrome observed in acute hepatitis B appears to be related to the deposition in tissue blood vessel walls of HBsAg-anti-HBs circulating immune complexes, leading to activation of the complement system and depressed serum complement levels.

In patients with chronic hepatitis B, other types of immune-complex disease may be seen. Glomerulonephritis with the nephritic syndrome is occasionally observed; HBsAg, immunoglobulin, and C3 deposition has been found in the glomerular basement membrane. While polyarteritis nodosa develops in considerably fewer than 1% of patients with chronic HBV infection, 20 to 30% of patients with polyarteritis nodosa have HBsAg in serum (Chap. 306). In these patients, the affected small and medium-sized arterioles have been shown to contain HBsAg, immunoglobulins, and complement components. Another extrahepatic manifestation of viral hepatitis, essential mixed cryoglobulinemia (EMC), was reported initially to be associated with hepatitis B. The disorder is characterized clinically by arthritis, cutaneous vasculitis (palpable purpura), and occasionally with glomerulonephritis and serologically by the presence of circulating cryoprecipitable immune complexes of more than one immunoglobulin class (Chaps. 264 and 306). Many patients with this syndrome have chronic liver disease, but the association with HBV infection is limited; instead, a substantial proportion have chronic HCV infection, with circulating immune complexes containing HCV RNA. Immune-complex glomerulonephritis is another recognized extrahepatic manifestation of chronic hepatitis C.

PATHOLOGY The typical morphologic lesions of all types of viral hepatitis are similar and consist of panlobular infiltration with mononuclear cells, hepatic cell necrosis, hyperplasia of Kupffer cells, and variable degrees of cholestasis. Hepatic cell regeneration is present, as evidenced by numerous mitotic figures, multinucleated cells, and "rosette" or "pseudoacinar" formation. The mononuclear infiltration consists primarily of small lymphocytes, although plasma cells and eosinophils occasionally are present. Liver cell damage consists of hepatic cell degeneration and necrosis, cell dropout, ballooning of cells, and acidophilic degeneration of hepatocytes (forming so-called Councilman or apoptotic bodies). Large hepatocytes with a ground-glass appearance of the cytoplasm may be seen in chronic but not in acute HBV infection; these cells contain HBsAg and can be identified histochemically with orcein or aldehyde fuchsin. In uncomplicated viral hepatitis, the reticulin framework is preserved.

In hepatitis C, the histologic lesion is often remarkable for a relative paucity of inflammation, a marked increase in activation of sinusoidal lining cells, lymphoid aggregates, the presence of fat (more frequent in genotype 3 and linked to increased fibrosis), and, occasionally, bile duct lesions in which biliary epithelial cells appear to be piled up without interruption of the basement membrane. Occasionally, microvesicular steatosis occurs in hepatitis D. In hepatitis E, a common histologic feature is marked cholestasis. A cholestatic variant of slowly resolving acute hepatitis A also has been described.

A more severe histologic lesion, *bridging hepatic necrosis*, also termed *subacute* or *confluent necrosis*, is occasionally observed in some patients with acute hepatitis. "Bridging" between lobules results from large areas of hepatic cell dropout, with collapse of the reticulin framework. Characteristically, the bridge consists of condensed reticulum, inflammatory debris, and degenerating liver cells that span adjacent portal areas, portal to central veins, or central vein to central vein. This lesion had been thought to have prognostic significance; in many of the originally described patients with this lesion, a subacute course terminated in death within several weeks to months or severe chronic hepatitis and postnecrotic cirrhosis developed. Subsequent investigations have failed to uphold the association between bridging necrosis and such a poor prognosis in patients with acute hepatitis. Therefore, although demonstration of this lesion in patients with chronic hepatitis has prognostic significance (Chap. 287), its demonstration during acute hepatitis is less meaningful, and liver biopsies to identify this lesion are no longer undertaken routinely in patients with acute hepatitis. In *massive hepatic necrosis* (fulminant hepatitis, acute yellow atrophy), the striking feature at postmortem examination is the finding of a small, shrunken, soft liver. Histologic examination reveals massive necrosis and dropout of liver cells of most lobules with extensive collapse and condensation of the reticulin framework. When histologic documentation is required in the management of fulminant or very severe hepatitis, a biopsy can be done by the angiographically guided transjugular route, which permits the performance of this invasive procedure in the presence of severe coagulopathy.

Immunohistochemical and electron-microscopic studies have localized HBsAg to the cytoplasm and plasma membrane of infected liver cells. In contrast, HBcAg predominates in the nucleus, but occasionally, scant amounts are also seen in the cytoplasm and on the cell membrane. HDV antigen is localized to the hepatocyte nucleus, while HAV, HCV, and HEV antigens are localized to the cytoplasm.

EPIDEMIOLOGY Before the availability of serologic tests for hepatitis viruses, all viral hepatitis cases were labeled either as "infectious" or "serum" hepatitis. Modes of transmission overlap, however, and *a clear distinction among the different types of viral hepatitis cannot be made solely on the basis of clinical or epidemiologic features* (Table 285-2). The most accurate means to distinguish the various types of viral hepatitis involves specific serologic testing.

Hepatitis A *This agent is transmitted almost exclusively by the fecal-oral route.* Person-to-person spread of HAV is enhanced by poor personal hygiene and overcrowding; large outbreaks as well as sporadic cases have been traced to contaminated food, water, milk, frozen raspberries and strawberries, and shellfish. Intrafamily and intrainstitutional spread are also common. Early epidemiologic observations suggested that there is a predilection for hepatitis A to occur in late fall and early winter. In temperate zones, epidemic waves have been recorded every 5 to 20 years as new segments of nonimmune population appeared; however, in developed countries, the incidence of hepatitis A has been declining, presumably as a function of improved sanitation, and these cyclic patterns are no longer being observed. No HAV carrier state has been identified after acute hepatitis A; perpetuation of the virus in nature depends presumably on nonepidemic, inapparent subclinical infection.

In the general population, anti-HAV, a marker for previous HAV infection, increases in prevalence as a function of increasing age and of decreasing socioeconomic status. In the 1970s, serologic evidence of prior hepatitis A infection occurred in about 40% of urban populations in the United States, most of whose members never recalled having had a symptomatic case of hepatitis. In subsequent decades, however, the prevalence of anti-HAV has been declining in the United States. In developing countries, exposure, infection, and subsequent immunity are almost universal in childhood. As the frequency of subclinical childhood infections declines in developed countries, a susceptible cohort of adults emerges. Hepatitis A tends to be more symptomatic in adults; therefore, paradoxically, as the frequency of HAV infection declines, the likelihood of clinically apparent, even severe, HAV illnesses increases in the susceptible adult population. Travel to endemic areas is a common source of infection for adults from nonendemic areas. More recently recognized epidemiologic foci of HAV infection include child-care centers, neonatal intensive care units, promiscuous homosexual men, and injection drug users. Although hepatitis A is rarely bloodborne, several outbreaks have been recognized in recipients of clotting factor concentrates.

Hepatitis B Percutaneous inoculation has long been recognized as a major route of hepatitis B transmission, but the outmoded designation "serum hepatitis" is an inaccurate label for the epidemiologic spectrum of HBV infection recognized today. As detailed below, most of the hepatitis transmitted by blood transfusion is not caused by HBV; moreover, in approximately two-thirds of patients with acute type B hepatitis, there is no history of an identifiable percutaneous exposure. We now recognize that many cases of hepatitis B result from less obvious modes of nonpercutaneous or covert percutaneous transmission.

TABLE 285-2 *Clinical and Epidemiologic Features of Viral Hepatitis*

Feature	HAV	HBV	HCV	HDV	HEV
Incubation (days)	15–45, mean 30	30–180, mean 60–90	15–160, mean 50	30–180, mean 60–90	14–60, mean 40
Onset	Acute	Insidious or acute	Insidious	Insidious or acute	Acute
Age preference	Children, young adults	Young adults (sexual and percutaneous), babies, toddlers	Any age, but more common in adults	Any age (similar to HBV)	Young adults (20–40 years)
Transmission					
Fecal-oral	+++	−	−	−	+++
Percutaneous	Unusual	+++	+++	+++	−
Perinatal	−	+++	±[a]	+	−
Sexual	±	++	±[a]	++	−
Clinical					
Severity	Mild	Occasionally severe	Moderate	Occasionally severe	Mild
Fulminant	0.1%	0.1–1%	0.1%	5–20%[b]	1–2%[e]
Progression to chronicity	None	Occasional (1–10%) (90% of neonates)	Common (50–70% chronic hepatitis; 80–90% chronic infection)	Common[d]	None
Carrier	None	0.1–30%[c]	1.5–3.2%	Variable[f]	None
Cancer	None	+ (neonatal infection)	+	±	None
Prognosis	Excellent	Worse with age, debility	Moderate	Acute, good Chronic, poor	Good
Prophylaxis	IG Inactivated vaccine	HBIG Recombinant vaccine	None	HBV vaccine (none for HBV carriers)	Unknown
Therapy	None	Interferon Lamivudine Adefovir	Pegylated interferon plus ribavirin	Interferon ±	None

[a] Primarily with HIV co-infection and high-level viremia in index case; risk ~5%.
[b] Up to 5% in acute HBV/HDV co-infection; up to 20% in HDV superinfection of chronic HBV infection.
[c] Varies considerably throughout the world and in subpopulations within countries; see text.
[d] In acute HBV/HDV co-infection, the frequency of chronicity is the same as that for HBV; in HDV superinfection, chronicity is invariable.
[e] 10–20% in pregnant women.
[f] Common in Mediterranean countries, rare in North America and western Europe.

HBsAg has been identified in almost every body fluid from infected persons, and at least some of these body fluids—most notably semen and saliva—are infectious, albeit less so than serum, when administered percutaneously or nonpercutaneously to experimental animals. Among the nonpercutaneous modes of HBV transmission, oral ingestion has been documented as a potential but inefficient route of exposure. By contrast, the two nonpercutaneous routes considered to have the greatest impact are intimate (especially sexual) contact and perinatal transmission.

In sub-Saharan Africa, intimate contact among toddlers is considered instrumental in contributing to the maintenance of the high frequency of hepatitis B in the population. Perinatal transmission occurs primarily in infants born to HBsAg carrier mothers or mothers with acute hepatitis B during the third trimester of pregnancy or during the early postpartum period. Perinatal transmission is uncommon in North America and western Europe but occurs with great frequency and is the most important mode of HBV perpetuation in the Far East and developing countries. Although the precise mode of perinatal transmission is unknown, and although approximately 10% of infections may be acquired in utero, epidemiologic evidence suggests that most infections occur approximately at the time of delivery and are not related to breast feeding. The likelihood of perinatal transmission of HBV correlates with the presence of HBeAg; 90% of HBeAg-positive mothers but only 10 to 15% of anti-HBe-positive mothers transmit HBV infection to their offspring. In most cases, acute infection in the neonate is clinically asymptomatic, but the child is very likely to become an HBsAg carrier.

The more than 350 million HBsAg carriers in the world constitute the main reservoir of hepatitis B in human beings. Serum HBsAg is infrequent (0.1 to 0.5%) in normal populations in the United States and western Europe. However, a prevalence of up to 5 to 20% has been found in the Far East and in some tropical countries; in persons with Down's syndrome, lepromatous leprosy, leukemia, Hodgkin's disease, polyarteritis nodosa; in patients with chronic renal disease on hemodialysis; and in injection drug users.

Other groups with high rates of HBV infection include spouses of acutely infected persons, sexually promiscuous persons (especially promiscuous men who have sex with men), health care workers exposed to blood, persons who require repeated transfusions especially with pooled blood product concentrates (e.g., hemophiliacs), residents and staff of custodial institutions for the developmentally handicapped, prisoners, and, to a lesser extent, family members of chronically infected patients. In volunteer blood donors, the prevalence of anti-HBs, a reflection of previous HBV infection, ranges from 5 to 10%, but the prevalence is higher in lower socioeconomic strata, older age groups, and persons—including those mentioned above—exposed to blood products.

Prevalence of infection, modes of transmission, and human behavior conspire to mold geographically different epidemiologic patterns of HBV infection. In the Far East and Africa, hepatitis B, a disease of the newborn and young children, is perpetuated by a cycle of maternal-neonatal spread. In North America and western Europe, hepatitis B is primarily a disease of adolescence and early adulthood, the time of life when intimate sexual contact as well as recreational and occupational percutaneous exposures tend to occur.

Hepatitis D   Infection with HDV has a worldwide distribution, but two epidemiologic patterns exist. In Mediterranean countries (northern Africa, southern Europe, the Middle East), HDV infection is endemic among those with hepatitis B, and the disease is transmitted predominantly by nonpercutaneous means, especially close personal contact. In nonendemic areas, such as the United States and northern Europe, HDV infection is confined to persons exposed frequently to blood and blood products, primarily injection drug users and hemophiliacs. HDV infection can be introduced into a population through drug users or by migration of persons from endemic to nonendemic areas. Thus, pat-

terns of population migration and human behavior facilitating percutaneous contact play important roles in the introduction and amplification of HDV infection. Occasionally, the migrating epidemiology of hepatitis D is expressed in explosive outbreaks of severe hepatitis, such as those that have occurred in remote South American villages as well as in urban centers in the United States. Ultimately, such outbreaks of hepatitis D—either of coinfections with acute hepatitis B or of superinfections in those already infected with HBV—may blur the distinctions between endemic and nonendemic areas. On a global scale, HDV infection is declining. Even in Italy, an HDV-endemic area, public health measures introduced to control HBV infection resulted during the 1990s in a 1.5%/year reduction in the prevalence of HDV infection.

Hepatitis C   Routine screening of blood donors for HBsAg and the elimination of commercial blood sources in the early 1970s reduced the frequency of, but did not eliminate, transfusion-associated hepatitis. During the 1970s, the likelihood of acquiring hepatitis after transfusion of voluntarily donated, HBsAg-screened blood was approximately 10% per patient (up to 0.9% per unit transfused); 90 to 95% of these cases were classified, based on serologic exclusion of hepatitis A and B, as "non-A, non-B" hepatitis. For patients requiring transfusion of pooled products, such as clotting factor concentrates, the risk was even higher, up to 20 to 30%.

During the 1980s, voluntary self-exclusion of blood donors with risk factors for AIDS and then the introduction of donor screening for anti-HIV reduced further the likelihood of transfusion-associated hepatitis to under 5%. During the late 1980s and early 1990s, the introduction first of "surrogate" screening tests for non-A, non-B hepatitis [alanine aminotransferase (ALT) and anti-HBc, both shown to identify blood donors with a higher likelihood of transmitting non-A, non-B hepatitis to recipients] and, subsequently, after the discovery of HCV, first-generation immunoassays for anti-HCV reduced the frequency of transfusion-associated hepatitis even further. A prospective analysis of transfusion-associated hepatitis conducted between 1986 and 1990 showed that the incidence of transfusion-associated hepatitis at one urban university hospital fell from a baseline of 3.8% per patient (0.45% per unit transfused) to 1.5% per patient (0.19% per unit) after the introduction of surrogate testing and to 0.6% per patient (0.03% per unit) after the introduction of first-generation anti-HCV assays. The introduction of second-generation anti-HCV assays reduced the frequency of transfusion-associated hepatitis C to almost imperceptible levels, 1 in 100,000, and these gains are being reinforced by the application of automated PCR testing of donated blood for HCV RNA.

In addition to being transmitted by transfusion, hepatitis C can be transmitted by other percutaneous routes, such as injection drug use. In addition, this virus can be transmitted by occupational exposure to blood, and the likelihood of infection is increased in hemodialysis units. Although the frequency of transfusion-associated hepatitis C fell as a result of blood donor screening, the overall frequency of hepatitis C remained the same until the early 1990s, when the overall frequency fell by 80%, in parallel with a reduction in the number of new cases in injection drug users. After the exclusion of anti-HCV-positive plasma units from the donor pool, rare, sporadic instances have occurred of hepatitis C among recipients of immune globulin (IG) preparations for intravenous (but not intramuscular) use.

Serologic evidence for HCV infection occurs in 90% of patients with a history of transfusion-associated hepatitis (almost all occurring before 1992, when second-generation HCV-screening tests were introduced), hemophiliacs and others treated with clotting factors, and injection drug users; 60 to 70% of patients with sporadic "non-A, non-B" hepatitis who lack identifiable risk factors; 0.5% of volunteer blood donors; and 1.8% of the general population in the United States, which translates into 4 million persons. Comparable frequencies of HCV infection occur in most countries around the world, with 170 million persons infected worldwide, but extraordinarily high prevalences of HCV infection occur in certain countries, such as Egypt, where more than 20% of the population in some cities is infected. The high frequency in Egypt is attributable to contaminated equipment used for medical procedures and unsafe injection practices. In the United States, African Americans and Mexican Americans have higher frequencies of HCV infection than whites, and 30- to 49-year-old adult males have the highest frequencies of infection. Hepatitis C accounts for 40% of chronic liver disease, is the most frequent indication for liver transplantation, and is estimated to account for 8000 to 10,000 deaths per year in the United States.

Most asymptomatic blood donors found to have anti-HCV and approximately 20 to 30% of persons with reported cases of acute hepatitis C do not fall into a recognized risk group; however, many such blood donors do recall risk-associated behaviors when questioned carefully.

As a bloodborne infection, HCV potentially can be transmitted sexually and perinatally; however, both of these modes of transmission are inefficient for hepatitis C. Although 10 to 15% of patients with acute hepatitis C report having potential sexual sources of infection, most studies have failed to identify sexual transmission of this agent. The chances of sexual and perinatal transmission have been estimated to be approximately 5%, well below comparable rates for HIV and HBV infections. Moreover, sexual transmission appears to be confined to such subgroups as persons with multiple sexual partners and sexually transmitted diseases; transmission of HCV infection is rare between stable, monogamous sexual partners. Breast feeding does not increase the risk of HCV infection between an infected mother and her infant. Infection of health workers is not dramatically higher than among the general population; however, health workers are more likely to acquire HCV infection through accidental needle punctures, the efficiency of which is ~3%. Infection of household contacts is rare as well.

Other groups with an increased frequency of HCV infection include patients who require hemodialysis and organ transplantation and those who require transfusions in the setting of cancer chemotherapy. In immunosuppressed individuals, levels of anti-HCV may be undetectable, and a diagnosis may require testing for HCV RNA. Although new acute cases of hepatitis C are rare, newly diagnosed cases are common among otherwise healthy persons who experimented briefly with injection drugs two or three decades earlier. Such instances usually remain unrecognized for years, until unearthed by laboratory screening for routine medical examinations, insurance applications, and attempted blood donation.

Hepatitis E This type of hepatitis, identified in India, Asia, Africa, and Central America, resembles hepatitis A in its primarily enteric mode of spread. The commonly recognized cases occur after contamination of water supplies such as after monsoon flooding, but sporadic, isolated cases occur. An epidemiologic feature that distinguishes HEV from other enteric agents is the rarity of secondary person-to-person spread from infected persons to their close contacts. Infections arise in populations that are immune to HAV and favor young adults. It is not known if hepatitis E occurs outside of recognized endemic areas, for example, in the United States, but preliminary studies suggest that HEV does not account for any of the sporadic "non-A, non-B" cases in nonendemic areas. Cases imported from endemic areas have been found in the United States. Several reports suggest a zoonotic reservoir for HEV in swine.

CLINICAL AND LABORATORY FEATURES ■ Symptoms and Signs Acute viral hepatitis occurs after an incubation period that varies according to the responsible agent. Generally, incubation periods for hepatitis A range from 15 to 45 days (mean 4 weeks), for hepatitis B and D from 30 to 180 days (mean 4 to 12 weeks), for hepatitis C from 15 to 160 days (mean 7 weeks), and for hepatitis E from 14 to 60 days (mean 5 to 6 weeks). The *prodromal symptoms* of acute viral hepatitis are systemic and quite variable. Constitutional symptoms of anorexia, nausea and vomiting, fatigue, malaise, arthralgias, myalgias, headache, photophobia, pharyngitis, cough, and coryza may precede the onset of jaundice by 1 to 2 weeks. The nausea, vomiting, and anorexia are frequently associated with alterations in olfaction and taste. A low-grade fever between 38 and 39°C (100 to 102°F) is more often present in hepatitis

A and E than in hepatitis B or C, except when hepatitis B is heralded by a serum sickness−like syndrome; rarely, a fever of 39.5 to 40°C (103 to 104°F) may accompany the constitutional symptoms. Dark urine and clay-colored stools may be noticed by the patient from 1 to 5 days before the onset of clinical jaundice.

With the onset of *clinical jaundice*, the constitutional prodromal symptoms usually diminish, but in some patients mild weight loss (2.5 to 5 kg) is common and may continue during the entire icteric phase. The liver becomes enlarged and tender and may be associated with right upper quadrant pain and discomfort. Infrequently, patients present with a cholestatic picture, suggesting extrahepatic biliary obstruction. Splenomegaly and cervical adenopathy are present in 10 to 20% of patients with acute hepatitis. Rarely, a few spider angiomas appear during the icteric phase and disappear during convalescence. During the *recovery phase*, constitutional symptoms disappear, but usually some liver enlargement and abnormalities in liver biochemical tests are still evident. The duration of the posticteric phase is variable, ranging from 2 to 12 weeks, and is usually more prolonged in acute hepatitis B and C. Complete clinical and biochemical recovery is to be expected 1 to 2 months after all cases of hepatitis A and E and 3 to 4 months after the onset of jaundice in three-quarters of uncomplicated cases of hepatitis B and C. In the remainder, biochemical recovery may be delayed. A substantial proportion of patients with viral hepatitis never become icteric.

Infection with HDV can occur in the presence of acute or chronic HBV infection; the duration of HBV infection determines the duration of HDV infection. When acute HDV and HBV infection occur simultaneously, clinical and biochemical features may be indistinguishable from those of HBV infection alone, although occasionally they are more severe. As opposed to patients with *acute* HBV infection, patients with *chronic* HBV infection can support HDV replication indefinitely. This can happen when acute HDV infection occurs in the presence of a nonresolving acute HBV infection. More commonly, acute HDV infection becomes chronic when it is superimposed on an underlying chronic HBV infection. In such cases, the HDV superinfection appears as a clinical exacerbation or an episode resembling acute viral hepatitis in someone already chronically infected with HBV. Superinfection with HDV in a patient with chronic hepatitis B often leads to clinical deterioration (see below).

In addition to superinfections with other hepatitis agents, acute hepatitis-like clinical events in persons with chronic hepatitis B may accompany spontaneous HBeAg−to−anti-HBe seroconversion or spontaneous reactivation, i.e., reversion from nonreplicative to replicative infection. Such reactivations can occur as well in therapeutically immunosuppressed patients with chronic HBV infection when cytotoxic-immunosuppressive drugs are withdrawn; in these cases, restoration of immune competence is thought to allow resumption of previously checked cell-mediated immune cytolysis of HBV-infected hepatocytes. Occasionally, acute clinical exacerbations of chronic hepatitis B may represent the emergence of a precore mutant (see "Virology and Etiology," above), and the subsequent course in such patients may be characterized by periodic exacerbations.

Laboratory Features The serum aminotransferases aspartate aminotransferase (AST) and ALT (previously designated SGOT and SGPT) show a variable increase during the prodromal phase of acute viral hepatitis and precede the rise in bilirubin level (Figs. 285-2 and 285-4). The acute level of these enzymes, however, does not correlate well with the degree of liver cell damage. Peak levels vary from 400 to 4000 IU or more; these levels are usually reached at the time the patient is clinically icteric and diminish progressively during the recovery phase of acute hepatitis. The diagnosis of anicteric hepatitis is based on clinical features and on aminotransferase elevations.

Jaundice is usually visible in the sclera or skin when the serum bilirubin value exceeds 43 μmol/L (2.5 mg/dL). When jaundice appears, the serum bilirubin typically rises to levels ranging from 85 to

TABLE 285-3 Commonly Encountered Serologic Patterns of Hepatitis B Infection

HBsAg	Anti-HBs	Anti-HBc	HBeAg	Anti-HBe	Interpretation
+	−	IgM	+	−	Acute hepatitis B, high infectivity
+	−	IgG	+	−	Chronic hepatitis B, high infectivity
+	−	IgG	−	+	1. Late acute or chronic hepatitis B, low infectivity 2. HBeAg-negative ("precore-mutant") hepatitis B (chronic or, rarely, acute)
+	+	+	+/−	+/−	1. HBsAg of one subtype and heterotypic anti-HBs (common) 2. Process of seroconversion from HBsAg to anti-HBs (rare)
−	−	IgM	+/−	+/−	1. Acute hepatitis B 2. Anti-HBc "window"
−	−	IgG	−	+/−	1. Low-level hepatitis B carrier 2. Hepatitis B in remote past
−	+	IgG	−	+/−	Recovery from hepatitis B
−	+	−	−	−	1. Immunization with HBsAg (after vaccination) 2. Hepatitis B in the remote past (?) 3. False-positive

340 μmol/L (5 to 20 mg/dL). The serum bilirubin may continue to rise despite falling serum aminotransferase levels. In most instances, the total bilirubin is equally divided between the conjugated and unconjugated fractions. Bilirubin levels >340 μmol/L (20 mg/dL) extending and persisting late into the course of viral hepatitis are more likely to be associated with severe disease. In certain patients with underlying hemolytic anemia, however, such as glucose-6-phosphate dehydrogenase deficiency and sickle cell anemia, a high serum bilirubin level is common, resulting from superimposed hemolysis. In such patients, bilirubin levels >513 μmol/L (30 mg/dL) have been observed and are not necessarily associated with a poor prognosis.

Neutropenia and lymphopenia are transient and are followed by a relative lymphocytosis. Atypical lymphocytes (varying between 2 and 20%) are common during the acute phase. Measurement of the prothrombin time (PT) is important in patients with acute viral hepatitis, for a prolonged value may reflect a severe hepatic synthetic defect, signify extensive hepatocellular necrosis, and indicate a worse prognosis. Occasionally, a prolonged PT may occur with only mild increases in the serum bilirubin and aminotransferase levels. Prolonged nausea and vomiting, inadequate carbohydrate intake, and poor hepatic glycogen reserves may contribute to hypoglycemia noted occasionally in patients with severe viral hepatitis. Serum alkaline phosphatase may be normal or only mildly elevated, while a fall in serum albumin is uncommon in uncomplicated acute viral hepatitis. In some patients, mild and transient steatorrhea has been noted as well as slight microscopic hematuria and minimal proteinuria.

A diffuse but mild elevation of the gamma globulin fraction is common during acute viral hepatitis. Serum IgG and IgM levels are elevated in about one-third of patients during the acute phase of viral hepatitis, but the serum IgM level is elevated more characteristically during acute hepatitis A. During the acute phase of viral hepatitis, antibodies to smooth muscle and other cell constituents may be present, and low titers of rheumatoid factor, nuclear antibody, and heterophil antibody can also be found occasionally. In hepatitis C and D, antibodies to LKM may occur; however, the species of LKM antibodies in the two types of hepatitis are different from each other as well as from the LKM antibody species characteristic of autoimmune chronic hepatitis type 2 (Chap. 287). The autoantibodies in viral hepatitis are nonspecific and can also be associated with other viral and systemic diseases. In contrast, virus-specific antibodies, which appear during and after hepatitis virus infection, are serologic markers of diagnostic importance.

As described above, serologic tests are available with which to establish a diagnosis of hepatitis A, B, D, and C. Tests for fecal or serum HAV are not routinely available. Therefore, a diagnosis of hepatitis A is based on detection of IgM anti-HAV during acute illness

(Fig. 285-2). Rheumatoid factor can give rise to false-positive results in this test.

A diagnosis of HBV infection can usually be made by detection of HBsAg in serum. Infrequently, levels of HBsAg are too low to be detected during acute HBV infection, even with the current generation of highly sensitive immunoassays. In such cases, the diagnosis can be established by the presence of IgM anti-HBc.

The titer of HBsAg bears little relation to the severity of clinical disease. Indeed, there may be an inverse correlation between the serum concentration of HBsAg and the degree of liver cell damage. For example, titers are highest in immunosuppressed patients, lower in patients with chronic liver disease (but higher in mild chronic than in severe chronic hepatitis), and very low in patients with acute fulminant hepatitis. These observations suggest that in hepatitis B the degree of liver cell damage and the clinical course are probably related to variations in the patient's immune response to HBV rather than to the amount of circulating HBsAg. In immunocompetent persons, however, there is a correlation between markers of HBV *replication* and liver injury (see below).

Another serologic marker that may be of value in patients with hepatitis B is HBeAg. Its principal clinical usefulness is as an indicator of relative infectivity. Because HBeAg is invariably present during early acute hepatitis B, HBeAg testing is indicated primarily during follow-up of chronic infection.

In patients with hepatitis B surface antigenemia of unknown duration, e.g., blood donors found to be HBsAg-positive and referred to a physician for evaluation, testing for IgM anti-HBc may be useful to distinguish between acute or recent infection (IgM anti-HBc-positive) and chronic HBV infection (IgM anti-HBc-negative, IgG anti-HBc-positive). A false-positive test for IgM anti-HBc may be encountered in patients with high-titer rheumatoid factor.

Anti-HBs is rarely detectable in the presence of HBsAg in patients with *acute* hepatitis B, but 10 to 20% of persons with *chronic* HBV infection may harbor low-level anti-HBs. This antibody is directed not against the common group determinant, *a*, but against the heterotypic subtype determinant (e.g., HBsAg of subtype *ad* with anti-HBs of subtype *y*). In most cases, this serologic pattern cannot be attributed to infection with two different HBV subtypes, and the presence of this antibody is not a harbinger of imminent HBsAg clearance. When such antibody is detected, its presence is of no recognized clinical significance (see "Virology and Etiology," above).

After immunization with hepatitis B vaccine, which consists of HBsAg alone, anti-HBs is the only serologic marker to appear. The commonly encountered serologic patterns of hepatitis B and their interpretations are summarized in Table 285-3. Tests for the detection of HBV DNA in liver and serum are now available. Like HBeAg, serum HBV DNA is an indicator of HBV replication, but tests for HBV DNA are more sensitive and quantitative. Hybridization assays for HBV DNA have a sensitivity of approximately 10^5 to 10^6 virions/mL, a relative threshold below which infectivity and liver injury are limited and HBeAg is usually undetectable. Currently, testing for HBV DNA has shifted from insensitive hybridization assays to amplification assays, e.g., the PCR-based assay, which can detect as few as 100 or 1000 virions/mL. With increased sensitivity, amplification assays remain reactive well below the threshold for infectivity and liver injury. These markers are useful in following the course of HBV replication in patients with chronic hepatitis B receiving antiviral chemotherapy, e.g., with interferon or lamivudine (Chap. 287). In immunocompetent persons, a general correlation does appear to exist between the level of HBV replication, as reflected by the level of HBV DNA in serum, and the degree of liver injury. High serum HBV DNA levels, increased expression of viral antigens, and necroinflammatory activity in the liver go hand in hand unless immunosuppression interferes with cytolytic T cell responses to virus-infected cells; reduction of HBV replication with antiviral drugs tends to be accompanied by an improvement in liver histology.

In patients with hepatitis C, an episodic pattern of aminotransferase elevation is common. A specific serologic diagnosis of hepatitis C can be made by demonstrating the presence in serum of anti-HCV. When a second- or third-generation immunoassay (that detects antibodies to nonstructural and nucleocapsid proteins) is used, anti-HCV can be detected in acute hepatitis C during the initial phase of elevated aminotransferase activity. This antibody may never become detectable in 5 to 10% of patients with acute hepatitis C, and levels of anti-HCV may become undetectable after recovery from acute hepatitis C. In patients with chronic hepatitis C, anti-HCV is detectable in >95% of cases. Nonspecificity can confound immunoassays for anti-HCV, especially in persons with a low prior probability of infection, such as volunteer blood donors, or in persons with circulating rheumatoid factor, which can bind nonspecifically to assay reagents. A supplementary recombinant immunoblot assay (RIBA), in which serum is incubated with a nitrocellulose strip containing viral protein bands, can be used to establish the specific viral proteins to which anti-HCV is directed (see "Virology and Etiology," above). Such RIBA determinations were used to confirm anti-HCV reactivity in blood donors, but determinations of HCV RNA have supplanted RIBA in most clinical settings. Assays for HCV RNA are the most sensitive tests for HCV infection and represent the "gold standard" in establishing a diagnosis of hepatitis C. HCV RNA can be detected even before acute elevation of aminotransferase activity and before the appearance of anti-HCV in patients with acute hepatitis C. In addition, HCV RNA remains detectable indefinitely, continuously in most but intermittently in some, in patients with chronic hepatitis C (even detectable in some persons with normal liver tests, i.e., asymptomatic carriers). In the small minority of patients with hepatitis C who lack anti-HCV, a diagnosis can be supported by detection of HCV RNA. If all these tests are negative and the patient has a well-characterized case of hepatitis after percutaneous exposure to blood or blood products, a diagnosis of hepatitis caused by another agent, as yet unidentified, can be entertained.

Amplification techniques are required to detect HCV RNA, and two are available. One is a branched-chain complementary DNA (bDNA) assay, in which the detection signal (a colorimetrically detectable enzyme bound to a complementary DNA probe) is amplified. The other involves target amplification, i.e., synthesis of multiple copies of the viral genome. This can be done by PCR or TMA, in which the viral RNA is reverse transcribed to complementary DNA and then amplified by repeated cycles of DNA synthesis. Both can be used as quantitative assays and a measurement of relative "viral load"; PCR and TMA, with a sensitivity of 10^2 IU/mL, are more sensitive than bDNA, with a sensitivity of 10^5. Determination of viral load is not a reliable marker of disease severity or prognosis but is helpful in predicting relative responsiveness to antiviral therapy. The same is true for determinations of HCV genotype (Chap. 287).

A proportion of patients with hepatitis C have isolated anti-HBc in their blood, a reflection of a common risk in certain populations to multiple bloodborne hepatitis agents. The anti-HBc in such cases is almost invariably of the IgG class and usually represents HBV infection in the remote past, rarely current HBV infection with low-level virus carriage.

The presence of HDV infection can be identified by demonstrating intrahepatic HDV antigen or, more practically, an anti-HDV seroconversion (a rise in titer of anti-HDV or de novo appearance of anti-HDV). Circulating HDV antigen, also diagnostic of acute infection, is detectable only briefly, if at all. Because anti-HDV is often undetectable once HBsAg disappears, retrospective serodiagnosis of acute self-limited, simultaneous HBV and HDV infection is difficult. Early diagnosis of acute infection may be hampered by a delay of up to 30 to 40 days in the appearance of anti-HDV.

When a patient presents with acute hepatitis and has HBsAg and anti-HDV in serum, determination of the class of anti-HBc is helpful in establishing the relationship between infection with HBV and HDV. Although IgM anti-HBc does not distinguish *absolutely* between acute and chronic HBV infection, its presence is a reliable indicator of recent infection and its absence a reliable indicator of infection in the remote past. In simultaneous acute HBV and HDV infections, IgM anti-HBc will be detectable, while in acute HDV infection superimposed on chronic HBV infection, anti-HBc will be of the IgG class.

Tests for the presence of HDV RNA are useful for determining the presence of ongoing HDV replication and relative infectivity. Currently, probes for this marker are restricted to a limited number of research laboratories. Diagnostic tests for hepatitis E are commercially available in several countries outside the United States; in the United States, diagnostic assays can be performed at the Centers for Disease Control and Prevention.

Liver biopsy is rarely necessary or indicated in acute viral hepatitis, except when there is a question about the diagnosis or when there is clinical evidence suggesting a diagnosis of chronic hepatitis.

A diagnostic algorithm can be applied in the evaluation of cases of acute viral hepatitis. A patient with acute hepatitis should undergo four serologic tests, HBsAg, IgM anti-HAV, IgM anti-HBc, and anti-HCV (Table 285-4). The presence of HBsAg, with or without IgM anti-HBc, represents HBV infection. If IgM anti-HBc is present, the HBV infection is considered acute; if IgM anti-HBc is absent, the HBV infection is considered chronic. A diagnosis of acute hepatitis B can be made in the absence of HBsAg when IgM anti-HBc is detectable. A diagnosis of acute hepatitis A is based on the presence of IgM anti-HAV. If IgM anti-HAV coexists with HBsAg, a diagnosis of simultaneous HAV and HBV infections can be made; if IgM anti-HBc (with or without HBsAg) is detectable, the patient has simultaneous acute hepatitis A and B, and if IgM anti-HBc is undetectable, the patient has acute hepatitis A superimposed on chronic HBV infection. The presence of anti-HCV supports a diagnosis of acute hepatitis C. Occasionally, testing for HCV RNA or repeat anti-HCV testing later during the illness is necessary to establish the diagnosis. Absence of all serologic markers is consistent with a diagnosis of "non-A, non-B, non-C" hepatitis, if the epidemiologic setting is appropriate.

In patients with chronic hepatitis, initial testing should consist of HBsAg and anti-HCV. Anti-HCV supports and HCV RNA testing establishes the diagnosis of chronic hepatitis C. If a serologic diagnosis of chronic hepatitis B is made, testing for HBeAg and anti-HBe is indicated to evaluate relative infectivity. Testing for HBV DNA in such patients provides a more quantitative and sensitive measure of the level of virus replication and, therefore, is very helpful during antiviral therapy (Chap. 287). In patients with hepatitis B, testing for anti-HDV is useful under the following circumstances: patients with

TABLE 285-4 *Simplified Diagnostic Approach in Patients Presenting with Acute Hepatitis*

Serologic Tests of Patient's Serum				
HBsAg	IgM Anti-HAV	IgM Anti-HBc	Anti-HCV	Diagnostic Interpretation
+	−	+	−	Acute hepatitis B
+	−	−	−	Chronic hepatitis B
+	+	−	−	Acute hepatitis A superimposed on chronic hepatitis B
+	+	+	−	Acute hepatitis A and B
−	+	−	−	Acute hepatitis A
−	+	+	−	Acute hepatitis A and B (HBsAg below detection threshold)
−	−	+	−	Acute hepatitis B (HBsAg below detection threshold)
−	−	−	+	Acute hepatitis C

severe and fulminant diseases, patients with severe chronic disease, patients with chronic hepatitis B who have acute hepatitis-like exacerbations, persons with frequent percutaneous exposures, and persons from areas where HDV infection is endemic.

PROGNOSIS   Virtually all previously healthy patients with hepatitis A recover completely from their illness with no clinical sequelae. Similarly, in acute hepatitis B, 95 to 99% of previously healthy adults have a favorable course and recover completely. Certain clinical and laboratory features, however, suggest a more complicated and protracted course. Patients of advanced age and with serious underlying medical disorders may have a prolonged course and are more likely to experience severe hepatitis. Initial presenting features such as ascites, peripheral edema, and symptoms of hepatic encephalopathy suggest a poorer prognosis. In addition, a prolonged PT, low serum albumin level, hypoglycemia, and very high serum bilirubin values suggest severe hepatocellular disease. Patients with these clinical and laboratory features deserve prompt hospital admission. The case-fatality rate in hepatitis A and B is very low (approximately 0.1%) but is increased by advanced age and underlying debilitating disorders. Among patients ill enough to be hospitalized for acute hepatitis B, the fatality rate is 1%. Hepatitis C is less severe during the acute phase than hepatitis B and is more likely to be anicteric; fatalities are rare, but the precise case-fatality rate is not known. In outbreaks of waterborne hepatitis E in India and Asia, the case-fatality rate is 1 to 2% and up to 10 to 20% in pregnant women. Patients with simultaneous acute hepatitis B and hepatitis D do not necessarily experience a higher mortality rate than do patients with acute hepatitis B alone; however, in several recent outbreaks of acute simultaneous HBV and HDV infection among injection drug users, the case-fatality rate has been approximately 5%. In the case of HDV superinfection of a person with chronic hepatitis B, the likelihood of fulminant hepatitis and death is increased substantially. Although the case-fatality rate for hepatitis D has not been defined adequately, in outbreaks of severe HDV superinfection in isolated populations with a high hepatitis B carrier rate, the mortality rate has been recorded in excess of 20%.

COMPLICATIONS AND SEQUELAE   A small proportion of patients with hepatitis A experience *relapsing hepatitis* weeks to months after apparent recovery from acute hepatitis. Relapses are characterized by recurrence of symptoms, aminotransferase elevations, occasionally jaundice, and fecal excretion of HAV. Another unusual variant of acute hepatitis A is *cholestatic hepatitis*, characterized by protracted cholestatic jaundice and pruritus. Rarely, liver test abnormalities persist for many months, even up to a year. Even when these complications occur, hepatitis A remains self-limited and does not progress to chronic liver disease. During the prodromal phase of acute hepatitis B, a serum sickness–like syndrome characterized by arthralgia or arthritis, rash, angioedema, and rarely hematuria and proteinuria may develop in 5 to 10% of patients. This syndrome occurs before the onset of clinical jaundice, and these patients are often erroneously diagnosed as having rheumatologic diseases. The diagnosis can be established by measuring serum aminotransferase levels, which are almost invariably elevated, and serum HBsAg. As noted above, EMC is an immune-complex disease that can complicate chronic hepatitis C and is part of a spectrum of B cell lymphoproliferative disorders, which, in rare instances, can evolve to B cell lymphoma (Chap. 97). Attention has been drawn as well to associations between hepatitis C and such cutaneous disorders as porphyria cutanea tarda and lichen planus. A mechanism for these associations is unknown.

The most feared complication of viral hepatitis is *fulminant hepatitis* (massive hepatic necrosis); fortunately, this is a rare event. Fulminant hepatitis is primarily seen in hepatitis B and D, as well as hepatitis E, but rare fulminant cases of hepatitis A occur primarily in older adults and in persons with underlying chronic liver disease, including, according to some reports, chronic hepatitis B and C. Hepatitis B accounts for >50% of fulminant hepatitis cases, a sizable pro-

portion of which are associated with HDV infection and another proportion with underlying chronic hepatitis C. Fulminant hepatitis is seen rarely in hepatitis C, but hepatitis E, as noted above, can be complicated by fatal fulminant hepatitis in 1 to 2% of all cases and in up to 20% of cases occurring in pregnant women. Patients usually present with signs and symptoms of encephalopathy that may evolve to deep coma. The liver is usually small and the PT excessively prolonged. The combination of rapidly shrinking liver size, rapidly rising bilirubin level, and marked prolongation of the PT, even as aminotransferase levels fall, together with clinical signs of confusion, disorientation, somnolence, ascites, and edema, indicates that the patient has hepatic failure with encephalopathy. Cerebral edema is common; brainstem compression, gastrointestinal bleeding, sepsis, respiratory failure, cardiovascular collapse, and renal failure are terminal events. The mortality rate is exceedingly high (>80% in patients with deep coma), but patients who survive may have a complete biochemical and histologic recovery. If a donor liver can be located in time, liver transplantation may be life-saving in patients with fulminant hepatitis (Chap. 291).

It is particularly important to document the disappearance of HBsAg after apparent clinical recovery from acute hepatitis B. Before laboratory methods were available to distinguish between acute hepatitis and acute hepatitis–like exacerbations (*spontaneous reactivations*) of chronic hepatitis B, observations suggested that approximately 10% of patients remained HBsAg-positive for >6 months after the onset of clinically apparent acute hepatitis B. Half these persons cleared the antigen from their circulations during the next several years, but the other 5% remained chronically HBsAg-positive. More recent observations suggest that the true rate of chronic infection after clinically apparent acute hepatitis B is as low as 1% in normal, immunocompetent, young adults. Earlier, higher estimates may have been biased by inadvertent inclusion of acute exacerbations in chronically infected patients; these patients, chronically HBsAg-positive before exacerbation, were unlikely to seroconvert to HBsAg-negative thereafter. Whether the rate of chronicity is 10 or 1%, such patients have anti-HBc in serum; anti-HBs is either undetected or detected at low titer against the opposite subtype specificity of the antigen (see "Laboratory Features," above). These patients may (1) be inactive carriers; (2) have low-grade, mild chronic hepatitis; or (3) have moderate to severe chronic hepatitis with or without cirrhosis. The likelihood of becoming an HBsAg carrier after acute HBV infection is especially high among neonates, persons with Down's syndrome, chronically hemodialyzed patients, and immunosuppressed patients, including persons with HIV infection.

Chronic hepatitis is an important late complication of acute hepatitis B occurring in a small proportion of patients with acute disease but more common in those who present with chronic infection without having experienced an acute illness (Chap. 287). Certain clinical and laboratory features suggest progression of acute hepatitis to chronic hepatitis: (1) lack of complete resolution of clinical symptoms of anorexia, weight loss, and fatigue and the persistence of hepatomegaly; (2) the presence of bridging or multilobular hepatic necrosis on liver biopsy during protracted, severe acute viral hepatitis; (3) failure of the serum aminotransferase, bilirubin, and globulin levels to return to normal within 6 to 12 months after the acute illness; and (4) the persistence of HBeAg beyond 3 months or HBsAg beyond 6 months after acute hepatitis.

Although acute hepatitis D infection does not increase the likelihood of chronicity of simultaneous acute hepatitis B, hepatitis D has the potential for contributing to the severity of chronic hepatitis B. Hepatitis D superinfection can transform asymptomatic or mild chronic hepatitis B into severe, progressive chronic hepatitis and cirrhosis; it also can accelerate the course of chronic hepatitis B. Some HDV superinfections in patients with chronic hepatitis B lead to fulminant hepatitis. Although HDV and HBV infections are associated with severe liver disease, mild hepatitis and even asymptomatic carriage have been identified in some patients, and the disease may become indolent beyond the early years of infection. After acute HCV infection, the likelihood of remaining chronically *infected* approaches 85 to 90%. Although many patients with chronic hepatitis C have no symptoms, cirrhosis may develop in as many as 20% within 10 to 20 years of acute illness; in some series of cases, cirrhosis has been reported in as many as 50% of patients with chronic hepatitis C. Although chronic hepatitis C accounts for at least 40% of cases of chronic liver disease and of patients undergoing liver transplantation for end-stage liver disease in the United States and Europe, in the majority of patients with chronic hepatitis C, morbidity and mortality are limited during the initial 20 years after the onset of infection. Progression of chronic hepatitis C may be influenced by hepatitis C genotype, age of acquisition, duration of infection, immunosuppression, coexisting excessive alcohol use, other hepatitis virus infection, or HIV co-infection. In fact, instances of severe and rapidly progressive chronic hepatitis B and C are being recognized with increasing frequency in patients with HIV infection (Chap. 173). In contrast, neither HAV nor HEV causes chronic liver disease.

Rare complications of viral hepatitis include pancreatitis, myocarditis, atypical pneumonia, aplastic anemia, transverse myelitis, and peripheral neuropathy. Persons with chronic hepatitis B, particularly those infected in infancy or early childhood and especially those with HBeAg, have an enhanced risk of hepatocellular carcinoma. The risk of hepatocellular carcinoma is increased as well in patients with chronic hepatitis C, almost exclusively in patients with cirrhosis, and almost always after at least several decades, usually after three decades of disease (Chap. 78). In children, hepatitis B may present rarely with anicteric hepatitis, a nonpruritic papular rash of the face, buttocks, and limbs, and lymphadenopathy (papular acrodermatitis of childhood or Gianotti Crosti syndrome).

DIFFERENTIAL DIAGNOSIS Viral diseases such as infectious mononucleosis; those due to cytomegalovirus, herpes simplex, and coxsackieviruses; and toxoplasmosis may share certain clinical features with viral hepatitis and cause elevations in serum aminotransferase and less commonly in serum bilirubin levels. Tests such as the differential heterophile and serologic tests for these agents may be helpful in the differential diagnosis if HBsAg, anti-HBc, IgM anti-HAV, and anti-HCV determinations are negative. Aminotransferase elevations can accompany almost any systemic viral infection; other rare causes of liver injury confused with viral hepatitis are infections with *Leptospira*, *Candida*, *Brucella*, *Mycobacteria*, and *Pneumocystis*. A complete drug history is particularly important, for many drugs and certain anesthetic agents can produce a picture of either acute hepatitis or cholestasis (Chap. 286). Equally important is a past history of unexplained "repeated episodes" of acute hepatitis. This history should alert the physician to the possibility that the underlying disorder is chronic hepatitis. Alcoholic hepatitis must also be considered, but usually the serum aminotransferase levels are not as markedly elevated and other stigmata of alcoholism may be present. The finding on liver biopsy of fatty infiltration, a neutrophilic inflammatory reaction, and "alcoholic hyaline" would be consistent with alcohol-induced rather than viral liver injury. Because acute hepatitis may present with right upper quadrant abdominal pain, nausea and vomiting, fever, and icterus, it is often confused with acute cholecystitis, common duct stone, or ascending cholangitis. Patients with acute viral hepatitis may tolerate surgery poorly; therefore, it is important to exclude this diagnosis, and in confusing cases, a percutaneous liver biopsy may be necessary before laparotomy. Viral hepatitis in the elderly is often misdiagnosed as obstructive jaundice resulting from a common duct stone or carcinoma of the pancreas. Because acute hepatitis in the elderly may be quite severe and the operative mortality high, a thorough evaluation including biochemical tests, radiographic studies of the biliary tree, and even liver biopsy may be necessary to exclude primary parenchymal liver disease. Another clinical constellation that may mimic acute hepatitis is right ventricular failure with passive hepatic congestion or hypoperfusion syndromes, such as those associated with shock, severe hypotension, and severe left ventricular failure. Also included in this general category is any disorder that interferes with venous return to the heart, such as right atrial myxoma, constrictive pericarditis, hepatic vein occlusion (Budd-Chiari syndrome), or venoocclusive disease. Clinical features are usually sufficient to distinguish between these vascular disorders and viral hepatitis. Acute fatty liver of pregnancy, cholestasis of pregnancy, eclampsia, and the HELLP syndrome (hemolysis, elevated liver tests, and low platelets) can be confused with viral hepatitis during pregnancy. Very rarely, malignancies metastatic to the liver can mimic acute or even fulminant viral hepatitis. Occasionally, genetic or metabolic liver disorders (e.g., Wilson's disease, α_1-antitrypsin deficiency) as well as nonalcoholic fatty liver disease are confused with viral hepatitis.

℞ TREATMENT

Treatment of Acute Attack In hepatitis B, among previously healthy adults who present with clinically apparent acute hepatitis, recovery occurs in approximately 99%; therefore, antiviral therapy is not likely to improve the rate of recovery and is not required. In rare instances of severe acute hepatitis B, treatment with a nucleoside analogue, such as lamivudine, at the 100-mg/d oral dose used to treat chronic hepatitis B (Chap. 287), has been attempted successfully. However, clinical trials have not been done to establish the efficacy of this approach, severe acute hepatitis B is not an approved indication for therapy, and the duration of therapy has not been determined. In typical cases of acute hepatitis C, recovery is rare, progression to chronic hepatitis is the rule, and meta-analyses of small clinical trials suggest that antiviral therapy with interferon α monotherapy (3 million units subcutaneously three times a week) is beneficial, reducing the rate of chronicity considerably by inducing sustained responses in 30 to 70% of patients. In a German multicenter study of 44 patients with acute symptomatic hepatitis C, initiation of intensive interferon α therapy (5 million units subcutaneously daily for 4 weeks, then three times a week for another 20 weeks) within an average of 3 months after infection resulted in a sustained virologic response rate of 98%. Although treatment of acute hepatitis C is recommended, the optimum regimen, duration of therapy, and time to initiate therapy remain to be determined. Many authorities now opt for the best regimen identified for the treatment of chronic hepatitis C, long-acting pegylated interferon plus the nucleoside analogue ribavirin, the efficacy of which is superior to that of standard interferon monotherapy regimens (Chap. 287). Because of the marked reduction over the last two decades in the frequency of acute hepatitis C, opportunities to identify and treat patients with acute hepatitis C are rare indeed. Hospital epidemiologists, however, will encounter health workers who sustain hepatitis C–contaminated needle sticks; when monitoring for ALT elevations and HCV RNA after these accidents identifies acute hepatitis C, therapy should be initiated.

Notwithstanding these specific therapeutic considerations, in most cases of typical acute viral hepatitis, specific treatment generally is not necessary. Although hospitalization may be required for clinically severe illness, most patients do not require hospital care. Forced and prolonged bed rest is not essential for full recovery, but many patients will feel better with restricted physical activity. A high-calorie diet is desirable, and because many patients may experience nausea late in the day, the major caloric intake is best tolerated in the morning. Intravenous feeding is necessary in the acute stage if the patient has persistent vomiting and cannot maintain oral intake. Drugs capable of producing adverse reactions such as cholestasis and drugs metabolized by the liver should be avoided. If severe pruritus is present, the use of the bile salt–sequestering resin cholestyramine is helpful. Glucocorticoid therapy has no value in acute viral hepatitis, even in severe cases associated with *bridging necrosis*, and may be hazardous.

Physical isolation of patients with hepatitis to a single room and bathroom is rarely necessary except in the case of fecal incontinence for hepatitis A and E or uncontrolled, voluminous bleeding for hepatitis B (with or without concomitant hepatitis D) and hepatitis C. Because most patients hospitalized with hepatitis A excrete little if any

HAV, the likelihood of HAV transmission from these patients during their hospitalization is low. Therefore, burdensome *enteric precautions are no longer recommended*. Although gloves should be worn when the bedpans or fecal material of patients with hepatitis A are handled, these precautions do not represent a departure from sensible procedure for all hospitalized patients. For patients with hepatitis B and hepatitis C, emphasis should be placed on blood precautions, i.e., avoiding direct, ungloved hand contact with blood and other body fluids. Enteric precautions are unnecessary. The importance of simple hygienic precautions, such as hand washing, cannot be overemphasized. Universal precautions that have been adopted for all patients apply to patients with viral hepatitis.

Hospitalized patients may be discharged when there is substantial symptomatic improvement, a significant downward trend in the serum aminotransferase and bilirubin values, and a return to normal of the PT. Mild aminotransferase elevations should not be considered contraindications to the gradual resumption of normal activity.

In *fulminant hepatitis*, the goal of therapy is to support the patient by maintenance of fluid balance, support of circulation and respiration, control of bleeding, correction of hypoglycemia, and treatment of other complications of the comatose state in anticipation of liver regeneration and repair. Protein intake should be restricted, and oral lactulose or neomycin administered. Glucocorticoid therapy has been shown in controlled trials to be ineffective. Likewise, exchange transfusion, plasmapheresis, human cross-circulation, porcine liver cross-perfusion, and hemoperfusion have not been proven to enhance survival; however, the efficacy of extracorporeal liver-assist devices, involving hollow-fiber chambers containing hepatocytes, is being evaluated in clinical trials. Meticulous intensive care is the one factor that does appear to improve survival. Orthotopic liver transplantation is resorted to with increasing frequency, with excellent results, in patients with fulminant hepatitis (Chap. 291).

PROPHYLAXIS Because application of therapy for acute viral hepatitis is limited, and because antiviral therapy for chronic viral hepatitis is effective in only a proportion of patients (Chap. 287), emphasis is placed on prevention through immunization. The prophylactic approach differs for each of the types of viral hepatitis. In the past, immunoprophylaxis relied exclusively on passive immunization with antibody-containing globulin preparations purified by cold ethanol fractionation from the plasma of hundreds of normal donors. Currently, for hepatitis A and B, active immunization with vaccines is available as well.

Hepatitis A Both passive immunization with IG and active immunization with killed vaccines are available. All preparations of IG contain anti-HAV concentrations sufficient to be protective. When administered before exposure or during the early incubation period, IG is effective in preventing clinically apparent hepatitis A. For postexposure prophylaxis of intimate contacts (household, sexual, institutional) of persons with hepatitis A, the administration of 0.02 mL/kg is recommended as early after exposure as possible; it may be effective even when administered as late as 2 weeks after exposure. Prophylaxis is not necessary for casual contacts (office, factory, school, or hospital), for most elderly persons, who are very likely to be immune, or for those known to have anti-HAV in their serum. In day-care centers, recognition of hepatitis A in children or staff should provide a stimulus for immunoprophylaxis in the center and in the children's family members. By the time most common-source outbreaks of hepatitis A are recognized, it is usually too late in the incubation period for IG to be effective; however, prophylaxis may limit the frequency of secondary cases. For travelers to tropical countries, developing countries, and other areas outside standard tourist routes, IG prophylaxis had been recommended, before a vaccine became available. When such travel lasted less than 3 months, 0.02 mL/kg was given; for longer travel or residence in these areas, a dose of 0.06 mL/kg every 4 to 6 months was recommended. Administration of plasma-derived globulin is safe;

all contemporary lots of IG are subjected to viral inactivation steps and must be free of HCV RNA as determined by PCR testing. Administration of intramuscular lots of IG has not been associated with transmission of HBV, HCV, or HIV.

Formalin-inactivated vaccines made from strains of HAV attenuated in tissue culture have been shown to be safe, immunogenic, and effective in preventing hepatitis A. Hepatitis A vaccines are approved for use in persons who are at least 2 years old and appear to provide adequate protection 4 weeks after a primary inoculation. If it can be given within 4 weeks of an expected exposure, such as by travel to an endemic area, hepatitis A vaccine is the preferred approach to *preexposure* immunoprophylaxis. If travel is more imminent, IG (0.02 mL/kg) should be administered at a different injection site, along with the first dose of vaccine. Because vaccination provides long-lasting protection (protective levels of anti-HAV should last 20 years after vaccination), persons whose risk will be sustained (e.g., frequent travelers or those remaining in endemic areas for prolonged periods) should be vaccinated, and vaccine should supplant the need for repeated IG injections. Other groups who are candidates for hepatitis A vaccination include military personnel, populations with cyclic outbreaks of hepatitis A (e.g., Alaskan natives), employees of day-care centers, primate handlers, laboratory workers exposed to hepatitis A or fecal specimens, children in communities with a high frequency of hepatitis A, and patients with chronic liver disease. Because of an increased risk of fulminant hepatitis A—observed in some experiences but not confirmed in others—among patients with chronic hepatitis C, patients with chronic hepatitis C have been singled out as candidates for hepatitis A vaccination. Other populations whose recognized risk of hepatitis A is increased should be vaccinated, including men who have sex with men, injection drug users, and persons with clotting disorders who require frequent administration of clotting-factor concentrates. Recommendations for dose and frequency differ for the two approved vaccine preparations (Table 285-5); all injections are intramuscular. Hepatitis A vaccine has been reported to be effective in preventing secondary household cases of acute hepatitis A, but its role in other instances of postexposure prophylaxis remains to be demonstrated.

Hepatitis B Until 1982, prevention of hepatitis B was based on *passive* immunoprophylaxis either with standard IG, containing modest levels of anti-HBs, or hepatitis B immune globulin (HBIG), containing high-titer anti-HBs. The efficacy of standard IG has never been established and remains questionable; even the efficacy of HBIG, demonstrated in several clinical trials, has been challenged, and its contribution appears to be in reducing the frequency of clinical *illness*, not in preventing *infection*. The first vaccine for *active* immunization, introduced in 1982, was prepared from purified, noninfectious 22-nm spherical forms of HBsAg derived from the plasma of healthy HBsAg carriers. In 1987, the plasma-derived vaccine was supplanted by a genetically engineered vaccine derived from recombinant yeast. The latter vaccine consists of HBsAg particles that are nonglycosylated but are otherwise indistinguishable from natural HBsAg; two recombinant vaccines are licensed for use in the United States. Current recommendations can be divided into those for preexposure and postexposure prophylaxis.

For *preexposure* prophylaxis against hepatitis B in settings of frequent exposure (health workers exposed to blood; hemodialysis pa-

TABLE 285-5 *Hepatitis A Vaccination Schedules*

Age, years	No. of Doses	Dose	Schedule, months
HAVRIX (GLAXOSMITHKLINE)			
2–18	2	720 ELU[a] (0.5 mL)	0, 6–12
>18	2	1440 ELU (1.0 mL)	0, 6–12
VAQTA (MERCK)			
2–17	2	25 units (0.5 mL)	0, 6
>17	2	50 units (1.0 mL)	0, 6–18

[a] Enzyme-linked immunoassay units.

tients and staff; residents and staff of custodial institutions for the developmentally handicapped; injection drug users; inmates of long-term correctional facilities; persons with multiple sexual partners; persons such as hemophiliacs who require long-term, high-volume therapy with blood derivatives; household and sexual contacts of HBsAg carriers; persons living in or traveling extensively in endemic areas; unvaccinated children under the age of 18; and unvaccinated children who are Alaskan natives, Pacific Islanders, or residents in households of first-generation immigrants from endemic countries), three intramuscular (deltoid, not gluteal) injections of hepatitis B vaccine are recommended at 0, 1, and 6 months. Pregnancy is *not* a contraindication to vaccination. In areas of low HBV endemicity such as the United States, despite the availability of safe and effective hepatitis B vaccines, a strategy of vaccinating persons in high-risk groups has not been effective. The incidence of new hepatitis B cases continued to increase in the United States after introduction of vaccines; fewer than 10% of all targeted persons in high-risk groups have actually been vaccinated, and approximately 30% of persons with sporadic acute hepatitis B do not fall into any high-risk-group category. Therefore, to have an impact on the frequency of HBV infection in an area of low endemicity such as the United States, universal hepatitis B vaccination in childhood has been recommended. For unvaccinated children born after the implementation of universal infant vaccination, vaccination during early adolescence, at age 11 to 12 years, was recommended, and this recommendation has been extended to include all unvaccinated children age 0 to 18 years. In HBV-hyperendemic areas, e.g., Asia, universal vaccination of children has resulted in a marked 10- to 15-year decline in hepatitis B and its complications.

The two available recombinant hepatitis B vaccines are comparable, one containing 10 μg of HBsAg (Recombivax-HB) and the other containing 20 μg of HBsAg (Engerix-B), and recommended doses for each injection vary for the two preparations (Table 285-6).

For unvaccinated persons sustaining an exposure to HBV, *postexposure* prophylaxis with a combination of HBIG (for rapid achievement of high-titer circulating anti-HBs) and hepatitis B vaccine (for achievement of long-lasting immunity as well as its apparent efficacy in attenuating clinical illness after exposure) is recommended. For *perinatal* exposure of infants born to HBsAg-positive mothers, a single dose of HBIG, 0.5 mL, should be administered intramuscularly in the thigh *immediately after birth*, followed by a complete course of three injections of recombinant hepatitis B vaccine (see doses above) to be started within the first 12 h of life. For those experiencing a direct percutaneous inoculation or transmucosal exposure to HBsAg-positive blood or body fluids (e.g., accidental *needle stick*, other mucosal penetration, or ingestion), a single intramuscular dose of HBIG, 0.06 mL/kg, administered as soon after exposure as possible, is followed by a complete course of hepatitis B vaccine to begin within the first week. For those exposed by *sexual* contact to a patient with acute hepatitis B, a single intramuscular dose of HBIG, 0.06 mL/kg, should be given within 14 days of exposure, to be followed by a complete course of hepatitis B vaccine. When both HBIG and hepatitis B vaccine are recommended, they may be given at the same time but at separate sites.

The precise duration of protection afforded by hepatitis B vaccine is unknown; however, approximately 80 to 90% of immunocompetent vaccinees retain protective levels of anti-HBs for at least 5 years, and 60 to 80% for 10 years. Thereafter and even after anti-HBs becomes undetectable, protection persists against clinical hepatitis B, hepatitis B surface antigenemia, and chronic HBV infection. Currently, *booster* immunizations are not recommended routinely, except in immunosuppressed persons who have lost detectable anti-HBs or immunocompetent persons who sustain percutaneous HBsAg-positive inoculations after losing detectable antibody. Specifically, for hemodialysis patients, annual anti-HBs testing is recommended after vaccination; booster doses are recommended when anti-HBs levels fall below 10 mIU/mL. For people at risk of both hepatitis A and B, a combined vaccine is available containing 720 enzyme-linked immunoassay units of inactivated HAV and 20 μg of recombinant HBsAg (at 0, 1, and 6 months).

Hepatitis D Infection with hepatitis D can be prevented by vaccinating susceptible persons with hepatitis B vaccine. No product is available for immunoprophylaxis to prevent HDV superinfection in HBsAg carriers; for them, avoidance of percutaneous exposures and limitation of intimate contact with persons who have HDV infection are recommended.

Hepatitis C IG is ineffective in preventing hepatitis C and is no longer recommended for postexposure prophylaxis in cases of perinatal, needle stick, or sexual exposure. Although a prototype vaccine that induces antibodies to HCV envelope protein has been developed, currently, hepatitis C vaccination is not feasible practically. Genotype and quasispecies viral heterogeneity, as well as rapid evasion of neutralizing antibodies by this rapidly mutating virus, conspire to render HCV a difficult target for immunoprophylaxis with a vaccine. Prevention of transfusion-associated hepatitis C has been accomplished by the following successively introduced measures: Exclusion of commercial blood donors and reliance on a volunteer blood supply; screening donor blood with surrogate markers such as ALT (no longer recommended) and anti-HBc, markers that identify segments of the blood donor population with an increased risk of bloodborne infections; exclusion of blood donors in high-risk groups for AIDS and the introduction of anti-HIV screening tests; and progressively sensitive serologic screening tests for HCV infection. Chemical and heat treatment of blood products used for large-pool and concentrated blood derivates are being pursued.

In the absence of active or passive immunization, prevention of hepatitis C includes behavior changes and precautions to limit exposures to infected persons. Recommendations designed to identify patients with clinically inapparent hepatitis as candidates for medical management have as a secondary benefit the identification of persons whose contacts could be at risk of becoming infected. A so-called "look-back" program has been recommended to identify persons who were transfused before 1992 with blood from a donor found subsequently to have hepatitis C. In addition, anti-HCV testing is recommended for anyone who received a blood transfusion or a transplanted organ before the introduction of second-generation screening tests in 1992, people who ever used injection drugs, chronically hemodialyzed patients, persons with clotting disorders who received clotting factors made before 1987 from pooled blood products, persons with elevated aminotransferase levels, health workers exposed to HCV-positive blood or contaminated needles, and children born to HCV-positive mothers.

For stable, monogamous sexual partners, sexual transmission of hepatitis C is unlikely, and sexual barrier precautions are not recommended. For persons with multiple sexual partners or with sexually transmitted diseases, the risk of sexual transmission of hepatitis C is increased, and barrier precautions (latex condoms) are recommended.

TABLE 285-6 *Preexposure Hepatitis B Vaccination Schedules*

Target Group	No. of Doses	Dose	Schedule, months
RECOMBIVAX-HB (MERCK)			
Infants, children (<11 years)	3	5 μg (0.5 mL)	0–2, 1–4, 6–18
Adolescents (11–19 years)	3	5 μg (0.5 mL)	0–2, 1–4, 4–6
Adults (≥20 years)	3	10 μg (1.0 mL)	0–2, 1–4, 4–6
Hemodialysis patients[a]	3	40 μg (1.0 mL)	0, 1, 6
ENGERIX-B (GLAXOSMITHKLINE)			
Infants, children (<10 years)	3	10 μg (0.5 mL)	0–2, 1–4, 6–18
Adolescents (10–19 years)	3	10 μg (0.5 mL)	0–2, 1–4, 4–6
Adults (≥ 20 years)	3	20 μg (1.0 mL)	0–2, 1–4, 4–6
Hemodialysis patients[a]	3	40 μg (1.0 mL)	0, 1, 6

[a] Includes other immunocompromised persons.

A person with hepatitis C should avoid sharing such items as razors, toothbrushes, and nail clippers with sexual partners and family members. No special precautions are recommended for babies born to mothers with hepatitis C, and breast feeding does not have to be restricted.

Hepatitis E   Whether IG prevents hepatitis E remains undetermined. A recombinant vaccine has been developed and is undergoing clinical testing.

FURTHER READING

BRANCH AD, SEEFF LB (eds): Hepatitis C: State of the art at the millennium. Semin Liver Dis 20:1, 127, 2000

CENTERS FOR DISEASE CONTROL AND PREVENTION: Updated U.S. Public Health Service guidelines for the management of occupational exposures to HBV, HCV, and HIV and recommendations for postexposure prophylaxis. Morb Mort Week Rep 50(RR-11):1, 2001

————: General recommendations on immunization: Recommendations of the Advisory Committee on Immunization Practices and the American Academy of Family Physicians. Morb Mort Week Rep 51(RR-2):1, 2002

CHU C-J et al: Hepatitis B virus genotype B is associated with earlier HBeAg seroconversion compared with hepatitis B virus genotype C. Gastroenterology 122:1756, 2002

CONSENSUS STATEMENT: EASL International Consensus Conference on Hepatitis C. J Hepatol 30:956, 1999

EL-SERAG HB et al: Extrahepatic manifestation of hepatitis C among United States male veterans. Hepatology 36:1439, 2002

JAECKEL E et al: Treatment of acute hepatitis C with interferon alfa-2b. N Engl J Med 345:1452, 2001

KOFF RS et al: Hepatitis A. Lancet 341:1643, 1998

LAUER GM, WALKER BD: Medical progress: Hepatitis C virus infection. N Engl J Med 345:41, 2001

LOK ASF, McMAHON BJ: Chronic hepatitis B. Hepatology 34:1225, 2001

MARGOLIS HS et al (eds): *Viral Hepatitis and Liver Disease*. Atlanta/London: International Medical Press, 2002

ORLAND JR et al: Acute hepatitis C. Hepatology 33:321, 2001

PAWLOTSKY J-M: Molecular diagnosis of viral hepatitis. Gastroenterology 122:1554, 2002

SCHREIBER GB et al: The risk of transfusion-transmitted viral infection. N Engl J Med 334:1685, 1996

SEEFF LB (ed): Long-term mortality and morbidity of transfusion-associated non-A, non-B, and type C hepatitis: A National Heart, Lung, and Blood Institute collaborative study. Hepatology 33:455, 2001

THIMME R et al: Viral and immunological determinants of hepatitis C virus clearance, persistence, and disease. Proc Natl Acad Sci USA 99:15661, 2002

TONG MJ et al: Clinical outcomes after transfusion-associated hepatitis C. N Engl J Med 332:1463, 1995

YANG H-I et al: Hepatitis B e antigen and the risk of hepatocellular carcinoma. N Engl J Med 347:168, 2002

286 TOXIC AND DRUG-INDUCED HEPATITIS
Jules L. Dienstag, Kurt J. Isselbacher

Liver injury may follow the inhalation, ingestion, or parenteral administration of a number of pharmacologic and chemical agents. These include industrial toxins (e.g., carbon tetrachloride, trichloroethylene, and yellow phosphorus), the heat-stable toxic bicyclic octapeptides of certain species of *Amanita* and *Galerina* (hepatotoxic mushroom poisoning), and, more commonly, pharmacologic agents used in medical therapy. It is essential that any patient presenting with jaundice or altered biochemical liver tests be questioned carefully about exposure to chemicals used in work or at home, drugs taken by prescription or bought "over the counter," and herbal or alternative medicines. Hepatotoxic drugs can injure the hepatocyte directly, e.g., via a free-radical or metabolic intermediate that causes peroxidation of membrane lipids and that results in liver cell injury. Alternatively, the drug or its metabolite can distort cell membranes or other cellular molecules, activate apoptotic pathways, or block biochemical pathways or cellular integrity. Such injuries, in turn, may lead to necrosis of hepatocytes; injure bile ducts, producing cholestasis; or block pathways of lipid movement, inhibit protein synthesis, or impair mitochondrial oxidation of fatty acids, resulting in lactic acidosis and fat accumulation (steatosis). In some cases, drug metabolites sensitize hepatocytes to toxic cytokines, and differences between susceptible and nonsusceptible drug recipients may be attributable to polymorphisms in elaboration of competing, protective cytokines, as has been suggested for acetaminophen hepatotoxicity (see below). In addition, a role has been shown for activation of nuclear transporters, such as the constitutive androstane receptor (CAR), in the induction of drug hepatotoxicity. In general, two major types of chemical hepatotoxicity have been recognized: (1) direct toxic type and (2) idiosyncratic type.

Most drugs, which are water-insoluble, undergo a series of metabolic transformation steps, culminating in a water-soluble form appropriate for renal or biliary excretion. This process begins with oxidation or methylation initially mediated by the mixed-function oxygenases cytochrome P450 (phase I reaction), followed by glucuronidation or sulfation (phase II reaction) or inactivation by glutathione. Most drug hepatotoxicity is mediated by a phase I toxic metabolite, but glutathione depletion, precluding inactivation of harmful compounds by glutathione S-transferase, can contribute as well.

As shown in Table 286-1, direct toxic hepatitis occurs with predictable regularity in individuals exposed to the offending agent and is dose-dependent. The latent period between exposure and liver injury is usually short (often several hours), although clinical manifestations may be delayed for 24 to 48 h. Agents producing toxic hepatitis are generally systemic poisons or are converted in the liver to toxic metabolites. The direct hepatotoxins result in morphologic abnormalities

TABLE 286-1 *Some Features of Toxic and Drug-Induced Hepatic Injury*

| Features | Direct Toxic Effect[a] | | Idiosyncratic[a] | | | Other[a] |
	(Carbon Tetrachloride)	(Acetaminophen)	(Halothane)	(Isoniazid)	(Chlorpromazine)	(Oral Contraceptive Agents)
Predictable and dose-related toxicity	+	+	0	0	0	+
Latent period	Short	Short	Variable	Variable	Variable	Variable
Arthralgia, fever, rash, eosinophilia	0	0	+	0	+	0
Liver morphology	Necrosis, fatty infiltration	Centrilobular necrosis	Similar to viral hepatitis	Similar to viral hepatitis	Cholestasis *with* portal inflammation	Cholestasis *without* portal inflammation, vascular lesions

[a] The drugs listed are typical samples.

that are reasonably characteristic and reproducible for each toxin. For example, carbon tetrachloride and trichloroethylene characteristically produce a centrilobular zonal necrosis, whereas yellow phosphorus poisoning typically results in periportal injury. The hepatotoxic octapeptides of *Amanita phalloides* usually produce massive hepatic necrosis. The lethal dose of the toxin is about 10 mg, the amount found in a single deathcap mushroom. Tetracycline, when administered in intravenous doses >1.5 g daily, leads to microvesicular fat deposits in the liver. Liver injury, which is often only one facet of the toxicity produced by the direct hepatotoxins, may go unrecognized until jaundice appears.

In idiosyncratic drug reactions the occurrence of hepatitis is usually infrequent and unpredictable, the response is not dose-dependent, and it may occur at any time during or shortly after exposure to the drug. Adding to the difficulty of predicting or identifying idiosyncratic drug hepatotoxicity is the occurrence of mild, transient, nonprogressive serum aminotransferase elevations that resolve with continued drug use. Such "adaptation," the mechanism of which is unknown, occurs in such drugs as isoniazid, valproate, phenytoin, and HMG-CoA reductase inhibitors (statins). Extrahepatic manifestations of hypersensitivity, such as rash, arthralgias, fever, leukocytosis, and eosinophilia, occur in about one-quarter of patients with idiosyncratic hepatotoxic drug reactions; this observation and the unpredictability of idiosyncratic drug hepatototoxicity contributed to the hypothesis that this category of drug reactions is immunologically mediated. More recent evidence, however, suggests that, in most cases, even idiosyncratic reactions represent direct hepatotoxity but are caused by drug metabolites rather than by the intact compound. Even the prototypes of idiosyncratic hepatoxicity reactions, halothane hepatitis and isoniazid hepatotoxicity, associated frequently with hypersensitivity manifestations, are now recognized to be mediated by toxic metabolites that damage liver cells directly. Currently, most idiosyncratic reactions are thought to result from differences in metabolic reactivity to specific agents; host susceptibility is mediated by the kinetics of toxic metabolite generation, which differs among individuals. Occasionally, however, the clinical features of an allergic reaction (prominent tissue eosinophilia, autoantibodies, etc.) are difficult to ignore. In vitro models have been described in which lymphocyte cytotoxicity can be demonstrated against rabbit hepatocytes altered by incubation with the potential offending drug. Furthermore, several instances of drug hepatotoxicity are associated with the appearance of autoantibodies, including a class of antibodies to liver-kidney microsomes, anti-LKM2, directed against a cytochrome P450 enzyme. Similarly, in selected cases, a drug or its metabolite has been shown to bind to a host cellular component forming a hapten; the immune response to this "neoantigen" is postulated to play a role in the pathogenesis of liver injury. Therefore, some authorities subdivide idiosyncratic drug hepatotoxicity into hypersensitivity (allergic) and "metabolic" categories. Several unusual exceptions notwithstanding, true drug allergy is difficult to support in most cases of idiosyncratic drug-induced liver injury.

Idiosyncratic reactions lead to a morphologic pattern that is more variable than those produced by direct toxins; a single agent is often capable of causing a variety of lesions, although certain patterns tend to predominate. Depending on the agent involved, idiosyncratic hepatitis may result in a clinical and morphologic picture indistinguishable from that of viral hepatitis (e.g., halothane) or may simulate extrahepatic bile duct obstruction clinically with morphologic evidence of cholestasis. Drug-induced cholestasis ranges from mild to increasingly severe: (1) bland cholestasis with limited hepatocellular injury (e.g., estrogens, 17,α-substituted androgens); (2) inflammatory cholestasis (e.g., phenothiazines, amoxicillin–clavulanic acid, oxacillin, erythromcyin estolate); (3) sclerosing cholangitis (e.g., after intrahepatic infusion of the chemotherapeutic agent floxuridine for hepatic metastases from a primary colonic carcinoma); (4) disappearance of bile ducts, "ductopenic" cholestasis, similar to that observed in chronic rejection following liver transplantation (e.g., carbamazepine, chlorpromazine, tricyclic antidepressant agents). Cholestasis may result

from binding of drugs to canalicular membrane transporters, accumulation of toxic bile acids resulting from canalicular pump failure, or genetic defects in canalicular transporter proteins. Morphologic alterations may also include bridging hepatic necrosis (e.g., methyldopa), or, infrequently, hepatic granulomas (e.g., sulfonamides). Some drugs result in macrovesicular or microvesicular steatosis or steatohepatitis, which in some cases has been linked to mitochondrial dysfunction and lipid peroxidation. Severe hepatotoxicity associated with steatohepatitis, most likely a result of mitochondrial toxicity, is being recognized with increasing frequency among patients receiving antiretroviral therapy with reverse transcriptase inhibitors (e.g., zidovudine, didanosine) or protease inhibitors (e.g., indinavir, ritonavir) for HIV infection (Chap. 173). Generally, such mitochondrial hepatotoxicity of these antiretroviral agents is reversible, but dramatic, nonreversible hepatotoxicity associated with mitochondrial injury (inhibition of DNA polymerase γ) was the cause of acute liver failure encountered during early clinical trials of fialuridine, a fluorinated pyrimidine analogue with potent antiviral activity against hepatitis B virus. Another potential target for idiosyncratic drug hepatotoxicity is sinusoidal lining cells; when these are injured, such as by high-dose chemotherapeutic agents (e.g., cyclophosphamide, melphalan, busulfan) administered prior to bone marrow transplantation, venoocclusive disease can result.

Not all adverse hepatic drug reactions can be classified as either toxic or idiosyncratic in type. For example, oral contraceptives, which combine estrogenic and progestational compounds, may result in impairment of hepatic tests and occasionally in jaundice. However, they do not produce necrosis or fatty change, manifestations of hypersensitivity are generally absent, and susceptibility to the development of oral contraceptive–induced cholestasis appears to be genetically determined. Such estrogen-induced cholestasis is more common in women with cholestasis of pregnancy, a disorder linked to genetic defects in multidrug resistance–associated canalicular transporter proteins. Other instances of genetically determined drug hepatotoxicity have been identified. For example, approximately 10% of the population have an autosomally recessive trait associated with the absence of cytochrome P450 enzyme 2D6 and have impaired debrisoquine-4-hydroxylase enzyme activity. As a result, they cannot metabolize, and are at increased risk of hepatotoxicity resulting from, certain compounds such as desipramine, propranolol, and quinidine.

Some forms of drug hepatotoxicity are so rare, e.g., occurring in <1:10,000 recipients, that they do not become apparent during clinical trials, involving only several thousand recipients, conducted to obtain drug registration. An example of such rare, but serious, idiosyncratic drug hepatotoxicity followed the approval and generalized use of troglitazone, a peroxisomal, proliferator activator–receptor γ agonist, the first-introduced example of a thiazolidinedione insulin-sensitizing agent. This instance of drug hepatotoxicity was not recognized until well after the drug was introduced, underlining the importance of postmarketing surveillance in identifying toxic drugs and in leading to their withdrawal from use.

Because drug-induced hepatitis is often a presumptive diagnosis and many other disorders produce a similar clinicopathologic picture, evidence of a causal relationship between the use of a drug and subsequent liver injury may be difficult to establish. The relationship is most convincing for the direct hepatotoxins, which lead to a high frequency of hepatic impairment after a short latent period. Idiosyncratic reactions may be reproduced, in some instances, when rechallenge, after an asymptomatic period, results in a recurrence of signs, symptoms, and morphologic and biochemical abnormalities. Rechallenge, however, is often ethically unfeasible, because severe reactions may occur.

Generally, drug hepatotoxicity is not more frequent in persons with underlying chronic liver disease. Reported exceptions include hepatotoxicity of aspirin, methotrexate, isoniazid (only in certain experiences), and antiretroviral therapy for HIV infection.

Principal Morphologic Change	Class of Agent	Example
Cholestasis	Anabolic steroid	Methyl testosterone
	Anti-inflammatory	Sulindac
	Antithyroid	Methimazole
	Antibiotic	Erythromycin estolate, nitrofurantoin, rifampin, amoxicillin–clavulanic acid, oxacillin
	Oral contraceptive	Norethynodrel with mestranol
	Oral hypoglycemic	Chlorpropamide
	Tranquilizer	Chlorpromazine[b]
	Oncotherapeutic	Anabolic steroids, busulfan, tamoxifen
	Immunosuppressive	Cyclosporine
	Anticonvulsant	Carbamazepine
	Calcium channel blocker	Nifedipine, verapamil
Fatty liver	Antibiotic	Tetracycline
	Anticonvulsant	Sodium valproate
	Antiarrhythmic	Amiodarone
	Antiviral	Dideoxynucleosides (e.g., zidovudine) protease inhibitors (e.g., indinavir, ritonavir)
	Oncotherapeutic	Asparaginase, methotrexate
Hepatitis	Anesthetic	Halothane[c]
	Anticonvulsant	Phenytoin, carbamazepine
	Antihypertensive	Methyldopa,[c] captopril, enalapril
	Antibiotic	Isoniazid,[c] rifampin, nitrofurantoin
	Diuretic	Chlorothiazide
	Laxative	Oxyphenisatin[c]
	Antidepressant	Iproniazid, amitriptyline, imipramine, trazodone, venlafaxine
	Anti-inflammatory	Ibuprofen, indomethacin, diclofenac, sulindac, bomfenac
	Antifungal	Ketoconazole, fluconazole, itraconazole
	Antiviral	Zidovudine, didanosine, nevirapine
	Calcium channel blocker	Nifedipine, verapamil, diltiazem
	Cholinesterase inhibitor	Tacrine
	Oral hypoglycemic	Troglitazone
	Antiandrogen	Flutamide
Mixed hepatitis/ cholestatic	Immunosuppressive	Azathioprine
	Lipid-lowering	Nicotinic acid, lovastatin and other statins
	Antibiotic	Amoxicillin–clavulanic acid, trimethoprim-sulfamethoxazole
	Antifungal	Terbinafine
Toxic (necrosis)	Hydrocarbon	Carbon tetrachloride
	Metal	Yellow phosphorus
	Mushroom	*Amanita phalloides*
	Analgesic	Acetaminophen
	Solvent	Dimethylformamide
Granulomas	Anti-inflammatory	Phenylbutazone
	Antibiotic	Sulfonamides
	Xanthine oxidase inhibitor	Allopurinol
	Antiarrhythmic	Quinidine, diltiazem
	Anticonvulsant	Carbamazepine

[a] Several agents cause more than one type of liver lesion and appear under more than one category.
[b] Rarely associated with primary biliary cirrhosis–like lesion.
[c] Occasionally associated with chronic hepatitis or bridging hepatic necrosis or cirrhosis.

℞ TREATMENT

Treatment of toxic and drug-induced hepatic disease is largely supportive, except in acetaminophen hepatotoxicity (see below). In patients with fulminant hepatitis resulting from drug hepatotoxicity, liver transplantation may be life-saving (Chap. 291). Withdrawal of the suspected agent is indicated at the first sign of an adverse reaction. In the case of the direct toxins, liver involvement should not divert attention from renal or other organ involvement, which may also threaten survival. Glucocorticoids for drug hepatotoxicity with allergic features, silibinin for hepatotoxic mushroom poisoning, and ursodeoxycholic acid for cholestatic drug hepatotoxicity have never been shown to be effective and are not recommended.

In Table 286-2, several classes of chemical agents are listed, together with examples of the pattern of liver injury produced by them.

Certain drugs appear to be responsible for the development of chronic as well as acute hepatic injury. For example, oxyphenisatin, methyldopa, and isoniazid have been associated with moderate to severe chronic hepatitis, and halothane and methotrexate have been implicated in the development of cirrhosis. A syndrome resembling primary biliary cirrhosis has been described following treatment with chlorpromazine, methyl testosterone, tolbutamide, and other drugs. Portal hypertension in the absence of cirrhosis may result from alterations in hepatic architecture produced by vitamin A or arsenic intoxication, industrial exposure to vinyl chloride, or administration of thorium dioxide. The latter three agents have also been associated with angiosarcoma of the liver. Oral contraceptives have been implicated in the development of hepatic adenoma and, rarely, hepatocellular carcinoma and hepatic vein occlusion (Budd-Chiari syndrome). Another unusual lesion, peliosis hepatis (blood cysts of the liver), has been observed in some patients treated with anabolic steroids. The existence of these hepatic disorders expands the spectrum of liver injury induced by chemical agents and emphasizes the need for a thorough drug history in all patients with liver dysfunction.

The following are the patterns of adverse hepatic reactions for some prototypic agents.

ACETAMINOPHEN HEPATOTOXICITY (DIRECT TOXIN) Acetaminophen can cause severe centrilobular hepatic necrosis when ingested in large amounts in suicide attempts or accidentally by children. A single dose of 10 to 15 g, occasionally less, may produce clinical evidence of liver injury. Fatal fulminant disease is usually (although not invariably) associated with ingestion of ≥25 g. Blood levels of acetaminophen correlate with the severity of hepatic injury (levels >300 μg/mL 4 h after ingestion are predictive of the development of severe damage; levels <150 μg/mL suggest that hepatic injury is highly unlikely). Nausea, vomiting, diarrhea, abdominal pain, and shock are early manifestations occurring 4 to 12 h after ingestion. Then 24 to 48 h later, when these features are abating, hepatic injury becomes apparent. Maximal abnormalities and hepatic failure may not be evident until 4 to 6 days after ingestion, and aminotransferase levels approaching 10,000 units are not uncommon. Renal failure and myocardial injury may be present.

Acetaminophen is metabolized predominantly by a phase II reaction to innocuous sulfate and glucuronide metabolites; however, a small proportion of acetaminophen is metabolized by a phase I reaction to a hepatotoxic metabolite formed from the parent compound by the cytochrome P450 2E1. This metabolite, *N*-acetyl-benzoquinone-imide (NAPQI), is detoxified by binding to "hepatoprotective" glutathione to become harmless, water-soluble mercapturic acid, which undergoes renal excretion. When excessive amounts of NAPQI are formed, or when glutathione levels are low, glutathione levels are depleted and overwhelmed, permitting covalent binding to nucleophilic hepatocyte macromolecules. This process is believed to lead to hepatocyte necrosis; the precise sequence and mechanism are unknown. Hepatic injury may be potentiated by prior administration of alcohol, phenobarbital, or other drugs, by conditions that stimulate the mixed-function oxidase system, or by conditions such as starvation that reduce hepatic glutathione levels. The xenobiotic (environmental, exogenous substance) receptor CAR has been shown in a mouse model of acetaminophen hepatotoxicity to induce acetaminophen-metabolizing enzymes and, thereby, regulate and increase hepatotoxicity. Cimetidine, which inhibits P450 enzymes, has the potential to reduce generation of the toxic metabolite. Alcohol induces cytochrome P450 2E1; consequently, increased levels of the toxic metabolite NAPQI are produced in chronic alcoholics after acetaminophen ingestion. In addition, alcohol suppresses hepatic glutathione production. Therefore, in chronic alcoholics, the toxic dose of acetaminophen may be as low as 2 g, and alcoholic patients should be warned specifically about the dangers of even standard doses of this commonly used drug. Such "therapeutic misadventures" also occur occasionally in patients with severe, febrile illnesses or pain syndromes; in such a setting, several days of anorexia and near-fasting coupled with regular administration of extra-strength acetaminophen formulations result in a combination of glutathione depletion and relatively high NAPQI levels in the absence of a history of recognized acetaminophen overdose.

℞ TREATMENT

Treatment of acetaminophen overdosage includes gastric lavage, supportive measures, and oral administration of activated charcoal or cholestyramine to prevent absorption of residual drug. Neither of these agents appears to be effective if given >30 min after acetaminophen ingestion; if they are used, the stomach lavage should be done before other agents are administered orally. The chances of possible-, probable-, and high-risk hepatotoxicity can be derived from a nomogram plot (Fig. 286-1), readily available in emergency departments, of acetaminophen plasma levels as a function of hours after ingestion. In patients with high acetaminophen blood levels (>200 μg/mL mea-

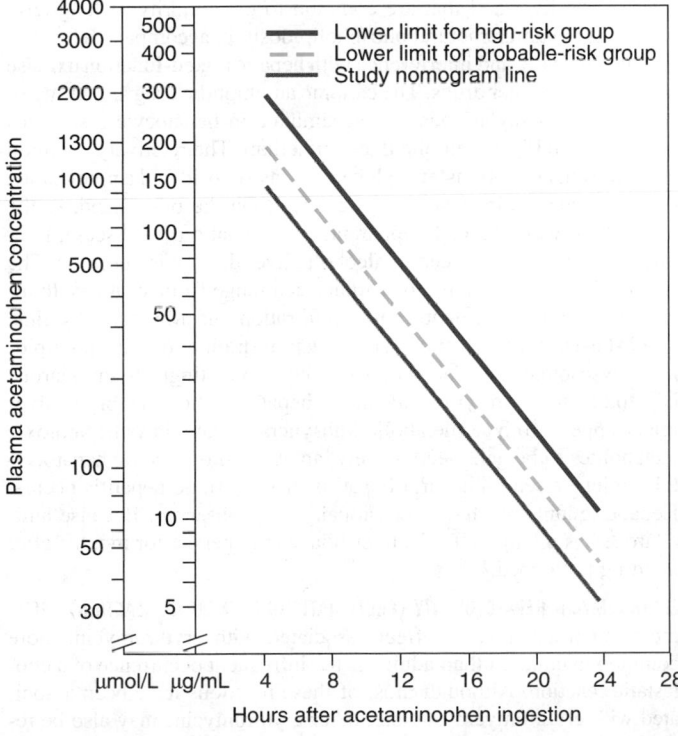

FIGURE 286-1 Nomogram to define risk of acetaminophen hepatotoxicity according to initial plasma acetaminophen concentration. (*After BH Rumack, H Matthew, Pediatrics 55:871, 1975.*)

sured at 4 h or >100 μg/mL at 8 h after ingestion), the administration of sulfhydryl compounds (e.g., cysteamine, cysteine, or N-acetylcysteine) appears to reduce the severity of hepatic necrosis. These agents appear to act by providing a reservoir of sulfhydryl groups to bind the toxic metabolites or by stimulating synthesis and repletion of hepatic glutathione. Therapy should be begun within 8 h of ingestion but may be effective even if given as late as 24 to 36 h after overdose. Later administration of sulfhydryl compounds is of uncertain value. Routine use of N-acetylcysteine has substantially reduced the occurrence of fatal acetaminophen hepatotoxicity. When given orally, N-acetylcysteine is diluted to yield a 5% solution. A loading dose of 140 mg/kg is given, followed by 70 mg/kg every 4 h for 15 to 20 doses. Whenever a patient with potential acetaminophen hepatotoxicity is encountered, a local poison control center should be contacted. Treatment can be stopped when plasma acetaminophen levels indicate that the risk of liver damage is low. If signs of hepatic failure (e.g., progressive jaundice, coagulopathy, confusion) occur despite N-acetylcysteine therapy for acetaminophen hepatotoxicity, liver transplantation may be the only option. Preliminary data suggest that early arterial blood lactate levels among such patients with acute liver failure may distinguish patients highly likely to require liver transplantation (lactate levels > 3.5 mmol/L) from those likely to survive without liver replacement.

Survivors of acute acetaminophen overdose usually have no evidence of hepatic sequelae. In a few patients, prolonged or repeated administration of acetaminophen in therapeutic doses appears to have led to the development of chronic hepatitis and cirrhosis.

HALOTHANE HEPATOTOXICITY (IDIOSYNCRATIC REACTION) Although currently quite rare, halothane hepatotoxicity was one of the prototypical, and most intensively studied, examples of idiosyncratic drug hepatotoxicity. Administration of halothane, a nonexplosive fluorinated hydrocarbon anesthetic agent that is structurally similar to chloroform, results in severe hepatic necrosis in a small number of individuals, many of whom have previously been exposed to this agent. The failure to produce similar hepatic lesions reliably in animals, the rarity of hepatic impairment in human beings, and the delayed appearance of hepatic injury suggest that halothane is not a direct hepatotoxin but rather a sensitizing agent. However, manifestations of hypersensitivity are seen in <25% of cases. A genetic predisposition leading to an idiosyncratic metabolic reactivity has been postulated and appears to be the most likely mechanism of halothane hepatotoxicity. Adults (rather than children), obese people, and women appear to be particularly susceptible. Fever, moderate leukocytosis, and eosinophilia may occur in the first week following halothane administration. Jaundice is usually noted 7 to 10 days after exposure but may occur earlier in previously exposed patients. Nausea and vomiting may precede the onset of jaundice. Hepatomegaly is often mild, but liver tenderness is common. The serum aminotransferase levels are elevated. The pathologic changes at autopsy are indistinguishable from massive hepatic necrosis resulting from viral hepatitis. The case-fatality rate of halothane hepatitis is not known but may vary from 20 to 40% in cases with severe liver involvement. Patients in whom unexplained spiking fever, especially delayed fever, or jaundice develops after halothane anesthesia should not receive this agent again. Because cross-reactions between halothane and methoxyflurane have been reported, the latter agent should not be used after halothane reactions. Later-generation halogenated hydrocarbon anesthetics, which have supplanted halothane except in rare instances (e.g., certain types of thoracic surgery), are felt to be associated with a lower risk of hepatotoxicity.

METHYLDOPA HEPATOTOXICITY (TOXIC AND IDIOSYNCRATIC REACTION) Minor alterations in liver tests are reported in about 5% of patients treated with this antihypertensive agent. These trivial abnormalities typically resolve despite continued drug administration. In <1% of patients, acute liver injury resembling viral or chronic hepatitis or, rarely, a cholestatic reaction is seen 1 to 20 weeks after methyldopa is started.

In 50% of cases the interval is <4 weeks. A prodrome of fever, anorexia, and malaise may be noted for a few days before the onset of jaundice. Rash, lymphadenopathy, arthralgia, and eosinophilia are rare. Serologic markers of autoimmunity are detected infrequently, and <5% of patients have a Coombs-positive hemolytic anemia. In about 15% of patients with methyldopa hepatotoxicity, the clinical, biochemical, and histologic features are those of moderate to severe chronic hepatitis, with or without bridging necrosis and macronodular cirrhosis. With discontinuation of the drug, the disorder usually resolves. Although methyldopa is currently used infrequently, its hepatotoxicity is very well characterized. Among the currently popular antihypertensive agents, angiotensin-converting enzyme (ACE) inhibitors, such as captopril and enalapril, have been blamed, albeit rarely, for hepatotoxicity (primarily cholestasis and cholestatic hepatitis, but also hepatocellular injury). Angiotensin-II receptor antagonists, such as losartan, are unlikely hepatotoxins, although rare reports of liver injury in their recipients have appeared.

ISONIAZID HEPATOTOXICITY (TOXIC AND IDIOSYNCRATIC REACTION)

In approximately 10% of adults treated with the antituberculosis agent isoniazid, elevated serum aminotransferase levels develop during the first few weeks of therapy; this appears to represent an adaptive response to a toxic metabolite of the drug. Whether or not isoniazid is continued, these values (usually <200 units) return to normal in a few weeks. In about 1% of treated patients, an illness develops that is indistinguishable from viral hepatitis; approximately half of these cases occur within the first 2 months of treatment, while in the remainder, clinical disease may be delayed for many months. Liver biopsy reveals morphologic changes similar to those of viral hepatitis or bridging hepatic necrosis. The disease may be severe, with a case-fatality rate of 10%. Important liver injury appears to be age-related, increasing substantially after age 35; the highest frequency is in patients over age 50, the lowest under the age of 20. Even for patients >50 years monitored carefully during therapy, hepatotoxicity occurs in only approximately 2%, well below the risk estimate derived from earlier experiences. Isoniazid hepatotoxicity is enhanced by alcohol, rifampin and pyrazinamide. Fever, rash, eosinophilia, and other manifestations of drug allergy are distinctly unusual. A reactive metabolite of acetylhydrazine, a metabolite of isoniazid, may be responsible for liver injury, and patients who are rapid acetylators would be more prone to such injury. Counterintuitively, in some reports, the opposite is true; slow acetylators are more likely to experience hepatotoxicity and more severe hepatotoxicity than rapid acetylators. Contrary to past reports, several recent studies suggest that hepatotoxicity due to isoniazid as well as to combination antituberculous therapy that includes isoniazid is more likely in patients with underlying chronic hepatitis B. A picture resembling chronic hepatitis has been observed in a few patients. Careful liver-test monitoring is advisable in patients being treated with isoniazid.

SODIUM VALPROATE HEPATOTOXICITY (TOXIC AND IDIOSYNCRATIC REACTION)

Sodium valproate, an anticonvulsant useful in the treatment of petit mal and other seizure disorders, has been associated with the development of severe hepatic toxicity and, rarely, fatalities, predominantly in children but also in adults. Asymptomatic elevations of serum aminotransferase levels have been recognized in as many as 45% of treated patients. These "adaptive" changes, however, appear to have no clinical importance, for major hepatotoxicity is not seen in the majority of patients despite continuation of drug therapy. In those rare patients in whom jaundice, encephalopathy, and evidence of hepatic failure are found, examination of liver tissue reveals microvesicular fat and bridging hepatic necrosis, predominantly in the centrilobular zone. Bile duct injury may also be apparent. It seems likely that sodium valproate is not directly hepatotoxic but that its metabolite, 4-pentenoic acid, may be responsible for hepatic injury. Valproate hepatotoxicity is more common in persons with mitochondrial enzyme deficiencies and may be ameliorated by administration of carnitine, which valproate therapy can deplete.

PHENYTOIN HEPATOTOXICITY (IDIOSYNCRATIC REACTION)

Phenytoin, formerly diphenylhydantoin, a mainstay in the treatment of seizure disorders, has been associated in rare instances with the development of severe hepatitis-like liver injury leading to fulminant hepatic failure. In many patients the hepatitis is associated with striking fever, lymphadenopathy, rash (Stevens-Johnson syndrome or exfoliative dermatitis), leukocytosis, and eosinophilia, suggesting an immunologically mediated hypersensitivity mechanism. Despite these observations, there is also evidence that metabolic idiosyncrasy may be responsible for hepatic injury. In the liver, phenytoin is converted by the cytochrome P450 system to metabolites, which include the highly reactive electrophilic arene oxides. These metabolites are normally metabolized further by epoxide hydrolases. A defect (genetic or acquired) in epoxide hydrolase activity could permit covalent binding of arene oxides to hepatic macromolecules, thereby leading to hepatic injury. Regardless of the mechanism, hepatic injury is usually manifest within the first 2 months after beginning phenytoin therapy. With the exception of an abundance of eosinophils in the liver, the clinical, biochemical, and histologic picture resembles that of viral hepatitis. In rare instances, bile duct injury may be the salient feature of phenytoin hepatotoxicity, with striking features of intrahepatic cholestasis. Asymptomatic elevations of aminotransferase and alkaline phosphatase levels have been observed in a sizable proportion of patients receiving long-term phenytoin therapy. These liver changes are believed by some authorities to represent the potent hepatic enzyme–inducing properties of phenytoin and are accompanied histologically by swelling of hepatocytes in the absence of necroinflammatory activity or evidence of chronic liver disease.

AMIODARONE HEPATOTOXICITY (TOXIC AND IDIOSYNCRATIC REACTION)

Therapy with this potent antiarrhythmic drug is accompanied in 15 to 50% of patients by modest elevations of serum aminotransferase levels that may remain stable or diminish despite continuation of the drug. Such abnormalities may appear days to many months after beginning therapy. A proportion of those with elevated aminotransferase levels have detectable hepatomegaly, and clinically important liver disease develops in <5% of patients. Features that represent a direct effect of the drug on the liver and that are common to the majority of long-term recipients are ultrastructural phospholipidosis, unaccompanied by clinical liver disease, and interference with hepatic mixed-function oxidase metabolism of other drugs. The cationic amphiphilic drug and its major metabolite desethylamiodarone accumulate in hepatocyte lysosomes and mitochondria and in bile duct epithelium. The relatively common elevations in aminotransferase levels are also considered a predictable, dose-dependent, direct hepatotoxic effect. On the other hand, in the rare patient with clinically apparent, symptomatic liver disease, liver injury resembling that seen in alcoholic liver disease is observed. The so-called pseudoalcoholic liver injury can range from steatosis, to alcoholic hepatitis-like neutrophilic infiltration and Mallory's hyaline, to cirrhosis. Electron-microscopic demonstration of phospholipid-laden lysosomal lamellar bodies can help to distinguish amiodarone hepatotoxicity from typical alcoholic hepatitis. This category of liver injury appears to be a metabolic idiosyncrasy that allows hepatotoxic metabolites to be generated. Rarely, an acute idiosyncratic hepatocellular injury resembling viral hepatitis or cholestatic hepatitis occurs. Hepatic granulomas have occasionally been observed. Because amiodarone has a long half-life, liver injury may persist for months after the drug is stopped.

ERYTHROMYCIN HEPATOTOXICITY (CHOLESTATIC IDIOSYNCRATIC REACTION)

The most important adverse effect associated with erythromycin, more common in children than adults, is the infrequent occurrence of a cholestatic reaction. Although most of these reactions have been associated with erythromycin estolate, other erythromycins may also be responsible. The reaction usually begins during the first 2 or 3 weeks of therapy and includes nausea, vomiting, fever, right upper quadrant abdominal pain, jaundice, leukocytosis, and moderately elevated aminotransferase levels. The clinical picture can resemble acute cholecystitis or bacterial cholangitis. Liver biopsy reveals variable cholestasis; portal inflammation comprising lymphocytes, polymorphonuclear leukocytes, and eosinophils; and scattered foci of hepatocyte necrosis. Symptoms and laboratory findings usually subside within a few days of drug withdrawal, and evidence of chronic liver disease has not been found on follow-up. The precise mechanism remains ill-defined.

ORAL CONTRACEPTIVE HEPATOTOXICITY (CHOLESTATIC REACTION) The administration of oral contraceptive combinations of estrogenic and progestational steroids leads to intrahepatic cholestasis with pruritus and jaundice in a small number of patients weeks to months after taking these agents. Especially susceptible seem to be patients with recurrent idiopathic jaundice of pregnancy, severe pruritus of pregnancy, or a family history of these disorders. With the exception of liver biochemical tests, laboratory studies are normal, and extrahepatic manifestations of hypersensitivity are absent. Liver biopsy reveals cholestasis with bile plugs in dilated canaliculi and striking bilirubin staining of liver cells. In contrast to chlorpromazine-induced cholestasis, portal inflammation is absent. The lesion is reversible on withdrawal of the agent. The two steroid components appear to act synergistically on hepatic function, although the estrogen may be primarily responsible. Oral contraceptives are contraindicated in patients with a history of recurrent jaundice of pregnancy. Primarily benign, but rarely malignant, neoplasms of the liver, hepatic vein occlusion, and peripheral sinusoidal dilatation have also been associated with oral contraceptive therapy. Focal nodular hyperplasia of the liver is not more frequent among users of oral contraceptives.

17,α-ALKYL-SUBSTITUTED ANABOLIC STEROIDS (CHOLESTATIC REACTION) In the majority of patients receiving these agents, used therapeutically mainly in the treatment of bone marrow failure but used surreptitiously and without medical indication by athletes to improve their performance, mild hepatic dysfunction develops. Impaired excretory function is the predominant defect, but the precise mechanism is uncertain. Jaundice, which appears to be dose-related, develops in only a minority of patients and may be the sole clinical manifestation of hepatotoxicity, although anorexia, nausea, and malaise may occur. Pruritus is not a prominent feature. Serum aminotransferase levels are usually <100 units, and serum alkaline phosphatase levels are normal, mildly elevated, or, in <5% of patients, three or more times the upper limit of normal. Examination of liver tissue reveals cholestasis without inflammation or necrosis. Hepatic sinusoidal dilatation and peliosis hepatis have been found in a few patients. The cholestatic disorder is usually reversible on cessation of treatment, although fatalities have been linked to peliosis. An association with hepatic adenoma and hepatocellular carcinoma has been reported.

TRIMETHOPRIM-SULFAMETHOXAZOLE HEPATOTOXICITY (IDIOSYNCRATIC REACTION) This antibiotic combination is used routinely for urinary tract infections in immunocompetent persons and for prophylaxis against and therapy of *Pneumocystis carinii* pneumonia in immunosuppressed persons (transplant recipients, patients with AIDS). With its increasing use, its occasional hepatotoxicity is being recognized with growing frequency. Its likelihood is unpredictable, but when it occurs, trimethoprim-sulfamethoxazole hepatotoxicity follows a relatively uniform latency period of several weeks and is often accompanied by eosinophilia, rash, and other features of a hypersensitivity reaction. Biochemically and histologically, acute hepatocellular necrosis predominates, but cholestatic features are quite frequent. Occasionally, cholestasis without necrosis occurs, and very rarely, a severe cholangiolytic pattern of liver injury is observed. In most cases, liver injury is self-limited, but rare fatalities have been recorded. The hepatotoxicity is attributable to the sulfamethoxazole component of the drug and is similar in features to that seen with other sulfonamides; tissue eosinophilia and granulomas may be seen. The risk of trimethoprim-sulfamethoxazole hepatotoxicity is increased in persons with HIV infection.

HMG-COA REDUCTASE INHIBITORS (STATINS) (IDIOSYNCRATIC MIXED HEPATOCELLULAR AND CHOLESTATIC REACTION) Between 1 and 2% of patients taking lovastatin, simvastatin, pravastatin, fluvastatin, or one of the newer statin drugs for the treatment of hypercholesterolemia experience asymptomatic, reversible elevations (> threefold) of aminotransferase activity. Acute hepatitis-like histologic changes, centrilobular necrosis, and centrilobular cholestasis have been described in several cases. In a larger proportion, minor aminotransferase elevations appear during the first several weeks of therapy. Careful laboratory monitoring can distinguish between patients with minor, transitory changes, who may continue therapy, and those with more profound and sustained abnormalities, who should discontinue therapy.

TOTAL PARENTERAL NUTRITION (STEATOSIS, CHOLESTASIS) Total parenteral nutrition (TPN) is often complicated by cholestatic hepatitis attributable to either steatosis, cholestasis, or gallstones (or gallbladder sludge). Steatosis or steatohepatitis may result from the excess carbohydrate calories in these nutritional supplements and is the predominant form of TPN-associated liver disorder in adults. The frequency of this complication has been reduced substantially by the introduction of balanced TPN formulas that rely on lipid as an alternative caloric source. Cholestasis and cholelithiasis, caused by the absence of stimulation of bile flow and secretion resulting from the lack of oral intake, is the predominant form of TPN-associated liver disease in infants, especially in premature neonates. Often, cholestasis in such neonates is multifactorial, contributed to by other factors such as sepsis, hypoxemia, and hypotension; occasionally, TPN-induced cholestasis in neonates culminates in chronic liver disease and liver failure. When TPN-associated liver test abnormalities occur in adults, balancing the TPN formula with more lipid is the intervention of first recourse. In infants with TPN-associated cholestasis, the addition of oral feeding may ameliorate the problem. Therapeutic interventions suggested, but not yet shown to be of proven benefit, include cholecystokinin, ursodeoxycholic acid, S-adenosyl methionine, and taurine.

"ALTERNATIVE MEDICINES" (IDIOSYNCRATIC HEPATITIS, STEATOSIS) The misguided popularity of herbal medications that are of scientifically unproven efficacy and that lack prospective safety oversight by regulatory agencies has resulted in occasional instances of hepatotoxicity. Included among the herbal remedies associated with toxic hepatitis are Jin Bu Huan (Chap. 10), xiao-chai-hu-tang, germander, chaparral, senna, mistletoe, skullcap, gentian, comfrey (containing pyrrolizidine alkaloids), Ma huang, bee pollen, valerian root, pennyroyal oil, kava, celandine, Impila (*Callilepsis laureaola*), LipoKinetix, and herbal teas. Recently well characterized are the acute hepatitis-like histologic lesions following Jin Bu Huan use: focal hepatocellular necrosis, mixed mononuclear portal tract infiltration, coagulative necrosis, apoptotic hepatocyte degeneration, tissue eosinophilia, and microvesicular steatosis. Megadoses of vitamin A can injure the liver, as can pyrrolizidine alkaloids, which often contaminate Chinese herbal preparations and can cause a venoocclusive injury leading to sinusoidal hepatic vein obstruction. Because some alternative medicines induce toxicity via active metabolites, alcohol and drugs that stimulate cytochrome P450 enzymes may enhance the toxicity of some of these products. Conversely, some alternative medicines also stimulate cytochrome P450 and may result in or amplify the toxicity of recognized drug hepatotoxins. Given the widespread use of such poorly defined herbal preparations, hepatotoxicity is likely to be encountered with increasing frequency; therefore, a drug history in patients with acute and chronic liver disease should include use of "alternative medicines" and other nonprescription preparations sold in so-called health food stores.

HIGHLY ACTIVE ANTIRETROVIRAL THERAPY (HAART) FOR HIV INFECTION (MITOCHONDRIAL TOXIC, IDIOSYNCRATIC, STEATOSIS; HEPATOCELLULAR, CHOLESTATIC, AND MIXED) The recognition of drug hepatotoxicity in persons with HIV infection is complicated in this population by the many alternative causes of liver injury (chronic viral hepatitis, fatty infiltration, infiltrative disorders, mycobacterial infection, etc.), but drug hepatotoxicity associated with HAART is an emerging and common type of liver injury in HIV-infected persons (Chap. 173). Although no one antiviral agent is recognized as a potent hepatotoxin, combination regimens including reverse transcriptase and protease inhibitors cause hepatotoxicity in ~10% of treated patients. Implicated most frequently are combinations including nucleoside analogue reverse transcriptase inhibitors zidovudine, didanosine, and, to a lesser extent, stavudine; protease inhibitors ritonavir and indinavir; and nonnucleoside reverse transcriptase inhibitors nevirapine and, to a lesser extent, efavirenz. These drugs cause predominantly hepatocellular injury but cholestatic injury as well, and prolonged (>6 months) use of reverse transcriptase inhibitors has been associated with mitochondrial injury, steatosis, and lactic acidosis. Distinguishing the impact of HAART hepatotoxicity in patients with HIV and hepatitis virus co-infection is made challenging by the following: (1) both chronic hepatitis B and hepatitis C can affect the natural history of HIV infection and the response to HAART, and (2) HAART can have an impact on chronic viral hepatitis. For example, immunologic reconstitution with HAART can result in immunologically mediated liver-cell injury in patients with chronic hepatitis B co-infection if lamivudine is withdrawn or if lamivudine resistance emerges. Infection with HIV, especially with low CD4+ T

cell counts, has been reported to increase the rate of hepatic fibrosis associated with chronic hepatitis C, and HAART therapy can increase levels of serum aminotransferases and hepatitis C virus RNA in patients with hepatitis C co-infection.

FURTHER READING

BISSELL DM et al: Drug-induced liver injury: Mechanisms and test systems. Hepatology 33:1009, 2001

FARRELL GC, LIDDLE C (guest eds.): Hepatotoxicity in the twenty-first century. Semin Liver Dis 22:109, 2002

MORGAN DJ, SMALLWOOD RA: Drug-induced liver disease. Curr Opin Gastroenterol 12:246, 1996

NOLAN CM et al: Hepatotoxicity associated with isoniazid preventive therapy. JAMA 281:1014, 1999

SCHMIDT LE et al: Acute versus chronic alcohol consumption in acetaminophen-induced hepatotoxicity. Hepatology 35:876, 2002

SULKOWSKI MS et al: Hepatotoxicity associated with antiretroviral therapy in adults infected with human immunodeficiency virus and the role of hepatitis C or B virus infection. JAMA 283:74, 2000

ZHANG J et al: Modulation of acetaminophen-induced hepatotoxicity by the xenobiotic receptor CAR. Science 298:422, 2002

ZIMMERMAN HJ et al: Drug-induced liver disease, in *Schiff's Diseases of the Liver*, 8th ed. E Schiff et al (eds). Philadelphia, Lippincott-Raven, 1999, p 973

287   CHRONIC HEPATITIS
Jules L. Dienstag, Kurt J. Isselbacher

Chronic hepatitis represents a series of liver disorders of varying causes and severity in which hepatic inflammation and necrosis continue for at least 6 months. Milder forms are nonprogressive or only slowly progressive, while more severe forms may be associated with scarring and architectural reorganization, which, when advanced, lead ultimately to cirrhosis. Several categories of chronic hepatitis have been recognized. These include chronic viral hepatitis (Chap. 285), drug-induced chronic hepatitis (Chap. 286), and autoimmune chronic hepatitis. In many cases, clinical and laboratory features are insufficient to allow assignment into one of these three categories; these "idiopathic" cases are also believed to represent autoimmune chronic hepatitis. Finally, clinical and laboratory features of chronic hepatitis are observed occasionally in patients with such hereditary/metabolic disorders as Wilson's disease (copper overload) and even occasionally in patients with alcoholic liver injury (Chap. 288). Although all types of chronic hepatitis share certain clinical, laboratory, and histopathologic features, chronic viral and chronic autoimmune hepatitis are sufficiently distinct to merit separate discussions.

CLASSIFICATION OF CHRONIC HEPATITIS   Common to all forms of chronic hepatitis are histopathologic distinctions based on localization and ex-

tent of liver injury. These vary from the milder forms, previously labeled chronic persistent hepatitis and chronic lobular hepatitis, to the more severe form, formerly called chronic active hepatitis. When first defined, these designations were felt to have prognostic implications, which have been challenged by more recent observations. Compared to the time three decades ago when the histologic designations chronic persistent, chronic lobular, and chronic active hepatitis were adopted, much more information is currently available about the causes, natural history, pathogenesis, serologic features, and therapy of chronic hepatitis. Therefore, categorization of chronic hepatitis based primarily upon histopathologic features has been replaced by a more informative classification based upon a combination of clinical, serologic, and histologic variables. Classification of chronic hepatitis is based upon (1) its *cause*, (2) its histologic activity, or *grade*, and (3) its degree of progression, or *stage*. Thus, neither clinical features alone nor histologic features—requiring liver biopsy—alone are sufficient to characterize and distinguish among the several categories of chronic hepatitis.

Classification by Cause   Clinical and serologic features allow the establishment of a diagnosis of *chronic viral hepatitis*, caused by hepatitis B, hepatitis B plus D, hepatitis C, or potentially other unknown viruses; *autoimmune hepatitis*, including several subcategories, types 1, 2, and 3, based on serologic distinctions; *drug-associated chronic hepatitis*; and a category of unknown cause, or *cryptogenic chronic hepatitis* (Table 287-1). These are addressed in more detail below.

Classification by Grade   Grade, a histologic assessment of necroinflammatory activity, is based upon examination of the liver biopsy. An assessment of important histologic features includes the degree of *periportal necrosis* and the disruption of the limiting plate of periportal hepatocytes by inflammatory cells (so-called *piecemeal necrosis* or *interface hepatitis*); the degree of confluent necrosis that links or forms bridges between vascular structures—between portal tract and portal tract or even more important bridges between portal tract and central vein—referred to as *bridging necrosis*; the degree of

TABLE 287-1   *Clinical and Laboratory Features of Chronic Hepatitis*

Type of Hepatitis	Diagnostic Test(s)	Autoantibodies	Therapy
Chronic hepatitis B	HBsAg, IgG anti-HBc, HBeAg, HBV DNA	Uncommon	IFN-α, lamivudine
Chronic hepatitis C	Anti-HCV, HCV RNA	Anti-LKM1[a]	PEG-IFN-α plus ribavirin
Chronic hepatitis D	Anti-HDV, HDV RNA, HBsAg, IgG anti-HBc	Anti-LKM3	IFN-α (?)
Autoimmune hepatitis	ANA[b] (homogeneous), anti-LKM1(±), hyperglobulinemia	ANA, anti-LKM1, anti-SLA[c]	Prednisone, azathioprine
Drug-associated	—	Uncommon	Withdraw drug
Cryptogenic	All negative	None	Prednisone (?), azathioprine (?)

[a] Antibodies to liver-kidney microsomes type 1 (autoimmune hepatitis type II and some cases of hepatitis C).

[b] Antinuclear antibody (autoimmune hepatitis type I).

[c] Antibodies to soluble liver antigen (autoimmune hepatitis type III).

Note: HBsAg, hepatitis B surface antigen; IFN-α, interferon α; PEG-IFN α, pegylated interferon α hepatocyte degeneration and focal necrosis within the lobule; and the degree of *portal inflammation*. Several scoring systems that take these histologic features into account have been devised, and the most popular is the numerical histologic activity index (HAI), based on the work of Knodell and Ishak (Table 287-2). Technically, the HAI, which is primarily a measure of *grade*, also includes an assessment of fibrosis, which is currently used to categorize *stage* of the disease, as described below. Based on the presence and degree of these features of histologic activity, chronic hepatitis can be graded as mild, moderate, or severe.

Classification by Stage The stage of chronic hepatitis, which reflects the level of progression of the disease, is based on the degree of fibrosis. When fibrosis is so extensive that fibrous septa surround parenchymal nodules and alter the normal architecture of the liver lobule, the histologic lesion is defined as cirrhosis. Staging is based on the degree of fibrosis as categorized by one of several numerical scales (Table 287-2).

Reconciliation between Histologic Classification and New Classification For historic purposes, and to provide the basis for navigating several decades worth of literature on chronic hepatitis, the histologic categories of chronic persistent hepatitis, chronic lobular hepatitis, and

TABLE 287-2 *Histologic Activity Index (HAI) (Knodell-Ishak Score) in Chronic Hepatitis*

Histologic Feature	HAI[a] Severity	HAI[a] Score	Modified HAI[b] Severity		Modified HAI[b] Score
1. Perioportal necrosis, including piecemeal necrosis (PN) and/or bridging necrosis (BN)	None	0	None		0
	Mild PN	1	Mild		1
	Moderate PN	3	Mild/moderate		2
	Marked PN	4	Moderate		3
	Moderate PN + BN	5	Severe		4
	Marked PN + BN	6			
	Multilobular necrosis	10			
2. Intralobular necrosis	None	0	Confluent	None	0
	Mild	1		Focal	1
	Moderate	3		Zone 3 some	2
	Marked	4		Zone 3 most	3
				Zone 3 + BN few	4
				Zone 3 + BN multiple	5
				Panacinar/multiacinar	6
			Focal	None	0
				≤ 1 focus/10× field	1
				2–4 foci/10× field	2
				5–10 foci/10× field	3
				>10 foci/10× field	4
3. Portal inflammation	None	0			0
	Mild	1			1
	Moderate	3			2
	Moderate/marked	3			3
	Marked	4			4
4. Fibrosis	None	0			0
	Portal fibrosis—some	1			1
	Portal fibrosis—most	1			2
	Bridging fibrosis—few	3			3
	Bridging fibrosis—many	3			4
	Incomplete cirrhosis	4			5
	Cirrhosis				6
Maximum score		22			Grade 18/Stage 6

[a] "Knodell Score," Hepatology 1:431, 1981 [b] "Ishak Score," Hepatology 24:289, 1996

chronic active hepatitis are correlated with their contemporary counterparts in Table 287-3. When the early classification was devised, chronic persistent and lobular hepatitis were felt to have a good prognosis, while chronic active hepatitis was considered a progressive disorder with a poor prognosis. The prognostic value of these histologic distinctions, however, was found to be limited, and this classification scheme has been supplanted by distinctions in grade and stage.

CHRONIC VIRAL HEPATITIS Both the enterically transmitted forms of viral hepatitis, hepatitis A and E, are self-limited and do not cause chronic hepatitis (rare reports notwithstanding in which acute hepatitis A serves as a trigger for the onset of autoimmune hepatitis in genetically susceptible patients). In contrast, the entire clinicopathologic spectrum of chronic hepatitis occurs in patients with chronic viral hepatitis B and C as well as in patients with chronic hepatitis D superimposed on chronic hepatitis B.

Chronic Hepatitis B The likelihood of chronicity after acute hepatitis B varies as a function of age. Infection at birth is associated with a clinically silent acute infection but a 90% chance of chronic infection, while infection in young adulthood in immunocompetent persons is typically associated with clinically apparent acute hepatitis but a risk of chronicity of only approximately 1%. Most cases of chronic hepatitis B among adults, however, occur in patients who never had a recognized episode of clinically apparent acute viral hepatitis. The degree of liver injury (grade) in patients with chronic hepatitis B is variable, ranging from none in inactive carriers, to mild, to severe. Among adults with chronic hepatitis B, histologic features are of prognostic importance. In one long-term study of patients with chronic hepatitis B, investigators found a 5-year survival of 97% for patients with mild chronic hepatitis, of 86% for patients with moderate to severe chronic hepatitis, and of only 55% for patients with chronic hepatitis and postnecrotic cirrhosis. The 15-year survival in these cohorts

were 77, 66, and 40%, respectively. On the other hand, more recent observations do not allow us to be so sanguine about the prognosis in patients with mild chronic hepatitis; among such patients followed for 1 to 13 years, progression to more severe chronic hepatitis and cirrhosis has been observed in more than a quarter of cases.

Probably more important to consider than histology alone in patients with chronic hepatitis B is the degree of hepatitis B virus (HBV) replication. As reviewed in Chap. 285, chronic hepatitis B can be divided into two phases based on the relative level of HBV replication. The relatively *replicative phase* is characterized by the presence in the serum of markers of HBV replication [hepatitis B e antigen (HBeAg) HBV DNA], by the presence in the liver of detectable intrahepatocyte nucleocapsid antigens [primarily hepatitis B core antigen (HBcAg)], by high infectivity, and by accompanying liver injury; HBV DNA can

TABLE 287-3 *Correlation Between Earlier and Contemporary Nomenclature of Chronic Hepatitis*

Old Classification	Contemporary Classification Grade (Activity)	Contemporary Classification Stage (Fibrosis)
Chronic persistent hepatitis[a]	Minimal or mild	None or mild
Chronic lobular hepatitis[b]	Mild or moderate	Mild
Chronic active hepatitis[c]	Mild, moderate, or severe	Mild, moderate, or severe

[a] Inflammatory infiltrate localized to, and confined within, portal tracts.
[b] Portal inflammation confined within portal tracts plus foci of necrosis and inflammation in the liver lobule, resembling slowly resolving acute hepatitis.
[c] Erosion of the limiting plate of periportal hepatocytes by inflammatory cells ("piecemeal necrosis" or "interface hepatitis"), usually with periportal connective tissue septa extending into the liver lobule. More severe instances involve hepatocellular dropout and collapse spanning liver lobules ("bridging necrosis"), and, in the most severe form, multilobular collapse, bridging necrosis, and collapse of lobules are extensive and associated with rapid clinical deterioration.

be detected in the liver but is extrachromosomal. In contrast, the relatively *nonreplicative phase* is characterized by the absence of conventional markers of HBV replication (HBeAg and HBV DNA detectable by hybridization) but an association with anti-HBe, the absence of intrahepatocytic HBcAg, limited infectivity, and minimal liver injury; HBV DNA can be detected in the liver but is integrated into the host genome. Those in the replicative phase tend to have more severe chronic hepatitis, while those in the nonreplicative phase tend to have minimal or mild chronic hepatitis or to be inactive hepatitis B carriers; however, distinctions in HBV replication and in histologic category do not always coincide. The likelihood of converting spontaneously from relatively replicative to nonreplicative chronic HBV infection is approximately 10 to 15% per year. As noted in Chap. 285, the conversion from replicative to nonreplicative chronic hepatitis B is associated with a transient elevation in aminotransferase activity resembling acute hepatitis; occasionally, spontaneous resumptions of replicative activity occur in nonreplicative infection; and occasionally, HBV variants occur in which serologic markers of replication (HBeAg) are absent, despite the presence of replicative infection (see below). Chronic HBV infection, especially when acquired at birth or in early childhood, is associated with an increased risk of hepatocellular carcinoma (Chap. 78). →*A discussion of the pathogenesis of liver injury in patients with chronic hepatitis B appears in Chap. 285.*

As noted in Chap. 285, *HBeAg-negative chronic hepatitis B*, i.e., chronic HBV infection with active virus replication, readily detectable HBV DNA (by insensitive hybridization assays with sensitivity thresholds of 10^5 to 10^6 virions/mL) but without HBeAg (anti-HBe-reactive), is more common than HBeAg-reactive chronic hepatitis B in Mediterranean and European countries and in Asia (and, correspondingly, in HBV genotypes other than A). Most such cases represent precore or core-promoter mutations acquired late in the natural history of the disease (mostly early-life onset; age range 40 to 55 years, older than that for HBeAg-reactive chronic hepatitis B); these mutations prevent translation of HBeAg from the precore component of the HBV genome (precore mutants) or are characterized by down-regulated transcription of precore mRNA (core-promoter mutants; Chap. 285). Although their levels of HBV DNA tend to be lower than among patients with HBeAg-reactive chronic hepatitis B, patients with HBeAg-negative chronic hepatitis B tend to have progressive liver injury (complicated more frequently by cirrhosis and hepatocellular carcinoma), to experience episodic reactivation of liver disease reflected in fluctuating levels of aminotransferase activity ("flares"), and, generally, to be more refractory to antiviral therapy (see below).

The spectrum of *clinical features* of chronic hepatitis B is broad, ranging from asymptomatic infection to debilitating disease or even end-stage, fatal hepatic failure. As noted above, the onset of the disease tends to be insidious in most patients, with the exception of the very few in whom chronic disease follows failure of resolution of clinically apparent acute hepatitis B. The clinical and laboratory features associated with progression from acute to chronic hepatitis B are discussed in Chap. 285. *Fatigue* is a common symptom, and persistent or intermittent *jaundice* is a common feature in severe or advanced cases. Intermittent deepening of jaundice and recurrence of malaise and anorexia, as well as worsening fatigue, are reminiscent of acute hepatitis; such exacerbations may occur spontaneously, often coinciding with evidence of virologic reactivation, may lead to progressive liver injury, and, when superimposed on well-established cirrhosis, may cause hepatic decompensation. Complications of cirrhosis occur in end-stage chronic hepatitis and include ascites, edema, bleeding gastroesophageal varices, hepatic encephalopathy, coagulopathy, or hypersplenism. Occasionally, these complications bring the patient to initial clinical attention. Extrahepatic complications of chronic hepatitis B, similar to those seen during the prodromal phase of acute hepatitis B, are associated with deposition of circulating hepatitis B antigen–antibody immune complexes. These include arthralgias and arthritis, which are

common, and the more rare purpuric cutaneous lesions (leukocytoclastic vasculitis), immune-complex glomerulonephritis, and generalized vasculitis (polyarteritis nodosa) (Chaps. 285 and 306).

Laboratory features of chronic hepatitis B do not distinguish adequately between histologically mild and severe hepatitis. Aminotransferase elevations tend to be modest for chronic hepatitis B but may fluctuate in the range of 100 to 1000 units. As is true for acute viral hepatitis B, alanine aminotransferase (ALT) tends to be more elevated than aspartate aminotransferase (AST); however, once cirrhosis is established, AST tends to exceed ALT. Levels of alkaline phosphatase activity tend to be normal or only marginally elevated. In severe cases, moderate elevations in serum bilirubin [51.3 to 171 μmol/L (3 to 10 mg/dL)] occur. Hypoalbuminemia and prolongation of the prothrombin time occur in severe or end-stage cases. Hyperglobulinemia and detectable circulating autoantibodies are distinctly absent in chronic hepatitis B (in contrast to autoimmune hepatitis). →*Viral markers of chronic HBV infection are discussed in Chap. 285.*

℞ TREATMENT

Although progression to cirrhosis is more likely in severe than in mild or moderate chronic hepatitis B, all forms of chronic hepatitis B can be progressive, and progression occurs primarily in patients with active HBV replication. Moreover, in populations of patients with chronic hepatitis B who are at risk for hepatocellular carcinoma (Chap. 78), the risk is highest for those with continued, high-level HBV replication. Therefore, management of chronic hepatitis B is directed at suppressing the level of virus replication. Early in its development, antiviral therapy for hepatitis B was confined to patients with HBeAg-reactive chronic hepatitis B; however, HBeAg-negative chronic hepatitis B has emerged as an important target for antiviral therapy as well. To date, three drugs have been approved for treatment of chronic hepatitis B: injectable interferon (IFN) α and two oral agents, lamivudine and adefovir dipivoxil; several other drugs are in the process of efficacy testing in clinical trials.

Interferon   Interferon-α was the first approved therapy for chronic hepatitis B. For immunocompetent adults with HBeAg-reactive chronic hepatitis B (who tend to have HBV DNA detectable by hybridization assay and histologic evidence of chronic hepatitis on liver biopsy), a 16-week course of IFN given subcutaneously at a daily dose of 5 million units, or three times a week at a dose of 10 million unit, results in a loss of HBeAg and hybridization-detectable HBV DNA (i.e., a reduction to levels below 10^5 to 10^6 virions/mL) in ~30% of patients, with a concomitant improvement in liver histology. Seroconversion from HBeAg to anti-HBe occurs in approximately 20%, and, in early trials, approximately 8% lost hepatitis B surface antigen (HBsAg). Successful interferon therapy and seroconversion are often accompanied by an acute hepatitis-like elevation in aminotransferase activity, which has been postulated to result from enhanced cytolytic T cell clearance of HBV-infected hepatocytes. Relapse after successful therapy is rare (1 or 2%). The likelihood of responding to IFN is higher in patients with lower levels of HBV DNA and substantial elevations of ALT. Although children can respond as well as adults, IFN therapy has not been effective in very young children infected at birth. Similarly, IFN therapy has not been effective in immunosuppressed persons, Asian patients with minimal-to-mild ALT elevations, or in patients with decompensated chronic hepatitis B (in whom such therapy can actually be detrimental, sometimes precipitating decompensation, often associated with severe adverse effects). Among patients with HBeAg loss during therapy, long-term follow-up has demonstrated that 80% experience eventual loss of HBsAg, i.e., all serologic markers of infection, and normalization of ALT over a 9-year posttreatment period. In addition, improved long-term and complication-free survival as well as a reduction in the frequency of hepatocellular carcinoma have been documented among interferon responders, supporting the conclusion that successful interferon therapy improves the natural history of chronic hepatitis B.

Retreatment of IFN nonresponders with another course of IFN may enhance response rates somewhat; however, currently, most would opt to address IFN nonresponders by offering them one of the newer, oral therapies.

Initial trials of brief-duration IFN therapy in patients with *HBeAg-negative chronic hepatitis B* were disappointing, suppressing HBV replication transiently during therapy but almost never resulting in sustained antiviral responses. In subsequent IFN trials among patients with HBeAg-negative chronic hepatitis B, however, more protracted courses, lasting up to a year and a half, have been reported to result in sustained remissions, with suppressed HBV DNA and aminotransferase activity, in ~20%.

Complications of IFN therapy include systemic "flulike" symptoms, marrow suppression, emotional lability (irritability commonly, depression rarely), autoimmune reactions (especially autoimmune thyroiditis), and miscellaneous side effects such as alopecia, rashes, diarrhea, and numbness and tingling of the extremities. With the possible exception of autoimmune thyroiditis, all these side effects are reversible upon dose lowering or cessation of therapy.

Whether or not IFN remains competitive with the newer generation of antivirals, it did represent the first successful antiviral approach, and it set the standard against which subsequent drugs are measured—the achievement of durable virologic, serologic, biochemical, and histologic responses; consolidation of virologic and biochemical benefit in the ensuing years after therapy; and improvement in the natural history of chronic hepatitis B. Indications for IFN therapy in patients with chronic hepatitis B are summarized in Table 287-4.

In patients with chronic hepatitis B, long-term therapy with glucocorticoids is not only ineffective but also detrimental. Short-term glucocorticoid therapy, however, which increases HBV replication and expression in hepatocytes but depresses cytolytic T cells, has been advocated as a potential antiviral approach. A brief course of glucocorticoids, followed by their abrupt withdrawal, permits steroid therapy–suppressed T cells to resume their function against hepatocytes enriched in HBV expression by the recent burst of steroid exposure. An acute hepatitis-like flare of aminotransferase activity follows and may be accompanied by a dramatic drop, or even loss of, HBV replication. Such glucocorticoid "priming" prior to interferon therapy has not been shown to be more effective than interferon alone and has been abandoned.

Lamivudine Several nucleoside analogues active against HBV are being evaluated and developed. The first of these to be approved, the dideoxynucleoside lamivudine, inhibits reverse transcriptase activity of both HIV and HBV and is a potent and effective agent for patients with chronic hepatitis B. Lamivudine suppresses HBV DNA by a median of four orders of magnitude at oral daily doses of 100 mg. In clinical trials, lamivudine therapy for 12 months was associated with almost universal suppression of HBV DNA detectable by hybridization assays; loss of HBeAg in 32 to 33%; HBeAg seroconversion (i.e., conversion from HBeAg-reactive to anti-HBe-reactive) in 16 to 20%;

normalization of ALT in approximately 40%; improvement in histology in over 50%; retardation in fibrosis in 20 to 30%; and prevention of progresstion to cirrhosis. HBeAg responses can occur even in subgroups who are resistant (e.g., those with high-level HBV DNA), or who failed in the past to respond, to IFN. As is true for IFN therapy of chronic hepatitis B, patients with near-normal ALT activity do not experience HBeAg responses (despite suppression of HBV DNA), and those with ALT levels exceeding five times the upper limit of normal can expect 1-year HBeAg seroconversion rates of 50 to 60%. Generally, HBeAg seroconversions are confined to patients who achieve suppression of HBV DNA to <10^4 genomes/mL. Among patients who undergo HBeAg responses during therapy, the response is sustained in the vast majority (~70 to 80%) for 4 to 6 months after cessation of therapy; therefore, the achievement of an HBeAg response represents a viable stopping point in therapy. Moreover, for patients with such several-month-sustained HBeAg responses, the durability of these responses over the next 2 years (the limit of follow-up monitoring in current trials) is ~80%, accompanied, at least in western patients, by a >20% HBsAg seroconversion rate, comparable to that seen at 2 years after IFN-induced HBeAg responses. If HBeAg is unaffected by lamivudine therapy, the current approach is to continue therapy until an HBeAg response occurs, but long-term therapy may be required to suppress HBV replication and, in turn, limit liver injury. Preliminary observations indicate that HBeAg seroconversions can increase to a level of 50% after 5 years of therapy. Histologic improvement continues to accrue with therapy beyond the first year; after a cumulative course of 3 years of lamivudine therapy, necroinflammatory activity is reduced in the majority of patients, and cirrhosis has been shown to regress to precirrhotic stages.

Losses of HBsAg have been few during the first year of lamivudine therapy, and this observation had been cited as an advantage of IFN over lamivudine; however, in head-to-head comparisons between IFN and lamivudine monotherapy, HBsAg losses were rare in both groups. Trials in which lamivudine and interferon were administered in combination failed to show a benefit of combination therapy over lamivudine monotherapy for either treatment-naive patients or prior interferon nonresponders; however, trials are currently underway to assess the potential value of combination lamivudine plus long-active pegylated IFN (developed for treatment of chronic hepatitis C, see below).

In patients with *HBeAg-negative chronic hepatitis B*, i.e., in those with precore and core-promoter HBV mutations, 1 year of lamivudine therapy results in HBV DNA suppression and normalization of ALT in three-quarters of patients and in histologic improvement in approximately two-thirds. Therapy has been shown to suppress HBV DNA to undetectable levels in 39%, as measured by sensitive polymerase chain reaction (PCR) amplification assays. Lacking HBeAg at the outset, patients with HBeAg-negative chronic hepatitis B cannot achieve an HBeAg response—a stopping point in HBeAg-reactive patients; invariably, when therapy is discontinued, reactivation is the rule. Therefore, these patients require long-term therapy; with successive years, the proportion with suppressed HBV DNA and normal ALT increases.

Clinical and laboratory side effects of lamivudine are negligible, indistinguishable from those observed in placebo recipients. During lamivudine therapy, transient ALT elevations, resembling those seen during IFN therapy and during spontaneous HBeAg-to-anti-HBe seroconversions, occur in a quarter of patients. These ALT elevations may result from restored cytolytic T cell activation permitted by suppression of HBV replication. Similar ALT elevations, however, occur at an identical frequency in placebo recipients, but ALT elevations associated with HBeAg seroconversion are confined to lamivudine-treated patients. When therapy is stopped after a year of therapy, two- to threefold ALT elevations occur in 20 to 30% of lamivudine-treated patients, representing renewed liver-cell injury as HBV replication returns. Although these posttreatment flares are almost always transient and mild, rare severe exacerbations, especially in cirrhotic patients,

TABLE 287-4 *Patients with Chronic Hepatitis B Who Are Candidates for Antiviral Therapy*

Clinical Feature	Interferon	Lamivudine	Adefovir
Detectable markers of HBV replication	Yes	Yes	Yes
Normal ALT activity	No	No	No
ALT <2 × upper limit of normal	No	No	No
ALT >2 × upper limit of normal	Yes	Yes	Yes
Immunocompetent	Yes	Yes	Yes
Immunocompromised	No	Yes	Yes
Adult acquisition (western)	Yes	Yes	Yes
Childhood acquisition (Asian)	No	Yes	Yes
Compensated liver disease	Yes	Yes	Yes
Decompensated liver disease	No	Yes	Yes
"Wild-type" HBeAg-reactive	Yes	Yes	Yes
HBeAg-negative chronic hepatitis	Yes	Yes	Yes
Interferon-refractory	No	Yes	Yes

Note: HBV, hepatitis B virus; ALT, alanine aminotransferase; HBeAg, hepatitis B e antigen.

have been observed, mandating close and careful clinical and virologic monitoring after discontinuation of treatment.

Long-term monotherapy with lamivudine is associated with methionine-to-valine or methionine-to-isoleucine mutations in the YMDD (tyrosine-methionine-aspartate-aspartate) motif of HBV DNA polymerase, analogous to mutations that occur in patients with HIV infection treated with this drug. During a year of therapy, YMDD mutations occur in 15 to 30% of patients; the frequency increases with each year of therapy, reaching 70% at year 5. Although transient elevations in ALT and HBV DNA levels occur when such variants emerge, YMDD-variant HBV appears to be less replicatively competent and a less robust pathogen. Even after YMDD mutations occur, HBV DNA and ALT levels as well as histologic scores tend to remain lower than baseline levels in immunocompetent patients. In immunosuppressed patients, a proportion of patients with YMDD mutations experience hepatic decompensation. Even in immunocompetent persons, ultimately, after 2 to 3 years, YMDD-variant HBV leads to a deterioration in histology. Therefore, if therapy is begun with lamivudine monotherapy, the emergence of a YMDD variant, reflected clinically by a breakthrough from suppressed levels of HBV DNA and ALT, is managed by adding another antiviral to which YMDD variants are sensitive (e.g., adefovir, see below).

Because lamivudine monotherapy can result universally in the rapid emergence of YMDD variants in persons with HIV infection, patients with chronic hepatitis B should be tested for anti-HIV prior to therapy; if HIV infection is identified, lamivudine monotherapy at the HBV daily dose of 100 mg is contraindicated. These patients should be treated with triple-drug antiretroviral therapy, including a lamivudine daily dose of 300 mg (Chap. 173). The safety of lamivudine during pregnancy has not been established.

Adefovir Dipivoxil The acyclic nucleotide analogue adefovir dipivoxil, the prodrug of adevovir, is a potent antiviral that, at an oral daily dose of 10 mg, reduces HBV DNA by approximately 3.5 to 4 logs and is equally effective in treatment-naïve patients and IFN nonresponders. In HBeAg-reactive chronic hepatitis B, a 48-week course of adefovir dipivoxil was shown to achieve histologic improvement (and reduce the progression of fibrosis) and normalization of ALT in half the patients, HBeAg seroconversion in 12%, HBeAg loss in 23%, and suppression to an undetectable level of HBV DNA in 21%, as measured by PCR. Similar to IFN and lamivudine, adefovir dipivoxil is more likely to achieve an HBeAg response in patients with high baseline ALT; for example, among adefovir-treated patients with ALT level >5 times the upper limit of normal, HBeAg seroconversions occurred in 25%. Although the durability of adefovir-induced HBeAg responses remains to be documented, expectations are that they will be as durable as those seen during lamivudine therapy and that HBeAg responses can be relied upon as a stopping point for adefovir therapy.

In patients with *HBeAg-negative chronic hepatitis B*, a 48-week course of 10 mg/d of adefovir dipivoxil resulted in histologic improvement in two-thirds, normalization of ALT in three-quarters, and suppression of HBV DNA to PCR-undetectable levels in half. As was true for lamivudine, because HBeAg responses—a potential stopping point—cannot be achieved in this group, reactivation is the rule when adefovir therapy is discontinued, and indefinite, long-term therapy is anticipated.

Adevofir contains a flexible acyclic linker instead of the L-nucleoside ring of lamivudine, avoiding steric hindrance by mutated amino acids. In addition, the molecular structure of phosphorylated adefovir is very similar to that of its natural substrate; therefore mutations to adefovir would also affect binding of the natural substrate, dATP. Hypothetically, these are among the reasons that resistance to adefovir dipivoxil has not been encountered in 1 year of clinical-trial therapy and in only 2.5% after 2 years of therapy, in both immunocompetent and immunocompromised patients. Among patients co-infected with HBV and HIV and who have normal CD4+ T cell counts, adefovir

dipivoxil is effective in suppressing HBV dramatically (in one study, by 5 logs). Moreover, adefovir dipivoxil is effective in lamivudine-associated YMDD-variant HBV and can be used when such lamivudine-induced variants emerge. When, in the past, this drug had been evaluated as therapy for HIV infection, doses of 60 to 120 mg were required to suppress HIV, and at these doses, the drug was nephrotoxic. Even at 30 mg/d, creatinine elevations of 44 μmol/L (0.5 mg/dL) occur in 10% of patients; however, at the HBV-effective dose of 10 mg, such elevations of creatinine are rarely encountered. If any nephrotoxicity does occur, it rarely appears before 6 to 8 months of therapy. Although renal tubular injury is a rare potential side effect, and although creatinine monitoring is recommended during treatment, the therapeutic index of adefovir dipivoxil is high, and the nephrotoxicity observed in clinical trials at higher doses was reversible. For patients with underlying renal disease, adefovir dipivoxil dose reductions are recommended: administration reduced to every 48 h for creatinine clearances of 20 to 49 mL/min, to every 72 h for creatinine clearances of 10 to 19 mL/min, and once a week, following dialysis, for patients undergoing hemodialysis. Adevofir dipivoxil is very well tolerated, and ALT elevations during and after withdrawal of therapy are similar to those observed and described above in clinical trials of lamivudine.

No treatment is recommended or available for inactive "nonreplicative" hepatitis B carriers. For patients with ALT levels less than twice the upper limit of normal, in whom sustained responses are not likely and who would require multiyear therapy, antiviral therapy is not currently recommended. For patients with ALT more than twice the upper limit, any one of the three available drugs is recommended, but in patients with HBeAg-negative chronic hepatitis B, the requirement for indefinite-duration therapy favors a drug such as adefovir dipivoxil, which is complicated only rarely by the emergence of resistance. Either lamivudine or adefovir is recommended for interferon-refractory patients. Whereas patients with decompensated chronic hepatitis B are not candidates for IFN therapy, they may respond to lamivudine or adefovir dipivoxil, with reversal of the signs of decompensation. Table 287-4 summarizes indications for antiviral therapy in patients with chronic hepatitis B. Interferon, lamivudine, and adefovir can each be used as first-line therapy (Table 287-5). Interferon requires only brief-duration therapy, too limited in duration to support viral variants, but requires subcutaneous injections and is associated with a high level of intolerability. Lamivudine requires long-term therapy in most patients and, when used alone, fosters the emergence of viral variants. On the other hand, lamivudine is taken orally, is very well tolerated, leads to improved histology even in the absence of HBeAg responses, and is effective even in patients who fail to respond to interferon. Adefovir, like lamivudine, is taken orally, is well tolerated, and is effective in IFN nonresponders. Its major advantage is the near absence of resistance. Although the drug is safe, creatinine monitoring is recommended. Although some prefer to begin with IFN, most physicians and patients prefer lamivudine or adefovir as first-line therapy.

For patients with end-stage chronic hepatitis B, liver transplantation is the only potential lifesaving intervention. In the absence of antiviral therapy, reinfection of the new liver is almost universal; however, the likelihood of liver injury associated with hepatitis B in the new liver is variable. The majority of patients become high-level viremic carriers with minimal liver injury. Unfortunately, an unpredictable proportion experience severe hepatitis B–related liver injury, sometimes a fulminant-like hepatitis, sometimes a rapid recapitulation of the original severe chronic hepatitis B (Chap. 291). Prevention of recurrent hepatitis B after liver transplantation has been achieved by *prophylaxis* with hepatitis B immune globulin and with the nucleoside analogues lamivudine and adefovir; in addition, nucleoside analogues have been used successfully to *reverse* posttransplantation liver injury associated with recurrent hepatitis B (Chap. 291).

Novel Antivirals and Strategies In addition to the three approved antiviral drugs for hepatitis B, several others are being evaluated in clinical trials, as listed in Table 287-6. Preliminary indications are that entecavir and is telbivudine can reduce HBV DNA levels by five and six logs, respectively, and that entecavir and is active against lamivudine-associated YMDD variants. Tenofovir, similar to adefovir, was developed for HIV infection but appears to have activity against wild-type and YMDD-variant HBV similar to that of adefovir; however, to date, it has not been studied extensively in patients with HBV infection.

Initial emphasis in the development of antiviral therapy for hepatitis B was placed on monotherapy; however, in the future, combination therapies will be studied. If combination therapies reduce HBV replication more substantially than monotherapies and avoid resistance, combination therapy regimens will become the norm.

Chronic Hepatitis D (Delta Hepatitis) The clinical and laboratory features of chronic hepatitis D virus (HDV) infection are summarized in Chap. 285. Chronic hepatitis D may follow acute co-infection with HBV but at a rate no higher than the rate of chronicity of hepatitis B. That is, although HDV co-infection can increase the severity of acute hepatitis B, HDV does not increase the likelihood of progression to chronic hepatitis B. However, when HDV superinfection occurs in a person who is already chronically infected with HBV, long-term HDV infection is the rule and a worsening of the liver disease the expected consequence. Except for severity, chronic hepatitis B plus D has similar clinical and laboratory features to those seen in chronic hepatitis B alone. Relatively severe chronic hepatitis, with or without cirrhosis, is the rule, and mild chronic hepatitis the exception. Occasionally, mild hepatitis, or even, rarely, inactive carriage, occurs in patients with chronic hepatitis B plus D, and recent observations suggest that the disease may become indolent after several years of infection. A distinguishing serologic feature of chronic hepatitis D is the presence in the circulation of antibodies to liver-kidney microsomes (anti-LKM); however, the anti-LKM seen in hepatitis D are designated anti-LKM3, are directed against uridine diphosphate glucuronosyltransferase, and are distinct from anti-LKM1 seen in patients with autoimmune hepatitis and in a subset of patients with chronic hepatitis C (see below).

Rx TREATMENT

Management is not well defined. Glucocorticoids are ineffective and are not used. Preliminary experimental trials of IFN-α suggested that conventional doses and durations of therapy lower levels of HDV RNA and aminotransferase activity only transiently during treatment but have no impact on the natural history of the disease. Although high-dose IFN-α (9 million units) three times a week for 12 months may be associated with a sustained loss of HDV replication and clinical improvement in up to 50% of patients, ultimately recurrent HDV replication becomes universal after cessation of therapy. Antiviral therapy for chronic hepatitis D remains the subject of experimental trials; lamivudine is not effective, but preliminary indications are that clevudine (L-FMAU) may be. In patients with end-stage liver disease secondary to chronic hepatitis D, liver transplantation has been effective. If hepatitis D recurs in the new liver without the expression of hepatitis B (an unusual serologic profile in immunocompetent persons,

TABLE 287-5 *Comparison of Interferon, Lamivudine, and Adefovir Dipivoxil Therapy for Chronic Hepatitis B[a]*

Feature	Interferon	Lamivudine	Adefovir
Route of administration	Injection	Oral	Oral
Duration of therapy[b]	4 months	≥52 weeks	≥48 weeks
Tolerability	Poorly tolerated	Well tolerated	Well tolerated
Nephrotoxicity	None	None	Creatinine monitoring recommended
HBeAg loss	33%	32–33%	23%
HBeAg seroconversion	18–20%	16–20%	12%
HBeAg seroconversion if ALT >5 × normal	Not reported	>50%	21%
Log$_{10}$ HBV DNA reduction	?	4	3.5–4
HBV DNA PCR-negative	Unlikely	~30% HBeAg+ 39% HBeAg−	21% HBeAg+ 51% HBeAg−
ALT normalization	Confined to HBeAg responders	>40% HBeAg+ >70% HBeAg−	50% HBeAg+ 72% HBeAg−
HBsAg loss during Rx	3–8%	2–4%	Unlikely
HBsAg loss after Rx	80% over 9 years	23% over 2 years	To be determined
Histologic improvement	Confined to HBeAg responders	>50% HBeAg+ >66% HBeAg−	>50% HBeAg+ >66% HBeAg−
Retardation of fibrosis	Not demonstrated	20–30%	20–30%
Viral resistance	None	15–30% @ 1 year 70% @ 5 years	None @ 1 year 2.5% @ 2 years
Natural history	Reduced mortality, decompensation, HCC	To be determined	To be determined
HBeAg-negative chronic hepatitis B	~20% sustained response after ≥1 year of Rx	>60–70% virologic and histologic response; relapse likely after Rx	Same as lamivudine
Candidate range[c]	Narrow	Broad	Broad
Cost (U.S. $)	~$5000/4 months	~$1700/year	~$5600/year

[a] Generally, these comparisons are based upon data on each drug tested individually versus placebo in registration clinical trials; because, with rare exception, these comparisons are not based on head-to-head testing of these drugs, relative advantages and disadvantages should be interpreted cautiously

[b] Duration of therapy in clinical efficacy trials; use in clinical practice may vary.

[c] See Table 287-4.

Note: HBeAg, hepatitis B e antigen; ALT, alanine aminotranferase; HBV, hepatitis B virus; PCR, polymerase chain reaction; HBsAg, hepatitis B surface antigen; HCC, hepatocellular carcinoma.

but common in transplant patients), liver injury is limited. In fact, the outcome of transplantation for chronic hepatitis D is superior to that for chronic hepatitis B (Chap. 291).

Chronic Hepatitis C Regardless of the epidemiologic mode of acquisition of hepatitis C virus (HCV) infection, chronic hepatitis follows acute hepatitis C in 50 to 70% of cases; even in those with a return to normal in aminotransferase levels after acute hepatitis C, chronic infection is common, adding up to an 85 to 90% likelihood of chronic HCV infection after acute hepatitis C. Furthermore, in patients with chronic transfusion-associated hepatitis followed for 10 to 20 years, progression to cirrhosis occurs in about 20%. Such is the case even for patients with relatively clinically mild chronic hepatitis, including those without symptoms, with only modest elevations of aminotransferase activity, and with mild chronic hepatitis on liver biopsy. Even in cohorts of well-compensated patients with chronic hepatitis C referred for clinical research trials (no complications of chronic liver

TABLE 287-6 *New Antiviral Drugs Being Developed for the Treatment of Chronic Hepatitis B*

Entecavir[a]
Telbivudine (L-dT)
Clevudine (L-FMAU)
Emtricitabine (FTC)
Pegylated alpha interferons

[a] Reported to have activity against lamivudine-associated YMDD-variant HBV.

Note: YMDD, tyrosine-methionine-aspartate-aspartate.

disease and with normal hepatic synthetic function), the prevalence of cirrhosis may be as high as 50%. Many cases of hepatitis C are identified in asymptomatic patients who have no history of acute hepatitis C, e.g., those discovered while attempting to donate blood or as a result of routine laboratory screening tests. The source of HCV infection in most of these cases is not defined, although a long-forgotten percutaneous exposure in the remote past can be elicited in a substantial proportion. Approximately a third of patients with chronic hepatitis C have normal or near-normal aminotransferase activity; although a third to a half of these patients have chronic hepatitis on liver biopsy, the grade of liver injury and stage of fibrosis tend to be mild in the vast majority. In some cases, more severe liver injury has been reported, even, rarely, cirrhosis, most likely the result of previous histologic activity. Among patients with persistent normal aminotransferase activity sustained over ≥5 years, histologic progression has been shown not to occur; however, approximately a quarter of patients with normal aminotransferase activity experience subsequent aminotransferase elevations, and histologic injury can be progressive once abnormal biochemical activity resumes. Therefore, continued clinical monitoring is indicated, even for patients with normal aminotransferase activity.

Despite this substantial rate of progression of chronic hepatitis C, and despite the fact that liver failure can result from end-stage chronic hepatitis C, the long-term prognosis for chronic hepatitis C in a majority of patients is relatively benign. Mortality over 10 to 20 years among patients with transfusion-associated chronic hepatitis C has been shown not to differ from mortality in a matched population of transfused patients in whom hepatitis C did not develop. Although death in the hepatitis group is more likely to result from liver failure, and although hepatic decompensation may occur in ~15% of such patients over the course of a decade, the majority (almost 60%) of patients remain asymptomatic and well compensated, with no clinical sequelae of chronic liver disease. Overall, then, chronic hepatitis C tends to be very slowly and insidiously progressive, if at all, in the vast majority of patients, while in approximately a quarter of cases, chronic hepatitis C will progress eventually to end-stage cirrhosis. Referral bias may account for the more severe outcomes described in cohorts of patients reported from tertiary-care centers versus the more benign outcomes in cohorts of patients monitored from initial blood-product-associated acute hepatitis. Still unexplained, however, are the wide ranges in reported progression to cirrhosis, from 2% over 17 years in a population of women with hepatitis C infection acquired from contaminated anti-D immune globulin to 30% over ≤11 years in recipients of contaminated intravenous immune globulin.

Progression of liver disease in patients with chronic hepatitis C has been reported to be more likely in patients with older age, longer duration of infection, advanced histologic stage and grade, genotype 1, more complex quasispecies diversity, and increased hepatic iron. Among these variables, however, duration of infection appears to be the most important, and many of the others probably reflect disease duration to some extent (e.g., quasispecies diversity, hepatic iron accumulation).

Perhaps the best prognostic indicator in chronic hepatitis C is liver histology. Patients with mild necrosis and inflammation as well as those with limited fibrosis have an excellent prognosis and limited progression to cirrhosis. In contrast, among patients with moderate to severe necroinflammatory activity or fibrosis, including septal or bridging fibrosis, progression to cirrhosis is highly likely over the course of 10 to 20 years. Among patients with compensated cirrhosis associated with hepatitis C, the 10-year survival is close to 80%; mortality occurs at a rate of 2 to 6% per year, decompensation at a rate of 4 to 5% per year, and hepatocellular carcinoma at a rate of 1 to 4% per year.

In addition, severity of chronic hepatitis is greater and progression of chronic liver disease is more accelerated in patients who have chronic hepatitis C as well as other liver processes, including alcoholic liver disease, chronic hepatitis B, HIV infection, hemochromatosis, and α_1-antitrypsin deficiency. No other epidemiologic or clinical features of chronic hepatitis C (e.g., severity of acute hepatitis, level of aminotransferase activity, level of HCV RNA, presence or absence of jaundice during acute hepatitis) are predictive of eventual outcome. Despite the relative benignity of chronic hepatitis C over time, cirrhosis following chronic hepatitis C has been associated with the late development, after several decades, of hepatocellular carcinoma (HCC) (Chap. 78). As noted above, the annual rate of HCC in cirrhotic patients with hepatitis C is 1 to 4%.

Clinical features of chronic hepatitis C are similar to those described above for chronic hepatitis B. Generally, *fatigue* is the most common symptom; jaundice is rare. Immune complex–mediated extrahepatic complications of chronic hepatitis C are less common than in chronic hepatitis B, with the exception of essential mixed cryoglobulinemia (Chap. 285). This is the case despite the fact that assays for immune complex–like activity are often positive in patients with chronic hepatitis C. In addition, chronic hepatitis C has been associated with extrahepatic complications unrelated to immune-complex injury. These include Sjögren's syndrome, lichen planus, and porphyria cutanea tarda. *Laboratory features* of chronic hepatitis C are similar to those in patients with chronic hepatitis B, but aminotransferase levels tend to fluctuate more (the characteristic episodic pattern of aminotransferase activity) and to be lower, especially in patients with long-standing disease. An interesting and occasionally confusing finding in patients with chronic hepatitis C is the presence of autoantibodies. Rarely, patients with autoimmune hepatitis (see below) and hyperglobulinemia have false-positive enzyme immunoassays for anti-HCV. On the other hand, some patients with serologically confirmable chronic hepatitis C have circulating anti-LKM. These antibodies are anti-LKM1, as seen in patients with autoimmune hepatitis *type 2* (see below), and are directed against a 33-amino-acid sequence of P450 IID6. The occurrence of anti-LKM1 in some patients with chronic hepatitis C may result from the partial sequence homology between the epitope recognized by anti-LKM1 and two segments of the HCV polyprotein. In addition, the presence of this autoantibody in some patients with chronic hepatitis C suggests that autoimmunity may be playing a role in the pathogenesis of chronic hepatitis C. →*Histopathologic features of chronic hepatitis C, especially those that distinguish hepatitis C from hepatitis B, are described in Chap. 285.*

℞ TREATMENT

Therapy for chronic hepatitis C has evolved substantially in the decade and a half since IFN-α was introduced for this indication. When first approved, IFN-α was administered via subcutaneous injection three times a week for 6 months but achieved a sustained virologic response (a reduction of HCV RNA to undetectable levels by PCR when measured ≥6 months after completion of therapy) below 10%. Doubling the duration of therapy—but not increasing the dose or changing IFN preparations—increased the sustained virologic response rate to ~20%, and addition to the regimen of daily ribavirin, an oral guanosine nucleoside, increased sustained virologic responses to 40%. When used alone, ribavirin is ineffective and does not reduce HCV RNA levels, but ribavirin enhances the efficacy of IFN by reducing the likelihood of virologic relapse after the achievement of an end-treatment response (response measured during, and maintained to the end of, treatment). Proposed mechanisms to explain the role of ribavirin include subtle direct reduction of HCV replication, immune modulation, and induction of virologic mutational catastrophe.

Many important lessons about antiviral therapy for chronic hepatitis C were learned from the experience with IFN monotherapy and combination IFN-ribavirin therapy. Even in the absence of biochemical and virologic responses, histologic improvement occurs in approximately three-quarters of all treated patients. Unlike the case in hepatitis B, in chronic hepatitis C, responses to therapy are not accompanied by transient, acute hepatitis–like aminotransferase elevations; instead, ALT levels fall precipitously during therapy. Up to 90% of virologic responses are achieved within the first 12 weeks of therapy; responses thereafter are rare. Sustained virologic responses are very durable; normal ALT, improved histology, and absence of HCV RNA in serum and liver have been documented 5 to 6 years after successful therapy, and "relapses" 2 years after sustained responses are almost unheard of. Thus, sustained virologic responses to antiviral therapy of chronic hepatitis C are tantamount to cures.

Patient variables that tend to correlate with sustained virologic responsiveness to IFN include low baseline HCV RNA level (<2 million copies/mL), histologically mild hepatitis and minimal fibrosis, favorable genotype (genotypes 2 and 3 as opposed to genotyptes 1 and 4), age <40, absence of obesity, and female gender. Patients with cirrhosis can respond, but they are less likely to do so. Studies of combination IFN-ribavirin therapy showed conclusively that, in patients with genotype 1, therapy should last a full year, while in those with genotypes 2 and 3, a 6-month course of therapy suffices. The response rate in African Americans is disappointingly low for reasons that remain obscure. Finally, the likelihood of a sustained response is best if adherence to the treatment regimen is high, i.e., if patients receive ≥80% of the IFN and ribavirin doses, and if they continue treatment for ≥80% of the anticipated duration of therapy. Other variables reported to correlate with increased responsiveness include brief duration of infection, low HCV quasispecies diversity, immunocompetence, and low liver iron levels. High levels of HCV RNA, more histologically advanced liver disease, and high quasispecies diversity all go hand in hand with advanced duration of infection, which may be the single most important variable determining IFN responsiveness. The ironic fact, then, is that patients whose disease is *least* likely to progress are the ones *most* likely to respond to interferon and vice versa. Finally, among patients with genotype 1b, responsiveness to IFN is enhanced in those with amino-acid-substitution mutations in the nonstructural protein 5A gene.

Side effects of IFN therapy are described above in the section on treatment of chronic hepatitis B. The most pronounced side effect of ribavirin therapy is hemolysis; a reduction in hemoglobin of up to 2 to 3 g or in hematocrit of 5 to 10% can be anticipated. A small, unpredictable proportion of patients experience profound, brisk hemolysis, resulting in symptomatic anemia; therefore, close monitoring of blood counts is crucial, and ribavirin should be avoided in patients with anemia or hemoglobinopathies and in patients with coronary artery disease or cerebrovascular disease, in whom anemia can precipitate an ischemic event. When symptomatic anemia occurs, ribavirin dose reductions or addition of erythropoietin to boost red blood cell levels may be required. In addition, ribavirin, which is renally excreted, should not be used in patients with renal insufficiency; the drug is teratogenic, precluding its use during pregnancy and mandating the use of efficient contraception during therapy.

Ribavirin can also cause nasal and chest congestion, pruritus, and precipitation of gout. Combination IFN-ribavirin therapy is more difficult to tolerate than IFN monotherapy. In one large clinical trial of combination therapy versus monotherapy, among those in the 1-year treatment group, 21% of the combination group (but only 14% of the monotherapy group) had to discontinue treatment, while 26% of the combination group (but only 9% of the monotherapy group) required dose reductions.

Studies of viral kinetics have shown that despite a virion half-life in serum of only 2 to 3 h, the level of HCV is maintained by a high replication rate of 10^{12} hepatitis C virions per day. IFN-α blocks virion production or release with an efficacy that increases with increasing drug doses; moreover, the calculated death rate for infected cells during IFN therapy is inversely related to viral load; patients with the most rapid death rate of infected hepatocytes are more likely to achieve undetectable HCV RNA at 3 months; achieving this landmark is predictive of a subsequent sustained response. Therefore, to achieve rapid viral clearance from serum and the liver, *high-dose induction therapy* has been advocated. In practice, however, high-dose induction therapy has not yielded higher sustained response rates.

Treatment of Choice For the treatment of chronic hepatitis C, standard IFNs have now been supplanted by "pegylated" IFNs, long-acting IFNs bound to polyethylene glycol (PEG). Such pegylated IFNs have elimination times up to sevenfold longer than standard IFNs, i.e., a substantially longer half-life, and achieve prolonged concentrations, permitting administration once, rather than three times, a week. Instead of the frequent drug peaks (linked to side effects) and troughs (when drug is absent) associated with frequent administration of short-acting IFNs, administration of pegylated IFNs results in drug concentrations that are more stable and sustained over time. Early studies showed that once-a-week pegylated IFN monotherapy is twice as effective as monotherapy with its standard IFN counterpart, approaches the efficacy of combination standard IFN plus ribavirin, and is as well tolerated as standard IFNs, without more difficult-to-manage thrombocytopenia and leukopenia than standard IFNs. The current standard of care, however, is a combination of pegylated IFN plus ribavirin.

Two pegylated IFNs are available, pegylated IFN-α2b and -α2a. In the registration trial for pegylated IFN-α2b plus ribavirin, the best regimen was 48 weeks of 1.5 μg per kilogram of pegylated IFN once a week plus 800 mg of ribavirin daily. A posthoc analysis suggested that weight-based dosing of ribavirin would have been more effective than the fixed 800-mg dose used in the study. In the first registration trial for pegylated IFN-α2a plus ribavirin, the best regimen was 48 weeks of 180 μg of pegylated IFN plus 1000 mg (for patients < 75 kg) to 1200 mg (for patients ≥ 75 kg) of ribavirin. Sustained virologic responses of 54% and 56% were reported in these two studies, respectively. A subsequent study of pegylated IFN-α2a plus ribavirin showed that, for patients with genotypes 2 and 3, a duration of 6 months and a ribavirin dose of 800 mg was sufficient. Among the three studies, for patients in the optimal treatment arm, sustained response rates for patients with genotype 1 were 42 to 51%, and for patients with genotypes 2 and 3 rates were 76 to 82%.

In the initial registration trials for combination pegylated IFN plus ribavirin, both combination pegylated IFN regimens were compared to standard IFN-α2b plus ribavirin. Side effects of the combination pegylated IFN-α2b regimen were comparable to those for the combination standard-IFN regimen; however, when the combination pegylated IFN-α2a regimen was compared to the combination standard IFN-α2b regimen, flulike symptoms and depression were less common in the combination pegylated IFN group. Although the two combination pegylated IFN regimens were not tested head-to-head, when each was tested against standard IFN-α2b plus ribavirin, combination pegylated IFN-α2a plus ribavirin appeared to be better tolerated. Recommended doses for the two pegylated IFNs plus ribavirin and other comparisons between the two therapies are shown in Table 287-7.

Unless ribavirin is contraindicated (see above), combination pegylated IFN plus ribavirin is the recommended course of therapy—24 weeks for genotypes 2 and 3 and 48 weeks for genotype 1. Measurement of quantitative HCV RNA levels at 12 weeks is helpful in guiding therapy; if a 2-log drop in HCV RNA has not been achieved by this time, chances for a sustained virologic response are negligible. If the goal of therapy is sustained virologic response, failure to achieve a 12-week 2-log drop in HCV RNA may be used as a signal to discontinue therapy, especially in those who do not tolerate the drugs well. Still, conceivably, some may achieve histologic benefit in the absence of a virologic response, and some clinicians choose to continue therapy even in the absence of a 2-log HCV RNA reduction at 12 weeks. Studies are underway to determine whether, even in the absence of a virologic response, maintenance therapy with pegylated IFN can slow histologic and clinical progression of hepatitis C.

Indications for Antiviral Therapy Patients with chronic hepatitis C who have elevated ALT levels, detectable HCV RNA, and chronic hepatitis of at least moderate grade and stage (portal or bridging fibrosis) are

TABLE 287-7

TABLE 287-7 *Comparison of Pegylated Interferon α2a and α2b for Chronic Hepatitis C*[a]

	PEG IFN-α2b	PEG IFN-α2a
PEG size	12 kDa linear	40 kDa branched
Mean terminal half-life	40 h	80 h
Mean clearance	94 mL/h per kg	22 mL/h per kg
Best-dose monotherapy	1.0 μg/kg (weight-based)	180 μg
Best-dose combination therapy	1.5 μg/kg (weight-based)	180 μg
Storage	Room temperature	Refrigerated
Ribavirin		
Genotype 1	800 mg[b]	1000–1200 mg[c]
Genotype 2/3	800 mg	800 mg
Duration of therapy		
Genotype 1	48 weeks	48 weeks
Genotype 2/3	48 weeks[d]	24 weeks
Efficacy of combination Rx	54%	56%
Genotype 1	42%	46–51%
Genotype 2/3	82%	76–78%
Side effects of pegylated interferon/ribavirin vs standard interferon/ribavirin[e]		
Fever	46% vs 33%	43% vs 56%
Myalgias	56% vs 50%	42% vs 50%
Rigors	48% vs 41%	24% vs 35%
Depression	31% vs 34%	22% vs 30%
Irritability	35% vs 34%	24% vs 28%

[a] These comparisons are based upon data on each drug tested individually versus other regimens in registration trials; because these comparisons are not based on head-to-head comparisons between the two drugs, and because the populations tested are not entirely analogous, relative advantages and disadvantages should be interpreted with caution.

[b] In the registration trial for pegylated IFN-α2b plus ribavirin, the optimal regimen was 1.5 μg of pegylated IFN plus 800 mg of ribavirin; however, a posthoc analysis of this study as well as data from other studies suggest that 1000 (for patients < 75 kg)–1200 (for patients ≥ 75 kg) mg of ribavirin might be better, certainly for genotype 1, and many clinicians prescribe the higher ribavirin doses.

[c] 1000 mg for patients < 75 kg; 1200 mg for patients ≥ 75 kg.

[d] In the registration trial for pegylated IFN-α2b plus ribavirin, all patients were treated for 48 weeks; however, data from other trials of standard IFNs and the other pegylated IFN suggest that 24 weeks should suffice for patients with genotypes 2 and 3.

[e] These comparisons show the frequency in registration trials of the listed side effects for the respective pegylated IFN plus ribavirin as compared to the listed side effects in comparitor groups who received standard IFN-α2b plus ribavirin. As noted above, these comparisons do not represent head-to-head tests of the two pegylated IFNs.

Note: PEG, polyethylene glycol; IFN, interferon.

candidates for antiviral therapy with pegylated IFN plus ribavirin, unless ribavirin is contraindicated (Table 287-8). Therapy with IFN has been shown to improve survival and complication-free survival and to slow progression of fibrosis. Prior to therapy, HCV genotype should be determined, and the genotype dictates the duration of therapy, 1 year (48 weeks) for patients with genotype 1 and 6 months (24 weeks) for those with genotypes 2 and 3. As noted above, the absence of a 2-log drop in HCV RNA at week 12 (an "early virologic response") weighs heavily against the likelihood of a sustained virologic response even if therapy is continued for the remainder of the planned full year; therefore, measuring HCV RNA at baseline and at 12 weeks is recommended routinely, especially for patients with genotype 1. The consensus view is that therapy can be discontinued if an early virologic response is not achieved; however, histologic benefit may occur even in the absence of a virologic response. In addition, if current trials show that maintenance therapy can slow the progression of chronic hepatitis C, early virologic nonresponders may be identified as candidates for maintenance therapy; the results of these trials are awaited. Although response rates are lower in patients with certain pretreatment variables, selection for treatment should not be based on symptoms, genotype, HCV RNA level, mode of acquisition of hepatitis C, or advanced hepatic fibrosis. Patients with cirrhosis can respond and should not be excluded as candidates for therapy.

Patients who have relapsed after a course of IFN monotherapy are candidates for retreatment with pegylated IFN plus ribavirin. For non-

responders to a prior course of IFN monotherapy, retreatment with IFN monotherapy or combination IFN plus ribavirin therapy is unlikely to achieve a sustained virologic response; however, a trial of combination pegylated IFN plus ribavirin may be worthwhile. End-treatment virologic responses as high as 40% can occur in this setting, but a sustained virologic response is the outcome in <20% of patients. Sustained virologic responses to retreatment of nonresponders are

TABLE 287-8 *Indications and Recommendations for Antiviral Therapy of Chronic Hepatitis C*

STANDARD INDICATIONS FOR THERAPY

Elevated ALT activity
Portal/bridging fibrosis or moderate to severe hepatitis on liver biopsy
Detectable HCV RNA

RETREATMENT RECOMMENDED

Relapsers after a previous course of standard IFN monotherapy or combination standard IFN/ribavirin therapy
  A course of pegylated IFN plus ribavirin
Nonresponders to a previous course of standard IFN monotherapy or combination standard IFN/ribavirin therapy
  A course of pegylated IFN plus ribavirin—more likely to achieve a sustained virologic response in Caucasian patients without previous ribavirin therapy, with low baseline HCV RNA levels, with a substantial reduction in HCV RNA during previous therapy, with genotypes 2 and 3, and without reduction in ribavirin dose.

ANTIVIRAL THERAPY NOT RECOMMENDED ROUTINELY BUT MANAGEMENT DECISIONS MADE ON AN INDIVIDUAL BASIS

Children (age <18 years)
Age >60
Normal ALT
Mild hepatitis on liver biopsy
Compensated cirrhosis
Patients with HIV infection and normal CD4+ counts

LONG-TERM MAINTENANCE THERAPY RECOMMENDED

Cutaneous vasculitis and glomerulonephritis associated with chronic hepatitis C

LONG-TERM MAINTENANCE THERAPY BEING ASSESSED IN CLINICAL TRIALS

Relapsers
Nonresponders

ANTIVIRAL THERAPY NOT RECOMMENDED

Decompensated cirrhosis

THERAPEUTIC REGIMENS

First-line treatment: Pegylated IFN subcutaneously once a week plus daily ribavirin orally
  1. HCV genotype 1—48 weeks of therapy
    Pegylated IFN-α2a, 180 μg, plus ribavirin, 1000 mg/d (weight <75 kg) to 1200 mg/d (weight ≥75 kg) *or*
    Pegylated IFN-α2b, 1.5 μg/kg, plus ribavirin, 800 mg/d (although higher, weight-based ribavirin doses above are preferred by many)
  2. HCV genotypes 2 and 3—24 weeks of therapy
    Pegylated IFN-α2a, 180 μg, plus ribavirin, 800 mg/d *or*
    Pegylated IFN-α2b, 1.5 μg/kg, plus ribavirin, 800 mg/d
Alternative regimen: Pegylated IFN (α2a, 180 μg, or α2b, 1.0 μg/kg) subcutaneously once a week (primarily for patients in whom ribavirin is contraindicated or not tolerated) for 24 (genotypes 2 and 3) or 48 (genotype 1) weeks

FEATURES ASSOCIATED WITH REDUCED RESPONSIVENESS

Advanced fibrosis (e.g., cirrhosis)
Long-duration disease
Genotype 1
High-level HCV RNA (>2 million copies/mL)
High HCV quasispecies diversity
Immunosuppression
African American
Obesity
Reduced adherence (lower drug doses and reduced duration of therapy)

Note: ALT, alanine aminotransferase; HCV, hepatitis C virus; IFN, interferon.

more frequent in those who had never received ribavirin in the past, in those with genotypes 2 and 3, in those with low pretreatment HCV RNA levels, but less frequent in African Americans, in those who failed to achieve a substantial reduction in HCV RNA during their previous course of therapy, and in those who required ribavirin-dose reductions.

Early treatment is indicated for persons with acute hepatitis C (Chap. 285). In patients with persistently normal or near-normal ALT levels, long-term monitoring studies have shown the absence of histologic progression, and the same applies to patients with histologically mild hepatitis C; however, patients with normal ALT and histologically mild hepatitis C respond just as well as those with elevated ALT and more histologically severe hepatitis to combination IFN plus ribavirin therapy (and, although not reported yet, probably to combination pegylated IFN plus ribavirin). Therefore, therapy for these patients should be considered and the decision made based upon such factors as patient motivation, genotype, stage of fibrosis, age, and comorbid conditions. A pretreatment liver biopsy is recommended in most cases to assess pretreatment histologic grade and stage.

Patients with compensated cirrhosis can respond to therapy, although their likelihood of a sustained response is lower than in noncirrhotics. Whether survival is improved after successful antiviral therapy in cirrhotics is controversial. Similarly, although several retrospective studies have suggested that antiviral therapy in cirrhotics with chronic hepatitis C reduces the frequency of HCC, less advanced disease in the treated cirrhotics, not treatment itself, may have accounted for the reduced frequency of HCC observed in the treated cohort; prospective studies to address this question are in progress. Patients with decompensated cirrhosis are not candidates for IFN-based antiviral therapy but should be referred for liver transplantation. After liver transplantation, recurrent hepatitis C is the rule, and the pace of disease progression is more accelerated than in immunocompetent patients (Chap. 291); current therapy with pegylated IFN and ribavirin is unsatisfactory in most patients, but attempts to minimize immunosuppression are beneficial. The cutaneous and renal vasculitis of HCV-associated essential mixed cryoglobulinemia (Chap. 285) may respond to antiviral therapy, but sustained responses are rare after discontinuation of therapy; therefore, prolonged, perhaps indefinite, therapy is recommended in this group.

Anecdotal reports suggest that antiviral therapy may be effective in porphyria cutanea tarda or lichen planus associated with hepatitis C. In patients with HCV/HIV co-infection, responses similar to those seen in other groups have been reported in patients with normal CD4+ T cell counts; careful monitoring for side effects of IFN/ribavirin and antiretroviral drugs is advisable. Persons with a history of injection-drug use and alcoholism can be treated successfully for chronic hepatitis C, preferably in conjunction with drug and alcohol treatment programs.

AUTOIMMUNE HEPATITIS ■ Definition Autoimmune hepatitis is a chronic disorder characterized by continuing hepatocellular necrosis and inflammation, usually with fibrosis, which tends to progress to cirrhosis and liver failure. When fulfilling criteria of severity, this type of chronic hepatitis may have a 6-month mortality of as high as 40%. The prominence of extrahepatic features of autoimmunity as well as seroimmunologic abnormalities in this disorder supports an autoimmune process in its pathogenesis; this concept is reflected in the labels "lupoid," plasma cell, or autoimmune hepatitis. Because autoantibodies and other typical features of autoimmunity do not occur in all cases, however, a broader, more appropriate designation for this type of chronic hepatitis is "idiopathic" or cryptogenic. Cases in which hepatotropic viruses, metabolic/genetic derangements, and hepatotoxic drugs have been excluded merit this designation and probably include a spectrum of heterogeneous liver disorders of unknown cause, a proportion of which have characteristic autoimmune features.

Immunopathogenesis The weight of evidence suggests that the progressive liver injury in patients with idiopathic/autoimmune hepatitis is the result of a cell-mediated immunologic attack directed against liver cells; in all likelihood, predisposition to autoimmunity is inherited, while the liver specificity of this injury is triggered by environmental (e.g., chemical or viral) factors. For example, patients have been described in whom apparently self-limited cases of acute hepatitis A or B led to autoimmune hepatitis, presumably because of genetic susceptibility or predisposition. Evidence to support an autoimmune pathogenesis in this type of hepatitis includes the following: (1) In the liver, the histopathologic lesions are composed predominantly of cytotoxic T cells and plasma cells; (2) circulating autoantibodies (nuclear, smooth muscle, thyroid, etc.; see below), rheumatoid factor, and hyperglobulinemia are common; (3) other autoimmune disorders—such as thyroiditis, rheumatoid arthritis, autoimmune hemolytic anemia, ulcerative colitis, proliferative glomerulonephritis, juvenile diabetes mellitus, and Sjögren's syndrome—occur with increased frequency in patients who have autoimmune hepatitis and in their relatives; (4) histocompatibility haplotypes associated with autoimmune diseases, such as HLA-B1, -B8, -DR3, and -DR4, are common in patients with autoimmune hepatitis; and (5) this type of chronic hepatitis is responsive to glucocorticoid/immunosuppressive therapy, effective in a variety of autoimmune disorders.

Cellular immune mechanisms appear to be important in the pathogenesis of autoimmune hepatitis. In vitro studies have suggested that in patients with this disorder, lymphocytes are capable of becoming sensitized to hepatocyte membrane proteins and of destroying liver cells. Abnormalities of immunoregulatory control over cytotoxic lymphocytes (impaired suppressor cell influences) may play a role as well. Studies of genetic predisposition to autoimmune hepatitis demonstrate that certain haplotypes are associated with the disorder, as enumerated above. The precise triggering factors, genetic influences, and cytotoxic and immunoregulatory mechanisms involved in this type of liver injury remain poorly defined.

Intriguing clues into the pathogenesis of autoimmune hepatitis come from the observation that circulating autoantibodies are prevalent in patients with this disorder. Among the autoantibodies described in these patients are antibodies to nuclei [so-called antinuclear antibodies (ANA), primarily in a homogeneous pattern] and smooth muscle (so-called anti-smooth-muscle antibodies, directed at actin), anti-LKM (see below), antibodies to "soluble liver antigen" (directed at a member of the glutathione S-transferase gene family), as well as antibodies to the liver-specific asialoglycoprotein receptor (or "hepatic lectin") and other hepatocyte membrane proteins. Although some of these provide helpful diagnostic markers, their involvement in the pathogenesis of autoimmune hepatitis has not been established.

Humoral immune mechanisms have been shown to play a role in the extrahepatic manifestations of autoimmune/idiopathic hepatitis. Arthralgias, arthritis, cutaneous vasculitis, and glomerulonephritis occurring in patients with autoimmune hepatitis appear to be mediated by the deposition in affected tissue vessels of circulating immune complexes, followed by complement activation, inflammation, and tissue injury. While specific viral antigen-antibody complexes can be identified in acute and chronic viral hepatitis, the nature of the immune complexes in autoimmune hepatitis has not been defined.

Many of the *clinical features* of autoimmune hepatitis are similar to those described for chronic viral hepatitis. The onset of disease may be insidious or abrupt; the disease may present initially like, and be confused with, acute viral hepatitis; a history of recurrent bouts of what had been labeled acute hepatitis is not uncommon. A subset of patients with autoimmune hepatitis has distinct features. Such patients are predominantly young to middle-aged women with marked hyperglobulinemia and high-titer circulating ANA. This is the group with positive LE preparations (initially labeled "lupoid" hepatitis) in whom other autoimmune features are common. Fatigue, malaise, anorexia, amenorrhea, acne, arthralgias, and jaundice are common. Occasionally, arthritis, maculopapular eruptions (including cutaneous vasculitis), erythema nodosum, colitis, pleurisy, pericarditis, anemia, azotemia, and sicca syndrome (keratoconjunctivitis, xerostomia) occur. In some patients, complications of cirrhosis, such as ascites and edema (associated with hypoalbuminemia), encephalopathy, hypersplenism, coagulopathy, or variceal bleeding may bring the patient to initial medical attention.

The course of autoimmune hepatitis may be variable. In those with mild disease or limited histologic lesions (e.g., piecemeal necrosis without bridging), progression to cirrhosis is limited. In those with severe symptomatic autoimmune hepatitis (aminotransferase levels >10 times normal, marked hyperglobulinemia, "aggressive" histologic lesions—bridging necrosis or multilobular collapse, cirrhosis), the 6-month mortality without therapy may be as high as 40%. Such severe disease accounts for only 20% of cases; the natural history of milder disease is variable, often accentuated by spontaneous remissions and exacerbations. Especially poor prognostic signs include multilobular collapse at the time of initial presentation and failure of the bilirubin to improve after 2 weeks of therapy. Death may result from hepatic failure, hepatic coma, other complications of cirrhosis (e.g., variceal hemorrhage), and intercurrent infection. In patients with established cirrhosis, hepatocellular carcinoma may be a late complication (Chap. 78).

Laboratory features of autoimmune hepatitis are similar to those seen in chronic viral hepatitis. Liver biochemical tests are invariably abnormal but may not correlate with the clinical severity or histopathologic features in individual cases. Many patients with autoimmune hepatitis have normal serum bilirubin, alkaline phosphatase, and globulin levels with only minimal aminotransferase elevations. Serum AST and ALT levels are increased and fluctuate in the range of 100 to 1000 units. In severe cases, the serum bilirubin level is moderately elevated [51 to 171 μmol/L (3 to 10 mg/dL)]. Hypoalbuminemia occurs in patients with very active or advanced disease. Serum alkaline phosphatase levels may be moderately elevated or near normal. In a small proportion of patients, marked elevations of alkaline phosphatase activity occur; in such patients, clinical and laboratory features overlap with those of primary biliary cirrhosis (Chap. 289). The prothrombin time is often prolonged, particularly late in the disease or during active phases.

Hypergammaglobulinemia (>2.5 g/dL) is common in autoimmune hepatitis. Rheumatoid factor is common as well. As noted above, circulating autoantibodies are also common. The most characteristic are ANA in a homogeneous staining pattern. Smooth-muscle antibodies are less specific, seen just as frequently in chronic viral hepatitis. Because of the high levels of globulins achieved in the circulation of some patients with autoimmune hepatitis, occasionally the globulins may bind nonspecifically in solid-phase binding immunoassays for viral antibodies. This has been recognized most commonly in tests for antibodies to hepatitis C virus, as noted above. In fact, studies of autoantibodies in autoimmune hepatitis have led to the recognition of new categories of autoimmune hepatitis. *Type I autoimmune hepatitis* is the classic syndrome occurring in young women, associated with marked hyperglobulinemia, lupoid features, and circulating ANA. *Type II autoimmune hepatitis*, often seen in children and more common in Mediterranean populations, is associated not with ANA but with anti-LKM. Actually, anti-LKM represent a heterogeneous group of antibodies. In type II autoimmune hepatitis, the antibody is anti-LKM1, directed against P450 IID6. This is the same anti-LKM seen in some patients with chronic hepatitis C. Anti-LKM2 is seen in drug-induced hepatitis, and anti-LKM3 is seen in patients with chronic hepatitis D. Type II autoimmune hepatitis has been subdivided by some authorities into two categories, one more typically autoimmune and the other associated with viral hepatitis type C. Autoimmune hepatitis type IIa is felt to be autoimmune, is more likely to occur in young women, is associated with hyperglobulinemia, is associated with high-titer anti-LKM1, responds to glucocorticoid therapy, and is seen commonly in western Europe and the United Kingdom. Type IIb autoimmune hepatitis is associated with HCV infection, tends to occur in older men, is associated with normal globulin levels and low-titer anti-

LKM1, responds to IFN, and occurs most commonly in Mediterranean countries. In addition, another type of autoimmune hepatitis has been recognized, *autoimmune hepatitis type III*. These patients lack ANA and anti-LKM1 and have circulating antibodies to soluble liver antigen, which are directed at hepatocyte cytoplasmic cytokeratins 8 and 18. Most of these patients are women and have clinical features similar to those of patients with type I autoimmune hepatitis.

Liver biopsy abnormalities are similar to those described for chronic viral hepatitis. Expanding portal tracts and extending beyond the plate of periportal hepatocytes into the parenchyma (designated "interface hepatitis" or "piecemeal necrosis") is a mononuclear cell infiltrate that, in autoimmune hepatitis, may include the presence of plasma cells. Necroinflammatory activity characterizes the lobular parenchyma, and evidence of hepatocellular regeneration is reflected by "rosette" formation, the occurrence of thickened liver cell plates, and regenerative "pseudolobules." Septal fibrosis, bridging fibrosis, and cirrhosis are frequent. Bile duct injury and granulomas are uncommon; however, a subgroup of patients with autoimmune hepatitis have histologic, biochemical, and serologic features overlapping those of primary biliary cirrhosis (Chap. 289).

Diagnostic Criteria   An international group has suggested a set of criteria for establishing a diagnosis of autoimmune hepatitis. Exclusion of liver disease caused by genetic disorders, viral hepatitis, drug hepatotoxicity, and alcohol are linked with such inclusive diagnostic criteria as hyperglobulinemia, autoantibodies, and characteristic histologic features. This international group has also suggested a comprehensive diagnostic scoring system that, rarely required for typical cases, may be helpful when typical features are not present. Factors that weigh in favor of the diagnosis include female gender; predominant aminotransferase elevation; presence and level of globulin elevation; presence of nuclear, smooth muscle, and LKM1 autoantibodies; concurrent other autoimmune diseases; characteristic histologic features (interface hepatitis, plasma cells, rosettes); HLA DR3 or DR4 markers; and response to treatment (see below). Weighing against the diagnosis are predominant alkaline phosphatase elevation, mitochondrial antibodies, markers of viral hepatitis, history of hepatotoxic drugs or excessive alcohol, histologic biliary changes, or such atypical histologic features as fatty infiltration, iron overload, and viral inclusions.

℞ TREATMENT

The mainstay of management in autoimmune or idiopathic (nonviral) hepatitis is glucocorticoid therapy. Several controlled clinical trials have documented that such therapy leads to symptomatic, clinical, biochemical, and histologic improvement as well as increased survival. A therapeutic response can be expected in up to 80% of patients. Unfortunately, therapy has not been shown to prevent ultimate progression to cirrhosis; however, instances of reversal of fibrosis and cirrhosis have been reported in patients responding to treatment. Although some advocate the use of prednisolone (the hepatic metabolite of prednisone), prednisone is just as effective and is favored by most authorities. Therapy may be initiated at 20 mg/d, but a popular regimen in the United States relies on an initiation dose of 60 mg/d. This high dose is tapered successively over the course of a month down to a maintenance level of 20 mg/d. An alternative but equally effective approach is to begin with half the prednisone dose (30 mg/d) along with azathioprine (50 mg/d). With azathioprine maintained at 50 mg/d, the prednisone dose is tapered over the course of a month down to a maintenance level of 10 mg/d. The advantage of the combination approach is a reduction, over the span of an 18-month course of therapy, in serious, life-threatening complications of steroid therapy from 66% down to under 20%. Azathioprine alone, however, is not effective in achieving remission, nor is alternate-day glucocorticoid therapy. Although therapy has been shown to be effective for severe autoimmune hepatitis (AST ≥ 10 times the upper limit of normal or ≥5 times the upper limit of normal in conjunction with serum globulin ≥ twice normal; bridging necrosis or multilobular necrosis on liver biopsy;

presence of symptoms), therapy is not indicated for mild forms of chronic hepatitis (which used to be labeled chronic persistent hepatitis or chronic lobular hepatitis), and the efficacy of therapy in mild or asymptomatic autoimmune hepatitis has not been established.

Improvement of fatigue, anorexia, malaise, and jaundice tends to occur within days to several weeks; biochemical improvement occurs over the course of several weeks to months, with a fall in serum bilirubin and globulin levels and an increase in serum albumin. Serum aminotransferase levels usually drop promptly, but improvements in AST and ALT alone do not appear to be a reliable marker of recovery in individual patients; histologic improvement, characterized by a decrease in mononuclear infiltration and in hepatocellular necrosis, may be delayed for 6 to 24 months. Still, if interpreted cautiously, aminotransferase levels are valuable indicators of relative disease activity, and many authorities do *not* advocate serial liver biopsies to assess therapeutic success or to guide decisions to alter or stop therapy. Therapy should continue for at least 12 to 18 months. After tapering and cessation of therapy, the likelihood of relapse is at least 50%, even if posttreatment histology has improved to show mild chronic hepatitis, and the majority of patients require therapy at maintenance doses indefinitely. Continuing azathioprine alone (2 mg per kg body weight daily) after cessation of prednisone therapy may reduce the frequency of relapse.

In medically refractory cases, an attempt should be made to intensify treatment with high-dose glucocorticoid monotherapy (60 mg daily) or combination glucocorticoid (30 mg daily) plus high-dose azathioprine (150 mg daily) therapy. After a month, doses of prednisone can be reduced by 10 mg a month, and doses of azathioprine can be reduced by 50 mg a month towards ultimate, conventional maintenance doses. Patients refractory to this regimen may be treated with cyclosporine, tacrolimus, or mycophenolate mofetil; however, to date, only limited anecdotal reports support these approaches. If medical therapy fails, or when chronic hepatitis progresses to cirrhosis and is associated with life-threatening complications of liver decompensation, liver transplantation is the only recourse (Chap. 291). Recurrence of autoimmune hepatitis in the new liver occurs rarely in most experiences but in as many as a third of cases in others.

DIFFERENTIAL DIAGNOSIS Early during the course of chronic hepatitis, the disease may resemble typical *acute viral hepatitis*. Without histologic assessment, severe chronic hepatitis cannot be readily distinguished based on clinical or biochemical criteria from mild chronic hepatitis. In adolescence, *Wilson's disease* may present with features of chronic hepatitis long before neurologic manifestations become apparent and before the formation of Kayser-Fleischer rings; in this age group, serum ceruloplasmin and serum and urinary copper determinations plus measurement of liver copper levels will establish the correct diagnosis. *Postnecrotic* or *cryptogenic cirrhosis* and *primary biliary cirrhosis* share clinical features with autoimmune hepatitis; biochemical, serologic, and histologic assessments are usually suffi-

cient to allow these entities to be distinguished from autoimmune hepatitis. Of course, the distinction between autoimmune ("idiopathic") and chronic viral hepatitis is not always straightforward, especially when viral antibodies occur in patients with autoimmune disease or when autoantibodies occur in patients with viral disease. Finally, the presence of extrahepatic features such as arthritis, cutaneous vasculitis, or pleuritis—not to mention the presence of circulating autoantibodies—may cause confusion with *rheumatologic disorders* such as rheumatoid arthritis and systemic lupus erythematosus. The existence of clinical and biochemical features of progressive necroinflammatory liver disease distinguishes chronic hepatitis from these other disorders, which are not associated with severe liver disease.

Finally, occasionally, features of autoimmune hepatitis overlap with features of autoimmune biliary disorders such as primary biliary cirrhosis, primary sclerosing cholangitis, or, even more rarely, mitochondrial-antibody-negative autoimmune cholangitis. Such overlap syndromes are difficult to categorize, and often response to therapy may be the distinguishing factor that establishes the diagnosis.

FURTHER READING

ALTER HJ, SEEFF LB: Recovery, persistence, and sequelae in hepatitis C virus infection: A perspective on long-term outcome. Semin Liver Dis 20:17, 2000

CZAJA AJ, FREESE DK: Diagnosis and treatment of autoimmune hepatitis. Hepatology 36:479, 2002

DIENSTAG JL et al: Histologic outcome during long-term lamivudine therapy. Gastroenterology 124:105, 2003

ESTEBAN R (guest ed): Advancing HBV therapy to overcome treatment challenges. Semin Liver Dis 22(Suppl 1):1, 2002

FRIED MV et al: Peginterferon alfa-2a plus ribavirin for chronic hepatitis C virus infection. N Engl J Med 347:975, 2002

GHANY MG et al: Progression of fibrosis in chronic hepatitis C. Gastroenterology 124:97, 2003

HADZIYANNIS SJ et al: Adefovir dipivoxil for the treatment of hepatitis B e antigen-negative chronic hepatitis B. N Engl J Med 348:800, 2003

MANNS MP (guest ed): Autoimmune hepatitis. Semin Liver Dis 22:1, 2002

MARCELLIN P et al: Adefovir dipivoxil for the treatment of hepatitis B e antigen-positive chronic hepatitis B. N Engl J Med 348:808, 2003

NATIONAL DIGESTIVE DISEASES INFORMATION CLEARINGHOUSE: *Chronic Hepatitis C: Current Disease Management*. NIH Publication No. 02-4230, 2002 (www.niddk.nih.gov/health/digest/pubs/chrnhepc.htm)

NATIONAL INSTITUTES OF HEALTH CONSENSUS DEVELOPMENT CONFERENCE: Management of hepatitis C. Hepatology 36(Suppl 1):1S, 2002

PAPATHEODORIDIS GV, HADZIYANNIS SJ: Diagnosis and management of pre-core mutant chronic hepatitis B. J Viral Hepatitis 8:311, 2001

POYNARD T et al: Impact of pegylated interferon alfa-2b and ribavirin on liver fibrosis in patients with chronic hepatitis C. Gastroenterology 122:1303, 2002

SULKOWSKI MS, THOMAS DL: Hepatitis C in the HIV-infected person. Ann Intern Med 138:197, 2003

YOSHIDA H et al: Interferon therapy prolonged life expectancy among chronic hepatitis C patients. Gastroenterology 123:483, 2002

288 ALCOHOLIC LIVER DISEASE
Mark E. Mailliard, Michael F. Sorrell

Chronic and excessive alcohol ingestion is one of the major causes of liver disease in the western world. The pathology of alcoholic liver injury comprises three major lesions, rarely existing in a pure form: (1) fatty liver, (2) alcoholic hepatitis, and (3) cirrhosis. Fatty liver is present in over 90% of binge and chronic drinkers. A much smaller percentage of heavy drinkers will progress to alcoholic hepatitis, thought to be a precursor to cirrhosis. The prognosis of severe alcoholic liver disease is dismal; the mortality of patients with alcoholic hepatitis concurrent with cirrhosis is nearly 60% at 4 years. Although alcohol is considered a direct hepatotoxin, only between 10 and 20% of alcoholics will develop alcoholic hepatitis. The explanation for this

apparent paradox is unclear but involves the interaction of facilitating and comorbid factors such as gender, heredity, and immunity.

ETIOLOGY AND PATHOGENESIS Quantity and duration of alcohol intake are the most important risk factors involved in the development of alcoholic liver disease (Table 288-1). The roles of beverage type and pattern of drinking are less clear. Progress of the hepatic injury beyond the fatty liver stage seems to require additional risk factors that remain incompletely defined. Women are more susceptible to alcoholic liver injury when compared to men. They develop advanced liver disease with substantially less alcohol intake. In general, the time it takes to develop liver disease is directly related to the amount of alcohol consumed. It is useful in estimating alcohol consumption to understand that one beer, four ounces of wine, or one ounce of 80% spirits all contain approximately 12 g of alcohol. The threshold for developing

TABLE 288-1 Risk Factors for Alcoholic Liver Disease

Risk Factor	Comment
Quantity	In men, 40–80 g/d of ethanol produces fatty liver; 160 g/d for 10–20 years causes hepatitis or cirrhosis. Only 15% of alcoholics develop alcoholic liver disease.
Gender	Women exhibit increased susceptibility to alcoholic liver disease at quantities >20 g/d; two drinks per day probably safe.
Hepatitis C	HCV infection concurrent with alcoholic liver disease is associated with younger age for severity, more advanced histology, decreased survival.
Genetics	Gene polymorphisms may include alcohol dehydrogenase, cytochrome P4502E1, and those associated with alcoholism (twin studies).
Malnutrition	Alcohol injury does not require malnutrition, but obesity and fatty liver from the effect of carbohydrate on the transcriptional control of lipid synthesis and transport may be factors. Patients should receive vigorous attention to nutritional support.

severe alcoholic liver disease in men is an intake of >60 to 80 g/d of alcohol for 10 years, while women are at increased risk for developing similar degrees of liver injury by consuming 20 to 40 g/d. Gender-dependent differences in the gastric and hepatic metabolism of alcohol, in addition to poorly understood hormonal factors, likely contribute to the increased susceptibility of women to alcohol-induced liver injury. Social, nutritional, immunologic, and host factors have all been postulated to play a part in the development of the pathogenic process.

Chronic infection with hepatitis C (HCV) (Chap. 287) is an important comorbidity in the progression of alcoholic liver disease to cirrhosis in chronic and excessive drinkers. Alcohol intake >50 g/d more than doubles the risk of cirrhosis in HCV-infected individuals. Patients with both alcoholic liver injury and HCV infection develop decompensated liver disease at a younger age and have poorer overall survival. As a consequence of the overlapping injurious processes secondary to alcohol abuse and HCV infection, patients can develop an increased liver iron burden and, rarely, porphyria cutanea tarda. In addition, alcohol intake in HCV-infected patients with cirrhosis increases the risk for the development of hepatocellular carcinoma.

Our understanding of the pathogenesis of alcoholic liver injury is incomplete. Alcohol is a direct hepatotoxin, but ingestion of alcohol initiates a variety of metabolic responses that influence the final hepatotoxic response. The initial concept of malnutrition as the major pathogenic mechanism has given way to the present understanding that the metabolism of alcohol by the hepatocyte initiates a pathogenic process involving production of protein-aldehyde adducts, lipid peroxidation, immunologic activity, and cytokine release (Fig. 288-1). The complex interaction of distinct hepatic cell types is crucial to alcohol-mediated liver injury. Stellate cell activation and collagen production are key events in hepatic fibrogenesis. The resulting fibrosis determines the extent of architectural derangement of the liver following chronic alcohol ingestion.

PATHOLOGY The liver has a limited repertoire in response to injury. Fatty liver is the initial and most common histologic response to hepatotoxic stimuli, including excessive alcohol ingestion. The accumulation of fat within the perivenular hepatocytes coincides with the location of alcohol dehydrogenase, the major enzyme responsible for alcohol metabolism. Continuing alcohol ingestion results in fat accumulation throughout the entire hepatic lobule. Despite extensive fatty change and distortion of the hepatocytes with macrovesicular fat, the cessation of drinking results in normalization of hepatic architecture and fat content within the liver. Alcoholic fatty liver has traditionally been regarded as entirely benign, but similar to the spectrum of nonalcoholic steatohepatitis, certain pathologic features such as giant mitochondria, perivenular fibrosis, and macrovesicular fat may be associated with progressive liver injury.

The transition between fatty liver and the development of alcoholic hepatitis is blurred. The hallmark of alcoholic hepatitis is hepatocyte injury characterized by ballooning degeneration, spotty necrosis, polymorphonuclear infiltrate, and fibrosis in the perivenular and perisinusoidal space of Disse. Mallory bodies are often present in florid cases but are neither specific nor necessary to establishing the diagnosis. Alcoholic hepatitis is thought to be a precursor to the development of cirrhosis. However, like fatty liver, it is potentially reversible with cessation of drinking. Cirrhosis is present in up to 50% of patients with biopsy-proven alcoholic hepatitis and its repair is difficult, even with abstention.

CLINICAL FEATURES The clinical manifestations of alcoholic fatty liver are subtle and characteristically detected as a consequence of the patient's visit for a seemingly unrelated matter. Previously unsuspected hepatomegaly is often the only clinical finding. Occasionally, patients with fatty liver will present with right upper quadrant discomfort, tender hepatomegaly, nausea, and jaundice. Differentiation of alcoholic fatty liver from nonalcoholic fatty liver is difficult unless an accurate drinking history is ascertained. Alcoholism does not respect social and economic class. In every instance where liver disease is present, a thoughtful and sensitive drinking history should be obtained. Alcoholic hepatitis is associated with a wide gamut of clinical features. Cytokine production is thought to be responsible for the systemic manifestations of alcoholic hepatitis. Fever, spider nevi, jaundice, and abdominal pain simulating an acute abdomen represent the extreme end of the spectrum, while many patients will be entirely asymptomatic. Recognition of the clinical features of alcoholic hepatitis is central to the initiation of an effective and appropriate diagnostic and therapeutic strategy.

CHRONIC ETHANOL INGESTION

FIGURE 288-1 Biomedical and cellular pathogenesis of liver injury secondary to chronic ethanol ingestion. MAA, malondialdehyde-acetaldehyde; TNF, tumor necrosis factor; TGF, transforming growth factor; IL, interleukin; PPAR, peroxisome proliferator-activated receptor; RXR, retinoid X receptor.

LABORATORY FEATURES Patients with alcoholic fatty liver are often identified through routine screening tests. The typical laboratory abnormalities are nonspecific and in-

TABLE 288-2 *Laboratory Diagnosis of Alcoholic Fatty Liver and Alcoholic Hepatitis*

Test	Comment
AST	Increased two- to sevenfold, less than 400 U/L, greater than ALT
ALT	Increased two- to sevenfold, less than 400 U/L
AST/ALT	Usually >1
GGTP	Not specific to alcohol, easily inducible, elevated in all forms of fatty liver
Bilirubin	May be markedly increased in alcoholic hepatitis despite modest elevation in alkaline phosphatase
PMN	If > 5500/μL, predicts severe alcoholic hepatitis when discriminant function > 32

Note: AST, aspartate aminotransferase; ALT, alanine aminotransferase; GGTP, gamma-glutamyl transpeptidase; PMN, polymorphonuclear cells.

clude modest elevations of the aspartate aminotransferase (AST), alanine aminotransferase (ALT), and gamma-glutamyl transpeptidase (GGTP), accompanied by hypertriglyceridemia, hypercholesterolemia, and occasionally hyperbilirubinemia. In alcoholic hepatitis and in contrast to other causes of fatty liver, the AST and ALT are usually elevated two- to sevenfold. They are rarely >400 IU, and the AST/ALT ratio >1 (Table 288-2). Hyperbilirubinemia is common and is accompanied by modest increases in the alkaline phosphatase level. Derangement in hepatocyte synthetic function indicates more serious disease. Hypoalbuminemia and coagulopathy are common in advanced liver injury. An increase in the circulating polymorphonuclear cell number >5500/μL parallels the occurrence of the lobular infiltration of neutrophils observed in the florid lesion of alcoholic hepatitis. Ultrasonography is useful in detecting fatty infiltration of the liver and determining liver size. The demonstration by ultrasound of portal vein flow reversal, ascites, and intraabdominal collaterals indicates serious liver injury with less potential for complete reversal of liver disease.

PROGNOSIS Critically ill patients with alcoholic hepatitis have short-term mortality rates approaching 70%. Severe alcoholic hepatitis is heralded by coagulopathy (prothrombin time > 5 s), anemia, serum albumin concentrations below <25 g/L (2.5 mg/dL), serum bilirubin levels > 137 μmol/L (8 mg/dL), renal failure, and ascites. A discriminant function calculated as 4.6 × [prothrombin time − control (seconds)] + serum bilirubin (mg/dL) can identify patients with a poor prognosis (discriminant function > 32). The presence of ascites, variceal hemorrhage, deep encephalopathy, or hepatorenal syndrome predicts a dismal prognosis. The pathologic stage of the injury can be helpful in predicting prognosis. Liver biopsy should be performed whenever possible to confirm the diagnosis, to establish potential

FIGURE 288-2 Effect of glucocorticoid therapy of severe alcoholic hepatitis on short-term survival: the result of a meta-analysis of individual data from three studies. Prednisolone, solid line; placebo, dotted line. *(Adapted from Mathurin et al., with permission from Elsevier Science)*

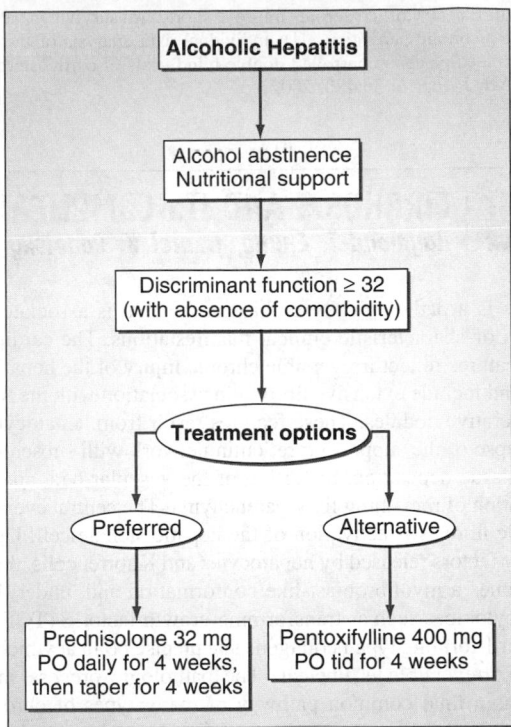

FIGURE 288-3 Treatment algorithm for alcoholic hepatitis. As identified by a calculated discriminant function > 32 (see text), patients with severe alcoholic hepatitis, without the presence of gastrointestinal bleeding or infection, would be candidates for either glucocorticoids or pentoxifylline administration.

reversibility of the liver disease, and to guide the therapeutic decisions.

℞ **TREATMENT**

Complete abstinence from alcohol is the cornerstone in the treatment of alcoholic liver disease. Improved survival and the potential for reversal of histologic injury regardless of the initial clinical presentation are associated with total avoidance of alcohol ingestion. Referral of patients to experienced alcohol counselors and/or alcohol treatment programs should be routine in the management of patients with alcoholic liver disease. Attention should be directed to the nutritional and psychosocial states during the evaluation and treatment periods. Because of data suggesting that the pathogenic mechanisms in alcoholic hepatitis involve cytokine release and the perpetuation of injury by immunologic processes, glucocorticoids have been extensively evaluated in the treatment of alcoholic hepatitis. Patients with severe alcoholic hepatitis, defined as a discriminant function > 32, were given prednisone, 40 mg/d, or prednisolone, 32 mg/d, for 4 weeks followed by a steroid taper (Fig. 288-2). Exclusion criteria included active gastrointestinal bleeding, sepsis, renal failure, or pancreatitis. Newer understanding of the role of cytokines in alcoholic liver injury and emerging experience with pharmacologic inhibition of tumor necrosis factor by pentoxifylline has led to the recent inclusion of this agent as an alternative to glucocorticoids in the therapy of severe alcoholic hepatitis (Fig. 288-3). Because of inordinate surgical mortality and the high rates of recidivism following transplantation, patients with alcoholic hepatitis are not candidates for immediate liver transplantation. The transplant candidacy of these patients should be reevaluated after a defined period of sobriety.

FURTHER READING

AKRIVIADIS E et al: Pentoxifylline improves short-term survival in severe acute alcoholic hepatitis: A double blind placebo controlled trial. Gastroenterology 119:1637, 2000

MATHURIN P et al: Corticosteroids improve short-term survival in patients with severe alcoholic hepatitis (AH): Individual data analysis of the last three randomized placebo controlled double blind trials of corticosteroids in severe AH. J Hepatol 36:480, 2002

PETERS MG, TERRAULT NA: Alcohol use and hepatitis C. Hepatology 36: S220, 2002

TELI MR et al: Determinants of progression to cirrhosis or fibrosis in pure alcoholic fatty liver. Lancet 346:987, 1995

TUYNS A, PEQUIGNOT G: Greater risk of ascitic cirrhosis in females in relation to alcohol consumption. Int J Epidemiol 13:53, 1984

289 | CIRRHOSIS AND ITS COMPLICATIONS
Raymond T. Chung, Daniel K. Podolsky

Cirrhosis is a pathologically defined entity that is associated with a spectrum of characteristic clinical manifestations. The cardinal pathologic features reflect irreversible chronic injury of the hepatic parenchyma and include extensive fibrosis in association with the formation of regenerative nodules. These features result from hepatocyte necrosis, collapse of the supporting reticulin network with subsequent connective tissue deposition, distortion of the vascular bed, and nodular regeneration of remaining liver parenchyma. The central event leading to hepatic fibrosis is activation of the hepatic stellate cell. Upon activation by factors released by hepatocytes and Kupffer cells, the stellate cell assumes a myofibroblast-like conformation and, under the influence of cytokines such as transforming growth factor β (TGF-β), produces fibril-forming type I collagen. The precise point at which fibrosis becomes irreversible is unclear. The pathologic process should be viewed as a final common pathway of many types of chronic liver injury. Clinical features of cirrhosis derive from the morphologic alterations and often reflect the severity of hepatic damage rather than the etiology of the underlying liver disease. Loss of functioning hepatocellular mass may lead to jaundice, edema, coagulopathy, and a variety of metabolic abnormalities; fibrosis and distorted vasculature lead to portal hypertension and its sequelae, including gastroesophageal varices and splenomegaly. Ascites and hepatic encephalopathy result from both hepatocellular insufficiency and portal hypertension.

Classification of the various types of cirrhosis based on either etiology or morphology alone is unsatisfactory. A single pathologic pattern may result from a variety of insults, while the same insult may produce several morphologic patterns. Nevertheless, most types of cirrhosis may be usefully classified by a mixture of etiologically and morphologically defined entities as follows: (1) alcoholic; (2) cryptogenic and posthepatitic; (3) biliary; (4) cardiac; and (5) metabolic, inherited, and drug-related. This chapter considers the various types of cirrhosis and their complications.

ALCOHOLIC CIRRHOSIS

Definition   *Alcoholic cirrhosis* is only one of many consequences resulting from chronic alcohol ingestion, and it often accompanies other forms of alcohol-induced liver injury, including alcoholic fatty liver and alcoholic hepatitis (Chap. 288). Alcoholic cirrhosis, historically referred to as *Laennec's cirrhosis*, is the most common type of cirrhosis encountered in North America and many parts of western Europe and South America. It is characterized by diffuse fine scarring, fairly uniform loss of liver cells, and small regenerative nodules, and therefore it is sometimes referred to as *micronodular cirrhosis*. However, micronodular cirrhosis may also result from other types of liver injury (e.g., following jejunoileal bypass), and thus alcoholic cirrhosis and micronodular cirrhosis are not necessarily synonymous. Conversely, alcoholic cirrhosis may progress to macronodular cirrhosis with time.

Etiology   See Chap. 288, "Alcoholic Liver Disease."

Pathology and Pathogenesis   With continued alcohol intake and destruction of hepatocytes, fibroblasts (including activated hepatic stellate cells that have transformed into myofibroblasts with contractile properties) appear at the site of injury and deposit collagen. Weblike septa of connective tissue appear in periportal and pericentral zones and eventually connect portal triads and central veins. This fine connective tissue network surrounds small masses of remaining liver cells, which regenerate and form nodules. Although regeneration occurs within the small remnants of parenchyma, cell loss generally exceeds replacement. With continuing hepatocyte destruction and collagen deposition, the liver shrinks in size, acquires a nodular appearance, and becomes hard as "end-stage" cirrhosis develops. Although alcoholic cirrhosis is usually a progressive disease, appropriate therapy and strict avoidance of alcohol may arrest the disease at most stages and permit functional improvement. In addition, there is strong evidence that concomitant chronic hepatitis C virus (HCV) infection significantly accelerates development of alcoholic cirrhosis.

Clinical Features ■ *SIGNS AND SYMPTOMS*   Alcoholic cirrhosis may be clinically silent, and many cases (10 to 40%) are discovered incidentally at laparotomy or autopsy. In many cases symptoms are insidious in onset, occurring usually after ≥10 years of excessive alcohol use and progressing slowly over subsequent weeks and months. Anorexia and malnutrition lead to weight loss and a reduction in skeletal muscle mass. The patient may experience easy bruising, increasing weakness, and fatigue. Eventually the clinical manifestations of hepatocellular dysfunction and portal hypertension ensue, including progressive jaundice, bleeding from gastroesophageal varices, ascites, and encephalopathy. The abrupt onset of one of these complications may be the first event prompting the patient to seek medical attention. In other cases, cirrhosis first becomes evident when the patient requires treatment of symptoms related to alcoholic hepatitis.

A firm, nodular liver may be an early sign of disease; the liver may be either enlarged, normal, or decreased in size. Other frequent findings include jaundice, palmar erythema, spider angiomas, parotid and lacrimal gland enlargement, clubbing of fingers, splenomegaly, muscle wasting, and ascites with or without peripheral edema. Men may have decreased body hair and/or gynecomastia and testicular atrophy, which, like the cutaneous findings, result from disturbances in hormonal metabolism, including increased peripheral formation of estrogen due to diminished hepatic clearance of the precursor androstenedione. Testicular atrophy may reflect hormonal abnormalities or the toxic effect of alcohol on the testes. In women, signs of virilization or menstrual irregularities may occasionally be encountered. Dupuytren's contractures resulting from fibrosis of the palmar fascia with resulting flexion contracture of the digits are associated with alcoholism but are not specifically related to cirrhosis.

Although the cirrhotic patient may stabilize if drinking is discontinued, over a period of years, the patient may become emaciated, weak, and chronically jaundiced. Ascites and other signs of portal hypertension may become increasingly prominent. Ultimately, most patients with advanced cirrhosis die in hepatic coma, commonly precipitated by hemorrhage from esophageal varices or intercurrent infection. Progressive renal dysfunction often complicates the terminal phase of the illness.

LABORATORY FINDINGS   In advanced alcoholic liver disease, abnormalities of laboratory tests are more common. Anemia may result from acute and chronic gastrointestinal blood loss, coexistent nutritional deficiency (notably of folic acid and vitamin B_{12}), hypersplenism, and a direct suppressive effect of alcohol on the bone marrow. Hemolytic anemia, presumably due to effects of hypercholesterolemia or erythrocyte membranes resulting in unusual spurlike projections (acanthocytosis), has been described in some alcoholics with cirrhosis. Mild or pronounced hyperbilirubinemia may be found, usually in association with varying elevations of serum alkaline phosphatase levels. Levels of serum AST (asparate aminotransferase) are frequently elevated, but levels >5 μkat (300 units) are unusual and should prompt one to look for other coincident or complicating factors. In contrast to viral hepatitis, the serum AST is usually disproportionately elevated relative to ALT (alanine aminotransferase), i.e., AST/ALT ratio >2. This discrepancy in alcoholic liver disease may result from the proportionally greater inhibition of ALT synthesis by ethanol, which may be partially reversed by pyridoxal phosphate.

The serum prothrombin time is frequently prolonged, reflecting reduced synthesis of clotting proteins, most notably the vitamin K−dependent factors (see "Coagulopathy," below). The serum albumin level is usually depressed, while serum globulins are increased. Hypoalbuminemia reflects in part overall impairment in hepatic protein synthesis, while hyperglobulinemia is thought to result from nonspecific stimulation of the reticuloendothelial system. Elevated blood ammonia levels in patients with hepatic encephalopathy reflect diminished hepatic clearance because of impaired liver function and shunting of portal venous blood around the cirrhotic liver into the systemic circulation (see "Hepatic Encephalopathy," below).

A variety of metabolic disturbances may be detected. Glucose intolerance due to endogenous insulin resistance may be present; however, clinical diabetes is uncommon. Central hyperventilation may lead to respiratory alkalosis in patients with cirrhosis. Dietary deficiency and increased urinary losses lead to hypomagnesemia and hypophosphatemia. In patients with ascites and dilutional hyponatremia, hypokalemia may occur from increased urinary potassium losses due in part to hyperaldosteronism. Prerenal azotemia is also observed in such patients.

Diagnosis Alcoholic cirrhosis should be strongly suspected in patients with a history of prolonged or excessive alcohol intake and physical signs of chronic liver disease. However, since only 10 to 15% of individuals with excessive alcohol intake develop cirrhosis, other causes and types of liver disease may have to be excluded. The clinical features and laboratory findings are usually sufficient to provide reasonable indication of the presence and extent of hepatic injury. Although a percutaneous needle biopsy of the liver is not usually necessary to confirm the typical findings of alcoholic hepatitis or cirrhosis, it may be helpful in distinguishing patients with less advanced liver disease from those with cirrhosis and in excluding other forms of liver injury such as viral hepatitis. Biopsy may also be helpful as a diagnostic tool in evaluating patients with clinical findings suggestive of alcoholic liver disease who deny alcohol intake. In patients with features of cholestasis, ultrasonography may be appropriate to exclude the presence of extrahepatic biliary obstruction. When the clinical status of an otherwise stable cirrhotic patient deteriorates without an obvious explanation, complicating conditions, such as infection, portal vein thrombosis, and hepatocellular carcinoma, should be sought.

Prognosis Abstinence from alcohol as well as early and appropriate medical care can decrease long-term morbidity and mortality and delay or prevent the appearance of further complications. Patients who have had a major complication of cirrhosis and who continue to drink have a 5-year survival of <50%. However, those patients who remain abstinent have a substantially better prognosis. In general, the overall outlook in patients with advanced liver disease remains poor; most of these patients eventually die as a result of massive variceal hemorrhage and/or profound hepatic encephalopathy.

℞ TREATMENT

Alcoholic cirrhosis is a serious illness that requires long-term medical supervision and careful management. Therapy of the underlying liver disease is largely supportive. Specific treatment is directed at particular complications such as variceal bleeding and ascites (see below). While some studies suggest that administration of glucocorticoids in moderately large doses for 4 weeks is helpful in patients with severe alcoholic hepatitis and encephalopathy, these drugs have no role in the treatment of established alcoholic cirrhosis. One study has suggested

survival benefit in alcoholic cirrhosis patients receiving S-adenosyl methionine, which may act to decrease proinflammatory cytokines.

The patient should be made to realize that there is no medication that will protect the liver against the effects of further alcohol ingestion. Therefore, alcohol should be absolutely forbidden. An important component of the complete care of such patients is encouragement to become involved in an appropriate alcohol counseling program.

All medicines must be administered with caution in the patient with cirrhosis, especially those eliminated or modified through hepatic metabolism or biliary pathways. In particular, care must be taken to avoid overzealous use of drugs that may directly or indirectly precipitate complications of cirrhosis. For example, vigorous treatment of ascites with diuretics may result in electrolyte abnormalities or hypovolemia, which can lead to coma. Similarly, even modest doses of sedatives can lead to deepening encephalopathy. Aspirin should be avoided in patients with cirrhosis because of its effects on coagulation and gastric mucosa. Acetaminophen should be used with caution and in doses of less than 2 g/d. Patients who drink alcohol are more sensitive to the hepatotoxic effects of acetaminophen, probably due to increased metabolism of the drug to toxic intermediates and decreased glutathione levels.

POSTHEPATITIC AND CRYPTOGENIC CIRRHOSIS

Definition Posthepatitic or postnecrotic cirrhosis represents the final common pathway of many types of chronic liver disease. *Coarsely nodular cirrhosis* and *multilobular cirrhosis* are terms synonymous with posthepatitic cirrhosis. The term *cryptogenic cirrhosis* has been used interchangeably with posthepatitic cirrhosis, but this designation should be reserved for those cases in which the etiology of cirrhosis is unknown (approximately 10% of all patients with cirrhosis).

Etiology Posthepatitic cirrhosis is a morphologic term referring to a defined stage of advanced chronic liver injury of either specific or unknown (cryptogenic) causes. Epidemiologic and serologic evidence suggest that in one-fourth to three-fourths of cases of posthepatitic cirrhosis, viral hepatitis (hepatitis B or hepatitis C) may be an antecedent factor. In areas where hepatitis B virus (HBV) infection is endemic (e.g., Southeast Asia, sub-Saharan Africa), up to 15% of the population may acquire the infection in early childhood, and cirrhosis may ultimately develop in one-fourth of these chronic carriers. Although HBV infection is much less prevalent in the United States, it is relatively common among certain high-risk groups (e.g., persons with multiple sexual partners, especially men who have sex with men, injection drug users) and contributes to an increased incidence of cirrhosis. In the United States, HCV infection accounts for many cases of cirrhosis following blood transfusions. Before routine screening of blood donors was introduced, hepatitis C occurred in 5 to 10% of blood recipients. Following infection, cirrhosis may ultimately develop in >20% of individuals after 20 years. Increasing recognition of the progressive nature of nonalcoholic fatty liver disease (NAFLD) has revealed that many cases previously designated cryptogenic cirrhosis may be attributable to this disorder (Chap. 290). Posthepatitic cirrhosis may also develop in patients with autoimmune hepatitis (Chap. 287).

The most common causes of cirrhosis in the United States that ultimately lead to liver transplantation include chronic HCV infection, alcohol, primary biliary cirrhosis, primary sclerosing cholangitis, and NAFLD. Less common causes of posthepatitic cirrhosis, including drugs and toxins, are listed in Table 289-1.

Pathology The posthepatitic liver is typically shrunken in size, distorted in shape, and composed of nodules of liver cells separated by dense and broad bands of fibrosis. The microscopic picture is consistent with the gross impression. Posthepatitic cirrhosis is characterized morphologically by (1) extensive confluent loss of liver cells, (2) stromal collapse and fibrosis resulting in broad bands of connective tissue containing the remains of many portal triads, and (3) irregular

TABLE 289-1   *Causes of Cirrhosis and/or Chronic Liver Disease*

Infectious Diseases	Drugs and Toxins (Chap. 286)
Brucellosis (Chap. 141)	Alcohol (Chap. 288)
Capillariasis (Chap. 201)	Amioradone
Echinococcosis (Chap. 240)	Arsenicals
Schistosomiasis (Chap. 203)	Oral contraceptives (Budd-Chiari)
Toxoplasmosis (Chap. 198)	Pyrrolidizine alkaloids and
Viral hepatitis [hepatitis B, C, D;	antineoplastic agents
cytomegalovirus; Epstein-Barr	(venoocclusive disease)
virus (Chaps. 285, 165, 166)]	

Inherited and Metabolic Disorders (Chap. 290)

Other Causes

α_1-Antitrypsin deficiency (Chap. 290)	Biliary obstruction (chronic) (Chap. 292)
Alagille's syndrome (Chap. 282)	Cystic fibrosis (Chap. 241)
Biliary atresia (Chap. 292)	Graft-versus-host disease (Chap. 100)
Familial intrahepatic cholestasis (FIC) types 1–3 (Chap. 292)	Jejunoileal bypass (Chap. 36)
Fanconi's syndrome (Chap. 340)	Nonalcoholic fatty liver disease (Chap. 290)
Galactosemia (Chap. 341)	Primary biliary cirrhosis (Chap. 289)
Gaucher's disease (Chap. 340)	
Glycogen storage disease (Chap. 341)	Primary sclerosing cholangitis (Chap. 292)
Hemochromatosis (Chap. 336)	Sarcoidosis (Chap. 309)
Hereditary fructose intolerance (Chap. 341)	
Hereditary tyrosinemia (Chap. 343)	
Wilson's disease (Chap. 339)	

nodules of regenerating hepatocytes, varying in size from microscopic to several centimeters in diameter.

Clinical Features   In patients with cirrhosis of known etiology in whom there is progression to a posthepatitic stage, the clinical manifestations are an extension of those resulting from the initial disease process. Usually clinical symptoms are related to portal hypertension and its sequelae, such as ascites, splenomegaly, hypersplenism, encephalopathy, and bleeding gastroesophageal varices. The hematologic and liver function abnormalities resemble those seen with other types of cirrhosis. In a few patients with posthepatitic cirrhosis, the diagnosis may be made incidentally at operation, at postmortem, or by a needle biopsy of the liver performed to investigate abnormal liver function tests or hepatomegaly.

Diagnosis and Prognosis   Posthepatitic cirrhosis should be suspected in patients with signs and symptoms of cirrhosis or portal hypertension. Needle or operative liver biopsies confirm the diagnosis, although nonuniformity of the pathologic process may result in sampling errors. The diagnosis of cryptogenic cirrhosis is reserved for those patients in whom no known etiology can be demonstrated. About 75% of patients have progressive disease despite supportive therapy and die within 1 to 5 years from complications, including variceal hemorrhage, hepatic encephalopathy, or superimposed hepatocellular carcinoma.

℞ TREATMENT

Management is usually limited to treatment of the complications of portal hypertension, including control of ascites, avoidance of drugs or excessive protein intake that may induce hepatic coma, and prompt treatment of infections (see below). In patients with asymptomatic cirrhosis, expectant management alone is appropriate. In those patients in whom posthepatitic cirrhosis has developed as a result of a treatable condition, therapy directed at the primary disorder may limit further progression (e.g., Wilson's disease, hemochromatosis).

BILIARY CIRRHOSIS

Biliary cirrhosis results from injury to or prolonged obstruction of either the intrahepatic or extrahepatic biliary system. It is associated with impaired biliary excretion, destruction of hepatic parenchyma, and progressive fibrosis. Primary biliary cirrhosis (PBC) is characterized by chronic inflammation and fibrous obliteration of intrahepatic bile ductules. Secondary biliary cirrhosis (SBC) is the result of longstanding obstruction of the larger extrahepatic ducts. Although primary and secondary biliary cirrhosis are separate pathophysiologic entities with respect to the initial insult, many clinical features are similar.

PRIMARY BILIARY CIRRHOSIS ■ **Etiology and Pathogenesis**   The cause of PBC remains unknown. Several observations suggest that a disordered immune response may be involved. PBC is frequently associated with a variety of disorders presumed to be autoimmune in nature, such as the syndrome of *c*alcinosis, *R*aynaud's phenomenon, *e*sophageal dysmotility, *s*clerodactyly, *t*elangiectasia (CREST); the sicca syndrome (dry eyes and dry mouth); autoimmune thyroiditis; type 1 diabetes mellitus; and IgA deficiency.

Most important, a circulating IgG antimitochondrial antibody (AMA) is detected in >90% of patients with PBC and only rarely in other forms of liver disease. It has been demonstrated that these autoantibodies recognize inner mitochondrial membrane proteins identified as enzymes of the pyruvate dehydrogenase complex (PDC), the branched chain–2-oxoacid dehydrogenase complex (BCOADC), and the 2-oxoglutarate dehydrogenase complex (OGDC). The major autoantigen in PBC (found in 90% of patients) has been identified as the 74-kDa E2 component of the PDC, dihydrolipoamide acetyltransferase. The antibodies are directed to a region essential for binding of a lipoic acid cofactor and inhibit the overall enzymatic activity of the PDC. Other AMA autoantibodies in PBC patients are directed to similar constituents of BCOADC and OGDC and also inhibit their enzymatic function. It remains unclear whether these properties have a direct pathogenetic role in the development of PBC. In addition to AMA, elevated serum levels of IgM and cryoproteins consisting of immune complexes capable of activating the alternative complement pathway are found in 80 to 90% of patients. Aberrant expression of major histocompatibility complex class II molecules has been found on biliary epithelium in association with PBC, suggesting that these cells may serve as antigen-presenting cells in this setting. Lymphocytes are prominent in the portal regions and surround damaged bile ducts. These histologic findings resemble those noted in graft-versus-host disease following bone marrow transplantation and suggest that damage to bile ducts may be immunologically mediated, perhaps reflecting a defect in a suppressor cell population. While it has been suggested that PBC may be initiated by molecular mimicry following infection or xenobiotic exposure, definitive evidence is lacking.

Pathology   PBC is divided into four stages based on morphologic findings. The earliest recognizable lesion (stage I), termed *chronic nonsuppurative destructive cholangitis*, is a necrotizing inflammatory process of the portal triads. It is characterized by destruction of medium and small bile ducts, a dense infiltrate of acute and chronic inflammatory cells, mild fibrosis, and occasionally, bile stasis. At times, periductal granulomas and lymph follicles are found adjacent to affected bile ducts. Subsequently, the inflammatory infiltrate becomes less prominent, the number of bile ducts is reduced, and smaller bile ductules proliferate (stage II). Progression over a period of months to years leads to a decrease in interlobular ducts, loss of liver cells, and expansion of periportal fibrosis into a network of connective tissue scars (stage III). Ultimately, cirrhosis, which may be micronodular or macronodular, develops (stage IV).

Clinical Features ■ *SIGNS AND SYMPTOMS*   Most patients with PBC are asymptomatic, and the disease is initially detected on the basis of elevated serum alkaline phosphatase levels during routine screening. The majority of such patients remain asymptomatic for prolonged periods, although many ultimately develop progressive liver injury.

Among patients with symptomatic disease, 90% are women age 35 to 60. Often the earliest symptom is pruritus, which may be either generalized or limited initially to the palms and soles. In addition, fatigue is commonly a prominent early symptom. After several months or years, jaundice and gradual darkening of the exposed areas of the skin (melanosis) may ensue. Other early clinical manifestations of PBC reflect impaired bile excretion. These include steatorrhea and the malabsorption of lipid-soluble vitamins. Protracted elevation of serum lipids, especially cholesterol, leads to subcutaneous lipid deposition around the eyes (xanthelasmas) and over joints and tendons (xanthomas). Over a period of months to years, the itching, jaundice, and hyperpigmentation slowly worsen. Eventually, signs of hepatocellular failure and portal hypertension develop and ascites appears. Progression may be quite variable. Whereas a proportion of asymptomatic patients may show no signs of progression for a decade or longer, in others, death due to hepatic insufficiency may occur within 5 to 10 years after the first signs of the illness. Such decompensation is often precipitated by uncontrolled variceal hemorrhage or infection.

Physical examination may be entirely normal in the early phase of the disease, when patients are asymptomatic or pruritus is the sole complaint. Later, there may be jaundice of varying intensity, hyperpigmentation of the exposed skin areas, xanthelasmas and tendinous and planar xanthomas, moderate to striking hepatomegaly, splenomegaly, and clubbing of the fingers. Bone tenderness, signs of vertebral compression, ecchymoses, glossitis, and dermatitis may all be noted. Clinical evidence of the sicca syndrome can be found in as many as 75% of patients, and serologic evidence of autoimmune thyroid disease in 25%. Other conditions encountered with increased frequency include rheumatoid arthritis, CREST syndrome, keratoconjunctivitis sicca, IgA deficiency, type 1 diabetes mellitus, scleroderma, pernicious anemia, and renal tubular acidosis. Bone disease is often a significant problem encountered over the course of the disease. While osteomalacia occurs due to diminished vitamin D absorption, accelerated osteoporosis in this patient population (the majority of whom are postmenopausal women) is even more common.

LABORATORY FINDINGS PBC is increasingly diagnosed at a presymptomatic stage, prompted by the finding of a twofold or greater elevation of the serum alkaline phosphatase during routine screening. Serum 5′-nucleotidase activity and γ-glutamyl transpeptidase levels are also elevated. In this setting, serum bilirubin is usually normal and aminotransferase levels minimally increased. The diagnosis is supported by a positive AMA test (titer > 1:40). The latter is both relatively specific and sensitive; a positive test is found in >90% of symptomatic patients and is present in <5% of patients with other liver diseases. As the disease evolves, the serum bilirubin level rises progressively and may reach 510 μmol/L (30 mg/dL) or more in the final stages. Serum aminotransferase values rarely exceed 2.5 to 3.3 μkat (150 to 200 units). Hyperlipidemia is common, and a striking increase of the serum unesterified cholesterol is often noted. An abnormal serum lipoprotein (lipoprotein X) may be present in PBC but is not specific and appears in other cholestatic conditions. A deficiency of bile salts in the intestine leads to moderate steatorrhea and impaired absorption of the fat-soluble vitamins and hypoprothrombinemia. Patients with PBC have elevated liver copper levels, but this finding is not specific and is found in all disorders in which there is prolonged cholestasis.

Diagnosis PBC should be considered in middle-aged women with unexplained pruritus or an elevated serum alkaline phosphatase and in whom there may be other clinical or laboratory features of protracted impairment of biliary excretion. Although a positive serum AMA determination provides important diagnostic evidence, false-positive results do occur; therefore, liver biopsy should be performed to confirm the diagnosis. Rarely, the AMA test may be negative in patients with histologic features of PBC. Frequently, patients have antibodies to the E2 protein in tests using these specific antigens. In some cases with histologic features of PBC and a negative AMA, antinuclear or smooth-muscle antibodies are present (as in autoimmune hepatitis), and the designation *autoimmune cholangitis* is applied. The natural history of this entity, however, appears to resemble that of PBC. If the AMA test is negative, the biliary tract should be evaluated to exclude primary sclerosing cholangitis and remediable extrahepatic biliary tract obstruction, especially in view of the frequent presence of co-existing cholelithiasis.

R̲x̲ TREATMENT

While there is no specific therapy for PBC, ursodiol has been shown to improve biochemical and histologic features and might improve survival, particularly liver transplantation–free survival (although this remains unproven). Ursodiol should be given in doses of 13 to 15 mg/kg per day, but lower doses are sometimes just as effective in reducing serum alkaline phosphatase and aminotransferase levels. Ursodiol should be given with food and can be taken in a single dose daily. Side effects are rare: gastrointestinal intolerance (diarrhea) and skin rashes occur but are uncommon. Isolated instances of severe exacerbation of pruritus have been reported in patients with advanced disease. Ursodiol probably works by replacing the endogenously produced hydrophobic bile acids with urosdeoxycholate, a hydrophilic and relatively nontoxic bile acid.

Unfortunately, ursodiol may not prevent ultimate progression of PBC, which is effectively predicted by the Mayo risk score, and the only established "cure" is liver transplantation. Results of liver transplantation for PBC are excellent, survival exceeding that for patients receiving transplantation for most other forms of end-stage liver disease. Recurrence of PBC after liver transplantation has been reported but is uncommon, and the recurrent disease is only slowly progressive. Most patients remain AMA positive after transplantation, and as many as 25% will have histologic features of PBC on liver biopsy after 5 years. Other therapies such as glucocorticoids, colchicine, methotrexate, azathioprine, cyclosporine, and tacrolimus have been reported as effective in small case series, but none have shown to be effective in adequately controlled trials.

Relief of symptoms is also an important part of management of PBC. As noted, ursodiol may be helpful in controlling symptoms and improving the patient's sense of well-being. Although the mechanism of the protracted pruritus is not entirely clear, cholestyramine, an oral bile salt–sequestering resin, may be helpful in doses of 12 to 16 g/d to decrease both pruritus and hypercholesterolemia. Rifampin, opiate antagonists (naloxone or naltrexone), ondansetron, plasmapheresis, and ultraviolet light have all been tried for control of pruritus, with varying results. Steatorrhea can be reduced by a low-fat diet and substituting medium-chain triglycerides for dietary long-chain triglycerides. Fat-soluble vitamins A, D, E, and K should be given at regular intervals. Zinc supplementation may be necessary if night blindness is refractory to vitamin A therapy. An important part of management of PBC and any cholestatic liver disease is assessment and treatment of osteoporosis and osteomalacia. Patients should be screened periodically by bone densitometry and treated as needed with calcium supplements (1500 mg/d), vitamin D (1000 IU/d), and/or bisphosphonate agents (e.g., alendronate) when osteoporosis is present. Progression of PBC leads to the typical complications of advanced liver disease (see below).

SECONDARY BILIARY CIRRHOSIS ■ Etiology SBC results from prolonged partial or total obstruction of the common bile duct or its major branches. In adults, obstruction is most frequently caused by postoperative strictures or gallstones, usually with superimposed infectious cholangitis. Chronic pancreatitis may lead to biliary stricture and secondary cirrhosis. SBC is also an important complication of primary sclerosing cholangitis, a progressive immunologic disorder of the intrahepatic and extrahepatic biliary tree (Chap. 292). Patients with malignant tumors of the common bile duct or pancreas rarely survive long enough to develop SBC. In children, congenital biliary atresia and cystic fibrosis are common causes of SBC. Choledochal cysts, if unrecognized, may also be a rare cause of SBC.

Pathology and Pathogenesis Unrelieved obstruction of the extrahepatic bile ducts leads to (1) bile stasis and focal areas of centrilobular necrosis followed by periportal necrosis, (2) proliferation and dilatation of the portal bile ducts and ductules, (3) sterile or infected cholangitis with accumulation of polymorphonuclear infiltrates around bile ducts, and (4) progressive expansion of portal tracts by edema and fibrosis. Extravasation of bile from ruptured interlobular bile ducts into areas of periportal necrosis leads to the formation of "bile lakes" surrounded by cholesterol-rich pseudoxanthomatous cells. As in other forms of cirrhosis, injury is accompanied by regeneration in residual parenchyma. These changes gradually lead to a finely nodular cirrhosis. In general, at least 3 to 12 months is required for biliary obstruction to result in cirrhosis. Relief of the obstruction is frequently accompanied by biochemical and morphologic improvement and may even ameliorate cirrhosis.

Clinical Features The symptoms, signs, and biochemical findings of SBC are similar to those of PBC. Jaundice and pruritus are usually the most prominent features. In addition, fever and/or right upper quadrant pain, reflecting bouts of cholangitis or biliary colic, are typical. The manifestations of portal hypertension are found only in advanced cases. SBC should be considered in any patient with clinical and laboratory evidence of prolonged obstruction to bile flow, especially when there is a history of previous biliary tract surgery or gallstones, bouts of ascending cholangitis, or right upper quadrant pain. Cholangiography (either percutaneous or endoscopic) usually demonstrates the underlying pathologic process. Liver biopsy, although not always necessary from a clinical standpoint, can document the development of cirrhosis.

℞ TREATMENT

Relief of obstruction to bile flow, by either endoscopic or surgical means, is the most important step in the prevention and therapy of SBC. Effective decompression of the biliary tract results in a significant improvement in both symptoms and survival, even in patients with established cirrhosis. When obstruction cannot be relieved, as in sclerosing cholangitis, antibiotics may be helpful acutely in controlling superimposed infection or, when administered on a chronic basis, as prophylactic therapy in suppressing recurring episodes of ascending cholangitis. Without relief of obstruction, there is a steady progression to end-stage cirrhosis and its terminal manifestations.

CARDIAC CIRRHOSIS

Definition Prolonged, severe right-sided congestive heart failure may lead to chronic liver injury and cardiac cirrhosis. The characteristic pathologic features of fibrosis and regenerative nodules distinguish cardiac cirrhosis from both reversible passive congestion of the liver due to acute heart failure and acute hepatocellular necrosis ("ischemic hepatitis" or "shock liver") resulting from systemic hypotension and hypoperfusion of the liver.

Etiology and Pathology In right-sided heart failure, retrograde transmission of elevated venous pressure via the inferior vena cava and hepatic veins leads to congestion of the liver. Hepatic sinusoids become dilated and engorged with blood, and the liver becomes tensely swollen. With prolonged passive congestion and ischemia from poor perfusion secondary to reduced cardiac output, necrosis of centrilobular hepatocytes ensues and leads to fibrosis in these central areas. Ultimately, centrilobular fibrosis develops, with collagen extending outward in a characteristic stellate pattern from the central vein. Gross examination of the liver shows alternating red (congested) and pale (fibrotic) areas, a pattern often referred to as "nutmeg liver." Improvement in management of cardiac disorders, particularly advances in surgical treatment, has reduced the frequency of cardiac cirrhosis.

Clinical Features A range of abnormalities of liver function tests may be found, though none is uniformly present. The serum bilirubin is usually only mildly increased and may be predominantly either conjugated or unconjugated. Mild to moderate elevation in alkaline phosphatase level and prothrombin time prolongation are sometimes present. The AST level is typically mildly elevated but may be transiently very high following a period of marked systemic hypotension

(shock liver), when the clinical picture can mimic acute viral or drug-induced hepatitis. In cases of tricuspid insufficiency the liver may be pulsatile, but this finding disappears as cirrhosis develops. With prolonged right-sided heart failure the liver becomes enlarged, firm, and usually nontender. The signs and symptoms of heart failure usually overshadow the liver disease. Bleeding from esophageal varices is rare, but chronic encephalopathy may be prominent, with a waxing and waning course reflecting variations in the severity of right-sided heart failure. Ascites and peripheral edema, often primarily related to the underlying cardiac dysfunction, may be worsened by the superimposed liver disease.

Diagnosis The presence of a firm, enlarged liver with signs of chronic liver disease in a patient with valvular heart disease, constrictive pericarditis, or cor pulmonale of long duration (>10 years) should suggest cardiac cirrhosis. Liver biopsy can confirm the diagnosis but is often contraindicated because of coagulopathy or ascites. Coexistent chronic heart and liver disease should also raise the possibility of hemochromatosis (Chap. 336), amyloidosis (Chap. 310), or other infiltrative diseases.

Budd-Chiari syndrome resulting from the occlusion of the hepatic veins or inferior vena cava may be confused with acute congestive hepatomegaly. In this condition the liver is grossly enlarged and tender, and severe intractable ascites is present. However, signs and symptoms of heart failure are notably absent. The most common cause is thrombosis of the hepatic veins, often in the setting of polycythemia rubra vera, myeloproliferative syndromes, paroxysmal nocturnal hemoglobinuria, oral contraceptive use, or other hypercoagulable states; it may also result from invasion of the inferior vena cava by tumor, such as renal cell or hepatocellular carcinoma. Idiopathic membranous obstruction of the inferior vena cava is the most common cause of this syndrome in Japan. Hepatic venography or liver biopsy showing centrilobular congestion and sinusoidal dilatation in the absence of right-sided heart failure establishes the diagnosis of Budd-Chiari syndrome. Venoocclusive disease affecting the sublobular branches of the hepatic veins and the hepatic venues may result from hepatic irradiation, treatment with certain antineoplastic agents as preparation for stem cell transplantation, or ingestion of pyrrolidizine alkaloids present in some herbal teas ("bush tea disease") and can mimic congestive hepatomegaly.

℞ TREATMENT

Prevention or treatment of cardiac cirrhosis depends on the diagnosis and therapy of the underlying cardiovascular disorder. Improvement in cardiac function frequently results in improvement of liver function and stabilization of the liver disease.

METABOLIC, HEREDITARY, DRUG-RELATED, AND OTHER TYPES OF CIRRHOSIS (See Table 289-1)

Cirrhosis or hepatitis may result from a wide variety of other processes encompassing the spectrum of etiologic factors listed in Table 289-2. Although some of these disorders have distinctive clinical or morphologic features, the manifestations of cirrhosis are largely independent of the underlying pathogenic mechanism.

NONCIRRHOTIC FIBROSIS OF THE LIVER

Several diseases, either congenital or acquired, may be associated with localized or generalized hepatic fibrosis. They are distinguished from

TABLE 289-2 *Some Causes of Noncirrhotic Hepatic Fibrosis*

Idiopathic portal hypertension (noncirrhotic portal fibrosis, Banti's syndrome); three variants:
    Intrahepatic phlebosclerosis and fibrosis
    Portal and splenic vein sclerosis
    Portal and splenic vein thrombosis
Schistosomiasis ("pipe-stem" fibrosis with presinusoidal portal hypertension)
Congenital hepatic fibrosis (may be associated with polycystic disease of liver and kidneys)

cirrhosis by the absence of hepatocellular damage and the lack of nodular regenerative activity. The clinical manifestations in such cases are largely secondary to portal hypertension. The different types of these disorders are indicated in Table 289-2; with the exception of schistosomiasis in some regions of the world, all these conditions are relatively rare.

MAJOR COMPLICATIONS OF CIRRHOSIS

The clinical course of patients with advanced cirrhosis is often complicated by a number of important sequelae that are independent of the etiology of the underlying liver disease. These include portal hypertension and its consequences (e.g., gastroesophageal varices and splenomegaly), ascites, hepatic encephalopathy, spontaneous bacterial peritonitis, hepatorenal syndrome, and hepatocellular carcinoma.

PORTAL HYPERTENSION ■ Definition and Pathogenesis Normal pressure in the portal vein is low (5 to 10 mmHg) because vascular resistance in the hepatic sinusoids is minimal. Portal hypertension (>10 mmHg) most commonly results from increased resistance to portal blood flow. Because the portal venous system lacks valves, resistance at any level between the right side of the heart and splanchnic vessels results in retrograde transmission of an elevated pressure. Increased resistance can occur at three levels relative to the hepatic sinusoids: (1) presinusoidal, (2) sinusoidal, and (3) postsinudoidal. Obstruction in the *presinusoidal* venous compartment may be anatomically outside the liver (e.g., portal vein thrombosis) or within the liver itself but at a functional level proximal to the hepatic sinusoids so that the liver parenchyma is not exposed to the elevated venous pressure (e.g., schistosomiasis).

Postsinusoidal obstruction may also occur outside the liver at the level of the hepatic veins (e.g., Budd-Chiari syndrome), the inferior vena cava, or, less commonly, within the liver (e.g., venoocclusive disease). When cirrhosis is complicated by portal hypertension, the increased resistance is usually *sinusoidal*. While distinctions between pre-, post-, and sinusoidal processes are conceptually appealing, functional resistance to portal flow in a given patient may occur at more than one level. Portal hypertension may also arise from increased blood flow (e.g., massive splenomegaly or arteriovenous fistulas), but the low outflow resistance of the normal liver makes this a rare clinical problem.

Cirrhosis is the most common cause of portal hypertension in the United States. Clinically significant portal hypertension is present in >60% of patients with cirrhosis. *Portal vein obstruction* is the second most common cause; it may be idiopathic or occur in association with cirrhosis, infection, pancreatitis, or abdominal trauma. Idiopathic portal vein thrombosis may develop in a variety of hypercoagulable states including polycythemia vera; essential thrombocythemia; deficiencies of protein C, protein S, or antithrombin III; resistance to activated protein C (factor V Leiden); and a mutation of the prothrombin gene (G20210A). Most of the remaining patients with idiopathic cases have a subclinical myeloproliferative disorder. Hepatic vein thrombosis (Budd-Chiari syndrome) and hepatic venoocclusive disease are relatively infrequent causes of portal hypertension (see above). Portal vein occlusion may result in massive hematemesis from gastroesophageal varices, but ascites is usually found only when cirrhosis is present. Noncirrhotic portal fibrosis (Table 289-2) accounts for only a few cases of portal hypertension.

Clinical Features The major clinical manifestations of portal hypertension include hemorrhage from gastroesophageal varices, splenomegaly with hypersplenism, ascites, and acute and chronic hepatic encephalopathy. These are related, at least in part, to the development of portal-systemic collateral channels. The absence of valves in the portal venous system facilitates retrograde (hepatofugal) blood flow from the high-pressure portal venous system to the lower-pressure systemic venous circulation. Major sites of collateral flow involve the veins around the cardioesophageal junction (esophagogastric varices), the rectum (hemorrhoids), retroperitoneal space, and the falciform ligament of the liver (periumbilical or abdominal wall collaterals). Abdominal wall

collaterals appear as tortuous epigastric vessels that radiate from the umbilicus toward the xiphoid and rib margins (caput medusae).

A frequent marker of the presence of cirrhosis in a patient being followed for chronic liver disease is a progressive decrease in platelet count. A low-normal platelet count can be the first clue to progression to cirrhosis. Ultimately, a marked decrease in platelets (to 30,000 to 60,000/μL) and white blood cells can occur.

Diagnosis In patients with known liver disease, the development of portal hypertension is usually revealed by the appearance of splenomegaly, ascites, encephalopathy, and/or esophageal varices. Conversely, the finding of any of these features should prompt evaluation of the patient for the presence of underlying portal hypertension and liver disease. Varices are most reliably documented by fiberoptic esophagoscopy; their presence lends indirect support to the diagnosis of portal hypertension. Magnetic resonance imaging and intravenous contrast computed tomography are also sensitive tools for detection of the collateral circulation of portal hypertension. Although rarely necessary, portal venous pressure may be measured directly by percutaneous transhepatic "skinny needle" catheterization or indirectly through transjugular cannulation of the hepatic veins. Both free and wedged hepatic vein pressure should be measured. While the latter is elevated in sinusoidal and postsinusoidal portal hypertension, including cirrhosis, this measurement is usually normal in presinusoidal portal hypertension. In patients in whom additional information is necessary (e.g., preoperative evaluation before portal-systemic shunt surgery) or when percutaneous catheterization is not feasible, mesenteric and hepatic angiography may be helpful. Particular attention should be directed to the venous phase to assess the patency of the portal vein and the direction of portal blood flow.

℞ TREATMENT

Although treatment is usually directed toward a specific complication of portal hypertension, attempts are sometimes made to reduce the pressure in the portal venous system. Surgical decompression procedures have been used for many years to lower portal pressure in patients with bleeding esophageal varices (see below). However, portal-systemic shunt surgery does not result in improved survival rates in patients with cirrhosis. Decompression can now be accomplished without surgery through the percutaneous placement of a portal-systemic shunt, termed a *transjugular intrahepatic portosystemic shunt* (TIPS). *β-Adrenergic blockade* with nonselective agents such as propranolol or nadolol reduces portal pressure through vasoconstrictive effects on both the splanchnic arterial bed and the portal venous system in combination with reduced cardiac output. Such therapy has been shown to be effective in preventing both a first variceal bleed and subsequent episodes after an initial bleed. Treatment of patients with clinically significant sequelae of portal hypertension, especially variceal bleeding, is titrated to reduce the hepatic venous pressure gradient (HVPG = wedged hepatic venous pressure − free hepatic venous pressure) to <12 mmHg or by 20% from baseline. When the HVPG is not available or feasible, reduction of resting pulse by 25% is reasonable if no contraindications to therapy exist.

Vigorous treatment of patients with alcoholic hepatitis and cirrhosis, chronic active hepatitis, or other liver diseases may lead to a fall in portal pressure and to a reduction in variceal size. In general, however, portal hypertension due to cirrhosis is not reversible. In appropriately selected patients, hepatic transplantation will be beneficial.

VARICEAL BLEEDING ■ Pathogenesis While vigorous hemorrhage may arise from any portal-systemic venous collaterals, bleeding is most common from varices in the region of the gastroesophageal junction. The factors contributing to bleeding from gastroesophageal varices are not entirely understood but include the degree of portal hypertension (>12 mmHg) and the size of the varices.

Clinical Features and Diagnosis Variceal bleeding often occurs without obvious precipitating factors and usually presents with painless but massive hematemesis with or without melena. Associated signs range from mild postural tachycardia to profound shock, depending on the extent of blood loss and degree of hypovolemia. Because patients with varices may bleed just as frequently from other gastrointestinal lesions (e.g., peptic ulcer, gastritis), exclusion of other bleeding sources is important even in patients with prior variceal hemorrhage. Endoscopy is the best approach to evaluate upper gastrointestinal hemorrhage in patients with known or suspected portal hypertension.

℞ TREATMENT

Management of Acute Bleeding (See Fig. 289-1) Variceal bleeding is a life-threatening emergency. Prompt estimation and vigorous replacement of blood loss to maintain intravascular volume are essential and take precedence over diagnostic studies and more specific intervention to stop the bleeding. However, excessive fluid administration can increase portal pressure with resultant further bleeding and should therefore be avoided. Replacement of clotting factors with fresh-frozen plasma is important in patients with coagulopathy. Patients are best managed in an intensive care unit and require close monitoring of central venous or pulmonary capillary wedge pressures, urine output, and mental status. When the patient is hemodynamically stable, attention should be directed toward specific diagnostic studies (especially endoscopy) and other therapeutic modalities to prevent further or recurrent bleeding.

About half of all episodes of variceal hemorrhage cease without intervention, although the risk of rebleeding is very high. The medical management of acute variceal hemorrhage includes the use of vasoconstrictors (somatostatin/octreotide or vasopressin), balloon tamponade, and endoscopic variceal ligation (EVL) or sclerosis of varices (sclerotherapy). Intravenous infusion of *vasopressin* at a rate of 0.1 to 0.4 U/min results in generalized vasoconstriction leading to diminished blood flow in the portal venous system. Intravenous infusion of vasopressin is as effective as selective intraarterial administration.

Control of bleeding can be achieved in up to 80% of cases, but bleeding recurs in more than half after the vasopressin is tapered and discontinued. Furthermore, a number of serious side effects, including cardiac and gastrointestinal tract ischemia, acute renal failure, and hyponatremia, may be associated with vasopressin therapy. Concurrent use of venodilators such as nitroglycerin as an intravenous infusion or isosorbide dinitrate sublingually may enhance the effectiveness of vasopressin and reduce complications. *Somatostatin* and its analogue, *octreotide*, are direct splanchnic vasoconstrictors. In some studies somatostatin, given as an initial 250-μg bolus followed by constant infusion (250 μg/h), has been found to be as effective as vasopressin. Octreotide at doses of 50 to 100 μg/h is also effective. These agents are preferable to vasopressin, offering equivalent efficacy with fewer complications. If bleeding is too vigorous or endoscopy is not available, *balloon tamponade* of the bleeding varices may be accomplished with a triple-lumen (Sengstaken-Blakemore) or four-lumen (Minnesota) tube with esophageal and gastric balloons. Because of the high risk of aspiration, endotracheal intubation should be performed prior to placing one of these tubes. After the tube is introduced into the stomach, the gastric balloon is inflated and pulled back into the cardia of the stomach. If bleeding does not stop, the esophageal balloon is inflated for additional tamponade. Complications occur in 15% or more of patients and include aspiration pneumonitis as well as esophageal rupture.

Where available, *endoscopic intervention* should be employed as the first-line treatment to control bleeding acutely (Chaps. 37 and 272). EVL, in which esophageal varices are ligated and strangulated by endoscopically placed small elastic O-rings, has generally supplanted endoscopic injection of sclerosants in the control of acute variceal bleeding. EVL controls acute bleeding in up to 90% of cases and should be repeated until obliteration of all varices is accomplished.

Surgical treatment of portal hypertension and variceal bleeding involves the creation of a portal-systemic shunt to permit decompression of the portal system. Two types of portal systemic shunts have been used: nonselective shunts, to decompress the entire portal system, and selective shunts, intended to decompress only the varices while maintaining blood flow to the liver itself. Nonselective shunts include end-to-side or side-to-side portacaval and proximal splenorenal anastomoses; selective shunts include the distal splenorenal shunt. Nonselective shunts are more likely to be complicated by encephalopathy than selective shunts. Emergency portal-systemic nonselective shunts may control acute hemorrhage, but such surgery is usually used only as a last resort because early operative mortality can be high.

In TIPS, a technique developed to create a portal-systemic shunt by a percutaneous approach, an expandable metal stent is advanced under angiographic guidance to the hepatic veins and then through the substance of the liver to create a direct portacaval channel. This technique offers an alternative to surgery for refractory bleeding due to portal hypertension. However, stents frequently undergo stenosis or become occluded over a period of months, necessitating revision, a second TIPS, or an alternative approach. Encephalopathy may occur after TIPS, just as in the surgical shunts, and is especially problematic in the elderly and those patients with preexisting encephalopathy. TIPS should be reserved for those individuals who fail endoscopic or medical management and are poor surgical risks. TIPS sometimes serves a useful role as a "bridge" for those patients with end-stage cirrhosis awaiting liver transplantation. Procedures such as esophageal transection have also been advocated for the management of acute variceal bleeding, but their efficacy remains unproven, and these procedures are usually considered a last resort.

The management of bleeding gastric fundal varices, found either alone or in conjunction with esophageal varices, is more problematic, since banding and sclerotherapy are generally not effective. Vasoactive pharmacologic therapy should be instituted, but TIPS or shunt surgery should be considered because of high failure and rebleeding rates. For isolated gastric varices, splenic vein thrombosis should be specifically sought, since splenectomy is curative.

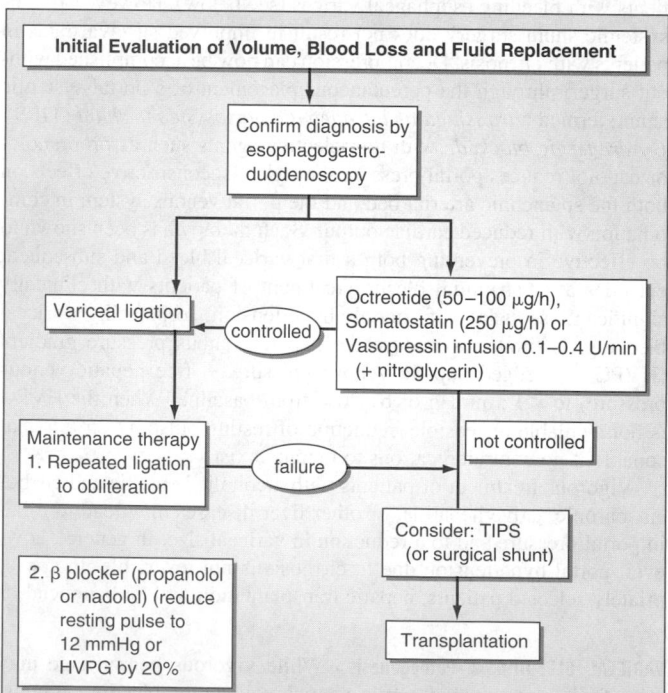

Initial Evaluation of Volume, Blood Loss and Fluid Replacement

Confirm diagnosis by esophagogastro-duodenoscopy

Variceal ligation — *controlled* — Octreotide (50–100 μg/h), Somatostatin (250 μg/h) or Vasopressin infusion 0.1–0.4 U/min (+ nitroglycerin)

Maintenance therapy
1. Repeated ligation to obliteration — *failure* — not controlled

2. β blocker (propanolol or nadolol) (reduce resting pulse to 12 mmHg or HVPG by 20%)

Consider: TIPS (or surgical shunt)

Transplantation

FIGURE 289-1 Approach to the patient with bleeding esophageal varices. Use of a beta blocker is the only intervention demonstrated to offer prophylactic benefit in a patient who has never bled. TIPS, transjugular intrahepatic portosystemic shunt; HVPG, hepatic venous pressure gradient.

Prevention of First Hemorrhage Prophylactic treatment with nonselective β-adrenergic antagonists (propranolol or nadolol) in patients with large ("high-risk") varices that have never bled appears to decrease the incidence of bleeding by 40 to 50% and prolong survival. Thus, endoscopic screening for varices in patients with cirrhosis is desirable; some have suggested this should be repeated every other year.

Although prophylactic banding of esophageal varices in the absence of proven bleeding cannot yet be recommended, one report suggests that banding may be more effective than beta-blockade in primary prevention of variceal bleeding in high-risk patients.

Prevention of Recurrent Hemorrhage Obliteration of varices by endoscopic band ligation reduces risk of recurrent hemorrhage by >50%. Pharmacologic agents also have demonstrated benefit. While the utility of beta blockers can be limited by concomitant hypotension, a number of studies demonstrate their value in secondary prevention of recurrent variceal hemorrhage. Pharmacologic and endoscopic therapy are comparable in overall reduction of rebleeding risk, but the subgroup of patients who achieve hemodynamic response to pharmacologic therapy appears to experience survival benefit.

Patients with portal hypertension in the absence of specific contraindications should be given propranolol or nadolol in doses that produce a 25% reduction in the resting heart rate or a reduction in the HVPG to 12 mmHg or 20% below baseline, where available. Propranolol may also prevent recurrent bleeding from severe portal hypertensive gastropathy in patients with cirrhosis. The optimal combination of endoscopic and pharmacologic therapy for prevention of recurrent hemorrhage remains to be established.

The role of portal-systemic shunt surgery after initial control of bleeding by nonoperative means is also uncertain. Surgically created shunts effectively reduce the risk of recurrent hemorrhage, but the overall mortality of patients undergoing such surgery is comparable to that of unoperated patients. Although patients who have undergone portal-systemic surgery succumb to recurrent bleeding less commonly than unoperated patients, this improvement is counterbalanced by increased morbidity from encephalopathy and death from progressive liver failure. Increasingly, therapeutic portal-systemic shunts have been reserved for patients who experience further bleeding despite serial endoscopic therapy.

Portal Hypertensive Gastropathy Although variceal hemorrhage is the most commonly encountered bleeding complication of portal hypertension, many patients will develop a congestive gastropathy due to the venous hypertension. In this condition, identified by endoscopic examination, the mucosa appears engorged and friable. Indolent mucosal bleeding occurs rather than the brisk hemorrhage typical of a variceal source. β-Adrenergic blockade with propranolol (reducing splanchnic arterial pressure as well as portal pressure) is sometimes effective in ameliorating this condition. Proton pump inhibitors or other agents useful in the treatment of peptic disease are usually not helpful.

SPLENOMEGALY ■ Definition and Pathogenesis Congestive splenomegaly is common in patients with severe portal hypertension. Rarely, massive splenomegaly from nonhepatic disease leads to portal hypertension due to increased blood flow in the splenic vein.

Clinical Features Although usually asymptomatic, splenomegaly may be massive and contribute to the thrombocytopenia or pancytopenia of cirrhosis. In the absence of cirrhosis, splenomegaly in association with variceal hemorrhage should suggest the possibility of splenic vein thrombosis.

℞ TREATMENT

Splenomegaly usually requires no specific treatment, although massive enlargement of the spleen may occasionally necessitate splenectomy at the time of shunt surgery. However, it should be noted that splenectomy without an accompanying shunt may actually increase portal pressure, and portal vein thrombosis may result from splenectomy.

Splenectomy may also be indicated if splenomegaly is the cause rather than the result of portal hypertension (as in splenic vein thrombosis). Thrombocytopenia alone is rarely severe enough to necessitate removal of the spleen. Splenectomy should be avoided in a patient eligible for liver transplantation.

ASCITES ■ Definition Ascites is the accumulation of excess fluid within the peritoneal cavity. It is most frequently encountered in patients with cirrhosis and other forms of severe liver disease, but a number of other disorders may lead to either transudative or exudative ascites (Chap. 39).

Pathogenesis The accumulation of ascitic fluid represents a state of total-body sodium and water excess, but the event that initiates this imbalance is unclear. Three theories have been proposed (Fig. 289-2). The "underfilling" theory suggests that the primary abnormality is inappropriate sequestration of fluid within the splanchnic vascular bed due to portal hypertension and a consequent decrease in effective circulating blood volume. According to this theory, an apparent decrease in intravascular volume (underfilling) is sensed by the kidney, which responds by retaining salt and water. The "overflow" theory suggests that the primary abnormality is inappropriate renal retention of salt and water in the absence of volume depletion. A third, more attractive theory, the peripheral arterial vasodilation hypothesis, may unify the earlier theories and accounts for the constellation of arterial hypotension and increased cardiac output in association with high levels of vasoconstrictor substances that are routinely found in patients with cirrhosis and ascites. Again, sodium retention is considered secondary to arterial vascular underfilling and the result of a disproportionate increase of the vascular compartment due to arteriolar vasodilation rather than from decreased intravascular volume. According to this theory, portal hypertension results in splanchnic arteriolar vasodilation, mediated by nitric oxide, and leading to underfilling of the arterial vascular space and baroreceptor-mediated stimulation of renin-angiotensin, sympathetic output, and antidiuretic hormone release.

Regardless of the initiating event, a number of factors contribute to accumulation of fluid in the abdominal cavity (Fig. 282-2). Elevated levels of serum epinephrine and norepinephrine have been well documented. *Increased central sympathetic outflow* is found in patients with cirrhosis and ascites but not in those with cirrhosis alone. Increased sympathetic output results in diminished natriuresis by acti-

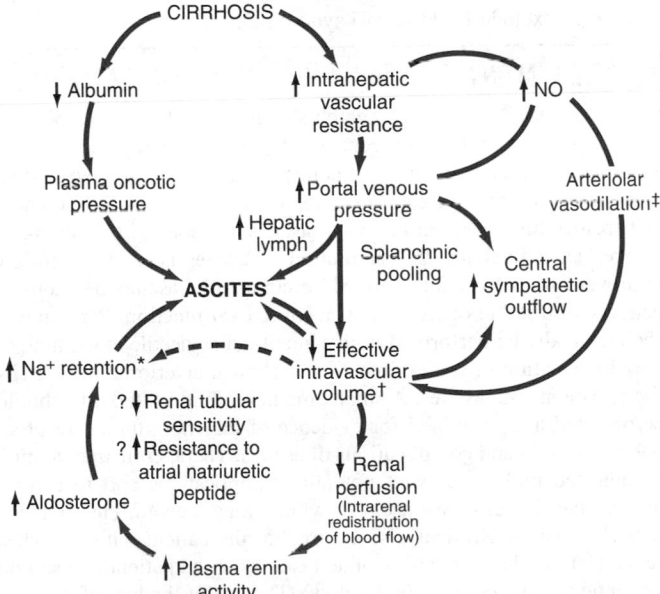

FIGURE 289-2 Multiple factors involved in development of ascites. Current concepts suggest that initiating factor may be primary sodium retention (*"overflow"), diminished effective intravascular volume (†"underfilling"), or arteriolar vasodilation (‡"vasodilation"). NO, nitric oxide.

vation of the renin-angiotensin system and diminished sensitivity to atrial natriuretic peptide. *Portal hypertension* plays an important role in the formation of ascites by raising hydrostatic pressure within the splanchnic capillary bed. *Hypoalbuminemia* and *reduced plasma oncotic pressure* also favor the extravasation of fluid from plasma to the peritoneal cavity, and thus ascites is infrequent in patients with cirrhosis unless both portal hypertension and hypoalbuminemia are present. Hepatic lymph may weep freely from the surface of the cirrhotic liver due to distortion and obstruction of hepatic sinusoids and lymphatics and contributes to ascites formation. In contrast to the contribution of transudative fluid from the portal vascular bed, hepatic lymph may weep into the peritoneal cavity even in the absence of marked hypoproteinemia because the endothelial lining of the hepatic sinusoids is discontinuous. This mechanism may account for the high protein concentration present in the ascitic fluid of some patients with venoocclusive disease or the Budd-Chiari syndrome.

Renal factors also play an important role in perpetuating ascites. Patients with ascites fail to excrete a water load in a normal fashion. They have increased renal sodium reabsorption by both proximal and distal tubules, the latter due largely to increased plasma renin activity and secondary hyperaldosteronism. Insensitivity to circulating atrial natriuretic peptide, often present in elevated concentrations in patients with cirrhosis and ascites, may be an important contributory factor in many patients. This insensitivity has been documented in those patients with the most severely impaired sodium excretion, who typically also exhibit low arterial pressure and marked overactivity of the renin-aldosterone axis. Renal vasoconstriction, perhaps resulting from increased serum prostaglandin or catecholamine levels, may also contribute to sodium retention. Recently a role for endothelin, a potent vasoconstrictor peptide, has been proposed. While elevated levels have been reported by some, this has not been observed by others.

Clinical Features and Diagnosis Usually ascites is first noticed by the patient because of increasing abdominal girth. More pronounced accumulation of fluid may cause shortness of breath because of elevation of the diaphragm. When peritoneal fluid accumulation exceeds 500 mL, ascites may be demonstrated on physical examination by the presence of shifting dullness, a fluid wave, or bulging flanks. Ultrasound examination, preferably with a Doppler study, can detect smaller quantities of ascites and should be performed when physical examination is equivocal or when the cause of the recent onset of ascites is not clear (e.g., exclude Budd-Chiari syndrome).

℞ TREATMENT

(See Fig. 289-3) A thorough search should be made for precipitating factors in the patient with recent onset of or worsening ascites, e.g., excessive salt intake, medication noncompliance, superimposed infection, worsening liver disease, portal vein thrombosis, or development of hepatocellular carcinoma. When ascites develops in the setting of severe, acute liver disease, resolution of ascites is likely to follow improvement in liver function. More commonly, ascites develops in patients with stable or steadily worsening liver function. Paracentesis should usually be performed with a small-gauge needle at the time of initial evaluation or at the time of any clinical deterioration of a cirrhotic patient with ascites. A small amount of fluid (<200 mL) should be obtained and examined for evidence of infection, tumor, or other possible causes and complications of ascites. Therapeutic intervention is indicated both to prevent potential complications and to control progressive increase in ascites, which may become pronounced enough to cause physical discomfort. For the patient with a modest accumulation, therapy can be undertaken as an outpatient and should be gentle and incremental (see below). The goal is the loss of no more than 1.0 kg/d if both ascites and peripheral edema are present and no more than 0.5 kg/d in patients with ascites alone. In some patients, particularly those with a large accumulation of fluid, it may be desirable to hospitalize the patient so that daily weights and frequent serum

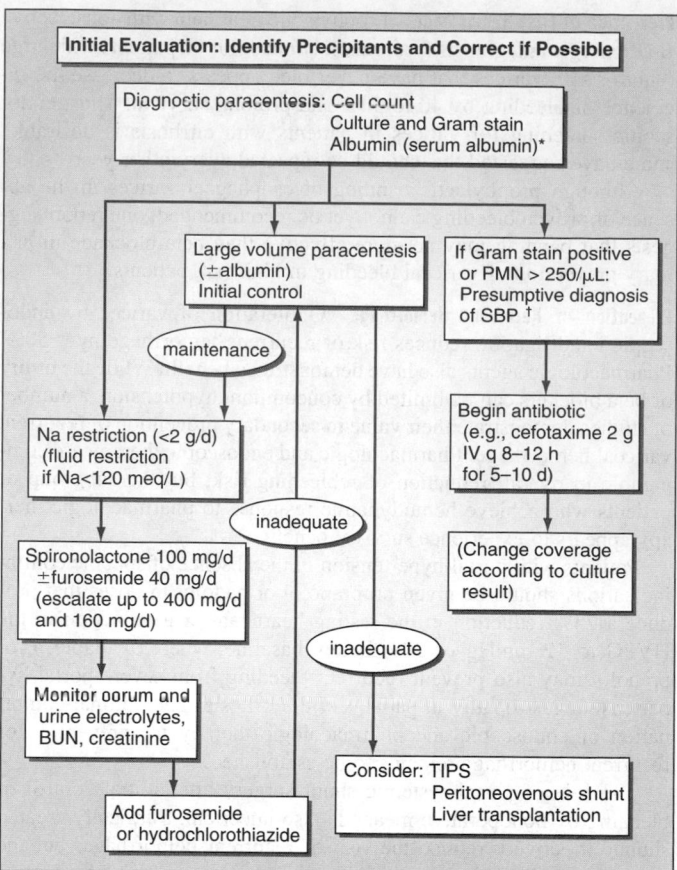

FIGURE 289-3 Approach to the patient with ascites [and spontaneous bacterial peritonitis (SBP)]. PMN, polymorphonuclear leukocytes; TIPS, transjugular intrahepatic portosystemic shunt. *Calculate SAAG [serum ascites albumin gradient = serum albumin − ascites albumin (g/dL)] to confirm high gradient (>1.1 g/dL) in portal hypertension. †If PMN >250/μL but culture is negative = culture negative neutrocytic ascites; begin empirical antibiotic and retap at 48 h; if culture is positive but PMN < 250/μL normal = monomicrobial nonneutrocytic bacterascites; retap; treat if PMN > 250/μL: if polymicrobial infection, exclude secondary peritonitis. U_{Na}, urinary sodium; U_{Ka}, urinary potassium; BUN, blood urea nitrogen.

electrolyte levels can be monitored and compliance ensured. Although abdominal girth measurements are frequently used as an index of fluid loss, they tend to be unreliable.

Salt restriction is the cornerstone of therapy. A diet containing 800 mg sodium (2 g NaCl) is often adequate to induce a negative sodium balance and permit diuresis. Response to salt restriction alone is more likely to occur if the ascites is of recent onset, the underlying liver disease is reversible, a precipitating factor can be corrected, or the patient has a high urinary sodium excretion (>25 mmol/d) and normal renal function. Fluid restriction of approximately 1000 mL/d does little to enhance diuresis but may be necessary to correct hyponatremia. If sodium restriction alone fails to result in diuresis and weight loss, diuretics should be prescribed. Because of the role of hyperaldosteronism in sustaining salt retention, spironolactone or other distal tubule–acting diuretics (triamterene, amiloride) are the drugs of choice. The development of azotemia or hyperkalemia may be limiting or even warrant a reduction in the dose of these medications. In some patients, diuresis does not occur despite maximal doses of distal tubule–acting agents because of avid proximal tubular sodium absorption. More potent, proximally acting diuretics (furosemide, bumetanide, torasemide) may be added to the regimen. Thus, spironolactone is initially given at a dose of 100 mg/d with or without furosemide, 40 mg/d, and both agents may be increased by 100- and 40-mg increments respectively: total dose should not exceed 400 mg/d and 160 mg/d, respectively. An indication of the minimum effective dose of spironolactone may be obtained by monitoring urinary electrolyte concentrations for a rise in sodium and fall in potassium concentrations, reflecting effective competitive inhibition of aldosterone. Great caution should be exercised to avoid plasma volume depletion, azotemia, and hypokalemia, which may lead to encephalopathy.

In patients with pronounced ascites, particularly those requiring hospitalization, large-volume paracentesis has proven to be an effective and less costly approach to initial management than prolonged bed rest and conventional diuretic treatment. In this approach, ascitic fluid is removed by peritoneal cannula using strict aseptic techniques and monitoring hemodynamic and renal function. This can be safely accomplished in a single session. Concomitant albumin replacement by intravenous infusion is prudent in the patient without peripheral edema, to avoid depleting the intravascular space and precipitating hypotension. Maintenance diuretic therapy in conjunction with sodium restriction may then be instituted to avoid recurrent ascites.

A minority of patients with advanced cirrhosis have "refractory ascites" or rapidly reaccumulate fluid after control by paracentesis. In some patients, a side-to-side *portacaval shunt* may result in improvement in ascites, although generally these patients are extremely poor surgical risks. In the past, intractable ascites has also been treated with the surgical implantation of a plastic *peritoneovenous shunt*, which has a pressure-sensitive, one-way valve allowing ascitic fluid to flow from the abdominal cavity to the superior vena cava. However, the usefulness of this technique is limited by a high rate of complications such as infection, disseminated intravascular coagulation, and thrombosis of the shunt. More recently, in selected patients, TIPS has been used effectively to control refractory ascites, although portal decompression, while mobilizing ascitic fluid, has precipitated severe hepatic encephalopathy in some patients. None of these shunts has been shown to extend life expectancy.

SPONTANEOUS BACTERIAL PERITONITIS (SBP)   Patients with ascites and cirrhosis may develop acute bacterial peritonitis without an obvious primary source of infection. Patients with advanced liver disease are particularly susceptible to SBP, which portends a poor prognosis (Chap. 112).

HEPATORENAL SYNDROME ■ Definition and Pathogenesis   Hepatorenal syndrome is a serious complication in the patient with cirrhosis and ascites and is characterized by worsening azotemia with avid sodium retention and oliguria in the absence of identifiable specific causes of renal dysfunction. The exact basis for this syndrome is not clear, but altered renal hemodynamics appear to be involved. There is evidence for inappropriate intense renal vasoconstriction, perhaps in response to the splanchnic vasodilation accompanying cirrhosis. The kidneys are structurally intact; urinalysis and pyelography are usually normal. Renal biopsy, although rarely needed, is also normal, and in fact, kidneys from such patients have been used successfully for renal transplantation.

Clinical Features and Diagnosis   Worsening azotemia, hyponatremia, progressive oliguria, and hypotension are the hallmarks of the hepatorenal syndrome. This syndrome, which is distinct from prerenal azotemia, may be precipitated by severe gastrointestinal bleeding, sepsis, or overly vigorous attempts at diuresis or paracentesis; it may also occur without an obvious cause. It is essential to exclude other causes of renal impairment often seen in these patients. These include prerenal azotemia or acute tubular necrosis due to hypovolemia (e.g., secondary to gastrointestinal bleeding or diuretic therapy) or an increased nitrogen load such as that seen as a result of bleeding. Drug nephrotoxicity is also often a consideration, particularly in the patient who has received agents such as aminoglycosides or contrast dye. The diagnosis rests on the finding of an elevated serum creatinine level [>133 μmol/L (>1.5 g/dL)] that fails to improve with volume expansion or withdrawal of diuretics, together with an unremarkable urine sediment. The diagnosis is supported by the demonstration of avid urinary sodium retention. Typically, the urine sodium concentration is <5 mmol/L, a concentration lower than that generally found in uncomplicated prerenal azotemia.

℞ TREATMENT

Treatment is usually unsuccessful. Although some patients with hypotension and decreased plasma volume may respond to infusions of salt-poor albumin, volume expansion must be undertaken with caution to avoid precipitating variceal bleeding. Vasodilator therapy, including intravenous infusions of low dose dopamine, is not effective. Evidence for the benefit of systemic vasoconstrictors alone or in combination with other agents such as terlipressin, norepinephrine with albumin, and octreotide with midodrine has emerged recently, but additional study is needed. While TIPS has been reported to improve renal function in some patients, its use cannot be recommended. In appropriate candidates, the treatment of choice for hepatorenal syndrome is liver transplantation. In patients with spontaneous bacterial peritonitis, early intravenous albumin infusion can prevent development of hepatorenal syndrome in some patients.

HEPATIC ENCEPHALOPATHY ■ Definition   Hepatic (portal systemic) encephalopathy is a complex neuropsychiatric syndrome characterized by disturbances in consciousness and behavior, personality changes, fluctuating neurologic signs, asterixis or "flapping tremor," and distinctive electroencephalographic changes. Encephalopathy may be *acute* and reversible or *chronic* and progressive. In severe cases, irreversible coma and death may occur. Acute episodes may recur with variable frequency.

Pathogenesis   The specific cause of hepatic encephalopathy is unknown. The most important factors in the pathogenesis are severe hepatocellular dysfunction and/or intrahepatic and extrahepatic shunting of portal venous blood into the systemic circulation so that the liver is largely bypassed. As a result of these processes, various toxic substances absorbed from the intestine are not detoxified by the liver and lead to metabolic abnormalities in the central nervous system (CNS). *Ammonia* is the substance most often incriminated in the pathogenesis of encephalopathy. Many, but not all, patients with hepatic encephalopathy have elevated blood ammonia levels, and recovery from encephalopathy is often accompanied by declining blood ammonia levels. Other compounds and metabolites that may contribute to the development of encephalopathy include mercaptans (derived from intestinal metabolism of methionine), short-chain fatty acids, and phenol. *False neurochemical transmitters* (e.g., octopamine), resulting in part from alterations in plasma levels of aromatic and branched-chain amino acids, may also play a role. An increase in the permeability of the blood-brain barrier to some of these substances may be an additional factor involved in the pathogenesis of hepatic encephalopathy. Several observations suggest that excessive concentrations of γ-aminobutyric acid (GABA), an inhibitory neurotransmitter, in the CNS are important in the reduced levels of consciousness seen in hepatic encephalopathy. Increased CNS GABA may reflect failure of the liver to extract precursor amino acids efficiently or to remove GABA produced in the intestine. In support of this, there is also evidence to suggest that endogenous benzodiazepines, which act through the GABA receptor, may contribute to the development of hepatic encephalopathy. This evidence includes isolation of 1,4-benzodiazepines from brain tissue of patients with fulminant hepatic failure as well as the partial response observed in some patients and experimental animals after administration of flumazenil, a benzodiazepine antagonist. However, the inconsistent effect of flumazenil in patients with encephalopathy, as well as potential methodologic pitfalls in the measurement of endogenous benzodiazepines, preclude definitive attribution of a role to these substances in the pathogenesis of hepatic encephalopathy. The finding of direct enhancement of GABA receptor activation by ammonia suggests that several of the factors described above may be operating via a final common pathway to produce the neuronal depression of hepatic encephalopathy. Finally, the observation of hyperintensity in the basal ganglia by magnetic resonance imaging in cirrhotic patients suggests that excessive *manganese dep-*

TABLE 289-3 *Common Precipitants of Hepatic Encephalopathy*

Increased nitrogen load	Drugs
Gastrointestinal bleeding	Narcotics, tranquilizers, sedatives
Excess dietary protein	Diuretics (see "Electrolyte
Azotemia	imbalance")
Constipation	Miscellaneous
Electrolyte and metabolic	Infection
imbalance	Surgery
Hypokalemia	Superimposed acute liver disease
Alkalosis	Progressive liver disease
Hypoxia	Portal-systemic shunts
Hyponatremia	
Hypovolemia	

osition may also contribute to the pathogenesis of hepatic encephalopathy. Further studies are needed to determine whether chelation therapy exerts long-term benefit.

In the patient with otherwise stable cirrhosis, hepatic encephalopathy often follows a clearly identifiable precipitating event (Table 289-3). Perhaps the most common predisposing factor is *gastrointestinal bleeding*, which leads to an increase in the production of ammonia and other nitrogenous substances, which are then absorbed. Similarly, *increased dietary protein* may precipitate encephalopathy as a result of increased production of nitrogenous substances by colonic bacteria. *Electrolyte disturbances*, particularly hypokalemic alkalosis secondary to overzealous use of diuretics, vigorous paracentesis, or vomiting, may precipitate hepatic encephalopathy. Systemic alkalosis causes an increase in the amount of nonionic ammonia (NH_3) relative to ammonium ions (NH_4). Only nonionic (uncharged) ammonia readily crosses the blood-brain barrier and accumulates in the CNS. Hypokalemia also directly stimulates renal ammonia production. Injudicious use of CNS-depressing drugs (e.g., barbiturates, benzodiazepines) and acute infection may trigger or aggravate hepatic encephalopathy, although the mechanisms involved are not clear. Other potential precipitating factors include superimposed acute viral hepatitis, alcoholic hepatitis, extrahepatic bile duct obstruction, constipation, surgery, and other coincidental medical complications.

Hepatic encephalopathy has protean manifestations, and any neurologic abnormality, including focal deficits, may be encountered. In patients with acute encephalopathy, neurologic deficits are completely reversible upon correction of underlying precipitating factors and/or improvement in liver function, but in patients with chronic encephalopathy, the deficits may be irreversible and progressive. Cerebral edema is frequently present and contributes to the clinical picture and overall mortality in patients with both acute and chronic encephalopathy.

The diagnosis of hepatic encephalopathy should be considered when four major factors are present: (1) acute or chronic hepatocellular disease and/or extensive portal-systemic collateral shunts (the latter may be either spontaneous, e.g., secondary to portal hypertension, or mechanically created, e.g., TIPS); (2) disturbances of awareness and mentation, which may progress from forgetfulness and confusion to stupor and finally coma; (3) shifting combinations of neurologic signs,

including asterixis, rigidity, hyperreflexia, extensor plantar signs, and rarely, seizures; and (4) a characteristic (but nonspecific) symmetric, high-voltage, triphasic slow-wave (2 to 5 per second) pattern on the electroencephalogram. Asterixis ("liver flap," "flapping tremor") is a nonrhythmic asymmetric lapse in voluntary sustained position of the extremities, head, and trunk. It is best demonstrated by having the patient extend the arms and dorsiflex the hands. Because elicitation of asterixis depends on sustained voluntary muscle contraction, it is not present in the comatose patient. Asterixis is nonspecific and also occurs in patients with other forms of metabolic brain disease. Disturbances of sleep with reversal of sleep/wake cycles are among the earliest signs of encephalopathy. Alterations in personality, mood disturbances, confusion, deterioration in self-care and handwriting, and daytime somnolence are additional clinical features of encephalopathy. *Fetor hepaticus*, a unique musty odor of the breath and urine believed to be due to mercaptans, may be noted in patients with varying stages of hepatic encephalopathy.

Grading or classifying the stages of hepatic encephalopathy is often helpful in following the course of the illness and assessing response to therapy. One useful classification is shown in Table 289-4.

The diagnosis of hepatic encephalopathy is usually one of exclusion. There are no diagnostic liver function test abnormalities, although an elevated serum ammonia level in the appropriate clinical setting is highly suggestive of the diagnosis. Examination of the cerebrospinal fluid is unremarkable, and computed tomography of the brain shows no characteristic abnormalities until late in stage IV when cerebral edema may supervene. A number of conditions, particularly disorders related to acute and chronic alcoholism, can mimic the clinical features of hepatic encephalopathy. These include acute alcohol intoxication, sedative overdose, delirium tremens, Wernicke's encephalopathy, and Korsakoff's psychosis (Chap. 361). Subdural hematoma, meningitis, and hypoglycemia or other metabolic encephalopathies must also be considered, especially in patients with alcoholic cirrhosis. In young patients with liver disease and neurologic abnormalities, Wilson's disease should be excluded.

R̲x̲ TREATMENT

(See Fig. 289-4) Early recognition and prompt treatment of hepatic encephalopathy are essential. Patients with acute, severe hepatic en-

TABLE 289-4 *Clinical Stages of Hepatic Encephalopathy*

Stage	Mental Status	Asterixis	EEG
I	Euphoria or depression, mild confusion, slurred speech, disordered sleep	+/−	Triphasic waves
II	Lethargy, moderate confusion	+	Triphasic waves
III	Marked confusion, incoherent speech, sleeping but arousable	+	Triphasic waves
IV	Coma; initially responsive to noxious stimuli, later unresponsive	−	Delta activity

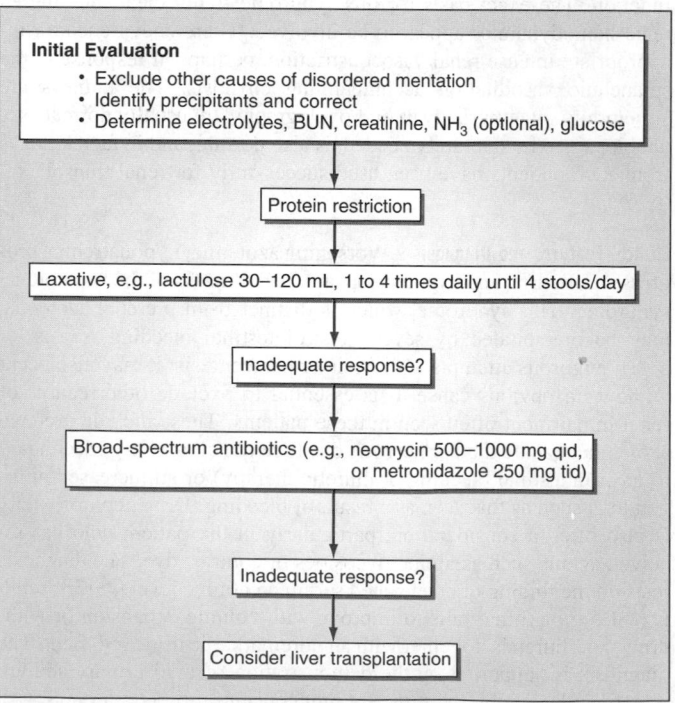

FIGURE 289-4 Approach to the patient with hepatic encephalopathy. BUN, blood urea nitrogen.

cephalopathy (stage IV) require the usual supportive measures for the comatose patient. Specific treatment of hepatic encephalopathy is aimed at (1) elimination or treatment of precipitating factors and (2) lowering of blood ammonia (and other toxin) levels by decreasing the absorption of protein and nitrogenous products from the intestine. In the setting of acute gastrointestinal bleeding, blood in the bowel should be promptly evacuated with laxatives (and enemas if necessary) in order to reduce the nitrogen load. Protein should be excluded from the diet, and constipation should be avoided. Ammonia absorption can be decreased by the administration of lactulose, a nonabsorbable disaccharide that acts as an osmotic laxative. Metabolism of lactulose by colonic bacteria may also result in an acid pH that favors conversion of ammonia to the poorly absorbed ammonium ion. In addition, lactulose may actually diminish ammonia production through its direct effects on bacterial metabolism. Acutely, lactulose syrup can be administered in a dose of 30 to 60 mL every hour until diarrhea occurs; thereafter the dose is adjusted (usually 15 to 30 mL three times daily) so that the patient has two to four soft stools daily. Intestinal ammonia production by bacteria can also be decreased by oral administration of a "nonabsorbable" antibiotic such as neomycin (0.5 to 1.0 g every 6 h). However, despite poor absorption, neomycin may reach sufficient concentrations in the bloodstream to cause renal toxicity. Equal benefits may be achieved with broad-spectrum antibiotics such as metronidazole. Flumazenil, a short-acting benzodiazepine antagonist, may have a role in management of hepatic encephalopathy precipitated by use of benzodiazepines, if there is a need for urgent therapy. Hemoperfusion to remove toxic substances and therapy directed primarily toward coincident cerebral edema in acute encephalopathy are also of unproven value. The efficacy of extracorporeal liver assist devices employing hepatocytes of porcine or human origin to bridge patients to recovery or transplantation is as yet unproven but is currently being studied.

Chronic encephalopathy may be effectively controlled by administration of lactulose. Management of patients with chronic encephalopathy should include dietary protein restriction (usually to 60 g/d) in combination with low doses of lactulose or neomycin. Nephrotoxicity or ototoxicity may be limiting in prolonged usage of neomycin. There are suggestions that vegetable protein may be preferable to animal protein.

OTHER SEQUELAE OF CIRRHOSIS ■ **Coagulopathy** Patients with cirrhosis often demonstrate a variety of abnormalities in both cellular and humoral clotting function. Thrombocytopenia may result from hypersplenism. In the alcoholic patient, there may be direct bone marrow suppression by ethanol. Diminished protein synthesis may lead to reduced production of fibrinogen (factor I), prothrombin (factor II), and factors V, VII, IX, and X. Reduction in levels of all factors except

factor V may be worsened by the coincident malabsorption of the fat-soluble cofactor vitamin K due to cholestasis (Chap. 275). Of these, factor VII appears to be pivotal. In cirrhosis, it is the first of the factors to become depleted and, because of its short half-life, replacement with plasma often fails to correct an elevated prothrombin time. Preliminary studies suggest that selective replacement of factor VII can correct the prothrombin time in patients with cirrhosis.

Hepatocellular Carcinoma   See Chap. 78.

HYPOXEMIA AND HEPATOPULMONARY SYNDROME ■ **Definition and Pathogenesis** Mild hypoxemia occurs in approximately one-third of patients with chronic liver disease. The hepatopulmonary syndrome is typically manifest by hypoxemia, platypnea, and orthodeoxia. Hypoxemia usually results from right-to-left intrapulmonary shunts through dilatations in intrapulmonary vessels that can be detected by contrast-enhanced echocardiography or a macroaggregated albumin lung perfusion scan. The mechanisms of shunt formation are unclear, but one animal model suggests that endothelin-1 levels and pulmonary nitric oxide, raised in cirrhosis, correlate with degree of shunting.

℞ TREATMENT

No specific treatment is consistently effective, though large arteriovenous shunts may be embolized. It is now increasingly recognized that liver transplantation may eventually lead to amelioration of the hepatopulmonary syndrome in cases that have not yet been complicated by advanced pulmonary hypertension.

FURTHER READING

DIXON JB et al: Nonalcoholic fatty liver disease: Predictors of nonalcoholic steatohepatitis and liver disease in the severely obese. Gastroenterology 121:91, 2001

DUVOUX C et al: Effects of noradrenaline and albumin in patients with type I hepatorenal syndrome: A pilot study. Hepatology 36:374, 2002

KAPLAN MM et al: Medical progress: Primary biliary cirrhosis. N Engl J Med 335:1570, 1996

MCCULLOUGH AJ, O'CONNOR JFB: Alcoholic liver disease: Recommendations for the American College of Gastroenterology. Am J Gastroenterol 93:2022, 1998

RIORDAN SM, WILLIAMS R: Treatment of hepatic encephalopathy. N Engl J Med 337:473, 1997

RUNYON BA et al: Management of adult patients with ascites caused by cirrhosis. Hepatology 27:264, 1998

SHARARA AI et al: Gastroesophageal variceal hemorrhage. N Engl J Med 345:669, 2001

VILLANUEVA C et al: Endoscopic ligation compared with combined treatment with nadolol and isosorbide mononitrate to prevent recurrent variceal bleeding. N Engl J Med 345:647, 2001

290 INFILTRATIVE, GENETIC, AND METABOLIC DISEASES AFFECTING THE LIVER
Daniel K. Podolsky

Many disseminated, systemic, or metabolic diseases involve the liver in a diffuse manner by the infiltration of abnormal cells or the accumulation of chemical substances or metabolites. Chemical accumulation may be extracellular or intracellular and may involve hepatocytes, Kupffer cells, or other elements of the reticuloendothelial system. Although infiltrative diseases may vary widely in cause and extrahepatic manifestations, the findings in the liver may be quite similar. Generalized enlargement and firmness of the liver, gradual and nonspecific deterioration of liver function, and, less often, signs of portal hypertension or ascites are typical features of this group of diseases. Differential diagnosis by clinical means may be difficult on occasion, but in patients in whom ancillary clinical findings do not establish the diagnosis, the diffusely infiltrated liver provides an excellent source of tissue for diagnostic purposes.

NONALCOHOLIC FATTY LIVER DISEASE (NAFLD), HEPATIC STEATOSIS (FATTY LIVER), AND NONALCOHOLIC STEATOHEPATITIS (NASH)

Slight to moderate enlargement of the liver due to a diffuse accumulation of neutral fat (triglycerides) in hepatocytes is an important clinical and pathologic finding. Imaging techniques such as computed tomography (CT), ultrasound, and magnetic resonance imaging (MRI) may each yield alterations suggesting increased fat in the liver. Several mechanisms can contribute to lipid accumulation in the liver. Fatty liver can be separated into two categories based on whether the fat droplets in the hepatocytes are macrovesicular or microvesicular (Table 290-1). In addition, fatty infiltration may be accompanied by necroinflammatory activity, a condition designated *nonalcoholic steatohepatitis*, a form of NAFLD. Although prospective data on natural history are limited, there is increasing evidence that patients may pro-

TABLE 290-1 *Causes of Hepatic Steatosis*

Macrovesicular (large fat droplets in hepatocytes)
    Alcohol, alcoholic liver disease[a]
    Insulin resistance
    Syndrome X (obesity, diabetes, hypertriglyceridemia, hypertension)
    Lipodystrophy
    Dysbetalipoproteinemias
    Protein-calorie malnutrition, starvation
    Total parenteral nutrition,[a] jejunoileal bypass
    Rapid weight loss
    Drugs,[a] e.g., methotrexate, aspirin, vitamin A, glucocorticoids,
        amiodarone, calcium channel blocker and synthetic estrogen,
        nucleoside analogues (ddI, AZT)
    Inflammatory bowel disease
Microvascular (small fat droplets in hepatocytes)
    Reye's syndrome
    Acute fatty liver of pregnancy
    Jamaican vomiting sickness
    Drugs, e.g., valproic acid, tetracycline, nucleoside analogues
    Environmental hepatotoxins (e.g., phosphorus, petrochemicals)

[a] May also be associated with necroinflammatory activity.

gress through several histologically distinct stages beginning with fatty liver and culminating in cirrhosis with intervening states of steatohepatitis and steatohepatitis with fibrosis (Fig. 290-1).

MACROVESICULAR FATTY LIVER   This is the most common type of fatty liver and is seen most frequently in alcoholism or alcoholic liver disease, diabetes mellitus, obesity, and prolonged parenteral nutrition. Hematoxylin and eosin-stained liver sections show hepatocytes with large, empty vacuoles with the nucleus "pushed" to the periphery of the cell. In general, fat in the liver is not damaging per se, and the fat will disappear with improvement or elimination of the predisposing condition.

Etiology   The major causes of fatty liver with macrovesicular fat depend on the age, geographic location, and metabolic-nutritional status of the patient population. *Chronic alcoholism* is the most common cause of hepatic steatosis in this country and in other countries with a high alcohol intake. The severity of fatty involvement is roughly proportional to the duration and degree of alcoholic excess. In addition, in western countries NAFLD/NASH is associated with obesity. Many of these patients (up to one-third) have type 2 diabetes and/or hyperlipidemia. The constellation of obesity, diabetes, hypertriglyceridemia, and hypertension has been designated *syndrome X* and has an especially strong association with progressive NAFLD. Age >45, obesity (body mass index ≥30), ratio of aspartate aminotransferase (AST)/to alanine aminotransferase (ALT) >1, and diabetes are all associated with increased risk for development of significant fibrosis. Inflammatory activity when present may reflect the combined effects of oxidative stress, subsequent lipid peroxidation, and abnormal cytokine expression, especially increased tumor necrosis factor.

Protein malnutrition, especially in infancy and early childhood, accounts for most cases of severe fatty liver in the tropical zones of

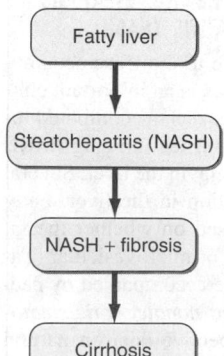

FIGURE 290-1 Hypothetical sequence of nonalcoholic fatty liver disease states. NASH, nonalcoholic steatohepatitis.

Africa, South America, and Asia. The hepatic changes may be associated with other clinical and pathologic features of kwashiorkor. *Jejunoileal bypass* for surgical treatment of morbid obesity was sometimes associated with severe fatty liver and hepatic failure that could be fatal. Ironically, patients with rapid weight loss or undergoing gastric bypass surgery for morbid obesity may also develop NAFLD. In patients with Cushing's syndrome and in those receiving large doses of glucocorticoids, fatty infiltration of the liver may occur. In many *chronic illnesses*, especially those complicated by impaired nutrition or malabsorption, increased fat is found in liver cells. For example, patients with severe ulcerative colitis, chronic pancreatitis, or protracted heart failure frequently have moderate hepatic steatosis at the time of death. Patients maintained on prolonged *total parenteral nutrition* may also develop a fatty liver. In some cases, fatty infiltration and steatohepatitis may occur in the absence of an identifiable cause.

Acute fatty liver is caused by a number of hepatotoxins and is frequently accompanied by signs and symptoms of liver failure. Carbon tetrachloride intoxication, DDT poisoning, and ingestion of substances containing yellow phosphorus result in severe hepatic steatosis. Acute and prolonged alcohol ingestion may also be considered in this category and may be associated with a rapidly enlarging and fat-laden liver.

Clinical Features   The signs and symptoms of hepatic steatosis are related to the degree of fat infiltration, the time course of its accumulation, and the underlying cause. The obese or diabetic patient with a chronic fatty liver is usually asymptomatic and has only mild tenderness over the enlarged liver. The liver function tests are normal or show mild elevations of alkaline phosphatase or aminotransferases. In contrast, the rapid accumulation of fat seen in the setting of hyperalimentation may lead to marked tenderness, presumably resulting from stretching of Glisson's capsule. Similarly, alcoholic patients with acute fatty liver following a bout of heavy drinking may have right upper quadrant pain and tenderness, often with laboratory evidence of cholestasis. The clinical presentation of fatty liver from hepatotoxins is similar to that of fulminant hepatic failure arising from any cause, with evidence of hepatic encephalopathy, marked elevations of prothrombin time and aminotransferases, and variable degrees of jaundice. Although steatohepatitis is generally thought to have a benign clinical course with improvement following elimination of the associated precipitant, in some individuals it may result in significant fibrosis and even cirrhosis. Recent studies indicate that substantial fibrosis or cirrhosis may be present in 15 to 50% of patients with NASH. In the only long-term follow-up study, 30% of patients with fibrosis had cirrhosis after 10 years. It is possible that some cases of "cryptogenic" cirrhosis are due to longstanding NASH and that the fat leaves the liver as end-stage liver disease develops.

Diagnosis   The findings of a firm, nontender, and generally enlarged liver with minimal hepatic dysfunction in a patient with chronic alcoholism, malnutrition, poorly controlled diabetes mellitus, or obesity should suggest hepatic steatosis. This can usually be detected by CT, MRI, or ultrasound. Modest elevations of aminotransferases are often found in association with hepatic steatohepatitis. A disproportional elevation in AST leading to an AST/ALT ratio >2 is generally associated with alcoholic hepatitis. When diagnostic uncertainty exists, needle biopsy of the liver will demonstrate the increased fat content, the presence of any fibrosis, and possibly the underlying primary disorder.

℞ TREATMENT

Adequate nutritional intake, removal of alcohol or offending toxins, and correction of any associated metabolic disorders usually result in recovery. There is no clinical rationale for the use of lipotropic agents such as choline. When indicated, attention should be directed to abstinence from alcohol, careful control of diabetes (by insulin therapy or use of oral hypoglycemic agents), weight loss, or correction of intestinal absorptive defects. In the alcoholic fatty liver, there is gradual disappearance of fat from the liver after 4 to 8 weeks of adequate diet and abstinence from alcohol. Similarly, fatty infiltration usually resolves within 2 weeks after discontinuation of parenteral hyperalimentation. Pilot studies in patients with NASH have suggested benefits from ursodiol, betaine (a precursor of S-adenosyl-methionine), and vitamin E and from phlebotomy. Troglitazone has shown some benefit in those patients with concomitant insulin resistance.

MICROVESICULAR FATTY LIVER This is the less common form of fatty liver. On microscopic examination, the fat is present in many small vacuoles. Although the droplets consist of triglycerides in both the macrovesicular and microvesicular forms, the reason for this difference in morphologic appearance is not clear.

Acute fatty liver of pregnancy (AFLP) is a syndrome that occurs late in pregnancy and is often associated with jaundice and hepatic failure. The liver is typically small. AFLP is more common when the mother is carrying a male fetus and may be associated with a deficiency of long-chain-3-hydroxy acyl COH dehydrogenase. AFLP usually necessitates termination of pregnancy due to the risk of rapid and fatal deterioration. Preeclampsia or the syndrome of *h*emolysis, *e*levated *l*iver enzymes, and *l*ow *p*latelet count (HELLP), which may complicate eclampsia, presents in a similar fashion and progresses to severe liver dysfunction, though typically with a normal size liver. Aminotransferase elevations are typically modest in all of these conditions (generally <500). If diagnosed in time, the disease usually resolves with termination of the pregnancy. Recurrence in subsequent pregnancies is rare.

Microvesicular fat accumulation also may be seen as a toxic reaction to valproic acid and with excessive doses of tetracycline. It is a typical finding in *Jamaican vomiting sickness*, which is caused by hypoglycin A present in unripened ackee fruit. The combination of lactic acidosis and severe liver injury with microvesicular fat has been described as a complication of nucleoside analogue therapy.

REYE'S SYNDROME (FATTY LIVER WITH ENCEPHALOPATHY) This acute illness is encountered exclusively in children <15 years. It is characterized clinically by vomiting and signs of progressive central nervous system damage, signs of hepatic injury, and hypoglycemia. Morphologically, there is extensive fatty vacuolization of the liver and renal tubules. There is mitochondrial dysfunction with decreased activity of hepatic mitochondrial enzymes. The cause is unknown, although viral agents and drugs, especially salicylates, have been implicated. Increased aspirin use and much higher serum salicylate levels in children with this illness than in the general population have been described during outbreaks of Reye's syndrome. Recognition of this relationship and reduced aspirin use in this setting may account for the decreasing incidence of Reye's syndrome. However, this illness may occur in the absence of exposure to salicylates. In fatal cases, the liver is enlarged and yellow with striking diffuse fatty microvacuolization of cells. Peripheral zonal hepatic necrosis has also been present in some cases. Fatty changes of the renal tubular cells, cerebral edema, and neuronal degeneration of the brain are the major extrahepatic changes. Electron-microscopic studies show structural alterations of mitochondria in liver, brain, and muscle.

The onset usually follows an upper respiratory tract infection, especially influenza or chickenpox. Within 1 to 3 days, persistent vomiting occurs, together with stupor, which usually progresses rapidly to generalized convulsions and coma. The liver is enlarged, but *jaundice is characteristically absent or minimal.* Elevations in serum aminotransferases and prothrombin time, hypoglycemia, metabolic acidosis, and elevated serum ammonia levels are the major laboratory findings. The mortality rate in Reye's syndrome is approximately 50%. Therapy consists of infusions of 20% glucose and fresh-frozen plasma, as well as intravenous mannitol to reduce the cerebral edema. Chronic liver disease has not been reported in survivors.

STORAGE DISEASES

Lipid storage diseases include the hereditary disorders of Gaucher's and Niemann-Pick diseases. Other rare diseases associated with increased fat in the liver include abetalipoproteinemia, Tangier disease, Fabry's disease, and types I and V hyperlipoproteinemia (Chap. 335).

Hepatic enlargement caused by distention of liver cells with glycogen is present in some poorly controlled diabetics and frequently in juvenile diabetes. More often, however, hepatomegaly is due to fatty infiltration (see above). Ketoacidosis and vigorous insulin therapy may further enhance hepatic enlargement.

HEPATIC MINERAL ACCUMULATION

WILSON'S DISEASE This is an uncommon inherited disorder of copper metabolism. Wilson's disease usually presents clinically in adolescence or young adulthood by which time there is excess copper accumulation in the liver and other tissues. Deficiency of the plasma copper protein ceruloplasmin is a characteristic feature. The accumulation appears to result from impaired copper excretion due to a mutation in a gene that encodes a P-type ATPase copper transporter. Clinically, patients may present in teenage or early adult years with chronic hepatitis, cirrhosis, or their complications. A small number of patients will present with fulminant hepatitis. Liver disease is often accompanied by softening and degeneration of the basal ganglia (hepatolenticular degeneration) due to copper deposition, which results in extrapyramidal neurologic and psychiatric symptoms. Brownish pigmentation of Descemet's membrane in the cornea (Kayser-Fleischer rings) is frequently present. Hemolytic anemia is also common, especially with fulminant disease. Liver biopsy may reveal findings ranging from fulminant hepatitis to chronic hepatitis and macronodular cirrhosis, in addition to excess copper levels. Typically, liver cells are ballooned and show increased glycogen with glycogen vacuolization in the nuclei. All patients under age 40 with unexplained chronic hepatitis or cirrhosis should be evaluated for possible Wilson's disease. Prompt diagnosis is important; treatment, which must be continued throughout life, can prevent progression of end-organ damage. →*For further discussion, see Chap. 339.*

HEMOCHROMATOSIS Hemochromatosis may be the most common genetic disorder of humans; it involves accumulation of abnormal amounts of iron due to inappropriate absorption from the intestine. Between 85 and 95% of patients with genetic hemochromatosis are homozygous for a point mutation (cystine to tyrosine at codon 282: C282). The liver, as a primary site of iron storage, is affected most directly. There is diffuse deposition of excess iron in hepatocytes, in contrast to the characteristic accumulation of iron in the reticuloendothelial compartment typical of secondary iron overload and hemosiderosis. Excess hepatic iron commonly results in hepatomegaly. Although liver function is initially well preserved, if the disease is untreated, progressive impairment is followed by the development of cirrhosis. Prompt diagnosis can permit the institution of effective lifelong therapy to reduce the iron load and halt progression of the disease. → *For further discussion, see Chap. 336.*

OTHER INFILTRATIVE AND METABOLIC DISEASES

α_1-**ANTITRYPSIN DEFICIENCY** Patients with homozygous deficiency of serum α_1-antitrypsin (α_1AT) are prone to develop emphysema in adult life. The disease is suggested by the absence of α_1-globulin on serum electrophoresis (α_1AT makes up 90% of this fraction normally) and confirmed by direct measurement of α_1AT. The exact phenotype can then be determined by electrophoresis. Although there are approximately 75 recognized alleles, only PiZ and PiS are associated with clinical disease. The molecular bases of these altered products have been related to single nucleic acid substitutions—e.g., PiZ is caused by a G (guanine) to A (adenine) transposition, which results in a substitution of a glutamic acid for lysine at residue 292 in the α_1AT protein. Hepatocytes of some patients with this deficiency contain globules positive with the periodic acid–Schiff reaction. Approximately 10% of children with homozygous deficiency (PiZZ phenotype) of α_1AT will develop significant liver disease, including neonatal hepatitis and progressive cirrhosis. It has been suggested that 15 to 20% of all chronic liver disease in infancy may be attributed to α_1AT deficiency. In adults, the most common manifestation of α_1AT deficiency is asymptomatic cirrhosis, which may progress from a micronodular to a macronodular state and may be complicated by the development of hepatocellular carcinoma. The occurrence of liver disease in these patients is not dependent on the development of lung disease. →*For further discussion, see Chap. 242.*

HURLER'S SYNDROME   This is an uncommon hereditary disease that is characterized by the widespread tissue deposition of mucopolysaccharide (chondroitin sulfate B and heparan sulfate) in many tissues. The liver is frequently enlarged and firm. Microscopically, Kupffer cells and other macrophages are enlarged and filled with metachromatic granular material. Cirrhosis may be a late complication. →*For further discussion, see Chap. 340.*

PORPHYRIAS   See Chap. 337.

RETICULOENDOTHELIAL DISORDERS (See also Chaps. 52 and 98)

Moderate to massive hepatomegaly and splenomegaly occur frequently in the various types of *leukemia* and *lymphoma*. Jaundice, when present, is usually slight and results from hemolysis, although cholestasis may occasionally be associated with lymphoma as a paraneoplastic syndrome. Deep and protracted jaundice is distinctly rare and is caused by obstruction of the intrahepatic or extrahepatic bile ducts by tumor. Liver biopsy specimens reveal portal and sinusoidal infiltrates in most cases of leukemia, but the cellular pattern may be mixed and nonspecific. Liver biopsy is diagnostic in only 5% of patients with *Hodgkin's disease*. This percentage is increased in those with advanced disease or splenomegaly. Directed biopsy at laparoscopy or laparotomy is more likely to be positive than "blind" needle biopsy. Nonspecific histologic changes in the liver have been described in patients with lymphoma and may contribute to the abnormal liver function tests.

Myeloid metaplasia and other myeloproliferative disorders associated with extramedullary hematopoiesis produce hepatomegaly which may reach huge proportions, especially following splenectomy. Serum alkaline phosphatase elevations are often found. Ascites and portal hypertension, resulting from diffuse involvement of portal venules and lymphatics, are rare complications.

GRANULOMATOUS INFILTRATIONS

Perhaps as a result of the large population of mononuclear phagocytes, a number of systemic granulomatous diseases involve the liver, including sarcoidosis, miliary tuberculosis, histoplasmosis, brucellosis, schistosomiasis, berylliosis, and drug reactions (Table 290-2). In addition, isolated granulomas of no diagnostic importance may be found occasionally in patients with various forms of cirrhosis and hepatitis. The liver infiltrated by granulomas may be slightly enlarged and firm,

TABLE 290-2   *Some Causes of Hepatic Granulomas*

SYSTEMIC DISEASE	
Sarcoidosis	Berylliosis
Hodgkin's and non-Hodgkin's lymphoma	Crohn's disease
	Wegener's granulomatosis
Primary biliary cirrhosis	Granulomatous hepatitis, idiopathic

INFECTIONS	
Bacterial	Parasitic
Tuberculosis	Schistosomiasis
Mycobacterium avium-intracellulare	Rickettsial
	Q fever
Brucellosis	Spirochetes
Leprosy	Syphilis
Viral	Drugs
Epstein-Barr virus	Sulfonamides
Cytomegalovirus	Isoniazid
Chicken pox	Allopurinol

but hepatic dysfunction is usually limited. Increases in serum alkaline phosphatase are common and may range from mild to marked. Occasionally, mild serum elevations in aminotransferases are also present. In a few patients with sarcoidosis or brucellosis, portal hypertension may develop, and extensive postnecrotic scarring or postnecrotic cirrhosis may follow healing of the granulomatous lesions, as in schistosomiasis.

Needle biopsy of the liver often provides the first definite evidence of a systemic or disseminated granulomatous disease. In patients with sarcoidosis who have neither clinical nor laboratory evidence of hepatic involvement, needle biopsy shows sarcoid granulomas in about 80% of cases. In cases of suspected miliary tuberculosis, a portion of the biopsy should be cultured and stained for mycobacteria. The organism can be detected in the majority of cases, particularly when caseating granulomas are present. Serial sections of the biopsy specimen should be examined if granulomas are not apparent. Individual granulomas are rarely specific in their microscopic appearance, and final diagnosis usually requires other clinical, laboratory, or histologic data.

In approximately 20% of patients, it is not possible to identify a cause for the granulomatous infiltration. When these infiltrates are accompanied by fever of unknown origin, the diagnosis of *granulomatous hepatitis* should be considered. This is an uncommon disorder of unknown cause and is diagnosed by exclusion. While granulomatous hepatitis invariably responds to moderate doses of glucocorticoids, relapses are frequent, and such therapy should never be undertaken unless tuberculous disease or other causes of granulomatous infiltration have been excluded. This may include an initial empirical trial of antituberculous therapy.

AMYLOIDOSIS   (See also Chap. 310)   Systemic amyloidosis, whether primary and idiopathic, familial, or secondary to chronic inflammatory or neoplastic diseases, often involves the liver. Grossly, the liver infiltrated with amyloid is enlarged and pale and rubbery in consistency. Microscopically, the birefringent amyloid deposits appear as homogeneous waxy material within the space of Disse, often being concentrated in the periportal areas and associated with atrophy of adjacent liver cell plates. Selective involvement of the walls of blood vessels, especially of the hepatic arterioles, may be a striking feature of primary amyloidosis. With this possible exception, however, the hepatic lesions are the same in all forms of amyloidosis and are present in 60 to 90% of cases.

An enlarged and firm liver is found in about 60% of patients, and ascites occurs in advanced stages of the disease in about 20%. Jaundice, portal hypertension, and other signs of chronic liver disease are usually absent. Liver function changes, although frequent, correlate poorly with the extent of liver infiltration. Hypoalbuminemia and elevated serum alkaline phosphatase are common. Hypoalbuminemia, however, may be related to the presence of nephrosis; the prothrombin time is usually normal. The diagnosis is established by biopsy of rectum, skin, liver, or other involved organs and demonstration of the characteristic Congo red–staining deposits by polarizing microscopy.

AIDS-RELATED LIVER DISEASE

Liver disease has become an important cause of morbidity and mortality in patients with HIV/AIDS, due largely to complications derived from chronic active hepatitis involving co-infection with hepatitis B and/or C viruses (Chaps. 173 and 285). This has become particularly evident in the era of highly active antiretroviral therapy (HAART), which has been successful in decreasing the levels of HIV viremia (Chap. 173). Patients are living longer due to the beneficial effects of HAART, and their liver disease and its complications have assumed a more important role in determining the ultimate clinical course of these patients. The approach to such patients is discussed in detail in Chaps. 173 and 285. Other important sources of liver damage in HIV-infected individuals are the direct hepatotoxic effects of antiretroviral drugs used in the HAART regimens. This is particularly true of the non-nucleoside analogue nevirapine (Chap. 173) as well as certain of the nucleoside analogues and protease inhibitors. Finally, patients with advanced HIV diseases commonly have evidence of secondary liver disease, generally mild, that is due to hepatic involvement with other systemic diseases. In these patients, hepatic granulomatous disease is often present and may be caused by opportunistic infections, with *Mycobacterium avium-intracellulare* being a common pathogen. Cytomegalovirus hepatitis and hepatic mycoses are less common. AIDS cholangiopathy is a well-recognized entity. It exhibits features similar to those found in primary sclerosing cholangitis and is typically associated with cryptosporidia, microsporidia, and/or cytomegalovirus infection in the biliary tree. Papillary stenosis is frequently present.

FURTHER READING

AMERICAN GASTROENTEROLOGICAL ASSOCIATION: Medical Position Statement: Nonalcoholic fatty liver disease. Gastroenterology 123:1702, 2002

ANGULO P: Nonalcoholic fatty liver disease. N Engl J Med 346:1221, 2002

KNOX TA, OLANS LB: Liver disease in pregnancy. N Engl J Med 335:569, 1996

SCRIVER CR et al (eds): *The Metabolic and Molecular Bases of Inherited Disease*, 8th ed. New York, McGraw-Hill, 2001

ZAKIM D, BOYER TD: *Hepatology: A Textbook of Liver Disease*, 3d ed. Philadelphia, Saunders, 1996

291 LIVER TRANSPLANTATION
Jules L. Dienstag

Liver transplantation—the replacement of the native, diseased liver by a normal organ (allograft)—has matured from an experimental procedure reserved for desperately ill patients to an accepted, lifesaving operation applied much earlier in the natural history of end-stage liver disease. The preferred and technically most advanced approach is *orthotopic transplantation*, in which the native organ is removed and the donor organ is inserted in the same anatomic location. Pioneered in the 1960s by Starzl at the University of Colorado and, later, at the University of Pittsburgh and by Calne in Cambridge, England, liver transplantation is now performed routinely by dozens of centers throughout North America and western Europe. Success measured as 1 year survival has improved from ~30% in the 1970s to >85% today. These improved prospects for prolonged survival, dating back to the early 1980s, resulted from refinements in operative technique, improvements in organ procurement and preservation, advances in immunosuppressive therapy, and, perhaps most influentially, more enlightened patient selection and timing. Despite the perioperative morbidity and mortality, the technical and management challenges of the procedure, and its costs, liver transplantation has become the approach of choice for selected patients whose chronic or acute liver disease is progressive, life-threatening, and unresponsive to medical therapy. Based on the current level of success, the number of liver transplants has continued to grow each year; in 2000 to 2002, approximately 4500 patients received liver allografts in the United States. Still, the demand for new livers continues to outpace availability; in the same period, >16,000 patients in the United States were on a waiting list for a donor liver. In response to this drastic shortage of donor organs, many transplantation centers have begun to supplement cadaver-organ liver transplantation with living-donor transplantation.

INDICATIONS Potential candidates for liver transplantation are children and adults who, in the absence of contraindications (see below), suffer from severe, irreversible liver disease for which alternative medical or surgical treatments have been exhausted or are unavailable. *Timing of the operation is of critical importance.* Indeed, improved timing and better patient selection are felt to have contributed more to the increased success of liver transplantation in the 1980s and beyond than all the impressive technical and immunologic advances combined. Although the disease should be advanced, and although opportunities for spontaneous or medically induced stabilization or recovery should be allowed, the procedure should be done sufficiently early to give the surgical procedure a fair chance for success. Ideally, transplantation should be considered in patients with end-stage liver disease who are experiencing or have experienced a life-threatening complication of hepatic decompensation, whose quality of life has deteriorated to unacceptable levels, or whose liver disease will result predictably in irreversible damage to the central nervous system (CNS). If this is done sufficiently early, the patient will not have developed any contraindications or extrahepatic systemic deterioration. Although patients with well-compensated cirrhosis can survive for many years, many patients

with quasi-stable chronic liver disease have much more advanced disease than may be apparent. As discussed below, the better the status of the patient prior to transplantation, the higher will be the anticipated success rate of transplantation. The decision about *when* to transplant is complex and requires the combined judgment of an experienced team of hepatologists, transplant surgeons, anesthesiologists, and specialists in support services, not to mention the well-informed consent of the patient and the patient's family.

Transplantation in Children Indications for transplantation in children are listed in Table 291-1. The most common is *biliary atresia. Inherited or genetic disorders of metabolism* associated with liver failure constitute another major indication for transplantation in children and adolescents. In Crigler-Najjar disease type I and in certain hereditary disorders of the urea cycle and of amino acid or lactate-pyruvate metabolism, transplantation may be the only way to prevent impending deterioration of CNS function, despite the fact that the native liver is structurally normal. Combined heart and liver transplantation has yielded dramatic improvement in cardiac function and in cholesterol levels in children with homozygous familial hypercholesterolemia; combined liver and kidney transplantation has been successful in patients with hereditary oxalosis. In hemophiliacs with transfusion-associated hepatitis and liver failure, liver transplantation has been associated with recovery of normal factor VIII synthesis.

Transplantation in Adults Liver transplantation is indicated for end-stage *cirrhosis* of all causes (Table 291-1). In sclerosing cholangitis and *Caroli's disease* (multiple cystic dilatations of the intrahepatic biliary tree), recurrent infections and sepsis associated with inflammatory and fibrotic obstruction of the biliary tree may be an indication for transplantation. Because prior biliary surgery complicates, and is a relative contraindication for, liver transplantation, surgical diversion of the biliary tree has been all but abandoned for patients with sclerosing cho-

TABLE 291-1 *Indications for Liver Transplantation*

Children	Adults
Biliary atresia	Primary biliary cirrhosis
Neonatal hepatitis	Secondary biliary cirrhosis
Congenital hepatic fibrosis	Primary sclerosing cholangitis
Alagille's disease[a]	Caroli's disease[c]
Byler's disease[b]	Cryptogenic cirrhosis
α_1-Antitrypsin deficiency	Chronic hepatitis with cirrhosis
Inherited disorders of metabolism	Hepatic vein thrombosis
Wilson's disease	Fulminant hepatitis
Tyrosinemia	Alcoholic cirrhosis
Glycogen storage diseases	Chronic viral hepatitis
Lysosomal storage diseases	Primary hepatocellular malignancies
Protoporphyria	Hepatic adenomas
Crigler-Najjar disease type I	
Familial hypercholesterolemia	
Hereditary oxalosis	
Hemophilia	

[a] Arteriohepatic dysplasia, with paucity of bile ducts, and congenital malformations, including pulmonary stenosis.
[b] Intrahepatic cholestasis, progressive liver failure, mental and growth retardation.
[c] Multiple cystic dilatations of the intrahepatic biliary tree.

langitis. In patients who undergo transplantation for *hepatic vein thrombosis (Budd-Chiari syndrome)*, postoperative anticoagulation is essential; underlying myeloproliferative disorders may have to be treated but are not a contraindication to liver transplantation. If a donor organ can be located quickly, before life-threatening complications—including cerebral edema—set in, patients with *fulminant hepatitis* are candidates for liver transplantation. Initially controversial but now routine candidates for liver transplantation are patients with *alcoholic cirrhosis, chronic viral hepatitis*, and *primary hepatocellular malignancies*. Although all three of these categories are considered to be high risk, liver transplantation can be offered to carefully selected patients, and, currently chronic hepatitis C and alcoholic liver disease are the most common indications for liver transplantation, accounting for 40% of all adult candidates for the procedure. Patients with alcoholic cirrhosis can be considered as candidates for transplantation if they meet strict criteria for abstinence and reform. Patients with chronic hepatitis C have early allograft and patient survival comparable to those of other subsets of patients after transplantation; however, reinfection in the donor organ is universal, recurrent hepatitis C is insidiously progressive, the impact of antiviral therapy is limited, and cirrhosis and late organ failure (beyond 5 years) are being recognized with increasing frequency. In patients with chronic hepatitis B, in the absence of measures to prevent recurrent hepatitis B, survival after transplantation is reduced by approximately 10 to 20%; however, prophylactic use of hepatitis B immune globulin (HBIg) during and after transplantation increases the success of transplantation to a level comparable to that seen in patients with nonviral causes of liver decompensation. The specific oral antiviral drugs lamivudine and adefovir dipivoxil (Chap. 287) can be used for both prophylaxis against, and treatment of, recurrent hepatitis B, facilitating further the management of patients undergoing liver transplantation for end-stage hepatitis B. Issues of disease recurrence are discussed in more detail below. Patients with nonmetastatic primary hepatobiliary tumors—primary hepatocellular carcinoma, cholangiocarcinoma, hepatoblastoma, angiosarcoma, epithelioid hemangioendothelioma, and multiple or massive hepatic adenomata—have undergone liver transplantation; however, for hepatobiliary malignancies, overall survival is significantly lower than that for other categories of liver disease. To minimize the very high likelihood of recurrent tumor after transplantation, some centers are evaluating experimental adjuvant chemotherapy protocols. Some transplantation centers have reported excellent long-term, recurrence-free survival in patients with unresectable hepatocellular carcinoma for single tumors <5 cm in diameter or for three or fewer lesions all <3 cm. Consequently, most centers restrict liver transplantation to patients whose hepatic malignancies are confined to these limits. Because the likelihood of recurrent cholangiocarcinoma is almost universal, this tumor is no longer considered an indication for transplantation.

CONTRAINDICATIONS   *Absolute contraindications* for transplantation include life-threatening systemic diseases, uncontrolled extrahepatic bacterial or fungal infections, preexisting advanced cardiovascular or pulmonary disease, multiple uncorrectable life-threatening congenital anomalies, metastatic malignancy, active drug or alcohol abuse, and HIV infection (Table 291-2). Because carefully selected patients in their sixties and even seventies have undergone transplantation successfully, advanced age per se is no longer considered an absolute contraindication; however, in older patients, a more thorough preoperative evaluation should be undertaken to exclude ischemic cardiac disease. Advanced age (>70 years), however, may be considered a *relative contraindication*—that is, a factor to be taken into account with other relative contraindications. Other relative contraindications include portal vein thrombosis, preexisting renal disease not associated with liver disease, intrahepatic or biliary sepsis, severe hypoxemia resulting from right-to-left intrapulmonary shunts, previous extensive hepatobiliary surgery, and any uncontrolled serious psychiatric disorder. Any one of these relative contraindications is insufficient in and

TABLE 291-2 *Contraindications to Liver Transplantation*

Absolute	Relative
Uncontrolled extrahepatobiliary infection	Age >70
Active, untreated sepsis	Prior extensive hepatobiliary surgery
Uncorrectable, life-limiting congenital anomalies	Portal vein thrombosis
Active substance or alcohol abuse	Renal failure
Advanced cardiopulmonary disease	Previous extrahepatic malignancy
Extrahepatobiliary malignancy	Severe obesity
Metastatic malignancy to the liver	Severe malnutrition/wasting
Cholangiocarcinoma	Medical noncompliance
AIDS	HIV seropositivity
Life-threatening systemic diseases	Intrahepatic sepsis
	Severe hypoxemia secondary to right-to-left intrapulmonary shunts
	Uncontrolled psychiatric disorder

of itself to preclude transplantation. For example, the problem of portal vein thrombosis can be overcome by constructing a graft from the donor liver portal vein to the recipient's superior mesenteric vein. Now that highly active antiretroviral therapy has dramatically improved the survival of persons with HIV infection (Chap. 173), and because chronic hepatitis C has emerged as a serious source of morbidity and mortality in the HIV-infected population, the applicability of liver transplantation to this previously excluded patient group is being reexamined. Clinical trials of liver transplantation for patients with HIV infection are in progress.

TECHNICAL CONSIDERATIONS   ■   **Cadaver Donor Selection** Cadaver donor livers for transplantation are procured primarily from victims of head trauma. Organs from brain-dead donors up to age 60 are acceptable if the following criteria are met: hemodynamic stability, adequate oxygenation, absence of bacterial or fungal infection, absence of abdominal trauma, absence of hepatic dysfunction, and serologic exclusion of hepatitis B and C viruses and HIV. Occasionally, organs from donors with hepatitis B and C are used, e.g., for recipients with prior hepatitis B and C, respectively. Donor organs with antibody to hepatitis B core antigen (anti-HBc) are used rarely, when the need is especially urgent, and recipients of these organs are treated prophylactically with HBIg and other antiviral drugs. Cardiovascular and respiratory functions are maintained artificially until the liver can be removed. Compatibility in ABO blood group and organ size between donor and recipient are important considerations in donor selection; however, ABO-incompatible or reduced-donor-organ transplants can be performed in emergency or marked donor-scarcity situations. Tissue typing for HLA matching is not required, and preformed cytotoxic HLA antibodies do not preclude liver transplantation. Following perfusion with cold electrolyte solution, the donor liver is removed and packed in ice. The use of University of Wisconsin (UW) solution, rich in lactobionate and raffinose, has permitted the extension of cold ischemic time up to 20 h; however, 12 h may be a more reasonable limit. Improved techniques for harvesting multiple organs from the same donor have increased the availability of donor livers, but the availability of donor livers is far outstripped by the demand. Currently, in the United States, all donor livers are distributed through a nationwide organ-sharing network [United Network of Organ Sharing (UNOS)] designed to allocate available organs based on regional considerations and recipient acuity. Recipients who require the highest level of care (intensive care) have the highest priority, but allocation strategies that balance highest urgency against best outcomes continue to evolve to distribute cadaver organs most effectively. Allocation based on the Child-Turcotte-Pugh (CTP) score, which uses five clinical variables (encephalopathy stage, ascites, bilirubin, albumin, and prothrombin time) and waiting time, has been supplanted by allocation based upon urgency alone, calculated by the Model for End-Stage Liver Disease (MELD) score. The MELD score is based upon a mathematical model that includes bilirubin, creatinine, and prothrombin time expressed as international normalized ratio (INR) (Table 291-3). Neither waiting time (except as a tie breaker between two potential recipients with the same MELD scores) nor posttransplantation outcome is taken into account, but the MELD score has been shown to be the best predictor of pretransplantation mortality, satisfies the prevailing view that medical need should be the decisive determinant, and eliminates both the subjectivity inherent in the CTP scoring system (presence and degree of ascites and hepatic encephalopathy) and the differences in waiting times among different regions of the country. Because candidates for liver transplantation who have hepatocellular carcinoma may not be sufficiently decompensated to compete for donor organs based upon urgency criteria alone, and because protracted waiting for cadaver donor organs results often in tumor growth beyond acceptable limits for transplantation, such patients are assigned extra MELD points (Table 291-3).

TABLE 291-3 *United Network for Organ Sharing (UNOS) Liver Transplantation Waiting List Criteria*

PREVIOUS ALLOCATION SCHEME (IN ORDER OF DESCENDING URGENCY)

Status 1	Fulminant hepatic failure (including primary graft nonfunction and hepatic artery thrombosis within 7 days after transplantation as well as acute decompensated Wilson's disease)[a]
Status 2A	Chronic liver disease with CTP[b] score $\geq$ 10, in intensive care unit, predicted <7 days to live, plus one of following: hepatic encephalopathy $\geq$ stage III, unresponsive variceal bleeding, heptorenal syndrome, refractory ascites or hepatic hydrothorax, coagulopathy with ongoing bleeding (cannot have extrahepatic sepsis, high-dose or double pressor dependency, or multiorgan failure)
Status 2B	Chronic liver disease with CTP score $\geq$ 10 or CTP score $\geq$ 7 plus one of following: variceal bleeding, heptorenal syndrome, history of spontaneous bacterial periotonitis, refractory ascites or hepatic hydrothorax, refractory bleeding
Status 3	CTP score $\geq$ 7
Status 7	Inactive

CURRENT ALLOCATION SCHEME

The Model for End-Stage Liver Disease (MELD) score, on a continuous scale,[c] determines allocation of donor organs. This model is based upon the following calculation:

$3.78 \times \log_e$ bilirubin (mg/100 mL) $+ 11.2 \times \log_e$ international normalized ratio (INR) $+ 9.57 \times \log_e$ creatinine (mg/100 mL) $+ 6.43$ ($\times$ 0 for alcoholic and cholestatic liver disease, $\times$ 1 for all other types of liver disease).[d,e,f]

Online calculators to determine MELD scores are available, such as *www.mayoclinic.org/gi-rst/mayomodel6.htm*

[a] For children < 18 years, status 1 includes acute or chronic liver failure plus hospitalization in an intensive care unit or inborn errors of metabolism.

[b] Child-Turcotte-Pugh (CTP) score components

Points	1	2	3
Encephalopathy	None	Stages I–II	Stages III–IV
Ascites	Absent	Slight, responsive	Moderate-severe
Bilirubin (mg/100 mL)	<2	2–3	>3
Albumin (g/100 mL)	>3.5	2.8–3.5	<2.8
Prothrombin time	<15 s	15–17 s	>17 s

The CTP score is calculated by assigning 1 point for any feature in column 1, 2 points for any feature in column 2, and 3 points for any feature in column 3. Class A = ≤6; class B = 7–9; class C = ≥10. For cholestatic disorders, such as primary biliary cirrhosis, primary sclerosing cholangitic, etc., the bilirubin categories are <4, 4–10, and >10.

[c] Instead of the 4 categories of severity in the previous system and 8 potential CTP scores between 7 and 15, the MELD scale is continuous, with 34 levels ranging between 6 and 40. The MELD scale replaces status 2A, 2B, and 3 (and 7), but status 1 is retained for those with the highest priority. Donor organs rarely become available unless the MELD score exceeds 20 to 30.

[d] Patients with hepatocellular carcinoma receive an extra 20 (for stage T1) or 24 (for stage T2) points. An α-fetoprotein level ≥ 500 ng/mL is considered as stage I hepatocellular carcinoma even without evidence for a tumor on imaging.

[e] Creatinine is included, because renal function is a validated predictor of survival in patients with liver disease. For adults undergoing dialysis twice a week, the creatinine in the equation is set to 4 mg/100 mL.

[f] For children <18 years, the Pediatric End-Stage Liver Disease (PELD) scale is used. This scale is based upon albumin, bilirubin, INR, growth failure, and age. Status 1 is retained, but the PELD replaces status 2 and 3.

Living-Donor Transplantation Occasionally, especially for liver transplantation in children, one cadaver organ can be split between two (one adult and one child) recipients. A more viable alternative, transplantation of the right lobe of the liver from a healthy adult into an adult recipient, is gaining increasing popularity. Living-donor transplantation of the left lobe (left lateral segment), introduced in the early 1990s to alleviate the extreme shortage of donor organs for small children, accounts currently for approximately a third of all liver transplantation procedures in children. Driven by the shortage of cadaver organs, living-donor transplantation involving the more sizable right lobe is being considered with increasing frequency in adults. More than 500 such procedures were done in 2001, representing >5% of all liver transplant operations done in the United States.

Living-donor transplantation can reduce waiting time and cold-ischemia time; is done under elective, rather than emergency, circumstances; and may be lifesaving in recipients who cannot afford to wait for a cadaver donor. The downside, of course, is the risk to the healthy donor (a mean of 10 weeks of medical disability; biliary complications in ~5%; postoperative complications such as wound infection, small-bowel obstruction, and incisional hernias in 9 to 19%; and, even, in 0.2 to 0.4%, death) as well as the increased frequency of biliary (15 to 32%) and vascular (10%) complications in the recipient. Potential donors must participate voluntarily without coercion, and transplantation teams should go to great lengths to exclude subtle coercive or inappropriate psychological factors as well as to outline carefully to both donor and recipient the potential benefits and risks of the procedure. Donors for the procedure should be 18 to 60 years old; have a compatible blood type with the recipient; have no chronic medical problems or history of major abdominal surgery; be related genetically or emotionally to the recipient; and pass an exhaustive series of clinical, biochemical, and serologic evaluations to unearth disqualifying medical disorders. The recipient should meet the same UNOS criteria for liver transplantation as recipients of a cadaver donor allograft.

Surgical Technique Removal of the recipient's native liver is technically difficult, particularly in the presence of portal hypertension with its associated collateral circulation and extensive varices, and even more so in the presence of scarring from previous abdominal operations. The combination of portal hypertension and coagulopathy (elevated prothrombin time and thrombocytopenia) may translate into large blood product transfusion requirements. After the portal vein and infrahepatic and suprahepatic inferior vena cavae are dissected, the hepatic artery and common bile duct are dissected. Then, the native liver is removed and the donor organ inserted. During the anhepatic phase, coagulopathy, hypoglycemia, hypocalcemia, and hypothermia are encountered and must be managed by the anesthesiology team. Caval, portal vein, hepatic artery, and bile duct anastomoses are performed in succession, the last by end-to-end suturing of the donor and recipient common bile ducts or by choledochojejunostomy to a Roux en Y loop if the recipient common bile duct cannot be used for reconstruction (e.g., in sclerosing cholangitis). A typical transplant operation lasts 8 h, with a range of 6 to 18 h. Because of excessive bleeding, large volumes of blood, blood products, and volume expanders may be required during surgery; however, blood requirements have fallen sharply with improvements in surgical technique and experience.

As noted above, emerging alternatives to orthotopic liver transplantation include split-liver grafts, in which one donor organ is divided and inserted into two recipients; and living-donor procedures, in which the left (for children) or the right (for adults) lobe of the liver is harvested from a living donor for transplantation into the recipient. In the adult procedure, once the right lobe is removed from the donor, the donor right hepatic vein is anastomosed to the recipient right hepatic vein remnant, followed by donor-to-recipient anastomoses of the portal vein and then the hepatic artery. Finally, the biliary anastomosis is performed, duct-to-duct if practical or via Roux-en-Y anastomosis. Heterotopic liver transplantation, in which the donor liver is inserted without removal of the native liver, has met with very limited success and acceptance, except in a very small number of centers. To support desperately ill patients until a suitable donor organ can be identified, several transplantation centers are studying extracorporeal perfusion with bioartificial liver cartridges constructed from hepatocytes bound to hollow fiber systems and used as temporary hepatic-assist devices, but their efficacy remains to be established. Areas of research with the potential to overcome the shortage of donor organs include hepatocyte transplantation and xenotransplantation with genetically modified organs of nonhuman origin (e.g., swine).

POSTOPERATIVE COURSE AND MANAGEMENT ■ Immunosuppressive Therapy

The introduction in 1980 of cyclosporine as an immunosuppressive agent contributed substantially to the improvement in survival after liver transplantation. Cyclosporine, a calcineurin inhibitor, blocks early activation of T cells and is specific for T cell functions that result from the interaction of the T cell with its receptor and that involve the calcium-dependent signal transduction pathway. As a result, the activity of cyclosporine leads to inhibition of lymphokine gene activation, blocking interleukins 2, 3, and 4, tumor necrosis factor α, as well as other lymphokines. Cyclosporine also inhibits B cell functions. This process occurs without affecting rapidly dividing cells in the bone marrow, which may account for the reduced frequency of posttransplantation systemic infections. The most common and important side effect of cyclosporine therapy is nephrotoxicity. Cyclosporine causes dose-dependent renal tubular injury and direct renal artery vasospasm. Following renal function, therefore, is important in monitoring cyclosporine therapy, perhaps even a more reliable indicator than blood levels of the drug. Nephrotoxicity is reversible and can be managed by dose reduction. Other adverse effects of cyclosporine therapy include hypertension, hyperkalemia, tremor, hirsutism, glucose intolerance, and gum hyperplasia.

Tacrolimus (originally labeled FK 506) is a macrolide lactone antibiotic isolated from a Japanese soil fungus, *Streptomyces tsukubaensis*. It has the same mechanism of action as cyclosporine but is 10 to 100 times more potent. Initially applied as "rescue" therapy for patients in whom rejection occurred despite the use of cyclosporine, tacrolimus was shown in two large, multicenter, randomized trials to be associated with a reduced frequency of acute rejection, refractory rejection, and chronic rejection. Although patient and graft survival are the same with these two drugs, the advantage of tacrolimus in minimizing episodes of rejection, reducing the need for additional glucocorticoid doses, and reducing the likelihood of bacterial and cytomegalovirus infection has simplified the management of patients undergoing liver transplantation. In addition, the oral absorption of tacrolimus is more predictable than that of cyclosporine, especially during the early postoperative period when T-tube drainage interferes with the enterohepatic circulation of cyclosporine. As a result, in most transplantation centers, tacrolimus has now supplanted cyclosporine for primary immunosuppression, and many centers rely on oral, rather than intravenous, administration from the outset. For transplantation centers that prefer cyclosporine, a new, better-absorbed, microemulsion preparation is now available.

Although tacrolimus is more potent than cyclosporine, it is also more toxic and more likely to be discontinued for adverse events. The toxicity of tacrolimus is similar to that of cyclosporine; nephrotoxicity and neurotoxicity are the most commonly encountered adverse effects, and neurotoxicity (tremor, seizures, hallucinations, psychoses, coma) is more likely and more severe in tacrolimus-treated patients. Both drugs can cause diabetes mellitus, but tacrolimus does not cause hirsutism or gingival hyperplasia. Because of overlapping toxicity between cyclosporine and tacrolimus, especially nephrotoxicity, and because tacrolimus reduces cyclosporine clearance, these two drugs should not be used together. Because 99% of tacrolimus is metabolized by the liver, hepatic dysfunction reduces its clearance; in primary graft nonfunction (when, for technical reasons or because of ischemic dam-

age prior to its insertion, the allograft is defective and does not function normally from the outset) tacrolimus doses have to be reduced substantially, especially in children. Both cyclosporine and tacrolimus are metabolized by the cytochrome P450 IIIA system, and, therefore, drugs that induce cytochrome P450 (e.g., phenytoin, phenobarbital, carbamazepine, rifampin) reduce available levels of cyclosporine and tacrolimus; drugs that inhibit cytochrome P450 (e.g., erythromycin, fluconazole, ketoconazole, clotrimazole, itraconazole, verapamil, diltiazem, nicardipine, cimetidine, danazol, metoclopramide, bromocriptine) increase cyclosporine and tacrolimus blood levels. Like azathioprine, cyclosporine and tacrolimus appear to be associated with a risk of lymphoproliferative malignancies (see below), which may occur earlier after cyclosporine or tacrolimus than after azathioprine therapy. Because of these side effects, combinations of cyclosporine or tacrolimus with prednisone and azathioprine—all at reduced doses—are preferable regimens for immunosuppressive therapy.

In patients with pretransplant renal dysfunction or renal deterioration that occurs intraoperatively or immediately postoperatively, tacrolimus or cyclosporine therapy may not be practical; under these circumstances, induction or maintenance of immunosuppression with monoclonal antibodies to T cells, OKT3, may be appropriate. Therapy with OKT3 has been especially effective in reversing acute rejection in the posttransplant period and is the standard treatment for acute rejection that fails to respond to methylprednisolone boluses. Intravenous infusions of OKT3 may be complicated by transient fever, chills, and diarrhea. When this drug is used to induce immunosuppression initially or to provide "rescue" in those who reject despite "conventional" therapy, the incidence of bacterial, fungal, and especially cytomegalovirus infections is increased during and after such therapy. In some centers, ganciclovir antiviral therapy is initiated prophylactically as a routine along with OKT3. Because OKT3 is such a potent immunosuppressive agent, its use is more likely to be complicated by opportunistic infection or lymphoproliferative disorders; therefore, and because of the availability of alternative immunosuppressive drugs, OKT3 is used less often nowadays. Another immunosuppressive drug being used for patients undergoing liver transplantation is mycophenolic acid, a nonnucleoside purine metabolism inhibitor derived as a fermentation product from several *Penicillium* species. Mycophenolate has been shown to be better than azathioprine, when used with other standard immunosuppressive drugs, in preventing rejection after renal transplantation and has been adopted as well for use in liver transplantation. The most common adverse effects of mycophenolate are leukopenia and gastrointestinal complaints. Rapamycin, an inhibitor of later events in T cell activation, is yet another drug undergoing evaluation as an immunosuppressive agent.

The most important principle of immunosuppression is that the ideal approach strikes a balance between immunosuppression and immunologic competence. Given sufficient immunosuppression, acute liver allograft rejection is always reversible; however, if the cumulative dose of immunosuppressive therapy is too large, the patient will succumb to opportunistic infection. Therefore, immunosuppressive drugs must be used judiciously, with strict attention to the infectious consequences of such therapy. In this vein, efforts have been made to minimize the use of glucocorticoids, a mainstay of immunosuppressive regimens, and, in some instances, steroid-free immunosuppression can be achieved.

Postoperative Complications Complications of liver transplantation can be divided into hepatic and nonhepatic categories (Tables 291-4 and 291-5). In addition, both immediately postoperative and late complications are encountered. Patients who undergo liver transplantation as a rule have been chronically ill for protracted periods and may be malnourished and wasted. The impact of such chronic illness and the multisystem failure that accompanies liver failure continues to require attention in the postoperative period. Because of the massive fluid losses and fluid shifts that occur during the operation, patients may remain fluid overloaded during the immediate postoperative period, straining cardiovascular reserve; this effect can be amplified in the face

TABLE 291-4 *Nonhepatic Complications of Liver Transplantation*

Fluid overload	
Cardiovascular instability	Arrhythmias
	Congestive heart failure
	Cardiomyopathy
Pulmonary compromise	Pneumonia
	Pulmonary capillary vascular permeability
	Fluid overload
Renal dysfunction	Prerenal azotemia
	Hypoperfusion injury (acute tubular necrosis)
	Drug nephrotoxicity
	$\downarrow$ Renal blood flow secondary to $\uparrow$ intraabdominal pressure
Hematologic	Anemia 2° to gastrointestinal and/or intraabdominal bleeding
	Hemolytic anemia, aplastic anemia
	Thrombocytopenia
Infection	Bacterial: early, common postoperative infections
	Fungal/parasitic: late, opportunistic infections
	Viral: late, opportunistic infections, recurrent hepatitis
Neuropsychiatric	Seizures
	Encephalopathy
	Depression
	Difficult psychosocial adjustment
Diseases of donor	Infectious
	Malignant
Malignancy	B-cell lymphoma (posttransplantation lymphoproliferative disorders)

venous line infections—rather than opportunistic infections; these infections may involve the biliary tree and liver as well. Beyond the first postoperative month, the toll of immunosuppression becomes evident, and opportunistic infections—cytomegalovirus, herpes viruses, fungal infections (*Aspergillus*, *Candida*, cryptococcal disease), mycobacterial infections, parasitic infections (*Pneumocystis*, *Toxoplasma*), bacterial infections (*Nocardia*, *Legionella*, and *Listeria*)—predominate. Rarely, early infections represent those transmitted with the donor liver, either infections present in the donor or infections acquired during procurement processing. De novo viral hepatitis infections acquired from the donor organ or, almost unheard of nowadays, from transfused blood products occur after typical incubation periods for these agents (well beyond the first month). Obviously, infections in an immunosuppressed host demand early recognition and prompt management; prophylactic antibiotic therapy is administered routinely in the immediate postoperative period. Use of sulfamethoxazole with trimethoprim reduces the incidence of postoperative *Pneumocystis carinii* pneumonia.

Neuropsychiatric complications include seizures (commonly associated with cyclosporine and tacrolimus toxicity), encephalopathy, depression, and difficult psychosocial adjustment. Rarely, diseases are transmitted by the allograft from the donor to the recipient. In addition to viral and bacterial infections, malignancies of donor origin have occurred. Posttransplantation lymphoproliferative disorders, especially B cell lymphoma, are a recognized complication associated with immunosuppressive drugs such as azathioprine, tacrolimus, and cyclosporine (see above). Epstein-Barr virus has been shown to play a contributory role in some of these tumors, which may regress when immunosuppressive therapy is reduced.

Long-term complications after liver transplantation attributable primarily to immunosuppressive medications include diabetes mellitus (associated with glucocorticoids) as well as hypertension, hyperlipidemia, and chronic renal insufficiency (associated with cyclosporine and tacrolimus). Monitoring and treating these disorders is a routine component of posttransplantation care; in some cases, they respond to changes in immunosuppressive regimen, while in others, specific treatment of the disorder is introduced.

Hepatic Complications Hepatic dysfunction after liver transplantation is similar to the hepatic complications encountered after major abdominal and cardiothoracic surgery; however, in addition, there may be complications such as primary graft failure, vascular compromise, failure or obstruction of the biliary anastomoses, and rejection. As in

of transient renal dysfunction and pulmonary capillary vascular permeability. Continuous monitoring of cardiovascular and pulmonary function, measures to maintain the integrity of the intravascular compartment and to treat extravascular volume overload, and scrupulous attention to potential sources and sites of infection are of paramount importance. Cardiovascular instability may also result from the electrolyte imbalance that may accompany reperfusion of the donor liver. Pulmonary function may be compromised further by paralysis of the right hemidiaphragm associated with phrenic nerve injury. The hyperdynamic state with increased cardiac output that is characteristic of patients with liver failure reverses rapidly after successful liver transplantation.

Other immediate management issues include renal dysfunction; prerenal azotemia, acute kidney injury associated with hypoperfusion (acute tubular necrosis), and renal toxicity caused by antibiotics, tacrolimus, or cyclosporine are frequently encountered in the postoperative period, sometimes necessitating dialysis. Occasionally, postoperative intraperitoneal bleeding may be sufficient to increase intraabdominal pressure, which, in turn, may reduce renal blood flow; this effect is rapidly reversible when abdominal distention is relieved by exploratory laparotomy to identify and ligate the bleeding site and to remove intraperitoneal clot. Anemia may also result from acute upper gastrointestinal bleeding or from transient hemolytic anemia, which may be autoimmune, especially when blood group O livers are transplanted into blood group A or B recipients. This autoimmune hemolytic anemia is mediated by donor intrahepatic lymphocytes that recognize red blood cell A or B antigens on recipient erythrocytes. Transient in nature, this process resolves once the donor liver is repopulated by recipient bone marrow–derived lymphocytes; the hemolysis can be treated by transfusing blood group O red blood cells and/or by administering higher doses of glucocorticoids. Transient thrombocytopenia is also commonly encountered. Aplastic anemia, a late occurrence, is rare but has been reported in almost 30% of patients who underwent liver transplantation for acute, severe hepatitis of unknown cause.

Bacterial, fungal, or viral infections are common and may be life-threatening postoperatively. Early after transplant surgery, common postoperative infections predominate—pneumonia, wound infections, infected intraabdominal collections, urinary tract infections, and intra-

TABLE 291-5 *Hepatic Complications of Liver Transplantation*

HEPATIC DYSFUNCTION COMMON AFTER MAJOR SURGERY	
Prehepatic	Pigment load
	Hemolysis
	Blood collections (hematomas, abdominal collections)
Intrahepatic	
Early	Hepatotoxic drugs and anesthesia
	Hypoperfusion (hypotension, shock, sepsis)
	Benign postoperative cholestasis
Late	Transfusion-associated hepatitis
	Exacerbation of primary hepatic disease
Posthepatic	Biliary obstruction
	$\downarrow$ Renal clearance of conjugated bilirubin (renal dysfunction)

HEPATIC DYSFUNCTION UNIQUE TO LIVER TRANSPLANTATION	
Primary graft nonfunction	
Vascular compromise	Portal vein obstruction
	Hepatic artery thrombosis
	Anastomotic leak with intraabdominal bleeding
Bile duct disorder	Stenosis, obstruction, leak
Rejection	
Recurrent primary hepatic disease	

nontransplant surgery, postoperative jaundice may result from prehepatic, intrahepatic, and posthepatic sources. *Prehepatic* sources represent the massive hemoglobin pigment load from transfusions, hemolysis, hematomas, ecchymoses, and other collections of blood. *Early intrahepatic* liver injury includes effects of hepatotoxic drugs and anesthesia; hypoperfusion injury associated with hypotension, sepsis, and shock; and benign postoperative cholestasis. *Late intrahepatic* sources of liver injury include posttransfusion hepatitis and exacerbation of primary disease. *Posthepatic* sources of hepatic dysfunction include biliary obstruction and reduced renal clearance of conjugated bilirubin. Hepatic complications unique to liver transplantation include primary graft failure associated with ischemic injury to the organ during harvesting; vascular compromise associated with thrombosis or stenosis of the portal vein or hepatic artery anastomoses; vascular anastomotic leak; stenosis, obstruction, or leakage of the anastomosed common bile duct; recurrence of primary hepatic disorder (see below); and rejection.

Transplant Rejection   Despite the use of immunosuppressive drugs, rejection of the transplanted liver still occurs in a proportion of patients, beginning 1 to 2 weeks after surgery. Clinical signs suggesting rejection are fever, right upper quadrant pain, and reduced bile pigment and volume. Leukocytosis may occur, but the most reliable indicators are increases in serum bilirubin and aminotransferase levels. Because these tests lack specificity, distinguishing among rejection and biliary obstruction, primary graft nonfunction, vascular compromise, viral hepatitis, cytomegalovirus infection, drug hepatotoxicity, and recurrent primary disease may be difficult. Radiographic visualization of the biliary tree and/or percutaneous liver biopsy often helps to establish the correct diagnosis. Morphologic features of acute rejection include portal infiltration, bile duct injury, and/or endothelial inflammation ("endothelialitis"); some of these findings are reminiscent of graft-versus-host disease and primary biliary cirrhosis. As soon as transplant rejection is suspected, treatment consists of intravenous methylprednisolone in repeated boluses; if this fails to abort rejection, many centers use antibodies to lymphocytes, such as OKT3, or polyclonal antilymphocyte globulin.

Chronic rejection is a relatively rare outcome that can follow repeated bouts of acute rejection or that occurs unrelated to preceding rejection episodes. Morphologically, chronic rejection is characterized by progressive cholestasis, focal parenchymal necrosis, mononuclear infiltration, vascular lesions (intimal fibrosis, subintimal foam cells, fibrinoid necrosis), and fibrosis. This process may be reflected as ductopenia—the vanishing bile duct syndrome. Some of the histologic hallmarks of chronic rejection may be so similar to those of chronic viral hepatitis that differentiation between the two may be difficult. Reversibility of chronic rejection is limited; in patients with therapy-resistant chronic rejection, retransplantation has yielded encouraging results.

OUTCOME ■ Survival   The survival rate for patients undergoing liver transplantation has improved steadily since 1983. One-year survival rates have increased from ~70% in the early 1980s to 85 to 90% in the late 1990s. Currently, the 5-year survival rate exceeds 60%. An important observation is the relation between clinical status before transplantation and outcome. For patients who undergo liver transplantation when their level of compensation is high (e.g., still working or only partially disabled), a 1-year survival rate of 85% is common. For those whose level of decompensation mandates continuous in-hospital care prior to transplantation, the 1-year survival rate is about 70%, while for those who are so decompensated that they require life support in an intensive care unit, the 1-year survival rate is ~50%. Indeed, the trend toward transplantation earlier in the natural history of end-stage liver disease is a major factor in the increased success of liver transplantation during the 1980s and 1990s. Another important distinction in survival has been drawn between high-risk and low-risk

patient categories. For patients who do not fit any "high-risk" designations, 1-year and 5-year survival rates of 85 and 80%, respectively, have been recorded. In contrast, among patients in high-risk categories—cancer, fulminant hepatitis, age >65, concurrent renal failure, respirator dependence, portal vein thrombosis, and history of a portacaval shunt or multiple right upper quadrant operations—survival statistics fall into the range of 60% at 1 year and 35% at 5 years. Survival after retransplantation for primary graft nonfunction is ~50%. Causes of failure of liver transplantation vary with time. Failures within the first 3 months result primarily from technical complications, postoperative infections, and hemorrhage. Transplant failures after the first 3 months are more likely to result from infection, rejection, or recurrent disease (such as malignancy or viral hepatitis).

Recurrence of Primary Disease   Features of autoimmune hepatitis, primary sclerosing cholangitis, and primary biliary cirrhosis overlap with those of rejection or posttransplantation bile-duct injury. Whether autoimmune hepatitis and sclerosing cholangitis recur after liver transplantation is controversial; data supporting recurrent autoimmune hepatitis (in up to a third of patients in some series) are more convincing than those supporting recurrent sclerosing cholangitis. Similarly, reports of recurrent primary biliary cirrhosis after liver transplantation have appeared; however, the histologic features of primary biliary cirrhosis and acute rejection are virtually indistinguishable and occur as frequently in patients with primary biliary cirrhosis as in patients undergoing transplantation for other reasons. Hereditary disorders such as Wilson's disease and α_1-antitrypsin deficiency have not recurred after liver transplantation; however, recurrence of disordered iron metabolism has been observed in some patients with hemochromatosis. Hepatic vein thrombosis (Budd-Chiari syndrome) may recur; this can be minimized by treating underlying lymphoproliferative disorders and by anticoagulation. Cholangiocarcinoma recurs almost invariably; therefore, few centers now offer transplantation to such patients. In patients with hepatocellular carcinoma, tumor recurrence in the liver is common after ~1 year, although better success has been reported (1- and 5-year survivals similar to those achieved in patients undergoing liver transplantation for nonmalignant diseases) in patients with an unresectable isolated lesion <5 cm or with three or fewer lesions all <3 cm. Trials are underway to assess the benefit of adjuvant chemotherapy.

Hepatitis A can recur after transplantation for fulminant hepatitis A, but such acute reinfection has no serious clinical sequelae. In fulminant hepatitis B, recurrence is not the rule; however, in the absence of any prophylactic measures, hepatitis B usually recurs after transplantation for end-stage chronic hepatitis B. Before the introduction of prophylactic antiviral therapy, immunosuppressive therapy sufficient to prevent allograft rejection led inevitably to marked increases in hepatitis B viremia, regardless of pretransplantation values. Overall graft and patient survival were poor, and some patients experienced a rapid recapitulation of severe injury—severe chronic hepatitis or even fulminant hepatitis—after transplantation. Also recognized in the era before availability of antiviral regimens was *fibrosing cholestatic hepatitis*, rapidly progressive liver injury associated with marked hyperbilirubinemia, substantial prolongation of the prothrombin time (both out of proportion to relatively modest elevations of aminotransferase activity), and rapidly progressive liver failure. This lesion has been suggested to represent a "choking off" of the hepatocyte by an overwhelming density of hepatitis B virus (HBV) proteins. Complications such as sepsis and pancreatitis were also observed more frequently in patients undergoing liver transplantation for hepatitis B prior to the introduction of antiviral therapy. The introduction of long-term prophylaxis with HBIg revolutionized liver transplantation for chronic hepatitis B. Neither preoperative hepatitis B vaccination, preoperative or postoperative interferon therapy, nor short-term (≤2 months) HBIg prophylaxis has been shown to be effective, but a retrospective analysis of data from several hundred European patients followed for 3 years after transplantation has shown that long-term (≥6 months) prophylaxis with HBIg is associated with a lowering of the risk of HBV reinfection from ~75% to 35% and a reduction in mortality from ~50% to 20%.

As a result of long-term HBIg use following liver transplantation for chronic hepatitis B, similar improvements in outcome have been observed in the United States, with 1-year survival rates between 75 and 90%. Currently, with HBIg prophylaxis, the outcome of liver transplantation for chronic hepatitis B is indistinguishable from that for chronic liver disease unassociated with chronic hepatitis B; essentially, medical concerns regarding liver transplantation for chronic hepatitis B have been eliminated. Passive immunoprophylaxis with HBIg is begun during the anhepatic stage of surgery, repeated daily for the first 6 postoperative days, then continued with infusions that are given either at regular intervals of 4 to 6 weeks or, alternatively, when anti-HBs levels fall below a threshold of 100 mIU/mL. The current approach in most centers is to continue HBIg indefinitely, which can add approximately $20,000 per year to the cost of care; some centers are evaluating regimens that shift to less frequent administration or to intramuscular administration in the late posttransplantation period. Still, occasionally, "breakthrough" HBV infection occurs.

Futher improving the outcome of liver transplantation for chronic hepatitis B is the current availability of such antiviral drugs as lamivudine and adefovir dipivoxil (Chap. 287). When lamivudine is administered to patients with decompensated liver disease, a proportion improve sufficiently to postpone imminent liver transplantation. In addition, lamivudine can be used to prevent recurrence of HBV infection when administered *prior* to transplantation, to treat hepatitis B that recurs *after* transplantation, including in patients who break through HBIg prophylaxis, and to reverse the course of otherwise fatal fibrosing cholestatic hepatitis. Clinical trials have shown that lamivudine monotherapy reduces the level of HBV replication substantially, sometimes even resulting in clearance of hepatitis B surface antigen (HBsAg); reduces alanine aminotransferase (ALT) levels; and improves histologic features of necrosis and inflammation. Long-term use of lamivudine is safe and effective, but, after several months, a proportion of patients become resistant to lamivudine, resulting from YMDD (tyrosine-methionine-aspartate-aspartate) mutations in the HBV polymerase motif (Chap. 287). In approximately half of such resistant patients, hepatic deterioration may ensue. Fortunately, adefovir dipivoxil is available as well and can be used to treat lamivudine-associated YMDD variants, effectively "rescuing" patients experiencing hepatic decompensation after lamivudine breakthrough. Currently, most liver transplantation centers combine HBIg plus lamivudine or adefovir, and additional antivirals are being introduced as well. Clinical trials are underway to define the optimal application of these antiviral agents in the management of patients undergoing liver transplantation for chronic hepatitis B; conceivably, in the future, combinations of oral antiviral drugs may supplant HBIg.

Prophylactic approaches applied to patients undergoing liver transplantation for chronic hepatitis B are being used as well for patients without hepatitis B who receive organs from donors with anti-HBc. Patients who undergo liver transplantation for chronic hepatitis B plus D are less likely to experience recurrent liver injury than patients undergoing liver transplantation for hepatitis B alone; still, such co-infected patients would also be offered standard posttransplantation prophylactic therapy for hepatitis B.

Accounting for up to 40% of all liver transplantation procedures, the most common indication for liver transplantation is end-stage liver disease resulting from chronic hepatitis C. Recurrence of hepatitis C virus (HCV) after liver transplantation can be documented in almost every patient, if sufficiently sensitive virus markers are used. Although acute and chronic liver injury occur after transplantation in patients with chronic hepatitis C, clinical consequences of recurrent hepatitis C are limited during the first 5 years after transplantation. Nonetheless, despite the relative clinical benignity of recurrent hepatitis C in the early years after liver transplantation, and despite the negligible impact

on patient survival during these early years, histologic studies have documented the presence of moderate to severe chronic hepatitis in more than half of all patients and bridging fibrosis or cirrhosis in ~10%. Moreover, progression to cirrhosis within 5 years is even more common, occurring in up to two-thirds of patients, after moderate hepatitis is detected in a 1-year biopsy. Ultimately, such histologic evidence of chronic hepatitis and cirrhosis will be expressed clinically as well, and the expectation is that the outcome beyond 10 years will not be as favorable as the 5-year statistics suggest. In a proportion of patients, even during the early posttransplantation period, recurrent hepatitis C may be sufficiently severe biochemically and histologically to merit antiviral therapy. Treatment with interferon monotherapy can *suppress* HCV-associated liver injury in approximately half of patients but rarely leads to *sustained* benefit. The addition of the nucleoside analogue ribavirin to interferon as well as the substitution of more effective and long-acting pegylated interferons for standard interferons (Chap. 287) have resulted in improved responses to antiviral therapy, and many centers have adopted some form of combination therapy for their patients with recurrent hepatitis C after liver transplantation. Overall, however, current approaches to antiviral therapy for hepatitis C after liver transplantation have been disappointing; sustained virologic responses are the exception, and reduced tolerability is often dose-limiting. Studies are underway to determine whether preemptive therapy immediately after transplantation provides any benefit over therapy introduced after clinical hepatitis occurs. Similarly, although interferon-based antiviral therapy is not recommended for patients with decompensated liver disease, some centers have experimented with pretransplantation antiviral therapy in an attempt to eradicate HCV replication prior to transplantation; preliminary results are promising. Initial trials of hepatitis C immune globulin preparations to prevent recurrent hepatitis C after liver transplantation have not been successful.

A small number succumb to early HCV-associated liver injury, and a syndrome reminiscent of fibrosing cholestatic hepatitis (see above) has been observed rarely. Because patients with more episodes of rejection receive more immunosuppressive therapy, and because immunosuppressive therapy enhances HCV replication, patients with severe or multiple episodes of rejection are more likely to experience early recurrence of hepatitis C after transplantation. Both HCV genotype 1b and high viral load have been linked to recurrent HCV-induced liver disease and to earlier disease recurrence after transplantation; however, the association between genotype and recurrence of HCV-associated liver injury has not been supported by more recent reports.

Patients who undergo liver transplantation for end-stage alcoholic cirrhosis are at risk of resorting to drinking again after transplantation, a potential source of recurrent alcoholic liver injury. Currently, alcoholic liver disease is one of the more common indications for liver transplantation, accounting for 20 to 25% of all liver transplantation procedures, and most transplantation centers screen candidates carefully for predictors of continued abstinence. Recidivism is more likely in patients whose sobriety prior to transplantation was <6 months. For abstinent patients with alcoholic cirrhosis, liver transplantation can be undertaken successfully, with outcomes comparable to those for other categories of patients with chronic liver disease, when coordinated by a team approach that includes substance abuse counseling.

Posttransplantation Quality of Life Full rehabilitation is achieved in the majority of patients who survive the early postoperative months and escape chronic rejection or unmanageable infection. Psychosocial maladjustment interferes with medical compliance in a small number of patients, but most manage to adhere to immunosuppressive regimens, which must be continued indefinitely. In one study, 85% of patients who survived their transplants returned to gainful activities. In fact, some women have conceived and carried pregnancies to term after transplantation without demonstrable injury to their infants.

FURTHER READING

BROWN RS JR et al: A survey of liver transplantation from living adult donors in the United States. N Engl J Med 348:818, 2003

CARITHERS RL JR: Liver transplantation. Liver Transpl 6:122, 2000

FISHMAN JA, RUBIN RH: Infection in organ-transplant recipients. N Engl J Med 338:1741, 1998

HOOFNAGLE JH et al: Liver transplantation for alcoholic liver disease: Executive statement and recommendations. Liver Transpl Surg 3:347, 1997

KEEFFE EB et al: Liver transplantation: Current status and novel approaches to liver replacement. Gastroenterology 120:749, 2001

SORRELL MF (Guest ed): Liver transplantation in the new millennium. Semin Liver Dis 20:409, 2000

VARGAS HE et al: A concise update on the status of liver transplantation for hepatitis B virus: The challenges in 2002. Liver Transpl 8:2, 2002

292 DISEASES OF THE GALLBLADDER AND BILE DUCTS
Norton J. Greenberger, Gustav Paumgartner

PHYSIOLOGY OF BILE PRODUCTION AND FLOW ▪ Bile Secretion and Composition Bile formed in the hepatic lobules is secreted into a complex network of canaliculi, small bile ductules, and larger bile ducts that run with lymphatics and branches of the portal vein and hepatic artery in portal tracts situated between hepatic lobules. These interlobular bile ducts coalesce to form larger septal bile ducts that join to form the right and left hepatic ducts, which in turn unite to form the common hepatic duct. The common hepatic duct is joined by the cystic duct of the gallbladder to form the common bile duct (CBD), which enters the duodenum (often after joining the main pancreatic duct) through the ampulla of Vater.

Hepatic bile is an isotonic fluid with an electrolyte composition resembling blood plasma. The electrolyte composition of gallbladder bile differs from that of hepatic bile because most of the inorganic anions, chloride and bicarbonate, have been removed by reabsorption across the gallbladder epithelium. As a result of water reabsorption, total solute concentration of bile increases from 3 to 4 g/dL in hepatic bile and 10 to 15 g/dL in gallbladder bile.

Major solute components of bile by moles percent include bile acids (80%), lecithin and traces of other phospholipids (16%), and unesterified cholesterol (4.0%). In the lithogenic state the cholesterol value can be as high as 8 to 10%. Other constituents include conjugated bilirubin, proteins (IgA, metabolites of hormones, and other proteins metabolized in the liver), electrolytes, mucus, and, often, drugs and their metabolites.

The total daily basal secretion of hepatic bile is approximately 500 to 600 mL. Many substances taken up or synthesized by the hepatocyte are secreted into the bile canalculi. The canalicular membrane forms microvilli and is associated with microfilaments of actin, microtubules, and other contractile elements. Prior to their secretion into the bile, many substances that are taken up into the hepatocyte are conjugated, while others such as phospholipids, a portion of primary bile acids, and some cholesterol are synthesized de novo in the hepatocyte. Three mechanisms are important in regulating bile flow: (1) active transport of bile acids from hepatocytes into the bile canalculi, (2) active transport of other organic anions, and (3) cholangiocellular secretion. The last is a secretin-mediated and cyclic AMP–dependent mechanism that results in the secretion of a sodium- and bicarbonate-rich fluid into the bile ducts.

Active vectorial secretion of biliary constituents from the portal blood into the bile canaliculi is driven by a distinct set of polarized transport systems at the basolateral (sinusoidal) and the canalicular plasma membrane domains of the hepatocyte. Two sinusoidal bile salt uptake systems have been cloned in humans, the Na$^+$/taurocholate cotransporter (NTCP) and the organic anion transporting proteins (OATPs), which also transport a large variety of non-bile salt organic anions. Several ATP-dependent canalicular transport systems ("export pumps") have been identified, the most important of which are: the bile salt export pump (BSEP); the conjugate export pump (MRP2), which mediates the canalicular excretion of various amphiphilic conjugates formed by phase II conjugation (e.g., bilirubin mono- and diglucuronides); the multidrug export pump (MDR1) for hydrophobic cationic compounds; and the phospholipid export pump (MDR3). Indirect evidence suggests that the two hemitransporters ABCG5/G8, functioning as a couple, constitute the principal canalicular cholesterol transporter. The canalicular membrane also contains ATP-independent transport systems such as the Cl$^-$/HCO$_3^-$ anion exchanger isoform 2 for canalicular bicarbonate secretion. For some of these transporters, genetic defects have been identified that are associated with various forms of cholestasis or defects of biliary excretion. BSEP is defective in progressive familial intrahepatic cholestasis (PFIC) type 2. Mutations of MRP2 cause the Dubin-Johnson syndrome, an inherited form of conjugated hyperbilirubinemia (Chap. 284). A defective MDR3 results in PFIC-3. ABCG5/G8, the canalicular half transporters for cholesterol and neutral sterols, are defective in sitosterolemia. The cystic fibrosis transmembrane regulator located on bile duct epithelial cells is defective in cystic fibrosis, which is associated with impaired cholangiocellular bile formation and chronic cholestatic liver disease.

The Bile Acids The primary bile acids, cholic acid and chenodeoxycholic acid (CDCA), are synthesized from cholesterol in the liver, conjugated with glycine or taurine, and excreted into the bile. Secondary bile acids, including deoxycholate and lithocholate, are formed in the colon as bacterial metabolites of the primary bile acids. However, lithocholic acid is much less efficiently absorbed from the colon than deoxycholic acid. Another secondary bile acid, found in low concentration, is ursodeoxycholic acid (UDCA), a stereoisomer of CDCA. In normal bile, the ratio of glycine to taurine conjugates is about 3:1.

Bile acids are detergent-like molecules that in aqueous solutions and above a critical concentration of about 2 mM form molecular aggregates called *micelles*. Cholesterol alone is sparingly soluble in aqueous environments, and its solubility in bile depends on both the total lipid concentration and the relative molar percentages of bile acids and lecithin. Normal ratios of these constituents favor the formation of solubilizing *mixed micelles*, while abnormal ratios promote the precipitation of cholesterol crystals in bile.

In addition to facilitating the biliary excretion of cholesterol, bile acids are necessary for the normal intestinal absorption of dietary fats, mainly cholesterol and fat-soluble vitamins, via a micellar transport mechanism (Chap. 275). Bile acids also serve as a major physiologic driving force for hepatic bile flow and aid in water and electrolyte transport in the small bowel and colon.

Enterohepatic Circulation Bile acids are efficiently conserved under normal conditions. Unconjugated, and to a lesser degree also conjugated, bile acids are absorbed by *passive diffusion* along the entire gut. Quantitatively much more important for bile salt recirculation, however, is the *active transport* mechanism for conjugated bile acids in the distal ileum (Chap. 275). The reabsorbed bile acids enter the portal bloodstream and are taken up rapidly by hepatocytes, reconjugated, and resecreted into bile (enterohepatic circulation).

The normal bile acid pool size is approximately 2 to 4 g. During digestion of a meal, the bile acid pool undergoes at least one or more enterohepatic cycles, depending on the size and composition of the meal. Normally, the bile acid pool circulates approximately 5 to 10 times daily. Intestinal absorption of the pool is about 95% efficient, so fecal loss of bile acids is in the range of 0.3 to 0.6 g/d. This fecal loss is compensated by an equal daily synthesis of bile acids by the liver, and thus the size of the bile acid pool is maintained. Bile acids returning to the liver suppress de novo hepatic synthesis of primary bile acids from cholesterol by inhibiting the rate-limiting enzyme cholesterol 7α-hydroxylase. While the loss of bile salts in stool is usually matched by increased hepatic synthesis, the maximum rate of synthesis is approximately 5 g/d, which may be insufficient to replete the bile acid pool size when there is pronounced impairment of intestinal bile salt reabsorption.

Gallbladder and Sphincteric Functions In the fasting state, the sphincter of Oddi offers a high-pressure zone of resistance to bile flow from the CBD into the duodenum. This tonic contraction serves to (1) prevent reflux of duodenal contents into the pancreatic and bile ducts and (2) promote bile filling of the gallbladder. The major factor controlling the evacuation of the gallbladder is the peptide hormone cholecystokinin (CCK), which is released from the duodenal mucosa in response to the ingestion of fats and amino acids. CCK produces (1) powerful contraction of the gallbladder, (2) decreased resistance of the sphincter of Oddi, and (3) enhanced flow of biliary contents into the duodenum.

Hepatic bile is "concentrated" within the gallbladder by energy-dependent transmucosal absorption of water and electrolytes. Almost the entire bile acid pool may be sequestered in the gallbladder following an overnight fast for delivery into the duodenum with the first meal of the day. The normal capacity of the gallbladder is about 30 mL of bile.

DISEASES OF THE GALLBLADDER

CONGENITAL ANOMALIES Anomalies of the biliary tract are not uncommon and include abnormalities in number, size, and shape (e.g., agenesis of the gallbladder, duplications, rudimentary or oversized "giant" gallbladders, and diverticula). *Phrygian cap* is a clinically innocuous entity in which a partial or complete septum (or fold) separates the fundus from the body. Anomalies of position or suspension are not uncommon and include left-sided gallbladder, intrahepatic gallbladder, retrodisplacement of the gallbladder, and "floating" gallbladder. The latter condition predisposes to acute torsion, volvulus, or herniation of the gallbladder.

GALLSTONES ■ Pathogenesis Gallstones are quite prevalent in most western countries. In the United States, autopsy series have shown gallstones in at least 20% of women and in 8% of men over the age of 40. It is estimated that at least 20 million persons in the United States have gallstones and that approximately 1 million new cases of cholelithiasis develop each year.

Gallstones are formed by concretion or accretion of normal or abnormal bile constituents. They are divided into two major types: cholesterol stones account for 80% of the total, with pigment stones comprising the remaining 20%. Cholesterol gallstones usually contain >50% cholesterol monohydrate plus an admixture of calcium salts, bile pigments, proteins, and fatty acids. Pigment stones are composed primarily of calcium bilirubinate; they contain <20% cholesterol.

CHOLESTEROL STONES AND BILIARY SLUDGE Cholesterol is essentially water insoluble and requires aqueous dispersion into either micelles or vesicles, both of which require the presence of a second lipid to solubilize the cholesterol. Cholesterol and phospholipids are secreted into bile as unilamellar bilayered vesicles, which are converted into mixed micelles consisting of bile acids, phospholipids, and cholesterol by the action of bile acids. If there is an excess of cholesterol in relation to phospholipids and bile acids, unstable cholesterol-rich vesicles remain, which aggregate into large multilamellar vesicles from which cholesterol crystals precipitate (Fig. 292-1).

There are several important mechanisms in the formation of lithogenic (stone-forming) bile. The most important is increased biliary secretion of cholesterol. This may occur in association with obesity, high-caloric and cholesterol-rich diets, or drugs (e.g., clofibrate) and may result from increased activity of HMG-CoA reductase, the rate-limiting enzyme of hepatic cholesterol synthesis, and increased hepatic uptake of cholesterol from blood. In patients with gallstones, dietary cholesterol *increases* biliary cholesterol secretion. This does not occur

FIGURE 292-1 Scheme showing pathogenesis of cholesterol gallstone formation. Conditions or factors that increase the ratio of cholesterol to bile acids and phospholipids (lecithin) favor gallstone formation. HMG-CoAR, hydroxymethylglutaryl–coenzyme A reductase; 7-α-OHase, cholesterol, 7α-hydroxylase; MDR3, multidrug resistance–associated protein 3, also called phospholipid export pump.

in non-gallstone patients on high-cholesterol diets. In addition to environmental factors such as high-caloric and cholesterol-rich diets, genetic factors play an important role in cholesterol hypersecretion and gallstone formation. A high prevalence of gallstones is found among first-degree relatives of gallstone carriers and in certain ethnic populations such as American Indians as well as Chilean Indians and Chilean Hispanics. A common genetic trait has been identified for some of these populations by mitochondrial DNA analysis. In some patients, impaired hepatic conversion of cholesterol to bile acids may also occur, resulting in an increase of the lithogenic cholesterol/bile acid ratio. Recently, a mutation in the *CYP7A1* gene has been described that results in a deficiency of the enzyme cholesterol 7α-hydroxylase, which catalyzes the initial step in cholesterol catabolism and bile acid synthesis. The homozygous state is associated with hypercholesterolemia and gallstones. Because the phenotype is expressed in the heterozygote state, mutations in the *CYP7A1* gene may contribute to the susceptibility to cholesterol gallstone disease in the population. Mutations in the *MDR3* gene, which encodes the phospholipid export pump in the canalicular membrane of the hepatocyte, may cause defective phospholipid secretion into bile, resulting in cholesterol supersaturation of bile and formation of cholesterol gallstones in the gallbladder and in the bile ducts. Thus an excess of biliary cholesterol in relation to bile acids and phospholipids is primarily due to hypersecretion of cholesterol, but hyposecretion of bile acids or phospholipids may contribute. An additional disturbance of bile acid metabolism that is likely to contribute to supersaturation of bile with cholesterol is enhanced conversion of cholic acid to deoxycholic acid, with replacement of the cholic acid pool by an expanded deoxycholic acid pool. It may result from enhanced dehydroxylation of cholic acid and increased absorption of newly formed deoxycholic acid. An increased deoxycholate secretion is associated with hypersecretion of cholesterol into bile.

While supersaturation of bile with cholesterol is an important prerequisite for gallstone formation, it is generally not sufficient by itself to produce cholesterol precipitation in vivo. Most people with supersaturated bile do not develop stones because the time required for cholesterol crystals to nucleate and grow is longer than the time bile spends in the gallbladder.

An important mechanism is *nucleation* of cholesterol monohydrate crystals, which is greatly accelerated in human lithogenic bile. Accelerated nucleation of cholesterol monohydrate in bile may be due to either an *excess of pronucleating factors* or a *deficiency of antinucleating factors*. Mucin and certain non-mucin glycoproteins appear to be pronucleating factors, while apolipoproteins AI and AII and other glycoproteins appear to be antinucleating factors. Cholesterol monohydrate crystal nucleation and crystal growth probably occur within the mucin gel layer. Vesicle fusion leads to liquid crystals, which, in turn, nucleate into solid cholesterol monohydrate crystals. Continued growth of the crystals occurs by direct nucleation of cholesterol molecules from supersaturated unilamellar or multilamellar biliary vesicles.

A third important mechanism in cholesterol gallstone formation is *gallbladder hypomotility*. If the gallbladder emptied all supersaturated or crystal-containing bile completely, stones would not be able to grow. A high percentage of patients with gallstones exhibits abnormalities of gallbladder emptying. Ultrasonographic studies show that gallstone patients have an increased gallbladder volume during fasting and also after a test meal (residual volume) and that fractional emptying after gallbladder stimulation is decreased. Gallbladder emptying is a major determinant of gallstone recurrence in patients who underwent biliary lithotripsy. Within 3 years, only 13% of patients with good but 53% of patients with poor gallbladder emptying form recurrent stones.

Biliary sludge is a thick mucous material that upon microscopic examination reveals lecithin-cholesterol crystals, cholesterol monohydrate crystals, calcium bilirubinate, and mucin thread or mucous gels. Biliary sludge typically forms a crescent-like layer in the most dependent portion of the gallbladder and is recognized by characteristic echoes on ultrasonography (see below). The presence of biliary sludge implies two abnormalities: (1) the normal balance between gallbladder mucin secretion and elimination has become deranged and (2) nucleation of biliary solutes has occurred. That biliary sludge may be a precursor form of gallstone disease is evident from several observations. In one study, 96 patients with gallbladder sludge were followed prospectively by serial ultrasound studies. In 18%, biliary sludge disappeared and did not recur for at least 2 years. In 60%, biliary sludge disappeared and reappeared; in 14%, gallstones (8% asymptomatic, 6% symptomatic) developed, and in 6%, severe biliary pain with or without acute pancreatitis occurred. In 12 patients, cholecystectomies were performed, 6 for gallstone-associated biliary pain and 3 in symptomatic patients with sludge but without gallstones who had prior attacks of pancreatitis; the latter did not recur after cholecystectomy. It should be emphasized that biliary sludge can develop with disorders that cause gallbladder hypomotility, i.e., surgery, burns, total parenteral nutrition, pregnancy, and oral contraceptives—all of which are associated with gallstone formation.

Two other conditions are associated with cholesterol stone or biliary sludge formation: pregnancy and very low calorie diet. There appear to be two key changes during pregnancy that contribute to a "cholelithogenic state": (1) a marked increase in cholesterol saturation during the third trimester and (2) sluggish gallbladder contraction in response to a standard meal, resulting in impaired gallbladder emptying. That these changes are related to pregnancy per se is supported by several studies that show reversal of these abnormalities after delivery. During pregnancy, gallbladder sludge develops in 20 to 30% of women and gallstones in 5 to 12%. While biliary sludge is a common finding during pregnancy, it is usually asymptomatic and often resolves spontaneously after delivery. Gallstones, which are less common than sludge and frequently associated with biliary colic, may also disappear after delivery because of spontaneous dissolution related to bile becoming unsaturated with cholesterol post partum.

Approximately 10 to 20% of people with rapid weight reduction achieved through very low calorie dieting develop gallstones. In a study involving 600 patients who completed a 16-week, 520-kcal/d diet, UDCA in a dosage of 600 mg/d proved highly effective in preventing gallstone formation; gallstones developed in only 3% of UDCA recipients compared to 28% of placebo-treated patients.

To summarize, cholesterol gallstone disease occurs because of several defects, which include (1) bile supersaturation with cholesterol, (2) nucleation of cholesterol monohydrate with subsequent crystal retention and stone growth, and (3) abnormal gallbladder motor function with delayed emptying and stasis. Other important factors known to predispose to cholesterol stone formation are summarized in Table 292-1.

PIGMENT STONES   Black pigment stones are composed of either pure calcium bilirubinate or polymer-like complexes with calcium and mucin glycoproteins. They are more common in patients who have chronic hemolytic states (with increased conjugated bilirubin in bile), liver

---

TABLE 292-1   *Predisposing Factors for Cholesterol and Pigment Gallstone Formation*

Cholesterol Stones
1. Demographic/genetic factors
   a. Prevalence highest in North American Indians, Chilean Indians, and Chilean Hispanics, greater in Northern Europe and North America than in Asia, lowest in Japan; familial disposition; hereditary aspects
2. Obesity
   a. Normal bile acid pool and secretion but increased biliary secretion of cholesterol
3. Weight loss
   a. Mobilization of tissue cholesterol leads to increased biliary cholesterol secretion while enterohepatic circulation of bile acids is decreased
4. Female sex hormones
   a. Estrogens stimulate hepatic lipoprotein receptors, increase uptake of dietary cholesterol, and increase biliary cholesterol secretion
   b. Natural estrogens, other estrogens, and oral contraceptives lead to decreased bile salt secretion and decreased conversion of cholesterol to cholesteryl esters
5. Increasing age
   a. Increased biliary secretion of cholesterol, decreased size of bile acid pool, decreased secretion of bile salts
6. Gallbladder hypomotility leading to stasis and formation of sludge
   a. Prolonged parenteral nutrition
   b. Fasting
   c. Pregnancy
   d. Drugs such as octreotide
7. Clofibrate therapy
   a. Increased biliary secretion of cholesterol
8. Decreased bile acid secretion
   a. Primary biliary cirrhosis
   b. Genetic defect of the *CYP7A1* gene
9. Decreased phospholipid secretion
   a. Genetic defect of the *MDR3* gene
10. Miscellaneous
    a. High-calorie, high-fat diet
    b. Spinal cord injury

Pigment Stones
1. Demographic/genetic factors: Asia, rural setting
2. Chronic hemolysis
3. Alcoholic cirrhosis
4. Pernicious anemia
5. Cystic fibrosis
6. Chronic biliary tract infection, parasite infections
7. Increasing age
8. Ileal disease, ileal resection or bypass

cirrhosis, Gilbert's syndrome, or cystic fibrosis. Gallbladder stones in patients with ileal diseases, ileal resection, or ileal bypass generally are also black pigment stones. Enthrohepatic recycling of bilirubin contributes to their pathogenesis. Brown pigment stones are composed of calcium salts of unconjugated bilirubin with varying amounts of cholesterol and protein. They are caused by the presence of increased amounts of unconjugated, insoluble bilirubin in bile that precipitates to form stones. Deconjugation of an excess of soluble bilirubin mono- and diglucuronides may be mediated by endogenous β-glucuronidase but may also occur by spontaneous alkaline hydrolysis. Sometimes, the enzyme is also produced when bile is chronically infected by bacteria. Pigment stone formation is especially prominent in Asians and is often associated with infections in the biliary tree (Table 292-1).

Diagnosis   Procedures of potential use in the diagnosis of cholelithiasis and other diseases of the gallbladder are detailed in Table 292-2. The plain abdominal film may detect gallstones containing sufficient calcium to be radiopaque (10 to 15% of cholesterol and approximately 50% of pigment stones). Plain radiography may also be of use in the diagnosis of emphysematous cholecystitis, porcelain gallbladder, limey bile, and gallstone ileus.

Ultrasonography of the gallbladder is very accurate in the identification of cholelithiasis and has several advantages over oral cholecystography (Fig. 292-2A). Stones as small as 2 mm in diameter may be confidently identified provided that firm criteria are used [e.g., acoustic "shadowing" of opacities that are within the gallbladder lumen and that change with the patient's position (by gravity)]. In major medical centers, the false-negative and false-positive rates for ultrasound in gallstone patients are about 2 to 4%. Biliary sludge is material of low echogenic activity that typically forms a layer in the most dependent position of the gallbladder. This layer shifts with postural changes but fails to produce acoustic shadowing; these two characteristics distinguish sludges from gallstones. Ultrasound can also be used to assess the emptying function of the gallbladder.

Oral cholecystography (OCG) is a useful procedure for the diagnosis of gallstones but has been largely replaced by ultrasound. It may be used to assess the patency of the cystic duct and gallbladder emptying function. Further, OCG can also delineate the size and number of gallstones and determine whether they are calcified.

Radiopharmaceuticals such as ^{99m}Tc-labeled N-substituted imino-

diacetic acids (HIDA, DIDA, DISIDA, etc.) are rapidly extracted from the blood and are excreted into the biliary tree in high concentration even in the presence of mild to moderate serum bilirubin elevations. Failure to image the gallbladder in the presence of biliary ductal visualization may indicate cystic duct obstruction, acute or chronic cholecystitis, or surgical absence of the organ. Such scans have their greatest application in the diagnosis of acute cholecystitis.

Symptoms of Gallstone Disease   Gallstones usually produce symptoms by causing inflammation or obstruction following their migration into the cystic duct or CBD. The most specific and characteristic symptom of gallstone disease is biliary colic. Obstruction of the cystic duct or CBD by a stone produces increased intraluminal pressure and distention of the viscus that cannot be relieved by repetitive biliary contractions. The resultant visceral pain is characteristically a severe, steady ache or fullness in the epigastrium or right upper quadrant (RUQ) of the abdomen with frequent radiation to the interscapular area, right scapula, or shoulder.

Biliary colic begins quite suddenly and may persist with severe intensity for 30 min to 5 h, subsiding gradually or rapidly. It is steady rather than intermittent as would be suggested by the word *colic*, which must be regarded as a misnomer, although in widespread use. An episode of biliary pain persisting beyond 5 h should raise the suspicion of acute cholecystitis (see below). Nausea and vomiting frequently accompany episodes of biliary pain. An elevated level of serum bilirubin and/or alkaline phosphatase suggests a common duct stone. Fever or chills (rigors) with biliary pain usually imply a complication, i.e., cholecystitis, pancreatitis, or cholangitis. Complaints of vague epigastric fullness, dyspepsia, eructation, or flatulence, especially following a fatty meal, should not be confused with biliary pain. Such symptoms are frequently elicited from patients with or without gallstone disease but are not specific for biliary calculi. Biliary colic may be precipitated by eating a fatty meal, by consumption of a large meal following a period of prolonged fasting, or by eating a normal meal; it is frequently nocturnal.

Natural History   Gallstone disease discovered in an asymptomatic patient or in a patient whose symptoms are not referable to cholelithiasis

TABLE 292-2   *Diagnostic Evaluation of the Gallbladder*

Diagnostic Advantages	Diagnostic Limitations	Comment
GALLBLADDER ULTRASOUND		
Rapid	Bowel gas	Procedure of choice for detection of stones
Accurate identification of gallstones (>95%)	Massive obesity	
	Ascites	
Simultaneous scanning of GB, liver, bile ducts, pancreas		
"Real-time" scanning allows assessment of GB volume, contractility		
Not limited by jaundice, pregnancy		
May detect very small stones		
RADIOISOTOPE SCANS (HIDA, DIDA, ETC.)		
Accurate identification of cystic duct obstruction	?Contraindicated in pregnancy	Indicated for confirmation of suspected acute cholecystitis; less sensitive and less specific in chronic cholecystitis; useful in diagnosis of acalculous cholecystopathy, especially if given with CCK to assess gallbladder emptying
Simultaneous assessment of bile ducts	Serum bilirubin >103–205 μmol/L (6–12 mg/dL)	
	Cholecystogram of low resolution	
PLAIN ABDOMINAL X-RAY		
Low cost	Relatively low yield	Pathognomonic findings in:
Readily available	?Contraindicated in pregnancy	Calcified gallstones
		Limey bile, porcelain GB
		Emphysematous cholecystitis
		Gallstone ileus
ORAL CHOLECYSTOGRAM		
		Largely replaced by GBUS

Note: GB, gallbladder; CCK, cholecystokinin; GBUS, gallbladder ultrasound.

FIGURE 292-2 Examples of ultrasound and radiologic studies of the biliary tract. *A.* An ultrasound study showing a distended gallbladder containing a single large stone (*arrow*) which casts an acoustic shadow. *B.* Endoscopic retrograde cholangiopancreatogram (ERCP) showing normal biliary tract anatomy. In addition to the endoscope and large vertical gallbladder filled with contrast dye, the common hepatic duct (chd), common bile duct (cbd), and pancreatic duct (pd) are shown. The arrow points to the ampulla of Vater. *C.* Endoscopic retrograde cholangiogram (ERC) showing choledocholithiasis. The biliary tract is dilatated and contains multiple radiolucent calculi. *D.* ERCP showing sclerosing cholangitis. The common bile duct shows areas that are strictured and narrowed.

is a common clinical problem. The natural history of "silent" or asymptomatic gallstones has occasioned much debate. A study of predominantly male silent gallstone patients suggests that the cumulative risk for the development of symptoms or complications is relatively low—10% at 5 years, 15% at 10 years, and 18% at 15 years. Patients remaining asymptomatic for 15 years were found to be unlikely to develop symptoms during further follow-up, and most patients who did develop complications from their gallstones experienced *prior* warning symptoms. Similar conclusions apply to diabetic patients with silent gallstones. Decision analysis has suggested that (1) the cumulative risk of death due to gallstone disease while on expectant management is small, and (2) prophylactic cholecystectomy is not warranted.

Complications requiring cholecystectomy are much more common in gallstone patients who have developed symptoms of biliary pain. Patients found to have gallstones at a young age are more likely to develop symptoms from cholelithiasis than are patients older than 60 years at the time of initial diagnosis. Patients with diabetes mellitus and gallstones may be somewhat more susceptible to septic complications, but the magnitude of risk of septic biliary complications in diabetic patients is incompletely defined.

℞ TREATMENT

Surgical Therapy In asymptomatic gallstone patients, the risk of developing symptoms or complications requiring surgery is quite small (in the range of 1 to 2% per year). Thus a recommendation for cholecystectomy in a patient with gallstones should probably be based on assessment of three factors: (1) the presence of symptoms that are frequent enough or severe enough to interfere with the patient's general routine; (2) the presence of a prior complication of gallstone disease, i.e., history of acute cholecystitis, pancreatitis, gallstone fistula, etc.; or (3) the presence of an underlying condition predisposing the patient to increased risk of gallstone complications (e.g., calcified or porcelain gallbladder and/or a previous attack of acute cholecystitis regardless of current symptomatic status). Patients with very large gallstones (>3 cm in diameter) and patients having gallstones in a congenitally anomalous gallbladder might also be considered for prophylactic cholecystectomy. Although young age is a worrisome factor in asymptomatic gallstone patients, few authorities would now recommend routine cholecystectomy in all young patients with silent stones. Laparoscopic cholecystectomy is a minimal-access approach for the removal of the gallbladder together with its stones. Its advantages include a markedly

shortened hospital stay as well as decreased cost, and it is the procedure of choice for most patients referred for elective cholecystectomy.

From several studies involving over 4000 patients undergoing laparoscopic cholecystectomy, the following key points emerge: (1) complications develop in about 4% of patients, (2) conversion to laparotomy occurs in 5%, (3) the death rate is remarkably low (i.e., <0.1%), and (4) bile duct injuries are unusual (i.e., 0.2 to 0.5%). These data indicate why laparoscopic cholecystectomy has become the "gold standard" for treating symptomatic cholelithiasis.

Medical Therapy—Gallstone Dissolution UDCA decreases cholesterol saturation of bile and also appears to produce a lamellar liquid crystalline phase in bile that allows a dispersion of cholesterol from stones by physical-chemical means. UDCA may also retard cholesterol crystal nucleation. In carefully selected patients with a functioning gallbladder and with radiolucent stones <10 mm in diameter, complete dissolution can be achieved in about 50% of patients within 6 months to 2 years with UDCA at a dose of 8 to 10 mg/kg per day. The highest success rate (i.e., >70%) occurs in patients with small (<5 mm) floating radiolucent gallstones. Probably no more than 10% of patients with *symptomatic* cholelithiasis are candidates for such treatment. However, in addition to the vexing problem of recurrent stones (30 to 50% over 3 to 5 years of follow-up), there is also the factor of taking an expensive drug for up to 2 years. The advantages and success of laparoscopic cholecystectomy have largely reduced the role of gallstone dissolution to patients who wish to avoid or are not candidates for elective cholecystectomy.

Gallbladder stones may be fragmented by extracorporeal shock waves. While such shock wave lithotripsy combined with medical litholytic therapy is safe and effective in carefully selected patients with gallbladder calculi (radiolucent, solitary stone <2 cm in well-contracting gallbladder), the procedure is employed infrequently because of the emergence of laparoscopic cholystectomy as the procedure of choice for symptomatic cholelithiasis, the recurrence of gallstones in 30% of patients within 5 years after lithotripsy combined with medical litholytic therapy, and the cost of taking UDCA for a variable period after the procedure.

ACUTE AND CHRONIC CHOLECYSTITIS ■ Acute Cholecystitis Acute inflammation of the gallbladder wall usually follows obstruction of the cystic duct by a stone. Inflammatory response can be evoked by three factors: (1) *mechanical inflammation* produced by increased intraluminal pressure and distention with resulting ischemia of the gallbladder mucosa and wall, (2) *chemical inflammation* caused by the release of lysolecithin (due to the action of phospholipase on lecithin in bile) and other local tissue factors, and (3) *bacterial inflammation*, which may play a role in 50 to 85% of patients with acute cholecystitis. The organisms most frequently isolated by culture of gallbladder bile in these patients include *Escherichia coli, Klebsiella* spp., *Streptococcus* spp., and *Clostridium* spp.

Acute cholecystitis often begins as an attack of biliary pain that progressively worsens. Approximately 60 to 70% of patients report having experienced prior attacks that resolved spontaneously. As the episode progresses, however, the pain of acute cholecystitis becomes more generalized in the right upper abdomen. As with biliary colic, the pain of cholecystitis may radiate to the interscapular area, right scapula, or shoulder. Peritoneal signs of inflammation such as increased pain with jarring or on deep respiration may be apparent. The patient is anorectic and often nauseated. Vomiting is relatively common and may produce symptoms and signs of vascular and extracellular volume depletion. Jaundice is unusual early in the course of acute cholecystitis but may occur when edematous inflammatory changes involve the bile ducts and surrounding lymph nodes.

A low-grade fever is characteristically present, but shaking chills or rigors are not uncommon. The RUQ of the abdomen is almost invariably tender to palpation. An enlarged, tense gallbladder is palpable in one-quarter to one-half of patients. Deep inspiration or cough during subcostal palpation of the RUQ usually produces increased pain and inspiratory arrest (Murphy's sign). A light thump delivered to the right subcostal area may elicit a marked increase in pain. Localized rebound tenderness in the RUQ is common, as are abdominal distention and hypoactive bowel sounds from paralytic ileus, but generalized peritoneal signs and abdominal rigidity are usually lacking, in the absence of perforation.

The diagnosis of acute cholecystitis is usually made on the basis of a characteristic history and physical examination. The triad of sudden onset of RUQ tenderness, fever, and leukocytosis is highly suggestive. Typically, leukocytosis in the range of 10,000 to 15,000 cells per microliter with a left shift on differential count is found. The serum bilirubin is mildly elevated [<85.5 μmol/L (5 mg/dL)] in fewer than half of patients, while about one-fourth have modest elevations in serum aminotransferases (usually less than a fivefold elevation). The radionuclide (e.g., HIDA) biliary scan may be confirmatory if bile duct imaging is seen without visualization of the gallbladder. Ultrasound will demonstrate calculi in 90 to 95% of cases.

Approximately 75% of patients treated medically have remission of acute symptoms within 2 to 7 days following hospitalization. In 25%, however, a complication of acute cholecystitis will occur despite conservative treatment (see below). In this setting, prompt surgical intervention is required. Of the 75% of patients with acute cholecystitis who undergo remission of symptoms, approximately one-quarter will experience a recurrence of cholecystitis within 1 year, and 60% will have at least one recurrent bout within 6 years. In view of the natural history of the disease, acute cholecystitis is best treated by early surgery whenever possible.

Mirrizzi's syndrome is a rare complication in which a gallstone becomes impacted in the cystic duct or neck of the gallbladder causing compression of the CBD, resulting in CBD obstruction and jaundice. Ultrasound shows gallstone(s) lying outside the hepatic duct. Endoscopic retrograde cholangiopancreatography (ERCP) or percutaneous transhepatic cholangiography (PTC) will usually demonstrate the characteristic extrinsic compression of the CBD. Surgery consists of removing the cystic duct, diseased gallbladder, and the impacted stone. The preoperative diagnosis of Mirrizzi's syndrome is important to avoid CBD injury.

ACALCULOUS CHOLECYSTITIS In 5 to 10% of patients with acute cholecystitis, calculi obstructing the cystic duct are not found at surgery. In over 50% of such cases, an underlying explanation for acalculous inflammation is not found. An increased risk for the development of acalculous cholecystitis is especially associated with serious trauma or

burns, with the postpartum period following prolonged labor, and with orthopedic and other nonbiliary major surgical operations in the postoperative period. It may possibly complicate periods of prolonged parenteral hyperalimentation. For some of these cases, biliary sludge in the cystic duct may be responsible. Other precipitating factors include vasculitis, obstructing adenocarcinoma of the gallbladder, diabetes mellitus, torsion of the gallbladder, "unusual" bacterial infections of the gallbladder (e.g., *Leptospira, Streptococcus, Salmonella*, or *Vibrio cholerae*), and parasitic infestation of the gallbladder. Acalculous cholecystitis may also be seen with a variety of other systemic disease processes (sarcoidosis, cardiovascular disease, tuberculosis, syphilis, actinomycosis, etc.) and may possibly complicate periods of prolonged parenteral hyperalimentation.

Although the clinical manifestations of acalculous cholecystitis are indistinguishable from those of calculous cholecystitis, the setting of acute gallbladder inflammation complicating severe underlying illness is characteristic of acalculous disease. Ultrasound, computed tomography (CT) scanning, or radionuclide examinations demonstrating a large, tense, static gallbladder without stones and with evidence of poor emptying over a prolonged period may be diagnostically useful in some cases. The complication rate for acalculous cholecystitis exceeds that for calculous cholecystitis. Successful management of acute acalculous cholecystitis appears to depend primarily on early diagnosis and surgical intervention, with meticulous attention to postoperative care.

ACALCULOUS CHOLECYSTOPATHY Disordered motility of the gallbladder can produce recurrent biliary pain in patients without gallstones. Infusion of an octapeptide of CCK can be used to measure the gallbladder ejection fraction during cholescintigraphy. CCK cholescintigraphy using ^{99}Tc-diisopropyl iminodiacetic acid (DIDA) or HIDA may document an abnormal gallbladder ejection fraction (<40% at 45 min). The surgical findings have included abnormalities such as chronic cholecystitis, gallbladder muscle hypertrophy, and/or a markedly narrowed cystic duct. Some of these patients may well have had antecedent gallbladder disease. The following criteria can be used to identify patients with acalculous cholecystopathy: (1) recurrent episodes of typical RUQ pain characteristic of biliary tract pain, (2) abnormal CCK cholescintigraphy demonstrating a gallbladder ejection fraction of <40%, and (3) infusion of CCK reproduces the patient's pain. An additional clue would be the identification of a large gallbladder on ultrasound examination. Finally, it should be noted that sphincter of Oddi dysfunction can also give rise to recurrent RUQ pain and CCK-scintigraphic abnormalities.

EMPHYSEMATOUS CHOLECYSTITIS So-called emphysematous cholecystitis is thought to begin with acute cholecystitis (calculous or acalculous) followed by ischemia or gangrene of the gallbladder wall and infection by gas-producing organisms. Bacteria most frequently cultured in this setting include anaerobes, such as *C. welchii* or *C. perfringens*, and aerobes, such as *E. coli*. This condition occurs most frequently in elderly men and in patients with diabetes mellitus. The clinical manifestations are essentially indistinguishable from those of nongaseous cholecystitis. The diagnosis is usually made on plain abdominal film by finding gas within the gallbladder lumen, dissecting within the gallbladder wall to form a gaseous ring, or in the pericholecystic tissues. The morbidity and mortality rates with emphysematous cholecystitis are considerable. Prompt surgical intervention coupled with appropriate antibiotics is mandatory.

Chronic Cholecystitis Chronic inflammation of the gallbladder wall is almost always associated with the presence of gallstones and is thought to result from repeated bouts of subacute or acute cholecystitis or from persistent mechanical irritation of the gallbladder wall by gallstones. The presence of bacteria in the bile occurs in more than one-quarter of patients with chronic cholecystitis. The presence of infected bile in a patient with *chronic* cholecystitis undergoing elective cholecystectomy probably adds little to the operative risk. Chronic cholecystitis may be asymptomatic for years, may progress to symptomatic gallbladder disease or to acute cholecystitis, or may present with complications (see below).

Complications of Cholecystitis ■ *EMPYEMA AND HYDROPS* Empyema of the gallbladder usually results from progression of acute cholecystitis with persistent cystic duct obstruction to superinfection of the stagnant bile with a pus-forming bacterial organism. The clinical picture resembles that of cholangitis with high fever, severe RUQ pain, marked leukocytosis, and often, prostration. Empyema of the gallbladder carries a high risk of gram-negative sepsis and/or perforation. Emergency surgical intervention with proper antibiotic coverage is required as soon as the diagnosis is suspected.

Hydrops or mucocele of the gallbladder may also result from prolonged obstruction of the cystic duct, usually by a large solitary calculus. In this instance, the obstructed gallbladder lumen is progressively distended, over a period of time, by mucus (mucocele) or by a clear transudate (hydrops) produced by mucosal epithelial cells. A visible, easily palpable, nontender mass sometimes extending from the RUQ into the right iliac fossa may be found on physical examination. The patient with hydrops of the gallbladder frequently remains asymptomatic, although chronic RUQ pain may also occur. Cholecystectomy is indicated, since empyema, perforation, or gangrene may complicate the condition.

GANGRENE AND PERFORATION Gangrene of the gallbladder results from ischemia of the wall and patchy or complete tissue necrosis. Underlying conditions often include marked distention of the gallbladder, vasculitis, diabetes mellitus, empyema, or torsion resulting in arterial occlusion. Gangrene usually predisposes to perforation of the gallbladder, but perforation may also occur in chronic cholecystitis without premonitory warning symptoms. *Localized perforations* are usually contained by the omentum or by adhesions produced by recurrent inflammation of the gallbladder. Bacterial superinfection of the walled-off gallbladder contents results in abscess formation. Most patients are best treated with cholecystectomy, but some seriously ill patients may be managed with cholecystostomy and drainage of the abscess. *Free perforation* is less common but is associated with a mortality rate of approximately 30%. Such patients may experience a sudden transient relief of RUQ pain as the distended gallbladder decompresses; this is followed by signs of generalized peritonitis.

FISTULA FORMATION AND GALLSTONE ILEUS *Fistulization* into an adjacent organ adherent to the gallbladder wall may result from inflammation and adhesion formation. Fistulas into the duodenum are most common, followed in frequency by those involving the hepatic flexure of the colon, stomach or jejunum, abdominal wall, and renal pelvis. Clinically "silent" biliary-enteric fistulas occurring as a complication of acute cholecystitis have been found in up to 5% of patients undergoing cholecystectomy. Asymptomatic cholecystoenteric fistulas may sometimes be diagnosed by finding gas in the biliary tree on plain abdominal films. Barium contrast studies or endoscopy of the upper gastrointestinal tract or colon may demonstrate the fistula. Treatment in the symptomatic patient usually consists of cholecystectomy, CBD exploration, and closure of the fistulous tract.

Gallstone ileus refers to mechanical intestinal obstruction resulting from the passage of a large gallstone into the bowel lumen. The stone customarily enters the duodenum through a cholecystoenteric fistula at that level. The site of obstruction by the impacted gallstone is usually at the ileocecal valve, provided that the more proximal small bowel is of normal caliber. The majority of patients do not give a history of either prior biliary tract symptoms or complaints suggestive of acute cholecystitis or fistulization. Large stones over 2.5 cm in diameter are thought to predispose to fistula formation by gradual erosion through the gallbladder fundus. Diagnostic confirmation may occasionally be found on the plain abdominal film (e.g., small-intestinal obstruction with gas in the biliary tree and a calcified, ectopic gallstone) or following an upper gastrointestinal series (cholecystoduo-

denal fistula with small-bowel obstruction at the ileocecal valve). Laparotomy with stone extraction (or propulsion into the colon) remains the procedure of choice to relieve obstruction. Evacuation of large stones within the gallbladder should also be performed. In general, the gallbladder and its attachment to the intestines should be left alone.

LIMEY (MILK OF CALCIUM) BILE AND PORCELAIN GALLBLADDER Calcium salts may be secreted into the lumen of the gallbladder in sufficient concentration to produce calcium precipitation and diffuse, hazy opacification of bile or a layering effect on plain abdominal roentgenography. This so-called limey bile, or milk of calcium bile, is usually clinically innocuous, but cholecystectomy is recommended, especially when it occurs in a hydropic gallbladder. In the entity called *porcelain gallbladder*, calcium salt deposition within the wall of a chronically inflamed gallbladder may be detected on the plain abdominal film. Cholecystectomy is advised in all patients with porcelain gallbladder because in a high percentage of cases this finding appears to be associated with the development of carcinoma of the gallbladder.

℞ TREATMENT

Medical Therapy Although surgical intervention remains the mainstay of therapy for acute cholecystitis and its complications, a period of in-hospital stabilization may be required before cholecystectomy. Oral intake is eliminated, nasogastric suction may be indicated, and extracellular volume depletion and electrolyte abnormalities are repaired. Meperidine or nonsteroidal anti-inflammatory drugs (NSAIDs) are usually employed for analgesia because they may produce less spasm of the sphincter of Oddi than drugs such as morphine. Intravenous antibiotic therapy is usually indicated in patients with severe acute cholecystitis even though bacterial superinfection of bile may not have occurred in the early stages of the inflammatory process. Antibiotic therapy is guided by the most common organisms likely to be present, which are *E. coli*, *Klebsiella* spp., and *Streptococcus* spp. Effective antibiotics include ureidopenicillins such as piperacillin or mezlocillin, ampicillin sulbactam, and third-generation cephalosporins. Anaerobic coverage by a drug such as metronidazole should be added if gangrenous or emphysematous cholecystitis is suspected. Similarly, combination therapy with an aminoglycoside and other antibiotics may be considered in diabetic or debilitated patients and in those with signs of gram-negative sepsis (Chap. 134). Postoperative complications of wound infection, abscess formation, or sepsis are reduced in antibiotic-treated patients.

Surgical Therapy The optimal timing of surgical intervention in patients with acute cholecystitis depends on stabilization of the patient. The clear trend is toward earlier surgery, and this is due in part to requirements for shorter hospital stays. Urgent (emergency) cholecystectomy or cholecystostomy is probably appropriate in most patients in whom a complication of acute cholecystitis such as empyema, emphysematous cholecystitis, or perforation is suspected or confirmed. In uncomplicated cases of acute cholecystitis, up to 30% of patients fail to resolve their symptoms on appropriate medical therapy, and progression of the attack or a supervening complication leads to the performance of early operation (within 24 to 72 h). The technical complications of surgery are not increased in patients undergoing early as opposed to delayed cholecystectomy. Delayed surgical intervention is probably best reserved for (1) patients in whom the overall medical condition imposes an unacceptable risk for early surgery and (2) patients in whom the diagnosis of acute cholecystitis is in doubt. Early cholecystectomy is the treatment of choice for most patients with acute cholecystitis. Mortality figures for emergency cholecystectomy in most centers approach 3%, while the mortality risk for elective or early cholecystectomy approximates 0.5% in patients under age 60. Of course, the operative risks increase with age-related diseases of other organ systems and with the presence of long- or short-term complications of gallbladder disease. Seriously ill or debilitated patients with cholecystitis may be managed with cholecystostomy and tube drainage of the gallbladder. Elective cholecystectomy may then be done at a later date.

Postcholecystectomy Complications Early complications following cholecystectomy include atelectasis and other pulmonary disorders, abscess formation (often subphrenic), external or internal hemorrhage, biliary-enteric fistula, and bile leaks. Jaundice may indicate absorption of bile from an intraabdominal collection following a biliary leak or mechanical obstruction of the CBD by retained calculi, intraductal blood clots, or extrinsic compression. Routine performance of intraoperative cholangiography during cholecystectomy has helped to reduce the incidence of these early complications.

Overall, cholecystectomy is a very successful operation that provides total or near-total relief of preoperative symptoms in 75 to 90% of patients. The most common cause of persistent postcholecystectomy symptoms is an overlooked symptomatic nonbiliary disorder (e.g., reflux esophagitis, peptic ulceration, pancreatitis, or—most often—irritable bowel syndrome). In a small percentage of patients, however, a disorder of the extrahepatic bile ducts may result in persistent symptomatology. These so-called postcholecystectomy syndromes may be due to (1) biliary strictures, (2) retained biliary calculi, (3) cystic duct stump syndrome, (4) stenosis or dyskinesia of the sphincter of Oddi, or (5) bile salt–induced diarrhea or gastritis.

CYSTIC DUCT STUMP SYNDROME In the absence of cholangiographically demonstrable retained stones, symptoms resembling biliary pain or cholecystitis in the postcholecystectomy patient have frequently been attributed to disease in a long (>1 cm) cystic duct remnant (cystic duct stump syndrome). Careful analysis, however, reveals that postcholecystectomy complaints are attributable to other causes in almost all patients in whom the symptom complex was originally thought to result from the existence of a long cystic duct stump. Accordingly, considerable care should be taken to investigate the possible role of other factors in the production of postcholecystectomy symptoms before attributing them to cystic duct stump syndrome.

PAPILLARY DYSFUNCTION, PAPILLARY STENOSIS, SPASM OF THE SPHINCTER OF ODDI, AND BILIARY DYSKINESIA Symptoms of biliary colic accompanied by signs of recurrent, intermittent biliary obstruction may be produced by papillary stenosis, papillary dysfunction, spasm of the sphincter of Oddi, and biliary dyskinesia. Papillary stenosis is thought to result from acute or chronic inflammation of the papilla of Vater or from glandular hyperplasia of the papillary segment. Five criteria have been used to define papillary stenosis: (1) upper abdominal pain, usually RUQ or epigastric; (2) abnormal liver tests; (3) dilatation of the common bile duct upon ERCP examination; (4) delayed (>45 min) drainage of contrast material from the duct; and (5) increased basal pressure of the sphincter of Oddi, a finding that may be of only minor significance. An alternative to ERCP is magnetic resonance cholangiography (MRC) if ERCP and/or biliary manometry are either unavailable or not feasible. In patients with papillary stenosis, quantitative hepatobiliary scintigraphy has revealed delayed transit from the common bile duct to the bowel, ductal dilatation, and abnormal time-activity dynamics. This technique can also be used before and after sphincterotomy to document improvement in biliary emptying. Treatment consists of endoscopic or surgical sphincteroplasty to ensure wide patency of the distal portions of both the bile and pancreatic ducts. The greater the number of the preceding criteria present, the greater the likelihood that a patient does have a degree of papillary stenosis sufficient to justify correction. The factors usually considered as indications for sphincterotomy include (1) prolonged duration of symptoms, (2) lack of response to symptomatic treatment, (3) presence of severe disability, and (4) the patient's choice of sphincterotomy over surgery (given a clear understanding on his or her part of the risks involved in both procedures).

Criteria for diagnosing dyskinesia of the sphincter of Oddi are even more controversial than those for papillary stenosis. Proposed mechanisms include spasm of the sphincter, denervation sensitivity resulting in hypertonicity, and abnormalities of the sequencing or frequency rates of sphincteric contraction waves. When thorough evaluation has failed to demonstrate another cause for the pain, and when cholangiographic and manometric criteria suggest a diagnosis of biliary dys-

kinesia, medical treatment with nitrites or anticholinergics to attempt pharmacologic relaxation of the sphincter has been proposed. Endoscopic biliary sphincterotomy (EBS) or surgical sphincteroplasty may be indicated in patients who fail to respond to a 2- to 3-month trial of medical therapy, especially if basal sphincter of Oddi pressures are elevated. EBS has become the procedure of choice for removing bile duct stones and for other biliary and pancreatic problems. A study of EBS found four key findings: (1) Dysfunction of the sphincter of Oddi was associated with an increased rise of complications, especially pancreatitis; (2) pancreatitis was more frequent in young patients; (3) difficulty in cannulating the bile duct and the use of "precut" sphincterotomy were important technique-related risk factors for complications; and (4) experience in the volume of procedures proved to be important; endoscopists who perform more than one EBS per week had lower complication rates than endoscopists who performed a smaller number of procedures.

Bile Salt–Induced Diarrhea and Gastritis Postcholecystectomy patients may develop symptoms of dyspepsia, which have been attributed to duodenogastric reflux of bile. However, firm data linking these symptoms to bile gastritis after surgical removal of the gallbladder are lacking. Cholecystectomy induces persistent changes in gut transit, and these changes effect a noticeable modification of bowel habits. Cholecystectomy shortens gut transit time by accelerating passage of the fecal bolus through the colon with marked acceleration in the right colon, thus causing an increase in colonic bile acid output and a shift in bile acid composition toward the more diarrheagenic secondary bile acids. Diarrhea that is severe enough, i.e., three or more watery movements per day, can be classified as postcholecystectomy diarrhea, and this occurs in 5 to 10% of patients undergoing elective cholecystectomy. Treatment with bile acid sequestering agents such as cholestyramine or colestipol is often effective in ameliorating troublesome diarrhea.

THE HYPERPLASTIC CHOLECYSTOSES The term *hyperplastic cholecystoses* is used to denote a group of disorders of the gallbladder characterized by excessive proliferation of normal tissue components.

Adenomyomatosis is characterized by a benign proliferation of gallbladder surface epithelium with glandlike formations, extramural sinuses, transverse strictures, and/or fundal nodule ("adenoma" or "adenomyoma") formation. Outpouchings of mucosa termed *Rokitansky-Aschoff sinuses* may be seen on oral cholecystography in conjunction with hyperconcentration of contrast medium. Characteristic dimpled filling defects also may be seen.

Cholesterolosis is characterized by abnormal deposition of lipid, especially cholesteryl esters within macrophages in the lamina propria of the gallbladder wall. In its diffuse form ("strawberry gallbladder"), the gallbladder mucosa is brick red and speckled with bright yellow flecks of lipid. The localized form shows solitary or multiple "cholesterol polyps" studding the gallbladder wall. Cholesterol stones of the gallbladder are found in nearly half the cases. Cholecystectomy is indicated in both adenomyomatosis and cholesterolosis when symptomatic or when cholelithiasis is present.

The prevalence of gallbladder polyps in the adult population is about 5%, with a marked male predominance. Few significant changes have been found over a 5-year period in asymptomatic patients with gallbladder polyps <10 mm in diameter. Cholecytstectomy is recommended in symptomatic patients, as well as in asymptomatic patients over 50 years of age, or in those whose polyps are >10 mm in diameter or associated with gallstones or polyp growth on serial ultrasonography.

DISEASES OF THE BILE DUCTS

CONGENITAL ANOMALIES ■ Biliary Atresia and Hypoplasia Atretic and hypoplastic lesions of the extrahepatic and major intrahepatic bile ducts are the most common biliary anomalies of clinical relevance encountered in infancy. The clinical picture is one of severe obstructive jaundice during the first month of life, with pale stools. When biliary atresia is suspected on the basis of clinical, laboratory, and imaging findings the diagnosis is confirmed by surgical exploration and operative cholangiography. The diagnosis is confirmed by surgical exploration with operative cholangiography. Approximately 10% of cases of biliary atresia are treatable with roux-en-Y choledochojejunostomy, with the Kasai procedure (hepatic portoenterostomy) being attempted in the remainder in an effort to restore some bile flow. Most patients, even those having successful biliary-enteric anastomoses, eventually develop chronic cholangitis, extensive hepatic fibrosis, and portal hypertension.

Choledochal Cysts   Cystic dilatation may involve the free portion of the CBD, i.e., choledochal cyst, or may present as diverticulum formation in the intraduodenal segment. In the latter situation, chronic reflux of pancreatic juice into the biliary tree can produce inflammation and stenosis of the extrahepatic bile ducts leading to cholangitis or biliary obstruction. Because the process may be gradual, approximately 50% of patients present with onset of symptoms after age 10. The diagnosis may be made by ultrasound, abdominal CT, MRC, or cholangiography. Only one-third of patients show the classic triad of abdominal pain, jaundice, and an abdominal mass. Ultrasonographic detection of a cyst separate from the gallbladder should suggest the diagnosis of choledochal cyst, which can be confirmed by demonstrating the entrance of extrahepatic bile ducts into the cyst. Surgical treatment involves excision of the "cyst" and biliary-enteric anastomosis. Patients with choledochal cysts are at increased risk for the subsequent development of cholangiocarcinoma.

Congenital Biliary Ectasia   Dilatation of intrahepatic bile ducts may involve either the major intrahepatic radicles (Caroli's disease), the inter- and intralobular ducts (congenital hepatic fibrosis), or both. In Caroli's disease, clinical manifestations include recurrent cholangitis, abscess formation in and around the affected ducts, and, often, gallstone formation within portions of ectatic intrahepatic biliary radicles. Ultrasound, MRC, and CT are of great diagnostic value in demonstrating cystic dilatation of the intrahepatic bile ducts. Treatment with ongoing antibiotic therapy is usually undertaken in an effort to limit the frequency and severity of recurrent bouts of cholangitis. Progression to secondary biliary cirrhosis with portal hypertension, extrahepatic biliary obstruction, cholangiocarcinoma, or recurrent episodes of sepsis with hepatic abscess formation is common.

CHOLEDOCHOLITHIASIS ■ Pathophysiology and Clinical Manifestations   Passage of gallstones into the CBD occurs in approximately 10 to 15% of patients with cholelithiasis. The incidence of common duct stones increases with increasing age of the patient, so that up to 25% of elderly patients may have calculi in the common duct at the time of cholecystectomy. Undetected duct stones are left behind in approximately 1 to 5% of cholecystectomy patients. The overwhelming majority of bile duct stones are cholesterol stones formed in the gallbladder, which then migrate into the extrahepatic biliary tree through the cystic duct. Primary calculi arising de novo in the ducts are usually pigment stones developing in patients with (1) hepatobiliary parasitism or chronic, recurrent cholangitis; (2) congenital anomalies of the bile ducts (especially Caroli's disease); (3) dilated, sclerosed, or strictured ducts; or (4) an *MDR3* gene defect leading to impaired biliary phospholipids secretion. Common duct stones may remain asymptomatic for years, may pass spontaneously into the duodenum, or (most often) may present with biliary colic or a complication.

Complications ■ CHOLANGITIS   Cholangitis may be acute or chronic, and symptoms result from inflammation, which usually requires at least partial obstruction to the flow of bile. Bacteria are present on bile culture in approximately 75% of patients with acute cholangitis early in the symptomatic course. The characteristic presentation of acute cholangitis involves biliary pain, jaundice, and spiking fevers with chills (Charcot's triad). Blood cultures are frequently positive, and

leukocytosis is typical. *Nonsuppurative acute cholangitis* is most common and may respond relatively rapidly to supportive measures and to treatment with antibiotics. In *suppurative acute cholangitis*, however, the presence of pus under pressure in a completely obstructed ductal system leads to symptoms of severe toxicity—mental confusion, bacteremia, and septic shock. Response to antibiotics alone in this setting is relatively poor, multiple hepatic abscesses are often present, and the mortality rate approaches 100% unless prompt endoscopic or surgical relief of the obstruction and drainage of infected bile are carried out. Endoscopic management of bacterial cholangitis is as effective as surgical intervention. ERCP with endoscopic sphincterotomy is safe and the preferred initial procedure for both establishing a definitive diagnosis and providing effective therapy.

OBSTRUCTIVE JAUNDICE   Gradual obstruction of the CBD over a period of weeks or months usually leads to initial manifestations of jaundice or pruritus without associated symptoms of biliary colic or cholangitis. Painless jaundice may occur in patients with choledocholithiasis, but this manifestation is much more characteristic of biliary obstruction secondary to malignancy of the head of the pancreas, bile ducts, or ampulla of Vater.

In patients whose obstruction is secondary to choledocholithiasis, associated chronic calculous cholecystitis is very common, and the gallbladder in this setting may be relatively indistensible. The absence of a palpable gallbladder in most patients with biliary obstruction from duct stones is the basis for *Courvoisier's law*, i.e., that the presence of a palpably enlarged gallbladder suggests that the biliary obstruction is secondary to an underlying malignancy rather than to calculous disease. Biliary obstruction causes progressive dilatation of the intrahepatic bile ducts as intrabiliary pressures rise. Hepatic bile flow is suppressed, and reabsorption and regurgitation of conjugated bilirubin into the bloodstream lead to jaundice accompanied by dark urine (bilirubinuria) and light-colored (acholic) stools.

CBD stones should be suspected in any patient with cholecystitis whose serum bilirubin level exceeds 85.5 μmol/L (5 mg/dL). The maximum bilirubin level is seldom over 256.5 μmol/L (15.0 mg/dL) in patients with choledocholithiasis unless concomitant hepatic disease or another factor leading to marked hyperbilirubinemia exists. Serum bilirubin levels of 342.0 μmol/L (20 mg/dL) or more should suggest the possibility of neoplastic obstruction. The serum alkaline phosphatase level is almost always elevated in biliary obstruction. A rise in alkaline phosphatase often precedes clinical jaundice and may be the only abnormality in routine liver function tests. There may be a two- to tenfold elevation of serum aminotransferases, especially in association with acute obstruction. Following relief of the obstructing process, serum aminotransferase elevations usually return rapidly to normal, while the serum bilirubin level may take 1 to 2 weeks to return to normal. The alkaline phosphatase level usually falls slowly, lagging behind the decrease in serum bilirubin.

PANCREATITIS   The most common associated entity discovered in patients with nonalcoholic acute pancreatitis is biliary tract disease. Biochemical evidence of pancreatic inflammation complicates acute cholecystitis in 15% of cases and choledocholithiasis in over 30%, and the common factor appears to be the passage of gallstones through the common duct. Coexisting pancreatitis should be suspected in patients with symptoms of cholecystitis who develop (1) back pain or pain to the left of the abdominal midline, (2) prolonged vomiting with paralytic ileus, or (3) a pleural effusion, especially on the left side. Surgical treatment of gallstone disease is usually associated with resolution of the pancreatitis.

SECONDARY BILIARY CIRRHOSIS   Secondary biliary cirrhosis may complicate prolonged or intermittent duct obstruction with or without recurrent cholangitis. Although this complication may be seen in patients with choledocholithiasis, it is more common in cases of prolonged obstruction from stricture or neoplasm. Once established, secondary biliary cirrhosis may be progressive even after correction of the obstructing process, and increasingly severe hepatic cirrhosis may lead to portal hypertension or to hepatic failure and death. Prolonged biliary obstruction may also be associated with clinically relevant deficiencies of the fat-soluble vitamins A, D, E, and K.

Diagnosis and Treatment   The diagnosis of choledocholithiasis is usually made by cholangiography (Table 292-3), either preoperatively by ERCP or intraoperatively at the time of cholecystectomy. As many as 15% of patients undergoing cholecystectomy will prove to have CBD stones. With the advent of laparoscopic cholecystectomy, the management of CBD stones in the presence of gallstones is gradually being

clarified. Preoperative ERCP with endoscopic papillotomy and stone extraction is the preferred approach. It not only provides stone clearance but also defines the anatomy of the biliary tree in relationship to the cystic duct. ERCP is indicated in gallstone patients who have any of the following risk factors: (1) a history of jaundice or pancreatitis, (2) abnormal tests of liver function, and (3) ultrasonographic evidence

TABLE 292-3   *Diagnostic Evaluation of the Bile Ducts*

Diagnostic Advantages	Diagnostic Limitations	Contraindications	Complications	Comment
HEPATOBILIARY ULTRASOUND				
Rapid Simultaneous scanning of GB, liver, bile ducts, pancreas Accurate identification of dilated bile ducts Not limited by jaundice, pregnancy Guidance for fine-needle biopsy	Bowel gas Massive obesity Ascites Barium Partial bile duct obstruction Poor visualization of distal CBD	None	None	Initial procedure of choice in investigating possible biliary tract obstruction
COMPUTED TOMOGRAPHY				
Simultaneous scanning of GB, liver, bile ducts, pancreas Accurate identification of dilated bile ducts, masses Not limited by jaundice, gas, obesity, ascites High-resolution image Guidance for fine-needle biopsy	Extreme cachexia Movement artifact Ileus Partial bile duct obstruction	Pregnancy	Reaction to iodinated contrast, if used	Indicated for evaluation of hepatic or pancreatic masses Procedure of choice in investigating possible biliary obstruction if diagnostic limitations prevent HBUS
MAGNETIC RESONANCE CHOLANGIOPANCREATOGRAPHY				
Useful modality for visualizing pancreatic and biliary ducts Has excellent sensitivity for bile duct dilatation, biliary stricture, and intraductal abnormalities Can identify pancreatic duct dilatation or stricture, pancreatic duct stenosis, and pancreas divisum	Cannot offer therapeutic intervention High cost	Claustrophobia Certain metals (iron)	None	
PERCUTANEOUS TRANSHEPATIC CHOLANGIOGRAM				
Extremely successful when bile ducts dilated Best visualization of proximal biliary tract Bile cytology/culture Percutaneous transhepatic drainage	Nondilated or sclerosed ducts	Pregnancy Uncorrectable coagulopathy Massive ascites ? Hepatic abscess	Bleeding Hemobilia Bile peritonitis Bacteremia, sepsis	Indicated when ERCP is contraindicated or failed
ENDOSCOPIC RETROGRADE CHOLANGIOPANCREATOGRAM				

Simultaneous pancreatography
Best visualization of distal biliary tract
Bile or pancreatic cytology
Endoscopic sphincterotomy and stone removal
Biliary manometry
	Gastroduodenal obstruction
	? Roux en Y biliary-enteric anastomosis
		Pregnancy
		? Acute pancreatitis
		? Severe cardiopulmonary disease
			Pancreatitis
			Cholangitis, sepsis
			Infected pancreatic pseudocyst
			Perforation (rare)
			Hypoxemia, aspiration
				Cholangiogram of choice in:
				  Absence of dilated ducts
				  ? Pancreatic, ampullary or gastroduodenal disease
				  Prior biliary surgery
				Endoscopic sphincterotomy a treatment possibility

ENDOSCOPIC ULTRASOUND				
Most sensitive method to detect ampullary stones				Can be used in pregnancy

Note: GB, gallbladder; CBD, common bile duct; HBUS, hepatobiliary ultrasound; ERCP, endoscopic retrograde cholangiopancreatography. Intravenous cholangiography is an obsolete technique because 40% of common duct stones are missed and there is poor reso-lution even with tomography. There are few indications for its use, especially since other cholangiographic techniques are usually available.

of a dilated CBD or stones in the duct. Alternatively, if intraoperative cholangiography reveals retained stones, postoperative ERCP can be carried out. The need for preoperative ERCP is expected to decrease further as laparoscopic techniques improve.

The widespread use of laparoscopic cholecystectomy and ERCP has decreased the incidence of complicated biliary tract disease and the need for choledocholithotomy and T-tube drainage of the bile ducts. EBS followed by spontaneous passage or stone extraction is the treatment of choice in the management of patients with common duct stones, especially in elderly or poor-risk patients.

TRAUMA, STRICTURES, AND HEMOBILIA Approximately 95% of benign strictures of the extrahepatic bile ducts result from surgical trauma and occur in about 1 in 500 cholecystectomies. Strictures may present with bile leak or abscess formation in the immediate postoperative period or with biliary obstruction or cholangitis as long as 2 years or more following the inciting trauma. The diagnosis is established by percutaneous or endoscopic cholangiography. Endoscopic brushing of biliary strictures may be helpful in establishing the nature of the lesion and is more accurate than bile cytology alone. When positive exfoliative cytology is obtained, the diagnosis of a neoplastic stricture is established. This procedure is especially important in patients with primary sclerosing cholangitis (PSC) who are predisposed to the development of cholangiocarcinomas. Successful operative correction of non-PSC bile duct strictures by a skillful surgeon with duct-to-bowel anastomosis is usually possible, although mortality rates from surgical complications, recurrent cholangitis, or secondary biliary cirrhosis are high.

Hemobilia may follow traumatic or operative injury to the liver or bile ducts, intraductal rupture of a hepatic abscess or aneurysm of the hepatic artery, biliary or hepatic tumor hemorrhage, or mechanical complications of choledocholithiasis or hepatobiliary parasitism. Diagnostic procedures such as liver biopsy, PTC, and transhepatic biliary drainage catheter placement may also be complicated by hemobilia. Patients often present with a classic triad of biliary pain, obstructive jaundice, and melena or occult blood in the stools. The diagnosis is sometimes made by cholangiographic evidence of blood clot in the biliary tree, but selective angiographic verification may be required. Although minor episodes of hemobilia may resolve without operative intervention, surgical ligation of the bleeding vessel is frequently required.

EXTRINSIC COMPRESSION OF THE BILE DUCTS Partial or complete biliary obstruction may sometimes be produced by extrinsic compression of the ducts. The most common cause of this form of obstructive jaundice is carcinoma of the head of the pancreas. Biliary obstruction may also occur as a complication of either acute or chronic pancreatitis or involvement of lymph nodes in the porta hepatis by lymphoma or metastatic carcinoma. The latter should be distinguished from cholestasis resulting from massive replacement of the liver by tumor.

HEPATOBILIARY PARASITISM Infestation of the biliary tract by adult helminths or their ova may produce a chronic, recurrent pyogenic cholangitis with or without multiple hepatic abscesses, ductal stones, or biliary obstruction. This condition is relatively rare but does occur in inhabitants of southern China and elsewhere in Southeast Asia. The organisms most commonly involved are trematodes or flukes, including *Clonorchis sinensis*, *Opisthorchis viverrini* or *O. felineus*, and *Fasciola hepatica*. The biliary tract also may be involved by intraductal migration of adult *Ascaris lumbricoides* from the duodenum or by intrabiliary rupture of hydatid cysts of the liver produced by *Echinococcus* spp. The diagnosis is made by cholangiography and the presence of characteristic ova on stool examination. When obstruction is present, the treatment of choice is laparotomy under antibiotic coverage, with common duct exploration and a biliary drainage procedure. It should be emphasized that in the Far East, one also sees cholangiohepatitis associated with pigment lithiasis, which may, in fact, be more common than cholangitis due to parasites.

SCLEROSING CHOLANGITIS Primary or idiopathic sclerosing cholangitis is characterized by a progressive, inflammatory, sclerosing, and obliterative process affecting the extrahepatic and/or the intrahepatic bile ducts. The disorder occurs in about 70% in association with inflammatory bowel disease, especially ulcerative colitis. It may also be associated (albeit rarely) with multifocal fibrosclerosis syndromes such as retroperitoneal, mediastinal, and/or periureteral fibrosis; Riedel's struma; or pseudotumor of the orbit.

Patients with primary sclerosing cholangitis often present with signs and symptoms of chronic or intermittent biliary obstruction: RUQ abdominal pain, pruritus, jaundice, or acute cholangitis. Late in the course, complete biliary obstruction, secondary biliary cirrhosis, hepatic failure, or portal hypertension with bleeding varices may occur. The diagnosis is usually established by finding multifocal, diffusely distributed strictures with intervening segments of normal or dilated ducts, producing a beaded appearance on cholangiography (Fig. 292-2D). The cholangiographic technique of choice in suspected cases is ERCP, since intrahepatic ductal involvement may make PTC difficult. When a diagnosis of sclerosing cholangitis has been established, a search for associated diseases, especially for chronic inflammatory bowel disease, should be carried out.

A recent study describes the natural history and outcome for 305 patients of Swedish descent with primary sclerosing cholangitis; 134 (44%) of the patients were asymptomatic at the time of diagnosis and, not surprisingly, had a significantly higher survival rate with a median follow-up time of 63 months. The independent predictors of a bad prognosis were age, serum bilirubin concentration, and liver histologic changes. Cholangiocarcinoma was found in 24 patients (8%). Inflammatory bowel disease was closely associated with primary sclerosing cholangitis and had a prevalence of 81% in this study population.

Small duct PSC is defined by the presence of chronic cholestasis and hepatic histology consistent with PSC but with normal findings on cholangiography. Small duct PSC is found in about 5% of patients with PSC and may represent an earlier stage of PSC associated with a significantly better long-term prognosis. However, such patients may progress to classic PSC and/or end-stage liver disease with consequent necessity of liver transplantation.

In patients with AIDS, cholangiopancreatography may demonstrate a broad range of biliary tract changes as well as pancreatic duct obstruction and occasionally pancreatitis (Chap. 173). Further, biliary tract lesions in AIDS include infection and cholangiopancreatographic changes similar to those of PSC. Changes noted include: (1) diffuse involvement of intrahepatic bile ducts alone, (2) involvement of both intra- and extrahepatic bile ducts, (3) ampullary stenosis, (4) stricture of the intrapancreatic portion of the common bile duct, and (5) pancreatic duct involvement. Associated infectious organisms include *Cryptosporidium*, *Mycobacterium avium-intracellulare*, cytomegalovirus, *Microsporidia*, and *Isospora*. In addition, acalculous cholecystitis occurs in up to 10% of patients. ERCP sphincterotomy, while not without risk, provides significant pain reduction in patients with AIDS-associated papillary stenosis. Secondary sclerosing cholangitis may occur as a long-term complication of choledocholithiasis, cholangiocarcinoma, operative or traumatic biliary injury, or contiguous inflammatory processes.

℞ **TREATMENT**

Therapy with cholestyramine may help control symptoms of pruritus, and antibiotics are useful when cholangitis complicates the clinical picture. Vitamin D and calcium supplementation may help prevent the loss of bone mass frequently seen in patients with chronic cholestasis. Glucocorticoids, methotrexate, and cyclosporine have not been shown to be efficacious in PSC. UDCA in high dosage (20 mg/kg) improves serum liver tests, but an effect on survival has not been documented. In cases where high-grade biliary obstruction (dominant strictures) has occurred, balloon dilatation or stenting may be appropriate. Only rarely is surgical intervention indicated. Efforts at biliary-enteric anastomosis or stent placement may, however, be complicated by recurrent cholangitis and further progression of the stenosing process. The prognosis is unfavorable, with a median survival of 9 to 12 years following the diagnosis, regardless of therapy. Four variables (age, serum bilirubin level, histologic stage, and splenomegaly) predict survival in patients with PSC and serve as the basis for a risk score. PSC is one of the most common indications for liver transplantation.

FURTHER READING

APSTEIN MD, CAREY MC: Pathogenesis of cholesterol gallstones: A parsimonious hypothesis. Eur J Clin Invest 26:343, 1996

BERR F et al: Disorders of bile acid metabolism in cholesterol gallstone disease. J Clin Invest 90:589, 1992

BROOME U et al: Natural history and outcome in 32 Swedish patients with small duct primary sclerosing cholangitis (PSC). J Hepatol 36:586, 2002

PAULETZKI J et al: Gallbladder emptying and gallstone formation: A prospective study on gallstone recurrence. Gastroenterology 111:765, 1996

PAUMPARTNER G: Nonsurgical management of gallstone disease, in *Sleisenger and Fordtran's Gastrointestinal and Liver Disease*, 7th ed, M Feldman et al (eds). Philadelphia, Saunders, 2002, 1107–1115

RANSOHOFF DF, GRACIE WA: Treatment of gallstones. Ann Intern Med 119: 606, 1993

ZACKS SL et al: A population-based cohort study comparing laparoscopic cholecystectomy and open cholecystectomy. Ann J Gastroenterol 97:334, 2002

Section 3 Disorders of the Pancreas

293 APPROACH TO THE PATIENT WITH PANCREATIC DISEASE
Phillip P. Toskes, Norton J. Greenberger

GENERAL CONSIDERATIONS

Inflammatory disease of the pancreas may be acute or chronic. Although good data exist concerning the frequency of acute pancreatitis (about 5000 new cases per year in the United States, with a mortality rate of about 10%), the number of patients who suffer with recurrent acute pancreatitis or chronic pancreatitis is largely undefined. Only one prospective study on the incidence of chronic pancreatitis is available; it showed an incidence of 8.2 new cases per 100,000 per year and a prevalence of 26.4 cases per 100,000. These numbers probably underestimate considerably the true incidence and prevalence, because non-alcohol-induced pancreatitis was largely ignored. At autopsy, the prevalence of chronic pancreatitis ranges from 0.04 to 5%. The relative inaccessibility of the pancreas to direct examination and the nonspecificity of the abdominal pain associated with pancreatitis make the diagnosis of pancreatitis difficult and usually dependent on elevation of blood amylase levels. Many patients with chronic pancreatitis do not have elevated blood amylase levels. Some patients with chronic pancreatitis develop signs and symptoms of pancreatic exocrine insufficiency, and thus objective evidence for pancreatic disease can be demonstrated. However, there is a very large reservoir of pancreatic exocrine function. More than 90% of the pancreas must be damaged before maldigestion of fat and protein is manifested. Even the secretin stimulation test, which is the most sensitive method of assessing pancreatic exocrine function, is probably abnormal only when >60% of exocrine function has been lost. Noninvasive, indirect tests of pancreatic exocrine function (fecal elastase, serum trypsinogen) are much more likely to give abnormal results in patients with obvious pancreatic disease, i.e., pancreatic calcification, steatorrhea, or diabetes mellitus, than in patients with occult disease. Thus, the number of patients who have subclinical exocrine dysfunction (<90% loss of function) is unknown.

The clinical manifestations of acute and chronic pancreatitis and pancreatic insufficiency are protean. Thus, patients may present with hypertriglyceridemia, vitamin B_{12} malabsorption, hypercalcemia, hypocalcemia, hyperglycemia, ascites, pleural effusions, and chronic abdominal pain with normal blood amylase levels. Indeed, if the clinician considers pancreatitis as a possible diagnosis only when presented with a patient having classic symptoms (i.e., severe, constant epigastric pain that radiates through to the back, along with an elevated blood amylase level), only a minority of patients with pancreatitis will be diagnosed correctly.

As emphasized in Chap. 294, the etiologies as well as the clinical manifestations of pancreatitis are quite varied. Although it is well appreciated that pancreatitis is frequently secondary to alcohol abuse and biliary tract disease, it can also be caused by drugs, trauma, and viral infections and is associated with metabolic and connective tissue disorders. In approximately 30% of patients with acute pancreatitis and 25 to 40% of patients with chronic pancreatitis, the etiology is obscure.

TESTS USEFUL IN THE DIAGNOSIS OF PANCREATIC DISEASE

Several tests have proved of value in the evaluation of pancreatic exocrine function. Examples of specific tests and their usefulness in the diagnosis of acute and chronic pancreatitis are summarized in Table 293-1 and Fig. 293-1. At most institutions, pancreatic function tests are performed if the diagnosis of pancreatic disease remains a possibility after noninvasive tests [ultrasound, computed tomography (CT)] and invasive tests [endoscopic retrograde cholangiopancreatography (ERCP)] have given normal or inconclusive results. In this regard, tests employing *direct* stimulation of the pancreas are the most sensitive.

PANCREATIC ENZYMES IN BODY FLUIDS The serum amylase level is widely used as a screening test for acute pancreatitis in the patient with acute abdominal pain or back pain. A value >65 U/L should raise the question of acute pancreatitis. Levels >130 U/L make the diagnosis more likely, and values greater than three times normal virtually clinch the diagnosis if gut perforation or infarction is excluded. In acute pancreatitis, the serum amylase is usually elevated within 24 h of onset and remains so for 1 to 3 days. Levels return to normal within 3 to 5 days unless there is extensive pancreatic necrosis, incomplete ductal obstruction, or pseudocyst formation. Approximately 85% of patients with acute pancreatitis have an elevated serum amylase level. This index may be normal, however, if (1) there is a delay (of 2 to 5 days) before blood samples are obtained, (2) the underlying disorder is chronic pancreatitis rather than acute pancreatitis, or (3) hypertriglyceridemia is present. Patients with hypertriglyceridemia and proven pancreatitis have been found to have spuriously low levels of amylase and perhaps lipase activity.

The serum amylase is often elevated in other conditions (Table 293-2), in part because the enzyme is found in many organs in addition to the pancreas (salivary glands, liver, small intestine, kidney, fallopian tube) and can be produced by various tumors (carcinomas of the lung, esophagus, breast, and ovary). An assay of serum trypsinogen (performed by several commercial laboratories) is quite helpful in this regard. Since this enzyme is secreted specifically by the pancreas, a normal serum trypsinogen level in a patient with minimal elevation of serum amylase essentially rules out acute pancreatitis. Urinary amylase measurements, including the amylase/creatinine clearance ratio, are no more sensitive or specific than blood amylase levels.

Elevation of ascitic fluid amylase occurs in acute pancreatitis as well as in (1) pancreatogenous ascites due to disruption of the main pancreatic duct or a leaking pseudocyst and (2) other abdominal disorders that simulate pancreatitis (e.g., intestinal obstruction, intestinal infarction, and perforated peptic ulcer). Elevation of pleural fluid am-

TABLE 293-1 Tests Useful in the Diagnosis of Acute and Chronic Pancreatitis and Pancreatic Tumors

Test	Principle	Comment
PANCREATIC ENZYMES IN BODY FLUIDS		
Amylase		
1. Serum	Pancreatic inflammation leads to increased enzyme levels	Simple; 20–40% false negatives and positives; reliable if test results are three times the upper limit of normal
2. Urine	Renal clearance of amylase is increased in acute pancreatitis	May be abnormal when serum levels normal; false negatives and positives
3. Ascitic fluid	Disruption of gland or main pancreatic duct leads to increased amylase concentration	Can establish diagnosis of pancreatitis; false positives occur with intestinal obstruction and perforated ulcer
4. Pleural fluid	Exudative pleural effusion with pancreatitis	False positives occur with carcinoma of the lung and esophageal perforation
5. Isoenzymes	P isoamylases arise from the pancreas; S isoamylases are from other sources	More specific than total serum amylase in diagnosis of acute pancreatitis; useful in identifying nonpancreatic causes of hyperamylasemia
Serum lipase	Pancreatic inflammation leads to increased enzyme levels	New methods have greatly simplified determination; positive in 70–85% of cases
Serum trypsinogen	Pancreatic inflammation leads to increased levels	*Elevated* in acute pancreatitis; *decreased* in chronic pancreatitis *with* steatorrhea; normal in chronic pancreatitis *without* steatorrhea and in steatorrhea with normal pancreatic function
STUDIES PERTAINING TO PANCREATIC STRUCTURE		
Radiologic and radionuclide tests		
1. Plain film of the abdomen	Abnormal in acute and chronic pancreatitis	Simple; normal in >50% of cases of both acute and chronic pancreatitis
2. Upper gastrointestinal x-rays	Abnormally thickened duodenal folds; displacement of stomach or widening of duodenal loop suggests a pancreatic mass (inflammatory, neoplastic, cystic)	Simple; frequently normal; largely superseded by US and CT scanning
3. Ultrasonography (US)	Can provide information on edema, inflammation, calcification, pseudocysts, and mass lesions	Simple, noninvasive; sequential studies quite feasible; useful in diagnosis of pseudocyst
4. CT scan	Permits detailed visualization of pancreas and surrounding structures	Useful in the diagnosis of pancreatic calcification, dilated pancreatic ducts, and pancreatic tumors; may not be able to distinguish between inflammatory and neoplastic mass lesions
5. Selective angiography	Can identify pancreatic neoplasms (1) by sheathing of celiac or superior mesenteric branches by tumor or (2) by tumor staining; displacement of vessels by tumor	Indicated (1) in suspected islet cell tumors and (2) before pancreatic or duodenal resection; most reliable features reflect nonresectable pancreatic cancer
6. Endoscopic retrograde cholangiopancreatography (ERCP)	Cannulation of pancreatic and common bile duct permits visualization of pancreatic-biliary ductal system	Provides diagnostic data in 60–85% of cases; differentiation of chronic pancreatitis from pancreatic carcinoma may be difficult
7. Endoscopic ultrasonography (EUS)	High-frequency transducer employed with EUS can produce very high resolution images and depict changes in the pancreatic duct and parenchyma with better detail	Exact role of EUS versus ERCP and CT not yet fully defined; sensitivity and specificity under study
8. Magnetic resonance cholangiopancreatography	Three-dimensional rendering has been used to produce very good images of the pancreatic duct by a noninvasive technique	May be used to evaluate patients judged to be at high risk for ERCP, such as the elderly; may replace ERCP as a diagnostic test, although large controlled studies need to be done
Pancreatic biopsy with US or CT guidance	Percutaneous biopsy with skinny needle and localization of lesion by US	High diagnostic yield; laparotomy avoided; requires special technical skills
TESTS OF EXOCRINE PANCREATIC FUNCTION		
Direct stimulation of the pancreas with analysis of duodenal contents		
1. Secretin-pancreozymin (CCK) test	Secretin leads to increased output of pancreatic juice and HCO_3^-; CCK leads to increased output of pancreatic enzymes; pancreatic secretory response is related to the functional mass of pancreatic tissue	Sensitive enough to detect occult disease; involves duodenal intubation and fluoroscopy; poorly defined normal enzyme response; overlap in chronic pancreatitis; large secretory reserve capacity of the pancreas
Measurement of intraluminal digestion products		
1. Microscopic examination of stool for undigested meat fibers and fat	Lack of proteolytic and lipolytic enzymes causes decreased digestion of meat fibers and triglycerides	Simple, reliable; not sensitive enough to detect milder cases of pancreatic insufficiency
2. Quantitative stool fat determination	Lack of lipolytic enzymes brings about impaired fat digestion	Reliable, reference standard for defining severity of malabsorption; does not distinguish between maldigestion and malabsorption
3. Fecal nitrogen	Lack of proteolytic enzymes leads to impaired protein digestion, resulting in an increase in stool nitrogen	Does not distinguish between maldigestion and malabsorption; low sensitivity

(continued)

TABLE 293-2— *(Continued)*

Test	Principle	Comment
Measurement of pancreatic enzymes in feces		
1. Elastase	Pancreatic secretion of proteolytic enzymes	Excellent specificity; sensitivity similar to that of serum trypsinogen
Miscellaneous tests		
1. Dual-labeled Schilling test	Intrinsic factor [57Co]cobalamin and Hog R protein [58Co]cobalamin are given together. Since proteases are necessary to cleave R protein, the ratio of labeled cobalamin excreted in urine is an index of exocrine dysfunction.	Time-consuming and expensive

ylase occurs in acute pancreatitis, chronic pancreatitis, carcinoma of the lung, and esophageal perforation.

Lipase may now be the single best enzyme to measure for the diagnosis of acute pancreatitis. Improvements in substrates and technology offer clinicians improved options, especially when a turbidimetric assay is used. The newer lipase assays have colipase as a cofactor and are fully automated.

An assay for trypsinogen (or for trypsin-like immunoreactivity) has a theoretical advantage over amylase and lipase determinations in that the pancreas is the only organ that contains this enzyme. The test appears to be useful in the diagnosis of both acute and chronic pancreatitis. Sensitivity and specificity are comparable to those of amylase and lipase determinations. Since trypsinogen is also excreted by the kidney, elevated serum values are found in renal failure, as is the case with serum amylase and lipase levels. *No single blood test is reliable for the diagnosis of acute pancreatitis in patients with renal failure.* Determining whether a patient with renal failure and abdominal pain has pancreatitis remains a difficult clinical problem. A recent study found that serum amylase levels were elevated in patients with renal dysfunction only when creatinine clearance was <50 mL/min. In such patients, the serum amylase level was invariably <500 IU/L in the absence of objective evidence of acute pancreatitis. In that study, serum lipase and trypsin levels paralleled serum amylase values.

A recent study evaluated the sensitivity and specificity of five assays used to diagnose acute pancreatitis: two for amylase, one for lipase, one for trypsin-like immunoreactivity (TLI), and one for pancreatic isoamylase. The data obtained (1) show that, if the best cutoff level is used, all these assays have similar specificities and (2) suggest that total serum amylase is as good an indicator of acute pancreatitis as any of the alternatives. However, inherent in many such studies is

the problem that the recognition and diagnosis of acute pancreatitis hinge on the finding of an elevated serum amylase level. The question arises as to whether any diagnostic test result can be proved superior to the total serum amylase level if hyperamylasemia is required for the diagnosis. In other studies, when "objective" confirmation of the clinical diagnosis of pancreatitis was required (ultrasonography, CT, laparotomy), the sensitivity of the serum amylase has been found to be as low as 68%. With these limitations in mind, the recommended screening tests for acute pancreatitis are *total serum amylase* and *serum lipase activities.* Serum amylase values greater than three times normal are highly specific.

STUDIES PERTAINING TO PANCREATIC STRUCTURE ■ Radiologic Tests Plain films of the abdomen provide useful information in 30 to 50% of patients with acute pancreatitis. The most frequent abnormalities include (1) a localized ileus, usually involving the jejunum ("sentinel loop"); (2) a generalized ileus with air-fluid levels; (3) the "colon cutoff sign," which results from isolated distention of the transverse colon; (4) duodenal distention with air-fluid levels; and (5) a mass, which is frequently a pseudocyst. In chronic pancreatitis, an important radiographic finding is pancreatic calcification, which characteristically is localized adjacent to and superimposed on the second lumbar vertebra (Fig. 294-3A).

TABLE 293-2 *Causes of Hyperamylasemia and Hyperamylasuria*

PANCREATIC DISEASE

I. Pancreatitis	II. Pancreatic trauma
A. Acute	III. Pancreatic carcinoma
B. Chronic: ductal obstruction	
C. Complications of pancreatitis	
1. Pancreatic pseudocyst	
2. Pancreatogenous ascites	
3. Pancreatic abscess	
4. Pancreatic necrosis	

NONPANCREATIC DISORDERS

I. Renal insufficiency	IV. Macroamylasemia
II. Salivary gland lesions	V. Burns
A. Mumps	VI. Diabetic ketoacidosis
B. Calculus	VII. Pregnancy
C. Irradiation sialadenitis	VIII. Renal transplantation
D. Maxillofacial surgery	IX. Cerebral trauma
III. "Tumor" hyperamylasemia	X. Drugs: morphine
A. Carcinoma of the lung	
B. Carcinoma of the esophagus	
C. Breast carcinoma, ovarian carcinoma	

OTHER ABDOMINAL DISORDERS

I. Biliary tract disease: cholecystitis, choledocholithiasis
II. Intraabdominal disease
  A. Perforated or penetrating peptic ulcer
  B. Intestinal obstruction or infarction
  C. Ruptured ectopic pregnancy
  D. Peritonitis
  E. Aortic aneurysm
  F. Chronic liver disease
  G. Postoperative hyperamylasemia

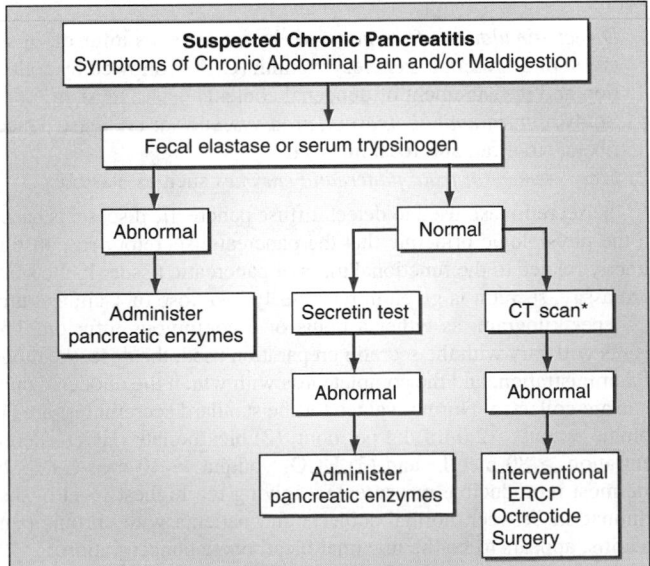

FIGURE 293-1 An approach to the patient with suspected chronic pancreatitis. EUS and MRCP are appropriate diagnostic alternatives.

Upper gastrointestinal x-rays may reveal displacement of the stomach by the retroperitoneal mass (Fig. 294-2*A*) or widening and effacement of the duodenal C loop, which also suggest the presence of a pancreatic mass, which could be inflammatory, cystic, or neoplastic. However, the use of x-ray films has been largely superseded by ultrasound.

Ultrasonography can provide important information in patients with acute pancreatitis, chronic pancreatitis, pancreatic calcification, pseudocyst, and pancreatic carcinoma. Echographic appearances can indicate the presence of edema, inflammation, and calcification (not obvious on plain films of the abdomen), as well as pseudocysts, mass lesions, and gallstones (Figs. 294-2*B* and 294-3*B*). In acute pancreatitis, the pancreas is characteristically enlarged. In pancreatic pseudocyst, the usual appearance is that of an echo-free, smooth, round fluid collection. Pancreatic carcinoma distorts the usual landmarks, and mass lesions >3.0 cm are usually detected as localized, echo-free solid lesions. Ultrasound is often the initial investigation for most patients with suspected pancreatic disease. However, obesity, excess small- and large-bowel gas, and recently performed barium contrast examinations can interfere with ultrasound studies.

CT is the best imaging study for initial evaluation of a suspected chronic pancreatic disorder and for the complications of acute and chronic pancreatitis. It is especially useful in the detection of pancreatic tumors, fluid-containing lesions such as pseudocysts and abscesses, and calcium deposits (Figs. 294-3*C* and 294-4*A*). Most lesions are characterized by (1) enlargement of the pancreatic outline, (2) distortion of the pancreatic contour, and/or (3) a fluid filling that has a different attenuation coefficient than normal pancreas. However, it is occasionally difficult to distinguish between inflammatory and neoplastic lesions. Oral water-soluble contrast agents may be used to opacify the stomach and duodenum during CT scans; this strategy permits more precise delineation of various organs as well as mass lesions. Dynamic CT (using rapid intravenous administration of contrast) is useful in estimating the degree of pancreatic necrosis and in predicting morbidity and mortality. Spiral (helical) CT provides clear images much more rapidly and essentially negates artifact caused by patient movement (Fig. 294-2*D*).

Endoscopic ultrasonography (EUS) produces high-resolution images of the pancreatic parenchyma and pancreatic duct with a transducer fixed to an endoscope that can be directed onto the surface of the pancreas through the stomach or duodenum. EUS is replacing ERCP for diagnostic purposes in many centers. EUS allows one to obtain information about the pancreatic duct as well as the parenchyma and has no complications associated with it, in contrast to the 5 to 20% of post-ERCP pancreatitis observed. EUS is also very good in detecting common bile duct stones. Pancreatic masses can be biopsied via EUS and one can deliver nerve blocks through EUS. Figures 294-2*A–C* show the value of EUS in demonstrating pancreatic calcification, pancreatic pseudocysts, and dilation of the main pancreatic duct. Although criteria for abnormalities on EUS in severe pancreatic disease have been developed, the true sensitivity and specificity of this procedure has yet to be determined. In particular, it is not clear whether EUS can detect early pancreatic disease before abnormalities appear on more conventional radiograph tests such as ultrasonography or CT. The exact role of EUS versus ERCP and CT has yet to be defined.

Magnetic resonance cholangiopancreatography (MRCP) is now being used to view both the bile duct and the pancreatic duct. Non-breath-holding and three-dimensional turbo spin-echo techniques are being utilized to produce superb MRCP images. The main pancreatic duct and common bile duct can be seen well, but there is still a question as to whether changes can be detected consistently in the secondary ducts. MRCP may be particularly useful to evaluate the pancreatic duct in high-risk patients such as the elderly because this is a noninvasive procedure.

Both EUS and MRCP may replace ERCP in some patients. As these techniques become more refined, they may well be the diagnostic

tests of choice to evaluate the pancreatic duct. ERCP is still needed to perform therapy of bile duct and pancreatic duct lesions.

Selective catheterization of the celiac and superior mesenteric arteries combined with superselective catheterization of others arteries, such as the hepatic, splenic, and gastroduodenal arteries, permits visualization of the pancreas and detection of pancreatic neoplasms and pseudocysts. Pancreatic neoplasms can be identified by the sheathing of blood vessels by a mass lesion (Fig. 294-1*D*). Hormone-producing pancreatic tumors are especially likely to exhibit increased vascularity and tumor staining. Angiographic abnormalities are noted in many patients with pancreatic carcinoma but are uncommon in patients without pancreatic disease. Angiography complements ultrasonography and ERCP in the study of patients with a suspected pancreatic lesion and may be carried out if ERCP is either unsuccessful or nondiagnostic.

ERCP may provide useful information on the status of the pancreatic ductal system and thus aid in the differential diagnosis of pancreatic disease (Figs. 294-1*C*, 294-3*D*, and 294-4*B*). Pancreatic carcinoma is characterized by stenosis or obstruction of either the pancreatic duct or the common bile duct; both ductal systems are often abnormal. In chronic pancreatitis, ERCP abnormalities include (1) luminal narrowing; (2) irregularities in the ductal system with stenosis, dilation, sacculation, and ectasia; and (3) blockage of the pancreatic duct by calcium deposits. The presence of ductal stenosis and irregularity can make it difficult to distinguish chronic pancreatitis from carcinoma. It is important to be aware that ERCP changes interpreted as indicating chronic pancreatitis actually may be due to the effects of aging on the pancreatic duct or to the fact that the procedure was performed within several weeks of an attack of acute pancreatitis. Although aging may cause impressive ductal alterations, it does not affect the results of pancreatic function tests (i.e., the secretin test). Elevated serum and/or urine amylase levels after ERCP have been reported in 25 to 75% of patients, but clinical pancreatitis is uncommon. If no lesion is found in the biliary and/or pancreatic ducts in a patient with repeated attacks of acute pancreatitis, manometric studies of the sphincter of Oddi may be indicated. Such studies, however, do increase the risk of post-ERCP/manometry acute pancreatitis. Such pancreatitis appears to be more common in patients with a nondilated pancreatic duct.

Pancreatic Biopsy with Radiologic Guidance Percutaneous aspiration biopsy of a pancreatic mass often distinguishes a pancreatic inflammatory mass from a pancreatic neoplasm.

TESTS OF EXOCRINE PANCREATIC FUNCTION

Pancreatic function tests (Table 293-1) can be divided into the following:

1. *Direct stimulation of the pancreas* by intravenous infusion of secretin or secretin plus cholecystokinin (CCK) followed by collection and measurement of duodenal contents
2. Study of *intraluminal digestion products*, such as undigested meat fibers, stool fat, and fecal nitrogen
3. *Measurement of fecal pancreatic enzymes* such as elastase

The secretin test, used to detect diffuse pancreatic disease, is based on the physiologic principle that the pancreatic secretory response is directly related to the functional mass of pancreatic tissue. In the standard assay, secretin is given intravenously in a dose of 1 clinical unit (CU) per kilogram, as either a bolus or a continuous infusion. The results will vary with the secretin preparation used, the dose, the mode of administration, and the completeness with which the duodenal contents are collected. Normal values for the standard secretin test are (1) volume output > 2.0 mL/kg per hour, (2) bicarbonate (HCO_3^-) concentration > 80 meq/L, and (3) HCO_3^- output > 10 meq/L in 1 h. The most reproducible measurement, giving the highest level of discrimination between normal subjects and patients with chronic pancreatitis, appears to be the maximal bicarbonate concentration.

The *combined secretin-CCK test* permits measurement of pancreatic amylase, lipase, trypsin, and chymotrypsin. Although there is overlap in the distributions of enzyme output in normal subjects and patients with pancreatitis in response to this test, markedly low enzyme outputs suggest advanced damage and destruction of acinar cells. With frank exocrine pancreatic insufficiency, there is usually an overall reduction in both HCO_3 concentration and output of several enzymes. However, with lesser degrees of pancreatic damage there may be a dissociation between HCO_3^- concentration and enzyme output. There may also be a dissociation between the results of the secretin test and those of tests of absorptive function. For example, patients with chronic pancreatitis often have abnormally low outputs of HCO_3^- after secretin but have normal fecal fat excretion. Thus the secretin test measures the secretory capacity of ductular epithelium, while fecal fat excretion indirectly reflects intraluminal lipolytic activity. Steatorrhea does not occur until intraluminal levels of lipase are markedly reduced, underscoring the fact that only small amounts of enzymes are necessary for intraluminal digestive activities. An abnormal secretin test result suggests only that chronic pancreatic damage is present; it will not consistently distinguish between chronic pancreatitis and pancreatic carcinoma.

Another test of exocrine pancreatic function is the *bentiromide test*.

This test is an indirect measure of pancreatic function and reflects intraluminal chymotrypsin activity. The test has excellent specificity but is not very sensitive. It no longer is available for clinical use in the United States.

The *serum trypsinogen level*, which is determined by radioimmunoassay, also has excellent specificity but is not very sensitive. It is a simple blood test that can detect severe damage to the exocrine pancreas. The normal values are 28 to 58 ng/mL, and any value <20 ng/mL reflects pancreatic steatorrhea.

Measurement of *intraluminal digestion products*, i.e., undigested muscle fibers, stool fat, and fecal nitrogen, is discussed in Chap. 275. The amount of elastase in stool reflects the pancreatic output of this proteolytic enzyme. Decreased elastase activity in stool has been reported in patients with chronic pancreatitis and cystic fibrosis. →*Tests useful in the diagnosis of exocrine pancreatic insufficiency and the differential diagnosis of malabsorption are also discussed in Chaps. 275 and 294.*

294 | ACUTE AND CHRONIC PANCREATITIS
Norton J. Greenberger, Phillip P. Toskes

BIOCHEMISTRY AND PHYSIOLOGY OF PANCREATIC EXOCRINE SECRETION

GENERAL CONSIDERATIONS The pancreas secretes 1500 to 3000 mL of isosmotic alkaline (pH > 8.0) fluid per day containing about 20 enzymes and zymogens. The pancreatic secretions provide the enzymes needed to effect the major digestive activity of the gastrointestinal tract and provide an optimal pH for the function of these enzymes.

REGULATION OF PANCREATIC SECRETION The exocrine pancreas is influenced by intimately interacting hormonal and neural systems. *Gastric acid* is the stimulus for the release of secretin, which stimulates the secretion of pancreatic juice rich in water and electrolytes. Release of cholecystokinin (CCK) from the duodenum and jejunum is largely triggered by long-chain fatty acids, certain essential amino acids (tryptophan, phenylalanine, valine, methionine), and gastric acid itself. CCK evokes an enzyme-rich secretion from the pancreas. The *parasympathetic nervous system* (via the vagus nerve) exerts significant control over pancreatic secretion. Secretion evoked by secretin and CCK depends on permissive roles of vagal afferent and efferent pathways. This is particularly true for enzyme secretion, whereas water and bicarbonate secretion is heavily dependent on the hormonal effects of secretin and CCK. Also, vagal stimulation effects the release of vasoactive intestinal peptide (VIP), a secretin agonist. Bile salts also stimulate pancreatic secretion, thereby integrating the functions of the biliary tract, pancreas, and small intestine.

Pancreatic exocrine secretion is influenced by inhibitory neuropeptides such as somatostatin, pancreatic polypeptide, peptide YY, neuropeptide Y, enkephalin, pancreastatin, calcitonin gene–related peptides, glucagon, and galanin. Although pancreatic polypeptide and peptide YY may act primarily on nerves outside the pancreas, somatostatin acts at multiple sites. Nitric oxide is also an important neurotransmitter. The mechanism of action of these various factors has not been fully defined.

WATER AND ELECTROLYTE SECRETION Bicarbonate is the ion of primary physiologic importance within pancreatic secretion. The ductal cells secrete bicarbonate predominantly derived from plasma (93%) rather than intracellular metabolism (7%). Bicarbonate enters through the sodium bicarbonate co-transporter with depolarization caused by chloride efflux through the cystic fibrosis transductance regulator (CFTR). Secretin and VIP, both of which increase intracellular cyclic AMP, act on the ductal cells opening the CFTR in promoting secretion. CCK, acting as a neuromodulator, markedly potentiates the stimulatory effects of secretin. Acetylcholine also plays an important role in ductal cell secretion. Bicarbonate helps neutralize gastric acid and creates the appropriate pH for the activity of pancreatic enzymes.

ENZYME SECRETION The acinar cell is highly compartmentalized and is concerned with the secretion of pancreatic enzymes. Proteins synthesized by the rough endoplasmic reticulum are processed in the Golgi and then targeted to the appropriate site, whether that be zymogen granules, lysosomes, or other cell compartments. The pancreas secretes amylolytic, lipolytic, and proteolytic enzymes. *Amylolytic enzymes*, such as amylase, hydrolyze starch to oligosaccharides and to the disaccharide maltose. The *lipolytic enzymes* include lipase, phospholipase A, and cholesterol esterase. Bile salts inhibit lipase in isolation; but colipase, another constituent of pancreatic secretion, binds to lipase and prevents this inhibition. Bile salts activate phospholipase A and cholesterol esterase. *Proteolytic enzymes* include endopeptidases (trypsin, chymotrypsin), which act on internal peptide bonds of proteins and polypeptides; exopeptidases (carboxypeptidases, aminopeptidases), which act on the free carboxyl- and amino-terminal ends of peptides, respectively; and elastase. The proteolytic enzymes are secreted as inactive precursors (zymogens). Ribonucleases (deoxyribonucleases, ribonuclease) are also secreted. *Enterokinase*, an enzyme found in the duodenal mucosa, cleaves the lysine-isoleucine bond of trypsinogen to form trypsin. Trypsin then activates the other proteolytic zymogens in a cascade phenomenon. All pancreatic enzymes have pH optima in the alkaline range. The nervous system initiates pancreatic enzyme secretion. The neurologic stimulation is cholinergic, involving extrinsic innervation by the vagus nerve and subsequent innervation by intrapancreatic cholinergic nerves. The stimulatory neurotransmitters are acetylcholine and gastrin-releasing peptides. These neurotransmitters activate calcium-dependent second messenger systems resulting in the release of zymogen granules. VIP is present in intrapancreatic nerves and potentiates the effect of acetylcholine. In contrast to other species, there are no CCK receptors on acinar cells in humans. CCK in physiologic concentrations stimulates pancreatic secretion by stimulating central vagal and intrapancreatic nerves.

AUTOPROTECTION OF THE PANCREAS Autodigestion of the pancreas is prevented by the packaging of proteases in precursor form and by the synthesis of protease inhibitors. These protease inhibitors are found in the acinar cell, the pancreatic secretions, and the α_1- and α_2-globulin fractions of plasma.

EXOCRINE-ENDOCRINE RELATIONSHIPS Insulin appears to be needed locally for secretin and CCK to promote exocrine secretion; thus, it acts in a permissive role for these two hormones.

ENTEROPANCREATIC AXIS AND FEEDBACK INHIBITION   Pancreatic enzyme secretion is controlled, at least in part, by a negative feedback mechanism induced by the presence of active serine proteases in the duodenum. To illustrate, perfusion of the duodenal lumen with phenylalanine causes a prompt increase in plasma CCK levels as well as increased secretion of chymotrypsin. However, simultaneous perfusion with trypsin blunts both responses. Conversely, perfusion of the duodenal lumen with protease inhibitors actually leads to enzyme hypersecretion. The available evidence supports the concept that the duodenum contains a peptide called *CCK-releasing factor* (CCK-RF) that is involved in stimulating CCK release. It appears that serine proteases inhibit pancreatic secretion by acting on a CCK-releasing peptide in the lumen of the small intestine. Thus the integrative result of both bicarbonate and enzyme secretion depends on a feedback process for both bicarbonate and pancreatic enzymes. Acidification of the duodenum releases secretin, which stimulates vagal-vagal and other neural pathways to activate pancreatic duct cells, which secrete bicarbonate. This bicarbonate then neutralizes the duodenal acid, and the feedback loop is completed. Duodenal proteins lead to a reduction in free proteases, thereby leading to an increase in free CCK-RF. CCK-RF is then released into the blood in physiologic concentrations, acting primarily through the neural pathways (vagal-vagal). This leads to acetylcholine-mediated pancreatic enzyme secretion. Proteases continue to be secreted from the pancreas until the protein within the duodenum and CCK-RF are digested. At this point, the free duodenal proteases rise again, thus completing this step in the feedback process.

ACUTE PANCREATITIS

GENERAL CONSIDERATIONS   Pancreatic inflammatory disease may be classified as (1) acute pancreatitis and (2) chronic pancreatitis. The pathologic spectrum of acute pancreatitis varies from *edematous pancreatitis*, which is usually a mild and self-limited disorder, to *necrotizing pancreatitis*, in which the degree of pancreatic necrosis correlates with the severity of the attack and its systemic manifestations. The term *hemorrhagic pancreatitis* is less meaningful in a clinical sense because variable amounts of interstitial hemorrhage can be found in pancreatitis as well as in other disorders such as pancreatic trauma, pancreatic carcinoma, and severe congestive heart failure.

The incidence of pancreatitis varies in different countries and depends on cause, e.g., alcohol, gallstones, metabolic factors, and drugs (Table 294-1). The estimated incidence in England is 5.4/100,000 per year; in the United States it is 79.8/100,000 per year, thus resulting in 185,000 new cases of acute pancreatitis annually.

ETIOLOGY AND PATHOGENESIS   There are many causes of acute pancreatitis (Table 294-1), but the mechanisms by which these conditions trigger pancreatic inflammation have not been identified. Gallstones continue to be the leading cause of acute pancreatitis in most series (30 to 60%). Alcohol is the second most common cause, responsible for 15 to 30% of cases in the United States. The incidence of pancreatitis in alcoholics is surprisingly low (5/100,000), indicating that in addition to the amount of alcohol ingested unknown factors affect a person's susceptibility to pancreatic injury. The mechanism of injury is not well understood. Hypertriglyceridemia is the cause of acute pancreatitis in 1.3 to 3.8% of cases; serum triglyceride levels are usually >11.3 mmol/L (>1000 mg/dL). Most patients with hypertriglyceridemia, when subsequently examined, show evidence of an underlying derangement in lipid metabolism, probably unrelated to pancreatitis. Patients with diabetes mellitus or who are on certain medications may also develop high triglyceride levels. Acute pancreatitis occurs in 5 to 20% of patients following endoscopic retrograde cholangiopancreatography (ERCP). Approximately 2 to 5% of cases of acute pancreatitis are drug-related. Drugs cause pancreatitis either by a hypersensitivity reaction or by the generation of a toxic metabolite, although in some cases it is not clear which of these mechanisms is operative. (Table 294-1).

TABLE 294-1   Causes of Acute Pancreatitis

Common Causes
- Gallstones (including microlithiasis)
- Alcohol (acute and chronic alcoholism)
- Hypertriglyceridemia
- Endoscopic retrograde cholangiopancreatography (ERCP), especially after biliary manometry
- Trauma (especially blunt abdominal trauma)
- Postoperative (abdominal and nonabdominal operations)
- Drugs (azathioprine, 6-mercaptopurine, sulfonamides, estrogens, tetracycline, valproic acid, anti-HIV medications)
- Sphincter of Oddi dysfunction

Uncommon causes
- Vascular causes and vasculitis (ischemic-hypoperfusion states after cardiac surgery)
- Connective tissue disorders and thrombotic thrombocytopenic purpura (TTP)
- Cancer of the pancreas
- Hypercalcemia
- Periampullary diverticulum
- Pancreas divisum
- Hereditary pancreatitis
- Cystic fibrosis
- Renal failure

Rare causes
- Infections (mumps, coxsackievirus, cytomegalovirus, echovirus, parasites)
- Autoimmune (e.g., Sjögren's syndrome)

Causes to consider in patients with recurrent bouts of acute pancreatitis without an obvious etiology
- Occult disease of the biliary tree or pancreatic ducts, especially microlithiasis, sludge
- Drugs
- Hypertriglyceridemia
- Pancreas divisum
- Pancreatic cancer
- Sphincter of Oddi dysfunction
- Cystic fibrosis
- Idiopathic

Autodigestion is one pathogenic theory, according to which pancreatitis results when proteolytic enzymes (e.g., trypsinogen, chymotrypsinogen, proelastase, and phospholipase A) are activated in the pancreas rather than in the intestinal lumen. A number of factors (e.g., endotoxins, exotoxins, viral infections, ischemia, anoxia, and direct trauma) are believed to activate these proenzymes. Activated proteolytic enzymes, especially trypsin, not only digest pancreatic and peripancreatic tissues but also can activate other enzymes, such as elastase and phospholipase.

Activation of Pancreatic Enzymes in the Pathogenesis of Acute Pancreatitis   Several recent studies have suggested that pancreatitis is a disease that evolves in three phases. The initial phase is characterized by intrapancreatic digestive enzyme activation and acinar cell injury. Zymogen activation appears to be mediated by lysosomal hydrolases such as cathepsin B which become co-localized with digestive enzymes in intracellular organelles; it is currently believed that acinar cell injury is the consequence of zymogen activation. The second phase of pancreatitis involves the activation, chemoattraction, and sequestration of neutrophils in the pancreas resulting in an intrapancreatic inflammatory reaction of variable severity. Neutrophil depletion induced by prior administration of an antineutrophil serum has been shown to reduce the severity of experimentally induced pancreatitis. There is also evidence to support the concept that neutrophil sequestration can activate trypsinogen. Thus, intrapancreatic acinar cell activation of trypsinogen could be a two-step process, i.e., with a neutrophil-independent and a neutrophil-dependent phase. The third phase of pancreatitis is due to the effects of activated proteolytic enzymes and mediators, released by the inflamed pancreas, on distant organs. Activated proteolytic enzymes, especially trypsin, not only digest pancreatic and peripancreatic tissues but also activate other enzymes such as elastase and phospholipase. The active enzymes then digest cellular membranes and cause proteolysis, edema, interstitial hemorrhage, vascular damage, coagulation necrosis, fat necrosis, and parenchymal cell necrosis. Cellular injury and death result in the liberation of bradykinin peptides, vasoactive substances, and histamine that can produce vasodilation, increased vascular permeability, and edema with profound effects on many organs, most notably the lung. The systemic inflammatory response syndrome (SIRS) and acute respiratory distress syndrome (ARDS) as well as multiorgan failure may occur as result of this cascade of local as well as distant effects.

CLINICAL FEATURES *Abdominal pain* is the major symptom of acute pancreatitis. Pain may vary from a mild and tolerable discomfort to severe, constant, and incapacitating distress. Characteristically, the pain, which is steady and boring in character, is located in the epigastrium and periumbilical region and often radiates to the back as well as to the chest, flanks, and lower abdomen. The pain is frequently more intense when the patient is supine, and patients often obtain relief by sitting with the trunk flexed and knees drawn up. Nausea, vomiting, and abdominal distention due to gastric and intestinal hypomotility and chemical peritonitis are also frequent complaints.

Physical examination frequently reveals a distressed and anxious patient. Low-grade fever, tachycardia, and hypotension are fairly common. Shock is not unusual and may result from (1) hypovolemia secondary to exudation of blood and plasma proteins into the retroperitoneal space (a "retroperitoneal burn"); (2) increased formation and release of kinin peptides, which cause vasodilation and increased vascular permeability; and (3) systemic effects of proteolytic and lipolytic enzymes released into the circulation. Jaundice occurs infrequently; when present, it usually is due to edema of the head of the pancreas with compression of the intrapancreatic portion of the common bile duct. Erythematous skin nodules due to subcutaneous fat necrosis may occur. In 10 to 20% of patients, there are pulmonary findings, including basilar rales, atelectasis, and pleural effusion, the latter most frequently left-sided. Abdominal tenderness and muscle rigidity are present to a variable degree, but, compared with the intense pain, these signs may be unimpressive. Bowel sounds are usually diminished or absent. A pancreatic pseudocyst may be palpable in the upper abdomen. A faint blue discoloration around the umbilicus (Cullen's sign) may occur as the result of hemoperitoneum, and a blue-red-purple or green-brown discoloration of the flanks (Turner's sign) reflects tissue catabolism of hemoglobin. The latter two findings, which are uncommon, indicate the presence of a severe necrotizing pancreatitis.

LABORATORY DATA The diagnosis of acute pancreatitis is usually established by the detection of an increased level of serum amylase. Values threefold or more above normal virtually clinch the diagnosis if overt salivary gland disease and gut perforation or infarction are excluded. However, there appears to be no definite correlation between the severity of pancreatitis and the degree of serum amylase elevation. After 48 to 72 h, even with continuing evidence of pancreatitis, total serum amylase values tend to return to normal. However, pancreatic isoamylase and lipase levels may remain elevated for 7 to 14 days. It will be recalled that amylase elevations in serum and urine occur in many conditions other than pancreatitis (Table 293-2). Importantly, patients with *acidemia* (arterial pH ≤ 7.32) may have spurious elevations in serum amylase. In one study, 12 of 33 patients with acidemia had elevated serum amylase, but only 1 had an elevated lipase value; in 9, salivary-type amylase was the predominant serum isoamylase. This finding explains why patients with diabetic ketoacidosis may have marked elevations in serum amylase without any other evidence of acute pancreatitis. Serum lipase activity increases in parallel with amylase activity, and measurement of both enzymes increases the diagnostic yield. An elevated serum lipase or trypsin value is usually diagnostic of acute pancreatitis; these tests are especially helpful in patients with nonpancreatic causes of hyperamylasemia (Table 293-2). Markedly increased levels of peritoneal or pleural fluid amylase [>1500 nmol/L (>5000 U/dL)] are also helpful, if present, in establishing the diagnosis.

Leukocytosis (15,000 to 20,000 leukocytes μL) occurs frequently.

Patients with more severe disease may show hemoconcentration with hematocrit values exceeding 50% because of loss of plasma into the retroperitoneal space and peritoneal cavity. *Hyperglycemia* is common and is due to multiple factors, including decreased insulin release, increased glucagon release, and an increased output of adrenal glucocorticoids and catecholamines. *Hypocalcemia* occurs in approximately 25% of patients, and its pathogenesis is incompletely understood. Although earlier studies suggested that the response of the parathyroid gland to a decrease in serum calcium is impaired, subsequent observations have failed to confirm this idea. Intraperitoneal saponification of calcium by fatty acids in areas of fat necrosis occurs occasionally, with large amounts (up to 6.0 g) dissolved or suspended in ascitic fluid. Such "soap formation" may also be significant in patients with pancreatitis, mild hypocalcemia, and little or no obvious ascites. *Hyperbilirubinemia* [serum bilirubin > 68 μmol/L (>4.0 mg/dL)] occurs in approximately 10% of patients. However, jaundice is transient, and serum bilirubin levels return to normal in 4 to 7 days. Serum alkaline phosphatase and aspartate aminotransferase (AST) levels are also transiently elevated and parallel serum bilirubin values. Markedly elevated serum lactic dehydrogenase (LDH) levels [>8.5 μmol/L (>500 U/dL)] suggest a poor prognosis. Serum albumin is decreased to ≤30 g/L (≤3.0 g/dL) in about 10% of patients; this sign is associated with more severe pancreatitis and a higher mortality rate (Table 294-2). *Hypertriglyceridemia* occurs in 15 to 20% of patients, and serum amylase levels in these individuals are often spuriously normal (Chap. 293). Approximately 25% of patients have *hypoxemia* (arterial P_{O_2} ≤ 60 mmHg), which may herald the onset of ARDS. Finally, the electrocardiogram is occasionally abnormal in acute pancreatitis with ST-segment and T-wave abnormalities simulating myocardial ischemia.

Although one or more radiologic abnormalities are found in >50% of patients, the findings are inconstant and nonspecific. The chief value of conventional x-rays [chest films; kidney, ureter, and bladder (KUB) studies] in acute pancreatitis is to help exclude other diagnoses, especially a perforated viscus. Upper gastrointestinal tract x-rays have been superseded by ultrasonography and computed tomography (CT). A CT scan may confirm the clinical impression of acute pancreatitis even in the face of normal serum amylase levels. Importantly, CT is quite helpful in indicating the severity of acute pancreatitis and the risk of morbidity and mortality (see below). Sonography and radionuclide scanning [N-p-isopropylacetanilide-iminodiacetic acid (PIPIDA) scan; hepatic 2,6-dimethyliminodiacetic acid (HIDA) scan] are useful in acute pancreatitis to evaluate the gallbladder and biliary tree. →*Radiologic studies useful in the diagnosis of acute pancreatitis are discussed in Chap. 293 and listed in Table 293-1.*

DIAGNOSIS Any severe acute pain in the abdomen or back should suggest acute pancreatitis. The diagnosis is usually entertained when a patient with a possible predisposition to pancreatitis presents with se-

---

TABLE 294-2 Risk Factors That Adversely Affect Survival in Acute Pancreatitis

1. Organ failure[a]
   a. Cardiovascular: hypotension (systolic blood pressure < 90 mmHg) or tachycardia > 130 beats/min
   b. Pulmonary: P_{O_2} < 60 mmHg
   c. Renal: oliguria (<50 mL/h) or increasing BUN or creatinine
   d. Gastrointestinal bleeding
2. Pancreatic necrosis[a] (see Table 294-4)
3. Obesity[a] (BMI > 29); age > 70
4. Hemoconcentration[a] (hematocrit > 44%)
5. C-Reactive protein > 150 mg/L
6. Trypsinogen activation peptide
   a. >3 Ranson criteria (not fully utilizable until 48 h)[b]
   b. Apache II score > 8 (cumbersome)[b]

[a] Most useful.
[b] Often cited, but less useful.

Note: BUN, blood urea nitrogen; BMI, body mass index.

vere and constant abdominal pain, nausea, emesis, fever, tachycardia, and abnormal findings on abdominal examination. Laboratory studies frequently reveal leukocytosis, an abnormal appearance on x-rays of the abdomen and chest, hypocalcemia, and hyperglycemia. The diagnosis is usually confirmed by the finding of an elevated level of serum amylase and/or lipase. Not all the above features have to be present for the diagnosis to be established.

The *differential diagnosis* should include the following disorders: (1) perforated viscus, especially peptic ulcer; (2) acute cholecystitis and biliary colic; (3) acute intestinal obstruction; (4) mesenteric vascular occlusion; (5) renal colic; (6) myocardial infarction; (7) dissecting aortic aneurysm; (8) connective tissue disorders with vasculitis; (9) pneumonia; and (10) diabetic ketoacidosis. A penetrating duodenal ulcer can usually be identified by upper gastrointestinal x-rays and/or endoscopy. A perforated duodenal ulcer is readily diagnosed by the presence of free intraperitoneal air. It may be difficult to differentiate acute cholecystitis from acute pancreatitis, since an elevated serum amylase may be found in both disorders. Pain of biliary tract origin is more right-sided and gradual in onset, and ileus is usually absent; sonography and radionuclide scanning are helpful in establishing the diagnosis of cholelithiasis and cholecystitis. Intestinal obstruction due to mechanical factors can be differentiated from pancreatitis by the history of colicky pain, findings on abdominal examination, and x-rays of the abdomen showing changes characteristic of mechanical obstruction. Acute mesenteric vascular occlusion is usually evident in elderly debilitated patients with brisk leukocytosis, abdominal distention, and bloody diarrhea, in whom paracentesis shows sanguineous fluid and arteriography shows vascular occlusion. Serum as well as peritoneal fluid amylase levels are increased, however, in patients with intestinal infarction. Systemic lupus erythematosus and polyarteritis nodosa may be confused with pancreatitis, especially since pancreatitis may develop as a complication of these diseases. Diabetic ketoacidosis is often accompanied by abdominal pain and elevated total serum amylase levels, thus closely mimicking acute pancreatitis. However, the serum lipase and pancreatic isoamylase levels are not elevated in diabetic ketoacidosis.

COURSE OF THE DISEASE AND COMPLICATIONS It is important to identify patients with acute pancreatitis who have an increased risk of dying. Multiple factor scoring systems (Ranson, Imrie, Apache II) are difficult to use, show poor predictive powers, and have not been uniformly embraced by clinicians. The key indicators of a severe attack of pancreatitis are listed in Table 294-2 and include age > 70 years, body mass index (BMI) > 30, hematocrit > 44%, admission C-reactive protein > 150 mg/L, and elevated levels of urine trypsinogen activation peptide (TAP). However, it is organ failure, in which respiratory failure (P_{O_2} < 60 mmHg) dominates, that determines outcome in the majority of difficult to manage cases. The presence of shock (systolic blood pressure < 90 mmHg or tachycardia > 130), renal failure [serum creatinine > 177 μmol/L (>2.0 mg/dL)], and gastrointestinal bleeding (>500 mL/24 h) are also key factors. The high mortality rate of such severely ill patients is due in large part to infection and warrants intensive radiologic intervention and monitoring and/or a combination of radiologic and surgical means, as discussed in detail below.

The local and systemic complications of acute pancreatitis are listed in Table 294-3. In the first 2 to 3 weeks after pancreatitis patients frequently develop an inflammatory mass, which may be due to pancreatic necrosis (with or without infection) or may represent an abscess or pseudocyst (see below). Systemic complications include pulmonary, cardiovascular, hematologic, renal, metabolic, and central nervous system abnormalities. Pancreatitis and hypertriglyceridemia constitute an association in which cause and effect remain incompletely understood. However, several reasonable conclusions can be drawn. First, hypertriglyceridemia can precede and apparently cause pancreatitis. Second, the vast majority (>80%) of patients with acute pancreatitis do not have hypertriglyceridemia. Third, almost all patients

with pancreatitis and hypertriglyceridemia have preexisting abnormalities in lipoprotein metabolism. Fourth, many of the patients with this association have persistent hypertriglyceridemia after recovery from pancreatitis and are prone to recurrent episodes of pancreatitis. Fifth, any factor (e.g., drugs or alcohol) that causes an abrupt increase in serum triglycerides to levels >11 mmol/L (1000 mg/dL) can precipitate a bout of pancreatitis that can be associated with significant complications and even become fulminant. To avert the risk of triggering pancreatitis, a fasting serum triglyceride measurement should be obtained before estrogen replacement therapy is begun in postmenopausal women. Fasting levels < 3.4 mmol/L (300 mg/dL) pose no risk, whereas levels >8.5 mmol/L (750 mg/dL) are associated with a high probability of developing pancreatitis. Finally, patients with a deficiency of apolipoprotein CII have an increased incidence of pancreatitis; apolipoprotein CII activates lipoprotein lipase, which is important in clearing chylomicrons from the bloodstream.

Purtscher's retinopathy, a relatively unusual complication, is manifested by a sudden and severe loss of vision in a patient with acute pancreatitis. It is characterized by a peculiar funduscopic appearance with cotton-wool spots and hemorrhages confined to an area limited by the optic disk and macula; it is believed to be due to occlusion of the posterior retinal artery with aggregated granulocytes.

The two most common causes of acute pancreatitis are biliary tract disease and alcoholism; other causes are listed in Table 294-1. The risk of acute pancreatitis in patients with at least one gallstone <5 mm in diameter is fourfold greater than that in patients with larger stones. However, after a conventional workup, a specific cause is not identified

---

TABLE 294-3 *Complications of Acute Pancreatitis*

LOCAL

Necrosis	Pancreatic ascites
Sterile	Disruption of main pancreatic
Infected	duct
Pancreatic fluid collections	Leaking pseudocyst
Pancreatic abscess	Involvement of contiguous
Pancreatic pseudocyst	organs by necrotizing
Pain	pancreatitis
Rupture	Massive intraperitoneal
Hemorrhage	hemorrhage
Infection	Thrombosis of blood vessels
Obstruction of gastrointestinal	(splenic vein, portal vein)
tract (stomach, duodenum,	Bowel infarction
colon)	Obstructive jaundice

SYSTEMIC

Pulmonary	Renal
Pleural effusion	Oliguria
Atelectasis	Azotemia
Mediastinal abscess	Renal artery and/or renal vein
Pneumonitis	thrombosis
Adult respiratory distress	Acute tubular necrosis
syndrome	Metabolic
Cardiovascular	Hyperglycemia
Hypotension	Hypertriglyceridemia
Hypovolemia	Hypocalcemia
Sudden death	Encephalopathy
Nonspecific ST-T changes in	Sudden blindness (Purtscher's
electrocardiogram simulating	retinopathy)
myocardial infarction	Central nervous system
Pericardial effusion	Psychosis
Hematologic	Fat emboli
Disseminated intravascular	Fat necrosis
coagulation	Subcutaneous tissues
Gastrointestinal hemorrhage[a]	(erythematous nodules)
Peptic ulcer disease	Bone
Erosive gastritis	Miscellaneous (mediastinum,
Hemorrhagic pancreatic necrosis	pleura, nervous system)
with erosion into major blood	
vessels	
Portal vein thrombosis, variceal	
hemorrhage	

[a] Aggravated by coagulation abnormalities (disseminated intravascular coagulation).

in about 30% of patients. It is important to note that ultrasound examinations fail to detect gallstones, especially microlithiasis and/or sludge, in 4 to 7% of patients. In one series of 31 patients diagnosed initially as having idiopathic acute pancreatitis, 23 were found to have occult gallstone disease. Thus, approximately two-thirds of patients with recurrent acute pancreatitis without an obvious cause actually have occult gallstone disease due to microlithiasis. Examination of duodenal aspirates in such cases often reveals cholesterol crystals, which confirm the diagnosis. Other diseases of the biliary tree and pancreatic ducts that can cause acute pancreatitis include choledochocele; ampullary tumors; pancreas divisum; and pancreatic duct stones, stricture, and tumor. Approximately 2 to 4% of patients with pancreatic carcinoma present with acute pancreatitis.

Recurrent Pancreatitis Approximately 25% of patients who have had an attack of acute pancreatitis have a recurrence. The two most common etiologic factors are alcohol and cholelithiasis. In patients with recurrent pancreatitis without an obvious cause the differential diagnosis should encompass occult biliary tract disease including microlithiasis, hypertriglyceridemia, drugs, pancreatic cancer, sphincter of Oddi dysfunction, pancreas divisum, cystic fibrosis, and pancreatic cancer (Table 294-1).

Pancreatitis in Patients with AIDS The incidence of acute pancreatitis is increased in patients with AIDS for two reasons: (1) the high incidence of infections involving the pancreas, such as infections with cytomegalovirus, *Cryptosporidium*, and the *Mycobacterium avium* complex; and (2) the frequent use by patients with AIDS of medications such as didanosine, pentamidine, and trimethoprim-sulfamethoxazole (Chap. 173).

℞ TREATMENT

In most patients (approximately 85 to 90%) with acute pancreatitis, the disease is self-limited and subsides spontaneously, usually within 3 to 7 days after treatment is instituted. Conventional measures include (1) analgesics for pain, (2) intravenous fluids and colloids to maintain normal intravascular volume, (3) no oral alimentation, and (4) nasogastric suction to decrease gastrin release from the stomach and prevent gastric contents from entering the duodenum. Recent controlled trials, however, have shown that nasogastric suction offers no clear-cut advantages in the treatment of mild to moderately severe acute pancreatitis. Its use, therefore, must be considered elective rather than mandatory.

It has been demonstrated that CCK-stimulated pancreatic secretion is almost abolished in four different experimental models of acute pancreatitis. This finding probably explains why drugs to block pancreatic secretion in acute pancreatitis have failed to have any therapeutic benefit. For this and other reasons, anticholinergic drugs are not indicated in acute pancreatitis. In addition to nasogastric suction and anticholinergic drugs, other therapies designed to "rest the pancreas" by inhibiting pancreatic secretion have not changed the course of the disease. Although antibiotics have been used in the treatment of acute pancreatitis, randomized, prospective trials have shown no benefit from their use in acute pancreatitis of mild to moderate severity.

However, current evidence favors the use of prophylactic antibiotics in necrotizing acute pancreatitis. A recent meta-analysis of controlled trials comparing antibiotic prophylaxis with no prophylaxis in patients with acute necrotizing pancreatitis showed significant reduction in sepsis by 21% [number needed to treat (NNT) = 5] and mortality by 12% (NNT = 8). Early antibiotic prophylaxis in patients with documented pancreatic necrosis is recommended; however, the optimal drug(s) and duration of therapy remain incompletely defined. The current recommendation is the use of a systemic antibiotic such as imipenem-cilastatin, 500 mg thrice daily for 2 weeks. In addition, because secondary infection of necrotic pancreatic tissue (abscess, pseudocyst or obstructed biliary passages, ascending cholangitis complicating choledocholithiasis) contributes to many of the late deaths from pancreatitis, appropriate antibiotic therapy of established infections is quite important.

Several other drugs have been evaluated by prospective controlled trials and found ineffective in the treatment of acute pancreatitis. The list, by no means complete, includes glucagon, H_2 blockers, protease inhibitors such as aprotinin, glucocorticoids, calcitonin, nonsteroidal anti-inflammatory drugs (NSAIDs), and lexiplafant, a platelet-activating factor inhibitor. A recent meta-analysis of somatostatin, ocreotide, and the antiprotease gabexate mesilate in therapy of acute pancreatitis suggested (1) a reduced mortality rate but no change in complications with octreotide, and (2) no effect on the mortality rate but reduced pancreatic damage with gabexate.

Intraabdominal *Candida* infection during acute necrotizing pancreatitis is increasing in frequency and is associated with an increased mortality rate. In one representatitve trial, intraabdominal *Candida* infection was found in 13 of 37 cases and was associated with a mortality rate fourfold greater than that associated with intraabdominal bacterial infection alone. Given the impact of *Candida* infection on the mortality rate in acute necrotizing pancreatitis and the apparent benefit of prophylactic chemotherapy, these data suggest earlier use of fungicides.

A CT scan, especially a contrast-enhanced dynamic CT (CECT) scan, provides valuable information on the severity and prognosis of acute pancreatitis (Fig. 294-1 and Table 294-4). In particular, a CECT scan allows estimation of the presence and extent of pancreatic necrosis. Recent studies suggest that the likelihood of prolonged pancreatitis or a serious complication is negligible when the CT severity index is 1 or 2 and low with scores of 3 to 6. However, patients with scores of 7 to 10 had a 92% morbidity rate and a 17% mortality rate. Necrosis is present in 20 to 30% of patients. Those with necrosis have a morbidity rate >20%, whereas those without necrosis have a morbidity rate <10% and a negligible mortality rate. A few retrospective studies have raised concern that the use of intravenous contrast early in the course of acute pancreatitis might intensify pancreatic necrosis. However, since prospective human studies are not available, it is reasonable to reserve CECT scans for patients with severe pancreatitis or suspected local septic complications. The patient with mild to moderate pancreatitis usually requires treatment with intravenous fluids, fasting, and possibly nasogastric suction for 2 to 4 days. A clear liquid diet is frequently started on the third to sixth day, and a regular diet by the fifth to seventh day. The decision to reintroduce oral intake is usually based on the following criteria: (1) a decrease in or resolution of abdominal pain; (2) the patient is hungry; and (3) organ dysfunction, if present, has improved. Elevation of serum amylase/lipase or persistent inflammatory changes seen on CT scans should not discourage feeding a hungry asymptomatic patient. In this regard, persistence of inflammatory changes on CT scans or persistent elevations in serum amylase/lipase may not normalize for weeks to months. The patient with unremitting *fulminant pancreatitis* usually requires inordinate amounts of fluid and close attention to complications such as cardiovascular collapse, respiratory insufficiency, and pancreatic infection. The latter should be managed by a combination of radiologic and surgical means (see below). While earlier uncontrolled studies suggested that *peritoneal lavage* through a percutaneous dialysis catheter was helpful in severe pancreatitis, subsequent studies indicate that this treatment does not influence the outcome of such attacks. Aggressive surgical pancreatic debridement (necrosectomy) should be undertaken soon after confirmation of the presence of infected necrosis, and multiple operations may be required. Since the mortality rate from sterile acute necrotizing pancreatitis is approximately 10%, laparotomy with adequate drainage and removal of necrotic tissue should be considered if conventional therapy does not halt the patient's deterioration. The use of parenteral nutrition makes it possible to give nutritional support to patients with severe, acute, or protracted pancreatitis who are unable to eat normally. Several studies have demonstrated that enteral feeding via a nasojejunal tube infused distal to the ligament of Treitz is associated with a decreased rate of complications, including infection, when compared to total parenteral nutrition. Patients with severe gallstone-induced pancreatitis may improve dramatically if papillotomy is

A

B

FIGURE 294-1 Acute pancreatitis: CT evolution. *A.* Contrast-enhanced CT scan of the abdomen performed on admission of a patient with clinical evidence of acute pancreatitis. Note the mildly decreased density of the body of the pancreas to the left of the midline (*arrow*). There are a few linear strands in the peripancreatic fat, suggesting inflammation (*open arrows*). A small amount of fluid is seen in the anterior pararenal space (*arrowhead*). *B.* Nine days after admission, there is a marked worsening with severe inflammation of the pancreas evidenced by anterior displacement of the posterior gastric wall (*arrows*), increased inflammation of the peripancreatic fat, and increased pancreatic effusion in the anterior perirenal space and around the splenic vein (*open arrows*). (*Courtesy of Dr. PR Ros, University of Florida College of Medicine.*)

carried out within the first 36 to 72 h of the attack. Studies indicate that only those patients with gallstone pancreatitis who are in the very severe group should be considered for urgent ERCP. Finally, the treatment for patients with hypertriglyceridemia-associated pancreatitis includes (1) weight loss to ideal weight, (2) a lipid-restricted diet, (3) exercise, (4) avoidance of alcohol and of drugs that can elevate serum triglycerides (i.e., estrogens, vitamin A, thiazides, and beta-blockers), and (5) control of diabetes.

INFECTED PANCREATIC NECROSIS, ABSCESS, AND PSEUDOCYST Infected pancreatic necrosis should be differentiated from pancreatic abscess. The former is a diffuse infection of an acutely inflamed, necrotic pancreas occurring in the first 1 to 2 weeks after the onset of pancreatitis. In contrast, a pancreatic abscess is an ill-defined, liquid collection of pus that evolves over a longer period, often 4 to 6 weeks. It tends to be less life-threatening and is associated with a lower rate of surgical mortality. Infected pancreatic necrosis should be treated by surgical debridement because the solid component of the infected pancreas is not amenable to effective radiologically guided percutaneous evacuation. Pancreatic abscess can be treated surgically or, in selected cases, by percutaneous drainage. The necrotic pancreas becomes secondarily infected in 40 to 60% of patients, most frequently with gram-negative bacteria of alimentary origin. Whether infection occurs depends on several factors, including the extent of pancreatic and peripancreatic necrosis, the degree of pancreatic ischemia and hypoperfusion, and the presence of organ or multiorgan failure.

The early diagnosis of pancreatic infection can be accomplished by CT-guided needle aspiration. In one study, 60 patients, representing 5% of all admissions for acute pancreatitis, were suspected of harboring a pancreatic infection on the basis of fever, leukocytosis, and an abnormal CT scan (pseudocyst or extrapancreatic fluid collection). Importantly, 60% of these patients had a pancreatic infection, and 55% of these infections developed in the first 2 weeks. These findings suggest that only guided aspiration can reliably distinguish sterile from infected pancreatic necrosis. The following are guidelines for patients meeting the above selection criteria: (1) Pseudocysts should be aspirated promptly, because more than half may be infected; (2) extrapancreatic fluid collections need not be aspirated promptly, because most are sterile; (3) if a necrotic pancreas is found initially to be sterile but fever and leukocytosis persist, several days of observation should be allowed to pass before reaspiration is considered, as clinical improve-

ment frequently occurs; and (4) if fever and leukocytosis recur after an interval of well-being, reaspiration should be considered.

Severe pancreatitis with the presence of key risk factors, postoperative pancreatitis, early oral feeding, early laparotomy, and perhaps injudicious use of antibiotics predispose to the development of pancreatic abscess, which occurs in 3 to 4% of patients with acute pancreatitis. Pancreatic abscess may also develop because of a communication between a pseudocyst and the colon, inadequate surgical drainage of a pseudocyst, or needling of a pseudocyst. The characteristic signs of abscess are fever, leukocytosis, ileus, and rapid deterioration in a patient previously recovering from pancreatitis. Sometimes, however, the only manifestations are persistent fever and signs of continuing pancreatic inflammation. Drainage of pancreatic abscesses by percutaneous catheter techniques, using CT guidance, has been only moderately successful (resolution in 50 to 60% of patients). Accordingly, laparotomy with radical sump drainage and possibly resection of necrotic tissue is usually required, because the mortality rate for undrained pancreatic abscess approaches 100%. Multiple abscesses are common, and reoperation is frequently necessary.

Pseudocysts of the pancreas are collections of tissue, fluid, debris, pancreatic enzymes, and blood which develop over a period of 1 to 4 weeks after the onset of acute pancreatitis; they form in approximately 15% of patients with acute pancreatitis. In contrast to true cysts, pseudocysts do not have an epithelial lining; their walls consist of necrotic tissue, granulation tissue, and fibrous tissue. Disruption of the pancre-

TABLE 294-4 *Severity Index in Acute Pancreatitis*

	Points
Grade of acute pancreatitis	
Normal pancreas	0
Pancreatic enlargement alone	1
Inflammation compared with pancreas and peripancreatic fat	2
One peripancreatic fluid collection	3
Two or more fluid collections	4
Degree of pancreatic necrosis	
No necrosis	0
Necrosis of one-third of pancreas	2
Necrosis of one-half of pancreas	4
Necrosis of more than one-half of pancreas	6
CT severity index (CTSI) = CT grade + necrosis score (0–10)	

atic ductal system is common. However, the subsequent course of this disruption varies widely, ranging from spontaneous healing to continuous leakage of pancreatic juice, which results in tense ascites. Pseudocysts are preceded by pancreatitis in 90% of cases and by trauma in 10%. Approximately 85% are located in the body or tail of the pancreas and 15% in the head. Some patients have two or more pseudocysts. Abdominal pain, with or without radiation to the back, is the usual presenting complaint. A palpable, tender mass may be found in the middle or left upper abdomen. The serum amylase level is elevated in 75% of patients at some point during their illness and may fluctuate markedly.

On x-ray examination, 75% of pseudocysts can be seen to displace some portion of the gastrointestinal tract (Fig. 294-2). Sonography, however, is reliable in detecting pseudocysts. Sonography also permits differentiation between an edematous, inflamed pancreas, which can give rise to a palpable mass, and an actual pseudocyst. Furthermore,

serial ultrasound studies will indicate whether a pseudocyst has resolved. CT complements ultrasonography in the diagnosis of pancreatic pseudocyst (Fig. 294-2), especially when the pseudocyst is infected.

In studies with sonography, pseudocysts were seen to resolve in 25 to 40% of patients. Pseudocysts that are >5 cm in diameter and that persist for >6 weeks should be considered for drainage. Recent natural history studies have suggested that noninterventional, expectant management is the best course in selected patients with minimal symptoms and no evidence of active alcohol use in whom the pseudocyst appears mature by radiography and does not resemble a cystic neoplasm. A significant number of these pseudocysts resolve spontaneously more than 6 weeks after their formation. Also, these studies demonstrate that large pseudocyst size is not an absolute indication for interven-

A

B

C

D

FIGURE 294-2 Pseudocyst of pancreas. *A.* Upper gastrointestinal x-ray showing displacement of stomach by pseudocyst. *B.* Sonogram showing pseudocyst (*cyst*). GB, gallbladder; MVP, portal vein. Behind the large pseudocyst is seen the calcified head of the pancreas. A dilated common bile duct (*asterisk*) is noted. *C.* CT scan showing pseudocyst. Note the large, lobulated fluid collection (*arrows*) surrounding the tail of the pancreas (*arrowheads*). Note also the dense, thin rim in the periphery representing the fibrous capsule of the pseudocyst. *D.* Spiral CT showing a pseudocyst (*small arrow*) with a pseudoaneurysm (light area in pseudocyst). Note the demonstration of the main pancreatic duct (*big arrow*), even though this duct is minimally dilated by ERCP. (*A, B courtesy of Dr. CE Forsmark, University of Florida College of Medicine; C, D courtesy of Dr. PR Ros, University of Florida College of Medicine.*)

tional therapy and that many peripancreatic fluid collections detected on CT in cases of acute pancreatitis resolve spontaneously. A pseudocyst that does not resolve spontaneously may lead to serious complications, such as (1) pain caused by expansion of the lesion and pressure on other viscera, (2) rupture, (3) hemorrhage, and (4) abscess. Rupture of a pancreatic pseudocyst is a particularly serious complication. Shock almost always supervenes, and mortality rates range from 14% if the rupture is not associated with hemorrhage to over 60% if hemorrhage has occurred. Rupture and hemorrhage are the prime causes of death from pancreatic pseudocyst. A triad of findings—an increase in the size of the mass, a localized bruit over the mass, and a sudden decrease in hemoglobin level and hematocrit without obvious external blood loss—should alert one to the possibility of hemorrhage from a pseudocyst. Thus, in patients who are stable and free of complications and in whom serial ultrasound studies show that the pseudocyst is shrinking, conservative therapy is indicated. Conversely, if the pseudocyst is expanding and is complicated by rupture, hemorrhage, or abscess, the patient should be operated on. With ultrasound or CT guidance, sterile chronic pseudocysts can be treated safely with single or repeated needle aspiration or more prolonged catheter drainage with a success rate of 45 to 75%. The success rate of these techniques for infected pseudocysts is considerably less (40 to 50%). Patients who do not respond to drainage require surgical therapy for internal or external drainage of the cyst.

Pseudoaneurysms develop in up to 10% of patients with acute pancreatitis at sites reflecting the distribution of pseudocysts and fluid collections (Fig. 294-2*D*). The splenic artery is most frequently involved, followed by the inferior and superior pancreatic duodenal arteries. This diagnosis should be suspected in patients with pancreatitis who develop upper gastrointestinal bleeding without an obvious cause or in whom thin-cut CT scanning reveals a contrast-enhanced lesion within or adjacent to a suspected pseudocyst. Arteriography is necessary to confirm the diagnosis.

PANCREATIC ASCITES AND PANCREATIC PLEURAL EFFUSIONS   Pancreatic ascites is usually due to disruption of the main pancreatic duct, often by an internal fistula between the duct and the peritoneal cavity or a leaking pseudocyst (Chap. 39). This diagnosis is suggested in a patient with an elevated serum amylase level in whom the ascites fluid has both increased levels of albumin [>30 g/L (>3.0 g/dL)] and a markedly elevated level of amylase. The fluid in true pancreatic ascites usually has an amylase concentration of >20,000 U/L as a result of the ruptured duct or leaking pseudocyst. Lower amylase elevations may be found in the peritoneal fluid of patients with acute pancreatitis. In addition, ERCP often demonstrates passage of contrast material from a major pancreatic duct or a pseudocyst into the peritoneal cavity. As many as 15% of patients with pseudocysts have concurrent pancreatic ascites. The differential diagnosis should include intraperitoneal carcinomatosis, tuberculous peritonitis, constrictive pericarditis, and Budd-Chiari syndrome.

If the pancreatic duct disruption is posterior, an internal fistula may develop between the pancreatic duct and the pleural space, producing a pleural effusion, which is usually left-sided and often massive. This complication often requires thoracentesis or chest tube drainage.

℞ TREATMENT

Treatment usually requires the use of nasogastric suction and parenteral alimentation to decrease pancreatic secretion. In addition, paracentesis is performed to keep the peritoneal cavity free of fluid and, it is hoped, to effect sealing of the leak. The long-acting somatostatin analogue octreotide, which inhibits pancreatic secretion, is useful in cases of pancreatic ascites and pleural effusion. If ascites continues to recur after 2 to 3 weeks of medical management, the patient should be operated on after pancreatography to define the anatomy of the abnormal duct. A disrupted main pancreatic duct can also be treated effectively by stenting. Patients in whom ERCP identifies two or more

sites of extravasation are unlikely to respond to conservative management and/or stenting.

CHRONIC PANCREATITIS AND PANCREATIC EXOCRINE INSUFFICIENCY

GENERAL AND ETIOLOGIC CONSIDERATIONS   Chronic inflammatory disease of the pancreas may present as episodes of acute inflammation in a previously injured pancreas or as chronic damage with persistent pain or malabsorption. The causes of relapsing chronic pancreatitis are similar to those of acute pancreatitis (Table 294-1), except that there is an appreciable incidence of cases of undetermined origin. In addition, the pancreatitis associated with gallstones is predominantly acute or relapsing-acute in nature. A cholecystectomy is almost always performed in patients after the first or second attack of gallstone-associated pancreatitis. Patients with chronic pancreatitis may present with persistent abdominal pain, with or without steatorrhea; some (~15%) present with steatorrhea and no pain.

Patients with chronic pancreatitis in whom there is extensive destruction of the pancreas (<10% of exocrine function remaining) have steatorrhea and azotorrhea. Among American adults, alcoholism is the most common cause of clinically apparent pancreatic exocrine insufficiency, while cystic fibrosis is the most frequent cause in children. In up to 25% of American adults with chronic pancreatitis, the cause is not known; that is, they have idiopathic chronic pancreatitis. Indeed, idiopathic chronic pancreatitis is the leading cause of nonalcoholic chronic pancreatitis in adults in the United States. In a recent series, genetic testing was done on 39 patients with idiopathic chronic pancreatitis. Seventeen patients had CFTR mutations and 9 had mutations in a trypsin inhibitor gene (PSTI). Pancreatitis risk was increased 14-fold by having the PSTI mutation, 40-fold by having two abnormal copies of CFTR, and 600-fold by having both. Thus, the risk of pancreatitis showed complex inheritance and was highest in individuals who had abnormalities in both the pancreatic ducts (CFTR) and acini (PSTI). These findings suggest that PSTI is a modifier gene for CFTR-related idiopathic chronic pancreatitis. Current knowledge indicates that about 15% of patients with idiopathic chronic pancreatitis have a genetic basis for this disorder. The therapeutic and prognostic implication of these findings remain to be determined. In other parts of the world, severe protein-calorie malnutrition is a common cause.

In certain countries, particularly Japan and Italy, there has been an increased interest in autoimmune chronic pancreatitis. The Japanese describe a distinct entity that is associated with the presence of autoantibodies in the blood, elevated levels of serum IgG, association with other autoimmune disorders such as primary biliary cirrhosis and inflammatory bowel disease, diffuse enlargement of the pancreas, and irregular narrowing of the main pancreatic duct. Symptoms are usually mild without acute relapsing attacks of pancreatitis, and patients usually experience a good therapeutic response to glucocorticoids. It is noteworthy that pancreatic pseudocysts and calcification within the pancreas are unusual. Although this kind of pancreatitis is not very common in the United States, all major medical centers are seeing examples of autoimmune chronic pancreatitis. Table 294-5 lists other causes of pancreatic exocrine insufficiency, but they are relatively uncommon.

PATHOPHYSIOLOGY   The events that initiate an inflammatory process in the pancreas are still not well understood, and the many hypotheses will not be reviewed here. In the case of alcohol-induced pancreatitis, it has been suggested that the primary defect may be the precipitation of protein (inspissated enzymes) in the ducts. The resulting ductal obstruction could lead to duct dilation, diffuse atrophy of the acinar cells, fibrosis, and eventual calcification of some of the protein plugs. However, the fact that some alcoholic patients with recurrent acute pancreatitis show no evidence of chronic pancreatitis does not support this hypothesis. In fact, experimental and clinical observations have shown that alcohol has direct toxic effects on the pancreas. While patients with alcohol-induced pancreatitis generally consume large amounts of alcohol, some consume very little (≤50 g/d). Thus prolonged consumption of "socially acceptable" amounts of alcohol is

TABLE 294-5 *Causes of Pancreatic Exocrine Insufficiency*

Alcohol, chronic alcoholism
Idiopathic pancreatitis
Cystic fibrosis
Hypertriglyceridemia
Severe protein-calorie malnutrition with hypoalbuminemia
    Tropical pancreatitis (Africa, Asia)
Pancreatic and duodenal neoplasms
Pancreatic resection
Gastric surgery
    Subtotal gastrectomy with Billroth I anastomosis
    Subtotal gastrectomy with Billroth II anastomosis
    Truncal vagotomy and pyloroplasty
Gastrinoma (Zollinger-Ellison syndrome)
Hereditary pancreatitis
Traumatic pancreatitis
Autoimmune pancreatitis
Abdominal radiotherapy
Hemochromatosis
Primary sclerosing cholangitis
Primary biliary cirrhosis
Shwachman's syndrome (pancreatic insufficiency and bone marrow
    dysfunction)
Trypsinogen deficiency
Enterokinase deficiency
Isolated deficiencies of amylase, lipase, or proteases
α_1-Antitrypsin deficiency

compatible with the development of pancreatitis. In addition, the finding of extensive pancreatic fibrosis in patients who died during their first attack of clinical acute alcohol-induced pancreatitis supports the concept that such patients already have chronic pancreatitis.

CLINICAL FEATURES Patients with relapsing chronic pancreatitis may present with symptoms identical to those of acute pancreatitis, but pain may be continuous, intermittent, or absent. The pathogenesis of this pain is poorly understood. Although the classic description is of epigastric pain radiating through the back, the pain pattern is often atypical; the pain may be worst in the right or left upper quadrant of the back or may be diffuse throughout the upper abdomen; it may even be referred to the anterior chest or flank. Characteristically it is persistent, deep-seated, and unresponsive to antacids. It often is worsened by ingestion of alcohol or a heavy meal (especially one rich in fat). Often the pain is severe enough to necessitate the frequent use of narcotics.

Weight loss, abnormal stools, and other signs or symptoms suggestive of malabsorption (Chap. 275) are common in chronic pancreatitis. However, clinically apparent deficiencies of fat-soluble vitamins are surprisingly rare. The physical findings in these patients are usually not impressive, so that there is a disparity between the severity of the abdominal pain and the physical signs (other than some abdominal tenderness and mild temperature elevation).

DIAGNOSTIC EVALUATION (See also Chap. 293) In contrast to relapsing acute pancreatitis, the serum amylase and lipase levels are usually not elevated in chronic pancreatitis. Elevations of serum bilirubin and alkaline phosphatase levels may indicate cholestasis secondary to chronic inflammation around the common bile duct (Fig. 294-3). Many patients demonstrate impaired glucose tolerance, and some have an elevated fasting blood glucose level.

The classic triad of pancreatic calcification, steatorrhea, and diabetes mellitus usually establishes the diagnosis of chronic pancreatitis and exocrine pancreatic insufficiency but is found in fewer than one-third of chronic pancreatitis patients. Accordingly, it is often necessary to perform an intubation test such as the *secretin stimulation test*, which usually gives abnormal results when 60% or more of pancreatic exocrine function has been lost. Approximately 40% of patients with chronic pancreatitis have *cobalamin (vitamin B$_{12}$)* malabsorption, which can be corrected by the administration of oral pancreatic enzymes. There is usually a marked excretion of fecal fat (Chap. 275), which can be reduced by the administration of oral pancreatic en-

zymes. The serum trypsinogen (Chap. 293) and the D-xylose urinary excretion test are useful in patients with "pancreatic steatorrhea," since the trypsinogen level will be abnormal, and D-xylose excretion is usually normal. A decreased serum trypsinogen (<20 ng/mL) or a fecal elastase level of <100 µg/mg of stool strongly suggests severe pancreatic exocrine insufficiency.

The radiographic hallmark of chronic pancreatitis is the presence of scattered calcification throughout the pancreas (Fig. 294-3). Diffuse pancreatic calcification indicates that significant damage has occurred and obviates the need for a secretin test. While alcohol is by far the most common cause, pancreatic calcification may also be seen in cases of severe protein-calorie malnutrition, hereditary pancreatitis, posttraumatic pancreatitis, hyperparathyroidism, islet cell tumors, and idiopathic chronic pancreatitis. A large prospective study has shown convincingly that pancreatic calcification decreases or even disappears spontaneously in one-third of patients with severe chronic pancreatitis; this outcome may also follow ductal decompression. Pancreatic calcification is a dynamic process that is incompletely understood.

Sonography, CT, and ERCP greatly aid the diagnosis of pancreatic disease. In addition to excluding pseudocysts and pancreatic cancer, sonography and CT may show calcification or dilated ducts associated with chronic pancreatitis (Fig. 294-4). ERCP and endoscopic ultrasound (EUS) are procedures that provide information about the main pancreatic duct and the smaller ducts. EUS is also useful in evaluating the pancreatic parenchyma. In patients with alcohol-induced pancreatitis, ERCP may reveal a pseudocyst missed by sonography or CT.

COMPLICATIONS OF CHRONIC PANCREATITIS The complications of chronic pancreatitis are protean. Cobalamin (vitamin B$_{12}$) malabsorption occurs in 40% of patients with alcohol-induced chronic pancreatitis and in virtually all with cystic fibrosis. It is consistently corrected by the administration of pancreatic enzymes (containing proteases). It may be due to excessive binding of cobalamin by cobalamin-binding proteins other than intrinsic factor, which ordinarily are destroyed by pancreatic proteases and therefore do not compete with intrinsic factor for cobalamin binding. Although most patients show impaired glucose tolerance, diabetic ketoacidosis and coma are uncommon. Similarly, end-organ damage (retinopathy, neuropathy, nephropathy) is also uncommon, and the appearance of these complications should raise the question of concomitant genetic diabetes mellitus. A nondiabetic retinopathy, peripheral in location and secondary to vitamin A and/or zinc deficiency, is common in these patients. Effusions containing high concentrations of amylase may occur into the pleural, pericardial, or peritoneal space. Gastrointestinal bleeding may occur from peptic ulceration, gastritis, a pseudocyst eroding into the duodenum, or ruptured varices secondary to splenic vein thrombosis due to inflammation of the tail of the pancreas. Icterus may occur, caused either by edema of the head of the pancreas, which compresses the common bile duct, or by chronic cholestasis secondary to a chronic inflammatory reaction around the intrapancreatic portion of the common bile duct (Fig. 294-3). The chronic obstruction may lead to cholangitis and ultimately to biliary cirrhosis. Subcutaneous fat necrosis may appear as tender red nodules on the lower extremities. Bone pain may be secondary to intramedullary fat necrosis. Inflammation of the large and small joints of the upper and lower extremities may occur. The incidence of pancreatic carcinoma is increased in patients with chronic pancreatitis who have been followed for 2 or more years. Twenty years after the diagnosis of chronic pancreatitis, the cumulative risk of pancreatic carcinoma is 4%. Perhaps the most common and troublesome complication is addiction to narcotics.

℞ TREATMENT

Therapy for patients with chronic pancreatitis is directed toward two major problems—pain and maldigestion. Patients with intermittent attacks of pain are treated essentially like those with acute pancreatitis

A

B

C

D

FIGURE 294-3 Radiologic abnormalities in chronic pancreatitis. *A.* Pancreatic calcification (*arrows*) and stenosis (tapering) of the intrahepatic portion of the common bile duct demonstrated by percutaneous transhepatic cholangiography. *B.* Pancreatic calcification (*large white arrow*) demonstrated by sonography. Note dilated pancreatic duct (*thin white arrow*) and splenic vein (*open arrow*). *C.* Pancreatic calcification (*vertical arrows*) and dilated pancreatic duct (*horizontal arrow*) demonstrated by CT scan. *D.* Endoscopic retrograde cholangiogram shows grossly dilated pancreatic ducts (*arrows*) in a patient with long-standing pancreatitis.

A

B

FIGURE 294-4 Chronic pancreatitis and pancreatic calculi: CT scan and ERCP appearance. *A.* In this contrast-enhanced CT scan of the abdomen, there is evidence of an atrophic pancreas with multiple calcifications (*arrows*). Note the markedly dilated pancreatic duct seen in this section through the body and tail (*open arrows*). *B.* ERCP in the same patient demonstrates the dilated pancreatic duct as well as an intrapancreatic duct calculus (*arrows*). These findings correlate nicely with the CT scan appearance.

(see above). Patients with severe and persistent pain should avoid alcohol completely and avoid large meals rich in fat. Since the pain is often severe enough to require frequent use of narcotics (and hence addiction), a number of surgical procedures have been developed for pain relief. ERCP allows the surgeon to plan the operative approach. If there is a stricture of the pancreatic duct, a local resection may ameliorate the pain. Unfortunately, isolated localized strictures are not common. In most patients with alcohol-induced disease, the pancreas is diffusely involved, and surgically correctible localized ductal disease is rare. When there is primary ductal obstruction and dilation, ductal decompression may provide effective pain palliation. Short-term pain relief may be achieved in up to 80% of patients, while long-term pain relief occurs in approximately 50%. In some of these patients, however, pain relief can be achieved only by resecting 50 to 95% of the gland. Although pain relief is achieved in three-quarters of these patients, they tend to develop pancreatic endocrine and exocrine insufficiency and must be treated with pancreatic enzyme replacement therapy. It is important to screen patients carefully, for such radical surgery is contraindicated in those who are severely depressed or suicidal or who continue to drink. Procedures such as splanchnicectomy, celiac ganglionectomy, and nerve blocks usually bring only temporary relief and are not recommended. Endoscopic treatment of chronic pancreatitis may involve sphincterotomy of the minor or major pancreatic sphincter, dilatation of strictures, removal of calculi, or stenting of the ventral or dorsal pancreatic duct. Although many of these techniques are technically impressive, none has been subjected to a randomized trial in patients with chronic pancreatitis. In addition, significant complications—acute pancreatitis, pancreatic abscess, damage to the pancreatic duct, and death—have occurred in up to 36% of patients after stent placement.

Three double-blind trials have demonstrated that administration of pancreatic enzymes decreases abdominal pain in selected patients with chronic pancreatitis. In these trials, approximately 75% of the patients evaluated experienced pain relief. The patients most likely to respond are those with mild to moderate exocrine pancreatic dysfunction, as evidenced by an abnormal secretin test, normal fat absorption, and minimal abnormalities on ERCP examination. These clinical observations seem to fit with data from humans and experimental animals demonstrating a negative feedback regulation for pancreatic exocrine secretion controlled by the amount of proteases within the lumen of the proximal small intestine. It seems reasonable to use the following approach for patients with severe, persistent, or continuous abdominal pain thought to be caused by chronic pancreatitis. After other causes of abdominal pain (peptic ulcer, gallstones, etc.) have been excluded, a pancreatic sonogram should be done. If no mass is found, a secretin test may be performed, because its results are usually abnormal in cases of chronic pancreatitis with pain. If the results are abnormal (i.e., decreased bicarbonate concentration or volume output), a 3- to 4-week trial of pancreatic enzyme administration is appropriate. Four to eight conventional tablets or capsules are taken at meals and at bedtime. There are a number of studies suggesting that patients may have small-duct chronic pancreatitis and chronic abdominal pain with a normal appearance on radiographic evaluations (ultrasound, CT, ERCP) but abnormal results on hormone stimulation tests (secretin test) and/or abnormal pancreatic histology. Such minimal-change chronic pancreatitis may respond well to pancreatic enzyme therapy (non-enteric-coated) for relief of abdominal pain. If no relief is obtained, and especially if the volume secreted during the secretin test is very low, ERCP or EUS should be performed. If a pseudocyst or a localized ductal obstruction is found, surgery should be considered. A patient who has dilated ducts may be a candidate for a surgical ductal decompression procedure. This procedure provides short-term relief in up to 80% of patients, although long-term results are closer to 50%. Some studies have shown octreotide to be effective in decreasing abdominal pain in patients with severe large-duct disease. If no surgically remediable lesion is found and severe pain continues despite abstinence from alcohol, subtotal pancreatic resection may be necessary.

The treatment of maldigestion rests on the use of pancreatic enzyme replacement therapy. Diarrhea and steatorrhea are usually improved by this treatment, although the steatorrhea may not be completely corrected. The major problem is delivering enough active enzyme into the duodenum. Steatorrhea could be abolished if 10% of the normal amount of lipase could be delivered to the duodenum at the proper time. This concentration of lipase cannot be achieved with the current preparations of pancreatic enzymes, even if the latter are given in large doses. The reason for these poor results may be that lipase is inactivated by gastric acid, that food empties from the stomach faster than do the pancreatic enzymes, and that batches of commercially available pancreatic extracts vary in enzyme activity.

For the usual patient, two or three enteric-coated capsules or eight conventional (non-enteric-coated) tablets of a potent enzyme preparation should be administered with meals. Some patients using conventional tablets require adjuvant therapy to improve enzyme replacement treatment. H_2 receptor antagonists, sodium bicarbonate, and proton pump inhibitors are effective adjuvants. Antacids containing calcium carbonate or magnesium hydroxide are not effective and may actually result in increased steatorrhea. Several publications have reported colonic strictures in patients with cystic fibrosis receiving extraordinarily high doses of high-potency pancreatic enzyme preparations. Such lesions have not been reported in adults with chronic pancreatitis.

Supportive measures include diet restriction and pain medications. The diet should be moderate in fat (30%), high in protein (24%), and low in carbohydrate (40%). Restriction of long-chain triglyceride intake can help patients who do not respond satisfactorily to pancreatic enzyme therapy. Use of foods containing mainly medium-chain fatty acids, which do not require lipase for digestion, may be beneficial. Nonnarcotic analgesics should be emphasized. Patients taking narcotic drugs for pain relief often become addicted and continue to have pain.

Patients with severe exocrine pancreatic insufficiency secondary to alcohol who continue to drink have a high mortality rate (in one series, 50% of patients who were followed for 5 to 12 years died during this period) and significant morbidity (weight loss, lassitude, vitamin deficiency, and narcotic addiction). Chronic pancreatitis carries significant medical and social costs. A recent study found that pancreatitis led to retirement in 11% of patients with the disease, accounting for 45% of all retirements. In 87% of patients with chronic pancreatitis unable to maintain gainful employment, alcoholism was a contributing factor. Patients with chronic pancreatitis also use substantial medical resources. In 1987 in the United States, this diagnosis accounted for 122,000 recorded outpatient visits and 56,000 hospital admissions. Pain may abate if progressive severe exocrine insufficiency continues. Patients who abstain from alcohol and use vigorous replacement therapy for maldigestion do reasonably well.

HEREDITARY PANCREATITIS Hereditary pancreatitis is a rare disease that is similar to chronic pancreatitis except for an early age of onset and evidence of hereditary factors (involving an autosomal dominant gene with incomplete penetrance). A genome-wide search using genetic linkage analysis identified the hereditary pancreatitis gene on chromosome 7. Mutations in ion codons 29 (exon 2) and 122 (exon 3) of the cationic trypsinogen gene cause autosomal dominant forms of hereditary pancreatitis. The codon 122 mutations lead to a substitution of the corresponding arginine with another amino acid, usually histidine. This substitution, when it occurs, eliminates a fail-safe trypsin self-destruction site necessary to eliminate trypsin that is prematurely activated within the acinar cell. These patients have recurring attacks of severe abdominal pain which may last from a few days to a few weeks. The serum amylase and lipase levels may be elevated during acute attacks but are usually normal. Patients frequently develop pancreatic calcification, diabetes mellitus, and steatorrhea, and, in addition, they have an increased incidence of pancreatic carcinoma, with the cumulative incidence being as high as 40% by age 70. Such patients often require ductal decompression for pain relief. Abdominal complaints in relatives of patients with hereditary pancreatitis should raise the question of pancreatic disease.

Pancreatic Secretory Trypsin Inhibitor (PSTI) Gene Mutations PSTI, or SPINK1, is a 56-amino-acid peptide that specifically inhibits trypsin by physically blocking its active site. SPINK1 acts as the first line of defense against prematurely activated trypsinogen in the acinar cell. Recently, it has been shown that the frequency of SPINK1 mutations in patients with idiopathic chronic pancreatitis is markedly increased, suggesting that these mutations may be associated with pancreatitis.

PANCREATIC ENDOCRINE TUMORS
→*Pancreatic endocrine tumors are discussed in Chap. 329.*

OTHER CONDITIONS
ANNULAR PANCREAS When the ventral pancreatic anlage fails to migrate correctly to make contact with the dorsal anlage, the result may be a ring of pancreatic tissue encircling the duodenum. Such an annular pancreas may cause intestinal obstruction in the neonate or the adult. Symptoms of postprandial fullness, epigastric pain, nausea, and vomiting may be present for years before the diagnosis is entertained. The radiographic findings are symmetric dilation of the proximal duodenum with bulging of the recesses on either side of the annular band, effacement but not destruction of the duodenal mucosa, accentuation of the findings in the right anterior oblique position, and lack of change on repeated examinations. The differential diagnosis should include duodenal webs, tumors of the pancreas or duodenum, postbulbar peptic ulcer, regional enteritis, and adhesions. Patients with annular pancreas have an increased incidence of pancreatitis and peptic ulcer. Because of these and other potential complications, the treatment is surgical even if the condition has been present for years. Retrocolic duodeno-jejunostomy is the procedure of choice, although some surgeons advocate Billroth II gastrectomy, gastroenterostomy, and vagotomy.

PANCREAS DIVISUM Pancreas divisum occurs when the embryologic ventral and dorsal pancreatic anlagen fail to fuse, so that pancreatic drainage is accomplished mainly through the accessory papilla. Pancreas divisum is the most common congenital anatomic variant of the human pancreas. Current evidence indicates that this anomaly does not predispose to the development of pancreatitis in the great majority of patients who harbor it. However, the combination of pancreas divisum and a small accessory orifice could result in dorsal duct obstruction. The challenge is to identify this subset of patients with dorsal duct pathology. Cannulation of the dorsal duct by ERCP is not as easily done as is cannulation of the ventral duct. Patients with pancreatitis and pancreas divisum demonstrated by ERCP should be treated with conservative measures. In many of these patients, pancreatitis is idiopathic and unrelated to the pancreas divisum. Endoscopic or surgical intervention is indicated only when the above methods fail. If marked dilation of the dorsal duct can be demonstrated, surgical ductal decompression should be performed. The appropriate therapy for patients without dilation of the dorsal duct is not yet defined. It should be stressed that the ERCP appearance of pancreas divisum—i.e., a small-caliber ventral duct with an arborizing pattern—may be mistaken as representing an obstructed main pancreatic duct secondary to a mass lesion.

MACROAMYLASEMIA In macroamylasemia, amylase circulates in the blood in a polymer form too large to be easily excreted by the kidney. Patients with this condition demonstrate an elevated serum amylase value, a low urinary amylase value, and a C_{am}/C_{cr} ratio of $<1\%$. The presence of macroamylase can be documented by chromatography of the serum. The prevalence of macroamylasemia is 1.5% of the nonalcoholic general adult hospital population. Usually macroamylasemia is an incidental finding and is not related to disease of the pancreas or other organs.

Macrolipasemia has now been documented in a few patients with cirrhosis or non-Hodgkin's lymphoma. In these patients, the pancreas appeared normal on ultrasound and CT examination. Lipase was shown to be complexed with immunoglobulin A. Thus, the possibility of *both* macroamylasemia and macrolipasemia should be considered in patients with elevated blood levels of these enzymes.

ACKNOWLEDGMENT
This chapter represents a revised version of the chapter by Dr. Norton J. Greenberger, Dr. Phillip P. Toskes, and Dr. Kurt J. Isselbacher that was in the previous editions of Harrison's.

FURTHER READING
DRAGANOV P, TOSKES PP: Chronic pancreatitis. Curr Opin Gastroenterol 18: 558, 2002

FORSMARK CE: The diagnosis of chronic pancreatitis. Gastrointest Endosc 52: 293, 2000

LOWENFELS AB et al: Prognosis of chronic pancreatitis: An international multicenter study. Am J Gastroenterol 89:1467, 1994

SOMOGYI L et al: Recurrent acute pancreatitis: An algorithmic approach to identification and elimination of inciting factors. Gastroenterology 120:708, 2001

YADAY Y et al: A critical evaluation of laboratory tests in acute pancreatitis. Am J Gastroenterol 97:1309, 2002

295 | INTRODUCTION TO THE IMMUNE SYSTEM
Barton F. Haynes, Anthony S. Fauci

DEFINITIONS

- *Adaptive immune system*—recently evolved system of immune responses mediated by T and B lymphocytes. Immune responses by these cells are based on specific antigen recognition by clonotypic receptors that are products of genes that rearrange during development and throughout the life of the organism. Additional cells of the adaptive immune system include various types of antigen-presenting cells (Table 295-9).

- *Antibody*—B cell–produced molecules encoded by genes that rearrange during B cell development consisting of immunoglobulin heavy and light chains that together form the central component of the B cell receptor for antigen. Antibody can exist as B cell surface antigen-recognition molecules or as secreted molecules in plasma and other body fluids (Table 295-10).

- *Antigens*—foreign or self molecules that are recognized by the adaptive and innate immune systems resulting in immune cell triggering, T cell activation, and/or B cell antibody production.

- *Antimicrobial peptides*—small peptides <100 amino acids in length that are produced by cells of the innate immune system and have anti-infectious agent activity (Table 295-2).

- *Apoptosis*—the process of *programmed cell death* whereby signaling through various "death receptors" on the surface of cells [e.g., tumor necrosis factor (TNF) receptors, CD95] leads to a signaling cascade that involves activation of the caspase family of molecules and leads to DNA cleavage and cell death. Apoptosis, which does not lead to induction of inordinate inflammation, is to be contrasted with *cell necrosis*, which does lead to induction of inflammatory responses.

- *B lymphocytes*—bone marrow–derived or bursal-equivalent lymphocytes that express surface immunoglobulin (the B cell receptor for antigen) and secrete specific antibody after interaction with antigen (Figs. 295-8, 295-10).

- *B cell receptor for antigen*—complex of surface molecules that rearrange during postnatal B cell development, made up of surface immunoglobulin (Ig) and associated Ig $\alpha\beta$ chain molecules that recognize nominal antigen via Ig heavy and light chain variable regions, and signal the B cell to terminally differentiate to make antigen-specific antibody (Figs. 295-7, 295-9).

- *CD classification of human lymphocyte differentiation antigens*—the development of monoclonal antibody technology led to the discovery of a large number of new leukocyte surface molecules. In 1982, the First International Workshop on Leukocyte Differentiation Antigens was held to establish a nomenclature for cell-surface molecules of human leukocytes. From this and subsequent leukocyte differentiation workshops has come the *cluster of differentiation (CD) classification* of leukocyte antigens (Table 295-1).

- *Complement*—cascading series of plasma enzymes and effector proteins whose function is to lyse pathogens and/or target them to be phagocytized by neutrophils and monocyte/macrophage lineage cells of the reticuloendothelial system (Fig. 295-4, Table 295-7).

- *Co-stimulatory molecules*—molecules of antigen-presenting cells (such as B7-1 and B7-2 or CD40) that lead to T cell activation when bound by ligands on activated T cells (such as CD28 or CD40 ligand) (Fig. 295-6).

- *Cytokines*—soluble proteins that interact with specific cellular receptors that are involved in the regulation of the growth and activation of immune cells and mediate normal and pathologic inflammatory and immune responses (Tables 295-5, 295-8).

- *Dendritic cells*—myeloid and/or lymphoid lineage antigen-presenting cells of the adaptive immune system. Immature dendritic cells, or dendritic cell precursors, are key components of the innate immune system by responding to infections with production of high levels of cytokines. Dendritic cells are key initiators both of innate immune responses via cytokine production and of adaptive immune responses via presentation of antigen to T lymphocytes (Figs. 295-10, 295-11, Table 295-4).

- *Innate immune system*—ancient immune recognition system of host cells bearing germ line–encoded pattern recognition receptors (PRRs) that recognize pathogens and trigger a variety of mechanisms of pathogen elimination. Cells of the innate immune system include natural killer (NK) cell lymphocytes, monocytes/macrophages, dendritic cells, neutrophils, basophils, eosinophils, tissue mast cells, and epithelial cells (Tables 295-2, 295-3, 295-4, 295-6, 295-7).

- *Large granular lymphocytes*—lymphocytes of the innate immune system with azurophilic cytotoxic granules that have NK cell activity capable of killing foreign and host cells with little or no self major histocompatibility complex (MHC) class I molecules (Fig. 295-3).

- *Natural killer cells*—large granular lymphocytes that kill target cells that express little or no HLA class I molecules, such as malignantly transformed cells and virally infected cells. NK cells express receptors that inhibit killer cell function when self MHC class I is present (Fig. 295-3).

- *Pathogen-associated molecular patterns* (PAMPs)—Invariant molecular structures expressed by large groups of microorganisms that are recognized by host cellular pattern recognition receptors in the mediation of innate immunity (Fig. 295-2).

- *Pattern recognition receptors* (PRRs)—germ line–encoded receptors expressed by cells of the innate immune system that recognize pathogen-associated molecular patterns (Table 295-3).

- *T cells*—thymus-derived lymphocytes that mediate adaptive cellular immune responses including T helper, T regulatory, and cytotoxic T lymphocyte effector cell functions (Figs. 295-5, 295-6, 295-10, 295-11).

- *T cell receptor for antigen*—complex of surface molecules that rearrange during postnatal T cell development made up of clonotypic T cell receptor (TCR) α and β chains that are associated with the CD3 complex composed of invariant γ, δ, ε, ζ, and η chains. The clonotypic TCR-α and -β chains recognize peptide fragments of protein antigen physically bound in antigen-presenting cell MHC class I or II molecules, leading to signaling via the CD3 complex to mediate effector functions (Fig. 295-6).

- *Tolerance*—B and T cell nonresponsiveness to antigens that results from encounter with foreign or self antigens by B and T lymphocytes in the absence of expression of antigen-presenting cell co-stimulatory molecules. Tolerance to antigens may be induced and maintained by multiple mechanisms either centrally (in the thymus) or peripherally at sites throughout the peripheral immune system.

Surface Antigen (Other Names)	Family	Molecular Mass, kDa	Distribution	Ligand(s)	Function
CD1a (T6, HTA-1)	Ig	49	CD, cortical thymocytes, Langerhans type of dendritic cells	TCRγδ T cells	CD1 molecules present lipid antigens of intracellular bacteria such as *M. leprae* and *M. tuberculosis* to TCRγδ T cells.
CD1b	Ig	45	CD, cortical thymocytes, Langerhans type of dendritic cells	TCRγδ T cells	
CD1c	Ig	43	DC, cortical thymocytes, subset of B cells, Langerhans type of dendritic cells	TCRγδ T cells	
CD1d	Ig	?	Cortical thymocytes, intestinal epithelium, Langerhans type of dendritic cells	TCRγδ T cells	
CD2 (T12, LFA-2)	Ig	50	T, NK	CD58, CD48, CD59, CD15	Alternative T cell activation, T cell anergy, T cell cytokine production, T- or NK-mediated cytolysis, T cell apoptosis, cell adhesion
CD3 (T3, Leu-4)	Ig	γ:23–28, δ:21–28, ε:20–25, η:21–22, ζ:16	T	Associates with the TCR	T cell activation and function; ζ is the signal transduction components of the CD3 complex
CD4 (T4, Leu-3)	Ig	55	T, myeloid	MHC-II, HIV, gp120, IL-16, SABP	T cell selection, T cell activation, signal transduction with p56*lck*, primary receptor for HIV
CD7 (3A1, Leu-9)	Ig	40	T, NK	K-12 (CD7L)	T and NK cell signal transduction and regulation of IFN-γ, TNF-α production
CD8 (T8, Leu-2)	Ig	34	T	MHC-I	T cell selection, T cell activation, signal transduction with p56*lck*
CD14 (LPS-receptor)	LRG	53–55	M, G (weak), not by myeloid progenitors	Endotoxin (lipopolysaccharide), lipoteichoic acid, PI	TLR4 mediates with LPS and other PAMP activation of innate immunity
CD19 B4	Ig	95	B (except plasma cells), FDC	Not known	Associates with CD21 and CD81 to form a complex involved in signal transduction in B cell development, activation, and differentiation
CD20 (B1)	Unassigned	33–37	B (except plasma cells)	Not known	Cell signaling, may be important for B cell activation and proliferation
CD21 (B2, CR2, EBV-R, C3dR)	RCA	145	Mature B, FDC, subset of thymocytes	C3d, C3dg, iC3b, CD23, EBV	Associates with CD19 and CD81 to form a complex involved in signal transduction in B cell development, activation, and differentiation; Epstein-Barr virus receptor
CD22 (BL-CAM)	Ig	130–140	Mature B	CDw75	Cell adhesion, signaling through association with p72*sky*, p53/56*lyn*, PI3 kinase, SHP1, fLCγ
CD23 (FcεRII, B6, Leu-20, BLAST-2)	C-type lectin	45	B, M, FDC	IgE, CD21, CD11b, CD11c	Regulates IgE synthesis, cytokine release by monocytes
CD28	Ig	44	T, plasma cells	CD80, CD86	Co-stimulatory for T cell activation; involved in the decision between T cell activation and anergy
CD40	TNFR	48–50	B, DC, EC, thymic epithelium, MP, cancers	CD154	B cell activation, proliferation, and differentiation, formation of GCs, isotype switching, rescue from apoptosis
CD45 (LCA, T200, B220)	PTP	180, 200, 210, 220	All leukocytes	Galectin-1, CD2, CD3, CD4	T and B activation, thymocyte development, signal transduction, apoptosis
CD45RA	PTP	210, 220	Subset T, medullary thymocytes, "naive" T	Galectin-1, CD2, CD3, CD4	Isoforms of CD45 containing exon 4 (A), restricted to a subset of T cells

(continued)

TABLE 295-1—(Continued)

Surface Antigen (Other Names)	Family	Molecular Mass, kDa	Distribution	Ligand(s)	Function
CD45RB	PTP	200, 210, 220	All leukocytes	Galectin-1, CD2, CD3, CD4	Isoforms of CD45 containing exon 5 (B)
CD45RC	PTP	210, 220	Subset T, medullary thymocytes, "naive" T	Galectin-1, CD2, CD3, CD4	Isoforms of CD45 containing exon 6 (C), restricted to a subset of T cells
CD45RO	PTP	180	Subset T, cortical thymocytes, "memory" T	Galectin-1, CD2, CD3, CD4	Isoforms of CD45 containing no differentially spliced exons, restricted to a subset of T cells
CD80 (B7-1, BB1)	Ig	60	Activated B and T, MP, DC	CD28, CD152	Co-regulator of T cell activation; signaling through CD28 stimulates and through CD152 inhibits T cell activation
CD86 (B7-2, B70)	Ig	80	Subset B, DC, EC, activated T, thymic epithelium	CD28, CD152	Co-regulator of T cell activation; signaling through CD28 stimulates and through CD152 inhibits T cell activation
CD95 (APO-1, Fas)	TNFR	135	Activated T and B	Fas ligand	Mediates apoptosis
CD152 (CTLA-4)	Ig	30–33	Activated T	CD80, CD86	Inhibits T cell proliferation
CD154 (CD40L)	TNF	33	Activated CD4+ T, subset CD8+ T, NK, M, basophil	CD40	Co-stimulatory for T cell activation, B cell proliferation and differentiation

Note: CTLA, cytotoxic T lymphocyte–associated protein; DC, dendritic cells; EBV, Epstein-Barr virus; EC, endothelial cells; ECM, extracellular matrix; FcγRIIIA, low-affinity IgG receptor isoform A; FDC, follicular dendritic cells; G, granulocytes; GC, germinal center; GPI, glycosyl phosphotidylinositol; HTA, human thymocyte antigen; IgG, immunoglobulin G; LCA, leukocyte common antigen; LPS, lipopolysaccharide; MHC-I, major histocompatibility complex class I; MP, macrophages; Mr, relative molecular mass; NK, natural killer cells; P, platelets; PBT, peripheral blood T cells; PI, phosphotidylinositol; PI3K, phosphotidylinositol 3-kinase; PLC, phospholipase C; PTP, protein tyrosine phos-phatase; TCR, T cell receptor; TNF, tumor necrosis factor; TNFR, tumor necrosis factor receptor. For an expanded list of cluster of differentiation (CD) human antigens, see Harrison's Online at *http://harrisons.accessmedicine.com*; and for a full list of CD human antigens from the most recent Human Workshop on Leukocyte Differentiation Antigens (VII), see *http//www.ncbi.nlm.nih.gov/prow/guide*.

Source: Compiled with permission from T Kishimoto et al (eds): *Leukocyte Typing VI*, New York, Garland Publishing 1997; R Brines et al: Immunology Today 18S:1, 1997; and S Shaw ed: *Protein Reviews on the Web* www.ncbi.nlm.nih.gov/prow/guide.

INTRODUCTION The human immune system has evolved over millions of years from both invertebrate and vertebrate organisms to develop sophisticated defense mechanisms to protect the host from microbes and their virulence factors. From invertebrates, humans have inherited the innate immune system, an ancient defense system that uses germ line–encoded proteins to recognize pathogens. Cells of the innate immune system, such as macrophages, dendritic cells, and NK lymphocytes, recognize pathogen molecular motifs that are highly conserved among many microbes (PAMPs) and use a diverse set of receptor molecules (PRRs). Important components of the recognition of microbes by the innate immune system are: (1) recognition by germ line–encoded host molecules, (2) recognition of key microbe virulence factors but not recognition of self molecules, and (3) nonrecognition of benign foreign molecules or microbes. Upon contact with pathogens, macrophages and NK cells may kill pathogens directly or may activate a series of events that both slows the infection and recruits the more recently evolved arm of the human immune system, the adaptive immune system.

Adaptive immunity is found only in vertebrates and is based on the generation of antigen receptors on T and B lymphocytes by germline gene rearrangements, such that individual T or B cells express unique antigen receptors on their surface capable of specifically recognizing diverse antigens of the myriad of infectious agents in the environment. Coupled with finely tuned specific recognition mechanisms that maintain tolerance (nonreactivity) to self antigens, T and B lymphocytes bring both *specificity* and *immune memory* to vertebrate host defenses.

This chapter describes the cellular components, molecules (Table 295-1), and mechanisms that make up the innate and adaptive immune systems, and describes how adaptive immunity is recruited to the defense of the host by innate immune responses. An appreciation of the cellular and molecular bases of innate and adaptive immune responses is critical to understanding the pathogenesis of inflammatory, autoimmune, infectious, and immunodeficiency diseases.

THE INNATE IMMUNE SYSTEM All multicellular organisms, including humans, have developed the use of a limited number of germ line–encoded molecules that recognize large groups of pathogens. Because of the myriad human pathogens, host molecules of the human innate immune system sense "danger signals" and either recognize PAMPs, the common molecular structures shared by many pathogens, or recognize host cell molecules produced in response to infection such as heat shock proteins and fragments of the extracellular matrix. PAMPs must be conserved structures vital to pathogen virulence and survival, such as bacterial endotoxin, so that pathogens cannot mutate molecules of PAMPs to evade human innate immune responses. PPRs are host proteins of the innate immune system that recognize PAMPs or host danger signal molecules (Tables 295-2, 295-3). Thus, recognition of pathogen molecules by hematopoietic and nonhematopoietic cell types leads to activation/production of the complement cascade, cytokines, and antimicrobial peptides as effector molecules. In addition, pathogen PAMPs and host danger signal molecules activate dendritic cells to mature and to express molecules on the dendritic cell surface that optimize antigen presentation to respond to foreign antigens.

PATTERN RECOGNITION Major PRR families of proteins include C-type lectins, leucine-rich proteins, macrophage scavenger receptor proteins, plasma pentraxins, lipid transferase, and integrins (Table 295-3). A major group of PRR collagenous glycoproteins with C-type lectin do-

TABLE 295-2 Major Components of the Innate Immune System

Pattern recognition receptors (PRR)	C type lectins, leucine-rich proteins, scavenger receptors, pentraxins, lipid transferases, integrins
Antimicrobial peptides	α-Defensins, β-defensins, cathelin, protegrin, granulysin, histatin, secretory leukoprotease inhibitor, and probiotics
Cells	Macrophages, dendritic cells, NK cells, NK-T cells, neutrophils, eosinophils, mast cells, basophils, and epithelial cells
Complement components	Classic and alternative complement pathway, and proteins that bind complement components
Cytokines	Autocrine, paracrine, endocrine cytokines that mediate host defense and inflammation, as well as recruit, direct, and regulate adaptive immune responses

Note: NK cells, natural killer cells.

TABLE 295-3 *Major Pattern Recognition Receptors (PRR) of the Innate Immune System*

PRR Protein Family	Sites of Expression	Examples	Ligands (PAMPs)	Functions of PRR
C-type lectins				
Humoral	Plasma proteins	Collectins, mannose-binding lectin	Bacterial and viral carbohydrates	Opsonization of bacteria and virus, activation of complement
Cellular	Macrophages, dendritic cell	Macrophage mannose receptor	Terminal mannose	Phagocytosis of pathogens
	Natural killer (NK) cells	NKG2-A	Carbohydrate on HLA molecules	Inhibits killing of host cells expressing HLA+ self peptides
Leucine-rich proteins	Macrophages, dendritic cells, epithelial cells	CD14	Lipopolysaccharide (LPS)	Binds LPS and Toll proteins
	Macrophages, dendritic cells, epithelial cells, many others	Toll-like receptors 1–9	Lipopolysaccharide	Binds multiple TLR ligands and activates the cell to produce cytokines to activate adaptive immunity. TLR ligands bind macrophages, dendritic cells, or B cell induces B7-1 (CD80) and B7-2 (CD86) co-stimulatory molecules that are required for T and B cell antigen presentation in adaptive immune responses
Scavenger receptors	Macrophage	Macrophage scavenger receptors	Bacterial cell walls	Phagocytosis of bacteria
Pentraxins	Plasma protein	C-creative proteins	Phosphatidyl choline	Opsonization of bacteria, activation of complement
	Plasma protein	Serum amyloid P	Bacterial cell walls	Opsonization of bacteria, activation of complement
Lipid transferases	Plasma protein	LPS binding protein	LPS	Binds LPS, transfers LPS to CD14
Integrins	Macrophages, dendritic cells, NK cells	CD11b,c; CD18	LPS	Signals cells, activates phagocytosis

Note: PAMPs, pathogen-associated molecular patterns.

Source: Adapted with permission from R Medzhitov, CA Janeway, Jr: Curr Opin Immunol 9:4, 1997a.

mains are termed *collectins* and include the serum protein, mannose-binding lectin (MBL). MBL and other collectins, as well as two other protein families—the pentraxins (such as C-reactive protein and serum amyloid P) and macrophage scavenger receptors—all have the property of opsonizing (coating) bacteria for phagocytosis by macrophages and can also activate the complement cascade to lyse bacteria. Integrins are cell-surface adhesion molecules that signal cells after cells bind bacterial lipopolysacchride (LPS) and activate phagocytic cells to ingest pathogens.

A series of recent discoveries has revealed the mechanisms of connection between the innate and adaptive immune systems; these include (1) the plasma protein, LPS-binding protein, which binds and transfers LPS to the macrophage LPS receptor, CD14; and (2) a human family of proteins called *Toll-like receptor proteins* (TLR), which are associated with CD14, bind LPS, and signal epithelial cells, dendritic cells, and macrophages to produce cytokines and upregulate cell-surface molecules that signal the initiation of adaptive immune responses (Fig. 295-1, Table 295-3, and Table 295-4). Proteins in the Toll family (TLR 1–9) can be expressed on macrophages, dendritic cells, and B cells as well as on a variety of non-hematopoietic cell types including respiratory epithelial cells. Upon ligation, these receptors activate a series of intracellular events that lead to the killing of bacteria- and virus-infected cells as well as to the recruitment and ultimate activation of antigen-specific T and B lymphocytes (Fig. 295-1). Importantly, signaling by massive amounts of LPS through TLR4 leads to the release of large amounts of cytokines that mediate LPS-induced shock. Mutations in TLR4 proteins in mice protect from LPS shock, and TLR mutations in humans protect from LPS-induced inflammatory diseases such as LPS-induced asthma (Fig. 295-2).

Cells of invertebrates and vertebrates produce antimicrobial small peptides containing fewer than 100 amino acids that can act as endogenous antibodies (Table 295-2). Some of these peptides are produced by epithelia that line various organs, while others are found in macrophages or neutrophils that ingest pathogens. Antimicrobial peptides have been identified that kill bacteria such as *Pseudomonas* spp., *Escherichia coli*, and *Mycobacterium tuberculosis*.

EFFECTOR CELLS OF INNATE IMMUNITY Cells of the innate immune system and their roles in the first line of host defense are described in Table 295-4. Equally important as their roles in the mediation of innate immune responses are the roles that each cell type plays in recruiting T and B lymphocytes of the adaptive immune system to engage in specific antipathogen responses.

Monocytes-Macrophages Monocytes arise from precursor cells within bone marrow (Fig. 295-2) and circulate with a half-life ranging from 1 to 3 days. Monocytes leave the peripheral circulation by marginating in capillaries and migrating into a vast extravascular pool. Tissue macrophages arise from monocytes that have migrated out of the circulation and by in situ proliferation of macrophage precursors in tissue. Common locations where tissue macrophages (and certain of their specialized forms) are found are lymph node, spleen, bone marrow, perivascular connective tissue, serous cavities such as the peritoneum, pleura, skin connective tissue, lung (alveolar macrophage), liver (Kupffer cell), bone (osteoclast), central nervous system (microglia), and synovium (type A lining cell).

In general, monocytes-macrophages are on the first line of defense associated with innate immunity; however, they also play a major role in recruitment of adaptive immune responses by mediation of functions such as binding LPS, the presentation of antigen to T lymphocytes, and the secretion of factors such as interleukin (IL) 1, TNF, IL-12, and IL-6, which are central to antigen-specific activation of T and B lymphocytes (Fig. 295-1). Although monocytes-macrophages were originally thought to be the major antigen-presenting cells (APCs) of the immune system, it is now clear that dendritic cells are the most potent and effective APCs in the body (see below). Monocytes-macrophages mediate innate immune effector functions such as destruction of antibody-coated bacteria, tumor cells, or even normal hematopoietic cells in certain types of autoimmune cytopenias. Monocytes-macrophages ingest bacteria or are infected by viruses, and in doing so, frequently undergo apoptosis. Macrophages that are "stressed" by intracellular infectious agents are recognized by dendritic cells as infected and apoptotic cells and are phagocytosed by dendritic cells. In this manner, dendritic cells "cross-present" infectious agent antigens of macrophages to T cells. Activated macrophages can also mediate antigen-nonspecific lytic activity and eliminate cell types such as tumor cells in the absence of antibody. This activity is largely mediated by cytokines (i.e., TNF-α and IL-1). Monocytes-macrophages express lineage-specific molecules (e.g., the cell-surface LPS receptor, CD14) as well as surface receptors for a number of molecules, including the Fc region of IgG, activated complement components, and various cytokines (Table 295-5). Finally, macrophage secretory products are more diverse than those of any other cell of the immune system. Among monocyte-macrophage-secreted products are hydrolytic enzymes, products of oxidative metabolism, TNF-α, IL-1, -6, -10, -12, -15, -18, and a number of chemoattractant cytokines (chemokines) involved in the orchestration of an immune response in tissues (Table 295-5).

Dendritic Cells Dendritic cells are bone marrow–derived APCs that are distinct from monocytes-macrophages and are derived from both lymphoid and myeloid lineages. They generally lack the standard T, B, NK, and monocyte cell markers but do express CD83 and other molecules that aid in their identification. They can be expanded in culture, and their function is enhanced by the cytokines granulocyte-macrophage colony-stimulating factor (GM-CSF), IL-1, IL-4, and TNF-α. They are distinguished by an exceptional ability to present antigen, by expression of high levels of MHC class II and co-stimulatory molecules, and by dendritic morphology with multiple thin membrane projections (veils).

Lymphoid dendritic cells are also called *plasmacytoid dendritic cells*. They express some lymphoid markers, are present in T cell zones of lymphoid organs, and circulate in blood. Plasmacytoid dendritic cells are the most potent producers of interferon (IFN)-α and are also important presenters of antigen to T cells. INF-α is a potent antiviral cytokine; it activates NK cells to kill virally infected cells and drives T_H1 helper T cell responses to respond to viral and bacterial infections (see below for T helper types of responses).

There are two types of myeloid dendritic cells: *interstitial dendritic cells* (also called *follicular dendritic cells*) and *Langerhans dendritic cells*. Myeloid interstitial dendritic cells express myeloid markers, secrete IL-12 and IL-10, and are important APCs for both T and B cells. They circulate in blood and are located in T cell zones of lymphoid organs; in germinal centers of B cell follicles; and in tissue interstices of lung, heart, and kidney. Interstitial, or follicular, dendritic cells have extensive, thin, finger-like projections that surround the B cells in the germinal centers, allowing for maximal exposure of trapped antigen. The retention of antigen on the surface of interstitial dendritic cell membranes is critical for the selection and growth of high-affinity

FIGURE 295-1 Role of Toll-like receptors (TLR) in the regulation of the response of macrophages to bacterial lipopolysaccharide (LPS). Lipopolysaccharide, a component of the cell wall of gram-negative bacteria, binds with high affinity to CD14, a glycosyl phosphatidylinositol–linked protein expressed on the surface of macrophages, and to TLR4 protein. This leads to activation of the transmembrane TLR4 protein, initiating an intracellular signaling cascade. Signaling through TLRs goes through the same signaling pathway as does interleukin (IL)1α and β signaling through the IL-1 receptor (R). The cytoplasmic domains of TRLs and IL-1R are highly homologous and are each called Toll-IL-1R cytoplasmic domains (TIR). Signaling by the TLR4 protein to the transcriptional regulatory complex of NF-κB and IκB occurs through the recruitment of MyD88 (a transcription factor) and the IL-1R-associated kinase (IRAK) and involves the adapter tumor necrosis factor receptor–associated factor 6 (TRAF-6) and the transcription factor NF-κB. Mitogen-activated protein kinase (MAPK) activates c-jun NH2-terminal kinase (Jnk), which in turn activates the nuclear transcription factor AP-1. AP-1 and NF-κB pass into the nucleus and bind to specific sequences in the promoter regions of immunomodulatory genes such as cytokine genes. This leads to the expression of immunomodulatory genes, including cytokines and co-stimulatory molecules. These gene products act on T and B cells to initiate the adaptive immune response. Under pathophysiologic conditions, high levels of immune system activation by bacterial LPS may lead to septic shock. (*Adapted from Modlin et al: N Engl J Med 340:1834, 1999; with permission.*)

clones of B cells and for the maintenance of B cell memory. Of note, HIV is trapped in large quantities on the processes of interstitial dendritic cells in lymphoid organs, allowing the lymphoid tissue to serve as a reservoir of virus and a source of infection for CD4+ T cells migrating into the area to provide help to B cells in the initiation and propagation of an HIV-specific humoral response (Chap. 173). Langerhans dendritic cells express the CD1a antigen in addition to myeloid markers; circulate in blood; and populate T cell zones of lymph node, the thymus medulla, and skin and gut epithelial layers. They produce IL-12 and are key APCs for T cell activation at epithelial and other sites.

When dendritic cells come in contact with bacterial products, viral proteins, or host proteins released as danger signals from distressed host cells (Fig. 295-2), they bind to various TLRs and activate dendritic cells to release cytokines that drive cells of the innate immune system to become activated to respond to the invading organism, and recruit T and B cells of the adaptive immune system to respond. TLR engagement on dendritic cells upregulates dendritic cell MHC class II, B7-1 (CD80), and B7-2 (CD86) that enhance specific antigen presentation and induce dendritic cell cytokine production (Table 295-1). Thus, plasmacytoid and myeloid dendritic cells are important bridges between early (innate) and later (adaptive) immunity.

Large Granular Lymphocytes/Natural Killer Cells Large granular lymphocytes (LGLs) account for ~5 to 10% of peripheral blood lymphocytes. LGLs are nonadherent, nonphagocytic cells with large azurophilic cytoplasmic granules. LGLs express surface receptors for the Fc portion of IgG (CD16) and for NCAM-I (CD56), and many LGLs express some T lineage markers, particularly CD8, and proliferate in response

Cell Type	Major Role in Innate Immunity	Major Role in Adaptive Immunity
Macrophages	Phagocytose and kill bacteria; produce antimicrobial peptides; bind lipopolysaccharide (LPS); produce inflammatory cytokines	Produce interleukin (IL) 1 and tumor necrosis factor (TNF) α to upregulate lymphocyte adhesion molecules and chemokines to attract antigen-specific lymphocytes; produce IL-12 to recruit T_H1 helper T cell responses; upregulate co-stimulatory and MHC molecules to facilitate T and B lymphocyte recognition and activation; macrophages and dendritic cells, after LPS signaling, upregulate co-stimulatory molecules B7-1 (CD80) and B7-2 (CD86) required for activation of antigen-specific antipathogen T cells; there are also Toll-like proteins on B cells and dendritic cells that after LPS ligation induce CD80 and CD86 on these cells for T cell antigen presentation.
Plasmacytoid dendritic cells (DCs) of lymphoid lineage	Produce large amounts of interferon (IFN)α, which has antitumor and antiviral activity, and are found in T cell zones of lymphoid organs; they circulate in blood	IFN-α is a potent activator of macrophage and mature DCs to phagocytose invading pathogens and present pathogen antigens to T and B cells
Myeloid dendritic cells are of two types: interstitial and Langerhans-derived	Interstitial DCs are strong producers of IL-12 and IL-10 and are located in T cell zones of lymphoid organs, circulate in blood, and are present in the interstices of the lung, heart, and kidney; Langerhans DCs are strong producers of IL-12; are located in T cell zones of lymph nodes, skin epithelia, and the thymic medulla; and circulate in blood	Interstitial DCs are potent antigen-presenting cells for T cells and are potent primers of B cell activation for antibody production; Langerhans DCs are potent antigen-presenting cells for T cell priming
Natural killer (NK) cells	Kill foreign and host cells that have low levels of MHC+ self peptides. Express NK receptors that inhibit NK function in the presence of high expression of self-MHC.	Produce TNF-α and IFN-γ that recruit T_H1 helper T cell responses
NK-T cells	Lymphocytes with both T cell and NK surface markers that recognize lipid antigens of intracellular bacteria such as *M. tuberculosis* by CD1 molecules and kill host cells infected with intracellular bacteria.	Produce IL-4 to recruit T_H2 helper T cell responses, IgG1 and IgE production
Neutrophils	Phagocytose and kill bacteria, produce antimicrobial peptides	Produce nitric oxide synthase and nitric oxide that inhibit apoptosis in lymphocytes and can prolong adaptive immune responses
Eosinophils	Kill invading parasites	Produce IL-5 that recruits Ig-specific antibody responses
Mast cells and basophils	Release TNF-α, IL-6, IFN-γ in response to a variety of bacterial PAMPs	Produce IL-4 that recruits T_H2 helper T cell responses and recruit IgG1- and IgE-specific antibody responses
Epithelial cells	Produce anti-microbial peptides; tissue specific epithelia produce mediator of local innate immunity, e.g. lung epithelial cells produce surfactant proteins (proteins within the collectin family) that bind and promote clearance of lung invading microbes	Produce TGF-β that triggers IgA-specific antibody responses

Note: MHC, major histocompatibility complex; PAMP, pathogen-associated molecular patterns.

Source: Adapted with permission from R Medzhitov, CA Janeway, Jr: Curr Opin Immunol 9:4, 1997a.

to IL-2. LGLs arise in both bone marrow and thymic microenvironments.

Functionally, LGLs share features with both monocytes-macrophages and neutrophils in that LGLs mediate both antibody-dependent cellular cytotoxicity (ADCC) and NK activity. ADCC is the binding of an opsonized (antibody-coated) target cell to an Fc receptor–bearing effector cell via the Fc region of antibody, resulting in lysis of the target by the effector cell. NK cell activity is the nonimmune (i.e., effector cell never having had previous contact with the target), MHC-unrestricted, non-antibody-mediated killing of target cells, which are usually malignant cell types, transplanted foreign cells, or virus-infected cells. Thus, LGLs that mediate NK cell activity may play an important role in immune surveillance and destruction of cells that spontaneously undergo malignant transformation in vivo. Subsets of NK cells may play a role in hematopoietic cell engraftment; some subsets stimulate bone marrow stem cells, and others stimulate engraftment. Lymphokine-activated killer (LAK) cells are NK lymphocytes that proliferate in vitro to high concentrations of IL-2 and

develop the ability to kill tumor cells more efficiently than unstimulated NK cells. Rare patients with complete absence of NK cells have been described who lack both NK cell activity and CD56+, CD16+ lymphocytes but have normal T and B cell function. NK cell hyporesponsiveness is also observed in patients with the *Chédiak-Higashi syndrome*, an autosomal recessive disease associated with fusion of cytoplasmic granules and defective degranulation of neutrophil lysosomes.

The ability of NK cells to kill target cells is inversely related to target cell expression of MHC class I molecules. Thus, NK cells kill target cells with low or no levels of MHC class I expression and are prevented from killing target cells with high levels of class I expression. Recent studies have demonstrated the presence of NK receptors (NK-Rs) or killer immunoglobulin-like receptors (KIRs) that bind to either classic MHC class I molecules in a polymorphic way or the MHC-class Ib molecule HLA-E (Fig. 295-3). In every person, NK cells express at least one NK-R that recognizes a self–MHC class I allele. NK-Rs of the Ig superfamily bind specific MHC class I molecules;

Lipoproteins
Lipoarabinomannan (MTB)
Lipopolysaccharide (LPS)
Leptospira
P. gingivalis
Peptidoglycan of gram-
positive organisms
Zymosan (yeast)
Glycophosphotidyl-
inositol anchor of
T.cruzi

LPS (gram-negative)
TAXOL (plant)
Respiratory
 syncytial virus
HSP60 (host)
Fibronectin (host)
Hyaluronan (host)

Flagellin of
gram-positive
bacteria

CpG DNA

TLR2   TLR6
        or
        TLR1

TLR4   MD-2   TLR5

TLR9

FIGURE 295-2 Toll-like receptors and their ligands. Certain pathogen-associated molecular patterns and host-derived products utilize Toll-like receptor (TLR) family members as critical signal transducers. TLR2 recognizes a variety of microbial products. TLR4 is essential for signaling via lipopolysaccharide (LPS) from Gram-negative bacteria; the exceptions are *Leptospira* and *Pseudomonas gingivalis*, the LPS of which is recognized by TLR2. TLR4 recognizes not only viral and plant products, but also endogenous host-derived products, such as heat shock protein 60 (HSP60) and fragments from fibronectin and hyaluronan. Compared with TLR2 and TLR4, recognition by TLR5 and TLR9 is more restricted and is required for flagellin and CpG DNA-mediated signaling, respectively. *(From S Akira et al: Nat Immunol 2:675, 2001; with permission.)*

e.g., the NK-R p140 binds HLA-A3, and NK-R p70 binds HLA-B27 (Fig. 295-3). A second NK-R of the C-type lectin family of proteins is termed *CD94/NKG2A* and binds the MHC-related protein HLA-E (Fig. 295-3). HLA-E has an MHC class I structure but exclusively binds the leader sequence peptides of classic MHC class I molecules in the HLA-E MHC-like "notch" (see "Molecular Basis of T Cell Recognition of Antigen," below). In this manner, CD94/NKG2A NK cell molecules survey and monitor the total level of classic MHC class I molecules on the surface of host cells. When cell-surface levels of host MHC class I molecules decrease, such as occurs during malignant transformation or viral infection of host cells, the altered host cell with diminished MHC class I expression is recognized by NK-Rs, and the NK cell is activated to kill the host tumor or virally infected cells. The ability of NK-Rs to bind to self-MHC and inhibit NK killing of normal host cells is a key protective mechanism for prevention of NK cell–mediated autoimmune disease. In addition, when HLA-E-positive cells become "stressed," such as occurs during viral infections, the leader sequence of heat shock protein-60 (HSP-60) is processed and inserted in the notch of HLA-E, yet this particular peptide/HLA-E complex is not recognized by NK cells. In this manner, NK cells can detect and recognize stressed virally infected cells for elimination.

Some NK cells express CD3 and are termed *NK/T cells*. NK/T cells can also express oligoclonal forms of the TCR for antigen that can recognize lipid molecules of intracellular bacteria when presented in the context of CD1 molecules on APCs. This mode of recognition of intracellular bacteria such as *Listeria monocytogenese* and *M. tuberculosis* by NK/T cells is thought to be an important defense mechanism against these organisms that, via usage of a clonal form of TCRs for antigen, incorporates components of both the innate and adaptive immune systems.

Neutrophils, Eosinophils, and Basophils Granulocytes are present in nearly all forms of inflammation and are amplifiers and effectors of innate immune responses. Unchecked accumulation and activation of granulocytes can lead to host tissue damage, as seen in neutrophil- and eosinophil-mediated *systemic necrotizing vasculitis*. Granulocytes are derived from stem cells in bone marrow. Each type of granulocyte (neutrophil, eosinophil, or basophil) is derived from a different subclass of progenitor cell, which is stimulated to proliferate by colony-stimulating factors (Table 295-5). During terminal maturation of

granulocytes, class-specific nuclear morphology and cytoplasmic granules appear that allow for histologic identification of granulocyte type.

Neutrophils express Fc receptors for IgG (CD16) and receptors for activated complement components (C3b or CD35). Upon interaction of neutrophils with opsonized bacteria or immune complexes, azurophilic granules (containing myeloperoxidase, lysozyme, elastase, and other enzymes) and specific granules (containing lactoferrin, lysozyme, collagenase, and other enzymes) are released, and microbicidal superoxide radicals (O_2^-) are generated at the neutrophil surface. The generation of superoxide leads to inflammation by direct injury to tissue and by alteration of macromolecules such as collagen and DNA.

Eosinophils express Fc receptors for IgG (CD32) and are potent cytotoxic effector cells for various parasitic organisms. In *Nippostrongylus brasiliensis* helminth infection, eosinophils are key cytotoxic effector cells in removal of these parasites. Key to regulation of eosinophil cytotoxicity to *N. brasiliensis* worms are antigen-specific T helper cells that produce IL-4, thus providing an example of regulation of innate immune responses by adaptive immunity antigen-specific T cells. Intracytoplasmic contents of eosinophils, such as major basic protein, eosinophil cationic protein, and eosinophil-derived neurotoxin, are capable of directly damaging tissues and may be responsible in part for the organ system dysfunction in the *hypereosinophilic syndromes* (Chap. 55). Since the eosinophil granule contains anti-inflammatory types of enzymes (histaminase, arylsulfatase, phospholipase D), eosinophils may homeostatically downregulate or terminate ongoing inflammatory responses.

The normal functions of basophils and tissue mast cells are not completely understood; they are potent reservoirs of cytokines such as IL-4. The capacity of basophil cytokines and mediators to increase local delivery of antibodies and complement by increasing vascular permeability is hypothetical. Thus, the basophil is identified principally with allergic reactions and some delayed cutaneous hypersensitivity states. Certainly, the promotion of increased vascular permeability by basophils is important in the genesis of inflammatory lesions in some vasculitis syndromes (Chap. 306). Basophils express high-affinity surface receptors for IgE (FcRI) and, upon cross-linking of basophil-bound IgE by antigen, release histamine, eosinophil chemotactic factor of anaphylaxis, and neutral protease—all mediators of immediate (anaphylaxis) hypersensitivity responses (Table 295-6). In addition, basophils express surface receptors for activated complement components (C3a, C5a), through which mediator release can be directly effected. →*For further discussion of tissue mast cells, see Chap. 298.*

THE COMPLEMENT SYSTEM The complement system, an important soluble component of the innate immune system, is a series of plasma enzymes, regulatory proteins, and proteins that are activated in a cascading fashion, resulting in cell lysis. There are four pathways of the complement system: the classic activation pathway activated by antigen/antibody immune complexes, the mannose-binding lectin (a serum collectin; Table 295-3) activation pathway activated by microbes with terminal mannose groups, the alternative activation pathway activated by microbes or tumor cells, and the terminal pathway that is common to the first three pathways and leads to the membrane attack complex that lyses cells (Fig. 295-4). The series of enzymes of the complement system are serine proteases.

Activation of the classic complement pathway via immune complex binding to C1q links the innate and adaptive immune systems via specific antibody in the immune complex. The alternative complement activation pathway is antibody-independent and is activated by binding of C3 directly to pathogens and "altered self" such as tumor cells. In the renal glomerular inflammatory disease, *IgA nephropathy*, IgA activates the alternative complement pathway and causes glomerular damage and decreased renal function. Activation of the classic complement pathway via C1, C4, and C2 and activation of the alternative pathway via factor D, C3, and factor B both lead to cleavage and

TABLE 295-5 *Cytokines and Cytokine Receptors*

Cytokine	Receptor	Cell Source	Cell Target	Biologic Activity
IL-1α,β	Type 1 IL-1R, type 2 IL-1R	Monocytes/macrophages, B cells, fibroblasts, most epithelial cells including thymic epithelium, endothelial cells	All cells	Upregulates adhesion molecule expression, neutrophil and macrophage emigration; mimics shock, fever; upregulates hepatic acute-phase protein production; facilitates hematopoiesis
IL-2	IL-2R α,β, common γ	T cells	T cells, B cells, NK cells, monocytes/macrophages	T cell activation and proliferation, B cell growth, NK cell proliferation and activation, enhanced monocyte/macrophage cytolytic activity
IL-3	IL-3R, common β	T cells, NK cells, mast cells	Monocytes/macrophages, mast cells, eosinophils, bone marrow progenitors	Stimulation of hematopoietic progenitors
IL-4	IL-4R α, common γ	T cells, mast cells, basophils	T cells, B cells, NK cells, monocytes/macrophages, neutrophils, eosinophils, endothelial cells, fibroblasts	Stimulates T$_H$2 helper T cell differentiation and proliferation; stimulates B cell Ig class switch to IgG1 and IgE; anti-inflammatory action on T cells, monocytes
IL-5	IL-5R α, common β	T cells, mast cells, and eosinophils	Eosinophils, basophils, murine B cells	Regulates eosinophil migration and activation
IL-6	IL-6R, gp130	Monocytes/macrophages, B cells, fibroblasts, most epithelium including thymic epithelium, endothelial cells	T cells, B cells, epithelial cells, hepatocytes, monocytes/macrophages	Induction of acute-phase protein production, T and B cell differentiation and growth, myeloma cell growth, osteoclast growth and activation
IL-7	IL-7R α, common γ	Bone marrow, thymic epithelial cells	T cells, B cells, bone marrow cells	Differentiation of B, T, and NK cell precursors, activation of T and NK cells
IL-8	CXCR1, CXCR2	Monocytes/macrophages, T cells, neutrophils, fibroblasts, endothelial cells, epithelial cells	Neutrophils, T cells, monocytes/macrophages, endothelial cells, basophils	Induces neutrophil, monocyte, and T cell migration; induces neutrophil adherance to endothelial cells and histamine release from basophils; stimulates angiogenesis; suppresses proliferation of hepatic precursors
IL-10	IL-10R	Monocytes/macrophages, T cells, B cells, keratinocytes, mast cells	Monocytes/macrophages, T cells, B cells, NK cells, mast cells	Inhibits macrophage proinflammatory cytokine production; downregulates cytokine class II antigen and B7-1 and B7-2 expression; inhibits differentiation of T$_H$1 helper T cells; inhibits NK cell function; stimulates mast cell proliferation and function and B cell activation and differentiation
IL-11	IL-11R, gp130	Bone marrow stromal cells	Megakaryocytes, B cells, hepatocytes	Induces megakaryocyte colony formation and maturation; enhances antibody responses; stimulates acute-phase protein production
IL-12 (35-kDa and 40-kDa subunits)	IL-12R	Activated macrophages, dendritic cells, neutrophils	T cells, NK cells	Induces T$_H$1 T helper cell formation and lymphokine-activated killer cell formation; increases CD8+ CTL activity
IL-13	IL-13/IL-4R	T cells (T$_H$2)	Monocytes/macrophages, B cells, endothelial cells, keratinocytes	Upregulation of VCAM-1 and C-C chemokine expression on endothelial cells; B cell activation and differentiation; inhibits macrophage proinflammatory cytokine production
IL-17	IL17R	CD4+ T cells	Fibroblasts, endothelium, epithelium	Enhanced cytokine secretion that promotes a predominant T$_H$1 response
IL-18	IL-18R (IL-1R-related protein)	Keratinocytes, macrophages	T cells, B cells, NK cells	Upregulated IFN-γ production, enhanced NK cell cytotoxicity
IFN-α	Type I interferon receptor	All cells	All cells	Antiviral activity; stimulates T cell, macrophage, and NK cell activity; direct antitumor effects; upregulates MHC class I antigen expression; used therapeutically in viral and autoimmune conditions

(continued)

TABLE 295-5—(Continued)

Cytokine	Receptor	Cell Source	Cell Target	Biologic Activity
IFN-β	Type I interferon receptor	All cells	All cells	Antiviral activity; stimulates T cell, macrophage, and NK cell activity; direct antitumor effects; upregulates MHC class I antigen expression; used therapeutically in viral and autoimmune conditions
IFN-γ	Type II interferon receptor	T cells, NK cells	All cells	Regulates macrophage and NK cell activation; stimulates immunoglobulin secretion by B cells; induction of class II histocompatibility antigens; T_H1 T cell differentiation
TNF-α	TNF-RI, TNF-RII	Monocytes/macrophages, mast cells, basophils, eosinophils, NK cells, B cells, T cells, keratinocytes, fibroblasts, thymic epithelial cells	All cells except erythrocytes	Fever, anorexia, shock, capillary leak syndrome, enhanced leukocyte cytotoxicity, enhanced NK cell function, acute-phase protein synthesis, proinflammatory cytokine induction
G-CSF	G-CSFR; gp130	Monocytes/macrophages, fibroblasts, endothelial cells, thymic epithelial cells, stromal cells	Myeloid cells, endothelial cells	Regulates myelopoiesis; enhances survival and function of neutrophils; clinical use in reversing neutropenia after cytotoxic chemotherapy
GM-CSF	GM-CSFR; common β	T cells, monocytes/macrophages, fibroblasts, endothelial cells, thymic epithelial cells	Monocytes/macrophages, neutrophils, eosinophils, fibroblasts, endothelial cells	Regulates myelopoiesis; enhances macrophage bactericidal and tumoricidal activity; mediator of dendritic cell maturation and function; upregulates NK cell function; clinical use in reversing neutropenia after cytotoxic chemotherapy
M-CSF	M-CSFR (c-*fms* proto-oncogene)	Fibroblasts, endothelial cells, monocytes/macrophages, T cells, B cells, epithelial cells including thymic epithelium	Monocytes/macrophages	Regulates monocyte/macrophage production and function
Fractalkine	CX3CR1	Activated endothelial cells	NK cells, T cells, monocytes/macrophages	Cell surface chemokine/mucin hybrid molecule that functions as a chemoattractant, leukocyte activator, and cell adhesion molecule

*Note:*1 CSF, colony-stimulating factor; CXCR, CXC-type chemokine receptor; G-CSF, granulocyte CSF; GM-CSF, granulocyte-macrophage CSF; IFN, interferon; IL, interleukin; IP, IFN-γ-inducible protein; M-CSF, macrophage CSF; MDC, macrophage-derived chemokine; MHC, major histocompatibility complex; NK, natural killer; PMBC, peripheral blood mononuclear cells; PF, platelet factor; SCF, stem cell factor; TNF, tumor necrosis factor; VCAM, vascular cell adhesion molecule. For an expanded list of cytokines, see Harrison's Online at *http://harrisons.accessmedicine.com.*

Source: From JS Sundy et al, in J Gallin and R Snyderman (eds): *Inflammation, Basic Principles and Clinical Correlates,* 3d ed. Philadelphia, Lippincott Williams & Wilkins, 1999, with permission.

activation of C3. C3 activation fragments, when bound to target surfaces such as bacteria and other foreign antigens, are critical for opsonization (coating by antibody and complement) in preparation for phagocytosis. The MBL pathway substitutes MBL-associated serine proteases (MASP) 1 and 2 for C1q, C1r, and C1s to activate C4. The MBL activation pathway is activated by mannose on the surface of bacteria and viruses.

The three pathways of complement activation all converge on the final common terminal pathway. C3 cleavage by each pathway results in activation of C5, C6, C7, C8, and C9 resulting in the membrane attack complex that physically inserts into the membranes of target cells or bacteria and lyses them.

Thus, complement activation is a critical component of innate immunity for responding to microbial infection. The functional consequences of complement activation by the three initiating pathways and the terminal pathway are shown in Fig. 295-4 and Table 295-7. In general the cleavage products of complement components facilitate microbe or damaged cell clearance (C1q, C4, C3), promote activation and enhancement of inflammation (anaphylatoxins, C3a, C5a), and promote microbe or opsonized cell lysis (membrane attack complex).

CYTOKINES Cytokines are soluble proteins produced by a wide variety of hematopoietic and nonhematopoietic cell types (Table 295-5). They are critical for both normal innate and adaptive immune responses, and

their expression may be perturbed in most immune, inflammatory, and infectious disease states.

Cytokines are involved in the regulation of the growth, development, and activation of immune system cells and in the mediation of the inflammatory response. In general, cytokines are characterized by considerable redundancy in that different cytokines have similar functions. In addition, many cytokines are pleiotropic in that they are capable of acting on many different cell types. This pleiotropism results from the expression on multiple cell types of receptors for the same cytokine (see below), leading to the formation of "cytokine networks." The action of cytokines may be: (1) autocrine when the target cell is the same cell that secretes the cytokine, (2) paracrine when the target cell is nearby, and (3) endocrine when the cytokine is secreted into the circulation and acts distal to the source.

Cytokines have been named based on presumed targets or based on presumed functions. Those cytokines that are thought to primarily target leukocytes have been named interleukins (IL-1, -2, -3, etc.). Many cytokines that were originally described as having a certain function have retained those names (granulocyte colony-stimulating factor or G-CSF, etc.). Cytokines belong in general to four major structural families, the four α-helix bundle family, the IL-1 family, the IL-17 family, and the chemokine family (Table 295-8). The four α-helix group is the largest family whose members have a three-dimensional core with four bundles of α-helices. Within this family are three sub-

FIGURE 295-3 A schematic representation of the human natural killer (NK) receptor repertoire. The NK cells of a given individual express clonally distributed NK-Rs for self-HLA class I molecules. In this representative donor (HLA haplotype: HLA-A1, A3; HLA-B7, B27; HLA-Cw3, Cw4), NK cells express at least one inhibitory receptor that interacts with self-HLA alleles. The NK-Rs depicted in white are those belonging to the Ig superfamily that recognize allelic forms of HLA class I molecules. CD94/NKG2A receptors (stippled blue) bind to the MHC class I-like molecules, HLA-E, that present leader sequence peptides of classic MHC class I molecules to CD94/NKG2A molecules. The receptors belonging to the Ig superfamily do not cover the whole set of HLA class I alleles and are not expressed by 100% of NK cells. CD94/NKG2A receptors play important roles in monitoring the total level of MHC class I molecules on viral and malignantly transformed cells. (*Adapted from A Moretta et al: Immunol Rev 155:105, 1997; with permission. For nomenclature, see EO Long et al: Protein Rev at www.ncbi.nlm.nih.gov/prow/guide 679664748_g.htm, 1999.*)

families, the IL-2, IFN, and IL-10 subfamilies. The second group of cytokines is the IL-1 family, made up of IL-1α, IL-1β, and IL-18, all of which share about 25% sequence homology to each other. Most of the IL-17 family of cytokines promote T_H1 types of T cell responses that lead to cytotoxic T cell effector function. Finally, chemokines are cytokines that regulate cell movement and trafficking. Chemokines act through G protein–coupled receptors and have a distinctive three-dimensional structure. IL-8 is the only chemokine that early on was named an interleukin.

TABLE 295-6 *Mediators Released from Human Mast Cells and Basophils*

Mediator	Actions
Histamine	Smooth-muscle contraction, increased vascular permeability
Slow-reacting substance of anaphylaxis (SRSA) (leukotriene C4, D4, E4)	Smooth-muscle contraction
Eosinophil chemotactic factor of anaphylaxis (ECF-A)	Chemotactic attraction of eosinophils
Platelet-activating factor	Activates platelets to secrete serotonin and other mediators: smooth-muscle contraction; induces vascular permeability
Neutrophil chemotactic factor (NCF)	Chemotactic attraction of neutrophils
Leukotactic activity (leukotriene B4)	Chemotactic attraction of neutrophils
Heparin	Anticoagulant
Basophil kallikrein of anaphylaxis (BK-A)	Cleaves kininogen to form bradykinin

FIGURE 295-4 The four pathways and the effector mechanisms of the complement system. Dashed arrows indicate the functions of pathway components. (*After BJ Morley, MJ Walport: The Complement Facts Books. London, Academic Press, Chap 2, 2000; with permission.*)

In general, cytokines exert their effects by influencing gene activation that results in cellular activation, growth, differentiation, functional cell-surface molecule expression, and cellular effector function. In this regard, cytokines can have dramatic effects on the regulation of immune responses and the pathogenesis of a variety of diseases. Indeed, T cells have been categorized on the basis of the pattern of cytokines that they secrete that results in either humoral immune response (T_H2) or a cell-mediated immune response (T_H1).

Cytokine receptors can be grouped into five general families based on similarities in their extracellular amino acid sequences and conserved structural domains. The *immunoglobulin (Ig) superfamily* represents a large number of cell-surface and secreted proteins. The IL-1 receptors (type 1, type 2) are examples of cytokine receptors with extracellular Ig domains.

TABLE 295-7 *Biologic Activities of Some Complement Components*

Component	Activity
C4a weak anaphylatoxin	Evokes histamine release from basophils and mast cells
C3a	Anaphylatoxin; evokes histamine release from basophils and mast cells
C5a	Anaphylatoxin; evokes histamine release from basophils and mast cells; potent chemoattractant for monocytes and neutrophils
C3b, C3bi	Enhancement of phagocytosis by neutrophils and monocytes; promotes immune-complex binding to cells within monocyte-macrophage system, as well as neutrophils; C3b with Bb forms alternative pathway C3 convertase and amplifies alternative pathway; promotes solubilization of immune complexes
C5–9	Membrane attack complex; forms transmembrane channels leading to cell destruction

Source: After S Ruddy, in WN Kelley et al (eds): *Textbook of Rheumatology*, 4th ed. Philadelphia, Saunders, 1993, with permission.

The hallmark of the *hematopoietic growth factor (type 1) receptor* family is that the extracellular regions of each receptor contain two conserved motifs. One motif located at the N terminus is rich in cysteine residues. The other motif is located at the C terminus proximal to the transmembrane region and comprises five amino acid residues, tryptophan-serine-X-tryptophan-serine (WSXWS). This family can be grouped on the basis of the number of receptor subunits they have and on the utilization of shared subunits. A number of cytokine receptors, i.e., IL-6, IL-11, IL-12, and leukemia inhibitory factor, are paired with gp130. There is also a common 150-kDa subunit shared by IL-3, IL-5, and GM-CSF receptors. The gamma chain (γ_c) of the IL-2 receptor is common to the IL-2, IL-4, IL-7, IL-9, and IL-15 receptors. Thus,

TABLE 295-8	*Four Major Structural Families of Cytokines*	
Four α-helix bundle family	Interleukin 2 (IL-2) Subfamily
	Interleukin:
	IL-2, IL-3, IL-4, IL-5, IL-6, IL-7, IL-9, IL-11, IL-12, IL-13, IL-15, IL-21, IL-23
	Not called interleukins:
	Colony-stimulating factor-1 (CSF1), granulocyte-macrophage colony-stimulating factor (CSF2), Flt-3 ligand, erythropoietin (EPO), thrombopoietin (THPO), leukocyte inhibitory factor (LIF)
	Not Interleukins:
	Growth hormone (GH1), prolactin (PRL), leptin (LEP), cardiotrophin (CTF1), ciliary neurotrophic factor (CNTF), cytokine receptor-like factor 1 (CLC or CLF)
	Interferon (IFN) subfamily
	IFN-β, IFN-α
	IL-10 subfamily
	IL-10, IL-19, IL-20, IL-22, IL-24 and IL-26
IL-1 Family	IL-1α (IL1A), IL-1β, (IL1B), IL-18 (IL-18), and paralogues
IL-17 Family	IL-17A, IL-17B, IL-17C, IL-17D, IL-17E, IL-17F
Chemokines	IL-8, MCP-1, MCP-2, MCP-3, MCP-4, eotaxin, TARC, LARC/MIP-3α, MDC, MIP-1α, MIP-1β, RANTES, MIP-3β, I-309, SLC, PARC, TECK, GROα, GROβ, NAP-2, IP-10, MIG, SDF-1, PF4

Note: GRO, growth-related peptide; IL, interleukin; IP, IFNδ-inducible protein; LARC, liver and activation-regulated chemokine; MCP, monocyte chemotactic protein; MDC, macrophage-derived chemokine; MIG, monoteine-induced by IFNδ; MIP, macrophage inflammatory protein; NAP, neutrophil-activating protein; PARC, pulmonary and activation-regulated chemokine; PF4, platelet factor; RANTES, regulated on activation normally T cell expressed and secreted; SDF, stromal-cell derived factor; SLC, secondary lymphoid tissue chemokine; TARC, thymus and activation-regulated chemokine; TECK, thymus-express chemokine.
Source: Adapted with permission from JW Schrader: Trends Immunol 23:573, 2002.

the specific cytokine receptor is responsible for ligand specific binding, while the subunits such as gp130, the 150-kDa subunit, and γ_c are important in signal transduction. The γ_c gene is on the X chromosome, and mutations in the γ_c protein result in the *X-linked form of severe combined immune deficiency syndrome (X-SCID)* (Chap. 297).

The members of the *interferon (type II) receptor* family include the receptors for IFN-γ, and -β, which share a similar 210-amino-acid binding domain with conserved cysteine pairs at both the amino and carboxy termini. The members of the *TNF (type III) receptor family* share a common binding domain composed of repeated cysteine-rich regions. Members of this family include the p55 and p75 receptors for TNF (TNFR1 and TNFR2, respectively); CD40 antigen, which is an important B cell–surface marker involved in immunoglobulin isotype switching; fas/Apo-1, whose triggering induces apoptosis; CD27 and CD30, which are found on activated T cells and B cells; and nerve growth factor receptor.

The common motif for the *seven transmembrane helix family* was originally found in receptors linked to GTP-binding proteins. This family includes receptors for chemokines, β-adrenergic receptors, and retinal rhodopsin. It is important to note that two members of the chemokine receptor family, CXC chemokine receptor type 4 (CXCR4) and β chemokine receptor type 5 (CCR5), have recently been found to serve as the two major coreceptors for binding and entry of HIV into CD4-expressing host cells (Chap. 173).

Significant advances have been made in defining the signaling pathways through which cytokines exert their effects intracellularly. The Janus family of protein tyrosine kinases (JAK) is a critical element involved in signaling via the hematopoietin receptors. Four JAK kinases, JAK1, JAK2, JAK3, and Tyk2, preferentially bind different cytokine receptor subunits. Cytokine binding to its receptor brings the cytokine receptor subunits into apposition and allows a pair of JAKs to transphosphorylate and activate one another. The JAKs then phosphorylate the receptor on the tyrosine residues and allow signaling molecules to bind to the receptor, where these molecules become phosphorylated. Signaling molecules bind the receptor because they have domains (SH2, or src homology 2 domains) that can bind phosphorylated tyrosine residues. There are a number of these important signaling molecules that bind the receptor, such as the adapter molecule SHC, which can couple the receptor to the activation of the mitogen-activated protein kinase pathway. In addition, an important class of substrate of the JAKs is the signal transducers and activators of transcription (STAT) family of transcription factors. STATs have SH2 domains that enable them to bind to phosphorylated receptors, where they are then phosphorylated by the JAKs. It appears that different STATs have specificity for different receptor subunits. The STATs then dissociate from the receptor and translocate to the nucleus, bind to DNA motifs that they recognize, and regulate gene expression. The STATs preferentially bind DNA motifs that are slightly different from one another and thereby control transcription of specific genes. The importance of this pathway is particularly relevant to lymphoid development. Mutations of JAK3 itself also result in a disorder identical to X-SCID; however, since JAK3 is found on chromosome 19 and not on the X chromosome, JAK3 deficiency occurs in boys and girls (Chap. 297).

THE ADAPTIVE IMMUNE SYSTEM Adaptive immunity is characterized by antigen-specific responses to a foreign antigen or pathogen. A key feature of adaptive immunity is that following the initial contact with antigen (*immunologic priming*), subsequent antigen exposure leads to more rapid and vigorous immune responses (*immunologic memory*). The adaptive immune system consists of dual limbs of cellular and humoral immunity. The principal effectors of cellular immunity are T lymphocytes, while the principal effectors of humoral immunity are B lymphocytes (Table 295-9). Both B and T lymphocytes derive from a common stem cell.

The proportion and distribution of immunocompetent cells in various tissues reflect cell traffic, homing patterns, and functional capabilities. Bone marrow is the major site of maturation of B cells, monocytes-macrophages, and granulocytes and contains pluripotent stem cells which, under the influence of various colony stimulating factors, are capable of giving rise to all hematopoietic cell types. T cell precursors also arise from hematopoietic stem cells and home to

TABLE 295-9	*Components of the Adaptive Immune System*

Cellular: Thymus-derived (T) lymphocytes—T cell precursors in the thymus; naive mature T lymphocytes before antigen exposure; memory T lymphocytes after antigen contact; helper T lymphocytes for B and T cell responses; cytotoxic T lymphocytes that kill pathogen-infected target cells

Humoral: Bone-marrow-derived (B) lymphocytes—B cell precursors in bone marrow; naive B cells prior to antigen recognition, memory B cells after antigen contact; plasma cells that secrete specific antibody

Cytokines: Soluble proteins that direct, focus, and regulate specific T versus B lymphocyte immune responses the thymus for maturation. Mature T lymphocytes, B lymphocytes, monocytes, and dendritic/Langerhans cells enter the circulation and home to peripheral lymphoid organs (lymph nodes, spleen) and the gut-associated lymphoid tissue (tonsil, Peyer's patches, and appendix) as well as the skin and mucous membranes and await activation by foreign antigen.

T Cells The pool of effector T cells is established in the thymus early in life and is maintained throughout life both by new T cell production in the thymus and by antigen-driven expansion of virgin peripheral T cells into "memory" T cells that reside in peripheral lymphoid organs. The thymus exports ~2% of the total number of thymocytes per day throughout life, with the total number of daily thymic emigrants decreasing by ~3% per year during the first four decades of life. Thymic emigrants can be identified by the expression of certain combinations of T cell surface markers and by the presence in nuclei of excised (deleted) pieces of rearranged TCR DNA, called *T cell receptor excision circles.*

Mature T lymphocytes constitute 70 to 80% of normal peripheral blood lymphocytes (only 2% of the total-body lymphocytes are contained in peripheral blood), 90% of thoracic duct lymphocytes, 30 to 40% of lymph node cells, and 20 to 30% of spleen lymphoid cells. In lymph nodes, T cells occupy deep paracortical areas around B cell germinal centers, and in the spleen, they are located in periarteriolar areas of white pulp (Chap. 54). T cells are the primary effectors of cell-mediated immunity, with subsets of T cells maturing into CD8+ cytotoxic T cells capable of lysis of virus-infected or foreign cells. In general, CD4+ T cells are also the primary regulatory cells of T and B lymphocyte and monocyte function by the production of cytokines and by direct cell contact. In addition, T cells regulate erythroid cell maturation in bone marrow, and through cell contact (CD40 ligand) have an important role in activation of B cells and induction of Ig isotype switching.

Human T cells express cell-surface proteins that mark stages of intrathymic T cell maturation or identify specific functional subpopulations of mature T cells. Many of these molecules mediate or participate in important T cell functions (Table 295-1; Fig. 295-5).

The earliest identifiable T cell precursors in bone marrow are CD34+ pro-T cells (i.e., cells in which TCR genes are neither rearranged nor expressed). In the thymus, CD34+ T cell precursors begin cytoplasmic (c) synthesis of components of the CD3 complex of TCR-associated molecules (Fig. 295-5.) Within T cell precursors, TCR for antigen gene rearrangement begins under the influence of IL-7 and yields two T cell lineages, expressing either TCRαβ chains or TCRγδ chains. T cells expressing the TCRαβ chains comprise the majority of peripheral T cells in blood, lymph node, and spleen and terminally differentiate into either CD4+ or CD8+ cells. Cells expressing TCRγδ chains circulate as a minor population in blood; their functions, although not fully understood, have been postulated to be those of immune surveillance at epithelial surfaces and cellular defenses against mycobacterial organisms and other intracellular bacteria (see below). Immature cortical thymocytes express both CD4 and CD8 (i.e., they are double positive); however, upon reaching functional maturity, T cell CD4 and CD8 are reciprocally expressed (i.e., T cells become single positive for either CD4 or CD8).

In the thymus, the recognition of self-peptides on thymic epithelial cells, thymic macrophages, and dendritic cells plays an important role in shaping the T cell repertoire to recognize foreign antigen (*positive selection*) and in eliminating highly autoreactive T cells (*negative selection*). As immature cortical thymocytes begin to express surface TCR for antigen, autoreactive thymocytes are destroyed (negative selection), thymocytes with TCRs capable of interacting with foreign antigen peptides in the context of self–MHC antigens are activated and develop to maturity (positive selection), and thymocytes with TCR that are incapable of binding to self–MHC antigens die of attrition (*no selection*). Mature thymocytes that are positively selected are either

FIGURE 295-5 Human T cell maturation. sCD3, surface CD3 expression; cCD3, cytoplasmic CD3 expression; TCR, T cell receptor.

CD4+ helper T cells or MHC class II–restricted cytotoxic (killer) T cells, or they are CD8+ T cells destined to become MHC class I–restricted cytotoxic T cells. *MHC class I– or class II–restricted* means that T cells recognize antigen peptide fragments only when they are presented in the antigen-recognition site of a class I or class II MHC molecule, respectively (see below).

After thymocyte maturation and selection, CD4 and CD8 thymocytes leave the thymus and migrate to the peripheral immune system. It is important to note that the adult thymus continues to function, albeit with decreasing output, well into adult life. Thus, the thymus continues to be a contributor to the peripheral immune system, both normally and when the peripheral T cell pool is damaged, such as occurs in AIDS and cancer chemotherapy.

MOLECULAR BASIS OF T CELL RECOGNITION OF ANTIGEN The TCR for antigen is a complex of molecules consisting of an antigen-binding heterodimer of either αβ or γδ chains noncovalently linked with five CD3 subunits (γ, δ, ε, ζ, and η) (Fig. 295-6). The CD3 ζ chains are either disulfide-linked homodimers (CD3-ζ₂) or disulfide-linked heterodimers composed of one ζ chain and one η chain. TCRαβ or TCRγδ molecules must be associated with CD3 molecules to be inserted into the T cell surface membrane, TCRα being paired with TCRβ and TCRγ being paired with TCRδ. Molecules of the CD3 complex mediate transduction of T cell activation signals via TCRs, while TCRα and -β or -γ and -δ molecules combine to form the TCR antigen-binding site.

The α, β, γ, and δ TCR for antigen molecules have amino acid sequence homology and structural similarities to immunoglobulin heavy and light chains and are members of the *immunoglobulin gene superfamily* of molecules. The genes encoding TCR molecules are encoded as clusters of gene segments that rearrange during the course of T cell maturation. This creates an efficient and compact mechanism for housing the diversity requirements of antigen receptor molecules. The TCRα chain is on chromosome 14 and consists of a series of V (variable), J (joining), and C (constant) regions. The TCRβ chain is on chromosome 7 and consists of multiple V, D (diversity), J, and C TCRβ loci. The TCRγ chain is on chromosome 7, and the TCRδ chain is in the middle of the TCRα locus on chromosome 14. Thus, molecules of the TCR for antigen have constant (framework) and variable regions, and the gene segments encoding the α, β, γ, and δ chains of these molecules are recombined and selected in the thymus, culminating in synthesis of the completed molecule. In both T and B cell precursors (see below), DNA rearrangements of antigen receptor genes involve the same enzymes, recombinase activating gene (RAG)1 and RAG2, both DNA-dependent protein kinases.

TCR diversity is created by the different V, (D), and J segments that are possible for each receptor chain by the many permutations of V, D, and J segment combinations, by "N-region diversification" due to the addition of nucleotides at the junction of rearranged gene segments, and the pairing of individual chains to form a TCR dimer. As T cells mature in the thymus, the repertoire of antigen-reactive T cells is modified by selection processes that eliminate many autoreactive T cells, enhance the proliferation of cells that function appropriately with self-MHC molecules and antigen, and allow T cells with nonproductive TCR rearrangements to die.

TCRαβ cells do not recognize native protein or carbohydrate antigens. Instead, T cells recognize only short (~9 to 13 amino acids) peptide fragments derived from protein antigens taken up or produced in APCs. Foreign antigens may be taken up by endocytosis into acidified intracellar vesicles or by phagocytosis and degraded into small peptides that associate with MHC class II molecules (exogenous antigen-presentation pathway). Other foreign antigens arise endogenously in the cytosol (such as from replicating viruses) and are broken down into small peptides that associate with MHC class I molecules (endogenous antigen-presenting pathway). Thus, APCs proteolytically degrade foreign proteins and display peptide fragments embedded in the MHC class I or II antigen-recognition site on the MHC molecule surface, where foreign peptide fragments are available to bind to TCRαβ or TCRγδ chains of reactive T cells. CD4 molecules act as an adhesive and, by direct binding to MHC class II (DR, DQ, or DP) molecules, stabilize the interaction of TCR with peptide antigen (Fig. 295-6). Similarly, CD8 molecules also act as adhesives to stabilize the TCR-antigen interaction by direct CD8 molecule binding to MHC class I (A, B, or C) molecules.

Antigens that arise in the cytosol and are processed via the endogenous antigen-presentation pathway are cleaved into small peptides by a 28-subunit complex of proteases called the *proteasome*. From the proteasome, antigen peptide fragments are transported from the cytosol into the lumen of the endoplasmic reticulum by a heterodimeric complex termed *transporters associated with antigen processing*, or TAP proteins. There, MHC class I molecules in the endoplasmic reticulum membrane physically associate with processed cytosolic peptides. Following peptide association with class I molecules, peptide–class I complexes are exported to the Golgi apparatus, and then to the cell surface, for recognition by CD8+ T cells.

Antigens taken up from the extracellular space via endocytosis into

Before MHC-peptide binding to T cell receptor

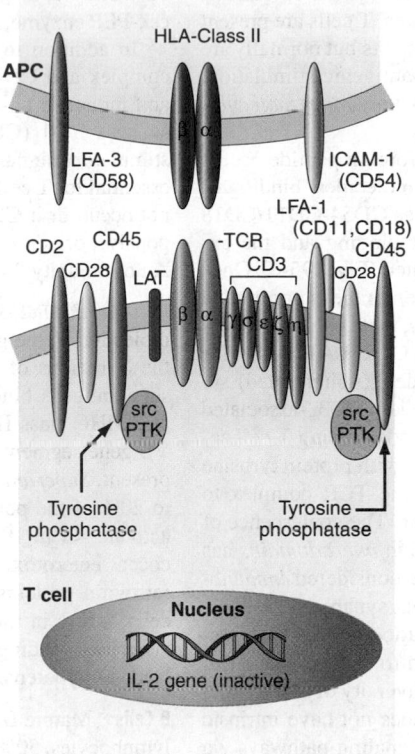

After MHC-peptide binding to T cell receptor

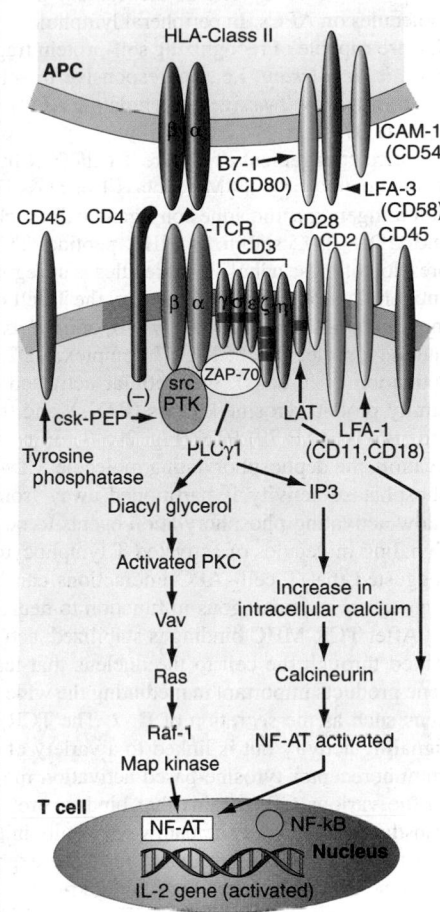

FIGURE 295-6 Molecules involved in human T cell recognition of antigen and in human T cell activation. *A.* Schematic arrangement of antigen-presenting cell (APC) molecules (top cell) and T cell molecules (bottom cell) before MHC-peptide binding to T cell receptor (TCR). *B.* The changes that occur in T cell and APC molecules after MHC-peptide binding to TCR. The black triangle at the tip of the αβ chains of MHC class II molecules represents a peptide fragment of "processed" protein antigen. After TCR ligation, src protein tyrosine kinase (PTK) is activated via dephosphorylation and the TCR complex is joined by CD4, CD2, and CD28 as well as the linker for activated T lymphocytes (LAT) in a lipid microdomain area (gray area). Activation signals are mediated via immunoreceptor tyrosine-based activation (ITAM) sequences in LAT and CD3 chains (blue bars) that bind to enzymes and transduce activation signals to the nucleus via the indicated intracellular activation pathways. See text for details of the activation and signal transduction process. *(Adapted from A Weiss and DR Littman: Cell 76:263, 1995; with permission.)*

intracellular acidified vesicles are degraded by vesicle proteases into peptide fragments. Intracellular vesicles containing MHC class II molecules fuse with peptide-containing vesicles, thus allowing peptide fragments to physically bind to MHC class II molecules. Peptide–MHC class II complexes are then transported to the cell surface for recognition by CD4+ T cells.

Whereas it is generally agreed that the TCRαβ receptor recognizes peptide antigens in the context of MHC class I or class II molecules, lipids in the cell wall of intracellular bacteria such as *M. tuberculosis* can also be presented to a wide variety of T cells, including subsets of CD4−, CD8− TCRαβ T cells, TCRγδ T cells, and a subset of CD8+ TCRαβ T cells. Importantly, bacterial lipid antigens are not presented in the context of MHC class I or II molecules, but rather are presented in the context of MHC-related CD1 molecules. Some γδ T cells that recognize lipid antigens via CD1 molecules have very restricted TCR usage, do not need antigen priming to respond to bacterial lipids, and may actually be a form of innate rather than acquired immunity to intracellular bacteria.

Just as foreign antigens are degraded and their peptide fragments presented in the context of MHC class I or class II molecules on APCs, endogenous self-proteins are also degraded and self-peptide fragments are presented to T cells in the context of MHC class I or class II molecules on APCs. In peripheral lymphoid organs, T cells are present that are capable of recognizing self-protein fragments but normally are *anergic* or *tolerant*, i.e., nonresponsive to self-antigenic stimulation, due to lack of self-antigen upregulating APC *co-stimulatory molecules* such as B7-1 and B7-2 (see below).

Once engagement of mature T cell TCR by foreign peptide occurs in the context of self–MHC class I or class II molecules, binding of non-antigen-specific adhesion ligand pairs such as CD54-CD11/CD18 and CD58-CD2 stabilizes MHC peptide–TCR binding and the expression of these adhesion molecules is upregulated (Fig. 295-6). Once antigen ligation of the TCR occurs, the T cell membrane is partitioned into *lipid membrane microdomains*, or *lipid rafts*, that coalesce the key signaling molecules TCR/CD3 complex, CD28, CD2, LAT (linker for activation of T cells), intracellular activated (dephosphorylated) src family protein tyrosine kinases (PTKs), and the key CD3ζ-associated protein-70 (ZAP-70) PTK (Fig. 295-7). Importantly, during T cell activation, the dephosphorylating molecule, CD45, with protein tyrosine phosphatase activity is partitioned away from the TCR complex to allow activating phosphorylation events to occur. The coalescence of signaling molecules of activated T lymphocytes in *microdomains* has suggested that T cell–APC interactions can be considered *immunologic synapses*, analogous in function to neuronal synapses.

After TCR-MHC binding is stabilized, activation signals are transmitted through the cell to the nucleus that lead to the expression of gene products important in mediating the wide diversity of T cell functions such as the secretion of IL-2. The TCR does not have intrinsic signaling activity but is linked to a variety of signaling pathways via immunoreceptor tyrosine-based activation motifs (ITAMs) expressed on the various CD3 chains that bind to proteins that mediate signal transduction. Each of the pathways results in the activation of particular transcription factors that control the expression of cytokine and cytokine receptor genes. Thus, antigen-MHC binding to the TCR induces the activation of the src family of PTKs, fyn and lck (lck is associated with CD4 or CD8 co-stimulatory molecules); phosphorylation of CD3ζ chain; activation of the related tyrosine kinases ZAP-70 and syk; and downstream activation of the calcium-dependent calcineurin pathway, the ras pathway, and the protein kinase C pathway. Each of these pathways leads to activation of specific families of transcription factors (including NF-AT, fos and jun, and rel/NF-κB) that form heteromultimers capable of inducing expression of IL-2, IL-2 receptor, IL-4, TNF-α, and other T cell mediators. The src family

kinases require dephosphorylation of an inactivation site by CD45 phosphatase before they can be phosphorylated on an activation site. Furthermore, the activity through the receptor is downregulated by the csk-PEP enzyme, a phosphatase that inactivates the src family kinases.

In addition to the signals delivered to the T cell from the TCR complex and CD4 and CD8, molecules on the T cell such as CD28 and inducible co-stimulator (ICOS) and molecules on dendritic cells such as B7-1 (CD80) and B7-2 (CD86) also deliver important co-stimulatory signals that upregulate T cell cytokine production and are essential for T cell activation. If signaling through CD28 or ICOS does not occur, or if CD28 is blocked, the T cell becomes *anergic* (nonresponsive, or *tolerant*) rather than activated (see "Immune Tolerance and Autoimmunity," below).

T CELL SUPERANTIGENS Conventional antigens bind to MHC class I or II molecules in the groove of the αβ heterodimer and bind to T cells via the V regions of the TCRα and -β chains (Fig. 295-6). In contrast, superantigens bind directly to the lateral portion of the TCRβ chain and MHC class II β chain and stimulate T cells based solely on the Vβ gene segment utilized independent of the D, J, and Vα sequences present. *Superantigens* are protein molecules capable of activating up to 20% of the peripheral T cell pool, whereas conventional antigens activate <1 in 10,000 T cells. T cell superantigens include staphylococcal enterotoxins, other bacterial products, and certain nonhuman retroviral proteins. Superantigen stimulation of human peripheral T cells occurs in the clinical setting of the *staphylococcal toxic shock syndrome*, leading to massive overproduction of T cell cytokines that leads to hypotension and shock (Chap. 120).

B Cells Mature B cells comprise 10 to 15% of human peripheral blood lymphocytes, 50% of splenic lymphocytes, and ~10% of bone marrow lymphocytes. B cells express on their surface intramembrane immunoglobulin (Ig) molecules that function as B cell receptors (BCRs) for antigen in a complex of Ig-associated α and β signaling molecules with properties similar to those described in T cells (Fig. 295-7). Unlike T cells, which recognize only processed peptide fragments of conventional antigens embedded in the notches of MHC class I and class II antigens of APCs, B cells are capable of recognizing and proliferating to whole unprocessed native antigens via antigen binding to B cell surface Ig (sIg) receptors. B cells also express surface receptors for the Fc region of IgG molecules (CD32) as well as receptors for activated complement components (C3d or CD21, C3b or CD35). The primary function of B cells is to produce antibodies. B cells also serve as APCs and are highly efficient at antigen processing. Their antigen-presenting function is enhanced by a variety of cytokines. Mature B cells are derived from bone marrow precursor cells that arise continuously throughout life (Figs. 295-2, 295-10).

B lymphocyte development can be separated into antigen-independent and antigen-dependent phases. Antigen-independent B cell development occurs in primary lymphoid organs and includes all stages of B cell maturation up to the sIg+ mature B cell. Antigen-dependent B cell maturation is driven by the interaction of antigen with the mature B cell sIg, leading to memory B cell induction, Ig class switching, and plasma cell formation. Antigen-dependent stages of B cell maturation occur in secondary lymphoid organs, including lymph node, spleen, and gut Peyer's patches. In contrast to the T cell repertoire that is generated intrathymically before contact with foreign antigen, the repertoire of B cells expressing diverse antigen-reactive sites is modified by further alteration of Ig genes after stimulation by antigen—a process called *somatic mutation*—which occurs in lymph node germinal centers.

During B cell development, diversity of the antigen-binding variable region of Ig is generated by an ordered set of Ig gene rearrangements that are similar to the rearrangements undergone by TCR α, β, γ, and δ genes. For the heavy chain, there is first a rearrangement of D segments to J segments, followed by a second rearrangement between a V gene segment and the newly formed D-J sequence; the C segment is aligned to the V-D-J complex to yield a functional Ig heavy chain gene (V-D-J-C). During later stages, a functional κ or λ light

FIGURE 295-7 The pre-B cell receptor and B-cell antigen receptor associate with the signal-transducing heterodimer Igα/Igβ. Solid horizontal bars in α and β chains denote the immunoreceptor tyrosine-based activation motif (ITAM). Signals from the antigen receptors are further propagated downstream by other signaling molecules such as the syk and the src family of tyrosine kinases (fyn, lyn, blk, and btk), as well as by the phosphatase, SHP-1. *(Adapted from K-P Lam, K Rajewsky: Inflammation: Basic Principles and Clinical Correlates, 3d ed., Philadelphia, Lippincott Williams & Wilkins, pp 151–166, 1999; with permission.)*

chain gene is generated by rearrangement of a V segment to a J segment, ultimately yielding an intact Ig molecule composed of heavy and light chains.

The process of Ig gene rearrangement is regulated and results in a single antibody specificity produced by each B cell, with each Ig molecule comprising one type of heavy chain and one type of light chain. Although each B cell contains two copies of Ig light and heavy chain genes, only one gene of each type is productively rearranged and expressed in each B cell, a process termed *allelic exclusion.*

There are ~300 V_κ genes and 5 J_κ genes, resulting in the pairing of V_κ and J_κ genes to create >1500 different light chain combinations. The number of distinct κ light chains that can be generated is increased by somatic mutations within the V_κ and J_κ genes, thus creating large numbers of possible specificities from a limited amount of germ-line genetic information. As noted above, in heavy chain Ig gene rearrangement, the VH domain is created by the joining of three types of germ-line genes called V_H, D_H, and J_H, thus allowing for even greater diversity in the variable region of heavy chains than of light chains.

The most immature B cell precursors (early pro-B cells) lack cytoplasmic Ig (cIg) and sIg (Fig. 295-8). The large pre-B cell is marked by the acquisition of the surface pre-BCR composed of μ heavy (H) chains and a pre-B light chain, termed ψLC (Fig. 295-7). ψLC is a surrogate light chain receptor encoded by the nonrearranged V pre-B and the λ5 light chain locus (the pre-BCR). Pro- and pre-B cells are driven to proliferate and mature by signals from bone marrow stroma, in particular, IL-7. Light chain rearrangement occurs in the small pre-B cell stage such that the full BCR is expressed at the immature B cell stage. Immature B cells have rearranged Ig light chain genes and express sIgM. As immature B cells develop into mature B cells, sIgD is expressed as well as sIgM. At this point, B lineage development in bone marrow is complete, and B cells exit into the peripheral circulation and migrate to secondary lymphoid organs to encounter specific antigens.

Random rearrangements of Ig genes occasionally generate self-reactive antibodies, and mechanisms must be in place to correct these mistakes. One such mechanism is BCR editing, whereby autoreactive BCRs are mutated to not react with self-antigens. If receptor editing is unsuccessful in eliminating autoreactive B cells, then autoreactive B cells undergo negative selection in the bone marrow through induction of apoptosis after BCR engagement of self-antigen.

After leaving the bone marrow, B cells populate peripheral B cell sites, such as lymph node and spleen, and await contact with foreign antigens that react with each B cell's clonotypic receptor. As antigen-driven B cell activation occurs through the BCR, a process known as *somatic hypermutation* takes place whereby point mutations in rearranged H- and L-genes give rise to mutant sIg molecules, some of which bind antigen better than the original sIg molecules. Somatic hypermutation, therefore, is a process whereby memory B cells in peripheral lymph organs have the best binding, or the highest affinity antibodies. This overall process of generating the best antibodies is called *affinity maturation of antibody.*

Lymphocytes that synthesize IgG, IgA, and IgE are derived from sIgM+, sIgD+ mature B cells. Ig class switching occurs in lymph node and other peripheral lymphoid tissue germinal centers. CD40 on B cells and CD40 ligand on T cells comprise a critical co-stimulatory receptor-ligand pair of immune-stimulatory molecules. Pairs of CD40+ B cells and CD40 ligand+ T cells bind and drive B cell Ig switching via T cell–produced cytokines such as IL-4 and transforming growth factor (TGF) β. IL-1, -2, -4, -5, and -6 synergize to drive mature B cells to proliferate and differentiate into Ig-secreting cells.

Humoral Mediators of Adaptive Immunity: Immunoglobulins   Immunoglobulins are the products of differentiated B cells and mediate the humoral arm of the immune response. The primary functions of antibodies are to bind specifically to antigen and bring about the inactivation or removal of the offending toxin, microbe, parasite, or other foreign substance from the body. The structural basis of Ig molecule function and Ig gene organization has provided insight into the role of antibodies in normal protective immunity, pathologic immune-mediated damage by immune complexes, and autoantibody formation against host determinants.

All immunoglobulins have the basic structure of two heavy and two light chains (Figs. 295-7 and 295-9). Immunoglobulin isotype (i.e., G, M, A, D, E) is determined by the type of Ig heavy chain present. IgG and IgA isotypes can be divided further into subclasses (G1, G2, G3, G4, and A1, A2) based on specific antigenic determinants on Ig heavy chains. The characteristics of human immunoglobulins are outlined in Table 295-10. The four chains are covalently linked by disulfide bonds. Each chain is made up of a V region and C regions (also called *domains*), themselves made up of units of ~110 amino

	Stem cell	Early pro-B cell	Late pro-B cell	Large pre-B cell	Small pre-B cell	Immature B cell	Mature B cell
H-chain genes	Germ line	DJ rearranged	VDJ rearranged	VDJ rearranged	VDJ rearranged	VDJ rearranged	VDJ rearranged
L-chain genes	Germ line	Germ line	Germ line	Germ line	VJ rearranged	VJ rearranged	VJ rearranged
Surface Ig	Absent	Absent	Absent	μ H-chain at surface as part of pre-β receptor	μ H-chain in cytoplasm and at surface	IgM expressed on cell surface	IgD and IgM made from alternatively spliced H-chain transcripts
Surface marker proteins	CD34	CD34 CD10 CD19 CD38	CD10 CD19 CD20 CD38 CD40	CD19 CD20 CD38 CD40	CD19 CD20 CD38 CD40	CD19 CD20 CD40	CD19 CD20 CD21 CD40

FIGURE 295-8   Developmental stages of B cells. Elements of the developing B cell receptor for antigen (BCR) are shown schematically. The classification into the various stages of B cell development is primarily defined by rearrangement of the immunoglobulin (Ig), heavy (H), and light (L) chain genes and by the absence or presence of specific surface markers. [*Adapted from CA Janeway et al (eds): Immunobiology. The Immune System in Health and Disease, 4th ed, New York, Garland, 1999; with permission.*]

FIGURE 295-9 Schematic structure of the immunoglobulin G (IgG) molecule.

acids. Light chains have one variable (V_L) and one constant (C_L) unit; heavy chains have one variable unit (V_H) and three or four constant (C_H) units, depending on isotype. As the name suggests, the constant, or C, regions of Ig molecules are made up of homologous sequences and share the same primary structure as all other Ig chains of the same isotype and subclass. Constant regions are involved in biologic functions of Ig molecules. The C_{H2} domain of IgG and the C_{H4} units of IgM are involved with the binding of the C1q portion of C1 during complement activation. The C_H region at the carboxy-terminal end of the IgG molecule, the Fc region (Fig. 295-9), binds to surface Fc receptors (CD16, CD32, CD64) of macrophages, LGLs, B cells, neutrophils, and eosinophils.

Variable regions (V_L and V_H) constitute the antibody-binding (Fab) region of the molecule. Within the V_L and V_H regions are hypervariable regions (extreme sequence variability) that constitute the antigen-binding site unique to each Ig molecule. The idiotype is defined as the specific region of the Fab portion of the Ig molecule to which antigen binds. Antibodies against the idiotype portion of an antibody molecule are called *anti-idiotype antibodies*. The formation of such antibodies in vivo during a normal B cell antibody response may generate a negative (or "off") signal to B cells to terminate antibody production.

IgG comprises ~75 to 85% of total serum immunoglobulin. The four IgG subclasses are numbered in order of their level in serum,

IgG1 being found in greatest amounts and IgG4 the least. IgG subclasses have clinical relevance in their varying ability to bind macrophage and neutrophil Fc receptors and to activate complement (Table 295-10). Moreover, selective deficiencies of certain IgG subclasses give rise to clinical syndromes in which the patient is inordinately susceptible to bacterial infections. IgG antibodies are frequently the predominant antibody made after rechallenge of the host with antigen (secondary antibody response).

IgM antibodies normally circulate as a 950-kDa pentamer with 160-kDa bivalent monomers joined by a molecule called the *J chain*, a 15-kDa nonimmunoglobulin molecule that also effects polymerization of IgA molecules. IgM is the first immunoglobulin to appear in the immune response (primary antibody response) and is the initial type of antibody made by neonates. Membrane IgM in the monomeric form also functions as a major antigen receptor on the surface of mature B cells (Fig. 295-9). IgM is an important component of immune complexes in autoimmune diseases. For example, IgM antibodies against IgG molecules (rheumatoid factors) are present in high titers in *rheumatoid arthritis*, other collagen diseases, and some infectious diseases (*subacute bacterial endocarditis*).

IgA comprises only 7 to 15% of total serum immunoglobulin but is the predominant class of immunoglobulin in secretions. IgA in secretions (tears, saliva, nasal secretions, gastrointestinal tract fluid, and human milk) is in the form of secretory IgA (sIgA), a polymer consisting of two IgA monomers, a joining molecule, again called the J chain, and a glycoprotein called the *secretory protein*. Of the two IgA subclasses, IgA1 is primarily found in serum, whereas IgA2 is more prevalent in secretions. IgA fixes complement via the alternative complement pathway and has potent antiviral activity in humans by prevention of virus binding to respiratory and gastrointestinal epithelial cells.

IgD is found in minute quantities in serum and, together with IgM, is a major receptor for antigen on the B cell surface. IgE, which is present in serum in very low concentrations, is the major class of immunoglobulin involved in arming mast cells and basophils by binding to these cells via the Fc region. Antigen cross-linking of IgE molecules on basophil and mast cell surfaces results in release of mediators of the immediate hypersensitivity response (Table 295-6).

TABLE 295-10   Physical, Chemical, and Biologic Properties of Human Immunoglobulins

Property	IgG	IgA	IgM	IgD	IgE
Usual molecular form	Monomer	Monomer, dimer	Pentamer, hexamer	Monomer	Monomer
Other chains	None	J chain, SC	J chain	None	None
Subclasses	G1, G2, G3, G4	A1, A2	None	None	None
Heavy chain allotypes	Gm (=30)	No A1, A2m (2)	None	None	None
Molecular mass, kDa	150	160, 400	950, 1150	175	190
Sedimentation constant, Sw20	6.6S	7S, 11S	19S	7S	8S
Carbohydrate content, %	3	7	10	9	13
Serum level in average adult, mg/mL	9.5–12.5	1.5–2.6	0.7–1.7	0.04	0.0003
Percentage of total serum Ig	75–85	7–15	5–10	0.3	0.019
Serum half-life, days	23	6	5	3	2.5
Synthesis rate, mg/kg per day	33	65	7	0.4	0.016
Antibody valence	2	2,4	10,12	2	2
Classical complement activation	+(G1, 2?, 3)	–	++	–	–
Alternate complement activation	+(G4)	+	–	+	–
Binding cells via Fc	Macrophages, neutrophils, large granular lymphocytes	Lymphocytes	Lymphocytes	None	Mast cells, basophils, B cells
Biologic properties	Placental transfer, secondary Ab for most antipathogen responses	Secretory immunoglobulin	Primary Ab responses	Marker for mature B cells	Allergy, antiparasite responses

Source: After L Carayannopoulos and JD Capra, in WE Paul (ed): *Fundamental Immunology*, 2d ed. New York, Raven, 1989; with permission.

CELLULAR INTERACTIONS IN REGULATION OF NORMAL IMMUNE RESPONSES The net result of activation of the humoral (B cell) and cellular (T cell) arms of the adaptive immune system by foreign antigen is the elimination of antigen directly by specific effector T cells or in concert with specific antibody. Figure 295-10 is a simplified schematic diagram of the T and B cell responses indicating some of these cellular interactions.

The expression of adaptive immune cell function is the result of a complex series of immunoregulatory events that occur in phases. Both T and B lymphocytes mediate immune functions, and each of these cell types, when given appropriate signals, passes through stages, from activation and induction through proliferation, differentiation, and ultimately effector functions. The effector function expressed may be at the end point of a response, such as secretion of antibody by a differentiated plasma cell, or it might serve a regulatory function that modulates other functions, such as is seen with CD4+ and CD8+ T lymphocytes that modulate both differentiation of B cells and activation of CD8+ cytotoxic T cells.

CD4 helper T cells can be subdivided on the basis of cytokines produced (Figs. 295-10 and 295-11). Activated T_H1-type helper T cells secrete IL-2, IFN-γ, IL-3, TNF-α, GM-CSF, and TNF-β, while activated T_H2-type helper T cells secrete IL-3, -4, -5, -6, -10, and -13. T_H1 CD4+ T cells, through elaboration of IFN-γ, have a central role in mediating intracellular killing by a variety of pathogens. T_H1 CD4+ T cells also provide T cell help for generation of cytotoxic T cells and some types of opsonizing antibody, and generally respond to antigens that lead to delayed hypersensitivity types of immune responses for many intracellular viruses and bacteria (such as HIV or *M. tuberculosis*). In contrast, T_H2 cells have a primary role in regulatory humoral immunity and isotype switching. In addition, T_H2 cells, through production of IL-4 and IL-10, have a regulatory role in limiting proinflammatory responses mediated by T_H1 cells (Table 295-5). In addition, T_H2 CD4+ T cells provide help to B cells for specific Ig production and respond to antigens that require high antibody levels for foreign antigen elimination (extracellular encapsulated bacteria such as *Streptococcus pneumoniae* and certain parasite infections). The type of T cell response generated in an immune response is determined by the microbe PAMPs presented to the dentritic cells, the TLRs on the dendritic cells that become activated, the types of dendritic cells that are activated, and the cytokines that are produced. Commonly, myeloid dendritic cells produce IL-12 and activate T_H1 T cell responses that result in IFN-γ and cytotoxic T cell induction, and plasmacytoid dendritic cells product IFN-α and lead to T_H2 responses that result in IL-4 production and enhanced antibody responses.

As shown in Figs. 295-10 and 295-11, upon activation by dendritic cells, T cell subsets that produce IL-2, IL-3, IFN-γ, and/or IL-4, -5, -6, -10, and -13 are generated that exert positive and negative influences on effector T and B cells. For B cells, trophic effects are mediated by a variety of cytokines, particularly T cell–derived IL-3, -4, -5, and -6, that act at sequential stages of B cell maturation, resulting in B cell proliferation, differentiation, and ultimately antibody secretion. For cytotoxic T cells, trophic factors include inducer T cell secretion of IL-2, IFN-γ, and IL-12. In addition, B cells themselves are capable of serving as APCs, processing and presenting antigens to T cells, and secreting TNF-α and IL-6.

An important type of immunomodulatory T cell that controls immune responses are *CD4+ and CD8+ T regulatory cells*. These cells constitutively express the α chain of the IL-2 receptor (CD25), produce large amounts of IL-10, and can suppress both T and B cell responses. T regulatory cells are induced by immature dendritic cells and play key roles in maintaining tolerance to self-antigens in the periphery. Loss of T regulatory cells is the cause of organ-specific autoimmune disease in mice such as autoimmune thyroiditis, adrenalitis, and oophoritis (see "Immune Tolerance and Autoimmunity," below). T regulatory cells also play key roles in controlling the magnitude and duration of immune responses to microbes. Normally, after the initial immune response to a microbe has eliminated the invader, T regulatory cells are activated to suppress the anti-microbe response and prevent host injury. Some microbes have adapted to induce T regulatory cell activation at the site of infection to promote parasite infection and survival. In *Leishmania* infection, the parasite locally induces T regulatory cell accumulation at skin infection sites that dampens anti-*Leishmania* T cell responses and prevents elimination of the parasite.

FIGURE 295-10 Schematic model of intercellular interactions of adaptive immune system cells. In this figure the arrows denote that cells develop from precursor cells or produce cytokines or antibodies; lines ending with bars indicate suppressive intercellular interactions. Stem cells differentiate into either T cells, antigen-presenting dendritic cells, natural killer cells, macrophages, granulocytes, or B cells. Foreign antigen is processed by dendritic cells, and peptide fragments of foreign antigen are presented to CD4+ and/or CD8+ T cells. CD8+ T cell activation leads to induction of cytotoxic T lymphocyte (CTL) or killer T cell generation, as well as induction of cytokine-producing CD8+ cytotoxic T cells. For antibody production against the same antigen, active antigen is bound to sIg within the B cell receptor complex and drives B cell maturation into plasma cells that secrete Ig. T_H1 or T_H2 CD4+ T cells producing interleukin (IL) 4, IL-5, or interferon (IFN) γ regulate the Ig class switching and determine the type of antibody produced. CD4+, CD25+ T regulatory cells produce IL-10 and downregulate T and B cell responses once the microbe has been eliminated. GM-CSF, granulocyte-macrophage colony stimulating factor; TNF, tumor necrosis factor.

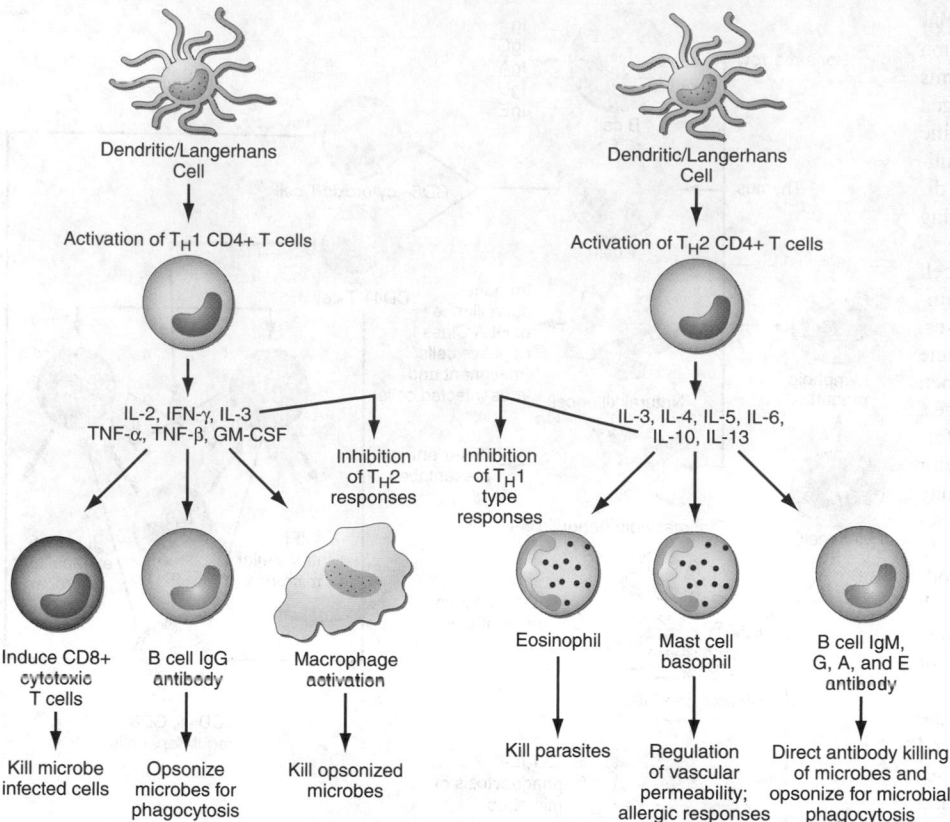

Immune tolerance is defined as the absence of activation of pathogenic autoreactivity. *Autoimmune diseases* are syndromes caused by the activation of T or B cells or both, with no evidence of other causes such as infections or malignancies (Chap. 299). Once thought to be mutually exclusive, immune tolerance and autoimmunity are now both recognized to be present normally in health, and when abnormal, represent extremes from the normal state. For example, it is now known that low levels of autoreactivity of T and B cells with self-antigens in the periphery are critical to their survival. Similarly, low levels of autoreactivity and thymocyte recognition of self-antigens in the thymus are the mechanisms whereby (1) normal T cells are positively selected to survive and leave the thymus to respond to foreign microbes in the periphery, and (2) T cells highly reactive to self-antigens are negatively selected and die to prevent overly self-reactive T cells from getting into the periphery (central tolerance). However, not all self-antigens are expressed in the thymus to delete highly self-reactive T cells, and there are mechanisms for peripheral tolerance induction of T cells as well. Unlike the presentation of microbial antigens by mature dendritic cells, the presentation of self-antigens by immature dendritic cells neither activates nor matures the dendritic cells to express high levels of co-stimulatory molecules such as B7-1 (CD80) or B7-2 (CD86). When

FIGURE 295-11 CD4+ helper T 1 (T$_H$1) cells and T$_H$2 T cells secrete distinct but overlapping sets of cytokines. T$_H$1 CD4+ cells are frequently activated in immune and inflammatory reactions against intracellular bacteria or viruses, while T$_H$2 CD4+ cells are frequently activated for certain types of antibody production against parasites and extracellular encapsulated bacteria; they are also activated in allergic diseases. GM-CSF, granulocyte-macrophage colony stimulating factor; IFN, interferon; IL, interleukin; TNF, tumor necrosis factor. [*Adapted from S Romagnani: CD4 effector cells, in J Gallin, R Snyderman (eds): Inflammation: Basic Principles and Clinical Correlates, 3d ed. Philadelphia, Lippincott Williams & Wilkins, 1999; with permission.*]

It is thought that many chronic infections such as by *M. tuberculosis* are associated with abnormal T regulatory cell activation that prevents elimination of the microbe.

Although B cells recognize native antigen via B cell surface Ig receptors, B cells require T cell help to produce high-affinity antibody of multiple isotypes that are the most effective in eliminating foreign antigen. This T cell dependence likely functions in the regulation of B cell responses and in protection against excessive autoantibody production. T cell–B cell interactions that lead to high-affinity antibody production require: (1) processing of native antigen by B cells and expression of peptide fragments on the B cell surface for presentation to T$_H$ cells, (2) the ligation of B cells both by the TCR complex and the CD40 ligand, (3) induction of the process termed *antibody isotype switching* in antigen-specific B cell clones, and (4) induction of the process of *affinity maturation* of antibody in the germinal centers of B cell follicles of lymph node and spleen.

Naive B cells express cell-surface IgD and IgM, and initial contact of naive B cells with antigen is via binding of native antigen to B cell–surface IgM. T cell cytokines, released following T$_H$2 cell contact with B cells or by a "bystander" effect, induce changes in Ig gene conformation that promote recombination of Ig genes. These events then result in the "switching" of expression of heavy chain exons in a triggered B cell, leading to the secretion of IgG, IgA, or, in some cases, IgE antibody with the same V region antigen specificity as the original IgM antibody, for response to a wide variety of extracellular bacteria, protozoa, and helminths. CD40 ligand expression by activated T cells is critical for induction of B cell antibody isotype switching and for B cell responsiveness to cytokines. Patients with mutations in T cell CD40 ligand have B cells that are unable to undergo isotype switching, resulting in lack of memory B cell generation and the immunodeficiency syndrome of *X-linked hyper-IgM syndrome* (Chap. 297).

peripheral T cells are stimulated by dendritic cells expressing self-antigens in the context of HLA molecules, sufficient stimulation of T cells occurs to keep them alive, but otherwise they remain anergic, or nonresponsive, until they contact a dendritic cell with high levels of co-stimulatory molecules expressing microbial antigens. In the latter setting, normal T cells then become activated to respond to the microbe. If B cells have high self-reactivity BCRs, they normally undergo receptor editing to express a less autoreactive receptor or are induced to die. Although many autoimmune diseases are characterized by the abnormal or pathogenic autoantibody production (Table 295-11), most autoimmune diseases are caused by a combination of excess T and B cell reactivity.

Multiple factors contribute to the genesis of clinical autoimmune disease syndromes including genetic susceptibility (Table 295-12), environmental immune stimulants such as drugs (e.g., procainamide and dilantin with drug-induced systemic lupus erythematosus), infectious agent triggers (such as Epstein-Barr virus and autoantibody production against red blood cells and platelets), and loss of T regulatory cells (leading to thyroiditis, adrenalitis, and oophoritis).

THE CELLULAR AND MOLECULAR CONTROL OF PROGRAMMED CELL DEATH The process of apoptosis (programmed cell death) plays a crucial role in regulating normal immune responses to antigen. In general, a wide variety of stimuli trigger one of several apoptotic pathways to eliminate microbe-infected cells, eliminate cells with damaged DNA, or eliminate activated immune cells that are no longer needed (Fig. 295-12). The largest known family of "death receptors" are the tumor necrosis factor receptor (TNF-R) family [TNF-R1, TNF-R2, Fas (CD95), death receptor 3 (DR3), death receptor 4 (TRAIL-R1), and death receptor 5 (DR5, TRAIL-R2)]; their ligands are all in the TNF-α family. Binding of ligands to these death receptors leads to a signaling cascade

Autoantigen	Autoimmune Diseases	Autoantigen	Autoimmune Diseases
CELL- OR ORGAN-SPECIFIC AUTOIMMUNITY			
Acetylcholine receptor	Myasthenia gravis	Insulin receptor	Type B insulin resistance, acanthosis, systemic lupus erythematosus (SLE)
Actin	Chronic active hepatitis, primary bilary cirrhosis	Intrinsic factor type 1	Pernicious anemia
Adenine nucleotide translator (ANT)	Dilated cardiomyopathy, myocarditis	Leukocyte function-associated antigen (LFA-1)	Treatment-resistant Lyme arthritis
β-Adrenoreceptor	Dilated cardiomyopathy	Myelin-associated glycoprotein (MAG)	Polyneuropathy
Aromatic L-amino acid decarboxylase	Autoimmune polyendocrine syndrome type 1 (APS-1)	Myelin-basic protein	Multiple sclerosis, demyelinating diseases
Asialoglycoprotein receptor	Autoimmune hepatitis	Myelin oligodendrocyte glycoprotein (MOG)	Multiple sclerosis
Bactericidal/permeability-increasing protein (Bpi)	Cystic fibrosis vasculitides	Myosin	Rheumatic fever
Calcium-sensing receptor	Acquired hypoparathyroidism	p-80-Collin	Atopic dermatitis
Cholesterol side-chain cleavage enzyme (CYPlla)	Autoimmune polyglandular syndrome-1	Pyruvate dehydrogenase complex-E2 (PDC-E2)	Primary biliary cirrhosis
Collagen type IV-α3-chain	Goodpasture syndrome	Sodium iodide symporter (NIS)	Graves' disease, autoimmune hypothyroidism
Cytochrome P450 2D6 (CYP2D6)	Autoimmune hepatitis	SOX-10	Vitiligo
Desmin	Crohn disease, coronary artery disease	Thyroid and eye muscle shared protein	Thyroid-associated ophthalmopathy
Desmoglein 1	Pemphigus foliaceus	Thyroglobulin	Autoimmune thyroiditis
Desmoglein 3	Pemphigus vulgaris	Thyroid peroxidase	Autoimmune Hashimoto thyroiditis
F-actin	Autoimmune hepatitis	Throtropin receptor	Graves' disease
GM gangliosides	Guillain-Barré syndrome	Tissue transglutaminase	Celiac disease
Glutamate decarboxylase (GAD65)	Type 1 diabetes, stiff man syndrome	Transcription coactivator p75	Atopic dermatitis
Glutamate receptor (GLUR)	Rasmussen encephalitis	Tryptophan hydroxylase	Autoimmune polyglandular syndrome-1
H/K ATPase	Autoimmune gastritis	Tyrosinase	Vitiligo, metastatic melanoma
17-α-Hydroxylase (CYP17)	Autoimmune polyglandular syndrome-1	Tyrosine hydroxylase	Autoimmune polyglandular syndrome-1
21-Hydroxylase (CYP21)	Addison disease		
IA-2 (ICA512)	Type 1 diabetes		
Insulin	Type 1 diabetes, insulin hypoglycemic syndrome (Hirata disease)		
SYSTEMIC AUTOIMMUNITY			
ACTH	ACTH deficiency	Histone H2A-H2B-DNA	SLE
Aminoacyl-tRAN histidyl synthetase	Myositis, dermatomyositis	IgE receptor	Chronic idiopathic urticaria
Aminoacyl-tRNA synthetase (several)	Polymyositis, dermatomyositis	Keratin	RA
Cardiolipin	SLE	Ku-DNA-protein kinase	SLE
Carbonic anhydrase II	SLE, Sjögren syndrome, systemic sclerosis	Ku-nucleoprotein	Connective tissue syndrome
Collagen (multiple types)	Rheumatoid arthritis (RA), SLE, progressive systemic sclerosis	La phosphoprotein (La 55-B)	Sjögren syndrome
Centromere-associated proteins	Systemic sclerosis	Myeloperoxidase	Necrotizing and crescentic glomerulonephritis (NCGN), systemic vasculitis
DNA-dependent nucleosine-stimulated ATPase	Dermatomyositis	Proteinase 3 (PR3)	Wegener granulomatosis, Churg-Strauss syndrome
Fibrillarin	Scleroderma	RNA polymerase I–III (RNP)	Systemic sclerosis, SLE
Fibronectin	SLE, RA, morphea	Signal recognition protein (SRP54)	Polymyositis
Glucose-6-phosphate isomerase	RA	Topoisomerase-1 (Scl-70)	Scleroderma, Raynaud syndrome
β2-Glycoprotein I (B2-GPI)	Primary antiphospholipid syndrome	Tublin	Chronic liver disease, visceral leishmaniasis
Golgin (95, 97, 160, 180)	Sjögren syndrome, SLE, RA	Vimentin	Systemic autoimmune disease
Heat shock protein	Various immune-related disorders		
Hemidesmosomal protein 180	Bullous pemphigoid, herpes gastationis, cicatricial pemphigoid		
PLASMA PROTEIN AND CYTOKINE AUTOIMMUNITY			
C1 inhibitor	Autoimmune C1 deficiency	Glycoprotein IIb/IIIg and Ib/IX	Autoimmune thrombocytopenia purpura
C1q	SLE, membrane proliferative glomerulonephritis (MPGN)	IgA	Immunodeficiency associated with SLE, pernicious anemia, thyroiditis, Sjögren's syndrome and chronic active hepatitis
Cytokines (IL-1α, IL-1β, IL-6, IL-10, LIF)	RA, systemic sclerosis, normal subjects		
Factor II, factor V, factor VII, factor VIII, factor IX, factor X, factor XI, thrombin vWF	Prolonged coagulation time	Oxidized LDL (OxLDL)	Atherosclerosis
CANCER AND PARANEOPLASTIC AUTOIMMUNITY			
Amphiphysin	Neuropathy, small-cell lung cancer	p62 (IGF-II mRNA-binding protein)	Hepatocellular carcinoma (China)
Cyclin B1	Hepatocellular carcinoma	Recoverin	Cancer-associated retinopathy
DNA topoisomerase II	Liver cancer	Ri protein	Paraneoplastic opsoclonus myoclonus ataxia
Desmoplakin	Paraneoplastic pemphigus		
Gephyrin	Paraneoplastic stiff man syndrome	βIV spectrin	Lower motor neuron syndrome
Hu proteins	Paraneoplastic encephalomyclitis	Synaptotagmin	Lambert-Eaton myasthenic syndrome
Neuronal nicotinic acetylcholine receptor	Subacute autonomic neuropathy, cancer	Voltage-gated calcium channels	Lambert-Eaton myasthenic syndrome
p53	Cancer, SLE	Yo protein	Paraneoplastic cerebellar degeneration

Source: From A Lernmark et al: J Clin Invest 108:1091, 2001; with permission.

TABLE 295-12 *Immune System Molecule Defects in Animals or Humans that Cause Autoimmune or Malignant Syndromes*

Protein	Defect	Disease or Syndrome	Observation in Animal Models or Humans
CYTOKINES AND SIGNALING PROTEINS			
Tumor necrosis factor (TNF) α	Overexpression	Inflammatory bowel disease (IBD), arthritis, vasculitis	Mice
TNF-α	Underexpression	Systemic lupus erythematosus (SLE)	Mice
Interleukin-1-receptor antagonist	Underexpression	Arthritis	Mice
IL-2	Overexpression	IBD	Mice
IL-7	Overexpression	IBD	Mice
IL-10	Overexpression	IBD	Mice
IL-2 receptor	Overexpression	IBD	Mice
IL-10 receptor	Overexpression	IBD	Mice
IL-3	Overexpression	Demyelinating syndrome	Mice
Interferon-δ	Overexpression in skin	SLE	Mice
STAT-3	Underexpression	IBD	Mice
STAT-4	Overexpression	IBD	Mice
Transforming growth factor (TGF) β	Underexpression	Systemic wasting syndrome and IBD	Mice
TGF-β receptor in T cells	Underexpression	SLE	Mice
Programmed death (PD-1)	Underexpression	SLE-like syndrome	Mice
Cytotoxic T lymphocyte, antigen-4 (CTLA-4)	Underexpression	Systemic lymphoproliferative disease	Mice
IL-10	Underexpression	IBD (mouse) Type 1 diabetes, thyroid disease, primary (human)	Mice and humans
MAJOR HISTOCOMPATIBILITY LOCUS MOLECULES[a]			
HLA B27	Allele expression or over-expression	Inflammatory bowel disease	Rats and humans
Complement deficiency of C1,2,3 or 4	Underexpression	See Table 305-13	Humans
LIGHT (TNF superfamily 14)	Overexpression	Systemic lymphoproliferative (mouse) and autoimmunity	Mice
HLA class II DQB10301, DQB10302	Allele expression	Juvenile-onset diabetes	Human
HLA class II DQB10401, DQB10402	Allele expression	Rheumatoid arthritis	Humans
HLA class I B27	Allele expression	Ankylosing spondylitis, IBD	Rats and humans
APOPTOSIS PROTEINS			
TNFactor receptor 1 (TNF-R1)	Underexpression	Familial periodic fever syndrome	Humans
Fas (CD95; Apo-1)	Underexpression	Autoimmune lymphoproliferative syndrome type 1 (ALPS 1); malignant lymphoma; bladder cancer	Humans
Fas ligand	Underexpression	SLE (only one case identified)	Humans
Perforin	Underexpression	Familial hemophagocytic lymphohistiocytosis (FHL)	Humans
Caspase 10	Underexpression	Autoimmune lymphoproliferative syndrome type II (ALPS II)	Humans
bcl-10	Underexpression	Non-Hodgkin's lymphoma	Humans
P53	Underexpression	Various malignant neoplasms	Humans
Bax	Underexpression	Colon cancer; hematopoietic malignancies	Humans
bcl-2	Underexpression	Non-Hodgkin's lymphoma	Humans
c-IAP2	Underexpression	Low-grade MALT lymphoma	Humans
NAIP1	Underexpression	Spinal muscular atrophy	Humans

[a] Many autoimmune diseases are associated with a myriad of major compatibility complex gene allele (HLA) types. There are presented here as examples.
Note: MALT, mucosa-associated lymphoid tissue.

Source: Adopted from L Mullauer et al: Mutat Res 488:211, 2001; A Davidson, B Diamond: N Engl J Med 345:340, 2001; with permission.

that involves activation of the *caspase* family of molecules that leads to DNA cleavage and cell death. Two other pathways of programmed cell death involve nuclear *p53* in the elimination of cells with abnormal DNA and *mitochondrial cytochrome c* to induce cell death in damaged cells (Fig. 295-12). A number of human diseases have now been described that result from, or are associated with, mutated apoptosis genes (Table 295-12). These include mutations in the TNF-R1 in *hereditary periodic fever (familial Mediterranean fever)* (Chap. 279), Fas and Fas ligand in autoimmune and lymphoproliferation syndromes, and multiple associations of mutations in genes in the apoptotic pathway with malignant syndromes.

MECHANISMS OF IMMUNE-MEDIATED DAMAGE TO MICROBES OR HOST TISSUES

Several responses by the host innate and adaptive immune systems to foreign microbes culminate in rapid and efficient elimination of microbes. In these scenarios, the classic weapons of the adaptive immune system (T cells, B cells) interface with cells (macrophages, dendritic cells, NK cells, neutrophils, eosinophils, basophils) and soluble products (microbial peptides, pentraxins, complement and coagulation systems) of the innate immune system (Chaps. 55 and 298).

There are five general phases of host defenses: (1) migration of leukocytes to sites of antigen localization; (2) antigen-nonspecific recognition of pathogens by macrophages and other cells and systems of the innate immune system; (3) specific recognition of foreign antigens mediated by T and B lymphocytes; (4) amplification of the inflammatory response with recruitment of specific and nonspecific effector cells by complement components, cytokines, kinins, arachidonic acid metabolites, and mast cell–basophil products; and (5) macrophage, neutrophil, and lymphocyte participation in destruction of antigen with ultimate removal of antigen particles by phagocytosis (by macrophages or neutrophils) or by direct cytotoxic mechanisms (involving macrophages, neutrophils, and lymphocytes). Under normal circumstances, orderly progression of host defenses through these phases results in a well-controlled immune and inflammatory response that protects the host from the offending antigen. However, dysfunction of any of the host defense systems can damage host tissue and produce clinical disease. Furthermore, for certain pathogens or antigens, the normal immune response itself might contribute substantially to the tissue damage. For example, the immune and inflammatory response in the brain to certain pathogens such as *M. tuberculosis* may be responsible for much of the morbidity of this disease in that organ system (Chap. 150). In addition, the morbidity associated with certain pneumonias such as that caused by *Pneumocystis carinii* may be associated more with inflammatory infiltrates than with the tissue destructive effects of the microorganism itself (Chap. 191).

The Molecular Basis of Lymphocyte–Endothelial Cell Interactions The control of lymphocyte circulatory patterns between the bloodstream and peripheral lymphoid organs operates at the level of lymphocyte–endothelial cell interactions to control the specificity of lymphocyte subset entry into organs. Similarly, lymphocyte–endothelial cell interactions regulate the entry of lymphocytes into inflamed tissue. Adhesion molecule expression on lymphocytes and endothelial cells regulates the retention and subsequent egress of lymphocytes within tissue sites of antigenic stimulation, delaying cell exit from tissue and preventing reentry into the circulating lymphocyte pool. All types of lymphocyte migration begin with lymphocyte attachment to specialized regions of vessels, termed *high endothelial venules* (HEVs). An important concept is that adhesion molecules do not generally bind their ligand until a conformational change (ligand activation) occurs in the adhesion molecule that allows ligand binding. Induction of a conformation-dependent determinant on an adhesion molecule can be accomplished by cytokines or via ligation of other adhesion molecules on the cell.

The first stage of lymphocyte–endothelial cell interactions, *attachment and rolling*, occurs when lymphocytes leave the stream of flowing blood cells in a postcapillary venule and roll along venule endothelial cells (Fig. 295-13). Lymphocyte rolling is mediated by the L-selectin molecule (LECAM-1, LAM-1, CD62L) and slows cell transit time through venules, allowing time for activation of adherent cells.

The second stage of lymphocyte–endothelial cell interactions, *firm adhesion with activation-dependent stable arrest*, requires stimulation of lymphocytes by chemoattractants or by endothelial cell–derived cytokines. Cytokines thought to participate in adherent cell activation include members of the IL-8 family, platelet-activation factor, leukotriene B$_4$, and C5a. Following activation by chemoattractants, lymphocytes shed L-selectin from the cell surface and upregulate cell CD11b/18 (MAC-1) or CD11a/18 (LFA-1) molecules, resulting in firm attachment of lymphocytes to HEVs.

Lymphocyte homing to peripheral lymph nodes involves adhesion of L-selectin to carbohydrate of peripheral node HEVs, whereas homing of lymphocytes to intestine Peyer's patches primarily involves adhesion of the $\alpha 4, \beta 7$ integrin to MAdCAM-1 oligosaccharides on the Peyer's patch HEVs. However, for migration to mucosal Peyer's patch lymphoid aggregates, naive lymphocytes primarily use L-selectin, whereas memory lymphocytes use $\alpha 4, \beta 7$ integrin. $\alpha 4, \beta 1$ integrin (CD49d/CD29, VLA-4)–VCAM-1 interactions are important in the initial

FIGURE 295-12 Scheme of major apoptosis pathways. DD, death domain; DED, death effector domain. (*From L Mullauer et al: Mutat Res 488:211, 2001; with permission.*)

interaction of memory lymphocytes with HEVs of multiple organs in sites of inflammation.

The third stage of leukocyte emigration in HEVs is *sticking and arrest*. Sticking of the lymphocyte to endothelial cells and arrest at the site of sticking are mediated predominantly by ligation of $\alpha L, \beta 2$ integrin LFA-1 to the integrin ligand ICAM-1 on HEVs. While the first three stages of lymphocyte attachment to HEVs takes only a few seconds, the fourth stage of lymphocyte emigration, *transendothelial migration*, takes ~10 min. Although the molecular mechanisms that control lymphocyte transendothelial migration are not fully characterized, the HEV CD44 molecule and molecules of the HEV glycocalyx (extracellular matrix) are thought to play important regulatory roles in this process (Fig. 295-13). Finally, expression of matrix metalloproteases capable of digesting the subendothelial basement membrane,

FIGURE 295-13 Schematic of the multistep model of leukocyte migration in high endothelial venules (HEV). The initial interaction of lymphocytes with HEV in peripheral lymph nodes is mediated by L-selectin (CD62L) that recognizes HEV mucin-like counterreceptors such as glycosylation-dependent cell adhesion molecule 1 (GlyCAM-1). Activation of lymphocyte adhesiveness occurs via G protein–coupled receptors (GPCR) that bind to chemokines anchored to endothelial cells by glycoaminoglycans (GAG). The integrin leukocyte function–associated molecule 1 (LFA-1) and very late antigen-4 (VLA-4) and their HEV counterreceptors, intercellular adhesion molecule 1 (ICAM-1; CD54) play a major role in lymphocyte arrest in HEV. The molecular mechanisms of lymphocyte extravasations are not completely worked out. (*From DD Patel, BF Haynes: Curr Dir Autoimmun 3:133, 2001; with permission.*)

rich in nonfibrillar collagen, appears to be required for the penetration of lymphoid cells into the extravascular sites.

Abnormal induction of HEV formation and use of the molecules discussed above have been implicated in the induction and maintenance of inflammation in a number of chronic inflammatory diseases. In animal models of type 1 diabetes mellitus, MAdCAM-1 and GlyCAM-1 have been shown to be highly expressed on HEVs in inflamed pancreatic islets, and treatment of these animals with inhibitors of L-selectin and $\alpha4$ integrin function blocked the development of type 1 diabetes mellitus (Chap. 323). A similar role for abnormal induction of the adhesion molecules of lymphocyte emigration has been suggested in *rheumatoid arthritis* (Chap. 301), *Hashimoto's thyroiditis* (Chap. 320), *Graves' disease* (Chap. 320), *multiple sclerosis* (Chap. 262), *Crohn's disease* (Chap. 276), and *ulcerative colitis* (Chap. 276).

Immune-Complex Formation Clearance of antigen by immune-complex formation between antigen and antibody is a highly effective mechanism of host defense. However, depending on the level of immune complexes formed and their physicochemical properties, immune complexes may or may not result in host and foreign cell damage. After antigen exposure, certain types of soluble antigen-antibody complexes freely circulate and, if not cleared by the reticuloendothelial system, can be deposited in blood vessel walls and in other tissues such as renal glomeruli and cause *vasculitis* or *glomerulonephritis* syndromes (Chaps. 264 and 306).

Immediate-Type Hypersensitivity Helper T cells that drive anti-allergen IgE responses are usually T_H2-type inducer T cells that secrete IL-4, IL-5, IL-6, and IL-10. Mast cells and basophils have high-affinity receptors for the Fc portion of IgE (FcRI), and cell-bound antiallergen IgE effectively "arms" basophils and mast cells. Mediator release is triggered by antigen (allergen) interaction with Fc receptor–bound IgE; the mediators released are responsible for the pathophysiologic changes of *allergic diseases* (Table 295-6). Mediators released from mast cells and basophils can be divided into three broad functional types: (1) those that increase vascular permeability and contract smooth muscle (histamine, platelet-activating factor, SRS-A, BK-A), (2) those that are chemotactic for or activate other inflammatory cells (ECF-A, NCF, leukotriene B$_4$), and (3) those that modulate the release of other mediators (BK-A, platelet-activating factor) (Chap. 298).

Cytotoxic Reactions of Antibody In this type of immunologic injury, complement-fixing (C1-binding) antibodies against normal or foreign cells or tissues (IgM, IgG1, IgG2, IgG3) bind complement via the classic pathway and initiate a sequence of events similar to that initiated by immune-complex deposition, resulting in cell lysis or tissue injury. Examples of antibody-mediated cytotoxic reactions include red cell lysis in *transfusion reactions*, *Goodpasture's syndrome* with anti-glomerular basement membrane antibody formation, and *pemphigus vulgaris* with antiepidermal antibodies inducing blistering skin disease.

Classic Delayed-Type Hypersensitivity Reactions Inflammatory reactions initiated by mononuclear leukocytes and not by antibody alone have been termed *delayed-type hypersensitivity reactions*. The term *delayed* has been used to contrast a secondary cellular response that appears 48 to 72 h after antigen exposure with an *immediate* hypersensitivity response generally seen within 12 h of antigen challenge and initiated by basophil mediator release or preformed antibody. For example, in an individual previously infected with *M. tuberculosis* organisms, intradermal placement of tuberculin purified-protein derivative as a skin test challenge results in an indurated area of skin at 48 to 72 h, indicating previous exposure to tuberculosis.

The cellular events that result in classic delayed-type hypersensitivity responses are centered around T cells (predominantly, though not exclusively, IFN-γ, IL-2, and TNF-α-secreting T_H1-type helper T cells) and macrophages. First, local immune and inflammatory responses at the site of foreign antigen upregulate endothelial cell adhesion molecule expression, promoting the accumulation of lymphocytes at the tissue site. In the general scheme outlined in Figs. 295-10 and 295-11, antigen is processed by dendritic cells and presented to small numbers of CD4+ T cells expressing a TCR specific for the antigen. IL-12 produced by APCs induces T cells to produce IFN-γ (T_H-1 response). Macrophages frequently undergo epithelioid cell transformation and fuse to form multinucleated giant cells in response to IFN-γ. This type of mononuclear cell infiltrate is termed *granulomatous inflammation*. Examples of diseases in which delayed-type hypersensitivity plays a major role are fungal infections (*histoplasmosis*; Chap. 183), mycobacterial infections (*tuberculosis, leprosy*; Chaps. 150 and 151), chlamydial infections (*lymphogranuloma venereum*; Chap. 160), helminth infections (*schistosomiasis*; Chap. 203), reactions to toxins (*berylliosis*; Chap. 238), and hypersensitivity reactions to organic dusts (*hypersensitivity pneumonitis*; Chap. 237). In addition, delayed-type hypersensitivity responses play important roles in tissue damage in autoimmune diseases such as *rheumatoid arthritis*, *temporal arteritis*, and *Wegener's granulomatosis* (Chaps. 301 and 306).

CLINICAL EVALUATION OF IMMUNE FUNCTION Clinical assessment of immunity requires investigation of the four major components of the immune system that participate in host defense and in the pathogenesis of autoimmune diseases: (1) humoral immunity (B cells); (2) cell-mediated immunity (T cells, monocytes); (3) phagocytic cells of the reticuloendothelial system (macrophages), as well as polymorphonuclear leukocytes; and (4) complement. Clinical problems that require an evaluation of immunity include chronic infections, recurrent infection, unusual infecting agents, and certain autoimmune syndromes. The type of clinical syndrome under evaluation can provide information regarding possible immune defects (Chap. 297). Defects in cellular immunity generally result in viral, mycobacterial, and fungal infections. An extreme example of deficiency in cellular immunity is *AIDS* (Chap. 173). Antibody deficiencies result in recurrent bacterial infections, frequently with organisms such as *S. pneumoniae* and *Haemophilus influenzae* (Chap. 297). Disorders of phagocyte function are frequently manifested by recurrent skin infections, often due to *Staphylococcus aureus* (Chap. 55). Finally, deficiencies of early and late complement components are associated with autoimmune phenomena and recurrent *Neisseria* infections (Table 295-13). →*For further discussion of useful initial screening tests of immune function, see Chap. 297.*

IMMUNOTHERAPY Most current therapies for autoimmune and inflammatory diseases involve the use of nonspecific immune-modulating or

TABLE 295-13 *Complement Deficiencies and Associated Diseases*

Component	Associated Diseases
CLASSIC PATHWAY	
C1q, C1r, C1s, C4	Immune-complex syndromes,[a] pyogenic infections
C2	Immune-complex syndromes,[a] few with pyogenic infections
C1 inhibitor	Rare immune-complex disease, few with pyogenic infections
C3 AND ALTERNATIVE PATHWAY C3	
C3	Immune-complex syndromes,[a] pyogenic infections
D	Pyogenic infections
Properdin	*Neisseria* infections
I	Pyogenic infections
H	Hemolytic uremic syndrome
MEMBRANE ATTACK COMPLEX	
C5, C6, C7, C8	Recurrent *Neisseria* infections, immune-complex disease
C9	Rare *Neisseria* infections

[a] Immune-complex syndromes include systemic lupus erythematosus (SLE) and SLE-like syndromes, glomerulonephritis, and vasculitis syndromes.
Source: After JA Schifferli and DK Peters, Lancet 88:957, 1983; with permission.

immunosuppressive agents such as glucocorticoids or cytotoxic drugs. The goal of development of new treatments for immune-mediated diseases is to design ways to specifically interrupt pathologic immune responses, leaving nonpathologic immune responses intact. Novel ways to interrupt pathologic immune responses that are under investigation include: the use of anti-inflammatory cytokines or specific cytokine inhibitors as anti-inflammatory agents; the use of monoclonal antibodies against T or B lymphocytes as therapeutic agents; the induction of anergy by administration of soluble CTLA-4 protein; the use of intravenous Ig for certain infections and immune complex–mediated diseases; the use of specific cytokines to reconstitute components of the immune system; and bone marrow transplantation to replace the pathogenic immune system with a more normal immune system (Table 295-14) (Chaps. 55, 297, and 173).

Cytokines and Cytokine Inhibitors Recently a humanized mouse anti-TNF-α monoclonal antibody (MAb) has been tested in both rheumatoid arthritis and ulcerative colitis. Use of anti-TNF-α antibody therapy has resulted in clinical improvement in patients with these diseases and has opened the way for targeting TNF-α to treat other severe forms of autoimmune and/or inflammatory disease. Blockage of TNF-α has been effective in *rheumatoid arthritis, psoriasis, Crohn's disease*, and

ankylosing spondylitis. Anti-TNF-α MAb (infliximab) has been approved for treatment of patients with rheumatoid arthritis.

Other cytokine inhibitors under investigation are recombinant soluble TNF-α receptor (R) fused to human Ig and soluble IL-1 receptor (termed *IL-1 receptor antagonist*, or IL-1 ra). Soluble TNF-αR (etanercept) and IL-1 ra act to inhibit the activity of pathogenic cytokines in rheumatoid arthritis, i.e., TNF-α and IL-1, respectively. Similarly, anti-IL-6, IFN-β, and IL-11 act to inhibit pathogenic proinflammatory cytokines. Anti-IL-6 inhibits IL-6 activity, while IFN-β and IL-11 decrease IL-1 and TNF-α production.

Recent studies have identified mutations in the IL-12 gene in patients susceptible to severe myobacterial infections. IL-12 is a critical cytokine for induction of IFN-γ and cytotoxic T lymphocytes (CTLs) against intracellular organisms; it is under study for treatment of severe infections such as that caused by *M. tuberculosis* and for treatment of various cancers. In this latter setting, IL-12 is being studied for its ability to enhance antitumor cellular immunity by enhancing the induction of antitumor CTL.

Of particular note has been the successful use of IFN-γ in the treat-

---

TABLE 295-14 *Current Status of Development of Immunomodulatory Agents*

Agents	Rationale	Status
CYTOKINES AND CYTOKINE INHIBITORS TO INHIBIT IMMUNE RESPONSES AND INFLAMMATION		
Anti-TNF-α monoclonal antibody: Humanized mouse chimeric MAb, infliximab Fully humanized MAb, adalimumab	Inhibit TNF-α	FDA approved for rheumatoid arthritis, Crohn's colitis (infliximab); FDA approved for rheumatoid arthritis (adalimumab)
Recombinant TNF-receptor-Ig fusion protein (etanercept)	Inhibit TNF-α	FDA approved for rheumatoid arthritis, juvenile rheumatoid arthritis, psoriasis
Recombinant IL-1 receptor antagonist (IL-1Ra) (anakinra)	Inhibit IL-1α and -β	FDA approved for rheumatoid arthritis
Anti-IL-6 monoclonal antibody	Inhibit IL-6	Tested in phase I trial in rheumatoid arthritis
Interferon-β	Inhibit IL-1, decrease synovial T cells	In trials for use in rheumatoid arthritis
Interferon-γ	Induce monocyte/macrophage activation	Effective in treating monocyte/macrophage phagocytic defects in chronic granulomatous disease
IL-11	Inhibit TNF-α and IL-1 production	In trials for Crohn's colitis
IL-12	Stimulate anti-tumor and anti-viral or bacterial cytotoxic T lymphocyte responses	Trials underway for use in cancer patients; trials planned in humans to prevent/treat severe infections
MONOCLONAL ANTIBODIES AGAINST T OR B CELLS		
Anti-CD3 anti-T cell monoclonal antibody	Inhibit T cell function; induce T cell lymphopenia	FDA approved for treatment of cardiac and renal allograft rejection
Anti-CD4 monoclonal antibody	Inhibit CD4+ T cell function	In trials for rheumatoid arthritis
Anti-CD40 ligand (CD154) monoclonal antibody	Inhibit CD40-CD40 ligand interaction; induces T cell tolerance	In primate trials for prevention of renal allograft rejection
SOLUBLE T CELL MOLECULE		
Soluble CTLA-4 protein	Inhibit CD28-B7-1 and B7-2 interactions; induce tolerance to organ grafts; inhibit autoimmune T cell reactivity in autoimmune diseases	In trials for preventing GVHD in bone marrow transplantation and for treatment of psoriasis
INTRAVENOUS IMMUNOGLOBULIN		
IVIg	Reticuloendothelial cell blockage; complement inhibition; regulation of idiotype/anti-idiotype antibodies; modulation of cytokine production; modulation of lymphocyte production	FDA approved for Kawasaki's disease and immune thrombocytopenia purpura; treatment of GVHD, multiple sclerosis, myasthenia gravis, Guillain-Barré syndrome, and chronic inflammatory demyelinating polyneuropathy supported by clinical trials
CYTOKINES FOR IMMUNE RECONSTITUTION		
IL-2	Induce proliferation of peripheral memory CD4+ and CD8+ T cells	In trial for treatment of HIV infection
IL-7	Induce renewed thymopoiesis	Under consideration for treatment of diseases associated with T cell deficiency
HEMATOPOIETIC STEM CELL TRANSPLANTATION		
Hematopoietic stem transplantation for immune reconstitution	Remove pathologic autoreactive immune system and replace with less autoreactive immunity	In clinical trials for systemic lupus erythematosus, multiple sclerosis, and scleroderma

Note: FDA, US Food and Drug Administration; GVHD, graft-versus-host disease.

ment of the phagocytic cell defect in *chronic granulomatous disease* (Chap. 55). Intermittent infusions of IL-2 in HIV-infected individuals in the early or intermediate stages of disease have resulted in substantial and sustained increases in CD4+ T cells.

Monoclonal Antibodies to T and B Cells The OKT3 MAb against human T cells has been used for several years as a T cell–specific immunosuppressive agent that can substitute for horse anti-thymocyte globulin (ATG) in the treatment of solid organ transplant rejection. OKT3 produces fewer allergic reactions than ATG but does induce human anti-mouse Ig antibody—thus limiting its use. Anti-CD4 MAb therapy has been used in trials to treat patients with rheumatoid arthritis. While inducing profound immunosuppression, anti-CD4 MAb treatment also induces susceptibility to severe infections. Treatment of patients with a MAb against the T cell molecule CD40 ligand (CD154) is under investigation to induce tolerance to organ transplants, with promising results reported in animal studies.

Tolerance Induction Specific immunotherapy has moved into a new era with the introduction of soluble CTLA-4 protein into clinical trials. Use of this molecule to block T cell activation via TCR/CD28 ligation during organ or bone marrow transplantation has showed promising results in animals and in early human clinical trials. Specifically, treatment of bone marrow with CTLA-4 protein reduces rejection of the graft in HLA mismatched bone marrow transplantation. In addition, promising results with soluble CTLA-4 have been reported in the downmodulation of autoimmune T cell responses in the treatment of psoriasis.

Intravenous Immunoglobulin (IVIg) IVIg has been used successfully to block reticuloendothelial cell function and immune complex clearance in various immune cytopenias such as immune thrombocytopenia (Chap. 101). In addition, IVIg is useful for prevention of tissue damage in certain inflammatory syndromes such as Kawasaki's disease (Chap. 306) and as Ig replacement therapy for certain types of immunoglobulin deficiencies (Chap. 297). In addition, controlled clinical trials support the use of IVIg in selected patients with graft-versus-host disease, multiple sclerosis, myasthenia gravis, Guillain-Barré syndrome, and chronic demyelinating polyneuropathy (Table 295-14).

Stem Cell Transplantation Hematopoietic stem cell transplantation (SCT) is now being comprehensively studied to treat several autoimmune diseases, including systemic lupus erythematosus, multiple sclerosis, and scleroderma. The goal of immune reconstitution in autoimmune disease syndromes is to replace a dysfunctional immune system with a normally reactive immune cell repertoire. Preliminary results in patients with scleroderma and lupus have showed encouraging results. Controlled clinical trials in these three diseases are now being launched in the United States and Europe to compare the toxicity and efficacy of conventional immunosuppression therapy with that of myeloablative autologous SCT.

Thus, a number of recent insights into immune system function have spawned a new field of interventional immunotherapy and have enhanced the prospect for development of specific and nontoxic therapies for immune and inflammatory diseases.

FURTHER READING

AKIRA S et al: Toll-like receptors: Critical proteins linking innate and acquired immunity. Nat Immunol 2:675, 2001

ARMITAGE RJ et al: CD40L: A multifunctional ligand. Semin Immunol 5:401, 1993

BENSCHOP RJ, CAMBIER JC: B cell development: Signal transduction by antigen receptors and their surrogates. Curr Opin Immunol 11:143, 1999

DAVIDSON A, DIAMOND B: Autoimmune diseases. N Engl J Med 345: 340, 2001

DIAMOND B et al: The immune tolerance network and rheumatic disease: Immune tolerance comes to the clinic. Arthritis Rheum 44:1730, 2001

GLEICH GJ: Eosinophils, basophils and mast cells. J Allergy Clin Immunol 84: 1024, 1989

HAYNES BF et al: The role of the thymus in immune reconstitution in aging bone marrow transplantation and AIDS. Ann Rev Immunol, 18:529, 2000

JANEWAY CA et al (eds): *Immunobiology. The Immune System in Health and Disease*, 4th ed. New York, Garland, 1999

KOPP EB, MEDZHITOV R: The Toll-receptor family and control of innate immunity. Curr Opin Immunol 11:13, 1999

LAM K-P, RAJEWSKY K: B cell development, in *Inflammation: Basic Principles and Clinical Correlates*, 3d ed. J Gallin, R Snyderman (eds). Philadelphia, Lippincott Williams & Wilkins, 1999, pp 151–166

LIU Y-J et al: Dendritic cell lineage, plasticity and cross-regulation. Nat Immunol 2:585:2001

LONG EO et al: KIR, in Protein Reviews on the Web, at *http://www.ncbi.nlm.nih.gov/prow/guide679664748_g.htm*, 1999

MEDZHITOV R, JANEWAY CA Jr.: Innate immunity: Impact on the adaptive immune response. Curr Opin Immunol 9:4, 1997a

———, ———: Innate immunity: The virtues of a nonclonal system of recognition. Cell 91:295, 1997b

MICHAELSSON J et al: A signal peptide derived from hsp60 binds HLA-E and interferes with CD94/NKG2A Recognition. J Exp Med 196:1403, 2002

MODLIN RL et al: The Toll of innate immunity on microbial pathogens. N Engl J Med 340:1834, 1999

MORETTA A et al: Major histocompatibility complex class I–specific receptors on human natural killer and T lymphocytes. Immunol Rev 155:105, 1997

MORLEY BJ, WALPORT MJ: *The Complement Facts Books*. London, Academic Press, Chap 2, 2000

PATEL DD, HAYNES BF: Leukocyte homing to synovium. Curr Dir Autoimmun 3:133, 2001

PULENDRAN B et al: Modulating the immune response with dendritic cells and their growth factors. Trends Immunol 22:41, 2001

SAKAGUCHI S: Regulatory T cells: Mediating compromises between host and parasite. Nature Immunol 4:10, 2003

SCHRADER JW: Interleukin is as interleukin does. Trends Immunol 23:573, 2002

SHEVACH EM: Regulatory T cells in autoimmunity. Annu Rev Immunol 18: 423, 2000

SHINKAI K et al: Helper T cells regulate type-2 innate immunity in vivo. Nature 420:825, 2002

296 THE MAJOR HISTOCOMPATIBILITY GENE COMPLEX
Gerald T. Nepom, Joel D. Taurog

THE HLA COMPLEX AND ITS PRODUCTS

The human major histocompatibility complex (MHC), commonly called the human leukocyte antigen (HLA) complex, is a 4-megabase (Mb) region on chromosome 6 (6p21.3) that is densely packed with expressed genes. The best known of these genes are the HLA class I and class II genes, whose products are critical for immunologic specificity and transplantation histocompatibility, and they play a major role in susceptibility to a number of autoimmune diseases. Many other genes in the HLA region are also essential to the innate and antigen-specific functioning of the immune system. The HLA region shows extensive conservation with the MHC of other mammals in terms of genomic organization, gene sequence, and protein structure and function. Much of our understanding of the MHC has come from investigation of the MHC in mice, which is termed the *H-2 complex*, and to a lesser degree from other species as well. Nonetheless, in this chapter discussion will be confined to information applicable to the MHC in humans.

The *HLA class I genes* are located in a 2-Mb stretch of DNA at the telomeric end of the HLA region (Fig. 296-1). The classic (MHC class Ia) HLA-A, -B, and -C loci, the products of which are integral participants in the immune response to intracellular infections, tumors, and allografts, are expressed in all nucleated cells and are highly polymorphic in the population. *Polymorphism* refers to a high degree of allelic variation within a genetic locus that leads to extensive variation between different individuals expressing different alleles. Over 260 alleles at HLA-A, 500 at HLA-B, and 125 at HLA-C have been identified in different human populations, making this the most highly polymorphic segment known within the human genome. Each of the alleles at these loci encodes a *heavy chain* (also called an α *chain*) that associates noncovalently with the nonpolymorphic light chain β₂-*microglobulin*, encoded on chromosome 15.

FIGURE 296-1 Physical map of the HLA region, showing the class I and class II loci, other immunologically important loci, and a sampling of other genes mapped to this region. Gene orientation is indicated by arrowheads. Scale is in kilobase (kb). The approximate genetic distance from DP to A is 3.2 cM. This includes 0.8 cM between A and B (including 0.2 cM between C and B), 0.4 to 0.8 cM between B and DR-DQ, and 1.6 to 2.0 cM between DR-DQ and DP.

The nomenclature of HLA genes and their products reflects the grafting of newer DNA sequence information on an older system based on serology. Among class I genes, alleles of the HLA-A, -B, and -C loci were originally identified in the 1950s, 1960s, and 1970s by alloantisera, derived primarily from multiparous women, who in the course of normal pregnancy produce antibodies against paternal antigens expressed on fetal cells. The serologic allotypes were designated by consecutive numbers, e.g., HLA-A1, HLA-B8. Currently, under World Health Organization (WHO) nomenclature, class I alleles are given a single designation that indicates locus, serologic specificity, and sequence-based subtype. For example, HLA-A*0201 indicates subtype 1 of the serologically defined allele HLA-A2. Subtypes that differ from each other at the nucleotide but not the amino acid sequence level are designated by an extra numeral, e.g., HLA-B*07021 and HLA-B*07022 are two variants of the HLA-B7 subtype of HLA-B*0702. The nomenclature of class II genes, discussed below, is made more complicated by the fact that both chains of a class II molecule are encoded by closely linked HLA-encoded loci, both of which may be polymorphic, and by the presence of differing numbers of isotypic DRB loci in different individuals. It has become clear that accurate HLA genotyping requires DNA sequence analysis, and the identification of alleles at the DNA sequence level has contributed greatly to the understanding of the role of HLA molecules as peptide-binding ligands, to the analysis of associations of HLA alleles with certain diseases, to the study of the populations genetics of HLA, and to a clearer understanding of the contribution of HLA differences to allograft rejection and graft-vs-host disease. Current databases of HLA class I and class II sequences can be accessed by internet (e.g., from the IMGT/HLA Database, *http://www.ebi.ac.uk/imgt/hla*), and frequent updates of HLA gene lists are published in several journals.

As shown in Fig. 296-2 and discussed below in detail, two characteristic structural features in particular define the functional properties of class I and class II HLA molecules. First is the *peptide-binding groove* that enables these molecules to form highly stable complexes with a wide array of peptide sequences that can be recognized as antigens by T cells. Second is a site for binding either the CD8 (in the case of class I HLA molecules) or the CD4 (in the case of HLA class II) molecules, which are expressed on mature T lymphocytes. In the case of class I molecules, peptide binding provides a display on the cell surface of peptides derived from intracellular proteins and thus serve as a readout to CD8+ T cells of the proteins being produced within somatic cells. The polymorphism at the loci encoding these molecules predominantly affects the amino acid residues that make up the peptide-binding groove, further amplifying the array of peptides that can be bound by different HLA molecules and generating important functional immune differences and transplantation incompatibility among different individuals.

The nonclassic, or class Ib, MHC molecules, HLA-E, -F, and -G, are much less polymorphic than MHC Ia and appear to have distinct functions. The HLA-E molecule, which has a peptide repertoire restricted to signal peptides cleaved from classic MHC class I molecules, is the major self-recognition target for the natural killer (NK) cell inhibitory receptors NKG2A or NKG2C paired with CD94 (see below and Chap. 295); four HLA-E alleles are known. HLA-G is expressed selectively in extravillous trophoblasts, the fetal cell population directly in contact with maternal tissues. It binds a wide array of peptides, is expressed in six different alternatively spliced forms, and provides inhibitory signals to both NK cells and T cells, presumably in the service of maintaining maternofetal tolerance. The function of HLA-F remains largely unknown. Although HLA-C is considered a classic class I molecule, its degree of polymorphism and level of surface expression are significantly lower than those of HLA-A and HLA-B. Moreover, unlike HLA-A and -B molecules, which function primarily by presenting antigen to CD8+ T cells expressing αβ T cell receptors, the primary function of HLA-C molecules appears to be to serve as targets of NK cell recognition (see below).

Additional class I–like genes have been identified, some HLA-linked and some encoded on other chromosomes, that show only distant homology to the class Ia and Ib molecules, but which share the three-dimensional class I structure. Those on chromosome 6p21 include MIC-A and MIC-B, which are encoded centromeric to HLA-B, and HLA-HFE, located 3 to 4 cM (centi-Morgan) telomeric of HLA-F. MIC-A and MIC-B do not bind peptide but are expressed on gut and other epithelium in a stress-inducible manner and serve as activation signals for certain γδ T cells, NK cells, CD8 T cells, and activated macrophages, acting through the activating NKG2D receptors. Fifty-four MIC-A and seventeen MIC-B alleles are known, and additional diversification comes from variable alanine repeat sequences in the transmembrane domain. HLA-HFE encodes the gene defective in hereditary hemochromatosis (Chap. 336). Among the non-HLA, class I–like genes, CD1 refers to a family of molecules that present glycolipids or other nonpeptide ligands to certain T cells, including T cells with NK activity; FcRn binds IgG within lysosomes and protects it from catabolism (Chap. 295); and Zn-α₂-glycoprotein 1 binds a nonpeptide ligand and promotes catabolism of triglycerides in adipose tissue. Like the HLA-A, -B, -C, -E, -F, and -G heavy chains, each of which forms a heterodimer with β₂-microglobulin (Fig. 296-2), the class I–like molecules, HLA-HFE, FcRn, and CD1 also bind to β₂-microglobulin, but MIC-A, MIC-B, and Zn-α₂-glycoprotein 1 do not.

The *HLA class II region* is also illustrated in Fig. 296-1. Multiple class II genes are arrayed within the centromeric 1 Mb of the HLA region, forming distinct haplotypes. A *haplotype* refers to an array of alleles at polymorphic loci along a chromosomal segment. Multiple class II genes are present on a single haplotype, clustered into three major subregions: HLA-DR, -DQ, and -DP. Each of these subregions contains at least one functional alpha (A) locus and one functional beta (B) locus. Together these encode proteins which form the α and β polypeptide chains of a mature class II HLA molecule. Thus, the DRA and DRB genes encode an HLA-DR molecule; products of the DQA1

MHC class I

Peptide-binding cleft

α_2 α_1

N

C

β_2-Microglobulin

α_3

A

α_1

Peptide-binding cleft

β Sheet

α Helix

C α_2

MHC class II

Peptide-binding cleft

β_1 α_1

N

C α_2

β_2

B

α_1

Peptide-binding cleft

β_1

D

FIGURE 296-2 Side (*A*, *B*) and top (*C*, *D*) views of the MHC class I and class II molecules. The α_1 and α_2 domains of class I and the α_1 and β_1 domains of class II form a β-sheet platform that forms the floor of the peptide-binding groove, and α helices that form the sides of the groove. The α_3 (*A*) and β_2 domains (*B*) project from the cell surface and form the contact sites for CD8 and CD4, respectively. (*Adapted from C. Janeway et al, Immunobiology Bookshelf, 2d ed., Garland Publishing, New York, 1997, with permission.*)

polymorphism, products of different DQA1 alleles can, with some limitations, pair with products of different DQB1 alleles through both *cis* and *trans* pairing to create combinatorial complexity and expand the number of expressed class II molecules. Because of the enormous allelic diversity in the general population, most individuals are heterozygous at all of the class I and class II loci. Thus, most individuals express six classic class I molecules (two each of HLA-A, -B, and -C) and around eight class II molecules—two DP, two DR (more in the case of haplotypes with additional functional DRB genes), and up to four DQ (two *cis* and two *trans*).

The localization of polymorphic residues in class II molecules is similar to that for class I, i.e, it is predominantly in sites that affect peptide binding (see below). In the case of class II molecules, the peptides displayed on the cell surface are primarily derived from proteins acquired from the extracellular environment, processed through the endosomal-lysosomal pathway, and presented to CD4+ T cells.

OTHER GENES IN THE MHC In addition to the class I and class II genes themselves, there are numerous genes interspersed among the HLA loci that have interesting and important immunologic functions. Our current concept of the function of MHC genes now encompasses many of these additional genes. As discussed in more detail below, TAP and LMP genes are also polymorphic and encode molecules that participate in intermediate steps in the HLA class I biosynthetic pathway. Another set of HLA genes, DMA and DMB, perform an analogous function for the class II pathway. These genes encode an intracellular molecule that facilitates the proper complexing of HLA class II molecules with antigen (see below). The *HLA class III region* is a name given to a cluster of genes between the class I and class II complexes, which includes genes for the two closely related cytokines tumor necrosis factor (TNF)-α and lymphotoxin (TNF-β); the complement components C2, C4, and Bf; heat shock protein (HSP)70; and the enzyme 21-hydroxylase.

The class I genes HLA-A, -B, and -C are expressed in all nucleated cells, although generally to a higher degree on leukocytes than on nonleukocytes. In contrast, the class II genes show a more restricted distribution: HLA-DR and HLA-DP genes are constitutively expressed on most cells of the myeloid cell lineage, whereas all three class II gene families (HLA-DR, -DQ, and -DP) are inducible by certain stimuli provided by inflammatory cytokines such as interferon γ. Within the lymphoid lineage, expression of these class II genes is constitutive on B cells and inducible on human T cells. Most endothelial and epithelial cells in the body, including the vascular endothelium and the intestinal epithelium, are also inducible for class II gene expression. Thus, while these somatic tissues normally express only class I and not class II genes, during times of local inflammation they are recruited by cytokine stimuli to express class II genes as well, thereby becoming active participants in ongoing immune responses. Class II expression is controlled largely at the transcriptional level through a conserved

and DQB1 genes form an HLA-DQ molecule; and the DPA1 and DPB1 genes encode an HLA-DP molecule. There are several DRB genes (DRB1, DRB2, DRB3, etc.), so that two expressed DR molecules are encoded on most haplotypes by combining the α-chain product of the DRA gene with separate β chains. More than 325 alleles have been identified at the HLA-DRB1 locus, with most of the variation occurring within limited segments encoding residues that interact with antigens. Detailed analysis of sequences and population distribution of these alleles strongly suggests that this diversity is actively selected by environmental pressures associated with pathogen diversity.

The class II region was originally termed the *D-region*. The allelic gene products were first detected by their ability to stimulate lymphocyte proliferation by *mixed lymphocyte reaction*, and were named Dw1, Dw2, etc. Subsequently, serology was used to identify gene products on peripheral blood B cells, and the antigens were termed *DR* (D-related). After additional class II loci were identified, these came to be known as DQ and DP. In the DQ region, both DQA1 and DQB1 are polymorphic, with 22 DQA1 alleles and >50 DQB1 alleles. The current nomenclature is largely analogous to that discussed above for class I, using the convention "locus * allele." Thus, for example, subtypes of the serologically defined specificity DR4, encoded by the DRB1 locus, are termed DRB1*0401, -0402, etc. In addition to allelic set of promoter elements that interact with a protein known as *CIITA*. Cytokine-mediated induction of CIITA is a principal method by which tissue-specific expression of HLA gene expression is controlled. Other HLA genes involved in the immune response, such as TAP and LMP, are also susceptible to upregulation by signals such as interferon γ. Sequence data for the entire HLA region can be accessed on the internet (e.g., *http://www.sanger.ac.uk/HGP/Chr6*). Many new genes have been discovered, the functions of which remain to be determined, as well as numerous microsatellite regions and other genetic elements. The gene density of the class II region is high, with approximately one protein encoded every 30 kb, and that of the class I and class III regions is even higher, with approximately one protein encoded every 15 kb.

LINKAGE DISEQUILIBRIUM In addition to extensive polymorphism at the class I and class II loci, another characteristic feature of the HLA complex is *linkage disequilibrium*. This is formally defined as a deviation from Hardy-Weinberg equilibrium for alleles at linked loci. This is reflected in the very low recombination rates between certain loci within the HLA complex. For example, recombination between DR and DQ loci is almost never observed in family studies, and characteristic haplotypes with particular arrays of DR and DQ alleles are found in every population. Similarly, the complement components C2, C4, and Bf are almost invariably inherited together, and the alleles at these loci are found in characteristic haplotypes. In contrast, there is a recombinational hotspot between DQ and DP, which are separated by 1 to 2 cM of genetic distance, despite their close physical proximity. Certain extended haplotypes encompassing the interval from DQ into the class I region are commonly found, the most notable being the haplotype DR3-B8-A1, which is found, in whole or in part, in 10 to 30% of northern European Caucasians. The genetic mechanisms that account for linkage disequilibrium in HLA have not been determined. It has been hypothesized that selective pressures may maintain certain haplotypes, but this remains to be determined. As discussed below under HLA and immunologic disease, one consequence of the phenomenon of linkage disequilibrium has been the resulting difficulty in assigning HLA-disease associations to a single allele at a single locus.

MHC STRUCTURE AND FUNCTION

Class I and class II molecules display a distinctive structural architecture, which contains specialized functional domains responsible for the unique genetic and immunologic properties of the HLA complex. The principal known function of both class I and class II HLA molecules is to bind antigenic peptides in order to present antigen to an appropriate T cell. The ability of a particular peptide to satisfactorily bind to an individual HLA molecule is a direct function of the molecular fit between the amino acid residues on the peptide with respect to the amino acid residues of the HLA molecule. The bound peptide forms a tertiary structure called the *MHC-peptide complex*, which communicates with T lymphocytes through binding to the T cell receptor (TCR) molecule. The first site of TCR-MHC-peptide interaction in the life of a T cell occurs in the thymus, where self-peptides are presented to developing thymocytes by MHC molecules expressed on thymic epithelium and hematopoietically derived antigen-presenting cells, which are primarily responsible for positive and negative selection, respectively (Chap. 295). Mature T cells encounter MHC molecules in the periphery both in the maintenance of tolerance (Chap. 299) and in the initiation of immune responses. Because most antibody responses and all T cell responses are T cell dependent (Chap. 295), the MHC-peptide-TCR interaction is the central event in the initiation of most antigen-specific immune responses, since it is the event that actually confers the specificity. Thus, the population of MHC–T cell complexes expressed in the thymus shapes the TCR repertoire. For potentially immunogenetic peptides, the ability of a given peptide to be generated and bound by an HLA molecule is a primary determinant of whether or not an immune response to that peptide can be generated, and the repertoire of peptides that a particular individual's HLA molecules can bind exerts a major influence over the specificity of that individual's immune response.

When a TCR molecule binds to an HLA-peptide complex, it forms intermolecular contacts with both the antigenic peptide and with the HLA molecule itself. The outcome of this recognition event depends on the density and duration of the binding interaction, accounting for a dual specificity requirement for activation of the T cell. That is, the TCR must be specific both for the antigenic peptide and for the HLA molecule. The polymorphic nature of the presenting molecules, and the influence that this exerts on the peptide repertoire of each molecule, results in the phenomenon of *MHC restriction* of the T cell specificity for a given peptide. The binding of CD8 or CD4 molecules to the class I or class II molecule, respectively, also contributes to the interaction between T cell and the HLA-peptide complex, by providing for the selective activation of the appropriate T cell.

CLASS I STRUCTURE (Fig. 296-2*A*) As noted above, MHC class I molecules provide a cell-surface display of peptides derived from intracellular proteins, and they also provide the signal for self-recognition by NK cells. Surface-expressed class I molecules consist of an MHC-encoded 44-kD glycoprotein heavy chain, a non-MHC-encoded 12-kD light chain β_2-microglobulin, and an antigenic peptide, typically 8 to 11 amino acids in length and derived from intracellularly produced protein. The heavy chain displays a prominent peptide-binding groove. In HLA-A and -B molecules, the groove is approximately 3 nm in length by 1.2 nm in maximum width (30 Å × 12 Å), whereas it is apparently somewhat wider in HLA-C. Antigenic peptides are noncovalently bound in an extended conformation within the peptide-binding groove, with both N- and C-terminal ends anchored in pockets within the groove (A and F pockets, respectively) and, in many cases, with a prominent kink, or arch, approximately one-third of the way from the N-terminus that elevates the peptide main chain off the floor of the groove.

A remarkable property of peptide binding by MHC molecules is the ability to form highly stable complexes with a wide array of peptide sequences. This is accomplished by a combination of peptide sequence–independent and peptide sequence–dependent bonding. The former consists of hydrogen bond and van der Waals interactions between conserved residues in the peptide-binding groove and charged or polar atoms along the peptide backbone. The latter is dependent upon the six side pockets that are formed by the irregular surface produced by protrusion of amino acid side chains from within the binding groove. The side chains lining the pockets interact with some of the peptide side chains. The sequence polymorphism among different class I alleles and isotypes predominantly affects the residues that line these pockets, and the interactions of these residues with peptide residues constitute the sequence-dependent bonding that confers a particular sequence "motif" on the range of peptides that can bind any given MHC molecule.

CLASS I BIOSYNTHESIS (Fig. 296-3*A*). The biosynthesis of the classic MHC class I molecules reflects their role in presenting endogenous peptides. The heavy chain is cotranslationally inserted into the membrane of the endoplasmic reticulum (ER), where it becomes glycosylated and associates sequentially with the chaperone proteins calnexin and ERp57. It then forms a complex with β_2-microglobulin, and this complex associates with the chaperone calreticulin and the MHC-encoded molecule tapasin, which physically links the class I complex to TAP, the MHC-encoded transporter associated with antigen processing. Meanwhile, peptides generated within the cytosol from intracellular proteins by the multisubunit, multicatalytic proteasome complex are actively transported into the ER by TAP, where they are trimmed by a peptidase known as *ERAAP* (ER aminopeptidase associated with antigen processing). At this point, peptides with appropriate sequence complementarity bind specific class I molecules to form complete, folded heavy chain–β_2-microglobulin–peptide trimer complexes. These are transported rapidly from the ER, through the *cis*- and *trans*-Golgi where the N-linked oligosaccharide is further processed, and thence to the cell surface.

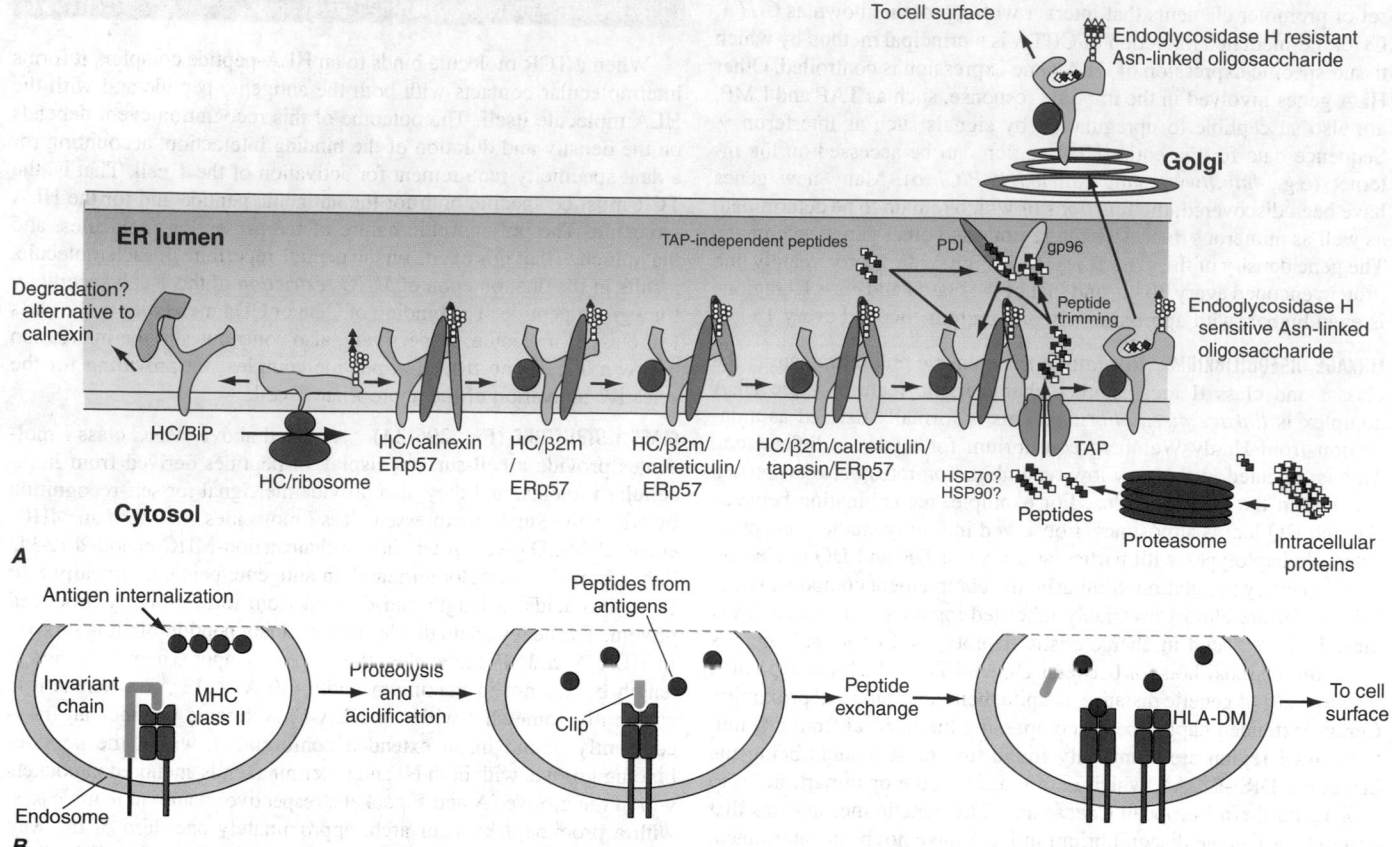

FIGURE 296-3 Biosynthesis of class I (*A*) and class II (*B*) molecules. *A.* Nascent heavy chain (HC) becomes associated with β_2-microglobulin (β2m) and peptide through interactions with a series of chaperones. Peptides generated by the proteasome are transported into the endoplasmic reticulum (ER) by TAP. Peptides undergo N-terminal trimming in the ER and become associated with chaperones, including gp96 and PDI. Once peptide binds to HC-β2m, the HC-β2m-peptide trimeric complex exits the ER and is transported by the secretory pathway to the cell surface. In the Golgi, the N- linked oligosaccharide undergoes maturation, with addition of sialic acid residues. Molecules are not necessarily drawn to scale. *B.* Pathway of HLA class II molecule assembly and antigen processing. After transport through the Golgi and post-Golgi compartment, the class II–invariant chain complex moves to an acidic endosome, where the invariant chain is proteolytically cleaved into fragments and displaced by antigenic peptides, facilitated by interactions with the DMA-DMB chaperone protein. This class II molecule–peptide complex is then transported to the cell surface.

Most of the peptides transported by TAP are produced in the cytosol by proteolytic cleavage of intracellular proteins by the multisubunit, multicatalytic protesasome, and inhibitors of the proteasome dramatically reduce expression of class I–presented antigenic peptides. A thiol-dependent oxidoreductase Erp57, which mediates disulfide bond rearrangements, also appears to play an important role in folding the class I–peptide complex into a stable multicomponent molecule. The MHC-encoded proteasome subunits LMP2 and LMP7 may influence the spectrum of peptides produced but are not essential for proteasome function.

CLASS I FUNCTION ■ Peptide Antigen Presentation On any given cell, a class I molecule occurs in 100,000 to 200,000 copies and binds several hundred to several thousand distinct peptide species. The vast majority of these peptides are self-peptides to which the host immune system is tolerant by one or more of the mechanisms that maintain tolerance, e.g., clonal deletion in the thymus or clonal anergy or clonal ignorance in the periphery (Chaps. 295 and 299). However, class I molecules bearing foreign peptides expressed in a permissive immunologic context activate CD8 T cells, which, if naïve, will then differentiate into cytolytic T lymphocytes (CTLs). These T cells and their progeny, through their $\alpha\beta$ TCRs, are then capable of Fas/CD95- and/or perforin-mediated cytotoxicity and/or cytokine secretion (Chap. 295) upon further encounter with the class I–peptide combination that originally activated it, and also with other combinations of class I molecule plus peptide that present a similar immunochemical stimulus to the TCR. As alluded to above, this phenomenon by which T cells recognize foreign antigens in the context of specific MHC alleles is termed *MHC restriction*, and the specific MHC molecule is termed the *restriction element*. The most common source of foreign peptides presented by class I molecules is viral infection, in the course of which peptides from viral proteins enter the class I pathway. The generation of a strong CTL response that destroys virally infected cells represents an important antigen-specific defense against many viral infections (Chap. 295). In the case of some viral infections—hepatitis B, for example—CTL-induced target cell apoptosis is thought to be a more important mechanism of tissue damage than any direct cytopathic effect of the virus itself. The importance of the class I pathway in the defense against viral infection is underscored by the identification of a number of viral products that interfere with the normal class I biosynthetic pathway and thus block the immunogenetic expression of viral antigens.

Other examples of intracellularly generated peptides that can be presented by class I molecules in an immunogenic manner include peptides derived from nonviral intracellular infectious agents (e.g., *Listeria*, *Plasmodium*), tumor antigens, minor histocompatibility antigens, and certain autoantigens. There are also situations in which cell surface–expressed class I molecules are thought to acquire and present exogenously derived peptides.

HLA Class I Receptors and NK Cell Recognition (Chap. 295) NK cells, which play an important role in innate immune responses, are activated to cytotoxicity and cytokine secretion by contact with cells that lack MHC class I expression, and NK cell activation is inhibited by cells that express MHC class I. In humans, the recognition of class I molecules by NK cells is carried out by three classes of receptor families, the killer cell–inhibitory cell receptor (KIR) family, the leukocyte Ig-like receptor (LIR) family, and the CD94/NKG2 family. The KIR family, also called CD158, is encoded on chromosome 19q13.4 and consists of glycoproteins of the immunoglobulin (Ig) superfamily, currently divided into two types, the inhibitor (L) and stimulatory (S)

KIRs. KIR molecules of the L class bind HLA class I molecules and inhibit NK cell–mediated cytotoxicity and are also expressed on subsets of T lymphocytes. An estimated 40 genes are divided into two subfamilies, 2DL and 3DL, which contain, respectively, either two or three Ig domains. The KIR2DL1 molecules primarily recognize alleles of HLA-C, which possess a lysine at position 80 (HLA-Cw2, -4, -7 and -8), while the KIR2DL2 and KIR2DL3 families primarily recognize alleles of HLA-C with asparagine at this position (HLA-Cw1, -3, -5 and -6). The KIR3D molecules predominantly recognize HLA-B alleles that fall into the HLA-Bw4 class determined by residues 77 to 83 in the α_1 domain of the heavy chain. Less is known about the stimulatory KIR receptors, and their primary specificity may be for nonclassic class I molecules or for related structures present on some pathogens. The most common KIR haplotype in Caucasians contains one activating KIR and six inhibitory KIR genes, although there is a great deal of diversity in the population, with at least 15 different haplotypes. It appears that most individuals have at least one inhibitory KIR for a self-HLA class I molecule, providing a structural basis for NK cell target specificity.

The LIR gene family (CD85, also called ILT) is encoded centromeric of the KIR locus on 19q13.4, and it encodes a variety of inhibitory immunoglobulin-like receptors expressed on many lymphocyte and other hematopoietic lineages. Interaction of LIR-1 (ILT2) with NK or T cells inhibits activation and cytotoxicity, mediated by many different HLA class I molecules, including HLA-G. HLA-F also appears to interact with LIR molecules, although the functional context for this is not understood.

The third family of NK receptors for HLA is encoded in the NK complex on chromosome 12p12.3-13.1 and consists of CD94 and five NKG2 genes, A/B, C, E/H, D, and F. These molecules are C-type (calcium-binding) lectins and most function as disulfide-bonded heterodimers between CD94 and one of the NKG2 glycoproteins. The principle ligand of CD94/NKG2A receptors is the HLA-E molecule, complexed to a peptide derived from the signal sequence of classic HLA class I molecules and HLA-G. Thus, analogous to the way in which KIR receptors recognize HLA-C, the NKG2 receptor monitors self–class I expression, albeit indirectly through peptide recognition in the context of HLA-E. NKG2C, -E, and -H appear to have similar specificities but act as activating receptors. NKG2D is expressed as a homodimer and functions as an activating receptor expressed on NK cells, $\gamma\delta$ TCR T cells, and activated CD8 T cells. When complexed with an adaptor called DAP10, NKG2D recognizes MIC-A and MIC-B molecules and activates the cytolytic response. NKG2D also binds a class of molecules known as *ULBP*, structurally related to class I molecules but not encoded in the MHC. →*The function of NK cells in immune responses is discussed in Chap. 295.*

CLASS II STRUCTURE (Fig. 296-2*B*)   A specialized functional architecture similar to that of the class I molecules can be seen in the example of a class II molecule depicted in Fig. 296-2*B*, with an antigen-binding cleft arrayed above a supporting scaffold that extends the cleft toward the external cellular environment. However, in contrast to the HLA class I molecular structure, β_2-microglobulin is not associated with class II molecules. Rather, the class II molecule is a heterodimer, composed of a 29-kD α chain and a 34-kD β chain. The amino-terminal domains of each chain form the antigen-binding elements which, like the class I molecule, cradle a bound peptide in a groove bounded by extended α-helical loops, one encoded by the A (α chain) gene and one by the B (β chain) gene. Like the class I groove, the class II antigen-binding groove is punctuated by pockets that contact the side chains of amino acid residues of the bound peptide, but unlike the class I groove, it is open at both ends. Therefore, peptides bound by class II molecules vary greatly in length, since both the N- and C-terminal ends of the peptides can extend through the open ends of this groove. Approximately 11 amino acids within the bound peptide form intimate contacts with the class II molecule itself, with backbone hydrogen bonds and specific side chain interactions combining to provide, respectively, stability and specificity to the binding (Fig. 296-4).

FIGURE 296-4   Top view of the HLA-DR1 molecule containing the peptide 296-318 from influenza hemagglutinin. The N terminus of the peptide is at left, and the peptide lies relatively flat within the peptide-binding groove in an extended conformation with a pronounced twist. Some 35% of the peptide surface is potentially available for interaction with the antigen receptor on T cells. Pockets in the peptide-binding site accommodate 5 of the 13 side chains of the bound peptide, manifesting the peptide specificity of HLA-DR1. Twelve hydrogen bonds between conserved HLA-DR1 residues and the main chain of the peptide provide a universal mode of peptide binding. The ends of the binding groove are open, and longer variants of the peptide can extend out from each end. In contrast, peptides bound to class I molecules are anchored into pockets at their N and C termini by conserved residues, and the middle portion of the peptide is typically kinked upwards out of the groove. (*Adapted from LJ Stern et al: Nature 368:215, 1994. Copyright 1994 Macmillan Magazines Ltd, with permission.*)

The genetic polymorphisms that distinguish different class II genes correspond to changes in the amino acid composition of the class II molecule, and these variable sites are clustered predominantly around the pocket structures within the antigen-binding groove. As with class I, this is a critically important feature of the class II molecule, which explains how genetically different individuals have functionally different HLA molecules.

As noted above, the class I–peptide complex is preferentially recognized by CD8 T cells, and the class II–peptide complex is preferentially recognized by CD4 T cells. These interactions provide an important signal for activation of specific T cell lineages during antigen-recognition events. The CD8 recognition site is located on the α_3 domain of the MHC class I molecule, and the CD4 recognition site is located on the β_2 domain of the class II molecule, in both cases remote from the peptide-binding site.

BIOSYNTHESIS AND FUNCTION OF CLASS II MOLECULES (Fig. 296-3*B*)   The intracellular assembly of class II molecules occurs within a specialized compartmentalized pathway that differs dramatically from the class I pathway described above. As illustrated in Fig. 296-3*B*, the class II molecule assembles in the ER in association with a chaperone molecule, known as the *invariant chain*. The invariant chain performs at least two roles. First, it binds to the class II molecule and blocks the peptide-binding groove, thus preventing antigenic peptides from binding. This role of the invariant chain appears to account for one of the important differences between class I and class II MHC pathways, since it can explain why class I molecules present endogenous peptides from proteins newly synthesized in the ER but class II molecules generally do not. Second, the invariant chain contains molecular localization signals that direct the class II molecule to traffic into post-Golgi compartments known as *endosomes*, which develop into specialized acidic compartments where proteases cleave the invariant chain, and antigenic peptides can now occupy the class II groove. The specificity and tissue distribution of these proteases appear to be an important way in which the immune system regulates access to the peptide-binding groove and T cells become exposed to specific self-antigens. Differences in protease expression in the thymus and in the periphery may in part determine which specific peptide sequences comprise the peripheral repertoire for T cell recognition. It is at this stage in the intracellular pathway, after cleavage of the invariant chain, that the MHC-encoded DM molecule catalytically facilitates the exchange of peptides within the class II groove to help optimize the specificity and stability of the MHC-peptide complex.

Once this MHC-peptide complex is deposited in the outer cell membrane it becomes the target for T cell recognition via a specific TCR expressed on lymphocytes. Because the endosome environment contains internalized proteins retrieved from the extracellular environment, the class II–peptide complex often contains bound antigens that were originally derived from extracellular proteins. In this way, the class II peptide–loading pathway provides a mechanism for immune surveillance of the extracellular space. This appears to be an important feature that permits the class II molecule to bind foreign peptides, distinct from the endogenous pathway of class I–mediated presentation.

ROLE OF HLA IN TRANSPLANTATION The development of modern clinical transplantation in the decades since the1950s provided a major impetus for elucidation of the HLA system, as allograft survival is highest when donor and recipient are HLA-identical. Although many molecular events participate in transplantation rejection, allogeneic differences at class I and class II loci play a major role. Class I molecules can promote T cell responses in several different ways. In the cases of allografts in which the host and donor are mismatched at one or more class I loci, host T cells can be activated by classic *direct alloreactivity*, in which the antigen receptors on the host T cells react with the foreign class I molecule expressed on the allograft. In this situation, the response of any given TCR may be dominated by the allogeneic MHC molecule, the peptide bound to it, or some combination of the two. Another type of host antigraft T cell response involves the uptake and processing of donor MHC antigens by host antigen-presenting cells and the subsequent presentation of the resulting peptides by host MHC molecules. This mechanism is termed *indirect alloreactivity*.

In the case of class I molecules on allografts that are shared by the host and the donor, a host T cell response may still be triggered because of peptides that are presented by the class I molecules of the graft but not of the host. The most common basis for the existence of these endogenous antigen peptides, called *minor histocompatibility antigens*, is a genetic difference between donor and host at a non-MHC locus encoding the structural gene for the protein from which the peptide is derived. These loci are termed *minor histocompatibility loci*, and nonidentical individuals typically differ at many such loci. CD4 T cells react to analogous class II variation, both direct and indirect, and class II differences alone are sufficient to drive allograft rejection.

ASSOCIATION OF HLA ALLELES WITH SUSCEPTIBILITY TO DISEASE It has long been postulated that infectious agents provide the driving force for the allelic diversification seen in the HLA system. An important corollary of this hypothesis is that resistance to specific pathogens may differ between individuals, based on HLA genotype. Observations of specific HLA genes associated with resistance to malaria or dengue fever, persistence of hepatitis B, and to disease progression in HIV infection are consistent with this model. Pathogen diversity is probably also the major selective pressure favoring HLA heterozygosity. The extraordinary scope of HLA allelic diversity increases the likelihood that most new pathogens will be recognized by some HLA molecules, helping to assure immune fitness to the host. However, another consequence of diversification is that some alleles may become preferentially selective for recognition of self-antigens as well. Indeed, particular HLA alleles are strongly associated with certain disease states, particularly for some common autoimmune diseases (Chap. 299). By comparing allele frequencies in patients with any particular disease and in control

populations, a large number of such associations have been identified, some of which are listed in Table 296-1. The strength of genetic association is reflected in the term *relative risk*, which is a statistical odds ratio representing the risk of disease for an individual carrying a particular genetic marker compared with the risk for individuals in that population without that marker. The nomenclature shown in Table 296-1 reflects both the HLA serotype (e.g., DR3, DR4) and the HLA genotype (e.g., DRB1*0301, DRB1*0401). It very likely the class I and class II alleles themselves are the true susceptibility alleles for most of these associations. However, as discussed below, because of the extremely strong linkage disequilibrium between the DR and DQ loci, in some cases it has been difficult to determine the specific locus or combination of class II loci involved. In some cases, the susceptibility gene may be one of the HLA-linked genes located near the class I or class II region, but not the HLA gene itself, and in other cases the susceptibility gene may be a non-HLA gene, such as TNF-α, which is nearby.

As might be predicted from the known function of the class I and class II gene products, almost all of the diseases associated with specific HLA alleles have an immunologic component to their pathogenesis. It should be stressed that even the strong HLA associations with disease (those associations with relative risk of ≥ 10) implicate normal, rather than defective, alleles. Most individuals who carry these susceptibility genes do not express the associated disease; in this way the particular HLA gene is permissive for disease but requires other environmental (e.g., the presence of specific antigens) or genetic factors for full penetrance. In each case studied, even in diseases with very strong HLA associations, the concordance of disease in monozygotic twins is higher than in HLA-identical dizygotic twins or other sibling pairs, indicating that non-HLA genes contribute to susceptibility and can significantly modify the risk attributable to HLA.

Another group of diseases is genetically linked to HLA, not because of the immunologic function of HLA alleles, but rather because they are caused by autosomal dominant or recessive abnormal alleles at loci that happen to reside in or near the HLA region. Examples of these are 21-hydroxylase deficiency (Chap. 321), hemochromatosis (Chap. 336), and spinocerebellar ataxia (Chap. 353).

CLASS I ASSOCIATIONS WITH DISEASE Although the associations of human disease with particular HLA alleles or haplotypes predominantly involve the class II region, there are also several prominent disease associations with class I alleles. These include the association of Behçet's disease (Chap. 307) with HLA-B51, psoriasis vulgaris (Chap. 47) with HLA-Cw6, and, most notably, the spondyloarthropathies (Chap. 305) with HLA-B27. Twenty-five HLA-B locus alleles, designated HLA-B*2701 to B*2725, encode the family of B27 class I molecules. All of the subtypes share a common B pocket in the peptide-binding groove, a deep, negatively charged pocket that shows a strong preference for binding the arginine side chain. In addition, B27 is among the most negatively charged of HLA class I heavy chains, and the overall preference is for positively charged peptides. HLA-B*2705 is the predominant subtype in Caucasians and most other non-Oriental populations, and this subtype is very highly associated with ankylosing spondylitis (AS) (Chap. 305), both in its idiopathic form and in association with chronic inflammatory bowel disease or psoriasis vulgaris. It is also associated with reactive arthritis (ReA) (Chap. 305), with other idiopathic forms of peripheral arthritis (undifferentiated spondyloarthropathy), and with recurrent acute anterior uveitis. B27 is found in 50 to 90% of individuals with these conditions, compared with a prevalence of ~7% in North American Caucasians. The prevalence of B27 in patients with idiopathic AS is 90%, and in AS complicated by iritis or aortic insufficiency it is close to 100%. The absolute risk of spondyloarthropathy in unselected B27+ individuals has been variously estimated at 2 to 13% and >20% if a B27+ first-degree relative is affected. The concordance rate of AS in identical twins is very high, at least 65%. It can be concluded that the B27 molecule itself is involved in disease pathogenesis, based on strong evidence from clinical epidemiology and on the occurrence of a spondyloarthropathy-like disease in HLA-B27 transgenic rats. Both AS and ReA are associated with the B27 subtypes B*2702, -04, and -05, and anecdotal association has been reported for subtypes B*2701, -03, -07, -08, -10, and -11.

The association of B27 with these diseases may derive from the specificity of a particular peptide or family of peptides bound to B27 or through another mechanism that is independent of the peptide specificity of B27. The first alternative can be further subdivided into mechanisms that involve T cell recognition of B27-peptide complexes and those that do not. A variety of other roles for B27 in disease pathogenesis have been postulated, including molecular or antigenic mimicry between B27 and certain bacteria and reduced killing of intracellular bacteria in cells expressing B27. HLA B27 has been shown to form heavy chain homodimers, utilizing the cysteine residue at position 67 of the B57 α chain. These homodimers are expressed on the surface of lymphocytes and monocytes from patients with AS, and receptors including KIR3DL1, KIR3DL2, and ILT4 are capable of binding to them. Whether these interactions contribute to disease susceptibility or pathogenesis is currently unknown.

CLASS II DISEASE ASSOCIATIONS As can be seen in Table 296-1, the majority of associations of HLA and disease are with class II alleles. Several diseases have complex HLA genetic associations.

Celiac Disease In the case of celiac disease (Chap. 275), it is probable that the HLA-DQ genes are the primary basis for the disease association. HLA-DQ genes present on both the celiac-associated DR3 and DR7 haplotypes include the DQB1*0201 gene, and further detailed studies have documented a specific class II $\alpha\beta$ dimer encoded by the DQA1*0501 and DQB1*0201 genes, which appears to account for the HLA genetic contribution to celiac disease susceptibility. This specific HLA association with celiac disease may have a straightforward explanation: peptides derived from the wheat gluten component gliaden are bound to the molecule encoded by DQA1*0501 and DQB1*0201 and presented to T cells. A gliaden-derived peptide that has been implicated in this immune activation binds the DQ class II dimer best when the peptide contains a glutamine to glutamic acid substitution. It has been proposed that tissue transglutaminase, an enzyme present at increased levels in the intestinal cells of celiac patients, converts glutamine to glutamic acid in gliadin, creating peptides that are capable of being bound by the DQ2 molecule and presented to T cells.

Pemphigus Vulgaris In the case of pemphigus vulgaris (Chap. 49), there are two HLA haplotypes associated with disease, DRB1*0402-DQB1*0302 and DRB1*1401-DQB1*0503. Peptides derived from epidermal autoantigens have been implicated that preferentially bind to the DRB1*0402-encoded molecule, suggesting that specific peptide binding by this disease-associated class II molecule is important in disease. However, there are no class II genes in common between the disease-associated DR4 and DR14 haplotypes, and there is no evidence for any interaction of the latter haplotype interacting with the epidermal peptides that bind the DRB1*0402-encoded molecule. Thus, the most likely interpretation is that each of these class II associations with pemphigus represents a different pathway to a comparable clinical outcome.

Juvenile Arthritis Pauciarticular juvenile arthritis (Chap. 301) is an autoimmune disease associated with genes at the DRB1 locus and also with genes at the DPB1 locus. Patients with both DPB1*0201 and a DRB1 susceptibility allele (usually DRB1*08 or -*05) have a higher relative risk than expected from the additive effect of those genes alone. In juvenile patients with rheumatoid factor−positive polyarticular disease, heterozygotes carrying both DRB1*0401 and -*0404 have a relative risk >100, reflecting an apparent synergy in individuals inheriting both of these susceptibility genes.

Type I Diabetes Mellitus There are several aspects of the genetics of type I diabetes (Chap. 323) that illustrate the complex nature of HLA associations with autoimmune diseases. First, type 1 (autoimmune) diabetes mellitus is associated with both DR3 and DR4 serotypes and

TABLE 296-1 *Significant HLA Class I and Class II Associations with Disease*[a]

	Marker	Gene	Strength of Association
SPONDYLOARTHROPATHIES			
Ankylosing spondylitis	B27	B*2702, -04, -05	++++
Reiter's syndrome	B27		++++
Acute anterior uveitis	B27		+++
Reactive arthritis (*Yersinia, Salmonella, Shigella, Chlamydia*)	B27		+++
Psoriatic spondylitis	B27		+++
COLLAGEN-VASCULAR DISEASES			
Juvenile arthritis, pauciarticular	DR8		++
	DR5		++
Rheumatoid arthritis	DR4	DRB1*0401, -04, -05	+++
Sjögren's syndrome	DR3		++
Systemic lupus erythematosus			
Caucasian	DR3		+
Japanese	DR2		++
AUTOIMMUNE GUT AND SKIN			
Gluten-sensitive enteropathy (celiac disease)	DR3	DQA1*0501 DQB1*0201	+++
Chronic active hepatitis	DR3		++
Dermatitis herpetiformis	DR3		+++
Psoriasis vulgaris	Cw6		++
Pemphigus vulgaris	DR4	DRB1*0402	+++
	DR6	DQB1*0503	
AUTOIMMUNE ENDOCRINE			
Type 1 diabetes mellitus	DR4	DQB1*0302	+++
	DR3		++
	DR2	DQB1*0602	—[b]
Hyperthyroidism (Graves')	B8		+
	DR3		+
Hyperthyroidism (Japanese)	B35		+
Adrenal insufficiency	DR3		++
AUTOIMMUNE NEUROLOGIC			
Myasthenia gravis	B8		+
	DR3		+
Multiple sclerosis	DR2	DRB1*1501 DRB5*0101	++
OTHER			
Behçet's disease	B51		++
Congenital adrenal hyperplasia	B47	21·OH (Cyp21B)	+++
Narcolepsy	DR2		++++
Goodpasture's syndrome (anti-GBM)	DR2		++

[a] Various diseases associated with HLA genes are listed, with the HLA serotype or linked marker most frequently found related to disease. Genes are listed for cases where specific alleles have been identified as responsible for this association. The strength of association reflects the likelihood of disease in individuals with the marker compared to individuals who do not carry the marker; ++++, relative risk > 10; +++, relative risk > 5; ++, relative risk > 3; +, relative risk > 1.5.
[b] Strong negative association, i.e., genetic association with protection from diabetes.

their corresponding genes. The presence of both the DR3 and DR4 haplotypes in one individual confers the highest known genetic risk for type 1 diabetes, and individuals carrying either of these haplotypes also carry some increased risk. Specific class II genes on each haplotype have been thoroughly studied, and the strongest association is with DQB1*0302, a specific gene on the diabetes-associated DR4 haplotypes. Thus, all DR4 haplotypes that carry a DQB1*0302 gene are associated with type 1 diabetes, whereas related DR4 haplotypes that carry a different DQB1 gene are not. The primary class II determinant of susceptibility, therefore, is HLA-DQB1*0302. However, the relative risk associated with inheritance of this gene can be modified, depending on other HLA genes present either on the same or a second haplotype. For example, just as the presence of a second haplotype containing DR3 is associated with increased diabetes risk, the presence of a DR2-positive haplotype containing a DQB1*0602 gene is associated with decreased risk. This gene, DQB1*0602, is considered "protective" for type 1 diabetes. Even some DRB1 genes that can occur on the same haplotype as DQB1*0302 may modulate risk, so that individuals with the DR4 haplotype that contains DRB1*0403 are less susceptible to type 1 diabetes than individuals with other DR4-DQB1*0302 haplotypes.

Although the presence of a DR3 haplotype in combination with the DR4-DQB1*0302 haplotype is a very high risk combination for diabetes susceptibility, the specific gene on the DR3 haplotype that is responsible for this synergy is not yet identified. This is because the predominant HLA-DR3 haplotype in Caucasians has very tight linkage with other genes within the MHC, including HLA-A1, -B8, -Cw7, and -C4A, as discussed above. Thus, any of a large variety of genes within the HLA region on this DR3 haplotype may be the primary gene(s) responsible for contributing to diabetes susceptibility. An example that more directly implicates other genes linked to DR3 is the association between HLA genes and systemic lupus erythematosus (SLE) (Chap. 300). The C4A null alleles that are present on the HLA-DR3 haplotypes in SLE are also often present in patients without DR3, notably those with HLA-DR2. This implicates the presence of a C4A silent allele, which is a defective structural gene for the C4 complement component, rather than the expression of any particular class II gene, as a potential susceptibility gene within HLA associated with SLE.

HLA and Rheumatoid Arthritis The HLA genes associated with rheumatoid arthritis (RA) (Chap. 301) are DRB1*0401 and DRB1*0404. These genes encode a distinctive sequence of amino acids from codons 67 to 74 of the DRβ molecule: RA-associated class II molecules carry the sequence LeuLeuGluGlnArgArgAlaAla or LeuLeuGlu-GlnLysArgAlaAla in this region, while non-RA-associated genes carry one or more differences in this region. These residues form a portion of the molecule that lies in the middle of the α-helical portion of the DRB1-encoded class II molecule, termed the *shared epitope.*

These DR4-positive RA-associated alleles are most frequent among patients with more severe, erosive disease. The frequency of these DR4-positive alleles is lower among rheumatoid factor–negative patients with RA, as well as among patients with nonerosive forms of the disease. It is important to note that, although the frequency of these DRB1 susceptibility alleles in RA patients is high, the same genes are also prevalent in the unaffected population, and thus the absolute risk associated with these susceptibility alleles is low. The highest risk for susceptibility to RA comes in individuals who carry both a DRB1*0401 and DRB1*0404 gene. Some forms of RA are associated with other HLA genes, such as DRB1*01, -*1001, and -*1402, which also carry the shared epitope sequence, strongly suggesting that this part of the class II molecule contributes directly to disease pathogenesis.

MOLECULAR MECHANISMS FOR HLA-DISEASE ASSOCIATIONS As noted above, HLA molecules play a key role in the selection and establishment of the antigen-specific T cell repertoire and a major role in the subsequent activation of those T cells during the initiation of an immune response. Precise genetic polymorphisms characteristic of individual alleles dictate the specificity of these interactions and thereby instruct and guide antigen-specific immune events. These same genetically determined pathways are therefore implicated in disease pathogenesis when specific HLA genes are responsible for autoimmune disease susceptibility.

The fate of developing T cells within the thymus is determined by the affinity of interaction between T cell receptor and HLA molecules bearing self-peptides, and thus the particular HLA types of each individual control the precise specificity of the T cell repertoire (Chap. 295). The primary basis for HLA-associated disease susceptibility may well lie within this thymic maturation pathway. The positive selection of potentially autoreactive T cells, based on the presence of specific HLA susceptibility genes, may establish the threshold for disease risk in a particular individual.

At the time of onset of a subsequent immune response, the primary role of the HLA molecule is to bind peptide and present it to antigen-specific T cells. The HLA complex can therefore be viewed as encoding genetic determinants of precise immunologic activation events. Antigenic peptides that bind particular HLA molecules are capable of stimulating T cell immune responses; peptides that do not bind are not presented to T cells and are not immunogenic. This genetic control of the immune response is mediated by the polymorphic sites within the HLA antigen–binding groove that interact with the bound peptides. In autoimmune and immune-mediated diseases, it is likely that specific tissue antigens that are targets for pathogenic lymphocytes are complexed with the HLA molecules encoded by specific susceptibility alleles. In autoimmune diseases with an infectious etiology, it is likely that immune responses to peptides derived from the initiating pathogen are bound and presented by particular HLA molecules to activate T lymphocytes that play a triggering or contributory role in disease pathogenesis. The concept that early events in disease initiation are triggered by specific HLA-peptide complexes offers some prospects for therapeutic intervention, since it may be possible to design compounds that interfere with the formation or function of specific HLA-peptide–T cell receptor interactions.

When considering mechanisms of HLA associations with immune response and disease, it is well to remember that just as HLA genetics are complex, so are the mechanisms likely to be heterogeneous. Immune-mediated disease is a multistep process in which one of the HLA-associated functions is to establish a repertoire of potentially reactive T cells, while another HLA-associated function is to provide the essential peptide-binding specificity for T cell recognition. For diseases with multiple HLA genetic associations, it is possible that both of these interactions occur and synergize to advance an accelerated pathway of disease.

FURTHER READING

BRAUD VM et al: Functions of nonclassical MHC and non-MHC-encoded class I molecules. Curr Opin Immunol 11:100, 1999

HAMMER J et al: HLA class II peptide binding specificity and autoimmunity. Adv Immunol 66:67, 1997

HILL AV: The immunogenetics of human infectious diseases. Annu Rev Immunol 16:593, 1998

NEPOM GT: Major histocompatibility complex–directed susceptibility to rheumatoid arthritis. Adv Immunol 68:315, 1998

———, KWOK WW: Molecular basis for HLA-DQ associations with IDDM. Diabetes 47:117, 1998

PAMER E, CRESSWELL P: Mechanisms of MHC class I–restricted antigen processing. Annu Rev Immunol 16:323, 1998

STERN LJ, WILEY DC: Antigenic peptide binding by class I and class II histocompatibility proteins. Structure 2:245, 1994

TAUROG JD et al: Inflammatory disease in HLA-B27 transgenic rats. Immunol Rev 169:209, 1999

Specific adaptive immune responses are mediated by developmentally independent, but functionally interacting, families of lymphocytes. T lymphocytes mediate cellular immunity, while B lymphocytes and their plasma cell progeny produce antibodies to provide humoral immunity. The activities of B and T cells and their products in host defense are closely integrated with innate immune functions of other cells of the reticuloendothelial system. Dendritic cells, Langerhans' cells in the skin, and macrophages play an important role in the trapping and presentation of antigens to T and B cells to initiate the immune response. Macrophages also become effector cells, especially when activated by cytokine products of lymphocytes. The scavenger activity of macrophages and polymorphonuclear leukocytes is directed and made specific by antibodies in concert with cytokines and the complement system. Natural killer (NK) cells, a population of granular lymphocytes with receptors specific for major histocompatibility complex (MHC) class I molecules, may spontaneously kill tumor and virus-infected cells, activities that are enhanced by the cytokine products of immune and inflammatory cells. Killing by NK cells can also be targeted by IgG antibodies for which NK cells have cell-surface receptors. The interaction of basophils and tissue mast cells with IgE antibodies in causation of immediate-type hypersensitivity is discussed in Chap. 298. Consideration of these interrelationships is an important part of the analysis of patients with suspected immune deficiency.

DIFFERENTIATION OF T AND B CELLS

The functional deficits that occur in both congenital and acquired immunodeficiencies are usefully viewed as being caused by defects at various points along the differentiation pathways of immunocompetent cells. Lymphoid progenitors derived from hematopoietic stem cells may migrate to the thymus to begin T cell development or remain in the fetal liver or bone marrow where they enter the B and NK cell pathways of development (Fig. 297-1). Immature T and B cells then migrate through the circulation to the spleen, lymph nodes, intestine, and other peripheral lymphoid organs. In these sites, they may encounter antigens presented by dendritic cells or macrophages and respond with proliferation, differentiation, and mediation of immune responses. →*Chap. 295 provides a general account of their roles in cellular and humoral immunity.*

Differentiation of T or B cells may be arrested at either the primary or secondary stages. Reflecting the complex cellular interactions involved in immune responses and the pivotal role played by T lymphocytes, immune deficiencies primarily involving T cells are usually also associated with abnormal B cell function.

CLINICAL DISEASE FEATURES COMMON TO IMMUNE DEFICIENCY

Immunodeficiency syndromes, whether congenital, spontaneously acquired, or iatrogenic, are characterized by unusual susceptibility to infection and not infrequently to autoimmune disease and lymphoreticular

malignancies. The types of infection often provide the first clue to the nature of the immunologic defect.

Patients with *defects in humoral immunity* have recurrent or chronic sinopulmonary infection, meningitis, and bacteremia, most commonly caused by pyogenic bacteria such as *Haemophilus influenzae*, *Streptococcus pneumoniae*, and *Staphylococcus aureus*. These and other pyogenic organisms also cause frequent infections in individuals who have either neutropenia or a deficiency of the pivotal third component of complement (C3). The tripartite collaboration of antibody, complement, and phagocytes in host defense against pyogenic organisms makes it important to assess all three systems in individuals with unusual susceptibility to bacterial infections.

Antibody-deficient patients in whom cell-mediated immunity is intact have an interesting response to viral infections. The clinical course of primary infection with viruses such as varicella zoster or rubeola, unless complicated by bacterial infection, does not differ significantly from that of the normal host. However, multiple bouts of chickenpox and measles may occur. Such observations suggest that intact T cells may be sufficient for control of established viral infections, while antibodies play an important role in limiting the initial dissemination of virus and in providing long-lasting protection. Exceptions to this generalization are becoming more widely recognized. Agammaglobulinemic patients fail to clear hepatitis B virus from their circulation and

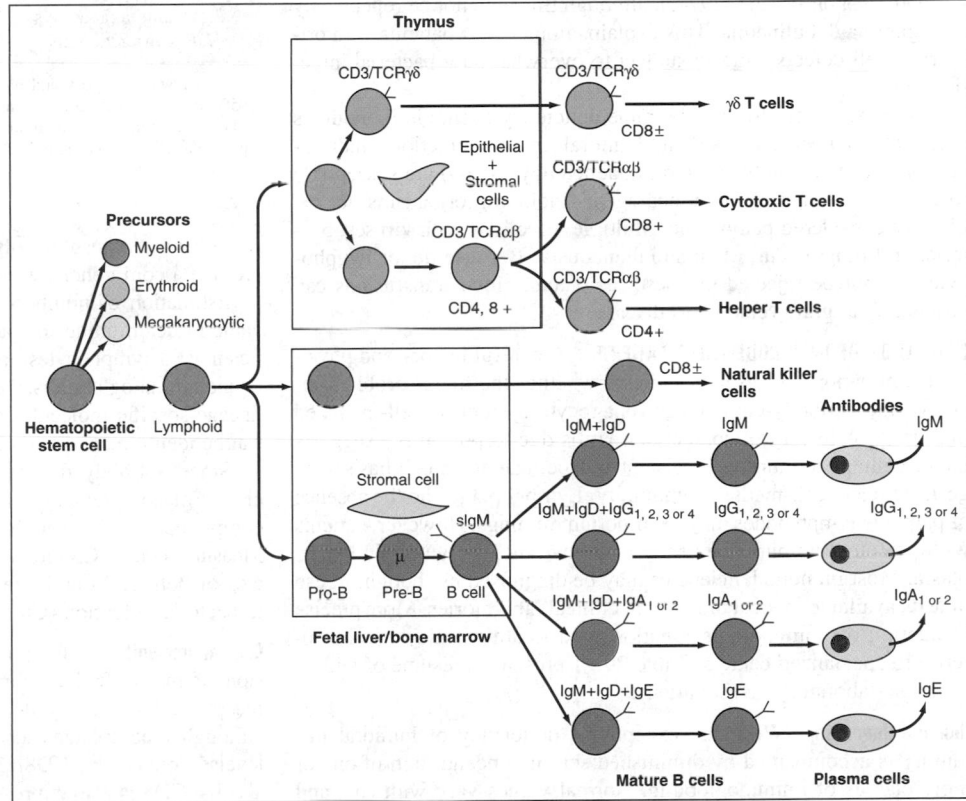

FIGURE 297-1 Hypothetical model outlining the differentiation of hematopoietic stem cells along T, B, and NK cell lineages. The antigen presenting dendritic cells, not shown here, are derived from both lymphoid and myeloid progenitors. Failure to develop T and B cells may result from defective stem cells or from inborn metabolic errors affecting both cell types. Rarely, other hematopoietic cell lines are also absent. Absence of either T or B cells suggests malfunction of central lymphoid tissues, including the thymus and the fetal liver–bone marrow complex. B cell deficiency may result from failure to generate pre-B cells from their stem cell precursors or from failure of pre-B cells to give rise to their B lymphocyte progeny. Similarly, differentiation may be arrested at several levels within the T cell lineage; arrests at the thymocyte level and failure to develop the helper subset have been observed in immunodeficient patients. Agammaglobulinemia and deficiencies of some T cell functions may occur despite the presence of normal numbers of B or T cells in the circulation. Failure of B lymphocytes to differentiate to plasma cells can be due to intrinsic cellular abnormalities or to faulty T cell regulation.

have a progressive, and often fatal, course. Poliomyelitis has occurred following live-virus vaccination in some patients. Chronic encephalitis, which may progress over a period of months to years, is a particular threat in congenitally agammaglobulinemic boys. Echoviruses and adenoviruses have been isolated from brain, spinal fluid, or other sites in such patients.

The occurrence of an unusually serious infection, for example, *H. influenzae* meningitis in an older child or adult, warrants consideration of humoral immune deficiency. Recurrent bacterial pneumonias also suggest this possibility. Chronic otitis media occurs frequently in patients with hypogammaglobulinemia and is significant because of its relative rarity in normal adults. Pansinusitis, although almost invariably present in immunoglobulin deficiency, is a less helpful finding because it is not rare in apparently normal people. Bacterial infections of the skin or urinary tract are less frequent problems in hypogammaglobulinemic patients. Infestation with the intestinal parasite *Giardia lamblia* is a frequent cause of diarrhea in antibody-deficient patients.

Abnormalities of cell-mediated immunity predispose to disseminated virus infections, particularly with latent viruses such as herpes simplex (Chap. 163), varicella zoster (Chap. 164), and cytomegalovirus (Chap. 166). In addition, patients so affected almost invariably develop mucocutaneous candidiasis and frequently acquire systemic fungal infections. Pneumonia caused by *Pneumocystis carinii* is also common (Chap. 191). Severe enteritis caused by *Cryptosporidium* infection may extend to the biliary tract to result in sclerosing cholangitis.

T cell deficiency is always accompanied by some abnormality of antibody responses (Fig. 297-1), although this may not be reflected by hypogammaglobulinemia. This explains in part why patients with primary T cell defects are also subject to overwhelming bacterial infection.

The most severe form of immune deficiency occurs in individuals who lack both cell-mediated and humoral immune functions. Individuals with severe combined immunodeficiency (SCID) are susceptible to the whole range of infectious agents including organisms not ordinarily considered pathogenic. Multiple infections with viruses, bacteria, and fungi occur, often simultaneously. Because donor lymphocytes cannot be rejected by these recipients, blood transfusions can produce fatal graft-versus-host disease.

EVALUATION OF IMMUNODEFICIENT PATIENTS   A careful history and physical examination will usually indicate whether the major problem involves the antibody-complement-phagocyte system or cell-mediated immunity. A history of contact dermatitis due to poison ivy suggests intact cellular immunity. Persistent mucocutaneous candidiasis suggests deficient cell-mediated immunity. Lymphopenia and the absence of palpable lymph nodes may be important findings. However, patients with profound immunodeficiency may have diffuse lymphoid hyperplasia. Most immunodeficiencies may be diagnosed by thoughtful use of tests available in local or regional clinical laboratories. More precise evaluation of immunologic functions and treatment may require referral to specialized centers. Table 297-1 presents a résumé of widely available laboratory investigations.

Humoral Immunity   With rare exceptions, deficiency of humoral immunity is accompanied by diminished serum concentration of one or more classes of immunoglobulin. Normal values vary with age, and adult concentrations of IgM (1.0 ± 0.4 g/L) are reached at about 1 year, of IgG (10.0 ± 3.0 g/L) at 5 to 6 years, and of IgA (2.5 ± 1.0 g/L) by puberty (Chap. 295). The wide range of values among normal adults creates difficulty in defining the lower limits of normal. Reasonable estimates for low values are below 0.4 g/L for IgM, 5 g/L for IgG, and 0.5 g/L for IgA. In the presence of borderline hypogammaglobulinemia, assessing the patient's capacity to produce specific antibodies becomes particularly important. Isohemagglutinins and "febrile agglutinins" are valuable standard assays, and measurements of pre- and postimmunization titers to tetanus toxoid, diphtheria toxoid,

TABLE 297-1   *Laboratory Evaluation of Host Defense Status*

Initial Screening Assays[a]
Complete blood count with differential smear
Serum immunoglobulin levels: IgM, IgG, IgA, IgD, IgE
Other Readily Available Assays
Quantification of blood mononuclear cell populations by
   immunofluorescence assays employing monoclonal antibody markers[b]
   T cells: CD3, CD4, CD8, $TCR\alpha\beta$, $TCR\gamma\delta$
   B cells: CD19, CD20, CD21, Ig(μ, δ, γ, α, κ, λ), Ig-associated
      molecules (α, β)
   Activation markers: HLA-DR, CD25, CD80 (B cells), CD154 (T cells)
   NK cells: CD16/CD56
   Monocytes: CD15
T cell functional evaluation
   1. Delayed hypersensitivity skin tests (PPD, *Candida*, histoplasmin,
      tetanus toxoid)
   2. Proliferative response to mitogens (anti-CD3 antibody,
      phytohemagglutinin, concanavalin A) and allogeneic cells (mixed
      lymphocyte response)
   3. Cytokine production
B cell functional evaluation
   1. Natural or commonly acquired antibodies: isohemagglutinins;
      antibodies to common viruses (influenza, rubella, rubeola) and
      bacterial toxins (diphtheria, tetanus)
   2. Response to immunization with protein (tetanus toxoid) and
      carbohydrate (pneumococcal vaccine, *H. influenzae B* vaccine)
      antigens
   3. Quantitative IgG subclass determinations
Complement
   1. CH_{50} assays (classic and alternative pathways)
   2. C3, C4, and other components
Phagocyte function
   1. Reduction of nitroblue tetrazolium
   2. Chemotaxis assays
   3. Bactericidal activity

[a] Together with a history and physical examination, these tests will identify more than 95% of patients with primary immunodeficiencies.
[b] The menu of monoclonal antibody markers may be expanded or contracted to focus on particular clinical questions.

H. influenzae capsular polysaccharide, and *S. pneumoniae* serotypes provide a comprehensive assessment of humoral responsiveness.

Estimation of numbers of circulating B and T lymphocytes is of value in determining the pathogenesis of certain types of immune deficiency. B lymphocytes are identified by the presence of membrane-bound immunoglobulins, their associated α- and β-chain units, and other lineage-specific molecules on the B cell surface (Table 297-1), which can be identified and enumerated by specific monoclonal antibodies.

Since antibody deficiency may be mimicked clinically by deficiency of complement components, measurement of total hemolytic complement (CH_{50}) should be a part of the evaluation of host defense. Measurement of C3 alone is inadequate for screening, since deficiencies of both early and late complement components may predispose to bacterial infection (Chap. 295).

Cellular Immunity   T lymphocytes may be enumerated by their expression of the TCR/CD3 complex of surface molecules (TCR; T cell receptor). The CD4 molecule serves as a marker for helper T cells, although macrophages also express this molecule in relatively low levels. Conversely, $CD8\alpha\beta$ heterodimers are expressed by cytotoxic T cells. CD8 is also expressed by some $\gamma\delta$ T cells and by NK cells as $CD8\alpha\alpha$ homodimeric molecules.

Normal levels of serum immunoglobulins and antibody responsiveness are reliable indices of intact helper T cell function. T lymphocyte function can be measured directly by delayed hypersensitivity skin testing using a variety of antigens to which the majority of older children and adults have been sensitized. A generally useful skin test antigen is a 1:5 dilution of tetanus toxoid injected intradermally, since almost all individuals will have been sensitized. Purified protein derivative (PPD), histoplasmin, mumps antigen, and extracts of *Candida* or *Trichophyton* also may be used.

T lymphocyte function may be estimated in vitro by the capacity of cells to proliferate in response to antigens to which the patient has been sensitized, to lymphocytes from an unrelated donor, to antibodies that cross-link the CD3/TCR complex, or to the T cell mitogens, such as phytohemagglutinin and concanavalin A. The response is usually quantified 3 days later by measurement of incorporation of radioactive thymidine into newly synthesized DNA. The production of cytokines (or interleukins) by activated T cells can be measured, as can the ability of T cells activated in mixed lymphocyte culture to lyse target cells. Finally, assays exist for detection of defects in T cell surface receptors and specific elements of their signal transduction pathways.

CLASSIFICATION *Primary immunodeficiencies* may be either congenital or manifested later in life and are currently classified according to mode of inheritance and whether the genetic defect affects T cells, B cells, or both (Table 297-2). The following discussion emphasizes three related concepts: (1) that immunodeficiencies are logically viewed as defects of cellular differentiation; (2) that these defects may involve either primary development of T or B cells or the antigen-dependent phase of their differentiation; and (3) that defects of B cell differentiation may in some instances reflect faulty T-B collaboration.

Secondary immunodeficiencies are those not caused by intrinsic

TABLE 297-2 *Primary Immunodeficiencies—Laboratory and Clinical Features*

| | Lymphocytes | | | Cellular Immunity | Humoral Immunity | | | | | Common Infections |
| | | | | | Serum Immunoglobulins | | | | Antibody Responses | |
	B	T	NK		M	G	A	E		
Severe combined immunodeficiency (SCID)										
Adenosine deaminse (ADA) deficiency	−	−	+	−	↓	↓	↓	↓	−	Bacteria, viruses, fungi
Artemis deficiency (SCIDA)	−	−	+	−	↓	↓	↓	↓	−	Bacteria, viruses, fungi
CD45 deficiency	+	−	−	−	↓	↓	↓	↓	−	Bacteria, viruses, fungi
Interleukin receptor γ chain deficiency (X-linked SCID)	+	−	−	−	N	↓	↓	↓	−	Bacteria, viruses, fungi
Janus-associated kinase 3 (JAK3) deficiency	+	−	−	−	N	↓	↓	↓	−	Bacteria, viruses, fungi
Recombinase activating gene (RAG 1/2) deficiency	−	−	+	−	↓	↓	↓	↓	−	Bacteria, viruses, fungi
Reticular dysgenesis	−	−	−	−	↓	↓	↓	↓	−	Bacteria, viruses, fungi
TAP-1 or TAP-2 deficiency (MHC class I deficiency)	+	±	+	−	N	N	N	N	+	Bacteria, viruses, fungi
Primary T Cell Deficiency										
CD8 deficiency	+	±	+	±	N	N	N	N	+	Bacteria
DiGeorge syndrome	+	−	+	−	N	N	N	N	±	Bacteria, viruses, fungi
MHC class II deficiency	+	±	+	+	N	↓	↓	↓	+	Bacteria, viruses, fungi
Nude syndrome (wing helix nude deficiency)	+	−	+	−	N	N/↓	N/↓	N/↓	±	Bacteria, viruses, fungi
Purine nucleotide phosphorylase (PNP) deficiency	+	−	+	−	N	↓	↓	↓	±	Bacteria, viruses, fungi
T cell receptor deficiency (CD3₋ or CD3ϵ deficiency)	+	+	+	−	N	N	N	N	±	Bacteria, viruses, fungi
Zap70 tyrosine kinase deficiency	+	±	+	−	N	N/↓	N/↓	N/↓	±	Bacteria, viruses, fungi
Predominantly antibody deficiency										
IgG subclass deficiency	+	+	+	+	N	N/↓	N/↓	N/↓	±	Bacteria
Autosomal recessive agammaglobulinemia (λ5, Igβ, or BLNK deficiency)	−	+	+	+	↓	↓	↓	↓	−	Bacteria, *Giardia lamblia*
Common variable immune deficiency	+	+	+	+	N/↓	↓	↓	↓	−	Bacteria, *Giardia lamblia*
Selective IgA deficiency	+	+	+	+	N	N	↓	N	±	Bacteria, *Giardia lamblia*
X-linked agammaglobulinemia	−	+	+	+	↓	↓	↓	↓	−	Bacteria, *Giardia lamblia*
Hyper IgM syndrome										
Activation-induced cytidine deaminase deficiency	+	+	+	+	N/↑	↓	↓	↓	±	Bacteria
X-linked CD40 ligand deficiency	+	+	+	+	N/↑	↓	N/↓	↓	±	Bacteria, viruses, fungi
X-linked IKK-gamma (NEMO) deficiency	+	+	+	+	N/↑	↓	↓	↓	±	Bacteria, viruses, fungi
CD40 deficiency	+	+	+	+	N/↑	↓	N/↓	↓	±	Bacteria, viruses, fungi
Other well-defined immunodeficiency syndromes										
Ataxia telangiectasia	+	+	+	+	N/↑	N/↓	N/↓	↓	±	Bacteria
Hyper IgE syndrome	+	+	+	+	N	N	N	↑↑↑	+	Bacteria
Immunodeficiency with thymoma	−	+	+	±	↓	↓	↓	↓	±	Bacteria
Wiskott-Aldrich syndrome	+	±	+	±	↓	N	↑	↑	±	Bacteria
Interferon γ receptor deficiency	+	+	+	+	N	N	N	N	+	Mycobacteria, viruses
Interleukin 12 and interleukin 12 receptor deficiency	+	+	+	+	N	N	N	N	+	Mycobacteria, *Salmonella*
X-linked lymphoproliferative syndrome	+	+	+	+	N	N/↓	N/↓	N/↓	±	Epstein-Barr virus

Note: B, B cells; T, T cells; NK, natural killer lymphocytes; +, normal levels; −, reduced or absent levels; N, ↑, ↓, normal, elevated, or reduced serum immunoglobulins.

abnormalities in development or function of T and B cells. The best known of these is AIDS, which may follow infection with the human immunodeficiency virus (Chap. 173). Other examples are immune deficiency associated with malnutrition, protein-losing enteropathy, and intestinal lymphangiectasia. Also considered secondary are immunodeficiencies resulting from hypercatabolic states such as occur in myotonic dystrophy; immunodeficiency associated with lymphoreticular malignancy; and immunodeficiency resulting from treatment with x-rays, antilymphocyte antibodies, or immunosuppressive drugs.

Incidence As a group, the primary immunodeficiencies are relatively common. The most frequent, isolated IgA deficiency, occurs in approximately 1 in 600 individuals in Europe and North America. Common variable immunodeficiency, a related disorder characterized by pan-hypogammaglobulinemia, is the next most common disorder. Both of these immunodeficiency states often become clinically evident in young adults.

The more severe forms of primary immunodeficiency are relatively rare, have their onset early in life, and all too frequently result in death during childhood. However, patients with congenital hypogammaglobulinemia may lead relatively healthy lives with adequate antibody-replacement therapy. In a referral center for patients with immunodeficiency diseases, approximately two-thirds of the immunodeficient patients will be adults.

Severe Combined Immunodeficiency The SCID syndrome is characterized by gross functional impairment of both humoral and cell-mediated immunity and by susceptibility to devastating fungal, bacterial, and viral infections. Inherited either as an X-linked or autosomal recessive defect, affected infants rarely survive beyond 1 year without treatment.

The overall incidence of SCID is 1 in 100,000 to 1 in 1,000,000. The syndrome has been associated with a diversity of defects in development of immunocompetent cells, which are caused by mutations in genes whose products are necessary for the normal differentiation of T, B, and, sometimes, NK cells.

In one autosomal recessive form of SCID characterized by severe lymphopenia, the failure in T and B cell development is due to mutations in the *RAG-1* or *RAG-2* genes, the combined activities of which are needed for V(D)J recombination. A function-loss mutation in either the DNA-dependent tyrosine kinase or the *Artemis* genes may cause SCID, since they also encode essential enzymes for the V(D)J gene rearrangement process. About half of patients with autosomal recessive SCID are deficient in an enzyme involved in purine metabolism, adenosine deaminase (ADA), due to mutations in the *ADA* gene. The abortive lymphoid differentiation associated with ADA deficiency is due to intracellular accumulation of adenosine and deoxyadenosine nucleotides that trigger apoptosis of immature T and B lineage cells.

SCID may also occur with an X-linked inheritance pattern. Aborted thymocyte differentiation and an absence of peripheral T cells and NK cells is seen in X-linked SCID. B lymphocytes are present in normal numbers but are functionally defective. The defective gene encodes a common γ chain of the receptors for interleukin (IL) 2, -4, -7, -9, and -15, thus disrupting the action of this important set of lymphokines. The same T⁻ NK⁻B⁺ SCID phenotype seen in X-linked SCID can be inherited as an autosomal recessive disease due to mutations in the gene for JAK3 protein kinase deficiency. This enzyme associates with the common γ chain of the receptors for IL-2, -4, -7, -9, and -15 to serve as a key element in their signal transduction pathways.

℞ TREATMENT

The cellular defects in SCID patients logically rest with the pluripotent hematopoietic stem cells or their lymphoid progenitor progeny. Accordingly, the immunologic deficits in all of the different types of SCID patients have been repaired by transplantation of histocompatible bone marrow as a source of stem cells, thereby implying that the stromal microenvironments of these individuals are intact and capable of supporting T and B cell development. However, antibody deficiency requiring immunoglobulin replacement therapy may persist for years in the γc-deficient and JAK3-deficient patients, unless the defective B cells are eliminated prior to bone marrow transplantation to allow their replacement with normal B cells of donor origin. *Ex vivo* insertion of a γc transgene into bone marrow progenitors has successfully corrected the immune deficiency of X-linked SCID patients. Notably, however, chance insertion of the γc transgene near a tumor-suppressor gene was associated with development of a γδ T cell lymphoproliferative disorder in two patients so treated. In ADA-deficient patients without histocompatible bone marrow donors, the administration of exogenous ADA (conjugated to polyethylene glycol to prolong its half-life) may improve immunologic function and clinical status. Hematopoietic stem cell gene therapy has also been used successfully in treating ADA-deficient SCID patients; myeloablative conditioning was required to clear a space in the bone marrow for the ADA transduced cells. Treatment of SCID patients should be performed in centers with a strong research interest in this problem. It is crucial that these patients be recognized and treated early. Live viral vaccines or blood transfusions must be avoided since they can cause fatal infections and graft-versus-host disease in SCID patients.

Primary T Cell Immunodeficiency Reflecting the diversity of T cell functions, abnormalities of T cell development may be responsible for a wide spectrum of immune deficiencies, including combined immunodeficiency, selective defects in cell-mediated immunity, and syndromes presenting as antibody deficiency. These defects may be acquired (Chap. 173) as well as congenital.

THE DIGEORGE SYNDROME This classic example of isolated T cell deficiency results from maldevelopment of thymic epithelial elements derived from the third and fourth pharyngeal pouches. The gene defect has been mapped to chromosome 22q11 in most patients with the DiGeorge syndrome, and to chromosome 10p in others. Defective development of organs dependent on cells of embryonic neural crest origin includes: congenital cardiac defects, particularly those involving the great vessels; hypocalcemic tetany, due to failure of parathyroid development; and absence of a normal thymus. Facial abnormalities may include abnormal ears, shortened philtrum, micrognathia, and hypertelorism. Serum immunoglobulin concentrations are frequently normal, but antibody responses, particularly of IgG and IgA isotypes, are usually impaired. T cell levels are reduced, whereas B cell levels are normal. Affected individuals usually have a small, histologically normal thymus located near the base of the tongue or in the neck, allowing most patients to develop functional T cells in numbers that may or may not be adequate for host defense.

THE NUDE SYNDROME The human disease counterpart to the *nude* mouse is caused by mutations of the *whn* (winged-helix-nude) gene that result in impairment of hair follicle and epithelial thymic development. The human *nude* phenotype is characterized by congenital baldness, nail dystrophy, and severe T cell immunodeficiency.

T CELL RECEPTOR DEFICIENCY Since the expression and function of antigen-specific TCRs is dependent on their signal transducing CD3γ, δ, ε, and ζ-η chains, defective genes for any of these receptor components can impair T cell development and function. Immunodeficiencies due to inherited CD3γ and CD3ε mutations have been identified. CD3γ mutations result in a selective deficit in CD8 T cells, whereas CD3ε mutations lead to a preferential reduction in CD4 T cells, thus implying differences in the signal transduction roles for each CD3 component.

MHC CLASS II DEFICIENCY Because T cells are required for B cell responses to most antigens, any gene defect (or acquired disorder) that interferes with T cell development and cell-mediated immunity will also compromise antibody production and humoral immunity. MHC class II deficiency results in one such immunodeficiency in that the TCRαβ must see protein antigens as peptide fragments held within the α helical grooves of class II and class I molecules encoded by the MHC. Antigen-presenting cells in individuals with this relatively rare disorder fail to express the class II molecules DP, DQ, and DR on their surface. Limited numbers of helper CD4 T cells are therefore generated in the thymus, and they fail to see antigen in the periphery. Affected individuals experience recurrent bronchopulmonary infections, chronic diarrhea, and severe viral infections that usually prove fatal before 4 years of age. The defect is caused by mutations in genes that encode essential transcriptional factors that bind to promoter elements for the MHC class II genes. The class II transactivator (*CIITA*) gene is mutated in one subgroup of MHC class II–deficient patients, whereas mutations in *RFX* genes encoding additional transcriptional factors for MHC class II genes are responsible for the defective development and function of CD4 T cells in other families: *RFXANK* in subgroup B, *RFX5* in subgroup C, and *RFXAP* in subgroup D.

ZAP70 TYROSINE KINASE DEFICIENCY Recurrent and opportunistic infections begin within the first year of life in individuals with a deficiency in ZAP70 tyrosine kinase, a pivotal component in the TCR/CD3 signal transduction cascade. The rare inheritance of mutations in both alleles of the *ZAP70* gene results in a selective deficiency of CD8 T cells and dysfunction of CD4 T cells, which are present in normal numbers. Severe immunodeficiency is the inevitable consequence.

PURINE NUCLEOSIDE PHOSPHORYLATION DEFICIENCY Function-loss mutations of the *purine nucleoside phosphorylase (PNP)* gene are associated with an often severe and selective deficiency of T lymphocyte function. This enzyme functions in the same purine salvage pathway as ADA; toxic effects of the PNP deficiency may result from the intracellular accumulation of deoxyguanosine triphosphate.

ATAXIA-TELANGIECTASIA Ataxia-telangiectasia (AT) is an autosomal recessive genetic disorder characterized by cerebellar ataxia, oculocutaneous telangiectasia, and immunodeficiency. The mutant *ATM* gene has sequence similarity to the phosphatidyl-inositol-3 kinases that are involved in signal transduction. The *ATM* gene belongs to a conserved family of genes that monitor DNA repair and coordinate DNA synthesis with cell division. The deleterious effects of the *ATM* gene are widespread. Truncal ataxia may become evident when walking begins and is progressive. Telangiectasia, primarily represented by dilated blood vessels in the ocular sclera, in a butterfly area of the face, and on the ears, is an early diagnostic feature. Immunodeficiency may be clinically manifest by recurrent and chronic sinopulmonary infection leading to bronchiectasis, although not all patients have overt immunodeficiency. Ovarian agenesis is a frequent occurrence. Persistence of very high serum levels of oncofetal proteins, including α fetoprotein and carcinoembryonic antigen, may be of diagnostic value. Frequent causes of death are chronic pulmonary disease and malignancy. Lymphomas are most common, although carcinomas also occur.

The immunologic abnormalities seem to be related to maldevelopment of the thymus. The markedly hypoplastic thymus is similar in appearance to an embryonic thymus. The peripheral T cell pool is reduced in size, especially in lymphoid tissue compartments. Cutaneous anergy and delayed rejection of skin grafts are common. Although B lymphocyte development is normal, most patients are deficient in serum IgE and IgA, and a smaller number have reduced serum levels of IgG, particularly of the IgG2, IgG4 subclasses.

The defect in DNA repair mechanisms in AT patients renders their cells highly susceptible to radiation-induced chromosomal damage and resultant tumor development. AT is a rare disorder, one in 10,000 to 100,000 incidence, but 1% of the population is heterozygous for an AT mutation. This is important because the heterozygous state also predisposes to enhanced cellular radiosensitivity and cancer, especially breast cancer in females (Chap. 353).

℞ TREATMENT

Therapeutic options other than symptomatic treatment are limited for this group of patients. Live vaccines and blood transfusions containing viable T cells should be assiduously avoided. Exposure to x-irradiation should also be avoided in patients with AT. Therapeutic intervention in the form of an epithelial thymic transplant should repair the T cell deficiency in patients with the *nude* syndrome and in the most severe

cases of the DiGeorge syndrome where T cells are absent. Treatment by bone marrow transplantation is sometimes successful after myeloablative conditioning in patients with PNP and MHC class II deficiencies. Preventive therapy for *P. carinii* in the form of trimethoprim-sulfamethoxazole should be considered. Immunoglobulin infusions are also recommended for those T cell–deficient individuals with severe antibody deficiency reflected by low serum levels of IgG.

Immunoglobulin Deficiency Syndromes ■ *X-LINKED AGAMMAGLOBULINEMIA* Males with this syndrome often begin to have recurrent bacterial infections in the first year of life when maternally derived immunoglobulins have disappeared. Although B cell progenitors are found in the bone marrow, affected individuals have very few immunoglobulin-bearing B lymphocytes in their circulation and lack primary and secondary lymphoid follicles. The developmental block is evident at the pre-B cell level (Fig. 297-1). Mutations of *Bruton's tyrosine kinase (Btk)* gene are responsible for X-linked agammaglobulinemia. B cells in heterozygous female carriers exclusively utilize the X chromosome with the normal *Btk* gene, while T cells and myeloid cells express either X chromosome. A variant disorder, *X-linked agammaglobulinemia with growth hormone deficiency*, has been associated with *Btk* mutations that result in truncated messages.

Agammaglobulinemia is a misnomer, since most of these patients synthesize some immunoglobulins. Within the same family, some affected males may have substantial levels of IgM, IgG, and IgA, while others are nearly agammaglobulinemic. Btk-deficient patients typically are very deficient in circulating B lymphocytes. The few B lymphocytes that escape the block in pre-B cell differentiation are impaired in their responsiveness to antigenic stimulation, making antibody replacement therapy essential in these patients.

Sinopulmonary bacterial infections constitute the most frequent clinical problem. *Mycoplasma* infections also cause arthritis in some of these patients. Chronic encephalitis of viral etiology, sometimes associated with dermatomyositis, can be a fatal complication. These complications are reduced by treatment with intravenous immunoglobulin.

AUTOSOMAL RECESSIVE AGAMMAGLOBULINEMIA This syndrome can result from mutations in a variety of genes whose products are required for B lineage differentiation. For example, signals induced via pre-B receptors are essential for pre-B cell development. Consequently, mutations in any of the genes coding pre-B receptor components—μ *heavy chain*, *surrogate light chain* (*VpreB* and $\lambda5/14.1$), *Igα*, and *Igβ*—can block B lineage differentiation. Congenital absence of B cells, agammaglobulinemia, and recurrent bacterial infections have been seen in children with function-loss mutations in both alleles of the μ *heavy chain* gene or the $\lambda5/14.1$ and *Igβ* genes. Disruption of B cell development may also occur as a consequence of mutations in genes coding transcription factors for pre-B receptor genes or for key elements in the pre-B receptor signaling pathway. For example, mutations in the *BLNK* gene can cause agammaglobulinemia because this gene encodes a cytoplasmic adaptor protein that is essential for B cell development.

TRANSIENT HYPOGAMMAGLOBULINEMIA OF INFANCY This diagnosis is reserved for those rare instances in which normal physiologic hypogammaglobulinemia of infancy is unusually prolonged and severe. IgG levels normally drop to 3.0 to 4.0 g/L between 3 and 6 months of age as maternally derived IgG is catabolized. The IgG levels subsequently rise, reflecting the infants' increased synthetic capacity. Periodic immunologic assessment is needed to differentiate transient hypogammaglobulinemia from other forms of antibody deficiency. Antibody replacement therapy is recommended only in the face of severe or recurrent infections.

IgA DEFICIENCY An inability to produce antibodies of the IgA1 and IgA2 subclasses occurs in approximately 1 in 600 individuals of European origin, a much higher incidence than is seen for other primary immunodeficiencies. IgA deficiency is much less common in people of

Asian and African origin. In Japan, for example, the incidence is approximately 1 in 18,500. While the precise genetic basis for this difference in incidence is unknown, IgA deficiency is frequently associated with certain MHC haplotypes that are more common in Caucasians.

Individuals with isolated IgA deficiency may appear healthy or present with an increased number of respiratory infections of varying severity, and a few have progressive pulmonary disease leading to bronchiectasis. Chronic diarrheal diseases also occur. Reductions in the IgG2 and IgG4 subclasses are associated with the increased infections in some IgA-deficient individuals. The incidence of asthma and other atopic diseases among IgA-deficient patients is high. Conversely, the incidence of IgA deficiency among atopic children has been found to be more than 20 times that in the normal population. IgA deficiency is also significantly associated with arthritis (Chap. 301) and systemic lupus erythematosus (Chap. 300). IgA-deficient patients frequently produce autoantibodies. Some of them produce antibodies to IgA, which make them vulnerable to severe anaphylactic reactions when transfused with normal blood or blood products containing IgA.

An accurate picture of the clinical consequences of IgA deficiency requires lifelong study of affected individuals. Among 204 healthy young adults whose IgA deficiency was identified when they served as blood donors, 80% were found to experience episodes of infections, drug allergy, autoimmune disorders, or atopic disease during the next 20 years of their life. They had an increased susceptibility to pneumonia, recurrent episodes of respiratory infections, and a higher incidence of autoimmune diseases, including vitiligo, autoimmune thyroiditis, and possibly rheumatoid arthritis.

IgA deficiency is often familial. It can also occur in association with congenital intrauterine infections, such as toxoplasmosis, rubella, and cytomegalovirus infection, or following treatment with phenytoin, penicillamine, or other medications in genetically susceptible individuals. The pathogenesis of IgA deficiency, whether genetic or triggered by environmental insult, involves a block in B cell differentiation that may reflect defective interaction between T and B cells.

Treatment of IgA deficiency is essentially symptomatic. IgA cannot be effectively replaced by exogenous immunoglobulin or plasma, and use of either can increase the risk of development of antibodies to IgA. IgA-deficient patients in need of transfusion should be screened for the presence of antibodies to IgA and ideally should be given blood only from IgA-deficient donors. Immunoglobulin infusions may benefit the exceptional IgA-deficient person in whom IgG2 and IgG4 subclass deficiencies are associated with severe infections, but the risk of anaphylactic reactions to contaminating IgA must always be considered in treating these patients.

IgG SUBCLASS DEFICIENCIES   Selective deficiencies in one or more of the four IgG subclasses are seen in some patients with repeated infections. The IgG subclass deficiency may easily go undetected when the total serum IgG level is measured, because IgG2, IgG3, and IgG4 together account for only 30 to 40% of the IgG antibodies. Even a deficiency in IgG1 may be masked by increases in the remaining IgG isotypes. However, the availability of subclass-specific monoclonal antibodies allows precise measurement of IgG subclass levels.

Homozygous deletions of genes encoding the constant region of the different γ chains are the basis for the IgG subclass deficiency in some individuals. For example, deletion of the $C_{\alpha 1}$, $C_{\gamma 2}$, $C_{\gamma 4}$, and C_{ϵ} genes in the heavy chain locus on both chromosomes 14 was responsible for one individual's inability to make IgA1, IgG2, IgG4, and IgE. Because other components of their immune system are intact, individuals with this and other patterns of C_H-gene deletions may not have unusual infections.

Most of the IgG subclass–deficient individuals with repeated infections appear to have regulatory defects that prevent normal B cell differentiation. The defect may extend to other isotypes. IgA deficiency may accompany IgG2 and IgG4 subclass deficiencies (see "IgA

Deficiency," above); an inability to produce IgM antibodies to polysaccharide antigens often reflects a broader defect in antibody responsiveness. While patients with IgG subclass deficiency may benefit from administration of immunoglobulin, a thorough assessment of humoral immunity is needed to identify the relatively few who need this therapy.

COMMON VARIABLE IMMUNODEFICIENCY   This diagnostic category includes a heterogeneous group, mostly adults, who have in common the clinical manifestations of deficient production of all the different classes of antibodies. The majority of these hypogammaglobulinemic patients have normal numbers of B lymphocytes that are clonally diverse but phenotypically immature. B lymphocytes in these patients are able to recognize antigens and can proliferate in response, but they largely fail to become memory B cells and mature plasma cells. This abortive differentiation pattern leads to the frequent occurrence of nodular B lymphocyte hyperplasia, resulting in splenomegaly and intestinal lymphoid hyperplasia, sometimes of massive proportion.

It is important to note that common variable immunodeficiency and IgA deficiency represent polar ends of a clinical spectrum due to the same underlying gene defect(s) in a large subset of these patients. The two disorders feature similar B cell differentiation arrests, differing only in the numbers of immunoglobulin classes involved. Over a period of years, IgA-deficient patients may progress to the pan-hypogammaglobulinemia phenotype characteristic of common variable immunodeficiency, and vice versa. Both disorders occur frequently within the same family, and the same MHC haplotypes are associated with both immunodeficiency patterns. Family studies suggest an underlying susceptibility gene in the MHC class III region for both disorders.

It is important to consider the diagnosis of common variable immunodeficiency in adults with chronic pulmonary infections, some of whom will present with bronchiectasis. Intestinal diseases—including chronic giardiasis, intestinal malabsorption, and atrophic gastritis with pernicious anemia—are common in this group of patients. Patients with common variable immunodeficiency may also present with signs and symptoms highly suggestive of lymphoid malignancy, including fever, weight loss, anemia, thrombocytopenia, splenomegaly, generalized lymphadenopathy, and lymphocytosis. Histologic examination of lymphoid tissues usually reveals germinal center hyperplasia that may be difficult to distinguish from nodular lymphoma (Chap. 97). Demonstration of a normal distribution of immunoglobulin isotypes and light chain classes for circulating and tissue B lymphocytes can serve to distinguish these patients from those having a monoclonal B cell malignancy with secondary hypogammaglobulinemia. The administration of intravenous immunoglobulin in adequate doses (see below) is an essential part of the prevention and treatment of all these complications.

X-LINKED IMMUNODEFICIENCY WITH HYPER IgM   In this syndrome, typically the IgG and IgA levels are very low, while IgM levels may be very high, normal, or even low. The development of B lymphocytes bearing IgM and IgD and the absence of IgG and IgA B lymphocytes indicate a defect in isotype switching. The defective *CD40L* gene in these patients encodes a transiently expressed molecule on activated T cells that is the ligand for the CD40 molecule on dendritic (D) cells and B cells. Gene mutations that preclude normal CD40 ligand expression prevent normal T and B cell cooperation, germinal center formation, V-region diversification by somatic hypermutation, and isotype switching. T cell responses are also compromised in these CD40 ligand–deficient patients because their T cells are deprived of an important activation stimulus as a consequence of the defective T, D, and B cell interactions (Chap. 295). Consequently, these patients experience more severe infections than those occurring with other hypogammaglobulinemic states. In addition to recurrent bacterial infections, pneumonia may be caused by *P. carinii*, cytomegalovirus, *Aspergillus*, *Cryptosporidium*, and other unusual organisms. Enteritis due to cryptosporidial infection may extend into the biliary tract to result in a sclerosing cholangitis and hepatic cirrhosis. Neutropenia is frequent in affected males and increases their vulnerability to infections.

Immunodeficiency with hyper IgM is also seen in patients of both sexes who lack mutations in their *CD40L* gene. One such hyper IgM syndrome is caused by deficiency of activation-induced cytidine deaminase (AID). Patients with AID mutations make IgM antibodies of relatively low affinity because this nuclear enzyme is essential for immunoglobulin isotype switching and somatic hypermutation. The non-X-linked form of immunodeficiency with hyper IgM can also be caused by *CD40* mutation or by mutations of genes coding components of the CD40/CD40L signaling pathways. Impaired signaling through the nuclear factor–kappa B (NF-kB) pathway due to *I Kappa–B kinase gamma IKBKG* mutations can cause an X-linked hyper-IgM and anhidrotic ectodermal dysplasia (XHM-ED) syndrome with or without osteopetrosis and lymphedema.

℞ TREATMENT

Replacement therapy with human immunoglobulin is the therapeutic cornerstone for antibody-deficient patients who have recurrent infections and who are deficient in IgG. Maintenance of serum IgG levels above 5.0 g/L will prevent most systemic infections in the patients. These serum levels can usually be achieved by intravenous administration of immunoglobulin, 400 to 500 mg/kg, at 3- to 4-week intervals. In patients with mild to moderate IgG deficiency (3.0 to 5.0 g/L) or isolated IgG subclass deficiencies, the decision to treat should be based on evaluation of clinical symptoms and antibody responses to antigenic challenge. Since immunoglobulin preparations are composed almost entirely of IgG antibodies, they are of no value for repairing deficiencies of immunoglobulins other than IgG. Infusions of immunoglobulin are also not benign. While HIV transmission has not been reported, previous epidemics of hepatitis C virus infections in hypogammaglobulinemic patients receiving contaminated immunoglobulin preparations have led to improved safety measures for current commercial preparations. Some antibody-deficient patients develop symptoms of diaphoresis, tachycardia, flank pain, and hypotension during immunoglobulin infusion. This reaction may be resolved by slowing the rate of immunoglobulin infusion. Thrombotic complications, including stroke, myocardial infarction, and pulmonary emboli, have also been reported to be associated with rapid immunoglobulin infusion. Serious anaphylactic reactions may occur as a consequence of antibodies produced by the patient against donor immunoglobulins, particularly IgA (Chap. 99). The potential for severe adverse reactions merits administration of the initial immunoglobulin infusion under medical supervision in a hospital or clinic setting.

A heightened index of suspicion of infection is essential for antibody-deficient patients. Identification of infectious agents in order to select appropriate antibiotic, antiparasitic, or antiviral therapy is also very important. Immunoglobulin infusions usually do not suffice to eliminate chronic sinopulmonary infections with *H. influenzae* and other microorganisms, and a prolonged course of antibiotic therapy may be required to treat these infections effectively and prevent progression to pulmonary fibrosis and bronchiectasis. Maintenance of good pulmonary toilet with regular postural drainage and chest percussion can be especially important in management of these patients. Infestation with *G. lamblia*, a common cause of chronic diarrhea in antibody-deficient patients, usually responds to therapy with metronidazole.

Cryptosporidial infections in CD40 ligand–deficient patients may respond to long-term treatment with amphotericin B and flucytosine. The neutropenia frequently associated with infections in these patients may or may not resolve with improvement of infections and antibody replacement therapy. Bone marrow transplantation following myeloablative pretransplantation therapy can be curative for boys with this devastating immunodeficiency. This treatment has a much greater chance of success when performed during childhood.

Miscellaneous Immunodeficiency Syndromes Infection with *Candida albicans* is the almost universal accompaniment of severe deficiencies in cell-mediated immunity. *Chronic mucocutaneous candidiasis* is dif-

ferent because superficial candidiasis is usually the only major manifestation of immunodeficiency in this syndrome. These patients rarely develop systemic infection with *Candida* or other fungal agents and are not unusually susceptible to virus or bacterial disease. No uniformity of immunologic defects has been identified in these patients, although defects of antibody formation have been detected occasionally. Humoral immunity, including ability to make specific anti-*Candida* antibodies, is usually normal. Many patients are anergic, some to a variety of antigens and some only to *Candida*. The syndrome is often congenital and may be associated with single or multiple endocrinopathies as well as iron deficiency. One well-defined genetic disorder, *autoimmune polyendocrinopathy-candidiasis-ectodermal dystrophy* (APECED) is caused by autoimmune regulator (*AIRE*) mutations. The AIRE transcription factor upregulates ectopic expression of many tissue-specific proteins in the thymus to promote the development of immunologic tolerance to self-antigens. Treatment of associated con-

TABLE 297-3 *Primary Immunodeficiencies Associated with or Secondadry to Other Diseases[a]*

Chromosomal instability or defective repair
  Bloom syndrome (*BLM* helicase)
  DNA ligase IV deficiency
  Fanconi anemia (multiple complementation groups)
  ICF syndrome (*DNMT3B* DNA methyltransferase)
  Nijmegen breakage syndrome (*Nibrin*)
  Seckel syndrome
  Xeroderma pigmentosum (multiple complementation groups)
Chromosomal defects
  Down syndrome (trisomy 21)
  Turner syndrome (X chromosome monosomy)
  Deletions or rings of chromosome 18 (18p- and 18q-)
Immunodeficiency with generalized growth retardation
  Schimke immuno-osseous dysplasia (*SMARCAL1*)
  Dubowitz syndrome
  Kyphomelic dysplasia with SCID
  Mulibrey nannism (*TRIM37*)
  Growth retardation, facial anomalies, and immunodeficiency
  Progeria (Hutchinson-Gilford syndrome)
  Thumb agenesis, short stature, and immunodeficiency
  X-linked agammaglobulinemia with growth hormone deficiency (*BTK*)
Immunodeficiency with dermatologic defects
  Dyskeratosis congenita
    Autosomal dominant (*TERC*)
    Autosomal recessive
    X-linked, Zinsser-Cole-Engman syndrome (*dyskerin*)
  Ectrodactyly-ectodermal dysplasia-clefting syndrome
  Erythroderma desquamative of Leiner
  Griscelli syndrome, partial albinism (*RAB27A*)
  Netherton syndrome (*SPINK5*)
  Omenn syndrome (*RAG 1/2*)
  Trichothiodystrophy, congenital ichthyosis (*ERCC2/XPD* or *ERCC3/XPB*)
Hereditary metabolic defects
  α-Mannosidosis (*MAN2B1*)
  Acrodermatitis enteropathica, zinc deficiency type (*SLC39A4*)
  Propionyl-CoA carboxylase, beta subunit, deficiency (*PCCB*)
  Glycogen storage disease, type 1b (*G6PT1*)
  Hyperzincemia with functional zinc depletion
  Oroticaciduria I (*UMPS*)
  Transcobalamin 2 deficiency (*TCN2*)
Hypercatabolism of immunoglobulin
  Familial hypercatabolism
  Intestinal lymphangiectasia
Other
  Chédiak-Higashi syndrome (*CHS1*)
  Cartilage-hair hypoplasia (endoribonuclease *RMRP*)
  Chronic mucocutaneous candidiasis
  Autoimmune polyendocrinopathy-candidiasis-ectodermal dystrophy (APECED)
  Hereditary or congenital hyposplenia or asplenia
  Ivemark syndrome

[a] Mutant genes indicated in parentheses.

TABLE 297-4 *Genes or Genetic Loci Associated with Primary Immunodeficiencies*

Disorder	Gene or Locus	Chromosome
Severe combined immunodeficiency (SCID)		
Adenosine deaminase deficiency	*ADA*	20q13.11
Artemis deficiency	*ARTEMIS*	10p
CD45 deficiency	*CD45*	1q31-32
DNA-dependent protein kinase deficiency	*PRKDC*	8q11
Interleukin receptor γ chain deficiency	*IL2RG*	Xq13
Janus-associated kinase 3 deficiency	*JAK3*	19p13.1
Recombinase activating gene deficiency	*RAG1, RAG2*	11p13
Primary T cell immunodeficiency		
Antigen peptide transporter deficiency	*TAP1, TAP2*	6p21.3
CD8 deficiency	*CD8*	2p12
DiGeorge syndrome	*DGCR1*	22q11
	DGCR2	10p13
Nude syndrome	*WHN*	17q11-q12
T cell receptor deficiency:		
CD3γ	*CD3G*	7q35
CD3ε	CD3E	11q23
MHC class II deficiency:		
MHC class II transactivator (group A)	*CIITA*	16p13
Regulatory factor X, ankyrin-repeat containing (group B)	*RFXANK*	19p12
Regulatory factor X, 5 (group C)	*RFX5*	1q21.1-q21.3
Regulatory factor X-associated protein (group D)	*RFXAP*	13q14
Zeta-chain-associated protein kinase deficiency	*ZAP70*	2q12
Purine nucleotide phosphorylase deficiency	*NP*	14q13.1
Predominantly antibody deficiencies		
Activation-induced cytidine deaminase deficiency	*HIGM2*	12p13
CD40 deficiency	*HIGM3*	20 q12-q13.2
IgA deficiency/common variable immunodeficiency	*MHC*	6p21.3
Immunoglobulin-associated beta (Igβ) deficiency	*CD79B*	17q23
Immunoglobulin heavy chain deficiencies	*IGHG11*	14q32.33
BLNK deficiency	*BLNK*	10q23.2
Surrogate light chain deficiency	*IGLL55*	22q11.21
X-linked agammaglobulinemia	*BTK*	Xq21.3-q22
X-linked hyper-IgM syndrome	*HIGM1*	Xq26
XHM with ectodermal dysplasia (XHM-ED)	*IKBKG*	Xq28
Other well-defined immunodeficiency syndromes		
Ataxia telangiectasia	*ATM*	11q22.3
Interferon γ receptor deficiency	*IFNGR1*	6q23-q24
	IFNGR2	21q22.1-22.2
Interleukin 12 deficiency	*IL12B*	5q31-q33
Interleukin 12 receptor deficiency	*IL12RB1*	19p13.1
Mannose binding lectin deficiency	*MBL2*	10q11.2-q21
Wiskott-Aldrich syndrome	*WAS*	Xp11.23-p11.22
X-linked lymphoproliferative syndrome	*SH2D1A/SAP*	Xq25

ditions may lead to improvement or even cure of *Candida* infection. In other patients, intensive treatment with amphotericin B coupled with surgical removal of infected nails has led to sustained improvement. Oral antifungal agents, such as fluconazole and itraconazole, may also be effective.

INTERFERON γ RECEPTOR DEFICIENCY This immunodeficiency is characterized by serious infections caused by bacille Calmette-Guérin vaccine and environmental non-tuberculous mycobacteria. Associated salmonella infections occur in a minority of the cases. This syndrome can be caused by mutations in the interferon γ receptor signal-transducing chain (*IFNGR2*). Two additional forms of this syndrome are caused by different types of mutations in the interferon γ receptor 1 (*IFNGR1*) gene that encodes the ligand binding chain of the interferon γ receptor. Null mutations in both *IFNGR1* alleles are responsible for a more severe autosomal recessive form. A less severe form, inherited in an autosomal dominant pattern, is caused by *IFNGR1* mutations in a small deletional hotspot that result in a truncated receptor chain lacking the cytoplasmic tail. Accumulation of the truncated receptor on the surface of macrophages compromises their response to interferon γ and the killing of ingested mycobacterium.

INTERLEUKIN 12 RECEPTOR DEFICIENCY Mutations in the gene coding the β₁ subunit of the IL-12 receptor can also result in disseminated mycobacterial infections attributable to bacille Calmette-Guérin and non-tuberculous mycobacteria, and in some cases non-typhi salmonella

infections. Although the clinical manifestations are usually less severe than in patients with complete IFNGR1 deficiency, IL-12 receptor deficiency may predispose individuals to clinical tuberculosis as well. Deficient interferon γ production by the otherwise normal NK and T cells is seen in IL-12 receptor deficient patients, and therapeutic use of interferon γ may cure their mycobacterial infection.

IMMUNODEFICIENCY WITH THYMOMA The association of hypogammaglobulinemia with spindle cell thymoma usually occurs relatively late in adult life. Bacterial infections and severe diarrhea often reflect the antibody deficiency, whereas fungal and viral infections are infrequent complications. T cell numbers and cell-mediated immunity are usually intact, but these patients are very deficient in circulating B lymphocytes and pre-B cells in the bone marrow. They also frequently have eosinopenia and may develop erythroid aplasia. Complete bone marrow failure sometimes occurs. The relationship between the usually benign thymoma and apparent abnormalities of hematopoietic stem cells remains conjectural, and treatment is limited to immunoglobulin administration and symptomatic therapy.

WISKOTT-ALDRICH SYNDROME This X-linked disease characterized by eczema, thrombocytopenia, and repeated infections is caused by mutations in the *WASP* gene. The WASP protein is expressed in cells of all hematopoietic lineages. It may serve a cytoskeletal organizing role for signaling elements that are particularly important in platelets and T cells. The platelets are small and have a shortened half-life. Affected male infants often present with bleeding, and most do not survive childhood, dying of complications of bleeding, infection, or lymphoreticular malignancy. The immunologic defects include low serum concentrations of IgM, while IgA and IgG are normal and IgE is frequently increased. The number and class distribution of B lymphocytes are usually normal. Functionally, these patients are unable to make antibodies to polysaccharide antigens normally; responses to protein antigens may also be impaired late in the course of the disease. Most patients eventually acquire T cell deficiencies. Affected boys frequently become anergic, and their T cells do not respond normally to antigenic challenge. This results in vulnerability to overwhelming infections with herpes simplex virus and other infectious agents.

Transplantation of histocompatible bone marrow from a sibling donor following myeloablative therapy can correct both the hematologic and immunologic abnormalities. In patients lacking a suitable donor, intravenous immunoglobulin infusions or splenectomy may improve platelet counts and reduce the risk of serious hemorrhage. Because of the increased risk of pneumococcal bacteremia, splenectomized patients should receive prophylactic penicillin.

X-LINKED LYMPHOPROLIFERATIVE SYNDROME This disease involves a selective impairment in immune elimination of Epstein-Barr virus (EBV). A fulminant and fatal outcome is the consequence of EBV infection in approximately half of the affected males. Hypogammaglobulinemia is the outcome in 30%, and B cell malignancies are acquired in approximately 25% of EBV-infected patients. The disease may be manifested from early childhood onward, depending on the time of EBV infection. Carrier females handle EBV infections normally. Cytotoxic T cells and NK appear to be primarily responsible for control of EBV infection in normal persons. In males with the X-linked lymphoproliferative syndrome, this process is impaired as a consequence of mutations in a gene coding a T cell and NK cell signaling element called SH2D1A or SAP. Intravenous immunoglobulins should be administered to affected males who develop hypogammaglobulinemia. Bone marrow transplantation from an HLA-matched donor may be curative, especially in younger children with this syndrome. However, myeloablative chemotherapy is a necessary prerequisite to successful bone marrow transplantation, thereby increasing the risk of this procedure.

HYPER-IgE SYNDROME The hyper IgE syndrome (Chap. 55) is characterized by recurrent abscesses involving skin, lungs, and other organs and very high IgE levels. IgE levels may decline with time to reach normal levels in approximately 20% of affected adults. Staphylococcal infection is common to all patients, but most have infections with other pyogenic organisms as well. Abnormal neutrophil chemotaxis is an inconsistent finding, and diminished antibody responses to secondary immunization have been noted. Non-immunologic features include impaired shedding of the primary teeth, recurrent bone fractures, hyperextensible joints, and scoliosis. Males and females are affected in an inheritance pattern suggesting an autosomal dominant defect with variable penetrance, but the gene defect has not been identified. Prophylaxis with penicillinase-resistant penicillins or cephalosporins is highly recommended to prevent staphylococcal infections. Pneumatoceles, a frequent complication of pneumonias, may require surgical excision.

Metabolic Abnormalities Associated with Immunodeficiency The relation of deficiencies of the purine salvage enzymes adenosine deaminase and purine nucleoside phosphorylase to immunodeficiency was discussed earlier. The syndrome of *acrodermatitis enteropathica* includes severe desquamating skin lesions, intractable diarrhea, bizarre neurologic symptoms, variable combined immunodeficiency, and an often fatal outcome. This disease is apparently caused by an inborn error of metabolism resulting in malabsorption of dietary zinc and can be treated effectively by parenteral or large oral doses of zinc. Zinc deficiency

might in part account for the immunodeficiency that accompanies severe malnutrition. Inherited *deficiency of transcobalamin II*, the serum carrier molecule responsible for transport of vitamin B_{12} to tissues, is associated with failure of immunoglobulin production as well as megaloblastic anemia, leukopenia, thrombocytopenia, and severe malabsorption. All abnormalities of this rare disorder are reversed by administration of vitamin B_{12}. Finally, primary immunodeficiencies are associated with or are secondary to a number of diverse diseases (Table 297-3).

CONCLUSION Defective genes have been identified for most of the primary immunodeficiency diseases that are currently recognized (Table 297-4). It can be anticipated that many different gene mutations will be identified in other individuals with increased susceptibility to infection. Identification of the mutant genes is the first step toward a better understanding of the pathogenesis of immunodeficiency disease and improved therapeutic strategies. Successful gene repair is the ultimate goal for these individuals.

FURTHER READING

AIUTI A et al: Correction of ADA-SCID by stem cell gene therapy combined with non-ablative conditioning. Science 296:2410, 2002

BUCKLEY RH: Primary cellular immunodeficiencies. J Allergy Clin Immunol 109:747, 2002

BURROWS PD, COOPER MD: IgA deficiency. Adv Immunol 65:245, 1997

FISCHER A: Primary immunodeficiency diseases: Natural mutant models for the study of the immune system. Scand J Immunol 55:238, 2002

GELFAND EW: Antibody-directed therapy: Past, present, and future. J Allergy Clin Immunol 108:S111, 2001

HACIEN-BEY AS et al: Sustained correction of X-linked severe combined immunodeficiency by *ex vivo* gene therapy. N Engl J Med 346:1185, 2002

OCHS HD et al: *Primary Immunodeficiency Diseases*. New York, Oxford University Press, 1999

ROSEN FS et al: Primary immunodeficiency diseases. Report of an IUIS Scientific Committee. Clin Exp Immunol 119(Suppl 1):1, 1999

Section 2   Disorders of Immune-Mediated Injury

298 ALLERGIES, ANAPHYLAXIS, AND SYSTEMIC MASTOCYTOSIS
K. Frank Austen

The term *atopic allergy* implies a familial tendency to manifest such conditions as asthma, rhinitis, urticaria, and eczematous dermatitis (atopic dermatitis) alone or in combination. However, individuals without an atopic background may also develop hypersensitivity reactions, particularly urticaria and anaphylaxis, associated with the same class of antibody, IgE, found in atopic individuals. Inasmuch as the mast cell is the key effector cell of the biologic response in allergic rhinitis, urticaria, anaphylaxis, and systemic mastocytosis, the introduction to these clinical problems will consider the developmental biology, activation pathway, product profile, and target tissues for this cell type.

The fixation of IgE to human mast cells and basophils, a process termed *sensitization*, prepares these cells for subsequent antigen-specific activation. The sensitization of the high-affinity Fc receptor for IgE, designated FcεRI, also stabilizes the cellular expression of the receptor. FcεRI is composed of one α, one β, and two disulfide-linked γ chains, which together cross the plasma membrane seven times. The α chain is responsible for IgE binding, and the β and γ chains provide for signal transduction that follows the aggregation of the sensitized tetrameric receptors by polymeric antigen. Signal transduction is initiated through the action of a *src* family–related tyrosine kinase, termed *Lyn*, that is constitutively associated with the β chain. Lyn transphosphorylates the canonical immunoreceptor tyrosine based ac-

tivation motifs (ITAMs) of the β and γ chains of the receptor, resulting in recruitment of more active Lyn to the β chain and of the Syk/zap-70 family tyrosine kinases. The phosphorylated tyrosines in the ITAMs function as binding sites for the tandem *src* homology two (SH2) domains within these kinases. Syk activates not only phospholipase Cγ but also phosphatidylinositol-3-kinase to provide phosphatidyl-3,4,5-triphosphate, which allows membrane targeting of the Tec family kinases (Btk and Itk) and their activation by Lyn. The phospholipase Cγ cleavage of the phospholipid membrane substrate provides inositol-1,4,5-triphosphate (IP$_3$) and 1,2-diacylglycerols (1,2-DAGs) so as to mobilize intracellular calcium and activate protein kinase C. The subsequent opening of calcium-regulated activated channels provides the sustained elevations of intracellular calcium required to recruit the mitogen-activated protein kinases, JNK and p38 (serine/threonine kinases), which provide cascades to augment arachidonic acid release and to mediate nuclear translocation of transcription factors for various cytokines. The calcium ion–dependent activation of phospholipases cleaves membrane phospholipids to generate lysophospholipids, which, like 1,2-DAG, are fusogenic and may facilitate the fusion of the secretory granule perigranular membrane with the cell membrane, a step that releases the membrane-free granules containing the preformed mediators of mast cell effects.

The secretory granule of the human mast cell has a crystalline structure, unlike mast cells of lower species. IgE-dependent cell activation results in solubilization and swelling of the granule contents within the first minute of receptor perturbation; this reaction is followed by the ordering of intermediate filaments about the swollen granule, movement of the granule toward the cell surface, and fusion of the perigranular membrane with that of other granules and with the plasmalemma to form extracellular channels for mediator release while maintaining cell viability.

In addition to exocytosis, aggregation of $Fc\epsilon RI$ initiates two other pathways for generation of bioactive products, namely, lipid mediators and cytokines. The biochemical steps involved in expression of such cytokines as tumor necrosis factor α (TNF-α), interleukin (IL) 6, IL-4, IL-5, IL-13, granulocyte-macrophage colony-stimulating factor (GM-CSF), and others have not been specifically defined for mast cells. Nonetheless, inhibition studies of cytokine production (IL-1β, TNF-α, and IL-6) in mouse mast cells with cyclosporine or FK506 reveal binding to the ligand-specific immunophilin and attenuation of the calcium ion– and calmodulin-dependent serine/threonine phosphatase, calcineurin.

Lipid mediator generation (Fig. 298-1) involves translocation of calcium ion–dependent cytosolic phospholipase A_2 to the outer nuclear membrane, with subsequent release of arachidonic acid for metabolic processing by the distinct prostanoid and leukotriene pathways. The constitutive prostaglandin endoperoxide synthase (PGHS-1/cyclooxygenase-1) and the de novo inducible PGHS-2 (cyclooxygenase-2) convert released arachidonic acid to the sequential intermediates, prostaglandins G_2 and H_2. The glutathione-dependent hematopoietic prostaglandin D_2 (PGD$_2$) synthase then converts PGH$_2$ to PGD$_2$, the predominant mast cell prostanoid.

For the leukotriene biosynthetic pathway, the released arachidonic acid is metabolized by 5-lipoxygenase (5-LO) in the presence of an integral nuclear membrane protein, the 5-LO activating protein (FLAP). The calcium ion–dependent translocation of 5-LO to the nuclear membrane converts the arachidonic acid to the sequential intermediates, 5-hydroperoxyeicosatetraenoic acid and leukotriene (LT)

A_4. LTA$_4$ is conjugated with reduced glutathione by LTC$_4$ synthase, an integral nuclear membrane protein homologous to FLAP. Intracellular LTC$_4$ is released by a carrier-specific export step for extracellular conversion to LTD$_4$ and LTE$_4$ by sequential removal of glutamic acid and glycine. Alternatively, cytosolic LTA$_4$ hydrolase converts some LTA$_4$ to the dihydroxy leukotriene LTB$_4$, which also undergoes specific export. Two receptors for LTB$_4$, LTB$_1$R and LTB$_2$R, mediate chemotaxis of human neutrophils. Two receptors for the cysteinyl leukotrienes, CysLT$_1$R and CysLT$_2$R, are present on smooth muscle of the airways and the microvasculature and on hematopoietic cells such as eosinophils and mast cells. Whereas CysLT$_1$R has a preference for LTD$_4$ and is blocked by the receptor antagonists in clinical use, CysLT$_2$R is equally responsive to LTC$_4$ and is unaffected by these antagonists. The lysophospholipid formed during release of arachidonic acid from 1-O-alkyl-2-acyl-sn-glyceryl-3-phosphorylcholine can be acetylated in the second position to form platelet-activating factor (PAF).

Unlike most other cells of bone marrow origin, mast cells leave the marrow and circulate as committed progenitors lacking their definitive secretory granules and characteristic $Fc\epsilon RI$. These committed progenitors express the receptor, c-*kit*, for stem cell factor (SCF), and unlike other lineages, they retain and increase its expression with maturation. The SCF interaction with c-*kit* is an absolute requirement for the development of constitutive tissue mast cells residing in skin and connective tissue sites and for the T cell–dependent comitogenesis providing mast cells to mucosal surfaces. Indeed, in clinical T cell deficiencies, mast cells are absent from the intestinal mucosa but are present in the submucosa. Based on the immunodetection of secretory granule neutral proteases, mast cells in the lung parenchyma and intestinal mucosa selectively express tryptase, and those in the intestinal and airway submucosa, skin, lymph nodes, and breast parenchyma express tryptase, chymase, and carboxypeptidase A (CPA). The secretory granules of mast cells selectively positive for tryptase exhibit closed scrolls with a periodicity suggestive of a crystalline structure by electron microscopy; whereas the secretory granules of mast cells with mutiple proteases are scroll-poor, with an amorphous or lattice-like appearance.

Mast cells are distributed at cutaneous and mucosal surfaces and in submucosal tissues about venules and could influence the entry of foreign substances by their rapid response capability (Fig. 298-2). Upon stimulus-specific activation and secretory granule exocytosis, histamine and acid hydrolases are solubilized, whereas the neutral proteases, which are cationic, remain largely complexed to the anionic protcoglycans, heparin and chrondroitin sulfate E, so as to function in concert. Histamine and the various lipid mediators (PGD$_2$, LTC$_4$/D$_4$/E$_4$, PAF) alter venular permeability, thereby allowing influx of plasma proteins such as complement and immunoglobulins, whereas LTB$_4$ mediates leukocyte–endothelial cell adhesion and subsequent directed migration (chemotaxis). The accumulation of leukocytes and plasma opsonins would facilitate defense of the microenvironment. The inflammatory response can also be detrimental, as in bronchial asthma, where the smooth-muscle constrictor activity of the cysteinyl leukotrienes is evident and much more potent than that of histamine.

The cellular component of the mast cell–mediated inflammatory response would be augmented and sustained by cytokines and chemokines of mast cell origin. IgE-dependent activation of human skin mast cells in situ elicits TNF-α production and release, which in turn induces endothelial cell responses favoring leukocyte adhesion. Similarly, activation of purified human lung mast cells or cord blood–derived cultured mast cells in vitro results in substantial production of proinflammatory (TNF-α) and immunomodulatory cytokines (IL-4, IL-5, IL-13) and chemokines. Bronchial biopsies of patients with bronchial asthma reveal that mast cells are immunohistochemically positive for IL-4 and IL-5, but that the predominant localization of IL-4, IL-5, and GM-CSF is to T cells, defined as T_H2 by this profile. IL-4 modulates the T cell phenotype to the T_H2 subtype, determines the isotype switch to IgE (as does IL-13), and upregulates $Fc\epsilon RI$-mediated expression of cytokines by mast cells.

FIGURE 298-1 Pathways for biosynthesis and release of membrane-derived lipid mediators from mast cells. In the 5-lipoxygenase pathway leukotriene A_4 (LTA$_4$) is the intermediate from which the terminal-pathway enzymes generate the distinct final products, leukotriene C_4 (LTC$_4$) and leukotriene B_4 (LTB$_4$), which leave the cell by separate saturable transport systems. Gamma glutamyl transpeptidase and a dipeptidase then cleave glutamic acid and glycine from LTC$_4$ to form LTD$_4$ and LTE$_4$, respectively. The only mast cell product of the cyclooxygenase system is PGD$_2$.

An immediate and late cellular phase of allergic inflammation can be induced in the skin, nose, or lung of some allergic humans with local allergen challenge. In the immediate phase of a local challenge, there is pruritus and watery discharge from the nose, bronchospasm and mucus secretion in the lungs, and a wheal-and-flare response with pruritus in the skin. The reduced nasal patency, reduced pulmonary function, or evident erythema with swelling at the skin site in a late-phase response at 6 to 8 h is associated with biopsy findings of infiltrating and activated T_H2 type T cells, eosinophils, basophils, and even some neutrophils. This allergic inflammation proceeding from early mast cell activation to late cellular infiltration has been used as an experimental surrogate of perennial rhinitis or bronchial asthma. However, in bronchial asthma there is a separate variable, intrinsic hyperreactivity of the airways.

Consideration of the mechanism of immediate-type hypersensitivity diseases in the human has focused largely on the IgE-dependent recognition of otherwise nontoxic substances. A region of chromosome 5 (5q23-31) contains genes implicated in the control of IgE levels including IL-4 and IL-13, as well as IL-3 and IL-9 involved in reactive mast cell hyperplasia and IL-5 and GM-CSF central to eosinophil development and their enhanced tissue viability. Genes with linkage to the specific IgE response to particular allergens include those encoding the major histocompatibility complex (MHC) and certain chains of the T cell receptor (TCR-$\alpha\delta$). The complexity of atopy and the associated diseases includes susceptibility, severity, and therapeutic responses, each of which is among the separate variables modulated by both innate and adaptive immune stimuli.

The induction of allergic disease requires sensitization of a predisposed individual to specific allergen. This sensitization can occur anytime in life, although the greatest propensity for the development of allergic disease appears to occur in childhood and early adolescence. Exposure of a susceptible individual to an allergen results in processing of the allergen by antigen-presenting cells of the monocytic lineage located throughout the body at surfaces that contact the outside environment, such as the nose, lungs, eyes, skin, and intestine. These antigen-presenting cells process the allergen protein and present the epitope-bearing peptides via their MHC to particular T cell helper subsets. The T cell response depends both on cognate recognition through various ligand/receptor interactions and on the cytokine microenvironment, with IL-4 directing a T_H2 response and interferon (IFN)γ a T_H1 profile. T cells can potentially induce several responses to an allergen, including those typical of contact dermatitis, known as the T_H1 type response, and those mediated by IgE, known as the T_H2 allergic response. The T_H2 response is associated with activation of specific B cells that can also present allergens or that transform into plasma cells for antibody production. Synthesis and release into the serum of allergen-specific IgE by plasma cells result in sensitization of IgE Fc receptor–bearing cells including mast cells and basophils, which subsequently are capable of becoming activated upon exposure to the specific allergen. In certain diseases, including those associated with atopy, the monocyte and eosinophil populations can express a trimeric high-affinity receptor, FcϵRI, which lacks the β chain, and yet respond to its aggregation.

ANAPHYLAXIS

DEFINITION The life-threatening anaphylactic response of a sensitized human appears within minutes after administration of specific antigen and is manifested by respiratory distress, laryngeal edema, and/or intense bronchospasm, often followed by vascular collapse or by shock without antecedent respiratory difficulty. Cutaneous manifestations exemplified by pruritus and urticaria with or without angioedema are characteristic of such systemic anaphylactic reactions. Gastrointestinal

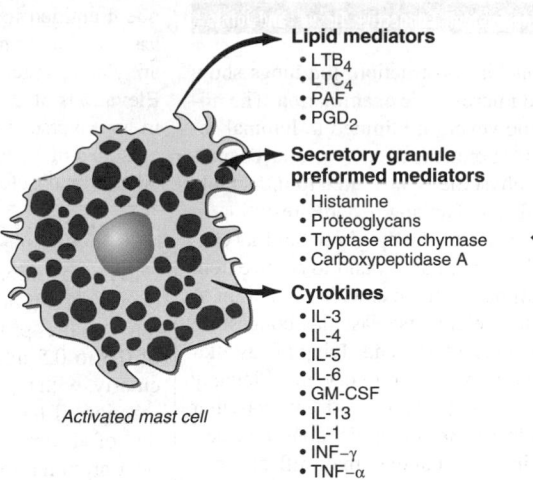

FIGURE 298-2 Bioactive mediators of three categories generated by IgE-dependent activation of murine mast cells can elicit common but sequential target cell effects leading to acute and sustained inflammatory responses. LT, leukotriene; PAF, platelet-activating factor; PGD$_2$, prostaglandin D$_2$; IL, interleukin; GM-CSF, granulocyte-macrophage colony-stimulating factor; INF, interferon; TNF, tumor necrosis factor.

manifestations include nausea, vomiting, crampy abdominal pain, and diarrhea.

PREDISPOSING FACTORS AND ETIOLOGY There is no convincing evidence that age, sex, race, occupation, or geographic location predisposes a human to anaphylaxis except through exposure to some immunogen. According to most studies, atopy does not predispose individuals to anaphylaxis from penicillin therapy or venom of a stinging insect but is a risk factor for allergens in food or latex.

The materials capable of eliciting the systemic anaphylactic reaction in humans include the following: heterologous proteins in the form of hormones (insulin, vasopressin, parathormone), enzymes (trypsin, chymotrypsin, penicillinase, streptokinase), pollen extracts (ragweed, grass, trees), nonpollen extracts (dust mites, dander of cats, dogs, horses, and laboratory animals), food (milk, eggs, seafood, nuts, grains, beans, gelatin in capsules), antiserum (antilymphocyte gamma globulin), occupation-related proteins (latex rubber products), and Hymenoptera venom (yellow jacket, yellow and baldfaced hornets, paper wasp, honey bee, imported fire ants); polysaccharides such as dextran and thiomerosal as a vaccine preservative; and most commonly drugs such as protamine and antibiotics (penicillins, cephalosporins, amphotericin B, nitrofurantoin, quinolones), local anesthetics (procaine, lidocaine), muscle relaxants (suxamethonium, gallamine, pancuronium), vitamins (thiamine, folic acid), diagnostic agents (sodium dehydrocholate, sulfobromophthalein), and occupation-related chemicals (ethylene oxide), which are considered to function as haptens that form immunogenic conjugates with host proteins. The conjugating hapten may be the parent compound, a nonenzymatically derived storage product, or a metabolite formed in the host.

PATHOPHYSIOLOGY AND MANIFESTATIONS Individuals differ in the time of appearance of symptoms and signs, but the hallmark of the anaphylactic reaction is the onset of some manifestation within seconds to minutes after introduction of the antigen, generally by injection or less commonly by ingestion. There may be upper or lower airway obstruction or both. Laryngeal edema may be experienced as a "lump" in the throat, hoarseness, or stridor, while bronchial obstruction is associated with a feeling of tightness in the chest and/or audible wheezing. Patients with bronchial asthma are predisposed to severe involvement of the lower airways. A characteristic feature is the eruption of well-circumscribed, discrete cutaneous wheals with erythematous, raised, serpiginous borders and blanched centers. These urticarial eruptions are intensely pruritic and may be localized or disseminated. They may coalesce to form giant hives, and they seldom persist beyond 48 h. A localized, nonpitting, deeper edematous cutaneous process, angioedema, may also be present. It may be asymptomatic or cause a burning or stinging sensation.

In fatal cases with clinical bronchial obstruction, the lungs show marked hyperinflation on gross and microscopic examination. The microscopic findings in the bronchi, however, are limited to luminal secretions, peribronchial congestion, submucosal edema, and eosinophilic infiltration, and the acute emphysema is attributed to intractable bronchospasm that subsides with death. The angioedema resulting in death by mechanical obstruction occurs in the epiglottis and larynx, but the process is also evident in the hypopharynx and to some extent in the trachea; on microscopic examination there is wide separation of the collagen fibers and the glandular elements; vascular congestion and eosinophilic infiltration are also present. Patients dying of vascular collapse without antecedent hypoxia from respiratory insufficiency have visceral congestion with a presumptive loss of intravascular blood volume. The associated electrocardiographic abnormalities, with or without infarction, noted in some patients may reflect a primary cardiac event or be secondary to a critical reduction in blood volume.

The angioedematous and urticarial manifestations of the anaphylactic syndrome have been attributed to release of endogenous histamine. A role for the cysteinyl leukotrienes in altering pulmonary mechanics by causing marked bronchiolar constriction seems likely. Vascular collapse without respiratory distress in response to experimental challenge with the sting of a hymenopteran was associated not only with marked and prolonged elevations in blood histamine but also with evidence of intravascular coagulation and kinin generation. The finding that patients with systemic mastocytosis and episodic hypotension proceeding to vascular collapse excrete large amounts of PGD_2 metabolites in addition to histamine suggests that PGD_2 is also of importance in the hypotensive anaphylactic reactions. The cysteinyl leukotrienes may be involved in the pathobiologic process in patients with myocardial ischemia without or with infarction.

DIAGNOSIS The diagnosis of an anaphylactic reaction depends largely on an accurate history revealing the onset of the appropriate symptoms and signs within minutes after the responsible material is encountered. When only a portion of the full syndrome is present, such as isolated urticaria, sudden bronchospasm in a patient with asthma, or vascular collapse after intravenous administration of an agent, it may be appropriate to consider a complement-mediated immune complex reaction, an idiosyncratic response to any of the nonsteroidal anti-inflammatory agents, or the direct effect of certain drugs or diagnostic agents on mast cells. Intravenous administration of a chemical mast cell–degranulating agent, including opiate derivatives and radiographic contrast media, may elicit generalized urticaria, angioedema, and a sensation of retrosternal oppression with or without clinically detectable bronchoconstriction or hypotension. Aspirin and other nonsteroidal anti-inflammatory agents such as indomethacin, aminopyrine, and mefenamic acid may precipitate a life-threatening episode of obstruction of upper or lower airways, especially in patients with asthma, that is clinically reminiscent of anaphylaxis but is not associated with a detectable IgE response. This syndrome, which is commonly associated with nasal polyposis, is due to inhibition of PGHS-1 with corresponding unregulated, amplified generation of the cysteinyl leukotrienes via the 5-LO/LTC$_4$ synthase pathway. In the transfusion anaphylactic reaction that occurs in patients with IgA deficiency, the responsible specificity resides in IgG or IgE anti-IgA; the mechanism of the reaction mediated by IgG anti-IgA is presumed to be complement activation with secondary mast cell participation.

The presence of specific IgE in the heart blood of patients dying of systemic anaphylaxis has been demonstrated at postmortem by passive transfer of the serum intradermally into a normal recipient, followed in 24 h by antigen challenge into the same site, with subsequent development of a wheal and flare, the *Prausnitz-Küstner reaction*. To avoid the hazards of transferring hepatitis or other infections to a recipient, it is preferable to use the serum to seek passive sensitization of a human leukocyte suspension enriched with basophils for subsequent antigen-induced histamine release. Furthermore, radioimmunoassays have demonstrated specific IgE antibodies in patients with anaphylactic reactions, but such approaches require purified antigens. Elevations of β-tryptase levels in serum implicate mast cell activation in an adverse systemic reaction and are particularly informative with episodes of hypotension during general anesthesia or when there has been a fatal outcome.

R_x TREATMENT

Early recognition of an anaphylactic reaction is mandatory, since death occurs within minutes to hours after the first symptoms. Mild symptoms such as pruritus and urticaria can be controlled by administration of 0.3 to 0.5 mL of 1:1000 epinephrine subcutaneously or intramuscularly, with repeated doses as required at 20-min intervals for a severe reaction. If the antigenic material was injected into an extremity, the rate of absorption may be reduced by prompt application of a tourniquet proximal to the reaction site, administration of 0.2 mL of 1:1000 epinephrine into the site, and removal without compression of an insect stinger, if present. An intravenous infusion should be initiated to provide a route for administration of 2.5 mL epinephrine, diluted 1:10,000, at 5- to 10-min intervals, volume expanders such as normal saline, and vasopressor agents such as dopamine if intractable hypotension occurs. Replacement of intravascular volume due to postcapillary venular leakage may require several liters of saline. Epinephrine provides both α- and β-adrenergic effects, resulting in vasoconstriction, bronchial smooth-muscle relaxation, and attenuation of enhanced venular permeability. Beta blockers are relatively contraindicated in persons at risk for anaphylactic reactions, especially those sensitive to Hymenoptera venom or those undergoing immunotherapy for respiratory system allergy. When epinephrine fails to control the anaphylactic reaction, hypoxia due to airway obstruction or related to a cardiac arrhythmia, or both, must be considered. Oxygen via a nasal catheter or intermittent positive-pressure breathing of oxygen with inhaled or nebulized albuterol may be helpful, but either endotracheal intubation or a tracheostomy is mandatory for oxygen delivery if progressive hypoxia develops. Ancillary agents such as the antihistamine diphenhydramine, 50 to 100 mg intramuscularly or intravenously, and aminophylline, 0.25 to 0.5 g intravenously, are appropriate for urticaria-angioedema and bronchospasm, respectively. Intravenous glucocorticoids are not effective for the acute event but may alleviate later recurrence of bronchospasm, hypotension, or urticaria. Furthermore, in a syndrome termed *idiopathic anaphylaxis* with recurrent angioedema of the upper airways, glucocorticoid administration may be beneficial by reducing the frequency of attacks and/or the severity of episodes.

PREVENTION Prevention of anaphylaxis must take into account the sensitivity of the recipient, the dose and character of the diagnostic or therapeutic agent, and the effect of the route of administration on the rate of absorption. If there is a definite history of a past anaphylactic reaction, even though mild, it is advisable to select another agent or procedure. A knowledge of cross-reactivity among agents is critical since, for example, cephalosporins share a common β-lactam ring with the penicillins. A prick or scratch skin test should precede an intradermal skin test, since the latter has a higher risk of causing anaphylaxis. These tests should be performed before the administration of certain materials that are likely to elicit anaphylactic reactions, such as allergenic extracts, or when the nature of the past adverse reaction is unknown. With regard to penicillin, two-thirds of patients with a positive reaction history and positive skin tests to benzylpenicilloyl-polylysine (BPL) and/or the minor determinant mixture (MDM) of benzylpenicillin products experience allergic reactions with treatment, and these are almost uniformly of the anaphylactic type in those patients with minor determinant reactivity. Even patients without a history of previous clinical reactions have a 2 to 6% incidence of positive skin tests to the two test materials, and about 3 per 1000 with a negative history experience anaphylaxis with therapy, with a mortality of about 1 per 100,000. Skin testing for antibiotics should be performed only on patients with a positive clinical history consistent with an IgE-mediated reaction and in imminent need of the antibiotic in question; skin testing is of no value for non-IgE-mediated eruptions. Desensitization with most antibiotics can proceed by the intravenous, subcutaneous, or oral route. Typically, graded quantities of the antibiotic are given by the selected route using double doses until a therapeutic dosage is achieved. Due to the risk of systemic anaphylaxis during the course of desensitization, such a procedure should be performed only in a setting in which resuscitation equipment is at hand and an intravenous line is in place. It is critical to give the therapeutic agent at regular intervals to prevent the reestablishment of a sensitized cell pool of large size.

A different form of protection involves the development of blocking antibody of the IgG class, which is protective against Hymenoptera venom–induced anaphylaxis by interacting with antigen so that less reaches the sensitized tissue mast cells; to be effective, this immunotherapy requires the use of specific or cross-reacting Hymenoptera venom. Because sensitization can be transient, the maximal risk for systemic anaphylactic reactions in persons with Hymenoptera sensitivity occurs in association with a currently positive skin test. Although there is only low-grade cross-reactivity between honey bee and yellow jacket venoms, there is a high degree of cross-reactivity between yellow jacket venom and the rest of the vespid venoms (yellow or bald-faced hornets and wasps). Prevention involves modification of outdoor activities to exclude bare feet, wearing perfumed toiletries, eating in areas attractive to insects, clipping hedges or grass, and hauling away trash or fallen fruit. As with each anaphylactic sensitivity, the individual should wear an informational bracelet and have immediate access to an unexpired epinephrine kit. The limitations of lifestyle and the psychological duress can be addressed by venom immunotherapy to achieve a venom-specific IgG titer. Although it has been recommended that venom therapy be continued indefinitely or until the skin and specific serum IgE tests are unremarkable, there is evidence that 5 years of treatment induces a state of resistance to sting reactions that is independent of serum levels of specific IgG or IgE. This contrasts with the definite relation of sting immunity to specific IgG earlier in the treatment regime. For children with a systemic reaction limited to skin, the likelihood of progression to more serious respiratory or vascular manifestations is low, and thus immunotherapy is not recommended.

URTICARIA AND ANGIOEDEMA

DEFINITION Urticaria and angioedema may appear separately or together as cutaneous manifestations of localized nonpitting edema; a similar process may occur at mucosal surfaces of the upper respiratory or gastrointestinal tract. *Urticaria* involves only the superficial portion of the dermis, presenting as well-circumscribed wheals with erythematous raised serpiginous borders with blanched centers that may coalesce to become giant wheals. *Angioedema* is a well-demarcated localized edema involving the deeper layers of the skin, including the subcutaneous tissue. Recurrent episodes of urticaria and/or angioedema of less than 6 weeks' duration are considered acute, whereas attacks persisting beyond this period are designated chronic.

PREDISPOSING FACTORS AND ETIOLOGY The occurrence of urticaria and angioedema is probably more frequent than usually described because of the evanescent, self-limited nature of such eruptions, which seldom require medical attention when limited to the skin. Although persons in any age group may experience acute or chronic urticaria and/or angioedema, these lesions increase in frequency after adolescence, with the highest incidence occurring in persons in the third decade of life; indeed, one survey of college students indicated that 15 to 20% had experienced a pruritic wheal reaction.

The classification of urticaria-angioedema presented in Table 298-1 focuses on the different mechanisms for eliciting clinical disease and can be useful for differential diagnosis; nonetheless, most cases of chronic urticaria are idiopathic. Urticaria and/or angioedema occurring

TABLE 298-1 *Classification of Urticaria and/or Angioedema*

1. IgE-dependent
   a. Specific antigen sensitivity (pollens, foods, drugs, fungi, molds, Hymenoptera venom, helminths)
   b. Physical: dermographism, cold, solar, cholinergic, vibratory, exercise-related
   c. Autoimmune
2. Bradykinin-mediated
   a. Hereditary angioedema: C1 inhibitor deficiency: null (type 1) and dysfunctional (type 2)
   b. Acquired angioedema: C1 inhibitor deficiency: anti-idiotype and anti-C1 inhibitor
   c. Angiotensin-converting enzyme inhibitors
3. Complement-mediated
   a. Necrotizing vasculitis
   b. Serum sickness
   c. Reactions to blood products
4. Nonimmunologic
   a. Direct mast cell–releasing agents (opiates, antibiotics, curare, D-tubocurarine, radiocontrast media)
   b. Agents that alter arachidonic acid metabolism (aspirin and nonsteroidal anti-inflammatory agents, azo dyes, and benzoates)
5. Idiopathic

during the appropriate season in patients with seasonal respiratory allergy or as a result of exposure to animals or molds is attributed to inhalation or physical contact with pollens, animal dander, and mold spores, respectively. However, urticaria and angioedema secondary to inhalation are relatively uncommon compared to urticaria and angioedema elicited by ingestion of fresh fruits, shellfish, fish, milk products, chocolate, legumes including peanuts, and various drugs that may elicit not only the anaphylactic syndrome with prominent gastrointestinal complaints but also chronic urticaria.

Additional etiologies include physical stimuli such as cold, heat, solar rays, exercise, and mechanical irritation. The physical urticarias can be distinguished by the precipitating event and other aspects of the clinical presentation. *Dermographism*, which occurs in 1 to 4% of the population, is defined by the appearance of a linear wheal at the site of a brisk stroke with a firm object or by any configuration appropriate to the eliciting event. Dermographism has a prevalence that peaks in the second to third decades. It is not influenced by an atopic diathesis and has a duration generally of less than 5 years. *Pressure urticaria*, which often accompanies dermographism or chronic idiopathic urticaria, presents in response to a sustained stimulus such as a shoulder strap or belt, running (feet), or manual labor (hands). *Cholinergic urticaria* is distinctive in that the pruritic wheals are of small size (1 to 2 mm) and are surrounded by a large area of erythema; attacks are precipitated by fever, a hot bath or shower, or exercise and are presumptively attributed to a rise in core body temperature. *Exercise-related anaphylaxis* can be precipitated by exertion alone or can be dependent on prior food ingestion. The clinical presentation can be limited to erythema and pruritic urticaria but may progress to angioedema of the face, oropharynx, larynx, or intestine or to vascular collapse; it is distinguished from cholinergic urticaria by presenting with wheals of conventional size and by not occurring with fever or a hot bath. *Cold urticaria*, either acquired or hereditary, is local at body areas exposed to low ambient temperature or cold objects (ice cube) but can progress to vascular collapse with immersion in cold water (swimming). *Solar urticaria* is subdivided into three groups by the response to specific portions of the light spectrum. *Vibratory angioedema* may occur after years of occupational exposure or can be idiopathic; it may be accompanied by cholinergic urticaria. Other rare forms of physical allergy, always defined by stimulus-specific elicitation, include *local heat urticaria*, *aquagenic urticaria* from contact with water of any temperature (sometimes associated with polycythemia vera), and *contact urticaria* from direct interaction with some chemical substance.

Angioedema without urticaria due to generation of bradykinin occurs with C1 inhibitor (C1INH) deficiency that may be inborn as an autosomal dominant characteristic or may be acquired. The angiotensin-converting enzyme (ACE) inhibitors can provoke a similar clinical presentation in 0.1 to 0.5% of hypertensive patients due to attenuated degradation of bradykinin. The urticaria and angioedema associated with classic serum sickness or with hypocomplementemic cutaneous necrotizing angiitis are believed to be immune-complex diseases. The drug reactions to mast cell granule–releasing agents and to nonsteroidal anti-inflammatory drugs may be systemic, resembling anaphylaxis, or limited to cutaneous sites.

PATHOPHYSIOLOGY AND MANIFESTATIONS Urticarial eruptions are distinctly pruritic, involve any area of the body from the scalp to the soles of the feet, and appear in crops of 24- to 72-h duration, with old lesions fading as new ones appear. The most common sites for urticaria are the extremities and face, with angioedema often being periorbital and in the lips. Although self-limited in duration, angioedema of the upper respiratory tract may be life-threatening due to laryngeal obstruction, while gastrointestinal involvement may present with abdominal colic, with or without nausea and vomiting, and may precipitate unnecessary surgical intervention. No residual discoloration occurs with either urticaria or angioedema unless there is an underlying process leading to superimposed extravasation of erythrocytes.

The pathology of urticaria and angioedema is usually characterized by edema of the dermis in urticaria and of the subcutaneous tissue as well as the dermis in angioedema. Collagen bundles in affected areas are widely separated, and the venules are sometimes dilated. The perivenular infiltrate may consist of lymphocytes, eosinophils, and neutrophils that are present in varying combination and number throughout the dermis.

Perhaps the best-studied example of IgE- and mast cell–mediated urticaria and angioedema is *cold urticaria*. Cryoglobulins may be recognized, but not in the majority of patients. Immersion of an extremity in an ice bath precipitates angioedema of the distal portion with urticaria at the air interface within minutes of the challenge. Histologic studies reveal marked mast cell degranulation with associated edema of the dermis and subcutaneous tissues. The venous effluent of the cold-challenged and angioedematous extremity reveals a marked rise in plasma content of histamine, whereas the venous effluent of the contralateral normal extremity contains no increment of this mediator. Elevated levels of histamine have been found in the plasma of venous effluent and in the fluid of suction blisters at experimentally induced lesional sites in patients with dermographism, pressure urticaria, vibratory angioedema, light urticaria, and heat urticaria. By ultrastructural analysis, the pattern of mast cell degranulation in cold urticaria resembles an IgE-mediated response with solubilization of granule contents, fusion of the perigranular and cell membranes, and discharge of granule contents, whereas in a dermographic lesion there is an additional superimposed zonal (piecemeal) degranulation. Elevations of plasma histamine levels with biopsy-proven mast cell degranulation have also been demonstrated with systemic attacks of *cholinergic urticaria* and *exercise-related anaphylaxis* precipitated experimentally in subjects exercising on a treadmill while wearing a wet suit; however, only in cholinergic urticaria is there a concomitant decrease in pulmonary function.

Up to one-third of patients with chronic urticaria have autoantibodies to IgE or to the α chain of the FcϵRI. In these patients, autologous serum injected into their own skin can induce a wheal and flare involving mast cell activation, but the relationship of such antibodies to the clinical course remains to be defined. In vitro studies reveal that these autoantibodies can mediate basophil degranulation with enhancement by serum as a source of the anaphylatoxic fragment, C5a.

Hereditary angioedema is an autosomal dominant disease due to a deficiency of C1INH (type 1) in about 85% of patients and to a dysfunctional protein (type 2) in the remainder. In the acquired form there

is excessive consumption of C1INH due either to immune complexes formed between anti-idiotypic antibody and monoclonal IgG presented by B cell lymphomas or to an autoantibody directed to C1INH. C1INH blocks the catalytic function of activated factor XII (Hageman factor) and of kallikrein, as well as the C1r/C1s components of C1. During clinical attacks of angioedema, C1INH-deficient patients have elevated plasma levels of bradykinin, particularly in the venous effluent of an involved extremity, and reduced levels of prekallikrein and high-molecular-weight kininogen, from which bradykinin is cleaved. The parallel decline in the complement substrates, C4 and C2, reflect the action of activated C1 during such attacks. Mice with targeted disruption of the gene for C1INH exhibit a chronic increase in vascular permeability. The pathobiology is aggravated by administration of an ACE inhibitor (captopril) and is attenuated by breeding the C1INH null strain to a bradykinin 2 receptor (Bk2R) null strain. As ACE is also described as kininase II, the use of blockers results in impaired bradykinin degradation and explains the angioedema occurring idiosyncratically in hypertensive patients with a normal C1INH.

DIAGNOSIS The rapid onset and self-limited nature of urticarial and angioedematous eruptions are distinguishing features. Additional characteristics are the occurrence of the urticarial crops in various stages of evolution and the asymmetric distribution of the angioedema. Urticaria and/or angioedema involving IgE-dependent mechanisms are often appreciated by historic considerations implicating specific allergens or physical stimuli, by seasonal incidence, and by exposure to certain environments. Direct reproduction of the lesion with physical stimuli is particularly valuable because it so often establishes the cause of the lesion. The diagnosis of an environmental allergen based on the clinical history can be confirmed by skin testing or assay for allergen-specific IgE in serum. IgE-mediated urticaria and/or angioedema may or may not be associated with an elevation of total IgE or with peripheral eosinophilia. Fever, leukocytosis, and an elevated sedimentation rate are absent.

The classification of urticarial and angioedematous states noted in Table 298-1 in terms of possible mechanisms necessarily includes some differential diagnostic points. Hypocomplementemia is not observed in IgE-mediated mast cell disease and may reflect either an acquired abnormality generally attributed to the formation of immune complexes or a genetic deficiency of C1INH. Chronic recurrent urticaria, generally in females, associated with arthralgias, an elevated sedimentation rate, and normo- or hypocomplementemia suggests an underlying cutaneous necrotizing angiitis. Vasculitic urticaria typically persists longer than 72 h, whereas conventional urticaria often has a duration of less than 24 to 48 h. Confirmation depends on a biopsy that reveals cellular infiltration, nuclear debris, and fibrinoid necrosis of the venules. The same pathobiologic process accounts for the urticaria in association with such diseases as systemic lupus erythematosus or viral hepatitis with or without an associated arteritis. Serum sickness per se or a similar clinical entity due to drugs includes not only urticaria but also pyrexia, lymphadenopathy, myalgia, and arthralgia or arthritis. Urticarial reactions to blood products or intravenous administration of immunoglobulin are defined by the event and generally are not progressive unless the recipient is IgA-deficient in the former case or the reagent is aggregated in the latter.

The diagnosis of hereditary angioedema is suggested not only by family history but also by the lack of pruritus and of urticarial lesions, the prominence of recurrent gastrointestinal attacks of colic, and episodes of laryngeal edema. Laboratory diagnosis depends on demonstrating a deficiency of C1INH antigen (type 1) or a nonfunctional protein (type 2) by a catalytic inhibition assay. While levels of C1 are normal, its substrates, C4 and C2, are chronically depleted and fall further during attacks due to the activation of additional C1. The acquired forms of C1INH deficiency have the same clinical manifestations but differ in the lack of a familial element and exhibit a reduction of C1 function and C1q protein as well as C1INH, C4, and C2. Inborn and acquired C1INH deficiency and ACE inhibitor–elicited angioedema are associated with elevated levels of bradykinin.

Urticaria and angioedema must be differentiated from contact sensitivity, a vesicular eruption that progresses to chronic thickening of the skin with continued allergenic exposure. They must also be differentiated from atopic dermatitis, a condition that may present as erythema, edema, papules, vesiculation, and oozing proceeding to a subacute and chronic stage in which vesiculation is less marked or absent and scaling, fissuring, and lichenification predominate in a distribution that characteristically involves the flexor surfaces. In cutaneous mastocytosis, the reddish brown macules and papules, characteristic of urticaria pigmentosa, urticate with pruritus upon trauma; and in systemic mastocytosis, without or with urticaria pigmentosa, there is an episodic systemic flushing with or without urticaria but no angioedema.

Rx TREATMENT

Identification of the etiologic factor(s) and their elimination provide the most satisfactory therapeutic program; this approach is feasible to varying degrees with IgE-mediated reactions to allergens or physical stimuli. For most forms of urticaria, H_1 antihistamines such as chlorpheniramine or diphenhydramine, and including the nonsedating class such as loratadine or cetirizine, are effective in attenuating both urtication and pruritus. Cyproheptadine and especially hydroxyzine have proven effective when H_1 antihistamines have been inadequate. Doxepin, a dibenzoxepin tricyclic compound with both H_1 and H_2 receptor antagonist activity, is yet another alternative. Terbutaline, an α-adrenergic agonist, or a $CysLT_1R$ antagonist may be added to the treatment regimen. Topical glucocorticoids are of no value, and systemic glucocorticoids are generally avoided in idiopathic, allergen-induced, or physical urticarias due to their long-term toxicity. Systemic glucocorticoids are useful in the management of patients with pressure urticaria, with vasculitic urticaria (especially with eosinophil prominence), with idiopathic angioedema with or without urticaria, or with chronic urticaria that responds poorly to conventional treatment. With persistent vasculitic urticaria, hydroxychloroquine or colchicine may be added to the regimen after hydroxyzine and before or along with systemic glucocorticoids.

The therapy of inborn C1INH deficiency has been simplified by the finding that attenuated androgens correct the biochemical defect and afford prophylactic protection; their efficacy is attributed to production by the normal gene of an amount of functional C1INH sufficient to control the spontaneous activation of C1. The antifibrinolytic agent ϵ-aminocaproic acid may be used for preoperative prophylaxis but is contraindicated in patients with thrombotic tendencies or ischemia due to arterial atherosclerosis. Infusion of isolated C1INH protein appears useful in prophylaxis and to ameliorate an attack.

SYSTEMIC MASTOCYTOSIS

DEFINITION *Systemic mastocytosis* is defined by mast cell hyperplasia that in most instances is indolent and nonneoplastic. The hyperplasia is generally recognized only in bone marrow and in the normal peripheral distribution sites of the cells, such as skin, gastrointestinal mucosa, liver, and spleen. Mastocytosis occurs at any age and has a slight preponderance in males. The prevalence of systemic mastocytosis is not known, a familial occurrence has not been established, and atopy is not increased.

CLASSIFICATION AND PATHOPHYSIOLOGY A recent consensus classification for mastocytosis recognizes cutaneous mastocytosis with variants and four systemic forms (Table 298-2). The form designated as *indolent systemic mastocytosis* (ISM) accounts for the majority of patients; it implies that there is no evidence of an associated hematologic disorder, liver disease, or lymphadenopathy and is not known to alter life expectancy. In *systemic mastocytosis associated with clonal hematologic non-mast cell lineage disease* (SM-AHNMD), the prognosis is determined by the nature of the associated disorder, which can range from dysmyelopoiesis to leukemia. In *aggressive systemic mastocytosis* (ASM), mast cell proliferation in parenchymal organs causing impaired liver function, hypersplenism, and/or malabsorption has a poor

TABLE 298-2 *Classification of Mastocytosis*

Cutaneous mastocytosis (CM)
   Urticaria pigmentosa (UP)/maculopapular cutaneous mastocytosis (MPCM)
      Variants: plaque form, nodular form; telangiectasia macularis eruptive perstans (TMEP); diffuse cutaneous mastocytosis (DCM)
   Solitary mastocytoma of skin
Indolent systemic mastocytosis (ISM)
Systemic mastocytosis with an associated clonal hematologic non-mast cell lineage disease (SM-AHNMD)
Aggressive systemic mastocytosis (ASM)
   Variant: lymphadenopathic mastocytosis with eosinophilia
Mast cell leukemia (MCL)
Mast cell sarcoma (MCS)

Source: Modified from P Valent et al, in ES Jaffee et al (eds): *World Health Organization Classification of Tumors: Pathology and Genetics in Tumors of Hematopoietic and Lymphoid Tissues*, Lyon, IARC Press, 2001.

prognosis in the absence of a hematologic disorder; a subset of these patients have prominent eosinophilia with hepatosplenomegaly and lymphadenopathy. *Mast cell leukemia* is the rarest form of the disease and is invariably fatal at present; the peripheral blood contains circulating, metachromatically staining, atypical mast cells.

A point mutation of A to T at codon 816 that causes an aspartic acid to valine substitution is found in multiple cell lineages in patients with mastocytosis, indicating a somatic gain-in-function mutation. This substitution, as well as others at 816, is characteristic of adults with SM-AHNMD but is also detected in patients with ISM and cutaneous mastocytosis, as might be anticipated because mast cells at any site are of bone marrow lineage. In infants and children with cutaneous manifestations, namely, urticaria pigmentosa or bullous lesions, visceral involvement is usually lacking, and resolution is common because gain-in-function mutations are infrequent.

CLINICAL MANIFESTATIONS The clinical manifestations of systemic mastocytosis, distinct from a leukemic complication, are due to tissue occupancy by the mast cell mass, the tissue response to that mass, and the release of bioactive substances acting at both local and distal sites. The pharmacologically induced manifestations are pruritus, flushing, palpitations and vascular collapse, gastric distress, lower abdominal crampy pain, and recurrent headache. The increase in cell burden is evidenced by the lesions of urticaria pigmentosa at skin sites, but it also contributes to bone pain and malabsorption. The mast cell–mediated fibrotic changes are limited to liver, spleen, and bone marrow and presumably relate to the functional characteristics of mast cells developing at those sites, as opposed to those at sites without fibrosis, such as the gastrointestinal tissue or skin. Immunofluorescent analysis of bone marrow and skin lesions in ISM and of spleen, lymph node, and skin in ASM has revealed only one mast cell phenotype, namely, scroll-poor cells expressing tryptase, chymase, and CPA.

The cutaneous lesions of urticaria pigmentosa are reddish-brown macules or papules that respond to trauma with urtication and erythema (Darier's sign). The apparent incidence of these lesions is $\geq 90\%$ in patients with ISM and $<50\%$ in those with SM-AHNMD or ASM. Approximately 1% of patients with ISM have skin lesions that appear as tan-brown macules with striking patchy erythema and associated telangiectasia (telangiectasia macularis eruptiva perstans). In the upper gastrointestinal tract, histamine-mediated hypersecretion is the most common problem, with resultant gastritis and peptic ulcer. In the lower intestinal tract, the occurrence of diarrhea and abdominal pain is attributed to increased motility due to mast cell mediators, and this can be aggravated by malabsorption with secondary nutritional insufficiency and osteomalacia. The periportal fibrosis associated with mast cell infiltration and a prominence of eosinophils may lead to portal hypertension and ascites. In some patients, flushing and recurrent vascular collapse are markedly aggravated by an idiosyncratic response to a minimal dosage of nonsteroidal anti-inflammatory agents. The neuropsychiatric disturbances are clinically most evident as impaired recent memory, decreased attention span, and "migraine-like" headaches. Patients in every category of systemic mastocytosis may experience exacerbation of a specific clinical sign or symptom with alcohol ingestion, use of mast cell–interactive narcotics, or ingestion of nonsteroidal anti-inflammatory agents.

DIAGNOSIS Although the diagnosis of mastocytosis is generally suspected on the basis of the clinical history and physical findings, and can be supported by laboratory procedures, it can be established only by a tissue diagnosis. By recent convention, the diagnosis of systemic mastocytosis is facilitated by bone marrow biopsy to meet the criteria of one major plus one minor or three minor findings (Table 298-3). The bone marrow provides the major criterion by revealing aggregates of mast cells, often in paratrabecular and perivascular locations with lymphocytes and eosinophils, as well as the minor criteria of an abnormal mast cell morphology, an aberrant mast cell membrane immunophenotype, or a codon 816 mutation in any cell type. A serum total tryptase level and/or a 24-h urine collection for measurement of histamine, histamine metabolites, or metabolites of PGD_2 are useful common noninvasive approaches to consider before bone marrow biopsy. The α form of tryptase is elevated in more than one-half of patients with systemic mastocytosis and provides a minor criterion; the β form is increased in patients undergoing an anaphylactic reaction. Additional studies directed by the presentation include a bone scan or skeletal survey; contrast studies of the upper gastrointestinal tract with small-bowel follow-through, computed tomography scan, or endoscopy; and a neuropsychiatric evaluation, including an electroencephalogram.

The differential diagnosis requires the exclusion of other flushing disorders. The 24-h urine assessment of 5-hydroxy-indoleacetic acid and metanephrines should exclude a carcinoid tumor or a pheochromocytoma. Most patients with recurrent anaphylaxis, including the idiopathic group, present with angioedema and/or wheezing, which are not manifestations of systemic mastocytosis.

℞ TREATMENT

The management of systemic mastocytosis uses a stepwise and symptom/sign–directed approach that includes an H_1 antihistamine for flushing and pruritus, an H_2 antihistamine or proton pump inhibitor for gastric acid hypersecretion, oral cromolyn sodium for diarrhea and abdominal pain, and aspirin for severe flushing with or without associated vascular collapse, despite use of H_1 and H_2 antihistamines, to block biosynthesis of PGD_2. Systemic glucocorticoids appear to alleviate the malabsorption. Headaches are generally managed with tricyclic antidepressants and other neurotransmitter-modifying agents. Ketotifen has been used to alleviate flushing in patients with gastric intolerance to nonsteroidal anti-inflammatory agents and in patients with bone pain or intractable headaches. The efficacy of IFN-α in ASM is controversial, and this may relate to dosage limitations due to side effects. Treatment with hydroxyurea to reduce the mast cell lineage progenitors may have merit in ASM. Chemotherapy is appropriate for the frank leukemias.

TABLE 298-3 *Diagnostic Criteria for Systemic Mastocytosis^a*

Major: Multifocal dense infiltrates of mast cells in bone marrow or other extracutaneous tissues with confirmation by immunodetection of tryptase or metachromasia

Minor: Abnormal mast cell morphology with a spindle shape and/or multilobed or eccentric nucleus

Aberrant mast cell surface phenotype with expression of CD25 and CD2 (IL-2 receptor) in addition to C117 (c-*kit*)

Detection of codon 816 mutation in peripheral blood cells, bone marrow cells, or lesional tissue

Total serum tryptase (mostly alpha) greater than 20 ng/mL

^{a} Diagnosis requires either major and one minor or three minor criteria.

ALLERGIC RHINITIS

DEFINITION Allergic rhinitis is characterized by sneezing; rhinorrhea; obstruction of the nasal passages; conjunctival, nasal, and pharyngeal itching; and lacrimation, all occurring in a temporal relationship to allergen exposure. Although commonly seasonal due to elicitation by airborne pollens, it can be perennial in an environment of chronic exposure. The incidence of allergic rhinitis in North America is about 7%, with the peak occurring in childhood and adolescence.

PREDISPOSING FACTORS AND ETIOLOGY Allergic rhinitis generally presents in atopic individuals, i.e., in persons with a family history of a similar or related symptom complex and a personal history of collateral allergy expressed as eczematous dermatitis, urticaria, and/or asthma (Chap. 236). Up to 40% of patients with rhinitis manifest asthma, whereas ~70% of individuals with asthma experience rhinitis. Symptoms generally appear before the fourth decade of life and tend to diminish gradually with aging, although complete spontaneous remissions are uncommon. A relatively small number of weeds that depend on wind rather than insects for cross-pollination, as well as grasses and some trees, produce sufficient quantities of pollen suitable for wide distribution by air currents to elicit seasonal allergic rhinitis. The dates of pollination of these species generally vary little from year to year in a particular locale but may be quite different in another climate. In the temperate areas of North America, trees typically pollinate from March through May, grasses in June and early July, and ragweed from mid-August to early October. Molds, which are widespread in nature because they occur in soil or decaying organic matter, may propagate spores in a pattern dependent on climatic conditions. Perennial allergic rhinitis occurs in response to allergens that are present throughout the year, including desquamating epithelium in animal dander, cockroach-derived proteins, mold spores, or dust, which has mites such as *Dermatophagoides farinae* and *D. pteronyssinus*. Dust mites are scavengers of flecks of human skin and coat the digestate with mite-specific protein for excretion. In up to one-half of patients with perennial rhinitis, no clear-cut allergen can be demonstrated as causative. The ability of allergens to cause rhinitis rather than lower respiratory symptoms may be attributed to their large size, 10 to 100 μm, and retention within the nose.

PATHOPHYSIOLOGY AND MANIFESTATIONS Episodic rhinorrhea, sneezing, obstruction of the nasal passages with lacrimation, and pruritus of the conjunctiva, nasal mucosa, and oropharynx are the hallmarks of allergic rhinitis. The nasal mucosa is pale and boggy, the conjunctiva congested and edematous, and the pharynx is generally unremarkable. Swelling of the turbinates and mucous membranes with obstruction of the sinus ostia and eustachian tubes precipitates secondary infections of the sinuses and middle ear, respectively. Nasal polyps, representing mucosal protrusions containing edema fluid with variable numbers of eosinophils, can arise concurrently with infection within the nasopharynx or sinuses and increase obstructive symptoms.

The nose presents a large mucosal surface area through the folds of the turbinates and serves to adjust the temperature and moisture content of inhaled air and to filter out particulate materials above 10 μm in size by impingement in a mucous blanket; ciliary action moves the entrapped particles toward the pharynx. Entrapment of pollen and digestion of the outer coat by mucosal enzymes such as lysozymes release protein allergens generally of 10,000 to 40,000 molecular weight. The initial interaction occurs between the allergen and intraepithelial mast cells and then proceeds to involve deeper perivenular mast cells, both of which are sensitized with specific IgE. During the symptomatic season when the mucosae are already swollen and hyperemic, there is enhanced adverse reactivity to the seasonal pollen as well as to antigenically unrelated pollens for which there is underlying hypersensitivity due to improved penetration of the allergens. Biopsy specimens of nasal mucosa during seasonal rhinitis show submucosal edema with infiltration by eosinophils, along with some basophils and neutrophils.

The mucosal surface fluid contains IgA that is present because of its secretory piece and also IgE, which apparently arrives by diffusion from plasma cells in proximity to mucosal surfaces. IgE fixes to mucosal and submucosal mast cells, and the intensity of the clinical response to inhaled allergens is quantitatively related to the naturally occurring pollen dose. In sensitive individuals, the introduction of allergen into the nose is associated with sneezing, "stuffiness," and discharge, and the fluid contains histamine, PGD_2, and leukotrienes. Thus the mast cells of the nasal mucosa and submucosa generate and release mediators through IgE-dependent reactions that are capable of producing tissue edema and eosinophilic infiltration.

DIAGNOSIS The diagnosis of seasonal allergic rhinitis depends largely on an accurate history of occurrence coincident with the pollination of the offending weeds, grasses, or trees. The continuous character of perennial allergic rhinitis due to contamination of the home or place of work makes historic analysis difficult, but there may be a variability in symptoms that can be related to exposure to animal dander, dust mite and/or cockroach allergens, or work-related allergens such as latex. Patients with perennial rhinitis commonly develop the problem in adult life, and manifest nasal congestion and a postnasal discharge, often associated with thickening of the sinus membranes demonstrated by radiography. The term *vasomotor rhinitis* designates a condition of enhanced reactivity of the nasopharynx in which a symptom complex resembling perennial allergic rhinitis occurs with nonspecific stimuli. Other entities to be excluded are structural abnormalities of the nasopharynx; exposure to irritants; upper respiratory infection; pregnancy with prominent nasal mucosal edema; prolonged topical use of α-adrenergic agents in the form of nose drops (rhinitis medicamentosa); and the use of certain therapeutic agents such as rauwolfia, β-adrenergic antagonists, or estrogens.

The nasal secretions of allergic patients are rich in eosinophils, and a modest peripheral eosinophilia is a common feature. Local or systemic neutrophilia implies infection. Total serum IgE is frequently elevated, but the demonstration of immunologic specificity for IgE is critical to an etiologic diagnosis. A skin test by the intracutaneous route (puncture or prick) with the allergens of interest provides a rapid and reliable approach to identifying allergen-specific IgE that has sensitized cutaneous mast cells. A positive intracutaneous skin test with 1:10 to 1:20 weight/volume of extract has a high predictive value for the presence of allergy. An intradermal test with a 1:500 to 1:1000 dilution of 0.05 mL may follow if indicated by history when the intracutaneous test is negative; but while more sensitive, it is less reliable due to the reactivity of some asymptomatic individuals at the test dose. Skin testing by the intracutaneous route for food allergens can be supportive of the clinical history. A double-blind, placebo-controlled challenge may document a food allergy, but such a procedure does bear the risk of an anaphylactic reaction. An elimination diet is safer but is tedious and less definitive. Food allergy is uncommon as a cause of allergic rhinitis.

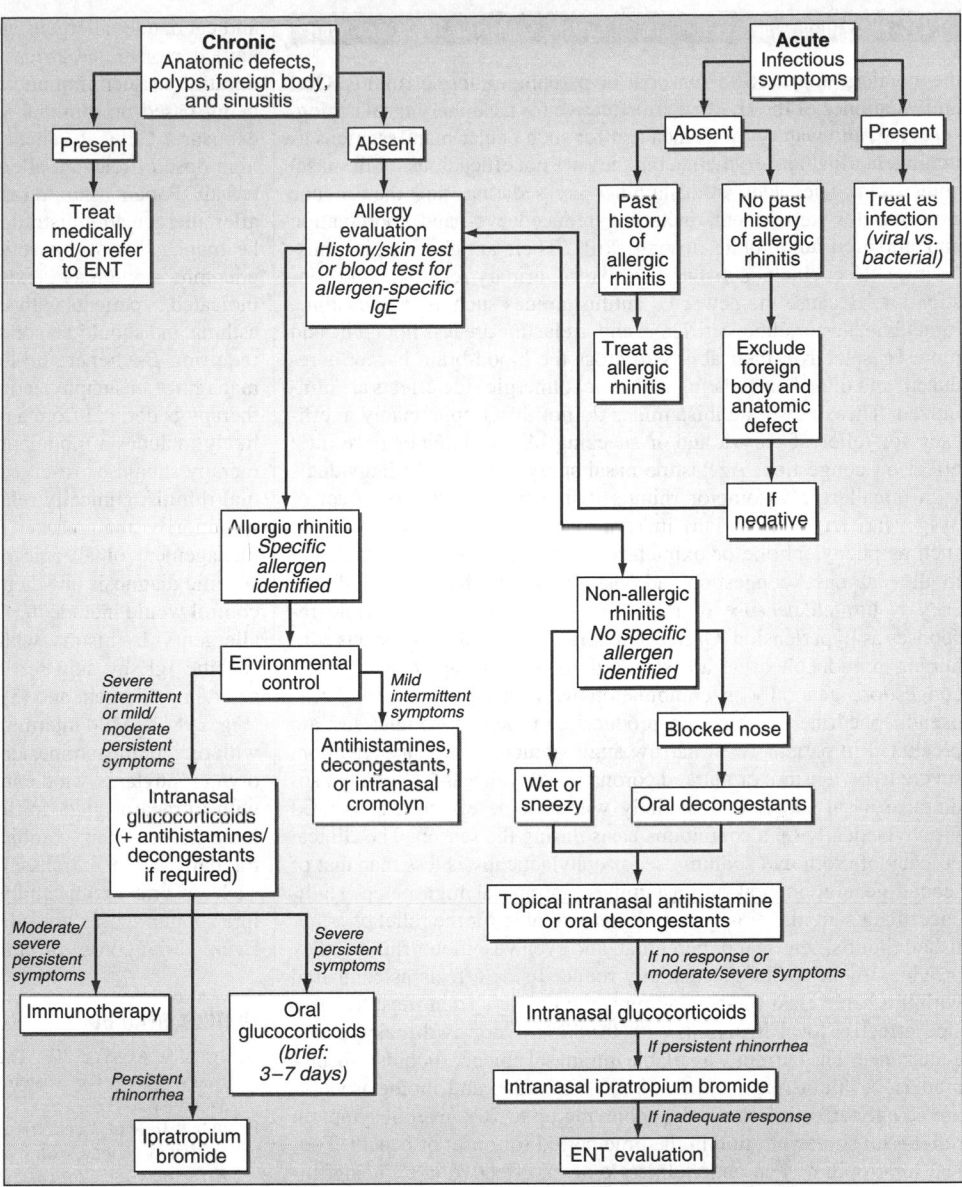

FIGURE 298-3 Algorithm for the diagnosis and management of rhinitis. ENT, ear, nose, and throat surgeon.

Newer methodology for detecting total IgE, including the development of enzyme-linked immunosorbent assays (ELISA) employing anti-IgE bound to either a solid-phase or a liquid-phase particle, provides rapid and cost-effective determinations. Measurements of specific anti-IgE in serum are obtained by its binding to an allergen and quantitation by subsequent uptake of labeled anti-IgE. As compared to the skin test, the assay of specific IgE in serum is less sensitive but has high specificity.

PREVENTION Avoidance of exposure to the offending allergen is the most effective means of controlling allergic diseases; removal of pets from the home to avoid animal danders, utilization of air filtration devices to minimize the concentrations of airborne pollens, elimination of cockroach-derived proteins by chemical destruction of the pest and careful food storage, travel to nonpollinating areas during the critical periods, and even a change of domicile to eliminate a mold spore problem may be necessary. Control of dust mites by allergen avoidance includes use of plastic-lined covers for mattresses, pillows, and comforters, and elimination of carpets and drapes.

℞ TREATMENT

Although allergen avoidance is the most cost-effective means of managing allergic rhinitis, treatment with pharmacologic agents represents the standard approach to seasonal or perennial allergic rhinitis. Oral antihistamines of the H_1 class are effective for nasopharyngeal itching, sneezing, and watery rhinorrhea and for such ocular manifestations as itching, tearing, and erythema, but they are not efficacious for the nasal congestion. The older antihistamines are sedating, and they induce psychomotor impairment, including reduced eye-hand coordination and impaired automobile driving skills. Their anticholinergic (muscarinic) effects include visual disturbance, urinary retention, and constipation. Because the newer H_1 antihistamines such as fexofenadine, loratadine, desloradine, cetirizine, and azelastine are less lipophilic and more H_1 selective, their ability to cross the blood-brain barrier is reduced, and thus their sedating and anticholinergic side effects are minimized. These newer antihistamines do not differ appreciably in efficacy for relief of coryza and/or sneezing. Antihistamines have little effect on congestion. Azelastine nasal spray may benefit individuals with nonallergic vasomotor rhinitis, but it has an adverse effect of dysgeusia (taste perversion) in some patients. α-Adrenergic agents such as phenylephrine or oximetazoline are generally used topically to alleviate nasal congestion and obstruction, but the duration of efficacy is limited because of rebound rhinitis and such systemic responses as hypertension. Oral α-adrenergic agonist decongestants containing pseudoephedrine are standard for the management of nasal congestion, generally in combination with an antihistamine. These pseudoephedrine combination products can cause insomnia and are precluded in patients with narrow angle glaucoma, urinary retention, severe hypertension, or marked coronary artery disease. Cromolyn sodium, a nasal spray, is essentially without side effects and is used prophylactically on a continuous basis during the season. The clinical efficacy of cromolyn sodium used prophylactically is less than that of second-generation oral antihistamines. Intranasal high-potency glucocorticoids are the most potent drugs available for the relief of established rhinitis, seasonal or perennial, and even vasomotor rhinitis; they provide efficacy with substantially reduced side effects as compared with this same class of agent administered orally. Their most frequent side effect is local irritation, with *Candida* overgrowth being a rare occurrence. The currently available intranasal glucocorticoids—beclomethasone, flunisolide, budesonide, fluticasone, and mometasone—are equally effective clinically, achieving up to 70% overall symptom relief with some variation in the time period for onset of benefit. Topical ipratropium is an anticholinergic agent effective in reducing rhinorrhea, including that in patients with perennial symptoms, and it can be additionally efficacious when combined with intranasal steroids. For systemic symptoms not related to the nasopharynx, such as allergic conjunctivitis, treatment may be local.

Immunotherapy, often termed *hyposensitization*, consists of repeated subcutaneous injections of gradually increasing concentrations of the allergen(s) considered to be specifically responsible for the symptom complex. Controlled studies of ragweed, grass, dust mite, and cat dander allergens administered for treatment of allergic rhinitis have demonstrated at least partial relief of symptoms and signs. The duration of such immunotherapy is 3 to 5 years, with discontinuation being based on minimal symptoms over two consecutive seasons of exposure. Clinical benefit appears related to the administration of a high dose of relevant allergen advancing from weekly to monthly intervals. Patients should remain at the treatment site for at least 20 min after allergen administration so that any anaphylactic consequence can be managed. Local reactions with erythema and induration are not uncommon and may persist for 1 to 3 days. Immunotherapy is contraindicated in patients with significant cardiovascular disease or unstable asthma and should be conducted with particular caution in any patient requiring β-adrenergic blocking therapy because of the difficulty in managing an anaphylactic complication. The response to immunotherapy is derived from a complex of cellular and humoral effects that likely includes a modulation in T cell cytokine production. Immunotherapy should be reserved for clearly documented seasonal or perennial rhinitis, clinically related to defined allergen exposure with confirmation by the presence of allergen-specific IgE. A sequence for the management of allergic or perennial rhinitis based on an allergen-specific diagnosis and stepwise management as required for symptom control would include the following: (1) identification of the offending allergen(s) by history with confirmation of the presence of allergen-specific IgE by skin test and/or serum assay; (2) avoidance of the offending allergen; and (3) medical management in a stepwise fashion (Fig. 298-3). Mild intermittent symptoms of allergic rhinitis are treated with oral antihistamines, intranasal antihistamines, or intranasal cromolyn prophylaxis. Moderate to more severe allergic rhinitis is managed with intranasal glucocorticoids plus oral antihistamines or antihistamine-decongestant combinations. Persistent allergic rhinitis requiring the daily use of intranasal glucocorticoids with add-on interventions such as oral antihistamines, decongestant combinations, or topical ipratropium merits consideration of allergen-specific immunotherapy. Even a brief course of oral prednisone can be indicated.

FURTHER READING

BOYCE JA, AUSTEN KF: The biology of the mast cell, in *Immunologic Diseases*, 6th ed, KF Austen et al (eds). Philadelphia, Lippincott Williams & Wilkins, 2001

PENROSE JF et al: Leukotrienes: Biosynthetic pathways, release, and receptor-mediated actions with relevance to disease states, in *Inflammation: Basic Principles and Clinical Correlates*, 3d ed, JI Gallin and R Snyderman (eds). Philadelphia, Lippincott Williams & Wilkins, 1999

SOTER NA, KAPLAN AP: Urticaria and angioedema, in *Fitzpatrick's Dermatology in General Medicine*, 6th ed, IM Freedberg et al (eds). New York, McGraw-Hill, 2003, pp 1129–1139

VALENTINE MD: Insect venom allergy, in *Immunologic Diseases*, 6th ed, KF Austen et al (eds). Philadelphia, Lippincott Williams & Wilkins, 2001

WOROBEC A, METCALFE DD: Anaphylactic syndrome, in *Immunologic Diseases*, 6th ed, KF Austen et al (eds). Philadelphia, Lippincott Williams & Wilkins, 2001

299 AUTOIMMUNITY AND AUTOIMMUNE DISEASES
Peter E. Lipsky, Betty Diamond

One of the classically accepted features of the immune system is the capacity to distinguish self from non-self. Although they are able to recognize and generate reactions to a vast array of foreign materials, most animals do not mount immune responses to self-antigens under ordinary circumstances and thus are tolerant to self. Whereas recognition of self plays an important role in shaping both the T cell and B cell repertoires of immune receptors and plays an essential role in the recognition of nominal antigen by T cells, the development of potentially harmful immune responses to self-antigens is, in general, precluded. Autoimmunity, therefore, represents the end result of the breakdown of one or more of the basic mechanisms regulating immune tolerance.

The essential feature of an autoimmune disease is that tissue injury is caused by the immunologic reaction of the organism with its own tissues. Autoimmunity, on the other hand, refers merely to the presence of antibodies or T lymphocytes that react with self-antigens and does not necessarily imply that the development of self-reactivity has pathogenic consequences.

Autoimmunity may be seen in normal individuals and in higher frequency in normal older people. In addition, autoreactivity may develop during various infectious conditions. The expression of autoimmunity may be self-limited, as occurs with many infectious processes, or persistent. When autoimmunity is induced by an inciting event, such as infection or tissue damage from trauma or infarction, there may or may not be ensuing pathology. Even in the presence of organ pathology, it may be difficult to determine whether the damage is mediated by autoreactivity. Thus, the presence of self-reactivity may be either the cause or a consequence of an ongoing pathologic process.

MECHANISMS OF AUTOIMMUNITY

Since Ehrlich first postulated the existence of mechanisms to prevent the generation of self-reactivity in 1900, ideas concerning the nature of this inhibition have developed in parallel with the progressive increase in understanding of the immune system. Burnet's clonal selection theory included the idea that interaction of lymphoid cells with their specific antigens during fetal or early postnatal life would lead to elimination of such "forbidden clones." This idea became untenable, however, when it was shown by a number of investigators that autoimmune diseases could be induced by simple immunization procedures, that autoantigen-binding cells could be demonstrated easily in the circulation of normal individuals, and that self-limited autoimmune phenomena frequently developed during infections. These observations indicated that clones of cells capable of responding to autoantigens were present in the repertoire of antigen-reactive cells in normal adults and suggested that mechanisms in addition to clonal deletion were responsible for preventing their activation.

Currently, three general processes are thought to be involved in the maintenance of selective unresponsiveness to autoantigens (Table 299-1): (1) sequestration of self-antigens, rendering them inaccessible to the immune system; (2) specific unresponsiveness (tolerance or anergy) of relevant T or B cells; and (3) limitation of potential reactivity by regulatory mechanisms.

Derangements of these normal processes may predispose to the development of autoimmunity (Table 299-2). In general, these abnormal responses relate to stimulation by exogenous agents, usually bacterial or viral, or endogenous abnormalities in the cells of the immune system. Microbial superantigens, such as staphylococcal protein A and staphylococcal enterotoxins, are substances that can stimulate a broad range of T and B cells based upon specific interactions with selected families of immune receptors irrespective of their antigen specificity. If autoantigen reactive T and/or B cells express these receptors, autoimmunity might develop. Alternatively, molecular mimicry or cross-reactivity between a microbial product and a self-antigen might lead to activation of autoreactive lymphocytes. One of the best examples of autoreactivity and autoimmune disease resulting from molecular mimicry is rheumatic fever, in which antibodies to the M protein of streptococci cross-react with myosin, laminin, and other matrix proteins. Deposition of these autoantibodies in the heart initiates an inflammatory response. Molecular mimicry between microbial proteins and host tissues has been reported in type 1 diabetes mellitus, rheumatoid arthritis, and multiple sclerosis. The capacity of nonspecific stimulation of the immune system to predispose to the development of autoimmunity has been explored in a number of models; one is provided by the effect of adjuvants on the production of autoimmunity. Autoantigens become much more immunogenic when administered with adjuvant. It is presumed that infectious agents may be able to overcome self-tolerance because they possess molecules, such as bacterial endotoxin, that have adjuvant-like effects on the immune system by stimulating cells through Toll-like receptors.

Endogenous derangements of the immune system may also contribute to the loss of immunologic tolerance to self-antigens and the development of autoimmunity (Table 299-2). Many autoantigens re-

TABLE 299-2 Mechanisms of Autoimmunity

I. Exogenous
  A. Molecular mimicry
  B. Superantigenic stimulation
  C. Microbial adjuvanticity
II. Endogenous
  A. Altered antigen presentation
    1. Loss of immunologic privilege
    2. Presentation of novel or cryptic epitopes (epitope spreading)
    3. Alteration of self-antigen
    4. Enhanced function of antigen-presenting cells
      a. Costimulatory molecule expression
      b. Cytokine production
  B. Increased T cell help
    1. Cytokine production
    2. Costimulatory molecules
  C. Increased B cell function
  D. Apoptotic defects
  E. Cytokine imbalance
  F. Altered immunoregulation

side in immunologically privileged sites, such as the brain or the anterior chamber of the eye. These sites are characterized by the inability of engrafted tissue to elicit immune responses. Immunologic privilege results from a number of events, including the limited entry of proteins from those sites into lymphatics, the local production of immunosuppressive cytokines such as transforming growth factor (TGF) β, and the local expression of molecules such as Fas ligand that can induce apoptosis of activated T cells. Lymphoid cells remain in a state of immunologic ignorance (neither activated nor anergized) to proteins expressed uniquely in immunologically privileged sites. If the privileged site is damaged by trauma or inflammation, or if T cells are activated elsewhere, proteins expressed at this site can become the targets of immunologic assault. Such an event may occur in multiple sclerosis and sympathetic ophthalmia, in which antigens uniquely expressed in the brain and eye, respectively, become the target of activated T cells.

Alterations in antigen presentation may also contribute to autoimmunity. This may occur by epitope spreading, in which protein determinants (epitopes) not routinely seen by lymphocytes (cryptic epitopes) are recognized as a result of immunologic reactivity to associated molecules. For example, animals immunized with one protein component of a multimolecular complex may be induced to produce antibodies to the other components of the complex. Finally, inflammation, drug exposure, or normal senescence may cause a primary chemical alteration in proteins, resulting in the generation of immune responses that cross-react with normal self-proteins. Alterations in the availability and presentation of autoantigens may be important components of immunoreactivity in certain models of organ-specific autoimmune diseases. In addition, these factors may be relevant in understanding the pathogenesis of various drug-induced autoimmune conditions. However, the diversity of autoreactivity manifest in non-organ-specific systemic autoimmune diseases suggests that these conditions might result from a more general activation of the immune system rather than from an alteration in individual self-antigens.

A number of experimental models have suggested that intense stimulation of T lymphocytes can produce nonspecific signals that bypass the need for antigen-specific helper T cells and lead to polyclonal B cell activation with the formation of multiple autoantibodies. For example, antinuclear, antierythrocyte, and antilymphocyte antibodies are produced during the chronic graft-versus-host reaction. In addition, true autoimmune diseases, including autoimmune hemolytic anemia and immune complex–mediated glomerulonephritis, can also be induced in this manner. While it is clear that such diffuse activation of helper T cell activity can cause autoimmunity, nonspecific stimulation of B lymphocytes can also lead to the production of autoantibodies. Thus, the administration of polyclonal B cell activators, such as bac-

TABLE 299-1 Mechanisms Preventing Autoimmunity

1. Sequestration of self-antigen
2. Generation and maintenance of tolerance
  a. Central deletion of autoreactive lymphocytes
  b. Peripheral anergy of autoreactive lymphocytes
  c. Receptor replacement by autoreactive lymphocytes
3. Regulatory mechanisms

TABLE 299-3 *Mechanisms of Tissue Damage in Autoimmune Disease*

Effector	Mechanism	Target	Disease
Autoantibody	Blocking or inactivation	α Chain of the nicotinic acetylcholine receptor	Myasthenia gravis
		Phospholipid–β_2-glycoprotein 1 complex	Antiphospholipid syndrome
		Insulin receptor	Insulin-resistant diabetes mellitus
		Intrinsic factor	Pernicious anemia
	Stimulation	TSH receptor (LATS)	Graves' disease
		Proteinase-3 (ANCA)	Wegener's granulomatosis
		Epidermal cadherin$_1$ Desmoglein 3	Pemphigus vulgaris
	Complement activation	α_3 Chain of collagen IV	Goodpasture's syndrome
	Immune-complex formation	Double-strand DNA	Systemic lupus erythematosus
		Ig	Rheumatoid arthritis
	Opsonization	Platelet GpIIb:IIIa	Autoimmune thrombocytopenic purpura
		Rh antigens, I antigen	Autoimmune hemolytic anemia
	Antibody-dependent cellular cytotoxicity	Thyroid peroxidase, thyroglobulin	Hashimoto's thyroiditis
T cells	Cytokine production	?	Rheumatoid arthritis, multiple sclerosis, type 1 diabetes mellitus
	Cellular cytotoxicity	?	Type 1 diabetes mellitus

Note: ANCA, antineutrophil cytoplasmic antibody; LATS, long-acting thyroid stimulator; TSH, thyroid-stimulating hormone.

terial endotoxin, to normal mice leads to the production of a number of autoantibodies, including those directed to DNA and IgG (rheumatoid factor).

Primary alterations in the activity of T and/or B cells, cytokine imbalances, or defective immunoregulatory circuits may also contribute to the emergence of autoimmunity. For example, decreased apoptosis, as can be seen in animals with defects in Fas (CD95) or Fas ligand or in patients with related abnormalities, can be associated with the development of autoimmunity. Similarly, diminished production of tumor necrosis factor (TNF) and interleukin (IL) 10 has been reported to be associated with the development of autoimmunity.

Autoimmunity may also result from an abnormality of immunoregulatory mechanisms. Observations made in both human autoimmune disease and animal models suggest that defects in the generation and expression of regulatory T cell activity may allow for the production of autoimmunity. Administration of normal regulatory T cells or factors derived from them can prevent the development of autoimmune disease in rodent models of autoimmunity.

It should be apparent that no single mechanism can explain all the varied manifestations of autoimmunity. Furthermore, genetic evaluation has shown that a number of abnormalities often need to converge to induce an autoimmune disease. Additional factors that appear to be important determinants in the induction of autoimmunity include age, sex (many autoimmune diseases are far more common in women), genetic background, exposure to infectious agents, and environmental contacts. How all of these disparate factors affect the capacity to develop self-reactivity is currently being intensively investigated.

GENETIC CONSIDERATIONS Evidence in humans that there are susceptibility genes for autoimmunity comes from family studies and especially from studies of twins. Studies in type 1 diabetes mellitus, rheumatoid arthritis, multiple sclerosis, and systemic lupus erythematosus (SLE) have shown that approximately 15 to 30% of pairs of monozygotic twins show disease concordance, compared with <5% of dizygotic twins. The occurrence of different autoimmune diseases within the same family has suggested that certain susceptibility genes may predispose to a variety of autoimmune diseases. Genetic mapping

has begun to identify chromosomal regions that predispose to specific autoimmune diseases. In addition to this evidence from humans, certain inbred mouse strains reproducibly develop specific spontaneous or experimentally induced autoimmune diseases, whereas others do not. These findings have led to an extensive search for genes that determine susceptibility to autoimmune disease.

The most consistent association for susceptibility to autoimmune disease has been with particular alleles of the major histocompatibility complex (MHC). It has been suggested that the association of MHC genotype with autoimmune disease relates to differences in the ability of different allelic variations of MHC molecules to present autoantigenic peptides to autoreactive T cells. An alternative hypothesis involves the role of MHC alleles in shaping the T cell receptor repertoire during T cell ontogeny in the thymus. Additionally, specific MHC gene products themselves may be the source of peptides that can be recognized by T cells. Cross-reactivity between such MHC peptides and peptides derived from proteins produced by common microbes may trigger autoimmunity by molecular mimicry. However, MHC genotype alone does not determine the development of autoimmunity. Identical twins are far more likely to develop the same autoimmune disease than MHC-identical nontwin siblings, suggesting that genetic factors other than the MHC also affect disease susceptibility. Recent studies of the genetics of type 1 diabetes, SLE, rheumatoid arthritis, and multiple sclerosis in humans and mice have shown that there are several independently segregating disease susceptibility loci in addition to the MHC.

There is evidence that several other genes are important in increasing susceptibility to autoimmune disease. In humans, inherited homozygous deficiency of the early proteins of the classic pathway of complement (C1, C4, or C2) is very strongly associated with the development of SLE. In mice and humans, abnormalities in the genes encoding proteins involved in the regulation of apoptosis, including Fas (CD95) and Fas ligand (CD95 ligand), are strongly associated with the development of autoimmunity. There is also evidence that inherited variation in the level of expression of certain cytokines, such as TNFα or IL-10, may also increase susceptibility to autoimmune disease.

A further important factor in disease susceptibility is the hormonal status of the patient. Many autoimmune diseases show a strong sex bias, which appears in most cases to relate to the hormonal status of women.

IMMUNOPATHOGENIC MECHANISMS IN AUTOIMMUNE DISEASES The mechanisms of tissue injury in autoimmune diseases can be divided into antibody-mediated and cell-mediated processes. Representative examples are listed in Table 299-3.

The pathogenicity of autoantibodies can be mediated through several mechanisms, including opsonization of soluble factors or cells, activation of an inflammatory cascade via the complement system, and interference with the physiologic function of soluble molecules or cells.

In autoimmune thrombocytopenic purpura, opsonization of platelets targets them for elimination by phagocytes. Likewise, in autoimmune hemolytic anemia, binding of immunoglobulin to red cell membranes leads to phagocytosis and lysis of the opsonized cell. Goodpasture's syndrome, a disease characterized by lung hemorrhage and severe glomerulonephritis, represents an example of antibody binding leading to local activation of complement and neutrophil accumulation and activation. The autoantibody in this disease binds to the α_3 chain of type IV collagen in the basement membrane. In SLE, activation of the complement cascade at sites of immunoglobulin deposition in renal glomeruli is considered to be a major mechanism of renal damage.

Autoantibodies can also interfere with normal physiologic functions of cells or soluble factors. Autoantibodies against hormone receptors can lead to stimulation of cells or to inhibition of cell function through interference with receptor signaling. For example, long-acting thyroid stimulators, which are autoantibodies that bind to the receptor for thyroid-stimulating hormone, are present in Graves' disease and function as agonists, causing the thyroid to respond as if there were an excess of thyroid-stimulating hormone. Alternatively, antibodies to the insulin receptor can cause insulin-resistant diabetes mellitus through receptor blockade. In myasthenia gravis, autoantibodies to the acetylcholine receptor can be detected in 85 to 90% of patients and are responsible for muscle weakness. The exact location of the antigenic epitope, the valence and affinity of the antibody, and perhaps other characteristics determine whether activation or blockade results from antibody binding.

Antiphospholipid antibodies are associated with thromboembolic events in primary and secondary antiphospholipid syndrome and have also been associated with fetal wastage. The major antibody is directed to the phospholipid–β_2-glycoprotein I complex and appears to exert a procoagulant effect. In pemphigus vulgaris, autoantibodies bind to a component of the epidermal cell desmosome, desmoglein 3, and play a role in the induction of the disease. They exert their pathologic effect by disrupting cell-cell junctions through stimulation of the production of epithelial proteases, leading to blister formation. Cytoplasmic antineutrophil cytoplasmic antibody (c-ANCA), found in Wegener's granulomatosis, is an antibody to an intracellular antigen, the 29-kDa serine protease (proteinase-3). In vitro experiments have shown that IgG anti-c-ANCA causes cellular activation and degranulation of primed neutrophils.

It is important to note that autoantibodies of a given specificity may cause disease only in genetically susceptible hosts, as has been shown in experimental models of myasthenia gravis. Finally, some autoantibodies seem to be markers for disease but have as yet no known pathogenic potential.

AUTOIMMUNE DISEASE Manifestations of autoimmunity are found in a large number of pathologic conditions. However, their presence does not necessarily imply that the pathologic process is an autoimmune disease. A number of attempts to establish formal criteria for the diagnosis of autoimmune diseases have been made, but none is universally accepted. One set of criteria is shown in Table 299-4; however, this should be viewed merely as a guide in consideration of the problem.

To classify a disease as autoimmune, it is necessary to demonstrate that the immune response to a self-antigen causes the observed pathology. Initially, the demonstration that antibodies against the affected tissue could be detected in the serum of patients suffering from various diseases was taken as evidence that these diseases had an autoimmune basis. However, such autoantibodies are also found when tissue damage is caused by trauma or infection, and the autoantibody is secondary to tissue damage. Thus, it is necessary to show that autoimmunity is pathogenic before classifying a disease as autoimmune.

If the autoantibodies are pathogenic, it may be possible to transfer disease to experimental animals by the administration of autoantibodies, with the subsequent development of pathology in the recipient similar to that seen in the patient from whom the antibodies were obtained. This has been shown, for example, in Graves' disease. Some autoimmune diseases can be transferred from mother to fetus and are observed in the newborn babies of diseased mothers. The symptoms of the disease in the newborn usually disappear as the levels of the

TABLE 299-4 *Human Autoimmune Disease: Presumptive Evidence for an Immunologic Pathogenesis*

Major Criteria
1. Presence of autoantibodies or evidence of cellular reactivity to self
2. Documentation of relevant autoantibody or lymphocytic infiltrate in the pathologic lesion.
3. Demonstration that relevant autoantibody or T cells can cause tissue pathology
   a. Transplacental transmission
   b. Adaptive transfer into animals
   c. In vitro impact on cellular function

Supportive Evidence
1. Reasonable animal model
2. Beneficial effect from immunosuppressive agents
3. Association with other evidence of autoimmunity
4. No evidence of infection or other obvious cause

maternal antibody decrease. An exception is congenital heart block, in which damage to the developing conducting system of the heart as a result of transfer of anti-Ro antibody from the mother results in permanent heart block.

In most situations, the critical factors that determine when the development of autoimmunity results in autoimmune disease have not been delineated. The relationship of autoimmunity to the development of autoimmune disease may relate to the fine specificity of the antibodies or T cells or their specific effector capabilities. In many circumstances a mechanistic understanding of the pathogenic potential of autoantibodies has not been established. In some autoimmune diseases, biased production of cytokines by helper T (T_H) cells may play a role in pathogenesis. In this regard, T cells can differentiate into specialized effector cells that predominantly produce interferon γ (T_H1) or IL-4 (T_H2) (Chap. 295). The former facilitate macrophage activation and classic cell-mediated immunity, whereas the latter are thought to have regulatory functions and are involved in the resolution of normal immune responses and also the development of responses to a variety of parasites. In a number of autoimmune diseases, such as rheumatoid arthritis, multiple sclerosis, type 1 diabetes mellitus, and Crohn's disease, there appears to be biased differentiation of T_H1 cells, with resultant organ damage.

ORGAN-SPECIFIC VERSUS SYSTEMIC AUTOIMMUNE DISEASES Autoimmune diseases form a spectrum, from those specifically affecting a single organ to systemic disorders with involvement of many organs (Table 299-5). Hashimoto's autoimmune thyroiditis is an example of an organ-specific autoimmune disease (Chap. 320). In this disorder, there is a specific lesion in the thyroid associated with infiltration of mono-

TABLE 299-5 *Some Autoimmune Diseases*

ORGAN SPECIFIC

Graves' disease	Autoimmune hemolytic anemia
Hashimoto's thyroiditis	
Autoimmune polyglandular syndrome	Autoimmune thrombocytopenic purpura
Type 1 diabetes mellitus	
Insulin-resistant diabetes mellitus	Pernicious anemia
Immune-mediated infertility	Myasthenia gravis
Autoimmune Addison's disease	Multiple sclerosis
Pemphigus vulgaris	Guillain-Barré syndrome
Pemphigus foliaceus	Stiff-man syndrome
Dermatitis herpetiformis	Acute rheumatic fever
Autoimmune alopecia	Sympathetic ophthalmia
Vitiligo	Goodpasture's syndrome

ORGAN NONSPECIFIC (SYSTEMIC)

Systemic lupus erythematosus	Wegener's granulomatosis
Rheumatoid arthritis	Antiphospholipid syndrome
Systemic necrotizing vasculitis	Sjögren's syndrome

nuclear cells and damage to follicular cells. Antibody to thyroid constituents can be demonstrated in nearly all cases. Other organ- or tissue-specific autoimmune disorders include pemphigus vulgaris, autoimmune hemolytic anemia, idiopathic thrombocytopenic purpura, Goodpasture's syndrome, myasthenia gravis, and sympathetic ophthalmia. One important feature of some organ-specific auto-immune diseases is the tendency for overlap, such that an individual with one specific syndrome is more likely to develop a second syndrome. For example, there is a high incidence of pernicious anemia in individuals with autoimmune thyroiditis. More striking is the tendency for individuals with an organ-specific autoimmune disease to develop multiple other manifestations of autoimmunity without the development of associated organ pathology. Thus, as many as 50% of individuals with pernicious anemia have non-cross-reacting antibodies to thyroid constituents, whereas patients with myasthenia gravis may develop antinuclear antibodies, antithyroid antibodies, rheumatoid factor, antilymphocyte antibodies, and polyclonal hypergammaglobulinemia. Part of the explanation for this may relate to the genetic elements shared by individuals with these different diseases.

Systemic autoimmune diseases differ from organ-specific diseases in that pathologic lesions are found in multiple, diverse organs and tissues. The hallmark of these conditions is the demonstration of associated relevant autoimmune manifestations that are likely to be etiologic in the organ pathology. SLE represents the prototype of these disorders because of its abundance of autoimmune manifestations.

SLE is a disease of protean manifestations that characteristically involves the kidneys, joints, skin, serosal surfaces, blood vessels, and central nervous system (Chap. 300). The disease is associated with a vast array of autoantibodies whose production appears to be a part of a generalized hyperreactivity of the humoral immune system. Other features of SLE include generalized B cell hyperresponsiveness, polyclonal hypergammaglobulinemia, and increased titers of antibodies to commonly encountered viral antigens.

℞ TREATMENT

Treatment of autoimmune diseases can focus on either suppressing the induction of autoimmunity, restoring normal regulatory mechanisms, or inhibiting the effector mechanisms. To eliminate autoreactive cells, immunosuppressive or ablative therapies are most commonly used. In recent years, cytokine blockade has been demonstrated to be effective in preventing immune activation in some diseases. New therapies are currently in clinical trials to target lymphoid cells more specifically, either by blocking a costimulatory signal needed for T or B cell activation, by eliminating the effector T cells or B cells, or by using autoantigen itself to induce tolerance. The major advance in inhibiting effector mechanisms has been the introduction of cytokine blockade, targeting at TNF or IL-1, that appears to limit organ damage in some diseases. Therapies that prevent target organ damage or support target organ function remain an important therapeutic approach to autoimmune disease.

FURTHER READING

DAVIDSON A, DIAMOND B: Autoimmune diseases. N Engl J Med 345:340, 2001

GREEN EA, FLAVELL RA: The initiation of autoimmune diabetes. Curr Opin Immunol 11.663, 1999

LIPSKY PE: Systemic lupus erythematosus: An autoimmune disease of B cell hyperactivity. Nat Immunol 2:764, 2001

MARRACK P et al: Autoimmune disease: Why and where it occurs. Nat Med 7:889, 2001

MCDEVITT HO: The role of MHC class II molecules in susceptibility and resistance to autoimmunity. Curr Opin Immunol 10:677, 1998

ROSE NR: The role of infection in the pathogenesis of autoimmune disease. Semin Immunol 10:5, 1998

SHEVACH EM: Suppressor T cells: Rebirth, function and homeostasis. Curr Biol 10:R572, 2000

300 | SYSTEMIC LUPUS ERYTHEMATOSUS
Bevra Hannahs Hahn

DEFINITION AND PREVALENCE Systemic lupus erythematosus (SLE) is an autoimmune disease in which organs, tissues, and cells undergo damage mediated by tissue-binding autoantibodies and immune complexes. Ninety percent of patients are women of child-bearing years; people of both genders, all ages, and all ethnic groups are susceptible. Prevalence of SLE in the United States is 15 to 50 per 100,000; the highest prevalence among ethnic groups is in African Americans.

PATHOGENESIS AND ETIOLOGY SLE is caused by interactions between susceptibility genes and environmental factors, resulting in abnormal immune responses. The immune responses include hyperreactivity and hypersensitivity of T and B lymphocytes and ineffective regulation of antigen availability and of ongoing antibody responses. Hyperreactivity of T and B cells is indicated by increased surface expression of molecules such as HLA-D and CD40L, showing that cells are easily activated by antigens that induce first-activating signals and by molecules that drive cells to full activation via second signals. The end result of these abnormalities is sustained production of pathogenic autoantibodies and formation of immune complexes that bind target tissues, resulting in (1) sequestration and destruction of Ig-coated circulating cells; (2) fixation and cleaving of complement proteins; and (3) release of chemotaxins, vasoactive peptides, and destructive enzymes into tissues. Many autoantibodies in persons with SLE are directed against DNA/protein or RNA/protein complexes such as nucleosomes, some nucleolar RNA, and spliceosomal RNA (Table 300-1). During apoptosis these antigens migrate to cell surfaces, where they are enclosed in blebs, and membrane phospholipids change orientation so that antigenic portions are near the surface. Intracellular molecules altered during cell activation or damage migrate to the cell surface. All these antigens near or in cell surfaces probably activate the immune system to produce autoantibodies. In individuals with SLE, phagocytosis and removal of apoptotic cells and of immune complexes are impaired. Thus, in SLE, antigens are available; they are presented in locations recognized by the immune system; and the antigens, autoantibodies, and immune complexes persist for prolonged periods of time, allowing tissue damage to accumulate to the point of clinical illness.

SLE is a multigenic disease. It is likely that alleles of multiple normal genes each contribute a small amount to the abnormal immune responses; if enough variations accumulate, disease results. Some predisposing genes are located in the HLA region (particularly HLA class II DR and DQ genes, and HLA class III genes encoding C'2 and C'4). The relevant HLA DR/DQ genes increase risk for SLE by approximately twofold if one susceptibility haplotype is present and by four- to sixfold if two or more are present. Some proteins important in clearing apoptotic cells play a role in genetic susceptibility; for example, homozygous deficiencies of early components of complement Clq, C'2, and C'4 and certain alleles of mannose-binding ligand increase the risk for SLE. Clq deficiency confers the highest genetic risk known but is rare. There are at least five chromosomal regions independent of HLA that contain susceptibility genes. Within one of these regions on chromosome 1 are alleles encoding Fcγ receptors that bind subsets of IgG (IgG1, -2, or -3): African Americans inheriting one allele of FcγRIIA have a receptor that binds the Ig in immune complexes weakly; those persons have increased risk for lupus nephritis. Caucasians and Asians in some populations with alleles of FcγRIIIA that bind Ig weakly are predisposed to SLE. A region on chromosome 16 contains genes that predispose to SLE, rheumatoid arthritis, psoriasis, and Crohn's disease, suggesting the presence of "autoimmunity genes" that, when interacting with other genes, predispose to different autoimmune diseases. Thus, SLE is modified by multiple susceptibility genes, some of which interact. There are likely to be protective gene alleles as well. These gene combinations influence immune responses to the external and internal environment; when such responses are too high and/or too prolonged, autoimmunity results.

Female gender is permissive for SLE; females of many mammalian species make higher antibody responses than males. Women exposed to estrogen-containing oral contraceptives or hormone replacement have an increased risk of developing SLE (approximately twofold). Estradiol binds to receptors on T and B lymphocytes, increasing activation and survival of those cells, thus favoring prolonged immune responses.

Several environmental stimuli may influence SLE. Exposure to ultraviolet light causes SLE flares in approximately 70% of patients, possibly by increasing apoptosis in keratinocytes and other cells or by altering DNA and intracellular proteins to make them antigenic. It is likely that various infections that stimulate immune responses (antibodies and activated T lymphocytes)

TABLE 300-1	Autoantibodies of SLE		
Antibody	Prevalence, %	Antigen Recognized	Clinical Utility
Antinuclear antibodies	98	Multiple nuclear	Best screening test; repeated negative tests make SLE unlikely
Anti-dsDNA	70	DNA (double-stranded)	High titers are SLE-specific and in some patients correlate with disease activity, nephritis, vasculitis
Anti-Sm	25	Protein complexed to 6 species of nuclear U1 RNA	Specific for SLE; no definite clinical correlations; most patients also have anti-RNP; more common in African Americans and Asians than Caucasians
Anti-RNP	40	Protein complexed to U1 RNAγ	Not specific for SLE; high titers associated with syndromes that have overlap features of several rheumatic syndromes including SLE; more common in African Americans than Caucasians
Anti-Ro (SS-A)	30	Protein complexed to hY RNA, primarily 60 kDa and 52 kDa	Not specific for SLE; associated with sicca syndrome, subacute cutaneous lupus, and neonatal lupus with congenital heart block; associated with decreased risk for nephritis
Anti-La (SS-B)	10	47-kDa protein complexed to hY RNA	Usually associated with anti-Ro; associated with decreased risk for nephritis
Antihistone	70	Histones associated with DNA (in nucleosome, chromatin)	More frequent in drug-induced lupus than in SLE
Antiphospholipid	50	Phospholipids, β_2 glycoprotein 1 cofactor, prothrombin	Three tests available—ELISAs for cardiolipin and B2G1, sensitive prothrombin time (DRVVT); predisposes to clotting, fetal loss, thrombocytopenia
Antierythrocyte	60	Erythrocyte membrane	Measured as direct Coombs' test; a small proportion develop overt hemolysis
Antiplatelet	30	Surface and altered cytoplasmic antigens in platelets	Associated with thrombocytopenia but sensitivity and specificity are not good; this is not a useful clinical test
Antineuronal	60	Neuronal and lymphocyte surface antigens	In some series a positive test in CSF correlate with active CNS lupus
Antiribosomal P	20	Protein in ribosomes	In some series a positive test in serum correlates with depression or psychosis due to CNS lupus

Note: ELISA, enzyme-linked immunosorbent assay; DRVVT, dilute Russell viper venom time; CSF, cerebrospinal fluid; CNS, central nervous system.

that cross-react with self or responses that, as they mature, develop the ability to recognize self can promote autoimmune responses that lead to SLE. The observation that children and adults with SLE are more likely to be infected by Epstein-Barr Virus (EBV) than age-, gender-, and ethnically matched controls without SLE is intriguing, because EBV activates B lymphocytes and also contains amino acid sequences that mimic sequences on human spliceosomes—a common autoantibody specificity in people with SLE. Thus, interplay between genetic susceptibility, gender, and environmental stimuli may result in autoimmunity.

For maximal production of harmful autoantibodies, B cells require help from T cells, and those functions of T and B cells are normally downregulated by several mechanisms. In murine SLE models, many downregulating networks are abnormal, including generation of multiple types of regulatory and natural killer T cells and of humoral idiotypic downregulating networks.

PATHOLOGY In SLE, biopsies of affected skin show deposition of Ig at the dermal-epidermal junction (DEJ), injury to basal keratinocytes, and inflammation dominated by T lymphocytes in the DEJ and around blood vessels and dermal appendages. Clinically unaffected skin may also show Ig deposition at the DEJ. In renal biopsies, the pattern of injury is important in diagnosis and in selecting the best therapy. The World Health Organization (WHO) has classified lupus nephritis as grade I (no histologic changes), II (proliferative changes confined to the mesangium), III (proliferative changes in tufts of 10 to 50% of glomeruli; higher proportions of glomeruli affected suggest worse

prognosis), IV [diffuse proliferative glomerulonephritis (DPGN) affecting >50% of glomeruli], V (predominantly membranous changes with various degrees of proliferation), and VI (end stage, scarred glomeruli). In addition, pathologists report the extent of inflammatory (potentially reversible) and chronic (irreversible scarring in glomeruli, renal tubules, and blood vessels) changes. In general, treatment for lupus nephritis is not recommended in patients with class I or II disease or with extensive irreversible changes. In contrast, aggressive immunosuppression is recommended for patients with class III, IV, or V inflammatory proliferative lesions because the majority of those individuals, if untreated, develop end-stage renal disease (ESRD) within 2 years. In children, a diagnosis of SLE can be established on the basis of renal histology without meeting additional diagnostic criteria (Table 300-2). Histologic abnormalities in blood vessels are not specific for SLE: leukocytoclastic vasculitis is most common (Chap. 306). Lymph node biopsies show nonspecific diffuse chronic inflammation.

DIAGNOSIS The diagnosis of SLE is based on characteristic clinical features and autoantibodies. Criteria for classification are listed in Table 300-2, and an algorithm for diagnosis and initial therapy is shown in Fig. 300-1. The criteria are intended for confirming the diagnosis of SLE in patients included in studies; the author uses them in individual patients for estimating the probability that a disease is SLE. Any combination of 4 or more of 11 criteria, well-documented at any time during a patient's history, makes it likely that the patient has SLE (specificity and sensitivity are ~95% and 75%, respectively). In many

TABLE 300-2   Classification Criteria for the Diagnosis of SLE[a]

Malar rash	Fixed erythema, flat or raised, over the malar eminences
Discoid rash	Erythematous circular raised patches with adherent keratotic scaling and follicular plugging; atrophic scarring may occur
Photosensitivity	Exposure to ultraviolet light causes rash
Oral ulcers	Includes oral and nasopharyngeal ulcers, observed by physician
Arthritis	Nonerosive arthritis of two or more peripheral joints, with tenderness, swelling, or effusion
Serositis	Pleuritis or pericarditis documented by ECG or rub or evidence of effusion
Renal disorder	Proteinuria >0.5 g/d or ≥3+, or cellular casts
Neurologic disorder	Seizures or psychosis without other causes
Hematologic disorder	Hemolytic anemia or leukopenia (<4000/μL) or lymphopenia (<1500/μL) or thrombocytopenia (<100,000/μL) in the absence of offending drugs
Immunologic disorder	Anti-dsDNA, anti-Sm, and/or anti-phospholipid
Antinuclear antibodies	An abnormal titer of ANA by immunofluorescence or an equivalent assay at any point in time in the absence of drugs known to induce ANAs

[a] If ≥4 of these criteria, well documented, are present at any time in a patient's history, the diagnosis is likely to be SLE. Specificity is ~95%: sensitivity is ~75%.
Note: ECG, electrocardiography; dsDNA, double-stranded DNA; ANA, antinuclear antibodies.
Source: Criteria published by EM Tan et al: Arthritis Rheum 25:1271, 1982; updated by MC Hochberg, Arthritis Rheum 40:1725, 1997.

patients, additional criteria accrue over time. Antinuclear antibodies (ANA) are positive in >95% of patients during the course of disease; repeated negative tests suggest that the diagnosis is not SLE. High-titer IgG antibodies to double-stranded DNA and antibodies to the Sm antigen are both specific for SLE and, therefore, favor the diagnosis in the presence of compatible clinical manifestations. The presence in an individual of multiple autoantibodies without clinical symptoms should not be considered diagnostic for SLE, although such persons are at increased risk.

INTERPRETATION OF CLINICAL MANIFESTATIONS   When a diagnosis of SLE is made, it is important to establish the severity and potential reversibility of the illness and estimate the possible consequences of various therapeutic interventions. In the following paragraphs, descriptions of some disease manifestations begin with relatively mild problems and progress to those more life-threatening.

Overview and Systemic Manifestations   At its onset, SLE may involve one or several organ systems; over time, additional manifestations of disease may occur (Table 300-3). Most of the autoantibodies characteristic of each person are present at the time clinical manifestations appear (Tables 300-1 and 300-2). Severity of SLE varies from mild and intermittent to severe and fulminant. Most patients experience exacerbations interspersed with periods of relative quiescence; however, permanent complete remissions (absence of symptoms with no treatment) are rare. Systemic symptoms, particularly fatigue and myalgias/arthralgias, are present most of the time. Severe systemic illness requiring glucocorticoid therapy can occur with fever, prostration, weight loss, and anemia in addition to any other organ-targeted manifestations.

Musculoskeletal Manifestations   Most people with SLE have intermittent polyarthritis, varying from mild to disabling, characterized by soft tissue swelling and tenderness in joints, most commonly in hands, wrists, and knees. Presence of visible synovitis suggests active systemic disease. Joint deformities (hands and feet) develop in only 10%. Erosions on joint x-rays are rare; their presence suggests a non-lupus inflammatory arthropathy such as rheumatoid arthritis (Chap. 301). If pain persists in a single joint, such as knee, shoulder, or hip, a diagnosis of ischemic necrosis of bone should be considered, particularly if there are no other manifestations of active SLE. The prevalence of ischemic necrosis of bone is increased in SLE, especially in patients treated with systemic glucocorticoids. Myositis with clinical muscle weakness, elevated creatine kinase levels, and biopsy evidence of muscle necrosis and inflammation can occur, although most patients have myalgias without frank myositis. Glucocorticoid and, rarely, antimalarial therapies can also cause muscle weakness; these adverse effects must be distinguished from active disease.

Cutaneous Manifestations   Lupus dermatitis can be classified as discoid lupus erythematosus (DLE), systemic rash, subacute cutaneous lupus erythematosus (SCLE), or "other." Discoid lesions are roughly circular with slightly raised, scaly hyperpigmented erythematous rims and depigmented, atrophic centers in which all dermal appendages are permanently destroyed. Lesions can be disfiguring, partic-

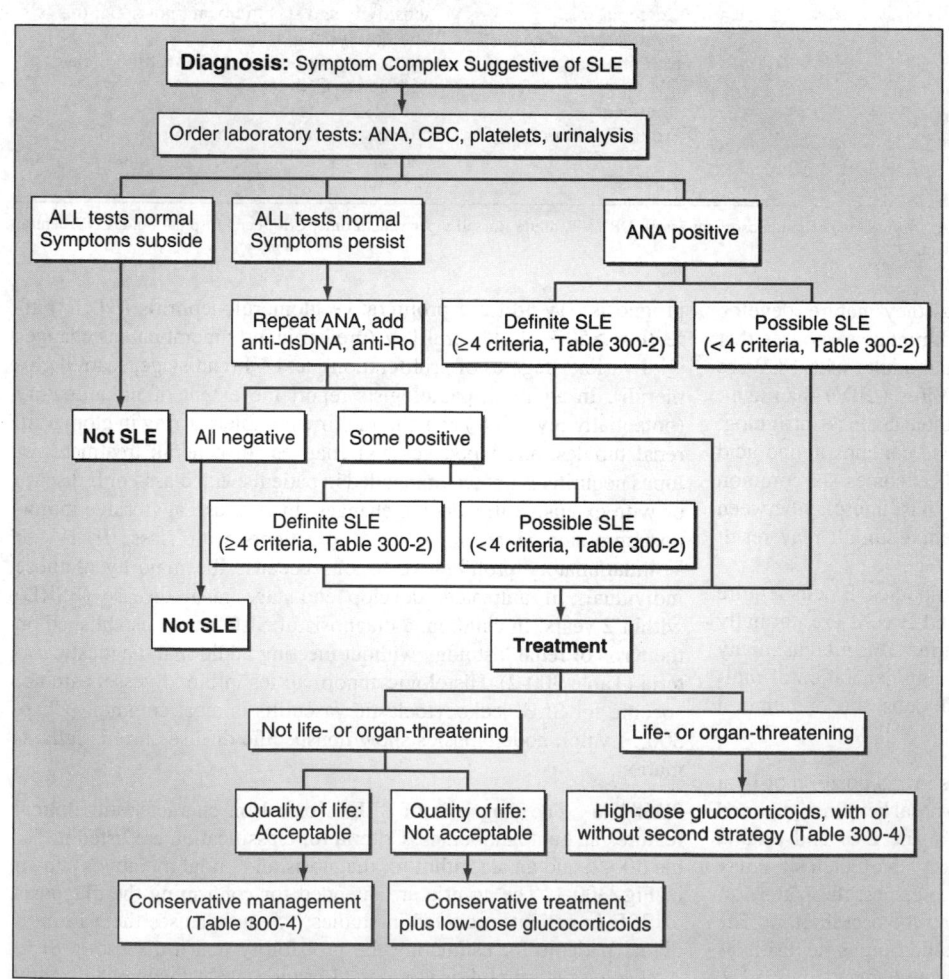

FIGURE 300-1 Algorithm for diagnosis and initial therapy of SLE. ANA, antinuclear antibodies; CBC, complete blood count.

TABLE 300-3 *Clinical Manifestations of SLE and Prevalence over the Entire Course of Disease*[a]

Systemic: Fatigue, malaise, fever, anorexia, weight loss	95
Musculoskeletal	95
Arthralgias/myalgias	95
Nonerosive polyarthritis	60
Hand deformities	10
Myopathy/myositis	25/5
Ischemic necrosis of bone	15
Cutaneous	80
Photosensitivity	70
Malar rash	50
Oral ulcers	40
Alopecia	40
Discoid rash	20
Vasculitis rash	20
Other (e.g., urticaria, subacute cutaneous lupus)	15
Hematologic	85
Anemia (chronic disease)	70
Leukopenia (<4000/μL)	65
Lymphopenia (<1500/μL)	50
Thrombocytopenia (<100,000/μL)	15
Lymphadenopathy	15
Splenomegaly	15
Hemolytic anemia	10
Neurologic	60
Cognitive disorder	50
Mood disorder	40
Headache	25
Seizures	20
Mono-, polyneuropathy	15
Stroke, TIA	10
Acute confusional state or movement disorder	2–5
Aseptic meningitis, myelopathy	<1
Cardiopulmonary	60
Pleurisy, pericarditis, effusions	30–50
Myocarditis, endocarditis	10
Lupus pneumonitis	10
Coronary artery disease	10
Interstitial fibrosis	5
Pulmonary hypertension, ARDS, hemorrhage	<5
Renal	30–50
Proteinuria >500 mg/24 h, cellular casts	30–50
Nephrotic syndrome	25
End-stage renal disease	5–10
Gastrointestinal	40
Nonspecific (nausea, mild pain, diarrhea)	30
Abnormal liver enzymes	40
Vasculitis	5
Thrombosis	15
Venous	10
Arterial	5
Ocular	15
Sicca syndrome	15
Conjunctivitis, episcleritis	10
Vasculitis	5

[a] Numbers indicate percent of patients who have the manifestation sometime during the course of illness.

Note: TIA, transient ischemic attack; ARDS, acute respiratory distress syndrome.

ularly on the face and scalp. Treatment consists primarily of local glucocorticoids and systemic antimalarials. Only 5% of people with DLE have SLE (although half have positive ANA); however, among people with SLE, as many as 20% have DLE. The most common SLE rash is a photosensitive, slightly raised erythema, occasionally scaly, on the face (particularly the cheeks and nose—the "butterfly" rash), ears, chin, V region of the neck, upper back, and extensor surfaces of the arms. Worsening of this rash often accompanies flare of systemic disease. SCLE consists of scaly red patches similar to psoriasis or attacks of circular red-rimmed lesions. Patients with these manifestations are exquisitely photosensitive; most have antibodies to Ro (SS-A). Many other rashes are seen less frequently in SLE, including recurring urticaria, lichen planus–like dermatitis, bullae, and panniculitis ("lupus profundus"). Rashes of SLE can be minor or very severe;

they may be the major disease manifestation. Small, painful ulcerations on the oral or nasal mucosa are common in SLE: the lesions resemble aphthous ulcers and usually indicate systemic disease activity.

Renal Manifestations Nephritis is usually the most serious manifestation of SLE, particularly since nephritis and infection are the leading causes of mortality in the first decade of disease. Since nephritis is asymptomatic in most lupus patients, urinalysis should be ordered in any person suspected of having SLE. The classification of lupus nephritis is primarily histologic (see "Pathology," above). Renal biopsy is useful in planning current and near-future therapies. Patients with dangerous proliferative forms of glomerular damage usually have microscopic hematuria and proteinuria (>500 mg per 24 h); approximately one-half develop nephrotic syndrome, and most develop hypertension. If DPGN is untreated, virtually all patients develop ESRD within 2 years of diagnosis. Therefore, aggressive immunosuppression is indicated (usually systemic glucocorticoids plus a cytotoxic drug), unless damage is irreversible. African-American individuals are more likely to develop ESRD than are Caucasians, even with the most current therapies. Overall in the United States, ~20% of individuals with DPGN die or develop ESRD within 10 years of diagnosis. Such individuals require aggressive control of SLE and of the complications of renal disease and of therapy. A small proportion of SLE patients with proteinuria (usually nephrotic) have membranous glomerular changes without proliferation on renal biopsy. Their outcome is better than for those with DPGN, but proteinuria is less likely to improve on lupus nephritis immunosuppressive therapies. Lupus nephritis tends to be an ongoing disease, with flares requiring re-treatment over many years. For most people with lupus nephritis, accelerated atherosclerosis becomes important after several years of disease; attention must be given to control of blood pressure, hyperlipidemia, and hyperglycemia.

Nervous System Manifestations There are many central nervous system (CNS) and peripheral nervous system manifestations of SLE; in some patients these are the major cause of morbidity and mortality. It is useful to approach this diagnostically by asking first whether the symptoms result from SLE or another condition (such as infection in immunosuppressed individuals). If symptoms are related to SLE, it should be determined whether they are caused by a diffuse process or vascular occlusive disease. The most common manifestation of diffuse CNS lupus is cognitive dysfunction, particularly difficulties with memory and reasoning. Headaches are also common; when excruciating, they often indicate SLE flare; when milder, they are difficult to distinguish from migraine or tension headaches. Seizures of any type may be caused by lupus; treatment often requires both anti-seizure and immunosuppressive therapies. Psychosis can be the dominant manifestation of SLE; it must be distinguished from glucocorticoid-induced psychosis. The latter usually occurs in the first weeks of glucocorticoid therapy, at doses of ≥40 mg of prednisone or equivalent; psychosis resolves over several days after glucocorticoids are decreased or stopped. Myelopathy is not rare and is often disabling; high-dose glucocorticoid therapy is recommended and should be started within hours or a few days of the onset of symptoms.

Vascular Occlusions The prevalence of transient ischemic attacks, strokes, and myocardial infarctions is increased in patients with SLE. These vascular events are increased in, but not exclusive to, SLE patients with antibodies to phospholipids (aPL). Ischemia in the brain can be caused by focal occlusion (either noninflammatory or associated with vasculitis) or by embolization from carotid artery plaque or from fibrinous vegetations of Libman-Sachs endocarditis. Appropriate tests for aPL (see below) and for sources of emboli should be ordered in such patients to estimate the need for, intensity of, and duration of anti-inflammatory and/or anticoagulant therapies. In SLE, myocardial infarctions are primarily manifestations of accelerated atherosclerosis. The increased risk for vascular events is as much as 50-fold in women with SLE <45 years old compared to healthy women. Characteristics associated with increased risk for atherosclerosis include older age, hypertension, dyslipidemia, aPL, repeated high scores for disease activity, and high cumulative doses of glucocorticoids. When it is most likely that an event results from clotting, long-term anticoagulation is the therapy of choice. Two processes can occur at once—vasculitis plus bland vascular occlusions—in which case it is appropriate to treat with anticoagulation plus immunosuppression.

Pulmonary Manifestations The most common pulmonary manifestation of SLE is pleuritis with or without pleural effusion. This manifestation, when mild, may respond to treatment with nonsteroidal anti-inflammatory drugs (NSAIDs); when more severe, patients require a brief course of glucocorticoid therapy. Pulmonary infiltrates also occur as a manifestation of active SLE and are difficult to distinguish from infection on imaging studies. Life-threatening pulmonary manifestations include interstitial inflammation, leading to fibrosis, and intraalveolar hemorrhage; both of these probably require aggressive immunosuppressive and supportive treatments early after their onset.

Cardiac Manifestations Pericarditis is the most frequent cardiac manifestation; it usually responds to anti-inflammatory therapy and infrequently leads to tamponade. More serious cardiac manifestations are myocarditis and fibrinous endocarditis of Libman-Sachs. The endocardial involvement can lead to valvular insufficiencies, most commonly of the mitral or aortic valves, or to embolic events. It has not been proved that glucocorticoid or other immunosuppressive therapies lead to improvement of lupus myocarditis or endocarditis, but it is usual practice to administer a trial of high-dose steroids along with appropriate supportive therapy for heart failure, arrhythmia, or embolic events. As discussed above, patients with SLE are at increased risk for myocardial infarction, usually due to accelerated atherosclerosis.

Hematologic Manifestations The most frequent hematologic manifestation of SLE is anemia, usually normochromic normocytic, reflecting chronic illness. Hemolysis can be rapid in onset and severe, requiring high-dose glucocorticoid therapy, which is effective in most patients. Leukopenia is also common and almost always consists of lymphopenia, not granulocytopenia; this rarely predisposes to infections and by itself usually does not require therapy. Thrombocytopenia may be a recurring problem. If platelet counts are $>40,000/\mu L$ and abnormal bleeding is absent, therapy may not be required. High-dose glucocorticoid therapy (e.g., 1 mg/kg per day of prednisone or equivalent) is usually effective for the first few episodes of severe thrombocytopenia. Recurring or prolonged hemolytic anemia or thrombocytopenia, or disease requiring an unacceptably high dose of daily glucocorticoids, should be treated with an additional strategy (see "Treatment," below).

Gastrointestinal Manifestations Nausea, sometimes with vomiting, and diarrhea can be manifestations of an SLE flare, as can diffuse abdominal pain caused by autoimmune peritonitis. Increases in serum AST and ALT are common when SLE is active. These manifestations usually improve promptly during systemic glucocorticoid therapy. Vasculitis involving the intestine may be life-threatening; perforations, ischemia, bleeding, and sepsis are frequent complications. Aggressive immunosuppressive therapy with high-dose glucocorticoids is recommended for short-term control; evidence of recurrence is an indication for additional therapies.

Ocular Manifestations Sicca syndrome (Sjögren's syndrome; Chap. 304) and nonspecific conjunctivitis are common in SLE and rarely threaten vision. In contrast, retinal vasculitis and optic neuritis are serious manifestations: blindness can develop over days to weeks. Aggressive immunosuppression is recommended, although there are no controlled trials to prove effectiveness. Complications of glucocorticoid therapy include cataracts (common) and glaucoma.

LABORATORY TESTS Laboratory tests serve (1) to establish or rule out the diagnosis; (2) to follow the course of disease, particularly to suggest that a flare is occurring or organ damage is developing; and (3) to identify adverse effects of therapies.

Tests for Autoantibodies (See Tables 300-1 and 300-2) Diagnostically, the most important autoantibodies to detect are ANA since the test is positive in >95% of patients, usually at the onset of symptoms. A few patients develop ANA within 1 year of symptom onset; repeated testing may then be useful. ANA-negative lupus exists but is very rare in adults and is usually associated with other autoantibodies (anti-Ro or anti-DNA). High-titer IgG antibodies to double-stranded DNA (dsDNA) (but not to single-stranded DNA) are specific for SLE. There is no international standardized test for ANA; variability between different service laboratories is high. Enzyme-linked immunosorbent assays (ELISA) and immunofluorescent reactions of sera with the dsDNA in the flagellate *Crithidia lucilliae* have ~60% sensitivity for SLE; identification of high-avidity anti-dsDNA in the Farr assay is not as sensitive but may correlate better with risk for nephritis. Titers of anti-dsDNA vary over time. In some patients, increase in quantities of anti-dsDNA herald a flare, particularly of nephritis or vasculitis. Antibodies to Sm are also specific for SLE and assist in diagnosis; anti-Sm antibodies do not usually correlate with disease activity or clinical manifestations. aPL are not specific for SLE, but their presence fulfills one classification criterion and they identify patients at increased risk for venous or arterial clotting, thrombocytopenia, and fetal loss. There are two widely accepted tests that measure different antibodies (anticardiolipin and the lupus anticoagulant): (1) ELISA for anticardiolipin (internationally standardized with good reproducibility) and (2) a sensitive phospholipid-based activated prothrombin time such as the dilute Russell venom viper test. Some centers also recommend measurement of antibodies to β_2 glycoprotein 1, a serum protein cofactor that is the target of most antibodies to cardiolipin and some lupus anticoagulants. High titers of IgG anticardiolipin (>50 IU) indicate high risk for a clinical episode of clotting. Quantities of aPL may vary markedly over time; repeated testing is justified if clinical manifestations of the antiphospholipid antibody syndrome (APS) appear. To make a diagnosis of APS, with or without SLE, requires the presence of clotting and/or repeated fetal losses plus at least two positive tests for aPL, at least 6 weeks apart.

An additional autoantibody test with predictive value (not used for diagnosis) detects anti-Ro, which indicates increased risk for neonatal lupus, sicca syndrome, and SCLE. Women with child-bearing potential and SLE should be screened for aPL and anti-Ro.

Standard Tests for Diagnosis Screening tests for complete blood count, platelet count, and urinalysis may detect abnormalities that contribute to the diagnosis and influence management decisions.

Tests for Following Disease Course It is useful to follow tests that indicate the status of organ involvement known to be present during SLE flares. These might include hemoglobin levels, platelet counts, urinalysis, and serum levels of creatinine or albumin. There is great interest in identification of additional markers of disease activity. Candidates include levels of anti-DNA antibodies, several components of complement (C'3 is most widely available), activated complement products, soluble interleukin (IL) 2, and urinary monocyte chemotactic protein 1. None are uniformly agreed upon as reliable indicators of response or flare. The physician should determine for each patient whether certain laboratory test changes predict flare. If so, altering therapy in response to these changes is acceptable to prevent flares. In addition, given the increased prevalence of atherosclerosis in SLE, it is advisable to follow the recommendations of the National Cholesterol Education Program for testing.

℞ TREATMENT

There is no cure for SLE, and complete sustained remissions are rare. Therefore, the physician should plan to control acute, severe flares then develop maintenance strategies that suppress symptoms to an acceptable level and prevent organ damage. Usually patients will endure some adverse effects of medications. Therapeutic choices depend on: (1) whether disease manifestations are life-threatening or likely to cause organ damage, justifying aggressive therapies; (2) whether manifestations are potentially reversible; and (3) the best approaches to preventing complications of disease and its treatments. Therapies, doses, and adverse effects are listed in (Table 300-4).

Conservative Therapies for Management of Non-Life-Threatening Disease Among patients with fatigue, pain, and autoantibodies of SLE, but without major organ involvement, management can be directed to suppression of symptoms. Analgesics and antimalarials are mainstays. NSAIDs are useful analgesics/anti-inflammatories, particularly for arthritis/arthralgias; however, SLE patients compared to the general population are at increased risk for NSAID-induced aseptic meningitis, elevated serum transaminases, hypertension, and renal dysfunction. Cyclooxygenase-2 specific inhibitors, compared to nonspecific

TABLE 300-4 *Medications for the Management of SLE*

Medication	Dose Range	Drug Interactions	Serious or Common Adverse Effects
NSAIDs, salicylates (Ecotrin[a] and St. Joseph's aspirin[a] approved by FDA for use in SLE)	Doses toward upper limit of recommended range usually required	A2R/ACE inhibitors, glucocorticoids, fluconazole, methotrexate, thiazides	NSAIDs: Higher incidence of aseptic meningitis, transaminitis, decreased renal function, vasculitis of skin; Salicylates: ototoxicity, tinnitus; Both: GI events and symptoms, allergic reactions, dermatitis, dizziness, acute renal failure, edema, hypertension
Topical glucocorticoids	Mid-potency for face; mid to high potency other areas	None known	Atrophy of skin, contact dermatitis, folliculitis, hypopigmentation, infection
Topical sunscreens	SPF 15 at least; 30+ preferred	None known	Contact dermatitis
Hydroxychloroquine[a] (quinacrine can be added or substituted)	200–400 mg qd (100 mg qd)	None known	Retinal damage, agranulocytosis, aplastic anemia, ataxia, cardiomyopathy, dizziness, myopathy, ototoxicity, peripheral neuropathy, pigmentation of skin, seizures, thrombocytopenia; Quinacrine usually causes diffuse yellow skin coloration
DHEA (dehydroepiandrosterone)	200 mg qd	Unclear	Acne, menstrual irregularities, high serum levels of testosterone
Methotrexate (for dermatitis, arthritis)	10–25 mg once a week, with folic acid; decrease dose if CrCl < 60 mL/min	Acitretin, leflunomide, NSAIDs and salicylates, penicillins, probenecid, sulfonamides, trimethoprim	Anemia, bone marrow suppression, leukopenia, thrombocytopenia, hepatotoxicity, nephrotoxicity, infections, neurotoxicity, pulmonary fibrosis, pneumonitis, severe dermatitis, seizures
Glucocorticoids, oral[a] (several specific brands are approved by FDA for use in SLE)	Prednisone, prednisolone: 0.5–1 mg/kg per day for severe SLE; 0.07–0.3 mg/kg per day or qod for milder disease	A2R/ACE antagonists, antiarrhythmics class III, β_2 cyclosporine, NSAIDs and salicylates, phenothiazines, phenytoins, quinolones, rifampin, risperidone, thiazides, sulfonylureas, warfarin	Infection, VZV infection, hypertension, hyperglycemia, hypokalemia, acne, allergic reactions, anxiety, aseptic necrosis of bone, Cushingoid changes, CHF, fragile skin, insomnia, menstrual irregularities, mood swings, osteoporosis, psychosis
Methylprednisolone sodium succinate, intravenous[a] (approved for lupus nephritis)	For severe disease, 1 g IV qd × 3 days	As for oral glucocorticoids	As for oral glucocorticoids (if used repeatedly); anaphylaxis
Cyclophosphamide[b] Intravenous	7–25 mg/kg q month × 6; consider mesna administration with dose	Allopurinol, bone marrow suppressants, colony-stimulating factors, doxorubicin, rituximab, succinylcholine, zidovudine	Infection, VZV infection, bone marrow suppression, leukopenia, anemia, thrombocytopenia, hemorrhagic cystitis (less with IV), carcinoma of the bladder, alopecia, nausea, diarrhea, malaise, malignancy, sterility
Oral	1.5–3 mg/kg per day; Decrease dose for CrCl < 25 mL/min		
Mycophenolate mofetil[b] (approved for lupus nephritis)	2–3 g/d PO	Acyclovir, antacids, azathioprine, bile acid–binding resins, ganciclovir, iron salts, probenecid, oral contraceptives	Infection, leukopenia, anemia, thrombocytopenia, lymphoma, lymphoproliferative disorders, malignancy; Alopecia, cough, diarrhea, fever, GI symptoms, headache, hypertension, hypercholesterolemia, hypokalemia, insomnia peripheral edema, transaminitis, tremor, rash
Azathioprine[b]	2–3 mg/kg per day PO; decrease frequency of dose if CrCl < 50 mL/min	ACE inhibitors, allopurinol, bone marrow suppressants, interferons, mycophenolate mofetil, rituximab, warfarin, zidovudine	Infection, VZV infection, bone marrow suppression, leukopenia, anemia, thrombocytopenia, pancreatitis, hepatotoxicity, malignancy, alopecia, fever, flulike illness, GI symptoms

[a] Indicates medication is approved for use in SLE by the U.S. Food and Drug Administration.
[b] Indicates the medication has been used with glucocorticoids in the trials showing efficacy.

Note: NSAIDs, nonsteroidal anti-inflammatory drugs; FDA, U.S. Food and Drug Administration; A2R, angiotensin 2 receptor; ACE, angiotensin-converting enzyme; GI, gastrointestinal; SPF, sun protection factor; CrCl, creatinine clearance; VZV, varicella-zoster virus; CHF, congestive heart failure.

NSAIDs, are no safer in this regard, although they may cause fewer adverse gastrointestinal events (studies are not available in SLE). Antimalarials (hydroxychloroquine, chloroquine, and quinacrine) often reduce dermatitis, arthritis, and fatigue; a randomized placebo-controlled prospective trial has shown that hydroxychloroquine reduces the number of disease flares. Because of potential retinal toxicity, patients receiving antimalarials should undergo opthalmologic examinations at least annually. A recent placebo-controlled prospective trial suggests that administration of dehydroepiandrosterone may reduce disease activity. If quality of life is inadequate in spite of these conservative measures, treatment with low doses of systemic glucocorticoids may be necessary.

Life-Threatening SLE: Proliferative Forms of Lupus Nephritis

The mainstay of treatment for any inflammatory life-threatening or organ-threatening manifestations of SLE is systemic glucocorticoids (0.5 to 2 mg/kg per day orally or 1000 mg of methylprednisolone sodium succinate intravenously daily for 3 days followed by 0.5–1 mg/kg of daily prednisone or equivalent). Evidence that glucocorticoid therapy is life-saving comes from retrospective studies from the predialysis era; survival is significantly better in people with DPGN treated with high-dose daily glucocorticoids (40 to 60 mg of prednisone daily for 4 to 6 months) versus lower doses. Currently, high doses are recommended for much shorter periods; recent trials of interventions for severe SLE employ 4 to 6 weeks of these doses. Thereafter, doses are tapered as rapidly as the clinical situation permits, usually to a maintenance dose varying from 5 to 10 mg of prednisone, prednisolone, or equivalent per day or 10 to 20 mg every other day. Most patients with an episode of severe lupus require many years of maintenance therapy with low-dose glucocorticoids, which can be increased to prevent or treat disease flares. However, frequent attempts to gradually reduce the glucocorticoid requirement are recommended because virtually everyone develops important adverse effects (Table 300-4). Prospective controlled trials in active lupus nephritis show that administration of high doses of glucocorticoids (1000 mg of methylprednisolone daily for 3 days) by intravenous routes compared to daily oral routes shortens the time to maximal improvement by a few weeks but does not result ultimately in better renal function. It has become standard practice to initiate therapy for active, potentially life-threatening SLE with high-dose intravenous glucocorticoid pulses, based on studies in lupus nephritis. This approach must be tempered by safety considerations, such as the presence of conditions adversely affected by glucocorticoids (infection, hyperglycemia, hypertension, osteoporosis, etc).

Cytotoxic drugs are another important class of drugs used to treat serious SLE. Almost all prospective controlled trials in SLE involving cytotoxic agents have been conducted in patients with lupus nephritis. The alkylating agent cyclophosphamide has become the standard drug used for controlling life-threatening active lupus nephritis, particularly in patients whose renal biopsies show WHO grades III, IV, and V proliferative or membranoproliferative forms of nephritis. All successful studies with cyclophosphamide have also used concomitant glucocorticoid therapy; cyclophosphamide responses begin 3 to 16 weeks after treatment is initiated, whereas glucocorticoid responses may begin within 24 h. Cyclophosphamide should be administered to patients whose severe lupus is likely to be reversible (Table 300-4); those with high serum creatinine levels [e.g., $\geq$265 μmol/L $\geq$3.0 mg/dL)] of many months duration and high chronicity scores on renal biopsy are not likely to respond. Prospective studies suggest that ESRD is significantly less frequent in patients treated with cyclophosphamide (intermittent intravenous or daily oral) compared to patients treated with glucocorticoids alone or azathioprine plus glucocorticoids. This benefit becomes measurable 5 years or more following initiation of therapy. Short-term results of any intervention (e.g., 1 to 2 years) are useful but may not adequately describe the overall utility of that approach. The recommended duration of cyclophosphamide therapy

is controversial; one prospective controlled trial (from the U.S. National Institutes of Health) comparing 6 months of intermittent intravenous treatment (monthly doses) to 30 months of treatment (6 monthly doses followed by quarterly doses) showed fewer disease flares in the 30-month group. However, a recent prospective controlled trial suggests that similar good improvement occurs if 6 monthly doses of intravenous cyclophosphamide (500 mg/m^2) plus 2 quarterly doses are followed by daily azathioprine for 2 years; equally effective was intravenous cyclophosphamide, 500 mg total, every 2 weeks for six doses, followed by daily azathioprine. Approximately 90% of this group were Caucasian. Response of lupus nephritis to cyclophosphamide and glucocorticoids is better in Caucasian groups than in African Americans. Therefore, interpretation of studies using different therapeutic approaches must include considerations of ethnicity as well as duration of follow-up and differences in inclusion and exclusion criteria for entry. The adverse effects most likely to influence patient choice against the use of cyclophosphamide are a high rate of irreversible ovarian or testicular failure with increasing cumulative doses, nausea and malaise that often accompany each intravenous dose, alopecia, and frequent infections.

Since glucocorticoid-plus-cyclophosphamide therapy has many adverse effects and is often disliked by patients, there has been a search for other cytotoxic agents and for different approaches that are less toxic. Azathioprine (a purine antagonist) added to glucocorticoids probably reduces the number of SLE flares and the maintenance glucocorticoid requirement; however, this approach requires several months to be effective, and cyclophosphamide is effective in a higher proportion of patients. Daily oral azathioprine may have fewer adverse effects than daily oral cyclophosphamide; intermittent intravenous cyclophosphamide probably has fewer adverse effects than daily oral cyclophosphamide. Mycophenolate mofetil (a relatively lymphocyte-specific inhibitor of inosine monophosphate dehydrogenase) is an effective cytotoxic agent in some patients with severe SLE. A recent prospective study in Chinese patients with lupus nephritis comparing daily oral mycophenolate plus prednisolone for 12 months to daily oral cyclophosphamide plus prednisolone for 6 months followed by oral daily azathioprine plus prednisolone showed good improvement in ~80% of patients in both groups at 1 year of follow-up and fewer adverse effects with mycophenolate. Chlorambucil is an alkylating agent that can be substituted for cyclophosphamide; the risk of irreversible bone marrow suppression may be greater with this agent. Methotrexate (a folinic acid antagonist) may have a role in the treatment of arthritis and dermatitis but probably not in life-threatening disease. The role of leflunomide, a relatively lymphocyte-specific pyrimidine antagonist, is being studied in patients with SLE. Cyclosporine, which inhibits production of IL-2 and inhibits T lymphocyte functions, has not been studied in prospective controlled trials in SLE but is nonetheless used by some clinicians. Since it has potential nephrotoxicity, but no bone marrow toxicity, the author uses it (in doses of 3 to 5 mg/kg per day orally) in patients with steroid-resistant cytopenias of SLE or in steroid-resistant patients who have developed bone marrow suppression from standard cytotoxic agents.

Special Conditions in SLE that May Require Additional or Different Therapies

■ *PREGNANCY AND LUPUS* Fertility rates for men and women with SLE are probably normal. However, rate of fetal loss is increased (approximately two- to threefold) in women with SLE. Fetal demise is higher in mothers with high disease activity, antiphospholipid antibodies, and/or nephritis. Suppression of disease activity can be achieved by administration of systemic glucocorticoids. A placental enzyme 11-β-dehydrogenase 2 deactivates glucocorticoids; it is more effective in deactivating prednisone and prednisolone than the fluorinated glucocorticoids dexamethasone and betamethasone. Therefore, maternal SLE should be controlled with prednisone/prednisolone at the lowest effective doses for the shortest time required. Adverse effects of prenatal glucocorticoid exposure (primarily betamethasone) on offspring may include low birth weight, developmental abnormalities in the

CNS, and predilection toward adult metabolic syndrome. In SLE patients with aPL (on at least two occasions) and prior fetal losses, treatment with heparin (standard or low-molecular-weight) plus low-dose aspirin has been shown in prospective controlled trials to increase significantly the proportion of live births. An additional potential problem for the fetus is the presence of antibodies to Ro, sometimes associated with neonatal lupus (rash and congenital heart block). The latter can be life-threatening; therefore the presence of anti-Ro requires vigilant monitoring of fetal heart rates with prompt intervention if distress occurs. Women with SLE usually tolerate pregnancy without disease flares. However, a small proportion develop severe flares requiring aggressive glucocorticoid therapy or early delivery. Poor maternal outcomes are highest in women with active nephritis or irreversible organ damage in kidneys, brain, or heart.

LUPUS AND APS Patients with SLE who have venous or arterial clotting, and/or repeated fetal losses, and at least two positive tests for aPL have APS and should be managed with long-term anticoagulation. A target INR of 3.0 is recommended, based on reduction of new clotting events in patients treated to this target INR compared to patients treated to lower INR levels, in retrospective analyses of cohorts with primary or secondary APS.

MICROVASCULAR THROMBOTIC CRISIS (THROMBOTIC THROMBOCYTOPENIC PURPURA, HEMOLYTIC UREMIC SYNDROME) This syndrome of hemolysis, thrombocytopenia, and microvascular thrombosis in kidneys, brain, and other tissues carries a high mortality rate and occurs most commonly in young individuals with lupus nephritis. The most useful laboratory tests are identification of schistocytes on peripheral blood smears and elevated serum levels of lactate dehydrogenase. Plasma exchange or extensive plasmapheresis is usually life-saving; there is no evidence that glucocorticoids or cytotoxic drugs are effective.

LUPUS DERMATITIS Patients with any form of lupus dermatitis should minimize exposure to ultraviolet light, employing appropriate clothing and sunscreens with a sun protection factor of at least 15. Topical glucocorticoids and antimalarials (such as hydroxychloroquine) are effective in reducing lesion severity in most patients and are relatively safe. Systemic treatment with retinoic acid is a useful strategy in patients with inadequate improvement on topical glucocorticoids and antimalarials; adverse effects are potentially severe (particularly fetal abnormalities). Extensive, pruritic, bullous, or ulcerating dermatitides usually improve promptly after institution of systemic glucocorticoids; tapering may be accompanied by flare of lesions, thus necessitating use of a second medication such as hydroxychloroquine, retinoids, or cytotoxic medications such as methotrexate or azathioprine. In therapy-resistant lupus dermatitis there are reports of success with topical tacrolimus or with systemic dapsone or thalidomide (the extreme danger of fetal deformities from thalidomide requires permission from and supervision by the supplier).

Preventive Therapies Prevention of complications of SLE and its therapy include providing appropriate vaccinations (the administration of influenza and pneumococcal vaccines has been studied in patients with SLE; flare rates are similar to those receiving placebo) and suppressing recurrent urinary tract infections. In addition, strategies to prevent osteoporosis should be initiated in most patients likely to require long-term glucocorticoid therapy and/or with other predisposing factors. Control of hypertension and appropriate prevention strategies for atherosclerosis, including monitoring and treatment of dyslipidemias, management of hyperglycemia, and obesity, are recommended.

Experimental Therapies Several new biologics and selective cytotoxic medications are in various phases of clinical trials in the United States. Most strategies target T or B lymphocytes, particularly those under-

going activation, rather than entire cell populations. These include LJP394 (may tolerize B cells making anti-DNA), antibodies to CD40L and CTLA4-Ig fusion protein (interrupt T/B second signals), antibody to complement C'5, and antibody to CD20 (depletes some B cells). Several studies have employed transplantation of hematopoietic stem cells for the treatment of severe and refractory SLE.

PATIENT OUTCOMES, PROGNOSIS, AND SURVIVAL Survival in patients with SLE is 90 to 95% at 2 years, 82 to 90% at 5 years, 71 to 80% at 10 years, and 63 to 75% at 20 years. Poor prognosis (approximately 50% mortality in 10 years) is associated with (at the time of diagnosis) high serum creatinine levels [>124 μmol/L (>1.4 mg/dL)], hypertension, nephrotic syndrome (24-h urine protein excretion >2.6 g), anemia [hemoglobin <124 g/L (<12.4 g/dL)], hypoalbuminemia, hypocomplementemia, and aPL. Prognosis is worse in African Americans than in Caucasians. Patients who require renal transplantation have a relatively high incidence of graft rejection (approximately twice that of patients with other causes of ESRD), but overall patient survival is comparable (85% at 2 years). Lupus nephritis occurs in 10% of transplanted kidneys. Disability in patients with SLE is common due primarily to chronic renal disease, fatigue, arthritis, and pain. As many as 25% of patients may experience remissions, sometimes for a few years, but these are rarely permanent. The leading causes of death in the first decade of disease are systemic disease activity, renal failure, and infections; subsequently, thromboembolic events become increasingly frequent causes of mortality.

DRUG-INDUCED LUPUS This is a syndrome of positive ANA associated with symptoms such as fever, malaise, arthritis or intense arthralgias/myalgias, serositis, and/or rash. The syndrome appears during therapy with certain medications and biologic agents, is predominant in Caucasians, has less female predilection than SLE, rarely involves kidneys or brain, is rarely associated with anti-dsDNA, is commonly associated with antibodies to histones, and usually resolves over several weeks after discontinuation of the offending medication. The list of substances that can induce lupus-like disease is long. Among the most frequent are the anti-arrhythmics procaineamide, disopyramide, propafenone; the antihypertensives hydralazine, several angiotensin-converting enzyme inhibitors and beta-blockers; the antithyroid propylthiouracil; the antipsychotics chlorpromazine and lithium; the anticonvulsants carbamazepine and phenytoin; the antibiotics isoniazid, minocycline, and macrodantin; the antirheumatic sulfasalazine; the diuretic hydrochlorothiazide; the antihyperlipidemics lovastatin and simvastatin; and the biologics interferons and tumor necrosis factor inhibitors. ANA usually appears before symptoms; however, many of the medications mentioned above induce ANA in patients who never develop symptoms of drug-induced lupus. It is appropriate to test for ANA at the first hint of relevant symptoms and to use test results to help decide whether to withdraw the suspect agent.

FURTHER READING

DAVIDSON A, DIAMOND B: Autoimmune diseases. N Engl J Med 354:340, 2001

GAFFNEY PM et al: Recent advances in the genetics of systemic lupus erythematosus. Rheum Dis Clin North Am 28:111, 2002

HAHN BH: Mechanisms of disease: Antibodies to DNA. N Engl J Med 338: 1359, 1998

HOUSSIAU FA et al: Immunosuppressive therapy in lupus nephritis: the Euro-Lupus Nephritis Trial, a randomized trial of low-dose versus high-dose cyclophosphamide therapy. Arthritis Rheum 46:2121, 2002

LEVINE JS et al: The antiphospholipid syndrome. N Engl J Med 346:752, 2002

WALLACE DJ, HAHN BH (eds): *Dubois' Lupus Erythematosus*, 6th ed. Philadelphia, Lippincott Williams & Wilkins, 2002

Rheumatoid arthritis (RA) is a chronic multisystem disease of unknown cause. Although there are a variety of systemic manifestations, the characteristic feature of RA is persistent inflammatory synovitis, usually involving peripheral joints in a symmetric distribution. The potential of the synovial inflammation to cause cartilage damage and bone erosions and subsequent changes in joint integrity is the hallmark of the disease. Despite its destructive potential, the course of RA can be quite variable. Some patients may experience only a mild oligoarticular illness of brief duration with minimal joint damage, whereas others will have a relentless progressive polyarthritis with marked functional impairment.

EPIDEMIOLOGY AND GENETICS The prevalence of RA is approximately 0.8% of the population (range 0.3 to 2.1%); women are affected approximately three times more often than men. The prevalence increases with age, and sex differences diminish in the older age group. RA is seen throughout the world and affects all races. However, the incidence and severity seem to be less in rural sub-Saharan Africa and in Caribbean blacks. The onset is most frequent during the fourth and fifth decades of life, with 80% of all patients developing the disease between the ages of 35 and 50. The incidence of RA is more than six times greater in 60- to 64-year-old women compared to 18- to 29-year-old women. Recent data indicate that the incidence of RA may be diminishing.

Family studies indicate a genetic predisposition. For example, severe RA is found at approximately four times the expected rate in first-degree relatives of individuals with disease associated with the presence of the autoantibody, rheumatoid factor; approximately 10% of patients with RA will have an affected first-degree relative. Moreover, monozygotic twins are at least four times more likely to be concordant for RA than dizygotic twins, who have a similar risk of developing RA as nontwin siblings. Only 15 to 20% of monozygotic twins are concordant for RA, however, implying that factors other than genetics play an important etiopathogenic role. Of note, the highest risk for concordance of RA is noted in twins who have two HLA-DRB1 alleles known to be associated with RA. The class II major histocompatibility complex allele HLA-DR4 (DRβ1*0401) and related alleles are known to be major genetic risk factors for RA. Early studies showed that as many as 70% of patients with classic or definite RA express HLA-DR4 compared with 28% of control individuals. An association with HLA-DR4 has been noted in many populations, including North American and European whites, Chippewa Indians, Japanese, and native populations in India, Mexico, South America, and southern China. In a number of groups, including Israeli Jews, Asian Indians, and Yakima Indians of North America, however, there is no association between the development of RA and HLA-DR4. In these individuals, there is an association between RA and the closely related HLA-DR1 (DRβ1*0101) in the former two groups and HLA-Dw16 (DRβ1*1402) in the latter. It has been estimated that the risk of developing RA in a person with DRβ1*0401 or the closely related DRβ1*0404 is 1 in 35 and 1 in 20, respectively, whereas the presence of both alleles puts persons at an even greater risk. In certain groups of patients, there does not appear to be a clear association between HLA-DR4–related epitopes and RA. Thus, nearly 75% of African-American RA patients do not have this genetic element. Moreover, there is an association with HLA-DR10 (DRβ1*1001) in Spanish and Italian patients, with HLA-DR9 (DRβ1*0901) in Chileans, and with HLA-DR3 (DRβ1*0301) in Arab populations.

Additional genes in the HLA-D complex may also convey altered susceptibility to RA. Certain HLA-DR alleles, including HLA-DR5 (DRβ1*1101), HLA-DR2 (DRβ1*1501), HLA-DR3 (DRβ1*0301), and HLA-DR7 (DRβ1*0701), may protect against the development of RA in that they tend to be found at lower frequency in RA patients than in controls. Moreover, the HLA-DQ alleles, DQβ1*0301 and DQβ1*0302, that are in linkage disequilibrium with HLA-DR4 and DQβ1*0501, have also been associated with RA. This has raised the possibility that HLA-DQ alleles may represent the actual RA susceptibility genes, whereas specific HLA-DR alleles may convey protection. In this model, the complement of HLA-DR and DQ alleles determines RA susceptibility. Disease manifestations have also been associated with HLA phenotype. Thus, early aggressive disease and extraarticular manifestations are more frequent in patients with DRβ1*0401 or DRβ1*0404, and more slowly progressive disease in those with DRβ1*0101. The presence of both DRβ1*0401 and DRβ1*0404 appears to increase the risk for both aggressive articular and extraarticular disease. It has been estimated that HLA genes contribute only a portion of the genetic susceptibility to RA. Thus genes outside the HLA complex also contribute. These include genes controlling the expression of the antigen receptor on T cells and both immunoglobulin heavy and light chains. Moreover, polymorphisms in the tumor necrosis factor (TNF) and the interleukin (IL) 10 genes are also associated with RA, as is a region on chromosome 3 (3q13). In addition, a number of other genetic regions appear to confer risk for RA.

Genetic risk factors do not fully account for the incidence of RA, suggesting that environmental factors also play a role in the etiology of the disease. This is emphasized by epidemiologic studies in Africa that have indicated that climate and urbanization have a major impact on the incidence and severity of RA in groups of similar genetic background.

ETIOLOGY The cause of RA remains unknown. It has been suggested that RA might be a manifestation of the response to an infectious agent in a genetically susceptible host. Because of the worldwide distribution of RA, it has been hypothesized that if an infectious agent is involved, the organism must be ubiquitous. A number of possible causative agents have been suggested, including *Mycoplasma*, Epstein-Barr virus (EBV), cytomegalovirus, parvovirus, and rubella virus, but convincing evidence that these or other infectious agents cause RA has not emerged. The process by which an infectious agent might cause chronic inflammatory arthritis with a characteristic distribution also remains a matter of controversy. One possibility is that there is persistent infection of articular structures or retention of microbial products in the synovial tissues that generates a chronic inflammatory response. Alternatively, the microorganism or response to the microorganism might induce an immune response to components of the joint by altering its integrity and revealing antigenic peptides. In this regard, reactivity to type II collagen and heat shock proteins has been demonstrated. Another possibility is that the infecting microorganism might prime the host to cross-reactive determinants expressed within the joint as a result of "molecular mimicry." Recent evidence of similarity between products of certain gram-negative bacteria and EBV and the HLA-DR4 molecule itself has supported this possibility. Finally, products of infecting microorganisms, such as superantigens, might induce the disease. Superantigens are proteins with the capacity to bind to HLA-DR molecules and particular V$_\beta$ segments of the heterodimeric T cell receptor and stimulate specific T cells expressing the V$_\beta$ gene products (Chap. 295). The role of superantigens in the etiology of RA remains speculative. Of all the potential environmental triggers, the only one clearly associated with the development of RA is cigarette smoking.

PATHOLOGY AND PATHOGENESIS Microvascular injury and an increase in the number of synovial lining cells appear to be the earliest lesions in rheumatoid synovitis. The nature of the insult causing this response is not known. Subsequently, an increased number of synovial lining cells is seen along with perivascular infiltration with mononuclear cells. Before the onset of clinical symptoms, the perivascular infiltrate is predominantly composed of myeloid cells, whereas in symptomatic arthritis, T cells can also be found, although their number does not appear to correlate with symptoms. As the process continues, the synovium becomes edematous and protrudes into the joint cavity as villous projections.

Light-microscopic examination discloses a characteristic constellation of features, which include hyperplasia and hypertrophy of the synovial lining cells; focal or segmental vascular changes, including microvascular injury, thrombosis, and neovascularization; edema; and infiltration with mononuclear cells, often collected into aggregates around small blood vessels (Fig. 301-1). The endothelial cells of the rheumatoid synovium have the appearance of high endothelial venules of lymphoid organs and have been altered by cytokine exposure to facilitate entry of cells into tissue. Rheumatoid synovial endothelial cells express increased amounts of various adhesion molecules involved in this process. Although this pathologic picture is typical of RA, it can also be seen in a variety of other chronic inflammatory arthritides. The mononuclear cell collections are variable in composition and size. The predominant infiltrating cell is the T lymphocyte. CD4+ T cells predominate over CD8+ T cells and are frequently found in close proximity to HLA-DR+ macrophages and dendritic cells. Increased numbers of a separate population of T cells expressing the γδ form of the T cell receptor have also been found in the synovium, although they remain a minor population there and their role in RA has not been delineated. The major population of T cells in the rheumatoid synovium is composed of CD4+ memory T cells that form the majority of cells aggregated around postcapillary venules. Scattered throughout the tissue are CD8+ T cells. Both populations express the early activation antigen, CD69. Besides the accumulation of T cells, rheumatoid synovitis is also characterized by the infiltration of variable numbers of B cells and antibody-producing plasma cells. In advanced disease, structures similar to germinal centers of secondary lymphoid organs may be observed in the synovium. Both polyclonal immunoglobulin and the autoantibody rheumatoid factor are produced within the synovial tissue, which leads to the local formation of immune complexes. Antibodies to synovial tissue components may also contribute to inflammation. Increased numbers of activated mast cells are also found in the rheumatoid synovium. Local release of the contents of their granules may contribute to inflammation. Finally, the synovial fibroblasts in RA manifest evidence of activation in that they produce a number of enzymes such as collagenase and cathepsins that can degrade components of the articular matrix. These activated fibroblasts are particularly prominent in the lining layer and at the interface with bone and cartilage. Osteoclasts are also prominent at sites of bone erosion. Activated mesenchymal stromal cells, similar to those found in normal bone marrow, can also be found in the rheumatoid synovium.

The rheumatoid synovium is characterized by the presence of a number of secreted products of activated lymphocytes, macrophages, and fibroblasts. The local production of these cytokines and chemokines appears to account for many of the pathologic and clinical manifestations of RA. These effector molecules include those that are derived from T lymphocytes, those originating from activated myeloid cells, and those secreted by other cell types in the synovium, such as fibroblasts and endothelial cells. The activity of these chemokines and cytokines appears to account for many of the features of rheumatoid synovitis, including the synovial tissue inflammation, synovial fluid inflammation, synovial proliferation, and cartilage and bone damage, as well as the systemic manifestations of RA. In addition to the production of effector molecules that propagate the inflammatory process, local factors are produced that tend to slow the inflammation, including specific inhibitors of cytokine action and additional cytokines, such as transforming growth factor (TGF-β), which inhibits many of the features of rheumatoid synovitis including T cell activation and proliferation, B cell differentiation, and migration of cells into the inflammatory site.

These findings have suggested that the propagation of RA is an immunologically mediated event, although the original initiating stimulus has not been characterized. One view is that the inflammatory process in the tissue is driven by the CD4+ T cells infiltrating the synovium. Evidence for this includes (1) the predominance of CD4+ T cells in the synovium; (2) the increase in soluble IL-2 receptors, a product of activated T cells, in blood and synovial fluid of patients with active RA; and (3) amelioration of the disease by removal of T cells by thoracic duct drainage or peripheral lymphapheresis or suppression of their proliferation or function by drugs, such as cyclosporine, leflunomide, or nondepleting monoclonal antibodies to CD4, or inhibitors of T cell activation, such as the T cell co-stimulation competitor, CTLA-4·Ig. In addition, the association of RA with certain HLA-DR or -DQ alleles, whose only known functions are to shape the repertoire of CD4+ T cells during ontogeny in the thymus and bind and present antigenic peptides to CD4+ T cells in the periphery, strongly implies a role for CD4+ T cells in the pathogenesis of the disease. Finally, patients with established RA who become infected with HIV have also been noted to improve, although this has not been a uniform finding. Within the rheumatoid synovium, the CD4+ T cells differentiate predominantly into T_H1-like effector cells producing the proinflammatory cytokine interferon (IFN) γ and appear to be deficient in differentiation into T_H2-like effector cells capable of producing the anti-inflammatory cytokine IL-4. As a result of the ongoing secretion of IFN-γ without the regulatory influences of IL-4, macrophages are activated to produce the proinflammatory cytokines IL-1 and TNF and also increase expression of HLA molecules. Direct contact between activated T cells and myeloid cells may also lead to the production of proinflammatory cytokines by the latter. Moreover, T lymphocytes express surface molecules such as CD154 (CD40 ligand) and also produce a variety of cytokines that promote B cell proliferation and differentiation into antibody-forming cells and therefore may also promote local B cell stimulation. The resultant production of immunoglobulin and rheumatoid factor can lead to immune-complex formation with consequent complement activation and exacerbation of the inflammatory process by the production of the anaphylatoxins, C3a and C5a, and the chemotactic factor C5a. In addition, antibodies may be produced to other self-antigens than can contribute to disease pathogenesis. The tissue inflammation is reminiscent of chronic inflammatory responses to persistent microorganisms, although it has become clear that the number of T cells producing cytokines such as IFN-γ is less than is found in typical delayed-type hypersensitivity reactions, perhaps owing to the large amount of reactive oxygen species produced locally in the synovium that can dampen T cell function. It remains unclear whether the persistent T cell activity represents a response to a persistent exogenous antigen or to altered autoantigens such as collagen, immunoglobulin, or one of the heat shock proteins, or perhaps both. Alternatively, it could represent persistent responsiveness to activated autologous cells such as might occur as a result

FIGURE 301-1 Histology of rheumatoid synovitis. *A.* The characteristic features of rheumatoid inflammation with hyperplasia of the lining layer (*arrow*) and mononuclear infiltrates in the sublining layer (*double arrow*). *B.* A higher magnification of the largely CD4+ T cell infiltrate around postcapillary venules (*arrow*).

of EBV infection or persistent response to a foreign antigen or super-antigen in the synovial tissue. Finally, rheumatoid inflammation could reflect persistent stimulation of T cells by synovial-derived antigens that cross-react with determinants introduced during antecedent exposure to foreign antigens or infectious microorganisms. The important contribution of B lymphocytes to the chronic inflammatory process has been emphasized by the observation that treatment with a monoclonal antibody to the B cell marker, CD20, caused prompt depletion of B lymphocytes and an amelioration of signs and symptoms of inflammation.

Overriding the chronic inflammation in the synovial tissue is an acute inflammatory process in the synovial fluid. The exudative synovial fluid contains more polymorphonuclear leukocytes than mononuclear cells. A number of mechanisms play a role in stimulating the exudation of synovial fluid. Locally produced antibodies to tissue components and immune complexes can activate complement and generate anaphylatoxins and chemotactic factors. Local production of chemokines and cytokines with chemotactic activity as well as inflammatory mediators such as leukotriene B$_4$ and products of complement activation can attract neutrophils. Moreover, many of these same agents can also stimulate the endothelial cells of postcapillary venules to become more efficient at binding circulating cells. The net result is the enhanced migration of polymorphonuclear leukocytes into the synovial site. In addition, vasoactive mediators such as histamine produced by the mast cells that infiltrate the rheumatoid synovium may also facilitate the exudation of inflammatory cells into the synovial fluid. Finally, the vasodilatory effects of locally produced prostaglandin E$_2$ may also facilitate entry of inflammatory cells into the inflammatory site. Once in the synovial fluid, the polymorphonuclear leukocytes can ingest immune complexes, with the resultant production of reactive oxygen metabolites and other inflammatory mediators, further adding to the inflammatory milieu. Locally produced cytokines and chemokines can additionally stimulate polymorphonuclear leukocytes. The production of large amounts of cyclooxygenase and lipoxygenase pathway products of arachidonic acid metabolism by cells in the synovial fluid and tissue further accentuates the signs and symptoms of inflammation.

The precise mechanism by which bone and cartilage destruction occurs has not been completely resolved. Although the synovial fluid contains a number of enzymes potentially able to degrade cartilage, the majority of destruction occurs in juxtaposition to the inflamed synovium, or pannus, that spreads to cover the articular cartilage. This vascular granulation tissue is composed of proliferating fibroblasts, small blood vessels, and a variable number of mononuclear cells and produces a large amount of degradative enzymes, including collagenase and stromelysin, that may facilitate tissue damage. The cytokines IL-1 and TNF play an important role by stimulating the cells of the pannus to produce collagenase and other neutral proteases. These same two cytokines also activate chondrocytes in situ, stimulating them to produce proteolytic enzymes that can degrade cartilage locally and also inhibiting synthesis of new matrix molecules. Finally, these two cytokines may contribute to the local demineralization of bone by activating osteoclasts that accumulate at the site of local bone resorption. Prostaglandin E$_2$ produced by fibroblasts and macrophages may also contribute to bone demineralization. The common final pathway of bone erosion is likely to involve the activation of osteoclasts that are present in large numbers at these sites. Systemic manifestations of RA can be accounted for by release of inflammatory effector molecules from the synovium. These include IL-1, TNF, and IL-6, which account for many of the manifestations of active RA, including malaise, fatigue, and elevated levels of serum acute-phase reactants. The importance of TNF in producing these manifestations is emphasized by the prompt amelioration of symptoms following administration of a monoclonal antibody to TNF or a soluble TNF receptor Ig construct to patients with RA. In addition, immune complexes produced within the synovium and entering the circulation may account for other features of the disease, such as systemic vasculitis.

As shown in Fig. 301-2, the pathology of RA evolves over the duration of this chronic disease. The earliest event appears to be a nonspecific inflammatory response initiated by an unknown stimulus and characterized by accumulation of macrophages and other mononuclear cells within the sublining layer of the synovium. The activity of these cells is demonstrated by the increased appearance of macrophage-derived cytokines, including TNF, IL-1β, and IL-6. Subsequently, activation and differentiation of memory CD4+ T cells is induced, presumably in response to antigenic peptides displayed by a variety of antigen-presenting cells in the synovial tissue. The activated memory T cells are capable of producing cytokines, especially IFN-γ, which amplify and perpetuate the inflammation. The presence of activated T cells expressing CD154 (CD40 ligand) can induce polyclonal B cell stimulation and differentiation of memory B cells and plasma cells that produce autoantibodies locally. The cascade of cytokines produced in the synovium activates a variety of cells in the synovium, bone, and cartilage to produce effector molecules that can cause tissue damage characteristic of chronic inflammation. It is important to emphasize that there is no current way to predict the progress from one stage of inflammation to the next, and once established, each can influence the other. Important features of this model include the following: (1) the major pathologic events vary with time in this chronic disease; (2) the time required to progress from one step to the next may vary in different patients, and the events, once established, may persist simultaneously; (3) once established, the major pathogenic events operative in an individual patient, may vary at different times; (4) the process is chronic and reiterative, with successive events stimulating progressive amplification of inflammation; and (5) once memory T cells and B cells have been generated, anti-inflammatory and anti-cytokine therapy may be capable of suppressing disease manifestations but not preventing recrudescence of disease activity once therapy is discontinued. These considerations have important implications with regard to appropriate treatment.

CLINICAL MANIFESTATIONS ■ Onset Characteristically, RA is a chronic polyarthritis. In approximately two-thirds of patients, it begins insidiously with fatigue, anorexia, generalized weakness, and vague musculoskeletal symptoms until the appearance of synovitis becomes apparent. This prodrome may persist for weeks or months and defy diagnosis. Specific symptoms usually appear gradually as several joints, especially those of the hands, wrists, knees, and feet, become affected in a symmetric fashion. In approximately 10% of individuals, the onset is more acute, with a rapid development of polyarthritis, often accompanied by constitutional symptoms, including fever, lymphadenopathy, and splenomegaly. In approximately one-third of patients, symptoms may initially be confined to one or a few joints. Although the pattern of joint involvement may remain asymmetric in a few patients, a symmetric pattern is more typical.

Signs and Symptoms of Articular Disease Pain, swelling, and tenderness may initially be poorly localized to the joints. Pain in affected joints, aggravated by movement, is the most common manifestation of established RA. It corresponds in pattern to the joint involvement but does not always correlate with the degree of apparent inflammation. Generalized stiffness is frequent and is usually greatest after periods of inactivity. Morning stiffness of greater than 1-h duration is an almost invariable feature of inflammatory arthritis and may serve to distinguish it from various noninflammatory joint disorders. Notably, however, the presence of morning stiffness may not reliably distinguish between chronic inflammatory and noninflammatory arthritides, as it is also found frequently in the latter. The majority of patients will experience constitutional symptoms such as weakness, easy fatigability, anorexia, and weight loss. Although fever to 40°C occurs on occasion, temperature elevation in excess of 38°C is unusual and suggests the presence of an intercurrent problem such as infection.

Clinically, synovial inflammation causes swelling, tenderness, and limitation of motion. Initially, impairment in physical function is caused by pain and inflammation, and disability owing to this is a frequent early feature of aggressive RA. Warmth is usually evident on examination, especially of large joints such as the knee, but erythema is infrequent. Pain originates predominantly from the joint capsule, which is abundantly supplied with pain fibers and is markedly sensitive to stretching or distention. Joint swelling results from accumulation of synovial fluid, hypertrophy of the synovium, and thickening of the joint capsule. Initially, motion is limited by pain. The inflamed joint is usually held in flexion to maximize joint volume and minimize distention of the capsule. Later, fibrous or bony ankylosis or soft tissue contractures lead to fixed deformities.

Although inflammation can affect any diarthrodial joint, RA most often causes symmetric arthritis with characteristic involvement of certain specific joints such as the proximal interphalangeal and metacarpophalangeal joints. The distal interphalangeal joints are rarely involved. Synovitis of the wrist joints is a nearly uniform feature of RA and may lead to limitation of motion, deformity, and median nerve entrapment (carpal tunnel syndrome). Synovitis of the elbow joint often leads to flexion contractures that may develop early in the disease. The knee joint is commonly involved with synovial hypertrophy, chronic effusion, and frequently ligamentous laxity. Pain and swelling behind the knee may be caused by extension of inflamed synovium into the popliteal space (Baker's cyst). Arthritis in the forefoot, ankles, and subtalar joints can produce severe pain with ambulation as well as a number of deformities. Axial involvement is usually limited to the upper cervical spine. Involvement of the lumbar spine is not seen, and lower back pain cannot be ascribed to rheumatoid inflammation. On occasion, inflammation from the synovial joints and bursae of the upper cervical spine leads to atlantoaxial subluxation. This usually presents as pain in the occiput but on rare occasions may lead to compression of the spinal cord.

With persistent inflammation, a variety of characteristic joint changes develop. These can be attributed to a number of pathologic events, including laxity of supporting soft tissue structures; damage or weakening of ligaments, tendons, and the joint capsule; cartilage degradation; muscle imbalance; and unopposed physical forces associated with the use of affected joints. Characteristic changes of the hand include (1) radial deviation at the wrist with ulnar deviation of the digits, often with palmar subluxation of the proximal phalanges ("Z" deformity); (2) hyperextension of the proximal interphalangeal joints, with compensatory flexion of the distal interphalangeal joints (swan-neck deformity); (3) flexion contracture of the proximal interphalangeal joints and extension of the distal interphalangeal joints (boutonnière deformity); and (4) hyperextension of the first interphalangeal joint and flexion of the first metacarpophalangeal joint with a consequent loss of thumb mobility and pinch. Typical joint changes may also develop in the feet, including eversion at the hindfoot (subtalar joint), plantar subluxation of the metatarsal heads, widening of the forefoot, hallux valgus, and lateral deviation and dorsal subluxation of the toes. Later in the disease, disability is more related to structural damage to articular structures.

Extraarticular Manifestations RA is a systemic disease with a variety of extraarticular manifestations. Although these occur frequently, not all of them have clinical significance. However, on occasion, they may be the major evidence of disease activity and source of morbidity and require management per se. As a rule, these manifestations occur in individuals with high titers of autoantibodies to the Fc component of immunoglobulin G (rheumatoid factors).

Rheumatoid nodules develop in 20 to 30% of persons with RA.

FIGURE 301-2 The progression of rheumatoid synovitis. This figure depicts the evolution of the pathogenic mechanisms and ultimate pathologic changes involved in the development of rheumatoid synovitis. The stages of rheumatoid arthritis are proposed to be an initiation phase of nonspecific inflammation, followed by an amplification phase resulting from T cell activation, and finally a stage of chronic inflammation with tissue injury. A variety of stimuli may initiate the initial phase of nonspecific inflammation, which may last for a protracted period of time with no or moderate symptoms. When activation of memory T cells in response to a variety of peptides presented by antigen-presenting cells occurs in genetically susceptible individuals, amplification of inflammation occurs with the promotion of local rheumatoid factor production and enhanced capacity to mediate tissue damage.

They are usually found on periarticular structures, extensor surfaces, or other areas subjected to mechanical pressure, but they can develop elsewhere, including the pleura and meninges. Common locations include the olecranon bursa, the proximal ulna, the Achilles tendon, and the occiput. Nodules vary in size and consistency and are rarely symptomatic, but on occasion they break down as a result of trauma or become infected. They are found almost invariably in individuals with circulating rheumatoid factor. Histologically, rheumatoid nodules consist of a central zone of necrotic material including collagen fibrils, noncollagenous filaments, and cellular debris; a midzone of palisading macrophages that express HLA-DR antigens; and an outer zone of granulation tissue. Examination of early nodules has suggested that the initial event may be a focal vasculitis. In some patients, treatment with methotrexate can increase the number of nodules dramatically.

Clinical weakness and atrophy of skeletal muscle are common. Muscle atrophy may be evident within weeks of the onset of RA and is usually most apparent in musculature approximating affected joints. Muscle biopsy may show type II fiber atrophy and muscle fiber necrosis with or without a mononuclear cell infiltrate.

Rheumatoid vasculitis (Chap. 306), which can affect nearly any organ system, is seen in patients with severe RA and high titers of circulating rheumatoid factor. Rheumatoid vasculitis is very uncommon in African Americans. In its most aggressive form, rheumatoid vasculitis can cause polyneuropathy and mononeuritis multiplex, cutaneous ulceration and dermal necrosis, digital gangrene, and visceral infarction. While such widespread vasculitis is very rare, more limited forms are not uncommon, especially in white patients with high titers of rheumatoid factor. Neurovascular disease presenting either as a mild distal sensory neuropathy or as mononeuritis multiplex may be the only sign of vasculitis. Cutaneous vasculitis usually presents as crops of small brown spots in the nail beds, nail folds, and digital pulp. Larger ischemic ulcers, especially in the lower extremity, may also develop. Myocardial infarction secondary to rheumatoid vasculitis has been reported, as has vasculitic involvement of lungs, bowel, liver, spleen, pancreas, lymph nodes, and testes. Renal vasculitis is rare.

Pleuropulmonary manifestations, which are more commonly observed in men, include pleural disease, interstitial fibrosis, pleuropulmonary nodules, pneumonitis, and arteritis. Evidence of pleuritis is found commonly at autopsy, but symptomatic disease during life is infrequent. Typically, the pleural fluid contains very low levels of glucose in the absence of infection. Pleural fluid complement is also low compared with the serum level when these are related to the total protein concentration. Pulmonary fibrosis can produce impairment of the diffusing capacity of the lung. Pulmonary nodules may appear singly or in clusters. When they appear in individuals with pneumoconiosis, a diffuse nodular fibrotic process (Caplan's syndrome) may develop. On occasion, pulmonary nodules may cavitate and produce a pneumothorax or bronchopleural fistula. Rarely, pulmonary hypertension secondary to obliteration of the pulmonary vasculature occurs. In addition to pleuropulmonary disease, upper airway obstruction from cricoarytenoid arthritis or laryngeal nodules may develop.

Clinically apparent heart disease attributed to the rheumatoid process is rare, but evidence of asymptomatic pericarditis is found at autopsy in 50% of cases. Pericardial fluid has a low glucose level and is frequently associated with the occurrence of pleural effusion. Although pericarditis is usually asymptomatic, on rare occasions death has occurred from tamponade. Chronic constrictive pericarditis may also occur.

RA tends to spare the central nervous system directly, although vasculitis can cause peripheral neuropathy. *Neurologic manifestations* may also result from atlantoaxial or midcervical spine subluxations. Nerve entrapment secondary to proliferative synovitis or joint deformities may produce neuropathies of median, ulnar, radial (interosseous branch), or anterior tibial nerves.

The rheumatoid process involves the *eye* in fewer than 1% of patients. Affected individuals usually have long-standing disease and nodules. The two principal manifestations are episcleritis, which is usually mild and transient, and scleritis, which involves the deeper layers of the eye and is a more serious inflammatory condition. Histologically, the lesion is similar to a rheumatoid nodule and may result in thinning and perforation of the globe (scleromalacia perforans). From 15 to 20% of persons with RA may develop Sjögren's syndrome with attendant keratoconjunctivitis sicca.

Felty's syndrome consists of chronic RA, splenomegaly, neutropenia, and, on occasion, anemia and thrombocytopenia. It is most common in individuals with long-standing disease. These patients frequently have high titers of rheumatoid factor, subcutaneous nodules, and other manifestations of systemic rheumatoid disease. Felty's syndrome is very uncommon in African Americans. It may develop after joint inflammation has regressed. Circulating immune complexes are often present, and evidence of complement consumption may be seen. The leukopenia is a selective neutropenia with polymorphonuclear leukocyte counts of <1500 cells/μL and sometimes <1000 cell/μL. Bone marrow examination usually reveals moderate hypercellularity with a paucity of mature neutrophils. However, the bone marrow may be normal, hyperactive, or hypoactive; maturation arrest may be seen. Hypersplenism has been proposed as one of the causes of leukopenia, but splenomegaly is not invariably found and splenectomy does not always correct the abnormality. Excessive margination of granulocytes caused by antibodies to these cells, complement activation, or binding of immune complexes may contribute to granulocytopenia. Patients with Felty's syndrome have increased frequency of infections usually associated with neutropenia. The cause of the increased susceptibility to infection is related to the defective function of polymorphonuclear leukocytes as well as the decreased number of cells.

Osteoporosis secondary to rheumatoid involvement is common and may be aggravated by glucocorticoid therapy. Glucocorticoid treatment may cause significant loss of bone mass, especially early in the course of therapy, even when low doses are employed. Osteopenia in RA involves both juxtaarticular bone and long bones distant from involved joints. RA is associated with a modest decrease in mean bone mass and a moderate increase in the risk of fracture. Bone mass appears to be adversely affected by functional impairment and active inflammation, especially early in the course of the disease.

RA is associated with an increased incidence of lymphoma, especially large B cell lymphoma. Notably, this is particularly observed in those with persistent inflammatory disease.

RA in the Elderly The incidence of RA continues to increase past age 60. It has been suggested that elderly-onset RA might have a poorer prognosis, as manifested by more persistent disease activity, more frequent radiographically evident deterioration, more frequent systemic involvement, and more rapid functional decline. Aggressive disease is largely restricted to those patients with high titers of rheumatoid factor. By contrast, elderly patients who develop RA without elevated titers of rheumatoid factor (seronegative disease) generally have less severe, often self-limited disease.

LABORATORY FINDINGS No tests are specific for diagnosing RA. However, rheumatoid factors, which are autoantibodies reactive with the Fc portion of IgG, are found in more than two-thirds of adults with the disease. Widely utilized tests largely detect IgM rheumatoid factors. The presence of rheumatoid factor is not specific for RA. Rheumatoid factor is found in 5% of healthy persons. The frequency of rheumatoid factor in the general population increases with age, and 10 to 20% of individuals over 65 years old have a positive test. In addition, a number of conditions besides RA are associated with the presence of rheumatoid factor. These include systemic lupus erythematosus, Sjögren's syndrome, chronic liver disease, sarcoidosis, interstitial pulmonary fibrosis, infectious mononucleosis, hepatitis B, tuberculosis, leprosy, syphilis, subacute bacterial endocarditis, visceral leishmaniasis, schistosomiasis, and malaria. In addition, rheumatoid factor may appear transiently in normal individuals after vaccination or transfusion and may also be found in relatives of individuals with RA.

The presence of rheumatoid factor does not establish the diagnosis of RA as the predictive value of the presence of rheumatoid factor in determining a diagnosis of RA is poor. Thus fewer than one-third of unselected patients with a positive test for rheumatoid factor will be found to have RA. Therefore, the rheumatoid factor test is not useful as a screening procedure. However, the presence of rheumatoid factor can be of prognostic significance because patients with high titers tend to have more severe and progressive disease with extraarticular manifestations. Rheumatoid factor is uniformly found in patients with nodules or vasculitis. In summary, a test for the presence of rheumatoid factor can be employed to confirm a diagnosis in individuals with a suggestive clinical presentation and, if present in high titer, to designate patients at risk for severe systemic disease. A number of additional autoantibodies may be found in patients with RA, including antibodies to filaggrin, citrullinated proteins, calpastatin, components of the spliceosome (RA-33), and an unknown antigen, Sa. Some of these may be useful in diagnosis in that they may occur early in the disease before rheumatoid factor is present or may be associated with aggressive disease.

Normochromic, normocytic anemia is frequently present in active RA. It is thought to reflect ineffective erythropoiesis; large stores of iron are found in the bone marrow. In general, anemia and thrombocytosis correlate with disease activity. The white blood cell count is usually normal, but a mild leukocytosis may be present. Leukopenia may also exist without the full-blown picture of Felty's syndrome. Eosinophilia, when present, usually reflects severe systemic disease.

The erythrocyte sedimentation rate is increased in nearly all patients with active RA. The levels of a variety of other acute-phase reactants including ceruloplasmin and C-reactive protein are also elevated, and generally such elevations correlate with disease activity and the likelihood of progressive joint damage.

Synovial fluid analysis confirms the presence of inflammatory arthritis, although none of the findings is specific. The fluid is usually turbid, with reduced viscosity, increased protein content, and a slightly decreased or normal glucose concentration. The white cell count varies between 5 and 50,000/μL; polymorphonuclear leukocytes predominate. A synovial fluid white blood cell count >2000/μL with more than 75% polymorphonuclear leukocytes is highly characteristic of inflammatory arthritis, although not diagnostic of RA. Total hemolytic complement, C3, and C4 are markedly diminished in synovial fluid relative to total protein concentration as a result of activation of the classic complement pathway by locally produced immune complexes.

RADIOGRAPHIC EVALUATION Early in the disease, radiographic evaluations of the affected joints are usually not helpful in establishing a diagnosis. They reveal only that which is apparent from physical examination, namely, evidence of soft tissue swelling and joint effusion. As the disease progresses, abnormalities become more pronounced, but none of the radiographic findings is diagnostic of RA. The diagnosis, however, is supported by a characteristic pattern of abnormalities, including the tendency toward symmetric involvement. Juxtaarticular osteopenia may become apparent within weeks of onset. Loss of articular cartilage and bone erosions develop after months of sustained activity. The primary value of radiography is to determine the extent of cartilage destruction and bone erosion produced by the disease, particularly when one is attempting to estimate the aggressive nature of the disease, monitoring the impact of therapy with disease-modifying drugs, or determining the need for surgical intervention. Other means of imaging bones and joints, including ^{99m}Tc bisphosphonate bone scanning and magnetic resonance imaging, may be capable of detecting early inflammatory changes that are not apparent from standard radiography but are rarely necessary in the routine evaluation of patients with RA.

CLINICAL COURSE AND PROGNOSIS The course of RA is quite variable and difficult to predict in an individual patient. Most patients experience persistent but fluctuating disease activity, accompanied by a variable degree of joint abnormalities and functional impairment. After 10 to 12 years, <20% of patients will have no evidence of disability or joint abnormalities. Within 10 years, ~50% of patients will have work disability. A number of features are correlated with a greater likelihood of developing joint abnormalities or disabilities. These include the presence of >20 inflamed joints, a markedly elevated erythrocyte sedimentation rate, radiographic evidence of bone erosions, the presence of rheumatoid nodules, high titers of serum rheumatoid factor, the presence of functional disability, persistent inflammation, advanced age at onset, the presence of comorbid conditions, low socioeconomic status or educational level, or the presence of HLA-DRβ1*0401 or -DRβ*0404. The presence of one or more of these implies the presence of more aggressive disease with a greater likelihood of developing progressive joint abnormalities and disability. Persistent elevation of the erythrocyte sedimentation rate, disability, and pain on longitudinal follow-up are good predictors of work disability. Patients who lack these features have more indolent disease with a slower progression to joint abnormalities and disability. The pattern of disease onset does not appear to predict the development of disabilities. Approximately 15% of patients with RA will have a short-lived inflammatory process that remits without major disability. These individuals tend to lack the aforementioned features associated with more aggressive disease.

Several features of patients with RA appear to have prognostic significance. Remissions of disease activity are most likely to occur during the first year. White females tend to have more persistent synovitis and more progressively erosive disease than males. Persons who present with high titers of rheumatoid factor, C-reactive protein, and haptoglobin also have a worse prognosis, as do individuals with subcutaneous nodules or radiographic evidence of erosions at the time of initial evaluation. Sustained disease activity of more than 1 year's duration portends a poor outcome, and persistent elevation of acute-phase reactants appears to correlate strongly with radiographic progression. A large proportion of inflamed joints manifest erosions within 2 years, whereas the subsequent course of erosions is highly variable; however, in general, radiographic damage appears to progress at a constant rate in patients with RA. Foot joints are affected more frequently than hand joints. Despite the decrease in the rate of progressive joint damage with time, functional disability, which develops early in the course of the disease, continues to worsen at the same rate, although the most rapid rate of functional loss occurs within the first 2 years of disease.

The median life expectancy of persons with RA is shortened by 3 to 7 years. Of the 2.5-fold increase in mortality rate, RA itself is a contributing feature in 15 to 30%. The increased mortality rate seems to be limited to patients with more severe articular disease and can be attributed largely to infection and gastrointestinal bleeding. Recent evidence has also shown an important role of cardiovascular disease in the increased mortality of RA patients, and this appears to diminish with effective anti-inflammatory therapy. Drug therapy may also play a role in the increased mortality rate seen in individuals with RA. Factors correlated with early death include disability, disease duration or severity, glucocorticoid use, age at onset, and low socioeconomic or educational status.

DIAGNOSIS The mean delay from disease onset to diagnosis is 9 months. This is often related to the nonspecific nature of initial symptoms. The diagnosis of RA is easily made in persons with typical established disease. In a majority of patients, the disease assumes its characteristic clinical features within 1 to 2 years of onset. The typical picture of bilateral symmetric inflammatory polyarthritis involving small and large joints in both the upper and lower extremities with sparing of the axial skeleton except the cervical spine suggests the diagnosis. Constitutional features indicative of the inflammatory nature of the disease, such as morning stiffness, support the diagnosis. Demonstration of subcutaneous nodules is a helpful diagnostic feature. Additionally, the presence of rheumatoid factor, inflammatory synovial fluid with increased numbers of polymorphonuclear leukocytes, and radiographic findings of juxtaarticular bone demineralization and erosions of the affected joints substantiate the diagnosis.

The diagnosis is somewhat more difficult early in the course when only constitutional symptoms or intermittent arthralgias or arthritis in an asymmetric distribution may be present. A period of observation may be necessary before the diagnosis can be established. A definitive diagnosis of RA depends predominantly on characteristic clinical features and the exclusion of other inflammatory processes. The isolated finding of a positive test for rheumatoid factor or an elevated erythrocyte sedimentation rate, especially in an older person with joint pains, should not itself be used as evidence of RA.

In 1987, the American College of Rheumatology developed revised criteria for the classification of RA (Table 301-1). These criteria demonstrate a sensitivity of 91 to 94% and a specificity of 89% when used

---

TABLE 301-1 *The 1987 Revised Criteria for the Classification of RA*

1. Guidelines for classification
   a. Four of seven criteria are required to classify a patient as having rheumatoid arthritis (RA).
   b. Patients with two or more clinical diagnoses are not excluded.
2. Criteria*
   a. Morning stiffness: Stiffness in and around the joints lasting 1 h before maximal improvement.
   b. Arthritis of three or more joint areas: At least three joint areas, observed by a physician simultaneously, have soft tissue swelling or joint effusions, not just bony overgrowth. The 14 possible joint areas involved are right or left proximal interphalangeal, metacarpophalangeal, wrist, elbow, knee, ankle, and metatarsophalangeal joints.
   c. Arthritis of hand joints: Arthritis of wrist, metacarpophalangeal joint, or proximal interphalangeal joint.
   d. Symmetric arthritis: Simultaneous involvement of the same joint areas on both sides of the body.
   e. Rheumatoid nodules: Subcutaneous nodules over bony prominences, extensor surfaces, or juxtaarticular regions observed by a physician.
   f. Serum rheumatoid factor: Demonstration of abnormal amounts of serum rheumatoid factor by any method for which the result has been positive in less than 5% of normal control subjects.
   g. Radiographic changes: Typical changes of RA on posteroanterior hand and wrist radiographs that must include erosions or unequivocal bony decalcification localized in or most marked adjacent to the involved joints.

*Criteria a–d must be present for at least 6 weeks. Criteria b–e must be observed by a physician.
Source: From FC Arnett et al: Arthritis Rheum 31:315, 1988.

to classify patients with RA compared with control subjects with rheumatic diseases other than RA. Although these criteria were developed as a means of disease classification for investigational purposes, they can be useful as guidelines for establishing the diagnosis. Failure to meet these criteria, however, especially during the early stages of the disease, does not exclude the diagnosis. Indeed, these criteria do not effectively differentiate patients with new-onset RA from those with a variety of other forms of early inflammatory arthritis. Moreover, in patients with early arthritis, the criteria do not discriminate effectively between patients who subsequently develop persistent, disabling, or erosive disease and those who do not.

℞ TREATMENT

General Principles The goals of therapy of RA are (1) relief of pain, (2) reduction of inflammation, (3) protection of articular structures, (4) maintenance of function, and (5) control of systemic involvement. Since the etiology of RA is unknown, the pathogenesis is not completely delineated, and the mechanisms of action of some of the therapeutic agents employed are uncertain, therapy remains somewhat empirical. None of the therapeutic interventions is curative, and therefore all must be viewed as palliative, aimed at relieving the signs and symptoms of the disease. The various therapies employed are directed at nonspecific suppression of the inflammatory or immunologic process in the hope of ameliorating symptoms and preventing progressive damage to articular structures.

Management of patients with RA involves an interdisciplinary approach, which attempts to deal with the various problems that these individuals encounter with functional as well as psychosocial interactions. A variety of physical therapy modalities may be useful in decreasing the symptoms of RA. Rest ameliorates symptoms and can be an important component of the total therapeutic program. In addition, splinting to reduce unwanted motion of inflamed joints may be useful. Exercise directed at maintaining muscle strength and joint mobility without exacerbating joint inflammation is also an important aspect of the therapeutic regimen. A variety of orthotic and assistive devices can be helpful in supporting and aligning deformed joints to reduce pain and improve function. Education of the patient and family is an important component of the therapeutic plan to help those involved become aware of the potential impact of the disease and make appropriate accommodations in life-style to maximize satisfaction and minimize stress on joints.

Medical management of RA involves five general approaches. The first is the use of aspirin, other nonsteroidal anti-inflammatory drugs (NSAIDs), and simple analgesics to control the symptoms and signs of the local inflammatory process. These agents are rapidly effective at mitigating signs and symptoms, but they appear to exert minimal effect on the progression of the disease. Recently, specific inhibitors of the isoform of cyclooxygenase (COX) that is upregulated at inflammatory sites (COX-2) have been developed. COX inhibitors (known as Coxibs), which selectively inhibit COX-2 and not COX-1, have been shown to be as effective as classic NSAIDs, which inhibit both isoforms of COX, but to cause significantly less gastroduodenal ulceration. The second line of therapy involves use of low-dose oral glucocorticoids. Although low-dose glucocorticoids have been widely used to suppress signs and symptoms of inflammation, recent evidence suggests that they may also retard the development and progression of bone erosions. Intraarticular glucocorticoids can often provide transient symptomatic relief when systemic medical therapy has failed to resolve inflammation. The third line of agents includes a variety of agents that have been classified as the disease-modifying or slow-acting antirheumatic drugs. These agents appear to have the capacity to decrease elevated levels of acute-phase reactants in treated patients and, therefore, are thought to modify the inflammatory component of RA and thus its destructive capacity. Recently, combinations of dis-

ease-modifying antirheumatic drugs (DMARDs) have shown promise in controlling the signs and symptoms of RA. A fourth group of agents are the cytokine-neutralizing agents, which have been shown to have a major impact on the signs and symptoms of RA and also to slow progressive damage to articular structures. A fifth group of agents are the immunosuppressive and cytotoxic drugs that have been shown to ameliorate the disease process in some patients. Additional approaches have been employed in an attempt to control the signs and symptoms of RA. Substituting omega-3 fatty acids such as eicosapentaenoic acid found in certain fish oils for dietary omega-6 essential fatty acids found in meat has also been shown to provide symptomatic improvement in patients with RA. A variety of nontraditional approaches have also been claimed to be effective in treating RA, including diets, plant and animal extracts, vaccines, hormones, and topical preparations of various sorts. Many of these are costly, and none has been shown to be effective. However, belief in their efficacy ensures their continued use by some patients.

Drugs ■ *NONSTEROIDAL ANTI-INFLAMMATORY DRUGS* Besides aspirin, many NSAIDs are available to treat RA. As a result of the capacity of these agents to block the activity of the COX enzymes and therefore the production of prostaglandins, prostacyclin, and thromboxanes, they have analgesic, anti-inflammatory, and antipyretic properties. In addition, the agents may exert other anti-inflammatory effects. These agents are all associated with a wide spectrum of toxic side effects. Some, such as gastric irritation, azotemia, platelet dysfunction, and exacerbation of allergic rhinitis and asthma, are related to the inhibition of cyclooxygenase activity, whereas a variety of others, such as rash, liver function abnormalities, and bone marrow depression, may not be. None of the NSAIDs has been shown to be more effective than aspirin in the treatment of RA. However, these nonaspirin drugs are associated with a lower incidence of gastrointestinal intolerance. None of the newer NSAIDs appears to show significant therapeutic advantages over the other available agents. In addition, there is no consistent advantage of any of these newer agents over the others with respect to the incidence or severity of toxic manifestations. Recent evidence indicates that two separate enzymes, COX-1 and -2, are responsible for the initial metabolism of arachidonic acid into various inflammatory mediators. The former is constitutively present in many cells and tissues, including the stomach and the platelet, whereas the latter is specifically induced in response to inflammatory stimuli and is absent from the normal stomach and platelet. Inhibition of COX-2 accounts for the anti-inflammatory effects of NSAIDs, whereas inhibition of COX-1 induces much of the mechanism-based toxicity. As the currently available NSAIDs inhibit both enzymes, therapeutic benefit and toxicity are intertwined. Coxibs have been approved for the treatment of RA. Clinical trials have shown that Coxibs suppress the signs and symptoms of RA as effectively as classic COX-nonspecific NSAIDs but are associated with a significantly reduced incidence of gastroduodenal ulceration and appear to reduce the incidence of gastrointestinal bleeding, perforations, and obstruction to a variable degree compared with classic NSAIDs. However, the use of Coxibs is associated with sodium retention, hypertension, and peripheral edema in a fraction of patients, and the use of some Coxibs may be associated with an increased frequency of myocardial infarction. This suggests that Coxibs might be considered instead of classic COX-nonspecific NSAIDs, especially in persons with increased risk of NSAID-induced major upper gastrointestinal side effects, including persons over 65, those with a history of peptic ulcer disease, persons receiving glucocorticoids or anticoagulants, or those requiring high doses of NSAIDs.

DISEASE-MODIFYING ANTIRHEUMATIC DRUGS Clinical experience has delineated a number of agents that appear to have the capacity to alter the course of RA. This group of agents includes methotrexate, gold compounds, D-penicillamine, the antimalarials, and sulfasalazine. Despite having no chemical or pharmacologic similarities, in practice these agents share a number of characteristics. They exert minimal direct nonspecific anti-inflammatory or analgesic effects, and therefore NSAIDs must be continued during their administration, except in a few cases when true remissions are induced with them. The appearance of benefit from DMARD therapy is usually delayed for weeks or months. As many as two-thirds of patients develop some clinical improvement as a result of therapy with any of these agents, although the induction of true remissions is unusual. In addition to clinical improvement, there is frequently an improvement in serologic evidence of disease activity, and titers of rheumatoid factor and C-reactive protein and the erythrocyte sedimentation rate frequently decline. Moreover, emerging evidence suggests that DMARDs actually retard the development of bone erosions or facilitate their healing. Furthermore, developing evidence suggests that early aggressive treatment with DMARDs may be effective at slowing the appearance of bone erosions.

Which DMARD should be the drug of first choice remains controversial, and trials have failed to demonstrate a consistent advantage of one over the other. Despite this, methotrexate has emerged as the DMARD of choice because of its relatively rapid onset of action, its capacity to effect sustained improvement with ongoing therapy, and the higher level of patient retention on therapy. Each of the DMARDs is associated with considerable toxicity, and therefore careful patient monitoring is necessary. Toxicity of the various agents also becomes important in determining the drug of first choice. Of note, failure to respond or development of toxicity to one DMARD does not preclude responsiveness to another. Thus, a similar percentage of RA patients who have failed to respond to one DMARD will respond to another when it is given as the second disease-modifying drug.

No characteristic features of patients have emerged that predict responsiveness to a DMARD. Moreover, the indications for the initiation of therapy with one of these agents are not well defined. Recently, evidence has emerged that the initiation of DMARD therapy early in the course of RA clearly has a major impact on the development of bone erosions and the progression to disability. It is now felt that DMARD therapy should be begun as soon as the diagnosis of RA is established, especially in those with any evidence of aggressive disease with a poor prognosis.

The folic acid antagonist methotrexate, given in an intermittent low dose (7.5 to 30 mg once weekly), is currently a frequently utilized DMARD. Most rheumatologists recommend use of methotrexate as the initial DMARD, especially in individuals with evidence of aggressive RA. Recent trials have documented the efficacy of methotrexate and have indicated that its onset of action is more rapid than other DMARDs, and patients tend to remain on therapy with methotrexate longer than they remain on other DMARDs because of better clinical responses and less toxicity. Long-term trials have indicated that methotrexate does not induce remission but rather suppresses symptoms while it is being administered. Maximal improvement is observed after 6 months of therapy, with little additional improvement thereafter. Major toxicity includes gastrointestinal upset, oral ulceration, and liver function abnormalities that appear to be dose-related and reversible and hepatic fibrosis that can be quite insidious, requiring liver biopsy for detection in its early stages. Drug-induced pneumonitis has also been reported. Liver biopsy is recommended for individuals with persistent or repetitive liver function abnormalities. Concurrent administration of folic acid or folinic acid may diminish the frequency of some side effects without diminishing effectiveness.

Glucocorticoid Therapy Systemic glucocorticoid therapy can provide effective symptomatic therapy in patients with RA. Low-dose (<7.5 mg/d) prednisone has been advocated as useful additive therapy to control symptoms. Moreover, recent evidence suggests that low-dose glucocorticoid therapy may retard the progression of bone erosions. Monthly pulses with high-dose glucocorticoids may be useful in some patients and may hasten the response when therapy with a DMARD is initiated.

Anti-Cytokine Agents Recently, biologic agents that bind and neutralize TNF have become available. One of these is a TNF type II receptor fused to IgG1 (etanercept), the second is a chimeric mouse/human monoclonal antibody to TNF (infliximab), and the third is a fully human antibody to TNF (adalimumab). Clinical trials have shown that parenteral administration of any of these TNF neutralizing agents is remarkably effective at controlling signs and symptoms of RA in patients who have failed DMARD therapy, as well as in DMARD naïve patients. Repetitive therapy with these agents is effective with or without concomitant methotrexate. These agents not only are effective in persistently controlling signs and symptoms of RA in a majority of patients, but they have also been shown to slow the rate of progression of joint damage assessed radiographically and to improve disability. Side effects include the potential for an increased risk of serious infections. Particularly notable is the capacity of TNF blockade to increase the risk of developing reactivation of dormant tuberculosis. It is prudent to carry out tuberculin skin testing and, if necessary, further evaluation with chest radiographs before beginning therapy with an anti-TNF agent to limit the chance of inciting reactivation of tuberculosis. TNF neutralizing therapy can also induce the development of anti-DNA antibodies, but rarely is there associated evidence of signs and symptoms of systemic lupus erythematosus. Other side effects include infusion or injection site reactions and rarely the development of demyelinating central nervous system disease. Although these side effects are uncommon, their occurrence mandates that TNF-neutralizing therapy be supervised by physicians with experience in their use.

Anakinra is a recombinant IL-1 receptor antagonist that competitively blocks the binding of IL-1β and IL-1α to the IL-1 receptor and thereby inhibits the activity of these two related proinflammatory cytokines. Anakinra has been shown to improve the signs and symptoms of RA, to decrease disability, and to slow progression of articular damage associated radiographically. It can be given as monotherapy or in combination with methotrexate. The major side effects are injection site reactions.

Immunosuppressive Therapy The immunosuppressive drugs azathioprine, leflunomide, cyclosporine, and cyclophosphamide have been shown to be effective in the treatment of RA and to exert therapeutic effects similar to those of the DMARDs. However, these agents appear to be no more effective than the DMARDs. Moreover, they cause a variety of toxic side effects, and cyclophosphamide appears to predispose the patient to the development of malignant neoplasms. Therefore, these drugs have been reserved for patients who have clearly failed therapy with DMARDs and anti-cytokine therapy. On occasion, extraarticular disease such as rheumatoid vasculitis may require cytotoxic immunosuppressive therapy.

Leflunomide is metabolized to an active metabolite that acts to inhibit dihydroorotate dehydrogenase, an essential enzyme in the pyrimidine biosynthetic pathway. Its predominant action is to inhibit the proliferation of T lymphocytes. Leflunomide has been shown to control the signs and symptoms of RA and to slow the progression of joint damage as effectively as methotrexate. Leflunomide can be given alone or with methotrexate and is the most frequently employed immunosuppressive agent used to treat patients with RA. It is used as monotherapy in patients who have had adverse reactions to methotrexate or inadequate responses to it. The major side effect is the associated increase in liver function enzymes that occurs in 5% of patients receiving leflunomide alone and in >50% of individuals taking leflunomide with methotrexate.

Surgery Surgery plays a role in the management of patients with severely damaged joints. Although arthroplasties and total joint replacements can be done on a number of joints, the most successful procedures are carried out on hips, knees, and shoulders. Realistic goals of these procedures are relief of pain and reduction of disability. Reconstructive hand surgery may lead to cosmetic improvement and some functional benefit. Open or arthroscopic synovectomy may be useful in some patients with persistent monarthritis, especially of the knee.

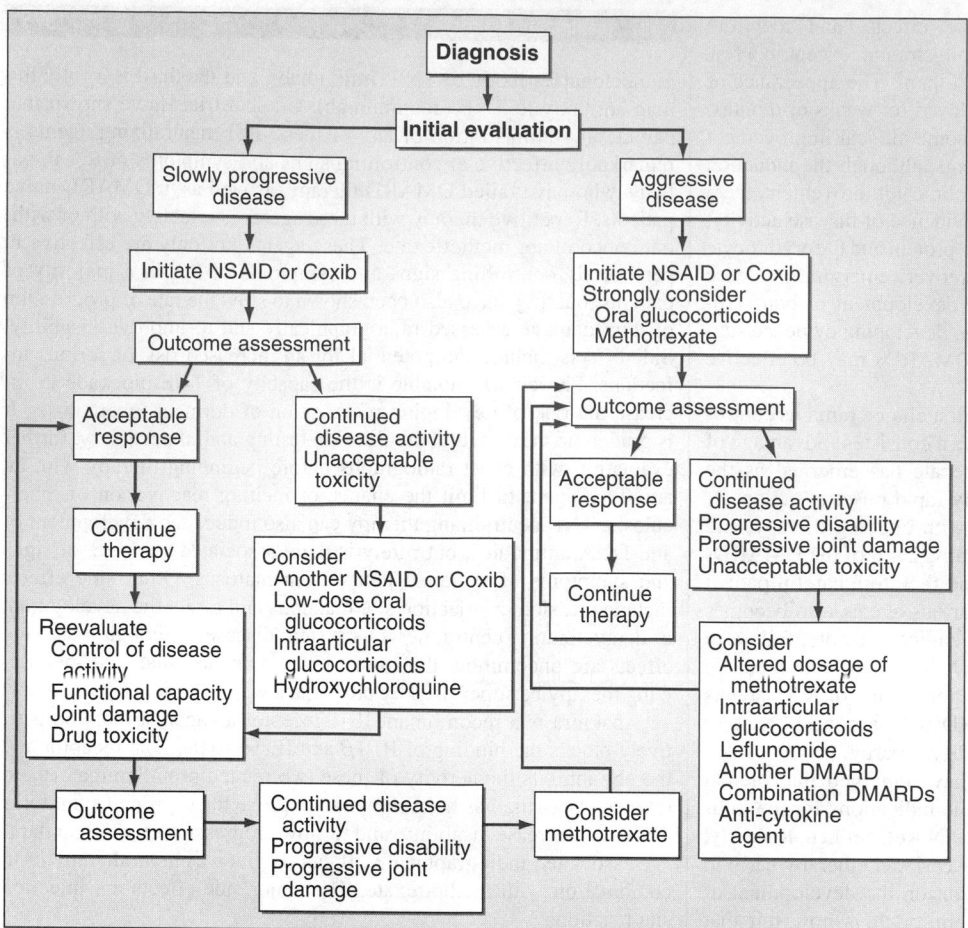

FIGURE 301-3 Algorithm for the medical management of rheumatoid arthritis. NSAID, nonsteroidal anti-inflammatory drug; Coxib, COX-2 inhibitors; DMARD, disease-modifying antirheumatic drug.

graphic evidence of cartilage loss is clear-cut evidence of the destructive potential of the inflammatory process and indicates the need for DMARD therapy. The other indications as outlined above, including persistent pain, joint swelling, or functional impairment, are much more subjective, however. As persistent inflammation, involvement of multiple joints, elevated levels of acute-phase reactants, and rheumatoid factor titers correlate with the development of disability and/or bony erosions, some have advocated the use of these prognostic indicators of aggressive disease in the decision to employ DMARDs early in the course of RA. The decision to begin use of a DMARD and/or low-dose oral glucocorticoids requires experience and clinical judgment as well as the ability to assess joint swelling and functional activity and the patient's pain tolerance and expectation of therapy accurately. In this setting, the fully informed patient must play an active role in the decision to begin DMARD and/or low-dose oral glucocorticoid therapy, after careful review of the therapeutic and toxic potential of the various drugs. If DMARD therapy, usually methotrexate, fails to control signs and symptoms of RA, a decision to add or switch to an anti-cytokine agent is considered. These are quite potent at controlling signs and symptoms of RA, slowing damage to articular structures, and limiting disability but are very expensive and associated with serious adverse events. The decision to employ these agents requires considerable experience, judgment, and the agreement of a fully informed patient.

If a patient responds to a DMARD, therapy is continued with careful monitoring to avoid toxicity. All DMARDs provide a suppressive effect and therefore require prolonged administration. Even with successful therapy, local injection of glucocorticoids may be necessary to diminish inflammation that may persist in a limited number of joints. In addition, NSAIDs or Coxibs may be necessary to mitigate symptoms. Even after inflammation has totally resolved, symptoms from loss of cartilage and supervening degenerative joint disease or altered joint function may require additional treatment. Surgery may also be necessary to relieve pain or diminish the functional impairment secondary to alterations in joint function. Recently an alternative approach to treat patients with RA has been suggested. This involves the initiation of therapy with multiple agents early in the course of disease in an attempt to control inflammation, followed by maintenance on one or more agents as necessary to control disease activity.

Although synovectomy may offer short-term relief of symptoms, it does not appear to retard bone destruction or alter the natural history of the disease. In addition, early tenosynovectomy of the wrist may prevent tendon rupture.

APPROACH TO THE PATIENT

An approach to the medical management of patients with RA is depicted in Fig. 301-3. The principles underlying care of these patients reflect the variability of the disease, the frequent persistent nature of the inflammation and its potential to cause disability, the relationship between sustained inflammation and bone erosions, and the need to reevaluate the patient frequently for symptomatic response to therapy, progression of disability and joint damage, and side effects of treatment. At the onset of disease it is difficult to predict the natural history of an individual patient's illness. Therefore, the usual approach is to attempt to alleviate the patient's symptoms with NSAIDs or Coxibs. Some patients may have mild disease that requires no additional therapy. However, if the patient has any evidence of aggressive disease, as described above, initiation of DMARD therapy should be considered as early as feasible. In RA patients there appears to be a window of opportunity early in the course of the disease, during which initiation of aggressive therapy can have a major impact on subsequent damage to articular structures and disability.

At some time during most patients' course, the possibility of initiating DMARD therapy and/or low-dose oral glucocorticoids is entertained. With aggressive disease this might occur sooner, often within 1 to 3 months of diagnosis, whereas in patients with more indolent disease, smoldering activity may not require such therapy for many years. The development of bone erosions or radio-

FURTHER READING

ARNETT FC et al: The American Rheumatism Association 1987 Revised Criteria for the Classification of Rheumatoid Arthritis. Arthritis Rheum 31: 315, 1988

CHOI HK et al: Methotrexate and mortality in patients with rheumatoid arthritis: A prospective study. Lancet 359:1173, 2002

DROSSAERS-BAKKER KW et al: Long-term outcome in rheumatoid arthritis: A simple algorithm of baseline parameters can predict radiographic damage, disability, and disease course at 12-year followup. Arthritis Rheum 47: 383, 2002

GOLDBACH-MANSKY R, LIPSKY PE: New concepts in the treatment of rheumatoid arthritis. Annu Rev Med 54:197, 2003

KWOH CK et al: Guidelines for the management of rheumatoid arthritis. 2002 Update. Arthritis Rheum 46:328, 2002

LIPSKY PE, DAVIS LS: The central involvement of T cells in rheumatoid arthritis. Immunologist 6:121, 1998

———— et al: Infliximab and methotrexate in the treatment of rheumatoid arthritis. Anti-Tumor Necrosis Factor Trial in Rheumatoid Arthritis with Concomitant Therapy Study Group. N Engl J Med 343:1594, 2000

VAN EVERDINGEN AA et al: Low-dose prednisone therapy for patients with early active rheumatoid arthritis: Clinical efficacy, disease-modifying properties, and side effects: A randomized, double-blind, placebo-controlled clinical trial. Ann Intern Med 136:1, 2002

302 RHEUMATIC FEVER
Edward L. Kaplan

In many parts of the world, especially in industrialized countries, acute rheumatic fever (ARF) is less common than it was during the early and mid-years of the twentieth century. In the late 1940s, patients with rheumatic fever (RF) and rheumatic heart disease accounted for more than half of schoolchildren recognized to have cardiovascular problems in the United States. During World War II, there were >20,000 cases of ARF in U.S. Navy personnel alone. The incidence of RF has declined remarkably in the industrialized countries of the world, where the disease has become rare. However, in many developing countries, which account for almost two-thirds of the world's population, streptococcal infections, RF, and rheumatic heart disease remain a very significant public health problem. The magnitude of the problem in these countries today is similar to that in North America 60 years ago.

The decreased incidence of ARF and the low prevalence of rheumatic heart disease in industrialized countries have led many physicians and public health authorities to the incorrect conclusion that these conditions are no longer a problem. However, starting in the 1980s, unexpected scattered outbreaks of ARF among both adults and children in North America have confirmed the capacity for this potentially serious illness to reappear and pose significant public health problems. As an example, >600 cases of ARF were seen in middle-class populations in Salt Lake City, Utah, between 1985 and the end of 2002. The disease continues to be a major public health problem in many developing countries of the world. Neither antimicrobial agents nor other public health measures have been totally effective in the control of RF in the industrialized or industrializing world.

EPIDEMIOLOGY The epidemiology of ARF is identical to that of group A streptococcal upper respiratory tract infections (Chap. 121). As is the case for streptococcal sore throat, ARF most often occurs in children; the peak age-related incidence is between 5 and 15 years. Most initial attacks in adults take place at the end of the second and beginning of the third decades of life. Rarely, initial attacks occur as late as the fourth decade, and recurrent attacks have been documented as late as the fifth decade.

Epidemiologic risk factors classically associated with individual attacks and especially with outbreaks of ARF include lower standards of living, especially crowding; the disease has been more common among socially and economically disadvantaged populations. However, the outbreaks in the United States in the late 1980s and early 1990s cannot be explained entirely by these factors. The large Utah outbreak of >600 cases during 17 years has affected primarily middle-class patients with ready access to medical care. Therefore, one can conclude that the organism itself as well as the degree of host/herd immunity to the prevalent M-types in an affected community are equally important risk factors.

Studies have shown that ~3% of individuals with untreated group A streptococcal pharyngitis will develop RF. The epidemiology of RF is also influenced by the serotypes of group A streptococci present in a population. The concept of "rheumatogenecity" of specific strains is largely based upon epidemiologic evidence associating certain serotypes with RF (serotypes 1, 3, 5, 6, 18, etc.). Mucoid isolates are frequently associated with virulence and with RF.

PATHOGENESIS More than half a century ago the pioneering studies of Lancefield differentiated β-hemolytic streptococci into serologic groups (Chap. 121). This ultimately led to the association of infection by the group A organism of the pharynx and tonsils (not of the skin) and the subsequent development of ARF. However, the mechanism(s) responsible for the development of RF after an infection remains incompletely defined. Historically, approaches to understanding the pathogenesis of RF have been grouped into three major categories: (1) direct infection by the group A streptococcus, (2) a toxic effect of streptococcal extracellular products on the host tissues, and (3) an abnormal or dysfunctional immune response to one or more as yet unidentified somatic or extracellular antigens produced by all (or perhaps only by some) group A streptococci ("antigenic mimicry.")

There is insufficient evidence to support direct infection of the heart as the inciting event. Additionally, while toxins such as streptolysin O and others have been postulated to have a pathogenetic role, there is relatively little convincing evidence of this at the present time. Major efforts have focused on an abnormal immune response by the human host to one or more group A streptococcal antigens.

The hypothesis of "antigenic mimicry" between human and group A streptococcal antigens has been studied extensively and has concentrated on two interactions. The first is the similarity between the group-specific carbohydrate of the group A streptococcus and the glycoprotein of heart valves; the second involves the molecular similarity among the streptococcal cell membrane, streptococcal M protein sarcolemma, and other moieties of the human myocardial cell. Investigators have studied tissue-specific antigens as well as major histocompatibility antigens in an attempt to define the pathogenesis.

The possibility of a predisposing genetic influence in some individuals is one of the most tantalizing of the incompletely understood factors that might contribute to susceptibility to RF. The precise genetic factors influencing the attack rate have never been adequately defined. Observations have been described that support the concept that this nonsuppurative sequel to a group A streptococcal upper respiratory tract infection results from an abnormal immune response by the human host. Thus, differences in immune responses to streptococcal antigens have been reported. Further, new data suggest that a unique surface marker on non-T lymphocytes in patients with RF and rheumatic heart disease may be associated with individuals who are susceptible to developing RF after a streptococcal infection because of abnormal immune responses; conclusive proof gained by prospective studies is not yet available.

DIAGNOSIS There is no specific laboratory test that can establish a diagnosis of RF. The diagnosis, therefore, is a clinical one but requires supporting evidence from the clinical microbiology and clinical immunology laboratories. Because of the variety of signs and symptoms associated with the RF syndrome, in 1944 Jones first proposed criteria to assist the clinician in standardizing the diagnosis of RF. The most recent modification of the *Jones criteria* (Updated Jones Criteria) was published in 1992 by a Special Writing Group of the American Heart Association (Table 302-1). A recent consideration of the Jones criteria by the American Heart Association has basically not resulted in change.

TABLE 302-1 *The Jones Criteria for Rheumatic Fever, Updated 1992*

Major Criteria	Minor Criteria
Carditis	Clinical
Migratory polyarthritis	Fever
Sydenham's chorea	Arthralgia
Subcutaneous nodules	Laboratory
Erythema marginatum	Elevated acute phase reactants
	Prolonged PR interval
plus	
Supporting evidence of a recent group A streptococcal infection (e.g., positive throat culture or rapid antigen detection test; and/or elevated or increasing streptococcal antibody test)	

Source: Modified from the Special Writing Group of the American Heart Association: JAMA 268:2069, 1992.

There are five criteria termed *major* because they are most commonly found in patients with RF: carditis, migratory polyarthritis, Sydenham's chorea, subcutaneous nodules, and erythema marginatum.

The *carditis* of ARF is a pancarditis involving the pericardium, myocardium, and endocardium. In most published series, between 40 and 60% of patients with ARF have evidence of carditis, which is characterized by one or more of the following: sinus tachycardia, the murmur of mitral regurgitation, an S_3 gallop, a pericardial friction rub, and cardiomegaly. The introduction of echocardiography has assisted in the identification of subtle abnormalities of the mitral valve, and these may be present in an additional 20% of patients who do not have an audible heart murmur. A prolonged PR interval and evidence of heart failure may be present as well, but these are nonspecific and may be found in a number of other diseases. Among the more controversial aspects of diagnosing RF has been the several reports of significant valvular (particularly of the mitral valve) involvement in the absence of audible murmurs. Although there are suggestions in the literature that echocardiographic criteria be included with the Jones criteria, the long-term follow-ups remain inadequate at the present time.

Healing of the rheumatic valvulitis may cause fibrous thickening and adhesion, resulting in the most serious complication of RF, i.e., valvular stenosis and/or regurgitation (Chap. 219). The mitral valve is involved most frequently, followed by the aortic valve. However, isolated aortic valve disease as a consequence of ARF is quite rare. In patients with aortic valve disease due to RF, the mitral valve is almost always simultaneously affected. Even minor degrees of rheumatic valvular involvement can lead to susceptibilities to infective endocarditis (Chap. 109). Although rheumatic pericarditis can cause a serous effusion, fibrin deposits, and even pericardial calcification, it does not lead to constrictive pericarditis.

A *migratory polyarthritis* is present in as many as 75% of cases, most often affecting the ankles, wrists, knees, and elbows over a period of days. It usually does not affect the small joints of the hands or feet and seldom involves the hip joints. Since salicylates and other anti-inflammatory drugs usually cause prompt resolution of joint symptoms, it is important that the clinician *not* prescribe these medications until it is determined whether the arthritis is migratory. The arthritis of ARF is extremely painful. Pain can be controlled with codeine or similar analgesics until the diagnosis is established. The difference between arthralgia (subjective joint pain) and arthritis (joint pain and swelling) must be understood. Too often, arthralgia is used (incorrectly) as a major criterion. An inflammatory reactive arthritis associated with streptococcal pharyngitis is often confused with the arthritis or arthralgias of ARF. Currently, several antibiotics have been promoted to be used in a <10-day course of therapy. The data at the present time are inconclusive as regards short-course therapy, and most recommendations at the present time recommend a full 10-day course of antibiotics orally for treatment of streptococcal pharyngitis.

Sydenham's chorea occurs in <10% of patients with RF. The latent period between the onset of the initiating streptococcal infection and the onset of Sydenham's chorea may be as long as several months. While differing from the other manifestations, this central nervous system disorder is a part of the RF complex and should be managed as such. Many patients who appear to have only chorea may present several decades later with evidence of typical rheumatic valvular disease. There is no definitive laboratory test for establishing a diagnosis of Sydenham's chorea, and the diagnosis is one of exclusion. Patients with Sydenham's chorea should be given secondary prophylaxis for prevention of recurrent attacks, even if they do not appear to have rheumatic heart disease.

Subcutaneous nodules and *erythema marginatum* are rare major manifestations, usually present in <10% of cases. Subcutaneous nodules are found over extensor surfaces of joints, are seen most often in patients with long-standing rheumatic heart disease, and are extremely rare in patients experiencing an initial attack. Erythema marginatum is an uncommon manifestation. It is an evanescent macular eruption with rounded borders—usually concentrated on the trunk.

The *minor criteria* (Table 302-1) are nonspecific and may be present in many clinical conditions.

To fulfill the Jones criteria, either two major criteria, or one major criterion and two minor criteria, *plus* evidence of an antecedent streptococcal infection are required. The latter may be provided by recovery of the organism on culture or by evidence of an immune response to one of the commonly measured group A streptococcal antibodies (e.g., anti-streptolysin O, anti-deoxyribonuclease B). Since the accurate diagnosis of RF has future medical and financial implications, the clinician is obligated to evaluate any patient completely until the suspected diagnosis is either established or excluded.

Both the clinical microbiology and the clinical immunology laboratories have important roles in confirming the diagnosis of RF. An attempt should be made to recover the organism from a throat culture, although group A streptococci can be recovered from the upper respiratory tract of only 25 to 40% of patients at the time the diagnosis is made. If a rapid antigen detection test is used but is negative, a confirmatory throat culture must be performed. It is helpful to obtain two or three cultures from the throat at the time the diagnosis is suspected, but before initiating antibiotic therapy, in order to confirm the presence of the organism.

At least 80% of patients with ARF have an elevated anti-streptolysin O titer at presentation. If one employs two additional streptococcal antibody tests such as the anti-DNAse B or anti-hyaluronidase test, the percentage of patients who show evidence of a preceding group A streptococcal infection will rise to >95%. While an initially elevated titer is convincing, being able to demonstrate a rise in titer from the acute to the convalescent phase is a more reliable means of documenting the recent infection. If three antibody tests are done and there is no evidence of a preceding infection, the diagnosis must be seriously reconsidered.

℞ TREATMENT

There are two necessary therapeutic approaches to patients with ARF: anti-streptococcal antibiotic therapy and therapy for the clinical manifestations of the disease. At the time of diagnosis, *all* patients with ARF should be treated as if they have a group A streptococcal infection, whether or not the organism is recovered by culture. In addition to the relatively large percentage of such patients who may have a negative throat culture at the time of diagnosis, others may have only a few organisms present in the throat. Conventional antibiotic treatment should be started immediately: a complete 10-day course in adults of either oral penicillin V (500 mg twice daily) or erythromycin (250 mg four times daily) for those with penicillin allergy. Many choose intramuscular benzathine penicillin G (a single intramuscular injection of 1.2 million units) for the treatment of the presumed streptococcal infection; this will also serve as the first dose of secondary prophylaxis for the prevention of recolonization of the upper respiratory tract in the future. Intramuscular benzathine penicillin G has been reported to result in a transient elevation of the erythrocyte sedimentation rate, which can prove confusing in the acute phase of the disease.

Following the initial anti-streptococcal therapy, secondary prophylaxis should be initiated to prevent subsequent infection of the upper respiratory tract with group A streptococci. Recommendations of the American Heart Association and of the World Health Organization are for intramuscular injection of 1.2 million units of benzathine penicillin G every 4 weeks or for oral penicillin V (250 mg twice daily) or oral sulfadiazine (1.0 g daily). Recent studies have shown that in those individuals who are at high risk for recurrence of RF, intramuscular benzathine penicillin G given every 3 weeks is more effective in reducing the risk of recurrence. Since it is known that the risk of recurrence of RF is highest during the first 5 years after the attack, secondary prophylaxis is always given for at least this period. After that the decision to continue or discontinue secondary prophylaxis is dependent upon whether the patient has documented rheumatic heart disease and whether the patient is at high risk of exposure to streptococci (e.g., students, school teachers, medical and military personnel). Many believe that those with documented recurrences and/or documented rheumatic valvular heart disease should receive secondary prophylaxis for life. The duration of prophylaxis is often individualized for specific patients.

Medical therapy for the manifestations of RF depends on the clinical status of the patient. For adult patients with the arthritis of RF, salicylates in doses escalating to 2 g four times daily are very effective and will result in marked clinical improvement, often within 12 h. When this prompt relief does not occur, one should reexamine the original diagnosis. Salicylates may be given for 4 to 6 weeks and gradually tapered so as to prevent a rebound. The erythrocyte sedimentation rate is one method for determining the rate of taper for salicylates. Usually this requires at least 2 weeks. There are no conclusive data to support using nonsteroidal anti-inflammatory drugs for ARF. There is no indication for the use of steroids (usually prednisone) solely for the treatment of the arthritis of RF.

Most experienced physicians believe that there is a role for steroids in patients with severe carditis accompanied by congestive heart failure. However, neither salicylates nor glucocorticoids influence the future development of valvular heart disease. In adults, prednisone can be started in doses as high as 30 mg four times daily in especially severe cases, and, as the patient improves, salicylates can be added during the tapering of the steroid dose; this may require 4 to 6 weeks.

In the presence of congestive heart failure, conventional medical measures (Chap. 216) are indicated. In the past, patients with ARF were kept at complete bed rest for months. This is inappropriate unless there is a specific reason such as persistent active carditis or severe heart failure. Patients with arthritis will begin to feel better very soon after anti-inflammatory therapy with salicylates is begun. They may be released from bed rest but should not resume full activity until signs of inflammatory process have abated and the acute-phase reactants have returned to normal.

FURTHER READING

BISNO AL et al: Practice guidelines for the diagnosis and management of group A streptococcal pharyngitis. (Infectious Disease Society of America.) Clin Infect Dis 35:113, 2002

COMMITTEE ON RHEUMATIC FEVER, ENDOCARDITIS AND KAWASAKI DISEASE OF THE COUNCIL ON CARDIOVASCULAR DISEASE IN THE YOUNG OF THE AMERICAN HEART ASSOCIATION: Treatment of acute streptococcal pharyngitis and prevention of rheumatic fever: A statement for health professionals. Pediatrics 96:758, 1995

DAJANI A: Rheumatic fever, in Braunwald's Heart Disease, 7th ed, DP Zipes et al (eds). Philadelphia, Saunders, 2005

FERRIERI P et al: Proceedings of the Jones Criteria Workshop. Special writing group of the American Heart Association. Circulation 106:2521, 2002

SHET A, KAPLAN EL: The clinical use and interpretation of group A streptococcal antibody tests: A practical approach for the pediatrician or primary care physician. Pediatr Infect Dis J 21:420, 2002

STEVENS DL, KAPLAN EL (eds): Streptococcal Infections: Clinical Aspects, Microbiology, and Molecular Pathogenesis. New York, Oxford Univ Press, 2000

303 SYSTEMIC SCLEROSIS (SCLERODERMA) AND RELATED DISORDERS
Bruce C. Gilliland

DEFINITION   Systemic sclerosis (SSc) is a chronic multisystem disorder of unknown etiology characterized clinically by thickening of the skin caused by accumulation of connective tissue and by structural and functional abnormalities of visceral organs, including the gastrointestinal tract, lungs, heart, and kidneys. Classification of SSc and scleroderma-like disorders is shown in Table 303-1. Vascular damage, immune activation, and excessive synthesis and deposition of extracellular matrix are prominent features of SSc. The degree and rate of skin and internal organ involvement vary among patients. Two subsets, however, can be identified, even though there is some overlap (Table 303-2). One subset is referred to as *diffuse cutaneous scleroderma* and is characterized by the rapid development of symmetric skin thickening of proximal and distal extremities, face, and trunk. These patients are at greater risk for developing kidney and other visceral disease early in their course. The other subset is *limited cutaneous scleroderma*, which is defined by symmetric skin thickening limited to distal extremities and face. This subset frequently has features of the *CREST syndrome*, standing for *c*alcinosis, *R*aynaud's phenomenon, *e*sophageal dysmotility, *s*clerodactyly, and *t*elangiectasia. The prognosis in limited cutaneous scleroderma is better except for those patients who, after many years, develop pulmonary arterial hypertension or biliary cirrhosis. Involvement of visceral organs may also occur in the absence of any skin involvement, which is referred to as *systemic sclerosis sine scleroderma*. Survival is determined by the severity of visceral disease, especially involving the lungs, heart, and/or kidneys.

TABLE 303-1 Classification of Scleroderma/Systemic Sclerosis and Scleroderma-Like Disorders

Systemic sclerosis
  Limited cutaneous disease
  Diffuse cutaneous disease
  Sine scleroderma
  Undifferentiated connective tissue disease
  Overlap syndromes
Localized scleroderma
  Morphea
  Linear scleroderma
  En coup de sabre
Chemically induced scleroderma-like disorders
  Toxic-oil syndrome
  Vinyl chloride–induced disease
  Bleomycin-induced fibrosis
  Pentazocine-induced fibrosis
  Epoxy- and aromatic hydrocarbons–induced fibrosis
  Eosinophilia-myalgia syndrome
Other scleroderma-like disorders
  Scleredema adultorum of Buschke
  Scleromyxedema
  Chronic graft-vs.-host disease
  Eosinophilic fasciitis
  Digital sclerosis in diabetes
  Primary amyloidosis and amyloidosis associated with multiple myeloma

TABLE 303-2 *Subsets of Systemic Sclerosis*

	Diffuse	Limited[a]
Skin involvement	Distal and proximal extremities, face, trunk	Distal to elbows, face
Raynaud's phenomenon	Onset within 1 year or at time of skin changes	May precede skin disease by years
Organ involvement	Pulmonary (interstitial fibrosis); renal (renovascular hypertensive crisis); gastrointestinal; cardiac	Gastrointestinal; pulmonary arterial hypertension after 10–15 years of disease in <10% of patients; biliary cirrhosis
Nail fold capillaries	Dilatation and dropout	Dilatation without significant dropout
Antinuclear antibodies	Anti-topoisomerase 1	Anticentromere

a Also referred to as CREST (*c*alcinosis, *R*aynaud's, *e*sophageal dysmotility, *s*clerodactyly, *t*elangiectasia).

Preliminary criteria for the classification of systemic sclerosis were developed by the American Rheumatism Association (now called the American College of Rheumatology) for the purpose of uniformity in clinical studies. A major criterion was the presence of sclerodermatous involvement proximal to the digits, affecting proximal portions of the extremities, face, neck, or trunk usually in a bilateral and symmetrical pattern. Sclerodactyly was almost always present. This single major criterion was present in 91% if SSc patients and in less than 1% of comparison disorders. Minor criteria were sclerodactyly, digital pitting scars or tissue loss of the volar pads of the fingertips, and bibasilar pulmonary fibrosis. The diagnosis of SSc was based on the presence of the major criterion or two or more minor criteria. The sensitivity of these criteria was 97%, and the specificity 98%. These criteria are not, however, applicable to clinical practice as some patients with limited cutaneous SSc do not meet these criteria. These patients may have esophageal and/or bowel dysmotility or pulmonary arterial hypertension without pulmonary fibrosis. Scleroderma can also occur in a localized form limited to the skin, subcutaneous tissue, and muscle and without systemic involvement. Localized scleroderma occurs most often in children and young women but can affect any age group. The two localized forms are *morphea*, which occurs as single or multiple plaques of skin induration, and *linear scleroderma*, which involves an extremity or the face. Linear scleroderma of one side of the forehead and scalp produces a disfiguration referred to as *en coup de sabre* because it resembles a wound from a sword. It may be associated with hemiatrophy of the same side of the face.

SSc also occurs in association with features of other connective tissue diseases. The term *overlap syndrome* has been used to describe such patients. Undifferentiated connective tissue disease has been suggested as a designation for patients who do not have diagnostic criteria for any one connective tissue disease. *Mixed connective tissue disease* (MCTD), a syndrome involving features of systemic lupus erythematosus (SLE), SSc, polymyositis, and rheumatoid arthritis and very high titers of circulating antibody to nuclear ribonucleoprotein (RNP) antigen, will be discussed later in the chapter. *Eosinophilic fasciitis* and the *eosinophilia-myalgia syndrome* (EMS) associated with contaminated L-tryptophan ingestion (Chap. 369) are scleroderma-like illnesses and will also be discussed in this chapter.

EPIDEMIOLOGY SSc has a worldwide distribution and affects all races. The onset of disease is unusual in childhood and young men. The incidence increases with age, peaking in the third to fifth decade. Women overall are affected approximately three times as often as men and even more often during the mid to late childbearing years (≥8:1). African Americans are affected approximately twice as frequently, have a lower age of onset, and more often have diffuse cutaneous involvement and pulmonary fibrosis than Caucasians. Hispanics and Native Americans may also have more severe disease than Caucasians. The annual incidence has been estimated to be 19 cases per million population. The reported prevalence of SSc is between 19 and 75 per 100,000 persons. An exceptionally high prevalence of SSc (469 per 100,000 persons) has been noted in the Choctaw Native Americans in Oklahoma—the highest found to date in any ethnic group. Both incidence and prevalence may be underestimated because patients with early and atypical disease may be overlooked in surveys. Genetic factors play a role in the susceptibility and expression of SSc. Familial aggregation for SSc has been reported in ~1.5% of SSc families. SSc in a first-degree relative is a very strong relative risk factor for SSc. There is also an increased incidence of other autoimmune diseases, including SLE and rheumatoid arthritis, as well as antinuclear antibodies in first-degree relatives of SSc patients. In a recent study, the rate of concordance of SSc in monozygotic twins was only 4.7%, the same as in dizygotic twins. The concordance for the presence of antinuclear antibodies was significantly greater in monozygotic twins (90%) than in dizygotic twins (40%). SSc-associated serum autoantibodies (see Laboratory Findings below) were found only in twins with SSc. The finding of antinuclear antibodies in spouses of SSc patients suggests that environmental factors are also involved in the development of antinuclear antibodies. Studies have not shown a strong association between human leukocyte antigens (HLA) and susceptibility to SSc. C4A null alleles (C4AQ0) and HLA-DQA2 have been reported by some investigators to be markers for disease susceptibility. In a recent study, the frequency of HLA-DQA1*0501 was increased in Caucasian men with SSc over healthy controls from the same geographic area. No one HLA type has been shown to be associated with disease susceptibility in all ethnic groups. A more consistent relationship has been found between certain HLA types and the occurrence of specific autoantibodies in SSc patients. Anticentromere antibodies have been shown to be associated with HLA-DRβ1*0101 and -DQβ1*0501 in Caucasians, African Americans, and Hispanics. Antitopoisomerase 1 antibodies, on the other hand, are associated most frequently with HLA-DRβ1*1101, *1104 and -DQβ1*0301 in Caucasians and African Americans, -DRβ1*1502 in Japanese, and -DRβ1*1602 in Chocktaw Native Americans.

Stronger evidence for a genetic role in SSc comes from studies of the Chocktaw Native Americans in Oklahoma who have a very high incidence of SSc. Affected individuals have in common diffuse cutaneous disease, pulmonary fibrosis, and antitopoisomerase antibodies. These autoantibodies are associated with the haplotype DQ 7, DR2 (DRβ1*1602) in this population of Native Americans. The association is stronger for the presence of antitopoisomerase antibodies than for the presence of SSc, as many individuals with autoantibodies do not have SSc. The extracellular fibrillin-1 matrix gene, FBN1, has also been found to be strongly associated with SSc in Chocktaw Native Americans. Not all SSc-affected individuals express the gene, and vice versa. The majority of Chocktaws were shown to produce autoantibodies to recombinant fibrillin-1 proteins. Of interest is that a tandem duplication of the murine gene, *fbn1*, in the tight-skin mouse (murine model of SSc) is thought to be responsible for the tight-skin mouse phenotype.

Infectious agents may play a role in the pathogenesis of SSc in the genetically susceptible individual. Latent cytomegalovirus (CMV) infection has been implicated in the vascular injury of SSc either by direct vascular injury or by immune-mediated mechanisms involving molecular mimicry in which viral and host proteins share similar amino acid sequences. Sera from SSc patients were shown to have antibodies that recognized an epitope contained within human CMV late protein UL94. This epitope is similar to a protein expressed in human endothelial cells. Incubation of SSc serum containing this antibody with endothelial cells was shown to induce apoptosis of endothelial cells, which is a feature of the vascular pathology observed in SSc. Parvovirus B19 has also been implicated in the development of SSc. In one study parvovirus B19 was detected in the bone marrow of >50% of SSc patients, compared to none in normal controls. Also, the frequency of anti-parvovirus B19 antibody was shown to be increased in SSc patients. The actual role of this virus or other micro-organisms in the pathogenesis of SSc awaits further studies.

Several environmental factors have been associated with the development of SSc and scleroderma-like illnesses. SSc appears to be more common in coal and gold miners, especially in those with more extensive exposure, suggesting that silica dust may be a predisposing factor. Workers exposed to polyvinyl chloride may develop Raynaud's phenomenon, acroosteolysis, scleroderma-like skin lesions, pulmonary fibrosis, and nail fold capillary abnormalities similar to those observed in SSc. These workers may also develop hepatic fibrosis and angiosarcoma. The observation that individuals exposed to similar amounts of vinyl chloride do not develop the same degree of disease suggests that a genetic factor may determine susceptibility and disease severity. The development of scleroderma has also been associated with exposure to epoxy resins and aromatic hydrocarbons such as benzine, toluene, and trichloroethylene. In 1981, in Spain, a multisystem disease resembling scleroderma occurred following the ingestion of aniline-adulterated cooking oil (rapeseed oil). Approximately 20,000 people were affected. The patients initially developed interstitial pneumonitis, eosinophilia, arthralgias, arthritis, and myositis, followed subsequently by joint contractures, skin thickening, Raynaud's phenomenon, pulmonary hypertension, sicca syndrome, and resorption of the distal fingertips. Extensive sclerosis of the dermis and subcutaneous tissue has been noted in patients receiving pentazocine, a nonnarcotic analgesic agent. Bleomycin, an anticancer agent, produces fibrotic skin nodules, linear hyperpigmentation, alopecia, Raynaud's phenomenon, gangrene of fingers, and pulmonary fibrosis affecting mainly the lower lobes. Scleroderma and other connective tissue diseases have been reported in women who have had silicone breast implants. Recent studies have not shown that women with these implants carry an increased risk for developing scleroderma or other connective tissue diseases. Localized fibrosis, however, can occur around the implant. While environmental factors or undefined infectious agents may be of etiologic significance, the cause of SSc remains unknown.

PATHOGENESIS The outstanding feature of SSc is overproduction and accumulation of collagen and other extracellular matrix proteins, including fibronectin, tenascin, fibrillin-1, and glycosaminoglycans, in skin and other organs. The disease process involves immunologic mechanisms, vascular endothelial cell activation and/or injury, and activation of fibroblasts resulting in production of excessive collagen (Fig. 303-1).

An early event in SSc that precedes fibrosis is vascular injury involving small arteries, arterioles, and capillaries in the skin, gastrointestinal tract, kidneys, heart, and lungs. Raynaud's phenomenon, the initial symptom of SSc in the majority of patients, is a clinical expression of the abnormal regulation of blood flow resulting from vascular injury. Injury to endothelial cells and basal lamina occurs early and is followed by proliferation of the intima and smooth-muscle cells, with deposition of matrix and perivascular fibrosis leading to narrowing of the lumen and eventual obliteration of the vessel. As vascular damage progresses, the microvascular bed in the skin and other sites is diminished, producing a state of chronic ischemia. Vascular abnormalities can be observed in the nail folds by wide-field microscopy, which shows drop-out of capillaries with dilatation and tortuosity of remaining ones. In the skin, remaining capillaries may proliferate and dilate to become visible telangiectasia. Endothelial cell damage is reflected in elevated levels of factor VIII/von Willebrand factor in the sera of some patients with SSc.

Several mechanisms for endothelial injury or activation have been proposed in SSc. Any or all of these mechanisms may be involved in a given patient; some evidence for each exists. A cytotoxic factor for endothelium has been identified in some patients that degrades the basal lamina, releasing fragments of type IV collagen and laminin. This factor, a type IV collagenase, is secreted by activated T cells and is referred to as *granzyme 1* because of its location in cytolytic T cells. Type IV collagen and laminin fragments may stimulate an immune response to the basal lamina. Both antibodies and cell-mediated immunity to type IV collagen and laminin have been observed in some SSc patients and may be involved in endothelial injury or may be an epiphenomenon. Anti-endothelial cell antibodies (AECA) may be another mechanism for microvascular damage. In 25% of SSc patients, AECA have been shown to mediate antibody-dependent cell cytotoxicity against human endothelial cells. Circulating AECA in general have been reported in the sera of SSc patients in amounts ranging from 21 to 85%. This wide variation reflects patient selection, type of assay, and the source of endothelium. These antibodies are not specific for SSc and are found in other connective tissue diseases. The frequency of AECA is higher in patients with diffuse cutaneous SSc. They have also been shown to be associated with digital infarcts, pulmonary hypertension, and impaired alveolocapillary diffusion. Studies have shown that AECA initiate programmed cell death (apoptosis) of endothelial cells, which may be an important event in the pathogenesis of SSc. These antibodies also induce expression of vascular cell adhesion molecule-1 (VCAM-1), intercellular adhesion molecule-1 (ICAM-1), E-selectin, and P-selectin on endothelial cells in SSc and stimulate the production of chemoattractants [interleukin (IL) 1, IL-8, monocyte chemotactic protein (MCP)], leading to the binding of T and B cells, natural killer cells, and monocytes to the endothelium and their migration into the perivascular tissue. Elevated serum levels of VCAM-1, ICAM-1, and P-selectin are observed in early stages of SSc.

The injury to the endothelium leads to a state favoring vasoconstriction and tissue ischemia. The damaged endothelium produces decreased amounts of prostacylin, which is an important vasodilator and inhibitor of platelet aggregation. Platelets are activated on binding to the damaged endothelium and release thromboxane, a potent vasoconstrictor. Activated platelets also release platelet-derived growth factor (PDGF), which is chemotactic and mitogenic for both smooth-muscle cells and fibroblasts, and transforming growth factor (TGF) β, which stimulates fibroblast collagen synthesis. These and other cytokines stimulate intimal fibrosis and, with their passage through the injured endothelium, may produce adventitial and perivascular fibrosis. Endothelin-1, a vasoconstricting factor released from endothelial cells on cold exposure, is also increased in SSc patients. In addition, it stimulates fibroblasts and smooth-muscle cells. The vasoconstriction action of endothelin-1 is normally opposed by endothelium-derived relaxation factor (EDRF, nitric oxide), also secreted by endothelial cells. The normal compensatory increase in EDRF is not seen in some patients with SSc, suggesting impairment of its synthesis. An increased α_2 adrenergic–mediated vasoconstriction has been demonstrated in SSc dermal arterioles. A deficiency of vasodilatory neuropeptides resulting from sensory system nerve damage may also produce a

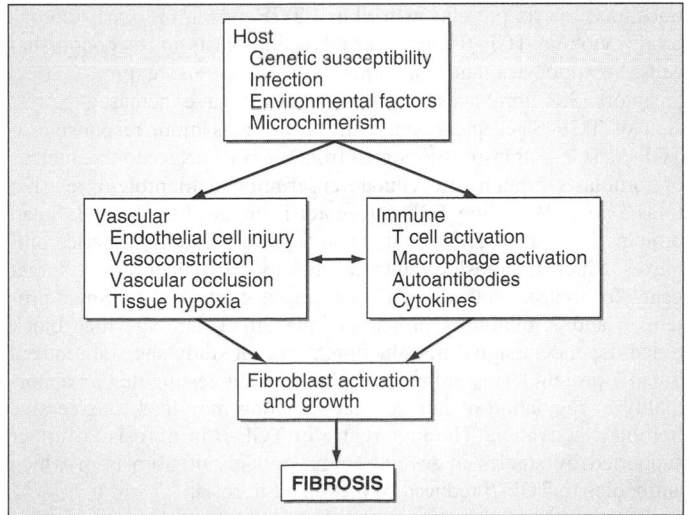

FIGURE 303-1 Algorithm for the multifactorial pathogenic mechanisms of systemic sclerosis.

condition favoring vasoconstriction. Vasoconstriction itself also contributes to endothelial damage through a mechanism of reperfusion injury. Following hypoxic endothelial injury from vasoconstriction, reperfusion can lead to release of oxygen free radicals, causing further tissue damage.

Existing evidence indicates that cell-mediated immunity plays a central role in the development of fibrosis in SSc. T cells, macrophages, endothelial cells, and other cells along with cytokines and growth factors interact in a complex manner to stimulate fibrosis. The vascular endothelium has been proposed as a target for cell-mediated immunity. Laminin and type IV collagen, components of the subendothelial basement membrane, induce in vitro transformation of lymphocytes from SSc patients. In the early stages of SSc, a mononuclear cell infiltrate consisting predominantly of activated helper-inducer T cells (T_H2 type) surrounds small blood vessels in the dermis. Subsequently, mononuclear cell infiltrates are found in macroscopically normal-appearing skin adjacent to areas of fibrosis. T cell hyperactivity is reflected by increased serum levels of CD4+ T cells. The ratio of CD4+ to CD8+ T cells is also increased. Elevated circulating levels of IL-2, a product of activated T cells, and IL-2 receptors have been shown to be associated with active fibrosis. In addition, serum levels of IL-4 are increased in SSc patients. IL-4, a product of activated T cells, stimulates fibroblast chemotaxis and proliferation and collagen production. In a recent study, CD8+ T cells isolated from bronchoalveolar lavage fluid from SSc patients made IL-4 and/or IL-5 mRNA. SSc patients with these type 2 cytokines were more likely to have alveolitis and a lower forced vital capacity. Although larger studies are needed, the findings suggest that these cytokines are involved in the pathogenesis of interstitial pulmonary fibrosis. Another cytokine, interferon γ, is produced by activated T cells (T_H1 type) and stimulates macrophages but inhibits collagen synthesis by fibroblasts. Reduced serum levels of interferon γ are found in some SSc patients. In vitro stimulation of T cells from SSc patients did not show an increased production of interferon γ compared to normal individuals, suggesting an inability in SSc patients to suppress fibrosis normally.

Macrophages are present in increased numbers in the infiltrates of SSc lesions, including the pulmonary alveoli. Activated macrophages secrete several important products involved in the pathogenesis of SSc including IL-1, IL-6, tumor necrosis factor (TNF) α, TGF-β, and PDGF. IL-1 has been shown to stimulate fibroblast proliferation and collagen synthesis. The important role for IL-6 may be in stimulating the local release of tissue inhibitor of metalloproteinase (TIMP) by fibroblasts and thereby limiting the breakdown of collagen. The role of TGF-β and PDGF secreted by macrophages and other cells is discussed below. In addition to the above cytokines, macrophages secrete *fibronectin*, a large matrix protein that is increased in SSc lesions. Fibronectin is also secreted by fibroblasts. Fibronectin interacts with collagen in the SSc lesions where it binds fibroblasts and mononuclear cells through receptors called *integrins*. Fibronectin functions as a chemoattractant and mitogen for fibroblasts.

Additional support for involvement of cell-mediated immunity in the pathogenesis of SSc is the appearance of scleroderma-like lesions in patients with graft-versus-host disease (GVHD) after bone marrow transplantation and in a murine model of chronic GVHD, conditions known to be associated with activated T cells. GVHD and SSc are both associated with progressive skin induration, joint contractures, and gastrointestinal and pulmonary involvement and are frequently accompanied by Sjögren's syndrome. Antinuclear antibodies are present in both diseases. Raynaud's phenomenon and kidney involvement are infrequent in GVHD.

Mast cells may also be involved in the development of fibrosis. Increased numbers of mast cells are found in the dermis in both involved and uninvolved skin. Mast cell degranulation has been noted in skin that subsequently became fibrosed. Interaction with T cells may be one mechanism for mast cell degranulation resulting in release of tryptase that stimulates fibroblast collagen synthesis. Release of histamine from mast cells may also contribute to edema observed in early disease.

Fibroblast growth and synthesis of collagen, fibronectin, and glycosaminoglycans are increased in SSc. The number of α-smooth muscle actin-positive fibroblasts is greatly increased in SSc lesions. Fibroblasts from SSc appear to have aberrant regulation of growth compared with fibroblasts from normal persons. When fibroblasts from affected SSc skin are removed and cultured in vitro, they continue to produce excessive quantities of collagen. The collagen is biochemically normal, and the proportion of type I to type III is the same as in normal skin. Fibroblasts from SSc patients appear to be in a state of permanent activation, due in part to autocrine and paracrine stimulation by TGF-β and connective tissue growth factor (CTGF). These activated cells are thought to represent an expanded subpopulation of fibroblasts that inherently express increased matrix genes. Studies have revealed a subpopulation of SSc fibroblasts that produces two to three times more collagen than other cells from the same tissue. Fibroblasts with a high-collagen-producing phenotype may be clonally selected by cytokines or other immune stimuli. Another explanation for the subpopulation of high-collagen-producing fibroblasts is that fibroblasts with low-collagen-producing phenotype may be selectively removed by apoptosis. Fibroblasts expressing elevated levels of mRNA for types I and III collagen have been demonstrated by in situ hybridization, particularly around dermal blood vessels in affected SSc skin. Collagen deposition is also initially perivascular in other organs including myocardium, muscle, and kidney. A small number of fibroblasts express increased levels of mRNA for types VI and VII collagen. Type VII collagen is normally found at the dermal-epidermal basement membrane zone and is the major component of anchoring fibrils that act to stabilize the attachment of the basement membrane to the underlying dermis. In SSc patients, type VII collagen is found throughout the dermis and may account for the indurated, tightly bound skin in this disease. PDGF receptors are expressed on SSc fibroblasts not only from affected areas but also from macroscopically normal-appearing skin. Fibroblasts from normal persons lack expression of these receptors. TGF-β has been shown to upregulate the expression of these receptors in SSc fibroblasts but not in normal cells and, in conjunction with PDGF, stimulates SSc fibroblast proliferation. Macrophages and fibroblasts are capable of secreting PDGF and TGF-β, and activated T cells release TGF-β. TGF-β also induces the synthesis of CTGF by fibroblasts, which further stimulates fibroblast proliferation and extracellular matrix proteins including collagen synthesis. CTGF mRNA and protein expression in SSc tissue are increased, and serum levels of CTGF have been found to be elevated in SSc and correlate with the degree of dermal and pulmonary fibrosis.

TGF-β is considered to play an essential role in mediating fibrosis in SSc. TGF-β stimulates fibroblast proliferation and synthesis of extracellular matrix proteins as well as CTGF, which in turn is a profibrotic cytokine. TGF-β is synthesized by fibroblasts and by endothelial cells, keratinocytes, and inflammatory cells that also express TGF-β receptors. SSc fibroblasts have been shown to have increased expression of TGF-β receptors, rendering these cells more responsive to TGF-β. TGF-β transmits its signal from the cell surface to the nucleus of fibroblasts through intracellular transcription factor proteins referred to as *Smads*. When the TGF-β receptor is engaged by TGF-β, Smad proteins 2, 3, and 4 are activated and assemble into multimeric complexes, which are translocated to the nucleus where they activate target genes for matrix synthesis. This pathway is controlled by Smad proteins 6 and 7, inhibitory proteins of the Smad family, which block Smad-dependent signal transduction. A recent study showed reduced Smad 7 protein levels in involved SSc skin, suggesting that an abnormality in regulation of intracellular signaling may lead to excessive fibroblast activation. The importance of TGF-β in fibrosis is further supported by studies in several animal models of fibrosis in which antibodies to TGF-β reduced or prevented fibrosis.

Recent studies have suggested that microchimerism may be involved in the pathogenesis of SSc. Microchimerism in SSc is of interest because of the clinical similarities between SSc and GVHD after allogeneic bone marrow transplantation. Also relevant are the predilection for women in SSc and the increased incidence of SSc in women after the childbearing years. Fetal progenitor cells can persist in the serum of normal women for many years after childbirth. Microchimerism can also occur in nulligravid women and in men with SSc as non-host cells may come from blood transfusion, engraftment of cells from a twin, or from maternal cells in utero. Two-directional traffic of cells occurs during pregnancy. Compared to normal controls, both the quantity and frequency of immune fetal cells have been found to be increased in the serum of SSc patients. The mechanism by which microchimerism is involved in the pathogenesis is not known, but it is conceivable that these small numbers of non-host cells alter immune regulation, leading to autoimmunity.

Chromosomal abnormalities have been noted in >90% of SSc patients. These acquired abnormalities include chromatid breaks, acentric fragments, and ring chromosomes and are found in ~30% of mitotic cells. A chromosomal breakage factor has been found in the serum of SSc patients and their first-degree relatives. The significance of these chromosomal abnormalities is unknown.

PATHOLOGY ■ **Skin** In the skin, a thin epidermis overlies compact bundles of collagen that lie parallel to the epidermis. Fingerlike projections of collagen extend from the dermis into the subcutaneous tissue and bind the skin to the underlying tissue. Dermal appendages are atrophied, and rete pegs are lost. In early stages of disease, a mononuclear cell infiltrate of predominantly T cells surrounds small dermal blood vessels. Increased numbers of T cells, monocytes, plasma cells, and mast cells are found, particularly in the lower dermis of involved skin.

Gastrointestinal Tract In the lower two-thirds of the esophagus, the histologic findings consist of a thin mucosa and increased collagen in the lamina propria, submucosa, and serosa. The degree of fibrosis is less than in the skin. Atrophy of the muscularis in the esophagus and throughout the involved portions of the gastrointestinal tract is more prominent than the amount of fibrotic replacement of muscle. Ulceration of the mucosa is often present and may be due to either SSc or superimposed peptic esophagitis. Chronic esophageal reflux can lead to metaplasia of the lower esophagus (Barrett's esophagus), which is a premalignant lesion. Striated muscles in the upper third of the esophagus are relatively spared. Similar changes may be found throughout the gastrointestinal tract, especially in the second and third portions of the duodenum, in the jejunum, and in the large intestine. Atrophy of the muscularis of the large intestine may lead to the development of large-mouth diverticula. In the later stages of the disease, the involved portions of the gastrointestinal tract become dilated. Infiltration of lymphocytes and plasma cells in the lamina propria is also present.

Lung With pulmonary involvement, diffuse interstitial fibrosis, thickening of the alveolar membrane, and peribronchial and pleural fibrosis are observed. Bronchiolar epithelial proliferation accompanies the pulmonary fibrosis. Rupture of septa produces small cysts and areas of bullous emphysema. Small pulmonary arteries and arterioles show intimal thickening, fragmentation of the elastica, and muscular hypertrophy; this may occur without interstitial pulmonary fibrosis and produce pulmonary hypertension, particularly in a subset of patients with limited cutaneous SSc.

Musculoskeletal System The synovium in patients with arthritis is similar to that seen in early rheumatoid arthritis and shows edema with infiltration of lymphocytes and plasma cells. A characteristic finding is a thick layer of fibrin overlying and within the synovium. Later in the disease the synovium may become fibrotic. Fibrinous deposits appear on the surfaces of tendon sheaths and in the overlying fascia and may lead to audible creaking over moving tendons.

Histologic features of primary myopathy consist of interstitial and perivascular lymphocytic infiltrations, degeneration of muscle fibers, and interstitial fibrosis. Arterioles may be thickened, and capillaries may be decreased in number. Pathologic and electrophysiologic findings of polymyositis in proximal muscles are present in the few pa-

tients who are considered to have the overlap syndrome of SSc and polymyositis.

Heart Cardiac involvement consists of degeneration of myocardial fibers and irregular areas of interstitial fibrosis that are most prominent around blood vessels. Intermittent spasm of blood vessels may result in contraction band necrosis, similar to changes observed in myocardial infarction in patients with atherosclerotic coronary artery disease. Fibrosis also involves the conduction system, leading to atrioventricular conduction defects and arrhythmias. The wall of smaller coronary arteries may be thickened. Fibrinous pericarditis and pericardial effusions are found in some patients.

Kidney Renal involvement is found in over half the patients and consists of intimal hyperplasia of the interlobular arteries; fibrinoid necrosis of the afferent arterioles, including the glomerular tuft; and thickening of the glomerular basement membrane. Small cortical infarctions and glomerulosclerosis may be present. The renal pathologic change is often indistinguishable from that observed in malignant hypertension. Renal vascular lesions, however, may be present in the absence of hypertension. Immunofluorescence studies of kidney have shown IgM, complement components, and fibrinogen in the walls of affected vessels. Angiographic renal studies in patients with SSc may show constriction of the interlobular arteries, a finding that simulates the vasospasm of the digital arteries observed in Raynaud's phenomenon. Cold-induced Raynaud's phenomenon has been shown to decrease renal blood flow.

Other Organs Primary liver involvement is not common. Primary biliary cirrhosis occurs in some patients, particularly in those with the limited cutaneous form of SSc. Fibrosis of the thyroid gland may develop in the presence or absence of autoimmune thyroiditis.

Thickening of the periodontal membrane with replacement of the lamina dura is demonstrated radiographically as widening of the periodontal space and may cause gingivitis and loosening of the teeth. The decreased oral aperture and mucosal dryness make eating and oral hygiene difficult.

CLINICAL MANIFESTATIONS (See Table 303-3) ■ **Raynaud's Phenomenon** SSc usually begins insidiously; the first symptoms are frequently Raynaud's phenomenon and puffy fingers. Some 95% of patients will experience Raynaud's phenomenon, which is defined as episodic vasoconstriction of small arteries and arterioles of fingers, toes, and sometimes the tip of the nose and earlobes. Episodes are brought on by cold exposure, vibration, or emotional stress. Patients experience pallor and/or cyanosis followed by rubor on rewarming. Pallor and/or cyanosis are usually associated with coldness and numbness of fingers and/or toes, and rubor with pain and tingling. Not all patients appreciate the three color phases. A history of digit pallor appears to be the most reliable symptom for the presence of Raynaud's phenomenon.

TABLE 303-3 *Clinical Features of Systemic Sclerosis*

Clinical Feature	% Patients during Course of Disease	
	Limited[a]	Diffuse[a]
Raynaud's phenomenon	95–100	90–95
Skin thickening	98[b]	100
Subcutaneous calcinosis	50	10
Telangiectasia	85	40
Arthralgias/arthritis	40	70
Myopathy	5	50
Esophageal dysmotility	80	80
Pulmonary fibrosis	35	40
Isolated pulmonary arterial hypertension	<10	<1
Congestive heart failure	<1	30
Renal crisis	<1	15

[a] Limited cutaneous and diffuse cutaneous subsets of SSc.
[b] 2% or fewer of patients have SSc sine scleroderma.

FIGURE 303-2 Swollen hands and fingers in early systemic sclerosis. Swelling may also involve forearms, distal lower extremities, and face. Edematous phase may last weeks to months or even longer.

Raynaud's phenomenon may precede skin changes by several months or even years in those patients who subsequently develop the limited cutaneous form of SSc. In diffuse cutaneous SSc, skin changes are seen typically within a year of the onset of Raynaud's phenomenon. After 2 or more years of Raynaud's phenomenon, few patients who have this as their only symptom will subsequently develop SSc.

Skin Features　In early disease, fingers and hands are swollen (Fig. 303-2). Swelling may also involve forearms, feet, lower legs, and face. However, lower extremities are relatively spared. This edematous phase may last for a few weeks, months, or even longer. The edema may be pitting or nonpitting and accompanied by erythema. The skin changes begin distally in the extremities and advance proximally. The skin gradually becomes firm, thickened, and eventually tightly bound to underlying subcutaneous tissue (indurative phase). In patients with diffuse cutaneous scleroderma, skin changes will become generalized, involving initially the extremities, followed by the face and trunk over a period of time, varying from months to a few years. In some patients, the skin changes may develop gradually over several years. Rapid progression of these changes over a 1- to 3-year period is associated with a greater risk of visceral disease, particularly of the lungs, heart, or kidneys. Also in diffuse cutaneous SSc, the skin changes usually peak in 3 to 5 years and then slowly improve. On the other hand, patients with limited cutaneous scleroderma will usually have a more gradual progression of skin changes, which are restricted to fingers or distal extremity and face and may continue to worsen. In both subsets of SSc, skin thickening is usually greater in the distal extremity. After many years of disease, the skin may soften and return to normal thickness or become thin and atrophic.

In the extremities, the taut skin over fingers gradually limits full extension, and flexion contractures develop (Fig. 303-3). Ulcers may appear on the volar pads of the fingertips and over bony prominences such as elbows, malleoli, and the extensor surface of the proximal interphalangeal joints of the hands. These ulcers may become secondarily infected. The volar pads of the fingertips develop pitting scars and lose soft tissue. In some instances, resorption of the terminal phalanges occurs. Skin over the extremities, face, and trunk may become darkly pigmented, even without exposure to the sun. Hyperpigmentation of the skin may occur over superficial blood vessels and tendons. Areas of hypopigmentation may also develop, similar to vitiligo, involving the eyebrows, scalp, and trunk. The sparing of pigment around hair follicles gives the skin a "salt-and-pepper" appearance. Other patients may develop a diffuse tanning of the skin. The skin loses hair, oil, and sweat glands and so becomes dry and coarse. Vaginal dryness occurs and may cause dyspareunia.

In some patients, particularly those with the limited cutaneous form of disease, calcific deposits develop in intracutaneous and subcutaneous tissue. The sites commonly involved are periarticular tissue, digital

pads, olecranon and prepatellar bursae, and skin along the extensor surface of the forearms. The overlying skin may break down, with drainage of calcific material. Involvement of the face results in thinning of the lips, loss of skin wrinkles and facial expression, as well as microstomia, which may make eating and dental hygiene difficult (Fig. 303-4). The nose takes on a pinched or beaklike appearance. Wrinkles appear around the mouth perpendicular to the lips. Small telangiectatic mats may appear on the fingers, face, lips, tongue, and buccal mucosa after several years. They are seen more frequently in patients with limited cutaneous SSc but are also observed in patients with long-standing diffuse cutaneous SSc. The capillary beds of nail folds of the fingers may show enlargement of capillaries with little or no capillary loss, usually indicative of limited cutaneous scleroderma. In diffuse cutaneous scleroderma, there is disorganization of the capillary beds with dilated capillaries interspersed with areas where capillaries have disappeared (Fig. 303-5). These capillary changes, which are observed by wide-angle microscopy or with an ophthalmoscope used as a magnifier, are not found in patients who have only Raynaud's phenomenon.

Musculoskeletal Features　More than half the patients with SSc complain of pain, swelling, and stiffness of the fingers and knees. A symmetric polyarthritis resembling rheumatoid arthritis may be seen. In more advanced stages of the disease, leathery crepitation can be palpated over moving joints, especially the knee. Extensive fibrotic thickening of the tendon sheaths in the wrist can produce a carpal tunnel syndrome. Muscle weakness is usually present in patients with severe skin involvement and, in most cases, is due to disuse atrophy. There is a distinctive histologic myopathy that accompanies SSc that is not associated with muscle enzyme abnormalities. A few patients develop a myositis characterized by proximal muscle weakness and muscle enzyme elevations that are identical to polymyositis (overlap syndrome). In addition to terminal phalanges, resorption of bone may involve ribs, clavicle, and angle of mandible.

Gastrointestinal Features　The majority of patients from both subsets of SSc have gastrointestinal involvement. Symptoms attributable to esophageal involvement are present in >50% of patients and include epigastric fullness, burning pain in the epigastric or retrosternal regions, and regurgitation of gastric contents. These symptoms, most noticeable when the patient is lying flat or bending over, are due to the reduced tone of the gastroesophageal sphincter and to dilatation of the distal esophagus. Peptic esophagitis frequently occurs and may lead to strictures and narrowing of the lower esophagus. However, it seldom results in bleeding. Barrett's metaplasia may develop, but transition to adenocarcinoma is uncommon. Dysphagia, particularly of solid foods, may occur independent of other esophageal symptoms and is caused by loss of esophageal motility due to neuromuscular dys-

FIGURE 303-3 Flexion deformities of the fingers and sclerodactlyly. The skin over the fingers and hands is taunt and indurated. There is shortening and bony resorption of distal phalanges of the second and third fingers. Ulcers may develop over the distal phalanges and dorsal surfaces of the metacarpal phalangeal and proximal interphalangeal joints.

FIGURE 303-4 Skin over cheeks and forehead is tight and shiny with loss of wrinkles and facial expression. There are furrows around the mouth perpendicular to the lips and the lips are thin. The nose has a pinched appearance.

function. Manometry or cineradiography reveals decreased amplitude or disappearance of peristaltic waves in the lower two-thirds of the esophagus. Raynaud's phenomenon in the absence of a connective tissue disease is also associated with esophageal dysmotility. Later in the course of the illness, dilatation and atony of the lower portion of the esophagus as well as reflux are seen. With gastric involvement, barium studies show dilatation, atony, and delayed gastric emptying. Patients may complain of early satiety. Gastric outlet obstruction can also occur.

Hypomotility of the small intestine produces symptoms of bloating and abdominal pain and may suggest an intestinal obstruction or paralytic ileus (pseudoobstruction). Malabsorption syndrome with weight loss, diarrhea, and anemia is due to bacterial overgrowth in the atonic intestine or possibly to obliteration of lymphatics by fibrosis. Roentgenographic features of the second and third portions of the duodenum and of the jejunum include dilatation, loss of the usual feathery pattern, and delayed disappearance of barium. Pneumatosis intestinalis occasionally occurs and appears as radiolucent cysts or linear streaks within the wall of the small intestine. Benign pneumoperitoneum may result from the rupture of these cysts. Involvement of the large intestine may cause chronic constipation and fecal impaction with episodes of bowel obstruction. A segment of atonic bowel may act as a fulcrum for intussuception to occur. Barium studies of the large intestine may show dilatation, atony, and large-mouth diverticula. Laxity of the anal sphincter may cause incontinence or rarely anal prolapse. Some patients may have gastrointestinal features of SSc with little or no cutaneous or other organ involvement, referred to as *SSc sine*

FIGURE 303-5 Nail fold capillaries in normal person (*left panel*) and in scleroderma patient (*right panel*). Capillary loops are found just proximal to the cuticle using a wide angle microscope, a dermatoscope, or an opthalmoscope serving as a magnifier. Immersion oil is placed over the nail fold to reduce reflection of light. *Left panel*: Capillary loops are small and well organized being parallel to each other and perpendicular to the nail. *Right panel*: Enlarged dilated capillary loops are interspersed with areas where capillaries have disappeared.

scleroderma. Vascular ectasia may develop in the stomach and intestine and can be the source of gastrointestinal bleeding. These dilated submucosal capillaries in the stomach appear on endoscopy as broad stripes—hence the term *watermelon stomach*.

Pulmonary Features Pulmonary involvement occurs in at least two-thirds of SSc patients and is now the leading cause of death in SSc, replacing renal disease, which can usually be treated effectively. The most common symptom is exertional dyspnea, often accompanied by a dry, nonproductive cough. Bilateral basilar rales may be present. In the majority of patients, symptoms usually correlate with radiologic evidence of pulmonary fibrosis and with restrictive lung disease on pulmonary function tests.

Pulmonary function tests are frequently abnormal and show a reduction in vital capacity and decreased lung compliance. Impairment of gas exchange is reflected by a low diffusing capacity and low P_{O_2} with exercise. These abnormalities may be present even when the chest radiograph is normal. Chest film may show a pattern of linear densities, mottling, and honeycombing involving most prominently the lower two-thirds of the lung. Early interstitial pulmonary disease can be detected by high-resolution computed tomography (HRCT) and bronchoalveolar lavage (BAL). Active inflammatory alveolitis gives a "ground glass" appearance on HRCT. The recovery by BAL of increased numbers of cells, mostly alveolar macrophages accompanied by neutrophils or eosinophils, is evidence for alveolitis.

Both interstitial fibrosis and vascular lesions are found in the lungs of patients with SSc. Interstitial pulmonary fibrosis may be the predominant lesion in patients with diffuse or limited cutaneous SSc. Patients with diffuse cutaneous involvement who have antitopoisomerase 1 antibodies are particularly at risk of developing severe pulmonary fibrosis. In the absence of significant interstitial fibrosis, a severe form of pulmonary arterial hypertension may develop after many years of disease in a subset of patients with limited cutaneous SSc. Fewer than 10% of patients will develop this complication, which is caused by narrowing and obliteration of pulmonary arteries and arterioles by intimal fibrosis and medial hypertrophy. Pulmonary hypertension is manifested initially by exertional dyspnea and eventually by the appearance of right-sided heart failure. Pulmonary artery pressure can be measured noninvasively by two-dimensional echocardiography. The prognosis is extremely poor with the development of pulmonary hypertension; the mean duration of survival is ~2 years.

A less common pulmonary problem is aspiration pneumonia resulting from gastric reflux due to lower esophageal atony. Restriction of chest movement caused by extensive fibrotic skin involvement of the thorax rarely occurs. Superimposed bacterial or viral infection can be a serious complication in patients with pulmonary fibrosis. An increased frequency of alveolar cell and bronchogenic carcinoma is seen in patients with pulmonary fibrosis.

Cardiac Features Primary cardiac involvement in SSc includes pericarditis with or without effusions, heart failure, and varying degrees of heart block or arrhythmias. The majority of patients with diffuse cutaneous SSc have cardiac abnormalities. Cardiomyopathy attributable to myocardial fibrosis appears in <10% of patients and involves primarily those patients with diffuse cutaneous scleroderma. Radionuclide studies have shown abnormalities of left ventricular function due to myocardial fibrosis. Cold-induced vasospasm of the hands produces defects in myocardial thallium perfusion. The characteristic pathologic feature of contraction band necrosis results from cardiac muscle damage caused by intermittent vasospasm of coronary vessels. Patients may experience angina pectoris even though coronary angiograms are normal. Patients can also develop left ventricular failure secondary to systemic hypertension or cor pulmonale secondary to pulmonary arterial hypertension.

Renal Features Renal failure was the leading cause of death in SSc until the advent of effective treatment. Significant renal disease occurs mostly in those patients with diffuse cutaneous scleroderma. A high risk of renal crisis is present in those patients who have rapidly progressive widespread skin thickening in their first 2 to 3 years of disease. Renal crisis is characterized by malignant hypertension, which can progress rapidly to renal failure. These patients manifest hypertensive encephalopathy, severe headache, retinopathy, seizures, and left ventricular failure. Hematuria and proteinuria are followed by oliguria and renal failure. The mechanism for the hypertensive crisis is activation of the renin-angiotensin system. Before the advent of effective antihypertensive drugs, the majority of these patients died within 6 months. A small number of patients may develop renal crises in the absence of hypertension. Renal failure can also develop insidiously later in the course of disease in the setting of mild to moderate hypertension and proteinuria. In these patients or those with clinically unrecognized renal disease, reduction of renal plasma flow secondary to heart failure or volume depletion resulting from overdiuresis may precipitate renal crisis. An indicator of impending renal failure is microangiopathic anemia, which may occur in a normotensive patient. The presence of a large chronic pericardial effusion may also herald subsequent renal failure.

Other Features   Symptoms of dry eyes and/or dry mouth are frequently present in patients with SSc. Lip biopsy may show lymphocytic infiltration of minor salivary glands characteristic of Sjögren's syndrome or intraglandular or periglandular fibrosis secondary to SSc. Antibodies to SS-A (Ro) and/or SS-B (La) are found in those patients with lip biopsies consistent with Sjögren's syndrome (overlap syndrome-SSc and Sjögren's syndrome) and not in those with salivary gland fibrosis.

Hypothyroidism occurs in a significant number of patients and may be associated with high levels of antithyroid antibodies. Fibrosis of the thyroid gland may be present but also occurs in the absence of autoimmune thyroiditis. Other manifestations of SSc include trigeminal neuralgia and male impotence secondary to decreased penile tumescence. These men have normal serum levels of testosterone and gonadotropins. Pathogenesis of this abnormality has been considered to be caused by vascular and/or autonomic nervous system abnormalities. Biliary cirrhosis is occasionally observed in patients with limited cutaneous SSc.

LABORATORY FINDINGS   The erythrocyte sedimentation rate may be elevated. Hypoproliferative anemia related to chronic inflammation is the most common cause of anemia in SSc. Anemia may also be caused by iron deficiency secondary to gastrointestinal bleeding. Bacterial overgrowth due to atony of the small bowel may lead to vitamin B_{12} and/or folic acid–deficiency anemia. Microangiopathic hemolytic anemia is most often associated with renal involvement and is caused by the presence of intravascular fibrin in renal arterioles. Polyclonal hypergammaglobulinemia, consisting mostly of IgG, is found in approximately half the patients. Rheumatoid factor, in low titer, is present in 25% of patients. Cryoglobulins may be present in the serum. Antinuclear antibodies detected by using a cultured human laryngeal carcinoma cell line (HEp-2) substrate are present in 95% of patients (Table 303-4). Antinuclear antibodies that have a high specificity for SSc are antitopoisomerase 1 (Scl-70), antinucleolar, and anticentromere. Antitopoisomerase 1, originally called anti-Scl-70, recognizes the nuclear enzyme DNA topoisomerase 1, a nuclear enzyme involved in the unwinding of DNA for replication and RNA transcription. These antibodies are found in ~20% of all SSc patients and in ~40% of those with diffuse cutaneous SSc. They are associated with diffuse cutaneous involvement, interstitial pulmonary disease, and renal and other visceral organ involvement. A very high frequency of these antibodies has been reported in Choctaw Native Americans in association with diffuse cutaneous SSc. They are seldom present in other disorders or in conjunction with anticentromere antibodies. Anticentromere antibodies react with protein antigens located in the kinetochore region of chromosomes and are present in 40 to 80% of patients with limited cutaneous scleroderma or CREST syndrome. Anticentromere antibod-

TABLE 303-4 *Autoantibodies in Systemic Sclerosis*

Autoantibody	Clinical Association	Percent[a]
Anti-topoisomerase 1	Diffuse cutaneous SSc	40
Anticentromere	Limited cutaneous SSc	60–80
Anti-RNA polymerase I, II, III	Diffuse cutaneous SSc	5–40
Anti-Th RNP	Limited cutaneous SSc	14
Anti-U$_1$ RNP	Limited cutaneous SSc	5–10
	Mixed connective tissue disease	95–100
Anti-U$_3$ RNP[b]	Diffuse and limited cutaneous SSc, skeletal myopathy, pulmonary arterial hypertension	5
Anti-PM/Scl	Overlap (SSc, polymyositis)	25

[a] Approximate percentages for the predominant clinical association.
[b] Anti-fibrillarin.

ies are found in only about 2 to 5% of patients with diffuse cutaneous scleroderma and rarely in other connective tissue diseases. They are found occasionally in patients with only Raynaud's phenomenon and may indicate subsequent development of limited cutaneous disease. Antinucleolar antibodies are relatively specific for SSc and are present in ~20 to 30% of patients. Several antinucleolar antibodies have been associated with SSc: Anti-RNA polymerases I, II, and III are found in patients with diffuse cutaneous SSc who have a higher prevalence of renal and cardiac involvement. Anti-Th RNP has been found in patients with limited cutaneous SSc, and anti-PM-Scl, formerly referred to as anti-PM1, along with anti-Ku, may be found in a subset of patients with overlapping features of limited cutaneous SSc and polymyositis. Anti-U$_3$ RNP (anti-fibrillarin) is also highly specific for SSc and may be associated with skeletal muscle disease, bowel involvement, and pulmonary arterial hypertension. Anti-U$_1$ RNP is found in ~5 to 10% of SSc patients and in 95 to 100% of those patients with the overlap syndrome of MCTD. The titers in MCTD are usually high (see below). Anti-SS-A (Ro) and/or anti-SS-B (La) are present in those patients with overlap syndrome of SSc and Sjögren's syndrome.

DIAGNOSIS   The diagnosis of SSc presents no difficulty in the presence of Raynaud's phenomenon, with typical skin lesions and visceral involvement. Although Raynaud's phenomenon may be the first symptom of SSc, most patients with Raynaud's phenomenon alone do not develop a connective tissue disease. Other causes of Raynaud's phenomenon include thoracic outlet (scalenus anticus and cervical rib) syndromes, shoulder-hand syndrome, trauma (jackhammer or vibratory machine operators), previous cold injury, vinyl chloride exposure, and circulating cryoglobulins or cold agglutinins. Linear scleroderma and morphea are localized forms of scleroderma that can usually be distinguished clinically. In early disease, SSc may initially be confused with rheumatoid arthritis, SLE, or polymyositis when articular or muscle involvement is prominent. SSc without cutaneous involvement should be considered in patients with unexplained pulmonary fibrosis, pulmonary hypertension, cardiomyopathies, heart block, dysphagia, or malabsorption syndrome. Several conditions have scleroderma-like features but lack the visceral involvement. Scleredema (scleredema adultorum of Buschke) occurs predominantly in children and is characterized by painless edematous induration involving the face, scalp, neck, trunk, and proximal portions of the extremities. Involvement of the hands and feet usually does not occur. Scleredema may be associated with previous streptococcal infection and is usually self-limited, resolving in 6 to 12 months. Histology reveals accumulation of mucopolysaccharides in the dermis and skeletal muscle. A rare entity, scleromyxedema is manifested by yellowish or pale red papules in association with diffuse skin thickening that may involve the face and hands. Acid mucopolysaccharide deposits are found in the dermis. Monoclonal IgG may be detected in some of these patients. Patients with insulin-dependent diabetes mellitus may develop digital sclerosis and contractures (prayer hand deformity). Primary amyloidosis and amyloidosis associated with multiple myeloma may involve the skin of the extremities and face diffusely to give the appearance of scleroderma. Biopsy will clearly differentiate these entities.

COURSE AND PROGNOSIS The course of SSc is quite variable. Until the disease differentiates into recognizable subsets, prognosis in early disease is difficult to predict. Patients with limited cutaneous scleroderma, especially those with anticentromere antibodies, have a good prognosis, with the notable exception of those few patients, <10%, who after ≥10 to 20 years develop pulmonary arterial hypertension. Malabsorption syndrome and primary biliary cirrhosis are the causes of morbidity and mortality in some patients with limited cutaneous disease. On the other hand, the prognosis is generally worse in patients with diffuse cutaneous disease, particularly when the onset occurs at an older age. In addition, males have a worse prognosis. Renal and other visceral organ disease may develop early in the course of those patients with rapidly progressive generalized skin thickening. Death occurs most often from pulmonary, cardiac, and renal involvement. With the advent of effective therapy for renal crisis along with renal dialysis for those patients with renal failure, survival has greatly improved. In patients with diffuse cutaneous disease, the 5-year cumulative survival rate is ~70% and the 10-year is ~55%. In limited cutaneous disease the 5-year is ~90% and the 10-year is ~75%.

Skin may spontaneously soften after years of disease. Softening occurs in the reverse order of original skin involvement, beginning with the trunk and followed by the proximal and then the distal extremities. Sclerodactyly and flexion contractures may persist. Skin thickness may eventually approach normal; however, the skin may be atrophic.

℞ TREATMENT

Even though SSc cannot be cured, treatment of involved organ systems can relieve symptoms and improve function. The doctor-patient relationship is extremely important in caring for patients with this chronic debilitating illness. Once the diagnosis of SSc has been made, the patient and family should be instructed about this disorder. The patient will need repeated explanations and reassurances throughout his or her illness. Depending on the severity of illness, the patient will require monitoring of blood pressure, blood counts, urinalysis, and monitoring of renal and pulmonary function on a regular basis.

Effectiveness of drug therapy in SSc is difficult to evaluate because of the variable course and severity of disease especially within its subsets. Controlled drug studies have been difficult to achieve because of this variability and the relative few number of SSc patients. Several drugs with antifibrotic, immunosuppressive, or both properties have been tried in the treatment of SSc without any consistent or prolonged benefit. These drugs have included D-penicillamine, colchicine, IFN-γ, IFN-α, and recombinant human relaxin. In the past, high-dose D-penicillamine (750–1000 mg/d) has been used in patients with early diffuse cutaneous SSc, but a recent study showed no benefit of high versus low doses of this drug (see below). The rationale for using D-penicillamine was that it interfered with inter- and intramolecular cross-linking of collagen and was also thought to be immunosuppressive. Several earlier uncontrolled studies with D-penicillamine showed a reduction in skin thickening and prevention of significant internal organ involvement when compared to historic controls. Five-year cumulative survival rates of 80% had been reported in D-penicillamine–treated patients. A recent study did not show an advantage of high-dose D-penicillamine treatment in SSc. The results of a 2-year double-blind randomized study comparing high-dose D-penicillamine (750–1000 mg/d) with low-dose D-penicillamine (125 mg every other day) in patients with early diffuse cutaneous SSc did not show a significant difference between the groups as to the degree of skin thickening, occurrence of renal crises, other organ involvement and mortality. The majority of adverse or toxic effects occurred in the high dosage group. This study, however, did not compare patients on low-dose D-penicillamine versus placebo. It is possible that this drug in low dose might have some beneficial effect in SSc. Its therapeutic value, however, in SSc remains in question. Open uncontrolled trials with colchicine showed skin improvement, but other studies were negative. Randomized controlled multicenter trials with recombinant human IFN-γ demonstrated modest improvement in skin sclerosis. Worsening of Raynaud's phenomenon and development of renal crisis as well as influenza-like symptoms were noted in patients treated with recombinant human IFN-γ, and follow-up studies have not been done. IFN-α in a controlled trial showed no benefit. In a randomized, double-blind, placebo-controlled trial, recombinant human relaxin given by continuous subcutaneous infusion for 24 weeks was associated with reduced skin thickening and improved mobility in patients with moderate to severe diffuse cutaneous scleroderma. A subsequent follow-up, however, did not demonstrate any significant benefit. It is unlikely that further studies with this agent will be done.

Several immunosuppressive agents have been tried in SSc. The rationale for using these agents is based on the cellular and humoral immunologic abnormalities that have been demonstrated in SSc. The results of immunosuppressive therapy have been disappointing and, as of now, no agent has been clearly shown in a controlled prospective study to fully suppress or reverse the disease process of SSc. A controlled randomized, double-blind trial with chlorambucil versus control was negative. Earlier reports of benefit with azathioprine have not been confirmed in controlled studies. Cyclosporine was shown to decrease skin induration without improvement in pulmonary or cardiac manifestations. Concern regarding nephrotoxicity has limited its use in SSc. Randomized controlled trials of methotrexate in early diffuse cutaneous SSc have shown mixed results, with one study showing improvement and others showing marginal, if any, clinical benefit. Extracorporeal photopheresis employing ultraviolet A irradiation after the patient has received oral 6-methoxypsoralen has been tried in SSc with the initial report showing skin improvement. The methodology of this study has been challenged and other studies did not show efficacy. Treatment with 5-fluorouracil led to some skin improvement but caused significant gastrointestinal toxicity. Several uncontrolled studies using cyclophosphamide in treating early sclerodermal interstitial lung disease have shown improvement or stabilization of pulmonary function. Improvement of skin induration was also noted in some patients. A controlled study in patients with early and active alveolitis is currently in progress. Because of the poor prognosis in SSc patients who have a rapid onset of diffuse cutaneous disease and early visceral organ involvement (pulmonary, cardiac, or renal), clinical trials are in progress using high-dose immunosuppressive therapy followed by autologous stem cell transplantation. The rationale is that high doses of an immunosuppressive drug such as cyclophosphamide may reverse or modify the disease course. The autologous stem cell transplantation permits the rapid reconstitution of hematopoiesis. Initial results of a multicenter study involving 19 patients with poor prognoses showed improvement of skin and disability scores exceeding those reported with other therapies. Internal organ function was the same or slightly worse following treatment. Four patients had progressive or nonresponsive disease. Two patients died of treatment complications and one of progressive SSc. The role of high-dose immunosuppressive therapy in SSc needs further evaluation in prospective controlled studies before its clinical efficacy can be determined. This treatment is at present experimental.

Several other agents including minocycline, thalidomide and etanercept have been reported to improve skin involvement in small uncontrolled studies. Randomized controlled studies will need to be performed to know whether these agents are effective.

Antiplatelet therapy may play a role in the treatment of SSc, since the biologic products of platelets affect blood vessels. Low doses of aspirin block the formation of thromboxane A_2, a powerful vasoconstrictor and platelet aggregator. In addition, dipyridamole, 200 to 400 mg in divided daily doses, also decreases platelet adhesion to damaged vessel walls. While these drugs have a reasonable therapeutic rationale, a 2-year double-blind study did not show any benefit from their use.

Glucocorticoids are not effective in improving or preventing skin induration and the progression of SSc. They can be beneficial in certain situations. Short courses of low-dose prednisone (10 mg/d or less) may decrease edema associated with the edematous phase of early skin involvement and may also be useful in relieving joint and tendon pain. Higher doses of a glucocorticoid such as prednisone 20–30 mg/d are indicated in only those patients with inflammatory myositis, pericarditis, and possibly in patients with early active alveolitis. The dose should be reduced as soon as possible to the lowest effective dose, which in some patients may require the addition of a steroid-sparing agent such as methotrexate or azathioprine. Glucocorticoids should not be used for the indolent primary form of muscle disease of SSc (see Musculoskeletal System, above). Glucocorticoids have been associated with the development of renal crisis. A retrospective case-control study in patients with early diffuse cutaneous SSc showed a significant association between prior high-dose glucocorticoids (prednisone $\geq$ 15 mg/d) and the development of scleroderma renal crisis. For this reason, glucocorticoids should be used cautiously in SSc.

The management of Raynaud's phenomenon is directed at control of vasospasm. Patients should be advised to dress warmly and wear mittens and socks, not to smoke, to remove causes of external stress, and to avoid drugs such as amphetamine and ergotamine. Cold drafts should be avoided. Air-conditioned rooms in warm climates can also be a problem for patients with Raynaud's phenomenon. Beta-blocking drugs may make Raynaud's phenomenon worse. Warmth of the central body induces peripheral vasodilatation. Drugs that block sympathetic vasoconstriction, such as reserpine, α-methyldopa, phenoxybenzamine, and prazosin, may be useful in the treatment of Raynaud's phenomenon, but their side effects often curtail extended use. The calcium channel blockers nifedipine, diltiazem, and the longer acting amlodipine can be effective in alleviating Raynaud's phenomenon, but side effects of light-headedness and palpitations may limit their use. The sustained-release form of nifedipine is better tolerated; the dose is 30 mg/d up to 60 or 90 mg/d as required to control symptoms. Nitroglycerin paste, applied to an affected digit, may improve local blood flow. Sildenafil, a phosphodiesterase inhibitor used primarily for erectile dysfunction, is a vasodilator and may be helpful in treating Raynaud's phenomenon. In a 12-week pilot study, losartan (50 mg/d), a specific nonpeptide angiotensen II type 1 receptor antagonist, reduced the severity and frequency of Raynaud's phenomenon episodes. Ketanserin (40 mg TID), an oral serotonin antagonist, has also been shown to be effective. Selective serotonin reuptake inhibitors (e.g., fluoxetine, 20 mg/d) may be beneficial in some patients. These drugs decrease platelet 5-hydroxytryptamine, which is thought to play a role in the pathogenesis of Raynaud's phenomenon. Studies with intravenous iloprost, a prostacyclin analogue, have shown a decrease in frequency and severity of Raynaud's phenomenon and healing of digital ulcers in some patients. Iloprost is still not available in the United States for general use. Intravenous alprostadil, a prostaglandin, can be effective in treating severe Raynaud's phenomenon with digital ulcers. Intravenous epoprostenol and oral Bosentan, an endothelin-1 receptor antagonist, used in the treatment of pulmonary hypertension, also improves Raynaud's phenomenon. Pentoxifylline (400 mg TID) may also improve perfusion by increasing the deformability of the red cell plasma membranes. Techniques of biofeedback have also been used with variable success for teaching patients to control the temperature of their hands. Stellate ganglion blockage may be useful in temporarily alleviating severe ischemic pain in the fingers. Surgical cervical sympathectomy usually provides only temporary improvement, and it, along with other forms of therapy, does not prevent progression of the vascular lesion. Digital sympathectomy can be effective in some patients. The response to any therapy for Raynaud's phenomenon is limited by the degree of existing structural narrowing of digital arteries. In patients with severe Raynaud's phenomenon and refractory digital ulcers, distal ulnar artery occlusion should be considered. A positive Allen test is suggestive, and the diagnosis is confirmed by angiogra-

phy. When ulnar artery occlusion is present, revascularization and a digital sympathectomy may be beneficial. Gangrene of distal digits may occur and require surgical amputation.

Skin care is very important in SSc. Dryness of the skin may be reduced by avoiding frequent use of detergent soaps and by regularly applying hydrophilic ointments and bath oils. Regular exercise helps to maintain flexibility of extremities and pliability of skin. Massaging the skin several times a day may also be beneficial. Fingertip ulcerations can be protected by applying a guard or cage over the end of the finger. The use of an occlusive dressing, such as the hydrocolloid duoDERM or other membranes, over a noninfected ulcer may promote healing and protect the finger. Skin ulcers should be kept clean by soaking or by surgical or chemical debridement. Sympatholytic drugs or local nitroglycerin paste applied to or adjacent to the ulcer may be beneficial in promoting healing. Infected ulcers can usually be treated with topical antibiotics but may require systemic antibiotics, especially when there is a question of underlying osteomyelitis. The development of calcinosis cannot be prevented, nor can deposits be dissolved. Warfarin has been reported to reduce calcinosis in a few patients.

In patients experiencing dry mouth, frequent sips of water help to relieve symptoms. Pilocarpine hydrochloride tablets may increase salivary secretions in some patients. Patients with dry eyes should use artificial tears regularly.

Patients with reflux esophagitis are treated with small, frequent meals, antacids between meals, and elevation of the head of the bed. Patients should be advised not to lie down for a few hours after a meal and to avoid coffee, tea, alcohol, peppermint, and chocolate, which reduce the pressure of the lower esophageal sphincter. Fatty foods and late-evening snacks should be avoided. Cimetidine, ranitidine, or other newer H_2 blockers may be beneficial. Gastric acid (proton) pump inhibitors are more effective in treating erosive esophagitis than are H_2 blockers. Metoclopramide does not significantly improve esophageal motility; it increases lower esophageal sphincter tone and promotes gastric emptying and can be of help in some patients. The dose is 10 mg given 15–20 min before each meal up to 4 times a day. Nifedipine and, to a lesser extent, diltiazem reduce lower esophageal sphincter tone resulting in esophageal reflux. Patients with dysphagia should be instructed to chew their food thoroughly and wash it down with fluids. Malabsorption syndrome due to duodenal hypomotility and bacterial overgrowth causes bloating and diarrhea, which may improve with intermittent use of appropriate antibiotics. Antibiotics are rotated every 2 weeks. Commonly used antibiotics are metronidazole, vancomycin, erythromycin, ciprofloxacin, neomycin, and tetracycline. Patients with severe debilitating malabsorption may benefit from parenteral hyperalimentation. Patients with chronic intestinal pseudoobstruction might respond to octreotide. Stool softeners and mild laxatives are usually adequate for treating constipation caused by hypomotility of the colon.

Articular symptoms are treated with nonsteroidal anti-inflammatory agents. Low-dose prednisone ($\leq$10 mg/d) may improve symptoms in those not responding to these agents. Physical therapy may help to reduce the loss of joint mobility that occurs in SSc.

In patients with diffuse cutaneous SSc, the early recognition of alveolitis as previously described (see "Pulmonary Features") may allow treatment that might slow or prevent the development of pulmonary fibrosis. Cyclophosphamide has been reported in uncontrolled studies to be beneficial, and a controlled study is presently being done. The role of glucocorticoids in preventing progression of interstitial lung disease is not clear but may be of benefit in early disease. *N* acetylcysteine has been used as an antioxidant to reduce lung damage in patients with respiratory distress syndromes and may help in SSc lung disease. Pulmonary fibrosis is not reversible, and therefore treatment is directed at symptoms or complications. Pulmonary infection requires prompt treatment with antibiotics. Hypoxia necessitates giving low concentrations of oxygen. Patients should receive polyvalent pneumoccal vaccine (Pneumovax) and yearly influenza immunizations.

For patients with limited cutaneous SSc who develop isolated pulmonary arterial hypertension, treatment is limited. The usual treatment is supplemental oxygen, anticoagulation, and the administration of a vasodilator. A calcium channel blocker such as nifedipine lowers pulmonary arterial resistance and improves cardiac function, but in most patients this is only for a short period of time. Few patients survive more than 5 years. Heart-lung or single-lung transplantation may be a therapeutic option only in those patients without other significant systemic involvement. Intravenous epoprostenol (prostacyclin) is now given to treat SSc-associated pulmonary hypertension. Epoprostenol is infused continuously via a central line with a portable pump. Improvement in symptoms of right heart failure and exercise tolerance occurred. Also hemodynamic tests showed a decrease in the pulmonary vascular resistance and pulmonary artery pressure both in the short term and in a few patients after 1 or 2 years. Bosentan, an orally administered endothelin-1 receptor antagonist, has been shown to improve exercise capacity and cardiopulmonary hemodynamics in patients with pulmonary arterial hypertension, both primary and secondary to SSc. In some treated SSc patients, Raynaud's phenomenon also improved.

Recognition of early signs of renal hypertensive crisis is important in order to preserve renal function and prevent hypertensive encephalopathy. Renal involvement is often accompanied by hypertension and mild to moderate proteinuria. An occasional patient may be normotensive. Antihypertensive agents are often effective in lowering blood pressure and stabilizing or reversing renal failure. These drugs include propranolol, clonidine, and minoxidil. Particularly effective are the angiotensin-converting enzyme inhibitors, which include captopril, enalapril, and lisinopril. Dialysis may be required in patients with progressive renal failure. Some patients, however, have a slow return of renal function after several months and may no longer require dialysis. Patients are usually not candidates for kidney transplantation because of the other systemic manifestations of SSc.

Patients with cardiac failure require careful monitoring of digitalis and diuretic administration. Noninflammatory pericardial effusions may also improve with diuretics. Care should be taken to avoid overdiuresis, which may lead to decreased renal blood flow, decreased cardiac output, and renal failure.

MIXED CONNECTIVE TISSUE DISEASE

MCTD is an overlap syndrome characterized by combinations of clinical features of SLE (Chap. 300), SSc, polymyositis (Chap. 370), and rheumatoid arthritis (Chap. 301) and the presence of very high titers of circulating autoantibodies to nuclear RNP antigen. This antibody in high titer, now referred to as *anti U₁ RNP*, has been a justification for considering MCTD as a distinct clinical entity. MCTD has been challenged as a distinct disorder by those who consider it as a subset of SLE or scleroderma. Others prefer to classify MCTD as an undifferentiated connective tissue disease. MCTD occurs worldwide and in all races. The peak onset of disease is in the second and third decades, but MCTD is seen in children and the elderly. Women are predominantly affected. The pathogenic mechanisms in MCTD reflect the disorders making up this syndrome.

Clinical Features The presenting symptoms of MCTD are most often Raynaud's phenomenon, puffy hands, arthralgias, myalgias, and fatigue. Occasionally, patients may present with the acute onset of high fever, polymyositis, arthritis, and neurologic features such as trigeminal neuralgia and aseptic meningitis. The various features of the connective tissue disorders making up MCTD develop over months and years.

The fingers as well as the entire hand may be puffy, followed later by sclerodactyly. Sclerodermal changes are usually limited to the distal extremities and sometimes the face but spare the trunk. Telangiectasia and calcinosis may develop. Some patients have mucocutaneous features of SLE including a classic malar rash, photosensitivity, discoid lesions, alopecia, and painful oral ulcerations. An erythematous rash over the knuckles, elbows, and knees and heliotropic eyelids, typical of dermatomyositis, are uncommon.

Joint pain, stiffness, and swelling involving the peripheral joints occur frequently. Deformities of the hands similar to those of rheumatoid arthritis may develop but usually without bony erosions. A destructive polyarthritis is occasionally observed. Myalgias are a frequent symptom. Some patients develop typical symptoms of polymyositis with proximal muscle weakness, abnormal electromyographic findings, elevated levels of muscle enzymes, and inflammatory changes on muscle biopsy.

Approximately 85% of patients have pulmonary involvement, which is often asymptomatic. Diffusing capacity for carbon monoxide may be the only abnormality. Pleurisy commonly occurs but is seldom associated with large pleural effusions. Some patients develop interstitial lung disease. Pulmonary arterial hypertension is the most common cause of death in MCTD.

Approximately 25% of patients develop renal disease. Membranous glomerulonephritis is most common and usually mild but can cause nephrotic syndrome. Diffuse proliferative glomerulonephritis is unusual in MCTD, perhaps because of the protective role believed to be played by the high titers of anti-U₁ RNP. Renal crisis secondary to malignant renovasculature hypertension, as occurs in scleroderma, is seen in a few patients.

Gastrointestinal involvement is seen in ~70% of patients. The most common manifestations are esophageal dysmotility, lower esophageal sphincter laxity, and gastroesophageal reflux. Bowel manifestations mimic those of scleroderma bowel disease.

Pericarditis occurs in 30% of patients. Other cardiac features include myocarditis, arrhythmia, conduction disturbances, and mitral valve prolapse. Other clinical features of MCTD include trigeminal neuropathy, peripheral neuropathy, aseptic meningitis, lymphadenopathy, and Sjögren's syndrome. The majority of patients have developed, or will develop within 5 years of presentation, diagnostic clinical criteria for one of the overlapping connective tissue diseases, most often SLE or SSc.

Laboratory Findings Anemia of chronic inflammation is seen in the majority of patients. A positive direct Coombs' test is found in many patients, but hemolytic anemia is unusual. Leukopenia, thrombocytopenia, or both are present in some patients. Hypergammaglobulinemia is common, and rheumatoid factor is present in 50% of patients.

All patients, by definition of MCTD, have antibodies to U₁ RNP. The specificity of this antibody is to the 70-kDa protein complexed to small nuclear RNA. The anti-U₁ RNP antibodies are associated with HLA-DR4 but not with -DR2 and -DR3 as found in SLE. Molecular mimicry has been demonstrated between U₁ RNP and retroviral antigens by some laboratories.

℞ TREATMENT

The treatment of MCTD is essentially the same as would be indicated for the respective connective tissue diseases defining this syndrome. More than half the patients have a favorable course. The 10-year survival rate overall is ~80% but varies depending on the connective tissue disease that may eventually develop.

EOSINOPHILIC FASCIITIS

Eosinophilic fasciitis is a scleroderma-like syndrome of unknown cause characterized by inflammation followed later by sclerosis of the dermis, subcutis, and deep fascia. The disease affects adults and often occurs after strenuous physical activity. Patients do not have Raynaud's phenomenon or internal organ involvement. Several immunologic abnormalities have been associated with eosinophilic fasciitis and include aplastic anemia, myelodysplastic syndrome, and thrombocytopenia. Patients usually have the abrupt onset of symmetric tenderness and swelling of the extremities, rapidly followed by induration of the skin and subcutaneous tissue. The skin takes on a cobblestone or puckered appearance. Carpal tunnel syndrome appears early in the course, and flexion contractures develop later. A low-grade myositis is often present, but creatinine kinase levels are usually normal. A marked eosinophilia is found in the early stage of disease and subsequently decreases. Increased levels of polyclonal IgG and immune complexes are often present in the serum. A full-thickness biopsy consisting of skin, fascia, and superficial muscle shows perivascular infiltration of histiocytes, eosinophils, lymphocytes, and plasma cells. Biopsies later in the course show sclerosis. Spontaneous improvement and occasionally complete remission may occur after 2 to 5 years of disease. Some patients have persistent disease, while others are left with flexion contractures. Administration of glucocorticoids may provide symptomatic improvement and will decrease the eosinophilia. Improvement has been reported with the use of the H_2 blocker cimetidine.

EOSINOPHILIA-MYALGIA SYNDROME

In 1989, reports of patients with scleroderma-like skin changes, myalgias, and eosinophilia dramatically increased. Most, but not all, of these cases were associated with ingestion of L-tryptophan manufactured by a single Japanese company. Batches of L-tryptophan implicated in EMS were found to contain trace amounts of a contaminant identified as a dimer of L-tryptophan that appeared in 1988 after changes were made in the method of manufacturing this drug. It is not clear whether this chemical contaminant is the etiologic agent or whether another unidentified substance is responsible. *L-Tryptophan products were taken off the market in 1990.* The onset of EMS can be either abrupt or insidious. In the early phases of the disease, clinical manifestations include low-grade fever, fatigue, dyspnea, cough, arthralgias/arthritis, evanescent erythematous rashes, muscle cramping, and severe myalgias. Pulmonary infiltrates may be present. Over the next 2 to 3 months, scleroderma-like skin changes appear. Some patients develop a peripheral neuropathy, which may persist. An ascending polyneuropathy may lead to paralysis and respiratory failure requiring ventilatory assistance. Cognitive dysfunction with impairment of memory and concentration has been recognized in this syndrome. Myocarditis and cardiac arrhythmias occur in some patients, and a few patients develop pulmonary hypertension. Approximately a third of patients have features of eosinophilic fasciitis. EMS most closely resembles toxic oil syndrome; however, Raynaud's phenomenon does not occur, and there is a lower prevalence of pulmonary hypertension and thromboembolic disease. The peripheral eosinophil count is $>1000/\mu L$ in most patients. The histologic findings on biopsy of skin, fascia, and superficial muscle are similar to those found in eosinophilic fasciitis. The clinical features of EMS may persist after L-tryptophan has been discontinued. EMS may run a chronic course, and response to therapy has been variable. Treatment has included glucocorticoids, antimalarial drugs, immunosuppressive drugs, and plasmapheresis. Prednisone was beneficial during the acute inflammatory phase of the disease in the majority of patients and resulted in resolution of pulmonary infiltrates, peripheral edema, and eosinophilia. In the later phase of the illness, no treatment was found to be of particular value. The pathogenesis of this disease is not known. A followup of patients 2 years after their onset of illness showed that most symptoms and physical findings had resolved or improved except for cognitive dysfunction, which became worse in approximately one-third of the patients, and peripheral neuropathy, which remained unchanged (Chap. 370).

FURTHER READING

CLEMENTS PJ et al: High-dose versus low-dose D-penicillamine in early diffuse systemic sclerosis: Analysis of a two-year, double-blind, randomized, controlled clinical trial. Arthritis Rheum 42:1194, 1999

DEMARCO PJ et al: Predictors and outcomes of scleroderma renal crisis: The high-dose versus low-dose D-penicillamine in early diffuse system sclerosis trial. Arthritis Rheum 46.2836, 2002

FEGHALI-BOSTWICK C et al: Analysis of systemic sclerosis in twins reveals low concordance for disease and high concordance for the presence of antinuclear antibodies. Arthritis Rheum 48:1956, 2003

HAMAMDZIC D et al: Role of infectious agents in the pathogenesis of systemic sclerosis. Curr Opin Rheumatol 14:694, 2002

HERTZMAN PA et al: The eosinophilia-myalgia syndrome: Status of 205 patients and results of treatment 2 years after onset. Ann Intern Med 122:851, 1995

MCSWEENEY PA et al: High-dose immunosuppressive therapy for severe systemic sclerosis: Initial outcomes. Blood 100:1602, 2002

NELSON JL et al: Microchimerism and human autoimmune disease. Lupus 11: 651, 2002

ROSE S et al: Gastrointestinal manifestations of scleroderma. Gastroenterol Clin North Am 27:563, 1998

RUBIN LJ et al: Bosentan therapy for pulmonary arterial hypertension. N Engl J Med 346:896, 2002

STEEN VD, MEDSGER TA: Case-control study of corticosteroids and other drugs that either precipitate or protect from the development of scleroderma renal crisis. Arthritis Rheum 41:1613, 1998

304 | SJÖGREN'S SYNDROME
Haralampos M. Moutsopoulos

DEFINITION

Sjögren's syndrome is a chronic, slowly progressive autoimmune disease characterized by lymphocytic infiltration of the exocrine glands resulting in xerostomia and dry eyes. Approximately one-third of patients present with systemic manifestations. A small but significant number of patients may develop malignant lymphoma. The disease can be seen alone (primary Sjögren's syndrome) or in association with other autoimmune rheumatic diseases (secondary Sjögren's syndrome) (Table 304-1).

INCIDENCE AND PREVALENCE

The disease affects predominantly middle-age women (female-to-male ratio 9:1), although it occurs in all ages, including childhood. The prevalence of primary Sjögren's syndrome is approximately 0.5 to 1.0%. In addition, 30% of patients with autoimmune rheumatic diseases suffer from secondary Sjögren's syndrome.

PATHOGENESIS

Sjögren's syndrome is characterized by lymphocytic infiltration of the exocrine glands and B lymphocyte hyperreactivity, as illustrated by circulating autoantibodies. In one-fourth of the patients, it is accompanied by an oligomonoclonal B cell process, which is characterized by cryoprecipitable monoclonal immunoglobulins with rheumatoid factor activity.

Sera of patients with Sjögren's syndrome often contain a number of autoantibodies directed against non-organ-specific antigens such as immunoglobulins (rheumatoid factors) and extractable nuclear and cytoplasmic antigens (Ro/SS-A, La/SS-B). Ro/SS-A autoantigen consists of two polypeptides (52 and 60 kDa) in conjunction with cytoplasmic RNAs, whereas the 48-kDa La/SS-B protein is bound to RNA III polymerase transcripts. Autoantibodies to Ro/SS-A and La/SS-B antigens are usually detected at the time of diagnosis and are associated with earlier disease onset, longer disease duration, salivary gland enlargement, severity of lymphocytic infiltration of minor salivary glands, and certain extraglandular manifestations. Antibodies to α-fodrin (120 kDa), a salivary gland–specific protein, have been found

TABLE 304-1 *Association of Sjögren's Syndrome with Other Autoimmune Diseases*

Rheumatoid arthritis	Primary biliary cirrhosis
Systemic lupus erythematosus	Vasculitis
Scleroderma	Chronic active hepatitis
Mixed connective tissue disease	

TABLE 304-2 *Incidence of Extraglandular Manifestations in Primary Sjögren's Syndrome*

Clinical Manifestation	Percent
Arthralgias/arthritis	60
Raynaud's phenomenon	37
Lymphadenopathy	14
Lung involvement	14
Vasculitis	11
Kidney involvement	9
Liver involvement	6
Lymphoma	6
Splenomegaly	3
Peripheral neuropathy	2
Myositis	1

in sera of patients with Sjögren's syndrome. The major infiltrating cells in the affected exocrine glands are activated B and T lymphocytes. Macrophages and natural killer cells are rarely detected. In chronic lesions, a small but persistent number of dendritic cells are apparent in lymphoid follicle–like formations. In contrast to the infiltrating lymphocytes, the glandular epithelial cells undergo apoptotic death. Ductal and acinar epithelial cells appear to play a significant role in the initiation and perpetuation of the autoimmune injury since they inappropriately produce proinflammatory cytokines and lympho-attractant chemokines and express on their surface nuclear autoantigens. Further, they express class II major histocompatibility complex (MHC) and co-stimulatory molecules and are able to provide the second signal for lymphocyte activation. Redistribution of the water-channel protein aquaporin-5 from the apical membranes to the cytoplasm of acinar epithelial cells has also been observed.

Immunogenetic studies have demonstrated that HLA-B8, -DR3, and -DRw52 are prevalent in patients with primary Sjögren's syndrome as compared with the normal control population. Molecular analysis of HLA class II genes has revealed that patients with Sjögren's syndrome, regardless of their ethnic origin, are highly associated with the HLA DQA1*0501 allele.

CLINICAL MANIFESTATIONS

The majority of Sjögren's syndrome patients have symptoms related to diminished lacrimal and salivary gland function. In most patients, the primary syndrome runs a slow and benign course. The initial manifestations can be mucosal dryness or nonspecific, and 8 to 10 years

TABLE 304-3 *Differential Diagnosis of Sicca Symptoms*

Xerostomia	Dry Eye	Bilateral Parotid Gland Enlargement
Viral infections	Inflammation	Viral infections
Drugs	Stevens-Johnson	Mumps
Psychotherapeutic	syndrome	Influenza
Parasympatholytic	Pemphigoid	Epstein-Barr
Antihypertensives	Chronic conjunctivitis	Coxsackievirus A
Psychogenic	Chronic blepharitis	Cytomegalovirus
Irradiation	Sjögren's syndrome	HIV
Diabetes mellitus	Toxicity	Sarcoidosis
Trauma	Burns	Amyloidosis
Sjögren's	Drugs	Sjögren's syndrome
syndrome	Neurologic conditions	Metabolic
	Impaired lacrimal	Diabetes mellitus
	gland function	Hyperlipoprotein-
	Impaired eyelid	emias
	function	Chronic
	Miscellaneous	pancreatitis
	Trauma	Hepatic cirrhosis
	Hypovitaminosis A	Endocrine
	Blink abnormality	Acromegaly
	Lid scarring	Gonadal
	Anesthetic cornea	hypofunction
	Epithelial irregularity	

TABLE 304-4 *Differential Diagnosis of Sjögren's Syndrome*

HIV Infection and Sicca Syndrome	Sjögren's Syndrome	Sarcoidosis
Predominant in young males	Predominant in middle-aged women	Invariable
Lack of autoantibodies to Ro/SS-A and/or La/SS-B	Presence of autoantibodies	Lack of autoantibodies to Ro/SS-A and/or La/SS-B
Lymphoid infiltrates of salivary glands by CD8+ lymphocytes	Lymphoid infiltrates of salivary glands by CD4+ lymphocytes	Granulomas in salivary glands
Association with HLA-DR5	Association with HLA-DR3 and -DRw52	Unknown
Positive serologic tests for HIV	Negative serologic tests for HIV	Negative serologic tests for HIV

elapse from the initial symptoms to full-blown development of the disease.

The principal oral symptom of Sjögren's syndrome is dryness (xerostomia). Patients complain of difficulty in swallowing dry food, inability to speak continuously, a burning sensation, increase in dental caries, and problems in wearing complete dentures. Physical examination shows a dry, erythematous, sticky oral mucosa. There is atrophy of the filiform papillae on the dorsum of the tongue, and saliva from the major glands is either not expressible or cloudy. Enlargement of the parotid or other major salivary glands occurs in two-thirds of patients with primary Sjögren's syndrome but is uncommon in those with the secondary syndrome. Diagnostic tests include sialometry, sialog-

TABLE 304-5 *Revised International Classification Criteria for Sjögren's Syndrome[a,b,c]*

  I. Ocular symptoms: a positive response to at least one of three validated questions.
    1. Have you had daily, persistent, troublesome dry eyes for more than 3 months?
    2. Do you have a recurrent sensation of sand or gravel in the eyes?
    3. Do you use tear substitutes more than three times a day?
  II. Oral symptoms: a positive response to at least one of three validated questions.
    1. Have you had a daily feeling of dry mouth for more than 3 months?
    2. Have you had recurrent or persistently swollen salivary glands as an adult?
    3. Do you frequently drink liquids to aid in swallowing dry foods?
  III. Ocular signs: objective evidence of ocular involvement defined as a positive result to at least one of the following two tests:
    1. Shirmer's I test, performed without anesthesia ($\leq$5 mm in 5 min)
    2. Rose Bengal score or other ocular dye score ($\geq$4 according to van Bijsterveld's scoring system)
  IV. Histopathology: In minor salivary glands focal lymphocytic sialoadenitis, with a focus score $\geq$ 1.
  V. Salivary gland involvement: objective evidence of salivary gland involvement defined by a positive result to at least one of the following diagnostic tests:
    1. Unstimulated whole salivary flow ($\leq$1.5 mL in 15 min)
    2. Parotid sialography
    3. Salivary scintigraphy
  VI. Antibodies in the serum to Ro/SS-A or La/SS-B antigens, or both

[a] Exclusion criteria: Past head and neck radiation treatment, hepatitis C infection, AIDS, preexisting lymphoma, sarcoidosis, graft versus host disease, use of anticholinergic drugs.
[b] Primary Sjögren's syndrome: any four of the six items, as long as item IV (histopathology) or VI (serology) is positive, or any three of the four objective criteria items (items III, IV, V, VI).
[c] In patients with a potentially associated disease (e.g., another well-defined connective tissue disease), the presence of item I or item II plus any two from among items III, IV, and V may be considered as indicative of secondary Sjögren's syndrome.
Source: From Vitali C et al.

FIGURE 304-1 Treatment algorithm for Sjögren's syndrome.

raphy, and scintigraphy. The labial minor salivary gland biopsy permits histopathologic confirmation of the focal lymphocytic infiltrates.

Ocular involvement is the other major manifestation of Sjögren's syndrome. Patients usually complain of a sandy or gritty feeling under the eyelids. Other symptoms include burning, accumulation of thick strands at the inner canthi, decreased tearing, redness, itching, eye fatigue, and increased photosensitivity. These symptoms are attributed to the destruction of corneal and bulbar conjunctival epithelium, defined as *keratoconjunctivitis sicca*. Diagnostic evaluation of keratoconjunctivitis sicca includes measurement of tear flow by Schirmer's I test and tear composition as assessed by the tear breakup time or tear lysozyme content. Slit-lamp examination of the cornea and conjunctiva after rose Bengal staining reveals punctate corneal ulcerations and attached filaments of corneal epithelium.

Involvement of other exocrine glands occurs less frequently and includes a decrease in mucous gland secretions of the upper and lower respiratory tree, resulting in dry nose, throat, and trachea (xerotrachea), and diminished secretion of the exocrine glands of the gastrointestinal tract, leading to esophageal mucosal atrophy, atrophic gastritis, and subclinical pancreatitis. Dyspareunia due to dryness of the external genitalia and dry skin may also occur.

Extraglandular (systemic) manifestations are seen in one-third of patients with Sjögren's syndrome (Table 304-2), while they are very

rare in patients with Sjögren's syndrome associated with rheumatoid arthritis. These patients complain more often of easy fatigability, low-grade fever, Raynaud's phenomenon, myalgias, and arthralgias. Most patients with primary Sjögren's syndrome experience at least one episode of nonerosive arthritis during the course of their disease. Manifestations of pulmonary involvement are frequent but rarely important clinically. Dry cough is the major manifestation that is attributed to small airway disease. Renal involvement includes interstitial nephritis, clinically manifested by hyposthenuria and renal tubular dysfunction with or without acidosis. Untreated acidosis may lead to nephrocalcinosis. Glomerulonephritis is a rare finding that occurs in patients with mixed cryoglobulinemia, or systemic lupus erythematosus overlapping with Sjögren's syndrome. Vasculitis affects small and medium-sized vessels. The most common clinical features are purpura, recurrent urticaria, skin ulcerations, glomerulonephritis, and mononeuritis multiplex. Sensorineural hearing loss was found in one-half of patients with Sjögren's syndrome and correlated with the presence of anticardiolipin antibodies.

It has been suggested that primary Sjögren's syndrome with vasculitis may also present with multifocal, recurrent, and progressive nervous system disease, such as hemiparesis, transverse myelopathy, hemisensory deficits, seizures, and movement disorders. Aseptic meningitis and multiple sclerosis have also been reported in these patients.

Lymphoma is a well-known manifestation of Sjögren's syndrome that usually presents later in the illness. Persistent parotid gland enlargement, purpura, leukopenia, cryoglobulinemia, and low C4 complement levels are manifestations suggesting the development of lymphoma. Most lymphomas are extranodal, marginal zone B cell, and low grade. Usually the low-grade lymphomas are detected incidentally upon evaluating the labial biopsy.

The affected lymph nodes are usually peripheral. Survival is decreased in patients with B symptoms, lymph node mass >7 cm in diameter, and high or intermediate histologic grade.

Routine laboratory tests reveal mild normochromic, normocytic anemia. An elevated erythrocyte sedimentation rate is found in approximately 70% of patients.

DIAGNOSIS AND DIFFERENTIAL DIAGNOSIS

The diagnosis of primary Sjögren's syndrome is obtained if the patient presents with eye and/or mouth dryness, the eye tests disclose keratoconjunctivitis sicca, the mouth evaluation reveals the classic manifestations of the syndrome, and the patient's serum reacts with Ro/SS-A and/or La/SS-B autoantigens. Labial biopsy is needed when the diagnosis is uncertain or to rule out conditions that may cause dry mouth or eyes or parotid gland enlargement (Tables 304-3, 304-4). Validated diagnostic criteria have been established by a European study and have now been further improved by a European-American study group (Table 304-5).

℞ TREATMENT

Treatment of Sjögren's syndrome is aimed at symptomatic relief and limiting the damaging local effects of chronic xerostomia and keratoconjunctivitis sicca by substituting or simulating the missing secretions (Fig. 304-1).

To replace deficient tears, there are several readily available ophthalmic preparations (Tearisol; Liquifilm; 0.5% methylcellulose; Hypo Tears). If corneal ulcerations are present, eye patching and boric acid ointments are recommended. Certain drugs that may increase lacrimal and salivary hypofunction such as diuretics, antihypertensive drugs, and antidepressants should be avoided.

For xerostomia the best replacement is water. Propionic acid gels may be used to treat vaginal dryness. To stimulate secretions, pilocarpine (5 mg thrice daily) or cevimeline (30 mg thrice daily) administered orally appears to improve sicca manifestations and both are well tolerated. Hydroxychloroquine (200 mg) is helpful for arthralgias.

Patients with renal tubular acidosis should receive sodium bicar-bonate orally (0.5 to 2.0 mmol/kg in four divided doses). Glucocorticoids (1 mg/kg per day) and/or immunosuppressive agents (e.g., cyclophosphamide) are indicated only for the treatment of systemic vasculitis.

FURTHER READING

IOANNIDIS JP et al: Long-term risk of mortality and lymphoproliferative disease and predictive classification of primary Sjögren's syndrome. Arthritis Rheum 46:741, 2002

MANOUSSAKIS MN, MOUTSOPOULOS HM: Sjögren's syndrome: Current concepts. Adv Intern Med 47:191, 2001

MOUTSOPOULOS NM, MOUTSOPOULOS HM: Therapy of Sjögren's syndrome. Springer Semin Immunopathol 23:131, 2001

SKOPOULI FN et al: Clinical evolution, and morbidity and mortality of primary Sjögren's syndrome. Semin Arthritis Rheum 29:296, 2000

VITALI C et al: Classification criteria for Sjögren's syndrome: A revised version of the European criteria proposed by the American-European Consensus Group. Ann Rheum Dis 61:554, 2002

---

305 THE SPONDYLOARTHRITIDES
Joel D. Taurog

The spondyloarthritides are a group of disorders that share certain clinical features and an association with the HLA-B27 allele. These disorders include ankylosing spondylitis, reactive arthritis, psoriatic arthritis and spondylitis, enteropathic arthritis and spondylitis, juvenile-onset spondyloarthritis, and undifferentiated spondyloarthritis. The similarities in clinical manifestations and genetic predisposition suggest that these disorders share pathogenic mechanisms.

ANKYLOSING SPONDYLITIS

Ankylosing spondylitis (AS) is an inflammatory disorder of unknown cause that primarily affects the axial skeleton; peripheral joints and extraarticular structures may also be involved. The disease usually begins in the second or third decade; the male to female prevalence is approximately 3:1. Older names include *Marie-Strümpell disease* or *Bechterew's disease*.

EPIDEMIOLOGY AS shows a striking correlation with the histocompatibility antigen HLA-B27 and occurs worldwide roughly in proportion to the prevalence of this antigen (Chap. 296). In North American Caucasians, the general prevalence of B27 is 7%, whereas >90% of patients with AS have inherited this antigen. The association with B27 is independent of disease severity.

In population surveys, 1 to 6% of adults inheriting B27 have been found to have AS. In contrast, in families of patients with AS, the prevalence is 10 to 30% among adult first-degree relatives inheriting B27. The concordance rate in identical twins is approximately 65%. It is currently believed that susceptibility to AS is determined almost entirely by genetic factors, with B27 comprising about one-third of the genetic component.

PATHOLOGY The enthesis, the site of ligamentous attachment to bone, is thought to be the primary site of pathology in AS, particularly in the lesions around the pelvis and spine. Enthesitis is associated with prominent edema of the adjacent bone marrow and is often characterized by erosive lesions that eventually undergo ossification.

Sacroiliitis is usually one of the earliest manifestations of AS, with features of both enthesitis and synovitis. The early lesions consist of subchondral granulation tissue, infiltrates of lymphocytes and macrophages in ligamentous and periosteal zones, and subchondral bone marrow edema. Synovitis follows and may progress to pannus formation with islands of new bone formation. The eroded joint margins are gradually replaced by fibrocartilage regeneration and then by ossification. Ultimately, the joint may be totally obliterated.

In the spine, early in the process there is inflammatory granulation tissue at the junction of the annulus fibrosus of the disk cartilage and the margin of vertebral bone. The outer annular fibers are eroded and eventually replaced by bone, forming the beginning of a bony syndesmophyte, which then grows by continued enchondral ossification, ultimately bridging the adjacent vertebral bodies. Ascending progression of this process leads to the "bamboo spine" observed radiographically. Other lesions in the spine include diffuse osteoporosis, erosion of vertebral bodies at the disk margin, "squaring" of vertebrae, and inflammation and destruction of the disk-bone border. Inflammatory arthritis of the apophyseal joints is common, with erosion of cartilage by pannus, often followed by bony ankylosis.

Bone mineral density is significantly diminished in the spine and proximal femur early in the course of the disease, before the advent of significant immobilization.

Peripheral arthritis in AS can show synovial hyperplasia, lymphoid infiltration, and pannus formation, but the process lacks the exuberant synovial villi, fibrin deposits, ulcers, and accumulations of plasma cells seen in rheumatoid arthritis (RA) (Chap. 301). Central cartilaginous erosions caused by proliferation of subchondral granulation tissue are common in AS but rare in RA.

PATHOGENESIS The pathogenesis of AS is incompletely understood but is almost certainly immune mediated. The dramatic response of all aspects of the disease to therapeutic blockade of tumor necrosis factor α (TNF-α) indicates that this cytokine plays a central role in the immunopathogenesis of AS. The inflamed sacroiliac joint is infiltrated with CD4+ and CD8+ T cells and macrophages and shows high levels of TNF-α. No specific event or exogenous agent that triggers the onset of disease has been identified, although overlapping features with reactive arthritis and inflammatory bowel disease (IBD) suggest that enteric bacteria may play a role. Elevated serum titers of antibodies to certain enteric bacteria are common in AS patients, but no role for these antibodies in the pathogenesis of AS has been identified. Evidence that B27 plays a direct role is provided by the finding that rats transgenic for B27 spontaneously develop spondylitis, along with colitis, peripheral arthritis, and other lesions characteristic of the spondyloarthritides.

Some evidence has accumulated for autoimmunity to the cartilage proteoglycan aggrecan. Sharing of proteoglycan antigenic epitopes may be a possible explanation for the distribution of pathologic sites in AS.

CLINICAL MANIFESTATIONS The symptoms of the disease are usually first noticed in late adolescence or early adulthood; the median age in western countries is 23. In 5% of patients, symptoms begin after age 40.

The initial symptom is usually dull pain, insidious in onset, felt deep in the lower lumbar or gluteal region, accompanied by low-back morning stiffness of up to a few hours' duration that improves with activity and returns following periods of inactivity. Within a few months of onset, the pain has usually become persistent and bilateral. Nocturnal exacerbation of pain that forces the patient to rise and move around may be frequent.

In some patients, bony tenderness (presumably reflecting enthesitis) may accompany back pain or stiffness, while in others it may be the predominant complaint. Common sites include the costosternal junctions, spinous processes, iliac crests, greater trochanters, ischial tuberosities, tibial tubercles, and heels. Occasionally, bony chest pain is the presenting complaint. Arthritis in the hips and shoulders ("root" joints) occurs in 25 to 35% of patients, in many cases early in the disease course. Arthritis of peripheral joints other than the hips and shoulders, usually asymmetric, occurs in up to 30% of patients and can occur at any stage of the disease. Neck pain and stiffness from involvement of the cervical spine are usually relatively late manifestations. Occasional patients, particularly in the older age group, present with predominantly constitutional symptoms such as fatigue, anorexia, fever, weight loss, or night sweats.

AS often has a juvenile onset in developing countries. In these individuals, peripheral arthritis and enthesitis usually predominate, with axial symptoms supervening in late adolescence.

Initially, physical findings mirror the inflammatory process. The most specific findings involve loss of spinal mobility, with limitation of anterior and lateral flexion and extension of the lumbar spine and of chest expansion. Limitation of motion is usually out of proportion to the degree of bony ankylosis, reflecting muscle spasm secondary to pain and inflammation. Pain in the sacroiliac joints may be elicited either with direct pressure or with maneuvers that stress the joints. In addition, there is commonly tenderness upon palpation at the sites of symptomatic bony tenderness and paraspinous muscle spasm.

The Schober test is a useful measure of lumbar spine flexion. The patient stands erect, with heels together, and marks are made directly over the spine 5 cm below and 10 cm above the lumbosacral junction (identified by a horizontal line between the posterosuperior iliac spines.) The patient then bends forward maximally, and the distance between the two marks is measured. The distance between the two marks increases by ≥5 cm in the case of normal mobility and by <4 cm in the case of decreased mobility. Chest expansion is measured as the difference between maximal inspiration and maximal forced expiration in the fourth intercostal space in males or just below the breasts in females. Normal chest expansion is ≥5 cm.

Limitation or pain with motion of the hips or shoulders is usually present if either of these joints is involved. It should be emphasized that early in the course of mild cases, symptoms may be subtle and nonspecific, and the physical examination may be completely normal.

The course of the disease is extremely variable, ranging from the individual with mild stiffness and radiographically equivocal sacroiliitis to the patient with a totally fused spine and severe bilateral hip arthritis, possibly accompanied by severe peripheral arthritis and extraarticular manifestations. Pain tends to be persistent early in the disease and then becomes intermittent, with alternating exacerbations and quiescent periods. In a typical severe untreated case with progression of the spondylitis to syndesmophyte formation, the patient's posture undergoes characteristic changes, with obliterated lumbar lordosis, buttock atrophy, and accentuated thoracic kyphosis. There may be a forward stoop of the neck or flexion contractures at the hips, compensated by flexion at the knees. The progression of the disease may be followed by measuring the patient's height, chest expansion, Schober test, and occiput-to-wall distance. Occasional individuals are encountered with advanced physical findings who report having never had significant symptoms.

In some but not all studies, onset of the disease in adolescence correlates with a worse prognosis. Early severe hip involvement is an indication of progressive disease. The disease in women tends to progress less frequently to total spinal ankylosis, although there is some evidence for an increased prevalence of isolated cervical ankylosis and peripheral arthritis in women. In industrialized countries, peripheral arthritis (distal to hips and shoulders) occurs overall in about 25% of patients, usually as a late manifestation, whereas in developing countries, the prevalence is much higher, with onset typically early in the disease course. Pregnancy has no consistent effect on AS, with symptoms improving, remaining the same, or deteriorating in about one-third of pregnant patients, respectively.

The most serious complication of the spinal disease is spinal fracture, which can occur with even minor trauma to the rigid, osteoporotic spine. The cervical spine is most commonly involved. These fractures are often displaced and cause spinal cord injury.

The most common extraarticular manifestation is acute anterior uveitis, which occurs in 30% of patients and can antedate the spondylitis. Attacks are typically unilateral, causing pain, photophobia, and increased lacrimation. These tend to recur, often in the opposite eye. Cataracts and secondary glaucoma are not uncommon sequelae. Up to 60% of patients have inflammation in the colon or ileum. This is usually asymptomatic, but in 5 to 10% of patients with AS, frank IBD will develop. Aortic insufficiency, sometimes producing symptoms of congestive heart failure, occurs in a few percent of patients, occasionally early in the course of the spinal disease but usually after prolonged disease. Third-degree heart block may occur alone or together with aortic insufficiency. Subclinical pulmonary lesions and cardiac dysfunction may be relatively common. Cauda equina syndrome and slowly progressive upper pulmonary lobe fibrosis are rare complications of long-standing AS. Retroperitoneal fibrosis is a rare associated condition. Prostatitis has been reported to have an increased prevalence in men with AS. Amyloidosis is rare (Chap. 310).

Several validated measures of disease activity and functional outcome have recently been developed for AS. Despite the persistence of the disease, most patients remain gainfully employed. The effect of AS on survival is controversial. Some, but not all, studies have suggested that AS shortens life span, compared with the general population. Mortality attributable to AS is largely the result of spinal trauma, aortic insufficiency, respiratory failure, amyloid nephropathy, or complications of therapy such as upper gastrointestinal hemorrhage.

LABORATORY FINDINGS No laboratory test is diagnostic of AS. In most ethnic groups, B27 is present in approximately 90% of patients with AS. Erythrocyte sedimentation rate (ESR) and C-reactive protein (CRP) are often, but not always, elevated. Mild anemia may be present. Patients with severe disease may show an elevated alkaline phosphatase level. Elevated serum IgA levels are common. Rheumatoid factor and antinuclear antibodies are largely absent unless caused by a coexistent disease. Synovial fluid from peripheral joints in AS is nonspecifically inflammatory. In cases with restriction of chest wall motion, decreased vital capacity and increased functional residual capacity are common, but airflow measurements are normal and ventilatory function is usually well maintained.

RADIOGRAPHIC FINDINGS Radiographically demonstrable sacroiliitis is usually present in AS. The earliest changes by standard radiography are blurring of the cortical margins of the subchondral bone, followed by erosions and sclerosis. Progression of the erosions leads to "pseudowidening" of the joint space; as fibrous and then bony ankylosis supervene, the joints may become obliterated. The changes and progression of the lesions are usually symmetric.

In the lumbar spine, progression of the disease leads to straightening, caused by loss of lordosis, and reactive sclerosis, caused by osteitis of the anterior corners of the vertebral bodies with subsequent erosion, leading to "squaring" of the vertebral bodies. Progressive ossification leads to eventual formation of marginal syndesmophytes, visible on plain films as bony bridges connecting successive vertebral bodies anteriorly and laterally.

In mild cases, years may elapse before unequivocal sacroiliac abnormalities are evident on plain radiographs. Computed tomography

(CT) and magnetic resonance imaging (MRI) can detect abnormalities reliably at an earlier stage than plain radiography. MRI is highly sensitive and specific for identifying early intraarticular inflammation, cartilage changes, and underlying bone marrow edema in sacroiliitis (Fig. 305-1). In suspected cases in which conventional radiography does not reveal definite sacroiliac abnormalities or is undesirable (e.g., in young women or children), dynamic MRI is the procedure of choice for establishing a diagnosis of sacroiliitis.

Reduced bone mineral density can be detected by dual-energy x-ray absorptiometry of the femoral neck and the lumbar spine. Falsely elevated readings related to spinal ossification can be avoided by using a lateral projection of the L3 vertebral body.

DIAGNOSIS It is important to establish the diagnosis of early AS before the development of irreversible deformity. Modified New York criteria (1984) are widely used for diagnosis. These consist of the following: (1) a history of inflammatory back pain (see below); (2) limitation of motion of the lumbar spine in both the sagittal and frontal planes; (3) limited chest expansion, relative to standard values for age and sex; and (4) definite radiographic sacroiliitis. The presence of radiographic sacroiliitis plus any one of the other three criteria is sufficient for a diagnosis of definite AS. The use of MRI to demonstrate sacroiliitis significantly increases the sensitivity of these criteria (Fig. 305-1).

The presence of B27 is neither necessary nor sufficient for the diagnosis, but the B27 test can be helpful in patients with suggestive clinical findings who have not yet developed radiographic sacroiliitis. Moreover, the absence of B27 in a typical case of AS significantly increases the probability of coexistent IBD.

AS must be differentiated from numerous other causes of low-back pain, some of which are far more common than AS. The inflammatory back pain of AS is usually distinguished by the following five features: (1) age of onset below 40, (2) insidious onset, (3) duration >3 months before medical attention is sought, (4) morning stiffness, and (5) improvement with exercise or activity. The most common causes of back pain other than AS are primarily mechanical or degenerative rather than inflammatory and do not show these features. Less common metabolic, infectious, and malignant causes of back pain must also be differentiated from AS. Ochronosis can produce a phenotype that is clinically and radiographically similar to AS.

Marked calcification and ossification of paraspinous ligaments occur in *diffuse idiopathic skeletal hyperostosis* (DISH). Ligamentous calcification and ossification are usually most prominent in the anterior spinal ligament and give the appearance of "flowing wax" on the anterior bodies of the vertebrae. Intervertebral disk spaces are preserved, and sacroiliac and apophyseal joints appear normal, helping to differentiate DISH from spondylosis and from AS, respectively.

DISH occurs in the middle-aged and elderly. Patients are frequently asymptomatic but may have stiffness. Radiographic changes are generally much more dramatic than symptoms.

Rx TREATMENT

The publication in 2000 of dramatic responses to anti-TNF-α therapy heralded a revolution in the management of AS and other spondyloarthritides. Patients with AS treated with either infliximab (chimeric human/mouse anti-TNF-α monoclonal antibody) or etanercept (soluble p75 TNF-α receptor–IgG fusion protein) have shown rapid, profound, and sustained reductions in all clinical and laboratory measures of disease activity. Patients with long-standing disease and even complete spinal ankylosis have shown striking improvement in both objective and subjective indicators of disease activity and function, including morning stiffness, pain, spinal mobility, peripheral joint swelling, CRP, and ESR. MRI studies indicate substantial resolution of bone marrow edema, enthesitis, and joint effusions in the sacroiliac joints, spine, and peripheral joints. Overall, 10 studies published from 2000 to 2002 (9 with infliximab, 1 with etanercept; 7 open label, 3 randomized controlled trials; duration 8 to 54 weeks) have reported a median 60% reduction in the Bath Ankylosing Spondylitis Disease Activity Index (BASDAI), the most commonly used measure of disease activity (range 45 to 93%, vs. 3 to 10% in the three placebo groups). At present, it is not definitely known whether this therapy will halt the progression of the disease, but it seems likely to do so. Whether this therapy can reverse ankylosis or other damage is less clear but also not improbable.

The administration of these agents to AS patients has been similar to that in RA. Infliximab is given as an intravenous infusion, typically at a dose of 5 mg per kg body weight, and then repeated 2 weeks later, again 6 weeks later, and then at 8-week intervals. Etanercept is given in a dose of 25 mg by subcutaneous injection twice weekly.

Although these potent immunosuppressive agents have so far been remarkably safe, six types of side effects have been seen: (1) serious infections, including disseminated tuberculosis; (2) hematologic disorders such as pancytopenia; (3) demyelinating disorders; (4) exacerbation of congestive heart failure; (5) systemic lupus erythematosus–related autoantibodies and clinical features; and (6) hypersensitivity infusion or injection site reactions. Increased incidence of malignancy is of theoretical concern.

Although serious complications have been uncommon, neither the incidence of side effects nor the long-term effects of these agents are yet known. Moreover, the currently available anti-TNF-α agents are quite expensive. Thus, uncertainty remains as to which patients with AS and other spondyloarthritides should be given this form of therapy. Previously, the mainstay of treatment for AS was nonsteroidal anti-inflammatory drug (NSAID) therapy with drugs such as indomethacin or more recently COX-2 inhibitors, combined with exercise programs designed to maintain posture and range of motion. Sulfasalazine, in doses of 2 to 3 g/d, and methotrexate, in doses of 10 to 25 mg/wk, have been shown to be of modest benefit, primarily for peripheral arthritis. No therapeutic role for gold or oral glucocorticoids has been documented in AS. Recent studies suggest potential benefit in AS from three diverse agents: the bisphosphonate pamidronate, at

FIGURE 305-1 Early sacroiliitis of ankylosing spondylitis. Magnetic resonance imaging of the sacroiliac joints of a 23-year-old woman with progressive right-sided inflammatory back pain of 6 months' duration. Conventional radiographs were normal. A fat-suppressed image employing a short tau inversion recovery (STIR) sequence shows acute sacroiliitis on the right side, with edema in the juxtaarticular bone marrow (*asterisks*), in the region of the synovium and joint capsule (*thin arrow*), and in the region of the interosseous ligaments (*thick arrow*). Early chronic changes, including cortical erosions and joint space widening, were evident in the right sacroiliac joint in T1-, contrast-enhanced T1-, and T2*-weighted images (not shown). The patient subsequently developed radiographically evident bilateral sacroiliitis, fulfilling the criteria for ankylosing spondylitis. (*Photo provided by Dr. Jürgen Braun; previously published in Zeitschrift für Rheumatologie 58.61, 1999. Reproduced with permission.*)

a dose of 60 mg given monthly by intravenous infusion; thalidomide, 200 mg/d, perhaps also acting through inhibition of TNF-α; and the α-emitting isotope ^{224}Ra, at a dose of 1 MBq given weekly by intravenous infusion.[1]

AS is a chronic progressive disease with a significant impact on productivity and quality of life. Although there are patients with mild AS whose pain is well controlled with NSAID therapy and whose disease shows little radiographic progression, many, if not most, patients have axial pain, stiffness, and disease progression despite conventional therapy. Thus, should anti-TNF-α agents, or similarly potent biologicals, prove reasonably safe and continuously effective, it can be predicted that eventually these agents will become standard therapy for most patients with AS.

The most common indication for surgery in patients with AS is severe hip joint arthritis, the pain and stiffness of which are usually dramatically relieved by total hip arthroplasty. A small number of patients may benefit from surgical correction of extreme flexion deformities of the spine or of atlantoaxial subluxation.

Attacks of uveitis are usually managed effectively with local glucocorticoid administration in conjunction with mydriatic agents, although systemic glucocorticoids or even immunosuppressive drugs may be required in some cases. The response of uveitis to anti-TNF-α therapy has not been as predictable as that of other features of AS. Coexistent cardiac disease may require pacemaker implantation and/or aortic valve replacement. Management of osteoporosis of the axial skeleton is at present similar to that used for primary osteoporosis, since data specific for AS are not available.

REACTIVE ARTHRITIS

Reactive arthritis (ReA) refers to acute nonpurulent arthritis complicating an infection elsewhere in the body. In recent years, the term has been used primarily to refer to spondyloarthritides following enteric or urogenital infections and occurring predominantly in individuals with the histocompatibility antigen HLA-B27. In the setting of HIV infection, the association with B27 is not necessarily found. →*Other forms of reactive and infection-related arthritis not associated with B27 and showing a different spectrum of clinical features, such as rheumatic fever or Lyme disease, are discussed in Chaps. 302 and 157.*

HISTORIC BACKGROUND The association of acute arthritis with episodes of diarrhea or urethritis has been recognized for centuries. A large number of cases during World Wars I and II focused attention on the triad of arthritis, urethritis, and conjunctivitis, which became known as *Reiter's syndrome*, often occurring with additional mucocutaneous lesions. This eponym is now of historic interest only.

The identification of bacterial species capable of triggering the clinical syndrome and the finding that up to 85% of the patients possess the B27 antigen have led to the unifying concept of ReA as a clinical syndrome triggered by specific etiologic agents in a genetically susceptible host. A similar spectrum of clinical manifestations can be triggered by enteric infection with any of several *Shigella*, *Salmonella*, *Yersinia*, and *Campylobacter* species; by genital infection with *Chlamydia trachomatis*; and possibly by other agents as well. The triad of arthritis, urethritis, and conjunctivitis represents one part of the spectrum of the clinical manifestations of ReA, particularly that induced by *Shigella* or *Chlamydia*. For the purposes of this chapter, the use of the term *ReA* will be restricted to those cases of spondyloarthritis in which there is at least presumptive evidence for a related antecedent infection. Patients with clinical features of ReA who lack evidence of an antecedent infection will be considered to have *undifferentiated spondyloarthritis*, discussed below.

---

[1]Azathioprine, methotrexate, sulfasalazine, infliximab, etanercept, pamidronate, thalidomide, and ^{224}Ra have not been approved for this purpose by the U.S. Food and Drug Administration at the time of publication.

EPIDEMIOLOGY Outside the setting of HIV infection, ReA occurs predominantly in individuals who have inherited the B27 gene; in most series in which *Shigella*, *Yersinia*, or *Chlamydia* are the triggering infectious agents, 60 to 85% of patients are B27 positive. The prevalence of B27 tends to be much lower ($\leq$50%) in ReA triggered by *Salmonella* and even lower for *Campylobacter*. The disease is most common in individuals 18 to 40 years of age, but it can occur both in children over 5 years of age and in older adults.

The sex ratio in ReA following enteric infection is nearly 1:1, whereas venereally acquired ReA occurs predominantly in men. The overall prevalence and incidence of ReA are difficult to assess because of the variable prevalence of the triggering infections and genetic susceptibility factors in different populations. The spondyloarthritides were previously almost unknown in sub-Saharan Africa, where <1% of the population carries B27. However, ReA and other peripheral spondyloarthritides have now become the most common rheumatic diseases in Africans in the wake of the AIDS epidemic, with no association to B27. Spondyloarthritis in Africans with HIV infection usually occurs in individuals with stage I disease (as classified by the World Health Organization). It is often the first manifestation of infection and often remits with disease progression. In contrast, western Caucasian patients with HIV and spondyloarthritis are predominantly B27 positive, and the arthritis flares as AIDS advances.

PATHOLOGY Synovial histology is similar to that of other inflammatory arthropathies. Enthesitis shows increased vascularity and macrophage infiltration of fibrocartilage. Microscopic histopathologic evidence of inflammation has occasionally been noted in the colon and ileum of patients with postvenereal ReA, but much less commonly than in postenteric ReA. The skin lesions of keratoderma blennorrhagica, which is associated mainly with venereally acquired ReA, are histologically indistinguishable from psoriatic lesions.

ETIOLOGY AND PATHOGENESIS Of the four *Shigella* species *S. sonnei*, *S. boydii*, *S. flexneri*, and *S. dysenteriae*, *S. flexneri* has most often been implicated in cases of ReA, both sporadic and epidemic. *S. sonnei*, although responsible for the majority of cases of shigellosis in the United States, has only rarely been implicated in cases of ReA.

Other bacteria identified definitively as triggers of ReA include several *Salmonella* spp., *Y. enterocolitica*, *C. jejuni*, and *C. trachomatis*. There is evidence implicating several other microorganisms, including *Y. pseudotuberculosis*, *Clostridium difficile*, and *Ureaplasma urealyticum*. There are also numerous isolated reports of acute arthritis preceded by other bacterial, viral, or parasitic infections, but whether the microorganisms involved are actual triggers of ReA remains to be determined.

It has not been determined whether ReA occurs by the same pathogenic mechanism following infection with each of these microorganisms, nor has the mechanism been fully elucidated in the case of any one of the known bacterial triggers. Most, if not all, of the triggering organisms produce lipopolysaccharide (LPS) and share a capacity to attack mucosal surfaces, to invade host cells, and to survive intracellularly. Antigens from *Chlamydia*, *Yersinia*, *Salmonella*, and *Shigella* have been shown to be present in the synovium and/or synovial fluid leukocytes of patients with ReA for long periods following the acute attack. In ReA triggered by *Y. enterocolitica*, bacterial LPS and heat shock protein antigens have been found in peripheral blood cells years after the triggering infection. In the case of *C. trachomatis*, synovial persistence of microbial DNA and RNA suggests the presence of viable organisms, despite uniform failure to culture the organism from these specimens. ReA, at least in some cases, thus may be a form of chronic infection, rather than solely "reactive." T cells that specifically respond to antigens of the inciting organism have been found in inflamed synovium but not in peripheral blood of patients with ReA. These T cells are predominantly CD4+, but CD8+ B27-restricted bacteria-specific cytolytic T cells have also been isolated in *Yersinia*- and *C. trachomatis*-induced ReA. A unique conserved T cell antigen receptor sequence has been identified in B27-restricted synovial T cells in ReA. Unlike the synovial CD4 T cells in RA, which are predominantly of the T_H1 phenotype, those in ReA also show a T_H2 phenotype. It is likely that antigen-specific T cells play an important role in the pathogenesis of ReA, but the mechanisms remain to be determined.

The role of HLA-B27 in ReA also remains to be determined. The presence of HLA-B27 significantly prolongs the intracellular survival of *Y. enterocolitica* and *S. enteritidis* in human and mouse cell lines. Prolonged intracellular bacterial survival, promoted by B27, other factors, or both, may permit trafficking of infected leukocytes from the site of primary infection to joints, where a T cell response to persistent bacterial antigens may then promote arthritis.

CLINICAL FEATURES   The clinical manifestations of ReA constitute a spectrum that ranges from an isolated, transient monarthritis to severe multisystem disease. Usually, a careful history will elicit evidence of an antecedent infection 1 to 4 weeks before onset of symptoms of the reactive disease. However, in a sizable minority, no clinical or laboratory evidence of an antecedent infection can be found. In many cases of presumed venereally acquired reactive disease, there is a history of a recent new sexual partner, even in the absence of laboratory evidence of infection.

Constitutional symptoms are common, including fatigue, malaise, fever, and weight loss. The musculoskeletal symptoms are usually acute in onset. Arthritis is usually asymmetric and additive, with involvement of new joints occurring over a period of a few days to 1 to 2 weeks. The joints of the lower extremities, especially the knee, ankle, and subtalar, metatarsophalangeal, and toe interphalangeal joints, are the most common sites of involvement, but the wrist and fingers can be involved as well. The arthritis is usually quite painful, and tense joint effusions are not uncommon, especially in the knee. Patients often cannot walk without support. Dactylitis, or "sausage digit," a diffuse swelling of a solitary finger or toe, is a distinctive feature of ReA and other peripheral spondyloarthritides but can be seen in polyarticular gout and sarcoidosis. Tendinitis and fasciitis are particularly characteristic lesions, producing pain at multiple insertion sites (entheses), especially the Achilles insertion, the plantar fascia, and sites along the axial skeleton. Spinal and low-back pain are quite common and may be caused by insertional inflammation, muscle spasm, acute sacroiliitis, or, presumably, arthritis in intervertebral articulations.

Urogenital lesions may occur throughout the course of the disease. In males, urethritis may be marked or relatively asymptomatic and may be either an accompaniment of the triggering infection or a result of the reactive phase of the disease. Prostatitis is also common. Similarly, in females, cervicitis or salpingitis may be caused either by the infectious trigger or by the sterile reactive process.

Ocular disease is common, ranging from transient, asymptomatic conjunctivitis to an aggressive anterior uveitis that occasionally proves refractory to treatment and may result in blindness.

Mucocutaneous lesions are frequent. Oral ulcers tend to be superficial, transient, and often asymptomatic. The characteristic skin lesions, *keratoderma blenorrhagica*, consist of vesicles that become hyperkeratotic, ultimately forming a crust before disappearing. They are most common on the palms and soles but may occur elsewhere as well. In patients with HIV infection, these lesions are often extremely severe and extensive, to the point of dominating the clinical picture (Chap. 173). Lesions on the glans penis, termed *circinate balanitis*, are common; these consist of vesicles that quickly rupture to form painless superficial erosions, which in circumcised individuals can form crusts similar to those of keratoderma blenorrhagica. Nail changes are common and consist of onycholysis, distal yellowish discoloration, and/or heaped-up hyperkeratosis.

Less frequent or rare manifestations of ReA include cardiac conduction defects, aortic insufficiency, central or peripheral nervous system lesions, and pleuropulmonary infiltrates.

Long-term follow-up studies suggest that some joint symptoms persist in 30 to 60% of patients with ReA. Recurrences of the acute syndrome are common, and as many as 25% of patients either become unable to work or are forced to change occupations because of persistent joint symptoms. Chronic heel pain is often particularly distressing. Some aspects of AS are also common sequelae. In most studies, HLA-B27-positive patients have shown a worse outcome than B27-negative patients. The extent to which the long-term prognosis varies with different inciting agents is not known. However, patients with *Yersinia*-induced arthritis appear to have less chronic disease than those whose initial episode follows epidemic shigellosis.

LABORATORY AND RADIOGRAPHIC FINDINGS   The ESR is usually elevated during the acute phase of the disease. Mild anemia may be present, and acute-phase reactants tend to be increased. Synovial fluid is nonspecifically inflammatory. In most ethnic groups, 50 to 85% of the patients are B27 positive, although the prevalence of B27 can be much lower in cases triggered by *Campylobacter* or *Salmonella* infections. It is unusual for the triggering infection to persist at the site of primary mucosal infection through the time of onset of the reactive disease, but it may occasionally be possible to culture the organism, e.g., in the case of *Yersinia*- or *Chlamydia*-induced disease. Serologic evidence of a recent infection may be present, such as a marked elevation of antibodies to *Yersinia*, *Salmonella*, or *Chlamydia*.

In early or mild disease, radiographic changes may be absent or confined to juxtaarticular osteoporosis. With long-standing persistent disease, marginal erosions and loss of joint space can be seen in affected joints. Periostitis with reactive new bone formation is characteristic of the disease, as it is with all the spondyloarthritides. Spurs at the insertion of the plantar fascia are common.

Sacroiliitis and spondylitis may be seen as late sequelae. The sacroiliitis is more commonly asymmetric than in AS, and the spondylitis, rather than ascending symmetrically from the lower lumbar segments, can begin anywhere along the lumbar spine. The syndesmophytes may be coarse and nonmarginal, arising from the middle of a vertebral body, a pattern rarely seen in primary AS. Progression to spinal fusion is uncommon.

DIAGNOSIS   ReA is a clinical diagnosis, there being no definitively diagnostic laboratory test or radiographic finding. The diagnosis should be entertained in any patient with an acute inflammatory, asymmetric, additive arthritis or tendinitis. The evaluation should include questioning regarding possible triggering events such as an episode of diarrhea or dysuria. On physical examination, attention must be paid to the distribution of the joint and tendon involvement and to possible sites of extraarticular involvement, such as the eyes, mucous membranes, skin, nails, and genitalia. Synovial fluid analysis may be helpful in excluding septic or crystal-induced arthritis. Culture, serology, or molecular methods may help to identify a triggering infection.

Although typing for B27 is not needed to secure the diagnosis in clear-cut cases, it may have prognostic significance in terms of severity, chronicity, and the propensity for spondylitis and uveitis. Furthermore, it can be helpful diagnostically in atypical cases, a positive test increasing and a negative test decreasing the probability of ReA. HIV testing is often indicated and may be necessary in order to select appropriate therapy.

It is important to differentiate ReA from disseminated gonococcal disease (Chap. 128), both of which can be venereally acquired and associated with urethritis. Unlike ReA, gonococcal arthritis and tenosynovitis tend to involve both upper and lower extremities equally, to lack back symptoms, and to be associated with characteristic vesicular skin lesions. A positive gonococcal culture from the urethra or cervix does not exclude a diagnosis of ReA; however, culturing gonococci from blood, skin lesion, or synovium establishes the diagnosis of disseminated gonococcal disease. Polymerase chain reaction (PCR) assay for *Neisseria gonorrheae* and *C. trachomatis* may be helpful. Occasionally, only a therapeutic trial of antibiotics can distinguish the two.

ReA shares many features in common with psoriatic arthropathy. However, psoriatic arthritis is usually gradual in onset; the arthritis tends to affect primarily the upper extremities; there is less associated periarthritis; and there are usually no associated mouth ulcers, urethritis, or bowel symptoms.

℞ TREATMENT

Most patients with ReA are benefitted to some degree by NSAIDs, although rarely are symptoms of the acute arthritis completely ameliorated, and some patients fail to respond at all. Indomethacin, 75 to 150 mg/d in divided doses, is the initial treatment of choice. Other NSAIDs may be tried, with phenylbutazone, 100 mg tid or qid, being the NSAID of last resort, to be used only in severe, refractory cases because of its potentially serious side effects. There are no published data on the use of selective COX-2 inhibitors, but these may be tried in patients who do not tolerate conventional NSAIDs.

Several controlled trials have failed to demonstrate any benefit for antibiotic therapy in ReA. However, prompt, appropriate antibiotic treatment of acute chlamydial urethritis may prevent subsequent ReA.

Multicenter trials have suggested that sulfasalazine, up to 3 g/d in divided doses, may be beneficial to patients with persistent ReA.[1] Patients with persistent disease may respond to azathioprine, 1 to 2 mg/kg per day, or to methotrexate, 7.5 to 15 mg per week. Although no trials of anti-TNF-α in ReA have been reported, anecdotal evidence supports the use of these agents in severe chronic cases, although lack of response has also been observed.

Tendinitis and other enthesitic lesions may benefit from intralesional glucocorticoids. Uveitis may require aggressive treatment with glucocorticoids to prevent serious sequelae. Skin lesions ordinarily require only symptomatic treatment. In patients with HIV infection and ReA, many of whom have severe skin lesions, the skin lesions in particular respond to anti-retroviral therapy. Cardiac complications are managed conventionally; management of neurologic complications is symptomatic.

Comprehensive management includes counseling of patients in the avoidance of sexually transmitted disease and exposure to enteropathogens, as well as appropriate use of physical therapy, vocational counseling, and continued surveillance for long-term complications such as ankylosing spondylitis.

PSORIATIC ARTHRITIS

Psoriatic arthritis (PsA) refers to an inflammatory arthritis that characteristically occurs in individuals with psoriasis.

HISTORIC BACKGROUND The association between arthritis and psoriasis was noted in the nineteenth century. In the 1960s, on the basis of epidemiologic and clinical studies, it became clear that unlike RA the arthritis associated with psoriasis was usually seronegative, often involved the distal interphalangeal (DIP) joints of the fingers and the spine and sacroiliac joints, had distinctive radiographic features, and showed considerable familial aggregation. In the 1970s, PsA was included in the broader category of the spondyloarthritides because of features similar to those of AS and ReA.

EPIDEMIOLOGY A recent consensus has emerged that, among individuals with psoriasis, the prevalence of PsA is about 5 to 10%, but figures as high as 30% continue to be reported. In Caucasian populations, psoriasis is estimated to have a prevalence of 1 to 3%. Psoriasis and PsA are less common in other races in the absence of HIV infection. First-degree relatives of PsA patients have an elevated risk for psoriasis, for PsA itself, and for other forms of spondyloarthritis. Of patients with psoriasis, 30% have an affected first-degree relative. In monozygotic twins, the concordance for psoriasis is ≥65%, and for PsA ≥30%. A variety of HLA associations have been found. HLA-Cw6 is highly associated with psoriasis, particularly familial juvenile onset (type I) psoriasis. HLA-B27 is highly associated with psoriatic spondylitis (see below). HLA-DR7, -DQ3, and -B57 are associated with PsA because of linkage disequilibrium with Cw6. Other associations include HLA-B13, -B37, -B38, -B39, and DR4. The MIC-A-A9 allele at the HLA-B-linked MIC-A locus has also recently been reported associated with PsA, as have certain killer immunoglobulin-like receptor (KIR) alleles. The complex inheritance patterns of psoriasis and PsA suggest that several unlinked allelic loci are required for susceptibility. However, only the MHC has shown consistent linkage from study to study.

PATHOLOGY The inflamed synovium in PsA resembles that of RA, although with somewhat less hyperplasia and cellularity than in RA, and somewhat greater vascularity. Some studies have indicated a higher tendency to synovial fibrosis in PsA. Unlike RA, PsA shows prominent enthesitis, with histology similar to that of the other spondyloarthritides.

PATHOGENESIS PsA is almost certainly immune mediated, although the mechanism is as yet not well understood. PsA synovium shows infiltration with T cells, B cells, and macrophages, and upregulation of leukocyte homing receptors. CD8+ T cells are more frequent in PsA. Cytokine production in the synovium in PsA resembles that in psoriatic skin lesions and in RA synovium, having predominantly a T_H1 pattern. Interleukin (IL) 2, interferon γ, TNF-α, and IL-1β, -6, -8, -10, -12, -13, and -15 are found in PsA synovium or synovial fluid. Differences between PsA and RA in this regard are primarily quantitative, not qualitative.

CLINICAL FEATURES In 60 to 70% of cases, psoriasis precedes joint disease. In 15 to 20%, the two manifestations appear within 1 year of each other. In about 15 to 20% of cases, the arthritis precedes the onset of psoriasis and can present a diagnostic challenge. The frequency in men and women is almost equal, although the frequency of disease patterns differs somewhat in the two sexes. The disease can begin in childhood or late in life, but typically begins in the fourth or fifth decade, at an average age of 37 years.

The spectrum of arthropathy associated with psoriasis is quite broad. Several classification schemes have been proposed, but the most widely accepted is that of Wright and Moll, who described five patterns: (1) arthritis of the DIP joints; (2) asymmetric oligoarthritis; (3) symmetric polyarthritis similar to RA; (4) axial involvement (spine and sacroiliac joints); and (5) arthritis mutilans, a highly destructive form of disease. These patterns are not fixed, and in many patients the pattern that persists chronically differs from that of the initial presentation.

Nail changes in the fingers or toes occur in 90% of patients with PsA, compared with 40% of psoriatic patients without arthritis, and pustular psoriasis is said to be associated with more severe arthritis. Several articular features distinguish PsA from other joint disorders. Dactylitis occurs in >30%; enthesitis and tenosynovitis are also common, and are probably present in most patients, although often not appreciated on physical examination. Shortening of digits because of underlying osteolysis is particularly characteristic of PsA, and there is a much greater tendency than in RA for both fibrous and bony ankylosis of small joints. Rapid ankylosis of one or more PIP joints early in the course of disease is not uncommon. Back and neck pain and stiffness are also common in PsA.

Arthropathy confined to the DIP joints predominates in about 15% of cases. Accompanying nail changes in the affected digits are almost always present. These joints are also often affected in the other patterns of PsA. Approximately 30% of patients have asymmetric oligoarthritis. This pattern commonly involves a knee or another large joint with a few small joints in the fingers or toes, often with dactylitis. Symmetric polyarthritis occurs in about 40% of PsA patients. It may be indistinguishable from RA in terms of the joints involved, but other features characteristic of PsA are usually also present. In general, peripheral joints in PsA tend to be somewhat less tender than in RA, although signs of inflammation are usually present. Almost any peripheral joint can be involved. Axial arthropathy without peripheral involvement is found in about 5% of PsA patients. It may be indistinguishable from idiopathic AS, although more neck involvement and less thoracolumbar spinal involvement is characteristic, and nail changes are not found in idiopathic AS. About 5% of PsA patients have arthritis mutilans, in which there can be widespread shortening of digits ("telescoping"), sometimes coexisting with ankylosis and contractures in other digits.

Six patterns of nail involvement are identified: pitting, horizontal ridging, onycholysis, yellowish discoloration of the nail margins, dystrophic hyperkeratosis, and combinations of these findings. Other extraarticular manifestations of the spondyloarthritides are common. Eye involvement, either conjunctivitis or uveitis, is reported in 7 to 33% of PsA patients. Unlike the uveitis associated with AS, the uveitis in PsA shows more tendency to be bilateral, chronic, and/or posterior. Aortic valve insufficiency has been found in <4% of patients, usually after long-standing disease.

Widely varying estimates of clinical outcome have been reported in PsA. At its worst, severe PsA with arthritis mutilans is at least as crippling and ultimately fatal as severe RA. Unlike RA, however, many patients with PsA experience temporary remissions. Overall, erosive disease develops in the majority of patients, progressive disease with deformity and disability is common, and in some large published series mortality was found to be significantly increased compared with the general population.

The psoriasis and associated arthropathy seen in individuals infected with HIV both tend to be severe and can occur in populations with very little psoriasis in noninfected individuals. Severe enthesopathy, dactylitis, and rapidly progressive joint destruction are seen, but axial involvement is very rare. This condition is prevented by or responds well to anti-retroviral therapy.

LABORATORY AND RADIOGRAPHIC FINDINGS   There are no diagnostic laboratory tests for PsA. ESR and CRP are often, but not always, elevated. A small percentage of patients may have low titers of rheumatoid factor or antinuclear antibodies. Uric acid may be elevated in the presence of extensive psoriasis. HLA-B27 is found in 50 to 70% of patients with axial disease, but in ≤15 to 20% in patients with only peripheral joint involvement.

The peripheral and axial arthropathies in PsA show a number of radiographic features that distinguish them from RA and AS, respectively. Characteristics of peripheral PsA include DIP involvement, including the classic "pencil-in-cup" deformity; marginal erosions with adjacent bony proliferation ("whiskering"); small joint ankylosis; osteolysis of phalangeal and metacarpal bone, with telescoping of digits; and periostitis and proliferative new bone at sites of enthesitis. Characteristics of axial PsA include asymmetric sacroiliitis; compared with idiopathic AS, less zygoapophyseal joint arthritis; fewer and less symmetric and delicate syndesmophytes; fluffy hyperperiostosis on anterior vertebral bodies; severe cervical spine involvement, with a tendency to atlantoaxial subluxation but relative sparing of the thoracolumbar spine; and paravertebral ossification. Ultrasound and MRI both readily demonstrate enthesitis and tendon sheath effusions that can be difficult to assess on physical examination.

DIAGNOSIS   The diagnosis of PsA is primarily clinical and can be challenging when the arthritis precedes psoriasis, the psoriasis is undiagnosed or obscure, or the joint involvement closely resembles another form of arthritis. A high index of suspicion is needed in any patient with an undiagnosed inflammatory arthropathy. The history should include inquiry about psoriasis in the patient and family members. Patients should be asked to disrobe for the physical examination, and psoriasiform lesions should be sought in the scalp, ears, umbilicus, and gluteal folds in addition to more accessible sites, and the finger and toe nails should be carefully examined. Axial symptoms or signs, dactylitis, enthesitis, ankylosis, the pattern of joint involvement, and characteristic radiographic changes can be helpful clues. The differential diagnosis of isolated DIP involvement is short. Osteoarthritis (Heberden's nodes) is usually not inflammatory; gout involving more than one DIP joint often involves other sites and is accompanied by

tophi; the very rare entity multicentric reticulohistiocytosis involves other joints and has characteristic small pearly periungual skin nodules; and the uncommon entity inflammatory osteoarthritis, like the others, lacks the nail changes of PsA. Radiography can be helpful in all of these cases and in distinguishing between psoriatic spondylitis and idiopathic AS. A history of trauma to an affected joint preceding the onset of arthritis is said to occur more frequently in PsA than in other types of arthritis, perhaps reflecting the Koebner phenomenon in which psoriatic skin lesions can arise at sites of the skin trauma.

℞ TREATMENT

Ideally, coordinated therapy is directed at both the skin and joints in PsA. As described above for AS, use of the anti-TNF-α agents promises to revolutionize the treatment of PsA. Prompt and dramatic resolution of both arthritis and skin lesions has been observed in at least five trials of etanercept and infliximab. Many of the responding patients had long-standing disease that was resistant to all previous therapy, as well as extensive skin disease. Although the effect on disease progression has not yet been reported, the clinical response is even more dramatic than in RA, in which both etanercept and infliximab have been shown to halt the progression of joint erosions.

Other treatment for PsA has been based on drugs that have efficacy in RA and/or in psoriasis. Although methotrexate in doses of 15 to 25 mg/wk and sulfasalazine (usually given in doses of 2 to 3 g/d) have each been found to have clinical efficacy in controlled trials, neither effectively halts progression of erosive joint disease. Other agents with efficacy in psoriasis reported to benefit PsA are cyclosporine, retinoic acid derivatives, and psoralen plus ultraviolet light (PUVA). There is controversy regarding the efficacy in PsA of gold and antimalarials, which have been widely used in RA. The new antirheumatic agent leflunomide is currently being evaluated.

All of these treatments require careful monitoring. Use of immunosuppressive therapy, including anti-TNF-α agents, methotrexate, and cyclosporine, is largely contraindicated in HIV-associated PsA.

In one large prospective series, 7% of patients with PsA required musculoskeletal surgery beginning at a mean of 13 years' disease duration. Indications for surgery are similar to those in RA, although there is an impression that outcomes in PsA may be less satisfactory.

SAPHO SYNDROME

The syndrome of synovitis, acne, pustulosis, hyperostosis, and osteitis (SAPHO) is characterized by a variety of skin and musculoskeletal manifestations. Dermatologic manifestations include palmoplantar pustulosis, acne conglobata, acne fulminans, and hidradenitis suppurativa. The main musculoskeletal findings are sternoclavicular and spinal hyperostosis, chronic recurrent foci of sterile osteomyelitis, and occasionally peripheral arthritis. Cases with one or a few manifestations are probably the rule. Granulomas may be present on bone biopsy. The ESR is usually elevated, sometimes dramatically. In some series, B27 is present in about 30% of the cases. Either bone scan or CT scan is helpful diagnostically. Therapy has been inadequate, with high dose NSAIDs, including phenylbutazone, providing the most relief from bone pain. Response to pamidronate and to anti-TNF-α therapy has been observed anecdotally.

UNDIFFERENTIATED AND JUVENILE-ONSET SPONDYLOARTHRITIS

Many patients, usually young adults, present with some features of one or more of the spondyloarthritides discussed above but lack criteria for these diagnoses. For example, a patient may present with inflammatory synovitis of one knee, Achilles tendinitis, and dactylitis of one digit, or sacroiliitis in the absence of other criteria for AS. Such patients are said to have undifferentiated spondyloarthritis, or simply spondyloarthritis, as defined by the European Spondyloarthropathy Study Group (ESSG criteria, Fig. 305-2). Some of these patients may

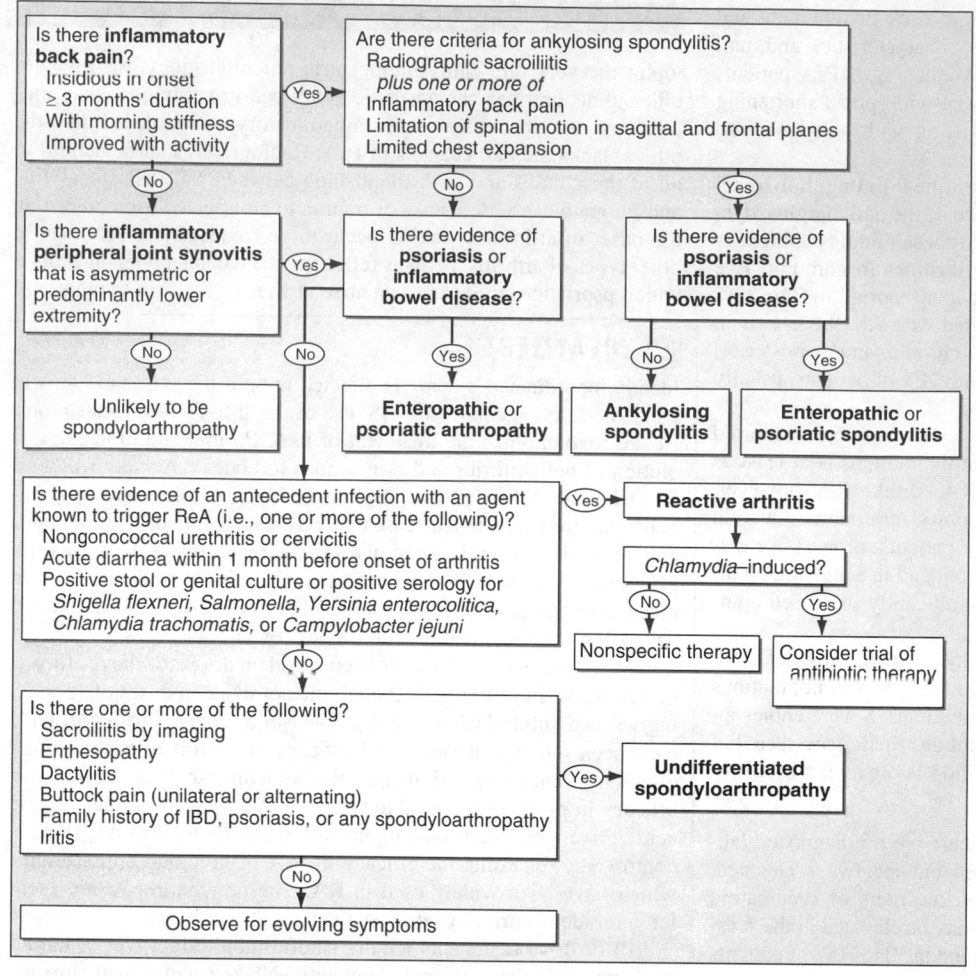

FIGURE 305-2 Algorithm for diagnosis of the spondyloarthritides, adapted from the European Spondyloarthropathy Study Group criteria. If a diagnosis of psoriatic arthropathy, reactive arthritis, or undifferentiated spondyloarthritis is made on the basis of peripheral arthropathy, then HIV infection needs to be considered.

have ReA in which the triggering infection remains clinically silent. In some other cases, the patient subsequently develops IBD or psoriasis or the process eventually meets criteria for AS. Approximately half the patients with undifferentiated spondyloarthritis are HLA-B27 positive, and thus the absence of B27 is not useful in establishing or excluding the diagnosis. In familial cases, which are almost always B27 positive, there is often eventual progression to AS.

In juvenile-onset spondyloarthritis, which begins between ages 7 and 16, most commonly in boys (60 to 80%), an asymmetric, predominantly lower extremity oligoarthritis and enthesitis without extraarticular features is the typical mode of presentation. The prevalence of B27 in this condition, which has been termed the seronegative, enthesopathy, arthropathy (SEA) syndrome, is approximately 80%. Many, but not all, of these patients go on to develop AS in late adolescence or adulthood.

Management of undifferentiated spondyloarthritis is similar to that of the other spondyloarthritides. Response to anti-TNF-α therapy has been documented, and this therapy is indicated in severe, persistent cases not responsive to other treatment. Current pediatric textbooks and journals should be consulted for information on management of juvenile-onset spondyloarthritis. An algorithm for the diagnosis of the spondyloarthritides in adults is presented in Fig. 305-2.

ENTEROPATHIC ARTHRITIS

HISTORIC BACKGROUND A relationship between arthritis and IBD was observed in the 1930s. The relationship was further defined by the epidemiologic studies in the 1950s and '60s and included in the concept of the spondyloarthritides in the 1970s.

EPIDEMIOLOGY Both of the common forms of IBD, ulcerative colitis (UC) and Crohn's disease (CD) (Chap. 276), are associated with spondyloarthritis. UC and CD both have an estimated prevalence of 0.05 to 0.1%, and the incidence of each is thought to have increased in recent decades. AS and peripheral arthritis are both associated with UC and with CD. Wide variations have been reported in the estimated frequencies of these associations. In three recent European series encompassing almost 2000 patients with IBD for a median 5 to 10 years, overall, AS was diagnosed in 2%, inflammatory back pain in 9%, enthesopathy in 7%, and peripheral arthritis in 10%, with somewhat higher frequencies found in CD than in UC. The combined total frequency of spondyloarthritis was 19%. These figures are somewhat lower than earlier estimates. Asymptomatic radiographic sacroiliitis was found in an additional 5%.

The prevalence of UC or CD in patients with AS is thought to be 5 to 10%. However, investigation of unselected spondyloarthritis patients by ileocolonoscopy has revealed that from one-third to two-thirds of patients with AS have subclinical intestinal inflammation that is evident either macroscopically or histologically. These lesions have also been found in patients with undifferentiated spondyloarthritis or ReA (both enterically and urogenitally acquired).

Both UC and CD have a tendency to familial aggregation, more so for CD. HLA associations have been weak and inconsistent. HLA-B27 is found in about 70% of patients with IBD and AS, but in ≤15% of patients with IBD and peripheral arthritis or IBD alone. Certain alleles of the *NOD2/CARD15* gene on chromosome 16 have recently been found in up to half of patients with CD. It appears that these alleles are not associated with the spondyloarthritides, either occurring alone or in association with CD, but the data are not yet conclusive.

PATHOLOGY Available data for IBD-associated peripheral arthritis suggest a nonspecific inflammatory synovitis, although one study found granulomas associated with CD. Association with arthropathy does not affect the gut histology of UC or CD (Chap. 276). The subclinical inflammatory lesions in the colon and distal ileum associated with spondyloarthritis have been classified as either acute or chronic. The former resemble acute bacterial enteritis, with largely intact architecture and neutrophilic infiltration in the lamina propria. The latter resemble the lesions of CD, with distortion of villi and crypts, aphthoid ulceration, and mononuclear cell infiltration in the lamina propria.

PATHOGENESIS Both IBD and the spondyloarthropathies are immune mediated, but the specific pathogenic mechanisms are poorly understood, and the connection between the two is obscure. IBD is a common phenotype in a number of rodent lines with transgenic overexpression or targeted deletion of genes involved in immune processes. Arthritis is an accompanying prominent feature in two of these IBD models, HLA-B27 transgenic rats and mice with constitutive overexpression of TNF-α, and immune dysregulation is prominent in both. Several lines of evidence indicate trafficking of leukocytes between the gut and the joint. Mucosal leukocytes from IBD patients have been shown to bind avidly to synovial vasculature through several different adhesion molecules, and T cells with identical antigen receptor sequences have been isolated from both the gut and the synovium in the same patient. Macrophages expressing CD163 are prominent in the inflammatory lesions of both gut and synovium in the spondyloarthritides.

CLINICAL FEATURES AS associated with IBD is clinically indistinguishable from idiopathic AS. It runs a course independent of the bowel disease, and in many patients it precedes the onset of IBD, sometimes by many years. In contrast, peripheral arthritis has generally been reported to parallel the activity of the bowel disease, although it not infrequently begins before onset of overt bowel disease. A recent large study classified the peripheral arthritis of IBD patients into two types. Type 1 involved fewer than five joints, was associated with acute self-limited attacks, and often coincided with relapses of IBD. Type 2 involved five or more joints, tended to be symmetric, and ran a chronic course independent of IBD. The patterns of joint involvement were similar in UC and CD. Type 1 arthritis involved primarily the knee and ankle, whereas type 2 involved these joints but also tended to involve joints in the hand and upper extremity. This dichotomy has yet to be confirmed, but both types are characteristic of the spectrum of peripheral arthritis previously described in IBD. In general, erosions and deformities are infrequent in IBD-associated peripheral arthritis, and joint surgery is rarely required. Dactylitis and enthesopathy are occasionally found. In addition to the ~20% of IBD patients with spondyloarthritis, a comparable percentage have arthralgias or fibromyalgia symptoms.

Other extraintestinal manifestations of IBD are seen in addition to arthropathy, including uveitis, pyoderma gangrenosum, erythema nodosum, and finger clubbing, all somewhat more common in CD than UC. The uveitis shares the features described above for PsA-associated uveitis.

LABORATORY AND RADIOGRAPHIC FINDINGS Laboratory findings reflect the inflammatory and metabolic manifestations of IBD. Joint fluid is usually at least mildly inflammatory. Of patients with AS and IBD, about 70% carry the HLA-B27 gene, compared with >90% of patients with AS alone and 50 to 70% of those with AS and psoriasis. Hence, definite or probable AS in a B27-negative individual in the absence of psoriasis should prompt a search for occult IBD. Radiographic changes in the axial skeleton are the same as in uncomplicated AS. Erosions are uncommon in peripheral arthritis but may occur, particularly in the metatarsophalangeal joints. Isolated destructive hip disease has been described.

DIAGNOSIS Diarrhea and arthritis are both common conditions that can coexist for a variety of reasons. When etiopathogenically related, reactive arthritis and IBD-associated arthritis are the most common causes. Rare causes include celiac disease, blind loop syndromes, and Whipple's disease. In most cases, diagnosis depends upon investigation of the bowel disease.

℞ **TREATMENT**

As with the spondyloarthritides, treatment of CD is being revolutionized by therapy with infliximab, particularly in patients with fistulas or refractory disease. Recent anecdotal evidence suggests that associated arthritis responds promptly to infliximab. It is of interest that the spondyloarthritides respond to both infliximab and etaner-

cept, whereas only infliximab has efficacy in CD and neither agent is effective in UC. Other treatment for IBD, including sulfasalazine and related drugs, systemic glucocorticoids, and immunosuppressive drugs, are also usually of benefit for associated peripheral arthritis. NSAIDs are generally helpful and well tolerated, but they can precipitate flares of IBD.

WHIPPLE'S DISEASE

Whipple's disease (Chap. 275) is a rare chronic bacterial infection, mostly of middle-aged Caucasian men, caused by *Tropheryma whippelii*. At least 75% of affected individuals develop an oligo- or polyarthritis. The joint manifestations usually precede other symptoms of the disease by 5 years or more; they are particularly important because antibiotic therapy is curative, whereas the untreated disease is fatal. Large and small peripheral joints and sacroiliac joints may be involved. The arthritis is abrupt in onset, migratory, usually lasts hours to a few days and then resolves completely. Chronic polyarthritis and joint space loss, visible on x-ray, can occur but are not typical. Eventually, prolonged diarrhea, malabsorption, and weight loss occur. Other manifestations of systemic disease include fever, edema, serositis, endocarditis, pneumonia, hypotension, lymphadenopathy, hyperpigmentation, subcutaneous nodules, clubbing, and uveitis. Central nervous system involvement eventually develops in 80% of untreated patients, with cognitive changes, headache, diplopia, and papilledema, and may be appreciated by abnormalities on MRI. Oculomasticatory and oculo-facial-skeletal myorhythmia, accompanied by supranuclear vertical gaze palsy, are said to be pathognomonic. Laboratory abnormalities include anemia and changes from malabsorption. There may be a weak association with HLA-B27. Synovial fluid is usually inflammatory. Radiography rarely shows joint erosions but may show sacroiliitis. Abdominal CT may reveal lymphadenopathy. Foamy macrophages containing PAS-staining bacterial remnants can be seen in biopsies of small intestine, synovium, lymph node, and other tissues. Diagnosis is established by PCR amplification of the 16S ribosomal gene sequences of *T. whippelii* in biopsied tissue. The organism has recently been isolated, and serologic tests may become available. The syndrome responds best to therapy with penicillin (or ceftriaxone) and streptomycin for 2 weeks followed by trimethoprim-sulfamethoxazole for 1 to 2 years. Monitoring for central nervous system relapse is critical.

FURTHER READING

BOWNESS P: HLA B27 in health and disease: A double-edged sword? Rheumatology (Oxford) 41:857, 2002

BRANDT J et al: Successful short term treatment of severe undifferentiated spondyloarthropathy with the anti-tumor necrosis factor-alpha monoclonal antibody infliximab. J Rheumatol 29:118, 2002

BRAUN J et al: Treatment of active ankylosing spondylitis with infliximab: A randomised controlled multicentre trial. Lancet 359:1187, 2002

BROWN MA et al: Genetic aspects of susceptibility, severity, and clinical expression in ankylosing spondylitis. Curr Opin Rheumatol 14:354, 2002

DOUGADOS M et al: The European Spondyloarthropathy Study Group preliminary criteria for the classification of spondyloarthropathy. Arthritis Rheum 34:1218, 1991

GLADMAN DD: Current concepts in psoriatic arthritis. Curr Opin Rheumatol 14:361, 2002

GORMAN JD et al: Treatment of ankylosing spondylitis by inhibition of tumor necrosis factor alpha. N Engl J Med 346:1349, 2002

306 THE VASCULITIS SYNDROMES
Michael C. Sneller, Carol A. Langford, Anthony S. Fauci

DEFINITION *Vasculitis* is a clinicopathologic process characterized by inflammation of and damage to blood vessels. The vessel lumen is usually compromised, and this is associated with ischemia of the tissues supplied by the involved vessel. A broad and heterogeneous group of syndromes may result from this process, since any type, size, and location of blood vessel may be involved. Vasculitis and its consequences may be the primary or sole manifestation of a disease; alternatively, vasculitis may be a secondary component of another primary disease. Vasculitis may be confined to a single organ, such as the skin, or it may simultaneously involve several organ systems.

CLASSIFICATION A major feature of the vasculitic syndromes as a group is the fact that there is a great deal of heterogeneity at the same time as there is considerable overlap among them. This heterogeneity and overlap in addition to a lack of understanding of the pathogenesis of these syndromes have been major impediments to the development of a coherent classification system for these diseases. Table 306-1 lists the major vasculitis syndromes. The distinguishing and overlapping features of these syndromes are discussed below.

PATHOPHYSIOLOGY AND PATHOGENESIS Generally, most of the vasculitic syndromes are assumed to be mediated at least in part by immunopathogenic mechanisms that occur in response to certain antigenic stimuli (Table 306-2). However, evidence supporting this hypothesis is for the most part indirect and may reflect epiphenomena as opposed to true causality. Furthermore, it is unknown why some individuals might develop vasculitis in response to certain antigenic stimuli, whereas others do not. It is likely that a number of factors are involved in the ultimate expression of a vasculitic syndrome. These include the genetic predisposition, environmental exposures, and the regulatory mechanisms associated with immune response to certain antigens.

Pathogenic Immune-Complex Formation Vasculitis is generally considered within the broader category of *immune-complex diseases* that include serum sickness and certain of the connective tissue diseases, of which systemic lupus erythematosus (Chap. 300) is the prototype. Although deposition of immune complexes in vessel walls is the most widely accepted pathogenic mechanism of vasculitis, the causal role of immune complexes has not been clearly established in most of the vasculitic syndromes. Circulating immune complexes need not result in deposition of the complexes in blood vessels with ensuing vasculitis, and many patients with active vasculitis do not have demonstrable circulating or deposited immune complexes. The actual antigen contained in the immune complex has only rarely been identified in vasculitic syndromes. In this regard, hepatitis B antigen has been identified in both the circulating and deposited immune complexes in

TABLE 306-2 *Potential Mechanisms of Vessel Damage in Vasculitis Syndromes*

Pathogenic immune complex formation and/or deposition
    Henoch-Schönlein purpura
    Vasculitis associated with collagen vascular diseases
    Serum sickness and cutaneous vasculitis syndromes
    Hepatitis C–associated essential mixed cryoglobulinemia
    Hepatitis B–associated polyarteritis nodosa
Production of antineutrophilic cytoplasmic antibodies
    Wegener's granulomatosis
    Churg-Strauss syndrome
    Microscopic polyangiitis
Pathogenic T lymphocyte responses and granuloma formation
    Giant cell arteritis
    Takayasu's arteritis
    Wegener's granulomatosis
    Churg-Strauss syndrome

Source: Adapted from Sneller and Fauci.

a subset of patients with systemic vasculitis, most notably in polyarteritis nodosa (see below). The syndrome of essential mixed cryoglobulinemia is strongly associated with hepatitis C virus infection; hepatitis C virions and hepatitis C virus antigen-antibody complexes have been identified in the cryoprecipitates of these patients (see below).

The mechanisms of tissue damage in immune complex–mediated vasculitis resemble those described for serum sickness. In this model, antigen-antibody complexes are formed in antigen excess and are deposited in vessel walls whose permeability has been increased by vasoactive amines such as histamine, bradykinin, and leukotrienes released from platelets or from mast cells as a result of IgE-triggered mechanisms. The deposition of complexes results in activation of complement components, particularly C5a, which is strongly chemotactic for neutrophils. These cells then infiltrate the vessel wall, phagocytose the immune complexes, and release their intracytoplasmic enzymes, which damage the vessel wall. As the process becomes subacute or chronic, mononuclear cells infiltrate the vessel wall. The common denominator of the resulting syndrome is compromise of the vessel lumen with ischemic changes in the tissues supplied by the involved vessel. Several variables may explain why only certain types of immune complexes cause vasculitis and why only certain vessels are affected in individual patients. These include the ability of the reticuloendothelial system to clear circulating complexes from the blood, the size and physicochemical properties of immune complexes, the relative degree of turbulence of blood flow, the intravascular hydrostatic pressure in different vessels, and the preexisting integrity of the vessel endothelium.

Antineutrophil Cytoplasmic Antibodies (ANCA) ANCA are antibodies directed against certain proteins in the cytoplasmic granules of neutrophils and monocytes. These autoantibodies are present in a high percentage of patients with certain systemic vasculitis syndromes, particularly Wegener's granulomatosis and microscopic polyangiitis, and in patients with necrotizing and crescentic glomerulonephritis. There are two major categories of ANCA based on different targets for the antibodies. The terminology of *cytoplasmic ANCA* (c-ANCA) refers to the diffuse, granular cytoplasmic staining pattern observed by immunofluorescence microscopy when serum antibodies bind to indicator neutrophils. Proteinase-3, the 29-kDa neutral serine proteinase present in neutrophil azurophilic granules, is the major c-ANCA antigen. More than 90% of patients with typical active Wegener's granulomatosis have detectable antibodies to proteinase-3 (see below). The terminology of *perinuclear ANCA* (p-ANCA) refers to the more localized perinuclear or nuclear staining pattern of the indicator neutrophils. The major target for p-ANCA is the enzyme myeloperoxidase; other targets that can produce a p-ANCA pattern of staining include elastase, cathepsin G, lactoferrin, lysozyme, and bactericidal/permeability-increasing protein. However, only antibodies to myeloperoxi-

TABLE 306-1 *Vasculitis Syndromes*

Primary Vasculitis Syndromes	Secondary Vasculitis Syndromes
Wegener's granulomatosis	Drug-induced vasculitis
Churg-Strauss syndrome	Serum sickness
Polyarteritis nodosa	Vasculitis associated with other
Microscopic polyangiitis	primary diseases
Giant cell arteritis	Infection
Takayasu's arteritis	Malignancy
Henoch-Schönlein purpura	Rheumatic disease
Idiopathic cutaneous vasculitis	
Essential mixed cryoglobulinemia	
Behçet's syndrome	
Isolated vasculitis of the central	
nervous system	
Cogan's syndrome	
Kawasaki disease	

dase have been convincingly associated with vasculitis. Antimyeloperoxidase antibodies have been reported to occur in variable percentages of patients with microscopic polyangiitis, Churg-Strauss syndrome, crescentic glomerulonephritis, Goodpasture's syndrome, and Wegener's granulomatosis (see below). A p-ANCA pattern of staining that is not due to antimyeloperoxidase antibodies has been associated with nonvasculitic entities such as rheumatic and nonrheumatic autoimmune diseases, inflammatory bowel disease, certain drugs, and infections such as endocarditis and bacterial airway infections in patients with cystic fibrosis.

It is unclear why patients with these vasculitis syndromes develop antibodies to myeloperoxidase or proteinase-3, whereas such antibodies are rare in other inflammatory diseases and autoimmune diseases. There are a number of in vitro observations that suggest possible mechanisms whereby these antibodies can contribute to the pathogenesis of the vasculitis syndromes. Proteinase-3 and myeloperoxidase reside in the azurophilic granules and lysosomes of resting neutrophils and monocytes, where they are apparently inaccessible to serum antibodies. However, when neutrophils or monocytes are primed by tumor necrosis factor (TNF) α or interleukin (IL) 1, proteinase-3 and myeloperoxidase translocate to the cell membrane where they can interact with extracellular ANCA. The neutrophils then degranulate and produce reactive oxygen species that can cause tissue damage. Furthermore, ANCA-activated neutrophils can adhere to and kill endothelial cells in vitro. Activation of neutrophils and monocytes by ANCA also induces the release of proinflammatory cytokines such as IL-1 and IL-8. Recent adoptive transfer experiments in genetically engineered mice provide further evidence for a direct pathogenic role of ANCA in vivo. In contradiction, however, a number of clinical and laboratory observations argue against a primary pathogenic role for ANCA. Patients may have active Wegener's granulomatosis in the absence of ANCA; the absolute height of the antibody titers does not correlate well with disease activity; and patients with Wegener's granulomatosis in remission may continue to have high antiproteinase-3 (c-ANCA) titers for years (see below). Thus, the role of these autoantibodies in the pathogenesis of systemic vasculitis remains unclear.

Pathogenic T Lymphocyte Responses and Granuloma Formation In addition to the classic immune complex–mediated mechanisms of vasculitis as well as ANCA, other immunopathogenic mechanisms may be involved in damage to vessels. The most prominent of these are delayed hypersensitivity and cell-mediated immune injury as reflected in the histopathologic feature of granulomatous vasculitis. However, immune complexes themselves may induce granulomatous responses. Vascular endothelial cells can express HLA class II molecules following activation by cytokines such as interferon (IFN) γ. This allows these cells to participate in immunologic reactions such as interaction with CD4+ T lymphocytes in a manner similar to antigen-presenting macrophages. Endothelial cells can secrete IL-1, which may activate T lymphocytes and initiate or propagate in situ immunologic processes within the blood vessel. In addition, IL-1 and TNF-α are potent inducers of endothelial-leukocyte adhesion molecule 1 (ELAM-1) and vascular cell adhesion molecule 1 (VCAM-1), which may enhance the adhesion of leukocytes to endothelial cells in the blood vessel wall. Other mechanisms such as direct cellular cytotoxicity, antibody directed against vessel components, or antibody-dependent cellular cytotoxicity have been suggested in certain types of vessel damage. However, there is no convincing evidence to support their causal contribution to the pathogenesis of any of the recognized vasculitic syndromes.

APPROACH TO THE PATIENT

The diagnosis of vasculitis is often considered in any patient with an unexplained systemic illness. However, there are certain clinical abnormalities that when present alone or in combination should suggest a diagnosis of vasculitis. These include palpable purpura, pulmonary infiltrates and microscopic hematuria, chronic inflammatory sinusitis, mononeuritis multiplex, unexplained ischemic

events, and glomerulonephritis with evidence of multisystem disease. A number of nonvasculitic diseases may also produce some or all of these abnormalities. Thus, the first step in the workup of a patient with suspected vasculitis is to exclude other diseases that produce clinical manifestations that can mimic vasculitis (Table 306-3). It is particularly important to exclude infectious diseases with features that overlap those of vasculitis, especially if the patient's clinical condition is deteriorating rapidly and empirical immunosuppressive treatment is being contemplated.

Once diseases that mimic vasculitis have been excluded, the workup should follow a series of progressive steps that establish the diagnosis of vasculitis and determine, where possible, the category of the vasculitis syndrome (Fig. 306-1). This approach is of considerable importance since several of the vasculitis syndromes require aggressive therapy with glucocorticoids and cytotoxic agents, while other syndromes usually resolve spontaneously and require symptomatic treatment only. The definitive diagnosis of vasculitis is made upon biopsy of involved tissue. The yield of "blind" biopsies of organs with no subjective or objective evidence of involvement is very low and should be avoided. When syndromes such as polyarteritis nodosa, Takayasu's arteritis, or isolated central nervous system vasculitis are suspected, angiogram of organs with suspected involvement should be performed. However, angiograms should not be performed routinely when patients present with localized cutaneous vasculitis with no clinical indication of visceral involvement.

The constellation of clinical, laboratory, biopsy, and radiographic findings usually allows proper categorization to a specific syndrome, and therapy where appropriate should be initiated according to this information (see individual syndromes below). If an offending antigen that precipitates the vasculitis is recognized, the antigen should be removed where possible. If the vasculitis is associated with an underlying disease such as an infection, neoplasm, or connective tissue disease, the underlying disease should be treated. If the syndrome does not resolve following removal of an offending antigen or treatment of an underlying disease, or if there is no recognizable underlying disease, treatment should be initiated according to the category of the vasculitis syndrome.

TABLE 306-3 Conditions That Can Mimic Vasculitis

Infectious diseases
  Bacterial endocarditis
  Disseminated gonococcal infection
  Pulmonary histoplasmosis
  Coccidioidomycosis
  Syphilis
  Lyme disease
  Rocky Mountain spotted fever
  Whipple's disease
Coagulopathies/thrombotic microangiopathies
  Antiphospholipid antibody syndrome
  Thrombotic thrombocytopenic purpura
Neoplasms
  Atrial myxoma
  Lymphoma
  Carcinomatosis
Drug toxicity
  Cocaine
  Amphetamines
  Ergot alkaloids
  Methysergide
  Arsenic
Sarcoidosis
Atheroembolic disease
Goodpasture's syndrome
Amyloidosis
Migraine
Cryofibrinogenemia

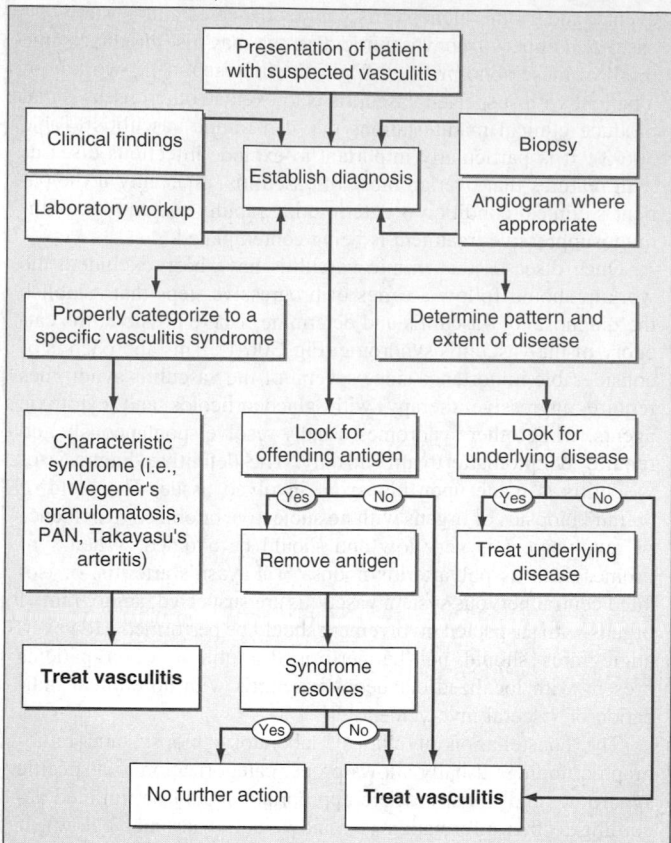

FIGURE 306-1   Algorithm for the approach to a patient with suspected diagnosis of vasculitis.

Treatment options will be considered under the individual syndromes (see below), and general principles of therapy will be considered at the end of the chapter.

WEGENER'S GRANULOMATOSIS

DEFINITION   *Wegener's granulomatosis* is a distinct clinicopathologic entity characterized by granulomatous vasculitis of the upper and lower respiratory tracts togcthcr with glomerulonephritis. In addition, variable degrees of disseminated vasculitis involving both small arteries and veins may occur.

INCIDENCE AND PREVALENCE   Wegener's granulomatosis is an uncommon disease with an estimated prevalence of 3 per 100,000. It is extremely rare in blacks compared with whites; the male-to-female ratio is 1:1. The disease can be seen at any age; approximately 15% of patients are <19 years of age, but only rarely does the disease occur before adolescence; the mean age of onset is approximately 40 years.

PATHOLOGY AND PATHOGENESIS   The histopathologic hallmarks of Wegener's granulomatosis are necrotizing vasculitis of small arteries and veins together with granuloma formation, which may be either intravascular or extravascular (Fig. 306-2). Lung involvement typically appears as multiple, bilateral, nodular cavitary infiltrates (Fig. 306-3), which on biopsy almost invariably reveal the typical necrotizing granulomatous vasculitis. Upper airway lesions, particularly those in the sinuses and nasopharynx, typically reveal inflammation, necrosis, and granuloma formation, with or without vasculitis.

In its earliest form, renal involvement is characterized by a focal and segmental glomerulitis that may evolve into a rapidly progressive crescentic glomerulonephritis. Granuloma formation is only rarely seen on renal biopsy. In contrast to other forms of glomerulonephritis, evidence of immune complex deposition is not found in the renal lesion of Wegener's granulomatosis. In addition to the classic triad of

FIGURE 306-2   Lung biopsy in a patient with Wegener's granulomatosis. Biopsy revealed necrotizing vasculitis with granuloma formation. This section demonstrates several well-formed multinucleated giant cells in an area of granulomatous inflammation.

disease of the upper and lower respiratory tracts and kidney, virtually any organ can be involved with vasculitis, granuloma, or both.

The immunopathogenesis of this disease is unclear, although the involvement of upper airways and lungs with granulomatous vasculitis suggests an aberrant cell-mediated immune response to an exogenous or even endogenous antigen that enters through or resides in the upper airway. Chronic nasal carriage of *Staphylococcus aureus* has been reported to be associated with a higher relapse rate of Wegener's gran-

FIGURE 306-3   Computed tomography scan of a patient with Wegener's granulomatosis. The patient developed multiple, bilateral, and cavitary infiltrates.

ulomatosis; however, there is no evidence for a role of this organism in the pathogenesis of the disease.

Peripheral blood mononuclear cells obtained from patients with Wegener's granulomatosis manifest increased secretion of IFN-γ but not of IL-4, IL-5, or IL-10 compared to normal controls. In addition, TNF-α production from peripheral blood mononuclear cells and CD4+ T cells is elevated. Furthermore, monocytes from patients with Wegener's granulomatosis produce increased amounts of IL-12. These findings indicate an unbalanced T_H1-type T-cell cytokine pattern in this disease that may have pathogenic and perhaps ultimately therapeutic implications.

A high percentage of patients with Wegener's granulomatosis develop ANCA and these autoantibodies may play a role in the pathogenesis of this disease (see above).

CLINICAL AND LABORATORY MANIFESTATIONS Involvement of the upper airways occurs in 95% of patients with Wegener's granulomatosis. Patients often present with severe upper respiratory tract findings such as paranasal sinus pain and drainage and purulent or bloody nasal discharge, with or without nasal mucosal ulceration (Table 306-4). Nasal septal perforation may follow, leading to saddle nose deformity. Serous otitis media may occur as a result of eustachian tube blockage. Subglottic tracheal stenosis resulting from active disease or scarring occurs in approximately 16% of patients and may result in severe airway obstruction.

Pulmonary involvement may be manifested as asymptomatic infiltrates or may be clinically expressed as cough, hemoptysis, dyspnea, and chest discomfort. It is present in 85 to 90% of patients. Endo-

bronchial disease, either in its active form or as a result of fibrous scarring, may lead to obstruction with atelectasis.

Eye involvement (52% of patients) may range from a mild conjunctivitis to dacryocystitis, episcleritis, scleritis, granulomatous sclerouveitis, ciliary vessel vasculitis, and retroorbital mass lesions leading to proptosis.

Skin lesions (46% of patients) appear as papules, vesicles, palpable purpura, ulcers, or subcutaneous nodules; biopsy reveals vasculitis, granuloma, or both. Cardiac involvement (8% of patients) manifests as pericarditis, coronary vasculitis, or, rarely, cardiomyopathy. Nervous system manifestations (23% of patients) include cranial neuritis, mononeuritis multiplex, or, rarely, cerebral vasculitis and/or granuloma.

Renal disease (77% of patients) generally dominates the clinical picture and, if left untreated, accounts directly or indirectly for most of the mortality in this disease. Although it may smolder in some cases as a mild glomerulitis with proteinuria, hematuria, and red blood cell casts, it is clear that once clinically detectable renal functional impairment occurs, rapidly progressive renal failure usually ensues unless appropriate treatment is instituted.

While the disease is active, most patients have nonspecific symptoms and signs such as malaise, weakness, arthralgias, anorexia, and weight loss. Fever may indicate activity of the underlying disease but more often reflects secondary infection, usually of the upper airway.

Characteristic laboratory findings include a markedly elevated erythrocyte sedimentation rate (ESR), mild anemia and leukocytosis, mild hypergammaglobulinemia (particularly of the IgA class), and mildly elevated rheumatoid factor. Thrombocytosis may be seen as an acute-phase reactant. Approximately 90% of patients with active Wegener's granulomatosis have a positive antiproteinase-3 ANCA. However, in the absence of active disease, the sensitivity drops to approximately 60 to 70%. A small percentage of patients with Wegener's granulomatosis may have antimyeloperoxidase rather than antiproteinase-3 antibodies.

DIAGNOSIS The diagnosis of Wegener's granulomatosis is made by the demonstration of necrotizing granulomatous vasculitis on tissue biopsy in a patient with compatible clinical features. Pulmonary tissue offers the highest diagnostic yield, almost invariably revealing granulomatous vasculitis. Biopsy of upper airway tissue usually reveals granulomatous inflammation with necrosis but may not show vasculitis. Renal biopsy can confirm the presence of pauci-immune glomerulonephritis.

The specificity of a positive antiproteinase-3 ANCA for Wegener's granulomatosis is very high, especially if active glomerulonephritis is present. However, the presence of ANCA should be adjunctive and, with very rare exceptions, should not substitute for a tissue diagnosis. False-positive ANCA titers have been reported in certain infectious and neoplastic diseases.

In its typical presentation, the clinicopathologic complex of Wegener's granulomatosis usually provides ready differentiation from other disorders. However, if all the typical features are not present at once, it needs to be differentiated from the other vasculitides, Goodpasture's syndrome (Chap. 264), tumors of the upper airway or lung, and infectious diseases such as histoplasmosis (Chap. 183), mucocutaneous leishmaniasis (Chap. 196), and rhinoscleroma (Chap. 27) as well as noninfectious granulomatous diseases.

Of particular note is the differentiation from *midline granuloma* and *upper airway neoplasms*, which are part of the spectrum of *midline destructive diseases*. These diseases lead to extreme tissue destruction and mutilation localized to the midline upper airway structures including the sinuses; erosion through the skin of the face commonly occurs, a feature that is extremely rare in Wegener's granulomatosis. Although blood vessels may be involved in the intense inflammatory reaction and necrosis, primary vasculitis is seen rarely. When systemic involvement occurs, it usually declares itself as a neoplastic process.

TABLE 306-4 *Wegener's Granulomatosis: Frequency of Clinical Manifestations in 158 Patients Studied at the National Institutes of Health*

Manifestation	Percent at Disease Onset	Percent Throughout Course of Disease
Kidney		
Glomerulonephritis	18	77
Ear/nose/throat	73	92
Sinusitis	51	85
Nasal disease	36	68
Otitis media	25	44
Hearing loss	14	42
Subglottic stenosis	1	16
Ear pain	9	14
Oral lesions	3	10
Lung	45	85
Pulmonary infiltrates	25	66
Pulmonary nodules	24	58
Hemoptysis	12	30
Pleuritis	10	28
Eyes		
Conjunctivitis	5	18
Dacryocystitis	1	18
Scleritis	6	16
Proptosis	2	15
Eye pain	3	11
Visual loss	0	8
Retinal lesions	0	4
Corneal lesions	0	1
Iritis	0	2
Other[a]		
Arthralgias/arthritis	32	67
Fever	23	50
Cough	19	46
Skin abnormalities	13	46
Weight loss (>10% body weight)	15	35
Peripheral neuropathy	1	15
Central nervous system disease	1	8
Pericarditis	2	6
Hyperthyroidism	1	3

[a] Fewer than 1% had parotid, pulmonary artery, breast, or lower genitourinary (urethra, cervix, vagina, testicular) involvement.

Source: Hoffman et al.

In this regard, it is likely that midline granuloma is part of the spectrum of *angiocentric immunoproliferative lesions*. The latter are considered to represent a spectrum of postthymic T cell proliferative lesions and should be treated as such (Chap. 97). The term *idiopathic* has been applied to midline granuloma when extensive diagnostic workup including multiple biopsies has failed to reveal anything other than inflammation and necrosis. Under these circumstances, it is possible that the tumor cells were masked by the intensive inflammatory response. Such cases have responded to local irradiation with 50 Gy (5000 rad). Upper airway lesions should never be irradiated in Wegener's granulomatosis.

Wegener's granulomatosis must also be differentiated from *lymphomatoid granulomatosis*, which is an Epstein-Barr virus–positive B cell proliferation that is associated with an exuberant T cell reaction. Lymphomatoid granulomatosis is characterized by lung, skin, central nervous system, and kidney involvement in which atypical lymphocytoid and plasmacytoid cells infiltrate nonlymphoid tissue in an angioinvasive manner. In this regard, it clearly differs from Wegener's granulomatosis in that it is not an inflammatory vasculitis in the classic sense but an infiltration of vessels with atypical mononuclear cells; granuloma may be present in involved tissues. Up to 50% of patients may develop a true malignant lymphoma

---

℞ TREATMENT

Wegener's granulomatosis was formerly universally fatal, usually within a few months after the onset of clinically apparent renal disease. Glucocorticoids alone led to some symptomatic improvement, with little effect on the ultimate course of the disease. It has been well established that the most effective therapy in this disease is cyclophosphamide given in doses of 2 mg/kg per day orally together with glucocorticoids. The leukocyte count should be monitored closely during therapy, and the dosage of cyclophosphamide should be adjusted in order to maintain the count above $3000/\mu L$, which generally maintains the neutrophil count at approximately $1500/\mu L$. With this approach, clinical remission can usually be induced and maintained without causing severe leukopenia with its associated risk of infection. As it was originally studied, cyclophosphamide was continued for 1 year following the induction of complete remission and gradually tapered and discontinued thereafter.

At the initiation of therapy, glucocorticoids should be administered together with cyclophosphamide. This can be given as prednisone, 1 mg/kg per day initially (for the first month of therapy) as a daily regimen, with gradual conversion to an alternate-day schedule followed by tapering and discontinuation after approximately 6 months.

Using the above regimen, the prognosis of this disease is excellent; marked improvement is seen in >90% of patients, and complete remissions are achieved in 75% of patients. A number of patients who developed irreversible renal failure but who achieved subsequent remission on appropriate therapy have undergone successful renal transplantation.

Despite the dramatic remissions induced by the therapeutic regimen described above, long-term follow-up of patients has revealed that approximately 50% of remissions are later associated with one or more relapses. Reinduction of remission is almost always achieved; however, a high percentage of patients ultimately have some degree of morbidity from irreversible features of their disease, such as varying degrees of renal insufficiency, hearing loss, tracheal stenosis, saddle nose deformity, and chronically impaired sinus function. The determination of relapse should be based on objective evidence of disease activity taking care to rule out other features that may have a similar appearance such as infection, medication toxicity, or chronic disease sequelae. The ANCA titer can be misleading. Many patients who achieve remission continue to have elevated titers for years. In addition, one study found that >40% of patients who were in remission and had a fourfold increase in ANCA titer did not have a relapse in disease. Patients who relapse may not do so until many months or years after the rise in ANCA titer. Thus, a rise in ANCA titer by itself is not a harbinger of immediate disease relapse and should not lead to reinstitution or increase in immunosuppressive therapy. However, such a finding should prompt the clinician to examine the patient carefully for any objective evidence of active disease and to monitor that patient closely.

Certain types of morbidity are related to toxic side effects of treatment. Glucocorticoid-related side effects can include diabetes mellitus, cataracts, life-threatening infectious disease complications, serious osteoporosis, and severe cushingoid features. The risk of such toxicities can be reduced with the use of an alternate-day glucocorticoid regimen as outlined in the preceding regimen. Cyclophosphamide-related toxicities are more frequent and severe. Cystitis to varying degrees occurs in at least 30% of patients, bladder cancer in 6%, myelodysplasia in 2%, and there is a high risk of permanent infertility in both men and women.

Some reports have indicated therapeutic success with less frequent and severe toxic side effects using intermittent boluses of intravenous cyclophosphamide ($1\ g/m^2$ per month) in place of daily administration. However, we and others have found an increased rate of relapse with bolus intravenous cyclophosphamide. We therefore strongly recommend that the drug be given as daily oral therapy.

In patients with immediately life-threatening disease, such as rapidly progressive glomerulonephritis, a regimen of daily cyclophosphamide and glucocorticoids is clearly the treatment of choice to induce remission. However, after patients have achieved remission, consideration can be given to stopping cyclophosphamide and beginning methotrexate or azathioprine for remission maintenance. This approach is aimed at lessening the toxicity associated with chronic cyclophosphamide therapy. Methotrexate is administered orally starting at a dosage of 0.3 mg/kg as a single weekly dose, not to exceed 15 mg/week. If the treatment is well tolerated after 1 to 2 weeks, the dosage should be increased by 2.5 mg weekly up to a dosage of 20 to 25 mg/week and maintained at that level. This regimen is given for 2 years past remission, after which time it is tapered by 2.5 mg each month until discontinuation. To lessen toxicity, methotrexate is often given together with folic acid, 1 mg daily, or folinic acid, 5 to 10 mg once a week 24 h following methotrexate. Azathioprine, 2 mg/kg per day, has also proven effective in some patients in maintaining remission following induction with daily cyclophosphamide. There have been no studies to date comparing methotrexate to azathioprine for remission maintenance. In the absence of such data, the choice of agent is often based on toxicity profile, as methotrexate cannot be given to patients with renal insufficiency or chronic liver disease.

For selected patients whose disease is not immediately life threatening or in those patients who have experienced significant cyclophosphamide toxicity, methotrexate together with glucocorticoids given at the dosages described above may be considered as an alternative for initial therapy.

Although certain reports have indicated that trimethoprim-sulfamethoxazole (TMP-SMX) may be of benefit in the treatment of Wegener's granulomatosis, there are no firm data to substantiate this, particularly in patients with serious renal and pulmonary disease. In a study examining the effect of trimethoprim-sulfamethoxazole on relapse, decreased relapses were shown only with regard to upper airway disease, and no differences in major organ relapses were observed. Trimethoprim-sulfamethoxazole alone should never be used to treat active Wegener's granulomatosis outside of the upper airway.

Not all manifestations of Wegener's granulomatosis require or respond to cytotoxic therapy. In managing non-major organ disease, such as that isolated to the sinus, joints, or skin, the risks of treatment should be carefully weighed against the benefits. Given the potential toxicities of this agent, treatment with cyclophosphamide is rarely if ever justified for the treatment of isolated sinus disease in Wegener's granulomatosis. Although patients with non-major organ disease may be effectively treated without cytotoxic therapy, these individuals must be monitored closely for the development of disease activity affecting the lungs, kidneys, or other major organs. Subglottic tracheal stenosis and endobronchial stenosis are examples of disease manifestations that do not typically respond to systemic immunosuppressive treatment.

CHURG-STRAUSS SYNDROME

DEFINITION Churg-Strauss syndrome, also referred to as *allergic angiitis and granulomatosis,* was described in 1951 by Churg and Strauss and is characterized by asthma, peripheral and tissue eosinophilia, extravascular granuloma formation, and vasculitis of multiple organ systems.

INCIDENCE AND PREVALENCE Churg-Strauss syndrome is an uncommon disease with an estimated annual incidence of 1 to 3 per million. The disease can occur at any age with the possible exception of infants. The mean age of onset is 48 years, with a female-to-male ratio of 1.2:1.

PATHOLOGY AND PATHOGENESIS The necrotizing vasculitis of Churg-Strauss syndrome involves small and medium-sized muscular arteries, capillaries, veins, and venules. A characteristic histopathologic feature of Churg-Strauss syndrome are granulomatous reactions that may be present in the tissues or even within the walls of the vessels themselves. These are usually associated with infiltration of the tissues with eosinophils. This process can occur in any organ in the body; lung involvement is predominant, with skin, cardiovascular system, kidney, peripheral nervous system, and gastrointestinal tract also commonly involved. Although the precise pathogenesis of this disease is uncertain, its strong association with asthma and its clinicopathologic manifestations, including eosinophilia, granuloma, and vasculitis, point to aberrant immunologic phenomena.

CLINICAL AND LABORATORY MANIFESTATIONS Patients with Churg-Strauss syndrome often exhibit nonspecific manifestations such as fever, malaise, anorexia, and weight loss, which are characteristic of a multisystem disease. The pulmonary findings in Churg-Strauss syndrome clearly dominate the clinical picture with severe asthmatic attacks and the presence of pulmonary infiltrates. Mononeuritis multiplex is the second most common manifestation and occurs in up to 72% of patients. Allergic rhinitis and sinusitis develop in up to 61% of patients and are often observed early in the course of disease. Clinically recognizable heart disease occurs in approximately 14% of patients and is an important cause of mortality. Skin lesions occur in approximately 51% of patients and include purpura in addition to cutaneous and subcutaneous nodules. The renal disease in Churg-Strauss syndrome is less common and generally less severe than that of Wegener's granulomatosis and microscopic polyangiitis.

The characteristic laboratory finding in virtually all patients with Churg-Strauss syndrome is a striking eosinophilia, which reaches levels >1000 cells/μL in >80% of patients. Evidence of inflammation as evidenced by elevated ESR, fibrinogen, or α_2-globulins can be found in 81% of patients. The other laboratory findings reflect the organ systems involved. Approximately 48% of patients with Churg-Strauss syndrome have circulating ANCA that is usually antimyeloperoxidase.

DIAGNOSIS Although the diagnosis of Churg-Strauss syndrome is optimally made by biopsy in a patient with the characteristic clinical manifestations (see above), histologic confirmation can be challenging as the pathognomonic features often do not occur simultaneously. In order to be diagnosed with Churg-Strauss syndrome, a patient should have evidence of asthma, peripheral blood eosinophilia, and clinical features consistent with vasculitis.

Rx TREATMENT

The prognosis of untreated Churg-Strauss syndrome is poor, with a reported 5-year survival of 25%. With treatment, prognosis is favorable, with one study finding a 78-month actuarial survival rate of 72%. Myocardial involvement is the most frequent cause of death and is responsible for 39% of patient mortality. Glucocorticoids alone appear to be effective in many patients. Dosage tapering is often limited by

asthma, and many patients require low-dose prednisone for persistent asthma many years after clinical recovery from vasculitis. In glucocorticoid failure or in patients who present with fulminant multisystem disease, the treatment of choice is a combined regimen of daily cyclophosphamide and prednisone (see "Wegener's Granulomatosis" for a detailed description of this therapeutic regimen).

POLYARTERITIS NODOSA

DEFINITION *Polyarteritis nodosa* (PAN), also referred to as *classic PAN,* was described in 1866 by Kussmaul and Maier. It is a multisystem, necrotizing vasculitis of small and medium-sized muscular arteries in which involvement of the renal and visceral arteries is characteristic. PAN does not involve pulmonary arteries, although bronchial vessels may be involved; granulomas, significant eosinophilia, and an allergic diathesis are not observed.

INCIDENCE AND PREVALENCE It is difficult to establish an accurate incidence of PAN because previous reports have included PAN and microscopic polyangiitis as well as other related vasculitides. PAN as currently defined, is felt to be a very uncommon disease.

PATHOLOGY AND PATHOGENESIS The vascular lesion in PAN is a necrotizing inflammation of small and medium-sized muscular arteries. The lesions are segmental and tend to involve bifurcations and branchings of arteries. They may spread circumferentially to involve adjacent veins. However, involvement of venules is not seen in PAN and, if present, suggests microscopic polyangiitis (see below). In the acute stages of disease, polymorphonuclear neutrophils infiltrate all layers of the vessel wall and perivascular areas, which results in intimal proliferation and degeneration of the vessel wall. Mononuclear cells infiltrate the area as the lesions progress to the subacute and chronic stages. Fibrinoid necrosis of the vessels ensues with compromise of the lumen, thrombosis, infarction of the tissues supplied by the involved vessel, and, in some cases, hemorrhage. As the lesions heal, there is collagen deposition, which may lead to further occlusion of the vessel lumen. Aneurysmal dilatations up to 1 cm in size along the involved arteries are characteristic of PAN. Granulomas and substantial eosinophilia with eosinophilic tissue infiltrations are not characteristically found and suggest Churg-Strauss syndrome (see above).

Multiple organ systems are involved, and the clinicopathologic findings reflect the degree and location of vessel involvement and the resulting ischemic changes. As mentioned above, pulmonary arteries are not involved in PAN, and bronchial artery involvement is uncommon. The pathology in the kidney in classic PAN is that of arteritis without glomerulonephritis. In patients with significant hypertension, typical pathologic features of glomerulosclerosis may be seen alone or superimposed on lesions of glomerulonephritis. In addition, pathologic sequelae of hypertension may be found elsewhere in the body.

The presence of hepatitis B antigenemia in approximately 10 to 30% of patients with systemic vasculitis, particularly of the PAN type, together with the isolation of circulating immune complexes composed of hepatitis B antigen and immunoglobulin, and the demonstration by immunofluorescence of hepatitis B antigen, IgM, and complement in the blood vessel walls, strongly suggest the role of immunologic phenomena in the pathogenesis of this disease. Hairy cell leukemia can be associated with PAN; the pathogenic mechanisms of this association are unclear.

CLINICAL AND LABORATORY MANIFESTATIONS Nonspecific signs and symptoms are the hallmarks of PAN. Fever, weight loss, and malaise are present in over one-half of cases. Patients usually present with vague symptoms such as weakness, malaise, headache, abdominal pain, and myalgias that can rapidly progress to a fulminant illness. Specific complaints related to the vascular involvement within a particular organ system may also dominate the presenting clinical picture as well as the entire course of the illness (Table 306-5). In PAN, renal involvement most commonly manifests as hypertension, renal insufficiency, or hemorrhage due to microaneurysms.

TABLE 306-5 *Clinical Manifestations Related to Organ System Involvement in Classic Polyarteritis Nodosa*

Organ System	Percent Incidence	Clinical Manifestations
Renal	60	Renal failure, hypertension
Musculoskeletal	64	Arthritis, arthralgia, myalgia
Peripheral nervous system	51	Peripheral neuropathy, mononeuritis multiplex
Gastrointestinal tract	44	Abdominal pain, nausea and vomiting, bleeding, bowel infarction and perforation, cholecystitis, hepatic infarction, pancreatic infarction
Skin	43	Rash, purpura, nodules, cutaneous infarcts, livedo reticularis, Raynaud's phenomenon
Cardiac	36	Congestive heart failure, myocardial infarction, pericarditis
Genitourinary	25	Testicular, ovarian, or epididymal pain
Central nervous system	23	Cerebral vascular accident, altered mental status, seizure

Source: From TR Cupps, AS Fauci: *The Vasculitides*. Philadelphia, Saunders, 1981.

There are no diagnostic serologic tests for PAN. In >75% of patients, the leukocyte count is elevated with a predominance of neutrophils. Eosinophilia is seen only rarely and, when present at high levels, suggests the diagnosis of Churg-Strauss syndrome. The anemia of chronic disease may be seen, and an elevated ESR is almost always present. Other common laboratory findings reflect the particular organ involved. Hypergammaglobulinemia may be present, and up to 30% of patients have a positive test for hepatitis B surface antigen. Antibodies against myeloperoxidase or proteinase-3 (ANCA) are rarely found in patients with PAN.

DIAGNOSIS The diagnosis of PAN is based on the demonstration of characteristic findings of vasculitis on biopsy material of involved organs. In the absence of easily accessible tissue for biopsy, the angiographic demonstration of involved vessels, particularly in the form of aneurysms of small and medium-sized arteries in the renal, hepatic, and visceral vasculature, is sufficient to make the diagnosis. Aneurysms of vessels are not pathognomonic of PAN; furthermore, aneurysms need not always be present, and angiographic findings may be limited to stenotic segments and obliteration of vessels. Biopsy of symptomatic organs such as nodular skin lesions, painful testes, and nerve/muscle provides the highest diagnostic yields.

℞ TREATMENT

The prognosis of untreated PAN is extremely poor, with a reported 5-year survival rate between 10 and 20%. Death usually results from gastrointestinal complications, particularly bowel infarcts and perforation, and cardiovascular causes. Intractable hypertension often compounds dysfunction in other organ systems, such as the kidneys, heart, and central nervous system, leading to additional late morbidity and mortality in PAN. With the introduction of treatment, survival rate has increased substantially. Favorable therapeutic results have been reported in PAN with the combination of prednisone and cyclophosphamide (see "Wegener's Granulomatosis" for a detailed description of this therapeutic regimen). In less severe cases of PAN, glucocorticoids alone have resulted in disease remission. Favorable results have also been reported in the treatment of PAN related to hepatitis B virus with IFN-α in combination with glucocorticoids and plasma exchange. Careful attention to the treatment of hypertension can lessen the acute and late morbidity and mortality associated with renal, cardiac, and central nervous system complications of PAN. Following successful treatment, relapse of PAN has been estimated to occur in only 10% of patients.

MICROSCOPIC POLYANGIITIS

DEFINITION The term *microscopic polyarteritis* was introduced into the literature by Davson in 1948 in recognition of the presence of glomerulonephritis in patients with PAN. In 1992, the Chapel Hill Consensus Conference on the Nomenclature of Systemic Vasculitis adopted the term *microscopic polyangiitis* to connote a necrotizing vasculitis with few or no immune complexes affecting small vessels (capillaries, venules, or arterioles). Glomerulonephritis is very common in microscopic polyangiitis, and pulmonary capillaritis often occurs. The absence of granulomatous inflammation in microscopic polyangiitis is said to differentiate it from Wegener's granulomatosis.

INCIDENCE AND PREVALENCE The incidence of microscopic polyangiitis has not yet been reliably established due to its previous inclusion as part of PAN. The mean age of onset is approximately 57 years of age, and males are slightly more frequently affected than females.

PATHOLOGY AND PATHOGENESIS The vascular lesion in microscopic polyangiitis is histologically similar to that in PAN. Unlike PAN, the vasculitis seen in microscopic polyangiitis has a predilection to involve capillaries and venules in addition to small and medium-sized arteries. Immunohistochemical staining reveals a paucity of immunoglobulin deposition in the vascular lesion of microscopic polyangiitis, suggesting that immune complex formation does not play a role in the pathogenesis of this syndrome. The renal lesion seen in microscopic polyangiitis is identical to that of Wegener's granulomatosis. Like Wegener's granulomatosis, microscopic polyangiitis is highly associated with the presence of ANCA, which may play a role in pathogenesis of this syndrome (see above).

CLINICAL AND LABORATORY MANIFESTATIONS Because of its predilection to involve the small vessels, microscopic polyangiitis and Wegener's granulomatosis share similar clinical features. Disease onset may be gradual with initial symptoms of fever, weight loss, and musculoskeletal pain; however, it is often acute. Glomerulonephritis occurs in at least 79% of patients and can be rapidly progressive, leading to renal failure. Hemoptysis may be the first symptom of alveolar hemorrhage, which occurs in 12% of patients. Other manifestations include mononeuritis multiplex and gastrointestinal tract and cutaneous vasculitis. Upper airways disease and pulmonary nodules are not typically found in microscopic polyangiitis and, if present, suggest Wegener's granulomatosis.

Features of inflammation may be seen, including an elevated ESR, anemia, leukocytosis, and thrombocytosis. ANCA are present in 75% of patients with microscopic polyangiitis, with antimyeloperoxidase antibodies being the predominant ANCA associated with this disease.

DIAGNOSIS The diagnosis is based on histologic evidence of vasculitis or pauci-immune glomerulonephritis in a patient with compatible clinical features of multisystem disease. Although microscopic polyangiitis is strongly ANCA-associated, no studies have as yet established the sensitivity and specificity of ANCA in this disease.

℞ TREATMENT

The 5-year survival rate for patients with treated microscopic polyangiitis is 74% with disease-related mortality occurring from alveolar hemorrhage or gastrointestinal, cardiac, or renal disease. To date there has been limited disease-specific information on the treatment of microscopic polyangiitis. Available data together with a predilection for this disease to affect the small vessels support a therapeutic approach similar to that used in Wegener's granulomatosis. Patients with immediately life-threatening disease should be treated with the combination of prednisone and daily cyclophosphamide (see "Wegener's Granulomatosis" for a detailed description of this therapeutic regimen). Disease relapse has been observed in at least 34% of patients. Treatment for such relapses would be similar to that used at the time of initial presentation and based upon site and severity of disease.

GIANT CELL ARTERITIS

DEFINITION *Giant cell arteritis*, also referred to as *cranial arteritis* or *temporal arteritis*, is an inflammation of medium- and large-sized arteries. It characteristically involves one or more branches of the carotid artery, particularly the temporal artery. However, it is a systemic disease that can involve arteries in multiple locations.

INCIDENCE AND PREVALENCE Giant cell arteritis occurs almost exclusively in individuals >50 years. It is more common in women than in men and is rare in blacks. The incidence of giant cell arteritis varies widely in different studies and in different geographic regions. A high incidence has been found in Scandinavia and in regions of the United States with large Scandinavian populations, compared to a lower incidence in southern Europe. The annual incidence rates in individuals ≥50 years range from 6.9 to 32.8 per 100,000 population. Familial aggregation has been reported, as has an association with HLA-DR4. In addition, genetic linkage studies have demonstrated an association of temporal arteritis with alleles at the HLA-DRB1 locus, particularly HLA-DRB1*04 variants. The disease is closely associated with *polymyalgia rheumatica*, which is more common than giant cell arteritis. In Olmsted County, Minnesota, the annual incidence of polymyalgia rheumatica in individuals ≥50 years is 58.7 per 100,000 population.

PATHOLOGY AND PATHOGENESIS Although the temporal artery is most frequently involved in this disease, patients often have a systemic vasculitis of multiple medium- and large-sized arteries, which may go undetected. Histopathologically, the disease is a panarteritis with inflammatory mononuclear cell infiltrates within the vessel wall with frequent giant cell formation. There is proliferation of the intima and fragmentation of the internal elastic lamina. Pathophysiologic findings in organs result from the ischemia related to the involved vessels. Distinct cytokine patterns as well as T lymphocytes expressing specific antigen receptors have been described, suggesting the involvement of immunopathogenic mechanisms in temporal arteritis. IL-6 and IL-1β expression have been detected in a majority of circulating monocytes of patients with temporal arteritis and polymyalgia rheumatica. T cells recruited to vasculitic lesions in patients with temporal arteritis produce predominantly IL-2 and IFN-γ, and the latter has been suggested to be involved in the progression to overt arteritis. Sequence analysis of the T cell receptor of tissue-infiltrating T cells in lesions of temporal arteritis indicates restricted clonal expansion, suggesting that an antigen residing in the arterial wall is recognized by a small fraction of T cells.

CLINICAL AND LABORATORY MANIFESTATIONS The disease is characterized clinically by the complex of fever, anemia, high ESR, and headaches in a patient over the age of 50 years. Other manifestations include malaise, fatigue, anorexia, weight loss, sweats, and arthralgias. The polymyalgia rheumatica syndrome is characterized by stiffness, aching, and pain in the muscles of the neck, shoulders, lower back, hips, and thighs.

In patients with involvement of the temporal artery, headache is the predominant symptom and may be associated with a tender, thickened, or nodular artery, which may pulsate early in the disease but may become occluded later. Scalp pain and claudication of the jaw and tongue may occur. A well-recognized and dreaded complication of giant cell arteritis, particularly in untreated patients, is ischemic optic neuropathy, which may lead to serious visual symptoms, even sudden blindness in some patients. However, most patients have complaints relating to the head or eyes before visual loss. Attention to such symptoms with institution of appropriate therapy (see below) will usually avoid this complication. Claudication of the extremities, strokes, myocardial infarctions, and infarctions of visceral organs have been reported. Of note, giant cell arteritis is associated with an increased risk of aortic aneurysm, which is usually a late complication and may lead to dissection and death.

Characteristic laboratory findings in addition to the elevated ESR include a normochromic or slightly hypochromic anemia. Liver function abnormalities are common, particularly increased alkaline phosphatase levels. Increased levels of IgG and complement have been reported. Levels of enzymes indicative of muscle damage such as serum creatine kinase are not elevated.

DIAGNOSIS The diagnosis of giant cell arteritis and its associated clinicopathologic syndrome can often be suggested clinically by the demonstration of the complex of fever, anemia, and high ESR with or without symptoms of polymyalgia rheumatica in a patient >50 years. The diagnosis is confirmed by biopsy of the temporal artery. Since involvement of the vessel may be segmental, positive yield is increased by obtaining a biopsy segment of 3 to 5 cm together with serial sectioning of biopsy specimens. Ultrasonography of the temporal artery has been reported to be helpful in diagnosis. A temporal artery biopsy should be obtained as quickly as possible in the setting of ocular signs and symptoms, and under these circumstances therapy should not be delayed pending a biopsy. In this regard, it has been reported that temporal artery biopsies may show vasculitis even after more than 14 days of glucocorticoid therapy. A dramatic clinical response to a trial of glucocorticoid therapy can further support the diagnosis.

℞ TREATMENT

Disease-related mortality from giant cell arteritis is very uncommon with fatalities occurring from cerebrovascular events, myocardial infarction, or aortic aneurysms. The goals of treatment are to reduce symptoms and, most importantly, to prevent visual loss. Giant cell arteritis and its associated symptoms are exquisitely sensitive to glucocorticoid therapy. Treatment should begin with prednisone, 40 to 60 mg/d for approximately 1 month, followed by a gradual tapering. When ocular signs and symptoms occur, it is important that therapy be initiated or adjusted to control them. Although the optimal duration of glucocorticoid therapy has not been established, most series have found that patients require treatment for ≥2 years. The ESR can serve as a useful indicator of inflammatory disease activity in monitoring and tapering therapy and can be used to judge the pace of the tapering schedule. However, minor increases in the ESR can occur as glucocorticoids are being tapered and do not necessarily reflect an exacerbation of arteritis, particularly if the patient remains symptom-free. Under these circumstances, the tapering should continue with caution. Glucocorticoid toxicity occurs in 35 to 65% of patients and represents an important cause of patient morbidity. The use of weekly methotrexate as a glucocorticoid-sparing agent has been examined in two randomized placebo-controlled trials that reached conflicting conclusions.

TAKAYASU'S ARTERITIS

DEFINITION *Takayasu's arteritis* is an inflammatory and stenotic disease of medium- and large-sized arteries characterized by a strong predilection for the aortic arch and its branches. For this reason, it is often referred to as the *aortic arch syndrome*.

INCIDENCE AND PREVALENCE Takayasu's arteritis is an uncommon disease with an estimated annual incidence rate of 1.2 to 2.6 cases per million. It is most prevalent in adolescent girls and young women. Although it is more common in Asia, it is neither racially nor geographically restricted.

PATHOLOGY AND PATHOGENESIS The disease involves medium- and large-sized arteries, with a strong predilection for the aortic arch and its branches; the pulmonary artery may also be involved. The most commonly affected arteries seen by angiography are listed in Table 306-6. The involvement of the major branches of the aorta is much more marked at their origin than distally. The disease is a panarteritis with inflammatory mononuclear cell infiltrates and occasionally giant cells. There are marked intimal proliferation and fibrosis, scarring and vascularization of the media, and disruption and degeneration of the elastic lamina. Narrowing of the lumen occurs with or without thrombosis. The vasa vasorum are frequently involved. Pathologic changes in various organs reflect the compromise of blood flow through the involved vessels.

Immunopathogenic mechanisms, the precise nature of which is uncertain, are suspected in this disease. As with several of the vasculitis

TABLE 306-6 *Frequency of Arteriographic Abnormalities and Potential Clinical Manifestations of Arterial Involvement in Takayasu's Arteritis*

Artery	Percent of Arteriographic Abnormalities	Potential Clinical Manifestations
Subclavian	93	Arm claudication, Raynaud's phenomenon
Common carotid	58	Visual changes, syncope, transient ischemic attacks, stroke
Abdominal aorta[a]	47	Abdominal pain, nausea, vomiting
Renal	38	Hypertension, renal failure
Aortic arch or root	35	Aortic insufficiency, congestive heart failure
Vertebral	35	Visual changes, dizziness
Coeliac axis[a]	18	Abdominal pain, nausea, vomiting
Superior mesenteric[a]	18	Abdominal pain, nausea, vomiting
Iliac	17	Leg claudication
Pulmonary	10–40	Atypical chest pain, dyspnea
Coronary	<10	Chest pain, myocardial infarction

[a] Arteriographic lesions at these locations are usually asymptomatic but may potentially cause these symptoms.

Source: Kerr et al.

syndromes, circulating immune complexes have been demonstrated, but their pathogenic significance is unclear.

CLINICAL AND LABORATORY MANIFESTATIONS Takayasu's arteritis is a systemic disease with generalized as well as vascular symptoms. The generalized symptoms include malaise, fever, night sweats, arthralgias, anorexia, and weight loss, which may occur months before vessel involvement is apparent. These symptoms may merge into those related to vascular compromise and organ ischemia. Pulses are commonly absent in the involved vessels, particularly the subclavian artery. The frequency of arteriographic abnormalities and the potentially associated clinical manifestations are listed in Table 306-6. Hypertension occurs in 32 to 93% of patients and contributes to renal, cardiac, and cerebral injury.

Characteristic laboratory findings include an elevated ESR, mild anemia, and elevated immunoglobulin levels.

DIAGNOSIS The diagnosis of Takayasu's arteritis should be suspected strongly in a young woman who develops a decrease or absence of peripheral pulses, discrepancies in blood pressure, and arterial bruits. The diagnosis is confirmed by the characteristic pattern on arteriography, which includes irregular vessel walls, stenosis, poststenotic dilatation, aneurysm formation, occlusion, and evidence of increased collateral circulation. Complete aortic arteriography should be obtained, unless this is renally contraindicated, in order to fully delineate the distribution and degree of arterial disease. Histopathologic demonstration of inflamed vessels adds confirmatory data; however, tissue is rarely readily available for examination.

℞ TREATMENT

The long-term outcome of patients with Takayasu's arteritis has varied widely between studies. Although two North American reports found overall survival to be ≥94%, or the 5-year mortality rate from other studies has ranged from 0 to 35%. Disease-related mortality most often occurs from congestive heart failure, cerebrovascular events, myocardial infarction, aneurysm rupture, or renal failure. Even in the absence of life-threatening disease Takayasu's arteritis can be associated with significant morbidity. The course of the disease is variable, and although spontaneous remissions may occur, Takayasu's arteritis is most often chronic and relapsing. Although glucocorticoid therapy in doses of 40 to 60 mg prednisone per day alleviates symptoms, there are no convincing studies that indicate that they increase survival. The combination of glucocorticoid therapy for acute signs and symptoms and an aggressive surgical and/or angioplastic approach to stenosed vessels has markedly improved outcome and decreased morbidity by lessening

the risk of stroke, correcting hypertension due to renal artery stenosis, and improving blood flow to ischemic viscera and limbs. Unless it is urgently required, surgical correction of stenosed arteries should be undertaken only when the vascular inflammatory process is well controlled with medical therapy. In individuals who are refractory to or unable to taper glucocorticoids, methotrexate in doses up to 25 mg per week has yielded encouraging results.

HENOCH-SCHÖNLEIN PURPURA

DEFINITION *Henoch-Schönlein purpura*, also referred to as *anaphylactoid purpura*, is a distinct systemic vasculitis syndrome that is characterized by palpable purpura (most commonly distributed over the buttocks and lower extremities), arthralgias, gastrointestinal signs and symptoms, and glomerulonephritis. It is a small-vessel vasculitis.

INCIDENCE AND PREVALENCE Henoch-Schönlein purpura is usually seen in children; most patients range in age from 4 to 7 years; however, the disease may also be seen in infants and adults. It is not a rare disease; in one series it accounted for between 5 and 24 admissions per year at a pediatric hospital. The male-to-female ratio is 1.5:1. A seasonal variation with a peak incidence in spring has been noted.

PATHOLOGY AND PATHOGENESIS The presumptive pathogenic mechanism for Henoch-Schönlein purpura is immune-complex deposition. A number of inciting antigens have been suggested including upper respiratory tract infections, various drugs, foods, insect bites, and immunizations. IgA is the antibody class most often seen in the immune complexes and has been demonstrated in the renal biopsies of these patients.

CLINICAL AND LABORATORY MANIFESTATIONS In pediatric patients, palpable purpura is seen in virtually all patients; most patients develop polyarthralgias in the absence of frank arthritis. Gastrointestinal involvement, which is seen in almost 70% of pediatric patients, is characterized by colicky abdominal pain usually associated with nausea, vomiting, diarrhea, or constipation and is frequently accompanied by the passage of blood and mucus per rectum; bowel intussusception may occur. Renal involvement occurs in 10 to 50% of patients and is usually characterized by mild glomerulonephritis leading to proteinuria and microscopic hematuria, with red blood cell casts in the majority of patients (Chap. 264); it usually resolves spontaneously without therapy. Rarely, a progressive glomerulonephritis will develop. In adults, presenting symptoms are most frequently related to the skin and joints, while initial complaints related to the gut are less common. Although certain studies have found that renal disease is more frequent and more severe in adults, this has not been a consistent finding. However, the course of renal disease in adults may be more insidious and thus requires close follow-up. Myocardial involvement can occur in adults but is rare in children.

Laboratory studies generally show a mild leukocytosis, a normal platelet count, and occasionally eosinophilia. Serum complement components are normal, and IgA levels are elevated in about one-half of patients.

DIAGNOSIS The diagnosis of Henoch-Schönlein purpura is based on clinical signs and symptoms. Skin biopsy specimen can be useful in confirming leukocytoclastic vasculitis with IgA and C3 deposition by immunofluorescence. Renal biopsy is rarely needed for diagnosis but may provide prognostic information in some patients.

℞ TREATMENT

The prognosis of Henoch-Schönlein purpura is excellent. Mortality is exceedingly rare, and 1 to 5% of children progress to end-stage renal disease. Most patients recover completely, and some do not require therapy. Treatment is similar for adults and children. When glucocorticoid therapy is required, prednisone, in doses of 1 mg/kg per day and tapered according to clinical response, has been shown to be useful in decreasing tissue edema, arthralgias, and abdominal discomfort; however, it has not proven beneficial in the treatment of skin or renal disease and does not appear to shorten the duration of active disease or lessen the chance of recurrence. Patients with rapidly progressive glomerulonephritis have been anecdotally reported to benefit from intensive plasma exchange combined with cytotoxic drugs. Disease recurrences have been reported in 10 to 40% of patients.

IDIOPATHIC CUTANEOUS VASCULITIS

DEFINITION The term *cutaneous vasculitis* is defined broadly as inflammation of the blood vessels of the dermis. Due to its heterogeneity, cutaneous vasculitis has been described by a variety of terms including *hypersensitivity vasculitis* and *cutaneous leukocytoclastic angiitis*. However, cutaneous vasculitis is not one specific disease but a manifestation that can be seen in a variety of settings. In >70% of cases, cutaneous vasculitis occurs either as part of a primary systemic vasculitis or as a secondary vasculitis related to an inciting agent or an underlying disease (see "Secondary Vasculitis"). In the remaining 30% of cases, cutaneous vasculitis occurs idiopathically.

INCIDENCE AND PREVALENCE Cutaneous vasculitis represents the most commonly encountered vasculitis in clinical practice. The exact incidence of idiopathic cutaneous vasculitis has not been determined due to the predilection for cutaneous vasculitis to be associated with an underlying process and the variability of its clinical course.

PATHOLOGY AND PATHOGENESIS The typical histopathologic feature of cutaneous vasculitis is the presence of vasculitis of small vessels. Postcapillary venules are the most commonly involved vessels; capillaries and arterioles may be involved less frequently. This vasculitis is characterized by a *leukocytoclasis*, a term that refers to the nuclear debris remaining from the neutrophils that have infiltrated in and around the vessels during the acute stages. In the subacute or chronic stages, mononuclear cells predominate; in certain subgroups, eosinophilic infiltration is seen. Erythrocytes often extravasate from the involved vessels, leading to palpable purpura.

CLINICAL AND LABORATORY MANIFESTATIONS The hallmark of idiopathic cutaneous vasculitis is the predominance of skin involvement. Skin lesions may appear typically as palpable purpura; however, other cutaneous manifestations of the vasculitis may occur, including macules, papules, vesicles, bullae, subcutaneous nodules, ulcers, and recurrent or chronic urticaria. The skin lesions may be pruritic or even quite painful, with a burning or stinging sensation. Lesions most commonly occur in the lower extremities in ambulatory patients or in the sacral area in bedridden patients due to the effects of hydrostatic forces on the postcapillary venules. Edema may accompany certain lesions, and hyperpigmentation often occurs in areas of recurrent or chronic lesions.

There are no specific laboratory tests diagnostic of idiopathic cutaneous vasculitis. A mild leukocytosis with or without eosinophilia is characteristic, as is an elevated ESR. Laboratory studies should be aimed towards ruling out features to suggest an underlying disease or a systemic vasculitis.

DIAGNOSIS The diagnosis of cutaneous vasculitis is made by the demonstration of vasculitis on biopsy. An important diagnostic principle in patients with cutaneous vasculitis is to search for an etiology of the vasculitis—be it an exogenous agent, such as a drug or an infection, or an endogenous condition, such as an underlying disease (Fig. 306-1). In addition, a careful physical and laboratory examination should be performed to rule out the possibility of systemic vasculitis. This should start with the least invasive diagnostic approach and proceed to the more invasive only if clinically indicated.

℞ TREATMENT

When an antigenic stimulus is recognized as the precipitating factor in the cutaneous vasculitis, it should be removed; if this is a microbe, appropriate antimicrobial therapy should be instituted. If the vasculitis is associated with another underlying disease, treatment of the latter often results in resolution of the former. In situations where disease is apparently self-limited, no therapy, except possibly symptomatic therapy, is indicated. When cutaneous vasculitis persists and when there is no evidence of an inciting agent, an associated disease, or an un-

derlying systemic vasculitis, the decision to treat should be based on weighing the balance between the degree of symptoms and the risk of treatment. Some cases of idiopathic cutaneous vasculitis resolve spontaneously, while others remit and relapse. In those patients with persistent vasculitis, a variety of therapeutic regimens have been tried with variable results. In general, the treatment of idiopathic cutaneous vasculitis has not been satisfactory. Fortunately, since the disease is generally limited to the skin, this lack of consistent response to therapy usually does not lead to a life-threatening situation. Glucocorticoids are often used in the treatment of idiopathic cutaneous vasculitis. Therapy is usually instituted as prednisone, 1 mg/kg per day, with rapid tapering where possible, either directly to discontinuation or by conversion to an alternate-day regimen followed by ultimate discontinuation. In cases that prove refractory to glucocorticoids, a trial of a cytotoxic agent may be indicated. Patients with chronic vasculitis isolated to cutaneous venules rarely respond dramatically to any therapeutic regimen, and cytotoxic agents should be used only as a last resort in these patients. Methotrexate and azathioprine have been used in such situations in anecdotal reports. Although cyclophosphamide is the most effective therapy for the systemic vasculitides, it should almost never be used for idiopathic cutaneous vasculitis because of the potential toxicity. Other agents with which there have been anecdotal reports of success include dapsone, colchicine, and nonsteroidal anti-inflammatory agents.

ESSENTIAL MIXED CRYOGLOBULINEMIA

DEFINITION Cryoglobulins are cold-precipitable monoclonal or polyclonal immunoglobulins. Cryoglobulinemia may be associated with a systemic vasculitis characterized by palpable purpura, arthralgias, weakness, neuropathy, and glomerulonephritis. Although this can be observed in association with a variety of underlying disorders including multiple myeloma, lymphoproliferative disorders, connective tissue diseases, infection, and liver disease, in many instances it appeared to be idiopathic. Because of the apparent absence of an underlying disease and the presence of cryoprecipitate containing oligoclonal/polyclonal immunoglobulins, this entity was referred to as *essential mixed cryoglobulinemia*. Since the discovery of hepatitis C, it has been established that in the vast majority of patients, essential mixed cryoglobulinemia is related to an aberrant immune response to chronic hepatitis C infection.

INCIDENCE AND PREVALENCE The incidence of essential mixed cryoglobulinemia has not been established. It has been estimated, however, that 5% of patients with chronic hepatitis C will develop the syndrome of essential mixed cryoglobulinemia.

PATHOLOGY AND PATHOGENESIS Skin biopsies in essential mixed cryoglobulinemia reveal an inflammatory infiltrate surrounding and involving blood vessel walls, with fibrinoid necrosis, endothelial cell hyperplasia, and hemorrhage. Deposition of immunoglobulin and complement is common. Abnormalities of uninvolved skin including basement membrane alterations and deposits in vessel walls may be found. Membranoproliferative glomerulonephritis is responsible for 80% of all renal lesions in essential mixed cryoglobulinemia.

The association between hepatitis C and essential mixed cryoglobulinemia has been supported by the high frequency of documented hepatitis C infection, the presence of hepatitis C RNA and anti–hepatitis C antibodies in serum cryoprecipitates, evidence of hepatitis C antigens in vasculitic skin lesions, and the effectiveness of antiviral therapy (see below). Current evidence suggest that in the majority of cases, essential mixed cryoglobulinemia occurs when an aberrant immune response to hepatitis C infection leads to the formation of immune complexes consisting of hepatitis C antigens, polyclonal hepatitis C–specific IgG, and monoclonal IgM rheumatoid factor. The deposition of these immune complexes in blood vessel walls triggers an inflammatory cascade that results in the clinical syndrome of essential mixed cryoglobulinemia.

CLINICAL AND LABORATORY MANIFESTATIONS The most common clinical manifestations of essential mixed cryoglobulinemia are cutaneous vasculitis, arthritis, peripheral neuropathy, and glomerulonephritis. Renal disease develops in 10 to 30% of patients. Life-threatening rapidly progressive glomerulonephritis or vasculitis of the central nervous system, gastrointestinal tract, or heart occurs infrequently.

The presence of circulating cryoprecipitates is the fundamental finding in essential mixed cryoglobulinemia. Rheumatoid factor is almost always found and may be a useful clue to the disease when cryoglobulins are not detected. Hypocomplementemia occurs in 90% of patients. An elevated ESR and anemia occur frequently. Evidence for hepatitis C infection must be sought in all patients by testing for hepatitis C antibodies and hepatitis C RNA.

℞ TREATMENT

Acute mortality from essential mixed cryoglobulinemia is uncommon, but the presence of glomerulonephritis is a poor prognostic sign for overall outcome. In such patients, 15% progress to end-stage renal disease with 40% later experiencing fatal cardiovascular disease, infection, or liver failure. As indicated above, the majority of cases are associated with hepatitis C infection. In such patients, treatment with IFN-α and ribavirin (Chap. 285) can prove beneficial. Clinical improvement with IFN-α and ribavirin is dependent on the virologic response. Patients who clear hepatitis C from the blood have objective improvement in their vasculitis along with significant reductions in levels of circulating cryoglobulins, IgM, and rheumatoid factor. However, substantial portions of patients with hepatitis C do not have a sustained virologic response to such therapy, and the vasculitis typically relapses with the return of viremia. While transient improvement can be observed with glucocorticoids, a complete response is seen in only 7% of patients. Plasmapheresis and cytotoxic agents have been used in anecdotal reports. These observations have not been confirmed, and such therapies carry significant risks.

BEHÇET'S SYNDROME

Behçet's Syndrome is a clinicopathologic entity characterized by recurrent episodes of oral and genital ulcers, iritis, and cutaneous lesions. The underlying pathologic process is a leukocytoclastic venulitis, although vessels of any size and in any organ can be involved. →*This disorder is described in detail in Chap. 307.*

ISOLATED VASCULITIS OF THE CENTRAL NERVOUS SYSTEM

Isolated vasculitis of the central nervous system is an uncommon clinicopathologic entity characterized by vasculitis restricted to the vessels of the central nervous system without other apparent systemic vasculitis. Although the arteriole is most commonly affected, vessels of any size can be involved. The inflammatory process is usually composed of mononuclear cell infiltrates with or without granuloma formation.

Patients may present with severe headaches, altered mental function, and focal neurologic defects. Systemic symptoms are generally absent. Devastating neurologic abnormalities may occur depending on the extent of vessel involvement. The diagnosis is generally made by demonstration of characteristic vessel abnormalities on angiography (Fig. 306-4) and confirmed by biopsy of the brain parenchyma and leptomeninges. In the absence of a brain biopsy, care should be taken not to misinterpret as true primary vasculitis angiographic abnormalities that might actually be related to another cause. The differential diagnosis includes infection, atherosclerosis, emboli, connective tissue disease, sarcoidosis, malignancy, vasospasm, and drug-associated causes. The prognosis of this disease is poor; however, some reports indicate that glucocorticoid therapy, alone or together with cyclophosphamide administered as described above, has induced sustained clinical remissions in a small number of patients.

COGAN'S SYNDROME

Cogan's syndrome is characterized by interstitial keratitis together with vestibuloauditory symptoms. It may be associated with a systemic

FIGURE 306-4 Cerebral angiogram from a 32-year-old male with central nervous system vasculitis. Dramatic beading (*arrow*) typical of vasculitis is seen.

vasculitis, particularly aortitis with involvement of the aortic valve. Glucocorticoids are the mainstay of treatment. Initiation of treatment as early as possible after the onset of hearing loss improves the likelihood of a favorable outcome.

KAWASAKI DISEASE

Kawasaki disease, also referred to as *mucocutaneous lymph node syndrome*, is an acute, febrile, multisystem disease of children. Some 80% of cases occur prior to the age of 5, with the peak incidence occurring at ≤2 years. It is characterized by nonsuppurative cervical adenitis and changes in the skin and mucous membranes such as edema; congested conjunctivae; erythema of the oral cavity, lips, and palms; and desquamation of the skin of the fingertips. Although the disease is generally benign and self-limited, it is associated with coronary artery aneurysms in approximately 25% of cases, with an overall case-fatality rate of 0.5 to 2.8%. These complications usually occur between the third and fourth weeks of illness during the convalescent stage. Vasculitis of the coronary arteries is seen in almost all the fatal cases that have been autopsied. There is typical intimal proliferation and infiltration of the vessel wall with mononuclear cells. Beadlike aneurysms and thromboses may be seen along the artery. Other manifestations include pericarditis, myocarditis, myocardial ischemia and infarction, and cardiomegaly.

Apart from the up to 2.8% of patients who develop fatal complications, the prognosis of this disease for uneventful recovery is excellent. High-dose intravenous γ globulin (2 g/kg as a single infusion over 10 h) together with aspirin (100 mg/kg per day for 14 days followed by 3 to 5 mg/kg per day for several weeks) have been shown to be effective in reducing the prevalence of coronary artery abnormalities when administered early in the course of the disease.

POLYANGIITIS OVERLAP SYNDROMES

Some patients with systemic vasculitis manifest clinicopathologic characteristics that do not fit precisely into any specific disease but have overlapping features of different vasculitides. Active systemic vasculitis in such settings has the same potential for causing irreversible organ system damage as when it occurs in one of the defined syndromes listed in Table 306-1. The diagnostic and therapeutic considerations as well as the prognosis for these patients depend on the sites and severity of active vasculitis. Patients with vasculitis that could potentially cause irreversible damage to a major organ system should be treated as described under "Wegener's granulomatosis."

Drug-Induced Vasculitis Vasculitis associated with drug reactions usually presents as palpable purpura that may be generalized or limited to the lower extremities or other dependent areas; however, urticarial lesions, ulcers, and hemorrhagic blisters may also occur (Chap. 50). Signs and symptoms may be limited to the skin, although systemic manifestations such as fever, malaise, and polyarthralgias may occur. Although the skin is the predominant organ involved, systemic vasculitis may result from drug reactions. Drugs that have been implicated in vasculitis include allopurinol, thiazides, gold, sulfonamides, phenytoin, and penicillin (Chap. 50).

An increasing number of drugs have been reported to cause vasculitis associated with antimyeloperoxidase ANCA. Of these, the best evidence of causality exists for hydralazine and propylthiouracil. The clinical manifestations in ANCA-positive drug-induced vasculitis can range from cutaneous lesions to glomerulonephritis and pulmonary hemorrhage. Outside of drug discontinuation, treatment should be based on the severity of the vasculitis. Patients with immediately life-threatening small-vessel vasculitis should initially be treated with glucocorticoids and cyclophosphamide as described for Wegener's granulomatosis. Following clinical improvement, consideration may be given for tapering such agents along a more rapid schedule.

Serum Sickness and Serum Sickness–Like Reactions These reactions are characterized by the occurrence of fever, urticaria, polyarthralgias, and lymphadenopathy 7 to 10 days after primary exposure and 2 to 4 days after secondary exposure to a heterologous protein (classic serum sickness) or a nonprotein drug such as penicillin or sulfa (serum sickness–like reaction). Most of the manifestations are not due to a vasculitis; however, occasional patients will have typical cutaneous venulitis that may progress rarely to a systemic vasculitis.

Vasculitis Associated with Other Underlying Primary Diseases Certain *infections* may directly trigger an inflammatory vasculitic process. For example, rickettsias can invade and proliferate in the endothelial cells of small blood vessels causing a vasculitis (Chap. 158). In addition, the inflammatory response around blood vessels associated with certain systemic fungal diseases such as histoplasmosis (Chap. 183) may mimic a primary vasculitic process. A leukocytoclastic vasculitis predominantly involving the skin with occasional involvement of other organ systems may be a minor component of many other infections. These include *subacute bacterial endocarditis*, *Epstein-Barr virus infection*, *HIV infection*, as well as a number of other infections.

Vasculitis can be associated with certain *malignancies*, particularly lymphoid or reticuloendothelial neoplasms. Leukocytoclastic venulitis confined to the skin is the most common finding; however, widespread systemic vasculitis may occur. Of particular note is the association of *hairy cell leukemia* (Chap. 97) with PAN.

A number of *connective tissue diseases* have vasculitis as a secondary manifestation of the underlying primary process. Foremost among these are *systemic lupus erythematosus* (Chap. 300), *rheumatoid arthritis* (Chap. 301), *inflammatory myositis* (Chap. 370), *relapsing polychondritis* (Chap. 308), and *Sjögren's syndrome* (Chap. 304). The most common form of vasculitis in these conditions is the small-vessel venulitis isolated to the skin. However, certain patients may develop a fulminant systemic necrotizing vasculitis.

Secondary vasculitis has also been observed in association with *ulcerative colitis*, *congenital deficiencies of various complement components*, *retroperitoneal fibrosis*, *primary biliary cirrhosis*, α_1-antitrypsin deficiency, and *intestinal bypass surgery*.

PRINCIPLES OF TREATMENT

Once a diagnosis of vasculitis has been established, a decision regarding therapeutic strategy must be made (Fig. 306-1). The vasculitis syndromes represent a wide spectrum of diseases with varying degrees of severity. Since the potential toxic side effects of certain therapeutic regimens may be substantial, the risk-versus-benefit ratio of any therapeutic approach should be weighed carefully. Specific therapeutic regimens are discussed above for the individual vasculitis syndromes; however, certain general principles regarding therapy should be considered. On the one hand, glucocorticoids and/or cytotoxic therapy should be instituted immediately in diseases where irreversible organ system dysfunction and high morbidity and mortality have been clearly established. Wegener's granulomatosis is the prototype of a severe systemic vasculitis requiring such a therapeutic approach (see above). On the other hand, when feasible, aggressive therapy should be avoided for vasculitic manifestations that rarely result in irreversible organ system dysfunction and that usually do not respond to such therapy. For example, idiopathic cutaneous vasculitis usually resolves with symptomatic treatment, and prolonged courses of glucocorticoids uncommonly result in clinical benefit. Cytotoxic agents have not proved to be beneficial in idiopathic cutaneous vasculitis, and their toxic side effects generally outweigh any potential beneficial effects. Glucocorticoids should be initiated in those systemic vasculitides that cannot be specifically categorized or for which there is no established standard therapy; cytotoxic therapy should be added in these diseases only if an adequate response does not result or if remission can only be achieved and maintained with an unacceptably toxic regimen of glucocorticoids. When remission is achieved, one should continually attempt to taper glucocorticoids to an alternate-day regimen and discontinue when possible. When using cytotoxic regimens, one should base the choice of agent upon the available therapeutic data supporting efficacy in that disease, the site and severity of organ involvement, and the toxicity profile of the drug.

Physicians should be thoroughly aware of the toxic side effects of therapeutic agents employed (Table 306-7). Many of the side effects of glucocorticoid therapy are markedly decreased in frequency and duration in patients on alternate-day regimens compared to daily regimens. When cyclophosphamide is administered chronically in doses of 2 mg/kg per day for substantial periods of time (one to several years), the incidence of cystitis is at least 30% and the incidence of bladder cancer is at least 6%. Bladder cancer can occur several years after discontinuation of cyclophosphamide therapy; therefore, monitoring for bladder cancer should continue indefinitely in patients who have received prolonged courses of daily cyclophosphamide. Instructing the patient to take cyclophosphamide all at once in the morning with a large amount of fluid throughout the day in order to maintain

TABLE 306-7 *Major Toxic Side Effects of Drugs Commonly Used in the Treatment of Systemic Vasculitis*

GLUCOCORTICOIDS	
Osteoporosis	Growth suppression in children
Cataracts	Hypertension
Glaucoma	Avascular necrosis of bone
Diabetes mellitus	Myopathy
Electrolyte abnormalities	Alterations in mood
Metabolic abnormalities	Psychosis
Suppression of inflammatory and immune responses leading to opportunistic infections	Pseudotumor cerebri
	Peptic ulcer diathesis
	Pancreatitis
Cushingoid features	
CYCLOPHOSPHAMIDE	
Bone marrow suppression	Hypogammaglobulinemia
Cystitis	Pulmonary fibrosis
Bladder carcinoma	Myelodysplasia
Gonadal suppression	Oncogenesis
Gastrointestinal intolerance	
METHOTREXATE	
Gastrointestinal intolerance	Pneumonitis
Stomatitis	Teratogenicity
Neutropenia	Opportunistic infections
Hepatotoxicity (may lead to fibrosis or cirrhosis)	

a dilute urine can reduce the risk of bladder injury. Significant alopecia is unusual in the chronically administered, low-dose regimen. Permanent infertility can occur in both men and women. Bone marrow suppression is an important toxicity of cyclophosphamide and can be observed during glucocorticoid tapering or over time, even after periods of stable measurements. Monitoring of the complete blood count every 1 to 2 weeks for as long as the patient receives cyclophosphamide can effectively prevent cytopenias. When the white blood count (WBC) is maintained at $>3000/\mu L$, and the patient is not receiving daily glucocorticoids, the incidence of life-threatening opportunistic infections is low. However, the WBC is not an accurate predictor of risk of all opportunistic infections; and infections with *Pneumocystis carinii* and certain fungi can be seen in the face of WBCs that are within normal limits, particularly in patients receiving glucocorticoids. All vasculitis patients who are not allergic to sulfa and who are receiving daily glucocorticoids in combination with a cytotoxic drug should receive trimethoprim-sulfamethoxazole as prophylaxis against *P. carinii* infection.

Finally, it should be emphasized that each patient is unique and requires individual decision-making. The above outline should serve as a framework to guide therapeutic approaches; however, flexibility should be practiced in order to provide maximal therapeutic efficacy with minimal toxic side effects in each patient.

FURTHER READING

GUILLEVIN L et al: Microscopic polyangiitis. Clinical and laboratory findings in eighty-five patients. Arthritis Rheum 42:421, 1999
HOFFMAN GS SPECKS U: Antineutrophil cytoplasmic antibodies. Arthritis Rheum 41:1521, 1998
——— et al: Wegener's granulomatosis: An analysis of 158 patients. Ann Intern Med 116:488, 1992
JENNETTE JC et al: Nomenclature of systemic vasculitis. Proposal of an international consensus conference. Arthritis Rheum 37:187, 1994
KERR G et al: Takayasu arteritis. Ann Intern Med 120:919, 1994
LANGFORD CA et al: Use of cytotoxic agents and cyclosporine in the treatment of autoimmune disease. Part 2: Inflammatory bowel disease, systemic vasculitis, and therapeutic toxicity. Ann Intern Med 129:49, 1998
——— et al: A staged approach to the treatment of Wegener's granulomatosis: Induction of remission with glucocorticoids and daily cyclophosphamide switching to methotrexate for remission maintenance. Arthritis Rheum 42: 2666, 1999
LUDVIKSSON BR et al: Active Wegener's granulomatosis is associated with HLA-DR+ CD4+ T cells exhibiting an unbalanced Th-1 type T cell cytokine pattern: Reversal with IL-10. J Immunol 160:3602, 1998
SNELLER MC, FAUCI AS: Pathogenesis of vasculitis syndromes. Med Clin North Am 81:221, 1997

307 | BEHÇET'S SYNDROME
Haralampos M. Moutsopoulos

DEFINITION

Behçet's syndrome is a multisystem disorder presenting with recurrent oral and genital ulcerations as well as ocular involvement. Internationally agreed diagnostic criteria have been proposed (Table 307-1).

PREVALENCE, PATHOGENESIS, AND PATHOLOGY

The syndrome affects young males and females from the Mediterranean region, the Middle East, and the Far East, suggesting a link with the ancient Silk Route. Males and females are affected equally, but males often have more severe disease. Blacks are not affected.

The etiology and pathogenesis of this syndrome remain obscure; vasculitis is the main pathologic lesion with a tendency to venous thrombus formation, and circulating autoantibodies to human oral mucous membranes are found in approximately 50% of the patients. In endemic areas the syndrome is associated with HLA-B5 (B51) alloantigen, and approximately 1 in 10 patients has an affected relative.

CLINICAL FEATURES

The recurrent aphthous ulcerations are a sine qua non for the diagnosis. The ulcers are usually painful, shallow or deep with a central yellowish necrotic base, appear singly or in crops, and are located anywhere in the oral cavity. The ulcers persist for 1 to 2 weeks and subside without leaving scars. The genital ulcers are less common, more specific, do not affect the glans penis or urethra, and produce scrotal scars.

Skin involvement includes folliculitis, erythema nodosum, an acne-like exanthem, and infrequently vasculitis. Nonspecific skin inflammatory reactivity to any scratches or intradermal saline injection (pathergy test) is a common and specific manifestation.

TABLE 307-1 *Diagnostic Criteria of Behçet's Disease*

Recurrent oral ulceration plus two of the following:
  Recurrent genital ulceration
  Eye lesions
  Skin lesions
  Pathergy test

Eye involvement with scarring, bilateral panuveitis is the most dreaded complication, since it occasionally progresses rapidly to blindness. The eye disease is usually present at the onset but may also develop within the first few years. In addition to iritis, posterior uveitis, retinal vessel occlusions, and optic neuritis can be seen in some patients with the syndrome. Hypopyon uveitis, a specific but rare manifestation, is a layer of inflammatory cells visible because of the effects of gravity; it usually indicates severe retinal vascular disease.

The arthritis of Behçet's syndrome is not deforming and affects the knees and ankles.

Superficial or deep peripheral vein thrombosis is seen in one-fourth of the patients. Pulmonary emboli are a rare complication. The superior vena cava is obstructed occasionally, producing a dramatic clinical picture. Arterial involvement occurs infrequently and presents with aortitis or peripheral arterial aneurysm and arterial thrombosis. Pulmonary artery vasculitis presenting with dyspnea, cough, chest pain, hemoptysis, and infiltrates on chest roentgenograms has been reported recently in 5% of patients.

Neurologic involvement (5 to 10%) appears mainly in the parenchymal form (80%); it is associated with brain stem involvement and has a serious prognosis. Dural sinus thrombi (20%) are associated with headache and increased intracranial pressure.

Gastrointestinal involvement consists of mucosal ulcerations of the gut.

Laboratory findings are mainly nonspecific indices of inflammation, such as leukocytosis and elevated erythrocyte sedimentation rate, as well as C-reactive protein levels; antibodies to the human oral mucosa are also found.

Rx | TREATMENT

The severity of the syndrome usually abates with time. Apart from the patients with parenchymal neurologic involvement, the life expectancy seems to be normal, and the only serious complication is blindness.

Mucous membrane involvement may respond to topical glucocorticoids in the form of mouthwash or paste. In more serious cases thalidomide (100 mg/d) is effective. Thrombophlebitis is treated with aspirin, 325 mg/d. Colchicine or interferon α can be beneficial for the mucocutaneous manifestations of the syndrome. Uveitis and central nervous system involvement require systemic glucocorticoid therapy (prednisone, 1 mg/kg per day) and azathioprine, 2 to 3 mg/kg per day, or cyclosporine, 5 to 10 mg/kg per day. Preliminary data suggest that anti-tumor necrosis factor block may be an alternative therapeutic modality for panuveitis. Early initiation of azathioprine tends to favorably affect the long-term prognosis of Behçet's syndrome.

FURTHER READING

MEADOR R et al: Behçet's disease: Immunopathologic and therapeutic aspects. Curr Rheumatol Rep 4:47, 2002

SFIKAKIS PP. Behçet's disease: a new target for anti-tumour necrosis factor treatment. Ann Rheum Dis 61 (Suppl 2):51, 2002
YAZICI H et al: Behçet's disease. Curr Opin Rheumatol 13:18, 2001
———— et al: Behçet's syndrome: Where do we stand? Am J Med 112:75, 2002

308 RELAPSING POLYCHONDRITIS
Bruce C. Gilliland

Relapsing polychondritis is an uncommon inflammatory disorder of unknown cause characterized by an episodic and generally progressive course affecting predominantly the cartilage of the ears, nose, and laryngotracheobronchial tree. Other manifestations include scleritis, neurosensory hearing loss, polyarthritis, cardiac abnormalities, skin lesions, and glomerulonephritis. The peak age of onset is between the ages of 40 to 50 years, but relapsing polychondritis may affect children and the elderly. It is found in all races, and both sexes are equally affected. No familial tendency is apparent. A significantly higher frequency of HLA-DR4 has been found in patients with relapsing polychondritis than in normal individuals. A predominant subtype allele(s) of HLA-DR4 was not found. Approximately 30% of patients with relapsing polychondritis will have another rheumatologic disorder, the most frequent being systemic vasculitis, followed by rheumatoid arthritis, systemic lupus erythematosus (SLE), Sjögren's syndrome, or ankylosing spondylitis. Nonrheumatic disorders associated with relapsing polychondritis include inflammatory bowel disease, primary biliary cirrhosis, and myelodysplastic syndrome (Table 308-1).

Diagnostic criteria were suggested over 20 years ago by McAdam et al. and modified by Damiani and Levine a few years later. These criteria continue to be generally used in clinical practice. McAdam et al. proposed the following: (1) recurrent chondritis of both auricles; (2) nonerosive inflammatory arthritis; (3) chondritis of nasal cartilage; (4) inflammation of ocular structures including conjunctivitis, keratitis, scleritis/episcleritis, and/or uveitis; (5) chondritis of the laryngeal and/or tracheal cartilages; and (6) cochlear and/or vestibular damage manifested by neurosensory hearing loss, tinnitus, and/or vertigo. The diagnosis is certain when three or more of these features are present along with a positive biopsy from the ear, nasal, or respiratory cartilage. Damiani and Levine later suggested that the diagnosis could be made when one or more of the above features and a positive biopsy were present, when two or more separate sites of cartilage inflammation were present that responded to glucocorticoids or dapsone, or when three or more of the above features were present. A biopsy is not necessary in most patients with clinically evident disease.

PATHOLOGY AND PATHOPHYSIOLOGY   The earliest abnormality of hyaline and elastic cartilage noted histologically is a focal or diffuse loss of basophilic staining indicating depletion of proteoglycan from the cartilage matrix. Inflammatory infiltrates are found adjacent to involved cartilage and consist predominantly of mononuclear cells and occasional plasma cells. In acute disease, polymorphonuclear white cells may also be present. Destruction of cartilage begins at the outer edges and advances centrally. There is lacunar breakdown and loss of chondrocytes. Degenerating cartilage is replaced by granulation tissue and later by fibrosis and focal areas of calcification. Small loci of cartilage regeneration may be present. Immunofluorescence studies have shown immunoglobulins and complement at sites of involvement. Extracellular granular material observed in the degenerating cartilage matrix by electron microscopy has been interpreted to be enzymes, immunoglobulins, or proteoglycans.

Immunologic mechanisms play a role in the pathogenesis of relapsing polychondritis. Immunoglobulin and complement deposits are found at sites of inflammation. In addition, antibodies to type II collagen and to matrilin-1 and immune complexes are detected in the sera of some patients. The possibility that an immune response to type II collagen may be important in the pathogenesis is supported experimentally by the occurrence of auricular chondritis in rats immunized with type II collagen. Antibodies to type II collagen are found in the sera of these animals, and immune deposits are detected at sites of ear inflammation. Humoral immune responses to type IX and type XI collagen, matrilin-1, and cartilage oligomeric matrix protein have been demonstrated in some patients. In a study, rats immunized with matrilin-1 were found to develop severe inspiratory stridor and swelling of the nasal septum. The rats had severe inflammation with erosions of the involved cartilage, which was characterized by increased numbers of CD 4+ and CD 8+ T cells in the lesions. The cartilage of the joints and ear pinna was not involved. All had IgG antibodies to matrilin-1. Matrilin-1 is a noncollagenous protein present in the extracellular matrix in cartilage. It is present in high concentrations in the trachea and is also present in the nasal septum but not in articular cartilage. A subsequent study demonstrated serum anti-matrilin-1 antibodies in approximately 13% of patients with relapsing polychondritis; approximately 70 of these patients had respiratory symptoms. Cell-mediated immunity may also be operative in causing tissue injury, since lymphocyte transformation can be demonstrated when lymphocytes of patients are exposed to cartilage extracts. T cells specific for type II collagen have been found in some patients, and CD 4+ T cells have been observed at sites of cartilage inflammation. The accumulating data strongly suggest that both humoral and cell-mediated immunity play an important role in the pathogenesis of relapsing polychondritis.

Dissolution of cartilage matrix can be induced by the intravenous injection of crude papain, a proteolytic enzyme, into young rabbits, which results in collapse of their normally rigid ears within 4 h. Reconstitution of the matrix occurs in about 7 days. In relapsing polychondritis, loss of cartilage matrix also most likely results from action of proteolytic enzymes released from chondrocytes, polymorphonuclear white cells, and monocytes that have been activated by inflammatory mediators.

CLINICAL MANIFESTATIONS   The onset of relapsing polychondritis is frequently abrupt with the appearance of one or two sites of cartilagenous inflammation. Fever, fatigue, and weight loss occur and may precede the clinical signs of relapsing polychondritis by several weeks. Relapsing polychondritis may go unrecognized for several months or even years in patients who only initially manifest intermittent joint pain and/or swelling, or who have unexplained eye inflammation, hearing loss, valvular heart disease, or pulmonary symptoms. The pattern of cartilagenous involvement and the frequency of episodes vary widely among patients.

TABLE 308-1   Disorders Associated with Relapsing Polychondritis[a]

Systemic vasculitis	Behçet's syndrome
Rheumatoid arthritis	Inflammatory bowel disease
Systemic lupus erythematosus	Primary biliary cirrhosis
Sjögren's syndrome	Myelodysplastic syndrome
Spondyloarthropathies	

[a] Systemic vasculitis is the most common association followed by rheumatoid arthritis, systemic lupus erythematosus, and Sjögren's syndrome.

Source: Modified from Michet.

TABLE 308-2   Clinical Manifestations of Relapsing Polychondritis

Clinical Feature	Frequency, %	
	Presenting	Cumulative
Auricular chondritis	40	85
Hearing loss	10	30
Nasal chondritis	25	55
Saddle nose deformity	20	30
Ocular deformities	20	50
Respiratory disease	25	50
Arthritis	35	50
Aortic regurgitation	—	5
Vasculitis	3	10

Source: Modified from Isaak et al.

Auricular chondritis is the most frequent presenting manifestation of relapsing polychondritis in 40% of patients and eventually affects about 85% of patients (Table 308-2). One or both ears are involved, either sequentially or simultaneously. Patients experience the sudden onset of pain, tenderness, and swelling of the cartilaginous portion of the ear (Fig. 308-1). Earlobes are spared because they do not contain cartilage. The overlying skin has a beefy red or violaceous color. Prolonged or recurrent episodes result in a flabby or droopy ear as a sequela of cartilage destruction. Swelling may close off the eustachian tube (causing otitis media) or the external auditory meatus, either of which can impair hearing. Inflammation of the internal auditory artery or its cochlear branch produces hearing loss, vertigo, ataxia, nausea, and vomiting. Vertigo is almost always accompanied by hearing loss. The cartilage of the nose becomes inflamed during the first or subsequent attacks. Approximately 50% of patients will eventually have nose involvement. Patients may experience nasal stuffiness, rhinorrhea, and epistaxis. The bridge of the nose becomes red, swollen, and tender and may collapse, producing a saddle deformity (Fig. 308-2). In some patients, the saddle deformity develops insidiously without overt inflammation. Saddle nose is observed more frequently in younger patients, especially in women.

Arthritis is the presenting manifestation in relapsing polychondritis in approximately one-third of patients and may be present for several months before other features appear. Eventually, more than half the patients will have arthritis. The arthritis is usually asymmetric and oligo- or polyarticular, and involves both large and small peripheral joints. An episode of arthritis lasts from a few days to several weeks and resolves spontaneously without residual joint deformity. Attacks

FIGURE 308-2   Saddle nose results from destruction and collapse of the nasal cartilage. (*Reprinted from the Clinical Slide Collection on the Rheumatic Diseases, © 1991, 1995, 1997, 1998, 1999. Used by permission of the American College of Rheumatology.*)

of arthritis may not be temporally related to other manifestations of relapsing polychondritis. The joints are warm, tender, and swollen. Joint fluid has been reported to be noninflammatory. In addition to peripheral joints, inflammation may involve the costochondral, sternomanubrial, and sternoclavicular cartilages. Destruction of these cartilages may result in a pectus excavatum deformity or even a flail anterior chest wall. Relapsing polychondritis may occur in patients with preexisting rheumatoid arthritis, Reiter's syndrome, psoriatic arthritis, or ankylosing spondylitis.

Eye manifestations occur in more than half of patients and include conjunctivitis, episcleritis, scleritis, iritis, and keratitis. Eye involvement is seldom the presenting feature. Ulceration and perforation of the cornea may occur and cause blindness. Other manifestations include eyelid and periorbital edema, proptosis, cataracts, optic neuritis, extraocular muscle palsies, retinal vasculitis, and renal vein occlusion.

Laryngotracheobronchial involvement occurs in ~50% of patients. Symptoms include hoarseness, a nonproductive cough, and tenderness over the larynx and proximal trachea. Mucosal edema, strictures, and/or collapse of laryngeal or tracheal cartilage may cause stridor and life-threatening airway obstruction necessitating tracheostomy. Collapse of cartilage in bronchi leads to pneumonia and, when extensive, to respiratory insufficiency.

Aortic regurgitation occurs in about 5% of patients and is due to progressive dilation of the aortic ring or to destruction of the valve cusps. Mitral and other heart valves are less often affected. Other cardiac manifestations include pericarditis, myocarditis, and conduction abnormalities. Aneurysms of the proximal, thoracic, or abdominal aorta may occur even in the absence of active chondritis and occasionally rupture.

Systemic vasculitis may occur in association with relapsing polychondritis. Vasculitides include leukocytoclastic vasculitis, polyarteritis, temporal arteritis, and Takayasu's arteritis (Chap. 306). Neurologic abnormalities usually occur as a result of underlying vasculitis, manifesting as seizures, strokes, ataxia, and peripheral and cranial nerve neuropathies. Cranial nerves II, III, VI, and VII are most often involved. Approximately 25% of patients have skin lesions, none of which is characteristic for relapsing polychondritis, that reflect associated vasculitis. These include purpura, erythema nodosum, erythema multiforme, angioedema/urticaria, livedo reticularis, and panniculitis. Segmental necrotizing glomerulonephritis with crescent formation has been noted in some patients, usually in association with microscopic polyangiitis, but may occur in the absence of systemic vasculitis.

FIGURE 308-1   *Left.* The pinna is erythematous, swollen, and tender. Not shown is the ear lobule that is spared as there is no underlying cartilage. *Right.* The pinna is thickened and deformed. The destruction of the underlying cartilage results in a floppy ear. (*Reprinted from the Clinical Slide Collection on the Rheumatic Diseases, © 1991, 1995, 1997, 1998, 1999. Used by permission of the American College of Rheumatology.*)

The course of disease is highly variable, with episodes lasting from a few days to several weeks and then subsiding spontaneously. Attacks may recur at intervals varying from weeks to months. In other patients, the disease has a chronic, smoldering course. In a few patients, the disease may be limited to one or two episodes of cartilage inflammation. In one study, the 5-year estimated survival rate was 74% and the 10-year survival rate 55%. In contrast to earlier series, only about half the deaths could be attributed to relapsing polychondritis or complications of treatment. Pulmonary complications accounted for only 10% of all fatalities. In general, patients with more widespread disease have a worse prognosis.

LABORATORY FINDINGS Mild leukocytosis and normocytic, normochromic anemia are often present. Eosinophilia is observed in 10% of patients. The erythrocyte sedimentation rate and C-reactive protein are usually elevated. Rheumatoid factor and antinuclear antibody tests are occasionally positive in low titers. Antibodies to type II collagen are present in fewer than half the patients and are specific. Circulating immune complexes may be detected, especially in patients with early active disease. Elevated levels of γ globulin may be present. Antineutrophil cytoplasmic antibodies (ANCA), either cytoplasmic (C-ANCA) or perinuclear (P-ANCA), are found in some patients with active disease. The upper and lower airways can be evaluated by imaging techniques such as linear tomography, laryngotracheography, and computed tomography, and by bronchoscopy. Magnetic resonance imaging (MRI) is helpful in evaluation of the larynx and trachea. Bronchography is performed to demonstrate bronchial narrowing. Intrathoracic airway obstruction can also be evaluated by inspiratory-expiratory flow studies. The chest film may show narrowing of the trachea and/or the main bronchi, widening of the ascending or descending aorta due to an aneurysm, and cardiomegaly when aortic insufficiency is present. MRI can be used in assessing aortic aneurysmal dilatation. Radiographs may show calcification at previous sites of cartilage damage involving ear, nose, larynx, or trachea.

DIAGNOSIS Diagnosis is based on recognition of the typical clinical features. Biopsies of the involved cartilage from the ear, nose, or respiratory tract will confirm the diagnosis but are only necessary when clinical features are not typical. Patients with Wegener's granulomatosis may have a saddle nose and pulmonary involvement but can be distinguished by the absence of auricular involvement and the presence of granulomatous lesions in the tracheobronchial tree. Patients with Cogan's syndrome have interstitial keratitis and vestibular and auditory abnormalities, but this syndrome does not involve the respiratory tract or ears. Reiter's syndrome may initially resemble relapsing polychondritis because of oligoarticular arthritis and eye involvement, but it is distinguished in time by the appearance of urethritis and typical mucocutaneous lesions and the absence of nose or ear cartilage

involvement. Rheumatoid arthritis may initially suggest relapsing polychondritis because of arthritis and eye inflammation. The arthritis in rheumatoid arthritis, however, is erosive and symmetric. In addition, rheumatoid factor titers are usually high compared with those in relapsing polychondritis. Bacterial infection of the pinna may be mistaken for relapsing polychondritis but differs by usually involving only one ear, including the earlobe. Auricular cartilage may also be damaged by trauma or frostbite.

Relapsing polychondritis may develop in patients with a variety of autoimmune disorders, including SLE, rheumatoid arthritis, Sjögren's syndrome, and vasculitis. In most cases, these disorders antedate the appearance of polychondritis, usually by months or years. It is likely that these patients have an immunologic abnormality that predisposes them to development of this group of autoimmune disorders.

℞ TREATMENT

In patients with active chondritis, prednisone, 40 to 60 mg/d, is often effective in suppressing disease activity; it is tapered gradually once disease is controlled. In some patients, prednisone can be stopped, while in others low doses in the range of 10 to 15 mg/d are required for continued suppression of disease. Dapsone instead of prednisone has been effective in suppressing inflammation in some patients. Immunosuppressive drugs such as methotrexate, cyclophosphamide, azathioprine, or cyclosporine should be reserved for patients who fail to respond to prednisone or who require high doses for control of disease activity. Patients with significant ocular inflammation often require intraocular steroids as well as high doses of prednisone. Heart valve replacement or repair of an aortic aneurysm may be necessary. In patients with early subglottic disease, intralesional injection of glutocorticoids may be beneficial. When obstruction is severe, tracheostomy is required. Stents may be necessary in patients with tracheobronchial collapse.

FURTHER READING

HOCHBERG MC: Relapsing polychondritis, in *Kelley's Textbook of Rheumatology*, 6th ed, S Ruddy et al (eds). Philadelphia, Saunders, 2001, pp 1463–1467

ISAAK BL et al: Ocular and systemic findings in relapsing polychondritis. Ophthalmology 93:681, 1986

LETKO E et al: Relapsing polychondritis: A clinical review. Semin Arthritis Rheum 31:384, 2002

MICHET CT: Relapsing polychondritis, in *Arthritis and Allied Conditions*, 14th ed, WJ Koopman (ed). Philadelphia, Lippincott Williams & Wilkins, 2001, pp 1774–1783

ZEUNER M et al: Relapsing polychondritis: Clinical and immunogenic analysis of 62 patients. J Rheumatol 24:96, 1997

---

309 SARCOIDOSIS
Ronald G. Crystal

DEFINITION Sarcoidosis is a chronic, multisystem disorder of unknown cause characterized in affected organs by an accumulation of T lymphocytes and mononuclear phagocytes, noncaseating epithelioid granulomas, and derangements of the normal tissue architecture. Although there are usually skin anergy and depressed cellular immune processes in the blood, sarcoidosis is characterized at the sites of disease by exaggerated T helper 1 (T_H1) lymphocyte immune processes. All parts of the body can be involved, but the organ most frequently affected is the lung. Involvement of the skin, eye, liver, and lymph nodes is also common. The disease is often acute or subacute and self-limiting, but in many individuals it is chronic, waxing and waning over many years.

ETIOLOGY The cause of sarcoidosis is unknown. Various infectious and noninfectious agents have been implicated, but there is no proof that

any specific agent is responsible. However, all available evidence is consistent with the concept that the disease results from an exaggerated cellular immune response (acquired, inherited, or both) to a limited class of persistent antigens or self-antigens.

INCIDENCE AND PREVALENCE Sarcoidosis is a relatively common disease affecting individuals of both sexes and almost all ages, races, and geographic locations. Females appear to be slightly more susceptible than males. Cases of sarcoidosis have been described in all of the major races, and the disease is found throughout the world. It has been suggested that sarcoidosis is more common in certain geographic areas such as the southeastern part of the United States, but when case-matched controls have been used, these geographic differences are less convincing. There is a remarkable diversity of the prevalence of sarcoidosis among certain ethnic and racial groups, with a range of <1 to 64 per 100,000 worldwide. The prevalence of sarcoidosis is from 10 to 40 per 100,000 in the United States and Europe. In the United States, most patients are black, with a ratio of blacks to whites ranging from 10:1 to 17:1. In Europe, however, the disease affects mostly whites. Furthermore, while the prevalence per 100,000 in Sweden is 64, in France it is 10, in Poland 3, yet for Irish females living in London it is 200. In contrast, the disease is very rare among Inuit, Canadian Indians, New Zealand Maoris, and Southeast Asians.

Most patients present with sarcoidosis between the ages of 20 and 40, but the disease can occur in children and in the elderly. Several hundred kindred groups with familial sarcoidosis have been described, and the disease has been observed in twins, more commonly in monozygotic than in dizygotic pairs. There have also been several instances of husband-wife pairs identified, and geographic foci of sarcoidosis among unrelated individuals living closely within a community, arguing for some environmental factors in the pathogenesis of the disease. Although the disease is believed to result from exaggerated cellular immune responses to a limited class of antigens, no clear patterns in any HLA locus have emerged. Unlike many diseases in which the lung is involved, sarcoidosis favors nonsmokers.

PATHOPHYSIOLOGY AND IMMUNOPATHOGENESIS The first manifestation of the disease is an accumulation of mononuclear inflammatory cells, mostly CD4+ T_H1 lymphocytes and mononuclear phagocytes, in affected organs. This inflammatory process is followed by the formation of granulomas, aggregates of macrophages and their progeny, epithelioid cells, and multinucleated giant cells. The typical sarcoid granuloma is a compact structure composed of an aggregate of mononuclear phagocytes surrounded by a rim of CD4+ T lymphocytes and, to a far lesser extent, B lymphocytes. The overall structure is relatively discrete and is interspersed with fine collagen fibrils, presumably remnants of the underlying connective tissue matrix. The giant cells within the granuloma can be of the Langhans' or foreign-body variety and often contain inclusions such as Schaumann bodies (conchlike struc-

tures), asteroid bodies (stellate-like structures), and residual bodies (refractile calcium-containing inclusions).

Together the accumulated T cells, mononuclear phagocytes, and granulomas represent the active disease. Other than the fact that they take up space and thus their bulk modifies the local architecture, for all except late-stage cases, there is no evidence that the mononuclear inflammatory cells dispersed in the tissue or in the granuloma injure the affected organ by releasing mediators that damage the normal parenchymal cells or the extracellular matrix. Rather, organ dysfunction in sarcoidosis results mostly from the accumulated inflammatory cells distorting the architecture of the affected tissue; if a sufficient number of structures vital to the function of the tissue are involved, the disease becomes clinically apparent in that organ. Thus, while autopsy series show that, to some extent, sarcoidosis involves most organs in the majority of patients, the disease manifests clinically only in organs where it affects function (such as the lung and eye) or in organs where it is readily observed (such as the skin or, by x-ray, the hilar nodes). For example, in the lung, the inflammatory cells and granulomas distort the walls of the alveoli, bronchi, and blood vessels (Fig. 309-1A), thus altering the intimate relationships between air and blood necessary for normal gas exchange. When a sufficient amount of pulmonary tissue is involved, it is sensed by the individual as dyspnea. In contrast, most individuals with sarcoidosis have granulomatous mononuclear cell inflammation in the liver but usually do not have symptoms or significant functional derangements referable to that organ, likely because the disease process does not modify the local structures sufficiently to affect function.

If the disease is suppressed, either spontaneously or with therapy, the mononuclear inflammation is reduced in intensity and the number of granulomas is reduced. The granulomas resolve either by dispersion of the cells or by centripetal proliferation of fibroblasts from the periphery of the granuloma inward, to form a small scar. In chronic cases,

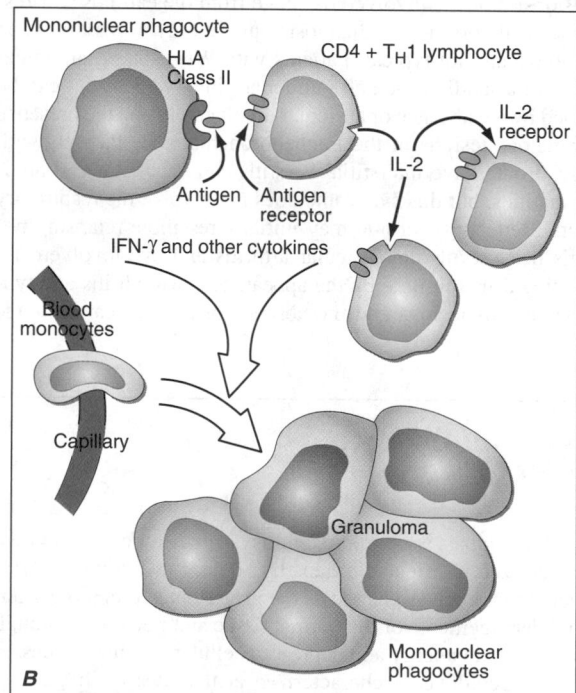

FIGURE 309-1 Pathogenesis of sarcoidosis. *A.* Histologic abnormalities. Normal alveoli (*top*) and alveoli in active sarcoidosis (*bottom*). The latter are distorted by the accumulated CD4+ T_H1 lymphocytes, alveolar macrophages, and macrophages aggregated into granulomas. There is mild damage to alveolar epithelial and endothelial cells. *B.* The exaggerated processes of T_H1 lymphocytes in affected organs result in the accumulation of these cells along with macrophages and macrophages aggregated into granulomas. The trigger for the T_H1 lymphocytes is unknown. It may be a limited class of antigens or self-antigens presented in the context of class II HLA surface molecules by mononuclear phagocytes to the T_H1 lymphocyte. The antigen class II HLA complex is identified by the T cell antigen receptor, and the T cell is activated. Consequent to this process the immune response is exaggerated and skewed to produce activated T_H1 lymphocytes that release IL-2, which drives the accumulation of more T lymphocytes. The activated T_H1 lymphocytes also release interferon γ (INF-γ). Together with cytokines such as IL-12, macrophage inflammatory protein 1α and granulocyte-macrophage colony-stimulating factor released in the local milieu, there is recruitment and activation of blood monocytes and subsequent granuloma formation.

the mononuclear cell inflammation persists for years. If the intensity of the inflammation is sufficiently high for a sufficiently long period, the derangements to the affected tissues result in extensive damage, the development of fibrosis, and permanent loss of organ function.

The available evidence suggests that active sarcoidosis results from an exaggerated cellular immune response to a variety of antigens or self-antigens, in which the process of T lymphocyte triggering, proliferation, and activation is skewed in the direction of CD4+ T_H1 lymphocyte processes (Fig. 309-1B). The result is an exaggerated T_H1 T lymphocyte response and thus the accumulation of large numbers of activated T_H1 cells in the affected organs. Since the activated T_H1 lymphocyte releases mediators that attract and activate mononuclear phagocytes, it is likely that the process of granuloma formation is a secondary phenomenon that is a consequence of the exaggerated T_H1 cell process. In this context, the current hypotheses of the cause of sarcoidosis, not mutually exclusive, include the following: (1) The disease is caused by a class of persistent antigens, nonself or self, that trigger only the T_H1 cell arm of the immune response; (2) the disease results from an inadequate suppressor arm of the immune response, such that T_H1 cell processes cannot be shut down in a normal fashion; or (3) the disease results from inherited (and/or acquired) differences in immune response genes, such that the response to a variety of antigens is an exaggerated, T_H1 cell process.

Independent of the inciting agent(s) or the reason why there is an exaggerated T_H1 cell response, there is a general understanding of the processes responsible for the maintenance of the inflammation and the development of the granuloma. The T_H1 lymphocytes accumulate at the sites of disease, at least in part, because they proliferate in these sites at an exaggerated rate. This T cell proliferation is maintained by the spontaneous release of interleukin (IL) 2, the T cell growth factor, by activated T_H1 cells in the local milieu. In this regard, sarcoidosis is a remarkable example of compartmentalization of the immune system and a dramatic illustration of why disease activity of sarcoidosis cannot be assessed by evaluating the immune system only in the blood. Whereas the T_H1 cells in the involved organs are releasing IL-2 and proliferating at an enhanced rate, the T cells in other sites, such as blood, are quiescent. Furthermore, while there is a marked enhancement of the number of T_H1 cells at the sites of disease, the numbers of T_H1 cells in the blood are normal or slightly reduced. In the involved organs, the ratio of CD4+ to CD8+ T cells may be as high as 10:1 compared to the ratio of 2:1 found in normal tissues or in the blood of affected individuals.

In addition to driving other T_H1 cells in the affected organs to proliferate, the T_H1 cells at the sites of disease are activated and release mediators that both recruit and activate mononuclear phagocytes. The activated T_H1 cells accomplish this by releasing a variety of mediators (lymphokines) including proteins capable of recruiting blood monocytes to the local milieu of the activated T cells and interferon γ, a protein that, among its many actions, activates mononuclear phagocytes. Together with cytokines such as IL-12 and others released locally, these mediators recruit blood monocytes to the affected organs and activate them, providing the building blocks for the formation of the granuloma.

In addition to these exaggerated cellular immune processes, active sarcoidosis is also characterized by hyperglobulinemia. Included among the immunoglobulins are antibodies against a variety of infectious agents as well as IgM anti-T cell antibodies. However, there is no evidence that any of these antibodies plays a role in the pathogenesis of the disease, and they are thought to result from the nonspecific polyclonal stimulation of B cells by the activated T cells at the site of disease.

If the damage in the affected organs is sufficiently extensive that the remaining parenchymal cells cannot reestablish the normal tissue architecture, the usual result is fibrosis, the proliferation of mesenchymal cells, and deposition of their connective tissue products. There is convincing evidence that the fibroblast proliferation is directed by tissue macrophages spontaneously releasing growth signals for fibroblasts, including platelet-derived growth factor, fibronectin, and

insulin-like growth factor 1. It is not known, however, why this fibrotic process occurs only in a relatively small proportion of individuals with sarcoidosis.

CLINICAL MANIFESTATIONS   Sarcoidosis is a systemic disease, and thus the clinical manifestations may be generalized or focused on one or more organs. However, because the lung is almost always involved, most patients have symptoms referable to the respiratory system. Independent of the site, the clinical manifestations of the disease relate directly to the exaggerated T_H1 lymphocyte–mononuclear phagocyte granulomatous inflammatory process itself or to the sequelae resulting from the permanent damage caused by this process.

Sarcoidosis is occasionally discovered in a completely asymptomatic individual, but more commonly it presents abruptly over 1 to 2 weeks or the affected individual develops symptoms insidiously over several months. Independent of the mode of presentation, ~75% of all cases present in individuals younger than 40 years.

The asymptomatic form is usually detected by a routine examination, such as a chest film. In the United States, this form represents about 10 to 20% of all cases, but in countries where chest films are mandatory in preemployment screening programs, the proportion of asymptomatic patients is higher.

So-called acute or subacute sarcoidosis develops abruptly over a period of a few weeks and represents 20 to 40% of all cases. These individuals usually have constitutional symptoms such as fever, fatigue, malaise, anorexia, or weight loss. These symptoms are usually mild, but in ~25% of the acute cases the constitutional complaints are extensive. Many patients have respiratory symptoms, including cough, dyspnea, a vague retrosternal chest discomfort, and/or polyarthritis. Two syndromes have been identified in the acute group. *Löfgren's syndrome*, frequent in Scandinavian, Irish, and Puerto Rican females, includes the complex of erythema nodosum (Fig. 309-2) and x-ray findings of bilateral hilar adenopathy, often accompanied by joint symptoms, including arthritis at the ankles, knees, wrists, or elbows. The *Heerfordt-Waldenström syndrome* describes individuals with fever, parotid enlargement, anterior uveitis, and facial nerve palsy.

The insidious form of sarcoidosis develops over months and is usually associated with respiratory complaints without constitutional symptoms. In the United States, 40 to 70% of all patients with sarcoidosis patients are in this category. About 10% of these individuals have symptoms referable to organs other than the lung. It is the individuals who present with the insidious form of sarcoidosis who most commonly go on to develop chronic sarcoidosis, with permanent damage to the lung and other organs.

FIGURE 309-2 Erythema nodosum is a panniculitis characterized by tender deep-seated nodules and plaques usually located on the lower extremities.

Despite the fact that sarcoidosis is a systemic disease and some evidence of inflammation can be detected in most organs in the majority of patients, sarcoidosis is important clinically because of the pulmonary abnormalities and, to a lesser extent, lymph node, skin, liver, and eye involvement. Far less commonly, other organs are involved significantly.

Lung Of individuals with sarcoidosis, 90% have abnormal findings on chest x-ray at some time during their course (Fig. 309-3A). Overall, ~50% develop permanent pulmonary abnormalities, and 5 to 15% have progressive fibrosis of the lung parenchyma. Sarcoidosis of the lung is primarily an interstitial lung disease (Chap. 243) in which the inflammatory process involves the alveoli, small bronchi, and small blood vessels. These individuals typically have symptoms of dyspnea, particularly with exercise, and a dry cough. In acute and subacute cases, physical examination usually reveals dry rales. Hemoptysis is rare, as is production of sputum. Occasionally, the large airways are involved to a degree sufficient to cause dysfunction. Distal atelectasis can result from endobronchial sarcoidosis or from external compression from enlarged intrathoracic nodes. Rarely, wheezing is heard, incorrectly suggesting asthma. Large-vessel pulmonary granulomatous arteritis is common, but it rarely causes major problems. If it dominates the pulmonary lesions, it is sometimes called *necrotizing sarcoidal granulomatosis*. The pleura is involved in 1 to 5% of cases, almost always manifesting as a unilateral pleural effusion with characteristics of an exudate containing lymphocytes. The effusions usually clear within a few weeks, but chronic pleural thickening can result. Pneumothorax or hydropneumothorax is observed in sarcoid but is very rare.

Lymph Nodes Lymphadenopathy is very common in sarcoidosis. Intrathoracic nodes are enlarged in 75 to 90% of all patients; usually this involves the hilar nodes, but the paratracheal nodes are commonly involved ((Fig. 309-3A). Less frequently, there is enlargement of subcarinal, anterior mediastinal, or posterior mediastinal nodes. Peripheral lymphadenopathy is very common, particularly involving the cervical, axillary, epitrochlear, and inguinal nodes. The nodes in the retroperitoneal area and in the mesenteric chain also can enlarge. All these nodes are nonadherent, with a firm, rubbery texture. Palpation causes no pain. Unlike nodes in tuberculosis, the nodes do not ulcerate. The lymphadenopathy rarely causes a problem for the affected individual; however, if it is massive, it can be disfiguring and can impinge on other organs and lead to functional impairment.

Skin Sarcoidosis involves the skin in ~25% of patients. The most common lesions are erythema nodosum (Fig. 309-2), plaques, maculopapular eruptions, subcutaneous nodules, and lupus pernio (Fig. 309-4). Erythema nodosum, comprising bilateral, tender red nodules on the anterior surface of the legs, is not specific for sarcoidosis but is common, particularly in acute sarcoidosis, in combination with systemic symptoms and polyarthralgias. Treatment is not required, since the lesions resolve spontaneously in 2 to 4 weeks. Erythema nodosum is much more common among patients with sarcoidosis in Europe than in the United States. Skin plaques associated with sarcoidosis are purple, indolent lesions, often raised, and usually occur on the face, buttocks, and extremities. The maculopapular eruptions occur on the face around the eyes and nose, on the back, and on the extremities. These are elevated lesions <1 cm in diameter with a flat, waxy top. Subcutaneous nodules are most common on the trunk and extremities. Lupus pernio is characterized by indurated blue-purple, swollen, shiny lesions on the nose, cheeks, lips, ears, fingers, and knees. The lesions on the tip of the nose cause a bulbous appearance, sometimes associated with varicosities. The nasal mucosa is usually involved, and underlying bone can be destroyed. Sarcoidosis can also involve old surgical scars and tattoos. Although it may be disfiguring, cutaneous sarcoidosis rarely causes major problems. Clubbing of the fingers is occasionally observed in sarcoidosis, usually in association with extensive pulmonary fibrosis.

Eye Eye involvement occurs in ~25% of patients with sarcoidosis, and it can cause blindness. The usual lesions involve the uveal tract, iris, ciliary body, and choroid. Of those patients with eye involvement, ~75% have anterior uveitis and 25 to 35% have posterior uveitis. There is blurred vision, tearing, and photophobia. The uveitis can develop rapidly and may clear spontaneously over a 6- to 12-month period. It also can develop insidiously and be chronic. The uveitis often occurs in association with retinal vasculitis. Conjunctival involvement is also common, usually with small, yellow nodules. When the lacrimal gland is involved, a keratoconjunctivitis sicca syndrome, with dry, sore eyes, can result.

FIGURE 309-3 Common laboratory findings of sarcoidosis. *A.* Schematic view of the abnormal findings on the chest x-ray. Shown are changes observed with the average frequency of occurrence. *B.* Typical gallium-67 scan of an individual with active sarcoidosis. The isotope has accumulated in the lung parenchyma (LP), liver (L), spleen (S), parotid (P), hilar nodes (HN), and pelvic nodes (PN). *C.* Cells recovered by bronchoalveolar lavage of an individual with active pulmonary sarcoidosis. The lavage analysis reflects the inflammation in the tissue. Shown are alveolar macrophages (*large cells*) and lymphocytes (*small cells*). The cell population is dominated by the T_H1 subset of CD4+ lymphocytes, in contrast to normal individuals, in whom lymphocytes represent <20% of the cell population.

FIGURE 309-4 Sarcoid. *A.* Infiltrated papules and plaques of variable color are seen in a typical paranasal and periorbital location. *B.* Infiltrated, hyperpigmented, and erythematous coalescent papules and plaques on the upper area.

Upper Respiratory Tract The nasal mucosa is involved in up to 20% of patients, usually presenting with nasal stuffiness. Any of the structures of the mouth can be involved, particularly the tonsils but also the tongue. Sarcoidosis involves the larynx in ~5% of patients. The epiglottis and areas around the true vocal cords are usually involved, but the cords themselves are not. These individuals are usually hoarse, and they have dyspnea, wheezing, and stridor; complete obstruction can occur.

Bone Marrow and Spleen Sarcoidosis of the marrow is reported in 15 to 40% of patients, but it rarely causes hematologic abnormalities other than a mild anemia, neutropenia, eosinophilia, and occasionally, thrombocytopenia. Although splenomegaly occurs in only 5 to 10% of patients, celiac angiography or splenic biopsy reveals involvement in 50 to 60% of patients. The presentation and complications of splenomegaly in sarcoidosis are similar to those of splenomegaly in general.

Liver Although liver biopsy reveals liver involvement in 60 to 90% of patients, liver dysfunction is usually not important clinically. Sarcoidosis generally involves the periportal areas. Isolated granulomatous hepatitis can occur. Approximately 20 to 30% have hepatomegaly and/or biochemical evidence of liver involvement. Usually these changes reflect a cholestatic pattern and include an elevated alkaline phosphatase level; the bilirubin and aminotransferase levels are only mildly elevated, and jaundice is rare. Rarely, portal hypertension can develop, as can intrahepatic cholestasis with cirrhosis. There are several reports of the development of sarcoidosis in association of the treatment of chronic hepatitis C with interferon α.

Kidney Clinically apparent primary renal involvement in sarcoidosis is rare, although tubular, glomerular, and renal artery diseases have been reported. More commonly, but still in only 1 to 2% of all patients, there is a disorder of calcium metabolism with hypercalciuria, with or without hypercalcemia. If chronic, nephrocalcinosis and nephrolithiasis can result. It is believed that the calcium abnormalities are associated with enhanced calcium absorption in the gut, which is related to an abnormally high level of circulating 1,25-dihydroxyvitamin D produced by mononuclear phagocytes in the granulomas.

Nervous System All components of the nervous system can be involved in sarcoidosis. Neurologic findings are observed in about 5% of patients. Seventh nerve involvement with unilateral facial paralysis is most common. It occurs suddenly and is usually transient. Other common manifestations of neurosarcoid include optic nerve dysfunction, papilledema, palate dysfunction, hearing abnormalities, hypothalamic and pituitary abnormalities, chronic meningitis, and, occasionally, space-occupying lesions. Psychiatric disturbances have been described, and seizures can occur. Rarely, multiple lesions occur that mimic multiple sclerosis, spinal cord abnormalities, and peripheral neuropathy.

Musculoskeletal System The bones, joints, and/or muscles can be involved in sarcoidosis. Bone lesions are observed in 3 to 13% of patients and include variable-sized cysts in areas of expanded bone, with well-defined, round, punched-out lesions or lattice-like changes, often at the ends of the affected bones. The lesions are cortical, with the periostium preserved. Hand and foot bones are the common sites, but most bones can be involved. Occasionally, the bone lesions are tender and painful. Dactylitis with soft tissue swelling can be present over the affected digit. Joint involvement is more common, with an incidence of 25 to 50% in known cases of sarcoidosis. Arthralgias and frank arthritis occur mostly in large joints; they can be migratory and are usually transient, but they can be chronic and result in deformities. Although muscle biopsy frequently demonstrates granulomatous inflammation, muscle dysfunction is rare. However, nodules, polymyositis, and chronic myopathy have been described.

Heart Approximately 5% of patients have significant heart involvement, with clinical evidence of cardiac dysfunction. Left ventricular wall involvement is common. Arrhythmias are frequent, and serious conduction disturbances, including complete heart block, can occur. Sudden death has been associated with cardiac sarcoid. Papillary muscle dysfunction, pericarditis, and congestive heart failure are also observed. Cor pulmonale secondary to chronic pulmonary fibrosis may occur but is uncommon.

Endocrine and Reproductive System The hypothalamic-pituitary axis is the part of the endocrine system most commonly involved; this condition usually presents as diabetes insipidus. Anterior pituitary dysfunction is also seen, manifesting as a deficiency in one or more pituitary hormones. Complete hypopituitarism is rare. Much less frequently, sarcoidosis can cause primary dysfunction of other endocrine glands. Adrenal cortical involvement resulting in Addison's syndrome has been described. The reproductive organs may be involved, but infertility is rare. Pregnancy is not affected by sarcoidosis, and women with sarcoidosis who become pregnant usually improve during pregnancy. However, the disease may flare post partum; presumably this variation results from fluctuations in endogenous glucocorticoid production.

Exocrine Glands Parotid enlargement is a classic feature of sarcoidosis, but clinically apparent parotid involvement occurs in <10% of patients. Bilateral involvement is the rule. The gland is usually nontender, firm, and smooth. Xerostomia can occur; other exocrine glands are affected only rarely.

Gastrointestinal Tract Although sarcoidosis involvement of the gastrointestinal tract is found occasionally at autopsy, it rarely has clinical importance. Occasionally, patients have esophageal or gastric symptoms. Rarely, the peritoneum is involved with accompanying ascites.

Sarcoid can present as an isolated pancreatic lesion mimicking pancreatic carcinoma.

COMPLICATIONS The respiratory tract abnormalities cause most of the morbidity and mortality associated with sarcoidosis. The major problems are those characteristic of interstitial lung disease (Chap. 243), particularly dyspnea and insufficient oxygen delivery to vital organs. Respiratory failure with carbon dioxide retention is rare. In some patients, lung destruction results in formation of bullae that may harbor mycetomas, which are usually aspergillomas; erosion into the parenchyma can result in massive bleeding. The most common complications apart from the lung are associated with the eye; however, with therapy, blindness is rare. Complications of other organs include a gamut of abnormalities. The most serious are central nervous system (CNS) lesions or cardiac involvement leading to congestive heart failure or sudden death.

LABORATORY ABNORMALITIES Common abnormalities in the blood include lymphocytopenia, an occasional mild eosinophilia, an increased erythrocyte sedimentation rate, hyperglobulinemia, and an elevated level of angiotensin-converting enzyme (ACE). False-positive tests for rheumatoid factor or antinuclear antibodies can be observed. Hypercalcemia is rare. Other serum abnormalities relate to involvement of specific organs such as liver, kidney, or endocrine glands.

Because the lung is involved so commonly, the routine chest film is almost always abnormal (Fig. 309-3A). The three classic x-ray patterns of pulmonary sarcoidosis are type I—bilateral hilar adenopathy with no parenchymal abnormalities; type II—bilateral hilar adenopathy with diffuse parenchymal changes; and type III—diffuse parenchymal changes without hilar adenopathy. The type III pattern is sometimes split into two categories, with films that show fibrosis and upper lobe retraction classified separately. Although patients with type I x-ray patterns tend to have the acute or subacute, reversible form of the disease while those with types II and III often have the chronic, progressive disease, these patterns do not represent consecutive "stages" of sarcoidosis. Thus, except for epidemiologic purposes, this x-ray categorization is mostly of historic interest. The hilar adenopathy is almost always bilateral, but unilateral node enlargement can be seen. Nodes are also common in the paratracheal region. The diffuse parenchymal changes are typically reticulonodular infiltrates, but an acinar pattern is observed occasionally. Large nodules, similar to those of metastatic disease, are unusual but can occur. When there is massive fibrosis, the hila are pulled upward and there are conglomerate masses in the midlung zones. Some of the unusual chest x-ray findings in sarcoidosis include "egg shell" calcification of hilar nodes, pleural effusions, cavitation, atelectasis, pulmonary hypertension, pneumothorax, and cardiomegaly. Computed tomography of the chest is rarely helpful for either diagnosis or prognosis but can identify early fibrosis. A "ground-glass" appearance is often associated with an active alveolitis but more likely results from the granulomas.

The lung function abnormalities of sarcoidosis are typical for interstitial lung disease (Chap. 243) and include decreased lung volumes and diffusing capacity with a normal or supernormal ratio of the forced expiratory volume in 1 s to the forced vital capacity. Occasionally there is evidence of airflow limitation. There is usually mild hypoxemia and a mild, compensated hypocarbia.

The gallium-67 lung scan is usually abnormal, showing a pattern of diffuse uptake. If present, enlarged nodes are detected in these scans, as is inflammation in a variety of extrathoracic sites that usually have no clinical importance (Fig. 309-3B). Bronchoalveolar lavage typically demonstrates an increased proportion of lymphocytes, most of which are members of the activated T$_H$1 subset of CD4+ T lymphocytes (Fig. 309-3C). The remaining cells are mostly alveolar macrophages. In patients with significant fibrosis, a few neutrophils are also found. Eosinophils are rare.

The other laboratory features of sarcoidosis depend on the specific organ involved.

DIAGNOSIS For a typical case, the diagnosis of sarcoidosis is made by a combination of clinical, radiographic, and histologic findings (Fig. 309-5A). In a young adult with constitutional complaints, respiratory symptoms, erythema nodosum, blurred vision, and bilateral hilar adenopathy, the diagnosis is almost always sarcoidosis. Commonly, however, the findings are more subtle. Because sarcoidosis can occur in almost any place in the body, like tuberculosis or syphilis, it can be confused with many other disorders. In this context, the differential diagnosis of sarcoidosis must cover a wide range. However, it is confused most commonly with neoplastic diseases such as lymphoma or with disorders also characterized by a mononuclear cell granulomatous inflammatory process, such as the mycobacterial and fungal disorders.

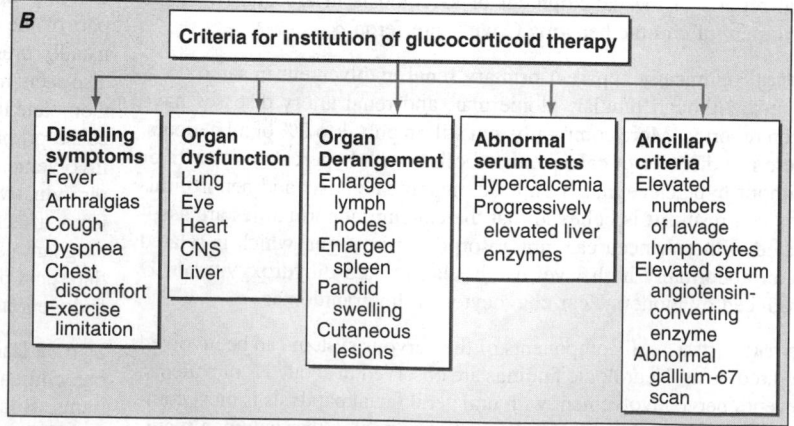

FIGURE 309-5 Diagnostic and therapeutic algorithms relevant to sarcoidosis. *A.* Diagnosis of sarcoidosis. If the history and physical examination suggest sarcoidosis, the diagnosis is made by a combination of history, physical examination, and diagnostic test. No tests are definitive for sarcoidosis; the diagnosis is made by a combination of findings. The major diagnostic tests carry the most weight, with biopsy and histologic assessment of the relevant organ the most important. Assessment of function of the organ systems that appear to be affected help with diagnosis and decisions about therapy. *B.* Therapy of sarcoidosis. Once the definitive diagnosis is made, the decision to not treat or to institute treatment with glucocorticoids is based on the presence or absence of disabling symptoms, organ dysfunction, organ derangement, and results of various tests of disease activity. Any organ can be threatened by sarcoidosis, but lung, eye, heart, liver, and central nervous system are at greatest risk. The disease can wax and wane, and periodic assessments at 3- to 6-month intervals are used to reevaluate decisions regarding therapy.

The presence of skin anergy is typical but not diagnostic of sarcoidosis. Individuals with sarcoidosis who develop active tuberculosis react strongly to skin tests with purified protein derivative. The Kveim-Siltzbach skin test, the intradermal injection of a heat-treated suspension of a sarcoidosis spleen extract which is biopsied 4 to 6 weeks later, yields sarcoidosis-like lesions in 70 to 80% of individuals with sarcoidosis, with <5% false-positive results. The Kveim-Siltzbach material is no longer available, and with the use of the transbronchial biopsy to obtain lung parenchyma for diagnostic purposes, the Kveim-Siltzbach test is only of historic interest.

No blood findings are diagnostic of the disease. Serum levels of ACE are elevated in approximately two-thirds of patients with sarcoidosis. Approximately 5% of all positive tests are not sarcoidosis and are seen in a variety of disorders, including asbestosis, silicosis, berylliosis, fungal infection, granulomatous hepatitis, hypersensitivity pneumonitis, leprosy, lymphoma, and tuberculosis. Hypercalcemia or an elevated 24-h urine calcium level is consistent with the diagnosis but is not specific.

The chest x-ray cannot be used as the sole criterion for the diagnosis of sarcoidosis. While the finding of bilateral hilar adenopathy is the hallmark of this disease, a similar pattern is occasionally observed in lymphoma, tuberculosis, coccidioidomycosis, brucellosis, and bronchogenic carcinoma.

The pattern of the gallium-67 scan is not diagnostic for sarcoidosis, nor is the finding of an increased proportion of lymphocytes among the cells recovered by bronchoalveolar lavage. However, the typical patterns of these tests (Fig. 309-3*B* and *C*) put the diagnosis in the general category of granulomatous lung disorders.

Whether or not the presentation is "classic," biopsy evidence of a mononuclear cell granulomatous inflammatory process is mandatory to make a definitive diagnosis of sarcoidosis. Because the lung is involved so frequently, it is the most common site to be biopsied, usually through a fiberoptic bronchoscope. Less common, but acceptable, sites for biopsy are the hilar nodes (by mediastinoscopy), the skin, conjunctiva, or lip. Rarely, the spleen, intraabdominal nodes, muscle, parotid or other salivary glands, upper respiratory tract, or the heart is biopsied for diagnostic purposes. At any of these sites, the findings must include the typical noncaseating granulomas. However, although histologic evidence is mandatory for a definitive diagnosis of sarcoidosis, the histologic findings are not sufficiently specific to make the diagnosis by themselves, since noncaseating granulomas are found in a number of other diseases, including infections and malignancy. Furthermore, although the liver or scalene nodes often reveal "positive" biopsies in cases of sarcoidosis, noncaseating granulomas from other causes are so frequent in these sites that they are not considered acceptable sites for establishing the diagnosis. Thus the definitive diagnosis of sarcoidosis is based on the biopsy in the context of the history, physical examination, blood tests, x-ray, lung function, and, if available, gallium-67 scan and bronchoalveolar lavage. Patients with HIV infection commonly have lymphocytopenia, chest x-ray abnormalities, positive gallium-67 chest scans, and increased proportions of lavage lymphocytes (early in the course of the disease), and they can have lung granulomas; thus, serologic testing for HIV infection should always be done in individuals suspected of having sarcoidosis.

PROGNOSIS Overall, the prognosis in sarcoidosis is good. Most individuals who present with the acute disease are left with no significant sequelae. Approximately half of all patients have some permanent organ dysfunction, but for most this is mild, stable, and progresses rarely. In ~15 to 20% of patients, the disease remains active or recurs intermittently. Death is attributable directly to the disease in ~10% of all those affected.

℞ **TREATMENT**

The therapy of choice for sarcoidosis is glucocorticoids (Fig. 309-5*B*). Methotrexate is usually the second-line medication. Various other drugs have been used in refractory cases, including indomethacin, oxyphenbutazone, chloroquine, hydroxychloroquine, thalidomide, infliximab, etanercept, pentoxifylline, tacrolimus, *p*-aminobenzoate, allopurinol, levamisole, azothioprine, and cyclophosphamide; but there is no evidence, apart from anecdotal, uncontrolled reports, to support their efficacy. Cyclosporine is ineffective for the pulmonary manifestations of the disease; anecdotal reports suggest that it may be useful in extrathoracic sarcoid not responding to glucocorticoids.

The major problem in treating sarcoidosis is in deciding when to treat. Because the disease clears spontaneously in ~50% of patients, and because the permanent organ derangements often do not improve with glucocorticoid treatment, there is controversy among clinicians as to the criteria for treatment. However, there is no question that glucocorticoids effectively suppress the activated T_H1 lymphocyte processes occurring at the sites of disease. Thus, the major problem in making decisions concerning therapy in sarcoidosis is to determine the extent and activity of the inflammatory process in the organs at greatest risk, such as the lung, eye, heart, and CNS.

For the lung, this is based on a combination of history, physical findings, chest x-ray, and pulmonary function tests. Centers that see large numbers of these individuals sometimes use criteria based on gallium-67 lung scans and bronchoalveolar lavage findings to help define active disease. Computed tomography is not usually helpful in treatment decisions. The serum level of ACE has been suggested as a criterion for disease activity, but it is not specific for the lung. Unless the respiratory impairment is devastating, active pulmonary sarcoidosis is observed usually without therapy for 2 to 3 months; if the inflammation does not subside spontaneously, therapy is instituted. For the eye, decisions concerning therapy are based on slit-lamp examination and tests for visual acuity. For the heart and CNS, decisions are based on an estimate of the severity of the involvement; patients with minor dysfunction are usually observed, while patients with significant cardiac or neurologic abnormalities are treated. Usually, it is not necessary to treat the systemic symptoms, but occasionally the extent of the fevers, fatigue, and/or weight loss necessitate therapy.

The usual therapy for sarcoidosis is prednisone, 1 mg/kg, for 4 to 6 weeks, followed by a slow taper over 2 to 3 months. This regimen is repeated if the disease again becomes active. Alternate-day therapy is used by some clinicians, but there is no evidence that it is as effective. High-dose bolus intravenous glucocorticoids are used occasionally but are probably not as effective as oral therapy. There is no evidence that inhaled glucocorticoids are efficacious. Mild ocular disease responds usually to local therapy, but suppression of the uveitis often requires systemic glucocorticoids. Methotrexate, 5 to 15 mg/week in a single oral dose, is often used when glucocorticoids are contraindicated or in refractory cases, but there is a cumulative risk for side effects, particularly hepatotoxicity. There is often a 6-month time lag before improvement is seen with methotrexate. Lung transplant, usually unilateral, is reserved for end-stage disease. The presence of mycetomas is usually a contraindication for transplant. There is a 30 to 80% incidence of recurrence of sarcoid in the transplanted lung, but it is rarely significant.

FURTHER READING

BAUGHMAN RP et al:: Sarcoidosis. Lancet 361, 1111, 2003

CRYSTAL RG: Interstitial lung disease of unknown etiology: Disorders characterized by chronic inflammation of the lower respiratory tract. N Engl J Med 310:154, 235, 1984

JOHNS CJ, MICHELE TM: The clinical management of sarcoidosis. A 50-year experience at the Johns Hopkins Hospital. Medicine 78:65, 1999

ROBINSON DS et al: Granulomatous processes, in *The Lung: Scientific Foundations*, 2d ed, RG Crystal et al (eds). Philadelphia, Lippincott-Raven, 1996, pp 2395–2410

ZIEGENHAGEN MW, MÜLLER-QUERNHEIM J: The cytokine network in sarcoidosis and its clinical relevance. J Intern Med 253:18, 2003

DEFINITION AND CLASSIFICATION *Amyloidosis* results from a sequence of changes in protein folding that leads to the deposition of insoluble amyloid fibrils, mainly in the extracellular spaces of organs and tissues. Depending upon the biochemical nature of the amyloid precursor protein, amyloid fibrils can be deposited locally or may involve virtually every organ system of the body. Amyloid fibril deposition may have no apparent clinical consequences or may be associated with severe pathophysiologic changes. Named by Virchow in 1854 on the basis of color after staining with iodine and sulfuric acid, all amyloid fibrils share an identical secondary structure, the β-pleated sheet conformation, and a unique ultrastructure. All amyloid deposits contain the pentraxin serum amyloid P (SAP) and glycosaminoglycans. Abnormal protein folding and assembly can also result in protein deposition (e.g., in brain or kidney) that lacks the classic fibrillar morphology of amyloid and the presence of SAP.

The amyloidoses are classified according to the identity of the fibril-forming protein (Table 310-1). *Systemic amyloidoses* are neoplastic, inflammatory, genetic, or iatrogenic in origin, while *localized amyloidoses* or *organ-limited amyloidoses* are associated with aging and diabetes and occur in isolated organs without evidence of systemic involvement.

Despite their biochemical and clinical differences, the various amyloidoses share common pathophysiologic features: (1) an amyloidogenic precursor in appropriate concentration; (2) appropriate host genetic background; (3) abnormalities in proteolysis of fibril precursors and nascent amyloid fibrils; and (4) alterations in extracellular matrix constituents such as glycosaminoglycans and Apo E. The guidelines for nomenclature and classification of amyloid and amyloidosis were updated in 2001 by the Nomenclature Committee of the International Society of Amyloidosis (Table 310-1). Amyloid deposits should be classified using the capital letter A as the first letter of designation followed by the protein designation without any open space; for example, AL for amyloidosis involving immunoglobulin light chains.

ETIOLOGY AND PATHOGENESIS OF THE SYSTEMIC AMYLOIDOSES ▪ Light Chain Amyloidosis (AL) The most common form of systemic amyloidosis seen in current clinical practice is AL (primary idiopathic amyloidosis, or that associated with multiple myeloma) resulting from fibril formation by fragments of monoclonal antibody light chains in primary amyloidosis and in some cases of multiple myeloma (Chap. 98). Fewer than 20% of patients with AL have myeloma. The rest have other monoclonal gammopathies, light chain disease, or even agammaglobulinemia (producing light chains, but not intact immunoglobulin). About 15 to 20% of patients with myeloma have amyloidosis. A monoclonal population of bone marrow plasma cells is present and consistently produces either small lambda or kappa fragments or immunoglobulins that are processed (cleaved) in an abnormal fashion by macrophage enzymes to produce the partially degraded light chains responsible for AL amyloidosis. Lambda chain class predominates over kappa in AL by a 2:1 ratio, whereas in multiple myeloma and normal immunoglobulin synthesis, the reverse is true. Indeed, almost all lambda VI family chains have been associated with amyloid. The primary structure of each amyloid-forming light chain is unique, reflecting the features of the B cell clone that produced it. Also, nonfibrillar deposition diseases have been described. There are three forms of human light chain–associated renal and systemic diseases: AL amyloidosis, cast nephropathy, and light chain deposition disease. Rarely, heavy chain amyloid deposition (AH) has been reported.

Amyloid A Amyloidosis (AA) AA amyloidosis (secondary, reactive, or acquired amyloidosis) occurs most frequently as a complication of chronic inflammatory disease. Effective treatment of the underlying inflammatory condition has reduced incidence in developed countries. In the past in the United States, tuberculosis (Chap. 150), osteomyelitis (Chap. 111), and leprosy (Chap. 151) were the most common precipitating diseases, and they remain so in developing countries. During inflammation, the cytokines interleukin (IL) 1, IL-6, and tumor necrosis factor (TNF) stimulate hepatic synthesis of serum amyloid A, the AA fibril precursor. Thus, effective treatment of the underlying inflammatory disorder blocks the stimulus for precursor synthesis. Familial deposition of the AA protein occurs in patients with the hereditary periodic fever syndromes familial Mediterranean fever (FMF), TNF receptor–associated periodic syndrome (TRAPS), Muckle-Wells syndrome (MWS), and familial cold uticaria (FCU) (Chap. 279). Colchicine treatment effectively blocks attacks of FMF and reduces the incidence of AA amyloidosis in association with FMF. FMF is an autosomal recessive disorder subdivided into phenotype I, with irregularly occurring fever and abdominal, chest, or joint pain, preceding or accompanying renal amyloid; and phenotype

TABLE 310-1 *Amyloid Fibril Proteins and Their Precursors*

Amyloid Protein	Precursor	Systemic (S) or Localized (L)	Syndrome or Involved Tissues
AL	Immunoglobulin light chain	S, L	Primary
			Myeloma-associated
AH	Immunoglobulin heavy chain	S, L	Primary
			Myeloma-associated
ATTR	Transthyretin	S	Familial
			Senile systemic
		L?	Tenosynovium
Aβ_2M	β_2-microglobulin	S	Hemodialysis
		L?	Joints
AA	(Apo)serum AA	S	Secondary, reactive
AApoAI	Apolipoprotein AI	S	Familial
		L	Aortic
AApoAII	Apolipoprotein AII	S	Familial
AGel	Gelsolin	S	Familial
ALys	Lysozyme	S	Familial
AFib	Fibrinogen α-chain	S	Familial
ACys	Cystatin C	S	Familial
ABri[a]	ABriPP	L, S?	Familial dementia, British
ADan[a]	*ADanPP*	L	*Familial dementia, Danish*
Aβ	Aβ protein precursor (AβPP)	L	Alzheimer's disease, aging
APrP	Prion protein	L	Spongiform encephalopathies
ACal	(Pro)calcitonin	L	C-cell thyroid tumors
AIAPP	Islet amyloid polypeptide	L	Islets of Langerhans
			Insulinomas
AANF	Atrial natriuretic factor	L	Cardiac atria
APro	Prolactin	L	Aging pituitary
			Prolactinomas
AIns	Insulin	L	Iatrogenic
AMed	Lactadherin	L	Senile aortic, media
AKer	Kerato-epithelin	L	Cornea; familial
A(tbn)[b]	*tbn[b]*	*L*	*Pindborg tumors*
ALac	*Lactoferrin*	*L*	*Cornea; familial*

[a] ADan is coming from the same gene as ABri and has identical N-terminal sequence. It will be a matter of further discussion whether ADan should be included in the nomenclature as a separate protein (see text)
[b] To be named.
Note: Proteins in italics are preliminary.
Source: Reprinted from P Westermark et al: Amyloid 9:197, 2002, with permission.

II, in which renal amyloidosis is the first or only manifestation of the disease (Chap. 279). FMF is caused by mutations (17 identified to date) in the gene designated *MEFV* that encodes a 781-amino-acid protein named *pyrin* that appears to be a transcription factor. There is a strong correlation between the M694V mutation in MEFV and development of amyloidosis. TRAPS is an autosomal dominant disorder characterized by mutations in the TNF receptor that lead to defective shedding of the receptor and thus an impediment to the return to homeostasis. Remarkably, AA amyloidosis is not seen as a complication of the hyper IgD periodic fever syndrome (HIDS) that is associated with mutations in the mevalonate kinase gene.

Heredofamilial Amyloidoses   There are a number of types of familial amyloidosis that are dominantly transmitted in association with a mutation that enhances protein misfolding and fibril formation. The protein precursors and the amyloidoses are: transthyretin (ATTR), apolipoprotein AI (AApoAI), apolipoprotein AII (AApoAII), cystatin C (ACys), gelsolin (AGel), fibrinogen alpha chain (AFib), and lysozyme (ALys). The mutant proteins, although present from birth, are associated with a delayed onset of disease symptoms, usually after three to seven decades of life. The familial amyloidoses present as neuropathy, nephropathy, cardiomyopathy, hepatomegaly, visceral pathology, lattice corneal dystrophy, and dementia. The familial amyloidoses are less commonly seen in clinical practice than AL amyloidosis, but the overlap in clinical symptoms and organ involvement makes the chemical identification of the fibril-forming protein imperative.

ATTR   The most frequently occurring form of familial amyloidosis involves transthyretin (TTR), a 14-kDa protein originally described as prealbumin, that transports thyroxine and retinol-binding protein in the blood. The first mutation to be identified in Portuguese families and in families of Swedish origin was a single amino acid substitution, methionine for valine at position 30 (V30M). To date, more than 80 TTR variants have been defined, most of which are amyloidogenic. Variant TTR gene carriers exhibit clinically heterogeneous amyloidoses according to the nature of the amino acid substitution. Patients with the V30M mutation are symptomatic in the third to fifth decades of life with progressive polyneuropathy, postural hypotension, and little myocardial infiltration. Patients with the T60A mutation are symptomatic at an older age than V30M patients and exhibit peripheral and autonomic peripheral neuropathies and progressive myocardial amyloid infiltration. Nearly 4% of the African-American population carries the V122I allele that is associated with infiltrative cardiomyopathy and carpal tunnel syndrome. The disease is late in onset, and recognition requires a high degree of clinical suspicion.

AApoAI   Deposition of apolipoprotein AI variants (G26R, W50R, L60R, L75P, L90P, L174S, and deletion mutations) can be associated with peripheral neuropathy that is clinically similar to the type of familial amyloidosis that is caused by variants of TTR. In some kindreds, the clinical presentation is kidney or liver failure without neurologic symptoms.

AApoAII   A variant of apolipoprotein AII with an extension of the coding region that results in a 25% larger molecule than the wild-type protein is associated with a familial amyloidosis with involvement of kidney glomeruli.

AGel   Two mutations, D187N and D187Y, within the actin-binding region of gelsolin lead to deposition of a 71-residue fragment encompassing the mutation in blood vessels and basement membrane. AGel has been reported primarily in Finland, but also in Denmark, Japan, the Netherlands, and the United States. Clinical manifestations of lattice corneal dystrophy and cranial neuropathy are followed by peripheral neuropathy, dystrophic skin changes, and involvement of other organs.

ALys   Hereditary nonneuropathic systemic amyloidosis has been described in English and French families in which lysozyme is the major fibril protein. Three mutations have been described—I56T, W64R, and D67H. Clinical manifestations include visceral involvement and, in some kindreds, nephropathy.

AFib   Hereditary nonneuropathic renal amyloidosis has been described in families with one of three mutations in the fibrinogen A α chains, R524L, E526V, or R554L.

Aβ₂M   In long-term hemodialysis, amyloidosis is now well recognized as a serious bone and joint complication. β_2-microglobulin is the major constituent of the amyloid fibrils, and formation of advanced glycation end products of β_2-microglobulin has been implicated in the pathogenesis of $A\beta_2M$.

ETIOLOGY AND PATHOGENESIS OF THE LOCALIZED AMYLOIDOSES ■ Polypeptide Hormone–Derived Amyloidosis   Amyloid deposits are common in polypeptide hormone–producing tissues and tumors. Calcitonin is deposited in the hereditary amyloid syndrome, medullary carcinoma of the thyroid (ACal) (Chap. 320). Prolactin is commonly deposited in the aging pituitary (APro). In AIAPP, islet amyloid polypeptide, also referred to as amylin, is deposited as amyloid fibrils in 90% of individuals with type 2 diabetes (Chap. 323), in endocrine tumors (Chap. 329), and in insulinoma (Chap. 329). AIAPP is thought to play an important role in the beta cell failure associated with type 2 diabetes. Human insulin does not naturally form amyloid fibrils, although fibrils of porcine insulin, AIns, are sometimes found as subcutaneous nodules at sites of insulin injection in diabetic individuals. The form of amyloid that occurs in Pindborg tumors, odontogenic tumors, has been identified as a fragment of a protein of unknown function (FLJ20513) and is thus designated as an amyloid to be named A(*tbn*) (Table 310-1).

Localized Corneal Amyloid   AKer (kerato-epithelin) is deposited as a corneal amyloid fibril protein in association with mutations in the *BIGH3* gene. Lactoferrin, without significant size truncation, is apparently deposited as corneal amyloid with trichiasis.

Localized Cardiovascular Amyloid   Localized deposits of AApoAI in atheromatous plaques, AMed (derived from medin, a fragment of aortic smooth muscle cell–derived lactoadherin) in the aortic media and AANF (atrial natriuretic factor–derived amyloid) in cardiac atria, were initially thought to be clinically insignificant but are now being viewed as potentially pathogenic.

Amyloidosis Associated with Alzheimer's Disease   A novel protein, β-amyloid protein ($A\beta$), is the major fibril protein in the amyloid deposits of the cerebrovascular walls and the cores of the neuritic plaques of Alzheimer's disease (AD) patients and also in individuals with Down's syndrome (Chap. 57). The intracellular neurofibrillary tangles (ATau) are composed of paired helical filaments arranged in a twisted conformation and have as their major component an abnormally phosphorylated τ-protein, a microtubule-associated protein. $A\beta$ varies in length from 39 to 43 amino acids and is derived from a large transmembrane glycoprotein called amyloid β-precursor protein (AβPP). Mutations in AβPP are associated with familial AD and also with a different type of amyloidosis, hereditary cerebral hemorrhage with amyloidosis (Dutch type). Other forms of familial AD are associated with mutations in genes that encode presenilin proteins. Familial dementias have also been found to be associated with deposition of a newly characterized amyloid fibril protein in families of British and Danish origin (Table 310-1). The 40-amino-acid residue fibril protein is composed of the 22 C-terminal amino acids of the wild-type protein and a 12-amino-acid extension that is due to a mutation in the stop codon.

Prion Diseases   Prions are a unique class of infectious proteins associated with a group of neurodegenerative diseases, the transmissible spongiform encephalopathies. In humans, these diseases include kuru, Creutzfeldt-Jakob disease, Gerstmann-Straussler-Scheinker syndrome, and fatal familial insomnia (Chap. 363); in animals, scrapie and bovine spongiform encephalopathy (mad cow disease). PrP^Sc is a pathogenic, transmissible spongiform encephalopathy–specific form of the host-encoded prion protein (PrP); PrP^Sc differs from PrP in that it contains a high amount of β-pleated sheet structure and is insoluble and resistant to proteolytic enzymes. PrP^{Sc} deposits either consist of or can be readily converted to amyloid fibrils. APrP is similar to Aβ and ATTR in that both familial and sporadic forms occur. In addition, infectious prion diseases have resulted from the transmission of PrP^{Sc} by ritualistic cannibalism, corneal transplantation, treatment with cadaveric human growth hormone, and a variety of neurosurgical procedures. It has been suggested that the earlier onset familial forms of amyloidosis are due to accelerated fibril formation from mutant precursors, whereas in sporadic cases, amyloid fibrils are formed more slowly from normal precursor molecules. The mutant PrP molecules are nearer the thermodynamic threshold for transition to the amyloidogenic PrP^{Sc} conformation than are the normal. The transition from normal to amyloidogenic PrP^{Sc} is essentially irreversible but very slow. The disease progresses because, once formed, amyloidogenic PrP^{Sc} can seed the conversion of normal molecules into an amyloidogenic form.

Localized Deposition of Systemic Amyloid Proteins The AL and ATTR forms of amyloidosis are usually systemic but are also observed in localized deposits. For example, AL is found in skin, lung, and other sites of the body. Cardiac amyloidosis involving wild-type TTR is considered to be localized but in some cases also to have a systemic component with predominant cardiac involvement, i.e., senile systemic amyloidosis.

CLINICAL MANIFESTATIONS The clinical manifestations of amyloidosis are varied and depend entirely on the biochemical nature of the fibril protein (Table 310-2). Proteinuria is often the first symptom associated with systemic amyloidosis, particularly of the AA and AL type; peripheral neuropathies are associated with familial amyloidoses, and dementia and cognitive dysfunction with amyloid deposits in brain. Organ enlargement, especially of the liver, kidney, spleen, and heart, may be prominent in the case of AL and AA amyloidosis; however, this does not occur in familial amyloidosis, AD, or PrP diseases.

Kidney Renal involvement may consist of mild proteinuria or frank nephrosis (Chaps. 40 and 261). In some cases, the urinary sediment may show a few red blood cells. The renal lesion is usually not reversible and in time leads to progressive azotemia and death. The

prognosis does not appear to be related to the degree of the proteinuria; when azotemia finally develops, the prognosis is grave. Treatment by peritoneal dialysis or hemodialysis or kidney transplantation improves the prognosis considerably (Chaps. 262 and 263). Hypertension is rare, except in long-standing amyloidosis. Renal tubular acidosis or renal vein thrombosis may occur. Localized accumulation of amyloid may be noted in the ureter, bladder, or other parts of the genitourinary tract.

Heart Cardiac amyloidosis can present as intractable heart failure (Chap. 216). Electrocardiographic abnormalities include a low-voltage QRS complex and abnormalities in atrioventricular and intraventricular conduction, often resulting in varying degrees of heart block (Chap. 210). Owing to their propensity to develop conduction defects and arrhythmias, patients with cardiac amyloidosis appear to be especially sensitive to digitalis, and this drug should be used with caution.

With respect to systemic amyloidoses, cardiac amyloidosis is common in primary (AL) and heredofamilial amyloidosis and very rare in the secondary (AA) form. With respect to localized amyloidosis, cardiac amyloidosis of the wild type or nonvariant TTR type is common after 80 years of age; also AANF may be present in the atria and AMed in the aortic media. In systemic amyloidosis, cardiac manifestations consist primarily of congestive failure and cardiomegaly (with or without murmurs) and a variety of arrhythmias and are comparable in AL and the familial amyloidoses, the predominant forms with cardiomyopathy (Chap. 221). Although these manifestations predominantly reflect diffuse myocardial amyloid, the endocardium, valves, and pericardium may also be involved. Pericarditis with effusion is rare, although the differential diagnosis of constrictive pericarditis versus restrictive cardiomyopathy frequently arises. Echocardiography has demonstrated symmetric thickening of the left ventricular wall, hypokinesia and decreased systolic contraction and thickening of the interventricular septum and left ventricular posterior wall, and left ventricular cavities of small to normal size (Chap. 211). Two-dimensional echocardiography produces the characteristic findings of thickened right and left ventricles, a normal left ventricular cavity, and, especially, a diffuse hyperrefractile "granular sparkling" appearance. Hearts that are heavily infiltrated with amyloid may or may not show an enlarged silhouette. Fluoroscopy usually shows decreased mobility of the ventricular wall; angiographic studies usually demonstrate thickened ventricular wall, decreased ventricular mobility, and absence of rapid ventricular filling in early diastole.

Liver While hepatic involvement is common except in heredofamilial amyloidosis of the TTR type, liver function abnormalities are minimal and occur late in the disease (Chap. 290). Portal hypertension occurs but is uncommon. Intrahepatic cholestasis has been noted in about 5% of patients with AL (primary) amyloidosis. Hepatomegaly is common, and AL hepatic amyloid is usually accompanied by the nephrotic syndrome and congestive heart failure with poor prognosis. Amyloidosis of the spleen characteristically is not associated with leukopenia and anemia.

Skin Involvement of the skin is one of the most characteristic manifestations of primary (AL) amyloidosis (Chap. 48). Other forms of amyloidosis such as lichen amyloidosis are thought to involve forms of keratin. In AL amyloidosis, the usually nonpruritic lesions may consist of slightly raised, waxy papules or plaques that are usually clustered in the folds of the axillae, anal, or inguinal regions; the face and neck; or mucosal areas such as ear or tongue. Periorbital ecchymoses ("black eye" or "raccoon syndrome") have been reported.

Gastrointestinal Tract Gastrointestinal symptoms are common in all systemic types of amyloidosis either from direct involvement of the gastrointestinal tract at any level or from infiltration of the autonomic nervous system with amyloid (Chap. 271). Symptoms include obstruction, ulceration, malabsorption, hemorrhage, protein loss, and diarrhea (Chap. 275). Infiltration of the tongue is characteristic of primary amyloidosis (AL) or amyloidosis accompanying multiple myeloma and occasionally leads to macroglossia. When not enlarged, the tongue

TABLE 310-2 *Clinical Presentation of Systemic Amyloidosis*

Disease	Symptoms
AL (primary)	Monoclonal immunoglobulin in urine or serum plus any of the following: Unexplained nephrotic syndrome Hepatomegaly Carpal tunnel syndrome Macroglossia Malabsorption or unexplained diarrhea or constipation Peripheral neuropathy Cardiomyopathy
AA (secondary)	Chronic infection (osteomyelitis, tuberculosis) or chronic inflammation (rheumatoid arthritis, granulomatous ileitis) plus development of any of the following: Proteinuria Hepatomegaly Unexplained gastrointestinal disease
Hereditary amyloidosis	Family history of neuropathy plus any of the following: Early sensorimotor disassociation Vitreous opacities Renal disease Autonomic nervous system symptoms Cardiovascular disease Gastrointestinal disease No family history of neuropathy but Idiopathic cardiomyopathy Idiopathic renal disease

may become stiffened and firm to palpation. Gastrointestinal bleeding may occur from any of a number of sites, notably the esophagus, stomach, or large intestine, and may be severe. Amyloid infiltration of the esophagus may lead to an incompetent or nonrelaxing lower esophageal sphincter, nonspecific motility disorders of the esophageal body, or rarely achalasia. Small-bowel lesions may lead to clinical and x-ray changes of obstruction. A malabsorption syndrome is common. Amyloidosis (AA or secondary) may also develop in association with other entities involving the gastrointestinal tract, especially tuberculosis (Chap. 150), granulomatous enteritis (Chap. 276), lymphoma (Chap. 97), and Whipple's disease (Chap. 275); differentiation of these conditions, which give rise to secondary amyloidosis, from diffuse primary amyloidosis of the small bowel may be difficult. Similarly, amyloidosis of the stomach may closely mimic gastric carcinoma, with obstruction, achlorhydria, and the radiologic appearance of tumor masses.

Nervous System Neurologic manifestations, especially prominent in the heredofamilial amyloidoses, may include peripheral neuropathy, postural hypotension, inability to sweat, Adies's pupil, hoarseness, and sphincter incompetence (Chaps. 22 and 364). The cranial nerves are generally spared, except in the Finnish hereditary amyloidosis (AGcl). Carpal tunnel syndrome may be caused by several amyloidoses, especially primary (AL) and chronic hemodialysis ($A\beta_2M$) amyloid. Peripheral neuropathy is frequent in the former type. $A\beta$ amyloid occurs in the central nervous system as a component of senile plaques and in blood vessels ("congophilic angiopathy") (Chap. 351). The protein concentration in the cerebrospinal fluid may be increased. Infiltrates of the cornea or vitreous body may be present in hereditary amyloid syndromes and give rise to a bilateral scalloping appearance of the pupil.

Endocrine Amyloid may infiltrate the thyroid or other endocrine glands but rarely causes endocrine dysfunction. Local amyloid deposits almost invariably accompany medullary carcinoma of the thyroid (Chap. 320). Amyloid is often found in the adrenal gland, pituitary gland, and pancreas. Pancreatic islet amyloid as a complication of type 2 diabetes is especially prominent and is caused by the islet amyloid polypeptide (IAPP, amylin). Clinical dysfunction is present when there is significant replacement of the gland by amyloid (Chap. 323).

Joints and Muscles Amyloid can directly, although rarely, involve articular structures by its presence in the synovial membrane and synovial fluid or in the articular cartilage. In these cases it is almost always of the AL type and associated with multiple myeloma (Chap. 98). Amyloid arthritis can mimic a number of the rheumatic diseases because it can present as a symmetric arthritis of small joints with nodules, morning stiffness, and fatigue (Chap. 311). The synovial fluid usually has a low white blood cell count, a good to fair mucin clot, a predominance of mononuclear cells, and no crystals. Studies of surgical specimens suggest a significant incidence of amyloid in cartilage, capsule, and synovium in osteoarthritis (Chap. 312). Amyloid infiltration of muscle may lead to a pseudomyopathy. Shoulder muscle infiltration can produce the "shoulder pad" sign. Amyloid is

TABLE 310-3	Diagnosis of Amyloidosis

BIOPSY

Common sites	Rare sites
Subcutaneous abdominal fat aspirate	Kidney
Rectum	Liver
Skin	Bone marrow
Gingiva	Synovium
Occasional sites	Spleen
Small intestine	
Muscle	
Nerve	

APPROPRIATE STAIN

Congo red, viewed by polarization microscopy
Thioflavin (less specific)
Potassium permanganate pretreatment, then Congo red stain
Other:
  Cotton dyes (comparable with Congo red)
  Crystal violet (less sensitive)

PROTEIN OR DNA STUDIES

Mutant protein identification
Immunocytochemistry: immunofluorescent or immunoperoxidase stains with specific antisera

found in muscle inclusion body disease, where $A\beta$ and/or PrP have been identified.

Deposition of β_2-microglobulin as amyloid fibrils in the musculoskeletal systems is a serious complication of long-term hemodialysis. $A\beta_2M$ presents as the carpal tunnel syndrome, cystic bone lesions, and even destructive spondyloarthropathy. Carpal tunnel syndrome is also associated with AL and ATTR (Chap. 262).

Respiratory System The nasal sinuses, larynx, and trachea may be involved by accumulation of AL amyloid, which blocks the ducts, in the case of the sinuses, or the air passages. Amyloidosis of the lung

FIGURE 310-1 Microscopic tissue appearance of amyloid. *A.* Congo red–stained section of amyloidotic kidney. *B.* Polarization microscopy of section *A* showing green birefringence of glomeruli and blood vessels. *C.* Congo red–stained section of uterus. *D.* Polarization microscopy of section *C* showing the vascular amyloid as well as amyloid in the muscle wall.

TABLE 310-4 *Symptoms, Diagnosis, and Treatment of Systemic Amyloidosis*

AL (Primary)	AA (Secondary)	Familial Amyloidosis
SYMPTOMS		
Unexplained nephropathy, cardiomyopathy, neuropathy Hepatomegaly syndrome Macroglossia Malabsorption or unexplained diarrhea or constipation Any of the above *plus* monoclonal immunoglobulin in urine	Proteinuria Hepatomegaly and/or splenomegaly *plus* Chronic infection (osteomyelitis, tuberculosis) or chronic inflammation (rheumatoid arthritis, granulomatous ileitis)	Family history of peripheral neuropathy, nephropathy *plus* any of following: Carpal tunnel syndrome Vitreous opacities Renal disease Autonomic nervous system symptoms Cardiovascular disease Gastrointestinal disease Sensorimotor disassociation
LABORATORY DIAGNOSIS		
Serum, urine immunofixation electrophoresis Bone marrow biopsy with kappa and lambda light chain immunohistochemistry	Elevated serum amyloid A (SAA) Positive immunohistochemical staining for AA protein in tissue specimen	Identification of protein variant in serum DNA-based test for mutant gene
TREATMENT OPTIONS		
Depending upon cardiac involvement or stage of disease Cyclic oral melphalan and prednisolone High dose IV melphalan with stem cell rescue	Aggressive treatment underlying inflammatory condition (monitor SAA) Surgical excision infection (bone resection, cholecystectemy) Colchicine for prevention and treatment of AA amyloidosis in FMF	Organ transplantation (liver) (ATTR)

Note: FMF, familial Mediterranean fever.

involves the bronchi and alveolar septa diffusely. The lower respiratory tract is affected most frequently in primary (AL) amyloidosis and in the disease associated with dysproteinemia. Pulmonary symptoms attributable to amyloid are present in about 30% of cases. Amyloid may be localized in the bronchi or pulmonary parenchyma and may resemble a neoplasm. In these cases, local excision should be attempted and, when successful, may be followed by prolonged remissions.

Hematopoietic System Hematologic changes may include fibrinogenopenia, increased fibrinolysis, and selective deficiency of clotting factors (Chap. 53). Deficient factor X seems to be due to nonspecific calcium-dependent binding to the polyanionic amyloid fibrils. Splenectomy in the patient with such a factor X deficiency can relieve the deficiency and the associated bleeding disorder, since factor X has been shown to bind to the large masses of splenic amyloid. Endothelial damage together with the clotting abnormalities lead to a propensity toward abnormal bleeding.

DIAGNOSIS Amyloid fibrils are identified in biopsy or necropsy tissue sections (Table 310-3). The systemic amyloidoses offer a choice of biopsy sites; abdominal fat aspirates or renal or rectal biopsies are often performed. Microscopically, amyloid deposits stain pink with the hematoxylin-eosin stain and show metachromasia with crystal violet. The widely used and useful Congo red stain imparts a unique green birefringence when stained tissue sections are viewed using the polarizing microscope (Fig. 310-1). Fluorescent dyes such as thioflavin are sensitive screening stains for amyloid deposits in brain and other tissues; however, specificity should be confirmed. After amyloid has been identified by staining, it should be chemically classified by genomic DNA and protein studies and by immunohistochemistry. In the case of heredofamilial amyloidosis, the presence of mutant TTR (or gelsolin, Apo AI, etc.) establishes the specific diagnosis of the disease. Isoelectric focusing is used as a simple screening test for variant transthyretins associated with familial TTR amyloidosis. In order to establish the relationship of immunoglobulin-related amyloid

to multiple myeloma, electrophoretic and immunoelectrophoretic studies on serum and urine should be performed when the biopsy reveals amyloid deposition. Most of these patients will have only relatively small paraprotein components, and only a few will have frank multiple myeloma. If AL and familial amyloidosis have been ruled out, AA amyloidosis should be suspected in patients with renal amyloid and a chronic inflammatory condition (Table 310-4).

PROGNOSIS Generalized amyloidosis is usually a slowly progressive disease that leads to death if untreated. The average survival in most large series of AL amyloid is ~12 months and in familial amyloidosis is ~7 to 15 years. A number of individuals with amyloid have been followed 5 to 10 years and longer. The course of amyloidosis is difficult to document, because dating the time of origin of the disease is rarely possible. When amyloidosis deops in patients with rheumatoid arthritis, it seldom becomes evident when the arthritis is of less than 2 years' duration. When amyloidosis develops in patients with multiple myeloma, manifestations leading to initial hospitalization are more apt to be related to amyloid disease than to myeloma. In these cases, prognosis is very poor, and life expectancy is usually less than 6 months.

Rx TREATMENT

Rational therapy should be directed at (1) reducing precursor production, (2) inhibiting the extracellular deposition of amyloid fibrils, and (3) promoting lysis or mobilization of existing amyloid deposits. There are new specific therapies for the various amyloidoses. In certain of the heredofamilial amyloidoses, genetic counseling is an important aspect of treatment, and the removal of the site of synthesis of the mutant protein by liver transplantation has proven remarkably successful. Liver transplantation has been carried out since 1990 for ATTR patients in Sweden, the United States, Portugal, Spain, and other countries. It appears that disease progression is halted and that there is some improvement in autonomic nervous system function. The utilization of chronic hemodialysis and of kidney transplantation has clearly improved the prognosis of renal amyloid.

In the case of AL amyloid, the fact that immunoglobulin light chain is made by plasma cells has led to the use of alkylating agents. However, these agents are toxic and not very effective. The most effective form of treatment currently is stem cell transplantation and immunosuppressive drugs (melphalan). Several long-term remissions have been reported, but serious complications, even death, can occur. A novel anthracycline, iododoxorubicin (IDOX), has been shown to bind to AL amyloid (similar to Congo red) in vivo and promote amyloid resorption. A subset of AL patients responds transiently to this experimental agent; and it is thought that IDOX may prove useful in combination with other forms of treatment. Cardiac tranplantation in selected cases of AL or heredofamilial amyloidosis has its advocates and has been successful.

Colchicine has been shown to be effective in preventing acute attacks and amyloidosis in patients with FMF (Chap. 279). Several clinical trials are in progress for AD.

The major causes of death are heart disease and renal failure. Sudden death, presumably due to arrhythmias, is common. Occasionally, gastrointestinal hemorrhage, respiratory failure, intractable heart failure, and superimposed infections are the terminal events.

FURTHER READING

BENSON MD: Amyloidosis, in *The Metabolic and Molecular Bases of Inherited Disease*, 8th ed, CR Scriver et al (eds). New York, McGraw-Hill, 2000, pp 5345–5378.

COHEN AS, SIPE JD: Amyloidosis, in *Clinical Immunology*, 2d ed, RR Rich et al (eds). St. Louis, Mosby Year Book, 2001, Chap. 71, pp 1–8

FALK RH et al: The systemic amyloidoses. N Engl J Med 337:898, 1997

PICKEN MM: The changing concepts of amyloid. Arch Pathol Lab Med 125:38, 2001

ROCKEN C, SHAKESPEARE A: Pathology, diagnosis and pathogenesis of AA amyloidosis. Virchows Archiv 440:111, 2002

SIPE JD: Amyloidosis. Crit Rev Clin Lab Sci 31:325, 1994

Section 3   Disorders of the Joints and Adjacent Tissues

311   APPROACH TO ARTICULAR AND MUSCULOSKELETAL DISORDERS
John J. Cush, Peter E. Lipsky

Musculoskeletal complaints account for more than 315 million outpatient visits per year. Recent surveys by the Centers for Disease Control and Prevention suggest that 33% (69.9 million) of the U.S. population is affected by arthritis or joint disorders. Many of these are self-limited conditions requiring minimal evaluation and only symptomatic therapy and reassurance. However, in some patients, musculoskeletal symptoms may herald a more serious condition that requires further evaluation or additional laboratory testing to confirm the suspected diagnosis or document the extent and nature of the pathologic process. The initial goal of the clinician is to formulate a differential diagnosis that leads to an accurate diagnosis and timely therapy, while avoiding excessive diagnostic testing and unnecessary treatment (Table 311-1). There are several urgent conditions that must be diagnosed promptly to avoid significant morbid or mortal sequelae. These "red flag" diagnoses include septic arthritis, acute crystal-induced arthritis (e.g., gout), and fracture. Each of these may be suspected by an acute onset with a monoarticular or focal presenting complaint (see below).

Individuals with musculoskeletal complaints should be evaluated in a uniform, logical manner with a thorough history, a comprehensive physical examination, and, if appropriate, laboratory testing. The goals of the initial encounter are to determine whether the musculoskeletal complaint is (1) *articular* or *nonarticular* in origin, (2) *inflammatory* or *noninflammatory* in nature, (3) *acute* or *chronic* in duration, and (4) *localized* or *widespread* (*systemic*) in distribution.

With such an approach and an understanding of the pathophysiologic processes that underlie musculoskeletal complaints, an adequate diagnosis can be made in the vast majority of individuals. However, some patients will not fit immediately into an established diagnostic category. Many musculoskeletal disorders resemble each other at the outset, and some may take weeks or months to evolve into a readily recognizable diagnostic entity. This consideration should temper the desire to establish a definitive diagnosis at the first encounter.

ARTICULAR VERSUS NONARTICULAR   The musculoskeletal evaluation must discriminate the anatomic site(s) of origin of the patient's complaint. For example, ankle pain can result from a variety of pathologic conditions involving disparate anatomic structures, including gonococcal arthritis, calcaneal fracture, Achilles tendinitis, cellulitis, and peripheral neuropathy. Distinguishing between articular and nonarticular conditions requires a careful and detailed examination. Articular structures include the synovium, synovial fluid, articular cartilage, intraarticular ligaments, joint capsule, and juxtaarticular bone. Nonarticular (or periarticular) structures, such as supportive extraarticular ligaments, tendons, bursae, muscle, fascia, bone, nerve, and overlying skin, may be involved in the pathologic process. Articular disorders may be characterized by deep or diffuse pain, limited range of motion on active and passive movement, swelling (caused by synovial proliferation, effusion, or bony enlargement), crepitation, instability, "locking," or deformity. By contrast, nonarticular disorders tend to be painful on active but not passive range of motion, demonstrate point or focal tenderness in regions distinct from articular structures, and have physical findings remote from the joint capsule. Moreover, nonarticular disorders seldom demonstrate crepitus, instability, or deformity.

INFLAMMATORY VERSUS NONINFLAMMATORY DISORDERS   In the course of a musculoskeletal evaluation, the examiner should elicit symptoms and signs that will narrow or establish the diagnosis. A primary objective is to identify the nature of the underlying pathologic process. Musculoskeletal disorders are generally classified as inflammatory or noninflammatory. Inflammatory disorders may be infectious (infection with *Neisseria gonorrhoea* or *Mycobacterium tuberculosis*), crystal-induced (gout, pseudogout), immune-related [rheumatoid arthritis (RA), systemic lupus erythematosus (SLE)], reactive (rheumatic fever, Reiter's syndrome), or idiopathic. Inflammatory disorders may be identified by the presence of all or some of the four cardinal signs of inflammation (erythema, warmth, pain, or swelling), systemic symptoms (prolonged morning stiffness, fatigue, fever, weight loss), or laboratory evidence of inflammation [elevated erythrocyte sedimentation rate (ESR) or C-reactive protein, thrombocytosis, anemia of chronic disease, or hypoalbuminemia]. Articular stiffness commonly accompanies chronic musculoskeletal disorders. However, the chronology and magnitude of stiffness may be diagnostically important. Morning stiffness related to inflammatory disorders (such as RA) is precipitated by prolonged rest, is often several hours in duration, and may improve with activity and anti-inflammatory medications. By contrast, intermittent stiffness associated with noninflammatory conditions (such as osteoarthritis) is precipitated by brief periods of rest, usually lasts <60 min, and is exacerbated by activity. Fatigue may accompany inflammation (as seen in RA and polymyalgia rheumatica) and can also be a feature of fibromyalgia (a noninflammatory disorder), anemia, cardiac failure, endocrinopathy, poor nutrition, poor sleep, or psychiatric disorders. Noninflammatory disorders may related to trauma (rotator cuff tear), ineffective repair (osteoarthritis), neoplasm (pigmented villonodular synovitis), or pain amplification (fibromyalgia). Noninflammatory disorders are often characterized by pain without swelling or

---

TABLE 311-1   *Evaluation of Patients with Musculoskeletal Complaints*

Goals
  Accurate diagnosis
  Timely provision of therapy
  Avoidance of unnecessary diagnostic testing
Approach
  Anatomic localization of complaint (articular vs. nonarticular)
  Determination of the nature of the pathologic process (inflammatory vs. noninflammatory)
  Determination of the extent of involvement (monarticular, polyarticular, focal, widespread)
  Determination of chronology (acute vs. chronic)
  Formulation of a differential diagnosis

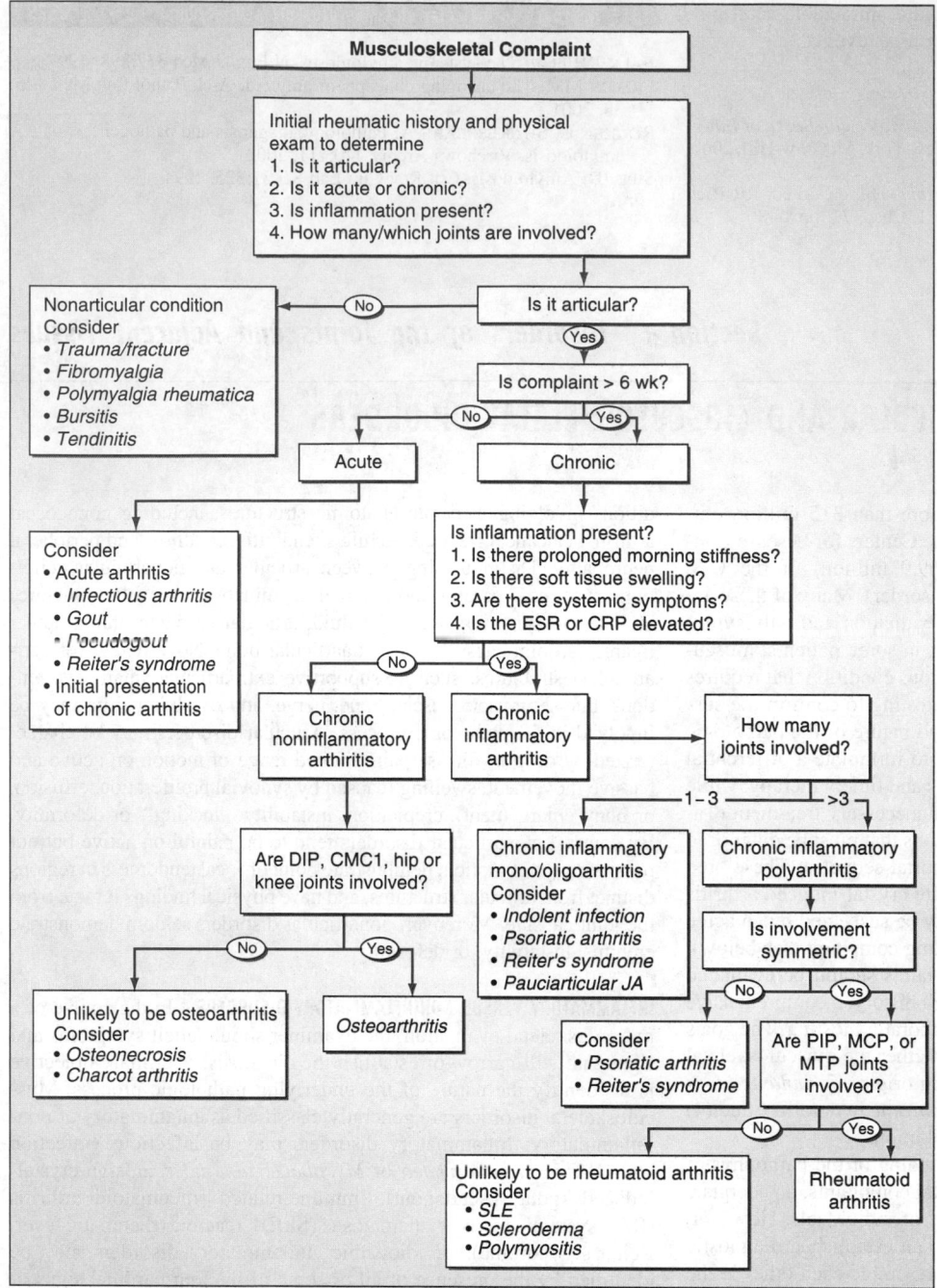

Musculoskeletal Complaint

↓

Initial rheumatic history and physical exam to determine
1. Is it articular?
2. Is it acute or chronic?
3. Is inflammation present?
4. How many/which joints are involved?

↓

Is it articular? — No → Nonarticular condition
Consider
- *Trauma/fracture*
- *Fibromyalgia*
- *Polymyalgia rheumatica*
- *Bursitis*
- *Tendinitis*

Yes ↓

Is complaint > 6 wk?

No → Acute   Yes → Chronic

Acute → Consider
- Acute arthritis
  - *Infectious arthritis*
  - *Gout*
  - *Pseudogout*
  - *Reiter's syndrome*
- Initial presentation of chronic arthritis

Chronic → **Is inflammation present?**
1. Is there prolonged morning stiffness?
2. Is there soft tissue swelling?
3. Are there systemic symptoms?
4. Is the ESR or CRP elevated?

No → Chronic noninflammatory arthiritis
Yes → Chronic inflammatory arthritis

Chronic noninflammatory arthiritis → **Are DIP, CMC1, hip or knee joints involved?**

No → Unlikely to be osteoarthritis
Consider
- *Osteonecrosis*
- *Charcot arthritis*

Yes → *Osteoarthritis*

Chronic inflammatory arthritis → **How many joints involved?**

1–3 → Chronic inflammatory mono/oligoarthritis
Consider
- *Indolent infection*
- *Psoriatic arthritis*
- *Reiter's syndrome*
- *Pauciarticular JA*

>3 → Chronic inflammatory polyarthritis

Chronic inflammatory polyarthritis → **Is involvement symmetric?**

No → Consider
- *Psoriatic arthritis*
- *Reiter's syndrome*

Yes → **Are PIP, MCP, or MTP joints involved?**

No → Unlikely to be rheumatoid arthritis
Consider
- *SLE*
- *Scleroderma*
- *Polymyositis*

Yes → Rheumatoid arthritis

FIGURE 311-1 Algorithm for the diagnosis of musculoskeletal complaints. An approach to formulating a differential diagnosis (shown in italics). (ESR, erythrocyte sedimentation rate; CRP, C-reactive protein; DIP, distal interphalangeal; CMC, carpometacarpal; PIP, proximal interphalangeal; MCP, metacarpophalangeal; MTP, metatarsophalangeal; PMR, polymyalgia rheumatica; SLE, systemic lupus erythematosus; JA, juvenile arthritis.)

warmth, absence of inflammatory or systemic features, minimal or absent morning stiffness, and normal (for age) or negative laboratory investigations.

Identification of the nature of the underlying process and the site of the complaint will enable the examiner to narrow the diagnostic considerations and to assess the need for immediate diagnostic or therapeutic intervention, or for continued observation. Figure 311-1 presents a logical approach to the evaluation of patients with musculoskeletal complaints.

CLINICAL HISTORY   Additional historic features may be helpful in establishing the nature and extent of the pathologic process and may provide important clues to the diagnosis. Aspects of the patient profile, including age, sex, race, and family history, can provide important information. Certain diagnoses are more frequent in different *age* groups

(Fig. 311-2). SLE, rheumatic fever, and Reiter's syndrome occur more frequently in the young, whereas fibromyalgia is most frequent in middle age and osteoarthritis and polymyalgia rheumatica are more prevalent among the elderly. Diagnostic clustering is also evident when *sex* and *race* are considered. Gout and the spondyloarthropathies (e.g., ankylosing spondylitis, Reiter's syndrome) are more common in men, whereas RA and fibromyalgia are more frequent in women. *Racial predilections* are noted with certain disorders. Thus, polymyalgia rheumatica, giant cell arteritis, and Wegener's granulomatosis commonly affect whites, whereas sarcoidosis and SLE more commonly affects African Americans. *Familial aggregation* may be seen in disorders such as ankylosing spondylitis, gout, RA, and Heberden's nodes of osteoarthritis.

The chronology of the complaint is an important diagnostic feature and can be divided into the *onset*, *evolution*, and *duration*. The onset of disorders such as septic arthritis or gout tends to be abrupt, whereas osteoarthritis, RA, and fibromyalgia may have more indolent presentations. The evolution of patients' complaints may also provide useful information. Disorders should be classified as either chronic (osteoarthritis), intermittent (gout), migratory (rheumatic fever, gonococcal or viral arthritis), or additive (RA, Reiter's syndrome). Musculoskeletal disorders are typically classified as acute or chronic based upon a disease duration that is either less than or greater than 6 weeks, respectively. Acute arthropathies tend to be infectious, crystal-induced, or reactive. Chronic arthritides often include noninflammatory and immunologic disorders such as osteoarthritis or RA, respectively. The duration of patients' complaints may alter the diagnostic considerations. For example, the musculoskeletal signs and symptoms of hepatitis B virus infection may be identical with those of early RA at the onset but rarely persist beyond 3 weeks.

The *number* and *distribution* of involved articulations should be noted. Articular disorders are classified based on the number of joints involved, as either *monarticular* (one joint), *oligoarticular* or *pauciarticular* (two to four joints), or *polyarticular* (more than 4 joints). Nonarticular disorders may be classified as either focal or widespread. Complaints secondary to trauma and gout are typically focal or monarticular, whereas others, such as polymyositis, RA, and fibromyalgia, are more diffuse or polyarticular in their presentation. Joint involvement in RA tends to be symmetric, whereas the spondyloarthropathies and gout are often asymmetric. The upper extremities are frequently involved in RA, whereas lower extremity arthritis is characteristic of Reiter's syndrome and gout at their onset. Involvement of the axial skeleton is common in osteoarthritis and ankylosing spondylitis but is infrequent in RA, with the notable exception of the cervical spine.

The clinical history should also identify *precipitating events*, such

FIGURE 311-2 Age at onset for common rheumatic conditions; ranked by prevalence estimates in the United States in 1998. *Estimates vary. (RA, rheumatoid arthritis; PMR, polymyalgia rheumatica; SLE, systemic lupus erythematosus; JRA, juvenile rheumatoid arthritis; DM, dermatomyositis; PM, polymyositis.)

as trauma, drug administration (Table 311-2), or antecedent or intercurrent illnesses, that may have contributed to the patient's complaint. Lastly, a thorough *rheumatic review of systems* may disclose associated features outside the musculoskeletal system and provide useful diagnostic information. A variety of musculoskeletal disorders may be associated with systemic features such as fever (SLE, infection), rash (SLE, Reiter's syndrome, dermatomyositis), myalgias, weakness (polymyositis, polymyalgia rheumatica), or morning stiffness (inflammatory arthritis). In addition, some conditions are associated with involvement of other organ systems including the eyes (Behçet's disease, sarcoidosis, Reiter's syndrome), gastrointestinal tract (scleroderma, inflammatory bowel disease), genitourinary tract (Reiter's syndrome, gonococcemia), or the nervous system (Lyme disease, vasculitis).

PHYSICAL EXAMINATION The goal of the physical examination is to ascertain the structures involved, the nature of the underlying pathology,

the extent and functional consequences of the process, and the presence of systemic or extraarticular manifestations. A knowledge of topographic anatomy is necessary to identify the primary site(s) of involvement and differentiate articular from nonarticular disorders. The musculoskeletal examination depends largely on careful inspection, palpation, and a variety of specific physical maneuvers to elicit diagnostic signs (Table 311-3). Although most articulations of the appendicular skeleton can be examined in this manner, adequate inspection and palpation are not possible for many axial (e.g., zygapophyseal) and inaccessible (e.g., sacroiliac or hip) joints. For such joints, there is a greater reliance upon specific maneuvers and imaging for assessment.

Examination of involved and uninvolved joints will determine whether *pain, warmth, erythema,* or *swelling* is present. The locale and level of pain elicited by palpation or movement should be quantified. For example, the number of tender joints on palpation or the patients' report of pain intensity (on a scale of 1 to 10) may be noted. The examination should distinguish true articular swelling caused by synovial effusion or synovial proliferation from nonarticular or periarticular involvement, which usually extends beyond the normal joint margins or full extent of the synovial space. Synovial effusion can be distinguished from synovial hypertrophy or bony hypertrophy by palpation or specific maneuvers. For example, small to moderate knee effusions may be identified by the "bulge sign" or "ballottement of the patellae." Bursal effusions (e.g., effusions of the olecranon or prepatellar bursa) overlie bony prominences and are fluctuant with sharply defined borders. Joint *stability* can be assessed by palpation and by the application of manual stress. *Subluxation* or *dislocation,* which may be secondary to traumatic, mechanical, or inflammatory causes, can be assessed by inspection and palpation. Joint *volume* can be assessed by palpation. Distention of the articular capsule usually causes pain. The patient will attempt to minimize the pain by maintaining the joint in the position of least intraarticular pressure and greatest volume, usually partial flexion. For this reason, inflammatory effusions may give rise to flexion contractures. Clinically, this may be detected as obvious swelling, voluntary or fixed flexion deformities, or diminished range of motion—especially on extension, when joint volumes are decreased. Active and passive *range of motion* should be assessed in all planes, with contralateral comparison. Serial evaluations of joint

TABLE 311-2 *Drug-Induced Musculoskeletal Conditions*

Arthralgias
Quinidine, amphotericin B, cimetidine, quinolones, chronic acyclovir, interferon, IL-2, nicardipine, vaccines, rifabutin

Myalgias/myopathy
Glucocorticoids, penicillamine, hydroxychloroquine, AZT, lovastatin, simvastatin, pravastatin, clofibrate, interferon, IL-2, alcohol, cocaine, taxol, docetaxel, colchicine, quinolones

Gout
Diuretics, aspirin, cytotoxics, cyclosporine, alcohol, moonshine, ethambutol

Drug-induced lupus
Hydralazine, procainamide, quinidine, phenytoin, methyldopa, isoniazid, chlorpromazine, lithium, penicillamine, tetracycline, infliximab

Osteonecrosis
Glucocorticoids, alcohol, radiation

Osteopenia
Glucocorticoids, chronic heparin, phenytoin, methotrexate

Scleroderma
Vinyl chloride, bleomycin, pentazocine, organic solvents, carbidopa, tryptophan, rapeseed oil

Vasculitis
Allopurinol, amphetamines, cocaine, thiazides, penicillamine, propylthiouracil

Note: IL-2, interleukin 2.

TABLE 311-3 *Glossary of Musculoskeletal Terms*

Crepitus
A palpable (less commonly audible) vibratory or crackling sensation elicited with joint motion; fine joint crepitus is common and often insignificant in large joints; coarse joint crepitus indicates advanced cartilaginous and degenerative changes (as in osteoarthritis).

Subluxation
Alteration of joint alignment such that articulating surfaces incompletely approximate each other

Dislocation
Abnormal displacement of articulating surfaces such that the surfaces are not in contact

Range of motion
For diarthrodial joints, the arc of measurable movement through which the joint moves in a single plane

Contracture
Loss of full movement resulting from a fixed resistance due either to tonic spasm of muscle (reversible) or to fibrosis of periarticular structures (permanent)

Deformity
Abnormal shape or size of a structure; may result from bony hypertrophy, malalignment of articulating structures, or damage to periarticular supportive structures

Enthesitis
Inflammation of the entheses (tendinous or ligamentous insertions on bone)

Epicondylitis
Infection or inflammation involving an epicondyle

motion may be recorded with a goniometer to quantify the arc of movement. Each joint should be passively manipulated through its full range of motion (including, as appropriate, flexion, extension, rotation, abduction, adduction, lateral bending, inversion, eversion, supination, pronation, and medial or lateral deviation, or bending). Limitation of motion is frequently caused by effusion, pain, deformity, or contracture. If passive motion exceeds active motion, a periarticular process (e.g., tendon rupture or myopathy) should be considered. *Contractures* may reflect antecedent synovial inflammation or trauma. Joint *crepitus* may be felt during palpation or maneuvers and may be prominent or coarse in osteoarthritis. Joint *deformity* usually indicates a long-standing or aggressive pathologic process. Deformities may result from ligamentous destruction, soft tissue contracture, bony enlargement, ankylosis, erosive disease, or subluxation. Examination of the musculature will document strength, atrophy, pain, or spasm. Muscle weakness should be characterized as proximal or distal. Muscle strength is graded on a 5-point scale: 0 for no movement; 1 for trace movement or twitch; 2 for movement with gravity eliminated; 3 for movement against gravity only; 4 for movement against gravity and resistance; and 5 for normal strength. The examiner should assess carefully for nonarticular or periarticular involvement, especially when articular complaints are not supported by objective findings referable to the joint capsule. The identification of musculoskeletal pain of soft tissue origin (nonarticular pain) will prevent unwarranted and often expensive additional evaluations. Specific maneuvers may reveal nonarticular abnormalities, such as a carpal tunnel syndrome (which can be identified by Tinel's or Phalen's sign). Other examples of soft tissue abnormalities include olecranon bursitis, epicondylitis (e.g., tennis elbow), enthesitis (e.g., Achilles tendinitis), and trigger points associated with fibromyalgia.

LABORATORY INVESTIGATIONS The vast majority of musculoskeletal disorders can be easily diagnosed by a complete history and physical examination. An additional objective of the initial encounter is to determine whether additional investigations or immediate therapy are required. A number of features indicate the need for additional evaluation. Monarticular conditions require additional evaluation, as do traumatic or inflammatory conditions and conditions accompanied by neurologic changes or systemic manifestations of serious disease. Finally, individuals with chronic symptoms (>6 weeks), especially when there has been a lack of response to symptomatic measures, are candidates for additional evaluation. The extent and nature of the additional investigation should be dictated by the clinical features and suspected pathologic process. Laboratory tests should be used to confirm a specific clinical diagnosis and not be used as a tool to screen or evaluate patients with vague rheumatic complaints. Indiscriminate use of broad batteries of diagnostic tests and radiographic procedures is rarely useful or cost-effective means to establish a diagnosis.

Besides a complete blood count, including a white blood cell (WBC) and differential count, the routine evaluation should include a determination of an acute-phase reactant such as the ESR or C-reactive protein, which can be useful in discriminating inflammatory from non-inflammatory musculoskeletal disorders. Both are inexpensive and easily obtained and may be elevated with infections, inflammatory arthritis, autoimmune disorders, neoplasia, pregnancy, and advanced age. Serum uric acid determinations are useful only when gout has been diagnosed and therapy contemplated.

Serologic tests for rheumatoid factor, antinuclear antibodies (ANA), complement levels, Lyme and antineutrophil cytoplasmic antibodies, or antistreptolysin O titer should be carried out only when there is clinical evidence to suggest a relevant associated diagnosis, as these have poor predictive value when used for screening, especially when the pretest probability is low. Although, 4 to 5% of a healthy population will have positive tests for rheumatoid factor and ANA, only 1% and 0.4% of the population will have RA or SLE, respectively. IgM rheumatoid factor (autoantibodies against the Fc portion

of IgG) is found in 80% of patients with RA and may also be seen in low titers in patients with chronic infections (*tuberculosis*, leprosy); other autoimmune diseases (SLE, Sjögren's syndrome); and chronic pulmonary, hepatic, or renal diseases. ANAs are found in nearly all patients with SLE and may also be seen in patients with other auto-immune diseases (polymyositis, scleroderma, antiphospholipid syndrome), drug-induced lupus (resulting from hydralazine, procainamide, or quinidine), chronic hepatitic, or renal disorders. The interpretation of a positive ANA may depend on the magnitude of the titer and the pattern observed under immunofluorescence microscopy. Diffuse and speckled patterns are least specific, whereas a peripheral, or rim, pattern is highly specific and suggestive of autoantibodies against double-stranded (native) DNA. This pattern is seen only in patients with SLE.

Aspiration and analysis of synovial fluid are always indicated in acute monarthritis or when an infectious or crystal-induced arthropathy is suspected. Synovial fluid analysis may be crucial in distinguishing between noninflammatory and inflammatory processes. This distinction can be made on the basis of the appearance, viscosity, and cell count of the synovial fluid. Tests for synovial fluid glucose, protein, lactate dehydrogenase, lactic acid, or autoantibodies are not recommended as they are insensitive or have little discriminatory value. Normal synovial fluid is clear or a pale straw color and is viscous, primarily because of the high levels of hyaluronate. Noninflammatory synovial fluid is clear, viscous, and amber-colored, with a white blood cell count of $<2000/\mu L$ and a predominance of mononuclear cells. The viscosity of synovial fluid is assessed by expressing fluid from the syringe one drop at a time. Normally there is a stringing effect, with a long tail behind each synovial drop. Effusions caused by osteoarthritis or trauma usually have normal viscosity. Inflammatory fluid is turbid and yellow, with an increased white cell count (2000 to $50,000/\mu L$) and a polymorphonuclear leukocyte predominance. Inflammatory fluid has reduced viscosity, diminished hyaluronate, and little or no tail following each drop of synovial fluid. Such effusions are found in RA, gout, other inflammatory arthritides, and septic arthritis. Infectious fluid is opaque, and purulent, with a white cell count usually $>50,000/\mu L$, a predominance of polymorphonuclear leukocytes (>75%), and low viscosity. Such effusions are typical of septic arthritis, but they occur rarely with sterile inflammatory arthritides such as RA or gout. In addition, hemorrhagic synovial fluid may be seen with trauma, hemarthrosis, or neuropathic arthritis. An algorithm for synovial fluid aspiration and analysis is shown in Fig. 311-3. Synovial fluid should be analyzed immediately for appearance, viscosity, and cell count. Cellularity and the presence of crystals may be assessed by either light or polarizing microscopy. Monosodium urate crystals, seen in gouty effusions, are long, needle-shaped, negatively birefringent, and usually intracellular, whereas calcium pyrophosphate dihydrate crystals, found in chondrocalcinosis and pseudogout, are usually short, rhomboid-shaped, positively birefringent crystals. Whenever infection is suspected, synovial fluid should be Gram-stained and cultured appropriately. If gonococcal arthritis is suspected, immediate plating of the fluid on appropriate culture medium is indicated. Synovial fluid from patients with chronic monarthritis should also be cultured for *M. tuberculosis* and fungi. Last, it should be noted that crystal-induced arthritis and infection occasionally occur together in the same joint.

DIAGNOSTIC IMAGING IN JOINT DISEASES Conventional radiography has been a valuable tool in the diagnosis and staging of articular disorders. Plain x-rays are most appropriate when there is a history of trauma, suspected chronic infection, progressive disability, or monarticular involvement; when therapeutic alterations are considered; or when a baseline assessment is desired for what appears to be a chronic process. However, in most inflammatory disorders, early radiography is rarely helpful in establishing a diagnosis and may only reveal soft tissue swelling or juxtaarticular demineralization. As the disease progresses, calcification (of soft tissues, cartilage, or bone), joint space narrowing, erosions, bony ankylosis, new bone formation (sclerosis, osteophytes,

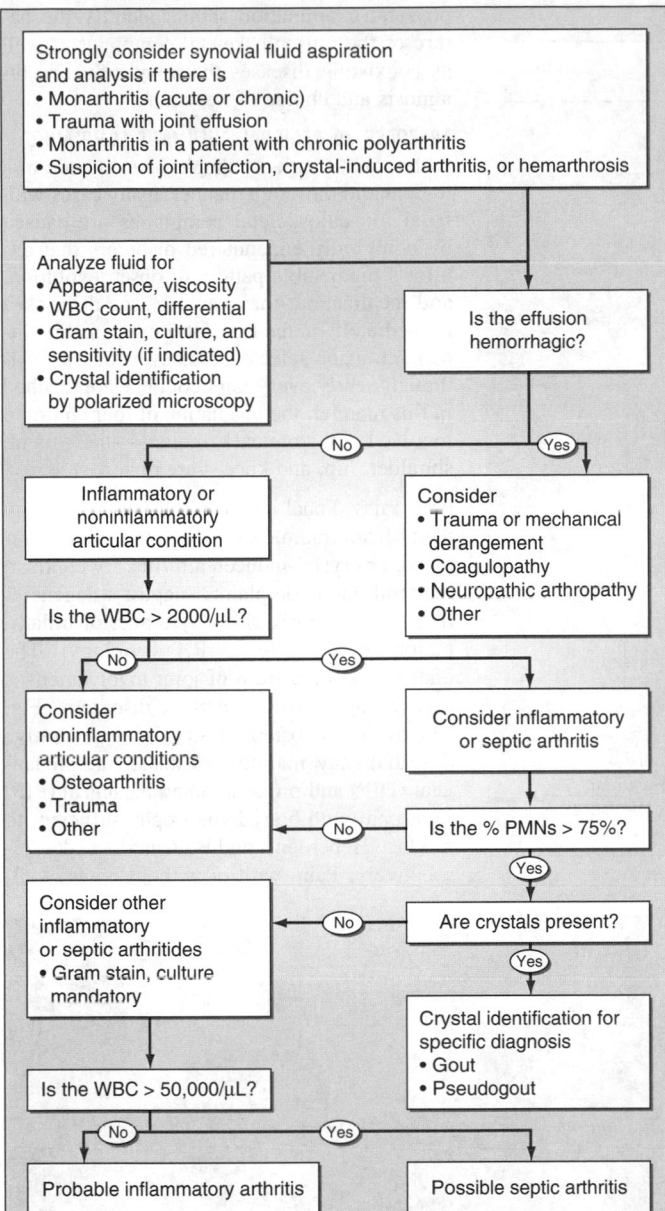

FIGURE 311-3 Algorithmic approach to the use and interpretation of synovial fluid aspiration and analysis. [WBC, white blood cell (count); PMNs, polymorphonuclear (leukocytes).]

or periostitis), or subchondral cysts may develop and suggest specific clinical entities. Consultation with a radiologist will help define proper imaging modality, technique, and positioning and prevent the need for further studies.

Additional imaging techniques may possess greater diagnostic sensitivity and facilitate early diagnosis in a limited number of articular disorders and in selected circumstances and are indicated when conventional radiography is not adequate (Table 311-4). *Ultrasonography* is useful in the detection of soft tissue abnormalities that cannot be fully appreciated by clinical examination. Although inexpensive and easily performed, in only a limited number of circumstances is it the preferred method of evaluation. The foremost application of ultrasound is in the diagnosis of synovial (Baker's) cysts, although rotator cuff tears and various tendon injuries may be evaluated with ultrasound by an experienced operator. *Radionuclide scintigraphy* provides useful information regarding the metabolic status of bone and, along with radiography, is well suited for total-body assessment of the extent and distribution of musculoskeletal involvement. Radionuclide imaging is a very sensitive, but poorly specific, means of detecting inflammatory

or metabolic alterations in bone or periarticular soft tissue structures. The limited tissue contrast resolution of scintigraphy may obscure the distinction between a bony or periarticular process and may necessitate the additional use of other imaging modalities. Scintigraphy, using ^{99m}Tc, ^{67}Ga, or ^{111}In-labeled WBCs has been applied to a variety of articular disorders with variable success (Table 311-4). [^{99m}Tc] pertechnate or diphosphate scintigraphy may be useful in identifying infection, neoplasia, inflammation, increased blood flow, bone remodeling, heterotopic bone formation, or avascular necrosis (Fig. 311-4). The poor specificity of ^{99m}Tc scanning has limited its use to investigational and serial assessments of joint or bone involvement, inflammatory or infectious processes, and surveys for bone metastases. ^{67}Ga binds to serum and cellular transferrin and lactoferrin and is preferentially taken up by neutrophils, macrophages, bacteria, and tumor tissue (e.g., lymphoma) and is useful in the identification of infection and malignancies. Scanning with ^{111}In-labeled WBCs has been used to detect both infectious and inflammatory arthritis. Although both have been used with success, ^{111}In-labeled WBC scanning is superior to ^{67}Ga in the early diagnosis of osteomyelitis and infected prosthetic joints. Prior treatment with antibiotics may reduce the diagnostic sensitivity of both ^{67}Ga and ^{111}In-labeled WBC scintigraphy.

Computed tomography (CT) provides rapid reconstruction of sagittal, coronal, and axial images and spatial relationships among anatomic structures. It has proved to be most useful in the assessment of the axial skeleton because of its ability to visualize in the axial plane. Articulations previously considered difficult to visualize using conventional radiography, such as the zygapophyseal, sacroiliac, sternoclavicular, and hip joints, can be effectively evaluated using CT. CT has been demonstrated to be useful in the diagnosis of low back pain syndromes, sacroiliitis, osteoid osteoma, tarsal coalition, osteomyelitis, intraarticular osteochondral fragments, and advanced osteonecrosis. Helical or spiral CT (with or without contrast angiography) is a novel technique that is rapid, cost effective, and sensitive in diagnosing pulmonary embolism or obscure fractures, often in the setting of initially equivocal findings. High-resolution CT can be advocated in the evaluation of suspected or established infiltrative lung disease (e.g., scleroderma or rheumatoid lung).

Magnetic resonance imaging (MRI) has significantly advanced the ability to image musculoskeletal structures. MRI has the advantages of providing multiplanar images with fine anatomic detail and contrast resolution (Fig. 311-5). Other advantages are the lack of ionizing radiation and adverse effects and the superior ability to visualize bone marrow and soft tissue periarticular structures, which have led to the increased use of this modality. The advantages of MRI are counterbalanced by high cost and long procedural time, factors that have limited its use in the evaluation of musculoskeletal disorders. MRI should be used only when it will provide necessary information that cannot be obtained by less expensive and noninvasive means.

MRI can image fascia, vessels, nerve, muscle, cartilage, ligaments, tendons, pannus, synovial effusions, and bone marrow. Visualization of particular structures can be enhanced by altering the pulse sequence to produce either T1- or T2-weighted spin echo, gradient echo, or inversion recovery [including short tau inversion recovery (STIR)] images. Because of its sensitivity to changes in marrow fat, MRI is a sensitive but nonspecific means of detecting osteonecrosis and osteomyelitis (Fig. 311-5). Because of its enhanced soft tissue resolution, MRI is more sensitive than arthrography or CT in the diagnosis of soft tissue injuries (e.g., meniscal and rotator cuff tears); intraarticular derangements; and spinal cord damage, subluxation, or synovitis.

RHEUMATOLOGIC EVALUATION OF THE ELDERLY The incidence of rheumatic diseases rises with age, and so ~58% of those >65 will have joint complaints. Musculoskeletal disorders in elderly patients are often not diagnosed because the signs and symptoms may be insidious, chronic, or overshadowed by comorbidities. These difficulties are compounded by the diminished reliability of laboratory testing in the elderly, who

TABLE 311-4 *Diagnostic Imaging Techniques for Musculoskeletal Disorders*

Method	Imaging Time, h	Cost[a]	Current Indications
Ultrasound[b]	<1	+	Synovial cysts
			Rotator cuff tears
			Tendon injury
Radionuclide scintigraphy			
^{99m}Tc	1–4	++	Metastatic bone survey
			Evaluation of Paget's disease
			Quantitative joint assessment
			Acute infection
			Acute and chronic osteomyelitis
^{111}In-WBC	24	+++	Acute infection
			Prosthetic infection
			Acute osteomyelitis
^{67}Ga	24–48	++++	Acute and chronic infection
			Acute osteomyelitis
Computed tomography	<1	+++	Herniated intervertebral disk
			Sacroiliitis
			Spinal stenosis
			Spinal trauma
			Osteoid osteoma
			Tarsal coalition
Magnetic resonance imaging	1/2–2	+++++	Avascular necrosis
			Osteomyelitis
			Intraarticular derangement and soft tissue injury
			Derangements of axial skeleton and spinal cord
			Herniated intervertebral disk
			Pigmented villonodular synovitis
			Inflammatory and metabolic muscle pathology

[a] Relative cost for imaging study.   [b] Results depend on operator.

physical examination should identify the nature of the musculoskeletal complaint as well as coexisting diseases that may influence diagnosis and choice of treatment.

APPROACH TO REGIONAL RHEUMATIC COMPLAINTS

Although all patients should be evaluated in a logical and thorough manner, many cases with focal musculoskeletal complaints are caused by commonly encountered disorders that exhibit a predictable pattern of onset, evolution, and localization; they can often be diagnosed immediately on the basis of limited historic information and selected maneuvers or tests. Although nearly every joint could be approached in this manner, the evaluation of four common involved anatomical regions—the hand, shoulder, hip, and knee—are reviewed here.

Hand Pain Focal or unilateral hand pain may result from trauma, overuse, infection, or a reactive or crystal-induced arthritis. By contrast, bilateral hand complaints suggest a degenerative (e.g., osteoarthritis), systemic, or inflammatory/immune (e.g., RA) etiology. The distribution or pattern of joint involvement is highly suggestive of certain disorders (Fig. 311-6). Thus, osteoarthritis (or degenerative arthritis) may manifest as distal interphalangeal (DIP) and proximal interphalangeal (PIP) joint pain with bony hypertrophy sufficient to produce Heberden's and Bouchard's nodes, respectively. Pain, with or without bony swell-

often manifest nonpathologic abnormal results. For example, the ESR may be misleadingly elevated, and low-titer positive tests for rheumatoid factor and ANAs may be seen in up to 15% of elderly patients. Although nearly all rheumatic disorders afflict the elderly, certain diseases and drug-induced disorders (Table 311-2) are more common in this age group. The elderly should be approached in the same manner as other patients with musculoskeletal complaints, but with additional inquiries to exclude common geriatric musculoskeletal disorders. An emphasis on identifying the rheumatic consequences of intercurrent medical conditions and therapies is extremely important. Osteoarthritis, osteoporosis, gout, pseudogout, polymyalgia rheumatica, vasculitis, drug-induced lupus erythematosus, and chronic salicylate toxicity are all more common in the elderly than in other individuals. The

FIGURE 311-5 Superior sensitivity of magnetic resonance imaging in the diagnosis of osteonecrosis of the femoral head. A 45-year-old woman receiving high-dose glucocorticoids developed right hip pain. Conventional x-rays (*top*) demonstrated only mild sclerosis of the right femoral head. T1-weighted MRI (*bottom*) demonstrated low density signal in the right femoral head, diagnostic of osteonecrosis.

FIGURE 311-4 [^{99m}Tc]diphosphonate scintigraphy of the feet of a 33-year-old black male with Reiter's syndrome, manifested by sacroiliitis, urethritis, uveitis, asymmetric oligoarthritis, and enthesitis. This bone scan demonstrates increased uptake indicative of enthesitis involving the insertions of the left Achilles tendon, plantar aponeurosis, and right tibialis posterior tendon as well as arthritis of the right first interphalangeal joint.

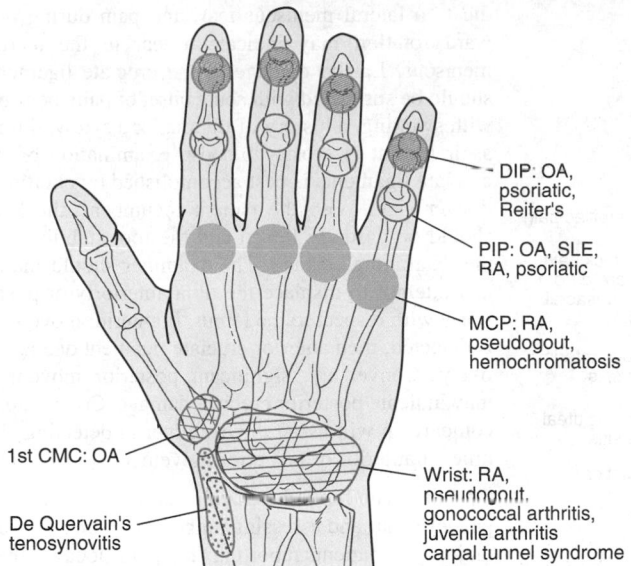

DIP: OA, psoriatic, Reiter's

PIP: OA, SLE, RA, psoriatic

MCP: RA, pseudogout, hemochromatosis

1st CMC: OA

De Quervain's tenosynovitis

Wrist: RA, pseudogout, gonococcal arthritis, juvenile arthritis carpal tunnel syndrome

FIGURE 311-6 Sites of hand or wrist involvement and their potential disease associations. (DIP, distal interphalangeal; OA, osteoarthritis; PIP, proximal interphalangeal; SLE, systemic lupus erythematosus; RA, rheumatoid arthritis; MCP, metacarpophalangeal; CMC, carpometacarpal.) *(From JJ Cush, AF Kavanaugh: Rheumatology: Diagnosis and Therapeutics. Baltimore, Lippincott Williams & Wilkins, 1999; with permission.)*

ing, involving the base of the thumb (first carpometacarpal joint) is also highly suggestive of osteoarthritis. By contrast, RA tends to involve the PIP, metacarpophalangeal, intercarpal, and carpometacarpal joints (wrist) with pain, prolonged stiffness, and palpable synovial tissue hypertrophy. Psoriatic arthritis may also involve the DIP and PIP joints and the carpus with inflammatory pain, stiffness, and synovitis. Moreover, the diagnosis of psoriatic arthritis can be suggested by nail pitting or onycholysis. Soft tissue swelling may also be noted over the dorsum of the hand and wrist and may suggest an inflammatory extensor tendon tenosynovitis possibly caused by gonococcal infection, gout, or inflammatory arthritis. The diagnosis of tenosynovitis may be suggested by local warmth and edema and is confirmed when pain is induced by maintaining the wrist in a fixed, neutral position and flexing the digits distal to the metacarpophalangeal joints to stretch the extensor tendon sheaths.

Focal wrist pain localized to the radial aspect may be caused by DeQuervains tenosynovitis resulting from inflammation of the tendon sheath(s) involving the abductor pollicis longus or extensor pollicis brevis (Fig. 311-6). This commonly results from overuse or follows pregnancy and may be diagnosed with Finkelstein's test. A positive result is present when local wrist pain is induced after the thumb is flexed across the palm and placed inside a clenched fist and the patient actively deviates the hand downward with ulnar deviation at the wrist. Carpal tunnel syndrome is another common disorder of the upper extremity and results from compression of the median nerve within the carpal tunnel. Manifestations include paresthesia in the thumb, second, third, and radial half of the fourth finger and, at times, atrophy of thenar musculature. Carpal tunnel syndrome is commonly associated with pregnancy, edema, trauma, osteoarthritis, inflammatory arthritis, and infiltrative disorders (e.g., amyloidosis). The diagnosis is suggested by a positive Tinel's or Phalen's sign. With each test, paresthesia in a median nerve distribution is induced or increased by either "thumping" the volar aspect of the wrist (Tinel's sign) or pressing the extensor surfaces of both flexed wrists against each other (Phalen's sign).

Shoulder Pain   During the evaluation of shoulder disorders, the examiner should carefully note any history of trauma, infection, inflammatory disease, occupational hazards, or previous cervical disease. In addition, the patient should be questioned as to the activities or movement(s) that elicit shoulder pain. Shoulder pain is frequently referred from the cervical spine but may also be referred from intrathoracic

lesions (e.g., a Pancoast tumor) or from gall bladder, hepatic, or diaphragmatic disease. The shoulder should be put through its full range of motion both actively and passively (with examiner assistance): forward flexion, extension, abduction, adduction, and rotation. Manual inspection of the periarticular structures will often provide important diagnostic information. The examiner should apply direct manual pressure over the subacromial bursa that lies lateral to and immediately beneath the acromion. Subacromial bursitis is a frequent cause of shoulder pain. Anterior to the subacromial bursa, the bicipital tendon traverses the bicipital groove. This tendon is best identified by palpating it in its groove as the patient rotates the humerus internally and externally. Direct pressure over the tendon may reveal pain indicative of bicipital tendinitis. Palpation of the acromioclavicular joint may disclose local pain, bony hypertrophy, or, uncommonly, synovial swelling. Whereas osteoarthritis and RA commonly affect the acromioclavicular joint, osteoarthritis seldom involves the glenohumeral joint, unless there is a traumatic or occupational cause. The glenohumeral joint is best palpated anteriorly by placing the thumb over the humeral head (just medial and inferior to the coracoid process) and having the patient rotate the humerus internally and externally. Pain localized to this region is indicative of glenohumeral pathology. Synovial effusion or tissue is seldom palpable but, if present, may suggest infection, RA, or an acute tear of the rotator cuff.

Rotator cuff tendinitis or tear is a very common cause of shoulder pain. The rotator cuff is formed by the tendons of the supraspinatus, infraspinatus, teres minor, and subscapularis muscles. Rotator cuff tendinitis is suggested by pain on active abduction (but not passive abduction), pain over the lateral deltoid muscle, night pain, and evidence of the impingement sign. This maneuver is performed by the examiner raising the patient's arm into forced flexion while stabilizing and preventing rotation of the scapula. A positive sign is present if pain develops before 180° of forward flexion. A complete tear of the rotator cuff is more common in the elderly and often results from trauma; it may manifest in the same manner as tendinitis but is less common. The diagnosis is also suggested by the drop arm test in which the patient is unable to maintain his or her arm outstretched once it is passively abducted. If the patient is unable to hold the arm up once 90° of abduction is reached, the test is positive. Tendinitis or tear of the rotator cuff can be confirmed by MRI or arthrography.

Knee Pain   A careful history should delineate the chronology of the knee complaint and whether there are predisposing conditions, trauma, or medications that might underlie the complaint. For example, patellofemoral disease (e.g., osteoarthritis) may cause anterior knee pain that worsens with climbing stairs. Observation of the patient's gait is also important. The knee should be carefully inspected in the upright (weight-bearing) and prone positions for swelling, erythema, contusion, laceration, or malalignment. The most common form of malalignment in the knee is *genu varum* (bowlegs) and *genu valgum* (knock knees). Bony swelling of the knee joint commonly results from hypertrophic osseous changes seen with disorders such as osteoarthritis and neuropathic arthropathy. Swelling caused by hypertrophy of intrasynovial structures (i.e., synovium or synovial effusion) may manifest as a fluctuant, ballotable, or soft tissue enlargement in the suprapatellar pouch (superior reflection of the synovial cavity) or lateral and medial to the patella. Synovial effusions may also be detected by balloting the patella downward toward the femoral groove or by eliciting a "bulge sign." With the the knee extended the examiner should manually compress, or "milk," synovial fluid down from the suprapatellar pouch and lateral to the patellae. The application of manual pressure lateral to the patella may cause an observable shift in synovial fluid (bulge) to the medial aspect. The examiner should note that this maneuver is only effective in detecting small to moderate effusions (<100 mL). Inflammatory disorders such as RA, gout, and Reiter's syndrome may involve the knee joint and produce significant pain, stiffness, swelling, or warmth. A popliteal or *Baker's cyst* is best palpated with

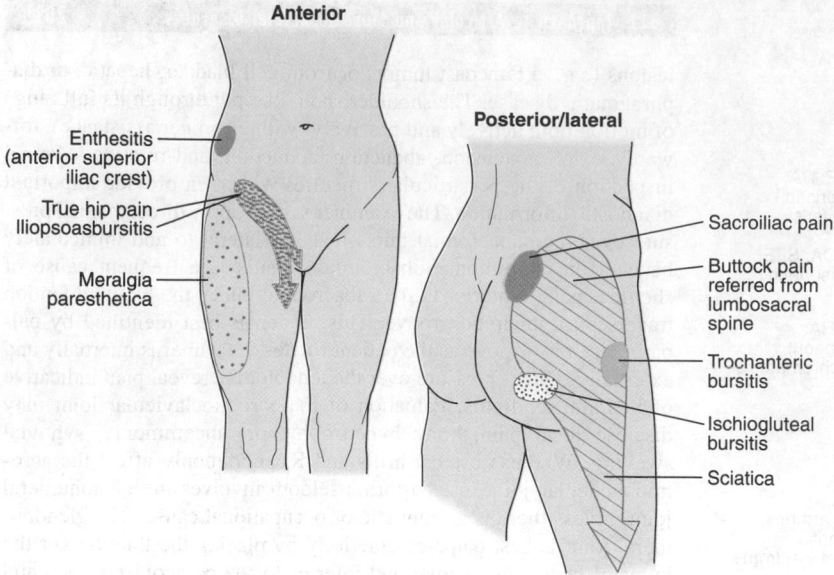

FIGURE 311-7 Origins of hip pain. *(From JJ Cush, AF Kavanaugh: Rheumatology: Diagnosis and Therapeutics. Baltimore, Lippincott Williams & Wilkins, 1999; with permission.)*

the knee partially flexed and is best seen with the patient standing and knees fully extended to visualize popliteal swelling or fullness from a posterior view.

Anserine bursitis is an often missed periarticular cause of knee pain in adults. The pes anserine bursa underlies the semimembranosus tendon and may become inflamed and painful following trauma, overuse, or inflammation. It is often tender in patients with fibromyalgia. Anserine bursitis manifests primarily as point tenderness inferior and medial to the patella and overlies the medial tibial plateau. Swelling and erythema may not be present. Other forms of bursitis may also present as knee pain. The prepatellar bursa is superficial and is located over the inferior portion of the patella. The infrapatellar bursa is deeper and lies beneath the patellar ligament before its insertion on the tibial tubercle.

Internal derangement of the knee may result from trauma or degenerative processes. Damage to the meniscal cartilage (medial or lateral) frequently presents as chronic or intermittent knee pain. Such an injury should be suspected when there is a history of trauma or athletic activity and when the patient relates symptoms of "locking," clicking, or "giving way" of the joint. Pain may be detected during direct palpation over the medial or lateral joint line. The diagnosis may also be suggested by ipsilateral joint line pain when the knee is stressed laterally or medially. A positive McMurray test may indicated a meniscal tear. To perform this test, the knee is first flexed at 90°, and the leg is then extended while simultaneously the lower extremity is torqued medially or laterally. A painful click during inward rotation may in-

dicate a lateral meniscus tear, and pain during outward rotation may indicate a tear in the medial meniscus. Lastly, damage to the cruciate ligaments should be suspected with acute onset of pain, possibly with swelling, a history of trauma, or a synovial fluid aspirate that is grossly bloody. Examination of the cruciate ligaments is best accomplished by eliciting a drawer sign. With the patient recumbent, the knee should be partially flexed and the foot stabilized on the examining surface. The examiner should manually attempt to displace the tibia anteriorly or posteriorly with respect to the femur. If anterior movement is detected, then anterior cruciate ligament damage is likely. Conversely, significant posterior movement may indicate posterior cruciate damage. Contralateral comparison will assist the examiner in detecting significant anterior or posterior movement.

Hip Pain   The hip is best evaluated by observing the patient's gait and assessing range of motion. The vast majority of patients reporting "hip pain" localize their pain unilaterally to the posterior or gluteal musculature (Fig. 311-7). Such pain may or may not be associated with low back pain and tends to radiate down the posterolateral aspect of the thigh. This presentation frequently results from degenerative arthritis of the lumbosacral spine and commonly follows a dermatomal distribution with involvement of nerve roots between L5 and S1. Some individuals instead localize their "hip pain" laterally to the area overlying the trochanteric bursa. Because of the depth of this bursa, swelling and warmth are usually absent. Diagnosis of trochanteric bursitis can be confirmed by inducing point tenderness over the trochanteric bursa. Range of movement may be limited by pain. Pain in the hip joint is less common and tends to be located anteriorly, over the inguinal ligament; it may radiate medially to the groin or along the anteromedial thigh. Uncommonly, iliopsoas bursitis may mimic true hip joint pain. Diagnosis of iliopsoas bursitis may be suggested by a history of trauma or inflammatory arthritis. Pain associated with an iliopsoas bursitis is localized to the groin or anterior thigh and tends to worsen with hyperextension of the hip; many patients prefer to flex and externally rotate the hip to reduce the pain from a distended bursa.

FURTHER READING

BROWER AC: Imaging techniques and modalities, in *Arthritis in Black and White*, AC Brower (ed). Philadelphia, Saunders, 1998, p 1

KAVANAUGH A: The utility of immunologic laboratory tests in patients with rheumatic diseases. Arthritis Rheum 44:2221, 2001

SCHUMACHER HR JR: Arthritis of recent onset: A guide to evaluation and initial therapy for primary care physicians. Postgrad Med 97:52, 1995

SHMERLING RH et al: Synovial fluid tests: What should be ordered? JAMA 264:1009, 1990

312 | OSTEOARTHRITIS
Kenneth D. Brandt

Osteoarthritis (OA), also erroneously called degenerative joint disease, represents failure of the diarthrodial (movable, synovial-lined) joint. In idiopathic (primary) OA, the most common form of the disease, no predisposing factor is apparent. Secondary OA is pathologically indistinguishable from idiopathic OA but is attributable to an underlying cause (Table 312-1).

EPIDEMIOLOGY AND RISK FACTORS   OA is the most common joint disease of humans. Among the elderly, knee OA is the leading cause of chronic disability in developed countries; some 100,000 people in the United

States are unable to walk independently from bed to bathroom because of OA of the knee or hip.

In those <55 years, the joint distribution of OA in men and women is similar; in older individuals, hip OA is more common in men, while OA of interphalangeal joints and the thumb base is more common in women. Similarly, radiographic evidence of knee OA, and especially of *symptomatic* knee OA, is more common in women than in men (Table 312-2).

Racial differences exist in both the prevalence of OA and the pattern of joint involvement. The Chinese in Hong Kong have a lower incidence of hip OA than whites; OA is more frequent in Native Americans than in whites. Interphalangeal joint OA and especially hip OA are much less common in South African blacks than in whites in the same population. Whether these differences are genetic or due to

TABLE 312-1   Classification of Osteoarthritis

312 Osteoarthritis   2037

I. Idiopathic
  A. Localized OA
    1. Hands: Heberden's and Bouchard's nodes (nodal), erosive interphalangeal arthritis (nonnodal), 1st carpometacarpal joint
    2. Feet: hallux valgus, hallux rigidus, contracted toes (hammer/cock-up toes), talonavicular
    3. Knee:
      a. Medial compartment
      b. Lateral compartment
      c. Patellofemoral compartment
    4. Hip:
      a. Eccentric (superior)
      b. Concentric (axial, medial)
      c. Diffuse (coxae senilis)
    5. Spine:
      a. Apophyseal joints
      b. Intervertebral joints (disks)
      c. Spondylosis (osteophytes)
      d. Ligamentous (hyperostosis, Forestier's disease, diffuse idiopathic skeletal hyperstosis)
    6. Other single sites, e.g., glenohumoral, acromioclavicular, tibiotalar, sacroiliac, temporomandibular
  B. Generalized includes 3 or more of the areas listed above (Kellgren-Moore)
II. Secondary
  A. Trauma
    1. Acute
    2. Chronic (occupational, sports)
  B. Congenital or developmental
    1. Localized diseases: Legg-Calvé-Perthes, congenital hip dislocation, slipped epiphysis
    2. Mechanical factors: unequal lower extremity length, valgus/varus deformity, hypermobility syndromes
    3. Bone dysplasias: epiphyseal dysplasia, spondyloepiphyseal dysplasia, osteonychodystrophy
  C. Metabolic
    1. Ochronosis (alkaptonuria)
    2. Hemochromatosis
    3. Wilson's disease
    4. Gaucher's disease
  D. Endocrine
    1. Acromegaly
    2. Hyperparathyroidism
    3. Diabetes mellitus
    4. Obesity
    5. Hypothyroidism
  E. Calcium deposition diseases
    1. Calcium pyrophosphate dihydrate deposition
    2. Apatite arthropathy
  F. Other bone and joint diseases
    1. Localized: fracture, avascular necrosis, infection, gout
    2. Diffuse: rheumatoid (inflammatory) arthritis, Paget's disease, osteopetrosis, osteochondritis
  G. Neuropathic (Charcot joints)
  H. Endemic
    1. Kashin-Beck
    2. Mseleni
  I. Miscellaneous
    1. Frostbite
    2. Caisson's disease
    3. Hemoglobinopathies

Source: From HJ Mankin et al: J Rheumatol 13:1127, 1986, with permission.

differences in joint usage related to life-style or occupation is unknown.

In some cases, the relation of heredity to OA is less ambiguous. Thus, the mother and sister of a woman with distal interphalangeal (DIP) joint OA (Heberden's nodes) are, respectively, two to three times as likely to exhibit OA in these joints as the mother and sister of an unaffected woman. Association analyses have identified several candidate genes encoding structural proteins of the extracellular matrix of cartilage and bone and implicated in regulation of bone density. However, no mutation has been identified in the common primary (i.e.,

idiopathic) form of OA. Most of the mutations identified are associated with relatively rare syndromes, a feature of which can be classified as secondary OA. Mutations in COL2A1 genes, for example, have been associated with clinical phenotypes ranging from mild spondyloepiphyseal dysplasia to severe generalized OA, with onset at an early age. It is likely that classifications of "common OA" will eventually be developed based on causative gene defect rather than on variable clinical phenotypes. This could permit the development of tests permitting the diagnosis of molecular defects and, ideally, prophylactic therapy.

Age is the most powerful risk factor for OA. In a radiographic survey of women <45 years, only 2% had OA; between the ages of 45 and 64 years, however, the prevalence was 30%, and for those >65 years it was 68%. In males, the figures were similar, but somewhat lower, in the older age groups.

Major trauma and repetitive joint use are also important risk factors for OA. Anterior cruciate ligament insufficiency or meniscus damage (and meniscectomy) may lead to knee OA. Although damage to the articular cartilage may occur at the time of injury or subsequently, with use of the affected joint, even normal cartilage will degenerate if the joint is unstable. A person with a trimalleolar fracture will almost certainly develop ankle OA. The pattern of joint involvement in OA is influenced by prior vocational or avocational overload. Thus, although ankle OA is common in ballet dancers, elbow OA in baseball pitchers, and metacarpophalangeal joint OA in prize fighters, OA is not very common at any of these sites in the general population.

Given the growing participation of the population of the United States in cardiovascular fitness programs, it is important to note that, if major trauma is excluded, there are no convincing data to support an association between specific nonprofessional athletic activities and arthritis. Neither long-distance running nor jogging has been shown to cause OA. This apparent lack of association may, however, be due to the lack of good long-term studies, the difficulty in retrospective assessment of activities, and selection bias, i.e., early discontinuation of the activity by those incurring joint damage. In contrast, vocational activities, such as those performed by jackhammer operators, cotton mill and shipyard workers, and coal miners, may lead to OA in the joints exposed to repetitive occupational use. Men whose jobs required knee bending and at least moderate physical demands had a higher rate of radiographic evidence of knee OA, and more severe radiographic changes, than men whose jobs required neither.

Obesity is a risk factor for both knee and hand OA. For those in the highest quintile for body mass index at baseline examination, the relative risk for developing knee OA in the ensuing 36 years was 1.5 for men and 2.1 for women. For *severe* knee OA, the relative risk rose to 1.9 for men and 3.2 for women, suggesting that obesity plays an even larger role in the etiology of the most serious cases of knee OA. Obese subjects who have not yet developed OA can reduce their risk: A weight loss of only 5 kg was associated with a 50% reduction in the odds of developing symptomatic knee OA.

The correlation between the pathologic severity of OA and symptoms is poor. Many people with radiographic changes of advanced OA have no symptoms. The risk factors for *pain and disability* in affected individuals are poorly understood. Disability in subjects with knee OA is more strongly associated with quadriceps muscle weakness than with joint pain or radiographic severity. For the same degree of path-

TABLE 312-2   Risk Factors for OA

Age	Repetitive stress, e.g., vocational[a]
Female sex	Obesity[a]
Race	Congenital/developmental defects[a]
Genetic factors	Prior inflammatory joint disease
Major joint trauma[a]	Metabolic/endocrine disorders

[a] Potentially modifiable.

Source: Adapted from M Hochberg: J Rheumatol 18:1438, 1991, with permission.

FIGURE 312-1 *A.* Normal articular cartilage. Note the intact surface and even distribution of chondrocytes. Mitotic figures are not present in normal adult articular cartilage. *B.* Osteoarthritic cartilage. Note the disruption of surface integrity, with vertical fissures (fibrillation) and irregular distribution of cells. Many of the chondrocytes have replicated and exist in clusters. Stained with safranin-O, which binds to the sulfated glycosaminoglycan chains of proteoglycans. Note patchy areas of diminished staining (pale extracellular matrix) due to proteoglycan depletion.

ologic severity, women are more likely to be symptomatic than men, those on welfare more likely than those who are working, and those who are divorced more likely than those who are married. For patients who had poor social support, periodic phone calls from a trained lay interviewer were as effective as a nonsteroidal anti-inflammatory drug (NSAID) in reducing joint pain, emphasizing the importance of psychosocial factors as determinants of pain.

PATHOLOGY Although the cardinal pathologic feature of OA is a progressive loss of articular cartilage, OA is not a disease of only the cartilage but a disease of an *organ*, the synovial joint, in which all of the tissues are affected: subchondral bone, synovium, meniscus, ligaments, and supporting neuromuscular apparatus as well as the cartilage.

The most striking morphologic changes in OA are usually seen in load-bearing areas of the articular cartilage. In the early stages the cartilage is thicker than normal, but with progression of OA the joint surface thins, the cartilage softens, the integrity of the surface is breached, and vertical clefts develop (fibrillation) (Fig. 312-1). Deep cartilage ulcers, extending to bone, may appear. Areas of fibrocartilaginous repair may develop, but these are inferior to pristine hyaline articular cartilage in their ability to withstand mechanical stress. All of the cartilage is metabolically active and the chondrocytes replicate, forming clusters (clones). Later, however, the cartilage becomes hypocellular.

Remodeling and hypertrophy of bone are major features of OA. Appositional bone growth occurs in the subchondral region, leading to the bony "sclerosis" seen radiographically. The abraded bone under a cartilage ulcer may take on the appearance of ivory (eburnation). Growth of cartilage and bone at the joint margins leads to osteophytes (spurs), which alter the contour of the joint and may restrict movement. A patchy chronic synovitis and thickening of the joint capsule may further restrict movement. Periarticular muscle wasting is common and may play a major role in symptoms and, as indicated above, in disability.

PATHOGENESIS The main load on articular cartilage—the major target tissue in OA—is generated by the contraction of the muscles that stabilize or move the joint. Although cartilage is an excellent shock absorber in terms of its bulk properties, at most sites it is only 1 to 2 mm thick—too thin to serve as the sole shock-absorbing structure in the joint. Additional protective mechanisms are provided by the subchondral bone and periarticular muscles.

Articular cartilage serves two essential functions within the joint, both of which are mechanical. First, it provides a remarkably smooth bearing surface, so that the bones glide effortlessly over each other with joint movement. With synovial fluid as lubricant, the coefficient of friction for cartilage rubbed against cartilage, even under physiologic loading, is 15 times lower than that of two ice cubes passed across each other! Second, articular cartilage prevents the concentration of stresses so the bones do not shatter when the joint is loaded.

OA develops in either of two settings: (1) the biomaterial properties of the articular cartilage and subchondral bone are normal, but excessive loading of the joint causes the tissues to fail; or (2) the applied load is reasonable, but the material properties of the cartilage or bone are inferior.

Although articular cartilage is highly resistant to wear under conditions of repeated oscillation, repetitive impact loading soon leads to joint failure. This fact accounts for the high prevalence of OA at specific sites related to vocational or avocational overloading. In general, the earliest changes occur at the sites in the joint that are subject to the greatest compressive loads. Some cases of so-called idiopathic OA of the hip may be due to subtle congenital or developmental defects, such as congenital subluxation/dislocation, acetabular dysplasia, Legg-Calvé-Perthes disease, or slipped capital femoral epiphysis, which increase joint congruity and concentrate the dynamic load.

Clinical conditions that reduce the ability of the cartilage or subchondral bone to deform are associated with development of OA. In ochronosis, for example, accumulation of homogentisic acid polymers leads to stiffening of the cartilage; in osteopetrosis, stiffness of the subchondral trabeculae occurs. In both conditions, severe generalized OA is usually apparent by the age of 40 years. If the subchondral bone is stiffened experimentally, repetitive impact loading soon leads to breakdown of the overlying cartilage. Conversely, osteoporosis, in which the bone is abnormally soft, may protect against OA.

The Extracellular Matrix of Normal Articular Cartilage Articular cartilage is composed of two major macromolecular species: proteoglycans (PGs), which are responsible for the compressive stiffness of the tissue and its ability to withstand load, and collagen, which provides tensile strength and resistance to shear. Although lysomal proteases (cathepsins) have been demonstrated within the cells and matrix of normal articular cartilage, their low pH optimum makes it likely that the proteoglycanase activity of these enzymes will be confined to intracellular sites or the immediate pericellular area. However, cartilage also contains a family of matrix metalloproteinases (MMPs), including stromelysin, collagenase, and gelatinase, which can degrade all the components of the extracellular matrix at neutral pH. Each is secreted by the chondrocyte as a latent proenzyme that must be activated by proteolytic cleavage of its N-terminal sequence. The level of MMP activity in the cartilage at any given time represents the balance between activation of the proenzyme and inhibition of the active enzyme by tissue inhibitors. Much of the total tissue pool of aggrecan, the major PG in articular cartilage, is degraded by a proteinase, which cleaves the protein core of the molecule at a site distinct from the cleavage site of the MMP. The enzyme responsible for this cleavage is referred to as *aggrecanase*.

The turnover of normal cartilage is affected through a degradative cascade; the driving force appears to be interleukin (IL) 1, a cytokine produced by mononuclear cells (including synovial lining cells) and synthesized by chondrocytes. IL-1 stimulates the synthesis and secretion of the latent MMPs and of tissue plasminogen activator. Plasminogen, the substrate for the latter enzyme, may be synthesized by the chondrocyte or may enter the cartilage from the synovial fluid. Both plasminogen and stromelysin may play a role in activation of the latent MMPs. In addition to its catabolic effect on cartilage, IL-1 suppresses PG synthesis by the chondrocyte, inhibiting matrix repair (see below). The major proteinases involved in degradation of matrix of human articular cartilage appear to be collagenase-3 (MMP-13) and aggrecanase-1 (ADAMTS4). Control of MMP-13 activity appears to be exerted via transcriptional activation by cytokines and activation of the pro-form at the cell surface. The transcriptional activity is mediated primarily through the p38 mitogen-activated protein kinase pathway, but also involves nuclear factor kappa B. Interest currently exists in the inhibition of cartilage matrix degradation by therapeutic agents that block the p38-dependant transcriptional activity of MMP-13 expression or control extracellular activation of the secreted form of ADAMTS4.

The balance of the system lies with inhibitors of matrix degrading enzymes, e.g., tissue inhibitor of metalloproteinase (TIMP) and plasminogen activator inhibitor-1 (PAI-1), which are synthesized by the chondrocyte and limit the degradative activity of MMPs and plasminogen activator, respectively. If TIMP or PAI-1 is destroyed or present in concentrations that are insufficient relative to those of active enzymes, stromelysin and plasmin are free to act on matrix substrates. Stromelysin can degrade the protein core of the PG and activate latent collagenase. Conversion of latent stromelysin to an active, highly destructive protease by plasmin provides a second mechanism for matrix degradation.

Polypeptide mediators, e.g., insulin-like growth factor-1 (IGF-1) and transforming growth factor β (TGF-β), stimulate biosynthesis of PGs. They regulate matrix metabolism in normal cartilage and may play a role in matrix repair in OA. These growth factors modulate catabolic as well as anabolic pathways of chondrocyte metabolism; by down-regulating chondrocyte receptors for IL-1, they may decrease PG degradation. In addition to its responsiveness to cytokines and a variety of other biologic mediators, chondrocyte metabolism in normal cartilage can be modulated directly by mechanical loading. Whereas static loading inhibits synthesis of PGs and protein, loads of relatively brief duration may stimulate matrix biosynthesis.

Pathophysiology of Cartilage Changes in OA Most investigators feel that the primary changes in OA begin in the cartilage. A change in the arrangement and size of the collagen fibers is apparent. Biochemical data are consistent with the presence of a defect in the collagen network of the matrix, perhaps due to disruption of the "glue" that binds adjacent fibers. This is among the earliest matrix changes observed and appears to be irreversible.

Although "wear" may be a factor in the loss of cartilage, strong evidence supports the concept that MMPs account for much of the loss of cartilage matrix in OA. Whether their synthesis and secretion are stimulated by IL-1 or by other factors (e.g., mechanical stimuli), MMPs, plasmin, and cathepsins all appear to be involved in the breakdown of articular cartilage in OA. TIMP and PAI-1 may work to stabilize the system, at least temporarily, while growth factors such as IGF-1 and TGF-β are implicated in repair processes that may heal the lesion or, at least, stabilize the process. A stoichiometric imbalance exists between the levels of active enzyme and the level of TIMP, which may be only modestly increased.

Nitric oxide (NO) may play a significant role in articular cartilage damage in OA insofar as NO stimulates synthesis of MMPs by chondrocytes. Chondrocytes are a major source of NO, the synthesis of which is stimulated by IL-1 and tumor necrosis factor and by shear stress. In an experimental model of OA, treatment with a selective inhibitor of inducible NO synthase reduced the severity of cartilage damage.

The chondrocytes in OA cartilage undergo active cell division and are very active metabolically, producing increased quantities of DNA, RNA collagen, PG, and noncollagenous proteins. For this reason, it is inaccurate to call OA *degenerative* joint disease. Prior to cartilage loss and PG depletion, this marked biosynthetic activity may lead to an increase in PG concentration, which may be associated with thickening

of the cartilage and a stage of homeostasis referred to as *compensated OA.* These mechanisms may maintain the joint in a reasonably functional state for years. The repair tissue, however, often does not hold up as well under mechanical stresses as does normal hyaline cartilage and eventually, at least in some cases, the rate of PG synthesis falls and "end-stage" OA develops, with full-thickness loss of cartilage.

Traumatic joint injury is a risk factor for secondary OA (Table 312-1). Mechanical injury to articular cartilage in vitro results in swelling, alteration in biomechanical properties, cell death, changes in biosynthesis of matrix macromolecules, loss of PGs, degradation of collagen, and an increase in MMP gene expression.

The extent to which the above changes are due to direct mechanical damage versus cell-mediated degradation is unclear. Injury may result in increased responsiveness of the chondrocyte to stimulation by cytokines. On the other hand, it may facilitate diffusion of cytokines into the matrix. In contrast to knee cartilage, glycosaminoglycan loss from ankle cartilage is not increased after mechanical injury of the tissue and exposure to cytokines. Chondrocytes in articular cartilage from some joints may react differently to cytokines, mechanical forces, and growth factors than to those in other joints, perhaps accounting for the lower incidence of OA in some joints than in others, e.g., ankle vs. knee.

CLINICAL FEATURES The joint pain of OA is often described as a deep ache localized to the involved joint. Typically, it is aggravated by joint use and relieved by rest but, as the disease progresses, it may become persistent. Nocturnal pain, interfering with sleep, is seen particularly in advanced OA of the hip and may be enervating. Stiffness of the involved joint after a period of inactivity (e.g., a night's sleep or automobile ride) may be prominent but usually lasts <20 min. Systemic manifestations are not a feature of primary OA.

Because articular cartilage is aneural, the joint pain in OA must arise from other structures (Table 312-3). In some cases it may be due to stretching of nerve endings in the periosteum covering osteophytes; in others, to microfractures in subchondral bone or medullary hypertension caused by distortion of blood flow by thickened subchondral trabeculae. Joint instability, leading to stretching of the joint capsule, and muscle spasm may also be sources of pain.

In some patients with OA, joint pain may be due to synovitis. In advanced OA, histologic evidence of synovial inflammation may be as marked as that in synovium of a patient with rheumatoid arthritis (Chap. 301). Synovitis in OA may be due to phagocytosis of shards of cartilage and bone from the abraded joint surface (wear particles), release from the cartilage of soluble matrix macromolecules, or crystals of calcium pyrophosphate or hydroxyapatite. In other cases, immune complexes, containing antigens derived from cartilage matrix, may be sequestered in collagenous tissues of the joint, leading to low-grade chronic synovitis. In contrast, in the earlier stages of OA, synovial inflammation may be absent, suggesting that the joint pain is due to one of the other factors mentioned above.

Physical examination of the OA joint may reveal localized tenderness and bony or soft tissue swelling. Bony crepitus (the sensation of bone rubbing against bone, evoked by joint movement) is characteristic. Synovial effusions, if present, are usually not large. Palpation may reveal some warmth over the joint. Periarticular muscle atrophy may be due to disuse or reflex inhibition of muscle contraction. In the

TABLE 312-3 *Causes of Joint Pain and Patients with OA*

Source	Mechanism
Synovium	Inflammation
Subchondral bone	Medullary hypertension, microfractures
Osteophyte	Stretching of periosteal nerve endings
Ligaments	Stretch
Capsule	Inflammation, distention
Muscle	Spasm

advanced stages of OA, there may be gross deformity, bony hypertrophy, subluxation, and marked loss of joint motion. The notion that OA is inexorably progressive, however, is incorrect. In many patients, the disease stabilizes; in some, regression of joint pain and even of radiographic changes occur.

Although the diagnosis of OA is often straightforward, because of the high prevalence of radiographic changes of OA in asymptomatic individuals, it is important to ensure that joint pain in a patient with radiographic evidence of OA is not due to some other cause, such as soft tissue rheumatism (e.g., anserine bursitis at the knee, trochanteric bursitis at the hip), radiculopathy, referral of pain from another joint (25% of patients with hip disease have pain referred to the knee), entrapment neuropathy, vascular disease (claudication), or some other type of arthritis (e.g., crystal-induced synovitis, septic arthritis). It is usually not difficult to differentiate OA from a systemic rheumatic disease, such as rheumatoid arthritis, because joint involvement in the latter disease is usually symmetric and polyarticular, with arthritis in wrists and metacarpophalangeal joints (sites not usually involved in OA), and constitutional features, such as prolonged morning stiffness, fatigue, weight loss, or fever, may be seen.

LABORATORY AND RADIOGRAPHIC FINDINGS The diagnosis of OA is usually based on clinical and radiographic features. In the early stages, the radiograph may be normal but joint space narrowing becomes evident as articular cartilage is lost. Other characteristic findings include subchondral bone sclerosis, subchondral cysts, and osteophytosis. A change in the contour of the joint, due to bony remodeling, and subluxation may be seen. Although tibiofemoral joint space narrowing has been considered to be a radiographic surrogate for articular cartilage thinning, joint space narrowing alone does not accurately indicate the status of the articular cartilage in patients with early OA who do not have radiographic evidence of bony changes (e.g., subchondral sclerosis or cysts, osteophytes). Similarly, osteophytosis alone, in the absence of other radiographic features of OA, may be due to aging rather than OA. As indicated above, there is often great disparity between the severity of radiographic findings, severity of symptoms, and functional ability in OA; while >90% of persons over age 40 have some radiographic changes of OA in weight-bearing joints, only 30% are symptomatic.

No laboratory studies are diagnostic for OA, but laboratory testing may help identify an underlying causes of secondary OA. Because primary OA is not systemic, the erythrocyte sedimentation rate, serum chemistry determinations, blood counts, and urinalysis are normal. Synovial fluid analysis reveals mild leukocytosis (<2000 white blood cells per microliter), with a predominance of mononuclear cells. Synovial fluid analysis is of particular value in excluding other conditions, such as calcium pyrophosphate dihydrate deposition disease (Chap. 313), gout (Chap. 313) or septic arthritis (Chap. 314).

Prior to the appearance of radiographic changes, the ability to clinically diagnose OA without an invasive procedure (e.g., arthroscopy) is limited. Magnetic resonance imaging and ultrasonography have not been sufficiently validated to justify their routine clinical use for diagnosis of OA or monitoring disease progression.

OA AT SPECIFIC JOINT SITES ■ Interphalangeal Joints Heberden's nodes (bony enlargement of the DIP joint) are the most common form of idiopathic OA (Fig. 312-2). A similar process at the proximal interphalangeal joints leads to Bouchard's nodes. Often, these nodes develop gradually, with little or no discomfort, and usually do not interfere significantly with function. However, they may present acutely with pain, redness, and swelling, sometimes triggered by minor trauma. Gelatinous dorsal cysts may develop at the insertion of the digital extensor tendon into the base of the distal phalanx.

EROSIVE OA In erosive OA, DIP and/or proximal interphalangeal joints of the hand are most prominently affected. Erosive OA is more destructive than typical nodal OA; x-ray evidence of collapse of the subchondral plate is characteristic, and bony ankylosis may occur. De-

FIGURE 312-2 Nodal osteoarthritis. Note bony enlargement of distal and proximal interphalangeal joints (Heberden's nodes and Bouchard's nodes, respectively). *(Reprinted from the Clinical Slide Collection on the Rheumatic Diseases, 1991, 1995. Reproduced with permission of the American College of Rheumatology.)*

formity and functional impairment may be severe. The synovium is much more extensively infiltrated with mononuclear cells than in other forms of OA.

GENERALIZED OA Generalized OA is characterized by involvement of three or more joints or groups of joints (DIP and proximal interphalangeal joints are counted as one group each). Heberden's and Bouchard's nodes are prominent. "Flare-ups" of inflammation may be marked by soft tissue swelling, redness, and warmth. The erthryocyte sedimentation rate may be elevated, but serum rheumatoid factor tests are negative.

Thumb Base The second most frequent area of involvement in OA is the thumb base. Swelling, tenderness, and crepitus on movement of the joint and loss of motion and strength are common. Osteophytes may lead to a "squared" appearance (Fig. 312-3). Pain with pinch leads to adduction of the thumb and contracture of the first web space, often resulting in compensatory hyperextension of the first metacarpophalangeal joint and swan-neck deformity of the thumb.

Hip Congenital or developmental defects of the hip (e.g., acetabular dysplasia, Legg-Calvé-Perthes disease, slipped capital epiphysis) can lead to OA. Pain from hip OA is generally referred to the inguinal area but may be referred to the buttock or proximal thigh. Less commonly, hip OA presents as knee pain. Pain can be evoked by putting the involved hip through its range of motion. Flexion may be painless initially, but internal rotation will exacerbate pain. Loss of internal rotation occurs early, followed by loss of extension, adduction, and flexion due to capsular fibrosis and/or buttressing osteophytes.

Knee OA of the knee may involve the medial or lateral femorotibial compartment and/or the patellofemoral compartment. Palpation may

FIGURE 312-3 Osteoarthritis of the first carpometacarpal joint. Note the squared appearance of the thumb base, due to bony enlargement and remodeling of the joint.

reveal bony hypertrophy (osteophytes) and tenderness. Effusions, if present, are generally small. Joint movement commonly elicits bony crepitus. OA in the medial compartment may result in a varus (bow-leg) deformity; OA in the lateral compartment may produce a valgus (knock-knee) deformity. A positive "shrug" sign (pain with manual compression of the patella against the femur during quadriceps contraction) may be a sign of patellofemoral OA.

Chondromalacia patellae, which is also characterized by anterior knee pain and a positive shrug sign, is a syndrome of patellofemoral pain in teenagers and young adults. It is more common in females. It may be caused by a variety of factors (e.g., abnormal quadriceps angle, patella alta, trauma). Although exploration of the knee may reveal softening and fibrillation of cartilage on the posterior aspect of the patella, this change is usually not progressive; chondromalacia patellae is usually not a precursor of OA. In most cases, analgesics or NSAIDs and physical therapy are effective; in some, pain may be relieved by surgical correction of patellar malalignment.

Spine OA of the spine can involve the apophyseal joints, intervertebral disks, and paraspinous ligaments. *Spondylosis* refers to degenerative disk disease. The diagnosis of spinal OA should be reserved for patients with involvement of the apophyseal joints, and not only disk degeneration. Symptoms of spinal OA include localized pain and stiffness. Nerve root compression by an osteophyte blocking a neural foramen, prolapse of a degenerated disk, or subluxation of an apophyseal joint may cause radicular pain and motor weakness.

Marked calcification and ossification of paraspinous ligaments occur in diffuse idiopathic skeletal hyperostosis (DISH), which must be distinguished from OA. Although DISH is often categorized as a variant of OA, the diarthrodial joints are not involved. In radiographs, ligamentous calcification and ossification in the anterior spinal ligaments give the appearance of "flowing wax" on the anterior vertebral bodies. However, a radiolucency may be seen between the newly deposited bone and the vertebral body, differentiating DISH from the marginal osteophytes in spondylosis. Intervertebral disk spaces are preserved, and sacroiliac and apophyseal joints appear normal, helping to differentiate DISH from spondylosis and from ankylosing spondylitis, respectively. DISH occurs in the middle-aged and elderly and is more common in men than in women. Patients are frequently asymptomatic but may have musculoskeletal stiffness. The radiographic changes are generally much more severe than might be predicted from the mild symptoms.

℞ TREATMENT

Treatment of OA is aimed at reducing pain, maintaining mobility, and minimizing disability. The vigor of the therapeutic intervention should be dictated by the severity of the condition in the individual patient. For those with only mild disease, reassurance, instruction in joint protection, and an occasional analgesic may be all that is required; for those with more severe OA, especially of knee or hip, a comprehensive program comprising a spectrum of nonpharmacologic measures supplemented by an analgesic and/or NSAID is appropriate.

Nonpharmacologic Measures ■ *REDUCTION OF JOINT LOADING* OA may be caused or aggravated by poor body mechanics. Correction of poor posture and a support for excessive lumbar lordosis can be helpful. Excessive loading of the involved joint should be avoided. Patients with knee or hip OA should avoid prolonged standing, kneeling, and squatting. Obese patients should be counseled to lose weight. In patients with medial compartment knee OA, a wedged insole may decrease joint pain.

Rest periods during the day may be of benefit, but complete immobilization of the painful joint is rarely indicated, except in cases of hand OA. For DIP joint OA that is so painful that it interferes with hand function, a custom-molded thermoplastic splint that blocks flexion can reduce pain, improve overall hand function, and reduce muscle spasm. Splinting can also be very effective for trapeziometacarpal joint and pantrapezial OA. Rigid immobilization is not an acceptable long-term option for pain in the proximal interphalangeal joints, however,

because it limits hand function and can result in shortening of the collateral ligaments. In patients with unilateral OA of the hip or knee, a cane, held in the contralateral hand, may reduce joint pain by reducing the joint contact forces. Bilateral disease may necessitate use of crutches or a walker.

PATELLAR TAPING OA of the patellofemoral compartment can cause severe pain, especially with kneeling, squatting, or climbing stairs. Medial taping of the patella can significantly reduce pain in such cases. The taping procedure is simple and inexpensive and patients can learn to apply their own tape after minimal instruction. The prompt relief of symptoms that may be achieved by taping may be maintained by isometric exercises to strengthen the vastus medialis obliquus component of the quadriceps muscle, facilitating realignment of the patella on a long-term basis.

WEDGED INSOLES/ORTHOSES In patients with medial compartment knee OA, pain severity has been shown to be related to the magnitude of the external adduction moment (a measure of the varus torque on the knee during gait). Wedged insoles may be useful in conservative treatment of OA of the medial tibial femoral compartment. Their use may change the spatial position of the lower limb so that the mechanical axis becomes more nearly vertical and the calcaneal axis is shifted to a valgus position with respect to the tibiotalar joint, reducing excessive loading on the medial compartment of the knee and strain on the lateral collateral ligament. Use of lateral wedged insoles may result in a significant decrease in NSAID consumption by patients with knee OA. A polypropylene mesh insole is practical, inexpensive, and washable and may last about 2 years, i.e., approximately twice as long as a leather insole.

THERMAL MODALITIES Application of heat to the OA joint may reduce pain and stiffness. A variety of modalities are available; often, the least expensive and most convenient is a hot shower or bath. Occasionally, better analgesia may be obtained with ice than with heat.

EXERCISE Those who exercise regularly live longer and are healthier than those who are sedentary. Because OA of weight-bearing joints limits physical activity and the amount of exercise that an individual can perform, persons with this condition are at increased risk for hypertension, obesity, diabetes, and cardiovascular disease, i.e., diseases related to their inactivity. Only 24% of individuals with arthritis report a level of physical activity sufficient to achieve health; 75% do nothing or are not sufficiently active. Arthritis is *the* major reason that elderly individuals are not active or limit their activity and is a greater factor in limiting activity than heart disease, hypertension, blindness, or diabetes. Studies of cardiovascular health have shown that the aerobic capacity (cardiovascular fitness) of men with severe knee OA is >30% lower than that of controls who do not have OA. Even at slow speed, individuals with knee OA expend more energy (measured as oxygen consumption) in walking than age- and sex-matched controls.

Disability in patients with OA may have more to do with their ability to remain active and physically fit and maintain normal body weight than with pathologic changes in the OA joint. Even if we cannot cure OA, we can cure inactivity. Men in their forties who were not performing sufficient physical activity and had low scores on a treadmill test were found to have remarkably higher death rates than those who were fit. However, among those who were not fit at the outset but who *became* fit, the risk of mortality decreased by 44%.

The amount of *aerobic conditioning* (e.g., walking, cycling, aquatic exercise) necessary for cardiovascular fitness is not so great that it cannot be achieved by people with OA. Patients with OA of lower extremity joints who are able to perform moderate to vigorous exercise at least 3 days per week (i.e., 70 to 85% of maximal heart rate)—an intensity that permits an individual to talk while exercising continuously for 20 to 60 min—improve their fitness and health without exacerbating their joint pain or increasing their need for analgesic drugs. Persons with OA who exercise consistently at this level report decreases in joint pain and disability while improving their cardiovascular muscular fitness (strength and endurance). They also report improvement in function and quality of life and exhibit improved gait and walking speed. Patients with hip or knee OA can participate safely in conditioning exercises to improve fitness and health without increasing their joint pain or need for analgesics or NSAIDs.

Disuse of the OA joint because of pain will lead to muscle atrophy. Because periarticular muscles play a major role in protecting the articular cartilage from stress, strengthening exercises are important. In patients with knee OA, strengthening of the periarticular muscles may result, within weeks, in a decrease in joint pain as great as that seen with NSAIDs. Most of the information available about the benefits of *therapeutic exercise* relates to strength training. However, the benefits of therapeutic exercise go far beyond muscle strengthening. In studies that employed 4 to 10 instructional sessions followed by self-directed home exercise in which patients initially exercised up to 5 days per week, with recommendations to decrease the frequency over the next 6 months to 2 days per week, compliance was excellent. The results showed that pain, anxiety, and depression decreased, while lower extremity strength, endurance, proprioception, and functional status improved and disability was reduced. With fairly minimal intervention and self directed exercise, patients with OA can achieve and maintain important gains.

PATIENT EDUCATION For effective management of many patients with OA, encouragement, reassurance, advice about exercise, and recommendation of measures to unload the arthritic joint (such as a cane and proper footwear) may be all that is required. Patient education programs offer benefits beyond those that can be achieved with an NSAID in symptomatic treatment of patients with OA. Patient education interventions provide an additive benefit 20 to 30% as great as that of NSAID treatment alone. Relevant education for the patient with OA is not education about joint anatomy or the definition of an osteophyte but is education in *self-management* that emphasizes the central role of the patient in managing the disease; furthermore, it teaches the skills required to permit patients to manage medically and emotionally and to maintain their role in society.

A variety of self-management programs have been developed for patients with OA, such as the Arthritis Self-Management Program that is sponsored in the United States by the Arthritis Foundation. Participation in a structured community-based education intervention, led by trained lay leaders, can result in significant decreases in pain, disability, and depression. Patients who participate in such programs report greater performance of self-management behaviors, e.g., taking their medication properly, communicating with their healthcare providers. Furthermore, the benefits may endure for years, even with no reinforcement of the intervention.

TIDAL IRRIGATION OF THE KNEE Copious irrigation of the OA knee through a large-bore needle, flushing out fibrin, cartilage shards, and other debris, has been reported to provide months of comfort for some patient whose joint pain has been refractory to analgesics, NSAIDs, and intraarticular glucocorticoid injections. However, results of a randomized controlled trial of patients with knee OA that included a sham-irrigation procedure led to the conclusion that the bulk of the benefit from this procedure is attributable to the placebo effect.

ARTHROSCOPIC DEBRIDEMENT AND LAVAGE Arthroscopic surgery can be helpful in alleviating knee pain and improving function in the subgroup of patients with knee OA in whom loose bodies, flaps of cartilage, or disruption of the meniscus (e.g., a bucket handle tear) cause mechanical symptoms, such as locking, giving way of the limb, or catching. Although arthroscopic debridement, e.g., smoothing of the surface of fibrillated articular cartilage or meniscus, trimming of osteophytes, and removal of inflamed synovium, is employed widely in patients with symptomatic knee OA who do not have mechanical symptoms, but who have not benefited from pharmacologic therapy,

this therapeutic modality appears to be of no greater symptomatic benefit than placebo in such patients.

Pharmacologic Therapy ■ *NSAIDs AND ACETAMINOPHEN (N-ACETYL-p-AMINOPHENOL, APAP)* Drug therapy for OA today is palliative; no pharmacologic agent has been shown to prevent, delay the progression of, or reverse the pathologic changes of OA in humans. Although claims have been made that some NSAIDs slow the rate of cartilage damage, adequately controlled clinical trials in humans with OA to support this view are lacking.

In management of OA pain, pharmacologic agents should be used as adjuncts to nonpharmacologic measures, such as those described above. The latter are the *keystone* of OA treatment. Although NSAIDs often decrease joint pain and improve mobility in OA, the magnitude of improvement is generally modest—on average, about 30% reduction in pain and 15% improvement in function. Many patients taking a full therapeutic dose of NSAIDs continue to experience a significant level of residual joint pain. On the other hand, low (i.e., analgesic) doses of NSAIDs may be as effective as anti-inflammatory doses; 30 to 40% of patients with OA may find APAP—an analgesic recommended for treatment of mild-moderate pain—as effective as an NSAID. Even in patients with clinical signs of joint inflammation (synovial effusion, tenderness), relief of joint pain by APAP may be as effective as that achieved with an NSAID. Nonetheless, if simple analgesics are inadequate, it is reasonable to prescribe an NSAID for the patient with OA.

However, concern over the use of NSAIDs in OA has grown in recent years because of the adverse effects of these agents, especially those related to the gastrointestinal tract. Those at greatest risk for OA, i.e., the elderly, appear to be at greater risk than younger individuals for gastrointestinal symptoms, ulceration, hemorrhage, and death as a result of NSAID use. The annual rate of hospitalization for peptic ulcer disease among elderly current NSAID users was 16 per 1000, i.e., four times greater than that for persons not taking an NSAID. Among people age ≥65, as many as 30% of all hospitalizations and deaths related to peptic ulcer disease have been attributed to NSAID use. Risk factors for hemorrhage and other ulcer complications associated with NSAID use include, in addition to age, a history of peptic ulcer disease or of upper gastrointestinal bleeding, concomitant use of glucocorticoids or anticoagulants, and, possibly, smoking and alcohol consumption (Table 312-4).

SELECTIVE COX-2 INHIBITORS In patients who carry risk factors for an NSAID-associated gastrointestinal catastrophe, a cyclooxygenase (COX)-2 selective NSAID may be preferable to even a low dose of a nonselective COX inhibitor. In contrast to the nonselective NSAIDs, all of which inhibit COX-1 as well as COX-2, selective COX-2 inhibitors, e.g., celecoxib, rofecoxib, valdecoxib, are now available. These exhibit no greater efficacy than nonselective NSAIDs, but endoscopic studies show that they are associated with a lower incidence of gastroduodenal ulcer than nonselective NSAIDs. Of additional advantage with respect to the issue of upper gastrointestinal bleeding, selective COX-2 inhibitors do not have a clinically significant effect on platelet aggregation or bleeding time.

Results of two large-size gastrointestinal safety studies, the CLASS trial and VIGOR study, have been published (Table 312-5). Both were designed to ascertain whether treatment with celecoxib or rofecoxib, respectively, resulted in a lower incidence of clinically important NSAID-associated ulcers and ulcer complications than that seen with

TABLE 312-4 *Risk Factors for Upper Gastrointestinal Adverse Events in Patients Taking NSAIDs*

Increasing age	History of upper gastrointestinal
Comorbidity (poor or fair general	bleeding
health)	Anticoagulation
Oral glucocorticoids	Combination NSAID therapy
History of peptic ulcer	Increasing NSAID dose

Note: NSAID, nonsteroidal anti-inflammatory drug.

nonselective NSAIDs. In the VIGOR trial, a clear reduction in the incidence of upper gastrointestinal events was apparent in the rofecoxib treatment arm, in comparison with the naproxen arm. The risk of all clinical upper gastrointestinal events was reduced by some 54% ($p < .01$), of complicated upper gastrointestinal events by 57% ($p = .005$), and of any gastrointestinal bleeding by 62% ($p < .01$). In the CLASS study, the annualized incidence rates of ulcer complications (the primary outcome measure) with celecoxib was not significantly different from that and with the comparator nonselective NSAIDs after 6 months of treatment, although the difference for ulcer complications combined with symptomatic ulcers was significant (2.08% vs 3.54%, respectively, $p = .02$). Although a significant reduction in ulcer complications was seen with celecoxib, use of low-dose aspirin for cardiovascular prophylaxis appeared to mitigate the gastroprotective effect of celecoxib. (Although only 22% of subjects in the CLASS study were taking low-dose aspirin, as many as 60% of patients with OA >60 years old may do so in clinical practice.) Furthermore, the superiority of celecoxib observed among nonaspirin users during the first 6 months was not sustained in patients treated for 12 months.

Unexpectedly, the incidence of myocardial infarction (MI) in the VIGOR study was fourfold greater among patients treated with rofecoxib than with naproxen. Although (1) the absolute number of MIs was small; (2) the study was not powered to compare the effects of the two treatments on MI; (3) the comparability of the treatment groups with respect to the prevalence of risk factors for MI (e.g., obesity, smoking, hypercholesterolemia, diabetes mellitus) was unknown; (4) the dose of rofecoxib was two to four times greater than that used for treatment of OA; and (5) the trial was conducted in patients with rheumatoid arthritis, in which the incidence of MI is about twice as great as that in OA. The rofecoxib label contains a caveat about use of this drug in patients predisposed to ischemic heart disease.

GLUCOCORTICOID INJECTION Systemic glucocorticoids have no place in the treatment of OA. However, intra- or periarticular injection of a depot glucocorticoid preparation may provide marked symptomatic relief for weeks to months. Because studies in animal models have suggested that glucocorticoids may produce cartilage damage, and frequent injections of large amounts of steroids have been associated with joint breakdown in humans, the injection should generally not be repeated in a given joint more often than every 4 to 6 months.

INTRAARTICULAR INJECTION OF HYALURONAN Intraarticular injection of hyaluronan has been approved for treatment of patients with knee OA who have failed a program of nonpharmacologic therapy and simple analgesics. Because the duration of benefit following treatment may exceed by many months the synovial half-life of exogenous hyaluronan, the mechanism of action is unclear. However, the placebo response to intraarticular injection of hyaluronan is often large and sustained. For example, the pivotal clinical trial of Hyalgan failed to demonstrate superiority of oral naproxen, 500 mg bid, over intraarticular injections of saline. Furthermore, intraarticular injection of a preparation of the high-molecular-weight hylan (Synvisc) which had been denatured to eliminate its viscoelasticity, was no less efficacious than injection of the intact hylan or non-cross-linked lower molecular weight hyaluronan. Consistent with this observation, no difference in efficacy was observed in a randomized placebo-controlled trial of Synvisc, a lower molecular weight hyaluronan formulation, and placebo.

OPIOIDS Health professionals and patients hold concerns about tolerance and physical and psychological dependence, and many physicians

TABLE 312-5 *Comparison of Study Designs for Rofecoxib (VIGOR) and Celecoxib (CLASS) Gastrointestinal (GI)*

Parameter	Trial	
	VIGOR	CLASS
Number of subjects	8076	7982
Mean age	~58 years	~60 years; ~38% >65 years
Underlying disease	Rheumatoid arthritis	Osteoarthritis 73%, rheumatoid arthritis 27%
Duration of follow-up	Median, 9 months Maximum, 13 months	Median, 9 months Maximum, 13 months
Type of analysis	Intention to treat (includes events within 14 days of last dose of study drug)	Excludes events on day 0–2 and >6 months
Dose of Coxib	Rofecoxib, 50 mg/d	Celecoxib, 400 mg/d
Comparator NSAID	Naproxen, 1000 mg/d	Ibuprofen, 2400 mg/d or diclofenac, 150 mg/d
Low-dose aspirin	Not permitted	22%
Concurrent steroid use	56%	30%
Primary end point	Clinical upper GI events	Complicated ulcers
Secondary end point	Complicated upper GI events	Symptomatic + complicated ulcers

Note: NSAID, nonsteroidal anti-inflammatory drug.
Source: Derived from VIGOR: Bombardier C et al: N Engl J Med 343:1520, 2000, with permission; CLASS: Silverstein F et al: JAMA 284:1247, 2000.

hesitate to prescribe opioids for patients with nonmalignant chronic pain because of concerns about legal action by governmental regulatory authorities. However, the prevalence of narcotic abuse among older people is low: <1% of patients attending methadone maintenance programs are ≥60 years.

For acute flares of OA pain, when APAP or an NSAID does not provide adequate pain relief or is not well tolerated, a weak opioid, e.g., oral codeine, deserves consideration. Because codeine, when taken alone in a dose of 60 mg, is no more effective than 650 mg of aspirin or APAP, it is used in combination with these drugs to treat moderate or moderately severe OA pain.

Opioids may also be useful for chronic OA pain. The major problem associated with the use of chronic opioid therapy for OA pain is the side effects of these agents, e.g., nausea, vomiting, constipation, urinary retention, mental confusion, drowsiness, and respiratory depression. In the elderly, the central nervous system effects of opioids (e.g., dizziness) may have particularly serious consequences. Prescription of either codeine or propoxyphene may increase the risk of hip fracture by 60%. Concurrent use of these opioids and a psychotropic drug (e.g., sedative, antidepressant, antipsychotic) carries a fracture risk 2.6 times as high as that in nonusers of either drug class.

Tramadol hydrochloride is a centrally acting analgesic with a dual mechanism of action: the molecule is a μ-opioid agonist and also inhibits reuptake of norepinephrine and serotonin. Although the affinity of binding to the μ-opioid regimen is some 6000 times lower than that of morphine, the opioid and nonopioid activities are synergistic. In contrast to NSAIDs, tramadol does not inhibit prostaglandin synthesis and has no adverse effects on the gastric mucosa, kidney, or platelet. It is a useful adjunct in patients with OA in whom APAP or a low dose of NSAID is ineffective or contraindications exist to the use of an NSAID. Improvement with tramadol, 200 to 400 mg/d, is comparable to that with ibuprofen, 1200 to 2400 mg/d, in patients with chronic joint pain. Because development of tolerance or dependence appears to be uncommon with long-term administration, tramadol has not been scheduled as a controlled substance. In general, its efficacy and adverse event profile are comparable to those of APAP/codeine. The latter, however, is considerably less expensive.

The frequency and severity of side effects of tramadol may be reduced considerably if treatment is initiated at a very low dose (e.g., 25 mg/d), which can then be increased gradually every few days. However, this "start low, go slow" approach limits the usefulness of the drug in management of acute pain. Because it inhibits the reuptake of serotonin and norepinephrine, tramadol should not generally be given to patients receiving a tricyclic antidepressant, selective serotonin reuptake inhibitor, or monoamine oxidase inhibitor. These combinations have been reported to cause convulsions. Even in the absence of concomitant therapy with the above agents, however, seizures may occasionally occur in some patients taking tramadol.

A combination of tramadol and APAP in a 37.5 mg/325 mg tablet (ULTRACET) has recently become available. It has a more rapid onset of action than tramadol alone and longer duration of action than APAP alone. In subjects with an acute flare of hip or knee OA, who received 1 or 2 tablets of tramadol/APAP qid for 10 days in addition to their usual NSAID therapy, tramadol/APAP was significantly superior to placebo with respect to improvement in joint pain and global assessment by subjects and physicians. However, treatment-related adverse events (e.g., nausea, dizziness, vomiting) were reported in nearly 25% of the tramadol/APAP group, but in only 8% of the placebo group. Furthermore, the above figures may understate the true incidence of adverse events with this formulation, because subjects were excluded from the study if they had previously failed tramadol therapy or had discontinued tramadol because of an adverse event.

RUBEFACIENTS/CAPSAICIN Because use of systemic analgesics and NSAIDs is often accompanied by adverse effects and older individuals with OA often require medication for comorbid conditions (e.g., hypertension, heart disease, diabetes mellitus) and are at increased the risk of serious drug interactions with NSAIDs, topical therapy for management of OA has appeal.

Application of topical irritants to painful joints and muscles and the local heat provided by rubefacients may be beneficial. However, although topical medications are widely used in the United States as over-the-counter preparations, they are not often prescribed for OA in this country, chiefly because evidence of their efficacy is limited. Except for formulations of salicylate, topical NSAIDs have not been approved for use in the United States. It is unclear whether the benefit attributed to their use is mediated through a pharmacologic action, placebo effect, or their action as a rubefacient. Capsaicin cream, which depletes local sensory nerve endings of substance P, may reduce joint pain and tenderness when applied topically by patients with hand or knee OA, even when used as monotherapy, i.e., without NSAIDs or systemic analgesics.

Glucosamine, Chondroitin Sulfate Glucosamine and chondroitin sulfate have recently enjoyed striking popularity for treatment of OA. They are sold widely in pharmacies, supermarkets, and health food stores but are not approved for use in OA by the U.S. Food and Drug Administration. Several studies have shown glucosamine to be superior to placebo and comparable to NSAIDs with respect to efficacy in patients with knee OA, and to have a better safety profile than NSAIDs. However, the efficacy of neither glucosamine nor chondroitin sulfate has been examined in large, well-designed placebo-controlled trials. In a meta-analysis of randomized, double-blind, placebo-controlled studies of glucosamine and chondroitin sulfate, moderate symptomatic benefit was demonstrated for both agents, relative to placebo. In studies of chondroitin sulfate, symptomatic improvement was apparent as long as 12 months after the onset of treatment. However, when only high-quality or large-size trials were considered, the effect sizes for glucosamine and chondroitin sulfate were diminished, i.e., the better the study design, the smaller the therapeutic benefit. In three recent randomized, double-blind trials in which the manufacturer did not have access to the raw data and was not involved in data analysis, glucosamine was no more effective than placebo.

The question arises whether glucosamine is "chondroprotective." Results of two recent randomized clinical trials have led to the suggestion that glucosamine not only improves joint pain in patients with knee OA, but protects against articular cartilage damage, based upon analyses of changes in joint space width in the standing anteroposterior (AP) knee radiograph. However, concern has been expressed about the interpretation of the results of these studies because of limitations of the radiographic methods employed. A multicenter study supported by the National Institutes of Health, the Glucosamine Chondroitin Arthritis Intervention Trial (GAIT), is in progress which is comparing glucosamine, chondroitin sulfate, the combination, and celecoxib with placebo in patients with knee OA. Although the primary outcome measure is joint pain after 6 months of treatment, approximately 50% of the subjects will be maintained on treatment for 2 years and radiographs obtained at baseline will be compared with those obtained after 1 year and 2 years of treatment.

Orthopedic Surgery Joint replacement surgery should be reserved for patients with advanced OA in whom aggressive medical management has failed. In such cases total joint arthroplasty may be remarkably effective in relieving pain and increasing mobility. Osteotomy, which is surgically more conservative than arthroplasty, can eliminate the concentration of peak dynamic loads and may provide effective pain relief in patients with hip or knee OA. It is of greatest benefit when the disease is only moderately advanced.

Cartilage Regeneration Chondroplasty (abrasion arthroplasty) has enjoyed some popularity as treatment for OA, but well-controlled studies of its efficacy are lacking and the fibrocartilage that resurfaces the abraded bone is inferior to normal hyaline cartilage in its ability to withstand mechanical loads. In one study, knee pain and function were not related to the extent of cartilage regeneration 2 years later in patients who had undergone tibial osteotomy for medial compartment knee OA. Autologous chondrocyte transplantation and attempts at cartilage repair using mesenchymal stem cells and autologous osteochondral plugs are currently being used experimentally for repair of focal chondral defects, but have not been proved to be effective in treatment of OA.

A Rational Approach to the Nonsurgical Management of OA Nonpharmacologic management, as described above, is the foundation of treatment of OA pain and is as important, or more important, than drug treatment, which plays an adjunctive or complementary role in management of this disease. Figure 312-4 provides an algorithm that might be applied to treatment of a newly diagnosed patient with knee OA. The progressive levels of treatment are associated with increasing cost, decreasing convenience for the patient, and increasing risk of side effects. The scheme should not be interpreted dogmatically as a fixed progression of steps. Treatment of OA must be individualized, and the treatment program flexible. For example, in some patients it may be reasonable to institute patellar taping or to prescribe a wedged insole on the initial visit, or an intraarticular glucocorticoid injection on a later visit. Maintaining regular contact with the patient, e.g., via periodic telephone calls, may reduce joint pain to a level beyond that which can be achieved with an NSAID alone and this, or some surrogate measure, warrants incorporation into the treatment program.

It is reasonable to prescribe APAP initially, in a dose up to 4000 mg/d, because of its low cost, excellent safety profile, and the fact that it is as efficacious as NSAIDs in many patients with OA when an analgesic is required for treatment of OA pain. If this does not control joint symptoms within a reasonable period of time, a *low dose* of NSAID (e.g., ibuprofen, 1200 mg/d; naproxen, 500 mg/d) may be substituted for, or added to, the APAP. In patients with significant risk factors for a serious upper gastrointestinal adverse event, if a nonselective NSAID is used, even in a low dose, it is reasonable to recommend coadministration of a gastroprotective agent, such as misoprostol or a proton pump inhibitor, which have been shown by endoscopy to be effective in treating and preventing NSAID gastropathy. Because the risk of an NSAID-associated gastrointestinal catastrophe is dose-dependent, the lowest effective dose of NSAID should be employed. Salsalate and other nonacetylated salicylates, which have only minimal effect on prostaglandin synthase, are as effective as other NSAIDs and have a lower rate of serious gastrointestinal side effects. However, ototoxicity and central nervous system toxicity may limit their use.

When NSAIDs are required, they may be prescribed on an "as needed" basis, rather than in a fixed daily dose; pain control has been shown to be comparable and the risk of toxicity will be reduced. Once treatment with an NSAID or simple analgesic is initiated, the need for

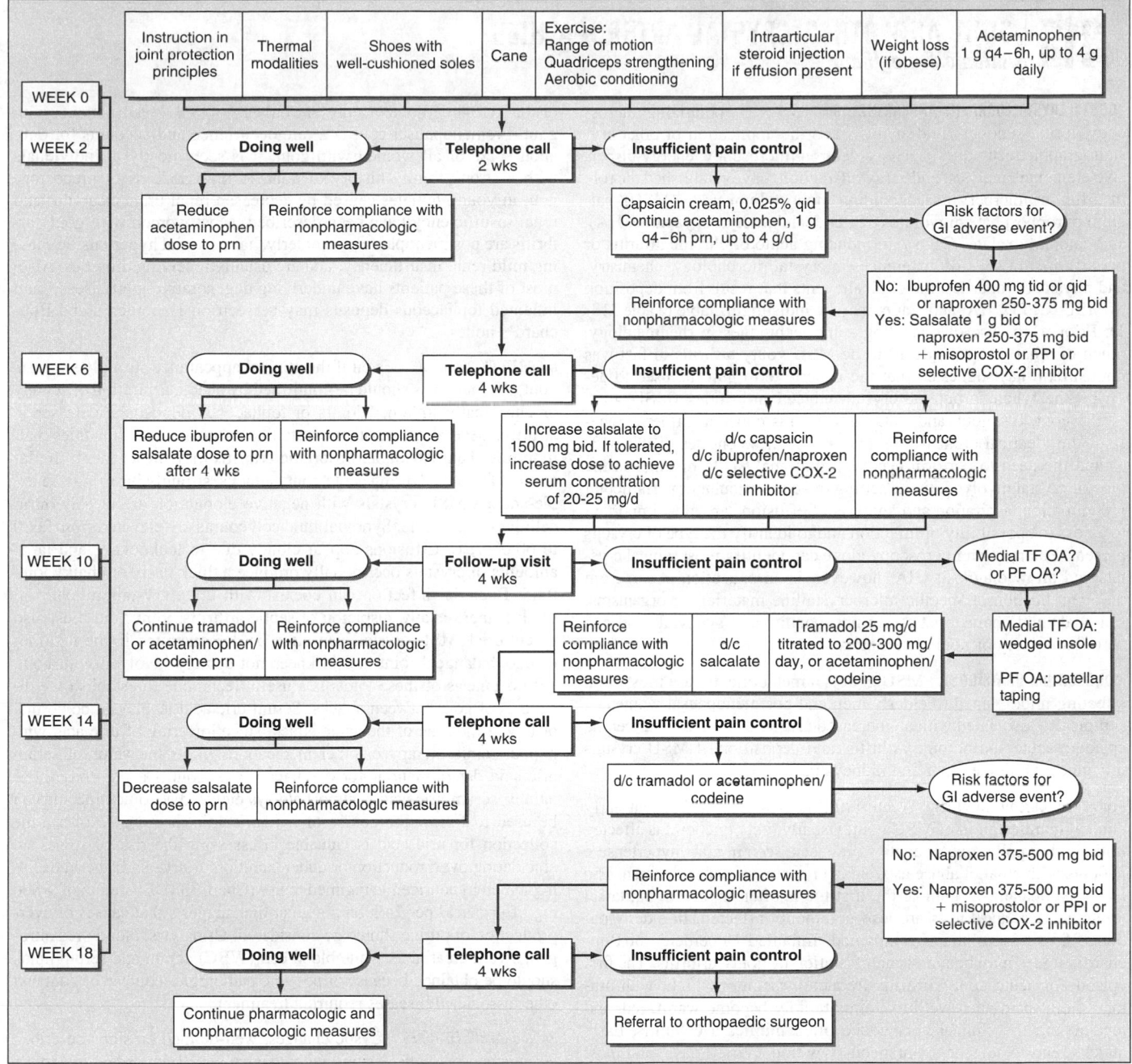

FIGURE 312-4 Algorithm for management of a newly diagnosed patient with knee OA. TF, tibiofemoral; PF, patellofemoral; PPI, proton pump inhibitor; d/c, discontinue.

(Modified from KD Brandt: Diagnosis and Nonsurgical Management of Osteoarthritis, 2d ed, Professional Communications, Inc., Caddo, OK, 2000, pp 1–304)

continuation of that treatment requires ongoing assessment. For many patients with OA, it will be possible eventually to reduce the dose of drug or to use the agent only intermittently during exacerbations of joint pain.

FURTHER READING

BOMBARDIER C et al: Comparison of upper gastrointestinal toxicity of rofecoxib and naproxen in patients with rheumatoid arthritis. N Engl J Med 343:1520, 2000

BRANDT KD, BRADLEY JD: Should the initial drug used to treat osteoarthritis pain be a nonsteroidal antiinflammatory drug? J Rheumatol 28:467, 2001

FELSON DT: Epidemiology of osteoarthritis, in *Osteoarthritis*, 2nd ed, KD Brandt et al (eds). Oxford, Oxford University Press, 2003, pp 9–16

JÜNI P et al: Are selective COX-2 inhibitors superior to traditional nonsteroidal anti-inflammatory drugs? Adequate analysis of the CLASS trial indicates that this may not be the case. BMJ 324:1287, 2002

MCALINDON T: An evaluation of glucosamine for the treatment of OA, in KD Brandt et al (eds): Proceedings of Symposium: Controversies and Practical Issues in the Management of Osteoarthritis. J Clin Rheum, 95(Suppl):S27, 2003

MINOR MA: The utility and importance of non-pharmacologic therapy for the patient with OA, in KD Brandt et al (eds): Proceedings of Symposium: Controversies and Practical Issues in the Management of Osteoarthritis. J Clin Rheum, 9(Suppl):S19, 2003

MOSELEY JB et al: A controlled trial of arthroscopic surgery for osteoarthritis of the knee. N Engl J Med 347:81, 2002

SILVERSTEIN FE et al: Gastrointestinal toxicity with celecoxib vs nonsteroidal anti-inflammatory drugs for osteoarthritis and rheumatoid arthritis. The CLASS Study: A randomized controlled trial. JAMA 284:1247, 2000

"GOUT" CRYSTALLOGRAPHY AND ARTHRITIS The use of polarizing microscopy during synovial fluid analysis and the application of other crystallographic techniques, such as electron microscopy, energy-dispersive elemental analysis, and x-ray diffraction, have established the role of different microcrystals, including monosodium urate (MSU), calcium pyrophosphate dihydrate (CPPD), calcium hydroxyapatite (HA), and calcium oxalate (CaOx), in inducing acute or chronic arthritis or periarthritis. In spite of differences in crystal morphology, chemistry, and physical properties, the clinical events that result from deposition of MSU, CPPD, HA, and CaOx may be indistinguishable (Table 313-1). Prior to the use of crystallographic techniques in rheumatology, much of what was considered to be MSU gouty arthritis in fact was not. Simkin has suggested that the generic term *gout* be used to describe the whole group of crystal-induced arthritides (MSU gout, CPPD gout, HA gout, and CaOx gout). This concept further emphasizes the identical clinical presentations of these entities (Table 313-1) and the need to perform synovial fluid analysis to distinguish the type of crystal involved. In the setting of acute articular or periarticular inflammation, aspiration and analysis of effusions are most important to assess the possibility of infection and to identify the type of crystals present. Polarization microscopy alone can identify most typical crystals and allow diagnosis. HA, however, is an exception. Apart from the identification of specific microcrystalline materials or organisms, synovial fluid characteristics are nonspecific, and synovial fluid can be inflammatory or noninflammatory.

MONOSODIUM URATE GOUT MSU gout is a metabolic disease most often affecting middle-aged to elderly men and postmenopausal women. It is typically associated with an increased uric acid pool, hyperuricemia, episodic acute and chronic arthritis, and deposition of MSU crystals in connective tissue tophi and kidneys (Chap. 338).

Acute and Chronic Arthritis Acute arthritis is the most frequent early clinical manifestation of MSU gout. Usually, only one joint is affected initially, but polyarticular acute gout is also seen in male hypertensive patients with ethanol abuse as well as in postmenopausal women. The metatarsophalangeal joint of the first toe is often involved, but tarsal joints, ankles, and knees are also commonly affected. In elderly patients, finger joints may be inflamed. Inflamed Heberden's or Bouchard's nodes may be a first manifestation of gouty arthritis. The first episode of acute gouty arthritis frequently begins at night with dramatic joint pain and swelling. Joints rapidly become warm, red, and tender, and the clinical appearance often mimics a cellulitis. Early attacks tend to subside spontaneously within 3 to 10 days, and most of the patients do not have residual symptoms until the next episode. Several events may precipitate acute gouty arthritis: dietary excess, trauma, surgery, excessive ethanol ingestion, adrenocorticotropic hormone (ACTH) and glucocorticoid withdrawal, hypouricemic therapy, and serious medical illnesses such as myocardial infarction and stroke.

After many acute mono- or oligoarticular attacks, a proportion of gouty patients may present with a chronic nonsymmetric synovitis, causing potential confusion with rheumatoid arthritis (Chap. 301). Less commonly, chronic gouty arthritis will be the only manifestation and, more rarely, the disease will manifest as inflamed or noninflamed periarticular tophaceous deposits in the absence of chronic synovitis

(Table 313-1). Women represent only 5 to 17% of all patients with gout. Premenopausal gout is a rare occurrence and accounts for only about 17% of all women with gout; it is seen mostly in individuals with a strong family history of gout. A few kindreds of precocious gout in young females caused by decreased renal urate clearance and renal insufficiency have been described. Most women with gouty arthritis are postmenopausal and elderly, have arterial hypertension causing mild renal insufficiency, and are usually receiving diuretics. Also, most of these patients have underlying degenerative joint disease, and inflamed tophaceous deposits may be seen on Heberden's and Bouchard's nodes.

LABORATORY DIAGNOSIS Even if the clinical appearance strongly suggests gout, the diagnosis should be confirmed by needle aspiration of acutely or chronically inflamed joints or tophaceous deposits. Acute septic arthritis, several of the other crystalline-associated arthropathies, palindromic rheumatism, and psoriatic arthritis may present with similar clinical features. During acute gouty attacks, strongly birefringent needle-shaped MSU crystals with negative elongation are largely intracellular (Fig. 313-1). Synovial fluid cell counts are elevated from 2000 to 60,000/μL. Effusions appear cloudy due to leukocytes, and large amounts of crystals occasionally produce a thick pasty or chalky joint fluid. Bacterial infection can coexist with urate crystals in synovial fluid; if there is any suspicion of septic arthritis, joint fluid must also be cultured. MSU crystals can often be demonstrated in the first metatarsophalangeal joint and in knees not acutely involved with gout. Arthrocentesis of these joints is a useful technique to establish the diagnosis of gout between attacks. Serum uric acid levels can be normal or low at the time of the acute attack, since lowering of uric acid with hypouricemic therapy or other medications limits the value of serum uric acid determinations for the diagnosis of gout. Despite these limitations, serum uric acid is almost always elevated at some time and can be used to follow the course of hypouricemic therapy. A 24-h urine collection for uric acid is valuable in assessing the risk of stones, in elucidating overproduction or underexcretion of uric acid, and in deciding which hypouricemic regimen to use (Chap. 338). Excretion of >800 mg of uric acid per 24 h on a regular diet suggests that causes of overproduction of purine should be considered. Urinalysis, blood urea nitrogen, serum creatinine, white blood cell (WBC) count, and serum lipids should be obtained because of possible pathologic sequelae of gout and other associated diseases requiring treatment.

RADIOGRAPHIC FEATURES Cystic changes, well-defined erosions described as punched-out lytic lesions with overhanging bony edges [Martel's sign, or G sign (G for gout)], associated with soft tissue calcified masses are characteristic radiographic features of chronic tophaceous gout. However, similar radiographic signs can also be observed in erosive osteoarthritis, destructive apatite arthropathies, and rheumatoid arthritis.

TABLE 313-1 *Musculoskeletal Manifestations of Crystal-Induced Arthritis*

Acute mono- or polyarthritis	Destructive arthropathies
Bursitis	Pseudo-rheumatoid arthritis
Tendinitis	Pseudo-ankylosing spondylitis
Enthesitis	Spinal stenosis
Tophaceous deposits	Crown dens syndrome
Peculiar type of osteoarthritis	Carpal tunnel syndrome
Synovial osteochondromatosis	Tendon rupture

℞ TREATMENT

Acute Gouty Arthritis The mainstay of treatment during an acute attack is the administration of an anti-inflammatory drug such as colchicine, nonsteroidal anti-inflammatory drugs (NSAIDs), or glucocorticoids depending on the age of the patient and comorbid conditions. Both colchicine and NSAIDs may be quite toxic in the elderly, particularly in the presence of renal insufficiency and gastrointestinal disorders. In elderly patients, one may favor the use of intraarticular glucocorticoid injections for attacks involving one or two larger joints or ice pack applications along with lower oral doses of colchicine for gouty synovitis affecting small joints. Colchicine given orally is a traditional and effective treatment, if used early in the attack, in at least 85% of patients. One tablet (0.6 mg) is given every hour until relief of symptoms or gastrointestinal toxicity occurs, or a total of four to eight tablets may be given in accordance with the age of the patient. The drug must be stopped promptly at the first sign of loose stools, and symptomatic treatment must be given for the diarrhea. Intravenous colchicine is sometimes used and can reduce, though not eliminate, the gastrointestinal side effects. Intravenous colchicine is most reliable for pre- or postoperative prophylaxis in 1- to 2-mg doses when patients cannot take medications orally. Life-threatening colchicine toxicity and sudden death have been described with the administration of >4 mg/d intravenously. The intravenous dose for acute gouty arthritis is 1 to 2 mg given slowly through an established venous line over 10 min in a soluset, and two additional doses of 1 mg each may be given at 6-h intervals, but the total dose should never exceed 4 mg. NSAIDs are affective in ~90% of patients, and the resolution of signs and symptoms usually occurs in 5 to 7 days. The most effective drugs are those with a short half-life and include indomethacin, 25 to 50 mg tid, ibuprofen, 800 mg tid, or diclofenac, 50 mg tid. Cyclooxygenase-2 highly selective inhibitors arc probably equally effective but with less short-term gastrointestinal toxicity. Oral glucocorticoids such as prednisone, 30 to 50 mg/d as the initial dose and tapered over 5 to 7 days, a single intravenous dose of methylprednisolone, 7 mg of betametasone, or 20 to 40 mg of intraarticular triamcinolone acetonide have been equally effective. ACTH as an intramuscular injection of 40 to 80 IU in a single dose or every 12 h for 1 to 2 days is effective in patients with acute polyarticular refractory gout or with a contraindication for using colchicine or NSAIDs.

Hypouricemic Therapy Attempts to normalize serum uric acid to <300 μmol/L (5.0 mg/dL) to prevent recurrent gouty attacks and eliminate tophaceous deposits entail a commitment to long-term hypouricemic regimens and medications that generally arc required for life. Hy pouricemic therapy should be considered when the hyperuricemia cannot be corrected by simple means (control of body weight, low-purine diet, increase in liquid ingestion, limitation of ethanol intake, and avoidance of diuretic use). The decision to initiate hypouricemic therapy is usually made taking into consideration the number of acute attacks, family history of gout, presence of MSU tophaceous deposits, uric acid excretion >800 mg per 24 hours, presence of uric acid stones, and risk for acute uric acid nephropathy during chemotherapy for myeloproliferative disorders. Uricosuric agents, such as probenecid, can be used in patients with good renal function who underexcrete uric acid, with <600 mg in a 24-hour urine sample. Urine volume must be maintained by ingestion of 1500 mL of water every day. Probenecid can be started at a dosage of 200 mg twice daily and increased gradually as needed up to 2 g in order to maintain a serum uric acid level <300 μmol/L (5 mg/dL). Probenecid is the drug of choice to treat elderly patients with hypertension and thiazide dependence; however, probenecid is not effective with a renal creatinine clearance <1 mL/s. These patients may require allopurinol or benzbromarone (not available in the United States), which is another uricosuric drug that is effective in patients with renal failure and who are receiving diuretics. Allopurinol is the best drug to lower serum urate in overproducers, stone formers, and patients with advanced renal failure. It can be given in a single morning dose, 300 mg initially and increasing up to 800 mg if needed. In most patients, it is not necessary to start at a lower dose; however, in patients with renal failure, the dosage should be adjusted depending on the serum creatinine concentration in order to minimize side effects. Patients with frequent acute attacks may require lower initial doses to prevent exacerbations. Toxicity of allopurinol has been recognized increasingly in patients with renal failure who use thiazide diuretics and in those patients allergic to penicillin and ampicillin. The most serious side effects include skin rash with progression to life-threatening toxic epidermal necrolysis, systemic vasculitis, bone marrow suppression, granulomatous hepatitis, and renal failure. Urate-lowering drugs should

FIGURE 313-1 Extracellular and intracellular monosodium urate crystals, as seen in a fresh preparation of synovial fluid, illustrate needle- and rod-shaped strongly negative birefringent crystals (compensated polarized light microscopy; 400×).

not be initiated during acute attacks. This is especially important in patients who have refractory acute arthritis or who had a flare-up previously with hypouricemic drugs. Colchicine prophylaxis in doses of 0.6 mg one to two times daily is usually continued, along with hypouricemic therapy, until the patient is normouricemic and without gouty attacks for 3 months. However, prophylactic colchicine treatment may be necessary as long as tophi are present. Recombinant urate oxidase uricase can be used in the short-term prophylaxis and treatment of chemotherapy-associated hyperuricemia in patients with lymphoproliferative and myeloproliferative disorders.

CPPD DEPOSITION DISEASE ■ Pathogenesis The deposition of CPPD crystals in articular tissues is most common in the elderly, affecting 10 to 15% of persons 65 to 75 years old and 30 to 60% of those >85 years old. In most cases this process is asymptomatic, and the cause of CPPD deposition is uncertain. Because >80% of patients are more than 60 years old and 70% have preexisting joint damage from other conditions, it is likely that biochemical changes in aging cartilage favor crystal nucleation. Examples of such chemical alterations include the following. There is an increased production of inorganic pyrophosphate and decreased levels of pyrophosphatases in cartilage extracts from patients with CPPD arthritis. This condition, which increases inorganic pyrophosphate and promotes CPPD crystal formation, may also inhibit hydroxyapatite formation. The increase in pyrophosphate production appears to be related to enhanced activity of ATP pyrophosphohydrolase and 5′-nucleotidase, which catalyze the reaction of ATP to adenosine and pyrophosphate. This pyrophosphate could combine with calcium to form CPPD crystals in matrix vesicles or on collagen fibers. There is a diminution in the levels of cartilage glycosaminoglycans that normally inhibit and regulate crystal nucleation. These deficiencies may lead to increased crystal deposition. In vitro studies have demonstrated that transforming growth factor β1 and epidermal growth factor both stimulate the production of pyrophosphate by articular cartilage and thus may contribute to the deposition of CPPD crystals. The release of CPPD crystals into the joint space is followed by the phagocytosis of these crystals by neutrophils, which respond by releasing inflammatory substances. In addition, neutrophils release a glycopeptide that is chemotactic for other neutrophils, thus augmenting the inflammatory events. The same substance is present in MSU gout.

A minority of patients with CPPD arthropathy have metabolic abnormalities or hereditary CPPD disease (Table 313-2). These associations suggest that a variety of different metabolic products may enhance CPPD deposition. Included among these conditions are the

TABLE 313-2 *Conditions Associated with Calcium Pyrophosphate Dihydrate Disease*

Aging
Disease-associated
   Primary hyperparathyroidism
   Hemochromatosis
   Hypophosphatasia
   Hypomagnesemia
   Chronic tophaceous gout
   Postmeniscectomy
Epiphyseal dysplasias
Hereditary: Slovakian-Hungarian, Spanish, Spanish-American (Argentinian,[a] Colombian, and Chilean), French,[a] Swedish, Dutch, Canadian, Mexican-American, Italian-American,[a] German-American, Japanese, Tunisian, Jewish, English[a]

[a] Mutations in the ANKH gene.

"four H's" of hyperparathyroidism, hemochromatosis, hypophosphatasia, and hypomagnesemia. Hemochromatosis and hyperparathyroidism are good examples. Ferrous ions and hypercalcemia may either directly alter cartilage or inhibit inorganic pyrophosphatases, leading to enhanced susceptibility to CPPD deposition. The presence of CPPD arthritis in individuals <50 years old should lead to consideration of these metabolic disorders and inherited forms of disease, including those identified in a variety of ethnic groups (Table 313-2). Genomic DNA studies performed on five different kindreds have shown a possible location of the genetic defects on chromosome 8q in one, and on chromosome 5p in the other four in a region that expresses the gene of a membrane pyrophosphate channel (*ANK* gene). A defective gene described in the *ank/ank* mice causes elevation of the intracellular pyrophosphate and reduction of the extracellular pyrophosphate and promotes apatite deposition. Mutations described in the human *ANK* gene in four kindreds with CPPD arthritis might increase extracellular pyrophosphate and induce CPPD crystal formation (Fig. 313-2). Identification of these genes will help elucidate the pathogenesis of both the familial and the more common sporadic form of the disease. Investigation should include inquiry for evidence of familial aggregation and evaluation of serum calcium, phosphorus, alkaline phosphatase, magnesium, serum ferritin, and transferritin saturation.

Clinical Manifestations CPPD arthropathy may be asymptomatic, acute, subacute, or chronic or cause acute synovitis superimposed on chronically involved joints. Acute CPPD arthritis was originally termed *pseudogout* by McCarty and coworkers because of its striking similarity to MSU gout. Other clinical manifestations of CPPD deposition include (1) induction or enhancement of peculiar forms of osteoarthritis; (2) induction of severe destructive disease that may radiographically mimic neuropathic arthritis; (3) production of symmetric proliferative synovitis, clinically similar to rheumatoid arthritis and frequently seen in familial forms with early onset; (4) intervertebral disk and ligament calcification with restriction of spine mobility, mimicking ankylosing spondylitis (also seen in hereditary forms); and (5) rarely spinal stenosis (most commonly seen in the elderly) (Table 313-1).

The knee is the joint most frequently affected in CPPD arthropathy.

FIGURE 313-2 Mutations in *ANKH* gene associated with familial CPPD gout. CMD, cranial metaphyseal dysplasia.

FIGURE 313-3 Intracellular and extracellular calcium pyrophosphate dihydrate crystals, as seen in a fresh preparation of synovial fluid, illustrate rectangular, rod-shaped, and rhomboid weakly positive birefringent crystals (compensated polarized light microscopy; 400×).

Other sites include the wrist, shoulder, ankle, elbow, and hands. Rarely, the temporomandibular joint and ligamentum flavum of the spinal canal are involved. Clinical and radiographic evidence indicates that CPPD deposition is polyarticular in at least two-thirds of patients. When the clinical picture resembles that of slowly progressive osteoarthritis, diagnosis may be more difficult. Joint distribution may provide important clues suggesting CPPD disease. For example, primary osteoarthritis rarely involves a metacarpophalangeal, wrist, elbow, shoulder, or ankle joint. If radiographs reveal punctate and/or linear radiodense deposits in fibrocartilaginous joint menisci or articular hyaline cartilage (chondrocalcinosis), the diagnostic certainty of CPPD is further enhanced. *Definitive diagnosis* requires demonstration of typical crystals in synovial fluid or articular tissue (Fig. 313-3). In the absence of joint effusion or indications to obtain a synovial biopsy, chondrocalcinosis is presumptive of CPPD deposition. One exception is chondrocalcinosis due to CaOx in some patients with chronic renal failure.

Acute attacks of CPPD arthritis may be precipitated by trauma, arthroscopy, or hyaluronate injections. Rapid diminution of serum calcium concentration, as may occur in severe medical illness or after surgery (especially parathyroidectomy), can also lead to pseudogout attacks.

In as many as 50% of cases, CPPD gout is associated with low-grade fever and, on occasion, temperatures as high as 40°C. Whether or not radiographic proof of chondrocalcinosis is evident in the involved joint(s), synovial analysis with microbial cultures is essential to rule out the possibility of infection. In fact, infection in a joint with any microcrystalline deposition process can lead to crystal shedding and subsequent synovitis from both crystals and microorganisms. Synovial fluid in acute CPPD gout has inflammatory qualities. The WBC count can range from several thousand cells to 100,000 cells/μL, the mean being about 24,000 cells/μL and the predominant cell being the neutrophil. Polarization microscopy usually reveals rhomboid crystals with weak positive birefringence inside fibrin clots and in neutrophils (Fig. 313-3).

℞ TREATMENT

Untreated acute attacks may last a few days to as long as a month. Treatment by joint aspiration and NSAIDs, or colchicine, or intraarticular glucocorticoid injection may result in return to prior status in ≤10 days. For patients with frequent recurrent attacks of CPPD gout, daily prophylactic treatment with low doses of colchicine may be helpful in decreasing the frequency of the attacks. Severe polyarticular attacks usually require short courses of glucocorticoids. Unfortunately, there is no effective way to remove CPPD deposits from cartilage and synovium. Uncontrolled studies suggest that radioactive synovectomy (with yttrium 90) or the administration of antimalarial agents may be helpful in controlling persistent synovitis. Patients with progressive destructive large-joint arthropathy usually require joint replacement.

CALCIUM HYDROXYAPATITE DEPOSITION DISEASE ■ Pathogenesis

HA is the primary mineral of bone and teeth. Abnormal accumulation can occur in areas of tissue damage (dystrophic calcification), in hypercalcemic or hyperparathyroid states (metastatic calcification), and in certain conditions of unknown cause (Table 313-3). In chronic renal failure, hyperphosphatemia enhances HA deposition

FIGURE 313-4 *A.* Cytoplasmic round inclusions inside synovial fluid cells represent aggregates of apatite crystals (fresh preparation, ordinary light microscopy; 288×). *B.* An electron micrograph demonstrates a cluster of dark apatite crystals within a synovial fluid mononuclear cell (21,600×).

both in and around joints. Familial aggregation is rarely seen, but no association with human *ANK* mutations have been described thus far.

HA may be released from exposed bone and cause the acute synovitis occasionally seen in chronic stable osteoarthritis (e.g., "hot" Heberden's nodes). HA deposition is also an important factor in an extremely destructive chronic arthropathy of the elderly that occurs most often in knees and shoulders (Milwaukee shoulder). Joint destruction is associated with attenuation or rupture of supporting structures, leading to instability and deformity. Progression tends to be indolent, and synovial fluid WBC counts are usually <2000/μL. Symptoms range from minimal to severe pain and disability that may lead to joint replacement surgery. Whether severely affected patients merely represent an extreme synovial tissue response to the HA crystals that are so common in osteoarthritis is uncertain. Synovial membrane tissue cultures exposed to HA (or CPPD) crystals markedly increased the release of collagenases and neutral proteases, underscoring the destructive potential of abnormally stimulated synovial lining cells.

Clinical Manifestations Periarticular and articular deposits may coexist and be associated with acute and/or chronic damage to the joint capsule, tendons, bursa, or articular surfaces. The most common sites of HA deposition include bursae and tendons in and/or around the knees, shoulders, hips, and fingers. Clinical manifestations include asymptomatic radiographic abnormalities, acute synovitis, bursitis, tendinitis,

and chronic destructive arthropathy. Most patients with HA arthropathy are elderly. Although the true incidence of HA arthritis is not known, 30 to 50% of patients with osteoarthritis have HA microcrystals in their synovial fluid. Such crystals can frequently be identified in clinically stable osteoarthritic joints, but they are more likely to come to attention in persons experiencing acute or subacute worsening of joint pain and swelling. The synovial fluid WBC count in HA arthritis is usually low (<2000/μL) but may at times have as many as 50,000/μL. Most synovial fluid analyses reveal a predominance of mononuclear cells. Occasionally, neutrophils may dominate.

Diagnosis Radiographic findings in HA arthropathy are not diagnostic. Intra- and/or periarticular calcifications with or without erosive, destructive, or hypertrophic changes may be present.

Definitive diagnosis of HA arthropathy depends on identification of crystals from synovial fluid or tissue (Fig. 313-4). Individual crystals are very small, nonbirefringent, and can only be seen by electron microscopy. Clumps of crystals may appear as 1- to 20-μm shiny intra- or extracellular globules that stain purplish with Wright's stain and bright red with alizarin red S. Absolute identification depends on electron microscopy with energy-dispersive elemental analysis, x-ray diffraction, or infrared spectroscopy.

℞ TREATMENT

Treatment of HA arthritis is nonspecific. Acute attacks of bursitis or synovitis may be self-limiting, resolving in from days to several weeks. Aspiration of effusions and the use of either NSAIDs or oral colchicine for 2 weeks or intra- or periarticular injection of glucocorticoid salts appears to shorten the duration and intensity of symptoms. In patients with underlying severe destructive articular changes, response to medical therapy is usually less rewarding.

CaOx DEPOSITION DISEASE ■ Pathogenesis

Primary oxalosis is a rare hereditary metabolic disorder (Chap. 343). Enhanced production of oxalic acid may result from at least two different enzyme defects, leading to hyperoxalemia and deposition of calcium oxalate crystals in tissues. Nephrocalcinosis, renal failure, and death usually occur before age 20. Acute and/or chronic CaOx arthritis and periarthritis may complicate primary oxalosis during later years of illness.

Secondary oxalosis is more common than the primary disorder. It is one of the many metabolic abnormalities that complicate end-stage renal disease (ESRD). In ESRD, calcium oxalate deposits have long been recognized in visceral organs, blood vessels, bones, and even cartilage. However, it was not until 1982 that such deposits were demonstrated to be one of the causes of arthritis in chronic renal failure. Thus far, reported patients have been dependent on long-term hemodialysis or peritoneal dialysis (Chap. 262), and many had received

TABLE 313-3 *Conditions Associated with Hydroxyapatite Deposition Disease*

Aging
Osteoarthritis
Hemorrhagic shoulder effusions in the elderly (Milwaukee shoulder)
Destructive arthropathy
Tendinitis, bursitis
Tumoral calcinosis (sporadic cases)
Disease-associated
  Hyperparathyroidism
  Milk-alkali syndrome
  Renal failure/long-term dialysis
  Connective tissue diseases (e.g., progressive systemic sclerosis, CREST syndrome, idiopathic myositis, SLE)
  Heterotopic calcification following neurologic catastrophes (e.g., stroke, spinal cord injury)
Hereditary
  Bursitis, arthritis
  Tumoral calcinosis
  Fibrodysplasia ossificans progressiva

Note: CREST, calcinosis cutis, Raynaud's phenomenon, esophageal dysmotility, sclerodactyly, telangiectasia; SLE, systemic lupus erythematosus.

FIGURE 313-5 Bipyramidal and small polymorphic calcium oxalate crystals (ordinary light microscopy; 400×).

ascorbic acid supplements. Ascorbic acid is metabolized to oxalate, which is inadequately cleared in uremia and by dialysis. Such supplements are now usually avoided in dialysis programs because of the risk of enhancing hyperoxalosis and its sequelae.

Clinical Manifestations and Diagnosis As was noted for the other calcium salts, CaOx aggregates can be found in bone, articular cartilage, synovium, and periarticular tissues. From these sites, crystals may be shed, causing acute synovitis. Persistent aggregates of CaOx may, like HA and CPPD, stimulate synovial proliferation and enzyme release, resulting in progressive articular destruction. Deposits have been documented in fingers, wrists, elbows, knees, ankles, and feet.

Each of the known microcrystalline arthropathies may be a complication of ESRD, and rare patients have more than one type of crystal present in a joint effusion. The advent of crystallographic techniques has made it clear that most arthritic problems in ESRD are not, as was once believed, due to MSU gout. Clinical features of acute CaOx arthritis may not be distinguishable from those due to sodium urate, CPPD, or HA. Radiographs may reveal chondrocalcinosis, a feature of either CPPD or CaOx deposition. CaOx-induced synovial effusions are usually noninflammatory, with <2000 leukocytes/μL. Neutrophils or mononuclear cells have predominated. CaOx crystals have a variable shape and variable birefringence to polarized light. The most easily recognized forms are bipyramidal and have strong positive birefringence (Fig. 313-5).

℞ TREATMENT

Treatment of CaOx arthropathy with NSAIDs, colchicine, intraarticular glucocorticoids, and/or an increased frequency of dialysis has produced only slight improvement. In primary oxalosis, liver transplantation has induced a significant reduction in crystal deposits (Chap. 343).

FURTHER READING

FAM AG: Difficult gout and new approaches for control of hyperuricemia in the allopurinol-allergic patient. Curr Rheumatol Rep 3:29, 2001

MALDONADO I et al: Familial calcium crystal diseases: What have we learned? Curr Opin Rheumatol 13:225, 2001

REGINATO AJ et al: Familial and clinical aspects of calcium pyrophosphate deposition disease. Curr Rheumatol Rep 1:112, 1999

SCHLESINGER N, SCHUMACHER HR JR: Gout: Can management be improved? Curr Opin Rheumatol 13:240, 2001

SCHUMACHER HR JR et al: Randomized double-blind trial of etoricoxib and indomethacin in treatment of acute gouty arthritis. BMJ 324:458, 2002

314 INFECTIOUS ARTHRITIS
Lawrence C. Madoff, Scott J. Thaler, James H. Maguire

INTRODUCTION AND APPROACH TO THE PATIENT Although *Staphylococcus aureus*, *Neisseria gonorrhoeae*, and other bacteria are the most common causes of infectious arthritis, various mycobacteria, spirochetes, fungi, and viruses also infect joints. Since acute bacterial infection can rapidly destroy articular cartilage, all inflamed joints must be evaluated without delay to exclude noninfectious processes and to determine appropriate antimicrobial therapy and drainage procedures. For more detailed information on infectious arthritis due to specific organisms, the reader is referred to the chapters on those organisms.

Acute bacterial infection typically involves a single joint or a few joints. Subacute or chronic monarthritis or oligoarthritis suggests mycobacterial or fungal infection; episodic inflammation is seen in syphilis, Lyme disease, and the reactive arthritis that follows enteric infections and chlamydial urethritis (Table 314-1). Acute polyarticular inflammation occurs as an immunologic reaction during the course of endocarditis, rheumatic fever, disseminated neisserial infection, and acute hepatitis B. Bacteria and viruses occasionally infect multiple joints, the former most commonly in persons with rheumatoid arthritis.

Aspiration of synovial fluid—an essential element in the evaluation of potentially infected joints—can be performed without difficulty in most cases by the insertion of a large-bore needle into the site of maximal fluctuation or tenderness or by the route of easiest access. Ultrasonography or fluoroscopy may be used to guide aspiration of difficult-to-localize effusions of the hip and, occasionally, the shoulder and other joints. Normal synovial fluid contains <180 cells (predominantly mononuclear cells) per microliter. Synovial cell counts averaging 100,000/μL (range, 25,000 to 250,000/μL), with >90% neutro-

phils, are characteristic of acute bacterial infections. Crystal-induced, rheumatoid, and other noninfectious inflammatory arthritides are usually associated with <30,000 to 50,000 cells/μL; cell counts of 10,000 to 30,000/μL, with 50 to 70% neutrophils and the remainder lymphocytes, are common in mycobacterial and fungal infections. Definitive diagnosis of an infectious process relies on identification of the pathogen in stained smears of synovial fluid, isolation of the pathogen from cultures of synovial fluid and blood, or detection of microbial nucleic acids and proteins by polymerase chain reaction (PCR)–based assays and immunologic techniques.

ACUTE BACTERIAL ARTHRITIS ■ Pathogenesis Bacteria enter the joint from the bloodstream; from a contiguous site of infection in bone or soft tissue; or by direct inoculation during surgery, injection, or trauma. In hematogenous infection, bacteria escape from synovial capillaries, which have no limiting basement membrane, and within hours provoke neutrophilic infiltration of the synovium. Neutrophils and bacteria enter the joint space; later, bacteria adhere to articular cartilage. Degradation of cartilage begins within 48 h as a result of increased intraarticular pressure, release of proteases and cytokines from chondrocytes and synovial macrophages, and invasion of the cartilage by bacteria and inflammatory cells. Histologic studies reveal bacteria lining the synovium and cartilage as well as abscesses extending into the synovium, cartilage, and—in severe cases—subchondral bone. Synovial proliferation results in the formation of a pannus over the cartilage, and thrombosis of inflamed synovial vessels develops. Bacterial factors that appear important in the pathogenesis of infective arthritis include various surface-associated adhesins in *S. aureus* that permit adherence to cartilage and endotoxins that promote chondrocyte-mediated breakdown of cartilage.

Microbiology The hematogenous route of infection is the most common route in all age groups, and nearly every bacterial pathogen is capable of causing septic arthritis. In infants, group B streptococci, gram-negative enteric bacilli, and *S. aureus* are the usual pathogens. Since the advent of the *Haemophilus influenzae* vaccine, *S. aureus*, *Streptococcus pyogenes* (group A *Streptococcus*), and (in some centers) *Kingella kingae* have predominated among children <5 years of age. Among young adults and adolescents, *N. gonorrhoeae* is the most commonly implicated organism. *S. aureus* accounts for most nongonococcal isolates in adults of all ages; gram-negative bacilli, pneumococci, and β-hemolytic streptococci—particularly groups A and B, but also groups C, G, and F—are involved in up to one-third of cases in older adults, especially those with underlying comorbid illnesses.

Infections following surgical procedures or penetrating injuries are due most often to *S. aureus* and occasionally to other gram-positive bacteria or gram-negative bacilli. Infections with coagulase-negative staphylococci are unusual except after the implantation of prosthetic joints or arthroscopy. Anaerobic organisms, often in association with aerobic or facultative bacteria, are found after human bites and when decubitus ulcers or intraabdominal abscesses spread into adjacent joints. Polymicrobial infections complicate traumatic injuries with extensive contamination. Bites and scratches from cats and other animals may introduce *Pasteurella multocida* into joints.

Nongonococcal Bacterial Arthritis ■ *EPIDEMIOLOGY* Although hematogenous infections with virulent organisms such as *S. aureus*, *H. influenzae*, and pyogenic streptococci occur in healthy persons, there is an underlying host predisposition in many cases of septic arthritis. Patients with rheumatoid arthritis have the highest incidence of infective arthritis (most often secondary to *S. aureus*) because of chronically inflamed joints; glucocorticoid therapy; and frequent breakdown of rheumatoid nodules, vasculitic ulcers, and skin overlying deformed joints. Diabetes mellitus, glucocorticoid therapy, hemodialysis, and malignancy all carry an increased risk of infection with *S. aureus* and gram-negative bacilli. Tumor necrosis factor (TNF) inhibitors (etanercept and infliximab), increasingly used for the treatment of rheumatoid arthritis, predispose to mycobacterial infections and possibly to other pyogenic bacterial infections and could be associated with septic arthritis in this population. Pneumococcal infections complicate alcoholism, deficiencies of humoral immunity, and hemoglobinopathies. Pneumococci, *Salmonella*, and *H. influenzae* cause septic arthritis in persons infected with HIV. Persons with primary immunoglobulin deficiency are at risk for mycoplasmal arthritis, which results in permanent joint damage if treatment with tetracycline and intravenous (IV) immunoglobulin replacement is not administered promptly. Intravenous drug users acquire staphylococcal and streptococcal infections from their own flora and acquire pseudomonal and other gram-negative infections from drugs and injection paraphernalia.

CLINICAL MANIFESTATIONS Some 90% of patients present with involvement of a single joint—most commonly the knee, less frequently the hip, and still less often the shoulder, wrist, or elbow. Small joints of the hands and feet are more likely to be affected after direct inoculation or a bite. Among IV drug users, infections of the spine, sacroiliac joints, or sternoclavicular joints are more common than infections of the appendicular skeleton. Polyarticular infection is most common among patients with rheumatoid arthritis and may resemble a flare of the underlying disease.

The usual presentation consists of moderate to severe pain that is uniform around the joint, effusion, muscle spasm, and decreased range of motion. Fever in the range of 38.3° to 38.9°C (101° to 102°F) and sometimes higher is common but may be lacking, especially in persons with rheumatoid arthritis, renal or hepatic insufficiency, or conditions

TABLE 314-1 *Differential Diagnosis of Arthritis Syndromes*

Acute Monarticular Arthritis	Chronic Monarticular Arthritis	Polyarticular Arthritis
Staphylococcus aureus	*Mycobacterium tuberculosis*	*Neisseria meningitidis*
Streptococcus pneumoniae		*N. gonorrhoeae*
β-Hemolytic streptococci	Nontuberculous mycobacteria	Nongonococcal bacterial arthritis
Gram-negative bacilli		Bacterial endocarditis
Neisseria gonorrhoeae	*Borrelia burgdorferi*	*Candida* species
Candida species	*Treponema pallidum*	Poncet's disease (tuberculous rheumatism)
Crystal-induced arthritis	*Candida* species	Hepatitis B virus
Fracture	*Sporothrix schenckii*	Parvovirus B19
Hemarthrosis	*Coccidioides immitis*	HIV
Foreign body	*Blastomyces dermatitidis*	Human T-lymphotropic virus type I
Osteoarthritis	*Aspergillus* species	Rubella virus
Ischemic necrosis	*Cryptococcus neoformans*	Arthropod-borne viruses
Monarticular rheumatoid arthritis	*Nocardia* species	Sickle cell disease flare
	Brucella species	Reactive arthritis
	Legg-Calvé-Perthes disease	Serum sickness
	Osteoarthritis	Acute rheumatic fever
		Inflammatory bowel disease
		Systemic lupus erythematosus
		Rheumatoid arthritis/Still's disease
		Other vasculitides
		Sarcoidosis

requiring immunosuppressive therapy. The inflamed, swollen joint is usually evident on examination except in the case of a deeply situated joint, such as the hip, shoulder, or sacroiliac joint. Cellulitis, bursitis, and acute osteomyelitis, which may produce a similar clinical picture, should be distinguished from septic arthritis by their greater range of motion and less-than-circumferential swelling. A focus of extraarticular infection, such as a boil or pneumonia, should be sought. Peripheral-blood leukocytosis with a left shift and elevation of the erythrocyte sedimentation rate or C-reactive protein level are common.

Plain radiographs show evidence of soft tissue swelling, joint-space widening, and displacement of tissue planes by the distended capsule. Narrowing of the joint space and bony erosions indicate advanced infection and a poor prognosis. Ultrasound is useful for detecting effusions in the hip, and computed tomography or magnetic resonance imaging can demonstrate infections of the sacroiliac joint, the sternoclavicular joint, and the spine very well.

LABORATORY FINDINGS Specimens of peripheral blood and synovial fluid should be obtained before antibiotics are administered. Blood cultures are positive in up to 50% of *S. aureus* infections but are less frequently positive in infections due to other organisms. The synovial fluid is turbid, serosanguineous, or frankly purulent. Gram-stained smears confirm the presence of large numbers of neutrophils. Levels of total protein and lactate dehydrogenase in synovial fluid are elevated, and the glucose level is depressed; however, these findings are not specific for infection, and measurement of these levels is not necessary to make the diagnosis. The synovial fluid should be examined for crystals, because gout and pseudogout can resemble septic arthritis clinically, and infection and crystal-induced disease occasionally occur together. Organisms are seen on synovial fluid smears in nearly three-quarters of infections with *S. aureus* and streptococci and in 30 to 50% of infections due to gram-negative and other bacteria. Cultures of synovial fluid are positive in >90% of cases. Inoculation of synovial fluid into bottles containing liquid media for blood cultures increases the yield of culture, especially if the pathogen is a fastidious organism or the patient is taking an antibiotic. Although not yet widely available, PCR-based assays for bacterial DNA will also be useful for the diagnosis of partially treated or culture-negative bacterial arthritis.

℞ **TREATMENT**

Prompt administration of systemic antibiotics and drainage of the involved joint can prevent destruction of cartilage, postinfectious degenerative arthritis, joint instability, or deformity. Once samples of blood and synovial fluid have been obtained for culture, empirical antibiotics should be given that are directed against bacteria visualized on smears or against the pathogens that are likely, given the patient's age and risk factors. Initial therapy should consist of the IV administration of bactericidal agents; direct instillation of antibiotics into the joint is not necessary to achieve adequate levels in synovial fluid and tissue. An IV third-generation cephalosporin such as cefotaxime (1 g every 8 h) or ceftriaxone (1 to 2 g every 24 h) provides adequate empirical coverage for most community-acquired infections in adults when smears show no organisms. Either oxacillin or nafcillin (2 g every 4 h) is used if there are gram-positive cocci on the smear. If methicillin-resistant *S. aureus* is a possible pathogen (e.g., in hospitalized patients), IV vancomycin (1 g every 12 h) should be given. In addition, an aminoglycoside or third-generation cephalosporin should be given to IV drug users or other patients in whom *Pseudomonas aeruginosa* may be the responsible agent.

Definitive therapy is based on the identity and antibiotic susceptibility of the bacteria isolated in culture. Infections due to staphylococci are treated with oxacillin, nafcillin, or vancomycin for 4 weeks. Pneumococcal and streptococcal infections due to penicillin-susceptible organisms respond to 2 weeks of therapy with penicillin G (2 million units IV every 4 h); infections caused by *H. influenzae* and by strains of *S. pneumoniae* that are resistant to penicillin are treated with cefotaxime or ceftriaxone for 2 weeks. Most enteric gram-negative infections can be cured in 3 to 4 weeks by a second- or third-generation cephalosporin given intravenously or by a fluoroquinolone, such as levofloxacin (500 mg IV or orally every 24 h). *P. aeruginosa* infection should be treated for at least 2 weeks with a combination regimen of an aminoglycoside plus either an extended-spectrum penicillin, such as mezlocillin (3 g IV every 4 h), or an antipseudomonal cephalosporin, such as ceftazidime (1 g IV every 8 h). If tolerated, this regimen is continued for an additional 2 weeks; alternatively, a fluoroquinolone, such as ciprofloxacin (750 mg orally bid), is given by itself or with the penicillin or cephalosporin in place of the aminoglycoside.

Timely drainage of pus and necrotic debris from the infected joint is required for a favorable outcome. Needle aspiration of readily accessible joints such as the knee may be adequate if loculations or particulate matter in the joint does not prevent its thorough decompression. Arthroscopic drainage and lavage may be employed initially or within several days if repeated needle aspiration fails to relieve symptoms, decrease the volume of the effusion and the synovial white cell count, and clear bacteria from smears and cultures. In some cases, arthrotomy is necessary to remove loculations and debride infected synovium, cartilage, or bone. Septic arthritis of the hip is best managed with arthrotomy, particularly in young children, in whom infection threatens the viability of the femoral head. Septic joints do not require immobilization except for pain control before symptoms are alleviated by treatment. Weight bearing should be avoided until signs of inflammation have subsided, but frequent passive motion of the joint is indicated to maintain full mobility. While addition of glucocorticoids to antibiotic treatment improves the outcome of *S. aureus* arthritis in experimental animals, no clinical trials have yet evaluated this approach in humans.

Gonococcal Arthritis ■ *EPIDEMIOLOGY* Although its incidence has declined in recent years, gonococcal arthritis (Chap. 128) has accounted for up to 70% of episodes of infectious arthritis in persons <40 years of age in the United States. Arthritis due to *N. gonorrhoeae* is a consequence of bacteremia arising from gonococcal infection or, more frequently, from asymptomatic gonococcal mucosal colonization of the urethra, cervix, or pharynx. Women are at greatest risk during menses and during pregnancy and overall are two to three times more likely than men to develop disseminated gonoccal infection (DGI) and arthritis. Persons with complement deficiencies, especially of the terminal components, are prone to recurrent episodes of gonococcemia. Strains of gonococci that are most likely to cause DGI include those

that produce transparent colonies in culture, have the type IA outer-membrane protein, or are of the AUH-auxotroph type.

CLINICAL MANIFESTATIONS AND LABORATORY FINDINGS The most common manifestation of DGI is a syndrome of fever, chills, rash, and articular symptoms. Small numbers of papules that progress to hemorrhagic pustules develop on the trunk and the extensor surfaces of the distal extremities. Migratory arthritis and tenosynovitis of the knees, hands, wrists, feet, and ankles are prominent. The cutaneous lesions and articular findings are believed to be the consequence of an immune reaction to circulating gonococci and immune-complex deposition in tissues. Thus, cultures of synovial fluid are consistently negative, and blood cultures are positive in <45% of patients. Synovial fluid may be difficult to obtain from inflamed joints and usually contains only 10,000 to 20,000 leukocytes/μL.

True gonococcal septic arthritis is less common than the DGI syndrome and always follows DGI, which is unrecognized in one-third of patients. A single joint, such as the hip, knee, ankle, or wrist, is usually involved. Synovial fluid, which contains >50,000 leukocytes/μL, can be obtained with ease; the gonococcus is only occasionally evident in gram-stained smears, and cultures of synovial fluid are positive in <40% of cases. Blood cultures are almost always negative.

Because it is difficult to isolate gonococci from synovial fluid and blood, specimens for culture should be obtained from potentially infected mucosal sites. Cultures and gram-stained smears of skin lesions are occasionally positive. All specimens for culture should be plated onto Thayer-Martin agar directly or in special transport media at the bedside and transferred promptly to the microbiology laboratory in an atmosphere of 5% CO_2, as generated in a candle jar. PCR-based assays are extremely sensitive in detecting gonococcal DNA in synovial fluid. A dramatic alleviation of symptoms within 12 to 24 h after the initiation of appropriate antibiotic therapy supports a clinical diagnosis of the DGI syndrome if cultures are negative.

℞ TREATMENT

Initial treatment consists of ceftriaxone (1 g IV or intramuscularly every 24 h) to cover possible penicillin-resistant organisms. Once local and systemic signs are clearly resolving and if the sensitivity of the isolate permits, the 7-day course of therapy can be completed with an oral agent such as ciprofloxacin (500 mg twice daily). Ciprofloxacin (500 mg orally/400 mg IV twice daily) may also be used as initial therapy in areas where resistance has not become prevalent; if penicillin-susceptible organisms are isolated, amoxicillin (500 mg three times daily) may be used. Suppurative arthritis usually responds to needle aspiration of involved joints and 7 to 14 days of antibiotic treatment. Arthroscopic lavage or arthrotomy is rarely required. Patients with disseminated gonococcal infection should be treated for *Chlamydia trachomatis* infection unless this infection is ruled out by appropriate testing.

It is noteworthy that arthritis symptoms similar to those seen in DGI occur in meningococcemia. A dermatitis-arthritis syndrome, purulent monarthritis, and reactive polyarthritis have been described. All respond to treatment with IV penicillin.

SPIROCHETAL ARTHRITIS ■ **Lyme Disease** Lyme disease (Chap. 157) due to infection with the spirochete *Borrelia burgdorferi* causes arthritis in up to 70% of persons who are not treated. Intermittent arthralgias and myalgias—but not arthritis—occur within days or weeks of inoculation of the spirochete by the *Ixodes* tick. Later, there are three patterns of joint disease: (1) Fifty percent of untreated persons experience intermittent episodes of monarthritis or oligoarthritis involving the knee and/or other large joints. The symptoms wax and wane without treatment over months, and each year 10 to 20% of patients report loss of joint symptoms. (2) Twenty percent of untreated persons develop a pattern of waxing and waning arthralgias. (3) Ten percent of untreated patients develop chronic inflammatory synovitis resulting in erosive lesions and destruction of the joint. Serologic tests for IgG antibodies to *B. burgdorferi* are positive in >90% of persons with Lyme arthritis, and a PCR-based assay detects *Borrelia* DNA in 85%.

℞ TREATMENT

Lyme arthritis generally responds well to therapy. A regimen of oral doxycycline (100 mg twice daily for 30 days), oral amoxicillin (500 mg four times daily for 30 days), or parenteral ceftriaxone (2 g/d for 2 to 4 weeks) is recommended. Patients who do not respond to a total of 2 months of oral therapy or 1 month of parenteral therapy are unlikely to benefit from additional antibiotic therapy and are treated with anti-inflammatory agents or synovectomy. Failure of therapy is associated with host features such as the HLA-DR4 genotype, persistent reactivity to OspA (outer-surface protein A), and the presence of hLFA-1 (human leukocyte function–associated antigen 1), which cross-reacts with OspA.

Syphilitic Arthritis Articular manifestations occur in different stages of syphilis (Chap. 153). In early congenital syphilis, periarticular swelling and immobilization of the involved limbs (Parrot's pseudoparalysis) complicate osteochondritis of long bones. Clutton's joint, a late manifestation of congenital syphilis that typically develops between the ages of 8 and 15 years, is caused by chronic painless synovitis with effusions of large joints, particularly the knees and elbows. Secondary syphilis may be associated with arthralgias; with symmetric arthritis of the knees and ankles and occasionally of the shoulders and wrists; and with sacroiliitis. The arthritis follows a subacute to chronic course with a mixed mononuclear and neutrophilic synovial-fluid pleocytosis (typical cell counts, 5000 to 15,000/μL). Immunologic mechanisms may contribute to the arthritis, and symptoms usually improve rapidly with penicillin therapy. In tertiary syphilis, Charcot's joint is a result of sensory loss due to tabes dorsalis. Penicillin is not helpful in this setting.

MYCOBACTERIAL ARTHRITIS Tuberculous arthritis (Chap. 150) accounts for ~1% of all cases of tuberculosis and for 10% of extrapulmonary cases. The most common presentation is chronic granulomatous monarthritis. An unusual syndrome, Poncet's disease, is a reactive symmetric form of polyarthritis that affects persons with visceral or disseminated tuberculosis. No mycobacteria are found in the joints, and symptoms resolve with antituberculous therapy.

Unlike tuberculous osteomyelitis (Chap. 111), which typically involves the thoracic and lumbar spine (50% of cases), tuberculous arthritis primarily involves the large weight-bearing joints, in particular the hips, knees, and ankles, and only occasionally involves smaller non-weight-bearing joints. Progressive monarticular swelling and pain develop over months to years, and systemic symptoms are seen in only half of all cases. Tuberculous arthritis occurs as part of a disseminated primary infection or through late reactivation, often in persons with HIV infection or other immunocompromised hosts. Coexistent active pulmonary tuberculosis is unusual.

Aspiration of the involved joint yields fluid with an average cell count of 20,000/μL, with ~50% neutrophils. Acid-fast staining of the fluid yields positive results in fewer than one-third of cases, and cultures are positive in 80%. Culture of synovial tissue taken at biopsy is positive in ~90% of cases and shows granulomatous inflammation in most. DNA amplification methods such as PCR can shorten the time to diagnosis to 1 or 2 days. Radiographs reveal peripheral erosions at the points of synovial attachment, periarticular osteopenia, and eventually joint-space narrowing. Therapy for tuberculous arthritis is the same as that for tuberculous pulmonary disease, requiring the administration of multiple agents for 6 to 9 months. Therapy is more prolonged in immunosuppressed individuals, such as those infected with HIV.

Various atypical mycobacteria (Chap. 152) found in water and soil may cause chronic indolent arthritis. Such disease results from trauma and direct inoculation associated with farming, gardening, or aquatic activities. Smaller joints, such as the digits, wrists, and knees, are usually involved. Involvement of tendon sheaths and bursae is typical. The mycobacterial species involved include *Mycobacterium marinum*, *M. avium-intracellulare*, *M. terrae*, *M. kansasii*, *M. fortuitum*, and *M. chelonae*. In persons who have HIV infection or are receiving immunosuppressive therapy, hematogenous spread to the joints has been reported for *M. kansasii*, *M. avium-intracellulare*, and *M. haemophilum*. Diagnosis usually requires biopsy and culture, and therapy is based on antimicrobial susceptibility patterns.

FUNGAL ARTHRITIS Fungi are an unusual cause of chronic monarticular arthritis. Granulomatous articular infection with the endemic dimorphic fungi *Coccidioides immitis*, *Blastomyces dermatitidis*, and (less commonly) *Histoplasma capsulatum* results from hematogenous seeding or direct extension from bony lesions in persons with disseminated disease. Joint involvement is an unusual complication of sporotrichosis (infection with *Sporothrix schenckii*) among gardeners and other persons who work with soil or sphagnum moss. Articular sporotrichosis is six times more common among men than among women, and alcoholics and other debilitated hosts are at risk for polyarticular infection.

Candida infection involving a single joint—usually the knee, hip, or shoulder—results from surgical procedures, intraarticular injections, or (among critically ill patients with debilitating illnesses, such as diabetes mellitus or hepatic or renal insufficiency, and patients receiving immunosuppressive therapy) hematogenous spread. *Candida* infections in IV drug users typically involve the spine, sacroiliac joints, or other fibrocartilaginous joints. Unusual cases of arthritis due to *Aspergillus* species, *Cryptococcus neoformans*, *Pseudallescheria boydii*, and the dematiaceous fungi have also resulted from direct inoculation or disseminated hematogenous infection in immunocompromised persons.

The synovial fluid in fungal arthritis usually contains 10,000 to 40,000 cells/μL, with ~70% neutrophils. Stained specimens and cultures of synovial tissue often confirm the diagnosis of fungal arthritis when studies of synovial fluid give negative results. Treatment consists of drainage and lavage of the joint and systemic administration of an antifungal agent directed at a specific pathogen. The doses and duration of therapy are the same as for disseminated disease (see Part VI, Section 16). Intraarticular instillation of amphotericin B has been used in addition to IV therapy.

VIRAL ARTHRITIS Viruses produce arthritis by infecting synovial tissue during systemic infection or by provoking an immunologic reaction that involves joints. As many as 50% of women report persistent arthralgias and 10% report frank arthritis within 3 days of the rash that follows natural infection with rubella virus and within 2 to 6 weeks after receipt of live-virus vaccine. Episodes of symmetric inflammation of fingers, wrists, and knees uncommonly recur for >1 year, but a syndrome of chronic fatigue, low-grade fever, headaches, and myalgias can persist for months or years. Intravenous immunoglobulin has been helpful in selected cases. Self-limited monarticular or migratory polyarthritis may develop within 2 weeks of the parotitis of mumps; this sequela is more common among men than among women. Approximately 10% of children and 60% of women develop arthritis after infection with parvovirus B19. In adults, arthropathy sometimes occurs without fever or rash. Pain and stiffness, with less prominent swelling (primarily of the hands but also of the knees, wrists, and ankles), usually resolve within weeks, although a small proportion of patients develop chronic arthropathy.

About 2 weeks before the onset of jaundice, up to 10% of persons with acute hepatitis B develop an immune complex–mediated, serum sickness–like reaction with maculopapular rash, urticaria, fever, and arthralgias. Less common developments include symmetric arthritis involving the hands, wrists, elbows, or ankles and morning stiffness that resembles a flare of rheumatoid arthritis. Symptoms resolve at the time jaundice develops. Many persons with chronic hepatitis C infection report persistent arthralgia or arthritis, both in the presence and in the absence of cryoglobulinemia. Painful arthritis involving larger joints often accompanies the fever and rash of several arthropod-borne viral infections, including those caused by chikungunya, O'nyong-nyong, Ross River, Mayaro, and Barmah Forest viruses. Symmetric arthritis involving the hands and wrists may occur during the convalescent phase of infection with lymphocytic choriomeningitis virus. Patients infected with an enterovirus frequently report arthralgias, and echovirus has been isolated from patients with acute polyarthritis.

Several arthritis syndromes are associated with HIV infection. Reiter's syndrome with painful lower-extremity oligoarthritis often follows an episode of urethritis in HIV-infected persons. HIV-associated Reiter's syndrome appears to be extremely common among persons with the HLA-B27 haplotype, but sacroiliac joint disease is unusual and is seen mostly in the absence of HLA-B27. Up to one-third of HIV-infected persons with psoriasis develop psoriatic arthritis. Painless monarthropathy and persistent symmetric polyarthropathy occasionally complicate HIV infection. Chronic persistent oligoarthritis of the shoulders, wrists, hands, and knees occurs in women infected with human T-cell lymphotropic virus type I. Synovial thickening, destruction of articular cartilage, and leukemic-appearing atypical lymphocytes in synovial fluid are characteristic, but progression to T cell leukemia is unusual.

PARASITIC ARTHRITIS Arthritis due to parasitic infection is rare. The guinea worm *Dracunculus medinensis* may cause destructive joint lesions in the lower extremities as migrating gravid female worms invade joints or cause ulcers in adjacent soft tissues that become secondarily infected. Hydatid cysts infect bones in 1 to 2% of cases of infection with *Echinococcus granulosus*. The expanding destructive cystic lesions may spread to and destroy adjacent joints, particularly the hip and pelvis. In rare cases, chronic synovitis has been associated with the presence of schistosomal eggs in synovial biopsies. Monarticular arthritis in children with lymphatic filariasis appears to respond to therapy with diethylcarbamazine, even in the absence of microfilariae in synovial fluid. Reactive arthritis has been attributed to hookworm, *Strongyloides*, *Cryptosporidium*, and *Giardia* infection in case reports, but confirmation is required.

POSTINFECTIOUS OR REACTIVE ARTHRITIS Reiter's syndrome, a reactive polyarthritis, develops several weeks after ~1% of cases of nongonococcal urethritis and 2% of enteric infections, particularly those due to *Yersinia enterocolitica*, *Shigella flexneri*, *Campylobacter jejuni*, and *Salmonella* species. Only a minority of these patients have the other findings of classic Reiter's syndrome, including urethritis, conjunctivitis, uveitis, oral ulcers, and rash. Studies have identified microbial DNA or antigen in synovial fluid or blood, but the pathogenesis of this condition is poorly understood.

Reiter's syndrome is most common among young men (except after *Yersinia* infection) and has been linked to the HLA-B27 locus as a potential genetic predisposing factor. Patients report painful, asymmetric oligoarthritis affecting mainly the knees, ankles, and feet. Low-back pain is common, and radiographic evidence of sacroiliitis is found in patients with long-standing disease. Most patients recover within 6 months, but prolonged recurrent disease is more common in cases following chlamydial urethritis. Anti-inflammatory agents help to relieve symptoms, but the role of prolonged antibiotic therapy in eliminating microbial antigen from the synovium is controversial.

Migratory polyarthritis and fever constitute the usual presentation of acute rheumatic fever in adults (Chap. 302). This presentation is distinct from that of poststreptococcal reactive arthritis, which also follows infections with group A *Streptococcus* but is not migratory, lasts beyond the typical 3-week maximum of acute rheumatic fever, and responds poorly to aspirin.

INFECTIONS IN PROSTHETIC JOINTS Infection complicates 1 to 4% of total joint replacements. The majority of infections are acquired intraoperatively or immediately postoperatively as a result of wound breakdown or infection; less commonly, these joint infections develop later after joint replacement and are the result of hematogenous spread or direct inoculation. The presentation may be acute, with fever, pain, and local signs of inflammation, especially in infections due to *S. aureus*, pyogenic streptococci, and enteric bacilli. Alternatively, infection may persist for months or years without causing constitutional symptoms when less virulent organisms, such as coagulase-negative staphylococci or diphtheroids, are involved. Such indolent infections are usually acquired during joint implantation and are discovered during evaluation of chronic unexplained pain or after a radiograph shows loosening of the prosthesis; the erythrocyte sedimentation rate and C-reactive protein level are usually elevated in such cases.

The diagnosis is best made by needle aspiration of the joint; accidental introduction of organisms during aspiration must be meticulously avoided. Synovial fluid pleocytosis with a predominance of polymorphonuclear leukocytes is highly suggestive of infection, since other inflammatory processes uncommonly affect prosthetic joints. Culture and Gram's stain usually yield the responsible pathogen. Use of special media for unusual pathogens such as fungi, atypical mycobacteria, and *Mycoplasma* may be necessary if routine and anaerobic cultures are negative.

R̲x̲ TREATMENT

Treatment includes surgery and high doses of parenteral antibiotics, which are given for 4 to 6 weeks because bone is usually involved. In most cases, the prosthesis must be replaced to cure the infection. Implantation of a new prosthesis is best delayed for several weeks or months because relapses of infection occur most commonly within this time frame. In some cases, reimplantation is not possible, and the patient must manage without a joint, with a fused joint, or even with amputation. Cure of infection without removal of the prosthesis is occasionally possible in cases that are due to streptococci or pneumococci and that lack radiologic evidence of loosening of the prosthesis. In these cases, antibiotic therapy must be initiated within several days of the onset of infection, and the joint should be drained vigorously either by open arthrotomy or arthroscopically. In selected patients who prefer to avoid the high morbidity associated with joint removal and reimplantation, suppression of the infection with antibiotics may be a reasonable goal. A high cure rate with retention of the prosthesis has been reported when the combination of oral rifampin and ciprofloxacin is given for 3 to 6 months to persons with staphylococcal prosthetic joint infection of short duration. This approach, which is based on the ability of rifampin to kill organisms adherent to foreign material and in the stationary growth phase, requires confirmation in prospective trials.

Prevention To avoid the disastrous consequences of infection, candidates for joint replacement should be selected with care. Rates of infection are particularly high among patients with rheumatoid arthritis, persons who have undergone previous surgery on the joint, and persons with medical conditions requiring immunosuppressive therapy. Perioperative antibiotic prophylaxis, usually with cefazolin, and measures to decrease intraoperative contamination, such as laminar flow, have lowered the rates of perioperative infection to <1% in many centers. After implantation, measures should be taken to prevent or rapidly treat extraarticular infections that might give rise to hematogenous spread to the prosthesis. The effectiveness of prophylactic antibiotics for the prevention of hematogenous infection following dental procedures has not been demonstrated; in fact, viridans streptococci and other components of the oral flora are extremely unusual causes of prosthetic joint infection. Accordingly, the American Dental Association and the American Academy of Orthopaedic Surgeons do not recommend antibiotic prophylaxis for most dental patients with total joint replacements. They do, however, recommend prophylaxis for patients who may be at high risk of hematogenous infection, including those with inflammatory arthropathies, immunosuppression, type 1 diabetes mellitus, joint replacement within 2 years, previous prosthetic joint infection, malnourishment, or hemophilia. The recommended regimen is amoxicillin (2 g orally) 1 h before dental procedures associated with a high incidence of bacteremia. Clindamycin (600 mg orally) is suggested for patients allergic to penicillin.

FURTHER READING

BARDIN T: Gonococcal arthritis. Best Pract Res Clin Rheumatol 17:201, 2003

DONATTO KC: Orthopedic management of septic arthritis. Rheum Dis Clin North Am 24:275, 1998

GOLDENBERG DL: Septic arthritis. Lancet 351:197, 1998

HARRINGTON JT: Mycobacterial and fungal arthritis. Curr Opin Rheumatol 10:335, 1998

MEDINA RODRIGUEZ F: Rheumatic manifestations of human immunodeficiency virus infection. Rheum Dis Clin North Am 29:145, 2003

MEEHAN AM et al: Outcome of penicillin-susceptible streptococcal prosthetic joint infection treated with debridement and retention of the prosthesis. Clin Infect Dis 36:845, 2003

STENGEL D et al: Systematic review and meta-analysis of antibiotic therapy for bone and joint infections. Lancet Infect Dis 1:175, 2001

YTTERBERG SR: Viral arthritis. Curr Opin Rheumatol 11:275, 1999

315 FIBROMYALGIA, ARTHRITIS ASSOCIATED WITH SYSTEMIC DISEASE, AND OTHER ARTHRITIDES
Bruce C. Gilliland

FIBROMYALGIA

Fibromyalgia is a commonly encountered disorder characterized by chronic widespread musculoskeletal pain, stiffness, paresthesia, disturbed sleep, and easy fatigability along with multiple painful tender points, which are widely and symmetrically distributed. Fibromyalgia affects predominantly women in a ratio of 9 to 1 compared to men. This disorder is found in most countries, in most ethnic groups, and in all types of climates. The prevalence of fibromyalgia in the general population of a community in the United States using the 1990 American College of Rheumatology (ACR) classification criteria (see below) was reported to be 3.4% in women and 0.5% in men. Contrary to some previous reports, fibromyalgia was not found to be present mainly in young women but, rather, to be most prevalent in women ≥50 years. The prevalence increased with age, being 7.4% in women between the ages of 70 and 79. Although not common, fibromyalgia also occurs in children. The reported prevalence of fibromyalgia in some rheumatology clinics has been as high as 20%. Most patients present with fibromyalgia between the ages of 30 to 50 years.

Pathogenesis Several causative mechanisms for fibromyalgia have been postulated to explain abnormal pain perception. Several abnormalities of the central nervous system have been suggested. Disturbed sleep has been implicated as a factor in the pathogenesis. Nonrestorative sleep or awakening unrefreshed has been observed in most patients with fibromyalgia. Sleep electroencephalographic studies in patients with fibromyalgia have shown disruption of normal stage 4 sleep [non–rapid eye movement (NREM) sleep] by many repeated α-wave intrusions. The idea that stage 4 sleep deprivation has a role in causing this disorder was supported by the observation that symptoms of fibromyalgia developed in normal subjects whose stage 4 sleep was disrupted artificially by induced α-wave intrusions. This sleep disturbance, however, has been demonstrated in healthy individuals; in emotionally distressed individuals; and in patients with sleep apnea, fever, osteoarthritis, or rheumatoid arthritis. Low levels of serotonin metabolites have been reported in the cerebrospinal fluid (CSF) of patients with fibromyalgia, suggesting that a deficiency of serotonin, a neurotransmitter that regulates pain and NREM sleep, might also be involved in the pathogenesis of fibromyalgia. Drugs that affect serotonin metabolism have not had a dramatic effect on fibromyalgia, however. Fibromyalgia patients as a group have been reported by some investigators to have reduced levels of growth hormone, which is important for muscle repair and strength. Growth hormone is secreted normally during stage 4 sleep, which is disturbed in patients with fibromyalgia. The reduction of growth hormone may explain the extended periods of muscle pain following exertion in these patients. The level of the neurotransmitter substance P has been reported to be increased in the CSF of fibromyalgia patients and may play a role in spreading muscle pain. Patients with fibromyalgia have a decreased cortisol response to stress. Low urinary free cortisol and a diminished cortisol response to

corticotropin-releasing hormone suggest an abnormal hypothalamic-pituitary-adrenal axis. Autonomic dysfunction has also been suggested to play a role in the pathogenesis of fibromyalgia. Some patients experience orthostatic hypotension on tilt table testing and may have increased resting supine heart rates. Disturbances of the autonomic and peripheral nervous system may also account for the dry eyes and mouth and the cold sensitivity and Raynaud's-like symptoms seen in patients with fibromyalgia. Single photon emission computed tomography (SPECT) imaging has demonstrated reduced blood flow to the thalamus, caudate nucleus, and pontine tectum, which are areas in the brain involved in the signaling, integration, and modulation of pain. Patients with fibromyalgia have been shown to perceive stimuli such as heat or pressue as painful with less degree of stimulation than normal individuals. The actual threshold for detecting stimuli appears to be similar in both patients and normal subjects.

Many patients with fibromyalgia have psychological abnormalities; there has been disagreement as to whether some of these abnormalities represent reactions to the chronic pain or whether the symptoms of fibromyalgia are a reflection of psychiatric disturbance. Approximately 30% of patients fit a psychiatric diagnosis, the most common being depression, anxiety, somatization, and hypochondriases. Studies have also shown a high prevalence of sexual and physical abuse and eating disorders. However, fibromyalgia also occurs in patients without significant psychiatric problems.

Since patients experience pain from muscle and musculotendinous sites, many studies have been done to examine muscle, both structurally and physiologically. Inflammation or diagnostic muscle abnormalities have not been found. Evidence indicates deconditioning of muscles, and patients experience a greater degree of postexertional pain than do unaffected persons. A better understanding of fibromyalgia awaits further studies.

Clinical Manifestations Symptoms are generalized musculoskeletal aching and stiffness and fatigue. Patients may complain of low back pain, which may radiate into the buttocks and legs. Others complain of pain and tightness in the neck and across the upper posterior shoulders. Patients complain of muscle pain after even mild exertion and some degree of pain is always present. The pain has been described as a burning or gnawing pain or as soreness, stiffness, or aching. Pain may begin in one region, such as the shoulders, neck, or lower back (see "Myofascial Pain Syndrome," below) before it eventually becomes widespread. Patients may complain of joint pain and perceive that their joints are swollen; however, joint examination yields normal findings. Stiffness is usually present on arising in the morning; usually it improves during the day, but in some patients it lasts all day. Patients may complain of numbness of their hands and feet. They may also feel colder overall than others in the home, and some may experience Raynaud's-like phenomena or actual Raynaud's phenomenon. Patients complain of feeling fatigued and exhausted and wake up tired. They also awaken frequently at night and have trouble falling back to sleep.

FIGURE 315-1 Tender points in fibromyalgia. Suboccipital muscle insertion at base of skull; anterior aspect of intertransverse process spaces at C5–7; midpoint of upper border of trapezius muscle; above scapular spine near medial border of scapula; second costochondral junction; lateral epicondyle; upper outer quadrant of buttocks; posterior aspect of trochanteric prominence; medial fat pad of knee (all bilateral). *(From the brochure "Fibromyalgia," Arthritis Information, Advise and Guidance, Disease Series. Used by permission of the Arthritis Foundation.)*

Patients may experience cognitive impairment with difficulty thinking and loss of short-term memory. Headaches, including migraine type, are also common symptons. Others experience episodes of light-headedness, dizziness, anxiety, or depression. Symptoms are made worse by stress or anxiety, cold, damp weather, and overexertion. Patients often feel better during warmer weather and vacations.

The characteristic feature on physical examination is the demonstration of specific sites or points, which are more tender or painful than the same sites in normal individuals. The ACR Criteria for Fibromyalgia defines 18 tender points (Fig. 315-1). These points of tenderness are remarkably constant in location. A moderate and consistent degree of pressure should be used in digital palpation of these tender points. As a guideline to reduce variability in the interpretation of point tenderness, the amount of force applied should be 4 kg (~9 lb), which is the degree of force required to just blanch the examiner's thumbnail. This amount of pressure does not produce significant tenderness or pain in normal subjects. Some workers recommend that the tender site be palpated using a rolling motion, which may be more effective in eliciting the tenderness. The tender sites can also be examined using a dolorimeter, which is a spring-loaded pressure gauge; however, digital palpation appears to be as effective and accurate. Some investigators have quantitated the degree of tenderness or pain, but the number of tender point sites is more diagnostic. Some patients are tender all over although still more tender or painful at the specific tender point sites.

Skinfold tenderness may be present, particularly over the upper scapular region. Subcutaneous nodules may be felt at sites of tenderness. Nodules in similar locations are present in normal persons but are not tender.

Fibromyalgia may be triggered by emotional stress, infections and other medical illness, surgery, hypothyroidism, and trauma. It has appeared in some patients with hepatitis C infection, HIV infection, parvovirus B19 infection, or Lyme disease. In the latter situation, fibromyalgia may persist despite adequate antibiotic treatment for Lyme disease, and especially anxious patients may believe that they still have Lyme disease. Disorders commonly associated with fibromyalgia include irritable bowel syndrome, irritable bladder, headaches (including migraine headaches), dysmenorrhea, premenstrual syn-

drome, restless leg syndrome, temporomandibular joint pain, non-cardiac chest pain, Raynaud's phenomenon, and sicca syndrome.

The course of fibromyalgia is variable. Symptoms wax and wane in some patients, while in others pain and fatigue are persistent regardless of therapy. Studies from tertiary medical centers indicate a poor prognosis for most patients. The prognosis may be better in community-treated patients. In a community-based study reported after 2 years of treatment, 24% of patients were in remission, and 47% no longer fulfilled the ACR criteria for fibromyalgia.

Diagnosis Fibromyalgia is diagnosed by a history of widespread musculoskeletal pain present for at least 3 months and the demonstration of significant tenderness or pain in at least 11 of the 18 tender point sites on digital palpation (Fig. 315-1). The ACR criteria are useful for standardizing the diagnosis; however, not all patients with fibromyalgia meet these criteria (Table 315-1). Some patients have fewer tender sites and more regional pain and may be considered to have fibromyalgia.

The musculoskeletal and neurologic examinations are normal in fibromyalgia patients, and there are no laboratory abnormalities. Fibromyalgia may occur in patients with rheumatoid arthritis, systemic lupus erythematosus (SLE), other connective tissue diseases, or other medical illness. A distinction is no longer made between primary and secondary fibromyalgia (concomitant with other disease), as the signs and symptoms are similar. Fibromyalgia and chronic fatigue syndrome have many similarities (Chap. 370). Both are associated with fatigue, abnormal sleep, musculoskeletal pain, impaired memory and concentration, and psychiatric conditions such as less severe forms of depression and anxiety. Patients with chronic fatigue syndrome, however, are more likely to have symptoms suggesting a viral illness. These include mild fever, sore throat, and pain in the axillary and anterior and posterior cervical lymph nodes. The onset of chronic fatigue syndrome is usually sudden; patients are usually able to date the onset. While many patients with chronic fatigue syndrome have tender or painful points, the diagnosis does not require their presence. Patients with fibromyalgia may be misdiagnosed with SLE or Sjögren's syndrome as these disorders have in common symptoms of musculoskeletal pain, dry eyes, cold hands, and fatigue. The antinuclear antibody (ANA) test may also be positive. The frequency of a positive ANA

TABLE 315-1 The American College of Rheumatology 1990 Criteria for the Classification of Fibromyalgia[a]

1. History of widespread pain. Pain is considered widespread when all of the following are present:
   a. Pain in the left side of the body
   b. Pain in the right side of the body
   c. Pain above the waist
   d. Pain below the waist
   e. Axial skeletal pain (cervical spine or anterior chest or thoracic spine or low back)
2. Pain on digital palpation in at least 11 of the following 18 tender point sites (see Fig. 315-1):
   a. Occiput: bilateral, at the suboccipital muscle insertion
   b. Low cervical: bilateral, at the anterior aspect of the intertransverse spaces at C5–7
   c. Trapezius: bilateral, at the midpoint of the upper border
   d. Supraspinatus: bilateral, at the origin, above the scapular spine near the medial border
   e. Second rib: bilateral, at the second costochondral junction, just lateral to the junction on the upper surface
   f. Lateral epicondyle: bilateral, 2 cm distal to the epicondyle
   g. Gluteal: bilateral, in the upper outer quadrant of the buttock
   h. Greater trochanter: bilateral, posterior to the trochanteric prominence
   i. Knee: bilateral, at the medial fat pad proximal to the joint line

Digital palpation should be performed with a moderate degree of pressure. For a tender point to be considered positive, the subject must state that the palpation was painful. "Tender" is not to be considered painful.

[a] For purposes of classification, patients will be said to have fibromyalgia if both criteria are satisfied. Widespread pain must have been present for at least 3 months. The presence of a second clinical disorder does not exclude the diagnosis of fibromyalgia.
Source: Modified from F Wolfe et al: Arthritis Rheum 33:171, 1990.

test in fibromyalgia patients, however, is the same as sex- and aged-matched normal controls. The predictive value of a positive ANA test in patients without characteristic symptoms and objective features of a connective tissue disease is quite low. Discretion is advised before ordering an ANA test. Patients with fibromyalgia may complain of muscle weakness, but on muscle strength testing, they have "give-away" weakness secondary to pain. Proximal muscle weakness and elevated muscle enzymes distinguish patients with polymyositis. Polymyalgia rheumatica is distinguished from fibromyalgia in an elderly patient by the presence of more proximal muscle stiffness and pain and an elevated erythrocyte sedimentation rate. Patients should be evaluated for hypothyroidism, which may have symptoms similar to fibromyalgia or may accompany fibromyalgia. Disturbed sleep, musculoskeletal pain, and fatigue occur in patients with sleep apnea and restless leg syndrome. A distinguishing feature of sleep apnea is the presence of significant daytime somnolence. These patients should be referred to a sleep laboratory for evaluation and treatment. Myofascial pain syndrome, which involves an area such as the shoulder or neck, may represent a localized form of fibromyalgia (see "Myofascial Pain Syndrome" below). Some patients with this syndrome progress to fibromyalgia.

The diagnosis of fibromyalgia has taken on a more complex significance in regard to labor and industry issues. This has become a significant issue since it has been reported that 10 to 25% of patients are not able to work in any capacity, while others require modification of their work. Disability evaluation in fibromyalgia is controversial. The diagnosis of fibromyalgia is not accepted by all. It is hard to evaluate patients' perceptions of their inability to function. The determination of tender points can also be subjective, on the part of both the physician and the patient, particularly when issues of compensation are pending. Patients also encounter difficulty in having their illness recognized as a disability. Physicians have been placed in the inappropriate role of assessing the patient's disability. Physicians are not in a position to quantitate disability at the workplace; that is better done by a work evaluation specialist. Better instruments are clearly needed for measuring disability, particularly in patients with fibromyalgia.

℞ TREATMENT

Patients should be informed that they have a condition that is not crippling, deforming, or degenerative, and that treatment is available. The initial step in treatment is to improve the quality of sleep. The use of tricyclics such as amitriptyline (10 to 50 mg), nortriptyline (10 to 75 mg), and doxepin (10 to 25 mg) or a pharmacologically similar drug, cyclobenzaprine (10 to 40 mg), 1 to 2 h before bedtime will give the patient restorative sleep (stage 4 sleep), resulting in clinical improvement. Patients should be started on a low dose, which is increased gradually as needed. Side effects of these tricyclics and cyclobenzaprine limit their use; these include constipation, dry mouth, weight gain, drowsiness, and difficulty thinking. Trazodone or zolpidem also improves sleep quality. In patients with restless leg syndrome, clonazepam may be effective. Depression and anxiety should next be treated with appropriate drugs and, when indicated, with psychiatric counseling. Fluoxetine, sertraline, paroxetine, citalopram, or other newer selective serotonin reuptake inhibitors can be used as antidepressants. Other useful antidepressants are trazodone and venlafaxine. Alprazolam and lorazepam are effective for anxiety. Patients may also benefit by regular aerobic exercises, which are started after patients begin to have improved sleep and less pain and fatigue. Exercise should be of a low-impact type and begun at a low level. Eventually, the patient should be exercising 20 to 30 min 3 to 4 days a week. Regular stretching exercises are also very important. Salicylates or other nonsteroidal anti-inflammatory drugs (NSAIDs) only partially improve symptoms. Glucocorticoids have been of little benefit and should not be used in these patients. Opiate analgesics should be avoided. For pain, acetaminophen or tramadol may be useful. Also gabapentin (300 to 1200 mg/d in divided doses) may reduce pain. Local measures such as heat, massage, injection of tender sites with steroids or lidocaine, and acupuncture provide only temporary relief of symptoms. Other therapies that may help to varying degrees including biofeedback, behavioral modification, hypnotherapy, and stress management and relaxation response training. Life stresses should be identified and discussed with the patient, and the patient should be provided with help on how to cope with these stresses. Patients may benefit from a multidisciplinary team approach involving a mental health professional, a physical therapist, and a physical medicine and rehabilitation specialist. Group therapy may be beneficial. Patients should be well educated about their disorder and taught the importance of self help. There are patient support groups in many communities. While treatment of fibromyalgia is effective in some patients, others continue to have chronic disease, which is relieved only partially if at all.

ARTHRITIS ASSOCIATED WITH SYSTEMIC DISEASE

ARTHROPATHY OF ACROMEGALY Acromegaly is the result of excessive production of growth hormone by an adenoma in the anterior pituitary gland (Chap. 318). Middle-aged persons are most often affected. The excessive secretion of growth hormone along with insulin-like growth factor I stimulates proliferation of cartilage, periarticular connective tissue, and bone, resulting in several musculoskeletal abnormalities, including osteoarthritis, back pain, muscle weakness, and carpal tunnel syndrome.

An arthropathy resembling osteoarthritis is a common feature, affecting most often the knees, shoulders, hips, and hands. Single or multiple joints may be affected. The overgrowth of cartilage initially produces widening of the joint space. The newly synthesized cartilage is not developed in an organized manner, making it susceptible to fissuring, ulceration, and destruction. Ligamental laxity of the joint resulting from the growth of connective tissue also contributes to the development of osteoarthritis. With breakdown and loss of cartilage, the joint space narrows, and subchondral sclerosis and osteophytes appear on radiographs. Joint examination reveals marked crepitus and hypermobility. Joint fluid is noninflammatory. Calcium pyrophosphate dihydrate crystals are found in the cartilage in some cases of acromegaly arthropathy and, when shed into the joint, can produce attacks of pseudogout. Chondrocalcinosis may also be observed radiographically. Approximately half of the patients with acromegaly experience back pain, which is predominantly lumbosacral. Hypermobility of the spine may be a contributing factor in back pain. Radiograph of the spine shows normal or increased intervertebral disk spaces, hypertrophic anterior osteophytes, and ligamental calcification. These changes are similar to those observed in patients with diffuse idiopathic skeletal hyperostosis. Dorsal kyphosis in conjunction with elongation of the ribs contributes to the development of the barrel chest seen in acromegalic patients. The hands and feet become enlarged owing to soft tissue proliferation. The fingers are thickened and have spadelike distal tufts. One-third of patients have a thickened heel pad. Approximately 25% of patients have Raynaud's phenomenon.

Carpal tunnel syndrome occurs in about half of patients. The median nerve is compressed by the excessive growth of connective tissue in the carpal tunnel. The median nerve also becomes enlarged. Patients with acromegaly also develop proximal muscle weakness, which is thought to be caused by the effect of growth hormone on muscle. Results of muscle enzyme assays and electromyography are normal. Muscle biopsy specimens show muscle fibers of varying size and no inflammatory changes.

ARTHROPATHY OF HEMOCHROMATOSIS Hemochromatosis is a disorder of iron storage. Excessive amounts of iron are absorbed from the intestine, leading to iron deposition in parenchymal cells, which results in tissue damage and impairment of organ function (Chap. 336). Symptoms of hemochromatosis usually begin between the ages of 40 and 60 but can occur earlier. Arthritis, which occurs in 20 to 40% of patients, usually begins after the age of 50 and may be the first clinical feature of hemochromatosis. The arthropathy is an osteoarthritis-like disorder affecting the small joints of the hands, followed later by larger joints such as knees, ankles, shoulders, and hips. The second and third metacarpophalangeal joints of both hands are often the first joints affected; they can provide an important clue to the possibility of hemochromatosis. Patients experience stiffness and pain. Morning stiffness usually lasts less than half an hour. The affected joints are enlarged and mildly tender. Synovial tissue is not appreciatively increased. Radiographs show irregular narrowing of the joint space, subchondral sclerosis, and subchondral cysts. There is juxtaarticular proliferation of bone, with frequent hooklike osteophytes. The synovial fluid is noninflammatory. The synovium shows mild to moderate proliferation of lining cells, fibrosis, and a low number of inflammatory cells, which are mononuclear. In approximately half of patients, there is evidence of calcium pyrophosphate deposition disease (CPDD), and patients may experience episodes of pseudogout. Iron can be demonstrated in the lining cells of the synovium and also in chondrocytes.

Iron may damage the articular cartilage in several ways. Iron catalyzes superoxide-dependent lipid peroxidation, which may play a role in joint damage. In animal models, ferric iron has been shown to interfere with collagen formation. Iron has also been shown to increase the release of lysosomal enzymes from cells in the synovial membrane. Iron may also play a role in the development of chondrocalcinosis. Iron inhibits synovial tissue pyrophosphatase in vitro and, therefore, may inhibit pyrophosphatase in vivo, resulting in chondrocalcinosis. Iron in synovial cells may also inhibit the clearance of calcium pyrophosphate from the joint.

℞ TREATMENT

The treatment of hemochromatosis is repeated phlebotomy. Unfortunately, this treatment has little effect on the arthritis, which, along with chondrocalcinosis, usually continues to progress. Treatment of the arthritis consists of administration of acetaminophen and NSAIDs. Acute pseudogout attacks are treated with higher doses of an NSAID or a short cause of glucocorticoids. Placement of a hip or knee prosthesis has been successful in advanced disease.

HEMOPHILIC ARTHROPATHY Hemophilia is a sex-linked recessive genetic disorder characterized by the absence or deficiency of factor VIII (hemophilia A, or classic hemophilia) or factor IX (hemophilia B, or Christmas disease) (Chap. 102). Hemophilia A is by far the more common type, constituting 85% of cases. Spontaneous hemarthrosis is a common problem with both types of hemophilia and can lead to a chronic deforming arthritis. The frequency and severity of hemarthrosis are related to the degree of clotting factor deficiency. Hemarthrosis is not common in other inherited disorders of coagulation, such as von Willebrand's disease or factor V deficiency.

Hemarthrosis becomes evident after 1 year of age, when the child begins to walk and run. In order of frequency, the joints most commonly affected are the knees, ankles, elbows, shoulders, and hips. Small joints of the hands and feet are occasionally involved.

In the initial stage of arthropathy, hemarthrosis produces a warm, tensely swollen, and painful joint. The patient holds the affected joint in flexion and guards against any movement. Blood in the joint remains liquid because of the absence of intrinsic clotting factors and the absence of tissue thromboplastin in the synovium. The blood in the joint space is resorbed over a period of a week or longer, depending on the size of the hemarthrosis. Joint function usually returns to normal or baseline in about 2 weeks.

Recurrent hemarthrosis leads to the development of a chronic arthritis. The involved joints remain swollen, and flexion deformities develop. In the later stages of arthropathy, joint motion is restricted and function is severely limited. Joint ankylosis, subluxation, and laxity are features of end-stage disease.

Bleeding into muscle and soft tissue also causes musculoskeletal

disorders. When bleeding into the iliopsoas muscle occurs, the hip is held in flexion because of the pain, resulting in a hip flexion contracture. Rotation of the hip is preserved, which distinguishes this problem from intraarticular hemorrhage. Expansion of the hematoma may place pressure on the femoral nerve, resulting in a femoral neuropathy. Another problem is shortening of the heel cord secondary to bleeding into the gastrocnemius. Hemorrhage into a closed compartment space, such as the volar compartment in the forearm, can result in muscle necrosis, neuropathy and flexion deformities of the wrist and fingers. When bleeding involves periosteum or bone, a pseudotumor forms. These occur distal to the elbows or knees in children and improve with treatment of the hemophilia. Surgical removal is indicated if the pseudotumor continues to enlarge. In adults, they occur in the femur and pelvis and are usually refractory to treatment. When bleeding occurs in muscle, cysts may develop within the muscle. Needle aspiration of a cyst is contraindicated because it can induce bleeding.

Septic arthritis can occur in hemophilia and is difficult at times to distinguish from acute hemarthrosis on physical examination. Whenever there is suspicion of an infected joint, the joint should be aspirated immediately, the fluid cultured, and the patient started on antibiotics that provide broad coverage until the results of the culture are known. The patient should be infused with the deficient clotting factor before the joint is tapped to decrease the risk of further bleeding.

Radiographs of joints reflect the stage of disease. In early stages there is only capsule distention; later, juxtaarticular osteopenia, marginal erosions, and subchondral cysts develop. In late disease, the joint space is narrowed and there is bony overgrowth. The changes are similar to those observed in osteoarthritis. Unique features of hemophilic arthropathy are widening of the femoral intercondylar notch, enlargement of the proximal radius, and squaring of the distal end of the patella.

Recurrent hemarthrosis produces synovial hyperplasia and hypertrophy. A pannus covers the cartilage. Cartilage is damaged by collagenase and other degradative enzymes released by mononuclear cells in the overlying synovium. Hemosiderin is found in synovial lining cells, the subsynovium, and chondrocytes and may also play a role in cartilage destruction.

℞ TREATMENT

The treatment of hemarthrosis is initiated with the immediate infusion of factor VIII or IX at the first sign of joint or muscle hemorrhage. The patient is placed at bed rest, with the involved joint in as much extension as the patient can tolerate. Analgesic doses of an NSAID and local icing may help with the pain. NSAIDs can be given safely for short periods even though they have a stabilizing effect on platelets. Studies have shown no significant abnormalities in platelet function or bleeding time in hemophiliacs receiving ibuprofen. The cyclooxygenase-2 inhibitors celecoxib, rofecoxib, and kaldecoxib do not interfere with platelet function and can be safely given for pain. Synovectomy, open or arthroscopic, may be indicated in patients with chronic synovial proliferation and recurrent hemarthrosis. Hypertrophied synovium is very vascular and subject to bleeding. Both types of synovectomy reduce the number of hemarthroses and slow the roentgenographic progression of hemophilic arthropathy. Open surgical synovectomy, however, is associated with some loss of range of motion. Radiosynovectomy with either yttrium 90 silicate or phosphorus 31 colloid has also been effective and may be a useful alternative when surgical synovectomy is not practical. Total joint replacement is indicated for severe joint destruction and incapacitating pain. Because of the young age of hemophilic patients, total-joint prostheses may need to be replaced more than once during their lives.

ARTHROPATHIES ASSOCIATED WITH HEMOGLOBINOPATHIES ■ Sickle Cell Disease Sickle cell disease (Chap. 91) is associated with several musculoskeletal abnormalities (Table 315-2). Children under the age of 5 may develop diffuse swelling, tenderness, and warmth of the hands and feet lasting from 1 to 3 weeks. The condition, referred to as *sickle cell dactylitis* or *hand-foot syndrome*, has also been observed in sickle cell

TABLE 315-2 *Musculoskeletal Abnormalities in Sickle Cell Disease*

Sickle cell dactylitis	Avascular necrosis
Joint effusions in sickle cell crises	Bone changes secondary to marrow
Osteomyelitis	hyperplasia
Infarction of bone	Septic arthritis
Infarction of bone marrow	Gouty arthritis

disease and sickle cell thalassemia. Dactylitis is believed to result from infarction of the bone marrow and cortical bone leading to periostitis and soft tissue swelling. Radiographs show periosteal elevation, subperiosteal new bone formation, and areas of radiolucency and increased density involving the metacarpals, metatarsals, and proximal phalanges. These bone changes disappear after several months. The syndrome leaves little or no residual damage. Because hematopoiesis ceases in the small bones of hands and feet with age, the syndrome is rarely seen after age 4 or 5 and does not occur in adults.

Sickle cell crisis is often associated with periarticular pain and joint effusions. The joint and periarticular area are warm and tender. Knees and elbows are most often affected, but other joints can be involved. Joint effusions are noninflammatory, with white cell counts <1000/μL; mononuclear cells predominate. There have been a few reports of sterile inflammatory effusion with high cell counts consisting of mostly polymorphonuclear white cells. Synovial biopsies have shown mild lining cell proliferation and microvascular thrombosis. Scintigraphic studies have shown decreased marrow uptake adjacent to the involved joint. The joint effusion and periarticular pain are considered to be the result of ischemia and infarction of the synovium and adjacent bone and bone marrow. The treatment is that for sickle cell crisis (Chap. 91).

Patients with sickle cell disease may also develop osteomyelitis, which commonly involves the long tubular bones (Chap. 111). These patients are particularly susceptible to bacterial infections, especially *Salmonella* infections, which are found in more than half of cases. The most common isolate is *S. typhimurium* (Chap. 137). Radiographs of the involved site show periosteal elevation initially, followed by disruption of the cortex. Treatment of the infection results in healing of the bone lesion. Sickle cell disease is also associated with bone infarction resulting from thrombosis secondary to the sickling of red cells. Bone infarction also occurs in hemoglobin S-C disease and sickle cell thalassemia (Chap. 91). The bone pain in sickle cell crisis is due to bone and bone marrow infarction. In children, infarction of the epiphyseal growth plate interferes with normal growth of the affected extremity. Radiographically, infarction of the bone cortex results in periosteal elevation and irregular thickening of the bone cortex. Infarction in the bone marrow leads to lysis, fibrosis, and new bone formation.

Avascular necrosis of the head of the femur is seen in ~5% of patients. It also occurs in the humeral head and less commonly in the distal femur, tibial condyles, distal radius, vertebral bodies, and other juxtaarticular sites. The mechanism for avascular necrosis is most likely the same as for bone infarction. Subchondral hemorrhage may play a role in the deterioration of articular cartilage. Irregularity of the femoral head or of other bone surfaces affected by avascular necrosis eventually results in degenerative joint disease. Radiograph of the affected joint may show patchy radiolucency and density followed by flattening of the bone. Magnetic resonance imaging (MRI) is a sensitive technique for detecting early avascular necrosis as well as bone infarction elsewhere. Total hip replacement and placement of prostheses in other joints may improve function and relieve pain in those patients with severe joint destruction.

Septic arthritis is occasionally encountered in sickle cell disease (Chap. 314). Multiple joints may be infected. Joint infection may result from hematogenous spread or from spread of contiguous osteomyelitis. Microorganisms identified include *Staphylococcus aureus*, *Streptococcus*, *Escherichia coli*, and *Salmonella*. The latter is not seen as frequently in septic arthritis as it is in osteomyelitis. Acute gouty arthritis is uncommon in sickle cell disease, even though 40% of patients

are hyperuremic. Hyperuricemia is due to overproduction of uric acid secondary to increased red cell turnover. Attacks may be polyarticular.

The bone marrow hyperplasia in sickle cell disease results in widening of the medullary cavities, thinning of the cortices, and coarse trabeculations and central cupping of the vertebral bodies. These changes are also seen to a lesser degree in hemoglobin S-C disease and sickle cell thalassemia. In normal individuals, red marrow is located mostly in the axial skeletal, but in sickle cell disease, red marrow is found in the bones of the extremities and even in the tarsal and carpal bones. Vertebral compression may lead to dorsal kyphosis, and softening of the bone in the acetabulum may result in protrusio acetabuli.

Thalassemia β-Thalassemia is a congenital disorder of hemoglobin synthesis characterized by impaired production of β chains (Chap. 91). Bone and joint abnormalities occur in β-thalassemia, being most common in the major and intermedia groups. In one study, ~50% of patients with β-thalassemia had evidence of symmetric ankle arthropathy, characterized by a dull aching pain aggravated by weight bearing. The onset was most often in the second or third decade of life. The degree of ankle pain in these patients varied. Some patients experienced self-limited ankle pain, which occurred only after strenuous physical activity and lasted several days to weeks. Other patients had chronic ankle pain, which became worse with walking. Symptoms eventually abated in a few patients. Compression of the ankle, calcaneus, or forefoot was painful in some patients. Synovial fluid from two patients was noninflammatory. Radiographs of ankle showed osteopenia, widened medullary spaces, thin cortices, and coarse trabeculations. These findings were largely the result of bone marrow expansion. The joint space was preserved. Specimens of bone from three patients revealed osteomalacia, osteopenia, and microfractures. Increased osteoblasts as well as increased foci of bone resorption were present on the bone surface. Iron staining was found in the bone trabeculae, in osteoid, and in the cement line. Synovium showed hyperplasia of lining cells, which contained deposits of hemosiderin. This arthropathy was considered to be related to the underlying bone pathology. The role of iron overload or abnormal bone metabolism in the pathogenesis of this arthropathy is not known. The arthropathy was treated with analgesics and splints. Patients were also transfused to decrease hematopoiesis and bone marrow expansion.

Patients with β-thalassemia major and intermedia also have involvement of other joints, including the knees, hips, and shoulders. Acquired hemochromatosis with arthropathy has been described in a patient with thalassemia. Gouty arthritis and septic arthritis can occur. Avascular necrosis is not a feature of thalassemia because there is no sickling of red cells leading to thrombosis and infarction.

β-Thalassemia minor (trait) is also associated with joint manifestations. Chronic seronegative oligoarthritis affecting predominantly ankles, wrists, and elbows has been described. These patients had mild persistent synovitis without large effusions. Joint erosions were not seen. Recurrent episodes of an acute asymmetric arthritis have also been reported; episodes last less than a week and may affect knees, ankles, shoulders, elbows, wrists, and metacarpal phalangeal joints. The mechanism for this arthropathy is unknown. Treatment with nonsteroidal drugs was not particularly effective.

MUSCULOSKELETAL DISORDERS ASSOCIATED WITH HYPERLIPIDEMIA (See also Chap. 335) Musculoskeletal manifestations may be the first indication of a hereditary disorder of lipoprotein metabolism. Patients with familial hypercholesterolemia (previously referred to as type II hyperlipoproteinemia) may have recurrent migratory polyarthritis involving knees and other large peripheral joints and, to a lesser degree, peripheral small joints. In a few patients, the arthritis is monarticular. Fever may accompany the arthritis. Pain ranges from moderate to very severe to incapacitating. The involved joints can be warm, erythematous, swollen, and tender. Arthritis usually has a sudden onset, lasts from a few days to 2 weeks, and does not cause joint damage. Episodes may suggest acute gout attacks. Several attacks occur a year. Synovial fluid from involved joints is not inflammatory and contains few white cells and no crystals. Joint involvement may actually represent inflammatory periarthritis or peritendinitis and not intraarticular disease. The recurrent, transient nature of the arthritis may suggest rheumatic fever, especially since patients with hyperlipoproteinemia have an elevated erythrocyte sedimentation rate and a falsely elevated antistreptolysin O titer. Patients may also experience Achilles tendinitis, which can be very painful. Attacks of tendinitis come on gradually and last only a few days. Fever is not present. Patients may be asymptomatic between attacks. During an attack the Achilles tendon is warm, erythematous, swollen, and tender to palpation. Achilles tendinitis and other joint manifestations often precede the appearance of xanthomas and may be the first clinical indication of hyperlipoproteinemia. Attacks of tendinitis may occur following treatment with a lipid-lowering drug. Patients also have tendinous xanthomas in the Achilles, patellar, and extensor tendons of the hands over the knuckles and feet. Xanthomas have also been reported in the peroneal tendon, the plantar aponeurosis, and the periosteum overlying the distal tibia. These xanthomas are located within tendon fibers. Tuberous xanthomas are soft subcutaneous masses located over the extensor surfaces of the elbows, knees, and hands, as well as on the buttocks. They appear in childhood in homozygous patients and after the age of 30 in heterozygous patients. Patients with elevated plasma levels of very low density lipoprotein (VLDL) and triglyceride (previously referred to as type IV hyperlipoproteinemia) may also have a mild inflammatory arthritis affecting large and small peripheral joints, usually in an asymmetric pattern with only a few joints involved at a time. The onset of arthritis is usually in middle age. Arthritis may be persistent or recurrent, with episodes lasting a few days to weeks. Joint pain is severe in some patients. Patients may experience morning stiffness. Joint tenderness and periarticular hyperesthesia may also be present, as may synovial thickening. Joint fluid is usually noninflammatory and without crystals but may have increased white blood cell counts with predominantly mononuclear cells. The fluid is occasionally lactescent. Radiographs may show juxtaarticular osteopenia and cystic lesions. Large bone cysts have been noted in a few patients. Xanthoma and bone cysts are also observed in other lipoprotein disorders. The pathogenesis of arthritis in patients with familial hypercholesterolemia or with elevated levels of VLDL and triglyceride is not well understood. Salicylates, other NSAIDs, or analgesics usually provide relief of symptoms. Clinical improvement may also occur in patients treated with lipid lowering agents; however, patients treated with a HMG CoA reductase agent may experience myalgias, and a few patients may develop polymyositis or even rhabdomyolysis. Myositis has also been reported with the use of niacin (Chap. 370).

OTHER ARTHRITIDES

NEUROPATHIC JOINT DISEASE Neuropathic joint disease (Charcot's joint) is a progressive destructive arthritis associated with loss of pain sensation, proprioception, or both. In addition, normal muscular reflexes that modulate joint movement are decreased. Without these protective mechanisms, joints are subjected to repeated trauma, resulting in progressive cartilage and bone damage. Neuropathic arthropathy was first described by Jean-Martin Charcot in 1868 in patients with tabes dorsalis. The term *Charcot joint* is commonly used interchangeably with *neuropathic joint*. Today, diabetes mellitus is the most frequent cause of neuropathic joint disease. A variety of other disorders are associated with neuropathic arthritis including leprosy, yaws, syringomyelia, meningomyelocoele, congenital indifference to pain, peroneal muscular atrophy (Charcot-Marie-Tooth disease), and amyloidosis. An arthritis resembling neuropathic joint disease is seen in patients who have received frequent intraarticular glucocorticoid injections into a weight-bearing joint and in patients with CPDD. The distribution of joint involvement depends on the underlying neurologic disorder (Table 315-3). In tabes dorsalis, knees, hips, and ankles are most com-

TABLE 315-3   Disorders Associated with Neuropathic Joint Disease

Diabetes mellitus	Amyloidosis
Tabes dorsalis	Leprosy
Meningomyelocele	Congenital indifference to pain
Syringomyelia	Peroneal muscular atrophy

monly affected; in syringomyelia, the glenohumeral joint, elbow, and wrist; and in diabetes mellitus, the tarsal and tarsometatarsal joints.

Pathology and Pathophysiology The pathologic changes in the neuropathic joint are similar to those found in the severe osteoarthritic joint. There is fragmentation and eventual loss of articular cartilage with eburnation of the underlying bone. Osteophytes are found at the joint margins. With more advanced disease, erosions are present on the joint surface. Fractures, devitalized bone, and intraarticular loose bodies may be present. Microscopic fragments of cartilage and bone are seen in the synovial tissue.

At least two underlying mechanisms are believed to be involved in the pathogenesis of neuropathic arthritis. An abnormal autonomic nervous system is thought to be responsible for the increased blood flow to the joint and subsequent resorption of bone. Loss of bone, particularly in the diabetic foot, may be the initial manifestation. With the loss of deep pain, proprioception, and protective neuromuscular reflexes, the joint is subjected to repeated injuries including ligamental tears and bone fractures. The mechanism of injury that occurs following frequent intraarticular glucocorticoid injections is thought to be due to the analgesic effect of glucocorticoids leading to overuse of an already damaged joint, which results in accelerated cartilage damage. It is not understood why only a few patients with neuropathies develop neuropathic arthritis.

Clinical Manifestations Neuropathic joint disease usually begins in a single joint and then progresses to involve other joints, depending on the underlying neurologic disorder. The involved joint progressively becomes enlarged from bony overgrowth and synovial effusion. Loose bodies may be palpated in the joint cavity. Joint instability, subluxation, and crepitus occur as the disease progresses. Neuropathic joints may develop rapidly, and a totally disorganized joint with multiple bony fragments may evolve in a patient within weeks or months. The amount of pain experienced by the patient is less than would be anticipated based on the degree of joint involvement. Patients may experience sudden joint pain from intraarticular fractures of osteophytes or condyles.

Neuropathic arthritis is encountered most often in patients with diabetes mellitus, with the incidence estimated in the range of 0.5%. The usual age of onset is ≥50 years following several years of diabetes, but exceptions occur. The tarsal and tarsometatarsal joints are most often affected, followed by the metatarsophalangeal and talotibial joints. The knees and spine are occasionally involved. In about 20%, neuropathic arthritis may be present in both feet. Patients often attribute the onset of foot pain to antecedent trauma such as twisting their foot. Neuropathic changes may develop rapidly following a foot fracture or dislocation. Swelling of the foot and ankle are often present. Downward collapse of the tarsal bones leads to convexity of the sole, referred to as a "rocker foot." Large osteophytes may protrude from the top of the foot. Calluses frequently form over the metatarsal heads and may lead to infected ulcers and osteomyelitis. Radiographs may show resorption and tapering of the distal metatarsal bones. The term *Lisfranc fracture-dislocation* is sometimes used to describe the destructive changes at the tarsometatarsal joints.

Diagnosis The diagnosis of neuropathic arthritis is based on the clinical features and characteristic radiographic findings in a patient with an underlying sensory neuropathy. The differential diagnosis of neuropathic arthritis includes osteomyelitis, osteonecrosis, advanced osteoarthritis, stress fractures, and CPDD. Radiographs in neuropathic arthritis initially show changes of osteoarthritis with joint space narrowing, subchondral bone sclerosis, osteophytes, and joint effusions followed later by marked destructive and hypertrophic changes. Soft tissue swelling, bone resorption, fractures, large osteophytes, extraarticular bone fragments, and subluxation are present with advanced arthropathy. The radiographic findings of neuropathic arthritis may be difficult to differentiate from those of osteomyelitis, especially in the diabetic foot. The joint margins in a neuropathic joint tend to be distinct, while in osteomyelitis, they are blurred. Imaging studies and cultures of fluid and tissue from the joint are often required to exclude osteomyelitis. MRI is helpful in differentiating these disorders. Another useful study is a bone scan using indium 111–labeled white blood cells or indium 111–labeled immunoglobulin G, which will show an increased uptake in osteomyelitis but not in a neuropathic joint. A technetium bone scan will not distinguish osteomyelitis from neuropathic arthritis as increased uptake is observed in both. The joint fluid in neuropathic arthritis is noninflammatory; may be xanthochromic or even bloody; and may contain fragments of synovium, cartilage, and bone. The finding of calcium pyrophosphate dihydrate crystals suggests the diagnosis of a crystal-associated neuropathic-like arthropathy. In the absence of such crystals, the presence of increased number of leukocytes may indicate osteomyelitis.

℞ TREATMENT

The primary focus of treatment is to provide stabilization of the joint. Treatment of the underlying disorder, even if successful, does not usually alter the joint disease. Braces and splints are helpful. Their use requires close surveillance, since patients may be unable to appreciate pressure from a poorly adjusted brace. In the diabetic patient, early recognition and treatment of a Charcot's foot by prohibiting weight bearing of the foot for at least 8 weeks may possibly prevent severe disease from developing. Fusion of a very unstable joint may improve function, but nonunion is frequent, especially when immobilization of the joint is inadequate.

HYPERTROPHIC OSTEOARTHROPATHY AND CLUBBING Hypertrophic osteoarthropathy (HOA) is characterized by clubbing of digits and, in more advanced stages, by periosteal new bone formation and synovial effusions. HOA occurs in primary or familial form and usually begins in childhood. The secondary form of HOA is associated with intrathoracic malignancies, suppurative lung disease, congenital heart disease, and a variety of other disorders and is more common in adults. Clubbing is almost always a feature of HOA but can occur as an isolated manifestation (Fig. 315-2). The presence of clubbing in isolation is generally considered to represent either an early stage or an element in the spectrum of HOA. The presence of only clubbing in a patient usually has the same clinical significance as HOA.

Pathology and Pathophysiology In HOA, the bone changes in the distal extremities begin as periostitis followed by new bone formation. At this stage, a radiolucent area may be observed between the new periosteal bone and subjacent cortex. As the process progresses, multiple layers of new bone are deposited, which become contiguous with the cortex and result in cortical thickening. The outer portion of bone is laminated in appearance, with an irregular surface. Initially, the process of periosteal new bone formation involves the proximal and distal diaphyses of the tibia, fibula, radius, and ulna and, less frequently, the femur, humerus, metacarpals, metatarsals, and phalanges. Occasionally, scapulae, clavicles, ribs, and pelvic bones are also affected. In long-standing disease, these changes extend to involve metaphyses and musculotendinous insertions. The adjacent interosseous membranes may become ossified. The distribution of the bone manifestations is usually bilateral and symmetric. The soft tissue overlying the distal third of the arms and legs may be thickened. Mononuclear cell infiltration may be present in the adjacent soft tissue. Proliferation of connective tissue occurs in the nail bed and volar pad of digits, giving the distal phalanges a clubbed appearance. Small blood vessels in the clubbed digits are dilated and have thickened walls. In addition, the number of arteriovenous anastomoses is increased. The synovia of involved joints show edema, varying degrees of synovial cell proliferation, thickening of the subsynovium, vascular congestion, vascular obliteration with thrombi, and small numbers of lymphocyte infiltrates.

Several theories have been suggested for the pathogenesis of HOA. Most have either been disproved or have not explained the development in all clinical disorders associated with HOA. Previously proposed neurogenic and humoral theories are no longer considered likely explanations for HOA. The neurogenic theory was based on the observation that vagotomy resulted in symptomatic improvement in a small number of patients with lung tumors and HOA. It was postulated that vagal stimuli from the tumor site led via a neural reflex to efferent nerve impulses to the distal extremities, resulting in HOA. This theory, however, did not explain HOA in conditions where vagal stimulation did not occur, as in cyanotic congenital heart disease or arterial aneurysms. The humoral theory postulated that soluble substances that are normally inactivated or removed during passage through the lung reached the systemic circulation in an active form and stimulated the changes of HOA. Substances proposed included prostaglandins, ferritin, bradykinin, estrogen, and growth hormone. These substances seemed unlikely candidates, since their blood levels in HOA patients overlapped those in individuals without HOA. Furthermore, these substances did not explain the development of localized HOA associated with arterial aneurysms or infected arterial grafts.

Recent studies have suggested a role for platelets in the development of HOA. It has been observed that megakaryocytes and large platelet particles, present in venous circulation, were fragmented in their passage through normal lung. In patients with cyanotic congenital heart disease and in other disorders associated with right-to-left shunts, these large platelet particles bypass the lung and reach the distal extremities, where they can interact with endothelial cells. Platelet clumps have been demonstrated to form on an infected heart valve in bacterial endocarditis, in the wall of arterial aneurysms, and on infected arterial grafts. These platelet particles may also reach the distal extremities and interact with endothelial cells. Platelet-endothelial activation in the distal portion of extremities would then result in the release of platelet-derived growth factor (PDGF) and other factors leading to the proliferation of connective tissue and periosteum. Stimulation of fibroblasts by PDGF and transforming growth factor β results in cell growth and collagen synthesis. Elevated plasma levels of von Willebrand factor antigen have been found in patients with both primary and secondary forms of HOA, indicating endothelial activation or damage. Abnormalities of collagen synthesis have been demonstrated in the involved skin of patients with primary HOA. Fibroblasts from affected skin were shown to have increased collagen synthesis, increased $\alpha 1(I)$ procollagen mRNA, and evidence for up-regulation of collagen transcription. Other factors are undoubtedly involved in the pathogenesis of HOA, and further studies are needed to better understand this disorder.

FIGURE 315-2 Clubbing of fingers. *(Reprinted from the Clinical Slide Collection on the Rheumatic Diseases, Copyright 1991, 1995. Used by permission of the American College of Rheumatology.)*

Clinical Manifestations Primary or familial HOA, also referred to as *pachydermoperiostitis* or *Touraine-Solente-Golé syndrome*, usually begins insidiously at puberty. In a smaller number of patients, the onset is in the first year of life. The disorder is inherited as an autosomal dominant trait with variable expression and is nine times more common in boys than in girls. Approximately one-third of patients have a family history of primary HOA.

Primary HOA is characterized by clubbing, periostitis, and unusual skin features. A small number of patients with this syndrome do not express clubbing. The skin changes and periostitis are prominent features of this syndrome. The skin becomes thickened and coarse. Deep nasolabial folds develop, and the forehead may become furrowed. Patients may have heavy-appearing eyelids and ptosis. The skin is often greasy, and there may be excessive sweating of the hands and feet. Patients may also experience acne vulgaris, seborrhea, and folliculitis. In a few patients, the skin over the scalp becomes very thick and corrugated, a feature that has been descriptively termed *cutis verticis gyrata*. The distal extremities, particularly the legs, become thickened owing to proliferation of new bone and soft tissue; when the process is extensive, the distal lower extremities resemble those of an elephant. The periostitis is usually not painful, as it may be in secondary HOA. Clubbing of the fingers may be extensive, producing large, bulbous deformities and clumsiness. Clubbing also affects the toes. Patients may experience articular and periarticular pain, especially in the ankles and knees, and joint motion may be mildly restricted owing to periarticular bone overgrowth. Noninflammatory effusions occur in the wrists, knees, and ankles. Synovial hypertrophy is not found. Associated abnormalities observed in patients with primary HOA include hypertrophic gastropathy, bone marrow failure, female escutcheon, gynecomastia, and cranial suture defects. In patients with primary HOA, the symptoms disappear when adulthood is reached.

HOA secondary to an underlying disease occurs more frequently than primary HOA. It accompanies a variety of disorders and may precede clinical features of the associated disorder by months. Clubbing is more frequent than the full syndrome of HOA in patients with associated illnesses. Because clubbing evolves over months and is usually asymptomatic, it is often recognized first by the physician and not the patient. Patients may experience a burning sensation in their fingertips. Clubbing is characterized by widening of the fingertips, enlargement of the distal volar pad, convexity of the nail contour, and the loss of the normal 15° angle between the proximal nail and cuticle. The thickness of the digit at the base of the nail is greater than the thickness at the distal interphalangeal joint. An objective measurement of finger clubbing can be made by determining the diameter at the base of the nail and at the distal interphalangeal joint of all 10 digits. Clubbing is present when the sum of the individual digit ratios is >10. At the bedside, clubbing can be appreciated by having the patient place the dorsal surface of the distal phalanges of the fourth fingers together with the nails of the fourth fingers opposing each other. Normally, an open area is visible between the bases of the opposing fingernails; when clubbing is present, this open space is no longer visible. The base of the nail feels spongy when compressed, and the nail can be easily rocked on its bed. Marked periungual erythema is usually present. When clubbing is advanced, the finger may have a drumstick appearance, and the distal interphalangeal joint can be hyperextended. Periosteal involvement in the distal extremities may produce a burning or deep-seated aching pain. The pain can be quite incapacitating and is aggravated by dependency and relieved by elevation of the affected limbs. The overlying soft tissue may be swollen, and the skin slightly erythematous. Pressure applied over the distal forearms and legs may be quite painful.

Patients may also experience joint pain, most often in the ankles, wrists, and knees. Joint effusions may be present; usually they are small and noninflammatory. The small joints of the hands are rarely affected. Severe joint or bone pain may be the presenting symptom of an underlying lung malignancy and may precede the appearance of

TABLE 315-4 *Disorders Associated with Hypertrophic Osteoarthropathy*

Pulmonary	Cardiovascular
Bronchogenic carcinoma and other neoplasms	Cyanotic congenital heart disease
Lung abscesses, empyema, bronchiectasis	Subacute bacterial endocarditis
Chronic interstitial pneumonitis	Infected arterial grafts[a]
Cystic fibrosis	Aortic aneurysm[b]
Chronic obstructive lung disease	Aneurysm of major extremity artery[a]
Sarcoidosis	Patent ductus arteriosus[b]
Gastrointestinal	Arteriovenous fistula of major extremity vessel[a]
Inflammatory bowel disease	
Sprue	Thyroid (thyroid acropathy)
Neoplasms: esophagus, liver, bowel	Hyperthyroidism (Graves' disease)

[a] Unilateral involvement.
[b] Bilateral lower extremity involvement.

clubbing. In addition, the progression of HOA tends to be more rapid when associated with malignancies, most notably bronchogenic carcinoma. Unlike primary HOA, excessive sweating and oiliness of the skin and thickening of the facial skin are uncommon in secondary HOA.

HOA occurs in 5 to 10% of patients with intrathoracic malignancies, the most common being bronchogenic carcinoma and pleural tumors (Table 315-4). Lung metastases infrequently cause HOA. HOA is also seen in patients with intrathoracic infections, including lung abscesses, empyema, bronchiectasis, chronic obstructive lung disease, and, uncommonly, pulmonary tuberculosis. HOA may also accompany chronic interstitial pneumonitis, sarcoidosis, and cystic fibrosis. In the latter, clubbing is more common than the full syndrome of HOA. Other causes of clubbing include congenital heart disease with right-to-left shunts, bacterial endocarditis, Crohn's disease, ulcerative colitis, sprue, and neoplasms of the esophagus, liver, and small and large bowel. In patients with congenital heart disease with right-to-left shunts, clubbing alone occurs more often than the full syndrome of HOA.

Unilateral clubbing has been found in association with aneurysms of major extremity arteries, infected arterial grafts, and with arteriovenous fistulas of brachial vessels. Clubbing of the toes but not fingers has been associated with an infected abdominal aortic aneurysm and patent ductus arteriosus. Clubbing of a single digit may follow trauma and has been reported in tophaceous gout and sarcoidosis. While clubbing occurs more commonly than the full syndrome in most diseases, periostitis in the absence of clubbing has been observed in the affected limb of patients with infected arterial grafts.

Hyperthyroidism (Graves' disease), treated or untreated, is occasionally associated with clubbing and periostitis of the bones of the hands and feet. This condition is referred to as *thyroid acropathy*. Periostitis is asymptomatic and occurs in the midshaft and diaphyseal portion of the metacarpal and phalangeal bones. The long bones of the extremities are seldom affected. Elevated levels of long-acting thyroid stimulator are found in the serum of these patients.

Laboratory Findings The laboratory abnormalities reflect the underlying disorder. The synovial fluid of involved joints has <500 white cells per microliter, and the cells are predominantly mononuclear. Radiographs show a faint radiolucent line beneath the new periosteal bone along the shaft of long bones at their distal end. These changes are observed most frequently at the ankles, wrists, and knees. The ends of the distal phalanges may show osseous resorption. Radionuclide studies show pericortical linear uptake along the cortical margins of long bones that may be present before any radiographic changes.

℞ TREATMENT

The treatment of HOA is to identify the associated disorder and treat it appropriately. The symptoms and signs of HOA may disappear completely with removal or effective chemotherapy of a tumor or with antibiotic therapy and drainage of a chronic pulmonary infection. Vagotomy or percutaneous block of the vagus nerve leads to symptomatic relief in some patients. Aspirin, other nonsteroidal anti-inflammatory drugs (NSAIDs), or analgesics may help control symptoms of HOA.

REFLEX SYMPATHETIC DYSTROPHY SYNDROME The reflex sympathetic dystrophy syndrome is now referred to as *complex regional pain syndrome, type 1*, by the new Classification of the International Association for the Study of Pain. It is characterized by pain and swelling, usually of a distal extremity, accompanied by vasomotor instability, trophic skin changes, and the rapid development of bony demineralization. →*Reflex sympathetic dystrophy syndrome, including its treatment, is covered in greater detail in Chap. 355.*

TIETZE'S SYNDROME AND COSTOCHONDRITIS Tietze's syndrome is manifested by painful swelling of one or more costochondral articulations. The age of onset is usually before 40, and both sexes are affected equally. In most patients only one joint is involved, usually the second or third costochondral joint. The onset of anterior chest pain may be sudden or gradual. The pain may radiate to the arms or shoulders and is aggravated by sneezing, coughing, deep inspirations, or twisting motions of the chest. The term *costochondritis* is often used interchangeably with *Tietze's syndrome*, but some workers restrict the former term to pain of the costochondral articulations without swelling. Costochondritis is observed in patients over age 40; tends to affect the third, fourth, and fifth costochondral joints; and occurs more often in women. Both syndromes may mimic cardiac or upper abdominal causes of pain. Rheumatoid arthritis, ankylosing spondylitis, and Reiter's syndrome may involve costochondral joints but are distinguished easily by their other clinical features. Other skeletal causes of anterior chest wall pain are xiphoidalgia and the slipping rib syndrome, which usually involves the tenth rib. Malignancies such as breast cancer, prostate cancer, plasma cell cytoma, and sarcoma can invade the ribs, thoracic spine, or chest wall and produce symptoms suggesting Tietze's syndrome. They should be easily distinguishable by radiographs and biopsy. Analgesics, anti-inflammatory drugs, and local glucocorticoid injections usually relieve symptoms.

MYOFASCIAL PAIN SYNDROME

Myofascial pain syndrome is characterized by localized musculoskeletal pain and tenderness in association with trigger points. The pain is deep and aching and may be accompanied by a burning sensation. Myofascial pain may follow trauma, overuse, or prolonged static contraction of a muscle or muscle group, which may occur when reading or writing at a desk or working at a computer. In addition, this syndrome may be associated with underlying osteoarthritis of the neck or low back. Trigger points are a diagnostic feature of this syndrome. Pain is referred from trigger points to defined areas distant from the original tender points. Palpation of the trigger point reproduces or accentuates the pain. The trigger points are usually located in the center of a muscle belly, but they can occur at other sites, such as costosternal junctions, the xyphoid process, ligamentous and tendinous insertions, fascia, and fatty areas. Trigger point sites in muscle have been described as feeling indurated and taut, and palpation may cause the muscle to twitch. These findings, however, have been shown not to be unique for myofascial pain syndrome, since in a controlled study they were also present in fibromyalgia patients and normal subjects. Myofascial pain most often involves the posterior neck, low back, shoulders, and chest. Chronic pain in the muscles of the posterior neck may involve referral of pain from the trigger point in the erector neck muscle or upper trapezius to the head, leading to persistent headaches, which may last for days. Trigger points in the paraspinal muscles of the low back may refer pain to the buttock. Pain may be referred down the leg from a trigger point in the gluteus medius and can mimic sciatica. A trigger point in the infraspinatus muscle may produce local and referred pain over the lateral deltoid and down the outside of the arm into the hand. Injection of a local anesthetic such as 1% lidocaine into the trigger point site often results in pain relief. Another useful technique is first to spray from the trigger point toward the area of referred pain with an agent such as ethyl chloride and then to stretch

the muscle. This maneuver may need to be repeated several times. Massage and application of ultrasound to the affected area may also be beneficial. Patients should be instructed in methods to prevent muscle stresses related to work and recreation. Posture and resting positions are important in preventing muscle tension. The prognosis in most patients is good. In some patients, myofascial pain syndrome may evolve into fibromyalgia. Patients at risk for developing fibromyalgia are thought to be those with anxiety, depression, nonrestorative sleep, and fatigue.

TUMORS OF JOINTS Primary tumors and tumor-like disorders of synovium are uncommon but should be considered in the differential diagnosis of monarticular joint disease. In addition, metastases to bone and primary bone tumors adjacent to a joint may produce joint symptoms. →*For further discussion, see Chap. 84.*

Pigmented villonodular synovitis is characterized by the slowly progressive, exuberant, benign proliferation of synovial tissue, usually involving a single joint. The most common age of onset is in the third decade, and women are affected slightly more often than men. The cause of this disorder is unknown.

The synovium has a brownish color and numerous large, finger-like villi that fuse to form pedunculated nodules. There is marked hyperplasia of synovial cells in the stroma of the villi. Hemosiderin granules and lipids are found in the cytoplasm of macrophages and in the interstitial tissue. Multinucleated giant cells may be present. The proliferative synovium grows into the subsynovial tissue and invades adjacent cartilage and bone.

The clinical picture of pigmented villonodular synovitis is characterized by the insidious onset of swelling and pain in one joint, most commonly the knee. Other joints affected include the hips, ankles, calcaneocuboid joints, elbows, and small joints of the fingers or toes. The disease may also involve the common flexor sheath of the hands or fingers. Less commonly, tendon sheaths in the wrist, ankle, or foot may be involved. Symptoms may be mild and intermittent and may be present for years before the patient seeks medical attention. Radiographs may show joint space narrowing, erosions, and subchondral cysts. The joint fluid contains blood and is dark red or almost black in color. Lipid-containing macrophages may be present in the fluid. The joint fluid may be clear if hemorrhages have not occurred.

The treatment of pigmented villonodular synovitis is complete synovectomy. With incomplete synovectomy, the villonodular synovitis recurs, and the rate of tissue growth may be faster than originally. Irradiation of the involved joint has been successful in some patients.

Synovial chondromatosis is a disorder characterized by multiple focal metaplastic growths of normal-appearing cartilage in the synovium or tendon sheath. Segments of cartilage break loose and continue to grow as loose bodies. When calcification and ossification of loose bodies occur, the disorder is referred to as *synovial osteochondromatosis*. The disorder is usually monarticular and affects young to middle-aged individuals. The knee is most often involved, followed by hip, elbow, and shoulder. Symptoms are pain, swelling, and decreased motion of the joint. Radiographs may show several rounded calcifications within the joint cavity. Treatment is synovectomy; however, the tumor may recur.

Hemangiomas occur in synovium and in tendon sheaths. The knee is affected most commonly. Recurrent episodes of joint swelling and pain usually begin in childhood. The joint fluid is bloody. Treatment is excision of the lesion. *Lipomas* occur most often in the knee, originating in the subsynovial fat on either side of the patellar tendon. Lipomas also appear in tendon sheaths of the hands, wrists, feet, and ankles. In some instances, surgical removal is necessary.

Synovial sarcoma is a malignant neoplasm often found near a large joint of both upper and lower extremities, being more common in the lower extremity. It seldom arises within the joint itself. Synovial sarcomas comprise 10% of soft tissue sarcomas. The tumor is believed to arise from primitive mesenchymal tissue that differentiates into epithelial cells and/or spindle cells. Small foci of calcification may be present in the tumor mass. It occurs most often in young adults and is more common in men. The tumor presents as a slowly growing deep seated mass near a joint, without much pain. The area of the knee is the most common site, followed by the foot, ankle, elbow, and shoulder. Other primary sites include the buttocks, abdominal wall, retroperitoneum, and mediastinum. The tumor spreads along tissue planes. The most common site of visceral metastasis is lung. The diagnosis is made by biopsy. Treatment is wide resection of the tumor including adjacent muscle and regional lymph nodes, followed by chemotherapy and radiation therapy. Currently used chemotherapeutic agents are doxorubicin, ifosfamide, and cisplatin. Amputation of the involved distal extremity may be required. Chemotherapy may be beneficial in some patients with metastatic disease. Isolated pulmonary metastasis can be surgically removed. The 5-year survival with treatment is variable depending on the staging

of the tumor ranging from approximately 25 to 60% or higher. Synovial sarcomas tend to recur locally and eventually metastasize to regional lymph nodes, lungs, and skeleton.

FURTHER READING

ALTMAN RD, TENENBAUM J: Hypertrophic osteoarthropathy, in *Kelley's Textbook of Rheumatology*, 6th ed, S Ruddy et al (eds). Philadelphia, Saunders, 2001, pp 1589–1594

CRONIN ME: Rheumatic aspects of endocrinopathies, in *Arthritis and Allied Conditions*, 14th ed, WJ Koopman (ed). Philadelphia, Lippincott Williams & Wilkins, 2001, pp 2530–2547

GOLDENBERG DL: Fibromyalgia syndrome a decade later: What have we learned? Arch Intern Med 159:777, 1999

HECK LW JR: Arthritis associated with hematologic disorders, storage diseases, disorders of lipid metabolism, and dysproteinemias, in *Arthritis and Allied Conditions*, 14th ed, WJ Koopman (ed). Philadelphia, Lippincott Williams & Wilkins, 2001, pp 1903–1924

WOLFE F et al: The prevalence and characteristics of fibromyalgia in the general population. Arthritis Rheum 38:19, 1995

316 PERIARTICULAR DISORDERS OF THE EXTREMITIES
Bruce C. Gilliland

A number of periarticular disorders have become increasingly common over the past two to three decades, due in part to greater participation in recreational sports by individuals of a wide range of ages. This chapter discusses some of the more common periarticular disorders of the extremities.

BURSITIS Bursitis is inflammation of a bursa, which is a thin-walled sac lined with synovial tissue. The function of the bursa is to facilitate movement of tendons and muscles over bony prominences. Excessive frictional forces from overuse, trauma, systemic disease (e.g., rheumatoid arthritis, gout), or infection may cause bursitis. *Subacromial bursitis* (subdeltoid bursitis) is the most common form of bursitis. The subacromial bursa, which is contiguous with the subdeltoid bursa, is located between the undersurface of the acromion and the humeral head, and is covered by the deltoid muscle. Bursitis is caused by repetitive overhead motion and often accompanies rotator cuff tendinitis. Another frequently encountered form is *trochanteric bursitis*, which involves the bursa around the insertion of the gluteus medius onto the greater trochanter of the femur. Patients experience pain over the lateral aspect of the hip and upper thigh and have tenderness over the posterior aspect of the greater trochanter. External rotation and resisted abduction of the hip elicit pain. *Olecranon bursitis* occurs over the posterior elbow, and when the area is acutely inflamed, infection or gout should be excluded by aspirating the bursa and performing a Gram stain and culture on the fluid as well as examining the fluid for urate crystals. *Achilles bursitis* involves the bursa located above the insertion of the tendon to the calcaneus and results from overuse and wearing tight shoes. *Retrocalcaneal bursitis* involves the bursa that is located between the calcaneus and posterior surface of the Achilles tendon. The pain is experienced at the back of the heel, and swelling appears on the medial and/or lateral side of the tendon. It occurs in association with spondyloarthropathies, rheumatoid arthritis, gout, or trauma. *Ischial bursitis* (weaver's bottom) affects the bursa separating the gluteus medius from the ischial tuberosity and develops from prolonged sitting and pivoting on hard surfaces. *Iliopsoas bursitis* affects the bursa that lies between the iliopsoas muscle and hip joint and is lateral to the femoral vessels. Pain is experienced over this area and is made worse by hip extension and flexion. *Anserine bursitis* is an inflammation of the sartorius bursa located over the medial side of the tibia just below the knee and under the conjoint tendon and is manifested by pain on climbing stairs. Tenderness is present over the insertion of the conjoint tendon of the sartorius, gracilis, and semitendinosus. *Prepatellar bursitis* (housemaid's knee) occurs in the bursa situated between the patella and overlying skin and is caused by kneel-

ing on hard surfaces. Gout or infection may also occur at this site. Treatment of bursitis consists of prevention of the aggravating situation, rest of the involved part, administration of a nonsteroidal antiinflammatory drug (NSAID), or local glucocorticoid injection.

ROTATOR CUFF TENDINITIS AND IMPINGEMENT SYNDROME Tendinitis of the rotator cuff is the major cause of a painful shoulder and is currently thought to be caused by inflammation of the tendon(s). The rotator cuff consists of the tendons of the supraspinatus, infraspinatus, subscapularis, and teres minor muscles, and inserts on the humeral tuberosities. Of the tendons forming the rotator cuff, the supraspinatus tendon is the most often affected, probably because of its repeated impingement (impingement syndrome) between the humeral head and the undersurface of the anterior third of the acromion and coracoacromial ligament above as well as the reduction in its blood supply that occurs with abduction of the arm (Fig. 316-1). The tendon of the infraspinatus and that of the long head of the biceps are less commonly involved. The process begins with edema and hemorrhage of the rotator cuff, which evolves to fibrotic thickening and eventually to rotator cuff degeneration with tendon tears and bone spurs. Subacromial bursitis also accompanies this syndrome. Symptoms usually appear

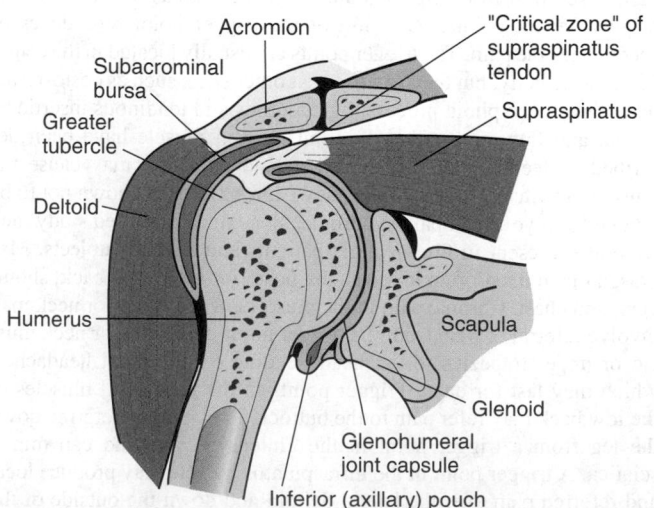

FIGURE 316-1 Coronal section of the shoulder illustrating the relationships of the glenohumeral joint, the joint capsule, the subacromial bursa, and the rotator cuff (supraspinatus tendon). [*From F Kozin, in WI Koopman (ed): Arthritis and Allied Conditions, 13th ed. Baltimore, Williams & Wilkins, 1997, with permission.*]

after injury or overuse, especially with activities involving elevation of the arm with some degree of forward flexion. Impingement syndrome occurs in persons participating in baseball, tennis, swimming, or occupations that require repeated elevation of the arm. Those over age 40 are particularly susceptible. Patients complain of a dull aching in the shoulder, which may interfere with sleep. Severe pain is experienced when the arm is actively abducted into an overhead position. The arc between 60 and 120° is especially painful. Tenderness is present over the lateral aspect of the humeral head just below the acromion. NSAIDs, local glucocorticoid injection, and physical therapy may relieve symptoms. Surgical decompression of the subacromial space may be necessary in patients refractory to conservative treatment.

Patients may tear the supraspinatus tendon acutely by falling on an outstretched arm or lifting a heavy object. Symptoms are pain, along with weakness of abduction and external rotation of the shoulder. Atrophy of the supraspinatus muscles develops. The diagnosis is established by arthrogram, ultrasound or magnetic resonance imaging. Surgical repair may be necessary in patients who fail to respond to conservative measures. In patients with moderate to severe tears and functional loss, surgery is indicated.

CALCIFIC TENDINITIS This condition is characterized by deposition of calcium salts, primarily hydroxyapatite, within a tendon. The exact mechanism of calcification is not known but may be initiated by ischemia or degeneration of the tendon. The supraspinatus tendon is most often affected because it is frequently impinged on and has a reduced blood supply when the arm is abducted. The condition usually develops after age 40. Calcification within the tendon may evoke acute inflammation, producing sudden and severe pain in the shoulder. However, it may be asymptomatic or not related to the patient's symptoms.

BICIPITAL TENDINITIS AND RUPTURE Bicipital tendinitis, or tenosynovitis, is produced by friction on the tendon of the long head of the biceps as it passes through the bicipital groove. When the inflammation is acute, patients experience anterior shoulder pain that radiates down the biceps into the forearm. Abduction and external rotation of the arm are painful and limited. The bicipital groove is very tender to palpation. Pain may be elicited along the course of the tendon by resisting supination of the forearm with the elbow at 90° (Yergason's supination sign). Acute rupture of the tendon may occur with vigorous exercise of the arm and is often painful. In a young patient, it should be repaired surgically. Rupture of the tendon in an older person may be associated with little or no pain and is recognized by the presence of persistent swelling of the biceps ("Popeye" muscle) produced by the retraction of the long head of the biceps. Surgery is usually not necessary in this setting.

DE QUERVAINS' TENOSYNOVITIS In this condition, inflammation involves the abductor pollicis longus and the extensor pollicis brevis as these tendons pass through a fibrous sheath at the radial styloid process. The usual cause is repetitive twisting motion of the wrist. It may occur in pregnancy, and it also occurs in mothers from holding their babies with the thumb outstretched. Patients experience pain on grasping with their thumb such as with pinching. Swelling and tenderness are often present over the radial styloid process. The Finkelstein sign is positive, which is elicited by having the patient place the thumb in the palm and close the fingers over it. The wrist is then ulnarly deviated resulting in pain over the involved tendon sheath in the area of the radial styloid. Treatment consists initially of splinting the wrist and an NSAID. When severe or refractory to conservative treatment, glucocorticoid injections can be very effective.

PATELLAR TENDINITIS (JUMPER'S KNEE) Tendinitis involves the patellar tendon at its attachment to the lower pole of the patella. Patients may experience pain when jumping during basketball or volleyball, going up stairs, or when doing deep knee squats. Tenderness is noted on examination over the lower pole of the patella. Treatment consists of rest, icing, and NSAIDS, followed by strengthening and increasing flexibility.

ADHESIVE CAPSULITIS Often referred to as "frozen shoulder," adhesive capsulitis is characterized by pain and restricted movement of the shoulder, usually in the absence of intrinsic shoulder disease. Night pain is often present in the affected shoulder. Adhesive capsulitis, however, may follow bursitis or tendinitis of the shoulder or be associated with systemic disorders such as chronic pulmonary disease, myocardial infarction, and diabetes mellitus. Prolonged immobility of the arm contributes to the development of adhesive capsulitis, and reflex sympathetic dystrophy is thought to be a pathogenic factor. The capsule of the shoulder is thickened, and a mild chronic inflammatory infiltrate and fibrosis may be present.

Adhesive capsulitis occurs more commonly in women after age 50. Pain and stiffness usually develop gradually over several months to a year but progress rapidly in some patients. Pain may interfere with sleep. The shoulder is tender to palpation, and both active and passive movement are restricted. Radiographs of the shoulder show osteopenia. The diagnosis is confirmed by arthrography, in that only a limited amount of contrast material, usually <15 mL, can be injected under pressure into the shoulder joint.

In most patients, the condition improves spontaneously 1 to 3 years after onset. While pain usually improves, most patients are left with some limitation of shoulder motion. Early mobilization of the arm following an injury to the shoulder may prevent the development of this disease. Slow but forceful injection of contrast material into the joint may lyse adhesions and stretch the capsule, resulting in improvement of shoulder motion. Manipulation under anesthesia may be helpful in some patients. Once the disease is established, therapy may have little effect on its natural course. Local injections of glucocorticoids, NSAIDs, and physical therapy may provide relief of symptoms.

LATERAL EPICONDYLITIS (TENNIS ELBOW) Lateral epicondylitis, or tennis elbow, is a painful condition involving the soft tissue over the lateral aspect of the elbow. The pain originates at or near the site of attachment of the common extensors to the lateral epicondyle and may radiate into the forearm and dorsum of the wrist. This painful condition is thought to be caused by small tears of the extensor aponeurosis resulting from repeated resisted contractions of the extensor muscles. The pain usually appears after work or recreational activities involving repeated motions of wrist extension and supination against resistance. Most patients with this disorder injure themselves in activities other than tennis, such as pulling weeds, carrying suitcases or briefcases, or using a screwdriver. The injury in tennis usually occurs when hitting a backhand with the elbow flexed. Shaking hands and opening doors can reproduce the pain. Striking the lateral elbow against a solid object may also induce pain.

The treatment is usually rest along with administration of an NSAID. Ultrasound, icing, and friction massage may also help relieve pain. When pain is severe, the elbow is placed in a sling or splinted at 90° of flexion. When the pain is acute and well localized, injection of a glucocorticoid using a small-gauge needle may be effective. Following injection, the patient should be advised to rest the arm for at least 1 month and avoid activities that would aggravate the elbow. Once symptoms have subsided, the patient should begin rehabilitation to strengthen and increase flexibility of the extensor muscles before resuming physical activity involving the arm. A forearm band placed 2.5 to 5.0 cm (1 to 2 in.) below the elbow may help to reduce tension on the extensor muscles at their attachment to the lateral epicondyle. The patient should be advised to restrict activities requiring forcible extension and supination of the wrist. Improvement may take several months. The patient may continue to experience mild pain but, with care, can usually avoid the return of debilitating pain. In an occasional patient, surgical release of the extensor aponeurosis may be necessary.

MEDIAL EPICONDYLITIS Medial epicondylitis is an overuse syndrome resulting in pain over the medial side of the elbow with radiation into the forearm. The cause of this syndrome is considered to be repetitive resisted motions of wrist flexion and pronation, which lead to micro-tears and granulation tissue at the origin of the pronator teres and forearm flexors, particularly the flexor carpi radialis. This overuse syndrome is usually seen in patients >35 years and is much less common than lateral epicondylitis. It occurs most often in work-related repetitive activities but also occurs with recreational activities such as swinging a golf club (golfer's elbow) or throwing a baseball. On physical examination, there is tenderness just distal to the medial epicondyle over the origin of the forearm flexors. Pain can be reproduced by resisting wrist flexion and pronation with the elbow extended. Radiographs are usually normal. The differential diagnosis of patients with medial elbow symptoms include tears of the pronator teres, acute medial collateral ligament tear, and medial collateral ligament instability. Ulnar neuritis has been found in 25 to 50% of patients with medial epicondylitis and is associated with tenderness over the ulnar nerve at the elbow as well as hypesthesia and paresthesia on the ulnar side of the hand.

The initial treatment of medial epicondylitis is conservative, involving rest, NSAIDs, friction massage, ultrasound, and icing. Some patients may require splinting. Injections of glucocorticoids at the painful site may also be effective. Patients should be instructed to rest at least 1 month. Also, patients should be started on physical therapy once the pain has subsided. In patients with chronic debilitating medial epicondylitis that remains unresponsive after at least a year of treatment, surgical release of the flexor muscle at its origin may be necessary and is often successful.

FURTHER READING

GISPEN JG: Painful shoulder and the reflex sympathetic dystrophy syndrome, in *Arthritis and Allied Conditions*, 14th ed, WJ Koopman (ed). Philadelphia, Lippincott Williams & Wilkins, 2001, pp 2095–2142

LINTNER SA et al: Sports medicine, in *Kelley's Textbook of Rheumatology*, 6th ed, S Ruddy et al (eds). Philadelphia, Saunders, 2001, pp 439–456

MATSEN FA III, ARNTZ CT: Subacromial impingement, in *The Shoulder*, CA Rockwood Jr (ed). Philadelphia, Saunders, 1990, pp 623–646

NEER CS II: Impingement lesions. Clin Orthop 173:70, 1983

317 PRINCIPLES OF ENDOCRINOLOGY
J. Larry Jameson

The management of endocrine disorders requires an understanding of such disparate areas as intermediary metabolism, reproductive physiology, bone metabolism, and growth. Accordingly, the practice of endocrinology is intimately linked to a conceptual framework for understanding hormone secretion, hormone action, and principles of feedback control systems. The endocrine system is evaluated primarily by measuring hormone concentrations, thereby arming the clinician with valuable diagnostic information. Most disorders of the endocrine system are amenable to effective treatment, once the correct diagnosis is determined. Endocrine deficiency disorders are treated with physiologic hormone replacement; hormone excess conditions, usually due to benign glandular adenomas, are managed by removing tumors surgically or by reducing hormone levels medically.

SCOPE OF ENDOCRINOLOGY

The specialty of endocrinology encompasses the study of glands and the hormones they produce. The term *endocrine* was coined by Starling to contrast the actions of hormones secreted internally (endocrine) with those secreted externally (*exocrine*) or into a lumen, such as the gastrointestinal tract. The term *hormone*, derived from a Greek phrase meaning "to set in motion," aptly describes the dynamic actions of hormones as they elicit cellular responses and regulate physiologic processes through feedback mechanisms.

Unlike many other specialties in medicine, it is not possible to define endocrinology strictly along anatomic lines. The classic endocrine glands—pituitary, thyroid, parathyroid, pancreatic islets, adrenal, and gonads—communicate broadly with other organs through the nervous system, hormones, cytokines, and growth factors. In addition to its traditional synaptic functions, the brain produces a vast array of peptide hormones, spawning the discipline of neuroendocrinology. Through the production of hypothalamic releasing factors, the central nervous system exerts a major regulatory influence over pituitary hormone secretion (Chap. 318). The peripheral nervous system modulates adrenal medulla and pancreatic islet hormone production. The immune and endocrine systems are also intimately intertwined. The adrenal glucocorticoid, cortisol, is a powerful immunosuppressant. Cytokines and interleukins (ILs) have profound effects on the functions of the pituitary, adrenal, thyroid, and gonads. Common endocrine diseases, such as autoimmune thyroid disease and type 1 diabetes mellitus, are caused by dysregulation of immune surveillance and tolerance. Less common diseases such as polyglandular failure, Addison's disease, and lymphocytic hypophysitis also have an immunologic basis.

The interdigitation of endocrinology with physiologic processes in other specialties sometimes blurs the role of hormones. For example, hormones play an important role in maintenance of blood pressure, intravascular volume, and peripheral resistance in the cardiovascular system. Vasoactive substances such as catecholamines, angiotensin II, endothelin, and nitric oxide are involved in dynamic changes of vascular tone, in addition to their multiple roles in other tissues. The heart is the principal source of atrial natriuretic peptide, which acts in classic endocrine fashion to induce natriuresis at a distant target organ (the kidney). Erythropoietin, a traditional circulating hormone, is made in the kidney and stimulates erythropoiesis in the bone marrow (Chap. 52). The kidney is also integrally involved in the renin-angiotensin axis (Chap. 321) and is a primary target of several hormones including parathyroid hormone (PTH), mineralocorticoids, and vasopressin. The gastrointestinal tract produces a surprising number of peptide hormones such as cholecystokinin, ghrelin, gastrin, secretin, and vasoactive intestinal peptide, among many others. Carcinoid and islet tumors can secrete excessive amounts of these hormones, leading to specific clinical syndromes (Chap. 329). Many of these gastrointestinal hormones are also produced in the central nervous system, where their functions remain poorly understood. As new hormones such as inhibin, ghrelin, and leptin are discovered, they become integrated into the science and practice of medicine on the basis of their functional roles rather than their tissues of origin or their structures or mechanisms of action.

Characterization of hormone receptors frequently reveals unexpected relationships to factors in nonendocrine disciplines. The growth hormone (GH) receptor, for example, is a member of the cytokine receptor family. The G protein–coupled receptors (GPCRs), which mediate the actions of many peptide hormones, are used in numerous physiologic processes including vision, smell, and neurotransmission.

It is apparent that hormones and growth factors play an important functional role in all organ systems. Though endocrinologists are not usually involved in the administration of the hormones or growth factors used to treat diseases in other specialties (e.g., cardiology, hematology), the principles of endocrinology can be applied in these cases, thus emphasizing the impact of endocrinology across multiple disciplines.

NATURE OF HORMONES

Hormones can be divided into five major classes: (1) *amino acid derivatives* such as dopamine, catecholamines, and thyroid hormone; (2) *small neuropeptides* such as gonadotropin-releasing hormone (GnRH), thyrotropin-releasing hormone (TRH), somatostatin, and vasopressin; (3) *large proteins* such as insulin, luteinizing hormone (LH), and PTH produced by classic endocrine glands; (4) *steroid hormones* such as cortisol and estrogen that are synthesized from cholesterol-based precursors; and (5) *vitamin derivatives* such as retinoids (vitamin A) and vitamin D. A variety of *peptide growth factors*, most of which act locally, share actions with hormones. As a rule, amino acid derivatives and peptide hormones interact with cell-surface membrane receptors. Steroids, thyroid hormones, vitamin D, and retinoids are lipid-soluble and interact with intracellular nuclear receptors.

HORMONE AND RECEPTOR FAMILIES

Many hormones and receptors can be grouped into families, reflecting their structural similarities (Table 317-1). The evolution of these families generates diverse but highly selective pathways of hormone action. Recognizing these relationships allows extrapolation of information gleaned from one hormone or receptor to other family members.

The glycoprotein hormone family, consisting of thyroid-stimulating hormone (TSH), follicle-stimulating hormone (FSH), LH, and human chorionic gonadotropin (hCG), illustrates many features of related hormones. The glycoprotein hormones are heterodimers that share the α subunit in common; the β subunits are distinct and confer specific biologic actions. The overall three-dimensional architecture of the β subunits is similar, reflecting the locations of conserved disulfide bonds that restrain protein conformation. The cloning of the β-subunit genes from multiple species suggests that this family arose from a common ancestral gene, probably by gene duplication and subsequent divergence to evolve new biologic functions.

As the hormone families enlarge and diverge, their receptors must co-evolve, if new biologic functions are to be derived. Related GPCRs, for example, have evolved for each of the glycoprotein hormones.

TABLE 317-1 *Membrane Receptor Families and Signaling Pathways*

Receptors	Effectors	Signaling Pathways
G protein–coupled seven-transmembrane (GPCR)		
β-Adrenergic	$G_s\alpha$, adenylate cyclase	Stimulation of cyclic AMP production, protein kinase A
LH, FSH, TSH	Ca^{2+} channels	
Glucagon		
PTH, PTHrP		Calmodulin, Ca^{2+}-dependent kinases
ACTH, MSH		
GHRH, CRH		
α-Adrenergic	$G_i\alpha$	Inhibition of cyclic AMP production
Somatostatin		Activation of K^+, Ca^{2+} channels
TRH, GnRH	G_q, G_{11}	Phospholipase C, diacylglycerol, IP_3, protein kinase C, voltage-dependent Ca^{2+} channels
Receptor tyrosine kinase		
Insulin, IGF-I	Tyrosine kinases, IRS-1 to IRS-4	MAP kinases, PI 3-kinase, RSK
EGF, NGF	Tyrosine kinases, ras	Raf, MAP kinases, RSK
Cytokine receptor–linked kinase		
GH, PRL	JAK, tyrosine kinases	STAT, MAP kinase, PI 3-kinase, IRS 1, IRS 2
Serine Kinase		
Activin, TGF-β, MIS	Serine kinase	Smads

Note: IP_3, inositol triphosphate; IRS, insulin receptor substrates; MAP, mitogen-activated protein; MSH, melanocyte-stimulating hormone; NGF, nerve growth factor; PI, phosphatylinositol; RSK, ribosomal S6 kinase; TGF-β, transforming growth factor β. For all other abbreviations, see text.

These receptors are structurally similar, and each is coupled to the $G_s\alpha$ signaling pathway. However, there is minimal overlap of hormone binding. For example, TSH binds with high specificity to the TSH receptor but interacts minimally with the LH or the FSH receptor. Nonetheless, there can be subtle physiologic consequences of hormone cross-reactivity with other receptors. Very high levels of hCG during pregnancy stimulate the TSH receptor and increase thyroid hormone levels.

Insulin, insulin-like growth factor (IGF) I, and IGF-II share structural similarities that are most apparent when precursor forms of the proteins are compared. In contrast to the high degree of specificity seen with the glycoprotein hormones, there is moderate cross-talk among the members of the insulin/IGF family. High concentrations of an IGF-II precursor produced by certain tumors (e.g., sarcomas) can cause hypoglycemia, partly because of binding to insulin and IGF-I receptors (Chap. 86). High concentrations of insulin also bind to the IGF-I receptor, perhaps accounting for some of the clinical manifestations seen in severe insulin resistance.

Another important example of receptor cross-talk is seen with PTH and parathyroid hormone–related peptide (PTHrP) (Chap. 332). PTH is produced by the parathyroid glands, whereas PTHrP is expressed at high levels during development and by a variety of tumors (Chap. 86). These hormones share amino acid sequence similarity, particularly in their amino-terminal regions. Both hormones bind to a single PTH receptor that is expressed in bone and kidney. Hypercalcemia and hypophosphatemia may therefore result from excessive production of either hormone, making it difficult to distinguish hyperparathyroidism from hypercalcemia of malignancy solely on the basis of serum chemistries. However, sensitive and specific assays for PTH and PTHrP now allow these disorders to be separated more readily.

Based on their specificities for DNA binding sites, the nuclear receptor family can be subdivided into type 1 receptors (GR, MR, AR, ER, PR) that bind steroids and type 2 receptors (TR, VDR, RAR, PPAR) that bind thyroid hormone, vitamin D, retinoic acid, or lipid derivatives. Certain functional domains in nuclear receptors, such as the zinc finger DNA-binding domains, are highly conserved. However, selective amino acid differences within this domain confer DNA sequence specificity. The hormone-binding domains are more variable, providing great diversity in the array of small molecules that can bind to different nuclear receptors. With few exceptions, hormone binding is highly specific for a single type of nuclear receptor. One exception involves the highly related glucocorticoid and mineralocorticoid receptors. Because the mineralocorticoid receptor also binds glucocorticoids with high affinity, an enzyme (11β-hydroxysteroid dehydrogenase) located in renal tubular cells inactivates glucocorticoids, allowing selective responses to mineralocorticoids such as aldosterone. However, when very high glucocorticoid concentrations occur, as in Cushing's syndrome, the glucocorticoid degradation pathway becomes saturated, allowing excessive cortisol levels to exert mineralocorticoid effects (sodium retention, potassium wasting). This phenomenon is particularly pronounced in ectopic adrenocorticotropic hormone (ACTH) syndromes (Chap. 321). Another example of relaxed nuclear receptor specificity involves the estrogen receptor, which can bind an array of compounds, some of which share little structural similarity to the high-affinity ligand estradiol. This feature of the estrogen receptor makes it susceptible to activation by "environmental estrogens" such as resveratrol, octylphenol, and many other aromatic hydrocarbons. On the other hand, this lack of specificity provides an opportunity to synthesize a remarkable series of clinically useful antagonists (e.g., tamoxifen) and selective estrogen response modulators (SERMs), such as raloxifene. These compounds generate distinct conformations that alter receptor interactions with components of the transcription machinery (see below), thereby conferring their unique actions.

HORMONE SYNTHESIS AND PROCESSING

The synthesis of peptide hormones and their receptors occurs through a classic pathway of gene expression: transcription → mRNA → protein → posttranslational protein processing → intracellular sorting, membrane integration, or secretion (Chap. 56). Though endocrine genes contain regulatory DNA elements similar to those found in many other genes, their exquisite control by other hormones also necessitates the presence of specific hormone response elements. For example, the TSH genes are repressed directly by thyroid hormones acting through the thyroid hormone receptor, a member of the nuclear receptor family. Steroidogenic enzyme gene expression requires specific transcription factors such as steroidogenic factor-1 (SF-1), acting in conjunction with signals transmitted by trophic hormones (e.g., ACTH or LH). For some hormones, substantial regulation occurs at the level of translational efficiency. Insulin biosynthesis, while requiring ongoing gene transcription, is regulated primarily at the translational level in response to elevated levels of glucose or amino acids.

Many hormones are embedded within larger precursor polypeptides that are proteolytically processed to yield the biologically active hormone. Examples include: proopiomelanocortin (POMC) → ACTH; proglucagon → glucagon; proinsulin → insulin; pro-PTH → PTH, among others. In many cases, such as POMC and proglucagon, these precursors generate multiple biologically active peptides. It is provocative that hormone precursors are typically inactive, presumably adding an additional level of regulatory control. This is true not only for peptide hormones but also for certain steroids (testosterone → dihydrotestosterone) and thyroid hormone (T_4 → T_3).

Hormone precursor processing is intimately linked to intracellular sorting pathways that transport proteins to appropriate vesicles and enzymes, resulting in specific cleavage steps, followed by protein folding and translocation to secretory vesicles. Hormones destined for secretion are translocated across the endoplasmic reticulum under the guidance of an amino-terminal signal sequence that is subsequently cleaved. Cell-surface receptors are inserted into the membrane via short segments of hydrophobic amino acids that remain embedded within the lipid bilayer. During translocation through the Golgi and endoplasmic reticulum, hormones and receptors are also subject to a variety of posttranslational modifications, such as glycosylation and phosphorylation, which can alter protein conformation, modify circulating half-life, and alter biologic activity.

Synthesis of most steroid hormones is based on modifications of the precursor, cholesterol. Multiple regulated enzymatic steps are required for the synthesis of testosterone (Chap. 325), estradiol (Chap. 326), cortisol (Chap. 321), and vitamin D (Chap. 331). This large number of synthetic steps predisposes to multiple genetic and acquired disorders of steroidogenesis.

HORMONE SECRETION, TRANSPORT, AND DEGRADATION

The circulating level of a hormone is determined by its rate of secretion and its circulating half-life. After protein processing, peptide hormones (GnRH, insulin, GH) are stored in secretory granules. As these granules mature, they are poised beneath the plasma membrane for imminent release into the circulation. In most instances, the stimulus for hormone secretion is a releasing factor or neural signal that induces rapid changes in intracellular calcium concentrations, leading to secretory granule fusion with the plasma membrane and release of its contents into the extracellular environment and bloodstream. Steroid hormones, in contrast, diffuse into the circulation as they are synthesized. Thus, their secretory rates are closely aligned with rates of synthesis. For example, ACTH and LH induce steroidogenesis by stimulating the activity of *s*teroidogenic *a*cute *r*egulatory (StAR) protein (transports cholesterol into the mitochondrion) along with other rate-limiting steps (e.g., cholesterol side-chain cleavage enzyme, CYP11A1) in the steroidogenic pathway.

Hormone transport and degradation dictate the rapidity with which a hormonal signal decays. Some hormonal signals are evanescent (e.g., somatostatin), whereas others are longer lived (e.g., TSH). Because somatostatin exerts effects in virtually every tissue, a short half-life allows its concentrations and actions to be controlled locally. Structural modifications that impair somatostatin degradation have been useful for generating long-acting therapeutic analogues, such as octreotide (Chap. 318). On the other hand, the actions of TSH are highly specific for the thyroid gland. Its prolonged half-life accounts for relatively constant serum levels, even though TSH is secreted in discrete pulses.

An understanding of circulating hormone half-life is important for achieving physiologic hormone replacement, as the frequency of dosing and the time required to reach steady state are intimately linked to rates of hormone decay. T_4, for example, has a circulating half-life of 7 days. Consequently, >1 month is required to reach a new steady state, but single daily doses are sufficient to achieve constant hormone levels. T_3, in contrast, has a half-life of 1 day. Its administration is associated with more dynamic serum levels and it must be administered two to three times per day. Similarly, synthetic glucocorticoids vary widely in their half-lives; those with longer half-lives (e.g., dexamethasone) are associated with greater suppression of the hypothalamic-pituitary-adrenal (HPA) axis. Most protein hormones [e.g., ACTH, GH, prolactin (PRL); PTH, LH] have relatively short half-lives (<20 min), leading to sharp peaks of secretion and decay. The only accurate way to profile the pulse frequency and amplitude of these hormones is to measure levels in frequently sampled blood (every 10 min) over long durations (8 to 24 h). Because this is not practical in a clinical setting, an alternative strategy is to pool three to four samples drawn at about 30-min intervals, recognizing that pulsatile secretion makes it difficult to establish a narrow normal range. Rapid hormone decay is useful in certain clinical settings. For example, the short half-life of PTH allows the use of intraoperative PTH determinations to confirm successful removal of an adenoma. This is particularly valuable diagnostically when there is a possibility of multicentric disease or parathyroid hyperplasia, as occurs with multiple endocrine neoplasia (MEN) or renal insufficiency.

Many hormones circulate in association with serum-binding proteins. Examples include: (1) T_4 and T_3 binding to thyroxine-binding globulin (TBG), albumin, and thyroxine-binding prealbumin (TBPA); (2) cortisol binding to cortisol-binding globulin (CBG); (3) androgen and estrogen binding to sex hormone–binding globulin (SHBG) (also called testosterone-binding globulin, TeBG); (4) IGF-I and -II binding to multiple IGF-binding proteins (IGFBPs); (5) GH interactions with GH-binding protein (GHBP), a circulating fragment of the GH receptor extracellular domain; and (6) activin binding to follistatin. These interactions provide a hormonal reservoir, prevent otherwise rapid degradation of unbound hormones, restrict hormone access to certain sites (e.g., IGFBPs), and modulate the unbound, or "free," hormone concentrations. Although a variety of binding protein abnormalities have been identified, most have little clinical consequence, aside from creating diagnostic problems. For example, TBG deficiency can greatly reduce total thyroid hormone levels, but the free concentrations of T_4 and T_3 remain normal. Liver disease and certain medications can also influence binding protein levels (e.g., estrogen increases TBG) or cause displacement of hormones from binding proteins (e.g., salsalate displaces T_4 from TBG). Only unbound hormone is available to interact with receptors and thereby elicit a biologic response. Short-term perturbations in binding proteins change the free hormone concentration, which in turn induces compensatory adaptations through feedback loops. SHBG changes in women are an exception to this self-correcting mechanism. When SHBG decreases because of insulin resistance or androgen excess, the unbound testosterone concentration is increased, potentially leading to hirsutism (Chap. 44). The increased unbound testosterone level does not result in an adequate compensatory feedback correction because estrogen, and not testosterone, is the primary regulator of the reproductive axis.

HORMONE ACTION THROUGH RECEPTORS

Receptors for hormones are divided into two major classes—membrane and nuclear. *Membrane receptors* primarily bind peptide hormones and catecholamines. *Nuclear receptors* bind small molecules that can diffuse across the cell membrane, such as thyroid hormone, steroids, and vitamin D. Certain general principles apply to hormone-receptor interactions, regardless of the class of receptor. Hormones bind to receptors with specificity and a high affinity that generally coincides with the dynamic range of circulating hormone concentrations. Low concentrations of free hormone (usually 10^{-12} to 10^{-9} M) rapidly associate and dissociate from receptors in a bimolecular reaction, such that the occupancy of the receptor at any given moment is a function of hormone concentration and the receptor's affinity for the hormone. Receptor numbers vary greatly in different target tissues, providing one of the major determinants of specific cellular responses to circulating hormones. For example, ACTH receptors are located almost exclusively in the adrenal cortex, and FSH receptors are found only in the gonads. In contrast, insulin and thyroid hormone receptors are widely distributed, reflecting the need for metabolic responses in all tissues.

MEMBRANE RECEPTORS

Membrane receptors for hormones can be divided into several major groups: (1) seven transmembrane GPCRs, (2) tyrosine kinase receptors, (3) cytokine receptors, and (4) serine kinase receptors (Fig. 317-

FIGURE 317-1   Membrane receptor signaling. MAPK, mitogen-activated protein kinase; PKA, -C, protein kinase A, C; TGF, transforming growth factor. For other abbreviations, see text.

1). The *seven transmembrane GPCR family* binds a remarkable array of hormones including large proteins (e.g., LH, PTH), small peptides (e.g., TRH, somatostatin), catecholamines (epinephrine, dopamine), and even minerals (e.g., calcium). The extracellular domains of GPCRs vary widely in size and are the major binding site for large hormones. The transmembrane-spanning regions are composed of hydrophobic α-helical domains that traverse the lipid bilayer. Like some channels, these domains are thought to circularize and form a hydrophobic pocket into which certain small ligands fit. Hormone binding induces conformational changes in these domains, transducing structural changes to the intracellular domain, which is a docking site for G proteins.

The large family of *G proteins*, so named because they bind guanine nucleotides (GTP, GDP), provides great diversity for coupling signaling pathways to different receptors. G proteins form a heterotrimeric complex that is composed of various α and $\beta\gamma$ subunits. The α subunit contains the guanine nucleotide–binding site and hydrolyzes GTP $\rightarrow$ GDP. The $\beta\gamma$ subunits are tightly associated and modulate the activity of the α subunit, as well as mediating their own effector signaling pathways. G protein activity is regulated by a cycle that involves GTP hydrolysis and dynamic interactions between the α and $\beta\gamma$ subunits. Hormone binding to the receptor induces GDP dissociation, allowing Gα to bind GTP and dissociate from the $\beta\gamma$ complex. Under these conditions, the Gα subunit is activated and mediates signal transduction through various enzymes such as adenylate cyclase or phospholipase C. GTP hydrolysis to GDP allows reassociation with the $\beta\gamma$ subunits and restores the inactive state. As described below, a variety of endocrinopathies result from G protein mutations or from mutations in receptors that modify their interactions with G proteins.

There are more than a dozen isoforms of the Gα subunit. G$_s\alpha$ stimulates, whereas G$_i\alpha$ inhibits adenylate cyclase, an enzyme that generates the second messenger, cyclic AMP, leading to activation of protein kinase A (Table 317-1). G$_q$ subunits couple to phospholipase C, generating diacylglycerol and inositol triphosphate, leading to activation of protein kinase C and the release of intracellular calcium.

The *tyrosine kinase receptors* transduce signals for insulin and a variety of growth factors, such as IGF-I, epidermal growth factor (EGF), nerve growth factor, platelet-derived growth factor, and fibroblast growth factor. The cysteine-rich extracellular ligand-binding domains contain growth factor binding sites. After ligand binding, this class of receptors undergoes autophosphorylation, inducing interactions with intracellular adaptor proteins such as Shc and insulin receptor substrates 1 to 4. In the case of the insulin receptor, multiple kinases are activated including the Raf-Ras-MAPK and the Akt/protein kinase B pathways. The tyrosine kinase receptors play a prominent role in cell growth and differentiation as well as in intermediary metabolism.

The GH and PRL receptors belong to the *cytokine receptor* family (Chap. 295). Analogous to the tyrosine kinase receptors, ligand binding induces receptor interaction with intracellular kinases—the Janus kinases (JAKs), which phosphorylate members of the signal transduction and activators of transcription (STAT) family—as well as other signaling pathways (Ras, PI3-K, MAPK). The activated STAT proteins translocate to the nucleus and stimulate expression of target genes (Chap. 318).

The *serine kinase receptors* mediate the actions of activins, transforming growth factor β, müllerian-inhibiting substance (MIS, also known as anti-müllerian hormone, AMH), and bone morphogenic proteins (BMPs). This family of receptors (consisting of type I and II subunits) signal through proteins termed *smads* (fusion of terms for *Caenorhabditis elegans* sma + mammalian mad). Like the STAT proteins, the smads serve a dual role of transducing the receptor signal and acting as transcription factors. The pleomorphic actions of these growth factors dictate that they act primarily in a local (paracrine or autocrine) manner. Binding proteins, such as follistatin (which binds activin and other members of this family), function to inactivate the growth factors and restrict their distribution.

NUCLEAR RECEPTORS

The family of nuclear receptors has grown to nearly 100 members, many of which are still classified as orphan receptors because their ligands, if they exist, remain to be identified (Fig. 317-2). Otherwise, most nuclear receptors are classified based on the nature of their ligands. Though all nuclear receptors ultimately act to increase or decrease gene transcription, some (e.g., glucocorticoid receptor) reside primarily in the cytoplasm, whereas others (e.g., thyroid hormone receptor) are always located in the nucleus. After ligand binding, the cytoplasmically localized receptors translocate to the nucleus. There is growing evidence that certain nuclear receptors

Homodimer Steroid Receptors
ER, AR, PR, GR

Heterodimer Receptors
TR, VDR, RAR, PPAR

Orphan Receptors
SF-1, DAX-1, HNF4α

Ligands

DNA response elements

Ligand induces coactivator binding → Activated

Ligand dissociates corepressors and induces coactivator binding → Silenced → Activated

Constitutive activator or repressor binding → Activated

Gene Expression

Hormone (−/+) | Basal Hormone (−/+) | Receptor (−/+)

FIGURE 317-2   Nuclear receptor signaling. ER, estrogen receptor; AR, androgen receptor; PR, progesterone receptor; GR, glucocorticoid receptor; TR, thyroid hormone receptor; VDR, vitamin D receptor; RAR, retinoic acid receptor; PPAR, peroxisome proliferator activated receptor; SF-1, steroidogenic factor-1; DAX, *dosage sensitive sex-reversal, adrenal hypoplasia congenita, X-chromosome*; HNF4α, hepatic nuclear factor 4α.

(e.g., glucocorticoid, estrogen) can also activate or repress signal transduction pathways, providing a mechanism for cross-talk between membrane and nuclear receptors.

The structures of nuclear receptors have been extensively studied, including by x-ray crystallography. The DNA binding domain, consisting of two zinc fingers, contacts specific DNA recognition sequences in target genes. Most nuclear receptors bind to DNA as dimers. Consequently, each monomer recognizes an individual DNA motif, referred to as a "half-site." The steroid receptors, including the glucocorticoid, estrogen, progesterone, and androgen receptors, bind to DNA as homodimers. Consistent with this twofold symmetry, their DNA recognition half-sites are palindromic. The thyroid, retinoid, peroxisome proliferator activated, and vitamin D receptors bind to DNA preferentially as heterodimers in combination with retinoid X receptors (RXRs). Their DNA half-sites are arranged as direct repeats. Receptor specificity for DNA sequences is determined by (1) the sequence of the half-site, (2) the orientation of the half-sites (palindromic, direct repeat), and (3) the spacing between the half-sites. For example, vitamin D, thyroid, and retinoid receptors recognize similar tandemly repeated half-sites (TAAGTCA), but these DNA repeats are spaced by three, four, and five nucleotides, respectively.

The carboxy-terminal hormone-binding domain mediates transcriptional control. For type II receptors, such as thyroid hormone receptor (TR) and retinoic acid receptor (RAR), co-repressor proteins bind to the receptor in the absence of ligand and silence gene transcription. Hormone binding induces conformational changes, triggering the release of co-repressors and inducing the recruitment of coactivators that stimulate transcription. Thus, these receptors are capable of mediating dramatic changes in the level of gene activity. Certain disease states are associated with defective regulation of these events. For example, mutations in the TR prevent co-repressor dissociation, resulting in a dominant form of hormone resistance (Chap. 320). In promyelocytic leukemia, fusion of RARα to other nuclear proteins causes aberrant gene silencing and prevents normal cellular differentiation. Treatment with retinoic acid reverses this repression and allows cellular differentiation and apoptosis to occur (Chap. 96). Most type 1 steroid receptors do not interact with co-repressors, but ligand binding still mediates interactions with an array of coactivators. X-ray crystallography shows that various SERMs induce distinct receptor conformations. The tissue-specific responses caused by these agents in breast, bone, and uterus appear to reflect distinct interactions with coactivators. The receptor-coactivator complex stimulates gene transcription by several pathways including (1) recruitment of enzymes (histone acetyl transferases) that modify chromatin structure, (2) interactions with additional transcription factors on the target gene, and (3) direct interactions with components of the general transcription apparatus to enhance the rate of RNA polymerase II–mediated transcription.

FUNCTIONS OF HORMONES

The functions of individual hormones are described in detail in subsequent chapters. Nevertheless, it is useful to illustrate how most biologic responses require integration of several different hormonal pathways. The physiologic functions of hormones can be divided into three general areas: (1) growth and differentiation, (2) maintenance of homeostasis, and (3) reproduction.

GROWTH

Multiple hormones and nutritional factors mediate the complex phenomenon of growth (Chap. 318). Short stature may be caused by GH deficiency, hypothyroidism, Cushing's syndrome, precocious puberty, malnutrition or chronic illness, or genetic abnormalities that affect the epiphyseal growth plates (e.g., *FGFR3* or *SHOX* mutations). Many factors (GH, IGF-I, thyroid hormone) stimulate growth, whereas others (sex steroids) lead to epiphyseal closure. Understanding these hormonal interactions is important in the diagnosis and management of growth disorders. For example, delaying exposure to high levels of sex steroids may enhance the efficacy of GH treatment.

MAINTENANCE OF HOMEOSTASIS

Though virtually all hormones affect homeostasis, the most important among these are the following:

1. Thyroid hormone—controls about 25% of basal metabolism in most tissues
2. Cortisol—exerts a permissive action for many hormones in addition to its own direct effects
3. PTH—regulates calcium and phosphorus levels
4. Vasopressin—regulates serum osmolality by controlling renal free water clearance
5. Mineralocorticoids—control vascular volume and serum electrolyte (Na^+, K^+) concentrations
6. Insulin—maintains euglycemia in the fed and fasted states

The defense against hypoglycemia is an impressive example of integrated hormone action (Chap. 324). In response to the fasted state and falling blood glucose, insulin secretion is suppressed, resulting in decreased glucose uptake and enhanced glycogenolysis, lipolysis, proteolysis, and gluconeogenesis to mobilize fuel sources. If hypoglycemia develops (usually from insulin administration or sulfonylureas), an orchestrated counterregulatory response occurs—glucagon and epinephrine rapidly stimulate glycogenolysis and gluconeogenesis, whereas GH and cortisol act over several hours to raise glucose levels and antagonize insulin action.

Although free water clearance is primarily controlled by vasopressin, cortisol and thyroid hormone are also important for facilitating renal tubular responses to vasopressin (Chap. 319). PTH and vitamin D function in an interdependent manner to control calcium metabolism (Chap. 331). PTH stimulates renal synthesis of 1,25 dihydroxyvitamin D, which increases calcium absorption in the gastrointestinal tract and enhances PTH action in bone. Increased calcium, along with vitamin D, feeds back to suppress PTH, thereby maintaining calcium balance.

Depending on the severity of a given stress and whether it is acute or chronic, multiple endocrine and cytokine pathways are activated to mount an appropriate physiologic response (Chap. 318). In severe acute stress such as trauma or shock, the sympathetic nervous system is activated and catecholamines are released, leading to increased cardiac output and a primed musculoskeletal system. Catecholamines also increase mean blood pressure and stimulate glucose production. Multiple stress-induced pathways converge on the hypothalamus, stimulating several hormones including vasopressin and corticotropin-releasing hormone (CRH). These hormones, in addition to cytokines (tumor necrosis factor α, IL-2, IL-6), increase ACTH and GH production. ACTH stimulates the adrenal gland, increasing cortisol, which in turn helps to sustain blood pressure and dampen the inflammatory response. Increased vasopressin acts to conserve free water.

REPRODUCTION

The stages of reproduction include: (1) sex determination during fetal development (Chap. 328); (2) sexual maturation during puberty (Chaps. 325 and 326); (3) conception, pregnancy, lactation, and childrearing (Chap. 326); and (4) cessation of reproductive capability at menopause (Chap. 327). Each of these stages involves an orchestrated interplay of multiple hormones, a phenomenon well illustrated by the dynamic hormonal changes that occur during each 28-day menstrual cycle. In the early follicular phase, pulsatile secretion of LH and FSH stimulates the progressive maturation of the ovarian follicle. This results in gradually increasing estrogen and progesterone levels, leading to enhanced pituitary sensitivity to GnRH, which, when combined with accelerated GnRH secretion, triggers the LH surge and rupture of the mature follicle. Inhibin, a protein produced by the granulosa cells, enhances follicular growth and feeds back to the pituitary to selectively suppress FSH, without affecting LH. Growth factors such as EGF and IGF-I modulate follicular responsiveness to gonadotropins. Vascular endothelial growth factor and prostaglandins play a role in follicle vascularization and rupture.

During pregnancy, the increased production of prolactin, in combination with placentally derived steroids (e.g., estrogen and progesterone), prepares the breast for lactation. Estrogens induce the production of progesterone receptors, allowing for increased responsiveness to progesterone. In addition to these and other hormones involved in lactation, the nervous system and oxytocin mediate the suckling response and milk release.

HORMONAL FEEDBACK REGULATORY SYSTEMS

Feedback control, both negative and positive, is a fundamental feature of endocrine systems. Each of the major hypothalamic-pituitary-hormone axes is governed by negative feedback, a process that maintains hormone levels within a relatively narrow range (Chap. 318). Examples of hypothalamic-pituitary negative feedback include (1) thyroid hormones on the TRH-TSH axis, (2) cortisol on the CRH-ACTH axis, (3) gonadal steroids on the GnRH-LH/FSH axis, and (4) IGF-I on the growth hormone–releasing hormone (GHRH)-GH axis (Fig. 317-3). These regulatory loops include both positive (e.g., TRH, TSH) and negative components (e.g., T_4, T_3), allowing for exquisite control of hormone levels. As an example, a small reduction of thyroid hormone triggers a rapid increase of TRH and TSH secretion, resulting in thyroid gland stimulation and increased thyroid hormone production. When the thyroid hormone reaches a normal level, it feeds back to suppress TRH and TSH, and a new steady state is attained. Feedback regulation also occurs for endocrine systems that do not involve the pituitary gland, such as calcium feedback on PTH, glucose inhibition of insulin secretion, and leptin feedback on the hypothalamus. An understanding of feedback regulation provides important insights into endocrine testing paradigms (see below).

Positive feedback control also occurs but is not well understood. The primary example is estrogen-mediated stimulation of the midcycle LH surge. Though chronic low levels of estrogen are inhibitory, gradually rising estrogen levels stimulate LH secretion. This effect, which is illustrative of an endocrine rhythm (see below), involves activation of the hypothalamic GnRH pulse generator. In addition, estrogen-primed gonadotropes are extraordinarily sensitive to GnRH, leading to a 10- to 20-fold amplification of LH release.

PARACRINE AND AUTOCRINE CONTROL

The aforementioned examples of feedback control involve classic endocrine pathways in which hormones are released by one gland and act on a distant target gland. However, local regulatory systems, often involving growth factors, are increasingly recognized. *Paracrine regulation* refers to factors released by one cell that act on an adjacent cell in the same tissue. For example, somatostatin secretion by pancreatic islet δ cells inhibits insulin secretion from nearby β cells. *Autocrine regulation* describes the action of a factor on the same cell from which it is produced. IGF-I acts on many cells that produce it, including chondrocytes, breast epithelium, and gonadal cells. Unlike endocrine actions, paracrine and autocrine control are difficult to document because local growth factor concentrations cannot be readily measured.

Anatomic relationships of glandular systems also greatly influence hormonal exposure—the physical organization of islet cells enhances their intercellular communication; the portal vasculature of the hypothalamic-pituitary system exposes the pituitary to high concentrations of hypothalamic releasing factors; testicular seminiferous tubules gain exposure to high testosterone levels produced by the interdigitated Leydig cells; the pancreas receives nutrient information from the gastrointestinal tract; and the liver is the proximal target of insulin action because of portal drainage from the pancreas.

HORMONAL RHYTHMS

The feedback regulatory systems described above are superimposed on hormonal rhythms that are used for adaptation to the environment. Seasonal changes, the daily occurrence of the light-dark cycle, sleep, meals, and stress are examples of the many environmental events that affect hormonal rhythms. The *menstrual cycle* is repeated on average every 28 days, reflecting the time required to follicular maturation and ovulation (Chap. 326). Essentially all pituitary hormone rhythms are entrained to sleep and the *circadian cycle*, generating reproducible patterns that are repeated approximately every 24 h. The HPA axis, for example, exhibits characteristic peaks of ACTH and cortisol production in the early morning, with a nadir during the night. Recognition of these rhythms is important for endocrine testing and treatment. Patients with Cushing's syndrome characteristically exhibit increased midnight cortisol levels when compared to normal individuals (Chap. 321). In contrast, morning cortisol levels are similar in these groups, as cortisol is normally high at this time of day in normal individuals. The HPA axis is more susceptible to suppression by glucocorticoids administered at night as they blunt the early morning rise of ACTH. Understanding these rhythms allows glucocorticoid replacement that mimics diurnal production by administering larger doses in the morning than in the afternoon (Chap. 321). Disrupted sleep rhythms can alter hormonal regulation. For example, sleep deprivation causes mild insulin resistance and hypertension, which are reversible at least in the short term.

Other endocrine rhythms occur on a more rapid time scale. Many peptide hormones are secreted in discrete bursts every few hours. LH and FSH secretion are exquisitely sensitive to GnRH pulse frequency. Intermittent pulses of GnRH are required to maintain pituitary sensitivity, whereas continuous exposure to GnRH causes pituitary gonadotrope desensitization. This feature of the hypothalamic-pituitary-gonadotrope (HPG) axis forms the basis for using long-acting GnRH agonists to treat central precocious puberty or to decrease testosterone levels in the management of prostate cancer.

It is important to be aware of the pulsatile nature of hormone secretion and the rhythmic patterns of hormone production when relating serum hormone measurements to normal values. For some hormones, integrated markers have been developed to circumvent hormonal fluctuations. Examples include 24-h urine collections for cortisol, IGF-I as a biologic marker of GH action, and HbA1c as an index of long-term (weeks to months) blood glucose control.

Often, one must interpret endocrine data only in the context of other hormonal results. For example, PTH levels are typically assessed in combination with serum calcium concentrations. A high serum calcium level in association with elevated PTH is suggestive of hyperparathyroidism, whereas a suppressed PTH in this situation is more likely to be caused by hypercalcemia of malignancy or other causes of hypercalcemia. Similarly, TSH should be elevated when T_4 and T_3

FIGURE 317-3   Feedback regulation of endocrine axes. CNS, central nervous system.

concentrations are low, reflecting reduced feedback inhibition. When this is not the case, it is important to consider other abnormalities in the hormonal axis, such as secondary hypothyroidism, which is caused by a defect at the level of the pituitary.

PATHOLOGIC MECHANISMS OF ENDOCRINE DISEASE

Endocrine diseases can be divided into three major types of conditions: (1) hormone excess, (2) hormone deficiency, and (3) hormone resistance (Table 317-2).

CAUSES OF HORMONE EXCESS

Syndromes of hormone excess can be caused by neoplastic growth of endocrine cells, autoimmune disorders, and excess hormone administration. Benign endocrine tumors, including parathyroid, pituitary, and adrenal adenomas, often retain the capacity to produce hormones, perhaps reflecting the fact that they are relatively well differentiated. Many endocrine tumors exhibit subtle defects in their "set points" for feedback regulation. For example, in Cushing's disease, impaired feedback inhibition of ACTH secretion is associated with autonomous function. However, the tumor cells are not completely resistant to feedback, as evidenced by ACTH suppression by higher doses of dexamethasone (e.g., high-dose dexamethasone test) (Chap. 321). Similar

set point defects are also typical of parathyroid adenomas and autonomously functioning thyroid nodules.

The molecular basis of some endocrine tumors, such as the MEN syndromes (MEN 1, 2A, 2B), have provided important insights into tumorigenesis (Chap. 330). MEN 1 is characterized primarily by the triad of parathyroid, pancreatic islet, and pituitary tumors. MEN 2 predisposes to medullary thyroid carcinoma, pheochromocytoma, and hyperparathyroidism. The *MEN1* gene, located on chromosome 11q13, encodes a putative tumor-suppressor gene, menin. Analogous to the paradigm first described for retinoblastoma, the affected individual inherits a mutant copy of the *MEN1* gene, and tumorigenesis ensues after a somatic "second hit" leads to loss of function of the normal *MEN1* gene (through deletion or point mutations).

In contrast to inactivation of a tumor-suppressor gene, as occurs in MEN 1 and most other inherited cancer syndromes, MEN 2 is caused by activating mutations in a single allele. In this case, activating mutations of the *RET* proto-oncogene, which encodes a receptor tyrosine kinase, leads to thyroid C-cell hyperplasia in childhood before the development of medullary thyroid carcinoma. Elucidation of the pathogenic mechanism has allowed early genetic screening for *RET* mutations in individuals at risk for MEN 2, permitting identification of those who may benefit from prophylactic thyroidectomy and biochemical screening for pheochromocytoma and hyperparathyroidism.

Mutations that activate hormone receptor signaling have been identified in several GPCRs. For example, activating mutations of the LH receptor cause a dominantly transmitted form of male-limited precocious puberty, reflecting premature stimulation of testosterone synthesis in Leydig cells (Chap. 325). Activating mutations in these GPCRs are predominantly located in the transmembrane domains and induce receptor coupling to $G_s\alpha$, even in the absence of hormone. Consequently, adenylate cyclase is activated and cyclic AMP levels increase in a manner that mimics hormone action. A similar phenomenon results from activating mutations in $G_s\alpha$. When these occur early in development, they cause McCune-Albright syndrome. When they occur only in somatotropes, the activating $G_s\alpha$ mutations cause GH-secreting tumors and acromegaly (Chap. 318).

In autoimmune Graves' disease, antibody interactions with the TSH receptor mimic TSH action, leading to hormone overproduction (Chap. 320). Analogous to the effects of activating mutations of the TSH receptor, these stimulating autoantibodies induce conformational changes that release the receptor from a constrained state, thereby triggering receptor coupling to G proteins.

CAUSES OF HORMONE DEFICIENCY

Most examples of hormone deficiency states can be attributed to glandular destruction caused by autoimmunity, surgery, infection, inflammation, infarction, hemorrhage, or tumor infiltration (Table 317-2). Autoimmune damage to the thyroid gland (Hashimoto's thyroiditis) and pancreatic islet β cells (type 1 diabetes mellitus) is a prevalent cause of endocrine disease. Mutations in a number of hormones, hormone receptors, transcription factors, enzymes, and channels can also lead to hormone deficiencies.

HORMONE RESISTANCE

Most severe hormone resistance syndromes are due to inherited defects in membrane receptors, nuclear receptors, or in the pathways that transduce receptor signals. These disorders are characterized by defective hormone action, despite the presence of increased hormone levels. In complete androgen resistance, for example, mutations in the androgen receptor cause genetic (XY) males to have a female phenotypic appearance, even though LH and testosterone levels are increased (Chap. 328). In addition to these relatively rare genetic disorders, more common acquired forms of functional hormone resistance include insulin resistance in type 2 diabetes mellitus, leptin resistance in obesity, and GH resistance in catabolic states. The pathogenesis of functional resistance involves receptor downregulation and

---

TABLE 317-2 *Causes of Endocrine Dysfunction*

Type of Endocrine Disorder	Examples
Hyperfunction	
Neoplastic	
Benign	Pituitary adenomas, hyperparathyroidism, autonomous thyroid or adrenal nodules, pheochromocytoma
Malignant	Adrenal cancer, medullary thyroid cancer, carcinoid
Ectopic	Ectopic ACTH, SIADH secretion
Multiple endocrine neoplasia	MEN1, MEN2
Autoimmune	Graves' disease
Iatrogenic	Cushing's syndrome, hypoglycemia
Infectious/inflammatory	Subacute thyroiditis
Activating receptor mutations	LH, TSH, Ca^{2+} and PTH receptors, $G_s\alpha$
Hypofunction	
Autoimmune	Hashimoto's thyroiditis, type 1 diabetes mellitus, Addison's disease, polyglandular failure
Iatrogenic	Radiation-induced hypopituitarism, hypothyroidism, surgical
Infectious/inflammatory	Adrenal insufficiency, hypothalamic sarcoidosis
Hormone mutations	GH, LHβ, FSHβ, vasopressin
Enzyme defects	21-Hydroxylase deficiency
Developmental defects	Kallmann syndrome, Turner syndrome, transcription factors
Nutritional/vitamin deficiency	Vitamin D deficiency, iodine deficiency
Hemorrhage/infarction	Sheehan's syndrome, adrenal insufficiency
Hormone resistance	
Receptor mutations	
Membrane	GH, vasopressin, LH, FSH, ACTH, GnRH, GHRH, PTH, leptin, Ca^{2+}
Nuclear	AR, TR, VDR, ER, GR, PPAR$_\gamma$
Signaling pathway mutations	Albright's hereditary osteodystrophy
Postreceptor	Type 2 diabetes mellitus, leptin resistance

Note: AR, androgen receptor; ER, estrogen receptor; GR, glucocorticoid receptor; PPAR, peroxisome proliferator activated receptor; SIADH, syndrome of inappropriate antidiuretic hormone; TR, thyroid hormone receptor; VDR, vitamin D receptor. For all other abbreviations, see text.

Disorder	Approx. Prevalence in Adults[a]	Screening/Testing Recommendations[b]	Specific Guidelines	Chapter
Obesity	23% BMI > 30 50% BMI > 25	Calculate BMI Measure waist circumference Exclude secondary causes Consider comorbid complications	NHLBI Clinical Guidelines on the Identification, Evaluation, and Treatment of Overweight and Obesity	64

Type 2 diabetes mellitus	>6%	Test every 3 years or more often in high-risk groups:
		  Fasting plasma glucose (FPG) > 126 mg/dL
		  Random plasma glucose > 200 mg/dL
		An elevated HbA1c
		Consider comorbid complications
			Expert Committee on the Diagnosis and Classification of Diabetes Mellitus	323

Hyperlipidemia	15–20%	Cholesterol screening at least every 5 years; more often in high-risk groups Lipoprotein analysis (LDL, HDL) for increased cholesterol, CAD, diabetes Consider secondary causes	Expert Panel of the National Cholesterol Education Program (NCEP)	335
Hypothyroidism	5–10%, women 0.5–2%, men	TSH; confirm with free T_4 Screen women after age 35 and every 5 years thereafter	American Thyroid Association	320
Graves' disease	1–3%, women 0.1%, men	TSH, free T_4		320
Thyroid nodules and neoplasia	5%	Physical examination of thyroid Fine-needle aspiration biopsy	American Thyroid Association	320
Osteoporosis	5%, women 1%, men	Bone mineral density measurements in women >65 years or in postmenopausal women or men at risk Exclude secondary causes	World Health Organization National Osteoporosis Foundation	333
Hyperparathyroidism	0.1–0.5%, women > men	Serum calcium PTH, if calcium is elevated Assess comorbid conditions	NIH Consensus Conference on Diagnosis and Management of Asymptomatic Primary Hyperparathyroidism	332
Infertility	10%, couples	Investigate both members of couple Semen analysis in male Assess ovulatory cycles in female Specific tests as indicated		45
Polycystic ovarian syndrome	4–7% women	Free testosterone, DHEAS Consider comorbid conditions		326
Hirsutism	Variable	Free testosterone, DHEAS Exclude secondary causes Additional tests as indicated		44
Menopause	Median age, 51	FSH		327
Hyperprolactinemia	Common in women with amenorrhea or galactorrhea	PRL level MRI, if not medication-related		318
Erectile dysfunction	10–15%	PRL, testosterone Consider secondary causes (e.g., diabetes)		43
Gynecomastia	Common in older men	Often, no tests are indicated Consider Klinefelter syndrome Consider medications, hypogonadism, liver disease		325
Klinefelter syndrome	0.2%, men	Karyotype Testosterone		328
Turner syndrome	0.03%, women	Karyotype Consider comorbid conditions		328

[a] The prevalence of most disorders varies among ethnic groups and with aging.
[b] See individual chapters for additional information on evaluation and treatment. Early testing is indicated in patients with signs and symptoms of disease or in those at increased risk.

Note: BMI, body mass index; CAD, coronary artery disease; DHEAS, dehydroepiandrosterone; HDL, high-density lipoprotein; LDL, low-density lipoprotein. For other abbreviations, see text.

postreceptor desensitization of signaling pathways; functional forms of resistance are generally reversible.

APPROACH TO THE PATIENT

Because endocrinology interfaces with numerous physiologic systems, there is no standard endocrine history and examination. Moreover, because most glands are relatively inaccessible, the examination usually focuses on the manifestations of hormone excess or deficiency, as well as direct examination of palpable glands, such as the thyroid and gonads. For these reasons, it is important to evaluate patients in the context of their presenting symptoms, review of systems, family and social history, and exposure to medications that may affect the endocrine system. Astute clinical skills are required to detect subtle symptoms and signs suggestive of underlying endocrine disease. For example, a patient with Cushing's syndrome may manifest specific findings, such as central fat redistribution, striae, and proximal muscle weakness, in addition to features seen commonly in the general population, such as obesity, plethora, hypertension, and glucose intolerance. Similarly, the insidious onset of hypothyroidism—with mental slowing, fatigue, dry skin, and other features—can be difficult to distinguish from similar, nonspecific findings in the general population. Clinical judgment, based on knowledge of disease prevalence and pathophysiology, is required to decide when to embark on more extensive evaluation of these disorders. Laboratory testing plays an essential role in endocrinology by allowing quantitative assessment of hormone levels and dynamics. Radiologic imaging tests, such as computed tomography (CT) scan, magnetic resonance imaging (MRI), thyroid scan, and ultrasound, are also used for the diagnosis of endocrine disorders. However, these tests are generally employed only after a hormonal abnormality has been established by biochemical testing.

HORMONE MEASUREMENTS AND ENDOCRINE TESTING Radioimmunoassays are the most important diagnostic tool in endocrinology, as they allow sensitive, specific, and quantitative determination of steady-state and dynamic changes in hormone concentrations. Radioimmunoassays use antibodies to detect specific hormones. For many peptide hormones, these measurements are now configured as immunoradiometric assays (IRMAs), which use two different antibodies to increase binding affinity and specificity. There are many variations of these assays—a common format involves using one antibody to capture the antigen (hormone) onto an immobilized surface and a second antibody, labeled with a fluorescent or radioactive tag, to detect the antigen. These assays are sensitive enough to detect plasma hormone concentrations in the picomolar to nanomolar range, and they can readily distinguish structurally related proteins, such as PTH from PTHrP. A variety of other techniques are used to measure specific hormones, including mass spectroscopy, various forms of chromatography, and enzymatic methods; bioassays are now rarely used.

Most hormone measurements are based on plasma or serum samples. However, urinary hormone determinations remain useful for the evaluation of some conditions. Urinary collections over 24 h provide an integrated assessment of the production of a hormone or metabolite, many of which vary during the day. It is important to assure complete collections of 24-h urine samples; simultaneous measurement of creatinine provides an internal control for the adequacy of collection and can be used to normalize some hormone measurements. A 24-h urine free cortisol measurement largely reflects the amount of unbound cortisol, thus providing a reasonable index of biologically available hormone. Other commonly used urine determinations include: 17-hydroxycorticosteroids, 17-ketosteroids, vanillylmandelic acid (VMA), metanephrine, catecholamines, 5-hydroxyindoleacetic acid (5-HIAA), and calcium.

The value of quantitative hormone measurements lies in their correct interpretation in a clinical context. The normal range for most hormones is relatively broad, often varying by a factor of two- to tenfold. The normal ranges for many hormones are gender- and age-specific. Thus, using the correct normative database is an essential part of interpreting hormone tests. The pulsatile nature of hormones, and factors that can affect their secretion such as sleep, meals, and medications, must also be considered. Cortisol values increase fivefold between midnight and dawn; reproductive hormone levels vary dramatically during the female menstrual cycle.

For many endocrine systems, much information can be gained from basal hormone testing, particularly when different components of an endocrine axis are assessed simultaneously. For example, low testosterone and elevated LH levels suggest a primary gonadal problem, whereas a hypothalamic-pituitary disorder is likely if both LH and testosterone are low. Because TSH is a sensitive indicator of thyroid function, it is generally recommended as a first-line test for thyroid disorders. An elevated TSH level is almost always the result of primary hypothyroidism, whereas a low TSH is most often caused by thyrotoxicosis. These predictions can be confirmed by determining the free thyroxine level. Elevated calcium and PTH levels suggest hyperparathyroidism, whereas PTH is suppressed in hypercalcemia caused by malignancy or granulomatous diseases. A suppressed ACTH in the setting of hypercortisolemia, or increased urine free cortisol, is seen with hyperfunctioning adrenal adenomas.

It is not uncommon, however, for baseline hormone levels associated with pathologic endocrine conditions to overlap with the normal range. In this circumstance, dynamic testing is useful to further separate the two groups. There are a multitude of dynamic endocrine tests, but all are based on principles of feedback regulation, and most responses can be remembered based on the pathways that govern endocrine axes. *Suppression tests* are used in the setting of suspected endocrine hyperfunction. An example is the dexamethasone suppression test used to evaluate Cushing's syndrome (Chaps. 318 and 321). *Stimulation tests* are generally used to assess endocrine hypofunction. The ACTH stimulation test, for example, is used to assess the adrenal gland response in patients with suspected adrenal insufficiency. Other stimulation tests use hypothalamic-releasing factors such as TRH, GnRH, CRH, and GHRH to evaluate pituitary hormone reserve (Chap. 318). Insulin-induced hypoglycemia evokes pituitary ACTH and GH responses. Stimulation tests based on reduction or inhibition of endogenous hormones are now used infrequently. Examples include metyrapone inhibition of cortisol synthesis and clomiphene inhibition of estrogen feedback.

SCREENING AND ASSESSMENT OF COMMON ENDOCRINE DISORDERS Because many endocrine disorders are prevalent in the adult population (Table 317-3), most are diagnosed and managed by general internists, family practitioners, or other primary health care providers. The high prevalence and clinical impact of certain endocrine diseases justifies vigilance for features of these disorders during routine physical examinations; laboratory screening is indicated in selected high-risk populations.

FURTHER READING

LEO CP et al: Hormonal genomics. Endocr Rev 23:369, 2002

McDONNELL DP et al: Definition of the molecular and cellular mechanisms underlying the tissue-selective agonist/antagonist activities of selective estrogen receptor modulators. Recent Prog Horm Res 57:295, 2002

McKENNA NJ, O'MALLEY BW: Combinatorial control of gene expression by nuclear receptors and coregulators. Cell 108:465, 2002

NAKAE J et al: Distinct and overlapping functions of insulin and IGF-I receptors. Endocr Rev 22:818, 2001

WEINSTEIN LS et al: Endocrine manifestations of stimulatory G protein alpha-subunit mutations and the role of genomic imprinting. Endocr Rev 22:675, 2001

The anterior pituitary is often referred to as the "master gland" because, together with the hypothalamus, it orchestrates the complex regulatory functions of multiple other endocrine glands. The anterior pituitary gland produces six major hormones: (1) prolactin (PRL), (2) growth hormone (GH), (3) adrenocorticotropin hormone (ACTH), (4) luteinizing hormone (LH), (5) follicle-stimulating hormone (FSH), and (6) thyroid-stimulating hormone (TSH) (Table 318-1). Pituitary hormones are secreted in a pulsatile manner, reflecting stimulation by an array of specific hypothalamic releasing factors. Each of these pituitary hormones elicits specific responses in peripheral target tissues. The hormonal products of these peripheral glands, in turn, exert feedback control at the level of the hypothalamus and pituitary to modulate pituitary function (Fig. 318-1). Pituitary tumors cause characteristic hormone excess syndromes. Hormone deficiency may be inherited or acquired. Fortunately, efficacious treatments exist for the various pituitary hormone excess and deficiency syndromes. Nonetheless, these diagnoses are often elusive, emphasizing the importance of recognizing subtle clinical manifestations and performing the correct laboratory diagnostic tests. →*For discussion of disorders of the posterior pituitary, or neurohypophysis, see Chap. 319.*

ANATOMY AND DEVELOPMENT

ANATOMY The pituitary gland weighs ~600 mg and is located within the sella turcica ventral to the diaphragma sella; it comprises anatomically and functionally distinct anterior and posterior lobes. The sella is contiguous to vascular and neurologic structures, including the cavernous sinuses, cranial nerves, and optic chiasm. Thus, expanding intrasellar pathologic processes may have significant central mass effects in addition to their endocrinologic impact.

Hypothalamic neural cells synthesize specific releasing and inhibiting hormones that are secreted directly into the portal vessels of the pituitary stalk. Blood supply of the pituitary gland is derived from the superior and inferior hypophyseal arteries (Fig. 318-2). The hypothalamic-pituitary portal plexus provides the major blood source for the anterior pituitary, allowing reliable transmission of hypothalamic peptide pulses without significant systemic dilution; consequently, pituitary cells are exposed to sharp spikes of releasing factors and in turn release their hormones as discrete pulses (Fig. 318-3).

The posterior pituitary is supplied by the inferior hypophyseal arteries. In contrast to the anterior pituitary, the posterior lobe is directly innervated by hypothalamic neurons (supraopticohypophyseal and tuberohypophyseal nerve tracts) via the pituitary stalk (Chap. 319). Thus, posterior pituitary production of vasopressin (antidiuretic hormone; ADH) and oxytocin is particularly sensitive to neuronal damage by lesions that affect the pituitary stalk or hypothalamus.

PITUITARY DEVELOPMENT The embryonic differentiation and maturation of anterior pituitary cells have been elucidated in considerable detail. Pituitary development from Rathke's pouch involves a complex interplay of lineage-specific transcription factors expressed in pluripotential stem cells and gradients of locally produced growth factors (Table 318-1). The transcription factor Pit-1 determines cell-specific expression of GH, PRL, and TSH in somatotropes, lactotropes, and thyrotropes. Expression of high levels of estrogen receptors in cells that contain Pit-1 favors PRL expression, whereas thyrotrope embronic factor (TEF) induces TSH expression. Pit-1 binds to GH, PRL, and TSH gene regulatory elements, as well as to recognition sites on its own promoter, providing a mechanism for perpetuating selective pituitary phenotypic stability. The transcription factor Prop-1 induces the pituitary development of Pit-1-specific lineages, as well as gonadotropes. Gonadotrope cell development is further defined by the cell-specific expression of the nuclear receptors, steroidogenic factor (SF-1) and DAX-1. Development of corticotrope cells, which express the proopiomelanocortin (POMC) gene, requires corticotropin upstream transcription element (CUTE) and the PTX-1 transcription factor. Abnormalities of pituitary development caused by mutations of Pit-1, Prop-1, SF-1, and DAX-1 result in a series of rare, selective or combined, pituitary hormone deficits.

TABLE 318-1 *Anterior Pituitary Hormone Expression and Regulation*

Cell	Corticotrope	Somatotrope	Lactotrope	Thyrotrope	Gonadotrope
Tissue-specific transcription factor	PTX-1, CUTE	Prop-1, Pit-1	Prop-1, Pit-1	Prop-1, Pit-1, TEF	SF-1, DAX-1
Fetal appearance	6 weeks	8 weeks	12 weeks	12 weeks	12 weeks
Hormone	POMC	GH	PRL	TSH	FSH LH
Chromosomal locus	2p	17q	6	α −6q; β-1p	β-11p; β-19q
Protein	Polypeptide	Polypeptide	Polypeptide	Glycoprotein α, β subunits	Glycoprotein α, β subunits
Amino acids	266 (ACTH 1–39)	191	199	211	210 204
Stimulators	CRH, AVP, gp-130 cytokines	GHRH, GHRP	Estrogen, TRH, VIP	TRH	GnRH, activins, estrogen
Inhibitors	Glucocorticoids	Somatostatin, IGF-I	Dopamine	T_3, T_4, dopamine, somatostatin, glucocorticoids	Sex steroids, inhibin
Target gland	Adrenal	Liver, other tissues	Breast, other tissues	Thyroid	Ovary, testis
Trophic effect	Steroid production	IGF-I production, growth induction, insulin antagonism	Milk production	T_4 synthesis and secretion	Sex steroid production, follicle growth, germ cell maturation
Normal range	ACTH, 4–22 pg/L	<0.5 μg/L[a]	M < 15; F <20 μg/L	0.1–5 mU/L	M, 5–20 IU/L, F (basal), 5–20 IU/L

[a] Hormone secretion integrated over 24 h.
Note: M, male; F, female. For other abbreviations, see text.

Source: Adapted from I Shimon, S Melmed, in P Conn, S Melmed (eds): *Endocrinology: Basic and Clinical Principles.* Totowa, NJ, Humana, 1996.

FIGURE 318-1 Diagram of pituitary axes. Hypothalamic hormones regulate anterior pituitary trophic hormones that, in turn, determine target gland secretion. Peripheral hormones feed back to regulate hypothalamic and pituitary hormones. For abbreviations, see text.

HYPOTHALAMIC AND ANTERIOR PITUITARY INSUFFICIENCY

Hypopituitarism results from impaired production of one or more of the anterior pituitary trophic hormones. Reduced pituitary function can result from inherited disorders; more commonly, it is acquired and reflects the mass effects of tumors or the consequences of inflammation or vascular damage. These processes may also impair synthesis or secretion of hypothalamic hormones, with resultant pituitary failure (Table 318-2).

DEVELOPMENTAL AND GENETIC CAUSES OF HYPOPITUITARISM ■ **Pituitary Dysplasia** Pituitary dysplasia may result in aplastic, hypoplastic, or ectopic pituitary gland development. Because pituitary development requires midline cell migration from the nasopharyngeal Rathke's pouch, midline craniofacial disorders may be associated with pituitary dysplasia. Acquired pituitary failure in the newborn can also be caused by birth trauma, including cranial hemorrhage, asphyxia, and breech delivery.

SEPTO-OPTIC DYSPLASIA Hypothalamic dysfunction and hypopituitarism may result from dysgenesis of the septum pellucidum or corpus callosum. Affected children have mutations in the *HESX1* gene, which is involved in early development of the ventral prosencephalon. These children exhibit variable combinations of cleft palate, syndactyly, ear deformities, hypertelorism, optic atrophy, micropenis, and anosmia. Pituitary dysfunction leads to diabetes insipidus, GH deficiency and short stature, and, occasionally, TSH deficiency.

Tissue-Specific Factor Mutations Several pituitary cell–specific transcription factors, such as Pit-1 and Prop-1, are critical for determining the development and function of specific anterior pituitary cell lineages. Autosomal dominant or recessive Pit-1 mutations cause combined GH, PRL, and TSH deficiencies. These patients present with growth failure and varying degrees of hypothyroidism. The pituitary may appear hypoplastic on magnetic resonance imaging (MRI).

Prop-1 is expressed early in pituitary development and appears to be required for Pit-1 function. Familial and sporadic *PROP1* mutations result in combined GH, PRL, TSH, and gonadotropin deficiency, with preservation of ACTH. Over 80% of these patients have growth retardation and, by adulthood, all are deficient in TSH and gonadotropins. Because of gonadotropin deficiency, they do not enter puberty spontaneously. In some cases, the pituitary gland is enlarged.

Developmental Hypothalamic Dysfunction ■ *KALLMANN SYNDROME* This syndrome results from defective hypothalamic gonadotropin-releasing hormone (GnRH) synthesis and is associated with anosmia or hyposmia due to olfactory bulb agenesis or hypoplasia (Chap. 325). The syndrome may also be associated with color blindness, optic atrophy, nerve deafness, cleft palate, renal abnormalities, cryptorchidism, and neurologic abnormalities such as mirror movements. Defects in the *KAL* gene, which maps to chromosome Xp22.3, prevent embryonic migration of GnRH neurons from the hypothalamic olfactory placode to the hypothalamus. Genetic abnormalities, in addition to *KAL* mutations, can also cause isolated GnRH deficiency, as autosomal recessive and dominant modes of transmission have been described. GnRH deficiency prevents progression through puberty. Males present with delayed puberty and pronounced hypogonadal features, including micropenis, probably the result of low testosterone levels during infancy. Female patients present with primary amenorrhea and failure of secondary sexual development.

Kallmann syndrome and other causes of congenital GnRH deficiency are characterized by low LH and FSH levels and low concentrations of sex steroids (testosterone or estradiol). In sporadic cases of isolated gonadotropin deficiency, the diagnosis is often one of exclusion after eliminating other causes of hypothalamic-pituitary dysfunction. Repetitive GnRH administration restores normal pituitary gonadotropin responses, pointing to a hypothalamic defect.

Long-term treatment of males with human chorionic gonadotropin

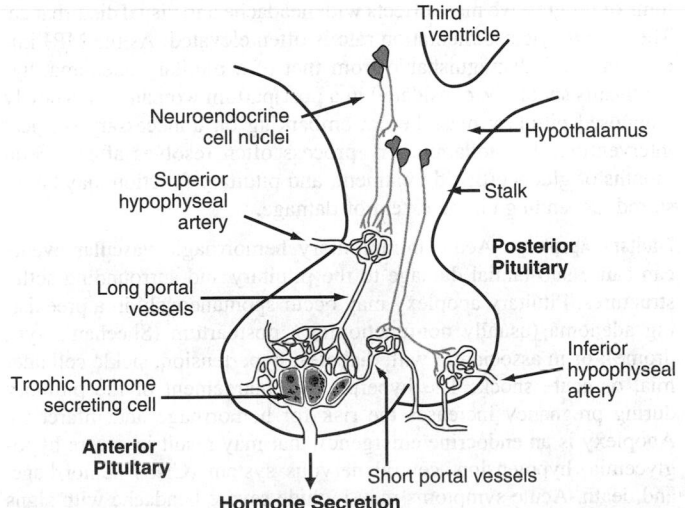

FIGURE 318-2 Diagram of hypothalamic-pituitary vasculature: The hypothalamic nuclei produce hormones that traverse the portal system and impinge on anterior pituitary cells to regulate pituitary hormone secretion. Posterior pituitary hormones are derived from direct neural extensions.

FIGURE 318-3 Hypothalamic gonadotropin-releasing hormone (GnRH) pulses induce secretory pulses of luteinizing hormone (LH).

TABLE 318-2 *Etiology of Hypopituitarism*[a]

Development/structural
   Transcription factor defect
   Pituitary dysplasia/aplasia
   Congenital CNS mass, encephalocele
   Primary empty sella
   Congenital hypothalamic disorders (septo-optic dysplasia, Prader-Willi
     syndrome, Laurence-Moon-Biedl syndrome, Kallmann syndrome)
Traumatic
   Surgical resection
   Radiation damage
   Head injuries
Neoplastic
   Pituitary adenoma
   Parasellar mass (meningioma, germinoma, ependymoma, glioma)
   Rathke's cyst
   Craniopharyngioma
   Hypothalamic hamartoma, gangliocytoma
   Pituitary metastases (breast, lung, colon carcinoma)
   Lymphoma and leukemia
   Meningioma
Infiltrative/inflammatory
   Hemochromatosis
   Lymphocytic hypophysitis
   Sarcoidosis
   Histiocytosis X
   Granulomatous hypophysitis
Vascular
   Pituitary apoplexy
   Pregnancy-related (infarction with diabetes; postpartum necrosis)
   Sickle cell disease
   Arteritis
Infections
   Fungal (histoplasmosis)
   Parasitic (toxoplasmosis)
   Tuberculosis
   Pneumocystis carinii

[a] Trophic hormone failure associated with pituitary compression or destruction usually occurs sequentially GH > FSH > LH > TSH > ACTH. During childhood, growth retardation is often the presenting feature, and in adults hypogonadism is the earliest symptom.

(hCG) or testosterone restores pubertal development and secondary sex characteristics; females can be treated with cyclic estrogen and progestin. Fertility may also be restored by the administration of gonadotropins or by using a portable infusion pump to deliver subcutaneous, pulsatile GnRH.

LAURENCE-MOON-BARDET-BIEDL SYNDROME This rare autosomal recessive disorder is characterized by mental retardation; obesity; and hexadactyly, brachydactyly, or syndactyly. Central diabetes insipidus may or may not be associated. GnRH deficiency occurs in 75% of males and half of affected females. Retinal degeneration begins in early childhood, and most patients are blind by age 30.

FRÖHLICH SYNDROME (ADIPOSE GENITAL DYSTROPHY) A broad spectrum of hypothalamic lesions may be associated with hyperphagia, obesity, and central hypogonadism. Decreased GnRH production in these patients results in attenuated pituitary FSH and LH synthesis and release. Deficiencies of leptin, or its receptor, cause these clinical features (Chap. 64).

Prader-Willi Syndrome Chromosome 15q deletions are associated with hypogonadotropic hypogonadism, hyperphagia-obesity, chronic muscle hypotonia, mental retardation, and adult-onset diabetes mellitus (Chap. 57). Multiple somatic defects also involve the skull, eyes, ears, hands, and feet. Diminished hypothalamic oxytocin- and vasopressin-producing nuclei have been reported. Deficient GnRH synthesis is suggested by the observation that chronic GnRH treatment restores pituitary LH and FSH release.

ACQUIRED HYPOPITUITARISM Hypopituitarism may be caused by accidental or neurosurgical trauma; vascular events such as apoplexy;

pituitary or hypothalamic neoplasms such as pituitary adenomas, craniopharyngiomas, or metastatic tumors; inflammatory disease such as lymphocytic hypophysitis; infiltrative disorders such as sarcoidosis, hemochromatosis (Chap. 336), and tuberculosis; or irradiation.

Hypothalamic Infiltration Disorders These disorders—including sarcoidosis, histiocytosis X, amyloidosis, and hemochromatosis—frequently involve both hypothalamic and pituitary neuronal and neurochemical tracts. Consequently, diabetes insipidus occurs in half of patients with these disorders. Growth retardation is seen if attenuated GH secretion occurs before pubertal epiphyseal closure. Hypogonadotropic hypogonadism and hyperprolactinemia are also common.

Inflammatory Lesions Pituitary damage and subsequent dysfunction can be seen with chronic infections such as tuberculosis, opportunistic fungal infections associated with AIDS, and in tertiary syphilis. Other inflammatory processes, such as granulomas or sarcoidosis, may mimic a pituitary adenoma. These lesions may cause extensive hypothalamic and pituitary damage, leading to trophic hormone deficiencies.

Cranial Irradiation Cranial irradiation may result in long-term hypothalamic and pituitary dysfunction, especially in children and adolescents, as they are more susceptible to damage following whole-brain or head and neck therapeutic irradiation. The development of hormonal abnormalities correlates strongly with irradiation dosage and the time interval after completion of radiotherapy. Up to two-thirds of patients ultimately develop hormone insufficiency afer a median dose of 50 Gy (5000 rad) directed at the skull base. The development of hypopituitarism occurs over 5 to 15 years and usually reflects hypothalamic damage rather than absolute destruction of pituitary cells. Though the pattern of hormone loss is variable, GH deficiency is most common, followed by gonadotropin and ACTH deficiency. When deficiency of one or more hormones is documented, the possibility of diminished reserve of other hormones is likely. Accordingly, anterior pituitary function should be evaluated over the long term in previously irradiated patients, and replacement therapy instituted when appropriate (see below).

Lymphocytic Hypophysitis This occurs mainly in pregnant or post-partum women; it usually presents with hyperprolactinemia and MRI evidence of a prominent pituitary mass resembling an adenoma, with mildly elevated PRL levels. Pituitary failure caused by diffuse lymphocytic infiltration may be transient or permanent but requires immediate evaluation and treatment. Rarely, isolated pituitary hormone deficiencies have been described, suggesting a selective autoimmune process targeted to specific cell types. Most patients manifest symptoms of progressive mass effects with headache and visual disturbance. The erythrocyte sedimentation rate is often elevated. As the MRI image may be indistinguishable from that of a pituitary adenoma, hypophysitis should be considered in a post-partum woman with a newly diagnosed pituitary mass before embarking on unnecessary surgical intervention. The inflammatory process often resolves after several months of glucocorticoid treatment, and pituitary function may be restored, depending on the extent of damage.

Pituitary Apoplexy Acute intrapituitary hemorrhagic vascular events can cause substantial damage to the pituitary and surrounding sellar structures. Pituitary apoplexy may occur spontaneously in a preexisting adenoma (usually nonfunctioning); postpartum (Sheehan's syndrome); or in association with diabetes, hypertension, sickle cell anemia, or acute shock. The hyperplastic enlargement of the pituitary during pregnancy increases the risk for hemorrhage and infarction. Apoplexy is an endocrine emergency that may result in severe hypoglycemia, hypotension, central nervous system (CNS) hemorrhage, and death. Acute symptoms may include severe headache with signs of meningeal irritation, bilateral visual changes, ophthalmoplegia, and, in severe cases, cardiovascular collapse and loss of consciousness. Pituitary computed tomography (CT) or MRI may reveal signs of intratumoral or sellar hemorrhage, with deviation of the pituitary stalk and compression of pituitary tissue.

Patients with no evident visual loss or impaired consciousness can be observed and managed conservatively with high-dose glucocorticoids. Those with significant or progressive visual loss or loss of consciousness require urgent surgical decompression. Visual recovery after surgery is inversely correlated with the length of time after the acute event. Therefore, severe ophthalmoplegia or visual deficits are indications for early surgery. Hypopituitarism is very common after apoplexy.

Empty Sella A partial or apparently totally empty sella is often an incidental MRI finding. These patients usually have normal pituitary function, implying that the surrounding rim of pituitary tissue is fully functional. Hypopituitarism, however, may develop insidiously. Pituitary masses may undergo clinically silent infarction with development of a partial or totally empty sella by cerebrospinal fluid (CSF) filling the dural herniation. Rarely, functional pituitary adenomas may arise within the rim of pituitary tissue, and these are not always visible on MRI.

PRESENTATION AND DIAGNOSIS The clinical manifestations of hypopituitarism depend on which hormones are lost and the extent of the hormone deficiency. GH deficiency causes growth disorders in children and leads to abnormal body composition in adults (see below). Gonadotropin deficiency causes menstrual disorders and infertility in women and decreased sexual function, infertility, and loss of secondary sexual characteristics in men. TSH and ACTH deficiency usually develop later in the course of pituitary failure. TSH deficiency causes growth retardation in children and features of hypothyroidism in children and in adults. The secondary form of adrenal insufficiency caused by ACTH deficiency leads to hypocortisolism with relative preservation of mineralocorticoid production. PRL deficiency causes failure of lactation. When lesions involve the posterior pituitary, polyuria and polydipsia reflect loss of vasopressin secretion. Epidemiologic studies have documented an increased mortality rate in patients with long-standing pituitary damage, primarily from increased cardiovascular and cerebrovascular disease.

LABORATORY INVESTIGATION Biochemical diagnosis of pituitary insufficiency is made by demonstrating low levels of trophic hormones in the setting of low target hormone levels. For example, low free thyroxine in the setting of a low or inappropriately normal TSH level suggests secondary hypothyroidism. Similarly, a low testosterone level without elevation of gonadotropins suggests hypogonadotropic hypogonadism. Provocative tests may be required to assess pituitary reserve (Table 318-3). GH responses to insulin-induced hypoglycemia, arginine, L-dopa, growth hormone–releasing hormone (GHRH), or growth hormone–releasing peptides (GHRPs) can be used to assess GH reserve. PRL and TSH responses to thyrotropin-releasing hormone (TRH) reflect lactotrope and thyrotrope function. Corticotropin-

---

TABLE 318-3 *Tests of Pituitary Insufficiency*

Hormone	Test	Blood Samples	Interpretation
Growth hormone	Insulin tolerance test: Regular insulin (0.05–0.15 U/kg IV)	−30, 0, 30, 60, 120 min for glucose and GH	Glucose < 40 mg/dL; GH should be >3 μg/L
	GHRH test: 1 μg/kg IV	0, 15, 30, 45, 60, 120 min for GH	Normal response is GH >3 μg/L
	L-Arginine test: 30 g IV over 30 min	0, 30, 60, 120 min for GH	Normal response is GH >3 μg/L
	L-dopa test: 500 mg PO	0, 30, 60, 120 min for GH	Normal response is GH >3 μg/L
Prolactin	TRH test: 200–500 μg IV	0, 20, and 60 min for TSH and PRL	Normal prolactin is >2 μg/L and increase >200% of baseline
ACTH	Insulin tolerance test: Regular insulin (0.05–0.15 U/kg IV)	−30, 0, 30, 60, 90 min for glucose and cortisol	Glucose <40 mg/dL Cortisol should increase by >7 μg/dL or to >20 μg/dL
	CRH test: 1 μg/kg ovine CRH IV at 0800 h	0, 15, 30, 60, 90, 120 min for ACTH and cortisol	Basal ACTH increases 2- to 4-fold and peaks at 20–100 pg/mL Cortisol levels >20–25 μg/dL
	Metyrapone test: Metyrapone (30 mg/kg) at midnight	Plasma 11-deoxycortisol and cortisol at 8 A.M.; ACTH can also be measured	Plasma cortisol should be <4 μg/dL to assure an adequate response Normal response is 11-deoxycortisol >7.5 μg/dL or ACTH >75 pg/mL
	Standard ACTH stimulation test: ACTH 1-24 (Cosyntropin), 0.25 mg IM or IV	0, 30, 60 min for cortisol and aldosterone	Normal response is cortisol >21 μg/dL and aldosterone response of >4 ng/dL above baseline
	Low-dose ACTH test: ACTH 1-24 (Cosyntropin), 1 μg IV	0, 30, 60 min for cortisol	Cortisol should be >21 μg/dL
	3-day ACTH stimulation test consists of 0.25 mg ACTH 1-24 given IV over 8 h each day		Cortisol >21 μg/dL
TSH	Basal thyroid function tests: T₄, T₃, TSH	Basal tests	Low free thyroid hormone levels in the setting of TSH levels that are not appropriately increased
	TRH test: 200–500 μg IV	0, 20, 60 min for TSH and PRL	TSH should increase by >5 mU/L unless thyroid hormone levels are increased
LH, FSH	LH, FSH, testosterone, estrogen	Basal tests	Basal LH and FSH should be increased in postmenopausal women Low testosterone levels in the setting of low LH and FSH
	GnRH test: GnRH (100 μg) IV	0, 30, 60 min for LH and FSH	In most adults, LH should increase by 10 IU/L and FSH by 2 IU/L Normal responses are variable
Multiple hormones	Combined anterior pituitary test: GHRH (1 μg/kg), CRH (1 μg/kg), GnRH (100 μg), TRH (200 μg) are given IV	−30, 0, 15, 30, 60, 90, 120 min for GH, ACTH, cortisol, LH, FSH, and TSH	Combined or individual releasing hormone responses must be elevated in the context of basal target gland hormone values and may not be diagnostic (see text)

Note: For abbreviations, see text.

Trophic Hormone Deficit	Hormone Replacement
ACTH	Hydrocortisone (10–20 mg A.M.; 10 mg P.M.)
	Cortisone acetate (25 mg A.M.; 12.5 mg P.M.)
	Prednisone (5 mg A.M.; 2.5 mg P.M.)
TSH	L-Thyroxine (0.075–0.15 mg daily)
FSH/LH	Males
	Testosterone enanthate (200 mg IM every 2 weeks)
	Testosterone skin patch (5 mg/d)
	Females
	Conjugated estrogen (0.65–1.25 mg qd for 25 days)
	Progesterone (5–10 mg qd) on days 16–25
	Estradiol skin patch (0.5 mg, every other day)
	For fertility: Menopausal gonadotropins, human chorionic gonadotropins
GH	Adults: Somatotropin (0.3–1.0 mg SC qd)
	Children: Somatotropin [0.02–0.05 (mg/kg per day)]
Vasopressin	Intranasal desmopressin (5–20 μg twice daily)
	Oral 300–600 μg qd

[a] All doses shown should be individualized for specific patients and should be reassessed during stress, surgery, or pregnancy. Male and female fertility requirements should be managed as discussed in Chap. 45.

Note: For abbreviations, see text.

releasing hormone (CRH) administration induces ACTH release, and administration of synthetic ACTH (cortrosyn) evokes adrenal cortisol release as an indirect indicator of pituitary ACTH reserve (Chap. 321). ACTH reserve is most reliably assessed during insulin-induced hypoglycemia. However, this test should be performed cautiously in patients with suspected adrenal insufficiency because of increased risk of hypoglycemia and hypotension. Insulin-induced hypoglycemia is contraindicated in patients with coronary heart disease or seizure disorders.

TREATMENT

Hormone replacement therapy, including glucocorticoids, thyroid hormone, sex steroids, growth hormone, and vasopressin, is usually free of complications. Treatment regimens that mimic physiologic hormone production allow for maintenance of satisfactory clinical homeostasis. Effective dosage schedules are outlined in Table 318-4. Patients in need of glucocorticoid replacement require careful dose adjustments during stressful events such as acute illness, dental procedures, trauma, and acute hospitalization (Chap. 321).

HYPOTHALAMIC, PITUITARY, AND OTHER SELLAR MASSES

PITUITARY TUMORS Pituitary adenomas are the most common cause of pituitary hormone hypersecretion and hyposecretion syndromes in adults. They account for ~10% of all intracranial neoplasms. At autopsy, up to a quarter of all pituitary glands harbor an unsuspected microadenoma (<10 mm diameter). Similarly, pituitary imaging detects small pituitary lesions in at least 10% of normal individuals.

Pathogenesis Pituitary adenomas are benign neoplasms that arise from one of the five anterior pituitary cell types. The clinical and biochemical phenotype of pituitary adenomas depend on the cell type from which they are derived. Thus, tumors arising from lactotrope (PRL), somatotrope (GH), corticotrope (ACTH), thyrotrope (TSH), or gonadotrope (LH, FSH) cells hypersecrete their respective hormones (Table 318-5). Plurihormonal tumors that express combinations of GH, PRL, TSH, ACTH, and the glycoprotein hormone α subunit may be diagnosed by careful immunocytochemistry or may manifest as clinical syndromes that combine features of these hormonal hypersecretory syndromes. Morphologically, these tumors may arise from a single polysecreting cell type or consist of cells with mixed function within the same tumor.

Hormonally active tumors are characterized by autonomous hormone secretion with diminished responsiveness to the normal physiologic pathways of inhibition. Hormone production does not always correlate with tumor size. Small hormone-secreting adenomas may cause significant clinical perturbations, whereas larger adenomas that produce less hormone may be clinically silent and remain undiagnosed (if no central compressive effects occur). About one-third of all adenomas are clinically nonfunctioning and produce no distinct clinical hypersecretory syndrome. Most of these arise from gonadotrope cells and may secrete small amounts of α- and β-glycoprotein hormone subunits or, very rarely, intact circulating gonadotropins. True pituitary carcinomas with documented extracranial metastases are exceedingly rare.

Almost all pituitary adenomas are monoclonal in origin, implying the acquisition of one or more somatic mutations that confer a selective growth advantage. In addition to direct studies of oncogene mutations, this idea is supported by X-chromosomal inactivation analyses of tumors in female patients heterozygous for X-linked genes. Consistent with their clonal origin, complete surgical resection of small pituitary adenomas usually cures hormone hypersecretion. Nevertheless, hypothalamic hormones, such as GHRH or CRH, also enhance the mitotic activity of their respective pituitary target cells, in addition to their role in pituitary hormone regulation. Thus, patients harboring rare abdominal or chest tumors elaborating ectopic GHRH or CRH may present with somatotrope or corticotrope hyperplasia.

Several etiologic genetic events have been implicated in the development of pituitary tumors. The pathogenesis of sporadic forms of acromegaly has been particularly informative as a model of tumorigenesis. GHRH, after binding to its G protein–coupled somatotrope receptor, utilizes cyclic AMP as a second messenger to stimulate GH secretion and somatotrope proliferation. A subset (~35%) of GH-secreting pituitary tumors contain sporadic mutations in Gsα (Arg 201 → Cys or His; Gln 227 → Arg). These mutations inhibit intrinsic GTPase activity, resulting in constitutive elevation of cyclic AMP, Pit-1 induction, and activation of cyclic AMP response element binding protein (CREB), thereby promoting somatotrope cell proliferation.

Adenoma Cell Origin	Hormone Product	Clinical Syndrome
Lactotrope	PRL	Hypogonadism, galactorrhea
Gonadotrope	FSH, LH, subunits	Silent or hypogonadism
Somatotrope	GH	Acromegaly/gigantism
Corticotrope	ACTH	Cushing's disease
Mixed growth hormone and prolactin cell	GH, PRL	Acromegaly, hypogonadism, galactorrhea
Other plurihormonal cell	Any	Mixed
Acidophil stem cell	PRL, GH	Hypogonadism, galactorrhea, acromegaly
Mammosomatotrope	PRL, GH	Hypogonadism, galactorrhea, acromegaly
Thyrotrope	TSH	Thyrotoxicosis
Null cell	None	Pituitary failure
Oncocytoma	None	Pituitary failure

[a] Hormone-secreting tumors are listed in decreasing order of frequency. All tumors may cause local pressure effects, including visual disturbances, cranial nerve palsy, and headache.

Note: For abbreviations, see text.

Source: Adapted from S Melmed, in JL Jameson (ed): *Principles of Molecular Medicine*, Totowa, Humana Press, 1998.

Characteristic loss of heterozygosity (LOH) in various chromosomes has been documented in large or invasive macroadenomas, suggesting the presence of putative tumor suppressor genes at these loci. LOH of chromosome region on 11q13, 13, and 9 is present in up to 20% of sporadic pituitary tumors including GH-, PRL-, and ACTH-producing adenomas and in some nonfunctioning tumors.

Compelling evidence also favors growth factor promotion of pituitary tumor proliferation. Basic fibroblast growth factor (bFGF) is abundant in the pituitary and has been shown to stimulate pituitary cell mitogenesis. Other factors involved in initiation and promotion of pituitary tumors include loss of negative-feedback inhibition (as seen with primary hypothyroidism or hypogonadism) and estrogen-mediated or paracrine angiogenesis. Growth characteristics and neoplastic behavior may also be influenced by several activated oncogenes, including *RAS* and pituitary tumor transforming gene (*PTTG*).

Genetic Syndromes Associated with Pituitary Tumors   Several familial syndromes are associated with pituitary tumors, and the genetic mechanisms for some of these have been unraveled.

Multiple endocrine neoplasia (MEN) 1 is an autosomal dominant syndrome characterized primarily by a genetic predisposition to parathyroid, pancreatic islet, and pituitary adenomas (Chap. 330). MEN1 is caused by inactivating germline mutations in *MENIN*, a constitutively expressed tumor-suppressor gene located on chromosome 11q13. Loss of heterozygosity, or a somatic mutation of the remaining normal *MENIN* allele, leads to tumorigenesis. About half of affected patients develop prolactinomas; acromegaly and Cushing's syndrome are less commonly encountered.

Carney syndrome is characterized by spotty skin pigmentation, myxomas, and endocrine tumors including testicular, adrenal, and pituitary adenomas. Acromegaly occurs in about 20% of patients. A subset of patients have mutations in the R1α regulatory subunit of protein kinase A (*PRKAR1A*).

McCune-Albright syndrome consists of polyostotic fibrous dysplasia, pigmented skin patches, and a variety of endocrine disorders, including GH-secreting pituitary tumors, adrenal adenomas, and autonomous ovarian function (Chap. 326). Hormonal hypersecretion is due to constitutive cyclic AMP production caused by inactivation of the GTPase activity of Gsα. The Gsα mutations occur postzygotically, leading to a mosaic pattern of mutant expression.

Familial acromegaly is a rare disorder in which family members may manifest either acromegaly or gigantism. The disorder is associated with LOH at a chromosome 11q13 locus distinct from that of *MENIN*.

OTHER SELLAR MASSES   *Craniopharyngiomas* are derived from Rathke's pouch. They arise near the pituitary stalk and commonly extend into the suprasellar cistern. These tumors are often large, cystic, and locally invasive. Many are partially calcified, providing a characteristic appearance on skull x-ray and CT images. More than half of all patients present before age 20, usually with signs of increased intracranial pressure, including headache, vomiting, papilledema, and hydrocephalus. Associated symptoms include visual field abnormalities, personality changes and cognitive deterioration, cranial nerve damage, sleep difficulties, and weight gain. Anterior pituitary dysfunction and diabetes insipidus are common. About half of affected children present with growth retardation.

Treatment usually involves transcranial or transsphenoidal surgical resection followed by postoperative radiation of residual tumor. This approach can result in long-term survival and ultimate cure, but most patients require lifelong pituitary hormone replacement. If the pituitary stalk is uninvolved and can be preserved at the time of surgery, the incidence of subsequent anterior pituitary dysfunction is significantly diminished.

Developmental failure of Rathke's pouch obliteration may lead to *Rathke's cysts*, which are small (<5 mm) cysts entrapped by squamous epithelium; these cysts are found in about 20% of individuals at autopsy. Although Rathke's cleft cysts do not usually grow and are often diagnosed incidentally, about a third present in adulthood with com-

pressive symptoms, diabetes insipidus, and hyperprolactinemia due to stalk compression. Rarely, internal hydrocephalus develops. The diagnosis is suggested preoperatively by visualizing the cyst wall on MRI, which distinguishes these lesions from craniopharyngiomas. Cyst contents range from CSF-like fluid to mucoid material. *Arachnoid cysts* are rare and generate an MRI image isointense with cerebrospinal fluid.

Sella chordomas usually present with bony clival erosion, local invasiveness, and, on occasion, calcification. Normal pituitary tissue may be visible on MRI, distinguishing chordomas from aggressive pituitary adenomas. Mucinous material may be obtained by fine-needle aspiration.

Meningiomas arising in the sellar region may be difficult to distinguish from nonfunctioning pituitary adenomas. Meningiomas typically enhance on MRI and may show evidence of calcification or bony erosion. Meningiomas may cause compressive symptoms.

Histiocytosis X comprises a variety of syndromes associated with foci of eosinophilic granulomas. Diabetes insipidus, exophthalmos, and punched-out lytic bone lesions (*Hand-Schüller-Christian disease*) are associated with granulomatous lesions visible on MRI, as well as a characteristic axillary skin rash. Rarely, the pituitary stalk may be involved.

Pituitary metastases occur in ~3% of cancer patients. Blood-borne metastatic deposits are found almost exclusively in the posterior pituitary. Accordingly, diabetes insipidus can be a presenting feature of lung, gastrointestinal, breast, and other pituitary metastases. About half of pituitary metastases originate from breast cancer; about 25% of patients with breast cancer have such deposits. Rarely, pituitary stalk involvement results in anterior pituitary insufficiency. The MRI diagnosis of a metastatic lesion may be difficult to distinguish from an aggressive pituitary adenoma; the diagnosis may require histologic examination of excised tumor tissue. Primary or metastatic lymphoma, leukemias, and plasmacytomas also occur within the sella.

Hypothalamic hamartomas and *gangliocytomas* may arise from astrocytes, oligodendrocytes, and neurons with varying degrees of differentiation. These tumors may overexpress hypothalamic neuropeptides including GnRH, GHRH, or CRH. In GnRH-producing tumors, children present with precocious puberty, psychomotor delay, and laughing-associated seizures. Medical treatment of GnRH-producing hamartomas with long-acting GnRH analogues effectively suppresses gonadotropin secretion and controls premature pubertal development. Rarely, hamartomas are also associated with craniofacial abnormalities; imperforate anus; cardiac, renal, and lung disorders; and pituitary failure (*Pallister-Hall syndrome*). Hypothalamic hamartomas are often contiguous with the pituitary, and preoperative MRI diagnosis may not be possible. Histologic evidence of hypothalamic neurons in tissue resected at transsphenoidal surgery may be the first indication of a primary hypothalamic lesion.

Hypothalamic gliomas and *optic gliomas* occur mainly in childhood and usually present with visual loss. Adults have more aggressive tumors; about a third are associated with neurofibromatosis.

Brain germ-cell tumors may arise within the sellar region. These include *dysgerminomas*, which are frequently associated with diabetes insipidus and visual loss. They rarely metastasize. *Germinomas, embryonal carcinomas, teratomas,* and *choriocarcinomas* may arise in the parasellar region and produce hCG. These germ-cell tumors present with precocious puberty, diabetes insipidus, visual field defects, and thirst disorders. Many patients are GH-deficient with short stature.

METABOLIC EFFECTS OF HYPOTHALAMIC LESIONS   Lesions involving the anterior and preoptic hypothalamic regions cause paradoxical vasoconstriction, tachycardia, and hyperthermia. Acute hyperthermia is usually due to a hemorrhagic insult, but poikilothermia may also occur. Central disorders of thermoregulation result from posterior hypothalamic damage. The *periodic hypothermia syndrome* comprises episodic attacks of rectal temperatures <30°C, sweating, vasodilation, vomiting, and bradycardia (Chap. 19). Damage to the ventromedial nuclei by craniopharyngiomas, hypothalamic trauma, or inflammatory disorders may be associated with *hyperphagia* and *obesity*. This region appears to contain an energy-satiety center where melanocortin receptors are influenced by leptin, insulin, POMC products, and gastrointestinal peptides (Chap. 64). Hypothalamic gliomas in early childhood may be associated with a diencephalic syndrome characterized by progressive severe emaciation and growth failure. Polydipsia and hypodipsia are associated with damage to central osmo-receptors located in preoptic nuclei (Chap. 319). Slow-growing hypothalamic lesions can cause increased somnolence and disturbed sleep cycles as well as obesity, hypothermia, and emotional outbursts. Lesions of the central hypothalamus may stimulate sympathetic neurons, leading to elevated serum catecholamine and cortisol levels. These patients are predisposed to cardiac arrhythmias, hypertension, and gastric erosions.

EVALUATION ■ Local Mass Effects

Clinical manifestations of sellar lesions vary, depending on the anatomic location of the mass and direction of its extension (Table 318-6). The dorsal roof of the sella presents the least resistance to soft tissue expansion from within the confines of the sella; consequently, pituitary adenomas frequently extend in a suprasellar direction. Bony invasion may ultimately occur as well.

Headaches are common features of small intrasellar tumors, even with no demonstrable suprasellar extension. Because of the confined nature of the pituitary, small changes in intrasellar pressure stretch the dural plate; however, the severity of the headache correlates poorly with adenoma size or extension.

Suprasellar extension can lead to visual loss by several mechanisms, the most common being compression of the optic chiasm, but direct invasion of the optic nerves or obstruction of CSF flow leading to secondary visual disturbances also occurs. Pituitary stalk compression by a hormonally active or inactive intrasellar mass may compress the portal vessels, disrupting pituitary access to the hypothalamic hormones and dopamine; this results in hyperprolactinemia and concurrent loss of other pituitary hormones. This "stalk section" phenomenon may also be caused by trauma, whiplash injury with posterior clinoid stalk compression, or skull base fractures. Lateral mass invasion may impinge on the cavernous sinus and compress its neural contents, leading to cranial nerve III, IV, and VI palsies as well as effects on the ophthalmic and maxillary branches of the fifth cranial nerve (Chap. 355). Patients may present with diplopia, ptosis, ophthalmoplegia, and decreased facial sensation, depending on the extent of neural damage. Extension into the sphenoid sinus indicates that the pituitary mass has eroded through the sellar floor. Aggressive tumors rarely invade the palate roof and cause nasopharyngeal obstruction, infection, and CSF leakage. Both temporal and frontal lobes may be invaded, leading to uncinate seizures, personality disorders, and anosmia. Direct hypothalamic encroachment by an invasive pituitary mass may cause important metabolic sequelae, precocious puberty or hypogonadism, diabetes insipidus, sleep disturbances, dysthermia, and appetite disorders.

MRI Sagittal and coronal T1-weighted spin-echo MRI imaging, before and after administration of gadolinium, allow precise visualization of the pituitary gland with clear delineation of the hypothalamus, pituitary stalk, pituitary tissue and surrounding suprasellar cisterns, cavernous sinuses, sphenoid sinus, and optic chiasm. Pituitary gland height ranges from 6 mm in children to 8 mm in adults; during pregnancy and puberty, the height may reach 10 to 12 mm. The upper aspect of the adult pituitary is flat or slightly concave, but in adolescent and pregnant individuals, this surface may be convex, reflecting physiologic pituitary enlargement. The stalk should be vertical. CT scan is indicated to define the extent of bony erosion or the presence of calcification.

The soft tissue consistency of the pituitary gland is slightly heterogeneous on MRI. Anterior pituitary signal intensity resembles that of brain matter on T1-imaging (Fig. 318-4). Adenoma density is usually lower than that of surrounding normal tissue on T1-weighted imaging, and the signal intensity increases with T2-weighted images. The high phospholipid content of the posterior pituitary results in a "pituitary bright spot."

Sellar masses are commonly encountered as incidental findings on MRI, and most of these are pituitary adenomas (incidentalomas). In the absence of hormone hypersecretion, these small lesions can be safely monitored by MRI, which is performed annually and then less often if there is no evidence of growth. Resection should be considered for incidentally discovered macroadenomas, as about one-third become invasive or cause local pressure effects. If hormone hypersecretion is evident, specific therapies are indicated. When larger masses (>1 cm) are encountered, they should also be distinguished from non-adenomatous lesions. Meningiomas are often associated with bony hyperostosis; craniopharyngiomas may be calcified and are usually hypodense, whereas gliomas are hyperdense on T2-weighted images.

Impacted Structure	Clinical Impact
Pituitary	Hypogonadism
	Hypothyroidism
	Growth failure and adult hyposomatotropism
	Hypoadrenalism
Optic chiasm	Loss of red perception
	Bitemporal hemianopia
	Superior or bitemporal field defect
	Scotoma
	Blindness
Hypothalamus	Temperature dysregulation
	Appetite and thirst disorders
	Obesity
	Diabetes insipidus
	Sleep disorders
	Behavioral dysfunction
	Autonomic dysfunction
Cavernous sinus	Opthalmoplegia ± ptosis or diplopia
	Facial numbness
Frontal lobe	Personality disorder
	Anosmia
Brain	Headache
	Hydrocephalus
	Psychosis
	Dementia
	Laughing seizures

TABLE 318-6 *Features of Sellar Mass Lesions*[a]

[a] As the intrasellar mass expands, it first compresses intrasellar pituitary tissue, then usually invades dorsally through the dura to lift the optic chiasm or laterally to the cavernous sinuses. Bony erosion is rare, as is direct brain compression. Microadenomas may present with headache.

FIGURE 318-4 Pituitary adenoma. Coronal T1-weighted postcontrast MR image shows a homogeneously enhancing mass (*arrowheads*) in the sella turcica and suprasellar region compatible with a pituitary adenoma; the small arrows outline the carotid arteries.

Ophthalmologic Evaluation Because optic tracts may be contiguous to an expanding pituitary mass, reproducible visual field assessment that uses perimetry techniques should be performed on all patients with sellar mass lesions that abut the optic chiasm (Chap. 25). Bitemporal hemianopia or superior bitemporal defects are classically observed, reflecting the location of these tracts within the inferior and posterior part of the chiasm. Homonymous cuts are postchiasmal and monocular field cuts are prechiasmal. Loss of red perception is an early sign of optic tract pressure. Early diagnosis reduces the risk of blindness, scotomas, or other visual disturbances.

Laboratory Investigation The presenting clinical features of functional pituitary adenomas (e.g., acromegaly, prolactinomas, or Cushing's disease) should guide the laboratory studies (Table 318-7). However, for a sellar mass with no obvious clinical features of hormone excess, laboratory studies are geared towards determining the nature of the tumor and assessing the possible presence of hypopituitarism. When a pituitary adenoma is suspected based on MRI, initial hormonal evaluation usually includes: (1) basal PRL; (2) insulin-like growth factor (IGF) I; (3) 24-h urinary free cortisol (UFC) and/or overnight oral dexamethasone (1 mg) suppression test; (4) α-subunit, FSH, and LH levels; and (5) thyroid function tests. Additional hormonal evaluation may be indicated based on the results of these tests. Pending more detailed assessment of hypopituitarism, a menstrual history, testosterone level, 8 A.M. cortisol, and thyroid function tests usually identify patients with pituitary hormone deficiencies that require hormone replacement before further testing or surgery.

Histologic Evaluation Immunohistochemical staining of pituitary tumor specimens obtained at transsphenoidal surgery confirms clinical and laboratory studies and provides a histologic diagnosis when hormone studies are equivocal and in cases of clinically nonfunctioning tumors. Occasionally, ultrastructural assessment by electron microscopy is required for diagnosis.

℞ TREATMENT

OVERVIEW Successful management of sellar masses requires accurate diagnosis as well as selection of optimal therapeutic modalities. Most pituitary tumors are benign and slow-growing. Clinical features result from local mass effects and hormonal hypo- or hypersecretion syndromes caused directly by the adenoma or as a consequence of treatment. Thus, lifelong management and follow-up are necessary for these patients.

MRI technology with gadolinium enhancement for pituitary visualization, new advances in transsphenoidal surgery and in stereotactic

radiotherapy (including gamma-knife radiotherapy), and novel therapeutic agents have improved pituitary tumor management. The goals of pituitary tumor treatment include normalization of excess pituitary secretion, amelioration of symptoms and signs of hormonal hypersecretion syndromes, and shrinkage or ablation of large tumor masses with relief of adjacent structure compression. Residual anterior pituitary function should be preserved and can sometimes be restored by removing tumor mass. Ideally, adenoma recurrence should be prevented.

TRANSSPHENOIDAL SURGERY Transsphenoidal rather than transfrontal resection is the desired surgical approach for pituitary tumors, except for the rare invasive suprasellar mass surrounding the frontal or middle fossa, the optic nerves, or invading posteriorly behind the clivus. Intraoperative microscopy facilitates visual distinction between adenomatous and normal pituitary tissue, as well as microdissection of small tumors that may not be visible by MRI (Fig. 318-5). Transsphenoidal surgery also avoids the cranial invasion and manipulation of brain tissue required by subfrontal surgical approaches. Endoscopic techniques with three-dimensional intraoperative localization have improved visualization and access to tumor tissue. The endoscopic approach is also less traumatic, as the technique is endonasal and does not require a transsphenoidal retractor.

In addition to correction of hormonal hypersecretion, pituitary surgery is indicated for mass lesions that impinge on surrounding structures. Surgical decompression and resection are required for an expanding pituitary mass accompanied by persistent headache, progressive visual field defects, cranial nerve palsies, internal hydrocephalus, and, occasionally, intrapituitary hemorrhage and apoplexy. Transsphenoidal surgery is sometimes used for pituitary tissue biopsy and histologic diagnosis.

FIGURE 318-5 Transsphenoidal resection of pituitary mass via the endonasal approach. (*Adapted from Fahlbusch R: Endocrinol Metab Clin 21:669, 1992.*)

TABLE 318-7	Screening Tests for Functional Pituitary Adenomas	
	Test	**Comments**
Acromegaly	Serum IGF-I	Interpret IGF-I relative to age- and gender-matched controls
	Oral glucose tolerance test with GH obtained at 0, 30, and 60 min	Normal subjects should suppress growth hormone to <1 μg/L
Prolactinoma	Exclude medications	MRI of the sella should be ordered if prolactin is elevated
Cushing's disease	24-h urinary free cortisol	Ensure urine collection is total and accurate
	Dexamethasone (1 mg) at 11 P.M. and fasting plasma cortisol measured at 8 A.M.	Normal subjects suppress to <5 μg/dL
	ACTH assay	Distinguishes adrenal adenoma (ACTH suppressed) from ectopic ACTH or Cushing's disease (ACTH normal or elevated)

Note: For abbreviations, see text.

Whenever possible, the pituitary mass lesion should be selectively excised; normal tissue should be manipulated or resected only when critical for effective dissection. Nonselective hemihypophysectomy or total hypophysectomy may be indicated if no mass lesion is clearly discernible, multifocal lesions are present, or the remaining nontumorous pituitary tissue is obviously necrotic. This strategy increases the likelihood of hypopituitarism and the need for lifelong hormonal replacement.

Preoperative local compression signs, including visual field defects or compromised pituitary function, may be reversed by surgery, particularly when these deficits are not long-standing. For large and invasive tumors, it is necessary to determine the optimal balance between maximal tumor resection and preservation of anterior pituitary function, especially for preserving growth and reproductive function in younger patients. Similarly, tumor invasion outside of the sella is rarely amenable to surgical cure; the surgeon must judge the risk: benefit ratio of extensive tumor resection.

Side Effects   Tumor size and the degree of invasiveness largely determine the incidence of surgical complications. Operative mortality is about 1%. Transient diabetes insipidus and hypopituitarism occur in up to 20% of patients. Permanent diabetes insipidus, cranial nerve damage, nasal septal perforation, or visual disturbances may be encountered in up to 10% of patients. CSF leaks occur in 4% of patients. Less common complications include carotid artery injury, loss of vision, hypothalamic damage, and meningitis. Permanent side effects are rarely encountered after surgery for microadenomas.

RADIATION   Radiation is used either as a primary therapy for pituitary or parasellar masses or, more commonly, as an adjunct to surgery or medical therapy. Focused megavoltage irradiation is achieved by precise MRI localization, using a high-voltage linear accelerator and accurate isocentric rotational arcing. A major determinant of accurate irradiation is to reproduce the patient's head position during multiple visits and to maintain absolute head immobility. A total of <50 Gy (5000 rad) is given as 180-cGy (180 rad) fractions split over about 6 weeks. Stereotactic radiosurgery delivers a large single high-energy dose from a cobalt 60 source (gamma knife), linear accelerator, or cyclotron. Long-term effects of gamma-knife surgery are as yet unknown.

The role of radiation therapy in pituitary tumor management depends on multiple factors including the nature of the tumor, age of the patient, and the availability of surgical and radiation expertise. Because of its relatively slow onset of action, radiation therapy is usually reserved for postsurgical management. As an adjuvant to surgery, radiation is used to treat residual tumor and in an attempt to prevent regrowth. Irradiation offers the only effective means for ablating significant residual tumor tissue derived from nonfunctioning tumors. PRL-, GH-, and ACTH-secreting tumor tissues are also amenable to medical therapy.

Side Effects   In the short term, radiation may cause transient nausea and weakness. Alopecia and loss of taste and smell may be more long-lasting. Failure of pituitary hormone synthesis is common in patients who have undergone head and neck or pituitary-directed irradiation. More than 50% of patients develop failure of GH, ACTH, TSH, and/or gonadotropin secretion within 10 years, usually due to hypothalamic damage. Lifelong follow-up with testing of anterior pituitary hormone reserve is therefore necessary after radiation treatment. Optic nerve damage with impaired vision due to optic neuritis is reported in about 2% of patients who undergo pituitary irradiation. Cranial nerve damage is uncommon now that radiation doses are ≤2 Gy (200 rad) at any one treatment session and the maximum dose is <50 Gy (5000 rad). The advent of stereotactic radiotherapy may reduce damage to adjacent structures. The cumulative risk of developing a secondary tumor after conventional radiation is 1.3% after 10 years and 1.9% after 20 years.

MEDICAL   Medical therapy for pituitary tumors is highly specific and depends on tumor type. For prolactinomas, dopamine agonists are the treatment of choice. For acromegaly and TSH-secreting tumors, somatostatin analogues and, occasionally, dopamine agonists are indicated. ACTH-secreting tumors and nonfunctioning tumors are generally not responsive to medication and require surgery and/or irradiation.

PROLACTIN

SYNTHESIS   PRL consists of 198 amino acids and has a molecular mass of 21,500 kDa; it is weakly homologous to GH and human placental lactogen (hPL), reflecting the duplication and divergence of a common GH-PRL-hPL precursor gene on chromosome 6. PRL is synthesized in lactotropes, which comprise about 20% of anterior pituitary cells. Lactotropes and somatotropes are derived from a common precursor cell that may give rise to a tumor secreting both PRL and GH. Marked lactotrope cell hyperplasia develops during the last two trimesters of pregnancy and the first few months of lactation. These transient adaptive changes in the lactotrope population are induced by estrogen.

SECRETION   Normal adult serum PRL levels are about 10 to 25 μg/L in women and 10 to 20 μg/L in men. PRL secretion is pulsatile, with the highest secretory peaks occurring during rapid eye movement sleep. Peak serum PRL levels (up to 30 μg/L) occur between 4:00 and 6:00 A.M. The circulating half-life of PRL is about 50 min.

PRL is unique among the pituitary hormones in that the predominant central control mechanism is inhibitory, reflecting dopamine-mediated suppression of PRL release. This regulatory pathway accounts for the spontaneous PRL hypersecretion that occurs after pituitary stalk section, often a consequence of mass lesions at the skull base. Pituitary, dopamine type 2 (D_2) receptors mediate PRL inhibition. Targeted disruption (gene knockout) of the murine D_2 receptor results in hyperprolactinemia and lactotrope proliferation. As discussed below, dopamine agonists play a central role in the management of hyperprolactinemic disorders.

TRH (pyro Glu-His-Pro-NH2) is a hypothalamic tripeptide that releases prolactin within 15 to 30 min after intravenous injection. The physiologic relevance of TRH for PRL regulation is unclear, as it appears primarily to regulate TSH (Chap. 320). *Vasoactive intestinal peptide* (VIP) also induces PRL release, whereas glucocorticoids and thyroid hormone weakly suppress PRL secretion.

Serum PRL levels rise after exercise, meals, sexual intercourse, minor surgical procedures, general anesthesia, acute myocardial infarction, and other forms of acute stress. PRL levels also increase significantly (~tenfold) during pregnancy and decline rapidly within 2 weeks of parturition. If breastfeeding is initiated, basal PRL levels remain elevated; suckling stimulates reflex increases in PRL levels that last for about 30 to 45 min. Breast suckling activates neural afferent pathways in the hypothalamus that induce PRL release. With time, the suckling-induced responses diminish and interfeeding PRL levels return to normal.

ACTION   The PRL receptor is a member of the type I cytokine receptor family that also includes GH and interleukin (IL) 6 receptors. Ligand binding leads to receptor dimerization followed by intracellular signaling mediated by Janus kinase (JAK) and components of the signal transduction and activators of transcription (STAT) family that translocate to the nucleus, where they act as transcription factors on target genes. In the breast, the lobuloalveolar epithelium proliferates in response to PRL, placental lactogens, estrogen, progesterone, and local paracrine growth factors.

PRL acts to induce and maintain lactation, decrease reproductive function, and suppress sexual drive. These functions are geared towards ensuring that maternal lactation is sustained and not interrupted by pregnancy. PRL inhibits reproductive function by suppressing hypothalamic GnRH and pituitary gonadotropin secretion and by impairing gonadal steroidogenesis in both female and male subjects. In the ovary, PRL blocks folliculogenesis and inhibits granulosa cell aromatase activity, leading to hypoestrogenism and anovulation. PRL also has a luteolytic effect, generating a shortened, or inadequate, luteal phase of the menstrual cycle. In males, attenuated LH secretion leads to low testosterone levels and decreased spermatogenesis. These hormonal changes decrease libido and reduce fertility in patients with hyperprolactinemia.

HYPERPROLACTINEMIA ■ Etiology

Hyperprolactinemia is the most common pituitary hormone hypersecretion syndrome in both males and females. PRL-secreting pituitary adenomas (prolactinomas) are the most common cause of PRL levels >100 μg/L (see below). Less pronounced PRL elevation can also be seen with microprolactinomas but is more commonly caused by drugs, pituitary stalk compression, hypothyroidism, or renal failure (Table 318-8).

Pregnancy and lactation are the important physiologic causes of hyperprolactinemia. Sleep-associated hyperprolactinemia reverts to normal within an hour of awakening. Nipple stimulation and sexual orgasm may also cause acute PRL increases. Chest wall stimulation or trauma (including chest surgery and herpes zoster) invoke the reflex suckling arc with resultant hyperprolactinemia. Chronic renal failure elevates PRL by decreasing peripheral PRL clearance. Primary hypothyroidism is associated with mild hyperprolactinemia, probably because of enhanced TRH secretion.

Lesions of the hypothalamic-pituitary region that disrupt hypothalamic dopamine synthesis, portal vessel delivery, or lactotrope responses are associated with hyperprolactinemia. Thus, hypothalamic tumors, cysts, infiltrative disorders, and radiation-induced damage cause elevated PRL levels, usually in the range of 30 to 100 μg/L. Plurihormonal adenomas (including GH and ACTH tumors) may directly hypersecrete PRL. Clinically nonfunctioning pituitary tumors commonly compress the pituitary stalk to cause hyperprolactinemia.

Drug-induced inhibition or disruption of dopaminergic receptor function is a common cause of hyperprolactinemia (Table 318-8). Thus, many antipsychotics and antidepressants cause hyperprolactinemia. Methyldopa inhibits dopamine synthesis and verapamil blocks dopamine release, also leading to hyperprolactinemia. Hormonal agents that induce PRL include estrogens, antiandrogens, and TRH.

Presentation and Diagnosis

Amenorrhea, galactorrhea, and infertility are the hallmarks of hyperprolactinemia in women. If hyperprolactinemia develops prior to the menarche, primary amenorrhea results. More commonly, hyperprolactinemia develops later in life and leads to oligomenorrhea and, ultimately, to amenorrhea. If hyperprolactinemia is sustained, vertebral bone mineral density can be reduced compared to age-matched controls, particularly when associated with pronounced hypoestrogenemia. Galactorrhea is present in up to 80% of hyperprolactinemic women. Though usually bilateral and spontaneous, it may be unilateral or only expressed manually. Patients may also complain of decreased libido, weight gain, and mild hirsutism.

In men with hyperprolactinemia, diminished libido or visual loss (from optic nerve compression) are the usual presenting symptoms. Gonadotropin suppression leads to reduced testosterone, impotence, and oligospermia. True galactorrhea is uncommon in men with hyperprolactinemia. If the disorder is longstanding, secondary effects of hypogonadism are evident, including osteopenia, reduced muscle mass, and decreased beard growth.

The diagnosis of idiopathic hyperprolactinemia is made by exclusion of known causes of hyperprolactinemia in the setting of a normal pituitary MRI. Some of these patients may have small microadenomas below MRI sensitivity (~2 mm).

Laboratory Investigation

Basal, fasting morning PRL levels (normally <20 μg/L) should be measured to assess hypersecretion. Because hormone secretion is pulsatile and levels vary widely in some individuals with hyperprolactinemia, it may be necessary to measure levels on several different occasions when clinical suspicion is high. Both false positive and false-negative results may be encountered. In patients with markedly elevated PRL levels (>1000 μg/L), results may be falsely lowered because of assay artifacts; sample dilution is required to measure these high values accurately. Falsely elevated values may be caused by aggregated forms of circulating PRL, which are biologically inactive (macroprolactinemia). Hypothyroidism should be excluded by measuring TSH and T_4 levels.

℞ TREATMENT

Treatment of hyperprolactinemia depends on the cause of elevated PRL levels. Regardless of the etiology, however, treatment should be aimed at normalizing PRL levels to alleviate suppressive effects on gonadal function, halt galactorrhea, and preserve bone mineral density. Dopamine agonists are effective for many different causes of hyperprolactinemia (see "Treatment" for "Prolactinoma," below).

If the patient is taking a medication known to cause hyperprolactinemia, the drug should be withdrawn, if possible. For psychiatric patients who require neuroleptic agents, dose titration or the addition of a dopamine agonist can help restore normoprolactinemia and alleviate reproductive symptoms. However, dopamine agonists sometimes worsen the underlying psychiatric condition, especially at high doses. Hyperprolactinemia usually resolves after adequate thyroid hormone replacement in hypothyroid patients or after renal transplantation in patients receiving dialysis. Resection of hypothalamic or sellar mass lesions can reverse hyperprolactinemia caused by reduced dopamine tone. Granulomatous infiltrates occasionally respond to glucocorticoid administration. In patients with irreversible hypothalamic damage, no treatment may be warranted. In up to 30% of patients with hyperprolactinemia—with or without a visible pituitary microadenoma—the condition resolves spontaneously.

GALACTORRHEA

Galactorrhea, the inappropriate discharge of milk-containing fluid from the breast, is considered abnormal if it persists for longer than 6 months after childbirth or discontinuation of breast-feeding. Post-partum galactorrhea associated with amenorrhea is a self-limiting disorder usually associated with moderately elevated PRL levels. Galactorrhea may occur spontaneously, or be elicited by nipple pressure. In both males and females, galactorrhea may vary in color and consistency (transparent, milky, or bloody) and arise either unilaterally or bilaterally. Mammography or ultrasound is indicated for

---

TABLE 318-8 Etiology of Hyperprolactinemia^a

I. Physiologic hypersecretion	IV. Systemic disorders
A. Pregnancy	A. Chronic renal failure
B. Lactation	B. Hypothyroidism
C. Chest wall stimulation	C. Cirrhosis
D. Sleep	D. Pseudocyesis
E. Stress	E. Epileptic seizures
II. Hypothalamic–pituitary stalk damage	V. Drug-induced hypersecretion
A. Tumors	A. Dopamine receptor blockers
1. Craniopharyngioma	1. Phenothiazines: chlorpromazine, perphenazine
2. Suprasellar pituitary mass extension	2. Butyrophenones: haloperidol
3. Meningioma	3. Thioxanthenes
4. Dysgerminoma	4. Metoclopramide
5. Metastases	B. Dopamine synthesis inhibitors
B. Empty sella	1. α-Methyldopa
C. Lymphocytic hypophysitis	C. Catecholamine depletors
D. Adenoma with stalk compression	1. Reserpine
E. Granulomas	D. Opiates
F. Rathke's cyst	E. H_2 antagonists
G. Irradiation	1. Cimetidine, ranitidine
H. Trauma	F. Imipramines
1. Pituitary stalk section	1. Amitriptyline, amoxapine
2. Suprasellar surgery	G. Serotonin-reuptake inhibitors
III. Pituitary hypersecretion	1. Fluoxetine
A. Prolactinoma	H. Calcium channel blockers
B. Acromegaly	1. Verapamil
	I. Hormones
	1. Estrogens
	2. Antiandrogens

Note: Hyperprolactinemia >100 μg/L almost invariably is indicative of a prolactin-secreting pituitary adenoma. Physiologic causes, hypothyroidism, and drug-induced hyperprolactinemia should be excluded before extensive evaluation.

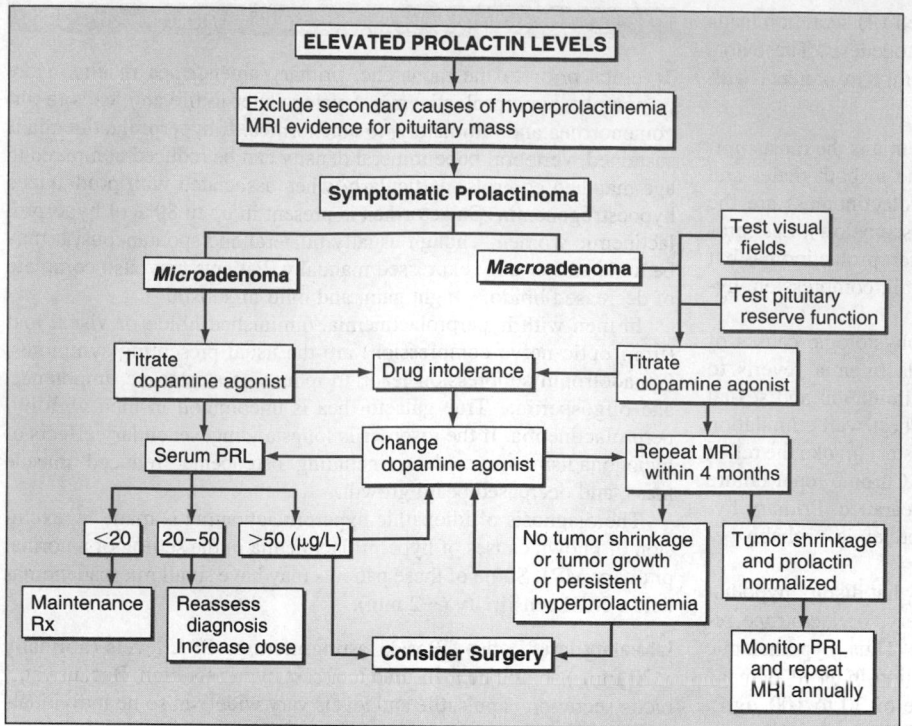

FIGURE 318-6 Management of prolactinoma. (MRI, magnetic resonance imaging; PRL, prolactin.)

bloody discharges (particularly from a single duct), which may be caused by breast cancer. Galactorrhea is commonly associated with hyperprolactinemia caused by any of the conditions listed in Table 318-8. Acromegaly is associated with galactorrhea in about one-third of patients. Treatment of galactorrhea usually involves managing the underlying disorder (e.g., replacing T_4 for hypothyroidism; discontinuing a medication; treating prolactinoma).

PROLACTINOMA ■ **Etiology and Prevalence** Tumors arising from lactotrope cells account for about half of all functioning pituitary tumors, with an annual incidence of ~3/100,000 population. Mixed tumors secreting combinations of GH and PRL, ACTH and PRL, and rarely TSH and PRL, are also seen. These plurihormonal tumors are usually recognized by immunohistochemistry, without apparent clinical manifestations from the production of additional hormones. Microadenomas are classified as <1 cm in diameter and do not usually invade the parasellar region. Macroadenomas are >1 cm in diameter and may be locally invasive and impinge on adjacent structures. The female:male ratio for microprolactinomas is 20:1, whereas the gender ratio is near 1:1 for macroadenomas. Tumor size generally correlates directly with PRL concentrations; values >100 μg/L are usually associated with macroadenomas. Males tend to present with larger tumors than females, possibly because the features of hypogonadism are less readily evident. PRL levels remain stable in most patients, reflecting the slow growth of these tumors. About 5% of microadenomas progress in the long term to macroadenomas. Hyperprolactinemia resolves spontaneously in about 30% of microadenomas.

Presentation and Diagnosis Women usually present with amenorrhea, infertility, and galactorrhea. If the tumor extends outside of the sella, visual field defects or other mass effects may be seen. Men often present with impotence, loss of libido, infertility, or signs of central CNS compression including headaches and visual defects. Assuming that known physiologic and medication-induced causes of hyperprolactinemia are excluded (Table 318-8), the diagnosis of prolactinoma is likely with a PRL level >100 μg/L. PRL levels <100 μg/L may be caused by microadenomas, other sellar lesions that decrease dopamine inhibition, or nonneoplastic causes of hyperprolactinemia. For this reason, an MRI should be performed in all patients with hyperprolactinemia. It is important to remember that hyperprolactinemia caused by the mass effects of nonlactotrope lesions is also corrected by treatment with dopamine agonists. Consequently, PRL suppression by dopamine agonists does not necessarily indicate that the lesion is a prolactinoma.

℞ TREATMENT

As microadenomas rarely progress to become macroadenomas, no treatment may be needed if fertility is not desired. Estrogen replacement is indicated to prevent bone loss and other consequences of hypoestrogenemia and does not appear to increase the risk of tumor enlargement. These patients should be monitored by regular serial PRL and MRI measurements.

For symptomatic microadenomas, therapeutic goals include control of hyperprolactinemia, reduction of tumor size, restoration of menses and fertility, and improvement of galactorrhea. Dopamine agonists should be titrated to achieve maximal PRL suppression and restoration of reproductive function (Fig. 318-6). A normalized PRL level does not assure reduced tumor size. However, tumor shrinkage is not usually seen in those who do not respond with lowered PRL levels. For macroadenomas, formal visual field testing should be performed before initiating dopamine agonists. MRI and visual fields should be assessed at 6- to 12-month intervals until the mass shrinks and annually thereafter until maximum size reduction has occurred.

MEDICAL Oral dopamine agonists (cabergoline or bromocriptine) are the mainstay of therapy for patients with micro- or macroprolactinomas. Dopamine agonists suppress PRL secretion and synthesis as well as lactotrope cell proliferation. About 20% of patients are resistant to dopaminergic treatment; they may have decreased D_2 dopamine receptor numbers or a postreceptor defect. D_2 receptor gene mutations in the pituitary have not been reported.

Cabergoline An ergoline derivative, cabergoline is a long-acting dopamine agonist with high D_2 receptor affinity. The drug effectively suppresses PRL for >14 days after a single oral dose and induces prolactinoma shrinkage in most patients. Cabergoline (0.5 to 1.0 mg twice weekly) achieves normoprolactinemia and resumption of normal gonadal function in ~80% of patients with microadenomas; galactorrhea improves or resolves in 90% of patients. Cabergoline normalizes PRL and shrinks ~70% of macroprolactinomas. Mass effect symptoms, including headaches and visual disorders, usually improve dramatically within days after cabergoline initiation; improvement of sexual function requires several weeks of treatment but may occur before complete normalization of prolactin levels. Drug withdrawal usually results in recurrent hyperprolactinemia and tumor reexpansion, with the risk of visual compromise. After initial control of PRL levels has been achieved, cabergoline should be reduced to the lowest effective maintenance dose. In ~5% of treated patients, hyperprolactinemia may resolve and not recur when dopamine agonists are discontinued after long-term treatment. Cabergoline may also be effective in patients resistant to bromocriptine. Adverse effects and drug intolerance are encountered less commonly than with bromocriptine.

Bromocriptine The ergot alkaloid bromocriptine mesylate is a dopamine receptor agonist that suppresses prolactin secretion. Because it is short-acting, the drug is preferred when pregnancy is desired. In microadenomas the drug rapidly lowers serum prolactin levels to normal in up to 70% of patients, decreases tumor size, and restores gonadal function. In patients with macroadenomas, prolactin levels are also normalized in 70% of patients and tumor mass shrinkage (≥50%) is achieved in up to 40% of patients.

Therapy is initiated by administering a low bromocriptine dose (0.625 to 1.25 mg) at bedtime with a snack, followed by gradually increasing the dose. Most patients are successfully controlled with a daily dose of ≤7.5 mg (2.5 mg tid).

Nausea, vomiting, and postural hypotension with faintness may occur in ~25% of patients after the initial dose. These symptoms may persist in some patients.

Other Dopamine Agonists These include *pergolide mesylate*, an ergot derivative with dopaminergic properties; *lisuride*, an ergot derivative; and *quinagolide* (CV 205-502, Norprolac), a nonergot oral dopamine agonist with specific D_2 receptor activity.

Side Effects Side effects of dopamine agonists include constipation, nasal stuffiness, dry mouth, nightmares, insomnia, and vertigo; decreasing the dose usually alleviates these problems. For the approximately 15% of patients who are intolerant of oral bromocriptine, dostinex may be better tolerated. Intravaginal administration of bromocriptine is often efficacious. Auditory hallucinations, delusions, and mood swings have been reported in up to 5% of patients and may be due to the dopamine agonist properties or to the lysergic acid derivative of the compounds. Rare reports of leukopenia, thrombocytopenia, pleural fibrosis, cardiac arrhythmias, and hepatitis have been described with bromocriptine.

Surgery Indications for surgical debulking include dopamine resistance or intolerance or the presence of an invasive macroadenoma with compromised vision that fails to improve rapidly after drug treatment. Initial PRL normalization is achieved in about 70% of microprolactinomas after surgical resection, but only 30% of macroadenomas can be successfully resected. Follow-up studies have shown that recurrence of hyperprolactinemia occurs in up to 20% of patients within the first year after surgery; long-term recurrence rates exceed 50% for macroadenomas. Radiotherapy for prolactinomas is reserved for patients with aggressive tumors that do not respond to maximally tolerated dopamine agonists and/or surgery.

PREGNANCY The pituitary increases in size during pregnancy, reflecting the stimulatory effects of estrogen and perhaps other growth factors. About 5% of microadenomas significantly increase in size, but 15 to 30% of macroadenomas grow during pregnancy. Bromocriptine has been used for over 25 years to restore fertility in women with hyperprolactinemia, without evidence of untoward teratogenic effects. Nonetheless, most authorities recommend strategies to minimize fetal exposure to the drug. For women taking bromocriptine who desire pregnancy, mechanical contraception should be used through three regular menstrual cycles to allow for conception timing. When pregnancy is confirmed, bromocriptine should be discontinued and PRL levels followed serially, especially if headaches or visual symptoms occur. For women harboring macroadenomas, regular visual field testing is recommended, and the drug should be reinstituted if tumor growth is apparent. Although pituitary MRI may be safe during pregnancy, this procedure should be reserved for symptomatic patients with severe headache and/or visual field defects. Alternatively, surgical decompression may be indicated if vision is threatened. Though comprehensive data support the efficacy and relative safety of bromocriptine-facilitated fertility, patients should be advised of potential unknown deleterious effects and the risk of tumor growth during pregnancy. As cabergoline is long-acting with a high D_2-receptor affinity, it is not approved for routine use when fertility is desired.

GROWTH HORMONE

SYNTHESIS GH is the most abundant anterior pituitary hormone, and GH-secreting somatotrope cells constitute up to 50% of the total anterior pituitary cell population. Mammosomatotrope cells, which coexpress PRL with GH, can be identified using double immunostaining techniques. Somatotrope development and GH transcription are determined by expression of the cell-specific Pit-1 nuclear transcription factor. Five distinct genes on chromosome 17q22 encode GH and re-

lated proteins. The pituitary GH gene (*hGH-N*) produces two alternatively spliced products that give rise to 22-kDa GH (191 amino acids) and a less abundant, 20-kDa GH molecule, with similar biologic activity. Placental syncytiotrophoblast cells express a GH variant (*hGH-V*) gene; the related hormone human chorionic somatotropin (HCS) is expressed by distinct members of the gene cluster.

SECRETION GH secretion is controlled by complex hypothalamic and peripheral factors. *GHRH* is a 44 amino acid hypothalamic peptide that stimulates GH synthesis and release. Ghrelin, or octonoylated gastric-derived peptide, as well as synthetic agonists of the *GHRP* receptor stimulate GHRH and also directly stimulate GH release. *Somatostatin* [somatotropin-release inhibiting factor (SRIF)] is synthesized in the medial preoptic area of the hypothalamus and inhibits GH secretion. GHRH is secreted as discrete spikes that elicit GH pulses, whereas SRIF sets basal GH tone. SRIF is also expressed in many extrahypothalamic tissues, including the CNS, gastrointestinal tract, and pancreas, where it also acts to inhibit islet hormone secretion. *IGF-I*, the peripheral target hormone for GH, feeds back to inhibit GH; estrogen induces GH, whereas glucocorticoid excess suppresses GH release.

Surface receptors on the somatotrope regulate GH synthesis and secretion. The GHRH receptor is a G protein–coupled receptor (GPCR) that signals through the intracellular cyclic AMP pathway. Activation of this receptor stimulates somatotrope cell proliferation as well as hormone production. Inactivating mutations of the GHRH receptor cause profound dwarfism (see below). A distinct surface receptor for ghrelin, a gastric-derived GH secretogogue, is expressed in the hypothalamus and pituitary. Somatostatin binds to five distinct receptor subtypes (SSTR1 to SSTR5); SSTR2 and SSTR5 subtypes preferentially suppress GH (and TSH) secretion.

GH secretion is pulsatile, with greatest levels at night, generally correlating with the onset of sleep. GH secretory rates decline markedly with age so that hormone production in middle age is about 15% of production during puberty. These changes are paralleled by an age-related decline in lean muscle mass. GH secretion is also reduced in obese individuals, though IGF-I levels are usually preserved, suggesting a change in the setpoint for feedback control. Elevated GH levels occur within an hour of deep sleep onset as well as after exercise, physical stress, trauma, and during sepsis. Integrated 24-h GH secretion is higher in women and is also enhanced by estrogen replacement. Using standard assays, random GH measurements are undetectable in ~50% of daytime samples obtained from healthy subjects and are undetectable in most obese and elderly subjects. Thus, single random GH measurements do not distinguish patients with adult GH deficiency from normal persons.

GH secretion is profoundly influenced by nutritional factors. Using newer ultrasensitive chemiluminescence-based GH assays with a sensitivity of 0.002 μg/L, a glucose load can be shown to suppress GH to <0.7 μg/L in female and to <0.07 μg/L in male subjects. Increased GH pulse frequency and peak amplitudes occur with chronic malnutrition or prolonged fasting. GH is stimulated by high-protein meals and by L-arginine. GH secretion is induced by dopamine and apomorphine (a dopamine receptor agonist), as well as by α-adrenergic pathways. β-Adrenergic blockage induces basal GH and enhances GHRH- and insulin-evoked GH release.

ACTION The pattern of GH secretion may affect tissue responses. The higher GH pulsatility observed in males, as compared to the relatively continuous GH secretion in females, may be an important biologic determinant of linear growth patterns and liver enzyme induction.

The 70-kDa peripheral GH receptor protein shares structural homology with the cytokine/hematopoietic superfamily. A fragment of the receptor extracellular domain generates a soluble GH binding protein (GHBP) that interacts with GH in the circulation. The liver contains the greatest number of GH receptors. GH binding induces receptor dimerization, followed by signaling through the JAK/STAT pathway. The activated STAT proteins translocate to the nucleus, where they modulate expression of GH-regulated target genes. GH analogues that bind to the receptor, but are incapable of mediating receptor dimerization, are potent antagonists of GH action and are being investigated for potential use in the treatment of acromegaly and diabetic microangiopathy.

GH induces protein synthesis and nitrogen retention and impairs glucose tolerance by antagonizing insulin action. GH also stimulates lipolysis, leading to increased circulating fatty acid levels, reduced omental fat mass, and enhanced lean body mass. GH promotes sodium, potassium, and water retention and elevates serum levels of inorganic phosphate. Linear bone growth occurs as a result of complex hormonal and growth factor actions, including those of IGF-I. GH stimulates epiphyseal prechondrocyte differentiation. These precursor cells produce IGF-I locally and are also responsive to the growth factor.

INSULIN-LIKE GROWTH FACTORS Though GH exerts direct effects in target tissues, many of its physiologic effects are mediated indirectly through IGF-I, a potent growth and differentiation factor. The major source of circulating IGF-I is hepatic in origin. Peripheral tissue IGF-I exerts local paracrine actions that appear to be both dependent and independent of GH. Thus, GH administration induces circulating IGF-I as well as stimulating IGF-I expression in multiple tissues.

Both IGF-I and -II are bound to high-affinity circulating IGF-binding proteins (IGFBPs) that regulate IGF bioactivity. Levels of IGFBP3 are GH-dependent, and it serves as the major carrier protein for circulating IGF-I. GH deficiency and malnutrition are associated with low IGFBP3 levels. IGFBP1 and -2 regulate local tissue IGF action but do not bind appreciable amounts of circulating IGF-I.

Serum IGF-I concentrations are profoundly affected by various physiologic factors. Levels increase during puberty, peak at 16 years, and subsequently decline by >80% during the aging process. IGF-I concentrations are higher in females than in males. Because GH is the major determinant of hepatic IGF-I synthesis, abnormalities of GH synthesis or action (e.g., pituitary failure, GHRH receptor defect, or GH receptor defect) reduce IGF-I levels. Hypocaloric states are associated with GH resistance; IGF-I levels are therefore low with cachexia, malnutrition, and sepsis. In acromegaly, IGF-I levels are invariably high and reflect a log-linear relationship with GH concentrations.

IGF-I Physiology Though IGF-I is not an approved drug, investigational studies provide insight into its physiologic effects. Injected IGF-I (100 μg/kg) induces hypoglycemia, and lower doses improve insulin sensitivity in patients with severe insulin resistance and diabetes. In cachectic subjects, IGF-I infusion (12 μg/kg per hour) enhances nitrogen retention and lowers cholesterol levels. Longer-term subcutaneous IGF-I injections exert a marked anabolic effect with enhanced protein synthesis. Although bone formation markers are induced, bone turnover may also be stimulated by IGF-I.

IGF-I side effects are dose-dependent, and overdose may result in hypoglycemia, hypotension, fluid retention, temporomandibular jaw pain, and increased intracranial pressure, all of which are reversible. Avascular femoral head necrosis has been reported. Chronic excess IGF-I would presumably result in features of acromegaly.

DISORDERS OF GROWTH AND DEVELOPMENT ■ **Skeletal Maturation and Somatic Growth** The growth plate is dependent on a variety of hormonal stimuli including GH, IGF-I, sex steroids, thyroid hormones, paracrine growth factors, and cytokines. The growth-promoting process also requires caloric energy, amino acids, vitamins, and trace metals and consumes about 10% of normal energy production. Malnutrition impairs chondrocyte activity and reduces circulating IGF-I and IGFBP3 levels.

Bone age is delayed in patients with all forms of true GH deficiency or GH receptor defects that result in attenuated GH action. Rarely, GH excess accelerates growth, particularly in the setting of delayed bone age from concomitant hypogonadism. Bone age is delayed by thyroid hormone deficiency. Consequently, congenital or acquired hypothyroidism is associated with stunted growth, which is partially reversed by thyroid hormone replacement (Chap. 320). Elevated pubertal sex steroid levels (especially estrogen) induce the GHRH-GH-IGF-I axis and also directly stimulate epiphyseal growth. High doses of estrogen lead to epiphyseal closure. A mutation of the estrogen receptor α prevented epiphyseal closure, confirming the important role of this pathway in bone maturation. Several pathologic conditions accompanied by increased levels of sex steroids, including precocious puberty, androgen exposure (exogenous or endogenous), congenital adrenal hyperplasia, and obesity, are associated with accelerated bone maturation. Thus, children with these conditions have accelerated early growth, but end up with reduced final height. In contrast to sex steroids, glucocorticoid excess inhibits linear growth.

Linear bone growth rates are very high in infancy and are pituitary-dependent. Mean growth velocity is ~6 cm/year in later childhood and is usually maintained within a given range on a standardized percentile chart. Peak growth rates occur during midpuberty when bone age is 12 (girls) or 13 (boys). Secondary sexual development is associated with elevated sex steroids that cause progressive epiphyseal growth plate closure.

Short stature may occur as a result of constitutive intrinsic growth defects or because of acquired extrinsic factors that impair growth. In general, delayed bone age in a child with short stature is suggestive of a hormonal or systemic disorder, whereas normal bone age in a short child is more likely to be caused by a genetic cartilage dysplasia or growth plate disorder (Chap. 342).

GH Deficiency in Children ■ *GH DEFICIENCY* Isolated GH deficiency is characterized by short stature, micropenis, increased fat, high-pitched voice, and a propensity to hypoglycemia. Familial modes of inheritance are seen in one-third of these individuals and may be autosomal dominant, recessive, or X-linked. About 10% of children with GH deficiency have mutations in the *GH-N* gene, including gene deletions and a wide range of point mutations. Mutations in transcription factors Pit-1 and Prop-1, which control somatotrope development, cause GH deficiency in combination with other pituitary hormone deficiencies, which may only become manifest in adulthood. The diagnosis of *idiopathic GH deficiency* (IGHD) should be made only after known molecular defects have been excluded.

GHRH RECEPTOR MUTATIONS Recessive mutations of the GHRH receptor gene in subjects with severe proportionate dwarfism are associated with low basal GH levels that cannot be stimulated by exogenous GHRH, GHRP, or insulin-induced hypoglycemia. The syndrome exemplifies the importance of the GHRH receptor for somatotrope cell proliferation and hormonal responsiveness.

GROWTH HORMONE INSENSITIVITY This is caused by defects of GH receptor structure or signaling. Homozygous or heterozygous mutations of the GH receptor are associated with partial or complete GH insensitivity and growth failure (*Laron syndrome*). The diagnosis is based on normal or high GH levels, with decreased circulating GHBP, and low IGF-I levels. Very rarely, defective IGF-I, IGF-I receptor, or IGF-I signaling defects are also encountered.

NUTRITIONAL SHORT STATURE Caloric deprivation and malnutrition, uncontrolled diabetes, and chronic renal failure represent secondary causes of abrogated GH receptor function. These conditions also stimulate production of proinflammatory cytokines, which can block GH-mediated signal transduction. Children with these conditions typically exhibit features of acquired short stature with elevated GH and low IGF-I levels. Circulating GH receptor antibodies may rarely cause peripheral GH insensitivity.

PSYCHOSOCIAL SHORT STATURE Emotional and social deprivation lead to growth retardation accompanied by delayed speech, discordant hyperphagia, and attenuated response to administered GH. A nurturing environment restores growth rates.

Presentation and Diagnosis Short stature is commonly encountered in clinical practice, and the decision to evaluate these children requires clinical judgement in association with auxologic data and family history. Short stature should be comprehensively evaluated if a patient's height is >3 SD below the mean for age or if the growth rate has decelerated. Skeletal maturation is best evaluated by measuring a radiologic bone age, which is based mainly on the degree of growth plate fusion. Final height can be predicted using standardized scales (Bayley-Pinneau or Tanner-Whitehouse) or estimated by adding 6.5 cm (boys) or subtracting 6.5 cm (girls) from the midparental height.

Laboratory Investigation Because GH secretion is pulsatile, GH deficiency is best assessed by examining the response to provocative stimuli including exercise, insulin-induced hypoglycemia, and other pharmacologic tests which normally increase GH to >7 μg/L in children. Random GH measurements do not distinguish normal children from those with true GH deficiency. Adequate adrenal and thyroid hormone replacement should be assured before testing. Age- and gender-matched IGF-I levels are not sufficiently sensitive or specific to make the diagnosis but can be useful to confirm GH deficiency. Pituitary MRI may reveal pituitary mass lesions or structural defects.

℞ TREATMENT

Replacement therapy with recombinant GH (0.02 to 0.05 mg/kg per day subcutaneously) restores growth velocity in GH-deficient children to ~10 cm/year. If pituitary insufficiency is documented, other associated hormone deficits should be corrected—especially adrenal steroids. GH treatment is also moderately effective for accelerating growth rates in children with Turner syndrome and chronic renal failure.

In patients with GH insensitivity and growth retardation due to mutations of the GH receptor, treatment with IGF-I bypasses the dysfunctional GH receptor. Growth rates have been maintained for several years, and this therapy now portends improved final adult stature in this group of patients.

ADULT GH DEFICIENCY (AGHD) This disorder is usually caused by hypothalamic or pituitary somatotrope damage. Acquired pituitary hormone deficiency follows a typical sequential pattern whereby loss of adequate GH reserve foreshadows subsequent hormone deficits. The sequential order of hormone loss is usually GH → FSH/LH → TSH → ACTH.

Presentation and Diagnosis The clinical features of AGHD include changes in body composition, lipid metabolism, and quality of life and cardiovascular dysfunction (Table 318-9). Body composition changes are common and include reduced lean body mass, increased fat mass

TABLE 318-9 Features of Adult Growth Hormone Deficiency

Clinical	Imaging
Impaired quality of life	Pituitary: Mass or structural damage
Decreased energy and drive	Bone: Reduced bone mineral density
Poor concentration	Abdomen: Excess omental adiposity
Low self-esteem	Laboratory
Social isolation	Evoked GH <3 ng/mL
Body composition changes	IGF-I and IGFBP3 low or normal
Increased body fat mass	Increased LDL-cholesterol
Central fat deposition	Concomitant gonadotropin, TSH,
Increased waist-hip ratio	and/or ACTH reserve deficits may
Decreased lean body mass	be present
Reduced exercise capacity	
Reduced maximum O$_2$ uptake	
Impaired cardiac function	
Reduced muscle mass	
Cardiovascular risk factors	
Impaired cardiac structure and	
function	
Abnormal lipid profile	
Decreased fibrinolytic activity	
Atherosclerosis	
Omental obesity	

Note: LDL, low-density lipoprotein; for other abbreviations, see text.

with selective deposition of intraabdominal visceral fat, and increased waist-to-hip ratio. Hyperlipidemia, left ventricular dysfunction, hypertension, and increased plasma fibrinogen levels may also be present. Bone mineral content is reduced, with resultant increased fracture rates. Patients may experience social isolation, depression, and difficulty in maintaining gainful employment. Adult hypopituitarism is associated with a threefold increased cardiovascular mortality rate in comparison to age- and sex-matched controls, and this may be due to GH deficiency.

Laboratory Investigation AGHD is rare, and in light of the nonspecific nature of associated clinical symptoms, patients appropriate for testing should be carefully selected on the basis of well-defined criteria. With few exceptions, testing should be restricted to patients with the following predisposing factors: (1) pituitary surgery, (2) pituitary or hypothalamic tumor or granulomas, (3) cranial irradiation, (4) radiologic evidence of a pituitary lesion, (5) childhood requirement for GH replacement therapy, or, rarely, (6) unexplained low age- and sex-matched IGF-I level. The transition of the GH-deficient adolescent to adulthood requires retesting to document adult GH deficiency. Up to 20% of patients treated for childhood-onset GH deficiency are found to be GH-sufficient on repeat testing as adults.

A significant proportion (~25%) of truly GH-deficient adults have low-normal IGF-I levels. Thus, as in the evaluation of GH deficiency in children, valid age- and gender-matched IGF-I measurements provide a useful index of therapeutic responses but are not sufficiently sensitive for diagnostic purposes. The most validated test to distinguish pituitary-sufficient patients from those with AGHD is insulin-induced (0.05 to 0.1 U/kg) hypoglycemia. After glucose reduction to ~40 mg/dL, most individuals experience neuroglycopenic symptoms (Chap. 324), and peak GH release occurs at 60 min and remains elevated for up to 2 h. About 90% of healthy adults exhibit GH responses >5 μg/L; AGHD is defined by a peak GH response to hypoglycemia of <3 μg/L. Although insulin-induced hypoglycemia is safe when performed under appropriate supervision, it is contraindicated in patients with diabetes, ischemic heart disease, cerebrovascular disease, or epilepsy, and in elderly patients. Alternative stimulatory tests include intravenous arginine (30 g), GHRH (1 μg/kg), and GHRP-6 (90 μg). Combinations of these tests may evoke GH secretion in subjects not responsive to a single test.

℞ TREATMENT

Once the diagnosis of AGHD is unequivocally established, replacement of GH may be indicated. Contraindications to therapy include the presence of an active neoplasm, intracranial hypertension, or uncontrolled diabetes and retinopathy. The starting dose of 0.15 to 0.3 mg/d should be titrated (up to a maximum of 1.25 mg/d) to maintain IGF-I levels in the mid-normal range for age- and gender-matched controls (Fig. 318-7). Women require higher doses than men, and elderly patients require less GH. Long-term GH maintenance sustains normal IGF-I levels and is associated with persistent body composition changes (e.g., enhanced lean body mass and lower body fat). High-density lipoprotein cholesterol increases, but total cholesterol and insulin levels do not change significantly. Lumbar spine bone mineral density increases, but this response is gradual (>1 year). Many patients note significant improvement in quality of life when evaluated by standardized questionnaires. The effect of GH replacement on mortality rates in GH-deficient patients is currently the subject of long-term prospective investigation.

About 30% of patients exhibit reversible dose related fluid retention, joint pain, and carpal tunnel syndrome, and up to 40% exhibit myalgias and paresthesia. Patients receiving insulin require careful monitoring for dosing adjustments, as GH is a potent counterregulatory hormone for insulin action. Patients with type 2 diabetes mellitus initially develop further insulin resistance. However, glycemic control improves with the sustained loss of abdominal fat associated with

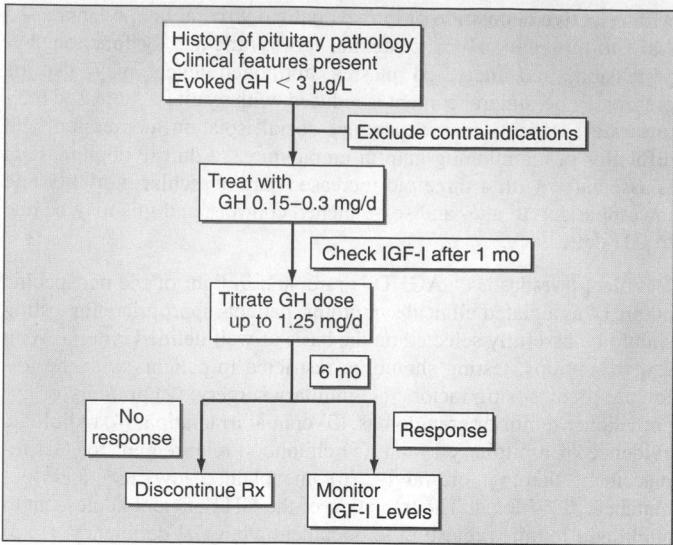

History of pituitary pathology
Clinical features present
Evoked GH < 3 μg/L

→ Exclude contraindications

Treat with
GH 0.15–0.3 mg/d

→ Check IGF-I after 1 mo

Titrate GH dose
up to 1.25 mg/d

→ 6 mo

No response   Response

Discontinue Rx   Monitor
IGF-I Levels

FIGURE 318-7 Management of adult growth hormone (GH) deficiency. (IGF, insulin-like growth factor.)

long-term GH replacement. Headache, increased intracranial pressure, hypertension, atrial fibrillation, and tinnitus occur rarely. Prevalence of pituitary tumor regrowth and potential progression of skin lesions are currently being assessed in long-term surveillance programs. To date, development of these potential side effects does not appear significant.

ACROMEGALY ■ Etiology GH hypersecretion is usually the result of somatotrope adenomas but is also rarely caused by extrapituitary lesions (Table 318-10). In addition to typical GH-secreting somatotrope adenomas, mixed mammosomatotrope tumors and acidophilic stem-cell adenomas can secrete both GH and PRL. In patients with acidophilic stem-cell adenomas, features of hyperprolactinemia (hypogonadism and galactorrhea) predominate over the less clinically evident signs of acromegaly. Occasionally, mixed plurihormonal tumors are encountered that secrete ACTH, the glycoprotein hormone α subunit, or TSH, in addition to GH. Patients with partially empty sella may present with GH hypersecretion due to a small GH-secreting adenoma within the compressed rim of pituitary tissue; some of these may reflect the spon-

TABLE 318-10 *Causes of Acromegaly*

	Prevalence, %
Excess growth hormone secretion	
Pituitary	98
Densely or sparsely granulated GH cell adenoma	60
Mixed GH cell and PRL cell adenoma	25
Mammosomatotrope cell adenoma	10
Plurihormonal adenoma	
GH cell carcinoma or metastases	
Multiple endocrine neoplasia-1 (GH cell adenoma)	
McCune-Albright syndrome	
Ectopic sphenoid or parapharyngeal sinus pituitary adenoma	
Extrapituitary tumor	
Pancreatic islet cell tumor	<1
Excess growth hormone–releasing hormone secretion	
Central	<1
Hypothalamic hamartoma, choristoma, ganglioneuroma	<1
Peripheral	<1
Bronchial carcinoid, pancreatic islet cell tumor, small cell lung cancer, adrenal adenoma, medullary thyroid carcinoma, pheochromocytoma	

Source: Adapted from S Melmed: N Engl J Med 322:966, 1990. Copyright © 1990, Massachusetts Medical Society. All rights reserved.

taneous necrosis of tumors that were previously larger. GH-secreting tumors rarely arise from ectopic pituitary tissue remnants in the nasopharynx or midline sinuses.

There are case reports of ectopic GH secretion by tumors of pancreatic, ovarian, or lung origin. Excess GHRH production may cause acromegaly because of chronic stimulation of somatotropes. These patients present with classic features of acromegaly, elevated GH levels, pituitary enlargement on MRI, and pathologic characteristics of pituitary hyperplasia. The most common cause of GHRH-mediated acromegaly is a chest or abdominal carcinoid tumor. Although these tumors usually express positive GHRH immunoreactivity, clinical features of acromegaly are evident in only a minority of patients with carcinoid disease. Excessive GHRH may also be elaborated by hypothalamic tumors, usually choristomas or neuromas.

Presentation and Diagnosis Protean manifestations of GH and IGF-I hypersecretion are indolent and often are not clinically diagnosed for 10 years or more. Acral bony overgrowth results in frontal bossing, increased hand and foot size, mandibular enlargement with prognathism, and widened space between the lower incisor teeth. In children and adolescents, initiation of GH hypersecretion prior to epiphyseal long bone closure is associated with the development of pituitary gigantism (Fig. 318-8). Soft tissue swelling results in increased heel pad thickness, increased shoe or glove size, ring tightening, characteristic coarse facial features, and a large fleshy nose. Other commonly encountered clinical features include hyperhidrosis, deep and hollow-sounding voice, oily skin, arthropathy, kyphosis, carpal tunnel syndrome, proximal muscle weakness and fatigue, acanthosis nigricans, and skin tags. Generalized visceromegaly occurs, including cardiomegaly, macroglossia, and thyroid gland enlargement.

The most significant clinical impact of GH excess occurs with respect to the cardiovascular system. Coronary heart disease, cardiomyopathy with arrhythmias, left ventricular hypertrophy, decreased diastolic function, and hypertension occur in about 30% of patients. Upper airway obstruction with sleep apnea occurs in about 60% of patients and is associated with both soft tissue laryngeal airway obstruction and central sleep dysfunction. Diabetes mellitus develops in 25% of patients with acromegaly, and most patients are intolerant of a glucose load (as GH counteracts the action of insulin). Acromegaly is associated with an increased risk of colon polyps and colonic malignancy; polyps are diagnosed in up to one-third of acromegalic patients. Overall mortality is increased about threefold and is due primarily to cardiovascular and cerebrovascular disorders, malignancy, and respiratory disease. Unless GH levels are controlled, survival is reduced by an average of 10 years compared with an age-matched control population.

Laboratory Investigation Age- and gender-matched serum IGF-I levels are elevated in acromegaly. Consequently, an IGF-I level provides a useful laboratory screening measure when clinical features raise the possibility of acromegaly. Due to the pulsatility of GH secretion, measurement of a single random GH level is not useful for the diagnosis or exclusion of acromegaly and does not correlate with disease severity. The diagnosis of acromegaly is confirmed by demonstrating the failure of GH suppression to < 1 μg/L within 1 to 2 h of an oral glucose load (75 g). About 20% of patients exhibit a paradoxical GH rise after glucose. About 60% of patients with GH-secreting tumors may exhibit paradoxical GH responses to TRH administration. PRL should be measured as it is elevated in ~25% of patients with acromegaly. Thyroid function, gonadotropins, and sex steroids may be attenuated because of tumor mass effects. Because most patients will undergo surgery with glucocorticoid coverage, tests of ACTH reserve in asymptomatic patients are more efficiently deferred until after surgery.

℞ TREATMENT

Surgical resection of GH-secreting adenomas is the initial treatment for most patients (Fig. 318-9). Somatostatin analogues are used as adjuvant treatment for preoperative shrinkage of large invasive macroadenomas, immediate relief of debilitating symptoms, and reduction of GH hypersecretion, in elderly patients experiencing morbidity, in patients who decline surgery, or, when surgery fails, to achieve biochemical control. Irradiation or repeat surgery may be required for patients who cannot tolerate or do not respond to adjunctive medical therapy. The high rate of late hypopituitarism and the slow rate (5 to 15 years) of biochemical response are the main disadvantages of radiotherapy. Irradiation is relatively ineffective in normalizing IGF-I levels. Stereotactic ablation of GH-secreting adenomas by gamma-knife radiotherapy is promising, but long-term results are not available and the side effects have not been clearly delineated. Somatostatin analogues may be given while awaiting the full effect of radiotherapy. Systemic sequelae of acromegaly, including cardiovascular disease, diabetes, and arthritis, should also be managed aggressively. Maxillofacial surgery for mandibular repair may also be indicated.

FIGURE 318-8 Features of acromegaly/gigantism. A 22-year-old man with gigantism due to excess growth hormone is shown to the left of his identical twin. The increased height and prognathism (*A*) and enlarged hand (*B*) and foot (*C*) of the affected twin are apparent. Their clinical features began to diverge at the age of approximately 13 years. (*Reproduced from R Gagel, IE McCutcheon: N Engl J Med 324:524, 1999, with permission.*)

SURGERY Transsphenoidal surgical resection by an experienced surgeon is the preferred primary treatment for both microadenomas (cure rate ~70%) and macroadenomas (<50% cured). Soft tissue swelling improves immediately after tumor resection. GH levels return to normal within an hour, and IGF-I levels are normalized within 3 to 4 days. In ~10% of patients, acromegaly may recur several years after apparently successful surgery; hypopituitarism develops in up to 15% of patients.

SOMATOSTATIN ANALOGUES Somatostatin analogues exert their therapeutic effects through SSTR2 and -5 receptors, both of which are expressed by GH-secreting tumors. Octreotide acetate is an 8-amino-acid synthetic somatostatin analogue. In contrast to native somatostatin, the analogue is relatively resistant to plasma degradation. It has a 2-h serum half-life and possesses 40-fold greater potency than native somatostatin to suppress GH. Octreotide is administered by subcutaneous injection, beginning with 50 μg tid; the dose can be gradually increased up to 1500 μg/d. Fewer than 10% of patients do not respond to the analogue. Octreotide suppresses integrated GH levels to <5 μg/L in ~70% of patients and to <2 μg/L in up to 60% of patients. It normalizes IGF-I levels in ~75% of treated patients. Prolonged use of the analogue is not associated with desensitization, even after ≥10 years of treatment. Rapid relief of headache and soft tissue swelling occurs in ~75% of patients within days to weeks of treatment initiation. Subjective clinical benefits of octreotide therapy occur more frequently than biochemical remission, and most patients report symptomatic improvement, including amelioration of headache, perspiration, obstructive apnea, and cardiac failure. Modest pituitary tumor size reduction occurs in about 40% of patients, but this effect is reversed when treatment is stopped.

Two long-acting somatostatin depot formulations, octreotide and lanreotide, are becoming the preferred medical treatment for acromegalic patients. *Sando-statin-LAR* is a sustained-release, long-acting formulation of octreotide incorporated into microspheres that sustain drug levels for several weeks after intramuscular injection. GH suppression occurs for as long as 6 weeks after a 30-mg injection; long-term monthly treatment sustains GH and IGF-I suppression and reduction of pituitary tumor size. *Lanreotide*, a slow-release depot somatostatin preparation, is a cyclic somatostatin octapeptide analogue that suppresses GH and IGF-I hypersecretion for 10 to 14 days after a 30-mg intramuscular injection. Long-term administration controls GH hypersecretion in two-thirds of

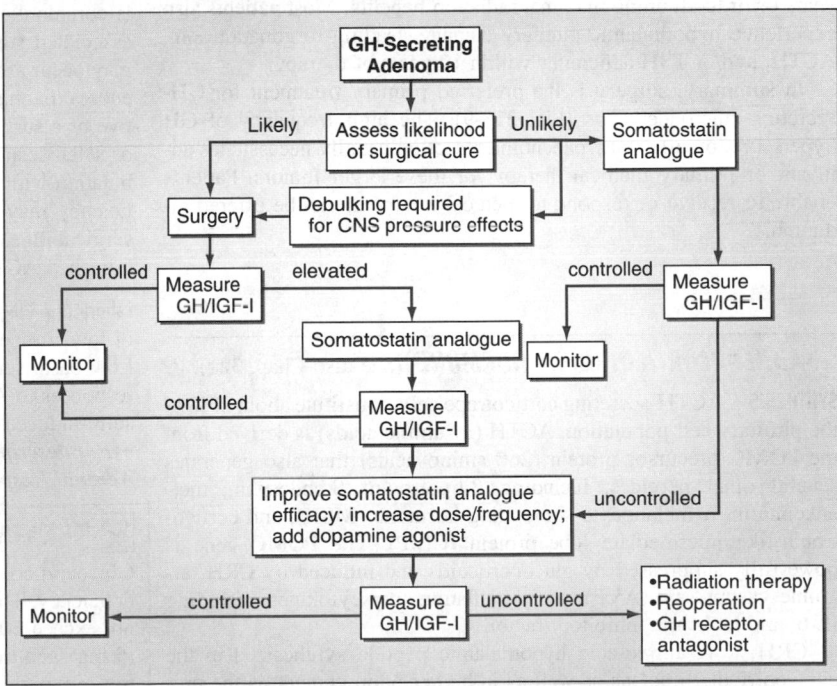

FIGURE 318-9 Management of acromegaly. (GH, growth hormone; CNS, central nervous system; IGF, insulin-like growth factor.) (*Adapted from S. Melmed et al: J Clin Endocrinol Metab 83:2646, 1998; © The Endocrine Society.*)

treated patients and improves patient compliance because of the long interval required between drug injections.

Side Effects Somatostatin analogues are well tolerated in most patients. Adverse effects are short-lived and mostly relate to drug-induced suppression of gastrointestinal motility and secretion. Nausea, abdominal discomfort, fat malabsorption, diarrhea, and flatulence occur in one-third of patients, though these symptoms usually remit within 2 weeks. Octreotide suppresses postprandial gallbladder contractility and delays gallbladder emptying; up to 30% of patients treated long-term develop echogenic sludge or asymptomatic cholesterol gallstones. Other side effects include mild glucose intolerance due to transient insulin suppression, asymptomatic bradycardia, hypothyroxinemia, and local pain at the injection site.

DOPAMINE AGONISTS Bromocriptine may suppress GH secretion in some acromegalic patients, particularly those with cosecretion of PRL. High doses (≥ 20 mg/d), administered as three to four daily doses, are usually required to lower GH, and therapeutic efficacy is modest. GH levels are suppressed to <5 μg/L in $\sim 20\%$ of patients, and IGF-I levels are normalized in only 10% of patients. Cabergoline also suppresses GH and decreases adenoma size when given at a relatively high dose of 0.5 mg/d. Combined treatment with octreotide and bromocriptine induces additive biochemical control compared to either drug alone.

GH ANTAGONISTS GH analogues (e.g., pegvisomant) antagonize endogenous GH action by blocking peripheral GH binding to its receptor. Consequently, serum IGF-I levels are suppressed, potentially reducing the deleterious effects of excess endogenous GH.

RADIATION External radiation therapy or high-energy stereotactic techniques are used as adjuvant therapy for acromegaly. An advantage of radiation is that patient compliance with long-term treatment is not required. Tumor mass is reduced, and GH levels are attenuated over time. However, 50% of patients require at least 8 years for GH levels to be suppressed to <5 μg/L; this level of GH reduction is achieved in about 90% of patients after 18 years but represents suboptimal GH suppression. Patients may require interim medical therapy for several years prior to attaining maximal radiation benefits. Most patients also experience hypothalamic-pituitary damage, leading to gonadotropin, ACTH, and/or TSH deficiency within 10 years of therapy.

In summary, surgery is the preferred primary treatment for GH-secreting microadenomas (Fig. 318-9). The high frequency of GH hypersecretion after macroadenoma resection usually necessitates adjuvant or primary medical therapy for these larger tumors. Patients unable to receive or respond to medical treatment can be offered radiation.

ADRENOCORTICOTROPIN HORMONE (See also Chap. 321)

SYNTHESIS ACTH-secreting corticotrope cells constitute about 20% of the pituitary cell population. ACTH (39 amino acids) is derived from the POMC precursor protein (266 amino acids) that also generates several other peptides, including β-lipotropin, β-endorphin, met-enkephalin, α melanocyte-stimulating hormone (MSH), and corticotropin-like intermediate lobe protein (CLIP). The POMC gene is powerfully suppressed by glucocorticoids and induced by CRH, arginine vasopressin (AVP), and proinflammatory cytokines, including IL-6, and leukemia inhibitory factor.

CRH, a 41-amino-acid hypothalamic peptide synthesized in the paraventricular nucleus as well as in higher brain centers, is the predominant stimulator of ACTH synthesis and release. The CRH receptor is a GPCR that is expressed on the corticotrope and induces POMC transcription.

SECRETION ACTH secretion is pulsatile and exhibits a characteristic circadian rhythm, peaking at 6 A.M. and reaching a nadir about midnight. Adrenal glucocorticoid secretion, which is driven by ACTH, follows a parallel diurnal pattern. ACTH circadian rhymicity is determined by variations in secretory pulse amplitude rather than changes in pulse frequency. Superimposed on this endogenous rhythm, ACTH levels are increased by AVP, physical stress, exercise, acute illness, and insulin-induced hypoglycemia.

Loss of cortisol feedback inhibition, as occurs in primary adrenal failure, results in extremely high ACTH levels. Glucocorticoid-mediated negative regulation of the hypothalamo-pituitary-adrenal (HPA) axis occurs as a consequence of both hypothalamic CRH suppression and direct attenuation of pituitary POMC gene expression and ACTH release.

Acute inflammatory or septic insults activate the HPA axis through the integrated actions of proinflammatory cytokines, bacterial toxins, and neural signals. The overlapping cascade of ACTH-inducing cytokines [tumor necrosis factor (TNF); IL-1, -2, and -6; and leukemia inhibitory factor] activates hypothalamic CRH and AVP secretion, pituitary POMC gene expression, and local paracrine pituitary cytokine networks. The resulting cortisol elevation restrains the inflammatory response and provides host protection. Concomitantly, cytokine-mediated central glucocorticoid receptor resistance impairs glucocorticoid suppression of the HPA. Thus, the neuroendocrine stress response reflects the net result of highly integrated hypothalamic, intrapituitary, and peripheral hormone and cytokine signals.

ACTION The major function of the HPA axis is to maintain metabolic homeostasis and to mediate the neuroendocrine stress response. ACTH induces cortical steroidogenesis by maintaining adrenal cell proliferation and function. The receptor for ACTH, designated *melanocortin-2 receptor*, is a GPCR that induces steroidogenesis by stimulating a cascade of steroidogenic enzymes (Chap. 321).

ACTH DEFICIENCY ■ **Presentation and Diagnosis** Secondary adrenal insufficiency occurs as a result of pituitary ACTH deficiency. It is characterized by fatigue, weakness, anorexia, nausea, vomiting, and, occasionally, hypoglycemia (due to diminished insulin counterregulation). In contrast to primary adrenal failure, hypocortisolism associated with pituitary failure is not usually accompanied by pigmentation changes or mineralocorticoid deficiency. ACTH deficiency is commonly due to glucocorticoid withdrawal following treatment-associated suppression of the HPA axis. Isolated ACTH deficiency may occur after surgical resection of an ACTH-secreting pituitary adenoma that has suppressed the HPA axis; this phenomenon is suggestive of a surgical cure. The mass effects of other pituitary adenomas or sellar lesions may lead to ACTH deficiency, but usually in combination with other pituitary hormone deficiencies. Partial ACTH deficiency may be unmasked in the presence of an acute medical or surgical illness, when clinically significant hypocortisolism reflects diminished ACTH reserve.

Laboratory Diagnosis Inappropriately low ACTH levels in the setting of low cortisol levels are characteristic of diminished ACTH reserve. Low basal serum cortisol levels are associated with blunted cortisol responses to ACTH stimulation and impaired cortisol response to insulin-induced hypoglycemia, or testing with metyrapone or CRH. →*For description of provocative ACTH tests, see "Tests of Pituitary-Adrenal Responsiveness" in Chap. 321.*

℞ TREATMENT

Glucocorticoid replacement therapy improves most features of ACTH deficiency. The total daily dose of hydrocortisone replacement should not exceed 30 mg daily, divided into two or three doses. Prednisone (5 mg each morning; 2.5 mg each evening) is longer acting and has fewer mineralocorticoid effects than hydrocortisone. Some authorities advocate lower maintenance doses in an effort to avoid cushingoid side effects. Doses should be increased several-fold during periods of acute illness or stress.

CUSHING'S DISEASE (ACTH-PRODUCING ADENOMA) (See also Chap. 321)

■ Etiology and Prevalence Pituitary corticotrope adenomas account for 70% of patients with endogenous causes of Cushing's syndrome. However, it should be recalled that iatrogenic hypercortisolism is the most common cause of cushingoid features. Ectopic tumor ACTH production, cortisol-producing adrenal adenomas, carcinoma, and hyperplasia account for the other causes; rarely, ectopic tumor CRH production is encountered.

ACTH-producing adenomas account for about 10 to 15% of all pituitary tumors. Because the clinical features of Cushing's syndrome often lead to early diagnosis, most ACTH-producing pituitary tumors are relatively small microadenomas. However, macroadenomas are also seen, and some ACTH-secreting adenomas are clinically silent. Cushing's disease is 5 to 10 times more common in women than in men. These pituitary adenomas exhibit unrestrained ACTH secretion, with resultant hypercortisolemia. However, they retain partial suppressibility in the presence of high doses of administered glucocorticoids, providing the basis for dynamic testing to distinguish pituitary and nonpituitary causes of Cushing's syndrome.

Presentation and Diagnosis The diagnosis of Cushing's syndrome presents two great challenges: (1) to distinguish patients with pathologic cortisol excess from those with physiologic or other disturbances of cortisol production; and (2) to determine the etiology of cortisol excess.

Typical features of chronic cortisol excess include thin, brittle skin, central obesity, hypertension, plethoric moon facies, purple striae and easy bruisability, glucose intolerance or diabetes mellitus, gonadal dysfunction, osteoporosis, proximal muscle weakness, signs of hyperandrogenism (acne, hirsutism), and psychologic disturbances (depression, mania, and psychoses) (Table 318-11). Hematopoietic features of hypercortisolism include leukocytosis, lymphopenia, and eosinopenia. Immune suppression includes delayed hypersensitivity. The protean manifestations of hypercortisolism make it challenging to decide which patients mandate formal laboratory evaluation. Certain features make pathologic causes of hypercortisolism more likely—these include characteristic central redistribution of fat, thin skin with striae and bruising, and proximal muscle weakness. In children and in young females, early osteoporosis may be particularly prominent. The primary cause of death is cardiovascular disease, but infections and risk of suicide are also increased.

Rapid development of features of hypercortisolism associated with skin hyperpigmentation and severe myopathy suggests the possibility of ectopic sources of ACTH. Hypertension, hypokalemic alkalosis, glucose intolerance, and edema are also more pronounced in these patients. Serum potassium levels <3.3 mmol/L are evident in ~70% of patients with ectopic ACTH secretion but are seen in <10% of patients with pituitary-dependent Cushing's disease.

Laboratory Investigation The diagnosis of Cushing's syndrome is based on laboratory documentation of endogenous hypercortisolism. Measurements of 24-h urine free cortisol (UFC) is a precise and cost-effective screening test. Alternatively, the failure to suppress plasma cortisol after an overnight 1-mg dexamethasone suppression test can be used to identify patients with hypercortisolism. As nadir levels of cortisol occur at night, elevated midnight samples of cortisol are suggestive of Cushing's syndrome. Basal plasma ACTH levels often distinguish patients with ACTH-independent (adrenal or exogenous glucocorticoid) from those with ACTH-dependent (pituitary, ectopic ACTH) Cushing's disease. Mean basal ACTH levels are about eight-fold higher in patients with ectopic ACTH secretion compared to those with pituitary ACTH-secreting adenomas. However, extensive overlap of ACTH levels in these two disorders precludes using ACTH to make the distinction. Instead, dynamic testing, based on differential sensitivity to glucocorticoid feedback, or ACTH stimulation in response to CRH or cortisol reduction is used to discriminate ectopic versus pituitary sources of excess ACTH (Table 318-12). Very rarely, circulating CRH levels are elevated, reflecting ectopic tumor-derived secretion of CRH and often ACTH. →*For discussion of dynamic testing for Cushing's syndrome, see Chap. 321.*

Most ACTH-secreting pituitary tumors are <5 mm in diameter, and about half are undetectable by sensitive MRI. The high prevalence of incidental pituitary microadenomas diminishes the ability to distinguish ACTH-secreting pituitary tumors accurately by MRI.

TABLE 318-11   *Clinical Features of Cushing's Syndrome (All Ages)*

Symptoms/Signs	Frequency, %
Obesity or weight gain (>115% ideal body weight)	80
Thin skin	80
Moon facies	75
Hypertension	75
Purple skin striae	65
Hirsutism	65
Abnormal glucose tolerance	55
Impotence	55
Menstrual disorders (usually amenorrhea)	60
Plethora	60
Proximal muscle weakness	50
Truncal obesity	50
Acne	45
Bruising	45
Mental changes	45
Osteoporosis	40
Edema of lower extremities	30
Hyperpigmentation	20
Hypokalemic alkalosis	15
Diabetes mellitus	15

Source: Adapted from MA Magiokou et al, in ME Wierman (ed), *Diseases of the Pituitary.* Totowa, NJ, Humana, 1997.

TABLE 318-12   *Differential Diagnosis of ACTH-Dependent Cushing's Syndrome*[a]

	ACTH-Secreting Pituitary Tumor	Ectopic ACTH Secretion
Etiology	Pituitary corticotrope adenoma	Bronchial, abdominal carcinoid
	Plurihormonal adenoma	Small cell lung cancer Thymoma
Gender	F > M	M > F
Clinical features	Slow onset	Rapid onset Pigmentation Severe myopathy
Serum potassium <3.3 μg/L	<10%	75%
24-h urinary free cortisol (UFC)	High	High
Basal ACTH level	Inappropriately high	Very high
Dexamethasone suppression 1 mg overnight		
Low dose (0.5 mg q6h)	Cortisol >5 μg/dL	Cortisol >5 μg/dL
High dose (2 mg q6h)	Cortisol >5 μg/dL	Cortisol >5 μg/dL
UFC > 80% suppressed	Microadenomas: 90% Macroadenomas: 50%	10%
Inferior petrosal sinus sampling (IPSS) Basal		
IPSS: peripheral	>2	<2
CRH-induced IPSS: peripheral	>3	<3

[a] ACTH-independent causes of Cushing's syndrome are diagnosed by suppressed ACTH levels and an adrenal mass in the setting of hypercortisolism. Iatrogenic Cushing's syndrome is excluded by history.

Note: ACTH, adrenocorticotropin hormone; F, female; M, male; CRH, corticotropin-releasing hormone.

Inferior Petrosal Venous Sampling Because pituitary MRI with gadolinium enhancement is insufficiently sensitive to detect small (<2 mm) pituitary ACTH-secreting adenomas, bilateral inferior petrosal sinus ACTH sampling before and after CRH administration may be required to distinguish these lesions from ectopic ACTH-secreting tumors that may have similar clinical and biochemical characteristics. Simultaneous assessment of ACTH concentrations in each inferior petrosal vein and in the peripheral circulation provides a strategy for confirming and localizing pituitary ACTH production. Sampling is performed at baseline and 2, 5, and 10 min after intravenous ovine CRH (1 μg/kg) injection. An increased ratio (>2) of inferior petrosal: peripheral vein ACTH confirms pituitary Cushing's disease. After CRH injection, peak petrosal:peripheral ACTH ratios of ≥3 confirm the presence of a pituitary ACTH-secreting tumor. The sensitivity of this test is >95%, with very rare false-positive results. False-negative results may be encountered in patients with aberrant venous anatomic drainage. Petrosal sinus catheterizations are technically difficult, and about 0.05% of patients develop neurovascular complications. The procedure should not be performed in patients with hypertension or in the presence of a well-visualized pituitary adenoma on MRI.

℞ TREATMENT

Selective transsphenoidal resection is the treatment of choice for Cushing's disease (Fig. 318-10). The remission rate for this procedure is ~80% for microadenomas but <50% for macroadenomas. After successful tumor resection, most patients experience a postoperative period of adrenal insufficiency that lasts for up to 12 months. This usually requires low-dose cortisol replacement, as patients experience steroid withdrawal symptoms as well as having a suppressed HPA axis. Biochemical recurrence occurs in approximately 5% of patients in whom surgery was initially successful.

When initial surgery is unsuccessful, repeat surgery is sometimes indicated, particularly when a pituitary source for ACTH is well documented. In older patients when growth and fertility are no longer important, hemi- or total hypophysectomy may be necessary if an adenoma is not recognized. Pituitary irradiation may be used after unsuccessful surgery, but it cures only about 15% of patients. Because radiation is slow and only partially effective in adults, steroidogenic inhibitors are used in combination with pituitary irradiation to block the adrenal effects of persistently high ACTH levels.

Ketoconazole, an imidazole derivative antimycotic agent, inhibits several P450 enzymes and effectively lowers cortisol in most patients with Cushing's disease when administered twice daily (600 to 1200 mg/d). Elevated hepatic transaminases, gynecomastia, impotence, gastrointestinal upset, and edema are common side effects. *Metyrapone* (2 to 4 g/d) inhibits 11β-hydroxylase activity and normalizes plasma cortisol in up to 75% of patients. Side effects include nausea and vomiting, rash, and exacerbation of acne or hirsutism. *Mitotane* (o, p'-DDD; 3 to 6 g/d orally in four divided doses) suppresses cortisol hypersecretion by inhibiting 11β-hydroxylase and cholesterol side-chain cleavage enzymes and by destroying adrenocortical cells. Side effects of mitotane include gastrointestinal symptoms, dizziness, gynecomastia, hyperlipidemia, skin rash, and hepatic enzyme elevation. It may also lead to hypoaldosteronism. Other agents include *aminoglutethimide* (250 mg tid), *trilostane* (200 to 1000 mg/d), *cyproheptadine* (24 mg/d), and IV *etomidate* (0.3 mg/kg per hour). Glucocorticoid insufficiency is a potential side effect of agents used to block steroidogenesis.

The use of steroidogenic inhibitors has decreased the need for bilateral adrenalectomy. Removal of both adrenal glands corrects hypercortisolism but may be associated with significant morbidity and necessitates permanent glucocorticoid and mineralocorticoid replacement. Adrenalectomy in the setting of residual corticotrope adenoma tissue predisposes to the development of *Nelson's syndrome*, a disorder characterized by rapid pituitary tumor enlargement and increased pigmentation secondary to high ACTH levels. Radiation therapy may be indicated to prevent the development of Nelson's syndrome after adrenalectomy.

GONADOTROPINS: FSH AND LH

SYNTHESIS AND SECRETION Gonadotrope cells comprise about 10% of anterior pituitary cells and produce two gonadotropins—LH and FSH. Like TSH and hCG, LH and FSH are glycoprotein hormones consisting of α and β subunits. The α subunit is common to these glycoprotein hormones; specificity is conferred by the β subunits, which are expressed by separate genes.

Gonadotropin synthesis and release are dynamically regulated. This is particularly true in females, in whom the rapidly fluctuating gonadal steroid levels vary throughout the menstrual cycle. Hypothalamic GnRH, a 10-amino-acid peptide, regulates the synthesis and secretion of both LH and FSH. GnRH is secreted in discrete pulses every 60 to 120 min, which in turn elicit LH and FSH pulses (Fig. 318-3). The pulsatile mode of GnRH input is essential to its action; pulses prime gonadotrope responsiveness, whereas continuous GnRH exposure induces desensitization. Based on this phenomenon, long-acting GnRH agonists are used to suppress gonadotropin levels in children with precocious puberty and in men with prostate cancer (Chap. 81) and are used in some ovulation-induction protocols to reduce endogenous gonadotropins (Chap. 45). Estrogens act at the hypothalamic and pituitary levels to control gonadotropin secretion. Chronic estrogen exposure is inhibitory, whereas rising estrogen levels, as occurs during the preovulatory surge, exert positive feedback to increase gonadotropin pulse frequency and amplitude. Progesterone slows GnRH pulse frequency but enhances gonadotropin responses to GnRH. Testosterone feedback in males also occurs at the hypothalamic and pituitary levels and partially reflects its conversion to estrogens.

Though GnRH is the main regulator of LH and FSH secretion, FSH synthesis is also under separate control by the gonadal peptides inhibin and activin, which are members of the transforming growth factor β (TGF-β) family. Inhibin selectively suppresses FSH, whereas activin stimulates FSH synthesis (Chap. 326).

ACTION The gonadotropin hormones interact with their respective GPCRs expressed in the ovary and testis, evoking germ-cell development and maturation and steroid hormone biosynthesis. In women, FSH regulates ovarian follicle development and stimulates ovarian estrogen production. LH mediates ovulation and maintenance of the cor-

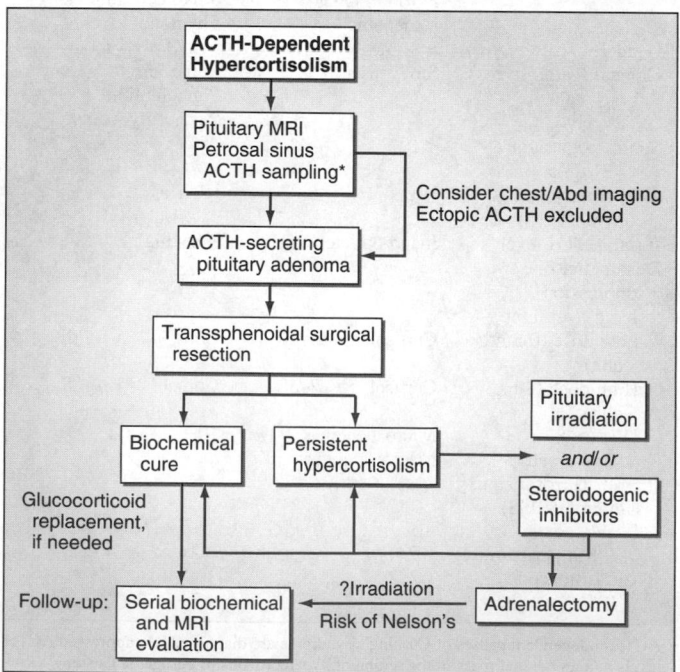

FIGURE 318-10 Management of Cushing's disease. (ACTH, adrenocorticotropin hormone; MRI, magnetic resonance imaging.) *, Not usually required.

pus luteum. In men, LH induces Leydig cell testosterone synthesis and secretion and FSH stimulates seminiferous tubule development and regulates spermatogenesis.

GONADOTROPIN DEFICIENCY Hypogonadism is the most common presenting feature of adult hypopituitarism, even when other pituitary hormones are also deficient. It is often a harbinger of hypothalamic or pituitary diseases that impair GnRH production or delivery through the pituitary stalk. As noted above, hypogonadotropic hypogonadism is a common presenting feature of hyperprolactinemia.

A variety of inherited and acquired disorders are associated with *isolated hypogonadotropic hypogonadism* (IHH) (Chap. 325). Hypothalamic defects associated with GnRH deficiency include two X-linked disorders, Kallmann syndrome (see above) and mutations in the *DAX1* gene. GnRH receptor mutations and inactivating mutations of the LH β and FSH β subunit genes are rare causes of selective gonadotropin deficiency. Acquired forms of GnRH deficiency leading to hypogonadotropism are seen in association with anorexia nervosa (Chap. 65), stress, starvation, and extreme exercise, but may also be idiopathic. Hypogonadotropic hypogonadism in these disorders is reversed by removal of the stressful stimulus.

Presentation and Diagnosis In premenopausal women, hypogonadotropic hypogonadism presents as diminished ovarian function leading to oligomenorrhea or amenorrhea, infertility, decreased vaginal secretions, decreased libido, and breast atrophy. In hypogonadal adult males, secondary testicular failure is associated with decreased libido and potency, infertility, decreased muscle mass with weakness, reduced beard and body hair growth, soft testes, and characteristic fine facial wrinkles. Osteoporosis occurs in both untreated hypogonadal females and males.

Laboratory Investigation Central hypogonadism is associated with low or inappropriately normal serum gonadotropin levels in the setting of low sex hormone concentrations (testosterone in males, estradiol in females). Three pooled serum samples drawn 20 min apart are used for accurate measurement of serum LH and FSH levels, thus allowing for the effects of hormone secretory pulses. Male patients have abnormal semen analysis.

Intravenous GnRH (100 μg) stimulates gonadotropes to secrete LH (which peaks within 30 min) and FSH (which plateaus during the ensuing 60 min). Normal responses vary according to menstrual cycle stage, age, and sex of the patient. Generally, LH levels increase about threefold, whereas FSH responses are less pronounced. In the setting of gonadotropin deficiency, a normal gonadotropin response to GnRH indicates intact gonadotrope function and suggests a hypothalamic abnormality. An absent response, however, cannot reliably distinguish pituitary from hypothalamic causes of hypogonadism. For this reason, GnRH testing usually adds little to the information gained from baseline evaluation of the hypothalamic-pituitary-gonadotrope axis, except in cases of isolated GnRH deficiency (e.g., Kallmann syndrome).

MRI examination of the sellar region and assessment of other pituitary functions are usually indicated in patients with documented central hypogonadism.

℞ TREATMENT

In males, testosterone replacement is necessary to achieve and maintain normal growth and development of the external genitalia, secondary sex characteristics, male sexual behavior, and androgenic anabolic effects including maintenance of muscle function and bone mass. Testosterone may be administered by intramuscular injections every 1 to 4 weeks or using patches that are replaced daily (Chap. 325). Testosterone creams are also available. Gonadotropin injections [hCG or human menopausal gonadotropin (hMG)] over 12 to 18 months are used to restore fertility. Pulsatile GnRH therapy (25 to 150 ng/kg every 2 h), administered by a subcutaneous infusion pump, is also effective for treatment of hypothalamic hypogonadism when fertility is desired.

In premenopausal women, cyclical replacement of estrogen and progesterone maintains secondary sexual characteristics and genitourinary tract integrity and prevents premature osteoporosis (Chap.

326). Gonadotropin therapy is used for ovulation induction. Follicular growth and maturation are initiated using hMG or recombinant FSH; hCG is subsequently injected to induce ovulation. As in men, pulsatile GnRH therapy can be used to treat hypothalamic causes of gonadotropin deficiency.

NONFUNCTIONING AND GONADOTROPIN-PRODUCING PITUITARY ADENOMAS ■
Etiology and Prevalence Nonfunctioning pituitary adenomas include those that secrete little or no pituitary hormones, as well as tumors that produce too little hormone to result in recognizable clinical features. They are the most common type of pituitary adenoma and are usually macroadenomas at the time of diagnosis because clinical features are inapparent until tumor mass effects occur. Based on immunohistochemistry, most clinically nonfunctioning adenomas can be shown to originate from gonadotrope cells. These tumors typically produce small amounts of intact gonadotropins (usually FSH) as well as uncombined α and LH β and FSH β subunits. Tumor secretion may lead to elevated α and FSH β subunits and, rarely, to increased LH β subunit levels. Some adenomas express α subunits without FSH or LH. TRH administration often induces an atypical increase of tumor-derived gonadotropins or subunits.

Presentation and Diagnosis Clinically nonfunctioning tumors may present with optic chiasm pressure and other symptoms of local expansion or be incidentally discovered on an MRI performed for another indication. Menstrual disturbances or ovarian hyperstimulation rarely occur in women with large tumors that produce FSH and LH. More commonly, adenoma compression of the pituitary stalk or surrounding pituitary tissue leads to attenuated LH and features of hypogonadism. PRL levels are usually slightly increased, also because of stalk compression. It is important to distinguish this circumstance from true prolactinomas, as most nonfunctioning tumors respond poorly to treatment with dopamine agonists.

Laboratory Investigation The goal of laboratory testing in clinically nonfunctioning tumors is to classify the type of the tumor, to identify hormonal markers of tumor activity, and to detect possible hypopituitarism. Free α subunit levels may be elevated in 10 to 15% of patients with nonfunctioning tumors. In female patients, peri- or postmenopausal basal FSH concentrations are difficult to distinguish from tumor-derived FSH elevation. Premenopausal women have cycling FSH levels, also preventing clear-cut diagnostic distinction from tumor-derived FSH. In men, gonadotropin-secreting tumors may be diagnosed because of slightly increased gonadotropins (FSH > LH) in the setting of a pituitary mass. Testosterone levels are usually low, despite the normal or increased LH level, perhaps reflecting reduced LH bioactivity or the loss of normal LH pulsatility. Because this pattern of hormone tests is also seen in primary gonadal failure and, to some extent, with aging (Chap. 325), the increased gonadotropins alone are insufficient for the diagnosis of a gonadotropin-secreting tumor. In the majority of patients with gonadotrope adenomas, TRH administration stimulates LH β subunit secretion; this response is not seen in normal individuals. GnRH testing is not helpful for making the diagnosis. For nonfunctioning and gonadotropin-secreting tumors, the diagnosis usually rests on immunohistochemical analyses of resected tumor tissue, as the mass effects of these tumors usually necessitate resection.

Although acromegaly or Cushing's syndrome usually presents with unique clinical features, clinically inapparent somatotrope or corticotrope adenomas can be excluded by a normal IGF-I value and normal 24-h urinary free cortisol levels. If PRL levels are <100 μg/L in a patient harboring a pituitary mass, a nonfunctioning adenoma causing pituitary stalk compression should be considered.

℞ TREATMENT

Asymptomatic small nonfunctioning adenomas with no threat to vision may be followed with regular MRI and visual field testing without immediate intervention. However, for larger macroadenomas, trans-

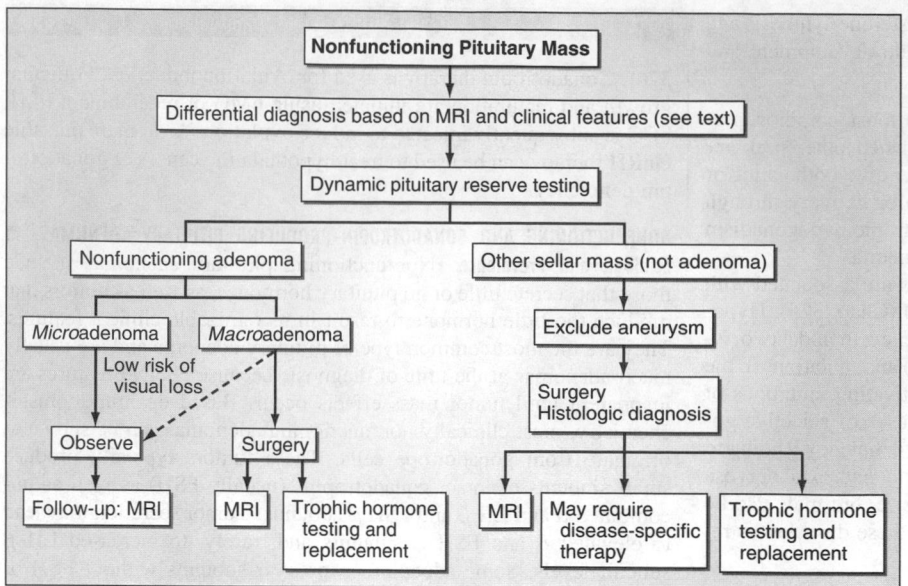

FIGURE 318-11 Management of a nonfunctioning pituitary mass.

sphenoidal surgery is the only effective way to reduce tumor size and relieve mass effects (Fig. 318-11). Although it is not usually possible to remove all adenoma tissue surgically, vision improves in 70% of patients with preoperative visual field defects. Preexisting hypopituitarism that results from tumor mass effects commonly improves or may resolve completely. Beginning about 6 months postoperatively, MRI scans should be performed yearly to detect tumor regrowth. Within 5 to 6 years following successful surgical resection, ~15% of nonfunctioning tumors recur. When substantial tumor remains after transsphenoidal surgery, adjuvant radiotherapy may be indicated to prevent tumor growth. Radiotherapy may be deferred if no postoperative residual mass is evident.

Nonfunctioning pituitary tumors respond poorly to dopamine agonist treatment, with modest tumor shrinkage occurring in <10% of patients. Although SSTR subtypes 2 and 5 have been identified on nonfunctioning pituitary adenomas, octreotide does not shrink these tumors and only modestly suppresses gonadotropin and α subunit levels. Visual improvement sometimes occurs without evident reduction of tumor size by MRI, presumably reflecting relief of pressure on the optic tracts. The selective GnRH antagonist, Nal-Glu GnRH, suppresses FSH hypersecretion but has no effect on adenoma size.

THYROID-STIMULATING HORMONE

SYNTHESIS AND SECRETION   TSH-secreting thyrotrope cells comprise 5% of the anterior pituitary cell population. TSH is structurally related to LH and FSH. It shares a common α subunit with these hormones but contains a specific TSH β subunit. TRH is a hypothalamic tripeptide (pyroglutamyl histidylprolinamide) that acts through a GPCR to stimulate TSH synthesis and secretion; it also stimulates the lactotrope cell to secrete PRL. TSH secretion is stimulated by TRH, whereas thyroid hormones, dopamine, SRIF, and glucocorticoids suppress TSH by overriding TRH induction.

The thyrotrope is stimulated by a release from the negative feedback inhibition by thyroid hormones. Thus, thyroid damage, (including surgical thyroidectomy), radiation-induced hypothyroidism, chronic thyroiditis, or prolonged goitrogen exposure are associated with increased TSH. Long-standing untreated hypothyroidism can lead to thyrotrope hyperplasia and pituitary enlargement, which may be evident on MRI.

ACTION   TSH is secreted in pulses, though the excursions are modest in comparison to other pituitary hormones because of the relatively low amplitude of the pulses and the relatively long half-life of

TSH. Consequently, single determinations of TSH suffice to assess its circulating levels. TSH binds to a GPCR on thyroid follicular cells to stimulate thyroid hormone synthesis and release (Chap. 320).

TSH DEFICIENCY   Features of central hypothyroidism, due to TSH deficiency, mimic those seen with primary hypothyroidism but are generally less severe. Pituitary hypothyroidism is characterized by low basal TSH levels in the setting of low free thyroid hormone. In contrast, patients with hypothyroidism of hypothalamic origin (presumably due to a lack of endogenous TRH) may exhibit normal or even slightly elevated TSH levels. There is evidence that the TSH produced in this circumstance has reduced biologic activity because of altered glycosylation.

TRH (200 μg) injected intravenously causes a two- to threefold increase in TSH (and PRL) levels within 30 min. Although TRH testing can be used to assess TSH reserve, abnormalities of the thyroid axis can usually be detected based on basal free T_4 and TSH levels, without the need for TRH testing.

Thyroid-replacement therapy should be initiated after establishing adequate adrenal function. Dose adjustment is based on thyroid hormone levels and clinical parameters rather than the TSH level.

TSH-SECRETING ADENOMAS   TSH-producing macroadenomas are rare but are often large and locally invasive when they occur. Patients usually present with thyroid goiter and hyperthyroidism, reflecting overproduction of TSH. Diagnosis is based on demonstrating elevated serum free T_4 levels, inappropriately normal or high TSH secretion, and MRI evidence of a pituitary adenoma.

It is important to exclude other causes of inappropriate TSH secretion, such as resistance to thyroid hormone, an autosomal dominant disorder caused by mutations in the thyroid hormone β receptor (Chap. 320). The presence of a pituitary mass and elevated α subunit levels are suggestive of a TSH-secreting tumor. Dysalbuminemic hyperthyroxinemia syndromes, caused by various mutations in serum thyroid hormone binding proteins, are also characterized by elevated thyroid hormone levels, but with normal rather than suppressed TSH levels. Moreover, free thyroid hormone levels are normal in these disorders, most of which are familial.

℞ TREATMENT

The initial therapeutic approach is to remove or debulk the tumor mass surgically, using either a transsphenoidal or subfrontal approach. Total resection is not often achieved as most of these adenomas are large and locally invasive. Normal circulating thyroid hormone levels are achieved in about two-thirds of patients after surgery. Thyroid ablation or antithyroid drugs (methimazole or propylthiouracil) can be used to reduce thyroid hormone levels. Dopamine agonists are rarely effective for suppressing TSH secretion from these tumors. However, somatostatin analogue treatment effectively normalizes TSH and α subunit hypersecretion, shrinks the tumor mass in 50% of patients, and improves visual fields in 75% of patients; euthyroidism is restored in most patients. In some patients, octreotide markedly suppresses TSH, causing biochemical hypothyroidism that requires concomitant thyroid hormone replacement. Lanreotide (30 mg intramuscularly), a long-acting somatostatin analogue (see above), effectively suppresses TSH and thyroid hormone in patients treated every 14 days.

DIABETES INSIPIDUS

→*See Chap. 319 for diagnosis and treatment of diabetes insipidus.*

FURTHER READING

ATTANUSIO AF et al: Human growth hormone replacement in adult hypopituitary patients. J Clin Endocrinol Metab 87:1600, 2002

MELMED S et al: Consensus. Guidelines for acromegaly management. J Clin Endocrinol Metab 87:4054, 2002

MOLITCH ME: Diagnosis and treatment of prolactinomas. Adv Intern Med 44: 117, 1999

NEWELL-PRICE J et al: The diagnosis and differential diagnosis of Cushing's syndrome and pseudo-Cushing's states. Endocr Rev 19:647, 1998

OLSON LE, ROSENFELD MG: Perspective: Genetic and genomic approaches in elucidating mechanisms of pituitary development. Endocrinology 143: 2007, 2002

319 DISORDERS OF THE NEUROHYPOPHYSIS
Gary L. Robertson

The neurohypophysis, or posterior pituitary gland, is formed by axons that originate in large cell bodies in the supraoptic and paraventricular nuclei of the hypothalamus. It produces two hormones: (1) arginine vasopressin (AVP), also known as antidiuretic hormone; and (2) oxytocin. AVP acts on the renal tubules to reduce water loss by concentrating the urine. Oxytocin stimulates postpartum milk letdown in response to suckling. AVP deficiency causes diabetes insipidus (DI), characterized by the production of large amounts of dilute urine. Excessive or inappropriate AVP production predisposes to hyponatremia if water intake is not reduced in parallel with urine output.

VASOPRESSIN

ACTION AVP is a nonapeptide composed of a six-membered disulfide ring and a tripeptide tail (Fig. 319-1). The most important, if not the only, physiologic action of AVP is to reduce water excretion by promoting concentration of urine. This antidiuretic effect is achieved by increasing the hydroosmotic permeability of cells that line the distal tubule and medullary collecting ducts of the kidney (Fig. 319-2). In the absence of AVP, these cells are impermeable to water and reabsorb little, if any, of the relatively large volume of dilute filtrate that enters from the proximal nephron. This results in the excretion of very large volumes (as much as 0.2 mL/kg per min) of maximally dilute urine (specific gravity and osmolarity ~1.000 and 50 mosmol/L, respectively), a condition known as a *water diuresis*. In the presence of AVP, these cells become selectively permeable to water, allowing it to diffuse back down the osmotic gradient created by the hypertonic renal medulla. As a result, the dilute fluid passing through the tubules is concentrated and the rate of urine flow decreases. The magnitude of this effect varies in direct proportion to the plasma AVP concentration and, at maximum levels, approximates a urine flow rate as low as 0.35 mL/min and a urine osmolarity as high as 1200 mosmol/L. AVP action is mediated via binding to G protein–coupled V_2 receptors on the serosal surface of the cell, activation of adenyl cyclase, and insertion into the luminal surface of water channels composed of a protein known as *aquaporin 2*.

At high concentrations, AVP also causes contraction of smooth muscle in blood vessels and in the gastrointestinal tract, induces glycogenolysis in the liver, and potentiates adrenocorticotropic hormone (ACTH) release by corticotropin-releasing factor. These effects are mediated by V_{1a} or V_{1b} receptors that are coupled to phospholipase C. Their role, if any, in human physiology/pathophysiology is still uncertain.

SYNTHESIS AND SECRETION AVP secretion is synthesized via a polypeptide precursor that includes AVP, neurophysin, and copeptin. After preliminary processing and folding, the precursor is packaged in neurosecretory vesicles where it is transported down the axon, further processed to AVP, and stored until the hormone and other components are released by exocytosis into peripheral blood.

AVP secretion is regulated primarily by the "effective" osmotic pressure of body fluids. This control is mediated by specialized hypothalamic cells, known as *osmoreceptors*, which are extremely sensitive to small changes in the plasma concentration of sodium and certain other solutes but are insensitive to other solutes such as urea or glucose. The osmoreceptors appear to include inhibitory as well as

stimulatory components that function in concert to form a threshold, or set point, control system for AVP release. Below this threshold, plasma AVP is suppressed to levels that permit the development of a maximum water diuresis. Above it, plasma AVP rises steeply in direct proportion to plasma osmolarity, quickly reaching levels sufficient to effect a maximum antidiuresis. The absolute levels of plasma osmolarity/sodium at which minimally and maximally effective levels of plasma AVP occur vary appreciably from person to person, owing apparently to genetic influences on the set and sensitivity of the system. However, the average threshold, or set point, for AVP release corresponds to a plasma osmolarity or sodium of about 280 mosmol/L or 135 meq/L, respectively; levels only 2 to 4% higher normally result in maximum antidiuresis. Though relatively stable in a healthy adult, the set of the osmoregulatory system can also be lowered by pregnancy, the menstrual cycle, and relatively large, acute reductions in blood pressure or volume.

The effects of acute changes in blood volume or pressure are mediated largely by neuronal afferents that originate in transmural pressure receptors of the heart and large arteries and project via the vagus and glossopharyngeal nerves to the brain stem, from whence postsynaptic projections ascend to the hypothalmus. These pathways maintain a tonic inhibitory tone that decreases when blood volume or pressure falls by >10 to 20%. This baroregulatory system is probably of minor importance in the physiology of AVP secretion because the hemodynamic changes required to affect it do not usually occur during normal activities. However, the baroregulatory system undoubtedly plays an important role in AVP secretion in patients with large, acute disturbances of hemodynamic function.

AVP secretion can also be stimulated by nausea, acute hypoglycemia, glucocorticoid deficiency, smoking, and, possibly, hyperangiotensinemia. The emetic stimuli are extremely potent since they typically elicit immediate, 50- to 100-fold increases in plasma AVP, even when the nausea is transient and unassociated with vomiting or other symptoms. They appear to act via the emetic center in the medulla and can be completely blocked by treatment with antiemetics such as fluphenazine. There is no evidence that pain or other noxious stresses have any affect on AVP unless they elicit a vasovagal reaction with its associated nausea and hypotension.

METABOLISM AVP distributes rapidly into a space roughly equal to the extracellular fluid volume. It is cleared irreversibly with a $t_{1/2}$ of 10 to 30 min. Most AVP clearance is due to degradation in the liver and kidneys. During pregnancy, the metabolic clearance of AVP is increased three- to fourfold due to placental production of an N-terminal peptidase.

THIRST Because AVP cannot reduce water loss below a certain minimum level obligated by urinary solute load and evaporation from skin

FIGURE 319-1 Primary structures of arginine vasopressin (AVP), oxytocin, and DDAVP.

FIGURE 319-2 Antidiuretic effect of arginine vasopressin (AVP) in the regulation of urine volume. In a typical 70-kg adult, the kidney filters about 180 L/d of plasma. Of this, approximately 144 L (80%) is reabsorbed isosmotically in the proximal tubule and another 8 L (4 to 5%) is reabsorbed without solute in the descending limb of Henle's loop. The remainder is diluted to an osmolarity of about 60 mmol/kg by selective reabsorption of sodium and chloride in the ascending limb. In the absence of AVP, the urine issuing from the loop passes largely unmodified through the distal tubules and collecting ducts, resulting in a maximum water diuresis. In the presence of AVP, solute-free water is reabsorbed osmotically through the principal cells of the collecting ducts, resulting in the excretion of a much smaller volume of concentrated urine. This antidiuretic effect is mediated via a G protein–coupled V_2 receptor that increases intracellular cyclic AMP, thereby inducing translocation of aquaporin 2 (AQP 2) water channels into the apical membrane. The resultant increase in permeability permits an influx of water that diffuses out of the cell through AQP 3 and AQP 4 water channels on the basal-lateral surface. The net rate of flux across the cell is determined by the number of AQP 2 water channels in the apical membrane and the strength of the osmotic gradient between tubular fluid and the renal medulla. Tight junctions on the lateral surface of the cells serve to prevent unregulated water flow.

and lungs, a mechanism for ensuring adequate intake is essential for preventing dehydration. This vital function is performed by the thirst mechanism. Like AVP, thirst is regulated primarily by an osmostat that is located in the anteromedial hypothalamus and is able to detect very small changes in the plasma concentration of sodium and certain other effective solutes. The thirst osmostat appears to be "set" about 5% higher than the AVP osmostat. This arrangement ensures that thirst, polydipsia, and dilution of body fluids do not occur until plasma osmolarity/sodium start to exceed the defensive capacity of the antidiuretic mechanism.

OXYTOCIN

Oxytocin is also a nonapeptide and differs from AVP only at positions 3 and 8 (Fig. 319-1). However, it has relatively little antidiuretic effect and seems to act mainly on mammary ducts to facilitate milk letdown during nursing. It may also help to initiate or facilitate labor by stimulating contraction of uterine smooth muscle, but it is not yet clear if this action is physiologic or necessary for normal delivery.

DEFICIENCIES OF VASOPRESSIN SECRETION AND ACTION

DIABETES INSIPIDUS ■ Clinical Characteristics Decreased secretion or action of AVP usually manifests as DI, a syndrome characterized by the production of abnormally large volumes of dilute urine. The 24-h urine volume is >50 mL/kg body weight and the osmolarity is <300 mosmol/L. The polyuria produces symptoms of urinary frequency, enuresis, and/or nocturia, which may disturb sleep and cause mild daytime fatigue or somnolence. It is also associated with thirst and a commensurate increase in fluid intake (polydipsia). Clinical signs of dehydration are uncommon unless fluid intake is impaired.

Etiology Deficient secretion of AVP can be primary or secondary. The primary form usually results from agenesis or irreversible destruction of the neurohypophysis and is variously referred to as *neurohypophyseal DI*, *pituitary DI*, or *central DI*. It can be caused by a variety of

congenital, acquired, or genetic disorders but almost half the time it is idiopathic (Table 319-1). The genetic form of neurohypophyseal DI is usually transmitted in an autosomal dominant mode and is caused by diverse mutations in the coding region of the AVP–neurophysin II (or AVP-NPII) gene. In this type, the AVP deficiency and DI begin several months to several years after birth and appear to be a result of selective degeneration of AVP-producing magnocellular neurons. An autosomal recessive form, due to inactivating mutations in the AVP gene, and an X-linked recessive form, due to an unidentified gene on Xq28, have also been described. A primary deficiency of plasma AVP can also result from increased metabolism by an N-terminal aminopeptidase produced by the placenta. It is referred to as *gestational DI* since the signs and symptoms manifest during pregnancy and usually remit several weeks after delivery. However, a subclinical deficiency in AVP secretion can often be demonstrated in the nonpregnant state, indicating that damage to the neurohypophysis may also contribute to the AVP deficiency. Finally, a primary deficiency of AVP can also result from malformation or destruction of the neurohypophysis by a variety of diseases or toxins (Table 319-1).

Secondary deficiencies of AVP result from inhibition of secretion by excessive intake of fluids. They are referred to as *primary polydipsia* and can be divided into three subcategories. One of them, called *dipsogenic DI*, is characterized by an inappropriate increase in thirst caused by a reduction in the "set" of the osmoregulatory mechanism. It sometimes occurs in association with multifocal diseases of the brain such as neurosarcoid, tuberculous meningitis, or multiple sclerosis but is often idiopathic. The second subtype, called *psychogenic polydipsia*, is not associated with thirst, and the polydipsia seems to be a feature of psychosis. The third subtype, which may be referred to as *iatrogenic polydipsia*, results from recommendations of health professionals or the popular media to increase fluid intake for its presumed preventive or therapeutic benefits for other disorders.

Primary deficiencies in the antidiuretic action of AVP result in *nephrogenic DI* (Table 319-1). It can be genetic, acquired, or caused by exposure to various drugs. The genetic form is usually transmitted in an X-linked mode and is caused by mutations in the coding region of the V_2 receptor gene. Autosomal recessive or dominant forms result from mutations in the gene encoding the aquaporin protein that forms the water channels in the distal nephron.

Secondary deficiencies in the antidiuretic response to AVP result from polyuria per se. They are caused by washout of the medullary concentration gradient and/or suppression of aquaporin function. They usually resolve 24 to 48 h after the polyuria is corrected but often complicate interpretation of tests commonly used for differential diagnosis.

Pathophysiology When the secretion or action of AVP is reduced to <80 to 85% of normal, urine concentration ceases and the rate of output increases to symptomatic levels. If the defect is primary (e.g., the patient has pituitary, gestational, or nephrogenic DI), the polyuria results in a small (1 to 2%) decrease in body water and a commensurate increase in plasma osmolarity and sodium concentration that stimulate thirst and a compensatory increase in water intake. As a result, *overt physical or laboratory signs of dehydration do not develop unless the patient also has a defect in thirst* (see below) *or fails to drink for some other reason.*

The severity of the antidiuretic defect varies markedly among patients with pituitary, gestational, or nephrogenic DI. In some, the deficiencies in AVP secretion or action are so severe that basal urine output approximates the maximum (10 to 15 mL/min); even an intense stimulus such as nausea or severe dehydration does not raise plasma AVP enough to concentrate the urine. In others, however, the deficiency in AVP secretion or action is incomplete, and a modest stimulus such as a few hours of fluid deprivation, smoking, or a vasovagal reaction increases plasma AVP sufficiently to produce a profound antidiuresis. The maximum urine osmolarity achieved in these patients is usually less than normal, largely because their maximal concentrating capacity is temporarily impaired by chronic polyuria. However, in a few patients with partial pituitary or nephrogenic DI, it can reach levels as high as 800 mosmol/L.

In primary polydipsia, the pathogenesis of the polydipsia and polyuria is the reverse of that in pituitary, nephrogenic, and gestational DI. Thus, the excessive intake of fluids slightly increases body water, thereby reducing plasma osmolarity, AVP secretion, and urinary concentration. The latter results in a compensatory increase in urinary free-water excretion that varies in direct proportion to intake. Therefore, clinically appreciable overhydration is uncommon unless the compensatory water diuresis is impaired by a drug or disease that stimulates or mimics endogenous AVP.

In the dipsogenic form of primary polydipsia, fluid intake is excessive because the osmotic threshold for thirst appears to be reset to the left, often well below that for AVP release. When deprived of fluids or subjected to some other acute osmotic or nonosmotic stimulus, these individuals invariably increase plasma AVP normally, but the resultant increase in urine concentration is usually subnormal because their renal capacity to concentrate the urine is also blunted by chronic polyuria. Thus, their antidiuretic response to these stimuli may be indistinguishable from that in patients with partial pituitary, partial gestational, or partial nephrogenic DI. Patients with psychogenic or iatrogenic polydipsia respond similarly to fluid restriction but do not complain of thirst and usually offer other explanations for their high fluid intake.

TABLE 319-1 Causes of Diabetes Insipidus

Pituitary diabetes insipidus	Nephrogenic diabetes insipidus
Acquired	Acquired
Head trauma (closed and penetrating)	Drugs
Neoplasms	Lithium
Primary	Demeclocycline
Craniopharyngioma	Methoxyflurane
Pituitary adenoma (suprasellar)	Amphotericin B
Dysgerminoma	Aminoglycosides
Meningioma	Cisplatin
Metastatic (lung, breast)	Rifampin
Hematologic (lymphoma, leukemia)	Foscarnet
Granulomas	Metabolic
Neurosarcoid	Hypercalcemia, hypercalciuria
Histiocytosis	Hypokalemia
Xanthoma disseminatum	Obstruction (ureter or urethra)
Infectious	Vascular
Chronic meningitis	Sickle cell disease and trait
Viral encephalitis	Ischemia (acute tubular necrosis)
Toxoplasmosis	Granulomas
Inflammatory	Neurosarcoid
Lymphocytic infundibuloneurohypophysitis	Neoplasms
Wegener's granulomatosis	Sarcoma
Lupus erythematosus	Infiltration
Scleroderma	Amyloidosis
Chemical toxins	Pregnancy
Tetrodotoxin	Idiopathic
Snake venom	Genetic
Vascular	X-linked recessive (AVP receptor-2 gene)
Sheehan's syndrome	Autosomal recessive (aquaporin-2 gene)
Aneurysm (internal carotid)	Autosomal dominant (aquaporin-2 gene)
Aortocoronary bypass	**Primary polydipsia**
Hypoxic encephalopathy	Acquired
Pregnancy (vasopressinase)	Psychogenic
Idiopathic	Schizophrenia
Congenital malformations	Obsessive-compulsive disorder
Septooptic dysplasia	Dipsogenic (abnormal thirst)
Midline craniofacial defects	Granulomas
Holoprosencephaly	Neurosarcoid
Hypogenesis, ectopia of pituitary	Infectious
Genetic	Tuberculous meningitis
Autosomal dominant (AVP-neurophysin gene)	Head trauma (closed and penetrating)
Autosomal recessive (AVP-neurophysin gene)	Demyelination
Autosomal recessive-Wolfram-(4p − WFS 1 gene)	Multiple sclerosis
X-linked recessive (Xq28)	Drugs
Deletion chromosome 7q	Lithium
	Carbamazepine
	Idiopathic
	Iatrogenic

Differential Diagnosis When symptoms of urinary frequency, enuresis, nocturia, and/or persistent thirst are present, the presence of polyuria should be verified by documenting a 24-h urine output > 50 mL/kg per day (>3500 mL in a 70-kg man). If the osmolarity of the 24-h urine is >300 mosmol/L, the polyuria is due to a solute diuresis and the patient should be evaluated for uncontrolled diabetes mellitus or other less common causes of excessive solute excretion. However, if the 24-h urine osmolarity is <300 mosmol/L, the patient has a water diuresis and should be evaluated further to determine which type of DI is present.

In differentiating between the various types of DI, the history, physical examination, and routine laboratory tests may be helpful but are rarely sufficient because few, if any, of the findings are pathognomonic. Except in the rare patient who is clearly dehydrated under basal conditions of *ad libitum* fluid intake, this evaluation should begin with a *fluid deprivation test*. To minimize patient discomfort, avoid excessive dehydration, and maximize the information obtained, the test should be started in the morning and water balance should be monitored closely with hourly measurements of body weight, plasma osmolarity and/or sodium concentration, and urine volume and osmolarity.

If fluid deprivation does not result in urine concentration (osmolarity >300 mosmol/L, specific gravity >1.010) before body weight decreases by 5% or plasma osmolarity/sodium exceed the upper limit of normal, primary polydipsia or a partial defect in AVP secretion or action are largely excluded. In these patients, severe pituitary or nephrogenic DI are the only remaining possibilities, and they can usually be distinguished by administering desmopressin (DDAVP, 0.03 μg/kg subcutaneously or intravenously) and repeating the measurement of urine osmolarity 1 to 2 h later. An increase of >50% indicates severe pituitary DI, whereas a smaller or absent response is strongly suggestive of nephrogenic DI.

However, in patients who concentrate their urine during fluid deprivation, the change in urine osmolarity after administration of desmopressin is not useful for differential diagnosis because the values vary widely and over the same range in primary polydipsia, partial pituitary DI, and partial nephrogenic DI. The best way to differentiate these three conditions is to measure plasma or urine AVP before and during the fluid deprivation test and analyze the result in relation to the concurrent plasma or urine osmolarity (Fig. 319-3). This approach invariably differentiates partial nephrogenic DI from partial pituitary DI and primary polydipsia. It also differentiates pituitary DI from primary polydipsia if the hormone is measured when plasma osmolarity or sodium is clearly above the normal range. However, the requisite level of hypertonic dehydration is difficult to produce by fluid deprivation alone when urine concentration occurs. Therefore, it is usually

FIGURE 319-3 Relationship of plasma AVP to urine osmolarity (*left*) and plasma osmolarity (*right*) before and during fluid deprivation–hypertonic saline infusion test in patients who are normal or have primary polydipsia (■), pituitary diabetes insipidus (■), or nephrogenic diabetes insipidus (■).

necessary to add an infusion of hypertonic (3%) saline and repeat the AVP measurements when plasma osmolarity rises to >300 mosmol/L (Na^+ > 145 mmol/L). This endpoint is usually reached within 30 to 120 min if the hypertonic saline is infused at a rate of 0.1 mL/kg per min and the fluid deprivation is maintained.

The differential diagnosis of DI may also be facilitated by magnetic resonance imaging (MRI) of the pituitary and hypothalamus. In most healthy adults and children, the posterior pituitary emits a hyperintense signal in T1 weighted mid-saggital images. This "bright spot" is almost invariably absent or abnormally small in patients with pituitary DI but is present in 80 to 90% of patients with primary polydipsia. Thus, the presence of a normal bright spot virtually excludes pituitary DI, whereas its absence supports but does not prove this diagnosis. Therefore, the MRI findings must be interpreted with caution and only in conjunction with other diagnostic studies based on assays of AVP or the differential responses to treatment.

℞ TREATMENT

The signs and symptoms of uncomplicated pituitary DI can be eliminated completely by treatment with DDAVP (Fig. 319-4). It is a synthetic analogue of AVP (Fig. 319-1) that acts selectively at V_2 receptors to increase urine concentration and decrease urine flow in a dose-dependent manner. It is also more resistant to degradation than AVP and has a three- to fourfold longer duration of action. DDAVP can be given by intravenous or subcutaneous injection, nasal inhalation, or oral tablet. The doses required to completely control pituitary DI vary widely, depending on the patient and the route of administration. However, they usually range from 1 to 2 μg qd or bid by injection, 10 to 20 μg bid or tid by nasal spray, or 100 to 400 μg bid or tid orally. The onset of action is rapid, ranging from as little as 15 min after injection to 60 min after oral administration. When given in doses sufficient to completely normalize urinary osmolarity and flow, desmopressin produces a slight (1 to 3%) increase in total-body water and a commensurate decrease in plasma osmolarity and sodium concentration that rapidly eliminate thirst and polydipsia. Consequently, water balance is maintained and hyponatremia does not develop unless the patient has an associated abnormality in the osmoregulation of thirst or ingests/receives excessive amounts of fluid for some other reason. Fortunately, abnormal thirst occurs in <10% of patients with pituitary DI, and the other causes of excessive intake can usually be eliminated by educating the patient about the risks of drinking for reasons other than thirst. Therefore, most patients with pituitary DI can take DDAVP in doses sufficient to maintain a normal urine output continuously and do not need to endure the inconvenience and discomfort of allowing intermittent escape to prevent water intoxication.

Pituitary DI can also be treated with chlorpropamide (Diabinese). The mechanism of its antidiuretic action is uncertain but may involve potentiation of the effect of small amounts of AVP or direct activation of the V_2 receptor. In patients with severe or partial pituitary DI, doses of chlorpropamide similar to those used in the treatment of diabetes mellitus (125 to 500 mg once daily) increase urine concentration and decrease urine flow, thirst, and polydipsia in a manner similar to desmopressin. The antidiuresis is almost always sufficient to reduce urine output by 30 to 70%. Moreover, its antidiuretic effect can be enhanced appreciably by co-treatment with a thiazide diuretic. Side effects of chlorpropamide include hypoglycemia, which can be precipitated by severe reductions in caloric intake or heavy exercise, and it may cause a disulfiram (Antabuse)-like reaction to ethanol. Chlorpropamide is contraindicated in the treatment of gestational DI because its teratogenicity is unknown.

Primary polydipsia cannot be treated with desmopressin because a sustained inhibition of the compensatory water diuresis almost invariably results in the development of water intoxication within 24 to 48 h. Iatrogenic polydipsia can often be corrected by patient counseling; however, there is no effective treatment for either psychogenic or dipsogenic DI. In the latter, nocturia or nocturnal enuresis can often be controlled safely by administering a single small dose of desmopressin at bedtime. If the dose is adjusted carefully to provide no more than 8 to 10 h of antidiuresis, it will not result in water intoxication, because patients with dipsogenic, as well as other forms of DI, tend to drink less fluid at night than during the day.

The symptoms and signs of nephrogenic DI are not affected by treatment with DDAVP or chlorpropamide but may be reduced by treatment with a thiazide diuretic and/or amiloride in conjunction with a low-sodium diet. Inhibitors of prostaglandin synthesis (e.g., indomethacin) are also effective in some patients.

FIGURE 319-4 Effect of desmopressin therapy on water balance in patient with uncomplicated pituitary diabetes insipidus. Note that treatment rapidly reduces thirst and fluid intake as well as urine output to normal, with only a slight increase in body water (weight) and decrease in plasma osmolarity/sodium. [*From Endocrinology and Metabolism, 4th ed, P Felig, L Frohman (eds). New York, McGraw-Hill, 2001, with permission.*]

SIC HYPERNATREMIA ■ Clinical Characteristics Adipsic hypernatre-
...is characterized by chronic or recurrent hypertonic dehydration
...a deficient AVP response to osmotic stimulation. Despite hyper-
...ic dehydration, these patients have little or no thirst and may even
...sist efforts to increase their oral intake of fluids. The hypernatremia
...ries in severity and usually is associated with commensurate signs
...f hypovolemia such as tachycardia, postural hypotension, azotemia,
...yperuricemia, and hypokalemia. Muscle weakness, pain, rhabdomy-
...olysis, hyperglycemia, hyperlipidemia, and acute renal failure may
also occur.

Pathophysiology Adipsic hypernatremia is caused by agenesis or destruction of the hypothalamic osmoreceptors that normally regulate
thirst and AVP secretion (Fig. 319-5). Lack of thirst and failure to
drink enough water to replenish renal and extrarenal losses decrease
total-body water and increase plasma osmolarity/sodium. Plasma renin
activity and aldosterone secretion also increase, and plasma potassium
falls due to increased urinary excretion. The osmoreceptor deficiency
can usually be traced to an identifiable congenital or acquired disease
in the hypothalamus but is sometimes idiopathic (Table 319-2). An
MRI typically shows a normal posterior pituitary bright spot, and the
AVP response to nonosmotic stimuli is also normal. Occasionally, the
neurohypophysis is also affected, resulting in a combined defect in
water balance that is particularly severe and difficult to manage.

Differential Diagnosis Adipsic hypernatremia should be distinguished
from the hypernatremia that results from various other causes. These

TABLE 319-2 *Causes of Adipsic Hypernatremia*

Acquired
  Vascular: Occlusion anterior communicating artery
  Tumors
    Primary
      Craniopharyngioma
      Pinealoma, germinoma
      Meningioma
      Glioma
    Metastatic (lung, breast)
  Granulomas: Neurosarcoid
              Histiocytosis
  Trauma: Closed
          Penetrating (pituitary-hypothalamic surgery)
  Psychogenic: Psychotic depression
  Other: Hydrocephalus
         Neurodegenerative
         AIDS, cytomegalovirus encephalitis
  Idiopathic
Congenital
  Midline malformation (septum and corpus callosum)
  Microcephaly
Genetic: Autosomal recessive (Schinzel-Giedion syndrome)

distinctions can usually be made from the history, physical examination, and routine laboratory tests. If a conscious patient denies thirst
and/or does not drink vigorously in the presence of significant hypernatremia, the diagnosis of hypodipsia or adipsia can be made with
confidence. This diagnosis is supported by physical laboratory evidence of hypovolemia (postural hypotension, azotemia, hypokalemia,
hyperuricemia, hyperreninemia) and a relative deficiency of plasma
AVP. During rehydration, patients may develop either DI or the syndrome of inappropriate antidiuretic hormone (SIADH) depending on
whether they have partial or total deficiency of the osmoregulation of
AVP (Fig. 319-5). If the patient is obtunded or otherwise unable to
answer questions or drink at the time of presentation, the possibility
of adipsic hypernatremia can be evaluated after rehydration by assessing the thirst and plasma AVP response to a controlled fluid deprivation–hypertonic saline infusion test similar to that described for
evaluation of DI.

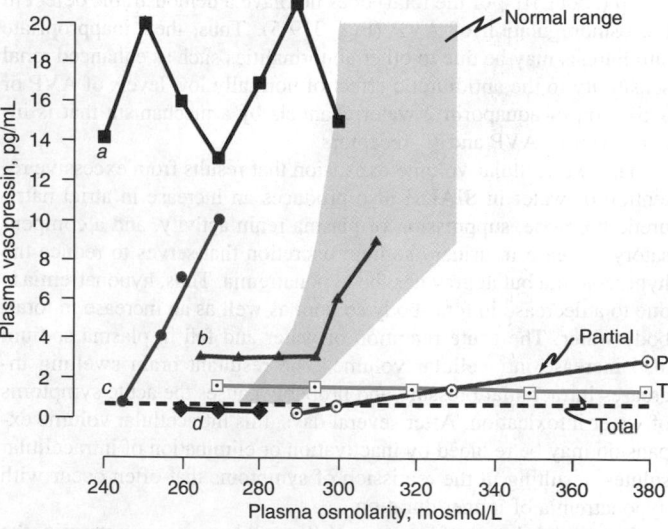

FIGURE 319-5 Heterogeneity of osmoregulatory dysfunction in adipsic hypernatremia (AH) and the syndrome of inappropriate antidiuretic hormone (SIADH). Each line
depicts schematically the relationship of plasma arginine vasopressin (AVP) to plasma
osmolarity during water loading and/or infusion of 3% saline in a patient with either
AH (open symbols) or SIADH (closed symbols). The shaded area indicates the normal
range of the relationship. The horizontal broken line indicates the plasma AVP level
below which the hormone is undetectable and urinary concentration usually does not
occur. Lines P and T represent patients with a selective deficiency in the osmoregulation
of thirst and AVP that is either partial (○) or total (□). In the latter, plasma AVP
does not change in response to increases or decreases in plasma osmolarity but remains
within a range sufficient to concentrate the urine even if overhydration produces hypotonic hyponatremia. In contrast, if the osmoregulatory deficiency is partial (○),
rehydration of the patient suppresses plasma AVP to levels that result in urinary dilution
and polyuria before plasma osmolarity and sodium are reduced to normal. Lines *a–d*
represent different defects in the osmoregulation of plasma AVP observed in patients
with SIADH. In *a* (■), plasma AVP is markedly elevated and fluctuates widely without
relation to changes in plasma osmolarity, indicating complete loss of osmoregulation.
In *b* (▲), plasma AVP remains fixed at a slightly elevated level until plasma osmolarity
reaches the normal range at which point it begins to rise appropriately, indicating a
selective defect in the inhibitory component of the osmoregulatory mechanism. In *c*
(●), plasma AVP rises in close correlation with plasma osmolarity before the latter
reaches the normal range, indicating downward resetting of the osmostat. In *d* (♦),
plasma AVP appears to be osmoregulated normally, suggesting that the inappropriate
antidiuresis is caused by some other abnormality.

TREATMENT

Adipsic hypernatremia should be treated by administering water by
mouth, if the patient is alert, or 0.45% saline intravenously, if the
patient is obtunded or uncooperative. The number of liters of free water
that will be required to correct the deficit (ΔFW) can be estimated from
body weight in kg (BW) and the serum sodium concentration in mmol/
L (S_{Na}) by the formula $\Delta FW = 0.5 BW \times [(S_{Na} - 140)/140]$. If serum
glucose (S_{Glu}) is elevated, the measured S_{Na} should be corrected ($S_{Na}*$)
by the formula $S_{Na}* = S_{Na} + [(S_{Glu} - 90)/36]$. This amount plus an
allowance for continuing insensible and urinary losses should be given
over a 24- to 48-h period. If DI is present or develops before rehydration is complete, desmopressin should also be given in standard doses
to minimize urinary losses. If hyperglycemia and/or hypokalemia are
present, insulin and/or potassium supplements should be given with
the expectation that both can be discontinued after rehydration is complete. These variables plus urine output and plasma urea/creatinine
should be monitored closely during treatment for signs of emerging
DI, SIADH, or acute renal failure.

Once the acute fluid and electrolyte imbalances are corrected, an
MRI of the brain and tests of anterior pituitary function should be
performed. A long-term management plan to prevent or minimize recurrence of the fluid and electrolyte imbalance should also be developed. This should include a practical method that the patient can use
to regulate fluid intake in accordance with day-to-day variations in
water balance. The most effective way to accomplish these objectives
is to prescribe desmopressin or chlorpropamide to completely control

DI, if it is present, and teach the patient how to use day-to-day changes in body weight as a guide for adjusting fluid intake. Prescribing a constant fluid intake is less satisfactory because it does not take into account the large, uncontrolled variations in insensible loss that inevitably occur.

EXCESS VASOPRESSIN SECRETION AND ACTION

HYPONATREMIA (See also Chap. 41) ■ **Clinical Characteristics** Excessive secretion or action of AVP results in the production of decreased volumes of more highly concentrated urine. If not accompanied by a commensurate reduction in fluid intake, the reduced suppressibility of AVP results in water retention and a decrease in plasma osmolarity/sodium. If the hyponatremia develops gradually or has been present for more than a few days, it may be asymptomatic. However, if it develops acutely, it is almost always accompanied by symptoms and signs of water intoxication that may include mild headache, confusion, anorexia, nausea, vomiting, coma, and convulsions. Severe hyponatremia may be lethal. Depending on the cause of the antidiuresis, osmotically inappropriate thirst and/or fluid intake and other disturbances of fluid and electrolyte balance may also be present.

Etiology Osmotically inappropriate antidiuresis can be caused by a primary defect in AVP secretion or action or can be secondary to a recognized nonosmotic stimulus such as hypovolemia, hypotension, or glucocorticoid deficiency. The primary forms are generally referred to as SIADH or euvolemic (type III) hyponatremia. They have many different causes, including ectopic production of AVP by lung cancer or other neoplasms, eutopic release by various diseases or drugs, and exogenous administration of AVP, desmopressin, or large doses of oxytocin (Table 319-3). The ectopic forms result from abnormal expression of the AVP-NPII gene by primary or metastatic malignancies. They do not usually remit unless the ectopic source is eliminated. The eutopic forms manifest most often in patients with acute infections or strokes, but the mechanisms by which these diseases disrupt osmoregulation are not known. A form of acute or chronic euvolemic hyponatremia very similar to SIADH can also result from stimulation of AVP secretion by protracted nausea or isolated glucocorticoid defi-

ciency. In these patients the excess AVP secretio[n] quickly and completely by specific treatments (an[d] corticoids) that are not useful in other forms of SIA[DH].

The secondary forms of osmotically inappropriat[e] usually divided into two groups: type I (hypervolem[ic]) (hypovolemic) hyponatremia. Type I occurs in so[dium]-edema-forming states such as congestive heart failure, nephrosis and is thought to be due to a reduction in "effe[ctive]" volume. Type II occurs in sodium-depleted states such as [gas]-troenteritis, diuretic abuse, or mineralocorticoid deficiency a[nd] ably a result of reduction in extracellular volume as well [as] volume and/or pressure.

Pathophysiology In SIADH, interference with the osmotic suppr[ession] of AVP release results in significant expansion and dilution of [body] fluids only if water intake exceeds the rate of insensible and uri[nary] output. The excess water intake often results from an associated de[fect] in the osmoregulation of thirst but can also be due to psychogenic [or] iatrogenic factors, including the administration of intravenous fluids[.]

In SIADH, the abnormal osmoregulation of antidiuretic function can take any of four distinct forms (Fig. 319-5). For example, AVP secretion remains fully responsive to changes in plasma osmolarity/sodium, but the threshold, or set point, of the osmoregulatory system is abnormally low. Patients with this type of downward resetting of the osmostat differ from those with the other types of osmoregulatory defect in that they are able to maximally suppress plasma AVP and dilute their urine if their fluid intake is high enough to reduce their plasma osmolarity/sodium to the new set point. Another, smaller subgroup (about 10% of the total) does not have a demonstrable defect in the osmoregulation of AVP (Fig. 319-5). Thus, their inappropriate antidiuresis may be due to other abnormalities such as enhanced renal sensitivity to the antidiuretic effect of normally low levels of AVP or activation of aquaporin 2 water channels by a mechanism that is independent of AVP and V_2 receptors.

The extracellular volume expansion that results from excessive retention of water in SIADH also produces an increase in atrial natriuretic hormone, suppression of plasma renin activity, and a compensatory increase in urinary sodium excretion that serves to reduce the hypervolemia but aggravates the hyponatremia. Thus, hyponatremia is due to a decrease in total-body sodium as well as an increase in total-body water. The acute retention of water and fall in plasma sodium also increase intracellular volume. The resultant brain swelling increases intracranial pressure and probably causes the acute symptoms of water intoxication. After several days, this intracellular volume expansion may be reduced by inactivation or elimination of intracellular solutes, resulting in the remission of symptoms that often occur with hyponatremia of longer duration.

In type I (edematous) or type II (hypovolemic) hyponatremia, the osmotic inhibition of AVP and urine concentration is counteracted by a hemodynamic stimulus that results from a substantial reduction in effective or absolute blood volume. In both cases, the reduced suppression of AVP appears to be due to downward resetting of the osmostat. The resultant antidiuresis is usually enhanced by decreased distal delivery of filtrate that results from increased reabsorption of sodium in proximal nephrons secondary to the hypovolemia. If it is not associated with a commensurate reduction in water intake, the marked reduction in urine output that ensues also leads to expansion and dilution of body fluids with symptoms of hyponatremia. This attenuates, but does not completely eliminate, the antidiuresis because the amount of water retained is usually insufficient to fully correct the effective or absolute hypovolemia. Unlike in SIADH, therefore, plasma renin activity is elevated, causing secondary hyperaldosteronism and hypokalemia. The disturbance in salt and water balance that underlies the hyponatremia also differs from SIADH in that total-body sodium and water are increased in type I but decreased in type II.

Differential Diagnosis SIADH is a diagnosis of exclusion that can usually be accomplished with routine historic, physical, and laboratory information. In a patient with hyponatremia, the possibility of simple

---

TABLE 319-3   *Causes of Syndrome of Inappropriate Antidiuretic Hormone (SIADH)*

Neoplasms	**Neurologic**
Carcinomas	Guillain-Barré syndrome
Lung	Multiple sclerosis
Duodenum	Delirium tremens
Pancreas	Amyotrophic lateral sclerosis
Ovary	Hydrocephalus
Bladder, ureter	Psychosis
Other neoplasms	Peripheral neuropathy
Thymoma	Congenital malformations
Mesothelioma	Agenesis corpus callosum
Bronchial adenoma	Cleft lip/palate
Carcinoid	Other midline defects
Gangliocytoma	**Metabolic**
Ewing's sarcoma	Acute intermittent porphyria
Head trauma (closed and penetrating)	**Pulmonary**
Infections	Asthma
Pneumonia, bacterial or viral	Pneumothorax
Abscess, lung or brain	Positive-pressure respiration
Cavitation (aspergillosis)	**Drugs**
Tuberculosis, lung or brain	Vasopressin or desmopressin
Meningitis, bacterial or viral	Chlorpropamide
Encephalitis	Oxytocin, high dose
AIDS	Vincristine
Vascular	Carbamazepine
Cerebrovascular occlusions,	Nicotine
hemorrhage	Phenothiazines
Cavernous sinus thrombosis	Cyclophosphamide
	Tricyclic antidepressants
	Monoamine oxidase inhibitors
	Serotonin reuptake inhibitors

dilution caused by an osmotically driven shift of water from the intracellular to the extracellular space should be excluded by measuring plasma glucose and/or plasma osmolarity. If the glucose is not elevated enough to account for the hyponatremia [serum sodium decreases ~1 meq/L for each rise in glucose 2.0 mmol/L (36 mg/dL)] and/or plasma osmolarity is reduced in proportion to sodium (each decrease in serum sodium of 1 meq/L should reduce plasma osmolarity by about 2 mosmol/L), the hyponatremia is "true" and can be typed or classified by standard clinical indicators of the extracellular fluid volume (Table 319-4). If these findings are ambiguous or contradictory, measuring the rate of urinary sodium excretion or plasma renin activity may be helpful. These measurements can be misleading, however, if SIADH is stable or resolving or if the patient has type II hyponatremia due to a primary defect in renal conservation of sodium, surreptitious diuretic abuse, or hyporeninemic hypoaldosteronism. The latter may be suspected if serum potassium is elevated instead of low as is usually seen in types I and II hyponatremia. Measurements of plasma AVP are currently of no diagnostic value since they exhibit the same wide variation in abnormalities in all three types of hyponatremia. In patients who fulfill the clinical criteria for type III (euvolemic) hyponatremia, plasma cortisol should also be measured to rule out unsuspected secondary adrenal insufficiency. If this is normal and there is no other obvious cause for SIADH, a careful search for occult lung cancer should also be undertaken.

TABLE 319-4 *Differential Diagnosis of Hyponatremia Based on Clinical Assessment of Extracellular Fluid Volume (ECFV)*

Clinical Findings	Type I, Hypervolemic	Type II, Hypovolemic	Type IIIA, Euvolemic	Type IIIB, Euvolemic (SIADH)
History				
CHF, cirrhosis, or nephrosis	Yes	No	No	No
Salt and water loss	No	Yes	No	No
ACTH–cortisol deficiency and/or nausea and vomiting	No	No	Yes	No
Physical examination				
Generalized edema, ascites	Yes	No	No	No
Postural hypotension	Maybe	Maybe	Maybe[a]	No
Laboratory				
BUN, creatinine	High-normal	High-normal	Low-normal	Low-normal
Uric acid	High-normal	High-normal	Low-normal	Low-normal
Serum potassium	Low-normal	Low-normal[b]	Normal[c]	Normal
Serum albumin	Low-normal	High-normal	Normal	Normal
Serum cortisol	Normal-high	Normal-high[d]	Low[e]	Normal
Plasma renin activity	High	High	Low[f]	Low
Urinary sodium (meq unit of time)[g]	Low	Low[h]	High[i]	High[i]

[a] Postural hypotension may occur in secondary (ACTH-dependent) adrenal insufficiency even though ECFV and aldosterone are usually normal.

[b] Serum potassium may be high if hypovolemia is due to aldosterone deficiency.

[c] Serum potassium may be low if vomiting causes alkalosis.

[d] Serum cortisol is low if hypovolemia is due to primary adrenal insufficiency (Addison's disease).

[e] Serum cortisol will be normal or high if the cause is nausea and vomiting rather than secondary (ACTH-dependent) adrenal insufficiency.

[f] Plasma renin activity may be high if the cause is secondary (ACTH) adrenal insufficiency.

[g] Urinary sodium should be expressed as the *rate of excretion* rather than the concentration. In a hyponatremic adult, an excretion rate > 25 meq/day (or 25 μeq/mg of creatinine) could be considered high.

[h] The rate of urinary sodium excretion may be high if the hypovolemia is due to diuretic abuse, primary adrenal insufficiency, or other causes of renal sodium wasting.

[i] The rate of urinary sodium excretion may be low if intake is curtailed by symptoms or treatment.

Note: SIADH, syndrome of inappropriate antidiuretic hormone; CHF, congestive heart failure; ACTH, adrenocorticotropic hormone; BUN, blood urea nitrogen.

TREATMENT

In acute SIADH, the keystone to treatment of hyponatremia is to restrict total fluid intake to less than the sum of insensible losses and urinary output. Total intake should include the water derived from food (300 to 500 mL/d). Because insensible losses in adults usually approximate 500 mL/d, total discretionary intake (all water in liquid form) should be at least 500 mL less than urinary output. If achieved, this deficit usually reduces body water and increases serum sodium by about 1 to 2% per day. If more rapid correction of the hyponatremia is desired to eliminate severe symptoms or signs, the fluid restriction can be supplemented by intravenous infusion of hypertonic (3%) saline. This treatment has the advantage of correcting the sodium deficiency that is partly responsible for the hyponatremia as well as producing a solute diuresis that serves to remove some of the excess water. However, if the hyponatremia has been present for more than 24 to 48 h, correction that is too rapid has the potential to produce central pontine myelinolysis, an acute, potentially fatal neurologic syndrome characterized by quadriparesis, ataxia, and abnormal extraocular movements. The following guidelines appear to minimize, if not eliminate, the risk of this complication: the 3% saline should be infused at a rate ≤0.05 mL/kg body weight per min; the effect should be monitored continuously by STAT measurements of serum sodium at least once every 2 h; and the infusion should be stopped as soon as serum sodium increases by 12 mmol/L or to 130 mmol/L, whichever comes first. Urinary output should also be monitored continuously since spontaneous remission of the SIADH can occur at any time and can result in an acute water diuresis that greatly accelerates the rate of rise in serum sodium produced by fluid restriction and 3% saline infusion.

In chronic SIADH, the hyponatremia can be corrected by treatment with demeclocycline, 150 to 300 mg orally three or four times a day, or fludrocortisone, 0.05 to 0.2 mg orally twice a day. The effect of the demeclocycline manifests in 7 to 14 days and is due to production of a reversible form of nephrogenic DI. Potential side effects include phototoxicity and azotemia. The effect of fludrocortisone also requires 1 to 2 weeks and is partly due to increased retention of sodium and possibly inhibition of thirst. It also increases urinary potassium excretion, which may require replacement through dietary adjustments or supplements. Fludrocortisone may induce hypertension, occasionally necessitating discontinuation of the treatment.

One or more nonpeptide AVP antagonists that block the antidiuretic effect of AVP may soon be approved for use in the United States. Preliminary studies with these antagonists in acute or chronic SIADH indicate that they produce a dose-dependent increase in urinary free-water excretion, which, if combined with a modest restriction of fluid intake, gradually reduces body water and corrects the hyponatremia without any recognized adverse effect. Thus, they may become the treatment of choice for those forms of SIADH in which there is inappropriate secretion of AVP that cannot be corrected by other, more specific therapy such as antiemetics or glucocorticoids.

When an SIADH-like syndrome is due to protracted nausea and vomiting or isolated glucocorticoid deficiency, all abnormalities can be corrected quickly and completely by giving an antiemetic or hydrocortisone. As with other treatments, care must be taken to ensure that serum sodium does not rise too quickly or too far.

In type I hyponatremia, the only treatment currently available is severe fluid restriction, administration of urea or mannitol to produce a solute diuresis, and/or administration of cardiotonics or serum albumin to correct the effective hypovolemia. None of these treatments is particularly effective, and some (e.g., administration of mannitol or albumin) carry significant risks. Infusion of hypertonic saline is contraindicated because it worsens the sodium retention and edema and may precipitate cardiovascular decompensation. However, preliminary studies indicate that the AVP antagonists may be almost as effective and safe in type I hyponatremia as they are in SIADH. Thus, they may become the treatment of choice for this form of hyponatremia also.

In type II hyponatremia, the defect in AVP secretion and water balance can usually be corrected easily and quickly by stopping the loss of sodium and water and/or replacing the deficits by mouth or intravenous infusion of normal or hypertonic saline. As with the treatment of other forms of hyponatremia, care must be taken to ensure that plasma sodium does not increase too rapidly. Fluid restriction or administration of AVP antagonists is contraindicated as they would only aggravate the underlying volume depletion and could result in cardiovascular decompensation.

FURTHER READING

ADROGUE HJ, MADIAS NE: Hyponatremia. N Engl J Med 342:1581, 2000

HANSEN LK et al: The genetic basis of familial neurohypophyseal diabetes insipidus. Trends Endocrinol Metab 8:363, 1997

ROBERTSON GL: Antidiuretic hormone: Normal and disordered function. Endocrinol Metab Clin North Am 30:671, 2001

VERBALIS JG: Vasopressin V$_2$ receptor antagonists. J Mol Endocrinol 29:1, 2002

WONG LL, VERBALIS JG: Systemic disease associated with disorders of water homeostasis. Endocrinol Metab Clin North Am 31:121, 2002

320   DISORDERS OF THE THYROID GLAND
J. Larry Jameson, Anthony P. Weetman

The thyroid gland produces two related hormones, thyroxine (T$_4$) and triiodothyronine (T$_3$) (Fig. 320-1). Acting through nuclear receptors, these hormones play a critical role in cell differentiation during development and help maintain thermogenic and metabolic homeostasis in the adult. Disorders of the thyroid gland result primarily from autoimmune processes that either stimulate the overproduction of thyroid hormones (*thyrotoxicosis*) or cause glandular destruction and hormone deficiency (*hypothyroidism*). In addition, benign nodules and various forms of thyroid cancer are relatively common and amenable to detection by physical examination.

ANATOMY AND DEVELOPMENT

The thyroid gland is located in the neck, anterior to the trachea, between the cricoid cartilage and the suprasternal notch. The thyroid (Greek *thyreos*, shield, plus *eidos*, form) consists of two lobes that are connected by an isthmus. It is normally 12 to 20 g in size, highly vascular, and soft in consistency. Four parathyroid glands, which produce parathyroid hormone (Chap. 332), are located in the posterior region of each pole of the thyroid. The recurrent laryngeal nerves traverse the lateral borders of the thyroid gland and must be identified during thyroid surgery to avoid vocal cord paralysis.

The thyroid gland develops from the floor of the primitive pharynx during the third week of gestation. The gland migrates from the foramen cecum, at the base of the tongue, along the thyroglossal duct to reach its final location in the neck. This feature accounts for the rare ectopic location of thyroid tissue at the base of the tongue (lingual thyroid), as well as for the presence of thyroglossal duct cysts along this developmental tract. Thyroid hormone synthesis normally begins at about 11 weeks' gestation.

The parathyroid glands migrate from the third (inferior glands) and fourth (superior glands) pharyngeal pouches and become embedded in the thyroid gland. Neural crest derivatives from the ultimobranchial body give rise to thyroid medullary C cells that produce calcitonin, a calcium-lowering hormone. The C cells are interspersed throughout the thyroid gland, although their density is greatest in the juncture of the upper one-third and lower two-thirds of the gland.

Thyroid gland development is controlled by a series of developmental transcription factors. Thyroid transcription factor (TTF) 1 (also known as NKX2A), TTF-2 (also known as FKHL15), and paired homeobox-8 (PAX-8) are expressed selectively, but not exclusively, in the thyroid gland. In combination, they orchestrate thyroid cell development and the induction of thyroid-specific genes such as thyroglobulin (Tg), thyroid peroxidase (TPO), the sodium iodide symporter (NIS), and the thyroid-stimulating hormone receptor (TSH-R). Mutations in these developmental transcription factors or their downstream target genes are rare causes of thyroid agenesis or dyshormonogenesis and can cause congenital hypothyroidism (Table 320-1). Congenital hypothyroidism is common enough (approximately 1 in 4000 newborns) that neonatal screening is performed in most industrialized countries (see below). Though the underlying causes of most cases of congenital hypothyroidism are unknown, early treatment with thyroid hormone replacement precludes potentially severe developmental abnormalities.

The mature thyroid gland contains numerous spherical follicles composed of thyroid follicular cells that surround secreted colloid, a proteinaceous fluid that contains large amounts of thyroglobulin, the protein precursor of thyroid hormones (Fig. 320-2). The thyroid follicular cells are polarized—the basolateral surface is apposed to the bloodstream and an apical surface faces the follicular lumen. Increased demand for thyroid hormone, usually signaled by thyroid-stimulating hormone (TSH) binding to its receptor on the basolateral surface of the follicular cells, leads to Tg reabsorption from the follicular lumen and proteolysis within the cell to yield thyroid hormones for secretion into the bloodstream.

REGULATION OF THE THYROID AXIS

TSH, secreted by the thyrotrope cells of the anterior pituitary, plays a pivotal role in control of the thyroid axis and serves as the most useful physiologic marker of thyroid hormone action. TSH is a 31-kDa hormone composed of α and β subunits; the α subunit is common to the other glycoprotein hormones [luteinizing hormone, follicle-stimulating hormone, human chorionic gonadotropin (hCG)], whereas the TSH β subunit is unique to TSH. The extent and nature of carbohydrate modification are modulated by thyrotropin-releasing hormone (TRH) stimulation and influence the biologic activity of the hormone.

The thyroid axis is a classic example of an endocrine feedback loop. Hypothalamic TRH stimulates pituitary production of TSH, which, in turn, stimulates thyroid hor-

FIGURE 320-1 Structures of thyroid hormones. Thyroxine (T$_4$) contains four iodine atoms. Deiodination leads to production of the potent hormone, triiodothyronine (T$_3$), or the inactive hormone, reverse T$_3$.

Thyroxine (T$_4$)
3,5,3',5'-Tetraiodothyronine

Deiodinase 1 or 2 (5'-Deiodination)   *Deiodinase 3 > 2* (5-Deiodination)

Tri-iodothyronine (T$_3$)
3,5,3'-Triiodothyronine

Reverse T$_3$ (rT$_3$)
3,3',5'-Triiodothyronine

mone synthesis and secretion. Thyroid hormones feed back negatively to inhibit TRH and TSH production (Fig. 320-2). The "set-point" in this axis is established by TSH. TRH is the major positive regulator of TSH synthesis and secretion. Peak TSH secretion occurs ~15 min after administration of exogenous TRH. Dopamine, glucocorticoids, and somatostatin suppress TSH but are not of major physiologic importance except when these agents are administered in pharmacologic doses. Reduced levels of thyroid hormone increase basal TSH production and enhance TRH-mediated stimulation of TSH. High thyroid hormone levels rapidly and directly suppress TSH and inhibit TRH-mediated stimulation of TSH, indicating that thyroid hormones are the dominant regulator of TSH production. Like other pituitary hormones, TSH is released in a pulsatile manner and exhibits a diurnal rhythm; its highest levels occur at night. However, these TSH excursions are modest in comparison to those of other pituitary hormones, in part because TSH has a relatively long plasma half-life (50 min). Consequently, single measurements of TSH are adequate for assessing its circulating level. TSH is measured using immunoradiometric assays that are highly sensitive and specific. These assays readily distinguish between normal and suppressed TSH values; thus, TSH can be used for the diagnosis of hyperthyroidism (low TSH) as well as hypothyroidism (high TSH).

TABLE 320-1 Genetic Causes of Congenital Hypothyroidism		
Defective Gene Protein	Inheritance	Consequences
PROP-1	Autosomal recessive	Combined pituitary hormone deficiencies with preservation of adrenocorticotropic hormone
PIT-1	Autosomal recessive Autosomal dominant	Combined deficiencies of growth hormone, prolactin, thyroid-stimulating hormone (TSH)
TSHβ	Autosomal recessive	TSH deficiency
TTF-1	Autosomal dominant	Variable thyroid hypoplasia, choreoathetosis, pulmonary problems
TTF-2	Autosomal recessive	Thyroid agenesis, choanal atresia, spiky hair
PAX-8	Autosomal dominant	Thyroid dysgenesis
TSH-receptor	Autosomal recessive	Resistance to TSH
$G_{s\alpha}$ (Albright hereditary osteodystrophy)	Autosomal dominant	Resistance to TSH
Na^+/I^- symporter	Autosomal recessive	Inability to transport iodide
THOX2	Autosomal dominant	Organification defect
Thyroid peroxidase	Autosomal recessive	Defective organification of iodide
Thyroglobulin	Autosomal recessive	Defective synthesis of thyroid hormone
Pendrin	Autosomal recessive	Pendred's syndrome: sensorineural deafness and partial organification defect in thyroid
Dehalogenase	Autosomal recessive	Loss of iodide reutilization

THYROID HORMONE SYNTHESIS, METABOLISM, AND ACTION

THYROID HORMONE SYNTHESIS Thyroid hormones are derived from Tg, a large iodinated glycoprotein. After secretion into the thyroid follicle, Tg is iodinated on selected tyrosine residues that are subsequently coupled via an ether linkage. Reuptake of Tg into the thyroid follicular cell initiates proteolysis and the release of newly synthesized T_4 and T_3.

Iodine Metabolism and Transport Iodide uptake is a critical first step in thyroid hormone synthesis. Ingested iodine is bound to serum proteins, particularly albumin. Unbound iodine is excreted in the urine. The thyroid gland extracts iodine from the circulation in a highly efficient manner. For example, 10 to 25% of radioactive tracer (e.g., ^{123}I) is taken up by the normal thyroid gland over 24 h; this value can rise to 70 to 90% in Graves' disease. Iodide uptake is mediated by the Na^+/I^- symporter (NIS), which is expressed at the basolateral membrane of thyroid follicular cells. NIS is most highly expressed in the thyroid gland but low levels are present in the salivary glands, lactating breast, and placenta. The iodide transport mechanism is highly regulated, allowing adaptation to variations in dietary supply. Low iodine levels increase the amount of NIS and stimulate uptake, whereas high iodine levels suppress NIS expression and uptake. The selective expression of the NIS in the thyroid allows isotopic scanning, treatment of hyperthyroidism, and ablation of thyroid cancer with radioisotopes of iodine, without significant effects on other organs. Mutation of the *NIS* gene is a rare cause of congenital hypothyroidism, underscoring its importance in thyroid hormone synthesis. Another iodine transporter, pendrin, is located on the apical surface of thyroid cells and mediates iodine efflux into the lumen. Mutation of the *PENDRIN* gene causes *Pendred syndrome*, a disorder characterized by defective organification of iodine, goiter, and sensorineural deafness.

Iodine deficiency is prevalent in many mountainous regions and in central Africa, central South America, and northern Asia. In areas of relative iodine deficiency, there is an increased prevalence of goiter and, when deficiency is severe, hypothyroidism and cretinism. *Cretin-*

ism is characterized by mental and growth retardation and occurs when children who live in iodine-deficient regions are not treated with iodine or thyroid hormone to restore normal thyroid hormone levels during early childhood. These children are often born to mothers with iodine deficiency, and it is likely that maternal thyroid hormone deficiency worsens the condition. Concomitant selenium deficiency may also contribute to the neurologic manifestations of cretinism. Iodine supplementation of salt, bread, and other food substances has markedly reduced the prevalence of cretinism. Unfortunately, however, iodine deficiency remains the most common cause of preventable mental deficiency, often because of resistance to the use of food additives or the cost of supplementation. In addition to overt cretinism, mild iodine deficiency can lead to subtle reduction of IQ. Oversupply of iodine,

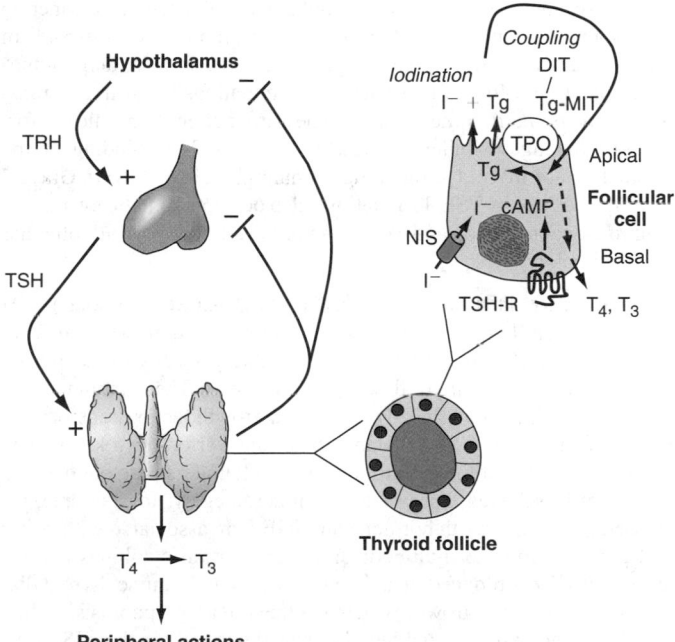

FIGURE 320-2 Regulation of thyroid hormone synthesis. *Left.* Thyroid hormones T_4 and T_3 feed back to inhibit hypothalamic production of thyrotropin-releasing hormone (TRH) and pituitary production of thyroid-stimulating hormone (TSH). TSH stimulates thyroid gland production of T_4 and T_3. *Right.* Thyroid follicles are formed by thyroid epithelial cells surrounding proteinaceous colloid, which contains thyroglobulin. Follicular cells, which are polarized, synthesize thyroglobulin and carry out thyroid hormone biosynthesis (see text for details). TSH-R, thyroid-stimulating hormone receptor; Tg, thyroglobulin; NIS, sodium-iodide symporter; TPO, thyroid peroxidase; DIT, di-iodotyrosine; MIT, monoiodotyrosine

through supplements or foods enriched in iodine (e.g., shellfish, kelp), is associated with an increased incidence of autoimmune thyroid disease. The recommended average daily intake of iodine is 150 μg/d for adults, 90 to 120 μg/d for children, and 200 μg/d for pregnant women. Urinary iodine is >10 μg/dL in iodine-sufficient populations.

Organification, Coupling, Storage, Release   After iodide enters the thyroid, it is trapped and transported to the apical membrane of thyroid follicular cells where it is oxidized in an organification reaction that involves TPO and hydrogen peroxide. The reactive iodine atom is added to selected tyrosyl residues within Tg, a large (660 kDa) dimeric protein that consists of 2769 amino acids. The iodotyrosines in Tg are then coupled via an ether linkage in a reaction that is also catalyzed by TPO. Either T_4 or T_3 can be produced by this reaction, depending on the number of iodine atoms present in the iodotyrosines. After coupling, Tg is taken back into the thyroid cell where it is processed in lysosomes to release T_4 and T_3. Uncoupled mono- and diiodotyrosines (MIT, DIT) are deiodinated by the enzyme dehalogenase, thereby recycling any iodide that is not converted into thyroid hormones.

Disorders of thyroid hormone synthesis are rare causes of congenital hypothyroidism. The vast majority of these disorders are due to recessive mutations in TPO or Tg, but defects have also been identified in the TSH-R, NIS, pendrin, hydrogen peroxide generation, and in dehalogenase. Because of the biosynthetic defect, the gland is incapable of synthesizing adequate amounts of hormone, leading to increased TSH and a large goiter.

TSH Action   TSH regulates thyroid gland function through the TSH-R, a seven-transmembrane G protein–coupled receptor (GPCR). The TSH-R is coupled to the α subunit of stimulatory G protein ($G_{s\alpha}$), which activates adenylyl cyclase, leading to increased production of cyclic AMP. TSH also stimulates phosphatidylinositol turnover by activating phospholipase C. The functional roles of the TSH-R are exemplified by the consequences of naturally occurring mutations. Recessive loss-of-function mutations are a rare cause of thyroid hypoplasia and congenital hypothyroidism. Dominant gain-of-function mutations cause sporadic or familial nonautoimmune hyperthyroidism that is characterized by goiter, thyroid cell hyperplasia, and autonomous function. Most of these activating mutations occur in the transmembrane domain of the receptor. They are thought to mimic conformational changes similar to those induced by TSH binding or the interactions of thyroid-stimulating immunoglobulins (TSI) in Graves' disease. Activating TSH-R mutations also occur as somatic events and lead to clonal selection and expansion of the affected thyroid follicular cell (see below).

Other Factors that Influence Hormone Synthesis and Release   Although TSH is the dominant hormonal regulator of thyroid gland growth and function, a variety of growth factors, most produced locally in the thyroid gland, also influence thyroid hormone synthesis. These include insulin-like growth factor I (IGF-I), epidermal growth factor, transforming growth factor β (TGF-β), endothelins, and various cytokines. The quantitative roles of these factors are not well understood, but they are important in selected disease states. In acromegaly, for example, increased levels of growth hormone and IGF-I are associated with goiter and predisposition to multinodular goiter. Certain cytokines and interleukins (ILs) produced in association with autoimmune thyroid disease induce thyroid growth, whereas others lead to apoptosis. Iodine deficiency increases thyroid blood flow and upregulates the NIS, stimulating more efficient uptake. Excess iodide transiently inhibits thyroid iodide organification, a phenomenon known as the *Wolff-Chaikoff effect*. In individuals with a normal thyroid, the gland escapes from this inhibitory effect and iodide organification resumes; the suppressive action of high iodide may persist, however, in patients with underlying autoimmune thyroid disease.

THYROID HORMONE TRANSPORT AND METABOLISM ■ **Serum Binding Proteins**
T_4 is secreted from the thyroid gland in at least 20-fold excess over T_3 (Table 320-2). Both hormones are bound to plasma proteins, including thyroxine-binding globulin (TBG), transthyretin (TTR), formerly known as thyroxine-binding prealbumin, or TBPA), and albumin. The plasma-binding proteins increase the pool of circulating hormone, delay hormone clearance, and may modulate hormone delivery to selected tissue sites. The concentration of TBG is relatively low (1 to 2 mg/dL), but because of its high affinity for thyroid hormones ($T_4 > T_3$), it carries about 80% of the bound hormones. Albumin has relatively low affinity for thyroid hormones but has a high plasma concentration (~3.5 g/dL), and it binds up to 10% of T_4 and 30% of T_3. TTR carries about 10% of T_4 but little T_3.

When the effects of the various binding proteins are combined, approximately 99.98% of T_4 and 99.7% of T_3 are protein-bound. Because T_3 is less tightly bound than T_4, the amount of unbound T_3 is greater than unbound T_4, even though there is less total T_3 in the circulation. The unbound, or free, concentrations of the hormones are ~2×10^{-11} M for T_4 and ~6×10^{-12} M for T_3, which roughly correspond to the thyroid hormone receptor binding constants for these hormones (see below). Only the unbound hormone is biologically available to tissues. Therefore, homeostatic mechanisms that regulate the thyroid axis are directed towards maintenance of normal concentrations of unbound hormones.

Dysalbuminemic Hyperthyroxinemia   A number of inherited and acquired abnormalities affect thyroid hormone binding proteins. X-linked TBG deficiency is associated with very low levels of total T_4 and T_3. However, because unbound hormone levels are normal, patients are euthyroid and TSH levels are normal. The importance of recognizing this disorder is to avoid efforts to normalize total T_4 levels, as this leads to thyrotoxicosis and is futile because of rapid hormone clearance in the absence of TBG. TBG levels are elevated by estrogen, which increases sialylation and delays TBG clearance. Consequently, in women who are pregnant or taking estrogen-containing contraceptives, elevated TBG increases total T_4 and T_3 levels; however, unbound T_4 and T_3 levels are normal. Mutations in TBG, TTR, and albumin that increase binding affinity for T_4 and/or T_3 cause disorders known as *euthyroid hyperthyroxinemia* or *familial dysalbuminemic hyperthyroxinemia* (FDH) (Table 320-3). These disorders result in increased total T_4 and/or T_3, but unbound hormone levels are normal. The familial nature of the disorders, and the fact that TSH levels are normal rather than suppressed, suggest this diagnosis. Unbound hormone levels (ideally measured by dialysis) are normal in FDH. The diagnosis can be confirmed by using tests that measure the affinities of radiolabeled hormone binding to specific transport proteins or by performing DNA sequence analyses of the abnormal transport protein genes.

Certain medications, such as salicylates and salsalate, can displace thyroid hormones from circulating binding proteins. Although these drugs transiently perturb the thyroid axis by increasing free thyroid hormone levels, TSH is suppressed until a new steady state is reached, thereby restoring euthyroidism. Circulating factors associated with acute illness may also displace thyroid hormone from binding proteins (see "Sick Euthyroid Syndrome," below).

TABLE 320-2 *Characteristics of Circulating T_4 and T_3*		
Hormone Property	T_4	T_3
Serum concentrations		
Total hormone	8 μg/dL	0.14 μg/dL
Fraction of total hormone in the free form	0.02%	0.3%
Free (unbound) hormone	21×10^{-12} M	6×10^{-12} M
Serum half-life	7 d	0.75 d
Fraction directly from the thyroid	100%	20%
Production rate, including peripheral conversion	90 μg/d	32 μg/d
Intracellular hormone fraction	~20%	~70%
Relative metabolic potency	0.3	1
Receptor binding	10^{-10} M	10^{-11} M

Deiodinases T_4 may be thought of as a precursor for the more potent T_3. T_4 is converted to T_3 by the deiodinase enzymes (Fig. 320-1). Type I deiodinase, which is located primarily in thyroid, liver, and kidney, has a relatively low affinity for T_4. Type II deiodinase has a higher affinity for T_4 and is found primarily in the pituitary gland, brain, brown fat, and thyroid gland. The presence of type II deiodinase allows it to regulate T_3 concentrations locally, a property that may be important in the context of levothyroxine (T_4) replacement. Type II deiodinase is also regulated by thyroid hormone—hypothyroidism induces the enzyme, resulting in enhanced $T_4 \rightarrow T_3$ conversion in tissues such as brain and pituitary. $T_4 \rightarrow T_3$ conversion is impaired by fasting, systemic illness or acute trauma, oral contrast agents, and a variety of medications (e.g., propylthiouracil, propranolol, amiodarone, glucocorticoids). Type III deiodinase inactivates T_4 and T_3 and is the most important source of reverse T_3 (rT_3). Massive hemangiomas that express type III deiodinase are a rare cause of hypothyroidism in infants.

THYROID HORMONE ACTION ■ Nuclear Thyroid Hormone Receptors

Thyroid hormones act by binding to nuclear *thyroid hormone receptors* (TRs) α and β. Both TRα and TRβ are expressed in most tissues, but their relative levels of expression vary among organs; TRα is particularly abundant in brain, kidney, gonads, muscle, and heart, whereas TRβ expression is relatively high in the pituitary and liver. Both receptors are variably spliced to form unique isoforms. The TRβ2 isoform, which has a unique amino terminus, is selectively expressed in the hypothalamus and pituitary, where it plays a role in feedback control of the thyroid axis. The TRα2 isoform contains a unique carboxy terminus that prevents thyroid hormone binding; it may function to block the action of other TR isoforms.

The TRs contain a central DNA-binding domain and a C-terminal ligand-binding domain. They bind to specific DNA sequences, termed *thyroid response elements* (TREs), in the promoter regions of target genes (Fig. 320-3). The receptors bind as homodimers or as heterodimers with retinoic acid X receptors (RXRs) (Chap. 317). The activated receptor can either stimulate gene transcription (e.g., myosin heavy chain α) or inhibit transcription (e.g., TSH β-subunit gene), depending on the nature of the regulatory elements in the target gene.

Thyroid hormones bind with similar affinities to TRα and TRβ. However, T_3 is bound with 10 to 15 times greater affinity than T_4, which explains its increased hormonal potency. Though T_4 is produced in excess of T_3, receptors are occupied mainly by T_3, reflecting $T_4 \rightarrow T_3$ conversion by peripheral tissues, greater T_3 bioavailability in the plasma, and receptors' greater affinity for T_3. After binding to TRs, thyroid hormone induces conformational changes in the receptors that modify its interactions with accessory transcription factors. In the absence of thyroid hormone binding, the aporeceptors bind to co-repressor proteins that inhibit gene transcription. Hormone binding dissociates the co-repressors and allows the recruitment of coactivators that enhance transcription. The discovery of TR interactions with co-repressors explains the fact that TR silences gene expression in the absence of hormone binding. Consequently, hormone deficiency has a profound effect on gene expression because it causes gene repression as well as loss of hormone-induced stimulation. This concept has been corroborated by the finding that targeted deletion of the TR genes in mice has a less pronounced phenotypic effect than hormone deficiency.

Thyroid Hormone Resistance Resistance to thyroid hormone (RTH) is an autosomal dominant disorder characterized by elevated thyroid hormone levels and inappropriately normal or elevated TSH. Individuals with RTH do not, in general, exhibit signs and symptoms that are typical of hypothyroidism because hormone resistance is partial and is compensated by increased levels of thyroid hormone. The clinical features of RTH can include goiter, attention deficit disorder, mild reduction in IQ, delayed skeletal maturation, tachycardia, and impaired metabolic responses to thyroid hormone.

The disorder is caused by mutations in the TRβ receptor gene. These mutations, located in restricted regions of the ligand-binding domain, cause loss of receptor function. However, because the mutant receptors retain the capacity to dimerize with RXRs, bind to DNA, and recruit co-repressor proteins, they function as antagonists of the remaining, normal TRβ and TRα receptors. This property, referred to as

TABLE 320-3 *Conditions Associated with Euthyroid Hyperthyroxinemia*

Disorder	Cause	Transmission	Characteristics
Familial dysalbuminemic hyperthyroxinemia (FDH)	Albumin mutations, usually R218H	AD	Increased T_4 Normal unbound T_4 Rarely increased T_3
TBG			
Familial excess	Increased TBG production	XL	Increased total T_4, T_3 Normal unbound T_4, T_3
Acquired excess	Medications (estrogen), pregnancy, cirrhosis, hepatitis	Acquired	Increased total T_4, T_3 Normal unbound T_4, T_3
Transthyretin[a]			
Excess	Islet tumors	Acquired	Usually normal T_4, T_3
Mutations	Increased affinity for T_4 or T_3	AD	Increased total T_4, T_3 Normal unbound T_4, T_3
Medications: propranolol, ipodate, iopanoic acid, amiodarone	Decreased $T_4 \rightarrow T_3$ conversion	Acquired	Increased T_4 Decreased T_3 Normal or increased TSH
Sick-euthyroid syndrome	Acute illness, especially psychiatric disorders	Acquired	Transiently increased unbound T_4 Decreased TSH T_4 and T_3 may also be decreased (see text)
Resistance to thyroid hormone (RTH)	Thyroid hormone receptor β mutations	AD	Increased unbound T_4, T_3 Normal or increased TSH Some patients clinically thyrotoxic

[a] Also known as thyroxine-binding prealbumin, TBPA.

Note: AD, autosomal dominant; TBG, thyroxine-binding globulin; TSH, thyroid-stimulating hormone; XL, X-linked.

FIGURE 320-3 Mechanism of thyroid hormone receptor action. The thyroid hormone receptor (TR) and retinoid X receptor (RXR) form heterodimers that bind specifically to thyroid hormone response elements (TRE) in the promoter regions of target genes. In the absence of hormone, TR binds co-repressor (CoR) proteins that silence gene expression. The numbers refer to a series of ordered reactions that occur in response to thyroid hormone: (1) T_4 or T_3 enters the nucleus; (2) T_3 binding dissociates CoR from TR; (3) Coactivators (CoA) are recruited to the T_3-bound receptor; (4) gene expression is altered.

as "dominant negative" activity, explains the autosomal dominant mode of transmission. The diagnosis is suspected when unbound thyroid hormone levels are increased without suppression of TSH. Similar hormonal abnormalities are found in other affected family members, although the TRβ mutation arises de novo in about 20% of patients. DNA sequence analysis of the TRβ gene provides a definitive diagnosis. RTH must be distinguished from other causes of euthyroid hyperthyroxinemia (e.g., FDH) and inappropriate secretion of TSH by TSH-secreting pituitary adenomas (Chap. 318). In most patients, no treatment is indicated; the importance of making the diagnosis is to avoid inappropriate treatment of mistaken hyperthyroidism and to provide genetic counseling.

PHYSICAL EXAMINATION

In addition to the examination of the thyroid itself, the physical examination should include a search for signs of abnormal thyroid function and the extrathyroidal features of ophthalmopathy and dermopathy (see below). Examination of the neck begins by inspecting the seated patient from the front and side, and noting any surgical scars, obvious masses, or distended veins. The thyroid can be palpated with both hands from behind or while facing the patient, using the thumbs to palpate each lobe. It is best to use a combination of these methods, especially when the nodules are small. The patient's neck should be slightly flexed to relax the neck muscles. After locating the cricoid cartilage, the isthmus can be identified and followed laterally to locate either lobe (normally the right lobe is slightly larger than the left). By asking the patient to swallow sips of water, thyroid consistency can be better appreciated as the gland moves beneath the examiner's fingers.

Features to be noted include thyroid size, consistency, nodularity, and any tenderness or fixation. An estimate of thyroid size (normally 12 to 20 g) should be made, and a drawing is often the best way to record findings. However, ultrasound is the method of choice when it is important to determine thyroid size accurately. The size, location, and consistency of any nodules should also be defined. A bruit over the gland indicates increased vascularity, as occurs in hyperthyroidism. If the lower borders of the thyroid lobes are not clearly felt, a goiter may be retrosternal. Large retrosternal goiters can cause venous distention over the neck and difficulty breathing, especially when the arms are raised (Pemberton's sign). With any central mass above the thyroid, the tongue should be extended, as thyroglossal cysts then move upward. The thyroid examination is not complete without assessment for lymphadenopathy in the supraclavicular and cervical regions of the neck.

LABORATORY EVALUATION

MEASUREMENT OF THYROID HORMONES   The enhanced sensitivity and specificity of *TSH assays* have greatly improved laboratory assessment of thyroid function. Because TSH levels change dynamically in response to alterations of T_4 and T_3, a logical approach to thyroid testing is to first determine whether TSH is suppressed, normal, or elevated. With rare exceptions (see below), a normal TSH level excludes a primary abnormality of thyroid function. This strategy depends on the use of immunoradiometric assays (IRMAs) for TSH that are sensitive enough to discriminate between the lower limit of the reference range and the suppressed values that occur with thyrotoxicosis. Extremely sensitive (fourth generation) assays can detect TSH levels ≤ 0.004 mU/L, but for practical purposes assays sensitive to ≤ 0.1 mU/L are sufficient. The widespread availability of the TSH IRMA has rendered the TRH stimulation test obsolete, as the failure of TSH to rise after an intravenous bolus of 200 to 400 μg TRH has the same implications as a suppressed basal TSH measured by IRMA.

The finding of an abnormal TSH level must be followed by measurements of circulating thyroid hormone levels to confirm the diagnosis of hyperthyroidism (suppressed TSH) or hypothyroidism (elevated TSH). Radioimmunoassays are widely available for serum *total*

T_4 and *total* T_3. T_4 and T_3 are highly protein-bound, and numerous factors (illness, medications, genetic factors) can influence protein binding. It is useful, therefore, to measure the free, or unbound, hormone levels, which correspond to the biologically available hormone pool. Two direct methods are used to measure *unbound thyroid hormones*: (1) unbound thyroid hormone competition with radiolabeled T_4 (or an analogue) for binding to a solid-phase antibody, and (2) physical separation of the unbound hormone fraction by ultracentrifugation or equilibrium dialysis. Though early unbound hormone immunoassays suffered from artifacts, newer assays correlate well with the results of the more technically demanding and expensive physical separation methods. An indirect method to estimate unbound thyroid hormone levels is to calculate the free T_3 or free T_4 index from the total T_4 or T_3 concentration and the *thyroid hormone binding ratio* (THBR). The latter is derived from the T_3-*resin uptake test*, which determines the distribution of radiolabeled T_3 between an absorbent resin and the unoccupied thyroid hormone binding proteins in the sample. The binding of the labeled T_3 to the resin is increased when there is reduced unoccupied protein binding sites (e.g., TBG deficiency) or increased total thyroid hormone in the sample; it is decreased under the opposite circumstances. The product of THBR and total T_3 or T_4 provides the *free T_3 or T_4 index*. In effect, the index corrects for anomalous total hormone values caused by abnormalities in hormone-protein binding.

Total thyroid hormone levels are *elevated* when TBG is increased due to estrogens (pregnancy, oral contraceptives, hormone replacement therapy, tamoxifen), and *decreased* when TBG binding is reduced (androgens, the nephrotic syndrome). Genetic disorders and acute illness can also cause abnormalities in thyroid hormone binding proteins, and various drugs (phenytoin, carbamazepine, salicylates, and nonsteroidal anti-inflammatory drugs) can interfere with thyroid hormone binding. Because unbound thyroid hormone levels are normal and the patient is euthyroid in all of these circumstances, assays that measure unbound hormone are preferable to those for total thyroid hormones.

For most purposes, the unbound T_4 level is sufficient to confirm thyrotoxicosis, but 2 to 5% of patients have only an elevated T_3 level (T_3 toxicosis). Thus, unbound T_3 levels should be measured in patients with a suppressed TSH but normal unbound T_4 levels.

There are several clinical conditions in which the use of TSH as a screening test may be misleading, particularly without simultaneous unbound T_4 determinations. Any severe nonthyroidal illness can cause abnormal TSH levels (see below). Although hypothyroidism is the most common cause of an elevated TSH level, rare causes include a TSH-secreting pituitary tumor (Chap. 318), thyroid hormone resistance, and assay artifact. Conversely, a suppressed TSH level, particularly <0.1 mU/L, usually indicates thyrotoxicosis but may also be seen during the first trimester of pregnancy (due to hCG secretion), after treatment of hyperthyroidism (because TSH remains suppressed for several weeks), and in response to certain medications (e.g., high doses of glucocorticoids or dopamine). Importantly, secondary hypothyroidism, caused by hypothalamic-pituitary disease, is associated with a variable (low to high-normal) TSH level, which is inappropriate for the low T_4 level. Thus, *TSH should not be used to assess thyroid function in patients with suspected or known pituitary disease*.

Tests for the end-organ effects of thyroid hormone excess or depletion, such as estimation of basal metabolic rate, tendon reflex relaxation rates, or serum cholesterol, are not useful as clinical determinants of thyroid function.

TESTS TO DETERMINE THE ETIOLOGY OF THYROID DYSFUNCTION   Autoimmune thyroid disease is detected most easily by measuring circulating antibodies against TPO and Tg. As antibodies to Tg alone are uncommon, it is reasonable to measure only TPO antibodies. About 5 to 15% of euthyroid women and up to 2% of euthyroid men have thyroid antibodies; such individuals are at increased risk of developing thyroid dysfunction. Almost all patients with autoimmune hypothyroidism, and up to 80% of those with Graves' disease, have TPO antibodies, usually at high levels.

TSI are antibodies that stimulate the TSH-R in Graves' disease. They can be measured in bioassays or indirectly in assays that detect antibody binding to the receptor. The main use of these assays is to predict neonatal thyrotoxicosis caused by high maternal levels of TSI in the last trimester of pregnancy.

Serum Tg levels are increased in all types of thyrotoxicosis except *thyrotoxicosis factitia* caused by self-administration of thyroid hormone. The main role for Tg measurement, however, is in the follow-up of thyroid cancer patients. After total thyroidectomy and radioablation, Tg levels should be undetectable; measurable levels (>1 to 2 ng/mL) suggest incomplete ablation or recurrent cancer.

RADIOIODINE UPTAKE AND THYROID SCANNING The thyroid gland selectively transports radioisotopes of iodine (^{123}I, ^{125}I, ^{131}I) and ^{99m}Tc pertechnetate, allowing thyroid imaging and quantitation of radioactive tracer fractional uptake.

Nuclear imaging of Graves' disease is characterized by an enlarged gland and increased tracer uptake that is distributed homogeneously. Toxic adenomas appear as focal areas of increased uptake, with suppressed tracer uptake in the remainder of the gland. In toxic multinodular goiter, the gland is enlarged—often with distorted architecture—and there are multiple areas of relatively increased or decreased tracer uptake. Subacute thyroiditis is associated with very low uptake because of follicular cell damage and TSH suppression. Thyrotoxicosis factitia is also associated with low uptake.

Although the use of fine-needle aspiration (FNA) biopsy has diminished the use of thyroid scans in the evaluation of solitary thyroid nodules, the functional features of thyroid nodules have some prognostic significance. So-called cold nodules, which have diminished tracer uptake, are usually benign. However, these nodules are more likely to be malignant (~5 to 10%) than so-called hot nodules, which are almost never malignant.

Thyroid scanning is also used in the follow-up of thyroid cancer. After thyroidectomy and ablation using ^{131}I, there is diminished radioiodine uptake in the thyroid bed, allowing the detection of metastatic thyroid cancer deposits that retain the ability to transport iodine. Whole-body scans using 111 to 185 MBq (3 to 5 mCi) ^{131}I are typically performed after thyroid hormone withdrawal to raise the TSH level or after the administration of recombinant human TSH.

THYROID ULTRASOUND Ultrasonography is used increasingly to assist in the diagnosis of nodular thyroid disease, a reflection of the limitations of the physical examination and improvements in ultrasound technology. Using 10-MHz instruments, spatial resolution and image quality are excellent, allowing the detection of nodules and cysts >3 mm. In addition to detecting thyroid nodules, ultrasound is useful for monitoring nodule size, for guiding FNA biopsies, and for the aspiration of cystic lesions. Ultrasound is also used in the evaluation of recurrent thyroid cancer, including possible spread to cervical lymph nodes.

HYPOTHYROIDISM

Iodine deficiency remains the most common cause of hypothyroidism worldwide. In areas of iodine sufficiency, autoimmune disease (Hashimoto's thyroiditis) and iatrogenic causes (treatment of hyperthyroidism) are most common (Table 320-4).

CONGENITAL HYPOTHYROIDISM ■ Prevalence Hypothyroidism occurs in about 1 in 4000 newborns. It may be transient, especially if the mother has TSH-R blocking antibodies or has received antithyroid drugs, but permanent hypothyroidism occurs in the majority. Neonatal hypothyroidism is due to thyroid gland dysgenesis in 80 to 85%, inborn errors of thyroid hormone synthesis in 10 to 15%, and is TSH-R antibody-

mediated in 5% of affected newborns. The developmental abnormalities are twice as common in girls. Mutations that cause congenital hypothyroidism are being increasingly recognized, but the vast majority remain idiopathic (Table 320-1).

Clinical Manifestations The majority of infants appear normal at birth, and <10% are diagnosed based on clinical features, which include prolonged jaundice, feeding problems, hypotonia, enlarged tongue, delayed bone maturation, and umbilical hernia. Importantly, permanent neurologic damage results if treatment is delayed. Typical features of adult hypothyroidism may also be present (Table 320-5). Other congenital malformations, especially cardiac, are four times more common in congenital hypothyroidism.

Diagnosis and Treatment Because of the severe neurologic consequences of untreated congenital hypothyroidism, neonatal screening programs have been established in developed countries. These are generally based on measurement of TSH or T_4 levels in heel-prick blood specimens. When the diagnosis is confirmed, T_4 is instituted at a dose of 10 to 15 μg/kg per day and the dosage is adjusted by close monitoring of TSH levels. T_4 requirements are relatively great during the first year of life, and a high circulating T_4 level is usually needed to normalize TSH. Early treatment with T_4 results in normal IQ levels, but subtle neurodevelopmental abnormalities may occur in those with the most severe hypothyroidism at diagnosis or when treatment is suboptimal.

TABLE 320-4 *Causes of Hypothyroidism*

Primary
  Autoimmune hypothyroidism: Hashimoto's thyroiditis, atrophic thyroiditis
  Iatrogenic: ^{131}I treatment, subtotal or total thyroidectomy, external irradiation of neck for lymphoma or cancer
  Drugs: iodine excess (including iodine-containing contrast media and amiodarone), lithium, antithyroid drugs, *p*-aminosalicyclic acid, interferon-α and other cytokines, aminoglutethimide
  Congenital hypothyroidism: absent or ectopic thyroid gland, dyshormonogenesis, TSH-R mutation
  Iodine deficiency
  Infiltrative disorders: amyloidosis, sarcoidosis, hemochromatosis, scleroderma, cystinosis, Riedel's thyroiditis
  Overexpression of type 3 deoiodinase in infantile hemangioma
Transient
  Silent thyroiditis, including postpartum thyroiditis
  Subacute thyroiditis
  Withdrawal of thyroxine treatment in individuals with an intact thyroid
  After ^{131}I treatment or subtotal thyroidectomy for Graves' disease
Secondary
  Hypopituitarism: tumors, pituitary surgery or irradiation, infiltrative disorders, Sheehan's syndrome, trauma, genetic forms of combined pituitary hormone deficiencies
  Isolated TSH deficiency or inactivity
  Bexarotene treatment
  Hypothalamic disease: tumors, trauma, infiltrative disorders, idiopathic

Note: TSH, thyroid-stimulating hormone; TSH-R, TSH receptor.

TABLE 320-5 *Signs and Symptoms of Hypothyroidism (Descending Order of Frequency)*

Symptoms	Signs
Tiredness, weakness	Dry coarse skin; cool peripheral extremities
Dry skin	
Feeling cold	Puffy face, hands, and feet (myxedema)
Hair loss	
Difficulty concentrating and poor memory	Diffuse alopecia
Constipation	Bradycardia
Weight gain with poor appetite	Peripheral edema
Dyspnea	Delayed tendon reflex relaxation
Hoarse voice	Carpal tunnel syndrome
Menorrhagia (later oligomenorrhea or amenorrhea)	Serous cavity effusions
Paresthesia	
Impaired hearing	

AUTOIMMUNE HYPOTHYROIDISM ■ Classification Autoimmune hypothyroidism may be associated with a goiter (Hashimoto's, or *goitrous thyroiditis*) or, at the later stages of the disease, minimal residual thyroid tissue (*atrophic thyroiditis*). Because the autoimmune process gradually reduces thyroid function, there is a phase of compensation when normal thyroid hormone levels are maintained by a rise in TSH. Though some patients may have minor symptoms, this state is called *subclinical hypothyroidism* or *mild hypothyroidism*. Later, free T_4 levels fall and TSH levels rise further; symptoms become more readily apparent at this stage (usually TSH > 10 mU/L), which is referred to as *clinical hypothyroidism* or *overt hypothyroidism*.

Prevalence The mean annual incidence rate of autoimmune hypothyroidism is up to 4 per 1000 women and 1 per 1000 men. It is more common in certain populations, such as the Japanese, probably because of genetic factors and chronic exposure to a high-iodine diet. The mean age at diagnosis is 60 years, and the prevalence of overt hypothyroidism increases with age. Subclinical hypothyroidism is found in 6 to 8% of women (10% over the age of 60) and 3% of men. The annual risk of developing clinical hypothyroidism is about 4% when subclinical hypothyroidism is associated with positive TPO antibodies.

Pathogenesis In Hashimoto's thyroiditis, there is a marked lymphocytic infiltration of the thyroid with germinal center formation, atrophy of the thyroid follicles accompanied by oxyphil metaplasia, absence of colloid, and mild to moderate fibrosis. In atrophic thyroiditis, the fibrosis is much more extensive, lymphocyte infiltration is less pronounced, and thyroid follicles are almost completely absent. Atrophic thyroiditis likely represents the end stage of Hashimoto's thyroiditis rather than a distinct disorder.

As with most autoimmune disorders, susceptibility to autoimmune hypothyroidism is determined by a combination of genetic and environmental factors, and the risk of either autoimmune hypothyroidism or Graves' disease is increased among siblings. HLA-DR polymorphisms are the best documented genetic risk factors for autoimmune hypothyroidism, especially HLA-DR3, -DR4, and -DR5 in Caucasians. A weak association also exists between polymorphisms in *CTLA-4*, a T cell–regulating gene, and autoimmune hypothyroidism. Both of these genetic associations are shared by other autoimmune diseases, which may explain the relationship between autoimmune hypothyroidism and other autoimmune diseases, especially type 1 diabetes mellitus, Addison disease, pernicious anemia, and vitiligo (Chap. 330). HLA-DR and *CTLA-4* polymorphisms account for approximately half of the genetic susceptibility to autoimmune hypothyroidism. The other contributory loci remain to be identified. A gene on chromosome 21 may be responsible for the association between autoimmune hypothyroidism and Down syndrome. The female preponderance of thyroid autoimmunity is most likely due to the effects of sex steroids on the immune response, but an X chromosome–related genetic factor is also possible, which may account for the high frequency of autoimmune hypothyroidism in Turner syndrome. Environmental susceptibility factors are also poorly defined at present. A high iodine intake may increase the risk of autoimmune hypothyroidism by immunologic effects or direct thyroid toxicity. There is no convincing evidence for a role of infection, except for the congenital rubella syndrome, in which there is a high frequency of autoimmune hypothyroidism. Viral thyroiditis does not induce subsequent autoimmune thyroid disease.

The thyroid lymphocytic infiltrate in autoimmune hypothyroidism is composed of activated CD4+ and CD8+ T cells, as well as B cells. Thyroid cell destruction is believed to be primarily mediated by the CD8+ cytotoxic T cells, which destroy their targets by either perforin-induced cell necrosis or granzyme B–induced apoptosis. In addition, local T cell production of cytokines, such as tumor necrosis factor (TNF), IL-1, and interferon (IFN) γ, may render thyroid cells more susceptible to apoptosis mediated by death receptors, such as Fas, which are activated by their respective ligands on T cells. These cytokines also impair thyroid cell function directly, and induce the expression of other proinflammatory molecules by the thyroid cells themselves, such as cytokines, HLA class I and class II molecules, adhesion molecules, CD40, and nitric oxide. Administration of high concentrations of cytokines for therapeutic purposes (especially IFN-α) is associated with increased autoimmune thyroid disease, possibly through mechanisms similar to those in sporadic disease.

Antibodies to Tg and TPO are clinically useful markers of thyroid autoimmunity, but any pathogenic effect is restricted to a secondary role in amplifying an ongoing autoimmune response. TPO antibodies fix complement, and complement membrane attack complexes are present in the thyroid in autoimmune hypothyroidism. However, transplacental passage of Tg or TPO antibodies has no effect on the fetal thyroid, which suggests that T cell–mediated injury is required to initiate autoimmune damage to the thyroid. Up to 20% of patients with autoimmune hypothyroidism have antibodies against the TSH-R, which, in contrast to TSI, do not stimulate the receptor but prevent the binding of TSH. These TSH-R-blocking antibodies therefore cause hypothyroidism and, especially in Asian patients, thyroid atrophy. Their transplacental passage may induce transient neonatal hypothyroidism. Rarely, patients have a mixture of TSI- and TSH-R-blocking antibodies, and thyroid function can oscillate between hyperthyroidism and hypothyroidism as one or the other antibody becomes dominant. Predicting the course of disease in such individuals is difficult, and they require close monitoring of thyroid function. Bioassays can be used to document that TSH-R-blocking antibodies reduce the cyclic AMP–inducing effect of TSH on cultured TSH-R-expressing cells, but these assays are difficult to perform. Assays that measure the binding of antibodies to the receptor by competition with radiolabeled TSH [TSH-binding inhibiting immunoglobulins (TBII)] do not distinguish between TSI- and TSH-R-blocking antibodies, but a positive result in a patient with spontaneous hypothyroidism is strong evidence for the presence of blocking antibodies. The use of these assays does not generally alter clinical management, although they may be useful to confirm the cause of transient neonatal hypothyroidism.

Clinical Manifestations The main clinical features of hypothyroidism are summarized in Table 320-5. The onset is usually insidious, and the patient may become aware of symptoms only when euthyroidism is restored. Patients with Hashimoto's thyroiditis may present because of goiter rather than symptoms of hypothyroidism. The goiter may not be large but is usually irregular and firm in consistency. It is often possible to palpate a pyramidal lobe, normally a vestigial remnant of the thyroglossal duct. Rarely, uncomplicated Hashimoto's thyroiditis is associated with pain.

Patients with atrophic thyroiditis, or the late stage of Hashimoto's thyroiditis, present with symptoms and signs of hypothyroidism. The skin is dry, and there is decreased sweating, thinning of the epidermis, and hyperkeratosis of the stratum corneum. Increased dermal glycosaminoglycan content traps water, giving rise to skin thickening without pitting (*myxedema*). Typical features include a puffy face with edematous eyelids and nonpitting pretibial edema (Fig. 320-4). There is pallor, often with a yellow tinge to the skin due to carotene accumulation. Nail growth is retarded, and hair is dry, brittle, difficult to manage, and falls out easily. In addition to diffuse alopecia, there is thinning of the outer third of the eyebrows, although this is not a specific sign of hypothyroidism.

Other common features include constipation and weight gain (despite a poor appetite). In contrast to popular perception, the weight gain is usually modest and due mainly to fluid retention in the myxedematous tissues. Libido is decreased in both sexes, and there may be oligomenorrhea or amenorrhea in long-standing disease, but menorrhagia is also common. Fertility is reduced and the incidence of miscarriage is increased. Prolactin levels are often modestly increased (Chap. 318) and may contribute to alterations in libido and fertility and cause galactorrhea.

Myocardial contractility and pulse rate are reduced, leading to a

FIGURE 320-4 Facial appearance in hypothyroidism. Note puffy eyes and thickened, pale skin.

reduced stroke volume and bradycardia. Increased peripheral resistance may be accompanied by hypertension, particularly diastolic. Blood flow is diverted from the skin, producing the cool extremities. Pericardial effusions occur in up to 30% of patients but rarely compromise cardiac function. Though alterations in myosin heavy chain isoform expression have been documented, cardiomyopathy is unusual. Fluid may also accumulate in other serous cavities and in the middle ear, giving rise to conductive deafness. Pulmonary function is generally normal, but dyspnea may be caused by pleural effusion, impaired respiratory muscle function, diminished ventilatory drive, or sleep apnea.

Carpal tunnel and other entrapment syndromes are common, as is impairment of muscle function with stiffness, cramps, and pain. On examination, there may be slow relaxation of tendon reflexes and pseudomyotonia. Memory and concentration are impaired. Rare neurologic problems include reversible cerebellar ataxia, dementia, psychosis, and myxedema coma. *Hashimoto's encephalopathy* is a rare and distinctive syndrome associated with myoclonus and slow-wave activity on electroencephalography, which can progress to confusion, coma, and death. It is steroid-responsive and may occur in the presence of autoimmune thyroiditis, without hypothyroidism. The hoarse voice and occasionally clumsy speech of hypothyroidism reflect fluid accumulation in the vocal cords and tongue.

The features described above are the consequence of thyroid hormone deficiency. However, autoimmune hypothyroidism may be associated with signs or symptoms of other autoimmune diseases, particularly vitiligo, pernicious anemia, Addison disease, alopecia areata, and type 1 diabetes mellitus. Less common associations include celiac disease, dermatitis herpetiformis, chronic active hepatitis, rheumatoid arthritis, systemic lupus erythematosus (SLE), and Sjögren's syndrome. Thyroid-associated ophthalmopathy, which usually occurs in Graves' disease (see below), occurs in about 5% of patients with autoimmune hypothyroidism.

Autoimmune hypothyroidism is uncommon in children and usually presents with slow growth and delayed facial maturation. The appearance of permanent teeth is also delayed. Myopathy, with muscle swelling, is more common in children than in adults. In most cases, puberty is delayed, but precocious puberty sometimes occurs. There may be intellectual impairment if the onset is before 3 years and the hormone deficiency is severe.

Laboratory Evaluation A summary of the investigations used to determine the existence and cause of hypothyroidism is provided in Fig. 320-5. A normal TSH level excludes primary (but not secondary) hypothyroidism. If the TSH is elevated, an unbound T_4 level is needed to confirm the presence of clinical hypothyroidism, but T_4 is inferior to TSH when used as a screening test, as it will not detect subclinical or mild hypothyroidism. Circulating unbound T_3 levels are normal in about 25% of patients, reflecting adaptive responses to hypothyroidism. T_3 measurements are therefore not indicated.

Once clinical or subclinical hypothyroidism is confirmed, the etiology is usually easily established by demonstrating the presence of TPO antibodies, which are present in 90 to 95% of patients with autoimmune hypothyroidism. TBII can be found in 10 to 20% of patients, but these determinations are not needed routinely. If there is any doubt about the cause of a goiter associated with hypothyroidism, FNA biopsy can be used to confirm the presence of autoimmune thyroiditis. Other abnormal laboratory findings in hypothyroidism may include increased creatine phosphokinase, elevated cholesterol and triglycerides, and anemia (usually normocytic or macrocytic). Except when accompanied by iron deficiency, the anemia and other abnormalities gradually resolve with thyroxine replacement.

Differential Diagnosis An asymmetric goiter in Hashimoto's thyroiditis may be confused with a multinodular goiter or thyroid carcinoma, in which thyroid antibodies may also be present. Ultrasound can be used to show the presence of a solitary lesion or a multinodular goiter, rather than the heterogeneous thyroid enlargement typical of Hashimoto's thyroiditis. FNA biopsy is useful in the investigation of focal nodules. Other causes of hypothyroidism are discussed below but rarely cause diagnostic confusion (Table 320-4).

OTHER CAUSES OF HYPOTHYROIDISM *Iatrogenic hypothyroidism* is a common cause of hypothyroidism and can often be detected by screening before symptoms develop. In the first 3 to 4 months after radioiodine treatment, transient hypothyroidism may occur due to reversible radiation damage rather than to cellular destruction. Low-dose thyroxine treatment can be withdrawn if recovery occurs. Because TSH levels are suppressed by hyperthyroidism, unbound T_4 levels are a better measure of thyroid function than TSH in the months following ra-

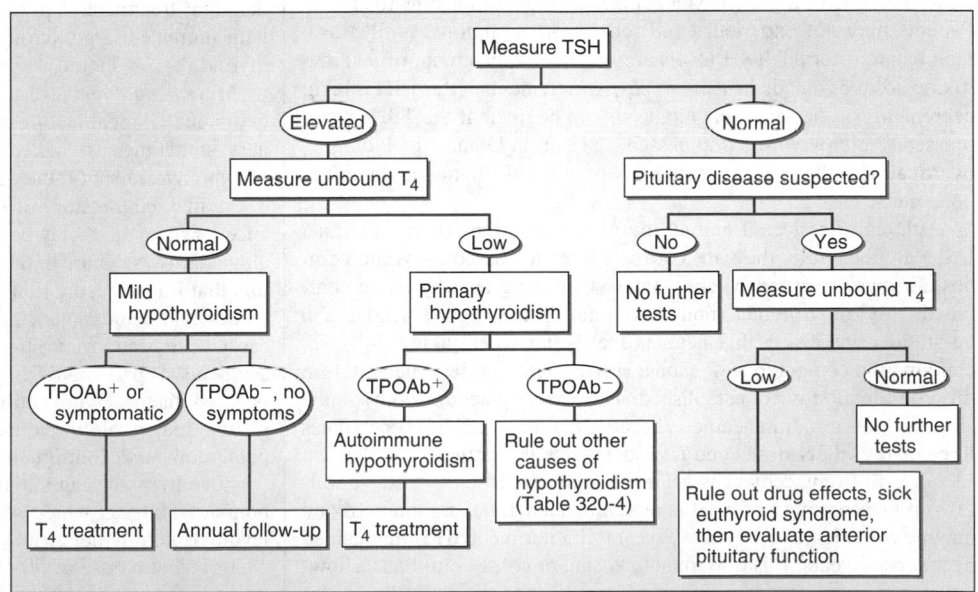

FIGURE 320-5 Evaluation of hypothyroidism. TPOAb⁺, thyroid peroxidase antibodies present; TPOAb⁻, thyroid peroxidase antibodies not present. TSH, thyroid-stimulating hormone.

dioiodine treatment. Mild hypothyroidism after subtotal thyroidectomy may also resolve after several months, as the gland remnant is stimulated by increased TSH levels.

Iodine deficiency is responsible for endemic goiter and cretinism but is an uncommon cause of adult hypothyroidism unless the iodine intake is very low or there are complicating factors, such as the consumption of thiocyanates in cassava or selenium deficiency. Though hypothyroidism due to iodine deficiency can be treated with thyroxine, public health measures to improve iodine intake should be advocated to eliminate this problem. Iodized salt or bread or a single bolus of oral or intramuscular iodized oil have all been used successfully.

Paradoxically, chronic iodine excess can also induce goiter and hypothyroidism. The intracellular events that account for this effect are unclear, but individuals with autoimmune thyroiditis are especially susceptible. Iodine excess is responsible for the hypothyroidism that occurs in up to 13% of patients treated with amiodarone (see below). Other drugs, particularly lithium, may also cause hypothyroidism. Transient hypothyroidism caused by thyroiditis is discussed below.

Secondary hypothyroidism is usually diagnosed in the context of other anterior pituitary hormone deficiencies; isolated TSH deficiency is very rare (Chap. 318). TSH levels may be low, normal, or even slightly increased in secondary hypothyroidism; the latter is due to secretion of immunoactive but bioinactive forms of TSH. The diagnosis is confirmed by detecting a low unbound T_4 level. The goal of treatment is to maintain unbound T_4 levels in the upper half of the reference range, as TSH levels cannot be used to monitor therapy.

℞ TREATMENT

Clinical Hypothyroidism If there is no residual thyroid function, the daily replacement dose of levothyroxine is usually 1.6 μg/kg body weight (typically 100 to 150 μg). In many patients, however, lower doses suffice until residual thyroid tissue is destroyed. In patients who develop hypothyroidism after the treatment of Graves' disease, there is often underlying autonomous function, necessitating lower replacement doses (typically 75 to 125 μg/d).

Adult patients under 60 without evidence of heart disease may be started on 50 to 100 μg levothyroxine (T_4) daily. The dose is adjusted on the basis of TSH levels, with the goal of treatment being a normal TSH, ideally in the lower half of the reference range. TSH responses are gradual and should be measured about 2 months after instituting treatment or after any subsequent change in levothyroxine dosage. The clinical effects of levothyroxine replacement are often slow to appear. Patients may not experience full relief from symptoms until 3 to 6 months after normal TSH levels are restored. Adjustment of levothyroxine dosage is made in 12.5- or 25-μg increments if the TSH is high; decrements of the same magnitude should be made if the TSH is suppressed. Patients with a suppressed TSH of any cause, including T_4 overtreatment, have an increased risk of atrial fibrillation and reduced bone density.

Although dessicated animal thyroid preparations (thyroid extract USP) are available, they are not recommended as potency and composition vary between batches. Interest in using levothyroxine combined with liothyronine (triiodothyronine, T_3) has been revived, based on studies suggesting that patients feel better when taking the T_4/T_3 combination compared to T_4 alone. However, a long-term benefit from this combination is not established. There is no place for liothyronine alone as long-term replacement, because the short half-life necessitates three or four daily doses and is associated with fluctuating T_3 levels.

Once full replacement is achieved and TSH levels are stable, follow-up measurement of TSH is recommended at annual intervals and may be extended to every 2 to 3 years, if a normal TSH is maintained over several years. It is important to ensure ongoing compliance, however, as patients do not feel any difference after missing a few doses of levothyroxine, this sometimes leads to self-discontinuation.

In patients of normal body weight who are taking ≥200 μg of levothyroxine per day, an elevated TSH level is often a sign of poor compliance. This is also the likely explanation for fluctuating TSH levels, despite a constant levothyroxine dosage. Such patients often have normal or high unbound T_4 levels, despite an elevated TSH, because they remember to take medication for a few days before testing; this is sufficient to normalize T_4, but not TSH, levels. It is important to consider variable compliance, as this pattern of thyroid function tests is otherwise suggestive of disorders associated with inappropriate TSH secretion (Table 320-3). Because T_4 has a long half-life (7 days), patients who miss doses can be advised to take up to three doses of the skipped tablets at once. Other causes of increased levothyroxine requirements must be excluded, particularly malabsorption (e.g., celiac disease, small-bowel surgery), estrogen therapy, and drugs that interfere with T_4 absorption or clearance such as cholestyramine, ferrous sulfate, calcium supplements, lovastatin, aluminum hydroxide, rifampicin, amiodarone, carbamazepine, and phenytoin.

Mild Hypothyroidism By definition, subclinical or mild hypothyroidism refers to biochemical evidence of thyroid hormone deficiency in patients who have few or no apparent clinical features of hypothyroidism. There are no universally accepted guidelines for the treatment of mild hypothyroidism. As long as excessive treatment is avoided, there is little risk in correcting a slightly increased TSH, and some patients likely derive modest clinical benefit from treatment. Moreover, there is some risk that patients will progress to overt hypothyroidism, particularly when the TSH level is >6 mU/L and TPO antibodies are present. Treatment is administered by starting with a low dose of levothyroxine (25 to 50 μg/d) with the goal of normalizing TSH. If thyroxine is not given, thyroid function should be evaluated annually.

Special Treatment Considerations Rarely, levothyroxine replacement is associated with pseudotumor cerebri in *children*. Presentation appears to be idiosyncratic and occurs months after treatment has begun. Women with a history or high risk of hypothyroidism should ensure that they are euthyroid prior to conception and during early pregnancy as maternal hypothyroidism may adversely affect fetal neural development. Thyroid function should be evaluated once pregnancy is confirmed and at the beginning of the second and third trimesters. The dose of levothyroxine may need to be increased by ≥50% during pregnancy and returned to previous levels after delivery. *Elderly* patients may require up to 20% less thyroxine than younger patients. In the elderly, especially patients with known coronary artery disease, the starting dose of levothyroxine is 12.5 to 25 μg/d with similar increments every 2 to 3 months until TSH is normalized. In some patients it may be impossible to achieve full replacement, despite optimal antianginal treatment. *Emergency surgery* is generally safe in patients with untreated hypothyroidism, although routine surgery in a hypothyroid patient should be deferred until euthyroidism is achieved.

Myxedema coma still has a high mortality rate, despite intensive treatment. Clinical manifestations include reduced level of consciousness, sometimes associated with seizures, as well as the other features of hypothyroidism (Table 320-5). Hypothermia can reach 23°C (74°F). There may be a history of treated hypothyroidism with poor compliance, or the patient may be previously undiagnosed. Myxedema coma almost always occurs in the elderly and is usually precipitated by factors that impair respiration, such as drugs (especially sedatives, anesthetics, antidepressants), pneumonia, congestive heart failure, myocardial infarction, gastrointestinal bleeding, or cerebrovascular accidents. Sepsis should also be suspected. Exposure to cold may also be a risk factor. Hypoventilation, leading to hypoxia and hypercapnia, plays a major role in pathogenesis; hypoglycemia and dilutional hyponatremia also contribute to the development of myxedema coma.

Levothyroxine can initially be administered as a single intravenous bolus of 500 μg, which serves as a loading dose. Although further levothyroxine is not strictly necessary for several days, it is usually continued at a dose of 50 to 100 μg/d. If suitable intravenous preparation is not available, the same initial dose of levothyroxine can be given by nasogastric tube (though absorption may be impaired in myxedema). An alternative is to give liothyronine (T_3) intravenously or via nasogastric tube, in doses ranging from 10 to 25 μg every 8 to 12 h. This treatment has been advocated because $T_4 \rightarrow T_3$ conversion is impaired in myxedema coma. However, excess liothyroxine has the potential to provoke arrhythmias. Another option is to combine levothyroxine (200 μg) and liothyronine (25 μg) as a single, initial intravenous bolus followed by daily treatment with levothyroxine (50 to 100 μg/d) and liothyronine (10 μg every 8 h).

Supportive therapy should be provided to correct any associated metabolic disturbances. External warming is indicated only if the temperature is <30°C, as it can result in cardiovascular collapse (Chap. 16). Space blankets should be used to prevent further heat loss. Parenteral hydrocortisone (50 mg every 6 h) should be administered, as there is impaired adrenal reserve in profound hypothyroidism. Any precipitating factors should be treated, including the early use of broad-spectrum antibiotics, pending the exclusion of infection. Ventilatory support with regular blood gas analysis is usually needed during the first 48 h. Hypertonic saline or intravenous glucose may be needed if there is hyponatremia or hypoglycemia; hypotonic intravenous fluids should be avoided because they may exacerbate water retention secondary to reduced renal perfusion and inappropriate vasopressin secretion. The metabolism of most medications is impaired, and sedatives should be avoided if possible or used in reduced doses. Medication blood levels should be monitored, when available, to guide dosage.

THYROTOXICOSIS

Thyrotoxicosis is defined as the state of thyroid hormone excess and is not synonymous with *hyperthyroidism*, which is the result of excessive thyroid function. However, the major etiologies of thyrotoxicosis are hyperthyroidism caused by Graves' disease, toxic multinodular goiter, and toxic adenomas. Other causes are listed in Table 320-6.

GRAVES' DISEASE ▪ Epidemiology Graves' disease accounts for 60 to 80% of thyrotoxicosis, but the prevalence varies among populations, depending mainly on iodine intake (high iodine intake is associated with an increased prevalence of Graves' disease). Graves' disease occurs in up to 2% of women but is one-tenth as frequent in men. The disorder rarely begins before adolescence and typically occurs between 20 and 50 years of age, but it also occurs in the elderly.

PATHOGENESIS As in autoimmune hypothyroidism, a combination of genetic factors, including HLA-DR and *CTLA-4* polymorphisms, and environmental factors contribute to Graves' disease susceptibility. The concordance for Graves' disease in monozygotic twins is 20 to 30%,

compared to <5% in dizygotic twins. Indirect evidence suggests that stress is an important environmental factor, presumably operating through neuroendocrine effects on the immune system. Smoking is a minor risk factor for Graves' disease and a major risk factor for the development of ophthalmopathy. Sudden increases in iodine intake may precipitate Graves' disease, and there is a threefold increase in the occurrence of Graves' disease in the postpartum period.

The hyperthyroidism of Graves' disease is caused by TSI that are synthesized in the thyroid gland as well as in bone marrow and lymph nodes. Such antibodies can be detected by bioassays or using the more widely available TBII assays. The presence of TBII in a patient with thyrotoxicosis is strong indirect evidence for the existence of TSI, and these assays are useful in monitoring pregnant Graves' patients in whom high levels of TSI can cross the placenta and cause neonatal thyrotoxicosis. Other thyroid autoimmune responses, similar to those in autoimmune hypothyroidism (see above), occur concurrently in patients with Graves' disease. In particular, TPO antibodies occur in up to 80% of cases and serve as a readily measurable marker of autoimmunity. Because T cell–mediated cytotoxicity can also affect thyroid function, there is no direct correlation between the level of TSI and thyroid hormone levels. In the long term, spontaneous autoimmune hypothyroidism may develop in up to 15% of Graves' patients.

Cytokines appear to play a major role in thyroid-associated ophthalmopathy. There is infiltration of the extraocular muscles by activated T cells; the release of cytokines such as IFN-γ, TNF, and IL-1 results in fibroblast activation and increased synthesis of glycosaminoglycans that trap water, thereby leading to characteristic muscle swelling. Late in the disease, there is fibrosis and only then do the muscle cells show evidence of injury. Orbital fibroblasts may be uniquely sensitive to cytokines, perhaps explaining the anatomic localization of the immune response. Though the pathogenesis of thyroid-associated ophthalmopathy remains unclear, there is mounting evidence that expression of the TSH-R may provide an important orbital autoantigen. In support of this idea, injection of TSH-R into certain strains of mice induces autoimmune hyperthyroidism, as well as features of ophthalmopathy. A variety of autoantibodies against orbital muscle and fibroblast antigens have been detected in patients with ophthalmopathy, but these antibodies most likely arise as a secondary phenomenon, dependent on T cell–mediated autoimmune responses. Similar mechanisms are involved in dermopathy.

Clinical Manifestations Signs and symptoms include features that are common to any cause of thyrotoxicosis (Table 320-7) as well as those specific for Graves' disease. The clinical presentation depends on the severity of thyrotoxicosis, the duration of disease, individual susceptibility to excess thyroid hormone, and the patient's age. In the elderly, features of thyrotoxicosis may be subtle or masked, and patients may present mainly with fatigue and weight loss, leading to *apathetic hyperthyroidism*.

Thyrotoxicosis may cause unexplained weight loss, despite an enhanced appetite, due to the increased metabolic rate. Weight gain occurs in 5% of patients, however, because of increased food intake.

TABLE 320-6 *Causes of Thyrotoxicosis*

Primary hyperthyroidism
Graves' disease
Toxic multinodular goiter
Toxic adenoma
Functioning thyroid carcinoma metastases
Activating mutation of the TSH receptor
Activating mutation of $G_{s\alpha}$ (McCune-Albright syndrome)
Struma ovarii
Drugs: iodine excess (Jod-Basedow phenomenon)
Thyrotoxicosis without hyperthyroidism
Subacute thyroiditis
Silent thyroiditis
Other causes of thyroid destruction: amiodarone, radiation, infarction of adenoma
Ingestion of excess thyroid hormone (thyrotoxicosis factitia) or thyroid tissue
Secondary hyperthyroidism
TSH-secreting pituitary adenoma
Thyroid hormone resistance syndrome: occasional patients may have features of thyrotoxicosis
Chorionic gonadotropin-secreting tumors[a]
Gestational thyrotoxicosis[a]

[a] Circulating TSH levels are low in these forms of secondary hyperthyroidism.
Note: TSH, thyroid-stimulating hormone.

TABLE 320-7 *Signs and Symptoms of Thyrotoxicosis (Descending Order of Frequency)*

Symptoms	Signs[a]
Hyperactivity, irritability, dysphoria	Tachycardia; atrial fibrillation in the elderly
Heat intolerance and sweating	Tremor
Palpitations	Goiter
Fatigue and weakness	Warm, moist skin
Weight loss with increased appetite	Muscle weakness, proximal myopathy
Diarrhea	Lid retraction or lag
Polyuria	Gynecomastia
Oligomenorrhea, loss of libido	

[a] Excludes the signs of ophthalmopathy and dermopathy specific for Graves' disease.

FIGURE 320-6 Features of Graves' disease. *A*. Facial appearance in Graves' disease; lid retraction, periorbital edema, and proptosis are marked. *B*. Thyroid dermopathy over the lateral aspects of the shins. *C*. Thyroid acropachy.

In Graves' disease the thyroid is usually diffusely enlarged to two to three times its normal size. The consistency is firm, but less so than in multinodular goiter. There may be a thrill or bruit due to the increased vascularity of the gland and the hyperdynamic circulation.

Lid retraction, causing a staring appearance, can occur in any form of thyrotoxicosis and is the result of sympathetic overactivity. However, Graves' disease is associated with specific eye signs that comprise *Graves' ophthalmopathy* (Fig. 320-6*A*). This condition is also called *thyroid-associated ophthalmopathy*, as it occurs in the absence of Graves' disease in 10% of patients. Most of these individuals have autoimmune hypothyroidism or thyroid antibodies. The onset of Graves' ophthalmopathy occurs within the year before or after the diagnosis of thyrotoxicosis in 75% of patients but can sometimes precede or follow thyrotoxicosis by several years, accounting for some cases of euthyroid ophthalmopathy.

Many patients with Graves' disease have little clinical evidence of ophthalmopathy. However, the enlarged extraocular muscles typical of the disease, and other subtle features, can be detected in almost all patients when investigated by ultrasound or computed tomography (CT) imaging of the orbits. Unilateral signs are found in up to 10% of patients. The earliest manifestations of ophthalmopathy are usually a sensation of grittiness, eye discomfort, and excess tearing. About a third of patients have proptosis, best detected by visualization of the sclera between the lower border of the iris and the lower eyelid, with the eyes in the primary position. Proptosis can be measured using an exophthalmometer. In severe cases, proptosis may cause corneal exposure and damage, especially if the lids fail to close during sleep. Periorbital edema, scleral injection, and chemosis are also frequent. In 5 to 10% of patients, the muscle swelling is so severe that diplopia results, typically but not exclusively when the patient looks up and laterally. The most serious manifestation is compression of the optic nerve at the apex of the orbit, leading to papilledema, peripheral field defects, and, if left untreated, permanent loss of vision.

Many scoring systems have been used to gauge the extent and activity of the orbital changes in Graves' disease. The "NO SPECS" scheme is an acronym derived from the following classes of eye change:

0 = <u>N</u>o signs or symptoms
1 = <u>O</u>nly signs (lid retraction or lag), no symptoms
2 = <u>S</u>oft tissue involvement (periorbital edema)
3 = <u>P</u>roptosis (>22 mm)
4 = <u>E</u>xtraocular muscle involvement (diplopia)
5 = <u>C</u>orneal involvement
6 = <u>S</u>ight loss

Although useful as a mnemonic, the NO SPECS scheme is inadequate to describe the eye disease fully, and patients do not necessarily progress from one class to another. When Graves' eye disease is active and severe, referral to an ophthalmologist is indicated and objective measurements are needed, such as lid fissure width; corneal staining with fluorescein; and evaluation of extraocular muscle function (e.g., Hess chart), intraocular pressure and visual fields, acuity, and color vision.

Thyroid dermopathy occurs in <5% of patients with Graves' dis-

Other prominent features include hyperactivity, nervousness, and irritability, ultimately leading to a sense of easy fatiguability in some patients. Insomnia and impaired concentration are common; apathetic thyrotoxicosis may be mistaken for depression in the elderly. Fine tremor is a frequent finding, best elicited by having patients stretch out their fingers and feeling the fingertips with the palm. Common neurologic manifestations include hyperreflexia, muscle wasting, and proximal myopathy without fasciculation. Chorea is a rare feature. Thyrotoxicosis is sometimes associated with a form of hypokalemic periodic paralysis; this disorder is particularly common in Asian males with thyrotoxicosis.

The most common cardiovascular manifestation is sinus tachycardia, often associated with palpitations, occasionally caused by supraventricular tachycardia. The high cardiac output produces a bounding pulse, widened pulse pressure, and an aortic systolic murmur and can lead to worsening of angina or heart failure in the elderly or those with preexisting heart disease. Atrial fibrillation is more common in patients >50 years. Treatment of the thyrotoxic state alone reverts atrial fibrillation to normal sinus rhythm in fewer than half of patients, suggesting the existence of an underlying cardiac problem in the remainder.

The skin is usually warm and moist, and the patient may complain of sweating and heat intolerance, particularly during warm weather. Palmar erythema; onycholysis; and, less commonly, pruritus, urticaria, and diffuse hyperpigmentation may be evident. Hair texture may become fine, and a diffuse alopecia occurs in up to 40% of patients, persisting for months after restoration of euthyroidism. Gastrointestinal transit time is decreased, leading to increased stool frequency, often with diarrhea and occasionally mild steatorrhea. Women frequently experience oligomenorrhea or amenorrhea; in men there may be impaired sexual function and, rarely, gynecomastia. The direct effect of thyroid hormones on bone resorption leads to osteopenia in long-standing thyrotoxicosis; mild hypercalcemia occurs in up to 20% of patients, but hypercalciuria is more common. There is a small increase in fracture rate in patients with a previous history of thyrotoxicosis.

ease (Fig. 320-6*B*), almost always in the presence of moderate or severe ophthalmopathy. Although most frequent over the anterior and lateral aspects of the lower leg (hence the term *pretibial myxedema*), skin changes can occur at other sites, particularly after trauma. The typical lesion is a noninflamed, indurated plaque with a deep pink or purple color and an "orange-skin" appearance. Nodular involvement can occur, and the condition can rarely extend over the whole lower leg and foot, mimicking elephantiasis. *Thyroid acropachy* refers to a form of clubbing found in <1% of patients with Graves' disease (Fig. 320-6*C*). It is so strongly associated with thyroid dermopathy that an alternative cause of clubbing should be sought in a Graves' patient without coincident skin and orbital involvement.

Laboratory Evaluation   Investigations used to determine the existence and cause of thyrotoxicosis are summarized in Fig. 320-7. In Graves' disease, the TSH level is suppressed and total and unbound thyroid hormone levels are increased. In 2 to 5% of patients (and more in areas of borderline iodine intake), only T_3 is increased (T_3 toxicosis). The converse state of T_4 toxicosis, with elevated total and unbound T_4 and normal T_3 levels, is occasionally seen when hyperthyroidism is induced by excess iodine, providing surplus substrate for thyroid hormone synthesis. Measurement of TPO antibodies is useful in differential diagnosis. Measurement of TBII or TSI will confirm the diagnosis but is not needed routinely. Associated abnormalities that may cause diagnostic confusion in thyrotoxicosis include elevation of bilirubin, liver enzymes, and ferritin. Microcytic anemia and thrombocytopenia may occur.

Differential Diagnosis   Diagnosis of Graves' disease is straightforward in a patient with biochemically confirmed thyrotoxicosis, diffuse goiter on palpation, ophthalmopathy, positive TPO antibodies, and often a personal or family history of autoimmune disorders. For patients with thyrotoxicosis who lack these features, the most reliable diagnostic method is a radionuclide (^{99m}Tc, ^{123}I, or ^{131}I) scan of the thyroid, which will distinguish the diffuse, high uptake of Graves' disease from nodular thyroid disease, destructive thyroiditis, ectopic thyroid tissue, and factitious thyrotoxicosis. In secondary hyperthyroidism due to a TSH-secreting pituitary tumor, there is also a diffuse goiter. The presence of a nonsuppressed TSH level and the finding of a pituitary tumor on CT or magnetic resonance imaging (MRI) scan readily identify such patients.

Clinical features of thyrotoxicosis can mimic certain aspects of other disorders including panic attacks, mania, pheochromocytoma, and the weight loss associated with malignancy. The diagnosis of thyrotoxicosis can be easily excluded if the TSH and T_3 levels are normal. A normal TSH also excludes Graves' disease as a cause of diffuse goiter.

Clinical Course   Clinical features generally worsen without treatment; mortality was 10 to 30% before the introduction of satisfactory therapy. Some patients with mild Graves' disease experience spontaneous relapses and remissions. Rarely, there may be fluctuation between hypo- and hyperthyroidism due to changes in the functional activity of TSH-R antibodies. About 15% of patients who enter remission after treatment with antithyroid drugs develop hypothyroidism 10 to 15 years later as a result of the destructive autoimmune process. The

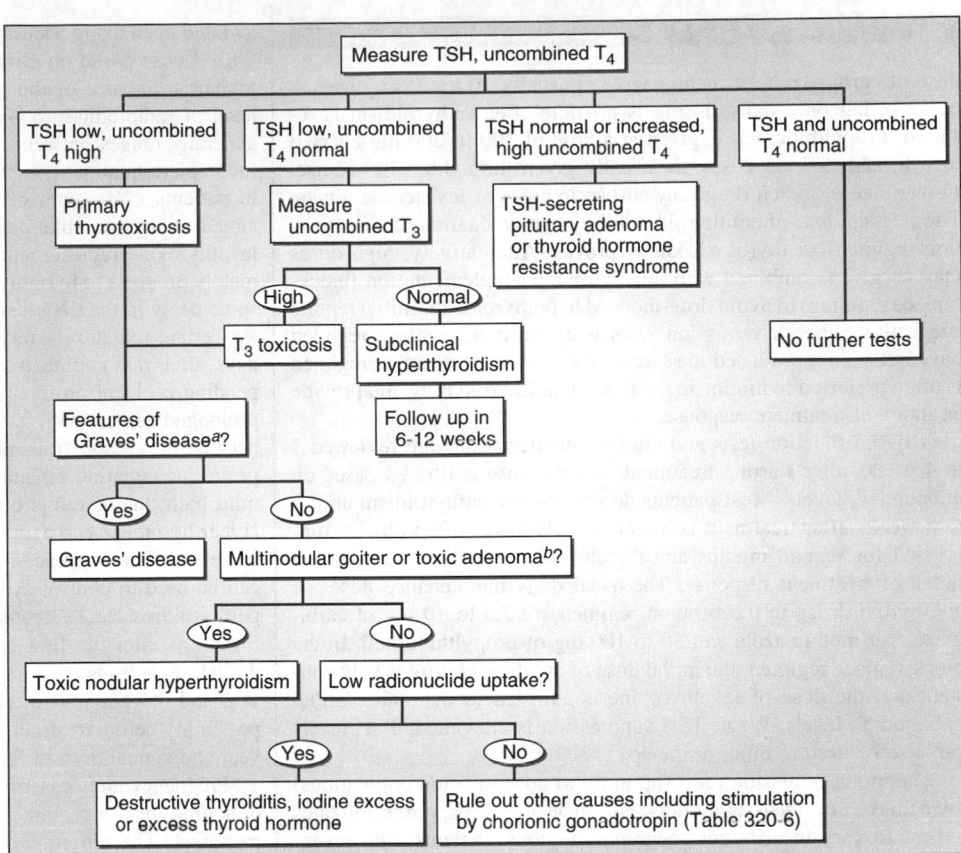

FIGURE 320-7   Evaluation of thyrotoxicosis. *ᵃDiffuse goiter, positive TPO antibodies, ophthalmopathy, dermopathy; ᵇcan be confirmed by radionuclide scan. TSH, thyroid-stimulating hormone.

clinical course of ophthalmopathy does not follow that of the thyroid disease. Ophthalmopathy typically worsens over the initial 3 to 6 months, followed by a plateau phase over the next 12 to 18 months, with spontaneous improvement, particularly in the soft tissue changes. However, the course is more fulminant in up to 5% of patients, requiring intervention in the acute phase if there is optic nerve compression or corneal ulceration. Diplopia may appear late in the disease due to fibrosis of the extraocular muscles. Some studies suggest that radioiodine treatment for hyperthyroidism worsens the eye disease in a small proportion of patients (especially smokers). Antithyroid drugs or surgery have no adverse effects on the clinical course of ophthalmopathy. Thyroid dermopathy, when it occurs, usually appears 1 to 2 years after the development of Graves' hyperthyroidism; it may improve spontaneously.

℞ TREATMENT

The *hyperthyroidism* of Graves' disease is treated by reducing thyroid hormone synthesis, using antithyroid drugs, or by reducing the amount of thyroid tissue with radioiodine (^{131}I) treatment or by subtotal thyroidectomy. Antithyroid drugs are the predominant therapy in many centers in Europe and Japan, whereas radioiodine is more often the first line of treatment in North America. These differences reflect the fact that no single approach is optimal and that patients may require multiple treatments to achieve remission.

The main *antithyroid drugs* are the thionamides, such as propylthiouracil, carbimazole, and the active metabolite of the latter, methimazole. All inhibit the function of TPO, reducing oxidation and organification of iodide. These drugs also reduce thyroid antibody levels by mechanisms that remain unclear, and they appear to enhance rates of remission. Propylthiouracil inhibits deiodination of $T_4 \rightarrow T_3$. However, this effect is of minor benefit, except in the most severe thyrotoxicosis, and is offset by the much shorter half-life of this drug (90 min) compared to methimazole (6 h).

There are many variations of antithyroid drug regimens. The initial dose of carbimazole or methimazole is usually 10 to 20 mg every 8 or 12 h, but once-daily dosing is possible after euthyroidism is restored. Propylthiouracil is given at a dose of 100 to 200 mg every 6 to 8 h, and divided doses are usually given throughout the course. Lower doses of each drug may suffice in areas of low iodine intake. The starting dose of antithyroid drugs can be gradually reduced (titration regimen) as thyrotoxicosis improves. Alternatively, high doses may be given combined with levothyroxine supplementation (block-replace regimen) to avoid drug-induced hypothyroidism. Initial reports suggesting superior remission rates with the block-replace regimen have not been reproduced in several other trials. The titration regimen is often preferred to minimize the dose of antithyroid drug and provide an index of treatment response.

Thyroid function tests and clinical manifestations are reviewed 3 to 4 weeks after starting treatment, and the dose is titrated based on unbound T_4 levels. Most patients do not achieve euthyroidism until 6 to 8 weeks after treatment is initiated. TSH levels often remain suppressed for several months and therefore do not provide a sensitive index of treatment response. The usual daily maintenance doses of antithyroid drugs in the titration regimen are 2.5 to 10 mg of carbimazole or methimazole and 50 to 100 mg of propylthiouracil. In the block-replace regimen, the initial dose of antithyroid drug is held constant and the dose of levothyroxine is adjusted to maintain normal unbound T_4 levels. When TSH suppression is alleviated, TSH levels can also be used to monitor therapy.

Maximum remission rates (up to 30 to 50% in some populations) are achieved by 18 to 24 months. For unclear reasons, remission rates appear to vary in different geographic regions. Patients with severe hyperthyroidism and large goiters are most likely to relapse when treatment stops, but outcome is difficult to predict. All patients should be followed closely for relapse during the first year after treatment and at least annually thereafter.

The common side effects of antithyroid drugs are rash, urticaria, fever, and arthralgia (1 to 5% of patients). These may resolve spontaneously or after substituting an alternative antithyroid drug. Rare but major side effects include hepatitis, an SLE-like syndrome, and, most importantly, agranulocytosis (<1%). It is essential that antithyroid drugs are stopped and not restarted if a patient develops major side effects. Written instructions should be provided regarding the symptoms of possible agranulocytosis (e.g., sore throat, fever, mouth ulcers) and the need to stop treatment pending a complete blood count to confirm that agranulocytosis is not present. Management of agranulocytosis is described in Chap. 94. It is not useful to monitor blood counts prospectively, as the onset of agranulocytosis is idiosyncratic and abrupt.

Propranolol (20 to 40 mg every 6 h) or longer acting beta blockers, such as atenolol, may be helpful to control adrenergic symptoms, especially in the early stages before antithyroid drugs take effect. The need for anticoagulation with warfarin should be considered in all patients with atrial fibrillation. If digoxin is used, increased doses are often needed in the thyrotoxic state.

Radioiodine causes progressive destruction of thyroid cells and can be used as initial treatment or for relapses after a trial of antithyroid drugs. There is a small risk of thyrotoxic crisis (see below) after radioiodine, which can be minimized by pretreatment with antithyroid drugs for at least a month before treatment. Antecedent treatment with antithyroid drugs should be considered for all elderly patients or for those with cardiac problems, to deplete thyroid hormone stores before administration of radioiodine. Antithyroid drugs must be stopped at least 3 days before radioiodine administration to achieve optimum iodine uptake.

Efforts to calculate an optimal dose of radioiodine that achieves euthyroidism, without a high incidence of relapse or progression to hypothyroidism, have not been successful. Some patients inevitably relapse after a single dose because the biologic effects of radiation vary between individuals, and hypothyroidism cannot be uniformly avoided even using accurate dosimetry. A practical strategy is to give a fixed dose based on clinical features, such as the severity of thyrotoxicosis, the size of the goiter (increases the dose needed), and the level of radioiodine uptake (decreases the dose needed). ^{131}I dosage generally ranges between 185 MBq (5 mCi) to 555 MBq (15 mCi). Incomplete treatment or early relapse is more common in males and in patients <40 years of age. Many authorities favor an approach aimed at thyroid ablation (as opposed to euthyroidism), given that levothyroxine replacement is straightforward and most patients ultimately progress to hypothyroidism over 5 to 10 years, frequently with some delay in the diagnosis of hypothyroidism.

Certain radiation safety precautions are necessary in the first few days after radioiodine treatment, but the exact guidelines vary depending on local protocols. In general, patients need to avoid close, prolonged contact with children and pregnant women for several days because of possible transmission of residual isotope and excessive exposure to radiation emanating from the gland. Rarely there may be mild pain due to radiation thyroiditis 1 to 2 weeks after treatment. Hyperthyroidism can persist for 2 to 3 months before radioiodine takes full effect. For this reason, β-adrenergic blockers or antithyroid drugs can be used to control symptoms during this interval. Persistent hyperthyroidism can be treated with a second dose of radioiodine, usually 6 months after the first dose. The risk of hypothyroidism after radioiodine depends on the dosage but is at least 10 to 20% in the first year and 5% per year thereafter. Patients should be informed of this possibility before treatment and require close follow-up during the first year and annual thyroid function testing.

Pregnancy and breast feeding are absolute contraindications to radioiodine treatment, but patients can conceive safely 6 months after treatment. The presence of severe ophthalmopathy requires caution, and some authorities advocate the use of prednisone, 40 mg/d, at the time of radioiodine treatment, tapered over 2 to 3 months to prevent exacerbation of ophthalmopathy. The overall risk of cancer after radioiodine treatment in adults is not increased, but many physicians avoid radioiodine in children and adolescents because of the theoretical risks of malignancy.

Subtotal thyroidectomy is an option for patients who relapse after antithyroid drugs and prefer this treatment to radioiodine. Some experts recommend surgery in young individuals, particularly when the goiter is very large. Careful control of thyrotoxicosis with antithyroid drugs, followed by potassium iodide (3 drops SSKI orally tid), is needed prior to surgery to avoid thyrotoxic crisis and to reduce the vascularity of the gland. The major complications of surgery—i.e., bleeding, laryngeal edema, hypoparathyroidism, and damage to the recurrent laryngeal nerves—are unusual when the procedure is performed by highly experienced surgeons. Recurrence rates in the best series are <2%, but the rate of hypothyroidism is only slightly less than that following radioiodine treatment.

The titration regimen of antithyroid drugs should be used to manage Graves' disease in *pregnancy*, as blocking doses of these drugs produce fetal hypothyroidism. Propylthiouracil is usually used because of relatively low transplacental transfer and its ability to block $T_4 \rightarrow T_3$ conversion. Also, carbimazole and methimazole have been associated with rare cases of fetal *aplasia cutis* and other defects, such as choanal atresia. The lowest effective dose of propylthiouracil should be given, and it is often possible to stop treatment in the last trimester since TSH-R antibodies tend to decline in pregnancy. Nonetheless, the transplacental transfer of these antibodies rarely causes *fetal thyrotoxicosis* or *neonatal thyrotoxicosis*. Poor intrauterine growth, a fetal heart rate of >160 beats/min, and high levels of maternal TSH-R antibodies in the last trimester may herald this complication. Antithyroid drugs given to the mother can be used to treat the fetus and may be needed for 1 to 3 months after delivery, until the maternal antibodies disappear from the baby's circulation. The postpartum period is a time of major risk for relapse of Graves' disease. Breast feeding is safe with low doses of antithyroid drugs. Graves' disease in *children* is best managed with antithyroid drugs, often given as a prolonged course of the titration regimen. Surgery may be indicated for severe disease. Radioiodine can also be used in children, although most experts defer this treatment until adolescence or later.

Thyrotoxic crisis, or *thyroid storm*, is rare and presents as a life-threatening exacerbation of hyperthyroidism, accompanied by fever, delirium, seizures, coma, vomiting, diarrhea, and jaundice. The mortality rate due to cardiac failure, arrhythmia, or hyperthermia is as high as 30%, even with treatment. Thyrotoxic crisis is usually precipitated by acute illness (e.g., stroke, infection, trauma, diabetic ketoacidosis), surgery (especially on the thyroid), or radioiodine treatment of a patient with partially treated or untreated hyperthyroidism. Management requires intensive monitoring and supportive care, identification and treatment of the precipitating cause, and measures that reduce thyroid hormone synthesis. Large doses of propylthiouracil (600-mg loading dose and 200 to 300 mg every 6 h) should be given orally or by nasogastric tube or per rectum; the drug's inhibitory action on $T_4 \rightarrow T_3$ conversion makes it the antithyroid drug of choice. One hour after the first dose of propylthiouracil, stable iodide is given to block thyroid hormone synthesis via the Wolff-Chaikoff effect (the delay allows the antithyroid drug to prevent the excess iodine from being incorporated into new hormone). A saturated solution of potassium iodide (5 drops SSKI every 6 h), or ipodate or iopanoic acid (0.5 mg every 12 h), may be given orally. (Sodium iodide, 0.25 g intravenously every 6 h is an alternative but is not generally available.) Propranolol should also be given to reduce tachycardia and other adrenergic manifestations (40 to 60 mg orally every 4 h; or 2 mg intravenously every 4 h). Although other β-adrenergic blockers can be used, high doses of propranolol decrease $T_4 \rightarrow T_3$ conversion, and the doses can be easily adjusted. Caution is needed to avoid acute negative inotropic effects, but controlling the heart rate is important, as some patients develop a form of high-output heart failure. Additional therapeutic measures include glucocorticoids (e.g., dexamethasone, 2 mg every 6 h), antibiotics if infection is present, cooling, oxygen, and intravenous fluids.

Ophthalmopathy requires no active treatment when it is mild or moderate, as there is usually spontaneous improvement. General measures include meticulous control of thyroid hormone levels, advice about cessation of smoking, and an explanation of the natural history of ophthalmopathy. Discomfort can be relieved with artificial tears (e.g., 1% methylcellulose) and the use of dark glasses with side frames. Periorbital edema may respond to a more upright sleeping position or a diuretic. Corneal exposure during sleep can be avoided by taping the eyelids shut. Minor degrees of diplopia improve with prisms fitted to spectacles. Severe ophthalmopathy, with optic nerve involvement or chemosis resulting in corneal damage, is an emergency requiring joint management with an ophthalmologist. Short-term benefit can be gained in about two-thirds of patients by the use of high-dose glucocorticoids (e.g., prednisone, 40 to 80 mg daily), sometimes combined with cyclosporine. Glucocorticoid doses are tapered by 5 mg every 1 to 2 weeks, but the taper often results in reemergence of congestive symptoms. Pulse therapy with intravenous methylprednisolone (1 g of methylprednisolone in 250 mL of saline infused over 2 h daily for 1 week) followed by an oral regimen is also used. Once the eye disease has stabilized, surgery may be indicated for relief of diplopia and correction of the appearance of the eyes. Orbital decompression can be achieved by removing bone from any wall of the orbit, thereby allowing displacement of fat and swollen extraocular muscles. The transantral route is used most often, as it requires no external incision. Proptosis recedes an average of 5 mm, but there may be residual or even worsened diplopia. Alternatively, retrobulbar tissue can be decompressed without the removal of bony tissue. External beam radiotherapy of the orbits has been used for many years, especially for ophthalmopathy of recent onset, but the objective evidence that this therapy is beneficial remains equivocal.

Thyroid dermopathy does not usually require treatment but can cause cosmetic problems or interfere with the fit of shoes. Surgical removal is not indicated. If necessary, treatment consists of topical, high-potency glucocorticoid ointment under an occlusive dressing. Octreotide may be beneficial.

OTHER CAUSES OF THYROTOXICOSIS Destructive thyroiditis (subacute or silent thyroiditis) typically presents with a short thyrotoxic phase due to the release of preformed thyroid hormones and catabolism of Tg (see "Subacute Thyroiditis," below). True hyperthyroidism is absent, as demonstrated by a low radionuclide uptake. Circulating Tg and IL-6 levels are usually increased. Other causes of thyrotoxicosis with low or absent thyroid radionuclide uptake include *thyrotoxicosis factitia*; iodine excess and, rarely, ectopic thyroid tissue, particularly teratomas of the ovary (*struma ovarii*); and functional metastatic follicular carcinoma. Whole-body radionuclide studies can demonstrate ectopic thyroid tissue, and thyrotoxicosis factitia can be distinguished from destructive thyroiditis by the clinical features and low levels of Tg. Amiodarone treatment is associated with thyrotoxicosis in up to 10% of patients, particularly in areas of low iodine intake.

TSH-secreting pituitary adenoma is a rare causes of thyrotoxicosis. It can be identified by the presence of an inappropriately normal or increased TSH level in a patient with hyperthyroidism, diffuse goiter, and elevated T_4 and T_3 levels (Chap. 318). Elevated levels of the α subunit of TSH, released by the TSH-secreting adenoma, support this diagnosis, which can be confirmed by demonstrating the pituitary tumor on CT or MRI scan. A combination of transsphenoidal surgery, sella irradiation, and octreotide may be required to normalize TSH, as many of these tumors are large and locally invasive at the time of diagnosis. Radioiodine or antithyroid drugs can be used to control thyrotoxicosis.

Thyrotoxicosis caused by *toxic multinodular goiter* and *hyperfunctioning solitary nodules* is discussed below.

THYROIDITIS

A clinically useful classification of thyroiditis is based on the onset and duration of disease (Table 320-8).

ACUTE THYROIDITIS Acute thyroiditis is rare and due to suppurative infection of the thyroid. In children and young adults, the most common cause is the presence of a piriform sinus, a remnant of the fourth branchial pouch that connects the oropharynx with the thyroid. Such sinuses are predominantly left sided. A long-standing goiter and degeneration in a thyroid malignancy are risk factors in the elderly. The patient presents with thyroid pain, often referred to the throat or ears, and a small, tender goiter that may be asymmetric. Fever, dysphagia, and erythema over the thyroid are common, as are systemic symptoms of a febrile illness and lymphadenopathy.

The differential diagnosis of *thyroid pain* includes subacute or, rarely, chronic thyroiditis, hemorrhage into a cyst, malignancy including lymphoma, and, rarely, amiodarone-induced thyroiditis or amyloidosis. However, the abrupt presentation and clinical features of acute thyroiditis rarely cause confusion. The erythrocyte sedimentation rate (ESR) and white cell count are usually increased, but thyroid

TABLE 320-8 *Causes of Thyroiditis*

Acute
   Bacterial infection: especially *Staphylococcus, Streptococcus*, and *Enterobacter*
   Fungal infection: *Aspergillus, Candida, Coccidioides, Histoplasma*, and *Pneumocystis*
   Radiation thyroiditis after ¹³¹I treatment
   Amiodarone (may also be subacute or chronic)
Subacute
   Viral (or granulomatous) thyroiditis
   Silent thyroiditis (including postpartum thyroiditis)
   Mycobacterial infection
Chronic
   Autoimmunity: focal thyroiditis, Hashimoto's thyroiditis, atrophic thyroiditis
   Riedel's thyroiditis
   Parasitic thyroiditis: echinococcosis, strongyloidiasis, cysticercosis
   Traumatic: after palpation

function is normal. FNA biopsy shows infiltration by polymorpho-nuclear leukocytes; culture of the sample can identify the organism. Caution is needed in immunocompromised patients as fungal, myco-bacterial, or *Pneumocystis* thyroiditis can occur in this setting. Anti-biotic treatment is guided initially by Gram stain and subsequently by cultures of the FNA biopsy. Surgery may be needed to drain an ab-scess, which can be localized by CT scan or ultrasound. Tracheal ob-struction, septicemia, retropharyngeal abscess, mediastinitis, and jug-ular venous thrombosis may complicate acute thyroiditis but are uncommon with prompt use of antibiotics.

SUBACUTE THYROIDITIS This is also termed *de Quervain's thyroiditis*, *granulomatous thyroiditis*, or *viral thyroiditis*. Many viruses have been implicated, including mumps, coxsackie, influenza, adenoviruses, and echoviruses, but attempts to identify the virus in an individual patient are often unsuccessful and do not influence management. The diag-nosis of subacute thyroiditis is often overlooked because the symptoms can mimic pharyngitis. The peak incidence occurs at 30 to 50 years, and women are affected three times more frequently than men.

Pathophysiology The thyroid shows a characteristic patchy inflamma-tory infiltrate with disruption of the thyroid follicles and multinucle-ated giant cells within some follicles. The follicular changes progress to granulomas accompanied by fibrosis. Finally, the thyroid returns to normal, usually several months after onset. During the initial phase of follicular destruction, there is release of Tg and thyroid hormones, leading to increased circulating T_4 and T_3 and suppression of TSH (Fig. 320-8). During this destructive phase, radioactive iodine uptake is low or undetectable. After several weeks, the thyroid is depleted of stored thyroid hormone and a phase of hypothyroidism typically oc-curs, with low unbound T_4 (and sometimes T_3) and moderately in-creased TSH levels. Radioactive iodine uptake returns to normal or is even increased as a result of the rise in TSH. Finally, thyroid hormone and TSH levels return to normal as the disease subsides.

Clinical Manifestations The patient usually presents with a painful and enlarged thyroid, sometimes accompanied by fever. There may be fea-tures of thyrotoxicosis or hypothyroidism, depending on the phase of the illness. Malaise and symptoms of an upper respiratory tract infec-tion may precede the thyroid-related features by several weeks. In other patients, the onset is acute, severe, and without obvious ante-cedent. The patient typically complains of a sore throat, and exami-nation reveals a small goiter that is exquisitely tender. Pain is often referred to the jaw or ear. Complete resolution is the usual outcome,

FIGURE 320-8 Clinical course of subacute thyroiditis. The release of thyroid hor-mones is initially associated with a thyrotoxic phase and suppressed thyroid-stimulating hormone (TSH). A hypothyroid phase then ensues, with low T_4 and TSH levels that are initially low but gradually increase. During the recovery phase, increased TSH levels combined with resolution of thyroid follicular injury leads to normalization of thyroid function, often several months after the beginning of the illness. ESR, erythrocyte sedimentation rate; UT$_4$, unbound T_4.

but permanent hypothyroidism can occur, particularly in those with coincidental thyroid autoimmunity. A prolonged course over many months, with one or more relapses, occurs in a small percentage of patients.

Laboratory Evaluation As depicted in Fig. 320-8, thyroid function tests characteristically evolve through three distinct phases over about 6 months: (1) thyrotoxic phase, (2) hypothyroid phase, and (3) recovery phase. In the thyrotoxic phase, T_4 and T_3 levels are increased, reflecting their discharge from the damaged thyroid cells, and TSH is suppressed. The T_4/T_3 ratio is greater than in Graves' disease or thyroid autonomy, in which T_3 is often disproportionately increased. The diagnosis is confirmed by a high ESR and low radioiodine uptake. Serum IL-6 levels increase during the thyrotoxic phase. The white blood cell count may be increased, and thyroid antibodies are negative. If the diagnosis is in doubt, FNA biopsy may be useful, particularly to distinguish unilateral involvement from bleeding into a cyst or neoplasm.

℞ TREATMENT

Relatively large doses of aspirin (e.g., 600 mg every 4 to 6 h) or nonsteroidal anti-inflammatory drugs are sufficient to control symp-toms in most cases. If this treatment is inadequate, or if the patient has marked local or systemic symptoms, glucocorticoids should be given. The usual starting dose is 40 to 60 mg prednisone, depending on se-verity. The dose is gradually tapered over 6 to 8 weeks, in response to improvement in symptoms and the ESR. If a relapse occurs during glucocorticoid withdrawal, treatment should be started again and with-drawn more gradually. In these patients, it is useful to wait until the radioactive iodine uptake normalizes before stopping treatment. Thy-roid function should be monitored every 2 to 4 weeks using TSH and unbound T_4 levels. Symptoms of thyrotoxicosis improve spontane-ously but may be ameliorated by β-adrenergic blockers; antithyroid drugs play no role in treatment of the thyrotoxic phase. Levothyroxine replacement may be needed if the hypothyroid phase is prolonged, but doses should be low enough (50 to 100 μg daily) to allow TSH-me-diated recovery.

SILENT THYROIDITIS *Painless thyroiditis*, or *"silent" thyroiditis*, occurs in patients with underlying autoimmune thyroid disease. It has a clin-ical course similar to that of subacute thyroiditis, except that there is little or no thyroid tenderness. The condition occurs in up to 5% of women 3 to 6 months after pregnancy and is then termed *postpartum thyroiditis*. Typically, patients have a brief phase of thyrotoxicosis, lasting 2 to 4 weeks, followed by hypothyroidism for 4 to 12 weeks, and then resolution; often, however, only one phase is apparent. The condition is associated with the presence of TPO antibodies antepar-tum, and is three times more common in women with type 1 diabetes mellitus. As in subacute thyroiditis, the radioactive iodine uptake is initially suppressed. In addition to the painless goiter, silent thyroiditis can be distinguished from subacute thyroiditis by the normal ESR and the presence of TPO antibodies. Glucocorticoid treatment is not in-dicated for silent thyroiditis. Severe thyrotoxic symptoms can be man-aged with a brief course of propranolol, 20 to 40 mg three or four times daily. Thyroxine replacement may be needed for the hypothyroid phase but should be withdrawn after 6 to 9 months, as recovery is the rule. Annual follow-up thereafter is recommended, as a proportion of these individuals develop permanent hypothyroidism.

DRUG-INDUCED THYROIDITIS Patients receiving IFN-α, IL-2, or amio-darone may develop painless thyroiditis. IFN-α, which is used to treat chronic hepatitis B or C, causes thyroid dysfunction in up to 5% of treated patients. It has been associated with painless thyroiditis, hy-pothyroidism, and Graves' disease. IL-2, which has been used to treat various malignancies, has also been associated with thyroiditis and hypothyroidism, though fewer patients have been studied. For discus-sion of amiodarone, see "Amiodarone Effects on Thyroid Function," below.

CHRONIC THYROIDITIS Focal thyroiditis is present in 20 to 40% of eu-thyroid autopsy cases and is associated with serologic evidence of autoimmunity, particularly the presence of TPO antibodies. These antibodies are 4 to 10 times more common in otherwise healthy women than men. The most common clinically apparent cause of chronic thyroiditis is *Hashimoto's thyroiditis*, an autoimmune disorder that often presents as a firm or hard goiter of variable size (see above). *Riedel's thyroiditis* is a rare disorder that typically occurs in middle-aged women. It presents with an insidious, painless goiter with local symptoms due to compression of the esophagus, trachea, neck veins, or recurrent laryngeal nerves. Dense fibrosis disrupts normal gland architecture and can extend outside the thyroid capsule. Despite these extensive histologic changes, thyroid dysfunction is uncommon. The goiter is hard, nontender, often asymmetric and fixed, leading to suspicion of a malignancy. Diagnosis requires open biopsy as FNA biopsy is usually inadequate. Treatment is directed to surgical relief of compressive symptoms. Tamoxifen may also be beneficial. There is an association between Riedel's thyroiditis and idiopathic fibrosis at other sites (retroperitoneum, mediastinum, biliary tree, lung, and orbit).

SICK EUTHYROID SYNDROME

Any acute, severe illness can cause abnormalities of circulating TSH or thyroid hormone levels in the absence of underlying thyroid disease, making these measurements potentially misleading. The major cause of these hormonal changes is the release of cytokines. Unless a thyroid disorder is strongly suspected, the routine testing of thyroid function should be avoided in acutely ill patients.

The most common hormone pattern in sick euthyroid syndrome (SES) is a decrease in total and unbound T_3 levels (low T_3 syndrome) with normal levels of T_4 and TSH. The magnitude of the fall in T_3 correlates with the severity of the illness. T_4 conversion to T_3 via peripheral deiodination is impaired, leading to increased reverse T_3 (rT_3). Despite this effect, decreased clearance rather than increased production is the major basis for increased rT_3. Also, T_4 is alternately metabolized to the hormonally inactive T_3 sulfate. It is generally assumed that this low T_3 state is adaptive, as it can be induced in normal individuals by fasting. Teleologically, the fall in T_3 may limit catabolism in starved or ill patients.

Very sick patients may exhibit a dramatic fall in total T_4 and T_3 levels (low T_4 syndrome). This state has a poor prognosis. A key factor in the fall in T_4 levels is altered binding to TBG. T_4 assays usually demonstrate a normal unbound T_4 level in such patients, depending on the assay method used. Fluctuation in TSH levels also creates challenges in the interpretation of thyroid function in sick patients. TSH levels may range from <0.1 to >20 mU/L; these alterations reverse after recovery, confirming the absence of underlying thyroid disease. A rise in cortisol or administration of glucocorticoids may provide a partial explanation for decreased TSH levels. However, the exact mechanisms underlying the subnormal TSH seen in 10% of sick patients and the increased TSH seen in 5% remain unclear.

Any severe illness can induce changes in thyroid hormone levels, but certain disorders exhibit a distinctive pattern of abnormalities. Acute liver disease is associated with an initial rise in total (but not unbound) T_3 and T_4 levels, due to TBG release; these levels become subnormal with progression to liver failure. A transient increase in total and unbound T_4 levels, usually with a normal T_3 level, is seen in 5 to 30% of acutely ill psychiatric patients. TSH values may be transiently low, normal, or high in these patients. In the early stage of HIV infection, T_3 and T_4 levels rise, even if there is weight loss. T_3 levels fall with progression to AIDS, but TSH usually remains normal. Renal disease is often accompanied by low T_3 concentrations, but with normal rather than increased rT_3 levels, due to an unknown factor that increases uptake of rT_3 into the liver.

The diagnosis of SES is challenging. Historic information may be limited, and patients often have multiple metabolic derangements. Useful features to consider include previous history of thyroid disease and thyroid function tests, evaluation of the severity and time course of the patient's acute illness, documentation of medications that may affect thyroid function or thyroid hormone levels, and measurements

of rT_3 together with unbound thyroid hormones and TSH. The diagnosis of SES is frequently presumptive, given the clinical context and pattern of laboratory values; only resolution of the test results with clinical recovery can clearly establish this disorder. Treatment of SES with thyroid hormone (T_4 and/or T_3) is controversial, but most authorities recommend monitoring the patient's thyroid function tests during recovery, without administering thyroid hormone, unless there is historic or clinical evidence suggestive of hypothyroidism. Sufficiently large randomized controlled trials using thyroid hormone are unlikely to resolve this therapeutic controversy in the near future, because clinical presentations and outcomes are highly variable.

AMIODARONE EFFECTS ON THYROID FUNCTION

Amiodarone is a commonly used type III antiarrhythmic agent (Chap. 214). It is structurally related to thyroid hormone and contains 39% iodine by weight. Thus, typical doses of amiodarone (200 mg/d) are associated with very high iodine intake, leading to >40-fold increases in plasma and urinary iodine levels. Moreover, because amiodarone is stored in adipose tissue, high iodine levels persist for >6 months after discontinuation of the drug. Amiodarone inhibits deiodinase activity, and its metabolites function as weak antagonists of thyroid hormone action. Amiodarone has the following effects on thyroid function: (1) acute, transient suppression of thyroid function; (2) hypothyroidism in patients susceptible to the inhibitory effects of a high iodine load; and (3) thyrotoxicosis that may be caused by at least three mechanisms—a Jod-Basedow effect from the iodine load in the setting of multinodular goiter, a thyroiditis-like condition, and possibly induction of autoimmune Graves' disease.

The initiation of amiodarone treatment is associated with a transient decrease of T_4 levels, reflecting the inhibitory effect of iodine on T_4 release. Soon thereafter, most individuals escape from iodide-dependent suppression of the thyroid (Wolff-Chaikoff effect), and the inhibitory effects on deiodinase activity and thyroid hormone receptor action become predominant. These events lead to the following pattern of thyroid function tests: increased T_4, decreased T_3, increased rT_3, and a transient increase of TSH (up to 20 mU/L). TSH levels normalize or are slightly suppressed by 1 to 3 months.

The incidence of hypothyroidism from amiodarone varies geographically, apparently correlating with iodine intake. Hypothyroidism occurs in up to 13% of amiodarone-treated patients in iodine-replete countries, such as the United States, but is less common (<6% incidence) in areas of lower iodine intake, such as Italy or Spain. The pathogenesis appears to involve an inability of the thyroid to escape from the high iodine load. Consequently, amiodarone-associated hypothyroidism is more common in women and individuals with positive TPO antibodies. It is usually unnecessary to discontinue amiodarone for this side effect, as levothyroxine can be used to normalize thyroid function. TSH levels should be monitored, because T_4 levels are often increased for the reasons described above.

The management of amiodarone-induced thyrotoxicosis (AIT) is complicated by the fact that there are several causes of thyrotoxicosis and because the increased thyroid hormone levels exacerbate underlying arrhythmias and coronary artery disease. Amiodarone treatment causes thyrotoxicosis in 10% of patients living in areas of low iodine intake and in 2% of patients in regions of high iodine intake. There are two major forms of AIT, although some patients have features of both. Type 1 AIT is associated with an underlying thyroid abnormality (preclinical Graves' disease or nodular goiter). Thyroid hormone synthesis becomes excessive as a result of increased iodine exposure (Jod-Basedow phenomenon). Type 2 AIT occurs in individuals with no intrinsic thyroid abnormalities and is the result of drug-induced lysosomal activation leading to destructive thyroiditis with histiocyte accumulation in the thyroid. Mild forms of type 2 AIT can resolve spontaneously or can occasionally lead to hypothyroidism. Color-flow doppler thyroid scanning shows increased vascularity in type 1 AIT but decreased vascularity in type 2 AIT. Thyroid scans are difficult to interpret in this setting, because the high endogenous iodine levels diminish tracer uptake. However, the presence of normal or increased uptake favors type 1 AIT.

In AIT the drug should be stopped, if possible, although this is often impractical because of the underlying cardiac disorder. Discontinuation of amiodarone will not have an acute effect because of its storage and prolonged half-life. High doses of antithyroid drugs can be used in type 1 AIT but are often ineffective. In type 2 AIT, oral contrast agents, such as sodium ipodate (500 mg/d) or sodium tyropanoate (500 mg, 1 to 2 doses/d), rapidly reduce T_4 and T_3 levels, decrease $T_4 \rightarrow T_3$ conversion, and may block tissue uptake of thyroid hormones. Potassium perchlorate, 200 mg every 6 h, has been used to reduce thyroidal iodide content. Perchlorate treatment has been associated with agranulocytosis, though the risk appears relatively low with short-term use. Glucocorticoids, administered as for subacute thyroiditis, are of variable benefit in type 2 AIT. Lithium blocks thyroid hormone release and can provide modest benefit. Near-total thyroidectomy rapidly decreases thyroid hormone levels and may be the most effective long-term solution, if the patient can undergo the procedure safely.

THYROID FUNCTION IN PREGNANCY

Four factors alter thyroid function in pregnancy: (1) the transient increase in hCG during the first trimester, which stimulates the TSH-R; (2) the estrogen-induced rise in TBG during the first trimester, which is sustained during pregnancy; (3) alterations in the immune system, leading to the onset, exacerbation, or amelioration of an underlying autoimmune thyroid disease (see above); and (4) increased urinary iodide excretion, which can cause impaired thyroid hormone production in areas of marginal iodine sufficiency. Women with a precarious iodine intake (<50 μg/d) are most at risk of developing a goiter during pregnancy, and iodine supplementation should be considered to prevent maternal and fetal hypothyroidism and the development of neonatal goiter.

The rise in circulating hCG levels during the first trimester is accompanied by a reciprocal fall in TSH that persists into the middle of pregnancy. This appears to reflect weak binding of hCG, which is present at very high levels, to the TSH-R. Rare individuals have been described with variant TSH-R sequences that enhance hCG binding and TSH-R activation. hCG-induced changes in thyroid function can result in transient gestational hyperthyroidism and/or *hyperemesis gravidarum*, a condition characterized by severe nausea and vomiting and risk of volume depletion. Antithyroid drugs are rarely needed, and parenteral fluid replacement usually suffices until the condition resolves.

Maternal hypothyroidism occurs in 2 to 3% of women of childbearing age and is associated with increased risk of developmental delay in the offspring. Thyroid hormone requirements are increased by 25 to 50 μg/d during pregnancy.

GOITER AND NODULAR THYROID DISEASE

Goiter refers to an enlarged thyroid gland. Biosynthetic defects, iodine deficiency, autoimmune disease, and nodular diseases can each lead to goiter, though by different mechanisms. Biosynthetic defects and iodine deficiency are associated with reduced efficiency of thyroid hormone synthesis, leading to increased TSH, which stimulates thyroid growth as a compensatory mechanism to overcome the block in hormone synthesis. Graves' disease and Hashimoto's thyroiditis are also associated with goiter. In Graves' disease, the goiter results mainly from the TSH-R-mediated effects of TSI. The goitrous form of Hashimoto's thyroiditis occurs because of acquired defects in hormone synthesis, leading to elevated levels of TSH and its consequent growth effects. Lymphocytic infiltration and immune system–induced growth factors also contribute to thyroid enlargement in Hashimoto's

thyroiditis. Nodular disease is characterized by the disordered growth of thyroid cells, often combined with the gradual development of fibrosis. Because the management of goiter depends on the etiology, the detection of thyroid enlargement on physical examination should prompt further evaluation to identify its cause.

Nodular thyroid disease is common, occurring in about 3 to 7% of adults when assessed by physical examination. Using more sensitive techniques, such as ultrasound, it is present in >25% of adults. Thyroid nodules may be solitary or multiple, and they may be functional or nonfunctional.

DIFFUSE NONTOXIC (SIMPLE) GOITER ■ Etiology and Pathogenesis When diffuse enlargement of the thyroid occurs in the absence of nodules and hyperthyroidism, it is referred to as a *diffuse nontoxic goiter*. This is sometimes called *simple goiter*, because of the absence of nodules, or *colloid goiter*, because of the presence of uniform follicles that are filled with colloid. Worldwide, diffuse goiter is most commonly caused by iodine deficiency and is termed *endemic goiter* when it affects >5% of the population. In nonendemic regions, *sporadic goiter* occurs, and the cause is usually unknown. Thyroid enlargement in teenagers is sometimes referred to as *juvenile goiter*. In general, goiter is more common in women than men, probably because of the greater prevalence of underlying autoimmune disease and the increased iodine demands associated with pregnancy.

In *iodine-deficient areas*, thyroid enlargement reflects a compensatory effort to trap iodide and produce sufficient hormone under conditions in which hormone synthesis is relatively inefficient. Somewhat surprisingly, TSH levels are usually normal or only slightly increased, suggesting increased sensitivity to TSH or activation of other pathways that lead to thyroid growth. Iodide appears to have direct actions on thyroid vasculature and may indirectly affect growth through vasoactive substances such as endothelins and nitric oxide. Endemic goiter is also caused by exposure to environmental *goitrogens* such as cassava root, which contains a thiocyanate, vegetables of the Cruciferae family (e.g., brussels sprouts, cabbage, and cauliflower), and milk from regions where goitrogens are present in grass. Though relatively rare, inherited defects in thyroid hormone synthesis lead to a diffuse nontoxic goiter. Abnormalities at each step in hormone synthesis, including iodide transport (NIS), Tg synthesis, organification and coupling (TPO), and the regeneration of iodide (dehalogenase), have been described.

CLINICAL MANIFESTATIONS AND DIAGNOSIS If thyroid function is preserved, most goiters are asymptomatic. Spontaneous hemorrhage into a cyst or nodule may cause the sudden onset of localized pain and swelling. Examination of a diffuse goiter reveals a symmetrically enlarged, nontender, generally soft gland without palpable nodules. Goiter is defined, somewhat arbitrarily, as a lateral lobe with a volume greater than the thumb of the individual being examined. If the thyroid is markedly enlarged, it can cause tracheal or esophageal compression. These features are unusual, however, in the absence of nodular disease and fibrosis. *Substernal goiter* may obstruct the thoracic inlet. *Pemberton's sign* refers to symptoms of faintness with evidence of facial congestion and external jugular venous obstruction when the arms are raised above the head, a maneuver that draws the thyroid into the thoracic inlet. Respiratory flow measurements and CT or MRI should be used to evaluate substernal goiter in patients with obstructive signs or symptoms.

Thyroid function tests should be performed in all patients with goiter to exclude thyrotoxicosis or hypothyroidism. It is not unusual, particularly in iodine deficiency, to find a low total T_4, with normal T_3 and TSH, reflecting enhanced $T_4 \rightarrow T_3$ conversion. A low TSH, particularly in older patients, suggests the possibility of thyroid autonomy or undiagnosed Graves' disease, causing subclinical thyrotoxicosis. TPO antibodies may be useful to identify patients at increased risk of autoimmune thyroid disease. Low urinary iodine levels (<10 μg/dL) support a diagnosis of iodine deficiency. Thyroid scanning is not generally necessary but will reveal increased uptake in iodine deficiency and most cases of dyshormonogenesis. Ultrasound is not generally indicated in the evaluation of diffuse goiter, unless a nodule is palpable on physical examination.

℞ TREATMENT

Iodine or thyroid hormone replacement induces variable regression of goiter in iodine deficiency, depending on how long it has been present and the degree of fibrosis that has developed. Because of the possibility of underlying thyroid autonomy, caution should be exercised when instituting suppressive thyroxine therapy in other causes of diffuse nontoxic goiter, particularly if the baseline TSH is in the low-normal range. In younger patients, the dose of levothyroxine can be started at 100 μg/d and adjusted to suppress the TSH into the low-normal but detectable range. Treatment of elderly patients should be initiated at 50 μg/d. The efficacy of suppressive treatment is greater in younger patients and for those with soft goiters. Significant regression is usually seen within 3 to 6 months of treatment; after this time it is unlikely to occur. In older patients, and in those with some degree of nodular disease or fibrosis, fewer than one-third demonstrate significant shrinkage of the goiter. Surgery is rarely indicated for diffuse goiter. Exceptions include documented evidence of tracheal compression or obstruction of the thoracic inlet, which are more likely to be associated with substernal multinodular goiters (see below). Subtotal or near-total thyroidectomy for these or cosmetic reasons should be performed by an experienced surgeon to minimize complication rates, which occur in up to 10% of cases. Surgery should be followed by mild suppressive treatment with levothyroxine to prevent regrowth of the goiter. Radioiodine reduces goiter size by about 50% in the majority of patients. It is rarely associated with transient acute swelling of the thyroid, which is usually inconsequential unless there is severe tracheal narrowing. If not treated with levothyroxine, patients should be followed after radioiodine treatment for the possible development of hypothyroidism.

NONTOXIC MULTINODULAR GOITER ■ **Etiology and Pathogenesis** Depending on the population studied, multinodular goiter (MNG) occurs in up to 12% of adults. MNG is more common in women than men and increases in prevalence with age. It is more common in iodine-deficient regions but also occurs in regions of iodine sufficiency, reflecting multiple genetic, autoimmune, and environmental influences on the pathogenesis.

There is typically wide variation in nodule size. Histology reveals a spectrum of morphologies ranging from hypercellular regions to cystic areas filled with colloid. Fibrosis is often extensive, and areas of hemorrhage or lymphocytic infiltration may be seen. Using molecular techniques, most nodules within a MNG are polyclonal in origin, suggesting a hyperplastic response to locally produced growth factors and cytokines. TSH, which is usually not elevated, may play a permissive or contributory role. Monoclonal lesions also occur within a MNG, reflecting mutations in genes that confer a selective growth advantage to the progenitor cell.

Clinical Manifestations Most patients with nontoxic MNG are asymptomatic and, by definition, euthyroid. MNG typically develops over many years and is detected on routine physical examination or when an individual notices an enlargement in the neck. If the goiter is large enough, it can ultimately lead to compressive symptoms including difficulty swallowing, respiratory distress (tracheal compression), or plethora (venous congestion), but these symptoms are uncommon. Symptomatic MNGs are usually extraordinarily large and/or develop fibrotic areas that cause compression. Sudden pain in a MNG is usually caused by hemorrhage into a nodule but should raise the possibility of invasive malignancy. Hoarseness, reflecting laryngeal nerve involvement, also suggests malignancy.

Diagnosis On examination, thyroid architecture is distorted and multiple nodules of varying size can be appreciated. Because many nodules are deeply embedded in thyroid tissue or reside in posterior or substernal locations, it is not possible to palpate all nodules. A TSH level should be measured to exclude subclinical hyper- or hypothy-

roidism, but thyroid function is usually normal. Tracheal deviation is common, but compression must usually exceed 70% of the tracheal diameter before there is significant airway compromise. Pulmonary function testing can be used to assess the functional effects of compression and to detect tracheomalacia, which characteristically causes inspiratory stridor. CT or MRI can be used to evaluate the anatomy of the goiter and the extent of substernal extension, which is often much greater than is apparent on physical examination. A barium swallow may reveal the extent of esophageal compression. MNG does not appear to predispose to thyroid carcinoma or to more aggressive carcinoma. For this reason, and because it is not possible to biopsy all nodular lesions, thyroid biopsies should be performed only if malignancy is suspected because of a dominant or enlarging nodule.

℞ TREATMENT

Most nontoxic MNGs can be managed conservatively. T_4 suppression is rarely effective for reducing goiter size and introduces the risk of thyrotoxicosis, particularly if there is underlying autonomy or if it develops during treatment. If levothyroxine is used, it should be started at low doses (50 μg) and advanced gradually while monitoring the TSH level to avoid excessive suppression. Contrast agents and other iodine-containing substances should be avoided because of the risk of inducing the *Jod-Basedow effect*, characterized by enhanced thyroid hormone production by autonomous nodules. Radioiodine is being used with increasing frequency because it often decreases goiter size and may selectively ablate regions of autonomy. Dosage of ^{131}I depends on the size of the goiter and radioiodine uptake but is usually about 3.7 MBq (0.1 mCi) per gram of tissue, corrected for uptake [typical dose, 370 to 1070 Mbq (10 to 29 mCi)]. Repeat treatment may be needed. It is possible to achieve a 40 to 50% reduction in goiter size in most patients. Earlier concerns about radiation-induced thyroid swelling and tracheal compression have diminished as recent studies have shown this complication to be rare. When acute compression occurs, glucocorticoid treatment or surgery may be needed. Radiation-induced hypothyroidism is less common than after treatment for Graves' disease. However, posttreatment autoimmune thyrotoxicosis may occur in up to 5% of patients treated for nontoxic MNG. Surgery remains highly effective but is not without risk, particularly in older patients with underlying cardiopulmonary disease.

TOXIC MULTINODULAR GOITER The pathogenesis of toxic MNG appears to be similar to that of nontoxic MNG; the major difference is the presence of functional autonomy in toxic MNG. The molecular basis for autonomy in toxic MNG remains unknown. As in nontoxic goiters, many nodules are polyclonal, while others are monoclonal and vary in their clonal origins. Genetic abnormalities known to confer functional autonomy, such as activating TSH-R or $G_{s\alpha}$ mutations (see below), are not usually found in the autonomous regions of toxic MNG goiter.

In addition to features of goiter, the clinical presentation of toxic MNG includes subclinical hyperthyroidism or mild thyrotoxicosis. The patient is usually elderly and may present with atrial fibrillation or palpitations, tachycardia, nervousness, tremor, or weight loss. Recent exposure to iodine, from contrast dyes or other sources, may precipitate or exacerbate thyrotoxicosis. The TSH level is low. The T_4 level may be normal or minimally increased; T_3 is often elevated to a greater degree than T_4. Thyroid scan shows heterogeneous uptake with multiple regions of increased and decreased uptake; 24-h uptake of radioiodine may not be increased.

℞ TREATMENT

The management of toxic MNG is challenging. Antithyroid drugs, often in combination with beta blockers, can normalize thyroid function and address clinical features of thyrotoxicosis. This treatment, however, often stimulates the growth of the goiter, and, unlike in

Graves' disease, spontaneous remission does not occur. Radioiodine can be used to treat areas of autonomy, as well as to decrease the mass of the goiter. Usually, however, some degree of autonomy remains, presumably because multiple autonomous regions emerge as soon as others are treated. Nonetheless, a trial of radioiodine should be considered before subjecting patients, many of whom are elderly, to surgery. Surgery provides definitive treatment of underlying thyrotoxicosis as well as goiter. Patients should be rendered euthyroid using antithyroid drugs before operation.

HYPERFUNCTIONING SOLITARY NODULE   A solitary, autonomously functioning thyroid nodule is referred to as *toxic adenoma*. The pathogenesis of this disorder has been unraveled by demonstrating the functional effects of mutations that stimulate the TSH-R signaling pathway. Most patients with solitary hyperfunctioning nodules have acquired somatic, activating mutations in the TSH-R (Fig. 320-9). These mutations, located primarily in the receptor transmembrane domain, induce constitutive receptor coupling to $G_{s\alpha}$, increasing cyclic AMP levels and leading to enhanced thyroid follicular cell proliferation and function. Less commonly, somatic mutations are identified in $G_{s\alpha}$. These mutations, which are similar to those seen in McCune-Albright syndrome (Chap. 326) or in a subset of somatotrope adenomas (Chap. 318), impair GTP hydrolysis, also causing constitutive activation of the cyclic AMP signaling pathway. In most series, activating mutations in either the TSH-R or the $G_{s\alpha}$ subunit genes are identified in >90% of patients with solitary hyperfunctioning nodules.

Thyrotoxicosis is usually mild. The disorder is suggested by the presence of the thyroid nodule, which is generally large enough to be palpable, and by the absence of clinical features suggestive of Graves' disease or other causes of thyrotoxicosis. A thyroid scan provides a definitive diagnostic test, demonstrating focal uptake in the hyperfunctioning nodule and diminished uptake in the remainder of the gland, as activity of the normal thyroid is suppressed.

℞ TREATMENT

Radioiodine ablation is usually the treatment of choice. Because normal thyroid function is suppressed, ^{131}I is concentrated in the hyperfunctioning nodule with minimal uptake and damage to normal thyroid tissue. Relatively large radioiodine doses [e.g., 370 to 1110 MBq (10 to 29.9 mCi)^{131}I] have been shown to correct thyrotoxicosis in about 75% of patients within 3 months. Hypothyroidism occurs in <10% of patients over the next 5 years. Surgical resection is also effective and is usually limited to enucleation of the adenoma or lobectomy, thereby preserving thyroid function and minimizing risk of hypoparathyroidism or damage to the recurrent laryngeal nerves. Medical therapy using antithyroid drugs and beta blockers can normalize thyroid function but is not an optimal long-term treatment. Ethanol injection under ultrasound guidance has been used successfully in some centers to ablate hyperfunctioning nodules. Repeated injections (often more than 5 sessions) are required to reduce nodule size. Normal thyroid function can be achieved in most patients using this technique.

BENIGN NEOPLASMS

The various types of benign thyroid nodules are listed in Table 320-9. These lesions are common (5 to 10% adults), particularly when assessed by sensitive techniques such as ultrasound. The risk of malignancy is very low for *macrofollicular adenomas* and *normofollicular adenomas*. Microfollicular, trabecular, and Hürthle cell variants raise greater concern, and the histology is more difficult to interpret. About one-third of palpable nodules are *thyroid cysts*. These may be recognized by their ultrasound appearance or based on aspiration of large amounts of pink or straw-colored fluid (colloid). Many are mixed cystic/solid lesions, in which case it is desirable to aspirate cellular components under ultrasound or harvest cells after cytospin of cyst fluid. Cysts frequently recur, even after repeated aspiration, and

FIGURE 320-9 Activating mutations of the TSH-R. Mutations (*) that activate the thyroid-stimulating hormone receptor (TSH-R) reside mainly in transmembrane 5 and intracellular loop 3, though mutations have occurred in a variety of different locations. The effect of these mutations is to induce conformational changes that mimic TSH binding, thereby leading to coupling to stimulatory G protein ($G_{s\alpha}$) and activation of adenylate cyclase (AC), an enzyme that generates cyclic AMP.

may require surgical excision if they are large or if the cytology is suspicious. Sclerosis has been used with variable success but is often painful and may be complicated by infiltration of the sclerosing agent.

The treatment approach for benign nodules is similar to that for MNG. TSH suppression with levothyroxine decreases the size of about 30% of nodules and may prevent further growth. The TSH level should

TABLE 320-9 Classification of Thyroid Neoplasms

BENIGN	
Follicular epithelial cell adenomas	
Macrofollicular (colloid)	
Normofollicular (simple)	
Microfollicular (fetal)	
Trabecular (embryonal)	
Hürtle cell variant (oncocytic)	

MALIGNANT	APPROXIMATE PREVALENCE, %
Follicular epithelial cell	
Well-differentiated carcinomas	
Papillary carcinomas	80–90
Pure papillary	
Follicular variant	
Diffuse sclerosing variant	
Tall cell, columnar cell variants	
Follicular carcinomas	5–10
Minimally invasive	
Widely invasive	
Hürthle cell carcinoma (oncocytic)	
Insular carcinoma	
Undifferentiated (anaplastic)	
carcinomas	
C cell (calcitonin-producing)	
Medullary thyroid cancer	10
Sporadic	
Familial	
MEN 2	
Other malignancies	
Lymphomas	1–2
Sarcomas	
Metastases	
Others	

Note: MEN, multiple endocrine neoplasia.

be suppressed into the low-normal range, assuming there are no contraindications; alternatively, nodule size can be monitored without suppression. If a nodule has not decreased in size after 6 to 12 months of suppressive therapy, treatment should be discontinued as little benefit is likely to accrue from long-term treatment.

THYROID CANCER

Thyroid carcinoma is the most common malignancy of the endocrine system. Malignant tumors derived from the follicular epithelium are classified according to histologic features. Differentiated tumors, such as papillary thyroid cancer (PTC) or follicular thyroid cancer (FTC), are often curable, and the prognosis is good for patients identified with early-stage disease. In contrast, anaplastic thyroid cancer (ATC) is aggressive, responds poorly to treatment, and is associated with a bleak prognosis.

The incidence of thyroid cancer (~9/100,000 per year) increases with age, plateauing after about age 50 (Fig. 320-10). Age is also an important prognostic factor—thyroid cancer at a young age (<20) or in older persons (>65) is associated with a worse prognosis. Thyroid cancer is twice as common in women as men, but male sex is associated with a worse prognosis. Additional important risk factors include a history of childhood head or neck irradiation, large nodule size (≥4 cm), evidence for local tumor fixation or invasion into lymph nodes, and the presence of metastases (Table 320-10).

Several unique features of thyroid cancer facilitate its management: (1) thyroid nodules are readily palpable, allowing early detection and biopsy by FNA; (2) iodine radioisotopes can be used to diagnose (^{123}I) and treat (^{131}I) differentiated thyroid cancer, reflecting the unique uptake of this anion by the thyroid gland; and (3) serum markers allow the detection of residual or recurrent disease, including the use of Tg levels for PTC and FTC and calcitonin for medullary thyroid cancer (MTC).

CLASSIFICATION   Thyroid neoplasms can arise in each of the cell types that populate the gland, including thyroid follicular cells, calcitonin-producing C cells, lymphocytes, and stromal and vascular elements, as well as metastases from other sites (Table 320-9). The American Joint Committee on Cancer (AJCC) has designated a staging system using the TNM classification (Table 320-11). Several other classification and staging systems are also widely used, some of which place greater emphasis on histologic features or risk factors such as age or gender.

PATHOGENESIS AND GENETIC BASIS ■ Radiation   Early studies of the pathogenesis of thyroid cancer focused on the role of external radiation, which predisposes to chromosomal breaks, presumably leading to genetic rearrangements and loss of tumor-suppressor genes. Exter-

TABLE 320-10   *Risk Factors for Thyroid Carcinoma in Patients with Thyroid Nodule*

History of head and neck irradiation	Family history of thyroid cancer or MEN 2
Age <20 or >70 years	Vocal cord paralysis, hoarse voice
Increased nodule size (>4 cm)	Nodule fixed to adjacent structures
New or enlarging neck mass	Suspected lymph node involvement
Male gender	Iodine deficiency (follicular cancer)

Note: MEN, multiple endocrine neoplasia.

nal radiation of the mediastinum, face, head, and neck region was administered in the past to treat an array of conditions including acne and enlargement of the thymus, tonsils, and adenoids. Radiation exposure increases the risk of benign and malignant thyroid nodules, is associated with multicentric cancers, and shifts the incidence of thyroid cancer to an earlier age group. Radiation from nuclear fallout also increases the risk of thyroid cancer. Children seem more predisposed to the effects of radiation than adults. Of note, radiation derived from ^{131}I therapy appears to contribute little, if any, increased risk of thyroid cancer.

TSH and Growth Factors   Thyroid growth is regulated primarily by TSH but also by a variety of growth factors and cytokines. Many differentiated thyroid cancers express TSH receptors and, therefore, remain responsive to TSH. This observation provides the rationale for T_4 suppression of TSH in patients with thyroid cancer. Residual expression of TSH receptors also allows TSH-stimulated uptake of ^{131}I therapy (see below).

Oncogenes and Tumor-Suppressor Genes   Thyroid cancers are monoclonal in origin, consistent with the idea that they originate as a consequence of mutations that confer a growth advantage to a single cell. In addition to increased rates of proliferation, some thyroid cancers exhibit impaired apoptosis and features that enhance invasion, angiogenesis, and metastasis. By analogy with the model of multistep carcinogenesis proposed for colon cancer (Chap. 68), thyroid neoplasms have been analyzed for a variety of genetic alterations, but without clear evidence of an ordered acquisition of somatic mutations as they progress from the benign to the malignant state. On the other hand, certain mutations are relatively specific for thyroid neoplasia, some of which correlate with histologic classification (Table 320-12). For example, activating mutations of the TSH-R and the $G_{s\alpha}$ subunit are associated with autonomously functioning nodules. Though these mutations induce thyroid cell growth, this type of nodule is almost always benign. A variety of rearrangements involving the *RET* gene on chromosome 10 bring this receptor tyrosine kinase under the control of other promoters, leading to receptor overexpression. *RET* rearrangements occur in 20 to

FIGURE 320-10   Age-associated incidence (—◆—) and mortality (—●—) rates for invasive thyroid cancer. [*Adapted from LAG Ries et al (eds): SEER Cancer Statistics Review, 1973–1996, Bethesda, National Cancer Institute, 1999.*]

TABLE 320-11   *American Joint Committee on Cancer Staging System for Thyroid Cancers Using the TNM Classification*[a]

Papillary or follicular thyroid cancers		
	<45 years	>45 years
Stage I	Any T, any N, M0	T1, N0, M0
Stage II	Any T, any N, M1	T2 or T3, N0, M0
Stage III	—	T4, N0, M0
		Any T, N1, M0
Stage IV	—	Any T, any N, M1
Anaplastic thyroid cancer		
Stage IV	All cases are stage IV	
Medullary thyroid cancer		
Stage I	T1, N0, M0	
Stage II	T2–T4, N0, M0	
Stage III	Any T, N1, M0	
Stage IV	Any T, any N, M1	

[a] Criteria include: T, the size and extent of the primary tumor (T1 ≤ 1 cm; 1 cm < T2 ≤ 4 cm; T3 > 4 cm; T4 direct invasion through the thyroid capsule); N, the absence (N0) or presence (N1) of regional node involvement; M, the absence (M0) or presence (M1) of metastases.

TABLE 320-12 *Genetic Alterations in Thyroid Neoplasia*

Gene/Protein	Type of Gene	Chromosomal Location	Genetic Abnormality	Tumor
TSH receptor	GPCR receptor	14q31	Point mutations	Toxic adenoma, differentiated carcinomas
$G_{s\alpha}$	G protein	20q13.2	Point mutations	Toxic adenoma, differentiated carcinomas
RET/PTC	Receptor tyrosine kinase	10q11.2	Rearrangements PTC1: (inv(10)q11.2q21) PTC2: (t(10;17)(q11.2;q23)) PTC3: ELE1/TK	PTC
RET	Receptor tyrosine kinase	10q11.2	Point mutations	MEN 2, medullary thyroid cancer
TRK	Receptor tyrosine kinase	1q23-24	Rearrangements	Multinodular goiter, papillary thyroid cancer
RAS	Signal transducing p21	Hras 11p15.5 Kras 12p12.1; Nras 1p13.2	Point mutations	Differentiated thyroid carcinoma, adenomas
p53	Tumor suppressor, cell cycle control, apoptosis	17p13	Point mutations Deletion, insertion	Anaplastic cancer
APC	Tumor suppressor, adenomatous polyposis coli gene	5q21-q22	Point mutations	Anaplastic cancer, also associated with familial polyposis coli
p16 (MTS1, CDKN2A)	Tumor suppressor, cell cycle control	9p21	Deletions	Differentiated carcinomas
p21/WAF	Tumor suppressor, cell cycle control	6p21.2	Overexpression	Anaplastic cancer
MET	Receptor tyrosine kinase	7q31	Overexpression	Follicular thyroid cancer
c-MYC	Receptor tyrosine kinase	8q24.12.-13	Overexpression	Differentiated carcinoma
PTEN	Phosphatase	10q23	Point mutations	PTC in Cowden's syndrome (multiple hamartomas, breast tumors, gastrointestinal polyps, thyroid tumors)
Loss of heterozygosity (LOH)	?Tumor suppressors	3p; 11q13 Other loci	Deletions	Differentiated thyroid carcinomas, anaplastic cancer
PAX8-PPARγ1	Transcription factor Nuclear receptor fusion	t(2;3)(q13;p25)	Translocation	Follicular adenoma or carcinoma

Note: TSH, thyroid-stimulating hormone; $G_{s\alpha}$, G-protein stimulating α-subunit; RET, rearranged during transfection proto-oncogene; PTC, papillary thyroid cancer; TRK, tyrosine kinase receptor; RAS, rat sarcoma proto-oncogene; p53, p53 tumor suppressor gene; MET, met proto-oncogene (hepatocyte growth factor receptor); c-MYC, cellular homologue of myelocytomatosis virus proto-oncogene; PTEN, phosphatase and tensin homologue; APC, adenomatous polyposis coli; MTS, multiple tumor suppressor; CDKN2A, cyclin-dependent kinase inhibitor 2A; P21, p21 tumor suppressor; WAF, wild-type p53 activated fragment; GPCR, G protein–coupled receptor; ELE1/TK, ret-activating gene ele1/tyrosine kinase; MEN 2, multiple endocrine neoplasia-2; PAX8, Paired domain transcription factor; PPARγ1, peroxisome-proliferator activated receptor γ1.
Source: Adapted with permission from P Kopp, JL Jameson, in JL Jameson (ed): *Principles of Molecular Medicine*. Totowa, NJ, Humana Press, 1998.

40% of PTCs in different series and were observed with increased frequency in tumors developing after the Chernobyl radiation disaster. Rearrangements in PTC have also been observed for another tyrosine kinase gene, *TRK1*, which is located on chromosome 1. To date, the identification of PTC with *RET* or *TRK1* rearrangements has not proven useful for predicting prognosis or treatment responses. Another rearrangement, linking the thyroid developmental transcription factor PAX8 to the nuclear receptor PPARγ, has been identified in a significance fraction of follicular adenomas and FTCs. *RAS* mutations are found in about 20 to 30% of thyroid neoplasms, including adenomas as well as PTC and FTC, suggesting that these mutations do not strongly affect tumor phenotype. Loss of heterozygosity, consistent with deletions of tumor-suppressor genes, is particularly common in FTC, often involving chromosomes 3p or 11q. Mutations of the tumor suppressor, p53, play an important role in the development of ATC. Because p53 plays a role in cell cycle surveillance, DNA repair, and apoptosis, its loss may contribute to the rapid acquisition of genetic instability as well as poor treatment responses (Chap. 69). The role of other tumor-suppressor genes in thyroid cancer is under investigation (Table 320-12).

MTC, when associated with multiple endocrine neoplasia (MEN) type 2, harbors an inherited mutation of the *RET* gene. Unlike the rearrangements of *RET* seen in PTC, the mutations in MEN2 are point mutations that induce constitutive activity of the tyrosine kinase (Chap. 330). MTC is preceded by hyperplasia of the C cells, raising the likelihood that as-yet-unidentified "second hits" lead to cellular transformation. A subset of sporadic MTC contain somatic mutations that activate *RET*.

WELL-DIFFERENTIATED THYROID CANCER ■ **Papillary** PTC is the most common type of thyroid cancer, accounting for 70 to 90% of well-differentiated thyroid malignancies. Microscopic PTC is present in up to 25% of thyroid glands at autopsy, but most of these lesions are very small (several millimeters) and are not clinically significant. Characteristic cytologic features of PTC help make the diagnosis by FNA or after surgical resection; these include psammoma bodies, cleaved nuclei with an "orphan-Annie" appearance caused by large nucleoli, and the formation of papillary structures.

PTC tends to be multifocal and to invade locally within the thyroid gland as well as through the thyroid capsule and into adjacent structures in the neck. It has a propensity to spread via the lymphatic system but can metastasize hematogenously as well, particularly to bone and lung. Because of the relatively slow growth of the tumor, a significant burden of pulmonary metastases may accumulate, sometimes with remarkably few symptoms. The prognostic implication of lymph node spread is debated. Lymph node involvement by thyroid cancer can be remarkably well tolerated but probably increases the risk of recurrence and mortality, particularly in older patients. The staging of PTC by the TNM system is outlined in Table 320-11. Most papillary cancers are identified in the early stages (>80% stages I or II) and have an excellent prognosis, with survival curves similar to expected survival (Fig. 320-11A). Mortality is markedly increased in stage IV disease (distant metastases), but this group comprises only about 1% of patients. The treatment of PTC is described below.

Follicular The incidence of FTC varies widely in different parts of the world; it is more common in iodine-deficient regions. FTC is difficult

FIGURE 320-11 Survival rates in patients with differentiated thyroid cancer. *A.* Papillary cancer, cohort of 1851 patients. I, 1107 (60%), II, 408 (22%), III, 312 (17%), IV, 24 (1%); *n* = 1185. *B.* Follicular cancer, cohort of 153 patients. I, 42 (27%), II, 82 (54%), III, 6 (4%); IV, 23 (15%); *n* = 153. *[Adapted from PR Larsen et al: William's Textbook of Endocrinology, 9th ed, JD Wilson et al (eds). Philadelphia, Saunders, 1998, pp 389–575; with permission.]*

to diagnose by FNA because the distinction between benign and malignant follicular neoplasms rests largely on evidence of invasion into vessels, nerves, or adjacent structures. FTC tends to spread by hematogenous routes leading to bone, lung, and central nervous system metastases. Mortality rates associated with FTC are less favorable than for PTC, in part because a larger proportion of patients present with stage IV disease (Fig. 320-11*B*). Poor prognostic features include distant metastases, age >50 years, primary tumor size >4 cm, Hürthle cell histology, and the presence of marked vascular invasion.

℞ TREATMENT

Surgery All well-differentiated thyroid cancers should be surgically excised. In addition to removing the primary lesion, surgery allows accurate histologic diagnosis and staging, and multicentric disease is commonly found in the contralateral thyroid lobe. Lymph node spread can also be assessed at the time of surgery, and involved nodes can be removed. Recommendations about the extent of surgery vary for stage I disease, as survival rates are similar for lobectomy and near-total thyroidectomy. Lobectomy is associated with a lower incidence of hypoparathyroidism and injury to the recurrent laryngeal nerves. However, it is not possible to monitor Tg levels or to perform whole-body ^{131}I scans in the presence of the residual lobe. Moreover, if final staging or subsequent follow-up indicates the need for radioiodine scanning or treatment, repeat surgery is necessary to remove the remaining thyroid tissue. Therefore, near-total thyroidectomy is preferable in almost all patients; complication rates are acceptably low if the surgeon is highly experienced in the procedure. This approach, in combination with postsurgical radioablation of the remnant thyroid tissue, facilitates the use of radioiodine scanning and Tg determinations to assess disease recurrence.

TSH Suppression Therapy As most tumors are still TSH-responsive, levothyroxine suppression of TSH is a mainstay of thyroid cancer treatment. Though TSH suppression clearly provides therapeutic benefit, there are no prospective studies that identify the optimal level of TSH suppression. A reasonable goal is to suppress TSH as much as possible without subjecting the patient to unnecessary side effects from excess thyroid hormone, such as atrial fibrillation, osteopenia, anxiety, and other manifestations of thyrotoxicosis. For patients at low risk of recurrence, TSH should be suppressed into the low but detectable range (0.1 to 0.5 IU/L). For patients at high risk of recurrence, or with known metastatic disease, complete TSH suppression is indicated, if there are no strong contraindications to mild thyrotoxicosis. In this instance, unbound T_4 must also be monitored to avoid excessive treatment.

Radioiodine Treatment Well-differentiated thyroid cancer still incorporates radioiodine, though less efficiently than normal thyroid follicular cells. Radioiodine uptake is determined primarily by expression of the NIS and is stimulated by TSH, requiring expression of the TSH-R. The retention time for radioactivity is influenced by the extent to which the tumor retains differentiated functions such as iodide trapping and organification. After near-total thyroidectomy, substantial thyroid tissue remains, particularly in the thyroid bed and surrounding the parathyroid glands. Consequently, ^{131}I ablation is necessary to eliminate remaining normal thyroid tissue and to treat residual tumor cells.

INDICATIONS The use of therapeutic doses of radioiodine remains an area of controversy in thyroid cancer management. Postoperative thyroid ablation and radiodine treatment of known residual PTC or FTC reduce recurrence rates. For tumors that take up iodine, ^{131}I treatment can reduce or eliminate residual disease with relatively little associated toxicity. However, it is not clear that prophylactic radioiodine treatment reduces mortality for patients at relatively low risk. Most patients with stage 1 PTC with primary tumors <1.5 cm in size can be managed safely with thyroxine suppression, without radiation treatment, as the risk of recurrence and mortality is very low. For patients with larger papillary tumors, spread to the adjacent lymph nodes, FTC, or evidence of metastases, thyroid ablation and radioiodine treatment are generally indicated.

^{131}I THYROID ABLATION AND TREATMENT As noted above, the decision to use ^{131}I for thyroid ablation should be coordinated with the surgical approach, as radioablation is much more effective when there is minimal remaining normal thyroid tissue. A typical strategy is to treat the patient for several weeks postoperatively with liothyronine (25 μg bid or tid), followed by thyroid hormone withdrawal. Ideally, the TSH level should increase to >50 IU/L over 3 to 4 weeks. The level to which TSH rises is dictated largely by the amount of normal thyroid tissue remaining postoperatively. A scanning dose of ^{131}I [usually 148 to 185 MBq (4 to 5 mCi)] will reveal the amount of residual tissue and provides guidance about the dose needed to accomplish ablation. A maximum outpatient ^{131}I dose is 1110 MBq (29.9 mCi) in the United States, though ablation is often more complete using greater doses [1850 to 2775 MBq (50 to 75 mCi)]. In patients with known residual cancer, the larger doses ensure thyroid ablation and may destroy remaining tumor cells. A whole-body scan following the high-dose radioiodine treatment is useful to identify possible metastatic disease.

FOLLOW-UP WHOLE-BODY THYROID SCANNING AND THYROGLOBULIN DETERMINATIONS An initial whole-body scan should be performed about 6 months after surgery and thyroid ablation. The strategy for follow-up management of thyroid cancer has been altered by the availability of recombinant human TSH (rhTSH) to stimulate ^{131}I uptake and by the improved sensitivity of Tg assays to detect residual or recurrent disease. A scheme for using either rhTSH or thyroid hormone withdrawal for thyroid scanning is summarized in Fig. 320-12. After thyroid ablation, rhTSH can be used to stimulate ^{131}I uptake without subjecting patients to thyroid hormone withdrawal and its associated symptoms of hypothyroidism and the risk of prolonged TSH-stimulated tumor growth.

FIGURE 320-12 Use of recombinant thyroid-stimulating hormone (TSH) in the follow-up of patients with thyroid cancer. Tg, thyroglobulin; rhTSH, recombinant human TSH.

This approach is recommended for patients predicted to be at low risk of disease recurrence, since rhTSH is not currently approved for use in conjunction with therapeutic doses of ^{131}I. Alternatively, in patients who are likely to require ^{131}I treatment, the traditional approach of thyroid hormone withdrawal can be used to increase TSH. This involves switching patients from levothyroxine (T$_4$) to the more rapidly cleared hormone, liothyronine (T$_3$), thereby allowing TSH to increase more quickly. If residual disease is detected on the initial whole-body scan [148 to 185 MBq (4 to 5 mCi)], a larger treatment dose, usually between 2775 and 5550 MBq (75 and 150 mCi), can be administered depending on the degree of residual uptake and assessment of cancer risk. Because TSH stimulates Tg levels, Tg measurements should be obtained after administration of rhTSH or when TSH levels have risen after thyroid hormone withdrawal. Investigational protocols are measuring Tg levels after rhTSH stimulation but without radioiodine scanning. If the initial whole-body scan is negative and Tg levels are low, a repeat scan should be performed 1 year later. If still negative, the patient can be managed with suppressive therapy and measurements of Tg every 6 to 12 months. If a second follow-up scan is negative, no further scanning may be necessary if the patient is at low risk and there is no clinical or laboratory evidence of recurrence. Many authorities advocate radioiodine treatment for scan-negative, Tg-positive (Tg >5 to 10 ng/mL) patients, as many derive therapeutic benefit from a large dose of ^{131}I.

In addition to radioiodine, external beam radiotherapy is also used to treat specific metastatic lesions, particularly when they cause bone pain or threaten neurologic injury (e.g., vertebral metastases).

ANAPLASTIC AND OTHER FORMS OF THYROID CANCER ■ Anaplastic Thyroid Cancer
As noted above, ATC is a poorly differentiated and aggressive cancer. The prognosis is poor, and most patients die within 6 months of diagnosis. Because of the undifferentiated state of these tumors, the up-

take of radioiodine is usually negligible, but it can be used therapeutically if there is residual uptake. Chemotherapy has been attempted with multiple agents, including anthracyclines and paclitaxel, but is usually ineffective. External radiation therapy can be attempted and continued if tumors are responsive.

Thyroid Lymphoma Lymphoma in the thyroid gland often arises in the background of Hashimoto's thyroiditis. A rapidly expanding thyroid mass suggests the possibility of this diagnosis. Diffuse large cell lymphoma is the most common type in the thyroid. Biopsies reveal sheets of lymphoid cells that can be difficult to distinguish from small cell lung cancer or ATC. These tumors are often highly sensitive to external radiation. Surgical resection should be avoided as initial therapy because it may spread disease that is otherwise localized to the thyroid. If staging indicates disease outside of the thyroid, treatment should follow guidelines used for other forms of lymphoma (Chap. 97).

MEDULLARY THYROID CARCINOMA MTC can be sporadic or familial and accounts for about 5 to 10% of thyroid cancers. There are three familial forms of MTC: MEN 2A, MEN 2B, and familial MTC without other features of MEN (Chap. 330). In general, MTC is more aggressive in MEN 2B than in MEN 2A, and familial MTC is more aggressive than sporadic MTC. Elevated serum calcitonin provides a marker of residual or recurrent disease. It is reasonable to test all patients with MTC for *RET* mutations, as genetic counseling and testing of family members can be offered to those individuals who test positive for mutations.

The management of MTC is primarily surgical. Unlike tumors derived from thyroid follicular cells, these tumors do not take up radioiodine. External radiation treatment and chemotherapy may provide palliation in patients with advanced disease (Chap. 330).

APPROACH TO THE PATIENT

Patient with a Thyroid Nodule Palpable thyroid nodules are found in about 5% of adults, but the prevalence varies considerably worldwide. Given this high prevalence rate, it is common for the practitioner to identify thyroid nodules. The main goal of this evaluation is to identify, in a cost-effective manner, the small subgroup of individuals with malignant lesions.

As described above, nodules are more common in iodine-deficient areas, in women, and with aging. Most palpable nodules are >1 cm in diameter, but the ability to feel a nodule is influenced by its location within the gland (superficial versus deeply embedded), the anatomy of the patient's neck, and the experience of the examiner. More sensitive methods of detection, such as thyroid ultrasound and pathologic studies, reveal thyroid nodules in >20% of glands. These findings have led to much debate about how to detect nodules and which nodules to investigate further. Most authorities still rely on physical examination to detect thyroid nodules, reserving ultrasound for monitoring nodule size or as an aid in thyroid biopsy.

It is important to distinguish whether a patient presents with a solitary thyroid nodule or a prominent nodule in the context of a MNG, as the incidence of malignancy is greater in solitary nodules. An approach to the evaluation of a solitary nodule is outlined in Fig. 320-13. Most patients with thyroid nodules have normal thyroid function tests. Nonetheless, thyroid function should be assessed by measuring a TSH level, which may be suppressed by one or more autonomously functioning nodules. If the TSH is suppressed, a radionuclide scan is indicated to determine if the identified nodule is "hot," as lesions with increased uptake are almost never malignant and FNA is unnecessary. Otherwise, FNA biopsy should be the first step in the evaluation of a thyroid nodule. FNA has good sensitivity and specificity when performed by physicians familiar with the procedure and when the results are interpreted by experienced cytopathologists. The technique is particularly accurate for detecting PTC. The distinction of benign and malignant follicular lesions is often not possible using cytology alone.

In several large studies, FNA biopsies yielded the following findings: 70% benign, 10% malignant or suspicious for malignancy, and 20% nondiagnostic or yielding insufficient material for diagnosis. Characteristic features of malignancy mandate surgery. A diagnosis of follicular neoplasm also warrants surgery, as benign and malignant lesions cannot be distinguished based on cytopathology or frozen section. The management of patients with benign lesions is more variable. Many authorities advocate TSH suppression, whereas others monitor nodule size without suppression. With either approach, thyroid nodule size should be monitored, either by palpation or ultrasound. Repeat FNA is indicated if a nodule enlarges, and a second biopsy should be performed within 2 to 5 years to confirm the benign status of the nodule.

Nondiagnostic biopsies occur for many reasons, including a fibrotic reaction with relatively few cells available for aspiration, a cystic lesion in which cellular components reside along the cyst margin, or a nodule that may be too small for accurate aspiration. For these reasons, ultrasound-guided FNA is useful when the FNA is repeated. Ultrasound is also increasingly used for initial biopsies in an effort to enhance nodule localization and the accuracy of sampling.

The evaluation of a thyroid nodule is stressful for most patients. They are concerned about the possibility of thyroid cancer, whether verbalized or not. It is constructive, therefore, to review the diagnostic approach and to reassure patients when malignancy is not found. When a suspicious lesion or thyroid cancer is identified, an explanation of the generally favorable prognosis and available treatment options should be provided.

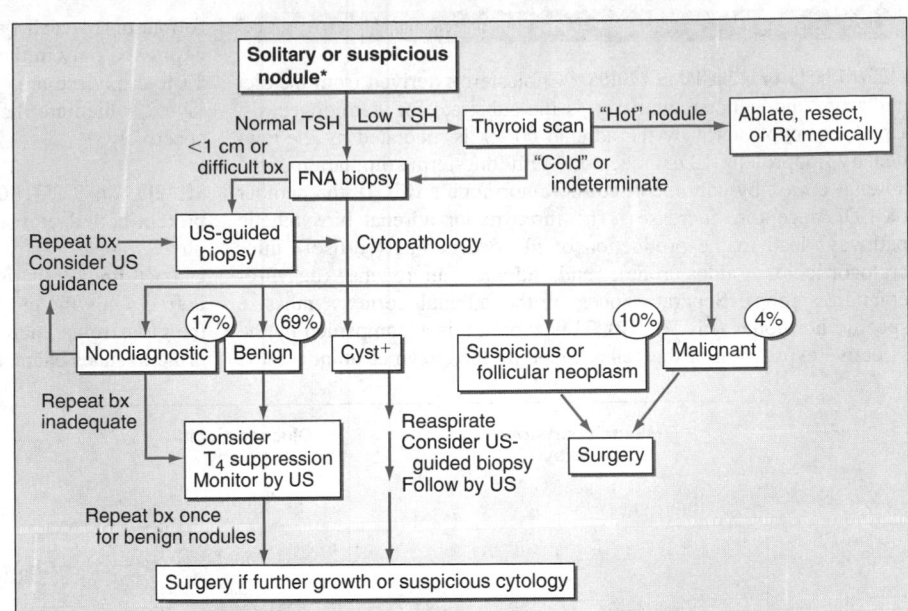

FIGURE 320-13   Approach to the patient with a thyroid nodule. *There are many exceptions to the suggested options. See text and references for details. †About one-third of nodules are cystic or mixed solid-cystic. US, ultrasound; TSH, thyroid-stimulating hormone; FNA, fine-needle aspiration.

FURTHER READING

DELANGE F et al: Iodine deficiency in the world: Where do we stand at the turn of the century? Thyroid 11:5, 2001

KOPP P: Perspective: Genetic defects in the etiology of congenital hypothyroidism. Endocrinology 143:2019, 2002

LADENSON PW et al: American Thyroid Association guidelines for detection of thyroid dysfunction. Arch Intern Med 160:1573, 2000

MAZZAFERRI EL et al: A concensus report of the role of serum thyroglobulin as a monitoring method for low-risk patients with papillary thyroid carcinoma. J Clin Endocrinol Metab 88:1433, 2003

WEETMAN AP: Graves' disease. N Engl J Med 343:1236, 2000

321 | DISORDERS OF THE ADRENAL CORTEX
Gordon H. Williams, Robert G. Dluhy

BIOCHEMISTRY AND PHYSIOLOGY

The adrenal cortex produces three major classes of steroids: (1) glucocorticoids, (2) mineralocorticoids, and (3) adrenal androgens. Consequently, normal adrenal function is important for modulating intermediary metabolism and immune responses through glucocorticoids; blood pressure, vascular volume, and electrolytes through mineralocorticoids; and secondary sexual characteristics (in females) through androgens. The adrenal axis plays an important role in the stress response by rapidly increasing cortisol levels. Adrenal disorders include hyperfunction (Cushing's syndrome) and hypofunction (adrenal insufficiency), as well as a variety of genetic abnormalities of steroidogenesis.

STEROID NOMENCLATURE   The basic structure of steroids is built upon a five-ring nucleus (Fig. 321-1). The carbon atoms are numbered in a sequence beginning with ring A. Adrenal steroids contain either 19 or 21 carbon atoms. The C_{19} steroids have methyl groups at C-18 and C-19. C_{19} steroids with a ketone group at C-17 are termed *17-ketosteroids*; C_{19} steroids have predominantly androgenic activity. The C_{21} steroids have a 2-carbon side chain (C-20 and C-21) attached at position 17 and methyl groups at C-18 and C-19; C_{21} steroids with a hydroxyl group at position 17 are termed *17-hydroxycorticosteroids*. The C_{21} steroids have either glucocorticoid or mineralocorticoid properties.

FIGURE 321-1   Basic steroid structure and nomenclature.

BIOSYNTHESIS OF ADRENAL STEROIDS Cholesterol, derived from the diet and from endogenous synthesis, is the substrate for steroidogenesis. Uptake of cholesterol by the adrenal cortex is mediated by the low-density lipoprotein (LDL) receptor. With long-term stimulation of the adrenal cortex by adrenocorticotropic hormone (ACTH), the number of LDL receptors increases. The three major adrenal biosynthetic pathways lead to the production of glucocorticoids (cortisol), mineralocorticoids (aldosterone), and adrenal androgens (dehydroepiandrosterone). Separate zones of the adrenal cortex synthesize specific hormones (Fig. 321-2). This zonation is accompanied by the selective expression of the genes encoding the enzymes unique to the formation of each type of steroid: aldosterone synthase is normally expressed only in the outer (glomerulosa) cell layer, whereas 21- and 17-hydroxylase are expressed in the (inner) faciculata-reticularis cell layers, which are the sites of cortisol and androgen biosynthesis, respectively.

STEROID TRANSPORT Cortisol circulates in the plasma as free cortisol, protein-bound cortisol, and cortisol metabolites. *Free cortisol* is a physiologically active hormone that is not protein-bound and therefore can act directly on tissue sites. Normally, <5% of circulating cortisol is free. Only the unbound cortisol and its metabolites are filterable at the glomerulus. Increased quantities of free steroid are excreted in the urine in states characterized by hypersecretion of cortisol, because the

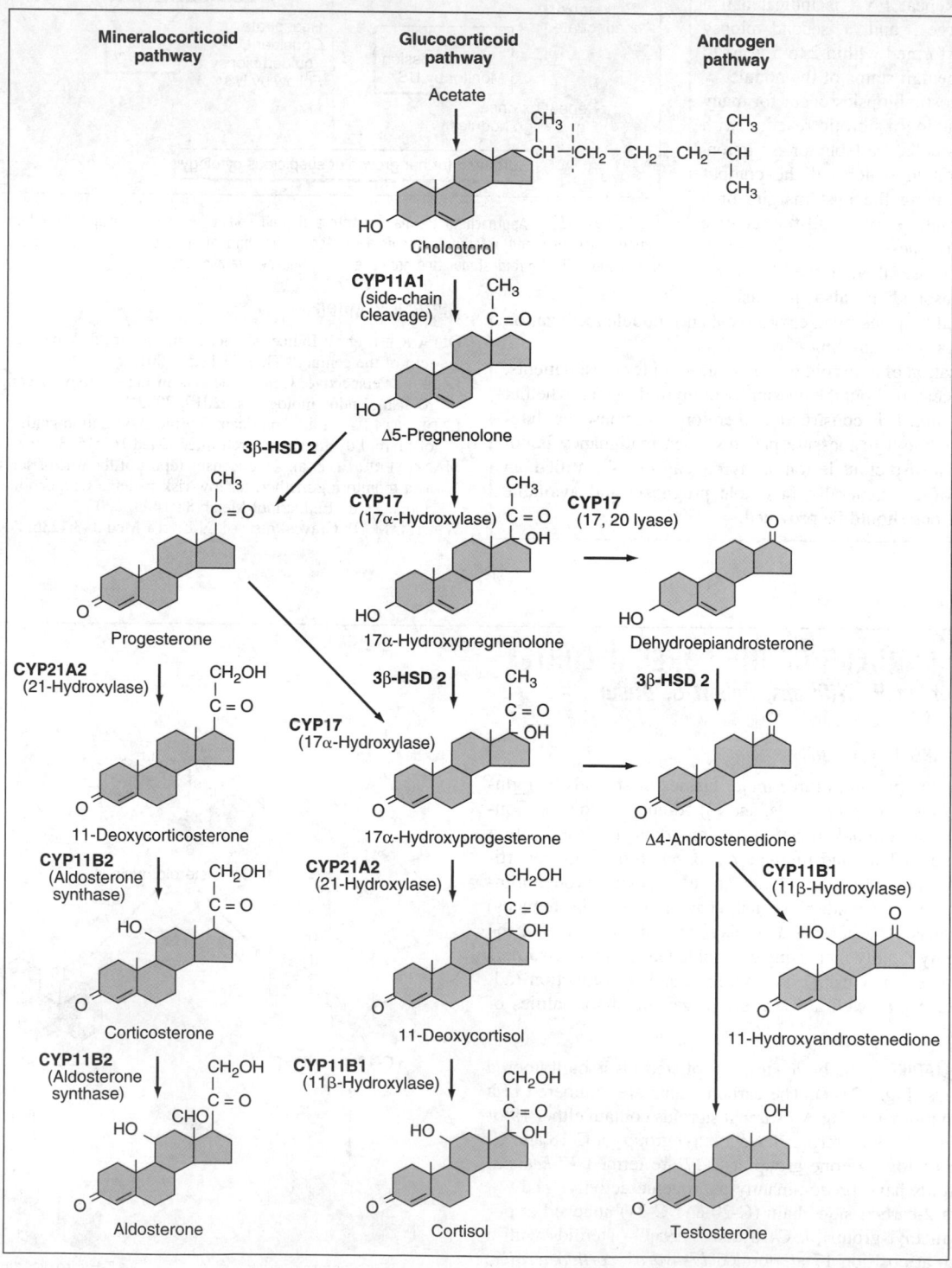

FIGURE 321-2 Biosynthetic pathways for adrenal steroid production; major pathways to mineralocorticoids, glucocorticoids, and androgens. 3β-HSD, 3β-hydroxysteroid dehydrogenase.

unbound fraction of plasma cortisol rises. Plasma has two cortisol-binding systems. One is a high-affinity, low-capacity α_2-globulin termed *transcortin* or *cortisol-binding globulin* (CBG), and the other is a low-affinity, high-capacity protein, *albumin*. Cortisol binding to CBG is reduced in areas of inflammation, thus increasing the local concentration of free cortisol. When the concentration of cortisol is >700 nmol/L (25 μg/dL), part of the excess binds to albumin, and a greater proportion than usual circulates unbound. CBG is increased in high-estrogen states (e.g., pregnancy, oral contraceptive administration). The rise in CBG is accompanied by a parallel rise in *protein-bound cortisol*, with the result that the total plasma cortisol concentration is elevated. However, the free cortisol level probably remains normal, and manifestations of glucocorticoid excess are absent. Most synthetic glucocorticoid analogues bind less efficiently to CBG (~70% binding). This may explain the propensity of some synthetic analogues to produce cushingoid effects at low doses. *Cortisol metabolites* are biologically inactive and bind only weakly to circulating plasma proteins.

Aldosterone is bound to proteins to a smaller extent than cortisol, and an ultrafiltrate of plasma contains as much as 50% of circulating aldosterone.

STEROID METABOLISM AND EXCRETION ■ Glucocorticoids The daily secretion of cortisol ranges between 40 and 80 μmol (15 and 30 mg; 8–10 mg/m²), with a pronounced circadian cycle. The plasma concentration of cortisol is determined by the rate of secretion, the rate of inactivation, and the rate of excretion of free cortisol. The liver is the major organ responsible for steroid inactivation. A major enzyme regulating cortisol metabolism is 11β-hydroxysteroid dehydrogenase (11β-HSD). There are two isoforms: 11β-HSD I is primarily expressed in the liver and acts as a reductase, converting the inactive cortisone to the active glucocorticoid, cortisol; the 11β-HSD II isoform is expressed in a number of tissues and converts cortisol to the inactive metabolite, cortisone. Mutations in the *11BHSD1* gene are associated with rapid cortisol turnover, leading to activation of the hypothalamic-pituitary-adrenal (HPA) axis and excessive adrenal androgen production in women. In animal models, excess omental expression of 11β-HSD I increases local glucocorticoid production and is associated with central obesity and insulin resistance. The oxidative reaction of 11β-HSD I is increased in hyperthyroidism. Mutations in the *11BHSD2* gene cause the syndrome of *apparent mineralocorticoid excess*, reflecting insufficient inactivation of cortisol in the kidney, allowing inappropriate cortisol activation of the mineralocorticoid receptor (see below).

Mineralocorticoids In individuals with normal salt intake, the average daily secretion of aldosterone ranges between 0.1 and 0.7 μmol (50 and 250 μg). During a single passage through the liver, >75% of circulating aldosterone is normally inactivated by conjugation with glucuronic acid. However, under certain conditions, such as congestive failure, this rate of inactivation is reduced.

Adrenal Androgens The major androgen secreted by the adrenal is dehydroepiandrosterone (DHEA) and its sulfuric acid ester (DHEAS). Approximately 15 to 30 mg of these compounds is secreted daily. Smaller amounts of androstenedione, 11β-hydroxyandrostenedione, and testosterone are secreted. DHEA is the major precursor of the urinary 17-ketosteroids. Two-thirds of the urine 17-ketosteroids in the male are derived from adrenal metabolites, and the remaining one-third comes from testicular androgens. In the female, almost all urine 17-ketosteroids are derived from the adrenal.

Steroids diffuse passively through the cell membrane and bind to intracellular receptors (Chap. 317). Glucocorticoids and mineralocorticoids bind with nearly equal affinity to the mineralocorticoid receptor (MR). However, only glucocorticoids bind to the glucocorticoid receptor (GR). After the steroid binds to the receptor, the steroid-receptor complex is transported to the nucleus, where it binds to specific sites on steroid-regulated genes, altering levels of transcription. Some actions of glucocorticoids (e.g., anti-inflammatory effects) are mediated by GR-mediated inhibition of other transcription factors, such as ac-

tivating protein-1 (AP-1) or nuclear factor kappa B (NFκB), which normally stimulate the activity of various cytokine genes. Because cortisol binds to the MR with the same affinity as aldosterone, mineralocorticoid specificity is achieved by local metabolism of cortisol to the inactive compound cortisone by 11β-HSD II. The glucocorticoid effects of other steroids, such as high-dose progesterone, correlate with their relative binding affinities for the GR. Inherited defects in the GR cause glucocorticoid resistance states. Individuals with GR defects have high levels of cortisol but do not have manifestations of hypercortisolism.

ACTH PHYSIOLOGY ACTH and a number of other peptides (lipotropins, endorphins, and melanocyte-stimulating hormones) are processed from a larger precursor molecule of 31,000 mol wt—proopiomelanocortin (POMC) (Chap. 318). POMC is made in a variety of tissues, including brain, anterior and posterior pituitary, and lymphocytes. The constellation of POMC-derived peptides secreted depends on the tissue. ACTH, a 39-amino-acid peptide, is synthesized and stored in basophilic cells of the anterior pituitary. The N-terminal 18-amino-acid fragment of ACTH has full biologic potency, and shorter N-terminal fragments have partial biologic activity. Release of ACTH and related peptides from the anterior pituitary gland is stimulated by corticotropin-releasing hormone (CRH), a 41-amino-acid peptide produced in the median eminence of the hypothalamus (Fig. 321-3). Urocortin, a neuropeptide related to CRH, mimics many of the central effects of CRH (e.g., appetite suppression, anxiety), but its role in ACTH reg-

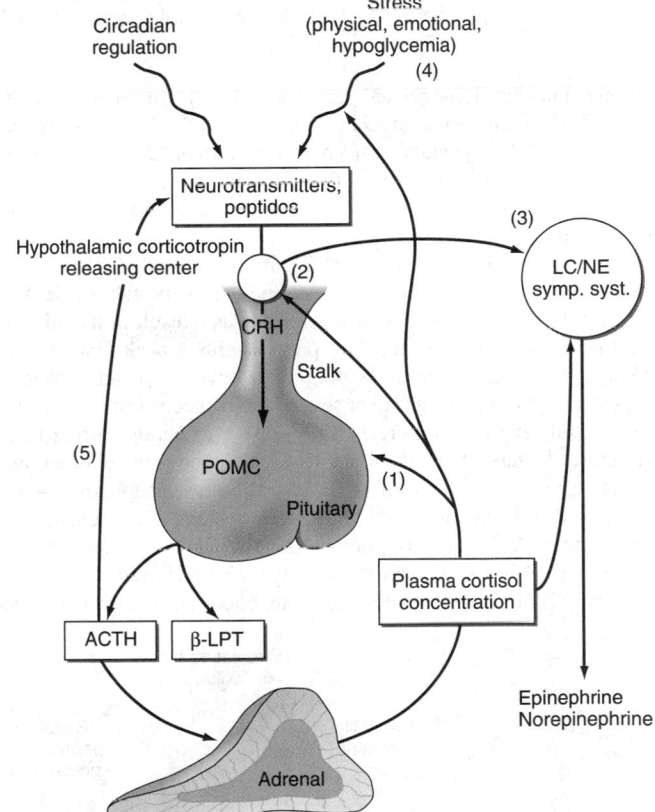

FIGURE 321-3 The hypothalamic-pituitary-adrenal axis. The main sites for feedback control by plasma cortisol are the pituitary gland (1) and the hypothalamic corticotropin-releasing center (2). Feedback control by plasma cortisol also occurs at the locus coeruleus/sympathetic system (3) and may involve higher nerve centers (4) as well. There may also be a short feedback loop involving inhibition of corticotropin-releasing hormone (CRH) by adrenocorticotropic hormone (ACTH) (5). Hypothalamic neurotransmitters influence CRH release; serotoninergic and cholinergic systems stimulate the secretion of CRH and ACTH; α-adrenergic agonists and γ-aminobutyric acid (GABA) probably inhibit CRH release. The opioid peptides β-endorphin and enkephalin inhibit, and vasopressin and angiotensin II augment, the secretion of CRH and ACTH. β-LPT, β-lipotropin; POMC, pro-opiomelanocortin; LC, locus coeruleus; NE, norepinephrine.

FIGURE 321-4 The immune-adrenal axis. Cortisol has anti-inflammatory properties that include effects on the microvasculature, cellular actions, and the suppression of inflammatory cytokines (the so-called immune-adrenal axis). A stress such as sepsis increases adrenal secretion, and cortisol in turn suppresses the immune response via this system. −, suppression; +, stimulation; CRH, corticotropin-releasing hormone; ACTH, adrenocorticotropic hormone; IL, interleukin; TNF, tumor necrosis factor; PAF, platelet activating factor.

ulation is unclear. Some related peptides such as β-lipotropin (β-LPT) are released in equimolar concentrations with ACTH, suggesting that they are cleaved enzymatically from the parent POMC before or during the secretory process. However, β-endorphin levels may or may not correlate with circulating levels of ACTH, depending on the nature of the stimulus.

The major factors controlling ACTH release include CRH, the free cortisol concentration in plasma, stress, and the sleep-wake cycle (Fig. 321-3). Plasma ACTH varies during the day as a result of its pulsatile secretion, and follows a circadian pattern with a peak just prior to waking and a nadir before sleeping. If a new sleep-wake cycle is adopted, the pattern changes over several days to conform to it. ACTH and cortisol levels also increase in response to eating. Stress (e.g., pyrogens, surgery, hypoglycemia, exercise, and severe emotional trauma) causes the release of CRH and arginine vasopressin (AVP) and activation of the sympathetic nervous system. These changes in turn enhance ACTH release, acting individually or in concert. For example, AVP release acts synergistically with CRH to amplify ACTH secretion; CRH also stimulates the locus coeruleus/sympathetic sys-

tem. Stress-related secretion of ACTH abolishes the circadian periodicity of ACTH levels but is, in turn, suppressed by prior high-dose glucocorticoid administration. The normal pulsatile, circadian pattern of ACTH release is regulated by CRH; this mechanism is the so-called open feedback loop. CRH secretion, in turn, is influenced by hypothalamic neurotransmitters including the serotoninergic and cholinergic pathways. The immune system also influences the HPA axis (Fig. 321-4). For example, inflammatory cytokines [tumor necrosis factor (TNF)-α, interleukin (IL) 1α, IL-1β, and IL-6] produced by monocytes increase ACTH release by stimulating secretion of CRH and/or AVP. Finally, ACTH release is regulated by the level of free cortisol in plasma. Cortisol decreases the responsiveness of pituitary corticotropic cells to CRH; the response of the POMC mRNA to CRH is also inhibited by glucocorticoids. In addition, glucocorticoids inhibit the locus coeruleus/sympathetic system and CRH release. The latter servomechanism establishes the primacy of cortisol in the control of ACTH secretion. The suppression of ACTH secretion that results in adrenal atrophy following *prolonged* glucocorticoid therapy is caused primarily by suppression of hypothalamic CRH release, as exogenous CRH administration in this circumstance produces a rise in plasma ACTH. Cortisol also exerts feedback effects on higher brain centers (hippocampus, reticular system, and septum) and perhaps on the adrenal cortex (Fig. 321-4).

The biologic half-life of ACTH in the circulation is <10 min. The action of ACTH is also rapid; within minutes of its release, the concentration of steroids in the adrenal venous blood increases. ACTH stimulates steroidogenesis via activation of adenyl cyclase. Adenosine-3′,5′-monophosphate (cyclic AMP), in turn, stimulates the synthesis of protein kinase enzymes, thereby resulting in the phosphorylation of proteins that activate steroid biosynthesis.

RENIN-ANGIOTENSIN PHYSIOLOGY Renin is a proteolytic enzyme that is produced and stored in the granules of the juxtaglomerular cells surrounding the afferent arterioles of glomeruli in the kidney. Renin acts on the basic substrate angiotensinogen (a circulating α₂-globulin made in the liver) to form the decapeptide angiotensin I (Fig. 321-5). Angiotensin I is then enzymatically transformed by angiotensin-converting enzyme (ACE), which is present in many tissues (particularly the pulmonary vascular endothelium), to the octapeptide angiotensin II by the removal of the two C-terminal amino acids. Angiotensin II is a potent pressor agent and exerts its action by a direct effect on arteriolar smooth muscle. In addition, angiotensin II stimulates production of aldosterone by the zona glomerulosa of the adrenal cortex; the heptapeptide angiotensin III may also stimulate aldosterone production. The two major classes of angiotensin receptors are termed *AT1* and *AT2*; AT1 may exist as two subtypes α and β. Most of the effects of angiotensins II and III are mediated by the AT1 receptor. Angiotensinases rapidly destroy angiotensin II (half-life, ~1 min), while the half-life of renin is more prolonged (10 to 20 min). In addition to circulating renin-angiotensin, many tissues have a local renin-angiotensin system and the ability to produce angiotensin II. These tissues include the uterus, placenta, vascular tissue, heart, brain, and, particularly, the adrenal cortex and kidney. Although the role of locally generated angiotensin II is not established, it may modulate the growth and function of the adrenal cortex and vascular smooth muscle.

The amount of renin released reflects the combined effects of four interdependent factors. The *juxtaglomerular cells*, which are specialized myoepithelial cells that cuff the afferent arterioles, act as miniature pressure transducers, sensing renal perfusion pressure and corresponding changes in afferent arteriolar perfusion pressures. For example, a reduction in circulating blood volume leads to a corresponding reduction in renal perfusion pressure and

FIGURE 321-5 The interrelationship of the volume and potassium feedback loops on aldosterone secretion. Integration of signals from each loop determines the level of aldosterone secretion.

afferent arteriolar pressure (Fig. 321-5). This change is perceived by the juxtaglomerular cells as a decreased stretch exerted on the afferent arteriolar walls, and the juxtaglomerular cells release more renin into the renal circulation. This results in the formation of angiotensin I, which is converted in the kidney and peripherally to angiotensin II by ACE. Angiotensin II influences sodium homeostasis via two major mechanisms: it changes renal blood flow so as to maintain a constant glomerular filtration rate, thereby changing the filtration fraction of sodium, and it stimulates the adrenal cortex to release aldosterone. Increasing plasma levels of aldosterone enhance renal sodium retention and thus result in expansion of the extracellular fluid volume, which, in turn, dampens the stimulus for renin release. In this context, the renin-angiotensin-aldosterone system regulates volume by modifying renal hemodynamics and tubular sodium transport.

A second control mechanism for renin release is centered in the *macula densa cells*, a group of distal convoluted tubular epithelial cells directly opposed to the juxtaglomerular cells. They may function as chemoreceptors, monitoring the sodium (or chloride) load presented to the distal tubule. Under conditions of increased delivery of filtered sodium to the macula densa, a signal is conveyed to decrease juxtaglomerular cell release of renin, thereby modulating the glomerular filtration rate and the filtered load of sodium.

The *sympathetic nervous system* regulates the release of renin in response to assumption of the upright posture. The mechanism is either a direct effect on the juxtaglomerular cell to increase adenyl cyclase activity or an indirect effect on either the juxtaglomerular or the macula densa cells via vasoconstriction of the afferent arteriole.

Finally, circulating factors influence renin release. Increased dietary intake of potassium decreases renin release, whereas decreased potassium intake increases it. The significance of these effects is unclear. Angiotensin II exerts negative feedback control on renin release that is independent of alterations in renal blood flow, blood pressure, or aldosterone secretion. *Atrial natriuretic peptides* also inhibit renin release. Thus, the control of renin release involves both *intrarenal* (pressor receptor and macula densa) and *extrarenal* (sympathetic nervous system, potassium, angiotensin, etc.) mechanisms. Steady-state renin levels reflect all these factors, with the intrarenal mechanism predominating.

GLUCOCORTICOID PHYSIOLOGY   The division of adrenal steroids into glucocorticoids and mineralocorticoids is arbitrary in that most glucocorticoids have some mineralocorticoid-like properties. The descriptive term *glucocorticoid* is used for adrenal steroids whose predominant action is on intermediary metabolism. Their overall actions are directed at enhancing the production of the high-energy fuel, glucose, and reducing all other metabolic activity not directly involved in that process. Sustained activation, however, results in a pathophysiologic state, e.g., Cushing's syndrome. The principal glucocorticoid is cortisol (hydrocortisone). The effect of glucocorticoids on intermediary metabolism is mediated by the GR. Physiologic effects of glucocorticoids include the regulation of protein, carbohydrate, lipid, and nucleic acid metabolism. Glucocorticoids raise the blood glucose level by antagonizing the secretion and actions of insulin, thereby inhibiting peripheral glucose uptake, which promotes hepatic glucose synthesis (gluconeogenesis) and hepatic glycogen content. The actions on protein metabolism are mainly catabolic, resulting in an increase in protein breakdown and nitrogen excretion. In large part, these actions reflect a mobilization of glycogenic amino acid precursors from peripheral supporting structures, such as bone, skin, muscle, and connective tissue, due to protein breakdown and inhibition of protein synthesis and amino acid uptake. Hyperaminoacidemia also facilitates gluconeogenesis by stimulating glucagon secretion. Glucocorticoids act directly on the liver to stimulate the synthesis of certain enzymes, such as tyrosine aminotransferase and tryptophan pyrrolase. Glucocorticoids regulate fatty acid mobilization by enhancing the activation of cellular lipase by lipid-mobilizing hormones (e.g., catecholamines and pituitary peptides).

The actions of cortisol on protein and adipose tissue vary in different parts of the body. For example, pharmacologic doses of cortisol can deplete the protein matrix of the vertebral column (trabecular bone), whereas long bones (which are primarily compact bone) are affected only minimally; similarly, peripheral adipose tissue mass decreases, whereas abdominal and interscapular fat expand.

Glucocorticoids have anti-inflammatory properties, which are probably related to effects on the microvasculature and to suppression of inflammatory cytokines. In this sense, glucocorticoids modulate the immune response via the so-called immune-adrenal axis (Fig. 321-4). This "loop" is one mechanism by which a stress, such as sepsis, increases adrenal hormone secretion, and the elevated cortisol level in turn suppresses the immune response. For example, cortisol maintains vascular responsiveness to circulating vasoconstrictors and opposes the increase in capillary permeability during acute inflammation. Glucocorticoids cause a leukocytosis that reflects release from the bone marrow of mature cells as well as inhibition of their egress through the capillary wall. Glucocorticoids produce a depletion of circulating eosinophils and lymphoid tissue, specifically T cells, by causing a redistribution from the circulation into other compartments. Thus, cortisol impairs cell-mediated immunity. Glucocorticoids also inhibit the production and action of the mediators of inflammation, such as the lymphokines and prostaglandins. Glucocorticoids inhibit the production and action of interferon by T lymphocytes and the production of IL-1 and IL-6 by macrophages. The antipyretic action of glucocorticoids may be explained by an effect on IL-1, which appears to be an endogenous pyrogen (Chap. 16). Glucocorticoids also inhibit the production of T cell growth factor (IL-2) by T lymphocytes. Glucocorticoids reverse macrophage activation and antagonize the action of migration-inhibiting factor (MIF), leading to reduced adherence of macrophages to vascular endothelium. Glucocorticoids reduce prostaglandin and leukotriene production by inhibiting the activity of phospholipase A$_2$, thus blocking release of arachidonic acid from phospholipids. Finally, glucocorticoids inhibit the production and inflammatory effects of bradykinin, platelet-activating factor, and serotonin. It is probably only at pharmacologic dosages that antibody production is reduced and lysosomal membranes are stabilized, the latter effect suppressing the release of acid hydrolases.

Cortisol levels respond within minutes to stress, whether physical (trauma, surgery, exercise), psychological (anxiety, depression), or physiologic (hypoglycemia, fever). The reasons why elevated glucocorticoid levels protect the organism under stress are not understood, but in conditions of glucocorticoid deficiency, such stresses may cause hypotension, shock, and death. Consequently, in individuals with adrenal insufficiency, glucocorticoid administration should be increased during stress.

Cortisol has major effects on body water. It helps regulate the extracellular fluid volume by retarding the migration of water into cells and by promoting renal water excretion, the latter effect mediated by suppression of vasopressin secretion, by an increase in the rate of glomerular filtration, and by a direct action on the renal tubule. The consequence is to prevent water intoxication by increasing solute-free water clearance. Glucocorticoids also have weak mineralocorticoid-like properties, and high doses promote renal tubular sodium reabsorption and increased urine potassium excretion. Glucocorticoids can also influence behavior; emotional disorders may occur with either an excess or a deficit of cortisol. Finally, cortisol suppresses the secretion of pituitary POMC and its derivative peptides (ACTH, β-endorphin, and β-LPT) and the secretion of hypothalamic CRH and vasopressin.

MINERALOCORTICOID PHYSIOLOGY   Mineralocorticoids modify function in two classes of cells—epithelial and nonepithelial.

Effects on Epithelia   Classically, mineralocorticoids are considered major regulators of extracellular fluid volume and are the major determinants of potassium metabolism. These effects are mediated by the binding of aldosterone to the MR in epithelial cells, primarily the principal cells in the renal cortical collecting duct. Because of its electrochemical gradient, sodium passively enters these cells from the urine via epithelial sodium channels located on the luminal membrane and is actively extruded from the cell via the Na/K-activated ATPase ("sodium pump") located on the basolateral membrane. The sodium pump also provides the driving force of potassium loss into the urine through potassium-selective luminal channels, again assisted by the electrochemical gradient for potassium in these cells. Aldosterone stimulates all three of these processes by increasing gene expression directly (for the sodium pump and the potassium channels) or via a complex process (for epithelial sodium channels) to increase both the number and activity of the sodium channels. Water passively follows the transported sodium, thus expanding intra- and extravascular volume.

Because the concentration of hydrogen ion is greater in the lumen than in the cell, hydrogen ion is also actively secreted. Mineralocorticoids also act on the epithelium of the salivary ducts, sweat glands, and gastrointestinal tract to cause reabsorption of sodium in exchange for potassium.

When normal individuals are given aldosterone, an initial period of sodium retention is followed by natriuresis, and sodium balance is reestablished after 3 to 5 days. As a result, edema does not develop. This process is referred to as the *escape phenomenon*, signifying an "escape" by the renal tubules from the sodium-retaining action of aldosterone. While renal hemodynamic factors may play a role in the escape, the level of atrial natriuretic peptide also increases. However, it is important to realize that there is no escape from the potassium-losing effects of mineralocorticoids.

Effect on Nonepithelial Cells The MR has been identified in a number of nonepithelial cells, e.g., neurons in the brain, myocytes, endothelial cells, and vascular smooth-muscle cells. In these cells, the actions of aldosterone differ from those in epithelial cells in several ways:

1. They do not modify sodium-potassium homeostasis.
2. The groups of regulated genes differ, although only a few are known; for example, in nonepithelial cells, aldosterone modifies the expression of several collagen genes and/or genes controlling tissue growth factors, e.g., transforming growth factor (TGF) β and plasminogen activator inhibitor, type 1 (PAI-1).
3. In some of these tissues (e.g., myocardium and brain), the MR is not protected by the 11β-HSD II enzyme. Thus, cortisol rather than aldosterone may be activating the MR. In other tissues (e.g., the vasculature), 11β-HSD II is expressed in a manner similar to that of the kidney. Therefore, aldosterone is activating the MR.
4. Some effects on nonepithelial cells may be via nongenomic mechanisms. These actions are too rapid—occurring within 1 to 2 min and peaking within 5 to 10 min—to be considered genomic, suggesting that they are secondary to activation of a cell-surface receptor. However, no cell-surface MR has been identified, raising the possibility that the same MR is mediating both genomic and nongenomic effects. Rapid, nongenomic effects have also been described for other steroids including estradiol, progesterone, thyroxine, and vitamin D.
5. Some of these tissues—the myocardium and vasculature—may also produce aldosterone, although this theory is controversial.

Regulation of Aldosterone Secretion Three primary mechanisms control adrenal aldosterone secretion: the renin-angiotensin system, potassium, and ACTH (Table 321-1). Whether these are also the primary regulatory mechanisms modifying nonadrenal production is uncertain. The renin-angiotensin system controls extracellular fluid volume via regulation of aldosterone secretion (Fig. 321-5). In effect, the renin-angiotensin system maintains the circulating blood volume constant by causing aldosterone-induced sodium retention during volume deficiency and by decreasing aldosterone-dependent sodium retention when volume is ample. There is an increasing body of evidence indicating that some tissues, in addition to the kidney, produce angiotensin II and may participate in the regulation of aldosterone secretion either from the adrenal or extraadrenal sources. Intriguingly, the ad-

TABLE 321-1 *Factors Regulating Aldosterone Biosynthesis*

Factor	Effect
Renin-angiotensin system	Stimulation
Sodium ion	Inhibition (?physiologic)
Potassium ion	Stimulation
Neurotransmitters	
Dopamine	Inhibition
Serotonin	Stimulation
Pituitary hormones	
ACTH	Stimulation
Non-ACTH pituitary hormones (e.g., growth hormone)	Permissive (for optimal response to sodium restriction)
β-Endorphin	Stimulation
γ-Melanocyte-stimulating hormone	Permissive
Atrial natriuretic peptide	Inhibition
Ouabain-like factors	Inhibition
Endothelin	Stimulation

Note: ACTH, adrenocorticotropic hormone.

renal itself is capable of synthesizing angiotensin II. What role(s) the extrarenal production of angiotensin II plays in normal physiology is still largely unknown. However, the tissue renin-angiotensin system is activated in utero in response to growth and development and/or later in life in response to injury.

Potassium ion directly stimulates aldosterone secretion, independent of the circulating renin-angiotensin system, which it suppresses (Fig. 321-5). In addition to a direct effect, potassium also modifies aldosterone secretion indirectly by activating the local renin-angiotensin system in the zona glomerulosa. This effect can be blocked by the administration of ACE inhibitors that reduce the local production of angiotensin II and thereby reduce the acute aldosterone response to potassium. An increase in serum potassium of as little as 0.1 mmol/L increases plasma aldosterone levels under certain circumstances. Oral potassium loading therefore increases aldosterone secretion, plasma levels, and excretion.

Physiologic amounts of ACTH stimulate aldosterone secretion acutely, but this action is not sustained unless ACTH is administered in a pulsatile fashion. Most studies relegate ACTH to a minor role in the control of aldosterone. For example, subjects receiving high-dose glucocorticoid therapy, and with presumed complete suppression of ACTH, have normal aldosterone secretion in response to sodium restriction.

Prior dietary intake of both potassium and sodium can alter the magnitude of the aldosterone response to acute stimulation. This effect results from a change in the expression and activity of aldosterone synthase. Increasing potassium intake or decreasing sodium intake sensitizes the response of the glomerulosa cells to acute stimulation by ACTH, angiotensin II, and/or potassium.

Neurotransmitters (dopamine and serotonin) and some peptides, such as atrial natriuretic peptide, γ-melanocyte-stimulating hormone (γ-MSH), and β-endorphin, also participate in the regulation of aldosterone secretion (Table 321-1). Thus, the control of aldosterone secretion involves both stimulatory and inhibitory factors.

ANDROGEN PHYSIOLOGY Androgens regulate male secondary sexual characteristics and can cause virilizing symptoms in women (Chap. 44). Adrenal androgens have a minimal effect in males whose sexual characteristics are predominantly determined by gonadal steroids (testosterone). In females, however, several androgen-like effects, e.g., sexual hair, are largely mediated by adrenal androgens. The principal adrenal androgens are DHEA, androstenedione, and 11-hydroxyandrostenedione. DHEA and androstenedione are weak androgens and exert their effects via conversion to the potent androgen testosterone in extraglandular tissues. DHEA also has poorly understood effects on the immune and cardiovascular systems. Adrenal androgen formation is regulated by ACTH, not by gonadotropins. Adrenal androgens are suppressed by exogenous glucocorticoid administration.

A basic assumption is that measurements of the plasma or urinary level of a given steroid reflect the rate of adrenal *secretion* of that steroid. However, urine *excretion* values may not truly reflect the secretion rate because of improper collection or altered metabolism. Plasma levels reflect the level of secretion only at the time of measurement. The plasma level (*PL*) depends on two factors: the secretion rate (*SR*) of the hormone and the rate at which it is metabolized, i.e., its metabolic clearance rate (*MCR*). These three factors can be related as follows:

$$PL = \frac{SR}{MCR} \quad \text{or} \quad SR = MCR \times PL$$

BLOOD LEVELS ■ Peptides The plasma levels of ACTH and angiotensin II can be measured by immunoassay techniques. Basal ACTH secretion shows a circadian rhythm, with lower levels in the early evening than in the morning. However, ACTH is secreted in a pulsatile manner, leading to rapid fluctuations superimposed on this circadian rhythm. Angiotensin II levels also vary diurnally and are influenced by dietary sodium and potassium intakes and posture. Both upright posture and sodium restriction elevate angiotensin II levels.

Most clinical determinations of the renin-angiotensin system, however, involve measurements of peripheral *plasma renin activity* (PRA) in which the renin activity is gauged by the generation of angiotensin I during a standardized incubation period. This method depends on the presence of sufficient angiotensinogen in the plasma as substrate. The generated angiotensin I is measured by radioimmunoassay. The PRA depends on the dietary sodium intake and on whether the patient is ambulatory. In normal humans, the PRA shows a diurnal rhythm characterized by peak values in the morning and a nadir in the afternoon. An alternative approach is to measure plasma active renin, which is easier and not dependent on endogenous substrate concentration. PRA and active renin correlate very well on low-sodium diets but less well on high-sodium diets.

Steroids Cortisol and aldosterone are both secreted episodically, and levels vary during the day, with peak values in the morning and low levels in the evening. In addition, the plasma level of aldosterone, but not of cortisol, is increased by dietary potassium loading, by sodium restriction, or by assumption of the upright posture. Measurement of the sulfate conjugate of DHEA may be a useful index of adrenal androgen secretion, as little DHEA sulfate is formed in the gonads and because the half-life of DHEA sulfate is 7 to 9 h. However, DHEA sulfate levels reflect both DHEA production and sulfatase activity.

URINE LEVELS For the assessment of glucocorticoid secretion, the urine 17-hydroxycorticosteroid assay has been replaced by measurement of urinary free cortisol. Elevated levels of urinary free cortisol correlate with states of hypercortisolism, reflecting changes in the levels of unbound, physiologically active circulating cortisol. Normally, the rate of excretion is higher in the daytime (7 A.M. to 7 P.M.) than at night (7 P.M. to 7 A.M.).

Urinary 17-ketosteroids originate in either the adrenal gland or the gonad. In normal women, 90% of urinary 17-ketosteroids is derived from the adrenal, and in men 60 to 70% is of adrenal origin. Urine 17-ketosteroid values are highest in young adults and decline with age.

A carefully timed urine collection is a prerequisite for all excretory determinations. Urinary creatinine should be measured simultaneously to determine the accuracy and adequacy of the collection procedure.

STIMULATION TESTS Stimulation tests are useful in the diagnosis of hormone deficiency states.

Tests of Glucocorticoid Reserve Within minutes after administration of ACTH, cortisol levels increase. This responsiveness can be used as an index of the functional reserve of the adrenal gland for production of cortisol. Under maximal ACTH stimulation, cortisol secretion increases tenfold, to 800 μmol/d (300 mg/d), but maximal stimulation can be achieved only with prolonged ACTH infusions.

A screening test (the so-called rapid ACTH stimulation test) involves the administration of 25 units (0.25 mg) of cosyntropin intravenously or intramuscularly and measurement of plasma cortisol levels before administration and 30 and 60 min after administration, the test can be performed at any time of the day. The most clear-cut criterion for a normal response is a stimulated cortisol level of >500 nmol/L (>18 μg/dL), and the minimal stimulated normal increment of cortisol is >200 nmol/L (>7 μg/dL) above baseline. Severely ill patients with elevated basal cortisol levels may show no further increases following acute ACTH administration.

Tests of Mineralocorticoid Reserve and Stimulation of the Renin-Angiotensin System Stimulation tests use protocols designed to create a programmed volume depletion, such as sodium restriction, diuretic administration, or upright posture. A simple, potent test consists of severe sodium restriction and upright posture. After 3 to 5 days of a 10-mmol/d sodium intake, rates of aldosterone secretion or excretion should increase two- to threefold over the control values. Supine morning plasma aldosterone levels are usually increased three- to sixfold, and they increase a further two- to fourfold in response to 2 to 3 h of upright posture.

When the dietary sodium intake is normal, stimulation testing requires the administration of a potent diuretic, such as 40 to 80 mg furosemide, followed by 2 to 3 h of upright posture. The normal response is a two- to fourfold rise in plasma aldosterone levels.

SUPPRESSION TESTS Suppression tests to document hypersecretion of adrenal hormones involve measurement of the target hormone response after standardized suppression of its tropic hormone.

Tests of Pituitary-Adrenal Suppressibility The ACTH release mechanism is sensitive to the circulating glucocorticoid level. When blood levels of glucocorticoid are increased in normal individuals, less ACTH is released from the anterior pituitary and less steroid is produced by the adrenal gland. The integrity of this feedback mechanism can be tested clinically by giving a glucocorticoid and judging the suppression of ACTH secretion by analysis of urine steroid levels and/or plasma cortisol and ACTH levels. A potent glucocorticoid such as dexamethasone is used, so that the agent can be given in an amount small enough not to contribute significantly to the pool of steroids to be analyzed.

The best *screening* procedure is the overnight dexamethasone suppression test. This involves the measurement of plasma cortisol levels at 8 A.M. following the oral administration of 1 mg dexamethasone the previous midnight. The 8 A.M. value for plasma cortisol in normal individuals should be <140 nmol/L (5 μg/dL).

The definitive test of adrenal suppressibility involves administering 0.5 mg dexamethasone every 6 h for two successive days while collecting urine over a 24-h period for determination of creatinine and free cortisol and/or measuring plasma cortisol levels. In a patient with a normal hypothalamic-pituitary ACTH release mechanism, a fall in the urine free cortisol to <80 nmol/d (30 μg/d) or of plasma cortisol to <140 nmol/L (5 μg/dL) is seen on the second day of administration.

A normal response to either suppression test implies that the glucocorticoid regulation of ACTH and its control of the adrenal glands is physiologically normal. However, an isolated abnormal result, particularly to the overnight suppression test, does not in itself demonstrate pituitary and/or adrenal disease.

Tests of Mineralocorticoid Suppressibility These tests rely on an expansion of extracellular fluid volume, which should decrease circulating plasma renin activity and decrease the secretion and/or excretion of aldosterone. Various tests differ in the rate at which extracellular fluid volume is expanded. One convenient suppression test involves the intravenous infusion of 500 mL/h of normal saline solution for 4 h, which normally suppresses plasma aldosterone levels to <220 pmol/L (<8 ng/dL) from a sodium-restricted diet or to <140 pmol/L (<5 ng/dL) from a normal sodium intake. Alternatively, a high-sodium diet can be administered for 3 days with 0.2 mg fludrocortisone twice daily. Aldosterone excretion is measured on the third day and should be <28 nmol/d (10 μg/d). These tests should not be performed in potassium-depleted individuals since they carry a risk of precipitating hypokalemia.

TESTS OF PITUITARY-ADRENAL RESPONSIVENESS Stimuli such as insulin-induced hypoglycemia, AVP, and pyrogens induce the release of ACTH from the pituitary by an action on higher neural centers or on the pituitary itself. Insulin-induced hypoglycemia is particularly useful, because it stimulates the release of both growth hormone and ACTH. In this test, regular insulin (0.05 to 0.1 U/kg body weight) is given intravenously as a bolus to reduce the fasting glucose level to at least 50% below basal. The normal cortisol response is a rise to >500 nmol/L (18 μg/dL). Glucose levels must be monitored during insulin-induced hypoglycemia, and it should be terminated by feeding or intravenous glucose, if subjects develop symptoms of hypoglycemia. This test is contraindicated in individuals with coronary artery disease or a seizure disorder.

Metyrapone inhibits 11β-hydroxylase in the adrenal. As a result, the conversion of 11-deoxycortisol (compound S) to cortisol is impaired, causing 11-deoxycortisol to accumulate in the blood and the blood level of cortisol to decrease (Fig. 321-2). The hypothalamic-pituitary axis responds to the declining cortisol blood levels by releasing more ACTH. Note that assessment of the response depends on both an intact hypothalamic-pituitary axis and an intact adrenal gland.

Although modifications of the original metyrapone test have been described, a commonly used protocol involves administering 750 mg of the drug by mouth every 4 h over a 24-h period and comparing the control and postmetyrapone plasma levels of 11-deoxycortisol, cortisol, and ACTH. In normal individuals, plasma 11-deoxycortisol levels should exceed 210 nmol/L (7 μg/dL) and ACTH levels should exceed 17 pmol/L (75 pg/mL) following metyrapone administration. The metyrapone test does not accurately reflect ACTH reserve if subjects are ingesting exogenous glucocorticoids or drugs that accelerate the metabolism of metyrapone (e.g., phenytoin).

A direct and selective test of the pituitary corticotrophs can be achieved with CRH. The bolus injection of ovine CRH (corticorelin ovine triflutate; 1 μg/kg body weight) stimulates secretion of ACTH and β-LPT in normal human subjects within 15 to 60 min. In normal individuals, the mean increment in ACTH is 9 pmol/L (40 pg/mL). However, the magnitude of the ACTH response is less than that produced by insulin-induced hypoglycemia, implying that additional factors (such as vasopressin) augment stress-induced increases in ACTH secretion.

The rapid ACTH test can often distinguish between primary and secondary adrenal insufficiency, because aldosterone secretion is preserved in secondary adrenal failure by the renin-angiotensin system and potassium. Cosyntropin (25 units) is given intravenously or intramuscularly, and plasma cortisol and aldosterone levels are measured before and at 30 and 60 min after administration. The cortisol response is abnormal in both groups, but patients with secondary insufficiency show an increase in aldosterone levels of at least 140 pmol/L (5 ng/dL). No aldosterone response is seen in patients in whom the adrenal cortex is destroyed. Alternatively, ACTH at a physiologic dose (1 μg), the so-called low-dose ACTH test, may be used to detect secondary adrenal insufficiency. An abnormal response is similar to that in the rapid ACTH test. However, levels need to be measured at 30 min, and the ACTH needs to be directly injected intravenously because it can be absorbed by plastic tubing. Because the use of a bolus of exogenous ACTH does not invariably exclude a diagnosis of secondary adrenocortical insufficiency, direct tests of pituitary ACTH reserve (metyrapone test, insulin-induced hypoglycemia) may be required in the appropriate clinical setting.

HYPERFUNCTION OF THE ADRENAL CORTEX

Excess cortisol is associated with Cushing's syndrome; excess aldosterone causes aldosteronism; and excess adrenal androgens cause adrenal virilism. These syndromes do not always occur in the "pure" form but may have overlapping features.

CUSHING'S SYNDROME ■ **Etiology** Cushing described a syndrome characterized by truncal obesity, hypertension, fatigability and weakness, amenorrhea, hirsutism, purplish abdominal striae, edema, glucosuria, osteoporosis, and a basophilic tumor of the pituitary. As awareness of this syndrome has increased, the diagnosis of Cushing's syndrome has been broadened into the classification shown in Table 321-2. Regardless of etiology, all cases of endogenous Cushing's syndrome are due to increased production of cortisol by the adrenal. In most cases the cause is *bilateral adrenal hyperplasia* due to hypersecretion of pituitary ACTH or ectopic production of ACTH by a nonpituitary source. The incidence of pituitary-dependent adrenal hyperplasia is three times greater in women than in men, and the most frequent age of onset is the third or fourth decade. Most evidence indicates that the primary defect is the de novo development of a pituitary adenoma, as tumors are found in >90% of patients with pituitary-dependent adrenal hyperplasia. Alternatively, the defect may occasionally reside in the hypothalamus or in higher neural centers, leading to release of CRH inappropriate to the level of circulating cortisol. This primary defect leads to hyperstimulation of the pituitary, resulting in hyperplasia or tumor formation. In surgical series, most individuals with hypersecretion of pituitary ACTH are found to have a microadenoma (<10 mm in diameter; 50% are ≤5 mm in diameter), but a pituitary macroadenoma (>10 mm) or diffuse hyperplasia of the corticotrope cells may be found. Traditionally, only an individual who has an ACTH-producing pituitary tumor is defined as having *Cushing's disease*, whereas Cushing's syndrome refers to all causes of excess cortisol: exogenous ACTH tumor, adrenal tumor, pituitary ACTH-secreting tumor, or excessive glucocorticoid treatment.

The *ectopic ACTH syndrome* is caused by nonpituitary tumors that secrete either ACTH and/or CRH and cause bilateral adrenal hyperplasia (Chap. 86). The ectopic production of CRH results in clinical, biochemical, and radiologic features indistinguishable from those caused by hypersecretion of pituitary ACTH. The typical signs and symptoms of Cushing's syndrome may be absent or minimal with ectopic ACTH production, and hypokalemic alkalosis is a prominent manifestation. Most of these cases are associated with the primitive small cell (oat cell) type of bronchogenic carcinoma or with carcinoid tumors of the thymus, pancreas, or ovary; medullary carcinoma of the thyroid; or bronchial adenomas. The onset of Cushing's syndrome may be sudden, particularly in patients with carcinoma of the lung, and this feature accounts in part for the failure of these patients to exhibit the classic manifestations. On the other hand, patients with carcinoid tumors or pheochromocytomas have longer clinical courses and usually exhibit the typical cushingoid features. The ectopic secretion of ACTH is also accompanied by the accumulation of ACTH fragments in plasma and by elevated plasma levels of ACTH precursor molecules.

TABLE 321-2 *Causes of Cushing's Syndrome*

Adrenal hyperplasia
  Secondary to pituitary ACTH overproduction
    Pituitary-hypothalamic dysfunction
    Pituitary ACTH-producing micro- or macroadenomas
  Secondary to ACTH or CRH-producing nonendocrine tumors
    (bronchogenic carcinoma, carcinoid of the thymus, pancreatic carcinoma, bronchial adenoma)
Adrenal macronodular hyperplasia (including ectopic expression of GIP receptors in the adrenal cortex)
Adrenal micronodular dysplasia
  Sporadic
  Familial (Carney's syndrome)
Adrenal neoplasia
  Adenoma
  Carcinoma
Exogenous, iatrogenic causes
  Prolonged use of glucocorticoids
  Prolonged use of ACTH

Note: ACTH, adrenocorticotropic hormone; CRH, corticotropin-releasing hormone; GIP, gastric inhibitory peptide.

Because such tumors may produce large amounts of ACTH, baseline steroid values are usually very high and increased skin pigmentation may be present.

Approximately 20 to 25% of patients with Cushing's syndrome have an adrenal neoplasm. These tumors are usually unilateral, and about half are malignant. Occasionally, patients have biochemical features both of pituitary ACTH excess and of an adrenal adenoma. These individuals may have *nodular hyperplasia* of both adrenal glands, often the result of prolonged ACTH stimulation in the absence of a pituitary adenoma. Two additional entities cause nodular hyperplasia: a familial disorder in children or young adults (so-called pigmented micronodular dysplasia; see below) and an abnormal cortisol response to gastric inhibitory polypeptide or luteinizing hormone, secondary to ectopic expression of receptors for these hormones in the adrenal cortex.

The most common cause of Cushing's syndrome is *iatrogenic* administration of steroids for a variety of reasons. Although the clinical features bear some resemblance to those seen with adrenal tumors, these patients are usually distinguishable on the basis of history and laboratory studies.

Clinical Signs, Symptoms, and Laboratory Findings   Many of the signs and symptoms of Cushing's syndrome follow logically from the known action of glucocorticoids (Table 321-3). Catabolic responses in peripheral supportive tissue causes muscle weakness and fatigability, osteoporosis, broad violaceous cutaneous striae, and easy bruisability. The latter signs are secondary to weakening and rupture of collagen fibers in the dermis. Osteoporosis may cause collapse of vertebral bodies and pathologic fractures of other bones. Decreased bone mineralization is particularly pronounced in children. Increased hepatic gluconeogenesis and insulin resistance can cause impaired glucose tolerance. Overt diabetes mellitus occurs in <20% of patients, who probably are individuals with a predisposition to this disorder. Hypercortisolism promotes the deposition of adipose tissue in characteristic sites, notably the upper face (producing the typical "moon" facies), the interscapular area (producing the "buffalo hump"), supraclavicular fat pads, and the mesenteric bed (producing "truncal" obesity) (Fig. 321-6). Rarely, episternal fatty tumors and mediastinal widening secondary to fat accumulation occur. The reason for this peculiar distribution of adipose tissue is not known, but it is associated with insulin resistance and/or elevated insulin levels. The face appears plethoric, even in the absence of any increase in red blood cell concentration. Hypertension is common, and emotional changes may be profound, ranging from irritability and emotional lability to severe depression, confusion, or even frank psychosis. In women, increased levels of adrenal androgens can cause acne, hirsutism, and oligomenorrhea or amenorrhea. Some signs and symptoms in patients with hypercortisolism—i.e., obesity, hypertension, osteoporosis, and diabetes—are nonspecific and therefore are less helpful in diagnosing the condition. On the other hand, easy bruising, typical striae, myopathy, and virilizing signs (although less frequent) are, if present, more suggestive of Cushing's syndrome (Table 321-3).

Except in iatrogenic Cushing's syndrome, plasma and urine cortisol levels are elevated. Occasionally, hypokalemia, hypochloremia, and metabolic alkalosis are present, particularly with ectopic production of ACTH.

Diagnosis   The diagnosis of Cushing's syndrome depends on the demonstration of increased cortisol production and failure to suppress cortisol secretion normally when dexamethasone is administered (Chap. 318). Once the diagnosis is established, further testing is designed to determine the etiology (Fig. 321-7 and Table 321-4).

For initial screening, the overnight dexamethasone suppression test is recommended (see above). In difficult cases (e.g., in obese or depressed patients), measurement of a 24-h urine free cortisol can also be used as a screening test. A level >140 nmol/d (50 μg/d) is suggestive of Cushing's syndrome. The definitive diagnosis is then established by failure of urinary cortisol to fall to less than <25 nmol/d (10 μg/d) or of plasma cortisol to fall to <140 nmol/L (5 μg/dL) after a

TABLE 321-3   *Frequency of Signs and Symptoms in Cushing's Syndrome*

Sign or Symptom	Percent of Patients
Typical habitus (centripetal obesity)[a]	97
Increased body weight	94
Fatigability and weakness	87
Hypertension (blood pressure >150/90)	82
Hirsutism[a]	80
Amenorrhea	77
Broad violaceous cutaneous striae[a]	67
Personality changes	66
Ecchymoses[a]	65
Proximal myopathy[a]	62
Edema	62
Polyuria, polydipsia	23
Hypertrophy of clitoris	19

[a] Features more specific for Cushing's syndrome.

standard low-dose dexamethasone suppression test (0.5 mg every 6 h for 48 h). Owing to circadian variability, plasma cortisol and, to a certain extent, ACTH determinations are not meaningful when performed in isolation, but the absence of the normal fall of plasma cortisol at midnight is consistent with Cushing's syndrome because there is loss of the diurnal cortisol rhythm.

The task of determining the etiology of Cushing's syndrome is complicated by the fact that all the available tests lack specificity and by the fact that the tumors producing this syndrome are prone to spontaneous and often dramatic changes in hormone secretion (periodic hormonogenesis). No test has a specificity >95%, and it may be necessary to use a combination of tests to arrive at the correct diagnosis.

Plasma ACTH levels can be useful in distinguishing the various causes of Cushing's syndrome, particularly in separating ACTH-dependent from ACTH-independent causes. In general, measurement of plasma ACTH is useful in the diagnosis of ACTH-independent etiologies of the syndrome, since most adrenal tumors cause low or undetectable ACTH levels [<2 pmol/L (10 pg/mL)]. Furthermore, ACTH-secreting pituitary macroadenomas and ACTH-producing nonendocrine tumors usually result in elevated ACTH levels. In the ectopic ACTH syndrome, ACTH levels may be elevated to >110 pmol/L (500 pg/mL), and in most patients the level is >40 pmol/L (200 pg/mL). In Cushing's syndrome as the result of a microadenoma or pituitary-hypothalamic dysfunction, ACTH levels range from 6 to 30 pmol/L (30 to 150 pg/mL) [normal, <14 pmol/L (<60 pg/mL)],

FIGURE 321-6 A woman with Cushing's syndrome due to a right adrenal cortical adenoma. *A.* One month prior to surgery, age 20. *B.* One year after surgery, age 21.

A   B

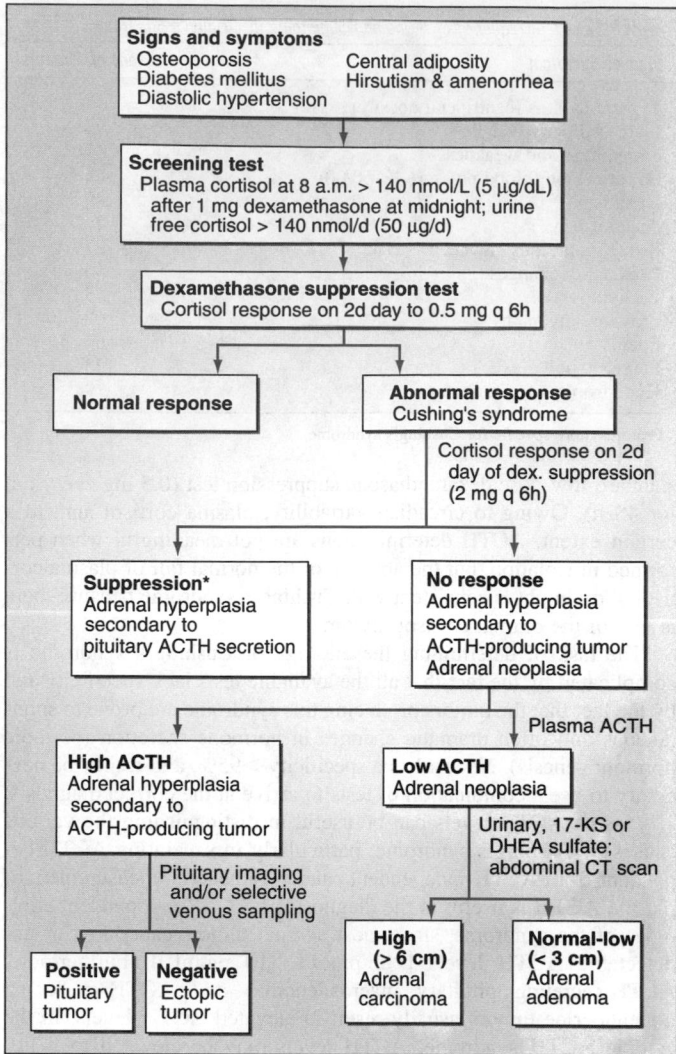

FIGURE 321-7 Diagnostic flowchart for evaluating patients suspected of having Cushing's syndrome. *This group probably includes some patients with pituitary-hypothalamic dysfunction and some with pituitary microadenomas. In some instances, a microadenoma may be visualized by pituitary magnetic resonance scanning. 17-KS, 17-ketosteroids; DHEA, dehydroepiandrosterone; ACTH, adrenocorticotropic hormone; CT, computed tomography.

with half of values falling in the normal range. However, the main problem with the use of ACTH levels in the differential diagnosis of Cushing's syndrome is that ACTH levels may be similar in individuals with hypothalamic-pituitary dysfunction, pituitary microadenomas, ectopic CRH production, and ectopic ACTH production (especially carcinoid tumors) (Table 321-4).

TABLE 321-4 *Diagnostic Tests to Determine the Type of Cushing's Syndrome*

Test	Pituitary Macro-adenoma	Pituitary Micro-adenoma	Ectopic ACTH or CRH Production	Adrenal Tumor
Plasma ACTH level	↑ to ↑↑	N to ↑	↑ to ↑↑↑	↓
Percent who respond to high-dose dexamethasone	<10	95	<10	<10
Percent who respond to CRH	>90	>90	<10	<10

Note: ACTH, adrenocorticotropic hormone; CRH, corticotropin-releasing hormone; N, normal; ↑, elevated; ↓, decreased. See text for definition of a response.

A useful step to distinguish patients with an ACTH-secreting pituitary microadenoma or hypothalamic-pituitary dysfunction from those with other forms of Cushing's syndrome is to determine the response of cortisol output to administration of high-dose dexamethasone (2 mg every 6 h for 2 days). An alternative 8-mg, overnight high-dose dexamethasone test has been developed; however, this test has a lower sensitivity and specificity than the standard test. When the diagnosis of Cushing's syndrome is clear-cut on the basis of baseline urinary and plasma assays, the high-dose dexamethasone suppression test may be used without performing the preliminary low-dose suppression test. The high-dose suppression test provides close to 100% specificity if the criterion used is suppression of urinary free cortisol by >90%. Occasionally, in individuals with bilateral nodular hyperplasia and/or ectopic CRH production, steroid output is also suppressed. Failure of low- and high-dose dexamethasone administration to suppress cortisol production (Table 321-4) can occur in patients with adrenal hyperplasia secondary to an ACTH-secreting pituitary macroadenoma or an ACTH-producing tumor of nonendocrine origin and in those with adrenal neoplasms.

Because of these difficulties, several additional tests have been advocated, such as the metyrapone and CRH infusion tests. The rationale underlying these tests is that steroid hypersecretion by an adrenal tumor or the ectopic production of ACTH will suppress the hypothalamic-pituitary axis so that inhibition of pituitary ACTH release can be demonstrated by either test. Thus, most patients with pituitary-hypothalamic dysfunction and/or a microadenoma have an increase in steroid or ACTH secretion in response to metyrapone or CRH administration, whereas most patients with ectopic ACTH-producing tumors do not. Most pituitary macroadenomas also respond to CRH, but their response to metyrapone is variable. However, false-positive and false-negative CRH tests can occur in patients with ectopic ACTH and pituitary tumors.

The main diagnostic dilemma in Cushing's syndrome is to distinguish those instances due to microadenomas of the pituitary from those due to ectopic sources (e.g., carcinoids or pheochromocytoma) that produce CRH and/or ACTH. The clinical manifestations are similar unless the ectopic tumor produces other symptoms, such as diarrhea and flushing from a carcinoid tumor or episodic hypertension from a pheochromocytoma. Sometimes, one can distinguish between ectopic and pituitary ACTH production by using metyrapone or CRH tests, as noted above. In these situations, computed tomography (CT) of the pituitary gland is usually normal. Magnetic resonance imaging (MRI) with the enhancing agent gadolinium may be better than CT for this purpose but demonstrates pituitary microadenomas in only half of patients with Cushing's disease. Because microadenomas can be detected in up to 10 to 20% of individuals without known pituitary disease, a positive imaging study does not prove that the pituitary is the source of ACTH excess. In those with negative imaging studies, selective petrosal sinus venous sampling for ACTH is now used in many referral centers. ACTH levels are measured at baseline, 2, 5, and 10 min after ovine CRH (1 μ/kg IV) injections. Peak petrosal:peripheral ACTH ratios of >3 confirm the presence of a pituitary ACTH-secreting tumor. In centers where petrosal sinus sampling is performed frequently, it has proved highly sensitive for distinguishing pituitary and nonpituitary sources of ACTH excess. However, the catheterization procedure is technically difficult, and complications have occurred.

The diagnosis of a *cortisol-producing adrenal adenoma* is suggested by low ACTH and disproportionate elevations in baseline urine free cortisol levels with only modest changes in urinary 17-ketosteroids or plasma DHEA sulfate. Adrenal androgen secretion is usually reduced in these patients owing to the cortisol-induced suppression of ACTH and subsequent involution of the androgen-producing zona reticularis.

The diagnosis of *adrenal carcinoma* is suggested by a palpable abdominal mass and by markedly elevated baseline values of both urine 17-ketosteroids and plasma DHEA sulfate. Plasma and urine cortisol levels are variably elevated. Adrenal carcinoma is usually resistant to both ACTH stimulation and dexamethasone suppression. Elevated adrenal androgen secretion often leads to virilization in the female. Estrogen-producing adrenocortical carcinoma usually presents with gynecomastia in men and dysfunctional uterine bleeding in women. These adrenal tumors secrete increased amounts of androstenedione, which is converted peripherally to the estrogens estrone and estradiol. Adrenal carcinomas that produce Cushing's syndrome are often associated with elevated levels of the intermediates of steroid biosynthesis (especially 11-deoxycortisol), suggesting inefficient conversion of the intermediates to the final product. This feature also accounts for the characteristic increase in 17-ketosteroids. Approximately 20% of adrenal carcinomas are not associated with endocrine syndromes and are presumed to be nonfunctioning or to produce biologically inactive steroid precursors. In addition, the excessive production of steroids is not always clinically evident (e.g., androgens in adult men).

FIGURE 321-8 Computed tomography (CT) is the preferred method for visualizing the adrenal glands (*arrows*). *A*. The normal right adrenal gland is adjacent to the inferior vena cava (V) where it emerges from the liver. Approximately 90% of right adrenal glands appear as linear structures extending posteriorly from the inferior vena cava into the space between the right lobe of the liver and the crus of the diaphragm. The normal left adrenal gland is lateral to the left crus of the diaphragm and below the stomach. Most left adrenal glands are shaped like an inverted V or Y. *B*. Adrenal CT scan of a patient with ectopic ACTH production. Both adrenal glands (*arrows*) are enlarged (compare with *A*). In contrast, only 50% of patients with bilateral adrenal hyperplasia secondary to pituitary ACTH hypersecretion show enlargement of the adrenals when imaged by CT scan. *C*. CT scan of a patient with Cushing's syndrome with biochemical evidence only of cortisol overproduction. The left adrenal has been replaced by a racquet-shaped 2-cm tumor (*arrow*). Attenuation of the tumor is low because of its high lipid content. *D*. CT scan in a patient with Cushing's syndrome and biochemical evidence of an adrenal carcinoma. In contrast to the tumor in *C*, the right-sided mass in this patient is large and has a heterogeneous appearance—usual characteristics of an adrenal carcinoma.

Differential Diagnosis ■ *PSEUDO-CUSHING'S SYNDROME* Problems in diagnosis include patients with obesity, chronic alcoholism, depression, and acute illness of any type. Extreme *obesity* is uncommon in Cushing's syndrome; furthermore, with exogenous obesity, the adiposity is generalized, not truncal. On adrenocortical testing, abnormalities in patients with exogenous obesity are usually modest. Basal urine steroid excretion levels in obese patients are also either normal or slightly elevated, and the diurnal pattern in blood and urine levels is normal. Patients with *chronic alcoholism* and those with *depression* share similar abnormalities in steroid output: modestly elevated urine cortisol, blunted circadian rhythm of cortisol levels, and resistance to suppression using the overnight dexamethasone test. In contrast to alcoholic subjects, depressed patients do not have signs and symptoms of Cushing's syndrome. Following discontinuation of alcohol and/or improvement in the emotional status, results of steroid testing usually return to normal. One or more of three tests have been used to differentiate mild Cushing's syndrome and pseudo-Cushing's syndrome. The serum cortisol level following the standard 2-day low-dose dexamethasone test has very high sensitivity and specificity. Although the CRH test alone is less useful, in combination with the low-dose dexamethasone test, there is nearly complete discrimination between these two conditions. Finally, a midnight cortisol level obtained in awake patients may have similar predictive value as the low-dose dexamethasone test if a cut-off of 210 nmol/L (7.5 μg/dL) is used. Patients with *acute illness* often have abnormal results on laboratory tests and fail to exhibit pituitary-adrenal suppression in response to dexamethasone, since major stress (such as pain or fever) interrupts the normal regulation of ACTH secretion. *Iatrogenic Cushing's syndrome*, induced by the administration of glucocorticoids or other steroids such as megestrol that bind to the glucocorticoid receptor, is indistinguishable by physical findings from endogenous adrenocortical hyperfunction. The distinction can be made, however, by measuring blood or urine cortisol levels in a basal state; in the iatrogenic syndrome these levels are low secondary to suppression of the pituitary-adrenal axis. The severity of iatrogenic Cushing's syndrome is related to the total steroid dose, the biologic half-life of the steroid, and the duration of therapy. Also, individuals taking afternoon and evening doses of glucocorticoids develop Cushing's syndrome more

readily and with a smaller total daily dose than do patients taking morning doses only.

Radiologic Evaluation for Cushing's Syndrome The preferred radiologic study for visualizing the adrenals is a CT scan of the abdomen (Fig. 321-8). CT is of value both for localizing adrenal tumors and for diagnosing bilateral hyperplasia. All patients believed to have hypersecretion of pituitary ACTH should have a pituitary MRI scan with gadolinium contrast. Even with this technique, small microadenomas may be undetectable; alternatively, false-positive masses due to cysts or nonsecretory lesions of the normal pituitary may be imaged. In patients with ectopic ACTH production, high-resolution chest CT is a useful first step.

Evaluation of Asymptomatic Adrenal Masses With abdominal CT scanning, many incidental adrenal masses (so-called incidentalomas) are discovered. This is not surprising, since 10 to 20% of subjects at autopsy have adrenocortical adenomas. The first step in evaluating such patients is to determine whether the tumor is functioning by means of appropriate screening tests, e.g., measurement of 24-h urine catecholamines and metabolites and serum potassium and assessment of adrenal cortical function by dexamethasone-suppression testing. However, 90% of incidentalomas are nonfunctioning. If an extra-adrenal malignancy is present, there is a 30 to 50% chance that the adrenal tumor is a metastasis. If the primary tumor is being treated and there are no other metastases, it is prudent to obtain a fine-needle aspirate of the adrenal mass to establish the diagnosis. In the absence of a known malignancy the next step is unclear. The probability of adrenal carcinoma is <0.01%, the vast majority of adrenal masses being benign adenomas. Features suggestive of malignancy include large size (a size > 4 to 6 cm suggests carcinoma); irregular margins;

and inhomogeneity, soft tissue calcifications visible on CT (Fig. 321-8), and findings characteristic of malignancy on a chemical-shift MRI image. If surgery is not performed, a repeat CT scan should be obtained in 3 to 6 months. Fine-needle aspiration is not useful to distinguish between benign and malignant primary adrenal tumors.

℞ TREATMENT

Adrenal Neoplasm   When an adenoma or carcinoma is diagnosed, adrenal exploration is performed with excision of the tumor. Adenomas may be resected using laparoscopic techniques. Because of the possibility of atrophy of the contralateral adrenal, the patient is treated pre- and postoperatively as if for total adrenalectomy, even when a unilateral lesion is suspected, the routine being similar to that for an Addisonian patient undergoing elective surgery (see Table 321-8).

Despite operative intervention, most patients with adrenal carcinoma die within 3 years of diagnosis. Metastases occur most often to liver and lung. The principal drug for the treatment of adrenocortical carcinoma is mitotane (*o,p′*-DDD), an isomer of the insecticide DDT. This drug suppresses cortisol production and decreases plasma and urine steroid levels. Although its cytotoxic action is relatively selective for the glucocorticoid-secreting zone of the adrenal cortex, the zona glomerulosa may also be inhibited. Because mitotane also alters the extraadrenal metabolism of cortisol, plasma and urinary cortisol levels must be assessed to titrate the effect. The drug is usually given in divided doses three to four times a day, with the dose increased gradually to tolerability (usually <6 g daily). At higher doses, almost all patients experience side effects, which may be gastrointestinal (anorexia, diarrhea, vomiting) or neuromuscular (lethargy, somnolence, dizziness). All patients treated with mitotane should receive long-term glucocorticoid maintenance therapy, and, in some, mineralocorticoid replacement is appropriate. In approximately one-third of patients, both tumor and metastases regress, but long-term survival is not altered. In many patients, mitotane only inhibits steroidogenesis and does not cause regression of tumor metastases. Osseous metastases are usually refractory to the drug and should be treated with radiation therapy. Mitotane can also be given as adjunctive therapy after surgical resection of an adrenal carcinoma, although there is no evidence that this improves survival. Because of the absence of a long-term benefit with mitotane, alternative chemotherapeutic approaches based on platinum therapy have been used. However, there are no data presently available indicating a prolongation of life.

BILATERAL HYPERPLASIA   Patients with hyperplasia usually have a relative or absolute increase in ACTH levels. Since therapy would logically be directed at reducing ACTH levels, the ideal primary treatment for ACTH- or CRH-producing tumors, whether pituitary or ectopic, is surgical removal. Occasionally (particularly with ectopic ACTH production) surgical excision is not possible because the disease is far advanced. In this situation, "medical" or surgical adrenalectomy may correct the hypercortisolism.

Controversy exists as to the proper treatment for bilateral adrenal hyperplasia when the source of the ACTH overproduction is not apparent. In some centers, these patients (especially those who suppress after the administration of a high-dose dexamethasone test) undergo surgical exploration of the pituitary via a transsphenoidal approach in the expectation that a microadenoma will be found (Chap. 318). However, in most circumstances selective petrosal sinus venous sampling is recommended, and the patient is referred to an appropriate center if the procedure is not available locally. If a microadenoma is not found at the time of exploration, total hypophysectomy may be needed. Complications of transsphenoidal surgery include cerebrospinal fluid rhinorrhea, diabetes insipidus, panhypopituitarism, and optic or cranial nerve injuries.

In other centers, total adrenalectomy is the treatment of choice. The cure rate with this procedure is close to 100%. The adverse effects include the certain need for lifelong mineralocorticoid and glucocor-

ticoid replacement and a 10 to 20% probability of a pituitary tumor developing over the next 10 years (Nelson's syndrome; Chap. 318). It is uncertain whether these tumors arise de novo or if they were present prior to adrenalectomy but were too small to be detected. Periodic radiologic evaluation of the pituitary gland by MRI as well as serial ACTH measurements should be performed in all individuals after bilateral adrenalectomy for Cushing's disease. Such pituitary tumors may become locally invasive and impinge on the optic chiasm or extend into the cavernous or sphenoid sinuses.

Except in children, pituitary irradiation is rarely used as primary treatment, being reserved rather for postoperative tumor recurrences. In some centers, high levels of gamma radiation can be focused on the desired site with less scattering to surrounding tissues by using stereotactic techniques. Side effects of radiation include ocular motor palsy and hypopituitarism. There is a long lag time between treatment and remission, and the remission rate is usually <50%.

Finally, in occasional patients in whom a surgical approach is not feasible, "medical" adrenalectomy may be indicated (Table 321-5). Inhibition of steroidogenesis may also be indicated in severely cushingoid subjects prior to surgical intervention. Chemical adrenalectomy may be accomplished by the administration of the inhibitor of steroidogenesis ketoconazole (600 to 1200 mg/d). In addition, mitotane (2 or 3 g/d) and/or the blockers of steroid synthesis aminoglutethimide (1 g/d) and metyrapone (2 or 3 g/d) may be effective either alone or in combination. Mitotane is slow to take effect (weeks). Mifepristone, a competitive inhibitor of the binding of glucocorticoid to its receptor, may be a treatment option. Adrenal insufficiency is a risk with all these agents, and replacement steroids may be required.

ALDOSTERONISM   Aldosteronism is a syndrome associated with hypersecretion of the mineralocorticoid aldosterone. In *primary* aldosteronism the cause for the excessive aldosterone production resides within the adrenal gland; in *secondary* aldosteronism the stimulus is extraadrenal.

Primary Aldosteronism   In the original descriptions of excessive and inappropriate aldosterone production, the disease was the result of an *aldosterone-producing adrenal adenoma* (Conn's syndrome). Most cases involve a unilateral adenoma, which is usually small and may occur on either side. Rarely, primary aldosteronism is due to an adrenal carcinoma. Aldosteronism is twice as common in women as in men, usually occurs between the ages of 30 and 50, and is present in ~1% of unselected hypertensive patients. However, the prevalence may be as high as 5%, depending on the criteria and study population. In many patients with clinical and biochemical features of primary aldosteronism, a solitary adenoma is not found at surgery. Instead, these patients have *bilateral cortical nodular hyperplasia*. In the literature, this disease is also termed *idiopathic hyperaldosteronism*, and/or *nodular hyperplasia*. The cause is unknown.

SIGNS AND SYMPTOMS   Hypersecretion of aldosterone increases the renal distal tubular exchange of intratubular sodium for secreted potassium and hydrogen ions, with progressive depletion of body potassium and development of hypokalemia. Most patients have diastolic hypertension, which may be very severe, and headaches. The hypertension is probably due to the increased sodium reabsorption and extracellular volume expansion. *Potassium depletion* is responsible for the muscle

---

TABLE 321-5   *Treatment Modalities for Patients with Adrenal Hyperplasia Secondary to Pituitary ACTH Hypersecretion*

Treatments to reduce pituitary ACTH production
  Transsphenoidal resection of microadenoma
  Radiation therapy
Treatments to reduce or eliminate adrenocortical cortisol secretion
  Bilateral adrenalectomy
  Medical adrenalectomy (metyrapone, mitotane, aminoglutethimide, ketoconazole)[a]

[a] Not curative but effective as long as chronically administered in selected patients.
Note: ACTH, adrenocorticotropic hormone.

weakness and fatigue and is due to the effect of potassium depletion on the muscle cell membrane. The polyuria results from impairment of urinary concentrating ability and is often associated with polydipsia. However, some individuals with mild disease, particularly the bilateral hyperplasia type, may have normal potassium levels and therefore have no symptoms associated with hypokalemia.

Electrocardiographic and roentgenographic signs of left ventricular enlargement are, in part, secondary to the hypertension. However, the left ventricular hypertrophy is disproportionate to the level of blood pressure when compared to individuals with essential hypertension, and regression of the hypertrophy occurs even if blood pressure is not reduced after removal of an aldosteronoma. Electrocardiographic signs of potassium depletion include prominent U waves, cardiac arrhythmias, and premature contractions. In the absence of associated congestive heart failure, renal disease, or preexisting abnormalities (such as thrombophlebitis), edema is characteristically absent. However, structural damage to the cerebral circulation, retinal vasculature, and kidney occurs more frequently than would be predicted based on the level and duration of the hypertension. Proteinuria may occur in as many as 50% of patients with primary aldosteronism, and renal failure occurs in up to 15%. Thus, it is probable that excess aldosterone production induces cardiovascular damage independent of its effect on blood pressure.

LABORATORY FINDINGS   Laboratory findings depend on both the duration and the severity of potassium depletion. An overnight concentration test often reveals impaired ability to concentrate the urine, probably secondary to the hypokalemia. Urine pH is neutral to alkaline because of excessive secretion of ammonium and bicarbonate ions to compensate for the metabolic alkalosis.

Hypokalemia may be severe (<3 mmol/L) and reflects body potassium depletion, usually >300 mmol. In mild forms of primary aldosteronism, potassium levels may be normal. *Hypernatremia* is infrequent but may be caused by sodium retention, concomitant water loss from polyuria, and resetting of the osmostat. Metabolic alkalosis and elevation of serum bicarbonate are caused by hydrogen ion loss into the urine and migration into potassium-depleted cells. The alkalosis is perpetuated by potassium deficiency, which increases the capacity of the proximal convoluted tubule to reabsorb filtered bicarbonate. If hypokalemia is severe, serum magnesium levels are also reduced.

DIAGNOSIS   The diagnosis is suggested by persistent hypokalemia in a nonedematous patient with a normal sodium intake who is not receiving potassium-wasting diuretics (furosemide, ethacrynic acid, thiazides). If hypokalemia occurs in a hypertensive patient taking a potassium-wasting diuretic, the diuretic should be discontinued and the patient should be given potassium supplements. After 1 to 2 weeks, the potassium level should be remeasured, and if hypokalemia persists, the patient should be evaluated for a mineralocorticoid excess syndrome (Fig. 321-9).

The criteria for the diagnosis of primary aldosteronism are (1) diastolic hypertension without edema, (2) hyposecretion of renin (as judged by low plasma renin activity levels) that fails to increase appropriately during volume depletion (upright posture, sodium depletion), and (3) hypersecretion of aldosterone that does not suppress appropriately in response to volume expansion.

Patients with primary aldosteronism characteristically *do not have edema*, since they exhibit an "escape" phenomenon from the sodium-retaining aspects of mineralocorticoids. Rarely, pretibial edema is present in patients with associated nephropathy and azotemia.

The estimation of plasma renin activity is of limited value in separating patients with primary aldosteronism from those with hypertension of other causes. Although failure of plasma renin activity to rise normally during volume-depletion maneuvers is a criterion for a diagnosis of primary aldosteronism, suppressed renin activity also occurs in ~25% of patients with essential hypertension.

Although a renin measurement alone lacks specificity, the ratio of serum aldosterone to plasma renin activity is a very useful screening

FIGURE 321-9   Diagnostic flowchart for evaluating patients with suspected primary aldosteronism. *Serum K+ may be normal in some patients with hyperaldosteronism who are taking potassium-sparing diuretics (spironolactone, triamterene) or who have a low sodium intake and a high potassium intake. †This step should not be taken if hypertension is severe (diastolic pressure > 115 mmHg) or if cardiac failure is present. Also, serum potassium levels should be corrected before the infusion of saline solution. Alternative methods that produce comparable suppression of aldosterone secretion include oral sodium loading (200 mmol/d) and the administration of fludrocortisone, 0.2 mg bid, for 3 days. ‡For example, Liddle's syndrome, apparent mineralocorticoid excess syndrome, or a deoxycorticosterone-secreting tumor. (GRA, glucocorticoid-remediable aldosteronism; CT, computed tomography; MRI, magnetic resonance imaging.)

test. A high ratio (>30), when aldosterone is expressed as ng/dL and plasma renin activity as ng/mL per hour, strongly suggests autonomy of aldosterone secretion. Aldosterone levels need to be >500 pmol/L (>15 ng/dL) when salt intake is not restricted. In some centers, the aldosterone/plasma renin activity ratio is used as a primary screen test in all normokalemic, difficult-to-control hypertensive patients, in addition to those with hypokalemia. Ultimately, it is necessary to demonstrate a lack of aldosterone suppression to diagnose primary aldosteronism (Fig. 321-9). The autonomy exhibited in these patients refers only to the resistance to suppression of secretion during volume expansion; aldosterone can and does respond in a normal or above-normal fashion to the stimulus of potassium loading or ACTH infusion.

Once hyposecretion of renin and failure of aldosterone secretion suppression are demonstrated, aldosterone-producing adenomas should be localized by abdominal CT scan, using a high-resolution scanner as many aldosteronomas are <1 cm in size. If the CT scan is negative, percutaneous transfemoral bilateral adrenal vein catheterization with adrenal vein sampling may demonstrate a two- to threefold increase in plasma aldosterone concentration on the involved side. In cases of hyperaldosteronism secondary to cortical nodular hyperplasia, no lateralization is found. It is important for samples to be obtained simultaneously if possible and for cortisol levels to be measured to ensure that false localization does not reflect dilution or an ACTH- or stress-induced rise in aldosterone levels. In a patient with an adenoma, the aldosterone/cortisol ratio lateralizes to the side of the lesion.

DIFFERENTIAL DIAGNOSIS Patients with hypertension and hypokalemia may have either primary or secondary hyperaldosteronism (Fig. 321-10). A useful maneuver to distinguish between these conditions is the measurement of plasma renin activity. Secondary hyperaldosteronism in patients with accelerated hypertension is due to elevated plasma renin levels; in contrast, patients with primary aldosteronism have suppressed plasma renin levels. Indeed, in patients with a serum potassium concentration of <2.5 mmol/L, a high ratio of plasma aldosterone to plasma renin activity in a random sample is usually sufficient to establish the diagnosis of primary aldosteronism without additional testing. Ectopic ACTH production should also be considered in patients with hypertension and severe hypokalemia.

Primary aldosteronism must also be distinguished from other *hypermineralocorticoid states*. Nonaldosterone mineralocorticoid states will have suppressed plasma renin activity but low aldosterone levels. The most common problem is to distinguish between hyperaldosteronism due to an adenoma and that due to idiopathic bilateral nodular hyperplasia. This distinction is important because hypertension associated with idiopathic hyperplasia does not usually benefit from bilateral adrenalectomy, whereas hypertension associated with aldosterone-producing tumors is usually improved or cured by removal of the adenoma. Although patients with idiopathic bilateral nodular hyperplasia tend to have less severe hypokalemia, lower aldosterone secretion, and higher plasma renin activity than do patients with primary aldosteronism, differentiation is impossible solely on clinical and/or biochemical grounds. An anomalous postural decrease in plasma aldosterone and elevated plasma 18-hydroxycorticosterone levels are present in most patients with a unilateral lesion. However, these tests are also of limited diagnostic value in the individual patient, because some adenoma patients have an increase in plasma aldosterone with upright posture, so-called renin-responsive aldosteronoma. A definitive diagnosis is best made by radiographic studies, including bilateral adrenal vein catheterization, as noted above.

In a few instances, hypertensive patients with hypokalemic alkalosis have adenomas that secrete deoxycorticosterone. Such patients have reduced plasma renin activity levels, but aldosterone levels are either normal or reduced, suggesting the diagnosis of mineralocorticoid excess due to a hormone other than aldosterone. Several inherited disorders have clinical features similar to those of primary aldosteronism (see below).

℞ TREATMENT

Primary aldosteronism due to an adenoma is usually treated by surgical excision of the adenoma. Where possible a laparoscopic approach is favored. However, dietary sodium restriction and the administration of an aldosterone antagonist—e.g., spironolactone—are effective in many cases. Hypertension and hypokalemia are usually controlled by doses of 25 to 100 mg spironolactone every 8 h. In some patients medical management has been successful for years, but chronic therapy in men is usually limited by side effects of spironolactone such as gynecomastia, decreased libido, and impotence.

When idiopathic bilateral hyperplasia is suspected, surgery is indicated only when significant, symptomatic hypokalemia cannot be controlled with medical therapy, i.e., by spironolactone, triamterene, or amiloride. Hypertension associated with idiopathic hyperplasia is usually not benefited by bilateral adrenalectomy.

Secondary Aldosteronism *Secondary aldosteronism* refers to an appropriately increased production of aldosterone in response to activation of the renin-angiotensin system (Fig. 321-10). The production rate of aldosterone is often higher in patients with secondary aldosteronism than in those with primary aldosteronism. Secondary aldosteronism usually occurs in association with the accelerated phase of hypertension or on the basis of an underlying edema disorder. Secondary aldosteronism in pregnancy is a normal physiologic response to estrogen-induced increases in circulating levels of renin substrate and plasma renin activity and to the anti-aldosterone actions of progestogens.

Secondary aldosteronism in hypertensive states is due either to a primary overproduction of renin (primary reninism) or to an overproduction of renin secondary to a decrease in renal blood flow and/or perfusion pressure (Fig. 321-10). Secondary hypersecretion of renin can be due to a narrowing of one or both of the major renal arteries by atherosclerosis or by fibromuscular hyperplasia. Overproduction of renin from both kidneys also occurs in severe arteriolar nephrosclerosis (malignant hypertension) or with profound renal vasoconstriction (the accelerated phase of hypertension). The secondary aldosteronism is characterized by hypokalemic alkalosis, moderate to severe increases in plasma renin activity, and moderate to marked increases in aldosterone levels.

Secondary aldosteronism with hypertension can also be caused by rare renin-producing tumors (primary reninism). In these patients, the biochemical characteristics are of renal vascular hypertension, but the primary defect is renin secretion by a juxtaglomerular cell tumor. The diagnosis can be made by demonstration of normal renal vasculature and/or demonstration of a space-occupying lesion in the kidney by radiographic techniques and documentation of a unilateral increase in renal vein renin activity. Rarely, these tumors arise in tissues such as the ovary.

Secondary aldosteronism is present in many forms of *edema*. The rate of aldosterone secretion is usually increased in patients with edema caused by either cirrhosis or the nephrotic syndrome. In congestive heart failure, elevated aldosterone secretion varies depending on the severity of cardiac failure. The stimulus for aldosterone release in these conditions appears to be *arterial hypovolemia* and/or hypotension. Thiazides and furosemide often exaggerate secondary aldosteronism via volume depletion; hypokalemia and, on occasion, alkalosis can then become prominent features. On occasion secondary hyperaldosteronism occurs without edema or hypertension (Bartter and Gitelman syndromes, see below).

Aldosterone and Cardiovascular Damage Although many studies have investigated the role of angiotensin II in mediating cardiovascular damage, additional evidence indicates that aldosterone has an important

Primary aldosteronism   **Secondary aldosteronism**

*Initiating event

FIGURE 321-10   Responses of the renin-aldosterone volume control loop in primary versus secondary aldosteronism role that is independent of angiotensin II. Patients with primary aldosteronism (in which angiotensin II levels are usually very low) have a higher incidence of left ventricular hypertrophy (LVH), albuminuria, and stroke than do patients with essential hypertension. Experimental animal models mimicking secondary aldosteronism (angiotensin infusion) or primary aldosteronism (aldosterone infusion) reveal a common pathophysiologic sequence. Within the first few days there is activation of proinflammatory molecules with a histologic picture of perivascular macrophage infiltrate and inflammation, followed by cellular death, fibrosis, and ventricular hypertrophy. These events are prevented if an aldosterone receptor antagonist is used or if adrenalectomy is performed initially. The same pathophysiologic sequence is seen in animals with average aldosterone levels and cardiovascular damage, i.e., diabetes mellitus, or genetic hypertensive rats. Importantly, the level of sodium intake is a critical co-factor. If salt intake is severely restricted, no damage occurs even though the aldosterone levels are markedly elevated. Thus, it is not the level of aldosterone per se that is responsible for the damage, but its level relative to the volume or sodium status of the individual.

Four clinical studies support these experimental results. In the RALES trial, patients with class II/IV heart failure were randomized to standard care or a low dose of the mineralocorticoid receptor antagonist, spironolactone. There was a 30% reduction in all-cause mortality and cardiovascular mortality and hospitalizations after 36 months. Two studies in hypertensive subjects addressed the question of the relative importance of a reduction of angiotensin II formation versus blockade of the MR in mediating cardiovascular damage. Subjects were randomized to eplerenone (an MR antagonist), enalapril (an ACE inhibitor), or both agents. In the first study the subjects had LVH, with the end point being a reduction in LVH. In the second, the subjects had diabetes mellitus and proteinuria, with the end point being a reduction in proteinuria. In both studies all three treatment arms substantially reduced the primary end point; however, the most potent effect occurred in the combination arms of the studies. In the monotherapy LVH arms, the reduction in LVH was similar, while in the proteinuria study, eplerenone produced a greater reduction than did enalapril. The final study was the EPHESUS trial, where individuals who developed congestive heart failure after an acute myocardial infarction were randomized to standard-of-care treatment with or without a small dose of eplerenone. Eplerenone administration produced a significantly greater reduction in mortality (15 to 17%) and in cardiovascular-related hospitalizations than the placebo arm. Thus, these four clinical studies provide strong support to the hypothesis that MR blockade has a significant added advantage over standard-of-care therapy in reducing cardiovascular mortality and surrogate end points. However, regulatory approval is pending.

SYNDROMES OF ADRENAL ANDROGEN EXCESS Adrenal androgen excess results from excess production of DHEA and androstenedione, which are converted to testosterone in extraglandular tissues; elevated testosterone levels account for most of the virilization. Adrenal androgen excess may be associated with the secretion of greater or smaller amounts of other adrenal hormones and may, therefore, present as "pure" syndromes of virilization or as "mixed" syndromes associated with excessive glucocorticoids and Cushing's syndrome. →*For further discussion of hirsutism and virilization, see Chap. 44.*

HYPOFUNCTION OF THE ADRENAL CORTEX

Cases of adrenal insufficiency can be divided into two general categories: (1) those associated with primary inability of the adrenal to elaborate sufficient quantities of hormone, and (2) those associated with a secondary failure due to inadequate ACTH formation or release (Table 321-6).

PRIMARY ADRENOCORTICAL DEFICIENCY (ADDISON'S DISEASE) The original description of Addison's disease—"general languor and debility, feebleness of the heart's action, irritability of the stomach, and a peculiar change of the color of the skin"—summarizes the dominant clinical

TABLE 321-6 *Classification of Adrenal Insufficiency*

PRIMARY ADRENAL INSUFFICIENCY

Anatomic destruction of gland (chronic or acute)
  "Idiopathic" atrophy (autoimmune, adrenoleukodystrophy)
  Surgical removal
  Infection (tuberculous, fungal, viral—especially in AIDS patients)
  Hemorrhage
  Invasion: metastatic
Metabolic failure in hormone production
  Congenital adrenal hyperplasia
  Enzyme inhibitors (metyrapone, ketoconazole, aminoglutethimide)
  Cytotoxic agents (mitotane)
ACTH-blocking antibodies
Mutation in ACTH receptor gene
Adrenal hypoplasia congenita

SECONDARY ADRENAL INSUFFICIENCY

Hypopituitarism due to hypothalamic-pituitary disease
Suppression of hypothalamic-pituitary axis
  By exogenous steroid
  By endogenous steroid from tumor

Note: ACTH, adrenocorticotropic hormone.

features. Advanced cases are usually easy to diagnose, but recognition of the early phases can be a real challenge.

Incidence Acquired forms of primary insufficiency are relatively rare, may occur at any age, and affect both sexes equally. Because of the common therapeutic use of steroids, secondary adrenal insufficiency is relatively common.

Etiology and Pathogenesis Addison's disease results from progressive destruction of the adrenals, which must involve >90% of the glands before adrenal insufficiency appears. The adrenal is a frequent site for chronic granulomatous diseases, predominantly tuberculosis but also histoplasmosis, coccidioidomycosis, and cryptococcosis. In early series, tuberculosis was responsible for 70 to 90% of cases, but the most frequent cause now is *idiopathic* atrophy, and an autoimmune mechanism is probably responsible. Rarely, other lesions are encountered, such as adrenoleukodystrophy, bilateral hemorrhage, tumor metastases, HIV, cytomegalovirus (CMV), amyloidosis, adrenomyeloneuropathy, familial adrenal insufficiency, or sarcoidosis.

Although half of patients with idiopathic atrophy have circulating adrenal antibodies, autoimmune destruction is probably secondary to cytotoxic T lymphocytes. Specific adrenal antigens to which autoantibodies may be directed include 21-hydroxylase (CYP21A2) and side chain cleavage enzyme, but the significance of these antibodies in the pathogenesis of adrenal insufficiency is unknown. Some antibodies cause adrenal insufficiency by blocking the binding of ACTH to its receptors. Some patients also have antibodies to thyroid, parathyroid, and/or gonadal tissue (Chap. 330). There is also an increased incidence of chronic lymphocytic thyroiditis, premature ovarian failure, type 1 diabetes mellitus, and hypo- or hyperthyroidism. The presence of two or more of these autoimmune endocrine disorders in the same person defines the polyglandular autoimmune syndrome type II. Additional features include pernicious anemia, vitiligo, alopecia, nontropical sprue, and myasthenia gravis. Within families, multiple generations are affected by one or more of the above diseases. Type II polyglandular syndrome is the result of a mutant gene on chromosome 6 and is associated with the HLA alleles B8 and DR3.

The combination of parathyroid and adrenal insufficiency and chronic mucocutaneous candidiasis constitutes type I polyglandular autoimmune syndrome. Other autoimmune diseases in this disorder include pernicious anemia, chronic active hepatitis, alopecia, primary hypothyroidism, and premature gonadal failure. There is no HLA association; this syndrome is inherited as an autosomal recessive trait. It is caused by mutations in the *a*utoimmune *p*olyendocrinopathy *c*andidiasis *e*ctodermal *d*ystrophy (APECED) gene located on chromosome 21q22.3. The gene encodes a transcription factor thought to be involved in lymphocyte function. The type I syndrome usually presents during childhood, whereas the type II syndrome is usually manifested in adulthood.

Clinical suspicion of adrenal insufficiency should be high in patients with AIDS (Chap. 173). CMV regularly involves the adrenal glands (so-called CMV necrotizing adrenalitis), and involvement with *Mycobacterium avium-intracellulare*, *Cryptococcus*, and Kaposi's sarcoma has been reported. Adrenal insufficiency in AIDS patients may not be manifest, but tests of adrenal reserve frequently give abnormal results. When interpreting tests of adrenocortical function, it is important to remember that medications such as rifampin, phenytoin, ketoconazole, megestrol, and opiates may cause or potentiate adrenal insufficiency. Adrenal hemorrhage and infarction occur in patients on anticoagulants and in those with circulating anticoagulants and hypercoagulable states, such as the antiphospholipid syndrome.

There are several rare genetic causes of adrenal insufficiency that present primarily in infancy and childhood (see below).

Clinical Signs and Symptoms Adrenocortical insufficiency caused by gradual adrenal destruction is characterized by an insidious onset of fatigability, weakness, anorexia, nausea and vomiting, weight loss, cutaneous and mucosal pigmentation, hypotension, and occasionally hypoglycemia (Table 321-7). Depending on the duration and degree of adrenal hypofunction, the manifestations vary from mild chronic fatigue to fulminating shock associated with acute destruction of the glands, as described by Waterhouse and Friderichsen.

Asthenia is the cardinal symptom. Early it may be sporadic, usually most evident at times of stress; as adrenal function becomes more impaired, the patient is continuously fatigued, and bed rest is necessary.

Hyperpigmentation may be striking or absent. It commonly appears as a diffuse brown, tan, or bronze darkening of parts such as the elbows or creases of the hand and of areas that normally are pigmented such as the areolae about the nipples. Bluish-black patches may appear on the mucous membranes. Some patients develop dark freckles, and irregular areas of vitiligo may paradoxically be present. As an early sign, tanning following sun exposure may be persistent.

Arterial hypotension with postural accentuation is frequent, and blood pressure may be in the range of 80/50 or less.

Abnormalities of gastrointestinal function are often the presenting complaint. Symptoms vary from mild anorexia with weight loss to fulminating nausea, vomiting, diarrhea, and ill-defined abdominal pain, which may be so severe as to be confused with an acute abdomen. Patients may have personality changes, usually consisting of excessive irritability and restlessness. Enhancement of the sensory modalities of taste, olfaction, and hearing is reversible with therapy. Axillary and pubic hair may be decreased in women due to loss of adrenal androgens.

Laboratory Findings In the early phase of gradual adrenal destruction, there may be no demonstrable abnormalities in the routine laboratory

TABLE 321-7 *Frequency of Symptoms and Signs in Adrenal Insufficiency*

Sign or Symptom	Percent of Patients
Weakness	99
Pigmentation of skin	98
Weight loss	97
Anorexia, nausea, and vomiting	90
Hypotension (<110/70)	87
Pigmentation of mucous membranes	82
Abdominal pain	34
Salt craving	22
Diarrhea	20
Constipation	19
Syncope	16
Vitiligo	9

parameters, but adrenal reserve is decreased—that is, while basal steroid output may be normal, a subnormal increase occurs after stress. Adrenal stimulation with ACTH uncovers abnormalities in this stage of the disease, eliciting a subnormal increase of cortisol levels or no increase at all. In more advanced stages of adrenal destruction, serum sodium, chloride, and bicarbonate levels are reduced, and the serum potassium level is elevated. The hyponatremia is due both to loss of sodium into the urine (due to aldosterone deficiency) and to movement into the intracellular compartment. This extravascular sodium loss depletes extracellular fluid volume and accentuates hypotension. Elevated plasma vasopressin and angiotensin II levels may contribute to the hyponatremia by impairing free water clearance. Hyperkalemia is due to a combination of aldosterone deficiency, impaired glomerular filtration, and acidosis. Basal levels of cortisol and aldosterone are subnormal and fail to increase following ACTH administration. Mild to moderate hypercalcemia occurs in 10 to 20% of patients for unclear reasons. The electrocardiogram may show nonspecific changes, and the electroencephalogram exhibits a generalized reduction and slowing. There may be a normocytic anemia, a relative lymphocytosis, and a moderate eosinophilia.

Diagnosis The diagnosis of adrenal insufficiency should be made only with ACTH stimulation testing to assess adrenal reserve capacity for steroid production (see above for ACTH test protocols). In brief, the best screening test is the cortisol response 60 min after 250 μg of cosyntropin given intramuscularly or intravenously. Cortisol levels should exceed 495 nmol/L (18 μg/dL). If the response is abnormal, then primary and secondary adrenal insufficiency can be distinguished by measuring aldosterone levels from the same blood samples. In secondary, but not primary, adrenal insufficiency the aldosterone increment will be normal [≥150 pmol/l (5 ng/dL)]. Furthermore, in primary adrenal insufficiency, plasma ACTH and associated peptides (β-LPT) are elevated because of loss of the usual cortisol-hypothalamic-pituitary feedback relationship, whereas in secondary adrenal insufficiency, plasma ACTH values are low or "inappropriately" normal (Fig. 321-11).

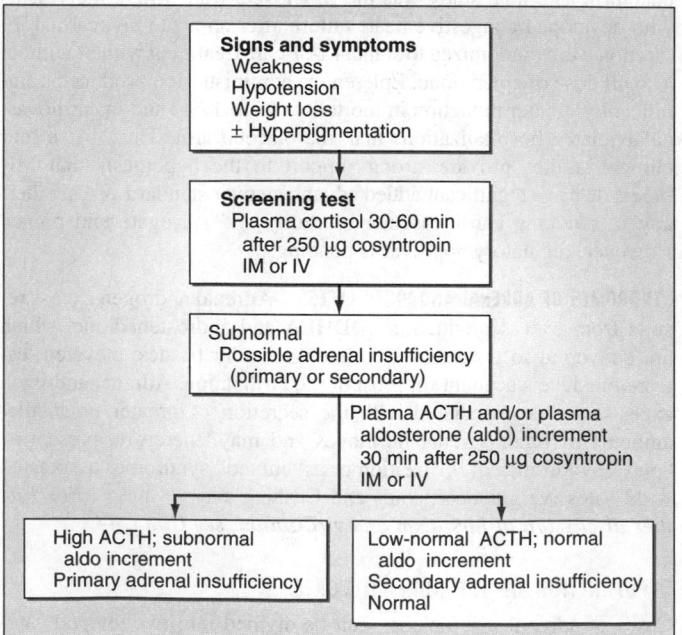

FIGURE 321-11 Diagnostic flowchart for evaluating patients with suspected adrenal insufficiency. Plasma adrenocorticotropic hormone (ACTH) levels are low in secondary adrenal insufficiency. In adrenal insufficiency secondary to pituitary tumors or idiopathic panhypopituitarism, other pituitary hormone deficiencies are present. On the other hand, ACTH deficiency may be isolated, as seen following prolonged use of exogenous glucocorticoids. Because the isolated blood levels obtained in these screening tests may not be definitive, the diagnosis may need to be confirmed by a continuous 24-h ACTH infusion. Normal subjects and patients with secondary adrenal insufficiency may be distinguished by insulin tolerance or metyrapone testing.

Differential Diagnosis Because weakness and fatigue are common, diagnosis of early adrenocortical insufficiency may be difficult. However, the combination of mild gastrointestinal distress, weight loss, anorexia, and a suggestion of increased pigmentation makes it mandatory to perform ACTH stimulation testing to rule out adrenal insufficiency, particularly before steroid treatment is begun. Weight loss is useful in evaluating the significance of weakness and malaise. Racial pigmentation may be a problem, but a *recent* and progressive *increase* in pigmentation is usually reported by the patient with gradual adrenal destruction. Hyperpigmentation is usually absent when adrenal destruction is rapid, as in bilateral adrenal hemorrhage. The fact that hyperpigmentation occurs with other diseases may also present a problem, but the appearance and distribution of pigment in adrenal insufficiency arc usually characteristic. When doubt exists, measurement of ACTH levels and testing of adrenal reserve with the infusion of ACTH provide clear-cut differentiation.

	Hydrocortisone Infusion, Continuous, mg/h	Hydrocortisone (Orally)		Fludrocortisone (Orally), 8 A.M.
		8 A.M.	4 P.M.	
Routine daily medication		20	10	0.1
Day before operation		20	10	0.1
Day of operation	10			
Day 1	5–7.5			
Day 2	2.5–5			
Day 3	2.5–5 *or*	40	20	0.1
Day 4	2.5–5 *or*	40	20	0.1
Day 5		40	20	0.1
Day 6		20	20	0.1
Day 7		20	10	0.1

[a] All steroid doses are given in milligrams. An alternative approach is to give 100 mg hydrocortisone as an intravenous bolus injection every 8 h on the day of the operation (see text).

RX TREATMENT

All patients with adrenal insufficiency should receive specific hormone replacement. These patients require careful education about the disease. Replacement therapy should correct both glucocorticoid and mineralocorticoid deficiencies. Hydrocortisone (cortisol) is the mainstay of treatment. The dose for most adults (depending on size) is 20 to 30 mg/d. Patients are advised to take glucocorticoids with meals or, if that is impractical, with milk or an antacid, because the drugs may increase gastric acidity and exert direct toxic effects on the gastric mucosa. To simulate the normal diurnal adrenal rhythm, two-thirds of the dose is taken in the morning, and the remaining one-third is taken in the late afternoon. Some patients exhibit insomnia, irritability, and mental excitement after initiation of therapy; in these, the dosage should be reduced. Other situations that may necessitate smaller doses are hypertension and diabetes mellitus. Obese individuals and those on anticonvulsive medications may require increased dosages. Measurements of plasma ACTH or cortisol or of urine cortisol levels do not appear to be useful in determining optimal glucocorticoid dosages.

Since the replacement dosage of hydrocortisone does not replace the mineralocorticoid component of the adrenal hormones, mineralocorticoid supplementation is usually needed. This is accomplished by the administration of 0.05 to 0.1 mg fludrocortisone per day by mouth. Patients should also be instructed to maintain an ample intake of sodium (3 to 4 g/d).

The adequacy of mineralocorticoid therapy can be assessed by measurement of blood pressure and serum electrolytes. Blood pressure should be normal and without postural changes; serum sodium, potassium, creatinine, and urea nitrogen levels should also be normal. Measurement of plasma renin levels may also be useful in titrating the dose.

In female patients with adrenal insufficiency, androgen levels are also low. Thus, some physicians believe that daily replacement with 25 to 50 mg of DHEA orally may improve quality of life and bone mineral density.

Complications of glucocorticoid therapy, with the exception of gastritis, are *rare* at the dosages recommended for treatment of adrenal insufficiency. Complications of mineralocorticoid therapy include hypokalemia, hypertension, cardiac enlargement, and even congestive heart failure due to sodium retention. Periodic measurements of body weight, serum potassium level, and blood pressure are useful. All patients with adrenal insufficiency should carry medical identification, should be instructed in the parenteral self-administration of steroids, and should be registered with a medical alerting system.

Special Therapeutic Problems During periods of intercurrent illness, especially in the setting of fever, the dose of hydrocortisone should be doubled. With severe illness it should be increased to 75 to 150 mg/d. When oral administration is not possible, parenteral routes should be employed. Likewise, before surgery or dental extractions, supplemental glucocorticoids should be administered. Patients should also be advised to increase the dose of fludrocortisone and to add salt to their otherwise normal diet during periods of strenuous exercise with sweating, during extremely hot weather, and with gastrointestinal upsets such as diarrhea. A simple strategy is to supplement the diet one to three times daily with salty broth (1 cup of beef or chicken bouillon contains 35 mmol of sodium). For a representative program of steroid therapy for the patient with adrenal insufficiency who is undergoing major surgery, see Table 321-8. This schedule is designed so that on the day of surgery it will mimic the output of cortisol in normal individuals undergoing prolonged major stress (10 mg/h, 250 to 300 mg/d). Thereafter, if the patient is improving and is afebrile, the dose of hydrocortisone is tapered by 20 to 30% daily. Mineralocorticoid administration is unnecessary at hydrocortisone doses >100 mg/d because of the mineralocorticoid effects of hydrocortisone at such dosages.

SECONDARY ADRENOCORTICAL INSUFFICIENCY ACTH deficiency causes *secondary* adrenocortical insufficiency; it may be a selective deficiency, as is seen following prolonged administration of excess glucocorticoids, or it may occur in association with deficiencies of multiple pituitary hormones (panhypopituitarism) (Chap. 318). Patients with secondary adrenocortical hypofunction have many symptoms and signs in common with those having primary disease but are *not hyperpigmented*, since ACTH and related peptide levels are low. In fact, plasma ACTH levels distinguish between primary and secondary adrenal insufficiency, since they are elevated in the former and decreased to absent in the latter. Patients with total pituitary insufficiency have manifestations of multiple hormone deficiencies. An additional feature distinguishing primary adrenocortical insufficiency is the *near-normal level of aldosterone secretion* seen in pituitary and/or isolated ACTH deficiencies (Fig. 321-11). Patients with pituitary insufficiency may have hyponatremia, which can be dilutional or secondary to a subnormal increase in aldosterone secretion in response to severe sodium restriction. However, severe *dehydration*, *hyponatremia*, and *hyperkalemia* are characteristic of severe mineralocorticoid insufficiency and favor a diagnosis of primary adrenocortical insufficiency.

Patients receiving long-term steroid therapy, despite physical findings of Cushing's syndrome, may develop adrenal insufficiency because of prolonged pituitary-hypothalamic suppression and adrenal atrophy secondary to the loss of endogenous ACTH. These patients have two deficits, a loss of adrenal responsiveness to ACTH and a failure of pituitary ACTH release. They are characterized by low blood cortisol and ACTH levels, a low baseline rate of steroid excretion, and abnormal ACTH and metyrapone responses. Most patients with steroid-induced adrenal insufficiency eventually recover normal HPA responsiveness, but recovery time varies from days to months. The rapid ACTH test provides a convenient assessment of recovery of HPA function. Because the plasma cortisol concentrations after injection of cosyntropin and during insulin-induced hypoglycemia are usually similar, the rapid ACTH test assesses the integrated HPA function (see "Tests of Pituitary-Adrenal Responsiveness," above). Some investigators suggest using the low-dose (1 μg) ACTH test for suspected secondary ACTH deficiency. Additional tests to assess pituitary ACTH reserve include the standard metyrapone and insulin-induced hypoglycemia tests.

Glucocorticoid therapy in patients with secondary adrenocortical insufficiency does not differ from that for the primary disorder. Mineralocorticoid therapy is usually not necessary, as aldosterone secretion is preserved.

ACUTE ADRENOCORTICAL INSUFFICIENCY Acute adrenocortical insufficiency may result from several processes. On the one hand, *adrenal crisis* may be a rapid and overwhelming intensification of chronic adrenal insufficiency, usually precipitated by sepsis or surgical stress. Alternatively, acute hemorrhagic destruction of both adrenal glands can occur in previously well individuals. In children, this event is usually associated with septicemia with *Pseudomonas* or meningococcemia (Waterhouse-Friderichsen syndrome). In adults, anticoagulant therapy or a coagulation disorder may result in bilateral adrenal hemorrhage. Occasionally, bilateral adrenal hemorrhage in the newborn results from birth trauma. Hemorrhage has been observed during pregnancy, following idiopathic adrenal vein thrombosis, and as a complication of venography (e.g., infarction of an adenoma). The third and most frequent cause of acute insufficiency is the rapid withdrawal of steroids from patients with adrenal atrophy owing to chronic steroid administration. Acute adrenocortical insufficiency may also occur in patients with congenital adrenal hyperplasia or those with decreased adrenocortical reserve when they are given drugs capable of inhibiting steroid synthesis (mitotane, ketoconazole) or of increasing steroid metabolism (phenytoin, rifampin).

Adrenal Crisis The long-term survival of patients with adrenocortical insufficiency depends largely on the prevention and treatment of adrenal crisis. Consequently, the occurrence of infection, trauma (including surgery), gastrointestinal upsets, or other stresses necessitates an immediate increase in hormone. In untreated patients, preexisting symptoms are intensified. Nausea, vomiting, and abdominal pain may become intractable. Fever may be severe or absent. Lethargy deepens into somnolence, and hypovolemic vascular collapse ensues. In contrast, patients previously maintained on chronic glucocorticoid therapy may not exhibit dehydration or hypotension until they are in a preterminal state, since mineralocorticoid secretion is usually preserved. In all patients in crisis, a precipitating cause should be sought.

℞ TREATMENT

Treatment is directed primarily toward repletion of circulating glucocorticoids and replacement of the sodium and water deficits. Hence an intravenous infusion of 5% glucose in normal saline solution should be started with a bolus intravenous infusion of 100 mg hydrocortisone followed by a continuous infusion of hydrocortisone at a rate of 10 mg/h. An alternative approach is to administer a 100-mg bolus of hydrocortisone intravenously every 6 h. However, only continuous infusion maintains the plasma cortisol constantly at stress levels [>830 nmol/L (30 μg/dL)]. Effective treatment of hypotension requires glucocorticoid replacement and repletion of sodium and water deficits. If the crisis was preceded by prolonged nausea, vomiting, and dehydration, several liters of saline solution may be required in the first few hours. Vasoconstrictive agents (such as dopamine) may be indicated in extreme conditions as adjuncts to volume replacement. With large doses of steroid, i.e., 100 to 200 mg hydrocortisone, the patient receives a maximal mineralocorticoid effect, and supplementary mineralocorticoid is superfluous. Following improvement, the steroid

dosage is tapered over the next few days to maintenance levels, and mineralocorticoid therapy is reinstituted if needed (Table 321-8).

ADRENAL CORTICOL INSUFFICIENCY IN ACUTELY ILL PATIENTS The physiology of the HPA axis is dramatically altered during critical illnesses such as trauma, surgery, sepsis, and shock. In such situations cortisol levels rise four- to sixfold, diurnal variation is abolished, and the unbound fractions of cortisol rise in the circulation and in target tissues. Inadequate cortisol production during critical illness can result in hypotension, reduced systemic vascular resistance, shock, and death.

A major area of controversy in presumably normal individuals is the correlation of clinical outcomes with the cortisol levels measured during critical illness. Subnormal cortisol production during acute severe illness has been termed "functional" or "relative" adrenal insufficiency. Conceptually, the elevated cortisol levels that are observed are viewed as insufficient to control the inflammatory response and maintain blood pressure. If such patients can be identified, treatment with supplementary cortisol could be beneficial.

A level of cortisol in a critically ill patient below which replacement glucocorticoids may improve prognosis is not firmly established, although many have accepted a level of ≤441 nmol/L (15 μg/dL). On the other hand, a random cortisol >938 nmol/L (34 μg/dL) in the setting of critical illness is unlikely to be associated with relative adrenal insufficiency. In patients who have random cortisol levels between 441 and 938 nmol/L (15 and 34 μg/dL), a cosyntropin stimulation test may identify patients with diminished adrenal reserve [increment <255 nmol/L (9 μg/dL)] who may benefit from supplementary cortisol treatment. If the diagnosis of relative or functional adrenal insufficiency is considered in an acutely ill, hypotensive patient, treatment with supplementary cortisol should be initiated promptly following the measurement of a random cortisol level and/or performing a cosyntropin stimulation test. Supplemental cortisol may be particularly beneficial in patients with septic shock where glucocorticoids have been reported to reduce mortality and the duration of vasopressor therapy. Such patients should be treated with 50 to 75 mg of intravenous hydrocortisone every 6 h as bolus treatment or the same amount as a continuous infusion. Treatment can be terminated if the cortisol levels obtained at the outset are normal. On the other hand, those patients with abnormal testing should be treated for 1 week and then tapered. In surviving patients, adrenal function should be reevaluated after resolution of the critical illness.

HYPOALDOSTERONISM

Isolated aldosterone deficiency accompanied by normal cortisol production occurs in association with hyporeninism, as an inherited biosynthetic defect, postoperatively following removal of aldosterone-secreting adenomas, during protracted heparin administration, in pretectal disease of the nervous system, and in severe postural hypotension.

The feature common to all forms of hypoaldosteronism is the inability to increase aldosterone secretion appropriately in response to salt restriction. Most patients have unexplained hyperkalemia, which is often exacerbated by restriction of dietary sodium intake. In severe cases, urine sodium wastage occurs at a normal salt intake, whereas in milder forms, excessive loss of urine sodium occurs only with salt restriction.

Most cases of isolated hypoaldosteronism occur in patients with a deficiency in renin production (so-called hyporeninemic hypoaldosteronism), most commonly in adults with diabetes mellitus and mild renal failure and in whom hyperkalemia and metabolic acidosis are out of proportion to the degree of renal impairment. Plasma renin levels fail to rise normally following sodium restriction and postural changes. The pathogenesis is uncertain. Possibilities include renal disease (the most likely), autonomic neuropathy, extracellular fluid volume expansion, and defective conversion of renin precursors to active renin. Aldosterone levels also fail to rise normally after salt restriction and volume contraction; this effect is probably related to the hyporeninism, since biosynthetic defects in aldosterone secretion usually cannot be demonstrated. In these patients, aldosterone secretion increases promptly after ACTH stimulation, but it is uncertain whether the magnitude of the response is normal. On the other hand, the level of aldosterone appears to be subnormal in relationship to the hyperkalemia.

Hypoaldosteronism can also be associated with high renin levels and low or elevated levels of aldosterone (see below). Severely ill patients may also have hyperreninemic hypoaldosteronism; such patients have a high mortality rate (80%). Hyperkalemia is not present. Possible explanations for the hypoaldosteronism include adrenal necrosis (uncommon) or a shift in steroidogenesis from mineralocorticoids to glucocorticoids, possibly related to prolonged ACTH stimulation.

Before the diagnosis of isolated hypoaldosteronism is considered for a patient with hyperkalemia, "pseudohyperkalemia" (e.g., hemolysis, thrombocytosis) should be excluded by measuring the *plasma* potassium level. The next step is to demonstrate a normal cortisol response to ACTH stimulation. Then, the response of renin and aldosterone levels to stimulation (upright posture, sodium restriction) should be measured. Low renin and aldosterone levels establish the diagnosis of hyporeninemic hypoaldosteronism. A combination of high renin levels and low aldosterone levels is consistent with an aldosterone biosynthetic defect or a selective unresponsiveness to angiotensin II. Finally, there is a condition that clinically and biochemically mimics hypoaldosteronism with elevated renin levels. However, the aldosterone levels are not low but high—so-called pseudohypoaldosteronism. This inherited condition is caused by a mutation in the epithelial sodium channel (see below).

℞ TREATMENT

The treatment is to replace the mineralocorticoid deficiency. For practical purposes, the oral administration of 0.05 to 0.15 mg fludrocortisone daily should restore electrolyte balance if salt intake is adequate (e.g., 150 to 200 mmol/d). However, patients with hyporeninemic hypoaldosteronism may require higher doses of mineralocorticoid to correct hyperkalemia. This need poses a potential risk in patients with hypertension, mild renal insufficiency, or congestive heart failure. An alternative approach is to reduce salt intake and to administer furosemide, which can ameliorate acidosis and hyperkalemia. Occasionally, a combination of these two approaches is efficacious.

GENETIC CONSIDERATIONS **Glucocorticoid Diseases** ■ *CONGENITAL ADRENAL HYPERPLASIA* Congenital adrenal hyperplasia (CAH) is the consequence of recessive mutations that cause one of several distinct enzymatic defects (see below). Because cortisol is the principal adrenal steroid regulating ACTH elaboration and because ACTH stimulates adrenal growth and function, a block in cortisol synthesis may result in the enhanced secretion of adrenal androgens and/or mineralocorticoids depending on the site of the enzyme block. In severe congenital virilizing hyperplasia, the adrenal output of cortisol may be so compromised as to cause adrenal deficiency despite adrenal hyperplasia.

CAH is the most common adrenal disorder of infancy and childhood (Chap. 328). Partial enzyme deficiencies can be expressed after adolescence, predominantly in women with hirsutism and oligomenorrhea but minimal virilization. Late-onset adrenal hyperplasia may account for 5 to 25% of cases of hirsutism and oligomenorrhea in women, depending on the population.

Etiology Enzymatic defects have been described in 21-hydroxylase (CYP21A2), 17α-hydroxylase/17,20-lyase (CYP17), 11β-hydroxylase (CYP11B1), and in (3β-HSD2) (Fig. 321-2). Although the genes encoding these enzymes have been cloned, the diagnosis of specific enzyme deficiencies with genetic techniques is not practical because of the large number of different deletions and missense mutations. CYP21A2 deficiency is closely linked to the HLA-B locus of chromosome 6 so that HLA typing and/or DNA polymorphism can be used to detect the heterozygous carriers and to diagnose affected individuals in some families (Chap. 296). The clinical expression in the different

disorders is variable, ranging from virilization of the female (CYP2/A2) to feminization of the male (3β-HSD2) (Chap. 328).

Adrenal virilization in the female at birth is associated with ambiguous external genitalia (*female pseudohermaphroditism*). Virilization begins after the fifth month of intrauterine development. At birth there may be enlargement of the clitoris, partial or complete fusion of the labia, and sometimes a urogenital sinus in the female. If the labial fusion is nearly complete, the female infant has external genitalia resembling a penis with hypospadias. In the *postnatal* period, CAH is associated with virilization in the female and isosexual precocity in the male. The excessive androgen levels result in accelerated growth, so that bone age exceeds chronologic age. Because epiphyseal closure occurs early, growth stops, but truncal development continues, the characteristic appearance being a short child with a well-developed trunk.

The most common form of CAH (95% of cases) is a result of impairment of CYP21A2. In addition to cortisol deficiency, aldosterone secretion is decreased in approximately one-third of the patients. Thus, with CYP21A2 deficiency, adrenal virilization occurs with or without a salt-losing tendency due to aldosterone deficiency (Fig. 321-2).

CYP11B1 deficiency causes a "hypertensive" variant of CAH. Hypertension and hypokalemia occur because of the impaired conversion of 11-deoxycorticosterone to corticosterone, resulting in the accumulation of 11-deoxycorticosterone, a potent mineralocorticoid. The degree of hypertension is variable. Steroid precursors are shunted into the androgen pathway.

CYP17 deficiency is characterized by hypogonadism, hypokalemia, and hypertension. This rare disorder causes decreased production of cortisol and shunting of precursors into the mineralocorticoid pathway with hypokalemic alkalosis, hypertension, and suppressed plasma renin activity. Usually, 11-deoxycorticosterone production is elevated. Because CYP17 hydroxylation is required for biosynthesis of both adrenal androgens and gonadal testosterone and estrogen, this defect is associated with sexual immaturity, high urinary gonadotropin levels, and low urinary 17-ketosteroid excretion. Female patients have primary amenorrhea and lack of development of secondary sexual characteristics. Because of deficient androgen production, male patients have either ambiguous external genitalia or a female phenotype (*male pseudohermaphroditism*). Exogenous glucocorticoids can correct the hypertensive syndrome, and treatment with appropriate gonadal steroids results in sexual maturation.

With 3β-HSD2 deficiency, conversion of pregnenolone to progesterone is impaired, so that the synthesis of both cortisol and aldosterone is blocked, with shunting into the adrenal androgen pathway via 17α-hydroxypregnenolone and DHEA. Because DHEA is a weak androgen, and because this enzyme deficiency is also present in the gonad, the genitalia of the male fetus may be incompletely virilized or feminized. Conversely, in the female, overproduction of DHEA may produce partial virilization.

Diagnosis The diagnosis of CAH should be considered in infants having episodes of acute adrenal insufficiency or salt-wasting or hypertension. The diagnosis is further suggested by the finding of hypertrophy of the clitoris, fused labia, or a urogenital sinus in the female or of isosexual precocity in the male. In infants and children with a CYP21A2 defect, increased urine 17-ketosteroid excretion and increased plasma DHEA sulfate levels are typically associated with an increase in the blood levels of 17-hydroxyprogesterone and the excretion of its urinary metabolite pregnanetriol. Demonstration of elevated levels of 17-hydroxyprogesterone in amniotic fluid at 14 to 16 weeks of gestation allows prenatal detection of affected female infants.

The diagnosis of a *salt-losing form* of CAH due to defects in CYP21A2 is suggested by episodes of acute adrenal insufficiency with hyponatremia, hyperkalemia, dehydration, and vomiting. These infants and children often crave salt and have laboratory findings indicating deficits in both cortisol and aldosterone secretion.

With the *hypertensive form* of CAH due to CYP11B1 deficiency, 11-deoxycorticosterone and 11-deoxycortisol accumulate. The diagnosis is confirmed by demonstrating increased levels of 11-deoxycortisol in the blood or increased amounts of tetrahydro-11-deoxycortisol in the urine. Elevation of 17-hydroxyprogesterone levels does not imply a coexisting CYP21A2 deficiency.

Very high levels of urine DHEA with low levels of pregnanetriol and of cortisol metabolites in urine are characteristic of children with 3β-HSD2 deficiency. Marked salt-wasting may also occur.

Adults with *late-onset adrenal hyperplasia* (partial deficiency of CYP21A2, CYP11B1, or 3β-HSD2) are characterized by normal or moderately elevated levels of urinary 17-ketosteroids and plasma DHEA sulfate. A high basal level of a precursor of cortisol biosynthesis (such as 17-hydroxyprogesterone, 17-hydroxypregnenolone, or 11-deoxycortisol), or elevation of such a precursor after ACTH stimulation, confirms the diagnosis of a partial deficiency. Measurement of steroid precursors 60 min after bolus administration of ACTH is usually sufficient. Adrenal androgen output is easily suppressed by the standard low-dose (2 mg) dexamethasone test.

℞ **TREATMENT**

Therapy in CAH patients consists of daily administration of glucocorticoids to suppress pituitary ACTH secretion. Because of its low cost and intermediate half-life, prednisone is the drug of choice except in infants, in whom hydrocortisone is usually used. In adults with late-onset adrenal hyperplasia, the smallest single bedtime dose of a long- or intermediate-acting glucocorticoid that suppresses pituitary ACTH secretion should be administered. The amount of steroid required by children with CAH is approximately 1 to 1.5 times the normal cortisol production rate of 27 to 35 μmol (10 to 13 mg) of cortisol per square meter of body surface per day and is given in divided doses two or three times per day. The dosage schedule is governed by repetitive analysis of the urinary 17-ketosteroids, plasma DHEA sulfate, and/or precursors of cortisol biosynthesis. Skeletal growth and maturation must also be monitored closely, as overtreatment with glucocorticoid replacement therapy retards linear growth.

Receptor Mutations *Isolated glucocorticoid deficiency* is a rare autosomal recessive disease secondary to a mutation in the ACTH receptor. Usually mineralocorticoid function is normal. Adrenal insufficiency is manifest within the first 2 years of life as hyperpigmentation, convulsions, and/or frequent episodes of hypoglycemia. In some patients the adrenal insufficiency is associated with achalasia and alacrima—Allgrove's, or triple A, syndrome. However, in some triple A syndrome patients, no mutation in the ACTH receptor has been identified, suggesting that a distinct genetic abnormality causes this syndrome. *Adrenal hypoplasia congenita* is a rare X-linked disorder caused by a mutation in the *DAX1* gene. This gene encodes an orphan nuclear receptor that plays an important role in the development of the adrenal cortex and also the hypothalamic-pituitary-gonadal axis. Thus, patients present with signs and symptoms secondary to deficiencies of all three major adrenal steroids—cortisol, aldosterone, and adrenal androgens—as well as gonadotropin deficiency. Finally a rare cause of hypercortisolism without cushingoid stigmata is *primary cortisol resistance* due to mutations in the glucocorticoid receptor. The resistance is incomplete because patients do not exhibit signs of adrenal insufficiency.

Miscellaneous Conditions Adrenoleukodystrophy causes severe demyelination and early death in children, and adrenomyeloneuropathy is associated with a mixed motor and sensory neuropathy with spastic paraplegia in adults; both disorders are associated with elevated circulating levels of very long chain fatty acids and cause adrenal insufficiency. Autosomal recessive mutations in the *s*teroidogenic *a*cute *r*egulatory (STAR) protein gene cause congenital lipoid adrenal hyperplasia (Chap. 328), which is characterized by adrenal insufficiency

and defective gonadal steroidogenesis. Because STAR mediates cholesterol transport into the mitochondrion, mutations in the protein cause massive lipid accumulation in steroidogenic cells, ultimately leading to cell toxicity.

MINERALOCORTICOID DISEASES Some forms of CAH have a mineralocorticoid component (see above). Others are caused by a mutation in other enzymes or ion channels important in mediating or mimicking aldosterone's action.

Hypermineralocorticoidism ■ *LOW PLASMA RENIN ACTIVITY* Rarely, hypermineralocorticoidism is due to a defect in cortisol biosynthesis, specifically 11- or 17-hydroxylation. ACTH levels are increased, with a resultant increase in the production of the mineralocorticoid 11-deoxycorticosterone. Hypertension and hypokalemia can be corrected by glucocorticoid administration. The definitive diagnosis is made by demonstrating an elevation of precursors of cortisol biosynthesis in the blood or urine or by direct demonstration of the genetic defect.

Glucocorticoid administration can also ameliorate hypertension or produce normotension even though a hydroxylase deficiency cannot be identified (Fig. 321-9). These patients have normal to slightly elevated aldosterone levels that do not suppress in response to saline but do suppress in response to 2 days of dexamethasone (2 mg/d). The condition is inherited as an autosomal dominant trait and is termed *glucocorticoid-remediable aldosteronism* (GRA). This entity is secondary to a chimeric gene duplication whereby the 11-β hydroxylase gene promoter (which is under the control of ACTH) is fused to the aldosterone synthase coding sequence. Thus, aldosterone synthase activity is ectopically expressed in the zona fasciculata and is regulated by ACTH, in a fashion similar to the regulation of cortisol secretion. Screening for this defect is best performed by assessing the presence or absence of the chimeric gene. Because the abnormal gene may be present in the absence of hypokalemia, its frequency as a cause of hypertension is unknown. Individuals with suppressed plasma renin levels and juvenile-onset hypertension or a history of early-onset hypertension in first-degree relatives should be screened for this disorder. Early hemorrhagic stroke also occurs in GRA-affected individuals.

GRA documented by genetic analysis may be treated with glucocorticoid administration or antimineralocorticoids, i.e., spironolactone, triamterene, or amiloride. Glucocorticoids should be used only in small doses to avoid inducing iatrogenic Cushing's syndrome. A combination approach is often necessary.

HIGH PLASMA RENIN ACTIVITY *Bartter syndrome* is characterized by severe hyperaldosteronism (hypokalemic alkalosis) with moderate to marked increases in renin activity and hypercalciuria, but normal blood pressure and no edema; this disorder usually begins in childhood. Renal biopsy shows juxtaglomerular hyperplasia. Bartter syndrome is caused by a mutation in the renal Na-K-2Cl co-transporter gene. The pathogenesis involves a defect in the renal conservation of sodium or chloride. The renal loss of sodium is thought to stimulate renin secretion and aldosterone production. Hyperaldosteronism produces potassium depletion, and hypokalemia further elevates prostaglandin production and plasma renin activity. In some cases, the hypokalemia may be potentiated by a defect in renal conservation of potassium.

Gitelman syndrome is an autosomal recessive trait characterized by renal salt wasting and as a result, as in Bartter syndrome, activation of the renin-angiotensin-aldosterone system. As a consequence affected individuals have low blood pressure, low serum potassium, low serum magnesium, and high serum bicarbonate. In contrast to Bartter syndrome, urinary calcium excretion is reduced. Gitelman syndrome results from loss-of-function mutations of the renal thiazide-sensitive Na-Cl co-transporter.

Increased Mineralocorticoid Action *Liddle syndrome* is a rare autosomal dominant disorder that mimicks hyperaldosteronism. The defect is in the genes encoding the β or η subunits of the epithelial sodium channel. Both renin and aldosterone levels are low, owing to the constitutively activated sodium channel and the resulting excess sodium reabsorption in the renal tubule.

TABLE 321-9 *A Checklist for Use Prior to the Administration of Glucocorticoids in Pharmacologic Doses*

Presence of tuberculosis or other chronic infection (chest x-ray, tuberculin test)
Evidence of glucose intolerance or history of gestational diabetes mellitus
Evidence of preexisting osteoporosis (bone density assessment in organ transplant recipients or postmenopausal patients)
History of peptic ulcer, gastritis, or esophagitis (stool guaiac test)
Evidence of hypertension or cardiovascular disease
History of psychological disorders

A rare autosomal recessive cause of hypokalemia and hypertension is 11β-HSD II deficiency, in which cortisol cannot be converted to cortisone and hence binds to the MR and acts as a mineralocorticoid. This condition, also termed *apparent mineralocorticoid excess syndrome*, is caused by a defect in the gene encoding the renal isoform of this enzyme, 11β-HSD II. Patients can be identified either by documenting an increased ratio of cortisol to cortisone in the urine or by genetic analysis. Patients with the 11β-HSD deficiency syndrome can be treated with small doses of dexamethasone, which suppresses ACTH and endogenous cortisol production but binds less well to the mineralocorticoid receptor than does cortisol.

The ingestion of candies or chewing tobacco containing certain forms of licorice produces a syndrome that mimics primary aldosteronism. The component of such agents that causes sodium retention is glycyrrhizinic acid, which inhibits 11β-HSD II and hence allows cortisol to act as a mineralocorticoid. The diagnosis is established or excluded by a careful history.

Decreased Mineralocorticoid Production or Action In patients with a deficiency in aldosterone biosynthesis, the transformation of corticosterone into aldosterone is impaired, owing to a mutation in the aldosterone synthase (CYP11B2) gene. These patients have low to absent aldosterone secretion, elevated plasma renin levels, and elevated levels of the intermediates of aldosterone biosynthesis (corticosterone and 18-hydroxycorticosterone).

Pseudohypoaldosteronism type I (PHA-I) is an autosomal recessive disorder that is seen in the neonatal period and is characterized by salt wasting, hypotension, hyperkalemia, and high renin and aldosterone levels. In contrast to the gain-of-function mutations in the epithelial sodium channel in Liddle syndrome, mutations in PHA-I result in loss of epithelial sodium channel function.

PHARMACOLOGIC CLINICAL USES OF ADRENAL STEROIDS

The widespread use of glucocorticoids emphasizes the need for a thorough understanding of the metabolic effects of these agents. Before adrenal hormone therapy is instituted, the expected gains should be weighed against undesirable effects. Several important questions should be addressed before initiating therapy. First, how serious is the disorder (the more serious, the greater the likelihood that the risk/benefit ratio will be positive)? Second, how long will therapy be required (the longer the therapy, the greater the risk of adverse side effects)? Third, does the individual have preexisting conditions that glucocorticoids may exacerbate (Table 321-9)? If so, then a careful risk/benefit assessment is required to ensure that the ratio is favorable given the increased likelihood of harm by steroids in these patients. Supplementary measures to minimize undesirable metabolic effects are shown in Table 321-10. Fourth, which preparation is best?

THERAPEUTIC CONSIDERATIONS The following considerations should be taken into account in deciding which steroid preparation to use:

1. *The biologic half-life.* The rationale behind alternate-day therapy is to decrease the metabolic effects of the steroids for a significant part of each 48 h period while still producing a pharmacologic effect durable enough to be effective. Too long a half-life would defeat the first purpose, and too short a half-life would defeat the second. In general, the more potent the steroid, the longer its biologic half-life.

TABLE 321-10 *Supplementary Measures to Minimize Undesirable Metabolic Effects of Glucocorticoids*

Monitor caloric intake to prevent weight gain.
Restrict sodium intake to prevent edema and minimize hypertension and potassium loss.
Provide supplementary potassium if necessary.
Provide antacid, H_2 receptor antagonist, and/or H^+,K^+-ATPase inhibitor therapy.
Institute alternate-day steroid schedule if possible. Patients receiving steroid therapy over a prolonged period should be protected by an appropriate increase in hormone level during periods of acute stress. A rule of thumb is to *double* the maintenance dose.
Minimize osteopenia by
 Administering gonadal hormone replacement therapy: 0.625–1.25 mg conjugated estrogens given cyclically with progesterone, unless the uterus is absent; testosterone replacement for hypogonadal men
Ensuring high calcium intake (should be approximately 1200 mg/d)
Administering supplemental vitamin D if blood levels of calciferol or 1,25(OH)$_2$ vitamin D are reduced
Administering bisphosphonate prophylactically, orally or parenterally, in high-risk patients

2. *The mineralocorticoid effects of the steroid.* Most synthetic steroids have less mineralocorticoid effect than hydrocortisone (Table 321-11).

3. *The biologically active form of the steroid.* Cortisone and prednisone have to be converted to biologically active metabolites before anti-inflammatory effects can occur. Because of this, in a condition for which steroids are known to be effective and when an adequate dose has been given without response, one should consider substituting hydrocortisone or prednisolone for cortisone or prednisone.

4. *The cost of the medication.* This is a serious consideration if chronic administration is planned. Prednisone is the least expensive of available steroid preparations.

5. *The type of formulation.* Topical steroids have the distinct advantage over oral steroids in reducing the likelihood of systemic side effects. In addition, some inhaled steroids have been designed to minimize side effects by increasing their hepatic inactivation if they are swallowed (Chap. 236). However, all topical steroids can be absorbed into the systemic circulation.

TABLE 321-11 *Glucocorticoid Preparations*

Commonly Used Name[a]	Estimated Potency[b]	
	Glucocorticoid	Mineralocorticoid
SHORT-ACTING		
Hydrocortisone	1	1
Cortisone	0.8	0.8
INTERMEDIATE-ACTING		
Prednisone	4	0.25
Prednisolone	4	0.25
Methylprednisolone	5	<0.01
Triamcinolone	5	<0.01
LONG-ACTING		
Paramethasone	10	<0.01
Betamethasone	25	<0.01
Dexamethasone	30–40	<0.01

[a] The steroids are divided into three groups according to the duration of biologic activity. Short-acting preparations have a biologic half-life <12 h; long-acting, >48 h; and intermediate, between 12 and 36 h. Triamcinolone has the longest half-life of the intermediate-acting preparations.

[b] Relative milligram comparisons with hydrocortisone, setting the glucocorticoid and mineralocorticoid properties of hydrocortisone as 1. Sodium retention is insignificant for commonly employed doses of methylprednisolone, triamcinolone, paramethasone, betamethasone, and dexamethasone.

ALTERNATE-DAY STEROID THERAPY The most effective way to minimize the cushingoid effects of glucocorticoids is to administer the total 48-h dose as a *single* dose of *intermediate-acting steroid* in the morning, *every other day*. If symptoms of the underlying disorder can be controlled by this technique, it offers distinct advantages. Three considerations deserve mention: (1) The alternate-day schedule may be approached through transition schedules that allow the patient to adjust gradually; (2) supplementary nonsteroid medications may be needed on the "off" day to minimize symptoms of the underlying disorder; and (3) many symptoms that occur during the off day (e.g., fatigue, joint pain, muscle stiffness or tenderness, and fever) may represent relative adrenal insufficiency rather than exacerbation of the underlying disease.

The alternate-day approach capitalizes on the fact that cortisol secretion and plasma levels normally are highest in the early morning and lowest in the evening. The normal pattern is mimicked by administering an intermediate-acting steroid in the morning (7 to 8 A.M.) (Table 321-11).

Initially, the steroid regimen often requires daily or more frequent doses of steroid to achieve the desired anti-inflammatory or immunity-suppressing action. *Only after this desired effect is achieved is an attempt made to switch to an alternate-day program.* A number of schedules can be used for transferring from a daily to an alternate-day program. The key points to be considered are flexibility in arranging a program and the use of supportive measures on the off day. One may attempt a gradual transition to the alternate-day schedule rather than an abrupt changeover. One approach is to keep the steroid dose constant on one day and gradually reduce it on the alternate day. Alternatively, the steroid dose can be increased on one day and reduced on the alternate day. In any case, it is important to anticipate that some increase in pain or discomfort may occur in the 36 to 48 h following the last dose.

WITHDRAWAL OF GLUCOCORTICOIDS FOLLOWING LONG-TERM USE It is possible to reduce a daily steroid dose gradually and eventually to discontinue it, but under most circumstances withdrawal of steroids should be initiated by first implementing an alternate-day schedule. Patients who have been on an alternate-day program for a month or more experience less difficulty during termination regimens. The dosage is gradually reduced and finally discontinued after a replacement dosage has been reached (e.g., 5 to 7.5 mg prednisone). Complications rarely ensue unless undue stress is experienced, and patients should understand that for ≥1 year after withdrawal from long-term high-dose steroid therapy, supplementary hormone should be given in the event of a serious infection, operation, or injury. A useful strategy in patients with symptoms of adrenal insufficiency on a tapering regimen is to measure plasma cortisol levels prior to the steroid dose. A level <140 nmol/L (5 μg/dL) indicates suppression of the pituitary-adrenal axis and implies that a more cautious tapering of steroids is indicated.

In patients on high-dose daily steroid therapy, it is advised to reduce dosage to ~20 mg prednisone daily as a single morning dose before beginning the transition to alternate-day therapy. If a patient cannot tolerate an alternate-day program, consideration should be given to the possibility that the patient has developed primary adrenal insufficiency.

FURTHER READING

BARZON L et al: Risk factors and long-term follow-up of adrenal incidentalomas. J Clin Endocrinol Metab 84:520, 1999

COOPER MS et al: Current concepts: Corticosteroid insufficiency in acutely ill patients. N Engl J Med 348: 727, 2003

NEWELL-PRICE J et al: Diagnosis and management of Cushing's syndrome. Lancet 353:2087, 1999

PITT B et al: Eplerenone, a selective aldosterone blocker, in patients with left ventricular dysfunction after myocardial infarction. N Engl J Med 348: 1309, 2003

YOUNG WF: Minireview: Primary aldosteronism—changing concepts in diagnosis and treatment. Endocrinology 144:2208, 2003

322 PHEOCHROMOCYTOMA
Lewis Landsberg, James B. Young

Pheochromocytomas produce, store, and secrete catecholamines. They are usually derived from the adrenal medulla but may develop from chromaffin cells in or about sympathetic ganglia (extraadrenal pheochromocytomas or paragangliomas). Related tumors that secrete catecholamines and produce similar clinical syndromes include chemodectomas derived from the carotid body and ganglioneuromas derived from the postganglionic sympathetic neurons.

The clinical features are due predominantly to the release of catecholamines and, to a lesser extent, to the secretion of other substances. Hypertension is the most common sign, and hypertensive paroxysms or crises, often spectacular and alarming, occur in over half the cases.

Pheochromocytoma occurs in approximately 0.1% of the hypertensive population but is, nevertheless, an important correctable cause of high blood pressure. Indeed, it is usually curable if diagnosed and treated, but it may be fatal if undiagnosed or mistreated. Postmortem series indicate that most pheochromocytomas are unsuspected clinically, even when the tumor is related to the fatal outcome.

PATHOLOGY ■ Location and Morphology In adults, approximately 80% of pheochromocytomas are unilateral and solitary, 10% are bilateral, and 10% are extraadrenal. In children, a fourth of tumors are bilateral, and an additional fourth are extraadrenal. Solitary lesions inexplicably favor the right side. Although pheochromocytomas may grow to large size (>3 kg), most weigh <100 g and are <10 cm in diameter. Pheochromocytomas are highly vascular.

The tumors are made up of large, polyhedral, pleomorphic chromaffin cells. Fewer than 10% of these tumors are malignant. As with several other endocrine tumors, malignancy cannot be determined from the histologic appearance; tumors that contain large numbers of aneuploid or tetraploid cells, as determined by flow cytometry, are more likely to recur. Local invasion of surrounding tissues or distant metastases indicate malignancy.

EXTRAADRENAL PHEOCHROMOCYTOMAS Extraadrenal pheochromocytomas usually weigh 20 to 40 g and are <5 cm in diameter. Most are located within the abdomen in association with the celiac, superior mesenteric, and inferior mesenteric ganglia. Approximately 10% are in the thorax, 1% are within the urinary bladder, and <3% are in the neck, usually in association with the sympathetic ganglia or the extracranial branches of the ninth or tenth cranial nerves.

Catecholamine Synthesis, Storage, and Release Pheochromocytomas synthesize and store catecholamines by processes resembling those of the normal adrenal medulla. Little is known about the mechanisms of catecholamine release from pheochromocytomas, but changes in blood flow and necrosis within the tumor may be the cause in some instances. These tumors are not innervated, and catecholamine release does not result from neural stimulation. Pheochromocytomas also store and secrete a variety of peptides, including endogenous opioids, adrenomedullin, endothelin, erythropoietin, parathyroid hormone–related protein, neuropeptide Y, and chromagranin A. These peptides contribute to the clinical manifestations in selected cases, as noted below.

EPINEPHRINE, NOREPINEPHRINE, AND DOPAMINE Most pheochromocytomas produce both norepinephrine and epinephrine, and the percentage of norepinephrine is usually greater than in the normal adrenal. Most extraadrenal pheochromocytomas secrete norepinephrine exclusively. Rarely, pheochromocytomas produce epinephrine alone, particularly in association with multiple endocrine neoplasia (MEN). Although epinephrine-producing tumors may cause a preponderance of metabolic and beta-receptor effects, in general the major catecholamine secreted cannot be predicted from the clinical presentation. Increased production of dopamine and homovanillic acid (HVA) is uncommon with benign lesions but may occur with malignant pheochromocytoma.

FAMILIAL PHEOCHROMOCYTOMA Pheochromocytoma may be inherited as an autosomal dominant trait either alone or in combination with other abnormalities such as MEN type 2A (Sipple's syndrome) or type 2B (mucosal neuroma syndrome) (Chap. 330), von Hippel–Lindau's (VHL) retinal cerebellar hemangioblastomosis, or von Recklinghausen's neurofibromatosis (type 1) and in association with paragangliomas of the neck. Recent evidence suggests that 25% of patients with pheochromocytoma may have an inherited form of the disease. Features that suggest familial disease include bilaterality, multicentricity (within the adrenal and at diverse sites), and age of onset <30 years.

GENETIC CONSIDERATIONS **MEN 2** The MEN 2A and 2B syndromes are associated with abnormalities in the *RET* protooncogene located in pericentromeric region of chromosome 10 (Chap. 330). These mutations result in the constitutive activation of the receptor tyrosine kinase, causing adrenal medullary chromaffin cell and thyroid parafollicular C cell hyperplasia and rendering the cells susceptible to malignant transformation. The *RET* mutations are located in the extracellular domain in MEN 2A and in the intracellular portion of the receptor in families with the MEN 2B syndrome. Mutations at specific sites in the *RET* protooncogene are highly predictive of pheochromocytoma. Pheochromocytomas in MEN 2 are multicentric and bilateral but not extraadrenal. Individuals at risk for MEN 2A and 2B should be screened periodically for pheochromocytoma by assay of a 24-h urine sample for catecholamines, including measurement of epinephrine. Pheochromocytoma should be excluded or removed before thyroid or parathyroid surgery.

VHL In the VHL syndrome, mutation of one copy of the VHL tumor-suppressor gene is associated with the development of tumors characteristic of the syndrome, including pheochromocytomas. Loss of function of the VHL tumor-suppressor gene promotes tumor formation by mechanisms that are incompletely understood but may involve alterations in mRNA transcript elongation. In the VHL syndrome, the frequency of pheochromocytoma varies considerably but may be as high as 60% in some kindreds. As in the MEN 2 syndromes, certain VHL mutations are highly associated with the development of pheochromocytoma. Of further interest is the recent finding that the VHL mutation has been identified in some kindreds with familial pheochromocytoma as the sole manifestation without other clinical evidence of the VHL syndrome. Missense mutations, as opposed to deletions, insertions, or nonsense mutations, appear to be more commonly associated with pheochromocytoma, which may be adrenal, extraadrenal, or multifocal. A high incidence of germ-line VHL mutations in patients with thoracic extraadrenal pheochromocytomas has also been reported.

Familial Paraganglioma Syndromes Mutations in the genes encoding succinate dehydrogenase subunit B (SDHB) and subunit D (SDHD) may occur in kindreds with inherited paraganglioma, usually located in the head or neck (glomus tumors) or carotid body. Paraganglioma in these syndromes are distinct from extraadrenal pheochromocytomas, which are also commonly referred to as *paragangliomas*. Adrenal or extraadrenal pheochromocytomas are often inherited in association with these paragangliomas.

Neurofibromatosis Type I Mutations in the *NF-I* gene predispose to the development of pheochromocytoma, although the association is not very common. It has been estimated that 1% of patients with pheochromocytoma have an *NF-I* mutation. Pheochromocytomas may occur in patients with minor clinical manifestations of neurofibromatosis such as a few café au lait spots, vertebral abnormalities, or kyphoscoliosis.

Nonsyndromic Familial Pheochromocytoma Patients presenting with a solitary adrenal pheochromocytoma, negative family history, and no evidence of associated disease may still have an inherited form of the disease. This is most common with the *SDHB* and *SDHD* mutations but also occurs with alterations in the *VHL* gene.

Screening for Genetic Disease Genetic screening for the *RET* mutation is available and of established utility in the evaluation of families for the MEN 2 syndromes. Genetic tests for the *SDH*, *NF-I*, and *VHL* mutations are not yet generally available. Screening in these kindreds therefore is dependent on a vigorous search for the associated diseases and a complete evaluation of family history.

CLINICAL FEATURES Pheochromocytoma occurs at all ages but is most common in young to midadult life. Some series show a slight female preponderance. Most patients come to medical attention as a result of hypertensive crisis, paroxysmal symptoms suggestive of seizure disorder or anxiety attacks, or hypertension that responds poorly to conventional treatment. Less commonly, unexplained hypotension or shock in association with surgery or trauma will suggest the diagnosis. Aberrant reactions to medications such as opioids or tricyclic antidepressants may bring the patient to clinical attention. In most patients the hypertension is associated with other symptoms, such as headaches, excessive sweating, and/or palpitations.

Hypertension Hypertension is the most common manifestation. In approximately 60% of cases the hypertension is sustained, although significant blood pressure lability is usually present, and half of patients with sustained hypertension have distinct crises or paroxysms. The other 40% have blood pressure elevations only during an attack. The hypertension is often severe, occasionally malignant, and may be resistant to treatment with standard antihypertensive drugs.

Paroxysms or Crises The paroxysm or crisis occurs in over half of patients. In an individual patient, the symptoms are often similar with each attack. The paroxysms may be frequent or sporadic, occurring at intervals as long as weeks or months. With time, the paroxysms usually increase in frequency, duration, and severity.

The attack usually has a sudden onset. It may last from a few minutes to several hours or longer. Headache, profuse sweating, palpitations, and apprehension, often with a sense of impending doom, are common. Pain in the chest or abdomen may be associated with nausea and vomiting. Either pallor or flushing may occur during the attack. The blood pressure is elevated, often to alarming levels, and the elevation is usually accompanied by tachycardia.

The paroxysm may be precipitated by any activity that displaces the abdominal contents. In some cases a particular stimulus may induce an attack in a characteristic fashion, but in others no clearly defined precipitating event can be found. Although anxiety may accompany the attacks, mental or psychological stress does not usually provoke a crisis.

Other Distinctive Clinical Features Symptoms and signs of an increased metabolic rate, such as profuse sweating and mild to moderate weight loss, are common. Orthostatic hypotension is a consequence of diminished plasma volume and blunted sympathetic reflexes. Both these factors predispose the patient with unsuspected pheochromocytoma to hypotension or shock during surgery or trauma. Secretion of the hypotensive peptide adrenomedullin may contribute to the hypotension in some patients.

CARDIAC MANIFESTATIONS Sinus tachycardia, sinus bradycardia, supraventricular arrhythmias, and ventricular premature contractions have all been noted. Angina and acute myocardial infarction may occur even in the absence of coronary artery disease. A catecholamine-induced increase in myocardial oxygen consumption and, perhaps, coronary spasm may play a role in these ischemic events. Electrocardiographic changes, including nonspecific ST-T wave changes, prominent U waves, left ventricular strain patterns, and right and left bundle branch blocks may be present in the absence of demonstrable ischemia or infarction. Cardiomyopathy, either congestive with myocarditis and myocardial fibrosis or hypertrophic with concentric or asymmetric hypertrophy, may be associated with heart failure and cardiac arrhythmias. Multiorgan system failure with noncardiogenic pulmonary edema may be the presenting manifestation. Elevated levels of amylase originating from damaged pulmonary endothelium and abdominal pain may suggest acute pancreatitis, although serum lipase levels are normal.

CARBOHYDRATE INTOLERANCE   Over half of patients have impaired carbohydrate tolerance due to suppression of insulin and stimulation of hepatic glucose output. The impaired glucose tolerance may require treatment with insulin and disappears after removal of the tumor.

HEMATOCRIT   An elevated hematocrit may be secondary to diminished plasma volume. Rarely, production of erythropoietin by the tumor may cause a true erythrocytosis.

OTHER MANIFESTATIONS   Hypercalcemia has been attributed to the ectopic secretion of parathyroid hormone–related protein. Fever and an elevated erythrocyte sedimentation rate have been reported in association with the production of interleukin 6. Elevated temperature more commonly reflects catecholamine mediated increases in metabolic rate and diminished heat dissipation secondary to vasoconstriction. Polyuria is an occasional finding, and rhabdomyolysis with myoglobinuric renal failure may result from extreme vasoconstriction with muscle ischemia. Ectopic production of adrenocorticotropic hormone and vasoactive intestinal peptide have been documented in association with the characteristic manifestations of inappropriate secretion of these hormones (Chap. 317).

PHEOCHROMOCYTOMA OF THE URINARY BLADDER   Pheochromocytoma in the wall of the urinary bladder may result in typical paroxysms in relation to micturition. The location in the bladder wall is responsible for the occurrence of symptoms while the tumors are quite small, and, consequently, catecholamine excretion may be normal or minimally elevated. Hematuria is present in over half of patients, and the tumor can often be visualized at cystoscopy.

Adverse Drug Interactions   Severe and occasionally fatal paroxysms have been induced by opiates, histamine, adrenocorticotropin, saralasin, and glucagon. These agents appear to release catecholamines directly from the tumor. Indirect-acting sympathomimetic amines, including methyldopa (when administered intravenously), may increase blood pressure by releasing catecholamines from the augmented stores within nerve endings. Drugs that block neuronal uptake of catecholamines, such as tricyclic antidepressants, may enhance the physiologic effects of circulating catecholamines. Indeed, all medications should be considered carefully and administered cautiously in patients with known or suspected pheochromocytoma.

DIAGNOSIS   The diagnosis is established by the demonstration of increased production of catecholamines or catecholamine metabolites. The diagnosis can usually be made by the analysis of a single 24-h urine sample, provided the patient is hypertensive or symptomatic at the time of collection.

Biochemical Tests   The assays employed include those for vanillylmandelic acid (VMA), the metanephrines, and unconjugated or "free" catecholamines. The VMA assay is both less sensitive and less specific than assays of metanephrines or catecholamines. Accuracy of diagnosis is improved when two of three determinations are employed. The following considerations apply to all the urinary tests: (1) Despite claims for the adequacy of determinations made on random urine samples, analysis of a full 24-h urine sample is preferable. Creatinine should also be determined to assess the adequacy of collection. (2) Where possible, the collection should be made when the patient is at rest, on no medication, and without recent exposure to radiographic contrast media. When it is not practical to discontinue all medications, drugs known specifically to interfere with these assays (as noted below) should be avoided. (3) The urine should be acidified and refrigerated during and after collection. (4) With high-quality assays, dietary restrictions are minimal and should be specified by the laboratory performing the analyses. (5) Although most patients with pheochromocytoma excrete increased amounts of catecholamines and catecholamine metabolites at all times, the yield is increased in patients with paroxysmal hypertension if a 24-h urine collection is initiated during a crisis.

FREE CATECHOLAMINES   The upper limit of normal for total urinary catecholamines is between 590 and 885 nmol (100 and 150 μg) per 24 h. In most patients with pheochromocytoma, values >1480 nmol (250 μg) per day are obtained. Measurement of epinephrine is often of value, since increased epinephrine excretion [>275 nmol (50 μg) per 24 h] is usually due to an adrenal lesion and may be the only abnormality in cases associated with MEN 2. False-positive increases in catecholamine excretion result from exogenous catecholamines and related drugs such as methyldopa, levodopa, labetalol, and sympathomimetic amines, which may elevate catecholamine excretion for up to 2 weeks. Endogenous catecholamines from stimulation of the sympathoadrenal system may also increase urinary catecholamine excretion. Relevant clinical situations that cause such increases include hypoglycemia, strenuous exertion, central nervous system disease with increased intracranial pressure, severe hypoxia, and clonidine withdrawal.

METANEPHRINES AND VMA   In most laboratories, the upper limit of normal is 7 μmol (1.3 mg) of total metanephrines and 35 μmol (7.0 mg) of VMA excretion per 24 h. In most patients with pheochromocytoma, the increase in these urinary metabolites is considerable, often to more than three times the normal range. Metanephrine excretion is increased by exogenous and endogenous catecholamines and by treatment with monoamine oxidase inhibitors; propranolol may cause a spurious increase in metanephrine excretion, since a propranolol metabolite interferes in the commonly used spectrophotometric assay. VMA is less affected by endogenous and exogenous catecholamines but is spuriously increased by a variety of drugs, including carbidopa. VMA excretion is decreased by monoamine oxidase inhibitors.

PLASMA CATECHOLAMINES   Measurement of plasma catecholamines has a limited application. The care required in obtaining basal levels and the satisfactory results with urinary determinations make measurement of plasma catecholamines unnecessary in most cases. Plasma catecholamine levels are affected by the same drugs and physiologic perturbations that increase urinary catecholamine excretion. In addition, α- and β-adrenergic receptor blocking agents may elevate plasma catecholamines by impairing clearance.

When the clinical features suggest pheochromocytoma and the urinary assay results are borderline, measurement of plasma catecholamines may be worthwhile. Markedly elevated basal levels of total catecholamines support the diagnosis, although approximately one-third of patients with pheochromocytoma have normal or slightly elevated basal values. The usefulness of plasma catecholamine determinations may be increased by agents that suppress sympathetic nervous system activity. Clonidine and ganglionic blocking agents reduce plasma catecholamine levels in normal subjects and in patients with essential hypertension. These drugs have little effect on catecholamine levels in patients with pheochromocytoma. In patients with elevated or borderline basal catecholamine values, failure to suppress plasma or urinary levels with clonidine supports the diagnosis of pheochromocytoma.

PLASMA METANEPHRINES   Measurement of free (unconjugated) total plasma metanephrines, fractionated into normetanephrine and metanephrine, is a highly sensitive technique for the diagnosis of pheochromocytoma. Questions of specificity, particularly among the elderly, as well as the availability of high-quality assays need to be addressed before plasma metanephrines replace the 24-h urinary measurement of free catecholamines and metanephrines as the screening test of choice.

Pharmacologic Tests Reliable methods for the measurement of catecholamines and catecholamine metabolites in urine have rendered obsolete both the provocative and adrenolytic tests, which are nonspecific and entail considerable risk. A modified version of the adrenolytic test may be of some use, however, as a therapeutic trial in a patient in hypertensive crisis with features suggestive of pheochromocytoma. A positive response to phentolamine (5-mg bolus following a test dose of 0.5 mg) is a reduction in blood pressure of at least 35/25 mmHg after 2 min that persists for 10 to 15 min. The pharmacologic response is never diagnostic, and biochemical confirmation is essential. Provocative tests in normotensive patients are potentially dangerous and rarely indicated. However, a glucagon provocative test may be of use in patients with paroxysmal hypertension and nondiagnostic basal catecholamine levels. Glucagon has a negligible effect on blood pressure or plasma catecholamine levels in normal or hypertensive subjects. In patients with pheochromocytoma, on the other hand, glucagon may increase both blood pressure and circulating catecholamine levels. The elevation in plasma catecholamine concentration, moreover, may occur without a blood pressure response. It must be emphasized, however, that life-threatening pressor crises have occurred after administration of glucagon to patients with pheochromocytoma, so the test should never be performed casually. Careful continuous monitoring of the blood pressure is required, intravenous access must be adequate, and phentolamine must be at hand to terminate the test if a significant pressor reaction ensues.

Differential Diagnosis Since the manifestations of pheochromocytoma can be protean, the diagnosis must be considered and excluded in many patients with suggestive clinical features. In patients with essential hypertension and "hyperadrenergic" features such as tachycardia, sweating, and increased cardiac output, and in patients with anxiety attacks associated with blood pressure elevations, analysis of a 24-h urine collection is usually decisive in excluding the diagnosis. Repeated determinations on urine collected during attacks may be necessary, however, before the diagnosis can be excluded with certainty. Pressor crises associated with clonidine withdrawal and the use of cocaine or monoamine oxidase inhibitors may mimic the paroxysms of pheochromocytoma. Factitious crises may be produced by self-administration of sympathomimetic amines in psychiatrically disturbed patients.

Intracranial lesions, particularly posterior fossa tumors or subarachnoid hemorrhage, may cause hypertension and increased excretion of catecholamines or catecholamine metabolites. While this is most common in patients with an obvious neurologic catastrophe, the possibility of subarachnoid or intracranial hemorrhage secondary to pheochromocytoma should be considered. Diencephalic or autonomic epilepsy may be associated with paroxysmal spells, hypertension, and increased plasma catecholamine levels. This rare entity may be difficult to distinguish from pheochromocytoma, but an aura, an abnormal electroencephalogram, and a beneficial response to anticonvulsant medications will often suggest this diagnosis.

℞ TREATMENT

Preoperative Management The induction of stable α-adrenergic blockade provides the foundation for successful surgical treatment. Once the diagnosis is established, the patient should be placed on phenoxybenzamine to induce a long-lasting, noncompetitive α-receptor blockade. The usual initial dose is 10 mg every 12 h, with increments of 10 to 20 mg added every few days until the blood pressure is controlled and the paroxysms disappear. Because of the long duration of action, the therapeutic effects are cumulative, and the optimal dose must be achieved gradually with careful monitoring of supine and upright blood pressures. Most patients require between 40 and 80 mg phenoxybenzamine per day, although ≥ 200 mg may be necessary. Phenoxybenzamine should be administered for at least 10 to 14 days prior to surgery. Over this time, the combination of α-receptor block-

ade and a liberal salt intake will restore the contracted plasma volume to normal. Before adequate α-adrenergic blockade with phenoxybenzamine is achieved, paroxysms may be treated with oral prazosin or intravenous phentolamine. Selective α_1 antagonists have been employed for preoperative preparation, but their role in preparative management should be limited to the treatment of individual paroxysms. They may be useful as antihypertensive agents in patients with suspected pheochromocytoma while workup is in progress, since they are usually better tolerated than phenoxybenzamine and will prevent serious pressor crises if pheochromocytoma is present. Nitroprusside, calcium channel blocking agents, and possibly angiotensin-converting enzyme inhibitors reduce blood pressure in patients with pheochromocytoma. Nitroprusside may also be useful in the treatment of pressor crises.

β-Adrenergic receptor blocking agents should be given only after alpha blockade has been induced, since administration of such agents by themselves may cause a paradoxic increase in blood pressure by antagonizing beta-mediated vasodilation in skeletal muscle. Beta blockade is usually initiated when tachycardia develops during the induction of α-adrenergic blockade. Low doses often suffice, and a reasonable starting dose is 10 mg propranolol three to four times per day, increased as needed to control the pulse rate. Beta blockade is effective for catecholamine-induced arrhythmias, particularly those potentiated by anesthetic agents.

Preoperative Localization of the Tumor Once pheochromocytoma is diagnosed, localization should be undertaken while the patient is being prepared for surgery. Computed tomography (CT) or magnetic resonance imaging (MRI) of the adrenals is usually successful in identifying intraadrenal lesions. Extraadrenal tumors within the chest can frequently be identified by conventional chest films or CT. MRI or positron emission tomography (PET) scanning with ^{18}F dopa is useful in identifying extraadrenal tumors. Abdominal aortography (once α-adrenergic blockade is complete) or venous sampling at different levels of the inferior and superior vena cava in search of catecholamine gradients has been useful in the past but are rarely necessary now. An additional localization technique involves a radionuclide scintiscan after administration of the radiopharmaceutical [131I]metaiodobenzylguanidine (MIBG). This agent is concentrated by the amine uptake process and produces an external scintigraphic image at the site of the tumor. This type of scanning may be useful in characterizing lesions discovered by CT when biochemical confirmation is indeterminate but is less useful at localizing extraadrenal pheochromocytomas than MRI or PET. Percutaneous fine-needle aspiration of chromaffin tumors is contraindicated; indeed, pheochromocytoma should be considered before adrenal lesions are aspirated.

Surgery Surgical treatment of pheochromocytoma is best performed in centers with experience in the preoperative, anesthetic, and intraoperative management of pheochromocytoma. Surgical mortality is <2 or 3%. Extensive experience with the laparoscopic approach over the past decade has demonstrated that in experienced hands pheochromocytoma can be safely and efficiently removed by this technique.

Monitoring during the surgical procedure should include continuous recording of arterial pressure and central venous pressure as well as electrocardiography; in the presence of cardiac disease or if congestive failure has been present, pulmonary capillary wedge pressure should be monitored. Adequate fluid replacement is crucial. Intraoperative hypotension responds better to volume replacement than to vasoconstrictors. Hypertension and cardiac arrhythmias are most likely during induction of anesthesia, intubation, and manipulation of the tumor. Intravenous phentolamine is usually sufficient to control the blood pressure, but nitroprusside may be required. Propranolol may be given in the treatment of tachycardia or ventricular ectopy.

PHEOCHROMOCYTOMA IN PREGNANCY Spontaneous labor and vaginal delivery in unprepared patients are usually disastrous for mother and fetus. In early pregnancy, the patient should be prepared with phenoxybenzamine, and the tumor should be removed as soon as the diagnosis is confirmed. The pregnancy need not be terminated, but the operative procedure itself may result in spontaneous abortion. In the third trimester, treatment with adrenergic blocking agents should be undertaken; when the fetus is of sufficient size, cesarean section may be followed by extirpation of the tumor. Although the safety of adrenergic blocking drugs in pregnancy is not established, these agents have been administered in several cases without obvious adverse effect. Antepartum diagnosis and treatment lowers the maternal death rate to that approaching nonpregnant pheochromocytoma patients; fetal death rate, however, remains elevated.

UNRESECTABLE AND MALIGNANT TUMORS   In cases of metastatic or locally invasive tumor in patients with intercurrent illness that precludes surgery, long-term medical management is required. When the manifestations cannot be adequately controlled by adrenergic blocking agents, the concomitant administration of metyrosine may be required. This agent inhibits tyrosine hydroxylase, diminishes catecholamine production by the tumor, and often simplifies chronic management. Malignant pheochromocytoma frequently recurs in the retroperitoneum, and it metastasizes most commonly to bone and lung. Although these malignant tumors are resistant to radiotherapy, combination chemotherapy is occasionally of some benefit. Use of ^{131}I-MIBG has had limited success in the treatment of malignant pheochromocytoma, due to poor uptake of the radioligand.

PROGNOSIS AND FOLLOW-UP   The 5-year survival rate after surgery is usually >95%, the recurrence rate is <10%. After successful surgery, catecholamine excretion returns to normal in about 2 weeks and should be measured to ensure complete tumor removal. Catecholamine excretion should be assessed at the reappearance of suggestive symptoms or yearly if the patient remains asymptomatic. For malignant pheochromocytoma, the 5-year survival rate is usually <50%, although long-term survival is occasionally noted.

Complete removal cures the hypertension in approximately three-fourths of patients. In the remainder, hypertension recurs but is usually well controlled by standard antihypertensive agents. In this group, either underlying essential hypertension or irreversible vascular damage induced by catecholamines may cause the persistence of the hypertension.

FURTHER READING

GILLAM MP, LANDSBERG L: Pheochromocytoma, in *Challenging Cases in Endocrinology*, M Molitch (ed). Humana Press 9:155–183, 2002

HARTMUT PH et al: Germ-line mutations in nonsyndromic pheochromocytoma. N Engl J Med 346:1459 2002

KERCHER KW et al: Laparoscopic adrenalectomy for pheochromocytoma. Surg Endosc 16:100, 2002

LENDERS JWM et al: Biochemical diagnosis of pheochromocytoma. JAMA 287:1427, 2002

SAWKA AM et al: A comparison of biochemical tests for pheochromocytoma: Measurement of fractionated plasma metanephrines compared with the combination of 24-h urinary metanephrines and catecholamines. J Clin Endocrinol Metab 88:553, 2003

323   DIABETES MELLITUS
Alvin C. Powers

Diabetes mellitus (DM) comprises a group of common metabolic disorders that share the phenotype of hyperglycemia. Several distinct types of DM exist and are caused by a complex interaction of genetics, environmental factors, and life-style choices. Depending on the etiology of the DM, factors contributing to hyperglycemia may include reduced insulin secretion, decreased glucose utilization, and increased glucose production. The metabolic dysregulation associated with DM causes secondary pathophysiologic changes in multiple organ systems that impose a tremendous burden on the individual with diabetes and on the health care system. In the United States, DM is the leading cause of end-stage renal disease (ESRD), nontraumatic lower extremity amputations, and adult blindness. With an increasing incidence worldwide, DM will be a leading cause of morbidity and mortality for the foreseeable future.

CLASSIFICATION

DM is classified on the basis of the pathogenic process that leads to hyperglycemia, as opposed to earlier criteria such as age of onset or type of therapy (Fig. 323-1). The two broad categories of DM are designated type 1 and type 2 (Table 323-1). Type 1A DM results from autoimmune beta cell destruction, which leads to insulin deficiency. Individuals with type 1B DM lack immunologic markers indicative of an autoimmune destructive process of the beta cells. However, they develop insulin deficiency by unknown mechanisms and are ketosis prone. Relatively few patients with type 1 DM are in the type 1B idiopathic category; many of these individuals are either African-American or Asian in heritage.

Type 2 DM is a heterogeneous group of disorders characterized by variable degrees of insulin resistance, impaired insulin secretion, and increased glucose production. Distinct genetic and metabolic defects

Type of Diabetes	Normal glucose tolerance	Hyperglycemia		
		Impaired fasting glucose or impaired glucose tolerance	Diabetes Mellitus		
			Not insulin requiring	Insulin required for control	Insulin required for survival
Type 1					
Type 2					
Other specific types					
Gestational Diabetes					
Time (years)					
FPG (mg/dL)	<110	110–125	≥126		
2-h PG (mg/dL)	<140	140–199	≥200		

FIGURE 323-1   Spectrum of glucose homeostasis and diabetes mellitus (DM). The spectrum from normal glucose tolerance to diabetes in type 1 DM, type 2 DM, other specific types of diabetes, and gestational DM is shown from left to right. In most types of DM, the individual traverses from normal glucose tolerance to impaired glucose tolerance to overt diabetes. Arrows indicate that changes in glucose tolerance may be bi-directional in some types of diabetes. For example, individuals with type 2 DM may return to the impaired glucose tolerance category with weight loss; in gestational DM diabetes may revert to impaired glucose tolerance or even normal glucose tolerance after delivery. The fasting plasma glucose (FPG) and 2-h plasma glucose (PG), after a glucose challenge for the different categories of glucose tolerance, are shown at the lower part of the figure. These values do not apply to the diagnosis of gestational DM. Some types of DM may or may not require insulin for survival, hence the dotted line. (Conventional units are used in the figure.) *(Adapted from American Diabetes Association, 2004.)*

in insulin action and/or secretion give rise to the common phenotype of hyperglycemia in type 2 DM (see below). Distinct pathogenic processes in type 2 DM have important potential therapeutic implications, as pharmacologic agents that target specific metabolic derangements

TABLE 323-1 *Etiologic Classification of Diabetes Mellitus*

I. Type 1 diabetes (β-cell destruction, usually leading to absolute insulin deficiency)
   A. Immune-mediated
   B. Idiopathic
II. Type 2 diabetes (may range from predominantly insulin resistance with relative insulin deficiency to a predominantly insulin secretory defect with insulin resistance)
III. Other specific types of diabetes
   A. Genetic defects of β-cell function characterized by mutations in:
      1. Hepatocyte nuclear transcription factor (HNF) 4α (MODY 1)
      2. Glucokinase (MODY 2)
      3. HNF-1α (MODY 3)
      4. Insulin promoter factor (IPF) 1 (MODY 4)
      5. HNF-1β (MODY 5)
      6. NeuroD1 (MODV6)
      7. Mitochondrial DNA
      8. Proinsulin or insulin conversion
   B. Genetic defects in insulin action
      1. Type A insulin resistance
      2. Leprechaunism
      3. Rabson-Mendenhall syndrome
      4. Lipodystrophy syndromes
   C. Diseases of the exocrine pancreas—pancreatitis, pancreatectomy, neoplasia, cystic fibrosis, hemochromatosis, fibrocalculous pancreatopathy
   D. Endocrinopathies—acromegaly, Cushing's syndrome, glucagonoma, pheochromocytoma, hyperthyroidism, somatostatinoma, aldosteronoma
   E. Drug- or chemical-induced—Vacor, pentamidine, nicotinic acid, glucocorticoids, thyroid hormone, diazoxide, β-adrenergic agonists, thiazides, phenytoin, α-interferon, protease inhibitors, clozapine, beta blockers
   F. Infections—congenital rubella, cytomegalovirus, coxsackie
   G. Uncommon forms of immune-mediated diabetes—"stiff-man" syndrome, anti-insulin receptor antibodies
   H. Other genetic syndromes sometimes associated with diabetes—Down's syndrome, Klinefelter's syndrome, Turner's syndrome, Wolfram's syndrome, Friedreich's ataxia, Huntington's chorea, Laurence-Moon-Biedl syndrome, myotonic dystrophy, porphyria, Prader-Willi syndrome
IV. Gestational diabetes mellitus (GDM)

Note: MODY, maturity onset of diabetes of the young.
Source: Adapted from American Diabetes Association, 2004.

have become available. Type 2 DM is preceded by a period of abnormal glucose homeostasis classified as impaired fasting glucose (IFG) or impaired glucose tolerance (IGT).

Two features of the current classification of DM diverge from previous classifications. First, the terms *insulin-dependent diabetes mellitus* (IDDM) and *noninsulin-dependent diabetes mellitus* (NIDDM) are obsolete. Since many individuals with type 2 DM eventually require insulin treatment for control of glycemia, the use of the term NIDDM generated considerable confusion. A second difference is that age is not a criterion in the classification system. Although type 1 DM most commonly develops before the age of 30, an autoimmune beta cell destructive process can develop at any age. It is estimated that between 5 and 10% of individuals who develop DM after age 30 have type 1A DM. Likewise, type 2 DM more typically develops with increasing age, but it also occurs in children, particularly in obese adolescents.

OTHER TYPES OF DM Other etiologies for DM include specific genetic defects in insulin secretion or action, metabolic abnormalities that impair insulin secretion, mitochondrial abnormalities, and a host of conditions that impair glucose tolerance (Table 323-1). *Maturity onset diabetes of the young* (MODY) is a subtype of DM characterized by autosomal dominant inheritance, early onset of hyperglycemia, and impairment in insulin secretion (discussed below). Mutations in the insulin receptor cause a group of rare disorders characterized by severe insulin resistance.

DM can result from pancreatic exocrine disease when the majority of pancreatic islets (>80%) are destroyed. Hormones that antagonize the action of insulin can lead to DM. Thus, DM is often a feature of endocrinopathies, such as acromegaly and Cushing's disease. Viral infections have been implicated in pancreatic islet destruction, but are an extremely rare cause of DM. Congenital rubella greatly increases the risk for DM; however, most of these individuals also have immunologic markers indicative of autoimmune beta cell destruction.

GESTATIONAL DIABETES MELLITUS (GDM) Glucose intolerance may develop during pregnancy. Insulin resistance related to the metabolic changes of late pregnancy increases insulin requirements and may lead to IGT. GDM occurs in approximately 4% of pregnancies in the United States; most women revert to normal glucose tolerance post-partum but have a substantial risk (30 to 60%) of developing DM later in life.

EPIDEMIOLOGY

The worldwide prevalence of DM has risen dramatically over the past two decades. Likewise, prevalence rates of IFG are also increasing. Although the prevalence of both type 1 and type 2 DM is increasing worldwide, the prevalence of type 2 DM is expected to rise more rapidly in the future because of increasing obesity and reduced activity levels. DM increases with aging. In 2000, the prevalence of DM was estimated to be 0.19% in people <20 years old and 8.6% in people >20 years old. In individuals >65 years the prevalence of DM was 20.1%. The prevalence is similar in men and women throughout most age ranges but is slightly greater in men >60 years.

There is considerable geographic variation in the incidence of both type 1 and type 2 DM. Scandinavia has the highest incidence of type 1 DM (e.g., in Finland, the incidence is 35/100,000 per year). The Pacific Rim has a much lower rate (in Japan and China, the incidence is 1 to 3/100,000 per year) of type 1 DM; Northern Europe and the United States share an intermediate rate (8 to 17/100,000 per year). Much of the increased risk of type 1 DM is believed to reflect the frequency of high-risk HLA alleles among ethnic groups in different geographic locations. The prevalence of type 2 DM and its harbinger, IGT, is highest in certain Pacific islands, intermediate in countries such as India and the United States, and relatively low in Russia and China. This variability is likely due to genetic, behavioral, and environmental factors. DM prevalence also varies among different ethnic populations within a given country. In 2000, the prevalence of DM in the United States was 13% in African Americans, 10.2% in Hispanic Americans, 15.5% in Native Americans (American Indians and Alaska natives), and 7.8% in non-Hispanic whites. The onset of type 2 DM occurs, on average, at an earlier age in ethnic groups other than non-Hispanic whites.

DIAGNOSIS

The National Diabetes Data Group and World Health Organization have issued diagnostic criteria for DM (Table 323-2) based on the following premises: (1) the spectrum of fasting plasma glucose (FPG) and the response to an oral glucose load varies among normal indi-

TABLE 323-2 *Criteria for the Diagnosis of Diabetes Mellitus*

- Symptoms of diabetes plus random blood glucose concentration $\geq$11.1 mmol/L (200 mg/dL)[a]   *or*
- Fasting plasma glucose $\geq$7.0 mmol/L (126 mg/dL)[b]   *or*
- Two-hour plasma glucose $\geq$11.1 mmol/L (200 mg/dL) during an oral glucose tolerance test[c]

[a] Random is defined as without regard to time since the last meal.
[b] Fasting is defined as no caloric intake for at least 8 h.
[c] The test should be performed using a glucose load containing the equivalent of 75 g anhydrous glucose dissolved in water; not recommended for routine clinical use.
Note: In the absence of unequivocal hyperglycemia and acute metabolic decompensation, these criteria should be confirmed by repeat testing on a different day.
Source: Modified from American Diabetes Association, 2004.

viduals, and (2) DM is defined as the level of glycemia at which diabetes-specific complications occur rather than on deviations from a population-based mean. For example, the prevalence of retinopathy in Native Americans (Pima Indian population) begins to increase at a FPG > 6.4 mmol/L (116 mg/dL) (Fig. 323-2).

Glucose tolerance is classified into three categories based on the FPG: (1) FPG < 5.6 mmol/L (100 mg/dL) is considered normal; (2) FPG ≥ 5.6 mmol/L (100 mg/dL) but <7.0 mmol/L (126 mg/dL) is defined as IFG; and (3) FPG ≥ 7.0 mmol/L (126 mg/dL) warrants the diagnosis of DM. IFG is comparable to IGT, which is defined as plasma glucose levels between 7.8 and 11.1 mmol/L (140 and 200 mg/dL) 2 h after a 75-g oral glucose load (Table 323-2). Individuals with IFG or IGT are at substantial risk for developing type 2 DM (40% risk over the next 5 years) and cardiovascular disease.

The revised criteria for the diagnosis of DM emphasize the FPG as a reliable and convenient test for diagnosing DM in asymptomatic individuals. A random plasma glucose concentration ≥11.1 mmol/L (200 mg/dL) accompanied by classic symptoms of DM (polyuria, polydipsia, weight loss) is sufficient for the diagnosis of DM (Table 323-2). Oral glucose tolerance testing, although still a valid mechanism for diagnosing DM, is not recommended as part of routine care.

Some investigators have advocated the hemoglobin A1c (A1C) as a diagnostic test for DM. Though there is a strong correlation between elevations in the plasma glucose and the A1C (discussed below), the relationship between the FPG and the A1C in individuals with normal glucose tolerance or mild glucose intolerance is less clear and thus the use of the A1C is not currently recommended for the diagnosis of diabetes.

The diagnosis of DM has profound implications for an individual from both a medical and financial standpoint. Thus, these diagnostic criteria must be satisfied before assigning the diagnosis of DM. Abnormalities on screening tests for diabetes should be repeated before making a definitive diagnosis of DM, unless acute metabolic derangements or a markedly elevated plasma glucose are present (Table 323-2). The revised criteria also allow for the diagnosis of DM to be withdrawn in situations where the FPG reverts to normal.

SCREENING Widespread use of the FPG as a screening test for type 2 DM is recommended because: (1) a large number of individuals who meet the current criteria for DM are asymptomatic and unaware that they have the disorder, (2) epidemiologic studies suggest that type 2

DM may be present for up to a decade before diagnosis, (3) as many as 50% of individuals with type 2 DM have one or more diabetes-specific complications at the time of their diagnosis, and (4) treatment of type 2 DM may favorably alter the natural history of DM. The American Diabetes Association (ADA) recommends screening all individuals >45 years every 3 years and screening individuals with additional risk factors (Table 323-3) at an earlier age. In contrast to type 2 DM, a long asymptomatic period of hyperglycemia is rare prior to the diagnosis of type 1 DM. A number of immunologic markers for type 1 DM are becoming available (discussed below), but their routine use is discouraged pending the identification of clinically beneficial interventions for individuals at high risk for developing type 1 DM.

INSULIN BIOSYNTHESIS, SECRETION, AND ACTION

BIOSYNTHESIS Insulin is produced in the beta cells of the pancreatic islets. It is initially synthesized as a single-chain 86-amino-acid precursor polypeptide, preproinsulin. Subsequent proteolytic processing removes the aminoterminal signal peptide, giving rise to proinsulin. Proinsulin is structurally related to insulin-like growth factors I and II, which bind weakly to the insulin receptor (Chap. 317). Cleavage of an internal 31-residue fragment from proinsulin generates the C peptide and the A (21 amino acids) and B (30 amino acids) chains of insulin, which are connected by disulfide bonds. The mature insulin molecule and C peptide are stored together and cosecreted from secretory granules in the beta cells. Because the C peptide is less susceptible than insulin to hepatic degradation, it is a useful marker of insulin secretion and allows discrimination of endogenous and exogenous sources of insulin in the evaluation of hypoglycemia (Chap. 324). Human insulin is now produced by recombinant DNA technology; structural alterations at one or more residues are useful for modifying its physical and pharmacologic characteristics (see below).

SECRETION Glucose is the key regulator of insulin secretion by the pancreatic beta cell, although amino acids, ketones, various nutrients, gastrointestinal peptides, and neurotransmitters also influence insulin secretion. Glucose levels >3.9 mmol/L (70 mg/dL) stimulate insulin synthesis, primarily by enhancing protein translation and processing. Glucose stimulation of insulin secretion begins with its transport into the beta cell by the GLUT2 glucose transporter (Fig. 323-3). Glucose phosphorylation by glucokinase is the rate-limiting step that controls glucose-regulated insulin secretion. Further metabolism of glucose-6-phosphate via glycolysis generates ATP, which inhibits the activity of an ATP-sensitive K+ channel. This channel consists of two separate proteins: one is the receptor for certain oral hypoglycemics (e.g., sulfonylureas, meglitinides); the other is an inwardly rectifying K+ channel protein. Inhibition of this K+ channel induces beta cell membrane depolarization, which opens voltage-dependent calcium channels (leading to an influx of calcium), and stimulates insulin secretion. Insulin secretory profiles reveal a pulsatile pattern of hormone release, with small secretory bursts occurring about every 10 min, superimposed upon greater amplitude oscillations of about 80 to 150 min. Meals or other major stimuli of insulin secretion induce large (four-

FIGURE 323-2 Relationship of diabetes-specific complication and glucose tolerance. This figure shows the incidence of retinopathy in Pima Indians as a function of the fasting plasma glucose (FPG), the 2-h plasma glucose after a 75-g oral glucose challenge (2-h PG), or glycated hemoglobin (A1C). Note that the incidence of retinopathy greatly increases at a fasting plasma glucose >116 mg/dL, or a 2-h plasma glucose of 185 mg/dL, or a A1C >6.0%. (Conventional units for blood glucose are used in the figure.) *(Copyright 2002, American Diabetes Association. From Diabetes Care 25(Suppl 1): S5 S20, 2002.)*

FPG (mg/dL)	70-	89-	93-	97-	100-	105-	109-	116-	136-	226-
2-h PG (mg/dL)	38-	94-	106-	116-	126-	138-	156-	185-	244-	364-
HbA1c (%)	3.4-	4.8-	5.0-	5.2-	5.3-	5.5-	5.7-	6.0-	6.7-	9.5-

TABLE 323-3   Risk Factors for Type 2 Diabetes Mellitus

- Family history of diabetes (i.e., parent or sibling with type 2 diabetes)
- Obesity (BMI ≥ 25 kg/m²)
- Habitual physical inactivity
- Race/ethnicity (e.g., African American, Hispanic American, Native American, Asian American, Pacific Islander)
- Previously identified IFG or IGT
- History of GDM or delivery of baby >4 kg (>9 lb)
- Hypertension (blood pressure ≥ 140/90 mmHg)
- HDL cholesterol level ≤ 35 mg/dL (0.90 mmol/L) and/or a triglyceride level ≥250 mg/dL (2.82 mmol/L)
- Polycystic ovary syndrome or acanthosis nigracans
- History of vascular disease

Note: BMI, body mass index; IFG, impaired fasting glucose; IGT, impaired glucose tolerance; GDM, gestational diabetes mellitus; HDL, high-density lipoprotein.
Source: Adapted from American Diabetes Association, 2004.

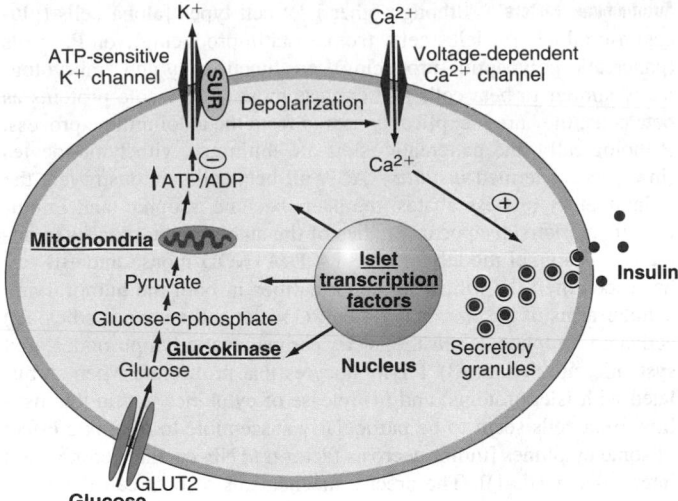

FIGURE 323-3 Diabetes and abnormalities in glucose-stimulated insulin secretion. Glucose and other nutrients regulate insulin secretion by the pancreatic beta cell. Glucose is transported by the GLUT2 glucose transporter; subsequent glucose metabolism by the beta cell alters ion channel activity, leading to insulin secretion. The SUR receptor is the binding site for drugs that act as insulin secretagogues. Mutations in the events or proteins underlined are a cause of maturity onset diabetes of the young (MODY) or other forms of diabetes. SUR, sulfonylurea receptor; ATP, adenosine triphosphate; ADP, adenosine diphosphate. (*Adapted from WL Lowe, in JL Jameson (ed): Principles of Molecular Medicine. Totowa, NI, Humana, 1998.*)

to fivefold increase versus baseline) bursts of insulin secretion that usually last for 2 to 3 h before returning to baseline. Derangements in these normal secretory patterns are one of the earliest signs of beta cell dysfunction in DM.

ACTION Once insulin is secreted into the portal venous system, ~50% is degraded by the liver. Unextracted insulin enters the systemic circulation where it binds to receptors in target sites. Insulin binding to its receptor stimulates intrinsic tyrosine kinase activity, leading to receptor autophosphorylation and the recruitment of intracellular signaling molecules, such as insulin receptor substrates (IRS) (Fig. 323-4). These and other adaptor proteins initiate a complex cascade of phosphorylation and dephosphorylation reactions, resulting in the widespread metabolic and mitogenic effects of insulin. As an example, activation of the phosphatidylinositol-3'-kinase (PI-3-kinase) pathway stimulates translocation of glucose transporters (e.g., GLUT4) to the cell surface, an event that is crucial for glucose uptake by skeletal muscle and fat. Activation of other insulin receptor signaling pathways induces glycogen synthesis, protein synthesis, lipogenesis, and regulation of various genes in insulin-responsive cells.

Glucose homeostasis reflects a precise balance between hepatic glucose production and peripheral glucose uptake and utilization. Insulin is the most important regulator of this metabolic equilibrium, but neural input, metabolic signals, and hormones (e.g., glucagon) result in integrated control of glucose supply and utilization (Chap. 324; see Fig. 324-1). In the fasting state, low insulin levels increase glucose production by promoting hepatic gluconeogenesis

and glycogenolysis. Glucagon also stimulates glycogenolysis and gluconeogenesis by the liver and renal medulla. Low insulin levels decrease glycogen synthesis, reduce glucose uptake in insulin-sensitive tissues, and promote mobilization of stored precursors. Postprandially, the glucose load elicits a rise in insulin and fall in glucagon, leading to a reversal of these processes. The major portion of postprandial glucose is utilized by skeletal muscle, an effect of insulin-stimulated glucose uptake. Other tissues, most notably the brain, utilize glucose in an insulin-independent fashion.

PATHOGENESIS

TYPE 1 DM Type 1A DM develops as a result of the synergistic effects of genetic, environmental, and immunologic factors that ultimately destroy the pancreatic beta cells. The temporal development of type 1A DM is shown schematically as a function of beta cell mass in Fig. 323-5. Individuals with a genetic susceptibility have normal beta cell mass at birth but begin to lose beta cells secondary to autoimmune destruction that occurs over months to years. This autoimmune process is thought to be triggered by an infectious or environmental stimulus and to be sustained by a beta cell–specific molecule. In the majority of individuals, immunologic markers appear after the triggering event but before diabetes becomes clinically overt. Beta cell mass then begins to decline, and insulin secretion becomes progressively impaired, although normal glucose tolerance is maintained. The rate of decline in beta cell mass varies widely among individuals, with some patients progressing rapidly to clinical diabetes and others evolving more slowly. Features of diabetes do not become evident until a majority of beta cells are destroyed (~80%). At this point, residual functional beta cells still exist but are insufficient in number to maintain glucose tolerance. The events that trigger the transition from glucose intolerance to frank diabetes are often associated with increased insulin requirements, as might occur during infections or puberty. After the initial clinical presentation of type 1A DM, a "honeymoon" phase may ensue during which time glycemic control is achieved with modest doses of insulin or, rarely, insulin is not needed. However, this fleeting phase of endogenous insulin production from residual beta cells disappears

FIGURE 323-4 Insulin signal transduction pathway in skeletal muscle. The insulin receptor has intrinsic tyrosine kinase activity and interacts with insulin receptor substrates (IRS and Shc) proteins. A number of "docking" proteins bind to these cellular proteins and initiate the metabolic actions of insulin [GrB-2, SOS, SHP-2, p65, p110, and phosphatidylinositol-3'-kinase (PI-3-kinase)]. Insulin increases glucose transport through PI-3-kinase and the Cbl pathway, which promotes translocation of intracellular vesicles containing GLUT4 glucose transporter to the plasma membrane. (*Adapted from WL Lowe, in Principles of Molecular Medicine, JL Jameson (ed). Totowa, NJ, Humana, 1998; A Virkamaki et al: J Clin Invest 103:931, 1999. For additional details see Saltiel and Kahn, 2001.*)

FIGURE 323-5   Temporal model for development of type 1 diabetes. Individuals with a genetic predisposition are exposed to an immunologic trigger that initiates an autoimmune process, resulting in a gradual decline in beta cell mass. The downward slope of the beta cell mass varies among individuals. This progressive impairment in insulin release results in diabetes when ~80% of the beta cell mass is destroyed. A "honeymoon" phase may be seen in the first 1 or 2 years after the onset of diabetes and is associated with reduced insulin requirements. *(Adapted from Medical Management of Type 1 Diabetes, 3d ed, JS Skyler (ed). Alexandria, VA, American Diabetes Association, 1998.)*

as the autoimmune process destroys the remaining beta cells, and the individual becomes completely insulin deficient.

GENETIC CONSIDERATIONS   Genetic susceptibility to type 1A DM involves multiple genes. The concordance of type 1A DM in identical twins ranges between 30 and 70%, indicating that additional modifying factors must be involved in determining whether diabetes develops. The major susceptibility gene for type 1A DM is located in the HLA region on chromosome 6. Polymorphisms in the HLA complex account for 40 to 50% of the genetic risk of developing type 1A DM. This region contains genes that encode the class II MHC molecules, which present antigen to helper T cells and thus are involved in initiating the immune response (Chap. 296). The ability of class II MHC molecules to present antigen is dependent on the amino acid composition of their antigen-binding sites. Amino acid substitutions may influence the specificity of the immune response by altering the binding affinity of different antigens for class II molecules.

Most individuals with type 1A DM have the HLA DR3 and/or DR4 haplotype. Refinements in genotyping of HLA loci have shown that the haplotypes DQA1*0301, DQB1*0302, DQA1*501, and DQB1*0201 are most strongly associated with type 1A DM. These haplotypes are present in 40% of children with type 1A DM as compared to 2% of the normal U.S. population.

In addition to MHC class II associations, at least 17 different genetic loci contribute susceptibility to type 1A DM. For example, polymorphisms in the promoter region of the insulin gene account for ~10% of the predisposition to type 1A DM. Genes that confer protection against the development of the disease also exist. The haplotype DQA1*0102, DQB1*0602 is present in 20% of the U.S. population but is extremely rare in individuals with type 1A DM (<1%).

The risk of developing type 1A DM is increased tenfold in relatives of individuals with the disease. Nevertheless, most individuals with predisposing haplotypes do not develop diabetes. In addition, most individuals with type 1A DM do not have a first-degree relative with this disorder.

Autoimmune Factors   Although other islet cell types [alpha cells (glucagon-producing), delta cells (somatostatin-producing), or PP cells (pancreatic polypeptide-producing)] are functionally and embryologically similar to beta cells and express most of the same proteins as beta cells, they are inexplicably spared from the autoimmune process. Pathologically, the pancreatic islets are infiltrated with lymphocytes (in a process termed *insulitis*). After all beta cells are destroyed, the inflammatory process abates, the islets become atrophic, and immunologic markers disappear. Studies of the autoimmune process in humans and animal models of type 1A DM (NOD mouse and BB rat) have identified the following abnormalities in both the humoral and cellular arms of the immune system: (1) islet cell autoantibodies; (2) activated lymphocytes in the islets, peripancreatic lymph nodes, and systemic circulation; (3) T lymphocytes that proliferate when stimulated with islet proteins; and (4) release of cytokines within the insulitis. Beta cells seem to be particularly susceptible to the toxic effect of some cytokines [tumor necrosis factor α (TNF-α), interferon γ, and interleukin-1 (IL-1)]. The precise mechanisms of beta cell death are not known but may involve formation of nitric oxide metabolites, apoptosis, and direct CD8+ T cell cytotoxicity. Islet autoantibodies are not thought to be involved in the destructive process, as these antibodies do not generally react with the cell surface of islet cells and are not capable of transferring diabetes mellitus to animals.

Pancreatic islet molecules targeted by the autoimmune process include insulin, glutamic acid decarboxylase (GAD, the biosynthetic enzyme for the neurotransmitter GABA), ICA-512/IA-2 (homology with tyrosine phosphatases), and phogrin (insulin secretory granule protein). Other less clearly defined autoantigens include an islet ganglioside and carboxypeptidase H. With the exception of insulin, none of the autoantigens are beta cell specific, which raises the question of how the beta cells are selectively destroyed. Current theories favor initiation of an autoimmune process directed at one beta cell molecule, which then spreads to other islet molecules as the immune process destroys beta cells and creates a series of secondary autoantigens. The beta cells of individuals who develop type 1A DM do not differ from beta cells of normal individuals, since transplanted islets are destroyed by a recurrence of the autoimmune process of type 1A DM.

Immunologic Markers   Islet cell autoantibodies (ICAs) are a composite of several different antibodies directed at pancreatic islet molecules such as GAD, insulin, IA-2/ICA-512, and an islet ganglioside and serve as a marker of the autoimmune process of type 1A DM. Assays for autoantibodies to GAD-65 are commercially available. Testing for ICAs can be useful in classifying the type of DM as type IA and in identifying nondiabetic individuals at risk for developing type 1A DM. ICAs are present in the majority of individuals (>75%) diagnosed with new-onset type 1A DM, in a significant minority of individuals with newly diagnosed type 2 DM (5 to 10%), and occasionally in individuals with GDM (<5%). ICAs are present in 3 to 4% of first-degree relatives of individuals with type 1A DM. In combination with impaired insulin secretion after intravenous glucose tolerance testing, they predict a >50% risk of developing type 1A DM within 5 years. Without this impairment in insulin secretion, the presence of ICAs predicts a 5-year risk of <25%. Based on these data, the risk of a first-degree relative developing type 1A DM is relatively low. At present, the measurement of ICAs in nondiabetic individuals is a research tool because no treatments have been approved to prevent the occurrence or progression of type 1A DM.

Environmental Factors   Numerous environmental events have been proposed to trigger the autoimmune process in genetically susceptible individuals; however, none have been conclusively linked to diabetes. Identification of an environmental trigger has been difficult because the event may precede the onset of DM by several years (Fig. 323-5). Putative environmental triggers include viruses (coxsackie and rubella most prominently), bovine milk proteins, and nitrosourea compounds.

Prevention of Type 1A DM   A number of interventions have successfully delayed or prevented diabetes in animal models. Some interventions have targeted the immune system directly (immunosuppression, selective T cell subset deletion, induction of immunologic tolerance to islet proteins), whereas others have prevented islet cell death by blocking cytotoxic cytokines or increasing islet resistance to the destructive process. Though results in animal models are promising, these interventions have not been successful in preventing type 1A DM in humans. The Diabetes Prevention Trial—type 1 recently concluded that administering insulin to individuals at high risk for developing type 1A DM did not prevent type 1A DM.

TYPE 2 DM Insulin resistance and abnormal insulin secretion are central to the development of type 2 DM. Although controversy remains regarding the primary defect, most studies support the view that insulin resistance precedes insulin secretory defects and that diabetes develops only if insulin secretion becomes inadequate.

GENETIC CONSIDERATIONS Type 2 DM has a strong genetic component. Major genes that predispose to this disorder have yet to be identified, but it is clear that the disease is polygenic and multifactorial. Various genetic loci contribute to susceptibility, and environmental factors (such as nutrition and physical activity) further modulate phenotypic expression of the disease. The concordance of type 2 DM in identical twins is between 70 and 90%. Individuals with a parent with type 2 DM have an increased risk of diabetes; if both parents have type 2 DM, the risk approaches 40%. Insulin resistance, as demonstrated by reduced glucose utilization in skeletal muscle, is present in many nondiabetic, first-degree relatives of individuals with type 2 DM. However, definition of the genetic susceptibility remains a challenge because the genetic defect in insulin secretion or action may not manifest itself unless an environmental event or another genetic defect, such as obesity, is superimposed. Mutations in various molecules involved in insulin action (e.g., the insulin receptor and enzymes involved in glucose homeostasis) account for a very small fraction of type 2 DM. Likewise, genetic defects in proteins involved in insulin secretion have not been found in most individuals with type 2 DM. Genome-wide scanning for mutations or polymorphisms associated with type 2 DM is being used in an effort to identify genes associated with type 2 DM. The gene for the protease, calpain 10, is associated with type 2 DM in Hispanic and some other populations.

Pathophysiology Type 2 DM is characterized by three pathophysiologic abnormalities: impaired insulin secretion, peripheral insulin resistance, and excessive hepatic glucose production. Obesity, particularly visceral or central (as evidenced by the hip-waist ratio), is very common in type 2 DM. Adipocytes secrete a number of biologic products (leptin, TFN-α, free fatty acids, resistin, and adiponectin) that modulate insulin secretion, insulin action, and body weight and may contribute to the insulin resistance. In the early stages of the disorder, glucose tolerance remains normal, despite insulin resistance, because the pancreatic beta cells compensate by increasing insulin output (Fig. 323-6). As insulin resistance and compensatory hyperinsulinemia progress, the pancreatic islets in certain individuals are unable to sustain the hyperinsulinemic state. IGT, characterized by elevations in postprandial glucose, then develops. A further decline in insulin secretion and an increase in hepatic glucose production lead to overt diabetes with fasting hyperglycemia. Ultimately, beta cell failure may ensue. Markers of inflammation such as IL-6 and C-reactive protein are often elevated in type 2 diabetes.

Metabolic Abnormalities ■ *INSULIN RESISTANCE* The decreased ability of insulin to act effectively on peripheral target tissues (especially muscle and liver) is a prominent feature of type 2 DM and results from a combination of genetic susceptibility and obesity. Insulin resistance is relative, however, since supernormal levels of circulating insulin will normalize the plasma glucose. Insulin dose-response curves exhibit a rightward shift, indicating reduced sensitivity, and a reduced maximal response, indicating an overall decrease in maximum glucose utilization (30 to 60% lower than normal individuals). Insulin resistance impairs glucose utilization by insulin-sensitive tissues and increases hepatic glucose output; both effects contribute to the hyperglycemia.

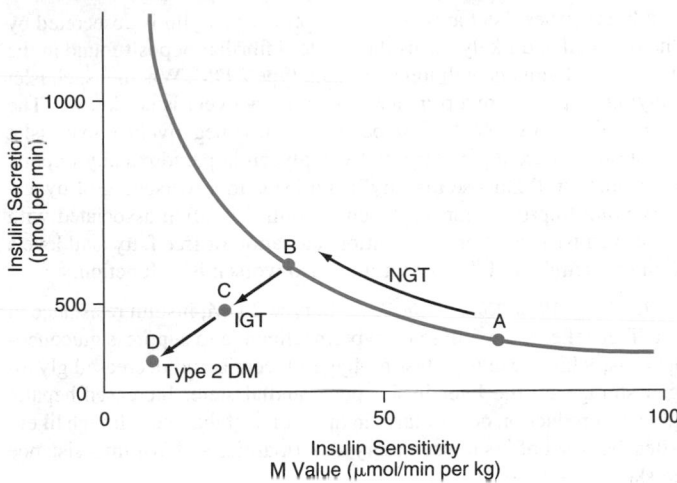

FIGURE 323-6 Metabolic changes during the development of type 2 diabetes mellitus (DM). Insulin secretion and insulin sensitivity are related, and as an individual becomes more insulin resistant (by moving from point A to point B), insulin secretion increases. A failure to compensate by increasing the insulin secretion results initially in impaired glucose tolerance (IGT; point C) and ultimately in type 2 DM (point D). *(Adapted from SE Kahn, J Clin Endocrinol Metab 86:4047, 2001; RN Bergman, M Ader, Trends Endocrinol Metab 11:351, 2000.)*

Increased hepatic glucose output predominantly accounts for increased FPG levels, whereas decreased peripheral glucose usage results in postprandial hyperglycemia. In skeletal muscle, there is a greater impairment in nonoxidative glucose usage (glycogen formation) than in oxidative glucose metabolism through glycolysis. Glucose metabolism in insulin-independent tissues is not altered in type 2 DM.

The precise molecular mechanism of insulin resistance in type 2 DM has not been elucidated. Insulin receptor levels and tyrosine kinase activity in skeletal muscle are reduced, but these alterations are most likely secondary to hyperinsulinemia and are not a primary defect. Therefore, postreceptor defects are believed to play the predominant role in insulin resistance (Fig. 323-4). Polymorphisms in IRS-1 may be associated with glucose intolerance, raising the possibility that polymorphisms in various postreceptor molecules may combine to create an insulin-resistant state. The pathogenesis of insulin resistance is currently focused on a PI-3-kinase signaling defect, which reduces translocation of GLUT4 to the plasma membrane, among other abnormalities. Of note, not all insulin signal transduction pathways are resistant to the effects of insulin [e.g., those controlling cell growth and differentiation and using the mitogen-activated protein (MAP) kinase pathway; Fig. 323-4]. Consequently, hyperinsulinemia may increase the insulin action through these pathways, potentially accelerating diabetes-related conditions such as atherosclerosis.

Another emerging theory proposes that elevated levels of free fatty acids, a common feature of obesity, may contribute to the pathogenesis of type 2 DM. Free fatty acids can impair glucose utilization in skeletal muscle, promote glucose production by the liver, and impair beta cell function.

IMPAIRED INSULIN SECRETION Insulin secretion and sensitivity are interrelated (Fig. 323-6). In type 2 DM, insulin secretion initially increases in response to insulin resistance to maintain normal glucose tolerance. Initially, the insulin secretory defect is mild and selectively involves glucose-stimulated insulin secretion. The response to other nonglucose secretagogues, such as arginine, is preserved. Eventually, the insulin secretory defect progresses to a state of grossly inadequate insulin secretion.

The reason(s) for the decline in insulin secretory capacity in type 2 DM is unclear. Despite the assumption that a second genetic defect—superimposed upon insulin resistance—leads to beta cell failure, intense genetic investigation has so far excluded mutations in islet candidate genes. Islet amyloid polypeptide or amylin is cosecreted by the beta cell and likely forms the amyloid fibrillar deposit found in the islets of individuals with long-standing type 2 DM. Whether such islet amyloid deposits are a primary or secondary event is not known. The metabolic environment of diabetes may also negatively impact islet function. For example, chronic hyperglycemia paradoxically impairs islet function ("glucose toxicity") and leads to a worsening of hyperglycemia. Improvement in glycemic control is often associated with improved islet function. In addition, elevation of free fatty acid levels ("lipotoxicity") and dietary fat may also worsen islet function.

INCREASED HEPATIC GLUCOSE PRODUCTION   In type 2 DM, insulin resistance in the liver reflects the failure of hyperinsulinemia to suppress gluconeogenesis, which results in fasting hyperglycemia and decreased glycogen storage by the liver in the postprandial state. Increased hepatic glucose production occurs early in the course of diabetes, though likely after the onset of insulin secretory abnormalities and insulin resistance in skeletal muscle.

Insulin Resistance Syndromes   The insulin resistance condition comprises a spectrum of disorders, with hyperglycemia representing one of the most readily diagnosed features. The *metabolic syndrome*, the *insulin resistance syndrome*, or *syndrome X* are terms used to describe a constellation of metabolic derangements that includes insulin resistance, hypertension, dyslipidemia [low high-density lipoprotein (HDL) and elevated triglycerides], central or visceral obesity, type 2 diabetes or IGT/IFG, and accelerated cardiovascular disease. This syndrome is very common. The Centers for Disease Control and Prevention (CDC) estimates that 20% of U.S. adults have this syndrome. Epidemiologic evidence supports hyperinsulinemia as a marker for coronary artery disease risk, though an etiologic role has not been demonstrated.

A number of relatively rare forms of severe insulin resistance include features of type 2 DM or IGT (Table 323-1). *Acanthosis nigricans* and signs of hyperandrogenism (hirsutism, acne, and oligomenorrhea in women) are also common physical features. Two distinct syndromes of severe insulin resistance have been described in adults: (1) type A, which affects young women and is characterized by severe hyperinsulinemia, obesity, and features of hyperandrogenism; and (2) type B, which affects middle-aged women and is characterized by severe hyperinsulinemia, features of hyperandrogenism, and autoimmune disorders. Individuals with the type A insulin resistance syndrome have an undefined defect in the insulin-signaling pathway; individuals with the type B insulin resistance syndrome have autoantibodies directed at the insulin receptor. These receptor autoantibodies may block insulin binding or may stimulate the insulin receptor, leading to intermittent hypoglycemia.

Polycystic ovary syndrome (PCOS) is a common disorder that affects premenopausal women and is characterized by chronic anovulation and hyperandrogenism (Chap. 326). Insulin resistance is seen in a significant subset of women with PCOS, and the disorder substantially increases the risk for type 2 DM, independent of the effects of obesity. Both metformin and the thiazolidinediones attenuate hyperinsulinemia, ameliorate hyperandrogenism, induce ovulation, and improve plasma lipids, but they are not approved for this indication.

Prevention   Type 2 DM is preceded by a period of IGT, and a number of life-style modifications and pharmacologic agents prevent or delay the onset of DM. The Diabetes Prevention Program (DPP) demonstrated that intensive changes in life-style (diet and exercise for 30 min/day five times/week) in individuals with IGT prevented or delayed the development of type 2 diabetes by 58% compared to placebo. This effect was seen in individuals regardless of age, sex, or ethnic group. In the same study, metformin prevented or delayed diabetes by 31% compared to placebo. The life-style intervention group lost 5 to 7% of their body weight during the 3 years of the study. Studies in Finnish and Chinese populations noted similar efficacy of diet and exercise in preventing or delaying type 2 DM; acarbose, metformin, and the thiazolidinediones prevent or delay type 2 DM, but are not approved for

this purpose. When administered to nondiabetic individuals for other reasons (cardiac, cholesterol lowering, etc.), two pharmacologic agents (ramipril, pravastatin) reduced the number of new cases of diabetes. Individuals with a strong family history, those at high risk for developing DM, or those with IFG or IGT should be strongly encouraged to maintain a normal body mass index (BMI) and engage in regular physical activity.

GENETICALLY DEFINED, MONOGENIC FORMS OF DIABETES MELLITUS

Several monogenic forms of DM have been identified. Five different variants of MODY, caused by mutations in genes encoding islet cell transcription factors or glucokinase (Fig. 323-3), have been identified so far, and all are transmitted as autosomal dominant disorders (Table 323-1). MODY 2 is the result of mutations in the glucokinase gene that lead to mild-to-moderate hyperglycemia. Glucokinase catalyzes the formation of glucose-6-phosphate from glucose, a reaction that is important for glucose sensing by the beta cells and for glucose utilization by the liver. As a result of glucokinase mutations, higher glucose levels are required to elicit insulin secretory responses, thus altering the set point for insulin secretion. Homozygous mutations in glucokinase cause severe, neonatal diabetes. MODY 1, MODY 3, and MODY 5 are caused by mutations in the hepatocyte nuclear transcription factors (HNF) 4α, HNF-1α, and HNF-1β, respectively. As their names imply, these transcription factors are expressed in the liver but also in other tissues, including the pancreatic islets and kidney (as a result, patients may also have renal absorption abnormalities and renal cysts). The mechanisms by which such mutations lead to DM is not well understood, but it is likely that these factors affect islet development or the transcription of genes that are important in stimulating insulin secretion. MODY 1 and 3 begin with mild hyperglycemia, but progressive impairment of insulin secretion requires treatment with oral agents or insulin. MODY 4 is a rare variant caused by mutations in the insulin promoter factor (IPF) 1, which is a transcription factor that regulates pancreatic development and insulin gene transcription. Homozygous inactivating mutations cause pancreatic agenesis, whereas heterozygous mutations result in DM. Studies of populations with type 2 DM suggest that mutations in the glucokinase gene and various islet cell transcription factors are very rare in ordinary type 2 DM.

ACUTE COMPLICATIONS OF DM

Diabetic ketoacidosis (DKA) and hyperglycemic hyperosmolar state (HHS) are acute complications of diabetes. DKA was formerly considered a hallmark of type 1 DM, but it also occurs in individuals who lack immunologic features of type 1A DM and who can subsequently be treated with oral glucose-lowering agents (these individuals with type 2 DM are often of Hispanic or African-American descent). HHS is primarily seen in individuals with type 2 DM. Both disorders are associated with absolute or relative insulin deficiency, volume depletion, and acid-base abnormalities. DKA and HHS exist along a continuum of hyperglycemia, with or without ketosis. The metabolic similarities and differences in DKA and HHS are highlighted in Table 323-4. Both disorders are associated with potentially serious complications if not promptly diagnosed and treated.

DIABETIC KETOACIDOSIS ■ **Clinical Features**   The symptoms and physical signs of DKA are listed in Table 323-5 and usually develop over 24 hours. DKA may be the initial symptom complex that leads to a diagnosis of type 1 DM, but more frequently it occurs in individuals with established diabetes. Nausea and vomiting are often prominent, and their presence in an individual with diabetes warrants laboratory evaluation for DKA. Abdominal pain may be severe and can resemble acute pancreatitis or ruptured viscous. Hyperglycemia leads to glucosuria, volume depletion, and tachycardia. Hypotension can occur because of volume depletion in combination with peripheral vasodilation. Kussmaul respirations and a fruity odor on the patient's breath (secondary to metabolic acidosis and increased acetone) are classic signs of the disorder. Lethargy and central nervous system depression may evolve into coma with severe DKA but should also prompt evaluation for other reasons for altered mental status (infection, hypoxia, etc.). Cerebral edema, an extremely serious complication of DKA, is seen most frequently in children. Signs of infection, which may precipitate DKA, should be sought on physical examination, even in the absence of fever. Tissue ischemia (heart, brain) can also be a precipitating factor.

Pathophysiology DKA results from relative or absolute insulin deficiency combined with counterregulatory hormone excess (glucagon, catecholamines, cortisol, and growth hormone). Both insulin deficiency and glucagon excess, in particular, are necessary for DKA to develop. The decreased ratio of insulin to glucagon promotes gluconeogenesis, glycogenolysis, and ketone body formation in the liver, as well as increases in substrate delivery from fat and muscle (free fatty acids, amino acids) to the liver.

The combination of insulin deficiency and hyperglycemia reduces the hepatic level of fructose-2,6-phosphate, which alters the activity of phosphofructokinase and fructose-1,6-bisphosphatase. Glucagon excess decreases the activity of pyruvate kinase, whereas insulin deficiency increases the activity of phosphoenolpyruvate carboxykinase. These changes shift the handling of pyruvate toward glucose synthesis and away from glycolysis. The increased levels of glucagon and catecholamines in the face of low insulin levels promote glycogenolysis. Insulin deficiency also reduces levels of the GLUT4 glucose transporter, which impairs glucose uptake into skeletal muscle and fat and reduces intracellular glucose metabolism (Fig. 323-4).

Ketosis results from a marked increase in free fatty acid release from adipocytes, with a resulting shift toward ketone body synthesis in the liver. Reduced insulin levels, in combination with elevations in catecholamines and growth hormone, increase lipolysis and the release of free fatty acids. Normally, these free fatty acids are converted to triglycerides or very low density lipoproteins (VLDL) in the liver. However, in DKA, hyperglucagonemia alters hepatic metabolism to favor ketone body formation, through activation of the enzyme carnitine palmitoyltransferase I. This enzyme is crucial for regulating fatty acid transport into the mitochondria, where beta oxidation and conversion to ketone bodies occur. At physiologic pH, ketone bodies exist as ketoacids, which are neutralized by bicarbonate. As bicarbonate stores are depleted, metabolic acidosis ensues. Increased lactic acid production also contributes to the acidosis. The increased free fatty acids increase triglyceride and VLDL production. VLDL clearance is also reduced because the activity of insulin-sensitive lipoprotein lipase in muscle and fat is decreased. Hypertriglyceridemia may be severe enough to cause pancreatitis.

DKA is initiated by inadequate levels of plasma insulin (Table 323-5). Most commonly, DKA is precipitated by increased insulin requirements, as might occur during a concurrent illness. Failure to augment insulin therapy often compounds the problem. Occasionally, complete omission of insulin by the patient or health care team (in a hospitalized patient with type 1 DM) precipitates DKA. Patients using insulin infusion devices with short-acting insulin are at increased risk of DKA, since even a brief interruption in insulin delivery (e.g., mechanical malfunction) quickly leads to insulin deficiency.

Laboratory Abnormalities and Diagnosis The timely diagnosis of DKA is crucial and allows for prompt initiation of therapy. DKA is characterized by hyperglycemia, ketosis, and metabolic acidosis (increased anion gap) along with a number of secondary metabolic derangements (Table 323-4). Occasionally, the serum glucose is only minimally elevated. Serum bicarbonate is frequently <10 mmol/L, and arterial pH ranges between 6.8 and 7.3, depending on the severity of the acidosis. Despite a total body potassium deficit, the serum potassium at presen-

TABLE 323-4 Laboratory Values in Diabetic Ketoacidosis (DKA) and Hyperglycemic Hyperosmolar State (HHS) (Representative Ranges at Presentation)

	DKA	HHS
Glucose,[a] μmol/L (mg/dL)	13.9–33.3 (250–600)	33.3–66.6 (600–1200)
Sodium, meq/L	125–135	135–145
Potassium,[a] meq/L	Normal to ↑[b]	Normal
Magnesium[a]	Normal[b]	Normal
Chloride[a]	Normal	Normal
Phosphate[a]	↓	Normal
Creatinine, μmol/L (mg/dL)	Slightly ↑	Moderately ↑
Osmolality (mOsm/mL)	300–320	330–380
Plasma ketones[a]	++++	+/−
Serum bicarbonate,[a] meq/L	<15 meq/L	Normal to slightly ↓
Arterial pH	6.8–7.3	>7.3
Arterial P_{CO_2},[a] mmHg	20–30	Normal
Anion gap[a] [Na − (Cl + HCO₃)], meq/L	↑	Normal to slightly ↑

[a] Large changes occur during treatment of DKA.
[b] Although plasma levels may be normal or high at presentation, total-body stores are usually depleted.

tation may be mildly elevated, secondary to the acidosis. Total-body stores of sodium, chloride, phosphorous, and magnesium are also reduced in DKA but are not accurately reflected by their levels in the serum because of dehydration and hyperglycemia. Elevated blood urea nitrogen (BUN) and serum creatinine levels reflect intravascular volume depletion. Interference from acetoacetate may falsely elevate the serum creatinine measurement. Leukocytosis, hypertriglyceridemia, and hyperlipoproteinemia are commonly found as well. Hyperamylasemia may suggest a diagnosis of pancreatitis, especially when accompanied by abdominal pain. However, in DKA the amylase is usually of salivary origin and thus is not diagnostic of pancreatitis. Serum lipase should be obtained if pancreatitis is suspected.

The measured serum sodium is reduced as a consequence of the hyperglycemia [1.6 mmol/L (1.6 meq) reduction in serum sodium for each 5.6 mmol/L (100 mg/dL) rise in the serum glucose]. A normal serum sodium in the setting of DKA indicates a more profound water deficit. In "conventional" units, the calculated serum osmolality [2 × (serum sodium + serum potassium) + plasma glucose (mg/dL)/18 + BUN/2.8] is mildly to moderately elevated, though to a lesser degree than that found in HHS (see below).

In DKA, the ketone body, β-hydroxybutyrate, is synthesized at a threefold greater rate than acetoacetate; however, acetoacetate is preferentially detected by a commonly used ketosis detection reagent (nitroprusside). Serum ketones are present at significant levels (usually positive at serum dilution of 1:8 or greater). The nitroprusside tablet, or stick, is often used to detect urine ketones; certain medications such as captopril or penicillamine may cause false-positive reactions. Serum or plasma assays for β-hydroxybutyrate more accurately reflect the true ketone body level.

The metabolic derangements of DKA exist along a spectrum, beginning with mild acidosis with moderate hyperglycemia evolving into more severe findings. The degree of acidosis and hyperglycemia do not necessarily correlate closely since a variety of factors determine

TABLE 323-5 Manifestations of Diabetic Ketoacidosis

Symptoms	Physical findings
Nausea/vomiting	Tachycardia
Thirst/polyuria	Dry mucous membranes/reduced skin turgor
Abdominal pain	
Shortness of breath	Dehydration / hypotension
Precipitating events	Tachypnea / Kussmaul respirations/respiratory distress
Inadequate insulin administration	
Infection (pneumonia/UTI/ gastroenteritis/sepsis)	Abdominal tenderness (may resemble acute pancreatitis or surgical abdomen)
Infarction (cerebral, coronary, mesenteric, peripheral)	Lethargy /obtundation / cerebral edema / possibly coma
Drugs (cocaine)	
Pregnancy	

Note: UTI, urinary tract infection.

the level of hyperglycemia (oral intake, urinary glucose loss). Keto-nemia is a consistent finding in DKA and distinguishes it from simple hyperglycemia. The differential diagnosis of DKA includes starvation ketosis, alcoholic ketoacidosis (bicarbonate >15 meq/L) and other in-creased anion gap acidosis (Chap. 42).

℞ TREATMENT

The management of DKA is outlined in Table 323-6. After initiating intravenous fluid replacement and insulin therapy, the agent or event that precipitated the episode of DKA should be sought and aggres-sively treated. If the patient is vomiting or has altered mental status, a nasogastric tube should be inserted to prevent aspiration of gastric contents. Central to successful treatment of DKA is careful monitoring and frequent reassessment to ensure that the patient and the metabolic derangements are improving. A comprehensive flow sheet should record chronologic changes in vital signs, fluid intake and output, and laboratory values as a function of insulin administered.

After the initial bolus of normal saline, replacement of the sodium and free water deficit is carried out over the next 24 h (fluid deficit is often 3 to 5 L). When hemodynamic stability and adequate urine out-put are achieved, intravenous fluids should be switched to 0.45% saline at a rate of 200 to 300 mL/h, depending on the calculated volume deficit. The change to 0.45% saline helps to reduce the trend toward hyperchloremia later in the course of DKA. Alternatively, initial use of lactated Ringer's intravenous solution may reduce the hyperchlo-remia that commonly occurs with normal saline.

A bolus of intravenous (0.15 units/kg) or intramuscular (0.4 units/kg) regular insulin should be administered immediately (Table 323-6), and subsequent treatment should provide continuous and adequate

---

TABLE 323-6   Management of Diabetic Ketoacidosis

1. Confirm diagnosis (↑ plasma glucose, positive serum ketones, meta-bolic acidosis).
2. Admit to hospital; intensive-care setting may be necessary for frequent monitoring or if pH < 7.00 or unconscious.
3. Assess: Serum electrolytes (K^+, Na^+, Mg^{2+}, Cl^-, bicarbonate, phos-phate)
   Acid-base status—pH, HCO_3^-, P_{CO_2}, β-hydroxybutyrate
   Renal function (creatinine, urine output)
4. Replace fluids: 2–3 L of 0.9% saline over first 1–3 h (5–10 mL/kg per hour); subsequently, 0.45% saline at 150–300 mL/h; change to 5% glucose and 0.45% saline at 100–200 mL/h when plasma glucose reaches 250 mg/dL (14 mmol/L).
5. Administer regular insulin: IV (0.1 units/kg) or IM (0.4 units/kg), then 0.1 units/kg per hour by continuous IV infusion; increase 2- to 10-fold if no response by 2–4 h. If initial serum potassium is < 3.3 mmol/L (3.3 meq/L), do not administer insulin until the potassium is corrected to > 3.3 mmol/L (3.3.meq/L).
6. Assess patient: What precipitated the episode (noncompliance, infec-tion, trauma, infarction, cocaine)? Initiate appropriate workup for pre-cipitating event (cultures, CXR, ECG).
7. Measure capillary glucose every 1–2 h; measure electrolytes (espe-cially K^+, bicarbonate, phosphate) and anion gap every 4 h for first 24 h.
8. Monitor blood pressure, pulse, respirations, mental status, fluid intake and output every 1–4 h.
9. Replace K^+: 10 meq/h when plasma K^+ < 5.5 meq/L, ECG normal, urine flow and normal creatinine documented; administer 40–80 meq/h when plasma K^+ <3.5 meq/L or if bicarbonate is given.
10. Continue above until patient is stable, glucose goal is 150–250 mg/dL, and acidosis is resolved. Insulin infusion may be decreased to 0.05–0.1 units/kg per hour.
11. Administer intermediate or long-acting insulin as soon as patient is eating. Allow for overlap in insulin infusion and subcutaneous insulin injection.

Note: CXR, chest x-ray; ECG, electrocardiogram.
Source: Adapted from M Sperling, in *Therapy for Diabetes Mellitus and Related Disor-ders*, American Diabetes Association, Alexandria, VA, 1998; and AE Kitabchi et al: Di-abetes Care 24:131, 2001.

---

levels of circulating insulin. Intravenous administration is preferred (0.1 units/kg per hour), because it assures rapid distribution and allows adjustment of the infusion rate as the patient responds to therapy. In-travenous regular insulin should be continued until the acidosis re-solves and the patient is metabolically stable. As the acidosis and in-sulin resistance associated with DKA resolve, the insulin infusion rate can be decreased (to 0.05 to 0.1 units/kg per hour). Intermediate or long-acting insulin, in combination with subcutaneous regular insulin, should be administered as soon as the patient resumes eating, as this facilitates transition to an outpatient insulin regimen and reduces length of hospital stay. It is crucial to continue the insulin infusion until adequate insulin levels are achieved by the subcutaneous route. Even relatively brief periods of inadequate insulin administration in this transition phase may result in DKA relapse.

Hyperglycemia usually improves at a rate of 4.2 to 5.6 mmol/L (75 to 100 mg/dL) per hour as a result of insulin-mediated glucose dis-posal, reduced hepatic glucose release, and rehydration. The latter re-duces catecholamines, increases urinary glucose loss, and expands the intravascular volume. The decline in the plasma glucose within the first 1 to 2 h may be more rapid and is mostly related to volume expansion. When the plasma glucose reaches 13.9 mmol/L (250 mg/dL), glucose should be added to the 0.45% saline infusion to maintain the plasma glucose in the 11.1 to 13.9 mmol/L (200 to 250 mg/dL) range, and the insulin infusion should be continued. Ketoacidosis be-gins to resolve as insulin reduces lipolysis, increases peripheral ketone body use, suppresses hepatic ketone body formation, and promotes bicarbonate regeneration. However, the acidosis and ketosis resolve more slowly than hyperglycemia. As ketoacidosis improves, β-hy-droxybutyrate is converted to acetoacetate. Ketone body levels may appear to increase if measured by laboratory assays that use the nitro-prusside reaction, which only detects acetoacetate and acetone. The improvement in acidosis and anion gap, a result of bicarbonate regen-eration and decline in ketone bodies, is reflected by a rise in the serum bicarbonate level and the arterial pH. Depending on the rise of serum chloride, the anion gap (but not bicarbonate) will normalize. A hy-perchloremic acidosis [serum bicarbonate of 15 to 18 mmol/L (15 to 18 meq/L)] often follows successful treatment and gradually resolves as the kidneys regenerate bicarbonate and excretes chloride.

Potassium stores are depleted in DKA [estimated deficit 3 to 5 mmol/kg (3 to 5 meq/kg)]. During treatment with insulin and fluids, various factors contribute to the development of hypokalemia. These include insulin-mediated potassium transport into cells, resolution of the acidosis (which also promotes potassium entry into cells), and urinary loss of potassium salts of organic acids. Thus, potassium re-pletion should commence as soon as adequate urine output and a nor-mal serum potassium are documented. If the initial serum potassium level is elevated, then potassium repletion should be delayed until the potassium falls into the normal range. Inclusion of 20 to 40 meq of potassium in each liter of intravenous fluid is reasonable, but additional potassium supplements may also be required. To reduce the amount of chloride administered, potassium phosphate or acetate can be sub-stituted for the chloride salt. The goal is to maintain the serum potas-sium >3.5 mmol/L (3.5 meq/L). If the initial serum potassium is less than 3.3 mmol/L (3.3 meq/L), do not administer insulin until the po-tassium is supplemented to >3.3 mmol/L (3.3 meq/L).

Despite a bicarbonate deficit, bicarbonate replacement is not usu-ally necessary. In fact, theoretical arguments suggest that bicarbonate administration and rapid reversal of acidosis may impair cardiac func-tion, reduce tissue oxygenation, and promote hypokalemia. The results of most clinical trials do not support the routine use of bicarbonate replacement, and one study in children found that bicarbonate use was associated with an increased risk of cerebral edema. However, in the presence of severe acidosis (arterial pH < 7.0 after initial hydration), the ADA advises bicarbonate [50 mmol/L (meq/L) of sodium bicar-bonate in 200 mL of 0.45% saline over 1 h if pH = 6.9 to 7.0; or 100 mmol/L (meq/L) of sodium bicarbonate in 400 mL of 0.45% saline over 2 h if pH 7 < 6.9]. Hypophosphatemia may result from increased glucose usage, but randomized clinical trials have not demonstrated that phosphate replacement is beneficial in DKA. If the serum phosphate is <0.32 mmol/L (1.0 mg/dL), then phosphate supplement should be considered and the serum calcium monitored. Hypomagnesemia may develop during DKA therapy and may also require supplementation.

With appropriate therapy, the mortality of DKA is low (<5%) and is related more to the underlying or precipitating event, such as infection or myocardial infarction. The major nonmetabolic complication of DKA therapy is cerebral edema, which most often develops in children as DKA is resolving. The etiology and optimal therapy for cerebral edema are not well established, but overreplacement of free water should be avoided. Venous thrombosis, upper gastrointestinal bleeding, and acute respiratory distress syndrome occasionally complicate DKA.

Following treatment, the physician and patient should review the sequence of events that led to DKA to prevent future recurrences. Foremost is patient education about the symptoms of DKA, its precipitating factors, and the management of diabetes during a concurrent illness. During illness or when oral intake is compromised, patients should: (1) frequently measure the capillary blood glucose; (2) measure urinary ketones when the serum glucose >16.5 mmol/L (300 mg/dL); (3) drink fluids to maintain hydration; (4) continue or increase insulin; and (5) seek medical attention if dehydration, persistent vomiting, or uncontrolled hyperglycemia develop. Using these strategies, early DKA can be prevented or detected and treated appropriately on an outpatient basis.

HYPERGLYCEMIC HYPEROSMOLAR STATE ■ Clinical Features The prototypical patient with HHS is an elderly individual with type 2 DM, with a several week history of polyuria, weight loss, and diminished oral intake that culminates in mental confusion, lethargy, or coma. The physical examination reflects profound dehydration and hyperosmolality and reveals hypotension, tachycardia, and altered mental status. Notably absent are symptoms of nausea, vomiting, and abdominal pain and the Kussmaul respirations characteristic of DKA. HHS is often precipitated by a serious, concurrent illness such as myocardial infarction or stroke. Sepsis, pneumonia, and other serious infections are frequent precipitants and should be sought. In addition, a debilitating condition (prior stroke or dementia) or social situation that compromises water intake may contribute to the development of the disorder.

Pathophysiology Relative insulin deficiency and inadequate fluid intake are the underlying causes of HHS. Insulin deficiency increases hepatic glucose production (through glycogenolysis and gluconeogenesis) and impairs glucose utilization in skeletal muscle (see above discussion of DKA). Hyperglycemia induces an osmotic diuresis that leads to intravascular volume depletion, which is exacerbated by inadequate fluid replacement. The absence of ketosis in HHS is not completely understood. Presumably, the insulin deficiency is only relative and less severe than in DKA. Lower levels of counterregulatory hormones and free fatty acids have been found in HHS than in DKA in some studies. It is also possible that the liver is less capable of ketone body synthesis or that the insulin/glucagon ratio does not favor ketogenesis.

Laboratory Abnormalities and Diagnosis The laboratory features in HHS are summarized in Table 323-4. Most notable are the marked hyperglycemia [plasma glucose may be >55.5 mmol/L (1000 mg/dL)], hyperosmolality (>350 mosmol/L), and prerenal azotemia. The measured serum sodium may be normal or slightly low despite the marked hyperglycemia. The corrected serum sodium is usually increased [add 1.6 meq to measured sodium for each 5.6-mmol/L (100 mg/dL) rise in the serum glucose]. In contrast to DKA, acidosis and ketonemia are absent or mild. A small anion gap metabolic acidosis may be present secondary to increased lactic acid. Moderate ketonuria, if present, is secondary to starvation.

Rx **TREATMENT**

Volume depletion and hyperglycemia are prominent features of both HHS and DKA. Consequently, therapy of these disorders shares sev-

eral elements (Table 323-6). In both disorders, careful monitoring of the patient's fluid status, laboratory values, and insulin infusion rate is crucial. Underlying or precipitating problems should be aggressively sought and treated. In HHS, fluid losses and dehydration are usually more pronounced than in DKA due to the longer duration of the illness. The patient with HHS is usually older, more likely to have mental status changes, and more likely to have a life-threatening precipitating event with accompanying comorbidities. Even with proper treatment, HHS has a substantially higher mortality than DKA (up to 15% in some clinical series).

Fluid replacement should initially stabilize the hemodynamic status of the patient (1 to 3 L of 0.9% normal saline over the first 2 to 3 h). Because the fluid deficit in HHS is accumulated over a period of days to weeks, the rapidity of reversal of the hyperosmolar state must balance the need for free water repletion with the risk that too rapid a reversal may worsen neurologic function. If the serum sodium is >150 mmol/L (150 meq/L), 0.45% saline should be used. After hemodynamic stability is achieved, the intravenous fluid administration is directed at reversing the free water deficit using hypotonic fluids (0.45% saline initially then 5% dextrose in water, D_5W). The calculated free water deficit (which averages 9 to 10 L) should be reversed over the next 1 to 2 days (infusion rates of 200 to 300 mL/h of hypotonic solution). Potassium repletion is usually necessary and should be dictated by repeated measurements of the serum potassium. In patients taking diuretics, the potassium deficit can be quite large and may be accompanied by magnesium deficiency. Hypophosphatemia may occur during therapy and can be improved by using KPO_4 and beginning nutrition.

As in DKA, rehydration and volume expansion lower the plasma glucose initially, but insulin is also required. A reasonable regimen for HHS begins with an intravenous insulin bolus of 5 to 10 units followed by intravenous insulin at a constant infusion rate (3 to 7 units/h). As in DKA, glucose should be added to intravenous fluid when the plasma glucose falls to 13.9 mmol/L (250 mg/dL), and the insulin infusion rate should be decreased to 1 to 2 units/h. The insulin infusion should be continued until the patient has resumed eating and can be transferred to a subcutaneous insulin regimen. The patient should be discharged from the hospital on insulin, though some patients can later switch to oral glucose-lowering agents.

CHRONIC COMPLICATIONS OF DM

The chronic complications of DM affect many organ systems and are responsible for the majority of morbidity and mortality associated with the disease. Chronic complications can be divided into vascular and nonvascular complications (Table 323-7). The vascular complications

---

TABLE 323-7 *Chronic Complications of Diabetes Mellitus*

Microvascular
  Eye disease
    Retinopathy (nonproliferative/proliferative)
    Macular edema
  Neuropathy
    Sensory and motor (mono- and polyneuropathy)
    Autonomic
  Nephropathy
Macrovascular
  Coronary artery disease
  Peripheral vascular disease
  Cerebrovascular disease
Other
  Gastrointestinal (gastroparesis, diarrhea)
  Genitourinary (uropathy/sexual dysfunction)
  Dermatologic
  Infectious
  Cataracts
  Glaucoma

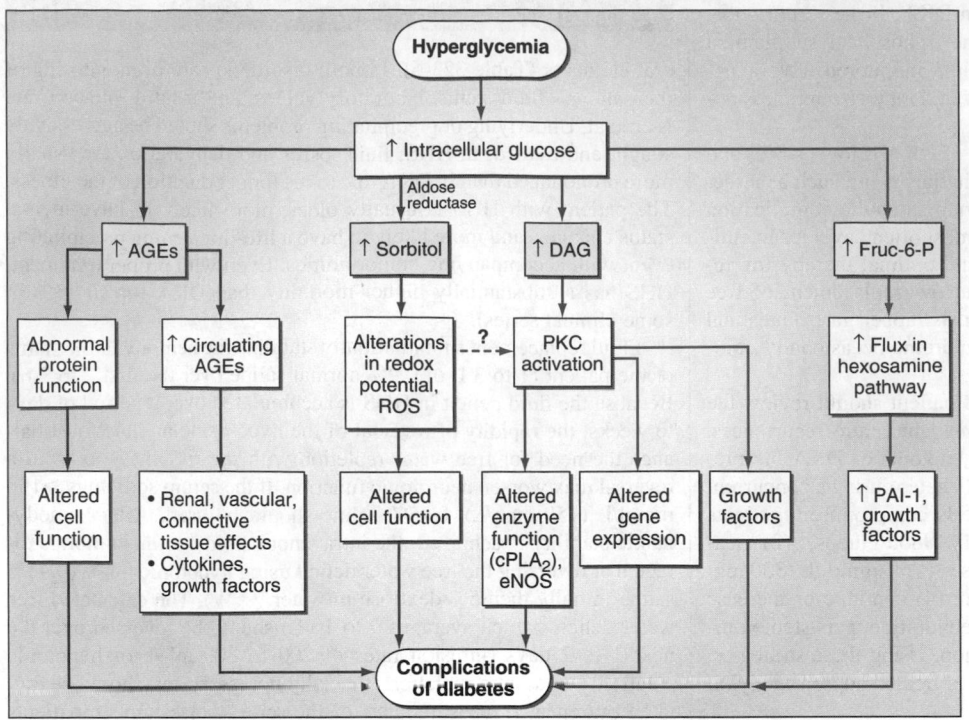

FIGURE 323-7 Possible molecular mechanisms of diabetes-related complications. AGEs, advanced glycation end products; PKC, protein kinase C; DAG, diacylglycerol; cPLA$_2$, phospholipase A$_2$; eNOS, endothelial nitric oxide synthase; ROS, reactive oxygen species; Fruc-6-P, fructose-6-phosphate; PAI-1, plasminogen activor inhibitor-1.

of DM are further subdivided into microvascular (retinopathy, neuropathy, nephropathy) and macrovascular complications (coronary artery disease, peripheral arterial disease, cerebrovascular disease). Nonvascular complications include problems such as gastroparesis, infections, and skin changes. The risk of chronic complications increases as a function of the duration of hyperglycemia; they usually become apparent in the second decade of hyperglycemia. Since type 2 DM often has a long asymptomatic period of hyperglycemia, many individuals with type 2 DM have complications at the time of diagnosis.

The microvascular complications of both type 1 and type 2 DM result from chronic hyperglycemia. Large, randomized clinical trials of individuals with type 1 or type 2 DM have conclusively demonstrated that a reduction in chronic hyperglycemia prevents or delays retinopathy, neuropathy, and nephropathy. Other incompletely defined factors may modulate the development of complications. For example, despite long-standing DM, some individuals never develop nephropathy or retinopathy. Many of these patients have glycemic control that is indistinguishable from those who develop microvascular complications, suggesting that there is a genetic susceptibility for developing particular complications.

Evidence implicating a causative role for chronic hyperglycemia in the development of macrovascular complications is less conclusive. However, coronary heart disease events and mortality are two to four times greater in patients with type 2 DM. These events correlate with fasting and postprandial plasma glucose levels as well as with the A1C. Other factors (dyslipidemia and hypertension) also play important roles in macrovascular complications.

MECHANISMS OF COMPLICATIONS Although chronic hyperglycemia is an important etiologic factor leading to complications of DM, the mechanism(s) by which it leads to such diverse cellular and organ dysfunction is unknown. Four prominent theories, which are not mutually exclusive, have been proposed to explain how hyperglycemia might lead to the chronic complications of DM (Fig. 323-7).

One theory is that increased intracellular glucose leads to the formation of advanced glycosylation end products (AGEs) via the nonenzymatic glycosylaton of intra- and extracellular proteins. Nonenzymatic glycosylation results from the interaction of glucose with amino groups on proteins. AGEs have been shown to cross-link proteins (e.g., collagen, extracellular matrix proteins), accelerate atherosclerosis, promote glomerular dysfunction, reduce nitric oxide synthesis, induce endothelial dysfunction, and alter extracellular matrix composition and structure. The serum level of AGEs correlates with the level of glycemia, and these products accumulate as glomerular filtration rate declines.

A second theory is based on the observation that hyperglycemia increases glucose metabolism via the sorbitol pathway. Intracellular glucose is predominantly metabolized by phosphorylation and subsequent glycolysis, but when increased, some glucose is converted to sorbitol by the enzyme aldose reductase. Increased sorbitol concentration alters redox potential, increases cellular osmolality, generates reactive oxygen species, and likely leads to other types of cellular dysfunction. However, testing of this theory in humans, using aldose reductase inhibitors, has not demonstrated significant beneficial effects on clinical endpoints of retinopathy, neuropathy, or nephropathy.

A third hypothesis proposes that hyperglycemia increases the formation of diacylglycerol leading to activation of protein kinase C (PKC). Among other actions, PKC alters the transcription of genes for fibronectin, type IV collagen, contractile proteins, and extracellular matrix proteins in endothelial cells and neurons.

A fourth theory proposes that hyperglycemia increases the flux through the hexosamine pathway, which generates fructose-6-phosphate, a substrate for O-linked glycosylation and proteoglycan production. The hexosamine pathway may alter function by glycosylation of proteins such as endothelial nitric oxide synthase or by changes in gene expression of transforming growth factor β (TGF-β) or plasminogen activator inhibitor-1 (PAI-1).

Growth factors appear to play an important role in DM-related complications, and their production is increased by most of these proposed pathways. Vascular endothelial growth factor (VEGF) is increased locally in diabetic proliferative retinopathy and decreases after laser photocoagulation. TGF-β is increased in diabetic nephropathy and stimulates basement membrane production of collagen and fibronectin by mesangial cells. Other growth factors, such as platelet-derived growth factor, epidermal growth factor, insulin-like growth factor I, growth hormone, basic fibroblast growth factor, and even insulin, have been suggested to play a role in DM-related complications. A possible unifying mechanism is that hyperglycemia leads to increased production of reactive oxygen species or superoxide in the mitochondria; these compounds may activate all for of the pathways described above. Although hyperglycemia serves as the initial trigger for complications of diabetes, it is still unknown whether the same pathophysiologic processes are operative in all complications or whether some pathways predominate in certain organs.

GLYCEMIC CONTROL AND COMPLICATIONS The Diabetes Control and Complications Trial (DCCT) provided definitive proof that reduction in chronic hyperglycemia can prevent many of the early complications of type 1 DM. This large multicenter clinical trial randomized over 1400 individuals with type 1 DM to either intensive or conventional diabetes management, and prospectively evaluated the development of retinopathy, nephropathy, and neuropathy. Individuals in the intensive diabetes management group received multiple administrations of insulin each day along with extensive educational, psychological, and medical support. Individuals in the conventional diabetes management group received twice-daily insulin injections and quarterly nutritional, educational, and clinical evaluation. The goal in the former group was normoglycemia; the goal in the latter group was prevention of symptoms of diabetes. Individuals in the intensive diabetes management group achieved a substantially lower hemoglobin A1C (A1C; 7.3%) than individuals in the conventional diabetes management group (A1C; 9.1%).

The DCCT demonstrated that improvement of glycemic control reduced nonproliferative and proliferative retinopathy (47% reduction), microalbuminuria (39% reduction), clinical nephropathy (54% reduction), and neuropathy (60% reduction). Improved glycemic control also slowed the progression of early diabetic complications. There was a nonsignificant trend in reduction of macrovascular events. The results of the DCCT predicted that individuals in the intensive diabetes management group would gain 7.7 additional years of vision, 5.8 additional years free from ESRD, and 5.6 years free from lower extremity amputations. If all complications of DM were combined, individuals in the intensive diabetes management group would experience 15.3 more years of life without significant microvascular or neurologic complications of DM, compared to individuals who received standard therapy. This translates into an additional 5.1 years of life expectancy for individuals in the intensive diabetes management group. The benefit of the improved glycemic control during the DCCT persisted even after the study concluded and glycemic control worsened.

The benefits of an improvement in glycemic control occurred over the entire range of A1C values (Fig. 323-8), suggesting that at any A1C level, an improvement in glycemic control is beneficial. Therefore, there is no threshold beneath which the A1C can be reduced and the complications of DM prevented. The clinical implication of this finding is that the goal of therapy is to achieve an A1C level as close to normal as possible, without subjecting the patient to excessive risk of hypoglycemia.

The United Kingdom Prospective Diabetes Study (UKPDS) studied the course of >5000 individuals with type 2 DM for >10 years. This study utilized multiple treatment regimens and monitored the effect of intensive glycemic control and risk factor treatment on the development of diabetic complications. Newly diagnosed individuals with type 2 DM were randomized to (1) intensive management using various combinations of insulin, a sulfonylurea, or metformin; or (2) conventional therapy using dietary modification and pharmacotherapy with the goal of symptom prevention. In addition, individuals were randomly assigned to different antihypertensive regimens. Individuals in the intensive treatment arm achieved an A1C of 7.0%, compared to a 7.9% A1C in the standard treatment group. The UKPDS demonstrated that each percentage point reduction in A1C was associated with a 35% reduction in microvascular complications. As in the

DCCT, there was a continuous relationship between glycemic control and development of complications. Improved glycemic control did not conclusively reduce (nor worsen) cardiovascular mortality but was associated with improvement with lipoprotein risk profiles, such as reduced triglycerides and increased HDL.

One of the major findings of the UKPDS was that strict blood pressure control significantly reduced both macro- and microvascular complications. In fact, the beneficial effects of blood pressure control were greater than the beneficial effects of glycemic control. Lowering blood pressure to moderate goals (144/82 mmHg) reduced the risk of DM-related death, stroke, microvascular end points, retinopathy, and heart failure (risk reductions between 32 and 56%). Despite concerns that insulin therapy is associated with weight gain and may worsen underlying insulin resistance and hyperinsulinemia, most available data support strict glycemic control in individuals with type 2 DM.

Similar reductions in the risks of retinopathy and nephropathy were also seen in a small trial of lean Japanese individuals with type 2 DM randomized to either intensive glycemic control or standard therapy with insulin (Kumamoto study). These results demonstrate the effectiveness of improved glycemic control in individuals of different ethnicity, and, presumably a different etiology of DM (i.e., phenotypically different from those in the DCCT and UKPDS).

The findings of the DCCT, UKPDS, and Kumamoto study support the idea that chronic hyperglycemia plays a causative role in the pathogenesis of diabetic microvascular complications. These landmark studies prove the value of metabolic control and emphasize the importance of (1) intensive glycemic control in all forms of DM, and (2) early diagnosis and strict blood pressure control in type 2 DM.

OPHTHALMOLOGIC COMPLICATIONS OF DIABETES MELLITUS   DM is the leading cause of blindness between the ages of 20 and 74 in the United States. The gravity of this problem is highlighted by the finding that individuals with DM are 25 times more likely to become legally blind than individuals without DM. Blindness is primarily the result of progressive diabetic retinopathy and clinically significant macular edema. Diabetic retinopathy is classified into two stages: nonproliferative and proliferative. *Nonproliferative diabetic retinopathy* usually appears late in the first decade or early in the second decade of the disease and is marked by retinal vascular microaneurysms, blot hemorrhages, and cotton wool spots (Fig. 323-9). Mild nonproliferative retinopathy progresses to more extensive disease, characterized by changes in venous vessel caliber, intraretinal microvascular abnormalities, and more numerous microaneurysms and hemorrhages. The pathophysiologic mechanisms invoked in nonproliferative retinopathy include loss of retinal pericytes, increased retinal vascular permeability, alterations in retinal blood flow, and abnormal retinal microvasculature, all of which lead to retinal ischemia.

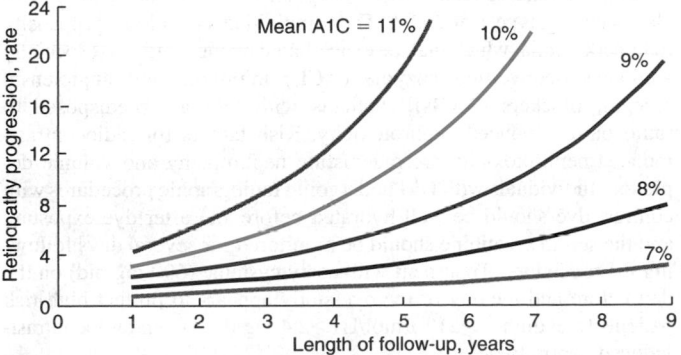

FIGURE 323-8   Relationship of glycemic control and diabetes duration to diabetic retinopathy. The progression of retinopathy in individuals in the Diabetes Control and Complications Trial is graphed as a function of the length of follow-up with different curves for different A1C values. *(Adapted from The Diabetes Control and Complications Trial Research Group, Diabetes 44:968, 1995.)*

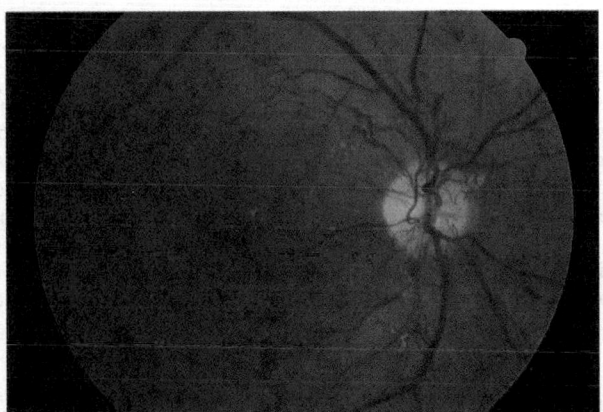

FIGURE 323-9   Diabetic retinopathy results in scattered hemorrhages and yellow exudates. This patient has neovascular vessels proliferating from the optic disc, requiring urgent pan retinal laser photocoagulation.

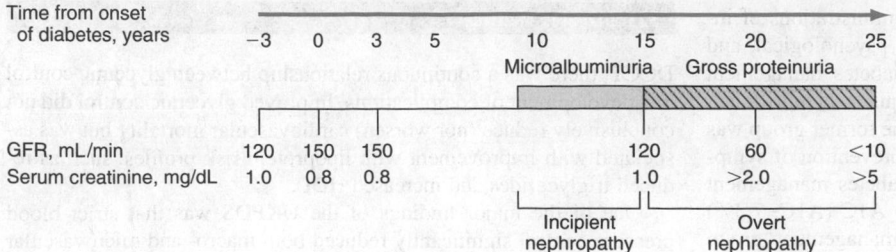

FIGURE 323-10 Time course of development of diabetic nephropathy. The relationship of time from onset of diabetes, the glomerular filtration rate (GFR), and the serum creatinine are shown. (*Adapted from RA DeFronzo, in Therapy for Diabetes Mellitus and Related Disorders, American Diabetes Association, Alexandria, VA, 1998.*)

The appearance of neovascularization in response to retinal hypoxia is the hallmark of *proliferative diabetic retinopathy*. These newly formed vessels appear near the optic nerve and/or macula and rupture easily, leading to vitreous hemorrhage, fibrosis, and ultimately retinal detachment. Not all individuals with nonproliferative retinopathy develop proliferative retinopathy, but the more severe the nonproliferative disease, the greater the chance of evolution to proliferative retinopathy within 5 years. This creates an important opportunity for early detection and treatment of diabetic retinopathy. *Clinically significant macular edema* can occur when only nonproliferative retinopathy is present. Fluorescein angiography is useful to detect macular edema, which is associated with a 25% chance of moderate visual loss over the next 3 years.

Duration of DM and degree of glycemic control are the best predictors of the development of retinopathy; hypertension is also a risk factor. Nonproliferative retinopathy is found in almost all individuals who have had DM for >20 years (25% incidence with 5 years, and 80% incidence with 15 years of type 1 DM). Although there is genetic susceptibility for retinopathy, it confers less influence than either the duration of DM or the degree of glycemic control.

℞ TREATMENT

The most effective therapy for diabetic retinopathy is prevention. Intensive glycemic and blood pressure control will delay the development or slow the progression of retinopathy in individuals with either type 1 or type 2 DM. Paradoxically, during the first 6 to 12 months of improved glycemic control, established diabetic retinopathy may transiently worsen. Fortunately, this progression is temporary, and in the long term, improved glycemic control is associated with less diabetic retinopathy. Individuals with known retinopathy are candidates for prophylactic photocoagulation when initiating intensive therapy. Once advanced retinopathy is present, improved glycemic control imparts less benefit, though adequate ophthalmologic care can prevent most blindness.

Regular, comprehensive eye examinations are essential for all individuals with DM. Most diabetic eye disease can be successfully treated if detected early. Routine, nondilated eye examinations by the primary care provider or diabetes specialist are *inadequate* to detect diabetic eye disease, which requires an ophthalmologist for optimal care of these disorders. Laser photocoagulation is very successful in preserving vision. Proliferative retinopathy is usually treated with pan-retinal laser photocoagulation, whereas macular edema is treated with focal laser photocoagulation. Although exercise has not been conclusively shown to worsen proliferative diabetic retinopathy, most ophthalmologists advise individuals with advanced diabetic eye disease to limit physical activities associated with repeated Valsalva maneuvers. Aspirin therapy (650 mg/d) does not appear to influence the natural history of diabetic retinopathy, but studies of other antiplatelet agents are under way.

RENAL COMPLICATIONS OF DIABETES MELLITUS Diabetic nephropathy is the leading cause of ESRD in the United States and a leading cause of DM-related morbidity and mortality. Proteinuria in individuals with DM is associated with markedly reduced survival and increased risk

of cardiovascular disease. Individuals with diabetic nephropathy almost always have diabetic retinopathy.

Like other microvascular complications, the pathogenesis of diabetic nephropathy is related to chronic hyperglycemia (Fig. 323-7). The mechanisms by which chronic hyperglycemia leads to ESRD, though incompletely defined, involve the effects of soluble factors (growth factors, angiotensin II, endothelin, AGEs), hemodynamic alterations in the renal microcirculation (glomerular hyperfiltration or hyperperfusion, increased glomerular capillary pressure), and structural changes in the glomerulus (increased extracellular matrix, basement membrane thickening, mesangial expansion, fibrosis). Some of these effects may be mediated through angiotensin II receptors. Smoking accelerates the decline in renal function.

The natural history of diabetic nephropathy is characterized by a fairly predictable sequence of events that was initially defined for individuals with type 1 DM but appears to be similar in type 2 DM (Fig. 323-10). Glomerular hyperperfusion and renal hypertrophy occur in the first years after the onset of DM and cause an increase of the glomerular filtration rate (GFR). During the first 5 years of DM, thickening of the glomerular basement membrane, glomerular hypertrophy, and mesangial volume expansion occur as the GFR returns to normal. After 5 to 10 years of type 1 DM, ~40% of individuals begin to excrete small amounts of albumin in the urine. *Microalbuminuria* is defined as 30 to 300 mg/d in a 24-h collection or 30 to 300 μg/mg creatinine in a spot collection (preferred method). The appearance of microalbuminuria (incipient nephropathy) in type 1 DM is an important predictor of progression to overt proteinuria (>300 mg/d) or overt nephropathy. Blood pressure may rise slightly at this point but usually remains in the normal range. Once overt proteinuria is present, there is a steady decline in GFR, and ~50% of individuals reach ESRD in 7 to 10 years. The early pathologic changes and albumin excretion abnormalities are reversible with normalization of plasma glucose. However, once overt nephropathy develops, the pathologic changes are likely irreversible.

The nephropathy that develops in type 2 DM differs from that of type 1 DM in the following respects: (1) microalbuminuria or overt nephropathy may be present when type 2 DM is diagnosed, reflecting its long asymptomatic period; (2) hypertension more commonly accompanies microalbuminuria or overt nephropathy in type 2 DM; and (3) microalbuminuria may be less predictive of diabetic nephropathy and progression to overt nephropathy in type 2 DM. Finally, it should be noted that albuminuria in type 2 DM may be secondary to factors unrelated to DM, such as hypertension, congestive heart failure, prostate disease, or infection. Diabetic nephropathy and ESRD secondary to this develop more commonly in African Americans, Native Americans, and Hispanic individuals than in Caucasians with type 2 DM.

Type IV renal tubular acidosis (hyporeninemic hypoaldosteronism) also occurs in type 1 or 2 DM. These individuals develop a propensity to hyperkalemia, which may be exacerbated by medications [especially angiotensin-converting enzyme (ACE) inhibitors and angiotensin receptor blockers (ARBs)]. Patients with DM are predisposed to radiocontrast-induced nephrotoxicity. Risk factors for radiocontrast-induced nephrotoxicity are preexisting nephropathy and volume depletion. Individuals with DM undergoing radiographic procedures with contrast dye should be well hydrated before and after dye exposure, and the serum creatinine should be monitored for several days following the procedure. Treatment with acetylcysteine (600 mg bid) on the day before and the day of the dye study appears to protect high-risk patients [creatinine, >212 μmol/L (>2.4 mg/dL)] from radiocontrast-induced nephrotoxicity.

℞ TREATMENT

The optimal therapy for diabetic nephropathy is prevention. As part of comprehensive diabetes care, microalbuminuria should be detected

FIGURE 323-11 Screening for microalbuminuria. *(Adapted from RA DeFronzo, In Therapy for Diabetes Mellitus and Related Disorders, American Diabetes Association, Alexandria, VA, 1998.)*

at an early stage when effective therapies can be instituted. The recommended strategy for detecting microalbuminuria is outlined in Fig. 323-11. Interventions effective in slowing progression from microalbuminuria to overt nephropathy include: (1) near normalization of glycemia, (2) strict blood pressure control, and (3) administration of ACE inhibitors or ARBs, and (4) treatment of dyslipidemia.

Improved glycemic control reduces the rate at which microalbuminuria appears and progresses in type 1 and type 2 DM. However, once overt nephropathy exists, it is unclear whether improved glycemic control will slow progression of renal disease. During the phase of declining renal function, insulin requirements may fall as the kidney is a site of insulin degradation. Furthermore, glucose-lowering medications (sulfonylureas and metformin) are contraindicated in advanced renal insufficiency.

Many individuals with type 1 or type 2 DM develop hypertension. Numerous studies in both type 1 and type 2 DM demonstrate the effectiveness of strict blood pressure control in reducing albumin excretion and slowing the decline in renal function. Blood pressure should be maintained at <130/80 mmHg in diabetic individuals without proteinuria. A slightly lower blood pressure (125/75) should be considered for individuals with microalbuminuria or overt nephropathy (see "Hypertension," below).

ACE inhibitors and ARBs reduce the progression of overt nephropathy in individuals with type 1 or type 2 DM and should be prescribed in individuals with type 1 or type 2 DM and microalbuminuria. After 2 to 3 months of therapy, measurement of proteinuria should be repeated and the drug dose increased until either the albuminuria disappears or the maximum dose is reached. If an ACE inhibitor has an unacceptable side-effect profile (hyperkalemia, cough, and renal insufficiency), ARBs can be used as alternatives. If use of either of these types of agents is not possible, then calcium channel blockers (nondihydropyridine class) can be used. However, their efficacy in slowing the fall in the GFR is not proven. Blood pressure control with any agent is extremely important, but a drug-specific benefit in diabetic nephropathy, independent of blood pressure control, has been shown only for ACE inhibitors in type 1 DM and ARBs in type 2 DM.

A consensus panel of the ADA suggests modest restriction of protein intake in diabetic individuals with microalbuminuria (0.8 g/kg per day) or overt nephropathy (<0.8 g/kg per day, which is the adult Recommended Daily Allowance, or about 10% of the daily caloric intake). Conclusive proof of the efficacy of protein restriction is lacking.

Nephrology consultation should be considered after the diagnosis

of early incipient nephropathy. Once overt nephropathy ensues, the likelihood of ESRD is very high. As compared to nondiabetic individuals, hemodialysis in patients with DM is associated with more frequent complications, such as hypotension (due to autonomic neuropathy or loss of reflex tachycardia), more difficult vascular access, and accelerated progression of retinopathy. Survival after the onset of ESRD is shorter in the diabetic population compared to nondiabetics with similar clinical features. Atherosclerosis is the leading cause of death in diabetic individuals on dialysis, and hyperlipidemia should be treated aggressively. Renal transplantation from a living-related donor is the preferred therapy but requires chronic immunosuppression. Combined pancreas-kidney transplant offers the promise of normoglycemia but requires substantial expertise.

NEUROPATHY AND DIABETES MELLITUS Diabetic neuropathy occurs in approximately 50% of individuals with long-standing type 1 and type 2 DM. It may manifest as polyneuropathy, mononeuropathy, and/or autonomic neuropathy. As with other complications of DM, the development of neuropathy correlates with the duration of diabetes and glycemic control; both myelinated and unmyelinated nerve fibers are lost. Because the clinical features of diabetic neuropathy are similar to those of other neuropathies, the diagnosis of *diabetic neuropathy* should be made only after other possible etiologies are excluded (Chap. 363).

Polyneuropathy/Mononeuropathy The most common form of diabetic neuropathy is distal symmetric *polyneuropathy*. It most frequently presents with distal sensory loss. Hyperesthesia, paresthesia, and dysesthesia also occur. Any combination of these symptoms may develop as neuropathy progresses. Symptoms include a sensation of numbness, tingling, sharpness, or burning that begins in the feet and spreads proximally. Neuropathic pain develops in some of these individuals, occasionally preceded by improvement in their glycemic control. Pain typically involves the lower extremities, is usually present at rest, and worsens at night. Both an acute (lasting <12 months) and a chronic form of painful diabetic neuropathy have been described. As diabetic neuropathy progresses, the pain subsides and eventually disappears, but a sensory deficit in the lower extremities persists. Physical examination reveals sensory loss, loss of ankle reflexes, and abnormal position sense.

Diabetic polyradiculopathy is a syndrome characterized by severe disabling pain in the distribution of one or more nerve roots. It may be accompanied by motor weakness. Intercostal or truncal radiculopathy causes pain over the thorax or abdomen. Involvement of the lumbar plexus or femoral nerve may cause pain in the thigh or hip and may be associated with muscle weakness in the hip flexors or extensors (diabetic amyotrophy). Fortunately, diabetic polyradiculopathies are usually self-limited and resolve over 6 to 12 months.

Mononeuropathy (dysfunction of isolated cranial or peripheral nerves) is less common than polyneuropathy in DM and presents with pain and motor weakness in the distribution of a single nerve. A vascular etiology has been suggested, but the pathogenesis is unknown. Involvement of the third cranial nerve is most common and is heralded by diplopia. Physical examination reveals ptosis and opthalmoplegia with normal pupillary constriction to light. Sometimes cranial nerves IV, VI, or VII (Bell's palsy) are affected. Peripheral mononeuropathies or simultaneous involvement of more than one nerve (mononeuropathy multiplex) may also occur.

Autonomic Neuropathy Individuals with long-standing type 1 or 2 DM may develop signs of autonomic dysfunction involving the cholinergic, noradrenergic, and peptidergic (peptides such as pancreatic polypeptide, substance P, etc.) systems. DM-related autonomic neuropathy can involve multiple systems, including the cardiovascular, gastrointestinal, genitourinary, sudomotor, and metabolic systems. Autonomic neuropathies affecting the cardiovascular system cause a resting tachycardia and orthostatic hypotension. Reports of sudden death have also been attributed to autonomic neuropathy. Gastroparesis and bladder-emptying abnormalities are often caused by the autonomic neuropathy seen in DM (discussed below). Hyperhidrosis of the upper extremities and anhidrosis of the lower extremities result from sympathetic nervous system dysfunction. Anhidrosis of the feet can promote dry skin with cracking, which increases the risk of foot ulcers. Autonomic neuropathy may reduce counterregulatory hormone release, leading to an inability to sense hypoglycemia appropriately (*hypoglycemia unawareness*; Chap. 324), thereby subjecting the patient to the risk of severe hypoglycemia and complicating efforts to improve glycemic control.

℞ TREATMENT

Treatment of diabetic neuropathy is less than satisfactory. Improved glycemic control should be pursued and will improve nerve conduction velocity, but the symptoms of diabetic neuropathy may not necessarily improve. Efforts to improve glycemic control may be confounded by autonomic neuropathy and hypoglycemia unawareness. Avoidance of neurotoxins (alcohol), supplementation with vitamins for possible deficiencies (B_{12}, B_6, folate; Chap. 61), and symptomatic treatment are the mainstays of therapy. Aldose reductase inhibitors do not offer significant symptomatic relief. Loss of sensation in the foot places the patient at risk for ulceration and its sequelae; consequently, prevention of such problems is of paramount importance. Since the pain of acute diabetic neuropathy may resolve over the first year, analgesics may be discontinued as progressive neuronal damage from DM occurs. Chronic, painful diabetic neuropathy is difficult to treat but may respond to tricyclic antidepressants (amitriptyline, desipramine, nortriptyline), gabapentin, nonsteroidal anti-inflammatory agents (avoid in renal dysfunction), and other agents (mexilitine, phenytoin, carbamazepine, capsaicin cream). Referral to a pain management center may be necessary.

Therapy of orthostatic hypotension secondary to autonomic neuropathy is challenging. A variety of agents have limited success (fludrocortisone, midodrine, clonidine, octreotide, and yohimbine) but each has significant side effects. Nonpharmacologic maneuvers (adequate salt intake, avoidance of dehydration and diuretics, and lower extremity support hose) may offer some benefit.

GASTROINTESTINAL/GENITOURINARY DYSFUNCTION   Long-standing type 1 and 2 DM may affect the motility and function of gastrointestinal (GI) and genitourinary systems. The most prominent GI symptoms are delayed gastric emptying (gastroparesis) and altered small- and large-bowel motility (constipation or diarrhea). *Gastroparesis* may present with symptoms of anorexia, nausea, vomiting, early satiety, and abdominal bloating. Nuclear medicine scintigraphy after ingestion of a radiolabeled meal is the best study to document delayed gastric emptying, but noninvasive "breath tests" following ingestion of a radiolabeled meal are under development. Though parasympathetic dysfunction secondary to chronic hyperglycemia is important in the development of gastroparesis, hyperglycemia itself also impairs gastric emptying. Nocturnal diarrhea, alternating with constipation, is a common feature of DM-related GI autonomic neuropathy. In type 1 DM, these symptoms should also prompt evaluation for celiac sprue because of its increased frequency. Esophageal dysfunction in long-standing DM is common but usually asymptomatic.

Diabetic autonomic neuropathy may lead to genitourinary dysfunction including cystopathy, erectile dysfunction, and female sexual dysfunction (reduced sexual desire, dyspareunia, reduced vaginal lubrication). Symptoms of diabetic cystopathy begin with an inability to sense a full bladder and a failure to void completely. As bladder contractility worsens, bladder capacity and the post-void residual increase, leading to symptoms of urinary hesitancy, decreased voiding frequency, incontinence, and recurrent urinary tract infections. Diagnostic evaluation includes cystometry and urodynamic studies.

Erectile dysfunction and retrograde ejaculation are very common

in DM and may be one of the earliest signs of diabetic neuropathy (Chap. 43). Erectile dysfunction, which increases in frequency with the age of the patient and the duration of diabetes, may occur in the absence of other signs of diabetic autonomic neuropathy.

℞ TREATMENT

Current treatments for these complications of DM are inadequate. Improved glycemic control should be a primary goal, as some aspects (neuropathy, gastric function) may improve. Smaller, more frequent meals that are easier to digest (liquid) and low in fat and fiber may minimize symptoms of gastroparesis. Cisapride (10 to 20 mg before each meal) is probably the most effective medication but has been removed from use in the United States except under special circumstances. Other agents with some efficacy include dopamine agonists (metoclopramide, 5 to 10 mg, and domperidone, 10 to 20 mg, before each meal) and bethanechol (10 to 20 mg before each meal). Erythromycin interacts with the motilin receptor and may promote gastric emptying. Diabetic diarrhea in the absence of bacterial overgrowth is treated symptomatically with loperamide but may respond to clonidine at higher doses (0.6 mg tid) or octreotide (50 to 75 μg tid subcutaneously). Treatment of bacterial overgrowth with antibiotics is sometimes useful (Chap. 275).

Diabetic cystopathy should be treated with timed voiding or self-catheterization. Medications (bethanechol) are inconsistently effective. The drug of choice for erectile dysfunction is sildenafil, but the efficacy in individuals with DM is slightly lower than in the nondiabetic population (Chap. 43). Sexual dysfunction in women may be improved with use of vaginal lubricants, treatment of vaginal infections, and systemic or local estrogen replacement.

CARDIOVASCULAR MORBIDITY AND MORTALITY   Cardiovascular disease is increased in individuals with type 1 or type 2 DM. The Framingham Heart Study revealed a marked increase in peripheral arterial disease, congestive heart failure, coronary artery disease, myocardial infarction (MI), and sudden death (risk increase from one- to fivefold) in DM. The American Heart Association recently designated DM as a major risk factor for cardiovascular disease (same category as smoking, hypertension, and hyperlipidemia). Type 2 diabetes patients without a prior MI have a similar risk for coronary artery–related events as nondiabetic individuals who have had a prior myocardial infarction. Because of the extremely high prevalence of underlying cardiovascular disease in individuals with diabetes (especially in type 2 DM), evidence of atherosclerotic vascular disease should be sought in an individual with diabetes who has symptoms suggestive of cardiac ischemia, peripheral or carotid arterial disease, a resting electrocardiogram indicative of prior infarction, plans to initiate an exercise program, proteinuria, or two other cardiac risk factors (ADA recommendations). The absence of chest pain ("silent ischemia") is common in individuals with diabetes, and a thorough cardiac evaluation is indicated in individuals undergoing major surgical procedures. The prognosis for individuals with diabetes who have coronary artery disease or myocardial infarction is worse than for nondiabetics. Coronary artery disease is more likely to involve multiple vessels in individuals with DM.

The increase in cardiovascular morbidity and mortality appears to relate to the synergism of hyperglycemia with other cardiovascular risk factors. For example, after controlling for all known cardiovascular risk factors, type 2 DM increases the cardiovascular death rate twofold in men and fourfold in women. Risk factors for macrovascular disease in diabetic individuals include dyslipidemia, hypertension, obesity, reduced physical activity, and cigarette smoking. Additional risk factors specific to the diabetic population include microalbuminuria, gross proteinuria, an elevation of serum creatinine, and abnormal platelet function. Insulin resistance, as reflected by elevated serum insulin levels, is associated with an increased risk of cardiovascular complications in individuals with and without DM. Individuals with insulin resistance and type 2 DM have elevated levels of plasminogen activator inhibitors (especially PAI-1) and fibrinogen, which enhances the coagulation process and impairs fibrinolysis, thus favoring the development of thrombosis. Diabetes is also associated with endothelial, vascular smooth muscle, and platelet dysfunction.

Proof that improved glycemic control reduces cardiovascular complications in DM is lacking; in fact, it is possible that macrovascular complications may be unaffected or even worsened by such therapy. Concerns about the atherogenic potential of insulin remain, since in nondiabetic individuals, higher serum insulin levels (indicative of insulin resistance) are associated with a greater risk of cardiovascular morbidity and mortality. In the DCCT, the number of cardiovascular events did not differ between the standard and intensively treated groups. However, the duration of DM in these individuals was relatively short, and the total number of events was very low. An improvement in the lipid profile of individuals in the intensive group [lower total and low-density lipoprotein (LDL) cholesterol, lower triglycerides] suggested that intensive therapy may reduce the risk of cardiovascular morbidity and mortality associated with DM. In the UKPDS, improved glycemic control did not conclusively reduce cardiovascular mortality. Importantly, treatment with insulin and the sulfonylureas did not appear to increase the risk of cardiovascular disease in individuals with type 2 DM, refuting prior claims about the atherogenic potential of these agents.

In addition to coronary artery disease, cerebrovascular disease is increased in individuals with DM (threefold increase in stroke). Individuals with DM have an increased incidence of congestive heart failure (diabetic cardiomyopathy). The etiology of this abnormality is probably multifactorial and includes factors such as myocardial ischemia from atherosclerosis, hypertension, and myocardial cell dysfunction secondary to chronic hyperglycemia.

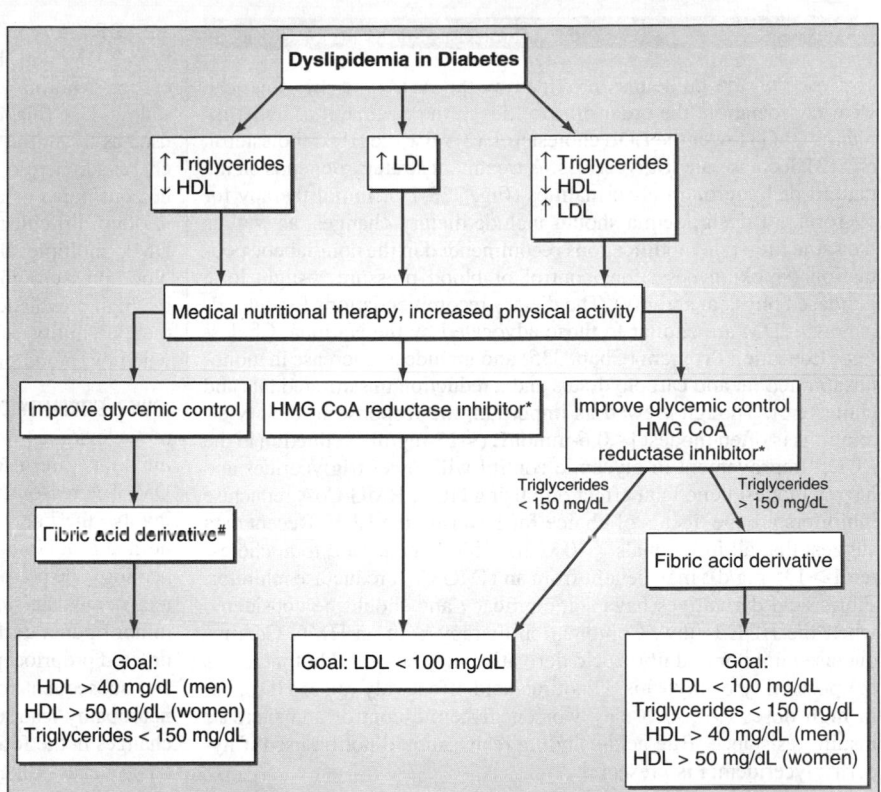

FIGURE 323-12 Dyslipidemia management in diabetes. *Second line treatment: fibric acid derivative or bile acid-binding resin. #Alternative treatment: high dose HMG CoA reductase inhibitor. The level of HDL in women should be 10 mg/dL higher. LDL, low-density lipoprotein; HDL, high-density lipoprotein.

℞ TREATMENT

In general, the treatment of coronary disease is no different in the diabetic individual (Chap. 226). Revascularization procedures for coronary artery disease, including percutaneous coronary interventions (PCI) and coronary artery bypass grafting (CABG), are less efficacious in the diabetic individual. Initial success rates of PCI in diabetic individuals are similar to those in the nondiabetic population, but diabetic patients have higher rates of restenosis and lower long-term patency and survival rates. The use of stents and a GPIIb/IIIa platelet inhibitor has improved the outcome in diabetic patients. Perioperative mortality from CABG is not altered in DM, but both short- and long-term survival are reduced. Recent trials indicate that diabetic individuals with multivessel coronary artery disease or recent Q-wave MI have better long-term survival with CABG than PCI.

The ADA has emphasized the importance of glycemic control and aggressive cardiovascular risk modification in all individuals with DM. Past trepidation about using beta blockers in individuals who have diabetes should not prevent use of these agents since they clearly benefit diabetic patients after MI. ACE inhibitors may also be particularly beneficial and should be considered in individuals with type 2 DM and other risk factors (smoking, dyslipidemia, history of cardiovascular disease, microalbuminuria).

Antiplatelet therapy reduces cardiovascular events in individuals with DM who have coronary artery disease. Current recommendations by the ADA include the use of aspirin for secondary prevention of coronary events. Although data demonstrating efficacy in primary prevention of coronary events in DM are lacking, antiplatelet therapy should be strongly considered, especially in diabetic individuals with other coronary risk factors such as hypertension, smoking, or dysli-

pidemia. The aspirin dose (81 to 325 mg) is the same as that in nondiabetic individuals. Aspirin therapy does not have detrimental effects on renal function or hypertension, nor does it influence the course of diabetic retinopathy.

Cardiovascular Risk Factors ▪ *DYSLIPIDEMIA* Individuals with DM may have several forms of dyslipidemia (Chap. 335). Because of the additive cardiovascular risk of hyperglycemia and hyperlipidemia, lipid abnormalities should be aggressively detected and treated as part of comprehensive diabetes care (Fig. 323-12). The most common pattern of dyslipidemia is hypertriglyceridemia and reduced HDL cholesterol levels. DM itself does not increase levels of LDL, but the small dense LDL particles found in type 2 DM are more atherogenic because they are more easily glycated and susceptible to oxidation. According to guidelines of the ADA and the American Heart Association, the target lipid values in diabetic individuals without cardiovascular disease should be: LDL < 2.6 mmol/L (100 mg/dL); HDL > 1.1 mmol/L (40 mg/dL) in men and >1.38 mmol/L (50 mg/dL) in women; and triglycerides < 1.7 mmol/L (150 mg/dL). The National Cholesterol Education Program Adult Treatment Panel III also recommends lowering the LDL to < 2.6 mmol/L (100 mg/dL) in diabetics. This is because the incidence of MI in type 2 DM is the same as that in patients without diabetes who have had a prior MI.

Almost all studies of diabetic dyslipidemia have been performed in individuals with type 2 DM because of the greater frequency of dyslipidemia in this form of diabetes. Interventional studies have shown that the beneficial effects of LDL reduction are similar in the diabetic and nondiabetic populations. Large prospective trials of primary and secondary intervention for coronary heart disease have included some individuals with type 2 DM, and subset analyses have consistently found that reductions in LDL reduce cardiovascular events and morbidity in individuals with DM. Most clinical trials used HMG CoA reductase inhibitors, although a fibric acid derivative has also shown to be beneficial. No prospective studies have addressed similar questions in individuals with type 1 DM.

Based on the guidelines provided by the ADA and the American Heart Association, the order of priorities in the treatment of hyperlipidemia is: (1) lower the LDL cholesterol, (2) raise the HDL cholesterol, and (3) decrease the triglycerides. A treatment strategy depends on the pattern of lipoprotein abnormalities (Fig. 323-11). Initial therapy for all forms of dyslipidemia should include dietary changes, as well as the same life-style modifications recommended in the nondiabetic population (smoking cessation, control of blood pressure, weight loss, increased physical activity). The dietary recommendations for individuals with DM are similar to those advocated by the National Cholesterol Education Program (Chap. 335) and include an increase in monounsaturated fat and carbohydrates and a reduction in saturated fats and cholesterol. Though viewed as important, the response to dietary alterations is often modest [<0.6-mmol/L (<25-mg/dL) reduction in the LDL]. Improvement in glycemic control will lower triglycerides and have a modest beneficial effect on raising HDL. HMG CoA reductase inhibitors are the agents of choice for lowering the LDL. Recent data suggest that all individuals >40 years with diabetes and total cholesterol >135 mg/dL may benefit from an HMG CoA reductase inhibitor. Fibric acid derivatives have some efficacy and should be considered when the HDL is low. Combination therapy with an HMG CoA reductase inhibitor and fibric acid derivative may be useful but increases the possibility of myositis. Nicotinic acid effectively raises HDL, but in high doses (>2 g/d) may worsen glycemic control and increase insulin resistance. Bile acid–binding resins should not be used if hypertriglyceridemia is present.

HYPERTENSION Hypertension can accelerate other complications of DM, particularly cardiovascular disease and nephropathy. Hypertension therapy should first emphasize life-style modifications such as weight loss, exercise, stress management, and sodium restriction. Antihypertensive agents should be selected based on the advantages and disadvantages of the therapeutic agent in the context of an individual patient's risk factor profile. DM-related considerations include the following:

1. ACE inhibitors are either glucose- and lipid-neutral or glucose- and lipid-beneficial and thus positively impact the cardiovascular risk profile. For example, captopril improves insulin resistance, reduces LDL slightly, and increases HDL slightly. α-Adrenergic blockers slightly improve insulin resistance and positively impact the lipid profile, whereas beta blockers and thiazide diuretics can increase insulin resistance and negatively impact the lipid profile. Calcium channel blockers, central adrenergic antagonists, and vasodilators are lipid- and glucose-neutral.

2. Beta blockers may slightly increase the risk of developing type 2 DM. Although often questioned because of the potential masking of hypoglycemic symptoms, beta blockers are safe in most patients with diabetes and reduce cardiovascular events. In one study of nondiabetic individuals, the ACE inhibitor ramipril reduced the risk of developing type 2 DM.

3. Sympathetic inhibitors and α-adrenergic blockers may worsen orthostatic hypotension in the diabetic individual with autonomic neuropathy.

4. Equivalent reduction in blood pressure by different classes of agents may not translate into equivalent protection from cardiovascular and renal endpoints. Thiazides, beta blockers, ACE inhibitors, and ARBs positively impact cardiovascular endpoints (MI or stroke). The cardiovascular protective effect of calcium channel blockers, central adrenergic antagonists, and α-adrenergic blockers is either controversial or not known. ACE inhibitors (in types 1 and 2 DM) and ARBs (in type 2 DM) slow the progression of diabetic renal disease; the effect of other classes of agents on diabetic nephropathy is not known.

5. Non-dihydropyridine calcium channel blockers (verapamil and diltiazem), rather than dihydropyridine agents (amlodipine and nifedipine), are preferred in diabetics.

If microalbuminuria or overt albuminuria is present, the optimal antihypertensive agent is an ACE inhibitor (in types 1 and 2 DM) or an ARB (in type 2 DM). Most prefer ARBs over ACE inhibitors in type 2 DM with hypertension and microalbuminuria. If albumin excretion is normal, then an ACE inhibitor is usually prescribed initially. A low-dose thiazide diuretic, beta blockers, or an ARB may also be used as the initial agent. Non-dihydropyridine calcium channel blockers, α-adrenergic blockers, and central adrenergic antagonists should be considered as additional or second-line agents. Since hypertension is often difficult to control with a single agent (especially in type 2 DM), multiple antihypertensive agents are usually required when blood pressure goals (<130/80 mmHg) are not achieved. Because of the high prevalence of atherosclerotic disease in individuals with DM, the possibility of renovascular hypertension should be considered when the blood pressure is not readily controlled.

LOWER EXTREMITY COMPLICATIONS DM is the leading cause of nontraumatic lower extremity amputation in the United States. Foot ulcers and infections are also a major source of morbidity in individuals with DM. The reasons for the increased incidence of these disorders in DM involve the interaction of several pathogenic factors: neuropathy, abnormal foot biomechanics, peripheral arterial disease, and poor wound healing. The peripheral sensory neuropathy interferes with normal protective mechanisms and allows the patient to sustain major or repeated minor trauma to the foot, often without knowledge of the injury. Disordered proprioception causes abnormal weight bearing while walking and subsequent formation of callus or ulceration. Motor and sensory neuropathy lead to abnormal foot muscle mechanics and to structural changes in the foot (hammer toe, claw toe deformity, prominent metatarsal heads, Charcot joint). Autonomic neuropathy results in anhidrosis and altered superficial blood flow in the foot, which promote drying of the skin and fissure formation. Peripheral arterial disease and poor wound healing impede resolution of minor breaks in the skin, allowing them to enlarge and to become infected.

Approximately 15% of individuals with DM develop a foot ulcer, and a significant subset will ultimately undergo amputation (14 to 24% risk with that ulcer or subsequent ulceration). Risk factors for foot ulcers or amputation include: male sex, diabetes >10 years' duration, peripheral neuropathy, abnormal structure of foot (bony abnormalities, callus, thickened nails), peripheral arterial disease, smoking, history of previous ulcer or amputation, and poor glycemic control.

℞ **TREATMENT**

The optimal therapy for foot ulcers and amputations is prevention through identification of high-risk patients, education of the patient, and institution of measures to prevent ulceration. High-risk patients should be identified during the routine foot examination performed on all patients with DM (see "Ongoing Aspects of Comprehensive Diabetes Care," below). Patient education should emphasize: (1) careful selection of footwear, (2) daily inspection of the feet to detect early signs of poor-fitting footwear or minor trauma, (3) daily foot hygiene to keep the skin clean and moist, (4) avoidance of self-treatment of foot abnormalities and high-risk behavior (e.g., walking barefoot), and (5) prompt consultation with a health care provider if an abnormality arises. Patients at high risk for ulceration or amputation may benefit from evaluation by a foot care specialist. Interventions directed at risk factor modification include orthotic shoes and devices, callus management, nail care, and prophylactic measures to reduce increased skin pressure from abnormal bony architecture. Attention to other risk factors for vascular disease (smoking, dyslipidemia, hypertension) and improved glycemic control are also important.

Despite preventive measures, foot ulceration and infection are common and represent a potentially serious problem. Due to the multifactorial pathogenesis of lower extremity ulcers, management of these lesions is multidisciplinary and often demands expertise in orthopedics, vascular surgery, endocrinology, podiatry, and infectious diseases. The plantar surface of the foot is the most common site of ulceration. Ulcers may be primarily neuropathic (no accompanying infection) or may have surrounding cellulitis or osteomyelitis. Cellulitis without ulceration is also frequent and should be treated with antibiotics that provide broad-spectrum coverage, including anaerobes (see below).

An infected ulcer is a clinical diagnosis, since superficial culture of any ulceration will likely find multiple possible bacterial pathogens. The infection surrounding the foot ulcer is often the result of multiple organisms (gram-positive and -negative organisms and anaerobes), and gas gangrene may develop in the absence of clostridial infection. Cultures taken from the debrided ulcer base or from purulent drainage are most helpful. Wound depth should be determined by inspection and probing with a blunt-tipped sterile instrument. Plain radiographs of the foot should be performed to assess the possibility of osteomyelitis in chronic ulcers that have not responded to therapy. Nuclear medicine bone scans may be helpful, but overlying subcutaneous infection is often difficult to distinguish from osteomyelitis. Indium-labeled white cell studies are more useful in determining if the infection involves bony structures or only soft tissue, but they are technically demanding. Magnetic resonance imaging of the foot may be the most specific modality, although distinguishing bony destruction due to osteomyelitis from destruction secondary to Charcot arthropathy is difficult. If surgical debridement is necessary, bone biopsy and culture may provide the answer.

Osteomyelitis is best treated by a combination of prolonged antibiotics (IV then oral) and possibly debridement of infected bone. The possible contribution of vascular insufficiency should be considered in all patients. Noninvasive blood-flow studies are often unreliable in DM, and angiography may be required, recognizing the risk of contrast-induced nephrotoxicity. Peripheral arterial bypass procedures are often effective in promoting wound healing and in decreasing the need for amputation of the ischemic limb.

A growing number of possible treatments for diabetic foot ulcers exist, but they have yet to demonstrate clear efficacy in prospective, controlled trials. A recent consensus statement from the ADA identified six interventions with demonstrated efficacy in diabetic foot wounds: (1) off-loading, (2) debridement, (3) wound dressings, (4) appropriate use of antibiotics, (5) revascularization, and (6) limited amputation. Off-loading is the complete avoidance of weight bearing on the ulcer, which removes the mechanical trauma that retards wound healing. Bed rest and a variety of orthotic devices or contact casting limit weight bearing on wounds or pressure points. Surgical debridement is important and effective, but clear efficacy of other modalities for wound cleaning (enzymes, soaking, whirlpools) is lacking. Dressings promote wound healing by creating a moist environment and protecting the wound. Antiseptic agents and topical antibiotics should be avoided. Referral for physical therapy, orthotic evaluation, and rehabilitation may be useful once the infection is controlled.

Mild or non-limb-threatening infections can be treated with oral antibiotics (cephalosporin, clindamycin, amoxicillin/clavulanate, and fluoroquinolones), surgical debridement of necrotic tissue, local wound care (avoidance of weight bearing over the ulcer), and close surveillance for progression of infection. More severe ulcers may require intravenous antibiotics as well as bed rest and local wound care. Urgent surgical debridement may be required. Intravenous antibiotics should provide broad-spectrum coverage directed toward *Staphylococcus aureus*, streptococci, gram-negative aerobes, and anaerobic bacteria. Initial antimicrobial regimens include cefotetan, ampicillin/sulbactam, or the combination of clindamycin and a fluoroquinolone. Severe infections, or infections that do not improve after 48 h of antibiotic therapy, require expansion of antimicrobial therapy to treat methicillin-resistant *S. aureus* (e.g., vancomycin) and *Pseudomonas aeruginosa*. If the infection surrounding the ulcer is not improving with intravenous antibiotics, reassessment of antibiotic coverage and reconsideration of the need for surgical debridement or revascularization are indicated. With clinical improvement, oral antibiotics and local wound care can be continued on an outpatient basis with close follow-up.

New information about wound biology has led to a number of new technologies (e.g., living skin equivalents and growth factors such as basic fibroblast growth factor) that may prove useful. Recombinant platelet-derived growth factor has some benefit and complement the therapies of off-loading, debridement, and antibiotics. Hyperbaric oxygen has been used, but rigorous proof of efficacy is lacking.

INFECTIONS Individuals with DM have a greater frequency and severity of infection. The reasons for this include incompletely defined abnormalities in cell-mediated immunity and phagocyte function associated with hyperglycemia, as well as diminished vascularization. Hyperglycemia aids the colonization and growth of a variety of organisms (*Candida* and other fungal species). Many common infections are more frequent and severe in the diabetic population, whereas several rare infections are seen almost exclusively in the diabetic population. Examples of this latter category includes rhinocerebral mucormycosis, emphysematous infections of the gall bladder and urinary tract, and "malignant" or invasive otitis externa. Invasive otitis externa is usually secondary to *P. aeruginosa* infection in the soft tissue surrounding the external auditory canal, usually begins with pain and discharge, and may rapidly progress to osteomyelitis and meningitis. These infections should be sought, in particular, in patients presenting with HHS.

Pneumonia, urinary tract infections, and skin and soft tissue infections are all more common in the diabetic population. In general, the organisms that cause pulmonary infections are similar to those found in the nondiabetic population; however, gram-negative organisms, *S. aureus*, and *Mycobacterium tuberculosis* are more frequent pathogens. Urinary tract infections (either lower tract or pyelonephritis) are the result of common bacterial agents such as *Escherichia coli*, though several yeast species (*Candida* and *Torulopsis glabrata*) are commonly observed. Complications of urinary tract infections include emphysematous pyelonephritis and emphysematous cystitis. Bacteriuria occurs frequently in individuals with diabetic cystopathy. Susceptibility to furunculosis, superficial candidal infections, and vulvovaginitis are increased. Poor glycemic control is a common denominator in individuals with these infections. Diabetic individuals have an increased rate of colonization of *S. aureus* in the skin folds and nares. Diabetic patients also have a greater risk of postoperative wound infections. Strict glycemic control reduces postoperative infections in diabetic individuals undergoing CABG and should be the goal in all diabetic patients with an infection.

DERMATOLOGIC MANIFESTATIONS The most common skin manifestations of DM are protracted wound healing and skin ulcerations. Diabetic dermopathy, sometimes termed *pigmented pretibial papules*, or "diabetic skin spots," begins as an erythematous area and evolves into an area of circular hyperpigmentation. These lesions result from minor mechanical trauma in the pretibial region and are more common in elderly men with DM. Bullous diseases (shallow ulcerations or erosions in the pretibial region) are also seen. *Necrobiosis lipoidica diabeticorum* is a rare disorder of DM that predominantly affects young women with type 1 DM, neuropathy, and retinopathy. It usually begins in the pretibial region as an erythematous plaque or papules that gradually enlarge, darken, and develop irregular margins, with atrophic centers and central ulceration. They may be painful. *Acanthosis nigricans* (hyperpigmented velvety plaques seen on the neck, axilla, or extensor surfaces) is sometimes a feature of severe insulin resistance and accompanying diabetes. Generalized or localized *granuloma annulare* (erythematous plaques on the extremities or trunk) and *scleredema* (areas of skin thickening on the back or neck at the site of previous superficial infections) are more common in the diabetic population. *Lipoatrophy* and *lipohypertrophy* can occur at insulin injection sites but are unusual with the use of human insulin. Xerosis and pruritus are common and are relieved by skin moisturizers.

APPROACH TO THE PATIENT

DM and its complications produce a wide range of symptoms and signs; those secondary to acute hyperglycemia may occur at any stage of the disease, whereas those related to chronic complications begin to appear during the second decade of hyperglycemia. Individuals with previously undetected type 2 DM may present with chronic complications of DM at the time of diagnosis. The history and physical examination should assess for symptoms or signs of acute hyperglycemia and should screen for the chronic complications and conditions associated with DM.

History A complete medical history should be obtained with special emphasis on DM-relevant aspects such as weight, family history of DM and its complications, risk factors for cardiovascular disease, exercise, smoking, and ethanol use. Symptoms of hyperglycemia include polyuria, polydipsia, weight loss, fatigue, weakness, blurry vision, frequent superficial infections (vaginitis, fungal skin infections), and slow healing of skin lesions after minor trauma. Metabolic derangements relate mostly to hyperglycemia (osmotic diuresis, reduced glucose entry into muscle) and to the catabolic state of the patient (urinary loss of glucose and calories, muscle breakdown due to protein degradation and decreased protein synthesis). Blurred vision results from changes in the water content of the lens and resolves as the hyperglycemia is controlled.

In a patient with established DM, the initial assessment should also include special emphasis on prior diabetes care, including the type of therapy, prior hemoglobin A1C levels, self-monitoring blood glucose results, frequency of hypoglycemia, presence of DM-specific complications, and assessment of the patient's knowledge about diabetes. The chronic complications may afflict several organ systems, and an individual patient may exhibit some, all, or none of the symptoms related to the complications of DM (see above). In addition, the presence of DM-related comorbidities should be sought (cardiovascular disease, hypertension, dyslipidemia).

Physical Examination In addition to a complete physical examination, special attention should be given to DM-relevant aspects such as weight or BMI, retinal examination, orthostatic blood pressure, foot examination, peripheral pulses, and insulin injection sites. Blood pressure > 130/80 mmHg is considered hypertension in individuals with diabetes. Careful examination of the lower extremities should seek evidence of peripheral neuropathy, calluses, superficial fungal infections, nail disease, and foot deformities (such as hammer or claw toes and Charcot foot) in order to identify sites of potential skin ulceration. Vibratory sensation (128-MHz tuning fork at the base of the great toe) and the ability to sense touch with a monofilament (5.07, 10-g monofilament) are useful to detect moderately advanced diabetic neuropathy. Since periodontal disease is more frequent in DM, the teeth and gums should also be examined.

Classification of DM in an Individual Patient The etiology of diabetes in an individual with new-onset disease can usually be assigned on the basis of clinical criteria. Individuals with type 1 DM tend to have the following characteristics: (1) onset of disease prior to age 30; (2) lean body habitus; (3) requirement of insulin as the initial therapy; (4) propensity to develop ketoacidosis; and (5) an increased risk of other autoimmune disorders such as autoimmune thyroid disease, adrenal insufficiency, pernicious anemia, and vitiligo. In contrast, individuals with type 2 DM often exhibit the following features: (1) develop diabetes after the age of 30; (2) are usually obese (80% are obese, but elderly individuals may be lean); (3) may not require insulin therapy initially; and (4) may have associated conditions such as insulin resistance, hypertension, cardiovascular disease, dyslipidemia, or PCOS. In type 2 DM, insulin resistance is often associated with abdominal obesity (as opposed to hip and thigh obesity) and hypertriglyceridemia. Although most individuals diagnosed with type 2 DM are older, the age of diagnosis is declining in some ethnic groups, and there is a marked increase among overweight children and adolescents. Some individuals with phenotypic type 2 DM present with DKA but lack autoimmune markers and may be later treated with oral glucose-lowering agents rather than insulin. On the other hand, some individuals (5–10%) with the phenotypic appearance of type 2 DM do not have absolute insulin deficiency but have autoimmune markers (ICA, GAD autoantibodies) suggestive of type 1A DM (termed *autoimmune diabetes not requiring insulin at diagnosis* or *latent autoimmune diabetes of the adult*). Such individuals are much more likely to require insulin treatment within 5 years. Thus, despite the revised classification of DM, it is remains difficult to categorize some patients unequivocally. Individuals who deviate from the clinical profile of type 1 and type 2 DM, or who have other associated defects such as deafness, pancreatic exocrine disease, and other endocrine disorders, should be classified accordingly (Table 323-1).

Laboratory Assessment The laboratory assessment should first determine whether the patient meets the diagnostic criteria for DM (Table 323-2) and then assess the degree of glycemic control (A1C, discussed below). In addition to the standard laboratory evaluation, the patient should be screened for DM-associated conditions (e.g., microalbuminuria, dyslipidemia, thyroid dysfunction). Individuals at high risk for cardiovascular disease should be screened for asymptomatic coronary artery disease by appropriate cardiac stress testing, when indicated.

The classification of the type of DM may be facilitated by laboratory assessments. Serum insulin or C-peptide measurements do not always distinguish type 1 from type 2 DM, but a low C-peptide level confirms a patient's need for insulin. Many individuals with new-onset type 1 DM retain some C-peptide production. Measurement of islet cell antibodies at the time of diabetes onset may be useful if the type of DM is not clear based on the characteristics described above.

LONG-TERM TREATMENT

OVERALL PRINCIPLES The goals of therapy for type 1 or type 2 DM are to: (1) eliminate symptoms related to hyperglycemia, (2) reduce or eliminate the long-term microvascular and macrovascular complications of DM, and (3) allow the patient to achieve as normal a life-style as possible. To reach these goals, the physician should identify a target level of glycemic control for each patient, provide the patient with the educational and pharmacologic resources necessary to reach this level, and monitor/treat DM-related complications. Symptoms of diabetes usually resolve when the plasma glucose is <11.1 mmol/L (200 mg/dL), and thus most DM treatment focuses on achieving the second and third goals.

The care of an individual with either type 1 or type 2 DM requires a multidisciplinary team. Central to the success of this team are the patient's participation, input, and enthusiasm, all of which are essential for optimal diabetes management. Members of the health care team include the primary care provider and/or the endocrinologist or diabetologist, a certified diabetes educator, and a nutritionist. In addition, when the complications of DM arise, subspecialists (including neurologists, nephrologists, vascular surgeons, cardiologists, ophthalmologists, and podiatrists) with experience in DM-related complications are essential.

A number of names are sometimes applied to different approaches to diabetes care, such as intensive insulin therapy, intensive glycemic control, and "tight control." The current chapter, however, will use the term *comprehensive diabetes care* to emphasize the fact that optimal diabetes therapy involves more than plasma glucose management. Though glycemic control is central to optimal diabetes therapy, comprehensive diabetes care of both type 1 and type 2 DM should also detect and manage DM-specific complications and modify risk factors for DM-associated diseases. In addition to the physical aspects of DM, social, family, financial, cultural, and employment-related issues may impact diabetes care.

PATIENT EDUCATION ABOUT DM, NUTRITION, AND EXERCISE   The patient with type 1 or type 2 DM should receive education about nutrition, exercise, care of diabetes during illness, and medications to lower the plasma glucose. Along with improved compliance, patient education allows individuals with DM to assume greater responsibility for their care. Patient education should be viewed as a continuing process with regular visits for reinforcement; it should *not* be a process that is completed after one or two visits to a nurse educator or nutritionist.

Diabetes Education   The diabetes educator is a health care professional (nurse, dietician, or pharmacist) with specialized patient education skills who is certified in diabetes education (e.g., American Association of Diabetes Educators). Education topics important for optimal diabetes care include self-monitoring of blood glucose; urine ketone monitoring (type 1 DM); insulin administration; guidelines for diabetes management during illnesses; management of hypoglycemia; foot and skin care; diabetes management before, during, and after exercise; and risk factor–modifying activities.

Nutrition   *Medical nutrition therapy* (MNT) is a term used by the ADA to describe the optimal coordination of caloric intake with other aspects of diabetes therapy (insulin, exercise, weight loss). Historically, nutrition education imposed restrictive, complicated regimens on the patient. Current practices have greatly changed, though many patients and health care providers still view the diabetic diet as monolithic and static. For example, MNT now includes foods with sucrose and seeks to modify other risk factors such as hyperlipidemia and hypertension rather than focusing exclusively on weight loss in individuals with type 2 DM. Like other aspects of DM therapy, MNT must be adjusted to meet the goals of the individual patient. Furthermore, MNT education is an important component of comprehensive diabetes care and should be reinforced by regular patient education. In general, the components of optimal MNT are similar for individuals with type 1 or type 2 DM (Table 323-8).

The goal of MNT in the individual with type 1 DM is to coordinate and match the caloric intake, both temporally and quantitatively, with the appropriate amount of insulin. MNT in type 1 DM and self-monitoring of blood glucose must be integrated to define the optimal insulin regimen. MNT must be flexible enough to allow for exercise, and the insulin regimen must allow for deviations in caloric intake. An important component of MNT in type 1 DM is to minimize the weight gain often associated with intensive diabetes management.

The goals of MNT in type 2 DM are slightly different and address the greatly increased prevalence of cardiovascular risk factors (hypertension, dyslipidemia, obesity) and disease in this population. The majority of these individuals are obese, and weight loss is strongly encouraged and should remain an important goal. Medical treatment of obesity is a rapidly evolving area and is discussed in Chap. 64. Hypocaloric diets and modest weight loss often result in rapid and dramatic glucose lowering in individuals with new-onset type 2 DM. Nevertheless, numerous studies document that long-term weight loss is uncommon. Current MNT for type 2 DM should emphasize modest caloric reduction, reduced fat intake, increased physical activity, and reduction of hyperlipidemia and hypertension. Increased consumption of soluble, dietary fiber may improve glycemic control in individuals with type 2 DM.

Exercise   Exercise has multiple positive benefits including cardiovascular risk reduction, reduced blood pressure, maintenance of muscle mass, reduction in body fat, and weight loss. For individuals with type 1 or type 2 DM, exercise is also useful for lowering plasma glucose (during and following exercise) and increasing insulin sensitivity.

Despite its benefits, exercise presents challenges for individuals with DM because they lack the normal glucoregulatory mechanisms (insulin falls and glucagon rises during exercise). Skeletal muscle is a major site for metabolic fuel consumption in the resting state, and the increased muscle activity during vigorous, aerobic exercise greatly increases fuel requirements. Individuals with type 1 DM are prone to either hyperglycemia or hypoglycemia during exercise, depending on the preexercise plasma glucose, the circulating insulin level, and the level of exercise-induced catecholamines. If the insulin level is too low, the rise in catecholamines may increase the plasma glucose excessively, promote ketone body formation, and possibly lead to ketoacidosis. Conversely, if the circulating insulin level is excessive, this relative hyperinsulinemia may reduce hepatic glucose production (decreased glycogenolysis, decreased gluconeogenesis) and increase glucose entry into muscle, leading to hypoglycemia.

To avoid exercise-related hyper- or hypoglycemia, individuals with type 1 DM should: (1) monitor blood glucose before, during, and after exercise; (2) delay exercise if blood glucose is >14 mmol/L (250 mg/dL), <5.5 mmol/L (100 mg/dL), or if ketones are present; (3) monitor glucose during exercise and ingest carbohydrate to prevent hypoglycemia; (4) decrease insulin doses (based on previous experience) before exercise and inject insulin into a nonexercising area; and (5) learn individual glucose responses to different types of exercise and increase food intake for up to 24 h after exercise, depending on intensity and duration of exercise. In individuals with type 2 DM, exercise-related hypoglycemia is less common but can occur in individuals taking either insulin or sulfonylureas.

Because asymptomatic cardiovascular disease appears at a younger age in both type 1 and type 2 DM, formal exercise tolerance testing may be warranted in diabetic individuals with any of the following: age >35 years, diabetes duration >15 years (type 1 DM) or >10 years (type 2 DM), microvascular complications of DM (retinopathy, microalbuminuria, or nephropathy), peripheral arterial disease, other risk factors of coronary artery disease, or autonomic neuropathy. Untreated proliferative retinopathy is a relative contraindication to vigorous exercise, as this may lead to vitreous hemorrhage or retinal detachment.

MONITORING THE LEVEL OF GLYCEMIC CONTROL   Optimal monitoring of glycemic control involves plasma glucose measurements by the patient and an assessment of long-term control by the physician (measurement of hemoglobin A1C and review of the patient's self-measurements of plasma glucose). These measurements are complementary: the patient's measurements provide a picture of short-term glycemic control, whereas the A1C reflects average glycemic control over the previous 2 to 3 months.

Self-Monitoring of Blood Glucose   Self-monitoring of blood glucose (SMBG) is the standard of care in diabetes management and allows the patient to monitor his or her blood glucose at any time. In SMBG, a small drop of blood and an easily detectable enzymatic reaction allow measurement of the capillary plasma glucose. A number of devices accurately measure glucose in blood obtained from the fingertip; al-

---

TABLE 323-8   Nutritional Recommendations for All Persons with Diabetes

- Protein to provide ~15–20% of kcal/d (~10% for those with nephropathy)
- Saturated fat to provide <10% of kcal/d (<7% for those with elevated LDL)
- Polyunsaturated fat to provide ~10% of kcal; avoid trans-unsaturated fatty acids
- 60–70% of calories to be divided between carbohydrate and monounsaturated fat, based on medical needs and personal tolerance; glycemic index of food not as important
- Use of caloric sweeteners, including sucrose, is acceptable.
- Fiber (20–35 g/d) and sodium (≤3000 mg/d) levels as recommended for the general healthy population
- Cholesterol intake ≤300 mg/d
- The same precautions regarding alcohol use in the general population also apply to individuals with diabetes. Alcohol may increase risk for hypoglycemia and therefore should be taken with food.

Note: LDL, low-density lipoprotein.
Source: Adapted from R Farkas-Hirsch, *Intensive Diabetes Management*, Alexandria, VA, American Diabetes Association, 1998; and American Diabetes Association: Diabetes Care 25:S1, 2002.

ternative testing sites (e.g., forearm) are less reliable. By combining glucose measurements with diet history, medication changes, and exercise history, the physician and patient can improve the treatment program.

The frequency of SMBG measurements must be individualized and adapted to address the goals of diabetes care. Individuals with type 1 DM should routinely measure their plasma glucose four to eight times per day to estimate and select mealtime boluses of short-acting insulin and to modify long-acting insulin doses. Most individuals with type 2 DM require less frequent monitoring, though the optimal frequency of SMBG has not been clearly defined. Individuals with type 2 DM who are on oral medications should utilize SMBG as a means of assessing the efficacy of their medication and the impact of diet. Since plasma glucose levels fluctuate less in these individuals, one to two SMBG measurements per day (or fewer) may be sufficient. Individuals with type 2 DM who are on insulin should utilize SMBG more frequently than those on oral agents. Urine glucose testing does not provide an accurate assessment of glycemic control.

Two devices for continuous blood glucose monitoring have been recently approved by the U.S. Food and Drug Administration (FDA). The Glucowatch uses iontophoresis to assess glucose in interstitial fluid, whereas the Minimed device uses an indwelling subcutaneous catheter to monitor interstitial fluid glucose. Both devices utilize immobilized glucose oxidase to generate electrons in response to changing glucose levels. Though clinical experience with these devices is limited, they perform well in clinical trials and appear to provide useful short-term information about the patterns of glucose changes as well as an enhanced ability to detect hypoglycemic episodes. These devices are not yet used routinely in diabetes management.

Ketones are an indicator of early diabetic ketoacidosis and should be measured in individuals with type 1 DM when the plasma glucose is consistently >16.7 mmol/L (300 mg/dL), during a concurrent illness; or with symptoms such as nausea, vomiting, or abdominal pain. Blood measurement of β-hydroxybutyrate is preferred over urine testing with nitroprusside-based assays that measure only acetoacetate and acetone.

Assessment of Long-Term Glycemic Control   Measurement of glycated hemoglobin is the standard method for assessing long-term glycemic control. When plasma glucose is consistently elevated, there is an increase in nonenzymatic glycation of hemoglobin; this alteration reflects the glycemic history over the previous 2 to 3 months, since erythrocytes have an average life span of 120 days. There are numerous laboratory methods for measuring the various forms of glycated hemoglobin, and these have significant interassay variations. Since glycated hemoglobin measurements are usually compared to prior measurements, it is essential for the assay results to be comparable. Depending on the assay methodology, hemoglobinopathies, anemias, and uremia may interfere with the A1C result.

Glycated hemoglobin or A1C should be measured in all individuals with DM during their initial evaluation and as part of their comprehensive diabetes care. As the primary predictor of long-term complications of DM, the A1C should mirror, to a certain extent, the short-term measurements of SMBG. These two measurements are complementary in that recent intercurrent illnesses may impact the SMBG measurements but not the A1C. Likewise, postprandial and nocturnal hyperglycemia may not be detected by the SMBG of fasting and preprandial capillary plasma glucose but will be reflected in the A1C. In standardized assays, the A1C approximates the following mean plasma glucose values: an A1C of 6% is 7.5 mmol/L (135 mg/dL), 7% is 9.5 mmol/L (170 mg/dL), 8% is 11.5 mmol/L (205 mg/dL), etc. [A 1% rise in the A1C translates into a 2.0-mmol/L (35 mg/dL) increase in the mean glucose.] In patients achieving their glycemic goal, the ADA recommends measurement of the A1C twice per year. More frequent testing (every 3 months) is warranted when glycemic control is inadequate, when therapy has changed, or in most patients

with type 1 DM. The degree of glycation of other proteins, such as albumin, has been used as an alternative indicator of glycemic control when the A1C is inaccurate (hemolytic anemia, hemoglobinopathies). The fructosamine assay (measuring glycated albumin) reflects the glycemic status over the prior 2 weeks. Current consensus statements do not favor the use of alternative assays of glycemic control, as there are no studies to indicate whether such assays accurately predict the complications of DM.

℞ TREATMENT

ESTABLISHMENT OF A TARGET LEVEL OF GLYCEMIC CONTROL   Because the complications of DM are related to glycemic control, normoglycemia or near normoglycemia is the desired, but often elusive, goal for most patients. However, normalization of the plasma glucose for long periods of time is extremely difficult, as demonstrated by the DCCT. Regardless of the level of hyperglycemia, improvement in glycemic control will lower the risk of diabetes complications (Fig. 323-8).

The target for glycemic control (as reflected by the A1C) must be individualized, and the goals of therapy should be developed in consultation with the patient after considering a number of medical, social, and life-style issues. Some important factors to consider include the patient's age, ability to understand and implement a complex treatment regimen, presence and severity of complications of diabetes, ability to recognize hypoglycemic symptoms, presence of other medical conditions or treatments that might alter the response to therapy, life-style and occupation (e.g., possible consequences of experiencing hypoglycemia on the job), and level of support available from family and friends.

The ADA has established suggested glycemic goals based on the premise that glycemic control predicts development of DM-related complications. In general, the target A1C should be <7.0% (Table 323-9). Other consensus groups (such as the Veterans Administration) have suggested A1C goals that take into account the patient's life expectancy at the time of diagnosis and the presence of microvascular complications. Such recommendations strive to balance the financial and personal costs of glycemic therapy with anticipated benefits (reduced health care costs, reduced morbidity). One limitation to this approach is that the onset of hyperglycemia in type 2 DM is difficult to ascertain and likely predates the diagnosis.

TYPE 1 DIABETES MELLITUS ■ **General Aspects**   The ADA recommendations for fasting and bedtime glycemic goals and A1C targets are summarized in Table 323-9. The goal is to design and implement insulin regimens that mimic physiologic insulin secretion. Because individuals with type 1 DM lack endogenous insulin production, administration of basal, exogenous insulin is essential for regulating glycogen breakdown, gluconeogenesis, lipolysis, and ketogenesis. Likewise, insulin replacement for meals should be appropriate for the carbohydrate intake and promote normal glucose utilization and storage.

Intensive Management   Intensive diabetes management has the goal of achieving euglycemia or near-normal glycemia. This approach requires multiple resources including thorough and continuing patient education, comprehensive recording of plasma glucose measurements and nutrition intake by the patient, and a variable insulin regimen that

---

TABLE 323-9   *Ideal Goals for Glycemic Control*[a]

Index	Goal
Preprandial plasma glucose, mmol/L (mg/dL)	5.0–7.2 (90–130)
Peak postprandial plasma glucose, mmol/L (mg/dL)	<10 (<180)
A1C, %	<7

[a] Plasma glucose values are 10–15% higher than whole blood values. The upper limit of the A1C reference range is 6.0% (mean 5.0%, with a standard deviation of 0.5%). These goals must be individualized for each patient and must consider the patient's age and other medical conditions.

Note: A1C, hemoglobin A1c.

Source: Adapted from American Diabetes Association, 2003.

TABLE 323-10 *Indications for Intensive Diabetes Management*

- Otherwise healthy adults with either type 1 or type 2 diabetes (selected adolescents and older children)
- Purposeful, therapeutic attempt to avoid or lessen microvascular complications
- All pregnant women with diabetes; all women with diabetes who are planning pregnancy
- Management of labile diabetes
- Availability of health care professionals with appropriate expertise
- Patients who have had kidney transplantation for diabetic nephropathy

Source: Adapted from R Farkas-Hirsch: *Intensive Diabetes Management*, Alexandria, VA American Diabetes Association, 1998.

matches glucose intake and insulin dose. Insulin regimens usually include multiple-component insulin regimens, multiple daily injections (MDI), or insulin infusion devices (each discussed below).

The benefits of intensive diabetes management and improved glycemic control include a reduction in the microvascular complications of DM and a possible delay or reduction in the macrovascular complications of DM. From a psychological standpoint, the patient experiences greater control over his or her diabetes and often notes an improved sense of well-being, greater flexibility in the timing and content of meals, and the capability to alter insulin dosing with exercise. In addition, intensive diabetes management in pregnancy reduces the risk of fetal malformations and morbidity. Intensive diabetes management is strongly encouraged in newly diagnosed patients with type 1 DM because it may prolong the period of C-peptide production, which may result in better glycemic control and a reduced risk of serious hypoglycemia.

Although intensive management confers impressive benefits, it is also accompanied by significant personal and financial costs and is therefore not appropriate for all individuals. Circumstances in which intensive diabetes management should be strongly considered are listed in Table 323-10.

Insulin Preparations Current insulin preparations are generated by recombinant DNA technology and consist of the amino acid sequence of human insulin or variations thereof. Animal insulin (beef or pork) is no longer used. Human insulin has been formulated with distinctive pharmacokinetics to mimic physiologic insulin secretion (Table 323-11). In the United States, all insulin is formulated as U-100 (100 units/mL), whereas in some other countries it is available in other units (e.g., U-40 = 40 units/mL). One short-acting insulin formulation, lispro, is an insulin analogue in which the 28th and 29th amino acids (lysine and proline) on the insulin B chain have been reversed by recombinant DNA technology. Insulin aspart is another genetically modified insulin analogue with very similar properties to lispro. These insulin analogues have full biologic activity but less tendency toward subcutaneous aggregation, resulting in more rapid absorption and onset of action and a shorter duration of action. These characteristics are particularly advantageous for allowing entrainment of insulin injection and action to rising plasma glucose levels following meals. The shorter duration of action also appears to be associated with a decreased number of hypoglycemic episodes, primarily because the decay of lispro action corresponds to the decline in plasma glucose after a meal. Insulin glargine is a long-acting biosynthetic human insulin that differs from normal insulin in that asparagine is replaced by glycine at amino acid 21, and two arginine residues are added to the C-terminus of the B chain. Compared to NPH insulin, the onset of insulin glargine action is later, the duration of action is longer (~24 h), and there is no pronounced

peak. A lower incidence of hypoglycemia, especially at night, has been reported with insulin glargine when compared to NPH insulin. Additional insulin analogues are currently under development.

Basal insulin requirements are provided by intermediate (NPH insulin or lente insulin) or long-acting (ultralente insulin or insulin glargine) insulin formulations. These are usually combined with short-acting insulin in an attempt to mimic physiologic insulin release with meals. Although mixing of intermediate and short-acting insulin formulations is common practice, this mixing may alter the insulin absorption profile (especially the short-acting insulins). For example, the absorption of regular insulin is delayed when mixed for even short periods of time (<5 min) with lente or ultralente insulin, but not when mixed with NPH insulin. Lispro absorption is delayed by mixing with NPH but not ultralente. Insulin glargine should not be mixed with other insulins and is not stable at room temperature. The miscibility of human regular and NPH insulin allows for the production of combination insulins that contain 70% NPH and 30% regular (70/30) or equal mixtures of NPH and regular (50/50). These combinations of insulin are more convenient for the patient but prevent adjustment of only one component of the insulin formulation. The alteration in insulin absorption when the patient mixes different insulin formulation should not discourage the patient from mixing insulin. However, the following guidelines should be followed: (1) mix the different insulin formulations in the syringe immediately before injection (inject within 2 min after mixing); (2) do not store insulin as a mixture; and (3) follow the same routine in terms of insulin mixing and administration to standardize the physiologic response to injected insulin. Several insulin formulations are available as insulin "pens," which may be more convenient for some patients.

Insulin Regimens Representations of the various insulin regimens that may be utilized in type 1 DM are illustrated in Fig. 323-13. Although the insulin profiles are depicted as "smooth," symmetric curves, there is considerable patient to patient variation in the peak and duration. In all regimens, intermediate- or long-acting insulins (NPH, lente, ultralente, or glargine insulin) supply basal insulin, whereas regular, insulin aspart, or lispro insulin provides prandial insulin. Lispro and insulin aspart should be injected just before or just after a meal; regular insulin is given 30 to 45 min prior to a meal.

A shortcoming of current insulin regimens is that injected insulin immediately enters the systemic circulation, whereas endogenous insulin is secreted into the portal venous system. Thus, exogenous insulin administration exposes the liver to subphysiologic insulin levels. No insulin regimen reproduces the precise insulin secretory pattern of

TABLE 323-11 *Pharmacokinetics of Insulin Preparations*

Preparation	Time of Action		
	Onset, h	Peak, h	Effective Duration, h
Short-acting			
Lispro	<0.25	0.5–1.5	3–4
Insulin aspart	<0.25	0.5–1.5	3–4
Regular	0.5–1.0	2–3	3–6
Intermediate-acting			
NPH	2–4	6–10	10–16
Lente	3–4	6–12	12–18
Long-acting			
Ultralente	6–10	10–16	18–20
Glargine	4	—[a]	24
Combinations			
75/25–75% protamine lispro, 25% lispro	0.5–1	Dual	10–14
70/30–70% NPH, 30% regular	0.5–1	Dual	10–16
50/50–50% NPH, 50% regular	0.5–1	Dual	10–16

[a] Glargine has minimal peak activity.
Source: Adapted from JS Skyler, *Therapy for Diabetes Mellitus and Related Disorders*, American Diabetes Association, Alexandria, VA, 1998.

FIGURE 323-13 Representative insulin regimens for the treatment of diabetes. For each panel, the y-axis shows the amount of insulin effect and the x-axis shows the time of day. B, breakfast; L, lunch; S, supper; HS, bedtime; CSII, continuous subcutaneous insulin infusion. *either lispro or insulin aspart can be used. The time of insulin injection is shown with a vertical arrow. The type of insulin is noted above each insulin curve. A. The injection of two shots of intermediate-acting insulin (NPH or lente) and short-acting insulin (lispro, insulin aspart, or regular). Only one formulation of short-acting insulin is used. B: A multiple-component insulin regimen consisting of one shot of glargine at bedtime to provide basal insulin coverage and three shots of lispro or insulin aspart to provide glycemic coverage for each meal. C: Insulin administration by insulin infusion device is shown with the basal insulin and a bolus injection at each meal. The basal insulin rate is decreased during the evening and increased slightly prior to the patient awakening in the morning. (*Adapted from Intensive Diabetes Management, 2d ed, R. Farkas-Hirsch (ed). Alexandria, VA, American Diabetes Association, 1998.*)

the pancreatic islet. However, the most physiologic regimens entail more frequent insulin injections, greater reliance on short-acting insulin, and more frequent capillary plasma glucose measurements. In general, individuals with type 1 DM require 0.5 to 1.0 U/kg per day of insulin divided into multiple doses. Initial insulin-dosing regimens should be conservative; approximately 40 to 50% of the insulin should be given as basal insulin. A single daily injection of insulin is not appropriate therapy in type 1 DM.

One commonly used regimen consists of twice-daily injections of an intermediate insulin (NPH or lente) mixed with a short-acting insulin before the morning and evening meal (Fig. 323-13A). Such regimens usually prescribe two-thirds of the total daily insulin dose in the morning (with about two-thirds given as intermediate-acting insulin and one-third as short-acting) and one-third before the evening meal (with approximately one-half given as intermediate-acting insulin and one-half as short-acting). The drawback to such a regimen is that it enforces a rigid schedule on the patient, in terms of daily activity and the content and timing of meals. Although it is simple and effective at avoiding severe hyperglycemia, it does not generate near-normal glycemic control in most individuals with type 1 DM. Moreover, if the patient's meal pattern or content varies or if physical activity is increased, hyperglycemia or hypoglycemia may result. Moving the intermediate insulin from before the evening meal to bedtime may avoid nocturnal hypoglycemia and provide more insulin as glucose levels rise in the early morning (so-called dawn phenomenon). The insulin dose in such regimens should be adjusted based on SMBG results with the following general assumptions: (1) the fasting glucose is primarily determined by the prior evening intermediate-acting insulin; (2) the pre-lunch glucose is a function of the morning short-acting insulin; (3) the pre-supper glucose is a function of the morning intermediate-acting insulin; and (4) the bedtime glucose is a function of the pre-supper, short-acting insulin.

Multiple-component insulin regimens refer to the combination of basal insulin; preprandial short-acting insulin; and changes in short-acting insulin doses to accommodate the results of frequent SMBG, anticipated food intake, and physical activity. Also referred to as MDI, such regimens offer the patient more flexibility in terms of life-style and the best chance for achieving near normoglycemia. One such regimen, shown in Fig. 323-13B, consists of a basal insulin with glargine at bedtime and preprandial lispro or insulin aspart. The lispro or insulin aspart dose is based on individualized algorithms that integrate the preprandial glucose and the anticipated carbohydrate intake. An alternative regimen is two equal doses of ultralente (breakfast and evening; 10 to 12 h apart) and preprandial lispro or insulin aspart. Another alternative multiple-component insulin regimen consists of bedtime intermediate insulin, a small dose of intermediate insulin at breakfast (20 to 30 % of bedtime dose), and preprandial short-acting insulin. There are numerous variations of these regimens that can be optimized for individual patients. Frequent SMBG (four to eight times per day) is absolutely essential for these types of insulin regimens.

Continuous subcutaneous insulin infusion (CSII) is another mul-

tiple-component insulin regimen (Fig. 323-13C). Sophisticated insulin infusion devices can accurately deliver small doses of insulin (microliters per hour). For example, multiple basal infusion rates can be programmed to: (1) accommodate nocturnal versus daytime basal insulin requirement, (2) alter infusion rate during periods of exercise, or (3) select different waveforms of insulin infusion. A preprandial insulin ("bolus") is delivered by the insulin infusion device based on instructions from the patient, which follow individualized algorithms that account for preprandial plasma glucose and anticipated carbohydrate intake. These devices require a health professional with considerable experience with insulin infusion devices and very frequent patient interactions with the diabetes management team. Insulin infusion devices present unique challenges, such as infection at the infusion site, unexplained hyperglycemia because the infusion set becomes obstructed, or diabetic ketoacidosis if the pump becomes disconnected. Since most physicians use lispro or insulin aspart in CSII, the extremely short half-life of these insulins quickly lead to insulin deficiency if the delivery system is interrupted. Essential to the safe use of infusion devices is thorough patient education about pump function and frequent SMBG.

TYPE 2 DIABETES MELLITUS ■ General Aspects The goals of therapy for type 2 DM are similar to those in type 1. While glycemic control tends to dominate the management of type 1 DM, the care of individuals with type 2 DM must also include attention to the treatment of conditions associated with type 2 DM (obesity, hypertension, dyslipidemia, cardiovascular disease) and detection/management of DM-related complications (Fig. 323-14). DM-specific complications may be present in up to 20 to 50% of individuals with newly diagnosed type 2 DM. Reduction in cardiovascular risk is of paramount importance as this is the leading cause of mortality in these individuals.

Diabetes management should begin with MNT (discussed above). An exercise regimen to increase insulin sensitivity and promote weight loss should also be instituted. After MNT and increased physical ac-

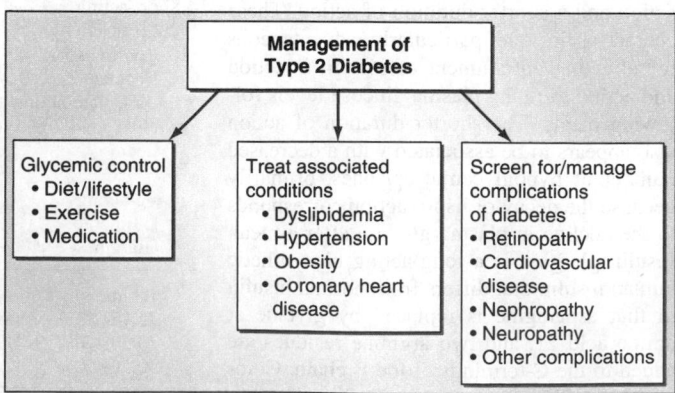

FIGURE 323-14 Essential elements in comprehensive diabetes care of type 2 diabetes.

tivity have been instituted, glycemic control should be reassessed; if the patient's glycemic target is not achieved after 3 to 4 weeks of MNT, pharmacologic therapy is indicated. Pharmacologic approaches to the management of type 2 DM include both oral glucose-lowering agents and insulin; most physicians and patients prefer oral glucose-lowering agents as the initial choice. Any therapy that improves glycemic control reduces "glucose toxicity" to the islet cells and improves endogenous insulin secretion. However, type 2 DM is a progressive disorder and ultimately requires multiple therapeutic agents and often insulin.

Glucose-Lowering Agents Advances in the therapy of type 2 DM have generated considerable enthusiasm for oral glucose-lowering agents that target different pathophysiologic processes in type 2 DM. Based on their mechanisms of action, oral glucose-lowering agents are subdivided into agents that increase insulin secretion, reduce glucose production, or increase insulin sensitivity (Table 323-12). Oral glucose-lowering agents (with the exception of α-glucosidase inhibitors) are ineffective in type 1 DM and should not be used for glucose management of severely ill individuals with type 2 DM. Insulin is sometimes the initial glucose-lowering agent.

INSULIN SECRETAGOGUES Insulin secretagogues stimulate insulin secretion by interacting with the ATP-sensitive potassium channel on the beta cell (Fig. 323-1). These drugs are most effective in individuals with type 2 DM of relatively recent onset (<5 years), who tend to be obese and have residual endogenous insulin production. At maximum doses, first-generation sulfonylureas are similar in potency to second-generation agents but have a longer half-life, a greater incidence of hypoglycemia, and more frequent drug interactions (Table 323-13). Thus, second-generation sulfonylureas are generally preferred. An advantage to a more rapid onset of action is better coverage of the postprandial glucose rise, but the shorter half-life of such agents requires more than once-a-day dosing. Sulfonylureas reduce both fasting and postprandial glucose and should be initiated at low doses and increased at 1- to 2-week intervals based on SMBG. In general, sulfonylureas increase

insulin acutely and thus should be taken shortly before a meal; with chronic therapy, though, the insulin release is more sustained. Repaglinide and nateglinide are not sulfonylureas but also interact with the ATP-sensitive potassium channel. Because of their short half-life, these agents are given with each meal or immediately before to reduce meal-related glucose excursions.

Insulin secretagogues are generally well tolerated. All of these agents, however, have the potential to cause profound and persistent hypoglycemia, especially in elderly individuals. Hypoglycemia is usually related to delayed meals, increased physical activity, alcohol intake, or renal insufficiency. Individuals who ingest an overdose of some agents develop prolonged and serious hypoglycemia and should be monitored closely in the hospital (Chap. 324). Most sulfonylureas are metabolized in the liver to compounds that are cleared by the kidney. Thus, their use in individuals with significant hepatic or renal dysfunction is not advisable. Weight gain, a common side effect of sulfonylurea therapy, results from the increased insulin levels and improvement in glycemic control. Some sulfonylureas have significant drug interactions with alcohol and some medications including warfarin, aspirin, ketoconazole, α-glucosidase inhibitors, and fluconazole. Despite prior concerns that use of sulfonylureas might increase cardiovascular risk, most recent trials have refuted this claim.

BIGUANIDES Metformin is representative of this class of agents. It reduces hepatic glucose production through an undefined mechanism and improves peripheral glucose utilization slightly (Table 323-12). Metformin reduces fasting plasma glucose and insulin levels, improves the lipid profile, and promotes modest weight loss. The initial starting dose of 500 mg once or twice a day can be increased to 1000 mg bid. An extended-release form and a combination formulation with glyburide and glipizid are available. Because of its relatively slow onset of action and gastrointestinal symptoms with higher doses, the dose

TABLE 323-12 *Oral Glucose-Lowering Therapies in Type 2 Diabetes*

	Mechanism of Action	Examples	Anticipated Reduction in A1C, %	Agent-Specific Advantages	Agent-Specific Disadvantages	Contraindications
Insulin secretagogues	↑ Insulin		1–2			
Sulfonylureas		See Table 323-13		Lower fasting blood glucose	Hypoglycemia weight gain, hyperinsulinemia	Renal/liver disease
Nonsulfonylureas		See Table 323-13		Short onset of action, lower postprandial glucose	Hypoglycemia	Renal/liver disease
Biguanides	↓ Hepatic glucose production, weight loss, ↑ glucose utilization, ↓ insulin resistance	Metformin	1–2	Weight loss, improved lipid profile, no hypoglycemia	Lactic acidosis, diarrhea, nausea	Serum creatinine >1.5 mg/dL (men), >1.4 mg/dL (women), radiographic contrast studies, seriously ill patients, acidosis
α-Glucosidase inhibitors	↓ Glucose absorption	Acarbose, miglitol	0.5–1.0	No risk of hypoglycemia	GI flatulence, ↑ liver function tests	Renal/liver disease
Thiazolidinediones	↓ Insulin resistance, ↑ glucose utilization	Rosiglitazone, pioglitazone	1–2	↓ Insulin and sulfonylurea requirements, ↓ triglycerides	Frequent hepatic monitoring for idiosyncratic hepatocellular injury (see text)	Liver disease, congestive heart failure
Medical nutrition therapy and physical activity	↓ Insulin resistance	Low-calorie, low-fat diet, exercise	1–2	Other health benefits	Compliance difficult, long-term success low	

Note: A1C, hemoglobin A1c.

TABLE 323-13   *Characteristics of Agents that Increase Insulin Secretion*

Generic Name	Approved Daily Dosage Range, mg	Duration of Action, h	Clearance
Sulfonylurea—first generation			
Chlorpropamide	100–500	>48	Renal
Tolazamide	100–1000	12–24	Hepatic, renal
Tolbutamide	500–3000	6–12	Hepatic
Sulfonylurea—second generation			
Glimepiride	1–8	24	Hepatic, renal
Glipizide	2.5–40	12–18	Hepatic
Glipizide (extended release)	5–10	24	Hepatic
Glyburide	1.25–20	12–24	Hepatic, renal
Glyburide (micronized)	0.75–12	12–24	Hepatic, renal
Nonsulfonylureas			
Repaglinide	0.5–16	2–6	Hepatic
Nateglinide	180–360	2–4	Renal

Source: Adapted from BR Zimmerman (ed): *Medical Management of Type 2 Diabetes*, 4th ed. Alexandria, VA, American Diabetes Association, 1998.

should be escalated every 2 to 3 weeks based on SMBG measurements. The major toxicity of metformin, lactic acidosis, can be prevented by careful patient selection. Metformin should not be used in patients with renal insufficiency [serum creatinine >133 μmol/L (1.5 mg/dL) in men or >124 μmol/L (1.4 mg/dL) in women, with adjustments for age], any form of acidosis, congestive heart failure, liver disease, or severe hypoxia. Metformin should be discontinued in patients who are seriously ill, in patients who can take nothing orally, and in those receiving radiographic contrast material. Insulin should be used until metformin can be restarted. Though well tolerated in general, some individuals develop gastrointestinal side effects (diarrhea, anorexia, nausea, and metallic taste) that can be minimized by gradual dose escalation. Because the drug is metabolized in the liver, it should not be used in patients with liver disease or heavy ethanol intake.

α-GLUCOSIDASE INHIBITORS   α-Glucosidase inhibitors (acarbose and miglitol) reduce postprandial hyperglycemia by delaying glucose absorption; they do not affect glucose utilization or insulin secretion (Table 323-12). Postprandial hyperglycemia, secondary to impaired hepatic and peripheral glucose disposal, contributes significantly to the hyperglycemic state in type 2 DM. These drugs, taken just before each meal, reduce glucose absorption by inhibiting the enzyme that cleaves oligosaccharides into simple sugars in the intestinal lumen. Therapy should be initiated at a low dose (25 mg of acarbose or miglitol) with the evening meal and may be increased to a maximal dose over weeks to months (50 to 100 mg for acarbose or 50 mg for miglitol with each meal). The major side effects (diarrhea, flatulence, abdominal distention) are related to increased delivery of oligosaccharides to the large bowel and can be reduced somewhat by gradual upward dose titration. α-Glucosidase inhibitors may increase levels of sulfonylureas and increase the incidence of hypoglycemia. Simultaneous treatment with bile acid resins and antacids should be avoided. These agents should not be used in individuals with inflammatory bowel disease, gastroparesis, or a serum creatinine >177 μmol/L (2.0 mg/dL). This class of agents is not as potent as other oral agents in lowering the hemoglobin A1C but is unique because it reduces the postprandial glucose rise even in individuals with type 1 DM. If hypoglycemia occurs while taking these agents, the patient should consume glucose since the degradation and absorption of complex carbohydrates will be retarded.

THIAZOLIDINEDIONES   Thiazolidinediones reduce insulin resistance. These drugs bind to the PPAR-γ (peroxisome proliferator-activated receptor-γ) nuclear receptor. The PPAR-γ receptor is found at highest levels in adipocytes but is expressed at lower levels in many other tissues. Agonists of this receptor promote adipocyte differentiation and may re-

duce insulin resistance indirectly because of enhanced fatty acid uptake and storage (Table 323-12). Circulating insulin levels decrease with use of the thiazolidinediones, indicating a reduction in insulin resistance. Although direct comparisons are not available, the two currently available thiazolidinediones appear to have similar efficacy; the therapeutic range for pioglitazone is 15 to 45 mg/d in a single daily dose and for rosiglitazone the total daily dose is 2 to 8 mg/d administered either once daily or twice daily in divided doses. The ability of thiazolidinediones to influence other features of the insulin resistance syndrome is under investigation.

The prototype of this class of drugs, troglitazone, was withdrawn from the U.S. market after reports of hepatotoxicity and an association with an idiosyncratic liver reaction that sometimes led to hepatic failure. Although rosiglitazone and pioglitazone do not appear to induce the liver abnormalities seen with troglitazone, the FDA recommends measurement of liver function tests prior to initiating therapy with a thiazolidinedione and at regular intervals (every 2 months for the first year and then periodically). The thiazolidinediones raise LDL and HDL slightly and lower triglycerides by 10 to 15%, but the clinical significance of these changes is not known. Thiazolidinediones are associated with minor weight gain (1 to 2 kg), a small reduction in the hematocrit, and a mild increase in plasma volume. Cardiac function is not affected, but peripheral edema CHF may occur and is more common in individuals treated with insulin. They are contraindicated in patients with liver disease or congestive heart failure (class III or IV). Thiazolidinediones have been shown to induce ovulation in premenopausal women with PCOS. Women should be warned about the risk of pregnancy, since the safety of thiazolidinediones in pregnancy is not established.

INSULIN THERAPY IN TYPE 2 DM   Insulin should be considered as the initial therapy in type 2 DM, particularly in lean individuals or those with severe weight loss, in individuals with underlying renal or hepatic disease that precludes oral glucose-lowering agents, or in individuals who are hospitalized or acutely ill. Insulin therapy is ultimately required by a substantial number of individuals with type 2 DM because of the progressive nature of the disorder and the relative insulin deficiency that develops in patients with long-standing diabetes.

Because endogenous insulin secretion continues and is capable of providing some coverage of mealtime caloric intake, insulin is usually initiated in a single dose of intermediate- or long-acting insulin (0.3 to 0.4 U/kg per day), given either before breakfast (NPH, lente, or ultralente) or just before bedtime (NPH, lente, ultralente, or glargine). Since fasting hyperglycemia and increased hepatic glucose production are prominent features of type 2 DM, bedtime insulin is more effective in clinical trials than a single dose of morning insulin. Some physicians prefer a relatively low, fixed starting dose of intermediate-acting insulin (~15 to 20 units in the morning and 5 to 10 units at bedtime) to avoid hypoglycemia. The insulin dose may then be adjusted in 10% increments as dictated by SMBG results. Both morning and bedtime intermediate insulin may be used in combination with oral glucose-lowering agents (biguanides, α-glucosidase inhibitors, or thiazolidinediones).

CHOICE OF INITIAL GLUCOSE-LOWERING AGENT   The level of hyperglycemia should influence the initial choice of therapy. Assuming maximal benefit of MNT and increased physical activity has been realized, patients with mild to moderate hyperglycemia [fasting plasma glucose <11.1 to 13.9 mmol/L (200 to 250 mg/dL)] often respond well to a single oral glucose-lowering agent. Patients with more severe hyperglycemia [fasting plasma glucose >13.9 mmol/L (250 mg/dL)] may respond partially but are unlikely to achieve normoglycemia with oral monotherapy. A stepwise approach that starts with a single agent and adds a second agent to achieve the glycemic target can be used (see "Combination Therapy," below). Insulin can be used as initial therapy in individuals with severe hyperglycemia [fasting plasma glucose >13.9 to 16.7 mmol/L (250 to 300 mg/dL)]. This approach is based on the rationale that more rapid glycemic control will reduce "glucose toxicity" to the islet cells, improve endogenous insulin secretion, and possibly allow oral glucose-lowering agents to be more effective. If this occurs, the insulin may be discontinued.

Insulin secretagogues, biguanides, α-glucosidase inhibitors, thiazolidinediones, and insulin are approved for monotherapy of type 2 DM. Although each class of oral glucose-lowering agents has unique advantages and disadvantages, certain generalizations apply: (1) insulin secretagogues, biguanides, and thiazolidinediones improve glycemic control to a similar degree (1 to 2% reduction in A1C) and are more effective than α-glucosidase inhibitors; (2) assuming a similar degree of glycemic improvement, no clinical advantage to one class of drugs has been demonstrated, and any therapy that improves glycemic control is likely beneficial; (3) insulin secretagogues and α-glucosidase inhibitors begin to lower the plasma glucose immediately, whereas the glucose-lowering effects of the biguanides and thiazolidinediones are delayed by several weeks to months; (4) not all agents are effective in all individuals with type 2 DM (primary failure); (5) biguanides, α-glucosidase inhibitors, and thiazolidinediones do not directly cause hypoglycemia; and (6) most individuals will eventually require treatment with more than one class of oral glucose-lowering agents or insulin, reflecting the progressive nature of type 2 DM.

Considerable clinical experience exists with sulfonylureas and metformin because they have been available for several decades. It is assumed that the α-glucosidase inhibitors and thiazolidinediones, which are newer classes of oral glucose-lowering drugs, will reduce DM-related complications by improving glycemic control, although long-term data are not yet available. The thiazolidinediones are theoretically attractive because they target a fundamental abnormality in type 2 DM, namely insulin resistance. However, these agents are currently more costly than others and require liver function monitoring.

A reasonable treatment algorithm for initial therapy proposes either a sulfonylurea or metformin as initial therapy because of their efficacy, known side-effect profile, and relatively low cost (Fig. 323-14). Metformin has the advantage that it promotes mild weight loss, lowers insulin levels, improves the lipid profile slightly, and may have a lower secondary failure rate. Metformin is the initial choice of many physicians for the treatment of the obese, type 2 diabetic. However, there is no difference in response rate or degree of glycemic control when metformin and sulfonylureas are compared in randomized, prospective clinical trials. Based on SMBG results and the A1C, the dose of either the sulfonylurea or metformin should be increased until the glycemic target is achieved. Thiazolidinediones are alternative, initial agents, but are much more expensive; α-glucosidase inhibitors are the least potent agents and not as desirable for monotherapy (Fig. 323-15).

Approximately one-third of individuals will reach their target glycemic goal using either a sulfonylurea or metformin as monotherapy. Approximately 25% of individuals will not respond to sulfonylureas or metformin; under these circumstances, the drug usually should be discontinued. Some individuals respond to one agent but not the other. The remaining individuals treated with either sulfonylureas or metformin alone will exhibit some improvement in glycemic control but will not achieve their glycemic target and should be considered for combination therapy.

COMBINATION THERAPY WITH GLUCOSE-LOWERING AGENTS A number of combinations of therapeutic agents are successful in type 2 DM, and the dosing of agents in combination is the same as when the agents are used alone. Because mechanisms of action of the first and second agents are different, the effect on glycemic control is usually additive. Commonly used regimens include: (1) insulin secretagogue with metformin or thiazolidinedione, (2) sulfonylurea with α-glucosidase inhibitor, and (3) insulin with metformin or thiazolidinedione. The combination of metformin and a thiazolidinedione is also effective and complementary. If adequate control is not achieved with two oral agents, bedtime insulin or a third oral agent may be added stepwise. However, long-term experience with any triple combination is lacking, and experience with two-drug combinations is relatively limited.

Insulin becomes required as type 2 DM enters the phase of relative insulin deficiency (as seen in long-standing DM) and is signaled by

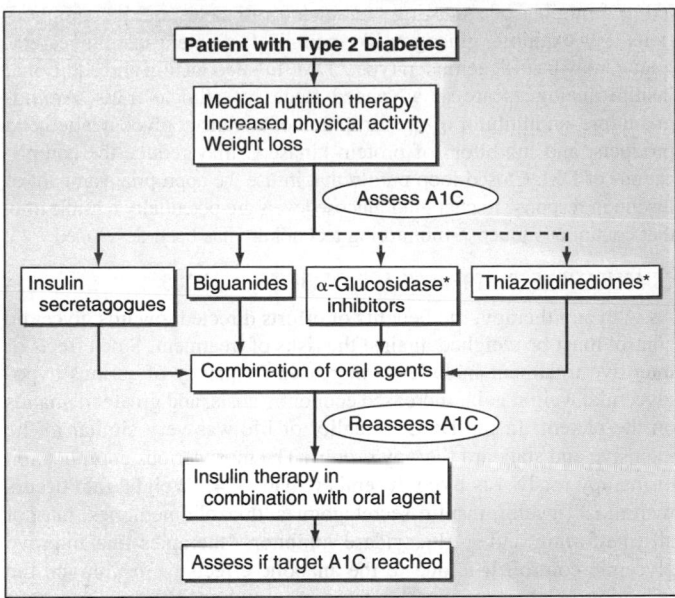

FIGURE 323-15 Glycemic management of type 2 diabetes. See text for discussion. *See text about use as monotherapy. The broken line indicates that biguanides or insulin secretagogues, but not α glucosidase inhibitors or thiazolidinediones, are preferred for initial therapy. A1C, hemoglobin A1c.

inadequate glycemic control with one or two oral glucose-lowering agents. Insulin can be used in combination with any of the oral agents in patients who fail to reach the glycemic target. For example, a single dose of intermediate- or long-acting insulin at bedtime is effective in combination with metformin. As endogenous insulin production falls further, multiple injections of intermediate-acting and short-acting insulin regimens are necessary to control postprandial glucose excursions. These combination regimens are identical to the intermediate-, long-acting, and short-acting combination regimens discussed above for type 1 DM. Since the hyperglycemia of type 2 DM tends to be more "stable," these regimens can be increased in 10% increments every 2 to 3 days using SMBG results. The daily insulin dose required can become quite large (1 to 2 units/kg per day) as endogenous insulin production falls and insulin resistance persists. Individuals who require >1 unit/kg per day of intermediate-acting insulin should be considered for combination therapy with metformin or a thiazolidinedione. The addition of metformin or a thiazolidinedione can reduce insulin requirements in some individuals with type 2 DM, while maintaining or even improving glycemic control.

Intensive diabetes management (Table 323-10) is a treatment option in type 2 patients who cannot achieve optimal glycemic control and are capable of implementing such regimens. A recent study from the Veterans Administration found that intensive diabetes management is not associated with a greater degree of side effects (hypoglycemia, weight gain) than standard insulin therapy. The effect of higher insulin levels associated with intensive diabetes management on the prognosis of diseases commonly associated with type 2 DM (cardiovascular disease, hypertension) is still debated. In selected patients with type 2 DM, insulin pumps improve glycemic control and are well tolerated.

EMERGING THERAPIES Whole pancreas transplantation (conventionally performed concomitantly with a renal transplant) may normalize glucose tolerance and is an important therapeutic option in type 1 DM, though it requires substantial expertise and is associated with the side effects of immunosuppression. Pancreatic islet transplantation has been plagued by limitations in pancreatic islet isolation and graft survival, but recent advances in specific immunomodulation have greatly improved the results. Islet transplantation is an area of active clinical investigation.

New insights into normal mechanisms of glucose homeostasis have led to a number of emerging therapies for diabetes and its complications. For example, glucagon-like peptide 1, a potent insulin secretagogue, may be efficacious in type 2 DM. Inhaled insulin and additional insulin analogues are in advanced stages of clinical trials. Aminoguanidine, an inhibitor of the formation of advanced glycosylation end products, and inhibitors of protein kinase C may reduce the complications of DM. Closed-loop pumps that infuse the appropriate amount of insulin in response to changing glucose levels are potentially feasible now that continuous glucose-monitoring technology has been developed.

COMPLICATIONS OF THERAPY FOR DIABETES MELLITUS

As with any therapy, the benefits of efforts directed towards glycemic control must be weighed against the risks of treatment. Side effects of intensive treatment include an increased frequency of serious hypoglycemia, weight gain, increased economic costs, and greater demands on the patient. In the DCCT, quality of life was very similar in the intensive and standard therapy groups. The most serious complication of therapy for DM is hypoglycemia (Chap. 324). Weight gain occurs with most (insulin, insulin secretagogues, thiazolidinediones) but not all (metformin and α-glucosidase inhibitors) therapies that improve glycemic control. It is due to the anabolic effects of insulin and the reduction in glucosuria without a corresponding decrease in caloric intake. In the DCCT, individuals with the greatest weight gain exhibited increases in LDL cholesterol and triglycerides as well as increases in blood pressure (both systolic and diastolic) similar to those seen in individuals with type 2 DM and insulin resistance. These effects could increase the risk of cardiovascular disease in intensively managed patients. As discussed previously, transient worsening of diabetic retinopathy or neuropathy sometimes accompanies improved glycemic control.

ONGOING ASPECTS OF COMPREHENSIVE DIABETES CARE

The morbidity and mortality of DM-related complications can be greatly reduced by timely and consistent surveillance procedures (Table 323-14). These screening procedures are indicated for all individuals with DM, but numerous studies have documented that most individuals with diabetes do not receive comprehensive diabetes care. Screening for dyslipidemia and hypertension should be performed annually. In addition to routine health maintenance, individuals with diabetes should also receive the pneumococcal and tetanus vaccines (at recommended intervals) and the influenza vaccine (annually). As discussed above, aspirin therapy should be considered in many patients with diabetes.

An annual comprehensive eye examination should be performed by a qualified optometrist or ophthalmologist. If abnormalities are detected, further evaluation and treatment require an ophthalmologist skilled in diabetes-related eye disease. Because many individuals with type 2 DM have had asymptomatic diabetes for several years before diagnosis, the ADA recommends the following ophthalmologic examination schedule: (1) individuals with onset of DM at <29 years should have an initial eye examination within 3 to 5 years of diagnosis, (2) individuals with onset of DM at >30 years should have an initial eye examination at the time of diabetes diagnosis, and (3) women with DM who are contemplating pregnancy should have an eye examination prior to conception and during the first trimester.

An annual foot examination should: (1) assess blood flow, sensation (monofilament testing), and nail care; (2) look for the presence of foot deformities such as hammer or claw toes and Charcot foot; and (3) identify sites of potential ulceration. Calluses and nail deformities should be treated by a podiatrist; the patient should be discouraged from self-care of even minor foot problems. The ADA advises a visual foot inspection for potential problems at each outpatient visit.

An annual microalbuminuria measurement (albumin-to-creatinine ratio in spot urine) is advised in individuals with type 1 or type 2 DM and no protein on a routine urinalysis (Fig. 323-10). If the urinalysis detects proteinuria, the amount of protein should be quantified by standard urine protein measurements. If the urinalysis was negative for protein in the past, microalbuminuria should be the annual screening examination. Routine urine protein measurements do not detect low levels of albumin excretion. Screening should commence 5 years after the onset of type 1 DM and at the time of onset of type 2 DM.

SPECIAL CONSIDERATIONS IN DIABETES MELLITUS

PSYCHOSOCIAL ASPECTS   As with any chronic, debilitating disease, the individual with DM faces a series of challenges that affect all aspects of daily life. The individual with DM must accept that he or she may develop complications related to DM. Even with considerable effort, normoglycemia can be an elusive goal, and solutions to worsening glycemic control may not be easily identifiable. The patient should view him- or herself as an essential member of the diabetes care team and not as someone who is cared for by the diabetes team. Emotional stress may provoke a change in behavior so that individuals no longer adhere to a dietary, exercise, or therapeutic regimen. This can lead to the appearance of either hyper- or hypoglycemia. Depression and eating disorders, including binge eating disorders, bulimia, and anorexia nervosa, appear to occur more frequently individuals with type 1 or type 2 DM (Chap. 65).

MANAGEMENT IN THE HOSPITALIZED PATIENT   Virtually all medical and surgical subspecialties may be involved in the care of hospitalized patients with diabetes. Hyperglycemia, whether in an individual with known diabetes or in one without diabetes, may be a predictor of poor outcome in hospitalized patients. General anesthesia, surgery, and concurrent illness raise the levels of counterregulatory hormones (cortisol, growth hormone, catecholamines, and glucagon), and infection may lead to transient insulin resistance and hyperglycemia. These factors increase insulin requirements by increasing glucose production and impairing glucose utilization and thus may worsen glycemic control. The concurrent illness or surgical procedure may lead to variable insulin absorption and also prevent the patient with DM from eating normally and may promote hypoglycemia. Glycemic control should be assessed (with A1C) and, if feasible, should be optimized prior to surgery. Electrolytes, renal function, and intravascular volume status should be assessed as well. The high prevalence of asymptomatic cardiovascular disease in individuals with DM (especially in type 2 DM) may require preoperative cardiovascular evaluation. Maintenance of a near normal glucose with insulin reduced the risk of postoperative infection after CABG, and in one study, reduced the morbidity and mortality in patients in a surgical intensive care unit.

The goals of diabetes management during hospitalization are avoidance of hypoglycemia, optimization of glycemic control and transition back to the outpatient diabetes treatment regimen. Optimal glycemic control in the hospitalized patient is <6.1 mmol/L (100 mg/dL, preprandial) and <10 mmol/L (180 mg/dL, postprandial). Attention to each stage in this process requires integrating information regarding the plasma glucose, diabetes treatment regimen, and clinical status of the patient. For example, some surgical procedures utilizing local anesthesia or epidural anesthesia may have minimal effects on glycemic control. If the patient is eating soon after the procedure and there is no disruption of the patient's regular meal plans, then glycemic control is usually maintained. A "consistent-carbohydrate diabetes meal plan" for hospital-

---

TABLE 323-14 *Guidelines for Ongoing Medical Care for Patients with Diabetes*

- Self-monitoring of blood glucose (individualized frequency)
- A1C testing (2–4 times/year)
- Patient education in diabetes management (annual)
- Medical nutrition therapy and education (annual)
- Eye examination (annual)
- Foot examination (1–2 times/year by physician; daily by patient)
- Screening for diabetic nephropathy (annual; see Fig. 323-11)
- Blood pressure measurement (quarterly)
- Lipid profile (annual)
- Influenza/pneumococcal immunizations
- Consider antiplatelet therapy (see text)

Note: A1C, hemoglobin A1c.

ized patients provides a similar amount of carbohydrate for a particular meal each day (but not necessarily the same amount for breakfast, lunch, and supper). The hospital diet should be determined by a nutritionist; terms such as "ADA diet" or "low sugar diet" are no longer used.

The physician caring for an individual with diabetes in the perioperative period, during times of infection or serious physical illness, or simply when fasting for a diagnostic procedure must monitor the plasma glucose vigilantly, adjust the diabetes treatment regimen, and provide glucose infusion as needed. Several different treatment regimens (intravenous or subcutaneous insulin regimens) can be employed successfully. Individuals with type 1 DM require continued insulin administration to maintain the levels of circulating insulin necessary to prevent DKA. Prolongation of a surgical procedure or delay in the recovery room is not uncommon and may result in periods of insulin deficiency. Even relatively brief periods without insulin may lead to mild DKA. Individuals with type 1 DM who are undergoing general anesthesia and surgery, or who are seriously ill, should receive continuous insulin, either through an intravenous insulin infusion or by subcutaneous administration of a reduced dose of long-acting insulin. Short-acting insulin alone is insufficient.

Perioperative Management Insulin infusions can effectively control plasma glucose in the perioperative period and when the patient is unable to take anything by mouth. The absorption of subcutaneous insulin may be variable in such situations because of changes in blood flow. The physician must consider carefully the clinical setting in which an insulin infusion will be utilized, including whether adequate ancillary personnel are available to monitor the plasma glucose frequently and whether they can adjust the insulin infusion rate, either based on an algorithm or in consultation with the physician. The initial rate for an insulin infusion may range from 0.5 to 5 units/h, depending on the degree of insulin resistance and the clinical situation. Based on hourly capillary glucose measurements, the insulin infusion rate is adjusted to maintain the plasma glucose within the optimal range. The insulin infusion can be temporarily discontinued if hypoglycemia occurs and may be resumed at a lower infusion rate once the plasma glucose exceeds 5.6 mmol/L (100 mg/dL).

Insulin infusion is the preferred method for managing patients with type 1 DM in the perioperative period or when serious concurrent illness is present (0.5 to 1.0 units/h of regular insulin). Insulin-infusion algorithms jointly developed and implemented by nursing and physician staff are advised. If the diagnostic or surgical procedure is brief and performed under local or regional anesthesia, a reduced dose of subcutaneous, long-acting insulin may suffice. This approach facilitates the transition back to the long-acting insulin after the procedure. The dose of long-acting insulin should be reduced by 30 to 40%, and short-acting insulin is either held or, likewise, reduced by 30 to 40%. Glucose may be infused to prevent hypoglycemia.

Individuals with type 2 DM can be managed with either regular insulin infusion 0.5 to 2 units/h or a reduced dose of subcutaneous intermediate- or long-acting insulin supplemented with short-acting insulin. Oral glucose-lowering agents are discontinued upon admission. Oral glucose-lowering agents are not useful in regulating the plasma glucose in clinical situations where the insulin requirements and glucose intake are changing rapidly. Moreover, these oral agents may be dangerous if the patient is fasting (e.g., hypoglycemia with sulfonylureas). Metformin should be withheld when radiographic contrast media will be given or if severe congestive heart failure, acidosis, or declining renal function is present.

Total Parenteral Nutrition (See also Chap. 63) Total parenteral nutrition (TPN) greatly increases insulin requirements. In addition, individuals not previously known to have DM may become hyperglycemic during TPN and require insulin treatment. Intravenous insulin infusion is the preferred treatment for hyperglycemia, and rapid titration to the required insulin dose is done most efficiently using a separate insulin infusion. After the total insulin dose has been determined, insulin may be added directly to the TPN solution or, preferably, given as a separate infusion. Often, individuals receiving either TPN or enteral nutrition

receive their caloric loads continuously and not at "meal times"; consequently, subcutaneous insulin regimens must be adjusted.

GLUCOCORTICOIDS Glucocorticoids increase insulin resistance, decrease glucose utilization, increase hepatic glucose production, and impair insulin secretion. These changes lead to a worsening of glycemic control in individuals with DM and may precipitate diabetes in other individuals ("steroid-induced diabetes"). The effects of glucocorticoids on glucose homeostasis are dose-related, usually reversible, and most pronounced in the postprandial period. If the fasting plasma glucose is near the normal range, oral diabetes agents (e.g., sulfonylureas, metformin) may be sufficient to reduce hyperglycemia. If the fasting plasma glucose >11.1 mmol/L (200 mg/dL), oral agents are usually not efficacious and insulin therapy is required. Short-acting insulin may be required to supplement long-acting insulin in order to control postprandial glucose excursions.

REPRODUCTIVE ISSUES Reproductive capacity in either men or women with DM appears to be normal. Menstrual cycles may be associated with alterations in glycemic control in women with DM. Pregnancy is associated with marked insulin resistance; the increased insulin requirements often precipitate DM and lead to the diagnosis of GDM. Glucose, which at high levels is a teratogen to the developing fetus, readily crosses the placenta, but insulin does not. Thus, hyperglycemia from the maternal circulation may stimulate insulin secretion in the fetus. The anabolic and growth effects of insulin may result in macrosomia. GDM complicates approximately 4% of pregnancies in the United States. The incidence of GDM is greatly increased in certain ethnic groups, including African Americans and Hispanic Americans, consistent with a similar increased risk of type 2 DM. Current recommendations advise screening for glucose intolerance between weeks 24 and 28 of pregnancy in women with high risk for GDM ($\geq$25 years; obesity; family history of DM; member of an ethnic group such as Hispanic American, Native American, Asian American, African American, or Pacific Islander). Therapy for GDM is similar to that for individuals with pregnancy-associated diabetes and involves MNT and insulin, if hyperglycemia persists. Oral glucose-lowering agents have not been approved for use during pregnancy. With current practices, the morbidity and mortality of the mother with GDM and the fetus are no different from those in the nondiabetic population. Individuals who develop GDM are at marked increased risk for developing type 2 DM in the future and should be screened periodically for DM. After delivery, glucose homeostasis should be reassessed in the mother. Most individuals with GDM revert to normal glucose tolerance, but some will continue to have overt diabetes or impairment of glucose tolerance. In addition, children of women with GDM appear to be at risk for obesity and glucose intolerance and have an increased risk of diabetes beginning in the later stages of adolescence.

Pregnancy in individuals with known DM requires meticulous planning and adherence to strict treatment regimens. Intensive diabetes management and normalization of the A1C are the standard of care for individuals with existing DM who are planning pregnancy. The most crucial period of glycemic control is soon after fertilization. The risk of fetal malformations is increased 4 to 10 times in individuals with uncontrolled DM at the time of conception and normal plasma glucose during the preconception period and throughout the periods of organ development in the fetus should be maintained.

LIPODYSTROPHIC DM Lipodystrophy, or the loss of subcutaneous fat tissue, may be generalized in certain genetic conditions such as leprechaunism. Generalized lipodystrophy is associated with severe insulin resistance and is often accompanied by acanthosis nigricans and dyslipidemia. Localized lipodystrophy associated with insulin injections has been reduced considerably by the use of human insulin.

Protease Inhibitors and Lipodystrophy Protease inhibitors used in the treatment of HIV disease (Chap. 173) have been associated with a centripetal accumulation of fat (visceral and abdominal area), accumulation of fat in the dorsocervical region, loss of extremity fat, decreased insulin sensitivity (elevations of the fasting insulin level and reduced glucose tolerance on intravenous glucose tolerance testing), and dyslipidemia. Although many aspects of the physical appearance of these individuals resemble Cushing's syndrome, increased cortisol levels do not account for this appearance. The possibility remains that this is related to HIV infection by some undefined mechanism, since some features of the syndrome were observed before the introduction of protease inhibitors. Therapy for HIV-related lipodystrophy is not well established.

FURTHER READING

AMERICAN DIABETES ASSOCIATION: Clinical practice recommendations 2002. Diabetes Care 27:51, 2004

CLEMENT S et al: Management of diabetes and hyperglycemia in hospitals. Diabetes Care 27:553, 2004

KIRPICHNIKOV D et al: Metformin: An update. Ann Intern Med 137:25, 2002

KNOWLER WC et al for the DIABETES PREVENTION PROGRAM RESEARCH GROUP: Reduction in the incidence of type 2 diabetes with lifestyle intervention or metformin. N Engl J Med 346:393, 2002

SALTIEL AR, KAHN CR: Insulin signalling and the regulation of glucose and lipid metabolism. Nature 414:799, 2001

THE WRITING TEAM FOR THE DIABETES CONTROL AND COMPLICATIONS TRIAL/EPIDEMIOLOGY OF THE DIABETES INTERVENTIONS AND COMPLICATIONS RESEARCH GROUP: Effect of intensive therapy on the microvascular complications of type 1 diabetes mellitus. JAMA 287:2563, 2002

UK PROSPECTIVE DIABETES STUDY GROUP: Intensive blood-glucose control with sulphonylureas or insulin compared with conventional treatment and risk of complications in patients with type 2 diabetes (UKPDS 33). Lancet 352:1998, 1998

324 HYPOGLYCEMIA
Philip E. Cryer

Hypoglycemia is most commonly the result of taking drugs used to treat diabetes mellitus or other drugs, including alcohol. However, a number of other disorders, including end-stage organ failure and sepsis, endocrine deficiencies, large mesenchymal tumors, insulinoma, and inherited metabolic disorders are also associated with hypoglycemia (Table 324-1). Hypoglycemia is sometimes defined as a plasma glucose level <2.5 to 2.8 mmol/L (<45 to 50 mg/dL). However, glucose thresholds for hypoglycemia-induced symptoms and physiologic responses vary widely, depending on the clinical setting. Therefore, an important framework for making the diagnosis of hypoglycemia is *Whipple's triad*: (1) symptoms consistent with hypoglycemia, (2) a low plasma glucose concentration, and (3) relief of symptoms after the plasma glucose level is raised. Hypoglycemia can cause significant morbidity and can be lethal, if severe and prolonged; it should be considered in any patient with confusion, altered level of consciousness, or seizures.

SYSTEMIC GLUCOSE BALANCE AND COUNTERREGULATION

Glucose is an obligate metabolic fuel for the brain under physiologic conditions. By contrast, other organs can use fatty acids, in addition to glucose, to generate energy. The brain cannot synthesize glucose and stores only a few minutes' supply as glycogen and therefore requires a continuous supply of glucose, which is delivered by facilitated diffusion from arterial blood. As the plasma glucose concentration falls below the physiologic range, blood-to-brain glucose transport becomes insufficient for adequate brain energy metabolism and functioning. Fortunately, redundant physiologic mechanisms prevent or rapidly correct hypoglycemia.

Plasma glucose levels are maintained within a narrow range, usually between 3.3 and 8.3 mmol/L (60 and 150 mg/dL), despite wide variation of food intake and activity level. This delicate balance requires dynamic regulation of glucose influx into the circulation as glucose utilization in various tissues can change rapidly. The diet is normally a major source of glucose. However, between meals or during fasting, plasma glucose levels are maintained primarily by the breakdown of glycogen and by gluconeogenesis (Fig. 324-1). In most persons, hepatic glycogen stores are sufficient to maintain plasma glucose levels for 8 to 12 h, but this time period can be shorter if glucose demand is increased by exercise or if glycogen stores are depleted by illness or starvation.

As glycogen stores are depleted, glucose is generated by gluconeogenesis, which occurs mainly in the liver but also in the kidneys. Gluconeogenesis requires a coordinated supply of precursors from

TABLE 324-1 *Causes of Hypoglycemia*

Drugs
  Especially insulin, sulfonylureas, ethanol
  Sometimes pentamidine, quinine
  Rarely salicylates, sulfonamides, and others
Critical illnesses
  Hepatic, renal, or cardiac failure
  Sepsis
  Starvation and inanition
Endocrine deficiencies
  Cortisol, growth hormone
  Glucagon and epinephrine (type 1 diabetes)
Non-β-cell tumors
  Fibrosarcoma, mesothelioma, rhabdomyosarcoma, liposarcoma, other sarcomas
  Hepatoma, adrenocortical tumors, carcinoid
  Leukemia, lymphoma, melanoma, teratoma
Endogenous hyperinsulinism
  Insulinoma
  Other β cell disorders
  Secretagogue (sulfonylurea)
  Autoimmune (autoantibodies to insulin, insulin receptor, β cell?)
  Ectopic insulin secretion
Disorders of infancy or childhood
  Transient intolerance of fasting
  Infants of diabetic mothers (hyperinsulinism)
  Congenital hyperinsulinism
  Inherited enzyme defects
Postprandial
  Reactive (after gastric surgery)
  Ethanol-induced
  Autonomic symptoms without true hypoglycemia
Factitious
  Insulin, sulfonylureas

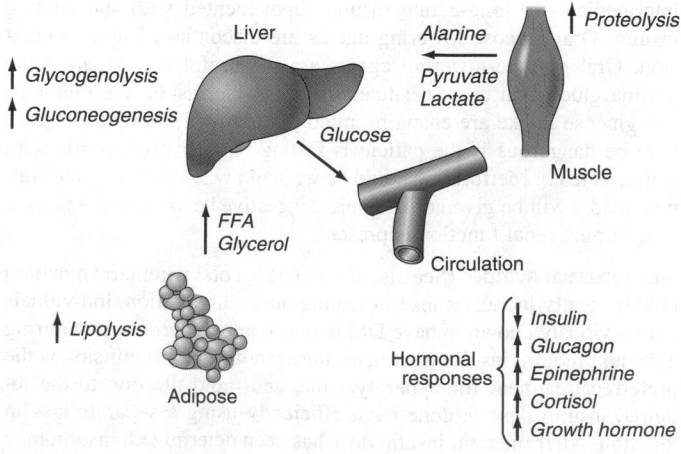

FIGURE 324-1 Overview of glucose metabolism and pathways of counterregulatory responses to fasting and hypoglycemia.

liver, muscle, and adipose tissue. Muscle provides lactate, pyruvate, alanine, and other amino acids. Triglycerides in adipose tissue are broken down into glycerol, which is a precursor for gluconeogenesis. Free fatty acids generate acetyl CoA for gluconeogenesis and provide an alternative fuel source to tissues other than the brain.

The balance of glucose production and its uptake and utilization in peripheral tissues are exquisitely regulated by a network of hormones, neural pathways, and metabolic signals (Chap. 323). Among the factors that control glucose production and utilization, insulin plays a dominant and pivotal role. In the fasting state, insulin is suppressed, allowing increased gluconeogenesis in the liver and the kidneys and enhancing glucose generation by the breakdown of liver glycogen. Low insulin levels also reduce glucose uptake and utilization in peripheral tissues and allow lipolysis and proteolysis to occur, which leads to the release of precursors for gluconeogenesis and provides alternative energy sources. In the fed state, insulin release from the pancreatic β cells reverses this process. Glycogenolysis and gluconeogenesis are inhibited, thereby reducing hepatic and renal glucose output; peripheral glucose uptake and utilization are enhanced; lipolysis and proteolysis are restrained; and energy storage is promoted by the conversion of substrates into glycogen, triglycerides, and proteins. Other hormones, such as glucagon, epinephrine, growth hormone, and cortisol, play less important roles in the control of glucose flux during normal physiologic circumstances. However, these hormones are critically important in the response to hypoglycemia.

As glucose levels approach, and ultimately enter, the hypoglycemic range, a characteristic sequence of *counterregulatory hormone responses* occurs. Glucagon is the first and most important of these responses. It promotes glycogenolysis and gluconeogenesis. Epinephrine can also play an important role in the acute response to hypoglycemia, particularly when glucagon is insufficient. It, too, stimulates glycogenolysis and gluconeogenesis and limits glucose utilization by insulin-sensitive tissues. When hypoglycemia is prolonged, growth hormone and cortisol also reduce glucose utilization and support its production.

The glucose thresholds at which various counterregulatory hormone responses occur are quite similar in healthy subjects (Table 324-2). Nevertheless, these thresholds are dynamic and can be influenced by recent metabolic events. A person with poorly controlled diabetes can have symptoms of hypoglycemia at higher-than-normal glucose levels. Recurrent hypoglycemia, which may occur in individuals with diabetes or an insulinoma, shifts thresholds for symptoms and counterregulatory responses to lower glucose levels.

CLINICAL MANIFESTATIONS

Symptoms of hypoglycemia can be divided into two categories, neuroglycopenic and neurogenic (or autonomic) responses. Neuroglycopenic symptoms are a direct result of central nervous system neuronal glucose deprivation. Symptoms include behavioral changes, confusion, fatigue, seizure, loss of consciousness, and, if hypoglycemia is severe and prolonged, death. Hypoglycemia-induced autonomic responses include adrenergic symptoms such as palpitations, tremor, and anxiety as well as cholinergic symptoms such as sweating, hunger, and paresthesia. Adrenergic symptoms are mediated by norepinephrine released from sympathetic postganglionic neurons and the release of epinephrine from the adrenal medullae. Increased sweating is mediated by cholinergic sympathetic nerve fibers. Patients with diabetes mellitus learn to recognize the characteristic symptoms of hypoglycemia, but

TABLE 324-2 *Physiologic Responses to Decreasing Plasma Glucose Concentrations*

Response	Glycemic Threshold, mmol/L (mg/dL)	Physiologic Effects	Role in the Prevention or Correction of Hypoglycemia (Glucose Counterregulation)
↓ Insulin	4.4–4.7 (80–85)	↑ R_a (↓R_d)	Primary glucose regulatory factor/first defense against hypoglycemia
↑ Glucagon	3.6–3.9 (65–70)	↑ R_a	Primary glucose counterregulatory factor
↑ Epinephrine	3.6–3.9 (65–70)	↑ R_a, ↓ R_d	Involved, critical when glucagon is deficient
↑ Cortisol and growth hormone	3.6–3.9 (65–70)	↑ R_a, ↓ R_d	Involved, not critical
Symptoms	2.8–3.1 (50–55)	↑ Exogenous glucose	Prompt behavioral defense (food ingestion)
↓ Cognition	< 2.8 (< 50)	—	(Compromises behavioral defense)

Note: R_a, rate of glucose appearance, glucose production by the liver and kidneys; R_d, rate of glucose disappearance, glucose utilization by insulin-sensitive tissues such as skeletal muscle. (R_d includes glucose utilization by the central nervous system, but the glucoregulatory hormones have no direct effects on that.)

these are less familiar to individuals with other causes of hypoglycemia. Symptoms may be less pronounced with repeated hypoglycemic episodes (see below).

Common signs of hypoglycemia include pallor and diaphoresis. Heart rate and the systolic blood pressure are typically raised, but these findings may not be prominent. The neuroglycopenic manifestations are valuable, albeit nonspecific, signs. Transient focal neurologic deficits occur occasionally.

CAUSES

Hypoglycemia is traditionally classified as *postprandial* or *fasting*. However, in the clinical setting, hypoglycemia is most commonly a result of diabetes treatment. This topic is therefore addressed before considering the other causes of hypoglycemia.

HYPOGLYCEMIA IN DIABETES

FREQUENCY AND IMPACT Were it not for hypoglycemia, diabetes would be rather easy to treat by administering enough insulin (or any effective drug) to lower plasma glucose concentrations to, or below, the normal range. But because current insulin-replacement regimens are imperfect, individuals with type 1 diabetes are at ongoing risk for periods of relative hyperinsulinemia with resultant hypoglycemia. Those attempting to achieve near-normal glycemic control may experience several episodes of asymptomatic or symptomatic hypoglycemia each week. Plasma glucose levels may be <2.8 mmol/L (<50 mg/dL) as often as 10% of the time. Such patients suffer an average of one episode of severe, temporarily disabling hypoglycemia, often with seizure or coma, in a given year. Although seemingly complete recovery from the latter is the rule, the possibility of persistent cognitive deficits has been raised, but permanent neurologic defects are rare. About 2 to 4% of deaths associated with type 1 diabetes are estimated to be a result of hypoglycemia. Fear of hypoglycemia can also lead to disabling psychosocial morbidity.

Hypoglycemia is a less frequent problem in type 2 diabetes but still occurs in those treated with insulin or sulfonylureas. Transient, mild hypoglycemia may be seen with the shorter-acting sulfonylureas and repaglinide or nateglinide, which also act by enhancing insulin secretion. Patients who take the long-acting sulfonylureas, chlorpropamide and glyburide, may experience episodes of severe hypoglycemia that last between 24 and 36 h.

CONVENTIONAL RISK FACTORS Insulin excess is the primary determinant of risk from iatrogenic hypoglycemia. Relative or absolute insulin excess occurs when: (1) insulin (or oral agent) doses are excessive, ill timed, or of the wrong type; (2) the influx of exogenous glucose is reduced (e.g., during an overnight fast or following missed meals or snacks); (3) insulin-independent glucose utilization is increased (e.g., during exercise); (4) insulin sensitivity is increased (e.g., with effective intensive therapy, in the middle of the night, late after exercise, or with increased fitness or weight loss); (5) endogenous glucose production is reduced (e.g., following alcohol ingestion); and (6) insulin clearance is reduced (e.g., in renal failure). However, analyses of the Diabetes Control and Complications Trial (DCCT) indicate that these conventional risk factors explain only a minority of episodes of severe iatrogenic hypoglycemia; other causes are involved in the majority of episodes.

HYPOGLYCEMIA-ASSOCIATED AUTONOMIC FAILURE It is now clear that inadequate physiologic counterregulatory and behavioral responses greatly compound the problem of hypoglycemia caused by insulin excess. Hypoglycemia-associated autonomic failure has two main components: (1) reduced counterregulatory hormone responses, which result in impaired glucose generation; and (2) hypoglycemia unawareness, which precludes appropriate behavioral responses, such as eating.

Defective Glucose Counterregulation The counterregulatory hormone response is fundamentally altered in patients with established (e.g., absent C peptide) type 1 diabetes. As insulin deficiency progresses over the first few months or years of the disease, circulating insulin levels are no longer tightly coordinated with glucose levels and are a passive function of administered insulin. Thus, insulin levels do not decline as glucose levels fall; the first defense against hypoglycemia is lost. Over the same time frame, the glucagon response to falling glucose levels diminishes, and the second defense against hypoglycemia is lost. The cause of defective glucagon production by the pancreatic islet α cells is unknown, but it is tightly linked to the loss of insulin production by the β cells. It is a functional abnormality rather than an absolute deficiency of glucagon, as responses to stimuli other than hypoglycemia are intact. The third defense against hypoglycemia is compromised when the epinephrine response to hypoglycemia is reduced. In contrast to the absent glucagon response, epinephrine deficiency is a threshold abnormality; an epinephrine response can still be elicited, but a lower plasma glucose concentration is required. This threshold shift is largely a result of recent antecedent hypoglycemia, although an additional anatomic component may also be present in patients affected by classic diabetic autonomic neuropathy. The development of a reduced epinephrine response is a critical pathophysiologic event. Prospective studies have shown that patients with combined deficiencies of glucagon and epinephrine suffer severe hypoglycemia at rates 25-fold or greater than individuals with absent glucagon but intact epinephrine responses.

Hypoglycemia Unawareness *Hypoglycemia unawareness* refers to a loss of the warning symptoms that alert individuals to the presence of hypoglycemia and prompt them to eat and abort the episode. Under these circumstances, the first manifestation of hypoglycemia is neuroglycopenia, when it is often too late for patients to treat themselves. Like defective counterregulation, the presence of hypoglycemia unawareness has been shown in prospective studies to be associated with a high frequency of severe hypoglycemia.

The interplay of factors involved in hypoglycemia-associated autonomic failure in type 1 diabetes, and consequent hypoglycemia unawareness, is summarized in Fig. 324-2. Periods of relative or absolute therapeutic insulin excess, in the setting of absent glucagon responses, lead to episodes of iatrogenic hypoglycemia. These episodes, in turn, cause reduced autonomic (including adrenomedullary) responses to falling glucose concentrations. These impaired autonomic responses result in reduced symptoms of impending hypoglycemia (e.g., hypoglycemia unawareness) because epinephrine responses are reduced in the setting of absent glucagon responses. Thus, a vicious cycle of recurrent hypoglycemia is created and perpetuated. The syndrome of hypoglycemia unawareness and the reduced epinephrine component of defective glucose counterregulation are reversible but require >2 weeks of scrupulous avoidance of hypoglycemia. This involves a shift of glycemic thresholds back to higher plasma glucose concentrations.

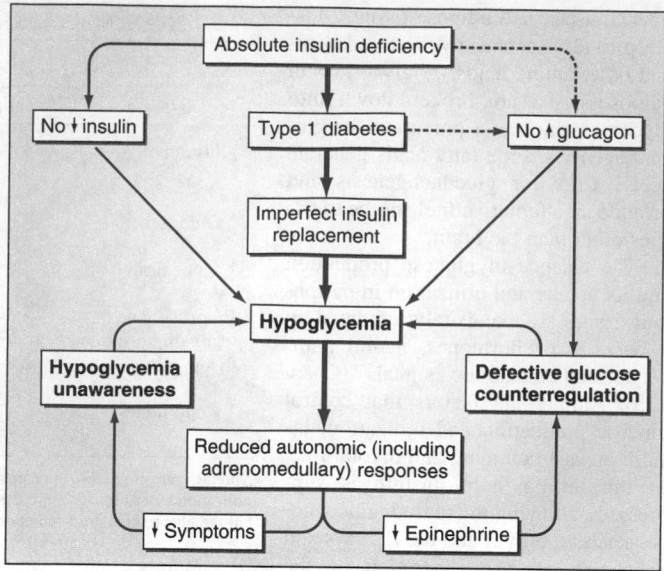

FIGURE 324-2 Hypoglycemia-associated autonomic failure and hypoglycemia unawareness in type 1 diabetes. (*PE Cryer: Diabetes 41:255, 1992.*)

HYPOGLYCEMIA RISK FACTOR REDUCTION A diagnosis of hypoglycemia unawareness can usually be made from the history. One should note that hypoglycemia unawareness implies that previous episodes of hypoglycemia have occurred, whether these are documented or not. If low glucose levels are not apparent from the patient's self-monitoring log, one should suspect hypoglycemia during the night. The presence of clinical hypoglycemia unawareness makes defective glucose counterregulation likely. It is possible to minimize the risk of hypoglycemia by applying the principles of modern therapy—patient education and empowerment, frequent self-monitoring of blood glucose, flexible insulin (and other drug) regimens, rational glycemic goals, and ongoing professional guidance and support. If hypoglycemia is a recognized problem, first consider each of the conventional risk factors summarized earlier and recommend the appropriate adjustments of medications, diet, and life-style. Nonselective beta blockers may attenuate the recognition of hypoglycemia and they impair glycogenolysis; a relatively selective β_1-antagonist (e.g., metoprolol or atenolol) is preferable when a beta blocker is indicated.

REACTIVE HYPOGLYCEMIA

Postprandial (reactive) hypoglycemia occurs only after meals and is self-limited. Postprandial hypoglycemia occurs in children with certain rare enzymatic defects in carbohydrate metabolism such as hereditary fructose intolerance and galactosemia (Chap. 341). Reactive hypoglycemia also occurs in some individuals who have undergone gastric surgery, which allows the rapid passage of food from the stomach to the small intestine. This type of *alimentary hypoglycemia* causes a rapid postprandial rise in plasma glucose levels and the release of gut incretins, which induce an exuberant insulin response and subsequent hypoglycemia. Administration of an α-glucosidase inhibitor, which delays carbohydrate digestion and thus glucose absorption from the intestine, can be considered for treatment of reactive hypoglycemia, although its efficacy remains to be established in controlled trials.

If postprandial symptoms occur as an idiopathic disorder, caution should be exercised before labeling a person with a diagnosis of hypoglycemia. Indeed, a self-diagnosis of hypoglycemia has often been reinforced by the finding of a "low" venous glucose concentration late after glucose ingestion. An oral glucose tolerance test should not be used in this setting. Plasma glucose falls as low as 2.4 mmol/L (43 mg/dL) after a 100-g glucose load in 5% of normal asymptomatic individuals, making it difficult to identify hypoglycemia based on the results of this test. The diagnosis of postprandial hypoglycemia requires documentation of Whipple's triad after a typical mixed meal. The cause of repetitive postprandial symptoms in certain individuals is unknown, but they may be particularly sensitive to the normal autonomic responses that follow ingestion of a meal.

FASTING HYPOGLYCEMIA

There are many causes of fasting hypoglycemia (Table 324-1). In addition to insulin and sulfonylureas used in the treatment of diabetes, ethanol use is a relatively common cause of hypoglycemia. Sepsis and renal failure are often complicated by hypoglycemia. Endocrine deficiencies, non-β-cell tumors, and endogenous hyperinsulinemia (including that caused by an insulinoma) are rare causes of hypoglycemia. Enzymatic metabolic errors that cause hypoglycemia are also rare but are being recognized more frequently in infants and children (Chaps. 341 and 343).

DRUGS In contrast to the sulfonylureas and rapid-acting insulin secretagogues (e.g., repaglinide, nateglinide), other oral hypoglycemic agents—biguanides (e.g., metformin), α-glucosidase inhibitors (e.g., acarbose, miglitol), and thiazolidinediones (e.g., rosiglitazone, pioglitazone)—do not act by stimulating insulin secretion. Therefore, with these agents, insulin levels usually decrease appropriately as plasma glucose levels fall. However, these drugs can contribute to hypoglycemia in other ways. Treatment with an α-glucosidase inhibitor alters the management of hypoglycemia; pure glucose should be used rather than ingestion of complex carbohydrates. Thiazolidinediones, as well as metformin, can predispose patients to hypoglycemia if they are receiving combined treatment with insulin or an insulin secretagogue.

Ethanol blocks gluconeogenesis but not glycogenolysis. Thus, alcohol-induced hypoglycemia typically occurs after a several-day ethanol binge during which the person eats little food, thereby causing glycogen depletion. Hypoglycemia in this setting can be profound, with mortality rates as high as 10%. Blood ethanol levels correlate poorly with plasma glucose concentrations at the time of diagnosis, as hypoglycemia occurs late in the sequence and often precludes further alcohol consumption.

Pentamidine, which is used to treat *Pneumocystis* pneumonia and other parasitic infections, is toxic to the pancreatic β cell. It causes insulin release initially, with hypoglycemia in about 10% of treated patients, and predisposes to the development of diabetes mellitus later. Quinine also stimulates insulin secretion. However, the relative contribution of hyperinsulinemia to the pathogenesis of hypoglycemia in quinine-treated patients who are critically ill with malaria is debated. Salicylates and sulfonamides can cause hypoglycemia, but do so rarely. There are reports of hypoglycemia attributed to nonselective β-adrenergic antagonists (e.g., propranolol) and a variety of other drugs.

CRITICAL ILLNESS Rapid and extensive hepatic destruction (e.g., severe toxic hepatitis) causes fasting hypoglycemia because the liver is the major site of endogenous glucose production. The mechanism of hypoglycemia reported in patients with cardiac failure is unknown but likely involves hepatic congestion. Although the kidneys are a source of glucose production, it is perhaps too simplistic to attribute hypoglycemia in persons with renal failure to this mechanism alone. The clearance of insulin is reduced substantially in renal failure, and reduced mobilization of gluconeogenic precursors has been reported.

Sepsis is sometimes complicated by hypoglycemia, which is multifactorial in origin. There is impaired endogenous glucose production, perhaps a result of hepatic hypoperfusion, and increased glucose utilization, which is induced by cytokines in macrophage-rich tissues such as the liver, spleen, and ileum and in muscle. Nutrition is also often inadequate in the setting of sepsis. Hypoglycemia can be seen with prolonged starvation, perhaps because of a loss of whole-body fat stores and the subsequent depletion of gluconeogenic precursors (e.g., amino acids), which necessitate increased glucose utilization.

ENDOCRINE DEFICIENCIES Neither cortisol nor growth hormone is critical to the prevention of acute hypoglycemia, at least in adults. However, hypoglycemia can occur with prolonged fasting in patients with untreated primary adrenocortical failure (Addison's disease) or hypopituitarism. Anorexia and weight loss are typical features of chronic

cortisol deficiency and likely result in glycogen depletion with increased reliance on gluconeogenesis. Cortisol deficiency is associated with low levels of gluconeogenic precursors, suggesting that substrate-limited gluconeogenesis, in the setting of glycogen depletion, is the cause of the impaired ability to tolerate fasting in cortisol-deficient individuals. Growth hormone deficiency can cause hypoglycemia in young children. In addition to extended fasting, high rates of glucose utilization (e.g., during exercise, pregnancy) or low rates of glucose production (e.g., following alcohol ingestion) can precipitate hypoglycemia in adults with hypopituitarism. Cortisol and growth hormone secretion should be evaluated in patients with fasting hypoglycemia when the history suggests pituitary or adrenal disease and when other causes of hypoglycemia are not apparent.

Hypoglycemia is not a feature of the epinephrine-deficient state that results from bilateral adrenalectomy when glucocorticoid replacement is adequate, nor does it occur during pharmacologic adrenergic blockage when other gluregulatory systems are intact. There are case reports of fasting hypoglycemia attributed to isolated glucagon or epinephrine deficiency, although hyperinsulinemia was not excluded convincingly in neonatal cases and other counterregulatory defects may have contributed in the adults. Thus, the regular assessment of glucagon and epinephrine secretion is not warranted.

NON-β-CELL TUMORS Fasting hypoglycemia, often termed *non-islet cell tumor hypoglycemia*, occurs in some patients with large mesenchymal or other tumors (e.g., hepatoma, adrenocortical tumors, carcinoids; Chap. 86. The glucose kinetic patterns resemble those of hyperinsulinism, but insulin secretion is suppressed appropriately during hypoglycemia. In most instances, hypoglycemia is due to overproduction of an incompletely processed form of insulin-like growth factor (IGF) II. Although total IGF-II levels are not consistently elevated, circulating free IGF-II levels are high. Hypoglycemia results from IGF-II actions through the insulin or IGF-I receptors.

ENDOGENOUS HYPERINSULINISM Hypoglycemia due to excessive endogenous insulin secretion can be caused by: (1) a primary pancreatic islet β cell disorder, typically a β cell tumor (insulinoma), sometimes multiple insulinomas, or, especially in infants or young children, a functional β cell disorder without an anatomic correlate; (2) a β cell secretagogue, often a sulfonylurea, and, theoretically, a β cell–stimulating autoantibody; (3) an autoantibody to insulin; or (4) ectopic insulin secretion. None of these disorders is common. Endogenous hyperinsulinism is more likely to occur in an overtly healthy individual without other apparent causes of hypoglycemia such as a relevant drug history, critical illness, endocrine deficiencies, or a non-β-cell tumor. Accidental, surreptitious, or even malicious administration of a sulfonylurea or insulin should also be considered in such individuals.

The fundamental pathophysiologic feature of endogenous hyperinsulinism is the failure of insulin secretion to fall to very low rates during hypoglycemia. This is assessed by measuring insulin, proinsulin, and C peptide, which is derived from the processing of proinsulin. Critical diagnostic findings are a plasma insulin concentration ≥ 36 pmol/L (≥ 6 μU/mL) and a plasma C-peptide concentration ≥ 0.2 mmol/L (≥ 0.6 ng/mL) when the plasma glucose concentration is ≤ 2.5 mmol/L (≤ 45 mg/dL) in the fasting state with symptoms of hypoglycemia. Insulin and C-peptide levels do not need to be absolutely increased (e.g., relative to euglycemic normal values) but only inappropriately increased in the setting of fasting hypoglycemia. Plasma proinsulin concentrations are also inappropriately elevated, particularly in patients with an insulinoma. Sulfonylureas, because they stimulate insulin secretion, result in a pattern of glucose, insulin, and C-peptide levels that is indistinguishable from that produced by a primary β cell disorder. The measurement of sulfonylureas in plasma or urine distinguishes these conditions. Antibodies to insulin produce *autoimmune hypoglycemia* following the transition from the postprandial to the postabsorptive state, as insulin slowly dissociates from the antibodies. Total and free plasma insulin concentrations are inappropri-

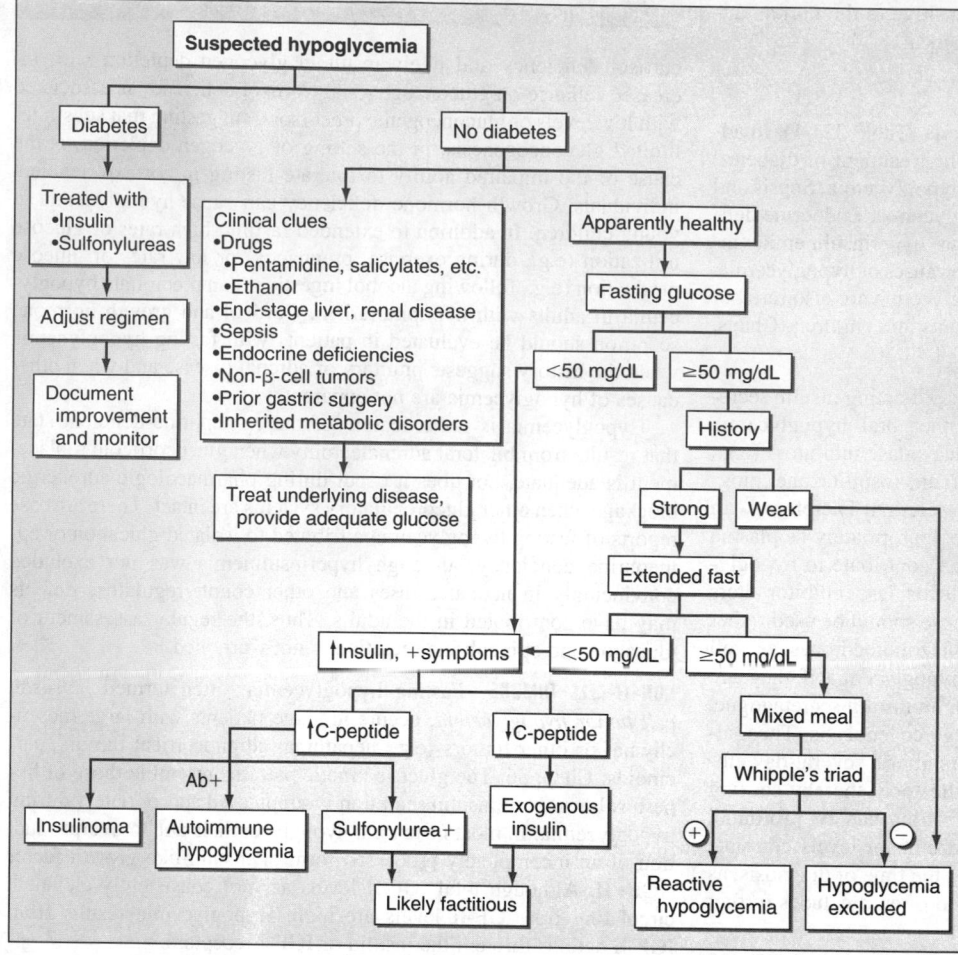

FIGURE 324-3 Diagnostic approach to a patient with suspected hypoglycemia based on a history of symptoms, a low plasma glucose concentration, or both.

The flowchart in Figure 324-3 contains the following elements:

Suspected hypoglycemia
→ Diabetes / No diabetes

Diabetes → Treated with • Insulin • Sulfonylureas → Adjust regimen → Document improvement and monitor

No diabetes →
- Clinical clues • Drugs • Pentamidine, salicylates, etc. • Ethanol • End-stage liver, renal disease • Sepsis • Endocrine deficiencies • Non-β-cell tumors • Prior gastric surgery • Inherited metabolic disorders → Treat underlying disease, provide adequate glucose
- Apparently healthy → Fasting glucose → <50 mg/dL / ≥50 mg/dL

≥50 mg/dL → History → Strong / Weak

Strong → Extended fast → ↑Insulin, +symptoms / <50 mg/dL / ≥50 mg/dL

↑Insulin, +symptoms → ↑C-peptide / ↓C-peptide

↑C-peptide → Ab+ → Insulinoma / Autoimmune hypoglycemia / Sulfonylurea+ → Likely factitious

↓C-peptide → Exogenous insulin

≥50 mg/dL → Mixed meal → Whipple's triad → (+) Reactive hypoglycemia / (−) Hypoglycemia excluded

---

phy has high sensitivity and may localize tumors not identified by palpation. Surgical resection of a solitary insulinoma is generally curative. Diazoxide, which inhibits insulin secretion, and the somatostatin analogue, octreotide, can be used to treat hypoglycemia in patients with unresectable insulinomas.

FACTITIOUS HYPOGLYCEMIA *Factitious hypoglycemia*, caused by malicious or self-administration of insulin or ingestion of a sulfonylurea, shares many clinical and laboratory features with insulinoma. It is most common among health care workers, patients with diabetes or their relatives, and people with a history of other factitious illnesses. When this diagnosis is suspected, it is useful to seek previous medical records, which may reveal admissions for similar episodes. In individuals taking exogenous insulin, factitious hypoglycemia can be distinguished from insulinoma by the presence of high insulin levels without a concomitant increase in the C-peptide level, which is suppressed by the exogenous insulin. As noted above, sulfonylureas stimulate endogenous insulin and can therefore be detected only by measuring drug levels in plasma or urine. Factitious or surreptitious hypoglycemia should be considered in every patient requiring a fasting test for hypoglycemia. In addition to laboratory tests, observing the patient's behavior may help make this diagnosis.

ately high. The distinguishing feature is the presence of circulating antibodies to insulin, but the need to measure these routinely is debated, since autoimmune hypoglycemia is rare. Autoantibodies to the insulin receptor are another rare cause of hypoglycemia and usually occur in the context of other autoimmune diseases. A few cases of ectopic insulin secretion (from a non-β-cell tumor) have been reported.

Insulinoma and Other Primary β Cell Disorders Insulinomas are uncommon, but because approximately 90% are benign, they are a treatable cause of potentially fatal hypoglycemia. The yearly incidence is estimated to be 1 in 250,000. About 60% of cases occur in women. The median age at presentation is 50 years in sporadic cases, but it usually presents in the third decade when associated with multiple endocrine neoplasia type 1 (Chap. 330). Insulinomas arise within the substance of the pancreas in >99% of cases and are usually small (1 to 2 cm). About 5 to 10% of insulinomas are malignant, as evidenced by the presence of metastases.

Insulinomas are almost always recognized because of hypoglycemia rather than mass effects. Unusually low plasma glucose concentrations may be required to produce symptoms and signs of hypoglycemia because recurrent hypoglycemia shifts the glycemic thresholds. Although symptomatic hypoglycemia can occur after an overnight fast, it often follows exercise. Rarely, symptomatic hypoglycemia occurs following meals, but most such patients have evidence of fasting hypoglycemia as well.

Octreotide scans localize approximately half of insulinomas. Arteriography has been used extensively in the past, but false-negative and false-positive results occur, and it is generally preferable to use less invasive computed tomography (CT) or magnetic resonance imaging (MRI) scans, which detect 45 to 75% of tumors. Preoperative ultrasound is valuable for some patients. Intraoperative ultrasonogra-

---

APPROACH TO THE PATIENT

In addition to recognition and documentation of hypoglycemia, and often urgent treatment, diagnosis of the hypoglycemic mechanism is critical for choosing a treatment that prevents, or at least minimizes, recurrent hypoglycemia. A diagnostic algorithm is shown in Fig. 324-3.

RECOGNITION AND DOCUMENTATION

Urgent treatment is often necessary in patients with suspected hypoglycemia. Blood should be drawn, whenever possible, before the administration of glucose to allow documentation of the plasma glucose level. Convincing documentation of hypoglycemia requires the fulfillment of Whipple's triad. Thus, *the ideal time to test the plasma glucose is during an episode associated with hypoglycemic symptoms.* A normal plasma glucose concentration measured when the patient is free of symptoms does not exclude hypoglycemia at the time of earlier symptoms. When the cause of hypoglycemia is obscure, additional assays should include glucose, insulin, C peptide, sulfonylurea levels, cortisol, and ethanol.

Hypoglycemia is sometimes detected serendipitously. A distinctly low plasma glucose measurement in a person without a history of corresponding symptoms raises the possibility of a laboratory error caused by ongoing metabolism of glucose by the formed elements of the blood after the sample is drawn. This type of artifactually low glucose level is particularly likely when leukocyte, erythrocyte, or platelet counts are abnormally high, but also if separation of the plasma or serum from the formed elements is delayed.

DIAGNOSIS OF THE HYPOGLYCEMIC MECHANISM

In an adult patient with documented hypoglycemia, a plausible hypoglycemic mechanism and further diagnostic evaluation can be guided by the history, physical examination, and available laboratory data (Fig. 324-3). In the absence of documented spontaneous hypoglycemia, overnight fasting, or food deprivation during observation in the outpatient setting, will sometimes elicit hypoglycemia and allow diagnostic evaluation. If there is a high degree of clinical suspicion, an extended fast lasting 48 to 72 h is often required to make the diagnosis. This procedure should be performed in the hospital with careful supervision and should be terminated if the plasma glucose drops to <2.5 mmol/L (<45 mg/dL) and the patient has symptoms. It is essential to draw blood samples for appropriate tests before administering glucose or allowing the patient to eat.

URGENT TREATMENT

Oral treatment with glucose tablets or glucose-containing fluids, candy, or food is appropriate if the patient is able and willing to take these. A reasonable initial dose is 20 g of glucose. If neuroglycopenia precludes oral feedings, parenteral therapy is necessary. Intravenous glucose (25 g) should be given using a 50% solution followed by a constant infusion of 5 or 10% dextrose. If intravenous therapy is not practical, subcutaneous or intramuscular glucagon can be used, particularly in patients with type 1 diabetes mellitus. Because it acts primarily by stimulating glycogenolysis, glucagon is ineffective in glycogen-depleted individuals (e.g., those with alcohol-induced hypoglycemia). It also stimulates insulin secretion and is therefore less useful in type 2 diabetes mellitus. These treatments raise plasma glucose concentrations only transiently, and patients should be encouraged to eat as soon as practical to replete glycogen stores.

PREVENTION OF RECURRENT HYPOGLYCEMIA

Prevention of recurrent hypoglycemia requires an understanding of the hypoglycemic mechanism. Offending drugs can be discontinued or their doses reduced. It should be remembered that hypoglycemia caused by sulfonylureas may recur after a period of several hours or days. Underlying critical illnesses can often be treated. Cortisol and growth hormone can be replaced if deficient. Surgical, radiotherapeutic, or chemotherapeutic reduction of a non-β-cell tumor can alleviate hypoglycemia, even if the tumor cannot be cured; glucocorticoid or growth hormone administration may also reduce hypoglycemic episodes in such patients. Surgical resection of an insulinoma is often curative; medical therapy with diazoxide or octreotide can be used if resection is not possible and in patients with a nontumor primary β cell disorder. The treatment of autoimmune hypoglycemia (e.g., with a glucocorticoid) is more problematic, but this disorder is often self-limited. Failing these treatments, frequent feedings and avoidance of fasting may be required. Uncooked cornstarch at bedtime or an overnight infusion of intragastric glucose may be necessary in some patients.

FURTHER READING

CRYER PE: *Hypoglycemia: Pathophysiology, Diagnosis and Treatment*. New York, Oxford Univ Press, 1997
———, CHILDS BP: Negotiating the barrier of hypoglycemia in diabetes. Diabetes Spectrum 15:20, 2001
SERVICE FJ: Hypoglycemic disorders. Endocrinol Metab Clin North Am 28: 467, 1999

325 DISORDERS OF THE TESTES AND MALE REPRODUCTIVE SYSTEM
Shalendar Bhasin, J. Larry Jameson

The male reproductive system regulates sexual differentiation, virilization, and the hormonal changes that accompany puberty, ultimately leading to spermatogenesis and fertility. Under the control of the pituitary hormones—luteinizing hormone (LH) and follicle-stimulating hormone (FSH)—the Leydig cells of the testes produce testosterone and germ cells are nurtured by Sertoli cells to divide, differentiate, and mature into sperm. During embryonic development, testosterone and dihydrotestosterone (DHT) induce the wolffian duct and virilization of the external genitalia. During puberty, testosterone promotes somatic growth and the development of secondary sexual characteristics. In the adult, testosterone is necessary for spermatogenesis and stimulation of libido and normal sexual function. This chapter focuses on the physiology of the testes and disorders associated with decreased androgen production, which may be caused by gonadotropin deficiency or by primary testis dysfunction. A variety of testosterone formulations now allow more physiologic androgen replacement. Infertility occurs in ~5% of men and is increasingly amenable to treatment by hormone replacement or by using sperm transfer techniques (Chap. 45). →*For further discussion of sexual dysfunction, disorders of the prostate, and testicular cancer, see Chaps. 43, 81, 82, respectively.*

DEVELOPMENT AND STRUCTURE OF THE TESTIS

The fetal testis develops from the undifferentiated gonad after expression of a genetic cascade that is initiated by the SRY (Sex-related gene on the Y chromosome) (Chap. 328). SRY induces differentiation of Sertoli cells, which surround germ cells, and together with peritubular myoid cells form testis cords that will later develop into seminiferous tubules. Fetal Leydig cells and endothelial cells migrate into the gonad from the adjacent mesonephros but may also arise from interstitial cells

that reside between testis cords. Leydig cells produce testosterone, which supports the growth and differentiation of wolffian duct structures that develop into the epididymus, vas deferens, and seminal vesicles. Testosterone is also converted to DHT (see below), which induces formation of the prostate and the external male genitalia including the penis, urethra, and scrotum. Testicular descent through the inguinal canal is controlled in part by Leydig cell production of insulin-like factor 3 (INSL3), which acts via a receptor termed *Great* (*G* protein–coupled *re*ceptor *a*ffecting *t*estis descent). Sertoli cells produce müllerian inhibiting substance (MIS), which causes regression of the müllerian structures including the fallopian tube, uterus, and upper segment of the vagina.

NORMAL MALE PUBERTAL DEVELOPMENT

Although puberty commonly refers to the maturation of the reproductive axis and the development of secondary sex characteristics, it involves a coordinated response of multiple hormonal systems including the adrenal gland and the growth hormone (GH) axis (Fig. 325-1). The development of secondary sexual characteristics is initiated by *adrenarche*, which usually occurs between 6 and 8 years of age when the adrenal gland begins to produce greater amounts of androgens from the zona reticularis, the principal site of dehydroepiandrosterone (DHEA) production. The sexual maturation process is greatly accelerated by the activation of the hypothalamic-pituitary axis and the production of gonadotropin-releasing hormone (GnRH). The so-called GnRH pulse generator in the hypothalamus is active during fetal life and early infancy but is quiescent until the early stages of puberty, when the sensitivity to steroid inhibition is gradually lost, causing reactivation of GnRH secretion. Leptin, a hormone produced by adi-

FIGURE 325-1　Pubertal events in males. Sexual maturity ratings for genitalia and pubic hair and divided into five stages. (*From WA Marshall, JM Tanner: Variations in the pattern of pubertal changes in boys. Arch Dis Child 45:13, 1970.*)

pose cells, may play a permissive role in this process, as leptin-deficient individuals fail to enter puberty (Chap. 64). Early puberty is characterized by nocturnal surges of LH and FSH. Growth of the testes is usually the first sign of puberty, reflecting an increase in seminiferous tubule volume. Increasing levels of testosterone deepen the voice and increase muscle growth. Conversion of testosterone to DHT leads to growth of the external genitalia and pubic hair. DHT also stimulates prostate and facial hair growth and initiates recession of the temporal hairline. The growth spurt occurs at a testicular volume of about 10 to 12 mL. GH increases early in puberty and is stimulated in part by the rise in gonadal steroids. GH increases the level of insulin-like growth factor 1 (IGF-1), which enhances linear bone growth. The prolonged pubertal exposure to gonadal steroids (mainly estradiol) ultimately causes epiphyseal closure and limits further bone growth.

REGULATION OF TESTICULAR FUNCTION

REGULATION OF THE HYPOTHALAMIC-PITUITARY-TESTIS AXIS IN ADULT MAN
Hypothalamic GnRH regulates the production of the pituitary gonadotropins, LH and FSH (Fig. 325-2). GnRH is released in discrete pulses approximately every 2 h, resulting in corresponding pulses of LH and FSH. These dynamic hormone pulses account in part for the wide variations in LH and testosterone, even within the same individual. LH acts primarily on the Leydig cell to stimulate testosterone synthesis. The regulatory control of androgen synthesis is mediated by testosterone and estrogen feedback on both the hypothalamus and the pituitary. FSH acts on the Sertoli cell to regulate spermatogenesis and the production of Sertoli products such as inhibin B, which acts to selectively suppress pituitary FSH. Despite these somewhat distinct Leydig and Sertoli cell–regulated pathways, testis function is integrated at several levels: GnRH regulates both gonadotropins; spermatogenesis requires high levels of testosterone; there are numerous paracrine interactions between Leydig and Sertoli cells that are necessary for normal testis function.

THE LEYDIG CELL: ANDROGEN SYNTHESIS
LH binds to its seven transmembrane, G protein–coupled receptor to activate the cyclic AMP pathway. Stimulation of the LH receptor induces *s*teroid *a*cute *r*egulatory (StAR) protein, along with several steroidogenic enzymes involved in androgen synthesis. LH receptor mutations cause Leydig cell hypoplasia or agenesis, underscoring the importance of this pathway for Leydig cell development and function. The rate-limiting process in testosterone synthesis is the delivery of cholesterol by the StAR protein to the inner mitochondrial membrane. Peripheral benzodiazepine receptor, a mitochondrial cholesterol-binding protein, is also an acute regulator of Leydig cell steroidogenesis. The five major enzymatic steps involved in testosterone synthesis are summarized in Fig. 325-3. After cholesterol transport into the mitochondrion, side chain cleavage by CYP11A1 to form pregnenolone is a limiting enzymatic step.

FIGURE 325-2　Human pituitary gonadotropin axis, structure of testis, seminiferous tubule. E$_2$, 17β estradiol; DHT, dihydrotestosterone.

The 17α-hydroxylase and the 17,20-lyase reactions are catalyzed by a single enzyme, CYP17; posttranslational modification (phosphorylation) of this enzyme and the presence of specific enzyme cofactors confer 17,20-lyase activity selectively in the testis and zona reticularis of the adrenal gland. Testosterone can be converted to the more potent DHT by 5α-reductase, or it can be aromatized to estradiol by CYP19 (aromatase).

Testosterone Transport and Metabolism　In males, 95% of circulating testosterone is derived from testicular secretion (3 to 10 mg/d). Direct secretion of testosterone by the adrenal and the peripheral conversion of androstenedione to testosterone collectively account for another 0.5 mg/d of testosterone. Only a small amount of DHT (70 μg/d) is secreted directly by the testis; most circulating DHT is derived from peripheral conversion of testosterone.

Circulating testosterone is bound to two plasma proteins: sex hormone–binding globulin (SHBG) and albumin (Fig. 325-4). SHBG binds testosterone with much greater affinity than albumin. Only 0.5 to 3% of testosterone is unbound. According to the "free hormone" hypothesis, only the unbound fraction is biologically active; however, albumin-bound hormone dissociates readily in the capillaries and may be bioavailable. SHBG concentrations are decreased by androgens, obesity, insulin, and nephrotic syndrome. Conversely, estrogen administration, hyperthyroidism, many chronic inflammatory illnesses, and aging are associated with high SHBG concentrations.

Testosterone is metabolized predominantly in the liver, although some degradation occurs in peripheral tissues, particularly the prostate and the skin. In the liver, testosterone is converted by a series of enzymatic steps into androsterone, etiocholanolone, DHT, and 3-α-androstanediol. These compounds undergo glucuronidation or sulfation before being excreted by the kidneys.

Mechanism of Androgen Action　The androgen receptor (AR) is homologous to other nuclear receptor proteins including the receptors for estrogen, glucocorticoids, and progesterone (Chap. 317). The AR is encoded by a gene on the long arm of the X chromosome and has a molecular mass of about 110 kDa. A polymorphic region in the amino

FIGURE 325-3 The biochemical pathway in the conversion of 27-carbon sterol cholesterol to androgens and estrogens.

FIGURE 325-4 Androgen metabolism and actions. SHBG, sex hormone–binding globulin.

terminus of the receptor, which contains a variable number of glutamine repeats, modifies the transcriptional activity of the receptor. The AR protein is distributed in both the cytoplasm and the nucleus. Androgen binding to the AR causes it to translocate into the nucleus where it binds to DNA or other transcription factors already bound to DNA. The ligand also induces conformational changes that allow the recruitment and assembly of tissue-specific cofactors. Thus, the AR is a ligand-regulated transcription factor. Some androgen effects may be mediated by nongenomic AR signal transduction pathways. Testosterone binds to AR with half the affinity of DHT. The DHT-AR complex also has greater thermostability, and a slower dissociation rate, than the testosterone-AR complex. However, the molecular basis for selective testosterone versus DHT actions remains incompletely explained.

THE SEMINIFEROUS TUBULES: SPERMATOGENESIS The seminiferous tubules are convoluted, closed loops with both ends emptying into the rete testis, a network of progressively larger efferent ducts that ultimately form the epididymis (Fig. 325-2). The seminiferous tubules total about 600 m in length and comprise about two-thirds of testis volume. The walls of the tubules are formed by polarized Sertoli cells that are apposed to peritubular myoid cells. Tight junctions between Sertoli cells create a blood-testis barrier. Germ cells comprise the majority of the seminiferous epithelium (~60%) and are intimately embedded within the cytoplasmic extensions of the Sertoli cells, which function as "nurse cells." Germ cells progress through characteristic morphologic stages of spermiogenesis, requiring ~24 days. A pool of type A spermatogonia serve as stem cells capable of self-renewal. Primary sper-

matocytes are derived from type B spermatogonia and undergo meiosis before progressing to spermatids that mature and are ultimately released from Sertoli cells as mature spermatozoa. Peristaltic-type action by peritubular myoid cells transports sperm into the efferent ducts. The normal adult testes produce >100 million sperm per day.

Naturally occurring mutations in the *FSHβ* gene and in the FSH receptor confirm an important, but not essential, role for this pathway in spermatogenesis. Females with these mutations are hypogonadal and infertile because ovarian follicles do not mature; males exhibit variable degrees of reduced spermatogenesis, presumably because of impaired Sertoli cell function. Because Sertoli cells produce inhibin B, an inhibitor of FSH, seminiferous tubule damage (e.g., by radiation) causes a selective increase of FSH. Androgens reach very high concentrations locally in the testis and are essential for spermatogenesis. Several cytokines and growth factors are also involved in the regulation of spermatogenesis by paracrine and autocrine mechanisms. A number of knockout mouse models exhibit impaired germ cell development or spermatogenesis, presaging possible mutations associated with male infertility. In humans, microdeletions of several Y chromosome azoospermia factor (*AZF*) genes (e.g., RNA-binding motif, *RBM*; deleted in azoospermia, *DAZ*) are associated with oligospermia or azoospermia.

CLINICAL AND LABORATORY EVALUATION OF MALE REPRODUCTIVE FUNCTION

HISTORY AND PHYSICAL EXAMINATION The history should focus on developmental stages such as puberty and growth spurts, as well as androgen-dependent events such as early morning erections, frequency and intensity of sexual thoughts, and frequency of masturbation or intercourse. Although libido and the overall frequency of sexual acts is decreased in androgen-deficient men, young hypogonadal men may achieve erections in response to visual erotic stimuli. Men with acquired androgen deficiency often report decreased energy and increased irritability.

The physical examination should focus on secondary sex characteristics such as hair growth, possible gynecomastia, testicular volume, prostate, and height and body proportions. Eunuchoidal proportions are defined as an arm span >2 cm greater than height and suggest that androgen deficiency occurred before epiphyseal fusion. Hair growth in the face, axilla, chest, and pubic regions is androgen-dependent;

however, changes may not be noticeable unless androgen deficiency is severe and prolonged. Ethnicity also influences the intensity of hair growth (Chap. 44). Testicular volume is best measured by using a Prader orchidometer. Testes range from 3.5 to 5.5 cm in length, which corresponds to a volume of 12 to 25 mL. Advanced age does not influence testicular size, although the consistency becomes less firm. Asian men generally have smaller testes than western Europeans, independent of differences in body size. Because of its possible role in infertility, the presence of varicocele should be sought by palpation while the patient is standing; it is more common on the left side. Patients with Klinefelter syndrome have markedly reduced testicular volumes (1 to 2 mL). In congenital hypogonadotropic hypogonadism, testicular volumes provide a good index for the degree of gonadotropin deficiency and the likelihood of response to therapy.

GONADOTROPIN AND INHIBIN MEASUREMENTS LH and FSH are measured using two-site immunoradiometric, immunofluorometric, or chemiluminescent assays, which have very low cross-reactivity with other pituitary glycoprotein hormones and human chorionic gonadotropin (hCG) and have sufficient sensitivity to measure the low levels present in patients with hypogonadotropic hypogonadism. In men with a low testosterone level, an LH level can distinguish hypergonadotropic (high LH) versus hypogonadotropic (low or inappropriately normal LH) hypogonadism. An elevated LH level indicates a primary defect at the testicular level, whereas a low or inappropriately normal LH level suggests a defect at the hypothalamic-pituitary level. LH pulses occur about every 1 to 3 h in normal men. Thus, gonadotropin levels fluctuate, and samples should be pooled or repeated when results are equivocal. FSH is less pulsatile than LH because it has a longer half-life. Increased FSH suggests damage to the seminiferous tubules. Inhibin B, a Sertoli cell product that suppresses FSH, is reduced with seminiferous tubule damage. Inhibin B is a dimer with α-β_B subunits and is measured by two-site immunoassays.

GnRH Stimulation Testing The GnRH test is performed by measuring LH and FSH concentrations at baseline and at 30 and 60 min after intravenous administration of 100 μg of GnRH. A minimally acceptable response is a twofold LH increase and a 50% FSH increase. In the prepubertal period or with severe GnRH deficiency, the gonadotrope may not respond to a single bolus of GnRH because it has not been primed by endogenous hypothalamic GnRH; in these patients, GnRH responsiveness may be restored by chronic, pulsatile GnRH administration. With the availability of sensitive and specific LH assays, GnRH stimulation testing is used rarely except to evaluate gonadotrope function in patients who have undergone pituitary surgery or have a space-occupying lesion in the hypothalamic-pituitary region.

TESTOSTERONE ASSAYS ■ Total Testosterone Total testosterone includes both unbound and protein-bound testosterone and is measured by radioimmunoassays or immunometric assays. A single random sample provides a good approximation of the average testosterone concentration with the realization that testosterone levels fluctuate in response to pulsatile LH. Testosterone is generally lower in the late afternoon and is reduced by acute illness. The testosterone concentration in healthy young men ranges from 300 to 1000 ng/dL in most laboratories. Alterations in SHBG levels due to aging, obesity, some types of medications, chronic illness, or on a congenital basis can affect total testosterone levels.

Measurement of Free Testosterone Levels Most circulating testosterone is bound to SHBG and to albumin; only 0.5 to 3% of circulating testosterone is unbound or "free." Free testosterone concentrations can be calculated from algorithms based on total testosterone and SHBG concentrations. The free fraction is best measured by equilibrium dialysis. Tracer analogue methods are relatively inexpensive and convenient but they are less reliable because changes in SHBG affect the results. Bioavailable testosterone refers to unbound testosterone plus testosterone that is loosely bound to albumin; it can be estimated by the ammonium sulfate precipitation method.

hCG Stimulation Test The hCG stimulation test is performed by administering a single injection of 1500 to 4000 IU of hCG intramuscularly and measuring testosterone levels at baseline and 24, 48, 72, and 120 h after hCG injection. An alternative regimen involves three injections of 1500 units of hCG on successive days, and measuring testosterone levels 24 h after the last dose. An acceptable response to hCG is a doubling of the testosterone concentration in adult men. In prepubertal boys, an increase in testosterone to >150 ng/dL indicates the presence of testicular tissue. No response may indicate an absence of testicular tissue or marked impairment of Leydig cell function. Measurement of MIS, a Sertoli cell product, is also used to detect the presence of testes in prepubertal boys with cryptorchidism.

SEMEN ANALYSIS Semen analysis is the most important step in the evaluation of male infertility (Chap. 45). Samples are collected by masturbation following a period of abstinence for 2 to 3 days. Semen volumes and sperm concentrations vary considerably among fertile men, and several samples may be needed before concluding that the results are abnormal. Analysis should be performed within an hour of collection. The normal ejaculate volume is 2 to 6 mL and contains sperm counts of >20 million/mL, with a motility of >50% and >15% normal morphology. Some men with low sperm counts are nevertheless fertile. A variety of tests for sperm function can be performed in specialized laboratories, but these add relatively little to the treatment options.

TESTICULAR BIOPSY Testicular biopsy is useful in some patients with oligospermia or azoospermia, as an aid in diagnosis and indication for the feasibility of treatment. Using local anesthesia, fine-needle aspiration biopsy is performed to aspirate tissue for histology. Alternatively, open biopsies can be performed under local or general anesthesia when more tissue is required. A normal biopsy in an azoospermic man with a normal FSH level suggests obstruction of the vas deferens, which may be correctable surgically. Biopsies are also used to harvest sperm for intracytoplasmic sperm injection (ICSI) and to classify disorders such as hypospermatogenesis (all stages present but in reduced numbers), germ cell arrest (usually at primary spermatocyte stage), and Sertoli cell–only syndrome (absent germ cells) or hyalinization (sclerosis with absent cellular elements).

DISORDERS OF SEXUAL DIFFERENTIATION
See Chap. 328

DISORDERS OF PUBERTY

PRECOCIOUS PUBERTY Puberty in boys before age 9 is considered precocious. *Isosexual precocity* refers to premature sexual development consistent with phenotypic sex and includes features such as the development of facial hair and phallic growth. Isosexual precocity is divided into gonadotropin-dependent and gonadotropin-independent causes of androgen excess (Table 325-1). *Heterosexual precocity* refers to the premature development of feminizing features in boys, such as breast development.

Gonadotropin-Dependent Precocious Puberty This disorder is also called *central precocious puberty* (CPP) and it is less common in boys than in girls. It is caused by premature activation of the GnRH pulse generator, sometimes because of central nervous system (CNS) lesions such as hypothalamic hamartomas, but it is often idiopathic. CPP is characterized by gonadotropin levels that are inappropriately elevated for age. Because pituitary priming has occurred, GnRH elicits LH and FSH responses typical of those seen in puberty or in adults. Magnetic resonance imaging (MRI) should be performed to exclude a mass, structural defect, or infectious or inflammatory process.

Gonadotropin-Independent Precocious Puberty This group of disorders includes hCG-secreting tumors; congenital adrenal hyperplasia; sex steroid–producing tumors of the testis, adrenal, and ovary; accidental or deliberate exogenous sex steroid administration; hypothyroidism; and

TABLE 325-1 *Causes of Precocious or Delayed Puberty in Boys*

I. Precocious puberty
  A. Gonadotropin-dependent
    1. Idiopathic
    2. Hypothalamic hamartoma or other lesions
    3. CNS tumor or inflammatory state
  B. Gonadotropin-independent
    1. Congenital adrenal hyperplasia
    2. hCG-secreting tumor
    3. McCune-Albright syndrome
    4. Activating LH receptor mutation
    5. Exogenous androgens
II. Delayed puberty
  A. Constitutional delay of growth and puberty
  B. Systemic disorders
    1. Chronic disease
    2. Malnutrition
    3. Anorexia nervosa
  C. CNS tumors and their treatment (radiotherapy and surgery)
  D. Hypothalamic-pituitary causes of pubertal failure (low gonadotropins)
    1. Congenital disorders (Table 325-2)
      a. Hypothalamic syndromes (e.g., Prader-Willi)
      b. Idiopathic hypogonadotropic hypogonadism
      c. Kallmann syndrome
      d. GnRH receptor mutations
      e. Adrenal hypoplasia congenita
      f. *PROP1* mutations
      g. Other mutations affecting pituitary development/function
    2. Acquired disorders
      a. Pituitary tumors
      b. Hyperprolactinemia
  E. Gonadal causes of pubertal failure (elevated gonadotropins)
    1. Klinefelter syndrome
    2. Bilateral undescended testes or anorchia
    3. Orchitis
    4. Chemotherapy or radiotherapy
  F. Androgen insensitivity

Note: CNS, central nervous system; hCG, human chronic gonadotropin; LH, luteinizing hormone; GnRH, gonadotropin-releasing hormone.

activating mutations of the LH receptor or $G_s\alpha$ subunit. In these cases, androgens from the testis or the adrenal are increased but gonadotropins are low.

FAMILIAL MALE-LIMITED PRECOCIOUS PUBERTY This is transmitted in an autosomal dominant manner. It is caused by activating mutations in the LH receptor, leading to constitutive stimulation of the cyclic AMP pathway and testosterone production. The disorder is also called *testotoxicosis*. Clinical features include premature virilization in boys, growth acceleration in early childhood, and advanced bone age followed by premature epiphyseal fusion. Testosterone is elevated and LH is suppressed. Treatment options include inhibitors of testosterone synthesis (e.g., ketoconazole), androgen receptor antagonists (e.g., flutamide), and aromatase inhibitors (e.g., anastrazole).

McCUNE-ALBRIGHT SYNDROME This is a sporadic disorder caused by somatic (postzygotic) activating mutations in the $G_s\alpha$ subunit that links G protein–coupled receptors to intracellular signaling pathways (Chap. 334). The mutations impair the guanosine triphosphatase activity of the $G_s\alpha$ protein, leading to constitutive activation of adenylyl cyclase. Like activating LH receptor mutations, this stimulates testosterone production and causes gonadotropin-independent precocious puberty. In addition to sexual precocity, affected individuals may have autonomy in the adrenals, pituitary, and thyroid glands. Café au lait spots are characteristic skin lesions that reflect the onset of the somatic mutations in melanocytes during embryonic development. Polyostotic fibrous dysplasia is caused by activation of the parathyroid hormone receptor pathway in bone. Treatment is similar to that in patients with activating LH receptor mutations. Bisphosphonates have been used to treat bone lesions.

CONGENITAL ADRENAL HYPERPLASIA Boys with congenital adrenal hyperplasia (CAH) who are not well controlled with glucocorticoid suppression

of adrenocorticotropic hormone (ACTH) can develop premature virilization because of excessive androgen production by the adrenal gland (Chaps. 321 and 328). LH is low and the testes are small. Rarely, adrenal rests may develop within the testis because of chronic ACTH stimulation.

Heterosexual Sexual Precocity Breast enlargement in prepubertal boys can result from familial aromatase excess, estrogen-producing tumors in the adrenal gland, Sertoli cell tumors in the testis, marijuana smoking, or estrogen use. Occasionally, germ cell tumors that secrete hCG can be associated with breast enlargement due to excessive stimulation of estrogen production (see "Gynecomastia," below).

APPROACH TO THE PATIENT

After verification of precocious development, serum LH and FSH levels should be measured to determine whether gonadotropins are increased in relation to chronologic age (gonadotropin-dependent) or whether sex steroid secretion is occurring independent of LH and FSH (gonadotropin-independent). In children with gonadotropin-dependent precocious puberty, CNS lesions should be excluded by history, neurologic examination, and MRI scan of the head. If organic causes are not found, one is left with the diagnosis of idiopathic central precocity. Patients with high testosterone but suppressed LH concentrations have gonadotropin-independent sexual precocity; in these patients, DHEA sulfate (DHEAS) and 17α-hydroxyprogesterone should be measured. High levels of testosterone and 17α-hydroxyprogesterone suggest the possibility of CAH due to 21α-hydroxylase or 11β-hydroxylase deficiency. If testosterone and DHEAS are elevated, adrenal tumors should be excluded by obtaining a computed tomography (CT) scan of the adrenal glands. Patients with elevated testosterone but without increased 17α-hydroxyprogesterone or DHEAS should undergo careful evaluation of the testis by palpation and ultrasound to exclude a Leydig cell neoplasm. Activating mutations of the LH receptor should be considered in children with gonadotropin-independent precocious puberty in whom CAH, androgen abuse, and adrenal and testicular neoplasms have been excluded.

℞ TREATMENT

In patients with a known cause (e.g., a CNS lesion or a testicular tumor), therapy should be directed towards the underlying disorder. In patients with idiopathic CPP, long-acting GnRH analogues can be used to suppress gonadotropins and decrease testosterone, halt early pubertal development, delay accelerated bone maturation, and prevent early epiphyseal closure. The treatment is most effective for increasing final adult height if it is initiated before age 6. Puberty resumes after discontinuation of the GnRH analogue. Counseling is an important aspect of the overall treatment strategy. In children with gonadotropin-independent precocious puberty, inhibitors of steroidogenesis, such as ketoconazole, and AR antagonists have been used empirically without data from clinical trials.

DELAYED PUBERTY Puberty is delayed in boys if it has not ensued by age 14, an age that is 2 to 2.5 standard deviations above the mean for healthy children. Delayed puberty is more common in boys than in girls. There are four main categories of delayed puberty: (1) Constitutional delay of growth and puberty (~60% of cases); (2) functional hypogonadotropic hypogonadism caused by systemic illness or malnutrition (~20% of cases); (3) hypogonadotropic hypogonadism caused by genetic or acquired defects in the hypothalamic-pituitary region (~10% of cases); and (4) hypergonadotropic hypogonadism secondary to primary gonadal failure (~15% of cases) (Table 325-1). Functional hypogonadotropic hypogonadism is more common in girls than in boys. Permanent causes of hypogonadotropic or hypergonadotropic hypogonadism are identified in <25% of boys with delayed puberty.

APPROACH TO THE PATIENT

Any history of systemic illness, eating disorders, excessive exercise, social and psychological problems, and abnormal patterns of linear growth during childhood should be verified. Boys with pubertal delay may have accompanying emotional and physical immaturity relative to their peers, which can be a source of anxiety. Physical examination should focus on height; arm span; weight; visual fields; and secondary sex characteristics including hair growth, testicular volume, phallic size, and scrotal reddening and thinning. Testicular size >2.5 cm generally indicates that the child has entered puberty.

The main diagnostic challenge is to distinguish those with constitutional delay, who will progress through puberty at a later age, from those with an underlying pathologic process. Constitutional delay should be suspected when there is a family history and when there are delayed bone age and short stature. Pituitary priming by pulsatile GnRH is required before LH and FSH are synthesized and secreted normally. Thus, blunted responses to exogenous GnRH can be seen in patients with constitutional delay, GnRH deficiency, or pituitary disorders (see "GnRH Stimulation Testing," above). On the other hand, low-normal basal gonadotropin levels or a normal response to exogenous GnRH is consistent with an early stage of puberty, which is often heralded by nocturnal GnRH secretion. Thus, constitutional delay is a diagnosis of exclusion that requires ongoing evaluation until the onset of puberty and the growth spurt.

℞ TREATMENT

If therapy is considered appropriate, it can begin with 25 to 50 mg testosterone enanthate or testosterone cypionate every 2 weeks, or by using a 2.5-mg testosterone patch or 25-mg testosterone gel. Because aromatization of testosterone to estrogen is obligatory for mediating androgen effects on epiphyseal fusion, concomitant treatment with aromatase inhibitors may allow attainment of greater final adult height. Testosterone treatment should be interrupted after 6 months to determine if endogenous LH and FSH secretion have ensued. Other causes of delayed puberty should be considered when there are associated clinical features or when boys do not enter puberty spontaneously after a year of observation or treatment.

Reassurance without hormonal treatment is appropriate for many individuals with presumed constitutional delay of puberty. However, the impact of delayed growth and pubertal progression on a child's social relationships and school performance is often underappreciated.

DISORDERS OF THE MALE REPRODUCTIVE AXIS DURING ADULTHOOD

HYPOGONADOTROPIC HYPOGONADISM Because LH and FSH are trophic hormones for the testes, impaired secretion of these pituitary gonadotropins results in secondary hypogonadism, which is characterized by low testosterone in the setting of low LH and FSH. Those with the most severe deficiency have complete absence of pubertal development, sexual infantilism and, in some cases, hypospadias and undescended testes. Patients with partial gonadotropin deficiency have delayed or arrested sexual development. The 24-h LH secretory profiles are heterogeneous in patients with hypogonadotropic hypogonadism, reflecting variable abnormalities of LH pulse frequency or amplitude. In severe cases, basal LH is low and there are no LH pulses. A smaller subset of patients has low-amplitude LH pulses or markedly reduced pulse frequency. Occasionally, only sleep-entrained LH pulses occur, reminiscent of the pattern seen in the early stages of puberty. Hypogonadotropic hypogonadism can be classified into congenital and acquired disorders. Congenital disorders most commonly involve GnRH deficiency, which leads to gonadotropin deficiency. Acquired disorders are much more common than congenital disorders and may result from a variety of sellar mass lesions or infiltrative diseases of the hypothalamus or pituitary.

Congenital Disorders Associated with Gonadotropin Deficiency Most cases of congenital hypogonadotropic hypogonadism are idiopathic, despite extensive endocrine testing and imaging studies of the sellar region. Among known causes, familial hypogonadotropic hypogonadism can be transmitted as an X-linked (20%), autosomal recessive (30%), or autosomal dominant (50%) trait. Some individuals with idiopathic hypogonadotropic hypogonadism (IHH) have sporadic mutations in the same genes that cause inherited forms of the disorder. *Kallmann syndrome* is an X-linked disorder caused by mutations in the *KAL1* gene, which encodes anosmin, a protein that mediates the migration of neural progenitors of the olfactory bulb and GnRH-producing neurons. These individuals have GnRH deficiency and variable combinations of anosmia or hyposmia, renal defects, and neurologic abnormalities including mirror movements. Gonadotropin secretion and fertility can be restored by administration of pulsatile GnRH or by gonadotropin replacement. Mutations in the *FGFR1* gene cause an autosomal dominant form of hypogonadotropic hypogonadism that clinically resembles Kallmann syndrome. The *FGFR1* gene product may be the receptor for the *KAL1* gene product, anosmin, thereby explaining the similarity in clinical features. Other autosomal dominant causes remain unexplained. X-linked hypogonadotropic hypogonadism also occurs in adrenal hypoplasia congenita, a disorder caused by mutations in the *DAX1* gene, which encodes a nuclear receptor in the adrenal gland and reproductive axis. *Adrenal hypoplasia congenita* is characterized by absent development of the adult zone of the adrenal cortex, leading to neonatal adrenal insufficiency. Puberty usually does not occur or is arrested, reflecting variable degrees of gonadotropin deficiency. Although sexual differentiation is normal, some patients have testicular dysgenesis and impaired spermatogenesis despite gonadotropin replacement. *GnRH receptor mutations* account for ~40% of autosomal recessive and 10% of sporadic cases of hypogonadotropic hypogonadism. These patients have decreased LH response to exogenous GnRH. Some receptor mutations alter GnRH binding affinity, allowing apparently normal responses to pharmacologic doses of exogenous GnRH. Mutations in the G protein–coupled receptor, GPR54, cause gonadotropin deficiency without anosmia. Patients retain responsiveness to exogenous GnRA, suggesting an abnormality in the neural pathways controlling GnRH release. Rarely, recessive mutations in the *LHβ* or *FSHβ* genes have been described in patients with selective deficiencies of these gonadotropins. Deletions or mutations of the *GnRH* gene have not been found in patients with hypogonadotropic hypogonadism.

A number of homeodomain transcription factors are involved in the development and differentiation of the specialized hormone-producing cells within the pituitary gland (Table 325-2). Patients with mutations of *PROP1* have combined pituitary hormone deficiency that includes GH, prolactin (PRL) thyroid-stimulating hormone (TSH), LH, and FSH, but not ACTH. *LHX3* mutations cause combined pituitary hormone deficiency in association with cervical spine rigidity. *HESX1* mutations cause septooptic dysplasia and combined pituitary hormone deficiency.

Prader-Willi syndrome is characterized by obesity, hypotonic musculature, mental retardation, hypogonadism, short stature, and small hands and feet. Prader-Willi syndrome is a genomic imprinting disorder caused by deletions of the proximal portion of paternally derived chromosome 15q or by uniparental disomy of the maternal alleles (Chap. 57). *Laurence-Moon syndrome* is an autosomal recessive disorder characterized by obesity, hypogonadism, mental retardation, polydactyly, and retinitis pigmentosa. Recessive mutations of leptin, or its receptor, cause severe obesity and pubertal arrest, apparently because of hypothalmic GnRH deficiency (Chap. 64).

Acquired Hypogonadotropic Disorders ■ *SEVERE ILLNESS, STRESS, MALNUTRITION, AND EXERCISE* These may cause reversible gonadotropin deficiency. Although gonadotropin deficiency and reproductive dysfunction are well documented in these conditions in women, men exhibit similar but less pronounced responses. Unlike women, most male runners and other endurance athletes have normal gonadotropin and sex steroid

TABLE 325-2 *Causes of Congenital Hypogonadotropic Hypogonadism*

Gene	Locus	Inheritance	Associated Features
KAL1	Xp22	X-linked	Anosmia, renal agenesis, synkinesia, cleft lip/palate, oculomotor/visuospatial defects, gut malrotations
FGFR1	8p11-p12	AD	Anosmia, cleft lip/palate, synkinesia, syndactyly
LEP	7q31	AR	Obesity
LEPR	1p31	AR	Obesity
PC1	5q15-21	AR	Obesity, diabetes mellitus, ACTH deficiency
HESX1	3p21	AR	Septooptic dysplasia, CPHD
		AD	Isolated GH insufficiency
LHX3	9q34	AR	CPHD (ACTH spared), cervical spine rigidity
PROP1	5q35	AR	CPHD (ACTH usually spared)
GPR54	19p13	AR	None
GNRHR	4q21	AR	None
FSHβ	11p13	AR	↑ LH
LHβ	19q13	AR	↑ FSH
SF1 (NR5A1)	9p33	AD/AR	Primary adrenal failure, XY sex reversal
DAX1 (NR0B1)	Xp21	X-linked	Primary adrenal failure, impaired spermatogenesis

Abbreviations: ACTH, adrenocorticotropic hormone; AD, autosomal dominant; AR, autosomal recessive; CPHD, combined pituitary hormone deficiency; KAL1, Interval-1 gene; FGFR1, fibroblast growth factor receptor 1; LEP, leptin; LEPR, leptin receptor; PC1, prohormone convertase 1; HESX1, homeo box gene expressed in embryonic stem cells 1; LHX3, LIM homeobox gene 3; PROP1, Prophet of Pit 1; GPR54, G protein–coupled receptor 54; GNRHR, gonadotropin-releasing hormone receptor; FSHβ, follicle-stimulating hormone β-subunit; LHβ, luteinizing hormone β-subunit; SF1, steroidogenic factor 1; DAX1, *d*osage-sensitive sex-reversal, *a*drenal hypoplasia congenita, *X*-chromosome.

levels, despite low body fat and frequent intensive exercise. Testosterone levels fall at the onset of illness and recover during recuperation. The magnitude of gonadotropin suppression generally correlates with the severity of illness. Although hypogonadotropic hypogonadism is the most common cause of androgen deficiency in patients with acute illness, some have elevated levels of LH and FSH, which suggest primary gonadal dysfunction. The pathophysiology of reproductive dysfunction during acute illness is unknown but likely involves a combination of cytokine and/or glucocorticoid effects. There is a high frequency of low testosterone levels in patients with chronic illnesses such as HIV infection, end-stage renal disease, chronic obstructive lung disease, and many types of cancer and in patients receiving glucocorticoids. Some 20% of HIV-infected men with low testosterone levels have elevated LH and FSH levels; these patients presumably have primary testicular dysfunction. The remaining 80% have either normal or low LH and FSH levels; these men have a central hypothalamic-pituitary defect or a dual defect involving both the testis and the hypothalamic-pituitary centers. Muscle wasting is common in chronic diseases associated with hypogonadism, which also leads to debility, poor quality of life, and adverse outcome of disease. There is great interest in exploring strategies that can reverse androgen deficiency or attenuate the sarcopenia associated with chronic illness.

Men who are heavy users of marijuana have decreased testosterone secretion and sperm production. The mechanism of marijuana-induced hypogonadism is decreased GnRH secretion. Gynecomastia observed in marijuana users can also be caused by plant estrogens in crude preparations.

OBESITY In men with mild to moderate obesity, SHBG levels decrease in proportion to the degree of obesity, resulting in lower total testosterone levels. However, free testosterone levels usually remain within the normal range. The decrease in SHBG levels is caused by increased circulating insulin, which inhibits SHBG production. Estradiol levels are higher in obese men compared to healthy, non-obese controls, because of aromatization of testosterone to estradiol in adipose tissue. Weight loss is associated with reversal of these abnormalities including an increase in total and free testosterone levels and a decrease in

estradiol levels. A subset of massively obese men may have a defect in the hypothalamic-pituitary axis as suggested by low free testosterone in the absence of elevated gonadotropins.

HYPERPROLACTINEMIA (See also Chap. 318) Elevated PRL levels are associated with hypogonadotropic hypogonadism. PRL inhibits hypothalamic GnRH secretion either directly or through modulation of tuberoinfundibular dopaminergic pathways. A PRL-secreting tumor may also destroy the surrounding gonadotropes by invasion or compression of the pituitary stalk. Treatment with dopamine agonists reverses gonadotropin deficiency, although there may be a delay relative to PRL suppression.

SELLAR MASS LESIONS Neoplastic and nonneoplastic lesions in the hypothalamus or pituitary can directly or indirectly affect gonadotrope function. In adults, pituitary adenomas constitute the largest category of space-occupying lesions affecting gonadotropin and other pituitary hormone production. Pituitary adenomas that extend into the suprasellar region can impair GnRH secretion and mildly increase PRL secretion (usually <50 μg/L) because of impaired tonic inhibition by dopaminergic pathways. These tumors should be distinguished from prolactinomas, which typically secrete higher PRL levels. The presence of diabetes insipidus suggests the possibility of a craniopharyngioma, infiltrative disorder, or other hypothalamic lesions (Chap. 319).

HEMOCHROMATOSIS (See also Chap. 336) Both the pituitary and testis can be affected by excessive iron deposition. However, the pituitary defect is the predominant lesion in most patients with hemochromatosis and hypogonadism. The diagnosis of hemochromatosis is suggested by the association of characteristic skin pigmentation, hepatic enlargement or dysfunction, diabetes mellitus, arthritis, cardiac conduction defects, and hypogonadism.

PRIMARY TESTICULAR CAUSES OF HYPOGONADISM Common causes of primary testicular dysfunction include Klinefelter syndrome, uncorrected cryptorchidism, cancer chemotherapy, radiation to the testes, trauma, torsion, infectious orchitis, HIV infection, anorchia syndrome, and myotonic dystrophy. Primary testicular disorders may be associated with impaired spermatogenesis, decreased androgen production, or both. →*See Chap. 328 for disorders of testis development, androgen synthesis, and androgen action.*

Klinefelter Syndrome (See also Chap. 328) Klinefelter syndrome is the most common chromosomal disorder associated with testicular dysfunction and male infertility. It occurs in about 1 in 1000 live-born males. Azoospermia is the rule in men with Klinefelter syndrome who have the 47,XXY karyotype; however, men with mosaicism may have germ cells, especially at a younger age. Testicular histology shows hyalinization of seminiferous tubules and absence of spermatogenesis. Although their function is impaired, the number of Leydig cells appears to increase. Testosterone is decreased and estradiol is increased, leading to clinical features of undervirilization and gynecomastia.

Cryptorchidism Cryptorchidism occurs when there is incomplete descent of the testis from the abdominal cavity into the scrotum. About 3% of full-term and 30% of premature male infants have at least one cryptorchid testis at birth, but descent is usually complete by the first few weeks of life. The incidence of cryptorchidism is <1% by 9 months of age. Cryptorchidism is associated with increased risk of malignancy and infertility. Unilateral cryptorchidism, even when corrected before puberty, is associated with decreased sperm counts, possibly reflecting unrecognized damage to the fully descended testis.

Acquired Testicular Defects *Viral orchitis* may be caused by the mumps virus, echovirus, lymphocytic choriomeningitis virus, and group B arboviruses. Orchitis occurs in as many as one-fourth of adult men with mumps; the orchitis is unilateral in about two-thirds, and bilateral in the remainder. Orchitis usually develops a few days after the onset of parotitis but may precede it. The testis may return to normal size and function or undergo atrophy. Semen analysis returns to normal for three fourths of men with unilateral involvement but normal for only one-third of men with bilateral orchitis. *Trauma*, including testicular torsion, can also cause secondary atrophy of the testes. The exposed position of the testes in the scrotum renders them susceptible to both thermal and physical trauma, particularly in men with hazardous occupations.

The testes are sensitive to *radiation damage*. Doses >200 mGy (20 rad) are associated with increased FSH and LH levels and damage to the spermatogonia. After ~800 mGy (80 rad), oligospermia or azoospermia develops, and higher doses may obliterate the germinal epithelium. Permanent androgen deficiency in adult men is uncommon after therapeutic radiation; however, most boys given direct testicular radiation therapy for acute lymphoblastic leukemia have permanently low testosterone levels. Sperm banking should be considered before patients undergo radiation treatment or chemotherapy.

Drugs interfere with testicular function by several mechanisms including inhibition of testosterone synthesis (e.g., ketoconazole), blockade of androgen action (e.g., spironolactone), increased estrogen (e.g., marijuana), or direct inhibition of spermatogenesis (e.g., chemotherapy). Cyclophosphamide causes azoospermia or extreme oligospermia within a few weeks after the initiation of therapy. In about half of patients, spermatogenesis returns within 3 years after cessation of therapy. Combination chemotherapy for acute leukemia, Hodgkin disease, and other malignancies may impair Leydig cell function. Alcohol, when consumed in excess for prolonged periods, decreases testosterone, independent of liver disease or malnutrition. Elevated estradiol and decreased testosterone levels may occur in men taking digitalis.

The occupational and recreational history should be carefully evaluated in all men with infertility because of the toxic effects of many *chemical agents* on spermatogenesis. Known environmental hazards include microwaves and ultrasound and chemicals such as nematocide dibromochloropropane, cadmium, and lead. In some populations, sperm density is said to have declined by as much as 40% in the past 50 years. Environmental estrogens or antiandrogens may be partly responsible.

Testicular failure also occurs as a part of *polyglandular autoimmune insufficiency* (Chap. 330). Sperm antibodies can cause isolated male infertility. In some instances, these antibodies are secondary phenomena resulting from duct obstruction or vasectomy. Granulomatous diseases can affect the testes, and testicular atrophy occurs in 10 to 20% of men with lepromatous leprosy because of direct tissue invasion by the mycobacteria. The tubules are involved initially, followed by endarteritis and destruction of Leydig cells.

Systemic disease can cause primary testis dysfunction in addition to suppressing gonadotropin production. In cirrhosis, a combined testicular and pituitary abnormality leads to decreased testosterone production independent of the direct toxic effects of ethanol. Impaired hepatic extraction of adrenal androstenedione leads to extraglandular conversion to estrone and estradiol, which partially suppresses LH. Testicular atrophy and gynecomastia are present in approximately one-half of men with cirrhosis. In chronic renal failure, androgen synthesis and sperm production decrease despite elevated gonadotropins. The elevated LH level is due to reduced clearance, but it does not restore normal testosterone production. About one-fourth of men with renal failure have hyperprolactinemia. Improvement in testosterone production with hemodialysis is incomplete, but successful renal transplantation may return testicular function to normal. Testicular atrophy is present in one-third of men with sickle cell anemia. The defect may be at either the testicular or the hypothalamic-pituitary level. Sperm density can decrease temporarily after acute febrile illness in the absence of a change in testosterone production. Infertility in men with celiac disease is associated with a hormonal pattern typical of androgen resistance, namely elevated testosterone and LH levels.

Neurologic diseases associated with altered testicular function include myotonic dystrophy, spinobulbar muscular atrophy, and paraplegia. In myotonic dystrophy, small testes may be associated with impairment of both spermatogenesis and Leydig cell function. Spinobulbar muscular atrophy is caused by an expansion of the glutamine repeat sequences in the amino-terminal region of the AR; this expansion impairs function of the AR, but it is unclear how the alteration is related to the neurologic manifestations. Men with spinobulbar muscular atrophy often have undervirilization and infertility as a late manifestation. Spinal cord lesions that cause paraplegia can lead to a temporary decrease in testosterone levels and may cause persistent defects in spermatogenesis; some patients retain the capacity for penile erection and ejaculation.

ANDROGEN INSENSITIVITY SYNDROMES   Mutations in the AR cause resistance to the action of testosterone and DHT. These X-linked mutations are associated with variable degrees of defective male phenotypic development and undervirilization (Chap. 328). Although not technically hormone insensitivity syndromes, two genetic disorders impair testosterone conversion to active sex steroids. Mutations in the *SRD5A2* gene, which encodes 5α-reductase type 2, prevent the conversion of testosterone to DHT, which is necessary for the normal development of the male external genitalia. Mutations in the *CYP19* gene, which encodes aromatase, prevent testosterone conversion to estradiol. Males with *CYP19* mutations have delayed epiphyseal fusion, tall stature, eunuchoidal proportions, and osteoporosis, consistent with evidence from an estrogen receptor–deficient individual that these testosterone actions are mediated indirectly via estrogen.

GYNECOMASTIA

Gynecomastia refers to enlargement of the male breast. It is caused by excess estrogen action and is usually the result of an increased estrogen/androgen ratio. True gynecomastia is associated with glandular breast tissue that is >4 cm in diameter and is often tender. Glandular tissue enlargement should be distinguished from excess adipose tissue; glandular tissue is firmer and contains fibrous-like cords. Gynecomastia occurs as a normal physiologic phenomenon in the newborn, during puberty, and with aging, but it can also result from pathologic conditions associated with androgen deficiency or estrogen excess. The prevalence of gynecomastia increases with age and body mass index (BMI), likely because of increased aromatase activity in adipose tissue. Medications that alter androgen metabolism or action may also cause gynecomastia. The relative risk of breast cancer is increased in men with gynecomastia, although the absolute risk is relatively small.

PATHOLOGIC GYNECOMASTIA   Any cause of *androgen deficiency* can lead to gynecomastia, reflecting an increased estrogen/androgen ratio, as estrogen synthesis still occurs by aromatization of residual adrenal and gonadal androgens. Gynecomastia is a characteristic feature of Klinefelter syndrome (Chap. 328). *Androgen insensitivity* disorders also cause gynecomastia. *Excess estrogen production* may be caused by tumors, including Sertoli cell tumors in isolation or in association with Peutz-Jegher syndrome or Carney complex. Tumors that produce hCG, including some testicular tumors, stimulate Leydig cell estrogen synthesis. *Increased conversion of androgens to estrogens* can be a result of increased availability of substrate (androstenedione) for extraglandular estrogen formation (CAH, hyperthyroidism, and most feminizing adrenal tumors) or to diminished catabolism of androstenedione (liver disease) so that estrogen precursors are shunted to aromatase in peripheral sites. Obesity is associated with increased aromatization of androgen precursors to estrogens. Extraglandular aromatase activity can also be increased in tumors of the liver or adrenal gland or rarely as an inherited disorder. Several families with *increased peripheral aromatase activity* inherited as an autosomal or as an X-linked disorder have been described. *Drugs* can cause gynecomastia by acting directly as estrogenic substances (e.g., oral contraceptives, phytoestrogens, digitalis), inhibiting androgen synthesis (e.g., ketoconazole), or action (e.g., spironolactone).

It is challenging to determine when to evaluate gynecomastia, since up to two-thirds of pubertal boys and half of hospitalized men have palpable glandular tissue (Fig. 325-5). In addition to the extent of gynecomastia, recent onset, rapid growth, tender tissue, and occur-

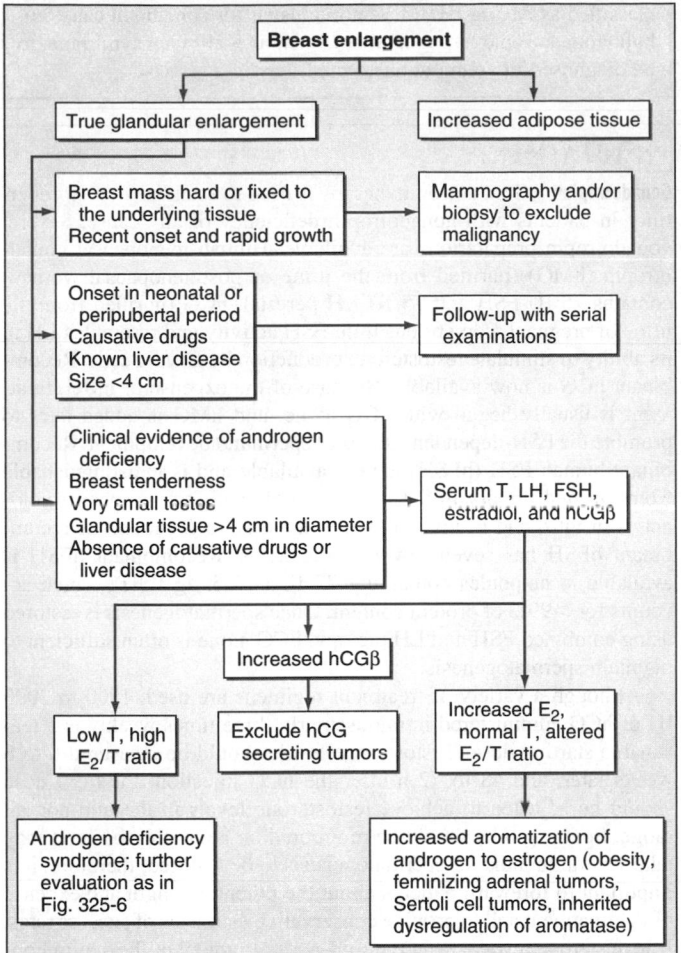

FIGURE 325-5 Evaluation of gynecomastia. T, testosterone; LH, luteinizing hormone; FSH, follicle-stimulating hormones; hCGβ, human chorionic gonadoltopin β; E₂, 17β-estradiol.

rence in a lean subject should prompt more extensive evaluation. This should include a careful drug history, measurement and examination of the testes, assessment of virilization, evaluation of liver function, and hormonal measurements including testosterone, estradiol, and androstenedione, LH, and hCG. If testes are small, a karyotype should be obtained to exclude Klinefelter syndrome. Despite this evaluation, the diagnosis is established in fewer than one-half of patients, probably because of subtle alterations of the estrogen/androgen ratio.

℞ TREATMENT

When the primary cause can be identified and corrected, breast enlargement usually subsides over several months. However, if gynecomastia is of long duration, surgery is the most effective therapy. Indications for surgery include severe psychologic and/or cosmetic problems, continued growth or tenderness, or suspected malignancy. In patients who have painful gynecomastia and who are not candidates for other therapy, treatment with antiestrogens such as tamoxifen (20 mg/d) reduces pain and breast tissue size in about two-thirds of patients. Aromatase inhibitors can be effective in the early proliferative phase of the disorder, although the experience is largely based on the use of testolactone, a relatively weak aromatase inhibitor; placebo-controlled trials with more potent aromatase inhibitors such as anastrazole, fadrozole, letrozole, or fromestane are needed.

AGING-RELATED CHANGES IN MALE REPRODUCTIVE FUNCTION

A number of cross-sectional and longitudinal studies (e.g., The Baltimore Longitudinal Study of Aging and the Massachusetts Male Aging Study) have established that testosterone concentrations decrease

with advancing age. This age-related decline starts in the third decade of life and progresses slowly; the rate of decline in testosterone concentrations is greater for men with chronic illness and for those taking medications than in healthy older men. Because SHBG concentrations are higher in older men than in younger men, free or bioavailable testosterone concentrations decline with aging to a greater extent than total testosterone concentrations. The age-related decline in testosterone is due to defects at all levels of the hypothalamic-pituitary-testicular axis: pulsatile GnRH secretion is attenuated, LH response to GnRH is reduced, and testicular response to LH is impaired. However, the gradual rise of LH with aging suggests that testis dysfunction is the main cause of declining androgen levels. The term *andropause* has been used to denote age-related decline in testosterone concentrations; this term is a misnomer because there is no discrete time when testosterone concentrations decline abruptly.

It is speculated that age-related decline in testosterone concentrations contributes to sexual dysfunction, loss of muscle mass and function, frailty, gain in fat mass, cognitive impairment, and loss of body hair. Initial studies of testosterone supplementation in older men with low or low normal testosterone levels have demonstrated a modest increase of fat-free mass and grip strength; a decrease in fat mass; an improved sense of well being, energy, visuo-spatial orientation, and verbal memory; and a modest increment in bone mineral density. However, the long-term risks of testosterone supplementation in older men remain largely unknown. In particular, physiologic testosterone replacement might increase the risk of prostate cancer or exacerbate cardiovascular disease. Population screening of all older men for low testosterone levels is not recommended, and testing should be restricted to men who have symptoms or physical features attributable to androgen deficiency. In men with documented androgen deficiency, testosterone replacement may be considered on an individualized basis and should be instituted after careful discussion of the risks and benefits (see "Testosterone Replacement," below).

Testicular morphology, semen production, and fertility are maintained up to a very old age in men. Although concern has been expressed about age-related increases in germ cell mutations and impairment of DNA repair mechanisms, the frequency of chromosomal aneuploidy or structural abnormalities does not increase in the sperm of older men. However, the incidence of autosomal dominant diseases, such as achondroplasia, polyposis coli, Marfan syndrome, and Apert syndrome, increases in the offspring of men who are advanced in age, consistent with transmission of sporadic missense mutations.

APPROACH TO THE PATIENT

Hypogonadism is often heralded by decreased sex drive, reduced frequency of sexual intercourse or inability to maintain erections, reduced beard growth, loss of muscle mass, decreased testicular size, and gynecomastia. Less than 10% of patients with erectile dysfunction alone have testosterone deficiency. Thus, it is useful to look for a constellation of symptoms and signs suggestive of androgen deficiency. Except when extreme, these clinical features may be difficult to distinguish from changes that occur with normal aging. Moreover, androgen deficiency may develop gradually. Population studies, such as the Massachusetts Male Aging Study, suggest that about 4% of men between the ages of 40 and 70 have testosterone levels <150 ng/dL. Thus, androgen deficiency is not uncommon. The changes for the clinician are (1) to decide when to evaluate a man for possible androgen deficiency, (2) to assess when there is laboratory evidence for androgen deficiency and determine its cause, and (3) to decide when and how to treat patients with androgen deficiency.

When symptoms or clinical features suggest possible androgen deficiency, the laboratory evaluation is initiated by the measurement of total testosterone, preferably in the morning (Fig. 325-6). A total testosterone level <200 ng/dL, in association with symp-

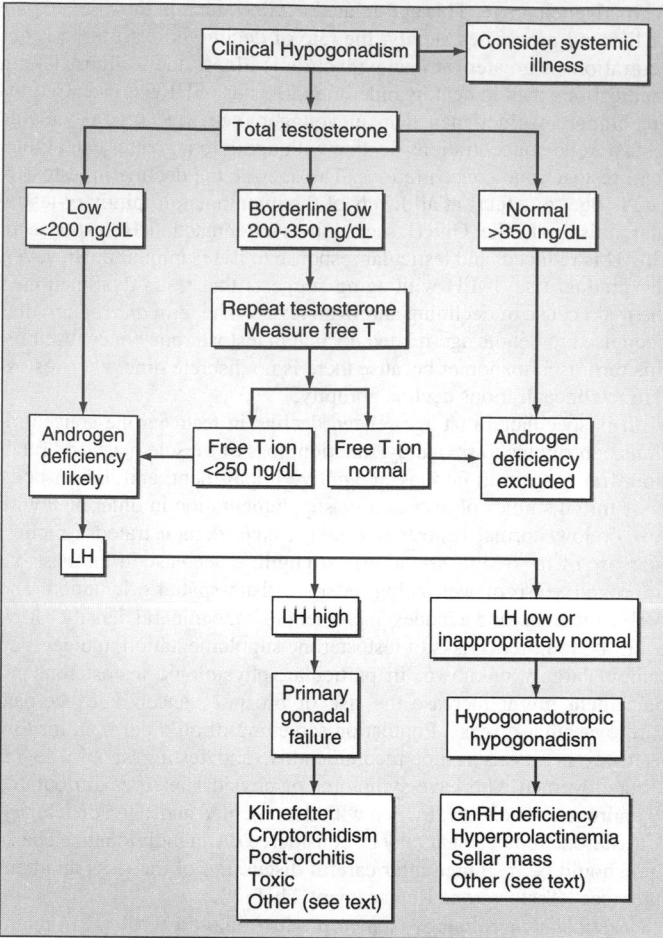

FIGURE 325-6 Evaluation of hypogonadism. T, testosterone; LH, luteinizing hormone; GnRH, gonadotropin-releasing hormone.

toms, is evidence of testosterone deficiency. An early-morning testosterone level >350 ng/dL makes the diagnosis of androgen deficiency unlikely. In men with testosterone levels between 200 and 350 ng/dL, the total testosterone level should be repeated and a free testosterone level should be measured. In older men and in patients with other clinical states that are associated with alterations in SHBG levels, a direct measurement of free testosterone level by equilibrium dialysis can be useful in unmasking testosterone deficiency.

When androgen deficiency has been confirmed by low testosterone concentrations, LH should be measured to classify the patient as having hypergonadotropic (high LH) or hypogonadotropic (low or inappropriately normal LH) hypogonadism. An elevated LH level indicates that the defect is at the testicular level. Common causes of primary testicular failure include Klinefelter syndrome, HIV infection, uncorrected cryptorchidism, cancer chemotherapeutic agents, radiation, surgical orchiectomy, or prior infectious orchitis. Unless causes of primary testicular failure are known, a karyotype should be performed in men with low testosterone and elevated LH to exclude Klinefelter syndrome. Men who have a low testosterone but "inappropriately normal" or low LH levels have hypogonadotropic hypogonadism; their defect resides at the hypothalamic-pituitary level. Common causes of acquired hypogonadotropic hypogonadism include space-occupying lesions of the sella, hyperprolactinemia, chronic illness, hemochromatosis, excessive exercise, and substance abuse. Measurement of PRL and MRI scan of the hypothalamic-pituitary region can help exclude the presence of a space-occupying lesion. Patients in whom known causes of hypogonadotropic hypogonadism have been excluded are

classified as having IHH. It is not unusual for congenital causes of hypogonadotropic hypogonadism, such as Kallmann syndrome, to be diagnosed in young adults.

℞ TREATMENT

Gonadotropins Gonadotropin therapy is used to establish or restore fertility in patients with gonadotropin deficiency of any cause. Several gonadotropin preparations are available. Human menopausal gonadotropin (hMG) (purified from the urine of postmenopausal women) contains 75 IU FSH and 75 IU LH per vial. hCG (purified from the urine of pregnant women) has little FSH activity and resembles LH in its ability to stimulate testosterone production by Leydig cells. Recombinant hCG is now available. Because of the expense of hMG, treatment is usually begun with hCG alone, and hMG is added later to promote the FSH-dependent stages of spermatid development. Recombinant human FSH (hFSH) is now available and is indistinguishable from purified urinary hFSH in its biologic activity and pharmacokinetics in vitro and in vivo, although the mature β subunit of recombinant hFSH has seven fewer amino acids. Recombinant hFSH is available in ampoules containing 75 IU (~7.5 μg FSH), which accounts for >99% of protein content. Once spermatogenesis is restored using combined FSH and LH therapy, hCG alone is often sufficient to maintain spermatogenesis.

Although a variety of treatment regimens are used, 1500 to 2000 IU of hCG administered intramuscularly three times weekly is a reasonable starting dose. Testosterone levels should be measured 6 to 8 weeks later, and 48 to 72 h after the hCG injection; the hCG dose should be adjusted to achieve testosterone levels in the mid-normal range. Sperm counts should be monitored on a monthly basis. It may take several months for spermatogenesis to be restored; therefore, it is important to forewarn patients about the potential length and expense of the treatment and to provide conservative estimates of success rates. If testosterone levels are in the mid-normal range but the sperm concentrations are low after 6 months of therapy with hCG alone, FSH should be added. This can be done by using hMG, highly purified urinary hFSH, or recombinant hFSH. The selection of FSH dose is empirical. A common practice is to start with the addition of 75 IU FSH three times each week in conjunction with the hCG injections. If sperm densities are still low after 3 months of combined treatment, the FSH dose should be increased to 150 IU. Occasionally, it may take ≥18 to 24 months for spermatogenesis to be restored.

The two best predictors of success using gonadotropin therapy in hypogonadotropic men are testicular volume at presentation and time of onset. In general, men with testicular volumes >8 mL have better response rates than those who have testicular volumes <4 mL. Patients who became hypogonadotropic after puberty experience higher success rates than those who have never undergone pubertal changes. Spermatogenesis can usually be reinitiated by hCG alone, with high rates of success for men with postpubertal onset of hypogonadotropism. The presence of a primary testicular abnormality, such as cryptorchidism, will attenuate testicular response to gonadotropin therapy. Prior androgen therapy does not affect subsequent response to gonadotropin therapy.

GnRH In patients with documented GnRH deficiency, both pubertal development and spermatogenesis can be successfully induced by pulsatile administration of low doses of GnRH. This response requires normal pituitary and testicular function. Therapy usually begins with an initial dose of 25 ng/kg per pulse administered subcutaneously every 2 h by a portable infusion pump. Testosterone, LH, and FSH levels should be monitored. The dose of GnRH is increased until testosterone levels reach the mid-normal range. Doses ranging from 25 to 200 ng/kg may be required to induce virilization. Once pubertal changes have been initiated, the dose of GnRH can often be reduced. Increased sperm counts and testicular volume have been reported in >70% of treated men, and improvements in sexual function and virilization can be induced in >90% of patients. Cutaneous infections occur but are infrequent and minor. Carrying a portable infusion device can be cumbersome, and follow-up of these patients requires physician supervision and laboratory monitoring. Some patients with IHH have cryptorchidism; men with this additional testicular defect may not respond to GnRH or gonadotropin therapy.

Comparative studies of gonadotropin therapy and pulsatile GnRH administration demonstrate that these two therapies are similar in terms of the time to first appearance of sperm or pregnancy rates; both approaches are equally effective in inducing spermatogenesis in men with hypogonadotropic hypogonadism caused by GnRH deficiency. However, most patients find intermittent gonadotropin injections preferable to wearing a continuous infusion pump.

Testosterone Replacement Androgen therapy is indicated to restore testosterone levels to normal to correct features of androgen deficiency. Testosterone replacement improves libido and overall sexual activity, increases energy, lean muscle mass, and bone density and provides the patient a better sense of well-being. The benefits of testosterone replacement therapy have only been proven in men who have documented androgen deficiency, as demonstrated by testosterone levels that are well below the lower limit of normal (<250 ng/dL).

Testosterone is available in a variety of formulations with distinct pharmacokinetics (Table 325-3). Testosterone serves as a prohormone and is converted to 17β-estradiol by aromatase and to 5α-dihydrotes-

terone by 5α-reductase. Therefore, when evaluating testosterone formulations, it is important to consider whether the formulation being used can achieve physiologic estradiol and DHT concentrations, in addition to normal testosterone concentrations. Although testosterone concentrations at the lower end of the normal male range can restore sexual function, it is not clear whether low-normal testosterone levels can maintain bone mineral density and muscle mass. The current recommendation is to restore testosterone levels to the mid-normal range.

ORAL DERIVATIVES OF TESTOSTERONE Testosterone is well-absorbed after oral administration but quickly degrades during the first pass through the liver. Therefore, it is not possible to achieve sustained blood levels of testosterone after oral administration of crystalline testosterone. 17α-alkylated derivatives of testosterone (e.g., 17α-methyl testosterone, oxandrolone, fluoxymesterone) are relatively resistant to hepatic degradation and can be administered orally; however, because of the potential for hepatotoxicity, including cholestatic jaundice, peliosis, and hepatoma, these formulations should not be used for testosterone replacement. Hereditary angioedema due to C1 esterase deficiency is the only exception to this general recommendation; in this condition, oral 17α-alkylated androgens are useful because they stimulate hepatic synthesis of the C1 esterase inhibitor.

TABLE 325-3 *Clinical Pharmacology of Testosterone Formulations*

Formulation	Regimen	Pharmacokinetics	DHT and Estradiol	Advantages	Disadvantages
Testosterone enanthate or cypionate	100 mg IM weekly or 200 mg IM every 2 weeks	After a single IM injection, testosterone levels rise into the supraphysiologic range and then decline gradually into the hypogonadal range by the end of the dosing interval	DHT and estradiol levels rise in proportion to the increase in testosterone levels; T:DHT and T:E$_2$ ratios do not change	Corrects symptoms of androgen deficiency Relatively inexpensive, if self-administered Flexibility of dosing	Requires IM injection Peaks and valleys in testosterone levels
Scrotal testosterone patch	One scrotal patch designed to deliver 6 mg over 24 h applied daily	Normalizes testosterone levels in many but not all androgen-deficient men	Estradiol levels are in the physiologic male range, but DHT levels rise into the supraphysiologic range	Corrects symptoms of androgen deficiency	To promote optimum adherence of the patch, scrotal skin needs to be shaved High DHT levels
Nongenital transdermal system	One or two patches, designed to deliver 5–10 mg testosterone over 24 h applied daily on nonpressure areas	Restores testosterone, DHT, and estradiol levels into the physiologic male range	T:DHT and T:estradiol levels are in the physiologic male range	Ease of application, corrects symptoms of androgen deficiency, and mimics the normal diurnal rhythm of testosterone secretion. Lesser increase in hemoglobin than injectable esters	Testosterone levels in some androgen-deficient men may be in the low-normal range; these men may need application of two patches daily Skin irritation at the application site in some patients
Testosterone gel	Testosterone gel containing 50 to 100 mg testosterone should be applied daily	Restores testosterone and estradiol levels into the physiologic male range	DHT levels and T:DHT ratios are lower in hypogonadal men treated with the testosterone gel than in healthy eugonadal men	Corrects symptoms of androgen deficiency, provides flexibility of dosing, ease of application, good skin tolerability	Potential of transfer to a female partner or child by direct skin-to-skin contact; moderately high DHT levels
17α-methyl testosterone	Orally active, 17α-alkylated compound that should not be used because of potential for liver toxicity	Orally active			Clinical responses variable; potential for liver toxicity; should not be used for treatment of androgen deficiency
Buccal adhesive testosterone	An adhesive, 10-mg tablet applied to buccal mucosa twice daily	Absorbed through buccal mucosa	Serum T and DHT in the normal male range	Ease of application	Limited experience, no evidence of liver toxicity, effects of food and brushing unclear

Note: DHT, dihydrotestosterone; T, testosterone, E$_2$, 17β-estradiol.

Source: Adapted from: American College of Physicians/American Society of Internal Medicine Disease Management Module on Male Hypogonadism.

INJECTABLE FORMS OF TESTOSTERONE The esterification of testosterone at the 17β-hydroxy position makes the molecule hydrophobic and extends its duration of action. The slow release of testosterone ester from an oily depot in the muscle accounts for its extended duration of action. The longer the side chain, the greater the hydrophobicity of the ester and longer the duration of action. Thus, testosterone enanthate and cypionate with longer side chains have longer duration of action than testosterone propionate. Within 24 h after intramuscular administration of 200 mg testosterone enanthate or cypionate, testosterone levels rise into the high-normal or supraphysiologic range and then gradually decline into the hypogonadal range over the next 2 weeks. A bimonthly regimen of testosterone enanthate or cypionate therefore results in peaks and troughs in testosterone levels that are accompanied by changes in a patient's mood, sexual desire, and energy level. The kinetics of testosterone enanthate and cypionate are similar. Estradiol and DHT levels are normal if testosterone replacement is physiologic.

TRANSDERMAL TESTOSTERONE Three transdermal testosterone patches are commercially available: a scrotal testosterone patch (Testoderm) and two nongenital patches (Androderm and Testoderm TTS). The scrotal transdermal testosterone patch, when applied daily to the scrotal skin, produces mid-normal testosterone levels in hypogonadal men 4 to 8 h after application followed by a gradual decrease in testosterone levels over the next 24 h. Estradiol levels are normal but DHT levels are increased due to the conversion of testosterone to DHT by the high amounts of 5α-reductase in scrotal skin. There was initial concern that exposure to high DHT levels might have deleterious effects on the prostate; however, long-term follow-up of men treated with the scrotal patch has not revealed an unexpected increase in prostate problems.

With nongenital testosterone patches, testosterone, DHT, and estradiol levels are in the mid-normal range 4 to 12 h after application. Sexual function and a sense of well-being are restored in androgen-deficient men treated with the nongenital patch. One 5-mg patch may not be sufficient to increase testosterone into the mid-normal male range in all hypogonadal men; some patients may need daily administration of two 5-mg patches to achieve the targeted testosterone concentrations. The transdermal systems are more expensive than testosterone esters. The use of nongenital patches may be associated with skin irritation in some individuals.

TESTOSTERONE GEL Two testosterone gels (Androgel) and Testim are available in 2.5- and 5-g unit doses that nominally deliver 25 and 50 mg of testosterone to the application site. Initial pharmacokinetic studies have demonstrated that 50-, 75-, and 100-mg doses applied daily to the skin can maintain total and free testosterone concentrations in the mid- to high-normal range in hypogonadal men. Total and free testosterone concentrations are uniform throughout the 24-h period. The current recommendations are to begin with a 50-mg dose and adjust the dose based on testosterone levels. The advantages of the testosterone gel are in its ease of application, its invisibility after application, and its flexibility of dosing. A major concern is the potential for inadvertent transfer of the gel to a sexual partner or to children who may come in close contact with the patient. The ratio of DHT to testosterone concentrations is higher in men treated with the testosterone gel.

A buccal adhesive testosterone tablet, which adheres to the buccal mucosa and releases testosterone as it is slowly dissolved, has been approved. After twice daily application of 10 to 20 mg tablets, serum testosterone levels are maintained within the normal male range in a majority of treated hypogonadal men. The adverse effects include buccal ulceration in a few subjects. The clinical experience with this formulation is limited, and the effects of food and brushing on absorption have not been studied in detail.

TESTOSTERONE FORMULATIONS NOT AVAILABLE IN THE UNITED STATES Testosterone undecanoate, when administered orally in oleic acid, is absorbed preferentially through the lymphatics into the systemic circulation and is spared the first-pass degradation in the liver. Doses of 40 to 80 mg orally, two or three times daily, are typically used. However, the clinical responses are variable and suboptimal. DHT-to-testosterone ratios are higher in hypogonadal men treated with oral testosterone undecanoate, as compared to eugonadal men.

Implants of crystalline testosterone can be inserted in the subcutaneous tissue by means of a trocar through a small skin incision. Testosterone is released by surface erosion of the implant and absorbed into the systemic circulation. Four to six 200-mg implants can maintain testosterone in the mid- to high-normal range for up to 6 months. Potential drawbacks include incising the skin for insertion and removal, and spontaneous extrusions and fibrosis at the site of the implant.

NOVEL ANDROGEN FORMULATIONS A number of androgen formulations with better pharmacokinetics or more selective activity profiles are under development. A biodegradable testosterone microsphere formulation provides physiologic testosterone levels for 10 to 11 weeks. Two long-acting esters, testosterone buciclate and testosterone undecanoate, when injected intramuscularly, can maintain circulating testosterone concentrations in the male range for 7 to 12 weeks. Initial clinical trials have demonstrated the feasibility of administering testosterone by the sublingual or buccal routes. 7α-methyl-19-nortestosterone is an androgen that cannot be 5α-reduced; therefore, compared to testosterone, it has relatively greater agonist activity in muscle and gonadotropin suppression but lesser activity on the prostate.

Analogous to the selective estrogen receptor modulators, such as raloxifene, it may be possible to develop selective androgen receptor modulators (SARMs) that exert the desired physiologic effects on muscle, bone, or sexual function but without adversely affecting the prostate and the cardiovascular system.

PHARMACOLOGIC USES OF ANDROGENS In addition to hypogonadism, androgens have been used to treat a variety of disorders with the hope that anabolic actions of the agents (such as increase in nitrogen retention and muscle mass, increased hemoglobin) would outweigh any deleterious (e.g., virilization) actions of the drugs. The most common nonreplacement uses of androgen have been attempts to improve nitrogen balance in catabolic states (e.g., AIDS), self-administration by athletes to increase muscle mass and/or athletic performance, attempts to enhance erythropoiesis in refractory anemias (including the anemia of renal failure), treatment of hereditary angioedema and endometriosis, and management of growth retardation of various etiologies. Most of the expected benefits in these disorders have not been realized. The modest pharmacologic doses of androgens have little physiologic effect in men when superimposed on normal testicular androgen; in women, the virilizing side effects of androgens are formidable.

The most pervasive form of androgen abuse is by male athletes with the expectation that it will improve muscle development and athletic performance. In controlled studies using modest pharmacologic doses (two to four times the usual replacement doses), these agents do not consistently improve performance. However, at the doses frequently taken by athletes (which sometimes exceed 10 times the replacement dose), androgens enhance nitrogen balance and muscle mass; since the drugs have multiple side effects at high doses, these benefits do not outweigh the risks associated with androgen abuse in men, while androgen use by female athletes is associated with disfiguring virilization. The only established indications for androgen therapy aside from male hypogonadism are in selected patients with anemia due to bone marrow failure (an indication largely supplanted by erythropoietin) or for hereditary angioedema.

RECOMMENDED REGIMENS FOR ANDROGEN REPLACEMENT Testosterone esters are administered weekly at doses of 75 to 100 mg intramuscularly, or 150 to 200 mg every 2 weeks. One 6-mg scrotal patch should be applied daily after shaving the scrotal skin. One or two 5-mg nongenital testosterone patches can be applied daily over the skin of the back, thigh, or upper arm away from pressure areas. Testosterone gel is typically applied over a covered area of skin at a dose of 50 to 100 mg daily; patients should wash their hands after gel application.

ESTABLISHING EFFICACY OF TESTOSTERONE REPLACEMENT THERAPY Because a clinically useful marker of androgen action is not available, restoration of testosterone levels into the mid-normal range remains the goal of therapy. Measurements of LH and FSH are not useful in assessing the adequacy of testosterone replacement. Testosterone should be measured 3 months after initiating therapy to assess adequacy of therapy. In patients who are treated with testosterone enanthate or cypionate, testosterone levels should be 350 to 600 ng/dL 1 week after the injection. If testosterone levels are outside this range, adjustments should be made to either the dose or the interval between injections. In men on transdermal patch or gel therapy, testosterone levels should be in the mid-normal range (500 to 800 ng/dL) 4 to 12 h after application. If testosterone levels are outside this range, the dose should be adjusted.

Restoration of sexual function, secondary sex characteristics, and energy level and one's sense of well being are important objectives of testosterone replacement therapy. The patient should also be asked about sexual desire and activity, the presence of early morning erections, and whether he is able to achieve and maintain erections that are adequate for sexual intercourse. Some hypogonadal men continue to complain about sexual dysfunction even after testosterone replacement has been instituted; these patients may benefit from counseling. The hair growth in response to androgen replacement is variable and depends on ethnicity. Hypogonadal men with prepubertal onset of androgen deficiency who begin testosterone therapy in their late 20s or 30s may find it difficult to adjust to their newly found sexuality and may benefit from counseling. If the patient has a sexual partner, the partner should be included in counseling because of the dramatic physical and sexual changes that occur with androgen treatment.

CONTRAINDICATIONS FOR ANDROGEN ADMINISTRATION Testosterone administration is contraindicated in men with a history of prostate cancer because androgens can promote tumor growth (Table 325-4). Testosterone should not be prescribed to men with severe symptoms of benign prostatic hypertrophy (AUA symptom score > 22), because even small increases in prostate volume may exacerbate obstructive symptoms. Testosterone replacement should not be administered to men with baseline hematocrit ≥52%. Testosterone can induce and exacerbate sleep apnea because of its neuromuscular effects on the upper airway.

MONITORING POTENTIAL ADVERSE EXPERIENCES The clinical effectiveness and safety of testosterone replacement therapy should be performed 3 and 6 months after initiating testosterone therapy and annually thereafter.

Hemoglobin Levels Administration of testosterone to androgen-deficient men is typically associated with a 3 to 5% increase in hemoglobin levels. Clinically significant erythrocytosis is uncommon in young hypogonadal men but can occur in men who have sleep apnea, a significant smoking history, chronic obstructive lung disease, or who are older in age. The magnitude of hemoglobin increase during testosterone therapy appears related to the peak testosterone levels. Transdermal testosterone replacement may produce a smaller hemoglobin increase than testosterone esters.

Digital Examination of the Prostate and Serum PSA Levels Testosterone replacement therapy increases prostate volume to the size seen in age-matched controls but should not increase prostate volume beyond that expected for age. There is no evidence that testosterone replacement causes prostate cancer. However, androgen administration can exacerbate pre-existing prostate cancer. Many older men harbor microscopic foci of cancer in their prostates. It is not known whether long-term testosterone administration will induce these microscopic foci to grow into clinically significant cancers.

Prostate-specific antigen (PSA) levels are lower in testosterone-deficient men and are restored to normal after testosterone replacement. There is considerable test-retest variability in PSA measurements; the average interassay coefficient of variation of PSA assays is 15%. The 95% confidence interval for the change in PSA values, measured 3 to 6 months apart, is 1.4 ng/mL. Increments in PSA levels after testosterone supplementation in androgen-deficient men are generally <0.5 ng/mL, and increments >1.0 ng/mL over a 3 to 6-month period are unusual. Nevertheless, administration of testosterone to men with baseline PSA levels between 2.5 and 4.0 ng/mL will cause PSA levels to exceed 4.0 ng/mL for some, and many of these men may undergo prostate biopsies. PSA velocity criterion can be used for patients who have sequential PSA measurements for >2 years; a change of >0.40 ng/mL per year merits closer urologic follow-up.

Cardiovascular Risk Assessment The long-term effects of testosterone supplementation on cardiovascular risk are unknown. Testosterone effects on lipids depend on the dose (physiologic or supraphysiologic), the route of administration (oral or parenteral), and the formulation (whether aromatizable or not). Physiologic testosterone replacement by an aromatizable androgen has a modest effect on high-density lipoprotein (HDL) or no effect at all. In middle-aged men with low testosterone levels, physiologic testosterone replacement has been shown to improve insulin sensitivity and reduce visceral obesity. In epidemiologic studies, testosterone concentrations are inversely related to waist-to-hip ratio and directly correlated with HDL cholesterol levels. These data suggest that physiologic testosterone concentrations is correlated with factors associated with reduced cardiovascular risk. However, no prospective studies have examined the effect on testosterone replacement on cardiovascular risk.

MALE SEXUAL DYSFUNCTION
See Chap. 43.

MALE INFERTILITY
See Chap. 45.

BENIGN AND MALIGNANT PROSTATE DISORDERS
See Chap. 81.

TESTICULAR NEOPLASMS
See Chap. 82.

ACKNOWLEDGMENT
We are grateful to James E. Griffin and Jean D. Wilson, authors of Disorders of the Testes in the 15th edition of Harrison's, for contributions to this chapter.

FURTHER READING

ACHERMANN JC et al: Inherited disorders of the gonadotropin hormones. Mol Cell Endocrinol 179:89, 2001

BHASIN S, BUCKWALTER JG: Testosterone supplementation of older men: A rational idea whose time has not yet come. J Androl 122:718, 2001

FELDMAN HA et al: Age trends in the level of serum testosterone and other hormones in middle-aged men: Longitudinal results from the Massachusetts male aging study. J Clin Endocrinol Metab 87:589, 2002

LIU PY et al: Androgens and cardiovascular disease. Endocr Rev 24:313, 2003

SEDLMEYER IL, PALMERT MR: Delayed puberty: Analysis of a large case series from an academic center. J Clin Endocrinol Metab 87:1613, 2002

TABLE 325-4   *Contraindications for Androgen Replacement*

- The presence or history of prostate cancer
- Baseline PSA ≥ 4 ng/mL or a palpable abnormality of the prostate without urologic evaluation to rule out prostate cancer
- Severe symptoms of lower urinary tract obstruction as indicated by IPSS or AUA symptom score of ≥22
- Baseline hematocrit > 52%
- Severe sleep apnea
- Class IV congestive heart failure

Note: PSA, prostate-specific antigen, IPSS, International Prostate Symptom Score; AUA, American Urological Association.

Normal female reproduction requires the integrated action of the central nervous system, the pituitary gland, and the ovary to orchestrate the monthly cycle of ovarian follicle development and the release of ova. The hormonal changes associated with the menstrual cycle prepare the uterus for implantation if fertilization occurs. After menopause, these cycles cease, and there is a marked reduction in sex steroid levels, leading to physiologic changes. Disorders of the female reproductive system may be developmental, structural, or hormonal in etiology. The reproductive tract is also susceptible to sexually transmitted diseases, which may cause active or chronic infections and predispose to infertility and neoplasia. Gynecologic malignancies, particularly of the ovary, uterus, and cervix, are relatively common. Although many women receive specialized care from obstetrician-gynecologists, a good understanding of the female reproductive system and its disorders is essential for comprehensive healthcare by internists and family practitioners.

DEVELOPMENT, STRUCTURE, AND FUNCTION OF THE OVARY

EMBRYOLOGY

The primordial germ cells migrate to the genital ridge adjacent to the mesonephric kidney by the fifth week of gestation and undergo mitotic division. The gonads exist in an undifferentiated state until the seventh week of fetal life, at which time the primitive ovary can be distinguished from the testis (Chap. 328). From the fifth month of fetal life, the primordial follicle consists of the primary oocyte arrested in meiosis, a single surrounding layer of granulosa cells, and a basement membrane that separates the primordial follicle from surrounding stromal (interstitial) tissues. The ovary contains a finite number of germ cells, the number peaking at about 7 million oogonia by the fifth to sixth month of gestation. Subsequently, the germ cells decrease in number through a process of atresia so that approximately 1 million remain at birth, 400,000 are present at menarche, and only a few remain at menopause.

PUBERTAL MATURATION

The final maturation of ovarian follicles commences during puberty. The two major hormones that regulate follicular development are the pituitary gonadotropins—follicle-stimulating hormone (FSH) and luteinizing hormone (LH) (Fig. 326-1). In the neonate, concomitant with the decrease in estrogen and progesterone levels caused by separation from the placenta, there is a rebound increase in gonadotropin secretion for the first few months of life. With continued maturation of the hypothalamic-pituitary system, the hypothalamic-pituitary axis (the so-called gonadostat) becomes exquisitely sensitive to negative feedback by low levels of circulating steroid hormones, and plasma gonadotropins again decrease. As the time of puberty nears, a decrease in the sensitivity of the gonadostat allows for increased secretion of FSH and LH, possibly secondary to increased episodic or pulsatile secretion of gonadotropin-releasing hormone (GnRH) by the hypothalamus (Chap. 318). The increase in estrogen secretion exerts a positive feedback, which leads to an exaggeration of the pulsatile release of LH and eventually to menarche and ovulation, after which plasma gonadotropin concentrations reach adult values but vary across the menstrual cycle. After the menopause, plasma gonadotropin levels rise, then plateau 5 to 10 years after menopause and remain fairly constant until the eighth to ninth decade of life, when the levels may fall. Although ovarian function is regulated primarily by LH and FSH, the ovary is a source of protein hormones and growth factors such as inhibin and activin that play an important role in ovarian function and regulation. The production of inhibin by the mature ovary accounts, in part, for the selective reduction in FSH that is seen during the reproductive years (Fig. 326-1).

At age 10 to 11, the first secondary sexual characteristics begin to appear in girls, namely, development of the breast buds (*thelarche*), followed by the development of pubic hair (*pubarche*), and later by the development of axillary hair (*adrenarche*). The growth of pubic and axillary hair is believed to be initiated by adrenal androgens, the levels of which begin to rise at approximately 6 to 8 years of age. A growth spurt ensues, and peak growth rate is attained by age 12.

The culmination of puberty is the onset of predictable, cyclic menses. The average time between the beginning of breast development and the onset of menses (*menarche*) is 2 years. During the first few years after menarche, menstrual cycles are often irregular and unpredictable due to anovulation. The age of menarche is variable and is influenced by socioeconomic and genetic factors and by general health. In the United States, the mean age of menarche is believed to have decreased at a rate of 3 to 4 months per decade over the past 100 years and is now approximately 12 years of age, a change believed to be due to improved nutrition. Leptin levels have been correlated with the onset of the pubertal process. A critical combination of total body weight and percent body fat is associated with development of hypothalamic insensitivity to feedback by steroids that leads to increased secretion of gonadotropins and finally to menarche. Obese girls have earlier menarche than girls with normal body weight. In contrast, active participation in sports or ballet, malnutrition, and chronic debilitating disease can delay menarche.

MATURE OVARY

MORPHOLOGY The anatomic components and function of the adult ovary are illustrated schematically in Fig. 326-2. Under the influence of gonadotropins, a group of primary follicles are recruited, and by day 6 to 8 of the menstrual cycle, one follicle becomes mature or "dominant," a process characterized by accelerated growth of granulosa cells and enlargement of the fluid-filled antrum. The follicles not destined to ovulate undergo degeneration, similar to the atresia that occurs during embryogenesis. Just prior to ovulation, meiosis resumes in the ovum of the dominant follicle, and the first meiotic division results in formation of the first polar body. The antrum rapidly enlarges (up to 10 to 25 mm in size), follicular fluid increases in amount, and the follicular surface thins and forms a conical stigma. Ovulation from the dominant follicle occurs 16 to 23 h after the LH peak and 24 to 38 h after the onset of the LH surge when the follicular wall ruptures in the area of the stigma. The ovum is then expelled together with a mass of surrounding granulosa cells called *cumulus cells*. The rupture is believed to result from the action of hydrolytic enzymes on the surface of the follicle, possibly under the control of prostaglandins. The second meiotic division occurs after the egg is fertilized by a sperm, and the second polar body is then extruded. The formation of the *corpus luteum* begins in the retained remnant of the

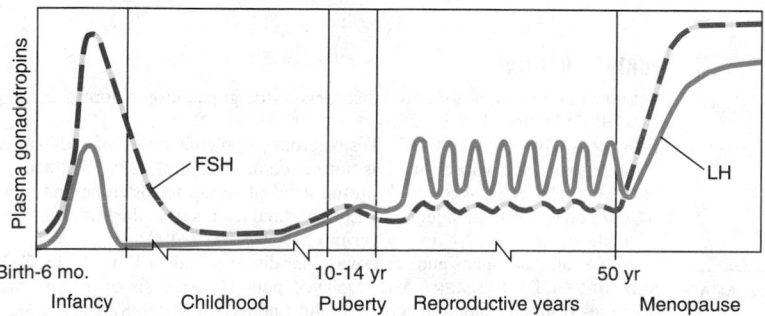

FIGURE 326-1 Pattern of gonadotropin secretion during different stages of life in women. FSH, follicle-stimulating hormone; LH, luteinizing hormone.

ovulated follicle; the remaining granulosa and theca cells increase in size and accumulate lipids and a yellow pigment, lutein, to become "luteinized." After a period of 14 ± 2 days (the functional life of the corpus luteum), the corpus luteum begins to atrophy, to be replaced in time by a fibrous scar, the *corpus albicans*. The factors that limit the life span of the human corpus luteum are not known, but if pregnancy occurs, the corpus luteum persists under the influence of placental chorionic gonadotropin, and progesterone is produced by the corpus luteum for the support of pregnancy.

HORMONE FORMATION ■ Steroid Hormones

Like other steroid hormones, ovarian steroids are derived from cholesterol (Fig. 326-3). The ovary can synthesize cholesterol de novo and can also utilize cholesterol obtained from circulating lipoproteins as substrate for steroid hormone formation. Virtually all ovarian cells are believed to possess the complete complement of enzymes required for the synthesis of estradiol from cholesterol (Fig. 326-3); however, different cell types in the ovary contain different amounts of these enzymes so that the main steroids produced vary in different compart-

FIGURE 326-2 Developmental changes in the adult ovary during a complete 28-day cycle.

ments. For example, the corpus luteum forms mainly progesterone and 17-hydroxyprogesterone, whereas theca and stromal cells convert cholesterol to androstenedione and testosterone. Granulosa cells are particularly rich in the aromatase enzyme responsible for estrogen synthesis and utilize as substrates for this process androgens synthesized in the adjacent theca cells.

LH acts primarily to regulate the early steps in steroid hormone biosynthesis, namely, the transport of cholesterol into the mitochondria by steroidogenic acute regulatory (StAR) protein and its conversion to pregnenolone. FSH acts mainly to regulate the final process by which androgens are aromatized to estrogens. As a consequence, LH enhances substrate flow and the formation of androgens and/or progesterone in the absence of FSH, whereas FSH action is impeded in the absence of LH because of diminished substrate for aromatization.

ESTROGENS   The principal estrogen secreted by the ovary and the most potent estrogen is estradiol. Estrone is also produced by the ovary, but most estrone is formed by extraglandular conversion of androstenedione in peripheral tissues. Estriol (16-hydroxyestradiol), the main estrogen in urine, arises from the 16-hydroxylation of estrone and estradiol. Catechol estrogens are formed by hydroxylation of estrogens at the C-2 or C-4 position and may act as the intracellular mediators of some estrogen action. Estrogens promote development of the secondary sexual characteristics in women and cause uterine growth, thickening of the vaginal mucosa, thinning of the cervical mucus, and development of the ductule system of the breasts. Estrogens also alter lipid profiles and exert effects on the vascular endothelium. The classic mechanism of estrogen action in target tissues is similar to that for other steroid hormones and involves binding to a nuclear steroid receptor—either estrogen receptor (ER)α or ERβ—and enhancement of the transcription of various target genes (Chap. 317). There is growing evidence that ERs also act through nonclassic mechanisms to alter signal transduction, independent of receptor binding to DNA. ERs have specific tissue site expression and bind various estrogens with different affinities, thereby conferring selective actions. The relatively promiscuous binding of synthetic and environmental estrogens by the ER has allowed the development of selective estrogen receptor modulators (SERMs), such as tamoxifen and raloxifene.

PROGESTERONE   Progesterone is the principal hormone secreted by the corpus luteum and is responsible for progestational effects, i.e., in-

duction of secretory activity in the endometrium of the estrogen-primed uterus in preparation for implantation of the fertilized egg. Progesterone also induces a decidual reaction in endometrium. Other effects include inhibition of uterine contractions, an increase in the viscosity of cervical mucus, glandular development of the breasts, and an increase in basal body temperature (thermogenic effect).

ANDROGENS   The ovary synthesizes a variety of 19-carbon steroids, including dehydroepiandrosterone, androstenedione, testosterone, and dihydrotestosterone, principally in stromal and thecal cells. The major ovarian 19-carbon steroid is androstenedione (Fig. 326-3), part of which is secreted into the plasma and part of which is converted to estrogen in granulosa cells or to testosterone in the interstitium. Androstenedione can also be converted to testosterone and estrogens in peripheral tissues. Only testosterone and dihydrotestosterone are true androgens that interact with the androgen receptor and induce virilizing signs in women (Chap. 44).

Other Hormones   *Inhibin* is secreted in two forms (A and B) by the follicle and inhibits the release of FSH by the hypothalamic-pituitary unit. *Activin* is also secreted by the follicle and may enhance FSH secretion as well as having local effects on ovarian steroidogenesis. *Follistatin* is an activin-binding protein that attenuates the actions of activin and other members of the transforming growth factor (TGF)β family.

Some ovarian hormones play an uncertain role in human physiology. *Relaxin*, a polypeptide hormone produced by the human corpus luteum and by the decidua, causes softening of the cervix and loosening of the symphysis pubis in preparation for parturition in animals. *Oxytocin, vasopressin*, and other hypothalamic and pituitary hormones are also present in granulosa and/or luteal cells, but their function in these cells is unknown. Granulosa cells secrete *oocyte maturation inhibitor* (OMI), a factor that prevents premature ovulation. In addition, in the gonads of both sexes a *meiosis-inducing substance* triggers the onset of meiosis, an event that occurs earlier in ovarian than in testicular development. Local growth factors [including insulin-like growth factors (IGFs) 1 and 2 and TGFα and -β] may also influence steroid secretion by the ovary.

THE NORMAL MENSTRUAL CYCLE   The menstrual cycle is divided into a follicular or proliferative phase and a luteal, or secretory, phase (Fig.

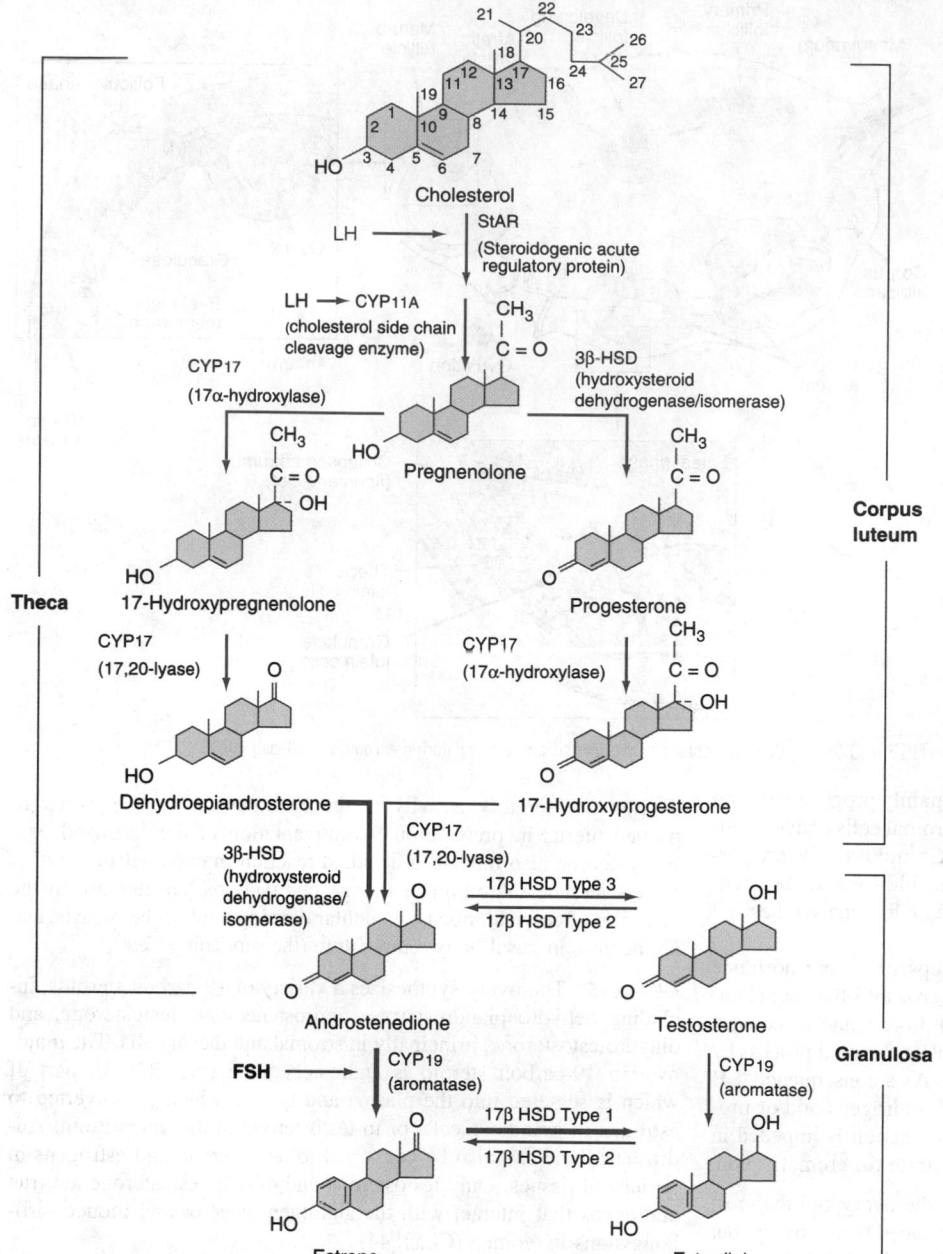

FIGURE 326-3 The principal pathway of steroid hormone biosynthesis in the ovary. The major enzyme complements for the corpus luteum, stroma, and granulosa cells are shown by the brackets; as a consequence, these cells produce predominantly progesterone and 17-OH progesterone, androgen, and estrogen, respectively. The major sites of action of luteinizing hormone (LH) and follicle-stimulating hormone (FSH) in mediating this pathway are shown in the horizontal arrows. The thin arrow emphasizes that the metabolism of 17-hydroxyprogesterone is limited in the human ovary. 17β HSD, 17β-hydroxysteroid dehydrogenase.

acterized by anovulation) occur at menarche and near the onset of menopause. At the end of a cycle, plasma levels of estrogen and progesterone fall and circulating levels of FSH increase. Under the influence of FSH, follicular recruitment results in development of the follicle that will be dominant during the next cycle.

After the onset of menses, follicular development continues, but FSH levels decrease. Approximately 8 to 10 days prior to the midcycle LH surge, plasma estradiol levels begin to rise as the result of estradiol formation by the granulosa cells of the dominant follicle. During the second half of the follicular phase, LH levels also begin to rise (owing to positive feedback). Just before ovulation, estradiol secretion reaches a peak and then falls. Immediately thereafter, a further rise in the plasma level of LH mediates the final maturation of the follicle, followed by follicular rupture and ovulation 16 to 23 h after the LH peak. The rise in LH is accompanied by a smaller increase in the level of plasma FSH, the physiologic significance of which is unclear. The plasma progesterone level also begins to rise just prior to midcycle and facilitates the positive feedback action of estradiol on LH secretion.

At the onset of the luteal phase, plasma gonadotropins decrease and plasma progesterone increases. A secondary rise in estrogens causes further gonadotropin suppression. Near the end of the luteal phase, progesterone and estrogen levels fall, and FSH levels begin to rise to initiate the development of the next follicle (usually in the contralateral ovary) and the next menstrual cycle. Inhibin A levels are low in the follicular phase but reach a peak in the luteal phase. Inhibin B levels, in contrast, are increased in the follicular phase and low in the luteal phase.

The endometrium lining the uterine cavity undergoes marked alterations in response to the changing plasma levels of ovarian hormones (Fig. 326-4). Concurrent with the decrease in plasma estrogen and progesterone and the decline of corpus luteum function in the late luteal phase, intense vasospasm occurs in the spiral arterioles supplying blood to the endometrium, causing ischemic necrosis, endometrial desquamation, and bleeding. This vasospasm is caused by locally synthesized prostaglandins. The onset of bleeding marks the first day of the menstrual cycle. By the fourth to fifth day, the endometrium is thin. During the proliferative phase, glandular growth of the endometrium is mediated by estrogen. After ovulation, increased progesterone levels lead to further thickening of the endometrium, but the rapid growth slows. The endometrium then enters the secretory phase, characterized by tortuosity of the glands, curling of the spiral arterioles, and glandular secretion. As corpus luteum function begins to wane in the absence of conception, the sequence of events leading to menstruation is again set into action.

326-4). The secretion of FSH and LH is fundamentally under negative feedback control by ovarian steroids (particularly estradiol) and by inhibin (which selectively suppresses FSH), but the response of gonadotropins to different levels of estradiol varies. FSH secretion is inhibited progressively as estrogen levels increase—typical negative feedback. In contrast, LH secretion is suppressed maximally by sustained low levels of estrogen and is enhanced by a rising level of estradiol—positive feedback. Feedback of estrogen involves both the hypothalamus and pituitary. Negative feedback suppresses GnRH and inhibits gonadotropin production. Positive feedback is associated with an increased frequency of GnRH secretion and enhanced pituitary sensitivity to GnRH.

The length of the menstrual cycle is defined as the time from the onset of one menstrual bleeding episode to onset of the next. In women of reproductive age, the cycle averages 28 ± 3 days and the mean duration of flow is 4 ± 2 days. Longer menstrual cycles (usually char-

Biphasic changes in basal body temperature are characteristic of the ovulatory cycle and are mediated by alterations in progesterone levels (Fig. 326-4). An increase in basal body temperature by 0.3 to 0.5°C begins after ovulation, persists during the luteal phase, and returns to the normal baseline (36.2 to 36.4°C) after the onset of the subsequent menses.

MENOPAUSE

The *menopause* is defined as the final episode of menstrual bleeding in women. Menopause is the consequence of exhaustion of ovarian follicles, a process that begins during fetal development. The median age of women at the time of cessation of menstrual bleeding is 50 to 51 years. Preceding the menopause, the pattern of menstrual cycles is variable, but the interval between menses usually becomes shorter, as follicular recruitment is hastened by increases in FSH. Day 3 FSH and 17β-estradiol (E_2) levels are often elevated. Ovulatory cycles continue for some period of time, then anovulation becomes common.

The ovaries of postmenopausal women are small and wrinkled, and the residual cells are predominantly stromal. Estrogen and androgen levels in plasma are reduced but not absent. Before the menopause, plasma androstenedione is derived almost equally from the adrenals and the ovaries; after menopause, the ovarian contribution ceases so that the plasma levels of androstenedione fall by 50%. However, the menopausal ovary continues to secrete testosterone, presumably formed in stromal cells. After menopause, extraglandular estrogen formation is the major pathway for estrogen synthesis. Because adipose tissue is a major site of extraglandular estrogen production, peripheral estrogen formation may actually be enhanced in obese postmenopausal women. The predominant estrogen formed is estrone rather than estradiol. →*For discussion of the management of menopause, see Chap. 327.*

FIGURE 326-4 The hormonal, ovarian, endometrial, and basal body temperature changes and relationships throughout the normal menstrual cycle.

LABORATORY AND CLINICAL ASSESSMENT OF HORMONAL STATUS

The hormonal status of women can usually be assessed by history and physical examination. In general, the presence of secondary sexual characteristics such as normal female breast development indicates adequate estrogen secretion in the past, and the presence of regular, predictable, cyclic menses implies that ovulation and the production of gonadotropins, estrogen, progesterone, and androgens are adequate and that the outflow tract is intact. Such a history may be more valuable than laboratory tests in evaluating ovarian hormone status. However, laboratory tests provide valuable ancillary information in the evaluation of women with endocrine dysfunction or infertility (Chap. 45).

PITUITARY GONADOTROPINS

Plasma gonadotropins are assessed by immunoassay. Because both FSH and LH are secreted in a pulsatile manner, the results obtained from a single serum sample may be difficult to interpret. Moreover, the values vary widely during the menstrual cycle, particularly at the time of the midcycle gonadotropin surge. Consequently, plasma gonadotropin measurements are of greatest use in evaluating women with suspected ovarian failure and in supporting the diagnosis of polycystic ovarian syndrome (PCOS) or hypogonadotropic hypogonadism. FSH levels that are persistently >40 IU/L are diagnostic of ovarian failure, and an LH value <0.8 IU/L suggests hypogonadotropic hypogonadism. In practice, however, gonadotropin values may be equivocal and must be interpreted in the context of other historic, physical, and laboratory findings.

OVARIAN HORMONES

ESTROGEN The presence of normal secondary sexual characteristics implies that estrogen production was adequate in the past. The current estrogen status can be estimated by pelvic examination. The presence of a moist, rugated vagina with copious, clear, thin cervical mucus that

can be stretched and that exhibits arborization or ferning when spread on a slide is strong evidence of adequate estrogen production. Cytologic demonstration of mature vaginal epithelial cells and abundant cornified squamous epithelial cells with pyknotic nuclei confirms the presence of adequate estrogen levels.

The progesterone-withdrawal test provides a functional assessment of the endometrium, outflow tract, and estrogen status. If menses appear within a week to 10 days after the end of a trial of medroxyprogesterone acetate (10 mg by mouth once or twice a day for 5 days) or after a single intramuscular injection of progesterone (100 mg), then prior estrogen priming was adequate to allow withdrawal bleeding.

Owing to its variable level in plasma during the normal cycle and the difficulty of estimating the day of the cycle in women with abnormal cycles, the measurement of estrogen levels in plasma or urine is of little use in the routine assessment of estrogen status. Measurement of plasma estradiol is useful during attempts to induce ovulation with gonadotropins to prevent the development of the ovarian hyperstimulation syndrome and is used along with ultrasound assessment to monitor follicular growth in women during in vitro fertilization.

PROGESTERONE Cyclic, predictable menses also imply that adequate progesterone is secreted during the luteal phase of the menstrual cycle. Assessment of progesterone is useful to detect ovulation and to evaluate the adequacy of the luteal phase in infertile women. Several functional assays of progesterone can be used. The least expensive and most useful is the daily measurement of basal body temperature throughout a cycle. Owing to the thermogenic properties of progesterone, a normal biphasic monthly curve showing a temperature elevation lasting for approximately 2 weeks after ovulation is a valid indication of progesterone secretion during the luteal phase (Fig. 326-4). The presence of viscous cervical mucus that does not stretch or fern and of predominantly intermediate cells on vaginal cytology or demonstration of a secretory epithelium in an endometrial biopsy during the luteal phase on days 20 to 22 of the cycle provides additional assessment of progesterone secretion. In addition, plasma progesterone can be measured to assess the function of the corpus luteum; a level

$> 10 \ \mu mol/L \ (> 3 \ ng/mL)$ suggests successful ovulation and adequate corpus luteum function.

ANDROGEN   Under normal conditions, the ovary secretes androstenedione, testosterone, and dehydroepiandrosterone. In conditions of androgen excess, hirsutism and/or virilization are common. The evaluation of androgen excess is discussed in Chap. 44.

DIAGNOSIS OF PREGNANCY

Pregnancy is usually recognized on the basis of history and physical examination. That is, a woman with previously cyclic, predictable menses develops amenorrhea accompanied by breast tenderness, malaise, lassitude, and nausea, and on physical examination the uterus is soft and enlarged.

Human chorionic gonadotropin (hCG) is secreted by the trophoblastic cells of the placenta into the maternal plasma and excreted in the urine. Plasma or urine assays of hCG make it possible to detect pregnancies 8 to 10 days after ovulation, before the first missed menstrual period and long before pregnancy can be diagnosed by clinical assessments. Sensitive and specific hCG-based pregnancy tests are now available for patients to use at home.

DISORDERS OF OVARIAN FUNCTION

PREPUBERTAL YEARS

Puberty is said to be *precocious* if breast budding begins before age 8 or if menarche occurs before age 9. Those disorders in which the developing sexual characteristics are appropriate for the genetic and gonadal sex—i.e., feminization in girls or virilization in boys—are termed *isosexual precocity*, whereas *heterosexual precocity* occurs when sexual characteristics are not in accord with the genetic sex, namely, virilization in girls or feminization in boys. Pubertal disorders of boys are described in Chap. 325.

ISOSEXUAL PRECOCIOUS PUBERTY   Isosexual precocious puberty in girls can be divided into three major categories (Table 326-1).

True Precocious Puberty   True precocious puberty (gonadotropin-dependent) is characterized by an early but otherwise normal sequence of pubertal development, including increased secretion of gonadotropins and ovulatory menstrual cycles. Constitutional or idiopathic precocious puberty accounts for 90% of cases. The disorder is more common in girls than boys. No cause for the premature maturation of the central nervous system–hypothalamic-pituitary axis can be identified, and the diagnosis is confirmed by finding an adult pattern of LH and FSH release on a GnRH stimulation test. Premature appearance of secondary sexual characteristics and of ovulatory cycles with the accompa-

TABLE 326-1   Differential Diagnosis of Sexual Precocity

I. Isosexual precocity
  A. True precocious puberty
    1. Constitutional
    2. Organic brain disease
    3. Congenital adrenal hyperplasia
  B. Precocious pseudopuberty
    1. Ovarian tumors
    2. Adrenal tumors
    3. McCune-Albright syndrome
    4. Hypothyroidism
    5. Russell-Silver syndrome
    6. Estrogen-containing medications
  C. Incomplete sexual precocity
    1. Premature thelarche
    2. Premature adrenarche
    3. Premature pubarche
II. Heterosexual precocity
  A. Ovarian tumors
  B. Adrenal tumors
  C. Congenital adrenal hyperplasia

nying risk of fertility may cause significant emotional disturbance. Therefore, prompt initiation of therapy is imperative. GnRH analogues suppress gonadotropins and inhibit estrogen synthesis, thereby blocking precocious puberty; they may also prevent premature closure of the epiphyses and the resulting short stature.

About 10% of cases are due to organic brain diseases, including brain tumors (hypothalamic gliomas, astrocytomas, ependymomas, germinomas, and hamartomas), encephalitis, meningitis, hydrocephalus, head injury, tuberous sclerosis, and neurofibromatosis. It is essential to distinguish this group of patients from those with the idiopathic disorder, and patients whose disorder is designated as idiopathic occasionally prove to have such tumors. Most patients with organic lesions serious enough to cause precocious puberty have obvious neurologic signs and symptoms. Evaluation of all patients with precocious puberty should include, at a minimum, computed tomography (CT) or magnetic resonance imaging (MRI) of the brain. The success of treatment depends on the nature of the lesion, but surgical and radiation treatment of well-localized tumors is occasionally successful.

A rare cause of isosexual precocity is congenital adrenal hyperplasia due to 21-hydroxylase deficiency in girls when treatment has been delayed until 4 to 8 years of age (Chap. 321). After initiation of glucocorticoid replacement, such individuals may undergo isosexual precocious puberty.

Precocious Pseudopuberty   Precocious pseudopuberty (gonadotropin-independent) occurs when girls undergo feminization as a consequence of enhanced estrogen formation but do not ovulate or develop cyclic menses. Ovarian cysts or tumors that secrete estrogen (granulosa-theca cell tumors) are the most frequent cause of precocious pseudopuberty. Granulosa-theca cell tumors associated with intestinal polyps and pigmentation of the mucous membranes occur in the Peutz-Jeghers syndrome. Other ovarian tumors that secrete estrogens (or androgens that can be converted to estrogens at extraglandular sites) include dysgerminomas, teratomas, cystadenomas, and ovarian carcinomas (Chap. 83). Ovarian tumors can usually be detected by rectoabdominal examination or by ultrasound, CT, MRI, and/or laparoscopy. Ovarian teratomas and choriocarcinomas and other carcinomas that secrete hCG do not cause precocious puberty in girls unless they also secrete estrogen (hCG or LH in the absence of FSH does not induce ovarian estrogen production). Rarely, feminizing tumors of the adrenal cause isosexual precocious puberty by direct formation of estrogens or by secretion of weak androgens, which are converted to estrogens in extraglandular tissues. The *McCune-Albright syndrome* (polyostotic fibrous dysplasia) is due to an activating mutation in the G protein, $G_{s\alpha}$, that occurs during embryogenesis, leading to a mosaic pattern of expression in various tissues. It is characterized by café au lait spots, cystic fibrous dysplasia of bones, and sexual precocity. In the ovary, the $G_{s\alpha}$ mutation mimics the action of FSH, leading to autonomous follicle development and estrogen formation. Occasionally, this disorder leads to true precocious puberty. *Primary hypothyroidism* is occasionally associated with enhanced secretion of FSH, inducing ovarian estrogen secretion. High levels of thyroid-stimulating hormone (TSH) caused by hypothyroidism may also stimulate the FSH receptor. The *Russell-Silver syndrome*, or congenital asymmetry, is associated with short stature and precocious feminization. *Estrogen-containing medications*, including use of estrogen-containing creams for diaper rash or the ingestion of meat from estrogen-treated animals or poultry or of any estrogen by mouth, can cause this disorder.

Incomplete Isosexual Precocity   This term is used to describe the premature development of a single pubertal event and encompasses several entities. Breast budding before age 7 (*premature thelarche*) without other evidence of estrogen secretion and without premature bone maturation is believed to be due to a transient increase in estrogen secretion or to increased sensitivity to the small amounts of circulating estrogens formed before puberty. Usually, the disorder is self-limited and resolves spontaneously. Occasionally, axillary hair and/or pubic hair (*premature adrenarche* and *premature pubarche*) appear without any other secondary sexual development. The phenomenon is associated with adrenal androgen secretion in the range of normal puberty and can be distinguished from syndromes of virilization by the absence of clitoromegaly. It requires no treatment, and patients enter puberty at about the average time.

HETEROSEXUAL PRECOCITY Virilization in a prepubertal female is usually due to congenital adrenal hyperplasia or to androgen secretion by an ovarian or adrenal tumor. The manifestations of virilization are described in Chap. 44. Virilization in girls with congenital adrenal hyperplasia usually occurs in a background of variable sexual ambiguity (Chap. 328).

EVALUATION OF SEXUAL PRECOCITY The evaluation of sexual precocity involves a careful history and physical examination, including rectoabdominal examination, abdominal sonography, determination of bone age, and GnRH stimulation test, and measurement of thyroid hormones, TSH, and gonadotropins (and androgen or estrogen levels when appropriate). MRI and/or CT scans should be obtained if a neurologic disorder is suspected and no evidence of an ovarian or adrenal tumor is found.

REPRODUCTIVE YEARS

DISORDERS OF THE MENSTRUAL CYCLE ■ Abnormal Uterine Bleeding Between menarche and the menopause, almost every woman experiences one or more episodes of abnormal uterine bleeding, here defined as any bleeding pattern that differs in frequency, duration, or amount from the pattern observed during a normal menstrual cycle. In normal women, the average menstrual cycle is 28 ± 3 days, the mean duration of menstrual flow is 4 ± 2 days, and the average blood loss is 35 to 80 mL. A variety of descriptive terms (such as *menorrhagia, metrorrhagia*, and *menometrorrhagia*) have been used to characterize patterns of abnormal uterine bleeding. A more logical approach is to divide abnormal uterine bleeding into those patterns associated with ovulatory cycles and those associated with anovulatory cycles.

Ovulatory Cycles Normal menstrual bleeding with ovulatory cycles is spontaneous, regular, cyclic, and predictable and is frequently associated with discomfort (*dysmenorrhea*). Deviations from this pattern associated with cycles that are still regular and predictable are most often due to organic disease of the outflow tract. For example, regular but prolonged and excessive bleeding episodes unassociated with bleeding dyscrasias (hypermenorrhea or menorrhagia) can result from abnormalities of the uterus such as submucous leiomyomas, adenomyosis, or endometrial polyps. Regular, cyclic, predictable menstruation characterized by spotting or light bleeding is termed *hypomenorrhea* and is due to obstruction of the outflow tract as from intrauterine synechiae or scarring of the cervix. Intermenstrual bleeding between episodes of regular, ovulatory menstruation is also often due to cervical or endometrial lesions. An exception to the association between organic disease and abnormal uterine bleeding is the occurrence of regular menstruation more frequently than 21 days apart (*polymenorrhea*). Such cycles may be a normal variant.

Anovulatory Cycles Dysfunctional uterine bleeding refers to bleeding that is unpredictable with respect to amount, onset, and duration and is usually painless. This disorder is not due to abnormalities of the uterus but rather to chronic anovulation and occurs when there is interruption of the normal sequence of follicular and luteal phases under the influence of a dominant follicle and its resulting corpus luteum. As discussed above, uterine bleeding in ovulatory cycles occurs because of progesterone withdrawal and requires that the endometrium first be primed with estrogen. (When castrates or postmenopausal women are given progesterone, withdrawal bleeding usually does not occur.)

Dysfunctional uterine bleeding can occur in women who have a transient disruption of the synchronous hypothalamic-pituitary-ovarian patterns necessary for ovulatory cycles, most often at the extremes of the reproductive life—in the early menarche and in the perimenopausal period—but also after temporary stress or intercurrent illness.

Primary dysfunctional uterine bleeding can result from three disorders.

1. *Estrogen withdrawal bleeding* occurs when estrogen is given to a castrated or postmenopausal woman and then withdrawn. As in other types of dysfunctional uterine bleeding, this form of menstrual bleeding is usually painless.
2. *Estrogen breakthrough bleeding* occurs when there is continuous estrogen stimulation of the endometrium not interrupted by cyclic progesterone secretion and withdrawal. This is the most common type of dysfunctional uterine bleeding and is usually due to anovulation associated with chronic acyclic estrogen production, as in women with PCOS. Such women may have histories of irregular, unpredictable menses; oligomenorrhea; or amenorrhea (see below). Alternatively, estrogen breakthrough bleeding can occur in hypogonadal women given estrogens chronically rather than intermittently and in women with estrogen-secreting tumors of the ovary. Estrogen breakthrough bleeding may be profuse and is unpredictable with respect to duration, amount of flow, and time of occurrence. The endometrium is typically thin because its repair between episodes of bleeding is incomplete.
3. *Progesterone breakthrough bleeding* occurs in the presence of abnormally high ratios of progesterone to estrogen, i.e., in women using continuous low-dose oral contraceptives.

The approach to a patient with dysfunctional uterine bleeding begins with a careful history of menstrual patterns and prior hormonal therapy. Since not all urogenital tract bleeding is from the uterus, rectal, bladder, and vaginal or cervical sources must be excluded by physical examination. If the bleeding is from the uterus, a pregnancy-related disorder such as abortion or ectopic pregnancy must be ruled out.

℞ TREATMENT

Once the diagnosis of dysfunctional uterine bleeding is established, a rational approach to management is as follows: During a first episode of dysfunctional bleeding, it is reasonable to observe the patient without intervention, provided the bleeding is not copious and no evidence of bleeding dyscrasia is present. If bleeding is moderately severe, control can be achieved with relatively high dose estrogen oral contraceptives for 3 weeks. Alternatively, a regimen of three or four low-dose oral contraceptive pills per day for 1 week followed by tapering to the usual dosage for up to 3 weeks is also effective. If uterine bleeding is more severe, hospitalization, bed rest, and intramuscular injections of estradiol valerate (10 mg) and hydroxyprogesterone caproate (500 mg) or intravenous or intramuscular conjugated estrogens (25 mg) usually control the bleeding. After initial treatment, iron replacement should be instituted, and recurrence can be prevented by cyclic oral contraceptives for 2 to 3 months (or more if pregnancy is not desired). Alternatively, menses can be induced every 2 to 3 months with medroxyprogesterone acetate, 10 mg taken orally once or twice a day for 10 days. If hormone therapy fails to control uterine bleeding, an endometrial biopsy, hysteroscopy, or dilatation and curettage may be required for diagnosis and therapy. Indeed, uterine sampling should be performed prior to hormone therapy in women at risk for endometrial cancer (e.g., in women who are approaching the age of menopause or who are massively obese); endometrial cancer is rare in ovulatory women of reproductive age.

Amenorrhea An acceptable definition of amenorrhea is failure of menarche by age 15, irrespective of the presence or absence of secondary sexual characteristics, or the absence of menstruation for 6 months in a woman with previous periodic menses. However, women who do not fulfill these criteria should be evaluated if (1) the patient and/or her family are greatly concerned, (2) no breast development has occurred by age 13, or (3) any sexual ambiguity or virilization is present. Amenorrhea is commonly categorized as either primary (the woman has never menstruated) or secondary (when menstruation has been present for a variable period of time in the past and has ceased). However, some disorders can cause either primary or secondary amenorrhea. For example, most women with gonadal dysgenesis have primary amenorrhea, but some have a few follicles and ovulate for short periods so that pregnancy occurs rarely. Furthermore, patients with chronic anovulation (PCOS) usually have secondary amenorrhea but on occasion have primary amenorrhea. For these reasons, categorization of amenorrhea into primary and secondary types is less helpful than a classification based on the underlying physiologic derangements: (1) anatomic defects, (2) ovarian failure, and (3) chronic anovulation with or without estrogen present.

ANATOMIC DEFECTS   Anatomic or structural defects of the genital tract can preclude menstrual bleeding. Starting from the caudal end of the female genital tract, labial fusion is often associated with disorders of sexual development, particularly female pseudohermaphroditism (congenital adrenal hyperplasia or exposure to maternal androgens in utero; Chap. 328). Congenital defects of the vagina, imperforate hymen, and transverse vaginal septae can also cause amenorrhea. These women frequently have accumulation of menstrual blood behind the obstruction and may have cyclic, predictable episodes of abdominal pain.

More severe müllerian anomalies include müllerian agenesis (the Mayer-Rokitansky-Küster-Hauser syndrome), second in frequency only to gonadal dysgenesis as a cause of primary amenorrhea. It can be caused by mutations in the genes encoding anti-müllerian hormone (AMH) or its receptor (AMHR). Women with this syndrome have a 46,XX karyotype, female secondary sex characteristics, and normal ovarian function, including cyclic ovulation, but have absence or hypoplasia of the vagina. The uterus usually consists of only rudimentary bicornuate cords, but if the uterus contains endometrium, cyclic abdominal pain and accumulation of blood may occur, as in other forms of outlet obstruction. One-third of women with this syndrome have abnormalities of the urogenital tract, and one-tenth have skeletal anomalies, usually involving the spine. The major diagnostic problem is distinguishing müllerian agenesis from complete androgen insensitivity syndrome, in which 46,XY genetic males with testes differentiate as phenotypic women but with a blind vaginal pouch and no uterus (Chap. 328). Androgen insensitivity can be diagnosed by demonstrating a male level of serum testosterone and a 46,XY karyotype, whereas demonstration of a 46,XX karyotype, the biphasic basal body temperature curve characteristic of ovulation, and elevated levels of progesterone during the luteal phase establish the diagnosis of müllerian agenesis.

Other abnormalities of the uterus that cause amenorrhea include obstruction due to scarring or stenosis of the cervix, often as a result of surgery, electrocautery, laser therapy, or cryosurgery. Such destruction of the endometrium (Asherman's syndrome) usually follows vigorous curettage for postpartum hemorrhage or after therapeutic abortion complicated by infection. This diagnosis is confirmed by hysterosalpingography or by direct visual examination of the endometrial scarring or synechiae using a hysteroscope.

Treatment of disorders of the outflow tract is surgical.

OVARIAN FAILURE   Primary ovarian failure is associated with elevated plasma gonadotropin levels and can result from several causes. The most frequent cause is *gonadal dysgenesis*, in which the germ cells are absent and the ovary is replaced by a fibrous streak (Chap. 328). A 45,X karyotype is found in about half of women with this disorder, and most have somatic defects, including short stature, webbed neck, shield chest, and cardiovascular defects, collectively termed the *Turner phenotype*. The remainder of women with X chromosome abnormalities have chromosomal mosaicism with or without associated structural abnormalities of the X. Approximately 90% of women with gonadal dysgenesis due to partial or complete deletion of the X never have menstrual bleeding, and the remaining 10% have sufficient follicles to experience menses and, rarely, fertility; the menstrual and reproductive lives of such individuals are invariably brief.

One-tenth of individuals identified as having bilateral streak gonads have a normal 46,XX or 46,XY karyotype and are said to have *pure gonadal dysgenesis*. These individuals have either normal or above-average stature, owing to failure of estrogen-mediated epiphyseal closure in the presence of a normal chromosomal constitution. Pure gonadal dysgenesis does not constitute a phenotypic or chromosomally homogeneous disorder.

Other causes of ovarian failure and amenorrhea include deficiency of the *CYP17* gene that encodes 17α-hydroxylase and 17,20-lyase activities, premature ovarian failure, the resistant-ovary syndrome, and ovarian failure secondary to chemotherapy or radiation therapy for malignancy. *17α-Hydroxylase deficiency* is a rare, autosomal recessive disorder characterized by primary amenorrhea, sexual infantilism, and hypertension, the latter due to increased production of desoxycorticosterone (DOC); women with *17,20-lyase deficiency* have primary amenorrhea and sexual infantilism with normal blood pressure. The diagnosis of *premature ovarian failure* or *premature menopause* applies to women who cease menstruating before age 40. The ovaries in such women are similar to those of postmenopausal women, containing few or no follicles as the result of accelerated follicular atresia. Premature ovarian failure due to ovarian antibodies may be one component of polyglandular failure, together with adrenal insufficiency, hypothyroidism, and other autoimmune disorders (Chap. 330). A rare form of ovarian failure is the *resistant-ovary syndrome*, in which the ovaries contain many follicles that are arrested in development prior to the antral stage, possibly because of resistance to the action of FSH in the ovary. A subset of these individuals have mutations in FSH or its receptor. To differentiate this disorder from the 46,XX variety of pure gonadal dysgenesis, which is also associated with sexual immaturity, it is necessary to perform ovarian biopsy or genetic testing. Women with ovarian failure who desire pregnancy have been treated with hormone replacement and transfer of donor embryos to the uterine cavity or fallopian tubes.

℞ TREATMENT

In women with decreased estrogen production, whether due to ovarian dysfunction or to hypogonadotropic hypogonadism, treatment with cyclic estrogens should be instituted to induce the development and maintenance of female secondary sexual characteristics and to prevent osteoporosis. The most commonly used medications are conjugated estrogens (0.625 to 1.25 mg/d by mouth) together with medroxyprogesterone acetate (2.5 mg/d or 5 to 10 mg during the last several days of monthly estrogen treatment to prevent development of endometrial hyperplasia). Alternatively, oral contraceptives may be given to premenopausal-age women (Chap. 45). Abnormal bleeding in women receiving estrogen replacement mandates histologic evaluation of the endometrium.

Chronic Anovulation   At least 80% or more of gynecologic endocrine disorders result from chronic anovulation. Women with chronic anovulation fail to ovulate spontaneously but may ovulate with appropriate therapy. The ovaries of such women do not secrete estrogen in a normal cyclic pattern. It is clinically useful to differentiate those women who produce enough estrogen to have withdrawal bleeding after progestogen therapy from those who do not; the latter often have hypothalamic-pituitary dysfunction.

CHRONIC ANOVULATION WITH ESTROGEN PRESENT   This disorder is most commonly caused by *polycystic ovarian syndrome*, which is characterized by infertility, hirsutism, obesity, insulin resistance, and amenorrhea or oligomenorrhea. When spontaneous uterine bleeding occurs in women with PCOS, it is unpredictable as to time of onset, duration, and amount; on occasion the bleeding can be severe.

PCOS, as originally described by Stein and Leventhal, was characterized by enlarged, polycystic ovaries, but it is now known to be associated with a variety of pathologic findings in the ovaries, only some of which result in enlargement and none of which are pathognomonic. The most common finding is a white, smooth, sclerotic ovary with a thickened capsule, multiple follicular cysts in various stages of atresia, a hyperplastic theca and stroma, and rare or absent corpora albicans. Other ovaries have hyperthecosis in which the ovarian stroma is hyperplastic and may contain lipid-laden luteal cells. Thus, the diagnosis of PCOS is a clinical one, based on the coexistence of chronic anovulation and varying degrees of androgen excess. The fundamental defect that causes PCOS is unknown, and it is likely to have several distinct causes.

In most women with PCOS, menarche occurs at the expected time, but oligomenorrhea ensues after a variable period. Signs of androgen excess (hirsutism) usually become evident soon after menarche. One scenario suggests that this disorder originates as an exaggerated adrenarche in obese girls (Fig. 326-5). The combination of elevated levels of adrenal androgens and obesity leads to increased formation of extraglandular estrogen. This estrogen exerts a positive feedback on LH secretion and negative feedback on FSH secretion, resulting in a ratio of LH to FSH levels in plasma that is characteristically greater than 2. The increased LH levels can then lead to hyperplasia of the ovarian stroma and theca cells and increased androgen production, which in turn provides more substrate for peripheral aromatization and perpetuates the chronic anovulation. In the advanced stage of the disorder, the ovary is the major site of androgen production, but the adrenal may continue to secrete excess androgen as well. Ovarian follicles from women with PCOS have low aromatase activity, but normal aromatase can be induced by treatment with FSH. An association exists between PCOS/hyperthecosis, virilization, acanthosis nigricans, and insulin resistance; in the ovary, insulin may interact via the insulin-like growth factor receptors to enhance androgen synthesis in insulin-resistant states. Women with PCOS have an increased incidence of impaired glucose tolerance and type 2 diabetes mellitus.

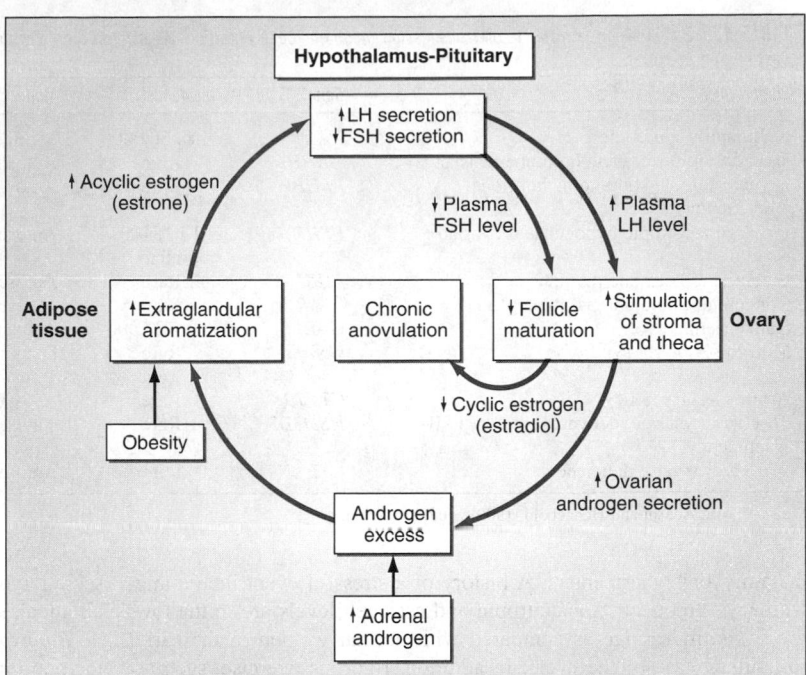

FIGURE 326-5 Proposed mechanism for the initiation and perpetuation of chronic anovulation in polycystic ovarian syndrome (PCOS). This cycle may be entered or initiated via adrenal androgen excess or obesity, both of which result in enhanced extraglandular formation of estrogens. The therapy of PCOS involves interruption of the cycle at any of several steps. [From SSC Yen et al (eds), Reproductive Endocrinology. Philadelphia, Saunders, 1999; and from U Goebelmann, in Reproductive Endocrinology, Infertility, and Contraception, 2d ed, DR Mishell Jr, V Davajan (eds), Philadelphia, Davis, 1986.]

Rx TREATMENT

Treatment of PCOS is directed toward interrupting the self-perpetuating cycle and can be accomplished in several ways, such as by decreasing ovarian androgen secretion (by wedge resection or the use of oral contraceptive agents), decreasing peripheral estrogen formation (by weight reduction), or enhancing FSH secretion [by administration of clomiphene, human menopausal gonadotropin (hMG), GnRH (gonadorelin) by portable infusion pump, or purified FSH (urofollitropin)]. The choice of therapy depends on the clinical findings and the needs of the patient. An attempt at weight reduction is appropriate in all who are obese. If the woman is not hirsute and does not desire pregnancy, periodic withdrawal menses can be induced with medroxyprogesterone acetate 10 days per month; such treatment prevents the development of endometrial hyperplasia. If the woman is hirsute and does not desire pregnancy, the ovarian (and possibly the adrenal) component of androgen production can be suppressed with combined estrogen-progestogen oral contraceptive agents. Combined oral contraceptives are also indicated if prolonged or excessive menstrual bleeding is present. Once androgen excess is controlled, treatment of previously existing hair growth by shaving, depilatories, or electrolysis may be indicated (Chap. 44). If pregnancy is desired, ovulation must be induced. Insulin-sensitizing drugs, such as metformin and the thiazolidinediones, improve fertility in women with PCOS. Clomiphene promotes ovulation in three-fourths of cases, or ovulation can be induced with hMG, urofollitropin, or gonadorelin (Chap. 45). Pretreatment with GnRH analogues prior to use of hMG, urofollitropin, or gonadorelin may improve the rates of ovulation and pregnancy. Women with PCOS are at increased risk of ovarian hyperstimulation after treatment with gonadotropins. They also experience increased rates of spontaneous abortion. An alternative therapy is ovarian drilling by laser or cautery performed at laparoscopy when hormonal therapy is not effective; however, the procedure is associated with a high incidence of ovarian adhesions.

Chronic anovulation with estrogen present may also occur with tumors of the ovary. These include granulosa-theca cell tumors, Brenner tumors, cystic teratomas, mucous cystadenomas, and Krukenberg tumors (Chap. 83). Such tumors can either secrete excess estrogen themselves or produce androgens that are aromatized in extraglandular sites. Chronic anovulation and the clinical features of PCOS result. Occasionally, areas of the ovary not involved with tumors show the characteristic histologic changes of PCOS. Other causes of chronic anovulation with estrogen present include adrenal production of excess androgen (usually adult-onset adrenal hyperplasia due to partial 21-hydroxylase deficiency) and hypothyroidism.

CHRONIC ANOVULATION WITH ESTROGEN ABSENT Women with chronic anovulation who have low or absent estrogen production and do not experience withdrawal bleeding after progestogen treatment usually have hypogonadotropic hypogonadism due to disease of either the pituitary or the central nervous system.

Isolated hypogonadotropic hypogonadism associated with defects of smell (olfactory bulb defects) is known as the *Kallmann syndrome* (Chap. 318), which is due to a single gene defect in the X-linked *KAL* gene. Affected women are sexually infantile and have a defect in the synthesis and/or release of GnRH. Hypothalamic lesions that impair GnRH production and cause hypogonadotropic hypogonadism include craniopharyngioma, germinoma (pinealoma), glioma, Hand-Schüller-Christian disease, teratomas, endodermal-sinus tumors, tuberculosis, sarcoidosis, and metastatic tumors that cause suppression or destruction of the hypothalamus. Central nervous system trauma and irradiation can also cause hypothalamic amenorrhea and deficiencies in secretion of growth hormone, adrenocorticotropic hormone (ACTH), vasopressin, and thyroid hormone. Rare, autosomal recessive defects in the GnRH receptor have also been described.

More commonly, gonadotropin deficiency leading to chronic anovulation is believed to arise from functional disorders of the hypo-

TABLE 326-2 *Incidence and Mode of Transmission of Single-Gene Mutations Associated with Reproductive Dysfunction in Women*

Phenotype	Gene	Incidence	Mode of Transmission
Kallmann's syndrome	KAL	1 in 50,000	X-linked
Gonadotropin-releasing hormone resistance	GNRHR	Rare	Autosomal recessive
Isolated follicle-stimulating hormone deficiency	FSHB	Rare	Autosomal recessive
Hypergonadotropic hypogonadal ovarian failure	FSHR	1 in 8300 (Finland)	Autosomal recessive
Luteinizing hormone resistance	LHR	Rare	Autosomal recessive
Congenital lipoid adrenal hyperplasia	STAR	Rare	Autosomal recessive
Galactosemia	GALT	1 in 187,000	Autosomal recessive
McCune-Albright syndrome	GNASI	Rare	Dominant postzygotic mutation
Aromatase deficiency	CYP19	Rare	Autosomal recessive
3β-Hydroxysteroid dehydrogenase type II deficiency	HSD3B2	Rare	Autosomal recessive
17α-Hydroxylase deficiency	CYP17	Rare	Autosomal recessive

Source: From Adashi and Hennebold, 1999, with permission.

thalamus or higher centers. A history of a stressful event in a young woman is frequent. Gonadotropin and estrogen levels are in the low to low-normal range as compared with normal women in the early follicular phase of the cycle. In addition, rigorous exercise, such as jogging or ballet, and diets that result in excessive weight loss may lead to chronic anovulation, particularly in girls with a history of prior menstrual irregularity. The amenorrhea in these women does not appear to be a result of weight loss alone but a combination of a decrease in body fat and chronic stress. An extreme form of weight loss with chronic anovulation occurs in anorexia nervosa (Chap. 65). In anorexia nervosa amenorrhea can precede, follow, or coincide with weight loss.

In addition, chronic debilitating diseases such as end-stage kidney disease, malignancy, inflammatory bowel disease, and malabsorption can lead to hypogonadotropic hypogonadism via a hypothalamic mechanism.

Treatment of chronic anovulation due to hypothalamic disorders includes ameliorating the stressful situation, decreasing exercise, and correcting weight loss, as appropriate. These women are susceptibleto the development of osteoporosis; estrogen replacement therapy is recommended to induce and maintain normal secondary sexual characteristics and prevent bone loss in those who do not desire pregnancy, and gonadotropin or gonadorelin therapy is indicated when pregnancy is desired. When appropriate, therapy is directed at the primary disease of the hypothalamus.

Disorders of the pituitary can lead to the estrogen-deficient form of chronic anovulation by at least two mechanisms—direct interference with gonadotropin secretion by lesions that either obliterate or interfere with the gonadotrope cells (chromophobe adenomas, Sheehan's syndrome) or inhibition of gonadotropin secretion in association with excess prolactin (prolactinoma). *Pituitary tumors* may secrete no hormone, one hormone, or more than one hormone (Chap. 318). Prolactin levels are elevated in 50 to 70% of patients with pituitary tumors, either because of prolactin secretion by the tumor itself (in the case of prolactinomas) or because the tumor mass interferes with the normal hypothalamic inhibition of prolactin secretion.

Prolactin excess associated with low levels of LH and FSH constitutes a specific subtype of hypogonadotropic hypogonadism. Onetenth or more of amenorrheic women have increased levels of prolactin, and more than half of women with both galactorrhea and amenorrhea have elevated prolactin levels. The amenorrhea is most often associated with decreased or absent estrogen production, but prolactin-secreting tumors on occasion are associated with normal ovulatory menses or chronic anovulation with estrogen present. In the latter half of pregnancy, prolactin-secreting pituitary tumors may expand, leading to headaches, compression of the optic chiasm, bitemporal hemianopia, and blindness. Therefore, before inducing ovulation for the purposes of achieving pregnancy, it is mandatory to exclude

the presence of a pituitary tumor. →*The evaluation, differential diagnosis, and management of hyperprolactinemia are described in Chap. 318.*

Large pituitary tumors such as null cell adenomas—whether or not hyperprolactinemia is present—are likely to be associated with deficiency of hormones in addition to gonadotropins (Chap. 318).

Craniopharyngiomas, which are thought to arise from remnants of Rathke's pouch, occur most frequently in the second decade of life and often extend into the suprasellar region. Many of these tumors calcify and can be diagnosed by conventional skull film or CT. Patients often present with sexual infantilism, delayed puberty, and amenorrhea due to gonadotropin deficiency; secretion of TSH, ACTH, growth hormone, and vasopressin may also be impaired.

Panhypopituitarism can be caused by mutations in transcription factors (Pit-1; Prop-1) involved in pituitary gland development, result from surgical or radiation treatment of pituitary adenomas, or develop after postpartum hemorrhage (Sheehan's syndrome) (Chap. 318). Table 326-2 outlines the incidence and mode of single gene mutations associated with reproductive dysfunction in women.

Evaluation of Amenorrhea A general scheme for the evaluation of women with amenorrhea is given in Fig. 326-6. On physical examination, attention should be given to three features: (1) the degree of maturation of the breasts, pubic and axillary hair, and external genitalia; (2) the current estrogen status; and (3) the presence or absence of a uterus. Pregnancy should be excluded in all women with amenorrhea; it is prudent to perform a suitable pregnancy screening test even when the history and physical examination are not suggestive. Once that is done, the cause of amenorrhea can frequently be diagnosed clinically. For example, Asherman's syndrome is suggested by a history of curettage in a woman who previously menstruated; in women with primary amenorrhea and sexual infantilism, the essential differential diagnosis is between gonadal dysgenesis and hypopituitarism; and the diagnosis of gonadal dysgenesis (Turner's syndrome) or of anatomic defects of the outflow tract (müllerian agenesis, testicular feminization, and cervical stenosis) is frequently suggested on the basis of physical findings. When a specific cause is suspected, it is appropriate to proceed directly to confirm the diagnosis (obtaining a chromosomal karyotype or measurement of plasma gonadotropins). It is also useful to measure serum prolactin and FSH levels during the initial evaluation.

Estrogen status is evaluated by determining if the vaginal mucosa is moist and rugated and if the cervical mucus can be stretched and shown to fern upon drying. If these criteria are indeterminate, a progestational challenge is indicated, most often the administration of 10 mg medroxyprogesterone acetate by mouth once or twice daily for 5 days or 100 mg progesterone in oil intramuscularly. (It should be emphasized that progestogen should never be administered until pregnancy is excluded.) If estrogen levels are adequate (and the outflow tract is intact), menstrual bleeding should occur within 1 week of ending the progestogen treatment. If withdrawal bleeding occurs, the diagnosis is chronic anovulation with estrogen present, usually caused by PCOS.

If no withdrawal bleeding or only minimal vaginal spotting occurs, the nature of the subsequent workup depends on the results of the initial prolactin assay. If plasma prolactin is elevated, or if galactorrhea is present, radiography of the pituitary should be undertaken. When the plasma prolactin level is normal in an anovulatory woman with estrogen absent and with elevated FSH levels, the diagnosis is ovarian failure. If the gonadotropins are in the low or normal range, the diagnosis is either hypothalamic-pituitary disorder or an anatomic defect of the outflow tract. As indicated previously, the diagnosis of outflow tract disorder is usually suspected or established on the basis of the history and physical findings. When the physical findings are not clear-cut, it is useful to administer cyclic estrogen plus progestogen (1.25 mg oral conjugated estrogens per day for 3 weeks, with 10 mg medroxyprogesterone acetate added for the last 7 to 10 days of estrogen treatment), followed by 10 days of observation. If no bleeding occurs, the diagnosis of Asherman's syndrome or another anatomic defect of the outflow tract is confirmed by hysterosalpingography or hysteroscopy. If withdrawal bleeding occurs following the estrogen-progestogen combination, the diagnosis of chronic anovulation with estrogen absent (functional hypothalamic amenorrhea) is suggested. Radiologic evaluations of the pituitary-hypothalamic areas may be indicated in the latter cases—irrespective of the prolactin level—because of the risk of overlooking a pituitary-hypothalamic tumor and because the diagnosis of functional hypothalamic amenorrhea is one of exclusion.

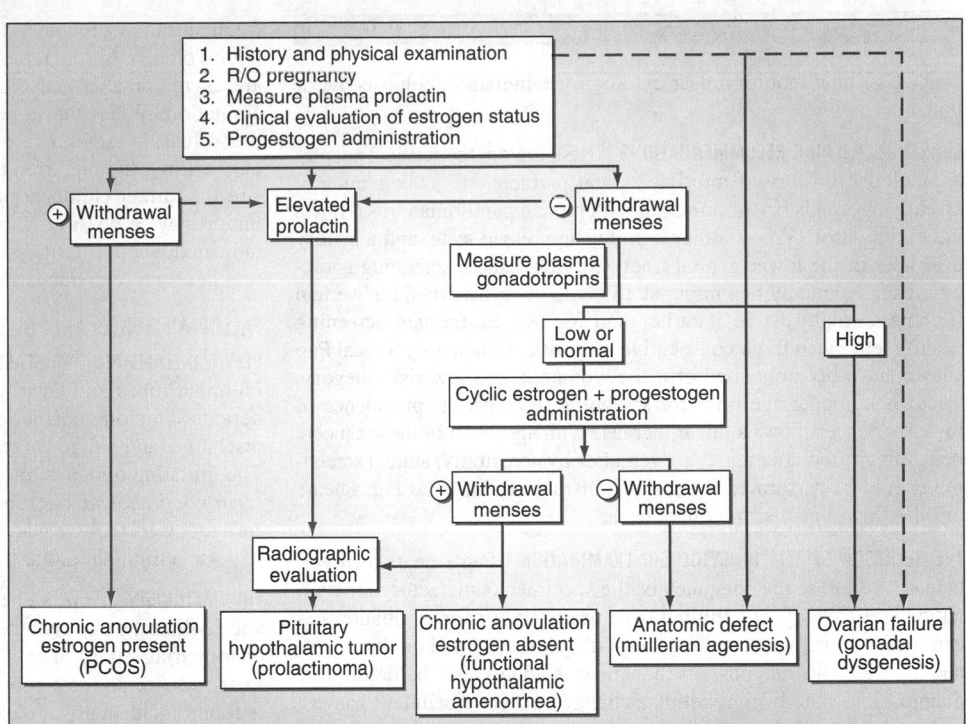

FIGURE 326-6 Flow diagram for the evaluation of women with amenorrhea. The most common diagnosis for each category is shown in parentheses. The dotted lines indicate that in some instances a correct diagnosis can be reached on the basis of history and physical examination alone. PCOS, polycystic ovarian syndrome.

INFERTILITY Infertility, the failure to become pregnant after 1 year of unprotected intercourse, affects approximately 10 to 15% of couples and is a common reason for seeking gynecologic assistance. Male factors account for at least 25% of infertility problems (Chap. 325). In women, failure of ovulation accounts for 40% of cases; pelvic factors, such as tubal disease or endometriosis, account for half. In 10 to 20% of infertile women no etiology is found. →*The evaluation and management of infertility are discussed in Chap. 45.*

PREGNANCY (See also Chap. 6) The possibility of pregnancy should be considered in all women of reproductive age who are evaluated for medical illness or considered for surgery. Procedures such as x-ray exposure, drugs, and anesthetics may be harmful to the developing fetus, and a variety of medical problems may worsen during pregnancy, including hypertension; diseases of the heart, lungs, kidney, and liver; and metabolic and endocrine disorders. Abnormal vaginal bleeding or amenorrhea during the reproductive years should prompt consideration of a complication of pregnancy, such as incomplete abortion, ectopic pregnancy, or trophoblastic disease (hydatidiform mole or choriocarcinoma). Women who present with these complications of pregnancy often have histories of abdominal pain and vaginal bleeding and may have evidence of intraabdominal hemorrhage.

Choriocarcinoma is a particular problem because of its protean manifestations. Half these malignancies follow pregnancies complicated by hydatidiform mole, and the remainder occur after spontaneous abortion, ectopic pregnancy, or normal deliveries. Patients may present with intraabdominal bleeding due to rupture of the uterus, liver, or ovary, with pulmonary manifestations (cough, hemoptysis, pleuritic pain, dyspnea, and respiratory failure) or gastrointestinal symptoms, usually chronic blood loss or melena. In addition, patients can present with cerebral metastases or renal involvement. The diagnosis can be established by demonstrating an elevated level of the β subunit of hCG in plasma. Treatment and cure are possible with chemotherapeutic agents (dactinomycin and/or methotrexate). →*The manifestations of choriocarcinoma in men are discussed in Chap. 82.*

OTHER DISORDERS OF THE FEMALE REPRODUCTIVE TRACT

VULVA

Most disorders of the vulva are a result of sexually transmitted diseases, most commonly syphilis (painless chancre), condylomata acuminata (venereal warts), and herpes vulvitis (painful ulcers; Chap. 115). All other lesions of the vulva, particularly in older women, must be biopsied. Early biopsy of cancer of the vulva is mandatory, because when it becomes symptomatic (pruritus and bleeding), it has often progressed to an advanced stage.

VAGINA

Infections of the vagina usually present as vaginal discharge and pruritus. The most frequent organisms are *Trichomonas*, *Candida albicans*, and *Gardnerella vaginalis* (Chap. 115). The diagnosis is made by microscopic examination of the discharge, and appropriate therapy can be instituted using vaginal or oral antibiotics.

Abnormalities of the vagina and cervix in female offspring of women given diethylstilbestrol during pregnancy include adenosis of the vagina and structural abnormalities of the vagina, cervix, and uterus; the risk of developing a rare vaginal cancer (adenocarcinoma, clear cell type) is increased (2 per 10,000 exposed women). Periodic examination of women at risk should begin at age 12 to 14, and reexamination should be done after any episode of abnormal bleeding.

CERVIX

Preinvasive lesions of the cervix (also known as *cervical intraepithelial neoplasia*) and invasive carcinoma of the cervix can be detected reliably by obtaining a Papanicolaou (Pap) smear.

EVALUATION OF THE PAP SMEAR The incidence of invasive cervical cancer has declined as a result of Pap smear screening. In the United States, approximately 2 to 3 million abnormal Pap smears are found each year. Most represent low-grade lesions but require appropriate follow-up. The follow-up of abnormal Pap smears requires an understanding of the Bethesda system for evaluating such smears (see below) and of the limitations of cytologic screening systems. Further evaluation may require repeat cytologic examination, colposcopy, or both.

CURRENT SCREENING RECOMMENDATIONS   Risk factors for cervical neoplasia include a history of multiple sexual partners, coitus beginning at an early age, a history of infection with human papilloma virus (HPV), infection with HIV or another immunosuppressed state, and a history of cancer of the lower genital tract. Cervical cancer screening is recommended annually beginning at 18 years of age or when the woman becomes sexually active, if earlier than age 18. Less frequent screening is sufficient when three consecutive, negative, satisfactory annual Pap smears have been obtained or if the woman is in a low-risk category. There is no upper age limit for screening, because the prevalence of invasive cancer shows a linear increase with age, most of these cancers being diagnosed after age 50. Even after hysterectomy, annual screening should be performed if there is a history of abnormal Pap smears or other lower genital tract neoplasia.

THE BETHESDA SYSTEM OF CYTOLOGIC EXAMINATION   Pap smears are evaluated in regard to the adequacy of the specimen (satisfactory for evaluation, satisfactory but limited, or unsatisfactory for evaluation because of a stated reason), the general diagnosis (normal or abnormal), and a descriptive diagnosis if the smear is abnormal. The descriptive diagnoses include benign cellular changes, reactive cellular changes, and epithelial cell abnormalities, the latter including (1) atypical squamous cells of undetermined significance (ASCUS); (2) low-grade squamous intraepithelial lesion (LSIL), which is further categorized to include HPV infection, cervical intraepithelial neoplasia (CIN 1), and high-grade squamous intraepithelial lesion (HSIL), which is itself subdivided into CIN 2 and CIN 3); and (3) squamous cell carcinoma.

GUIDELINES FOR THE MANAGEMENT OF WOMEN WITH ABNORMAL PAP SMEARS
For ASCUS smears that are unqualified or suggest a reactive process, a repeat smear should be obtained every 4 to 6 months for 2 years until three consecutive negative smears have been obtained. For ASCUS smears that are unqualified but have severe inflammation, any specific cause should be treated, and the smear should be repeated in 2 to 3 months; because invasive carcinoma can be obscured by severe inflammation, clinical evaluation is mandatory. For postmenopausal women not using hormone replacement, a course of topical estrogen should be applied before the test is repeated. For LSIL smears, the Pap test is repeated every 4 to 6 months for 2 years until three consecutive negative smears have been obtained; treatment of HPV is of no established benefit, and there is a high rate of regression of LSIL, so that in compliant, low-risk individuals, the outcome is usually favorable. If LSIL is persistent, colposcopy with directed biopsy is performed, and endocervical curettage is undertaken if a specific diagnosis is made by biopsy. Cervical cone biopsy or loop electrosurgical excision procedures are performed for higher-grade lesions such as HSIL. If cervical cancer is diagnosed by biopsy, clinical staging is performed, and the patient is treated with radiation therapy or surgery.

UTERUS

Only 40% of cases of endometrial adenocarcinoma are detected by Pap smear. In women at high risk for endometrial carcinoma (because of obesity, a history of chronic anovulatory cycles, diabetes mellitus, hypertension, or unopposed estrogen treatment), yearly endometrial sampling should be performed. Measurement of endometrial thickness by sonography can indicate which patients are at risk for endometrial pathology. Endometrial thickness <5 mm is rarely associated with either hyperplasia or cancer. Low-dose oral estrogen therapy rarely causes breakthrough or withdrawal bleeding in postmenopausal women. Therefore, irrespective of whether the patient is using estrogen therapy, the occurrence of postmenopausal bleeding makes it mandatory to obtain a tissue diagnosis by either endometrial sampling or curettage to exclude endometrial cancer.

One of the most common disorders of the uterus and the most

frequent tumor of women (one of four women affected) is the uterine leiomyoma, or fibroid tumor. Three-fourths of women with leiomyoma are asymptomatic, and the diagnosis is made on routine pelvic examination. When the tumor is associated with excessive menstrual blood loss, is large or fast-growing, or causes significant pelvic pain (see below), the preferred treatment is hysterectomy if there is no desire for further childbearing. Embolism of the vascular supply to the tumor may be possible. In young women, myomectomy is sometimes indicated when infertility or repeated fetal wastage is a manifestation or where future childbearing is desired.

FALLOPIAN TUBES AND OVARIES

PELVIC INFLAMMATORY DISEASE (PID)   This is a common disorder of the fallopian tubes and usually becomes symptomatic after a menstrual period; symptoms include fever, chills, abdominal pain, and vaginal discharge, and pelvic tenderness on physical examination is common. The initiating organism most often is *Chlamydia trachomatis* or *Neisseria gonorrhoeae*, but tuboovarian abscess and sterility are probably caused by mixed aerobic and anaerobic superinfections and require wide-spectrum antibiotic treatment (Chap. 115).

ENDOMETRIOSIS   This is a benign disorder characterized by the presence and proliferation of endometrial tissue (stroma and glands) outside the endometrial cavity. The clinical manifestations are variable. Endometriosis occurs most commonly between the ages of 30 and 40 and is found incidentally at the time of surgery in approximately one-fifth of all gynecologic operations. The fertility rate is reduced in affected women. The disorder usually involves the posterior cul-de-sac or the ovaries and it occasionally involves distant sites (lung, umbilicus). The major symptom is pelvic pain, characteristically dysmenorrhea (see below). However, the frequency and severity of symptoms correlate poorly with the extent of disease. Other manifestations include dyspareunia, pain with defecation, and infertility. The characteristic physical findings are multiple tender nodules palpable along the uterosacral ligament at the time of rectal-vaginal examination, a posteriorly fixed uterus, or enlarged, cystic ovaries. The diagnosis can be confirmed only by direct visualization, usually at diagnostic laparoscopy. Treatment depends on the degree of involvement and the desires of the patient and includes observation for mild disease with no associated infertility or pain, hormonal suppressive therapy, conservative surgery by laparoscopy or laparotomy if fertility is desired, or removal of the uterus, tubes, and ovaries in severe disease. Endometriosis is rare after the menopause.

Any adnexal mass that persists for more than 6 weeks or is larger than 6 cm must be evaluated. Although ovarian cysts and neoplasms are the most common pelvic adnexal masses, tumors of the fallopian tubes, uterus, gastrointestinal tract, or urinary tract should also be considered. Sonography or radiographic evaluation is often helpful in identifying the nature of the adnexal mass prior to surgical exploration. →*For a discussion of ovarian tumors, see Chap. 83.*

EVALUATION OF PELVIC PAIN

The evaluation of pelvic pain requires a careful history and pelvic examination. This often leads to the correct diagnosis and institution of appropriate treatment. Pelvic pain may originate in the pelvis or be referred from another region of the body. A pelvic source is suggested by the history (e.g., dysmenorrhea and dyspareunia) and physical findings, but a high index of suspicion must be entertained for extrapelvic disorders that refer to the pelvis, such as appendicitis, diverticulitis, cholecystitis, intestinal obstruction, and urinary tract infections. If the pain is severe and the diagnosis is unclear, the workup should follow that outlined for the acute abdomen (Chap. 13).

"PHYSIOLOGIC" PELVIC PAIN

PAIN ASSOCIATED WITH OVULATION ("MITTELSCHMERZ")   Many women experience low abdominal discomfort with ovulation, typically a dull aching pain at midcycle in one lower quadrant lasting from minutes to hours. It is rarely severe or incapacitating. The pain may result from peritoneal irritation by follicular fluid released into the peritoneal cavity at ovulation. The onset of discomfort at midcycle, and short duration of pain, suggest this diagnosis.

PREMENSTRUAL OR MENSTRUAL PAIN In normal ovulatory women, somatic symptoms during the few days prior to menses may be insignificant or disabling. Such symptoms include edema, breast engorgement, and abdominal bloating or discomfort. A symptom complex of cyclic irritability, depression, and lethargy is known as *premenstrual syndrome*, which appears to be caused by changes in gonadal steroid levels. Although there is no consensus about therapy, randomized, controlled trials suggest improvement in some women with the daily use of serotonin-reuptake inhibitors.

Severe or incapacitating uterine cramping during ovulatory menses and in the absence of demonstrable disorders of the pelvis is termed *primary dysmenorrhea*. Primary dysmenorrhea is caused by prostaglandin-induced uterine ischemia and is treated with nonsteroidal anti-inflammatory drugs and/or oral contraceptive agents.

PELVIC PAIN DUE TO ORGANIC CAUSES

Severe dysmenorrhea associated with disease of the pelvis is termed *secondary dysmenorrhea*. Organic causes of pelvic pain can be classified as (1) uterine, (2) adnexal, (3) vulvar or vaginal, and (4) pregnancy-associated.

UTERINE PAIN Pain of uterine etiology is often chronic and continuous and increases in intensity during menstruation and intercourse. Causes include leiomyomas of the uterus (particularly submucous and degenerating leiomyomas), adenomyosis, and cervical stenosis. Infections of the uterus associated with intrauterine manipulation following dilatation and curettage or with the insertion of intrauterine devices can also cause pelvic pain. Pelvic pain due to endometrial or cervical cancer is usually a late manifestation.

ADNEXAL PAIN The most common cause of pain in the adnexae (fallopian tubes and ovaries) is infection (Chap. 115). Acute salpingo-oophoritis presents as low abdominal pain, fever, and chills and begins a few days after a menstrual period. Chronic PID results from either a single episode or multiple episodes of infection and may present as infertility associated with chronic pelvic pain that increases in intensity with menses and intercourse. On physical examination, cervical motion tenderness, adnexal tenderness, and adnexal thickening and/or masses may be present. PID may become a surgical emergency if

peritonitis results from rupture of a tuboovarian abscess. Ovarian cysts or neoplasms may cause pelvic pain that becomes more severe with torsion or rupture of the mass, and ectopic pregnancy must be considered in the differential diagnosis. If there is a question of an adnexal mass or if the patient is so obese as to preclude a thorough pelvic examination, abdominal or vaginal ultrasound may be useful. Endometriosis involving fallopian tubes, ovaries, or peritoneum may cause both chronic low abdominal pain and infertility; the magnitude of tissue involvement does not always correlate with the severity of symptoms. Endometriosis pain typically increases with menstruation and, if the posterior ligaments of the uterus are involved, with intercourse.

VULVAR OR VAGINAL PAIN Pain in these areas is most often due to infectious vaginitis and is characteristically associated with vaginal discharge and pruritus. Herpetic vulvitis, other dermatologic conditions of the vulva, condyloma acumination, and cysts or abscesses of Bartholin's glands may also cause vulvar pain.

PREGNANCY-ASSOCIATED DISORDERS Pregnancy must be considered in the differential diagnosis of pelvic pain during the reproductive years. Threatened abortion or incomplete abortion often presents with uterine cramping, bleeding, or passage of tissue following a period of amenorrhea. Ectopic pregnancy may be insidious in presentation or result in abrupt intraperitoneal hemorrhage and maternal death. A culdocentesis may be indicated if a ruptured ectopic pregnancy is suspected. Serial hCG measurements may help in establishing a diagnosis of tubal pregnancy and are useful in determining if an intrauterine pregnancy is viable.

FURTHER READING

ADASHI EY, HENNEBOLD JD: Single-gene mutations resulting in reproductive dysfunction in women. N Engl J Med 340:709, 1999

BRADLEY LD et al: Radiographic imaging techniques for the diagnosis of abnormal uterine bleeding. Obstet Gynecol Clin North Am 27:245, 2000

HEWITT GD: Acute and chronic pelvic pain in female adolescents. Med Clin North Am 84:1009, 2000

HUTCHINS FL et al: Embolotherapy for myoma-induced menorrhagia. Obstet Gynecol Clin North Am 27:397, 2000

MCGEE EA, HSUEH AWJ: Initial and cyclic recruitment of ovarian follicles. Endocr Rev 21:200, 2000

SHANG Y et al: Cofactor dynamics and sufficiency in estrogen receptor–regulated transcription. Cell 103: 843, 2000

327 THE MENOPAUSE TRANSITION AND POSTMENOPAUSAL HORMONE THERAPY
JoAnn E. Manson, Shari S. Bassuk

Menopause is the permanent cessation of menstruation due to loss of ovarian follicular function. It is diagnosed retrospectively after 12 months of amenorrhea. The average age at menopause is 51 years among U.S. women. *Perimenopause* refers to the time period preceding menopause, when fertility wanes and menstrual cycle irregularity increases, until the first year after cessation of menses. The onset of perimenopause precedes the final menses by 2 to 8 years, with a mean duration of 4 years. Smoking accelerates the menopausal transition by 2 years.

Although the peri- and postmenopausal periods share many symptoms, the physiology and clinical management of the two periods differ. Low-dose oral contraceptives have become a therapeutic mainstay in perimenopause, whereas postmenopausal hormone therapy (HT) has been a common method of symptom alleviation after menstruation ceases.

PERIMENOPAUSE

PHYSIOLOGY Ovarian mass and fertility decline sharply after age 35 and even more precipitously during perimenopause; depletion of primary follicles, a process that begins before birth, occurs steadily until menopause (Chap. 326). In perimenopause, intermenstrual intervals shorten significantly (typically by 3 days) due to an accelerated follicular phase. Follicle-stimulating hormone (FSH) levels rise, due to altered folliculogenesis and reduced inhibin secretion. In contrast to the consistently high FSH and low estradiol levels seen in menopause, perimenopause is characterized by "irregularly irregular" hormone levels. The propensity for anovulatory cycles can produce a hyperestrogenic, hypoprogestagenic environment that may account for the increased incidence of endometrial hyperplasia or carcinoma, uterine polyps, and leiomyoma observed among women of perimenopausal age. Mean serum levels of selected ovarian and pituitary hormones during the menopausal transition are shown in Fig. 327-1. With transition into menopause, estradiol levels fall markedly, whereas estrone levels are relatively preserved, reflecting peripheral aromatization of adrenal and ovarian androgens. FSH levels increase more than those of luteinizing hormone (LH), presumably because of the loss of inhibin, as well as estrogen feedback.

FIGURE 327-1 Mean serum levels of ovarian and pituitary hormones during the menopausal transition. FSH, follicle-stimulating hormone; LH, luteinizing hormone. *(From JL Shifren, Schiff: The aging ovary. J Women's Health Gend-Based Med 9:5–3, 2000, with permission.)*

DIAGNOSTIC TESTS Because of their extreme intraindividual variability, FSH and estradiol levels are imperfect diagnostic indicators of perimenopause in menstruating women. However, a low FSH in the early follicular phase (days 2 to 5) of the menstrual cycle is inconsistent with a diagnosis of perimenopause. FSH measurement can also aid in assessing fertility; levels of <20 mIU/mL, 20 to <30 mIU/mL, and ≥30 mIU/mL measured on day 3 of the cycle indicate a good, fair, and poor likelihood of achieving pregnancy, respectively.

SYMPTOMS Anovulatory cycles may be associated with irregular bleeding. Some perimenopausal women experience classic postmenopausal symptoms such as hot flashes and night sweats, insomnia, vaginal dryness, mood swings, or depression. In one U.S. study, nearly 60% of women reported hot flashes in the 2 years before their final menses. Symptom intensity, duration, and frequency are highly variable.

℞ TREATMENT

For women with irregular or heavy menses or hormonally related symptoms that impair quality of life, low-dose combined oral contraceptives are a staple of therapy. Static doses of estrogen and progestin (e.g., 20 μg of ethinyl estradiol and 1 mg of norethindrone acetate daily for 21 days each month) can eliminate vasomotor symptoms and restore regular cyclicity. Oral contraceptives provide other benefits, including protection against ovarian and endometrial cancers and increased bone density, although it is not clear whether use during perimenopause decreases fracture risk later in life. Moreover, the contraceptive benefit is important, given that the unintentional pregnancy rate among women in their forties rivals that of adolescents. Contraindications to oral contraceptive use include cigarette smoking, liver disease, a history of thromboembolism or cardiovascular disease, breast cancer, or unexplained vaginal bleeding. Progestin-only formulations (e.g., 0.35 mg norethindrone daily) or medroxyprogesterone (Depo-Provera) injections (e.g., 150 mg intramuscularly every 3 months) may provide an alternative for the treatment of perimenopausal menorrhagia in women who smoke or have cardiovascular risk factors. Although progestins neither regularize cycles nor reduce the number of bleeding days, they reduce the volume of menstrual flow.

Nonhormonal strategies to reduce menstrual flow include use of nonsteroidal anti-inflammatory agents such as mefenamic acid (initial dose of 500 mg at start of menses, then 250 mg qid for 2 to 3 days) or, when medical approaches fail, endometrial ablation. It should be noted that menorrhagia requires an evaluation to rule out uterine disorders. Transvaginal ultrasound with saline enhancement is useful for detecting leiomyomata or polyps, and endometrial aspiration can identify hyperplastic changes.

TRANSITION TO MENOPAUSE For sexually active women using contraceptive hormones to alleviate perimenopausal symptoms, the question of when and if to switch to HT must be individualized. Estrogen and progestin doses in HT are lower than those in oral contraceptives and have not been documented to prevent pregnancy. Though a 1-year absence of spontaneous menses reliably indicates ovulation cessation, it is not possible to assess the natural menstrual pattern while a woman is taking an oral contraceptive. Women willing to switch to a barrier method of contraception should do so; if menses occur spontaneously, oral contraceptive use can be resumed. The average age of final menses among relatives can serve as a guide for when to initiate this process, which can be repeated yearly until menopause has occurred.

MENOPAUSE AND POSTMENOPAUSAL HORMONE THERAPY

One of the most complex health care decisions facing women is whether or not to use postmenopausal hormone therapy. HT, once prescribed primarily to relieve vasomotor symptoms, has been promoted as a strategy to forestall various disorders that accelerate after menopause, including osteoporosis and cardiovascular disease. More than 30% of postmenopausal women in the United States currently use HT. This widespread use is unwarranted given the paucity of conclusive data, until very recently, on the health consequences of such therapy. Although many women rely on their health care providers for a definitive answer to the question of whether to use postmenopausal hormones, balancing the benefits and risks for an individual patient is challenging.

Although observational studies suggest that HT prevents cardiovascular and other chronic diseases, the apparent benefits may result at least in part from differences between women who opt to take postmenopausal hormones and women who do not. Those choosing HT tend to be healthier, have greater access to medical care, are more compliant with prescribed treatments, and maintain a more health-promoting life-style. Randomized trials, which eliminate these confounding factors, have not consistently confirmed the benefits found in observational studies. Indeed, one arm of the largest trial of HT to date, the Women's Health Initiative (WHI), which examined more than 16,000 postmenopausal women for an average of 5.2 years, was stopped early because of an overall unfavorable risk-benefit ratio associated with estrogen-progestin therapy.

The following summary offers a decision-making guide based on a synthesis of currently available evidence. The decision is divided into one of short- (<5 years) or long-term (≥5 years) use of HT. Prevention of cardiovascular disease is eliminated from the equation due to lack of evidence for such benefits in recent randomized clinical trials.

BENEFITS AND RISKS OF POSTMENOPAUSAL HORMONE THERAPY (Table 327-1)

DEFINITE BENEFITS ■ *Symptoms of Menopause* Compelling evidence, including data from randomized clinical trials, indicates that estrogen therapy is highly effective for controlling vasomotor and genitourinary symptoms. Alternative approaches, including the use of antidepressants (such as venlafaxine, 75 to 150 mg/d), clonidine (0.1 to 0.2 mg/d), or vitamin E (400 to 800 IU/d) or the consumption of soy-based products or other phytoestrogens, may also alleviate vasomotor symptoms, although they are less effective than HT. For genitourinary symptoms, the efficacy of vaginal estrogen is similar to that of oral or transdermal estrogen.

Osteoporosis (see also Chap 333) ■ *BONE DENSITY* By reducing bone turnover and resorption rates, estrogen slows the aging-related bone loss experienced by most postmenopausal women. More than 50 randomized trials have demonstrated that postmenopausal estrogen therapy, with or without a progestin, rapidly increases bone mineral density at the spine by 4 to 6% and at the hip by 2 to 3%, and maintains those increases during treatment.

FRACTURES Data from observational studies indicate a 50 to 80% lower risk of vertebral fracture and a 25 to 30% lower risk of hip, wrist, and other peripheral fractures among current estrogen users; addition of a

TABLE 327-1 *Benefits and Risks of Postmenopausal Hormone Therapy (HT)*

Variable	Effect	Benefit or Risk — Relative	Benefit or Risk — Absolute	Sources of Evidence
DEFINITE BENEFITS				
Symptoms of menopause (vasomotor, genitourinary)	Definite improvement	>70 to 80% decrease		Observational studies and randomized trials
Osteoporosis	Definite increase in bone mineral density and decrease in fracture risk	2–5% increase in bone density; 25–50% decrease in risk of fractures	WHI: 50 fewer hip fractures (100 vs. 150) per 100,000 woman-years	Observational studies and randomized trials, including WHI
DEFINITE RISKS				
Endometrial cancer	Definite increase in risk with use of unopposed[a] estrogen; no increase with use of estrogen plus progestin	8- to 10-fold increased risk with use of unopposed estrogen for ≥10 yr; no excess risk with estrogen-progestin therapy	46 excess cases (52 vs. 6) per 100,000 woman-years of unopposed estrogen use (≥10 years of use); no excess with estrogen-progestin therapy	Observational studies and randomized trials
Venous thromboembolism	Definite increase in risk	≥2-fold increase	Secondary prevention: 390 excess cases per 100,000 woman-years	Randomized trial (HERS)
			Primary prevention: 180 excess cases per 100,000 woman-years	Observational studies and randomized trial (WHI)
Breast cancer	Increase in risk with long-term use (≥5 yr)	1.35-fold overall increase with HT use ≥5 yr	10–30 excess cases per 10,000 women using HT for 5 yr; 30–90 excess cases after 10 yr of use; 50–200 excess cases after 15 yr of use	Observational data (meta-analysis of 51 studies)
		25–30% increase with 5.2 yr of estrogen-progestin therapy; no increase with estrogen-only	WHI: 80 excess cases (300 vs. 380) per 100,000 woman-years of estrogen-progestin therapy	Randomized trials (WHI, HERS)
PROBABLE OR UNCERTAIN RISKS AND BENEFITS				
Cardiovascular disease Primary prevention	Probable increase in risk	WHI: 29% increase in CHD with estrogen-progestin; no apparent increase or decrease with estrogen-only	WHI: 70 excess cases (370 vs. 300) of CHD per 100,000 woman-years with estrogen-progestin	Observational studies suggest a 35–50% decrease in risk, while randomized trials show no effect or a harmful effect; most studies have assessed conjugated equine estrogen alone or in combination with medroxyprogesterone acetate
		40% increase in stroke with either estrogen-progestin or estrogen-only	80 excess cases (290 vs. 210) of stroke per 100,000 woman-years	
Secondary prevention	Probable early increase in risk	HERS: 50% increase in CHD in year 1; no overall effect over 4 years	Equal number of CHD cases over 4 years	Observational studies and randomized secondary prevention trials
Gallbladder disease	Probable increase in risk	1.4-fold increase	360 excess cases per 100,000 woman-years	Randomized trials (HERS)
Colorectal cancer	Probable decrease in risk	20–37% decrease with estrogen-progestin	24–60 fewer cases per 100,000 woman-years	Observational data, randomized trial (WHI)
Cognitive dysfunction	Unproven decrease in risk	Apparent increase in dementia after age 65	Uncertain	Inconsistent data from observational studies and randomized trials

[a] "Unopposed estrogen" refers to the use of estrogen without progestin.
Note: WHI, Women's Health Initiative; HERS, Heart and Estrogen/progestin Replacement Study; CHD, coronary heart disease.

Source: Adapted from Manson and Martin, with permission. Copyright © 2001 Massachusetts Medical Society. All rights reserved.

progestin does not appear to modify this benefit. Discontinuation of estrogen therapy leads to a diminution of protection. In the WHI, 5 to 6 years of either combined estrogen-progestin or estrogen-only was associated with a 30 to 40% reduction in hip fracture and 20 to 30% fewer total fractures among a population unselected for osteoporosis. Bisphosphonates (such as alendronate, 10 mg/d or 70 mg once per week or residronate, 5 mg/d or 35 mg once a week) and raloxifene (60 mg/d), a selective estrogen receptor modulator, have each been shown in randomized trials to increase bone mass density and decrease fracture rates. These agents, unlike estrogen, do not appear to have adverse effects on the endometrium or breast. Increased physical activity and adequate calcium (1000 to 1500 mg/d in two to three divided doses) and vitamin D (400 to 800 IU/d) intakes may also reduce the risk of osteoporosis-related fractures.

DEFINITE RISKS ■ Endometrial Cancer A combined analysis of 30 observational studies found a tripling of risk of endometrial cancer among short-term (1 to 5 years) users of unopposed estrogen and a nearly tenfold increased risk among users for 10 or more years. These findings are supported by results from the randomized Postmenopausal Estrogen/Progestin Interventions (PEPI) trial, in which 24% of women assigned to unopposed estrogen for 3 years developed atypical endometrial hyperplasia, a premalignant lesion, compared to only 1% of women assigned to placebo. Use of a progestin, which opposes the effects of estrogen on the endometrium, eliminates these risks.

Venous Thromboembolism A recent meta-analysis of 12 studies—8 case-control, 1 cohort, and 3 randomized trials—found that current estrogen use was associated with a doubling of risk for venous thromboembolism in postmenopausal women. Relative risks of thromboembolic events were even greater (2.7 to 5.1) in the three trials included in the meta-analysis. Results from the WHI indicate a twofold increase in risk of venous and pulmonary thromboembolism.

Breast Cancer An increased risk of breast cancer has been found among current or recent estrogen users in observational studies; this risk is directly related to duration of use. In a meta-analysis of 51 case-control and cohort studies, short-term use (<5 years) of postmenopausal hormone therapy did not appreciably elevate breast cancer incidence, whereas long-term use (≥5 years) was associated with a 35% increase in risk. In contrast to findings for endometrial cancer, combined estrogen-progestin regimens appear to increase breast cancer risk more than estrogen alone. Data from randomized trials also indicate that HT raises breast cancer risk. In the WHI, women assigned to receive combination therapy for an average of 5.2 years were 26% more likely to develop breast cancer than women assigned to placebo but estrogen-only did not increase risk. In the Heart and Estrogen/progestin Replacement Study (HERS), 4 years of combination therapy was associated with a 27% increase in breast cancer risk. Although the latter finding was not statistically significant, the totality of evidence strongly implicates estrogen-progestin therapy in breast carcinogenesis.

PROBABLE OR UNCERTAIN RISKS AND BENEFITS ■ Coronary Heart Disease/ Stroke Until recently, HT had been enthusiastically recommended as a possible cardioprotective agent. In the past three decades, multiple observational studies suggested, in the aggregate, that estrogen use leads to a 35 to 50% reduction in coronary heart disease incidence among postmenopausal women. The biologic plausibility of such an association is supported by data from randomized trials demonstrating that exogenous estrogen lowers plasma low-density lipoprotein (LDL) cholesterol and raises high-density lipoprotein (HDL) cholesterol levels by 10 to 15%. Administration of estrogen also favorably affects lipoprotein(a) levels, LDL oxidation, endothelial vascular function, and fibrinogen and plasminogen activator inhibitor-1. However, estrogen therapy also has unfavorable effects on other biomarkers of cardiovascular risk; it boosts triglyceride levels; promotes coagulation via factor VII, prothrombin fragments 1 and 2, and fibrinopeptide A elevations; and raises levels of the inflammatory marker C-reactive protein.

Randomized trials of estrogen or combined estrogen-progestin in women with preexisting cardiovascular disease have not confirmed the benefits reported in observational studies. In HERS, a secondary prevention trial designed to test the efficacy and safety of estrogen-progestin therapy on clinical cardiovascular outcomes, the 4-year incidence of coronary mortality and nonfatal myocardial infarction was similar in the active treatment and placebo groups, and a 50% increase in risk of coronary events was noted during the first year of the study among participants assigned to the active treatment group. Although it is possible that progestin may mitigate estrogen's benefits, the Estrogen Replacement and Atherosclerosis (ERA) trial indicated that angiographically determined progression of coronary atherosclerosis was unaffected by either opposed or unopposed estrogen treatment. Moreover, the Papworth Hormone Replacement Therapy Atherosclerosis

Study, a trial of transdermal estradiol with and without norethindone, the Women's Estrogen for Stroke Trial (WEST), a trial of oral 17β-estradiol, and the EStrogen in the Prevention of ReInfarction Trial (ESPRIT), a trial of oral estradiol valerate, found no cardiovascular benefits of the regimens studied. Thus, in clinical trials, HT has not proved effective for the secondary prevention of cardiovascular disease in postmenopausal women.

Primary prevention trials also suggest an early increase in cardiovascular risk and absence of cardioprotection with postmenopausal HT. Results from the large-scale WHI suggest a deleterious cardiovascular effect of hormone therapy. Women assigned to 5 years of estrogen-progestin therapy were 29% more likely to develop coronary heart disease and 41% more likely to suffer a stroke than those assigned to placebo. In the estrogen-only arm of the WHI, a similar increase in stroke and no effect on CHD were observed. Further research is needed on clinical characteristics as well as on biomarkers that predict increases or decreases in cardiovascular risk associated with exogenous hormone therapy. Whether different doses, formulations, or routes of administration of hormone therapy will produce different cardiovascular effects remains uncertain.

Gallbladder Disease Several large observational studies report a two- to threefold increased risk of gallstones or cholecystectomy among postmenopausal women taking estrogen. In HERS, women randomized to 4 years of estrogen-progestin therapy had a 38% greater risk of developing gallbladder disease than those assigned to placebo, a risk that climbed to 48% after 2.7 additional years of observational follow-up.

Colorectal Cancer Observational studies have suggested that HT reduces risks of colon and rectal cancer, although the estimated magnitudes of the relative benefits ranged from 8 to 33% in various meta-analyses. In the WHI, the only trial to examine the issue, estrogen-progestin therapy was associated with a significant 37% reduction in colorectal cancer over a 5-year period; no benefit was seen with estrogen-only.

Cognitive Decline and Dementia A meta-analysis of 10 case-control and 2 cohort studies suggested that postmenopausal HT is associated with a 33% decreased risk of dementia. Subsequent randomized trials, however, failed to demonstrate any benefit of estrogen therapy on the progression of mild to moderate Alzheimer's disease and indicated a potential adverse effect of estrogen-progestin therapy on the incidence of dementia.

Ovarian Cancer and Other Disorders On the basis of limited observational and randomized data, it has been hypothesized that HT increases the risk of ovarian cancer and reduces the risk of type 2 diabetes mellitus. These hypotheses require confirmation in additional clinical trials.

APPROACH TO THE PATIENT

The rational use of postmenopausal hormone therapy requires balancing the potential benefits and risks. Figure 327-2 provides one approach to decision making. The clinician should first determine whether the patient has an indication for initiating HT. Relief of menopausal symptoms and prevention of osteoporosis are the most valid reasons. The benefits and risks of such therapy should then be reviewed with the patient, giving more emphasis to absolute than to relative measures of effect, and pointing out uncertainties in clinical knowledge where relevant. Potential side effects—especially vaginal bleeding that may result from use of combined estrogen-progestin formulations recommended for women with an intact uterus—should be noted. The patient's own preference regarding therapy should be elicited and factored into the decision. Contraindications to HT should be assessed routinely and include unexplained vaginal bleeding, active liver disease, venous thromboembolism, or history of endometrial cancer (except stage 1 without deep invasion) or breast cancer. Relative contraindications include hypertriglyceridemia (>400 mg/dL) and active gallbladder disease (in such cases, transdermal estrogen is an option). Neither primary nor secondary prevention of heart disease should be viewed as an expected benefit of HT, and an increase in stroke and a small early increase in coronary artery disease risk should be considered. Nevertheless, such therapy may be appropriate, if the noncoronary benefits of treatment clearly outweigh risks. A woman who suffers an acute coronary event or stroke while on HT should stop therapy immediately.

Short-term use (<5 years) of HT is appropriate for relief of menopausal symptoms among women without contraindications to such use. However, such therapy should be avoided or considered only as a secondary option among women with preexisting heart disease or stroke due to their elevated baseline risk of future cardiovascular events. Women who have contraindications, or are opposed to HT, may derive benefit from the use of selective antidepressants, clonidine, or soy, and, for genitourinary symptoms, intravaginal estrogen creams or devices.

Long-term use (≥5 years) of HT is more problematic because a heightened risk of breast cancer must be factored into the decision. Reasonable candidates for such use include a small percentage of postmenopausal women and comprise those who have persistent severe vasomotor symptoms and/or have an increased risk of osteoporosis (e.g., those with osteopenia, a personal or family history of nontraumatic fracture, or a body mass index <22 kg/m²), who also have no personal or family history of breast cancer in a first-degree relative or other contraindications, and who have a strong personal preference for therapy. Poor candidates are women with cardiovascular disease, those at low risk of osteoporosis, and those at increased risk of breast cancer (e.g., women who have a first-degree relative with breast cancer, susceptibility genes such as *BRCA1* or *BRCA2*, or a personal history of cellular atypia detected by breast biopsy). Even in reasonable candidates, strategies to minimize dose and duration of use should be employed. For example, women using hormone replacement to relieve intense vasomotor symptoms in early postmenopause should consider discontinuing therapy before 5 years, resuming it only if vasomotor symptoms persist and/or an increased risk of osteoporosis is evident. In the latter situation, alternative therapies such as bisphosphonates or selective estrogen receptor modulators (SERMs) should be considered. Research on androgen-containing preparations has been limited, particularly in terms of long-term safety.

In addition to HT, control of symptoms and prevention of chronic disease can be accomplished by life-style choices, including smoking abstention, adequate physical activity, and a healthy diet. An expanding array of pharmacologic options—e.g., bisphosphonates or SERMs for osteoporosis, and cholesterol-lowering or antihypertensive agents for cardiovascular disease—should also reduce the widespread reliance on hormone use. However, short-term HT may still benefit some women.

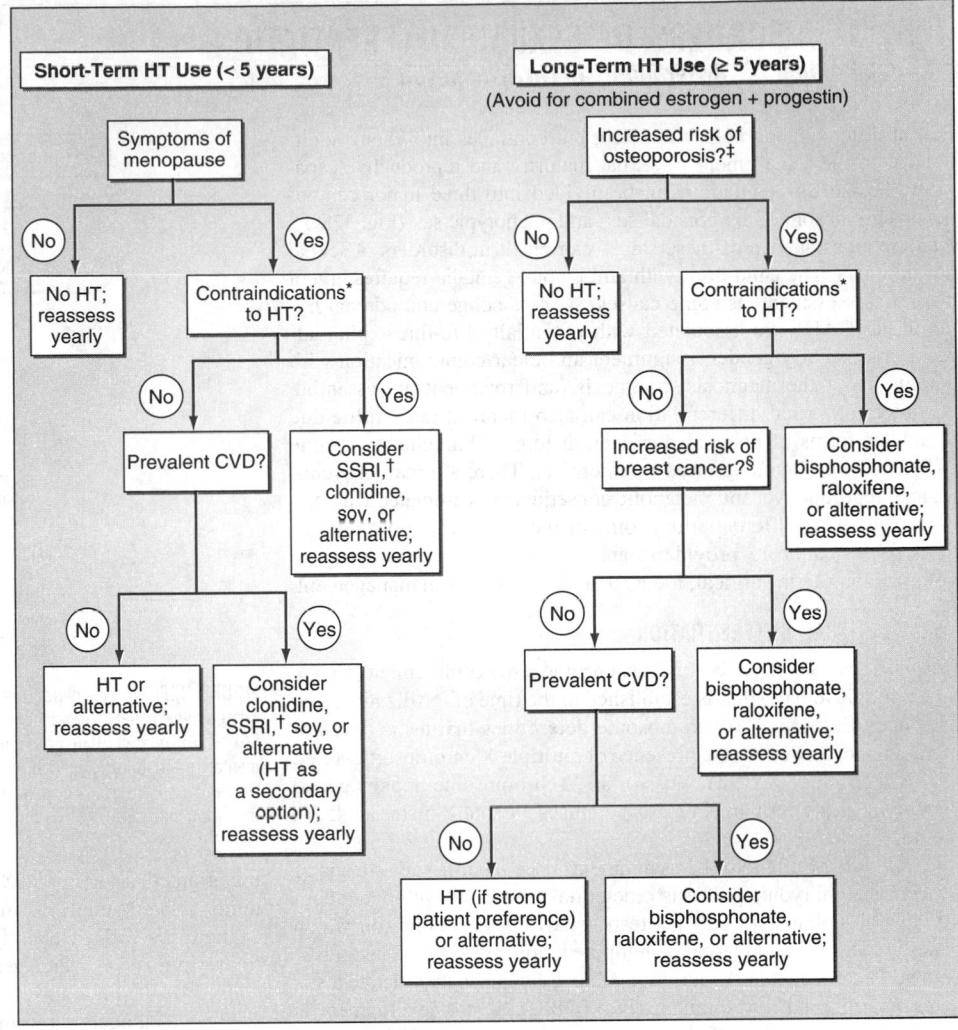

FIGURE 327-2 Flowchart for identifying appropriate candidates for short-term and long-term use of postmenopausal hormone therapy (HT). *Contraindications include unexplained vaginal bleeding, active liver disease, venous thromboembolism, or history of endometrial cancer (except stage 1 without deep invasion) or breast cancer. Relative contraindications include hypertriglyceridemia (>400 mg/dL) and active gallbladder disease (in such cases, transdermal estrogen is an option). †SSRI denotes selective serotonin reuptake inhibitor. ‡Increased risk of osteoporosis: documented osteopenia or osteoporosis, personal or family history of nontraumatic fracture, current smoking, or a body mass index <22 kg/m². §Increased risk of breast cancer: one or more first-degree relatives with breast cancer; susceptibility genes such as *BRCA1* or *BRCA2*; or a personal history of breast biopsy demonstrating atypia. CVD, cardiovascular disease. (*Adapted from Manson and Martin; with permission. Copyright © 2001 Massachusetts Medical Society. All rights reserved.*)

FURTHER READING

HULLEY S et al: Randomized trial of estrogen plus progestin for secondary prevention of coronary heart disease in postmenopausal women. Heart and Estrogen/progestin Replacement Study (HERS) Research Group. JAMA 280:605, 1998

MANSON JE, MARTIN KA: Clinical practice: Postmenopausal hormone-replacement therapy. N Engl J Med 345:34, 2001

NELSON HD et al: Postmenopausal hormone replacement therapy: Scientific review. JAMA 288:872, 2002

STEERING COMMITTEE FOR THE WOMEN'S HEALTH INITIATIVE: Effects of conjugated equine estrogen in postmenopausal women with hysterectomy: Principal results from the Women's Health Initiative randomized controlled trial. JAMA 2004, in press

WRITING GROUP FOR THE PEPI TRIAL: Effects of estrogen or estrogen/progestin regimens on heart disease risk factors in postmenopausal women. The Postmenopausal Estrogen/Progestin Interventions (PEPI) Trial. JAMA 273:199, 1995

WRITING GROUP FOR THE WOMEN'S HEALTH INITIATIVE INVESTIGATORS: Risks and benefits of estrogen plus progestin in healthy postmenopausal women. Principal results from the Women's Health Initiative randomized controlled trial. JAMA 288:321, 2002

Sexual differentiation begins in utero, but continues into young adulthood with the achievement of sexual maturity and reproductive capability. Sexual differentiation can be divided into three major components: chromosomal sex, gonadal sex, and phenotypic sex (Fig. 328-1). Abnormalities at each of these stages can result in disorders of sexual development. The child born with ambiguous genitalia requires urgent pediatric assessment, as some causes, such as congenital adrenal hyperplasia (CAH), are associated with potentially life-threatening adrenal crises. Early gender assignment and clear communication with parents about the diagnosis, prognosis, and treatment are essential. Disorders of sexual differentiation can also manifest later in life due to subtler forms of gonadal dysfunction [e.g., Klinefelter syndrome (KS)] and are often diagnosed by internists. There are many psychological, reproductive, and metabolic consequences associated with disorders of sexual differentiation; some of these patients avoid interactions with healthcare providers, and special effort is necessary to optimize long-term surgical, medical, and psychological management.

NORMAL SEXUAL DIFFERENTIATION

Chromosomal sex describes the sex chromosome complement (46,XY male; 46,XX female) that is established at the time of fertilization. The presence of a normal Y chromosome determines that testis development will occur, even in the presence of multiple X chromosomes (e.g., 47,XXY or 48,XXXY). The loss of an X chromosome impairs gonad development (45,X or 46,XY/45,X). Fetuses with no X material (45,Y) are not viable.

Gonadal sex refers to the assignment of gonadal tissue as testis or ovary. The embryonic gonad is bipotential, and can develop (at about 40 days gestation) into either a testis or ovary, depending on which genes are expressed. Ovarian development appears to be a constitutive pathway and occurs in the absence of specific genes that dictate testis determination and development (Fig. 328-2). Testis development is initiated by expression of the Y chromosome gene *SRY* (sex-determining region on the Y chromosome), which encodes an HMG box transcription factor. *SRY* is transiently expressed in cells destined to become Sertoli cells and serves as a pivotal switch to establish the testis lineage. Mutation of *SRY* prevents testis development in chromosomal 46,XY males, whereas translocation of *SRY* in 46,XX females is sufficient to induce testis development and a male phenotype. Other genes are necessary to continue testis development. *SOX9* (SRY-related HMG-box gene 9) is strikingly upregulated in the developing male gonad but is turned off in the female gonad. Transgenic expression of *SOX9* is sufficient to initiate testis formation in mice, and

FIGURE 328-1 Sexual differentiation can be divided into three major components: chromosomal sex, gonadal sex, and phenotypic sex. T, testosterone; DHT, dihydrotestosterone; MIS, müllerian-inhibiting substance; E₂, estradiol; P₄, progesterone.

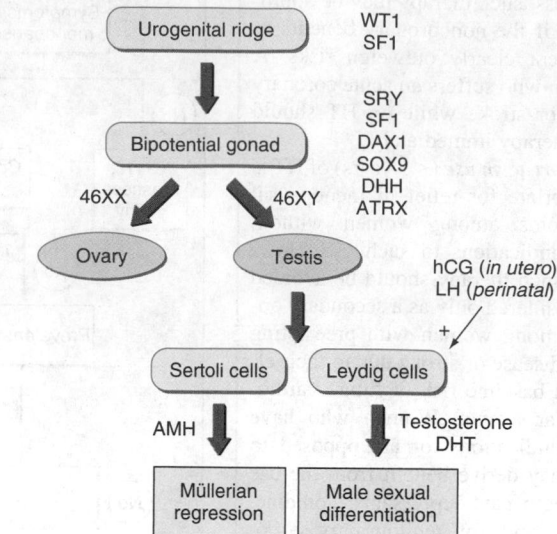

FIGURE 328-2 The genetic regulation of testis development. *WT1*, Wilms' tumor-related gene 1; *SF1*, steroidogenic factor 1; *SRY*, sex-related gene on the Y chromosome; *SOX9*, SRY-related HMG-box gene 9; *DHH*, desert hedgehog; *ATRX*, (α-thalassemia, mental retardation on the X); *DAX1*, dosage sensitive sex-reversal, adrenal hypoplasia congenita on the X chromosome, gene 1; *AMH*, anti-müllerian hormone (müllerian-inhibiting substance); DHT, dihydrotestosterone.

mutations that disrupt *SOX9* impair testis development. *WT1* (Wilms' tumor-related gene 1) is involved in renal and gonadal development. In the testis, *WT1* acts early in the genetic pathway and regulates the transcription of several genes including *SF1*, *DAX1*, and *AMH* (encoding *MIS*, müllerian-inhibiting substance). *SF1* (steroidogenic factor 1) encodes a nuclear receptor and is required for adrenal and gonadal development (both testis and ovary). It functions in cooperation with other transcription factors to regulate a large array of adrenal and gonadal genes, including many genes involved in steroidogenesis. The early expression pattern of *SF1* in the gonad parallels that of another orphan nuclear receptor, *DAX1* (dosage sensitive sex-reversal, adrenal hypoplasia congenita on the X chromosome, gene 1). In contrast to *SOX9*, *DAX1* is downregulated as the testis develops. Duplication of *DAX1* impairs testis development, possibly by antagonizing the function of SRY and SF1. Deletions or mutations of *DAX1*, on the other hand, lead to disordered formation of testis cords, revealing the exquisite sensitivity of the male sex-determining pathway to gene dosage effects. In addition to those mentioned above, human and murine mutations indicate that at least 10 other genes are also involved in gonadal differentiation and development as well as final positioning of the gonads.

It is unclear whether analogous "ovarian-determining genes" exist, or whether ovarian development only requires the absence of testis-determining genes. However, germ cells play a key role in supporting ovarian development and produce factors that inhibit the formation of testicular elements. This contrasts with the testis, which develops and undergoes steroidogenesis in the absence of germ cells. Once the ovary has formed, expression of a variety of specific genes is required for normal follicular development [e.g., follicle stimulating hormone (FSH) receptor, *GDF9*]. Steroidogenesis in the ovary requires the development of follicles containing granulosa cells and theca cells surrounding the oocytes (Chap. 326). Thus, there is minimal ovarian steroidogenesis until gonadotropins are produced at puberty.

Phenotypic sex refers to the structures of the external and internal genitalia, and secondary sex characteristics. The male phenotype requires the secretion of anti-müllerian hormone (AMH, müllerian-inhibiting substance) from Sertoli cells and testosterone from testicular

Leydig cells. AMH is a member of the TGF-β growth factor family and acts through specific receptors to cause regression of the müllerian structures (52 to 70 days gestation). At approximately 60 to 140 days gestation, testosterone supports the development of wolffian structures, including the epididymides, vasa deferentia, and seminal vesicles. Testosterone is also the precursor for dihydrotestosterone (DHT), a potent androgen that promotes development of the external genitalia, including the penis and scrotum (65–100 days, and beyond) (Fig. 328-3). The urogenital sinus develops into the prostate and prostatic urethra in the male and into the urethra and lower portion of the vagina in the female. The genital tubercle becomes the glans penis in the male and the clitoris in the female. The urogenital swellings form the scrotum or the labia majora, and the urethral folds fuse to form the shaft of the penis and the male urethra or the labia minora. In the female, wolffian ducts regress and the müllerian ducts form the fallopian tubes, uterus, and upper segment of the vagina. A normal female phenotype will develop in the absence of the gonad, but estrogen is needed for maturation of the uterus and breast at puberty.

DISORDERS OF CHROMOSOMAL SEX

Disorders of chromosomal sex result from abnormalities in the number or structure of the X or Y chromosomes (Table 328-1).

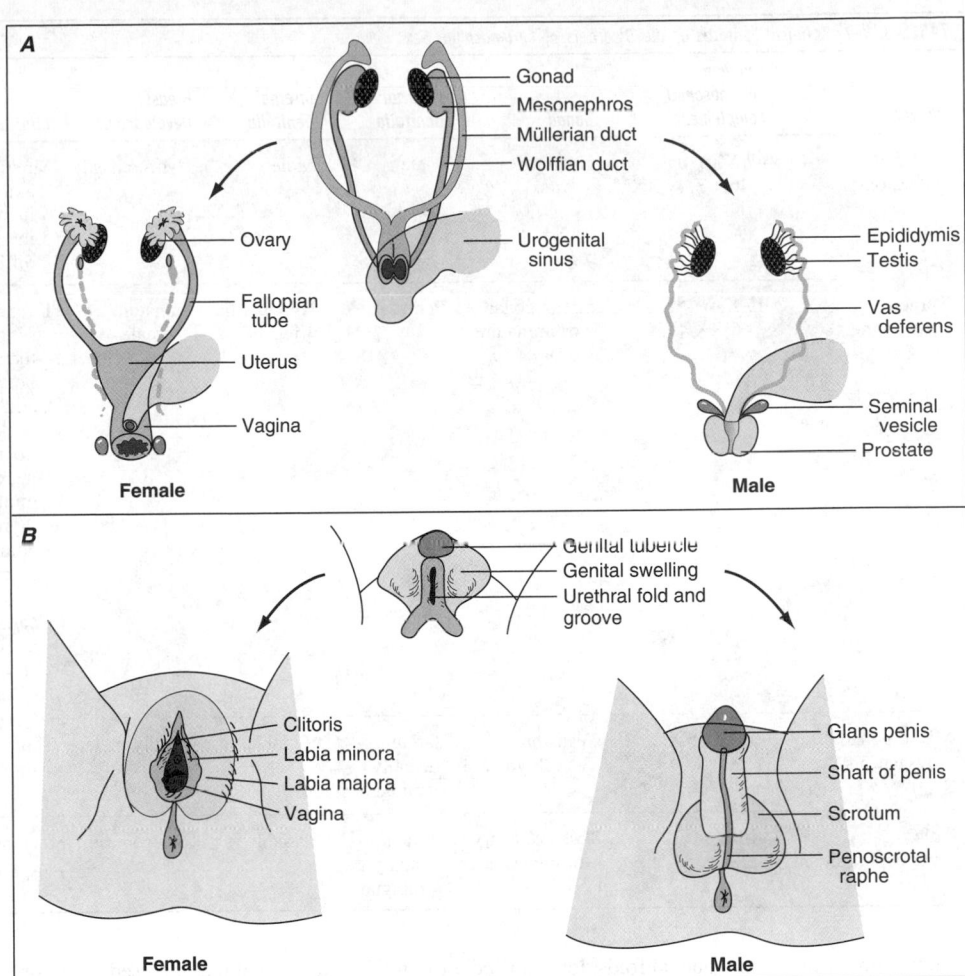

FIGURE 328-3   Normal sexual differentiation. *A.* Internal urogenital tract. *B.* External genitalia. [After JD Wilson, JE Griffin, in E Braunwald et al (eds): *Harrison's Principles of Internal Medicine*, 15th ed. New York, McGraw-Hill, 2001.]

KLINEFELTER SYNDROME (47,XXY AND MOSAIC VARIANTS) ■ Pathophysiology

The classic form of Klinefelter syndrome (KS) (47,XXY) occurs following meiotic nondisjunction of the sex chromosomes during gametogenesis (40% during spermatogenesis, 60% during oogenesis) (Chap. 57). Mosaic forms of KS (46,XY/47,XXY) are thought to result from chromosomal mitotic nondisjunction within the zygote, and occur in at least 10% of individuals with this condition. Other chromosomal variants of KS (e.g., 48,XXYY; 48,XXXY) have been reported but are less common.

Clinical Features   KS is characterized by small testes, infertility, gynecomastia, eunuchoid proportions, and poor virilization in phenotypic males. It has an incidence of 1 in 500 to 1000 men. In severe cases, individuals present prepubertally with small testes, or with impaired androgenization and gynecomastia at the time of puberty. Developmental delay and learning disabilities may be a feature. Later in life, eunuchoid features or infertility lead to the diagnosis. Testes are small and firm [median length 2.5 cm (4 mL volume); almost always <3.5 cm (12 mL)], and typically seem inappropriately small for the degree of androgenization. Biopsies are not usually necessary but reveal seminiferous tubule hyalinization and azoospermia. Other clinical features of KS are listed in Table 328-1. Plasma concentrations of follicle stimulating hormone (FSH) and luteinizing hormone (LH) are increased in most patients with 47,XXY (90 and 80%, respectively) and plasma testosterone is decreased (50–75%), reflecting primary gonadal failure. Estradiol is often increased because of chronic Leydig cell stimulation by LH and because of aromatization of androstenedione by adipose tissue; the increased ratio of estradiol/testosterone results in gynecomastia. Patients with mosaic forms of KS have less severe clinical features, larger testes, and sometimes achieve fertility.

℞ TREATMENT

Disfiguring gynecomastia should be treated by surgical reduction. Androgen supplementation (Chap. 325) improves virilization, libido, energy, and bone mineralization in underandrogenized men, but may worsen gynecomastia. Fertility has been achieved using in vitro fertilization in men with oligospermia, or with intracytoplasmic sperm injection when spermatids can be recovered from testicular biopsy. However, the risk of transmission of this chromosomal abnormality needs to be considered, and preimplantation screening may be desired.

TURNER SYNDROME (GONADAL DYSGENESIS) (45,X AND MOSAIC VARIANTS) ■

Pathophysiology   Approximately one-half of individuals with Turner syndrome (TS) have a 45,X karyotype, one-fourth have 46,XX/45,X mosaicism, and the remainder have structural abnormalities of the X chromosome such as X fragments, isochromosomes, or rings. The clinical features of TS result from haploinsufficiency of multiple X chromosomal genes (e.g., Short Stature Homeobox, *SHOX*). However, imprinted genes may also be affected when the inherited X has different parental origins.

Clinical Features   TS is characterized by bilateral streak gonads, primary amenorrhea, short stature, and multiple congenital anomalies in phenotypic females. It affects approximately 1 in 2500 women and is diagnosed at different ages depending on the dominant clinical features (Table 328-1). Prenatally, a diagnosis of TS is usually made incidentally after chorionic villous sampling or amniocentesis for unrelated reasons, such as advanced maternal age. Prenatal ultrasound findings include increased nuchal translucency and reduced fetal growth. The postnatal diagnosis of TS should be considered in female neonates or

TABLE 328-1 Clinical Features of the Disorders of Chromosomal Sex

Disorder	Common Chromosomal Complement	Gonad	External Genitalia	Internal Genitalia	Breast Development	Clinical Features
Klinefelter syndrome	47,XXY or 46,XY/47,XXY	Hyalinized testes	Male	Male	Gynecomastia	Small testes, azoospermia, decreased facial and axillary hair, decreased libido, tall stature & increased leg length, decreased penile length, increased risk of breast tumors, learning difficulties, obesity, varicose veins
Turner syndrome	45,X or 46,XX/45,X	Streak gonad or immature ovary	Female	Hypoplastic female	Immature female	Infancy: lymphedema, web neck, shield chest, low set hair line, cardiac defects and coarctation of the aorta, urinary tract malformations & horseshoe kidney Childhood: short stature, cubitus valgus, short neck, short 4th metacarpals, hypoplastic nails, micrognathia, scoliosis, otitis media & sensori-neural hearing loss, ptosis & amblyopia, multiple nevi & keloid formation, autoimmune thyroid disease, visuo-spatial learning difficulties Adulthood: pubertal failure & primary amenorrhea, hypertension, obesity, dyslipidemia, impaired glucose tolerance & insulin resistance, cardiovascular disease, aortic root dilatation, osteoporosis, inflammatory bowel disease, chronic hepatic dysfunction, increased risk of colon cancer, hearing loss
Mixed gonadal dysgenesis	46,XY/45,X	Testis or streak gonad	Variable— usually ambiguous	Variable	Usually male	Short stature, increased risk of gonadal tumors, some Turner syndrome features
True hermaphroditism	46,XY/46,XX	Testis & ovary or ovotestis	Variable— usually ambiguous	Variable	Gynecomastia	Increased risk of gonadal tumors

infants with lymphedema, nuchal folds, low hairline, or left-sided cardiac defects, and in girls with unexplained growth failure or pubertal delay. Although limited spontaneous pubertal development occurs in up to 30% of girls with TS (10%, 45,X; 30–40%, 45,X/46,XY), and approximately 2% reach menarche, the vast majority of women with TS develop complete ovarian failure. This diagnosis should be considered, therefore, in all women who present with primary or secondary amenorrhea and elevated gonadotropin levels.

℞ TREATMENT

The management of girls and women with TS requires a multidisciplinary approach because of the number of potentially involved organ systems. Detailed cardiac and renal evaluation should be performed at the time of diagnosis. Individuals with congenital heart defects (CHD) (30%) (bicuspid aortic valve, 30 to 50%; coarctation of the aorta, 30%; aortic root dilatation, 5%) require long-term follow-up by an experienced cardiologist, antibiotic prophylaxis for dental or surgical procedures, and serial imaging of aortic root dimensions, as progressive aortic root dilatation can occur. Individuals found to have congenital renal and urinary tract malformations (30%) are at risk for urinary tract infections, hypertension, and nephrocalcinosis. Hypertension can occur independent of cardiac and renal malformations, and should be monitored and treated as in other patients with essential hypertension. Clitoral enlargement or other evidence of virilization suggests the presence of covert, translocated Y chromosomal material and is associated with increased risk of gonadoblastoma, apparently the consequence of Y chromosomal genes distinct from SRY. Regular assessment of thyroid function, weight, dentition, hearing, speech, vision, and educational issues should be performed during childhood, and counseling about long-term growth and fertility issues should be provided. Patient support groups are active throughout the world.

The treatment of short stature in children with TS remains a challenge, as untreated final height rarely exceeds 150 cm. High-dose recombinant growth hormone stimulates growth rate in children with TS

and may be used alone or in combination with low doses of the non-aromatizable anabolic steroid oxandrolone (up to 0.05 mg/kg per d) in the older child (>8 years). However, final height increments are often modest (5–10 cm), and individualization of treatment regimens to response may be beneficial. Girls with evidence of gonadal failure require estrogen replacement to induce breast and uterine development, to support growth, and to maintain bone mineralization. Low-dose estrogen therapy (approximately one-sixth of the adult dose, 2 to 5 μg/d ethinylestradiol) is initiated between 12 to 14 years of age and increased gradually to induce feminization over a 2 to 3 year period. Progestins are later added to regulate withdrawal bleeds, and some women with TS have now achieved successful pregnancy after ovum donation and in vitro fertilization. Long-term follow-up of women with

TABLE 328-2 Disorders Causing Undervirilization in Karyotypic Males (46,XY)

Disorders of testis development
  True hermaphroditism (46,XY)
  Gonadal dysgenesis
  Absent testis syndrome
Disorders of androgen synthesis
  LH receptor mutations
  Smith-Lemli-Opitz syndrome
  Steroidogenic acute regulatory protein mutations
  Cholesterol side chain cleavage (CYP11A1) deficiency
  3β-Hydroxysteroid dehydrogenase 2 (HSD3B2) deficiency
  17α-Hydroxylase/17,20-lyase (CYP17) deficiency
  17β-Hydroxysteroid dehydrogenase 3 (HSD17B3) deficiency
  5α-Reductase 2 deficiency (SRD5A2)
  Aromatase overexpression
Disorders of androgen action
  Androgen Insensitivity Syndrome
  Androgen receptor cofactor defects
Other disorders of male reproductive tract
  Persistent müllerian duct syndrome
  Isolated hypospadias
  Cryptorchidism

TS involves careful surveillance of sex hormone replacement and reproductive function, bone mineralization, cardiac function and aortic root dimensions, blood pressure, weight and glucose tolerance, hepatic and lipid profiles, thyroid function, and hearing.

MIXED GONADAL DYSGENESIS (46,XY/45,X) Mixed gonadal dysgenesis typically results from 46,XY/45,X mosaicism. The phenotype of patients with this condition varies considerably, depending on the proportion and distribution of 46,XY cells. Although some patients have a predominantly female phenotype with somatic features of TS, streak gonads, and müllerian structures, other 46,XY/45,X individuals have a male phenotype and testes, and the diagnosis is made incidentally after amniocentesis or during investigation of infertility. In practice, most children who present to clinicians have ambiguous genitalia and variable somatic features. A female sex-of-rearing is often chosen (60%) if phallic development is poor, uterine structures are present, and if height potential is limited. However, gonadectomy is indicated to prevent further androgen secretion and to prevent development of gonadoblastoma (up to 25%). Individuals raised as males may require reconstructive surgery for hypospadias and removal of streak gonads. Scrotal testes can be preserved, but need regular examination for tumor development. Biopsy for carcinoma in situ is recommended in adolescence and testosterone supplementation may be required for virilization in puberty.

TRUE HERMAPHRODITISM (46,XY/46,XX) True hermaphroditism (TH) occurs when both an ovary and testis, or when an ovotestis, are found in one individual. For unclear reasons, gonadal asymmetry most often occurs with a testis on the right and an ovary on the left. True hermaphroditism due to 46,XY/46,XX mosaicism is rare and has a variable phenotype depending on the proportion of each cell line.

DISORDERS OF GONADAL AND PHENOTYPIC SEX

The clinical features of patients with disorders of gonadal and phenotypic sex are divided into the undervirilization of 46,XY males or inappropriate virilization of 46,XX females. These disorders comprise a spectrum of phenotypes ranging from complete "sex-reversal" (e.g., 46,XY phenotypic females or 46,XX males) to ambiguous genitalia.

UNDERVIRILIZED MALES (46,XY) (MALE PSEUDOHERMAPHRODITISM) Undervirilization of the male (46,XY) reflects defects in androgen production or action. It can result from disorders of testis development, defects of androgen synthesis, or resistance to testosterone and DHT (Table 328-2).

Disorders of Testis Development ■ *TESTICULAR DYSGENESIS* Patients with *pure gonadal dysgenesis* have streak gonads, müllerian structures (due to insufficient MIS secretion) and a complete absence of virilization.

TABLE 328-3 *Genetic Causes of Undervirilization of Karyotypic Males (46,XY)*

Gene	Inheritance	Gonad	Uterus	External Genitalia	Associated Features
DISORDERS OF TESTIS DEVELOPMENT					
WT1	AD	Dysgenetic testis	+/−	Female or ambiguous	Wilms' tumor, renal abnormalities, gonadal tumors (WAGR, Denys-Drash & Frasier syndromes)
SF1	AR/AD	Dysgenetic testis	+	Female or ambiguous	Primary adrenal failure
SRY	Y	Dysgenetic testis or ovary	+/−	Female or ambiguous	
SOX9	AD	Dysgenetic testis or ovary	+/−	Female or ambiguous	Campomelic dysplasia
DHH	AR	Testis/streak	+	Female	Minifascicular neuropathy
ATRX	X	Dysgenetic testis	−	Female or ambiguous	α-Thalassemia, developmental delay
ARX	X	Dysgenetic testis	−	Male or ambiguous	Mental retardation; X-linked lissencephaly
DAX1	dupXp21	Dysgenetic testis or ovary	+/−	Female or ambiguous	
WNT4	dup1p35	Dysgenetic testis	+	Ambiguous	
DISORDERS OF ANDROGEN SYNTHESIS					
LHR	AR	Testis	−	Female, ambiguous or micropenis	Leydig cell hypoplasia
DHCR7	AR	Testis	−	Variable	Smith-Lemli-Opitz syndrome: coarse facies, second-third toe syndactyly, failure to thrive, developmental delay, cardiac & visceral abnormalities
STAR	AR	Testis	−	Female	Congenital lipoid adrenal hyperplasia (primary adrenal failure)
CYP11A1	AR	Testis	−	Ambiguous	Congenital lipoid adrenal hyperplasia (primary adrenal failure)
HSD3B2	AR	Testis	−	Ambiguous	CAH, primary adrenal failure, partial virilization due to ↑ DHEA
CYP17	AR	Testis	−	Female or ambiguous	CAH, hypertension due to ↑ corticosterone & 11-deoxycorticosterone
HSD17B3	AR	Testis	−	Female or ambiguous	Partial virilization at puberty, ↑ androstenedione:testosterone ratio
SRD5A2	AR	Testis	−	Ambiguous	Partial virilization at puberty, ↑ testosterone:dihydrotestosterone ratio.
DISORDERS OF ANDROGEN ACTION					
Androgen receptor	X	Testis	−	Female, ambiguous, micropenis or normal male	Phenotypic spectrum from complete androgen insensitivity syndrome (female external genitalia) and partial androgen insensitivity (ambiguous) to normal male genitalia and infertility

Note: AR, autosomal recessive; AD, autosomal dominant; *WT1*, Wilms' tumor-related gene 1; *WAGR*, Wilms' tumor, aniridia, genitourinary anomalies, and mental retardation; *SF1*, steroidogenic factor 1; *SRY*, sex-related gene on the Y chromosome; *SOX9*, SRY-related HMG-box gene 9; *DHH*, desert hedgehog; *ATRX*, (α-thalassemia, mental retardation on the X); *ARX*, aristaless related homeobox, X-linked; *DAX1*, dosage sensitive sex-reversal, adrenal hypoplasia congenita on the X chromosome, gene 1; *WNT4*, wingless-type mouse mammary tumor virus integration site, 4; *LHR*, LH receptor; *DHCR7*, sterol 7δ reductase; *STAR*, steroidogenic acute regulatory protein; *CYP11A1*, P450 cholesterol side-chain cleavage; *HSD3B2*, 3β-hydroxysteroid dehydrogenase type 2; *CYP17*, 17α-hydroxylase and 17,20-lyase; *HSD17B3*, 17β-hydroxysteroid dehydrogenase type 3; *CYP19*, aromatase; *SRD5A2*, 5α-reductase type 2.

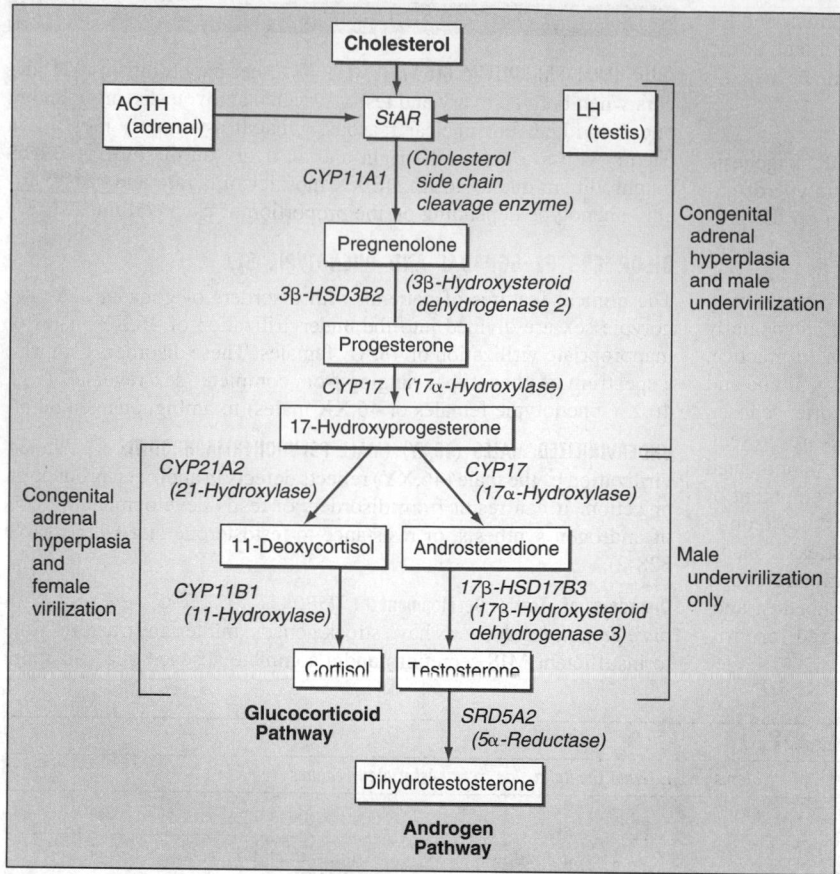

FIGURE 328-4 Pathways of glucocorticoid and androgen synthesis. Defects in *CYP21A2* and *CYP11B1* shunt steroid precursors into the androgen pathway and cause virilization of 46,XX females. Testosterone and dihydrotestosterone are synthesized in the testicular Leydig cells. Defects in enzymes involved in androgen synthesis result in undervirilization of 46,XY males. StAR, steroidogenic acute regulatory protein. [After JD Wilson, JE Griffin, in E Braunwald et al (eds): *Harrison's Principles of Internal Medicine*, 15th ed. New York, McGraw-Hill, 2001.]

Patients with *dysgenetic testes* produce enough MIS to regress the uterus and, sometimes, sufficient testosterone for partial virilization. Gonadal dysgenesis can result from mutations or deletions of testis-promoting genes (*WT1*, *SF1*, *SRY*, *SOX9*, *DAX1*, *DHH*, *ATRX*, *ARX*; also *DMRT*, and *SOX8* loci) or overexpression of factors that impair testis development when excessive (*WNT4*, *DAX1*) (Table 328-3). Associated clinical features may be present, reflecting additional functional roles for these genes. For example, renal dysfunction occurs in patients with specific *WT1* mutations (Denys-Drash and Frasier syndromes), primary adrenal failure occurs with *SF1* mutations, and severe cartilage abnormalities (campomelic dysplasia) are the predominant clinical feature of *SOX9* mutations. Dysgenetic testes should be removed to prevent malignancy, and estrogens can be used to induce secondary sex characteristics in 46,XY individuals raised as females. *Absent (vanishing) testis syndrome* reflects regression of the testis during development. The etiology is unknown but the absence of müllerian structures indicates adequate secretion of MIS in utero. Early testicular regression causes impaired virilization. Individuals raised as female should receive estrogen replacement at puberty. More frequently, late regression results in an otherwise normal male with anorchia. These individuals can be offered testicular prostheses and should receive androgen replacement in adolescence.

Disorders of Androgen Synthesis Defects in the pathway that regulates androgen synthesis (Fig. 328-4) cause undervirilization of the male fetus (Table 328-3). Müllerian regression is unaffected because Sertoli cell function is preserved.

LH RECEPTOR Mutations in the LH receptor cause Leydig cell hypoplasia and androgen deficiency. Defects of LH receptor synthesis or function preclude hCG (human chorionic gonadotropin) stimulation of

Leydig cells in utero, as well as LH stimulation of Leydig cells late in gestation and during the neonatal period. As a result, testosterone and DHT synthesis are insufficient for normal virilization of the internal and external genitalia, causing a spectrum of phenotypes that range from complete undervirilization to micropenis, depending on the severity of the mutation.

CONGENITAL ADRENAL HYPERPLASIA (CAH) Mutations in the genes that regulate cholesterol uptake and modification [*steroidogenic acute regulatory protein (StAR)*, *CYP11a*] affect both adrenal and gonadal steroidogenesis, and result in *congenital lipoid adrenal hyperplasia* (Chap. 321). Defects in *3β-hydroxysteroid dehydrogenase type 2 (HSD3B2)* also cause adrenal insufficiency, but the accumulation of dehydroepiandrosterone (DHEA) has a mild virilizing effect. Patients with congenital adrenal hyperplasia due to *17α-hydroxylase (CYP17) deficiency* have variable undervirilization and develop hypertension due to the potent salt-retaining effects of corticosterone and 11-deoxycorticosterone. Some mutations in *CYP17* selectively impair 17,20 lyase activity, without altering 17α-hydroxylase activity, leading to undervirilization without mineralocorticoid excess and hypertension.

SEX-STEROID PATHWAY ENZYMES Defects in *17β-hydroxysteroid dehydrogenase type 3 (HSD17B3)* and *5α-reductase type 2 (SRD5A2)* interfere with the synthesis of testosterone and DHT, respectively (Fig. 328-4). These conditions are characterized by minimal masculinization in childhood, but some phallic development can occur during adolescence due to the action of other enzyme isoforms. Individuals with *5α-reductase type 2* deficiency have normal wolffian structures and do not develop breast tissue. In some cultures, these individuals change gender role behavior from female to male at puberty, because the increase in testosterone induces muscle mass and other virilizing features. DHT cream can improve prepubertal phallic growth in patients raised as male. Individuals raised as female require gonadectomy, cosmetic surgery, and estrogen replacement.

Disorders of Androgen Action ■ *ANDROGEN INSENSITIVITY SYNDROME* Mutations in the androgen receptor (AR) cause resistance to androgen (testosterone, DHT) action or the *androgen insensitivity syndrome (AIS)*. AIS is a spectrum of disorders that affects at least 1 in 100,000 chromosomal males. Because the androgen receptor is X-linked, only males are affected and maternal carriers are phenotypically normal. XY individuals with *complete AIS (testicular feminization syndrome)* have a female phenotype, normal breast development, a short vagina but no uterus (because MIS production is normal), scanty pubic and axillary hair, and female psychosexual orientation. Gonadotropins and testosterone levels can be low, normal, or elevated, depending on the degree of androgen resistance and the contribution of estradiol to feedback inhibition of the hypothalamic-pituitary gonadal axis. Most patients present with inguinal herniae (containing testes) in childhood or with primary amenorrhea in adulthood. Gonadectomy is usually performed, as there is a low risk of malignancy, and estrogen replacement is prescribed. Surgical reconstruction or mechanical dilatation of the vagina permits sexual intercourse. *Partial AIS (Reifenstein syndrome)* results from less severe AR mutations. Patients often present in infancy with perineoscrotal hypospadias, small cryptorchid testes, and with gynecomastia at the time of puberty. Those individuals raised as males require hypospadias repair in childhood and breast reduction in adolescence. Supplemental androgens rarely improve virilization significantly, as endogenous androgens are already increased. More severely undervirilized patients present with clitoral enlargement and labial fusion, and may be raised as females. The surgical and psychosexual management of both these groups of patients is complex and requires

TABLE 328-4 Disorders Causing Virilization in Karyotypic Females (46,XX)

Ovarian transdifferentiation
    True hermaphroditism (46,XX)
    XX male
Increased androgen synthesis
    3β-Hydroxysteroid dehydrogenase 2 (HSD3B2) deficiency
    21-Hydroxylase (CYP21A2) deficiency
    11β-Hydroxylase (CYP11B1) deficiency
    Aromatase (CYP19) deficiency
    Glucocorticoid receptor mutations
Increased androgen exposure
    Maternal virilizing tumors (e.g., luteomas of pregnancy)
Androgenic drugs
Nonvirilizing disorders of the female reproductive tract
    Ovarian dysgenesis
    Müllerian agenesis
    Vaginal agenesis

active involvement of the parents and the patient during the appropriate stages of development. *Azoospermia* and male-factor infertility has also been described in association with mild loss of function mutations in the androgen receptor. Trinucleotide (CAG) repeat expansion, from a mean of 22 repeats to greater than 40 repeats, within a highly polymorphic region of the androgen receptor is associated with spinal and bulbar muscular atrophy (also known as Kennedy disease). These patients may show evidence of partial androgen insensitivity in adolescence or adulthood (e.g., gynecomastia).

OTHER DISORDERS AFFECTING MALES (46,XY) *Persistent Müllerian Duct syndrome* is the presence of a uterus in an otherwise normal male. This condition can result from mutations in AMH or its receptor (AMHR2). The uterus may be removed, but damage to vasa deferentia must be avoided. *Isolated hypospadias* occurs in approximately 1 in 200 males and is treated by surgical repair. Most cases are idiopathic, although evidence of penoscrotal hypospadias and bilateral cryptorchidism require investigation for an underlying genetic disorder (e.g., defect in testosterone action). *Cryptorchidism* (unilateral) affects up to 3% of boys at birth. Orchidopexy should be considered if the testis has not descended by early childhood. Bilateral cryptorchidism occurs less frequently, and should raise suspicion of gonadotropin deficiency or disorders of sexual development. A subset of patients with cryptorchidism have mutations in the insulin-like 3 (*INSL3*) gene or its receptor LGR8 (also known as *GREAT*), which mediates normal testicular descent.

VIRILIZED FEMALES (46,XX) (FEMALE PSEUDOHERMAPHRODITISM) Inappropriate virilization of females can occur when the gonad (ovary) con-

tains androgen-secreting testicular material, or after increased androgen exposure (Table 328-4).

Gonadal Transdifferentiation Testicular tissue can develop in 46,XX true hermaphrodites, and in 46,XX males with a translocation of *SRY* or duplication of *SOX9* (Table 328-5).

Increased Androgen Exposure ■ *21-HYDROXYLASE DEFICIENCY* The *classic form* of 21-hydroxylase deficiency has an incidence of between 1 in 5000 and 15,000 and is the most frequent cause of virilization in chromosomal 46,XX females (Table 328-5; Chap. 321). Affected individuals are homozygous or compound heterozygous for severe mutations in the enzyme 21-hydroxylase (*CYP21A2*). This mutation causes a block in adrenal glucocorticoid and mineralocorticoid synthesis, increasing 17-hydroxyprogesterone, and shunting steroid precursors into the androgen synthesis pathway (Fig. 328-4). Glucocorticoid insufficiency causes a compensatory elevation of adrenocorticotropin (ACTH), resulting in adrenal hyperplasia and additional synthesis of steroid precursors proximal to the enzymatic block. Increased androgen synthesis *in utero* causes virilization of the female fetus. Ambiguous genitalia are seen at birth, with varying degrees of clitoral enlargement and labial fusion. Infants with the *salt-wasting* form of 21-hydroxylase deficiency develop primary adrenal failure in the first few weeks of life. Thus, a diagnosis of 21-hydroxylase deficiency should be considered in any baby with ambiguous genitalia; a salt-wasting crisis is a potentially life-threatening event. Males with this syndrome have no genital abnormalities at birth but are equally susceptible to adrenal insufficiency and salt-losing crises. If untreated, males undergo premature virilization (pseudopuberty) because of increased androgen levels during childhood. Females with the *classic simple virilizing* form of this disorder also present with genital ambiguity, but do not develop salt loss.

The diagnosis of classic 21-hydroxylase deficiency is made by neonatal screening tests for increased 17-hydroxyprogesterone in some centers. In most cases, 17-hydroxyprogesterone is markedly increased. In adults, ACTH stimulation (0.25 mg cosyntropin IV) with assays for 17-hydroxyprogesterone at 0 and 30 min can be useful for detecting nonclassic 21-hydroxylase deficiency and heterozygotes (Chap. 321).

℞ **TREATMENT**

Glucocorticoids must be given to correct the cortisol insufficiency and to suppress ACTH stimulation, thereby preventing further virilization, rapid skeletal maturation, and the development of polycystic ovaries. Typically, hydrocortisone (10 to 20 mg/m² per d in divided doses) is used with a goal of suppressing 17-hydroxyprogesterone to <1000 ng/

TABLE 328-5 Genetic Causes of Virilization of Karyotypic Females (46,XX)

Gene	Inheritance	Gonad	Uterus	External Genitalia	Associated Features
OVARIAN TRANSDIFFERENTIATION					
SRY	translocation	Testis or ovotestis	−	Male or ambiguous	
SOX9	dup17q24	Unknown	−	Male or ambiguous	
INCREASED ANDROGEN SYNTHESIS					
HSD3B2	AR	Ovary	+	Ambiguous	CAH, primary adrenal failure, partial virilization due to ↑ DHEA
CYP21A2	AR	Ovary	+	Ambiguous	CAH, phenotypic spectrum from severe salt-losing forms associated with adrenal failure to simple virilizing forms with compensated adrenal function, ↑ 17-hydroxyprogesterone
CYP11B1	AR	Ovary	+	Ambiguous	CAH, hypertension due to ↑ 11-deoxycortisol & 11-deoxycorticosterone
CYP19	AR	Ovary	+	Ambiguous	Maternal virilization during pregnancy, absent breast development at puberty
Glucocorticoid receptor	AR	Ovary	+	Ambiguous	↑ ACTH, 17-hydroxyprogesterone and cortisol; failure of dexamethasone suppression

Note: AR, autosomal recessive; *SRY*, sex-related gene on the Y chromosome; *SOX9*, SRY-related HMG-box gene 9; CAH, congenital adrenal hyperplasia; *HSD3B2*, 3β-hydroxy-steroid dehydrogenase type 2; *CYP21A2*, 21-hydroxylase; *CYP11B1*, 11β-hydroxylase; *CYP19*, aromatase; ACTH, adrenocorticotropin.

dL. It is difficult, however, to fully suppress androgen production without using excessive glucocorticoid treatment, which can impair growth and predispose to obesity. Older adolescents and adults are often treated with dexamethasone at night to provide more complete ACTH suppression. In very severe cases, adrenalectomy has been advocated but incurs the risks of major surgery and total adrenal insufficiency. Salt-wasting conditions are treated with mineralocorticoid replacement. Infants usually need salt supplements up to the first year of life. Plasma renin activity and electrolytes are used to monitor mineralocorticoid replacement. Newer therapeutic approaches, such as antiandrogens and aromatase inhibitors (to block premature epiphyseal closure) are under evaluation. Parents and patients should be aware of the need for increased doses of steroids during sickness and patients should carry medic alert systems.

Girls with significant virilization usually undergo clitoral reduction (maintaining the glans and nerve supply) and vaginal reconstruction, but the optimal timing of these procedures is the subject of debate. Surgical revision or regular vaginal dilatation may be needed in adolescence or adulthood, and long-term psychological support and psychosexual counseling may be appropriate.

Prenatal treatment of 21-hydroxylase deficiency by the administration of dexamethasone to mothers has been shown to reduce the degree of virilization in affected female fetuses. However, treatment on the mother and child must be started before 9 weeks gestation and ideally before 6–7 weeks; long-term effects are still under evaluation.

OTHER CAUSES Increased androgen synthesis can also occur in CAH due to defects in *11β-hydroxylase (CYP11B1)* and *3β-hydroxysteroid dehydrogenase type 2 (HSD3B2)*, and with mutations in the genes encoding *aromatase (CYP19)* and the glucocorticoid receptor. Increased androgen exposure *in utero* can occur with maternal virilizing tumors and with ingestion of androgenic compounds.

OTHER DISORDERS AFFECTING FEMALES (46,XX) *Congenital absence of the vagina* occurs in association with *müllerian agenesis* or *hypoplasia* as part of the Mayer-Rokitansky-Kuster-Hauser syndrome. This diagnosis should be considered in otherwise phenotypically normal females with primary amenorrhea. Rarer associated features include renal (agenesis) and cervical spinal abnormalities.

ACKNOWLEDGMENT

We are grateful to JD Wilson and JE Griffin, the authors of Disorders of Sexual Differentiation *in the 15th edition of* Harrison's, *for contributions to this chapter.*

FURTHER READING

ACHERMANN JC et al: Genetic causes of human reproductive disease. J Clin Endocrinol Metab 87:2447, 2002

AHMED SF, HUGHES IA: The genetics of male undermasculinization. Clin Endocrinol 56:1, 2002

ELSHEIKH M et al: Turner's syndrome in adulthood. Endocr Rev 23:120, 2002

KOOPMAN P: The genetics and biology of vertebrate sex determination. Cell 105:843, 2001

TILMANN C, CAPEL B: Cellular and molecular pathways regulating mammalian sex determination. Recent Prog Horm Res 57:1, 2002

---

329 ENDOCRINE TUMORS OF THE GASTROINTESTINAL TRACT AND PANCREAS
Robert T. Jensen

Gastrointestinal neuroendocrine tumors (NETs) are tumors derived from the diffuse neuroendocrine system of the gastrointestinal (GI) tract, which is composed of amine- and acid-producing cells with different hormonal profiles, depending on the site of origin. The tumors they produce can be generally divided into carcinoid tumors and pancreatic endocrine tumors (PETs). These tumors were originally classified as APUDomas (for *amine precursor uptake and decarboxylation*), as were pheochromocytomas, melanomas, and medullary thyroid carcinomas because they share certain cytochemical features as well as various pathologic, biologic, and molecular features (Table 329-1). APUDomas were thought to have a similar embryonic origin from neural crest cells, but the peptide-secreting cells are not of neuroectodermal origin.

CLASSIFICATION/PATHOLOGY/TUMOR BIOLOGY OF NETS

NETs are composed of monotonous sheets of small round cells with uniform nuclei; mitoses are uncommon. They can be tentatively identified on routine histology; however, these tumors are principally recognized by their histologic staining patterns due to shared cellular proteins. Historically, silver staining was used and tumors were classified as showing an argentaffin reaction if they took up and reduced silver or as being argyrophilic if they did not reduce it. Immunocytochemical localization of chromogranins (A, B, C), neuron-specific enolase, or synaptophysin, which are all neuroendocrine cell markers, are now used (Table 329-1). Chromogranin A is the most widely used.

Ultrastructurally, these tumors possess electron-dense neurosecretory granules and frequently contain small clear vesicles that correspond to synaptic vesicles of neurons. NETs synthesize numerous peptides, growth factors, and bioactive amines that may be ectopically secreted, giving rise to a specific clinical syndrome (Table 329-2). The diagnosis of the specific syndrome requires the clinical features of the disease and cannot be made from the immunocytochemistry results only. The presence or absence of a specific clinical syndrome cannot be predicted from the immunocytochemistry (Table 329-1). Further-

more, pathologists cannot distinguish between benign and malignant NETs unless metastases or invasion are present.

Carcinoid tumors are frequently classified according to their anatomic area of origin (i.e., foregut, midgut, hindgut), because tumors with similar areas of origin share functional manifestations, histochemistry, and secretory products (Table 329-3). Foregut tumors generally have a low serotonin (5HT) content, are argentaffin-negative but argyrophilic, occasionally secrete adrenocorticotropic hormone (ACTH) or 5-hydroxytryptophan (5HTP) causing an atypical carcinoid syndrome (Fig. 329-1), are often multihormonal, and may metastasize to bone. They uncommonly produce a clinical syndrome due to secreted products. Midgut carcinoids are argentaffin-positive, have a high serotonin content, most frequently cause the typical carcinoid syndrome when they metastasize (Table 329-3, Fig. 329-1), release serotonin and tachykinins (substance P, neuropeptide K, substance K), rarely secrete 5HTP or ACTH, and uncommonly metastasize to bone. Hindgut carcinoids (rectum, transverse and descending colon) are argentaffin-negative, often argyrophilic, rarely contain serotonin or cause the carcinoid syndrome (Fig. 329-1, Table 329-3), rarely secrete 5HTP or ACTH, contain numerous peptides, and may metastasize to bone.

PETs can be classified into nine well-established specific functional syndromes, two possible specific functional syndromes (PETs secreting calcitonin or renin), and nonfunctional PETs [pancreatic polypeptide (PP)-secreting tumors; PPomas] (Table 329-2). Each of the functional syndromes is associated with symptoms due to the specific hormone released. In contrast, nonfunctional PETs release no products that cause a specific clinical syndrome. "Nonfunctional" is a misnomer in the strict sense because they frequently secrete a number of peptides (PP, chromogranin A, ghrelin, neurotensin); however, they cause no specific clinical syndrome. The symptoms caused by nonfunctional PETs are entirely due to the tumor per se.

Carcinoid tumors can occur in almost any GI tissue; however, at present most (70%) originate from one of three sites: bronchus, jejuno-

TABLE 329-1 *General Characteristics of GI Neuroendocrine Tumors [Carcinoids, Pancreatic Endocrine Tumors (PETs)]*

I. Share general neuroendocrine cell markers
  A. Chromogranins (A, B, C) are acidic monomeric soluble proteins found in the large secretory granules; chromogranin A is most widely used
  B. Neuron-specific enolase (NSE) is the γ-γ dimer of the enzyme enolase and is a cytosolic marker of neuroendocrine differentiation
  C. Synaptophysin is an integral membrane glycoprotein of 38,000 molecular weight found in small vesicles of neurons and neuroendocrine tumors

II. Pathologic similarities
  A. All are APUDomas showing *a*mine *p*recursor *u*ptake and *d*ecarboxylation
  B. Ultrastructurally they have dense-core secretory granules (>80 nm)
  C. Histologically appear similar with few mitoses and uniform nuclei
  D. Frequently synthesize multiple peptides/amines, which can be detected immunocytochemically but may not be secreted
  E. Presence or absence of clinical syndrome or type cannot be predicted by immunocytochemical studies
  F. Histologic classifications do not predict biologic behavior; only invasion or metastases establishes malignancy

III. Similarities of biologic behavior
  A. Generally slow growing, but a proportion are aggressive
  B. Secrete biologically active peptides/amines, which can cause clinical symptoms
  C. Generally have high densities of somatostatin receptors, which are used for both localization and treatment

IV. Similarities/differences in molecular abnormalities
  A. Similarities
    1. Uncommon—alterations in common oncogenes (*ras, jun, fos*, etc)
    2. Uncommon—alterations in common tumor-suppressor genes (p53, retinoblastoma).
    3. Alterations at MEN-1 gene locus (11q13) and p16^{INK4a} (9p21) occur in a proportion (10–30%).
  B. Differences
    1. PETs—loss of 3p (8–47%), 3q (8–41%), 11q (21–62%), 6q (18–68%); gains at 17q (10–55%), 7q (16–68%).
    2. Carcinoids—loss of 18q (38–67%) >18p (33–43%) >9p (21%); gains at 17q, 19p (57%).

Note: MEN, multiple endocrine neoplasia; PETs, pancreatic endocrine tumors.

ileum, or colon/rectum (Table 329-3). In the past, carcinoid tumors most frequently occurred in the appendix (i.e., 40%); however, the bronchus/lung and small intestine are now the most common sites. Overall, GI carcinoids are the most common site for these tumors, comprising 64%, with the respiratory tract a distant second at 28%.

The term *pancreatic endocrine tumor*, although widely used and therefore retained here, is also a misnomer because these tumors can occur either almost entirely in the pancreas (insulinomas, glucagonomas, nonfunctional PETs, PETs causing hypercalcemia) or at both pancreatic and extrapancreatic sites [gastrinomas, VIPomas (VIP, vasoactive intestinal peptide), somatostatinomas, GRFomas (GRF, growth hormone–releasing factor)]. PETs are also called *islet cell tumors*; however, this term is discouraged because many do not originate from the islets and they can occur at extrapancreatic sites.

The exact incidence of carcinoid tumors or PETs varies according to whether only symptomatic or all tumors are considered. The incidence of clinically significant carcinoids is 7 to 13 cases per million population per year, whereas any malignant carcinoids at autopsy are reported in 21 to 84 cases per million population per year. Clinically significant PETs have a prevalence of 10 cases per million population, with insulinomas, gastrinomas, and nonfunctional PETs having an incidence of 0.5 to 2 cases per million population per year (Table 329-2). VIPomas are 2- to 8-fold less common, glucagonomas are 17- to 30-fold less common, and somatostatinomas the least common. In autopsy studies 0.5 to 1.5% of all cases have a PET; however, in <1 in 1000 cases was a functional tumor present.

Both carcinoid tumors and PETs commonly show malignant behavior (Tables 329-2, 329-3). Except for insulinomas, in which <10% are malignant, 50 to 100% of PETs are malignant. The fraction of

carcinoid tumors showing malignant behavior varies in different locations. For the three most common sites of occurrence the incidence of metastases varies greatly: jejuno-ileum (58%) > lung/bronchus (6%) > rectum (4%). A number of factors influence survival and the aggressiveness of the tumor (Table 329-4). The presence of liver metastases is the single most important prognostic factor for both carcinoid tumors and PETs. Particularly important in the development of liver metastases is the size of the primary tumor. For small-intestinal carcinoids, the most frequent cause of the carcinoid syndrome due to metastatic disease in the liver, metastases occur in 15 to 25% if the tumor diameter is <1 cm, 58 to 80% if it is 1 to 2 cm, and >75% if >2 cm. Similar data exist for gastrinomas and other PETs. The presence of lymph node metastases, the depth of invasion, various histologic features (differentiation, mitotic rates, growth indices), and the presence of aneuploidy are all important prognostic factors for the development of metastatic disease (Table 329-4). For patients with carcinoid tumors, additional poor prognosis factors include the development of the carcinoid syndrome, older age, male gender, the presence of a symptomatic tumor, or increases in a number of tumor markers [5-hydroxyindolactic acid (5-HIAA), neuropeptide K, chromogranin A]. With PETs or gastrinomas, the best studied PET, a worse prognosis is associated with female gender, overexpression of the *Ha-Ras* oncogene or p53, the absence of multiple endocrine neoplasia (MEN) type 1, and higher levels of various tumor markers (i.e., chromogranin A, gastrin).

A number of genetic disorders are associated with an increased incidence of NETs (Table 329-5). Each is caused by a loss of a putative tumor-suppressor gene. The most important is MEN-1, which is an autosomal dominant disorder due to a defect in a 10-exon gene on 11q13 that encodes for a 610-amino-acid nuclear protein, menin (Chap. 330). In patients with MEN-1, 95 to 100% develop hyperparathyroidism due to parathyroid hyperplasia, 80 to 100% develop PETs, 54 to 80% develop pituitary adenomas, and bronchial carcinoids develop in 8%, thymic carcinoids in 8%, and gastric carcinoids in 13 to 30% of the patients with Zollinger-Ellison syndrome (ZES). In patients with MEN-1, 80 to 100% develop nonfunctional PETs; functional PETs occur in 80%, with 54% developing ZES, 21% insulinomas, 3% glucagonomas, and 1% VIPomas. MEN-1 is present in 20 to 25% of all patients with ZES, in 4% with insulinomas, and in a low percentage (<5%) of the other PETs.

Three phacomatoses associated with NETs are von Hippel–Lindau disease, von Recklinghausen's disease [neurofibromatosis (NF) type 1], and tuberous sclerosis (Bourneville's disease). Von Hippel–Lindau disease is an autosomal dominant disorder due to defects on chromosome 3p25, which encodes for a 213-amino-acid protein that interacts with the elongin family of proteins as a transcriptional regulator (Chap. 358). In addition to cerebellar hemangioblastomas, renal cancer, and pheochromocytomas, 10 to 17% of these patients develop a PET. Most are nonfunctional, although insulinomas and VIPomas are reported. Patients with NF-1 have defects in a gene on chromosome 17q11.2 encoding for a 2845-amino-acid protein, neurofibromin, which functions in normal cells as a suppressor of the ras signaling cascade (Chap. 358). Up to 12% of these patients develop an upper GI carcinoid tumor, characteristically in the periampullary region (54%). Many are classified as somatostatinomas because they contain somatostatin immunocytochemically; however, they uncommonly secrete somatostatin or produce a clinical somatostatinoma syndrome. NF-1 has rarely been associated with insulinomas and ZES. Tuberous sclerosis is caused by mutations that alter either the 1164-amino-acid protein, hamartin (TSC1), or the 1807-amino-acid protein, tuberin (TSC2) (Chap. 358). Both hamartin and tuberin interact in a pathway related to cytosolic G protein regulation. A few cases including nonfunctional and functional PETs (insulinomas and gastrinomas) have been reported in these patients.

In contrast to most common nonendocrine tumors such as carcinoma of the breast, colon, lung or stomach, PETs and carcinoid tumors

TABLE 329-2 GI Neuroendocrine Tumor Syndromes

Name	Biologically Active Peptide(s) Secreted	Incidence New Cases/10⁶ Population/Year	Tumor Location	Malignant, %	Associated with MEN-1, %	Main Symptoms/Signs
I. ESTABLISHED SPECIFIC FUNCTIONAL SYNDROME						
Carcinoid tumor						
Carcinoid syndrome	Serotonin, possibly tachykinins, motilin, prostaglandins	0.5–2	Midgut (75–87%) Foregut (2–33%) Hindgut (1–8%) Unknown (2–15%)	95–100	Rare	Diarrhea (32–84%) Flushing (63–75%) Pain (10–34%) Asthma (4–18%) Heart disease (11–41%)
Pancreatic endocrine tumor						
Zollinger-Ellison syndrome	Gastrin	0.5–1.5	Duodenum (70%) Pancreas (25%) Other sites (5%)	60–90	20–25	Pain (79–100%) Diarrhea (30–75%) Esophageal symptoms (31–56%)
Insulinoma	Insulin	1–2	Pancreas (>99%)	<10	4–5	Hypoglycemic symptoms (100%)
VIPoma (Verner-Morrison syndrome, pancreatic cholera, WDHA)	Vasoactive intestinal peptide	0.05–0.2	Pancreas (90%, adult) Other (10%, neural, adrenal, periganglionic)	40–70	6	Diarrhea (90–100%) Hypokalemia (80–100%) Dehydration (83%)
Glucagonoma	Glucagon	0.01–0.1	Pancreas (100%)	50–80	1–20	Rash (67–90%) Glucose intolerance (38–87%) Weight loss (66–96%)
Somatostatinoma	Somatostatin	Rare	Pancreas (55%) Duodenum-jejunum (44%)	>70	45	Diabetes mellitus (63–90%) Cholelithiasis (65–90%) Diarrhea (35–90%)
GRFoma	Growth hormone–releasing hormone	Unknown	Pancreas (30%) Lung (54%) Jejunum (7%) Other (13%)	>60	16	Acromegaly (100%)
ACTHoma	ACTH	Rare	Pancreas (4–16%, all ectopic Cushing's)	>95	Rare	Cushing's syndrome (100%)
PET causing carcinoid syndrome	Serotonin, ? tachykinins	Rare (43 cases)	Pancreas (<1% all carcinoids)	60–88	Rare	Same as carcinoid syndrome above
PET causing hypercalcemia	PTHrP, others unknown	Rare	Pancreas (rare cause of hypercalcemia)	84	Rare	Abdominal pain due to hepatic metastases
II. POSSIBLE SPECIFIC FUNCTIONAL SYNDROME						
PET secreting calcitonin	Calcitonin	Rare	Pancreas (rare cause of hypercalcitonemia)	>80	16	Diarrhea (50%)
PET secreting renin	Renin	Rare	Pancreas	Unknown	No	Hypertension
III. NO FUNCTIONAL SYNDROME						
PPoma/nonfunctional	None	1–2	Pancreas (100%)	>60	18–44	Weight loss (30–90%) Abdominal mass (10–30%) Pain (30–95%)

Note: MEN, multiple endocrine neoplasia; VIPoma, tumor-secreting vasoactive intestinal peptide; WDHA, watery diarrhea, hypokalemia, and achlorhydria syndrome; ACTH, adrenocorticotrophic hormone; PET, pancreatic endocrine tumor; PTHrP, parathyroid hormone–related peptide; PPoma, tumor secreting pancreatic polypeptide.

do not have alterations in common oncogenes (ras, myc, fos, src, jun) or common tumor-suppressor genes (p53, retinoblastoma susceptibility gene) (Table 329-1). Alterations that may be important in their pathogenesis including changes in the *MEN-1* gene, p16/MTS1 tumor-suppressor gene, and DPC 4/*Smad* 4 gene, amplification of the HER-2/*neu* protooncogene and growth factors and their receptors, and deletions of unknown tumor-suppressor genes as well as gains in other unknown genes. Comparative genomic hybridization and genome-wide allelotyping studies have shown genetic differences between PETs and carcinoids (Table 329-1), some of which have prognostic significance (Table 329-4). Mutations in the *MEN-1* gene are particularly important. Loss of heterozygosity at the MEN-1 locus on chromosome 11q13 occurs in 46% of sporadic PETs (those without MEN-1) and in 26 to 75% of sporadic carcinoid tumors. Mutations in the *MEN-1* gene are reported in 31 to 34% of sporadic gastrinomas. The presence of a number of these molecular alterations correlates with tumor growth, tumor size, and disease extent or invasiveness and may have prognostic significance.

CARCINOID TUMORS AND CARCINOID SYNDROME

GENERAL TUMOR CHARACTERISTICS OF THE MOST COMMON GI CARCINOID TUMORS ■ Appendiceal Carcinoids   These occur in 1 in every 200 to 300

appendectomies, usually in the appendiceal tip. Most are <1 cm in diameter without metastases; however, up to 35% have metastases (Table 329-3). Among 1570 appendiceal carcinoids, 62% were localized and 27% had regional and 8% had distant metastases. Of tumors 1 to 2 cm in diameter, half metastasized to lymph nodes. The percentage of larger carcinoids has decreased from 43.9% (1950 to 1969) to 2.4% (1992 to 1999).

Small Intestinal Carcinoids   These are frequently multiple; 70 to 80% are present in the ileum and 70% are within 60 cm (24 in.) of the ileocecal valve. Some 40% are <1 cm in diameter, 32% are 1 to 2 cm, and 29% are >2 cm. Between 35 and 70% are associated with metastases (Table 329-3). They characteristically cause a marked fibrotic reaction that can lead to intestinal obstruction. Distant metastases occur to liver in 36 to 60% of patients, to bone in 3%, and to lung in 4%. Even small carcinoid tumors of the small intestine (<1 cm) have metastases in 15 to 25%; the incidence increases to 58 to 100% for tumors 1 to 2 cm in diameter. Carcinoids also occur in the duodenum, with 31% having metastases. No duodenal tumor <1 cm metastasized, whereas 33% of those >2 cm had metastases. Small-intestinal carcinoids are the most common cause (60 to 87%) of the carcinoid syndrome (Table 329-6).

TABLE 329-3 *Carcinoid Tumor Location, Frequency of Metastases, and Association with the Carcinoid Syndrome*

	Location (% of Total)	Incidence of Metastases	Incidence of Carcinoid Syndrome
Foregut			
Esophagus	<0.1	—	—
Stomach	4.6	10	9.5
Duodenum	2.0	—	3.4
Pancreas	0.7	71.9	20
Gallbladder	0.3	17.8	5
Bronchus, lung, trachea	27.9	5.7	13
Midgut			
Jejunum	1.8	} 58.4	9
Ileum	14.9		9
Meckel's diverticulum	0.5		13
Appendix	4.8	38.8	<1
Colon	8.6	51	5
Liver	0.4	32.2	—
Ovary	1.0	32	50
Testis	<0.1	—	50
Hindgut			
Rectum	13.6	3.9	—

Source: Location is from the PAN-SEER data (1973–1999), and incidence of metastases from the SEER data (1992–1999), reported by IM Modlin et al: Cancer 97:934, 2003. Incidence of carcinoid syndrome is from 4349 cases studied from 1950–1971, reported by JD Godwin: Cancer 36:560, 1975.

Rectal Carcinoids Rectal carcinoids are found in 1 of every 2500 proctoscopies. Nearly all occur 4 to 13 cm above the dentate line. Most are small, with 66 to 80% being <1 cm in diameter; 5% metastasize. Tumors between 1 and 2 cm can metastasize in 5 to 30% of patients, and tumors >2 cm, which are uncommon, in >70%.

Bronchial Carcinoids Bronchial carcinoids are not related to smoking. A number of different classifications have been proposed. In some

TABLE 329-4 *Prognostic Factors in Neuroendocrine Tumors*

Both carcinoid tumors and PETs
  Presence of liver metastases ($p < .001$)
  Extent of liver metastases ($p < .001$)
  Presence of lymph node metastases ($p < .001$)
  Depth of invasion ($p < .001$)
  Primary tumor site ($p < .001$)
  Primary tumor size ($p < .005$)
  Various histologic features
    Tumor differentiation ($p < .001$)
    High growth indices (high Ki-67 index, PCNA expression)
    High mitotic counts ($p < .001$)
    Vascular or perineural invasion
    Flow cytometric features (i.e., aneuploidy)
Carcinoid tumors
  Presence of carcinoid syndrome
  Laboratory results [urinary 5-HIAA level ($p < .01$), plasma neuropeptide K ($p < .05$), serum chromogranin A ($p < .01$)]
  Presence of a secondary malignancy
  Male gender ($p < .001$)
  Older age ($p < .01$)
  Mode of discovery (incidental > symptomatic)
  Molecular findings [TGF-α expression ($p < .05$), chr 16q LOH or gain chr 4p ($p < .05$)]
PETs
  Ha-Ras oncogene or p53 overexpression
  Female gender
  MEN-1 syndrome absent
  Laboratory findings (increased chromogranin A in some studies; gastrinomas—increased gastrin level)
  Molecular findings [increased HER2/*neu* expression ($p = .032$), chr 1q, 3p,3q, or 6q LOH ($p = .0004$), EGF receptor overexpression ($p = .034$), gains in chr 7q, 17q, 17p, 20q]

Note: PET, pancreatic endocrine tumor; Ki-67, proliferation-associated nuclear antigen recognized by Ki-67 monoclonal antibody; PCNA, proliferating cell nuclear antigen; 5-HIAA, 5-hydroxy indolacetic acid; TGF-α, transforming growth factor α; chr, chromosome; LOH, loss of heterozygosity; MEN, multiple endocrine neoplasia; EGF, epidermal growth factor.

studies lung NETs are classified into four categories: typical carcinoid [also called bronchial carcinoid tumor, Kulchitsky cell carcinoma (KCC)-I]; atypical carcinoid (also called well-differentiated neuroendocrine carcinoma, KCC-II); intermediate small cell neuroendocrine carcinoma; and small cell neuroendocarcinoma (KCC-III). Another proposed classification includes three categories: benign or low-grade malignant (typical carcinoid); low-grade malignant (atypical carcinoid), and high-grade malignant (poorly differentiated carcinoma of the large cell or small cell type). These different categories of lung NETs have different prognoses varying from excellent for typical carcinoid to poor for small cell neuroendocrine carcinomas.

Gastric Carcinoids These account for 3 of every 1000 gastric neoplasms. Three different subtypes of gastric carcinoids are observed. Each originates from gastric enterochromaffin-like (ECL) cells in the gastric mucosa. Two subtypes are associated with hypergastrinemic states: (1) chronic atrophic gastritis (type I) (80% of all gastric carcinoids), or (2) ZES, almost always as part of the MEN-1 syndrome (type II) (6% of all cases). These tumors generally pursue a benign course, with 9 to 30% associated with metastases. They are usually multiple and small and infiltrate only to the submucosa. The third subtype of gastric carcinoid (type III) (sporadic) occurs without hypergastrinemia (14% of all carcinoids) and pursues an aggressive course, with 54 to 66% developing metastases. Sporadic carcinoids are usually single, large tumors, 50% have atypical histology, and they can be a cause of the carcinoid syndrome. Gastric carcinoids as a percentage of all carcinoids are increasing in frequency [1.96% (1969 to 1971), 3.6% (1973 to 1991), 5.8% (1991 to 1999)].

CARCINOID TUMORS WITHOUT THE CARCINOID SYNDROME The age of patients at diagnosis ranges from 10 to 93 years, with a mean age of 63 years for small intestine and 66 years for the rectum. The presentation

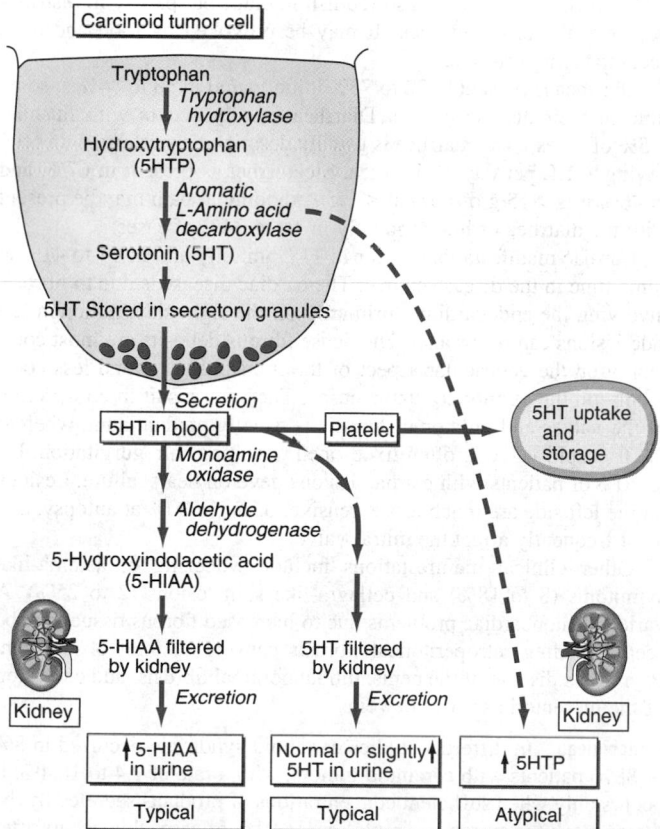

FIGURE 329-1 Synthesis, secretion, and metabolism of serotonin (5HT) in patients with typical and atypical carcinoid syndromes. Abbreviations: 5-HIAA, 5-hydroxyindolacetic acid.

TABLE 329-5 *Genetic Syndromes Associated with an Increased Incidence of Neuroendocrine Tumors [NETs: Carcinoids or Pancreatic Endocrine Tumors (PETs)]*

Syndrome	Location of Gene Mutation and Gene Product	NETs Seen/Frequency
Multiple endocrine neoplasia type 1 (MEN-1)	11q13 (encodes 610-amino-acid protein, menin)	80–100% develop PETs: (nonfunctional > gastrinoma > insulinoma) Carcinoids: gastric (13–30%), bronchial/thymic (8%)
von Hippel–Lindau disease	3q25 (encodes 213-amino-acid-protein)	12–17% develop PETs (almost always nonfunctional)
von Recklinghausen's disease [neurofibromatosis1 (NF-1)]	17q11.2 (encodes 2485-amino-acid protein, neurofibromin)	Duodenal somatostatinomas (usually nonfunctional) Rarely insulinoma, gastrinoma
Tuberous sclerosis	9q34 (TSCI) (encodes 1164-amino-acid protein, hamartin) 16p13 (TSC2) (encodes 1807-amino-acid protein, tuberin)	Uncommonly develop PETs [nonfunctional and functional (insulinoma, gastrinoma)]

is diverse and related to the site of origin and extent of malignant spread. In the appendix, carcinoid tumors are usually found incidentally during surgery for suspected appendicitis. Small-intestinal carcinoids in the jejunoileum present with periodic abdominal pain (51%), intestinal obstruction with ileus/invagination (31%), an abdominal tumor (17%), or GI bleeding (11%). Because of the vagueness of the symptoms the diagnosis is usually delayed about 2 years from onset of the symptoms, with a range up to 20 years. Duodenal, gastric, and rectal carcinoids are most frequently found by chance at endoscopy. The most common symptoms of rectal carcinoids are melena/bleeding (39%), constipation (17%), and diarrhea (12%). Bronchial carcinoids are frequently discovered as a lesion on a chest radiograph, and 31% of the patients are asymptomatic. Thymic carcinoids present as anterior mediastinal masses, usually on chest radiograph or computed tomography (CT) scan. Ovarian and testicular carcinoids usually present as masses discovered on physical examination or ultrasound. Metastatic carcinoid tumor in the liver frequently presents as hepatomegaly in a patient who may have minimal symptoms and near-normal liver function tests.

CARCINOID TUMORS WITH SYSTEMIC SYMPTOMS DUE TO SECRETED PRODUCTS
Carcinoid tumors immunocytochemically can contain numerous GI peptides: gastrin, insulin, somatostatin, motilin, neurotensin, tachykinins (substance K, substance P, neuropeptide K), glucagon, gastrin-releasing peptide, VIP, PP, other biologically active peptides (ACTH, calcitonin, growth hormone), prostaglandins, and bioactive amines (serotonin). These substances may or may not be released in sufficient

TABLE 329-6 *Clinical Characteristics in Patients with Carcinoid Syndrome*

	At Presentation	During Course of Disease
Symptoms/signs		
Diarrhea	32–73%	68–84%
Flushing	23–65%	63–74%
Pain	10%	34%
Asthma/wheezing	4–8%	3–18%
Pellagra	2%	5%
None	12%	22%
Carcinoid heart disease present	11%	14–41%
Demographics		
Male	46–59%	46–61%
Age		
Mean	57 yrs	52–54 yrs
Range	25–79 yrs	9–91 yrs
Tumor location		
Foregut	5–9%	2–33%
Midgut	78–87%	60–87%
Hindgut	1–5%	1–8%
Unknown	2–11%	2–15%

amounts to cause symptoms. In patients with carcinoid tumors, elevated serum levels of PP were found in 43%, motilin in 14%, gastrin in 15%, and VIP in 6%. Foregut carcinoids are more likely to produce various GI peptides than midgut carcinoids. Ectopic ACTH production causing Cushing's syndrome is increasingly seen with foregut carcinoids (respiratory tract primarily) and in some series was the most common cause of the ectopic ACTH syndrome, accounting for 64% of all cases. Acromegaly due to GRF release occurs with foregut carcinoids; the somatostatinoma syndrome with duodenal carcinoids. The most common systemic syndrome with carcinoid tumors is the carcinoid syndrome.

CARCINOID SYNDROME ■ Clinical Features The cardinal features at presentation and during the disease course are shown in Table 329-6. Flushing and diarrhea are the two most common symptoms, occurring in up to 73% initially and in up to 89% during the course of the disease. The characteristic flush is of sudden onset; it is a deep red or violaceous erythema of the upper body (especially the neck and face), often associated with a feeling of warmth, and occasionally associated with pruritus, lacrimation, diarrhea, or facial edema. Flushes may be precipitated by stress, alcohol, exercise, or certain foods such as cheese or by certain agents such as catecholamines, pentagastrin, and serotonin reuptake inhibitors. Flushing episodes may be brief, lasting 2 to 5 min, especially initially, or may last hours, especially later in the disease course. Flushing is usually seen with midgut carcinoids but can also occur with foregut carcinoids. With bronchial carcinoids the flushes are frequently prolonged for hours to days, reddish in color, and associated with salivation, lacrimation, diaphoresis, diarrhea, and hypotension. The flush associated with gastric carcinoids is also reddish in color but patchy in distribution over the face and neck. It may be provoked by food and have accompanying pruritus.

Diarrhea is present in 32 to 73% initially and in 68 to 84% at some time in their disease course. Diarrhea usually occurs with flushing (85% of cases). The diarrhea is usually described as watery, with 60% having <1 L per day of diarrhea. Steatorrhea is present in 67%, and in 46% it is >15 g/d (normal <7 g). Abdominal pain may be present with the diarrhea or independently in 10 to 34% of cases.

Cardiac manifestations occur in 11% initially and in 14 to 41% at some time in the disease course. The cardiac disease is due to fibrosis involving the endocardium, primarily on the right side, although left side lesions can occur also. The dense fibrous deposits are most commonly on the ventricular aspect of the tricuspid valve and less commonly on the pulmonary valve cusps. They can result in constriction of the valves and pulmonic stenosis is usually predominant, whereas the tricuspid valve is often fixed open, resulting in regurgitation. Up to 80% of patients with cardiac lesions develop heart failure. Lesions on the left side are much less extensive, occur in 30% at autopsy, and most frequently affect the mitral valve.

Other clinical manifestations include wheezing or asthma-like symptoms (8 to 18%) and pellagra-like skin lesions (2 to 25%). A variety of noncardiac problems due to increased fibrous tissue may be seen including retroperitoneal fibrosis causing urethral obstruction, Peyronie's disease of the penis, intraabdominal fibrosis, and occlusion of the mesenteric arteries or veins.

Pathobiology In different studies carcinoid syndrome occurred in 8% of 8876 patients with carcinoid tumors, with a rate of 1.4 to 18.4%. It occurs only when sufficient concentrations of products secreted by the tumor reach the systemic circulation. In 91% of cases this occurs after distant metastases to the liver. Rarely primary gut carcinoids with nodal metastases with extensive retroperitoneal invasion, pancreatic carcinoids with retroperitoneal lymph nodes, or carcinoids of the lung or ovary with direct access to the systemic circulation can cause the carcinoid syndrome without hepatic metastases. All carcinoid tumors do not have the same propensity to metastasize and cause the carcinoid syndrome (Table 329-3). Midgut carcinoids account for 60 to 67% of the cases of carcinoid syndrome, foregut tumors for 2 to 33%, hindgut for 1 to 8%, and an unknown primary location for 2 to 15% (Tables 329-2, 329-3).

One of the main secretory products of carcinoid tumors involved in the carcinoid syndrome is serotonin (Fig. 329-1), which is synthesized from tryptophan. Up to 50% of dietary tryptophan can be used in this synthetic pathway by tumor cells, which can result in inadequate supplies for conversion to niacin; thus, some patients (2.5%) develop pellagra-like lesions. Serotonin has numerous biologic effects including stimulating intestinal secretion, inhibition of absorption, increasing intestinal motility, and stimulating fibrogenesis. Serotonin overproduction is found in 56 to 88% of all carcinoid tumors; however, 12 to 26% of patients do not have the carcinoid syndrome. In 90 to 100% of patients with the carcinoid syndrome serotonin is overproduced. Through its effects on gut motility and intestinal secretion, serotonin is thought to be predominantly responsible for the diarrhea. Serotonin receptor antagonists (especially $5HT_3$ antagonists) relieve the diarrhea in most patients. However, prostaglandin E_2 and tachykinins may be important mediators of the diarrhea in some patients. Serotonin does not appear to be involved in the flushing, because flushing is not relieved by serotonin receptor antagonists. In patients with gastric carcinoids the red, patchy pruritic flush is likely due to histamine release, because it can be prevented by H_1 and H_2 receptor antagonists. Numerous studies show tachykinins are stored in carcinoid tumors and released during flushing. However, octreotide can relieve the flushing induced by pentagastrin in these patients without altering the stimulated increase in plasma substance P, suggesting other mediators must be involved in the flushing. Both histamine and serotonin may be responsible for the wheezing as well as the fibrotic reactions involving the heart, Peyronie's disease, and intraabdominal fibrosis. The exact mechanism of the heart disease is unclear. The valvular heart disease caused by the appetite-suppressant drug dexfenfluramine is histologically indistinguishable from that observed in carcinoid disease or after long exposure to $5HT_2$-preferring ergot drugs. Metabolites of fenfluramine have high affinity for $5HT_2$ receptors whose activation is known to cause fibroblast mitogenesis. High levels of $5HT_{2B}$ and $5HT_{2C}$ receptor transcripts are known to occur in heart valves. Studies on sheep aortic valve interstitial cells demonstrate serotonin interacts primarily with $5HT_{2A/2B}$ receptors and stimulates transforming growth factor-β and collagen biosynthesis. Thus, serotonin overproduction is important for the valvular changes, possibly by activating $5HT_2$ receptors in the endocardium. Both the magnitude of serotonin overproduction and prior chemotherapy are important predictors of progression of the heart disease. Atrial natriuretic peptide overproduction is also reported in patients with cardiac disease, but its role in the pathogenesis is unknown.

Patients may develop either a typical or atypical carcinoid syndrome (Fig. 329-1). In patients with the typical form, characteristically caused by a midgut carcinoid tumor, the conversion of tryptophan to 5HTP is the rate-limiting step. Once 5HTP is formed it is rapidly converted to 5HT and stored in secretory granules of the tumor or in platelets. A small amount remains in plasma and is converted to 5-HIAA, which appears in large amounts in the urine. These patients have an expanded serotonin pool size, increased blood and platelet serotonin, and increased urinary 5-HIAA. Some carcinoid tumors cause an atypical carcinoid syndrome thought due to a deficiency in the enzyme dopa decarboxylase in which 5HTP cannot be converted to 5HT (serotonin), and 5HTP is secreted into the bloodstream. In these patients plasma serotonin levels are normal but urinary levels may be increased because some 5HTP is converted to 5HT in the kidney. Characteristically, urinary 5HTP and 5HT are increased, but urinary 5-HIAA levels are only slightly elevated. Foregut carcinoids are the most likely to cause an atypical carcinoid syndrome.

One of the most life-threatening complications of the carcinoid syndrome is the development of a carcinoid crisis. This is more fre-

quent in patients who have intense symptoms from foregut tumors or have greatly increased urinary 5-HIAA levels (i.e., >200 mg/d). The crises may occur spontaneously or be provoked by stress, anesthesia, chemotherapy, or a biopsy. Patients develop intense flushing, diarrhea, abdominal pain, and cardiac abnormalities including tachycardia, hypertension, or hypotension. If not adequately treated it can be fatal.

Diagnosis of the Carcinoid Syndrome and Carcinoid Tumors The diagnosis of carcinoid syndrome relies on measurement of urinary or plasma serotonin or its metabolites in the urine. The measurement of 5-HIAA is most frequently used. False-positive elevations may occur if the patient is eating serotonin-rich foods, such as bananas, pineapple, walnuts, pecans, avocados, or hickory nuts, or taking certain medications (cough syrup containing guaifenesin, acetaminophen, salicylates, or L-dopa). The normal range in daily urinary 5-HIAA excretion is between 2 and 8 mg/d. 5-HIAA has 73% sensitivity and 100% specificity for carcinoid syndrome.

Most physicians use only the urinary 5-HIAA excretion rate; however, plasma and platelet serotonin levels, if available, may give additional information. Platelet serotonin levels are more sensitive than urinary 5-HIAA but are not generally available. Patients with foregut carcinoids may produce an atypical carcinoid syndrome. If this syndrome is suspected and the urinary 5-HIAA is minimally elevated or normal, other urinary metabolites of tryptophan such as 5HTP or 5HT should be measured (Fig. 329-1).

Flushing occurs in a number of other diseases including systemic mastocytosis or chronic myeloid leukemia with increased histamine release; in menopause; as a reaction to alcohol or glutamate; or as side effects of chlorpropamide, calcium channel blockers, and nicotinic acid. None of these conditions cause an increase in urinary 5-HIAA.

The diagnosis of carcinoid tumor can be suggested by the carcinoid syndrome, by recurrent abdominal symptoms in a healthy-appearing individual, or by discovering hepatomegaly or hepatic metastases associated with minimal symptoms. Ileal carcinoids, which make up 25% of all clinically detected carcinoids, should be suspected in patients with bowel obstruction, abdominal pain, flushing, or diarrhea.

Serum chromogranin A levels are elevated in 56 to 100% of patients with carcinoid tumors, and the level correlates with tumor bulk. Serum chromogranin A levels are not specific for carcinoid tumors because they are also elevated in patients with PETs and other NETs. Plasma neuron-specific enolase levels are also used as a marker of carcinoid tumors but are less sensitive than chromogranin A, being increased in only 17 to 47% of patients.

℞ TREATMENT

Carcinoid Syndrome Treatment includes avoiding conditions that precipitate flushing, dietary supplementation with nicotinamide, treatment of heart failure with diuretics, treatment of wheezing with oral bronchodilators, and controlling the diarrhea with antidiarrheal agents such as loperamide or diphenoxylate. If patients still have symptoms, serotonin receptor antagonists or somatostatin analogues (Fig. 329-2) are the drugs of choice.

There are 14 subclasses of serotonin (5HT) receptors; antagonists for most are not available. The $5HT_1$ and $5HT_2$ receptor antagonists methysergide, cyproheptadine, and ketanserin have all been used to control diarrhea but usually do not decrease flushing. The use of methysergide is limited because it can cause or enhance retroperitoneal fibrosis. Ketanserin diminishes diarrhea in 30 to 100% of patients. $5HT_3$ receptor antagonists (ondansetron, tropisetron, alosetron) can control diarrhea and nausea in up to 100% of patients and occasionally ameliorate the flushing. A combination of histamine H_1 and H_2 receptor antagonists (i.e., diphenhydramine and cimetidine or ranitidine) may control flushing in patients with foregut carcinoids.

Synthetic analogues of somatostatin (octreotide, lanreotide) are now the most widely used agents to control the symptoms of patients with carcinoid syndrome (Fig. 329-2). These drugs are effective at

FIGURE 329-2 Structure of somatostatin and synthetic analogues used for diagnostic or therapeutic indications.

trolling the symptoms of the carcinoid syndrome (61 to 85% of patients).

Short-term side effects occur in 40 to 60% of patients receiving subcutaneous somatostatin analogues. Pain at the injection site and side effects related to the GI tract (59% discomfort, 15% nausea, diarrhea) are the most common. They are usually short-lived and do not interrupt treatment. Important long-term side effects include gallstone formation, steatorrhea, and deterioration in glucose tolerance. The overall incidence of gallstones/biliary sludge is 52%, with 7% having symptomatic disease requiring surgical treatment.

Interferon-α controls symptoms of the carcinoid syndrome either alone or combined with hepatic artery embolization. The response rate to interferon-α alone is 42%, and when combined with hepatic artery embolization, diarrhea was controlled for 1 year in 43% and flushing in 86%.

Hepatic artery embolization alone or with chemotherapy (chemoembolization) has been used to control the symptoms of carcinoid syndrome. Embolization alone is reported to control symptoms in up to 76% of patients, and chemoembolization (5-fluorouracil, adriamycin, cisplatin, mitomycin) in 60 to 75% of patients. Hepatic artery embolization can have major side effects including nausea, vomiting, pain, and fever. The mortality rate is 5 to 7%.

Other drugs have been used successfully in small numbers of patients to control the symptoms of carcinoid syndrome. Parachlorophenylanine can inhibit tryptophan hydroxylase and therefore the conversion of tryptophan to 5HTP (Fig. 329-1). However, its severe side effects, including psychiatric disturbances, make it intolerable for long-term use. α-Methyldopa inhibits the conversion of 5HTP to 5HT; however, its effects are only partial.

Carcinoid Tumors (Nonmetastatic) Surgery is the only potentially curative therapy. Because the probability of metastatic disease increases with increasing primary tumor size, the extent of surgical resection is determined accordingly. With appendiceal carcinoids, simple appendectomy was curative in 103 patients followed for up to 35 years. With rectal carcinoids <1 cm, local resection is curative. With small-intestinal carcinoids <1 cm, consensus has not been reached. Because 15 to 69% of small-intestinal carcinoids this size have metastases in different studies, some recommend a wide resection with en bloc resection of the adjacent lymph-bearing mesentery. If the carcinoid tumor is >2 cm in rectal, appendiceal, or small-intestinal sites, a full cancer operation should be done. This includes a right hemicolectomy for appendiceal carcinoid, an abdominoperineal resection or low anterior resection for rectal carcinoid, and an en bloc resection of adjacent lymph nodes for small-intestinal carcinoids. For carcinoids 1 to 2 cm in the appendix, a simple appendectomy is proposed by some, whereas others favor a formal right hemicolectomy. For rectal carcinoids of 1 to 2 cm, a wide local full-thickness excision is recommended.

With type I or II gastric carcinoids, which are usually <1 cm, endoscopic removal is recommended. For type I or II gastric carcinoids >2 cm or locally invasive, some recommend total gastrectomy; others recommend antrectomy in type 1. For types I and III gastric carcinoids of 1 to 2 cm, some recommend endoscopic treatment, others surgical treatment. With type III gastric carcinoids >2 cm, excision and regional lymph node clearance are recommended. Most tumors <1 cm are treated endoscopically.

Resection of isolated or limited hepatic metastases may be beneficial (see below).

PANCREATIC ENDOCRINE TUMORS

Functional PETs usually present with symptoms due to hormone excess. Only late in the course of the disease does the tumor per se cause prominent symptoms such as abdominal pain. In contrast, all of the symptoms due to nonfunctional PETs are due to the tumor per se. The overall result is that some functional PETs may present with severe symptoms with a small or undetectable primary tumor, whereas nonfunctional tumors almost always present late in their disease course with large tumors that are usually metastatic. The mean delay between

relieving symptoms and decreasing urinary 5-HIAA levels in patients with carcinoid syndrome. Octreotide controls symptoms in >80% of patients, including the diarrhea and flushing, and produces a >50% decrease in urinary 5-HIAA excretion in 70% of patients. Patients with mild to moderate symptoms should initially be treated with 100 μg subcutaneously every 8 h. Individual responses vary; doses as high as 3000 μg/d have been given. About 40% of patients escape control after a median 4 months, and the dose may need to be increased. Similar results are reported with lanreotide.

In patients with carcinoid crises, somatostatin analogues are effective at both treating the condition as well as preventing its development during known precipitating events such as surgery, anesthesia, chemotherapy, or stress. Octreotide, 150 to 250 μg subcutaneously every 6 to 8 h, should be used 24 to 48 h before anesthesia and then continued throughout the procedure.

Sustained-release preparations of both octreotide [octreotide-LAR, (long-acting release)] and lanreotide [lanreotide-PR (prolonged release)] have been developed. Octreotide-LAR (30 mg/month) gives a plasma level ≥ 1 ng/mL for 25 days, whereas the non-sustained-release form would need to be injected three to six times a day to achieve this level. Lanreotide-PR is given intramuscularly every 10 to 14 days. Both sustained-release forms are highly effective at con-onset of continuous symptoms and diagnosis of a functional PET syndrome is 4 to 7 years. Therefore, the diagnoses are frequently missed for extended periods of time.

Treatment of PETs requires two different strategies. Treatment must be directed at the hormone excess state such as the gastric acid hypersecretion in gastrinomas or hypoglycemia in insulinomas. Ectopic hormone secretion usually causes the presenting symptoms and can cause life-threatening complications. Second, with all of the tumors except insulinomas, >50% are malignant (Table 329-2); therefore, treatment must also be directed against the tumor per se. Because these tumors are not frequently surgically curable due to the extent of disease, in many cases surgical resection for cure, which addresses both treatment aspects, is not possible.

GASTRINOMA (ZOLLINGER-ELLISON SYNDROME) A gastrinoma is a NET that secretes gastrin. The chronic hypergastrinemia results in marked gastric acid hypersecretion (ZES) and growth of the gastric mucosa, with increased numbers of parietal cells and proliferation of gastric ECL cells. The gastric acid hypersecretion characteristically causes peptic ulcer disease (PUD), often refractory and severe, as well as diarrhea. The most common presenting symptoms are abdominal pain (70 to 100%), diarrhea (37 to 73%), and gastroesophageal reflux disease (GERD) (30 to 35%), though 10 to 20% have diarrhea only. Although peptic ulcers may occur in unusual locations, most patients have a typical duodenal ulcer. Important observations that should suggest this diagnosis include PUD with diarrhea; PUD in an unusual location or with multiple lesions; and PUD that is refractory to treatment or persistent, associated with prominent gastric folds, associated with findings suggestive of MEN-1 (endocrinopathy, family history of ulcer or endocrinopathy, nephrolithiasis), or without *Helicobacter pylori* present. *H. pylori* is present in >90% of idiopathic peptic ulcers but is present in <50% of patients with gastrinomas. Chronic unexplained diarrhea should also suggest gastrinoma.

About 20 to 25% of patients have MEN-1, and in most cases the hyperparathyroidism is present before the gastrinoma. These patients are treated differently from those without MEN-1; therefore, MEN-1 should be sought in all patients by family history, by measuring plasma ionized calcium and prolactin levels and plasma hormone levels (parathormone, growth hormone).

Most gastrinomas (50 to 70%) are present in the duodenum, followed by the pancreas (20 to 40%) and other intraabdominal sites (mesentery, lymph nodes, biliary tract, liver, stomach, ovary). Rare cases may originate outside the abdominal cavity. In MEN-1 the gastrinomas are also usually in the duodenum (70 to 90%) or the pancreas (10 to 30%), and they are almost always multiple. Between 60 and 90% of gastrinomas are malignant (Table 329-2), with metastatic spread to lymph nodes and liver. Distant metastases to bone occur in 12 to 30% of patients with liver metastases.

Diagnosis The diagnosis of gastrinoma requires the demonstration of fasting hypergastrinemia and an increased basal gastric acid output (BAO) (hyperchlorhydria). Nearly all patients with gastrinomas have fasting hypergastrinemia, although in 40 to 60% the level may be elevated by less than a factor of 10. Therefore, when the diagnosis is suspected a fasting gastrin level should be determined first. Potent gastric acid–suppressant drugs such as proton pump inhibitors (omeprazole, pantoprazole, lansoprazole, rabeprazole) can suppress acid secretion sufficiently to cause hypergastrinemia; because of their prolonged duration of action, these drugs need to be discontinued for a week before the gastrin determination. If the gastrin level is elevated, gastric pH should be measured. If gastric pH < 2.0, the hypergastrinemia is not a physiologic response to achlorhydria (atrophic gastritis, pernicious anemia), another common cause of hypergastrinemia. If the fasting gastrin > 1000 μg/L (10 times increased) and the pH < 2.0, which occurs in 40 to 60% of patients with gastrinoma, the diagnosis is established after ruling out the possibility of retained antrum syndrome by history. In patients with hypergastrinemia with fasting gastrin < 1000 μg/L and gastric pH < 2.0, other conditions such as *H. pylori* infections, antral G cell hyperplasia/hyperfunction, gastric outlet

obstruction, or, rarely, renal failure can masquerade as a gastrinoma. To establish the diagnosis in this group, a determination of BAO and a secretin provocative test should be done. In patients with gastrinomas, BAO is usually (>80%) elevated (i.e., >15 meq/h) and the secretin provocative test is positive (i.e., >200 μg/L increase in serum gastrin level) (Chap. 274).

℞ TREATMENT

The gastric acid hypersecretion in patients with gastrinomas can be controlled in almost every case by oral gastric antisecretory drugs. Because of their long duration of action and potency, allowing once or twice a day dosing, the proton pump inhibitors (H^+, K^+-ATPase inhibitors) are the drugs of choice. Histamine H_2-receptor antagonists are also effective, although more frequent (every 4 to 8 h) and high doses are usually required. In patients with MEN-1 with hyperparathyroidism, correction of the hyperparathyroidism increases the sensitivity to gastric antisecretory drugs and decreases the BAO.

Although gastric acid secretion can be controlled, more than half the patients who are not cured (>60%) will die from tumor-related causes. Careful imaging studies are essential to localize the extent of the tumor (see below). About one-third of patients present with hepatic metastases; in <15% of those with hepatic metastases, the disease is limited so that surgical resection may be possible. Surgical cure is possible in 30 to 60% of all patients without MEN-1 or liver metastases (40% of all patients). In patients with MEN-1, surgical cure is rare because the tumors are multiple, frequently with lymph node metastases.

INSULINOMAS An insulinoma is an endocrine tumor of the pancreas derived from β cells that ectopically secrete insulin, which results in hypoglycemia. The average age of occurrence is in persons 40 to 50 years old. The most common clinical symptoms are due to the effect of the hypoglycemia on the central nervous system (neuroglycemic symptoms) and include confusion, headache, disorientation, visual difficulties, irrational behavior, or even coma. Also, most patients have symptoms due to excess catecholamine release secondary to the hypoglycemia including sweating, tremor, and palpitations. Characteristically these attacks are associated with fasting.

Insulinomas are generally small (>90% are <2 cm), usually not multiple (90%), and only 5 to 15% are malignant. They almost invariably occur only in the pancreas, distributed equally in the pancreatic head, body, and tail. Insulinomas should be suspected in all patients with hypoglycemia, especially those with attacks provoked by fasting or with a family history of MEN-1. Insulin is synthesized as proinsulin which consists of a 21-amino-acid α chain and a 30-amino-acid β chain connected by a 33-amino-acid connecting peptide (C peptide). In insulinomas, in addition to elevated plasma insulin levels, elevated plasma proinsulin levels are found and C-peptide levels can be elevated.

Diagnosis The diagnosis of insulinoma requires the demonstration of an elevated plasma insulin level at the time of hypoglycemia. Other causes of fasting hypoglycemia include the inadvertent or surreptitious use of insulin or oral hypoglycemic agents, severe liver disease, alcoholism, poor nutrition, or other extrapancreatic tumors. The most reliable test to diagnose insulinoma is a fast up to 72 h with serum glucose, C-peptide, and insulin measurements every 4 to 8 h. If at any point the patient becomes symptomatic or glucose levels are persistently <2.2 mmol/L (<40 mg/dL), the test should be terminated and repeat samples for the above studies obtained before glucose is given. Between 70 and 80% of patients with insulinoma will develop hypoglycemia during the first 24 h and 98% by 48 h. In nonobese normal subjects serum insulin levels should decrease to <43 pmol/L (<6 μU/mL) when blood glucose decreases to ≤2.2 mmol/L (<40 mg/dL) and the ratio of insulin to glucose is <0.3 (in mg/dL). In addition to having an insulin level > 6 μU/mL when blood glucose ≤ 40 mg/dL, some investigators also require an elevated C-peptide and serum proinsulin level and/or insulin:glucose ratio >0.3 for the diagnosis of insulinoma. Surreptitious use of insulin or hypoglycemic agents may be difficult to distinguish from the symptoms of insulinomas. The combination of proinsulin levels (normal in exogenous insulin/hypoglycemic agent users), C-peptide levels (low in exogenous insulin users), antibodies to insulin (positive in exogenous insulin users), and sulfonylurea levels in serum or plasma will allow the correct diagnosis to be made.

℞ TREATMENT

Only 5 to 15% of insulinomas are malignant; therefore, after appropriate imaging (see below), surgery should be performed. Some 75 to 95% of patients are cured by surgery. Before surgery, the hypoglycemia can be controlled by frequent small meals and the use of diazoxide (150 to 800 mg/d). Diazoxide is a benzothiadiazide whose hyperglycemic effect is attributed to inhibition of insulin release; 50 to 60% of patients respond to diazoxide. Its side effects are sodium retention and GI symptoms such as nausea. Other agents effective in some patients include verapamil and diphenylhydantoin. Long-acting somatostatin analogues such as octreotide are acutely effective in 40% of patients. However, octreotide needs to be used with care because it inhibits growth hormone secretion and can alter plasma glucagon levels and so worsen the hypoglycemia in some patients.

For the 5 to 15% of patients with malignant insulinomas, the above drugs or somatostatin analogues are used initially. If they are not effective, various antitumor treatments such as hepatic arterial embolization, chemoembolization, or chemotherapy have been used. These will be discussed below.

GLUCAGONOMAS   A glucagonoma is an endocrine tumor of the pancreas that secretes excessive amounts of glucagon, which causes a distinct syndrome characterized by dermatitis, glucose intolerance or diabetes, and weight loss. Glucagonomas occur in persons between 45 and 70 years of age and are clinically heralded by a characteristic dermatitis (migratory necrolytic erythema) (67 to 90%), accompanied by glucose intolerance (40 to 90%), weight loss (66 to 96%), anemia (33 to 85%), diarrhea (15 to 29%), and thromboembolism (11 to 24%). The characteristic rash usually starts as an annular erythema at intertriginous and periorificial sites, especially in the groin or buttock. It subsequently becomes raised, and bullae form and leave erosions when the bullae rupture. The lesions can wax and wane. A characteristic laboratory finding is hypoaminoacidemia, which occurs in 26 to 100% of patients.

Glucagonomas are generally large tumors at diagnosis, with average size of 5 to 10 cm. From 50 to 80% occur in the pancreatic tail, and from 50 to 82% have metastatic spread at presentation, usually to the liver. Glucagonomas are rarely extrapancreatic and usually occur singly.

Diagnosis   The diagnosis is confirmed by demonstrating an increased plasma glucagon level (normal is <150 μg/L). Plasma glucagon levels are >1000 μg/mL in 90%, are between 500 and 1000 μg/mL in 7%, and <500 μg/mL in 3%. A plasma glucagon level > 1000 μg/L is considered diagnostic of glucagonoma. Other diseases causing increased plasma glucagon levels include renal insufficiency, acute pancreatitis, hypercorticism, hepatic insufficiency, prolonged fasting, or familial hyperglucagonomia. These disorders do not increase plasma glucagon to >500 μg/L except cirrhosis.

℞ TREATMENT

In 50 to 80% of patients metastases are present at presentation, so curative surgical resection is not possible. Surgical debulking in patients with advanced disease or other antitumor treatments may be beneficial and will be discussed below. Long-acting somatostatin analogues such as octreotide or lanreotide improve the skin rash in 75%

of patients and may improve the weight loss, pain, and diarrhea, but usually do not improve the glucose intolerance.

SOMATOSTATINOMA SYNDROME   The somatostatinoma syndrome is due to a NET that secretes excessive amounts of somatostatin, which causes a distinct syndrome characterized by diabetes mellitus, gallbladder disease, diarrhea, and steatorrhea. Usually no distinction is made between a tumor that contains somatostatin-like immunoreactivity (somatostatinoma) and that does or does not produce a clinical syndrome (somatostatinoma syndrome) by secreting somatostatin (11 to 45% and 55 to 89%, respectively). In one review of 173 cases of somatostatinomas, only 11% were associated with the somatostatinoma syndrome. The mean age of patients is 51 years. Somatostatinomas occur primarily in the pancreas and small intestine, and the frequency of the symptoms differs in each. Each of the usual symptoms is more frequent in pancreatic than intestinal somatostatinomas: diabetes mellitus (95% vs. 21%), gallbladder disease (94% vs. 43%), diarrhea (92% vs. 38%), steatorrhea (83% vs. 12%), hypochlorhydria (86% vs. 12%), and weight loss (90% vs. 69%). Somatostatinomas occur in the pancreas in 56 to 74% of cases, with the primary location being in the pancreatic head. The tumors are usually solitary (90%) and large, with a mean size of 4.5 cm. Liver metastases are frequent (69 to 84% of patients).

Somatostatin is a tetradecapeptide (Fig. 329-2) that is widely distributed in the central nervous system and gastrointestinal tract, where it functions as a neurotransmitter or has paracrine and autocrine actions. It is a potent inhibitor of many processes, including release of almost all hormones, acid secretion, intestinal and pancreatic secretion, and intestinal absorption. Most of the clinical manifestations are directly related to these inhibitory actions.

Diagnosis   In most cases somatostatinomas have been found by accident either at the time of cholecystectomy or during endoscopy. The presence of psammoma bodies in a duodenal tumor should particularly raise suspicion. Duodenal somatostatin-containing tumors are increasingly associated with von Recklinghausen's disease. Most of these do not cause the somatostatinoma syndrome. The diagnosis of the somatostatinoma syndrome requires elevated plasma somatostatin levels.

℞ TREATMENT

Pancreatic tumors are frequently metastatic at presentation (70 to 92%), whereas 30 to 69% of small-intestinal somatostatinomas have metastases. Surgery is the treatment of choice for those without widespread hepatic metastases. Symptoms in patients with the somatostatinoma syndrome are also improved by octreotide treatment.

VIPOMAS   VIPomas are endocrine tumors that secrete excessive amounts of VIP, which causes a distinct syndrome characterized by large-volume watery diarrhea, hypokalemia, and dehydration. This syndrome is also called Verner-Morrison syndrome, pancreatic cholera, or WDHA syndrome for *w*atery *d*iarrhea, *h*ypokalemia, and *a*chlorhydria, which some patients develop. The mean age of patients is 49 years; however, it can occur in children, and when it does is usually caused by a ganglioneuroma or ganglioneuroblastoma.

The principal symptoms are large-volume diarrhea (100%) severe enough to cause hypokalemia (80 to 100%), dehydration (83%), hypochlorhydria (54 to 76%), and flushing (20%). The diarrhea is secretory in nature, persists during fasting, and is almost always >1 L/d and >3 L/d in 70%. Most patients do not have accompanying steatorrhea (16%), and the increased stool volume is due to increased excretion of sodium and potassium, which, with the anions, account for the osmolality of the stool. Patients frequently have hyperglycemia (25 to 50%) and hypercalcemia (25 to 50%).

VIP is a 28-amino-acid peptide that is an important neurotransmitter ubiquitously present in the central nervous system and GI tract. Its known actions include stimulation of small-intestinal chloride secretion and effects on smooth-muscle contractility, inhibition of acid secretion, and vasodilatory effects which explain most features of the clinical syndrome.

In adults 80 to 90% of VIPomas are pancreatic in location, with the rest due to VIP-secreting pheochromocytomas, intestinal carcinoids, and rarely ganglioneuromas. These tumors are usually not multiple, 50 to 75% are in the pancreatic tail, and 37 to 68% have hepatic metastases at diagnosis. In children <10 years, the syndrome is usually due to ganglioneuromas or ganglioblastomas, which are less malignant and account for 10% of VIPomas in adults.

Diagnosis The diagnosis requires the demonstration of an elevated plasma VIP level and the presence of large-volume diarrhea. A stool volume of <700 mL/d excludes the diagnosis of VIPoma. By fasting the patient, a number of causes can be excluded that can cause marked diarrhea. Other diseases that can give a secretory large-volume diarrhea include gastrinomas, chronic laxative abuse, carcinoid syndrome, systemic mastocytosis, rarely medullary thyroid cancer, diabetic diarrhea, and AIDS. Of these conditions, only VIPomas caused a marked increase in plasma VIP.

℞ **TREATMENT**

The most important initial treatment is to correct their dehydration, hypokalemia, and electrolyte losses with fluid and electrolyte replacement. These patients may require 5 L/d of fluid and >350 meq/d of potassium. Because 37 to 68% of adults with VIPomas have metastatic disease in the liver at presentation, a significant number of patients cannot be cured surgically. In these patients, long-acting somatostatin analogues such as octreotide or lanreotide are the drugs of choice.

Octreotide will control the diarrhea in 87% of patients. In nonresponsive patients, the combination of glucocorticoids and octreotide has proved helpful in a small number of patients. Other drugs reported to be helpful in small numbers of patients include prednisone (60 to 100 mg/d), clonidine, indomethacin, phenothiazines, loperamide, lidamidine, lithium, propranolol, and metochlorpramide.

Treatment of advanced disease with embolization, chemoembolization, and chemotherapy may also be helpful (see below).

NONFUNCTIONAL PANCREATIC ENDOCRINE TUMORS Nonfunctional PETs are endocrine tumors that originate in the pancreas and either secrete no products or their secreted products do not cause a specific clinical syndrome. The symptoms are due entirely to the tumor per se. Nonfunctional PETs almost always secrete chromogranin A (90 to 100%), chromogranin B (90 to 100%), PP (58%), α-human chorionic gonadotropin (hCG) (40%), and β-hCG (20%), but none cause a specific syndrome. Because the symptoms are due to the tumor per se, patients with nonfunctional PETs usually present late in their disease course with invasive tumors and hepatic metastases (64 to 92%), and the tumors are usually large (72% are >5 cm). These tumors are usually solitary except in patients with MEN-1, where they are multiple, and occur primarily in the pancreatic head. Even though these tumors do not cause a functional syndrome, immunocytochemical studies show that they synthesize numerous peptides and cannot be distinguished from functional tumors by immunocytochemistry.

The most common symptoms are abdominal pain (30 to 80%); jaundice (20 to 35%); and weight loss, fatigue, or bleeding; 10 to 15% are found incidentally. The average time from the beginning of symptoms to diagnosis is 5 years.

Diagnosis The diagnosis is established by histologic confirmation in a patient with a PET without either clinical symptoms or elevated plasma hormone levels of one of the established syndromes. Even though chromogranin A levels are elevated in almost every patient, this is not specific for this disease as it can be found in functional PETs, carcinoids, and other neuroendocrine disorders. Plasma PP is increased in 22 to 71% of patients and should strongly suggest the diagnosis in a patient with a pancreatic mass because it is usually normal in patients with pancreatic adenocarcinomas. Elevated plasma PP is not diagnostic of this tumor because it is elevated in a number of other conditions such as chronic renal failure, old age, inflammatory conditions, and diabetes.

℞ **TREATMENT**

Unfortunately, surgical curative resection can be considered only in the minority of patients because of the high frequency of metastatic disease. Treatment needs to be directed against the tumor per se (see below).

GRFOMAS GRFomas are endocrine tumors that secrete excessive amounts of GRF, which causes acromegaly. The true frequency of this syndrome is not known. GRF is a 44-amino-acid peptide, and 25 to 44% of PETs have GRF immunoreactivity, although it is uncommonly secreted. GRFomas are lung tumors in 47 to 54% of cases, PETs in 29 to 30%, and small-intestinal carcinoids in 8 to 10%, and up to 12% occur at other sites. Patients have a mean age of 38 years, and the symptoms are usually due to either acromegaly or the tumor per se. The acromegaly caused by GRFomas is indistinguishable from classic acromegaly. The pancreatic tumors are usually large (>6 cm) and liver metastases are present in 39%. They should be suspected in any patient with acromegaly and an abdominal tumor, in a patient with MEN-1 with acromegaly, or in a patient without a pituitary adenoma with acromegaly or associated with hyperprolactinemia, which occurs in 70% of GRFomas. GRFomas are an uncommon cause of acromegaly. The diagnosis is established by performing plasma assays for GRF and growth hormone. The normal level for GRF is <5 μg/L in men and <10 μg/L in women. Most GRFomas have a plasma GRF level ≥300 μg/L. Patients with GRFomas also have increased plasma insulin-like growth factor 1 levels similar to those in classic acromegaly. Surgery is the treatment of choice if diffuse metastases are not present. Long-acting somatostatin analogues such as octreotide or lanreotide are the agents of choice, with 75 to 100% of patients responding.

OTHER RARE PANCREATIC ENDOCRINE TUMOR SYNDROMES Cushing's (ACTHoma) due to a PET occurs in 4 to 16% of all ectopic Cushing's syndrome cases. It occurs in 5% of cases of sporadic gastrinomas, almost invariably in patients with hepatic metastases, and is an independent, poor prognostic factor. Paraneoplastic hypercalcemia due to PETs releasing parathyroid hormone–related peptide (PTHrP), a parathyroid hormone–like material, or unknown factor is rarely reported. The tumors are usually large, and liver metastases are usually present. Most (88%) appear to be due to release of PTHrP. PETs can occasionally cause the carcinoid syndrome. PETs secreting calcitonin appear to have a specific clinical syndrome. Half the patients have diarrhea, which disappears with resection of the tumor. That this could be a discrete syndrome is supported by finding that 25 to 42% of patients with medullary thyroid cancer with hypercalcitonemia develop diarrhea, likely secondary to a motility disorder. This is classified in Table 329-2 as a possible specific disorder because so few cases have been described. A renin-producing PET has been described in a patient presenting with hypertension (Table 329-2). Ghrelin is a 28-amino-acid peptide with growth hormone–releasing effect and a strong influence on appetite, among other functions. Even though it is detectable immunohistochemically in most PETs, only 1 in 24 patients (4%) with a PET had elevated plasma ghrelin levels and the patient was asymptomatic, suggesting that no specific syndrome is associated with release of ghrelin by a PET.

TUMOR LOCALIZATION

Localization of the primary tumor and determination of the extent of disease are essential to the proper management of all carcinoids and PETs. Without proper localization studies it is not possible (1) to determine whether the patient is a candidate for curative resection or cytoreductive surgery or requires antitumor treatment (2) or to predict the patient's prognosis.

Numerous tumor localization methods are used in both types of NETs including conventional imaging studies [CT scanning, magnetic resonance imaging (MRI), transabdominal ultrasound, selective angiography] and somatostatin receptor scintigraphy (SRS). In PETs, endoscopic ultrasound (EUS) and functional localization by measuring venous hormonal gradients are also useful. Bronchial carcinoids are usually detected by a standard chest radiograph and assessed by CT. Rectal, duodenal, colonic, and gastric carcinoids are usually detected by GI endoscopy.

PETs and carcinoid tumors frequently overexpress high-affinity somatostatin receptors in both their primary and their metastatic tumors. Of the five types of somatostatin receptors (sst_{1-5}), radiolabeled octreotide binds with high affinity to sst_2 and sst_5, lower for sst_3, and has a very low affinity for sst_1 and sst_4. Nearly all carcinoid tumors and PETs express sst_2, and many also have the other four sst subtypes. Interaction with these receptors can be used to localize NETs using [^{111}In-DTPA-D-Phe[1]]octreotide (Fig. 329-2) and radionuclide scanning (SRS) as well as for treatment of the hormone excess state with octreotide or lanreotide. Because of its sensitivity and ability to localize tumor throughout the body at one time, SRS is now the initial imaging modality of choice for localizing both primary NETs and metastases. SRS localizes tumor in 73 to 89% of patients with carcinoids and in 56 to 100% of patients with PETs, except for insulinomas. Insulinomas are usually small and have low densities of sst receptors, resulting in SRS being positive in only 12 to 50% of insulinomas. SRS has greater sensitivity than conventional imaging studies in localizing both the primary tumor and metastases. Figure 329-3 shows an example of the increased sensitivity of SRS in a patient with a gastrinoma. The CT scan (Fig. 329-3, *top*) did not show any disease after resection of the primary tumor; however, hypergastrinemia remained and the SRS demonstrated a metastasis in the liver (Fig. 329-3, *bottom*). Occasional

false-positive responses with SRS can occur (12% in one study) because numerous other normal tissues and diseases can have high densities of sst receptors including granulomas (sarcoid, tuberculosis, etc.), thyroid diseases (goiter, thyroiditis), and activated lymphocytes (lymphomas, wound infections). For PETs located in the pancreas, EUS is highly sensitive localizing 77 to 93% of insulinomas, which occur almost exclusively within the pancreas. EUS is less sensitive for extrapancreatic tumors. If liver metastases are identified by SRS, either a CT scan or MRI is then recommended to assess the size and exact location of the metastases because SRS does not give information on tumor size. Functional localization measuring hormone gradients after intraarterial calcium injections in insulinomas (insulin) or gastrin gradients after secretin injections in gastrinoma is a sensitive method, being positive in 80 to 100% of patients. However, this method gives only regional localization and is reserved for cases where the other imaging modalities are negative.

R_x TREATMENT

Advanced Disease (Diffuse Metastatic Disease) The single most important prognostic factor for survival is the presence of liver metastases (Fig. 329-4). For patients with foregut carcinoids without hepatic metastases, the 5-year survival is 95% and with distant metastases is 20% (Fig. 329-4, *bottom*). With gastrinomas the 5-year survival without liver metastases is 98%, with limited metastases in one hepatic lobe it is 78%, and with diffuse metastases it is 16% (Fig. 329-4, *top*). Therefore, treatment for advanced metastatic disease is important. A number of different modalities are effective, including cytoreductive surgery

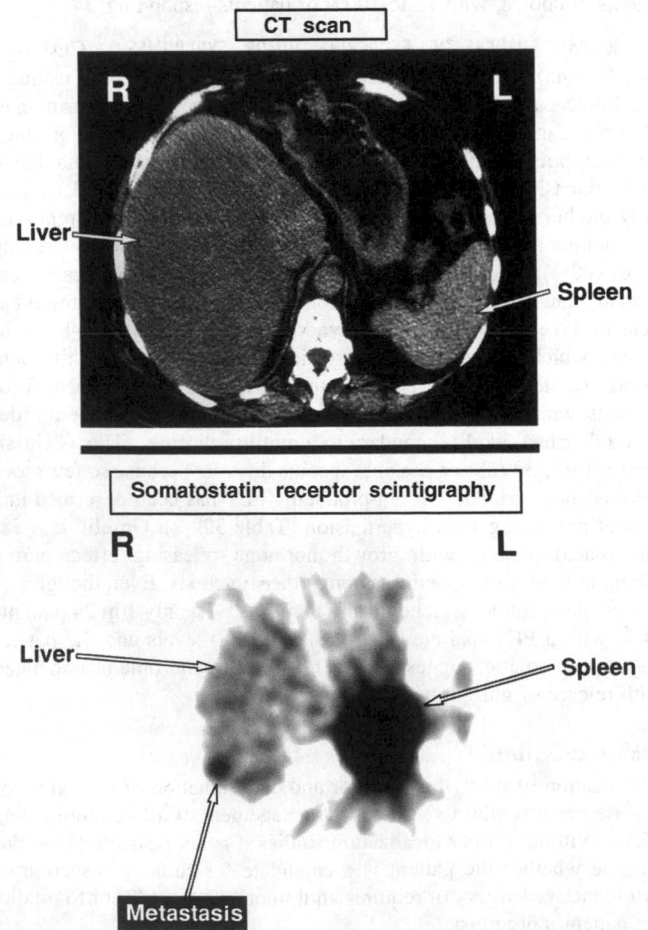

FIGURE 329-3 Ability of computed tomography (*top*) or somatostatin receptor scintigraphy (*bottom*) to localize metastatic gastrinoma in the liver in a patient with Zollinger-Ellison syndrome.

FIGURE 329-4 Effect of the presence and extent of liver metastases on survival in patients with gastrinomas (*top*) or carcinoid tumors (*bottom*). (*Top panel is drawn from data from 199 patients with gastrinomas modified from F Yu et al: J Clin Oncol 17:615, 1999. Bottom panel is drawn from data from 71 patients with foregut carcinoid tumors from EW McDermott et al: Br J Surg 81:1007, 1994; with permission.*)

(removal of all visible tumor), treatment with chemotherapy, somatostatin analogues, interferon α, hepatic embolization alone or with chemotherapy (chemoembolization), radiotherapy, and liver transplantation.

Specific Antitumor Treatments Cytoreductive surgery, unfortunately, is only possible in 9 to 22% of patients who present with limited hepatic metastases. Although no randomized studies have proven it extends life, results from a number of studies suggest it likely increases survival, and therefore it is recommended if possible.

Chemotherapy for metastatic carcinoid tumors has generally been disappointing, with response rates of 0 to 40% with various two- or three-drug combinations. Chemotherapy for PETs has been more successful with tumor shrinkage reported in 30 to 70% of patients. The current regimen of choice is streptozocin and doxorubicin.

Long-acting somatostatin analogues, such as octreotide and lanreotide, and interferon α rarely decrease tumor size (i.e., 0 to 17%); however, these drugs have tumoristatic effects, stopping additional growth in 26 to 95% of patients with NETs. How long tumor stabilization lasts or whether it prolongs survival has not been established. Somatostatin analogues can induce apoptosis in carcinoid tumors.

Hepatic embolization and chemoembolization (with dacarbazine, cisplatin, doxorubicin, 5-fluorouracil, or streptozocin) may decrease tumor bulk and help control the symptoms of the hormone-excess state. These modalities are generally reserved for cases in which treatment with somatostatin analogues, interferon (carcinoids), or chemotherapy (PETs) fails. Embolization, when combined with treatment with octreotide and interferon α, significantly reduces tumor progression compared to treatment with embolization and octreotide alone in patients with advanced midgut carcinoids.

Radiotherapy with radiolabeled somatostatin analogues (Fig. 329-2) that are internalized by the tumors is an approach being investigated.

Three different radionuclides are being used. High doses of [^{111}In-DTPA-D-Phe^1]octreotide (emits γ rays, internal conversion, and Auger electrons) and yttrium-90 (emits high energy β-particles) coupled by a DOTA-chelating group (Fig. 329-2) to octreotide or octreotate are being used as well as ^{177}Lu-coupled analogues (emit β- and γ-rays). In one study, treatment with the ^{111}In or ^{177}Lu compounds caused tumor stabilization in 41% and 40%, respectively, and a decrease in tumor size in 30% and 38%, respectively, in patients with advanced metastatic NETs. Hormone-directed radiation therapy may be helpful in patients with advanced, widespread metastatic disease.

The use of liver transplantation has been abandoned for treatment of most metastatic tumors to the liver. However, for metastatic NETs it is still a consideration. In a recent review of 103 cases of malignant NETs (48 PETs, 43 carcinoids) the 2- and 5-year survival rates were 60% and 47%, respectively. However, recurrence-free survival was low (<24%). For younger patients with metastatic NETs limited to the liver, liver transplantation may be justified.

FURTHER READING

CAPLIN ME et al: Carcinoid tumour. Lancet 352:799, 1998.

CORLETO VD et al: Molecular insights into gastrointestinal neuroendocrine tumors: Importance and recent advances. Dig Liver Dis 34:668, 2002

KULKE MH, MAYER RJ: Carcinoid tumors. N Engl J Med 340:858, 1999

KWEKKEBOOM D et al: Peptide receptor imaging and therapy. J Nucl Med 41: 1704, 2000

METZ DC, JENSEN RT: Endocrine tumors of the gastrointestinal tract, in AK Rustgi, JM Crawford (eds): *Gastrointestinal Cancers*. Edinburgh, Saunders, 2003, pp 681–720

MODLIN IM et al: A 5-decade analysis of 13,715 carcinoid tumors. Cancer 97: 934, 2003

330 DISORDERS AFFECTING MULTIPLE ENDOCRINE SYSTEMS
Steven I. Sherman, Robert F. Gagel

NEOPLASTIC DISORDERS AFFECTING MULTIPLE ENDOCRINE ORGANS

Several distinct genetic disorders predispose to endocrine gland neoplasia and cause hormone excess syndromes (Table 330-1). DNA-based genetic testing is now available for these disorders, but effective management requires an understanding of endocrine neoplasia and the range of clinical features that may be manifest in an individual patient.

MULTIPLE ENDOCRINE NEOPLASIA (MEN) TYPE 1 ■ Clinical Manifestations

MEN1, or Wermer's syndrome, is an autosomal dominant genetic syndrome characterized by neoplasia of parathyroid, pituitary, pancreatic islet, and other neuroendocrine cell types (Table 330-1). Each child born to an affected parent has a 50% probability of inheriting the gene. The variable penetrance of the several neoplastic components can make the differential diagnosis challenging.

Hyperparathyroidism is the most common manifestation of MEN1. Hypercalcemia may develop during the teenage years, and most individuals are affected by age 40 (Fig. 330-1). The neoplastic changes in hyperparathyroidism exemplify one of the cardinal features of endocrine tumors in MEN1—multicentricity. The neoplastic changes inevitably affect multiple parathyroid glands, making surgical cure difficult. Screening for hyperparathyroidism involves measurement of either an albumin-adjusted or ionized serum calcium level. The diagnosis is established by demonstrating elevated levels of serum calcium and inappropriately normal or high intact parathyroid hormone. Manifestations of hyperparathyroidism in MEN1 do not differ substantially from those in sporadic hyperparathyroidism and include calcium-containing kidney stones, bone abnormalities, and gastrointestinal and musculoskeletal complaints (Chap. 332).

Other familial disorders associated with hypercalcemia include familial isolated hyperparathyroidism, a broad categorization that includes at least two types, HRPT1 and HRPT2. The first type, HRPT1, includes familial parathyroid hyperplasia and adenomatosis. The second type, HRPT2, is associated with multiple cystic parathyroid ade-

TABLE 330-1 *Disease Associations in the Multiple Endocrine Neoplasia (MEN) Syndromes*

MEN1	MEN2	Mixed Syndromes
Parathyroid hyperplasia or adenoma	MEN2A	von Hippel–Lindau syndrome, pheochromocytoma, islet cell tumor, renal cell carcinoma, hemangioblastoma of central nervous system, retinal angiomas
Islet cell hyperplasia, adenoma, or carcinoma	MTC	
	Pheochromocytoma	
	Parathyroid hyperplasia or adenoma	
Pituitary hyperplasia or adenoma	Cutaneous lichen amyloidosis	
Other less common manifestations:	Hirschsprung disease	
foregut carcinoid,	Familial MTC	Neurofibromatosis with features of MEN 1 or 2
pheochromocytoma,	MEN2B	
subcutaneous or	MTC	Carney complex
visceral lipomas	Pheochromocytoma	Myxomas of heart, skin, and breast
	Mucosal and gastrointestinal neuromas	Spotty cutaneous pigmentation
	Marfanoid features	Testicular, adrenal, and GH-producing pituitary tumors
		Peripheral nerve schwannomas

Note: MTC, medullary thyroid carcinoma.

FIGURE 330-1 Age at onset of endocrine tumor expression in multiple endocrine neoplasia type 1 (MEN1). Data derived from retrospective analysis for each endocrine organ hyperfunction in 130 cases of MEN1. Age at onset is the age at first symptom or, with tumors not causing symptoms, age at the time of the first abnormal finding on a screening test. The rate of diagnosis of hyperparathyroidism increased sharply between ages 16 and 20 years. (*Reprinted with permission from S Marx et al: Ann Intern Med 129:484, 1998.*)

nomas and ossifying jaw fibromas. Inactivating mutations of the gene that encodes parafibromin were recently identified in nearly all families with HRPT2. Subsequent analysis of this gene in families with HRPT1 indicates that some patients with HRPT1 have mutations of the HRPT2 gene. Inactivating mutations of HRPT2 are also found commonly in sporadic parathyroid cancers. MEN2 (to be discussed below) should also be considered in the differential diagnosis. Another cause of familial hypercalcemia is familial hypercalcemic hypocalciuria (FHH), an autosomal dominant form of hypercalcemia caused by inactivating mutations of the calcium sensor, a transmembrane G protein–coupled receptor found in parathyroid tissue and kidney (Chap. 332). Hypercalcemia associated with MEN1, MEN2, HRPT1, and HRPT2 is characterized by increased urine calcium excretion (calcium/creatinine clearance ratio > 0.01) whereas in FHH it is associated with low urine calcium excretion (calcium/creatinine clearance ratio < 0.01). Another distinguishing feature is that the serum calcium level is rarely elevated at birth in patients with MEN1 but is frequently elevated in newborns with FHH.

Differentiation of hyperparathyroidism of MEN1 from other forms of familial primary hyperparathyroidism is usually based on family history, histologic features of resected parathyroid tissue, and, sometimes, long-term observation to determine whether other manifestations of MEN1 develop. Parathyroid hyperplasia is the most common cause of hyperparathyroidism in MEN1, although single and multiple adenomas have been described. Hyperplasia of one or more parathyroid glands is common in younger patients; adenomas are usually found in older patients or those with long-standing disease.

Neoplasia of the pancreatic islets is the second most common manifestation of MEN1 and tends to occur in parallel with hyperparathyroidism (Fig. 330-1). Increased pancreatic islet cell hormones include pancreatic polypeptide (75 to 85%), gastrin [60%; Zollinger-Ellison syndrome (ZES)], insulin (25 to 35%), vasoactive intestinal peptide (VIP) (3 to 5%; Verner-Morrison, or watery diarrhea, syndrome), glucagon (5 to 10%), and somatostatin (1 to 5%). The tumors rarely produce adrenocorticotropin (ACTH), corticotropin-releasing hormone (CRH), growth hormone–releasing hormone (GHRH), calcitonin gene products, neurotensin, gastric inhibitory peptide, and others. Many of the tumors produce more than one peptide. The pancreatic neoplasms differ from the other components of MEN1 in that approximately one-third of the tumors display malignant features, including hepatic metastases (Chap. 329).

Pancreatic islet cell tumors are diagnosed by identification of a characteristic clinical syndrome, hormonal assays with or without provocative stimuli, or radiographic techniques. One approach involves annual screening of individuals at risk with measurement of basal and meal-stimulated levels of pancreatic polypeptide to identify the tumors as early as possible; the rationale of this screening strategy is that surgical removal of islet cell tumors at an early stage will be curative. Other approaches to screening include measurement of serum gastrin and pancreatic polypeptide levels every 2 to 3 years, with the rationale that pancreatic neoplasms will be detected at a later stage but can be managed medically, if possible, or by surgery. High-resolution, early-phase computed tomography (CT) scanning or endoscopic ultrasound provides the best preoperative technique for identification of these tumors; intraoperative ultrasonography is the most sensitive method for detection of small tumors.

ZES is caused by excessive gastrin production and occurs in more than half of MEN1 patients with pancreatic islet cell tumors or small carcinoid-like tumors in the duodenal wall (Fig. 330-1) (Chap. 329). Approximately one-fourth of all ZES occurs in the context of MEN1. Clinical features include increased gastric acid production, recurrent peptic ulcers, diarrhea, and esophagitis. The ulcer diathesis is refractory to conservative therapy such as antacids. The diagnosis is made by finding increased gastric acid secretion, elevated basal gastrin levels in serum [generally >115 pmol/L (200 pg/mL)], and an exaggerated response of serum gastrin to either secretin or calcium. Other causes of elevated serum gastrin levels, such as achlorhydria, treatment with H_2 receptor antagonists or omeprazole, retained gastric antrum, small-bowel resection, gastric outlet obstruction, and hypercalcemia, should be excluded.

Insulinoma causes hypoglycemia in about one-third of MEN1 patients with pancreatic islet cell tumors (Fig. 330-1). The tumors may be benign or malignant (25%). The diagnosis can be established by documenting hypoglycemia during a short fast with simultaneous inappropriate elevation of serum insulin and C-peptide levels. More commonly, it is necessary to subject the patient to a supervised 12- to 72-h fast to provoke hypoglycemia (Chap. 324). Large insulinomas may be identified by CT scanning; small tumors not detected by radiographic techniques may be localized by selective arteriographic injection of calcium into each of the arteries that supply the pancreas and timed sampling of the hepatic vein for insulin to determine the anatomic region containing the tumor. Intraoperative ultrasonography can also be used to localize these tumors, but preoperative calcium injection data are helpful in guiding the appropriate pancreatic surgical procedure if multiple or no abnormalities are detected by intraoperative ultrasonography.

Glucagonoma in occasional MEN1 patients causes a syndrome of hyperglycemia, skin rash (necrolytic migratory erythema), anorexia, glossitis, anemia, depression, diarrhea, and venous thrombosis. In about half of these patients the plasma glucagon level is high, leading to its designation as the *glucagonoma syndrome*, although elevation of plasma glucagon level in MEN1 patients is not necessarily associated with these symptoms. Some patients with this syndrome also have elevated plasma ghrelin levels. The glucagonoma syndrome may represent a complex interaction between glucagon and ghrelin overproduction and the nutritional status of the patient.

The *Verner-Morrison syndrome*, or *watery diarrhea syndrome*, consists of watery diarrhea, hypokalemia, hypochlorhydria, and metabolic acidosis. The diarrhea can be voluminous and is almost always found in association with an islet cell tumor, prompting use of the term *pancreatic cholera*. However, the syndrome is not restricted to pancreatic islet tumors and has been observed with carcinoids or other tumors. This syndrome is believed to be due to overproduction of VIP, although plasma VIP levels are not always elevated. Hypercalcemia may be induced by the effects of VIP on bone as well as by hyperparathyroidism. The differential diagnosis includes other causes of chronic diarrhea, infectious or parasitic diseases, inflammatory bowel disease, or sprue or other endocrine causes such as ZES, carcinoid syndrome, or medullary thyroid carcinoma.

Pituitary tumors occur in more than half of patients with MEN1 and tend to be multicentric, making them difficult to resect (Chap. 318). Prolactinomas are most common (Fig. 330-1) and are diagnosed by finding serum prolactin levels >200 μg/L, with or without a pituitary mass evident by magnetic resonance imaging (MRI). Values <200 μg/L may be due to a prolactin-secreting neoplasm or to compression of the pituitary stalk by a different type of pituitary tumor. Acromegaly due to excessive growth hormone (GH) production is the second most common syndrome caused by pituitary tumors in MEN1 (Chap. 318) but is rarely caused by production of GHRH by an islet cell tumor (see above). Cushing's disease can be caused by ACTH-producing pituitary tumors or by ectopic production of ACTH or CRH by other components of MEN1 syndrome including islet cell or carcinoid tumors. Diagnosis of pituitary Cushing's disease is generally best accomplished by a high-dose dexamethasone suppression test or by petrosal venous sinus sampling for ACTH after intravenous injection of CRH (Chap. 318). Differentiation of a primary pituitary tumor from an ectopic CRH-producing tumor may be difficult because the pituitary is the source of ACTH in both disorders; documentation of CRH production by a pancreatic islet or carcinoid tumor may be the only method of proving ectopic CRH production. Adrenal cortical tumors are found in almost one-half of gene carriers but are rarely functional; malignancy in the cortical adenomas is uncommon.

Carcinoid tumors in MEN1 are of the foregut type and are derived from thymus, lung, stomach, or duodenum; they may metastasize or be locally invasive. These tumors usually produce serotonin, calcitonin, or CRH. The typical carcinoid syndrome with flushing, diarrhea, and bronchospasm is rare (Chap. 329). Mediastinal carcinoid tumors (an upper mediastinal mass) are more common in men; bronchial carcinoid tumors are more common in women. Carcinoid tumors are a late manifestation of MEN1; screening regularly for mediastinal carcinoid tumors by chest CT scans has been recommended because of the high rate of malignant transformation.

UNUSUAL MANIFESTATIONS OF MEN1 Subcutaneous or visceral lipomas and cutaneous leiomyomas may also be present but rarely undergo malignant transformation. Skin angiofibromas or collagenomas are seen in most patients with MEN1 when carefully sought.

GENETIC CONSIDERATIONS MEN1 is transmitted as an autosomal dominant trait, reflecting the fact that the gene that causes MEN1, located on chromosome 11q13, encodes a tumor-suppressor protein termed *menin* (Fig. 330-2). Affected individuals typically harbor a germline mutation in *MEN1* and acquire a "second hit" in the normal gene as a result of another mutation or, more commonly, loss of the portion of chromosome 11 that contains the MEN1 locus (Chap. 68). Though the function of menin is not well understood, it is a nuclear protein that interacts with at least two transcriptional factors, SMAD 3 and Jun D, suggesting a regulatory role in cell growth.

MEN1 gene mutations are found in >90% of families with the syndrome (Fig. 330-2). Genetic testing can be performed in individuals at risk for the development of MEN1 and is now commercially available in the United States and Europe. The major value of genetic testing in a kindred with an identifiable mutation is the assignment or exclusion of gene carrier status. In those identified as carrying the mutant gene, routine screening for individual manifestations of MEN1 should be performed as outlined above. Those with negative genetic test results (in a kindred with an identified mutation) can be excluded from further screening for MEN1. A significant percentage of sporadic

FIGURE 330-2 Schematic depiction of the MEN1 gene and the distribution of mutations. The shaded areas show coding sequence. The closed circles show the relative distribution of mutations, mostly inactivating, in each exon. Mutation data are derived from the Human Gene Mutation Database from which more detailed information can be obtained (*www.uwcm.ac.uk/uwcm/mg/hgmd0.html*). (*From M Krawczak, DN Cooper: Trends Genet 13:1321, 1998, with permission.*)

parathyroid, islet cell, and carcinoid tumors also have loss or mutation of *MEN1*. It is presumed that these mutations are somatic and occur in a single cell, leading to subsequent transformation.

R_x TREATMENT

Almost everyone who inherits a mutant *MEN1* gene develops at least one clinical manifestation of the syndrome. Most develop hyperparathyroidism, 80% develop pancreatic islet cell tumors, and more than half develop pituitary tumors. For most of these tumors, initial surgery is not curative and patients frequently require multiple surgical procedures on two or more endocrine glands during a lifetime. For this reason, it is essential to establish clear goals for management of these patients rather than to recommend surgery casually each time a tumor is discovered. Ranges for acceptable management are discussed below.

Hyperparathyroidism Individuals with serum calcium levels >3.0 mmol/L (12 mg/dL), evidence of calcium nephrolithiasis or renal dysfunction, neuropathic or muscular symptoms, or bone involvement (including osteopenia) should undergo parathyroid exploration. There is less agreement regarding the necessity for parathyroid exploration in individuals who do not meet these criteria, and observation may be appropriate in the MEN1 patient with asymptomatic hyperparathyroidism.

When parathyroid surgery is indicated in MEN1, all parathyroid tissue should be identified and removed at the time of primary operation, and parathyroid tissue should be implanted in the nondominant forearm. Thymectomy should also be performed because of the potential for later development of malignant carcinoid tumors. If reoperation for hyperparathyroidism is necessary at a later date, transplanted parathyroid tissue can be resected from the forearm under local anesthesia with titration of tissue removal to lower the intact parathyroid hormone (PTH) to <50% of basal.

A less desirable approach is to remove 3 to 3.5 parathyroid glands from the neck (leaving ~50 mg of parathyroid tissue), carefully marking the location of residual tissue so that the remaining tissue can be located easily during subsequent surgery. If this approach is utilized, intraoperative PTH measurements should be utilized to monitor adequacy of removal of parathyroid tissue with a goal of reducing postoperative serum intact PTH to ≤50% of basal values.

Pancreatic Islet Tumors (See Chap. 329 for discussion of pancreatic islet tumors not associated with MEN1.) Two features of pancreatic islet cell tumors in MEN1 complicate the management. First, the pancreatic islet cell tumors are multicentric, malignant about a third of the time, and cause death in 10 to 20% of patients. Second, removal of all pancreatic islets to prevent malignancy causes diabetes mellitus, a disease with significant long-term complications that include neuropathy, retinopathy, and nephropathy. These features make it difficult to formulate clear-cut guidelines, but some general concepts appear to be valid. First, islet cell tumors producing insulin, glucagon, VIP, GHRH, or CRH should be resected because medical therapy for the hormonal effects of these tumors is generally ineffective. Second, gastrin-producing islet cell tumors that cause ZES are frequently multicentric. Recent experience suggests that a high percentage of ZES in MEN1 is caused by duodenal wall tumors and that resection of these tumors improves the cure rate. Treatment with H_2 receptor antagonists (cimetidine or ranitidine) and the H^+,K^+-ATPase inhibitors (omeprazole or lansoprazole) provides an alternative, and some think preferable, therapy to surgery for control of ulcer disease in patients with multicentric tumors or with hepatic metastases. Third, total pancreatectomy at an early age may be justified to prevent malignancy for families who have a high incidence of malignant cell tumors that cause death.

Management of metastatic islet cell carcinoma is unsatisfactory. Hormonal abnormalities can sometimes be controlled. For example, ZES can be treated with H_2 receptor antagonists or H^+,K^+-ATPase inhibitors; the somatostatin analogues, octreotide or lanreotide, are useful in the management of carcinoid and the watery diarrhea syndrome. Bilateral adrenalectomy may be required for ectopic ACTH syndrome if medical therapy is ineffective (Chap. 321). Islet cell carcinomas frequently metastasize to the liver but may grow slowly. Hepatic artery embolization or chemotherapy (5-fluorouracil, streptozocin, chlorozotocin, doxorubicin, or dacarbazine) may reduce tumor mass, control symptoms of hormone excess, and prolong life; however, these treatments are never curative.

Pituitary Tumors Treatment of prolactinomas with dopamine agonists (bromocriptine, cabergoline, or quinagolide) usually returns the serum prolactin level to normal and prevents further tumor growth (Chap. 318). Surgical resection of a prolactinoma is rarely curative but may relieve mass effects. Transsphenoidal resection is appropriate for neoplasms that secrete ACTH, GH, or the α-subunit of the pituitary glycoprotein hormones. Octreotide reduces tumor mass in one-third of GH-secreting tumors and reduces GH and insulin-like growth factor I levels in >75% of patients. Pegvisomant, a GH receptor antagonist, rapidly lowers insulin-like growth factor levels 1/(IGF-1) and is now approved for treatment of acromegaly. Radiation therapy may be useful for large or recurrent tumors.

Advances in the management of MEN1, particularly islet cell and pituitary tumors, have improved outcome in these patients substantially. As a result, other neoplastic manifestations that develop later in the course of this disorder, such as carcinoid syndrome, are now seen with increased frequency.

MULTIPLE ENDOCRINE NEOPLASIA TYPE 2 ■ Clinical Manifestations Medullary thyroid carcinoma (MTC) and pheochromocytoma are associated in two major syndromes: MEN type 2A and MEN type 2B (Table 330-1). MEN2A is the combination of MTC, hyperparathyroidism, and pheochromocytoma. Three subvariants of MEN2A are familial medullary thyroid carcinoma (FMTC), MEN2A with cutaneous lichen amyloidosis, and MEN2A with Hirschsprung disease. MEN2B is the combination of MTC, pheochromocytoma, mucosal neuromas, intestinal ganglioneuromatosis, and marfanoid features.

MULTIPLE ENDOCRINE NEOPLASIA TYPE 2A MTC is the most common manifestation. This tumor usually develops in childhood, beginning as hyperplasia of the calcitonin-producing cells (C cells) of the thyroid. MTC is typically located at the junction of the upper one-third and lower two-thirds of each lobe of the thyroid, reflecting the high density of C cells in this location; tumors >1 cm in size are frequently associated with local or distant metastases. Measurement of the serum calcitonin level after calcium or pentagastrin injection makes it possible to diagnose this disorder at an early stage in its development (see below).

Pheochromocytoma occurs in ~50% of patients with MEN2A and causes hypertension with palpitations, nervousness, headaches, and sometimes sweating (Chap. 322). About half the tumors are bilateral. After unilateral adrenalectomy, >50% of patients develop a pheochromocytoma in the contralateral gland within a decade. A second feature of these tumors is a disproportionate increase in the secretion of epinephrine relative to norepinephrine. This characteristic differentiates the MEN2 pheochromocytomas from sporadic pheochromocytoma and those associated with von Hippel–Lindau (VHL) syndrome, hereditary paraganglioma, or neurofibromatosis. Capsular invasion is common, but metastasis is uncommon. Finally, the pheochromocytomas are almost always found in the adrenal gland, differentiating the pheochromocytomas in MEN2 from the extraadrenal tumors found in hereditary paraganglioma syndromes.

Hyperparathyroidism occurs in 15 to 20% of patients, with the peak incidence in the third or fourth decade. The manifestations of hyperparathyroidism do not differ from those in other forms of primary hyperparathyroidism (Chap. 332). Diagnosis is established by finding hypercalcemia, hypophosphatemia, hypercalciuria, and an inappropriately high serum level of intact PTH. Multiglandular parathyroid hyperplasia is the most common histologic finding, although with long-standing disease, adenomatous changes may be superimposed on hyperplasia.

The most common subvariant of MEN2A is familial MTC, an autosomal dominant syndrome in which MTC is the only manifestation (Table 330-1). The clinical diagnosis of FMTC is established by the identification of MTC in multiple generations without a pheochromocytoma. Since the penetrance of pheochromocytoma is 50% in MEN2A, it is possible that MEN2A could masquerade as FMTC in small kindreds. It is important to consider this possibility carefully before classifying a kindred as having FMTC; failure to do so could lead to death or serious morbidity from pheochromocytoma in an affected kindred member.

MULTIPLE ENDOCRINE NEOPLASIA TYPE 2B The association of MTC, pheochromocytoma, mucosal neuromas, and a marfanoid habitus is designated MEN2B. MTC in MEN2B develops earlier and is more aggressive than in MEN2A. Metastatic disease has been described prior to 1 year of age, and death commonly occurs in the second or third decade of life. However, the prognosis is not invariably bad even in patients with metastatic disease, as evidenced by a number of multigenerational families with this disease.

Pheochromocytoma occurs in more than half of MEN2B patients and does not differ from that in MEN2A. Hypercalcemia is rare in MEN2B, and there are no well-documented examples of hyperparathyroidism.

The mucosal neuromas and marfanoid body habitus are the most distinctive features and are recognizable in childhood. Neuromas are present on the tip of the tongue, under the eyelids, and throughout the gastrointestinal tract and are true neuromas, distinct from neurofibromas. The most common presentation in children relates to gastrointestinal symptomatology, including intermittent colic, pseudoobstruction, and diarrhea.

GENETIC CONSIDERATIONS Mutations of the *RET* proto-oncogene have been identified in most patients with MEN2 (Fig. 330-3). *RET* encodes a tyrosine kinase receptor that, in combination with a co-receptor, GDNF family-receptor alpha (GFRα), is normally activated by glial cell–derived neurotropic factor or other members of this transforming growth factor–like family of peptides including artemin, persephin, and neurturin. In the C cell there is evidence that persephin normally activates the RET/GFRα-4 receptor complex and is partially responsible for migration of the C cells into the thyroid gland, whereas in the gastrointestinal tract, glial cell–derived neurotrophic factor activates a RET/GFRα-1 complex. *RET* mutations induce constitutive activity of the receptor, explaining the autosomal dominant transmission of the disorder.

Naturally occurring mutations localize to two regions of the RET tyrosine kinase receptor. The first is a cysteine-rich extracellular domain; point mutations in the coding sequence for one of six cysteines (codons 609, 611, 618, 620, 630, or 634) cause amino acid substitutions that induce receptor dimerization and activation in the absence of its ligand. Codon 634 mutations occur in 80% of MEN2A kindreds and are most commonly associated with classic MEN2A features (Figs. 330-3 and 330-2); an arginine substitution at this codon accounts for half of all MEN2A mutations. All reported families with MEN2A and cutaneous lichen amyloidosis have a codon 634 mutation. Mutations of codons 609, 611, 618, or 620 occur in 10 to 15% of MEN2A kindreds and are more commonly associated with FMTC (Fig. 330-3). Mutations in codons 609, 618, and 620 have also been identified in a variant of MEN2A that includes Hirschsprung disease (Fig. 330-3).

The second region of the RET tyrosine kinase that is mutated in MEN2 is in the substrate recognition pocket at codon 918 (Fig. 330-3). This activating mutation is present in ~95% of patients with MEN2B and accounts for 5% of all *RET* proto-oncogene mutations in MEN2. Mutations of codons 883 and 922 have also been identified in a few patients with MEN2B.

Uncommon mutations (initially <5% of the total) include those of codons 533 (exon 8), 768, 790, 791, 804, 891, and 912. Mutations associated with only FMTC include codons 533, 768, V804M, and 912. A cautionary note is that rare mutations that were once associated with FMTC only (791, V804L, and 891) have been found in families with MEN2A as there are occasional reports of pheochromocytoma. At present it is reasonable to conclude that only kindreds with codon 533, 768, V804M, or 912 mutations are consistently associated with FMTC; in kindreds with all other *RET* mutations, pheochromocytoma is a possibility. Germline mutations occur in at least 6% of patients with apparently sporadic MTC, leading to the recommendation that all patients with MTC should be screened for these mutations. These findings mirror results in other malignancies where germline mutations of cancer-causing genes contribute to a greater percentage of apparently sporadic cancer than previously considered. The recognition of new mutations of *RET* almost 10 years following the initial discovery of *RET* mutations suggests that more will be identified in the future.

Somatic mutations (found only in the tumor and not transmitted in the germline) of the *RET* proto-oncogene have been identified in sporadic MTC; 25 to 35% of sporadic tumors have codon 918 mutations, and somatic mutations in codons 630, 768, and 804 have also been identified (Fig. 330-3).

FIGURE 330-3 Schematic diagram of the *RET* proto-oncogene showing mutations found in MEN type 2 and sporadic medullary thyroid carcinoma (MTC). The *RET* proto-oncogene is located on the proximal arm of chromosome 10q (10q11.2). Activating mutations of two functional domains of the RET tyrosine kinase receptor have been identified. The first affects a cysteine-rich (Cys-Rich) region in the extracellular portion of the receptor. Each germline mutation changes a cysteine at codons 609, 611, 618, 620, or 634 to another amino acid. The second region is the intracellular tyrosine kinase (TK) domain. Codon 634 mutations account for ~80% of all germline mutations. Mutations of codons 630, 768, 883, and 918 have been identified as somatic (nongermline) mutations that occur in a single parafollicular or C cell within the thyroid gland in sporadic MTC. A codon 918 mutation is the most common somatic mutation. Abbreviations: MEN2, multiple endocrine neoplasia type 2; CLA cutaneous lichen amyloidosis; FMTC, familial medullary thyroid carcinoma; Signal, the signal peptide; Cadherin, a cadherin-like region in the extracellular domain; TM, transmembrane domain; TK, tyrosine kinase domain.

TREATMENT

Screening for Multiple Endocrine Neoplasia Type 2 Death from MTC can be prevented by early thyroidectomy. The identification of *RET* proto-oncogene mutations and the application of DNA-based molecular diagnostic techniques to identify these mutations has simplified the screening process. During the initial evaluation of a kindred, a *RET* proto-oncogene analysis should be performed on an individual with proven MEN2A. Establishment of the specific germline mutation facilitates the subsequent analysis of other family members. Each family member at risk should be tested twice for the presence of the specific mutation; the second analysis should be performed on a new DNA sample and, ideally, in a second laboratory to exclude sample mix-up or technical error (see www.genetests.org for an up-to-date list of laboratory testing sites). Both false-positive and false-negative analyses have been described; a false-negative test result is of the greatest concern because calcitonin testing is now rarely performed as a diagnostic backup study; if there is a genetic test error, a child may present in the second or third decade with metastatic MTC. Individuals in a kindred with a known mutation who have two normal analyses can be excluded from further screening.

There is general consensus that children with codon 883, 918, and 922 mutations, those associated with MEN2B, should have a total thyroidectomy and central lymph node dissection (level VI) performed during the first months of life or soon after identification of the syndrome. If local metastasis is discovered, a more extensive lymph node dissection (levels II to V) is generally indicated. In children with codon 611, 618, 620, 630, 634, and 891 mutations, thyroidectomy should be performed before age 6 because of reports of local metastatic disease in children this age. Finally, there are kindreds with codon 609, 768, 790, 791, 804, and 912 mutations where the phenotype of MTC appears to be less aggressive. In kindreds with these mutations, two management approaches have been suggested: (1) perform a total thyroidectomy, with or without central node dissection, at some arbitrary age (perhaps 6 to 10 years of age); or (2) continue annual or biannual

calcitonin provocative testing with performance of total thyroidectomy, with or without central neck dissection, when the test becomes abnormal. The pentagastrin test involves measurement of serum calcitonin basally and at 2, 5, 10, and 15 min after a bolus injection of 5 μg pentagastrin per kilogram body weight. Before injection, patients should be warned of epigastric tightness, nausea, warmth, and tingling of extremities and reassured that the symptoms will last ~2 min. The recent unavailability of pentagastrin in the United States has led to use of a short calcium infusion, performed by obtaining a baseline serum calcitonin and then infusing 150 mg calcium salt intravenously over 10 min with measurement of serum calcium and calcitonin at 5, 10, 15, and 30 min after initiation of the infusion.

The *RET* proto-oncogene analysis should be performed in patients with suspected MEN2B to detect codon 883, 918, and 922 mutations, especially in newborn children where the diagnosis is suspected but the clinical phenotype is not fully developed. Other family members at risk for MEN2B should also be tested because the mucosal neuromas can be subtle and not always identified. Most MEN2B mutations represent de novo germline mutations derived from the paternal allele. In the rare families with proven germline transmission of MTC but no identifiable *RET* proto-oncogene mutation, annual pentagastrin or calcium-pentagastrin testing should be performed on members at risk.

Annual screening for pheochromocytoma in subjects with germline *RET* mutations should be performed by measuring basal plasma or 24-h urine catecholamines and metanephrines. The goal is to identify a pheochromocytoma before it causes significant symptoms or is likely to cause sudden death, an event most commonly associated with large tumors. Radiographic studies, such as MRI or CT scans, are generally reserved for individuals with abnormal screening tests or with symptoms suggestive of pheochromocytoma (Chap. 322). Women should be tested during pregnancy because undetected pheochromocytoma can cause maternal death during childbirth.

Measurement of serum calcium and parathyroid hormone levels every 2 to 3 years provides an adequate screen for hyperparathyroidism, except in those families in which hyperparathyroidism is a prominent component.

Medullary Thyroid Carcinoma Hereditary MTC is a multicentric disorder. Total thyroidectomy with a central lymph node dissection should be performed in children who carry the mutant gene. Incomplete thyroidectomy leaves the possibility of later transformation of residual C cells. The goal of early therapy is to cure, and a strategy that does not accomplish this goal is short-sighted. Long-term follow-up studies indicate an excellent outcome with ~90% of children free of disease 15 to 20 years after surgery. In contrast, 15 to 25% of patients whose diagnosis is based on a palpable thyroid nodule die from the disease within 15 to 20 years.

In adults with MTC >1 cm in size, metastases to regional lymph nodes are common (>75%). Total thyroidectomy with central lymph node dissection and selective dissection of other regional chains provide the best chance for cure. In patients with extensive local metastatic disease in the neck, external radiation may prevent local recurrence or reduce tumor mass but is not curative. Chemotherapy with combinations of adriamycin, vincristine, cyclophosphamide, and dacarbazine may provide palliation. The recent success of gleevec for treatment of chronic myelogenous leukemia and gastrointestinal stromal tumors has prompted efforts to develop inhibitors that target the RET tyrosine kinase. Preliminary in vitro studies have identified several promising agents, and human trials are forthcoming.

Pheochromocytoma The long-term goal for management of pheochromocytoma is to prevent death and cardiovascular complications. Improvements in radiographic imaging of the adrenals make direct examination of the apparently normal contralateral gland during surgery less important, and the rapid evolution of laparoscopic surgery has simplified management of early pheochromocytoma. The major question is whether to remove both adrenal glands or to remove only the affected adrenal at the time of primary surgery. Issues to be considered in this decision include the possibility of malignancy (<15 reported cases), the high probability of developing pheochromocytoma in the apparently unaffected gland over an 8- to 10-year period, and the risks of adrenal insufficiency caused by removal of both glands (at least two deaths related to adrenal insufficiency in MEN2 patients). Most clinicians recommend removing only the affected gland. If both adrenals are removed, glucocorticoid and mineralocorticoid replacement are mandatory. An alternative approach is to perform a cortical-sparing adrenalectomy, removing the pheochromocytoma and adrenal medulla, leaving the adrenal cortex behind. This approach is usually successful and eliminates the necessity for steroid hormone replacement in most patients, although the pheochromocytoma recurs in a small percentage.

Hyperparathyroidism Hyperparathyroidism has been managed by one of two approaches. Removal of 3.5 glands with maintenance of the remaining half gland in the neck is the usual procedure. In families in whom hyperparathyroidism is a prominent manifestation (almost always associated with a codon 634 *RET* mutation) and recurrence is common, total parathyroidectomy with transplantation of parathyroid tissue into the nondominant forearm is preferred. This approach is discussed above in the context of hyperparathyroidism associated with MEN1.

OTHER GENETIC ENDOCRINE TUMOR SYNDROMES A number of mixed syndromes exist in which the neoplastic associations differ from those in MEN1 or 2 (Table 330-1).

The cause of VHL syndrome, the association of central nervous system tumors, renal cell carcinoma, pheochromocytoma, and islet cell neoplasms, is a mutation in the *VHL* tumor-suppressor gene. Germline-inactivating mutations of the *VHL* gene cause tumor formation when there is additional loss or somatic mutation of the normal *VHL* allele in brain, kidney, pancreatic islet, or adrenal medullary cells. Missense mutations have been identified in >40% of VHL families with pheochromocytoma, suggesting that families with this type of mutation should be surveyed routinely for pheochromocytoma. A point that may be useful in differentiating VHL from MEN1 (overlapping features include islet cell tumor and rare pheochromocytoma) or MEN2 (overlapping feature is pheochromocytoma) is that hyperparathyroidism rarely occurs in VHL.

The molecular defect in type 1 neurofibromatosis inactivates neurofibromin, a cell membrane–associated protein that normally activates a GTPase. Inactivation of this protein impairs GTPase and causes continuous activation of p21 Ras and its downstream tyrosine kinase pathway. Endocrine tumors also form in less common neoplastic genetic syndromes. These include Cowden's disease, Carney complex, familial acromegaly, and familial carcinoid syndrome. Carney complex comprises myxomas of the heart, skin, and breast; peripheral nerve schwannomas; spotty skin pigmentation; and testicular, adrenal, and GH-secreting pituitary tumors. Linkage analysis has identified two loci: chromosome 2p in half of families and 17q in the others. The 17q gene has been identified as the regulatory subunit (type IA) of protein kinase A (PRKA1A).

IMMUNOLOGIC SYNDROMES AFFECTING MULTIPLE ENDOCRINE ORGANS

When immune dysfunction affects two or more endocrine glands and other nonendocrine immune disorders are present, the polyglandular autoimmune (PGA) syndromes should be considered. The PGA syndromes are classified as two main types: the type I syndrome starts in childhood and is characterized by mucocutaneous candidiasis, hypoparathyroidism, and adrenal insufficiency; the type II, or Schmidt syndrome, is more likely to present in adults and most commonly comprises adrenal insufficiency, thyroiditis, and type 1 diabetes mellitus (Table 330-2).

POLYGLANDULAR AUTOIMMUNE SYNDROME TYPE I PGA type I is usually recognized in the first decade of life and requires two of three components for diagnosis: mucocutaneous candidiasis, hypoparathyroidism, and adrenal insufficiency. Mineralocorticoids and glucocorticoids may be lost simultaneously or sequentially. This disorder is also called *autoimmune polyendocrinopathy-candidiasis-ectodermal dystrophy* (APECED). Other endocrine defects can include gonadal failure, hypothyroidism, anterior hypophysitis, and, less commonly, destruction of the β cells of the pancreatic islets and development of insulin-dependent (type 1) diabetes mellitus. Additional features include hypoplasia of the dental enamel, ungual dystrophy, tympanic membrane sclerosis, vitiligo, keratopathy, and gastric parietal cell dysfunction resulting in pernicious anemia. Some patients develop autoimmune hepatitis, malabsorption (variably attributed to intestinal lymphangiectasia, IgA deficiency, bacterial overgrowth, or hypoparathyroidism), asplenism, achalasia, and cholelithiasis (Table 330-2). At the outset, only one organ may be involved, but the number increases with time so that patients eventually manifest two to five components of the syndrome.

Most patients initially present with oral candidiasis in childhood; it is poorly responsive to treatment and relapses frequently. Chronic hypoparathyroidism usually occurs before adrenal insufficiency de-

TABLE 330-2 *Features of Polyglandular Autoimmune (PGA) Syndromes*

PGA I	PGA II
EPIDEMIOLOGY	
Autosomal recessive	Polygenic inheritance
Mutations in APECED gene	HLA-DR3 and HLA-DR4 associated
Childhood onset	Adult onset
Equal male:female ratio	Female predominance
DISEASE ASSOCIATIONS	
Mucocutaneous candidiasis	Adrenal insufficiency
Hypoparathyroidism	Hypothyroidism
Adrenal insufficiency	Graves' disease
Hypogonadism	Type 1 diabetes
Alopecia	Hypogonadism
Hypothyroidism	Hypophysitis
Dental enamel hypoplasia	Myasthenia gravis
Malabsorption	Vitiligo
Chronic active hepatitis	Alopecia
Vitiligo	Pernicious anemia
Pernicious anemia	Celiac disease

Note: APECED, autoimmune polyendocrinopathy-candidiasis-ectodermal dystrophy.

velops. More than 60% of postpubertal women develop premature hypogonadism. The endocrine components, including adrenal insufficiency and hypoparathyroidism, may not develop until the fourth decade, making continued surveillance necessary.

Type I PGA syndrome is usually inherited as an autosomal recessive trait. The responsible gene, designated as either *APECED* or *AIRE*, encodes a transcription factor that is expressed in thymus and lymph nodes; a variety of different mutations have been reported.

POLYGLANDULAR AUTOIMMUNE SYNDROME TYPE II PGA type II is characterized by two or more of the endocrinopathies listed in Table 330-2. Most often these include primary adrenal insufficiency, Graves' disease or autoimmune hypothyroidism, type 1 diabetes mellitus, and primary hypogonadism. Because adrenal insufficiency is relatively rare, it is frequently used to define the presence of the syndrome. Among patients with adrenal insufficiency, type 1 diabetes mellitus coexists in 52% and autoimmune thyroid disease occurs in 69%. However, many patients with antimicrosomal and antithyroglobulin antibodies never develop abnormalities of thyroid function. Thus, increased antibody titers alone are poor predictors of future disease. Other associated conditions include hypophysitis, celiac disease, atrophic gastritis, and pernicious anemia. Vitiligo, caused by antibodies against the melanocyte (see Fig. 46-12), and alopecia are less common than in the type I syndrome. Mucocutaneous candidiasis does not occur. A few patients develop a late-onset, usually transient hypoparathyroidism caused by antibodies that compete with parathyroid hormone for binding to the PTH receptor. Up to 25% of patients with myasthenia gravis, and an even higher percentage who have myasthenia and a thymoma, have PGA type II (Chap. 366).

The type II syndrome is familial in nature, often transmitted as an autosomal dominant trait with incomplete penetrance. Like many of the individual autoimmune endocrinopathies, certain HLA-DR3 and HLA-DR4 alleles increase disease susceptibility; several different genes probably contribute to the expression of this syndrome.

A variety of autoantibodies are seen in PGA type II, including antibodies directed against: (1) thyroid antigens such as thyroid peroxidase, thyroglobulin, or the thyroid-stimulating hormone (TSH) receptor; (2) adrenal side chain cleavage enzyme, steroid 21-hydroxylase, or ACTH receptor; and (3) pancreatic islet glutamic acid decarboxylase or the insulin receptor, among others.

DIAGNOSIS The clinical manifestations of adrenal insufficiency often develop slowly, may be difficult to detect, and can be fatal if not diagnosed and treated appropriately. Thus, prospective screening should be performed routinely in all patients and family members at risk for PGA types I and II. The most effective screening test for adrenal disease is a cosyntropin stimulation test (Chap. 321). A fasting blood glucose level can be obtained to screen for hyperglycemia. Additional screening tests should include measurements of TSH, luteinizing hormone, follicle-stimulating hormone, and, in men, testosterone levels. In families with suspected type I PGA syndrome, calcium and phosphorus levels should be measured. These screening studies should be performed every 1 to 2 years up to about age 50 in families with PGA type II syndrome and until about age 40 in patients with type I syndrome. Screening measurements of autoantibodies against potentially affected endocrine organs are of uncertain prognostic value. The differential diagnosis of PGA syndrome should include the DiGeorge syndrome (hypoparathyroidism due to glandular agenesis and mucocutaneous candidiasis), Kearns-Sayre syndrome (hypoparathyroidism, primary hypogonadism, type 1 diabetes mellitus, and panhypopituitarism), Wolfram's syndrome (congenital diabetes insipidus and diabetes mellitus), IPEX syndrome (*i*mmunodysregulation, *p*olyendocrinopathy, and *e*nteropathy, *X*-linked), and congenital rubella (type 1 diabetes mellitus and hypothyroidism).

℞ TREATMENT

With the exception of Graves' disease, the management of each of the endocrine components of the disease involves hormone replacement and is covered in detail in the chapters on adrenal, thyroid, gonadal,

and parathyroid disease (Chaps. 320, 321, 325, 326, and 332). One aspect of therapy deserves special emphasis. Namely, primary hypothyroidism can mask adrenal insufficiency by prolonging the half-life of cortisol; consequently, administration of thyroid hormone to a patient with unsuspected adrenal insufficiency can precipitate adrenal crisis. Thus, all patients with hypothyroidism in the context of PGA syndrome should be screened for adrenal disease and, if it is present, be treated with glucocorticoids prior to or concurrently with thyroid hormone therapy.

OTHER AUTOIMMUNE ENDOCRINE SYNDROMES ■ Insulin Receptor Antibodies Rare insulin-resistance syndromes occur in patients who develop antibodies that block the interaction of insulin with its receptor. Conversely, other classes of anti-insulin receptor antibodies can activate the receptor and can cause hypoglycemia; this disorder should be considered in the differential diagnosis of fasting hypoglycemia (Chap. 324).

Patients with insulin receptor antibodies and acanthosis nigricans are often middle-aged women who acquire insulin resistance in association with other autoimmune disorders such as systemic lupus erythematosus or Sjögren's syndrome. Vitiligo, alopecia, Raynaud's phenomenon, and arthritis may also be seen. Other autoimmune endocrine disorders, including thyrotoxicosis, hypothyroidism, and hypogonadism, occur rarely. Acanthosis nigricans, a velvety, hyperpigmented, thickened skin lesion, is prominent on the dorsum of the neck and other skin fold areas in the axillae or groin and often heralds the diagnosis in these patients. However, acanthosis nigricans also occurs in patients with obesity or polycystic ovarian syndrome, in which insulin resistance appears to be due to a postreceptor defect; thus acanthosis nigricans itself is not diagnostic of the immunologic form of insulin resistance.

Ataxia telangiectasia is an autosomal recessive disorder caused by mutations in *ATM*, a gene involved in cellular responses to ionizing radiation and oxidative damage (Chap. 352). This disorder is characterized by ataxia, telangiectasia, immune abnormalities, and an increased incidence of malignancies. Insulin-resistant diabetes mellitus occurs and is associated with anti-insulin antibodies.

Autoimmune Insulin Syndrome with Hypoglycemia This disorder typically occurs in patients with other autoimmune disorders and is caused by polyclonal insulin-binding autoantibodies that bind to endogenously synthesized insulin. If the insulin dissociates from the antibodies several hours or more after a meal, hypoglycemia can result. Most cases of the syndrome have been described in Japan, and there may be a genetic component. In plasma cell dyscrasias such as multiple myeloma, the plasma cells may produce monoclonal antibodies against insulin and cause hypoglycemia by a similar mechanism.

Antithyroxine Antibodies and Hypothyroidism Circulating autoantibodies against thyroid hormones in patients with both immune thyroid disease and plasma cell dyscrasias such as Waldenström's macroglobulinemia can bind thyroid hormones, decrease their biologic activity, and result in primary hypothyroidism. In other patients the antibodies simply interfere with thyroid hormone immunoassays and cause false elevations or decreases in measured hormone levels.

Crow-Fukase Syndrome The features of this syndrome are highlighted by an acronym that emphasizes its important features: *p*olyneuropathy, *o*rganomegaly, *e*ndocrinopathy, *M*-proteins, and *s*kin changes (POEMS). The most important feature is a severe, progressive sensorimotor polyneuropathy associated with a plasma cell dyscrasia. Localized collections of plasma cells (plasmacytomas) can cause sclerotic bone lesions and produce monoclonal IgG or IgA proteins. Endocrine manifestations include amenorrhea in women and impotence and gynecomastia in men, hypogonadism, hyperprolactinemia, type 2 diabetes mellitus, primary hypothyroidism, adrenal insufficiency, and hyperparathyroidism. Skin changes include hyperpigmentation, thickening of the dermis, hirsutism, and hyperhidrosis. Hepatomegaly and lymphadenopathy occur in about two-thirds of patients, and spleno-megaly is seen in about one-third. Other manifestations include increased cerebrospinal fluid pressure with papilledema, peripheral edema, ascites, pleural effusions, glomerulonephritis, and fever. Median survival may be >10 years, though shorter in patients with extravascular volume overload or clubbing.

The systemic nature of the disorder may cause confusion with other connective tissue diseases. The endocrine manifestations suggest an autoimmune basis of the disorder, but circulating antibodies against endocrine cells have not been demonstrated. Increased serum and tissue levels of interleukin 6, interleukin 1β, vascular endothelial growth factor, matrix metalloproteins, and tumor necrosis factor α are present, but the pathophysiologic basis for the POEMS syndrome is uncertain. Therapy directed against the plasma cell dyscrasia such as local radi-

ation of bony lesions, chemotherapy, thalidomide, plasmapheresis, bone marrow or stem cell transplantation, and treatment with all-*trans* retinoic acid may result in endocrine improvement.

FURTHER READING

BETTERLE C et al: Autoimmune adrenal insufficiency and autoimmune poly-endocrine syndromes: Autoantibodies, autoantigens, and their applicability in diagnosis and disease prediction. Endocr Rev 23:327, 2002

DISPENZIERI A et al: POEMS syndrome: Definitions and long-term outcome. Blood First Edition Paper, prepublished online November 27, 2002; DOI 10.1182/blood-2002-07-2299

HEINO M et al: Mutation analyses of North American APS-1 patients. Hum Mutat 13:69, 1999

MACHENS A et al: Early malignant progression of hereditary medullary thyroid carcinoma. N Engl J Med 349: 1517, 2003

PERHEENTUPA J: APS-1/APECED: The clinical disease and therapy. Endocrinol Metab Clin North Am 31:295, 2002

Section 2   Disorders of Bone and Mineral Metabolism

331 BONE AND MINERAL METABOLISM IN HEALTH AND DISEASE
F. Richard Bringhurst, Marie B. Demay, Stephen M. Krane, Henry M. Kronenberg

BONE STRUCTURE AND METABOLISM

Bone is a dynamic tissue that is remodeled constantly throughout life. The arrangement of compact and cancellous bone provides a strength and density suitable for mobility and protection. In addition, bone provides a reservoir for calcium, magnesium, phosphorus, sodium, and other ions necessary for homeostatic functions. The skeleton is highly vascular and receives about 10% of the cardiac output. Remodeling of bone is accomplished by two distinct cell types: osteoblasts produce bone matrix and osteoclasts resorb the matrix.

The extracellular components of bone consist of a solid mineral phase in close association with an organic matrix, of which 90 to 95% is type I collagen (Chap. 342). The noncollagenous portion of the

organic matrix is heterogeneous and contains serum proteins, such as albumin, as well as many locally produced proteins, whose functions are incompletely understood. These proteins include cell attachment/signaling proteins, such as thrombospondin, osteopontin, and fibronectin; calcium-binding proteins such as matrix gla protein and osteocalcin; and proteoglycans such as biglycan and decorin. Some of these proteins organize collagen fibrils; others initiate mineralization and binding of the mineral phase to the matrix.

The mineral phase is made up of calcium and phosphate and is best characterized as a poorly crystalline hydroxyapatite. The mineral phase of bone is deposited initially in intimate relation to the collagen fibrils and is found in specific locations in the "holes" between the collagen fibrils. This architectural arrangement of mineral and matrix results in a two-phase material well suited to withstand mechanical stresses. The organization of collagen influences the amount and type of mineral phase formed in bone. Although the primary structures of type I collagen in skin and bone tissues are similar, there are differences in posttranslational modifications and distribution of intermolecular cross-links. The holes in the packing structure of the collagen are larger in mineralized collagen of bone and dentin than in unmineralized collagens such as tendon. Single amino-acid substitutions in the helical portion of either the α1 (*COL1A1*) or α2 (*COL1A2*) chains of type I collagen disrupt the organization of bone in osteogenesis imperfecta. The severe skeletal fragility associated with these disorders highlights the importance of the fibrillar matrix in the structure of bone (Chap. 342).

Osteoblasts synthesize and secrete the organic matrix. They are derived from cells of mesenchymal origin (Fig. 331-1A). Active osteoblasts are found on the surface of newly forming bone. As an osteoblast secretes matrix, which is then mineralized, the cell becomes an *osteocyte*, still connected with its blood supply through a series of canaliculi. Osteocytes represent the vast majority of the cells in bone. They are thought to be the mechanosensors in bone that communicate signals to surface osteo-

A

Mesenchymal osteoblast progenitor → Osteoblast precursor (CBFA1+) → Active osteoblast

BMPs

PTH, Vit D
IGFs, BMPs, others

Collagen (I)
Alkaline phosphatase
Osteocalcin, osteopontin
Bone sialoprotein

B

Hematopoietic osteoclast progenitor → Commitment (M-CSF) → Osteoblast precursor (PU-1+) → Differentiation (RANK Ligand) → Mononuclear osteoclast (c-fos+ NFκB+ TRAF+) → Fusion (M-CSF RANK ligand IL-1, IL-6) → Quiescent osteoclast → (RANK Ligand IL-1) → Active osteoclast (c-src+ β3 integrin+ PYK2 kinase+ Cathepsin K+ TRAF+ Carbonic anhydrase II+)

FIGURE 331-1   Pathways regulating development of (A) osteoblasts and (B) osteoclasts. Hormones, cytokines, and growth factors that control cell proliferation and differentiation are shown above the arrows. Transcription factors and other markers specific for various stages of development are depicted below the arrows. BMPs, bone morphogenic proteins; PTH, parathyroid hormone; Vit D, vitamin D; IGFs, insulin-like growth factors; CBFA1, core binding factor A1; M-CSF, macrophage colony-stimulating factor; PU-1, a monocyte- and B lymphocyte–specific ets family transcription factor; NFκB, nuclear factor κB; TRAF, tumor necrosis factor–associated factors; RANK ligand, receptor activator of NFκB ligand; IL-1, interleukin-1; IL-6, interleukin-6. (*Modified from Suda et al, with permission.*)

blasts and their progenitors through the canalicular network. Mineralization of the matrix, both in trabecular bone and in osteones of compact cortical bone (*haversian systems*), begins soon after the matrix is secreted (primary mineralization) but is not completed for several weeks or even longer (secondary mineralization). While this mineralization takes advantage of the high concentrations of calcium and phosphate already near saturation in serum, mineralization is a carefully regulated process dependent on the activity of osteoblast-derived alkaline phosphatase, which probably works by hydrolyzing inhibitors of mineralization.

Genetic studies in humans and mice have identified several key genes that control osteoblast development. Core-binding factor A1 (*CBFA1*, also called *RUNX2*), is a transcription factor expressed specifically in chondrocyte (cartilage cells) and osteoblast progenitors, as well as in mature osteoblasts. *CBFA1* regulates the expression of several important osteoblast proteins including osterix (another transcription factor needed for osteoblast maturation), osteopontin, bone sialoprotein, type I collagen, osteocalcin, and receptor-activator of NFκB (RANK) ligand. *CBFA1* expression is regulated, in part, by bone morphogenic proteins (BMPs). *CBFA1*-deficient mice are devoid of osteoblasts, whereas mice with a deletion of only one allele (*CBFA1* +/−) exhibit a delay in formation of the clavicles and some cranial bones. The latter abnormalities are similar to those in the human disorder *cleidocranial dysplasia*, which is also caused by heterozygous inactivating mutations in *CBFA1*.

The paracrine signaling molecule, Indian hedgehog (Ihh), also plays a critical role in osteoblast development, as evidenced by Ihh-deficient mice that lack osteoblasts in bone formed on a cartilage mold (endochondral ossification). Signals originating from members of the wnt (wingless-type mouse mammary tumor virus integration site) family of paracrine factors are also important. Humans and mice missing a wnt-family co-receptor, LRP5 (lipoprotein receptor–related protein 5), have osteoporosis. Remarkably, humans with an overactive form of LPR5 have increased bone mass. Numerous other growth-regulatory factors affect osteoblast function, including the three closely related transforming growth factor βs, fibroblast growth factors (FGFs) 2 and 18, platelet-derived growth factor, and insulin-like growth factors (IGFs) I and II. Hormones, such as parathyroid hormone (PTH) and 1,25-dihydroxyvitamin D [1,25(OH)$_2$D] activate receptors expressed by osteoblasts to assure mineral homeostasis and to influence a variety of bone cell functions.

Resorption of bone is carried out mainly by *osteoclasts*, multinucleated cells that are formed by fusion of cells derived from the common precursor of macrophages and osteoclasts. Multiple factors regulating osteoclast development have been identified (Fig. 331-1*B*). Factors produced by osteoblasts or marrow stromal cells allow osteoblasts to control osteoclast development and activity. Macrophage colony-stimulating factor (M-CSF) plays a critical role during several steps in the pathway and ultimately leads to fusion of osteoclast progenitor cells to form multinucleated, active osteoclasts. RANK ligand, a member of the tumor necrosis factor (TNF) family, is expressed on the surface of osteoblast progenitors and stromal fibroblasts. In a process involving cell-cell interactions, RANK ligand binds to the RANK receptor on osteoclast progenitors, stimulating osteoclast differentiation and activation. Alternatively, a soluble decoy receptor, referred to as osteoprotegerin, can bind RANK ligand and inhibit osteoclast differentiation. Several growth factors and cytokines (including interleukins 1, 6, and 11; TNF; and interferon γ) modulate osteoclast differentiation and function. Most hormones that influence osteoclast function do not directly target this cell but instead influence M-CSF and RANK ligand signaling by osteoblasts. Both PTH and 1,25(OH)$_2$D increase osteoclast number and activity, whereas estrogen decreases osteoclast number and activity by this indirect mechanism. Calcitonin, in contrast, binds to its receptor on the basal surface of osteoclasts and directly inhibits osteoclast function.

Osteoclast-mediated resorption of bone takes place in scalloped spaces (*Howship's lacunae*) where the osteoclasts are attached through a specific $\alpha_v\beta_3$ integrin to components of the bone matrix such as osteopontin. The osteoclast forms a tight seal to the underlying matrix and secretes protons, chloride, and proteinases into a confined space likened to an extracellular lysosome. The active osteoclast surface forms a ruffled border that contains a specialized proton-pump ATPase, which secretes acid and solubilizes the mineral phase. Carbonic anhydrase (type II isoenzyme) within the osteoclast generates the needed protons. The bone matrix is resorbed in the acid environment adjacent to the ruffled border by proteases that act at low pH, such as cathepsin K.

In the embryo and in the growing child, bone develops by remodeling and replacing previously calcified cartilage (endochondral bone formation) or is formed without a cartilage matrix (intramembranous bone formation). Chondrocytes proliferate, secrete and mineralize a matrix, enlarge (hypertrophy), and then die, thereby enlarging bone and providing the matrix and factors that stimulate endochondral bone formation. This program is regulated by both local factors, such as IGF-I and -II, parathyroid hormone–related peptide (PTHrP), and FGFs, and by systemic hormones such as growth hormone, glucocorticoids, and estrogen.

New bone, whether formed in infants or in adults during repair, has a relatively high ratio of cells to matrix and is characterized by coarse fiber bundles of collagen that are interlaced and randomly dispersed (woven bone). In adults, the more mature bone is organized with fiber bundles regularly arranged in parallel or concentric sheets (lamellar bone). In long bones, deposition of lamellar bone in a concentric arrangement around blood vessels forms the haversian systems. Growth in length of bones is dependent on proliferation of cartilage cells and on the endochondral sequence at the growth plate. Growth in width and thickness is accomplished by formation of bone at the periosteal surface and by resorption at the endosteal surface, with the rate of formation exceeding that of resorption. In adults, after the growth plates close, growth in length and endochondral bone formation cease, except for some activity in the cartilage cells beneath the articular surface. Even in adults, however, remodeling of bone (within haversian systems as well as trabecular bone) continues throughout life. In adults, ~4% of the surface of trabecular bone (such as iliac crest) is involved in active resorption, whereas 10 to 15% of trabecular surfaces is covered with osteoid. Radioisotope studies indicate that as much as 18% of the total skeletal calcium is deposited and removed each year. Thus, bone is an active metabolizing tissue that requires an intact blood supply. The cycle of bone resorption and formation is a highly orchestrated process carried out by the basic multicellular unit, composed of a group of osteoclasts and osteoblasts (Fig. 331-2).

The response of bone to fractures, infection, and interruption of blood supply and to expanding lesions is relatively limited. Dead bone must be resorbed, and new bone must be formed, a process carried out in association with growth of new blood vessels into the involved area. In injuries that disrupt the organization of the tissue, such as a fracture in which apposition of fragments is poor or when motion exists at the fracture site, the progenitor stromal cells differentiate into cells with functional capacities different from those of osteoblasts, and varying amounts of fibrous tissue and cartilage are formed. When there is good apposition with fixation and little motion at the fracture site, repair occurs predominantly by formation of new bone without other scar tissue.

Remodeling of bone occurs along lines of force generated by mechanical stress. The signals from these mechanical stresses are sensed by osteocytes, which transmit signals to osteoclasts or osteoblasts, or their precursors. A bowing deformity increases new bone formation at the concave surface and resorption at the convex surface, seemingly designed to produce the strongest mechanical structure. Expanding lesions in bone, such as tumors, induce resorption at the surface in contact with the tumor, by producing ligands, such as PTHrP, that stimulate osteoclast differentiation and function. Even in a disorder as architecturally disruptive as Paget's disease, remodeling is dictated by mechanical forces. Thus, bone plasticity reflects the interaction of cells with each other and with the environment.

FIGURE 331-2 *Schematic representation of bone remodeling. The cycle of bone remodeling is carried out by the basic multicellular unit (BMU), comprising a group of osteoclasts and osteoblasts. In cortical bone, the BMUs tunnel through the tissue, whereas in cancellous bone, they move across the trabecular surface. The process of bone remodeling is initiated by contraction of the lining cells and the recruitment of osteoclast precursors. These precursors fuse to form multinucleated, active osteoclasts that mediate bone resorption. Osteoclasts adhere to bone and subsequently remove it by acidification and proteolytic digestion. As the BMU advances, osteoclasts leave the resorption site and osteoblasts move in to cover the excavated area and begin the process of new bone formation by secreting osteoid, which is eventually mineralized into new bone. After osteoid mineralization, osteoblasts flatten and form a layer of lining cells over new bone.*

The products of osteoblast and osteoclast activity can assist in the diagnosis and management of bone diseases. Osteoblast activity can be assessed by measuring serum bone-specific alkaline phosphatase. Similarly, osteocalcin, a protein secreted from osteoblasts, is made virtually only by osteoblasts. Osteoclast activity can be assessed by measurement of products of collagen degradation. Collagen molecules are covalently linked to each other in the extracellular matrix through the formation of hydroxypyridinium crosslinks (Chap. 342). These cross-linked peptides can be measured both in urine and in blood.

CALCIUM METABOLISM

Over 99% of the 1 to 2 kg of calcium present normally in the adult human body resides in the skeleton, where it provides mechanical stability and serves as a reservoir sometimes needed to maintain extracellular fluid (ECF) calcium concentration (Fig. 331-3). Skeletal calcium accretion first becomes significant during the third trimester of fetal life, accelerates throughout childhood and adolescence, reaches a peak in early adulthood, and gradually declines thereafter at rates that rarely exceed 1 to 2% per year. These slow changes in total skeletal calcium content contrast with relatively high daily rates of closely matched fluxes of calcium into and out of bone (approximately 250 to 500 mg each), a process mediated by coupled osteoblastic and osteoclastic activity. Another 0.5 to 1% of skeletal calcium is freely exchangeable (e.g., in chemical equilibrium) with that in the ECF.

The concentration of ionized calcium in the ECF must be maintained within a narrow range because of the critical role it plays in a

FIGURE 331-3 *Calcium homeostasis. Schematic illustration of calcium content of extracellular fluid (ECF) and bone as well as of diet and feces; magnitude of calcium flux per day as calculated by various methods is shown at sites of transport in intestine, kidney, and bone. Ranges of values shown are approximate and chosen to illustrate certain points discussed in text. In conditions of calcium balance, rates of calcium release from and uptake into bone are equal.*

wide array of cellular functions, especially those involved in neuromuscular activity, secretion, and signal transduction. Intracellular cytosolic free calcium levels are approximately 100 nmol/L and are 10,000-fold lower than ionized calcium concentration in the blood and ECF (1.1 to 1.3 mmol/L). This steep chemical gradient promotes rapid calcium influx through various membrane calcium channels that can be activated by hormones, metabolites, or neurotransmitters, swiftly changing cellular function. In blood, total calcium concentration is normally 2.2 to 2.6 mM (8.5 to 10.5 mg/dL), of which approximately 50% is ionized. The remainder is bound ionically to negatively charged proteins (predominantly albumin and immunoglobulins) or loosely complexed with phosphate, citrate, sulfate, or other anions. Alterations in serum protein concentrations directly affect the total blood calcium concentration, even if the ionized calcium concentration remains normal. An algorithm to correct for protein changes adjusts the total serum calcium (in mg/dL) upward by 0.8 times the deficit in serum albumin (g/dL) or by 0.5 times the deficit in serum immunoglobulin (in g/dL). Such corrections provide only rough approximations of actual free calcium concentrations, however, and may be misleading. Acidosis also alters ionized calcium by reducing its association with proteins. The best practice is to measure blood ionized calcium directly by a method that employs calcium-selective electrodes.

Control of the ionized calcium concentration in the ECF ordinarily is accomplished by adjusting the rates of calcium movement across intestinal and renal epithelia. These adjustments are mediated mainly via changes in blood levels of the hormones PTH and 1,25(OH)₂D. Blood ionized calcium directly suppresses PTH secretion by activating parathyroid calcium-sensing receptors (CaSRs). Also, ionized calcium indirectly affects PTH secretion via effects on 1,25(OH)₂D production. This active vitamin D metabolite inhibits PTH production by an incompletely understood mechanism of negative feedback (Chap. 332).

Normal dietary calcium intake in the United States varies widely, ranging from 10 to 37 mmol/d (400 to 1500 mg/d). Many individuals, in an effort to prevent osteoporosis, routinely supplement this further with oral calcium salts to a total intake of 37 to 50 mmol/d (1500 to 2000 mg/d). Intestinal absorption of ingested calcium involves both active (transcellular) and passive (paracellular) mechanisms. Passive calcium absorption is nonsaturable and approximates 5% of daily calcium intake, whereas the active mechanism, controlled principally by 1,25(OH)₂D, normally ranges from 20 to 70%. Active calcium transport occurs mainly in the proximal small bowel (duodenum and proximal jejunum), although some active calcium absorption occurs in most segments of the small intestine. Optimal rates of calcium absorption require gastric acid. This is especially true for weakly dissociable calcium supplements such as calcium carbonate. In fact, large boluses of calcium carbonate are poorly absorbed because of their neutralizing effect upon gastric acid. In achlorhydric subjects or for those taking drugs that inhibit gastric acid secretion, supplements should be taken with meals to optimize their absorption. Use of calcium citrate may be preferable in these circumstances. Calcium absorption may also be blunted in disease states such as pancreatic or biliary insufficiency, where ingested calcium remains bound to unabsorbed fatty acids or other food constituents. At high levels of calcium intake, synthesis of 1,25(OH)₂D is reduced, which decreases the rate of active intestinal calcium absorption. The opposite occurs with dietary calcium restriction. Some calcium, approximately 2.5 to 5.0 mmol/d (100 to 200 mg/d), is excreted as an obligate component of intestinal secretions and is not regulated by calciotropic hormones.

The feedback-controlled hormonal regulation of intestinal absorptive efficiency results in a relatively constant daily net calcium absorption of approximately 5 to 7.5 mmol/d (200 to 400 mg/d), despite large changes in daily dietary calcium intake. This daily load of absorbed calcium is excreted by the kidneys in a manner that is also tightly regulated by the concentration of ionized calcium in the blood. Approximately 8 to 10 g/d of calcium are filtered by the glomeruli, of which only 2 to 3% appears in the urine. Most filtered calcium (65%) is reabsorbed in the proximal tubules via a passive, paracellular route that is coupled to concomitant NaCl reabsorption and not specifically regulated. The cortical thick ascending limb of Henle's loop (cTAL) reabsorbs roughly another 20% of filtered calcium, also via a paracellular mechanism. Calcium reabsorption in the cTAL requires a tight-junctional protein called paracellin-1 and is inhibited by increased blood concentrations of calcium or magnesium, acting via the CaSR, which is highly expressed on basolateral membranes in this nephron segment. Operation of the renal CaSR provides a mechanism, independent of those engaged directly by PTH or 1,25(OH)$_2$D, whereby serum ionized calcium can control renal calcium reabsorption. Finally, ~10% of filtered calcium is reabsorbed in the distal convoluted tubules (DCT) by a transcellular mechanism. Calcium enters the luminal surface of the cell through specific apical calcium channels, whose number is regulated. It then moves across the cell in association with a specific calcium-binding protein (calbindin-D28k) that buffers cytosolic calcium concentrations from the large mass of transported calcium. Ca^{2+}-ATPases and Na/ Ca^{2+} exchangers actively extrude calcium across the basolateral surface and thereby maintain the transcellular calcium gradient. All of these steps are increased, directly or indirectly, by PTH. The DCT is also the site of action of thiazide diuretics, which lower urinary calcium excretion by blocking a NaCl transporter expressed on the apical surface of these cells. Conversely, dietary sodium loads, or increased distal sodium delivery caused by loop diuretics or saline infusion, reduce DCT calcium reabsorption by an action opposite to that of thiazides.

The homeostatic mechanisms that normally maintain a constant serum ionized calcium concentration may fail at extremes of calcium intake or when the hormonal systems or organs involved are compromised. Thus, even with maximal activity of the vitamin D–dependent intestinal active transport system, sustained calcium intakes <5 mmol/d (<200 mg/d) cannot provide enough net calcium absorption to replace obligate losses via the intestine, kidney, sweat, or other secretions. In this case, increased blood levels of PTH and 1,25(OH)$_2$D activate osteoclastic bone resorption to obtain needed calcium from bone, which leads to progressive bone loss and negative calcium balance. Increased PTH and 1,25(OH)$_2$D also enhance renal calcium reabsorption, and 1,25(OH)$_2$D enhances calcium absorption in the gut. At very high calcium intakes [> 100 mmol/d; > 4 g/d], passive intestinal absorption continues to deliver calcium into the ECF, despite maximally downregulated intestinal active transport and renal tubular calcium reabsorption. This can cause severe hypercalciuria, nephrocalcinosis, progressive renal failure, and hypercalcemia (e.g., "milk alkali syndrome"). Deficiency or excess of PTH or vitamin D, intestinal disease, and renal failure represent other commonly encountered challenges to normal calcium homeostasis (Chap. 332).

PHOSPHORUS METABOLISM

Although 85% of the ~600 g of body phosphorus is present in bone mineral, phosphorus is also a major intracellular constituent, both as the free anion(s) and as a component of numerous organophosphate compounds including structural proteins, enzymes, transcription factors, carbohydrate and lipid intermediates, high-energy stores (ATP, creatine phosphate), and nucleic acids. Unlike calcium, phosphorus exists intracellularly at concentrations close to those present in ECF (e.g., 1 to 2 mmol/L). In cells and in the ECF, phosphorus exists in several forms, predominantly as H$_2$PO$_4$$^-$ or NaHPO$_4$$^-$, with perhaps 10% as HPO$_4$$^{2-}$. This mixture of anions will be referred to here as "phosphate." In serum, about 12% of phosphorus is bound to proteins. Concentrations of phosphates in blood and ECF are generally expressed in terms of elemental phosphorus, the normal range in adults

being 0.75 to 1.45 mmol/L (2.5 to 4.5 mg/dL). Because the volume of the intracellular fluid compartment is twice that of the ECF, measurements of ECF phosphate may not accurately reflect phosphate availability within cells that follows even modest shifts of phosphate from one compartment to the other.

Phosphate is widely available in foods and is efficiently absorbed (65%) by the small intestine, even in the absence of vitamin D. On the other hand, phosphate absorptive efficiency may be further enhanced (to 85 to 90%) via active transport mechanisms that are stimulated by 1,25(OH)$_2$D. These involve activation of Na$^+$/PO$_4$$^{2-}$ co-transporters that move phosphate into intestinal cells against an unfavorable electrochemical gradient. Daily net intestinal phosphate absorption varies widely according to the composition of the diet but is generally in the range of 500 to 1000 mg/d. Phosphate absorption can be inhibited by large doses of calcium salts or by sevelamer hydrochloride (Renagel), strategies commonly used to control levels of serum phosphate in renal failure. Aluminum hydroxide antacids also reduce phosphate absorption but are less commonly used because of the potential for aluminum toxicity. Low serum phosphate directly stimulates renal proximal tubular synthesis of 1,25(OH)$_2$D.

Serum phosphate levels vary by as much as 50% on a normal day. This reflects the effect of food intake but also an underlying circadian rhythm that produces a nadir between 7 and 10 A.M. Carbohydrate administration, especially as intravenous dextrose solutions in fasting subjects, can decrease serum phosphate by >0.7 mmol/L (2 mg/dL) due to rapid uptake into, and utilization by, cells. A similar response is observed in the treatment of diabetic ketoacidosis and during metabolic or respiratory alkalosis. Because of this wide variation in serum phosphate, it is best to perform measurements in the basal, fasting state.

Control of serum phosphate is determined mainly by the rate of renal tubular reabsorption of the filtered load, which approximates 4 to 6 g/d. Because intestinal phosphate absorption is highly efficient, urinary excretion is not constant but varies directly with dietary intake. The fractional excretion of phosphate (ratio of phosphate to creatinine clearance) is generally in the range of 10 to 15%. The proximal tubule is the principal site at which renal phosphate reabsorption is regulated. This is accomplished by changes in the apical expression and activity of a specific Na$^+$/PO$_4$$^{2-}$ co-transporter (NaPi-2) in the proximal tubule. Apical expression of NaPi-2 is rapidly reduced by PTH, the major known hormonal regulator of renal phosphate excretion. FGF23 can dramatically impair phosphate reabsorption. Activating *FGF23* mutations cause the rare disorder autosomal dominant hypophosphatemic rickets. In contrast to PTH, this molecule also leads to reduced synthesis of 1,25(OH)$_2$D, which may worsen the resulting hypophosphatemia by lowering intestinal phosphate absorption. Renal reabsorption of phosphate is responsive to changes in dietary intake, such that experimental dietary phosphate restriction leads to a dramatic lowering of urinary phosphate within hours, preceding any decline in serum phosphate (e.g., filtered load). This physiologic renal adaptation to changes in dietary phosphate availability occurs independently of PTH. Findings in *FGF23*-knockout mice suggest that FGF23 normally acts to lower blood phosphate and 1,25(OH)$_2$D levels.

Renal phosphate reabsorption is impaired by hypocalcemia, hypomagnesemia, and severe hypophosphatemia. Phosphate clearance is enhanced by ECF volume expansion and impaired by dehydration. Phosphate retention is an important pathophysiologic feature of renal insufficiency (Chap. 261).

HYPOPHOSPHATEMIA ■ Causes Hypophosphatemia can occur by one or more of three primary mechanisms: (1) inadequate intestinal phosphate absorption, (2) excessive renal phosphate excretion, or (3) rapid redistribution of phosphate from the ECF into bone or soft tissue (Table 331-1). Because phosphate is so abundant in foods, inadequate intestinal absorption is almost never observed now that aluminum hydroxide antacids, which bind phosphate in the gut, are no longer commonly

TABLE 331-1 *Causes of Hypophosphatemia*

I. Reduced renal tubular phosphate reabsorption
  A. PTH/PTHrP-dependent
    1. Primary hyperparathyroidism
    2. Secondary hyperparathyroidism
      a. Vitamin D deficiency/resistance
      b. Calcium starvation/malabsorption
      c. Bartter syndrome
      d. Autosomal recessive renal hypercalciuria with hypomagnesemia
    3. PTHrP-dependent hypercalcemia of malignancy
    4. Familial hypocalciuric hypercalcemia
  B. PTH/PTHrP-independent
    1. Genetic hypophosphatemia
      a. X-linked hypophosphatemic rickets
      b. Dent disease
      c. Autosomal dominant hypophosphatemic rickets
      d. Fanconi syndrome(s)
      e. Cystinosis
      f. Wilson disease
      g. McCune-Albright syndrome (fibrous dysplasia)
      h. Idiopathic hypercalciuria (absorptive subtype)
      i. Hereditary hypophosphatemia with hypercalciuria (Bedouins)
    2. Tumor-induced osteomalacia
    3. Other systemic disorders
      a. Poorly controlled diabetes mellitus
      b. Alcoholism
      c. Hyperaldosteronism
      d. Hypomagnesemia
      e. Amyloidosis
      f. Hemolytic uremic syndrome
      g. Renal transplantation or partial liver resection
      h. Rewarming or induced hyperthermia
    4. Drugs or toxins
      a. Ethanol
      b. Acetazolamide, other diuretics
      c. High-dose estrogens or glucocorticoids
      d. Heavy metals (lead, cadmium)
      e. Toluene, *N*-methyl formamide
      f. Cisplatin, ifosfamide, foscarnet, rapamycin
      g. Calcitonin, pamidronate
II. Impaired intestinal phosphate absorption
  A. Aluminum-containing antacids
  B. Sevalamer
III. Shifts of extracellular phosphate into cells
  A. Intravenous glucose
  B. Insulin therapy of prolonged hyperglycemia or diabetic ketoacidosis
  C. Catecholamines (epinephrine, dopamine, albuterol)
  D. Acute respiratory alkalosis
  E. Gram-negative sepsis, toxic shock syndrome
  F. Recovery from starvation or acidosis
  G. Rapid cellular proliferation
    1. Leukemic blast crisis
    2. Intensive erythropoietin, other CSF therapy
IV. Accelerated net bone formation
  A. Following parathyroidectomy
  B. Treatment of vitamin D deficiency, Paget disease
  C. Osteoblastic metastases

Note: CSF, cerebrospinal fluid.

used. Fasting or starvation, however, may result in depletion of body phosphate and predispose to subsequent hypophosphatemia during refeeding, especially if this is accomplished with intravenous glucose alone.

Chronic hypophosphatemia usually signifies a persistent renal tubular phosphate-wasting disorder. Excessive activation of PTH/PTHrP receptors in the proximal tubule, because of primary or secondary hyperparathyroidism or because of the PTHrP-mediated hypercalcemia syndrome in malignancy (Chap. 332), is among the more common causes of renal hypophosphatemia, especially because of the high prevalence of vitamin D deficiency in older Americans. Familial hypocalciuric hypercalcemia and Jansen's chondrodystrophy are rare examples of genetic disorders in this category (Chap. 332). Several genetic diseases cause PTH/PTHrP-independent tubular phosphate wasting, with associated rickets and osteomalacia. The most common of these is X-linked hypophosphatemic rickets (XLHR), which results from inactivating mutations in an endopeptidase termed *PHEX* (phosphate-regulating gene with *h*omologies to *e*ndopeptidases on the *X* chromosome) that is most abundantly expressed on the surface of mature osteoblasts. It is believed that PHEX normally inactivates a phosphaturic hormone (phosphatonin) that impairs both renal tubular phosphate reabsorption and $1,25(OH)_2D$ synthesis in the proximal renal tubules. Disorders likely to share a related pathophysiology with XLHR are autosomal dominant hypophosphatemic rickets (ADHR) and tumor-induced osteomalacia (TIO). All of these manifest severe hypophosphatemia; renal phosphate wasting, sometimes accompanied by aminoaciduria; low blood levels of $1,25(OH)_2D$; low or low-normal serum levels of calcium; and evidence of impaired cartilage or bone mineralization. ADHR results from activating mutations in the gene encoding FGF23, which is phosphaturic when administered to mice. TIO is an acquired disorder in which tumors, usually of mesenchymal origin and generally histologically benign, secrete a phosphatonin-like molecule (Chap. 87). The hypophosphatemic syndrome resolves completely within hours to days following successful resection of the responsible tumor. Such tumors express large amounts of FGF23 mRNA, raising the possibility that FGF23 may be a phosphatonin. It is not yet clear if FGF23 is a physiologic substrate for PHEX, however. Dent's disease is an X-linked recessive disorder caused by inactivating mutations in CLCN5, a chloride transporter expressed in endosomes of the proximal tubule; features include hypercalciuria, hypophosphatemia, and recurrent kidney stones. Renal phosphate wasting is common among poorly controlled diabetics and alcoholics, who therefore are at risk for iatrogenic hypophosphatemia when treated with insulin or intravenous glucose, respectively. Diuretics and certain other drugs and toxins can cause defective renal tubular phosphate reabsorption (Table 331-1).

In hospitalized patients, hypophosphatemia is often attributable to massive redistribution of phosphate from the ECF into cells. Insulin therapy of diabetic ketoacidosis is a paradigm for this phenomenon, in which the severity of the hypophosphatemia is related to the extent of antecedent depletion of phosphate and other electrolytes (Chap. 323). The hypophosphatemia is usually greatest at a point many hours after initiation of insulin therapy and is difficult to predict from baseline measurements of serum phosphate at the time of presentation, when prerenal azotemia can obscure significant phosphate depletion. Other factors that may contribute to such acute redistributive hypophosphatemia include antecedent starvation or malnutrition, administration of intravenous glucose without other nutrients, elevated blood catecholamines (endogenous or exogenous), respiratory alkalosis, and recovery from metabolic acidosis.

Hypophosphatemia can also occur transiently (over weeks to months) during the phase of accelerated net bone formation following parathyroidectomy for severe primary hyperparathyroidism or during treatment of vitamin D deficiency or lytic Paget's disease. This is usually most prominent in patients who preoperatively have evidence of high bone turnover (e.g., high serum levels of alkaline phosphatase). Osteoblastic metastases can also lead to this syndrome.

Clinical and Laboratory Findings The clinical manifestations of severe hypophosphatemia reflect a generalized defect in cellular energy metabolism because of ATP depletion, a shift from oxidative phosphorylation toward glycolysis, and associated tissue or organ dysfunction. Acute, severe hypophosphatemia occurs mainly or exclusively in hospitalized patients with underlying serious medical or surgical illness and preexisting phosphate depletion due to excessive urinary losses, severe malabsorption, or malnutrition. Chronic hypophosphatemia tends to be less severe, with a clinical presentation dominated by musculoskeletal complaints such as bone pain, pseudofractures, and proximal muscle weakness or, in children, rickets and short stature.

Neuromuscular manifestations of severe hypophosphatemia are

variable but may include muscle weakness, lethargy, confusion, disorientation, hallucinations, dysarthria, dysphagia, oculomotor palsies, anisocoria, nystagmus, ataxia, cerebellar tremor, ballismus, hyporeflexia, impaired sphincter control, distal sensory deficits, paresthesia, hyperesthesia, generalized or Guillain Barré–like ascending paralysis, seizures, coma, and death. Serious sequelae such as paralysis, confusion, and seizures are likely only at phosphate concentrations <0.25 mmol/L (< 0.8 mg/dL). Rhabdomyolysis may develop during rapidly progressive hypophosphatemia. The diagnosis of hypophosphatemia-induced rhabdomyolysis may be overlooked, as up to 30% of patients with acute hypophosphatemia (< 0.7 mM) have creatine phosphokinase elevations that peak 1 to 2 days after the nadir in serum phosphate, when the release of phosphate from injured myocytes may have led to a near-normalization of circulating levels of phosphate.

Respiratory failure and cardiac dysfunction, reversible with phosphate treatment, may occur at serum phosphate levels of 0.5 to 0.8 mmol/L (1.5 to 2.5 mg/dL). Renal tubular defects, including tubular acidosis, glycosuria, and impaired reabsorption of sodium and calcium, may occur. Hematologic abnormalities correlate with reductions in intracellular ATP and 2,3-diphosphoglycerate and may include erythrocyte microspherocytosis and hemolysis; impaired oxyhemoglobin dissociation; defective leukocyte chemotaxis, phagocytosis, and bacterial killing; and platelet dysfunction with spontaneous gastrointestinal hemorrhage.

Rx TREATMENT

Severe hypophosphatemia [< 0.75 mmol/L (< 2 mg/dL)], particularly in the setting of underlying phosphate depletion, constitutes a dangerous electrolyte abnormality that should be corrected promptly. Unfortunately, the cumulative deficit in body phosphate cannot be easily predicted from knowledge of the circulating level of phosphate, and therapy must be approached empirically. The threshold for intravenous phosphate therapy and the dose administered should reflect consideration of renal function, the likely severity and duration of the underlying phosphate depletion, and the presence and severity of symptoms consistent with those of hypophosphatemia. In adults, phosphate may be safely administered intravenously as neutral mixtures of sodium and potassium phosphate salts at initial doses of 0.2 to 0.8 mmol/kg of elemental phosphorus over 6 h (e.g., 10 to 50 mmol over 6 h), with doses >20 mmol/6 h reserved for those who have serum levels <0.5 mmol/L (1.5 mg/dL) and normal renal function. A suggested approach is presented in Table 331-2. Serum levels of phosphate and calcium must be monitored closely (every 6 to 12 h) throughout treatment. It is necessary to avoid a serum calcium-phosphorus product >50 to reduce the risk of heterotopic calcification. Hypocalcemia, if present,

should be corrected before administering intravenous phosphate. Less severe hypophosphatemia, in the range of 0.5 to 0.8 mmol/L (1.5 to 2.5 mg/dL), can usually be treated with oral phosphate in divided doses of 750 to 2000 mg/d, as elemental phosphorus; higher doses can cause bloating and diarrhea.

Management of chronic hypophosphatemia requires knowing the cause(s) of the disorder. Hypophosphatemia related to the secondary hyperparathyroidism of vitamin D deficiency usually responds to treatment with vitamin D and calcium alone. XLHR, ADHR, TIO, and related renal tubular disorders are usually managed with divided oral doses of phosphate, often with calcium and 1,25(OH)$_2$D supplements to bypass the block in renal 1,25(OH)$_2$D synthesis and prevent secondary hyperparathyroidism caused by suppression of ECF calcium levels. Thiazide diuretics may be used to prevent nephrocalcinosis in patients who are managed this way. Complete normalization of hypophosphatemia is generally not possible in these conditions. Optimal therapy of TIO is extirpation of the responsible tumor, which may be localized by radiographic skeletal survey or bone scan (many are located in bone) or by radionuclide scanning using sestamibi or labeled octreotide. Successful treatment of TIO-induced hypophosphatemia with octreotide has been reported in a small number of patients.

HYPERPHOSPHATEMIA ■ Causes When the filtered load of phosphate and glomerular filtration rate (GFR) are normal, control of serum phosphate levels is achieved by adjusting the rate at which phosphate is reabsorbed by the proximal tubular NaPi-2 co-transporter. The principal hormonal regulator of NaPi-2 activity is PTH. Hyperphosphatemia, defined in adults as a fasting serum phosphate concentration >1.8 mmol/L (5.5 mg/dL), usually results from impaired glomerular filtration, hypoparathyroidism, excessive delivery of phosphate into the ECF (from bone, gut, or parenteral phosphate therapy), or some combination of these factors (Table 331-3). The upper limit of normal serum phosphate concentrations is higher in children and neonates [2.4 mmol/L (7 mg/dL)]. It is useful to distinguish hyperphosphatemia caused by impaired renal phosphate excretion from that which results from excessive delivery of phosphate into the ECF (Table 331-3).

TABLE 331-2 Intravenous Therapy of Hypophosphatemia

Consider
- Likely severity of underlying phosphate depletion
- Concurrent parenteral glucose administration
- Presence of neuromuscular, cardiopulmonary, or hematologic complications of hypophosphatemia
- Renal function [reduce dose by 50% if serum creatinine >220 μmol/L (>2.5 mg/dL)]
- Serum calcium level (correct hypocalcemia first; reduce dose by 50% in hypercalcemia)

Guidelines

Serum Phosphorus, mM(mg/dL)	Rate of Infusion, mmol/h	Duration, h	Total Administered, mmol
<0.8 (<2.5)	2.0	6	12
<0.5 (<1.5)	4.0	6	24
<0.3 (<1.0)	8.0	6	48

Rates shown are calculated for a 70-kg person; levels of serum calcium and phosphorus must be measured every 6 to 12 h during therapy; infusions can be repeated to achieve stable serum phosphorus levels > 0.8 mmol/L (>2.5 mg/dL); most formulations available in the United States provide 3 mmol/mL of sodium or potassium phosphate.

TABLE 331-3 Causes of Hyperphosphatemia

I. Impaired renal phosphate excretion
  A. Renal insufficiency
  B. Hypoparathyroidism
    1. Developmental
    2. Autoimmune
    3. After neck surgery or radiation
    4. Activating mutations of the calcium-sensing receptor
  C. Parathyroid suppression
    1. Parathyroid-independent hypercalcemia
      a. Vitamin D or vitamin A intoxication
      b. Sarcoidosis, other granulomatous diseases
      c. Immobilization, osteolytic metastases
      d. Milk-alkali syndrome
    2. Severe hypermagnesemia or hypomagnesemia
  D. Pseudohypoparathyroidism
  E. Acromegaly
  F. Tumoral calcinosis
  G. Heparin therapy
II. Massive extracellular fluid phosphate loads
  A. Rapid administration of exogenous phosphate (intravenous, oral, rectal)
  B. Extensive cellular injury or necrosis
    1. Crush injuries
    2. Rhabdomyolysis
    3. Hyperthermia
    4. Fulminant hepatitis
    5. Cytotoxic therapy
    6. Severe hemolytic anemia
  C. Transcellular phosphate shifts
    1. Metabolic acidosis
    2. Respiratory acidosis

In chronic renal insufficiency, reduced GFR leads to phosphate retention. Hyperphosphatemia, in turn, further impairs renal synthesis of 1,25(OH)₂D and stimulates PTH secretion and hypertrophy, both directly and indirectly (by lowering blood ionized calcium levels). Thus, hyperphosphatemia is a major cause of the secondary hyperparathyroidism of renal failure and must be addressed early in the course of the disease (Chaps. 261 and 332).

Hypoparathyroidism leads to hyperphosphatemia via increased expression of NaPi-2 co-transporters in the proximal tubule. Hypoparathyroidism, or parathyroid suppression, has multiple potential causes including autoimmune disease; developmental, surgical, or radiation-induced absence of functional parathyroid tissue; vitamin D intoxication or other causes of PTH-independent hypercalcemia; cellular PTH resistance (pseudohypoparathyroidism or hypomagnesemia); infiltrative disorders such as Wilson disease and hemochromatosis; and impaired PTH secretion caused by hypermagnesemia, severe hypomagnesemia, or activating mutations in the CaSR. Hypocalcemia may also contribute directly to impaired phosphate clearance, as calcium infusion can induce hyperphosphaturia in hypoparathyroid subjects. Increased tubular phosphate reabsorption also occurs in acromegaly, during heparin administration, and in tumoral calcinosis. Tumoral calcinosis is a rare genetic disorder in which elevated serum 1,25(OH)₂D, parathyroid suppression, increased intestinal calcium absorption, and focal hyperostosis with large, lobulated periarticular heterotopic ossifications (especially at shoulders or hips) are accompanied by hyperphosphatemia. In some forms of tumoral calcinosis serum phosphorus levels are normal.

When large amounts of phosphate are rapidly delivered into the ECF, hyperphosphatemia can occur despite normal renal function. Examples include overzealous intravenous phosphate therapy, oral or rectal administration of large amounts of phosphate-containing laxatives or enemas (especially in children), extensive soft tissue injury or necrosis (crush injuries, rhabdomyolysis, hyperthermia, fulminant hepatitis, cytotoxic chemotherapy), extensive hemolytic anemia, or transcellular phosphate shifts induced by severe metabolic or respiratory acidosis.

Clinical Findings The clinical consequences of acute, severe hyperphosphatemia are due mainly to the formation of widespread calcium phosphate precipitates and resulting hypocalcemia. Thus, tetany, seizures, accelerated nephrocalcinosis (with renal failure, hyperkalemia, hyperuricemia, and metabolic acidosis), and pulmonary or cardiac calcifications (including development of acute heart block) may occur. The severity of these complications relates to the elevation of serum phosphate levels, which can reach concentrations as high as 7 mmol/L (20 mg/dL) in instances of massive soft tissue injury or tumor lysis syndrome.

℞ TREATMENT

Therapeutic options for management of severe hyperphosphatemia are limited. Volume expansion may enhance renal phosphate clearance. Aluminum hydroxide antacids or sevalamer may be helpful in chelating and limiting absorption of offending phosphate salts present in the intestine. Hemodialysis is the most effective therapeutic strategy and should be considered early in the course of severe hyperphosphatemia, especially in the setting of renal failure and symptomatic hypocalcemia.

MAGNESIUM METABOLISM

Magnesium is the major intracellular divalent cation. Normal concentrations of extracellular magnesium and calcium are crucial for normal neuromuscular activity. Intracellular magnesium forms a key complex with ATP and is an important cofactor for a wide range of enzymes, transporters, and nucleic acids required for normal cellular function, replication, and energy metabolism. The concentration of magnesium in serum is closely regulated within the range of 0.7 to 1.0 mmol/L

(1.5 to 2.0 meq/L; 1.7 to 2.4 mg/dL), of which 30% is protein-bound and another 15% is loosely complexed to phosphate and other anions. Half of the 25 g (1000 mmol) of total body magnesium is located in bone, only half of which is insoluble in the mineral phase. Almost all extraskeletal magnesium is present within cells, where the total concentration is 5 mM, 95% of which is bound to proteins and other macromolecules. Because only 1% of body magnesium resides in the ECF, measurements of serum magnesium levels may not accurately reflect the level of total body magnesium stores.

Dietary magnesium content normally ranges from 6 to 15 mmol/d (140 to 360 mg/d), of which 30 to 40% is absorbed, mainly in the jejunum and ileum. Intestinal magnesium absorptive efficiency is stimulated by 1,25(OH)₂D and can reach 70% during magnesium deprivation. Urinary magnesium excretion normally matches net intestinal absorption and is approximately 4 mmol/d (100 mg/d). Regulation of serum magnesium concentrations is achieved mainly by control of renal magnesium reabsorption. Only 20% of filtered magnesium is reabsorbed in the proximal tubule, whereas 60% is reclaimed in the cTAL and another 5 to 10% in the DCT. Magnesium reabsorption in the cTAL occurs via a paracellular route that requires both a lumen-negative potential, created by NaCl reabsorption, and the tight-junction protein, paracellin-1. Magnesium reabsorption in the cTAL is increased by PTH but inhibited by hypercalcemia or hypermagnesemia, both of which activate the CaSR in this nephron segment.

HYPOMAGNESIA ■ Causes Hypomagnesemia usually signifies substantial depletion of body magnesium stores (0.5 to 1 mmol/kg). Hypomagnesemia can result from intestinal malabsorption; protracted vomiting, diarrhea, or intestinal drainage; defective renal tubular magnesium reabsorption; or rapid shifts of magnesium from the ECF into cells, bone, or third spaces (Table 331-4). Dietary magnesium deficiency is unlikely except possibly in the setting of alcoholism. A rare genetic disorder causing selective intestinal magnesium malabsorption has been described (primary infantile hypomagnesemia). Mal-

TABLE 331-4 Causes of Hypomagnesemia

I. Impaired intestinal absorption
  A. Primary infantile hypomagnesemia
  B. Malabsorption syndromes
  C. Vitamin D deficiency
II. Increased intestinal losses
  A. Protracted vomiting/diarrhea
  B. Intestinal drainage, fistulae
III. Impaired renal tubular reabsorption
  A. Genetic magnesium-wasting syndromes
    1. Gitelman syndrome
    2. Bartter syndrome
    3. Paracellin-1 mutations
    4. Na-K-ATPase g-subunit mutations (FXYD2)
    5. Autosomal dominant, with low bone mass
  B. Acquired renal disease
    1. Tubulointerstitial disease
    2. Postobstruction, ATN (diuretic phase)
    3. Renal transplantation
  C. Drugs and toxins
    1. Ethanol
    2. Diuretics (loop, thiazide, osmotic)
    3. Cisplatin
    4. Pentamidine, foscarnet
    5. Cyclosporine
    6. Aminoglycosides, amphotericin B
  D. Other
	IV. Extracellular fluid volume expansion
	  A. Hyperaldosteronism
	  B. SIADH
	  C. Diabetes mellitus
	  D. Hypercalcemia
	  E. Phosphate depletion
	  F. Metabolic acidosis
	  G. Hyperthyroidism
	V. Rapid shifts from extracellular fluid
	  A. Intracellular redistribution
	    1. Recovery from diabetic ketoacidosis
	    2. Refeeding syndrome
	    3. Correction of respiratory acidosis
	    4. Catecholamines
	  B. Accelerated bone formation
	    1. Post parathyroidectomy
	    2. Treatment of vitamin D deficiency
	    3. Osteoblastic metastases
	  C. Other
	    1. Pancreatitis, burns, excessive sweating
	    2. Pregnancy (3rd trimester) and lactation

Note: ATN, acute tubular necrosis; SIADH, syndrome of inappropriate anti-diuretic hormone.

absorptive states, often compounded by vitamin D deficiency, can critically limit magnesium absorption and produce hypomagnesemia, despite the compensatory effects of secondary hyperparathyroidism and of hypocalcemia and hypomagnesemia to enhance cTAL magnesium reabsorption. Diarrhea or surgical drainage fluid may contain ≥ 5 mmol/L of magnesium.

Several genetic magnesium-wasting syndromes are described, including inactivating mutations of genes encoding the DCT NaCl cotransporter (Gitelman syndrome), proteins required for cTAL Na-K-Cl$_2$ transport (Bartter syndrome), paracellin-1 (autosomal recessive renal hypomagnesemia with hypercalciuria), and a DCT Na-K-ATPase γ-subunit (autosomal dominant renal hypomagnesemia with hypocalciuria). ECF expansion, hypercalcemia, and severe phosphate depletion may impair magnesium reabsorption, as can various forms of renal injury, including those caused by drugs such as cisplatin, cyclosporine, aminoglycosides, and pentamidine (Table 331-4). A rising blood concentration of ethanol directly impairs tubular magnesium reabsorption, and persistent glycosuria with osmotic diuresis leads to magnesium wasting and likely contributes to the high frequency of hypomagnesemia in poorly controlled diabetics. Magnesium depletion is aggravated by metabolic acidosis, which causes intracellular losses as well.

Hypomagnesemia due to rapid shifts of magnesium from ECF into the intracellular compartment can occur during recovery from diabetic ketoacidosis, from starvation, or from respiratory acidosis. Less acute shifts may be seen during rapid bone formation after parathyroidectomy, with treatment of vitamin D deficiency, or with osteoblastic metastases. Large amounts of magnesium may be lost with acute pancreatitis, extensive burns, protracted and severe sweating, and during pregnancy and lactation.

Clinical and Laboratory Findings Hypomagnesemia may cause generalized alterations in neuromuscular function, including tetany, tremor, seizures, muscle weakness, ataxia, nystagmus, vertigo, apathy, depression, irritability, delirium, and psychosis. Patients are usually asymptomatic when serum magnesium concentrations are >0.5 mmol/L (1 meq/L; 1.2 mg/dL), although the severity of symptoms may not correlate with serum magnesium levels. Cardiac arrhythmias may occur, including sinus tachycardia, other supraventricular tachycardias, and ventricular arrhythmias. Electrocardiographic abnormalities may include prolonged PR or QT intervals, T-wave flattening or inversion, and ST straightening. Sensitivity to digitalis toxicity may be enhanced.

Other electrolyte abnormalities often seen with hypomagnesemia, including hypocalcemia (with hypocalciuria) and hypokalemia, may not be easily corrected unless magnesium is administered as well. The hypocalcemia may be a result of concurrent vitamin D deficiency, although hypomagnesemia can cause impaired synthesis of 1,25(OH)$_2$D, cellular resistance to PTH and, at very low serum magnesium [< 0.4 mmol/L (<0.8 meq/L; < 1 mg/dL)], a defect in PTH secretion; these abnormalities are reversible with therapy.

℞ TREATMENT

Mild, asymptomatic hypomagnesemia may be treated with oral magnesium salts [MgCl$_2$, MgO, Mg(OH)$_2$] in divided doses totaling 20 to 30 mmol/d (40 to 60 meq/d). Diarrhea may occur with larger doses. More severe hypomagnesemia should be treated parenterally, preferably with intravenous MgCl$_2$, which can be administered safely as a continuous infusion of 50 mmol/d (100 meq Mg^{2+}/d) if renal function is normal. If GFR is reduced, the infusion rate should be lowered by 50 to 75%. Use of intramuscular MgSO$_4$ is discouraged; the injections are painful and provide relatively little magnesium (2 mL of 50% MgSO$_4$ supplies only 4 mmol). MgSO$_4$ may be given intravenously instead of MgCl$_2$, although the sulfate anions may bind calcium in serum and urine and aggravate hypocalcemia. Serum magnesium should be monitored at intervals of 12 to 24 h during therapy, which may continue for several days because of impaired renal conservation of magnesium (only 50 to 70% of the daily intravenous magnesium dose is retained) and delayed repletion of intracellular deficits, which may be as high as 1 to 1.5 mmol/kg (2 to 3 meq/kg).

It is important to consider the need for calcium, potassium, and phosphate supplementation in patients with hypomagnesemia. Vitamin D deficiency frequently coexists and should be treated with oral or parenteral vitamin D or 25(OH)D [but not 1,25(OH)$_2$D, which may impair tubular magnesium reabsorption, possibly via PTH suppression]. In severely hypomagnesemic patients with concomitant hypocalcemia and hypophosphatemia, administration of intravenous magnesium alone may worsen hypophosphatemia, provoking neuromuscular symptoms or rhabdomyolysis, due to rapid stimulation of PTH secretion. This is avoided by administering both calcium and magnesium.

HYPERMAGNESEMIA ■ Causes Hypermagnesemia is rarely seen in the absence of renal insufficiency, as normal kidneys can excrete large amounts (250 mmol/d) of magnesium. Mild hypermagnesemia due to excessive reabsorption in the cTAL occurs with calcium-sensing receptor mutations in familial hypocalciuric hypercalcemia and has been described in some patients with adrenal insufficiency, hypothyroidism, or hypothermia. Massive exogenous magnesium exposures, usually via the gastrointestinal tract, can overwhelm renal excretory capacity and cause life-threatening hypermagnesemia (Table 331-5). A notable example of this is prolonged retention of even normal amounts of magnesium-containing cathartics in patients with intestinal ileus, obstruction, or perforation. Extensive soft tissue injury or necrosis can also deliver large amounts of magnesium into the ECF in patients who have suffered trauma, shock, sepsis, cardiac arrest, or severe burns.

Clinical and Laboratory Findings The most prominent clinical manifestations of hypermagnesemia are vasodilation and neuromuscular blockade, which may appear at serum magnesium concentrations >2 mmol/L (> 4 meq/L; > 4.8 mg/dL). Hypotension, refractory to vasopressors or volume expansion, may be an early sign. Nausea, lethargy, and weakness may progress to respiratory failure, paralysis, and coma, with hypoactive tendon reflexes, at serum magnesium levels >4 mmol/L. Other findings may include gastrointestinal hypomotility or ileus; facial flushing; pupillary dilation; paradoxical bradycardia; prolongation of PR, QRS, and QT intervals, heart block; and, at serum magnesium levels approaching 10 mmol/L, asystole.

Hypermagnesemia, acting via the CaSR, causes hypocalcemia and hypercalciuria due to both parathyroid suppression and impaired cTAL calcium reabsorption.

℞ TREATMENT

Successful treatment of hypermagnesemia generally involves identifying and interrupting the source of magnesium and employing measures to increase magnesium clearance from the ECF. Use of magnesium-free cathartics or enemas may be helpful in clearing ingested magnesium from the gastrointestinal tract. Vigorous intravenous hydration should be attempted, if appropriate. Hemodialysis is effective and may be required in patients with significant renal insufficiency. Calcium, administered intravenously in doses of 100 to 200 mg over 1 to 2 h, has been reported to provide temporary improvement in signs and symptoms of hypermagnesemia.

TABLE 331-5 *Causes of Hypermagnesemia*

Impaired Mg excretion	Rapid Mg mobilization from
Renal failure	soft tissues
Familial hypocalciuric	Trauma
hypercalcemia	Extensive burns
Excessive Mg intake	Shock, sepsis
Cathartics	Post cardiac arrest
Intestinal obstruction/perforation	Other disorders
following magnesium ingestion	Adrenal insufficiency
Parenteral magnesium administration	Hypothyroidism
Magnesium-rich urologic irrigants	Hypothermia

The final hydroxylation required for mature hormone formation occurs in the kidney (Fig. 331-5). The 25(OH)D-1α-hydroxylase is a tightly regulated cytochrome P450–like mixed function oxidase expressed in proximal convoluted tubule cells. PTH stimulates this microsomal enzyme, whereas calcium and the product of the enzyme's action, 1,25(OH)₂D, repress it. The 25(OH)D-1α-hydroxylase is also present in epidermal keratinocytes, but keratinocyte production of 1,25(OH)₂D is not thought to contribute to circulating levels of this hormone. The 1α-hydroxylase is present in the trophoblastic layer of the placenta and is produced in the granulomas of sarcoidosis, tuberculosis, and berylliosis as well as in lymphomas. In these latter pathologic states, the activity of the enzyme is induced by interferon γ and TNF but is not regulated by calcium or 1,25(OH)₂D; therefore, hypercalcemia may occur because of elevated levels of 1,25(OH)₂D. Treatment of sarcoidosis-associated hypercalcemia with glucocorticoids, ketoconazole, or chloroquine has been shown to lower serum 1,25(OH)₂D levels.

The major pathway for inactivation of vitamin D metabolites is an additional hydroxylation step by vitamin D–24-hydroxylase, an enzyme that is expressed in most tissues. 1,25(OH)₂D, the major inducer of vitamin D–24-hydroxylase, thus promotes its own inactivation, thereby limiting its biologic effects. Polar metabolites of 1,25(OH)₂D are secreted into the bile and reabsorbed via the enterohepatic circulation. Impairment of this circulation, seen with diseases of the terminal ileum, leads to accelerated losses of vitamin D metabolites.

ACTIONS OF 1,25(OH)₂D 1,25(OH)₂D mediates its biologic effects by binding to a member of the nuclear receptor superfamily, the vitamin D receptor (VDR). This receptor belongs to the subfamily that includes the thyroid hormone receptors, the retinoid receptors, and the peroxisome proliferator–activated receptors (Chap. 317). In contrast to the

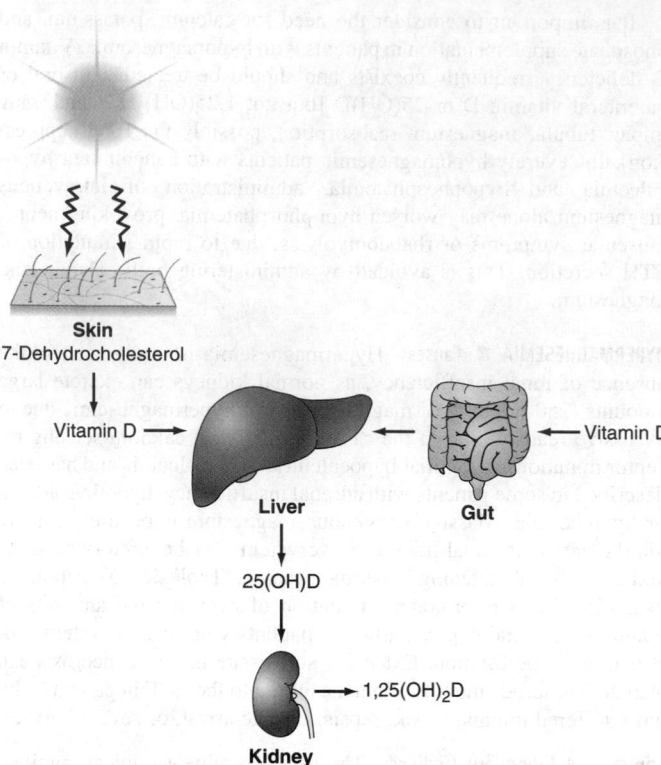

FIGURE 331-4   Vitamin D synthesis and activation. Vitamin D is synthesized in the skin in response to ultraviolet radiation and is also absorbed from the diet. It is then transported to the liver, where it undergoes 25-hydroxylation. This metabolite is the major circulating form of vitamin D. The final step in hormone activation, 1α-hydroxylation, occurs in the kidney.

VITAMIN D

SYNTHESIS AND METABOLISM   1,25-dihydroxyvitamin D [1,25(OH)₂D] is the major steroid hormone involved in mineral ion homeostasis regulation. Vitamin D and its metabolites are hormones and hormone precursors rather than vitamins, since in the proper biologic setting, they can be synthesized endogenously (Fig. 331-4). In response to ultraviolet radiation of the skin, a photochemical cleavage results in the formation of vitamin D from 7-dehydrocholesterol. Cutaneous production of vitamin D is decreased by melanin and high solar protection factor sunblocks, which effectively impair skin penetration of ultraviolet light. The increased use of sunblocks in North America and Western Europe and a reduction in the magnitude of solar exposure of the general population over the past several decades has led to an increased reliance on dietary sources of vitamin D. In the United States and Canada, these sources largely consist of fortified cereals and dairy products, in addition to fish oils and egg yolks. Vitamin D from plant sources is in the form of vitamin D₂, whereas that from animal sources is vitamin D₃. These two forms have equivalent biologic activity and are activated equally well by the vitamin D hydroxylases in humans. Vitamin D enters the circulation, whether absorbed from the intestine or synthesized cutaneously, bound to vitamin D–binding protein, an α-globulin synthesized in the liver. Vitamin D is subsequently 25-hydroxylated in the liver by cytochrome P450–like enzymes in the mitochondria and microsomes. The activity of this hydroxylase is not tightly regulated, and the resultant metabolite, 25-hydroxyvitamin D [25(OH)D], is the major circulating and storage form of vitamin D. Approximately 88% of 25(OH)D circulates bound to the vitamin D–binding protein, 0.03% is free, and the rest circulates bound to albumin. The half-life of 25(OH)D is approximately 2 to 3 weeks; however, it is dramatically shortened when vitamin D–binding protein levels are reduced, as can occur with increased urinary losses in the nephrotic syndrome.

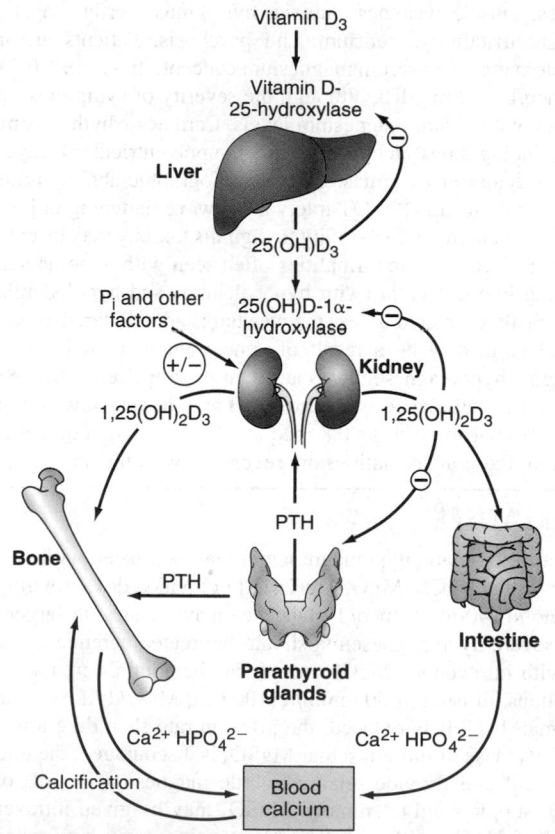

FIGURE 331-5   Schematic representation of the hormonal control loop for vitamin D metabolism and function. A reduction in the serum calcium below approximately 2.2 mmol/L (8.8 mg/dL) prompts a proportional increase in the secretion of parathyroid hormone (PTH) and so mobilizes additional calcium from the bone. PTH promotes the synthesis of 1,25(OH)₂D in the kidney, which, in turn, stimulates the mobilization of calcium from bone and intestine and regulates the synthesis of PTH by negative feedback.

other members of this subfamily, however, only one VDR isoform has been isolated. The VDR binds to target DNA sequences as a hetero-dimer with the retinoid X receptor, recruiting a series of coactivators that result in the induction of target gene expression. When the VDR causes repression of target gene expression, it either interferes with the action of activating transcription factors or recruits novel proteins to the VDR complex that cause transcriptional repression.

The affinity of the VDR for 1,25(OH)$_2$D is approximately three orders of magnitude higher than for the other vitamin D metabolites. Under normal physiologic circumstances, these other metabolites do not stimulate receptor-dependent actions. However, in states of vitamin D toxicity, the markedly elevated levels of 25(OH)D may lead to hypercalcemia by interacting directly with the VDR and by displacing 1,25(OH)$_2$D from serum vitamin D–binding protein, resulting in increased bioavailability of the active hormone.

The VDR is expressed in a wide range of cells and tissues. The molecular actions of 1,25(OH)$_2$D have been most extensively studied in tissues involved in the regulation of mineral ion homeostasis. This hormone is a major inducer of calbindin 9K, a calcium-binding protein expressed in the intestine, which is thought to play an important role in the active transport of calcium across the enterocyte. The two major calcium transporters expressed by intestinal epithelia, ECaC and ICaC, are also vitamin D responsive. By inducing the expression of these and other genes in the small intestine, 1,25(OH)$_2$D increases the efficiency of intestinal calcium absorption.

The VDR regulates the expression of several genes in osteoblasts. Target genes include the bone matrix proteins, osteocalcin and osteopontin, which are upregulated by 1,25(OH)$_2$D, in addition to type I collagen, which is transcriptionally repressed by 1,25(OH)$_2$D. 1,25(OH)$_2$D, as well as PTH, induces the expression of RANK ligand, which promotes osteoclast differentiation and increases osteoclast activity.

In the parathyroid gland, the VDR exerts antiproliferative effects on parathyroid cells and suppresses the transcription of the PTH gene. These effects of 1,25(OH)$_2$D on the parathyroid gland provide part of the rationale for current therapies directed at preventing and treating hyperparathyroidism associated with renal insufficiency.

The VDR is also expressed in tissues and organs that do not play a role in mineral ion homeostasis. Notable in this respect is the observation that 1,25(OH)$_2$D has an antiproliferative effect on several cell types, including keratinocytes, breast cancer cells, and prostate cancer cells. Alopecia is seen in humans and mice with mutant VDRs, but alopecia is not a feature of vitamin D deficiency, suggesting hormone-independent effects of the receptor.

VITAMIN D DEFICIENCY The mounting concern about the relationship between solar exposure and the development of skin cancer has led to increased reliance on dietary sources of vitamin D. Although the prevalence of vitamin D deficiency varies, the third National Health and Nutrition Examination Survey (NHANES III) revealed that vitamin D deficiency is common throughout the United States. The clinical syndrome of vitamin D deficiency can result from deficient production of vitamin D in the skin, lack of dietary intake, accelerated losses of vitamin D, impaired vitamin D activation, or resistance to the biologic effects of 1,25(OH)$_2$D (Table 331-6). The elderly and nursing home residents are particularly at risk for vitamin D deficiency, since both the efficiency of vitamin D synthesis in the skin and the absorption of vitamin D from the intestine decline with age.

Intestinal malabsorption of dietary fats can also lead to vitamin D deficiency. This is further exacerbated in the presence of terminal ileal disease, which results in impaired enterohepatic circulation of vitamin D metabolites. In addition to intestinal diseases, accelerated inactivation of vitamin D metabolites can be seen with drugs such as barbiturates, phenytoin, and rifampin, which induce hepatic cytochrome P450 mixed function oxidases. Impaired 25-hydroxylation, associated with severe liver disease or isoniazid, is an infrequent cause of vitamin D deficiency. Impaired 1α-hydroxylation is prevalent in the population with profound renal dysfunction, and therapeutic interventions should be considered in patients whose creatinine clearance is <0.5 mL/s (30 mL/min).

Mutations in the renal 1α-hydroxylase are the basis for the genetic disorder, pseudo-vitamin D–deficiency rickets. This autosomal recessive disorder presents with the syndrome of vitamin D deficiency in the first year of life. Affected children manifest growth retardation, rickets, and hypocalcemic seizures. Serum 1,25(OH)$_2$D levels are low, despite normal 25(OH)D levels and elevated PTH levels. Treatment with vitamin D metabolites that do not require 1α-hydroxylation corrects this disorder and must be continued throughout life. A second autosomal recessive disorder, hereditary vitamin D–resistant rickets, is caused by VDR mutations. Affected children present in a similar fashion during the first year of life, but alopecia often accompanies the disorder, demonstrating a functional role of the VDR in postnatal hair regeneration. Serum levels of 1,25(OH)$_2$D are dramatically elevated in these individuals, both because of increased production due to stimulation of 1α-hydroxylase activity as a consequence of secondary hyperparathyroidism and because of impaired inactivation, since induction of the 24-hydroxylase by 1,25(OH)$_2$D requires an intact VDR. Since the receptor mutation results in hormone resistance, daily calcium and phosphorus infusions may be required to bypass the defect in intestinal mineral ion absorption.

Regardless of the cause, the clinical manifestations of vitamin D deficiency are largely a consequence of impaired intestinal calcium absorption. Mild to moderate vitamin D deficiency is asymptomatic, whereas long-standing vitamin D deficiency results in hypocalcemia accompanied by secondary hyperparathyroidism, impaired mineralization of the skeleton (osteopenia on x-ray or decreased bone mineral density), and proximal myopathy. In the absence of an intercurrent illness, the hypocalcemia associated with long-standing vitamin D deficiency rarely presents with acute symptoms of hypocalcemia, such as numbness, tingling, or seizures. The concurrent development of hypomagnesemia, however, which impairs parathyroid gland function, or the administration of potent bisphosphonates, which impairs bone resorption, can lead to acute symptomatic hypocalcemia in vitamin D–deficient individuals.

RICKETS AND OSTEOMALACIA In children, prior to epiphyseal fusion, vitamin D deficiency results in growth retardation associated with an expansion of the growth plate known as *rickets*. Three layers of chondrocytes are present in the normal growth plate: the reserve zone, the proliferating zone, and the hypertrophic zone. Rickets, associated with impaired vitamin D action, is characterized by expansion of the hypertrophic chondrocyte layer. The expansion of the growth plate is thought to be a result of impaired apoptosis of the late hypertrophic chondrocytes, an event that precedes replacement of these cells by osteoblasts during endochondral bone formation. Investigations in mice lacking the VDR have demonstrated that maintenance of normal mineral ion homeostasis prevents the development of rickets. The observation that phosphate promotes chondrocyte apoptosis, combined with the presence of rickets in syndromes associated with renal phosphate wasting, suggests that hypophosphatemia, which in vitamin D deficiency is a consequence of secondary hyperparathyroidism, is a key etiologic factor in the development of the rachitic growth plate.

TABLE 331-6 Causes of Impaired Vitamin D Action	
Vitamin D deficiency	Impaired 1α-hydroxylation
Impaired cutaneous production	Hypoparathyroidism
Dietary absence	Renal failure
Malabsorption	Ketoconazole
Accelerated loss of vitamin D	1α-hydroxylase mutation
Increased metabolism (barbiturates, phenytoin, rifampin)	Oncogenic osteomalacia
	X-linked hypophosphatemic rickets
Impaired enterohepatic circulation	Target organ resistance
Impaired 25-hydroxylation	Vitamin D receptor mutation
Liver disease	Phenytoin
Isoniazid	

The hypocalcemia and hypophosphatemia that accompany vitamin D deficiency result in impaired mineralization of bone matrix, a condition known as *osteomalacia*. Osteomalacia is also a feature of long-standing hypophosphatemia, which may be a consequence of renal phosphate wasting or chronic use of etidronate or phosphate-binding antacids. This hypomineralized matrix is biomechanically inferior to normal bone and, as a result, patients with vitamin D deficiency are prone to bowing of weight-bearing extremities because of abnormal remodeling and to skeletal fractures. Vitamin D and calcium supplementation have been shown to decrease the incidence of hip fracture among ambulatory nursing home residents in France, suggesting that undermineralization of bone contributes significantly to morbidity in the elderly. Proximal myopathy is a striking feature of severe vitamin D deficiency, both in children and in adults. Rapid resolution of the myopathy is observed after vitamin D repletion.

Though vitamin D deficiency is the most common cause of rickets and osteomalacia, many disorders lead to inadequate mineralization of the growth plate and bone. Calcium deficiency without vitamin D deficiency, the disorders of vitamin D metabolism previously discussed, and hypophosphatemia can all lead to inefficient mineralization. Even in the presence of normal calcium and phosphate levels, chronic acidosis and drugs such as bisphosphonates can lead to osteomalacia. The inorganic calcium/phosphate mineral phase of bone cannot form at low pH, and bisphosphonates bind to and prevent mineral crystal growth. Since alkaline phosphatase is necessary for normal mineral deposition, probably because the enzyme can hydrolyze inhibitors of mineralization such as inorganic pyrophosphate, genetic inactivation of the alkaline phosphatase gene (hereditary hypophosphatasia) can also lead to rickets and osteomalacia in the setting of normal calcium and phosphate levels.

DIAGNOSIS OF VITAMIN D DEFICIENCY, RICKETS, AND OSTEOMALACIA The most specific screening test for vitamin D deficiency in otherwise healthy individuals is a serum 25(OH)D level. While the normal ranges vary, levels of 25(OH)D <37 nmol/L (<15 ng/mL) are associated with increasing PTH levels and lower bone density, suggesting the need to revise normative values. Vitamin D deficiency leads to impaired intestinal absorption of calcium, resulting in decreased serum total and ionized calcium levels. Hypocalcemia results in secondary hyperparathyroidism, a homeostatic response that initially maintains serum calcium levels at the expense of the skeleton. Alkaline phosphatase levels are often increased because of the PTH-induced increase in bone turnover. In addition to increasing bone resorption, PTH decreases urinary calcium excretion, while promoting phosphaturia. This results in hypophosphatemia, which exacerbates the mineralization defect in the skeleton. With prolonged vitamin D deficiency resulting in osteomalacia, calcium stores in the skeleton become relatively inaccessible, since osteoclasts cannot resorb unmineralized osteoid, and frank hypocalcemia ensues. Since PTH is a major stimulus for the renal 1α-hydroxylase, there is increased synthesis of the active hormone, 1,25(OH)$_2$D. Paradoxically, levels of this hormone may be normal in vitamin D deficiency. Measurements of 1,25(OH)$_2$D, therefore, do not provide an accurate index of vitamin D stores and should not be used to diagnose vitamin D deficiency in patients with normal renal function.

Radiologic features of vitamin D deficiency in children include a widened, expanded growth plate, characteristic of rickets. These findings are apparent not only in the long bones, but also at the costochondral junctions, where the expansion of the growth plate leads to swellings known as "rachitic rosaries." Impairment of intramembranous bone mineralization leads to delayed fusion of the calvarial sutures and a decrease in the radio-opacity of cortical bone in the long bones. If vitamin D deficiency occurs after epiphyseal fusion, the main radiologic finding is a decrease in cortical thickness and relative radiolucency of the skeleton. A specific radiologic feature of osteomalacia,

whether associated with phosphate wasting or vitamin D deficiency, is pseudofractures or Looser's zones (Fig. 331-6). These are radiolucent lines that occur where large arteries are in contact with the underlying skeletal elements; it is believed that the arterial pulsations lead to the radiolucencies. As a result, these pseudofractures are usually a few millimeters wide, several centimeters long, and are seen particularly in the scapula, the pelvis, and the femoral neck.

℞ TREATMENT

Daily intake of a multivitamin preparation that contains 400 IU of vitamin D is often insufficient to prevent vitamin D deficiency. Based on the observation that 800 IU of vitamin D, with calcium supplementation, decreases the risk of hip fractures in elderly women, 800 IU is considered to be a more appropriate daily dosage for prevention of vitamin D deficiency. The safety margin for vitamin D is large, and vitamin D toxicity is usually observed only in patients taking doses >40,000 IU daily. Treatment of vitamin D deficiency should be directed at the underlying disorder, if possible, and tailored to the severity of the condition. Vitamin D should always be repleted in conjunction with calcium supplementation since most, if not all, of the consequences of vitamin D deficiency are a result of impaired mineral ion homeostasis.

In patients whose 1α-hydroxylation is impaired, vitamin D analogues not requiring this activation step are preferred. These include dihydrotachysterol (DHT, 0.2 to 1.0 mg daily), 1,25(OH)$_2$D$_3$ [calcitriol (Rocaltrol), 0.25 to 0.5 μg daily], and 1α-hydroxyvitamin D$_2$ [doxercalciferol (Hectorol), 2.5 to 5 μg daily]. If the pathway required for activation of vitamin D is intact, severe vitamin D deficiency can be treated with pharmacologic repletion initially (50,000 IU weekly for 3 to 12 weeks), followed by maintenance therapy (800 IU daily). Pharmacologic doses may be required for maintenance therapy in patients who are taking drugs such as barbiturates or phenytoin that accelerate the metabolism of, or cause resistance to, 1,25-dihydroxyvitamin D. If intestinal malabsorption is a contributing factor, up to tenfold higher doses of vitamin D may be needed, or repletion can be performed with intramuscular vitamin D (250,000 IU biannually). Calcium supplementation should include 1.5 to 2.0 g of elemental calcium daily. Normocalcemia is usually observed within 1 week of institution of therapy, although increases in PTH and alkaline phosphatase levels may persist for 3 to 6 months.

FIGURE 331-6 Radiograph of the scapula of a 58-year-old woman with phosphaturia as a cause of osteomalacia. The presence of a pseudofracture or Looser's zone is indicated by an arrow.

The most efficacious methods to monitor treatment and resolution of vitamin D deficiency are serum and urinary calcium measurements. For patients who are vitamin D replete and are taking adequate calcium supplementation, the 24-h urinary calcium excretion should be in the range of 100 to 250 mg/24 h. Lower levels suggest problems with adhering to the treatment regimen or with absorption of calcium or vitamin D supplements. The 25(OH)D level can be remeasured to address the latter, although the half-life of this metabolite is long (3 weeks) and levels may continue to increase for many months on a stable regimen. Urinary calcium excretion >250 mg/24 h predisposes to nephrolithiasis and should prompt a reduction in vitamin D dosage and/or calcium supplementation.

FURTHER READING

MANOLAGAS SC: Birth and death of bone cells: Basic regulatory mechanisms and implications for the pathogenesis and treatment of osteoporosis. Endocr Rev 21:115, 2000

SHIMADA T et al: Cloning and characterization of FGF23 as a causative factor of tumor-induced osteomalacia. Proc Natl Acad Sci USA 98:6500, 2001

SUDA T et al: Modulation of osteoclast differentiation and function by the new members of the tumor necrosis factor receptor and ligand families. Endocr Rev 20:345, 1999

THOMAS MK, DEMAY MB: Vitamin D deficiency and disorders of vitamin D metabolism. Endocrinol Metab Clin North Am 29:611, 2000

WAGNER EF, KARSENTY G: Genetic control of skeletal development. Curr Opin Genet Dev 11:527, 2001

332 DISEASES OF THE PARATHYROID GLAND AND OTHER HYPER- AND HYPOCALCEMIC DISORDERS

John T. Potts, Jr

The four parathyroid glands are located posterior to the thyroid gland. They produce parathyroid hormone (PTH), which is the primary regulator of calcium physiology. PTH acts directly on bone, where it induces calcium resorption, and on the kidney, where it stimulates calcium reabsorption and synthesis of 1,25-dihydroxyvitamin D [1,25(OH)$_2$D], a hormone that stimulates gastrointestinal calcium absorption. Serum PTH levels are tightly regulated by a negative feedback loop. Calcium, acting through the calcium-sensing receptor, and vitamin D, acting through its nuclear receptor, inhibit PTH release and synthesis. Understanding the hormone pathways that regulate calcium levels and bone metabolism is essential for effective diagnosis and management of a wide array of hyper- and hypocalcemic disorders.

Hyperparathyroidism, characterized by excess production of PTH, is a common cause of hypercalcemia and is usually the result of autonomously functioning adenomas or hyperplasia. Surgery for this disorder is highly effective and has been shown to reverse some of the deleterious effects of long-standing PTH excess on bone density. Hypercalcemia of malignancy is also common and is usually due to the overproduction of parathyroid hormone–related peptide (PTHrP) by cancer cells. The similarities in the biochemical characteristics of hyperparathyroidism and hypercalcemia of malignancy, first noted by Albright in 1941, are now known to reflect the actions of PTH and PTHrP through the same G protein–coupled PTH/PTHrP receptor.

The genetic basis of multiple endocrine neoplasia (MEN) types 1 and 2, familial hypocalciuric hypercalcemia (FHH), the different forms of pseudohypoparathyroidism (PHP), Jansen's syndrome, disorders of vitamin D synthesis and action, and the molecular events associated with parathyroid gland neoplasia have provided new insights into calcium metabolism. The advent of new drugs, including bisphosphonates and selective estrogen receptor modulators (SERMs), offers new avenues for the treatment and prevention of metabolic bone disease. PTH analogues are promising therapeutic agents for the treatment of postmenopausal or senile osteoporosis, and calcimimetic agents, which act through the calcium-sensing receptor, may provide new approaches for PTH suppression.

PARATHYROID HORMONE

PHYSIOLOGY The primary function of PTH is to maintain the extracellular fluid (ECF) calcium concentration within a narrow normal range. The hormone acts directly on bone and kidney and indirectly on intestine through its effects on synthesis of 1,25(OH)$_2$D to increase serum calcium concentrations; in turn, PTH production is closely regulated by the concentration of serum ionized calcium. This feedback system is the critical homeostatic mechanism for maintenance of ECF calcium. Any tendency toward hypocalcemia, as might be in-

duced by calcium-deficient diets, is counteracted by an increased secretion of PTH. This in turn (1) increases the rate of dissolution of bone mineral, thereby increasing the flow of calcium from bone into blood; (2) reduces the renal clearance of calcium, returning more of the calcium filtered at the glomerulus into ECF; and (3) increases the efficiency of calcium absorption in the intestine by stimulating the production of 1,25(OH)$_2$D. Immediate control of blood calcium is due to PTH effects on bone and, to a lesser extent, on renal calcium clearance. Maintenance of steady-state calcium balance, on the other hand, probably results from the effects of 1,25(OH)$_2$D on calcium absorption (Chap. 331). The renal actions of the hormone are exerted at multiple sites and include inhibition of phosphate transport (proximal tubule), increased reabsorption of calcium (distal tubule), and stimulation of the renal 25(OH)D-1α-hydroxylase. As much as 12 mmol (500 mg) calcium is transferred between the ECF and bone each day (a large amount in relation to the total ECF calcium pool), and PTH has a major effect on this transfer. The homeostatic role of the hormone can preserve calcium concentration in blood at the cost of bone destruction.

PTH has multiple actions on bone, some direct and some indirect. PTH-mediated changes in bone calcium release can be seen within minutes. The chronic effects of PTH are to increase the number of bone cells, both osteoblasts and osteoclasts, and to increase the remodeling of bone; these effects are apparent within hours after the hormone is given and persist for hours after PTH is withdrawn. Continuous exposure to elevated PTH (as in hyperparathyroidism or long-term infusions in animals) leads to increased osteoclast-mediated bone resorption. However, the intermittent administration of PTH, elevating hormone levels for 1 to 2 h each day, leads to a net stimulation of bone formation rather than bone breakdown. Striking increases, especially in trabecular bone in the spine and hip, have been reported with the use of PTH in combination with estrogen. PTH as monotherapy caused a highly significant reduction in fracture incidence in a worldwide placebo-controlled trial.

Osteoblasts (or stromal cell precursors), which have PTH receptors, are crucial to this bone-forming effect of PTH; osteoclasts, which mediate bone breakdown, lack PTH receptors. PTH-mediated stimulation of osteoclasts is believed to be indirect, acting in part through cytokines released from osteoblasts to activate osteoclasts; in experimental studies of bone resorption in vitro, osteoblasts must be present for PTH to activate osteoclasts to resorb bone (Chap. 331).

STRUCTURE PTH is an 84-amino-acid single-chain peptide. The amino acid portion, PTH(1–34), is highly conserved and is critical for the biologic actions of the molecule. Modified synthetic fragments of the amino-terminal sequence as small as PTH(1–11) are sufficient to activate the major receptor (see below). The carboxyl-terminal region of

PTH binds to a separate receptor (cPTH-R), but it has not yet been cloned. Fragments shortened at the amino terminus bind to cPTH-R and inhibit the actions of the full-length PTH(1–84) or the PTH(1–34) active fragments.

BIOSYNTHESIS, SECRETION, AND METABOLISM ■ **Synthesis** Parathyroid cells have multiple methods of adapting to increased needs for PTH production. Most rapid (within minutes) is secretion of preformed hormone in response to hypocalcemia. Second, within hours, PTH mRNA expression is induced by sustained hypocalcemia. Finally, protracted challenge leads within days to cellular replication to increase gland mass.

PTH is initially synthesized as a larger molecule (preproparathyroid hormone, consisting of 115 amino acids), which is then reduced in size by a second cleavage (proparathyroid hormone, 90 amino acids) before secretion as the 84-amino-acid peptide. In one kindred with hypoparathyroidism, a mutation in the preprotein region of the gene interferes with hormone transport and secretion.

Transcriptional suppression of the PTH gene by calcium is nearly maximal at physiologic calcium concentrations. Hypocalcemia increases transcriptional activity within hours. $1,25(OH)_2D_3$ strongly suppresses PTH gene transcription. In patients with renal failure, intravenous administration of supraphysiologic levels of $1,25(OH)_2D_3$ or analogues of the active metabolite can dramatically suppress PTH overproduction, which is sometimes difficult to control due to severe secondary hyperparathyroidism. Regulation of proteolytic destruction of preformed hormone (posttranslational regulation of hormone production) is an important mechanism for mediating rapid (minutes) changes in hormone availability. High calcium increases and low calcium inhibits the proteolytic destruction of hormone stores.

Regulation of PTH Secretion PTH secretion increases steeply to a maximum value of five times the basal rate of secretion as calcium concentration falls from normal to the range of 1.9 to 2.0 mmol/L (7.5 to 8.0 mg/dL) (measured as total calcium). The ionized fraction of blood calcium is the important determinant of hormone secretion. Severe intracellular magnesium deficiency impairs PTH secretion (see below).

ECF calcium controls PTH secretion by interaction with a calcium sensor, a G protein–coupled receptor (GPCR) for which Ca^{2+} ions act as the ligand (see below). This receptor is a member of a distinctive subfamily of the GPCR superfamily that is characterized by a large extracellular domain suitable for "clamping" the small-molecule ligand. Stimulation of the receptor by high calcium levels suppresses PTH secretion. The receptor is present in parathyroid glands and the calcitonin-secreting cells (C cells) of the thyroid, as well as in other sites such as brain and kidney. Genetic evidence has revealed a key biologic role for the calcium-sensing receptor in parathyroid gland responsiveness to calcium and in renal calcium clearance. Point mutations associated with loss of function cause a syndrome FHH resembling hyperparathyroidism but with hypocalciuria. On the other hand, gain-of-function mutations cause a form of hypocalcemia resembling hypoparathyroidism (see below).

Metabolism The secreted form of PTH is indistinguishable by immunologic criteria and by molecular size from the 84-amino-acid peptide (PTH 1–84) extracted from glands. However, much of the immunoreactive material found in the circulation is smaller than the extracted or secreted hormone. The principal circulating fragments of immunoreactive hormone lack a portion of the critical amino-terminal sequence required for biologic activity and, hence, are biologically inactive fragments (so-called middle- and carboxyl-terminal fragments). Much of the proteolysis of hormone occurs in the liver and kidney. Peripheral metabolism of PTH does not appear to be regulated by physiologic states (high versus low calcium, etc.); hence peripheral metabolism of hormone, although responsible for rapid clearance of secreted hormone, appears to be a high-capacity, metabolically invariant catabolic process.

The rate of clearance of the secreted 84-amino-acid peptide from blood is more rapid than the rate of clearance of the biologically inactive fragment(s) corresponding to the middle- and carboxyl-terminal regions of PTH. Consequently, the interpretation of PTH immunoassays is influenced by the nature of the peptide fragments detected by the antibodies.

Although the problems inherent in PTH measurements have been largely circumvented by use of double-antibody assays that detect only the intact molecule, new evidence has revealed the existence of a hitherto unappreciated larger PTH fragment that may affect the interpretation of most currently available double-antibody assays. A large amino-terminally truncated form of PTH, possibly PTH(7–84), is present in normal and uremic individuals in addition to PTH(1–84). The concentration of the putative (7–84) fragment relative to that of intact PTH(1–84) is higher with induced hypercalcemia than in cucalcemic or hypocalcemic conditions and is higher in patients with renal failure. Growing evidence suggests that the PTH(7–84)-like amino-terminally truncated fragments can act as an inhibitor of PTH action and may be of clinical significance, particularly in renal failure. Efforts to prevent secondary hyperparathyroidism by a variety of measures (vitamin D analogues, higher calcium intake, and phosphate-lowering strategies) may have led to oversuppression of biologically active intact PTH since the amino-terminally truncated PTH reacts in many first-generation double-antibody PTH assays. The role, if any, of excessive PTH suppression due to inaccurate measurement of PTH in adynamic bone disease in renal failure (see below) is unknown. Newer assays with extreme amino-terminal epitopes that detect only full-length PTH(1–84) are being studied intensively.

PARATHYROID HORMONE–RELATED PROTEIN

The paracrine factor termed *PTHrP* is responsible for most instances of hypercalcemia of malignancy (Chap. 86), a syndrome that resembles hyperparathyroidism. Many different cell types produce PTHrP, including brain, pancreas, heart, lung, mammary tissue, placenta, endothelial cells, and smooth muscle. In fetal animals, PTHrP directs transplacental calcium transfer, and high concentrations of PTHrP are produced in mammary tissue and secreted into milk. Human and bovine milk contain very high concentrations of the hormone, the biologic significance of which is unknown. PTHrP may also play a role in uterine contraction and other biologic functions.

PTH and PTHrP, although distinctive products of different genes, exhibit considerable functional and structural homology (Fig. 332-1) and may have evolved from a shared ancestral gene. The structure of the gene for human PTHrP, however, is more complex than that of PTH, containing multiple exons and multiple sites for alternate splicing patterns during formation of the mature mRNA. Protein products of 141, 139, and 173 amino acids are produced, and other molecular forms may result from tissue-specific degradation at accessible internal cleavage sites. The biologic roles of these various molecular species and the nature of the circulating forms of PTHrP are unclear. It is uncertain whether PTHrP circulates at any significant level in adults; as a paracrine factor, PTHrP may be produced, act, and be destroyed locally within tissues. In adults PTHrP appears to have little influence on calcium homeostasis, except in disease states, when large tumors, especially of the squamous cell type, lead to massive overproduction of the hormone.

PTH AND PTHrP HORMONE ACTION Both PTH and PTHrP bind to and activate the PTH/PTHrP receptor. The 500-amino-acid PTH/PTHrP receptor (also known as the PTH-1 receptor, PTH1R) belongs to a subfamily of GPCRs that includes those for glucagon, secretin, and vasoactive intestinal peptide. The extracellular regions are involved in hormone binding, and the intracellular domains, after hormone activation, bind G protein subunits to transduce hormone signaling into cellular responses through stimulation of second messengers. A second receptor that binds PTH, termed the *PTH-2 receptor* (PTH2R), is expressed in brain, pancreas, and several other tissues. PTH1R responds equivalently to PTH and PTHrP, whereas PTH2R responds only to PTH. The endogenous ligand of this receptor is now believed to be a hPTH H-ALA VAL SER GLU ILE GLN LEU MET HIS ASN LEU GLY LYS HIS LEU –ASN SER MET GLU ARG VAL GLU TRP LEU ARG LYS LYS LEU GLN ASP

hPTHrp – – – – HIS – – LEU – ASP LYS – – SER ILE GLN ___ LEU ARG ___ ARG PHE PHE ___ HIS HIS LEU ILE ALA GLU

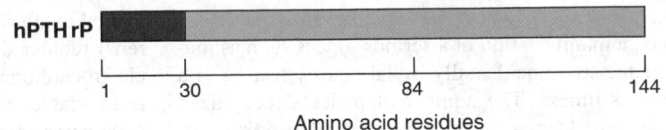

Amino acid residues   Amino acid residues

FIGURE 332-1 Schematic diagram to illustrate similarities and differences in structure of human parathyroid hormone (PTH) and human PTH-related peptide (PTHrP). Close structural (and functional) homology exists between the first 30 amino acids of hPTH and hPTHrP. The PTHrP sequence may be ≥144 amino acid residues in length. PTH is only 84 residues long; after residue 30, there is little structural homology between the two. Dashed lines in the PTHrP sequence indicate identity; underlined residues, although different from those of PTH, still represent conservative changes (charge or polarity preserved). Eleven amino acids are identical, and a total of 21 of 30 are homologues.

peptide distinct from PTH, a 39-amino-acid hypothalamic peptide (*tubular infundibular peptide*, TIP-39). PTH1R and PTH2R can be traced backward in evolutionary time to fish. Zebrafish PTH1R and PTH2R exhibit the same selective responses to PTH and PTHrP as do human PTH1R and PTH2R. The evolutionary conservation of structure and function suggests unique biologic roles for these receptors.

Studies using cloned PTH1R confirm that it can be coupled to more than one G protein and second-messenger kinase pathway, apparently explaining the multiplicity of pathways stimulated by PTH. Stimulation of protein kinases (A and C) and calcium transport channels is associated with a variety of hormone-specific tissue responses. These responses include inhibition of phosphate and bicarbonate transport, stimulation of calcium transport, and activation of renal 1α-hydroxylase in the kidney. The responses in bone include effects on collagen synthesis; increased alkaline phosphatase, ornithine decarboxylase, citrate decarboxylase, and glucose-6-phosphate dehydrogenase activities; DNA, protein, and phospholipid synthesis; and calcium and phosphate transport. Ultimately, these biochemical events lead to an integrated hormonal response in bone turnover and calcium homeostasis. PTH also activates Na^+/Ca^{2+} exchanges in renal distal tubular sites and stimulates translocation of preformed calcium transport channels, moving them from the interior to the apical surface to mediate increased tubular uptake of calcium. PTH-dependent stimulation of phosphate excretion (blocking reabsorption—the opposite effect from actions on calcium in the kidney) involves the sodium-dependent phosphate cotransporter, NPT-2, lowering its apical membrane content (and therefore function). Similar shifts may be involved in other renal tubular transport effects of PTH.

PTHrP exerts important developmental influences on fetal bone development and in adult physiology. A homozygous knockout of the PTHrP gene (or the gene for the PTH receptor) in mice causes a lethal deformity in which animals are born with severe skeletal deformities resembling chondrodysplasia (Fig. 332-2).

CALCITONIN (See also Chap. 330)

Calcitonin is a hypocalcemic peptide hormone that in several mammalian species acts as an antagonist to PTH. Calcitonin seems to be of limited physiologic significance in humans, however, at least in calcium homeostasis. It is of medical significance because of its role as a tumor marker in sporadic and hereditary cases of medullary carcinoma and its medical use as an adjunctive treatment in severe hypercalcemia and in Paget's disease of bone.

The hypocalcemic activity of calcitonin is accounted for primarily by inhibition of osteoclast-mediated bone resorption and secondarily by stimulation of renal calcium clearance. These effects are mediated by receptors on osteoclasts and renal tubular cells. Calcitonin exerts additional effects through receptors present in brain, gastrointestinal tract, and the immune system. The hormone, for example, exerts analgesic effects directly on cells in the hypothalamus and related structures, possibly by interacting with receptors for related peptide hormones, such as calcitonin gene–related peptide (CGRP) or amylin. The latter ligands have specific high-affinity receptors and can also bind to and trigger calcitonin receptors. The calcitonin receptors are homologous in structure to PTH1R.

The thyroid is the major source of the hormone, and the cells involved in calcitonin synthesis arise from neural crest tissue. During embryogenesis, these cells migrate into the ultimobranchial body, derived from the last branchial pouch. In submammalian vertebrates, the ultimobranchial body constitutes a discrete organ, anatomically separate from the thyroid gland; in mammals, the ultimobranchial gland fuses with and is incorporated into the thyroid gland.

The naturally occurring calcitonins consist of a peptide chain of 32 amino acids. There is considerable sequence variability among species. Calcitonin from salmon, which is used therapeutically, is 10 to 100 times more potent than mammalian forms in lowering serum calcium.

There are two calcitonin genes, α and β; the transcriptional control of these genes is complex. Two different mRNA molecules are transcribed from the α gene; one is translated into the precursor for calcitonin, and the other message is translated into an alternative product, CGRP. CGRP is synthesized wherever the calcitonin mRNA is expressed, e.g., in medullary carcinoma of the thyroid. The β, or CGRP-2, gene is transcribed into the mRNA for CGRP in the central nervous system (CNS); this gene does not produce calcitonin, however. CGRP has cardiovascular actions and may serve as a neurotransmitter or play a developmental role in the CNS.

The circulating level of calcitonin in humans is lower than that in many other species. In humans, even extreme variations in calcitonin production do not change calcium and phosphate metabolism; no definite effects are attributable to calcitonin deficiency (totally thyroidectomized patients receiving only replacement thyroxine) or excess (patients with medullary carcinoma of the thyroid, a calcitonin-secreting tumor) (Chap. 330). Calcitonin has been a useful pharmacologic agent to suppress bone resorption in Paget's disease (Chap. 334) and osteoporosis (Chap. 333) and in the treatment of hypercalcemia

FIGURE 332-2 Dual role for the actions of the PTH/PTHrP receptor (PTH1R). Parathyroid hormone (PTH; endocrine-calcium homeostasis) and PTH-related peptide (PTHrP; paracrine—multiple tissue actions including growth plate cartilage in developing bone) use the single receptor for their disparate functions mediated by the amino-terminal 30 residues of either peptide. Other regions of both ligands interact with other receptors (not shown).

of malignancy (see below). However, the physiologic role, if any, of calcitonin in humans is uncertain.

HYPERCALCEMIA

Hypercalcemia can be a manifestation of a serious illness such as malignancy or can be detected coincidentally by laboratory testing in a patient with no obvious illness. The number of patients recognized with asymptomatic hypercalcemia, usually hyperparathyroidism, increased in the late twentieth century but is now declining somewhat, perhaps due to decreased use of routine blood calcium measurements or for other unknown reasons.

Whenever hypercalcemia is confirmed, a definitive diagnosis must be established. Although hyperparathyroidism, a frequent cause of asymptomatic hypercalcemia, is a chronic disorder in which manifestations, if any, may be expressed only after months or years, hypercalcemia can also be the earliest manifestation of malignancy, the second most common cause of hypercalcemia in the adult. The causes of hypercalcemia are numerous (Table 332-1), but hyperparathyroidism and cancer account for 90% of cases.

Before undertaking a diagnostic workup, it is essential to be sure that true hypercalcemia, not a false-positive laboratory test, is present. A false-positive diagnosis of hypercalcemia is usually the result of inadvertent hemoconcentration during blood collection or elevation in serum proteins such as albumin. Hypercalcemia is a chronic problem, and it is cost-effective to obtain several serum calcium measurements; these tests need not be in the fasting state.

Clinical features are helpful in differential diagnosis. Hypercalcemia in an adult who is asymptomatic is usually due to primary hyperparathyroidism. In malignancy-associated hypercalcemia the disease is usually not occult; rather, symptoms of malignancy bring the patient to the physician, and hypercalcemia is discovered during the evaluation. In such patients the interval between detection of hypercalcemia and death is often <6 months. Accordingly, if an asymptomatic individual has had hypercalcemia or some manifestation of hypercalcemia, such as kidney stones, for >1 or 2 years, it is unlikely that malignancy is the cause. Nevertheless, differentiating primary hyperparathyroidism from *occult* malignancy can occasionally be difficult, and careful evaluation is required, particularly when the duration of the hypercalcemia is unknown. Hypercalcemia not due to hyperparathyroidism or malignancy can result from excessive vitamin D action, high bone turnover from any of several causes, or from renal

---

TABLE 332-1 *Classification of Causes of Hypercalcemia*

I. Parathyroid-related
   A. Primary hyperparathyroidism
      1. Solitary adenomas
      2. Multiple endocrine neoplasia
   B. Lithium therapy
   C. Familial hypocalciuric hypercalcemia
II. Malignancy-related
   A. Solid tumor with metastases (breast)
   B. Solid tumor with humoral mediation of hypercalcemia (lung, kidney)
   C. Hematologic malignancies (multiple myeloma, lymphoma, leukemia)
III. Vitamin D–related
   A. Vitamin D intoxication
   B. ↑ 1,25(OH)$_2$D; sarcoidosis and other granulomatous diseases
   C. Idiopathic hypercalcemia of infancy
IV. Associated with high bone turnover
   A. Hyperthyroidism
   B. Immobilization
   C. Thiazides
   D. Vitamin A intoxication
V. Associated with renal failure
   A. Severe secondary hyperparathyroidism
   B. Aluminum intoxication
   C. Milk-alkali syndrome

---

failure (Table 332-1). Dietary history and a history of ingestion of vitamins or drugs are often helpful in diagnosing some of the less frequent causes. PTH immunoassays based on double-antibody methods serve as the principal laboratory test in differential diagnosis.

Hypercalcemia from any cause can result in fatigue, depression, mental confusion, anorexia, nausea, vomiting, constipation, reversible renal tubular defects, increased urination, a short QT interval in the electrocardiogram, and, in some patients, cardiac arrhythmias. There is a variable relation from one patient to the next between the severity of hypercalcemia and the symptoms. Generally, symptoms are more common at calcium levels >2.9 to 3 mmol/L (11.5 to 12.0 mg/dL), but some patients, even at this level, are asymptomatic. When the calcium level is >3.2 mmol/L (13 mg/dL), calcification in kidneys, skin, vessels, lungs, heart, and stomach occurs and renal insufficiency may develop, particularly if blood phosphate levels are normal or elevated due to impaired renal function. Severe hypercalcemia, usually defined as ≥3.7 to 4.5 mmol/L (15 to 18 mg/dL), can be a medical emergency; coma and cardiac arrest can occur.

Acute management of the hypercalcemia is usually successful. The type of treatment is based on the severity of the hypercalcemia and the nature of associated symptoms, as outlined below.

PRIMARY HYPERPARATHYROIDISM ■ **Natural History and Incidence** Primary hyperparathyroidism is a generalized disorder of calcium, phosphate, and bone metabolism due to an increased secretion of PTH. The elevation of circulating hormone usually leads to hypercalcemia and hypophosphatemia. There is great variation in the manifestations. Patients may present with multiple signs and symptoms, including recurrent nephrolithiasis, peptic ulcers, mental changes, and, less frequently, extensive bone resorption. However, with greater awareness of the disease and wider use of multiphasic screening tests, including measurements of blood calcium, the diagnosis is frequently made in patients who have no symptoms and minimal, if any, signs of the disease other than hypercalcemia and elevated levels of PTH. The manifestations may be subtle, and the disease may have a benign course for many years or a lifetime. This milder form of the disease is usually termed *asymptomatic hyperparathyroidism*. Rarely, hyperparathyroidism develops or worsens abruptly and causes severe complications, such as marked dehydration and coma, so-called hypercalcemic parathyroid crisis.

The annual incidence of the disease is calculated to be as high as 0.2% in patients >60, with an estimated prevalence, including undiscovered asymptomatic patients, of ≥1%; some reports suggest the incidence may be declining, perhaps reflecting earlier overestimates. The disease has a peak incidence between the third and fifth decades but occurs in young children and in the elderly.

Etiology ■ *SOLITARY ADENOMAS* The cause of hyperparathyroidism is one or more hyperfunctioning glands. A single abnormal gland is the cause in ~80% of patients; the abnormality in the gland is usually a benign neoplasm or adenoma and rarely a parathyroid carcinoma. Some surgeons and pathologists report that the enlargement of multiple glands is common; double adenomas are reported. In ~15% of patients, all glands are hyperfunctioning; *chief cell parathyroid hyperplasia* is usually hereditary and frequently associated with other endocrine abnormalities.

MULTIPLE ENDOCRINE NEOPLASIA Hereditary hyperparathyroidism can occur without other endocrine abnormalities but is usually part of a *multiple endocrine neoplasia* syndrome (Chap. 330). MEN 1 (Wermer's syndrome) consists of hyperparathyroidism and tumors of the pituitary and pancreas, often associated with gastric hypersecretion and peptic ulcer disease (Zollinger-Ellison syndrome). MEN 2A is characterized by pheochromocytoma and medullary carcinoma of the thyroid, as well as hyperparathyroidism; MEN 2B has additional associated features such as multiple neuromas but usually lacks hyperparathyroidism. Each of these MEN syndromes is transmitted in an apparent autosomal dominant manner, although, as noted below, the genetic basis does not always involve a dominant allele.

Pathology Adenomas are most often located in the inferior parathyroid glands, but in 6 to 10% of patients, parathyroid adenomas may be located in the thymus, the thyroid, the pericardium, or behind the esophagus. Adenomas are usually 0.5 to 5 g in size but may be as large as 10 to 20 g (normal glands weigh 25 mg on average). Chief cells are predominant in both hyperplasia and adenoma. With chief cell hyperplasia, the enlargement may be so asymmetric that some involved glands appear grossly normal. If generalized hyperplasia is present, however, histologic examination reveals a uniform pattern of chief cells and disappearance of fat even in the absence of an increase in gland weight. Thus, microscopic examination of biopsy specimens of several glands is essential to interpret findings at surgery.

Parathyroid carcinoma is usually not aggressive. Long-term survival without recurrence is common if at initial surgery the entire gland is removed without rupture of the capsule. Recurrent parathyroid carcinoma is usually slow-growing with local spread in the neck, and surgical correction of recurrent disease may be feasible. Occasionally, however, parathyroid carcinoma is more aggressive, with distant metastases (lung, liver, and bone) found at the time of initial operation. It may be difficult to appreciate initially that a primary tumor is carcinoma; increased numbers of mitotic figures and increased fibrosis of the gland stroma may precede invasion. The diagnosis of carcinoma is often made in retrospect. Hyperparathyroidism from a parathyroid carcinoma may be indistinguishable from other forms of primary hyperparathyroidism; a potential clue to the diagnosis, however, is provided by the degree of calcium elevation. Calcium values of 3.5 to 3.7 mmol/L (14 to 15 mg/dL) are frequent with carcinoma and may alert the surgeon to remove the abnormal gland with care to avoid capsular rupture.

GENETIC CONSIDERATIONS **Defects Associated with Hyperparathyroidism** As in many other types of neoplasia, two fundamental types of genetic defects have been identified in parathyroid gland tumors: (1) overactivity of protooncogenes, and (2) loss of function of tumor-suppressor genes. The former, by definition, can lead to uncontrolled cellular growth and function by activation (gain-of-function mutation) of a single allele of the responsible gene, whereas the latter requires loss of function of both allelic copies.

Mutations in the *MENIN* gene locus on chromosome 11q13 are responsible for causing MEN 1; the normal allele of this gene fits the definition of a tumor-suppressor gene. A mutation of one allele is inherited; loss of the other allele via somatic cell mutation leads to monoclonal expansion and tumor development. In ~20% of sporadic parathyroid adenomas, the *MENIN* locus on chromosome 11 is deleted, implying that the same defect responsible for MEN 1 can also cause the sporadic disease (Fig. 332-3*A*). Consistent with the Knudson hypothesis for two-step neoplasia in certain inherited cancer syndromes (Chap. 68), the earlier onset of hyperparathyroidism in the hereditary syndromes reflects the need for only one mutational event to trigger the monoclonal outgrowth. In sporadic adenomas, typically occurring later in life, two different somatic events must occur before the *MENIN* gene is silenced.

Other presumptive antioncogenes involved in hyperparathyroidism include a gene mapped to chromosome 1p seen in 40% of sporadic parathyroid adenomas and a gene mapped to chromosome Xp11 in patients with secondary hyperparathyroidism and renal failure, who progressed to "tertiary" hyperparathyroidism, now known to reflect monoclonal outgrowths within previously hyperplastic glands.

The *Rb* gene, a tumor-suppressor gene located on chromosome 13q14, was initially associated with retinoblastomas but has since been implicated in many other forms of neoplasia including parathyroid carcinoma. Allelic deletion (with a presumed point mutation in the second allele) has been identified in all parathyroid carcinomas examined; there is also an abnormal staining pattern of the protein product of the gene. Allelic deletion is also seen in 10% of parathyroid adenomas, although the abnormal staining pattern of the Rb protein is not seen. Other gene loci on chromosome 13 may be involved in addition to the *Rb* locus.

There are two rare syndromes associated with hyperparathyroidism that involve one or more genes located on chromosome 1q. The he-

FIGURE 332-3 *A.* Schematic diagram indicating concept of autosomal recessive rather than autosomal dominant inheritance of tumor susceptibility. The patient with the hereditary abnormality (multiple endocrine neoplasia, or MEN) is envisioned as having one defective gene inherited from the affected parent on chromosome 11, but one copy of the normal gene is present from the other parent. In the monoclonal tumor (benign tumor), a somatic event, here partial chromosomal deletion, removes the remaining normal gene from a cell. In nonhereditary tumors, two successive somatic mutations must occur, a process that takes a longer time. By either pathway, the cell, deprived of growth-regulating influence from this gene, has unregulated growth and becomes a tumor. A different genetic locus also involving loss of a tumor-suppressor gene on chromosome 13 is involved in the pathogenesis of parathyroid carcinoma. *B.* Schematic illustration of the mechanism and consequences of gene rearrangement and overexpression of the PRAD 1 protooncogene (pericentromeric inversion of chromosome 11) in parathyroid adenomas. The excessive expression of PRAD 1 (a cell cycle control protein, cyclin D₁) by the highly active PTH gene promoter in the parathyroid cell contributes to excess cellular proliferation. [*From J Habener et al, in L DeGroot, JL Jameson (eds): Endocrinology, 4th ed. Philadelphia, Saunders, 2001, with permission.*]

reditary *hyperparathyroidism jaw tumor* (IIPT-JT) syndrome shows an autosomal dominant inheritance pattern; the jaw tumors are benign, but the parathyroid pathology may involve carcinoma as well as adenoma. Parathyroid carcinoma may also appear in the other syndrome, *familial isolated primary hyperparathyroidism* (FIPH). Both syndromes have been mapped through linkage studies to the chromosome 1q21-q31 region. Certain findings have led to speculation that this chromosome region might contain a protooncogene rather than a tumor-suppressor gene.

In some parathyroid adenomas, activation of a protooncogene has been identified (Fig. 332-3*B*). A reciprocal translocation involving chromosome 11 has been identified that juxtaposes the PTH gene promoter upstream of a gene product termed *PRAD-1*, a cyclin D protein that plays a key role in normal cell division. This translocation is found in as many as 15% of parathyroid adenomas, usually in larger tumors. Targeted overexpression of cyclin D_1 in the parathyroid glands of transgenic mice causes the development of hyperparathyroidism, consistent with the role of this cell cycle control protein in parathyroid neoplasia.

A mutated protooncogene, *RET*, is involved in each of the clinical variants of MEN 2 (Chap. 330). *RET* encodes a tyrosine kinase–type receptor; specific mutations lead to constitutive activity of the receptor, thereby explaining the autosomal dominant mode of transmission and the relatively early onset of neoplasia.

Signs and Symptoms   Half or more of patients with hyperparathyroidism are asymptomatic. In series in which patients are followed without operation, as many as 80% are classified as without symptoms. Manifestations of hyperparathyroidism involve primarily the kidneys and the skeletal system. Kidney involvement, due either to deposition of calcium in the renal parenchyma or to recurrent nephrolithiasis, was present in 60 to 70% of patients prior to 1970. With earlier detection, renal complications occur in <20% of patients in many large series. Renal stones are usually composed of either calcium oxalate or calcium phosphate. In occasional patients, repeated episodes of nephrolithiasis or the formation of large calculi may lead to urinary tract obstruction, infection, and loss of renal function. Nephrocalcinosis may also cause decreased renal function and phosphate retention.

The distinctive bone manifestation of hyperparathyroidism is *osteitis fibrosa cystica*, which occurred in 10 to 25% of patients in series reported 50 years ago. Histologically, the pathognomonic features are an increase in the giant multinucleated osteoclasts in scalloped areas on the surface of the bone (Howship's lacunae) and a replacement of the normal cellular and marrow elements by fibrous tissue. X-ray changes include resorption of the phalangeal tufts and replacement of the usually sharp cortical outline of the bone in the digits by an irregular outline (subperiosteal resorption). In recent years, osteitis fibrosa cystica is very rare in primary hyperparathyroidism, probably due to the earlier detection of the disease.

With the use of multiple markers of bone turnover, such as formation indices (bone-specific alkaline phosphatase, osteocalcin, and type I procollagen peptides) and bone resorption indices (including hydroxypyridinium collagen cross-links and telopeptides of type I collagen), increased skeletal turnover is detected in essentially all patients with established hyperparathyroidism.

Computed tomography (CT) scan and dual-energy x-ray absorptiometry (DEXA) of the spine provide reproducible quantitative estimates (within a few percent) of spinal bone density (Chap. 333). Similarly, bone density in the extremities can be quantified by densitometry of the hip or of the distal radius at a site chosen to be primarily cortical. Cortical bone density is reduced while cancellous bone density, especially in the spine, is relatively preserved. Serial studies in patients who choose to be followed without surgery have indicated that in the majority there is little further change over a number of years, consistent with laboratory data indicating relatively unchanged blood

calcium and PTH levels. After an initial loss of bone mass in patients with mild asymptomatic hyperparathyroidism, a new equilibrium may be reached, with bone density and biochemical manifestations of the disease remaining relatively unchanged.

In symptomatic patients, dysfunctions of the CNS, peripheral nerve and muscle, gastrointestinal tract, and joints also occur. It has been reported that severe neuropsychiatric manifestations may be reversed by parathyroidectomy; it remains unclear, in the absence of controlled studies, whether this improvement has a defined cause-and-effect relationship. Generally, the fact that hyperparathyroidism is common in elderly patients, in whom there are often other problems, suggests the possibility that such coexisting problems as hypertension, renal deterioration, and depression may not be parathyroid-related and suggests caution in recommending parathyroid surgery as a cure for these manifestations.

When present, neuromuscular manifestations may include proximal muscle weakness, easy fatigability, and atrophy of muscles and may be so striking as to suggest a primary neuromuscular disorder. The distinguishing feature is the complete regression of neuromuscular disease after surgical correction of the hyperparathyroidism.

Gastrointestinal manifestations are sometimes subtle and include vague abdominal complaints and disorders of the stomach and pancreas. Again, cause and effect are unclear. In MEN 1 patients with hyperparathyroidism, duodenal ulcer may be the result of associated pancreatic tumors that secrete excessive quantities of gastrin (Zollinger-Ellison syndrome). Pancreatitis has been reported in association with hyperparathyroidism, but the incidence and the mechanism are not established.

DIAGNOSIS   The diagnosis is typically made by detecting an elevated immunoreactive PTH level in a patient with asymptomatic hypercalcemia (see "Differential Diagnosis: Special Tests," below). Serum phosphate is usually low but may be normal, especially if renal failure has developed.

Many tests based on renal responses to excess PTH (renal calcium and phosphate clearance; blood phosphate, chloride, magnesium; urinary or nephrogenous cyclic AMP) were used in earlier decades. These tests have low specificity for hyperparathyroidism and are therefore not cost-effective; they have been replaced by PTH immunoassays.

℞ TREATMENT

Medical Surveillance versus Surgical Treatment   The critical management question is whether the disease should be treated surgically. If severe hypercalcemia [3.7 to 4.5 mmol/L (15 to 18 mg/dL)] is present, surgery is mandatory as soon as the diagnosis can be confirmed by a PTH immunoassay. However, in most patients with hyperparathyroidism, hypercalcemia is mild and does not require urgent surgical or medical treatment.

The National Institutes of Health (NIH) held a Consensus Conference on Management of Asymptomatic Hyperparathyroidism in 1990. *Asymptomatic hyperparathyroidism* was defined as documented (presumptive) hyperparathyroidism without signs or symptoms attributable to the disease. The consensus was that patients <50 should undergo surgery, given the long surveillance that would be required. Other considerations that favored surgery included concern that consistent follow-up would be unlikely or that coexistent illness would complicate management. Patients >50 were deemed appropriate for medical monitoring if certain criteria were met, the patients wished to avoid surgery, or the guidelines for recommending surgery were not present (Table 332-2). Careful evaluation of patients over the subsequent dozen years has both provided reassurance that in some patients medical monitoring rather than surgery is still prudent yet has promoted new questions about the natural history of the disease with or without surgery.

Data developed since the Consensus Conference indicated that a subgroup of patients had selective vertebral osteopenia out of proportion to bone loss at other sites and responded to surgery with striking restoration of bone mass (average >20%). In addition, as much as a

5% increase in bone mineral density in the spine and hip have been reported with alendronate use in asymptomatic hyperparathyroid patients. In light of this new information, the NIH convened a Workshop on Asymptomatic Hyperparathyroidism in 2002, and an independent (non-NIH) panel offered a revised set of recommendations. The changes reflect both practical considerations (such as the difficulty in creatinine clearance measurements and therefore substituting calculations based on serum creatinine) and concerns regarding potential deleterious skeletal effects in untreated patients (Tables 332-2 and 332-3). Accordingly, indication for surgical intervention was lowered (i.e., stricter serum calcium and bone density criteria). Asymptomatic patients should be monitored regularly. Surgical correction of hyperparathyroidism can always be undertaken when indicated, since the success rate is high (>90%), mortality is low, and morbidity is minimal. The goals of monitoring are early detection of worsening hypercalcemia, deteriorating bone or renal status, or other complications of hyperparathyroidism. No specific recommendations about medical therapy were made, but the promise of the newer agents was stressed, with the prediction that they would be used in clinical practice to increase bone mass in patients not electing surgery as further experience is gained. Neither panel recommended estrogen use in patients for whom surgery was not elected because there was insufficient cumulative experience with such therapy to balance theoretical risks (breast and endometrial cancer) versus benefits. Raloxifene (Evista), the first of the SERMS, has been shown to have many of the bone-protective effects of estrogen in osteoporotic subjects yet at the same time lowers the incidence of breast cancer; preliminary use of this agent in a small series of hyperparathyroid patients led to increased bone density. Experience with calcimimetics, drugs that selectively stimulate the calcium sensor and suppress PTH secretion, indicates that these agents decrease calcium levels to normal and lower PTH levels by at least 50% for >1 year of continuous use.

Surgical Treatment Parathyroid exploration is challenging and should be undertaken by an experienced surgeon. Certain features help in predicting the pathology (e.g., multiple abnormal glands in familial cases). However, some critical decisions regarding management can be made only during the operation.

As discussed above, there are many unresolved issues to consider in surgery for this disease. One surgical strategy is based on the view that typically only one gland (the adenoma) is abnormal. If an enlarged gland is found, a normal gland should be sought. In this view, if a biopsy of a normal-sized second gland confirms its histologic (and presumed functional) normality, no further exploration, biopsy, or excision is needed. At the other extreme is the minority viewpoint that all four glands be sought and that most of the total parathyroid tissue mass should be removed. The concern with the former approach is that the recurrence rate of hyperparathyroidism may be high if a second abnormal gland is missed; the latter approach could involve unnecessary surgery and an unacceptable rate of hypoparathyroidism. The majority viewpoint favors conservative surgery, i.e., removal of what is usually only one enlarged gland but only after four-gland exploration to eliminate the possibility that more than one gland is abnormal. When normal glands are found in association with one enlarged gland, excision of the single adenoma usually leads to cure or at least years free of symptoms. Long-term follow-up studies are limited to establish true rates of recurrence.

Recently, there has been growing experience with new surgical strategies that feature a minimally invasive approach guided by improved preoperative localization and intraoperative monitoring by PTH assays. Preoperative ^{99m}Tc sestamibi scans with positron emission computed tomography (SPECT) are used to predict the location of an abnormal gland and intraoperative sampling of PTH before and at 5-min intervals after removal of a suspected adenoma to confirm a rapid fall (>50%) to normal levels of PTH. In several centers, a combination of preoperative sestamibi imaging, cervical block anesthesia, minimal surgical incision, and intraoperative PTH measurements has allowed successful outpatient surgical management with a clear-cut cost benefit compared to general anesthesia and more extensive neck surgery. The use of these minimally invasive approaches requires clinical judgment to select patients unlikely to have multiple gland disease (e.g., MEN or secondary hyperparathyroidism). The growing acceptance of the technique and its relative ease for the patient has lowered the threshold for surgery.

When parathyroid carcinoma is encountered, the tissue should be widely excised; care must be taken to avoid rupture of the capsule to prevent local seeding of tumor cells.

Multiple gland hyperplasia, as predicted in familial cases, poses more difficult questions of surgical management. Once a diagnosis of hyperplasia is established, all the glands must be identified. Two schemes have been proposed for surgical management. One is to totally remove three glands with partial excision of the fourth gland; care is taken to leave a good blood supply for the remaining gland. Other surgeons advocate total parathyroidectomy with immediate transplantation of a portion of a removed, minced parathyroid gland into the muscles of the forearm, with the view that surgical excision is easier from the ectopic site in the arm if there is recurrent hyperfunction.

In a minority of cases, if no abnormal parathyroid glands are found in the neck, the issue of further exploration must be decided. There are documented cases of five or six parathyroid glands and of unusual locations for adenomas, such as in the mediastinum.

When a second parathyroid exploration is indicated, the minimally invasive techniques such as ultrasound, CT scan, and isotope scanning may be combined with venous sampling and/or selective digital arteriography in one of the centers specializing in these techniques. Intraoperative monitoring of PTH levels by rapid PTH immunoassays may be useful in guiding the surgery, especially in patients who are reexplored after an initial unsuccessful operation. At one center, long-term cures have been achieved with selective embolization or injection of large amounts of contrast material into the end-arterial circulation feeding the parathyroid tumor.

A decline in serum calcium occurs within 24 h after successful surgery; usually blood calcium falls to low-normal values for 3 to 5

TABLE 332-2 *Guidelines for Parathyroid Surgery in Asymptomatic Primary Hyperparathyroidism[a]*

Measurement	Guidelines, 1990	Guidelines, 2002
Serum calcium (above upper limit of normal)	0.3–0.4 mmol/L (1–6 mg/dL)	0.3 mmol/L (1.0 mg/dL)
24-h urinary calcium	>400 mg	>400 mg
Creatinine clearance	Reduced by 30%	Reduced by 30%
Bone mineral density	Z-score < −2.0 (forearm)	T-score < −2.5 at any site
Age	<50	<50

[a] Surgery is also indicated in patients for whom medical surveillance is neither desired nor possible.
Source: From JP Bilezikian et al: J Clin Endocrinol Metab 87:5353, 2002.

TABLE 332-3 *Management Guidelines for Patients with Aymptomatic Primary Hyperparathyroidism Who Do Not Undergo Parathyroid Surgery*

Measurement	Older Guidelines	New Guidelines
Serum calcium	Biannually	Biannually
24-h urinary calcium	Annually	Not recommended[a]
Creatinine clearance	Annually	Not recommended[a]
Serum creatinine	Annually	Annually[b]
Bone density	Annually (forearm)	Annually (lumbar spine, hip, forearm)
Abdominal x-ray (+/− ultrasound)	Annually	Not recommended[a]

[a] Except at the time of initial evaluation.
[b] If the serum creatinine concentration suggests a change in the creatinine clearance when the Cockroft-Gault equation is applied, further, more direct assessments of the creatinine clearance are recommended.
Source: From JP Bilezikian et al: J Clin Endocrinol Metab 87:5353, 2002.

days until the remaining parathyroid tissue resumes hormone secretion. Severe postoperative hypocalcemia is likely only if osteitis fibrosa cystica is present or if injury to all the normal parathyroid glands occurs during surgery. In general, patients with uncomplicated disease such as a single adenoma (the clear majority) who do not have symptomatic bone disease or a large deficit in bone mineral and who have good renal and gastrointestinal function have few problems with postoperative hypocalcemia. The extent of postoperative hypocalcemia varies with the surgical approach. If all glands are biopsied, hypocalcemia may be transiently symptomatic and more prolonged. Hypocalcemia is more likely to be symptomatic after second parathyroid explorations, particularly when normal parathyroid tissue was removed at the initial operation and when the manipulation and/or biopsy of the remaining normal glands is more extensive in the search for the missing adenoma.

Patients with hyperparathyroidism have efficient intestinal calcium absorption due to the increased levels of 1,25(OH)$_2$D stimulated by PTH excess. Once hypocalcemia signifies successful surgery, patients can be put on a high-calcium intake or be given oral calcium supplements. Despite mild hypocalcemia, most patients do not require parenteral therapy. If the serum calcium falls to <2 mmol/L (8 mg/dL), *and if the phosphate level rises simultaneously*, the possibility that surgery has caused hypoparathyroidism must be considered. With unexpected hypocalcemia, coexistent hypomagnesemia should be considered, as it interferes with PTH secretion and causes functional hypoparathyroidism (see below). Signs of hypocalcemia include symptoms such as muscle twitching, a general sense of anxiety, and positive Chvostek and Trousseau signs coupled with serum calcium consistently <2 mmol/L (8 mg/dL). Parenteral calcium replacement at a low level should be instituted when hypocalcemia is symptomatic. The rate and duration of intravenous therapy are determined by the severity of the symptoms and the response of the serum calcium to treatment. An infusion of 0.5 to 2 (mg/kg)/h or 30 to 100 mL/h of a 1-mg/mL solution usually suffices to relieve symptoms. Usually, parenteral therapy is required for only a few days. If symptoms worsen or if parenteral calcium is needed for >2 to 3 days, therapy with a vitamin D analogue and/or oral calcium (2 to 4 g/d) should be started (see below). It is cost-effective to use calcitriol (doses of 0.5 to 1.0 μg/d) because of the rapidity of onset of effect and prompt cessation of action when stopped, in comparison to other forms of vitamin D (see below). A rise in blood calcium after several months of vitamin D replacement may indicate restoration of parathyroid function to normal. It is also appropriate to monitor serum PTH serially to estimate gland function in such patients.

Magnesium deficiency may also complicate the postoperative course. Magnesium deficiency impairs the secretion of PTH, and so hypomagnesemia should be corrected whenever detected. Magnesium chloride is effective by mouth, but this compound is not widely available. Repletion is usually parenteral. Because the depressant effect of magnesium on central and peripheral nerve functions does not occur at levels <2 mmol/L (normal range 0.8 to 1.2 mmol/L), parenteral replacement can be given rapidly. A cumulative dose as great as 0.5 to 1 mmol/kg of body weight can be administered if severe hypomagnesemia is present; often, however, total doses of 20 to 40 mmol are sufficient. The magnesium is given either as an intravenous infusion over 8 to 12 h or in divided doses intramuscularly (magnesium sulfate, USP).

OTHER PARATHYROID-RELATED CAUSES OF HYPERCALCEMIA ■ Lithium Therapy Lithium, used in the management of bipolar depression and other psychiatric disorders, causes hypercalcemia in ~10% of treated patients. The hypercalcemia is dependent on continued lithium treatment, remitting and recurring when lithium is stopped and restarted. The parathyroid adenomas reported in some hypercalcemic patients with lithium therapy may reflect the presence of an independently occurring parathyroid tumor; a permanent effect of lithium on parathyroid gland growth need not be implicated as most patients have complete reversal of hypercalcemia when lithium is stopped. However, long-standing stimulation of parathyroid cell replication by lithium may predispose to development of adenomas (as is documented in secondary hyperparathyroidism and renal failure).

At the levels achieved in blood in treated patients, lithium can be shown in vitro to shift the PTH secretion curve to the right in response to calcium; i.e., higher calcium levels are required to lower PTH secretion, probably acting at the calcium sensor (see below); this effect can cause elevated PTH levels and consequent hypercalcemia in otherwise normal individuals. Fortunately, there are alternative medications for the underlying psychiatric illness. Parathyroid surgery should not be recommended unless hypercalcemia and elevated PTH levels persist after lithium is discontinued.

GENETIC DISORDERS CAUSING HYPERPARATHYROID-LIKE SYNDROMES ■ Familial Hypocalciuric Hypercalcemia FHH (also called *familial benign hypercalcemia*) is inherited as an autosomal dominant trait. Affected individuals are discovered because of asymptomatic hypercalcemia. This disorder and Jansen's disease (discussed below) are variants of hyperparathyroidism. FHH involves excessive secretion of PTH, whereas Jansen's disease is caused by excessive biologic activity of the PTH receptor in target tissues. Neither disorder, however, involves a primary growth disorder of the parathyroids.

The pathophysiology of FHH is now understood. The primary defect is abnormal sensing of the blood calcium by the parathyroid gland and renal tubule, causing inappropriate secretion of PTH and excessive renal reabsorption of calcium. The calcium sensor is a member of the third family of GPCRs (type C, or III). The receptor responds to the ECF calcium concentration, suppressing PTH secretion through second messenger signaling, thereby providing negative-feedback regulation of PTH secretion. Many different mutations in the calcium-sensing receptor have been identified in patients with FHH (Fig. 332-4). These mutations lower the capacity of the sensor to bind calcium, and the mutant receptors function as though blood calcium levels were low; excessive secretion of PTH occurs from an otherwise normal gland. Approximately two-thirds of patients with FHH have mutations within the protein-coding region of the gene. The remaining one-third of kindreds may have mutations in the gene promoter or may involve still unknown mechanisms in other regions of the genome identified through mapping studies (e.g., chromosome 19).

Even before elucidation of the pathophysiology of FHH, abundant clinical evidence served to separate the disorder from primary hyperparathyroidism. Patients with primary hyperparathyroidism have <99% renal calcium reabsorption, whereas most patients with FHH have >99% reabsorption. The hypercalcemia in FHH is often detectable in affected members of the kindreds in the first decade of life, whereas hypercalcemia rarely occurs in patients with primary hyperparathyroidism or the MEN syndromes who are <10. PTH may be elevated in FHH, but the values are usually normal or lower for the same degree of calcium elevation than in patients with primary hyperparathyroidism. Parathyroid surgery in a few patients with FHH led to permanent hypoparathyroidism, but hypocalciuria persisted nevertheless, establishing that hypocalciuria, therefore, is not PTH-dependent (now known to be due to the abnormal calcium sensor in the kidney).

Few clinical signs or symptoms are present in patients with FHH, and other endocrine abnormalities are not present. Most patients are detected as a result of family screening after hypercalcemia is detected in a proband. In those patients inadvertently operated upon, the parathyroids appeared normal or moderately hyperplastic. Parathyroid surgery is not appropriate, nor, in view of the lack of symptoms, does medical treatment seem needed to lower the calcium. Calcimimetic agents that bind to the calcium sensor and elevate the set point are under investigation.

One striking exception to the rule against parathyroid surgery in this syndrome is the occurrence, usually in consanguineous marriages (due to the rarity of the gene mutation), of a homozygous or compound heterozygote state, resulting in complete loss of the calcium sensor function. In this condition, neonatal severe hypercalcemia, total parathyroidectomy is mandatory.

Jansen's Disease Mutations in the PTH1R have been identified as responsible for this rare autosomal dominant syndrome (Fig. 332-4). Because the mutations lead to constitutive receptor function, one abnormal copy of the mutant receptor is sufficient to cause the disease, thereby accounting for its dominant mode of transmission. The disorder leads to short-limbed dwarfism due to abnormal regulation of the bone growth plate. In adult life, there are numerous abnormalities in bone, including multiple cystic resorptive areas resembling those seen in severe hyperparathyroidism. Hypercalcemia and hypophosphatemia with undetectable or low PTH levels are typically seen. The pathogenesis of the disease has been confirmed by transgenic experiments in which targeted expression of the mutant receptor to the growth plate emulated several features of the disorder.

MALIGNANCY-RELATED HYPERCALCEMIA ■ Clinical Syndromes and Mechanisms of Hypercalcemia Hypercalcemia due to malignancy is common (occurring with 10 to 15% of certain types of tumor, such as lung carcinoma), often severe and difficult to manage, and occasionally difficult to distinguish from primary hyperparathyroidism. Although malignancy is often clinically obvious or readily detectable by medical history, hypercalcemia can occasionally be due to an occult tumor. Previously, hypercalcemia associated with malignancy was thought to be due to local invasion and destruction of bone by tumor cells; many cases are now known to result from the elaboration by the malignant cells of humoral mediators of hypercalcemia. PTHrP is the responsible humoral agent in most solid tumors that cause hypercalcemia.

The histologic character of the tumor is more important than the extent of skeletal metastases in predicting hypercalcemia. Small-cell carcinoma (oat cell) and adenocarcinoma of the lung, although the most common lung tumors associated with skeletal metastases, rarely cause hypercalcemia. By contrast, as many as 10% of patients with squamous cell carcinoma of the lung develop hypercalcemia. Histologic studies of bone in patients with squamous cell or epidermoid carcinoma of the lung, in sites invaded by tumor as well as areas remote from tumor invasion, reveal increased bone remodeling, including osteoclastic and osteoblastic activity.

Two main mechanisms of hypercalcemia are operative in cancer hypercalcemia. Many solid tumors associated with hypercalcemia, particularly squamous cell and renal tumors, produce and secrete PTHrP that causes increased bone resorption and mediate the hypercalcemia through systemic actions on the skeleton. Alternatively, direct bone marrow invasion occurs with hematologic malignancies such as leukemia, lymphoma, and multiple myeloma. Lymphokines and cytokines produced by cells involved in the marrow response to the tumors promote resorption of bone through local destruction. Several hormones, hormone analogues, cytokines, and growth factors have been implicated as the result of clinical assays, in vitro tests, or chemical isolation. The etiologic factor produced by activated normal lymphocytes and by myeloma and lymphoma cells, termed *osteoclast activation factor*, now appears to represent the biologic action of several different cytokines, probably interleukin 1 and lymphotoxin or tumor necrosis factor. In some lymphomas, typically B cell lymphomas, there is a third mechanism, caused by an increased blood level of 1,25(OH)$_2$D, which is probably produced by lymphocytes.

The more common mechanism, usually termed *humoral hypercalcemia of malignancy*, solid tumors (cancers of the lung and kidney, in particular), in which bone metastases are absent, minimal, or not de-

FIGURE 332-4 Mutations in the calcium sensor receptor. The extracellular domain binds calcium, leading to conformational changes that stimulate Gq-coupled activation of the phospholipase C and suppression of PTH. The identified sequence alterations (X) cause loss of function and lead to inadequate suppression of parathyroid hormone release and, therefore, mild hypercalcemia (FHH); *, a gain-of-function mutation that causes hypocalcemia; •, conserved residues; ▲, acidic residues. (*From EM Brown et al: J Nutr 125:1965S, 1995, with permission.*)

tectable clinically, secrete PTHrP measurable by immunoassay. Secretion by the tumors of the PTH-like factor, PTHrP, activates the PTH1R, resulting in a pathophysiology closely resembling hyperparathyroidism. The clinical picture resembles primary hyperparathyroidism (hypophosphatemia accompanies hypercalcemia), and elimination or regression of the primary tumor leads to disappearance of the hypercalcemia.

As in hyperparathyroidism, patients with the humoral hypercalcemia of malignancy have elevated urinary nephrogenous cyclic AMP excretion, hypophosphatemia, and increased urinary phosphate clearance. However, in humoral hypercalcemia of malignancy, immunoreactive PTH is undetectable or suppressed, making the differential diagnosis easier. Other features of the disorder differ from those of true hyperparathyroidism. Patients may have high, rather than low, renal calcium clearance (relative to serum calcium when compared to true hyperparathyroidism, unlike the expected elevation) and low to normal levels of 1,25(OH)$_2$D. The reason that the humoral syndrome differs from hyperparathyroidism in these parameters is unclear since the biologic actions of PTH and PTHrP are presumably exerted through the same receptor. Other cytokines elaborated by the malignancy may be responsible for these variations from hyperparathyroidism. In some patients with the humoral hypercalcemia of malignancy, osteoclastic resorption is unaccompanied by an osteoblastic or bone-forming response, implying inhibition of the normal coupling of bone formation and resorption. Thus the interaction of more than one substance may determine whether hypercalcemia develops in a particular patient.

Several different assays (single- or double-antibody, different epitopes) have been developed to detect PTHrP. Most data indicate that circulating PTHrP levels are undetectable (or low) in normal individuals, elevated in most cancer patients with the humoral syndrome, and high in human milk. The etiologic mechanisms in cancer hypercalcemia may be multiple in the same patient. For example, in breast carcinoma (metastatic to bone) and in a distinctive type of T cell lymphoma/leukemia initiated by human T cell lymphotropic virus I, hypercalcemia is caused by direct local lysis of bone as well as by a humoral mechanism involving excess production of PTHrP.

Diagnostic Issues Levels of PTH measured by the double-antibody technique are undetectable or extremely low in tumor hypercalcemia, as would be expected with the mediation of the hypercalcemia by a factor other than PTH (the hypercalcemia suppresses the normal parathyroid glands). In a patient with minimal symptoms referred for hypercalcemia, low or undetectable PTH levels would focus attention on a possible occult malignancy.

Ordinarily, the diagnosis of cancer hypercalcemia is not difficult because tumor symptoms are prominent when hypercalcemia is detected. Indeed, hypercalcemia may be noted incidentally during the workup of a patient with known or suspected malignancy. Clinical suspicion that malignancy is the cause of the hypercalcemia is heightened when there are other paraneoplastic signs or symptoms, such as weight loss, fatigue, muscle weakness, or unexplained skin rash, or when symptoms specific for a particular tumor are present. Squamous cell tumors are most frequently associated with hypercalcemia, particularly tumors of the lung, kidney, head and neck, and urogenital tract. Radiologic examinations can focus on these areas when clinical evidence is unclear. Bone scans with technetium-labeled bisphosphonate are useful for detection of osteolytic metastases; the sensitivity is high, but specificity is low; results must be confirmed by conventional x-rays to be certain that areas of increased uptake are due to osteolytic metastases per se. Bone marrow biopsies are helpful in patients with anemia or abnormal peripheral blood smears.

R_x TREATMENT

Treatment of the hypercalcemia of malignancy is first directed to control of tumor; reduction of tumor mass usually corrects hypercalcemia. If a patient has severe hypercalcemia yet has a good chance for effective tumor therapy, treatment of the hypercalcemia should be vigorous while awaiting the results of definitive therapy. If hypercalcemia occurs in the late stages of a tumor that is resistant to anti-tumor therapy, the treatment of the hypercalcemia should be judicious as high calcium levels can have a mild sedating effect. Standard therapies for hypercalcemia (discussed below) are applicable to patients with malignancy.

VITAMIN D–RELATED HYPERCALCEMIA Hypercalcemia caused by vitamin D can be due to excessive ingestion or abnormal metabolism of the vitamin. Abnormal metabolism of the vitamin is usually acquired in association with a widespread granulomatous disorder. Vitamin D metabolism is carefully regulated, particularly the activity of renal 1α-hydroxylase, the enzyme responsible for the production of $1,25(OH)_2D$ (Chap. 331). The regulation of 1α-hydroxylase and the normal feedback suppression by $1,25(OH)_2D$ seem to work less well in infants than in adults and to operate poorly, if at all, in sites other than the renal tubule; these phenomena explain the occurrence of hypercalcemia secondary to excessive $1,25(OH)_2D_3$ production in infants with Williams' syndrome (see below) and in adults with sarcoidosis or lymphoma.

Vitamin D Intoxication Chronic ingestion of 50 to 100 times the normal physiologic requirement of vitamin D (amounts >50,000 to 100,000 U/d) is usually required to produce significant hypercalcemia in normal individuals. An upper limit of dietary intake of 2000 U/d (50 μg/d) in adults is now recommended because of concerns about potential toxic effects of cumulative supraphysiologic doses. Vitamin D excess increases intestinal calcium absorption and, if severe, also increases bone resorption.

Hypercalcemia in vitamin D intoxication is due to an excessive biologic action of the vitamin, perhaps the consequence of increased levels of $25(OH)D$ rather than merely increased levels of the active metabolite $1,25(OH)_2D$ (the latter may not be elevated in vitamin D intoxication). $25(OH)D$ has definite, if low, biologic activity in intestine and bone. The production of $25(OH)D$ is less tightly regulated than is the production of $1,25(OH)_2D$. Hence concentrations of $25(OH)D$ are elevated several-fold in patients with excess vitamin D intake.

The diagnosis is substantiated by documenting elevated levels of $25(OH)D$ >100 ng/mL. Hypercalcemia is usually controlled by restriction of dietary calcium intake and appropriate attention to hydration. These measures, plus discontinuation of vitamin D, usually lead to resolution of hypercalcemia. However, vitamin D stores in fat may be substantial, and vitamin D intoxication may persist for weeks after vitamin D ingestion is terminated. Such patients are responsive to glucocorticoids, which in doses of 100 mg/d of hydrocortisone or its equivalent, usually return serum calcium levels to normal over several days; severe intoxication may require intensive therapy.

Sarcoidosis and Other Granulomatous Diseases In patients with sarcoidosis and other granulomatous diseases, such as tuberculosis and fungal infections, excess $1,25(OH)_2D$ is synthesized in macrophages or other cells in the granulomas. Indeed, increased $1,25(OH)_2D$ levels have been reported in anephric patients with sarcoidosis and hypercalcemia. Macrophages obtained from granulomatous tissue convert $25(OH)D$ to $1,25(OH)_2D$ at an increased rate. There is a positive correlation in patients with sarcoidosis between $25(OH)D$ levels (reflecting vitamin D intake) and the circulating concentrations of $1,25(OH)_2D$, whereas normally there is no increase in $1,25(OH)_2D$ with increasing $25(OH)D$ levels due to multiple feedback controls on renal 1α-hydroxylase (Chap. 331). The usual regulation of active metabolite production by calcium or PTH does not operate in these patients; hypercalcemia does not lead to a reduction in the blood levels of $1,25(OH)_2D$ in patients with sarcoidosis. Clearance of $1,25(OH)_2D$ from blood may be decreased in sarcoidosis as well. PTH levels are usually low and $1,25(OH)_2D$ levels are elevated, but primary hyperparathyroidism and sarcoidosis may coexist in some patients.

Management of the hypercalcemia can often be accomplished by avoiding excessive sunlight exposure and limiting vitamin D and calcium intake. Presumably, however, the abnormal sensitivity to vitamin D and abnormal regulation of $1,25(OH)_2D$ synthesis will persist as long as the disease is active. Alternatively, glucocorticoids in the equivalent of ≤ 100 mg/d of hydrocortisone control hypercalcemia. Glucocorticoids appear to act by blocking excessive production of $1,25(OH)_2D$ as well as the response to it in target organs.

Idiopathic Hypercalcemia of Infancy This rare disorder, usually referred to as *Williams' syndrome*, is an autosomal dominant disorder characterized by multiple congenital development defects, including supravalvular aortic stenosis, mental retardation, and an elfin facies, in association with hypercalcemia due to abnormal sensitivity to vitamin D. The syndrome was first recognized in England after the fortification of milk with vitamin D. Levels of $1,25(OH)_2D$ are elevated, ranging from 46 to 120 nmol/L (150 to 500 pg/mL). The mechanism of the abnormal sensitivity to vitamin D and of the increased circulating levels of $1,25(OH)_2D$ is still unclear. Studies suggest that mutations involving the elastin locus and perhaps other genes on chromosome 7 may play a role in the pathogenesis.

HYPERCALCEMIA ASSOCIATED WITH HIGH BONE TURNOVER ■ **Hyperthyroidism** As many as 20% of hyperthyroid patients have high-normal or mildly elevated serum calcium concentrations; hypercalciuria is even more common. The hypercalcemia is due to increased bone turnover, with bone resorption exceeding bone formation. Severe calcium elevations are not typical, and the presence of such suggests a concomitant disease such as hyperparathyroidism. Usually, the diagnosis is obvious, but signs of hyperthyroidism may occasionally be occult, particularly in the elderly (Chap. 320). Hypercalcemia is managed by treatment of the hyperthyroidism.

Immobilization Immobilization is a rare cause of hypercalcemia in adults in the absence of an associated disease but may cause hypercalcemia in children and adolescents, particularly after spinal cord injury and paraplegia or quadriplegia. With resumption of ambulation, the hypercalcemia in children usually returns to normal.

The mechanism appears to involve a disproportion between bone formation and bone resorption. Hypercalciuria and increased mobilization of skeletal calcium can develop in normal volunteers subjected to extensive bed rest, although hypercalcemia is unusual. Immobilization of an adult with a disease associated with high bone turnover, however, such as Paget's disease, may cause hypercalcemia.

Thiazides Administration of benzothiadiazines (thiazides) can cause hypercalcemia in patients with high rates of bone turnover, such as patients with hypoparathyroidism treated with high doses of vitamin D. Traditionally, thiazides are associated with aggravation of hypercalcemia in primary hyperparathyroidism, but this effect can be seen in other high-bone-turnover states as well. The mechanism of thiazide action is complex. Chronic thiazide administration leads to reduction in urinary calcium; the hypocalciuric effect appears to reflect the enhancement of proximal tubular resorption of sodium and calcium in response to sodium depletion. Some of this renal effect is due to augmentation of PTH action and is more pronounced in individuals with intact PTH secretion. However, thiazides cause hypocalciuria in hypoparathyroid patients on high-dose vitamin D and oral calcium replacement if sodium intake is restricted. This finding is the rationale for the use of thiazides as an adjunct to therapy in hypoparathyroid patients, as discussed below. Thiazide administration to normal individuals causes a transient increase in blood calcium (usually within the high-normal range) that reverts to preexisting levels after a week or more of continued administration. If hormonal function and calcium and bone metabolism are normal, homeostatic controls are reset to counteract the calcium-elevating effect of the thiazides. In the presence of hyperparathyroidism or increased bone turnover from another cause, homeostatic mechanisms are ineffective. The abnormal effects of the thiazide on calcium metabolism disappear within days of cessation of the drug.

Vitamin A Intoxication Vitamin A intoxication is a rare cause of hypercalcemia and is most commonly a side effect of dietary faddism (Chap. 61). Calcium levels can be elevated into the 3 to 3.5 mmol/L (12 to 14 mg/dL) range after the ingestion of 50,000 to 100,000 units of vitamin A daily (10 to 20 times the minimum daily requirement). Typical features of severe hypercalcemia include fatigue, anorexia, and, in some, severe muscle and bone pain. Excess vitamin A intake is presumed to increase bone resorption.

The diagnosis can be established by history and by measurement of vitamin A levels in serum. Occasionally, skeletal x-rays reveal periosteal calcifications, particularly in the hands. Withdrawal of the vitamin is usually associated with prompt disappearance of the hypercalcemia and reversal of the skeletal changes. As in vitamin D intoxication, administration of 100 mg/d hydrocortisone or its equivalent leads to a rapid return of the serum calcium to normal.

HYPERCALCEMIA ASSOCIATED WITH RENAL FAILURE ■ Severe Secondary Hyperparathyroidism Secondary hyperparathyroidism occurs when partial resistance to the metabolic actions of PTH leads to excessive production of the hormone. Parathyroid gland hyperplasia occurs because resistance to the normal level of PTH leads to hypocalcemia, which, in turn, is a stimulus to parathyroid gland enlargement.

Secondary hyperparathyroidism occurs not only in patients with renal failure but also in those with osteomalacia due to multiple causes (Chap. 331), including deficiency of vitamin D action, and PHP (deficient response to PTH at the level of the receptor). Hypocalcemia seems to be the common denominator in initiating secondary hyperparathyroidism. Primary and secondary hyperparathyroidism can be distinguished conceptually by the autonomous growth of the parathyroid glands in primary hyperparathyroidism (presumably irreversible) and the adaptive response of the parathyroids in secondary hyperparathyroidism (typically reversible). In fact, reversal over weeks from an abnormal pattern of secretion, presumably accompanied by involution of parathyroid gland mass to normal, occurs in patients who have been treated effectively to reverse the resistance to PTH (such as with calcium and vitamin D in osteomalacia).

Patients with secondary hyperparathyroidism may develop bone pain, ectopic calcification, and pruritus. The bone disease seen in patients with secondary hyperparathyroidism and renal failure is termed *renal osteodystrophy*. Osteomalacia (predominantly due to vitamin D and calcium deficiency) and/or osteitis fibrosa cystica (excessive PTH action on bone) may occur.

Two other skeletal disorders are associated with long-term dialysis in patients with renal failure. Aluminum deposition (see below) is associated with an osteomalacia-like picture. The other entity is a low-bone-turnover state termed "aplastic" or "adynamic" bone disease; PTH levels are lower than in typical secondary hyperparathyroidism. It is believed that the condition is caused, at least in part, by excessive PTH suppression, which may be even greater than previously appreciated in light of evidence that some of the immunoreactive PTH detected by most commercially available PTH assays is not the full-length biologically active molecule (as discussed above).

℞ TREATMENT

Medical therapy to reverse secondary hyperparathyroidism includes reduction of excessive blood phosphate by restriction of dietary phosphate, the use of nonabsorbable antacids, and careful, selective addition of calcitriol (0.25 to 2.0 μg/d); calcium carbonate is preferred over aluminum-containing antacids to prevent aluminum toxicity. Intravenous calcitriol, administered as several pulses each week, helps control secondary hyperparathyroidism. Aggressive but carefully administered medical therapy can often, but not always, reverse hyperparathyroidism and its symptoms and manifestations.

Occasional patients develop severe manifestations of secondary hyperparathyroidism, including hypercalcemia, pruritus, extraskeletal calcifications, and painful bones, despite aggressive medical efforts to suppress the hyperparathyroidism. PTH hypersecretion no longer responsive to medical therapy, a state of severe hyperparathyroidism in patients with renal failure that requires surgery, has been referred to as *tertiary hyperparathyroidism*. Parathyroid surgery is necessary to control this condition. Based on genetic evidence from examination of tumor samples in these patients, the emergence of autonomous parathyroid function is due to a monoclonal outgrowth of one or more previously hyperplastic parathyroid glands. The adaptive response has become an independent contributor to disease; this finding seems to emphasize the importance of optimal medical management to reduce the proliferative response of the parathyroid cells that enables the irreversible genetic change.

Aluminum Intoxication Aluminum intoxication (and often hypercalcemia as a complication of medical treatment) may occur in patients on chronic dialysis; manifestations include acute dementia and unresponsive and severe osteomalacia. Bone pain, multiple nonhealing fractures, particularly of the ribs and pelvis, and a proximal myopathy may occur. Hypercalcemia develops when these patients are treated with vitamin D or calcitriol because of impaired skeletal responsiveness. Aluminum is present at the site of osteoid mineralization, osteoblastic activity is minimal, and calcium incorporation into the skeleton is impaired. Prevention is accomplished by avoidance of aluminum excess in the dialysis regimen; treatment of established disease involves mobilizing aluminum through the use of the chelating agent deferoxamine (Chap. 339).

Milk-Alkali Syndrome The milk-alkali syndrome is due to excessive ingestion of calcium and absorbable antacids such as milk or calcium carbonate. It is much less frequent since nonabsorbable antacids and other treatments became available for peptic ulcer disease. However, the increased use of calcium carbonate in the management of osteoporosis has led to reappearance of the syndrome. Several clinical presentations—acute, subacute, and chronic—have been described, all of which feature hypercalcemia, alkalosis, and renal failure. The chronic form of the disease, termed *Burnett's syndrome*, is associated with irreversible renal damage. The acute syndromes reverse if the excess calcium and absorbable alkali are stopped.

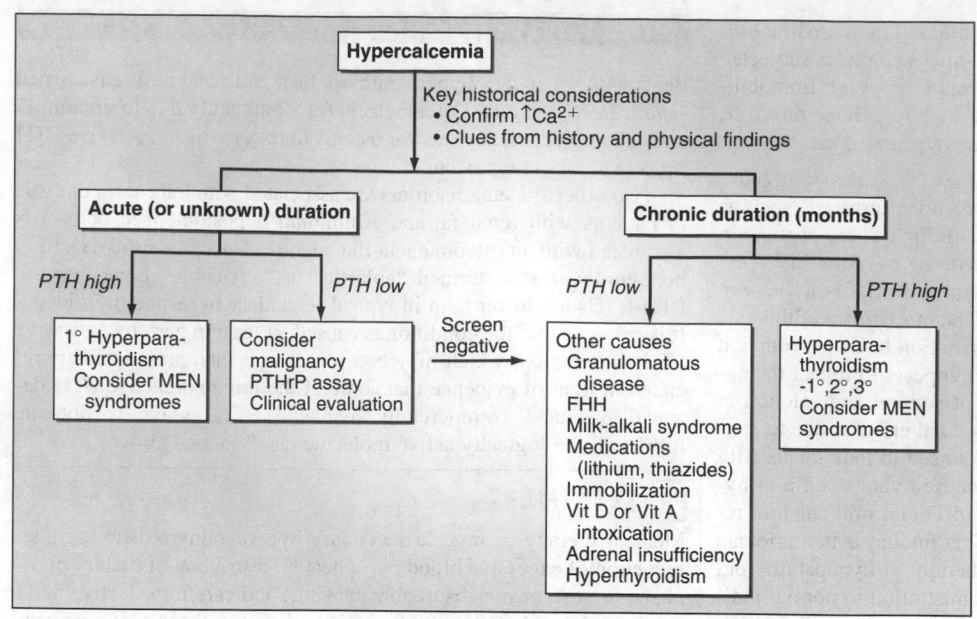

FIGURE 332-5 Algorithm for the evaluation of patients with hypercalcemia. See text for details. FHH, familial hypocalciuric hypercalcemia; MEN, multiple endocrine neoplasia; PTH, parathyroid hormone; PTHrP, parathyroid hormone–related peptide.

Individual susceptibility is important in the pathogenesis, as many patients are treated with calcium carbonate alkali regimens without developing the syndrome. One variable is the fractional calcium absorption as a function of calcium intake. Some individuals absorb a high fraction of calcium, even with intakes as high as 2 g or more of elemental calcium per day, instead of reducing calcium absorption with high intake, as occurs in most normal individuals. Resultant mild hypercalcemia after meals in such patients is postulated to contribute to the generation of alkalosis. Development of hypercalcemia causes increased sodium excretion and some depletion of total-body water. These phenomena and perhaps some suppression of endogenous PTH secretion due to mild hypercalcemia lead to increased bicarbonate resorption and to alkalosis in the face of continued calcium carbonate ingestion. Alkalosis per se selectively enhances calcium resorption in the distal nephron, thus aggravating the hypercalcemia. The cycle of mild hypercalcemia → bicarbonate retention → alkalosis → renal calcium retention → severe hypercalcemia perpetuates and aggravates hypercalcemia and alkalosis as long as calcium and absorbable alkali are ingested.

DIFFERENTIAL DIAGNOSIS: SPECIAL TESTS Differential diagnosis of hypercalcemia is best achieved by using clinical criteria, but the immunoassay for PTH is especially useful in distinguishing among major causes (Fig. 332-5). The clinical features that deserve emphasis are the presence or absence of symptoms or signs of disease and evidence of chronicity. If one discounts fatigue or depression, >90% of patients with primary hyperparathyroidism have *asymptomatic hypercalcemia*; symptoms of malignancy are usually present in cancer-associated hypercalcemia. Disorders other than hyperparathyroidism and malignancy cause <10% of cases of hypercalcemia, and some of the nonparathyroid causes are associated with clear-cut manifestations such as renal failure.

Hyperparathyroidism is the likely diagnosis in patients with *chronic hypercalcemia*. If hypercalcemia has been manifest for >1 year, malignancy can usually be excluded as the cause. A striking feature of malignancy-associated hypercalcemia is the rapidity of the course, whereby signs and symptoms of the underlying malignancy are evident within months of the detection of hypercalcemia. Although clinical considerations are helpful in arriving at the correct diagnosis of the cause of hypercalcemia, appropriate laboratory testing is essential for definitive diagnosis. The immunoassay for PTH should separate hyperparathyroidism from all other causes of hypercalcemia. Patients with hyperparathyroidism have elevated PTH levels despite hypercal-

cemia, whereas patients with malignancy and the other causes of hypercalcemia (except for disorders mediated by PTH such as lithium-induced hypercalcemia) have levels of hormone below normal or undetectable. Assays based on the double-antibody method for PTH exhibit very high sensitivity (especially if serum calcium is simultaneously evaluated) and specificity for the diagnosis of primary hyperparathyroidism (Fig. 332-6).

In summary, PTH values are elevated in >90% of parathyroid-related causes of hypercalcemia, undetectable or low in malignancy-related hypercalcemia, and undetectable or normal in vitamin D–related and high-bone-turnover causes of hypercalcemia. In view of the specificity of the PTH immunoassay and the high frequency of hyperparathyroidism in hypercalcemic patients, it is cost-effective to measure the PTH level in all hypercalcemic patients unless malignancy or a specific nonparathyroid disease is obvious. False-positive PTH assay results are rare. There are very rare reports of ectopic production of excess PTH by nonparathyroid tumors. Immunoassays for PTHrP are helpful in diagnosing certain types of malignancy-associated hypercalcemia. Although FHH is parathyroid-related, the disease should be managed distinctively from hyperparathyroidism. Clinical features and the low urinary calcium excretion can help make the distinction. Because the

FIGURE 332-6 Levels of immunoreactive parathyroid hormone (PTH) detected in patients with primary hyperparathyroidism, hypercalcemia of malignancy, and hypoparathyroidism. Boxed area represents the upper and normal limits of blood calcium and/or immunoreactive PTH. [*From SR Nussbaum, JT Potts, Jr, in L DeGroot, JL Jameson (eds): Endocrinology, 4th ed. Philadelphia, Saunders, 2001, with permission.*]

incidence of malignancy and hyperparathyroidism both increase with age, they can coexist as two independent causes of hypercalcemia.

1,25(OH)$_2$D levels are elevated in many (but not all) patients with primary hyperparathyroidism. In other disorders associated with hypercalcemia, concentrations of 1,25(OH)$_2$D are low or, at the most, normal. However, this test is of low specificity and is not cost-effective, as not all patients with hyperparathyroidism have elevated 1,25(OH)$_2$D levels, and not all nonparathyroid hypercalcemic patients have suppressed 1,25(OH)$_2$D. Measurement of 1,25(OH)$_2$D is, however, critically valuable in establishing the cause of hypercalcemia in sarcoidosis and certain B cell lymphomas.

A useful general approach is outlined in Fig. 332-5. If the patient is *asymptomatic* and there is evidence of *chronicity* to the hypercalcemia, hyperparathyroidism is almost certainly the cause. If PTH levels (usually measured at least twice) are elevated, the clinical impression is confirmed and little additional evaluation is necessary. If there is only a short history or no data as to the duration of the hypercalcemia, *occult malignancy* must be considered; if the PTH levels are not elevated, then a thorough workup must be undertaken for malignancy, including chest x-ray, CT of chest and abdomen, and bone scan. Immunoassays for PTHrP may be especially useful in such situations. Attention should also be paid to clues for underlying hematologic disorders such as anemia, increased plasma globulin, and abnormal serum immunoelectrophoresis; bone scans can be negative in some patients with metastases, such as in multiple myeloma. Finally, if a patient with chronic hypercalcemia is asymptomatic and malignancy therefore seems unlikely on clinical grounds, but PTH values are not elevated, it is useful to search for other chronic causes of hypercalcemia, such as occult sarcoidosis. A careful history of dietary supplements and drug use may suggest intoxication with vitamin D or vitamin A or the use of thiazides.

R_x TREATMENT

Hypercalcemic States The approach to medical treatment of hypercalcemia varies with its severity (Table 332-4). Mild hypercalcemia, <3.0 mmol/L (12 mg/dL), can be managed by hydration. More severe hypercalcemia [levels of 3.2 to 3.7 mmol/L (13 to 15 mg/dL)] must be managed aggressively; above that level, hypercalcemia can be life-threatening and requires emergency measures. By using a combination of approaches in severe hypercalcemia, the serum calcium concentration can be decreased by 0.7 to 2.2 mmol/L (3 to 9 mg/dL) within 24 to 48 h in most patients, enough to relieve acute symptoms, prevent death from hypercalcemic crisis, and permit diagnostic evaluation. Therapy can then be directed at the underlying disorder—the second priority.

TABLE 332-4 *Therapies for Severe Hypercalcemia*

Treatment	Onset of Action	Duration of Action	Advantages	Disadvantages
MOST USEFUL THERAPIES				
Hydration with saline	Hours	During infusion	Rehydration invariably needed	Volume overload, cardiac decompensation, intensive monitoring, electrolyte disturbance, inconvenience
Forced diuresis; saline plus loop diuretic	Hours	During treatment	Rapid action	
Bisphosphonates 1st generation: etidronate	1–2 days	5–7 days in doses used	First available bisphosphonate; intermediate onset of action	Less effective than other bisphosphonates
2d generation: pamidronate	1–2 days	10–14 days to weeks	High potency; intermediate onset of action	Fever in 20% hypophosphatemia, hypocalcemia, hypomagnesemia
3d generation: zolendronate	1–2 days	>3 weeks	High potency; rapid infusion; prolonged duration of action	Minor; fever, rarely hypocalcemia or hypophosphatemia
Calcitonin	Hours	1–2 days	Rapid onset of action; useful as adjunct in severe hypercalcemia	Rapid tachyphylaxis
SPECIAL USE THERAPIES				
Phosphate Oral	24 h	During use	Chronic management (with hypophosphatemia); low toxicity if P < 4 mg/dL	Limited use except as adjuvant or chronic therapy
Intravenous	Hours	During use and 24–48 h afterward	Rapid action, highly potent but *rarely used* except with severe hypercalcemia and cardiac and renal decompensation present	Ectopic calcification; renal damage, fatal hypocalcemia
Glucocorticoids	Days	Days, weeks	Oral therapy, antitumor agent	Active only in certain malignancies; glucocorticoid side effects
Dialysis	Hours	During use and 24–48 h afterward	Useful in renal failure; onset of effect in hours; can immediately reverse life-threatening hypercalcemia	Complex procedure, reserved for extreme or special circumstances

Hypercalcemia develops because of excessive skeletal calcium release, increased intestinal calcium absorption, or inadequate renal calcium excretion. Understanding the particular pathogenesis helps guide therapy. For example, hypercalcemia in patients with malignancy is primarily due to excessive skeletal calcium release and is, therefore, minimally improved by restriction of dietary calcium. On the other hand, patients with vitamin D hypersensitivity or vitamin D intoxication have excessive intestinal calcium absorption, and restriction of dietary calcium is beneficial. Decreased renal function or ECF depletion decreases urinary calcium excretion. In such situations, rehydration may rapidly reduce or reverse the hypercalcemia, even though increased bone resorption persists. As outlined below, the more severe the hypercalcemia, the greater the number of combined therapies that should be used. Rapid acting (hours) approaches—rehydration, forced diuresis, and calcitonin—can be used with the most effective antiresorptive agents, such as bisphosphonates (since severe hypercalcemia usually involves excessive bone resorption).

HYDRATION, INCREASED SALT INTAKE, MILD AND FORCED DIURESIS The first principle of treatment is to restore normal hydration. Many hypercalcemic patients are dehydrated because of vomiting, inanition, and/or hypercalcemia-induced defects in urinary concentrating ability. The resultant drop in glomerular filtration rate is accompanied by an additional decrease in renal tubular sodium and calcium clearance. Restoring a normal ECF volume corrects these abnormalities and increases urine calcium excretion by 2.5 to 7.5 mmol/d (100 to 300 mg/d). Increasing urinary sodium excretion to 400 to 500 mmol/d increases urinary calcium excretion even further than simple rehydration. After rehydration has been achieved, saline can be administered or furosemide or ethacrynic acid can be given twice daily to depress the tubular reabsorptive mechanism for calcium (care must be taken to prevent dehydration). The combined use of these therapies can increase urinary calcium excretion to ≥12.5 mmol/d (500 mg/d) in most hypercalcemic patients. Since this is a substantial percentage of the exchangeable calcium pool, the serum calcium concentration usually falls 0.25 to 0.75 mmol/L (1 to 3 mg/dL) within 24 h. Precautions should be taken to prevent potassium and magnesium depletion; calcium-containing renal calculi are a potential complication.

Under life-threatening circumstances, the preceding approach can be pursued more aggressively, giving as much as 6 L isotonic saline (900 mmol sodium) daily plus furosemide or equivalent in doses up to 100 mg every 1 to 2 h or ethacrynic acid in doses to 40 mg every 1 to 2 h. Urinary calcium excretion may exceed 25 mmol/d (1000 mg/d), and the serum calcium may decrease by ≥1 mmol/L (4 mg/dL) within 24 h. Depletion of potassium and magnesium is inevitable unless replacements are given; pulmonary edema can be precipitated. The potential complications can be reduced by careful monitoring of central venous pressure and plasma or urine electrolytes; catheterization of the bladder may be necessary. This treatment approach should be supplemented with agents to block bone resorption. Though these agents do not become effective for several days, forced diuresis is difficult to sustain even in patients with good cardiopulmonary and renal function.

BISPHOSPHONATES The bisphosphonates are analogues of pyrophosphate, with high affinity for bone, especially in areas of increased bone turnover, where they are powerful inhibitors of bone resorption. These bone-seeking compounds are stable in vivo because phosphatase enzymes cannot hydrolyze the central carbon-phosphorus-carbon bond. The bisphosphonates are concentrated in areas of high bone turnover and are taken up by and inhibit osteoclast action; the mechanism of action is complex. Bisphosphonates alter osteoclast proton pump function or impair the release of acid hydrolases into the extracellular lysosomes contiguous with mineralized bone. They may also inhibit the differentiation of monocyte-macrophage precursors into osteoclasts and possibly have effects on osteoblasts as well. The bisphosphonate molecules that contain amino groups in the side chain structure (see below) interfere with prenylation of proteins and can lead to cellular apoptosis. The highly active non-amino group–containing bisphosphonates are also metabolized to cytotoxic products.

The initial bisphosphonate widely used in clinical practice, etidronate, was effective but had several disadvantages, including the capacity to inhibit bone formation as well as blocking resorption. Subsequently, a number of second-generation compounds have become the mainstays of antiresorptive therapy for treatment of hypercalcemia and osteoporosis. The newer bisphosphonates have a highly favorable ratio of blocking resorption versus inhibiting bone formation; they inhibit osteoclast-mediated skeletal resorption yet do not cause mineralization defects at ordinary doses. Though the bisphosphonates have similar structures, the routes of administration, efficacy, toxicity, and side effects vary. The potency of the compounds for inhibition of bone resorption varies a thousandfold, increasing in the order of etidronate, tiludronate, pamidronate, alendronate, and risedronate. Oral alendronate and risedronate are approved for the therapy of osteoporosis in the United States, but in Europe only for the chronic treatment of hypercalcemia. Only the intravenous use of pamidronate is approved for the treatment of hypercalcemia in the United States; between 30 and 90 mg pamidronate, given as a single intravenous dose over a few hours, returns serum calcium to normal within 24 to 48 h with an effect that lasts for weeks in 80 to 100% of patients.

Even more potent third-generation bisphosphonates have been recently introduced into clinical practice. Zolendronate, said to be sev-eralfold more potent than second-generation compounds, is reported in preliminary trials to be superior in treatment of hypercalcemia, normalizing calcium faster and for longer periods of time after infusion. Doses of 1 to 4 mg can be given over a few minutes intravenously.

CALCITONIN Calcitonin acts within a few hours of its administration, through receptors on osteoclasts, to block bone resorption and, in addition, to increase urinary calcium excretion by inhibition of renal tubular calcium reabsorption. Results with calcitonin, particularly after 24 h of use, are variable, with minimal lowering of calcium. Tachyphylaxis, a known phenomenon with this drug, may explain the results. However, in life-threatening hypercalcemia, calcitonin can be used effectively within the first 24 h in combination with rehydration and saline diuresis while waiting for more sustained effects from a simultaneously administered bisphosphonate such as pamidronate. Usual doses of calcitonin are 2 to 8 U/kg of body weight intravenously, subcutaneously, or intramuscularly every 6 to 12 h.

OTHER THERAPIES Plicamycin (formerly mithramycin), which inhibits bone resorption, has been a useful therapeutic agent but is now seldom used because of its toxicity and the effectiveness of bisphosphonates. Plicamycin must be given intravenously, either as a bolus or by slow infusion; the usual dose is 25 μg/kg body weight. Gallium nitrate exerts a hypocalcemic action by inhibiting bone resorption and altering the structure of bone crystals. It is not often used now because of superior alternatives.

Glucocorticoids have utility, especially in hypercalcemia complicating certain malignancies. They increase urinary calcium excretion and decrease intestinal calcium absorption when given in pharmacologic doses, but they also cause negative skeletal calcium balance. In normal individuals and in patients with primary hyperparathyroidism, glucocorticoids neither increase nor decrease the serum calcium concentration. In patients with hypercalcemia due to certain osteolytic malignancies, however, glucocorticoids may be effective as a result of antitumor effects. The malignancies in which hypercalcemia responds to glucocorticoids include multiple myeloma, leukemia, Hodgkin's disease, other lymphomas, and carcinoma of the breast, at least early in the course of the disease. Glucocorticoids are also effective in treating hypercalcemia due to vitamin D intoxication and sarcoidosis. In all the preceding situations, the hypocalcemic effect develops over several days, and the usual glucocorticoid dosage is 40 to 100 mg prednisone (or its equivalent) daily in four divided doses. The side effects of chronic glucocorticoid therapy may be acceptable in some circumstances.

Dialysis is often the treatment of choice for severe hypercalcemia complicated by renal failure, which is difficult to manage medically. Peritoneal dialysis with calcium-free dialysis fluid can remove 5 to 12.5 mmol (200 to 500 mg) of calcium in 24 to 48 h and lower the serum calcium concentration by 0.7 to 3 mmol/L (3 to 12 mg/dL). Large quantities of phosphate are lost during dialysis, and serum inorganic phosphate concentrations usually fall, thus aggravating hypercalcemia. Therefore, the serum inorganic phosphate concentration should be measured after dialysis, and phosphate supplements should be added to the diet or to dialysis fluids if necessary.

Phosphate therapy, oral or intravenous, has a limited role in certain circumstances. Correcting hypophosphatemia lowers the serum calcium concentration by several mechanisms, including bone/calcium exchange. The usual oral treatment is 1 to 1.5 g phosphorus per day for several days, given in divided doses. It is generally believed, but not established, that toxicity does not occur if therapy is limited to restoring serum inorganic phosphate concentrations to normal.

Raising the serum inorganic phosphate concentration above normal decreases serum calcium levels, sometimes strikingly. Intravenous phosphate is one of the most dramatically effective treatments available for severe hypercalcemia but is toxic and even dangerous (fatal hypocalcemia). For these reasons, it is used rarely and only in severely hypercalcemic patients with cardiac or renal failure. A phosphate phosphorus dose of ≥1500 mg intravenously over 6 to 8 h leads to a prompt decrease in serum calcium of as much as 1.2 to 2.5 mmol/L (5 to 10 mg/dL) in patients with initially normal serum inorganic phosphate concentrations. This therapy should be employed only in extreme emergencies. Inorganic phosphate is commercially available for oral use in liquid, powder, and capsule form and as a liquid for intravenous use. If used, it is important to calculate doses in terms of phosphate phosphorus.

Summary The various therapies for hypercalcemia are listed in Table 332-4. The choice depends on the underlying disease, the severity of the hypercalcemia, the serum inorganic phosphate level, and the renal, hepatic, and bone marrow function. Mild hypercalcemia [≤3 mmol/L (12 mg/dL)] can usually be managed by hydration. Severe hypercalcemia [≥3.7 mmol/L (15 mg/dL)] requires rapid correction. Calcitonin should be given for its rapid, albeit short-lived, blockade of bone resorption, and intravenous pamidronate or zolendronate should be administered, although its onset of action is delayed for 1 to 2 days. In addition, for the first 24 to 48 h, aggressive sodium-calcium diuresis with intravenous saline and large doses of furosemide or ethacrynic acid following initial hydration should be initiated, but only if appropriate monitoring is available and cardiac and renal function are adequate. Otherwise, dialysis may be necessary. Intermediate degrees of hypercalcemia between 3.0 and 3.7 mmol/L (12 and 15 mg/dL) should be approached with vigorous hydration and then the most appropriate selection for the patient of the combinations used with severe hypercalcemia.

HYPOCALCEMIA

PATHOPHYSIOLOGY OF HYPOCALCEMIA: CLASSIFICATION BASED ON MECHANISM

Chronic hypocalcemia is less common than hypercalcemia; causes include chronic renal failure, hereditary and acquired hypoparathyroidism, vitamin D deficiency, PHP, and hypomagnesemia.

Acute rather than chronic hypocalcemia is seen in critically ill patients or as a consequence of certain medications and often does not require specific treatment. Transient hypocalcemia is seen with severe sepsis, burns, acute renal failure, and extensive transfusions with citrated blood. Although as many as half of patients in an intensive care setting are reported to have calcium concentrations <2.1 mmol/L (8.5 mg/dL), most do not have a reduction in ionized calcium. Patients with severe sepsis may have a decrease in ionized calcium (true hypocalcemia), but in other severely ill individuals, hypoalbuminemia is the primary cause of the reduced total calcium concentration. Alkalosis increases calcium binding to proteins, and in this setting direct measurements of ionized calcium should be made.

Medications such as protamine, heparin, and glucagon may cause transient hypocalcemia. These forms of hypocalcemia are usually not associated with tetany and resolve with improvement in the overall medical condition. The hypocalcemia after repeated transfusions of citrated blood usually resolves quickly.

Patients with *acute pancreatitis* have hypocalcemia that persists during the acute inflammation and varies in degree with the severity of the pancreatitis. The cause of hypocalcemia remains unclear. PTH values are reported to be low, normal, or elevated, and both resistance to PTH and impaired PTH secretion have been postulated. Occasionally, a chronic low total calcium and low ionized calcium concentration are detected in an elderly patient without obvious cause and with a paucity of symptoms; the pathogenesis is unclear.

Chronic hypocalcemia, however, is usually symptomatic and requires treatment. Neuromuscular and neurologic manifestations of chronic hypocalcemia include muscle spasms, carpopedal spasm, facial grimacing, and, in extreme cases, laryngeal spasm and convulsions. Respiratory arrest may occur. Increased intracranial pressure occurs in some patients with long-standing hypocalcemia, often in association with papilledema. Mental changes include irritability, depression, and psychosis. The QT interval on the electrocardiogram is prolonged, in contrast to its shortening with hypercalcemia. Arrhythmias occur, and digitalis effectiveness may be reduced. Intestinal cramps and chronic malabsorption may occur. Chvostek's or Trousseau's sign can be used to confirm latent tetany.

The classification of hypocalcemia shown in Table 332-5 is based on an organizationally useful premise that PTH is responsible for minute-to-minute regulation of plasma calcium concentration and, therefore, that the occurrence of hypocalcemia must mean a failure of the homeostatic action of PTH. Failure of the PTH response can occur if there is hereditary or acquired parathyroid gland failure, if PTH is ineffective in target organs, or if the action of the hormone is overwhelmed by the loss of calcium from the ECF at a rate faster than it can be replaced.

PTH ABSENT Whether hereditary or acquired, hypoparathyroidism has a number of common components. Symptoms of untreated hypocalcemia are shared by both types of hypoparathyroidism, although the onset of hereditary hypoparathyroidism is more gradual and is often associated with other developmental defects. Basal ganglia calcification and extrapyramidal syndromes are more common and earlier in onset in hereditary hypoparathyroidism. In earlier decades, acquired hypoparathyroidism secondary to surgery in the neck was more common than hereditary hypoparathyroidism, but the frequency of surgically induced parathyroid failure has diminished as a result of improved surgical techniques that spare the parathyroid glands and increased use of nonsurgical therapy for hyperthyroidism. PHP, an example of ineffective PTH action rather than a failure of parathyroid gland production, may share several features with hypoparathyroidism, including extraosseous calcification and extrapyramidal manifestations such as choreoathetotic movements and dystonia.

Papilledema and raised intracranial pressure may occur in both hereditary and acquired hypoparathyroidism, as do chronic changes in fingernails and hair and lenticular cataracts, the latter usually reversible with treatment of hypocalcemia. Certain skin manifestations, including alopecia and candidiasis, are characteristic of hereditary hypoparathyroidism associated with autoimmune polyglandular failure (Chap. 330).

Hypocalcemia associated with hypomagnesemia is associated with both deficient PTH release and impaired responsiveness to the hormone. Patients with hypocalcemia secondary to hypomagnesemia have absent or low levels of circulating PTH, indicative of diminished hormone release despite maximum physiologic stimulus by hypocalcemia. Plasma PTH levels return to normal with correction of the hypomagnesemia. Thus hypoparathyroidism with low levels of PTH in blood can be due to hereditary gland failure, acquired gland failure, or acute but reversible gland dysfunction (hypomagnesemia).

Genetic Abnormalities and Hereditary Hypoparathyroidism Hereditary hypoparathyroidism can occur as an isolated entity without other endocrine or dermatologic manifestations (idiopathic hypoparathyroidism).

TABLE 332-5 *Functional Classification of Hypocalcemia (Excluding Neonatal Conditions)*

PTH ABSENT	
Hereditary hypoparathyroidism Acquired hypoparathyroidism	Hypomagnesemia
PTH INEFFECTIVE	

Chronic renal failure
Active vitamin D lacking
  ↓ Dietary intake or sunlight
  Defective metabolism:
    Anticonvulsant therapy
    Vitamin D–dependent
    rickets type I
	Active vitamin D ineffective
	  Intestinal malabsorption
	  Vitamin D–dependent rickets
	    type II
	Pseudohypoparathyroidism

PTH OVERWHELMED	

Severe, acute hyperphosphatemia
  Tumor lysis
  Acute renal failure
  Rhabdomyolysis
	Osteitis fibrosa after
	  parathyroidectomy

Note: PTH, parathyroid hormone.

More typically, it occurs in association with other abnormalities such as defective development of the thymus or failure of other endocrine organs such as the adrenal, thyroid, or ovary (Chap. 330). Idiopathic and hereditary hypoparathyroidism are often manifest within the first decade but may appear later.

A rare form of hypoparathyroidism associated with defective development of both the thymus and the parathyroid glands is termed the *DiGeorge syndrome*, or the *velocardiofacial syndrome*. Congenital cardiovascular, facial, and other developmental defects are present, and most patients die in early childhood with severe infections, hypocalcemia and seizures, or cardiovascular complications. Some survive into adulthood, and milder, incomplete forms occur. Most cases are sporadic, but an autosomal dominant form involving microdeletions of chromosome 22q11.2 has been described. Smaller deletions in this region are seen in incomplete forms of the DiGeorge syndrome, appearing in childhood or adolescence, that are manifest primarily by parathyroid gland failure.

Hypoparathyroidism can occur in association with a complex hereditary autoimmune syndrome involving failure of the adrenals, the ovaries, the immune system, and the parathyroids in association with recurrent mucocutaneous candidiasis, alopecia, vitiligo, and pernicious anemia (Chap. 330). The responsible gene on chromosome 21q22.3 has been identified. The protein product, which resembles a transcription factor, has been termed the *autoimmune regulator*, or AIRE. A stop codon mutation occurs in many Finnish families with the disorder, commonly referred to as *polyglandular autoimmune type 1 deficiency*.

Gain-of-function mutations in the calcium-sensing receptor cause *autosomal dominant hypocalcemia*. These mutations induce constitutive receptor functions that lead to features that are the inverse of FHH. The activated receptor suppresses PTH secretion, leading to hypocalcemia; receptor activation in the kidney results in excessive renal calcium excretion. Recognition of the syndrome is important because efforts to treat the hypocalcemia of these patients with vitamin D analogues and increased oral calcium exacerbate the already excessive urinary calcium secretion (several grams or more per 24 h), leading to irreversible renal damage from stones and ectopic calcification.

Hypoparathyroidism is seen in two disorders associated with mitochondrial dysfunction and myopathy, one termed the *Kearns-Sayre syndrome* (KSS), with ophthalmaplegia and pigmentary retinopathy, and the other termed the *MELAS syndrome*, *m*itochondrial *e*ncephalopathy, *l*actic *a*cidosis, and *s*troke-like episodes. Mutations or deletions in mitochondrial genes have been identified.

The two other rare forms of hypoparathyroidism with other multisystem developmental abnormalities follow either an autosomal dominant pattern, with deafness and/or renal dysplasia, or an autosomal recessive pattern, with growth retardation and dysmorphic features.

Hereditary hypoparathyroidism occurs also as an isolated entity without any other defects. The pattern of inheritance varies and includes autosomal dominant, autosomal recessive, and X-linked inheritance patterns. In one family in which the disorder is transmitted as an autosomal dominant trait, a structural abnormality in the PTH gene has been identified. A defect in the signal sequence needed for processing of the hormone impairs PTH secretion. In another kindred with autosomal recessive inheritance, the mutant allele in the first intron of the PTH gene causes a splicing defect in mRNA production. An X-linked recessive form of hypoparathyroidism has been described in males and the defect has been localized to chromosome Xq26-q27.

Acquired Hypoparathyroidism *Acquired chronic hypoparathyroidism* is usually the result of inadvertent surgical removal of all the parathyroid glands; in some instances, not all the tissue is removed, but the remainder undergoes vascular supply compromise secondary to fibrotic changes in the neck after surgery. In the past, the most frequent cause of acquired hypoparathyroidism was surgery for hyperthyroidism. Hypoparathyroidism now usually occurs after surgery for hyperparathyroidism when the surgeon, facing the dilemma of removing too little tissue and thus not curing the hyperparathyroidism, removes too much. Parathyroid function may not be totally absent in all patients with postoperative hypoparathyroidism.

Even rarer causes of acquired chronic hypoparathyroidism include radiation-induced damage subsequent to radioiodine therapy of hyperthyroidism and glandular damage in patients with hemochromatosis or hemosiderosis after repeated blood transfusions. Infection may involve one or more of the parathyroids but usually does not cause hypoparathyroidism because all four glands are rarely involved.

Transient hypoparathyroidism is frequent following surgery for hyperparathyroidism. After a variable period of hypoparathyroidism, normal parathyroid function may return due to hyperplasia or recovery of remaining tissue. Occasionally, recovery occurs months after surgery.

℞ TREATMENT

Treatment of acquired and hereditary hypoparathyroidism involves replacement with vitamin D or $1,25(OH)_2D_3$ (calcitriol) combined with a high oral calcium intake. In most patients, blood calcium and phosphate levels are satisfactorily regulated, but some patients show resistance and a brittleness, with a tendency to alternate between hypocalcemia and hypercalcemia. For many patients, vitamin D in doses of 40,000 to 120,000 U/d (1 to 3 mg/d) combined with ≥1 g elemental calcium is satisfactory. The wide dosage range reflects the variation encountered from patient to patient; precise regulation of each patient is required. Compared to typical daily requirements in euparathyroid patients of 200 U/d, the high dose of vitamin D reflects the reduced conversion of vitamin D to $1,25(OH)_2D$. Many physicians now use 0.5 to 1.0 μg of calcitriol in management of such patients, especially if they are difficult to control. Because of its storage in fat, when vitamin D is withdrawn, weeks are required for the disappearance of the biologic effects, compared with a few days for calcitriol, which has a rapid turnover.

Oral calcium and vitamin D restore the overall calcium-phosphate balance but do not reverse the lowered urinary calcium reabsorption typical of hypoparathyroidism. Therefore, care must be taken to avoid excessive urinary calcium excretion after vitamin D and calcium replacement therapy; otherwise, kidney stones can develop. Thiazide diuretics lower urine calcium by as much as 100 mg/d in hypoparathyroid patients on vitamin D, provided they are maintained on a low-sodium diet. Use of thiazides seems to be of benefit in mitigating hypercalciuria and easing the daily management of these patients.

Hypomagnesemia Severe hypomagnesemia (<0.4 mmol/L; <0.8 meq/L) is associated with hypocalcemia (Chap. 331). Restoration of the total-body magnesium deficit leads to rapid reversal of hypocalcemia. There are at least two causes of the hypocalcemia—impaired PTH secretion and reduced responsiveness to PTH. →*For discussion of causes and treatment of hypomagnesemia, see Chap. 331.*

The effects of magnesium on PTH secretion are similar to those of calcium; hypermagnesemia suppresses and hypomagnesemia stimulates PTH secretion. The effects of magnesium on PTH secretion are normally of little significance, however, because the calcium effects dominate. Greater change in magnesium than in calcium is needed to influence hormone secretion. Nonetheless, hypomagnesemia might be expected to increase hormone secretion. It is therefore surprising to find that severe hypomagnesemia is associated with blunted secretion of PTH. The explanation for the paradox is that severe, chronic hypomagnesemia leads to intracellular magnesium deficiency, which interferes with secretion and peripheral responses to PTH. The mechanism of the cellular abnormalities caused by hypomagnesemia is unknown, although effects on adenylate cyclase (for which magnesium is a cofactor) have been proposed.

PTH levels are undetectable or inappropriately low in severe hypomagnesemia despite the stimulus of severe hypocalcemia, and acute repletion of magnesium leads to a rapid increase in PTH level. Serum phosphate levels are often not elevated, in contrast to the situation with acquired or idiopathic hypoparathyroidism, probably because phosphate deficiency is a frequent accompaniment of hypomagnesemia.

Diminished peripheral responsiveness to PTH also occurs in some patients, as documented by subnormal response in urinary phosphorus and urinary cyclic AMP excretion after administration of exogenous PTH to patients who are hypocalcemic and hypomagnesemic. Both blunted PTH secretion and lack of renal response to administered PTH can occur in the same patient. When acute magnesium repletion is undertaken, the restoration of PTH levels to normal or supranormal may precede restoration of normal serum calcium by several days.

℞ TREATMENT

Repletion of magnesium cures the condition. Repletion should be parenteral. Attention must be given to restoring the intracellular deficit, which may be considerable. After intravenous magnesium administration, serum magnesium may return transiently to the normal range, but unless replacement therapy is adequate serum magnesium will again fall. If the cause of the hypomagnesemia is renal magnesium wasting, magnesium may have to be given chronically to prevent recurrence (Chap. 331).

PTH INEFFECTIVE PTH is ineffective when the hormone receptor–guanyl nucleotide–binding protein complex is defective (PHP, discussed below), when PTH action to promote calcium absorption from the diet is impaired because of vitamin D deficiency or because vitamin D is ineffective (receptor or synthesis defects), or in chronic renal failure in which the calcium-elevating action of PTH is impaired.

Typically, hypophosphatemia is more severe than hypocalcemia in vitamin D deficiency states because of the increased secretion of PTH, which, although only partly effective in elevating blood calcium, is capable of promoting phosphaturia.

PHP, on the other hand, has a pathophysiology different from the other disorders of ineffective PTH action. PHP resembles hypoparathyroidism (in which PTH synthesis is deficient) and is manifested by hypocalcemia and hyperphosphatemia. The cause of the disorder is defective hormone activation of guanyl nucleotide–binding proteins, resulting in failure of PTH to increase intracellular cyclic AMP (see below).

Chronic Renal Failure Improved medical management of chronic renal failure now allows many patients to survive for years and hence time enough to develop features of renal osteodystrophy, which must be controlled to avoid its morbidity. Phosphate retention and impaired production of $1,25(OH)_2D$ are the principal factors that cause calcium deficiency, secondary hyperparathyroidism, and bone disease. Low levels of $1,25(OH)_2D$ due to hyperphosphatemia and destruction of renal tissue are critical in the development of hypocalcemia. The uremic state also causes impairment of intestinal absorption by mechanisms other than defects in vitamin D metabolism. Nonetheless, treatment with supraphysiologic amounts of vitamin D or calcitriol corrects the impaired calcium absorption.

Hyperphosphatemia in renal failure lowers blood calcium levels by several mechanisms, including extraosseous deposition of calcium and phosphate, impairment of the bone-resorbing action of PTH, and reduction in $1,25(OH)_2D$ production by remaining renal tissue.

℞ TREATMENT

Therapy of chronic renal failure (Chap. 261) involves appropriate management of patients prior to dialysis and adjustment of regimens once dialysis is initiated. Attention should be paid to restriction of phosphate in the diet; avoidance of aluminum-containing phosphate-binding antacids to prevent the problem of aluminum intoxication; provision of an adequate calcium intake by mouth, usually 1 to 2 g/d; and supplementation with 0.25 to 1.0 μg/d calcitriol. Each patient must be monitored closely. The aim of therapy is to restore normal calcium balance to prevent osteomalacia and secondary hyperparathyroidism and, in light of evidence of genetic changes and monoclonal outgrowths of parathyroid glands in renal failure patients, to prevent sec-

ondary from becoming autonomous hyperparathyroidism. Reduction of hyperphosphatemia and restoration of normal intestinal calcium absorption by calcitriol can improve blood calcium levels and reduce the manifestations of secondary hyperparathyroidism. Since adynamic bone disease can occur in association with low PTH levels, it is important to avoid excessive suppression of the parathyroid glands while recognizing the beneficial effects of controlling the secondary hyperparathyroidism. These patients should probably be closely monitored with PTH assays that detect only the full-length PTH(1–84) to ensure that biologically active PTH and not inactive, inhibitory PTH fragments are measured.

Vitamin D Deficiency Due to Inadequate Diet and/or Sunlight Vitamin D deficiency due to inadequate intake of dairy products enriched with vitamin D, lack of vitamin supplementation, and reduced sunlight exposure in the elderly, particularly during winter in northern latitudes, is more common in the United States than previously recognized. Diopsies of bone in elderly patients with hip fracture (documenting osteomalacia) and abnormal levels of vitamin D metabolites, PTH, calcium, and phosphate indicate that vitamin D deficiency may occur in as many as 25% of elderly patients, particularly in northern latitudes in the United States. Concentrations of 25(OH)D are low or low-normal in these patients. Quantitative histomorphometry of bone biopsy specimens reveals widened osteoid seams consistent with osteomalacia (Chap. 331). PTH hypersecretion compensates for the tendency for the blood calcium to fall but also induces renal phosphate wasting and results in osteomalacia.

Treatment involves adequate replacement with vitamin D and calcium until the deficiencies are corrected. Severe hypocalcemia rarely occurs in moderately severe vitamin D deficiency of the elderly, but vitamin D deficiency must be considered in the differential diagnosis of mild hypocalcemia.

Defective Vitamin D Metabolism ■ *ANTICONVULSANT THERAPY* Anticonvulsant therapy with any of several agents induces acquired vitamin D deficiency by increasing the conversion of vitamin D to inactive compounds. The more marginal the vitamin D intake in the diet, the more likely that anticonvulsant therapy will lead to abnormal mineral and bone metabolism →*For discussion of treatment, see Chap. 331.*

VITAMIN D–DEPENDENT RICKETS TYPE I Rickets can be due to *resistance to the action* of vitamin D as well as to vitamin D deficiency. Vitamin D–dependent rickets type I, previously termed *pseudo-vitamin D–resistant rickets*, differs from true vitamin D–resistant rickets (vitamin D-dependent rickets type II, see below) in that it is less severe and the biochemical and radiographic abnormalities can be reversed with appropriate doses of the vitamin or the active metabolite, $1,25(OH)_2D_3$. Physiologic amounts of calcitriol cure the disease (Chap. 331). This finding fits with the pathophysiology of the disorder, which is autosomal recessive, and is now known to be caused by mutations in the gene encoding $25(OH)D$-1α-hydroxylase. Both alleles are inactivated in all patients, and compount heterozygotes, harboring distinct mutations, are common.

Clinical features include hypocalcemia, often with tetany or convulsions, hypophosphatemia, secondary hyperparathyroidism, and osteomalacia, often associated with skeletal deformities and increased alkaline phosphatase. Treatment involves physiologic replacement doses of $1,25(OH)_2D_3$ (Chap. 331).

Vitamin D Ineffective ■ *INTESTINAL MALABSORPTION* Mild hypocalcemia, secondary hyperparathyroidism, severe hypophosphatemia, and a variety of nutritional deficiencies occur with gastrointestinal diseases. Hepatocellular dysfunction can lead to reduction in 25(OH)D levels, as in portal or biliary cirrhosis of the liver, and malabsorption of vitamin D and its metabolites, including $1,25(OH)_2D$, may occur in a variety of bowel diseases, hereditary or acquired. Hypocalcemia itself can lead to steatorrhea, due to deficient production of pancreatic enzymes and bile salts. Depending on the disorder, vitamin D or its

Type	Hypocalcemia, Hyperphosphatemia	Response of Urinary cAMP to PTH	Serum PTH	$G_{s\alpha}$ Subunit Deficiency	AHO	Resistance to Hormones in Addition to PTH
PHP-Ia	Yes	↓	↑	Yes	Yes	Yes
PHP-Ib	Yes	↓	↑	No	No	No
PHP-II	Yes	Normal	↑	No	No	No
PPHP	No	Normal	Normal	Yes	Yes	±

Note: ↓, decreased; ↑, increased; AHO, Albright's hereditary osteodystrophy; PTH, parathyroid hormone.

metabolites can be given parenterally, guaranteeing adequate blood levels of active metabolites.

VITAMIN D–DEPENDENT RICKETS TYPE II Vitamin D–dependent rickets type II results from end-organ resistance to the active metabolite $1,25(OH)_2D_3$. The clinical features resemble those of the type I disorder and include hypocalcemia, hypophosphatemia, secondary hyperparathyroidism, and rickets but also partial or total alopecia. Plasma levels of $1,25(OH)_2D$ are at least three times normal, in keeping with the refractoriness of the end organs. All of the genetically characterized phenotypes have mutations in the gene for the vitamin D receptor. Treatment is difficult, given the receptor defect (Chap. 331).

Pseudohypoparathyroidism PHP is a hereditary disorder characterized by symptoms and signs of hypoparathyroidism, typically in association with distinctive skeletal and developmental defects. The hypoparathyroidism is due to a deficient end-organ response to PTH. Hyperplasia of the parathyroids, a response to hormone resistance, causes elevation of PTH levels. Studies, both clinical and basic, have clarified some aspects of this syndrome, including the variable clinical spectrum, the pathophysiology, the genetic defects, and the inheritance.

A working classification of the various forms of PHP is given in Table 332-6. The classification scheme is based on the signs of ineffective PTH action (low calcium and high phosphate), urinary cyclic AMP response to exogenous PTH, the presence or absence of *Albright's hereditary osteodystrophy* (AHO), and assays of the concentration of the $G_{s\alpha}$ subunit of the adenylate cyclase enzyme. Using these criteria, there are four types: PHP type I, subdivided into a and b categories; PHP-II; and pseudopseudohypoparathyroidism (PPHP).

PHP-IA AND PHP-IB Individuals with PHP-I, the most common of the disorders, show a deficient urinary cyclic AMP response to administration of exogenous PTH. Patients with PHP-I are divided into type a, who have reduced amounts of $G_{s\alpha}$ in vitro assays with erythrocytes, and type b, with normal amounts of $G_{s\alpha}$ in erythrocytes. There is a third type (PHP-Ic, reported in a few patients) that differs from PHP-Ia only in having normal erythrocyte levels of $G_{s\alpha}$ despite having AHO, hypocalcemia, and decreased urinary cyclic AMP responses to PTH (presumably with a post-$G_{s\alpha}$ defect in adenyl cyclase stimulation).

Most patients show characteristic features of AHO, consisting of short stature, round face, skeletal anomalies (brachydactyly), and heterotopic calcification. Patients have low calcium and high phosphate levels, as with true hypoparathyroidism. PTH levels, however, are elevated, reflecting resistance to hormone action.

Amorphous deposits of calcium and phosphate are found in the basal ganglia in about half of patients. The defects in metacarpal and metatarsal bones are sometimes accompanied by short phalanges as well, possibly reflecting premature closing of the epiphyses. The typical findings are short fourth and fifth metacarpals and metatarsals. The defects are usually bilateral. Exostoses and radius curvus are frequent. Impairments in olfaction and taste and unusual dermatoglyphic abnormalities have been reported.

PPHP Multiple defects have now been identified in the *GNAS-1* gene in PHP-Ia and PPHP patients. This gene, which is located on chromosome 20q13, encodes the stimulatory G protein subunit $G_{s\alpha}$, among other products (see below). Mutations include abnormalities in splice junctions associated with deficient mRNA production and point mu-

tations that result in a protein with defective function as well as a 50% reduction in $G_{s\alpha}$ levels in erythrocytes.

Detailed analyses of disease transmission in affected kindreds have clarified many features of PHP-Ia, PPHP, and PHP-Ib (Fig. 332-7). The former two entities, traced through multiple kindreds, have an inheritance pattern consistent with gene imprinting—only females, not males, can transmit the full disease with hypocalcemia—and PHP and PPHP do not coexist in the same generation. The phenomenon of gene imprinting involves selective inactivation of either the maternal or the paternal allele (Chap. 56). In the case of the $G_{s\alpha}$ gene, it is paternally imprinted (silenced) so that the disease PHP-Ia is never inherited from the father carrying the defective allele but only from the mother. On the other hand, the defective allele is not imprinted or silenced in all tissues. It seems possible, therefore, that the AHO phenotype recognized in PPHP as well as PHP-Ia reflects haplotype insufficiency during embryonic development. In the renal cortex, however, it is postulated that only the maternal allele is normally active, such that lack of activity from a defective paternal allele is not of consequence. This explains the occurrence in PHP-Ia of hypocalcemia, hyperphosphatemia, and other stigmata such as variable resistance to other hormones (if similar tissue-specific imprinting occurs in other organs). Strong evidence favoring this overall hypothesis comes from gene knockout studies in the mouse (ablating exon 2 of the gene). Mice inheriting the mutant allele from the female had undetectable $G_{s\alpha}$ protein in renal cortex and were hypocalcemic and resistant to renal actions of PTH. Offspring inheriting the mutant allele from the male showed no evidence of PTH resistance or hypercalcemia.

The complex mechanisms that control the *GNAS-1* gene also contribute to challenges involved in unraveling the pathogenesis of these disorders. Alternative splicing patterns produce three different transcripts that encode distinct proteins. In addition to $G_{s\alpha}$, this gene encodes a second protein product with a unique NH_2-terminus (the XL exon); $XL_\alpha s$ includes exons 2–13. It is unknown whether this protein can function as a stimulatory G protein, but the mRNA encoding it is

FIGURE 332-7 Paternal imprinting of renal parathyroid hormone (PTH) resistance (*GNAS-1* gene for $G_{s\alpha}$ subunit) in pseudohypoparathyroidism (PHP). An impaired excretion of urinary cyclic AMP and phosphate is observed in patients with PHP. In the renal cortex, there is selective silencing of the paternal $G_{s\alpha}$ gene mRNA. The disease becomes manifest only in patients who inherit the defective gene from an obligate female carrier (*left*). If the genetic defect is inherited from an obligate male gene carrier, there is no biochemical abnormality; administration of PTH causes an appropriate increase in the urinary cyclic AMP and phosphate concentration [pseudo-PHP (PPHP); *right*]. Both patterns of inheritance lead to Albright's hereditary osteodystrophy (AHO), perhaps because of haplotype insufficiency—i.e., both copies of $G_{s\alpha}$ must be active in the fetus for normal bone development.

expressed in numerous endocrine tissues and is transcribed from only the paternal allele. A third transcript is transcribed from only the maternal allele and encodes the protein product, NESP55, which contains no homology with $XL_\alpha s$ or $G_s\alpha$.

PHP-Ib, lacking the AHO phenotype, shares with PHP-Ia the resistance to PTH action and a blunted urinary cyclic AMP response to administered PTH, a standard test for hormone resistance (Table 332-6). PHP-Ib patients, however, show normal levels of $G_s\alpha$ in erythrocytes. Bone responsiveness may be excessive rather than blunted in PHP-Ib compared to PHP-Ia patients, based on case reports that have emphasized an osteitis fibrosa–like pattern in some PHP patients who lack the AHO phenotype. The inheritance patterns in PHP-Ib kindreds are clearly consistent with paternal imprinting and lack male transmission of symptomatic disease; gene cloning studies have narrowed the responsible region to chromosome 20, close to—if not within—the *GNAS-1* gene locus. Elucidation of the responsible genetic and pathogenetic mechanisms in this disorder may further illuminate the function of the complex *GNAS-1* gene and the role of its products in hormonal signaling.

PHP-II refers to patients with hypocalcemia and hyperphosphatemia who have a normal urinary cyclic AMP response to PTH. These patients are assumed to have a defect in the response to PTH at a locus distal to cyclic AMP production, although at least some patients may instead have occult vitamin D deficiency.

The diagnosis of these hormone-resistant states can usually be made without difficulty when there is a positive family history for developmental defects and/or the presence of developmental anomalies, including brachydactyly, in association with the signs and symptoms of hypoparathyroidism. In all categories—PHP-Ia, -Ib, and -II—serum PTH levels are elevated, particularly when patients are hypocalcemic. However, patients with PHP-Ib or PHP-II do not have phenotypic abnormalities, only hypocalcemia with high PTH levels, confirming hormone resistance. In PHP-Ib, the response of urinary cyclic AMP to the administration of exogenous PTH is blunted. Levels of $G_s\alpha$ subunits in erythrocyte membranes are, however, normal in those with PHP-Ib. The diagnosis of PHP-II is more complex, in that cyclic AMP responses in urine are, by definition, normal. Since vitamin D deficiency itself can dissociate phosphaturic and urinary cyclic AMP responses to exogenous PTH, vitamin D deficiency must be excluded before the diagnosis of PHP-II can be entertained.

℞ TREATMENT

Treatment of PHP is similar to that of hypoparathyroidism, except that the doses of vitamin D and calcium are usually lower than those required in true hypoparathyroidism, presumably because the defect in PHP is only partial because of imprinting in specific tissues (renal cortex vs. renal medulla). Variability in response makes it necessary to establish the optimal regimen for each patient, based on maintaining the appropriate blood calcium level and urinary calcium excretion.

PTH Overwhelmed Occasionally, loss of calcium from the ECF is so severe that PTH cannot compensate. Such situations include acute pancreatitis and severe, acute hyperphosphatemia, often in association with renal failure, conditions in which there is rapid efflux of calcium from the ECF. Severe hypocalcemia can occur quickly; PTH rises in response to hypocalcemia but does not return blood calcium to normal.

Severe, Acute Hyperphosphatemia Severe hyperphosphatemia is associated with extensive tissue damage or cell destruction (Chap. 331). The combination of increased release of phosphate from muscle and impaired ability to excrete phosphorus because of renal failure causes moderate to severe hyperphosphatemia, the latter causing calcium loss from the blood and mild to moderate hypocalcemia. Hypocalcemia is usually reversed with tissue repair and restoration of renal function as phosphorus and creatinine values return to normal. There may even be a mild hypercalcemic period in the oliguric phase of renal function recovery. This sequence, severe hypocalcemia followed by mild hypercalcemia, reflects widespread deposition of calcium in muscle and

subsequent redistribution of some of the calcium to the ECF after phosphate levels return to normal.

Other causes of hyperphosphatemia include hypothermia, massive hepatic failure, and hematologic malignancies, either because of high cell turnover of malignancy or because of cell destruction by chemotherapy.

℞ TREATMENT

Treatment is directed toward lowering of blood phosphate by the administration of phosphate-binding antacids or dialysis, often needed for the management of renal failure. Although calcium replacement may be necessary if hypocalcemia is severe and symptomatic, calcium administration during the hyperphosphatemic period tends to increase extraosseous calcium deposition and aggravate tissue damage. The levels of $1,25(OH)_2D$ may be low during the hyperphosphatemic phase and return to normal during the oliguric phase of recovery.

Osteitis Fibrosis after Parathyroidectomy Severe hypocalcemia after parathyroid surgery is rare now that osteitis fibrosa cystica is an infrequent manifestation of hyperparathyroidism. When osteitis fibrosa cystica is severe, however, bone mineral deficits can be large. After parathyroidectomy, hypocalcemia can persist for days if calcium replacement is inadequate. Treatment may require parenteral administration of calcium; addition of calcitriol and oral calcium supplementation is sometimes needed for weeks to a month or two until bone defects are filled (which, of course, is of therapeutic benefit in the skeleton), making it possible to discontinue parenteral calcium and/or reduce the amount.

DIFFERENTIAL DIAGNOSIS OF HYPOCALCEMIA Care must be taken to ensure that true hypocalcemia is present; in addition, acute transient hypocalcemia can be a manifestation of a variety of severe, acute illnesses, as discussed above. *Chronic hypocalcemia*, however, can usually be ascribed to a few disorders associated with absent or ineffective PTH. Important clinical criteria include the duration of the illness, signs or symptoms of associated disorders, and the presence of features that suggest a hereditary abnormality. A nutritional history can be helpful in recognizing a low intake of vitamin D and calcium in the elderly, and a history of excessive alcohol intake may suggest magnesium deficiency.

Hypoparathyroidism and PHP are typically lifelong illnesses, usually (but not always) appearing by adolescence; hence a recent onset of hypocalcemia in an adult is more likely due to nutritional deficiencies, renal failure, or intestinal disorders that result in deficient or ineffective vitamin D. Neck surgery, even long past, however, can be associated with a delayed onset of postoperative hypoparathyroidism. A history of seizure disorder raises the issue of anticonvulsive medication. Developmental defects may point to the diagnosis of PHP. Rickets and a variety of neuromuscular syndromes and deformities may indicate ineffective vitamin D action, either due to defects in vitamin D metabolism or to vitamin D deficiency.

A pattern of *low calcium with high phosphorus* in the absence of renal failure or massive tissue destruction almost invariably means hypoparathyroidism or PHP. A *low calcium and low phosphorus* points to absent or ineffective vitamin D, thereby impairing the action of PTH on calcium metabolism (but not phosphate clearance). The relative ineffectiveness of PTH in calcium homeostasis in vitamin D deficiency, anticonvulsant therapy, gastrointestinal disorders, and hereditary defects in vitamin D metabolism leads to secondary hyperparathyroidism as a compensation. The excess PTH on renal tubule phosphate transport accounts for renal phosphate wasting and hypophosphatemia.

Exceptions to these patterns may occur. Most forms of hypomagnesemia are due to long-standing nutritional deficiency as seen in chronic alcoholics. Despite the fact that the hypocalcemia is principally due to an acute absence of PTH, phosphate levels are usually low, rather than elevated as in hypoparathyroidism. Chronic renal failure is often associated with hypocalcemia and hyperphosphatemia, despite secondary hyperparathyroidism.

Diagnosis is usually established by application of the PTH immunoassay, tests for vitamin D metabolites, and measurements of the urinary cyclic AMP response to exogenous PTH. In hereditary and acquired hypoparathyroidism and in severe hypomagnesemia, PTH is either undetectable or in the normal range. This finding in a hypocalcemic patient is supportive of hypoparathyroidism, as distinct from ineffective PTH action, in which even mild hypocalcemia is associated with elevated PTH levels. Hence a failure to detect elevated PTH levels establishes the diagnosis of hypoparathyroidism; elevated levels suggest the presence of secondary hyperparathyroidism, as found in many of the situations in which the hormone is ineffective due to associated abnormalities in vitamin D action. Assays for 25(OH)D and 1,25(OH)$_2$D can be helpful. Low or low normal 25(OH)D indicates vitamin D deficiency due to lack of sunlight, inadequate vitamin D intake, or intestinal malabsorption. A low level of 1,25(OH)$_2$D in the presence of elevated concentrations of PTH suggests ineffective PTH action in disorders such as chronic renal failure, severe vitamin D deficiency, vitamin D–dependent rickets type I, and PHP. Recognition that mild hypocalcemia, rickets, and hypophosphatemia are due to anticonvulsant therapy is made by history.

℞ TREATMENT

Hypocalcemic States   The management of hypoparathyroidism, PHP, chronic renal failure, and hereditary defects in vitamin D metabolism involves the use of vitamin D or vitamin D metabolites and calcium supplementation. Vitamin D itself is the least expensive form of vitamin D replacement and is frequently used in the management of uncomplicated hypoparathyroidism and some disorders associated with ineffective vitamin D action. When vitamin D is used prophylactically, as in the elderly or in those with chronic anticonvulsant therapy, there is a wider margin of safety than with the more potent metabolites. However, most of the conditions in which vitamin D is administered chronically for hypocalcemia require amounts 50 to 100 times the daily replacement dose because the formation of 1,25(OH)$_2$D is deficient. In such situations, vitamin D is no safer than the active metabolite because intoxication can occur with high-dose therapy (because of storage in fat). Calcitriol is more rapid in onset of action and also has a short biologic half-life.

Vitamin D [200 U (5 μg/d)] or calcifediol and lower doses of calcitriol (0.25 to 1.0 μg/d) are required to prevent rickets in normal individuals. In contrast, 40,000 to 12,000 U (1 to 3 mg) of vitamin D$_2$ or D$_3$ is typically required in hypoparathyroidism; doses of calcifediol are also high (several hundred micrograms per day). The dose of calcitriol is unchanged in hypoparathyroidism, since the defect is in hydroxylation by the 25(OH)D-1α-hydroxylase.

Patients with hypoparathyroidism should be given 2 to 3 g elemental calcium by mouth each day. The two agents, vitamin D or calcitriol and oral calcium, can be varied independently. If hypocalcemia alternates with episodes of hypercalcemia in more brittle patients with hypoparathyroidism, administration of calcitriol and use of thiazides, as discussed above, may make management easier.

FURTHER READING

BASTEPE M, JÜPPNER H: Pseudohypoparathyroidism: New insights into an old disease. Endocrinol Metab Clin North Am 29:569, 2000

BILEZIKIAN JP, POTTS JT JR: Asymptomatic primary hyperparathyroidism: New issues and new questions—bridging the past with the future. J Bone Min Res 17(Suppl 2):N57, 2002

CHEN H et al: Outpatient minimally invasive parathyroidectomy: A combination of sestamibi-SPECT localization, cervical block anesthesia, and intraoperative parathyroid hormone assay. Surgery 126:1021, 1999

REID R et al: Intravenous zoledronic acid in postmenopausal women with low bone mineral density. N Engl J Med 346:653, 2002

SILVERBERG SJ et al: Primary hyperparathyroidism: 10-year course with or without parathyroid surgery. N Engl J Med 332:1249, 1999

THAKKER RV: Molecular genetics of parathyroid disease. Curr Opin Endocrinol Diab 3:521, 1996

333   OSTEOPOROSIS
Robert Lindsay, Felicia Cosman

Osteoporosis, a condition characterized by decreased bone strength, is prevalent among postmenopausal women but also occurs in men and women with underlying conditions or major risk factors associated with bone demineralization. Its chief clinical manifestations are vertebral and hip fractures, although fractures can occur at any skeletal site. Osteoporosis affects >10 million individuals in the United States, but only a small proportion are diagnosed and treated.

DEFINITION   *Osteoporosis* is defined as a reduction of bone mass (or density) or the presence of a fragility fracture. Loss of bone tissue causes deterioration in the architecture of the skeleton, the combination leading to a markedly increased risk of fracture. Based on recommendation of a WHO committee, osteoporosis is defined operationally as a bone density that falls 2.5 standard deviations (SD) below the mean for young healthy adults of the same race and gender—also referred to as a *T-score* of −2.5. Those who fall at the lower end of the young normal range (a T-score of >1 SD below the mean) are defined as having low bone density and are considered to be at increased risk of osteoporosis.

EPIDEMIOLOGY   In the United States, as many as 8 million women and 2 million men have osteoporosis (T-score < −2.5), and an additional 18 million individuals have bone mass levels that put them at increased risk of developing osteoporosis (e.g., bone mass T-score < −1.0). Osteoporosis occurs more frequently with increasing age as bone tissue is progressively lost. In women, the loss of ovarian function at menopause (typically about age 50) precipitates rapid bone loss such that most women meet the diagnostic criteria for osteoporosis by age 70 to 80.

The epidemiology of fractures follows similar trends as bone density loss. Fractures of the distal radius increase in frequency before age 50 and plateau by age 60, with only a modest age-related increase thereafter. In contrast, incidence rates for hip fractures double every 5 years after age 70 (Fig. 333-1). This distinct epidemiology may be related to the way people fall as they age, with fewer falls on an outstretched hand and more directly on the hip. At least 1.5 million fractures occur each year in the United States as a consequence of osteoporosis. As the population continues to age, the total number of fractures will continue to escalate.

About 300,000 hip fractures occur each year in the United States, most of which require hospital admission and surgical intervention. The probability that a 50-year-old white individual will have a hip fracture during his or her lifetime is 14% for women and 5% for men; the risk for African Americans is lower (about half these rates). Hip fractures are associated with a high incidence of deep vein thrombosis and pulmonary embolism (20 to 50%) and a mortality rate between 5 and 20% during the year after surgery.

There are about 700,000 vertebral crush fractures per year in the United States. Only a fraction of these are recognized clinically, since many are relatively asymptomatic and are identified incidentally during radiography for other purposes (Fig. 333-2). Vertebral fractures rarely require hospitalization but are associated with long-term morbidity and a slight increase in mortality. Multiple fractures lead to height loss (often of several inches), kyphosis, and secondary pain and discomfort related to altered biomechanics of the back. Thoracic frac-

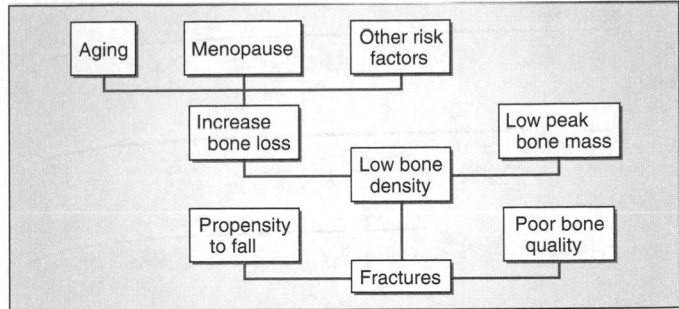

FIGURE 333-3 Factors leading to osteoporotic fractures.

FIGURE 333-1 Epidemiology of vertebral, hip, and Colles' fractures with age. [*Adapted from LJ Melton III, in BL Riggs, LJ Melton II (eds): Osteoporosis: Etiology, Diagnosis and Management, 2d ed. Rochester, MN, Mayo Foundation, 1995.*]

tures can be associated with restrictive lung disease, whereas lumbar fractures are associated with abdominal symptoms including distention, early satiety, and constipation.

Approximately 250,000 wrist fractures occur in the United States each year. Fractures of other bones (estimated to be about 300,000 per year) also occur with osteoporosis, which is not surprising given that bone loss is a systemic phenomenon. Fractures of the pelvis and proximal humerus are clearly associated with osteoporosis. Although some fractures are the result of major trauma, the threshold for fracture is reduced for an osteoporotic bone (Fig. 333-3). A list of common risk factors for osteoporotic fractures is summarized in Table 333-1. Prior fractures, a family history of osteoporotic fractures, and low body weight are each independent predictors of fracture. Chronic diseases that increase the risk of falling or frailty, including dementia, Parkinson's disease, and multiple sclerosis, also increase fracture risk.

In the United States and Europe, osteoporosis-related fractures are more common among women than men, presumably due to a lower peak bone mass as well as postmenopausal bone loss in women. However, this gender difference in bone density and age-related increase in hip fractures is not as apparent in some other cultures, possibly due to genetics, physical activity level, or diet.

PATHOPHYSIOLOGY ■ **Bone Remodeling** Osteoporosis results from bone loss due to normal age-related changes in bone remodeling as well as extrinsic and intrinsic factors that exaggerate this process. These changes may be superimposed on a low peak bone mass. Consequently, understanding the bone remodeling process is fundamental to understanding the pathophysiology of osteoporosis (Chap. 331). The skeleton increases in size by linear growth and by apposition of new bone tissue on the outer surfaces of the cortex (Fig. 333-4). This latter process is called *modeling*, a process that also allows the long bones to adapt in shape to the stresses placed upon them. Increased sex hormone production at puberty is required for skeletal maturation, which reaches maximum mass and density in early adulthood. Nutrition and life-style also play an important role in growth, though genetic factors are the major determinants of peak skeletal mass and density. Numerous genes control skeletal growth, peak bone mass, and body size, but it is likely that separate genes control skeletal structure and density. Heritability estimates of 50 to 80% for bone density and size have been derived based on twin studies. Though peak bone mass is often lower among individuals with a family history of osteoporosis, association studies of candidate genes [vitamin D receptor; type I collagen, the estrogen receptor (ER), interleukin (IL) 6; and insulin-like growth factor (IGF) I] and bone mass, bone turnover, and fracture prevalence have been inconsistent. Linkage studies suggest that a genetic locus on chromosome 11 is associated with high bone mass. Recently, a family with extremely high bone mass was identified with a point mutation in LRP 5, a low-density lipoprotein receptor–related protein.

Bone remodeling has two primary functions: (1) to repair microdamage within the skeleton to maintain skeletal strength, and (2) to supply calcium from the skeleton to maintain serum calcium. Remodeling may be activated by microdamage to bone as a result of excessive or accumulated stress. Acute demands for calcium involve osteoclast-mediated resorption as well as calcium transport by osteocytes.

Bone remodeling is also regulated by several circulating hormones, including estrogens, androgens, vitamin D, and parathyroid hormone (PTH), as well as locally produced growth factors such as IGF-I and -II, transforming growth factor (TGF) β, parathyroid hormone–related peptide (PTHrP), ILs, prostaglandins, and tumor necrosis factor

FIGURE 333-2 Lateral spine x-ray showing severe osteopenia and a severe wedge-type deformity (severe anterior compression).

TABLE 333-1 *Risk Factors for Osteoporosis Fracture*

Nonmodifiable	Estrogen deficiency
Personal history of fracture as	Early menopause (<45 years)
an adult	or bilateral ovariectomy
History of fracture in first-	Prolonged premenstrual amen-
degree relative	orrhea (>1 year)
Female sex	Low calcium intake
Advanced age	Alcoholism
Caucasian race	Impaired eyesight despite
Dementia	adequate correction
Potentially modifiable	Recurrent falls
Current cigarette smoking	Inadequate physical activity
Low body weight [<58 kg	Poor health/frailty
(127 lb)]	

FIGURE 333-4 Mechanism of bone remodeling. The basic molecular unit (BMU) moves along the trabecular surface at a rate of about 10 μm/d. The figure depicts remodeling over ~120 days. *A.* Origination of BMU-lining cells contract to expose collagen and attract preosteoclasts. *B.* Osteoclasts fuse into multinucleated cells that resorb a cavity. Mononuclear cells continue resorption and preosteoblasts are stimulated to proliferate. *C.* Osteoblasts align at bottom of cavity and start forming osteoid (black). *D.* Osteoblasts continue formation and mineralization. Previous osteoid starts to mineralize (horizontal lines). *E.* Osteoblasts begin to flatten. *F.* Osteoblasts turn into lining cells; bone remodeling at initial surface (left of drawing) is now complete, but BMU is still advancing (to the right). [*Adapted from: 5M Ott, in JP Bilezikian et al (eds): Principles of Bone Biology, vol. 18. San Diego, Academic Press, 1996, pp 231–241.*]

(TNF). The cytokine responsible for communication between the osteoblast and osteoclast has been identified as RANK or osteoprotegerin ligand (Chap. 331). The osteoclast receptor for this protein is referred to as RANK. A humoral decoy for RANK ligand is referred to as osteoprotegerin (Fig. 333-5). Modulation of osteoclast recruitment and activity appears to be related to the interplay among these three factors.

Additional influences include nutrition (particularly calcium intake) and physical activity level. The end result of this remodeling process is that the resorbed bone is replaced by an equal amount of new bone tissue. Thus, the mass of the skeleton remains constant after peak bone mass is achieved in adulthood. After age 30 to 45, however, the resorption and formation processes become imbalanced, and resorption exceeds formation. This imbalance may begin at different ages and varies at different skeletal sites; it becomes exaggerated in women after menopause. Excessive bone loss can be due to an increase in osteoclastic activity and/or a decrease in osteoblastic activity. In addition, an increase in remodeling activation frequency can magnify the small imbalance seen at each remodeling unit.

In trabecular bone, if the osteoclasts penetrate trabeculae, they leave no template for new bone formation to occur and, consequently, may cause rapid bone loss. In cortical bone, increased activation of remodeling creates more porous bone. The effect of this increased porosity on cortical bone strength may be modest if the overall diameter of the bone is not changed. However, decreased apposition of new bone on the periosteal surface coupled with increased endocortical resorption of bone decreases the biomechanical strength of long bones. Even a slight exaggeration in normal bone loss increases the risk of osteoporotic fracture.

Calcium Nutrition Peak bone mass may be impaired by inadequate calcium intake during growth among other nutritional factors (calories, protein, and other minerals), thereby leading to increased risk of osteoporosis later in life. During the adult phase of life, insufficient calcium intake induces secondary hyperparathyroidism and an increase in the rate of remodeling to maintain normal serum calcium levels. PTH stimulates the hydroxylation of vitamin D in the kidney, leading

to increased levels of 1,25-dihydroxyvitamin D [1,25(OH)$_2$D] and enhanced gastrointestinal calcium absorption. PTH also reduces renal calcium loss. Although these are appropriate short-term homeostatic responses for adjusting calcium economy, the long-term effects are detrimental to the skeleton because of the ongoing imbalance at remodeling sites.

Total daily calcium intakes of <400 mg are likely to be detrimental to the skeleton, but there are fewer data about intakes in the 600- to 800-mg range, which is the average intake among adults in the United States. The recommended daily required intake of 1000 to 1200 mg for adults accommodates population heterogeneity in controlling calcium balance (Chap. 60).

Vitamin D (See also Chap. 331) Severe vitamin D deficiency causes rickets in children or osteomalacia in adults. There is accumulating evidence that vitamin D deficiency may be more prevalent than previously thought, particularly among individuals at increased risk, such as the elderly; those living in northern latitudes; and in individuals with poor nutrition, malabsorption, or chronic liver or renal disease. Modest vitamin D deficiency [25-hydroxyvitamin D levels ≤50 nmol/L (20 ng/mL)] leads to compensatory secondary hyperparathyroidism and is an important risk factor for osteoporosis and fractures. Some studies have shown that >50% of inpatients on a general medical service exhibit biochemical features of vitamin D deficiency, including increased levels of PTH and alkaline phosphatase and lower levels of ionized calcium. In women living in northern latitudes, it has been shown that vitamin D levels decline during the winter months. This is associated with a striking seasonal bone loss, reflecting increased bone turnover. Even among healthy ambulatory individuals, mild vitamin D deficiency is increasing in prevalence. Treatment with vitamin D can return vitamin D levels to normal [>50 μmol/L (20 ng/mL)] and prevent the associated increase in bone remodeling, bone loss, and fractures. Reduced fracture rates have also been documented among individuals in northern latitudes who have greater vitamin D intake and have higher 25-hydroxyvitamin D [25(OH)D] levels (see below).

FIGURE 333-5 Steroid actions and interactions with growth factors/cytokines in bone cells at bone resorption and formation sites. Estrogen inhibits osteoclasts (OCL), cells that mediate bone resorption; estrogen stimulates osteoblasts (OB), cells that mediate bone formation. OBs produce many growth factors and cytokines that mediate estrogen action, some of which regulate the OCL indirectly. Estrogen deficiency stimulates OB production of IL-1, IL-6, and TNF-α (and inhibits apoptosis and extends the life span of OCLs). Estrogen deficiency decreases IL-1ra leading to enhanced OCL sensitivity to IL-1. Estrogen deficiency also decreases production of TGF-β and OPG-L, factors that mediate osteoclast apoptosis. Solid lines indicate well-documented pathways. Dashed lines indicate less well defined pathways. ER, estrogen receptor; AR, androgen receptor; OPG, osteoprotegerin; OPG-L, osteoprotegerin-ligand; IL, interleukin; IL-1ra, interleukin 1 receptor antagonist; TGF-β, transforming growth factor β; TNF-α, tumor necrosis factor α. (*Adapted from TC Spelsberg et al: Mol Endocrinol 13:819, 1999.*)

Estrogen Status Estrogen deficiency probably causes bone loss by two distinct but interrelated mechanisms: (1) activation of new bone remodeling sites, and (2) exaggeration of the imbalance between bone formation and resorption. The change in activation frequency causes a transient bone loss until a new steady state between resorption and formation is achieved. The remodeling imbalance, however, results in a permanent decrement in mass that can only be corrected by a remodeling event during which bone formation exceeds resorption. In addition, the very presence of more remodeling sites in the skeleton increases the probability that trabeculae will be penetrated, thereby eliminating the template upon which new bone can be formed and accelerating the loss of bony tissue.

The most frequent estrogen-deficient state is the cessation of ovarian function at the time of menopause, which occurs on average at the age of 51. Thus, with current life expectancy, an average woman will spend about 30 years without ovarian supply of estrogen. The mechanism by which estrogen deficiency causes bone loss is summarized in Fig. 333-5. Marrow cells (macrophages, monocytes, osteoclast precursors, mast cells) as well as bone cells (osteoblasts, osteocytes, osteoclasts) express ERs α and β. The net effect of estrogen deficiency is increased osteoclast recruitment and perhaps activity. Estrogen may also play an important role in determining the life span of bone cells by controlling the rate of apoptosis. Thus, in situations of estrogen deprivation, the life span of osteoblasts may be decreased whereas the longevity of osteoclasts is increased.

Since remodeling is initiated at the surface of bone, it follows that trabecular bone—which has a considerably larger surface area (80% of the total) than cortical bone—will be preferentially affected by estrogen deficiency. Fractures occur earliest at sites where trabecular bone contributes most to bone strength; consequently, vertebral fractures are the most common early consequence of estrogen deficiency.

Physical Activity Inactivity, such as prolonged bed rest or paralysis, results in significant bone loss. Concordantly, athletes have higher bone mass than the general population. These changes in skeletal mass are most marked when the stimulus begins during growth and before the age of puberty. Adults are less capable than children of increasing bone mass following restoration of physical activity. Epidemiologic data support the beneficial effects on the skeleton of chronic high levels of physical activity. Fracture risk is lower in rural communities and in countries where physical activity is maintained into old age. However, when exercise is initiated during adult life, the effects of moderate exercise are modest, with a bone mass increase of 1 to 2% in short-term studies of <2 years duration. It is argued that more active individuals are less likely to fall and are more capable of protecting themselves upon falling, thereby reducing fracture risk.

Chronic Disease Various genetic and acquired diseases are associated with an increase in the risk of osteoporosis (Table 333-2). Mechanisms that contribute to bone loss are unique for each disease and typically result from multiple factors including nutrition, reduced physical activity levels, and factors that affect bone-remodeling rates.

Medications A large number of medications used in clinical practice have potentially detrimental effects on the skeleton (Table 333-3). *Glucocorticoids* are the most common cause of medication-induced osteoporosis. It is often not possible to determine the extent to which osteoporosis is related to the glucocorticoid or to other factors, as treatment is superimposed on the effects of the primary disease, which may in itself be associated with bone loss (e.g., rheumatoid arthritis). Excessive doses of thyroid hormone can accelerate bone remodeling and result in bone loss.

Other medications have less detrimental effects upon the skeleton than pharmacologic doses of glucocorticoids. *Anticonvulsants* are thought to increase the risk of osteoporosis, although many affected individuals have concomitant vitamin D insufficiency, as some anticonvulsants induce the cytochrome P450 system and vitamin D metabolism. Patients undergoing transplantation are at high risk for rapid bone loss and fracture not only from glucocorticoids but also from treatment with other *immunosuppressants*, such as cyclosporine and

tacrolimus (FK506). In addition, these patients often have underlying metabolic abnormalities, such as hepatic or renal failure, that predispose to bone loss.

Cigarette Consumption The use of cigarettes over a long period has detrimental effects on bone mass. These effects may be mediated directly, by toxic effects on osteoblasts, or indirectly by modifying estrogen metabolism. On average, cigarette smokers reach menopause 1 to 2 years earlier than the general population. Cigarette smoking also produces secondary effects that can modulate skeletal status, including intercurrent respiratory and other illnesses, frailty, decreased exercise, poor nutrition, and the need for additional medications (e.g., glucocorticoids for lung disease).

MEASUREMENT OF BONE MASS Several noninvasive techniques are now available for estimating skeletal mass or density. These include dual-energy x-ray absorptiometry (DXA), single-energy x-ray absorptiometry (SXA), quantitative computed tomography (CT), and ultrasound.

DXA is a highly accurate x-ray technique that has become the standard for measuring bone density in most centers. Though it can be used for measurements of any skeletal site, clinical determinations are usually made of the lumbar spine and hip. Portable DXA machines have been developed that measure the heel (calcaneus), forearm (radius and ulna), or finger (phalanges). DXA can also be used to measure body composition. In the DXA technique, two x-ray energies are used to estimate the area of mineralized tissue, and the mineral content is divided by the area, which partially corrects for body size. However, this correction is only partial since DXA is a two-dimensional scanning technique and cannot estimate the depths or posteroanterior length of the bone. Thus, small people tend to have lower-than-average bone

TABLE 333-2 *Diseases Associated with an Increased Risk of Generalized Osteoporosis in Adults*

Hypogonadal states	Hematologic disorders/malignancy
Turner syndrome	Multiple myeloma
Klinefelter syndrome	Lymphoma and leukemia
Anorexia nervosa	Malignancy-associated parathyroid
Hypothalamic amenorrhea	hormone (PTHrP) production
Hyperprolactinemia	Mastocytosis
Other primary or secondary	Hemophilia
hypogonadal states	Thalassemia
Endocrine disorders	Selected inherited disorders
Cushing's syndrome	Osteogenesis imperfecta
Hyperparathyroidism	Marfan syndrome
Thyrotoxicosis	Hemochromatosis
Type 1 diabetes mellitus	Hypophosphatasia
Acromegaly	Glycogen storage diseases
Adrenal insufficiency	Homocystinuria
Nutritional and gastrointestinal	Ehlers-Danlos syndrome
disorders	Porphyria
Malnutrition	Menkes' syndrome
Parenteral nutrition	Epidermolysis bullosa
Malabsorption syndromes	Other disorders
Gastrectomy	Immobilization
Severe liver disease, espe-	Chronic obstructive pulmonary
cially biliary cirrhosis	disease
Pernicious anemia	Pregnancy and lactation
Rheumatologic disorders	Scoliosis
Rheumatoid arthritis	Multiple sclerosis
Ankylosing spondylitis	Sarcoidosis
	Amyloidosis

TABLE 333-3 *Drugs Associated with an Increased Risk of Generalized Osteoporosis in Adults*

Glucocorticoids	Excessive thyroxine
Cyclosporine	Aluminum
Cytotoxic drugs	Gonadotropin-releasing hormone agonists
Anticonvulsants	Heparin
Excessive alcohol	Lithium

mineral density (BMD). Bone spurs, which are frequent in osteoarthritis, tend to falsely increase bone density of the spine. Because DXA instrumentation is provided by several different manufacturers, the output varies in absolute terms. Consequently, it has become standard practice to relate the results to "normal" values using T-scores, which compare individual results to those in a young population that is matched for race and gender. Z-scores compare individual results to those of an age-matched population that is also matched for race and gender. Thus, a 60-year-old woman with a Z-score of −1 (1 SD below mean for age) has a T-score of −2.5 (2.5 SD below mean for a young control group) (Fig. 333-6).

CT is used primarily to measure the spine, and peripheral CT is used to measure bone in the forearm or tibia. Research into the use of CT for measurement of the hip is ongoing. The results obtained from CT are different from all others currently available since this technique specifically analyzes trabecular bone in vertebrae, eliminating posterior cortical elements of the spine, and can provide a true density (mass of bone per unit volume) measurement. However, CT remains expensive, involves greater radiation exposure, and is less reproducible.

Ultrasound is used to measure bone mass by calculating the attenuation of the signal as it passes through bone or the speed with which it traverses the bone. It is unclear whether ultrasound assesses bone quality, but this may be an advantage of the technique. Because of its relatively low cost and mobility, ultrasound is amenable for use as a screening procedure.

All of these techniques for measuring BMD have been approved by the U.S. Food and Drug Administration (FDA) based upon their capacity to predict fracture risk. The hip is the preferred site of measurement in most individuals, since it predicts the risk of hip fracture, the most important consequence of osteoporosis, better than any other bone density measurement site. When hip measurements are performed by DXA, the spine can be measured at the same time. In younger individuals, such as perimenopausal or early postmenopausal women, spine measurements may be the most sensitive indicator of bone loss.

When to Measure Bone Mass   Clinical guidelines developed by the National Osteoporosis Foundation recommend bone mass measurements in postmenopausal women, assuming they have risk factors for osteoporosis in addition to age, gender, and estrogen deficiency. The guidelines further recommend that bone mass measurement be considered in *all* women by age 65, a position ratified by the U.S. Preventive Health Services Task Force. Criteria approved for Medicare reimbursement of BMD are summarized in Table 333-4.

When to Treat Based Upon Bone Mass Results   Several guidelines suggest that patients be considered for treatment when BMD is >2.5 SD below the mean value for young adults (T-score ≤ −2.5). Treatment should also be considered in postmenopausal women with risk factors if BMD of the hip is <−2.0. Because the fracture risk increases continuously as T-scores decline, there is no critical threshold and treatment deci-

sions must be individualized. Clearly clinical status must be evaluated carefully, considering age, prior fracture history, weight, and family history of osteoporosis. Moreover, high bone turnover, particularly in older individuals, should be considered an independent risk factor for fracture and should prompt treatment at a higher BMD level.

APPROACH TO THE PATIENT

The perimenopausal transition is a good opportunity to initiate discussion about risk factors for osteoporosis and to consider indications for a BMD test. A careful history and physical examination should be performed to identify risk factors for osteoporosis. A low Z-score increases the suspicion of a secondary disease. Height loss >2.5 to 3.8 cm (>1 to 1.5 in.) is an indication for radiography to rule out asymptomatic vertebral fractures, as is the presence of significant kyphosis or back pain, particularly if it began after menopause. For patients who present with fractures, it is important to ensure that the fractures are not caused by an underlying malignancy. Usually this is clear on routine radiography, but on occasion, CT, magnetic resonance imaging, or radionuclide scans may be necessary.

Routine Laboratory Evaluation   There is no established algorithm for the evaluation of women presenting with osteoporosis. A general evaluation that includes complete blood count, serum calcium, and perhaps urine calcium is helpful for identifying selected secondary causes of low bone mass, particularly for women with fractures or very low Z-scores. An elevated serum calcium level suggests hyperparathyroidism or malignancy, whereas a reduced serum calcium level may reflect malnutrition and osteomalacia. In the presence of hypercalcemia, a serum PTH level differentiates between hyperparathyroidism (PTH↑) and malignancy (PTH↓), and a high PTHrP level can help document the presence of humoral hypercalcemia of malignancy (Chap. 332). A low urine calcium (<50 mg/24 h) suggests osteomalacia, malnutrition, or malabsorption; a high urine calcium (>300 mg/24 h) is indicative of hypercalciuria and must be investigated further. Hypercalciuria occurs primarily in three situations: (1) a renal calcium leak, which is more frequent in males with osteoporosis; (2) absorptive hypercalciuria, which can be idiopathic or associated with increased $1,25(OH)_2D$ in granulomatous disease; or (3) hematologic malignancies or conditions associated with excessive bone turnover such as Paget's disease, hyperparathyroidism, and hyperthyroidism.

Possible hyperthyroidism can be evaluated by measuring thyroid-stimulating hormone (TSH). When there is clinical suspicion of Cushing's syndrome, urinary free cortisol levels or a fasting serum cortisol should be measured after overnight dexamethasone. When bowel disease, malabsorption, or malnutrition is suspected, serum albumin, cholesterol, and a complete blood count should be checked. Asymptomatic malabsorption might be heralded by anemia (macrocytic-vitamin B_{12} or folate deficiency; or microcytic-iron deficiency) or low serum cholesterol or urinary calcium levels. If these or other features suggest malabsorption, further evaluation is required. Asymptomatic celiac disease with selective malabsorption is being found with increasing prevalence; the diagnosis can be made by testing for antigliadin, antiendomysial, or transglutam-

FIGURE 333-6   Relationship between Z-scores and T-scores in a 60-year-old woman (BMD, bone mineral density; SD, standard deviation).

TABLE 333-5 *Biochemical Markers of Bone Metabolism in Clinical Use*

Bone formation
    Serum bone-specific alkaline phosphatase
    Serum osteocalcin
    Serum propeptide of type I procollagen
Bone resorption
    Urine and serum cross-linked N-telopeptide
    Urine and serum cross-linked C-telopeptide
    Urine total free deoxypyridinoline
    Urine hydroxyproline
    Serum tartrate-resistant acid phosphatase
    Serum bone sialoprotein
    Urine hydroxylysine glycosides

inase antibodies but may require endoscopic biopsy. A trial of a gluten-free diet can be confirmatory (Chap. 275). When osteoporosis is found associated with symptoms of rash, multiple allergies, diarrhea, or flushing, mastocytosis should be excluded using 24-h urine histamine collection or serum tryptase.

Myeloma can masquerade as generalized osteoporosis, although it more commonly presents with bone pain and characteristic "punched-out" lesions on radiography. Serum and urine electrophoresis and evaluation for light chains in urine are required to exclude this diagnosis. A bone marrow biopsy may be required to rule out myeloma (in patients with equivocal electrophoretic results) and can also be used to exclude mastocytosis, leukemia, and other marrow infiltrative disorders, such as Gaucher's disease.

Bone Biopsy Tetracycline labeling of the skeleton allows determination of the rate of remodeling as well as evaluation for other metabolic bone diseases. The current use of BMD tests, in combination with hormonal evaluation and biochemical markers of bone remodeling, has largely replaced bone biopsy.

Biochemical Markers Several biochemical tests are now available that provide an index of the overall rate of bone remodeling (Table 333-5). Biochemical markers are usually characterized as those related primarily to *bone formation* or *bone resorption*. These tests measure the overall state of bone remodeling at a single point in time. Clinical use of these tests has been hampered by biologic variability (in part related to circadian rhythm) as well as to analytical variability.

For the most part, remodeling markers do not predict rates of bone loss well enough to use this information clinically. However, markers of bone resorption may help in the prediction of fracture risk, particularly in older individuals. In women ≥65 years, when bone density results are greater than the usual treatment thresholds noted above, a high level of bone resorption should prompt consideration of treatment. The primary use of biochemical markers is for monitoring the response to treatment. With the introduction of antiresorptive therapeutic agents, bone remodeling declines rapidly, with the fall in resorption occurring earlier than the fall in formation. Inhibition of bone resorption is maximal within 3 to 6 months. Thus, measurement of bone resorption prior to initiating therapy and 4 to 6 months after starting therapy provides an earlier estimate of patient response than does bone densitometry. A decline in resorptive markers can be ascertained after treatment with bisphosphonates or estrogen; this effect is less marked after treatment with either raloxifene or intranasal calcitonin. A biochemical marker response to therapy is particularly useful for asymptomatic patients and might help to ensure long-term compliance. Bone turnover markers are also useful in monitoring the effects of PTH, or teriparatide, which rapidly increases bone formation and later bone resorption.

℞ **TREATMENT**

Management of Osteoporotic Fractures Treatment of the patient with osteoporosis frequently involves management of acute fractures as well

as treatment of the underlying disease. Hip fractures almost always require surgical repair if the patient is to become ambulatory again. Depending on the location and severity of the fracture, condition of the neighboring joint, and general status of the patient, procedures may include open reduction and internal fixation with pins and plates, hemiarthroplasties, and total arthroplasties. These surgical procedures are followed by intense rehabilitation in an attempt to return patients to their prefracture functional level. Long bone fractures often require either external or internal fixation. Other fractures (e.g., vertebral, rib, and pelvic fractures) are usually managed with only supportive care, requiring no specific orthopedic treatment.

Only ~25 to 30% of vertebral compression fractures present with sudden-onset back pain. For acutely symptomatic fractures, treatment with analgesics is required, including nonsteroidal anti-inflammatory agents and/or acetaminophen, sometimes with the addition of a narcotic agent (codeine or oxycodone). A few small, randomized clinical trials suggest that calcitonin may reduce pain related to acute vertebral compression fracture. A recently developed technique involves percutaneous injection of artificial cement (polymethylmethacrylate) into the vertebral body (vertebroplasty or kyphoplasty); this has been reported to offer significant immediate pain relief in the majority of patients. Long-term effects are unknown, and conclusions are based on observational studies in patients with severe persistent back pain from acute or subacute vertebral fractures. There have been no randomized controlled trials of either vertebroplasty or kyphoplasty to date. Short periods of bed rest may be helpful for pain management, but, in general, early mobilization is recommended as it helps prevent further bone loss associated with immobilization. Occasionally, use of a soft elastic-style brace may facilitate earlier mobilization. Muscle spasms often occur with acute compression fractures and can be treated with muscle relaxants and heat treatments.

Severe pain usually resolves within 6 to 10 weeks. Chronic pain is probably not bony in origin; instead, it is related to abnormal strain on muscles, ligaments, and tendons and to secondary facet-joint arthritis associated with alterations in thoracic and/or abdominal shape. Chronic pain is difficult to treat effectively and may require analgesics, sometimes including narcotic analgesics. Frequent intermittent rest in a supine or semireclining position is often required to allow the soft tissues, which are under tension, to relax. Back-strengthening exercises (paraspinal) may be beneficial. Heat treatments help relax muscles and reduce the muscular component of discomfort. Various physical modalities, such as ultrasound and transcutaneous nerve stimulation, may be beneficial in some patients. Pain also occurs in the neck region, not as a result of compression fractures (which almost never occur in the cervical spine as a result of osteoporosis) but because of chronic strain associated from trying to elevate the head in a person with a severe thoracic kyphosis.

Multiple vertebral fractures are often associated with psychological symptoms, not always commonly appreciated. The changes in body configuration and back pain can lead to marked loss of self-image and a secondary depression. Altered balance, precipitated by the kyphosis and the anterior movement of the body's center of gravity, leads to a fear of falling, a consequent tendency to remain indoors, and the onset of social isolation. These symptoms can sometimes be alleviated by family support and/or psychotherapy. Medication may be necessary when depressive features are present.

Management of the Underlying Disease ▪ *RISK FACTOR REDUCTION* Patients should be thoroughly educated to reduce the likelihood of risk factors associated with bone loss and falling. Medications should be reviewed to ensure that any glucocorticoid medication is truly indicated and is being given in doses as low as possible. For those on thyroid hormone replacement, TSH testing should be performed to determine that an excessive dose is not being used, as thyrotoxicosis can be associated with increased bone loss. In patients who smoke, efforts should be made to facilitate smoking cessation. Reducing risk factors for falling also includes alcohol abuse treatment and a review of the medical regimen for any drugs that might be associated with orthostatic hypotension and/or sedation, including hypnotics and anxiolytics. If nocturia occurs, the frequency should be reduced, if possible (e.g., by decreasing or modifying diuretic use), as arising in the middle of sleep is a common precipitant of a fall. Patients should be instructed about environmental safety with regard to eliminating exposed wires, curtain strings, slippery rugs, and mobile tables. Avoiding stocking feet on wood floors, checking carpet condition (particularly on stairs), and providing good light in paths to bathrooms and outside the home are important preventive measures. Treatment for impaired vision is recommended, particularly a problem with depth perception, which is specifically associated with increased falling risk. Elderly patients with neurologic impairment (e.g., stroke, Parkinson's disease, Alzheimer's disease) are particularly at risk of falling and require specialized supervision and care.

NUTRITIONAL RECOMMENDATIONS ■ Calcium   A large body of data indicates that optimal calcium intake reduces bone loss and suppresses bone turnover. Recommended intakes from a recent report from the Institute of Medicine are shown in Table 333-6. The National Health and Nutritional Evaluation Studies (NHANES) have consistently documented that average calcium intakes fall considerably short of these recommendations. The preferred source of calcium is from dairy products and other foods, but many patients require calcium supplementation. Food sources of calcium are dairy products (milk, yogurt, and cheese) and fortified foods such as certain cereals, waffles, snacks, juices, and crackers. Some of these fortified foods contain as much calcium per serving as milk.

If a calcium supplement is required, it should be taken in doses ≤600 mg at a time, as the calcium absorption fraction decreases at higher doses. Calcium supplements should be calculated based on the elemental calcium content of the supplement, not the weight of the calcium salt (Table 333-7). Calcium supplements containing carbonate are best taken with food since they require acid for solubility. Calcium citrate supplements can be taken at any time.

Several controlled clinical trials of calcium plus vitamin D have confirmed reductions in clinical fractures, including fractures of the hip (~20 to 30% risk reduction). All recent studies of pharmacologic agents have been conducted in the context of calcium replacement (± vitamin D). Thus, it is standard practice to ensure an adequate calcium and vitamin D intake in patients with osteoporosis, whether they are receiving additional pharmacologic therapy or not.

Although side effects from supplemental calcium are minimal, individuals with a history of kidney stones should have a 24-h urine calcium determination before starting increased calcium to avoid hypercalciuria.

Vitamin D   Vitamin D is synthesized in skin under the influence of heat and ultraviolet light (Chap. 331). However, large segments of the population do not obtain sufficient vitamin D to maintain what is now considered an adequate supply [serum 25(OH)D consistently >50 μmol/L (20 ng/mL)]. Since vitamin D supplementation at doses that would achieve these serum levels is safe and inexpensive, the Institute of Medicine recommends daily intakes of 200 IU for adults <50 years of age, 400 IU for those from 50 to 70 years, and 600 IU for those >70 years. Multivitamin tablets usually contain 400 IU, and many calcium supplements also contain vitamin D. Some data suggest that higher doses may be required in the elderly and chronically ill.

Other Nutrients   Other nutrients such as salt and caffeine may have modest effects on calcium excretion or absorption. Adequate vitamin K status is required for optimal carboxylation of osteocalcin. States in which vitamin K nutrition or metabolism is impaired, such as with long-term warfarin therapy, have been associated with reduced bone mass.

Magnesium is abundant in foods, and magnesium deficiency is quite rare in the absence of a serious chronic disease. Magnesium supplementation may be warranted in patients with inflammatory bowel disease, celiac disease, chemotherapy, severe diarrhea, malnutrition, or alcoholism. Dietary phytoestrogens, which are derived primarily from soy products and legumes (e.g., garbanzo beans, chickpeas, and lentils), exert some estrogenic activity but are insufficiently potent to justify their use in place of a pharmacologic agent in the treatment of osteoporosis.

Patients with hip fracture are often frail and relatively malnourished. Some data suggest an improved outcome in such patients when they are provided calorie and protein supplementation. Excessive protein intake can increase renal calcium excretion but this can be corrected by an adequate calcium intake.

EXERCISE   Exercise in young individuals increases the likelihood that they will attain the maximal genetically determined peak bone mass. Meta-analyses of studies performed in postmenopausal women indicate that weight-bearing exercise prevents bone loss but does not appear to result in substantial gain of bone mass. This beneficial effect wanes if exercise is discontinued. Exercise also has beneficial effects on neuromuscular function, and it improves coordination, balance, and strength, thereby reducing the risk of falling. A walking program is a practical way to start. Other activities such as dancing, racquet sports, cross-country skiing, and use of gym equipment are also recommended, depending on the patient's personal preference. Even women who cannot walk benefit from swimming or water exercises, not so much for the effects on bone, which are quite minimal, but because of effects on muscle. Exercise habits should be consistent, optimally at least three times a week.

Pharmacologic Therapies   Until fairly recently, estrogen treatment, either by itself or in concert with a progestin, was the primary therapeutic agent for prevention or treatment of osteoporosis. Over the past 10 years, a number of new drugs have appeared, and more are expected in the near future. Some are agents that specifically treat osteoporosis (bisphosphonates, calcitonin, PTH); others, such as selective estrogen response modulators (SERMs), have broader effects. The availability of these drugs allows therapy to be tailored to the needs of an individual patient.

ESTROGENS   A large body of clinical trial data indicates that various types of estrogens (conjugated equine estrogens, estradiol, estrone, esterified estrogens, ethinyl estradiol, and mestranol) reduce bone turn-

TABLE 333-7 *Elemental Calcium Content of Various Oral Calcium Preparations*

Calcium Preparation	Elemental Calcium Content
Calcium citrate	60 mg/300 mg
Calcium lactate	80 mg/600 mg
Calcium gluconate	40 mg/500 mg
Calcium carbonate	400 mg/g
Calcium carbonate + 5 μg vitamin D₂ (OsCal 250)	250 mg/tablet
Calcium carbonate (Tums 500)	500 mg/tablet

Source: Adapted from SM Krane and MF Holick, Chap. 355 in HPIM, 14 ed, 1998.

TABLE 333-6 *Adequate Calcium Intake*

Life Stage Group	Estimated Adequate Daily Calcium Intake, mg/d
Young children (1–3 years)	500
Older children (4–8 years)	800
Adolescents and young adults (9–18 years)	1300
Men and women (19–50 years)	1000
Men and women (51 and older)	1200

Note: Pregnancy and lactation needs are the same as for nonpregnant women (e.g., 1300 mg/d for adolescents/young adult and 1000 mg/d for ≥19 years.)
Source: Adapted from the Standing Committee on the Scientific Evaluation of Dietary Reference Intakes. Food and Nutrition Board. Institute of Medicine. Washington, DC. 1997. National Academy Press.

over, prevent bone loss, and induce small increases in bone mass of the spine, hip, and total body. The effects of estrogen are seen in women with natural or surgical menopause and in late postmenopausal women with or without established osteoporosis. Estrogens are efficacious when administered orally or transdermally. For both oral and transdermal routes of administration, combined estrogen/progestin preparations are now available in many countries, obviating the problem of taking two tablets or using a patch and oral progestin. One large study, referred to as PEPI (Postmenopausal Estrogen/Progestin Intervention Trial), indicated that C-21 progestins alone do not augment the effect of standard estrogen doses on bone mass (Fig. 333-7).

Dose of Estrogen For oral estrogens, the standard recommended doses are 0.3 mg/d for esterified estrogens, 0.625 mg/d for conjugated equine estrogens, and 5 μg/d for ethinyl estradiol. For transdermal estrogen, the commonly used dose supplies 50 μg estradiol per day, but a lower dose may be appropriate for some individuals. Dose response data for conjugated equine estrogens indicate that lower doses are effective.

Fracture Data Epidemiologic databases indicate that women who take estrogen replacement have a 50% reduction, on average, of osteoporotic fractures, including hip fractures. The beneficial effect of estrogen is greatest among those who start replacement early and continue the treatment; the benefit declines after discontinuation such that there is no residual protective effect against fracture by 10 years after discontinuation. The first clinical trial evaluating fractures as secondary outcomes, the Heart and Estrogen-Progestin Replacement Study (HERS) trial, showed no effect of hormone therapy against hip or other clinical fractures in women with established coronary artery disease. These data made the results of the Women's Health Initiative (WHI) exceedingly important (Chap. 327). The estrogen-progestin arm of the WHI in >16,000 postmenopausal healthy women indicated that hormone therapy reduces the risk of hip fracture by 34% and all clinical fractures by 24%.

A few clinical trials have evaluated spine fracture occurrence as an outcome with estrogen therapy. One that used high doses of estrogen (2.5 mg/d conjugated equine estrogen) indicated marked vertebral fracture reduction in estrogen-treated women. Several other small studies, using lower estrogen doses, have consistently shown that estrogen treatment reduces the incidence of vertebral compression fracture.

The WHI has now provided a vast amount of data on the multisystemic effects of hormone therapy. Although earlier observational studies suggested that estrogen replacement might reduce heart disease, the WHI showed that combined estrogen-progestin treatment increased risk of fatal and nonfatal myocardial infarction by about 29%, confirming data from the HERS study. Other important relative risks included a 40% increase in stroke, 100% increase in venous thromboembolic disease, and a 26% increase in risk of breast cancer. Subsequent analyses have confirmed the increased risk of stroke and shown a twofold increase in dementia. Benefits other than the fracture reductions noted above included a 37% reduction in risk of colon cancer. These relative risks have to be interpreted in light of absolute risk (Fig. 333-8). For example, out of 10,000 women treated with estrogen-progestin for 1 year, there will be 8 excess heart attacks, 8 excess breast cancers, 18 excess venous thromboembolic events, 5 fewer hip fractures, 44 fewer clinical fractures, and 6 fewer colorectal cancers. These numbers must be multiplied by years of hormone treatment. There was no effect of hormone treatment on risk of uterine cancer or total mortality.

It is important to note that the WHI findings apply specifically to hormone treatment in the form of conjugated equine estrogen plus medroxyprogesterone acetate. Furthermore, the relative benefits and

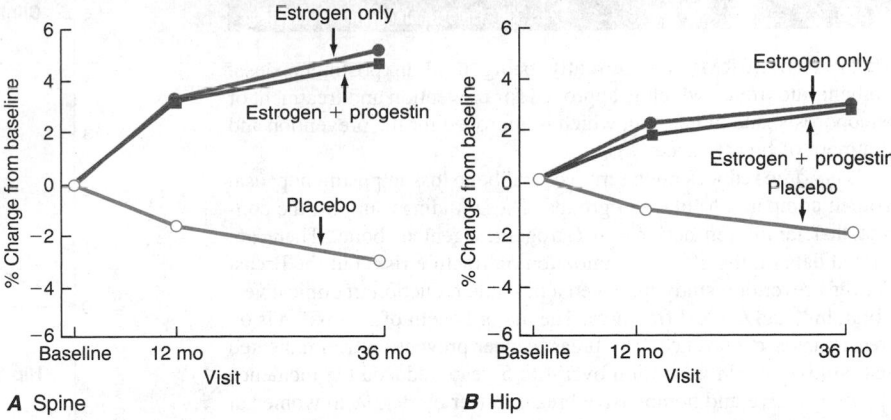

FIGURE 333-7 Results of hormone therapy regimens on bone mineral density (BMD) of the spine (*A*) and hip (*B*). Unadjusted mean percent change in BMD in the hip by treatment assignment and visit: adherent PEPI participants only. Results From the Postmenopausal Estrogen/Progestin Interventions (PEPI) Trial. Estrogen, conjugated equine estrogen 0.625 mg/d; progestin, medroxyprogesterone acetate 10 mg/d. (*Adapted from TL Bush et al: JAMA 276: 1389, 1996.*)

risks of unopposed estrogen in women who had hysterectomy are still being evaluated in the estrogen-only arm of the WHI.

Mode of Action Two subtypes of ERs, α and β, have been identified in bone and other tissues. Cells of monocyte lineage express both ERα and -β, as do osteoblasts. Estrogen-mediated effects vary depending on the receptor type. Using ER knockout mouse models, elimination of ERα produces a modest reduction in bone mass, whereas mutation of ERβ has less effect on bone. A male patient with a homozygous mutation of ERα had markedly decreased bone density as well as abnormalities in epiphyseal closure, confirming the important role of ERα in bone biology. The mechanism of estrogen action in bone is an area of active investigation (Fig. 333-5). Although data are conflicting, estrogens may inhibit osteoclasts directly. However, the majority of estrogen (and androgen) effects on bone resorption are mediated indirectly through paracrine factors produced by osteoblasts. These actions include: (1) increasing IGF-I and TGF-β, and (2) suppressing IL-1 (α and β), IL-6, TNF-α, and osteocalcin synthesis. The indirect estrogen actions primarily decrease bone resorption.

PROGESTINS In women with a uterus, daily progestin or cyclical progestins at least 12 days per month are prescribed in combination with estrogens to reduce the risk of uterine cancer. Medroxyprogesterone acetate and norethindrone acetate blunt the high-density lipoprotein response to estrogen, but micronized progesterone does not. Neither medroxyprogesterone acetate nor micronized progesterone appears to have an independent effect on bone; at lower doses, norethindrone acetate might have an additive benefit. On breast tissue, progestins may increase the risk of breast cancer.

FIGURE 333-8 Effects of hormone therapy on event rates (CHD, coronary heart disease; VTE, venous thromboembolic events). (*Adapted from: Women's Health Initiative. WHI HRT Update. Available at http://www.nhlbi.nih.gov/whi/hrtupd/upd20002.htm. 2002.*)

SERMS   Two SERMs are currently being used in postmenopausal women: raloxifene, which is approved for prevention and treatment of osteoporosis, and tamoxifen, which is approved for the prevention and treatment of breast cancer.

Tamoxifen reduces bone turnover and bone loss in postmenopausal women compared to placebo groups. These findings support the concept that tamoxifen acts as an estrogenic agent in bone. There are limited data on the effect of tamoxifen on fracture risk, but the Breast Cancer Prevention study indicated a possible reduction in clinical vertebral, hip, and Colles' fractures. The major benefit of tamoxifen is on breast cancer occurrence. The breast cancer prevention trial indicated that tamoxifen administration over 4 to 5 years reduced the incidence of new invasive and noninvasive breast cancer by ~45% in women at increased risk of breast cancer. The incidence of ER-positive breast cancers was reduced by 65%.

Raloxifene (60 mg/d) has effects on bone turnover and bone mass that are very similar to those of tamoxifen, indicating that this agent is also estrogenic on the skeleton. The effect of raloxifene on bone density (+1.4 to 2.8% versus placebo in the spine, hip, and total body) is somewhat less than that seen with standard doses of estrogens. Raloxifene reduces the occurrence of vertebral fracture by 30 to 50%, depending on the subpopulation; however, there are no data confirming that raloxifene can reduce the risk of nonvertebral fractures.

Raloxifene, like tamoxifen and estrogen, has effects in other organ systems. The most beneficial effect appears to be a reduction in invasive breast cancer (mainly decreased ER-positive) occurrence of about 65% in women who take raloxifene compared to placebo. In contrast to tamoxifen, raloxifene is not associated with an increase in the risk of uterine cancer or benign uterine disease. Raloxifene increases the occurrence of hot flashes but reduces serum total and low-density lipoprotein cholesterol, lipoprotein(a), and fibrinogen. In women at high risk of heart disease, preliminary data suggest that raloxifene may reduce the occurrence of heart disease and stroke outcomes by about 40%. A large ongoing pivotal study, called Raloxifene Use for the Heart (RUTH), will further evaluate vascular disease and breast cancer outcomes.

Mode of Action of SERMs   All SERMs bind to the ER, but each agent produces a unique receptor conformation. As a result, specific coactivator or co-repressor proteins are bound to the receptor (Chap. 317), resulting in differential effects on gene transcription that vary depending on other transcription factors present in the cell. Another aspect of selectivity is the affinity of each SERM for the different ERα and -β subtypes, which are expressed differentially in various tissues. These tissue-selective effects of SERMs offer the possibility of tailoring estrogen therapy to best meet the needs and risk factor profile of an individual patient.

BISPHOSPHONATES   Both alendronate and risedronate are approved for the prevention and treatment of postmenopausal osteoporosis and treatment of steroid-induced osteoporosis. Risedronate is also approved for the prevention of steroid-induced osteoporosis. Alendronate is approved for treatment of osteoporosis in men.

Alendronate has been shown to decrease bone turnover and increase bone mass in the spine by up to 8% versus placebo and by 6% versus placebo in the hip. Multiple trials have evaluated its effect on fracture occurrence. The Fracture Intervention Trial provided evidence in >2000 women with prevalent vertebral fractures that daily alendronate treatment (5 mg/d for 2 years and 10 mg/d for 9 months afterwards) reduces vertebral fracture risk by about 50%, multiple vertebral fractures by up to 90%, and hip fractures by up to 50% (Fig. 333-9). Several subsequent trials have confirmed these findings. For example, in a study of >1900 women with low bone mass treated with alendronate (10 mg/d) versus placebo, the incidence of all nonvertebral fractures was reduced by ~47% after only 1 year.

Trials comparing once-weekly alendronate, 70 mg, with daily 10-mg dosing have shown equivalence with regard to bone mass and bone

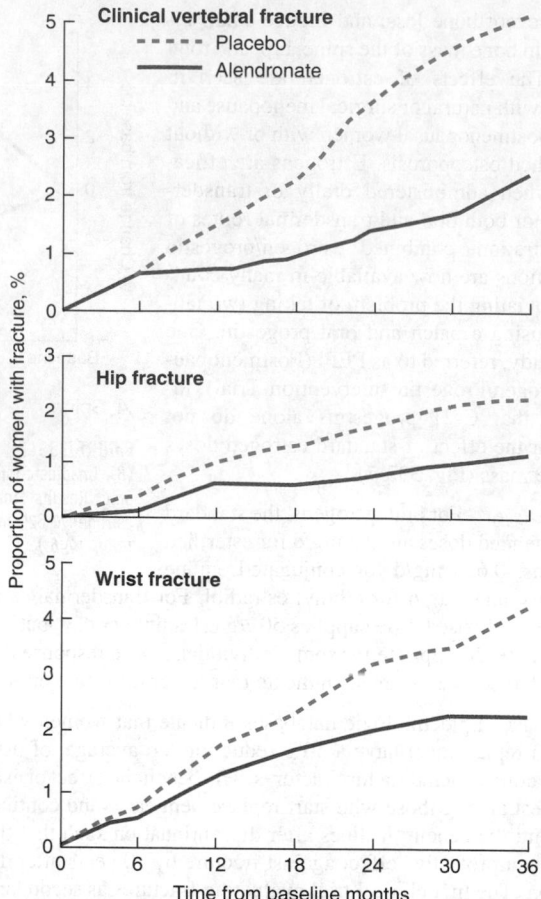

FIGURE 333-9   Cumulative proportions of women with osteoporosis who suffered clinical vertebral, hip, or wrist fracture during 3 years of treatment with alendronate or placebo (FIT 1). (*From DM Black et al: Lancet 348:1535, 1996.*)

turnover responses. Consequently, once-weekly therapy is generally preferred because of low incidence of gastrointestinal side effects and ease of administration. Alendronate should be given with a full glass of water before breakfast, as bisphosphonates are poorly absorbed. Because of the potential for esophageal irritation, alendronate is contraindicated in patients who have stricture or inadequate emptying of the esophagus. It is recommended that patients remain upright for at least 30 min after taking the medication to avoid esophageal irritation. Cases of esophagitis, esophageal ulcer, and esophageal stricture have been described, but the incidence appears to be low. In clinical trials, overall gastrointestinal symptomatology was no different with alendronate compared to placebo.

Risedronate also reduces bone turnover and increases bone mass. Controlled clinical trials have demonstrated 40 to 50% reduction in vertebral fracture risk over 3 years, accompanied by a 40% reduction in clinical nonspine fractures. The only clinical trial specifically designed to evaluate hip fracture outcome (HIP) indicated that risedronate reduced hip fracture risk in women in their 70s with confirmed osteoporosis by 40%. In contrast, risedronate was not effective at reducing hip fracture occurrence in older women without proven osteoporosis. Studies have shown that 35 mg of risedronate administered once weekly is therapeutically equivalent to 5 mg/d. Patients should take risedronate with a full glass of plain water [0.18 to 0.25 L (6 to 8 oz)], to facilitate delivery to the stomach, and should not lie down for 30 min after taking the drug. The incidence of gastrointestinal side effects in trials with risedronate was similar to that of placebo.

Etidronate was the first bisphosphonate to be approved, initially for use in Paget's disease and hypercalcemia. This agent has also been used in osteoporosis trials of smaller magnitude than those performed for alendronate and risedronate but is not approved by the FDA for treatment of osteoporosis. Etidronate probably has some efficacy against vertebral fracture when given as an intermittent cyclical regimen (2 weeks on, 2 1/2 months off). There has not been any study of its effectiveness against nonvertebral fractures.

Zoledronate and ibandronate are potent bisphosphonates with unique administration regimens (once yearly intravenously, once monthly orally) and are currently in clinical development.

Mode of Action   Bisphosphonates are structurally related to pyrophosphates, compounds that are incorporated into bone matrix. Bisphosphonates specifically impair osteoclast function and reduce osteoclast number, in part by the induction of apoptosis. Recent evidence suggests that the nitrogen-containing bisphosphonates also inhibit protein prenylation, one of the end products in the mevalonic acid pathway. This effect disrupts intracellular protein trafficking and may ultimately lead to apoptosis. Some bisphosphonates have very long retention in the skeleton and may exert long-term effects.

CALCITONIN   Calcitonin is a polypeptide hormone produced by the thyroid gland (Chap. 332). Its physiologic role is unclear as no skeletal disease has been described in association with calcitonin deficiency or calcitonin excess. Calcitonin preparations are approved by the FDA for Paget's disease, hypercalcemia, and osteoporosis in women >5 years past menopause.

Injectable calcitonin produces small increments in bone mass of the lumbar spine. However, difficulty of administration and frequent reactions, including nausea and facial flushing, make general use limited. In 1995, a nasal spray containing calcitonin (200 IU/d) was approved for treatment of osteoporosis in postmenopausal women. One study suggests that nasal calcitonin produces small increments in bone mass and a small reduction in new vertebral fractures in calcitonin-treated patients versus those on calcium alone. There has been no proven effectiveness against nonvertebral fractures.

Calcitonin is not indicated for prevention of osteoporosis and is not sufficiently potent to prevent bone loss in early postmenopausal women. As mentioned above, calcitonin might have an analgesic effect on bone pain, both in the subcutaneous and possibly the nasal form.

Mode of Action   Calcitonin suppresses osteoclast activity by direct action on the osteoclast calcitonin receptor. Osteoclasts exposed to calcitonin cannot maintain their active ruffled border, which normally maintains close contact with underlying bone.

PARATHYROID HORMONE   Endogenous PTH is an 84-amino-acid peptide that is largely responsible for calcium homeostasis (Chap. 332). Although chronic elevation of PTH, as occurs in hyperparathyroidism, is associated with bone loss (particularly cortical bone), PTH can also exert anabolic effects on bone. Consistent with this, some observational studies have indicated that mild elevations in PTH are associated with maintenance of trabecular bone mass. On the basis of these findings, preclinical and early clinical studies have been performed using an exogenous PTH analogue (1-34 PTH). The first randomized controlled trial in postmenopausal women showed that PTH, when superimposed on ongoing estrogen therapy, produced substantial increments in bone mass (13% over a 3-year period compared to estrogen alone) and reduced the risk of vertebral compression deformity. In one study (median 19 months' duration), 20 μg PTH(1-34) reduced vertebral fractures by 65% and nonvertebral fractures by 45% (Fig. 333-10). PTH(1-34) has now been approved by the FDA for treatment of patients with osteoporosis (both women and men) at high risk of fracture. Treatment is administered as a single daily injection given for a maximum of 2 years. Although there are no randomized controlled studies to confirm the need for an antiresorptive agent after PTH withdrawal, based on observational data and animal studies, it is likely that antiresorptive agents will be required to maintain PTH-induced benefits on bone mass and fracture. In contrast to combination

FIGURE 333-10   Number of incident vertebral deformities (15% and 20% reductions) in women with osteoporosis on hormone therapy (HT), compared to HT + PTH over 3 years. (HT, hormone therapy; PTH, parathyroid hormone.) (*From Cosman et al.*)

treatment with estrogen, there are no published data on use of PTH in combination with bisphosphonates or SERMs.

Side effects are generally mild and can include muscle pains, weakness, dizziness, headache, and nausea. Rodents given prolonged treatment with PTH in relatively high doses developed osteogenic sarcomas. It is not believed that this finding has any relevance to humans.

PTH use may be limited by its mode of administration; alternative modes of delivery are being investigated. The optimal frequency of administration also remains to be established, and it is possible that PTH might also be effective when used intermittently. Cost may also be a limiting factor.

Mode of Action   Exogenously administered PTH appears to have direct actions on osteoblast activity, with biochemical and histomorphometric evidence of de novo bone formation early in response to PTH, prior to activation of bone resorption. Subsequently, PTH activates bone remodeling but still appears to favor bone formation over bone resorption. PTH stimulates IGF-I and collagen production and appears to increase osteoblast number by stimulating replication, enhancing osteoblast recruitment, and inhibiting apoptosis. Unlike all other treatments, PTH produces a true increase in bone tissue and an apparent restoration of bone microarchitecture (Fig. 333-11).

FLUORIDE   Fluoride has been available for many years and is a potent stimulator of osteoprogenitor cells when studied in vitro. It has been used in multiple osteoporosis studies with conflicting results, in part related to use of varying doses and preparations. Despite increments

FIGURE 333-11   Effect of parathyroid hormone (PTH) treatment on bone microarchitecture. Paired biopsy specimens from a 64-year-old woman before (*A*) and after (*B*) treatment with PTH. (*From DW Dempster et al: J Bone Miner Res 16:1846, 2001.*)

in bone mass of up to 10%, there are no consistent effects of fluoride on vertebral or nonvertebral fracture, which might actually increase when high doses of fluoride are used. Fluoride remains an experimental agent, despite its long history and multiple studies.

OTHER POTENTIAL ANABOLIC AGENTS   Several small studies of growth hormone (GH), alone or in combination with other agents, have not shown consistent or substantial positive effects on skeletal mass. Many of these studies are relatively short-term, and the effects of GH, growth hormone–releasing hormone, and the IGFs are still under investigation. Anabolic steroids, mostly derivatives of testosterone, act primarily as antiresorptive agents to reduce bone turnover but may also stimulate osteoblastic activity. Effects on bone mass remain unclear but appear weak, in general, and use is limited by masculinizing side effects. Several recent observational studies suggest that the statin drugs, currently used to treat hypercholesterolemia, may be associated with increased bone mass and reduced fractures, but conclusions from clinical trials are mixed.

Nonpharmacologic Approaches   Protective pads worn around the outer thigh, which cover the trochanteric region of the hip can prevent hip fractures in elderly residents in nursing homes. The use of hip protectors is limited largely by compliance and comfort, but new devices are being developed that may circumvent these problems and provide adjunctive treatments.

Kyphoplasty and *vertebroplasty* are also useful nonpharmacologic approaches for the treatment of painful vertebral fractures. However, no long-term data are available.

Treatment Monitoring   There are currently no well-accepted guidelines for monitoring treatment of osteoporosis. Because most osteoporosis treatments produce small or moderate bone mass increments on average, it is reasonable to consider BMD as a monitoring tool. Changes must exceed ~4% in the spine and 6% in the hip to be considered significant in any individual. The hip is the preferred site due to larger surface area and greater reproducibility. Medication-induced increments may require several years to produce changes of this magnitude (if they do at all). Consequently, it can be argued that BMD should not be repeated at intervals <2 years. Only significant BMD reductions should prompt a change in medical regimen, as it is expected that many individuals will not show responses greater than the detection limits of the current measurement techniques.

Biochemical markers of bone turnover may prove useful for treatment monitoring, but there is currently little hard evidence to support this concept; it remains unclear which endpoint is most useful. If bone turnover markers are used, a determination should be made before starting therapy and repeated ≥4 months after therapy is initiated. In general, a change in bone turnover markers must be 30 to 40% lower than the baseline to be significant because of the biologic and technical variability in these tests. A positive change in biochemical markers and/or bone density can be useful to help patients adhere to treatment regimens.

GLUCOCORTICOID-INDUCED OSTEOPOROSIS

Osteoporotic fractures are a well-characterized consequence of the hypercortisolism associated with Cushing's syndrome. However, the therapeutic use of glucocorticoids is by far the most common form of glucocorticoid-induced osteoporosis. Glucocorticoids are widely used in the treatment of a variety of disorders, including chronic lung disorders, rheumatoid arthritis and other connective tissue diseases, inflammatory bowel disease, and posttransplantation. Osteoporosis and related fractures are serious side effects of chronic glucocorticoid therapy. Because the effects of glucocorticoids on the skeleton are often superimposed upon the consequences of aging and menopause, it is not surprising that women and the elderly are most frequently affected. The skeletal response to steroids is remarkably heterogeneous, however, and even young, growing individuals treated with glucocorticoids can present with fractures.

The risk of fractures depends on the dose and duration of gluco-

corticoid therapy, although recent data suggest that there may be no completely safe dose. Bone loss is more rapid during the early months of treatment, and trabecular bone is more severely affected than cortical bone. As a result, fractures have been shown to increase within 3 months of steroid treatment. There is an increase in fracture risk in both the axial and appendicular skeleton, including risk of hip fracture. Bone loss can occur with any route of steroid administration including high-dose inhaled glucocorticoids and intraarticular injections. Alternate-day delivery does not appear to ameliorate the skeletal effects of glucocorticoids.

Pathophysiology   Glucocorticoids increase bone loss by multiple mechanisms including: (1) inhibition of osteoblast function and an increase in osteoblast apoptosis, resulting in impaired synthesis of new bone; (2) stimulation of bone resorption, probably as a secondary effect; (3) impairment of the absorption of calcium across the intestine, probably by a vitamin D–independent effect; (4) increase of urinary calcium loss and induction of some degree of secondary hyperparathyroidism; (5) reduction of adrenal androgens and suppression of ovarian and testicular secretion of estrogens and androgens; and (6) induction of glucocorticoid myopathy, which may exacerbate effects on skeletal and calcium homeostasis as well as increase the risk of falls.

Evaluation of the Patient   Because of the prevalence of glucocorticoid-induced bone loss, it is important to evaluate the status of the skeleton in all patients starting or already receiving long-term glucocorticoid therapy. Modifiable risk factors should be identified, including those for falls. Examination should include height and muscle strength testing. Laboratory evaluation should include an assessment of 24-h urinary calcium. A task force of the American College of Rheumatology recommends that all patients on long-term (>6 months) glucocorticoids have measurement of bone mass at both the spine and hip using DXA. If only one skeletal site can be measured, it is best to assess the spine in individuals <60 years and the hip for those >60 years.

Prevention   Bone loss caused by glucocorticoids can be prevented, and the risk of fractures significantly reduced. Strategies must include using the lowest dose of glucocorticoid for disease management. Topical and inhaled routes of administration are preferred, where appropriate. Risk factor reduction is important, including smoking cessation, limitation of alcohol consumption, and participation in weight-bearing exercise, when appropriate. All patients should receive an adequate calcium and vitamin D intake from the diet or from supplements.

℞ TREATMENT

Only bisphosphonates have been demonstrated in large clinical trials to reduce the risk of fractures in patients being treated with glucocorticoids. Risedronate prevents bone loss and reduces vertebral fracture risk by about 70%. Similar beneficial effects are observed in studies of alendronate and etidronate. Controlled trials of hormone therapy have shown bone-sparing effects, and calcitonin also has some protective effect in the spine. Thiazides reduce urine calcium loss, but their role in prevention of fractures is unclear. PTH has also been studied in a small group of women with glucocorticoid-induced osteoporosis. Bone mass increased substantially, but no fracture data are available.

FURTHER READING

COSMAN F, LINDSAY R: Selective estrogen receptors modulators: Clinical spectrum. Endocr Rev 20:418, 1999

——— et al: Parathyroid hormone added to established hormone therapy: Effects on vertebral fracture and maintenance of bone mass after parathyroid hormone withdrawal. J Bone Miner Res 16:925, 2001

GUYATT G et al: Meta-analyses of therapies for postmenopausal osteoporosis. Endocr Rev 23:495, 2002

NEER RM et al: Effect of parathyroid hormone (1-34) on fractures and bone mineral density in postmenopausal women with osteoporosis. N Engl J Med 344:1434, 2001

WRITING GROUP FOR THE WOMEN'S HEALTH INITIATIVE INVESTIGATORS: Risks and benefits of estrogen plus progestin in healthy postmenopausal women: Principal results from the Women's Health Initiative randomized controlled trial. JAMA 288:321, 2002

PAGET DISEASE OF BONE

Paget disease is a localized bone disorder that often affects widespread areas of the skeleton through increased bone remodeling. The pathologic process is initiated by overactive osteoclastic bone resorption followed by a compensatory increase in osteoblastic new bone formation. New pagetic bone is structurally disorganized and more susceptible to deformities and fractures. Although most patients are asymptomatic, a variety of symptoms and complications may result directly from bony involvement or secondarily from the expansion of bone and subsequent compression of surrounding neural tissue.

EPIDEMIOLOGY There is a marked geographic variation in the frequency of Paget disease, with high prevalence in Western Europe (Great Britain, France, and Germany but not Switzerland or Scandinavia) and among those who have immigrated to Australia, New Zealand, South Africa, and North and South America. The disease is rare in native populations of the Americas, Africa, Asia, and the Middle East. The prevalence is greater in males and increases with age. Autopsy series reveal Paget disease in about 3% of those over age 40. Prevalence of positive skeletal radiographs in patients over age 55 is 2.5% for men and 1.6% for women. Elevated alkaline phosphatase (ALP) levels in asymptomatic patients has an age-adjusted incidence of 12.7 and 7 per 100,000 person-years in men and women, respectively. The frequency of diagnosis by either radiographic or biochemical criteria has decreased during the past 20 years.

ETIOLOGY The etiology of Paget disease of bone remains unknown, but evidence supports both genetic and viral etiologies. A positive family history is found in 5 to 25% of patients and, when present, raises the prevalence of the disease seven- to tenfold among first-degree relatives. Familial patterns of disease in several large kindred are consistent with an autosomal dominant pattern of inheritance with variable penetrance. A susceptibility locus for Paget disease has been mapped to chromosome 18q21-22, a region that contains the gene responsible for a rare Paget disease–like skeletal disorder known as familial expansile osteolysis. The gene encodes the receptor activator of nuclear factor-κB (RANK), a member of the tumor necrosis factor superfamily critical for osteoclast differentiation (Fig. 334-1). In other families, susceptibility loci have been mapped to loci on chromosomes 18q23, 6p21.3, 5q31, and 5q35. A homozygous deletion of the *TNFRSF11B* gene, which encodes osteoprotegrin (Fig. 334-1), causes juvenile Paget disease, a disorder characterized by uncontrolled osteoclastic differentiation and resorption. Thus, it is likely that Paget disease is genetically heterogeneous with divergent pathogenetic mechanisms in sporadic and familial forms.

Several lines of evidence suggest a viral etiology of Paget disease, including (1) the presence of cytoplasmic and nuclear inclusions resembling paramyxoviruses (measles and respiratory syncytial virus) in pagetic osteoclasts, and (2) viral mRNA in precursor and mature osteoclasts. The viral etiology is further supported by conversion of osteoclast precursors to pagetic-like osteoclasts by vectors containing the measles virus nucleocapsid or matrix genes. However, the viral etiology has been questioned by the inability to culture a live virus from pagetic bone and by failure to clone the full-length viral genes from material obtained from patients with Paget disease.

PATHOPHYSIOLOGY The principal abnormality in Paget disease is the increased number and activity of osteoclasts. Pagetic osteoclasts are large, increased 10- to 100-fold in number, and have a greater number of nuclei (as many as 100 compared to 3 to 5 nuclei in the normal osteoclast). The overactive osteoclasts create a sevenfold increase in resorptive surfaces and an erosion rate of 9 μg/d (normal is 1 μg/d). Several causes for the increased number and activity of pagetic osteoclasts have been identified: (1) osteoclastic precursors are hypersen

FIGURE 334-1 Diagram illustrating factors that promote differentiation and function of osteoclasts and osteoblasts and the role of the RANK pathway. Stromal bone marrow (mesenchymal) cells and differentiated osteoblasts produce multiple growth factors and cytokines, including macrophage colony-stimulating factor (M-CSF), to modulate osteoclastogenesis. RANKL (receptor activator of NFκB ligand) is produced by osteoblast progenitors and mature osteoblasts and can bind to a soluble decoy receptor known as OPG (osteoprotegrin) to inhibit RANKL action. Alternatively, a cell-cell interaction between osteoblast and osteoclast progenitors allows RANKL to bind to its membrane-bound receptor, RANK, thereby stimulating osteoclast differentiation and function. RANK binds intracellular proteins called TRAFS (tumor necrosis factor receptor-associated factors) that mediate receptor signaling through transcription factors such as NFκB. M-CSF binds to its receptor, c-fms, which is the cellular homologue of the *fms* oncogene. See text for the potential role of these pathways in disorders of osteoclast function such as Paget disease and osteopetrosis.

sitive to $1,25(OH)_2D_3$; (2) osteoclasts are hyperresponsive to RANK ligand (RANKL), the osteoclast stimulatory factor that mediates the effects of most osteotropic factors on osteoclast formation; (3) marrow stromal cells from pagetic lesions have increased RANKL expression; (4) osteoclast precursor recruitment is increased by interleukin (IL) 6, which is increased in the blood of patients with active Paget disease and is overexpressed in pagetic osteoclasts; (5) expression of the proto-oncogene c-*fos*, which increases osteoclastic activity, is increased; and (6) the antiapoptotic oncogene *Bcl*-2 in pagetic bone is overexpressed. Numerous osteoblasts are recruited to active resorption sites and produce large amounts of new bone matrix. As a result, bone turnover is high and bone mass is normal or increased, not reduced.

The characteristic feature of Paget disease is increased bone resorption accompanied by accelerated bone formation. An initial osteolytic phase involves prominent bone resorption and marked hypervascularization. Radiographically, this manifests as an advancing lytic wedge, or "blade of grass" lesion. The second phase is a period of very active bone formation and resorption that replaces normal lamellar bone with haphazard (woven) bone. The mosaic pattern of woven bone is structurally inferior and can bow and fracture more readily. At the same time, fibrous connective tissue may replace normal bone marrow. In the final sclerotic phase, bone resorption declines progressively and leads to a hard, dense, less vascular pagetic or mosaic bone, which represents the so-called burned-out phase of Paget disease. All three phases may be present at the same time at different skeletal sites.

CLINICAL MANIFESTATIONS Asymptomatic patients are often diagnosed by discovery of an elevated ALP level on routine blood chemistry testing or from an abnormality on a skeletal radiograph obtained for another indication. The skeletal sites most commonly involved are the pelvis, vertebral bodies, skull, femur, and tibia. Numerous active sites of skeletal involvement are more common in familial cases with an early presentation.

Pain is the most common presenting symptom. It results from in-

FIGURE 334-2   A 48-year-old woman with Paget disease of the skull. *Left.* Lateral radiograph showing areas of both bone resorption and sclerosis. *Right.* ⁹⁹ᵐTc HDP bone scan with anterior, posterior, and lateral views of the skull showing diffuse isotope uptake by the frontal, parietal, occipital, and petrous bones.

creased bony vascularity, expanding lytic lesions, fractures, bowing, or other deformities of the extremities. Bowing of the femur or tibia causes gait abnormalities and abnormal mechanical stresses with secondary osteoarthritis of the hip or knee joints. Long bone bowing also causes extremity pain by stretching the muscles attached to the bone softened by the pagetic process. Back pain results from enlarged pagetic vertebrae, vertebral compression fractures, spinal stenosis, degenerative changes of the joints, and altered body mechanics with kyphosis and forward tilt of the upper back. Rarely, spinal cord compression may result from bone enlargement or from the vascular steal syndrome. Skull involvement may cause headaches, symmetric or asymmetric enlargement of the parietal or frontal bones (frontal bossing), and increased head size. Cranial expansion may narrow cranial foramina and cause neurologic complications including hearing loss from cochlear nerve damage from temporal bone involvement, cranial nerve palsies, and softening of the base of the skull (*platybasia*) and the risk of brainstem compression. Pagetic involvement of the facial bones may cause facial deformity, loss of teeth and other dental conditions, and rarely, airway compression.

Fractures are serious complications of Paget disease and usually occur in long bones at areas of active or advancing lytic lesions. Common fracture sites are the femoral shaft and subtrochanteric regions. Neoplasms arising from pagetic bone are rare. The incidence of sarcoma appears to be decreasing, possibly because of earlier, more effective treatment with potent antiresorptive agents. The majority of tumors are osteosarcomas, which usually present with new pain in a long-standing pagetic lesion. Osteoclast-rich benign giant cell tumors may arise in areas adjacent to pagetic bone and respond to glucocorticoid therapy.

Cardiovascular complications may occur in patients with involvement of large (15 to 35%) portions of the skeleton and a high degree of disease activity (ALP four times above normal). The extensive arteriovenous shunting and marked increases in blood flow through the vascular pagetic bone lead to a high-output state and cardiac enlargement. However, high-output heart failure is relatively rare and usually develops in patients with concomitant cardiac pathology. In addition, calcific aortic stenosis and diffuse vascular calcifications have been associated with Paget disease.

DIAGNOSIS   The diagnosis may be suggested on clinical examination by the presence of enlarged skull with frontal bossing, bowing of an extremity, or short stature with simian posturing. An extremity with an area of warmth and tenderness to palpation may suggest an underlying pagetic lesion. Other findings include bony deformity of the pelvis, skull, spine and extremities; arthritic involvement of the joints adjacent to lesions; and leg length discrepancy resulting from deformities of the long bones.

Paget disease is usually diagnosed from radiologic and biochemical abnormalities. Radiographic findings typical of Paget disease include enlargement or expansion of an entire bone or area of a long bone, cortical thickening, coarsening of trabecular markings, and typical lytic and sclerotic changes. Skull radiographs (Fig. 334-2) reveal regions of "cotton wool," or osteoporosis circumscripta; thickening of diploic areas; and enlargement and sclerosis of a portion or all of one or more skull bones. Vertebral cortical thickening of the superior and inferior end plates creates a "picture frame" vertebra. Diffuse radiodense enlargement of a vertebra is referred to as "ivory vertebra." Pelvic radiographs may demonstrate disruption or fusion of the sacroiliac joints; porotic and radiodense lesions of the ilium with whorls of coarse trabeculation; thickened and sclerotic ileopectinal line (Brim sign); and softening with protrusio acetabuli, with axial migration of the hips and functional flexion contracture. Radiographs of long bones reveal bowing deformity and typical pagetic changes of cortical thickening and expansion and areas of lucency and sclerosis (Fig. 334-3). Radionuclide ⁹⁹ᵐTc bone scans are less specific but are more sensitive than standard radiographs for identifying sites of active skeletal lesions. Suspected areas of malignant transformation are best distinguished from pagetic bone by computed tomography (CT) or magnetic

FIGURE 334-3   Radiograph of a 73-year-old man with Paget disease of the right proximal femur. Note the coarsening of the trabecular pattern with marked cortical thickening and narrowing of the joint space consistent with osteoarthritis secondary to pagetic deformity of the right femur.

resonance imaging (MRI). Definitive diagnosis of malignancy requires bone biopsy.

Biochemical evaluation is useful in the diagnosis and management of Paget disease. The marked increase in bone turnover can be monitored using biochemical markers of bone formation and resorption. The parallel rise in serum ALP and urinary hydroxyproline levels, markers of bone formation and resorption, respectively, confirm the coupling of bone formation and resorption in Paget disease. The degree of bone marker elevation reflects the extent and severity of the disease. Patients with the highest elevation of ALP (10 times the upper limit of normal) typically have involvement of the skull and at least one other skeletal site. Lower values suggest less extensive involvement or a quiescent phase of the disease. For most patients, serum total ALP remains the test of choice both for diagnosis and assessing response to therapy. Occasionally, a symptomatic patient with evidence of progression at a single site may have a normal total ALP level but increased bone-specific ALP. Serum osteocalcin, a marker of bone formation, is not always elevated in patients with active Paget disease and is not recommended for use in diagnosis or management.

Urinary and serum deoxypyridinoline, N-telopeptide, and C-telopeptide levels are products of type I collagen degradation and are more specific for bone resorption than hydroxyproline. These newer bone resorption markers have distinct advantages over measurement of 24-h or second-morning void hydroxyproline/creatinine ratio, which requires control of dietary gelatin intake and precise urine collection and analysis. The new resorption markers decrease more rapidly in response to therapy than does ALP.

Serum calcium and phosphate levels are normal in Paget disease. Immobilization of a patient with active Paget disease may rarely cause hypercalcemia and hypercalciuria and increase the risk for nephrolithiasis. However, the discovery of hypercalcemia, even in the presence of immobilization, should prompt a search for another cause of hypercalcemia. In contrast, hypocalcemia or mild secondary hyperparathyroidism may develop in Paget patients with very active bone formation and insufficient dietary calcium intake. Hypocalcemia can occur during bisphosphonate therapy when bone resorption is rapidly suppressed and active bone formation continues. Hypocalcemia may be prevented by adequate calcium and vitamin D intake.

℞ TREATMENT

The development of effective and potent pharmacologic agents (Table 334-1) has changed the treatment philosophy from treating only symptomatic patients to treating asymptomatic patients who are at risk for complications. Pharmacologic therapy is indicated in the following circumstances: to control symptoms caused by metabolically active Paget disease such as bone pain, fracture, headache, pain from pagetic radiculopathy or arthropathy, or neurologic complications; to decrease local blood flow and minimize operative blood loss in patients undergoing surgery at an active pagetic site; to reduce hypercalciuria that may occur during immobilization; and to decrease the risk of complications when disease activity is high (elevated ALP) and when the site of involvement involves weight-bearing bones, areas adjacent to major joints, vertebral bodies, and skull. Whether early therapy prevents late complications remains to be determined. However, the restoration of normal bone architecture following suppression of pagetic activity suggests that treatment may prevent further deformities and complications.

Agents approved for treatment of Paget disease suppress the very high rates of bone resorption and secondarily decrease the high rates of bone formation (Table 334-1). As a result of decreasing bone turnover, pagetic structural patterns, including areas of poorly mineralized

TABLE 334-1 *Pharmacologic Agents Approved for Treatment of Paget Disease*

Name (Brand)	Potency[a]	Dose	Mode of Administration[b]
Etidronate (Didronel)	1	400 mg/d for 6 mos	Fasting with 6 oz tap water 2 h before or after a meal
Tiludronate (Skelid)	10	400 mg/d for 3 mos	Fasting with 6 oz tap water and wait 45 min before food, liquids are taken
Pamidronte (Aredia)	100	30 mg IV daily for 3 days or 60 to 90 mg IV at various intervals as determined by disease	
Alendronate (Fosamax)	700	40 mg/d for 6 mos	Fasting with 6 oz tap water and wait 45 min before food, liquids are taken
Risedronate (Actonel)	1000	30 mg/d for 2 mos	Fasting with 6 oz tap water and wait 45 min before food, liquids are taken
Calcitonin (Miacalcin)	NA	100 U sc daily	Dose may be reduced to 50 U qod for 6–18 mos

[a] Potency is relative to etidronate. For each tablet, etidronate strength is 400 mg; tiludronate is 200 mg; alendronate is 40 mg; and risedronate is 30 mg. Miacalcin nasal spray is not approved for use in Paget disease.
[b] 6 oz is 175 mL.

woven bone, are replaced by more normal cancellous or lamellar bone. The improvement in skeletal structure can be demonstrated on standard radiographs and ^{99m}Tc bone scans, which show decreased isotope accumulation in pagetic sites. Reduced bone turnover can be documented by a decline in urine or serum resorption markers (pyridinoline, deoxypyridinoline, N-telopeptide, C-telopeptide) and serum markers of bone formation (ALP, osteocalcin).

The potencies of various bisphosphonates are expressed relative to that of etidronate, the first clinically useful agent in this class. Etidronate use is now limited as the doses required to suppress bone resorption may impair mineralization. Thus, etidronate is administered in 6-month treatment cycles followed by a 6-month drug-free period. Failure to adhere to the cyclic regimen can produce osteomalacia manifested by bone pain and fractures. Etidronate should not be used in patients with advanced lytic lesions in weight-bearing bones. The major advantage of etidronate is that it is relatively well tolerated and only occasionally causes transient diarrhea or bone pain.

The second-generation oral bisphosphonates tiludronate, alendronate, and risedronate are more potent than etidronate in controlling bone turnover and thus induce a longer remission at a lower dose. The lower doses reduce the risks of impaired mineralization and osteomalacia. Oral bisphosphonates are poorly absorbed and have a potential to produce esophageal ulceration, reflux, and rarely, perforation. They should be taken first thing in the morning on an empty stomach, followed by maintenance of upright posture with no food or drink for 30 to 60 min. Other medications, liquids, and food should be delayed for at least 30 to 60 min after taking bisphosphonates to optimize absorption. Tiludronate daily for 3 months normalizes ALP in 24 to 35% of moderately affected patients. In patients with moderate to severe disease, alendronate for 6 months normalizes ALP in >67% of patients, with an overall fall in ALP of 79% compared to 44% with etidronate. In patients with moderately active disease, risedronate daily for 2 to 3 months reduces serum ALP by 80% and normalizes indices of bone turnover in 73% of patients compared to 15% of those receiving etidronate.

Pamidronate is the only bisphosphonate currently approved for intravenous use in Paget disease. The recommended dose is 30 mg dissolved in 500 mL of normal saline or dextrose intravenously over 4 h on three consecutive days. The dose can be adjusted to each patient's requirements. A single 60-mg dose of pamidronate intravenously may normalize bone turnover in patients with mild disease. In contrast, patients with moderate to severe disease (elevation of ALP of three to four times normal) may require two to four doses of pamidronate, 60 to 90 mg intravenously, every 1 to 2 weeks. Patients with very severe disease may require a total dose of pamidronate of 300 to 500 mg given weekly over several weeks. Although suppression of urinary bone markers occurs after a few days to weeks, normalization of serum ALP levels often requires at least 3 months. Consequently, the effects of pamidronate are best evaluated 3 months after the initial dose. Pamidronate is generally well tolerated; however, a small number of patients experience a flulike syndrome that may begin 24 h after the first infusion. In patients with high bone turnover, vitamin D (400 to 800 IU daily) and calcium (500 mg three times daily) should be provided to prevent hypocalcemia and secondary hyperparathyroidism. Indications for intravenous therapy include mild disease and normalization of bone turnover after a single infusion, previous prevention of disease progression, refractoriness to oral therapy, need for rapid response such for those with neurologic symptoms or with severe bone pain due to a lytic lesion, risk of an impending fracture, and as pretreatment prior to elective surgery in an area of active disease. Remission following pamidronate therapy may persist for as long as 1 year. Other bisphosphonate agents are in development.

The subcutaneous injectable form of salmon calcitonin is approved for the treatment of Paget disease. Intranasal calcitonin spray is approved for osteoporosis at a dose of 200 U/d; however, the efficacy of this dose in Paget disease has not been thoroughly studied. The usual starting dose of injectable calcitonin (100 U/d) reduces ALP by 50% and may relieve skeletal symptoms. The dose may be reduced to 50 U/day three times weekly after an initial favorable response to 100 U daily; however, the lower dose may require long-term use to sustain efficacy. The common side effects of calcitonin therapy are nausea and facial flushing. Secondary resistance after prolonged use may be due to either the formation of anti-calcitonin antibodies or downregulation of osteoclastic cell-surface calcitonin receptors. The lower potency and injectable mode of delivery make this agent a less attractive treatment option that should be reserved for patients who either do not tolerate or do not respond to bisphosphonates.

SCLEROSING BONE DISORDERS

OSTEOPETROSIS   *Osteopetrosis* refers to a group of disorders caused by severe impairment of osteoclast-mediated bone resorption. Other terms that are often used include marble bone disease, which captures the solid x-ray appearance of the involved skeleton, and Albers-Schonberg disease, which refers to the milder, adult form of osteopetrosis also known as autosomal dominant osteopetrosis type II. The major types of osteopetrosis include malignant (severe, infantile, autosomal recessive) osteopetrosis and benign (adult, autosomal dominant) osteopetrosis types I and II. A rare autosomal recessive intermediate form has a more benign prognosis. Autosomal recessive carbonic anhydrase (CA) II deficiency produces osteopetrosis of intermediate severity associated with renal tubular acidosis and cerebral calcification.

Etiology and Genetics   Naturally occurring and gene knockout animal models with phenotypes similar to those of the human disorders have been used to explore the genetic basis of osteopetrosis. The primary defect in osteopetrosis is the loss of osteoclastic bone resorption and preservation of normal osteoblastic bone formation. Osteoprotegerin (OPG) is a soluble decoy receptor that binds osteoblast-derived RANK ligand, which mediates osteoclast differentiation and activation (Fig. 334-1). Transgenic mice that overexpress OPG develop osteopetrosis, presumably by blocking RANK ligand. Mice deficient in RANK lack osteoclasts and develop severe osteopetrosis.

Recessive mutations of CA II prevent osteoclasts from generating an acid environment in the clear zone between its ruffled border and the adjacent mineral surface. Absence of CA II, therefore, impairs osteoclastic bone resorption. Other forms of human disease have less clear genetic defects. About one-half of the patients with malignant infantile osteopetrosis have a mutation in the *TCIRG1* gene encoding the osteoclast-specific subunit of the vacuolar proton pump, which mediates the acidification of the interface between bone mineral and the osteoclast ruffled border. Mutations in the *ClCN7* chloride channel gene cause autosomal dominant osteopetrosis type II.

Clinical Presentation   The incidence of autosomal recessive severe (malignant) osteopetrosis ranges from 1 in 200,000 to 1 in 500,000 live births. As bone and cartilage fail to undergo modeling, paralysis of one or more cranial nerves may occur due to narrowing of the cranial foramina. Failure of skeletal modeling also results in inadequate marrow space, leading to extramedullary hematopoiesis with hypersplenism and pancytopenia. Hypocalcemia due to lack of osteoclastic bone resorption may occur in infants and young children. The untreated infantile disease is fatal, often before age 5.

Adult (benign) osteopetrosis is an autosomal dominant disease that is usually diagnosed by the discovery of typical skeletal changes in young adults who undergo radiologic evaluation of a fracture. The prevalence is 1 in 100,000 to 1 in 500,000 adults. The course is not always benign, as fractures may be accompanied by loss of vision, deafness, psychomotor delay, mandibular osteomyelitis, and other complications usually associated with the juvenile form. In some kindred, nonpenetrance results in skip generations, while in other families severely affected children are born into families with benign disease. The milder form of the disease does not usually require treatment.

Radiography   Typically, there are generalized symmetric increases in bone mass with thickening of both cortical and trabecular bone. Diaphyses and metaphyses are broadened, and alternating sclerotic and lucent bands may be seen in the iliac crests, at the ends of long bones, and in vertebral bodies. The cranium is usually thickened, particularly at the base of the skull, and the paranasal and mastoid sinuses are underpneumatized.

Laboratory Findings   The only significant laboratory findings are elevated serum levels of osteoclast-derived tartrate-resistant acid phosphatase (TRAP) and the brain isoenzyme of creatine kinase. Serum calcium may be low in severe disease, and parathyroid hormone and 1,25-dihydroxyvitamin D levels may be elevated in response to hypocalcemia.

℞ TREATMENT

Allogenic HLA-identical bone marrow transplantation has been successful in some children. Following transplantation, the marrow contains progenitor cells and normally functioning osteoclasts. A cure is most likely when children are transplanted before age 4. Marrow transplantation from nonidentical HLA-matched donors has a much higher failure rate. Limited studies in small numbers of patients have suggested variable benefits following treatment with interferon gamma-1b, 1,25-dihydroxyvitamin D (which stimulates osteoclasts directly), methylprednisolone, and a low calcium/high-phosphate diet.

Surgical intervention is indicated to decompress optic or auditory nerve compression. Orthopedic management is required for the surgical treatment of fractures and their complications including malunion and post-fracture deformity.

PYKNODYSOSTOSIS   This is an autosomal recessive form of osteosclerosis that is believed to have affected the French impressionist painter Henri de Toulouse-Lautrec. The molecular basis involves mutations in the gene that encodes cathepsin K, a lysosomal metalloproteinase highly expressed in osteoclasts and important for bone matrix degradation. Osteoclasts are present but do not function normally. Pyknodysostosis is a form of short-limb dwarfism that presents with frequent fractures but usually normal life span. Clinical features include short stature; kyphoscoliosis and deformities of the chest; high arched palate; proptosis; blue sclerae; dysmorphic features including small face and chin, frontooccipital prominence, pointed beaked nose, large cranium, and obtuse mandibular angle; and small square hands with hypoplastic nails. Radiographs demonstrate a generalized increase in bone density, but in contrast to osteopetrosis, the long bones are normally shaped. Separated cranial sutures, including the persistent patency of the anterior fontanel, are characteristic of the disorder. There may also be hypoplasia of the sinuses, mandible, distal clavicles, and terminal phalanges. Persistence of deciduous teeth and sclerosis of the calvarium and base of the skull are also common. Histologic evaluation shows normal cortical bone architecture with decreased osteo-blastic and osteoclastic activities. Serum chemistries are normal, and unlike osteopetrosis, there is no anemia. There is no known treatment for this condition, and no reports of attempted bone marrow transplant.

PROGRESSIVE DIAPHYSEAL DYSPLASIA Also known as Camurati-Engel-man disease, progressive diaphyseal dysplasia is an autosomal domi-nant disorder that is characterized radiographically by diaphyseal hyperostosis and a symmetric thickening and increased diameter of the endosteal and periosteal surfaces of the diaphyses of the long bones, particularly the femur and tibia, and, less often, the fibula, radius, and ulna. The genetic defect responsible for the disease has been localized to the area of chromosome 19q13.2 encoding tumor growth factor (TGF)-β1. The mutation promotes activation of TGF-β1. The clinical severity is variable. The most common presenting symptoms are pain and tenderness of the involved areas, fatigue, muscle wasting, and gait disturbance. The weakness may be mistaken for muscular dystrophy. Characteristic body habitus includes thin limbs with little muscle mass yet prominent and palpable bones and, when the skull is involved, large head with prominent forehead and proptosis. Patients may also display signs of cranial nerve palsies, hydrocephalus, central hypo-gonadism, and Raynaud phenomenon. Radiographically, patchy pro-gressive endosteal and periosteal new bone formation is observed along the diaphyses of the long bones. Bone scintigraphy shows in-creased radiotracer uptake in involved areas.

Treatment with low-dose glucocorticoids relieves bone pain and may reverse the abnormal bone formation. Intermittent bisphosphonate therapy has produced clinical improvement in a limited number of patients.

HYPEROSTOSIS CORTICALIS GENERALISATA This is also known as Van Buchem disease; it is an autosomal recessive disorder characterized by endosteal hyperostosis in which osteosclerosis involves the skull, mandible, clavicles, and ribs. The major manifestations are due to narrowed cranial foramina with neural compressions that may result in optic atrophy, facial paralysis, and deafness. Adults may have an enlarged mandible. Serum ALP levels may be elevated, which reflects the uncoupled bone remodeling with high osteoblastic formation rates and low osteoclastic resorption. As a result, there is increased accu-mulation of normal bone. Endosteal hyperostosis with syndactyly, known as *sclerosteosis*, is a more severe form. The genetic defects for both sclerosteosis and van Buchem disease have been assigned to the same region of the chromosome 17q12-q21. It is possible that both conditions may have deactivating mutations in the *BEER* (bone-ex-pressed equilibrium regulator) gene.

MELORHEOSTOSIS Melorheostosis (Greek, "flowing hyperostosis") may occur sporadically or follow a pattern consistent with an autosomal recessive disorder. The major manifestation is progressive linear hy-perostosis in one or more bones of one limb, usually a lower extremity. The name comes from the radiographic appearance of the involved bone, which resembles melted wax that has dripped down a candle. Symptoms appear during childhood as pain or stiffness in the area of sclerotic bone. There may be associated ectopic soft tissue masses, composed of cartilage or osseous tissue, and skin changes overlying the involved bone, consisting of scleroderma-like areas and hypertri-chosis. The disease does not progress in adults, but pain and stiffness may persist. Laboratory tests are unremarkable. No specific etiology is known. There is no specific treatment. Surgical interventions to correct contractures are often unsuccessful.

OSTEOPOIKILOSIS The literal translation of osteopoikilosis is "spotted bones"; it is a benign autosomal dominant condition in which numer-ous small, variably shaped (usually round or oval) foci of bony scle-rosis are seen in the epiphyses and adjacent metaphyses. The lesions may involve any bone except the skull, ribs, and vertebrae. They may be misidentified as metastatic lesions. The main differentiating points are that bony lesions of osteopoikilosis are stable over time and do not accumulate radionucleotide on bone scanning. In some kindred, os-teopoikilosis is associated with connective tissue nevi known as *dermatofibrosis lenticularis disseminata*, also known as *Buschke-Ollendorf syndrome*. Histologic inspection reveals thickened but other-wise normal trabeculae and islands of normal cortical bone. No treatment is indicated.

DISORDERS ASSOCIATED WITH DEFECTIVE MINERALIZATION

HYPOPHOSPHATASIA This is a rare inherited disorder that presents as rickets in infants and children or osteomalacia in adults with paradox-ically low serum levels of ALP. The frequency of the severe neonatal and infantile forms is about 1 in 100,000 live births in Canada, where the disease is most common because of its high prevalence among Mennonites and Hutterites. It is rare in African Americans. The se-verity of the disease is remarkably variable, ranging from intrauterine death associated with profound skeletal hypomineralization at one ex-treme, to premature tooth loss as the only manifestation in some adults. Severe cases are inherited in an autosomal recessive manner, but the genetic patterns are less clear for the milder forms. The disease is caused by a deficiency of tissue nonspecific (bone/liver/kidney) ALP (*TNSALP*), which, although ubiquitous, results only in bone abnor-malities. Protein levels and functions of the other ALP isozymes (germ cell, intestinal, placental) are normal. Defective ALP permits accu-mulation of its major naturally occurring substrates including phos-phoethanolamine (PEA), inorganic pyrophosphate (PPi), and pyridoxal 5'-phosphate (PLP). The accumulation of PPi interferes with mineralization through its action as a potent inhibitor of hydroxyapa-tite crystal growth.

Perinatal hypophosphatasia becomes manifest during pregnancy and is often complicated by polyhydroamnios and intrauterine death. The infantile form becomes clinically apparent before age 6 months with failure to thrive, rachitic deformities, functional craniosynostosis despite widely open fontanels (which are actually hypomineralized areas of the calvarium), raised intracranial pressure, and flail chest and predisposition to pneumonia. Hypercalcemia and hypercalciuria are common. This form has a mortality rate of about 50%. Prognosis seems to improve for the children who survive infancy. Childhood hypophosphatasia has variable clinical presentation. Premature loss of deciduous teeth (before age 5 years) is the hallmark of the disease. Rickets causes delayed walking with waddling gait, short stature, and dolichocephalic skull with frontal bossing. The disease often improves during puberty but may recur in adult life. Adult hypophosphatasia presents during middle age with painful, poorly healing metatarsal stress fractures or thigh pain due to femoral pseudofractures.

Laboratory investigation reveals low ALP levels and normal or elevated levels of serum calcium and phosphorus despite clinical and radiologic evidence of rickets or osteomalacia. Serum parathyroid hor-mone, 25-hydroxyvitamin D, and 1,25-dihydroxyvitamin D levels are normal. The elevation of PLP is specific for the disease and may even be present in asymptomatic parents of severely affected children. As vitamin B$_6$ increases PLP levels, vitamin B$_6$ supplements should be discontinued 1 week before testing.

There is no established medical therapy. In contrast to other forms of rickets and osteomalacia, calcium and vitamin D supplementation should be avoided as they may aggravate hypercalcemia and hyper-calciuria. A low-calcium diet, glucocorticoids, and calcitonin have been used in a small number of patients with variable responses. Be-cause fracture healing is poor, placement of intramedullary rods is best for acute fracture repair and for prophylactic prevention of fractures.

AXIAL OSTEOMALACIA This is a rare disorder characterized by defective skeletal mineralization despite normal serum calcium and phosphate levels. Clinically, the disorder presents in middle-aged or elderly men with chronic axial skeletal discomfort. Cervical spine pain may also be present. Radiographic findings are mainly osteosclerosis due to coarsened trabecular patterns typical of osteomalacias. Spine, pelvis, and ribs are most commonly affected. Histologic changes show defec-tive mineralization and flat, inactive osteoblasts. The primary defect appears to be an acquired defect in osteoblast function. The course is benign and there is no established treatment. Calcium and vitamin D therapies are not effective.

FIBROGENESIS IMPERFECTA OSSIUM The is a rare condition of unknown etiology. It presents in both sexes, in middle age or later, with progressive, intractable skeletal pain and fractures, worsening immobilization, and a debilitating course. Radiographic evaluation reveals generalized osteomalacia, osteopenia, and occasional pseudofractures. Histologic features include a tangled pattern of collagen fibrils with abundant osteoblasts and osteoclasts. There is no effective treatment. Spontaneous remission has been reported in a small number of patients. Calcium and vitamin D have not been beneficial.

FIBROUS DYSPLASIA AND McCUNE ALBRIGHT SYNDROME

Fibrous dysplasia is a sporadic disorder characterized by the presence of one (monoostotic) or more (polyostotic) expanding fibrous skeletal lesions composed of bone-forming mesenchyme. The association of the polyostotic form with café-au-lait spots and hyperfunction of an endocrine system such as pseudo-precocious puberty of ovarian origin is known as *McCune-Albright syndrome* (MAS). A spectrum of the phenotypes is caused by activating mutations in the *GNAS1* gene, which encodes the α subunit of the stimulatory G protein ($G_s\alpha$). As the postzygotic mutations occur at different stages of early development, the extent and type of tissue affected are variable and explain the mosaic pattern of skin and bone changes. GTP binding activates the $G_s\alpha$ regulatory protein and mutations in regions of $G_s\alpha$ that selectively inhibit GTPase activity, which results in constitutive stimulation of the cyclic AMP–protein kinase A signal transduction pathway. Such mutations of the $G_s\alpha$ protein–coupled receptor may cause autonomous function in bone (parathyroid hormone receptor); skin (melanocyte-stimulating hormone receptor); and various endocrine glands including ovary (follicle-stimulating hormone receptor), thyroid (thyroid-stimulating hormone receptor), adrenal (adrenocorticotropic hormone receptor), and pituitary (growth hormone–releasing hormone receptor). The skeletal lesions are composed largely of mesenchymal cells that do not differentiate into osteoblasts, resulting in the formation of imperfect bone. In some areas of bone, fibroblast-like cells develop features of osteoblasts in that they produce extracellular matrix that organizes into woven bone. Calcification may occur in some areas. In other areas, cells have features of chondrocytes and produce cartilage-like extracellular matrix.

CLINICAL PRESENTATION Fibrous dysplasia occurs with equal frequency in both sexes, whereas MAS with precocious puberty is more common (10:1) in girls. The monoostotic form is the most common and is usually diagnosed in patients between 20 and 30 years of age without associated skin lesions. The polyostotic form typically manifests in children <10 years of age and may progress with age. Early-onset disease is generally more severe. Lesions may become quiescent in puberty and progress during pregnancy or with estrogen therapy. In polyostotic fibrous dysplasia, the lesions most commonly involve the maxilla and other craniofacial bones, ribs, and metaphyseal or diaphyseal portions of the proximal femur or tibia. Expanding bone lesions may cause pain, deformity, fractures, and nerve entrapment. Sarcomatous degeneration involving the facial bones or femur is infrequent (<1%). The risk of malignant transformation is increased by radiation, which has proven to be ineffective treatment. In rare patients with widespread lesions, renal phosphate wasting and hypophosphatemia may cause rickets or osteomalacia. Hypophosphatemia may be due to production of a phosphaturic factor by the abnormal fibrous tissue.

MAS patients may have café-au-lait spots, which are flat, hyperpigmented skin lesions that have rough borders ("coast of Maine") in contrast to the café-au-lait lesions of neurofibromatosis that have smooth borders ("coast of California"). The most common endocrinopathy is isosexual pseudo-precocious puberty in girls. Other less

common endocrine disorders include thyrotoxicosis, Cushing syndrome, acromegaly, hyperparathyroidism, hyperprolactinemia, and pseudo-precocious puberty in boys.

RADIOGRAPHIC FINDINGS In long bones, the fibrous dysplastic lesions are typically well-defined, radiolucent areas with thin cortices and a ground-glass appearance. Lesions may be lobulated with trabeculated areas of radiolucency (Fig. 334-4). Involvement of facial bones usually presents as radiodense lesions, which may create a leonine appearance (leontiasis osea). Expansile cranial lesions may narrow foramina and cause optic lesions, reduce hearing, and create other manifestations of cranial nerve compression.

LABORATORY RESULTS Serum ALP is occasionally elevated but calcium, parathyroid hormone, 25-hydroxyvitamin D, and 1,25-dihydroxyvitamin D levels are normal. Patients with extensive polyostotic lesions may have hypophosphatemia, hyperphosphaturia, and osteomalacia. Biochemical markers of bone turnover may be elevated.

℞ TREATMENT

Spontaneous healing of the lesions does not occur, and there is no established effective treatment. Improvement in bone pain and partial or complete resolution of radiographic lesions have been reported after intravenous bisphosphonate therapy. Surgical stabilization is used to prevent pathologic fracture or destruction of a major joint space, and to relieve nerve root or cranial nerve compression or sinus obstruction.

OTHER DYSPLASIAS OF BONE AND CARTILAGE

PACHYDERMOPERIOSTOSIS Pachydermoperiostosis, or hypertrophic osteoarthropathy (primary or idiopathic), is an autosomal dominant disorder characterized by periosteal new bone formation that involves the distal extremities. The lesions present as clubbing of the digits and hyperhydrosis and thickening of the skin, primarily of the face and forehead. The changes usually appear during adolescence, progress over the next decade, and then become quiescent. During the active phase, progressive enlargement of the hands and feet produces a paw-like appearance, which may be mistaken for acromegaly. Arthralgias, pseudogout, and limited mobility may also occur. The disorder must be differentiated from secondary hypertrophic osteopathy that develops during the course of serious pulmonary disorders. The two con-

FIGURE 334-4 Radiograph of a 16-year-old male with fibrous dysplasia of the right proximal femur. Note the multiple cystic lesions, including the large lucent lesion in the proximal mid-shaft with scalloping of the interior surface. The femoral neck contains two lucent cystic lesions.

ditions can be differentiated by standard radiography of the digits in which secondary pachydermoperiostosis has exuberant periosteal new bone formation and a smooth and undulating surface. In contrast, primary hypertrophic osteopathy has an irregular periosteal surface.

There are no diagnostic blood or urine tests. Synovial fluid does not have an inflammatory profile. There is no specific therapy, although a limited experience with colchicine suggests some benefit in controlling the arthralgias.

OSTEOCHONDRODYSPLASIAS These include several hundred heritable disorders of connective tissue. These primary abnormalities of cartilage manifest as disturbances in cartilage and bone growth. Selected growth plate chondrodysplasias are described here. →*For discussion of chondrodysplasias, see Chap. 342.*

Achondrodysplasia This is a relatively common form of short-limb dwarfism that occurs in 1 in 15,000 to 1 in 40,000 live births. The disease is caused by a mutation of the fibroblast growth factor receptor 3 (*FGFR3*) gene that results in a gain-of-function state. Most cases are sporadic mutations. However, when the disorder appears in families, the inheritance pattern is consistent with an autosomal dominant disorder. The primary defect is abnormal chondrocyte proliferation at the growth plate that causes development of short but proportionately thick long bones. Other regions of the long bones may be relatively unaffected. The disorder is manifest by the presence of short limbs (particularly the proximal portions), normal trunk, large head, saddle nose, and an exaggerated lumbar lordosis. Severe spinal deformity may lead to cord compression. The homozygous disorder is more serious than the sporadic form and may cause neonatal death. Pseudoachondroplasia clinically resembles achondroplasia but has no skull abnormalities.

Enchondromatosis This is also called dyschondroplasia, or Ollier disease; it is also a disorder of the growth plate in which the primary cartilage is not resorbed. Cartilage ossification proceeds normally but it is not resorbed normally, leading to cartilage accumulation. The changes are most marked at the ends of long bones where the highest growth rates occur. Chondrosarcoma develops infrequently. The association of enchondromatosis and cavernous hemangiomas of the skin and soft tissues is known as *Maffucci syndrome*. Both Ollier disease and Maffucci syndrome are associated with various malignancies, including granulosa cell tumor of the ovary and cerebral glioma.

Multiple Exostoses This is also called diaphyseal aclasis, or osteochondromatosis; it is a genetic disorder that follows an autosomal dominant pattern of inheritance. In this condition, areas of growth plates become displaced, presumably by growing through a defect in the perichondrium. The lesion begins with vascular invasion of the growth plate cartilage, resulting in a characteristic radiographic finding of a mass that is in direct communication with the marrow cavity of the parent bone. The underlying cortex is resorbed. The disease is caused by inactivating mutations of the *EXT1* and *EXT2* genes, whose products normally regulate processing of chondrocyte cytoskeletal proteins. The products of the *EXT* gene likely function as tumor suppressors, with the loss-of-function mutation resulting in abnormal proliferation of growth plate cartilage. Solitary or multiple lesions are located in the metaphyses of long bones. Although usually asymptomatic, the lesions may interfere with joint or tendon function or compress peripheral nerves. The lesions stop growing when growth ceases but may recur during pregnancy. There is a small risk for malignant transformation into chondrosarcoma.

EXTRASKELETAL (ECTOPIC) CALCIFICATION AND OSSIFICATION

Deposition of calcium phosphate crystals (*calcification*) or formation of true bone (*ossification*) in nonosseous soft tissue may occur by one of three mechanisms: (1) metastatic calcification due to a supranormal calcium x phosphate concentration product in extracellular fluid; (2) dystrophic calcification due to mineral deposition into metabolically impaired or dead tissue despite normal serum levels of calcium and phosphate; and (3) ectopic ossification, or true bone formation. Dis-

orders that may cause extraskeletal calcification or ossification are listed in Table 334-2.

METASTATIC CALCIFICATION Soft tissue calcification may complicate diseases associated with significant hypercalcemia, hyperphosphatemia, or both. In addition, vitamin D and phosphate treatments or calcium administration in the presence of mild hyperphosphatemia, such as during hemodialysis, may induce ectopic calcification. Calcium phosphate precipitation may complicate any disorder when the serum calcium × phosphate concentration product >75. The initial calcium phosphate deposition is in the form of small, poorly organized crystals, which subsequently organize into hydroxyapatite crystals. Calcifications that occur in hypercalcemic states with normal or low phosphate have a predilection for kidney, lungs, and gastric mucosa. Hyperphosphatemia with normal or low serum calcium may promote soft tissue calcification with predilection for the kidney and arteries. The disturbances of calcium and phosphate in renal failure and hemodialysis are common causes of soft tissue (metastatic) calcification.

TUMORAL CALCINOSIS This is a rare genetic disorder characterized by masses of metastatic calcifications in soft tissues around major joints, most often shoulders, hips, and ankles. Tumoral calcinosis differs from other disorders in that the periarticular masses contain hydroxyapatite crystals or amorphous calcium phosphate complexes, while in fibrodysplasia ossificans progressiva (below), true bone is formed in soft tissues. About one-third of tumoral calcinosis cases are familial, with both autosomal recessive and autosomal dominant modes of inheritance reported. The disease is also associated with a variably expressed abnormality of dentition marked by short bulbous roots, pulp calcification, and radicular dentin deposited in swirls. The primary defect responsible for the metastatic calcification appears to be hyperphosphatemia resulting from the increased capacity of the renal tubule to reabsorb filtered phosphate. Spontaneous soft tissue calcification is related to the elevated serum phosphate, which along with normal serum calcium exceeds the concentration product of 75.

All of the North American patients reported have been African-American. The disease usually presents in childhood and continues lifelong. The calcific masses are typically painless and grow at variable rates, sometimes becoming large and bulky. The masses are often located near major joints but remain extracapsular. Joint range of motion is not usually restricted unless the tumors are very large. Complications include compression of neural structures and ulceration of the overlying skin with drainage of chalky fluid and risk of secondary infection. Small deposits not detected by standard radiographs may be detected by ^{99m}Tc bone scanning. The most common laboratory findings are hyperphosphatemia and elevated serum 1,25-dihydroxyvitamin D levels. Serum calcium, parathyroid hormone, and ALP levels are usually normal. Renal function is also usually normal. Urine cal-

TABLE 334-2 *Diseases and Conditions Associated with Ectopic Calcification and Ossification*

Metastatic calcification	Dystrophic calcification
Hypercalcemic states	Inflammatory disorders
Primary hyperparathyroidism	Scleroderma
Sarcoidosis	Dermatomyositis
Vitamin D intoxication	Systemic lupus
Milk-alkali syndrome	erythematosus
Renal failure	Trauma-induced
Hyperphosphatemia	Ectopic ossification
Tumoral calcinosis	Myositis ossificans
Secondary hyperparathyroidism	Post surgery
Pseudohypoparathyroidism	Burns
Renal failure	Neurologic injury
Hemodialysis	Other trauma
Cell lysis following chemotherapy	Fibrodysplasia ossificans
Therapy with vitamin D and	progressiva
phosphate	

cium and phosphate excretions are low, and calcium and phosphate balances are positive.

An acquired form of the disease may occur with other causes of hyperphosphatemia, such as secondary hyperparathyroidism associated with hemodialysis, hypoparathyroidism, pseudohypoparathyroidism, and massive cell lysis following chemotherapy for leukemia. Tissue trauma from joint movement may contribute to the periarticular calcifications. Metastatic calcifications are also seen in conditions associated with hypercalcemia, such as in sarcoidosis, vitamin D intoxication, milk-alkali syndrome, and primary hyperparathyroidism. In these conditions, however, mineral deposits are more likely to occur in proton-transporting organs such as kidney, lungs, and gastric mucosa in which an alkaline milieu is generated by the proton pumps.

℞ TREATMENT

Therapeutic successes have been achieved with surgical removal of subcutaneous calcified masses, which tend not to recur if all calcification is removed from the site. Reduction of serum phosphate by chronic phosphorus restriction may be accomplished using low dietary phosphorus intake alone or in combination with oral phosphate binders. The addition of the phosphaturic agent acetazolamide may be useful. Limited experience using the phosphaturic action of calcitonin deserves further testing.

DYSTROPHIC CALCIFICATION Posttraumatic calcification may occur with normal serum calcium and phosphate levels and normal ion solubility product. The deposited mineral is either in the form of amorphous calcium phosphate or hydroxyapatite crystals. Soft tissue calcification complicating connective tissue disorders such as scleroderma, dermatomyositis, and systemic lupus erythematosus may involve localized areas of the skin or deeper subcutaneous tissue and is referred to as *calcinosis circumscripta*. Mineral deposition at sites of deeper tissue injury including periarticular sites is called *calcinosis universalis*.

ECTOPIC OSSIFICATION True extraskeletal bone formation that begins in areas of fasciitis following surgery, trauma, burns, or neurologic injury is referred to as *myositis ossificans*. The bone formed is organized as lamellar or trabecular, with normal osteoblasts and osteoclasts conducting active remodeling. Well-developed haversian systems and marrow elements may be present. A second cause of ectopic bone formation occurs in an inherited disorder, *fibrodysplasia ossificans progressiva*.

FIBRODYSPLASIA OSSIFICANS PROGRESSIVA This is also called *myositis ossificans progressiva*; it is a rare autosomal dominant disorder characterized by congenital deformities of the hands and feet and episodic soft tissue swellings that ossify. Ectopic bone formation occurs in fascia, tendons, ligaments, and connective tissue within voluntary muscles. Tender, rubbery induration, sometimes precipitated by trauma, develops in the soft tissue and gradually calcifies. Eventually, heterotopic bone forms at these sites of soft tissue trauma. Morbidity results from heterotopic bone interfering with normal movement and function of muscle and other soft tissues. Mortality is usually related to restrictive lung disease caused by an inability of the chest to expand. Laboratory tests are unremarkable.

There is no effective medical therapy. Bisphosphonates, glucocorticoids, and a low-calcium diet have largely been ineffective in halting progression of the ossification. Surgical removal of ectopic bone is not recommended, as the trauma of surgery may precipitate formation of new areas of heterotopic bone. Dental complications including frozen jaw may occur following injection of local anesthetics. Thus, CT imaging of the mandible should be undertaken to detect early sites of soft tissue ossification before they are appreciated by standard radiography.

ACKNOWLEDGMENT
The authors wish to acknowledge the contributions of Dr. Stephen M. Krane to this chapter in previous editions of Harrison's.

FURTHER READING

HOCKING LJ et al: Domain-specific mutations in sequestosome 1 (SQSTM1) cause familial and sporadic Paget disease. Hum Mol Genet 11:2735, 2002

HOFBAUER LC, HEUFELDER AE: Role of receptor activator of nuclear factor-kappa B ligand and osteoprotegerin in bone cell biology. J Mol Med 79: 243, 2001

SOBACCHI C et al: The mutational spectrum of human malignant autosomal recessive osteopetrosis. Hum Mol Genet 10:1767, 2001

WEINSTEIN LS et al: Endocrine manifestations of stimulatory G protein alpha-subunit mutations and the role of genomic imprinting. Endocrine Rev 22: 675, 2001

WHYTE MP et al: Osteoprotegrin deficiency and juvenile Paget disease. N Engl J Med 347:175, 2002

Section 3   Disorders of Intermediary Metabolism

335   DISORDERS OF LIPOPROTEIN METABOLISM
Daniel J. Rader, Helen H. Hobbs

Lipoproteins are complexes of lipids and proteins that are essential for the transport of cholesterol, triglycerides, and fat-soluble vitamins. Until recently, lipoprotein disorders were the purview of lipidologists, but the demonstration that lipid-lowering therapy significantly reduces the clinical complications of atherosclerotic cardiovascular disease (ASCVD) has brought the diagnosis and treatment of these disorders into the domain of the general internist. The metabolic consequences associated with changes in diet and lifestyle have increased the number of hyperlipidemic individuals who could benefit from lipid-lowering therapy. The development of safe, effective, and well-tolerated pharmacologic agents has greatly expanded the therapeutic armamentarium available to the physician to treat disorders of lipid metabolism. Therefore, the appropriate diagnosis and management of lipid disorders is critically important to the practice of medicine. This chapter reviews normal lipoprotein physiology, the pathophysiology of the known single-gene disorders of lipoprotein metabolism, the environmental factors that influence lipoprotein metabolism, and the practical approaches to their diagnosis and management.

LIPOPROTEIN METABOLISM

LIPOPROTEIN CLASSIFICATION AND COMPOSITION Lipoproteins are large, mostly spherical complexes that transport lipids (primarily triglycerides, cholesteryl esters, and fat-soluble vitamins) through body fluids (plasma, interstitial fluid, and lymph) to and from tissues. Lipoproteins play an essential role in the absorption of dietary cholesterol, long-chain fatty acids, and fat-soluble vitamins; the transport of triglycerides, cholesterol, and fat-soluble vitamins from the liver to peripheral tissues; and the transport of cholesterol from peripheral tissues to the liver.

Lipoproteins contain a core of hydrophobic lipids (triglycerides and cholesteryl esters) surrounded by hydrophilic lipids (phospholipids, unesterified cholesterol) and proteins that interact with body fluids.

The plasma lipoproteins are divided into five major classes based on their relative densities (Fig. 335-1 and Table 335-1): chylomicrons, very low density lipoproteins (VLDL), intermediate-density lipoproteins (IDL), low-density lipoproteins (LDL), and high-density lipoproteins (HDL). Each lipoprotein class comprises a family of particles that vary slightly in density, size, migration during electrophoresis, and protein composition. The density of a lipoprotein is determined by the amount of lipid and protein per particle. HDL is the smallest and most dense lipoprotein, whereas chylomicrons and VLDL are the largest and least dense lipoprotein particles. Most triglyceride is transported in chylomicrons or VLDL, and most cholesterol is carried as cholesteryl esters in LDL and HDL.

The apolipoproteins are required for the assembly and structure of lipoproteins (Table 335-2). Apolipoproteins also serve to activate enzymes important in lipoprotein metabolism and to mediate the binding of lipoproteins to cell-surface receptors. ApoA-I, which is synthesized in the liver and intestine, is found on virtually all HDL particles. ApoA-II is the second most abundant HDL apolipoprotein and is found on approximately two-thirds of all HDL particles. ApoB is the major structural protein of chylomicrons, VLDL, IDL, and LDL; one molecule of apoB, either apoB-48 (chylomicrons) or apoB-100 (VLDL, IDL, or LDL), is present on each lipoprotein particle. The human liver makes only apoB-100, and the intestine makes apoB-48, which is derived from the same gene by mRNA editing. ApoE is present in multiple copies on chylomicrons, VLDL, and IDL and plays a critical role in the metabolism and clearance of triglyceride-rich particles. Three apolipoproteins of the C-series (apoC-I, -II, and -III) also participate in the metabolism of triglyceride-rich lipoproteins. The other apolipoproteins are listed in Table 335-2.

TRANSPORT OF DIETARY LIPIDS (EXOGENOUS PATHWAY) The exogenous pathway of lipoprotein metabolism permits efficient transport of dietary lipids (Fig. 335-2). Dietary triglycerides are hydrolyzed by pancreatic lipases within the intestinal lumen and are emulsified with bile acids to form micelles. Dietary cholesterol and retinol are esterified (by the addition of a fatty acid) in the enterocyte to form cholesteryl esters and retinyl esters, respectively. Longer-chain fatty acids (>12 carbons) are incorporated into triglycerides and packaged with apoB-48, cholesteryl esters, retinyl esters, phospholipids, and cholesterol to form chylomicrons. Nascent chylomicrons are secreted into the intestinal lymph and delivered directly to the systemic circulation, where they are extensively processed by peripheral tissues before reaching the liver. The particles encounter lipoprotein lipase (LPL), which is anchored to proteoglycans that decorate the capillary endothelial surfaces of adipose tissue, heart, and skeletal muscle (Fig. 335-2). The triglycerides of chylomicrons are hydrolyzed by LPL, and free fatty acids are released; apoC-II, which is transferred to circulating chylomicrons, acts as a cofactor for LPL in this reaction. The released free fatty acids are taken up by adjacent myocytes or adipocytes and either oxidized or reesterified and stored as triglyceride. Some free fatty acids bind albumin and are transported to other tissues, especially the liver. The chylomicron particle progressively shrinks in size as the hydrophobic core is hydrolyzed and the hydrophilic lipids (cholesterol and phospholipids) on the particle surface are transferred to HDL. The resultant smaller, more cholesterol ester–rich particles are referred to as *chylomicron remnants*. The remnant particles are rapidly removed from the circulation by the liver in a process that requires apoE. Consequently, few, if any, chylomicrons are present in the blood after a 12-h fast, except in individuals with disorders of chylomicron metabolism.

TRANSPORT OF HEPATIC LIPIDS (ENDOGENOUS PATHWAY) The *endogenous pathway of lipoprotein metabolism* refers to the hepatic secretion and metabolism of VLDL to IDL and LDL (Fig. 335-2). VLDL particles resemble chylomicrons in protein composition but contain apoB-100 rather than apoB-48 and have a higher ratio of cholesterol to triglyceride (~1 mg of cholesterol for every 5 mg of triglyceride). The triglycerides of VLDL are derived predominantly from the esterification of long-chain fatty acids. The packaging of hepatic triglycerides with the other major components of the nascent VLDL particle (apoB-100, cholesteryl esters, phospholipids, and vitamin E) requires the action of the enzyme microsomal transfer protein (MTP). After secretion into the plasma, VLDL acquires multiple copies of apoE and apolipoproteins of the C series. The triglycerides of VLDL are hydrolyzed by LPL, especially in muscle and adipose tissue. As VLDL remnants undergo further hydrolysis, they continue to shrink in size and become *IDL*, which contain similar amounts of cholesterol and triglyceride. The liver removes approximately 40 to 60% of VLDL remnants and IDL by LDL receptor–mediated endocytosis via binding to apoE. The remainder of IDL is remodeled by hepatic lipase (HL) to form LDL; during this process, most of the triglyceride in the particle is hydrolyzed and all apolipoproteins except apoB-100 are transferred to other lipoproteins. The cholesterol in LDL accounts for ~70% of the plasma cholesterol in most individuals. Approximately 70% of circulating LDLs are cleared by LDL receptor–mediated endocytosis in the liver.

Lipoprotein	Density, g/mL[b]	Size nm[c]	Electrophoretic Mobility[d]	Apolipoproteins Major	Apolipoproteins Other	Other Constituents
Chylomicrons	0.930	75–1200	Origin	ApoB-48	A-I, A-IV, C-I, C-II, C-III	Retinyl esters
Chylomicron remnants	0.930–1.006	30–80	Slow pre-β	ApoB-48	E, A-I, A-IV, C-I, C-II, C-III	Retinyl esters
VLDL	0.930–1.006	30–80	Pre-β	ApoB-100	E, A-I, A-II, A-V, C-I, C-II, C-III	Vitamin E
IDL	1.006–1.019	25–35	Slow pre-β	ApoB-100	E, C-I, C-II, C-III	Vitamin E
LDL	1.019–1.063	18–25	β	ApoB-100		Vitamin E
HDL	1.063–1.210	5–12	Alpha	ApoA-I	A-II, A-IV, E, C-III	LCAT, CETP paroxonase
Lp(a)	1.050–1.120	25	Pre-β	ApoB-100	Apo(a)	

TABLE 335-1 *Major Lipoprotein Classes[a]*

[a] All of the lipoprotein classes contain phospholipids, esterified and unesterified cholesterol, and triglycerides to varying degrees.
[b] The density of the particle is determined by ultracentrifugation.
[c] The size of the particle is measured using gel electrophoresis.
[d] The electrophoretic mobility of the particle on agarose gel electrophoresis reflects the size and surface charge of the particle, with β being the position of LDL and α the position of HDL.
Note: VLDL, very low density lipoprotein; IDL, intermediate-density lipoprotein; LDL, low-density lipoprotein; HDL, high-density lipoprotein; Lp(a), lipoprotein A; LCAT, lecithin-cholesterol acyltransferase; CETP, cholesteryl ester transfer protein.

FIGURE 335-1 The density and size-distribution of the major classes of lipoprotein particles. Lipoproteins are classified by density and size, which are inversely related. VLDL, very low density lipoproteins; IDL, intermediate-density lipoproteins; LDL, low-density lipoproteins; HDL, high-density lipoproteins.

TABLE 335-2 *Major Apolipoproteins*

Apolipoprotein	Primary Source	Lipoprotein Association	Function
ApoA-I	Intestine, liver	HDL, chylomicrons	Structural protein for HDL; activates LCAT
ApoA-II	Liver	HDL, chylomicrons	Structural protein for HDL
ApoA-IV	Intestine	HDL, chylomicrons	Unknown
ApoA-V	Liver	VLDL	Unknown
ApoB-48	Intestine	Chylomicrons	Structural protein for chylomicrons
ApoB-100	Liver	VLDL, IDL, LDL, Lp(a)	Structural protein for VLDL, LDL, IDL, Lp(a); ligand for binding to LDL receptor
ApoC-I	Liver	Chylomicrons, VLDL, HDL	Unknown
ApoC-II	Liver	Chylomicrons, VLDL, HDL	Cofactor for LPL
ApoC-III	Liver	Chylomicrons, VLDL, HDL	Inhibits lipoprotein binding to receptors
ApoD	Spleen, brain, testes, adrenals	HDL	Unknown
ApoE	Liver	Chylomicron remnants, IDL, HDL	Ligand for binding to LDL receptor
ApoH	Liver	Chylomicrons, VLDL, LDL, HDL	B$_2$ glycoprotein I
ApoJ	Liver	HDL	Unknown
ApoL	Unknown	HDL	Unknown
Apo(a)	Liver	Lp(a)	Unknown

Note: HDL, high-density lipoprotein; LCAT, lecithin-cholesterol acyltransferase; VLDL, very low density lipoprotein; IDL, intermediate-density lipoprotein; LDL, low-density lipoprotein; Lp(a), lipoprotein A; LPL, lipoprotein lipase.

Lipoprotein(a) [Lp(a)] is a lipoprotein similar to LDL in lipid and protein composition, but it contains an additional protein called apolipoprotein(a) [apo(a)]. Apo(a) is synthesized in the liver and is attached to apoB-100 by a disulfide linkage. The mechanism by which Lp(a) is removed from the circulation is not known.

HDL METABOLISM AND REVERSE CHOLESTEROL TRANSPORT   All nucleated cells synthesize cholesterol but only hepatocytes can efficiently metabolize and excrete cholesterol from the body. The predominant route of cholesterol elimination is by excretion into the bile, either directly or after conversion to bile acids. Cholesterol in peripheral cells is transported from the plasma membranes of peripheral cells to the liver by an HDL-mediated process termed *reverse cholesterol transport* (Fig. 335-3).

Nascent HDL particles are synthesized by the intestine and the liver. The newly formed discoidal HDL particles contain apoA-I and phospholipids (mainly lecithin) but rapidly acquire unesterified cholesterol and additional phospholipids from peripheral tissues via transport by the membrane protein ATP-binding cassette protein A1 (ABCA1). Once incorporated in the HDL particle, cholesterol is esterified by lecithin-cholesterol acyltransferase (LCAT), a plasma enzyme associated with HDL. As HDL acquires more cholesteryl ester it becomes spherical, and additional apolipoproteins and lipids are transferred to the particles from the surfaces of chylomicrons and VLDL during lipolysis.

HDL cholesterol is transported to hepatoctyes by both an indirect and a direct pathway. HDL cholesteryl esters are transferred to apoB-containing lipoproteins in exchange for triglyceride by the cholesteryl ester transfer protein (CETP). The cholesteryl esters are then removed from the circulation by LDL receptor–mediated endocytosis. HDL cholesterol can also be taken up directly by hepatocytes via the scavenger receptor class BI (SR-BI), a cell-surface receptor that mediates the selective transfer of lipids to cells.

HDL particles undergo extensive remodeling within the plasma compartment as they transfer lipids and proteins to lipoproteins and cells. For example, after CETP-mediated lipid exchange, the triglyceride-enriched HDL becomes a substrate for HL, which hydrolyzes the triglycerides and phospholipids to generate smaller HDL particles.

DISORDERS OF LIPOPROTEIN METABOLISM

The identification and characterization of genes responsible for the genetic forms of hyperlipidemia have provided important molecular insight into the critical roles of apolipoproteins, enzymes, and receptors in lipid metabolism.

PRIMARY DISORDERS OF ApoB-CONTAINING LIPOPROTEIN BIOSYNTHESIS CAUSING LOW PLASMA CHOLESTEROL LEVELS (KNOWN ETIOLOGY)   The synthesis and secretion of apoB-containing lipoproteins in the enterocytes of the proximal small bowel and in the hepatocytes of the liver involve a complex series of events that coordinate the coupling of various lipids with apoB-48 and apoB-100, respectively.

Abetalipoproteinemia   Abetalipoproteinemia is a rare autosomal recessive disease caused by mutations in the gene encoding MTP, which transfers lipids to nascent chylomicrons and VLDL in the intestine and liver, respectively. Plasma cholesterol and triglyceride levels are extremely low in this disorder, and no chylomicrons, VLDL, LDL, or apoB are detectable. The parents of patients with abetalipoproteinemia (who are obligate heterozygotes) have normal plasma lipid and apoB levels. Abetalipoproteinemia usually presents in early childhood with diarrhea and failure to thrive and is characterized clinically by fat malabsorption, spinocerebellar degeneration, pigmented retinopathy, and acanthocytosis. The initial neurologic manifestations are loss of deep-tendon reflexes, followed by decreased distal lower extremity vibratory and proprioceptive sense, dysmetria, ataxia, and the development of a spastic gait, often by the third or fourth decade. Patients with abetalipoproteinemia also develop a progressive pigmented retinopathy presenting with decreased night and color vision, followed by reductions in daytime visual acuity and ultimately progressing to near blindness. The presence of spinocerebellar degeneration and pigmented retinopathy in this disease has resulted in misdiagnosis of Friedreich's ataxia. Rarely, patients with abetalipoproteinemia develop a cardiomyopathy with associated life-threatening arrhythmias.

Most clinical manifestations of abetalipoproteinemia result from defects in the absorption and transport of fat-soluble vitamins. Vitamin E and retinyl esters are normally transported from enterocytes to the liver by chylomicrons, and vitamin E is dependent on VLDL for transport out of the liver and into the circulation. Patients with abetalipoproteinemia are markedly deficient in vitamin E and are also mildly to moderately deficient in vitamin A and vitamin K. Treatment of abetalipoproteinemia consists of a low-fat, high-caloric, vitamin-enriched diet accompanied by large supplemental doses of vitamin E. It is imperative for treatment to be initiated as soon as possible to obviate the development of neurologic sequelae.

Familial Hypobetalipoproteinemia   Familial homozygous hypobetalipoproteinemia has a clinical picture similar to abetalipoproteinemia but is autosomal codominant in inheritance pattern. The disease can be differentiated from abetalipoproteinemia since the parents of the probands with this disorder have levels of plasma LDL-C and apoB that are less than half of the normal levels. Mutations in the gene encoding apoB-100 that interfere with protein synthesis are common causes of this disorder. These patients, like those with abetalipoproteinemia, should be referred to specialized centers for confirmation of the diagnosis and appropriate therapy.

PRIMARY DISORDERS OF ApoB-CONTAINING LIPOPROTEIN CATABOLISM CAUSING ELEVATED PLASMA CHOLESTEROL LEVELS (KNOWN ETIOLOGY)   Single-gene defects can result in the accumulation of specific classes of lipoprotein particles. Mutations in genes encoding key proteins in the metabolism and clearance of apoB-containing lipoproteins cause type I (chylomicronemia), type II (elevations in LDL) and type III (elevations in IDL) hyperlipoproteinemias (Table 335-3).

Lipoprotein Lipase and ApoC-II Deficiency (Familial Chylomicronemia Syndrome; Type I Hyperlipoproteinemia) LPL is required for the hydrolysis of triglycerides in chylomicrons and VLDL. ApoC-II is a cofactor for LPL (Fig. 335-2). Genetic deficiency of either LPL or apoC-II results in impaired lipolysis and profound elevations in plasma chylomicrons. These patients also have elevations in plasma VLDL, but chylomicronemia predominates. Normally chylomicrons are delipidated and removed from the circulation within 12 h of the last meal, but in LPL-deficient patients, the triglyceride-rich chylomicrons persist in the circulation for days. The fasting plasma is turbid, and if left at 4°C for a few hours, the chylomicrons float to the top and form a creamy supernatant. In these disorders, called *familial chylomicronemia syndromes*, fasting triglyceride levels are almost invariably >11.3 μmol/L (1000 mg/dL). Fasting cholesterol levels are also usually elevated, but to a much less severe degree.

LPL deficiency is autosomal recessive and has a population frequency of approximately one in a million. ApoC-II deficiency is also recessive in inheritance pattern and is even less common than LPL deficiency. Multiple mutations in the LPL and apoC-II genes cause these diseases. Obligate LPL heterozygotes have normal or mild to moderate elevations in plasma triglyceride levels, whereas individuals heterozygous for mutation in apoC-II are not hypertriglyceridemic.

Both LPL and apoC-II deficiency usually present in childhood with recurrent episodes of severe abdominal pain caused by acute pancreatitis. On fundoscopic examination the retinal blood vessels are opalescent (*lipemia retinalis*). Eruptive xanthomas, which are small yellowish-white papules, often appear in clusters on the back, buttocks, and extensor surfaces of the arms and legs. These typically painless skin lesions may become pruritic as they regress. Hepatosplenomegaly results from the uptake of circulating chylomicrons by reticuloendothelial cells in the liver and spleen. For reasons unknown, some patients with persistent and pronounced chylomicronemia never develop pancreatitis, eruptive xanthomas, or hepatosplenomegaly. Premature ASCVD has not been consistently demonstrated to be a feature of familial chylomicronemia syndromes.

The diagnoses of LPL and apoC-II deficiency are established enzymatically by assaying triglyceride lipolytic activity in post-heparin plasma. Blood is sampled after an intravenous heparin injection to release the endothelial-bound lipases. LPL activity is profoundly reduced in both LPL and apoC-II deficiency; in patients with apoC-II deficiency, the addition of normal pre-heparin plasma (a source of apoC-II) normalizes LPL activity, but this correction does not occur in patients with LPL deficiency.

The major therapeutic intervention in familial chylomicronemia syndromes is dietary fat restriction (to as little as 15 g/d) with fat-

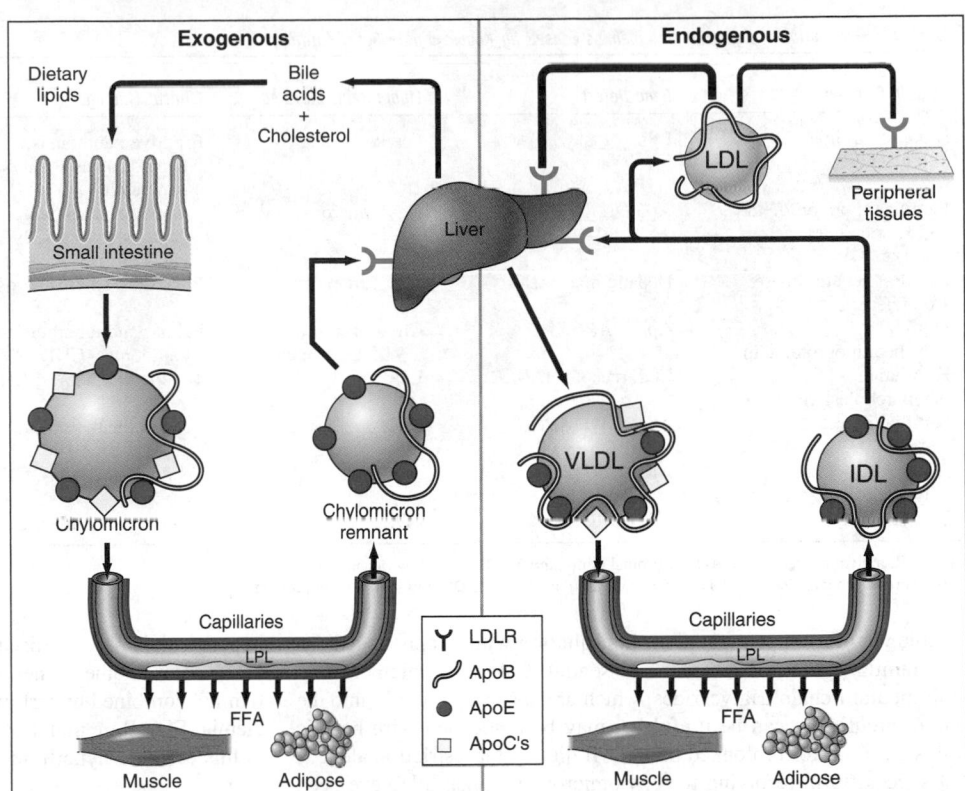

FIGURE 335-2 The exogenous and endogenous lipoprotein metabolic pathways. The exogenous pathway transports dietary lipids to the periphery and the liver. The exogenous pathway transports hepatic lipids to the periphery. LPL, lipoprotein lipase; FFA, free fatty acids; VLDL, very low density lipoproteins; IDL, intermediate-density lipoproteins; LDL, low-density lipoproteins; LDLR, low-density lipoprotein receptor.

FIGURE 335-3 HDL metabolism and reverse cholesterol transport. This pathway transports excess cholesterol from the periphery back to the liver for excretion in the bile. The liver and the intestine produce nascent HDL. Free cholesterol is acquired from macrophages and other peripheral cells and esterfied by LCAT, forming mature HDL. HDL cholesterol can be selectively taken up by the liver via SR-BI. Alternatively, HDL cholesteryl ester can be transferred by CETP from HDL to VLDL and chylomicrons, which can then be taken up by the liver. LCAT, lecithin-cholesterol acyltransferase; CETP, cholesteryl ester transfer protein; VLDL, very low density lipoproteins; IDL, intermediate-density lipoproteins; LDL, low-density lipoproteins; HDL, high-density lipoproteins; LDLR, low-density lipoprotein receptor; TG, triglycerides.

Genetic Disorder	Gene Defect	Lipoproteins Elevated	Clinical Findings	Genetic Transmission	Estimated Incidence
Lipoprotein lipase deficiency	LPL (*LPL*)	Chylomicrons	Eruptive xanthomas, hepatosplenomegaly pancreatitis	AR	1/1,000,000
Familial apolipoprotein C-II deficiency	ApoC-II (*APOC2*)	Chylomicrons	Eruptive xanthomas, hepatosplenomegaly pancreatitis	AR	<1/1,000,000
Familial hepatic lipase deficiency	Hepatic lipase (*LIPC*)	VLDL remnants	Premature atherosclerosis	AR	<1/1,000,000
Familial dysbetalipoproteinemia	ApoE (*APOE*)	Chylomicron and VLDL remnants	Palmar and tuberoeruptive xanthomas, CHD, PVD	AR AD	1/10,000
Familial hypercholesterolemia	LDL receptor (*LDLR*)	LDL	Tendon xanthomas, CHD	AD	1/500
Familial defective apoB-100	ApoB-100 (*APOB*) ($Arg_{3500} \rightarrow Gln$)	LDL	Tendon xanthomas, CHD	AD	1/1000
Autosomal recessive hypercholesterolemia	ARH (*ARH*)	LDL	Tendon xanthomas, CHD	AR	<1/1,000,000
Sitosterolemia	*ABCG5* or *ABCG8*	LDL	Tendon xanthomas, CHD	AR	<1/1,000,000

Note: AR, autosomal recessive; AD, autosomal dominant; VLDL, very low density lipoprotein; CHD, coronary heart disease; PVD, peripheral vascular disease; LDL, low-density lipoprotein.

soluble vitamin supplementation. Consultation with a registered dietician familiar with this disorder is essential. Caloric supplementation with medium-chain triglycerides, which are absorbed directly into the portal circulation, can be useful but may be associated with hepatic fibrosis if used for prolonged periods. If dietary fat restriction alone is not successful in resolving the chylomicronemia, fish oils have been effective in some patients. In patients with apoC-II deficiency, apoC-II can be provided by infusing fresh-frozen plasma to resolve the chylomicronemia. Management of patients with familial chylomicronemia syndrome is particularly challenging during pregnancy when VLDL production is increased. Plasmapheresis may be required if pancreatitis develops and the chylomicronemia is not responsive to diet therapy.

Hepatic Lipase Deficiency HL is a member of the same gene family as LPL and hydrolyzes triglycerides and phospholipids in remnant lipoproteins and HDL. HL deficiency is a very rare autosomal recessive disorder characterized by elevated plasma cholesterol and triglycerides (mixed hyperlipidemia) due to the accumulation of lipoprotein remnants. HDL-C is normal or elevated. The diagnosis is confirmed by measuring HL activity in post-heparin plasma. Due to the small number of patients with HL deficiency, the association of this genetic defect with ASCVD is not known, but lipid-lowering therapy is recommended.

Familial Dysbetalipoproteinemia (Type III Hyperlipoproteinemia) Like HL deficiency, familial dysbetalipoproteinemia (FDBL) (also known as *type III hyperlipoproteinemia* or *familial broad β disease*) is characterized by a mixed hyperlipidemia due to the accumulation of remnant lipoprotein particles. ApoE is present in multiple copies on chylomicron and VLDL remnants and mediates their removal via hepatic lipoprotein receptors (Fig. 335-2). FDBL is due to genetic variations in apoE that interfere with its ability to bind lipoprotein receptors. The *APOE* gene is polymorphic in sequence resulting in the expression of three common isoforms: apoE3, apoE2, and apoE4. Although associated with slightly higher LDL-C levels and increased coronary heart disease (CHD) risk, the apoE4 allele is not associated with FDBL. Patients with apoE4 have an increased incidence of late-onset Alzheimer disease. ApoE2 has a lower affinity for the LDL receptor. Therefore, chylomicron and VLDL remnants containing apoE2 are removed from plasma at a slower rate. Individuals who are homozygous for the E2 allele (the E2/E2 genotype) comprise the most common subset of patients with FDBL.

Approximately 1% of the general population are apoE2/E2 homozygotes but only a small minority of these individuals develop FDBL. In most cases an additional, identifiable factor precipitates the development of hyperlipoproteinemia. The most common precipitating factors are a high-caloric, high-fat diet, diabetes mellitus, obesity,

hypothyroidism, renal disease, estrogen deficiency, alcohol use, or the presence of another genetic form of hyperlipidemia, most commonly familial combined hyperlipidemia (FCHL) or familial hypercholesterolemia (FH). Rare mutations in apoE cause dominant forms of FDBL; in this case the hyperlipidemia is fully manifest in the heterozygous state.

Patients with FDBL usually present in adulthood with xanthomas and premature coronary and peripheral vascular disease. The disease seldom presents in women before menopause. Two distinctive types of xanthomas are seen in FDBL patients: tuberoeruptive and palmar xanthomas. *Tuberoeruptive xanthomas* begin as clusters of small papules on the elbows, knees, or buttocks and can grow to the size of small grapes. *Palmar xanthoma* (alternatively called *xanthomata striata palmaris*) are orange-yellow discolorations of the creases in the palms. In FDBL, the plasma cholesterol and triglyceride are elevated to a relatively similar degree until the triglyceride levels reach ~5.6 mol/L (~500 mg/dL), and then the triglycerides tends to be greater than cholesterol.

The traditional approach to diagnose this disorder is to use lipoprotein electrophoresis; in FDBL, the remnant lipoproteins accumulate in a broad β band. The preferred method to confirm the diagnosis of FDBL is to measure VLDL-C by ultracentrifugation and determine the ratio of VLDL-C to total plasma triglyceride; a ratio >0.30 is consistent with the diagnosis of FDBL. Protein methods (apoE phenotyping) or DNA-based methods (apoE genotyping) can be performed to confirm homozygosity for apoE2. However, absence of the apoE2/2 genotype does not rule out the diagnosis of FDBL, since other mutations in apoE can cause this condition.

Because FDBL is associated with increased risk of premature ASCVD, it should be treated aggressively. Other metabolic conditions that can worsen the hyperlipidemia (see above) should be actively treated. Patients with FDBL are typically very diet responsive and can respond dramatically to weight reduction and to low-cholesterol, low-fat diets. Alcohol intake should be curtailed. In postmenopausal women with FDBL, the dyslipidemia responds to estrogen-replacement therapy. HMG-CoA reductase inhibitors, fibrates, and niacin are all generally effective in the treatment of FDBL, and combination drug therapy is sometimes required.

Familial Hypercholesterolemia FH is an autosomal codominant disorder characterized by elevated plasma LDL-C with normal triglycerides, tendon xanthomas, and premature coronary atherosclerosis. FH is caused by >750 mutations in the LDL receptor gene and has a higher incidence in certain populations, such as Afrikaners, Christian Lebanese, and French Canadians, due to the founder effect. The elevated levels of LDL-C in FH are due to delayed catabolism of LDL and its precursor particles from the blood, resulting in increased rates of LDL production. There is a major gene dose effect, in that individuals with two mutated LDL receptor alleles (FH homozygotes) are much more affected than those with one mutant allele (FH heterozygotes).

Homozygous FH occurs in approximately 1 in 1 million persons world-wide. Patients with homozygous FH can be classified into one of two groups based on the amount of LDL receptor activity measured in their skin fibroblasts: those patients with <2% of normal LDL receptor activity (receptor negative) and those patients with 2 to 25% of normal LDL receptor activity (receptor defective). Most patients with homozygous FH present in childhood with cutaneous xanthomas on the hands, wrists, elbows, knees, heels, or buttocks. Arcus cornea is usually present and some patients have xanthelasmas. Total cholesterol levels are usually >12.93 mmol/L (500 mg/dL) and can be >25.86 mmol/L (1000 mg/dL). Accelerated atherosclerosis is a devastating complication of homozygous FH and can result in disability and death in childhood. Atherosclerosis often develops first in the aortic root and can cause aortic valvular or supravalvular stenosis and typically extends into the coronary ostia. Children with homozygous FH often develop symptomatic vascular disease before puberty, when symptoms can be atypical and sudden death is common. Untreated, receptor-negative patients with homozygous FH rarely survive beyond the second decade; patients with receptor-defective LDL receptor defects have a better prognosis but almost invariably develop clinically apparent atherosclerotic vascular disease by age 30, and often much sooner. Carotid and femoral disease develop later in life and are usually not clinically significant.

A careful family history should be taken, and plasma lipid levels should be measured in the parents and other first-degree relatives of patients with homozygous FH. The diagnosis can be confirmed by obtaining a skin biopsy and measuring LDL receptor activity in cultured skin fibroblasts or by quantifying the number of LDL receptors on the surfaces of lymphocytes using cell-sorting technology.

Combination therapy with an HMG-CoA reductase inhibitor and a bile acid sequestrant sometimes results in modest reductions in plasma LDL-C in the FH homozygote. Patients with homozygous FH invariably require additional lipid-lowering therapy. Since the liver is quantitatively the most important tissue for removing circulating LDL via the LDL receptor, liver transplantation is effective in decreasing plasma LDL-C levels in this disorder. Liver transplantation is, however, associated with substantial risks, including the requirement for long-term immunosuppression. The current treatment of choice for homozygous FH is LDL apheresis (a process where the LDL particles are selectively removed from the circulation), which can promote regression of xanthomas and may slow the progression of atherosclerosis. Initiation of LDL apheresis should be delayed until approximately 5 years of age except when evidence of atherosclerotic vascular disease is present.

Heterozygous FH is caused by the inheritance of one mutant LDL receptor allele and occurs in approximately 1 in 500 persons worldwide, making it one of the most common single gene disorders. It is characterized by elevated plasma LDL-C [usually 5.17 to 10.34 μmol/L (200 to 400 mg/dL)] and normal triglyceride levels. Patients with heterozygous FH have hypercholesterolemia from birth, although the disease is often not detected until adulthood, usually due to the detection of hypercholesterolemia on routine screening, the appearance of tendon xanthomas, or the premature development of symptomatic coronary atherosclerotic disease. Since the disease is codominant in inheritance and has a high penetrance (>90%), one parent and ~50% of the patient's siblings are usually hypercholesterolemic. The family history is frequently positive for premature ASCVD on one side of the family, particularly among male relatives. Corneal arcus is common, and tendon xanthomas involving the dorsum of the hands, elbows, knees, and especially the Achilles tendons are present in ~75% of patients. The age of onset of ASCVD is highly variable and depends in part on the molecular defect in the LDL receptor gene and other coexisting cardiac risk factors. FH heterozygotes with elevated plasma Lp(a) appear to be at greater risk for cardiovascular complications.

Untreated men with heterozygous FH have an ~50% chance of having a myocardial infarction before age 60. Although the age of onset of atherosclerotic heart disease is later in women with FH, coronary disease is significantly more common in women with FH than in the general female population.

No definitive diagnostic test for heterozygous FH is available. Although FH heterozygotes tend to have reduced levels of LDL receptor function in skin fibroblasts, there is significant overlap with the levels in normal fibroblasts. The clinical diagnosis is usually not problematic, but it is critical that hypothyroidism, nephrotic syndrome, and obstructive liver disease be excluded before initiating therapy.

FH patients should be treated aggressively to lower plasma levels of LDL-C. Initiation of a low-cholesterol, low-fat diet is recommended, but heterozygous FH patients inevitably require lipid-lowering drug therapy. HMG-CoA reductase inhibitors are especially effective in heterozygous FH, inducing upregulation of the normal LDL receptor allele in the liver. Many heterozygous FH patients can achieve desired LDL-C levels with HMG-CoA reductase inhibitor therapy alone, but combination drug therapy with the addition of a bile acid sequestrant or nicotinic acid is frequently required. Heterozygous FH patients who cannot be adequately controlled on combination drug therapy are candidates for LDL apheresis.

Familial Defective ApoB-100 Familial defective apoB-100 (FDB) is a dominantly inherited disorder that clinically resembles heterozygous FH. FDB occurs with a frequency of ~1 in 1000 in western populations. The disease is characterized by elevated plasma LDL-C levels with normal triglycerides, tendon xanthomas, and an increased incidence of premature ASCVD. FDB is caused by mutations in the LDL receptor–binding domain of apoB-100. Almost all patients with FDB have a substitution of glutamine for arginine at position 3500 in apoB-100, although other rarer mutations have been reported to cause this disease. As a consequence of the mutation in apoB-100, LDL binds the LDL receptor with reduced affinity and LDL is removed from the circulation at a reduced rate. Patients with FDB cannot be clinically distinguished from patients with heterozygous FH, although patients with FDB tend to have lower plasma LDL-C than FH heterozygotes. The apoB-100 gene mutation can be detected directly, but currently genetic diagnosis is not encouraged since the recommended management of FDB and heterozygous FH is identical.

Autosomal Recessive Hypercholesterolemia Autosomal recessive hypercholesterolemia (ARH) is a rare disorder (except in Sardinia) due to mutations in a protein (ARH) involved in LDL receptor–mediated endocytosis in the liver. ARH clinically resembles homozygous FH and is characterized by hypercholesterolemia, tendon xanthomas, and premature coronary artery disease. The hypercholesterolemia tends to be intermediate between the levels seen in FH homozygotes and FH heterozygotes. LDL receptor function in cultured fibroblasts is normal or only modestly reduced in ARH, whereas LDL receptor function in lymphocytes and the liver is negligible. Unlike FH homozygotes, the hyperlipidemia responds partially to treatment with HMG-CoA reductase inhibitors, but these patients usually require LDL apheresis to lower plasma LDL-C to recommended levels.

Wolman Disease and Cholesteryl Ester Storage Disease Wolman disease is an autosomal recessive disorder caused by complete deficiency of lysosomal acid lipase. After LDL is taken up from the cell surface by LDL receptor–mediated endocytosis, it is delivered from endosomes to lysosomes. In the acidic environment of the endosome, the particle dissociates from the receptor, which recycles to the cell surface. In the lysosome, apoB-100 is degraded and the cholesteryl esters and triglycerides of LDL are hydrolyzed by lysosomal acid lipase. Patients with Wolman disease fail to hydrolyze the neutral lipids, resulting in their accumulation within cells. The disease presents within the first weeks of life with hepatosplenomegaly, steatorrhea, adrenal calcification, and failure to thrive. The disease is usually fatal within the first year of life and can be diagnosed by measuring acid lipase activity in fibroblasts or liver tissue biopsy specimens. Cholesteryl ester storage disease is a less severe form of the same genetic disorder in which there is low, but detectable, acid lipase activity. Patients with this disorder sometimes present in childhood with hepatomegaly and a mixed hyperlipidemia, due to elevations in the levels of plasma LDL and VLDL. Other patients present later in life with hepatic fibrosis, portal hypertension, or with premature atherosclerosis.

Sitosterolemia Sitosterolemia is a rare autosomal recessive disease caused by mutations in one of two members of the adenosine triphosphate (ATP)-binding cassette transporter family, ABCG5 and ABCG8. These genes are expressed in the intestine and liver, where they form a functional complex to limit intestinal absorption and promote biliary excretion of plant- and animal-derived neutral sterols. In normal individuals, <5% of dietary plant sterols, of which sitosterol is the most plentiful, are absorbed by the proximal small intestine and delivered to the liver. Plant sterols in the liver are preferentially secreted into the bile, and plasma plant sterol levels are normally very low. In sitosterolemia, the intestinal absorption of plant sterols is increased and biliary excretion of the sterols is reduced, resulting in increased plasma levels of sitosterol and other plant sterols. The trafficking of cholesterol is also impaired. Patients with sitosterolemia can have either normal or elevated plasma levels of cholesterol. Irrespective of the plasma cholesterol level, these patients develop cutaneous and tendon xanthomas as well as premature atherosclerosis. Episodes of hemolysis, presumably secondary to the incorporation of plant sterols into the red blood cell membrane, are a distinctive clinical feature of this disease. The hypercholesterolemia in patients with sitosterolemia is unusually responsive to reductions in dietary cholesterol content. Sitosterolemia should be suspected when the plasma cholesterol level falls by >40% on a low-cholesterol diet (without associated weight loss).

Sitosterolemia is confirmed by demonstrating an elevated plasma sitosterol level. The hypercholesterolemia does not respond to HMG-CoA reductase inhibitors, but bile acid sequestrants and cholesterol-absorption inhibitors, such as ezetimibe, are effective in reducing plasma sterol levels in these patients.

PRIMARY DISORDERS OF ApoB-CONTAINING LIPOPROTEIN METABOLISM (UN-KNOWN ETIOLOGY) A large proportion of patients with elevated levels of apoB-containing lipoproteins have disorders in which the molecular defect has not been defined, largely because multiple other genetic and nongenetic factors contribute to the hyperlipidemia.

Familial Hypertriglyceridemia Familial hypertriglyceridemia (FHTG) is a relatively common (1 in 500) autosomal dominant disorder of unknown etiology characterized by moderately elevated plasma triglycerides accompanied by more modest elevations in cholesterol. VLDL is the major class of lipoproteins elevated in this disorder, which is

often referred to as type IV hyperlipoproteinemia (Frederickson classification, Table 335-4). The elevated plasma VLDL is due to increased VLDL production, impaired VLDL catabolism, or a combination of the two. Some patients with FHTG have a more severe form of hyperlipidemia in which both VLDL and chylomicrons are elevated (type V hyperlipidemia), as these two classes of lipoproteins compete for the same lipolytic pathway. Increased intake of simple carbohydrates, obesity, insulin resistance, alcohol use, or estrogen treatment, all of which increase VLDL synthesis, can precipitate the development of chylomicronemia. FHTG does not appear to be associated with increased risk of ASCVD in many families.

The diagnosis of FHTG is suggested by the triad of elevated plasma triglycerides [2.8 to 11.3 mmol/L (250 to 1000 mg/dL)], normal or only mildly increased cholesterol levels [<6.5 mmol/L (<250 mg/dL)], and reduced plasma HDL-C. Plasma LDL-C is generally not increased and is often reduced due to defective metabolism of the triglyceride-rich particles. The identification of other first-degree relatives with hypertriglyceridemia is useful in making the diagnosis. FDBL and FCHL should also be ruled out as these two conditions are associated with a significantly increased risk of ASCVD. The plasma apoB levels and the ratio of plasma cholesterol to triglyceride tend to be lower in FHTG than in either FDBL or FCHL.

It is important to exclude secondary causes of the hypertriglyceridemia before making the diagnosis of FHTG. Lipid-lowering drug therapy can frequently be avoided with appropriate dietary and lifestyle changes. Patients with plasma triglyceride levels >4.5 to 6.8 mmol/L (>400 to 600 mg/dL), after a trial of diet and exercise, should be considered for drug therapy to avoid the development of chylomicronemia and pancreatitis. A fibrate is a reasonable first line drug for FHTG, and niacin can also be considered in this condition.

Familial Combined Hyperlipidemia The molecular etiology of FCHL is unknown but is likely to involve defects in several different genes. FCHL is the most common primary lipid disorder, occurring in approximately 1 in 200 persons. Approximately 20% of patients who develop CHD before age 60 have FCHL.

FCHL is characterized by moderate elevation of plasma triglycerides and cholesterol and reduced plasma HDL-C. The disease is autosomal dominant, and affected family members typically have one of three possible phenotypes: (1) elevated plasma LDL-C, (2) elevated plasma triglycerides and VLDL-C, or (3) elevated plasma LDL-C and VLDL-C. A classic feature of FCHL is that the lipoprotein phenotype can switch among these phenotypes. FCHL can manifest in childhood but is sometimes not fully expressed until adulthood. Visceral obesity, glucose intolerance, insulin resistance, hypertension, and hyperuricemia are often present. These patients do not develop xanthomas.

Patients with FCHL almost always have significantly elevated plasma apoB. The levels of apoB are disproportionately high relative to plasma LDL-C due to the presence of small dense LDL particles,

TABLE 335-4 *Frederickson Classification of Hyperlipoproteinemias*

Phenotype	I	IIa	IIb	III	IV	V
Lipoprotein elevated	Chylomicrons	LDL	LDL and VLDL	Chylomicron and VLDL remnants	VLDL	Chylomicrons and VLDL
Triglycerides	++++	--	++	++ to +++	++	++++
Cholesterol	+ to ++	+++	++ to +++	++ to +++	-- to +	++ to +++
LDL-cholesterol	↓	+++	↑	↓	-- to +	++ to +++
HDL-cholesterol	↓↓↓	↑	↑	--	↓↓	↓↓↓
Plasma appearance	Lactescent	Clear	Clear	Turbid	Turbid	Lactescent
Xanthomas	Eruptive	Tendon, tuberous	None	Palmar, tuberoeruptive	None	Eruptive
Pancreatitis	+++	0	0	0	0	+++
Coronary atherosclerosis	0	+++	+++	+++	+/-	+/-
Peripheral atherosclerosis	0	+	+	++	+/-	+/-
Molecular defects	LPL and apoC-II	LDL receptor and apoB-100	Unknown	ApoE	Unknown	Unknown
Genetic nomenclature	FCS	FH, FDB	FCHL	FDBL	FHTG	FHTG

Note. LPL, lipoprotein lipase; apo, apolipoprotein; FCS, familial chylomicronemia syndrome; FH, familial hypercholesterolemia; FDB, familiar defective apoB; FCHL, familial combined hyperlipidemia; FDBL, familial dysbetalipoproteinemia; FHTG, familial hypertriglyceridemia.

which are characteristic of this syndrome and are highly atherogenic. *Hyperapobetalipoproteinemia* has been used as a term to describe the coupling of elevated plasma apoB with normal plasma cholesterol, and is probably a form of FCHL.

A mixed dyslipidemia [plasma triglyceride levels between 2.3 and 9.0 mmol/L (200 and 800 mg/dL), cholesterol levels between 5.2 and 10.3 mmol/L (200 and 400 mg/dL), and HDL-C levels <10.3 mmol/L (<40 mg/dL)] and a family history of hyperlipidemia and/or premature CHD suggests the diagnosis of FCHL. An elevated plasma apoB level or an increased number of small dense LDL particles in the plasma supports this diagnosis. FDBL should be considered and ruled out by beta-quantification in suspected patients with a mixed hyperlipidemia.

Individuals with FCHL should be treated aggressively due to significantly increased risk of premature CHD. Decreased dietary intake of saturated fat and simple carbohydrates, aerobic exercise, and weight loss have beneficial effects on the lipid profile. Patients with diabetes should be aggressively treated to maintain good glucose control. Most patients with FCHL require lipid-lowering drug therapy to reduce lipoprotein levels to the recommended range. HMG-CoA reductase inhibitors are very effective in lowering plasma levels of LDL-C and can also significantly reduce VLDL-C. Nicotinic acid decreases both LDL-C and VLDL-C, while raising plasma HDL-C, and is frequently effective for this condition when used in combination with HMG-CoA reductase inhibitors.

Polygenic Hypercholesterolemia　Polygenic hypercholesterolemia is characterized by hypercholesterolemia with a normal plasma triglyceride in the absence of secondary causes of hypercholesterolemia. Plasma LDL-C levels are not as elevated as they are in FH and FDB. Family studies are useful to differentiate polygenic hypercholesterolemia from the single-gene disorders described above; half of the first-degree relatives of patients with FH and FDB are hypercholesterolemic, whereas <10% of first-degree relatives of patients with polygenic hypercholesterolemia are hypercholesterolemic. Treatment of polygenic hypercholesterolemia is identical to that of other forms of hypercholesterolemia.

GENETIC DISORDERS OF HDL METABOLISM (KNOWN ETIOLOGY)　Mutations in certain genes encoding critical proteins in HDL synthesis and catabolism cause marked variations in plasma HDL-C levels. Unlike the genetic forms of hypercholesterolemia, which are invariably associated with premature coronary atherosclerosis, genetic forms of hypoalphalipoproteinemia (low HDL-C) are not always associated with accelerated atherosclerosis. Whereas high plasma LDL-C is invariably associated with increased atherosclerosis, the risk associated with low plasma levels of HDL-C depends on the underlying mechanism. Analysis of the genetic disorders of HDL metabolism has provided insights into the less well understood etiologic relationship between plasma HDL-C levels and atherosclerosis.

ApoA-I Deficiency and ApoA-I Mutations　Complete genetic deficiency of apoA-I due to mutations in the apoA-I gene result in the virtual absence of HDL from the plasma. The genes encoding apoA-I, apoC-III, apoA-IV, and apoA-V are clustered together on chromosome 11, and some patients with complete absence of apoA-I have deletions that include more than one of these genes. Because apoA-I is required for LCAT function, plasma and tissue levels of free cholesterol are increased, resulting in the development of corneal opacities and planar xanthomas. Clinically apparent coronary atherosclerosis typically appears between the fourth and seventh decade in the apoA-I-deficient patient.

Although missense mutations in the apoA-I gene have been identified in selected patients with low plasma HDL [usually 0.39 to 0.78 mmol/L (15 to 30 mg/dL)], they are very rare causes of low HDL-C levels in the general population. Patients with apoA-I$_{Milano}$ have very low plasma levels of HDL due to the rapid catabolism of the apolipoprotein, but these patients do not have an increased risk of premature CHD. Other than corneal opacities, most individuals with low plasma HDL-C levels due to missense mutations in apoA-I have no clinical sequelae. A few specific mutations in apoA-I cause systemic amyloi-

dosis, and the mutant apoA-I has been found as a component of the amyloid plaque.

Tangier Disease　Tangier disease is a rare autosomal codominant form of low plasma HDL-C caused by mutations in the gene encoding ABCA1, a cellular transporter that facilitates efflux of unesterified cholesterol and phospholipids from cells to apoA-I (Fig. 335-3). ABCA1 plays a critical role in the generation and stabilization of the mature HDL particle. In its absence, HDL is rapidly cleared from the circulation. Patients with Tangier disease have plasma HDL-C levels <0.13 mmol/L (<5 mg/dL) and extremely low circulating levels of apoA-I. The disease is associated with cholesterol accumulation in the reticuloendothelial system, resulting in hepatosplenomegaly and pathognomonic enlarged, grayish yellow or orange tonsils. An intermittent peripheral neuropathy (mononeuritis multiplex) or a sphingomyelia-like neurologic disorder can also be seen in this disorder. Tangier disease is associated with premature atherosclerotic disease, but the risk is not as high as might be anticipated given the markedly decreased plasma HDL-C and apoA-I. Plasma LDL-C is also low and this may attenuate the atherosclerotic risk. Obligate heterozygotes for ABCA1 mutations have moderately reduced plasma HDL-C levels and are also at increased risk of premature CHD.

LCAT Deficiency　LCAT deficiency is a rare disorder caused by mutations in lecithin:cholesterol acyltransferase (Fig. 335-3). LCAT is synthesized in the liver and secreted into the plasma, where it circulates associated with lipoproteins. Because the enzyme mediates the esterification of cholesterol, the proportion of free cholesterol in circulating lipoproteins is greatly increased (from ~25% to >70% of total plasma cholesterol). Lack of normal cholesterol esterification impairs the formation of mature HDL particles and leads to rapid catabolism of circulating apoA-I. Two genetic forms of LCAT deficiency have been described in humans—complete deficiency (also called *classic LCAT deficiency*) and partial deficiency (also called *fish-eye disease*). Progressive corneal opacification due to the deposition of free cholesterol in the lens, very low plasma HDL-C [usually <0.26 mmol/L (<10 mg/dL)], and variable hypertriglyceridemia are characteristic of both types. In partial LCAT deficiency, there are no other known clinical sequelae. In contrast, complete LCAT deficiency is characterized by a hemolytic anemia and progressive renal insufficiency that eventually leads to end-stage renal disease (ESRD). Despite the extremely low plasma levels of HDL-C and apoA-I, premature ASCVD is not a feature of either complete or partial LCAT deficiency, once again exemplifying the complex relationship between low plasma levels of HDL-C and the development of ASCVD. The diagnosis can be confirmed by assaying LCAT activity in the plasma.

CETP Deficiency　Mutations in the gene encoding cholesteryl ester transfer protein (CETP) cause a high HDL-C condition called *CETP deficiency*. CETP facilitates the transfer of cholesteryl esters among lipoproteins, especially from HDL to apoB containing lipoproteins in exchange for triglycerides (Fig. 335-3). Homozygous deficiency of CETP, which occurs predominantly in Japan, results in very high plasma HDL-C [>3.88 mmol/L (>150 mg/dL)] due to accumulation of large, cholesterol-rich HDL particles. Heterozygotes for CETP deficiency have only modestly elevated HDL-C. The relationship of CETP deficiency to risk of ASCVD remains a matter of debate.

PRIMARY DISORDERS OF HDL METABOLISM (UNKNOWN ETIOLOGY)　The gene defect in other individuals with either very high or very low plasma HDL-C is not known.

Primary Hypoalphalipoproteinemia　The most common inherited cause of low plasma HDL-C is termed *primary or familial hypoalphalipoproteinemia*. Hypoalphalipoproteinemia is defined as a plasma HDL-C level below the 10th percentile in the setting of relatively normal cholesterol and triglyceride levels, no apparent secondary causes of low plasma HDL-C, and no clinical signs of LCAT deficiency or Tangier disease. This syndrome is often referred to as "isolated low HDL." A family history of low HDL-C facilitates the diagnosis of an inherited condition, which usually follows an autosomal dominant pattern. The metabolic etiology of this disease appears to be primarily accelerated catabolism of HDL and its apolipoproteins. Several kindreds with primary hypoalphalipoproteinemia have been described in association with an increased incidence of premature ASCVD.

Familial Hyperalphalipoproteinemia Familial hyperalphalipoproteinemia has a dominant inheritance pattern. Plasma HDL-C is usually >2.07 mmol/L (80 mg/dL) in affected women and >1.81 mmol/L (70 mg/dL) in affected men. The genetic basis of primary hyperalphalipoproteinemia is not known, and the condition may be associated with decreased risk of CHD and increased longevity in some cases.

SECONDARY DISORDERS OF LIPOPROTEIN METABOLISM Significant changes in plasma levels of lipoproteins are seen in a variety of diseases. It is critical that secondary causes of hyperlipidemias (Table 335-5) are considered prior to initiation of lipid-lowering therapy.

Obesity Obesity is frequently, though not invariably, accompanied by hyperlipidemia. The increase in adipocyte mass and accompanying decrease in insulin sensitivity associated with obesity have multiple effects on lipid metabolism. More free fatty acids are delivered from the expanded adipose tissue to the liver where they are re-esterified in hepatocytes to form triglycerides, which are packaged into VLDL for secretion into the circulation. High dietary intake of simple carbohydrates also drives hepatic production of VLDL, leading to increases in VLDL and/or LDL in some obese individuals. Plasma HDL-C tends to be low in obesity. Weight loss is often associated with a reduction of plasma apoB-containing lipoproteins and an increase of plasma HDL-C.

Diabetes Mellitus Patients with type 1 diabetes mellitus are generally not hyperlipidemic if they are under good glycemic control. Diabetic ketoacidosis is frequently accompanied by hypertriglyceridemia due to increased hepatic influx of free fatty acids from adipose tissue. The hypertriglyceridemia responds dramatically to administration of insulin in the insulinopenic diabetic.

Patients with type 2 diabetes mellitus are usually dyslipidemic, even if under relatively good glycemic control. The high levels of insulin and insulin resistance associated with type 2 diabetes have multiple effects on fat metabolism: (1) a decrease in LPL activity resulting in reduced catabolism of chylomicrons and VLDL, (2) an in-

crease in the release of free fatty acid from the adipose tissue, (3) an increase in fatty acid synthesis in the liver, and (4) an increase in hepatic VLDL production. Patients with type 2 diabetes mellitus have several lipid abnormalities, including elevated plasma triglycerides (due to increased VLDL and lipoprotein remnants), elevated dense LDL, and decreased HDL-C. In some diabetic patients, especially those with a genetic defect in lipid metabolism, the triglycerides can be extremely elevated. Elevated plasma LDL-C levels are usually not a feature of diabetes mellitus and suggest the presence of an underlying lipoprotein abnormality or may indicate the development of diabetic nephropathy. Patients with lipodystrophy, who have profound insulin resistance, have markedly elevated VLDL and chylomicrons.

Thyroid Disease Hypothyroidism is associated with elevated plasma LDL-C due primarily to a reduction in hepatic LDL receptor function and delayed clearance of LDL. Conversely, plasma LDL-C is often reduced in the hyperthyroid patient. Hypothyroid patients may have increased circulating IDL, and some are mildly hypertriglyceridemic [<3.34 μmol/L (<300 mg/dL)]. Because hypothyroidism is easily overlooked, all patients presenting with elevated plasma LDL-C or IDL should be screened for hypothyroidism. Thyroid replacement therapy usually ameliorates the hypercholesterolemia.

Renal Disorders Nephrotic syndrome is associated with hyperlipoproteinemia, which is usually mixed but can manifest as hypercholesterolemia or hypertriglyceridemia alone. The hyperlipidemia of nephrotic syndrome appears to be due to a combination of increased hepatic production and decreased clearance of VLDL, with increased LDL production. Effective treatment of the underlying renal disease normalizes the lipid profile, but most patients with chronic nephrotic syndrome require lipid-lowering drug therapy.

ESRD is often associated with mild hypertriglyceridemia [<3.34 μmol/L (<300 mg/dL)] due to the accumulation of VLDL and remnant lipoproteins in the circulation. Triglyceride lipolysis and remnant clearance are both reduced in patients with renal failure. Because the risk of ASCVD is increased in hyperlipidemic patients with ESRD, they should be treated aggressively with lipid-lowering agents.

Patients with renal transplants are usually hyperlipidemic due to immunosuppression drugs (cyclosporine and glucocorticoids); they present a difficult management problem as HMG-CoA reductase inhibitors must be used cautiously in these patients.

Liver Disorders Because the liver is the principal site of formation and clearance of lipoproteins, it is not surprising that liver diseases can

TABLE 335-5 *Secondary Forms of Hyperlipidemia*

LDL		HDL					
Elevated	Reduced	Elevated	Reduced	VLDL Elevated	IDL Elevated	Chylomicrons Elevated	Lp(a) Elevated
Hypothyroidism	Severe liver	Alcohol	Smoking	Obesity	Multiple	Autoimmune	Renal
Nephrotic	disease	Exercise	DM type 2	DM type 2	myeloma	disease	insufficiency
syndrome	Malabsorption	Exposure to	Obesity	Glycogen storage	Monoclonal	Drugs:	Inflammation
Cholestasis	Malnutrition	chlorinated	Malnutrition	disease	gammopathy	Isotretinoin	Menopause
Acute	Gaucher disease	hydrocarbons	Gaucher	Hepatitis	Autoimmune		Orchidectomy
intermittent	Chronic infectious	Drugs:	disease	Alcohol	disease		Hypothyroidism
porphyria	disease	estrogen	Drugs:	Renal failure	Hypothyroidism		Acromegaly
Anorexia	Hyperthyroidisim		anabolic	Sepsis			Nephrosis
nervosa	Drugs: niacin		steroids,	Stress			Drugs: growth
Hepatoma	toxicity		beta	Cushing syndrome			hormone
Drugs:			blockers	Pregnancy			
thiazides,				Acromegaly			
cyclosporine,				Lipodystrophy			
tegretol				Drugs: estrogen, beta			
				blockers, furosemide,			
				glucocorticoids, bile			
				acid–binding			
				resins, retinoic			
				acid, HIV protease			
				inhibitors			

Note: LDL, low-density lipoprotein; HDL, high-density lipoprotein; VLDL, very low density lipoprotein; IDL, intermediate-density lipoprotein; Lp(a), lipoprotein A; DM, diabetes mellitus.

profoundly affect plasma lipid levels in a variety of ways. Hepatitis due to infection, drugs, or alcohol is often associated with increased VLDL synthesis and mild to moderate hypertriglyceridemia. Severe hepatitis and liver failure are associated with dramatic reductions in plasma cholesterol and triglycerides due to reduced lipoprotein biosynthetic capacity. Cholestasis is associated with hypercholesterolemia, which sometimes can be very severe. The major pathway by which cholesterol is excreted is via secretion into bile, either directly or after conversion to bile acids. Cholestasis blocks this critical excretory pathway. In cholestasis, free cholesterol coupled with phospholipids are secreted into the plasma as constituents of a lamellar particle called *Lp(X)*. These particles can deposit in skin folds, producing lesions resembling those seen in patients with FDBL (xanthomata strata palmaris). Planar and eruptive xanthomas can also be seen in patients with cholestasis.

Alcohol Regular alcohol consumption has a variable effect on plasma lipid levels. The most common effect of alcohol is to increase plasma triglyceride levels. Alcohol consumption stimulates hepatic secretion of VLDL, possibly by inhibiting the hepatic oxidation of free fatty acids, which then promote hepatic triglyceride synthesis and VLDL secretion. The usual lipoprotein pattern seen with alcohol consumption is type IV (increased VLDL), but persons with an underlying primary lipid disorder may develop severe hypertriglyceridemia (type V) if they drink alcohol. Regular alcohol use is also associated with a mild to moderate increase in plasma levels of HDL-C.

Estrogen Estrogen administration is associated with increased VLDL and HDL synthesis resulting in elevated plasma triglycerides and HDL-C. This lipoprotein pattern is distinctive since the levels of plasma triglyceride and HDL-C are typically inversely related. Estrogen treatment may convert a person with type IV to type V hyperlipidemia. Plasma triglyceride levels should be monitored when birth control pills or estrogen replacement therapy is initiated. Use of low-dose estrogen preparations or the estrogen patch can minimize the effect of exogenous estrogen on lipids.

Glycogen Storage Diseases Other rarer causes of secondary hyperlipidemias include glycogen storage diseases such as *von Gierke's disease*, which is caused by mutations in glucose-6-phosphatase. The inability to mobilize hepatic glucose during fasting results in hypoinsulinemia and increased release of free fatty acids from adipose tissue. Hepatic fatty acids synthesis is also increased, resulting in fat accumulation in the liver and increased VLDL secretion. The hyperlipidemia associated with this disease can be very severe but responds well to treatment of the underlying disorder.

Cushing Syndrome Glucocorticoid excess is associated with increased VLDL synthesis and hypertriglyceridemia. Patients with Cushing syndrome can also have mild elevations in plasma LDL-C.

Drugs Many drugs have a significant impact on lipid metabolism and can result in significant alterations in the lipoprotein profile (Table 335-5).

SCREENING Guidelines for the screening and management of lipid disorders have been provided by an expert Adult Treatment Panel (ATP) convened by the National Cholesterol Education Program (NCEP) of the National Heart Lung and Blood Institute. The NCEP ATPIII guidelines published in 2001 recommend that all adults over age 20 have plasma levels of cholesterol, triglyceride, LDL-C, and HDL-C measured after a 12-h overnight fast. In most clinical laboratories, the total cholesterol and triglycerides in the plasma are measured enzymatically and then the cholesterol in the supernatant is measured after precipitation of apoB-containing lipoproteins to determine the HDL-C. The LDL-C is estimated using the following equation:

$$LDL\text{-}C = total\ cholesterol - (triglycerides/5) - HDL\text{-}C$$

The VLDL-C is estimated by dividing the plasma triglyceride by 5, reflecting the ratio of cholesterol to triglyceride in VLDL particles. This formula is reasonably accurate if test results are obtained on fasting plasma and if the triglyceride level $<\sim4.0\ \mu mol/L$ (350 mg/dL).

The accurate determination of LDL-C levels in patients with triglyceride levels greater than this requires application of ultracentrifugation techniques (beta quantification), although direct assays for LDL-C are also available in some laboratories. →*For further discussion about screening, see Chap. 225.*

R̲x̲ TREATMENT

Multiple epidemiologic studies have demonstrated a strong relationship between serum cholesterol and CHD. Randomized controlled clinical trials have unequivocally documented that lowering plasma cholesterol reduces the risk of clinical events due to atherosclerosis (Chaps. 224 and 225). Although the proportional benefit accrued from reducing plasma LDL-C is similar over the entire range of LDL-C values, the absolute risk reduction depends on the baseline LDL-C, the presence of established CHD, and other cardiovascular risk factors.

Elevated plasma triglyceride levels are also associated with increased risk of CHD, but this relationship weakens considerably when statistical corrections are made for the plasma levels of LDL-C and HDL-C. Plasma levels of HDL-C are strongly and consistently inversely related to the prevalence and incidence of CHD, and yet no clinical trial data are available demonstrating that increasing plasma levels of HDL-C reduces the frequency of cardiovascular events. No pharmacologic agents are available that exclusively either lower plasma triglyceride levels or increase plasma HDL-C levels, contributing to the dearth of clinical trial data addressing the role of treatment of these lipid abnormalities in CHD prevention. Since both hypertriglyceridemia and low plasma levels of HDL-C confer higher ASCVD risk, the NCEP ATPIII recommends more aggressive therapy to lower the plasma LDL-C in patients with these dyslipidemias.

Nonpharmacologic Treatment ■ *DIET* Dietary modification is an important component in the management of hyperlipidemia. In the hypercholesterolemic patient, dietary saturated fat and cholesterol should be restricted. For patients who are hypertriglyceridemic, the intake of simple sugars should also be curtailed. For severe hypertriglyceridemia [>11.3 mmol/L (>1000 mg/dL)], restriction of total fat intake is critical. The most widely used diet to lower the LDL-C level is the "Step 1 diet" developed by the American Heart Association. Most patients have a relatively modest (<10%) decrease in plasma levels of LDL-C on a step I diet in the absence of any associated weight loss. Almost all persons experience a decrease in plasma HDL-C levels with a reduction in the amount of total and saturated fat in their diet.

FOODS AND ADDITIVES Certain foods and dietary additives are associated with modest reductions in plasma cholesterol levels. Plant stanol and sterol esters are available in a variety of foods such as spreads, salad dressings, and snack bars. They interfere with cholesterol absorption and reduce plasma LDL-C levels by ~10 to 15% when taken three times per day. The addition to the diet of psyllium, soy protein, or Chinese red yeast rice (which contains lovastatin) can have modest cholesterol-lowering effects. Other herbal approaches such as guggulipid require further study to assess their effectiveness.

WEIGHT LOSS AND EXERCISE The treatment of obesity, if present, can have a favorable impact on plasma lipid levels and should be actively encouraged. Plasma triglyceride and LDL-C levels tend to fall and HDL-C levels tend to increase in obese persons who lose weight. Aerobic exercise has a very modest elevating effect on plasma levels of HDL-C in most individuals but has cardiovascular benefits that extend beyond the effects on plasma lipid levels.

Pharmalogic Treatment The decision to use drug therapy depends on the cardiovascular risk (Chap. 225). An effective way to estimate absolute risk of a cardiovascular event over 10 years is to use a scoring system based on the Framingham Heart Study database. Patients with a 10-year absolute CHD risk of > 20% are considered "CHD risk equivalents." Current NCEP ATPIII guidelines call for drug therapy to reduce LDL-C to <2.6 mmol/L (<100 mg/dL) in patients with established

CHD, other ASCVD (aortic aneurysm, peripheral vascular disease, or cerebrovascular disease), diabetes mellitus, or CHD risk equivalents. Based on these guidelines, most CHD and CHD risk–equivalent patients require cholesterol-lowering drug therapy. Moderate risk patients with two or more risk factors and a 10-year absolute risk of 10 to 20% should be treated to a goal LDL-C of <3.4 mmol/L (<130 mg/dL). All other individuals have a goal of LDL-C <4.1 mmol/L (<160 mg/dL), but not all persons are candidates for drug therapy to achieve this goal.

Persons with markedly elevated plasma LDL-C levels [>4.9 mmol/L (>190 mg/dL)] should be considered for drug therapy even if their 10-year absolute CHD risk is not particularly elevated. The decision to initiate drug treatment in individuals with plasma LDL-C levels between 3.4 and 4.9 mmol/L (130 and 190 mg/dL) can be difficult. Although it is desirable to avoid drug treatment in patients who are unlikely to develop CHD, a very high proportion of patients who eventually develop CHD have plasma LDL-C levels that are in this range. Other clinical information can assist in the decision-making process. For example, a low plasma HDL-C [<1.0 mmol/L (<40 mg/dL) supports a decision in favor of more aggressive therapy. The diagnosis of the metabolic syndrome (Chap. 225) also identifies a higher risk individual who should be targeted for therapeutic life-style changes and might be a candidate for more aggressive drug therapy. Other laboratory tests, such as an elevated plasma Lp(a) or high-sensitivity C-reactive protein, may help to identify additional high-risk individuals. In persons at low risk, the emphasis should primarily be on dietary and life-style modification.

Drug treatment is also indicated in patients with triglycerides >11.3 mmol/L (>1000 mg/dL) who have been screened and treated for secondary causes of chylomicronemia. The goal is to reduce plasma triglycerides to <4.5 mmol/L (400 mg/dL) to prevent the risk of acute pancreatitis. Most major clinical end-point trials with statins have excluded persons with triglyceride levels >3.9 to 5.1 mmol/L (>350 to 450 mg/dL), and therefore there are few data regarding the effectiveness of statins in reducing cardiovascular risk in persons with triglycerides higher than this threshold. Combination therapy is often required for optimal control of mixed dyslipidemia.

HMG-COA REDUCTASE INHIBITORS 3-Hydroxy-3-methylglutaryl coenzyme A (HMG-CoA reductase) is the rate-limiting step in cholesterol bio-synthesis, and inhibition of this enzyme decreases cholesterol synthesis. By inhibiting cholesterol biosynthesis, HMG-CoA reductase inhibitors (statins) lead to increased hepatic LDL receptor activity and accelerated clearance of circulating LDL, resulting in a dose-dependent reduction in plasma LDL-C. There is wide interindividual variation in the initial response to a statin, but once a patient is on the medication, the doubling of the dose produces a 6% further reduction of plasma LDL-C. The HMG-CoA reductase inhibitors currently available differ in their LDL-C reducing effects (Table 335-6). HMG-CoA reductase inhibitors also reduce plasma triglycerides in a dose-dependent fashion, which is proportional to their LDL-C lowering effects [if the triglycerides are <3.9 mmol/L (<350 mg/dL)]. HMG-CoA reductase inhibitors have a modest HDL-raising effect (5 to 10%), and this effect is not dose-dependent.

HMG-CoA reductase inhibitors are well tolerated and can be taken in tablet form once a day. Potential side effects include dyspepsia, headaches, fatigue, and muscle or joint pains. Severe myopathy and even rhabdomyolysis occurs rarely. The risk of myopathy is increased by the presence of renal insufficiency and by coadministration of drugs that interfere with the metabolism of HMG-CoA reductase inhibitors, such as erythromycin and related antibiotics, antifungal agents, immunosuppressive drugs, and fibric acid derivatives. Severe myopathy can usually be avoided by careful patient selection, avoidance of interacting drugs, and by instructing the patient to contact the physician immediately in the event of unexplained muscle pain. In the event of muscle symptoms, the plasma creatine phosphokinase (CPK) level should be obtained to document the myopathy, but serum CPK levels do not need to be monitored on a routine basis as an elevated CPK in the absence of symptoms does not predict the development of myopathy and does not necessarily suggest the need for discontinuing the drug.

Another side effect of HMG-CoA reductase inhibitor therapy is hepatitis. Liver transaminases (ALT and AST) should be checked before starting therapy, at 8 weeks, and then every 6 months. Substantial (>3 × upper limit of normal) elevation in transaminases is relatively rare, and mild to moderate (1 to 3 × normal) elevation in transaminases in the absence of symptoms need not mandate discontinuing the medication. Severe clinical hepatitis associated with HMG-CoA reductase inhibitors is exceedingly rare, and the trend is toward less frequent monitoring of transaminases in patients taking HMG-CoA reductase inhibitors. The HMG-CoA reductase inhibitor–associated elevation in liver enzymes resolves after discontinuation of the medication.

TABLE 335-6 *Summary of the Major Drugs Used for the Treatment of Hyperlipidemia*

Drug	Major Indications	Starting Dose	Maximal Dose	Mechanism	Common Side Effects
HMG-CoA reductase inhibitors (statins)	Elevated LDL			↓ Cholesterol synthesis, ↓ hepatic LDL receptors, ↓ VLDL production	Myalgias, arthralgias, elevated transaminases, dyspepsia
Lovastatin		20 mg daily	80 mg daily		
Pravastatin		40 mg qhs	80 mg qhs		
Simvastatin		20 mg qhs	80 mg qhs		
Fluvastatin		20 mg qhs	80 mg qhs		
Atorvastatin		10 mg qhs	80 mg qhs		
Rosuvastatin		10 mg qhs	40 mg qhs		
Bile acid sequestrants	Elevated LDL			↑ Bile acid excretion and ↑ LDL receptors	Bloating, constipation, elevated triglycerides
Cholestyramine		4 g daily	32 g daily		
Colestipol		5 g daily	40 g daily		
Colesevelam		3750 mg daily	4375 mg daily		
Nicotinic acid	Elevated LDL, low HDL, elevated TG			↓ VLDL hepatic synthesis	Cutaneous flushing; GI upset; elevated glucose, uric acid, and liver function tests
Immediate-release		100 mg tid	2 g tid		
Sustained-release		250 mg bid	1.5 g bid		
Extended-release		500 mg qhs	2 g qhs		
Fibric acid derivatives	Elevated TG, elevated remnants			↑ LPL, ↓ VLDL synthesis	Dyspepsia, myalgia, gallstones, elevated transaminases
Gemfibrozil		600 mg bid	600 mg bid		
Fenofibrate		160 mg qd	160 mg qd		
Fish oils	Severely elevated TG	3 g daily	12 g daily	↓ Chylomicron and VLDL production	Dyspepsia, diarrhea, fishy odor to breath
Cholesterol absorption inhibitors				↓ Intestinal cholesterol absorption	Elevated transaminases
Ezetimibe	Elevated LDL	10 mg daily	10 mg daily		

Note: LDL, low-density lipoprotein; VLDL, very low density lipoprotein; HDL, high-density lipoprotein; TG, triglycerides; LPL, lipoprotein lipase.

Overall, HMG-CoA reductase inhibitors appear to be remarkably safe. Over 50,000 patients have been treated with HMG-CoA reductase inhibitors for over 5 to 6 years as a part of large randomized controlled clinical trials and no increase in any major noncardiac diseases have been seen in these individuals. HMG-CoA reductase inhibitors are the drug class of choice for LDL-C reduction and are by far the most widely used class of lipid-lowering drugs.

BILE ACID SEQUESTRANTS (RESINS) Bile acid sequestrants bind bile acids in the intestine and promote their excretion in the stool. In order to maintain an adequate bile acid pool, the liver diverts cholesterol to bile acid synthesis. The decreased hepatic intracellular cholesterol content upregulates the LDL receptor and enhances LDL clearance from the plasma. Bile acid sequestrants, including cholestyramine, colestipol, and colesevelam (Table 335-6), primarily reduce plasma LDL-C levels but can increase plasma triglycerides. Therefore, patients with hypertriglyceridemia should not be treated with bile acid–binding resins.

Cholestyramine and colestipol are insoluble resins that must be mixed with liquids. Colestipol is also available in large tablets but multiple tablets must be taken to achieve significant lowering of plasma LDL-C levels. The newest bile acid sequestrant, colesevelam, has greater bile acid–binding capacity than traditional resins. The colesevelam tablets are smaller, and fewer tablets per day are required. Most side effects of resins are limited to the gastrointestinal tract and include bloating and constipation. Bile acid sequestrants may bind other drugs (e.g., digoxin, warfarin) and interfere with their absorption. Therefore, all other medications should be taken either 1 h before or 4 h after the bile acid sequestrants.

Bile acid sequestrants are not systemically absorbed and are very safe. They are the cholesterol-lowering drug of choice in children and in women of childbearing age who are lactating, pregnant, or could become pregnant. These drugs can also be useful in young, well-motivated patients with moderate hypercholesterolemia who wish to avoid systemic drug therapy. This class of drugs is also useful in combination with HMG-CoA reductase inhibitors in patients who are unable to reach their LDL-C goal on HMG-CoA reductase inhibitor monotherapy and have relatively normal triglyceride levels.

NICOTINIC ACID (NIACIN) Nicotinic acid, or niacin, is a B-complex vitamin that reduces plasma triglyceride and LDL-C levels and raises the plasma HDL-C (Table 335-6) in high doses. Niacin is the only currently available lipid-lowering drug that significantly reduces plasma levels of Lp(a). If properly prescribed and monitored, niacin is a safe and effective lipid-lowering agent.

The cheapest form of niacin is immediate-release crystalline niacin. Niacin should be started at a low dose (100 mg three times a day) and taken with meals to delay absorption. The dose of niacin should be increased every 4 to 7 days by 100 mg until a dose of 500 mg tid is obtained. After 1 month on this dose, lipids and pertinent chemistries (glucose, uric acid, liver transaminases) should be measured. The dose can be further increased as needed up to a total dose of 6 g/d. The most frequent side effect is cutaneous flushing, but this improves with continued administration. In many patients, taking an aspirin 30 min prior to the niacin prevents flushing. Over-the-counter sustained-release forms of niacin are generally administered twice a day and are associated with less flushing, but some have been associated with rare cases of severe hepatitis. A clue to the development of niacin-induced hepatitis is a sudden, precipitous drop in the plasma lipid levels. A prescription form of extended-release niacin that is administered once daily at bedtime has not been associated with severe hepatic toxicity. Mild elevations in transaminases occur in up to 15% of patients treated with any form of niacin, but these elevations rarely require discontinuation of the medication. Niacin potentiates the effect of warfarin, and these two drugs should be prescribed together with caution. Acanthosis nigricans and maculopathy are infrequent side effects of niacin. Niacin is contraindicated in patients with peptic ulcer disease and can exacerbate the symptoms of esophageal reflux. Niacin can raise plasma levels of uric acid and precipitate gouty attacks in susceptible patients.

Niacin can raise fasting plasma glucose levels, but concerns regarding the use of niacin in diabetic patients have been allayed by the results of two studies. In one study, short-acting niacin treatment of dyslipidemia was associated with only a slight increase in fasting glucose and no significant change from baseline in the HbA1c. In the other, low-dose niacin was found to reduce triglycerides effectively and raise HDL-C in diabetics without adversely impacting glycemic control.

Successful therapy with niacin requires careful education and motivation of the patient. Its advantages are its low cost and long-term safety. It is the most effective drug currently available for raising HDL-C levels. It is particularly useful in patients with combined hyperlipidemia and low plasma levels of HDL-C and is effective in combination with statins.

FIBRIC ACID DERIVATIVES (FIBRATES) Fibric acid derivatives, or fibrates, are agonists of PPARα, a nuclear receptor involved in the regulation of carbohydrate and lipid metabolism. Fibrates stimulate LPL activity (enhancing triglyceride hydrolysis), reduce apoC-III synthesis (enhancing lipoprotein remnant clearance), and may reduce VLDL production. Fibrates are the most effective drugs available for reducing triglyceride levels, and they also raise HDL-C levels (Table 335-6). Fibrates have variable effects on LDL-C, and in hypertriglyceridemic patients can sometimes be associated with increases in plasma LDL-C levels.

Fibrates are generally very well tolerated. The most common side effect is dyspepsia. Myopathy and hepatitis occur rarely in the absence of other lipid-lowering agents. Fibrates promote cholesterol secretion into bile and are associated with an increased risk of gallstones. Importantly, fibrates can potentiate the effect of warfarin and certain oral hypoglycemic agents; the anticoagulation status and plasma glucose levels should be closely monitored in patients on these agents.

Fibrates are the drug class of choice in patients with severe hypertriglyceridemia [11.3 mmol/L (>1000 mg/dL)] and are a reasonable consideration in patients with moderate hypertriglyceridemia [4.5 to 11.3 mmol/L (400 to 1000 mg/dL)]. The Veterans Affairs High-Density Lipoprotein Intervention Trial study also suggests that they may have a role in high-risk patients with well-controlled LDL-C levels but elevated plasma triglyceride levels and low plasma levels of HDL-C. The relative indications of fibrates vs. statins and the role of combined therapy will be determined by ongoing and future trials.

Omega-3 Fatty Acids (Fish Oils) N-3 polyunsaturated fatty acids (PUFAs) are present in high concentration in fish and in flax seeds. The most widely used n-3 PUFAs for the treatment of hyperlipidemias are the two active molecules in fish oil, eicosapentanoic acid (EPA) and decohexanoic acid (DHA). N-3 PUFAs have been concentrated into tablets and in doses of 3 to 6 g/d decrease fasting and postprandial triglycerides. At least 6 g/d is usually required for a substantial triglyceride-lowering effect, and many patients require 9 to 12 g/d. Fish oil treatment of hypertriglyceridemia can be associated with a significant increase in plasma LDL-C levels. Fish oil supplements can be used in combination with fibrates, niacin, or statins to treat hypertriglyceridemia. In general, fish oils are well tolerated and appear to be safe, at least at doses up to 3 g. The large number of capsules required for a therapeutic effect, the associated dyspepsia, and fishy aftertaste have limited the clinical use of these agents. Although fish oil administration is associated with a prolongation in the bleeding time, no increase in bleeding has been seen in clinical trials.

CHOLESTEROL ABSORPTION INHIBITORS A new mechanism of cholesterol-lowering is the inhibition of intestinal cholesterol absorption. Ezetimibe (Table 335-6) inhibits the absorption of dietary and biliary cholesterol from the intestinal lumen. It reduces LDL-C cholesterol levels by ~18% as monotherapy or in combination with a statin. Cholesterol absorption inhibitors are particularly useful in combination with a statin in patients unable to reach their LDL-C goal on statin monotherapy.

COMBINATION DRUG THERAPY Combination drug therapy is frequently used in the following situations: (1) patients unable to reach their LDL-C goal on a single drug, (2) patients with combined hypertriglyceridemia and hypercholesterolemia that cannot be adequately controlled with a single drug, and (3) patients with elevated LDL-C and low HDL-C levels. Inability to achieve LDL-C goal is not uncommon on statin monotherapy. If the patient has a normal plasma triglyceride level, a bile acid sequestrant can be added. A cholesterol absorption inhibitor can also be used in this setting. Combination of niacin with a statin is an attractive option for high-risk patients who do not attain their target LDL-C level on statin monotherapy and who have an HDL-C <10.3 mmol/L (<40 mg/dL). One product currently available offers the combination of lovastatin and extended-release niacin in a single tablet.

Patients with combined hyperlipidemia frequently have persistent hypertriglyceridemia on statin monotherapy. Addition of niacin or a fibrate can reduce the plasma triglyceride level in these patients. Conversely, hypertriglyceridemic patients treated with a fibrate often fail to reach their LDL-C goal and are therefore candidates for the addition of a statin. Coadministration of statins and fibrates has obvious appeal in patients with combined hyperlipidemia, but no clinical trials have assessed the effectiveness of a statin-fibrate combination compared with either a statin or a fibrate alone in reducing cardiovascular events and the long-term safety of this combination is not known. Statin-fibrate combinations are known to be associated with an increased incidence of severe myopathy (up to 2.5%) and rhabdomyolysis, and patients treated with these two drugs must be carefully counseled and monitored. This combination of drugs should be used cautiously in patients with underlying renal or hepatic insufficiency; in the elderly, frail, and chronically ill; and in those on multiple medications.

Other Approaches Occasionally, patients cannot tolerate any of the existing lipid-lowering drugs at doses required for adequate control of their lipid levels. Some patients, mostly those with genetic lipid disorders, remain significantly hypercholesterolemic despite combination drug therapy. These patients are at high risk for development or progression of CHD and clinical CHD events.

LDL APHERESIS The preferred option for management of patients with refractory or drug-resistant hypercholesterolemia is LDL apheresis. In this process, the patient's plasma is passed over a column that selectively removes the LDL, and the LDL-depleted plasma is returned to the patient. Patients on maximally tolerated combination drug therapy who have CHD and a plasma LDL-C level >5.2 mmol/L (>200 mg/dL) or no CHD and a plasma LDL-C level >7.8 mmol/L (>300 mg/dL), are candidates for every-other-week LDL apheresis.

PARTIAL ILEAL BYPASS Partial ileal bypass interrupts the enterohepatic circulation of bile acids, resulting in upregulation of the hepatic LDL receptor and reduction in plasma LDL-C levels. Diarrhea is a common side effect, and the incidence of kidney stones, gallstones, and intestinal obstruction is increased after ileal bypass surgery. The clinical utility of partial ileal bypass at this time is limited to severely hypercholesterolemic patients with normal triglycerides who cannot tolerate existing lipid-lowering medications and do not have access to LDL apheresis. Partial ileal bypass has not been proven effective in patients with severe hypercholesterolemia who have not responded adequately to statins.

Management of Low HDL-C Severely reduced plasma HDL-C [<0.5 mmol/L (<20 mg/dL)] accompanied by triglycerides <4.5 mmol/L (<400 mg/dL) usually indicates the presence of a genetic disorder, such as a mutation in apoA-I, LCAT deficiency, or Tangier disease. HDL-C levels <0.5 mmol/L (<20 mg/dL) are common in the setting of severe hypertriglyceridemia, in which case the primary focus should be on the management of the triglycerides. Secondary causes of more moderate reductions in plasma HDL [0.5 to 10.3 mmol/L (20 to 40 mg/dL)] should be considered (Table 335-5). Smoking should be discontinued, obese persons should be encouraged to lose weight, sedentary persons should be encouraged to exercise, and diabetes should be optimally controlled. When possible, medications associated with reduced plasma levels of HDL-C should be discontinued. The presence of an isolated low plasma HDL-C level in a patient with a borderline plasma LDL-C should prompt consideration of LDL-lowering drug therapy in high-risk individuals. Statins increase plasma levels of HDL-C only modestly (~5 to 10%). Fibrates also have a modest effect on plasma HDL-C levels (increasing levels ~5 to 15%) except in patients with coexisting hypertriglyceridemia, where they can be more effective. Niacin is the most effective therapeutic agent and can increase plasma HDL-C levels by up to ~30%.

The issue of whether pharmacologic intervention should be used to specifically raise HDL-C levels has not been adequately addressed in clinical trials. Pending these studies, it may be reasonable to initiate therapy (with a fibrate or niacin) directed specifically at reducing plasma triglyceride levels and raising the plasma HDL-C level in persons with established CHD and low HDL-C levels whose plasma LDL-C levels are at or below the goal.

FURTHER READING

Executive Summary of the Third Report of the National Cholesterol Education Program (NCEP) expert panel on detection, evaluation, and treatment of high blood cholesterol in adults (Adult Treatment Panel III). JAMA 285: 2486, 2001

GOLDSTEIN JL et al: Familial hypercholesterolemia, in *The Metabolic and Molecular Bases of Inherited Disease*, 8th ed, CR Scriver et al (ed). New York, McGraw-Hill, 2001, pp 2863–2913

GRUNDY SM (ed): *Cholesterol-Lowering Therapy: Evaluation of Clinical Trial Evidence*. New York, Marcel Dekker, 2000

HEART PROTECTION STUDY COLLABORATIVE GROUP: MRC/BHF Heart Protection Study of cholesterol lowering with simvastatin in 20,536 high-risk individuals: A randomised placebo-controlled trial. Lancet 360:7, 2002

MULDOON MF et al: Cholesterol reduction and non-illness mortality: Meta-analysis of randomised clinical trials. BMJ 322:11, 2001

WILSON PWF et al: Prediction of coronary heart disease using risk factor categories. Circulation 97:1837, 1998

---

336 HEMOCHROMATOSIS
Lawrie W. Powell

DEFINITION

Hemochromatosis is a common disorder of iron storage in which an inappropriate increase in intestinal iron absorption results in deposition of excessive amounts of iron in parenchymal cells with eventual tissue damage and impaired function of organs. The iron-storage pigment in tissues was called *hemosiderin* because it was believed to be derived from the blood. The term *hemosiderosis* is used to describe the presence of stainable iron in tissues, but tissue iron must be quantified to assess body iron status accurately (see below and Chap. 90). *Hemochromatosis* implies potentially severe progressive iron overload leading to fibrosis and organ failure. Cirrhosis of the liver, diabetes mellitus, arthritis, cardiomyopathy, and hypogonadotrophic hypogonadism are common manifestations.

Although there is debate about definitions, it seems logical to use the following terminology:

1. *Hereditary hemochromatosis* or *genetic hemochromatosis*: This disorder is most often caused by inheritance of a mutant gene, termed *HFE*, which is tightly linked to the HLA-A locus on chromosome 6p (see below). Rarer forms of non-*HFE* hemochromatosis due to mutation in other key genes involved in iron metabolism have recently been described (Table 336-1). The disease can be recognized during its early stages when iron overload and organ damage are min-

TABLE 336-1 *Classification of Iron Overload States*

HEREDITARY HEMOCHROMATOSIS

Hemochromatosis, *HFE*-related (type 1)
 C282Y homozygosity
 C282Y/H63D compound heterozygosity
Hemochromatosis non-*HFE*-related
 Juvenile hemochromatosis (type 2)
 Mutated transferrin receptor 2 *TFR2* (type 3)
 Mutated ferroportin 1 (Ireg1) gene, *SLC11A3* (type 4)
 Mutated H Ferritin IRE (type 5)
 Solomon Island hemochromatosis (?defect) (type 6)

ACQUIRED IRON OVERLOAD

Iron-loading anemias	Chronic liver disease
Thalassemia major	Hepatitis C
Sideroblastic anemia	Alcoholic cirrhosis, especially
Chronic hemolytic	when advanced
anemias	Nonalcoholic steatohepatitis
Transfusional and	Porphyria cutanea tarda
parenteral iron	Dysmetabolic iron overload
overload	syndrome
Dietary iron overload	Post portacaval shunting

MISCELLANEOUS

Iron overload in sub-Sahara Africa
Neonatal iron overload
Aceruloplasminemia
Congenital atransferrinemia

imal. At this stage the disease is best referred to as *early hemochromatosis* or *precirrhotic hemochromatosis*.

2. *Secondary iron overload*: Tissue injury usually occurs secondary to an iron-loading anemia such as thalassemia or sideroblastic anemia, in which increased erythropoiesis is ineffective. In the acquired iron-loading disorders, massive iron deposits in parenchymal tissues can lead to the same clinical and pathologic features as in hemochromatosis.

PREVALENCE

HFE-associated hemochromatosis is one of the most common genetic diseases, although its prevalence varies in different ethnic groups. It is most common in populations of northern European extraction in whom approximately 1 in 10 persons are heterozygous carriers and 0.3 to 0.5% are homozygotes. However, expression of the disease is modified by several factors, especially alcohol consumption and dietary iron intake, blood loss associated with menstruation and pregnancy, and blood donation. The clinical expression of the disease is 5 to 10 times more frequent in men than in women. Nearly 70% of affected patients develop the first symptoms between ages 40 and 60. The disease is rarely evident before age 20, although with family screening (see below) and periodic health examinations, asymptomatic subjects with iron overload can be identified, including young menstruating women. Recent studies in European non-blood bank populations have revealed that 30% or more of homozygous individuals do not have evidence of iron overload. Thus, the penetrance of the mutation is variable.

GENETIC BASIS AND MODE OF INHERITANCE

The *HFE* gene involved in the most common form of hemochromatosis was cloned in 1996. A homozygous G → A mutation resulting in a cysteine to tyrosine substitution at position 282 (C282Y) is the most common mutation. It is identified in 85 to 100% of patients with hereditary hemochromatosis in populations of northern European descent but is found in only 60% of cases from Mediterranean populations (e.g., southern Italy). A second, relatively common *HFE* mutation has also been identified. This results in an amino acid substitution of histidine to aspartic acid at position 63 (H63D). Homozygosity for H63D is not associated with clinically significant iron overload. Some compound heterozygotes (e.g., one copy each of C282Y and H63D) have mild to moderately increased body iron stores. Thus, *HFE*-

associated hemochromatosis is inherited as an autosomal recessive trait; heterozygotes have no, or minimal, increase in iron stores. However, in some cases this slight increase in hepatic iron acts as a cofactor that aggravates other diseases such as porphyria cutanea tarda (PCT) and nonalcoholic steatohepatitis.

Mutations in other genes are responsible for non-*HFE* associated hemochromatosis, including juvenile hemochromatosis, which affects persons in the second and third decade of life (Table 336-1).

PATHOGENESIS

Normally, the body iron content of 3 to 4 g is maintained such that intestinal mucosal absorption of iron is equal to iron loss. This amount is approximately 1 mg/d in men and 1.5 mg/d in menstruating women. In hemochromatosis, mucosal absorption is inappropriate to body needs and amounts to 4 mg/d or more. The progressive accumulation of iron causes an early elevation in plasma iron, an increased saturation of transferrin, and progressive elevation of plasma ferritin level (Fig. 336-1). A liver protein, hepcidin, is proposed to increase *HFE*-mediated reticuloendothelial cell iron retention and to decrease intestinal iron uptake, thereby linking body stores with intestinal iron absorption.

The *HFE* gene encodes a 343-amino-acid protein that is structurally related to MHC class I proteins. The basic defect in hemochromatosis is a lack of cell surface expression of HFE (due to the C282Y mutation). The normal (wild type) HFE protein forms a complex with β_2-microglobulin and transferrin, and the C282Y mutation completely abrogates this interaction. As a result, the mutant HFE protein remains trapped intracellularly, reducing transferrin receptor–mediated iron uptake by the intestinal crypt cell. This is postulated to upregulate the divalent metal transporter (DMT-1) on the brush border of the villus cells, leading to inappropriately increased intestinal iron absorption (Fig. 336-2). In advanced disease, the body may contain 20 g or more of iron that is deposited mainly in parenchymal cells of the liver, pancreas, and heart. Iron may be increased 50- to 100-fold in the liver and pancreas and 5- to 25-fold in the heart. Iron deposition in the pituitary causes hypogonadotropic hypogonadism in both men and women. Tis-

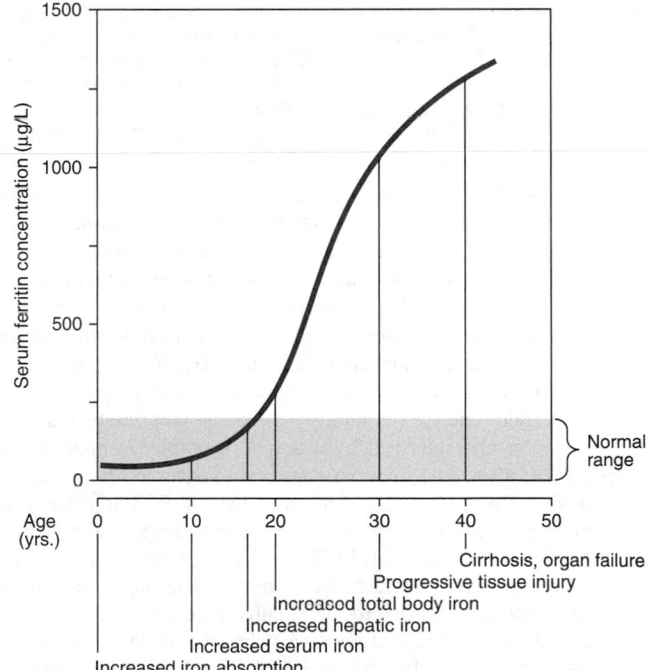

FIGURE 336-1 Sequence of events in genetic hemochromatosis and their correlation with the serum ferritin concentration. Increased iron absorption is present throughout life. Overt, symptomatic disease usually develops between ages 40 and 60, but latent disease can be detected long before this.

FIGURE 336-2 Pathways of normal iron homeostasis. Iron is absorbed in the proximal intestine after conversion from the ferric (Fe^{3+}) to the ferrous (Fe^{2+}) state by duodenal cytochrome D (DcytD), a ferrireductase. At the apical membrane of the mature villus cell, iron is imported by the divalent metal transporter (DMT1). Iron may be stored within the cell as ferritin or transferred across the basolateral membrane by the transporter, IREG1 (ferroportin-1), and is reoxidized by hephaestin (Heph) before binding to the transport protein, transferrin (Tf). Circulating iron is acquired by the liver primarily through the classic transferrin receptor-1 (TfR1) and by the related transferrin receptor-2 (TfR2). Reticuloendothelial macrophages acquire iron mainly by phagocytosis of senescent erythrocytes, and the iron is released via the iron export protein, IREG1. The released iron is oxidized to the ferric state by ceruloplasmin (Cp) before binding to transferrin. In response to increased iron, the liver produces hepcidin, which appears to communicate the level of iron stores to intestinal cells and reticuloendothelial (RE) cells. Hepcidin deficiency mimics hemochromatosis, as it is associated with increased intestinal iron absorption and decreased iron uptake in reticuloendothelial cells. HFE is a MHC class 1 molecule that forms a complex with β_2 microglobulin (β_2-M) and binds to TfR1.

Patients with hereditary hemochromatosis (HH) caused by *HFE* mutations fail to express a functional β_2-M:HFE:TfR complex. In addition, they have decreased hepatic expression of hepcidin. Although the pathogenesis of HH is incompletely understood, decreased expression of HFE in the intestine is thought to result in low iron levels in the crypt cells, leading to inappropriate upregulation of DMT1 and IREG1. This causes increased intestinal iron absorption, leading to increased tissue iron stores, with paradoxical sparing of iron loading in the RE system, perhaps because iron is efficiently exported by IREG1. Hb, hemoglobin. Also, a decreased expression of HFE in the liver may result in decreased hepcidin synthesis and upregulation of iron absorption.

sue injury may result from disruption of iron-laden lysosomes, from lipid peroxidation of subcellular organelles by excess iron, or from stimulation of collagen synthesis by activated stellate cells.

Secondary iron overload with deposition in parenchymal cells occurs in chronic disorders of erythropoiesis, particularly in those due to defects in hemoglobin synthesis or ineffective erythropoiesis such as sideroblastic anemia and thalassemia (Chap. 91). In these disorders, the absorption of iron is increased. Moreover, these patients require blood transfusions and are frequently treated inappropriately with iron. PCT, a disorder characterized by a defect in porphyrin biosynthesis (Chap. 337), is also sometimes associated with excessive parenchymal iron deposits. The magnitude of the iron load in PCT is usually insufficient to produce tissue damage. However, recent reports have found that many patients with PCT also have mutations in the *HFE* gene, and some have associated hepatitis C infection. Although the relationship among these disorders remains to be clarified, iron overload accentuates the inherited enzyme deficiency in PCT and should be avoided along with other agents (alcohol, estrogens, haloaromatic compounds) that may exacerbate PCT. Another cause of hepatic parenchymal iron overload is hereditary aceruloplasminemia. In this disorder, impairment of iron mobilization due to deficiency of ceruloplasmin (a ferroxidase) causes iron overload in hepatocytes. End-stage liver disease may also be associated with iron overload of the degree seen in hemochromatosis. The mechanism is uncertain, although hemolysis plays a role. Hemochromatosis in a heavy drinker can be distinguished from alcoholic liver disease by the presence of the C282Y mutation.

Excessive iron ingestion over many years rarely results in hemochromatosis. An important exception has been reported in South Africa among groups who brew fermented beverages in vessels made of iron. Hemochromatosis has been described in apparently normal persons who have taken medicinal iron over many years, but such individuals probably had a genetic disorder.

The common denominator in all patients with hemochromatosis is *excessive amounts of iron in parenchymal tissues.* Parenteral administration of iron in the form of blood transfusions or iron preparations results predominantly in reticuloendothelial cell iron overload. This appears to lead to less tissue damage than iron loading of parenchymal cells.

PATHOLOGY

At autopsy, the enlarged nodular liver and pancreas are rusty in color. Histologically, iron is increased in many organs, particularly in the liver, heart, and pancreas, and to a lesser extent in the endocrine glands.

The epidermis of the skin is thin, and melanin is increased in the cells of the basal layer. Deposits of iron are present around the synovial lining cells of the joints.

In the liver of patients with hemochromatosis, parenchymal iron is in the form of ferritin and hemosiderin. In the early stages these deposits are seen in the periportal parenchymal cells, especially within lysosomes in the pericanalicular cytoplasm of the hepatocytes. This stage progresses to perilobular fibrosis and eventually to deposition of iron in bile duct epithelium, Kupffer cells, and fibrous septa due to activation of stellate cells. In the advanced stage, a macronodular or mixed macro- and micronodular cirrhosis develops.

CLINICAL MANIFESTATIONS

Initial symptoms include weakness, lassitude, change in skin color, abdominal pain, loss of libido, and symptoms of diabetes mellitus. Hepatomegaly, increased pigmentation, spider angiomas, splenomegaly, arthropathy, ascites, cardiac arrhythmias, congestive heart failure, loss of body hair, testicular atrophy, and jaundice are prominent in advanced disease.

The *liver* is usually the first organ to be affected, and hepatomegaly is present in more than 95% of symptomatic patients. Hepatic enlargement may exist in the absence of symptoms or of abnormal liver function tests. Indeed, over half of patients with symptomatic hemochromatosis have little laboratory evidence of functional impairment of the liver, in spite of hepatomegaly and fibrosis. Loss of body hair, palmar erythema, testicular atrophy, and gynecomastia are common. Manifestations of portal hypertension and esophageal varices occur less commonly than in cirrhosis from other causes. Hepatocellular carcinoma develops in about 30% of patients with cirrhosis, and it is the most common cause of death in treated patients; hence the importance of early diagnosis and therapy. Its incidence increases with age, is more common in men, and occurs almost exclusively in cirrhotic patients. Splenomegaly occurs in approximately half of symptomatic cases.

Excessive skin pigmentation is present in over 90% of symptomatic patients at the time of diagnosis. The characteristic metallic or slate gray hue is sometimes referred to as bronzing and results from increased melanin and iron in the dermis. Pigmentation usually is diffuse and generalized, but it may be more pronounced on the face, neck, extensor aspects of the lower forearms, dorsa of the hands, lower legs, genital regions, and in scars.

Diabetes mellitus occurs in about 65% of patients and is more likely to develop in those with a family history of diabetes, suggesting that direct damage to the pancreatic islets by iron deposition occurs in combination with a genetic predisposition. The management is similar to that of other forms of diabetes, although pronounced insulin resistance is more common in association with hemochromatosis. Late complications are the same as seen in other causes of diabetes mellitus.

Arthropathy develops in 25 to 50% of patients. It usually occurs after age 50, but may occur as a first manifestation, or long after therapy. The joints of the hands, especially the second and third metacarpophalangeal joints, are usually the first joints involved, a feature that helps to distinguish the chondrocalcinosis associated with hemochromatosis from the idiopathic form (Chap. 313). A progressive polyarthritis involving wrists, hips, ankles, and knees may also ensue. Acute brief attacks of synovitis may be associated with deposition of calcium pyrophosphate (chondrocalcinosis or pseudogout), mainly in the knees. Radiologic manifestations include cystic changes of the subchondral bones, loss of articular cartilage with narrowing of the joint space, diffuse demineralization, hypertrophic bone proliferation, and calcification of the synovium. The arthropathy tends to progress despite removal of iron by phlebotomy. Although the relation of these abnormalities to iron metabolism is not known, the fact that similar changes occur in other forms of iron overload suggests that iron is directly involved.

Cardiac involvement is the presenting manifestation in about 15% of patients. The most common manifestation is congestive heart fail-

ure, which occurs in about 10% of young adults with the disease, especially those with juvenile hemochromatosis. Symptoms of congestive failure may develop suddenly, with rapid progression to death if untreated. The heart is diffusely enlarged and may be misdiagnosed as idiopathic cardiomyopathy if other overt manifestations are absent. Cardiac arrhythmias include premature supraventricular beats, paroxysmal tachyarrhythmias, atrial flutter, atrial fibrillation, and varying degrees of atrioventricular block.

Hypogonadism occurs in both sexes and may antedate other clinical features. Manifestations include loss of libido, impotence, amenorrhea, testicular atrophy, gynecomastia, and sparse body hair. These changes are primarily the result of decreased production of gonadotropins due to impairment of hypothalamic-pituitary function by iron deposition; however, primary testicular dysfunction may be seen in some cases. Adrenal insufficiency, hypothyroidism, and hypoparathyroidism may also occur.

DIAGNOSIS

The association of (1) hepatomegaly, (2) skin pigmentation, (3) diabetes mellitus, (4) heart disease, (5) arthritis, and (6) hypogonadism should suggest the diagnosis. However, a parenchymal iron overload of comparatively short duration or modest degree may exist with none or only some of these manifestations [e.g., in young patients (Fig. 336-1)]. Therefore, a high index of suspicion is needed to make the diagnosis early. Treatment before there is permanent organ damage can reverse the iron toxicity and restore life expectancy to normal.

The history should be particularly detailed in regard to disease in other family members, alcohol ingestion, iron intake, and ingestion of large doses of ascorbic acid, which promotes iron absorption (Chap. 61). Appropriate tests should be performed to exclude iron deposition due to hematologic disease. The presence of liver, pancreatic, cardiac, and joint disease should be confirmed by physical examination, roentgenography, and standard function tests of these organs. The degree of increase in total-body iron stores should be assessed with particular attention to an increase in parenchymal iron concentration, with or without tissue damage.

The methods available for assessing parenchymal iron stores include (1) measurement of serum iron and the percent saturation of transferrin (or the unsaturated iron-binding capacity); (2) measurement of serum ferritin concentration; (3) liver biopsy with measurement of the iron concentration and calculation of the hepatic iron index (Table 336-2), (4) estimation of chelatable iron stores following the administration of deferoxamine; and (5) computed tomography (CT) and/or magnetic resonance imaging (MRI) of the liver. Each has its advantages and limitations. The serum iron level and percent saturation of transferrin are elevated early in the course, but their specificity is reduced by significant false-positive and false-negative rates. For example, serum iron concentration may be increased in patients with alcoholic liver disease without iron overload; in this situation, however, the hepatic iron index is usually not increased as in hemochromatosis (Table 336-1). In otherwise healthy persons, a fasting serum transferrin saturation greater than 50% is abnormal and suggests homozygosity for hemochromatosis.

The serum ferritin concentration is usually a good index of body iron stores, whether decreased or increased. In fact, an increase of 1 μg/L in serum ferritin level reflects an increase of about 65 mg in body stores. In most untreated patients with hemochromatosis, the serum ferritin level is greatly increased (Fig. 336-1 and Table 336-1). However, in patients with inflammation and hepatocellular necrosis, serum ferritin levels may be elevated out of proportion to body iron stores due to increased release from tissues. A repeat determination of serum ferritin should therefore be carried out after acute hepatocellular damage has subsided, e.g., in alcoholic liver disease. Ordinarily, the combined measurements of the percent transferrin saturation and serum ferritin level provide a simple and reliable screening test for hemochromatosis, including the precirrhotic phase of the disease. If ei-

TABLE 336-2 *Representative Iron Values in Normal Subjects, Patients with Hemochromatosis, and Patients with Alcoholic Liver Disease*

Determination	Normal	Symptomatic Hemochromatosis	Homozygotes with Early, Asymptomatic Hemochromatosis	Heterozygotes	Alcoholic Liver Disease
Plasma iron, μmol/L (μg/dL)	9–27 (50–150)	32–54 (180–300)	Usually elevated	Elevated or normal	Often elevated
Total iron-binding capacity, μmol/L (μg/dL)	45–66 (250–370)	36–54 (200–300)	36–54 (200–300)	Elevated or normal	45–66 (250–370)
Transferrin saturation, percent	22–46	50–100	50–100	Normal or elevated	27–60
Serum ferritin, μg/L	10–200	900–6000	200–500	Usually <500	10–500
Urinary iron,[a] mg/24 h	0–2	9–23	2–5	2–5	Usually <5
Liver iron, μg/g dry wt	300–1400	6000–18,000	2000–4000	300–3000	300–2000
Hepatic iron index $\dfrac{(\mu g/g\ dry\ wt)}{56 \times age}$	<1.0	>2	Usually >2	<2	<2

[a] After intramuscular administration of 0.5 g deferoxamine.

ther of these tests is abnormal, genetic testing for hemochromatosis should be performed (Fig. 336-3).

The role of liver biopsy in the diagnosis and management of hemochromatosis has been reassessed as a result of the widespread availability of genetic testing for the C282Y mutation. The absence of severe fibrosis can be accurately predicted in most patients using clinical and biochemical variables. Thus, there is virtually no risk of severe fibrosis in a C282Y homozygous subject with: (1) serum ferritin level less than 1000 μg/L; (2) normal serum alanine amino transaminase values; (3) no hepatomegaly; and (4) no excess alcohol intake. However, it should be emphasized that liver biopsy is the only reliable method for establishing or excluding the presence of hepatic cirrhosis, which is the critical factor determining prognosis and the risk of developing hepatocellular carcinoma. Biopsy also permits histochemical estimation of tissue iron and measurement of hepatic iron concentration. Increased density of the liver due to iron deposition can be demonstrated by CT or MRI. A retrospective assessment of body iron storage is also provided by performing weekly phlebotomy and calculating the amount of iron removed before iron stores are exhausted (1 mL blood = approximately 0.5 mg iron).

SCREENING FOR HEMOCHROMATOSIS

When the diagnosis of hemochromatosis is established, it is important to counsel and screen other family members (Chap. 58). Asymptomatic as well as symptomatic family members with the disease usually have an increased saturation of transferrin and an increased serum ferritin concentration. These changes occur even before the iron stores are greatly increased (Fig. 336-1). All first-degree relatives of patients with hemochromatosis should be tested for the C282Y and H63D mutations and advised appropriately. In affected individuals, it is important to confirm or exclude the presence of cirrhosis and begin therapy as early as possible. When children of a proband are affected, a homozygote-heterozygote mating is most likely.

The role of population screening for hemochromatosis is controversial. Hemochromatosis fulfills the criteria established by the World Health Organization for population screening, and DNA testing could, in principle, be performed along with other neonatal tests. However, because iron overload does not develop until the second, third, or fourth decades, and the degree of penetrance is still uncertain, screening for phenotypic expression in adults is more practical at present (Fig. 336-3).

℞ TREATMENT

The therapy of hemochromatosis involves removal of the excess body iron and supportive treatment of damaged organs. Iron removal is best begun by weekly or twice-weekly phlebotomy of 500 mL. Although there is an initial modest decline in the volume of packed red blood cells to about 35 mL/dL, the level stabilizes after several weeks. The plasma transferrin saturation remains increased until the available iron stores are depleted. In contrast, the plasma ferritin concentration falls progressively, reflecting the gradual decrease in body iron stores. Since one 500-mL unit of blood contains 200 to 250 mg iron and about 25 g iron should be removed, weekly phlebotomy may be required for 1 or 2 years. When the transferrin saturation and ferritin level become normal, phlebotomies are performed at appropriate intervals to maintain levels within the normal range. The measurements promptly become abnormal with iron reaccumulation. Usually one phlebotomy every 3 months will suffice.

Chelating agents such as deferoxamine, when given parenterally, remove 10 to 20 mg iron per day, which is much less than that mobilized by once-weekly phlebotomy. Phlebotomy is also less expensive, more convenient, and safer for most patients. However, chelating agents are indicated when anemia or hypoproteinemia is severe enough to preclude phlebotomy. Subcutaneous infusion of deferoxamine using a portable pump is the most effective means of administration.

Alcohol consumption should be severely curtailed or eliminated as it increases the risk of cirrhosis in hereditary hemochromatosis nearly tenfold. The management of hepatic failure, cardiac failure, and diabetes mellitus is similar to conventional therapy for these conditions. Loss of libido and change in secondary sex characteristics are partially

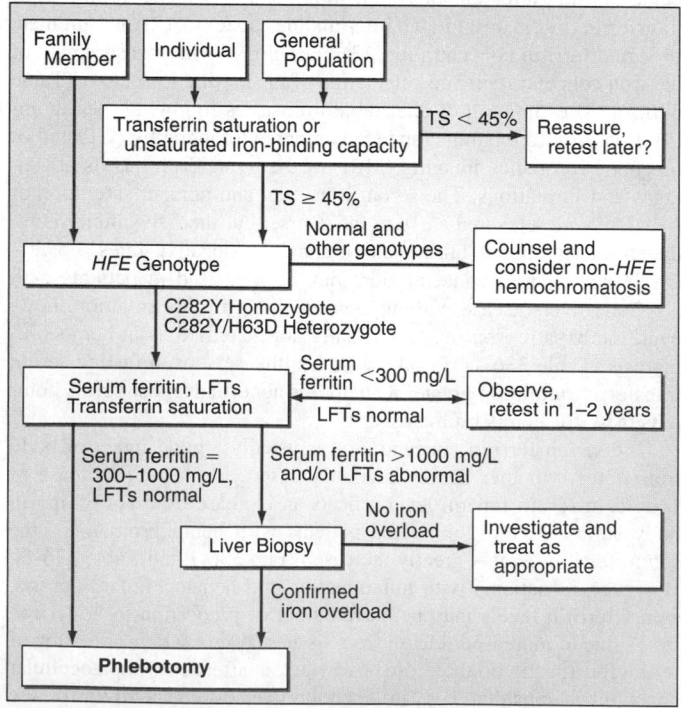

FIGURE 336-3 Algorithm for screening for *HFE*-associated hemochromatosis. LFT, liver function tests; TS, transferrin saturation. (*With permission from The Canadian Journal of Gastroenterology.*)

relieved by parenteral testosterone or gonadotropin therapy (Chap. 325).

PROGNOSIS

The principal causes of death are cardiac failure (30%), hepatocellular failure or portal hypertension (25%), and hepatocellular carcinoma (30%).

Life expectancy is improved by removal of the excessive stores of iron and maintenance of these stores at near-normal levels. The 5-year survival rate with therapy increases from 33 to 89%. With repeated phlebotomy, the liver and spleen decrease in size, liver function improves, pigmentation of skin decreases, and cardiac failure may be reversed. Diabetes improves in about 40%, but removal of excess iron has little effect on hypogonadism or arthropathy. Hepatic fibrosis may decrease, but cirrhosis is irreversible. End-stage liver disease can be treated with orthotopic liver transplantation, but the results are suboptimal unless excess iron stores are first corrected. Hepatocellular carcinoma usually occurs as a late sequela in patients who are cirrhotic at presentation. The apparent increase in its incidence in treated patients is probably related to their increased life span. Hepatocellular carcinoma does not appear to develop if the disease is treated in the precirrhotic stage. Indeed, the life expectancy of homozygotes treated before the development of cirrhosis is normal.

The importance of family screening and early therapy cannot be emphasized too strongly. Asymptomatic individuals detected by family studies should have phlebotomy therapy if iron stores are moderately to severely increased. Assessment of iron stores at appropriate intervals is also important. With this management approach, most manifestations of the disease can be prevented.

ACKNOWLEDGMENT
The author acknowledges the contribution of Dr. Kurt J. Isselbacher to this chapter in previous editions of Harrison's.

FURTHER READING

BEUTLER E et al: Penetrance of 845G → A (C282Y) *HFE* hereditary haemochromatosis mutation in the USA. Lancet 359:211, 2002

BRIDLE KR et al: Disrupted hepcidin regulation in HFE-associated haemochromatosis and the liver as a regulator of body iron homeostasis. Lancet 361:669, 2003

EDWARDS CQ et al: Prevalence of hemochromatosis among 11,065 presumably healthy blood donors. N Engl J Med 318:1355, 1988

FLEMING RE, SLY WS: Mechanisms of iron accumulation in hereditary hemochromatosis. Annu Rev Physiol 64:663, 2002

NICOLAS G et al: Lack of hepcidin expression and severe tissue iron overload in upstream stimulatory factor 2 (USF2) knockout mice. Proc Natl Acad Sci USA 98:8780, 2001

OLYNYK JK et al: A population based study of the clinical expression of the hemochromatosis gene. N Engl J Med 341:718, 1999

337 THE PORPHYRIAS
Robert J. Desnick

The porphyrias are inherited disorders, each involving a specific enzyme in the heme biosynthetic pathway (Fig. 337-1). These disorders are classified as either *hepatic* or *erythropoietic* depending on the primary site of overproduction and accumulation of the porphyrin precursor or porphyrin (Tables 337-1 and 337-2), although some have overlapping features. The major manifestations of the hepatic porphyrias are neurologic, including neuropathic abdominal pain, neuropathy, and mental disturbances, whereas the erythropoietic porphyrias characteristically cause cutaneous photosensitivity. The reason for neurologic involvement in the hepatic porphyrias is poorly understood. Cutaneous sensitivity to sunlight is due to long-wave ultraviolet light excitation of excess porphyrins in the skin, leading to cell damage, scarring, and deformation. Steroid hormones, drugs, and nutrition influence the production of porphyrin precursors and porphyrins, thereby precipitating or increasing the severity of some porphyrias. Thus, the porphyrias are ecogenetic disorders in which environmental, physiologic, and genetic factors interact to cause disease.

Because many symptoms of the porphyrias are nonspecific, diagnosis is often delayed. Laboratory testing is required to confirm or exclude the various types of porphyria (Table 337-2). Urinary δ-aminolevulinic acid (ALA) and porphobilinogen (PBG) are easily quantitated by chemical methods; the urinary porphyrin isomers can be separated and quantitated by high-performance liquid chromatography. The diagnostic profile of accumulated precursors and/or porphyrins in each disorder can also be defined by extraction and thin-layer chromatography of fecal porphyrins. However, a definite diagnosis requires demonstration of the specific enzyme deficiency or gene defect. The isolation and characterization of the cDNAs encoding the heme biosynthetic enzymes have permitted identification of the genetic basis of each porphyria. Molecular genetic analyses now make it possible to provide precise heterozygote identification and prenatal diagnoses in families with known mutations.

HEME BIOSYNTHESIS The first and last three enzymes in the heme biosynthetic pathway are located in the mitochondrion, whereas the other four are cytosolic (Fig. 337-1). The first enzyme, δ-aminolevulinate synthase (ALA-synthase), catalyzes the condensation of glycine, activated by pyridoxal phosphate and succinyl coenzyme A, to form ALA. In the liver, this rate-limiting enzyme can be induced by a variety of drugs, steroids, and other chemicals. Distinct erythroid-specific and nonerythroid (e.g., housekeeping) forms of ALA-synthase are encoded by separate genes; defects in the erythroid form cause X-linked sideroblastic anemia (XLSA).

The second enzyme, δ-aminolevulinate dehydratase (ALA-dehydratase), catalyzes the condensation of two molecules of ALA to form PBG. Four molecules of PBG condense to form the tetrapyrrole uroporphyrinogen (URO) III by a two-step process catalyzed by hydroxymethylbilane (HMB) synthase (also known as PBG-deaminase or URO I synthase) and URO III synthase. HMB synthase catalyzes the head-to-tail condensation of four PBG molecules by a series of deaminations to form the linear tetrapyrrole, HMB. URO-synthase catalyzes the rearrangement and rapid cyclization of HMB to form the asymmetric, physiologic, octacarboxylate porphyrinogen URO III isomer.

The fifth enzyme in the pathway, URO-decarboxylase, catalyzes the sequential removal of the four carboxyl groups from the acetic acid side chains of URO III to form coproporphyrinogen (COPRO) III, a tetracarboxylate porphyrinogen. This compound then enters the mitochondrion, where COPRO-oxidase, the sixth enzyme, catalyzes the decarboxylation of two of the four propionic acid groups to form the two vinyl groups of protoporphyrinogen (PROTO) IX, a dicarboxylate porphyrinogen. Next, PROTO-oxidase oxidizes PROTO IX to protoporphyrin IX by the removal of six hydrogen atoms. The product of the reaction is a porphyrin (oxidized form), in contrast to the preceding tetrapyrrole intermediates, which are porphyrinogens (reduced forms). Finally, ferrous iron is inserted into protoporphyrin IX to form heme, a reaction catalyzed by the eighth enzyme in the pathway, ferrochelatase (also known as heme synthetase or protoheme ferrolyase).

Mutations causing their respective porphyria have been identified in each of these genes. Thus, molecular diagnosis is now available for each porphyria, which is important in many cases where the diagnosis by other methods may be difficult.

REGULATION OF HEME BIOSYNTHESIS About 85% of the heme produced in the body is synthesized in erythroid cells to provide heme for hemoglobin; most of the remainder is produced in the liver, where the

MITOCHONDRIA

Succinyl COA

ALA-SYNTHASE

Glycine

FEEDBACK REPRESSION

Heme

FERROCHELATASE

$2 H^+$
Fe^{++}

Protoporphyrin IX

$6H$

PROTO-OXIDASE

Protoporphyrinogen IX

COPRO-OXIDASE

$2CO_2$ $2 H$

CYTOPLASM

ALA-DEHYDRATASE

δ-Aminolevulinic acid

H_2O

Porphobilinogen

HMB-SYNTHASE

$4 NH_3$

Hydroxymethylbilane

URO-SYNTHASE

H_2O

Uroporphyrinogen III

URO-DECARBOXYLASE

$4 H$
$4 CO_2$

Coproporphyrinogen III

FIGURE 337-1 The human heme biosynthetic pathway.

biosynthetic pathway is under negative feedback control. "Free" heme in the liver regulates the synthesis and mitochondrial translocation of the housekeeping form of ALA-synthase. Heme represses the synthesis of the ALA-synthase mRNA and interferes with the transport of the enzyme from the cytosol into mitochondria. ALA-synthase is increased by many of the same chemicals that induce the cytochrome P450 enzymes in the endoplasmic reticulum of the liver. Because most of the heme in the liver is used for the synthesis of cytochrome P450 enzymes, hepatic ALA-synthase and the cytochrome P450s are regulated in a coordinated fashion.

Different regulatory mechanisms control the production of heme for hemoglobin. The erythroid-specific ALA-synthase is encoded on the X-chromosome and it is expressed at higher levels than the hepatic

enzyme. An erythroid-specific control mechanism regulates iron transport into erythroid cells. During erythroid differentiation, the activities of the heme biosynthetic enzymes are increased.

THE HEPATIC PORPHYRIAS

The acute hepatic porphyrias are characterized by the rapid onset of neurologic manifestations. During the acute attack, individuals have markedly elevated plasma and urinary concentrations of the porphyrin precursors ALA and PBG, which originate from the liver.

ALA-DEHYDRATASE–DEFICIENT PORPHYRIA

This is a rare autosomal recessive disorder that has been described in only a few patients. Onset and severity of the disease are variable, presumably depending on the amount of residual ALA-dehydratase activity. Clinical features include abdominal pain and neuropathy, resembling acute intermittent porphyria (AIP; see below). Patients have increased urinary levels of ALA and coproporphyrin. ALA-dehydratase activity in erythrocytes is <5% of normal. Lead intoxication and hereditary tyrosinemia (fumarylacetoacetase deficiency) should be considered in the differential diagnosis of ALA-dehydratase–deficient porphyria, as they can inhibit ALA-dehydratase. DNA analyses reveal a variety of missense mutations that result in the amino acid substitutions in ALA-dehydratase. Heterozygotes are clinically asymptomatic and do not excrete increased levels of ALA, but they can be detected by demonstration of intermediate levels of erythrocyte ALA-dehydratase activity or by demonstrating a specific mutation in the *ALA-dehydratase* gene. Prenatal diagnosis of this disorder has not been achieved but should be possible by determination of the ALA-dehydratase activity and/or gene mutation in cultured chorionic villi or amniocytes. Treatment and prevention of the neurologic complications are the same as for other acute porphyrias (see below).

ACUTE INTERMITTENT PORPHYRIA
This hepatic porphyria is an autosomal dominant condition resulting from the half-normal level of HMB-synthase activity. The disease is widespread but is especially common in Scandinavia and Great Britain. The enzyme deficiency can be demonstrated in most heterozygous individuals, but clinical expression is highly variable. Activation of the disease is related to environmental or hormonal factors, such as drugs, diet, and steroid hormones, which can precipitate the manifestations. Attacks can be prevented by avoiding known precipitating factors.

Clinical Features Most heterozygotes remain clinically asymptomatic (latent) unless exposed to factors that increase the production of porphyrins. Endogenous and exogenous gonadal steroids, porphyrinogenic drugs, alcohol ingestion, and low-calorie diets, usually instituted for weight loss, are common precipitating factors. Table 337-3 provides a partial list of the major drugs that are harmful in AIP [and also in hereditary coproporphyria (HCP) and variegate porphyria (VP)] and some drugs and anesthetic agents known to be safe. More extensive lists of drugs considered harmful or safe are available (Anderson et al., 2001), but information is incomplete for many of them. Attacks also can be provoked by infections and surgery.

Because the neurovisceral symptoms rarely occur before puberty and are often nonspecific, a high index of suspicion is required to make the diagnosis. The disease can be disabling but is rarely fatal. Abdominal pain, the most common symptom, is usually steady and poorly localized but may be due to cramps. Ileus, abdominal distention, and decreased bowel sounds are common. However, increased bowel sounds and diarrhea may occur. Abdominal tenderness, fever, and leukocytosis are usually absent or mild because the symptoms are neurologic rather than inflammatory. Nausea, vomiting, constipation, tachycardia, hypertension, mental symptoms, pain in the limbs, head, neck, or chest, muscle weakness, sensory loss, dysuria, and urinary retention are characteristic. Tachycardia, hypertension, restlessness, tremors, and excess sweating are due to sympathetic overactivity.

The peripheral neuropathy is due to axonal degeneration (rather than demyelinization) and primarily affects motor neurons. Significant neuropathy does not occur with all acute attacks; abdominal symptoms are usually more prominent. Motor neuropathy affects the proximal muscles initially, more often in the shoulders and arms. The course and degree of involvement are variable. Deep tendon reflexes may be normal or hyperactive but are usually decreased or absent with advanced neuropathy. Motor weakness can be asymmetric and focal and may involve cranial nerves. Sensory changes such as paresthesia and loss of sensation are less prominent. Progressive muscle weakness can lead to respiratory and bulbar paralysis and death when diagnosis and treatment are delayed. Sudden death may result from sympathetic overactivity and cardiac arrhythmia.

Mental symptoms such as anxiety, insomnia, depression, disorientation, hallucinations, and paranoia can occur in acute attacks. Seizures can be due to neurologic effects or to hyponatremia. Treatment of seizures is difficult because virtually all antiseizure drugs (except bromides) may exacerbate AIP (clonazepam may be safer than phenytoin or barbiturates). Hyponatremia results from hypothalamic involvement and inappropriate vasopressin secretion or from electrolyte depletion due to vomiting, diarrhea, poor intake, or excess renal sodium loss. Persistent hypertension and impaired renal function may occur. When an attack resolves, abdominal pain may disappear within hours, and paresis begins to improve within days and may continue to improve over several years.

Diagnosis ALA and PBG levels are increased in plasma and urine during acute attacks. Urinary PBG excretion is usually 220 to 880 μmol/d (50 to 200 mg/d) [normal, 0 to 18 μmol/d (0 to 4 mg/d)], and urinary ALA excretion is 150 to 760 μmol/d (20 to 100 mg/d) [normal, 8 to 53 μmol/d (1 to 7 mg/d)]. The excretion of these compounds generally decreases with clinical improvement, particularly after hematin infusions (see below). A normal urinary PBG level effectively excludes AIP as a cause for current symptoms. Fecal porphyrins are usually normal or minimally increased in AIP, in contrast to HCP and VP. Most asymptomatic ("latent") heterozygotes with HMB-synthase deficiency have normal urinary excretion of ALA and PBG. Therefore, measurement of HMB-synthase in erythrocytes, or better, the detection of the family's HMB-synthase mutation, will diagnose asymptomatic family members.

The enzyme deficiency is detectable in erythrocytes from most AIP heterozygotes (*classic AIP*). Note that the activity is higher in young erythrocytes and may increase into the normal range in AIP when erythropoiesis is increased due to a concurrent condition. However, patients with the rare erythroid form of AIP (*erythroid, or variant, AIP*) have normal enzyme levels in erythrocytes and deficient activity in nonerythroid tissues (see below). The erythroid and housekeeping forms of HMB-synthase are encoded by a single gene, which has two promoters: one promoter generates the ubiquitously expressed housekeeping mRNA; the other promoter transcribes the erythroid-specific mRNA. Several deletions and >175 different mutations have been

TABLE 337-1 Classification of the Human Porphyrias

Type/Porphyria	Deficient Enzyme	Inheritance[a]	Photosensitivity	Neurovisceral Symptoms
HEPATIC PORPHYRIAS				
ALA-dehydratase deficiency (ADP)	ALA-dehydratase	AR	−	+
Acute intermittent porphyria (AIP)	HMB-synthase	AD	−	+
Porphyria cutanea tarda (PCT)	URO-decarboxylase	AD	+++	−
Hereditary coproporphyria (HCP)	COPRO-oxidase	AD	+	+
Variegate porphyria (VP)	PROTO-oxidase	AD	+	+
ERYTHROPOIETIC PORPHYRIAS				
X-linked sideroblastic anemia (XLSA)	ALA-synthase	XLR	−	−
Congenital erythropoietic porphyria (CEP)	URO-synthase	AR	+++	−
Erythropoietic protoporphyria (EPP)	Ferrochelatase	AD	+	−

[a] AR, autosomal recessive; AD, autosomal dominant; XLR, X-linked recessive.
Note: ALA, δ-aminolevulinic acid; HMB, hydroxymethylbilane; URO, uroporphyrinogen; COPRO, coproporphyrinogen; PROTO, protoporphyrinogen.

TABLE 337-2 The Major Metabolites Accumulated in the Human Porphyrias

Type/Porphyria	Increased Erythrocyte Porphyrins	Porphyrin Excretion	
		Urine	Stool
HEPATIC PORPHYRIAS			
ALA-dehydratase deficiency (ADP)	Zn-protoporphyrins	ALA, Coproporphyrin III	—
Acute intermittent porphyria (AIP)	—	ALA, PBG	—
Porphyria cutanea tarda (PCT)	—	Uroporphyrin I, 7-Carboxylate Porphyrin	Isocoproporphyrin
Hereditary coproporphyria (HCP)	—	ALA, PBG, Coproporphyrin III	Coproporphyrin III
Variegate porphyria (VP)	—	ALA, PBG Coproporphyrin III	Protoporphyrin IX 5-Carboxylate Porphyrin
ERYTHROPOIETIC PORPHYRIAS			
X-linked sideroblastic anemia (XLSA)	—	—	—
Congenital erythropoietic porphyria (CEP)	Uroporphyrin I	Uroporphyrin I	Coproporphyrin I, Uroporphyrin I
Erythropoietic protoporphyria (EPP)	Protoporphyrin IX	—	Protoporphyrin IX

Note: ALA, δ-aminolevulinic acid; PBG, porphobilinogen

TABLE 337-3 *Categories of Unsafe and Safe Drugs in AIP, HCP, and VP*

Unsafe	Safe
Barbiturates	Narcotic analgesics
Sulfonamide antibiotics	Aspirin
Meprobamate	Acetaminophen
Glutethimide	Phenothiazines
Methyprylon	Penicillin and derivatives
Ethchlorvynol	Streptomycin
Mephenytoin	Glucocorticoids
Succinimides	Bromides
Carbamazepine	Insulin
Valproic acid	Atropine
Pyrazolones	
Griseofulvin	
Ergots	
Synthetic estrogens and progestogens	
Danazol	
Alcohol	

found in the coding region of the gene in unrelated AIP families. These mutations alter the kinetic properties and/or stability of the mutant enzymes or create premature termination codons. Mutations that cause erythroid AIP variants with half-normal enzyme in nonerythroid tissues, but normal activity in erythrocytes, include point mutations in the initiation methionine codon (which prevent translation) and in the 5' donor splice site of intron 1 (which cause abnormal splicing of the HMB-synthase transcript) and a mutation in the housekeeping promoter. The prenatal diagnosis of a fetus at risk can be made with cultured amniotic cells or chorionic villi.

℞ TREATMENT

During acute attacks, narcotic analgesics may be required for abdominal pain, and phenothiazines are useful for nausea, vomiting, anxiety, and restlessness. Chloral hydrate can be given for insomnia, and benzodiazepines are probably safe in low doses, if a minor tranquilizer is required. Although intravenous glucose (at least 300 g/d) can be effective in acute attacks of porphyria, a more complete parenteral nutritional regimen may be beneficial if oral feeding is not possible for a prolonged period. However, intravenous heme is more effective than glucose in reducing porphyrin precursor excretion and probably leads to more rapid recovery. The response to heme therapy is reduced if delayed. Therefore, 3 to 4 mg of heme, in the form of hematin (Abbott Laboratories), heme albumin, or heme arginate (Leiras Oy, Turku, Finland), may be infused daily for 4 days beginning as soon as possible after onset of an attack. Heme arginate and heme albumin are chemically stable and are less likely than hematin to produce phlebitis or an anticoagulant effect. The rate of recovery from an acute attack depends on the degree of neuronal damage and may be rapid (1 to 2 days) with prompt therapy. Recovery from severe motor neuropathy may require months or years. Identification and avoidance of inciting factors can hasten recovery from an attack and prevent future attacks. Multiple inciting factors may contribute to a symptomatic episode. Frequent clear-cut cyclical attacks occur in some women and can be prevented with a long-acting gonadotropin-releasing hormone analogue (this indication is not approved by the U.S. Food and Drug Administration).

PORPHYRIA CUTANEA TARDA
Porphyria cutanea tarda (PCT), the most common of the porphyrias, can be sporadic (type I) or familial (types II and III) and can also develop after exposure to halogenated aromatic hydrocarbons. Hepatic URO-decarboxylase is deficient in all types of PCT; however, in types I and III PCT, URO-decarboxylase activity is normal in erythrocytes. In type II PCT, an autosomal dominant disorder, the enzyme is deficient in erythrocytes and other tissues. In type III PCT, deficiency of the enzyme is limited to the liver. Deficient hepatic URO-decarboxylase and a porphyrin pattern resembling PCT

can be produced by exposure of normal individuals to a number of halogenated aromatic hydrocarbons. Hepatoerythropoietic porphyria (HEP) is an autosomal recessive form of porphyria that results from marked systemic deficiency of URO-decarboxylase activity.

Clinical Features Cutaneous photosensitivity is the major clinical feature. Neurologic manifestations are not observed. Fluid-filled vesicles and bullae develop on sun-exposed areas such as the face, the dorsa of the hands and feet, the forearms, and the legs. The skin in these areas is friable, and minor trauma may lead to the formation of bullae. The appearance of small white plaques, termed *milia*, may precede or follow vesicle formation. Bullae and denuded skin heal slowly and are subject to infection. Other features include hypertrichosis and hyperpigmentation, especially of the face, and thickening, scarring, and calcification resembling the cutaneous changes of systemic sclerosis.

A number of factors contribute to the development of hepatic URO-decarboxylase deficiency, including excess alcohol, iron, and estrogens. The importance of excess hepatic iron as a precipitating factor is underscored by the finding that the incidence of the common hemochromatosis-causing mutations, *HFE* C282Y and H63D, are increased in patients with types I and II PCT (Chap. 336). Various chemicals can also induce PCT; an epidemic of PCT occurred in eastern Turkey in the 1950s as a consequence of wheat contaminated with the fungicide hexachlorobenzene. PCT also occurs after exposure to other chemicals, including di- and trichlorophenols and 2,3,7,8-tetrachlorodibenzo-(*p*)-dioxin (TCDD, dioxin). Patients with PCT characteristically have liver damage and are at risk for hepatocellular carcinoma. These carcinomas do not produce porphyrins.

HEP resembles congenital erythropoietic porphyria (CEP) and usually presents with blistering skin lesions, hypertrichosis, scarring, and red urine in infancy or childhood.

Diagnosis Porphyrins are increased in the liver, plasma, urine, and stool. The urinary ALA level may be slightly increased, but the PBG level is normal. Urinary porphyrins consist mostly of uroporphyrin and 7-carboxylate porphyrin, with lesser amounts of coproporphyrin and 5- and 6-carboxylate porphyrins. Plasma porphyrins are also increased in a pattern that resembles that in urine. Isocoproporphyrins are increased in feces and sometimes in plasma and urine. The finding of increased isocoproporphyrins is diagnostic for hepatic URO-decarboxylase deficiency.

Type II PCT and HEP can be distinguished from types I and III by finding decreased URO-decarboxylase in erythrocytes. URO-decarboxylase activity in liver, erythrocytes, and cultured skin fibroblasts in type II PCT is approximately 50% of normal in affected individuals and in family members with latent disease. In HEP, the URO-decarboxylase activity is markedly deficient, with typical levels of 3 to 10% of normal. Over 50 mutations have been identified in the coding region of the *URO-decarboxylase* gene from unrelated type II PCT and HEP patients. Excess hepatic iron contributes to development of sporadic and familial forms of PCT. As noted above, coinheritance of *HFE* mutations that cause hemochromatosis increases susceptibility to PCT-precipitating factors. In the familial forms (types II and III), iron inhibits the residual normal enzyme, so that enzymatic activity in liver is <50% of normal. In type I PCT the decreased hepatic URO-decarboxylase activity is not accompanied by a decrease in the amount of enzyme protein, suggesting that the enzyme is present in an inactive form; hepatic URO-decarboxylase activity gradually increases after a remission is induced by phlebotomy.

℞ TREATMENT

Alcohol, estrogens, iron supplements, and, if possible, any drugs that may exacerbate the disease should be discontinued, but this step does not always lead to improvement. A complete response can almost always be achieved by repeated phlebotomy to reduce hepatic iron. A unit (450 mL) of blood can be removed every 1 to 2 weeks. Because iron overload is not marked in most cases, remission may occur after only five or six phlebotomies. Hemoglobin levels and serum ferritin should be followed closely to prevent development of iron deficiency and anemia. After remission, continued phlebotomy may not be needed even if ferritin levels return to normal. Relapses are treated by additional phlebotomy.

PCT can also be treated with chloroquine or hydroxychloroquine, both of which form a complex with the excess porphyrins and promote their excretion. Small doses (e.g., 125 mg chloroquine phosphate twice weekly) should be given, because standard doses can induce transient, sometimes marked increases in photosensitivity and hepatocellular damage. Hepatic imaging can diagnose or exclude complicating hepatocellular carcinoma. Treatment of PCT in patients with end-stage renal disease is facilitated by administration of erythropoietin.

HEREDITARY COPROPORPHYRIA   HCP is an autosomal dominant form of hepatic porphyria that results from half-normal levels of COPRO-oxidase activity. Photosensitivity may occur. A few cases of homozygous HCP have been reported.

Clinical Features   HCP is influenced by the same factors that cause attacks in AIP. The disease is latent before puberty, and symptoms are more common in women. Neurovisceral symptoms and other manifestations are virtually identical to those of AIP. Photosensitivity may resemble that in PCT and VP. Cutaneous lesions may begin in childhood in rare homozygous cases.

Diagnosis   Coproporphyrin is markedly increased in the urine and feces in symptomatic disease and sometimes when there are no symptoms. Urinary ALA and PBG levels are increased during acute attacks but may return to normal when symptoms resolve. Although the diagnosis can be confirmed by measuring COPRO-oxidase activity, these assays are not widely available and require cells other than erythrocytes. Since the *COPRO-oxidase* gene has been cloned and >30 mutations, two-thirds of which are missense, have been identified in unrelated patients, DNA diagnosis of suspected patients is also available.

℞ TREATMENT

Neurologic symptoms are treated as in AIP (see above). Phlebotomy and chloroquine are ineffective when cutaneous lesions are present.

VARIEGATE PORPHYRIA   VP, a hepatic porphyria that results from the deficient activity of PROTO-oxidase, is transmitted in an autosomal dominant manner and can present with neurologic symptoms, photosensitivity, or both.

Clinical Features   Neurovisceral signs and symptoms develop after puberty and are similar to those of AIP or HCP (see above). Attacks are provoked by the same drugs, steroids, and nutritional factors that are detrimental in AIP. Skin manifestations are more common than in HCP but usually occur apart from the neurovisceral symptoms. Because the skin lesions in VP, HCP, and PCT are not distinguishable by clinical examination or biopsy, these conditions are diagnosed by assay of porphyrins and porphyrin precursors in blood, urine, and feces.

VP is particularly common in South Africa, where 3 of every 1000 whites have the disorder. Most are descendants of a couple who emigrated from Holland to South Africa in 1688. Homozygous VP is associated with photosensitivity, neurologic symptoms, and developmental disturbances, including growth retardation in infancy or childhood; all cases had increased erythrocyte levels of zinc protoporphyrin, a characteristic finding in all homozygous porphyrias so far described.

Dual porphyria, the simultaneous occurrence of VP and familial PCT, has been documented in several kindreds. *Chester porphyria* was described in a large British family in which individuals had acute porphyric attacks and deficiency of both PROTO-oxidase and HMB-synthase. Photosensitivity was not observed. It is unclear whether Chester porphyria is a variant of VP or AIP.

Diagnosis   When VP is symptomatic, levels of fecal protoporphyrin and coproporphyrin and of urinary coproporphyrin are increased. Urinary ALA and PBG levels are increased during acute attacks. Plasma levels of porphyrins are increased, particularly when there are cuta-

neous lesions. VP can be distinguished rapidly from all other porphyrias by examining the fluorescence emission spectrum of porphyrins in plasma at neutral pH. This test is particularly useful for differentiating VP from PCT.

Assays of PROTO-oxidase activity in cultured fibroblasts or lymphocytes are not widely available. Some latent cases of VP can be diagnosed by measurement of fecal porphyrins in relatives of VP patients. Over 90 mutations have been found in the *PROTO-oxidase* gene; 52% are missense mutations and 30% are small deletions or insertions.

℞ TREATMENT

Acute attacks are treated with hematin as in AIP. Other than avoiding sun exposure, there are few effective measures for treating the skin lesions. β-Carotene, phlebotomy, and chloroquine are not helpful.

THE ERYTHROPOIETIC PORPHYRIAS

In the erythropoietic porphyrias, porphyrins from bone marrow erythrocytes and plasma are deposited in the skin and lead to cutaneous photosensitivity.

X-LINKED SIDEROBLASTIC ANEMIA   XLSA results from the deficient activity of the erythroid form of ALA-synthase and is associated with ineffective erythropoiesis, weakness, and pallor.

Clinical Features   Typically, males with XLSA develop refractory hemolytic anemia, pallor, and weakness during infancy. They have secondary hypersplenism, become iron overloaded, and can develop hemosiderosis. The severity depends on the level of residual erythroid ALA-synthase activity and on the responsiveness of the specific mutation to pyridoxal 5′-phosphate supplementation (see below). Peripheral blood smears reveal a hypochromic, microcytic anemia with striking anisocytosis, poikilocytosis, and polychromasia; the leukocytes and platelets appear normal. Hemoglobin content is reduced, and the mean corpuscular volume and mean corpuscular hemoglobin concentration are decreased. Patients with milder, late-onset disease have been reported.

Diagnosis   Bone marrow examination reveals hypercellularity with a left shift and megaloblastic erythropoiesis with abnormal maturation. A variety of Prussian blue–staining sideroblasts are observed. Levels of urinary porphyrin precursors and of both urinary and fecal porphyrins are normal. The level of erythroid ALA-synthase is decreased in bone marrow, but this enzyme is difficult to measure in the presence of the normal ALA-synthase housekeeping enzyme. Definitive diagnosis requires the demonstration of mutations in the *erythroid ALA-synthase* gene.

℞ TREATMENT

The severe anemia may respond to pyridoxine supplementation. This cofactor is essential for ALA-synthase activity, and mutations in the pyridoxine-binding site of the enzyme have been found in several responsive patients. Cofactor supplementation may make it possible to eliminate or reduce the frequency of transfusion. Unresponsive patients may be transfusion-dependent and require chelation therapy.

CONGENITAL ERYTHROPOIETIC PORPHYRIA   CEP (also known as *Gunther's disease*) is an autosomal recessive disorder due to markedly deficient activity of URO-synthase; it is associated with hemolytic anemia and cutaneous lesions. CEP is characterized by accumulation of uroporphyrin I and coproporphyrin I isomers.

Clinical Features   Severe cutaneous photosensitivity begins in early infancy. The skin over sun-exposed areas is friable, and bullae and vesicles are prone to rupture and infection. Skin thickening, focal hypo- and hyperpigmentation, and hypertrichosis of the face and extremities are characteristic. Secondary infection of the cutaneous lesions can lead to disfigurement of the face and hands. Porphyrins are deposited in teeth and in bones. As a result, the teeth are reddish-brown and fluoresce on exposure to long-wave ultraviolet light. Hemolysis is probably due to the marked increase in erythrocyte porphyrins and leads to splenomegaly. Adults with a milder form of the disease have been described.

Diagnosis Uroporphyrin and coproporphyrin (mostly type I isomers) accumulate in the bone marrow, erythrocytes, plasma, urine, and feces. The diagnosis should be confirmed by demonstration of markedly deficient URO-synthase activity. The disease can be detected in utero by measuring porphyrins in amniotic fluid and URO-synthase activity in cultured amniotic cells or chorionic villi. Molecular analyses of the mutant alleles have revealed multiple different mutations, including four mutations in the recently discovered erythroid-specific promoter of the *URO-synthase* gene.

℞ TREATMENT

The transfusion of sufficient blood to suppress erythropoiesis is effective but results in iron overload. Splenectomy may reduce hemolysis and decrease transfusion requirements. Protection from sunlight and minor skin trauma is important. β-Carotene may be of some value. Complicating bacterial infections should be treated promptly. Recently, bone marrow transplantation has proven effective in several transfusion-dependent children, providing the rationale for stem-cell gene therapy.

ERYTHROPOIETIC PROTOPORPHYRIA Erythropoietic protoporphyria (EPP) is an autosomal dominant disorder due to the partial deficiency of ferrochelatase activity. Protoporphyrin accumulates in erythroid cells and plasma and is excreted in bile and feces. EPP is the most common erythropoietic porphyria and, after PCT, the second most common porphyria.

Clinical Features Skin photosensitivity usually begins in childhood. The skin manifestations differ from those of other porphyrias. Vesicular lesions are uncommon. Redness, swelling, burning, and itching can develop within minutes of sun exposure and resemble angioedema. Symptoms may seem out of proportion to the visible skin lesions. Sparse vesicles and bullae occur in 10% of cases. Chronic skin changes may include lichenification, leathery pseudovesicles, labial grooving, and nail changes. Severe scarring is rare, as are pigment changes, friability, and hirsutism.

The primary source of excess protoporphyrin is the bone marrow reticulocyte. Erythrocyte protoporphyrin is free (not complexed with zinc) and is mostly bound to hemoglobin. In plasma, protoporphyrin is bound to albumin. Hemolysis and anemia are usually absent or mild.

Liver function is usually normal, but in some patients accumulation of protoporphyrin causes chronic liver disease that can progress to liver failure and death. The hepatic complications are often preceded by

increasing levels of erythrocyte and plasma protoporphyrin and probably result, in part, from protoporphyrin accumulation in the liver. Protoporphyrin is insoluble, forms crystalline structures in liver cells, and can decrease hepatic bile flow. Gallstones composed at least in part of protoporphyrin occur in some patients.

Some obligate heterozygotes are asymptomatic and have little or no increase in erythrocyte protoporphyrin. Thus there is phenotypic variation in this disease.

Diagnosis Protoporphyrin levels are increased in bone marrow, circulating erythrocytes, plasma, bile, and feces. Urinary levels of porphyrin and porphyrin precursors are normal. Ferrochelatase activity in cultured lymphocytes or fibroblasts is decreased. DNA diagnosis by mutation analysis is possible, and multiple missense and nonsense mutations have been identified in the *ferrochelatase* gene.

℞ TREATMENT

Oral β-carotene (120 to 180 mg/d) improves tolerance to sunlight in many patients. The dosage may need to be adjusted to maintain serum carotene levels in the recommended range of 10 to 15 μmol/L (600 to 800 μg/dL). Mild skin discoloration due to carotenemia is the only significant side effect. The beneficial effects of β-carotene may involve quenching of singlet oxygen or free radicals. Unfortunately, this drug is less effective in other forms of porphyria associated with photosensitivity.

Treatment of hepatic complications is difficult. However, cholestyramine and other porphyrin absorbents such as activated charcoal may interrupt the enterohepatic circulation of protoporphyrin and promote its fecal excretion, leading to some improvement. Splenectomy may be helpful when the disease is accompanied by hemolysis and significant splenomegaly. Caloric restriction and drugs or hormones that may induce the heme pathway or impair hepatic excretory function should be avoided. Iron deficiency should be prevented or treated. Transfusions or intravenous heme therapy may suppress erythroid and hepatic protoporphyrin production and are sometimes beneficial. Liver transplantation has been carried out in some patients with severe liver complications.

FURTHER READING

ANDERSON KE et al: Disorders of heme biosynthesis: X-linked sideroblastic anemia and the porphyrias, in *The Metabolic and Molecular Bases of Inherited Disease*, 8th ed, CR Scriver et al (eds). New York, McGraw-Hill, 2001, p 2991

DESNICK RJ, ASTRIN KH: Congenital erythropoietic porphyria: Advances in pathogenesis and treatment. Br J Hematol 117:779, 2002

GROSS U et al: Erythropoietic and hepatic porphyria. J Inherit Metab Dis 23: 641, 2002

LAMBRECT RW, BONKOVSKY HL: Hemachromatosis and porphyria. Semin Gastrointest Dis 13:109, 2002

SARKANY RPE: The management of porphyria cutanea tarda. Clin Exp Dermatol 26:225, 2001

338 DISORDERS OF PURINE AND PYRIMIDINE METABOLISM
Robert L. Wortmann

Purines (adenine and guanine) and pyrimidines (cytosine, thymine, uracil) serve fundamental roles in the replication of genetic material, gene transcription, protein synthesis, and cellular metabolism. Disorders that involve abnormalities of nucleotide metabolism range from relatively common diseases such as hyperuricemia and gout, in which there is increased production or impaired excretion of a metabolic end product of purine metabolism (uric acid), to rare enzyme deficiencies that affect purine and pyrimidine synthesis or degradation. Understanding these biochemical pathways has led, in some instances, to the development of specific forms of treatment, such as the use of allopurinol to reduce uric acid production.

URIC ACID METABOLISM

Uric acid is the final breakdown product of purine degradation in humans. It is a weak acid with pK_as of 5.75 and 10.3. Urates, the ionized forms of uric acid, predominate in plasma extracellular fluid and synovial fluid, with approximately 98% existing as monosodium urate at pH 7.4. Monosodium urate is easily dialyzed from plasma. Binding of urate to plasma proteins has little physiologic significance.

Plasma is saturated with monosodium urate at a concentration of 415 μmol/L (6.8 mg/dL) at 37°C. At higher concentrations, plasma is therefore supersaturated, creating the potential for urate crystal precipitation. However, precipitation sometimes does not occur even at plasma urate concentrations as high as 4800 μmol/L (80 mg/dL), perhaps because of the presence of solubilizing substances in plasma.

Uric acid is more soluble in urine than in water, possibly because of the presence of urea, proteins, and mucopolysaccharides. The pH of urine greatly influences its solubility. At pH 5.0, urine is saturated with uric acid at concentrations ranging from 360 to 900 μmol/L (6 to 15 mg/dL). At pH 7.0, saturation is reached at concentrations between 9480 and 12,000 μmol/L (158 and 200 mg/dL). Ionized forms of uric acid in urine include mono- and disodium, potassium, ammonium, and calcium urates.

Although purine nucleotides are synthesized and degraded in all tissues, urate is produced only in tissues that contain xanthine oxidase, primarily the liver and small intestine. Urate production varies with the purine content of the diet and the rates of purine biosynthesis, degradation, and salvage (Fig. 338-1). Normally, two-thirds to three-fourths of urate is excreted by the kidneys, and most of the remainder is eliminated through the intestines. A four-component model describes the renal handling of uric acid in humans: (1) glomerular filtration, (2) tubular reabsorption, (3) secretion, and (4) postsecretory reabsorption (Fig. 338-2). Approximately 8 to 12% of urate filtered by the glomeruli is excreted in the urine as uric acid. After filtration, 98 to 100% of the urate is reabsorbed; about half of the reabsorbed urate is secreted back into the proximal tubule, and about 40% of that is again reabsorbed.

Serum urate levels vary with age and sex. Most children have serum urate concentrations of 180 to 240 μmol/L (3.0 to 4.0 mg/dL). Levels begin to rise in males during puberty but remain low in females until menopause. Mean serum urate values of adult men and premenopausal women are 415 and 360 μmol/L (6.8 and 6.0 mg/dL), respectively. After menopause, values for women increase to approximate those of men. In adulthood, concentrations rise steadily over time and vary with height, body weight, blood pressure, renal function, and alcohol intake.

HYPERURICEMIA

Hyperuricemia can result from increased production or decreased excretion of uric acid or from a combination of the two processes. Sustained hyperuricemia predisposes some individuals to develop clinical manifestations including gouty arthritis (Chap. 313), urolithiasis, and renal dysfunction (see below).

Hyperuricemia is defined as a plasma (or serum) urate concentration >420 μmol/L (7.0 mg/dL). The risk of developing gouty arthritis or urolithiasis increases with higher urate levels and escalates in proportion to the degree of elevation. Hyperuricemia is present in between

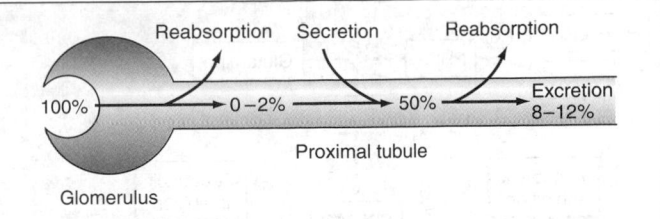

FIGURE 338-2 Schematic for handling of uric acid by the kidney. Components are illustrated with the percentage of filtered urate.

2.0 and 13.2% of ambulatory adults and is even more frequent in hospitalized individuals.

CAUSES OF HYPERURICEMIA Hyperuricemia may be classified as primary or secondary depending on whether the cause is innate or is the result of an acquired disorder. However, it is more useful to classify hyperuricemia in relation to the underlying pathophysiology, i.e., whether it results from increased production, decreased excretion, or a combination of the two (Fig. 338-1, Table 338-1).

Increased Urate Production Diet contributes to the serum urate in proportion to its purine content. Strict restriction of purine intake reduces the mean serum urate level by about 60 μmol/L (1.0 mg/dL) and urinary uric acid excretion by approximately 1.2 mmol/d (200 mg/d). Foods high in nucleic acid content include liver, "sweetbreads" (i.e., thymus and pancreas), kidney, and anchovy.

Endogenous sources of purine production also influence the serum urate level (Fig. 338-3). De novo purine biosynthesis is an 11-step process that forms inosine monophosphate (IMP). The rates of purine biosynthesis and urate production are determined, for the most part, by amidophosphoribosyltransferase (amidoPRT), which combines phosphoribosylpyrophosphate (PRPP) and glutamine. AmidoPRT is regulated by the substrate PRPP, which drives the reaction forward, and by the end products of biosynthesis (IMP and other ribonucleotides), which provide feedback inhibition. A secondary regulatory pathway is the salvage of purine bases by hypoxanthine phosphoribosyltransferase (HPRT). HPRT catalyzes the combination of the purine bases hypoxanthine and guanine with PRPP to form the respective ribonucleotides IMP and guanosine monophosphate (GMP). Increased

FIGURE 338-1 The total-body urate pool is the net result between urate production and excretion. Urate production is influenced by dietary intake of purines and the rates of de novo biosynthesis of purines from nonpurine precursors, nucleic acid turnover, and salvage by phosphoribosyltransferase activities. The formed urate is normally excreted by urinary and intestinal routes. Hyperuricemia can result from increased production, decreased excretion, or a combination of both mechanisms. When hyperuricemia exists, urate can precipitate and deposit in tissues as tophi.

TABLE 338-1 *Classification of Hyperuricemia by Pathophysiology*

URATE OVERPRODUCTION

Primary idiopathic	Myeloproliferative	Rhabdomyolysis
HPRT deficiency	diseases	Exercise
PRPP synthetase	Polycythemia vera	Alcohol
overactivity	Psoriasis	Obesity
Hemolytic processes	Paget's disease	Purine-rich diet
Lymphoproliferative	Glycogenosis III, V,	
diseases	and VII	

DECREASED URIC ACID EXCRETION

Primary idiopathic	Starvation ketosis	Drug ingestion
Renal insufficiency	Berylliosis	Salicylates (>2 g/d)
Polycystic kidney	Sarcoidosis	Diuretics
disease	Lead intoxication	Alcohol
Diabetes insipidus	Hyperparathyroidism	Levodopa
Hypertension	Hypothyroidism	Ethambutol
Acidosis	Toxemia of pregnancy	Pyrazinamide
Lactic acidosis	Bartter's syndrome	Nicotinic acid
Diabetic	Down syndrome	Cyclosporine
ketoacidosis		

COMBINED MECHANISM

Glucose-6-phosphatase	Fructose-1-phosphate	Alcohol
deficiency	aldolase deficiency	Shock

Note: HPRT, hypoxanthine phosphoribosyltransferase; PRPP, phosphoribosylpyrophosphate.

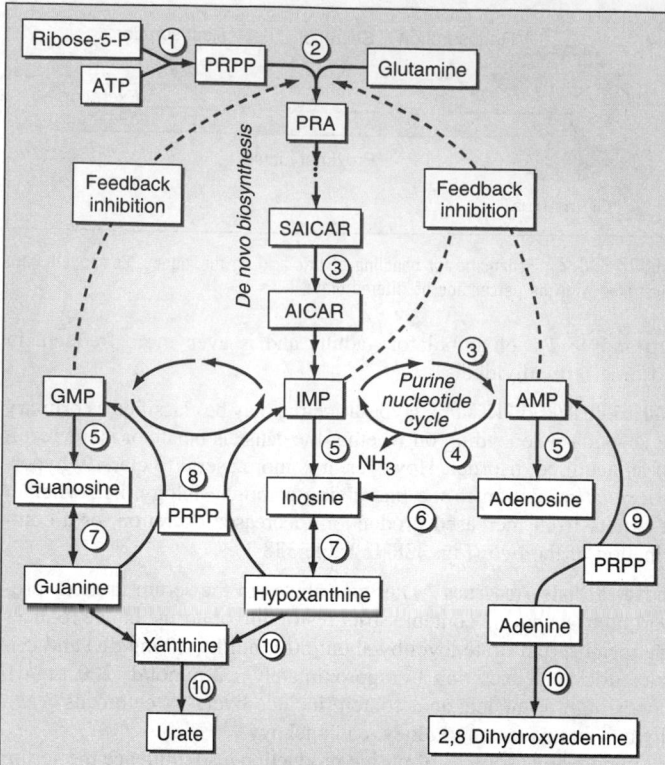

FIGURE 338-3 Abbreviated scheme of purine metabolism. (1) Phosphoribosylpyrophosphate (PRPP) synthetase, (2) amidophosphoribosyltransferase (amidoPRT), (3) adenylosuccinate lyase, (4) adenylate (AMP) deaminase, (5) 5'-nucleotidase, (6) adenosine deaminase, (7) purine nucleoside phosphorylase, (8) hypoxanthine phosphoribosyltransferase (HPRT), (9) adenine phosphoribosyltransferase (APRT), and (10) xanthine oxidase. PRA, phosphoribosylamine; SAICAR, succinylaminoimidazole carboxamide ribotide; AICAR, aminoimidazole carboxamide ribotide; GMP, guanylate; IMP, inosine monophosphate.

salvage activity thus retards de novo synthesis by reducing PRPP levels and increasing concentrations of inhibitory ribonucleotides.

Serum urate levels are closely coupled to the rates of de novo purine biosynthesis, which is driven in part by the level of PRPP, as evidenced by two X-linked inborn errors of purine metabolism. Both increased PRPP synthetase activity and HPRT deficiency are associated with overproduction of purines, hyperuricemia, and hyperuricaciduria (see below for clinical descriptions).

Accelerated purine nucleotide degradation can also cause hyperuricemia, i.e., with conditions of rapid cell turnover, proliferation, or cell death, as in leukemic blast crises, cytotoxic therapy for malignancy, hemolysis, or rhabdomyolysis. Hyperuricemia can result from excessive degradation of skeletal muscle ATP after strenuous physical exercise or status epilepticus and in glycogen storage diseases types III, V, and VII (Chap. 341). The hyperuricemia of myocardial infarction, smoke inhalation, and acute respiratory failure may also be related to accelerated breakdown of ATP.

Decreased Uric Acid Excretion Over 90% of individuals with sustained hyperuricemia have a defect in the renal handling of uric acid. Gouty individuals excrete approximately 40% less uric acid than nongouty individuals for any given plasma urate concentration. Uric acid excretion increases in gouty and nongouty individuals when plasma urate levels are raised by purine ingestion or infusion, but in those with gout, plasma urate concentrations must be 60 to 120 μmol/L (1 to 2 mg/dL) higher than normal to achieve equivalent uric acid excretion rates.

Altered uric acid excretion could theoretically result from decreased glomerular filtration, decreased tubular secretion, or enhanced tubular reabsorption. Decreased urate filtration does not appear to cause primary hyperuricemia but does contribute to the hyperuricemia of renal insufficiency. Although hyperuricemia is invariably present in chronic renal disease, the correlation between serum creatinine, urea nitrogen, and urate concentration is poor. Uric acid excretion per unit of glomerular filtration rate increases progressively with chronic renal insufficiency, but tubular secretory capacity tends to be preserved, tubular reabsorptive capacity is reduced, and extrarenal clearance of uric acid increases as renal damage becomes more severe.

Decreased tubular secretion of urate causes the secondary hyperuricemia of acidosis. Diabetic ketoacidosis, starvation, ethanol intoxication, lactic acidosis, and salicylate intoxication are accompanied by accumulations of organic acids (β-hydroxybutyrate, acetoacetate, lactate, or salicylates) that compete with urate for tubular secretion. Hyperuricemia may be due to enhanced reabsorption of uric acid distal to the site of secretion. This mechanism is known to be responsible for the hyperuricemia of extracellular volume depletion that occurs with diabetes insipidus or diuretic therapy.

Alcohol promotes hyperuricemia because of increased urate production and decreased uric acid excretion. Excessive alcohol consumption accelerates hepatic breakdown of ATP to increase urate production. Alcohol consumption can also induce hyperlacticacidemia, which blocks uric acid secretion. The higher purine content in some alcoholic beverages such as beer may also be a factor.

EVALUATION OF HYPERURICEMIA Hyperuricemia does not necessarily represent a disease, nor is it a specific indication for therapy. The decision to treat depends on the cause and the potential consequences of the hyperuricemia in each individual.

Quantification of uric acid excretion can be used to determine whether hyperuricemia is caused by overproduction or decreased excretion. On a purine-free diet, men with normal renal function excrete <3.6 mmol/d (600 mg/d). Thus, the hyperuricemia of individuals who excrete uric acid above this level while on a purine-free diet is due to purine overproduction; for those who excrete lower amounts on the purine-free diet, it is due to decreased excretion. If the assessment is performed while the patient is on a regular diet, the level of 4.2 mmol/d (800 mg/d) can be used as the discriminating value.

Pyrazinamide, which has a suppressive action on tubular secretion, can be used to investigate presecretory reabsorption of uric acid. Probenecid, an agent that inhibits postsecretory reabsorption, can be used to evaluate tubular secretion and postsecretory reabsorption.

COMPLICATIONS OF HYPERURICEMIA The most recognized complication of hyperuricemia is *gouty arthritis*. In the general population the prevalence of hyperuricemia ranges between 2.0 and 13.2%, and the prevalence of gout is between 1.3 and 3.7%. The higher the serum urate level, the more likely an individual is to develop gout. In one study, the incidence of gout was 4.9% for individuals with serum urate concentrations >540 μmol/L (9.0 mg/dL) compared with 0.5% for those with values between 415 and 535 μmol/L (7.0 and 8.9 mg/dL). The complications of gout correlate with both the duration and severity of hyperuricemia. →*For further discussion of gout, see Chap. 313.*

Hyperuricemia also causes several renal problems: (1) nephrolithiasis; (2) urate nephropathy, a rare cause of renal insufficiency attributed to monosodium urate crystal deposition in the renal interstitium; and (3) uric acid nephropathy, a reversible cause of acute renal failure resulting from deposition of large amounts of uric acid crystals in the renal collecting ducts, pelvis, and ureters.

Nephrolithiasis Uric acid nephrolithiasis occurs most commonly, but not exclusively, in individuals with gout. In gout, the prevalence of nephrolithiasis correlates with the serum and urinary uric acid levels, reaching approximately 50% with serum urate levels of 770 μmol/L (13 mg/dL) or urinary uric acid excretion >6.5 mmol/d (1100 mg/d).

Uric acid stones can develop in individuals with no evidence of arthritis, only 20% of whom are hyperuricemic. Uric acid can also play a role in other types of kidney stones. Some nongouty individuals with calcium oxalate or calcium phosphate stones have hyperuricemia or hyperuricaciduria. Uric acid may act as a nidus on which calcium oxalate can precipitate or lower the formation product for calcium oxalate crystallization.

Urate Nephropathy Urate nephropathy, sometimes referred to as *urate nephrosis*, is a late manifestation of severe gout and is characterized histologically by deposits of monosodium urate crystals surrounded by a giant cell inflammatory reaction in the medullary interstitium and pyramids. The disorder is now rare and cannot be diagnosed in the absence of gouty arthritis. The lesions may be clinically silent or cause proteinuria, hypertension, and renal insufficiency.

Uric Acid Nephropathy This reversible cause of acute renal failure is due to precipitation of uric acid in renal tubules and collecting ducts that causes obstruction to urine flow. Uric acid nephropathy develops following sudden urate overproduction and marked hyperuricaciduria. Factors that favor uric acid crystal formation include dehydration and acidosis. This form of acute renal failure occurs most often during an aggressive "blastic" phase of leukemia or lymphoma prior to or coincident with cytolytic therapy but has also been observed in individuals with other neoplasms, following epileptic seizures, and after vigorous exercise with heat stress. Autopsy studies have demonstrated intraluminal precipitates of uric acid, dilated proximal tubules, and normal glomeruli. The initial pathogenic events are believed to include obstruction of collecting ducts with uric acid and obstruction of distal renal vasculature.

If recognized, uric acid nephropathy is potentially reversible. Appropriate therapy has reduced the mortality from about 50% to practically nil. Serum levels cannot be relied on for diagnosis because this condition has developed in the presence of urate concentrations varying from 720 to 4800 μmol/L (12 to 80 mg/dL). The distinctive feature is the urinary uric acid concentration. In most forms of acute renal failure with decreased urine output, urinary uric acid content is either normal or reduced, and the ratio of uric acid to creatinine is <1. In acute uric acid nephropathy the ratio of uric acid to creatinine in a random urine sample or 24-h specimen is >1, and a value that high is essentially diagnostic.

HYPERURICEMIA AND SYNDROME X Syndrome X is characterized by abdominal obesity with visceral adiposity, impaired glucose tolerance due to insulin resistance with hyperinsulinemia, hypertriglyceridemia, increased low-density lipoprotein cholesterol, decreased high-density lipoprotein cholesterol, and hyperuricemia. Hyperinsulinemia reduces the renal excretion of uric acid and sodium. Not surprisingly, hyperuricemia resulting from euglycemic hyperinsulinemia may precede the onset of type 2 diabetes, hypertension, coronary artery disease, and gout in individuals with syndrome X.

℞ TREATMENT

ASYMPTOMATIC HYPERURICEMIA Hyperuricemia is present in approximately 5% of the population and in up to 25% of hospitalized individuals. The vast majority are at no clinical risk. Hyperuricemia does not appear to have a causal role in the development of coronary heart disease or death from cardiovascular disease. In the past, the association of hyperuricemia with cardiovascular disease and renal failure led to the use of urate-lowering agents for people with asymptomatic hyperuricemia. This practice is no longer recommended except for individuals receiving cytolytic therapy for neoplastic disease, in which treatment is given in an effort to prevent uric acid nephropathy. Because hyperuricemia can be a component of syndrome X, its presence is an indication to screen for and aggressively treat any accompanying obesity, hyperlipidemia, diabetes mellitus, or hypertension.

Hyperuricemic individuals are at risk to develop gouty arthritis, especially those with higher serum urate levels. However, most hyperuricemic persons never develop gout and prophylactic treatment is not indicated. Furthermore, neither structural kidney damage nor tophi are identifiable before the first attack. Reduced renal function cannot be attributed to asymptomatic hyperuricemia, and treatment of asymp-

tomatic hyperuricemia does not alter the progression of renal dysfunction in patients with renal disease. Increased risk of stone formation in people with asymptomatic hyperuricemia is not established.

Thus, because treatment with antihyperuricemic agents entails inconvenience, cost, and potential toxicity, routine treatment of asymptomatic hyperuricemia cannot be justified other than for prevention of acute uric acid nephropathy. In addition, routine screening for asymptomatic hyperuricemia is not recommended. If hyperuricemia is diagnosed, however, the cause should be determined. Causal factors should be corrected if the condition is secondary, and associated problems such as hypertension, hypercholesterolemia, diabetes mellitus, and obesity should be treated.

Symptomatic Hyperuricemia ■ *NEPHROLITHIASIS* (See Chap. 313 for treatment of gout.) Antihyperuricemic therapy is recommended for the individual who has both gouty arthritis and either uric acid– or calcium-containing stones, both of which may occur in association with hyperuricaciduria. Regardless of the nature of the calculi, fluid ingestion should be sufficient to produce a daily urine volume >2 L. Alkalinization of the urine with sodium bicarbonate or acetazolamide may be justified to increase the solubility of uric acid. Specific treatment of uric acid calculi requires reducing the urine uric acid concentration with allopurinol. Allopurinol administration decreases the serum urate concentration and the urinary excretion of uric acid in the first 24 h, with a maximum reduction occurring within 2 weeks. The average effective dose of allopurinol is 300 mg/d. Allopurinol can be given once a day because of the long half-life (18 h) of its active metabolite oxypurinol. The drug is effective in patients with renal insufficiency, but the dose should be reduced. Allopurinol is also useful in reducing the recurrence of calcium oxalate stones in gouty patients and in nongouty individuals with hyperuricemia or hyperuricaciduria. Potassium citrate (30 to 80 mmol/d orally in divided doses) is an alternative therapy for patients with uric acid stones alone or mixed calcium/uric acid stones. Allopurinol is also indicated for the treatment of 2,8-dihydroxyadenine kidney stones.

URIC ACID NEPHROPATHY Uric acid nephropathy is often preventable, and immediate, appropriate therapy has greatly reduced the mortality rate. Vigorous intravenous hydration and diuresis with furosemide dilute the uric acid in the tubules and promote urine flow to ≥100 mL/h. The administration of acetazolamide, 240 to 500 mg every 6 to 8 h, and sodium bicarbonate, 89 mmol/L, intravenously enhances urine alkalinity and thereby solubilizes more uric acid. It is important to ensure that the urine pH remains >7.0 and to watch for circulatory overload. In addition, antihyperuricemic therapy in the form of allopurinol in a single dose of 8 mg/kg is administered to reduce the amount of urate that reaches the kidney. If renal insufficiency persists, subsequent daily doses should be reduced to 100 to 200 mg because oxypurinol, the active metabolite of allopurinol, accumulates in renal failure. Despite these measures, hemodialysis may be required.

TABLE 338-2 Medications with Uricosuric Activity

Acetohexamide	Glyceryl guaiacolate
ACTH	Glycopyrrolate
Ascorbic acid	Halofenate
Azauridine	Meclofenamate
Benzbromarone	Phenolsulfonphthalein
Calcitonin	Phenylbutazone
Chlorprothixene	Probenecid
Citrate	Radiographic contrast agents
Dicumarol	Salicylates (>2 g/2d)
Diflunisal	Sulfinpyrazone
Estrogens	Tetracycline that is outdated
Glucocorticoids	Zoxazolamine

TABLE 338-3 Inborn Errors of Purine Metabolism

Enzyme	Activity	Inheritance	Clinical Features
Hypoxanthine phosphoribosyl-transferase	Complete deficiency	X-linked	Self-mutilation, choreoathetosis, hyperuricemia, gout, and uric acid lithiasis
	Partial deficiency	X-linked	Hyperuricemia, gout, and uric acid lithiasis
Phosphoribosyl-pyrophosphate synthetase	Overactivity	X-linked	Hyperuricemia, gout, uric acid lithiasis, and deafness
Adenine phosphoribosyl-transferase	Deficiency	Autosomal recessive	2,8-Dihydroxyadenine lithiasis
Xanthine oxidase	Deficiency	Autosomal recessive	Xanthinuria and xanthine lithiasis
Adenylosuccinate lyase	Deficiency	Autosomal recessive	Autism and psychomotor retardation
Myoadenylate deaminase	Deficiency	Autosomal recessive	Myopathy with exercise intolerance or asymptomatic
Adenosine deaminase	Deficiency	Autosomal recessive	Severe combined immunodeficiency disease and chrondro-osseous dysplasia
Purine nucleoside phosphorylase	Deficiency	Autosomal recessive	T cell–mediated immunodeficiency

HYPOURICEMIA

Hypouricemia, defined as a serum urate concentration <120 μmol/L (2.0 mg/dL) can result from decreased production of urate, increased excretion of uric acid, or a combination of both mechanisms. It occurs in <0.2% of the general population and <0.8% of hospitalized individuals. Hypouricemia causes no symptoms or pathology and therefore requires no therapy.

Most hypouricemia results from increased renal uric acid excretion. The finding of normal amounts of uric acid in a 24-h urine collection in an individual with hypouricemia is evidence for a renal cause. Medications with uricosuric properties (Table 338-2) include aspirin (at doses >2.0 g/d), x-ray contrast materials, and glycerylguaiacholate. Total parenteral hyperalimentation can also cause hypouricemia, possibly a result of the high glycine content of the infusion formula. Other causes of increased urate clearance include conditions such as neo-plastic disease, hepatic cirrhosis, diabetes mellitus, and inappropriate secretion of vasopressin; defects in renal tubular transport such as primary Fanconi syndrome and Fanconi syndromes caused by Wilson's disease, cystinosis, multiple myeloma, and heavy metal toxicity; and isolated congenital defects in the bidirectional transport of uric acid. Hypouricemia can also be caused by inherited forms of decreased urate production.

SELECTED INBORN ERRORS OF PURINE METABOLISM

(See also Table 338-3, Fig. 338-3)

HPRT DEFICIENCY The HPRT gene is located on the X chromosome. Affected males are hemizygous for the mutant gene; carrier females are asymptomatic. A complete deficiency of HPRT, the Lesch-Nyhan syndrome, is characterized by hyperuricemia, self-mutilative behavior, choreoathetosis, spasticity, and mental retardation. A partial deficiency of HPRT, the Kelley-Seeg-miller syndrome, is associated with hyperuricemia but no central nervous system manifestations. In both disorders, the hyperuricemia results from urate overproduction and can cause uric acid crystalluria, nephrolithiasis, obstructive uropathy, and gouty arthritis. Early diagnosis and appropriate therapy with allopurinol can prevent or eliminate all the problems attributable to hyperuricemia but have no effect on the behavioral or neurologic abnormalities.

INCREASED PRPP SYNTHETASE ACTIVITY Like the HPRT deficiency states, PRPP synthetase overactivity is X-linked and results in gouty arthritis and uric acid nephrolithiasis. Nerve deafness occurs in some families.

ADENINE PHOSPHORIBOSYLTRANSFERASE (APRT) DEFICIENCY APRT deficiency is inherited as an autosomal recessive trait. Affected individuals develop kidney stones composed of 2,8-dihydroxyadenine. Caucasians with the disorder have a complete deficiency (type I), whereas Japanese subjects have some measurable enzyme activity (type II). Expression of the defect is similar in the two populations, as is the frequency of the heterozygous state (0.4 to 1.1 per 100). Allopurinol treatment prevents stone formation.

HEREDITARY XANTHINURIA A deficiency of xanthine oxidase causes all purine in the urine to occur in the form of hypoxanthine and xanthine. About two-thirds of deficient individuals are asymptomatic. The remainder develop kidney stones composed of xanthine.

MYOADENYLATE DEAMINASE DEFICIENCY Primary (inherited) and secondary (acquired) forms of myoadenylate deaminase deficiency have been described. The primary form is inherited as an autosomal recessive trait. Clinically, some may have relatively mild myopathic symptoms with exercise or other triggers, but most individuals with this defect are asymptomatic. Therefore, another explanation for the myopathy should be sought in symptomatic patients with this deficiency. The acquired deficiency occurs in association with a wide variety of neuromuscular disease, including muscular dystrophies, neuropathies, inflammatory myopathies, and collagen vascular diseases.

ADENYLOSUCCINATE LYASE DEFICIENCY Deficiency of this enzyme is due to an autosomal recessive trait and

FIGURE 338-4 Abbreviated scheme of pyrimidine metabolism. (1) thymidine kinase, (2) dihydropyrimidine dehydrogenase, (3) thymidylate synthase, (4) UMP synthase, (5) 5'-nucleotidase. CMP, cytidine-5'-monophosphate; UMP, uridine-5'-monophosphate; UDP, uridine-5'-diphosphate; dUMP, deoxyuridine-5'-monophosphate; dTMP, deoxythymidine-5'monophosphate.

causes profound psychomotor retardation, seizures, and other movement disorders. All individuals with this deficiency are mentally retarded, and most are autistic.

ADENOSINE DEAMINASE DEFICIENCY AND PURINE NUCLEOSIDE PHOSPHORYLASE DEFICIENCY See Chap. 297.

PYRIMIDINE DISORDERS

The pyrimidine, cytidine, is found in both DNA and RNA; it is a complementary base pair for guanine. Thymidine is found only in DNA where it is paired with adenine. Uridine is found only in RNA and can pair with either adenine or guanine in RNA secondary structures. Pyrimidines can be synthesized by a de novo pathway (Fig. 338-4) or reused in a salvage pathway. Although more than 25 different enzymes are involved in pyrimidine metabolism, disorders of these pathways are rare. Seven disorders of pyrimidine metabolism have been discovered (Table 338-4), three of which are discussed below.

OROTIC ACIDURIA Hereditary orotic aciduria is caused by mutations in a bifunctional enzyme, uridine-5'-monophosphate (UMP) synthase, which converts orotic acid to UMP in the de novo synthesis pathway (Fig. 338-4). The disorder is characterized by hypochromic megaloblastic anemia that is unresponsive to vitamin B_{12} and folic acid, growth retardation, and neurologic abnormalities. Increased excretion of orotic acid causes crystalluria and obstructive uropathy. Replacement of uridine (100 to 200 mg/kg per day) corrects the anemia, reduces orotic acid excretion, and improves the other sequelae of the disorder.

PYRIMIDINE 5'-NUCLEOTIDASE DEFICIENCY Pyrimidine 5'-nucleotidase catalyzes the removal of the phosphate group from pyrimidine ribonucleoside monophosphates (cytidine-5'-monophosphate or UMP) (Fig. 338-4). An inherited deficiency of this enzyme causes hemolytic anemia with prominent basophilic stippling of erythrocytes. The accumulation of pyrimidines or cytidine diphosphate choline (CDPC) is thought to induce hemolysis. There is no specific treatment. Acquired pyrimidine 5'nucleotidase deficiency has been reported in lead poisoning and in thalassemia.

DIHYDROPYRIMIDINE DEHYDROGENASE DEFICIENCY Dihydropyrimidine dehydrogenase (DPD) is the rate-limiting enzyme in the pathway of uracil and thymine degradation (Fig. 338-4). Deficiency of this enzyme causes excessive urinary excretion of uracil and thymine. DPD deficiency causes nonspecific cerebral dysfunction with convulsive disorders, motor retardation, and mental retardation. No specific treatment is available.

TABLE 338-4 *Inborn Errors of Pyrimidine Metabolism*

Enzyme	Activity	Inheritance	Clinical Features
Uridine-5'-monophosphate synthetase	Deficiency	Autosomal recessive	Aortic acid crystalluria; obstructive uropathy, hypochromic megaloblastic anemia
Pyrimidine 5'-nucleotidase	Deficiency	Autosomal recessive	Hemolytic anemia
Pyrimidine 5'-nucleotidase	Superactivity	Uncertain	Developmental delay, seizures, ataxia, language deficit
Thymidine phosphorylase	Deficiency	Autosomal recessive	Mitochondrial neurogastrointestinal encephalopathy
Dihydropyrimidine dehydrogenase	Deficiency	Autosomal recessive	Seizures, motor and mental retardation
Dihydropyrimidinase	Deficiency	Uncertain	Seizures, mental retardation
Ureidopropionase	Deficiency	Uncertain	Hypotonia, dystonia, developmental delay

MEDICATION EFFECTS ON PYRIMIDINE METABOLISM A variety of medications can influence pyrimidine metabolism. The anticancer agents fluorodeoxyuridine and 5-fluorouracil (5-FU) and the antimicrobial agent fluorocytosine cause cytotoxicity when converted to fluorodeoxyuridylate (FdUMP), a specific suicide inhibitor of thymidylate synthase. Fluorocytosine must be converted to 5-FU to be effective. This conversion is catalyzed by cytosine deaminase activity. Fluorocytosine's action is selective because cytosine deaminase is present in bacteria and fungi but not in human cells.

DPD is involved in the degradation of 5-FU. Consequently, deficiency of this enzyme is associated with 5-FU neurotoxicity.

Leflunomide, which is used to treat rheumatoid arthritis, inhibits de novo pyrimidine synthesis by inhibiting dihydroorotate dehydrogenase, resulting in an antiproliferative effect on T cells. Allopurinol, which is used to block xanthine oxidase and purine synthesis, also inhibits orotidine-5'-phosphate decarboxylase, a step in UMP synthesis. Consequently, allopurinol use is associated with increased excretion of orotidine and orotic acid; there are no known clinical effects of this inhibition.

FURTHER READING

BECKER MA: Hyperuricemia and gout, in *The Metabolic and Molecular Bases of Inherited Disease*, 8th ed, CR Scriver et al (eds). New York, McGraw-Hill, 2001, pp 2513–2535

CULLETON BF et al: Serum uric acid risk for cardiovascular disease and death: The Framingham heart study. Ann Intern Med 131:7, 1999

FAM AG: Gout, diet, and the insulin resistance syndrome. J Rheumatol 29: 1350, 2002

WEBSTER DR et al: Hereditary orotic aciduria and other disorders of pyrimidine metabolism, in *The Metabolic and Molecular Bases of Inherited Disease*, 8th ed, CR Scriver et al (eds). New York, McGraw-Hill, 2001, pp 2663–2702

WORTMANN RL, KELLEY WN: Gout and hyperuricemia, in *Kelly's Textbook of Rheumatology*, 6th ed, ED Harris, Jr, S Ruddy, CB Sledge (eds). Philadelphia, Saunders, 2001, pp 1339–1376

339 WILSON DISEASE
George J. Brewer

Wilson disease is an autosomal recessive disorder caused by mutations in the *ATP7B* gene, a membrane-bound copper-transporting ATPase. Clinical manifestations are caused by copper toxicity and primarily involve the liver and the brain. Because effective treatment is available, it is important to make this diagnosis early.

GENETIC CONSIDERATIONS The frequency of Wilson disease in most populations is about 1 in 40,000, and the frequency of carriers of *ATP7B* mutations is about 1%. Based on these gene frequencies, the risk of Wilson disease in the children of an affected patient is about 1 in 200. Because a large number of inactivating mutations have been reported in the *ATP7B* gene, mutation screening is not practical, but DNA haplotype analysis can be used to genotype siblings of an affected patient.

PATHOGENESIS ATP7B protein deficiency impairs biliary copper excretion, resulting in positive copper balance, hepatic copper accumulation, and copper toxicity from oxidant damage. Excess hepatic copper is initially bound to metallothionein, but as this storage capacity is exceeded, liver damage begins as early as 3 years of age. Defective copper incorporation into apoceruloplasmin leads to excess catabolism and low blood levels of ceruloplasmin. Serum copper levels are usually lower than normal because of low blood ceruloplasmin, which normally binds >90% of serum copper. As the disease progresses, non-

TABLE 339-1 Useful Diagnosis Tests for Wilson Disease

Test	Usefulness[a]	Normal Value	Heterozygous Carriers	Wilson Disease
Serum ceruloplasmin	+	180–350 mg/L (18–35 mg/dL)	Low in 20%	Low in 85%
KF rings	++	Absent	Absent	Present in 99% + if neurologic or psychiatric symptoms present Present in 30–50% in hepatic presentation and presymptomatic state
24-h urine Cu	+++	0.3–0.8 μmol (20–50 μg)	Normal to 1.3 μmol (80 μg)	>1.6 μmol (>100 μg) in symptomatic patients 0.9 to >1.6 μmol (60 to >100 μg) in presymptomatic patients
Liver Cu	++++	0.3–0.8 μmol/g (20–50 μg) tissue	Normal to 2.0 μmol (125 μg)	>3.1 μmol (200 μg) (obstructive liver disease can cause false-positive results)
Haplotype analysis	++++ (Siblings only)	0 Matches	1 Match	2 Matches

[a] Usefulness: +, somewhat useful, to ++++, very useful.
Abbreviations: KF, Kayser-Fleischer; Cu, copper.

ceruloplasmin serum copper ("free" copper) levels increase, resulting in copper buildup in other parts of the body, such as the brain, leading to neurologic and psychiatric disease.

CLINICAL PRESENTATION ■ Hepatic Wilson disease may present as hepatitis, cirrhosis, or as hepatic decompensation, typically in the mid- to late-teenage years in western countries, although the age of presentation is quite broad and extends into the fourth decade of life. In India and countries in the Far East, the hepatic presentation may occur much earlier, often in children only five or six years of age.

An episode of hepatitis may occur, with elevated blood transaminase enzymes, with or without jaundice, and then spontaneously regress. Hepatitis often reoccurs, and most of these patients eventually develop cirrhosis.

Hepatic decompensation is associated with elevated serum bilirubin, reduced serum albumin and coagulation factors, ascites, peripheral edema, and hepatic encephalopathy. In severe hepatic failure, hemolytic anemia may occur because large amounts of copper are released into the bloodstream. The association of hemolysis and liver disease makes Wilson disease a likely diagnosis.

Neurologic The neurologic manifestations of Wilson disease typically occur in patients in their early twenties, although the age of onset extends from the second to the fifth decades of life. Magnetic resonance imaging and computed tomography scans reveal damage in the basal ganglia and occasionally in the pons, medulla, thalamus, cerebellum, and subcortical areas. The three main neurologic problems are of a movement disorder type: dystonia, incoordination, and tremor. Dysarthria and dysphagia are common. In some patients, the clinical picture closely resembles that of Parkinson's disease. Dystonia can involve any part of the body and eventually leads to grotesque positions of the limbs, neck, and trunk. Tremor, which is common, can be of any type. Autonomic disturbances may include orthostatic hypotension and sweating abnormalities as well as bowel, bladder, and sexual dysfunction. Memory loss, migraine-type headaches, and seizures may occur. Patients have difficulties focusing on tasks, but cognition is not usually grossly impaired. Sensory abnormalities and muscular weakness are not features of the disease.

Psychiatric A history of behavioral disturbances, with onset in the five years before diagnosis, is present in half of patients with neurologic disease. The features are diverse and may include loss of emotional control (temper tantrums, crying bouts), depression, hyperactivity, or loss of sexual inhibition.

Other Manifestations Some female patients have repeated spontaneous abortions, and most become amenorrheic prior to diagnosis. Cholelithiasis and nephrolithiasis occur with increased frequencies. Some patients may have osteoarthritis, particularly of the knee. Microscopic hematuria is common, and increased urinary excretion of phosphates, amino acids, glucose, or urates may occur; however, a full-blown Fanconi syndrome is rare. Sunflower cataracts and Kayser-Fleischer rings (copper deposits in the outer rim of the cornea) may be seen. Electrocardiographic and other cardiac abnormalities have been reported but are not common.

DIAGNOSIS Diagnostic tests for Wilson disease are listed in Table 339-1. Serum ceruloplasmin levels should be used only to affect the index of suspicion, because they are not always low in affected patients and are reduced in 20% of carriers. Kayser-Fleischer rings can only be diagnosed definitively by an ophthalmologist using a slit lamp. They are present in >99% of patients with neurologic/psychiatric forms of the disease and have been described very rarely in the absence of Wilson disease. Kayser-Fleischer rings are present in only about 30 to 50% of patients diagnosed in the hepatic or presymptomatic state; thus, the absence of rings does not exclude the diagnosis.

Symptomatic patients invariably have urine copper levels > 1.6 μmol (>100 μg) per 24 h. Heterozygotes never have values >1.6 μmol (>100 μg) per 24 h. About half of presymptomatic patients who are ultimately diagnosed as affected have urine copper values in an intermediate range between 0.9 and 1.6 μmol (60 and 100 μg) per 24 h. Because heterozygotes may have values up to 1.3 μmol (80 μg) per 24 h, patients in this range may require a liver biopsy for definitive diagnosis.

The "gold standard" for diagnosis remains liver biopsy with quantitative copper assays. Affected patients have values >3.1 μmol/g

TABLE 339-2 Recommended Anticopper Treatments for Wilson Disease

Disease Status	First Choice	Second Choice
Initial hepatic		
Hepatitis or cirrhosis without decompensation	Zinc[a]	Trientine
Hepatic decompensation		
Mild	Trientine[b] and zinc	Penicillamine[b] and zinc
Moderate	Trientine and zinc	Hepatic transplantation
Severe	Hepatic transplantation	Trientine and zinc
Initial neurologic/psychiatric	Tetrathiomolybdate[c] and zinc	Trientine and zinc
Maintenance	Zinc	Trientine
Presymptomatic	Zinc	Trientine
Pediatric	Zinc	Trientine
Pregnant	Zinc	Trientine

[a] Zinc acetate is supplied as Galzin. Recommended adult dose for all the above indications is 50 mg of elemental zinc three times daily, each dose separated from food and beverages other than water by at least 1 h, and separated from trientine or penicillamine doses by at least 1 h.

[b] Trientine is supplied as Syprine and penicillamine as Cuprimine. Recommended adult dosage for both drugs is 500 mg twice daily, each dose at least ½ h before or 2 h after meals.

[c] Tetrathiomolybdate is not yet commercially available but is expected to be marketed in the near future.

(>200 µg/g) dry weight of liver. Copper stains are not reliable. False-positive results can occur with long-standing obstructive liver disease, which can elevate hepatic and urine copper and rarely causes Kayser-Fleischer rings.

℞ TREATMENT

Recommended anticopper treatments are listed in Table 339-2. Penicillamine was previously the primary anticopper treatment but now plays a minor role because of its toxicity and because it worsens existing neurologic disease if used as initial therapy. If penicillamine is given, it should always be accompanied by 25 mg/d of pyridoxine. Trientine is a less toxic chelator and has largely supplanted penicillamine.

For patients with hepatitis or cirrhosis, without evidence of hepatic decompensation other than a mildly elevated bilirubin level and without neurologic or psychiatric symptoms from Wilson disease, zinc is the therapy of choice, although some advocate therapy with trientene. Zinc has proven efficacy in Wilson disease and is essentially nontoxic. It produces a negative copper balance by blocking intestinal absorption of copper, and it induces hepatic metallothionein synthesis, which sequesters additional toxic copper. All presymptomatic patients should be treated prophylactically, since the disease is close to 100% penetrant.

The first step in evaluating patients presenting with hepatic decompensation is to establish disease severity, which can be estimated using the Nazer prognostic index (Table 339-3). Patients with scores ≤6 can usually be managed with medical therapy. Patients with scores ≥10 should be considered immediately for liver transplantation, and those with scores between 7 and 9 require clinical judgment as to whether to recommend transplantation or medical therapy. A combination of trientine and zinc has been used to treat patients with Nazer scores as high as 9, but such patients should be watched carefully for indications of hepatic deterioration, which mandates transplantation.

For initial medical therapy of patients with hepatic decompensation, a chelator (trientine is preferred) plus zinc is recommended (Table 339-2). Zinc should not, however, be ingested simultaneously with trientine, as it will chelate zinc and form therapeutically ineffective complexes; the two drugs should be separated by at least 1 h. Hepatic transplantation is necessary for patients with severe hepatic decompensation.

For initial neurologic therapy, tetrathiomolybdate is emerging as the drug of choice because of its rapid action, preservation of neurologic function, and low toxicity. However, until tetrathiomolybdate is commercially available, trientine and zinc are recommended for 8 weeks, at which time the trientine can be stopped, and zinc continued for maintenance therapy. Although hepatic transplantation may improve neurologic symptoms, it does so only by removing copper, which can be done more safely and inexpensively with anticopper drugs.

Anticopper therapy must be lifelong. With treatment, liver function usually recovers after about a year, although residual liver damage is usually present. Neurologic and psychiatric symptoms usually improve between 6 and 24 months of treatment.

TABLE 339-3 *Prognostic Index of Nazer*

Laboratory Measurement	Normal Value	Score (in Points)				
		0	1	2	3	4
Serum bilirubin*	0.2–1.2 mg/dl	<5.8	5.8–8.8	8.8–11.7	11.7–17.5	>17.5
Serum aspartate transferase (AST)	10–35 IU/L	<100	100–150	151–200	201–300	>300
Prolongation of prothrombin time (seconds)	—	<4	4–8	9–12	13–20	>20

* If hemolysis is present, the serum bilirubin cannot be used as a measure of liver function until the hemolysis subsides.
Source: Modified with permission from Nazer H et al: Wilson's disease: Clinical presentation and use of prognostic index. *Gut* 1986; 27:1377–81.

Monitoring Anticopper Therapy When first using trientine or penicillamine, it is necessary to monitor for drug toxicity, particularly bone marrow suppression and proteinuria. Complete blood counts, standard biochemical profiles, and a urinalysis should be performed at weekly intervals for a month, then at 2-weekly intervals for 2 to 3 months, then at monthly intervals for 3 or 4 months, and at 4- to 6-monthly intervals thereafter.

The anticopper effects of trientine and penicillamine can be monitored by following 24-h "free" serum copper. Changes in urine copper are more difficult to interpret because excretion reflects the effect of the drug, as well as body loading with copper. Free serum copper is calculated by subtracting the ceruloplasmin copper from the total serum copper. Each 10 mg/L (mg/dL) of ceruloplasmin contributes 0.5 µmol/L (3.0 µg/dL) of serum copper. The normal free copper value is 1.6 to 2.4 µmol/L (10 to 15 µg/dL), and it often is as high as 7.9 µmol/L (50 µg/dL) in untreated Wilson disease. With treatment, free copper should be <3.9 µmol/L (<25 µg/dL).

Zinc treatment does not require blood or urine monitoring for toxicity. Its only significant side effect is gastric burning or nausea in about 10% of patients, usually with the first morning dose. This can be mitigated by taking the first dose an hour after breakfast or taking the zinc with a small amount of protein. Because zinc mainly affects stool copper, 24-h urine copper can be used to reflect body loading. The typical value in untreated symptomatic patients is >3.1 µmol (>200 µg) per 24 h. This level should decrease during the first 1 to 2 years of therapy to <2.0 µmol (<125 µg) per 24 h. A normal value [0.3 to 0.8 µmol (20 to 50 µg)] is rarely reached during the first decade of therapy and should raise concern about overtreatment (copper deficiency), the first sign of which is anemia and/or leukopenia.

FURTHER READING

BREWER GJ: Recognition, diagnosis and management of Wilson's disease. Proc Soc Ex Biol Med 223:39, 2000

BREWER GJ et al: Treatment of Wilson disease with ammonium tetrathiomolybdate: III. Initial therapy in 55 neurologically affected patients and follow-up with zinc therapy. Arch Neurol 60:379, 2003

———: Treatment of Wilson's disease with zinc: XV. Long-term follow-up studies. J Lab Clin Med 132:264, 1998

BULL PC et al: The Wilson disease gene is a putative copper transporting P-type ATPase similar to the Menkes gene. Nature Genet 5:327, 1993

COX DW, ROBERTS EA: Wilson Disease. GeneClinics, University of Washington, Seattle. Online. Available at *http://www.geneclinics.org/profiles/wilson/details.html*

SCHILSKY ML et al: Liver transplantation for Wilson's disease: Indications and outcome. Hepatology 19:583, 1994

---

340 LYSOSOMAL STORAGE DISEASES
Robert J. Hopkin, Gregory A. Grabowski

Lysosomes are heterogeneous subcellular organelles containing specific hydrolyases that allow targeted processing or degradation of proteins, nucleic acids, carbohydrates, and lipids. There are >30 different lysosomal storage diseases and these are classified based on the nature of the stored material (Table 340-1). The most prevalent among these disorders in adults will be reviewed here, including Fabry disease, Gaucher disease, and Niemann-Pick disease. Lysosomal storage diseases should be considered in the differential diagnosis of patients with neurologic, renal, or muscular degeneration and unexplained hepatomegaly, splenomegaly, cardiomyopathy, or skeletal dysplasias and deformations. Physical findings are disease-specific, and definitive diagnosis is made by enzyme assays.

TABLE 340-1 *Selected Lysosomal Storage Diseases*

Disorder[a]	Enzyme Deficiency	Stored Material	Clinical Types (Onset)	Inheritance	Neurologic
MUCOPOLYSACCHARIDOSES (MPS)					
MPS I H, Hurler (136)	α-L-Iduronidase	Dermatan sulfate Heparan sulfate	Infantile	AR	Mental retardation
MPS I H/S, Hurler/Scheie MPS I S, Scheie			Intermediate Adult		Mental retardation None
MPS II, Hunter (136)	Iduronate sulfatase	Dermatan sulfate Heparan sulfate	Severe infantile Mild juvenile	X-linked	Mental retardation, less in mild form
MPS III A, Sanfilippo A (136)	Heparan-N-sulfatase	Heparan sulfate	Late infantile	AR	Severe mental retardation
MPS III B, Sanfilippo B	N-Acctyl-α-glucosaminidase	Heparan sulfate	Late infantile	AR	Severe mental retardation
MPS III C, Sanfilippo C	Acetyl-CoA: α-glucosaminide N-acetyltransferase	Heparan sulfate	Late infantile	AR	Severe mental retardation
MPS III D, Sanfilippo D	N-Acetylglucosamine-6-sulfate sulfatase	Heparan sulfate	Late infantile	AR	Severe mental retardation
MPS IV A, Morquio (136)	N-Acetylgalactosamine-6-sulfate sulfatase	Keratan sulfate Chondroitin-6 sulfate	Childhood	AR	None
MPS VI B, Morquio (136)	β-Galactosidase		Childhood	AR	None
MPS VI, Maroteaux-Lamy (136)	Arylsulfatase B	Dermatan sulfate	Late infantile	AR	None
MPS VII (136)	β-Glucuronidase	Dermatan sulfate Heparan sulfate	Neonatal Infantile Adult	AR	Mental retardation, absent in some adults
GM₂ GANGLIOSIDOSES					
Tay-Sachs' disease (153)	β-Hexosaminidase A	GM_2 gangliosides	Infantile Juvenile	AR	Mental retardation, seizures, later juvenile form
Sandhoff's disease (153)	β-Hexosaminidases A and B	GM_2 gangliosides	Infantile	AR	Mental retardation, seizures
NEUTRAL GLYCOSPHINGOLIPIDOSES					
Fabry disease (150)	α-Galactosidase A	Globotriaosylceramide	Childhood	X-linked	Painful acroparesthesias
Gaucher disease (146)	Acid β-glucosidase	Glucosylceramide	Type 1 Type 2 Type 3	AR	None ++++ ++
Niemann-Pick disease (144) A and B	Sphingomyelinase	Sphingomyelin	Neuronopathic, type A Nonneuronopathic, type B	AR	Mental retardation and seizures
GLYCOPROTEINOSES					
Fucosidosis (140)	α-Fucosidase	Glycopeptides, oligosaccharides	Infantile Juvenile	AR	Mental retardation
α-Mannosidosis (140)	α-Mannosidase	Oligosaccharides	Infantile Milder variant	AR	Mental retardation
β-Mannosidosis (140)	β-Mannosidase	Oligosaccharides		AR	Seizures, mental retardation
Aspartylglucosaminuria (140)	Aspartylglucosaminidase	Aspartylglucosamine, glycopeptides	Young adult onset	AR	Mental retardation
Sialidosis (140)	Neuraminidase	Sialyloligosaccharides	Type I, congenital Type II, infantile and juvenile forms	AR	Myoclonus, mental retardation
MUCOLIPIDOSES (ML)					
ML-II, I-cell disease (138)	UDP-N-Acetylglucosamine-1-phosphotransferase	Glycoprotein, glyco-lipids	Infantile	AR	Mental retardation
ML-III, pseudo-Hurler polydystrophy (138)	UDP-N-Acetylglucosamine-1-phosphotransferase	Glycoprotein, glyco-lipids	Late infantile	AR	Mild mental retardation
LEUKODYSTROPHIES					
Krabbe's disease (147)	Galactosylceramidase	Galactosylceramide, Galactosyl sphingosine	Infantile	AR	Mental retardation
Metachromatic leukodystrophy (148)	Arylsulfatase A	Cerebroside sulfate	Infantile Juvenile Adult	AR	Mental retardation, dementia, and psychosis in adult
Multiple sulfatase deficiency (149)	Active site cysteine to C_α-formylglycine-converting enzyme	Sulfatides, mucopolysaccharides	Late infantile	AR	Mental retardation
DISORDERS OF NEUTRAL LIPIDS					
Wolman disease (142)	Acid lysosomal lipase	Cholesterol esters, triglycerides	Infantile	AR	Mild mental retardation
Cholesteryl ester storage disease (142)	Acid lysosomal lipase	Cholesteryl esters	Childhood	AR	None
Farber disease (142)	Acid ceramidase	Ceramide	Infantile Juvenile	AR	Occasional mental retardation

[a] Numbers in parentheses refer to the chapters in Scriver et al, 8th edition, for detailed reviews.   ***Note:*** AR, autosomal recessive.

Liver Spleen Enlargement	Skeletal Disease	Ophthalmologic	Hematologic	Unique Features
+++	++++	Corneal clouding	Vacuolated lymphocytes	Coarse facies, cardiovascular involvement, joint stiffness
+++	++++	Retinal degeneration, no corneal clouding	Granulated lymphocytes	Coarse facies, cardiovascular, joint stiffness, distinctive pebbly skin lesions
+	+	None	Granulated lymphocytes	Mild coarse facies
+	+	None	Granulated lymphocytes	Mild coarse facies
+	+	None	Granulated lymphocytes	Mild coarse facies
+	+	None	Granulated lymphocytes	Mild coarse facies
+	++++	Corneal clouding	Granulated neutrophils	Distinctive skeletal deformity, odontoid hypoplasia, aortic valve disease
±	++++		Granulated neutrophils and lymphocytes	Coarse facies, valvular heart disease
++	++++	Corneal clouding	Granulated neutrophils and lymphocytes	Coarse facies, valvular heart disease
+++	+++	Corneal clouding	Granulated neutrophils	Coarse facies, vascular involvement, hydrops fetalis in neonatal form
None	None	Cherry red spot in infantile form	None	Macrocephaly, hyperacusis in infantile form
++	±	Cherry red spot	None	Macrocephaly, hyperacusis
None	None	Corneal dystrophy, vascular lesions	None	Cutaneous angiokeratomas, hypohydrosis
++++	++++	None	Gaucher cells in bone marrow, cytopenias	Adult form highly variable
+++	+	Eye movements		
++++	++++	Eye movements		
++++	None	Macular degeneration	Foam cells in bone marrow	Pulmonary infiltrates
	Osteoporosis			Lung failure
++	++	None	Vacuolated lymphocytes, foam cells	Coarse facies, angiokeratomas in juvenile form
+++	++	Cataracts, corneal clouding	Vacuolated lymphocytes, granulated neutrophils	Coarse facies, enlarged tongue
	++	None	Vacuolated lymphocytes, foam cells	Angiokeratomas
±	++	None	Vacuolated lymphocytes, foam cells	Coarse facies
++, less in type I	++ less in type I	Cherry red spot	Vacuolated lymphocytes	MPS phenotype in type II
±	++++	Corneal clouding	Vacuolated and granulated neutrophils	Coarse facies, absence of mucopolysacchariduria, gingival hypoplasia
None	+++	Corneal clouding, mild retinopathy, hyperopic astigmatism		Coarse facies, stiffness of hands and shoulders
None	None	None	None	White matter globoid cells
None	None	Optic atrophy	None	Gait abnormalities in late infantile form
+	++	Retinal degeneration	Vacuolated and granulated cells	Absent activity of all known cellular sulfatases
+++	None	None	None	Adrenal calcification
Hepatomegaly	None	None	None	Cirrhosis
+/−	None	Macular degeneration	None	Arthropathy, subcutaneous nodules

PATHOGENESIS OF LYSOSOMAL STORAGE DISEASES

Lysosomal biogenesis involves ongoing synthesis of lysosomal hydrolases, membrane constitutive proteins, and new membranes. Lysosomes originate from the fusion of *trans*-Golgi network (TGN) vesicles with late endosomes. Progressive vesicular acidification accompanies the maturation of TGN vesicles, and this gradient facilitates the pH-dependent dissociation of receptors and ligands, as well as activating lysosomal hydrolases.

Abnormalities at any biosynthetic step can impair enzyme activation and lead to a lysosomal storage disorder. Following leader sequence clipping, complex oligosaccharide modifications occur during transit through the Golgi, including the mannose-6-phosphate modification of high-mannose oligosaccharide chains of many soluble lysosomal hydrolases. Lysosomal integral or associated membrane proteins are sorted to the membrane or interior of the lysosome by several different signals. Phosphorylation, sulfation, additional proteolytic processing, and macromolecular assembly of heteromers occur concurrently. These are critical to enzyme function, and defects can result in multiple enzyme/protein deficiencies.

The final common pathway for lysosomal storage diseases is the accumulation of specific macromolecules within tissues and cells that normally have a high flux of these substrates. The majority of lysosomal enzyme deficiencies result from point mutations or genetic rearrangements at a locus that encodes a single lysosomal hydrolase. However, some mutations cause deficiencies of several different lysosomal hydrolases by altering the enzymes/proteins involved in targeting, active site modifications, or macromolecular association or trafficking. All are inherited as autosomal recessive disorders, except Hunter (mucopolysaccharidosis, type II) and Fabry diseases, which are X-linked. Substrate accumulation leads to lysosomal distortion, which has significant pathologic consequences. In addition, abnormal amounts of metabolites may also have pharmacologic effects important to disease pathophysiology.

For many lysosomal diseases, the accumulated substrates are endogenously synthesized within particular tissue sites of pathology. Other diseases have greater exogenous substrate supplies. For example, they are delivered by low-density lipoprotein receptor–mediated uptake in Fabry and cholesteryl ester storage diseases or by phagocytosis in Gaucher disease type 1. The *threshold hypothesis* refers to a level of enzyme activity below which disease develops. Consequently, small changes in enzyme activity near the threshold can lead to or prevent disease. A critical element of this model is that enzymatic activity can be challenged by changes in substrate flux based on genetic background, cell turnover, recycling, or metabolic demands. Thus, a set level of residual enzyme may be adequate for substrate in some tissues or cells, but not in others.

SELECTED DISORDERS

TAY-SACHS DISEASE   About 1 in 30 Ashkenazi Jews is a carrier for Tay-Sachs disease, which is caused by total hexosaminidase A (Hex A) deficiency. The infantile form is a fatal neurodegenerative disease with macrocephaly, loss of motor skills, increased startle reaction, and a macular cherry red spot. The juvenile-onset form presents with ataxia and dementia, with death by age 10 to 15 years. The adult-onset disorder is characterized by clumsiness in childhood; progressive motor weakness in adolescence; and additional spinocerebellar, lower motor neuron symptoms, and dysarthria in adulthood. Intelligence declines slowly, and psychosis is common. Screening for Tay-Sachs disease carriers is recommended in the Ashkenazi Jewish population. *Sandhoff disease* is nearly identical to Tay-Sachs disease, but hepatosplenomegaly and bony dysplasias are also present.

FABRY DISEASE   Fabry disease is an X-linked disorder that results from mutations in the α-galactosidase gene. The estimated prevalence of hemizygous males is 1/40,000. Clinically, the disease manifests with angiokeratomas (telangiectatic skin lesions); hypohidrosis; corneal and lenticular opacities; acroparesthesia; and small-vessel disease of the kidney, heart, and brain.

The angiokeratomas and acroparesthesia may appear in childhood and lead to early diagnosis, if suspected. Angiokeratomas are punctate, dark red to blue-black, flat or slightly raised, usually symmetric, and do not blanch with pressure. They range from barely visible to several millimeters in diameter and have a tendency to increase in size and number with age. They usually are most dense between the umbilicus and knees—"the bathing suit area"—but may occur anywhere, including the mucosal surfaces. Angiokeratomas also occur in Fordyce scrotal angiokeratoma and several other lysosomal storage diseases. Corneal and lenticular lesions, detectable on slit-lamp examination, may help in establishing a diagnosis. Debilitating episodic burning pain of the hands, feet, and proximal extremities, acroparesthesia, can last from minutes to days and can be precipitated by changes in temperature, exercise, fatigue, or fever. Abdominal pain can resemble that from appendicitis or renal colic. Proteinuria, isosthenuria, and progressive renal dysfunction occur in the second to fourth decades. Hypertension, left ventricular hypertrophy, anginal chest pain with or without myocardial ischemia or infarction, and congestive heart failure can occur in the third to fourth decades. Leg lymphedema without hypoproteinemia and episodic diarrhea also occur. Death is due to renal failure or cardiovascular or cerebrovascular disease in untreated patients. Variants with residual α-galactosidase activity may have late-onset manifestations limited to the cardiovascular system that resemble hypertrophic cardiomyopathy. Up to 70% of heterozygous females may exhibit clinical manifestations, including central nervous system (CNS) and cardiac disease, but usually do not develop renal failure.

Phenytoin and carbamazepine diminish the chronic and episodic acroparesthesia. Chronic hemodialysis or kidney transplantation can be lifesaving in patients with renal failure. Enzyme therapy clears stored lipids from a variety of cells, particularly those of the renal, cardiac, and skin vascular endothelium. Renal insufficiency appears irreversible. Early institution of enzyme therapy likely will prevent or slow the progression of the life-threatening complications.

GAUCHER DISEASE   Gaucher disease is an autosomal recessive disorder that results from defective activity of acid β-glucosidase; >175 mutations have been described. Disease variants are classified based on the absence or presence and severity of neuronopathic involvement.

Type 1 Gaucher disease is a nonneuronopathic disease that can present in childhood to adulthood with slowly to rapidly progressive visceral disease. The average age at diagnosis is ~20 years in Caucasian populations and somewhat younger in other groups. This pattern of presentation is distinctly bimodal, with peaks at <10 to 15 years and at ~25 years. Younger patients tend to have a greater degree of hepatosplenomegaly and accompanying blood cytopenias. In contrast, the older group has a greater tendency for chronic bone disease. Hepatosplenomegaly occurs in virtually all symptomatic patients and can be minor or massive. Accompanying anemia and thrombocytopenia are variable and are not linearly related to liver or spleen volume. Severe liver dysfunction is unusual. Splenic infarctions can resemble an acute abdomen. Pulmonary hypertension and alveolar Gaucher cell accumulation are uncommon, but life-threatening, and can occur at any age.

All patients with Gaucher disease have nonuniform infiltration of bone marrow by lipid-laden macrophages, termed *Gaucher cells*. This can lead to marrow packing with subsequent infarction, ischemia, necrosis, and cortical bone destruction. Bone marrow involvement spreads from proximal to distal in the limbs and can involve the axial skeleton extensively, causing vertebral collapse. In addition to bone marrow involvement, bone remodeling is defective, with loss of total bone calcium leading to osteopenia, osteonecrosis, avascular infarction, and vertebral compression fractures and spinal cord involvement. Aseptic necrosis of the femoral head is common, as is fracture of the femoral neck. The mechanism by which diseased bone marrow macrophages interact with osteoclasts and/or osteoblasts to cause bone disease is not well understood. Chronic, ill-defined bone pain can be debilitating and poorly correlated with radiographic findings. "Bone crises" are associated with localized, excruciating pain, and, on occasion, local erythema, fever, and leukocytosis. Some patients have frequent crises, whereas other patients experience only one. These crises represent acute infarctions of bone, as evidenced in nuclear scans by localized absent uptake of pyrophosphate agents. Osteomyelitis should be excluded by appropriate cultures.

Decreased acid β-glucosidase activity (0 to 20% of normal) in nucleated cells makes the diagnosis. The enzyme is not present in bodily fluids. The sensitivity of enzyme testing is poor for heterozygote detection; molecular testing is preferred when the mutations are known. The disease frequency varies from about 1 in 1000 in Ashkenazi Jews to <1 in 100,000 in other populations. About 1 in 12 to 15 Ashkenazi Jews carries a Gaucher disease allele. Four common mutations account for ~90 to 95% of the mutations in affected patients: N370S (1226G), 84GG (a G insertion at cDNA position 84), L444P (1448C), and IVS-2 (an intron 2 splice junction mutation).

Genotype/phenotype studies indicate a significant correlation, though not absolute, between disease type and severity and the acid β-glucosidase genotype. The most common mutation in the Ashkenazi Jewish population (N370S) shares a 100% association with nonneuronopathic type 1 Gaucher disease. The N370S/N370S and N370S/other mutant allele genotypes are associated with later onset/less severe and with earlier onset/severe disease, respectively. As many as 50 to 60% of patients with the N370S/N370S genotype are discovered as asymptomatic family members. The other alleles are L444P (very low activity), 84GG (null), or IVS-2 (null), and rare/private or uncharacterized alleles. The L444P/L444P patients almost always have life-threatening to very severe/early-onset disease, and many, though not all, develop CNS involvement in the first two decades of life.

Symptomatic management of the blood cytopenias and joint replacement surgeries continue to have important roles in management. However, enzyme therapy is currently the treatment of choice in significantly affected patients and is highly efficacious and safe in diminishing the hepatosplenomegaly and improving bone marrow involvement and hematologic findings. The bone disease is decreased but not eliminated by enzyme replacement therapy. Adult patients may benefit from adjunctive treatment with bisphosphonates, which improves bone mineralization.

Type 2 Gaucher disease is a rare, severe CNS disease that leads to death by 2 years of age. *Type 3 Gaucher disease* has highly variable manifestations in the CNS and viscera. It can present in early childhood with rapidly progressive, massive visceral disease and slowly progressive to static CNS involvement; in adolescence with dementia; or in early adulthood with rapidly progressive, uncontrollable myoclonic seizures and mild visceral disease. Visceral disease in type 3 is nearly identical to that in type 1 but is generally more severe. Early CNS findings may be limited to defects in lateral gaze tracking, which may remain static for decades. Mental retardation can be slowly progressive or static. This variant is most frequent among individuals of Swedish descent.

NIEMANN-PICK DISEASE This is an autosomal recessive disorder that results from defects in acid sphingomyelinase. Types A and B are distinguished by an early age of onset and progressive CNS disease in type A. Type A typically has onset in the first 6 months, with rapidly progressive CNS deterioration, spasticity, failure to thrive, and massive hepatosplenomegaly. In contrast, B has a later, more variable onset and progression of hepatosplenomegaly, with eventual development of cirrhosis and hepatic replacement by foam cells. Affected patients develop progressive pulmonary disease with dyspnea, hypoxemia, and a reticular infiltrative pattern on chest x-ray. Foam cells are present in alveoli, lymphatic vessels, and pulmonary arteries. Progressive hepatic or lung disease lead to demise in adolescence to early adulthood.

The diagnosis is established by markedly decreased (1 to 10% of normal) sphingomyelinase activity in nucleated cells. There is no specific treatment for Neimann-Pick disease. The efficacy of hepatic or bone marrow transplantation has not been proven. Clinical trials using enzyme therapy are anticipated in the near future.

FURTHER READING

RISCH N: *Molecular epidemiology of Tay-Sachs disease.* Adv Genet 44:233, 2001

SCHIFFMANN R, BRADY RO: *New prospects for the treatment of lysosomal storage diseases.* Drugs 62:733, 2002

SCRIVER CR et al (eds): *The Metabolic and Molecular Bases of Inherited Diseases,* 8th ed. New York, McGraw-Hill, 2001

ZHAO H, GRABOWSKI GA: *Gaucher disease: Perspectives on a prototype lysosomal disease.* Cell Mol Life Sci 59:694, 2002

341 GLYCOGEN STORAGE DISEASES AND OTHER INHERITED DISORDERS OF CARBOHYDRATE METABOLISM
Yuan-Tsong Chen

Carbohydrate metabolism plays a vital role in cellular function by providing the energy required for most metabolic processes. The relevant biochemical pathways involved in the metabolism of these carbohydrates are shown in Fig. 341-1. Glucose is the principle substrate of energy metabolism in humans. Metabolism of glucose generates ATP via glycolysis and mitochondrial oxidative phosphorylation. Dietary sources of glucose are obtained by ingesting polysaccharides, primarily starch, and disaccharides including lactose, maltose, and sucrose. Galactose and fructose are two other monosaccharides that provide fuel for cellular metabolism; however, their role as fuel sources is much less significant than that of glucose. Galactose is derived from lactose (galactose + glucose), which is found in milk products, and is an important component for certain glycolipids, glycoproteins, and glycosaminoglycans. The two dietary sources of fructose are sucrose (fructose + glucose), a commonly used sweetener, and fructose itself, which is found in fruits, vegetables, and honey.

Glycogen, the storage form of glucose in animal cells, is composed of glucose residues joined in straight chains by $\alpha 1$-4 linkages and branched at intervals of 4 to 10 residues by $\alpha 1$-6 linkages. Glycogen forms a treelike molecule and can have a molecular weight of many millions; it may aggregate to form structures recognizable by electron microscopy. Defects in glycogen metabolism typically cause an accumulation of glycogen in the tissues; hence, the name *glycogen storage diseases*. The defects in gluconeogenesis or glycolytic pathways, including galactose and fructose metabolism, do not usually result in glycogen accumulation.

Clinical manifestations of the various disorders of carbohydrate metabolism differ markedly. The symptoms range from harmless to lethal. Unlike disorders of lipid metabolism, mucopolysaccharidoses, or other storage diseases, dietary therapy has been effective in many of the carbohydrate disorders. All of the genes responsible for the inherited defects of carbohydrate metabolism have been cloned, and mutations have been identified. Advances in our understanding of the molecular basis of these diseases are being used to improve diagnosis and management, and some of these disorders are candidates for enzyme replacement and early trials of gene therapy.

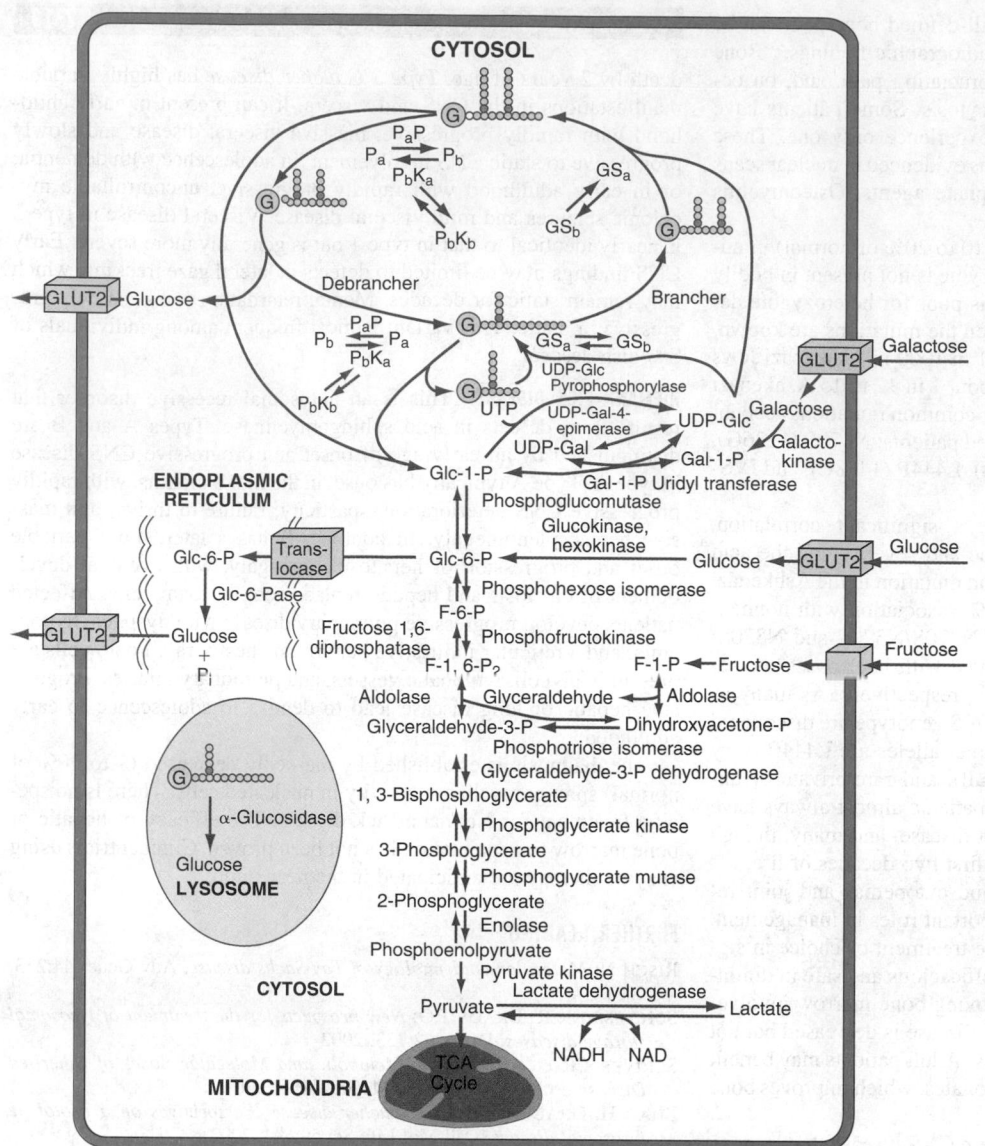

FIGURE 341-1 Metabolic pathways related to glycogen storage diseases and galactose and fructose disorders. Nonstandard abbreviations are as follows: GS$_a$, active glycogen synthase; GS$_b$, inactive glycogen synthase; P$_a$, active phosphorylase; P$_b$, inactive phosphorylase; P$_a$P, phosphorylase a phosphatase; P$_b$K$_a$, active phosphorylase b kinase; P$_b$K$_b$, inactive phosphorylase b kinase; G, glycogenin, the primer protein for glycogen synthesis. [Modified from AR Beaudet, in KJ Isselbacher et al (eds): Harrison's Principles of Internal Medicine, 13th ed. New York, McGraw-Hill, 1994, p 1855.]

Historically, the glycogen storage diseases were categorized numerically in the order in which the enzymatic defects were identified. They are also classified by the organs involved and clinical manifestations, the system followed in this chapter (Table 341-1). The overall frequency of all forms of glycogen storage disease is approximately 1 in 20,000 live births; most are inherited as autosomal recessive traits, but phosphoglycerate kinase deficiency and one form of phosphorylase kinase deficiency are X-linked disorders. The most common childhood disorders are glucose-6-phosphatase deficiency (type I), lysosomal acid α-glucosidase deficiency (type II), debrancher deficiency (type III), and liver phosphorylase kinase deficiency (type IX). The most common adult disorder is myophosphorylase deficiency (type V, or McArdle disease).

SELECTED LIVER GLYCOGENOSES

DISORDERS WITH HEPATOMEGALY AND HYPOGLYCEMIA ■ Type I Glycogen Storage Disease (Glucose-6-Phosphatase or Translocase Deficiency, von Gierke Disease)
Type I glycogen storage disease is an autosomal recessive disorder that causes glucose-6-phosphatase deficiency in liver, kidney, and intestinal mucosa. It can be divided into two subtypes: type Ia, in which the glucose-6-phosphatase enzyme is defective, and type Ib,

which is due to a defect in the translocase that transports glucose-6-phosphate across the microsomal membrane. The defects in both subtypes lead to inadequate conversion in the liver of glucose-6-phosphate to glucose and thus make affected individuals susceptible to fasting hypoglycemia.

CLINICAL AND LABORATORY FINDINGS Persons with type I disease may develop hypoglycemia and lactic acidosis during the neonatal period, but, more commonly, they present at 3 to 4 months of age with hepatomegaly. Hypoglycemia and lactic acidosis can develop after a short fast. These children often have doll-like faces with fat cheeks, relatively thin extremities, short stature, and a protuberant abdomen that is due to massive hepatomegaly; the kidneys are enlarged, but the spleen and heart are of normal size. The hepatocytes are distended by glycogen and fat with large and prominent lipid vacuoles. Despite hepatomegaly, liver enzymes are usually normal or near normal. Easy bruising and epistaxis are associated with a prolonged bleeding time as a result of impaired platelet aggregation/adhesion. Hyperuricemia is present. Hyperlipidemia includes elevation of triglycerides, cholesterol, and phospholipids.

LONG-TERM COMPLICATIONS Gout usually becomes symptomatic around puberty as a result of the long-term hyperuricemia. Puberty is often delayed. Virtually all females have ultrasound findings consistent with polycystic ovaries; however, the other clinical features of polycystic ovary syndrome, such as acne and hirsutism, are not seen. Secondary to the lipid abnormalities, there is an increased risk of pancreatitis. The dyslipidemia together with elevated erythrocyte aggregation predispose these patients to atherosclerosis. Frequent fractures and radiographic evidence of osteopenia are not uncommon in adult patients, and radial bone mineral content is significantly reduced in prepubertal patients. By the second or third decade of life, most patients with type I glycogen storage disease develop hepatic adenomas that can hemorrhage and, in some cases, become malignant. Renal disease is a serious late complication. Almost all patients older than 20 years have proteinuria and many have hypertension, kidney stones, nephrocalcinosis, and altered creatinine clearance. In some patients, renal function deteriorates and progresses to failure, requiring dialysis or transplantation.

DIAGNOSIS The diagnosis of type I disease can be suspected on the basis of clinical presentation and abnormal plasma lactate and lipid values. Before the glucose-6-phosphatase and glucose-6-phosphate translocase genes were cloned, a definitive diagnosis required a liver biopsy to demonstrate a deficiency. Gene-based mutation analysis now provides a noninvasive way of diagnosis for most patients with types Ia and Ib disease.

℞ **TREATMENT**

Treatment is designed to maintain normal blood glucose levels and is achieved by continuous nasogastric infusion of glucose or oral admin-

TABLE 341-1 *Features of Glycogen Storage Diseases and Galactose and Fructose Disorders*

Type/Common Name	Basic Defect	Clinical Features	Comments
LIVER GLYCOGENOSES			
Disorders with hepatomegaly and hypoglycemia			
Ia/von Gierke	Glucose-6-phosphatase	Growth retardation, enlarged liver and kidney, hypoglycemia, elevated blood lactate, cholesterol, triglycerides, and uric acid	Common, severe hypoglycemia Late complications in adulthood
Ib	Glucose-6-phosphate translocase	As for Ia, with additional findings of neutropenia and neutrophil dysfunction	~10% of type I
IIIa/Cori or Forbes	Liver and muscle debranching enzyme	Childhood: Hepatomegaly, growth retardation, muscle weakness, hypoglycemia, hyperlipidemia, elevated liver transaminases; liver symptoms improve with age Adulthood: muscle atrophy and weakness; onset: third to fourth decades; variable cardiomyopathy	Common, intermediate severity of hypoglycemia Liver cirrhosis can occur
IIIb	Liver debranching enzyme (normal muscle debrancher activity)	Liver symptoms same as in type IIIa; no muscle symptoms	~15% of type III
VI/Hers	Liver phosphorylase	Hepatomegaly, mild hypoglycemia, hyperlipidemia and ketosis; symptoms improve with age	Rare, "benign" glycogenosis
IX/phosphorylase kinase deficiency	Liver phosphorylase kinase α subunit	As for VI	Common, "benign glycogenosis," X-linked
0/glycogen synthase deficiency	Glycogen synthase	Fasting hypoglycemia and ketosis, elevated lactic acid and hyperglycemia after glucose load	Decreased glycogen stores
XI/Fanconi-Bickel	Glucose transporter-2	Failure to thrive, rickets, hepatomegaly, proximal renal tubular dysfunction, impaired glucose and galactose utilization	Rare, consanguinity in 70%
Disorders with liver cirrhosis			
IV/Andersen	Branching enzyme	Failure to thrive, hypotonia, hepatomegaly, splenomegaly, progressive liver cirrhosis and failure (death usually before fifth year); some without progression	One of the rarer glycogenoses; other neuromuscular variants exist
MUSCLE GLYCOGENOSES			
Disorders with muscle-energy impairment			
V/McArdle	Muscle phosphorylase	Exercise intolerance, muscle cramps, myoglobinuria on strenuous exercise, increased CK	Common, male predominance
VII/Tarui	Phosphofructokinase—M subunit	As for type V, with additional findings of a compensated hemolysis	Prevalent in Ashkenazi Jews and Japanese
Phosphoglycerate kinase deficiency	Phosphoglycerate kinase	As for type V, with additional findings of a hemolytic anemia and CNS dysfunction	Rare, X-linked
Phosphoglycerate mutase deficiency	Phosphoglycerate mutase—M subunit	As for type V	Rare; most patients are African American
Lactate dehydrogenase deficiency	Lactic acid dehydrogenase—M subunit	As for type V, with additional findings of erythematous skin eruption and uterine stiffness resulting in childbirth difficulty in female	Rare
Fructose 1,6-bisphosphate aldolase A deficiency	Fructose 1,6-bisphosphate aldolase A	As for type V, with additional finding of hemolytic anemia	Rare
Pyruvate kinase deficiency	Pyruvate kinase—muscle isozyme	Muscle cramps and/or fixed muscle weakness	Rare
Muscle phosphorylase kinase deficiency	Muscle-specific phosphorylase kinase	As for type V, some patients may have muscle weakness and atrophy	Rare, autosomal recessive
β-enolase deficiency	Muscle β-enolase	Exercise intolerance	Rare
Disorders with progressive skeletal myopathy and/or cardiomyopathy			
II/Pompe	Lysosomal acid α-glucosidase	Infantile: hypotonia, muscle weakness, cardiac enlargement and failure, fatal early Juvenile and adult: progressive skeletal muscle weakness and atrophy, proximal muscle and respiratory muscle are seriously affected	Common, undetectable, or very low level of enzyme activity in infantile form; residual enzyme activity in late-onset
Cardiac phosphorylase kinase deficiency	Cardiac-specific phosphorylase kinase	Severe cardiomyopathy and early heart failure	Very rare
GALACTOSE DISORDERS			
Galactosemia with uridyl transferase deficiency	Galactose 1-phosphate uridyl transferase	Vomiting, hepatomegaly, jaundice, cataracts, amino aciduria, failure to thrive	Long-term complications exist despite early diagnosis and treatment
Galactokinase deficiency	Galactokinase	Cataracts	Benign
Uridine diphosphate galactose 4-epimerase deficiency	Uridine diphosphate galactose 4-epimerase	Similar to transferase deficiency with additional findings of hypotonia and nerve deafness	Benign variant exists
FRUCTOSE DISORDERS			
Essential fructosuria	Fructokinase	Asymptomatic, positive urine reducing substance	Benign
Hereditary fructose intolerance	Fructose 1-phosphate aldolase B	Vomiting, lethargy, failure to thrive, hepatic failure	Prognosis good with early diagnosis and fructose restriction
Fructose 1,6-diphosphatase deficiency	Fructose 1,6-diphosphatase	Episodic hypoglycemia and lactic acidosis	Avoid fasting, good prognosis

Note: CK, creatine kinase; M, muscle; CNS, central nervous system.

istration of uncooked cornstarch. Uncooked cornstarch acts as a slow-release form of glucose and can be given at a dose of 1.6 g/kg every 4 h for infants younger than 2 years. As the child grows older, the cornstarch regimen can be changed to every 6 h, and can be given by mouth as a liquid (1:2, weight:volume) at a dose of 1.75 to 2.5 g/kg of body weight. Because fructose and galactose cannot be converted to free glucose, their dietary intake should be restricted. Dietary supplements of multivitamins and calcium are required. Allopurinol is given to lower uric acid levels. The hyperlipidemia can be reduced with lipid-lowering drugs such as HMG-CoA reductase inhibitors and fibric acids. Preliminary studies of treating microalbuminuria, an early indicator of renal dysfunction in these patients, have also shown angiotensin-converting enzyme (ACE) inhibitors to be beneficial. Citrate supplement may be beneficial in preventing or ameliorating nephrocalcinosis and development of urinary calculi.

Type III Glycogen Storage Disease (Debrancher Deficiency, Limit Dextrinosis)

Type III glycogenoses are autosomal recessive disorders caused by a deficiency of glycogen debranching enzyme. Debranching enzyme and phosphorylase are responsible for complete degradation of glycogen; when debranching enzyme is defective, glycogen breakdown is incomplete and an abnormal glycogen accumulates that has short outer chains and resembles limit dextrin.

CLINICAL AND LABORATORY FINDINGS Deficiency of glycogen debranching enzyme causes hepatomegaly, hypoglycemia, short stature, variable skeletal myopathy, and cardiomyopathy. The disorder usually involves both liver and muscle and is termed *type IIIa glycogen storage disease.* However, in about 15% of patients, the disease appears to involve only the liver and is classified as *type IIIb.* Remarkably, hepatomegaly and hepatic symptoms in most patients with type III disease improve with age and usually disappear after puberty.

Hypoglycemia, hyperlipidemia, and elevated liver transaminases occur in children. In contrast to type I disease, fasting ketosis is prominent, and blood lactate and uric acid concentrations are usually normal. Serum creatine kinase levels can sometimes be used to identify patients with muscle involvement, but normal levels do not rule out muscle enzyme deficiency.

DIAGNOSIS In type IIIa glycogen storage disease, deficient debranching enzyme activity can be demonstrated in liver, skeletal muscle, and heart. In contrast, patients with type IIIb have debranching enzyme deficiency in the liver but not in muscle. In the past, definitive assignment of subtype required enzyme assays in both liver and muscle. DNA-based analyses now provide a noninvasive way of subtyping these disorders in most patients.

℞ TREATMENT

Dietary management of type III disease is less demanding than that of type I. If hypoglycemia is present, frequent high-carbohydrate meals with cornstarch supplements or nocturnal gastric drip feedings are usually effective. A high-protein diet during the day plus overnight protein enteral infusion may be tried in patients with myopathy, but it is not established whether such a regimen is effective.

Type VI Glycogen Storage Disease [Liver Phosphorylase Deficiency (Hers Disease)]

These patients present with hepatomegaly and growth retardation early in childhood. Hypoglycemia, hyperlipidemia, and hyperketosis are usually mild, if present. Plasma lactic acid and uric acid levels are normal. The heart and skeletal muscles are not involved. The hepatomegaly and growth retardation improve with age and usually disappear at puberty. Treatment is symptomatic. A high-carbohydrate diet and frequent feeding are effective in preventing hypoglycemia, but most patients require no specific treatment.

Type IX Glycogen Storage Disease (Liver Phosphorylase Kinase Deficiency)

Defects of phosphorylase kinase cause a heterogeneous group of glycogenoses. The phosphorylase kinase enzyme complex consists of four subunits (α, β, γ, and δ), each encoded by different genes (X chromosome as well as autosomes) that are differentially expressed in various tissues. Phosphorylase kinase deficiency can be divided into several subtypes on the basis of the gene/subunit involved, the tissues that are primarily affected, and the mode of inheritance. The most common subtype is X-linked liver phosphorylase kinase deficiency, which is also one of the most common liver glycogenoses. Phosphorylase kinase activity may also be deficient in erythrocytes and leukocytes but is normal in muscle. Typically, a child between the ages of 1 and 5 presents with growth retardation and hepatomegaly. Levels of cholesterol, triglycerides, and liver enzymes are mildly elevated. Ketosis may occur after fasting. Lactic and uric acid levels are normal. Hypoglycemia is mild, if present. Hepatomegaly and abnormal blood chemistries gradually return to normal with age. Most adults achieve a normal final height and are practically asymptomatic, despite a persistent phosphorylase kinase deficiency.

Treatment is symptomatic. A high-carbohydrate diet and frequent feedings are effective in preventing hypoglycemia; some patients require no specific treatment. Prognosis is usually good; adult patients have normal stature and minimal hepatomegaly.

Other subtypes of Type IX include an autosomal recessive form of liver and muscle phosphorylase kinase deficiency, an autosomal recessive form of liver phosphorylase kinase deficiency that often develops into liver cirrhosis, a muscle-specific phosphorylase kinase deficiency that causes cramps and myoglobinuria with exercise, and a cardiac-specific phosphorylase kinase deficiency that is lethal during infancy because of massive glycogen deposition in the myocardium.

Other Liver Glycogenoses with Hepatomegaly and Hypoglycemia

These disorders include glycogen synthase deficiency (type 0) and hepatic glycogenosis with renal Fanconi syndrome (type XI). The latter is caused by defects in the facilitative glucose transporter 2 (GLUT-2), which transports glucose in and out of hepatocytes, pancreatic cells, and the basolateral membranes of intestinal and renal epithelial cells. The disease is characterized by proximal renal tubular dysfunction, impaired glucose and galactose utilization, and accumulation of glycogen in liver and kidney.

SELECTED MUSCLE GLYCOGENOSES

DISORDERS WITH MUSCLE-ENERGY IMPAIRMENT ■ Type V Glycogen Storage Disease (Muscle Phosphorylase Deficiency, McArdle Disease)

Type V glycogen storage disease is an autosomal recessive disorder caused by deficiency of muscle phosphorylase. McArdle disease is a prototypical muscle energy disorder as the enzyme deficiency limits ATP generation by glycogenolysis and results in glycogen accumulation.

CLINICAL AND LABORATORY FINDINGS Symptoms usually develop first in adulthood and are characterized by exercise intolerance with muscle cramps. Two types of activity tend to cause symptoms: (1) brief exercise of great intensity, such as sprinting or carrying heavy loads; and (2) less intense but sustained activity, such as climbing stairs or walking uphill. Moderate exercise, such as walking on level ground, can be performed by most patients for long periods. About half of patients report burgundy-colored urine after exercise, the consequence of myoglobinuria secondary to rhabdomyolysis. Intense myoglobinuria after vigorous exercise may cause renal failure. In rare cases, electromyography (EMG) findings may suggest an inflammatory myopathy, and the diagnosis can be confused with polymyositis.

The level of serum creatine kinase is usually elevated at rest and increases after exercise. Exercise also increases the levels of blood ammonia, inosine, hypoxanthine, and uric acid. The latter abnormalities are attributed to accelerated recycling of muscle purine nucleotides in the face of insufficient ATP production.

DIAGNOSIS Lack of an increase in blood lactate and exaggerated blood ammonia elevations after an ischemic exercise test are indicative of muscle glycogenosis and suggest a defect in the conversion of glycogen or glucose to lactate. The abnormal exercise response, however, is not limited to type V disease and can occur with other defects in glycogenolysis or glycolysis, such as deficiencies of muscle phosphofructokinase or debranching enzyme (when the test is done after fasting). Definitive diagnosis is made by enzymatic assay in muscle tissue or by mutation analysis of the myophosphorylase gene.

℞ TREATMENT

In general, avoidance of strenuous exercise can prevent major episodes of rhabdomyolysis; however, regular and moderate exercise is recommended to improve exercise capacity. A high-protein diet may increase exercise endurance, and creatine supplement has been shown to improve muscle function in some patients. In general, longevity does not appear to be affected.

DISORDERS WITH PROGRESSIVE SKELETAL MUSCLE MYOPATHY AND/OR CARDIOMYOPATHY ■ Type II Glycogen Storage Disease (Acid α-1,4 Glucosidase Deficiency, Pompe Disease) Type II disease is an autosomal recessive disorder caused by a deficiency of lysosomal acid α-1,4 glucosidase (acid maltase), an enzyme responsible for the degradation of glycogen in lysosomal vacuoles. It is characterized by the accumulation of glycogen in lysosomes as opposed to its accumulation in cytoplasm as in the other glycogenoses.

CLINICAL AND LABORATORY FINDINGS The disorder encompasses a range of phenotypes, each including myopathy but differing in age of onset, organ involvement, and clinical severity. The most severe is the infantile-onset disease with cardiomegaly, hypotonia, and death before age 1. Infants appear normal at birth but soon develop generalized muscle weakness with feeding difficulties, macroglossia, hepatomegaly, and congestive heart failure due to a hypertrophic cardiomyopathy.

The juvenile, or late-childhood, form is characterized by skeletal muscle manifestations, usually without cardiac involvement, and a slowly progressive course. The juvenile form typically presents as delayed motor milestones (if age of onset is early enough) and difficulty in walking. These manifestations are followed by swallowing difficulties, proximal muscle weakness, and respiratory muscle involvement. Death may occur before the end of the second decade.

An adult form of type II disease presents as a slowly progressive myopathy without cardiac involvement and has its onset between the second and seventh decades. The clinical picture is dominated by slowly progressive proximal muscle weakness with truncal involvement. The pelvic girdle, paraspinal muscles, and the diaphragm are most seriously affected. The initial symptoms may be respiratory insufficiency manifested by somnolence, morning headache, orthopnea, and exertional dyspnea.

Laboratory findings include elevated levels of serum creatine kinase, aspartate transaminase, and lactate dehydrogenase, particularly in infants. Muscle biopsy shows the presence of vacuoles that stain positively for glycogen, and muscle acid phosphatase is increased, presumably from a compensatory increase of lysosomal enzymes. EMG reveals myopathic features with irritability of muscle fibers and pseudomyotonic discharges. Serum creatine kinase is not always elevated in adults and, depending on the muscle biopsied or tested, muscle histology or EMG may not be abnormal. It is prudent to examine affected muscle.

DIAGNOSIS Diagnosis can be established by demonstration of the absence or reduced levels of acid α-glucosidase activity in muscle or cultured skin fibroblasts. Deficiency is usually more severe in the infantile form than in the juvenile and adult disorders.

℞ TREATMENT

Definitive therapy is not currently available; a high-protein diet may be useful for the juvenile and adult forms. Nocturnal ventilatory support in late-onset patients improves the quality of life and is beneficial during a period of respiratory decompensation. Clinical trials of enzyme replacement therapy have begun. Preliminary data have shown that recombinant acid α-glucosidase is capable of improving cardiac and skeletal muscle function in these patients.

SELECTED DISORDERS OF GALACTOSE METABOLISM

"Classic" *galactosemia* is due to galactose 1-phosphate uridyl transferase deficiency. It is a serious disease with an early onset of symptoms; the incidence is 1 in 60,000. The newborn infant normally receives up to 20% of caloric intake as lactose, which consists of glucose and galactose. Without the transferase, the infant is unable to metabolize galactose 1-phosphate (Fig. 341-1), the accumulation of which results in injury to parenchymal cells of the kidney, liver, and brain.

Widespread newborn screening for galactosemia has identified these infants early and allowed them to be placed on dietary restriction. Elimination of galactose from the diet reverses growth failure and renal and hepatic dysfunction and improves the prognosis. However, on long-term follow-up, these patients still have ovarian failure manifest as primary or secondary amenorrhea, as well as developmental delay and learning disabilities, which increase in severity with age. In addition, most patients have speech disorders, and a smaller number demonstrate poor growth and impaired motor function and balance (with or without overt ataxia). The treatment of galactosemia to prevent long-term complications remains a challenge.

Deficiency of *galactokinase* (Fig. 341-1) causes cataracts. Deficiency of *uridine diphosphate galactose 4-epimerase* can be benign when the enzyme deficiency is limited to blood cells but can be as severe as "classic" galactosemia when the enzyme deficiency is generalized.

SELECTED DISORDERS OF FRUCTOSE METABOLISM

Fructokinase deficiency (Fig. 341-1) causes a benign condition that is usually an incidental finding made through the detection of fructose as a reducing substance in the urine.

Deficiency of *fructose 1,6-bisphosphate aldolase* (aldolase B, hereditary fructose intolerance) is a serious disease of infants because of a defect in gluconeogenesis. These patients are healthy and asymptomatic until fructose or sucrose (table sugar) is ingested (usually from fruit, fruit juice, or sweetened cereal). Clinical manifestations may include jaundice, hepatomegaly, vomiting, lethargy, irritability, and convulsions. Laboratory findings include prolonged clotting time, hypoalbuminemia, elevation of bilirubin and transaminases, and proximal renal tubular dysfunction. If the disease is not diagnosed and intake of the noxious sugar persists, hypoglycemic episodes recur, and liver and kidney failure progress, eventually leading to death. Treatment consists of the complete elimination of all sources of sucrose, fructose, and sorbitol from the diet. With this treatment, liver and kidney dysfunction improve, and catch-up growth is common. Intellectual development is usually unimpaired. As the patient matures, symptoms become milder, even after fructose ingestion, and the long-term prognosis is good.

Fructose 1,6-diphosphatase deficiency is characterized by childhood life-threatening episodes of acidosis, hypoglycemia, hyperventilation, convulsions, and coma. These episodes are triggered by febrile infections and gastroenteritis when oral food intake decreases. Laboratory findings include low blood glucose, high lactate and uric acid levels, and metabolic acidosis. In contrast to hereditary fructose intolerance, there is usually no aversion to sweets, and renal tubular and liver functions are normal. Treatment of acute attacks consists of correction of hypoglycemia and acidosis by intravenous infusion. Later, avoidance of fasting and elimination of fructose and sucrose from the diet prevent further episodes. For long-term prevention of hypoglycemia, a slowly released carbohydrate such as cornstarch is useful. Prognosis is good as patients who survive childhood develop normally.

FURTHER READING

AMALFITANO A et al: Recombinant human acid-α-glucosidase enzyme therapy for infantile glycogen storage disease type II: Results of a phase I/II clinical trial. Genet Med 3:132, 2001

DIMAURO S, LAMPERTI C: Muscle glycogenoses. Muscle Nerve 24:984, 2001

SCRIVER CR et al (Eds): *The Metabolic and Molecular Bases of Inherited Disease*, 8th ed, New York, McGraw-Hill, 2001

SHEN J-J, CHEN Y-T: Molecular characterization of glycogen storage disease type III. Curr Mol Med 2:167, 2002

Heritable disorders that involve the major connective tissues of the body such as bone, skin, cartilage, blood vessels, and basement membranes are among the most common genetic diseases in human beings. Here we will focus primarily on those disorders that can have severe manifestations, are relatively common, and are sufficiently understood at the molecular level to provide useful paradigms: osteogenesis imperfecta (OI), the Ehlers-Danlos syndrome (EDS), chondrodysplasias (CDs), the Marfan syndrome (MFS), epidermolysis bullosa (EB), and the Alport syndrome (AS).

THE CHALLENGE OF CLASSIFYING THE DISEASES The original classification of connective tissue diseases was based on the pattern of inheritance, the cluster of signs and symptoms, the histologic changes in tissues, and limited information about the molecular defects involved. This classification included about a dozen types and subtypes for OI, about the same number for the EDS, and over 150 for the CDs. Several limitations in these original classifications are now apparent. One is that the same mutation does not always produce the same disease phenotype in terms of severity of the condition or its clinical course. Such phenotypic variation occurs in many genetic diseases, including the connective tissue disorders, in which some members of a family are severely affected, whereas others with the same mutation have a mild disorder.

Most patients with classic features of a severe connective tissue disease have a mutation in a gene, or genes, coding for a single protein.

For example, the majority of patients with OI have a mutation in one of the two genes coding for type I procollagen. Similarly, most patients with MFS have mutations in a gene for fibrillin. For other disease categories, the situation is more complex. In EDS, for example, the type IV variant is usually caused by mutations in the gene for type III procollagen, the type VI variant by defects in the gene for lysyl hydroxylase, and the type VII variant by defects in a gene required for processing type I procollagen to type I collagen.

Classifications of these disorders also tend to overemphasize the etiologic differences between severe genetic diseases that are apparent in infants and the more common diseases that appear much later in life. Single-gene defects can cause subsets of late-onset diseases such as osteoporosis, aneurysms, and osteoarthritis. For example, a small subset of patients with postmenopausal osteoporosis have mutations in the genes for procollagen I similar to the mutations in the same genes that produce lethal variants of OI. Likewise, a subset of patients with familial aortic aneurysms have mutations in the gene for procollagen III similar to the mutations in the same gene that cause lethal variants of type IV EDS, and occasional patients with osteoarthritis have mutations in the gene for procollagen II similar to the mutations in the same gene that cause lethal CDs.

DEFINITION AND COMPOSITION OF CONNECTIVE TISSUES The distinguishing feature of connective tissues is that it consists of complex macromolecules that are assembled into an insoluble extracellular matrix (Table 342-1). The macromolecules include at least 25 different types of collagens, the related fibrous proteins known as *elastin* and *fibrillin*, a series of proteoglycans, and other components whose structure and function are only partially defined. Differences in the connective tissues of bone, skin, and cartilage are partially explained by differences in the content of specific components (Table 342-1). For example, tendons and ligaments consist primarily of type I collagen fibrils and small amounts of other components that help organize the type I fibrils into thick fibers and fiber bundles. Cartilage consists primarily of fibrils of type II collagen in the form of arcades that are distended by highly charged proteoglycans. The extracellular matrix of the aorta contains collagens that provide tensile strength and elastin that provides elasticity. Differences among the connective tissues also depend on the three-dimensional organization of the molecular components. The type I collagen fibrils in tendon are packed into thick, parallel bundles of fibers, whereas type I collagen fibrils in skin are randomly oriented. In cortical bone, type I collagen fibrils form helical arrays around haversian canals.

BIOSYNTHESIS OF CONNECTIVE TISSUE Connective tissues form primarily by a process of self-assembly, in which a molecule of the correct size, shape, and surface property binds to other molecules with the same or similar structure in a spontaneous and precisely ordered manner. The molecular mechanisms and driving forces are similar to those involved in crystal formation.

Collagen Synthesis Collagens have a triple-helical conformation, because each of the three α chains has a simple, repetitive amino acid se-

TABLE 342-1 *Constituents of Connective Tissues in Various Tissues*

Connective Tissue	Major Constituents	Approximate Amounts, % dry wt	Characteristics or Functions
Dermis, ligaments, tendons	Type I collagen	80	Bundles of fibrils
	Type III collagen	5–15	Thin fibrils
	Type IV collagen, laminin, nidogen	<5	In basal laminae under epithelium and endothelium
	Types V, VI, and VII collagens	<5	VII forms anchoring fibrils; others unknown
	Elastin, fibrillin	<5	Provides elasticity
	Fibronectin	<5	Associated with collagen fibers and cell surfaces
	Proteoglycans,[a] hyaluronate	0.5	Provide resiliency
Bone (demineralized)	Type I collagen	90	Complex fibril network
	Type VI collagen	1–2	Function unclear
	Proteoglycans[a]	1	Function unclear
	Osteonectin, osteopontin, osteocalcin, α2-glycoprotein, sialoproteins	1–5	May regulate mineralization
Aorta	Type I collagen	20–40	Fibril network
	Type III collagen	20–40	Thin fibrils
	Elastin, fibrillin	20–40	Provide elasticity
	Type IV collagen, laminin, nidogen	<5	Form basal lamina
	Types V and VI collagens	<2	Functions unclear
	Proteoglycans[a]	<3	Provide resiliency
Cartilage	Type II collagen	40–50	Arcades of thin fibrils
	Type IX collagen	5–10	Links type II fibrils
	Type X collagen	5–10	Surrounds hypertrophic cells
	Type XI collagen	<10	Function unclear
	Proteoglycans,[a] hyaluronate	15–50	Provides resiliency

[a] As discussed in text, >30 proteoglycans have now been identified. They differ in the structures of their core proteins and their contents of glycosaminoglycan side chains of chondroitin-4-sulfate, chondroitin-6-sulfate, dermatan sulfate, and keratin sulfate. Basal lamina contain a proteoglycan with a side chain of heparan sulfate that resembles heparin.

quence of about 1000 amino acids in which glycine (Gly) appears as every third amino acid. Therefore, the sequence of each α chain can be designated as $(\text{-Gly-X-Y-})_{333}$, where X and Y represent amino acids other than glycine. To fold into a triple helix, every third amino acid in an α chain must be glycine, the smallest amino acid, since this residue must fit in a sterically restricted space where the three chains of the triple helix come together. Many of the X- and Y-position amino acids are proline and hydroxyproline, which, because of their ring structure, provide rigidity to the triple helix.

Twenty-five different collagens have been identified. Many are minor constituents that probably have highly specialized functions. The fibrillar collagens are abundant proteins that are found in tissues as long, highly ordered fibrils with a characteristic banding pattern revealed by electron microscopy. Type I collagen, the most abundant, is composed of two identical α chains called $\alpha1(I)$ and a third called $\alpha2(I)$. Type II collagen, the fibrillar collagen of cartilage, is composed of three identical α chains called $\alpha1(II)$. Type III collagen is found in small amounts in many tissues that contain type I collagen and in large amounts in large blood vessels; it is composed of three identical chains called $\alpha1(III)$. Type IV collagen in basement membranes self-assembles into a complex three-dimensional network that provides a diffusion barrier in the renal glomerulus, pulmonary alveolus, and other tissues.

Collagens are first synthesized as larger and more soluble precursors called *procollagens* that are composed of proα chains. As the proα chains of procollagen are synthesized on ribosomes, the free ends move into the cisternae of the rough endoplasmic reticulum (Fig. 342-1). Hydrophobic signal peptides at the N termini are cleaved, and additional posttranslational reactions begin. Proline residues in the Y position of the repeating -Gly-X-Y- sequences are converted to hydroxyproline by prolyl hydroxylase. The requirement for ascorbic acid as cofactor in the hydroxylation of prolyl residues explains why wounds fail to heal in scurvy (Chap. 61). If sufficient proline residues are not converted to hydroxyproline, collagen cannot fold into a triple helix that is stable at body temperature. The abnormal protein accumulates in the cisternae of the rough endoplasmic reticulum and is slowly degraded. Lysine residues in the Y position are similarly hydroxylated to hydroxylysine by lysyl hydroxylase. Many of the hydroxylysine residues are glycosylated with galactose or with galactose and glucose. A large mannose-rich oligosaccharide is assembled on the C-terminal propeptide of each chain.

After secretion, procollagen is processed to collagen by cleavage of the N-propeptides by procollagen N-proteinase and of the C-propeptides by procollagen C-proteinase. The processing converts the precursor to type I collagen and thereby decreases the solubility of the protein about 1000-fold. The entropic energy that is released drives the spontaneous self-assembly of the collagen into fibrils. Self-assembled collagen fibers have considerable tensile strength, which is increased by cross-linking reactions that form covalent bonds between α chains in one molecule and α chains in adjacent molecules. The first step in cross-linking is oxidation by lysyl oxidase of amino groups on a few lysine or hydroxylysine residues to form aldehydes that interact to form stable covalent bonds.

During growth and development, the collagen fibrils in all tissues undergo repeated synthesis, degradation, and resynthesis. The degradation of collagen fibers in tissues is initiated by specific collagenases. Collagen fibers in most tissues of normal adults undergo very little metabolic turnover. One exception to this is the collagen fibrils that are degraded and resynthesized as part of the continual remodeling of bone. Also, although the collagen in many adult tissues is metabolically stable, the rate of turnover increases under some circumstances. In starvation, a large fraction of the collagen in skin and other con-

FIGURE 342-1 Schematic representation of synthesis of a type I collagen fibril by a fibroblast. *A.* Intracellular steps in the assembly of the procollagen molecule. Hydroxylations and glycosylations of the proα chains begin soon after the amino termini pass into the cisternae of the rough endoplasmic reticulum and continue after the three chains associate through their carboxy-terminal propeptides and become disulfide linked. *B.* Cleavage of procollagen to collagen, self-assembly of the collagen molecule into quarter-staggered fibrils, and cross-linking of the molecules in the fibrils. Cleavage of the propeptides may occur within crypts of the fibroblast, as shown here, or some distance from the cell. Mutations (depicted by X) cause the synthesis of structurally abnormal pro$\alpha1(I)$ or pro$\alpha2(I)$ chains of type I procollagen by interfering either with protein assembly (procollagen suicide) (*A*) or with processing to normal collagen fibrils (*B*). (*From DJ Prockop et al, Am J Med Genet 34:60, 1989, with permission.*)

nective tissues is degraded, thus providing amino acids for gluconeogenesis. Large losses of collagen also occur in most connective tissues during immobilization or prolonged periods of low-gravitational stress. In rheumatoid arthritis, pannus invasion causes a rapid degradation of collagen in the articular cartilage. Glucocorticoids decrease the collagen content of most connective tissues, including bone, by decreasing the rate of collagen synthesis. Decreases in collagen weaken tissues. In many pathologic states, however, collagen is deposited in excess. With injury to tissue, inflammation is usually followed by increased deposition primarily of type I collagen fibrils in the form of fibrotic tissue and scars. The deposition of collagen fibrils during the repair process is largely irreversible and is a major feature of the pathologic changes in hepatic cirrhosis, pulmonary fibrosis, atherosclerosis, and nephrosclerosis and in the scarring of skin and ligaments after surgery or trauma.

Elastin Synthesis Elastin assembly appears to be closely related to that of collagen, since a few of the prolines in the protein are hydroxylated to hydroxyproline by prolyl hydroxylase. The elastin monomer, however, is a single polypeptide that does not fold into a defined three-dimensional structure and is not synthesized as a larger precursor molecule. Instead, it is slowly secreted from cells into extracellular compartments, where it forms amorphous deposits around previously deposited microfibrils. The elastin deposits then become covalently cross-linked through oxidation of lysine residues to aldehydes by the same lysyl oxidase that initiates the cross-linking of collagen. The microfibrils in elastin deposits are largely composed of fibrillin, a large protein that forms beadlike strands.

Proteoglycan Synthesis The synthesis of proteoglycans begins in the cisternae of the rough endoplasmic reticulum with assembly of a core protein that then undergoes sequential additions of sugars to generate large side chains of glycosaminoglycans. At least 30 proteoglycans have been identified by differences in the structures of their core proteins and their side chains. The major proteoglycan of cartilage, called

FIGURE 342-2 Examples of single-base mutations found in type I procollagen in patients with osteogenesis imperfecta (OI) and osteoporosis. Mild refers to type I OI, severe to type II OI, and moderate to type III or type IV OI.

aggrecan, has a core protein of about 2000 amino acids, which are bound multiple side chains of chondroitin sulfate and keratin sulfate, polysaccharides consisting of highly charged and repetitive disaccharide sequences. The highly charged proteoglycan aggregate binds water and small ions that distend the collagen network and thereby make the tissue resilient to pressure.

MUTATIONS THAT PRODUCE DISEASES OF CONNECTIVE TISSUES The most complete data on mutations causing heritable disorders of connective tissue are available on OI. Most patients with OI have mutations in either the gene for the proα1(I) chain or the gene for the proα2(I) chain of type I procollagen (the COL1A1 and COL1A2 genes). Most of the mutations in patients with severe OI cause synthesis of a structurally abnormal but partially functional proα chain. They include partial gene deletions, partial gene duplications, and RNA splicing mutations. The most common mutations, however, cause the substitution of single amino acids with bulky side chains for the glycine residues that appear as every third amino acid in the triple-helical domain of a proα chain (Fig. 342-2). The structurally abnormal proα chains exert their effects primarily through one of three mechanisms (Fig. 342-1). First, the presence of an abnormal proα chain in a procollagen molecule containing two normal proα chains can prevent folding of the protein into a triple-helical conformation and lead to degradation of the whole molecule in a process called *procollagen suicide*. Similar dominant negative mutations are seen with other multisubunit proteins. The net result of procollagen suicide is accumulation of the unfolded protein in the rough endoplasmic reticulum of cells and a reduction in the amount of collagen available for fibril assembly. Second, the presence of one abnormal proα chain in a procollagen molecule can interfere with cleavage of the N-propeptide from the protein. The persistence of the N-propeptide on a fraction of the molecules interferes with the self-assembly of normal collagen so that thin and irregular collagen fibrils are formed. Third, the substitution of a bulkier amino acid for glycine can produce a change in the conformation of the mol-

ecule and result in the assembly of collagen fibrils that are abnormally branched or abnormally thick and short.

Over 500 mutations in the two genes for type I procollagen have been found in patients with OI (Fig. 342-2). The data on mutations in type I procollagen that cause OI have been used as a paradigm for defining other mutations in other collagen and procollagen genes that cause other disorders of connective tissue.

Several generalizations can be made about mutations in collagen genes. One is that unrelated patients rarely have the same mutation in the same gene. Another is that mutations that cause the most severe disease are usually new mutations in one allele that occur either during the generation of the germline in one of the parents or during meiosis in the fertilized egg (Chap. 56). Another general trend is that similar mutations in different regions of the same gene can produce different disease syndromes in both severity and the major tissues involved. One reason for heterogeneity in pathologic manifestations is that different regions of a large molecule may be more important for its function in some connective tissues than in others. For example, some regions of the type I collagen molecule may be essential for the binding of mineralizing proteins in bone so that mutations in these regions cause fragile bones but do not impair function in skin and other nonmineralizing tissues. It is more difficult, however, to explain how the same mutation can produce a severe phenotype in some and a mild phenotype in other members of the same family. Such phenotypic variation appears to be characteristic of OI, where some subjects are short and have multiple fractures from minor trauma, whereas others in the same family can be of normal stature and free of fractures. In the past, such phenotypic variation was explained by undefined variations in the genetic background of different family members. Studies in transgenic mice, however, demonstrated similar phenotypic variation with expression of a mutated collagen gene in an inbred strain of mice whose genetic background was uniform. Therefore, the phenotypic variation is probably caused by undefined stochastic or chance events during embryonic and fetal development. Although dramatic phenotypic variations are relatively rare in OI and related disorders, it is important to consider in counseling families about the consequences of inherited mutations.

SPECIFIC DISORDERS

OSTEOGENESIS IMPERFECTA OI causes a generalized decrease in bone mass (osteopenia) and makes the bones brittle. The disorder is frequently associated with blue sclerae, dental abnormalities (dentinogenesis imperfecta), progressive hearing loss, and a positive family history. The most severe forms cause death in utero, at birth, or shortly thereafter. The course of mild and moderate forms is more variable. Some patients appear normal at birth and become progressively worse. Some have multiple fractures in infancy and childhood, improve after puberty, and fracture more frequently later in life. Women are particularly prone to fracture during pregnancy and after menopause. A few women from families with mild variants of OI do not develop fractures until after menopause, and their disease may be difficult to distinguish from postmenopausal osteoporosis.

Classification The most common classification for OI was developed by Sillence (Table 342-2). Type I, the mildest form, is inherited as an

TABLE 342-2 *Classification of Osteogenesis Imperfecta (OI)*

Type	Bone Fragility	Blue Sclerae	Abnormal Dentition	Hearing Loss	Inheritance[a]
I	Mild	Present	Present in some	Present in most	AD
II	Extreme	Present	Present in some	Unknown	S, rarely AR
III	Severe	Bluish at birth	Present in some	High incidence	AD, rarely AR
IV	Variable	Absent	Absent in IVA, present in IVB	High incidence	AD

[a] AD, autosomal dominant; AR, autosomal recessive; S, sporadic.

autosomal dominant trait. Most patients have distinctly blue sclerae. Type II is lethal in utero or shortly after birth. Types III and IV are intermediate in severity between types I and II. They differ from type I because they are greater in severity and because blue sclerae are absent or only slightly bluish in infancy and white in adulthood. Type III differs from type IV because it tends to become more severe with age. The distinction between type IV and type III OI may not be helpful. Therefore, it may be sufficient to classify patients simply as mild (type I), lethal (type II), and moderately severe (type III).

Incidence   Type I OI has a frequency of about 1 in 30,000. Type II OI has a reported incidence at birth of about 1 in 60,000, but the combined incidence of the three severe forms that are recognizable at birth (types II, III, and IV) may be much higher.

Skeletal Changes   In type I OI, the fragility of bones may be severe enough to limit physical activity or so mild that individuals are unaware of any disability. Radiographs of the skull in patients with mild disease may show a mottled appearance because of small islands of irregular ossification. In type II OI, bones and other connective tissues are so fragile that massive injuries can occur in utero or during delivery. Ossification of many bones is frequently incomplete. Continuously beaded or broken ribs and crumpled long bones (accordina femora) may be present. For unclear reasons, the long bones may be either thick or thin. In types III and IV, multiple fractures from minor physical stress can produce severe deformities. Kyphoscoliosis can impair respiration, cause cor pulmonale, and predispose to pulmonary infections. On radiographs the appearance of "popcorn-like" deposits of mineral on the ends of long bones is an ominous sign. Progressive neurologic symptoms may result from basilar compression and communicating hydrocephalus.

In all forms of OI, bone mineral density in unfractured bone is decreased. However, the degree of osteopenia may be difficult to evaluate because recurrent fractures limit exercise and thereby worsen the decrease in bone mass. Surprisingly, fractures appear to heal normally.

Ocular Changes   The sclerae can be normal, slightly bluish, or bright blue. The color is probably caused by a thinness of the collagen layers of the sclerae that allows the choroid layers to be seen. Blue sclerae, however, are an inherited trait in some families who do not have increased bone fragility.

Dentinogenesis Imperfecta   The teeth may be normal, moderately discolored, or grossly abnormal. The enamel generally appears normal, but the teeth may have a characteristic amber, yellowish brown, or translucent bluish gray color because of improper deposition or deficiency of dentin. The deciduous teeth are usually smaller than normal, whereas permanent teeth are frequently bell-shaped and restricted at the base. In some patients, the teeth readily fracture and need to be extracted. The defect in dentin is directly attributable to the fact that normal dentin is rich in type I collagen. Similar tooth defects, however, can be inherited without any evidence of OI.

Hearing Loss   Hearing loss usually begins during the second decade of life and occurs in more than 50% of individuals over age 30. The loss can be conductive, sensorineural, or mixed and varies in severity. The middle ear usually exhibits maldevelopment, deficient ossification, persistence of cartilage in areas that are normally ossified, and abnormal calcium deposits.

Associated Features   Changes in other connective tissues can include thin skin that scars extensively, joint laxity with permanent dislocations indistinguishable from those of EDS, and, occasionally, cardiovascular manifestations such as aortic regurgitation, floppy mitral valves, mitral incompetence, and fragility of large blood vessels. For reasons unknown, some patients develop a hypermetabolic state with elevated serum thyroxine levels, hyperthermia, and excessive sweating.

Molecular Defects   Most patients with OI have mutations in one of the two genes that encode type I procollagen. Over 90% of patients with type I OI and blue sclerae have mutations in the proα1(I) gene that

decrease the steady-state levels of the mRNA for proα1(I) chains and decrease the rates of synthesis of proα1(I) chains relative to those for proα2(I) chains. In more severe forms (types II, III, and IV), the effects of mutations that cause synthesis of abnormal proα chains are amplified by the three mechanisms discussed above (Fig. 342-1). Mutations that change the structure of the protein near the N-proteinase cleavage site cause accumulation of a partially processed procollagen and produce lax joints similar to those in type VII EDS that is caused by mutations in the gene for the N-proteinase. Mutations that change the structure in the middle or near the C terminus of the molecule tend to cause severe or lethal variants of OI. It is difficult, however, to correlate the site or nature of the mutation with the clinical phenotype (Fig. 342-2). Most patients are heterozygotes with mutations in a single allele, but rare patients are homozygotes with two mutated alleles for proα1(I) or proα2(I) chains.

Mosaicism in Germ-Line Cells and in Somatic Cells   Most lethal OI is the result of new autosomal dominant mutations. The frequency of a second child with lethal OI in the same family, however, is about 7% because of germ-line mosaicism in one of the parents. The presence of germ-line mosaicism has been indicated in several fathers of patients with type II OI by demonstrating the mutated gene in a fraction of their sperm. Because of the possibility for germ-line mosaicism, asymptomatic parents of a child with severe OI should be counseled that recurrence can occur.

Diagnosis   Diagnosis is usually made on the basis of clinical criteria. The presence of fractures together with blue sclerae, dentinogenesis imperfecta, or family history of the disease is usually sufficient to make the diagnosis. Other causes of pathologic fractures must be excluded, including the battered child syndrome, nutritional deficiencies, malignancies, and other inherited disorders such as CDs and hypophosphatasia. The absence of superficial bruises can be helpful in distinguishing OI from battered child syndrome. X-rays usually reveal a decrease in bone density that can be verified by photon or x-ray absorptiometry. There is no consensus, however, as to whether the diagnosis can be made by microscopy of bone. A molecular defect in type I procollagen can be demonstrated in at least half of patients by incubating skin fibroblasts with radioactive amino acids and then analyzing the proα chains by polyacrylamide gel electrophoresis. The analysis detects decreases in the rate of synthesis of proα1(I) chains relative to proα2(I) chains, abnormally long proα chains, abnormally short proα chains, and proα chains with excessive posttranslational modification because of an amino acid substitution that impairs folding of the triple helix. The mutations themselves can be defined in most patients by the sequencing of genomic DNA. Because each proband and family usually has a "private" mutation, extensive analysis of about 10,000 bases in each of the two genes is required to identify the exact mutation. After a mutation in a type I procollagen gene is identified, a simple test based on the polymerase chain reaction can be used to screen family members at risk and for prenatal diagnosis.

℞ TREATMENT

Many patients with OI have successful careers despite severe deformities. Those with mild disorder may need little treatment when fractures decrease after puberty, but women require special attention during pregnancy and after menopause, when fractures again increase. More severely affected children require a comprehensive program of physical therapy, surgical management of fractures and skeletal deformities, and vocational education.

Many of the fractures are only slightly displaced and have little soft tissue swelling. Therefore, they can be treated with minimal support or traction for a week or two followed by a light cast. If fractures are relatively painless, physical therapy can be initiated early. A judicious amount of exercise prevents loss of bone mass secondary to physical inactivity. Some physicians advocate insertion of steel rods into long bones to correct limb deformities; the risk/benefits and cost/

benefits of such procedures are difficult to evaluate. Aggressive conventional intervention is usually warranted for pneumonia and cor pulmonale. For severe hearing loss, stapedectomy or replacement of the stapes with a prosthesis may be successful. Moderately to severely affected patients should be evaluated periodically to anticipate possible neurologic problems. About half of children have a substantial increase in growth when given growth hormone. Treatment with bisphosphonates to decrease bone loss has been introduced on an experimental basis. Initial results are promising, but the long-term effects of decreasing bone resorption are unknown. Also, a clinical trial has been initiated to use stromal cells from bone marrow that can differentiate into osteoblasts after systemic infusion. In the first phase of the trial, four children with severe OI (type III) showed clinical improvement after marrow ablation and transplantation of whole bone marrow from an HLA-compatible sibling.

Counseling and emotional support are important for patients and their parents; and lay organizations in some countries provide help in these areas. Prenatal ultrasonography will detect severely affected fetuses at about 16 weeks of pregnancy. Diagnosis by demonstrating synthesis of abnormal proα chains or by DNA sequencing can be carried out in chorionic villa biopsies at 8 to 12 weeks of pregnancy.

EHLERS-DANLOS SYNDROME   EDS is characterized by hyperelasticity of the skin and hypermobile joints.

Classification   Nine types of EDS were initially defined primarily based on the extent to which the skin, joints, and other tissues are involved. Type I is the classic, severe form of the disease, with both severe joint hypermobility and skin that is velvety in texture, hyperextensible, and easily scarred. Type II is similar to type I but milder. In type III, joint hypermobility is more prominent than skin changes. In type IV, the skin changes are more prominent than joint changes. However, type IV patients are predisposed to sudden death from rupture of large blood vessels or other hollow organs. Type V is similar to type II but is inherited as an X-linked trait. Type VI is characterized by scoliosis, ocular fragility, and a cone-shaped deformity of the cornea (keratoconus). Type VII is characterized by marked joint hypermobility that is difficult to distinguish from type III except by the specific molecular defects in the processing of type I procollagen to collagen. Type VIII is distinguished by prominent periodontal changes. Types IX, X, and XI were defined on the basis of preliminary biochemical and clinical data, but these classifications have not proven to be useful. Because of overlapping signs and symptoms, many patients and families with some of the features of EDS cannot be assigned to any of the defined types.

Incidence   The incidence of EDS is difficult to establish, largely because patients with mild skin or joint symptoms rarely seek medical attention. It is also difficult to define the normal range of variation for joint mobility or skin elasticity. The incidence may be about 1 in 5000 births, although a higher value has been reported for blacks. Types I, II, and III account for most diagnoses.

Skin   The changes vary from thin and velvety skin to skin that is either dramatically hyperextensible ("rubber man" syndrome) or easily torn or scarred. Type I patients develop characteristic "cigarette-paper" scars. In type IV extensive scars and hyperpigmentation develop over bony prominences, and the skin may be so thin that subcutaneous blood vessels are visible. In type VIII the skin is more fragile than hyperextensible, and it heals with atrophic, pigmented scars. Easy bruisability occurs in several types of EDS.

Ligament and Joint Changes   Laxity and hypermobility of joints vary from mild to unreducible dislocations of hips and other large joints. In mild forms, patients learn to reduce dislocations by limiting physical activity. In more severe forms, surgical repair may be required. Some patients have progressive difficulty with age, but severe joint laxity is compatible with a normal life span.

Associated Changes   Mitral valve prolapse and hernias occur, particularly with type I. Pes planus and mild to moderate scoliosis are common. Extreme joint laxity and repeated dislocations may lead to degenerative arthritis. In type VI, the eye may rupture with minimal trauma, and kyphoscoliosis can cause respiratory impairment. Also, sclerae may be blue.

Molecular Defects   Mutations in two of the three genes for type V collagen have been found in patients with types I and II EDS. Mutations in both the α1(V) and α2(V) chain are found in patients with type I EDS, but to date only mutations in the α1(V) chain have been found in patients with type II EDS.

Most patients with type IV EDS have a defect either in the synthesis or structure of type III procollagen, a finding consistent with the fact that these patients are prone to spontaneous rupture of the aorta and intestines, tissues rich in type III collagen. The thinness and scarring of skin are more difficult to explain, since type III constitutes a small fraction of the collagen in skin (Table 342-1). Most of the 500 or more mutations in the type III procollagen gene lead to synthesis of abnormal but partially functional proα1(III) chains that produce procollagen suicide or alter fibril formation by the same mechanisms that amplify the effects of mutations in the genes for type I procollagen. Similar mutations in type III procollagen can cause aortic aneurysms in some individuals without other evidence of EDS type IV, MFS, or other inherited disorders of connective tissue.

Type VI EDS is caused by mutations in the gene that encodes lysyl hydroxylase. In one series, all the patients were homozygous or compound heterozygotes for the mutated genes, and all the mutations caused profound deficiency of lysyl hydroxylase, a decrease in the hydroxylysine content of collagen, and a decrease in the cross-links in collagen fibers. The decrease in cross-links is explained by the observation that some cross-links are less stable if formed from lysine instead of hydroxylysine.

Type VII EDS occurs because of a defect in the conversion of procollagen to collagen caused either by mutations that make type I procollagen resistant to cleavage by procollagen N-proteinase or by mutations that decrease the activity of the enzyme. The type VIIA mutations alter the cleavage site in the proα1(I) chain, and the type VIIB mutations alter the cleavage site in the proα2(I) chain. Both types are dominantly inherited. Type VIIC is caused by mutations that decrease the activity of procollagen N-proteinase and is inherited as an autosomal recessive trait. In all three forms of type VII EDS, the persistence of the N-propeptide causes the formation of collagen fibrils that are thin and irregular. Since most patients do not have clinical osteopenia, the thin and irregular fibrils apparently suffice for the structural integrity of bone but do not provide the necessary tensile strength for ligaments and joint capsules. However, some patients fracture easily, and their disorder is difficult to distinguish from variants of OI.

The cause of type VIII EDS is unknown. Type IX is a disorder of copper transport. The syndrome, also referred to as *Menkes' syndrome*, is due to an X-linked defect and is associated with cutis laxa, hypopigmentation, unusual hair ("kinky"), vascular aneurysms, neurologic degeneration, and mental retardation. Mutations in a gene coding for a copper-transporting ATPase cause the disease (Chaps. 339 and 344). Type X EDS may be caused by defects in fibronectin, but no specific mutations have been defined.

Diagnosis   The diagnosis is based on clinical criteria. Biochemical assays and gene analyses for known molecular defects in EDS are difficult and time-consuming, but specific diagnostic tests should be available in the future for families in whom the genes at fault have been defined.

℞ TREATMENT

There is no specific therapy. Surgical repair and tightening of joint ligaments require careful evaluation of individual patients, as the ligaments frequently do not hold sutures. Patients with easy bruisability should be evaluated for other bleeding disorders. Patients with type IV EDS and members of their families should probably be evaluated at regular intervals by sonography and related techniques for early detection of aneurysms. Surgical repair of aneurysms may be difficult because of increased friability of tissues, and there is limited experience with elective surgery in such patients. Also, women with type IV EDS should be counseled about the increased risk of uterine rupture, bleeding, and other complications of pregnancy.

CHONDRODYSPLASIAS (See also Chap. 334.) The CDs are inherited skeletal disorders that cause dwarfism and abnormal body proportions. The category also includes some individuals with normal stature and body proportions who have features such as ocular changes or cleft palate that are common in more severe CDs. Many patients develop degenerative joint changes, and mild CD in adults may be difficult to differentiate from primary generalized osteoarthritis. Some authors refer to the disorders as "skeletal dysplasias," but CD is a more widely used term.

Classification Over 150 distinct types and subtypes have been defined based on criteria such as "bringing death" (thanatophoric), causing "twisted" bones (diastrophic), affecting metaphyses (metaphyseal), affecting epiphyses (epiphyseal), and producing histologic changes such as an apparent increase in the fibrous material in the epiphyses (fibrochondrogenesis). Also, a number of eponyms are based on the first or most comprehensive case reports. Severe forms of the diseases produce gross distortions of most cartilaginous structures and of the eye. Mild forms are more difficult to classify. Among the features are cataracts, degeneration of the vitreous and retinal detachment, high forehead, hypoplastic facies, cleft palate, short extremities, and gross distortions of the epiphyses, metaphyses, and joint surfaces.

Incidence Data on the frequency of most CDs are not available, but the incidence of the Stickler syndrome may be as high as 1 in 10,000. Therefore, the diseases are probably among the more common heritable disorders of connective tissue.

Molecular Defects The first mutations shown to cause CDs were in the COL2A1 gene for type II collagen, the most abundant protein in cartilage. A number of mutations in this gene have now been reported in variants of CD ranging from mild to lethal. A large fraction of patients with lethal CDs, a smaller number of patients with moderately severe CDs, and about 2% of families with early-onset generalized osteoarthritis have mutations in the same gene. However, similar phenotypes can also be caused by mutations in other genes, including genes for three other collagens, additional components of the cartilage matrix, growth factors, growth factor receptors, and transcription factors. The number of mutated genes reported does not necessarily reflect the incidence of such mutations in the diseases themselves but rather the complexity of the genes and the technical difficulties in searching the complete gene for mutations. Also, it reflects the availability of large families for DNA linkage analysis and the vigor with which investigators have pursued their interest in a given gene. It is likely that mutations in additional genes will be found.

Mutations in the COL2A1 gene were first found in patients with severe CDs characterized by gross deformities of bones and cartilage such as spondyloepiphyseal dysplasia congenita, hypochondrogenesis/achondrogenesis II, and the Kniest syndrome. However, mutations in the COL2A1 gene have been found in a few families where few if any symptoms are present in childhood, but joint stiffness, joint pain, and degenerative changes of osteoarthritis develop in midlife. The mutations in the COL2A1 gene are similar to the mutations in the genes for types I and III procollagens, and the correlations between genotype and the severity of the phenotype are equally difficult. Stickler syndrome and related syndromes are caused by mutations in three different genes: the COL2AI gene for type II collagen and the COL11A1 and COL11A2 genes for type XI collagen. A series of mutations that introduce premature terminal signals in the COL2A1 gene lead to classic Stickler syndrome. However, some patients with classic Stickler syndrome have glycine substitutions in COL11A1. RNA splicing mutations in the COL11A1 gene are found in patients with the Marshall syndrome, which is similar to classic Stickler syndrome but with milder eye changes and more severe hearing loss.

Many individuals with the Schmid metaphyseal CD, characterized by short stature, *coxa vara*, flaring metaphyses, and waddling gait, have mutations in the gene for the type X collagen, a short, network-forming collagen found primarily in the hypertrophic zone of endochondral cartilage.

Mutations in the receptor for fibroblast growth factor (FGFR3) are present in most patients with achondroplasia, the most common cause of short-limbed dwarfism accompanied by macrocephaly and dysplasias of the metaphyses of long bones. The same single-base mutation in the gene that converts glycine to arginine at position 380 is present in >90% of patients. Most patients represent sporadic new mutations, and this nucleotide change must be one of the most common recurring mutations in the human genome. The mutation causes unregulated signal transduction through the receptor and inappropriate development of cartilage. Mutations that alter other domains of FGFRE3 have been found in patients with the more severe disorders hypochondroplasia and thanatophoric dysplasia and in a few families with a variant of craniosynostosis. However, most patients with craniosynostosis appear to have mutations in the related *FGFR2 gene*.

Mutations in the gene for the cartilage oligomeric matrix protein (COMP) have been found in patients with multiple epiphyseal dysplasia or pseudoachondroplasia and in related syndromes characterized by short limbs and degenerative arthritis. However, some families with multiple epiphyseal dysplasia had a mutation in the gene for the $\alpha1$(IX), $\alpha2$(IX), or $\alpha3$(IX) chain of type IX collagen (COL9A1, COL9A2, and COL9A3), or matrilin-3. All the known mutations in these two type IX collagen genes in patients with multiple epiphyseal dysplasia cause splicing out of the codons in the same domain. One predisposing mutation in COL9A2 and one predisposing mutation in COL9A3 were found in Finnish patients with the common condition of sciatica and herniations of vertebral discs.

Diagnosis The diagnosis of severe forms of CD is made on the basis of the physical appearance, x-ray findings, histologic changes, and clinical course.

℞ TREATMENT

No definitive therapy is available. Symptomatic treatment is directed to secondary features such as degenerative arthritis. Many patients require joint replacement surgery and corrective surgery for cleft palate. The eyes should be monitored carefully for the development of cataracts and the need for laser therapy to prevent retinal detachment. Patients should probably be advised to avoid obesity and contact sports. Counseling for the psychological problems of short stature is critical, and support groups have formed in many countries. Ultrasonography is sometimes successful for prenatal diagnosis but is less successful than for OI. Specific DNA tests are available for the CDs caused by mutations in most of the genes identified to date.

MARFAN SYNDROME MFS is characterized by a triad of features: (1) long, thin extremities frequently associated with other skeletal changes, such as loose joints and arachnodactyly; (2) reduced vision as the result of dislocations of the lenses (ectopia lentis); and (3) aortic aneurysms that typically begin at the base of the aorta.

Classification The clinical diagnosis is frequently problematic because some affected members of families with MFS present with only one or two features of the typical clinical triad. Also, many patients present with one or two of the features of MFS without a family history, apparently because they represent sporadic mutations. Therefore, it is frequently difficult to determine whether a patient with ectopia lentis or the characteristic body habitus of MFS is at risk for developing a life-threatening aortic aneurysm on the basis of clinical data alone. The new DNA diagnostic tests for mutations in the fibrillin-1 and fibrillin-2 genes can probably resolve most, but not all, of these problems. Most patients who are prone to develop an aortic aneurysm as a component of MFS can be identified by detection of mutations in the fibrillin-1 gene. Some of these patients develop aortic aneurysms because of a mutation in the fibrillin-1 gene without the skeletal or ocular changes characteristic of MFS. Patients with the rarer form of MFS, which is characterized by contractural arachnodactyly instead of loose joints, can usually be identified by detection of a mutation in the fibrillin-2 gene that is similar in structure to the gene for fibrillin-1. Preliminary data suggest that patients with mutations in the fibrillin-2 gene are not prone to develop aneurysms. However, affected members of some rare families with a mutation in the fibrillin-1 gene also do not develop aortic aneurysms, even though they may show the skeletal or ocular changes. Therefore, the DNA tests are most helpful if: (1) a mutation is detected in either of the two genes, and (2) informative data are available on the clinical symptoms that the same mutation produces in the patient's family or in other families with similar clinical features.

Incidence and Inheritance MFS has an incidence of about 1 in 10,000 in most racial and ethnic groups. The disorder is inherited as an autosomal dominant trait; at least one-fourth of patients do not have an affected parent, and therefore probably represent new mutations.

Skeletal Changes Patients have long limbs and are usually tall compared to other members of the same family. The ratio of the upper segment (top of the head to the top of the pubic ramus) to the lower segment (top of the pubic ramus to the floor) is usually 2 SDs below mean for age, race, and sex. The fingers and hands are long and slender and have a spider-like appearance (arachnodactyly). Many patients have severe chest deformities, including depression (pectus excavatum), protrusion (pectus carinatum), or asymmetry. Scoliosis is frequent and usually accompanied by kyphosis. High-arched palate and high pedal arches or pes planus are common. A few patients have severe joint hypermobility similar to EDS.

Cardiovascular Changes Cardiovascular abnormalities are the major source of morbidity and mortality (Chap. 231). Mitral valve prolapse develops early in life and in about one-quarter of patients progresses to mitral valve regurgitation of increasing severity because of redundancy of the leaflets, stretching of the chordae tendineae, and dilatation of the valvulae annulus. Dilatation of the root of the aorta and the sinuses of Valsalva are characteristic and ominous features of the disease that can develop at any age and in rare instances may be detected by echocardiography in utero. The rate of dilatation is unpredictable, but it can lead to aortic regurgitation, dissection of the aorta, and rupture. Dilatation is probably accelerated by physical and emotional stress, as well as by pregnancy.

Ocular Changes Dislocations of the lens may be readily apparent, but diagnosis usually requires pupillary dilatation and slit-lamp examination. The displacement is usually not progressive but may contribute to the formation of cataracts. The ocular globe is frequently elongated; most patients are myopic, and some develop retinal detachment. A few patients have lattice degeneration and retinal tears; most have adequate vision.

Associated Changes Striae may occur over the shoulders and buttocks. Otherwise the skin is normal. A number of patients develop spontaneous pneumothorax. Inguinal and incisional hernias are common. Marked dilatation of the dural sac is seen frequently in computed tomography scans, but the condition is usually asymptomatic. Patients are typically thin with little subcutaneous fat, but adults may develop centripetal obesity.

Molecular Defects Most patients with the classic features of MFS are heterozygotes for mutations in a gene on chromosome 15 that encodes fibrillin-1, a glycoprotein of 350 kDa that is a major component of elastin-associated microfibrils. These microfibrils are abundant in large blood vessels and the suspensory ligaments of the lens. Mutations in

the fibrillin-1 gene include missense, nonsense, in-frame deletions, and RNA splicing mutations. Many of the mutations are single amino acid substitutions in the epidermal growth factor-like domains of the molecule that may be involved in calcium binding. Mutations in the fibrillin-2 gene that cause the MFS variant characterized by contractures appear to follow a similar pattern. As with most genetic diseases, the nature and location of mutations in the genes are only an approximate guide to the severity of the phenotype unless the same mutation has been seen in other members of the same family or in similar unrelated patients. However, there is a clustering of mutations in the middle portion of the molecule of fibrillin-1 encoded by exons 23 to 32 that causes the most severe phenotype, referred to as *neonatal MFS*. The function of fibrillin has not been defined, but the data suggest that fibrillin self-assembles into a fibrillar structure and that the conformation and surface properties of the entire molecule are critical for normal assembly. Therefore, the functional consequences of mutations that change the amino acid sequence of fibrillin may be similar to the effects of mutations that change the conformation of a fibrillar collagen.

Diagnosis The diagnosis is easily established if the patient and other members of the family have dislocated lenses, aortic dilatation, and long and thin extremities together with kyphoscoliosis or other chest deformities. The diagnosis is frequently made if ectopia lentis and an aneurysm of the ascending aorta occur in the absence of a Marfan habitus or a positive family history. All patients with suspected diagnosis should have a slit-lamp examination and an echocardiogram. Also, homocystinuria should be ruled out by a negative cyanide-nitroprusside test for disulfides in the urine (Chap. 343). A few patients with types I, II, and III EDS have ectopia lentis but lack the Marfan habitus and instead have characteristic skin changes not present in MFS. Patients with familial aortic aneurysms tend to develop aneurysms at the base of the abdominal aorta. The location of the aneurysms, however, is somewhat variable, and the high incidence of aortic aneurysms in the general population (1 in 100) makes the differential diagnosis difficult unless other features of MFS are clearly present. A few families with familial aortic aneurysms have mutations in the gene for type III procollagen.

℞ TREATMENT

There is no established treatment, but several investigators have recommended use of propranolol or other β-adrenergic blocking agents to lower blood pressure and thereby delay or prevent aortic dilatation. Surgical correction of the aorta, aortic valve, and mitral valve has been successful in some patients; all patients should be followed carefully with echocardiography and other techniques for evaluation of cardiovascular changes (Chap. 231). Patients should probably be advised of the risks of severe physical and emotional stress and of pregnancy.

The scoliosis tends to be progressive and should be treated by mechanical bracing and physical therapy if >20° or by surgery if it progresses to >45°. Dislocated lenses rarely require surgical removal, but patients should be followed closely for retinal detachment.

Diagnostic tests based on detection of fibrillin defects in cultured skin fibroblasts or DNA analysis of the gene are now available from several laboratories.

DISEASES RELATED TO ELASTIN As may be expected from the role of elastin in maintaining the elasticity of skin, mutations in the elastin gene cause *cutis laxa*, a rare and heterogeneous group of disorders characterized by skin that is both lax and inelastic.

EPIDERMOLYSIS BULLOSA EB consists of a group of similar disorders in which the skin and related epithelial tissues break and blister as the result of minor trauma. As with most heritable disorders of connective tissues, the clinical manifestations range from lethal to mild.

Classification Four types of EB are defined on the basis of the level at which blistering occurs: EB simplex for blistering in the epidermis, EB hemidesmosomal for fissures between keratinocytes and the basal lamina, EB junctional for blistering in the dermal-epidermal junction, and EB dystrophica for blistering in the dermis.

Incidence The incidence of EB in the United States is estimated to be 1 in 50,000.

Molecular Defects The molecular basis of several specific variants of EB has been defined. A series of patients with EB simplex were found to have mutations in either keratin 14 or keratin 5, two of the major keratins in basal epithelial cells. Patients with the related syndrome, epidermolytic icthyosis, have mutations in keratin 1 and keratin 10. The new disease phenotype of hemidesmosomal EB has three clinical variants that are caused by mutations in one of four genes: (1) A generalized atrophic and benign form of EB is caused by mutations in the COL17A1 gene for type XVII collagen; (2) a variant with EB associated with pyloric atresia and other intestinal abnormalities is caused by mutations in either the gene for the α6 integrin (ITG A6) or the gene for the β4 integrin (ITG B4); and (3) another variant characterized by relatively mild blistering at birth but associated with late-onset muscular dystrophy is caused by mutations in the gene for plectin (PLEC-1). Junctional EB is caused by mutations in any one of three genes for laminin (LAMA-3, LAMB-3, LAMC-2). The most severe dystrophic form of EB is caused by mutations in the gene for type VII collagen (COL7A1) that forms the anchoring fibers binding the epidermis to the dermis.

Diagnosis The diagnosis is based on skin that readily breaks and forms blisters. Also, DNA diagnostic tests are available. EB simplex and EB hemidesmosomal are generally milder than EB junctional or EB dystrophica. EB dystrophica variants usually cause large and prominent scars. Precise classification within subtypes usually requires electron microscopy. The treatment is symptomatic.

ALPORT SYNDROME AS is an inherited disorder characterized by hematuria. Four forms of the disease are now recognized: (1) classic AS, which is inherited as an X-linked disorder with hematuria, sensorineural deafness, and conical deformation of the anterior surface of the lens (lenticonus); (2) a subtype of the X-linked form associated with diffuse leiomyomatosis; (3) an autosomal recessive form; and (4) an autosomal dominant form. The two autosomal forms can cause renal disease without deafness or lenticonus.

Incidence The incidence of AS is about 1 in 10,000 in the general population and as high as 1 in 5000 in some ethnic groups. About 80% of AS patients have the X-linked variant.

Molecular Defects Electron microscopy of kidneys from patients with classic AS demonstrates that the glomerular basement membrane is up to five times thicker than normal and the lamina densa is distorted and split. The X-linked and autosomal recessive forms are caused primarily by mutations in genes for the α3(IV), α4(IV), α5(IV), or α6(IV) chains of type IV collagen, a major component of basement membranes. The genes for the proteins are arranged in tandem pairs on different chromosomes in a head-to-head orientation and with overlapping promoters, i.e., the α1(IV) and α2(IV) genes are head-to-head on chromosome 13q34, the α3(IV) and α4(IV) genes are on chromosome 2q35-37, and the α5(IV) and α6(IV) genes are on chromosome Xq22. An X-linked variant is caused by mutations in the COL4A5 gene, and the X-linked variant associated with leiomyomatosis is caused by deletions that involve both the COL4A5 gene and the nearby COL4A6 gene. The autosomal recessive variants are caused by mutations in either the COL4A3 or COL4A4 genes. The mutations responsible for the autosomal dominant variants are still unknown, but they have been mapped to the same locus as the COL4A3 and COL4A4 genes.

Diagnosis The diagnosis of classic AS is based on X-linked inheritance of hematuria, sensorineural deafness, and lenticonus. Because of the X-linked transmission, women are generally underdiagnosed and are usually less severely affected than men. The hematuria progresses to nephritis and may cause renal failure in late adolescence in affected males and at older ages in some women. The sensorineural deafness is primarily in the high-tone range. It can frequently be detected only by an audiogram and is usually not progressive. The lenticonus can occur without nephritis but is generally considered to be pathognomonic of classic ASR. Renal transplantation is usually successful.

ACKNOWLEDGMENT
The authors acknowledge the contributions of Helena Kuivaniemi and Gerard Tromp to this chapter in previous editions of Harrison's.

FURTHER READING

INTERNATIONAL WORKING GROUP ON CONSTITUTIONAL DISEASES OF BONE: International nomenclature and classification of the osteochondrodysplasias (1997). Am J Med Genet 79:376, 1998

KUIVANIEMI H et al: Mutations in the fibrillar collagens (types I, II, III, IX and XI), and fibril-associated collagen, and the network-forming collagen (type X) cause a spectrum of diseases of bone, cartilage and blood vessels. Hum Mutat 9:300, 1997

MARINI JC: Osteogenesis imperfecta. Comprehensive management. Adv Pediatr 35:391, 1988

PEPIN M et al: Clinical and genetic features of Ehlers-Danlos syndrome type IV, the vascular type. N Engl J Med 342:673, 2000

RAMIREZ F et al: Marfan syndrome: New clues to genotype-phenotype correlations. Ann Med 31:202, 1999

343 INHERITED DISORDERS OF AMINO ACID METABOLISM PRESENTING IN ADULTS
Nicola Longo

Amino acids are not only the building blocks of proteins but also serve as neurotransmitters (glycine, glutamate, γ-aminobutyric acid) or as precursors of hormones, coenzymes, pigments, purines, or pyrimidines. Eight amino acids, referred to as *essential*, cannot be synthesized by humans and must be obtained from dietary sources. The others are formed endogenously. Each amino acid has a unique degradative pathway by which its nitrogen and carbon components are used for the synthesis of other amino acids, carbohydrates, and lipids. Disorders of amino acid metabolism and transport (Chap. 344) are individually rare—the incidences range from 1 in 10,000 for cystinuria or phenylketonuria to 1 in 200,000 for homocystinuria or alkaptonuria—but collectively they affect perhaps 1 in 1000 newborns. Almost all are transmitted as autosomal recessive traits.

The features of inherited disorders of amino acid catabolism are summarized in Table 343-1. In general, these disorders are named for the compound that accumulates to highest concentration in blood (-*emias*) or urine (-*urias*). For many conditions (often called *aminoacidopathies*), the parent amino acid is found in excess; for others, generally referred to as *organic acidemias*, products in the catabolic pathway accumulate. Which compound(s) accumulates depends, of course, on the site of the enzymatic block, the reversibility of the reactions proximal to the lesion, and the availability of alternative pathways of metabolic "runoff." Biochemical and genetic heterogeneity are common. Five distinct forms of hyperphenylalaninemia, seven forms of homocystinuria, and seven types of methylmalonic acidemia are recognized. Such heterogeneity reflects the presence of an even larger array of molecular defects.

The manifestations of these conditions differ widely (Table 343-1). Some, such as sarcosinemia, produce no clinical consequences. At the other extreme, complete deficiency of ornithine transcarbamylase is lethal in the untreated neonate. Central nervous system (CNS) dysfunction, in the form of developmental retardation, seizures, alterations

TABLE 343-1 *Inherited Disorders of Amino Acid Metabolism*

Aminoacid(s)	Condition	Enzyme Defect	Clinical Findings	Inheritance[a]
Phenylalanine	Phenylketonuria type I	Phenylalanine hydroxylase	Mental retardation, microcephaly, hypopigmented skin and hairs, eczema, "mousy" odor	AR
	Phenylketonuria type II	Dihydropteridine reductase	Mental retardation, hypotonia, spasticity, myoclonus	AR
	Phenylketonuria type III	6-Pyruvoyl-tetrahydropterin synthase	Dystonia, neurologic deterioration, seizures, mental retardation	AR
	GTP cyclohydrolase I deficiency	GTP cyclohydrolase I	Mental retardation, seizures, dystonia, temperature instability	AR
	Carbinolamine dehydratase deficiency	Pterin-4α-carbinolamine dehydratase	Transient hyperphenylalaninemia (benign)	AR
Tyrosine	Tyrosinemia type I (hepatorenal)	Fumarylacetoacetate hydrolase	Liver failure, cirrhosis, rickets, failure to thrive, peripheral neuropathy, "boiled cabbage" odor	AR
	Tyrosinemia type II (oculocutaneous)	Tyrosine transaminase	Palmoplantar keratosis, painful corneal erosions with photophobia, mental retardation (?)	AR
	Tyrosinemia type III	4-Hydroxyphenylpyruvate dioxygenase	Hypertyrosinemia with normal liver function, occasional mental delay	AR
	Hawkinsinuria	4-Hydroxyphenylpyruvate dioxygenase	Transient failure to thrive, metabolic acidosis in infancy	AD
	Alkaptonuria	Homogentisic acid oxidase	Ochronosis, arthritis, cardiac valve involvement, coronary artery calcification	AR
	Albinism (oculocutaneous)	Tyrosinase	Hypopigmentation of hair, skin, and optic fundus; visual loss; photophobia	AR
	Albinism (ocular)	Different enzymes or transporters	Hypopigmentation of optic fundus, visual loss	AR, XL
	DOPA-responsive dystonia	Tyrosine hydroxylase	Rigidity, truncal hypotonia, tremor, mental retardation	AR
GABA	4-Hydroxybutyric aciduria	Succinic semialdehyde dehydrogenase	Seizures, mental retardation, ataxia	AR
Tryptophan	Tryptophanuria	Unknown	Mental retardation, ataxia, skin photosensitivity	AR
	Hydroxykinureninuria	Kynureninase	Mental retardation, spasticity	AR
Histidine	Histidinemia	Histidine-ammonia lyase	Benign	AR
	Urocanic aciduria	Urocanase	Benign	AR
	Formiminoglutamic aciduria	Formiminotransferase	Occasional mental retardation	AR
Glycine	Glycine encephalopathy	Glycine cleavage (4 enzymes)	Infantile seizures, lethargy, apnea, profound mental retardation	AR
	Sarcosinemia	Sarcosine dehydrogenase	Benign	AR
	Hyperoxaluria type I	Alanine:glyoxylate aminotransferase	Calcium oxalate nephrolithiasis, renal failure	AR
	Hyperoxaluria type II	D-Glyceric acid dehydrogenase/glyoxylate reductase	Calcium oxalate nephrolithiasis, renal failure	AR
Serine	Phosphoglycerate dehydrogenase deficiency	Phosphoglycerate dehydrogenase	Seizures, microcephaly, mental retardation	AR
Proline	Hyperprolinemia type I	Proline oxidase	Benign	AR
	Hyperprolinemia type II	Δ^1-Pyrroline-5-carboxylate dehydrogenase	Febrile seizures, mental retardation	AR
	Hyperhydroxyprolinemia	Hydroxyproline oxidase	Benign	AR
	Prolidase deficiency	Prolidase	Mild mental retardation, chronic dermatitis	AR
Methionine	Hypermethioninemia	Methionine adenosyltransferase	Usually benign	AR
Homocystine	Homocystinuria	Cystathionine β-synthase	Lens dislocation, thrombotic vascular disease, mental retardation, osteoporosis	AR
	Homocystinuria	5,10-Methylene-tetrahydrofolate reductase	Mental retardation, gait and psychiatric abnormalities, recurrent strokes	AR
	Homocystinuria	Methionine synthase (CblE, -G)	Mental retardation, hypotonia, seizures, megaloblastic anemia	AR
	Homocystinuria and methylmalonic acidemia	Vitamin B_{12} lysosomal efflux and metabolism (CblC, -D, -F)	Mental retardation, lethargy, failure to thrive, hypotonia, seizures, megaloblastic anemia	AR
Cystathionine	Cystathioninuria	γ-Cystathioninase	Benign	AR
Cystine	Cystinosis	Cystinosin CTNS (lysosomal efflux)	Renal Fanconi syndrome, rickets, photophobia, hypotonia, renal failure	AR
S-Sulfo-L-cysteine	Sulfocysteinuria	Sulfate oxidase or molibdenum cofactor deficiency	Seizures, mental retardation, dislocated lenses	AR
Lysine	Hyperlysinemia, saccharopinuria	α-Aminoadipic semialdehyde synthase	Benign	AR
Lysine, tryptophan	α-Ketoadipic acidemia	α-Ketoadipic acid dehydrogenase	Benign	?
	Glutaric acidemia type I	Glutaryl-CoA dehydrogenase	Progressive severe dystonia and athetosis, mild mental retardation	AR
	Glutaric acidemia type II	Electron transfer flavoprotein, ETF ubiquinone oxidoreductase	Hypoglycemia, metabolic acidosis, "sweaty feet" odor, hypotonia, cardiomyopathy	AR

(continued)

TABLE 343-1—(Continued)

Aminoacid(s)	Condition	Enzyme Defect	Clinical Findings	Inheritance[a]
Ornithine	Gyrate atrophy of the choroid and retina	Ornithine-δ-aminotransferase	Myopia, night blindness, loss of peripheral vision, cataracts, chorioretinal degeneration	AR
Urea cycle	Carbamylphosphate synthase deficiency	Carbamylphosphate synthase I	Lethargy progressing to coma, protein aversion, mental retardation, hyperammonemia	AR
	N-Acetylglutamate synthase deficiency	N-Acetylglutamate synthase	Lethargy progressing to coma, protein aversion, mental retardation, hyperammonemia	AR
	Ornithine transcarbamylase deficiency	Ornithine transcarbamylase	Lethargy progressing to coma, protein aversion, mental retardation, hyperammonemia	XL
	Citrullinemia type I	Argininosuccinate synthase	Lethargy progressing to coma, protein aversion, mental retardation, hyperammonemia	AR
	Argininosuccinic acidemia	Argininosuccinate lyase	Lethargy progressing to coma, protein aversion, mental retardation, hyperammonemia	AR
	Arginase deficiency	Arginase	Spastic tetraparesis, mental retardation, mild hyperammonemia	AR
	Hyperornithinemia, hyperammonemia, homocitrullinuria	Mitochondrial ornithine carrier ORNT1	Vomiting, lethargy, failure to thrive, mental retardation, episodic confusion, hyperammonemia, protein intolerance	AR
	Citrullinemia type II	Mitochondrial aspartate/ glutamate carrier CTLN2	Neonatal intrahepatic cholestasis, adult presentation with sudden behavioral changes and stupor, coma, hyperammonemia	AR
Valine	Hypervalinemia	Valine aminotransferase	Vomiting, fever, failure to thrive, hypotonia	AR
Leucine, isoleucine	Hyperleucine-isoleucinemia	Leucine-isoleucine aminotransferase	Seizures, failure to thrive, mental retardation	?
Valine, leucine, isoleucine	Maple syrup urine disease (defective E1α, E1β, E2, E3)	Branched-chain ketoacid dehydrogenase	Lethargy, vomiting, encephalopathy, seizures, mental retardation, "maple syrup" odor, protein intolerance	AR
Leucine	Isovaleric acidemia	Isovaleryl-CoA dehydrogenase	Acidosis, ketosis, vomiting, coma, hyperammonemia, "sweaty feet" odor, protein intolerance	AR
	3-Methylcrotonyl glycinuria	3-Methylcrotonyl-CoA carboxylase	Stress-induced metabolic acidosis, hypotonia, hypoglycemia, "cat's urine" odor	AR
	3-Methylglutaconic aciduria type I	3-Methylglutaconyl-CoA hydratase deficiency	Stress-induced acidosis, mental retardation, hypotonia, hepatomegaly	AR
	3-Hydroxy-3-methylglutaric aciduria	3-Hydroxy-3-methylglutaryl-CoA lyase	Stress-induced hypoketotic hypoglycemia and acidosis, encephalopathy, hyperammonemia	AR
Isoleucine	3-Oxothiolase deficiency	3-Oxothiolase	Fasting-induced acidosis and ketosis, vomiting, lethargy	AR
Valine, isoleucine, methionine, threonine	Propionic acidemia (pccA, -B,-C)	Propionyl-CoA carboxylase (pcc)	Metabolic ketoacidosis, hyperammonemia, hypotonia, lethargy, coma, protein intolerance, mental retardation, hyperglycinemia	AR
	Multiple carboxylase/ biotinidase deficiency	Holocarboxylase synthase or biotinidase	Metabolic ketoacidosis, diffuse rash, alopecia, seizures, mental retardation	AR
	Methylmalonic acidemia (mutase, CblA, -B)	Methylmalonyl-CoA mutase or cobalamin reductase/ adenosyltransferase	Metabolic ketoacidosis, hyperammonemia, hypertonia, lethargy, coma, protein intolerance, mental retardation, hyperglycinemia	AR

[a] AR, autosomal recessive; XL, X-linked, AD, autosomal dominant.

Note: GTP, guanosine 5'-triphosphate; DOPA, dihydroxyphenylalanine; GABA, γ-aminobutyric acid; Cbl, cobalamin.

in sensorium, or behavioral disturbances, is present in more than half the disorders. Protein-induced vomiting, neurologic dysfunction, and hyperammonemia occur in many disorders of urea cycle intermediates. Metabolic ketoacidosis, often accompanied by hyperammonemia, is a frequent presenting finding in disorders of branched-chain amino acid metabolism. Some disorders produce focal tissue or organ involvement such as liver disease, renal failure, cutaneous abnormalities, or ocular lesions.

The analysis of plasma amino acids (by ion-exchange chromatography) and urine organic acids (by gas chromatography/mass spectrometry) is commonly used to diagnose and monitor most of these disorders. The diagnosis is confirmed by enzyme assay on cells or tissues from the patients or by DNA testing. The clinical manifestations in many of these conditions can be prevented or mitigated if a diagnosis is achieved early and appropriate treatment (i.e., dietary protein or amino acid restriction or vitamin supplementation) is instituted promptly. For this reason, several of these disorders are routinely screened for in newborns. Selected disorders that illustrate the principles, properties, and problems presented by the disorders of amino acid metabolism are discussed in this chapter.

THE HYPERPHENYLALANINEMIAS

The hyperphenylalaninemias (Table 343-1) result from impaired conversion of phenylalanine to tyrosine. The most common and clinically important is *phenylketonuria* (frequency 1:10,000), which is an autosomal recessive disorder characterized by an increased concentration of phenylalanine and its by-products in body fluids and by severe mental retardation if untreated in infancy. It results from reduced activity of phenylalanine hydroxylase (phenylketonuria type I). The accumulation of phenylalanine inhibits the transport of other amino acids required for protein or neurotransmitter synthesis, reduces synthesis and increases degradation of myelin, and leads to inadequate formation of norepinephrine and serotonin. Phenylalanine is a competitive inhibitor of tyrosinase, a key enzyme in the pathway of melanin synthesis, and accounts for the hypopigmentation of hair and skin. Untreated children with classic phenylketonuria are normal at birth, but fail to attain early developmental milestones, develop microcephaly, and demonstrate progressive impairment of cerebral function. Hyperactivity, seizures, and severe mental retardation are major clinical problems later in life. Electroencephalographic abnormalities; "mousy" odor of skin, hair, and urine (due to phenylacetate accumulation); and a ten dency to hypopigmentation and eczema complete the devastating clinical picture. In contrast, affected children who are detected and treated at birth show none of these abnormalities. To prevent mental retardation, diagnosis and initiation of dietary treatment of classic phenylketonuria must occur before the child is 3 weeks of age. For this reason, most newborns in North America and Europe are screened by determinations of blood phenylalanine levels. Abnormal values are confirmed using quantitative analysis of plasma amino acids. Dietary phenylalanine restriction is usually instituted if blood phenylalanine levels are >250 μmol/L (4 mg/dL). Treatment consists in a special diet low in phenylalanine and supplemented with tyrosine, since tyrosine becomes an essential amino acid in phenylalanine hydroxylase deficiency. With therapy, plasma phenylalanine concentrations should be maintained between 120 and 360 μmol/L (2 and 6 mg/dL). Dietary restriction should be continued and monitored indefinitely. Some patients with milder forms of phenylketonuria (phenylalanine <1200 μm at presentation) show increased tolerance to dietary proteins and improved metabolic control when treated with tetrahydrobiopterin (20 mg/kg per day), an essential cofactor of phenylalanine hydroxylase.

A number of women with phenylketonuria who have been treated since infancy will have reached adulthood and become pregnant. If maternal phenylalanine levels are not strictly controlled before and during pregnancy, their offspring are at increased risk for congenital defects and microcephaly (*maternal phenylketonuria*). After birth, these children have severe mental and growth retardation. Pregnancy risks can be minimized by continuing lifelong phenylalanine-restricted diets and assuring strict phenylalanine restriction 2 months prior to conception and throughout gestation.

THE HOMOCYSTINURIAS (HYPERHOMOCYSTEINEMIAS)

The homocystinurias are seven biochemically and clinically distinct disorders (Table 343-1) characterized by increased concentration of the sulfur-containing amino acid homocystine in blood and urine.

Classic homocystinuria, the most common (frequency 1:200,000), results from reduced activity of cystathionine β-synthase, the pyridoxal phosphate–dependent enzyme that condenses homocysteine with serine to form cystathionine. Most patients present between 3 and 5 years of age with dislocated optic lenses and mental retardation (in about half of cases). Some patients develop a marfanoid habitus and radiologic evidence of osteoporosis. Life-threatening vascular complications (affecting coronary, renal, and cerebral arteries) can occur during the first decade of life and are the major cause of morbidity and mortality. Classic homocystinuria can be diagnosed with analysis of plasma amino acids, showing elevated methionine and presence of free homocystine. Total plasma homocysteine is also extremely elevated (usually >100 μM). Treatment consists in a special diet restricted in protein and methionine and supplemented with cystine. In approximately half of patients, oral pyridoxine (25 to 500 mg/d) produces a fall in plasma methionine and homocystine concentration in body fluids. Folate deficiency should be prevented by adequate supplementation. Betaine is also effective in reducing homocystine levels in pyridoxine-unresponsive patients.

The other forms of homocystinuria are the result of impaired remethylation of homocysteine to methionine. This can be caused by defective methionine synthase or reduced availability of two essential cofactors, 5-methyltetrahydrofolate and methylcobalamin (methylvitamin B$_{12}$).

Hyperhomocysteinemia refers to increased total plasma concentration of homocysteine with or without an increase in free homocystine (disulfide form). Hyperhomocysteinemia, in the absence of significant homocystinuria, is found in some heterozygotes for the genetic defects noted above or in homozygotes for milder variants. Changes of homocysteine levels are also observed with increasing age; in postmenopausal women; in patients with renal failure, hypothyroidism, leukemias, or psoriasis; and during therapy with drugs such as methotrexate, nitrous oxide, isoniazid, and some antiepileptic agents. Homocysteine acts as an atherogenic and thrombophilic agent. An increase in total plasma homocysteine represents an independent risk factor for coronary, cerebrovascular, and peripheral arterial disease as well as for deep-vein thrombosis (Chap. 224). Homocysteine is synergistic with hypertension and smoking, and it is additive with other risk factors that predispose to peripheral arterial disease. In addition, hyperhomocysteinemia and folate and vitamin B$_{12}$ deficiency have been associated with an increased risk of neural tube defects in pregnant women. Vitamin supplements are effective in reducing plasma homocysteine levels in these cases.

ALKAPTONURIA

Alkaptonuria is a rare (frequency 1:200,000) disorder of tyrosine catabolism in which deficiency of homogentisate 1,2-dioxygenase (also known as *homogentisic acid oxidase*) leads to excretion of large amounts of homogentisic acid in urine and accumulation of oxidized homogentisic acid pigment in connective tissues (*ochronosis*). Alkaptonuria may go unrecognized until middle life when degenerative joint disease develops. Prior to this time, about half of the patients might be diagnosed for the presence of dark urine. Foci of gray-brown scleral pigment and generalized darkening of the concha, anthelix, and, finally, helix of the ear usually develop after age 30. Low back pain usually starts between 30 and 40 years of age. *Ochronotic arthritis* is heralded by pain, stiffness, and some limitation of motion of the hips, knees, and shoulders. Acute arthritis may resemble rheumatoid arthritis, but small joints are usually spared. Pigmentation of heart valves, larynx, tympanic membranes, and skin occurs, and occasional patients develop pigmented renal or prostatic calculi. Degenerative cardiovascular disease is increased in older patients. The diagnosis should be suspected in a patient whose urine darkens to blackness. Homogentistic acid in urine is identified by urine organic acid analysis or by a specific colorimetric test. Ochronotic arthritis is treated symptomatically (Chap. 312). Ascorbic acid and protein restriction are not effective in reducing homogentisic acid production. By contrast, nitisone [2-(2-nitro-4-trifluoromethylbenzoyl)-1,3-cyclohexanedione], a drug used in tyrosinemia type I, reduces urinary excretion of homogentisic acid and, in conjunction with a low-protein diet, might prevent the long-term complications of alkaptonuria.

FURTHER READING

MONTAU AC et al: Tetrahydrobiopterin as an alternative treatment for mild phenylketonuria. N Engl J Med 347:2122, 2002

MUDD SH et al: Disorders of transulfuration, in *The Molecular & Metabolic Bases of Inherited Disease*, 8th ed., CR Scriver et al (eds). New York, McGraw-Hill, 2001, pp 2007–2056

NYHAN WL, OZAND PT: *Atlas of Metabolic Diseases*. London, Chapman & Hall Medical, 1998

PHORNPHUTKUL C et al: One hundred years later: Alkaptonuria in the twenty-first century. N Engl J Med, 347:2111, 2002

Specific membrane transporters mediate the passage of a wide variety of substances across cellular membranes. Classes of substrates include amino acids, sugars, cations, anions, vitamins, and water. The number of inherited disorders of membrane transport continues to increase with the identification of new transporters and the clarification of the molecular basis of diseases with previously unknown pathophysiology. The first transport disorders identified affected the gut or the kidney, but transport processes are now proving essential for the normal function of every organ. Mutations in transporter molecules demonstrate in disorders of the heart, muscle, brain, and endocrine and sensory organs (Table 344-1). Inherited defects impairing the transport of selected amino acids that can present in adults are discussed here as examples of the abnormalities encountered; others are considered elsewhere in this text.

CYSTINURIA Cystinuria (frequency of 1 in 10,000 to 1 in 15,000) is an autosomal recessive disorder caused by defective transporters in the apical brush border of proximal renal tubule and small intestinal cells. It is characterized by impaired reabsorption and excessive urinary excretion of the dibasic amino acids lysine, arginine, ornithine, and cystine. Because cystine is poorly soluble, its overexcretion predisposes to the formation of renal, ureteral, and bladder stones. Such stones are responsible for the signs and symptoms of the disorder.

There are two variants of cystinuria. Homozygotes for both variants have high urinary excretion of cystine, lysine, arginine, and ornithine. Type I heterozygotes have normal urinary amino, whereas non-type I (formerly type II and type III) heterozygotes have moderately increased urinary excretion of each of the four amino acids. The gene for type I cystinuria (*SLC3A1*, chromosome 2p16.3) encodes a membrane glycoprotein. Non-type I cystinuria is caused by mutations in *SLC7A9* (chromosome 19q13) that encodes the $b^{0,+}$ amino acid transporter. The glycoprotein encoded by *SLC3A1* favors the correct processing of the $b^{0,+}$ membrane transporter, and explains why mutations in two different genes cause a similar disease.

Cystine stones account for 1 to 2% of all urinary tract calculi but are the most common cause of stones in children. Cystinuria homozygotes regularly excrete 2400 to 7200 μmol (600 to 1800 mg) of cystine daily. Since the maximum solubility of cystine in the physiologic urinary pH range of 4.5 to 7.0 is about 1200 μmol/L (300 mg/L), cystine needs to be diluted to 2.5 to 7 L of water to prevent crystalluria. Stone formation usually manifests in the second or third decade but may occur in the first year of life. Symptoms and signs are those typical of urolithiasis: hematuria, flank pain, renal colic, obstructive uropathy, and infection (Chap. 268). Recurrent urolithiasis may lead to progressive renal insufficiency.

Cystinuria is suspected after observing typical hexagonal crystals in the sediment of acidified, concentrated, chilled urine or after performing a urinary nitroprusside test. Quantitative urine amino acid analysis confirms the diagnosis of cystinuria by showing selective overexcretion of cystine, lysine, arginine, and ornithine. Quantitation is important for differentiating heterozygotes from homozygotes and for following free cystine excretion during therapy.

Management is aimed at preventing cystine crystal formation by increasing urinary volume and by maintaining an alkaline urine pH. Fluid ingestion in excess of 4 L/d is essential, and 5 to 7 L/d is optimal. Urinary cystine concentration should be <1000 μmol/L (250 mg/L). The daily fluid ingestion necessary to maintain this dilution of excreted cystine should be spaced over 24 h, with one-third of the total volume ingested between bedtime and 3 A.M. Cystine solubility rises sharply above pH 7.5, and urinary alkalinization (with bicarbonate or polycitrates) can be therapeutic. Penicillamine (1 to 3 g/d) and tiopronin (α-mercaptopropionylglycine, 800 to 1200 mg/d in four divided doses) undergo sulfhydryl-disulfide exchange with cystine to form mixed disulfides. Since these disulfides are much more soluble than cystine, pharmacologic therapy can prevent and promote dissolution of calculi. Penicillamine can have significant side effects and should be reserved for patients who fail to respond to hydration alone or who are in a high-risk category (one remaining kidney, renal insufficiency). When medical management fails, urologic surgery is required but should be a last resort as cystine stones reform more easily in scarred epithelium. Occasional patients progress to renal failure and require kidney transplantation.

DIBASIC AMINOACIDURIA This disorder is characterized by a defect in renal tubular reabsorption of the three dibasic amino acids lysine, arginine, and ornithine but *not* cystine. There are two variants, transmitted as autosomal recessive traits. In the common form of dibasic aminoaciduria (type II), also known as *lysinuric protein intolerance*, homozygotes show defective intestinal transport of dibasic amino acids as well as exaggerated renal losses. It is most common in Finland (1 in 60,000) and is rare elsewhere. The transport defect affects basolateral rather than luminal membrane transport and is associated with impairment of the urea cycle. The defective gene (*SLC7A7*, chromosome 14q11.2) encodes a unique membrane transporter, y$^+$LAT, which associates with the cell-surface glycoprotein 4F2 heavy chain to form the complete sodium-independent transporter y$^+$L.

Manifestations are related to the losses of ornithine, arginine, and lysine. Affected patients present in childhood with hepatosplenomegaly, protein intolerance, and episodic ammonia intoxication. Older patients may present with severe osteoporosis, impairment of kidney function, or interstitial changes in the lungs. Plasma concentrations of lysine, arginine, and ornithine are reduced, whereas urinary excretion of lysine and orotic acid are increased. Hyperammonemia may develop after the ingestion of protein loads or with infections, probably because of insufficient amounts of arginine and ornithine to maintain proper function of the urea cycle. The clinical features have been attributed to the hyperammonemia, to insufficient amounts of lysine to support protein synthesis during growth, and to decreased production of nitric oxide caused by arginine deficiency.

Therapy consists of dietary protein restriction and supplementation of citrulline (2 to 8 g/d), a neutral amino acid that fuels the urea cycle when metabolized to arginine and ornithine. Pulmonary disease responds to glucocorticoids or bronchoalveolar lavage in some patients.

HARTNUP DISEASE Hartnup disease (frequency 1 in 24,000) is an autosomal recessive disorder characterized by pellagra-like skin lesions, variable neurologic manifestations, and neutral and aromatic aminoaciduria. Alanine, serine, threonine, valine, leucine, isoleucine, phenylalanine, tyrosine, tryptophan, glutamine, asparagine, and histidine are excreted in urine in quantities 5 to 10 times normal, and intestinal transport of these same amino acids is defective. The clinical manifestations result from nutritional deficiency of the essential amino acid tryptophan, caused by its intestinal and renal malabsorption, and of niacin, which derives in part from tryptophan metabolism. Only a small fraction of patients with the chemical findings of this disorder develop a pellagra-like syndrome, implying that manifestations depend on other factors in addition to the transport defect. The diagnosis of Hartnup disease should be suspected in any patient with clinical features of pellagra who does not have a history of dietary niacin deficiency (Chap. 61). The neurologic and psychiatric manifestations range from attacks of cerebellar ataxia to mild emotional lability to frank delirium and are usually accompanied by exacerbations of the erythematous, eczematoid skin rash. Fever, sunlight, stress, and sulfonamide therapy provoke clinical relapses. Diagnosis is made by detection of the neutral aminoaciduria, which does not occur in dietary niacin deficiency. Treatment is directed at niacin repletion and includes a high-protein diet and daily nicotinamide supplementation (50 to 250 mg).

TABLE 344-1 *Genetic Disorders of Membrane Transport (Selected Examples)*

Class of Substance and Disorder	Individual Substrates	Tissues Manifesting Transport Defect	Proposed Molecular Basis of Defect	Major Clinical Manifestations	Inheritance
AMINO ACIDS					
Classic cystinuria	Cystine, lysine, arginine, ornithine	Proximal renal tubule, jejunal mucosa	Shared dibasic-cystine transport protein SLC3A1, SLC7A9	Cystine nephrolithiasis	AR
Dibasic amino-aciduria	Lysine, arginine, ornithine	Proximal renal tubule, jejunal mucosa	Dibasic transport protein SLC7A7	Type I: Benign Type II: Protein intolerance, hyperammonemia, retardation	AR
Hypercystinuria	Cystine	Proximal renal tubule	Cystine transport protein	Some risk of cystine nephrolithiasis	AR
Lysinuria	Lysine	Proximal renal tubule, jejunal mucosa	Lysine transport protein	Seizures, physical and mental retardation	Probable AR
Hartnup disease	Neutral amino acids	Proximal renal tubule, jejunal mucosa	Shared neutral amino acid transport protein	Constant neutral aminoaciduria, intermittent symptoms of pellagra	AR
Tryptophan malabsorption	Tryptophan	Jejunal mucosa	Tryptophan transport protein	Induloria, ?hypercalcemia, ?nephrocalcinosis	Probable AR
Methionine malabsorption	Methionine	Jejunal mucosa	Methionine transport protein	White hair, mental retardation, convulsions, hyperpneic attacks, edema	Probable AR
Histidinuria	Histidine	Proximal renal tubule, jejunal mucosa	Histidine transport protein	Mental retardation	AR
Iminoglycinuria	Glycine, proline, hydroxyproline	Proximal renal tubule, jejunal mucosa	Shared glycine–imino acid transport protein	None	AR
Dicarboxylic-aminoaciduria	Glutamic acid, aspartic acid	Proximal renal tubule, jejunal mucosa	Shared dicarboxylic amino acid transport protein	None	Probable AR
Cystinosis	Cystine	Lysosomal membranes	Cystine transport protein	Renal failure, hypothyroidism, blindness	AR
HEXOSES					
Glucose-galactose malabsorption	D-Glucose D-Galactose	Jejunal mucosa, proximal renal tubule	Shared Na$^+$-dependent glucose-galactose transport protein SGLT1	Watery diarrhea on feeding glucose, lactose, sucrose, or galactose	AR
Glucose-transport defect	D-Glucose	Ubiquitous	Facilitative glucose transporter GLUT1	Seizures, mental retardation	AD
Fanconi-Bickel syndrome	D-Glucose	Liver, kidney, pancreas, intestine	Facilitative glucose transporter GLUT2	Growth retardation, rickets, hepatorenal glycogenosis, hypo- and hyperglycemia	AR
URATE					
Hypouricemia	Uric acid	Proximal renal tubule	Urate transport protein SLC22A12	Hypouricemia, hyperuricosuria, ?hypercalciuria	AR
ANIONS					
Congenital chloridorrhea	Chloride, sulfate	Ileal and colonic mucosa	Cl$^-$/HCO$_3^-$ exchange pump carrier protein (DRA)	Hydramnios, watery diarrhea, elevated fecal chloride, metabolic alkalosis with volume depletion, hyperaldosteronism	AR
Dent disease, X-linked recessive hypophosphatemic rickets and nephrocalcinosis	Chloride, phosphate	Proximal renal tubule	Voltage-gated Cl$^-$ channel CLCN5	Proteinuria, hypercalciuria, nephrocalcinosis, nephrolithiasis, rickets	XL
CATIONS					
Nesidioblastosis of pancreas	Potassium	Pancreatic β cell	Sulfonylurea receptor SUR1, K$^+$ channel KCNJ11	Neonatal hypoglycemia, hyperinsulinemia	AR
Benign familial neonatal epilepsy	Potassium	Brain	Voltage-gated K$^+$ channels KCNQ2, KCNQ3	Neonatal convulsions, normal development	AD

(continued)

TABLE 344-1 *(Continued)*

Class of Substance and Disorder	Individual Substrates	Tissues Manifesting Transport Defect	Proposed Molecular Basis of Defect	Major Clinical Manifestations	Inheritance
WATER					
Nephrogenic diabetes insipidus	Water	Collecting tubule	Aquaporin 2 (water channel)	Polyuria, dehydration, hyposthenuria	AR, AD
VITAMINS					
Rogers' syndrome	Thiamine	Ubiquitous	Thiamine transporter SLC19A2	Megaloblastic anemia, diabetes, deafness	AR
OTHER					
Carnitine deficiency	Carnitine	Muscle, kidney, fibroblasts	High-affinity carnitine transporter OCTN2	Hypoketotic hypoglycemia, cardiomyopathy, hypotonia	AR
Benign recurrent and progressive familial intrahepatic cholestasis	Bile salts	Liver	Phosphatidylcholine transporter MDR3, phospholipid transporter ATP8B1, bile salt export pump BSEP	Cholestasis, hepatomegaly, cirrhosis, liver failure	AR

Note: AR, autosomal recessive; AD, autosomal dominant; XL, X-linked recessive.

FURTHER READING

BROER S, WAGNER CA: *Membrane Transporter Diseases. Molecular Bases of Inherited Transport Defects*. Kluver Academic/Plenum, New York, 2003, in press

LEVY HL: Hartnup disorder, in *The Molecular and Metabolic Bases of Inherited Disease*, 8th ed, CR Scriver et al (eds). New York, McGraw-Hill, 2001, pp 4957–4969

PALACIN M et al: Cystinuria, in *The Molecular and Metabolic Bases of Inherited Disease*, 8th ed, CR Scriver et al (eds). New York, McGraw-Hill, 2001, pp 4909–4932

———: The molecular bases of cystinuria and lysinuric protein intolerance. Curr Opin Genet Dev 11:328, 2001

345 | NEUROBIOLOGY OF DISEASE
Stephen L. Hauser, M. Flint Beal

The human nervous system is the organ of consciousness, cognition, ethics, and behavior; as such, it is the most intricate structure known to exist. One-third of the 35,000 genes encoded in the human genome are expressed in the nervous system. Each mature brain is composed of 100 billion neurons, several million miles of axons and dendrites, and $>10^{15}$ synapses. Neurons exist within a dense parenchyma of multifunctional glial cells that synthesize myelin, preserve homeostasis, and regulate immune responses. Measured against this background of complexity, the achievements of molecular neuroscience have been extraordinary. Advances in cell biology and genetics have provided new tools to explore the pathophysiology of nervous system diseases, clarifying their underlying causes, revealing new unanticipated groupings, and raising realistic hope that novel therapies and prevention strategies will be possible. This chapter reviews selected themes in neurobiology that provide a context for understanding fundamental mechanisms underlying neurologic disorders.

ION CHANNELS AND CHANNELOPATHIES   The resting potential of neurons and the action potentials responsible for impulse conduction are generated by ion currents and ion channels. Most ion channels are gated, meaning that they can transition between conformations that are open or closed to ion conductance. Individual ion channels are distinguished by the specific ions they conduct; by their kinetics; and by whether they directly sense voltage, are linked to receptors for neurotransmitters or other ligands such as neurotrophins, or are activated by second messengers. The diverse characteristics of different ion channels provide a means by which neuronal excitability can be exquisitely modulated at both the cellular and the subcellular levels. Mutations in ion channels—channelopathies—are responsible for a growing list of human neurologic disorders (Table 345-1). One example is epilepsy, a syndrome of diverse causes characterized by repetitive, synchronous firing of neuronal action potentials. Action potentials are normally generated by the opening of sodium channels and the inward movement of sodium ions down the intracellular concentration gradient. Depolarization of the neuronal membrane opens potassium channels, resulting in outward movement of potassium ions, repolarization, closure of the sodium channel, and hyperpolarization. Sodium or potassium channel subunit genes have long been considered candidate disease genes in inherited epilepsy syndromes, and recently such mutations have been identified (Chap. 348). These mutations appear to alter the normal gating function of these channels, increasing the inherent excitability of neuronal membranes in regions where the abnormal channels are expressed.

Whereas the specific clinical manifestations of channelopathies are quite variable, one common feature is that manifestations tend to be intermittent or paroxysmal, such as occurs in epilepsy, migraine, ataxia, myotonia, or periodic paralysis. Exceptions are clinically progressive channel disorders such as autosomal dominant hearing impairment. The neurologic channelopathies identified to date are all uncommon disorders caused by obvious mutations in channel genes. As the full repertoire of human ion channels and related proteins are identified, it is likely that additional channel-

opathies will be discovered. In addition to rare disorders that result from obvious mutations, it is possible that subtle allelic variations in channel genes or in their pattern of expression might underlie susceptibility to some common forms of epilepsy, migraine, or other disorders.

NEUROTRANSMITTERS AND NEUROTRANSMITTER RECEPTORS   Synaptic neurotransmission is the predominant means by which neurons communicate with each other. Classic neurotransmitters are synthesized in the presynaptic region of the nerve terminal; stored in vesicles; and released into the synaptic cleft, where they bind to receptors on the postsynaptic cell. Secreted neurotransmitters are eliminated by reuptake into the presynaptic neuron (or glia), by diffusion away from the synaptic cleft, and/or by specific inactivation. In addition to the classic neurotransmitters, many neuropeptides have been identified as definite or probable neurotransmitters; these include substance P, neurotensin, enkephalins, β-endorphin, histamine, vasoactive intestinal polypeptide, cholecystokinin, neuropeptide Y, and somatostatin. Peptide neurotransmitters are synthesized in the cell body rather than the nerve terminal and may colocalize with classic neurotransmitters in single neurons. Nitric oxide and carbon monoxide are gases that appear also to function as neurotransmitters, in part by signaling in a retrograde fashion from the postsynaptic to the presynaptic cell.

Neurotransmitters modulate the function of postsynaptic cells by binding to specific neurotransmitter receptors, of which there are two major types. *Ionotropic receptors* are direct ion channels that open after engagement by the neurotransmitter. *Metabotropic receptors* interact with G proteins, stimulating production of second messengers and activating protein kinases, which modulate a variety of cellular events. Ionotropic receptors are multiple subunit structures, whereas metabotropic receptors are composed of single subunits only. One important difference between ionotropic and metabotropic receptors is that the kinetics of ionotropic receptor effects are fast (generally <1 ms) because neurotransmitter binding directly alters the electrical properties of the postsynaptic cell, whereas metabotropic receptors function over longer time periods. These different properties contribute to the potential for selective and finely modulated signaling by neurotransmitters.

Neurotransmitter systems are perturbed in a large number of clinical disorders, examples of which are highlighted in Table 345-2. One example is the involvement of dopaminergic neurons originating in the substantia nigra of the midbrain and projecting to the striatum

TABLE 345-1   *Examples of Neurologic Channelopathies*

Category	Disorder	Channel Type	Gene	Chap. Ref.
Ataxias	Episodic ataxia-1	K	*KCNAI*	352
	Episodic ataxia-2	Ca	*CACNLIAd*	
	Spinocerebellar ataxia-6	Ca	*CACNLIAd*	
Migraine	Familial hemiplegic migraine	Ca	*CACNLIAd*	14
Epilepsy	Benign neonatal familial convulsions	K	*KCNQ2, KCNQ3*	348
	Generalized epilepsy with febrile convulsions plus	Na	*SCNIβ*	
Periodic paralysis	Hyperkalemic periodic paralysis	Na	*SCN4A*	368
	Hypokalemic periodic paralysis	Ca	*CACNLIA3*	
Myotonia	Myotonia congenita	Cl	*CLCN1*	368
	Paramyotonia congenita	Na	*SCN4A*	
Deafness	Jorvell and Lange-Nielsen syndrome (deafness, prolonged QT interval, and arrythmia)	K	*KCNQ1, KCNE1*	26
	Autosomal dominant progressive deafness	K	*KCNQ4*	

(nigrostriatal pathway) in Parkinson's disease (Chap. 351) and in heroin addicts after the ingestion of the toxin MPTP (1-methyl-4-phenyl-1,2,5,6-tetrahydropyridine).

A second important dopaminergic system arising in the midbrain is the mediocorticolimbic pathway, which is implicated in the pathogenesis of addictive behaviors including drug reward. Its key components include the midbrain ventral tegmental area (VTA), median forebrain bundle, and nucleus accumbens (Fig. 345-1). *Addictive drugs share the property of increasing dopamine release in the nucleus accumbens.* Amphetamine increases intracellular release of dopamine from vesicles and reverses transport of dopamine through the dopamine transporters. Patients prone to addiction show increased activation of the nucleus accumbens following administration of amphetamine. Cocaine binds to dopamine transporters and inhibits dopamine reuptake. Ethanol inhibits inhibitory neurons in the VTA, leading to increased dopamine release in the nucleus accumbens. Opioids also disinhibit these dopaminergic neurons by binding to μ receptors expressed by GABA-containing interneurons in the VTA. Nicotine increases dopamine release by activating nicotinic acetylcholine receptors on cell bodies and nerve terminals of dopaminergic VTA neurons. Tetrahydrocannabinol, the active ingredient of cannabis, also increases dopamine levels in the nucleus accumbens. Blockade of dopamine in the nucleus accumbens can terminate the rewarding effects of addictive drugs.

Not all cell-to-cell communication in the nervous system occurs via neurotransmission. Gap junctions provide for direct neuron-neuron electrical conduction and also create openings for the diffusion of ions and metabolites between cells. In addition to neurons, gap junctions

TABLE 345-2   *Principal Classic Neurotransmitters*

Neurotransmitter	Anatomy	Clinical Aspects
Acetylcholine (ACh) $$CH_3-\overset{\overset{O}{\|}}{C}-O-CH_2-CH_2-N-(CH_3)_3$$	Motor neurons in spinal cord → neuromuscular junction	Acetylcholinesterases (nerve gases) Myasthenia gravis (antibodies to ACh receptor) Congenital myasthenic syndromes (mutations in ACh receptor subunits) Lambert-Eaton syndrome (antibodies to Ca channels impair ACh release) Botulism (toxin disrupts ACh release by exocytosis)
	Basal forebrain → widespread cortex	Alzheimer's disease (selective cell death) Autosomal dominant frontal lobe epilepsy (mutations in CNS ACh receptor)
	Interneurons in striatum Autonomic nervous system (preganglionic and postganglionic sympathetic)	Parkinson's disease (tremor)
Dopamine [structure: catechol ring with HO, HO substituents and $-CH_2-CH_2-NH_3$ side chain]	Substantia nigra → striatum (nigrostriatal pathway)	Parkinson's disease (selective cell death) MPTP parkinsonism (toxin transported into neurons)
	Substantia nigra → limbic system and widespread cortex	Addiction, behavioral disorders
	Arcuate nucleus of hypothalamus → anterior pituitary (via portal veins)	Inhibits prolactin secretion
Norepinephrine (NE) [structure: catechol ring with HO, HO substituents and $-CH-CH_2-NH_2$ side chain with OH]	Locus coeruleus (pons) → limbic system, hypothalamus, cortex Medulla → locus coeruleus, spinal cord Postganglionic neurons of sympathetic nervous system	Mood disorders (MAOA inhibitors and tricyclics increase NE and improve depression) Anxiety Orthostatic tachycardia syndrome (mutations in NE transporter)
Serotonin [indole structure with HO and $-CH_2-CH_2-NH_2$ side chain, N–H]	Pontine raphe nuclei → widespread projections Medulla/pons → dorsal horn of spinal cord	Mood disorders (SSRIs improve depression) Migraine pain pathway Pain pathway
γ-Aminobutyric acid (GABA) $$H_2N-CH_2-CH_2-CH_2-COOH$$	Major inhibitory neurotransmitter in brain; widespread cortical interneurons and long projection pathways	Stiff person syndrome (antibodies to glutamic acid decarboxylase, the biosynthetic enzyme for GABA) Epilepsy (gabapentin and valproic acid increase GABA)
Glycine $$H_2N-CH_2-COOH$$	Major inhibitory neurotransmitter in spinal cord	Spasticity Hyperekplexia (myoclonic startle syndrome) due to mutations in glycine receptor
Glutamate $$H_2N-\underset{\underset{COOH}{\|}}{CH}-CH_2-CH_2-COOH$$	Major excitatory neurotransmitter; located throughout CNS, including cortical pyramidal cells	Seizures due to ingestion of domoic acid (a glutamate analogue) Rasmussen's encephalitis (antibody against glutamate receptor 3) Excitotoxic cell death

Note: CNS, central nervous system; MPTP, 1-methyl-4-phenyl-1,2,3,6-tetrahydropyridine; MAOA, monoamine oxidase A; SSRI, selective serotonin reuptake inhibitor.

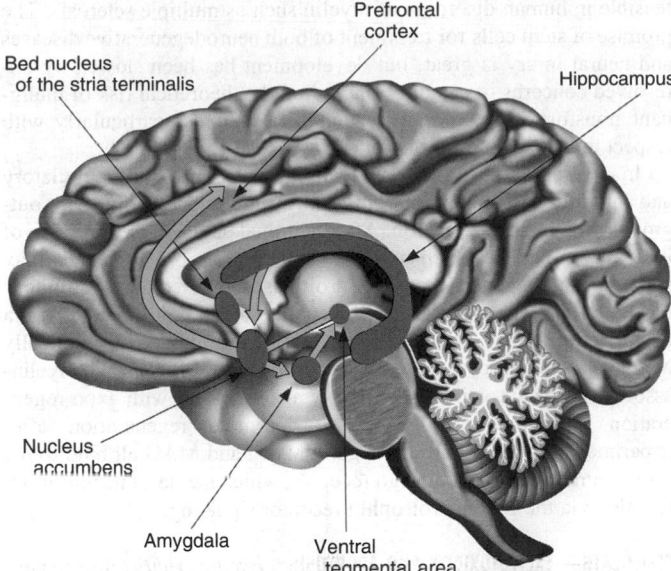

FIGURE 345-1 Mid-sagittal section of the human brain demonstrating limbic structures involved in brain reward pathways.

are also widespread in glia, creating a syncytium that protects neurons by removing glutamate and potassium from the extracellular environment. Gap junctions consist of membrane-spanning proteins, termed *connexins*, that pair across adjacent cells. Mechanisms that involve gap junctions have been related to a variety of neurologic disorders. Mutations in connexin 32, a gap junction protein expressed by Schwann cells, are responsible for the X-linked form of Charcot-Marie-Tooth disease (Chap. 364). Mutations in either of two gap junction proteins expressed in the inner ear—connexin 26 and connexin 31—result in autosomal dominant progressive hearing loss (Chap. 26). Glial calcium waves mediated through gap junctions also appear to explain the phenomenon of spreading depression associated with migraine auras and the march of epileptic discharges. Spreading depression is a neural response that follows a variety of different stimuli and is characterized by a circumferentially expanding negative potential that propagates at a characteristic speed of 20 m/s and is associated with an increase in extracellular potassium.

SIGNALING PATHWAYS AND GENE TRANSCRIPTION

The fundamental issue of how memory, learning, and thinking are encoded in the nervous system is likely to be clarified by identifying the signaling pathways involved in neuronal differentiation, axon guidance, and synapse formation, and by understanding how these pathways are modulated by experience. Many families of transcription factors, each comprising multiple individual components, are expressed in the nervous system. Elucidation of these signaling pathways has already begun to provide insights into the cause of a variety of neurologic disorders, including inherited disorders of cognition such as X-linked mental retardation. This problem affects approximately 1 in 500 males, and linkage studies in different families suggest that as many as 60 different X-chromosome encoded genes may be responsible. Rett syndrome, a common cause of (dominant) X-linked progressive mental retardation in females, is due to a mutation in a gene (*MECP2*) encoding a DNA-

binding protein involved in transcriptional repression. As the X chromosome comprises only ~3% of germline DNA, then by extrapolation the number of genes that potentially contribute to clinical disorders affecting intelligence in humans must be potentially very large. As discussed below, there is increasing evidence that abnormal gene transcription may play a role in neurodegenerative diseases such as Huntington's disease in which proteins with polyglutamine expansions bind to and sequester transcription factors. A critical transcription factor for neuronal survival is CREB (cyclic adenosine monophosphate responsive element-binding) protein, which also plays an important role in memory in the hippocampus.

MYELIN Myelin is the multilayered insulating substance that surrounds axons and speeds impulse conduction by permitting action potentials to jump between naked regions of axons (nodes of Ranvier) and across myelinated segments. A single oligodendrocyte usually ensheaths multiple axons in the central nervous system (CNS), whereas in the peripheral nervous system (PNS) each Schwann cell typically myelinates a single axon. Myelin is a lipid-rich material formed by a spiraling process of the membrane of the myelinating cell around the axon, creating multiple membrane bilayers that are tightly apposed (compact myelin) by charged protein interactions. A number of clinically important neurologic disorders are caused by inherited mutations in myelin proteins of the CNS or PNS. Constituents of myelin also have a propensity to be targeted as autoantigens in autoimmune demyelinating disorders (Fig. 345-2).

NEUROTROPHIC FACTORS Neurotrophic factors (Table 345-3) are secreted proteins that modulate neuronal growth, differentiation, repair, and survival; some have additional functions, including roles in neurotransmission and in the synaptic reorganization involved in learning and memory. The neurotrophin (NT) family contains nerve growth factor (NGF), brain-derived neurotrophic factor (BDNF), NT3, and NT4/5. The neurotrophins act at TrK and p75 receptors to promote survival of neurons. Because of their survival-promoting and anti-

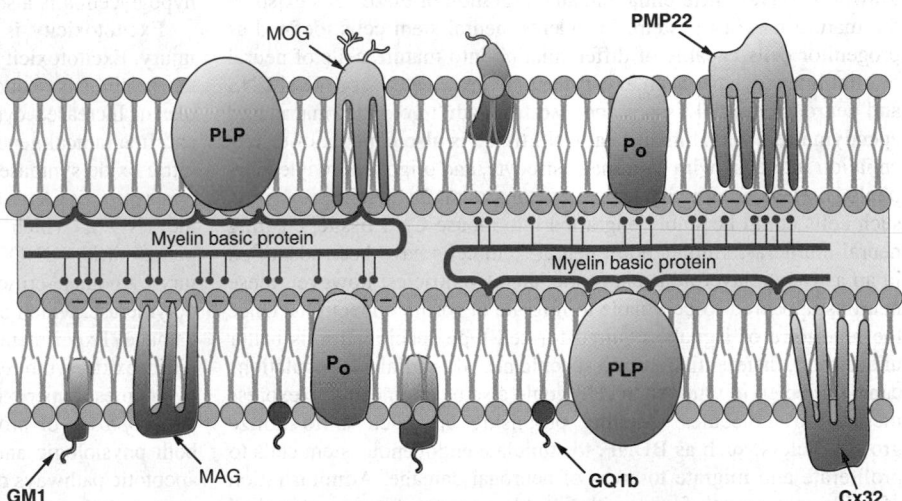

FIGURE 345-2 The molecular architecture of the myelin sheath illustrating the most important disease-related proteins. The illustration represents a composite of CNS and PNS myelin. Proteins restricted to CNS myelin are shown in green, proteins of PNS myelin are lavender, and proteins present in both CNS and PNS are red. In the CNS, the X-linked allelic disorders, Pelizaeus Merzbacher disease and one variant of familial spastic paraplegia, are caused by mutations in the gene for proteolipid protein (PLP) that normally promotes extracellular compaction between adjacent myelin lamellae. The homologue of PLP in the PNS is the P_0 protein, mutations in which cause the neuropathy Charcot-Marie-Tooth disease (CMT) type 1D. The most common form of CMT is the 1A subtype caused by a duplication of the *PMP22* gene; deletions in *PMP22* are responsible for another inherited neuropathy termed hereditary liability to pressure palsies (Chap. 364).

In multiple sclerosis (MS), myelin basic protein (MBP) and the quantitatively minor CNS protein, myelin oligodendrocyte glycoprotein (MOG), are likely T cell and B cell antigens, respectively (Chap. 359). The location of MOG at the outermost lamella of the CNS myelin membrane may facilitate its targeting by autoantibodies. In the PNS, autoantibodies against myelin gangliosides are implicated in a variety of disorders, including GQ1b in the Fisher variant of Guillain-Barré syndrome, GM1 in multifocal motor neuropathy, and sulfatide constituents of myelin-associated glycoprotein (MAG) in peripheral neuropathies associated with monoclonal gammopathies (Chap. 365).

TABLE 345-3 *Neurotrophic Factors*

Neurotrophin family	Transforming growth factor β
Nerve growth factor	family
Brain-derived neurotrophic	Glial-derived neurotrophic family
factor	Neurturin
Neurotrophin-3	Persephin
Neurotrophin-4	Fibroblast growth factor family
Neurotrophin-6	Hepatocyte growth factor
Cytokine family	Insulin-like growth factor (IGF)
Ciliary neurotrophic factor	family
Leukemia inhibitory factor	IGF-1
Interleukin-6	IGF-2
Cardiotrophin-1	

apoptotic effects, neurotrophic factors are in theory outstanding candidates for therapy of disorders characterized by premature death of neurons such as occurs in amyotrophic lateral sclerosis (ALS) and other degenerative motor neuron disorders. Knockout mice lacking receptors for ciliary neurotrophic factor (CNTF) or BDNF show loss of motor neurons, and experimental motor neuron death can be rescued by treatment with various neurotrophic factors including CNTF and BDNF. However, in phase 3 clinical trials, growth factors were ineffective in human ALS. The growth factor glial-derived neurotrophic factor (GDNF) is important for survival of dopaminergic neurons. It has shown promising neurorestorative effects in experimental models of Parkinson's disease and in early stage human clinical trials.

STEM CELLS AND TRANSPLANTATION The nervous system is traditionally considered to be a nonmitotic organ, in particular with respect to neurons. These concepts have been challenged by the finding that neural progenitor or stem cells exist in the adult CNS that are capable of differentiation, migration over long distances, and extensive axonal arborization and synapse formation with appropriate targets. These capabilities also indicate that the repertoire of factors required for growth, survival, differentiation, and migration of these cells exists in the mature nervous system. In rodents, neural stem cells, defined as progenitor cells capable of differentiating into mature cells of neural or glial lineage, have been experimentally propagated from fetal CNS and neuroectodermal tissues and also from adult germinal matrix and ependyma regions. Human fetal CNS tissue is also capable of differentiation into cells with neuronal, astrocyte, and oligodendrocyte morphology when cultured in the presence of growth factors. Impressively, such cells could be stably engrafted into mouse CNS tissue, creating neural chimeras. Human adult neural stem cells have been identified in an astrocyte layer adjacent to the lateral ventricles; however, these neurons appeared to be unable to migrate or form connections. Once the repertoire of signals required for cell type specification is better understood, differentiation into specific neural or glial subpopulations can be directed in vitro; such cells could also be engineered to express therapeutic molecules. Another promising approach is to utilize growth factors, such as BDNF, to stimulate endogenous stem cells to proliferate and migrate to areas of neuronal damage. Administration of epidermal growth factor with fibroblast growth factor replenished up to 50% of hippocampal CA1 neurons a month after global ischemia in rats. The new neurons made connections and improved performance in a memory task.

Experimental transplantation of human fetal dopaminergic neurons in patients with Parkinson's disease has shown that these transplanted cells can survive within the host striatum; however, some patients developed disabling dyskinesias and this approach is no longer in clinical development. Studies of transplantation for patients with Huntington's disease have also reported encouraging, although very preliminary, results. Oligodendrocyte precurser cells transplanted into mice with a dysmyelinating disorder effectively migrated in the new environment, interacted with axons, and mediated myelination; such experiments raise hope that similar transplantation strategies may be feasible in human disorders of myelin such as multiple sclerosis. The promise of stem cells for treatment of both neurodegenerative diseases and neural injury is great, but development has been slowed by unresolved concerns over safety (including the theoretical risk of malignant transformation of transplanted cells), ethics (particularly with respect to use of fetal tissue), and efficacy.

In developing brain, the extracellular matrix provides stimulatory and inhibitory signals that promote neuronal migration, neurite outgrowth, and axonal extension. After neuronal damage, reexpression of inhibitory molecules such as chondroitin sulfate proteoglycans may prevent tissue regeneration. Chondroitinase degraded these inhibitory molecules and enhanced axonal regeneration and motor recovery in a rat model of spinal cord injury. Several myelin proteins, specifically Nogo, oligodendrocyte myelin glycoprotein (OMGP), and myelin-associated glycoprotein (MAG), may also interfere with axon regeneration. Antibodies against Nogo promote regeneration after experimental focal ischemia. Nogo, OMGP, and MAG all bind to the same neural receptor, the Nogo receptor, which mediates its inhibitory function via the p75 neurotrophin receptor signaling.

CELL DEATH—EXCITOTOXICITY AND APOPTOSIS *Excitotoxicity* refers to neuronal cell death caused by activation of excitatory amino acid receptors (Fig. 345-3). Compelling evidence for a role of excitotoxicity, especially in ischemic neuronal injury, is derived from experiments in animal models. Experimental models of stroke are associated with increased extracellular concentrations of the excitatory amino acid neurotransmitter glutamate, and neuronal damage is attenuated by denervation of glutamate-containing neurons or the administration of glutamate receptor antagonists. The distribution of cells sensitive to ischemia corresponds closely with that of N-methyl-D-aspartate (NMDA) receptors (except for cerebellar Purkinje cells, which are vulnerable to hypoxia-ischemia but lack NMDA receptors); and competitive and noncompetitive NMDA antagonists are effective in preventing focal ischemia. In global cerebral ischemia, non-NMDA receptors (kainic acid and AMPA) are activated, and antagonists to these receptors are protective. Experimental brain damage induced by hypoglycemia is also attenuated by NMDA antagonists.

Excitotoxicity is not a single event but rather a cascade of cell injury. Excitotoxicity causes influx of calcium into cells, and much of the calcium is sequestered in mitochondria rather than in the cytoplasm. Increased cytoplasmic calcium causes metabolic dysfunction and free radical generation; activates protein kinases, phospholipases, nitric oxide synthase, proteases, and endonucleases; and inhibits protein synthesis. Activation of nitric oxide synthase generates nitric oxide (NO$^{\cdot}$), which can react with superoxide (O$_2^{\cdot}$) to generate peroxynitrite (ONOO$^-$), which may play a direct role in neuronal injury. Another critical pathway is activation of poly-ADP-ribose polymerase, which occurs in response to free radical–mediated DNA damage. Experimentally, mice with knockout mutations of neuronal nitric oxide synthase or poly-ADP-ribose polymerase, or those that overexpress superoxide dismutase, are resistant to focal ischemia.

Apoptosis, or programmed cell death, plays an important role in both physiologic and pathologic conditions. During embryogenesis, apoptotic pathways operate to destroy neurons that fail to differentiate appropriately or reach their intended targets. There is mounting evidence for an increased rate of apoptotic cell death in a variety of acute and chronic neurologic diseases. Apoptosis is characterized by neuronal shrinkage, chromatin condensation, and DNA fragmentation, whereas necrotic cell death is associated with cytoplasmic and mitochondrial swelling followed by dissolution of the cell membrane. Apoptotic and necrotic cell death can coexist or be sequential events, depending on the severity of the initiating insult. Cellular energy reserves appear to have an important role in these two forms of cell death, with apoptosis favored under conditions in which ATP levels are preserved. Evidence of DNA fragmentation has been found in a number of degenerative neurologic disorders, including Alzheimer's disease, Huntington's disease, and ALS. The best characterized genetic neurologic disorder related to apoptosis is infantile spinal muscular atrophy (Werdnig-Hoffmann disease), in which two genes thought to be involved in the apoptosis pathways are causative.

Mitochondria are essential in controlling specific apoptosis pathways. The redistribution of cytochrome c, as well as apoptosis-inducing factor (AIF), from mitochondria during apoptosis leads to the activation of a cascade of intracellular proteases known as caspases. Caspase-independent apoptosis occurs after DNA damage, activation of poly-ADP-ribose polymerase, and translocation of AIF into the nucleus. Redistribution of cytochrome c is prevented by overproduction of the apoptotic protein BCL2 and is promoted by the proapoptotic protein BAX. These pathways may be triggered by activation of a large pore in the mitochondrial inner membrane known as the *permeability transition pore*, although in other circumstances they occur independently. Recent studies suggest that blocking the mitochondrial pore reduces both hypoglycemic and ischemic cell death.

PROTEIN AGGREGATION AND NEURODEGENERATION

The possibility that protein aggregation plays a role in the pathogenesis of neurodegenerative diseases is a major focus of current research. Protein aggregation is a major histopathologic hallmark of neurodegenerative diseases. Deposition of β-amyloid is strongly implicated in the pathogenesis of Alzheimer's disease. Genetic mutations in familial Alzheimer's disease produce increased amounts of β-amyloid with 42 amino acids, which has an increased propensity to aggregate, as compared to β-amyloid with 40 amino acids. Mutations in genes encoding the microtubule-associated protein tau lead to altered splicing of tau and the production of neurofibrillary tangles in frontotemporal dementia and progressive supranuclear palsy. Familial Parkinson's disease is associated with mutations in α-synuclein, parkin, and the ubiquitin carboxy-terminal hydrolase. Parkin, which causes autosomal recessive early-onset Parkinson's disease, is a ubiquitin ligase. The characteristic histopathologic feature of Parkinson's disease is the Lewy body, an eosinophilic cytoplasmic inclusion that contains both neurofilaments and α-synuclein. Huntington's disease and cerebellar degenerations are associated with expansions of polyglutamine repeats in proteins, which aggregate to produce neuronal intranuclear inclusions. Familial ALS is associated with superoxide dismutase mutations and cytoplasmic inclusions containing superoxide dismutase. In autosomal dominant neurohypophyseal diabetes insipidus, mutations in vasopressin result in abnormal protein processing, accumulation in the endoplasmic reticulum, and cell death (Chap. 319).

The current major scientific question is whether protein aggregates contribute to neuronal death or whether they are merely secondary bystanders. Protein aggregates are usually ubiquinated, which targets them for degradation by the 26S component of the proteosome. An inability to degrade protein aggregates could lead to cellular dysfunction, impaired axonal transport, and cell death by apoptotic mechanisms.

In experimental models of Huntington's disease and cerebellar degeneration, protein aggregates are not well correlated with neuronal death. A substantial body of evidence suggests that the mutant proteins with polyglutamine expansions in these diseases bind to transcription factors and that this contributes to disease pathogenesis. Agents that upregulate gene transcription are neuroprotective in animal models of these diseases. A number of compounds have been developed to block β-amyloid production and/or aggregation, and these agents are being studied in early clinical trials in humans.

NEUROIMMUNOLOGY

The nervous system is traditionally considered to be an immunologically privileged organ, a concept originally derived from observations that tissue grafts implanted in the brain were not rejected efficiently. In this context, immune privilege of the CNS may be maintained by a variety of mechanisms, including the lack of an efficient surveillance function by T cells; the absence of a traditional lymphoid system; limited expression of major histocompatibility complex (MHC) molecules required for T cell recognition of antigen; effects of regulatory cytokines secreted spontaneously or in response to mediators such as NGF, creating an immunosuppressive milieu; and also from expression of fas ligand that can induce apoptosis of fas-expressing immune cells that enter the brain. The blood-brain barrier (BBB) partially isolates the brain from the peripheral environment and contributes to immune privilege. Anatomically, the barrier is created by the presence of impermeable tight junctions between endothelial cells and by a relative absence of transendothelial conduits for the passive diffusion of soluble molecules. The BBB serves to preserve CNS homeostasis by excluding neuroactive substances present in the serum, such as neurotransmitters and neurotrophic factors. Because of the BBB, lipid-insoluble molecules must utilize either ion channels or

FIGURE 345-3 Involvement of mitochondria in cell death. A severe excitotoxic insult (A) results in cell death by necrosis, whereas a mild excitotoxic insult (B) results in apoptosis. After a severe insult (such as ischemia), there is a large increase in glutamate activation of NMDA receptors, an increase in intracellular Ca²⁺ concentrations, activation of nitric oxide synthase (NOS), and increased mitochondrial Ca²⁺ and superoxide generation followed by the formation of ONOO⁻. This sequence results in damage to cellular macromolecules including DNA, leading to activation of poly-ADP-ribose polymerase (PARS). Both mitochondrial accumulation of Ca²⁺ and oxidative damage lead to activation of the permeability transition pore (PTP) that is linked to excitotoxic cell death. A mild excitotoxic insult can occur due either to an abnormality in an excitotoxicity amino acid receptor, allowing more Ca²⁺ flux, or to impaired functioning of other ionic channels or of energy production, which may allow the voltage-dependent NMDA receptor to be activated by ambient concentrations of glutamate. This event can then lead to increased mitochondrial Ca²⁺ and free radical production, yet relatively preserved ATP generation. The mitochondria may then release cytochrome c (Cytc), caspase 9, apoptosis-inducing factor (Aif), and perhaps other mediators that lead to apoptosis. The precise role of the PTP in this mode of cell death is still being clarified, but there does appear to be involvement of the adenine nucleotide transporter that is a key component of the PTP.

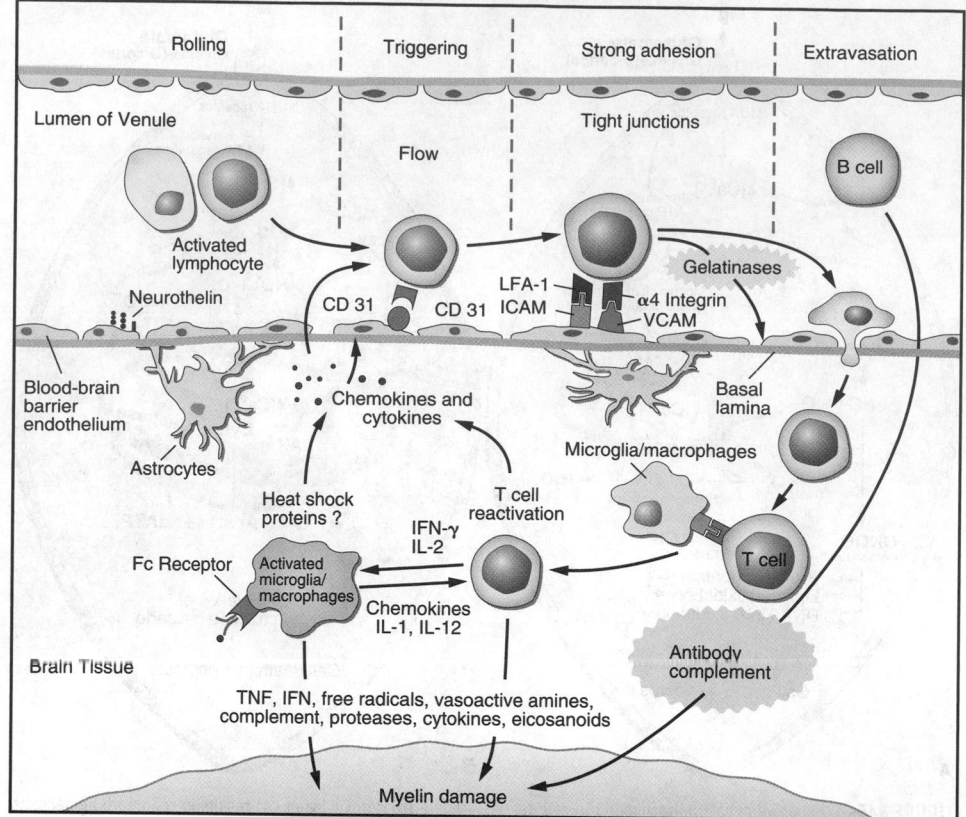

FIGURE 345-4 A model for experimental allergic encephalomyelitis (EAE). Crucial steps for disease initiation and progression include peripheral activation of preexisting autoreactive T cells; homing to the CNS and extravasation across the blood-brain barrier; reactivation of T cells by exposed autoantigens; secretion of cytokines; activation of microglia and astrocytes and recruitment of a secondary inflammatory wave; and immune-mediated myelin destruction. ICAM, intercellular adhesion molecule; LFA-1, leukocyte function-associated antigen-1; VCAM, vascular cell adhesion molecule; IFN, interferon; IL, interleukin; TNF, tumor necrosis factor.

specific transport systems (for glucose or various amino acids) to gain entry to the CNS. Astrocyte foot processes that encircle the subendothelial basal surface of small blood vessels in the brain contribute to development and maintenance of the BBB.

The concept of immune privilege is at odds with clinical experience that vigorous immune reactions readily occur in the nervous system in response to infections and that autoimmune diseases of the nervous system are relatively common. Although primary (sensitizing) immune responses are not easily generated in the CNS for the reasons outlined above, this is not the case for secondary immune responses. When sensitization to nervous system antigens occurs *outside* the nervous system (e.g., in a regional lymph node), activated autoreactive T lymphocytes are easily generated, and these cells readily cross the BBB and induce immune-mediated injury. The paradigm for this mechanism of T cell–mediated CNS disease is experimental allergic encephalomyelitis (EAE), a laboratory model for the human autoimmune

demyelinating disorders multiple sclerosis and acute disseminated encephalomyelitis; the sequence of events in EAE is illustrated in Fig. 345-4.

Under normal circumstances the BBB is impermeable to antibodies. For autoantibodies to reach the CNS, the BBB must first be disrupted. In inflammatory conditions it is thought that this disruption most often occurs via actions of proinflammatory cytokines elaborated within the brain consequent to interactions between pathogenic T cells and antigen-presenting cells (APCs). In contrast to the BBB, in the PNS the blood-nerve barrier is incomplete. Endothelial tight junctions are lacking, and the capacity of charged molecules, including antibodies, to cross the barrier appears to be greatest in two regions of the PNS: proximally in the spinal roots and distally at neuromuscular junctions. This anatomic feature is likely to contribute to the propensity of antibody mediated autoimmune disorders of the PNS to target proximal nerves (Guillain-Barré syndrome) or the neuromuscular junction (myasthenia gravis, Eaton-Lambert syndrome).

The major APCs in the CNS are microglial cells and macrophages; both cell types express MHC class 2 molecules as well as co-stimulatory molecules required for antigen presentation. Neurons do not express MHC class 2 molecules; however, some neurons express MHC class 1 proteins, which may be further increased in response to neuronal activity. Neuronal MHC class 1 molecules may function as retrograde postsynaptic signaling molecules that interact with presynaptic CD3 molecules to stabilize active synapses and transynaptically modulate neuronal function. A role of microglial activation as a contributor to cell death in neurodegenerative and chronic neuroinflammatory diseases is likely and is being actively investigated.

FURTHER READING

DAWSON TM, DAWSON VL: Rare genetic mutations shed light on the pathogenesis of Parkinson's disease. J Clin Invest 111:145, 2003

GAGE FH: Neurogenesis in the adult brain. J Neurosci 22:612, 2002

SANAI N et al: Unique astrocyte ribbon in adult human brain contains neural stem cells but lacks chain migration. Nature 427:740, 2004

SOTO C: Unfolding the role of protein misfolding in neurodegenerative diseases. Nature Rev Neurosci 4:49, 2003

WATKINS TA, BARRES BA: Nerve regeneration: Regrowth stumped by shared receptor. Curr Biol 12:654, 2002

346 APPROACH TO THE PATIENT WITH NEUROLOGIC DISEASE
Joseph B. Martin, Daniel H. Lowenstein, Stephen L. Hauser

Neurologic diseases are common and costly. According to one estimate, 180 million Americans suffer from a nervous system disorder, resulting in an annual cost of $634 billion (Table 346-1). Globally, these disorders are responsible for 28% of all years lived with a disability. Most patients with neurologic symptoms seek care from internists and other generalists rather than from neurologists, and this situation is likely to continue as primary care–based health care systems become increasingly prevalent. Because useful therapies now ex-

ist for these disorders, a skillfull approach to diagnosis is essential. Many errors result from an overreliance on costly neuroimaging procedures and laboratory tests, which, while useful, do not substitute for an adequate history and examination. The proper approach to the patient with a neurologic illness begins with the patient and focuses the clinical problem first in anatomic and then in pathophysiologic terms; only then should a specific diagnosis be entertained. The direct evaluation of the patient also informs the subsequent workup and ensures

TABLE 346-1 *Impact of Neurologic and Psychiatric Diseases in the U.S.*

Disorder	Patients, Millions	Cost, Billion $
Addiction	17.5	160
Alzheimer's disease	4	100
Blindness/vision loss	13	38.4
Deafness/hearing loss	28	56
Depression/manic depressive illness	17.5	47.3
Developmental disorders	8.6	30
Epilepsy	2.5	3.5
Head injury	2	25
Huntington's disease	0.03	—
Multiple sclerosis	0.3	2.5
Pain	80	100
Parkinson's disease	1	6
Schizophrenia	2	30
Spinal cord injury	0.25	5
Stroke	3	30
Total	180	634

Source: Modified from Dana Alliance for Brain Initiatives.

that technology is judiciously applied, a correct diagnosis is established in an efficient manner, and treatment is promptly initiated.

THE NEUROLOGIC METHOD ■ Locate the Lesion(s) The first priority is to identify the region of the nervous system that is likely to be responsible for the symptoms. Can the disorder be mapped to one specific location, is it multifocal, or is a diffuse process present? Are the symptoms restricted to the nervous system, or do they arise in the context of a systemic illness? Is the problem in the central nervous system (CNS), the peripheral nervous system (PNS), or both? If in the CNS, is the cerebral cortex, basal ganglia, brainstem, cerebellum, or spinal cord responsible? Are the pain-sensitive meninges involved? If in the PNS, could the disorder be located in peripheral nerves and, if so, are motor or sensory nerves primarily affected, or is a lesion in the neuromuscular junction or muscle more likely?

The first clues to defining the anatomic area of involvement appear in the history, and the examination is then directed to confirm or rule out these impressions and to clarify uncertainties suggested by the history. A more detailed examination of a particular region of the CNS or PNS is often indicated. For example, the examination of a patient who presents with a history of ascending paresthesias and weakness should be directed toward deciding, among other things, if the location of the lesion is in the spinal cord or peripheral nerves. Focal back pain, a spinal cord sensory level, and incontinence suggest a spinal cord origin, whereas a stocking-glove pattern of sensory loss suggests peripheral nerve disease; areflexia usually indicates peripheral neuropathy but may also be present with spinal shock in acute spinal cord disorders.

Deciding "where the lesion is" accomplishes the task of limiting the possible etiologies to a manageable, finite number. In addition, this strategy safeguards against making tragic errors. Symptoms of recurrent vertigo, diplopia, and nystagmus should not trigger "multiple sclerosis" as an answer (etiology) but "brainstem" or "pons" (location); then a diagnosis of brainstem arteriovenous malformation will not be missed for lack of consideration. Similarly, the combination of optic neuritis and spastic ataxic paraparesis should initially suggest optic nerve and spinal cord disease; multiple sclerosis, CNS syphilis, and vitamin B_{12} deficiency are treatable disorders that can produce this syndrome. Once the question, "Where is the lesion?" is answered, then the question, "What is the lesion?" can be addressed.

Define the Pathophysiology Clues to the pathophysiology of the disease process may also be present in the history. Primary neuronal (gray matter) disorders may present as early cognitive disturbances, movement disorders, or seizures, whereas white matter involvement produces predominantly "long tract" disorders of motor, sensory, visual, and cerebellar pathways. Progressive and symmetric symptoms often have a metabolic or degenerative origin; in such cases lesions are usu-

ally not sharply circumscribed. Thus, a patient with paraparesis and a clear spinal cord sensory level is unlikely to have vitamin B_{12} deficiency as the explanation. A Lhermitte symptom (electric shock–like sensations evoked by neck flexion) is due to ectopic impulse generation in white matter pathways and occurs with demyelination in the cervical spinal cord. Symptoms that worsen after exposure to heat or exercise may indicate conduction block in demyelinated axons, as occurs in multiple sclerosis. A patient with recurrent episodes of diplopia and dysarthria associated with exercise or fatigue may have a disorder of neuromuscular transmission such as myasthenia gravis. Slowly advancing visual scotoma with luminous edges, termed *fortification spectra*, indicates spreading cortical depression, typically with migraine.

THE NEUROLOGIC HISTORY As in all other aspects of clinical medicine, attention to the description of the symptoms experienced by the patient and substantiated by family members and others often permits an accurate localization and determination of the probable cause of the complaints, even before the neurologic examination is performed. Furthermore, a careful analysis of the history is a necessary prerequisite for bringing a focus to the neurologic examination that follows. Each complaint should be pursued as far as possible to elucidate the location of the lesion, the likely underlying pathophysiology, and potential etiologies. For example, a patient complains of weakness of the right arm. What are the associated features? Does the patient have difficulty with brushing hair or reaching upward (proximal) or buttoning buttons or opening a twist-top bottle (distal)? Also, negative associations may also be crucial. A patient with a right hemiparesis without a language deficit likely has a lesion (internal capsule, brainstem, or spinal cord) different from that of a patient with a right hemiparesis and aphasia (left hemisphere). Additional features of the history include the following:

1. *Temporal course of the illness.* It is important to determine the precise time of appearance and rate of progression of the symptoms experienced by the patient. The rapid onset of a neurologic complaint, occurring within seconds or minutes, usually indicates a vascular event, a seizure, or migraine. The onset of sensory symptoms located in one extremity that spread over a few seconds to adjacent portions of that extremity and then to the other regions of the body suggests a seizure. A more gradual onset and less well localized symptoms point to the possibility of a transient ischemic attack (TIA). A similar but slower temporal march of symptoms accompanied by headache, nausea, or visual disturbance suggests migraine. The presence of "positive" sensory symptoms (e.g., tingling or sensations that are difficult to describe) or involuntary motor movements suggests a seizure; in contrast, transient loss of function (negative symptoms) suggests a TIA. A stuttering onset where symptoms appear, stabilize, and then progress over hours or days also suggests cerebrovascular disease; an additional history of transient remission or regression indicates that the process is more likely due to ischemia rather than hemorrhage. A gradual evolution of symptoms over hours or days suggests a toxic, metabolic, infectious, or inflammatory process. Progressing symptoms associated with the systemic manifestations of fever, stiff neck, and altered level of consciousness imply an infectious process. Relapsing and remitting symptoms involving different levels of the nervous system suggest multiple sclerosis or other inflammatory processes; these disorders can occasionally produce new symptoms that are rapidly progressive over hours. Slowly progressive symptoms without remissions are characteristic of neurodegenerative disorders, chronic infections, gradual intoxications, and neoplasms.

2. *Patients' descriptions of the complaint.* The same words often mean different things to different patients. "Dizziness" may imply impending syncope, a sense of disequilibrium, or true spinning vertigo. "Numbness" may mean a complete loss of feeling, a positive sensation such as tingling, or paralysis. "Blurred vision" may be used to describe unilateral visual loss, as in transient monocular blindness, or diplopia.

The interpretation of the true meaning of the words used by patients to describe symptoms becomes even more complex when there are differences in primary languages and cultures.

3. *Corroboration of the history by others.* It is almost always helpful to obtain additional information from family, friends, or other observers to corroborate or expand the patient's description. Memory loss, aphasia, loss of insight, intoxication, and other factors may impair the patient's capacity to communicate normally with the examiner or prevent openness about factors that have contributed to the illness. Episodes of loss of consciousness necessitate that details be sought from observers to ascertain precisely what has happened during the event.

4. *Family history.* Many neurologic disorders have an underlying genetic component. The presence of a Mendelian disorder, such as Huntington's disease or Charcot-Marie-Tooth neuropathy, is often obvious if family data are available. More detailed questions about family history are often necessary in polygenic disorders such as multiple sclerosis, migraine, and many types of epilepsy. It is important to elicit family history about all illnesses, in addition to neurologic and psychiatric disorders. A familial propensity to hypertension or heart disease is relevant in a patient who presents with a stroke. There are numerous inherited neurologic diseases that are associated with multisystem manifestations that may provide clues to the correct diagnosis (e.g., neurofibromatosis, Wilson's disease, neuro-ophthalmic syndromes).

5. *Medical illnesses.* Many neurologic diseases occur in the context of systemic disorders. Diabetes mellitus, hypertension, and abnormalities of blood lipids predispose to cerebrovascular disease. A solitary mass lesion in the brain may be an abscess in a patient with valvular heart disease, a primary hemorrhage in a patient with a coagulopathy, a lymphoma or toxoplasmosis in a patient with AIDS, or a metastasis in a patient with underlying cancer. Patients with malignancy may also present with a paraneoplastic syndrome (Chap. 87) or complications from chemotherapy or radiotherapy. Marfan's syndrome and related collagen disorders predispose to dissection of the cranial arteries and aneurysmal subarachnoid hemorrhage; the latter may also occur with polycystic kidney disease. A recent onset of asthma suggests the possibility of polyarteritis nodosa. Various neurologic disorders occur with dysthyroid states or other endocrinopathies. It is especially important to look for the presence of systemic diseases in patients with peripheral neuropathy. Most patients with coma in a hospital setting have a metabolic, toxic, or infectious cause.

6. *Drug use and abuse and toxin exposure.* It is essential to inquire about the history of drug use, both prescribed and illicit. Aminoglycoside antibiotics may exacerbate symptoms of weakness in patients with disorders of neuromuscular transmission, such as myasthenia gravis, and may cause dizziness secondary to ototoxicity. Vincristine and other antineoplastic drugs can cause peripheral neuropathy, and immunosuppressive agents such as cyclosporine can produce encephalopathy. Excessive vitamin ingestion can lead to disease; for example vitamin A and pseudotumor cerebri, or pyridoxine and peripheral neuropathy. Many patients are unaware that over-the-counter sleeping pills, cold preparations, and diet pills are actually drugs. Alcohol, the most prevalent neurotoxin, is often not recognized as such by patients, and other drugs of abuse such as cocaine and heroin can cause a wide range of neurologic abnormalities. A history of environmental or industrial exposure to neurotoxins may provide an essential clue; consultation with the patient's co-workers or employer may be required.

7. *Formulating an impression of the patient.* Use the opportunity while taking the history to form an impression of the patient. Is the information forthcoming, or does it take a circuitous course? Is there evidence of anxiety, depression, hypochondriasis? Are there any clues to defects in language, memory, insight, or inappropriate behavior? The neurologic assessment begins as soon as the patient comes into the room and the first introduction is made.

THE NEUROLOGIC EXAMINATION   The neurologic examination is challenging and complex; it has many components and includes a number of skills that can be mastered only through repeated use of the same techniques on a large number of individuals with and without neurologic disease. Mastery of the complete neurologic examination is usually important only for physicians in neurology and associated specialties. However, knowledge of the basics of the examination, especially those components that are effective in screening for neurologic dysfunction, is essential for all clinicians, especially generalists.

There is no single, universally accepted sequence of the examination that must be followed, but most clinicians begin with assessment of mental status followed by the cranial nerves, motor system, sensory system, coordination, and gait. Whether the examination is basic or comprehensive, it is essential that it be performed in an orderly and systematic fashion to avoid errors and serious omissions. Thus, the best way to learn and gain expertise in the examination is to choose one's own approach and practice it frequently and do it in the same exact sequence each time.

The detailed description of the neurologic examination that follows describes the more commonly used parts of the examination, with a particular emphasis on the components that are considered most helpful for the assessment of common neurologic problems. Each section also includes a brief description of the minimal examination necessary for adequate screening for abnormalities in a patient who has no symptoms suggesting neurologic dysfunction. A screening examination done in this way can be completed in 3 to 5 min.

Several additional points about the examination are worth noting. First, in recording observations, it is important to describe what is found rather than to apply a poorly defined medical term (e.g., "patient groans to sternal rub" rather than "obtunded"). Second, subtle CNS abnormalities are best detected by carefully comparing a patient's performance on tasks that require simultaneous activation of both cerebral hemispheres (e.g., eliciting a pronator drift of an outstretched arm with the eyes closed; extinction on one side of bilaterally applied light touch, also with eyes closed; or decreased arm swing or a slight asymmetry when walking). Third, if the patient's complaint is brought on by some activity, reproduce the activity in the office. If the complaint is of dizziness when the head is turned in one direction, have the patient do this and look for associated signs on examination (e.g., nystagmus or dysmetria). If pain occurs after walking two blocks, have the patient leave the office and walk this distance and immediately return, and repeat the relevant parts of the examination. Finally, the use of tests that are individually tailored to the patient's problem can be of value in assessing changes over time. Tests of walking a 7.5-m (25-ft) distance (normal, 5 to 6 s; note assistance, if any), repetitive finger or toe tapping (normal, 20 to 25 taps in 5 s), or handwriting are examples.

Mental Status Examination (See also Chaps. 23, 257, and 350)

- *The bare minimum: During the interview, look for difficulties with communication and determine whether the patient has recall and insight into recent and past events.*

The mental status examination is underway as soon as the physician begins observing and talking with the patient. If the history raises any concern for abnormalities of higher cortical function or if cognitive problems are observed during the interview, then detailed testing of the mental status is indicated. The patient's ability to understand the language used for the examination, cultural background, educational experience, sensory or motor problems, or co-morbid conditions need to be factored into the applicability of the tests and interpretation of results.

The Folstein mini-mental status examination (MMSE) (Table 350-4) is a standardized screening examination of cognitive function that is extremely easy to administer and takes <10 min to complete. Using age-adjusted values for defining normal performance, the test is ~85% sensitive and 85% specific for making the diagnosis of dementia that is moderate or severe, especially in educated patients. When there is sufficient time available, the MMSE is one of the best methods for documenting the current mental status of the patient, and this is especially useful as a baseline assessment to which future scores of the MMSE can be compared.

Individual elements of the mental status examination can be subdivided into level of consciousness, orientation, speech and language, memory, fund of information, insight and judgment, abstract thought, and calculations.

Level of consciousness is the patient's relative state of awareness of the self and the environment, and ranges from fully awake to comatose. When the patient is not fully awake, the examiner should describe the responses to the minimum stimulus necessary to elicit a reaction, ranging from verbal commands to a brief, painful stimulus such as a squeeze of the trapezius muscle. Responses that are directed toward the stimulus and signify some degree of intact cerebral function (e.g., opening the eyes and looking at the examiner or reaching to push away a painful stimulus) must be distinguished from reflex responses of a spinal origin (e.g., triple flexion response—flexion at the ankle, knee, and hip in response to a painful stimulus to the foot). *Orientation* is tested by asking the person to state his or her name, location, and time (day of the week and date); time is usually the first to be affected in a variety of conditions. *Speech* is assessed by observing articulation, rate, rhythm, and prosody (i.e., the changes in pitch and accentuation of syllable and words). *Language* is assessed by observing the content of the patient's verbal and written output, response to spoken commands, and ability to read. A typical testing sequence is to ask the patient to name successively more detailed components of clothing, a watch or a pen; repeat the phrase "No ifs, ands, or buts"; follow a three-step, verbal command; write a sentence; and read and respond to a written command. *Memory* should be analyzed according to three main time scales: (1) immediate memory can be tested by saying a list of three items and having the patient repeat the list immediately, (2) short-term memory is assessed by asking the patient to recall the same three items 5 and 15 min later, and (3) long-term memory is evaluated by determining how well the patient is able to provide a coherent chronologic history of his or her illness or personal events. *Fund of information* is assessed by asking questions about major historic or current events, with special attention to educational level and life experiences. Abnormalities of *insight and judgment* are usually detected during the patient interview; a more detailed assessment can be elicited by asking the patient to describe how he or she would respond to situations having a variety of potential outcomes (e.g., "What would you do if you found a wallet on the sidewalk?"). *Abstract thought* can be tested by asking the patient to describe similarities between various objects or concepts (e.g., apple and orange, desk and chair, poetry and sculpture) or to list items having the same attributes (e.g., a list of four-legged animals). *Calculation ability* is assessed by having the patient carry out a computation that is appropriate to the patient's age and education (e.g., serial subtraction of 7 from 100 or 3 from 20; or word problems involving simple arithmetic).

Cranial Nerve Examination (See also Chaps. 25, 26, and 355)

- *The bare minimum: Check the fundi, visual fields, pupil size and reactivity, extraocular movements, and facial movements.*

The cranial nerves (CN) are best examined in numerical order, except for grouping together CN III, IV, and VI because of their similar function.

CN I (OLFACTORY) Testing is usually omitted unless there is suspicion for inferior frontal lobe disease (e.g., meningioma). With eyes closed, ask the patient to sniff a mild stimulus such as toothpaste or coffee and identify the odorant.

CN II (OPTIC) Check visual acuity (with eyeglasses or contact lens correction) using a Snellen chart or similar tool. Test the visual fields by confrontation, i.e., by comparing the patient's visual fields to your own. As a screening test, it is usually sufficient to examine the visual fields of both eyes simultaneously; individual eye fields should be tested if there is any reason to suspect a problem of vision by the history or other elements of the examination, or if the screening test

reveals an abnormality. Face the patient at a distance of approximately 0.6 to 1.0 m (2 to 3 ft) and place your hands at the periphery of your visual fields in the plane that is equidistant between you and the patient. Instruct the patient to look directly at the center of your face and to indicate when and where he or she sees one of your fingers moving. Beginning with the two inferior quadrants and then the two superior quadrants, move your index finger of the right hand, left hand, or both hands simultaneously and observe whether the patient detects the movements. A single small-amplitude movement of the finger is sufficient for a normal response. Focal perimetry and tangent screen examinations should be used to map out visual field defects fully or to search for subtle abnormalities. Optic fundi should be examined with an ophthalmoscope, and the color, size, and degree of swelling or elevation of the optic disc noted, as well as the color and texture of the retina. The retinal vessels should be checked for size, regularity, arterial-venous nicking at crossing points, hemorrhage, exudates, etc.

CN III, IV, VI (OCULOMOTOR, TROCHLEAR, ABDUCENS) Describe the size and shape of pupils and reaction to light and accommodation (i.e., as the eyes converge while following your finger as it moves toward the bridge of the nose). To check extraocular movements, ask the patient to keep his or her head still while tracking the movement of the tip of your finger. Move the target slowly in the horizontal and vertical planes; observe any paresis, nystagmus, or abnormalities of smooth pursuit (saccades, oculomotor ataxia, etc.). If necessary, the relative position of the two eyes, both in primary and multidirectional gaze, can be assessed by comparing the reflections of a bright light off both pupils. However, in practice it is typically more useful to determine whether the patient describes diplopia in any direction of gaze; true diplopia should almost always resolve with one eye closed. Horizontal nystagmus is best assessed at 45° and not at extreme lateral gaze (which is uncomfortable for the patient); the target must often be held at the lateral position for at least a few seconds to detect an abnormality.

CN V (TRIGEMINAL) Examine sensation within the three territories of the branches of the trigeminal nerve (ophthalmic, maxillary, and mandibular) on each side of the face. As with other parts of the sensory examination, testing of two sensory modalities derived from different anatomic pathways (e.g., light touch and temperature) is sufficient for a screening examination. Testing of other modalities, the corneal reflex, and the motor component of CN V (jaw clench—masseter muscle) is indicated when suggested by the history.

CN VII (FACIAL) Look for facial asymmetry at rest and with spontaneous movements. Test eyebrow elevation, forehead wrinkling, eye closure, smiling, and cheek puff. Look in particular for differences in the lower versus upper facial muscles; weakness of the lower two-thirds of the face with preservation of the upper third suggests an upper motor neuron lesion, whereas weakness of an entire side suggests a lower motor neuron lesion.

CN VIII (VESTIBULOCOCHLEAR) Check the patient's ability to hear a finger rub or whispered voice with each ear. Further testing for air versus mastoid bone conduction (Rinne) and lateralization of a 512-Hz tuning fork placed at the center of the forehead (Weber) should be done if an abnormality is detected by history or examination. Any suspected problem should be followed up with formal audiometry. →*For further discussion of assessing vestibular nerve function in the setting of dizziness or coma, see Chaps. 20 and 257, respectively.*

CN IX, X Observe the position and symmetry of the palate and uvula at rest and with phonation ("aah"). The pharyngeal ("gag") reflex is evaluated by stimulating the posterior pharyngeal wall on each side with a sterile, blunt object (e.g., tongue blade), but the reflex is often absent in normal individuals.

CN XI Check shoulder shrug (trapezius muscle) and head rotation to each side (sternocleidomastoid) against resistance.

CN XII Inspect the tongue for atrophy or fasciculations, position with protrusion, and strength when extended against the inner surface of the cheeks on each side.

Motor Examination (See also Chap. 21)

- *The bare minimum: Look for muscle atrophy and check extremity tone. Assess upper extremity strength by checking for pronator drift and strength of wrist or finger extensors. Tap the biceps, patellar, and Achilles reflexes. Test for lower extremity strength by having the patient walk normally and on heels and toes.*

The motor examination includes observations of muscle appearance, tone, strength, and reflexes. Although gait is in part a test of motor function, it is usually evaluated separately at the end of the examination.

APPEARANCE Inspect and palpate muscle groups under good light and with the patient in a comfortable and symmetric position. Check for muscle fasciculations, tenderness, and atrophy or hypertrophy. Involuntary movements may be present at rest (e.g., tics, myoclonus, choreoathetosis), during maintained posture (pill-rolling tremor of Parkinson's disease), or with voluntary movements (intention tremor of cerebellar disease or familial tremor).

TONE Muscle tone is tested by measuring the resistance to passive movement of a relaxed limb. Patients often have difficulty relaxing during this procedure, so it is useful to distract the patient to minimize active movements. In the upper limbs, tone is assessed by rapid pronation and supination of the forearm and flexion and extension at the wrist. In the lower limbs, while the patient is supine the examiner's hands are placed behind the knees and rapidly raised; with normal tone the ankles drag along the table surface for a variable distance before rising, whereas increased tone results in an immediate lift of the heel off the surface. Decreased tone is most commonly due to lower motor neuron or peripheral nerve disorders. Increased tone may be evident as spasticity (resistance determined by the angle and velocity of motion; corticospinal tract disease), rigidity (similar resistance in all angles of motion; extrapyramidal disease), or paratonia (fluctuating changes in resistance; frontal lobe pathways or normal difficulty in relaxing). Cogwheel rigidity, in which passive motion elicits jerky interruptions in resistance, is seen in parkinsonism.

STRENGTH Testing for pronator drift is an extremely useful method for screening upper limb weakness. The patient is asked to hold both arms fully extended and parallel to the ground with eyes closed. This position should be maintained for ~10 s; any flexion at the elbow or fingers or pronation of the forearm, especially if asymmetric, is a sign of potential weakness. Muscle strength is further assessed by having the patient exert maximal effort for the particular muscle or muscle group being tested. It is important to isolate the muscles as much as possible, i.e., hold the limb so that only the muscles of interest are active. It is also helpful to palpate accessible muscles as they contract. Grading muscle strength and evaluating the patient's effort is an art that takes time and practice. Muscle strength is traditionally graded using the following scale:

    0 = no movement
    1 = flicker or trace of contraction but no associated movement
        at a joint
    2 = movement with gravity eliminated
    3 = movement against gravity but not against resistance
    4− = movement against a mild degree of resistance
    4 = movement against moderate resistance
    4+ = movement against strong resistance
    5 = full power

However, in many cases it is more practical to use the following terms:

Paralysis = no movement
Severe weakness = movement with gravity eliminated

Moderate weakness = movement against gravity but not against mild resistance
Mild weakness = movement against moderate resistance
Full strength

Noting the pattern of weakness is as important as assessing the magnitude of weakness. Unilateral or bilateral weakness of the upper limb extensors and lower limb flexors ("pyramidal weakness") suggests a lesion of the pyramidal tract, bilateral proximal weakness suggests myopathy, and bilateral distal weakness suggests peripheral neuropathy.

REFLEXES ■ *Muscle Stretch Reflexes* Those that are typically assessed include the biceps (**C5**, C6), brachioradialis (C5, **C6**), and triceps (**C7**, C8) reflexes in the upper limbs and the patellar or quadriceps (**L3**, L4) and Achilles (**S1**, S2) reflexes in the lower limbs. The patient should be relaxed and the muscle positioned midway between full contraction and extension. Reflexes may be enhanced by asking the patient to voluntarily contract other, distant muscle groups (Jendrassik maneuver). For example, upper limb reflexes may be reinforced by voluntary teeth-clenching, and the Achilles reflex by hooking the flexed fingers of the two hands together and attempting to pull them apart. For each reflex tested, the two sides should be tested sequentially, and it is important to determine the smallest stimulus required to elicit a reflex rather than the maximum response. Reflexes are graded according to the following scale:

    0 = absent   3 = exaggerated
    1 = present but diminished   4 = clonus
    2 = normoactive

Cutaneous Reflexes The plantar reflex is elicited by stroking, with a noxious stimulus such as a tongue blade, the lateral surface of the sole of the foot beginning near the heel and moving across the ball of the foot to the great toe. The normal reflex consists of plantar flexion of the toes. With upper motor neuron lesions above the S1 level of the spinal cord, a paradoxical extension of the toe is observed, associated with fanning and extension of the other toes (termed an *extensor plantar response*, or *Babinski sign*). Superficial abdominal reflexes are elicited by gently stroking the abdominal surface near the umbilicus in a diagonal fashion with a sharp object (e.g., the wooden end of a cotton-tipped swab) and observing the movement of the umbilicus. Normally, the umbilicus will pull toward the stimulated quadrant. With upper motor neuron lesions, these reflexes are absent. They are most helpful when there is preservation of the upper (spinal cord level T9) but not lower (T12) abdominal reflexes, indicating a spinal lesion between T9 and T12, or when the response is asymmetric. Other useful cutaneous reflexes include the cremasteric (ipsilateral elevation of the testicle following stroking of the medial thigh; mediated by L1 and L2) and anal (contraction of the anal sphincter when the perianal skin is scratched; mediated by S2, S3, S4) reflexes. It is particularly important to test for these reflexes in any patient with suspected injury to the spinal cord or lumbosacral roots.

Primitive Reflexes With disease of the frontal lobe pathways, several primitive reflexes not normally present in the adult may appear. The suck response is elicited by lightly touching the center of the lips, and the root response the corner of the lips, with a tongue blade; the patient will move the lips to suck or root in the direction of the stimulus. The grasp reflex is elicited by touching the palm between the thumb and index finger with the examiner's fingers; a positive response is a forced grasp of the examiner's hand. In many instances stroking the back of the hand will lead to its release. The palmomental response is contraction of the mentalis muscle (chin) ipsilateral to a scratch stimulus diagonally applied to the palm.

Sensory Examination (See also Chap. 22)

- *The bare minimum: Ask whether the patient can feel light touch and the temperature of a cool object in each distal extremity. Check double simultaneous stimulation using light touch on the hands.*

Evaluating sensation is usually the most unreliable part of the examination, because it is subjective and is difficult to quantify. In the compliant and discerning patient, the sensory examination can be extremely helpful for the precise localization of a lesion. With patients who are uncooperative or lack an understanding of the tests, it may be useless. The examination should be focused on the suspected lesion. For example, in spinal cord, spinal root, or peripheral nerve abnormalities, all major sensory modalities should be tested while looking for a pattern consistent with a spinal level and dermatomal or nerve distribution. In patients with lesions at or above the brainstem, screening the primary sensory modalities in the distal extremities along with tests of "cortical" sensation is usually sufficient.

The five primary sensory modalities—light touch, pain, temperature, vibration, and joint position—are tested in each limb. Light touch is assessed by stimulating the skin with single, very gentle touches of the examiner's finger or a wisp of cotton. Pain is tested using a new pin, and temperature is assessed using a metal object (e.g., tuning fork) that has been immersed in cold and warm water. Vibration is tested using a 128-Hz tuning fork applied to the distal phalynx of the great toe or index finger just below the nailbed. By placing a finger on the opposite side of the joint being tested, the examiner compares the patient's threshold of vibration perception with his or her own. For joint position testing, the examiner grasps the digit or limb laterally and distal to the joint being assessed; small 1- to 2-mm excursions can usually be sensed. The Romberg maneuver is primarily a test of proprioception. The patient is asked to stand with the feet as close together as necessary to maintain balance while the eyes are open, and the eyes are then closed. A loss of balance with the eyes closed is an abnormal response.

"Cortical" sensation is mediated by the parietal lobes and represents an integration of the primary sensory modalities; testing cortical sensation is only meaningful when primary sensation is intact. Double simultaneous stimulation is especially useful as a screening test for cortical function; with the patient's eyes closed, the examiner lightly touches one or both hands and asks the patient to identify the stimuli. With a parietal lobe lesion, the patient may be unable to identify the stimulus on the contralateral side when both hands are touched. Other modalities relying on the parietal cortex include the discrimination of two closely placed stimuli as separate (two-point discrimination), identification of an object by touch and manipulation alone (stereognosis), and the identification of numbers or letters written on the skin surface (graphesthesia).

Coordination Examination (See also Chap. 21)

- *The bare minimum: Test rapid alternating movements of the fingers and feet, and the finger-to-nose maneuver.*

Coordination refers to the orchestration and fluidity of movements. Even simple acts require cooperation of agonist and antagonist muscles, maintenance of posture, and complex servomechanisms to control the rate and range of movements. Part of this integration relies on normal function of the cerebellar and basal ganglia systems. However, coordination also requires intact muscle strength and kinesthetic and propioceptive information. Thus, if the examination has disclosed abnormalities of the motor or sensory systems, the patient's coordination should be assessed with these limitations in mind.

Rapid alternating movements in the upper limbs are tested separately on each side by having the patient make a fist, partially extend the index finger, and then tap the index finger on the distal thumb as quickly as possible. In the lower limb, the patient rapidly taps the foot against the floor or the examiner's hand. Finger-to-nose testing is primarily a test of cerebellar function; the patient is asked to touch his or her index finger repetitively to the nose and then to the examiner's outstretched finger, which moves with each repetition. A similar test in the lower extremity is to have the patient raise the leg and touch the examiner's finger with the great toe. Another cerebellar test in the lower limbs is the heel-knee-shin maneuver; in the supine position the patient is asked to slide the heel of each foot from the knee down the shin of the other leg. For all these movements, the accuracy, speed, and rhythm are noted.

Gait Examination (See also Chap. 21)

- *The bare minimum: Observe the patient while walking normally, on the heels and toes, and along a straight line.*

Watching the patient walk is the most important part of the neurologic examination. Normal gait requires that multiple systems—including strength, sensation, and coordination—function in a highly integrated fashion. Unexpected abnormalities may be detected that prompt the examiner to return, in more detail, to other aspects of the examination. The patient should be observed while walking and turning normally, walking on the heels, walking on the toes, and walking heel-to-toe along a straight line. The examination may reveal decreased arm swing on one side (corticospinal tract disease), a stooped posture and short-stepped gait (parkinsonism), a broad-based unstable gait (ataxia), scissoring (spasticity), or a high-stepped, slapping gait (posterior column or peripheral nerve disease), or the patient may appear to be stuck in place (apraxia with frontal lobe disease).

NEUROLOGIC DIAGNOSIS   The clinical data obtained from the history and the examination are interpreted in terms of neuroanatomy and neurophysiology and assembled into one of the known syndromes (see Table 346-2; online). From the syndrome the physician should be able to determine the anatomic localization that best explains the clinical findings, to narrow the list of diagnostic possibilities, and to select the laboratory tests most likely to be informative. The laboratory assessment may include (1) serum electrolytes; complete blood count; and renal, hepatic, endocrine, and immune studies; (2) cerebrospinal fluid examination; (3) focused neuroimaging studies (Chap. 347); or (4) electrophysiologic studies (Chaps. 348 and 363). The anatomic localization, mode of onset and course of illness, other medical data, and laboratory findings are then integrated to establish an etiologic diagnosis.

It should be emphasized that the neurologic examination may be normal even in patients with a serious neurologic disease, such as seizures, chronic meningitis, or a TIA. A comatose patient may arrive with no available history, and in such cases the approach is as described in Chap. 257. In other patients, an inadequate history may be overcome by a succession of examinations from which the course of the illness can be inferred. In perplexing cases it is useful to remember that uncommon presentations of common diseases are more likely than rare etiologies. Thus, even in tertiary care settings, multiple strokes are usually due to emboli and not vasculitis, and dementia with myoclonus is usually Alzheimer's disease and not a prionopathy or a paraneoplastic disorder. Finally, the most important task of a primary care physician faced with a patient who has a new neurologic complaint is to assess the urgency of referral to a specialist. Here, the imperative is to rapidly identify patients likely to have nervous system infections, acute strokes, and spinal cord compression or other treatable mass lesions and arrange for immediate care.

FURTHER READING

BLUMENTHAL H: *Neuroanatomy Through Clinical Cases.* Sinauer Associates, 2002

DANA ALLIANCE FOR BRAIN INITIATIVES: *Delivery Results: A Progress Report on Brain Research.* New York, Dana Press, 1996

VICTOR M et al: *Principles of Neurology,* 7th Ed. New York, McGraw-Hill, 2001

The clinician caring for patients with neurologic symptoms is faced with an expanding number of imaging options, including computed tomography (CT), CT angiography (CTA), perfusion CT (pCT), magnetic resonance imaging (MRI), MR angiography (MRA), functional MRI (fMRI), MR spectroscopy (MRS), MR neurography, and perfusion MRI (pMRI). In addition, an increasing number of interventional neuroradiologic techniques are available including angiography; embolization and stenting of vascular structures; and spine interventions such as discography, selective nerve root injection, and epidural injections. Recent developments, such as multidetector CT angiography and gadolinium-enhanced MRA, have narrowed the indications for conventional angiography, which is now reserved for patients in whom small-vessel detail is essential for diagnosis or for whom interventional therapies are planned (Table 347-1).

In general, MRI is more sensitive than CT for the detection of lesions affecting the central nervous system (CNS), particularly those of the spinal cord, cranial nerves, and posterior fossa structures. Diffusion MR, a sequence that detects reduction of microscopic motion of water, is the most sensitive technique for detecting acute ischemic stroke and is useful in the detection of encephalitis, abscesses, and prion diseases. CT, however, can be quickly obtained and is widely available, making it a pragmatic choice for the initial evaluation of patients with suspected acute stroke, hemorrhage, and intracranial or spinal trauma. CT is also more sensitive than MRI for visualizing fine osseous detail and is indicated in the initial evaluation of conductive hearing loss as well as lesions affecting the skull base and calvarium.

COMPUTED TOMOGRAPHY ■ Technique
The CT image is a cross-sectional representation of anatomy created by a computer-generated analysis of the attenuation of x-ray beams passed through a section of the body. As the x-ray beam, collimated to the desired slice width, rotates around the patient, it passes through selected regions in the body. X-rays that are not attenuated by the body are detected by sensitive x-ray detectors aligned 180° from the x-ray tube. A computer calculates a "back projection" image from the 360° x-ray attenuation profile. Greater x-ray attenuation, e.g., as caused by bone, results in areas of high "density," while soft tissue structures, which have poor attenuation of x-rays, are lower in density. The resolution of an image depends on the radiation dose, the collimation (slice thickness), the field of view, and the matrix size of the display. A modern CT scanner is capable of obtaining sections as thin as 0.5 to 1 mm with submillimeter resolution at a speed of 0.5 to 1 s per section; complete studies of the brain can be completed in 20 to 60 s.

Helical CT is a type of scanner in which continuous CT information is obtained while the patient moves through the x-ray beam. In the helical scan mode, the table moves continuously through the rotating x-ray beam, generating a "helix" of information that can be reformatted into various slice thicknesses. Single or multiple (from 4 to 32) detectors positioned 180 degrees to the x-ray source may result in multiple slices per revolution of the beam around the patient. These "multidetector" scanners have further decreased the time per examination and permit rapid assessment of vascular anatomy as well as perfusion characteristics of brain parenchyma (Figs. 347-1 and 347-2). Advantages of multidetector scanning include shorter scan times, reduced patient and organ motion, and the ability to acquire images dynamically during the infusion of intravenous contrast that can be used to construct CT angiograms of vascular structures and CT perfusion images (Figs. 347-1B and 347-2). CTA images may be processed later for display in three dimensions to yield angiogram-like images (Figs. 347-1C and 349-12). CTA has proven useful in assessing the carotid bifurcation and intracranial arterial and venous anatomy.

Intravenous contrast is often administered prior to or during a CT study to identify vascular structures and to detect defects in the blood-brain barrier (BBB), which are associated with disorders such as tumors, infarcts, and infections. In the normal CNS, only vessels and structures lacking a BBB (e.g., the pituitary gland, choroid plexus, and dura) enhance after contrast administration. The use of iodinated contrast agents carries a risk of allergic reaction and adds additional expense and radiation dose. While helpful in characterizing mass lesions as well as essential for the acquisition of CTA studies, the decision to use contrast material should always be considered carefully.

Indications CT is the primary study of choice in the evaluation of acute trauma to the brain and spine, suspected subarachnoid hemorrhage, and conductive hearing loss (Table 347-1). CT is complementary to MR in the evaluation of the skull base, orbit, and osseous structures of the spine. In the spine, CT is useful in evaluating patients with osseous spinal stenosis and spondylosis, but MRI is often preferred in those with neurologic deficits. CT can also be obtained following intrathecal contrast injection to evaluate the intracranial cisterns (*CT cisternography*) for cerebrospinal fluid (CSF) fistula, as well as the spinal subarachnoid space (*CT myelography*).

Complications CT is safe, fast, and reliable. Radiation exposure is between 3 and 5 cGy per study. Care must be taken to reduce exposure when imaging children. The most frequent complications are associ-

---

TABLE 347-1 Guidelines for the Use of CT, Ultrasound, and MRI

Condition	Recommended Technique
Hemorrhage	
Acute parenchymal	CT > MR
Subacute/chronic	MRI
Subarachnoid hemorrhage	CT, CTA, lumbar puncture → angiography
Aneurysm	Angiography > CTA, MRA
Ischemic infarction	
Hemorrhagic infarction	CT
Bland infarction	MRI > CT
Carotid or vertebral dissection	MRI/MRA
Vertebral basilar insufficiency	CTA, MRI/MRA
Carotid stenosis	CTA > Doppler ultrasound, MRA
Suspected mass lesion	
Neoplasm, primary or metastatic	MRI + contrast
Infection/abscess	MRI + contrast
Immunosuppressed with focal findings	MRI + contrast
Vascular malformation	MRI +/− angiography
White matter disorders	MRI
Demyelinating disease	MRI +/− contrast
Dementia	MRI
Trauma	
Acute trauma	CT (noncontrast)
Shear injury/chronic hemorrhage	MRI
Headache/migraine	CT (noncontrast) / MRI
Seizure	
First time, no focal neurologic deficits	?CT as screen
Partial complex/refractory	MRI with coronal T2W imaging
Cranial neuropathy	MRI with contrast
Meningeal disease	MRI with contrast
SPINE	
Low back pain	
No neurologic deficits	MRI or CT after 4 weeks
With focal deficits	MRI > CT
Spinal stenosis	MRI or CT
Cervical spondylosis	MRI or CT myelography
Infection	MRI + contrast, CT
Myelopathy	MRI + contrast > myelography
Arteriovenous malformation	MRI, myelography/angiography

Note: CT, computed tomography; MRI, magnetic resonance imaging; MRA, MR angiography; CTA, CT angiography; T2W, T2-weighted.

ated with use of intravenous contrast agents. Two broad categories of contrast media, ionic and nonionic, are in use. Although ionic agents are relatively safe and inexpensive, they are associated with a higher incidence of reactions and side effects. As a result, ionic agents have been largely replaced by safer nonionic compounds (Table 347-2).

Contrast nephropathy may result from hemodynamic changes, renal tubular obstruction and cell damage, or immunologic reactions to contrast agents. A rise in serum creatinine of at least 85 μmol/L (1 mg/dL) within 48 h of contrast administration is often used as a definition of contrast nephropathy, although other causes of acute renal failure must be excluded. The prognosis is usually favorable, with serum creatinine levels returning to baseline within 1 to 2 weeks. Risk factors for contrast nephropathy include advanced age, preexisting renal disease, diabetes, dehydration, and high contrast dose. Patients with diabetes and those with mild renal failure should be well hydrated prior to the administration of contrast agents, although careful consideration should be given to alternative imaging techniques, such as MR imaging. Nonionic, low-osmolar media produce fewer abnormalities in renal blood flow and less endothelial cell damage but should still be used carefully in patients at risk (Table 347-3).

Other side effects are rare but include a sensation of warmth throughout the body and a metallic taste during intravenous administration of iodinated contrast media. Anaphylactic reactions to intravenous contrast media, while rare, are the most serious side effects and range from mild hives to bronchospasm, acute anaphylaxis, and death. The pathogenesis of these allergic reactions is not fully understood, but it is thought to include the release of mediators such as histamine, antibody-antigen reactions, and complement activation. Severe allergic reactions occur in ~0.04% of patients receiving nonionic media, sixfold fewer than with ionic media. Risk factors include a history of prior contrast reaction, food allergies to shellfish, and atopy (asthma and hay fever). In such patients, a noncontrast CT or MRI procedure should be considered as an alternative to contrast administration. If iodinated contrast is absolutely required, a nonionic agent should be used in conjunction with pretreatment with glucocorticoids and antihistamines (Table 347-4). Patients with allergic reactions to iodinated contrast material do not usually react to gadolinium-based MR contrast material, although it would be wise to pretreat patients with a prior allergic history to MR contrast administration in a similar fashion.

MAGNETIC RESONANCE IMAGING ■ **Technique** Magnetic resonance is a complex interaction between hydrogen protons in biologic tissues, a static magnetic field (the magnet), and energy in the form of radiofrequency (Rf) waves of a specific frequency introduced by coils placed next to the body part of interest. Spatial localization is achieved by magnetic gradients surrounding the main magnet, which impart slight changes in magnetic field throughout the imaging volume. The energy state of the hydrogen protons is transiently excited by the Rf, which is administered at a frequency specific for the field strength of the magnet. The subsequent return to equilibrium energy state (*relaxation*) of the protons results in a release of Rf energy (the *echo*), which is detected by the coils that delivered the Rf pulses. The echo is trans-

FIGURE 347-1 CT angiography (CTA) of ruptured anterior cerebral artery aneurysm. A 45-year-old man presents with acute headache. *A.* Noncontrast CT demonstrates intraventricular, subarachnoid, and frontal lobe hemorrhage. *B.* A partition from CT angiography demonstrates a suspicious enlargement of the anterior cerebral cerebral artery (*arrow*). *C.* 3D surface reconstruction using a workstation confirms the anterior cerebral aneurysm and demonstrates its orientation and relationship to nearby vessels (*arrow*). CTA image is produced by 1-mm helical CT scans performed during a rapid bolus infusion of intravenous contrast medium.

formed by Fourier analysis into the information used to form an MR image. The MR image thus consists of a map of the distribution of hydrogen protons, with signal intensity imparted by both density of hydrogen protons as well as differences in the relaxation time (see below) of hydrogen protons on different molecules.

T1 AND T2 RELAXATION TIMES The rate of return to equilibrium of perturbed protons is called the *relaxation rate*. The relaxation rate varies among normal and pathologic tissues. The relaxation rate of a hydrogen proton in a tissue is influenced by local interactions with surrounding molecules and atomic neighbors. Two relaxation rates, T1 and T2, influence the signal intensity of the image. The T1 relaxation time is the time, measured in milliseconds, for 63% of the hydrogen protons to return to their normal equilibrium state, while the T2 relaxation is the time for 63% of the protons to become dephased owing to interactions among nearby protons. The intensity of the signal within various tissues and image contrast can be modulated by altering acquisition parameters, such as the interval between Rf pulses (TR) and the time between the Rf pulse and the signal reception (TE). So-called T1-weighted (T1W) images are produced by keeping the TR and TE relatively short. T2-weighted (T2W) images are produced by using longer TR and TE times. Fat and subacute hemorrhage have short T1 relaxation rates and a high signal intensity on T1W images. Structures containing more water, such as CSF and edema, have long T1 and T2 relaxation rates, a low signal intensity on T1W images, and a high signal intensity on T2W images (Table 347-5). Gray matter contains 10 to 15% more water than white matter, which accounts for much of its contrast on MRI (Fig. 347-3). T2W images are more sensitive than T1W images to edema, demyelination, infarction, and chronic hemorrhage, while T1-weighted imaging is more sensitive to subacute hemorrhage and fat-containing structures.

A   B   C

D   E

FIGURE 347-2 A 49-year-old man with acute neck pain and right hemiparesis. *A.* Axial noncontrast CT scan demonstrates high density within the right middle cerebral artery (*arrow*) associated with subtle low density involving the right putamen (*arrowheads*). *B.* Mean transit time map calculated from a CT perfusion study obtained with a 40-cc contrast injection during which 45 images were obtained at the same slice location. Prolongation of the mean transit time is visible throughout the right hemisphere (*arrows*). *C.* Axial maximum intensity projection from CTA study through the Circle of Willis demonstrates an abrupt occlusion of the proximal right middle cerebral artery (*arrow*). Reconstitution of flow via collaterals is seen distal to the occlusion, however, the patient sustained a right basal ganglia infarction. *D.* Sagittal reformation through the right internal carotid artery. Low-density lipid laden plaque (*arrows*) narrows the lumen of the internal carotid artery (*black arrows*). The internal jugular vein is shown (*white arrows*). *E.* 3D surface CTA images (different patient) demonstrate calcification and narrowing of the right internal carotid artery, consistent with atherosclerotic disease.

Many different MR pulse sequences exist, and each can be obtained in various planes (Figs. 347-3, 4, 5). The selection of a proper protocol that will best answer a clinical question depends on an accurate clinical history and indication for the examination. Fluid-attenuated inversion recovery (FLAIR) is a useful pulse sequence that produces T2W images in which the normally high signal intensity of CSF is suppressed

TABLE 347-3 *Indications for Use of Nonionic Contrast Media*

- Prior adverse reaction to contrast media, with the exception of heat, flushing, or an episode of nausea or vomiting
- Asthma or other serious lung disease
- History of atopic allergies (pretreatment with steroid/antihistamines recommended)
- Children under the age of 2 years
- Renal failure or creatinine >177 μmol/L (>2.0 mg/dL)
- Cardiac dysfunction, including recent or imminent cardiac decompensation, severe arrhythmias, unstable angina pectoris, recent myocardial infarction, and pulmonary hypertension
- Diabetes
- Severe debilitation

TABLE 347-2 *Guidelines for Use of Intravenous Contrast in Patients with Impaired Renal Function*

Serum Creatinine, μmol/L (mg/dL)[a]	Recommendation
<133 (<1.5)	Use either ionic or nonionic at 2 mL/kg to 150 mL total
133–177 (1.5–2.0)	Nonionic; hydrate diabetics 1 mL/kg per hour × 10 h
>177 (>2.0)	Consider noncontrast CT or MRI; nonionic contrast if required
177–221 (2.0–2.5)	Nonionic only if required (as above); contraindicated in diabetics
>265 (>3.0)	Nonionic IV contrast given only to patients undergoing dialysis within 24 h

[a] Risk is greatest in patients with rising creatinine levels.
Note: CT, computed tomography; MRI, magnetic resonance imaging.

TABLE 347-4 *Guidelines for Premedication of Patients with Prior Contrast Allergy*

12 h prior to examination:
   Prednisone, 40 mg PO *or* methylprednisolone, 32 mg PO
2 h prior to examination:
   Prednisone, 40 mg PO *or* methylprednisolone, 32 mg PO *and*
   Cimetidine, 300 mg PO *or* ranitidine, 150 mg PO
Immediately prior to examination:
   Benadryl, 50 mg IV (alternatively, can be given PO 2 h prior to exam)

TABLE 347-5 *Some Common Intensities on T1- and T2-Weighted MRI Sequences*

Image	TR	TE	CSF	Fat	Brain	Edema
			\multicolumn{4}{c}{Signal Intensity}		
T1W	Short	Short	Low	High	Low	Low
T2W	Long	Long	High	Low	High	High

Note: TR, interval between radiofrequency (Rf) pulses; TE, interval between Rf pulse and signal reception; CSF, cerebrospinal fluid; T1W and T2W, T1- and T2-weighted.

(Fig. 347-5*A*). FLAIR images are more sensitive than standard spine echo images for the detection of lesions within or adjacent to CSF. Gradient echo imaging is most sensitive to magnetic susceptibility as seen with blood, calcium, and air, and is indicated in patients with traumatic brain injury. MR images can be generated in sagittal, coronal, axial, or oblique planes without changing the patient's position. Each plane obtained requires a separate sequence lasting 1 to 10 min. Three-dimensional volumetric imaging is also possible with MRI, resulting in a volume of data that can be reformatted in any orientation on a workstation to highlight certain disease processes.

MR CONTRAST MATERIAL The heavy-metal element gadolinium forms the basis of all currently approved intravenous MR contrast agents. Gadolinium is a paramagnetic substance, which means that it reduces the T1 and T2 relaxation times of nearby water protons, resulting in a high signal on T1W images and a low signal on T2W images (the latter requires a sufficient local concentration, usually in the form of a bolus). Unlike iodinated contrast agents, the effect of MR contrast agents depends on the presence of local hydrogen protons on which it must act to achieve the desired effect. Gadolinium is chelated to DTPA (diethylenetriaminepentaacetic acid), which allows safe renal excretion. Approximately 0.2 mL/kg body weight is administered intravenously; the cost is ~$60 per dose. Gadolinium-DTPA does not cross the intact BBB but will enhance lesions lacking a BBB (Fig. 347-4*A*) and areas of the brain that normally are devoid of the BBB. The agent is well tolerated, and severe allergic reactions to gadolinium are rare but have been reported. The adverse reaction rate in patients with a prior history of atopy or asthma is 3.7%; however, the reaction rate increases to 6.3% in those patients with a prior history of unspecified allergic reaction to iodinated contrast. These agents can be administered safely to children as well as adults. Renal failure does not occur.

Complications and Contraindications From the patient's perspective, an MRI examination can be intimidating, and a higher level of cooperation is required than with CT. The patient lies on a table that is moved into a long, narrow gap within the magnet. Approximately 5% of the population experiences severe claustrophobia in the MR environment. This can be reduced by mild sedation but remains a problem for some. Unlike CT, movement of the patient during an MR sequence distorts all the images; therefore, uncooperative patients should either be sedated for the MR study or scanned with CT. Generally, children under the age of 10 years usually require conscious sedation in order to complete the MR examination without motion degradation.

MRI is considered safe for patients, even at very high field strengths (>3 to 4 T). Serious injuries have been caused, however, by attraction of ferromagnetic objects into the magnet, which act as missiles if brought too close to the magnet. Likewise, ferromagnetic implants, such as aneurysm clips, may torque within the magnet, causing damage to vessels and even death. Metallic foreign bodies in the eye have moved and caused intraocular hemorrhage; screening for ocular metallic fragments is indicated in those with a history of metal work or ocular metallic foreign bodies. Implanted cardiac pacemakers are a contraindication to MRI owing to the risk of induced arrhythmias. All health care personnel and patients must be screened and educated thoroughly to prevent such disasters as the magnet is always "on." Table 347-6 lists common contraindications for MRI.

MAGNETIC RESONANCE ANGIOGRAPHY On routine spin echo MR sequences, moving protons (e.g., flowing blood, CSF) exhibit complex MR signals that range from high to low signal intensity relative to background stationary tissue. Fast-flowing blood returns no signal (flow void) on routine T1W or T2W spin echo MR images. Slower flowing blood, as occurs in veins or distal to arterial stenoses, may appear high in signal. However, using special pulse sequences called *gradient echo sequences*, it is possible to increase the signal intensity of moving protons in contrast to the low signal background intensity of stationary tissue. This creates angiography-like images, which can be manipulated in three dimensions to highlight vascular anatomy and relationships.

Two MRA techniques, time-of-flight (TOF) and phase-contrast, are routinely used. TOF, currently the technique used most frequently, relies on the suppression of nonmoving tissue to provide a low-intensity background for the high signal intensity of flowing blood entering the section; arterial or venous structures may be highlighted. A typical TOF angiography sequence results in a series of contiguous thin MR sections (0.9 mm thick), which can be viewed as a stack and manipulated to create an angiographic image data set that can be reformatted

A

B

FIGURE 347-3 *A.* Axial echo-planar diffusion-weighted MR image demonstrates a large area of reduced diffusion consistent with acute cerebral ischemia (*arrows*) located in the right posterior frontotemporal lobe. Reduced diffusion is consistent with cytotoxic edema and is most commonly associated with acute cerebral infarction. *B.* Time-of-flight MR angiography through the circle of Willis demonstrates a high-grade stenosis at the left middle cerebral artery bifurcation (*arrows*).

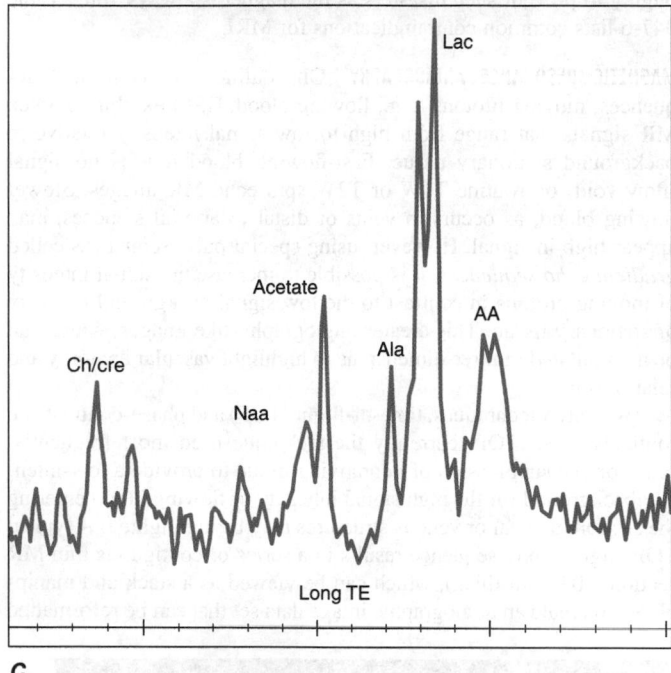

FIGURE 347-4 Middle age woman with fever and right hemiparesis. *A.* Coronal postcontrast T1-weighted image demonstrates a ring enhancing mass in the left frontal lobe (*arrows*). *B.* Axial diffusion weighted image demonstrates restricted diffusion (high signal intensity) within the lesion. Restricted diffusion in such a setting is highly suggestive of cerebral abscess. *C.* Single voxel proton spectroscopy obtained with a TE of 288 ms. In addition to the reduced Naa peak, abnormal peaks including acetate, alanine (Ala), lactate (Lac), and amino acids (AA) are visualized. These are highly suggestive of cerebral abscess. At biopsy a streptococcal abscess was identified.

MRA is lower in spatial resolution compared with conventional film-based angiography, and therefore the detection of small-vessel detail, such as is required in the workup of vasculitis, is problematic. MRA is also less sensitive to slowly flowing blood and thus may not reliably differentiate complete from near-complete occlusions. Motion, either by the patient or by anatomic structures, may distort the MRA images, creating artifacts. These limitations notwithstanding, MRA has proved useful in evaluation of the extracranial carotid and vertebral circulation as well as of larger-caliber intracranial arteries and dural sinuses. It has also proved useful in the noninvasive detection of intracranial aneurysms and vascular malformations.

ECHO-PLANAR MR IMAGING Recent improvements in gradients, software, and high-speed computer processors now permit extremely rapid MRI of the brain. With echo-planar MRI (EPI), fast gradients are switched on and off at high speeds to create the information used to form an image. In routine spin echo imaging, images of the brain can be obtained in 5 to 10 min. With EPI, all of the information required for processing an image is accumulated in 50 to 150 ms, and the information for the entire brain is obtained in 1 to 2 min, depending on the degree of resolution required or desired. Fast MRI reduces patient and organ motion, permitting diffusion imaging (Figs. 347-3, 4, 5 and Fig. 349-13), perfusion imaging during contrast infusion fMRI, and kinematic motion studies.

Perfusion and diffusion imaging are EPI techniques that are useful in early detection of ischemic injury of the brain and may be useful together to demonstrate infarcted tissue as well as ischemic but potentially viable tissue at risk of infarction (e.g., the ischemic penumbra). Diffusion-weighted imaging (DWI) assesses microscopic motion of water; restriction of motion appears as relative high signal intensity on diffusion-weighted images. DWI is the most sensitive technique for detection of acute cerebral infarction of <7 days' duration and is also sensitive to encephalitis and abscess formation, all of which demonstrate reduced diffusion or high signal.

Perfusion MRI involves the acquisition of EPI images during a rapid bolus of contrast material. Relative perfusion abnormalities can be identified. The relative cerebral blood volume, mean transit time,

and viewed in various planes and angles, much like that seen with conventional angiography (Fig. 347-3*B*). Noncontrast enhanced MRA provides a vascular flow map rather than the anatomic map shown by conventional angiography.

Phase-contrast MRA has a longer acquisition time than TOF MRA, but in addition to providing anatomic information similar to that of TOF imaging, it can be used to reveal the velocity and direction of blood flow in a given vessel. Through the selection of different imaging parameters, differing blood velocities can be highlighted; selective venous and arterial MRA images can thus be obtained. One advantage of phase-contrast MRA is the excellent suppression of high signal intensity background structures.

MRA can also be acquired during infusion of contrast material. Recently, contrast-enhanced MRA has become the standard for extracranial vascular MRA. This technique entails rapid imaging using coronal three-dimensional TOF sequences during a bolus infusion of 15 to 20 mL of gadolinium-DTPA. Proper technique and timing of acquisition relative to bolus arrival are critical for success. Advantages include a reduction in the time of acquisition (1 to 2 min vs. 10 min) and flow-related artifacts.

A   **B**

FIGURE 347-5   Herpes encephalitis. A 40-year-old man presents with altered mental status and fever. *A.* Coronal T2-weighted FLAIR image demonstrates expansion and high signal intensity involving the left medial temporal lobe, insular cortex, and left cingulate gyrus. *B.* Diffusion weighted image demonstrates high signal intensity indicative of restricted diffusion involving the left medial temporal lobe and hippocampus (*arrows*). This is most consistent with neuronal destruction and can be seen in acute infarction as well as infectious and inflammatory encephalitis. PCR evaluation of the CSF confirmed Herpes encephalitis. (*Case courtesy of Howard Rowley, MD, University of Wisconsin.*)

and cerebral blood flow throughout the image can be calculated within regions of interest. Delay in mean transit time and reduction in cerebral blood volume and cerebral blood flow are typically seen in infarction. Elevated or normal cerebral blood volume in a setting of reduced blood flow may indicate tissue that is at risk of infarction. pMRI imaging can also be used in the assessment of brain tumors where it has been shown to be helpful in differentiating intraaxial primary tumors from extraaxial tumors or metastasis.

Diffusion tract imaging (DTI) is a special diffusion technique that is capable of demonstrating white matter tracts and their relationship to lesions of the brain. Preferential microscopic motion of water along white matter tracts is detected by diffusion MR, which can also indicate the direction of white matter fiber tracts. This new technique has great potential in the assessment of brain maturation as well as disease entities that undermine the integrity of the white matter architecture.

fMRI of the brain is an EPI technique that localizes regions of activity in the brain following task activation. Neuronal activity elicits an increase in the delivery of oxygenated blood flow to a specific region of the brain, resulting in a slight alteration in the balance of oxyhemoglobin and deoxyhemoglobin, which yields a 2 to 3% increase in signal intensity within draining veins. Further work will determine whether these techniques are cost effective or clinically useful, but currently preoperative somatosensory and auditory cortex localization is possible. This technique has proved useful to neuroscientists interested in interrogating the localization of certain brain functions.

MAGNETIC RESONANCE NEUROGRAPHY   MR neurography is an MR technique that shows promise in detecting increased signal in irritated, inflamed, or infiltrated nerves. These images are obtained with fat-suppressed fast spin echo imaging or short inversion recovery sequences, and they may indicate nerves that are responsible for pain syndromes more precisely. Irritated or infiltrated nerves will demonstrate high signal on T2W imaging.

POSITRON EMISSION TOMOGRAPHY (PET)   PET relies on the detection of positrons emitted during the decay of a radionuclide that has been injected into a patient. The most frequently used moiety is 2-[¹⁸F]fluoro-2-deoxy-D-glucose (FDG), which is an analogue of glucose and is taken up by cells competitively with 2-deoxyglucose. Multiple images of glucose uptake activity are formed after 45 to 60 min. Images reveal differences in regional glucose activity among normal and pathologic brain structures. A lower activity of FDG in the parietal lobes has been associated with Alzheimer's disease. FDG PET is used primarily for the detection of extracranial metastatic disease. PET is no longer used primarily for differentiation of tumor from radiation necrosis.

MYELOGRAPHY ◼ **Technique**   Myelography involves the intrathecal instillation of specially formulated water-soluble iodinated contrast medium into the lumbar or cervical subarachnoid space. CT scanning is usually performed after myelography (*CT myelography*) to better demonstrate the spinal cord and roots, which appear as filling defects in the opacified subarachnoid space. *Low-dose CT myelography*, in which CT is performed after the subarachnoid injection of a small amount of relatively dilute contrast material, has replaced conventional myelography for many indications, thereby reducing exposure to radiation and contrast media. Newer multidetector scanners now obtain CT studies quickly so that reformations in sagittal and coronal planes, equivalent to traditional myelography projections, are now routine.

Indications   Myelography has been largely replaced by CT myelography and MRI for diagnosis of diseases of the spinal canal and cord (Table 347-1). Remaining indications for conventional plain film myelography include the evaluation of suspected meningeal or arachnoid cysts and the localization of spinal dural arteriovenous or CSF fistulas. Conventional myelography and CT myelography provide the most precise information in patients with prior spinal fusion and spinal fixation hardware.

Contraindications   Myelography is relatively safe; however, it should be performed with caution in any patient with elevated intracranial pressure or a history of allergic reaction to intrathecal contrast media. In patients with a suspected spinal block, MR is the preferred technique. If myelography is necessary, only a small amount of contrast medium should be instilled below the lesion in order to minimize the risk of neurologic deterioration. Lumbar puncture is to be avoided in patients with bleeding disorders, including patients receiving anticoagulant therapy, as well as in those with infections of the soft tissues.

Complications   Headache, nausea, and vomiting are the most frequent complications of myelography, occurring in up to 38% of patients. These symptoms are thought to result from neurotoxic effects of the contrast agent, persistent leakage of CSF at the puncture site, or psy-

TABLE 347-6 *Common Contraindications to MR Imaging*

Cardiac pacemaker or permanent pacemaker leads	Omniphase penile implant
Internal defibrillatory device	Swan-Ganz catheter
Cochlear prostheses	Magnetic stoma plugs
Bone growth stimulators	Magnetic dental implants
Spinal cord stimulators	Magnetic sphincters
Electronic infusion devices	Ferromagnetic IVC filters, coils, stents—safe 6 weeks after implantation
Intracranial aneurysm clips (some but not all)	
Ocular implants (some) or ocular metallic foreign body	Tattooed eyeliner (contains ferromagnetic material and may irritate eyes)
McGee stapedectomy piston prosthesis	

chological reactions to the procedure. Vasovagal syncope may occur during lumbar puncture; it is accentuated by the upright position used during lumbar myelography. Adequate hydration before and after myelography will reduce the incidence of this complication. Postural headache (post–lumbar puncture headache) is generally due to leakage of CSF from the puncture site, resulting in CSF hypotension; management is discussed in Chap. 14. Hearing loss is a rare complication of myelography. It may result from a direct toxic effect of the contrast medium or from an alteration of the pressure equilibrium between CSF and perilymph in the inner ear. Puncture of the spinal cord is a rare but serious complication of cervical (C1-2) and high lumbar puncture. The risk of cord puncture is greatest in patients with spinal stenosis or conditions that reduce CSF volume. In these settings, a low-dose lumbar injection followed by thin-section CT or MRI is a safer alternative to cervical puncture. Intrathecal contrast reactions are rare, but aseptic meningitis and encephalopathy may occur. The latter is usually dose-related and associated with contrast entering the intracranial subarachnoid space. Seizures occur following myelography in 0.1 to 0.3% of patients. Risk factors include a preexisting seizure disorder and the use of a total iodine dose of >4500 mg. Other reported symptoms include hyperthermia, hallucinations, depression, and anxiety states. These side effects have been reduced by the development of nonionic, water-soluble contrast agents, as well as by head elevation and generous hydration following myelography.

SPINE INTERVENTIONS ■ Discography The evaluation of back pain and radiculopathy may require diagnostic procedures that attempt either to reproduce the patient's pain or relieve it, indicating its correct source. Discography is performed by fluoroscopic placement of a 22- to 25-gauge needle into the intervertebral disc and subsequent injection of 1 to 3 mL of contrast media. The intradiscal pressure is recorded, as is an assessment of the patient's response to the injection of contrast material. Typically little or no pain is felt during injection of a normal disc, which does not accept much more than 1 mL of contrast material, even at pressures as high as 415 to 690 kPa (60 to 100 lb/in²). CT and plain films are obtained following the procedure.

Selective Nerve Root and Epidural Spinal Injections Percutaneous selective nerve root and epidural blocks with glucocorticoid and anesthetic mixtures may be both therapeutic as well as diagnostic, especially if a patient's pain is relieved. Typically 1 to 2 mL of an equal mixture of a long-acting glucocorticoid such as betamethasone and a long-acting anesthetic such as bupivicain 0.75% is instilled under CT or fluoroscopic guidance in the intraspinal epidural space or adjacent to an existing nerve root.

ANGIOGRAPHY ■ Technique Catheter angiography is indicated in the evaluation of patients with vascular pathology, particularly of smaller intracranial vessels. However, it carries the greatest risk of morbidity of all diagnostic imaging procedures, owing to the necessity of inserting a catheter into a blood vessel, directing the catheter to the required location, injecting contrast material to visualize the vessel, and removing the catheter while maintaining hemostasis. Therapeutic

transcatheter procedures (see below) have become important options for the treatment of some cerebrovascular diseases. The decision to undertake a diagnostic or therapeutic angiographic procedure requires careful assessment of the goals of the investigation and its attendant risks.

To improve tolerance to contrast agents, patients undergoing angiography should be well hydrated before and after the procedure. Since the femoral route is used most commonly, the femoral artery must be compressed after the procedure to prevent a hematoma from developing. The puncture site and distal pulses should be evaluated carefully after the procedure; complications can include thigh hematoma or lower extremity emboli.

Indications Table 347-1 lists some of the indications for conventional angiography. Angiography has been replaced for many indications by CT/CTA or MRI/MRA; however, angiography is still used for evaluating intracranial small-vessel pathology (such as vasculitis), for assessing vascular malformations and aneurysms, and in endovascular therapeutic procedures.

Complications A common femoral arterial puncture provides retrograde access via the aorta to the aortic arch and great vessels. The most feared complication of cerebral angiography is stroke. Thrombus can form on or inside the tip of the catheter, and atherosclerotic thrombus or plaque can be dislodged by the catheter or guidewire or by the force of injection and can embolize distally in the cerebral circulation. Risk factors for ischemic complications include limited experience on the part of the angiographer, atherosclerosis, vasospasm, low cardiac output, decreased oxygen-carrying capacity, advanced age, and possibly migraine. The risk of a neurologic complication varies but is ~4% for transient ischemic attack and stroke, 1% for permanent deficit, and <0.1% for death.

Ionic contrast material injected into the cerebral vasculature can be neurotoxic if the BBB is breached, either by an underlying disease or by the injection of hyperosmolar contrast agent. Ionic contrast media are less well tolerated than nonionic media, probably because they can induce changes in cell membrane electrical potentials. Patients with dolichoectasia of the basilar artery can suffer reversible brainstem dysfunction and acute short-term memory loss during angiography, owing to the slow percolation of the contrast material and the consequent prolonged exposure of the brain. Rarely, an intracranial aneurysm ruptures during an angiographic contrast injection, causing subarachnoid hemorrhage, perhaps as a result of injection under high pressure.

Spinal Angiography Spinal angiography may be indicated to evaluate vascular malformations and tumors and to identify the artery of Adamkiewicz (Chap. 356) prior to aortic aneurysm repair. The procedure is lengthy and requires the use of relatively large volumes of contrast; the incidence of serious complications, including paraparesis, subjective visual blurring, and altered speech, is ~2%. Gadolinium-enhanced MRA has been used successfully in this setting and has promise for replacing diagnostic spinal angiography for some indications.

INTERVENTIONAL NEURORADIOLOGY This rapidly developing field is providing new therapeutic options for patients with difficult neurovascular problems. Available procedures include detachable coil therapy for aneurysms, particulate or liquid adhesive embolization of arteriovenous malformations, balloon angioplasty and stenting of arterial stenosis or vasospasm, transarterial or transvenous embolization of dural arteriovenous fistulas, balloon occlusion of carotid-cavernous and vertebral fistulas, endovascular treatment of vein-of-Galen malformations, preoperative embolization of tumors, and thrombolysis of acute arterial or venous thrombosis. Many of these disorders place the patient at high risk of cerebral hemorrhage, stroke, or death.

The highest complication rates are found with the therapies designed to treat the highest-risk diseases. In a large series of surgically difficult intracranial aneurysms treated with detachable balloons, Higashida and colleagues reported a 7.4% incidence of stroke and a 9.8% death rate. These figures must be considered in light of the high morbidity and mortality associated with untreated and surgically unap-

proachable aneurysms (Chap. 349). The advent of the electrolytically detachable coil has reduced these rates and ushered in a new era in the treatment of cerebral aneurysms. One recent double-blind trial (ISAT) found a 28% reduction of morbity and mortality at 1 year among those treated for anterior circulation aneurysm with detachable coils versus neurosurgical clipping. It remains to be determined what the role of coils will be relative to surgical options, but in many centers, coiling of aneurysms has become standard therapy for many aneurysms.

Section 2 Diseases of the Central Nervous System

348 SEIZURES AND EPILEPSY
Daniel H. Lowenstein

A *seizure* (from the Latin *sacire*, "to take possession of") is a paroxysmal event due to abnormal, excessive, hypersynchronous discharges from an aggregate of central nervous system (CNS) neurons. Depending on the distribution of discharges, this abnormal CNS activity can have various manifestations, ranging from dramatic convulsive activity to experiential phenomena not readily discernible by an observer. Although a variety of factors influence the incidence and prevalence of seizures, ~5 to 10% of the population will have at least one seizure, with the highest incidence occurring in early childhood and late adulthood.

The meaning of the term seizure needs to be carefully distinguished from that of epilepsy. *Epilepsy* describes a condition in which a person has *recurrent* seizures due to a chronic, underlying process. This definition implies that a person with a single seizure, or recurrent seizures due to correctable or avoidable circumstances, does not necessarily have epilepsy. Epilepsy refers to a clinical phenomenon rather than a single disease entity, since there are many forms and causes of epilepsy. However, among the many causes of epilepsy there are various *epilepsy syndromes* in which the clinical and pathologic characteristics are distinctive and suggest a specific underlying etiology.

Using the definition of epilepsy as two or more unprovoked seizures, the incidence of epilepsy is ~0.3 to 0.5% in different populations throughout the world, and the prevalence of epilepsy has been estimated at 5 to 10 persons per 1000.

CLASSIFICATION OF SEIZURES

Determining the type of seizure that has occurred is essential for focusing the diagnostic approach on particular etiologies, selecting the appropriate therapy, and providing potentially vital information regarding prognosis. In 1981, the International League Against Epilepsy (ILAE) published a modified version of the International Classification of Epileptic Seizures that has continued to be a useful classification system (Table 348-1). This system is based on the clinical features of seizures and associated electroencephalographic findings. Other potentially distinctive features such as etiology or cellular substrate are not considered in this classification system, although this will undoubtedly change in the future as more is learned about the pathophysiologic mechanisms that underlie specific seizure types.

A fundamental principle is that seizures may be either partial (synonymous with focal) or generalized. *Partial seizures* are those in which the seizure activity is restricted to discrete areas of the cerebral cortex. *Generalized seizures* involve diffuse regions of the brain simultaneously. Partial seizures are usually associated with structural abnormalities of the brain. In contrast, generalized seizures may result from cellular, biochemical, or structural abnormalities that have a more widespread distribution.

PARTIAL SEIZURES Partial seizures occur within discrete regions of the brain. If consciousness is fully preserved during the seizure, the clinical manifestations are considered relatively simple and the seizure is termed a *simple partial seizure*. If consciousness is impaired, the symptomatology is more complex and the seizure is termed a *complex partial seizure*. An important additional subgroup comprises those seizures that begin as partial seizures and then spread diffusely throughout the cortex, i.e., *partial seizures with secondary generalization*.

Simple Partial Seizures Simple partial seizures cause motor, sensory, autonomic, or psychic symptoms without an obvious alteration in consciousness. For example, a patient having a partial motor seizure arising from the right primary motor cortex in the vicinity controlling hand movement will note the onset of involuntary movements of the contralateral, left hand. These movements are typically clonic (i.e., repetitive, flexion/extension movements) at a frequency of ~2 to 3 Hz; pure tonic posturing may be seen as well. Since the cortical region controlling hand movement is immediately adjacent to the region for facial expression, the seizure may also cause abnormal movements of the face synchronous with the movements of the hand. The electroencephalogram (EEG) recorded with scalp electrodes during the seizure (i.e., an ictal EEG) may show abnormal discharges in a very limited region over the appropriate area of cerebral cortex if the seizure focus involves the cerebral convexity. Seizure activity occurring within deeper brain structures is often not recorded by the standard EEG, however, and may require intracranial electrodes for its detection.

Three additional features of partial motor seizures are worth noting. First, in some patients the abnormal motor movements may begin in a very restricted region such as the fingers and gradually progress (over seconds to minutes) to include a larger portion of the extremity. This phenomenon, described by Hughlings Jackson and known as a "Jacksonian march," represents the spread of seizure activity over a progressively larger region of motor cortex. Second, patients may experience a localized paresis (Todd's paralysis) for minutes to many hours in the involved region following the seizure. Third, in rare instances the seizure may continue for hours or days. This condition, termed *epilepsia partialis continua*, is often refractory to medical therapy.

Simple partial seizures may also manifest as changes in somatic sensation (e.g., paresthesias), vision (flashing lights or formed hallucinations), equilibrium (sensation of falling or vertigo), or autonomic function (flushing, sweating, piloerection). Simple partial seizures arising from the temporal or frontal cortex may also cause alterations in hearing, olfaction, or higher cortical function (psychic symptoms). This includes the sensation of unusual, intense odors (e.g., burning rubber or kerosene) or sounds (crude or highly complex sounds), or an epigastric sensation that rises from the stomach or chest to the head. Some patients describe odd, internal feelings such as fear, a sense of

TABLE 348-1 Classification of Seizures

1. Partial seizures
   a. Simple partial seizures (with motor, sensory, autonomic, or psychic signs)
   b. Complex partial seizures
   c. Partial seizures with secondary generalization
2. Primarily generalized seizures
   a. Absence (petit mal)
   b. Tonic-clonic (grand mal)
   c. Tonic
   d. Atonic
   e. Myoclonic
3. Unclassified seizures
   a. Neonatal seizures
   b. Infantile spasms

impending change, detachment, depersonalization, déjà vu, or illusions that objects are growing smaller (micropsia) or larger (macropsia). When such symptoms precede a complex partial or secondarily generalized seizure, these simple partial seizures serve as a warning, or *aura*.

Complex Partial Seizures Complex partial seizures are characterized by focal seizure activity accompanied by a transient impairment of the patient's ability to maintain normal contact with the environment. The patient is unable to respond appropriately to visual or verbal commands during the seizure and has impaired recollection or awareness of the ictal phase. The seizures frequently begin with an aura (i.e., a simple partial seizure) that is stereotypic for the patient. The start of the ictal phase is often a sudden behavioral arrest or motionless stare, which marks the onset of the period of amnesia. The behavioral arrest is usually accompanied by *automatisms*, which are involuntary, automatic behaviors that have a wide range of manifestations. Automatisms may consist of very basic behaviors such as chewing, lip smacking, swallowing, or "picking" movements of the hands, or more elaborate behaviors such as a display of emotion or running. The patient is typically confused following the seizure, and the transition to full recovery of consciousness may range from seconds up to an hour. Examination immediately following the seizure may show an anterograde amnesia or, in cases involving the dominant hemisphere, a postictal aphasia.

The routine, interictal (i.e., between seizures) EEG in patients with complex partial seizures is often normal or may show brief discharges termed *epileptiform spikes*, or *sharp waves*. Since complex partial seizures can arise from the medial temporal lobe or inferior frontal lobe, i.e., regions distant from the scalp, the EEG recorded during the seizure may be nonlocalizing. However, the seizure focus is often detected using sphenoidal or surgically placed intracranial electrodes.

The range of potential clinical behaviors linked to complex partial seizures is so broad that extreme caution is advised before concluding that stereotypic episodes of bizarre or atypical behavior are not due to seizure activity. In such cases additional, detailed EEG studies may be helpful.

Partial Seizures with Secondary Generalization Partial seizures can spread to involve both cerebral hemispheres and produce a generalized seizure, usually of the tonic-clonic variety (discussed below). Secondary generalization is observed frequently following simple partial seizures, especially those with a focus in the frontal lobe, but may also be associated with partial seizures occurring elsewhere in the brain. A partial seizure with secondary generalization is often difficult to distinguish from a primarily generalized tonic-clonic seizure, since bystanders tend to emphasize the more dramatic, generalized convulsive phase of the seizure and overlook the more subtle, focal symptoms present at onset. In some cases, the focal onset of the seizure becomes apparent only when a careful history identifies a preceding aura (i.e., simple partial seizure). Often, however, the focal onset is not clinically evident and may be established only through careful EEG analysis. Nonetheless, distinguishing between these two entities is extremely important, as there may be substantial differences in the evaluation and treatment of partial versus generalized seizure disorders.

GENERALIZED SEIZURES By definition, generalized seizures arise from both cerebral hemispheres simultaneously. However, it is currently impossible to exclude entirely the existence of a focal region of abnormal activity that initiates the seizure prior to rapid secondary generalization. For this reason, generalized seizures may be practically defined as bilateral clinical and electrographic events without any detectable focal onset. Fortunately, several types of generalized seizures have distinctive features that facilitate clinical diagnosis.

Absence Seizures (Petit Mal) Absence seizures are characterized by sudden, brief lapses of consciousness without loss of postural control. The seizure typically lasts for only seconds, consciousness returns as sud-

denly as it was lost, and there is no postictal confusion. Although the brief loss of consciousness may be clinically inapparent or the sole manifestation of the seizure discharge, absence seizures are usually accompanied by subtle, bilateral motor signs such as rapid blinking of the eyelids, chewing movements, or small-amplitude, clonic movements of the hands.

Absence seizures usually begin in childhood (ages 4 to 8) or early adolescence and are the main seizure type in 15 to 20% of children with epilepsy. The seizures can occur hundreds of times per day, but the child may be unaware of or unable to convey their existence. The patient may be constantly piecing together experiences that have been interrupted by the seizures. Since the clinical signs of the seizures are subtle, especially to new parents, it is not surprising that the first clue to absence epilepsy is often unexplained "daydreaming" and a decline in school performance recognized by a teacher.

The electrophysiologic hallmark of typical absence seizures is a generalized, symmetric, 3-Hz spike-and-wave discharge that begins and ends suddenly, superimposed on a normal EEG background. Periods of spike-and-wave discharges lasting more than a few seconds usually correlate with clinical signs, but the EEG often shows many more brief bursts of abnormal cortical activity than were suspected clinically. Hyperventilation tends to provoke these electrographic discharges and even the seizures themselves and is routinely used when recording the EEG.

Typical absence seizures are often associated with generalized, tonic-clonic seizures, but patients usually have no other neurologic problems and respond well to treatment with specific anticonvulsants. Although estimates vary, ~60 to 70% of such patients will have a spontaneous remission during adolescence.

Atypical Absence Seizures Atypical absence seizures have features that deviate both clinically and electrophysiologically from typical absence seizures. For example, the lapse of consciousness is usually of longer duration and less abrupt in onset and cessation, and the seizure is accompanied by more obvious motor signs that may include focal or lateralizing features. The EEG shows a generalized, slow spike-and-wave pattern with a frequency of ≤2.5/s, as well as other abnormal activity. Atypical absence seizures are usually associated with diffuse or multifocal structural abnormalities of the brain and therefore may accompany other signs of neurologic dysfunction such as mental retardation. Furthermore, the seizures are less responsive to anticonvulsants compared to typical absence seizures.

Generalized, Tonic-Clonic Seizures (Grand Mal) Primarily generalized, tonic-clonic seizures are the main seizure type in ~10% of all persons with epilepsy. They are also the most common seizure type resulting from metabolic derangements and are therefore frequently encountered in many different clinical settings. The seizure usually begins abruptly without warning, although some patients describe vague premonitory symptoms in the hours leading up to the seizure. This prodrome is distinct from the stereotypic auras associated with focal seizures that secondarily generalize. The initial phase of the seizure is usually tonic contraction of muscles throughout the body, accounting for a number of the classic features of the event. Tonic contraction of the muscles of expiration and the larynx at the onset will produce a loud moan or "ictal cry." Respirations are impaired, secretions pool in the oropharynx, and cyanosis develops. Contraction of the jaw muscles may cause biting of the tongue. A marked enhancement of sympathetic tone leads to increases in heart rate, blood pressure, and pupillary size. After to 20 s, the tonic phase of the seizure typically evolves into the clonic phase, produced by the superimposition of periods of muscle relaxation on the tonic muscle contraction. The periods of relaxation progressively increase until the end of the ictal phase, which usually no more than 1 min. The postictal phase is characterized by unresponsiveness, muscular flaccidity, and excessive salivation that can cause stridorous breathing and partial airway obstruction. Bladder incontinence may occur at this point. Patients gradually regain consciousness over minutes to hours, and during this transition there is typically a period of postictal confusion. Patients

plain of headache, fatigue, and muscle ache that can last for many hours. The duration of impaired consciousness in the postictal phase can be extremely long, i.e., many hours, in patients with prolonged seizures or underlying CNS diseases such as alcoholic cerebral atrophy.

The EEG during the tonic phase of the seizure shows a progressive increase in generalized low-voltage fast activity, followed by generalized high-amplitude, polyspike discharges. In the clonic phase, the high-amplitude activity is typically interrupted by slow waves to create a spike-and-wave pattern. The postictal EEG shows diffuse slowing that gradually recovers as the patient awakens.

There are many variants of the generalized tonic-clonic seizure, including pure tonic and pure clonic seizures. Brief tonic seizures lasting only a few seconds are especially noteworthy since they are usually associated with specific epileptic syndromes having mixed seizure phenotypes, such as the Lennox-Gastaut syndrome (discussed below).

Atonic Seizures Atonic seizures are characterized by sudden loss of postural muscle tone lasting 1 to 2 s. Consciousness is briefly impaired, but there is usually no postictal confusion. A very brief seizure may cause only a quick head drop or nodding movement, while a longer seizure will cause the patient to collapse. This can be extremely dangerous, since there is a substantial risk of direct head injury with the fall. The EEG shows brief, generalized spike-and-wave discharges followed immediately by diffuse slow waves that correlate with the loss of muscle tone. Similar to pure tonic seizures, atonic seizures are usually seen in association with known epileptic syndromes.

Myoclonic Seizures Myoclonus is a sudden and brief muscle contraction that may involve one part of the body or the entire body. A normal, common physiologic form of myoclonus is the sudden jerking movement observed while falling asleep. Pathologic myoclonus is most commonly seen in association with metabolic disorders, degenerative CNS diseases, or anoxic brain injury (Chap. 21). Although the distinction from other forms of myoclonus is imprecise, myoclonic seizures are considered to be true epileptic events since they are caused by cortical (versus subcortical or spinal) dysfunction. The EEG may show bilaterally synchronous spike-and-wave discharges synchronized with the myoclonus, although these can be obscured by movement artifact. Myoclonic seizures usually coexist with other forms of generalized seizure disorders but are the predominant feature of juvenile myoclonic epilepsy (discussed below).

UNCLASSIFIED SEIZURES Not all seizure types can be classified as partial or generalized. This appears to be especially true of seizures that occur in neonates and infants. The distinctive phenotypes of seizures at these early ages likely result, in part, from differences in neuronal function and connectivity in the immature versus mature CNS.

EPILEPSY SYNDROMES

Epilepsy syndromes are disorders in which epilepsy is a predominant feature, and there is sufficient evidence (e.g., through clinical, EEG, radiologic, or genetic observations) to suggest a common underlying mechanism. Three important epilepsy syndromes are listed below; additional examples with a known genetic basis are shown in Table 348-2.

JUVENILE MYOCLONIC EPILEPSY Juvenile myoclonic epilepsy (JME) is a generalized seizure disorder of unknown cause that appears in early adolescence and is usually characterized by bilateral myoclonic jerks that may be single or repetitive. The myoclonic seizures are most frequent in the morning after awakening and can be provoked by sleep deprivation. Consciousness is preserved unless the myoclonus is especially severe. Many patients also experience generalized tonic-clonic seizures, and up to one-third have absence seizures. The condition is otherwise benign, and although complete remission is uncommon, the seizures respond well to appropriate anticonvulsant medication. There is often a family history of epilepsy, and genetic linkage studies suggest a polygenic cause.

LENNOX-GASTAUT SYNDROME Lennox-Gastaut syndrome occurs in children and is defined by the following triad: (1) multiple seizure types (usually including generalized tonic-clonic, atonic, and atypical absence seizures); (2) an EEG showing slow (<3 Hz) spike-and-wave discharges and a variety of other abnormalities; and (3) impaired cognitive function in most but not all cases. Lennox-Gastaut syndrome is associated with CNS disease or dysfunction from a variety of causes, including developmental abnormalities, perinatal hypoxia/ischemia, trauma, infection, and other acquired lesions. The multifactorial nature of this syndrome suggests that it is a nonspecific response of the brain to diffuse neural injury. Unfortunately, many patients have a poor prognosis due to the underlying CNS disease and the physical and psychosocial consequences of severe, poorly controlled epilepsy.

MESIAL TEMPORAL LOBE EPILEPSY SYNDROME Mesial temporal lobe epilepsy (MTLE) is the most common syndrome associated with complex partial seizures and is an example of a symptomatic, partial epilepsy with distinctive clinical, electroencephalographic, and pathologic features (Table 348-3). High-resolution magnetic resonance imaging (MRI) can detect the characteristic hippocampal sclerosis that appears to be essential in the pathophysiology of MTLE for many patients (Fig. 348-1). Recognition of this syndrome is especially important because it tends to be refractory to treatment with anticonvulsants but responds extremely well to surgical intervention. Advances in the understanding of basic mechanisms of epilepsy have come through studies of experimental models of MTLE, discussed below.

THE CAUSES OF SEIZURES AND EPILEPSY

Seizures are a result of a shift in the normal balance of excitation and inhibition within the CNS. Given the numerous properties that control neuronal excitability, it is not surprising that there are many different ways to perturb this normal balance, and therefore many different causes of both seizures and epilepsy. Three clinical observations emphasize how a variety of factors determine why certain conditions may cause seizures or epilepsy in a given patient.

1. *The normal brain is capable of having a seizure under the appropriate circumstances, and there are differences between individuals in the susceptibility or threshold for seizures.* For example, seizures may be induced by high fevers in children who are otherwise normal and who never develop other neurologic problems, including epilepsy. However, febrile seizures occur only in a relatively small proportion of children. This implies there are various underlying, *endogenous factors* that influence the threshold for having a seizure. Some of these factors are clearly genetic, as it has been shown that a family history of epilepsy will influence the likelihood of seizures occurring in otherwise normal individuals. Normal development also plays an important role, since the brain appears to have different seizure thresholds at different maturational stages.

2. *There are a variety of conditions that have an extremely high likelihood of resulting in a chronic seizure disorder.* One of the best examples of this is severe, penetrating head trauma, which is associated with up to a 50% risk of subsequent epilepsy. The high propensity for severe traumatic brain injury to lead to epilepsy suggests that the injury results in a long-lasting, pathologic change in the CNS that transforms a presumably normal neural network into one that is abnormally hyperexcitable. This process is known as *epileptogenesis*, and the specific changes that result in a lowered seizure threshold can be considered *epileptogenic factors*. Other processes associated with epileptogenesis include stroke, infections, and abnormalities of CNS development. Likewise, the genetic abnormalities associated with epilepsy likely involve processes that trigger the appearance of specific sets of epileptogenic factors.

3. *Seizures are episodic.* Patients with epilepsy have seizures intermittently and, depending on the underlying cause, many patients are completely normal for months or even years between seizures. This implies there are important provocative or *precipitating factors* that

TABLE 348-2 *Examples of Genes Associated with Epilepsy Syndromes*[a]

Gene (Locus)	Function of Gene	Clinical Syndrome	Comments
CHRNA4 (20q13.2) CHRNB2 (1q21.3)	Nicotinic acetylcholine receptor subunit; mutations cause alterations in Ca^{2+} flux through the receptor; this may reduce amount of GABA release in presynaptic terminals	Autosomal dominant nocturnal frontal lobe epilepsy (ADNFLE); childhood onset; brief, nighttime seizures with prominent motor movements; often misdiagnosed as primary sleep disorder	Rare; first identified in a large Australian family; other families found to have mutations in CHRNA2 or CHRNB2, and some families appear to have mutations at other loci
KCNQ2 (20q13.3) KCNQ3 (8q24)	Voltage-gated potassium channel subunits; mutation in pore regions may cause a 20–40% reduction of potassium currents, which will lead to impaired repolarization	Benign familial neonatal convulsions (BFNC); autosomal dominant inheritance; onset in 1st week of life in infants who are otherwise normal; remission usually within weeks to months; long-term epilepsy in 10–15%	Rare; sequence and functional homology to KCNQ1, mutations of which cause long QT syndrome and a cardiac-auditory syndrome
SCN1B (19q12.1)	β-subunit of a voltage-gated sodium channel; mutation disrupts disulfide bridge that is crucial for structure of extracellular domain; mutated β-subunit leads to slower sodium channel inactivation	Generalized epilepsy with febrile seizures plus (GEFS+); autosomal dominant inheritance; presents with febrile seizures at median 1 year, which may persist >6 years, then variable seizure types not associated with fever	Incidence uncertain; GEFS+ identified in other families with mutations in other sodium channel subunits (SCN1A and SCN2A) and $GABA_A$ receptor subunit (GABRG2); significant phenotypic heterogeneity within same family, including members with febrile seizures only
LGI1 (10q24)	Leucine-rich glioma-inactivated gene; previous evidence for role in glial tumor progression; likely to be involved in nervous system development	Autosomal dominant partial epilepsy with auditory features (ADPEAF), temporal lobe epilepsy with wide range of auditory and other sensory symptoms as major manifestation; age of onset usually between 10 and 25 years	Rare; at least one family with similar syndrome has mutation(s) elsewhere, LGI1 mutation is the only known mutation identified in temporal lobe epilepsy and the only non-ion-channel gene mutation known in idiopathic epilepsy
CSTB (21q22.3)	Cystatin B, a noncaspase cysteine protease inhibitor; normal protein may block neuronal apoptosis by inhibiting caspases directly or indirectly (via cathepsins), or controlling proteolysis	Progressive myoclonus epilepsy (PME) (Unverricht-Lundborg disease); autosomal recessive inheritance; age of onset between 6–15 years, myoclonic seizures, ataxia, and progressive cognitive decline; brain shows neuronal degeneration	Overall rare, but relatively common in Finland and Western Mediterranean (>1 in 20,000); precise role of cystatin B in human disease unknown, although mice with null mutations of cystatin B have similar syndrome
EPM2A (6q24)	Laforin, a protein tyrosine phosphatase (PTP); may influence glycogen metabolism, which is known to be regulated by phosphatases	Progressive myoclonus epilepsy (Lafora's disease); autosomal recessive inheritance; onset age 6–19 years, death within 10 years; brain degeneration associated with polyglucosan intracellular inclusion bodies in numerous organs	Most common PME in Southern Europe, Middle East, Northern Africa, and Indian subcontinent; genetic heterogeneity; unknown whether seizure phenotype due to degeneration or direct effects of abnormal laforin expression.
Doublecortin (Xq21-24)	Doublecortin, expressed primarily in frontal lobes; function unknown; potentially an intracellular signalling molecule	Classic lissencephaly associated with severe mental retardation and seizures in males; subcortical band heterotopia with more subtle findings in females (presumably due to random X-inactivation); X-linked dominant	Relatively rare but of uncertain incidence, recent increased ascertainment due to improved imaging techniques; relationship between migration defect and seizure phenotype unknown

[a] The first four syndromes listed in the table (ADNFLE, BFNC, GEFS+, and ADPEAF) are examples of idiopathic generalized epilepsies associated with identified gene mutations. The last three syndromes are examples of the numerous Mendelian disorders in which seizures are one part of the phenotype.

Note: GABA, γ-aminobutyric acid.

induce seizures in patients with epilepsy. Similarly, precipitating factors are responsible for causing the single seizure in someone without epilepsy. Precipitants include those due to intrinsic physiologic processes, such as psychological or physical stress, sleep deprivation, or hormonal changes associated with the menstrual cycle. They also include exogenous factors such as exposure to toxic substances and certain medications.

These observations emphasize the concept that the many causes of seizures and epilepsy result from a dynamic interplay between endogenous factors, epileptogenic factors, and precipitating factors. The potential role of each needs to be carefully considered when determining the appropriate management of a patient with seizures. For example, the identification of predisposing factors (e.g., family history of epilepsy) in a patient with febrile seizures may increase the necessity for closer follow-up and a more aggressive diagnostic evaluation. Finding an epileptogenic lesion may help in the estimation of seizure recurrence and duration of therapy. Finally, removal or modification of a precipitating factor may be an effective and safer method for preventing further seizures than the prophylactic use of anticonvulsant drugs.

CAUSES ACCORDING TO AGE In practice, it is useful to consider the etiologies of seizures based on the age of the patient, as age is one of the most important factors determining both the incidence and likely causes of seizures or epilepsy (Table 348-4). During the *neonatal period and early infancy*, potential causes include hypoxic-ischemic encephalopathy, trauma, CNS infection, congenital CNS abnormalities, and metabolic disorders. Babies born to mothers using neurotoxic drugs such as cocaine, heroin, or ethanol are susceptible to drug-withdrawal seizures in the first few days after delivery. Hypoglycemia and hypocalcemia, which can occur as secondary complications of peri-

TABLE 348-3   *Characteristics of the Mesial Temporal Lobe Epilepsy Syndrome*

History
- History of febrile seizures
- Family history of epilepsy
- Early onset
- Rare secondarily generalized seizures
- Seizures may remit and reappear
- Seizures often intractable

Clinical observations
- Aura common
- Behavioral arrest/stare
- Complex automatisms
- Unilateral posturing
- Postictal disorientation, memory loss, dysphasia (with focus in dominant hemisphere)

Laboratory studies
- Unilateral or bilateral anterior temporal spikes on EEG
- Hypometabolism on interictal PET
- Hypoperfusion on interictal SPECT
- Material-specific memory deficits on intracranial amobarbital (Wada) test
- MRI findings
  - Small hippocampus with increased signal on T2-weighted sequences
  - Small temporal lobe
  - Enlarged temporal horn
- Pathologic findings
  - Highly selective loss of specific cell populations within hippocampus in most cases

Note: EEG, electroencephalogram; PET, positron emission tomography; SPECT, single photon emission computed tomography.

FIGURE 348-1   Mesial temporal lobe epilepsy. The EEG suggested a right temporal lobe focus. Coronal high-resolution T2-weighted fast spin echo magnetic resonance image obtained through the body of the hippocampus demonstrates abnormal high signal intensity in the right hippocampus (white arrows; compare with the normal hippocampus on the left, black arrows) consistent with mesial temporal sclerosis.

natal injury, are also causes of seizures early after delivery. Seizures due to inborn errors of metabolism usually present once regular feeding begins, typically 2 to 3 days after birth. Pyridoxine (vitamin B$_6$) deficiency, an important cause of neonatal seizures, can be effectively treated with pyridoxine replacement. The idiopathic or inherited forms of benign neonatal convulsions are also seen during this time period.

The most common seizures arising in *late infancy and early childhood* are febrile seizures, which are seizures associated with fevers but without evidence of CNS infection or other defined causes. The overall prevalence is 3 to 5% and even higher in some parts of the world, such as Asia. Patients often have a family history of febrile seizures or epilepsy. Febrile seizures usually occur between 3 months and 5 years of age and have a peak incidence between 18 and 24 months. The typical scenario is a child who has a generalized, tonic-clonic seizure during a febrile illness in the setting of a common childhood infection such as otitis media, respiratory infection, or gastroenteritis. The seizure is likely to occur during the rising phase of the temperature curve (i.e., during the first day) rather than well into the course of the illness. A *simple* febrile seizure is a single, isolated event, brief, and symmetric in appearance. *Complex* febrile seizures are characterized by repeated seizure activity, duration >15 min, or have focal features. Approximately one-third of patients with febrile seizures will have a recurrence, but <10% have three or more episodes. Recurrences are much more likely when the febrile seizure occurs in the first year of life. Simple febrile seizures are not associated with an increase in the risk of developing epilepsy, while complex febrile seizures have a risk of 2 to 5%; other risk factors include the presence of preexisting neurologic deficits and a family history of nonfebrile seizures.

Childhood marks the age at which many of the well-defined epilepsy syndromes present. Some children who are otherwise normal develop idiopathic, generalized tonic-clonic seizures without other features that fit into specific syndromes. Temporal lobe epilepsy usually presents in childhood and may be related to mesial temporal lobe sclerosis (as part of the MTLE syndrome) or other focal abnormalities such as cortical dysgenesis. Other types of partial seizures, including those with secondary generalization, may be the relatively late manifestation of a developmental disorder, an acquired lesion such as head trauma, CNS infection (especially viral encephalitis), or very rarely a CNS tumor.

The period of *adolescence and early adulthood* is one of transition during which the idiopathic or genetically based epilepsy syndromes, including JME and juvenile absence epilepsy, become less common, while epilepsies secondary to acquired CNS lesions begin to predominate. Seizures that begin in patients in this age range may be associated with head trauma, CNS infections (including parasitic infections such as cysticercosis), brain tumors, congenital CNS abnormalities, illicit drug use, or alcohol withdrawal.

TABLE 348-4   *Causes of Seizures*

Neonates (<1 month)	Perinatal hypoxia and ischemia
	Intracranial hemorrhage and trauma
	Acute CNS infection
	Metabolic disturbances (hypoglycemia, hypocalcemia, hypomagnesemia, pyridoxine deficiency)
	Drug withdrawal
	Developmental disorders
	Genetic disorders
Infants and children (>1 mo and <12 years)	Febrile seizures
	Genetic disorders (metabolic, degenerative, primary epilepsy syndromes)
	CNS infection
	Developmental disorders
	Trauma
	Idiopathic
Adolescents (12–18 years)	Trauma
	Genetic disorders
	Infection
	Brain tumor
	Illicit drug use
	Idiopathic
Young adults (18–35 years)	Trauma
	Alcohol withdrawal
	Illicit drug use
	Brain tumor
	Idiopathic
Older adults (>35 years)	Cerebrovascular disease
	Brain tumor
	Alcohol withdrawal
	Metabolic disorders (uremia, hepatic failure, electrolyte abnormalities, hypoglycemia)
	Alzheimer's disease and other degenerative CNS diseases
	Idiopathic

Note: CNS, central nervous system.

Head trauma is a common cause of epilepsy in adolescents and adults. The head injury can be caused by a variety of mechanisms, and the likelihood of developing epilepsy is strongly correlated with the severity of the injury. A patient with a penetrating head wound, depressed skull fracture, intracranial hemorrhage, or prolonged posttraumatic coma or amnesia has a 40 to 50% risk of developing epilepsy, while a patient with a closed head injury and cerebral contusion has a 5 to 25% risk. Recurrent seizures usually develop within 1 year after head trauma, although intervals of ≥10 years are well known. In controlled studies, mild head injury, defined as a concussion with amnesia or loss of consciousness of <30 min, was found to be associated with only a slightly increased likelihood of epilepsy. Nonetheless, most epileptologists know of patients who have partial seizures within hours or days of a mild head injury and subsequently develop chronic seizures of the same type; such cases may represent rare examples of chronic epilepsy resulting from mild head injury.

The causes of seizures in *older adults* include cerebrovascular disease, trauma (including subdural hematoma), CNS tumors, and degenerative diseases. Cerebrovascular disease may account for ~50% of new cases of epilepsy in patients older than 65. Acute seizures (i.e., occurring at the time of the stroke) are seen more often with embolic rather than hemorrhagic or thrombotic stroke. Chronic seizures typically appear months to years after the initial event and are associated with all forms of stroke.

Metabolic disturbances such as electrolyte imbalance, hypo- or hyperglycemia, renal failure, and hepatic failure may cause seizures at any age. Similarly, endocrine disorders, hematologic disorders, vasculitides, and many other systemic diseases may cause seizures over a broad age range. A wide variety of medications and abused substances are known to precipitate seizures as well (Table 348-5).

BASIC MECHANISMS

MECHANISMS OF SEIZURE INITIATION AND PROPAGATION

Partial seizure activity can begin in a very discrete region of cortex and then spread to neighboring regions, i.e., there is a *seizure initiation* phase and a *seizure propagation* phase. The initiation phase is characterized by two concurrent events in an aggregate of neurons: (1) high-frequency bursts of action potentials, and (2) hypersynchronization. The bursting activity is caused by a relatively long-lasting depolarization of the neuronal membrane due to influx of extracellular calcium (Ca^{2+}), which leads to the opening of voltage-dependent sodium (Na^+) channels, influx of Na^+, and generation of repetitive action potentials. This is followed by a hyperpolarizing afterpotential mediated by γ-aminobutyric acid (GABA) receptors or potassium (K^+) channels, depending on the cell type. The synchronized bursts from a sufficient number of neurons result in a so-called spike discharge on the EEG.

Normally, the spread of bursting activity is prevented by intact hyperpolarization and a region of surrounding inhibition created by inhibitory neurons. With sufficient activation there is a recruitment of surrounding neurons via a number of mechanisms. Repetitive discharges lead to the following: (1) an increase in extracellular K^+, which blunts hyperpolarization and depolarizes neighboring neurons; (2) accumulation of Ca^{2+} in presynaptic terminals, leading to enhanced neurotransmitter release; and (3) depolarization-induced activation of the N-methyl-D-aspartate (NMDA) subtype of the excitatory amino acid receptor, which causes Ca^{2+} influx and neuronal activation. The recruitment of a sufficient number of neurons leads to a loss of the surrounding inhibition and propagation of seizure activity into contiguous areas via local cortical connections, and to more distant areas via long commissural pathways such as the corpus callosum.

Many factors control neuronal excitability, and thus there are many potential mechanisms for altering a neuron's propensity to have bursting activity. Mechanisms *intrinsic* to the neuron include changes in the conductance of ion channels, response characteristics of membrane receptors, cytoplasmic buffering, second-messenger systems, and protein expression as determined by gene transcription, translation, and posttranslational modification. Mechanisms *extrinsic* to the neuron include changes in the amount or type of neurotransmitters present at the synapse, modulation of receptors by extracellular ions and other molecules, and temporal and spatial properties of synaptic and nonsynaptic input. Nonneural cells, such as astrocytes and oligodendrocytes, have an important role in many of these mechanisms as well.

Certain recognized causes of seizures are explained by these mechanisms. For example, accidental ingestion of domoic acid, which is an analogue of glutamate (the principal excitatory neurotransmitter in the brain), causes profound seizures via direct activation of excitatory amino acid receptors throughout the CNS. Penicillin, which can lower the seizure threshold in humans and is a potent convulsant in experimental models, reduces inhibition by antagonizing the effects of GABA at its receptor. The basic mechanisms of other precipitating factors of seizures, such as sleep deprivation, fever, alcohol withdrawal, hypoxia, and infection, are not as well understood but presumably involve analogous perturbations in neuronal excitability. Similarly, the endogenous factors that determine an individual's seizure threshold may relate to these properties as well.

Knowledge of the mechanisms responsible for initiation and propagation of most generalized seizures (including tonic-clonic, myoclonic, and atonic types) remains rudimentary and reflects the limited understanding of the connectivity of the brain at a systems level. Much more is understood about the origin of generalized spike-and-wave discharges in absence seizures. These appear to be related to oscillatory rhythms normally generated during sleep by circuits connecting the thalamus and cortex. This oscillatory behavior involves an interaction between $GABA_B$ receptors, T-type Ca^{2+} channels, and K^+ channels located within the thalamus. Pharmacologic studies indicate that modulation of these receptors and channels can induce absence seizures, and there is speculation that the genetic forms of absence epilepsy may be associated with mutations of components of this system.

MECHANISMS OF EPILEPTOGENESIS

Epileptogenesis refers to the transformation of a normal neuronal network into one that is chronically hyperexcitable. There is often a delay of months to years between an initial CNS injury such as trauma, stroke, or infection and the first seizure. The injury appears to initiate a process that gradually lowers the seizure threshold in the affected region until a spontaneous seizure occurs. In many genetic and idiopathic forms of epilepsy, epileptogenesis is presumably determined by developmentally regulated events.

Pathologic studies of the hippocampus from patients with temporal lobe epilepsy have led to the suggestion that some forms of epileptogenesis are related to *structural changes in neuronal networks*. For example, many patients with MTLE have a highly selective loss of neurons that may contribute to inhibition of the main excitatory neurons within the dentate gyrus. There is also evidence that, in response to the loss of neurons, there is reorganization or "sprouting" of sur-

TABLE 348-5 *Drugs and Other Substances That Can Cause Seizures*	
Antimicrobials/antivirals	Psychotropics
β-lactam and related compounds	Antidepressants
Quinolones	Antipsychotics
Acyclovir	Lithium
Isoniazid	Radiographic contrast agents
Ganciclovir	Theophylline
Anesthetics and analgesics	Sedative-hypnotic drug
Meperidine	withdrawal
Tramadol	Alcohol
Local anesthetics	Barbiturates
Immunomodulatory drugs	Benzodiazepines
Cyclosporine	Drugs of abuse
OKT3 (monoclonal antibodies to	Amphetamine
T cells)	Cocaine
Tacrolimus (FK-506)	Phencyclidine
Interferons	Methylphenidate
	Flumazenil[a]

[a] In benzodiazepine-dependent patients.

viving neurons in a way that affects the excitability of the network. Some of these changes can be seen in experimental models of prolonged electrical seizures or traumatic brain injury. Thus, an initial injury such as head injury may lead to a very focal, confined region of structural change that causes local hyperexcitability. The local hyperexcitability leads to further structural changes that evolve over time until the focal lesion produces clinically evident seizures. Similar models have also provided strong evidence for long-term alterations in *intrinsic, biochemical properties of cells* within the network, such as chronic changes in glutamate receptor function.

GENETIC CAUSES OF EPILEPSY The most important recent progress in epilepsy research has been the identification of genetic mutations associated with a variety of epilepsy syndromes (Table 348-2). Although all of the mutations identified to date cause rare forms of epilepsy, their discovery has led to extremely important conceptual advances. For example, it appears that many of the inherited, idiopathic epilepsies (i.e., the relatively "pure" forms of epilepsy in which seizures are the phenotypic abnormality and brain structure and function are otherwise normal) are due to mutations affecting ion channel function. These syndromes are therefore part of the larger group of channelopathies causing paroxysmal disorders such as cardiac arrhythmias, episodic ataxia, periodic weakness, and familial hemiplegic migraine. In contrast, gene mutations observed in symptomatic epilepsies (i.e., disorders in which other neurologic abnormalities, such as cognitive impairment, coexist with seizures) are proving to be associated with pathways influencing CNS development or neuronal homeostasis. A current challenge is to identify the multiple susceptibility genes that underlie the more common forms of idiopathic epilepsies.

MECHANISMS OF ACTION OF ANTIEPILEPTIC DRUGS Antiepileptic drugs appear to act primarily by blocking the initiation or spread of seizures. This occurs through a variety of mechanisms that modify the activity of ion channels or neurotransmitters, and in most cases the drugs have pleiotropic effects. The mechanisms include inhibition of Na^+-dependent action potentials in a frequency-dependent manner (e.g., phenytoin, carbamazepine, lamotrigine, topiramate, zonisamide), inhibition of voltage-gated Ca^{2+} channels (phenytoin), decrease of glutamate release (lamotrigine), potentiation of GABA receptor function (benzodiazepines and barbiturates), and increase in the availability of GABA (valproic acid, gabapentin, tiagabine). The two most effective drugs for absence seizures, ethosuximide and valproic acid, probably act by inhibiting T-type Ca^{2+} channels in thalamic neurons.

In contrast to the relatively large number of antiepileptic drugs that can attenuate seizure activity, there are currently no drugs known to prevent the formation of a seizure focus following CNS injury. The eventual development of such "antiepileptogenic" drugs will provide an important means of preventing the emergence of epilepsy following injuries such as head trauma, stroke, and CNS infection.

EVALUATION OF THE PATIENT WITH A SEIZURE

When a patient presents shortly after a seizure, the first priorities are attention to vital signs, respiratory and cardiovascular support, and treatment of seizures if they resume (see "Treatment"). Life-threatening conditions such as CNS infection, metabolic derangement, or drug toxicity must be recognized and managed appropriately.

When the patient is not acutely ill, the evaluation will initially focus on whether there is a history of earlier seizures (Fig. 348-2). If this is the first seizure, then the emphasis will be to (1) establish whether the reported episode was a seizure rather than another paroxysmal event, (2) determine the cause of the seizure by identifying risk factors and precipitating events, and (3) decide whether anticonvulsant therapy is required in addition to treatment for any underlying illness.

In the patient with prior seizures or a known history of epilepsy, the evaluation is directed toward (1) identification of the underlying cause and precipitating factors, and (2) determination of the adequacy of the patient's current therapy.

HISTORY AND EXAMINATION The first goal is to determine whether the event was truly a seizure. An in-depth history is essential, for in many cases the diagnosis of a seizure is based solely on clinical grounds—the examination and laboratory studies are often normal. Questions should be focused on the symptoms before, during, and after the episode in order to discriminate a seizure from other paroxysmal events (see "Differential Diagnosis of Seizures"). Seizures frequently occur out-of-hospital, and the patient may be unaware of the ictal and immediate postictal phases; thus witnesses to the event should be interviewed carefully.

The history should also focus on risk factors and predisposing events. Clues for a predisposition to seizures include a history of febrile seizures, earlier auras or brief seizures not recognized as such, and a family history of seizures. Epileptogenic factors such as prior head trauma, stroke, tumor, or vascular malformation should be identified. In children, a careful assessment of developmental milestones may provide evidence for underlying CNS disease. Precipitating factors such as sleep deprivation, systemic diseases, electrolyte or metabolic derangements, acute infection, drugs that lower the seizure threshold (Table 348-5), or alcohol or illicit drug use should also be identified.

The general physical examination includes a search for signs of infection or systemic illness. Careful examination of the skin may reveal signs of neurocutaneous disorders, such as tuberous sclerosis or neurofibromatosis, or chronic liver or renal disease. A finding of organomegaly may indicate a metabolic storage disease, and limb asymmetry may provide a clue to brain injury early in development. Signs of head trauma and use of alcohol or illicit drugs should be sought. Auscultation of the heart and carotid arteries may identify an abnormality that predisposes to cerebrovascular disease.

All patients require a complete neurologic examination, with particular emphasis on eliciting signs of cerebral hemispheric disease (Chap. 346). Careful assessment of mental status (including memory, language function, and abstract thinking) may suggest lesions in the anterior frontal, parietal, or temporal lobes. Testing of visual fields will help screen for lesions in the optic pathways and occipital lobes. Screening tests of motor function such as pronator drift, deep tendon reflexes, gait, and coordination may suggest lesions in motor (frontal) cortex, and cortical sensory testing (e.g., double simultaneous stimulation) may detect lesions in the parietal cortex.

LABORATORY STUDIES Routine blood studies are indicated to identify the more common metabolic causes of seizures, such as abnormalities in electrolytes, glucose, calcium, or magnesium, and hepatic or renal disease. A screen for toxins in blood and urine should also be obtained from all patients in appropriate risk groups, especially when no clear precipitating factor has been identified. A lumbar puncture is indicated if there is any suspicion of meningitis or encephalitis and is mandatory in all patients infected with HIV, even in the absence of symptoms or signs suggesting infection.

Electroencephalography All patients who have a possible seizure disorder should be evaluated with an EEG as soon as possible. The EEG measures electrical activity of the brain by recording from electrodes placed on the scalp. The potential difference between pairs of electrodes is amplified and displayed on a computer monitor, oscilloscope, or paper. The characteristics of the normal EEG depend on the patient's age and level of arousal. The recorded activity represents the postsynaptic potentials of vertically oriented pyramidal cells in the cerebral cortex and is characterized by its frequency. In normal awake adults lying quietly with the eyes closed, an 8- to 13-Hz alpha rhythm is seen posteriorly in the EEG, intermixed with a variable amount of generalized faster beta activity (>13 Hz), and it is attenuated when the eyes are opened (Fig. 348-3). During drowsiness, the alpha rhythm is also attenuated; with light sleep, slower activity in the theta (4 to 7 Hz) and delta (<4 Hz) ranges becomes more apparent.

The EEG is best recorded from several different electrode arrangements (montages) in turn, and activating procedures are usually performed in an attempt to provoke abnormalities. Such procedures com-

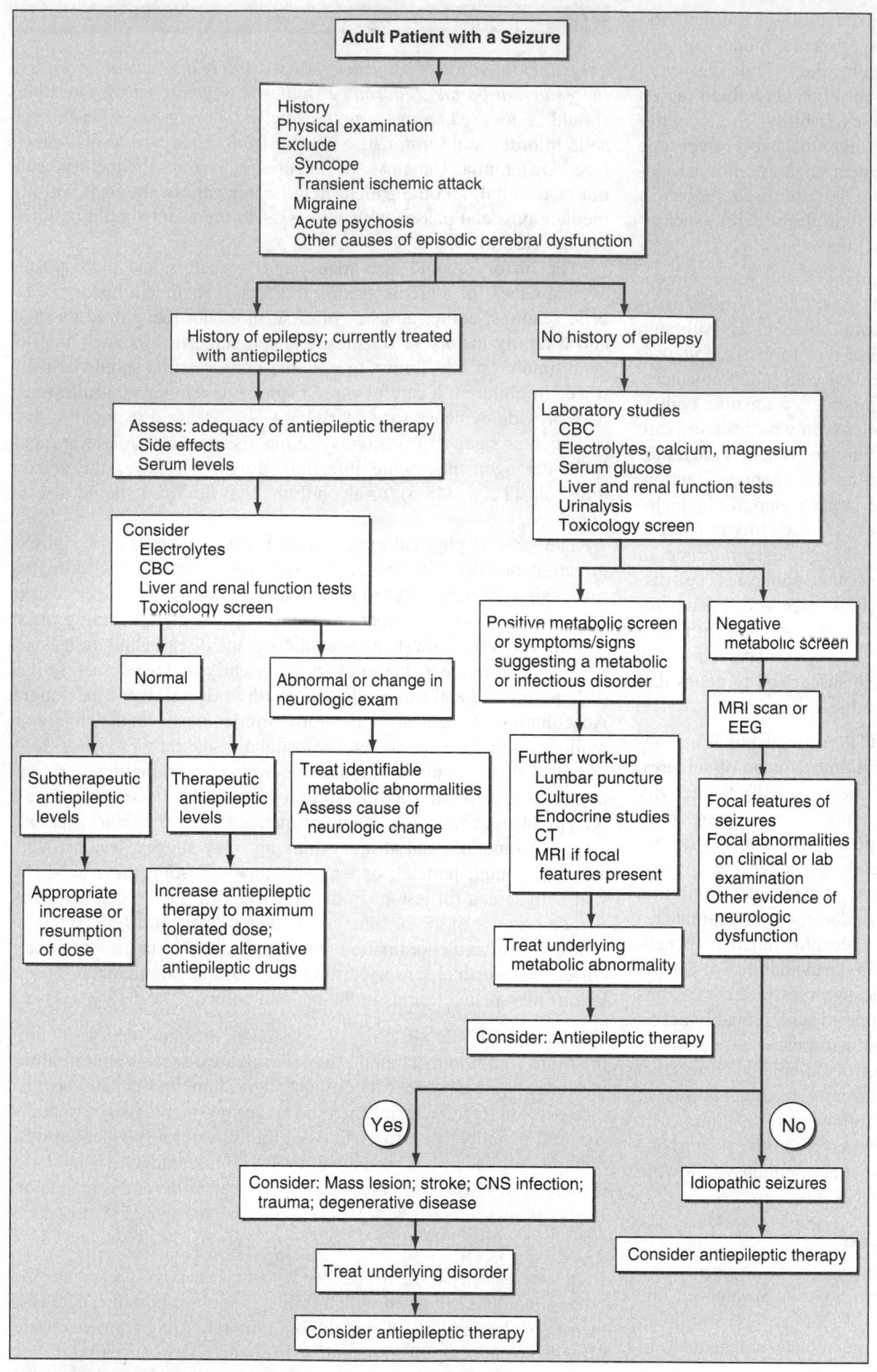

FIGURE 348-2 Evaluation of the adult patient with a seizure. CBC, complete blood count; CT, computed tomography; MRI, magnetic resonance imaging; EEG, electroencephalogram; CNS, central nervous system.

monly include hyperventilation (for 3 or 4 min), photic stimulation, sleep, and sleep deprivation on the night prior to the recording.

In the evaluation of a patient with suspected epilepsy, the presence of *electrographic seizure activity* during the clinically evident event, i.e., of abnormal, repetitive, rhythmic activity having an abrupt onset and termination, clearly establishes the diagnosis. The absence of electrographic seizure activity does not exclude a seizure disorder, however, because simple or complex seizures may originate from a region of cortex that is not within range of the scalp electrodes. The EEG is always abnormal during generalized tonic-clonic seizures. Since sei-

zures are typically infrequent and unpredictable, it is often not possible to obtain the EEG during a clinical event. Continuous monitoring for prolonged periods in video-EEG telemetry units for hospitalized patients or the use of portable equipment to record the EEG continuously on cassettes for ≥24 h in ambulatory patients has made it easier to capture the electrophysiologic accompaniments of clinical events.

The EEG may also be helpful in the interictal period by showing certain abnormalities that are highly supportive of the diagnosis of epilepsy. Such *epileptiform activity* consists of bursts of abnormal discharges containing spikes or sharp waves. The presence of epileptiform activity is not specific for epilepsy, but it has a much greater prevalence in patients with epilepsy than in normal individuals. However, even in an individual who is known to have epilepsy, the initial routine interictal EEG may be normal up to 60% of the time. Thus, the EEG cannot establish the diagnosis of epilepsy in many cases.

The EEG is also used for classifying seizure disorders and aiding in the selection of anticonvulsant medications. For example, episodic generalized spike-wave activity is usually seen in patients with typical absence epilepsy and may be seen with other generalized epilepsy syndromes. Focal interictal epileptiform discharges would support the diagnosis of a partial seizure disorder such as temporal lobe epilepsy or frontal lobe seizures, depending on the location of the discharges.

The routine scalp-recorded EEG may also be used to assess the prognosis of seizure disorders; in general, a normal EEG implies a better prognosis, whereas an abnormal background or profuse epileptiform activity suggests a poor outlook. Unfortunately, the EEG has not proved to be useful in predicting which patients with predisposing conditions, such as head injury or brain tumor, will go on to develop epilepsy, because in such circumstances epileptiform activity is commonly encountered regardless of whether seizures occur.

Brain Imaging Almost all patients with new-onset seizures should have a brain imaging study to determine whether there is an underlying structural abnormality that is responsible. The only potential exception to this rule is children who have an unambiguous history and examination suggestive of a benign, generalized seizure disorder such as absence epilepsy. MRI has been shown to be superior to computed tomography (CT) for the detection of cerebral lesions associated with epilepsy. In some cases MRI will identify lesions such as tumors, vascular malformations, or other pathologies that need immediate therapy. The use of newer MRI methods, such as fluid-attenuated inversion recovery (FLAIR), has increased the sensitivity for detection of abnormalities of cortical architecture, including hippocampal atrophy associated with mesial temporal sclerosis, and abnormalities of cortical neuronal migration. In such cases the findings may not lead to immediate therapy, but they do provide an explanation for the patient's seizures and point to the need for chronic anticonvulsant therapy or possible surgical resection.

In the patient with a suspected CNS infection or mass lesion, CT scanning should be performed emergently when MRI is not immediately available. Otherwise, it is usually appropriate to obtain an MRI study within a few days of the initial evaluation. Functional imaging procedures such as positron emission tomography (PET) and single photon emission computed tomography (SPECT) are also used to evaluate certain patients with medically refractory seizures (discussed below).

DIFFERENTIAL DIAGNOSIS OF SEIZURES

Disorders that may mimic seizures are listed in Table 348-6. In most cases seizures can be distinguished from other conditions by meticulous attention to the history and relevant laboratory studies. On occasion, additional studies, such as video-EEG monitoring, sleep studies, tilt table analysis, or cardiac electrophysiology, may be required to reach a correct diagnosis. Two of the more common nonepileptic syndromes in the differential diagnosis are detailed below.

Syncope (See also Chap. 20) The diagnostic dilemma encountered most frequently is the distinction between a generalized seizure and syncope. Observations by the patient and bystanders that can help discriminate between the two are listed in Table 348-7. Characteristics of a seizure include the presence of an aura, cyanosis, unconsciousness, motor manifestations lasting >30 s, postictal disorientation, muscle soreness, and sleepiness. In contrast, a syncopal episode is more likely if the event was provoked by acute pain or anxiety or occurred immediately after arising from the lying or sitting position. Patients with syncope often describe a stereotyped transition from consciousness to unconsciousness that includes tiredness, sweating, nausea, and tunneling of vision, and they experience a relatively brief loss of consciousness. Headache or incontinence usually suggests a seizure but may on occasion also occur with syncope. A brief period (i.e., 1 to 10 s) of convulsive motor activity is frequently seen immediately at the onset of a syncopal episode, especially if the patient remains in an upright posture after fainting (e.g., in a dentist's chair) and therefore has a sustained decrease in cerebral perfusion. Rarely, a syncopal episode can induce a full tonic-clonic seizure. In such cases the evaluation must focus on both the cause of the syncopal event as well as the possibility that the patient has a propensity for recurrent seizures.

Psychogenic Seizures Psychogenic seizures are nonepileptic behaviors that resemble seizures. They are often part of a conversion reaction precipitated by underlying psychological distress. Certain behaviors, such as side-to-side turning of the head, asymmetric and large-amplitude shaking movements of the limbs, twitching of all four extremities without loss of consciousness, and pelvic thrusting are more commonly associated with psychogenic rather than epileptic seizures. Psychogenic seizures often last longer than epileptic seizures and may wax and wane over minutes to hours. However, the distinction is sometimes difficult on clinical grounds alone, and there are many examples

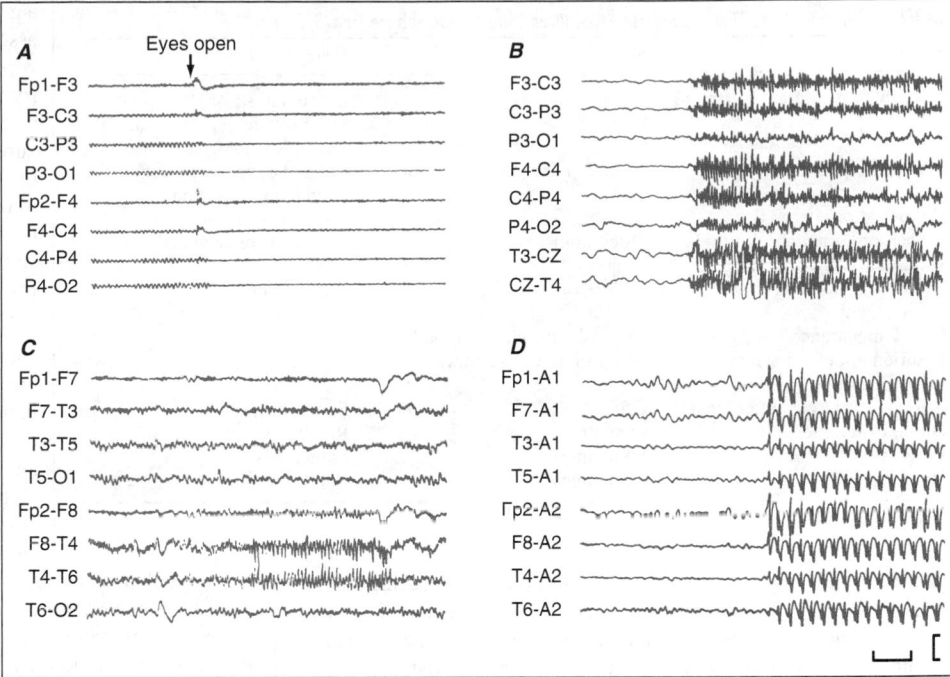

FIGURE 348-3 *A.* A normal EEG showing a posteriorly situated 9-Hz alpha rhythm that attenuates with eye opening. *B.* Onset of a tonic seizure showing generalized repetitive sharp activity with synchronous onset over both hemispheres. *C.* Burst of repetitive spikes in the right temporal region during a clinical spell suggestive of a complex partial seizure. *D.* Generalized 3-Hz spike-wave activity occurring synchronously over both hemispheres during an absence seizure. Horizontal calibration: 1s; vertical calibration: 200 μV in *A* and *C*, 400 μV in *B*, and 750 μV in *D*. Electrode placements are indicated at the left of each panel in accord with the international 10:20 system. A, earlobe; C, central; F, frontal; Fp, frontal polar; P, parietal; T, temporal; O, occipital. Right-sided placements are indicated by even numbers, left-sided placements by odd numbers, and midline placements by Z. [*From MJ Aminoff (ed): Electrodiagnosis in Clinical Neurology, 4th ed. New York, Churchill Livingstone, 1999.*]

of diagnostic errors made by experienced epileptologists. This is especially true for psychogenic seizures that resemble complex partial seizures, since the behavioral manifestations of complex partial seizures (especially of frontal lobe origin) can be extremely unusual, and in both cases the routine surface EEG may be normal. Video-EEG monitoring is often useful when historic features are nondiagnostic. Generalized tonic-clonic seizures always produce marked EEG abnormalities during and after the seizure. For suspected complex partial seizures of temporal lobe origin, the use of additional electrodes beyond the standard scalp locations (e.g., sphenoidal electrodes) may be required to localize a seizure focus. Measurement of serum prolactin levels may also help to discriminate between organic and psychogenic seizures, since most generalized seizures and many complex partial

TABLE 348-6 *Differential Diagnosis of Seizures*

Syncope	Transient ischemic attack (TIA)
Vasovagal syncope	Basilar artery TIA
Cardiac arrhythmia	Sleep disorders
Valvular heart disease	Narcolepsy/cataplexy
Cardiac failure	Benign sleep myoclonus
Orthostatic hypotension	Movement disorders
Psychological disorders	Tics
Psychogenic seizure	Nonepileptic myoclonus
Hyperventilation	Paroxysmal choreoathetosis
Panic attack	Special considerations in children
Metabolic disturbances	Breath-holding spells
Alcoholic blackouts	Migraine with recurrent
Delirium tremens	abdominal pain and cyclic
Hypoglycemia	vomiting
Hypoxia	Benign paroxysmal vertigo
Psychoactive drugs (e.g.,	Apnea
hallucinogens)	Night terrors
Migraine	Sleepwalking
Confusional migraine	
Basilar migraine	

Features	Seizure	Syncope
Immediate precipitating factors	Usually none	Emotional stress, Valsalva, orthostatic hypotension, cardiac etiologies
Premonitory symptoms	None or aura (e.g., odd odor)	Tiredness, nausea, diaphoresis, tunneling of vision
Posture at onset	Variable	Usually erect
Transition to unconsciousness	Often immediate	Gradual over seconds[a]
Duration of unconsciousness	Minutes	Seconds
Duration of tonic or clonic movements	30–60 s	Never more than 15 s
Facial appearance during event	Cyanosis, frothing at mouth	Pallor
Disorientation and sleepiness after event	Many minutes to hours	<5 min
Aching of muscles after event	Often	Sometimes
Biting of tongue	Sometimes	Rarely
Incontinence	Sometimes	Sometimes
Headache	Sometimes	Rarely

[a] May be sudden with certain cardiac arrhythmias.

seizures are accompanied by rises in serum prolactin (during the immediate 30-min postictal period), whereas psychogenic seizures are not. The diagnosis of psychogenic seizures does not exclude a concurrent diagnosis of epilepsy, since the two often coexist

℞ TREATMENT

Therapy for a patient with a seizure disorder is almost always multimodal and includes treatment of underlying conditions that cause or contribute to the seizures, avoidance of precipitating factors, suppression of recurrent seizures by prophylactic therapy with antiepileptic medications or surgery, and addressing a variety of psychological and social issues. Treatment plans must be individualized, given the many different types and causes of seizures as well as the differences in efficacy and toxicity of antiepileptic medications for each patient. In almost all cases a neurologist with experience in the treatment of epilepsy should design and oversee implementation of the treatment strategy. Furthermore, patients with refractory epilepsy or those who require polypharmacy with antiepileptic drugs should remain under the regular care of a neurologist.

Treatment of Underlying Conditions If the sole cause of a seizure is a metabolic disturbance such as an abnormality of serum electrolytes or glucose, then treatment is aimed at reversing the metabolic problem and preventing its recurrence. Therapy with antiepileptic drugs is usually unnecessary unless the metabolic disorder cannot be corrected promptly and the patient is at risk of having further seizures. If the apparent cause of a seizure was a medication (e.g., theophylline) or illicit drug use (e.g., cocaine), then appropriate therapy is avoidance of the drug; there is usually no need for antiepileptic medications unless subsequent seizures occur in the absence of these precipitants.

Seizures caused by a structural CNS lesion such as a brain tumor, vascular malformation, or brain abscess may not recur after appropriate treatment of the underlying lesion. However, despite removal of the structural lesion, there is a risk that the seizure focus will remain in the surrounding tissue or develop de novo as a result of gliosis and other processes induced by surgery, radiation, or other therapies. Most patients are therefore maintained on an antiepileptic medication for at least 1 year, and an attempt is made to withdraw medications only if the patient has been completely seizure-free. If seizures are refractory to medication, the patient may benefit from surgical removal of the epileptic brain region (see below).

Avoidance of Precipitating Factors Unfortunately, little is known about the specific factors that determine precisely when a seizure will occur in a patient with epilepsy. Some patients can identify particular situations that appear to lower their seizure threshold; these situations should be avoided. For example, a patient who has seizures in the setting of sleep deprivation should obviously be advised to maintain a normal sleep schedule. Many patients note an association between alcohol intake and seizures, and they should be encouraged to modify their drinking habits accordingly. There are also relatively rare cases of patients with seizures that are induced by highly specific stimuli such as a video game monitor, music, or an individual's voice ("reflex epilepsy"). If there is an association between stress and seizures, stress reduction techniques such as physical exercise, meditation, or counseling may be helpful.

Antiepileptic Drug Therapy Antiepileptic drug therapy is the mainstay of treatment for most patients with epilepsy. The overall goal is to completely prevent seizures without causing any untoward side effects, preferably with a single medication and a dosing schedule that is easy for the patient to follow. Seizure classification is an important element in designing the treatment plan, since some antiepileptic drugs have different activities against various seizure types. However, there is considerable overlap between many antiepileptic drugs, such that the choice of therapy is often determined more by specific needs of the patient, especially the patient's assessment of side effects.

WHEN TO INITIATE ANTIEPILEPTIC DRUG THERAPY Antiepileptic drug therapy should be started in any patient with recurrent seizures of unknown etiology or a known cause that cannot be reversed. Whether to initiate therapy in a patient with a single seizure is controversial. Patients with a single seizure due to an identified lesion such as a CNS tumor, infection, or trauma, in which there is strong evidence that the lesion is epileptogenic, should be treated. The risk of seizure recurrence in a patient with an apparently unprovoked or idiopathic seizure is uncertain, with estimates ranging from 31 to 71% in the first 12 months after the initial seizure. This uncertainty arises from differences in the underlying seizure types and etiologies in various published epidemiologic studies. Generally accepted risk factors associated with recurrent seizures include the following: (1) an abnormal neurologic examination, (2) seizures presenting as status epilepticus, (3) postictal Todd's paralysis, (4) a strong family history of seizures, or (5) an abnormal EEG. Most patients with one or more of these risk factors should be treated. Issues such as employment or driving may influence the decision whether or not to start medications as well. For example, a patient with a single, idiopathic seizure whose job depends on driving may prefer taking antiepileptic drugs rather than risk a seizure recurrence and the potential loss of driving privileges.

SELECTION OF ANTIEPILEPTIC DRUGS Antiepileptic drugs available in the United States are shown in Table 348-8, and the main pharmacologic characteristics of commonly used drugs are listed in Table 348-9. Older medications such as phenytoin, valproic acid, carbamazepine, and ethosuximide are generally used as first-line therapy for most seizure disorders since, overall, they are as effective as recently marketed drugs and significantly less expensive. Most of the new drugs that have become available in the past decade are used as add-on or alternative therapy.

In addition to efficacy, factors influencing the choice of an initial medication include the convenience of dosing (e.g., once daily versus three or four times daily) and potential side effects. Almost all of the commonly used antiepileptic drugs can cause similar, dose-related side effects such as sedation, ataxia, and diplopia. Close follow-up is required to ensure these are promptly recognized and reversed. Most of the drugs can also cause idiosyncratic toxicity such as rash, bone marrow suppression, or hepatotoxicity. Although rare, these side effects should be considered during drug selection, and patients require laboratory tests (e.g., complete blood count and liver function tests) prior to the institution of a drug (to establish baseline values) and during initial dosing and titration of the agent.

Antiepileptic Drug Selection for Partial Seizures Carbamazepine, phenytoin, or lamotrigine is currently the initial drug of choice for the treatment of partial seizures, including those that secondarily generalize. Overall they have very similar efficacy, but differences in pharmacokinetics and toxicity are the main determinants for use in a given patient. Phenytoin has a relatively long half-life and offers the advantage of once or twice daily dosing compared to two or three times daily dosing for carbamazepine (although a more expensive, extended-release form of carbamazepine is now available) and lamotrigine. An advantage of carbamazepine is that its metabolism follows first-order pharmacokinetics, and the relationship between drug dose, serum levels, and toxicity is linear. By contrast, phenytoin shows properties of saturation kinetics, such that small increases in phenytoin doses above a standard maintenance dose can precipitate marked side effects. This is one of the main causes of acute phenytoin toxicity. Long-term use of phenytoin is associated with untoward cosmetic effects (e.g., hirsutism, coarsening of facial features, and gingival hypertrophy), and effects on bone metabolism, so it is often avoided in young patients who are likely to require the drug for many years. Carbamazepine can cause leukopenia, aplastic anemia, or hepatotoxicity and would therefore be contraindicated in patients with predispositions to these problems. A major concern with lamotrigine is the occurrence of skin rash during the initiation of therapy. This can be extremely severe and lead to Stevens-Johnson syndrome if unrecognized and if the medication is not discontinued immediately. This risk can be reduced by slow introduction and titration. Lamotrigine must be started slowly when used as add-on therapy with valproic acid, since valproic acid can inhibit its metabolism, thereby substantially prolonging its half-life.

Valproic acid is an effective alternative for some patients with partial seizures, especially when the seizures secondarily generalize. Gastrointestinal side effects are fewer when using the valproate semisodium formulation (Depakote). Valproic acid also rarely causes reversible bone marrow suppression and hepatotoxicity, and laboratory testing is required to monitor toxicity. This drug should generally be avoided in patients with preexisting bone marrow or liver disease. Irreversible, fatal hepatic failure appearing as an idiosyncratic rather than dose-related side effect is a relatively rare complication; its risk is highest in children <2 years old, especially those taking other antiepileptic drugs or with inborn errors of metabolism.

Topiramate, tiagabine, levetiracetam, zonisamide, gabapentin, and oxcarbazepine are additional drugs currently used for the treatment of partial seizures with or without secondary generalization. Until recently, phenobarbital and other barbiturate compounds were commonly used as first-line therapy for many forms of epilepsy. However, the barbiturates frequently cause sedation in adults, hyperactivity in children, and other more subtle cognitive changes; thus, their use should be limited to situations in which no other suitable treatment alternatives exist.

Antiepileptic Drug Selection for Generalized Seizures Valproic acid is currently considered the best initial choice for the treatment of primarily generalized, tonic-clonic seizures. Lamotrigine, followed by carbamazepine and phenytoin, are suitable alternatives. Valproic acid is also particularly effective in absence, myoclonic, and atonic seizures and is therefore the drug of choice in patients with generalized epilepsy syndromes having mixed seizure types. Importantly, both carbamazepine and phenytoin can worsen certain types of generalized seizures, including absence, myoclonic, tonic, and atonic seizures. Ethosuximide is a particularly effective drug for the treatment of uncomplicated absence seizures, but it is not useful for tonic-clonic or partial seizures. Ethosuximide rarely causes bone marrow suppression, so that periodic monitoring of blood cell counts is required. Although approved for

TABLE 348-8 Selection of Antiepileptic Drugs

	Primary Generalized Tonic-Clonic	Partial[a]	Absence	Atypical Absence, Myoclonic, Atonic
First-Line	Valproic acid Lamotrigine	Carbamazepine Phenytoin Lamotrigine Valproic acid	Valproic acid Ethosuximide	Valproic acid
Alternatives	Phenytoin Carbamazepine Topiramate[b] Zonisamide[b] Felbamate Primidone Phenobarbital	Topiramate[b] Levetiracetam[b] Tiagabine[b] Zonisamide[b] Gabapentin[b] Primidone Phenobarbital	Lamotrigine Clonazepam	Lamotrigine Topiramate[b] Clonazepam Felbamate

[a] Includes simple partial, complex partial, and secondarily generalized seizures.
[b] As adjunctive therapy.

use in partial seizure disorders, lamotrigine appears to be effective in epilepsy syndromes with mixed, generalized seizure types such as JME and Lennox-Gastaut syndrome. Topiramate, zonisamide, and felbamate may have similar broad efficacy. Clinical trials are underway to establish the usefulness of levetiracetam in generalized seizure syndromes.

INITIATION AND MONITORING OF THERAPY Because the response to any antiepileptic drug is unpredictable, patients should be carefully educated about the approach to therapy. The goal is to prevent seizures and minimize the side effects of therapy; determination of the optimal dose is often a matter of trial and error. This process may take months or longer if the baseline seizure frequency is low. Most anticonvulsant drugs need to be introduced relatively slowly to minimize side effects, and patients should expect that minor side effects such as mild sedation, slight changes in cognition, or imbalance will typically resolve within a few days. Starting doses are usually the lowest value listed under the dosage column in Table 348-9. Subsequent increases should be made only after achieving a steady state with the previous dose (i.e., after an interval of five or more half-lives).

Monitoring of serum antiepileptic drug levels can be very useful for establishing the initial dosing schedule. However, the published therapeutic ranges of serum drug concentrations are only an approximate guide for determining the proper dose for a given patient. The key determinants are the clinical measures of seizure frequency and presence of side effects, not the laboratory values. Conventional assays of serum drug levels measure the total drug (i.e., both free and protein-bound). However, it is the concentration of free drug that reflects extracellular levels in the brain and correlates best with efficacy. Thus, patients with decreased levels of serum proteins (e.g., decreased serum albumin due to impaired liver or renal function) may have an increased ratio of free to bound drug, yet the concentration of free drug may be adequate for seizure control. These patients may have a "subtherapeutic" drug level, but the dose should be changed only if seizures remain uncontrolled, not just to achieve a "therapeutic" level. It is also useful to monitor free drug levels in such patients. In practice, other than during the initiation or modification of therapy, monitoring of antiepileptic drug levels is most useful for documenting compliance.

If seizures continue despite gradual increases to the maximum tolerated dose and documented compliance, then it becomes necessary to switch to another antiepileptic drug. This is usually done by maintaining the patient on the first drug while a second drug is added. The dose of the second drug should be adjusted to decrease seizure frequency without causing toxicity. Once this is achieved, the first drug can be gradually withdrawn (usually over weeks unless there is significant toxicity). The dose of the second drug is then further optimized based on seizure response and side effects. Monotherapy should be the goal whenever possible.

WHEN TO DISCONTINUE THERAPY Overall, about 70% of children and 60% of adults who have their seizures completely controlled with antiepi-

Generic Name	Trade Name	Principal Uses	Typical Dose; Dose Interval	Half-Life	Therapeutic Range	Adverse Effects Neurologic	Adverse Effects Systemic	Drug Interactions
Phenytoin (diphenyl-hydantoin)	Dilantin	Tonic-clonic (grand mal) Focal-onset	300–400 mg/d (3–6 mg/kg, adult; 4–8 mg/kg, child); qd-bid	24 h (wide variation, dose-dependent)	10–20 µg/mL	Dizziness Diplopia Ataxia Incoordination Confusion	Gum hyperplasia Lymphade-nopathy Hirsutism Osteomalacia Facial coarsening Skin rash	Level increased by isoniazid, sulfonamides, fluoxetine Level decreased by enzyme-inducing drugs[a] Altered folate metabolism
Carbamaze-pine	Tegretol Carbatrol	Tonic-clonic Focal-onset	600–1800 mg/d (15–35 mg/kg, child); bid-qid	10–17 h	6–12 µg/mL	Ataxia Dizziness Diplopia Vertigo	Aplastic anemia Leukopenia Gastrointestinal irritation Hepatotoxicity Hyponatremia	Level decreased by enzyme-inducing drugs[a] Level increased by erythromy-cin, propoxy-phene, isonia-zid, cimetidine, fluoxetine
Valproic acid	Depakene Depakote	Tonic-clonic Absence Atypical absence Myoclonic Focal-onset	750–2000 mg/d (20–60 mg/kg), bid-qid	15 h	50–150 µg/mL	Ataxia Sedation Tremor	Hepatotoxicity Thrombocy-topenia Gastrointestinal irritation Weight gain Transient alopecia Hyperam-monemia	Level decreased by enzyme-inducing drugs[a]
Lamotrigine	Lamictal	Focal-onset Tonic-clonic Atypical absence Myoclonic Lennox-Gastaut syndrome	150–500 mg/d; bid	25 h 14 h (with enzyme-inducers) 59 h (with valproic acid)	Not established	Dizziness Diplopia Sedation Ataxia Headache	Skin rash Stevens-Johnson syndrome	Level decreased by enzyme-inducing drugs[a] Level increased by valproic acid
Ethosuxi-mide	Zarontin	Absence (petit mal)	750–1250 mg/d (20-40 mg/kg); qd-bid	60 h, adult 30 h, child	40–100 µg/mL	Ataxia Lethargy Headache	Gastrointestinal irritation Skin rash Bone marrow suppression	
Gabapentin	Neurontin	Focal-onset	900–2400 mg/d; tid-qid	5–9 h	Not established	Sedation Dizziness Ataxia Fatigue	Gastrointestinal irritation Weight gain Edema	No known significant interactions
Topiramate	Topamax	Focal-onset Tonic-clonic Lennox-Gastaut syndrome	200–400 mg/d; bid	20–30 h	Not established	Psychomotor slowing Sedation Speech or language problems Fatigue Paresthesias	Renal stones (avoid use with other carbonic anhydrase inhibitors) Weight loss	Level decreased by enzyme-inducing drugs[a]
Tiagabine	Gabitril	Focal-onset Tonic-clonic	32–56 mg/d; bid-qid	7–9 h	Not established	Confusion Sedation Depression Dizziness Speech or language problems Paresthesias Psychosis	Gastrointestinal irritation	Level decreased by enzyme-inducing drugs[a]

(continued)

TABLE 348-9—(Continued)

Generic Name	Trade Name	Principal Uses	Typical Dose; Dose Interval	Half-Life	Therapeutic Range	Adverse Effects Neurologic	Adverse Effects Systemic	Drug Interactions
Phenobarbital	Luminol	Tonic-clonic Focal-onset	60–180 mg/d (1–4 mg/kg, adult); (3–6 mg/kg, child); qd	90 h (70 h in children)	10–40 µg/mL	Sedation Ataxia Confusion Dizziness Decreased libido Depression	Skin rash	Level increased by valproic acid, phenytoin
Primidone	Mysoline	Tonic-clonic Focal-onset	750–1000 mg/d (10–25 mg/kg); bid-tid	Primidone, 8–15 h Phenobarbital, 90 h	Primidone, 4–12 µg/mL Phenobarbital, 10–40 µg/mL	Same as phenobarbital		
Clonazepam	Klonopin	Absence Atypical absence Myoclonic	1–12 mg/d (0.1–0.2 mg/kg); qd-tid	24–48 h	10–70 ng/mL	Ataxia Sedation Lethargy	Anorexia	Level decreased by enzyme-inducing drugs[a]
Felbamate	Felbatol	Focal-onset Lennox-Gastaut syndrome	2400–3600 mg/d, (45 mg/kg, child); tid-qid	16–22 h	Not established	Insomnia Dizziness Sedation Headache	Aplastic anemia Hepatic failure Weight loss Gastrointestinal irritation	Increases phenytoin, valproic acid, active carbamazepine metabolite
Levetiracetam	Keppra	Focal-onset	1000–3000 mg/d; bid	6–8 h	Not established	Sedation Fatigue Incoordination Psychosis	Anemia Leukopenia	None known
Zonisamide	Zonegran	Focal-onset	200–400 mg/d; qd-bid	50–68 h	Not established	Sedation Dizziness Confusion Headache Psychosis	Anorexia Renal stones	Level decreased by enzyme-inducing drugs[a]
Oxcarbazepine	Trileptal	Focal-onset	900–2400 mg/d (30–45 mg/kg, child); bid	10–17 h (for active metabolite)	Not established	Fatigue Ataxia Dizziness Diplopia Vertigo Headache	See carbamazepine	Level decreased by enzyme-inducing drugs[a] May increase phenytoin

[a] Phenytoin, carbamazepine, phenobarbital.

leptic drugs can eventually discontinue therapy. The following patient profile yields the greatest chance of remaining seizure-free after drug withdrawal: (1) complete medical control of seizures for 1 to 5 years; (2) single seizure type, either partial or generalized; (3) normal neurologic examination, including intelligence; and (4) normal EEG. The appropriate seizure-free interval is unknown and undoubtedly varies for different forms of epilepsy. However, it seems reasonable to attempt withdrawal of therapy after 2 years in a patient who meets all of the above criteria, is motivated to discontinue the medication, and clearly understands the potential risks and benefits. In most cases it is preferable to reduce the dose of the drug gradually over 2 to 3 months. Most recurrences occur in the first 3 months after discontinuing therapy, and patients should be advised to avoid potentially dangerous situations such as driving or swimming during this period.

TREATMENT OF REFRACTORY EPILEPSY Approximately one-third of patients with epilepsy do not respond to treatment with a single antiepileptic drug, and it becomes necessary to try a combination of drugs to control seizures. Patients who have focal epilepsy related to an underlying structural lesion or those with multiple seizure types and developmental delay are particularly likely to require multiple drugs. There are currently no clear guidelines for rational polypharmacy, although in theory a combination of drugs with different mechanisms of action may be most useful. In most cases the initial combination therapy combines first-line drugs, i.e., carbamazepine, phenytoin, valproic acid, and lamotrigine. If these drugs are unsuccessful, then the addition of a newer drug such as topiramate or levetiracetam is indicated. Patients with myoclonic seizures resistant to valproic acid may benefit from the addition of clonazepam, and those with absence seizures may respond to a combination of valproic acid and ethosuximide. The same principles concerning the monitoring of therapeutic response, toxicity, and serum levels for monotherapy apply to polypharmacy, and potential drug interactions need to be recognized. If there is no improvement, a third drug can be added while the first two are maintained. If there is a response, the less effective or less well-tolerated of the first two drugs should be gradually withdrawn.

Surgical Treatment of Refractory Epilepsy Approximately 20% of patients with epilepsy are resistant to medical therapy despite efforts to find an effective combination of antiepileptic drugs. For some, surgery can be extremely effective in substantially reducing seizure frequency and even providing complete seizure control. Understanding the potential value of surgery is especially important when, at the time of diagnosis, a patient has an epilepsy syndrome that is considered likely to be drug-resistant. Rather than submitting the patient to years of unsuccessful medical therapy and the psychosocial trauma and increased mortality associated with ongoing seizures, the patient should have an efficient but relatively brief attempt at medical therapy and then be referred for surgical evaluation.

The most common surgical procedure for patients with temporal lobe epilepsy involves resection of the anteromedial temporal lobe (temporal lobectomy) or a more limited removal of the underlying hippocampus and amygdala (amygdalohippocampectomy). Focal seizures arising from extratemporal regions may be abolished by a focal neocortical resection with precise removal of an identified lesion (lesionectomy). When the cortical region cannot be removed, multiple subpial transection, which disrupts intracortical connections, is sometimes used to prevent seizure spread. Hemispherectomy or multilobar resection is useful for some patients with severe seizures due to hemispheric abnormalities such as hemimegaloencephaly or other dysplastic abnormalities, and corpus callosotomy has been shown to be effective for disabling tonic or atonic seizures, usually when they are part of a mixed-seizure syndrome (e.g., Lennox-Gastaut syndrome).

Presurgical evaluation is designed to identify the functional and structural basis of the patient's seizure disorder. Inpatient video-EEG monitoring is used to define the anatomic location of the seizure focus and to correlate the abnormal electrophysiologic activity with behavioral manifestations of the seizure. Routine scalp or scalp-sphenoidal recordings are usually sufficient for localization, and advances in neuroimaging have made the use of invasive electrophysiologic monitoring such as implanted depth electrodes or subdural electrodes less common. A high-resolution MRI scan is routinely used to identify structural lesions. Functional imaging studies such as SPECT and PET are adjunctive tests that may help verify the localization of an apparent epileptogenic region. Once the presumed location of the seizure onset is identified, additional studies, including neuropsychological testing and the intracarotid amobarbital test (Wada test) may be used to assess language and memory localization and to determine the possible functional consequences of surgical removal of the epileptogenic region. In some cases, the exact extent of the resection to be undertaken is determined by performing cortical mapping at the time of the surgical procedure, allowing for a tailored resection. This involves electrocorticographic recordings made with electrodes on the surface of the brain to identify the extent of epileptiform disturbances. If the region to be resected is within or near brain regions suspected of having sensorimotor or language function, electrical cortical stimulation mapping is performed in the awake patient to determine the function of cortical regions in question in order to avoid resection of so-called eloquent cortex, and thereby minimize postsurgical deficits.

Advances in presurgical evaluation and microsurgical techniques have led to a steady increase in the success of epilepsy surgery. Clinically significant complications of surgery are <5%, and the use of functional mapping procedures has markedly reduced the neurologic sequelae due to removal or sectioning of brain tissue. For example, about 70% of patients treated with temporal lobectomy will become seizure-free, and another 15 to 25% will have at least a 90% reduction in seizure frequency. Marked improvement is also usually seen in patients treated with hemispherectomy for catastrophic seizure disorders due to large hemispheric abnormalities. Postoperatively, patients generally need to remain on antiepileptic drug therapy, but the marked reduction of seizures following surgery can have a very beneficial effect on quality of life.

Vagus Nerve Stimulation (VNS)   VNS is a new treatment option for patients with medically refractory epilepsy who are not candidates for resective brain surgery. The procedure involves placement of a bipolar electrode on the midcervical portion of the left vagus nerve. The electrode is connected to a small, subcutaneous generator located in the infraclavicular region, and the generator is programmed to deliver intermittent electrical pulses to the vagus nerve. Unlike medications, there may be a delay between the initiation of VNS and the appearance of antiseizure effects. The precise mechanism of action of VNS is unknown, although experimental studies have shown that stimulation of vagal nuclei leads to widespread activation of cortical and subcortical pathways and an associated increased seizure threshold. In practice, the efficacy of VNS appears to be no greater than recently introduced anticonvulsant medications. Adverse effects of the surgery are rare, and stimulation-induced side effects, including transient hoarseness, cough, and dyspnea, are usually mild and well tolerated.

STATUS EPILEPTICUS   Status epilepticus refers to continuous seizures or repetitive, discrete seizures with impaired consciousness in the interictal period. The duration of seizure activity sufficient to meet the definition of status epilepticus has traditionally been specified as 15 to 30 min. However, a more practical definition is to consider status epilepticus as a situation in which the duration of seizures prompts the acute use of anticonvulsant therapy, typically when seizures last beyond 5 min.

Status epilepticus is an emergency and must be treated immediately, since cardiorespiratory dysfunction, hyperthermia, and metabolic derangements can develop as a consequence of prolonged seizures, and these can lead to irreversible neuronal injury. Furthermore, CNS injury can occur even when the patient is paralyzed with neuromuscular blockade but continues to have electrographic seizures. The most common causes of status epilepticus are anticonvulsant withdrawal or noncompliance, metabolic disturbances, drug toxicity, CNS infection, CNS tumors, refractory epilepsy, and head trauma.

Generalized status epilepticus is obvious when the patient is having overt convulsions. However, after 30 to 45 min of uninterrupted seizures, the signs may become increasingly subtle. Patients may have mild clonic movements of only the fingers, or fine, rapid movements of the eyes. There may be paroxysmal episodes of tachycardia, hypertension, and pupillary dilation. In such cases, the EEG may be the only method of establishing the diagnosis. Thus, if the patient stops having overt seizures, yet remains comatose, an EEG should be performed to rule out ongoing status epilepticus.

The first step in the management of a patient in status epilepticus is to attend to any acute cardiorespiratory problems or hyperthermia, perform a brief medical and neurologic examination, establish venous access, and send samples for laboratory studies to identify metabolic abnormalities. Anticonvulsant therapy should then begin without delay; a treatment approach is shown in Fig. 348-4.

BEYOND SEIZURES: OTHER MANAGEMENT ISSUES

Interictal Behavior   The adverse effects of epilepsy often go beyond the occurrence of clinical seizures, and the extent of these effects depends largely upon the etiology of the seizure disorder, the degree to which the seizures are controlled, and the presence of side effects from antiepileptic therapy. Many patients with epilepsy are completely normal between seizures and able to live highly successful and productive lives. In contrast, patients with seizures secondary to developmental abnormalities or acquired brain injury may have impaired cognitive function and other neurologic deficits. Frequent interictal EEG abnormalities have been shown to be associated with subtle dysfunction of memory and attention. Patients with many seizures, especially those emanating from the temporal lobe, often note an impairment of short-term memory that may progress over time.

Patients with epilepsy are at risk of developing a variety of psychiatric problems including depression, anxiety, and psychosis. This risk varies considerably depending on many factors, including the etiology, frequency, and severity of seizures and the patient's age and previous history. Depression occurs in ~20% of patients, and the incidence of suicide is higher in epileptic patients than in the general population. Depression should be treated through counseling or medication. The selective serotonin reuptake inhibitors typically have no effect on seizures, while the tricyclic antidepressants may lower the seizure threshold. Anxiety can appear as a manifestation of a seizure, and anxious or psychotic behavior can sometimes be observed as part of a postictal delirium. Postictal psychosis is a rare phenomenon that typically occurs after a period of increased seizure frequency. There is usually a brief lucid interval lasting up to a week, followed by days to weeks of agitated, psychotic behavior. The psychosis will usually resolve spontaneously but may require treatment with antipsychotic or anxiolytic medications.

There is ongoing controversy as to whether some patients with epilepsy (especially temporal lobe epilepsy) have a stereotypical "interictal personality." The predominant view is that the unusual or abnormal personality traits observed in such patients are, in most cases, not due to epilepsy but result from an underlying structural brain lesion, the effects of antiepileptic drugs, or psychosocial factors related to suffering from a chronic disease.

Mortality of Epilepsy Patients with epilepsy have a risk of death that is roughly two to three times greater than expected in a matched population without epilepsy. Most of the increased mortality is due to the underlying etiology of epilepsy, e.g., tumors or strokes in older adults. However, a significant number of patients die from accidents, status epilepticus, and a syndrome known as *sudden unexpected death in epileptic patients* (SUDEP), which usually affects young people with convulsive seizures and tends to occur at night. The cause of SUDEP is unknown; it may result from brainstem-mediated effects of seizures on cardiac rhythms or pulmonary function.

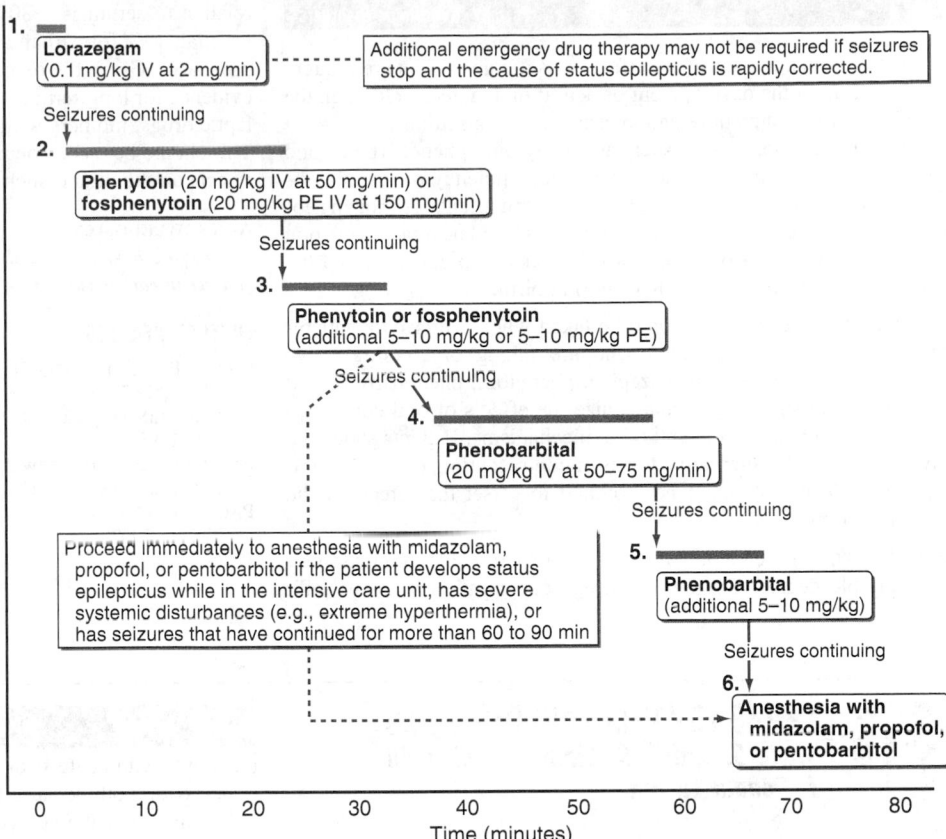

FIGURE 348-4 Pharmacologic treatment of generalized tonic-clonic status epilepticus in adults. IV, intravenous; PE, phenytoin equivalents. The horizontal bars indicate the approximate duration of drug infusions.

Psychosocial Issues There continues to be a cultural stigma about epilepsy, although it is slowly declining in societies with effective health education programs. Many patients with epilepsy harbor fears, such as the fear of becoming mentally retarded or dying during a seizure. These issues need to be carefully addressed by educating the patient about epilepsy and by ensuring that family members, teachers, fellow employees, and other associates are equally well informed. The Epilepsy Foundation of America (1-800-EFA-1000) is a patient advocacy organization and a useful source of educational material.

Employment and Driving Many patients with epilepsy face difficulty in obtaining or maintaining employment, even when their seizures are well controlled. Federal and state legislation is designed to prevent employers from discriminating against patients with epilepsy, and patients should be encouraged to understand and claim their legal rights. Patients in these circumstances also benefit greatly from the assistance of health providers who act as strong patient advocates.

Loss of driving privileges is one of the most disruptive social consequences of epilepsy. Physicians should be very clear about local regulations concerning driving and epilepsy, since the laws vary considerably among states and countries. In all cases, it is the physician's responsibility to warn patients of the danger imposed on themselves and others while driving if their seizures are uncontrolled (unless the seizures are not associated with impairment of consciousness or motor control). In general, most states allow patients to drive after a seizure-free interval (on or off medications) between 3 months and 2 years.

SPECIAL ISSUES RELATED TO WOMEN AND EPILEPSY

Catamenial Epilepsy Some women experience a marked increase in seizure frequency around the time of menses. This is thought to reflect either the effects of estrogen and progesterone on neuronal excitability or changes in antiepileptic drug levels due to altered protein binding. Acetazolamide (250 to 500 mg/d) may be effective as adjunctive therapy in some cases when started 7 to 10 days prior to the onset of

menses and continued until bleeding stops. Some patients may benefit from increases in antiepileptic drug dosages during this time or from control of the menstrual cycle through the use of oral contraceptives. Natural progestins may be of benefit to a subset of women.

Pregnancy Most women with epilepsy who become pregnant will have an uncomplicated gestation and deliver a normal baby. However, epilepsy poses some important risks to a pregnancy. Seizure frequency during pregnancy will remain unchanged in ~50% of women, increase in 30%, and decrease in 20%. Changes in seizure frequency are attributed to endocrine effects on the CNS, variations in antiepileptic drug pharmacokinetics (such as acceleration of hepatic drug metabolism or effects on plasma protein binding), and changes in medication compliance. It is useful to see patients at frequent intervals during pregnancy and monitor serum antiepileptic drug levels. Measurement of the unbound drug concentrations may be useful if there is an increase in seizure frequency or worsening of side effects of antiepileptic drugs.

The overall incidence of fetal abnormalities in children born to mothers with epilepsy is 5 to 6%, compared to 2 to 3% in healthy women. Part of the higher incidence is due to teratogenic effects of antiepileptic drugs, and the risk increases with the number of medications used (e.g., 10% risk of malformations with three drugs). A syndrome comprising facial dysmorphism, cleft lip, cleft palate, cardiac defects, digital hypoplasia, and nail dysplasia was originally ascribed to phenytoin therapy, but it is now known to occur with other first-line antiepileptic drugs (i.e., valproic acid and carbamazepine) as well. Also, valproic acid and carbamazepine are associated with a 1 to 2% incidence of neural tube defects compared with a baseline of 0.5 to 1%. Little is currently known about the safety of newer drugs.

Since the potential harm of uncontrolled seizures on the mother and fetus is considered greater than the teratogenic effects of antiepileptic drugs, it is currently recommended that pregnant women be maintained on effective drug therapy. When possible, it seems prudent to have the patient on monotherapy at the lowest effective dose, especially during the first trimester. Patients should also take folate (1 to 4 mg/d), since the antifolate effects of anticonvulsants are thought to play a role in the development of neural tube defects, although the benefits of this treatment remain unproved in this setting.

Enzyme-inducing drugs such as phenytoin, phenobarbital, and primidone cause a transient and reversible deficiency of vitamin K–dependent clotting factors in ~50% of newborn infants. Although neonatal hemorrhage is uncommon, the mother should be treated with oral vitamin K (20 mg daily) in the last 2 weeks of pregnancy, and the infant should receive vitamin K (1 mg) at birth.

Contraception Special care should be taken when prescribing antiepileptic medications for women who are taking oral contraceptive agents. Drugs such as carbamazepine, phenytoin, phenobarbital, and topiramate can significantly antagonize the effects of oral contraceptives via enzyme induction and other mechanisms. Patients should be advised to consider alternative forms of contraception, or their contraceptive medications should be modified to offset the effects of the antiepileptic medications.

Breast Feeding Antiepileptic medications are excreted into breast milk to a variable degree. The ratio of drug concentration in breast milk

relative to serum is ~80% for ethosuximide, 40 to 60% for phenobarbital, 40% for carbamazepine, 15% for phenytoin, and 5% for valproic acid. Given the overall benefits of breast feeding and the lack of evidence for long-term harm to the infant by being exposed to antiepileptic drugs, mothers with epilepsy can be encouraged to breast feed. This should be reconsidered, however, if there is any evidence of drug effects on the infant, such as lethargy or poor feeding.

ACKNOWLEDGMENT
The editors acknowledge the contributions of Michael J. Aminoff to this chapter in earlier editions of Harrison's.

FURTHER READING

CHANG B, LOWENSTEIN D: Mechanisms of disease: Epilepsy. N Engl J Med 349:1257, 2003
LOWENSTEIN DH, ALLDREDGE BK: Status epilepticus. N Engl J Med 338: 970, 1998
NOEBELS J: Exploring new gene discoveries in idiopathic generalized epilepsy. Epilepsia 44(Suppl 2):16, 2003
PACK AM, MORRELL MJ: Treatment of women with epilepsy. Semin Neurol 22:289, 2002
WIEBE S et al: A randomized, controlled trial of surgery for temporal-lobe epilepsy. N Engl J Med 345:311, 2001

349 CEREBROVASCULAR DISEASES
Wade S. Smith, S. Claiborne Johnston, J. Donald Easton

Cerebrovascular diseases include some of the most common and devastating disorders: ischemic stroke, hemorrhagic stroke, and cerebrovascular anomalies such as intracranial aneurysms and arteriovenous malformations (AVMs). They cause ~200,000 deaths each year in the United States and are a major cause of disability. The incidence of cerebrovascular diseases increases with age, and the number of strokes is projected to increase as the elderly population grows, with a doubling in stroke deaths in the United States by 2030. Most cerebrovascular diseases are manifest by the abrupt onset of a focal neurologic deficit, as if the patient was "struck by the hand of God". A stroke, or cerebrovascular accident, is defined by this abrupt onset of a neurologic deficit that is attributable to a focal vascular cause. Thus, the definition of stroke is clinical, and laboratory studies including brain imaging are used to support the diagnosis. The clinical manifestations of stroke are highly variable because of the complex anatomy of the brain and its vasculature. *Cerebral ischemia* is caused by a reduction in blood flow that lasts longer than several seconds. Neurologic symptoms are manifest within seconds because neurons lack glycogen, so energy failure is rapid. When blood flow is quickly restored, brain tissue can recover fully and the patient's symptoms are only transient: this is called a *transient ischemic attack* (TIA). Typically the neurologic signs and symptoms of a TIA last for 5 to 15 min but, by definition, must last <24 h. If the cessation of flow lasts for more than a few minutes, *infarction* or death of brain tissue results. Stroke has occurred if the neurologic signs and symptoms last for >24 h. A generalized reduction in cerebral blood flow due to systemic hypotension (e.g., cardiac arrhythmia, myocardial infarction, or hemorrhagic shock) usually produces syncope (Chap. 20). If low cerebral blood flow persists for a longer duration, then infarction in the border zones between the major cerebral artery distributions may develop. In more severe instances, *global hypoxia-ischemia* causes widespread brain injury; the constellation of cognitive sequelae that ensue is called *hypoxic-ischemic encephalopathy* (Chap. 258). *Focal ischemia* or infarction, on the other hand, is usually caused by thrombosis of the cerebral vessels themselves or by emboli from a proximal arterial source or the heart. *Cerebral hemorrhage* produces neurologic symptoms by producing a mass effect on neural structures or from the toxic effects of blood itself.

APPROACH TO THE PATIENT

Patients with acute stroke often do not seek medical assistance on their own, both because they are rarely in pain, as well as because they may lose the appreciation that something is wrong (**anosagnosia**). It is often a family member or a bystander who calls for help. The rapid evaluation of patients is essential for use of time-sensitive treatments such as thrombolysis. Patients at risk for stroke should be counseled to call emergency medical services immediately if they experience the sudden onset of any of the following: loss of sensory and/or motor function on one side of the body (nearly 85% of ischemic stroke patients have hemiparesis); change in vision, gait, or ability to speak or understand; or if they experience a sudden, severe headache.

There are several common causes of sudden-onset neurologic symptoms that may mimic stroke. An adequate history from an observer that no convulsive activity occurred at the onset reasonably excludes seizure. Tumors may present with acute neurologic symptoms due to hemorrhage, seizure, or hydrocephalus. Surprisingly, migraine can mimic cerebral ischemia, even in patients without a significant migraine history. When it develops without head pain (*acephalgic migraine*), the diagnosis may remain elusive. Patients without any prior history of complicated migraine may develop acephalgic migraine even after age 65. A sensory disturbance is often prominent, and the sensory deficit, as well as any motor deficits, tends to migrate slowly across a limb over minutes. The diagnosis of migraine becomes more secure as the cortical disturbance begins to cross vascular boundaries or if typical visual symptoms are present, such as scintillating scotomata (Chap. 14). At times it may be difficult to make the diagnosis until multiple episodes have occurred leaving behind no residual stroke or magnetic resonance imaging (MRI) changes consistent with stroke. Classically, metabolic encephalopathies produce fluctuating mental status without focal neurologic findings. However, in the setting of prior stroke or brain injury, a patient with fever or sepsis may manifest hemiparesis, which clears rapidly when the infection is remedied. The metabolic process serves to "unmask" a prior deficit. Once the diagnosis of stroke is made, a brain imaging study is necessary to determine if the cause of stroke is ischemia or hemorrhage (Fig. 349-1). Computed tomography (CT) imaging of the brain is the standard imaging modality to detect the presence or absence of intracranial hemorrhage (see "Imaging Studies," below). If the stroke is ischemic, administration of tissue plasminogen activator

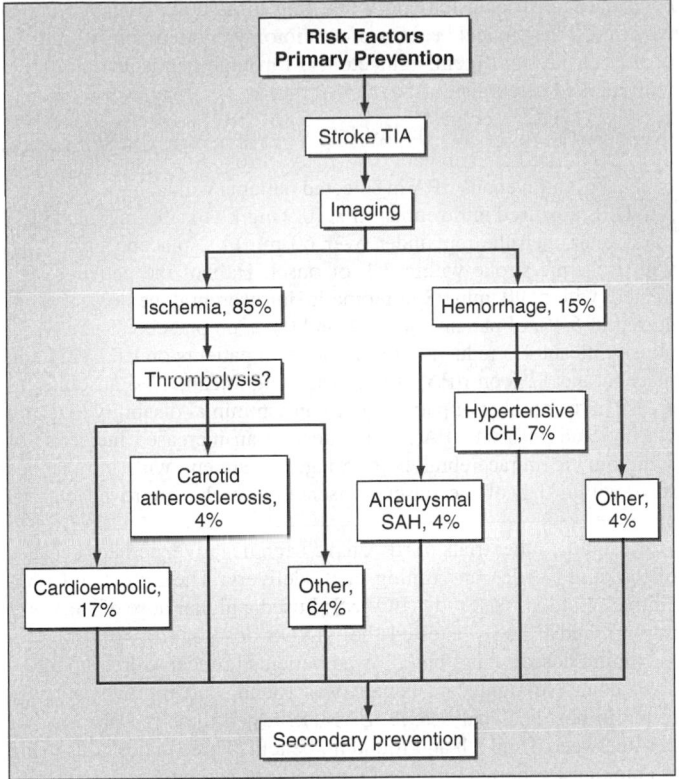

FIGURE 349-1 Schematic approach to acute stroke. Numbers are percentage of all strokes. Abbreviations: TIA, transient ischemic attack; SAH, subarachnoid hemorrhage; ICH, intracerebral hemorrhage.

(tPA) may be beneficial in restoring cerebral perfusion (see "Treatment" below). Medical management to reduce the risk of complications becomes the next priority, followed by plans for secondary prevention. For ischemic stroke, several strategies can reduce the risk of subsequent stroke in all patients, while other strategies are effective for patients with specific causes of stroke such as cardiac embolus and carotid atherosclerosis. For hemorrhagic stroke, aneurysmal subarachnoid hemorrhage (SAH) is the most important treatable condition followed by hypertensive intracranial hemorrhage.

ISCHEMIC STROKE

PATHOPHYSIOLOGY OF ISCHEMIC STROKE Acute occlusion of an intracranial vessel causes reduction in blood flow to the brain region it supplies. The magnitude of flow reduction is a function of collateral blood flow and this depends on individual vascular anatomy and the site of occlusion. A fall in cerebral blood flow to zero causes death of brain tissue within 4 to 10 min; values <16 to 18 mL/100 g tissue per min cause infarction within an hour; and values <20 mL/100 g tissue per min cause ischemia without infarction unless prolonged for several hours or days. If blood flow is restored prior to a significant amount of cell death, the patient may experience only transient symptoms, i.e., a TIA. Tissue surrounding the core region of infarction is ischemic but reversibly dysfunctional and is referred to as the *ischemic penumbra*. The penumbra may be imaged by using perfusion-diffusion imaging with MRI (see below and Fig. 349-13). The ischemic penumbra will eventually infarct if no change in flow occurs, and hence saving the ischemic penumbra

is the goal of thrombolytic therapy and newer therapies under investigation.

The complex processes that are involved in focal cerebral infarction are summarized in Fig. 349-2. Cellular death occurs via two distinct pathways: (1) a necrotic pathway in which cellular cytoskeletal breakdown is rapid, due principally to energy failure of the cell; and (2) an apoptotic pathway in which cells become programmed to die. Ischemia produces necrosis by starving neurons of glucose which in turn results in failure of mitochondria to produce ATP. Without ATP, membrane ion pumps stop functioning and neurons depolarize, allowing intracellular calcium to rise. Cellular depolarization also causes glutamate release from synaptic terminals; excess extracellular glutamate produces neurotoxicity by agonizing postsynaptic glutamate receptors that increase neuronal calcium influx. Free radicals are produced by membrane lipid degradation and mitochondrial dysfunction. Free radicals cause catalytic destruction of membranes and likely damage other vital functions of cells. Lesser degrees of ischemia, as are seen within the ischemic penumbra, favor apoptotic cellular death causing cells to die days to weeks later. There are no clinically proven strategies that alter these ischemic cascades despite extensive clinical study. It is clear, however, that fever dramatically worsens ischemia, as does hyperglycemia [glucose > 11.1 to 16.7 mmol/L (200 to 300 mg/dL)], so it is reasonable to suppress fever and prevent hyperglycemia as much as possible. Hypothermia and other neuroprotective strategies are subjects of continuing clinical research.

℞ TREATMENT

Acute Ischemic Stroke After the clinical diagnosis of stroke is made, an orderly process of evaluation and treatment should follow (Table 349-1). The first goal is to prevent or reverse brain injury. After initial stabilization, an emergency noncontrast head CT scan should be performed to differentiate ischemic from hemorrhagic stroke; there are no reliable clinical findings that conclusively separate ischemia from hemorrhage, although a more depressed level of consciousness and higher initial blood pressure favor hemorrhage, and a deficit that remits suggests ischemia. Treatments designed to reverse or lessen the amount of tissue infarction fall within five categories: (1) medical support, (2) thrombolysis, (3) anticoagulation, (4) antiplatelet agents, and (5) neuroprotection.

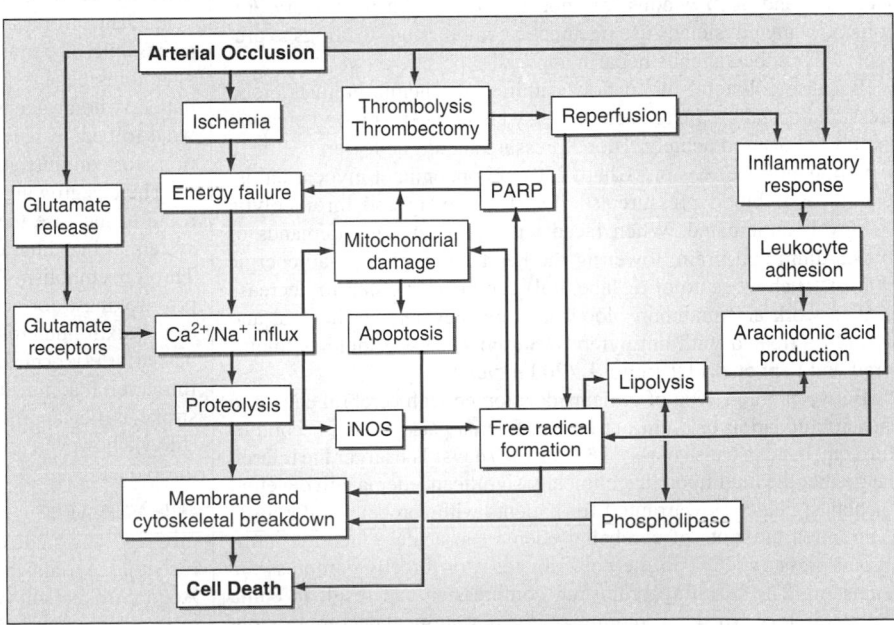

FIGURE 349-2 Major steps in the cascade of cerebral ischemia. See text for details. Abbreviations: PARP, poly-A ribose polymerase; iNOS, inducible nitric oxide synthase.

TABLE 349-1   *Clinical Management of Acute Stroke*

New onset of neurologic deficit: Stroke or TIA?	Differential diagnosis of new focal deficit
	Stroke or TIA
	Seizure with postictal Todd's paresis
	Tumor
	Migraine
	Metabolic encephalopathy
	  Fever/infection and old stroke
	  Hyperglycemia
	  Hypercalcemia
	  Hepatic encephalopathy

Initial assessment and management	ABCs, serum glucose
	Noncontrast head CT
	  Hemorrhage
	    Medical and surgical management
	  Tumor or other CNS process
	    Treat as indicated
	  Normal or hypodense area consistent with
	    acute ischemic stroke
	    Consider thrombolysis, aspirin
	    Maintain blood pressure and hydrate
	    Admit patient to appropriate level of care
	      depending on concomitant medical
	      problems and airway

Subsequent hospital management	Establish cause of stroke and risk factors
	Plan for secondary prophylaxis (drugs, risk
	  factor modifications)
	Obtain physical, occupational, and speech
	  therapy consultation and social work as
	  appropriate
	Provide nutrition
	Plan for discharge, including prescriptions for
	  risk factor reduction, including when to
	  institute antihypertensive treatment, and
	  antithrombotic medication prophylaxis

Note: ABCs, airway management, breathing, cardiac status; CNS, central nervous system; CT, computed tomography; TIA, transient ischemic attack.

MEDICAL SUPPORT When cerebral infarction occurs, the immediate goal is to optimize cerebral perfusion in the surrounding ischemic penumbra. Attention is also directed toward preventing the common complications of bedridden patients—infections (pneumonia, urinary tract, and skin) and deep venous thrombosis (DVT) with pulmonary embolism. Many physicians use pneumatic compression stockings to prevent DVT; subcutaneous heparin appears to be safe as well.

Because collateral blood flow within the ischemic brain is blood pressure dependent, there is controversy about whether blood pressure should be lowered acutely. Blood pressure should be lowered if there is malignant hypertension (Chap. 230) or concomitant myocardial ischemia or if blood pressure is >185/110 mmHg and thrombolytic therapy is anticipated. When faced with the competing demands of myocardium and brain, lowering the heart rate with a β_1-adrenergic blocker (such as esmolol or labetolol) can be a first step to decrease cardiac work and maintain blood pressure. Fever is detrimental and should be treated with antipyretics. Serum glucose should be monitored and kept at <11.1 mmol/L (200 mg/dL).

Between 5 and 10% of patients develop enough cerebral edema to cause obtundation or brain herniation. Edema peaks on the second or third day but can cause mass effect for ~10 days. The larger the infarct, the greater the likelihood that clinically significant edema will develop. Special vigilance is warranted for patients with cerebellar infarction. Even small amounts of cerebellar edema can acutely increase intracranial pressure (ICP) in the posterior fossa or directly compress the brainstem. The resulting brainstem compression can result in coma and respiratory arrest and require emergency surgical decompression. Water restriction and intravenous mannitol may be used to raise the scrum osmolarity, but hypovolemia should be avoided as this may

contribute to hypotension and worsening infarction. Trials are under way to test the clinical benefits of craniotomy and temporary removal of part of the skull (hemicraniectomy) for large hemispheric infarcts with marked cerebral edema.

THROMBOLYSIS The National Institute of Neurological Disorders and Stroke (NINDS) recombinant tPA (rtPA) Stroke Study showed a clear benefit for intravenous rtPA in selected patients with acute stroke. The NINDS study used intravenous rtPA (0.9 mg/kg to a 90-mg max; 10% as a bolus, then the remainder over 60 min) vs. placebo in patients with ischemic stroke within 3 h of onset. Half of the patients were treated within 90 min. Symptomatic intracerebral hemorrhage occurred in 6.4% of patients on rtPA and 0.6% on placebo. There was a nonsignificant 4% reduction in mortality in patients on rtPA (21% on placebo and 17% on rtPA); there was a significant 12% absolute increase in the number of patients with only minimal disability (32% on placebo and 44% on rtPA.) Thus, despite an increased incidence of symptomatic intracerebral hemorrhage, treatment with intravenous rtPA within 3 h of the onset of ischemic stroke improved clinical outcome.

Results of other trials of rtPA have been negative, perhaps because of the dose of rtPA and timing of its delivery. The European Cooperative Acute Stroke Study (ECASS) I used a higher dose of rtPA (1.2 mg/kg), and ECASS-II tested the NINDS dose of rtPA (0.9 mg/kg; maximum dose, 90 mg) but allowed patients to receive drug up to the sixth hour. No significant benefit was found, but improvement was found in post hoc analyses. ATLANTIS tested the NINDS dosing of rtPA between 3 and 5 h and found no benefit. Three major trials using streptokinase reported increased mortality for patients receiving streptokinase. Early administration of the fibrinolytic agent ancrod appears to improve outcomes for patients with acute ischemic stroke; although the drug has not been approved for clinical use, its efficacy provides further evidence that thrombolytics should have a role in treatment of acute ischemic stroke.

Because of the marked differences in trial design, including drug and dose used, time to thrombolysis, and severity of stroke, the precise efficacy of intravenous thrombolytics for acute ischemic stroke remains unclear. The risk of intracranial hemorrhage appears to rise with larger strokes, longer times from onset of symptoms, and higher doses of rtPA administered. The established dose of 0.9 mg/kg administered intravenously within 3 h of stroke onset appears safe. Many hospitals have developed expert stroke teams to facilitate this treatment. The drug is now approved in the United States, Canada, and Europe for acute stroke when given within 3 h from the time the stroke symptoms began, and efforts should be made to give it as early in this 3-h window as possible. The time of stroke onset is defined as the time the patient's symptoms began or the time the patient was last seen as normal. A patient who awakens with stroke has the onset defined as when they went to bed. Table 349-2 summarizes eligibility criteria and instructions for administration of rtPA.

There is growing interest in using thrombolytics via an intraarterial route to increase the concentration of drug at the clot and minimize systemic bleeding complications. The Prolyse in Acute Cerebral Thromboembolism (PROACT) II trial found benefit for intraarterial pro-urokinase for acute middle cerebral artery (MCA) occlusions up to the sixth hour following onset of stroke. Intraarterial treatment of basilar artery occlusions may also be beneficial for selected patients. Intraarterial administration of a thrombolytic agent for acute ischemic stroke is not approved by the U.S. Food and Drug Administration (FDA); however, many stroke centers offer this treatment based on these data.

ANTIPLATELET AGENTS Aspirin is the only antiplatelet agent that has been prospectively studied for the treatment of acute ischemic stroke. The recent large trials, the International Stroke Trial (IST) and the Chinese Acute Stroke Trial (CAST), found that the use of aspirin within 48 h of stroke onset reduced both stroke recurrence risk and mortality minimally. Among 19,435 patients in IST, those allocated to aspirin, 300 mg/d, had slightly fewer deaths within 14 days (9.0 vs. 9.4%), signif-

TABLE 349-2 *Administration of Intravenous Recombinant Tissue Plasminogen Activator (rtPA) for Acute Ischemic Stroke[a]*

Indication	Contraindication
Clinical diagnosis of stroke	Sustained BP > 185/110 despite treatment
Onset of symptoms to time of drug administration ≤3 h	Platelets < 100,000; HCT < 25%; glucose < 50 or > 400 mg/dL
CT scan showing no hemorrhage or edema of >⅓ of the MCA territory	Use of heparin within 48 h and prolonged PTT, or elevated INR
Age ≥18 years	Rapidly improving symptoms
Consent by patient or surrogate	Prior stroke or head injury within 3 months; prior intracranial hemorrhage
	Major surgery in preceding 14 days
	Minor stroke symptoms
	Gastrointestinal bleeding in preceding 21 days
	Recent myocardial infarction
	Coma or stupor

Administration of rtPA

Intravenous access with two peripheral IV lines (avoid arterial or central line placement)
Review eligibility for rtPA
Administer 0.9 mg/kg intravenously (maximum 90 mg) IV as 10% of total dose by bolus, followed by remainder of total dose over 1 h
Frequent cuff blood pressure monitoring
No other antithrombotic treatment for 24 h
For decline in neurologic status or uncontrolled blood pressure, stop infusion, give cryoprecipitate, and reimage brain emergently
Avoid urethral catheterization for ≥2 h

[a] See Activase (tissue plasminogen activator) package insert for complete list of contraindications and dosing.

Note: BP, blood pressure; CT, computed tomography; HCT, hematocrit; INR, international normalized ratio; MCA, middle cerebral artery; PTT, partial thromboplastin time.

icantly fewer recurrent ischemic strokes (2.8 vs. 3.9%), no excess of hemorrhagic strokes (0.9 vs. 0.8%), and a trend towards a reduction in death or dependence at 6 months (61.2 vs. 63.5%). In CAST, 21,106 patients with ischemic stroke received 160 mg/d of aspirin or a placebo for up to 4 weeks. There were very small reductions in the aspirin group in early mortality (3.3 vs. 3.9%), recurrent ischemic strokes (1.6 vs. 2.1%), and dependency at discharge or death (30.5 vs. 31.6%). These trials demonstrate that the use of aspirin in the treatment of acute ischemic stroke is safe and produces a small net benefit. For every 1000 acute strokes treated with aspirin, about 9 deaths or non-fatal stroke recurrences will be prevented in the first few weeks and ~13 fewer patients will be dead or dependent at 6 months.

Agents that act at the glycoprotein IIb/IIIa receptor are undergoing clinical trials in acute stroke treatment. Early results show that intravenous abciximab can be used safely within 6 h of stroke onset and suggest that it may be effective.

Anticoagulation The role of anticoagulation in atherothrombotic cerebral ischemia is uncertain. Several trials have investigated antiplatelet versus anticoagulant medications given within 12 to 24 h of the initial event. The U.S. Trial of Organon 10172 in Acute Stroke Treatment (TOAST), an investigational low-molecular-weight heparin, failed to show any benefit over aspirin. Use of subcutaneous unfractionated heparin versus aspirin was tested in IST. Heparin given subcutaneously afforded no additional benefit over aspirin and increased bleeding rates. Several trials of low-molecular-weight heparins have also shown no consistent benefit in acute ischemic stroke. Therefore, trials do not support the use of heparin or other anticoagulants for patients with atherothrombotic stroke.

In spite of the absence of evidence, heparin is still used frequently to treat stroke and TIA, primarily based on beliefs about its impact on pathophysiology. Theoretically, heparin may prevent propagation of clot within a thrombosed vessel or may prevent more emboli from occurring. Heparin is widely used for crescendo TIAs (TIAs that increase in frequency), despite the absence of data from controlled studies regarding this indication. In ~20% of patients with acute stroke,

deficits will progress over several hours to 1 to 2 days. Some physicians heparinize all patients with recent mild ischemic stroke in order to prevent some of this worsening, but this practice is discouraged. The bleeding complication rate for 7 days of heparin is about 10%, with a serious bleed rate of ~2%. Clearly the value of this approach must be clarified. Heparinization is generally accomplished by beginning an infusion without bolus and is monitored to maintain the activated partial thromboplastin time (PTT) at approximately twice normal.

Neuroprotection Neuroprotection is the concept of providing a treatment that prolongs the brain's tolerance to ischemia. Hypothermia is a powerful neuroprotective treatment in patients with cardiac arrest, but it has not been adequately studied in patients with stroke. Drugs that block the excitatory amino acid pathways have been shown to protect neurons and glia in animals, but despite multiple clinical trials, they have not yet been proven to be beneficial in humans. Even so, interest in neuroprotection continues because of the potential for agents to have limited risk, even when administered in the pre-hospital setting or in conjunction with thrombolytic agents.

Stroke Centers and Rehabilitation Patient care in comprehensive stroke units followed by rehabilitation services improves neurologic outcomes and reduces mortality. Use of clinical pathways and staff dedicated to the stroke patient can improve care. Stroke teams that provide emergency 24-h evaluation of acute stroke patients for acute medical management and consideration of thrombolysis are important.

Proper rehabilitation of the stroke patient includes early physical, occupational, and speech therapy. It is directed toward educating the patient and family about the patient's neurologic deficit, preventing the complications of immobility (e.g., pneumonia, DVT and pulmonary embolism, pressure sores of the skin, and muscle contractures), and providing encouragement and instruction in overcoming the deficit. The goal of rehabilitation is to return the patient to home and to maximize recovery by providing a safe, progressive regimen suited to the individual patient. Additionally, the use of restraint therapy has been shown to improve hemiparesis following stroke, even years following the stroke, suggesting that physical therapy can recruit unused neural pathways. This finding suggests that the human nervous system is more adaptable than originally thought and has stimulated active research into physical and pharmacologic strategies that can enhance long-term neural recovery.

ETIOLOGY OF ISCHEMIC STROKE (Table 349-3) Although the initial management of acute ischemic stroke often does not depend on the etiology, establishing a cause is essential in reducing the risk of recurrence. The clinical presentation and examination findings often establish the cause of stroke or narrow the possibilities to a few. Judicious use of laboratory testing and imaging studies completes the initial evaluation. Nevertheless, nearly 30% of strokes remain unexplained despite extensive evaluation.

Clinical examination should be focused on the peripheral and cervical vascular system (carotid auscultation for bruits, blood pressure, and pressure comparison between arms), the heart (dysrhythmia, murmurs), extremities (peripheral emboli), and retina [effects of hypertension and cholesterol emboli (Hollenhorst plaques)]. A complete neurologic examination is performed to localize the site of stroke. An imaging study of the brain is nearly always performed and is required for patients being considered for thrombolysis. A chest x-ray, electrocardiogram (ECG), urinalysis, complete blood count, erythrocyte sedimentation rate, serum electrolytes, blood urea nitrogen, creatinine, blood sugar, serologic test for syphilis, serum lipid profile, prothrombin time, and PTT are often useful and should be considered in all patients. An ECG may demonstrate conduction abnormalities and arrhythmias or reveal evidence of recent myocardial infarction (MI).

Cardioembolic Stroke Cardioembolism is responsible for ~20% of all ischemic strokes. Stroke caused by heart disease is primarily due to embolism of thrombotic material forming on the atrial or ventricular

TABLE 349-3 *Causes of Ischemic Stroke*

Common Causes	Uncommon Causes
Thrombosis	Hypercoagulable disorders
Lacunar stroke (small	Protein C deficiency
vessel)	Protein S deficiency
Large vessel thrombosis	Antithrombin III deficiency
Dehydration	Antiphospholipid syndrome
Embolic occlusion	Factor V Leiden mutation[a]
Artery-to-artery	Prothrombin G20210 mutation[a]
Carotid bifurcation	Systemic malignancy
Aortic arch	Sickle cell anemia
Arterial dissection	β-Thalassemia
Cardioembolic	Polycythemia vera
Atrial fibrillation	Systemic lupus erythematosus
Mural thrombus	Homocysteinemia
Myocardial infarction	Thrombotic thrombocytopenic
Dilated cardiomyopathy	purpura
Valvular lesions	Disseminated intravascular
Mitral stenosis	coagulation
Mechanical valve	Dysproteinemias
Bacterial endocarditis	Nephrotic syndrome
Paradoxical embolus	Inflammatory bowel disease
Atrial septal defect	Oral contraceptives
Patent foramen ovale	Venous sinus thrombosis[b]
Atrial septal aneurysm	Fibromuscular dysplasia
Spontaneous echo	Vasculitis
contrast	Systemic vasculitis (PAN, Wegner's,
	Takayasu's, giant cell arteritis)
	Primary CNS vasculitis
	Meningitis (syphilis, tuberculosis,
	fungal, bacterial, zoster
	Cardiogenic
	Mitral valve calcification
	Atrial myxoma
	Intracardiac tumor
	Marantic endocarditis
	Libman-Sacks endocarditis
	Subarachnoid hemorrhage vasospasm
	Drugs: cocaine, amphetamine
	Moyamoya disease
	Eclampsia

[a] Chiefly cause venous sinus thrombosis.
[b] May be associated with any hypercoagulable disorder.
Note: CNS, central nervous system; PAN, polyarteritis nodosa.

wall or the left heart valves. These thrombi then detach and embolize into the arterial circulation. The thrombus may fragment or lyse quickly, producing only TIA. Alternatively, the arterial occlusion may last longer, producing stroke. Embolic strokes tend to be sudden in onset, with maximum neurologic deficit at once. With reperfusion following more prolonged ischemia, petechial hemorrhage can occur within the ischemic territory. This is usually of no clinical significance and should be distinguished from frank intracranial hemorrhage into a region of ischemic stroke where the mass effect from the hemorrhage can cause a decline in neurologic function.

Emboli from the heart most often lodge in the MCA, the posterior cerebral artery (PCA), or one of their branches; infrequently, the anterior cerebral artery (ACA) territory is involved. Emboli large enough to occlude the stem of the MCA (3 to 4 mm) lead to large infarcts that involve both deep gray and white matter and some portions of the cortical surface and its underlying white matter. A smaller embolus may occlude a small cortical or penetrating arterial branch. The location and size of an infarct within a vascular territory depend on the extent of the collateral circulation.

The most significant causes of cardioembolic stroke in most of the world are nonrheumatic (often called nonvalvular) atrial fibrillation, MI, prosthetic valves, rheumatic heart disease, and ischemic cardiomyopathy (Table 349-3). Cardiac disorders causing brain embolism are discussed in the respective chapters on heart diseases. A few pertinent aspects are highlighted here.

Nonrheumatic atrial fibrillation is the most common cause of cerebral embolism overall. The presumed stroke mechanism is thrombus formation in the fibrillating atrium or atrial appendage, with subsequent embolization. Patients with atrial fibrillation have an average annual risk of stroke of ~5%. The risk varies according to the presence of certain risk factors, including older age, hypertension, poor left ventricular function, prior cardioembolism, diabetes, and thyrotoxicosis. Patients younger than 60 with none of these risk factors have an annual risk for stroke of ~0.5%, while those with most of the factors have a rate of ~15% per year. Left atrial enlargement and congestive heart failure are additional risk factors for formation of atrial thrombi. Rheumatic heart disease usually causes ischemic stroke when there is prominent mitral stenosis or atrial fibrillation. Guidelines for the use of warfarin and aspirin for secondary prevention are based on risk factors (Table 349-4).

Recent MI may be a source of emboli, especially when transmural and involving the anteroapical ventricular wall, and prophylactic anticoagulation following MI has been shown to reduce stroke risk. Mitral valve prolapse is not usually a source of emboli unless the prolapse is severe.

Paradoxical embolization occurs when venous thrombi migrate to the arterial circulation, usually via a patent foramen ovale or atrial septal defect. Bubble-contrast echocardiography (intravenous injection of agitated saline coupled with either transthoracic or transesophageal echocardiography) can demonstrate a cardiac right-to-left shunt, revealing the conduit for paradoxical embolization. Alternatively, a right-to-left shunt is implied if immediately following intravenous injection of agitated saline, high-intensity transients are observed during transcranial Doppler insonation of the MCA. Both techniques are highly sensitive for detection of right-to-left shunts. Besides venous clot, fat and tumor emboli, bacterial endocarditis, intravenous air, and amniotic fluid emboli associated with delivery may occasionally be responsible for paradoxical embolization. The importance of right-to-left shunt as a cause of stroke is debated, particularly because such shunts occur in ~15% of the general population. Some studies have suggested that the risk is only elevated in the presence of a coexisting atrial septal aneurysm. The presence of a venous source of embolus, most commonly a deep venous thrombus, may provide confirmation of the importance of a right-to-left shunt in a particular case.

Bacterial endocarditis can cause valvular vegetations that can give rise to multiple septic emboli (Chap. 109). The appearance of multifocal symptoms and signs in a patient with stroke makes bacterial endocarditis more likely. Infarcts of microscopic size occur, and large septic infarcts may evolve into brain abscesses or cause hemorrhage into the infarct, which generally precludes use of anticoagulation or thrombolytics. Mycotic aneurysms caused by septic emboli give rise to SAH or intracerebral hemorrhage.

Artery-to-Artery Embolic Stroke Thrombus formation on atherosclerotic plaques may embolize to intracranial arteries producing an artery-to-artery embolic stroke. Alternatively, a diseased vessel may acutely thrombose; the resulting blockage causes stroke by producing ischemia within the region of brain it supplied. Unlike the myocardial vessels, artery-to-artery embolism appears to be the dominant vascular mech-

TABLE 349-4 *Consensus Recommendation for Antithrombotic Prophylaxis in Atrial Fibrillation*

Age	Risk Factors[a]	Recommendation
Age ≤65	≥1	Warfarin INR 2–3
	0	Aspirin or no treatment
Age 65–75	≥1	Warfarin INR 2–3
	0	Warfarin INR 2–3 or aspirin
Age >75		Warfarin INR 2–3

[a] Risk factors include previous transient ischemic attack or stroke, hypertension, heart failure, diabetes, clinical coronary artery disease, mitral stenosis, prosthetic heart valves, or thyrotoxicosis.
Source: Modified from GW Albers et al: Antithrombotic therapy in atrial fibrillation. Chest 119:194S, 2001; with permission.

anism causing ischemia rather than thrombosis. The most common source of embolism is the carotid bifurcation, but any diseased vessel may be a source, including the aortic arch and common carotid, internal carotid, vertebral, and basilar arteries. Carotid bifurcation atherosclerosis is the most common source of artery-to-artery embolus, and specific treatments have proven efficacy in reducing risk.

CAROTID ATHEROSCLEROSIS Atherosclerosis within the carotid artery occurs most frequently within the common carotid bifurcation and proximal internal carotid artery. Additionally, the carotid siphon (portion within the cavernous sinus) is also vulnerable to atherosclerosis. Male gender, older age, smoking, hypertension, diabetes, and hypercholesterolemia are risk factors for carotid disease, as they are for stroke in general (Table 349-5). Carotid atherosclerosis produces an estimated 5% of ischemic stroke, and the risk of stroke rises the higher the degree of carotid narrowing. →*For further discussion of the pathogenesis of atherosclerosis, see Chap. 224.*

Carotid disease can be classified by whether the stenosis is symptomatic or asymptomatic and by the degree of stenosis (percent narrowing of the narrowest segment compared to a more distal internal carotid segment). Symptomatic carotid disease implies that the patient has experienced a stroke or TIA within the vascular distribution of the artery, and it is associated with a greater risk of subsequent stroke than asymptomatic stenosis, in which the patient is symptom free and the stenosis is detected through screening. Greater degrees of arterial narrowing are generally associated with a greater risk of stroke.

℞ TREATMENT

Surgical Therapy Surgery for atherosclerotic occlusive disease is largely limited to *carotid endarterectomy* for plaques located at the origin of the internal carotid artery in the neck.

Symptomatic carotid stenosis was studied in the North American Symptomatic Carotid Endarterectomy Trial (NASCET) and the European Carotid Surgery Trial (ECST). Both showed a substantial benefit for surgery in patients with a stenosis of >70%. In NASCET, the average cumulative ipsilateral stroke risk at 2 years was 26% for patients treated medically and 9% for those receiving the same medical treatment plus a carotid endarterectomy. This 17% *absolute* reduction in the surgical group is a 65% *relative* risk reduction favoring surgery (Table 349-5). NASCET also showed a significant benefit for patients with 50 to 70% stenosis, although less robust. ECST found harm for patients with stenosis in the 0 to 30% range treated surgically.

A patient's risk of stroke and possible benefit from surgery are related to the presence of retinal versus hemispheric symptoms, degree of arterial stenosis, extent of associated medical conditions, institutional surgical morbidity and mortality, and other factors. A patient with multiple atherosclerosis risk factors, symptomatic hemispheric ischemia, high-grade stenosis in the appropriate internal carotid artery, and an institutional perioperative morbidity and mortality rate of ≤6% generally should undergo carotid endarterectomy. If the perioperative stroke rate is >6% for any particular surgeon, however, the benefits of carotid endarterectomy are questionable.

The indications for surgical treatment of *asymptomatic carotid disease* have been clarified by the results of the Asymptomatic Carotid Atherosclerosis Study (ACAS), which randomized patients with ≥60% stenosis to medical treatment with aspirin or the same medical treatment plus carotid endarterectomy. The surgical group had a risk over 5 years for ipsilateral stroke (and any perioperative stroke or death) of 5.1%, compared to a risk in the medical group of 11%. While

this demonstrates a 53% *relative* risk reduction, the *absolute* risk reduction is only 5.9% over 5 years, or 1.2% annually (Table 349-5). The perioperative complication rate was higher in women, so they received only a 17% relative risk reduction over 5 years. Nearly half of the strokes in the surgery group were caused by preoperative angiograms.

The natural history of asymptomatic stenosis is an ~2% per year stroke rate, while symptomatic patients experience a 13% per year risk of stroke. Whether to recommend carotid revascularization for an asymptomatic patient remains controversial and depends on many factors including patient preference, age, and comorbidities. Medical therapy for reduction of atherosclerosis risk factors, including statins and aspirin, is generally recommended for patients with asymptomatic carotid stenosis. As with atrial fibrillation, it is imperative to counsel the patient about TIAs so their therapy can be revised if they become symptomatic.

Balloon angioplasty coupled with stenting is being used with increasing frequency to open stenotic carotid arteries and maintain their patency. This method has not yet been compared prospectively with endarterectomy, except in high-risk patients where one small trial suggested less morbidity with stenting compared with endarterectomy. Concern exists about distal embolization of plaque during vessel dilation, and many new devices designed to prevent distal embolization are undergoing clinical trials. Extracranial to intracranial (EC-IC) bypass surgery has been proven ineffective for atherosclerotic stenoses that are inaccessible to conventional carotid endarterectomy. However, using more functional techniques [positron emission tomography (PET) imaging] to select patients who may benefit from EC-IC bypass is currently being studied.

OTHER CAUSES OF ARTERY-TO-ARTERY EMBOLIC STROKE Intracranial atherosclerosis produces stroke either by an embolic mechanism or by in-situ thrombosis of a diseased vessel and is more common in patients of Asian and African-American descent. It is estimated that following a stroke or TIA from intracranial atherosclerosis the risk of a second stroke is ~15% per year. There is no proven superior treatment for stroke prevention in this disorder. Warfarin sodium and aspirin are being compared in a U.S. based prospective trial. Many neurointerventional centers are using intracranial angioplasty coupled with intracranial stenting, but this has not been compared with antithrombotic strategies for stroke prevention.

Dissection of the internal carotid or vertebral arteries or even vessels beyond the circle of Willis is a common source of embolic stroke in young (age <60 years) patients. The dissection is usually painful and precedes the stroke by several hours or days. Extracranial dissections rarely cause hemorrhage because of the tough adventitia of these vessels. Intracranial dissections, on the other hand, may produce SAH because the adventitia of intracranial vessels is thin and pseudoaneu-

TABLE 349-5 *Risk Factors for Stroke*

Risk Factor	Relative Risk	Relative Risk Reduction with Treatment	Number Needed to Treat[a] Primary Prevention	Number Needed to Treat[a] Secondary Prevention
Hypertension	2–5	38%	100–300	50–100
Atrial fibrillation	1.8–2.9	68% warfarin 21% aspirin	20–83	13
Diabetes	1.8–6	No proven effect		
Smoking	1.8	50% at 1 year, baseline risk at 5 years post cessation		
Hyperlipidemia	1.8–2.6	10–29%		—
Asymptomatic carotid stenosis	2.0	53%	85	N/A
Symptomatic carotid stenosis (70–99%)		65% at 2 years	N/A	12
Symptomatic carotid stenosis (50–69%)		29% at 5 years	N/A	77

[a] Number needed to treat to prevent one stroke annually. Prevention of other cardiovascular outcomes is not considered here.
Note: N/A, not applicable.

rysms may form, requiring treatment to prevent rerupture. The cause of dissection is usually unknown and recurrence is rare. Ehlers-Danlos type IV, Marfan's disease, cystic medial necrosis, and fibromuscular dysplasia are associated with dissections. Trauma (usually a motor vehicle accident or a sports injury) can cause carotid and vertebral artery dissections. Spinal manipulative therapy is independently associated with vertebral artery dissection and stroke. Most dissections heal spontaneously, and stroke or TIA is uncommon beyond 2 weeks. Although there are no trials comparing anticoagulation to antiplatelet agents, many physicians treat with anticoagulants for 3 to 6 months then convert to antiplatelet therapy after demonstration of vascular recanalization.

Small-Vessel Stroke   The term *lacunar infarction* refers to infarction following atherothrombotic or lipohyalinotic occlusion of a small artery (30 to 300 μm) in the brain. The term *small-vessel stroke* denotes occlusion of such a small penetrating artery and is now the preferred term. Small-vessel strokes account for ~20% of all strokes.

PATHOPHYSIOLOGY   The MCA stem, the arteries comprising the circle of Willis (A1 segment, anterior and posterior communicating arteries, and P1 segment), and the basilar and vertebral arteries all give rise to 30- to 300-μm branches that penetrate the deep gray and white matter of the cerebrum or brainstem (Fig. 349-3). Each of these small branches can occlude either by atherothrombotic disease at its origin or by the development of lipohyalinotic thickening. Thrombosis of these vessels causes small infarcts that are referred to as *lacunes* (Latin for "lake" of fluid noted at autopsy). They range in size from 3 mm to 2 cm. Hypertension and age are the principal risk factors.

CLINICAL MANIFESTATIONS   The most common *lacunar syndromes* are the following: (1) Pure motor hemiparesis from an infarct in the posterior

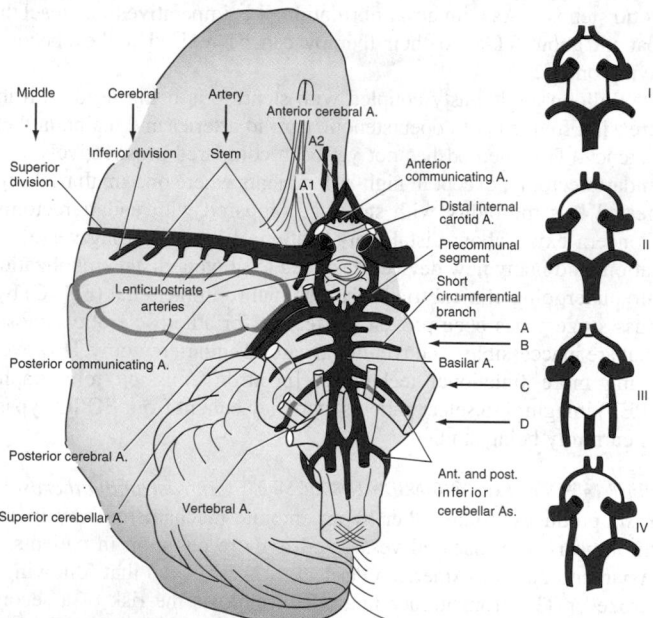

FIGURE 349-3   Diagram of the brainstem, cerebellum, inferior right frontal lobe, and transected temporal lobe. Principal branches of the vertebral basilar arterial system are pictured. The stem of the middle cerebral artery with its small, deep penetrating lenticulostriate arteries and the circle of Willis with its small, deep penetrating branches are shown. Roman numerals I, II, III, and IV represent some of the possible variations of the circle of Willis. A, B, C, and D arrows indicate the four levels of the brainstem diagrammed below (A, Fig. 349-11; B, Fig. 349-10; C, Fig. 349-9; D, Fig. 349-8). Although typical vascular syndromes of the pons and medulla have been designated by the shaded areas in Figs. 349-8 to 349-11, the shading is approximate only. Great variability in infarct size and location occurs when the basilar or vertebral arteries or one of their penetrating branches becomes occluded. This variability is because of variation in arterial anatomic location and available collateral circulation. Thus the stroke syndromes produced are often atypical, incomplete, or merge with one another. (*Courtesy of CM Fisher, MD.*)

limb of the internal capsule or basis pontis; the face, arm, and leg are almost always involved; (2) pure sensory stroke from an infarct in the ventrolateral thalamus; (3) ataxic hemiparesis from an infarct in the base of the pons; (4) dysarthria and a clumsy hand or arm due to infarction in the base of the pons or in the genu of the internal capsule; and (5) pure motor hemiparesis with "motor (Broca's) aphasia" due to thrombotic occlusion of a lenticulostriate branch supplying the genu and anterior limb of the internal capsule and adjacent white matter of the corona radiata.

Transient symptoms (small vessel TIAs) may herald a small-vessel infarct; they may occur several times a day and last only a few minutes. Recovery from a small-vessel stroke often begins within hours or days, and over weeks or months may be nearly complete; in some cases, however, there is severe permanent disability. Often, institution of combined antithrombotic treatments does not prevent eventual stroke in "stuttering lacunes."

A large-vessel source (either thrombosis or embolism) may manifest initially as a lacunar syndrome with small-vessel infarction. Therefore, the search for embolic sources (carotid and heart) should not be completely abandoned in the evaluation of these patients. Secondary prevention of lacunar stroke involves risk factor modification, specifically reduction in blood pressure (see "Primary and Secondary Prevention," below).

LESS COMMON CAUSES OF STROKE (Table 349-3)   *Hypercoagulable disorders* (Chap. 53) primarily cause increased risk of venous thrombosis and therefore may cause venous sinus thrombosis. Protein S deficiency and homocysteinemia may cause arterial thromboses as well. Systemic lupus erythematosus with Liebman-Sacks endocarditis can be a cause of embolic stroke. These conditions overlap with the antiphospholipid syndrome, which probably requires long-term anticoagulation to prevent further stroke.

Venous sinus thrombosis of the lateral or sagittal sinus or of small cortical veins (cortical vein thrombosis) occurs as a complication of pregnancy and the postpartum period, sepsis, and intracranial infections (meningitis). It is also seen with increased incidence in patients with laboratory-confirmed thrombophilia (Table 349-3) including polycythemia, sickle cell anemia, proteins C and S deficiency, factor V Leiden mutation (resistance to activated protein C), antithrombin III deficiency, homocysteinemia, and the prothrombin G20210 mutation. Women who take oral contraceptives and have the prothrombin G20210 mutation may be at high risk for sinus thrombosis. Patients present with headache, focal neurologic signs (especially paraparesis), and seizures. Often, CT imaging is normal unless an intracranial venous hemorrhage has occurred, but the venous sinus occlusion is readily visualized using magnetic resonance (MR) venography or conventional x-ray angiography. With greater degrees of sinus thrombosis, the patient may develop signs of increased ICP and coma. Intravenous heparin, regardless of the presence of intracranial hemorrhage, has been shown to reduce morbidity and mortality, and the long-term outcome is generally good. Heparin prevents further thrombosis and reduces venous hypertension and ischemia. If an underlying hypercoagulable state is not found, many physicians treat with warfarin sodium for 3 to 6 months then convert to aspirin, depending on the degree of resolution of the venous sinus thrombus. Anticoagulation is often continued indefinitely if thrombophilia is diagnosed.

Fibromuscular dysplasia affects the cervical arteries and occurs mainly in women. The carotid or vertebral arteries show multiple rings of segmental narrowing alternating with dilatation. Occlusion is usually incomplete. The process is often asymptomatic but occasionally is associated with an audible bruit, TIAs, or stroke. The cause and natural history of fibromuscular dysplasia is unknown (Chap. 232). TIA or stroke generally occurs only when the artery is severely narrowed or dissects. Anticoagulation or antiplatelet therapy may be helpful.

Temporal (giant cell) arteritis (Chap. 306) is a relatively common affliction of elderly persons in which the external carotid system, particularly the temporal arteries, becomes the site of a subacute granulomatous inflammation with giant cells. Occlusion of posterior ciliary arteries derived from the ophthalmic artery results in blindness in one or both eyes and can be prevented with glucocorticoids. It rarely causes stroke as the internal carotid artery is usually not inflamed. Idiopathic giant cell arteritis involving the great vessels arising from the aortic arch (*Takayasu's arteritis*) may cause carotid or vertebral thrombosis; it is rare in the western hemisphere.

Necrotizing (or granulomatous) arteritis, occurring alone or in association with generalized polyarteritis nodosa or Wegener's granulomatosis, involves the distal small branches (<2 mm diameter) of the main intracranial arteries and produces small ischemic infarcts in the brain, optic nerve, and spinal cord. The cerebrospinal fluid often shows pleocytosis, and the protein level is elevated. *Primary central nervous system vasculitis* is rare; small or medium-sized vessels are usually affected. Brain biopsy or high-resolution conventional x-ray angiography is usually required to make the diagnosis. Patients with any form of vasculitis may present with insidious progression of combined white and gray matter infarctions, prominent headache, and cognitive decline. Aggressive immunosuppression with glucocorticoids, and often cyclophosphamide, is usually necessary to prevent progression. Depending upon the duration of the disease, many patients can make an excellent recovery.

Drugs, in particular amphetamines and perhaps cocaine, may cause stroke on the basis of acute hypertension and drug-induced vasculitis. Abstinence appears to be the best treatment, as no data exist on use of any treatment. Phenylpropanolamine has been linked with intracranial hemorrhage as has cocaine, perhaps related to a drug-induced vasculitis. Arteritis can also occur as a consequence of bacterial, tuberculous, and syphilitic meningitis.

Moyamoya disease is a poorly understood occlusive disease involving large intracranial arteries, especially the distal internal carotid artery and the stem of the middle and anterior cerebral arteries. Vascular inflammation is absent. The lenticulostriate arteries develop a rich collateral circulation around the occlusive lesion, which gives the impression of a "puff of smoke" (*moyamoya* in Japanese) on conventional x-ray angiography. Other collaterals include transdural anastomoses between the cortical surface branches of the meningeal and scalp arteries. The disease occurs mainly in Asian children or young adults, but the appearance may be identical in adults who have atherosclerosis. The etiology of the childhood form is unknown. Because of the occurrence of intracranial hemorrhage from rupture of the transdural and pial anastomotic channels, anticoagulation is risky. Breakdown of dilated lenticulostriate arteries may produce parenchymal hemorrhage, and progressive occlusion of large surface arteries can occur, producing large-artery distribution strokes. Bypass of extracranial carotid arteries to the dura or MCAs may prevent stroke and hemorrhage.

Reversible posterior leukoencephalopathy can occur in head injury, migraine, sympathomimetic drug use, eclampsia, and the postpartum period. The etiology is unclear but likely involves widespread cerebral segmental vasoconstriction. Patients complain of headache and manifest fluctuating neurologic symptoms and signs, especially visual symptoms. Sometimes cerebral infarction ensues. Conventional x-ray angiography is the only means of establishing the diagnosis, but because angiography itself can cause spasm of vessels, even the existence of this vascular entity is debated.

Binswanger's disease (chronic progressive subcortical encephalopathy) is a rare condition in which infarction of the subcortical white matter occurs subacutely. CT or MRI scans detect periventricular white matter infarcts and gliosis. There is lipohyalinosis in the small arteries of the deep white matter, as in hypertension. There are usually associated lacunar infarcts. Binswanger's disease may represent a type of border zone ischemic infarction in the deep white matter between the penetrating arteries of the circle of Willis and of the cortex. The pathophysiologic basis of the disease is unclear, but it typically occurs in older patients with severe long-standing hypertension.

CADASIL (cerebral autosomal dominant arteriopathy with subcortical infarcts and leukoencephalopathy) is an inherited disorder that presents as small-vessel strokes, progressive dementia, and extensive symmetric white matter changes visualized by MRI. Approximately 40% of patients have migraine with aura, often manifest as transient motor or sensory deficits. Onset is usually in the fourth or fifth decade of life. This autosomal dominant condition is caused by one of several mutations in Notch-3, a member of a highly conserved gene family characterized by epidermal growth factor repeats in its extracellular domain. CADASIL is the only monogenic ischemic stroke syndrome so far described. Genetic testing is available.

TRANSIENT ISCHEMIC ATTACKS TIAs are episodes of stroke symptoms that last only briefly; the current definition of duration is <24 h, but the average duration of a TIA is ~12 min. The causes of TIA are similar to all causes of stroke, but because TIAs may herald stroke they are an important risk factor that should be considered separately. TIAs may arise from emboli to the brain or from in situ thrombosis of an intracranial vessel. With a TIA, the occluded blood vessel reopens and neurologic function is restored. However, infarcts of the brain do occur in 15 to 40% of TIAs even though neurologic signs and symptoms are absent.

In addition to the stroke syndromes discussed below, there are a few specific TIA symptoms that should receive special notice. *Amaurosis fugax*, or transient monocular blindness, occurs from emboli to the central retinal artery of one eye. This may indicate carotid stenosis as the cause or local ophthalmic artery disease.

The risk of stroke after a TIA is ~10% in the first 3 months, with most events occurring in the first 2 days. Therefore, urgent evaluation and treatment are justified. Since etiologies for stroke and TIA are identical, evaluation for TIA should parallel that of stroke (Tables 349-1 and 349-3). The improvement characteristic of TIA is a contraindication to thrombolysis. Acute antiplatelet therapy has not been tested specifically after TIA but is likely to be effective and is recommended. No large-scale trial has evaluated acute anticoagulation after TIA, a setting in which the risk of hemorrhage may be lower.

RISK FACTORS FOR ISCHEMIC STROKE Identification and control of modifiable risk factors is the best strategy to reduce the burden of stroke, as the total number of strokes could be reduced substantially by these means (Table 349-5).

PRIMARY AND SECONDARY PREVENTION ■ General Principles A number of medical and surgical interventions, as well as life-style modifications, are available for preventing stroke. Some of these can be widely applied because of their low cost and minimal risk; others are expensive and carry substantial risk but may be valuable for selected high-risk patients.

Evaluation of a patient's *clinical risk profile* can help determine which preventive treatments to offer. In addition to known risk factors for ischemic stroke (above), certain clinical characteristics also contribute to an increased risk of stroke (Table 349-5). NASCET found that even in patients with the same degree of carotid artery stenosis, specifically 70 to 99%, nine prospectively selected risk factors predicted the risk of vascular outcomes in the medically treated patients. The overall risk of stroke was much greater in a high-risk group (those with more than six risk factors) than in a low-risk group (those with fewer than six risk factors). Fully 39% of patients in the high-risk group treated medically experienced an ipsilateral stroke within 2 years. The rate for the low-risk group was less than half that but was still 17%.

Atherosclerosis Risk Factors The relationship of various factors to the risk of atherosclerosis is described in Chap. 225. Older age, family history of thrombotic stroke, diabetes mellitus, hypertension, tobacco smoking, abnormal blood cholesterol [particularly, low high-density lipoprotein (HDL) and/or high low-density lipoprotein (LDL), and other factors are either proven or probable risk factors for ischemic stroke, largely by their link to atherosclerosis. Risk of second stroke is strongly influenced by prior stroke or TIA, depending on cause.

Many cardiac conditions predispose to stroke, including atrial fibrillation and recent MI. Oral contraceptives may increase stroke risk, and certain inherited and acquired hypercoagulable states predispose to stroke. Hypertension is the most significant of the risk factors; in general, all hypertension should be treated. The presence of known cerebrovascular disease is not a contraindication to treatment aimed at achieving normotension. Also, the value of treating systolic hypertension in older patients has been clearly established. Lowering blood pressure to levels below those traditionally defining hypertension appears to reduce the risk of stroke even further. Data are particularly strong in support of angiotensin-converting enzyme inhibitors and angiotensin receptor blockers.

Several trials have confirmed that statin drugs reduce the risk of stroke even in patients without elevated LDL or low HDL. Although studies specifically targeting prevention of second stroke are still underway, results for patients with cardiovascular risk factors or dyslipidemia have been compelling, with a 20 to 30% relative risk reduction for stroke. Therefore, a statin should be considered in all patients with prior ischemic stroke. Tobacco smoking should be discouraged in all patients (Chap. 375). Whether or not tight control of blood sugar in patients with diabetes lowers stroke risk is uncertain.

Antiplatelet Agents *Platelet antiaggregation agents* can prevent atherothrombotic events, including TIA and stroke, by inhibiting the formation of intraarterial platelet aggregates. These can form on diseased arteries, induce thrombus formation, and occlude the artery or embolize into the distal circulation. Aspirin, clopidogrel, and the combination of aspirin plus extended-release dipyridamole are the antiplatelet agents most commonly used for this purpose. Ticlopidine has been largely abandoned because of its adverse effects.

Aspirin is the most widely studied antiplatelet agent. Aspirin acetylates platelet cyclooxygenase, which irreversibly inhibits the formation in platelets of thromboxane A_2, a platelet aggregating and vasoconstricting prostaglandin. This effect is permanent and lasts for the usual 8-day life of the platelet. Paradoxically, aspirin also inhibits the formation in endothelial cells of prostacyclin, an antiaggregating and vasodilating prostaglandin. This effect is transient. As soon as aspirin is cleared from the blood, the nucleated endothelial cells again produce prostacyclin. Aspirin in low doses given once daily inhibits the production of thromboxane A_2 in platelets without substantially inhibiting prostacyclin formation. The FDA recommends 50 to 325 mg of aspirin daily for stroke prevention.

Ticlopidine and clopidogrel block the ADP receptor on platelets and thus prevent the cascade resulting in activation of the glycoprotein IIb/IIIa receptor that leads to fibrinogen binding to the platelet and consequent platelet aggregation. Ticlopidine is more effective than aspirin; however, it has the disadvantage of causing diarrhea, skin rash, a low incidence of neutropenia, and thrombotic thrombocytopenic purpura. Clopidogrel is not associated with these important side effects. However, the CAPRIE (Clopidogrel versus Aspirin in Patients at Risk of Ischemic Events) trial, which led to FDA approval, found that it was only marginally more effective than aspirin in reducing risk of stroke. Studies of clopidogrel in combination with aspirin are in progress in both cerebrovascular and cardiovascular patients.

Dipyridamole is an antiplatelet agent that inhibits the uptake of adenosine by a variety of cells, including those of the vascular endothelium. The accumulated adenosine is an inhibitor of aggregation. At least in part through its effects on platelet and vessel wall phosphodiesterases, dipyridamole also potentiates the antiaggregatory effects of prostacyclin and nitric oxide produced by the endothelium and acts by inhibiting platelet phosphodiesterase, which is responsible for the breakdown of cyclic AMP. The resulting elevation in cyclic AMP inhibits aggregation of platelets. Dipyridamole has a controversial history in stroke prevention. The European Stroke Prevention Study-2 showed efficacy of both 50 mg daily of aspirin and extended-release dipyridamole in preventing stroke, and a significantly better risk re-

duction when the two agents were combined. A combination capsule of extended-release dipyridamole and aspirin is approved for prevention of stroke.

Many large clinical trials have demonstrated clearly that most antiplatelet agents reduce the risk of all important vascular atherothrombotic events (i.e., ischemic stroke, MI, and death due to all vascular causes) in patients at risk for these events. The overall *relative* reduction in risk of nonfatal stroke is about 25 to 30% and of all vascular events is about 25%. The *absolute* reduction varies considerably depending on the particular patient's risk. Individuals at very low risk for stroke seem to experience the same relative reduction, but their risk may be so low that the "benefit" is meaningless. On the other hand, individuals with a 10 to 15% risk of vascular events per year experience a reduction to about 7.5 to 11%.

Aspirin is inexpensive, can be given in low doses, and could be recommended for all adults to prevent both stroke and MI. However, it causes epigastric discomfort, gastric ulceration, and gastrointestinal hemorrhage, which may be asymptomatic or life-threatening. Consequently, not every 40- or 50-year-old should be advised to take aspirin regularly because the risk of atherothrombotic stroke is extremely low and is outweighed by the risk of adverse side effects. Conversely, every patient who has experienced an atherothrombotic stroke or TIA and has no contraindication should be taking an antiplatelet agent regularly because the average annual risk of another stroke is 8 to 10%; another few percent will experience a MI or vascular death. Clearly, the likelihood of benefit far outweighs the risks of treatment.

The choice of antiplatelet agent and dose must balance the risk of stroke, the expected benefit, and the risk and cost of treatment. However, there are no definitive data, and opinions vary. Many authorities believe low-dose (30 to 75 mg daily) and high-dose (650 to 1300 mg daily) aspirin are about equally effective. Some advocate very low doses to avoid adverse effects, and still others advocate very high doses to be sure the benefit is maximal. Most physicians in North America recommend 81 to 325 mg daily, while most Europeans recommend 50 to 100 mg. Similarly, the choice of aspirin, clopidogrel, or dipyridamole plus aspirin must balance the fact that the latter are more effective than aspirin but the cost is higher.

Anticoagulation Therapy and Noncardiogenic Stroke There are few data to support the use of long-term warfarin for preventing atherothrombotic stroke, either intracranially or extracranially. The WARSS study found no benefit of warfarin sodium (INR, 2 to 3) over aspirin, 325 mg, for secondary prevention of stroke but did find a slightly higher bleeding rate in the warfarin group. A prospective trial is ongoing to study warfarin versus aspirin in secondary stroke prevention for intracranial atherosclerosis.

Anticoagulation Therapy and Embolic Stroke Several trials have shown that anticoagulation (INR range, 2 to 3) in patients with chronic nonvalvular (nonrheumatic) atrial fibrillation prevents cerebral embolism and is safe. For primary prevention and for patients who have experienced stroke or TIA, anticoagulation with warfarin reduces the risk by about 67% which clearly outweighs the 1% risk per year of a major bleeding complication.

The decision to use anticoagulation for primary prevention is based primarily on risk factors (Table 349-4). The presence of any risk factor tips the balance in favor of anticoagulation.

Because of the high annual stroke risk in untreated rheumatic heart disease, primary prophylaxis against stroke has not been studied in a double-blind fashion. These patients generally receive long-term anticoagulation.

Anticoagulation also reduces the risk of embolism in acute MI. Most clinicians recommend a 3-month course of anticoagulation when there is anterior Q-wave infarction, substantial left ventricular dysfunction, congestive heart failure, mural thrombosis, or atrial fibrillation. Warfarin is recommended long-term if atrial fibrillation persists. Warfarin is currently being studied in patients with congestive heart failure.

Thromboembolism is one of the most serious complications of

prosthetic heart valve implantation. Anticoagulation has been proven effective for preventing strokes in this situation, while antiplatelet therapy alone has not. However, coupled with warfarin anticoagulation, aspirin adds substantial benefit. A greater degree of anticoagulation (INR of 3 to 4, depending on valve type) is recommended for some patients with prosthetic heart valves.

If the embolic source cannot be eliminated, anticoagulation should in most cases be continued indefinitely. Many neurologists recommend combining antiplatelet agents with anticoagulants for patients who "fail" one form of therapy (i.e., have another stroke or TIA). This empirical approach subjects the patient to an increased bleeding risk.

Other Causes of Stroke ■ *CAROTID DISEASE* Surgical or endovascular repair of carotid atherosclerosis is preferred over medical therapy for symptomatic carotid artery disease (see section above). Anticoagulation has not been directly compared with antiplatelet therapy for carotid disease.

DURAL SINUS THROMBOSIS Limited evidence exists to support short-term usage of anticoagulants, regardless of the presence of intracranial hemorrhage for venous infarction following sinus thrombosis

STROKE SYNDROMES A careful history and neurologic examination can often localize the region of brain dysfunction; if this region corresponds to a particular arterial distribution, the possible causes responsible for the syndrome can be narrowed. This is of particular importance when the patient presents with a TIA and a normal examination. For example, if a patient develops language loss and a right homonymous hemianopia, a search for causes of left middle cerebral emboli should be performed. A finding of an isolated stenosis of the right internal carotid artery in that patient, for example, suggests an asymptomatic carotid stenosis, and the search for other causes of stroke should continue. The following sections describe the clinical findings of cerebral ischemia associated with cerebral vascular territories depicted in Figs. 349-3 through 349-11. Stroke syndromes are divided into: (1) large-vessel stroke within the anterior circulation, (2) large-vessel stroke within the posterior circulation, and (3) small-vessel disease of either vascular bed.

Stroke Within the Anterior Circulation The internal carotid artery and its branches comprise the anterior circulation of the brain. These vessels can be occluded by intrinsic disease of the vessel (e.g., atherosclerosis or dissection) or by embolic occlusion from a proximal source as discussed above. Occlusion of each major intracranial vessel has distinct clinical manifestations.

MIDDLE CEREBRAL ARTERY Occlusion of the proximal MCA or one of its major branches is most often due to an embolus (artery-to-artery, cardiac, or of unknown source) rather than intracranial atherothrombosis. Atherosclerosis of the proximal MCA may cause distal emboli to the

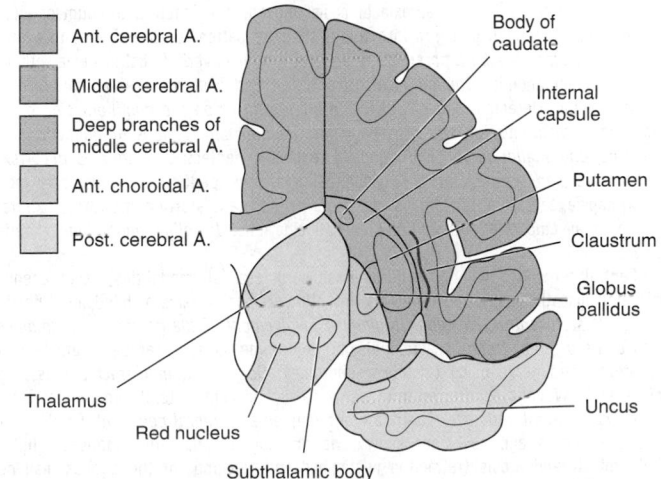

FIGURE 349-4 Diagram of a cerebral hemisphere in coronal section showing the territories of the major cerebral vessels. *(Courtesy of CM Fisher, MD.)*

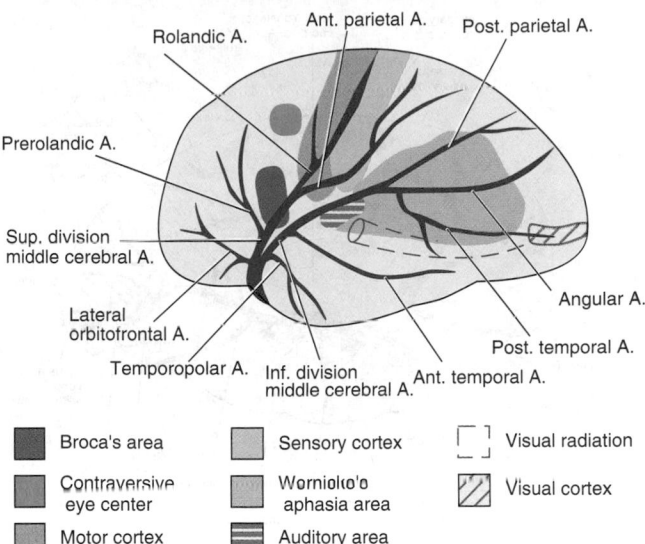

FIGURE 349-5 Diagram of a cerebral hemisphere, lateral aspect, showing the branches and distribution of the middle cerebral artery and the principal regions of cerebral localization. Note the bifurcation of the middle cerebral artery into a superior and inferior division. *(Courtesy of CM Fisher, MD.)*

Signs and symptoms: *Structures involved*

Paralysis of the contralateral face, arm, and leg; sensory impairment over the same area (pinprick, cotton touch, vibration, position, two-point discrimination, stereognosis, tactile localization, barognosis, cutaneographia): *Somatic motor area for face and arm and the fibers descending from the leg area to enter the corona radiata and corresponding somatic sensory system*

Motor aphasia: *Motor speech area of the dominant hemisphere*

Central aphasia, word deafness, anomia, jargon speech, sensory agraphia, acalculia, alexia, finger agnosia, right-left confusion (the last four comprise the Gerstmann syndrome): *Central, suprasylvian speech area and parietooccipital cortex of the dominant hemisphere*

Conduction aphasia: *Central speech area (parietal operculum)*

Apractognosia of the nondominant hemisphere, anosognosia, hemiasomatognosia, unilateral neglect, agnosia for the left half of external space, dressing "apraxia," constructional "apraxia," distortion of visual coordinates, inaccurate localization in the half field, impaired ability to judge distance, upside-down reading, visual illusions (e.g., it may appear that another person walks through a table): *Nondominant parietal lobe (area corresponding to speech area in dominant hemisphere); loss of topographic memory is usually due to a nondominant lesion, occasionally to a dominant one*

Homonymous hemianopia (often homonymous inferior quadrantanopia): *Optic radiation deep to second temporal convolution*

Paralysis of conjugate gaze to the opposite side: *Frontal contraversive field or projecting fibers*

middle cerebral territory or, less commonly, may produce low-flow TIAs. Collateral formation via leptomeningeal vessels often prevents MCA stenosis from becoming symptomatic.

The cortical branches of the MCA supply the lateral surface of the hemisphere except for (1) the frontal pole and a strip along the superomedial border of the frontal and parietal lobes supplied by the ACA, and (2) the lower temporal and occipital pole convolutions supplied by the PCA (Figs. 349-4, 349-6, and 349-7).

The proximal MCA (M1 segment) gives rise to penetrating branches (termed *lenticulostriate arteries*) that supply the putamen, outer globus pallidus, posterior limb of the internal capsule, the adjacent corona radiata, and most of the caudate nucleus. In the sylvian fissure, the MCA in most patients divides into *superior* and *inferior* divisions (M2 branches). Branches of the inferior division supply the inferior parietal and temporal cortex, and those from the superior division supply the frontal and superior parietal cortex (Fig. 349-5).

If the entire MCA is occluded at its origin (blocking both its penetrating and cortical branches) and the distal collaterals are limited, the clinical findings are contralateral hemiplegia, hemianesthesia, homonymous hemianopia, and a day or two of gaze preference to the ipsilateral side. Dysarthria is common because of facial weakness.

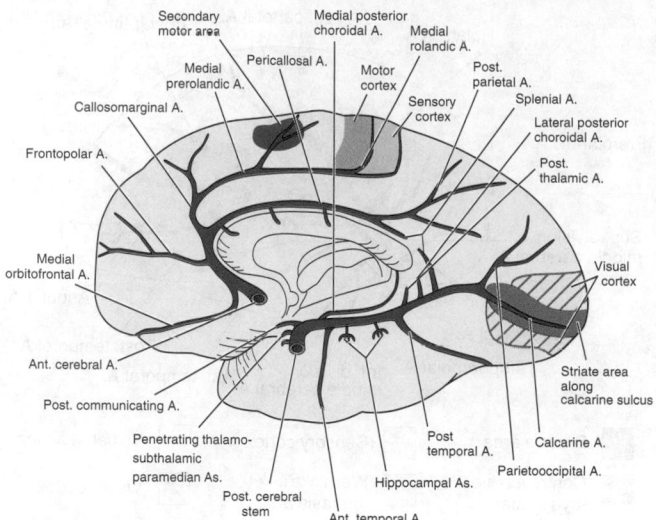

FIGURE 349-6 Diagram of a cerebral hemisphere, medial aspect, showing the branches and distribution of the anterior cerebral artery and the principal regions of cerebral localization. (*Courtesy of CM Fisher, MD.*)

Signs and symptoms: *Structures involved*

Paralysis of opposite foot and leg: *Motor leg area*

A lesser degree of paresis of opposite arm: *Arm area of cortex or fibers descending to corona radiata*

Cortical sensory loss over toes, foot, and leg: *Sensory area for foot and leg*

Urinary incontinence: *Sensorimotor area in paracentral lobule*

Contralateral grasp reflex, sucking reflex, gegenhalten (paratonic rigidity): *Medial surface of the posterior frontal lobe (?) supplemental motor area*

Abulia (akinetic mutism), slowness, delay, intermittent interruption, lack of spontaneity, whispering, reflex distraction to sights and sounds: *Uncertain localization—probably cingulate gyrus and medial inferior portion of frontal, parietal, and temporal lobes*

Impairment of gait and stance (gait apraxia): *Frontal cortex near leg motor area*

Dyspraxia of left limbs, tactile aphasia in left limbs: *Corpus callosum*

When the dominant hemisphere is involved, global aphasia is present also, and when the nondominant hemisphere is affected, anosognosia, constructional apraxia, and neglect are found (Chap. 23).

Complete MCA syndromes occur most often when an embolus occludes the stem of the artery. Cortical collateral blood flow and differing arterial configurations are probably responsible for the development of many partial syndromes. Partial syndromes may also be due to emboli that enter the proximal MCA without complete occlusion, occlude distal MCA branches, or fragment and move distally.

Partial syndromes due to embolic occlusion of a single branch include hand, or arm and hand, weakness alone (brachial syndrome) or facial weakness with nonfluent (Broca) aphasia (Chap. 23), with or without arm weakness (frontal opercular syndrome). A combination of sensory disturbance, motor weakness, and nonfluent aphasia suggests that an embolus has occluded the proximal superior division and infarcted large portions of the frontal and parietal cortices (Fig. 349-5). If a fluent (Wernicke's) aphasia occurs without weakness, the inferior division of the MCA supplying the posterior part (temporal cortex) of the dominant hemisphere is probably involved. Jargon speech and an inability to comprehend written and spoken language are prominent features, often accompanied by a contralateral, homonymous superior quadrantanopia. Hemineglect or spatial agnosia without weakness indicates that the inferior division of the MCA in the nondominant hemisphere is involved.

Occlusion of a lenticulostriate vessel produces small-vessel (lacunar) stroke within the internal capsule. This produces pure motor stroke or sensory-motor stroke contralateral to the lesion. Ischemia within the genu of the internal capsule causes primarily facial weakness followed by arm then leg weakness as the ischemia moves posterior within the capsule. Alternatively, the contralateral hand may become ataxic and dysarthria will be prominent (clumsy hand, dys-

arthria lacunar syndrome). Lacunar infarction affecting the globus pallidus and putamen often has few clinical signs, but parkinsonism and hemiballismus have been reported.

ANTERIOR CEREBRAL ARTERY   The ACA is divided into two segments: the precommunal (A1) circle of Willis, or stem, which connects the internal carotid artery to the anterior communicating artery, and the postcommunal (A2) segment distal to the anterior communicating artery (Figs. 349-3 and 349-7). The A1 segment gives rise to several deep penetrating branches that supply the anterior limb of the internal capsule, the anterior perforate substance, amygdala, anterior hypothalamus, and the inferior part of the head of the caudate nucleus (Fig. 349-4).

Occlusion of the proximal ACA is usually well tolerated because of collateral flow through the anterior communicating artery and collaterals through the MCA and PCA. Occlusion of a single A2 segment results in the contralateral symptoms noted in Fig. 349-6. If both A2 segments arise from a single anterior cerebral stem (contralateral A1

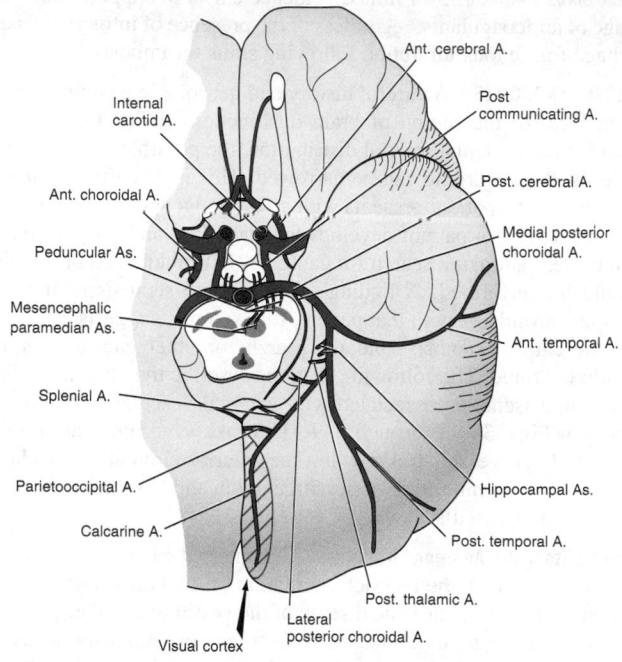

FIGURE 349-7 Inferior aspect of the brain with the branches and distribution of the posterior cerebral artery and the principal anatomic structures shown. (*Courtesy of CM Fisher, MD.*)

Signs and symptoms: *Structures involved*

Peripheral territory (see also Fig. 349-11). Homonymous hemianopia (often upper quadrantic): *Calcarine cortex or optic radiation nearby.* Bilateral homonymous hemianopia, cortical blindness, awareness or denial of blindness; tactile naming, achromatopia (color blindness), failure to see to-and-fro movements, inability to perceive objects not centrally located, apraxia of ocular movements, inability to count or enumerate objects, tendency to run into things that the patient sees and tries to avoid: *Bilateral occipital lobe with possibly the parietal lobe involved.* Verbal dyslexia without agraphia, color anomia: *Dominant calcarine lesion and posterior part of corpus callosum.* Memory defect: *Hippocampal lesion bilaterally or on the dominant side only.* Topographic disorientation and prosopagnosia: *Usually with lesions of nondominant, calcarine, and lingual gyrus.* Simultagnosia, hemivisual neglect: *Dominant visual cortex, contralateral hemisphere.* Unformed visual hallucinations, peduncular hallucinosis, metamorphopsia, teleopsia, illusory visual spread, palinopsia, distortion of outlines, central photophobia: *Calcarine cortex.* Complex hallucinations: *Usually nondominant hemisphere.*

Central territory. Thalamic syndrome: sensory loss (all modalities), spontaneous pain and dysesthesias, choreoathetosis, intention tremor, spasms of hand, mild hemiparesis: *Posteroventral nucleus of thalamus; involvement of the adjacent subthalamic body or its afferent tracts.* Thalamoperforate syndrome: crossed cerebellar ataxia with ipsilateral third nerve palsy (Claude's syndrome): *Dentatothalamic tract and issuing third nerve.* Weber's syndrome: third nerve palsy and contralateral hemiplegia: *Third nerve and cerebral peduncle.* Contralateral hemiplegia: *Cerebral peduncle.* Paralysis or paresis of vertical eye movement, skew deviation, sluggish pupillary responses to light, slight miosis and ptosis (retraction nystagmus and "tucking" of the eyelids may be associated): *Supranuclear fibers to third nerve, interstitial nucleus of Cajal, nucleus of Darkschewitsch, and posterior commissure.* Contralateral rhythmic, ataxic action tremor; rhythmic postural or "holding" tremor (rubral tremor): *Dentatothalamic tract (?).*

plegia, hemianesthesia (hypesthesia), and homonymous hemianopia. However, because this territory is also supplied by penetrating vessels of the proximal MCA and the posterior communicating and posterior choroidal arteries, minimal deficits may occur, and patients frequently recover substantially. Anterior choroidal strokes are usually the result of in situ thrombosis of the vessel, and the vessel is particularly vulnerable to iatrogenic occlusion during surgical clipping of aneurysms arising from the internal carotid artery.

INTERNAL CAROTID ARTERY   The clinical picture of internal carotid occlusion varies depending on whether the cause of ischemia is propagated thrombus, embolism, or low flow. The cortex supplied by the MCA territory is affected most often. With a competent circle of Willis, occlusion may go unnoticed. If the thrombus propagates up the internal carotid artery into the MCA or embolizes it, symptoms are identical to proximal MCA occlusion (see above). Sometimes there is massive infarction of the entire deep white matter and cortical surface. When the origins of both the ACA and MCA are occluded at the top of the carotid artery, abulia or stupor occurs with hemiplegia, hemianes-

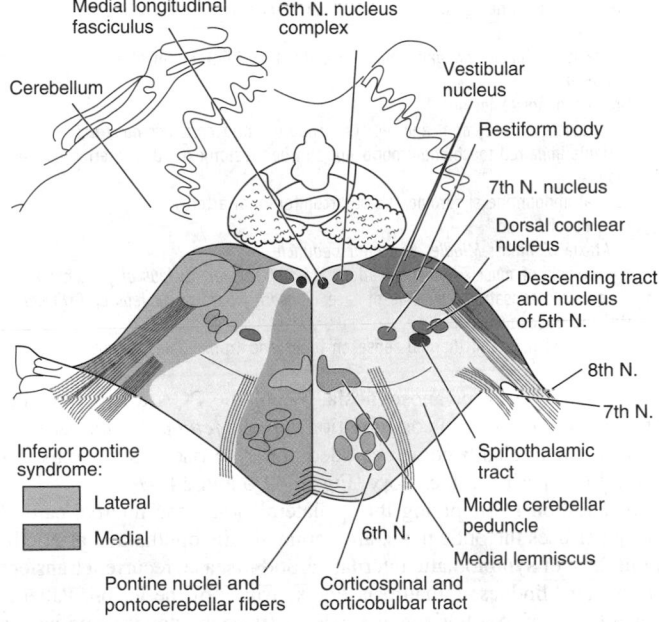

FIGURE 349-8   *(Courtesy of CM Fisher, MD.)*
Signs and symptoms: *Structures involved*

1. Medial medullary syndrome (occlusion of vertebral artery or of branch of vertebral or lower basilar artery)
   On side of lesion
       Paralysis with atrophy of half the tongue: *Ipsilateral twelfth nerve*
   On side opposite lesion
       Paralysis of arm and leg, sparing face; impaired tactile and proprioceptive sense over half the body: *Contralateral pyramidal tract and medial lemniscus*
2. Lateral medullary syndrome (occlusion of any of five vessels may be responsible—vertebral, posterior inferior cerebellar, superior, middle, or inferior lateral medullary arteries)
   On side of lesion
       Pain, numbness, impaired sensation over half the face: *Descending tract and nucleus fifth nerve*
       Ataxia of limbs, falling to side of lesion: *Uncertain—restiform body, cerebellar hemisphere, cerebellar fibers, spinocerebellar tract (?)*
       Nystagmus, diplopia, oscillopsia, vertigo, nausea, vomiting: *Vestibular nucleus*
       Horner's syndrome (miosis, ptosis, decreased sweating): *Descending sympathetic tract*
       Dysphagia, hoarseness, paralysis of palate, paralysis of vocal cord, diminished gag reflex: *Issuing fibers ninth and tenth nerves*
       Loss of taste: *Nucleus and tractus solitarius*
       Numbness of ipsilateral arm, trunk, or leg: *Cuneate and gracile nuclei*
   On side opposite lesion
       Impaired pain and thermal sense over half the body, sometimes face: *Spinothalamic tract*
3. Total unilateral medullary syndrome (occlusion of vertebral artery): Combination of medial and lateral syndromes
4. Lateral pontomedullary syndrome (occlusion of vertebral artery): Combination of lateral medullary and lateral inferior pontine syndrome
5. Basilar artery syndrome (the syndrome of the lone vertebral artery is equivalent): A combination of the various brainstem syndromes plus those arising in the posterior cerebral artery distribution.
       Bilateral long tract signs (sensory and motor; cerebellar and peripheral cranial nerve abnormalities): *Bilateral long tract; cerebellar and peripheral cranial nerves*
       Paralysis or weakness of all extremities, plus all bulbar musculature: *Corticobulbar and corticospinal tracts bilaterally*

segment atresia), the occlusion may affect both hemispheres. Profound abulia (a delay in verbal and motor response) and bilateral pyramidal signs with paraparesis and urinary incontinence result.

ANTERIOR CHOROIDAL ARTERY   This artery arises from the internal carotid artery and supplies the posterior limb of the internal capsule and the white matter posterolateral to it, through which pass some of the geniculocalcarine fibers (Figs. 349-4 and 349-7). The complete syndrome of anterior choroidal artery occlusion consists of contralateral hemi-

FIGURE 349-9   *(Courtesy of CM Fisher, MD.)*
Signs and symptoms: *Structures involved*

1. Medial inferior pontine syndrome (occlusion of paramedian branch of basilar artery)
   On side of lesion
       Paralysis of conjugate gaze to side of lesion (preservation of convergence): *Center for conjugate lateral gaze*
       Nystagmus: *Vestibular nucleus*
       Ataxia of limbs and gait: *Middle cerebellar peduncle (?)*
       Diplopia on lateral gaze: *Abducens nerve*
   On side opposite lesion
       Paralysis of face, arm, and leg: *Corticobulbar and corticospinal tract in lower pons*
       Impaired tactile and proprioceptive sense over half of the body: *Medial lemniscus*
2. Lateral inferior pontine syndrome (occlusion of anterior inferior cerebellar artery)
   On side of lesion
       Horizontal and vertical nystagmus, vertigo, nausea, vomiting, oscillopia: *Vestibular nerve or nucleus*
       Facial paralysis: *Seventh nerve*
       Paralysis of conjugate gaze to side of lesion: *Center for conjugate lateral gaze*
       Deafness, tinnitus: *Auditory nerve or cochlear nucleus*
       Ataxia: *Middle cerebellar peduncle and cerebellar hemisphere*
       Impaired sensation over face: *Descending tract and nucleus fifth nerve*
   On side opposite lesion
       Impaired pain and thermal sense over half the body (may include face): *Spinothalamic tract*

FIGURE 349-10 *(Courtesy of CM Fisher, MD.)*
Signs and symptoms: *Structures involved*

1. Medial midpontine syndrome (paramedian branch of midbasilar artery)
   On side of lesion
       Ataxia of limbs and gait (more prominent in bilateral involvement): *Pontine nuclei*
   On side opposite lesion
       Paralysis of face, arm, and leg: *Corticobulbar and corticospinal tract*
   Variable impaired touch and proprioception when lesion extends posteriorly: *Medial lemniscus*
2. Lateral midpontine syndrome (short circumferential artery)
   On side of lesion
       Ataxia of limbs: *Middle cerebellar peduncle*
       Paralysis of muscles of mastication: *Motor fibers or nucleus of fifth nerve*
       Impaired sensation over side of face: *Sensory fibers or nucleus of fifth nerve*
   On side opposite lesion
       Impaired pain and thermal sense on limbs and trunk: *Spinothalamic tract*

thesia, and aphasia or anosognosia. When the PCA arises from the internal carotid artery (a configuration called a *fetal posterior cerebral artery*), it may also become occluded and give rise to symptoms referable to its peripheral territory (Figs. 349-6 and 349-7).

In addition to supplying the ipsilateral brain, the internal carotid artery perfuses the optic nerve and retina via the ophthalmic artery. In about 25% of symptomatic internal carotid disease, recurrent transient monocular blindness (amaurosis fugax) warns of the lesion. Patients typically describe a horizontal shade that sweeps down or up across the field of vision. They may also complain that their vision was blurred in that eye or that the upper or lower half of vision disappeared. In most cases, these symptoms last only a few minutes. Rarely, ischemia or infarction of the ophthalmic artery or central retinal arteries occurs at the time of cerebral TIA or infarction.

A high-pitched prolonged carotid bruit fading into diastole is often associated with tightly stenotic lesions. As the stenosis grows tighter and flow distal to the stenosis becomes reduced, the bruit becomes fainter and may disappear when occlusion is imminent.

COMMON CAROTID ARTERY All symptoms and signs of internal carotid occlusion may also be present with occlusion of the common carotid artery. Bilateral common carotid artery occlusions at their origin may occur in Takayasu's arteritis (Chap. 306).

Stroke Within the Posterior Circulation The posterior circulation is composed of the paired vertebral arteries, the basilar artery, and the paired posterior cerebral arteries. The vertebral arteries join to form the basilar artery at the pontomedullary junction. The basilar artery divides into two posterior cerebral arteries in the interpeduncular fossa (Fig. 349-3). These major arteries give rise to long and short circumferential branches and to smaller deep penetrating branches that supply the cerebellum, medulla, pons, midbrain, subthalamus, thalamus, hippocampus, and medial temporal and occipital lobes. Occlusion of each vessel produces its own distinctive syndrome.

POSTERIOR CEREBRAL ARTERY In 75% of cases, both PCAs arise from the bifurcation of the basilar artery; in 20%, one has its origin from the ipsilateral internal carotid artery via the posterior communicating artery; in 5%, both originate from the respective ipsilateral internal carotid arteries (Fig. 349-3). The precommunal, or P1, segment of the true posterior cerebral artery is atretic in such cases.

PCA syndromes usually result from atheroma formation or emboli that lodge at the top of the basilar artery; posterior circulation disease may also be caused by dissection of either vertebral artery and fibromuscular dysplasia.

Two clinical syndromes are commonly observed with occlusion of the PCA: (1) *P1 syndrome*: midbrain, subthalamic, and thalamic signs, which are due to disease of the proximal P1 segment of the PCA or its penetrating branches (thalamogeniculate, Percheron, and posterior choroidal arteries); and (2) *P2 syndrome*: cortical temporal and occipital lobe signs, due to occlusion of the P2 segment distal to the junction of the PCA with the posterior communicating artery.

P1 Syndromes Infarction usually occurs in the ipsilateral subthalamus and medial thalamus and in the ipsilateral cerebral peduncle and midbrain (Fig. 349-7). A third nerve palsy with contralateral ataxia (Claude's syndrome) or with contralateral hemiplegia (Weber's syndrome) may result. The ataxia indicates involvement of the red nucleus or dentatorubrothalamic tract; the hemiplegia is localized to the cerebral peduncle. If the subthalamic nucleus is involved, contralateral

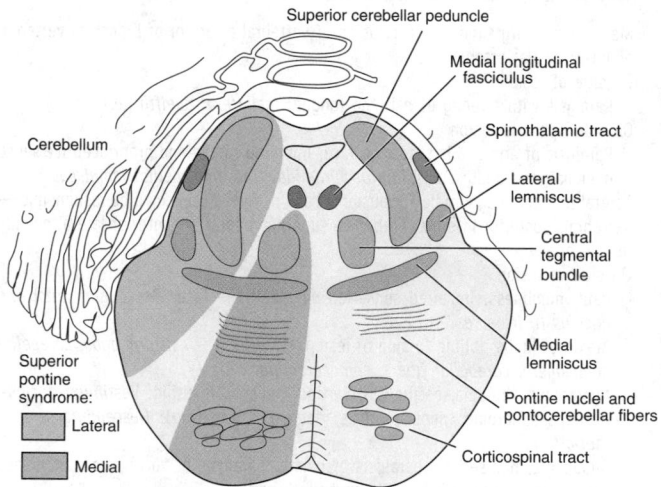

FIGURE 349-11 *(Courtesy of CM Fisher, MD.)*
Signs and symptoms: *Structures involved*

1. Medial superior pontine syndrome (paramedian branches of upper basilar artery)
   On side of lesion
       Cerebellar ataxia (probably): *Superior and/or middle cerebellar peduncle*
       Internuclear ophthalmoplegia: *Medial longitudinal fasciculus*
       Myoclonic syndrome, palate, pharynx, vocal cords, respiratory apparatus, face, oculomotor apparatus, etc.: *Localization uncertain—central tegmental bundle (?), dentate projection (?), inferior olivary nucleus (?)*
   On side opposite lesion
       Paralysis of face, arm, and leg: *Corticobulbar and corticospinal tract*
       Rarely touch, vibration, and position are affected: *Medial lemniscus*
2. Lateral superior pontine syndrome (syndrome of superior cerebellar artery)
   On side of lesion
       Ataxia of limbs and gait, falling to side of lesion: *Middle and superior cerebellar peduncles, superior surface of cerebellum, dentate nucleus*
       Dizziness, nausea, vomiting; horizontal nystagmus: *Vestibular nucleus*
       Paresis of conjugate gaze (ipsilateral): *Pontine contralateral gaze*
       Skew deviation: *Uncertain*
       Miosis, ptosis, decreased sweating over face (Horner's syndrome): *Descending sympathetic fibers*
       Tremor: *Dentate nucleus (?), superior cerebellar peduncle (?)*
   On side opposite lesion
       Impaired pain and thermal sense on face, limbs, and trunk: *Spinothalamic tract*
       Impaired touch, vibration, and position sense, more in leg than arm (there is a tendency to incongruity of pain and touch deficits): *Medial lemniscus (lateral portion)*

hemiballismus may occur. Occlusion of the artery of Percheron produces paresis of upward gaze and drowsiness, and often abulia. Extensive infarction in the midbrain and subthalamus occurring with bilateral proximal PCA occlusion presents as coma, unreactive pupils, bilateral pyramidal signs, and decerebrate rigidity.

Occlusion of the penetrating branches of thalamic and thalamogeniculate arteries produces less extensive thalamic and thalamocapsular lacunar syndromes. The *thalamic Déjerine-Roussy syndrome* consists of contralateral hemisensory loss followed later by an agonizing, searing or burning pain in the affected areas. It is persistent and responds poorly to analgesics. Anticonvulsants (carbamazepine or gabapentin) or tricyclic antidepressants may be beneficial.

P2 Syndromes (See also Fig. 349-7) Occlusion of the distal PCA causes infarction of the medial temporal and occipital lobes. Contralateral homonymous hemianopia with macula sparing is the usual manifestation. Occasionally, only the upper quadrant of visual field is involved. If the visual association areas are spared and only the calcarine cortex is involved, the patient may be aware of visual defects. Medial temporal lobe and hippocampal involvement may cause an acute disturbance in memory, particularly if it occurs in the dominant hemisphere. The defect usually clears because memory has bilateral representation. If the dominant hemisphere is affected and the infarct extends to involve the splenium of the corpus callosum, the patient may demonstrate alexia without agraphia. Visual agnosia for faces, objects, mathematical symbols, and colors and anomia with paraphasic errors (amnestic aphasia) may also occur in this setting, even without callosal involvement. Occlusion of the posterior cerebral artery can produce *peduncular hallucinosis* (visual hallucinations of brightly colored scenes and objects).

Bilateral infarction in the distal PCAs produces cortical blindness (blindness with preserved pupillary light reaction). The patient is often unaware of the blindness or may even deny it (*Anton's syndrome*). Tiny islands of vision may persist, and the patient may report that vision fluctuates as images are captured in the preserved portions. Rarely, only peripheral vision is lost and central vision is spared, resulting in "gun-barrel" vision. Bilateral visual association area lesions may result in *Balint's syndrome*, a disorder of the orderly visual scanning of the environment (Chap. 23), usually resulting from infarctions secondary to low flow in the "watershed" between the distal posterior and middle cerebral artery territories, as occurs after cardiac arrest. Patients may experience persistence of a visual image for several minutes despite gazing at another scene (*palinopia*). Embolic occlusion of the top of the basilar artery can produce any or all of the central or peripheral territory symptoms. The hallmark is the sudden onset of bilateral signs, including ptosis, pupillary asymmetry or lack of reaction to light, and somnolence.

VERTEBRAL AND POSTERIOR INFERIOR CEREBELLAR ARTERIES The vertebral artery, which arises from the innominate artery on the right and the subclavian artery on the left, consists of four segments. The first (V1) extends from its origin to its entrance into the sixth or fifth transverse vertebral foramen. The second segment (V2) traverses the vertebral foramina from C6 to C2. The third (V3) passes through the transverse foramen and circles around the arch of the atlas to pierce the dura at the foramen magnum. The fourth (V4) segment courses upward to join the other vertebral artery to form the basilar artery; only the fourth segment gives rise to branches that supply the brainstem and cerebellum. The posterior inferior cerebellar artery (PICA) in its proximal segment supplies the lateral medulla and, in its distal branches, the inferior surface of the cerebellum.

Atherothrombotic lesions have a predilection for V1 and V4 segments of the vertebral artery. The first segment may become diseased at the origin of the vessel and may produce posterior circulation emboli; collateral flow from the contralateral vertebral artery or the ascending cervical, thyrocervical, or occipital arteries is usually sufficient to prevent low-flow TIAs or stroke. When one vertebral artery is atretic and an atherothrombotic lesion threatens the origin of the other, the collateral circulation, which may also include retrograde

flow down the basilar artery, is often insufficient (Figs. 349-3 and 349-7). In this setting, low-flow TIAs may occur, consisting of syncope, vertigo, and alternating hemiplegia; this state also sets the stage for thrombosis. Disease of the distal fourth segment of the vertebral artery can promote thrombus formation manifest as embolism or with propagation as basilar artery thrombosis. Stenosis proximal to the origin of the posterior inferior cerebellar artery can threaten the lateral medulla and posterior inferior surface of the cerebellum.

If the subclavian artery is occluded proximal to the origin of the vertebral artery, there is a reversal in the direction of blood flow in the ipsilateral vertebral artery. Exercise of the ipsilateral arm may increase demand on vertebral flow, producing posterior circulation TIAs, or "subclavian steal."

Although atheromatous disease rarely narrows the second and third segments of the vertebral artery, this region is subject to dissection, fibromuscular dysplasia, and, rarely, encroachment by osteophytic spurs within the vertebral foramina.

Embolic occlusion or thrombosis of a V4 segment causes ischemia of the lateral medulla. The constellation of vertigo, numbness of the ipsilateral face and contralateral limbs, diplopia, hoarseness, dysarthria, dysphagia, and ipsilateral Horner's syndrome is called the lateral medullary (or Wallenberg's) syndrome (Fig. 349-8). Most cases result from ipsilateral vertebral artery occlusion; in the remainder, PICA occlusion is responsible. Occlusion of the medullary penetrating branches of the vertebral artery or PICA results in partial syndromes. *Hemiparesis is not a feature of vertebral artery occlusion.*

Rarely, a *medial medullary syndrome* occurs with infarction of the pyramid and contralateral hemiparesis of the arm and leg, sparing the face. If the medial lemniscus and emerging hypoglossal nerve fibers are involved, contralateral loss of joint position sense and ipsilateral tongue weakness occur.

Cerebellar infarction with edema can lead to *sudden respiratory arrest* due to raised ICP in the posterior fossa. Drowsiness, Babinski signs, dysarthria, and bifacial weakness may be absent, or present only briefly, before respiratory arrest ensues. Gait unsteadiness, headache, dizziness, nausea, and vomiting may be the only early symptoms and signs and should arouse suspicion of this impending complication, which may require neurosurgical decompression, often with an excellent outcome. Separating these symptoms from those of viral labrynthitis can be a challenge, but headache, neck stiffness, and unilateral dysmetria favor stroke.

BASILAR ARTERY Branches of the basilar artery supply the base of the pons and superior cerebellum and fall into three groups: (1) paramedian, 7 to 10 in number, which supply a wedge of pons on either side of the midline; (2) short circumferential, 5 to 7 in number, which supply the lateral two-thirds of the pons and middle and superior cerebellar peduncles; and (3) bilateral long circumferential (superior cerebellar and anterior inferior cerebellar arteries), which course around the pons to supply the cerebellar hemispheres.

Atheromatous lesions can occur anywhere along the basilar trunk but are most frequent in the proximal basilar and distal vertebral segments. Typically, lesions occlude either the proximal basilar and one or both vertebral arteries. The clinical picture varies depending on the availability of retrograde collateral flow from the posterior communicating arteries. Rarely, dissection of a vertebral artery may involve the basilar artery and, depending on the location of true and false lumen, may produce multiple penetrating artery strokes.

Although atherothrombosis occasionally occludes the distal portion of the basilar artery, emboli from the heart or proximal vertebral or basilar segments are more commonly responsible for "top of the basilar" syndromes.

Because the brainstem contains many structures in close apposition, a diversity of clinical syndromes may emerge with ischemia, reflecting involvement of the corticospinal and corticobulbar tracts, ascending sensory tracts, and cranial nerve nuclei (Figs. 349-9, 349-10, and 349-11).

The symptoms of transient ischemia or infarction in the territory of the basilar artery often do not indicate whether the basilar artery itself or one of its branches is diseased, yet this distinction has important implications for therapy. *The picture of complete basilar occlusion, however, is easy to recognize as a constellation of bilateral long tract signs (sensory and motor) with signs of cranial nerve and cerebellar dysfunction.* A "locked-in" state of preserved consciousness with quadriplegia and cranial nerve signs suggests complete pontine and lower midbrain infarction. The therapeutic goal is to identify *impending* basilar occlusion before devastating infarction occurs. A series of TIAs and a slowly progressive, fluctuating stroke are extremely significant as they often herald an atherothrombotic occlusion of the distal vertebral or proximal basilar artery.

TIAs in the proximal basilar distribution may produce dizziness (often described by patients as "swimming," "swaying," "moving," "unsteadiness" or "light-headedness"). Other symptoms that warn of basilar thrombosis include diplopia, dysarthria, facial or circumoral numbness, and hemisensory symptoms. In general, symptoms of basilar branch TIAs affect one side of the brainstem, whereas symptoms of basilar artery TIAs usually affect both sides, though a "herald" hemiparesis has been emphasized as an initial symptom of basilar occlusion. Most often TIAs, whether due to impending occlusion of the basilar artery or a basilar branch, are short-lived (5 to 30 min) and repetitive, occurring several times a day. The pattern suggests intermittent reduction of flow. Many neurologists treat with heparin to prevent clot propagation.

Atherothrombotic occlusion of the basilar artery with infarction usually causes *bilateral* brainstem signs. A gaze paresis or internuclear ophthalmoplegia associated with ipsilateral hemiparesis may be the only manifestation of bilateral brainstem ischemia. More often, unequivocal signs of bilateral pontine disease are present. Complete basilar thrombosis carries a high mortality.

Occlusion of a branch of the basilar artery usually causes *unilateral* symptoms and signs involving motor, sensory, and cranial nerves. As long as symptoms remain unilateral, concern over pending basilar occlusion should be reduced.

Occlusion of the superior cerebellar artery results in severe ipsilateral cerebellar ataxia, nausea and vomiting, dysarthria, and contralateral loss of pain and temperature sensation over the extremities, body, and face (spino- and trigeminothalamic tract). Partial deafness, ataxic tremor of the ipsilateral upper extremity, Horner's syndrome, and palatal myoclonus may occur rarely. Partial syndromes occur frequently (Fig. 349-11). With large strokes, swelling and mass effects may compress the midbrain or produce hydrocephalus; these symptoms may evolve rapidly. Neurosurgical intervention may be lifesaving in such cases.

Occlusion of the anterior inferior cerebellar artery produces variable degrees of infarction because the size of this artery and the territory it supplies vary inversely with those of the PICA. The principal symptoms include: (1) ipsilateral deafness, facial weakness, vertigo, nausea and vomiting, nystagmus, tinnitus, cerebellar ataxia, Horner's syndrome, and paresis of conjugate lateral gaze; and (2) contralateral loss of pain and temperature sensation. An occlusion close to the origin of the artery may cause corticospinal tract signs (Fig. 349-9).

Occlusion of one of the short circumferential branches of the basilar artery affects the lateral two-thirds of the pons and middle or superior cerebellar peduncle, whereas occlusion of one of the paramedian branches affects a wedge-shaped area on either side of the medial pons (Figs. 349-9 through 349-11).

IMAGING STUDIES (See also Chap. 347)   ■   **Computed Tomographic Scans** CT radiographic images identify or exclude hemorrhage as the cause of stroke, and they identify extraparenchymal hemorrhages, neoplasms, abscesses, and other conditions masquerading as stroke. Scans obtained in the first several hours after an infarction generally show

no abnormality, and the infarct may not be seen reliably for 24 to 48 h. CT may fail to show small ischemic strokes in the posterior fossa because of bone artifact; small infarcts on the cortical surface may also be missed.

Contrast-enhanced CT scans add specificity by showing contrast enhancement of subacute infarcts and allow visualization of venous structures. Coupled with newer generation scanners, CT angiography (CTA) can be performed with administration of intravenous iodinated contrast allowing visualization of the cervical and intracranial arteries. Carotid disease and intracranial vascular occlusions are readily identified with this method (Fig. 349-12). After an intravenous bolus of contrast, deficits in brain perfusion produced by vascular occlusion can also be demonstrated (Fig. 349-12 *C*). CT imaging is also sensitive for detecting subarachnoid hemorrhage, and CTA can readily identify intracranial aneurysms (see below). Because of its speed and wide availability, noncontrast head CT is the imaging modality of choice in patients with acute stroke (Fig. 349-1), and CTA and CT perfusion imaging may also be useful and convenient adjuncts.

Magnetic Resonance Imaging (MRI)   MRI reliably documents the extent and location of infarction in all areas of the brain, including the posterior fossa and cortical surface. It also identifies intracranial hemorrhage and other abnormalities but is less sensitive than CT for detecting acute blood. MRI scanners with magnets of higher field strength produce more reliable and precise images. Diffusion-weighted imaging is more sensitive for early brain infarction than standard MR sequences (Fig. 349-13), as is FLAIR (fluid-attenuated inversion recovery) imaging (Chap. 347). Using intravenous administration of gadolinium contrast, MR perfusion studies can be performed. Brain regions showing poor perfusion but no abnormality on diffusion are considered equivalent to the ischemic penumbra (see "Pathophysiol-

FIGURE 349-12   *A.* Computed tomography (CT) scan of the brain of a patient with a left middle cerebral artery (MCA) stroke of 3 h duration. As an earliest indicator of infarction, the "insular ribbon sign" is caused by edema (darker signal) within the left insular cortex and basal ganglia (*arrow*). *B.* Embolic occlusion of the MCA imaged with CT angiography during the acute stroke (*arrow*). *C.* Cerebral blood flow measured with CT perfusion; blood flow is reduced over a wider region of brain than appeared edematous in *A*. *D.* CT angiogram of a carotid artery showing high-grade stenosis (*arrow*) from atheroma in another patient.

FIGURE 349-13 Magnetic resonance imaging of acute stroke. *A.* Perfusion defect within this right hemisphere (bright signal) imaged after administration of an intravenous bolus of gadolinium contrast. *B.* Cerebral blood flow measured at the same time as in *A;* darker signal reflects decreased blood flow. *C.* Diffusion-weighted image obtained 5 h after onset of a right middle cerebral artery stroke; bright signal indicates regions of restricted diffusion that will progress to infarction. The discrepancy between the region of poor perfusion shown in *A* and *B* and the diffusion deficit, is called *diffusion-perfusion mismatch* and is a measure of the ischemic penumbra. Without specific therapy the region of infarction expands to match the perfusion deficit, as shown in the diffusion weighted image in *D* obtained 5 days later. *(Courtesy of Gregory Albers and Vincent Thijs, MD, Stanford University)*

ogy of Ischemic Stroke," above), and patients showing large regions of mismatch may be better candidates for acute revascularization. MR angiography is highly sensitive for stenosis of extracranial internal carotid arteries and of large intracranial vessels. With higher degrees of stenosis, MR angiography tends to overestimate the degree of stenosis when compared to conventional x-ray angiography. MRI with fat saturation is an imaging sequence used to visualize extra- or intracranial arterial dissection. This sensitive technique images clotted blood within the dissected vessel wall.

MRI is less sensitive for acute blood products than CT and is more expensive and time consuming and less readily available. Claustrophobia also limits its application. Most acute stroke protocols use CT because of these limitations. However, MRI may be useful outside the acute period by more clearly defining the extent and possible source of a stroke.

Cerebral Angiography Conventional x-ray cerebral angiography is the "gold standard" for identifying and quantifying atherosclerotic stenoses of the cerebral arteries and for identifying and characterizing other pathologies, including aneurysm, vasospasm, intraluminal thrombi, fibromuscular dysplasia, arteriovenous fistula, vasculitis, and collateral channels of blood flow. Endovascular techniques, which are evolving rapidly, can be used to deploy stents within delicate intracranial vessels, to perform balloon angioplasty of stenotic lesions, and to treat intracranial aneurysms by embolization. Recent studies have documented that intraarterial delivery of thrombolytic agents to patients with acute MCA stroke can effectively recanalize vessels and improve clinical outcomes. Although its use is investigational in many centers, cerebral angiography coupled with endovascular techniques for cerebral revascularization may become routine in the near future. Conven-

tional angiography carries risks of arterial damage, groin hemorrhage, embolic stroke, and renal failure from contrast nephropathy, so it should be reserved for situations where less invasive means are inadequate.

Ultrasound Techniques Stenosis at the origin of the internal carotid artery can be identified and quantified reliably by ultrasonography that combines a B-mode ultrasound image with a Doppler ultrasound assessment of flow velocity ("duplex" ultrasound). Transcranial Doppler (TCD) assessment of middle, anterior, and posterior cerebral artery flow and of vertebrobasilar flow is also useful. This latter technique can detect stenotic lesions in the large intracranial arteries because such lesions increase systolic flow velocity. In many cases, MR angiography combined with carotid and transcranial ultrasound studies eliminates the need for conventional x-ray angiography in evaluating vascular stenosis. Alternatively, CT angiography of the entire head and neck can be performed during the initial imaging of acute stroke. Because this images the entire arterial system relevant to stroke, with the exception of the heart, much of the clinician's stroke workup can be completed with one imaging study.

Perfusion Techniques Both xenon techniques (principally xenon-CT) and PET can quantify cerebral blood flow. These tools are generally used for research (Chap. 347) but can be useful for determining the significance of arterial stenosis and planning for revascularization surgery. Single photon emission tomography (SPECT), CT perfusion, and MR perfusion techniques report relative cerebral blood flow. Since CT imaging is used as the initial imaging modality for acute stroke, many centers now combine both CT angiography and CT perfusion imaging together with the noncontrast CT scan. CT perfusion imaging increases the sensitivity and improves accuracy in imaging ischemic brain. Alternatively, MR perfusion can be combined with MR diffusion imaging to identify the ischemic penumbra as the mismatch between these two imaging sequences (Fig. 349-13). The ability to image the ischemic penumbra allows more judicious selection of patients who may or may not benefit from acute interventions such as thrombolysis or investigational neuroprotective strategies.

INTRACRANIAL HEMORRHAGE

Hemorrhages are classified by their location and the underlying vascular pathology. Bleeding into subdural and epidural spaces is principally produced by trauma (Chap. 357). Intraparenchymal, intraventricular, and subarachnoid hemorrhage will be considered here.

DIAGNOSIS Intracranial hemorrhage is often discovered on noncontrast CT imaging of the brain during the acute evaluation of stroke. Since CT is more sensitive than routine MRI for acute blood, CT imaging is the preferred method for acute stroke evaluation (Fig. 349-1). The location of the hemorrhage narrows the differential diagnosis to a few entities. Table 349-6 lists the causes and anatomic spaces involved in hemorrhages.

EMERGENCY MANAGEMENT Close attention should be paid to airway management since a reduction in the level of consciousness is common. The initial blood pressure should be maintained until the results of the CT scan are reviewed. Patients with acute SAH should have blood pressure lowered to a normal range with nonvasodilating agents such as nicardipine, labetalol, or esmolol. Patients with cerebellar hemorrhages or with depressed mental status and radiographic evidence of hydrocephalus should undergo urgent neurosurgical evaluation. Based on the clinical examination and CT findings, further imaging studies may be necessary, including MRI or conventional x-ray angiography. Stuporous or comatose patients generally are treated presumptively for elevated ICP, with tracheal intubation and hyperventilation, mannitol administration, and elevation of the head of the bed while surgical consultation is obtained (Chap. 258).

SUBARACHNOID HEMORRHAGE Excluding head trauma, the most common cause of SAH is rupture of a saccular aneurysm. Other causes

TABLE 349-6 Causes of Intracranial Hemorrhage

Cause	Location	Comments
Head trauma	Intraparenchymal: frontal lobes, anterior temporal lobes; subarachnoid	Coup and contracoup injury during brain deceleration
Hypertensive hemorrhage	Putamen, globus pallidus, thalamus, cerebellar hemisphere, pons	Chronic hypertension produces hemorrhage from small (~100 μm) vessels in these regions
Transformation of prior ischemic infarction	Basal ganglion, subcortical regions, lobar	Occurs in 1–6% of ischemic strokes with predilection for large hemispheric infarctions
Metastatic brain tumor	Lobar	Lung, choriocarcinoma, melanoma, renal cell carcinoma, thyroid, atrial myxoma
Coagulopathy	Any	Uncommon cause; often associated with prior stroke or underlying vascular anomaly
Drug	Lobar, subarachnoid	Cocaine, amphetamine, phenylpropranolamine
Arteriovenous malformation	Lobar, intraventricular, subarachnoid	Risk is ~2–4% per year for bleeding
Aneurysm	Subarachnoid, intraparenchymal, rarely subdural	Mycotic and nonmycotic forms of aneurysms
Amyloid angiopathy	Lobar	Degenerative disease of intracranial vessels; linkage to Alzheimer's disease, rare in patients <60
Cavernous angioma	Intraparenchymal	Multiple cavernous angiomas linked to chromosome 7q
Dural arteriovenous fistula	Lobar, rarely subarachnoid	Produces bleeding by venous hypertension
Capillary telangiectasias	Usually brainstem	Rare cause of hemorrhage

include bleeding from a vascular anomaly and extension into the subarachnoid space from a primary intracerebral hemorrhage. Some idiopathic SAHs are localized to the perimesencephalic cisterns and are benign; they probably have a venous or capillary source, and angiography is unrevealing.

Saccular ("Berry") Aneurysm Autopsy and angiography studies have found that about 2% of adults harbor intracranial aneurysms, for a prevalence of 4 million persons in the United States; the aneurysm will rupture, producing SAH, in 25,000 to 30,000 cases per year. For patients who arrive alive at hospital, the mortality rate over the next month is about 45%. Of those who survive, more than half are left with major neurologic deficits as a result of the initial hemorrhage, cerebral vasospasm with infarction, or hydrocephalus. If the patient survives but the aneurysm is not obliterated, the rate of rebleeding is about 20% in the first 2 weeks and about 3% per year afterwards. Given these alarming figures, the major therapeutic emphasis is on preventing the predictable early complications of the SAH.

Unruptured, asymptomatic aneurysms are much less dangerous than a recently ruptured aneurysm. The annual risk of rupture for aneurysms <10 mm in size is ~0.1%, and for aneurysms ≥10 mm in size is ~0.5 to 1%; the surgical morbidity far exceeds these percentages. As more data become available, a true risk-benefit analysis for treating these aneurysms will result.

Giant aneurysms, those >2.5 cm in diameter, occur at the same sites (see below) as small aneurysms and account for 5% of cases. The three most common locations are the terminal internal carotid artery, MCA bifurcation, and top of the basilar artery. Their risk of rupture is about 6% in the first year after identification and may remain high indefinitely. They often cause symptoms by compressing the adjacent brain or cranial nerves.

Mycotic aneurysms are usually located distal to the first bifurcation of major arteries of the circle of Willis. Most result from infected emboli due to bacterial endocarditis causing septic degeneration of arteries and subsequent dilatation and rupture. Whether these lesions should be sought and repaired prior to rupture, or left to heal spontaneously, is controversial.

PATHOPHYSIOLOGY Saccular aneurysms occur at the bifurcations of the large to medium-sized intracranial arteries; rupture is into the subarachnoid space in the basal cisterns and often into the parenchyma of the adjacent brain. Approximately 85% of aneurysms occur in the anterior circulation, mostly on the circle of Willis. About 20% of patients have multiple aneurysms, many at mirror sites bilaterally. As an aneurysm develops, it typically forms a neck with a dome. The length of the neck and the size of the dome vary greatly and are factors that are important in planning neurosurgical obliteration or endovascular embolization. The arterial internal elastic lamina disappears at the base of the neck. The media thins, and connective tissue replaces smooth-muscle cells. At the site of rupture (most often the dome) the wall thins, and the tear that allows bleeding is often no more than 0.5 mm long. Aneurysm size and site are important in predicting risk of rupture. Those >7 mm in diameter and those at the top of the basilar artery and at the origin of the posterior communicating artery are at greater risk of rupture.

CLINICAL MANIFESTATIONS Most unruptured intracranial aneurysms are completely asymptomatic. Symptoms are usually due to rupture and resultant SAH. At the moment of aneurysmal rupture with major SAH, the ICP suddenly rises. This may account for the sudden transient loss of consciousness that occurs in nearly half of patients. Sudden loss of consciousness may be preceded by a brief moment of excruciating headache, but most patients first complain of headache upon regaining consciousness. In 10% of cases, aneurysmal bleeding is severe enough to cause loss of consciousness for several days. In about 45% of cases, severe headache associated with exertion is the presenting complaint. The patient often calls the headache "the worst headache of my life." Occasionally these ruptures may present as headache of only moderate intensity or as a change in the patient's usual headache pattern. The headache is usually generalized, often with neck stiffness, and vomiting is common.

Although sudden headache in the absence of focal neurologic symptoms is the hallmark of aneurysmal rupture, focal neurologic deficits may occur. Anterior communicating artery or MCA bifurcation aneurysms may rupture into the adjacent brain or subdural space and form a hematoma large enough to produce mass effect. The common deficits that result include hemiparesis, aphasia, and abulia.

Occasionally, prodromal symptoms suggest the location of a progressively enlarging unruptured aneurysm. A third cranial nerve palsy, particularly when associated with pupillary dilatation, loss of ipsilateral (but retained contralateral) light reflex, and focal pain above or behind the eye, may occur with an expanding aneurysm at the junction of the posterior communicating artery and the internal carotid artery. A sixth nerve palsy may indicate an aneurysm in the cavernous sinus, and visual field defects can occur with an expanding supraclinoid carotid or anterior cerebral artery aneurysm. Occipital and posterior cervical pain may signal a posterior inferior cerebellar artery or anterior inferior cerebellar artery aneurysm. Pain in or behind the eye and in the low temple can occur with an expanding MCA aneurysm. Thunderclap headache is a variant of migraine that simulates a SAH. Before concluding that a patient with sudden, severe headache has thunderclap migraine, a definitive workup for aneurysm or other intracranial pathology is required.

Aneurysms can undergo small ruptures and leaks of blood into the subarachnoid space, so-called sentinel bleeds. Sudden unexplained headache at any location should raise suspicion of SAH and be investigated, because a major hemorrhage may be imminent.

DELAYED NEUROLOGIC DEFICITS There are four major causes of delayed neurologic deficits: rerupture, hydrocephalus, vasospasm, and hyponatremia.

1. *Rerupture.* The incidence of rerupture of an untreated aneurysm in the first month following SAH is ~30%, with the peak in the first 7 days. Rerupture is associated with a 60% mortality and poor outcome. Early treatment eliminates this risk.

2. *Hydrocephalus.* Acute hydrocephalus can cause stupor and coma. More often, subacute hydrocephalus develops over a few days or weeks and causes progressive drowsiness or slowed mentation (abulia) with incontinence. Hydrocephalus is differentiated from cerebral vasospasm with a CT scan, TCD ultrasound, or conventional x-ray angiography. Hydrocephalus may clear spontaneously or require temporary ventricular drainage. Chronic hydrocephalus may develop weeks to months after SAH and manifest as gait difficulty, incontinence, or impaired mentation. Subtle signs may be a lack of initiative in conversation or a failure to recover independence.

3. *Vasospasm.* Narrowing of the arteries at the base of the brain following SAH causes symptomatic ischemia and infarction in ~30% of patients and is the major cause of delayed morbidity and death. Signs of ischemia appear 4 to 14 days after the hemorrhage, most often at 7 days. The severity and distribution of vasospasm determine whether infarction will occur.

Delayed vasospasm is believed to result from direct effects of clotted blood and its breakdown products on the artery. In general, the more blood that surrounds the arteries, the greater the chance of symptomatic vasospasm. Spasm of major arteries produces symptoms referable to the appropriate vascular territory (see "Stroke Syndromes," above). All of these focal symptoms may present abruptly, fluctuate, or develop over a few days. In most cases, focal spasm is preceded by a decline in mental status.

Vasospasm can be detected reliably with conventional x-ray angiography, but this invasive procedure is expensive and carries risk of stroke and other complications. TCD ultrasound is based on the principle that the velocity of blood flow within an artery will rise as the lumen diameter is narrowed. By directing the probe along the MCA and proximal ACA, carotid terminus, vertebral, and basilar arteries on a daily or every-other-day basis, vasospasm can be reliably detected and treatments initiated to prevent cerebral ischemia (see below). CT angiography is another method that can reliably detect vasospasm.

Severe cerebral edema in patients with infarction from vasospasm may increase the ICP enough to reduce cerebral perfusion pressure. Treatment is with mannitol and hyperventilation (Chap. 258).

4. *Hyponatremia.* Hyponatremia may be profound and develop quickly in the first 2 weeks following SAH. It usually results from inappropriate secretion of vasopressin (Chap. 319) and secretion of atrial and brain natriuretic factors, which produce a natriuresis. This "cerebral salt-wasting syndrome" clears over the course of 1 to 2 weeks and, in the setting of SAH, should not be treated with free-water restriction as this may increase the risk of stroke (see below).

LABORATORY EVALUATION AND IMAGING (Fig. 349-14) The hallmark of aneurysmal rupture is blood in the cerebrospinal fluid (CSF). More than 95% of cases have enough blood to be visualized on a high-quality noncontrast CT scan obtained within 72 h. If the scan fails to establish the diagnosis of SAH and no mass lesion or obstructive hydrocephalus is found, a lumbar puncture should be performed to establish the presence of subarachnoid blood. Lysis of the red blood cells and subsequent conversion of hemoglobin to bilirubin stains the spinal fluid yellow within 6 to 12 h of SAH. This xanthochromic spinal fluid peaks in intensity at 48 h and lasts for 1 to 4 weeks, depending on the amount of subarachnoid blood.

The extent and location of subarachnoid blood on noncontrast CT scan help locate the underlying aneurysm, identify the cause of any neurologic deficit, and predict delayed vasospasm. A high incidence of symptomatic vasospasm in the MCA and ACA has been found when early CT scans show subarachnoid clots >5 × 3 mm in the basal cisterns or layers of blood >1 mm thick in the cerebral fissures. CT scans less reliably predict vasospasm in the vertebral, basilar, or posterior cerebral arteries.

FIGURE 349-14 Subarachnoid hemorrhage. *A.* Computed tomography (CT) angiography revealing an aneurysm of the left superior cerebellar artery. *B.* Noncontrast CT scan at the level of the third ventricle revealing subarachnoid blood in the left sylvian fissure (bright) and within the left lateral ventricle. *C.* Conventional anteroposterior x-ray angiogram of the right vertebral and basilar artery showing the large aneurysm. *D.* Conventional angiogram following coil embolization of the aneurysm, whereby the aneurysm body is filled with platinum delivered through a microcatheter navigated from the femoral artery into the aneurysm neck.

Lumbar puncture prior to an imaging procedure is indicated only if a CT scan is not available at the time of the suspected SAH. Once the diagnosis of hemorrhage from a ruptured saccular aneurysm is suspected, four-vessel conventional x-ray angiography (both carotids and both vertebrals) is generally performed to localize and define the anatomic details of the aneurysm and to determine if other unruptured aneurysms exist (Fig. 349-14). CT angiography is an alternative method for locating the aneurysm and may be sufficient to plan definitive therapy. At some centers, the ruptured aneurysm can be treated using endovascular techniques at the time of the initial angiogram (see below).

The ECG frequently shows ST-segment and T-wave changes similar to those associated with cardiac ischemia. Prolonged QRS complex, increased QT interval, and prominent "peaked" or deeply inverted symmetric T waves are usually secondary to the intracranial hemorrhage. There is evidence that structural myocardial lesions produced by circulating catecholamines may occur after SAH, causing reversible cardiomyopathy sufficient to cause shock or congestive heart failure. Serious ventricular dysrhythmias are unusual.

Close monitoring (daily or twice daily) of electrolytes is important because hyponatremia can occur precipitously during the first 2 weeks following SAH (see above).

Rx TREATMENT

Early aneurysm repair prevents rerupture and allows the safe application of techniques to improve blood flow (e.g., induced hypertension and hypervolemia) should symptomatic vasospasm develop. An aneurysm can be "clipped" by a neurosurgeon or "coiled" by a neurointerventional radiologist. Surgical repair involves placing a metal clip across the aneurysm neck, thereby immediately eliminating the risk of rebleeding. This approach requires craniotomy and brain retraction, which is associated with neurologic morbidity. The newer endovascular technique involves placing platinum coils within the aneurysm via a catheter that is passed from the femoral artery. The aneurysm is packed tightly to enhance thrombosis and over time is walled-off from the circulation (Fig. 349-14). The only prospective randomized trial of surgery versus endovascular treatment for ruptured aneurysm, the International Study of Aneurysm Treatment (ISAT), was terminated early when 24% of patients treated with endovascular therapy were dead or dependent at 1 year compared to 31% treated with surgery, a 23% relative reduction. However, some aneurysms have a morphology that is not amenable to coiling, and only a few endovascular centers are available world-wide. Thus, surgery remains an important treatment option.

The medical management of SAH centers on protecting the airway, managing blood pressure before and after aneurysm treatment, preventing rebleeding prior to treatment, managing vasospasm, treating hydrocephalus, treating hyponatremia, and preventing pulmonary embolus.

Intracranial hypertension following aneurysmal rupture occurs secondary to subarachnoid blood, parenchymal hematoma, acute hydrocephalus, or loss of vascular autoregulation. Patients who are stuporous should undergo emergent ventriculostomy to prevent cerebral ischemia from high ICP. Medical therapies designed to combat raised ICP (e.g., mild hyperventilation, mannitol, and sedation) can also be used as needed (Chap. 258). High ICP refractory to treatment is a poor prognostic sign.

Prior to definitive treatment of the ruptured aneurysm, care is required to maintain adequate cerebral perfusion pressure while avoiding excessive elevation of arterial pressure. Occasionally an intracranial hematoma causing neurologic deterioration requires removal.

Because rebleeding is common, all patients who are not candidates for early aneurysm repair are put on bed rest in a quiet room and are given stool softeners to prevent straining. If headache or neck pain is severe, mild sedation and analgesia are prescribed. Extreme sedation is avoided because it can obscure changes in neurologic status. Adequate hydration is necessary to avoid a decrease in blood volume predisposing to brain ischemia.

Seizures are uncommon at the onset of aneurysmal rupture. The quivering, jerking, and extensor posturing that often accompany loss of consciousness are probably related to the sharp rise in ICP or, perhaps, acute generalized vasospasm. However, phenytoin is often given as prophylactic therapy since a seizure may promote rebleeding.

Glucocorticoids may help reduce the head and neck ache caused by the irritative effect of the subarachnoid blood. There is no good evidence that they reduce cerebral edema, are neuroprotective, or reduce vascular injury, and their routine use therefore is not recommended.

Antifibrinolytic agents are not routinely prescribed but may be considered in patients in whom aneurysm treatment cannot proceed immediately. They are associated with a reduced incidence of aneurysmal rerupture but are also associated with an increased incidence of delayed cerebral infarction and DVT.

Vasospasm remains the leading cause of morbidity and mortality following aneurysmal SAH and treatment of the aneurysm. Treatment with the calcium channel antagonist nimodipine (60 mg orally every 4 h) improves outcome, perhaps by preventing ischemic injury rather than reducing the risk of vasospasm. Nimodipine can cause significant hypotension in some patients, which may worsen cerebral ischemia in patients with vasospasm. Symptomatic cerebral vasospasm can also be treated by increasing the cerebral perfusion pressure by raising mean arterial pressure through plasma volume expansion and the judicious use of vasopressor agents, usually phenylephrine or dopamine. Raised perfusion pressure has been associated with clinical improvement in many patients, but high arterial pressure may promote rebleeding in unprotected aneurysms. Treatment with induced hypertension

and hypervolemia generally requires monitoring of arterial and central venous pressures. Volume expansion helps prevent hypotension, augments cardiac output, and reduces blood viscosity by reducing the hematocrit. This method is called "triple-H" (hypertension, hemodilution, and hypervolemic) therapy.

If symptomatic vasospasm persists despite optimal medical therapy, intraarterial vasodilators and percutaneous transluminal angioplasty are considered. Vasodilatation following angioplasty appears to be permanent, allowing triple-H therapy to be tapered sooner. The pharmacologic vasodilators (verapamil and nicardipine) do not last more than 8 to 24 h, and therefore multiple treatments may be required until the subarachnoid blood is reabsorbed.

Acute hydrocephalus can cause stupor or coma. It may clear spontaneously or require temporary ventricular drainage. When chronic hydrocephalus develops, ventricular shunting is the treatment of choice.

Free-water restriction is contraindicated in patients with SAH at risk for vasospasm because hypovolemia and hypotension may occur and precipitate cerebral ischemia. Many patients continue to experience a decline in serum sodium despite receiving parenteral fluids containing normal saline. Frequently, supplemental oral salt coupled with normal saline will mitigate hyponatremia, but often patients also require hypertonic saline. Care must be taken not to correct serum sodium too quickly in patients with marked hyponatremia of several days' duration, as central pontine myelinolysis (Chap. 258) may occur.

All patients should have pneumatic compression stockings applied to prevent pulmonary embolism. Systemic heparin is contraindicated in patients with ruptured and untreated aneurysms; it is a relative contraindication following craniotomy, and it may delay thrombosis of a coiled aneurysm.

INTRAPARENCHYMAL HEMORRHAGE Intraparenchymal hemorrhage is the most common type of intracranial hemorrhage. It accounts for about 10% of all strokes and is associated with a 50% case fatality rate. Incidence rates are particularly high in Asians and African Americans. Hypertension, trauma, and cerebral amyloid angiopathy cause the majority of these hemorrhages. Advanced age and heavy alcohol consumption increase the risk, and cocaine use is one of the most important causes in the young.

Hypertensive Intraparenchymal Hemorrhage ■ *PATHOPHYSIOLOGY* Hypertensive intraparenchymal hemorrhage (hypertensive hemorrhage or hypertensive intracerebral hemorrhage) usually results from spontaneous rupture of a small penetrating artery deep in the brain. The most common sites are the basal ganglia (putamen, thalamus, and adjacent deep white matter), deep cerebellum, and pons. When hemorrhages occur in other brain areas or in nonhypertensive patients, greater consideration should be given to hemorrhagic disorders, neoplasms, vascular malformations, and other causes. The small arteries in these areas seem most prone to hypertension-induced vascular injury. The hemorrhage may be small or a large clot may form and compress adjacent tissue, causing herniation and death. Blood may dissect into the ventricular space, which substantially increases morbidity and may cause hydrocephalus.

Most hypertensive intraparenchymal hemorrhages develop over 30 to 90 min, whereas those associated with anticoagulant therapy may evolve for as long as 24 to 48 h. Within 48 h macrophages begin to phagocytize the hemorrhage at its outer surface. After 1 to 6 months, the hemorrhage is generally resolved to a slitlike orange cavity lined with glial scar and hemosiderin-laden macrophages.

CLINICAL MANIFESTATIONS Although not particularly associated with exertion, intracerebral hemorrhages almost always occur while the patient is awake and sometimes when stressed. The hemorrhage generally presents as the abrupt onset of focal neurologic deficit. Seizures are uncommon. The focal deficit typically worsens steadily over 30 to 90 min and is associated with a diminishing level of consciousness and signs of increased ICP, such as headache and vomiting.

The putamen is the most common site for hypertensive hemorrhage, and the adjacent internal capsule is invariably damaged (Fig.

FIGURE 349-15   Transaxial noncontrast computed tomography scan through the region of the basal ganglia reveals a hematoma involving the left putamen in a patient with rapidly progressive onset of right hemiparesis. This is a typical hypertensive hemorrhage.

349-15). Contralateral hemiparesis is therefore the sentinel sign. When mild, the face sags on one side over 5 to 30 min, speech becomes slurred, the arm and leg gradually weaken, and the eyes deviate away from the side of the hemiparesis. The paralysis may worsen until the affected limbs become flaccid or extend rigidly. When hemorrhages are large, drowsiness gives way to stupor as signs of upper brainstem compression appear. Coma ensues, accompanied by deep, irregular, or intermittent respiration, a dilated and fixed ipsilateral pupil, and decerebrate rigidity. In milder cases, edema in adjacent brain tissue may cause progressive deterioration over 12 to 72 h.

Thalamic hemorrhages also produce a contralateral hemiplegia or hemiparesis from pressure on, or dissection into, the adjacent internal capsule. A prominent sensory deficit involving all modalities is usually present. Aphasia, often with preserved verbal repetition, may occur after hemorrhage into the dominant thalamus, and apractognosia or mutism occurs in some cases of nondominant hemorrhage. There may also be a homonymous visual field defect. Thalamic hemorrhages cause several typical ocular disturbances by virtue of extension medially into the upper midbrain. These include deviation of the eyes downward and inward so that they appear to be looking at the nose, unequal pupils with absence of light reaction, skew deviation with the eye opposite the hemorrhage displaced downward and medially, ipsilateral Horner's syndrome, absence of convergence, paralysis of vertical gaze, and retraction nystagmus. Patients may later develop a chronic, contralateral pain syndrome (Déjerine-Roussy syndrome).

In pontine hemorrhages, deep coma with quadriplegia usually occurs over a few minutes. There is often prominent decerebrate rigidity and "pin-point" (1 mm) pupils that react to light. There is impairment of reflex horizontal eye movements evoked by head turning (doll's-head or oculocephalic maneuver) or by irrigation of the ears with ice water (Chap. 257). Hyperpnea, severe hypertension, and hyperhidrosis are common. Death often occurs within a few hours, but small hemorrhages are compatible with survival.

Cerebellar hemorrhages usually develop over several hours and are characterized by occipital headache, repeated vomiting, and ataxia of gait. In mild cases there may be no other neurologic signs other than gait ataxia. Dizziness or vertigo may be prominent. There is often paresis of conjugate lateral gaze toward the side of the hemorrhage, forced deviation of the eyes to the opposite side, or an ipsilateral sixth nerve palsy. Less frequent ocular signs include blepharospasm, involuntary closure of one eye, ocular bobbing, and skew deviation. Dysarthria and dysphagia may occur. As the hours pass, the patient often becomes stuporous and then comatose from brainstem compression or

obstructive hydrocephalus; immediate surgical evacuation before brainstem compression occurs may be lifesaving. Hydrocephalus from fourth ventricle compression can be relieved by external ventricular drainage, but definitive hematoma evacuation is essential for survival. If the deep cerebellar nuclei are spared, full recovery is common.

Lobar Hemorrhage   Symptoms and signs appear over several minutes. Most lobar hemorrhages are small and cause a restricted clinical syndrome that simulates an embolus to an artery supplying one lobe. For example, the major neurologic deficit with an occipital hemorrhage is hemianopia; with a left temporal hemorrhage, aphasia and delirium; with a parietal hemorrhage, hemisensory loss; and with frontal hemorrhage, arm weakness. Large hemorrhages may be associated with stupor or coma if they compress the thalamus or midbrain. Most patients with lobar hemorrhages have focal headaches, and more than half vomit or are drowsy. Stiff neck and seizures are uncommon.

Other Causes of Intracerebral Hemorrhage   *Cerebral amyloid angiopathy* is a disease of the elderly in which arteriolar degeneration occurs and amyloid is deposited in the walls of the cerebral arteries. Amyloid angiopathy causes both single and recurrent lobar hemorrhages and is probably the most common cause of lobar hemorrhage in the elderly. It accounts for some intracranial hemorrhages associated with intravenous thrombolysis given for MI. This disorder can be suspected in patients who present with multiple hemorrhages (and infarcts) over several months or years, or in patients with "micro-bleeds" seen on brain MRI sequences sensitive for hemosiderin, but it is definitively diagnosed by demonstration of Congo red staining of amyloid in cerebral vessels. There is no specific therapy.

Cocaine is a frequent cause of stroke in young (age < 45) patients. Intracerebral hemorrhage, ischemic stroke, and SAH are all associated with cocaine use. Angiographic findings vary from completely normal arteries to large-vessel occlusion or stenosis, vasospasm, or changes consistent with vasculitis. The mechanism of cocaine-related stroke is not known, but cocaine enhances sympathetic activity causing acute, sometimes severe, hypertension, and this may lead to hemorrhage. Slightly more than half of cocaine-related intracranial hemorrhages are intracerebral, and the rest are subarachnoid. In cases of SAH, a saccular aneurysm is usually identified. Presumably, acute hypertension causes aneurysmal rupture.

Head injury often causes intracranial bleeding. The common sites are intracerebral (especially temporal and inferior frontal lobes) and into the subarachnoid, subdural, and epidural spaces. Trauma must be considered in any patient with an unexplained acute neurologic deficit (hemiparesis, stupor, or confusion), particularly if the deficit occurred in the context of a fall (Chap. 357).

Intracranial hemorrhages associated with *anticoagulant therapy* can occur at any location; they are often lobar or subdural. Anticoagulant-related intracerebral hemorrhages may evolve slowly, over 24 to 48 h. Coagulopathy should be reversed with fresh-frozen plasma or factor replacement and vitamin K to limit the volume of hemorrhage. When intracerebral hemorrhage is associated with thrombocytopenia (platelet count < 50,000/μL), transfusion of fresh platelets is indicated. Intracerebral hemorrhage associated with *hematologic disorders* (leukemia, aplastic anemia, thrombocytopenic purpura) can occur at any site and may present as multiple intracerebral hemorrhages. Skin and mucous membrane bleeding is usually evident and offers a diagnostic clue.

Hemorrhage into a *brain tumor* may be the first manifestation of neoplasm. Choriocarcinoma, malignant melanoma, renal cell carcinoma, and bronchogenic carcinoma are among the most common metastatic tumors associated with intracerebral hemorrhage. Glioblastoma multiforme in adults and medulloblastoma in children may also have areas of intracerebral hemorrhage.

Hypertensive encephalopathy is a complication of malignant hypertension. In this acute syndrome, severe hypertension is associated with headache, nausea, vomiting, convulsions, confusion, stupor, and coma. Focal or lateralizing neurologic signs, either transitory or permanent, may occur but are infrequent and therefore suggest some other vascular disease (hemorrhage, embolism, or atherosclerotic thrombosis). There are retinal hemorrhages, exudates, papilledema (hypertensive retinopathy), and evidence of renal and cardiac disease. In most cases ICP and CSF protein levels are elevated. The hypertension may be essential or due to chronic renal disease, acute glomerulonephritis, acute toxemia of pregnancy, pheochromocytoma, or other causes. Lowering the blood pressure reverses the process, but stroke can occur, especially if blood pressure is lowered too rapidly. Neuropathologic examination reveals multifocal to diffuse cerebral edema and hemorrhages of various sizes from petechial to massive. Microscopically, there are necrosis of arterioles, minute cerebral infarcts, and hemorrhages. The term *hypertensive encephalopathy* should be reserved for this syndrome and not for chronic recurrent headaches, dizziness, recurrent TIAs, or small strokes that often occur in association with high blood pressure.

Primary intraventricular hemorrhage is rare. It usually begins within the substance of the brain and dissects into the ventricular system without leaving signs of intraparenchymal hemorrhage. Alternatively, bleeding can arise from periependymal veins. Vasculitis, usually polyarteritis nodosa or lupus erythematosus, can produce hemorrhage into any region of the central nervous system; most hemorrhages are associated with hypertension, but the arteritis itself may cause bleeding by disrupting the vessel wall. *Sepsis* can cause small petechial hemorrhages throughout the cerebral white matter. *Moyamoya disease*, mainly an occlusive arterial disease that causes ischemic symptoms, may on occasion produce intraparenchymal hemorrhage, particularly in the young. Hemorrhages into the spinal cord are usually the result of an AVM or metastatic tumor. *Epidural spinal hemorrhage* produces a rapidly evolving syndrome of spinal cord or nerve root compression (Chap. 356). Spinal hemorrhages usually present with sudden back pain and some manifestation of myelopathy.

Laboratory and Imaging Evaluation The CT scan reliably detects acute focal hemorrhages in the supratentorial space. Small pontine hemorrhages may not be identified because of motion and bone-induced artifact that obscure structures in the posterior fossa. After the first 2 weeks, x-ray attenuation values of clotted blood diminish until they become isodense with surrounding brain. Mass effect and edema may remain. In some cases, a surrounding rim of contrast enhancement appears after 2 to 4 weeks and may persist for months. MRI, though more sensitive for delineating posterior fossa lesions, is generally not necessary in most instances. Images of flowing blood on MRI scan may identify AVMs as the cause of the hemorrhage. MRI, CT angiography, and conventional x-ray angiography are used when the cause of intracranial hemorrhage is uncertain, particularly if the patient is young or not hypertensive and the hematoma is not in one of the four usual sites for hypertensive hemorrhage. For example, hemorrhage into the temporal lobe suggests rupture of a MCA saccular aneurysm.

Since patients typically have focal neurologic signs and obtundation, and often show signs of increased ICP, a lumbar puncture should be avoided as it may induce cerebral herniation.

℞ TREATMENT

Acute Management Nearly 50% of patients with a hypertensive intracerebral hemorrhage die, but others may have a good to complete recovery if they survive the initial hemorrhage. The volume and location of the hematoma determine the prognosis. In general, supratentorial hematomas with volumes <30 mL have a good prognosis; 30 to 60 mL, an intermediate prognosis; and >60 mL, a poor prognosis during initial hospitalization. Extension into the ventricular system worsens the prognosis. Except in patients who are on therapeutic anticoagulation or who have a bleeding disorder, little can be done about the hemorrhage itself. Hematomas may expand for several hours following the initial hemorrhage, so treating severe hypertension seems reasonable to prevent hematoma progression.

Evacuation of the hematoma is usually not helpful, except in cerebellar hemorrhages. For cerebellar hemorrhages, a neurosurgeon should be consulted immediately to assist with the evaluation; most cerebellar hematomas >3 cm in diameter will require surgical evacuation. If the patient is alert without focal brainstem signs and if the hematoma is <1 cm in diameter, surgical removal is usually unnecessary. Patients with hematomas between 1 and 3 cm require careful observation for signs of impaired consciousness and precipitous respiratory failure.

Tissue surrounding hematomas is displaced and compressed but not necessarily infarcted. Hence, in survivors, major improvement commonly occurs as the hematoma is reabsorbed and the adjacent tissue regains its function. Careful management of the patient during the acute phase of the hemorrhage can lead to considerable recovery.

Surprisingly, despite large intraparenchymal hemorrhages, ICP is often not elevated. However, if the hematoma causes marked midline shift of structures with consequent obtundation, coma, or hydrocephalus, osmotic agents coupled with induced hyperventilation can be instituted to lower ICP (Chap. 258). These maneuvers will provide enough time to place a ventriculostomy or ICP monitor. Once ICP is recorded, further hyperventilation and osmotic therapy can be tailored to the individual patient. For example, if ICP is found to be high, CSF can be drained from the ventricular space and osmotic therapy continued; persistent or progressive elevation in ICP may prompt surgical evacuation of the clot or withdrawal of support. Alternately, if ICP is normal or only mildly elevated, induced hyperventilation can be reversed and osmotic therapy tapered. Since hyperventilation may actually produce ischemia by cerebral vasoconstriction, induced hyperventilation should be limited to acute resuscitation of the patient with presumptive high ICP and eliminated once other treatments (osmotic therapy or surgical treatments) have been instituted. Glucocorticoids are not helpful for the edema from intracerebral hematoma.

Prevention Hypertension is the leading cause of primary intracerebral hemorrhage. Prevention is aimed at reducing hypertension, excessive alcohol use, and use of illicit drugs such as cocaine and amphetamines.

VASCULAR ANOMALIES

Vascular anomalies can be divided into congenital vascular malformations and acquired vascular lesions.

CONGENITAL VASCULAR MALFORMATIONS True *arteriovenous malformations*, venous anomalies, and capillary telangiectasias are lesions that usually remain clinically silent through life. Although most AVMs are congenital, cases of acquired lesions have been reported.

True AVMs are congenital shunts between the arterial and venous systems that may present as headache, seizures, and intracranial hemorrhage. AVMs consist of a tangle of abnormal vessels across the cortical surface or deep within the brain substance. AVMs vary in size from a small blemish a few millimeters in diameter to a large mass of tortuous channels composing an arteriovenous shunt of sufficient magnitude to raise cardiac output. The blood vessels forming the tangle interposed between arteries and veins are usually abnormally thin and do not have a normal structure. AVMs occur in all parts of the cerebral hemispheres, brainstem, and spinal cord, but the largest ones are most frequently in the posterior half of the hemispheres, commonly forming a wedge-shaped lesion extending from the cortex to the ventricle.

Although the lesion is present from birth, bleeding or other symptoms are most common between the ages of 10 and 30, occasionally as late as the fifties. AVMs are more frequent in men, and rare familial cases have been described.

Headache (without bleeding) may be hemicranial and throbbing, like migraine, or diffuse. Focal seizures, with or without generalization, occur in about 30% of cases. Half of AVMs become evident as intracerebral hemorrhages. In most, the hemorrhage is mainly intraparenchymal with extension into the subarachnoid space in some cases. Blood is usually not deposited in the basal cisterns, and symptomatic cerebral vasospasm is rare. The risk of rerupture is about 18% per year and is particular high in the first few weeks. Hemorrhages may be massive, leading to death, or may be as small as 1 cm in diameter, leading to minor focal symptoms or no deficit. The AVM may be large enough to steal blood away from adjacent normal brain tissue or to increase venous pressure significantly to produce venous ischemia locally and in remote areas of the brain. This is seen most often with large AVMs in the territory of the MCA.

Large AVMs of the anterior circulation may be associated with a systolic and diastolic bruit (sometimes self-audible) over the eye, forehead, or neck and a bounding carotid pulse. Headache at the onset of AVM rupture is not generally as explosive as with aneurysmal rupture. MRI is better than CT for diagnosis, although contrast CT scanning sometimes detects calcification of the AVM.

Surgical treatment of symptomatic AVMs, often with preoperative embolization to reduce operative bleeding, is usually indicated for accessible lesions. Stereotaxic radiation, an alternative to surgery, can produce a slow sclerosis of arterial channels over 2 to 3 years.

Patients with asymptomatic AVMs have about a 2% per year risk for hemorrhage. Several angiographic features of the AVM can be used to help predict future bleeding risk. Paradoxically, smaller lesions seem to have a higher hemorrhage rate. The mortality rate with each bleed is about 15%. Given this natural history, surgical treatment is probably indicated for most AVMs that can be treated with reasonable surgical risk.

Venous anomalies are the result of development of anomalous cerebral, cerebellar, or brainstem drainage. These structures, unlike AVMs, are functional venous channels. They are of little clinical significance and should be ignored if found incidentally on brain imaging studies. Surgical resection of these anomalies may result in venous infarction and hemorrhage. Venous anomalies may be associated with cavernous malformations (see below), which do carry some bleeding risk. If resection of a cavernous malformation is attempted, the venous anomaly should not be disturbed.

Capillary telangiectasias are true capillary malformations that often form extensive vascular networks through an otherwise normal brain structure. The pons and deep cerebral white matter are typical locations, and these capillary malformations can be seen in patients with hereditary hemorrhagic telangiectasia (Osler-Rendu-Weber) syndrome. If bleeding does occur, it rarely produces mass effect or significant symptoms. No treatment options exist.

ACQUIRED VASCULAR LESIONS *Cavernous angiomas* are tufts of capillary sinusoids that form within the deep hemispheric white matter and brainstem with no normal intervening neural structures. The pathogenesis is unclear. Familial cavernous angiomas have been mapped to several different chromosomal loci; the gene responsible for the 7q-linked form encodes a protein that interacts with a member of the RAS family of GTPases. Cavernous angiomas are typically <1 cm in diameter and are often associated with a venous anomaly. Bleeding is usually of small volume, causing slight mass effect only. The bleeding

risk for single cavernous malformations is 0.7 to 1.5% per year and may be higher for patients with prior clinical hemorrhage or multiple malformations. Seizures may occur if the malformation is located near the cerebral cortex. Surgical resection eliminates bleeding risk and may reduce seizure risk, but it is reserved for those malformations that form near the brain surface. Radiation treatment has not been shown to be of benefit.

Dural arteriovenous fistulas are acquired connections usually from a dural artery to a dural sinus. Patients may complain of a pulse-synchronous cephalic bruit ("pulsatile tinnitus") and headache. Depending on the magnitude of the shunt, venous pressures may rise high enough to cause cortical ischemia or venous hypertension and hemorrhage. Surgical and endovascular techniques are usually curative. These fistulas may form because of trauma, but most are idiopathic. There is an association between fistulas and dural sinus thrombosis. Fistulas have been observed to appear months to years following venous sinus thrombosis, suggesting that angiogenesis factors elaborated from the thrombotic process may cause these anomalous connections to form. Alternatively, dural arteriovenous fistulas can produce venous sinus occlusion over time, perhaps from the high pressure and high flow through a venous structure.

FURTHER READING

ADAMS HP et al: Guidelines for the early management of patients with ischemic stroke: A scientific statement from the Stroke Council of the American Stroke Association. Stroke 34:1056, 2003

JOHNSTON SC: Clinical practice. Transient ischemic attack. N Engl J Med 347:1687, 2002

———— et al: Recommendations for the endovascular treatment of intracranial aneurysms: A statement for healthcare professionals from the Committee on Cerebrovascular Imaging of the American Heart Association Council on Cardiovascular Radiology. Stroke. 33:2536, 2002

MAS JL et al: Recurrent cerebrovascular events associated with patent foramen ovale, atrial septal aneurysm, or both. N Engl J Med 345:1740, 2001

MOHR JP et al: A comparison of warfarin and aspirin for the prevention of recurrent ischemic stroke. N Engl J Med. 345:1444, 2001

MOLYNEUX A: International Subarachnoid Aneurysm Trial (ISAT) of neurosurgical clipping versus endovascular coiling in 2143 patients with ruptured intracranial aneurysms: A randomised trial. Lancet 360:1267, 2002

OGILVY CS et al: AHA Scientific Statement: Recommendations for the management of intracranial arteriovenous malformations: A statement for healthcare professionals from a special writing group of the Stroke Council, American Stroke Association. Stroke 32:1458, 2001

PROGRESS COLLABORATIVE GROUP: Randomised trial of a perindopril-based blood-pressure-lowering regimen among 6105 individuals with previous stroke or transient ischaemic attack. Lancet 358:1033, 2001

ROTHWELL PM et al: Analysis of pooled data from the randomised controlled trials of endarterectomy for symptomatic carotid stenosis. Lancet 361:107, 2003

STAESSEN JA et al: Hypertension prevalence and stroke mortality across populations. JAMA 289:2420, 2003

350 | ALZHEIMER'S DISEASE AND OTHER DEMENTIAS
Thomas D. Bird, Bruce L. Miller

Dementia, a syndrome of many causes, affects >4 million Americans and results in a total health care cost of >$100 billion annually. It is defined as an acquired deterioration in cognitive abilities that impairs the successful performance of activities of daily living. Memory is the most common cognitive ability lost with dementia; 10% of persons over age 70 and 20 to 40% of individuals over age 85 have clinically identifiable memory loss. In addition to memory, other mental faculties are also affected in dementia, such as language, visuospatial ability, calculation, judgment, and problem solving. Neuropsychiatric and social deficits develop in many dementia syndromes resulting in depression, withdrawal, hallucinations, delusions, agitation, insomnia, and

disinhibition. The common forms of dementia are progressive, but some dementing illnesses are static or fluctuate dramatically from day to day.

MEMORY

Memory is a complex function of the brain that uses several storage buffers of differing capacity and duration. It can be divided into three major types: working, episodic, and long-term, or remote, memory. Working memory lasts for <30 s and has a limited storage capacity. Normal individuals can hold seven (plus or minus two) bits of information in working memory where these bits can be manipulated and either discarded or retained as a more permanent memory store. Working memory is highly vulnerable to distraction, requiring attention and vigilance for its maintenance. It is tested by asking the patient to recall digits backwards. The reticular activating system and prefrontal and parietal lobe networks are activated during working memory tasks.

Episodic memory lasts for minutes to many months or even years and binds information about "what," "where," and "when." Normal individuals lay down multiple episodic memories throughout the day, which allow them to move through life connected to previous experiences. On entering this memory buffer, information undergoes a process of consolidation. Significant events are more likely to be consolidated as a more permanent trace. Episodic memory is commonly tested by asking a patient to recall three words after 3 to 5 min. Other simple ways to test episodic memory include determining whether patients can remember what they had for breakfast, how they got to the office, or who examined them earlier in the day. The hippocampal complex is critical for episodic memory, and physiologic changes in synapses in this brain region accompany new episodic memories. Eventually episodic memories become independent of the hippocampal complex and move to neocortex.

Remote, or long-term, memory stores information lasting weeks to a lifetime and contains most of our personal experiences and knowledge. Some information appears to be stored accurately for an indefinite time, whereas other items fade or become distorted. More permanent stores of words, dates, historic facts, or names require the left anterior temporal cortex. The specific localization of other types of long-term memories is unknown, although the neocortex appears to be particularly important. Animal experiments have shown that long-term memory requires new protein synthesis, and the stabilization process probably involves physical changes at neuronal synapses.

Memory function includes *registration* (encoding or acquisition), *retention* (storage or consolidation), *stabilization* (consolidation), and *retrieval* (decoding or recall). Registration and retrieval are conscious processes. The process of encoding is dependent upon the frontal lobes and hippocampal complex, while the process of retrieval requires the frontal lobes. The hippocampal complex is vulnerable to metabolic insults such as seizures, hypoglycemia, hypoxia, and neurodegenerative processes, which explains why episodic memory deficits are the most common cognitive deficits that follow these varied disorders.

Several additional terms for memory types are sometimes used. *Amnesia* is a term used to describe an impairment in memory function. *Semantic memory* contains unchanging facts, principles, associations, and rules (for example, the number of days in a week). Injury to the anterior temporal neocortex will lead to loss of semantic memory. *Declarative (explicit) memory* refers to facts about the world and past personal events that must be consciously retrieved to be remembered. Episodic memory is the prototypical declarative, or explicit, memory. *Procedural (implicit) memory* is involved in learning and retaining a skill or procedure such as riding a bicycle, getting dressed, or driving a car. Abilities stored in procedural memory become automatic and do not require conscious implementation.

Finally, the term *executive function* refers to mental activity involved in planning, initiating, and regulating behavior. It is considered the central organizing function of the brain that results in systematic, goal-directed activity and is highly dependent upon working memory. Executive functions are active in situations where reflex or automatic behavior is not adequate. Executive functions are presumed to involve the frontal lobes (Chap. 23). Deficits in executive function occur frequently in patients with dementia.

FUNCTIONAL ANATOMY OF THE DEMENTIAS

Dementia results from disorders of cerebral neuronal circuits and is a result of the total quantity of neuronal loss combined with the specific location of such loss (Chap. 23). Episodic memory requires the dorsomedial nucleus of the thalamus (damaged in Korsakoff's syndrome due to thiamine deficiency) and the medial temporal lobes. Unilateral temporal lobe lesions produce mild to moderate amnesia for either verbal or nonverbal material, while bilateral lesions produce a severe anterograde learning disorder, i.e., an inability to store new memories, often with retained ability to recall old ones.

The components of the medial temporal lobe memory system include the hippocampus and adjacent cortex, including the entorhinal, perirhinal, and parahippocampal regions (Fig. 350-1). This includes a circular pathway of neurons from the entorhinal cortex to the dentate gyrus, CA3 and CA1 neurons of the hippocampus to the subiculum, and back to the entorhinal cortex; this pathway is heavily damaged in Alzheimer's disease (AD). This system is fast, has limited capacity, and performs a crucial function at the time of learning and establishing declarative memory and semantic associations. Its role continues after learning during a lengthy period of reorganization and consolidation, whereby memory stored in neocortex eventually becomes independent of the medial temporal lobe memory system. This process, by which the burden of long-term (permanent) memory storage is gradually assumed by neocortex, ensures that the medial temporal lobe system is constantly available for the acquisition of new information.

Functional imaging studies indicate that learning and memory involve many of the same regions of the cortex that process sensory information and control motor output. The forms of perceptual and motor learning that can occur without conscious recollections are mediated in part by contractions and expansions of representations in the sensory and motor cortex. One study, for example, has shown that the cortical representation of the fingers of the left hand of musical string players is larger than that in controls, suggesting that the representation of different parts of the body in the primary somatosensory cortex of humans depends on use and changes to conform to the current needs and experiences of the individual. Discrete cortical regions exist in the anterior temporal lobes in which object knowledge (such as words related to color, animals, tools, or action) is organized as a distributed system. Here the attributes of an object are stored close to the regions of the cortex that mediate perception of those attributes.

Procedural (implicit) memory appears to involve centers outside the hippocampus such as amygdala, basal ganglia, cerebellum, and sensory cortex. Different frontal regions are activated for different kinds of memory storage. Functional magnetic resonance imaging (MRI) studies show that the magnitude of focal activation in left prefrontal-temporal regions and right prefrontal-bilateral parahippocampal regions predicts how well verbal or visual stimuli, respectively, will be remembered.

FIGURE 350-1   The principal connections of the hippocampus. Afferent connections (*red arrows*) from the cingulate gyrus (cortical association fibers) and amygdala converge on the entorhinal cortex (part of the parahippocampal gyrus) and connect with the hippocampus via a polysynaptic circuit (*black arrows*) from dentate to CA3, CA1, and subiculum neurons with output back to the entorhinal cortex. Efferent connections (*broken arrows*) are principally via the fornix to the anterior nucleus of the thalamus, septal nucleus, and mammillary body.

The cholinergic system plays an important role in memory, and anticholinergic agents such as atropine and scopolamine interfere with memory. Choline acetyltransferase (the enzyme catalyzing the formation of acetylcholine) and cholinergic receptors are known to be deficient in the cortex of patients with AD. The brains of AD patients show severe neuronal loss in the nucleus basalis of Meynert, the major source of cholinergic input to the cerebral cortex. These findings form the basis for the use of cholinesterase inhibitors in the treatment of AD, with benefits thought to arise from increased available levels of acetylcholine. Behavior and mood are modulated by noradrenergic, serotonergic, and dopaminergic pathways, and norepinephrine has been shown to be reduced in the brainstem locus coeruleus in AD. Neurotrophins (Chap. 345) are also postulated to play a role in memory in part by preserving cholinergic neurons.

Long-term potentiation (LTP), which refers to a long-lasting enhancement of synaptic transmission resulting from repetitive stimulation of excitatory synapses, is presumed to be involved in memory acquisition and storage. LTP occurs in the hippocampus and is mediated by N-methyl-D-aspartate (NMDA) receptors as well as cyclic AMP-responsive element-binding (CREB) protein. Dementias have anatomically specific patterns of neuronal degeneration, which dictate the clinical symptomatology. AD begins in the entorhinal cortex, spreads to the hippocampus, then moves to posterior temporal and parietal neocortex and eventually causes a relatively diffuse degeneration throughout the cerebral cortex. Multi-infarct dementia is associated with focal damage in a random patchwork of cortical regions. Diffuse white matter damage may disrupt intracerebral connections and cause dementia syndromes similar to those associated with leukodystrophies, multiple sclerosis, and Binswanger's disease (see below). Subcortical structures including the caudate, putamen, thalamus, and substantia nigra also modulate cognition and behavior in ways that are not yet well understood. AD primarily presents as memory loss and is often associated with aphasia or other disturbance of language. In contrast, patients with frontal lobe or subcortical dementias such as frontotemporal dementia (FTD) or Huntington's disease are less likely to begin with memory and language problems and more likely to have difficulties with attention, judgment, awareness, and behavior.

Lesions of specific cortical-subcortical pathways will have important effects on behavior (Chap. 23). The dorsolateral prefrontal cortex has connections with the dorsolateral caudate, globus pallidus, and thalamus. Lesions of these pathways result in poor organization and planning, decreased cognitive flexibility, and impaired judgment. The lateral orbital frontal cortex connects with the ventromedial caudate, globus pallidus, and thalamus. Lesions of these connections cause irritability, impulsiveness, and distractibility. The anterior cingulate cortex connects with the nucleus accumbens, globus pallidus, and thalamus. Interruption of these connections produces apathy and poverty of speech or even akinetic mutism.

THE CAUSES OF DEMENTIA

The many causes of dementia are listed in Table 350-1. The frequency of each condition depends on the age group under study, the access of the group to medical care, the country of origin, and perhaps racial or

TABLE 350-1 *Differential Diagnosis of Dementia*

MOST COMMON CAUSES OF DEMENTIA

Alzheimer's disease	Alcoholism[a]
Vascular dementia	Parkinson's disease
Multi-infarct	Drug/medication intoxication[a]
Diffuse white matter disease (Binswanger's)	

LESS COMMON CAUSES OF DEMENTIA

Vitamin deficiencies	Toxic disorders
Thiamine (B$_1$): Wernicke's encephalopathy[a]	Drug, medication, and narcotic poisoning[a]
B$_{12}$ (pernicious anemia)[a]	Heavy metal intoxication[a]
Nicotinic acid (pellagra)[a]	Dialysis dementia (aluminum)
Endocrine and other organ failure	Organic toxins
Hypothyroidism[a]	Psychiatric
Adrenal insufficiency and Cushing's	Depression (pseudodementia)[a]
syndrome[a]	Schizophrenia[a]
Hypo- and hyperparathyroidism[a]	Conversion reaction[a]
Renal failure[a]	Degenerative disorders
Liver failure[a]	Huntington's disease
Pulmonary failure[a]	Pick's disease
Chronic infections	Dementia with Lewy bodies
HIV	Progressive supranuclear palsy (Steel-Richardson syndrome)
Neurosyphilis[a]	
Papovavirus (progressive multifocal leukoencephalopathy)	Multisystem degeneration (Shy-Drager syndrome)
Prion (Creutzfeldt-Jakob and Gerstmann-Sträussler-Scheinker diseases)	Hereditary ataxias (some forms)
Tuberculosis, fungal, and protozoal[a]	Motor neuron disease [amyotrophic lateral sclerosis (ALS); some forms]
Sarcoidosis[a]	Frontotemporal dementia
Whipple's disease[a]	Cortical basal degeneration
Head trauma and diffuse brain damage	Multiple sclerosis
Dementia pugilistica	Adult Down's syndrome with Alzheimer's
Chronic subdural hematoma[a]	ALS–Parkinson's–Dementia complex of Guam
Postanoxia	
Postencephalitis	Miscellaneous
Normal-pressure hydrocephalus[a]	Vasculitis[a]
Neoplastic	CADASIL
Primary brain tumor[a]	Acute intermittent porphyria[a]
Metastatic brain tumor[a]	Recurrent nonconvulsive seizures[a]
Paraneoplastic limbic encephalitis	Additional conditions in children or adolescents
	Hallervorden-Spatz disease
	Subacute sclerosing panencephalitis
	Metabolic disorders (e.g., Wilson's and Leigh's diseases, leukodystrophies, lipid storage diseases, mitochondrial mutations)

[a] Potentially reversible dementia.

ethnic background. AD is the most common cause of dementia in western countries, representing more than half of demented patients. Vascular disease is the second most common cause of dementia in the United States, representing 10 to 20%. In populations with limited access to medical care, where vascular risk factors are undertreated, the prevalence of vascular dementia can be much higher. Dementia associated with Parkinson's disease is the next most common category, and in many instances these patients suffer from dementia with Lewy bodies (DLB). Chronic intoxications including those resulting from alcohol and prescription drugs are an important, often treatable cause of dementia. Other disorders listed in the table are uncommon but important because many are reversible. The classification of dementing illnesses into two broad groups of reversible and irreversible disorders is a useful approach to the differential diagnosis of dementia.

In a study of 1000 persons attending a memory disorders clinic, 19% had a potentially reversible cause of the cognitive impairment and 23% had a potentially reversible concomitant condition. The three most common potentially reversible diagnoses were depression, hydrocephalus, and alcohol dependence.

The single strongest risk factor for dementia is increasing age. The prevalence of disabling memory loss increases with each decade over age 50 and is associated most often with the microscopic changes of AD at autopsy. Slow accumulation of mutations in neuronal mitochondria is also hypothesized to contribute to the increasing prevalence of dementia with age. Nonetheless, some centenarians have

TABLE 350-2 Evaluation of the Patient with Dementia

Routine Evaluation	Optional Focused Tests	Occasionally Helpful Tests
History	HIV	EEG
Physical examination	Chest x-ray	Parathyroid function
Laboratory tests	Lumbar puncture	Adrenal function
Thyroid function (TSH)	Liver function	Urine heavy metals
Vitamin B_{12}	Renal function	RBC sedimentation rate
Complete blood count	Urine toxin screen	Angiogram
Electrolytes	Psychometric testing	Brain biopsy
VDRL	Apolipoprotein E	SPECT
CT/MRI		

DIAGNOSTIC CATEGORIES

Reversible Causes	Irreversible/Degenerative Dementias	Psychiatric Disorders
Examples	Examples	Depression
Hypothyroidism	Alzheimer's	Schizophrenia
Thiamine deficiency	Frontotemporal dementia	Conversion reaction
Vitamin B_{12} deficiency	Huntington's	
Normal-pressure	Dementia with Lewy bodies	
hydrocephalus	Multi-infarct	
Chronic infection	Leukoencephalopathies	
Brain tumor	Parkinson's	
Drug intoxication		

Associated Treatable Conditions

Depression	Agitation
Seizures	Caregiver "burnout"
Insomnia	Drug side effects

intact memory function and no evidence of clinically significant dementia. Whether dementia is an inevitable consequence of normal human aging remains controversial.

Subtle cumulative decline in episodic memory is a natural part of aging. This frustrating experience, often the source of jokes and humor, is referred to as *benign forgetfulness of the elderly*. Benign means that it is not so progressive or serious that it impairs reasonably successful and productive daily functioning, although the distinction between benign and more significant memory loss can be difficult to make. At age 85 years the average person is able to remember approximately one-half the number of words that he or she could at age 18. A mild cognitive problem that has subtly begun to interfere with daily activities is referred to as *mild cognitive impairment* (MCI). A sizeable proportion of persons with MCI will progress to frank dementia, usually caused by AD. The conversion rate from MCI to AD is ~12% per year. It remains unclear why some individuals show progression and others do not. Factors that predict progression from MCI to AD include a memory deficit >1.5 standard deviations from the norm, family history of dementia, the presence of an apolipoprotein ε4 (Apo ε4) allele, and small hippocampal volumes.

The major degenerative dementias include AD, FTD and related disorders, DLB, and prion disorders including Creutzfeldt-Jakob disease (CJD). These disorders are all associated with the abnormal aggregation of a specific protein: $A\beta_{42}$ in AD, tau in FTD, α-synuclein in DLB, and PrP in CJD.

APPROACH TO THE PATIENT

(Tables 350-1 and 350-2) Three major issues should be kept in the forefront: (1) What is the most accurate diagnosis? (2) Is there a treatable or reversible component to the dementia? (3) Can the physician help to alleviate the burden on caregivers? The major degenerative dementias can usually be distinguished by the initial symptoms; neuropsychological, neuropsychiatric, and neurologic findings; and neuroimaging features (Table 350-3).

History The history should focus on the onset, duration, and tempo of progression of the dementia. An acute or subacute onset of confusion may represent delirium and should trigger the search for intoxication, infection, or metabolic derangement. An elderly person with slowly progressive memory loss over several years is likely to suffer from AD. Nearly 75% of AD patients begin with memory symptoms, but other early symptoms include difficulty with managing money, driving, shopping, following instructions, finding words, or navigating. A change in personality, disinhibition, gain of weight, or food obsession suggests FTD, not AD. FTD is also suggested by the finding of apathy, loss of executive function, progressive abnormalities in speech, or by a relative sparing of memory or spatial abilities. The diagnosis of DLB is suggested by the early presence of visual hallucinations, parkinsonism, delirium, rapid-eye-movement (REM) sleep disorder (the merging of dream states into wakefulness), or *Capgras syndrome*, the delusion that a familiar person has been replaced by an impostor.

A history of sudden stroke with an irregular stepwise progression suggests multi-infarct dementia. Multi-infarct dementia is also commonly seen in the setting of hyper-

TABLE 350-3 Clinical Differentiation of the Major Dementias

Disease	Initial Symptom	Mental Status	Neuropsychiatry	Neurology	Imaging
AD	Memory loss	Episodic memory loss	Initially normal	Initially normal	Entorhinal and hippocampal atrophy
Vascular	Often sudden; variable initial symptoms; apathy, falls, focal weakness	Frontal/executive cognitive slowing; can spare memory	Apathy, delusions, anxiety	Usually motor slowing, spasticity; can be normal	Cortical and/or subcortical infarctions, confluent white matter disease
FTD	Apathy; reduced judgment/ insight/speech/ language; hyperorality	Frontal/executive, language; spares drawing	Apathy, disinhibition, hyperorality, euphoria, depression	Vertical gaze palsy, axial rigidity, dystonia, alien hand (due to PSP/CBD overlap)	Frontal and/or temporal atrophy; spares posterior parietal lobe
DLB	Visual hallucinations, REM-sleep disorder, delirium, Capgras syndrome, parkinsonism	Drawing and frontal/ executive; spares memory; delirium prone	Visual hallucinations, depression, sleep disorder, delusions	Parkinsonism	Posterior parietal; hippocampi larger than in AD
Prion	Dementia, mood changes, anxiety, movement disorder	Variable, frontal/ executive, focal cortical, memory	Depression, anxiety	Myoclonus, rigidity, parkinsonism	Cortical ribboning and basal ganglia hyperintensities on diffusion/flare MRI

Note: AD, Alzheimer's disease; FTD, frontotemporal dementia; PSP, progressive supranuclear palsy; CBD, cortical basal degeneration; DLB, dementia with Lewy bodies; MRI, magnetic resonance imaging.

tension, atrial fibrillation, peripheral vascular disease, and diabetes. In patients suffering from cerebrovascular disease it can be difficult to determine whether the dementia is due to AD, multi-infarct dementia, or a mixture of the two. Rapid progression of the dementia in association with motor rigidity and myoclonus suggests a prion disease. Seizures may indicate strokes or neoplasm. Gait disturbance is commonly seen with multi-infarct dementia, Parkinson's disease, or normal-pressure hydrocephalus. Multiple sex partners or intravenous drug use should trigger a search for a central nervous system (CNS) infection, especially in persons with HIV. A history of recurrent head trauma could indicate chronic subdural hematoma, dementia pugilistica, or normal-pressure hydrocephalus. Alcoholism may suggest malnutrition and thiamine deficiency. A remote history of gastric surgery may result in loss of intrinsic factor and vitamin B_{12} deficiency. Certain occupations such as working in a battery or chemical factory might indicate heavy metal intoxication. A careful review of medications, especially of sedatives and tranquilizers, may raise the issue of chronic drug intoxication. A family history of dementia is found in Huntington's disease, familial AD, or familial FTD. Depressive signs such as insomnia or weight loss are often seen with pseudodementia due to depression, which can also be caused by the recent death of a loved one.

Physical and Neurologic Examination   A thorough examination is essential to document the dementia, look for other signs of nervous system involvement, and search for clues of a systemic disease that might be responsible for the cognitive disorder. AD does not affect motor systems until late in the course. In contrast, FTD patients often develop axial rigidity, supranuclear gaze palsy, or features of amyotrophic lateral sclerosis (ALS). In DLB, initial symptoms may be the new onset of a parkinsonian syndrome (resting tremor, cogwheel rigidity, bradykinesia, and festinating gait) with the dementia following later, or vice-versa. Corticobasal degeneration (CBD) is associated with dystonia and alien hand (unilateral involuntary movements of the upper limb resembling purposeful actions) and with asymmetric motor deficits or myoclonus. A presentation with unexplained falls, axial rigidity, and gaze deficits suggests progressive supranuclear palsy (PSP). CJD is suggested by diffuse rigidity, an akinetic state, and myoclonus.

Hemiparesis or other focal neurologic deficits may occur in multi-infarct dementia or brain tumor. Dementia with a myelopathy and peripheral neuropathy suggests vitamin B_{12} deficiency. A peripheral neuropathy could also indicate an underlying vitamin deficiency or heavy metal intoxication. Dry cool skin, hair loss, and bradycardia suggest hypothyroidism. Confusion associated with repetitive stereotyped movements may indicate ongoing seizure activity. Hearing impairment or visual loss may produce confusion and disorientation misinterpreted as dementia. Such sensory deficits are common in the elderly.

Cognitive and Neuropsychiatric Examination   Brief screening tools such as the mini-mental status examination (MMSE) help to confirm the presence of cognitive impairment and to follow the progression of dementia (Table 350-4). The MMSE is an easily administered 30-point test of cognitive function and contains tests of orientation, working and episodic memory, language comprehension, naming, and copying. In most patients with MCI and some with clinically apparent AD, the MMSE may be normal and a more rigorous set of neuropsychological tests will be required. Additionally, when the etiology for the dementia syndrome remains in doubt, a specially tailored evaluation should be performed that includes tasks of working and episodic memory, frontal executive tasks, language, visuospatial function, and perception. In AD the deficits involve episodic memory, category generation ("name as many animals as you can in one minute"), and visuoconstructive ability. Deficits in verbal or visual episodic memory are often the first neuropsychological abnormalities seen with AD, and tasks that require the patient to recall a long list of words or pictures after a predetermined

TABLE 350-4   *The Mini-Mental Status Examination*

	Points
Orientation	
Name: season/date/day/month/year	5 (1 for each name)
Name: hospital/floor/town/state/country	5 (1 for each name)
Registration	
Identify three objects by name and ask patient to repeat	3 (1 for each object)
Attention and calculation	
Serial 7s; subtract from 100 (e.g., 93–86–79–72–65)	5 (1 for each subtraction)
Recall	
Recall the three objects presented earlier	3 (1 for each object)
Language	
Name pencil and watch	2 (1 for each object)
Repeat "No ifs, ands, or buts"	1
Follow a 3-step command (e.g., "Take this paper, fold it in half, and place it on the table")	3 (1 for each command)
Write "close your eyes" and ask patient to obey written command	1
Ask patient to write a sentence	1
Ask patient to copy a design (e.g., intersecting pentagons)	1
TOTAL	30

delay will demonstrate deficits in most AD patients. In FTD the earliest deficits often involve frontal executive function or language (speech or naming). DLB patients have more severe deficits in visuospatial function but do better on episodic memory tasks than do patients with AD. Patients with vascular dementia often demonstrate a mixture of frontal executive and visuospatial deficits. In delirium, deficits tend to occur in the areas of attention, working memory, and frontal tasks.

A functional assessment should also be performed. The physician should determine the day-to-day impact of the disorder on the patient's memory, community affairs, hobbies, judgment, dressing, and eating. Knowledge of the patient's day-to-day function will help to organize a therapeutic approach with the family.

Neuropsychiatric assessment is important for diagnosis, prognosis, and treatment. In the early stages of AD mild depressive features, social withdrawal, and denial of illness are the most prominent psychiatric changes. However, patients often maintain their social skills into the middle stages of the illness when delusions, agitation, and sleep disturbance become more common. In FTD dramatic personality change, apathy, overeating, repetitive compulsions, disinhibition, euphoria, and loss of empathy are common. DLB shows visual hallucinations, delusions related to personal identity, and day-to-day fluctuation. Vascular dementia can present with psychiatric symptoms such as depression, delusions, disinhibition, or apathy.

Laboratory Tests   The choice of laboratory tests in the evaluation of dementia is not straightforward. A reversible or treatable cause must not be missed, yet no single etiology is common; thus a screen must employ multiple tests, each of which has a low yield. Cost/benefit ratios are difficult to assess, and many laboratory screening algorithms for dementia discourage multiple tests. Nevertheless, even a test with only a 1 to 2% positive rate is probably worth undertaking if the alternative is missing a treatable cause of dementia. The algorithm in Table 350-2 lists most screening tests for dementia. Recently the American Academy of Neurology recommended the routine measurement of thyroid function tests, a vitamin B_{12} level, and a neuroimaging study [computed tomography (CT) or MRI].

Neuroimaging studies will identify primary and secondary neoplasms, locate areas of infarction, reveal subdural hematomas, and suggest normal-pressure hydrocephalus or diffuse white matter disease. They also lend support to the diagnosis of AD, especially if there is hippocampal atrophy in addition to diffuse cortical atrophy. Focal frontal and/or anterior temporal atrophy suggest FTD. There is no specific pattern yet determined for DLB, although these patients tend to have less hippocampal atrophy than is seen in AD. Diffusion-weighted MRI will detect abnormalities in the cortical-ribbon and basal ganglia in the vast majority of patients with CJD. Large white matter abnormalities correlate with a vascular etiology for dementia. The role of functional imaging in the diagnosis of dementia is still under study. Single photon emission computed tomography (SPECT) and positron emission tomography (PET) scanning reveal temporal-parietal hypoperfusion or hypometabolism in AD, and frontotemporal hypoperfusion or hypometabolism in FTD, but most of these changes reflect atrophy. Recently, amyloid imaging has shown promise for the diagnosis of AD. Similarly, MRI perfusion and brain activation studies using functional MRI are under study as diagnostic tools.

Lumbar puncture need not be done routinely in the evaluation of dementia but is indicated if CNS infection is a serious consideration. Cerebrospinal fluid (CSF) levels of tau protein are increased and $A\beta_{42}$ amyloid decreased in some AD patients; however, the sensitivity and specificity of these measures are not sufficiently high to warrant routine measurement. Formal psychometric testing is not necessary in every patient but helps to document the severity of dementia, suggest psychogenic causes, and provide a semiquantitative method for following the disease course. An electroencephalogram (EEG) is rarely helpful except to suggest CJD (repetitive bursts of diffuse high-voltage sharp waves) or an underlying nonconvulsive seizure disorder (epileptiform discharges). Brain biopsy (including meninges) is not advised except to diagnose vasculitis, potentially treatable neoplasms, unusual infections, or systemic disorders such as vasculitis or sarcoid or in young persons where the diagnosis is uncertain. Angiography should be considered when cerebral vasculitis is a possible cause of the dementia.

SPECIFIC DEMENTIAS

ALZHEIMER'S DISEASE   AD is the most common cause of dementia in western countries. Approximately 10% of all persons over the age of 70 have significant memory loss, and in more than half the cause is AD. AD can occur, however, in any decade of adulthood. The annual cost of caring for a single AD patient in an advanced stage of the disease is estimated at $50,000. The disease also exacts a heavy emotional toll on family members and caregivers. AD most often presents with subtle onset of memory loss followed by a slowly progressive dementia that has a course of several years. Pathologically there is diffuse atrophy of the cerebral cortex with secondary enlargement of the ventricular system. Microscopically there are neuritic plaques containing $A\beta$ amyloid, silver-staining neurofibrillary tangles (NFTs) in neuronal cytoplasm, and accumulation of $A\beta$ amyloid in arterial walls of cerebral blood vessels. The identification of four different susceptibility genes has provided a foundation for rapid progress in understanding the biologic basis of AD.

Clinical Manifestations   The cognitive changes with AD tend to follow a characteristic pattern, beginning with memory impairment and spreading to language and visuospatial deficits. However, ~20% of AD patients present with nonmemory complaints such as word-finding, organizational, or navigational difficulty. In the early stages of the disease, the memory loss may go unrecognized or may be ascribed to benign forgetfulness. Once the memory loss begins to affect day-to-day activities or falls to <1.5 standard deviations from normal on standardized memory tasks, the disease is defined as MCI. Slowly the cognitive problems begin to interfere with daily activities, such as

keeping track of finances, following instructions on the job, driving, shopping, and housekeeping. Some patients are unaware of these difficulties (*anosognosia*), while others have considerable insight. Change of environment may be bewildering, and the patient may become lost on walks or while driving an automobile. In the middle stages of AD, the patient is unable to work, is easily lost and confused, and requires daily supervision. Social graces, routine behavior, and superficial conversation may be surprisingly retained. Language becomes impaired: first naming, then comprehension, and finally fluency. In some patients, *aphasia* is an early and prominent feature. Word-finding difficulties and circumlocution may be a problem even when formal testing demonstrates intact naming and fluency. *Apraxia* emerges and patients have trouble carrying out sequential motor tasks. Visuospatial deficits begin to interfere with dressing, eating, solving simple puzzles, and copying geometric figures. Patients may be unable to perform simple calculations or tell time.

In the late stages of the disease, some persons remain ambulatory but wander aimlessly. Loss of judgment, reason, and cognitive abilities occurs. Delusions are common, usually simple in quality, involving delusions of theft, infidelity, or misidentification. Approximately 10% of AD patients develop the Capgras syndrome, believing that a caregiver has been replaced by an impostor. In contrast to DLB where the Capgras syndrome is an early feature, in AD this syndrome emerges later in the course of the illness. Loss of inhibitions and aggression may alternate with passivity and withdrawal. Sleep-wake patterns are prone to disruption, and nighttime wandering becomes disturbing to the household. Some patients develop a shuffling gait, with generalized muscle rigidity associated with slowness and awkwardness of movement. Patients often look parkinsonian (Chap. 351) but rarely have tremor. In end-stage AD, patients become rigid, mute, incontinent, and bedridden. Help may be needed with the simplest tasks, such as eating, dressing, and toilet function. Hyperactive tendon reflexes may be noted. Myoclonic jerks (sudden brief contractions of various muscles or the whole body) may occur spontaneously or in response to physical or auditory stimulation. Myoclonus raises the possibility of a prion disease (Chap. 362), but the course of AD is much more prolonged. Generalized seizures may also occur. Often, death results from malnutrition, secondary infections, pulmonary emboli, or heart disease. The typical duration of AD is 8 to 10 years, but the course can range from 1 to 25 years. For unknown reasons, some AD patients show a steady downhill decline in function, while others have prolonged plateaus without major deterioration.

Diagnosis   Early in the disease course, other etiologies of dementia should be excluded (see above). Neuroimaging studies (CT and MRI) do not show a single specific pattern with AD and may be normal early in the course of the disease. As AD progresses, diffuse cortical atrophy becomes apparent, and MRI scans show atrophy of the hippocampus (Fig. 350-2A, B). Functional imaging studies in AD reveal hypoperfusion or hypometabolism in the posterior temporal-parietal cortex (Fig. 350-2C, D). The EEG is normal or shows nonspecific slowing. Routine spinal fluid examination is also normal. The use of blood Apo ε genotyping is discussed under "Genetic Considerations" below.

Slowly progressive decline in memory and orientation, normal results on laboratory tests, and an MRI or CT scan showing only diffuse or posteriorly predominant cortical and hippocampal atrophy are highly suggestive of AD. A clinical diagnosis of AD, reached after careful evaluation, is confirmed at autopsy ~90% of the time, with misdiagnosed cases usually representing one of the other dementing disorders (Table 350-3).

Epidemiology   The most important risk factors for AD are old age and a positive family history. The frequency of AD increases with each decade of adult life, reaching 20 to 40% of the population over the age of 85. A positive family history of dementia suggests a genetic cause of AD. Female gender may also be a risk factor independent of the greater longevity of women. Some AD patients have a past history of head trauma with concussion, but this appears to be a relatively minor risk factor. AD is more common in groups with lower educational attainment, but education influences test-taking ability, and it is clear that AD can affect persons of all intellectual levels. One study found that the capacity to express complex written language in early adulthood correlated with a decreased risk for AD. Numerous environmental factors, including aluminum, mercury, and viruses, have been proposed as causes of AD, but none has been demonstrated to play a significant role. Several studies suggest that the use of nonsteroidal anti-inflammatory agents is associated with a decreased risk of AD, but this has not been confirmed in large prospective studies. Vascular disease does not seem to be a direct cause of AD, but amyloid angiopathy can lead to ischemic infarctions or hemorrhages. Elevated homocysteine and cholesterol levels, hypertension, and insufficient exercise are all being explored as potential risk factors for AD.

Pathology The most severe pathology is usually found in the hippocampus, temporal cortex, and nucleus basalis of Meynert (lateral septum). The most important microscopic findings are neuritic "senile" plaques and NFTs. These lesions accumulate in small numbers during normal aging of the brain but occur in excess in AD. Neuritic plaques contain a central core that includes Aβ amyloid, proteoglycans, Apo ε4, α1 anti-chymotrypsin, and other proteins. Aβ amyloid is a protein of 39 to 42 amino acids that is derived proteolytically from a larger transmembrane protein, amyloid precursor protein (APP), which has neurotrophic and neuroprotective activity. The normal function of Aβ amyloid is unknown. Soluble amyloid fibrils may represent the initial pathologic event in AD leading to formation of neuritic plaques. The plaque core is surrounded by the debris of degenerating neurons, microglia, and macrophages. The accumulation of Aβ amyloid in cerebral arterioles, termed *amyloid angiopathy*, may lead to cerebral lobar hemorrhages. NFTs are silver-staining, twisted neurofilaments in neuronal cytoplasm that represent abnormally phosphorylated tau protein and appear as paired helical filaments by electron microscopy. Tau is a microtubule-associated protein that may function to assemble and stabilize the microtubules that convey cell organelles, glycoproteins, and other important materials through the neuron. A hyperphosphorylated state of tau impairs its capacity to bind to microtubules. AD is also associated with decreased levels of several proteins and neurotransmitters in the cerebral cortex, especially acetylcholine, its synthetic enzyme choline acetyltransferase, and nicotinic cholinergic receptors. Reduction of acetylcholine may result from degeneration of cholinergic neurons in the nucleus basalis of Meynert that project to many areas of the cortex. There is also reduction in norepinephrine levels in brainstem nuclei such as the locus coeruleus.

GENETIC CONSIDERATIONS Several genes have been found to play important roles in the pathogenesis of at least some cases of AD. The first to be identified was the *APP* gene on chromosome 21. Point mutations in *APP* produce early-onset, autosomal dominant AD. APP is a membrane-spanning protein that is subsequently processed into smaller units, including Aβ amyloid that is deposited in neuritic plaques. Aβ peptide results from cleavage of APP by β- and γ-secretases (Fig. 350-3). Only very rare families with AD-producing *APP* mutations have been identified. However, adults with trisomy 21 (Down's syndrome) who survive beyond age 40 consistently develop a progressive dementia superimposed upon their baseline mental retardation and accompanied by typical neuropathologic changes of AD. Presumably the extra dose of the *APP* gene on chromosome 21 is the initiating cause of AD in adult Down's syndrome and results in an excess of cerebral amyloid.

FIGURE 350-2 Alzheimer's disease. Axial T1-weighted MR images through the midbrain of a normal 86-year-old athletic individual (A) and a 77-year-old male (B) with Alzheimer's disease. Note that both individuals have prominent sulci and slight dilatation of the lateral ventricles. However, there is a reduction in the volume of the hippocampus of the patient with Alzheimer's disease (arrows) compared with that of the normal-for-age hippocampus of the older individual. Fluorodeoxyglucose positron emission tomographic scans of a normal control (C) and a patient with Alzheimer's disease (D). Note that the patient with Alzheimer's disease has decreased activity in the parietal lobes bilaterally (arrows), a typical finding in this condition. (*Images courtesy of TF Budinger, University of California.*)

Investigation of large families with multigenerational familial AD led to the discovery of two additional AD genes, termed the *presenilins*. Presenilin-1 (*PS-1*) is on chromosome 14 and encodes a protein called S182. Mutations in this gene cause an early-onset AD (onset before age 60 and often before age 50) transmitted in an autosomal dominant, highly penetrant fashion. More than 50 different mutations have been found in the *PS-1* gene in families from a wide range of ethnic backgrounds. Presenilin-2 (*PS-2*) is on chromosome 1 and encodes a protein called STM2. The two genes (*PS-1* and *PS-2*) are highly homologous and encode similar proteins that at first appeared to have seven transmembrane domains (hence the designation *STM*), but subsequent studies have suggested eight such domains with a ninth submembrane region. Both S182 and STM2 are cytoplasmic neuronal proteins that are widely expressed throughout the nervous system. They are homologous to a cell-trafficking protein, sel 12, found in the nematode *Coenorhabditis elegans*. Patients with mutations in these genes have elevated plasma levels of Aβ42 amyloid, suggesting a possible link between the presenilins and APP. There is evidence that *PS-1* is involved in the cleavage of APP at the γ-secretase site, and mutations in either gene (*PS-1* or *PS-2*) may disturb this function. Mutations in *PS-1* have thus far proved to be the most common cause of early-onset familial AD, representing 40 to 70% of this relatively rare syndrome. Mutations in *PS-1* tend to produce AD with an earlier age of onset (mean onset, 45 years) and a shorter, more rapidly pro-

Step 1: Cleavage by either α- or β-secretase

Step 2: Cleavage by γ-secretase

FIGURE 350-3 Amyloid precursor protein (APP) is catabolized by β-, α-, and γ-secretases. A key initial step is the digestion by either β-secretase (BASE) or α-secretase [(ADAM10 or ADAM17 (TACE))], producing smaller nontoxic products. Cleavage of the β-secretase product by γ-secretase (step 2) results in either the toxic Aβ$_{42}$ or the nontoxic Aβ$_{40}$ peptide; cleavage of the α-secretase product by γ-secretase produces the nontoxic P3 peptide. Excess production of Aβ$_{42}$ is a key initiator of cellular damage in Alzheimer's disease. Current AD research is focused on developing therapies designed to reduce accumulation of Aβ$_{42}$ by antagonizing β- or γ-secretases; promoting α-secretase; or clearing Aβ$_{42}$ that has already formed by use of specific antibodies.

gressive course (mean duration 6 to 7 years) than the disease caused by mutations in *PS-2* (mean onset 53 years; duration 11 years). Some carriers of uncommon *PS-2* mutations have had onset of dementia after the age of 70. Mutations in the *presenilins* are rarely involved in the more common sporadic cases of late-onset AD occurring in the general population. DNA testing for these uncommon mutations is now possible on a research basis, and mutation analysis of *PS-1* is commercially available. Such testing is likely to be positive only in early-onset familial cases of AD. Any testing of asymptomatic at-risk individuals should be done only in the context of formal genetic counseling.

A discovery of great importance has implicated the *Apo ε* gene on chromosome 19 in the pathogenesis of late-onset familial and sporadic forms of AD. *Apo ε* is involved in cholesterol transport (Chap. 335) and has three alleles, designated 2, 3, and 4. The Apo ε4 allele has a strong association with AD in the general population, including sporadic and late-onset familial cases. Approximately 40 to 65% of AD patients, compared to 24 to 30% of the nondemented Caucasian population, has at least one ε4 allele. Many AD patients have no ε4 allele, however, and individuals with ε4 may never develop AD. Nevertheless, it is clear that the Apo ε4 allele, especially in the homozygous 4/4 state, is an important risk factor for AD. It appears to act as a dose-dependent modifier of age of onset, with the earliest onset associated with the ε4/4 homozygous state. Apo ε may be involved with the clearance of amyloid; clearance is least efficient with Apo ε4. Apo ε is present in the neuritic amyloid plaques of AD, and it may be involved in NFT formation, because it binds to tau. Apo ε4 decreases neurite outgrowth in cultures of dorsal root ganglion neurons, perhaps indicating a deleterious role in the brain's response to injury. Some cognitively normal ε4 heterozygotes and homozygotes have also been found by PET to have decreased cerebral cortical metabolic rates, suggesting possible presymptomatic abnormalities compatible with the earliest stage of AD. Finally, there is suggestive evidence that the ε2 allele may be "protective."

Apo ε testing is not indicated as a predictive test for AD in normal persons. In demented persons who meet clinical criteria for AD, the finding of an ε4 allele increases the reliability of diagnosis; however, its absence does not eliminate the diagnosis of AD. Furthermore, all patients with dementia, including those with an ε4 allele, require a search for reversible causes of their cognitive impairment. The ε4 allele is not associated with FTD, DLB, or CJD.

Additional genes are also likely to be involved in AD. Potential candidate genes have been described on chromosomes 12 (α$_2$-macroglobulin) and 10.

℞ TREATMENT

AD cannot be cured, and no highly effective drug exists. The focus is on judicious use of cholinesterase inhibitor drugs; symptomatic management of behavioral problems; and building rapport with the patient, family members, and other caregivers.

Tacrine (tetrahydroaminoacridine), donepezil, rivastigmine, and galantamine are approved by the U.S. Food and Drug Administration (FDA) for treatment of AD. Their pharmacologic action is presumed to be inhibition of cholinesterase, with a resulting increase in cerebral levels of acetylcholine. Controlled studies indicate that cholinesterase inhibitors improve caregiver ratings of patients' functioning and decrease the rate of decline in cognitive test scores over periods of up to 3 years. The average patient on an anticholinesterase compound maintains his or her MMSE score at 1 year, whereas a placebo-treated patient declines two to three points over the same time period. Nevertheless, these compounds are only modestly efficacious and offer little or no benefit in the late stages of AD. Tacrine is expensive and may cause hepatotoxicity, thus it is rarely used. Donepezil avoids liver toxicity and can be administered once daily (5 to 10 mg), offering an advantage over the other cholinesterase inhibitors.

In a prospective observational study, the use of estrogen-replacement therapy appeared to protect—by ~50%—against development of AD in women. This study appeared to confirm the results of two earlier case-controlled studies. However, a prospective placebo-controlled study of a combined estrogen-progesterone therapy for asymptomatic postmenopausal women appeared to increase the prevalence of dementia. This study has markedly dampened enthusiasm for hormone treatments for the prevention of dementia. Additionally, no benefit has been found in the treatment of established AD with estrogen.

In patients with moderately advanced AD, a prospective trial of the antioxidants selegiline (Chap. 351), α-tocopherol (vitamin E), or both slowed institutionalization and progression to death. Because vitamin E has less potential for toxicity than selegiline and is inexpensive, the doses used in this study of 1000 IU twice daily are offered to many patients with AD. However, the beneficial effects of vitamin E are likely to be small.

A controlled trial of an extract of *Ginkgo biloba* found modest improvement in cognitive function in subjects with AD and vascular dementia. This study requires confirmation before *Ginkgo biloba* is considered an effective treatment for dementia because there was a high subject dropout rate and no improvement on a clinician's judgment scale.

One study of AD subjects in the mid-stages of disease showed a slowing of progression over a 28-week course in patients treated with memantine, an NMDA receptor antagonist.

There has been considerable enthusiasm for a strategy involving vaccination against the Aβ protein. This approach was highly effective in mouse models of AD; amyloid deposits were effectively cleared, and cognitive decline was arrested. The mechanism appears to involve generation of antibodies against Aβ, which cross the blood-brain barrier and eliminate neuritic plaques. Unfortunately, in human trials this approach led to life-threatening meningoencephalitis in some vaccinated individuals. Modifications of the vaccine approach are under development.

Several retrospective studies have suggested that nonsteroidal antiinflammatory agents and statins (HMG-CoA reductase inhibitors) may protect against dementia. Controlled prospective studies are under way. Other prospective studies designed to lower serum homocysteine levels are in progress, based upon epidemiologic studies that revealed an association of elevated homocysteine levels with dementia progression.

Mild to moderate depression, common in the early stages of AD, may respond to antidepressant or cholinesterase inhibitors. Selective serotonin reuptake inhibitors (SSRIs) are commonly used due to their low anticholinergic side effects. Generalized seizures should be treated with an appropriate anticonvulsant, such as phenytoin or carbamazepine. For management of behavioral disturbances and suggestions for caregivers, see "General Symptomatic Treatment of the Patient with Dementia," below.

VASCULAR DEMENTIA Dementia associated with cerebrovascular disease can be divided into two general categories: multi-infarct dementia and diffuse white matter disease (also called subcortical arteriosclerotic encephalopathy, or Binswanger's disease). Cerebrovascular disease appears to be a more common cause of dementia in Asia than in Europe and North America. Individuals who have had several strokes may develop chronic cognitive deficits, commonly called *multi-infarct dementia*. The strokes may be large or small (sometimes lacunar) and usually involve several different brain regions. The occurrence of dementia appears to depend partly on the total volume of damaged cortex, but it is also more common in individuals with left-hemisphere lesions, independent of any language disturbance. Patients typically report a history of discrete episodes of sudden neurologic deterioration. Many multi-infarct dementia patients have a history of hypertension, diabetes, coronary artery disease, or other manifestations of widespread atherosclerosis. Physical examination usually shows focal neurologic deficits such as hemiparesis, a unilateral Babinski reflex, a visual field defect, or pseudobulbar palsy. The recurrent strokes result in a stepwise progression of disease. Neuroimaging studies show multiple areas of infarction. Thus, the history and neuroimaging findings differentiate this condition from AD. However, both AD and multiple infarctions are common and sometimes occur together. With normal aging, there is also an accumulation of amyloid in cerebral blood vessels, leading to a condition called *cerebral amyloid angiopathy of aging* (not associated with dementia), which predisposes older persons to hemorrhagic lobar stroke. AD patients with amyloid angiopathy may be at increased risk of cerebral infarction.

Some individuals with dementia are discovered on MRI to have bilateral subcortical white matter abnormalities, termed *diffuse white matter disease* (or leukoaraiosis), often occurring in association with lacunar infarctions (Fig. 350-4). The dementia may be insidious in onset and progress slowly, features that distinguish it from multi-infarct dementia, although other patients can show a stepwise deterioration more typical of multi-infarct dementia. Early symptoms are mild confusion, apathy, changes in personality, depression, psychosis, and

FIGURE 350-4 Diffuse white matter disease (Binswanger's disease). Axial T2-weighted MR image through the lateral ventricles reveals multiple areas of abnormal high signal intensity involving the periventricular white matter as well as the corona radiata and lentiform nuclei (*arrows*). While seen in some individuals with normal cognition, this appearance is more pronounced in patients with dementia of a vascular etiology.

memory or executive deficits. Marked difficulties in judgment and orientation and dependence on others for daily activities develop later. Euphoria, elation, depression, or aggressive behaviors are common. Both pyramidal and cerebellar signs may be present in the same patient. A gait disorder appears in at least half of affected patients. With advanced disease, urinary incontinence and dysarthria with or without other pseudobulbar features (e.g., dysphagia, emotional lability) are frequent. Seizures and myoclonic jerks appear in a minority of patients. This disorder is a microangiopathy due to occlusive disease of small penetrating cerebral arteries and arterioles. The patients usually, but not always, have a history of hypertension, but any disease causing stenosis of small cerebral vessels may be the critical underlying factor. The term *Binswanger's disease* should be used with caution, because it does not really identify a single entity.

A dominantly inherited form of diffuse white matter disease is known as *cerebral autosomal dominant arteriopathy with subcortical infarcts and leukoencephalopathy* (CADASIL). Clinically there is a progressive dementia developing in the fifth to seventh decades in multiple family members who may also have a history of migraine and recurrent stroke without hypertension. Skin biopsy may show characteristic dense bodies in the media of arterioles. The disease is caused by mutations in the notch 3 gene, and there is a commercially available genetic test. The frequency of this disorder is unknown, and there are no known treatments. Mitochondrial disorders can present with strokelike episodes and can selectively injure basal ganglia or cortex. Many such patients show other findings suggestive of a neurologic or systemic disorder such as ophthalmoplegia, retinal degeneration, deafness, myopathy, neuropathy, or diabetes. Diagnosis is difficult, but serum, and especially CSF, levels of lactate and pyruvate may be abnormal, and biopsy of affected tissue is often diagnostic.

Treatment of vascular dementia must be focused on the underlying causes, such as hypertension, atherosclerosis, and diabetes. Recovery of lost cognitive function is not likely to occur, although fluctuations with periods of improvement are common. Anticholinesterase compounds appear to be useful, as in AD (see above).

FRONTOTEMPORAL DEMENTIA AND RELATED DISORDERS ■ **Frontotemporal Dementia** FTD often begins between 50 and 70 years of age, and in this age group its prevalence may approach that of AD. Men and women are equally affected. Unlike AD, behavioral symptoms often predominate in the early stages of FTD. FTD can be sporadic or familial. The clinical heterogeneity is remarkable; patients demonstrate combinations of disinhibition, dementia, apraxia, parkinsonism, and motor neuron disease. In many families with an autosomal dominant pattern of inheritance, mutations in the tau gene on chromosome 17 have been found; in others, the dementia has been linked to 17 but does not involve tau. In still other families, chromosomes 3 and 9 have been linked to FTD.

Early symptoms are divided between cognitive, behavioral, and sometimes motor abnormalities, reflecting degeneration of the anterior frontal and temporal regions, basal ganglia, and motor neurons. Cognitive presentations typically spare memory and involve planning, judgment, or language. Poor business decisions, difficulty organizing work plans, and speech and language deficits emerge. Insight into the disorder is often severely impaired. Common behavioral deficits associated with FTD include apathy, disinhibition, weight gain, food fetishes, compulsions, and euphoria.

Findings at the bedside are dictated by the anatomic localization of the disorder. Asymmetric left frontal cases present with nonfluent aphasias, while left anterior temporal degeneration is characterized by loss of words and concepts related to language (semantic dementia). Nonfluent patients quickly progress to mutism, while those with semantic dementia develop features of visual agnosia, losing the ability to recognize faces, objects, and words (Chap. 23). Copying, calculating, and navigation often remain normal into later in the illness. These left hemisphere presentations of FTD have been called *primary pro*

FIGURE 350-5 Frontotemporal dementia (FTD). Coronal MRI sections from one patient with frontally predominant FTD (*left*) and another with temporally predominant FTD (*right*). Prominent atrophy affecting the frontal gyri (*white arrows*) is present in frontally predominant FTD, particularly affecting the right frontal region; note also the thinning of the corpus callosum superior to the lateral ventricles. This patient presented with dysinhibition and antisocial behavior. In the temporally predominant patient, severe atrophy in the left temporal lobe (*open arrows*) and amygdala (*white arrowheads*) is present; this patient presented with progressive aphasia. (*Images courtesy of H Rosen and G Schauer, University of California at San Francisco.*)

gressive aphasia. In contrast, right frontal or temporal cases show profound alterations in social conduct with loss of empathy, disinhibition, and antisocial behaviors predominating. Memory and visuospatial skills are relatively spared in most FTD patients. There is a striking overlap between FTD and PSP, CBD, and motor neuron disease; ophthalmoplegia, dystonia, swallowing symptoms, and fasciculations are common at presentation of FTD or emerge during the course of the illness.

The anatomic hallmark of FTD is a marked atrophy of the temporal and/or frontal lobes, which can be visualized by neuroimaging studies (Figs. 350-5 and 350-6). The atrophy is sometimes remarkably asymmetric. A variety of pathologies have been associated with the clinical syndrome. The most consistent microscopic findings include gliosis and neuronal loss, and many cases show swollen or ballooned neurons containing cytoplasmic inclusions that in the majority of cases stain for tau. These aggregates sometimes resemble those found in PSP and CBD; tau is accepted as playing a major role in the pathogenesis of all three conditions. A toxic gain of function related to tau underlies the pathogenesis of many familial cases and is presumed to play a role in sporadic cases as well. Finally, many patients show no cellular inclusions, and the pathology remains bland with frontal and temporal gliosis, vacuolar changes, and neuronal loss the only evidence for disease. Nearly 80% of FTD patients show involvement of the basal ganglia at autopsy, and 15% go on to develop motor neuron disease, indicating the multisystem nature of this illness. Depletion of seratonergic and glutamatergic neurons is present in many patients. In contrast to AD, the cholinergic system is relatively spared in FTD.

Pick's disease was historically described as a progressive degenerative disorder of the anterior frontal and temporal neocortex accompanied by intracellular inclusions (*Pick's bodies*) that stain positive with silver (argyrophilic) and tau. Many of the τ-positive inclusions in FTD cases, however, are not labeled with silver stains. Although the nomenclature for these patients has remained controversial, the term *FTD* is increasingly used for all patients with frontotemporal degenerations, whereas Pick's disease is used to classify pathologically the subset of FTD cases that show Pick's bodies at autopsy.

The burden on caregivers of FTD patients is extremely high. Treatment is symptomatic, and there are currently no therapies known to slow progression or improve cognitive symptoms. Many of the behaviors that accompany FTD such as depression, hyperorality, compulsions, and irritability can be ameliorated with serotonin-modifying antidepressants. The co-association with motor disorders necessitates the careful use antipsychotics, which can exacerbate this problem.

Progressive Supranuclear Palsy PSP is a degenerative disease that usually begins with falls and a vertical supranuclear gaze paresis and progresses to symmetric rigidity and dementia. A stiff, unstable posture

with hyperextension of the neck and slow gait with frequent falls is characteristic. Early in the disease, patients have difficulty with downgaze and lose vertical opticokinetic nystagmus on downward movement of a target. Although patients have very limited voluntary eye movements, oculocephalic reflexes (doll's head maneuver) are retained; thus, the eye movement disorder is supranuclear. Frequent unexplained and sometimes spectacular falls are common secondary to a combination of axial rigidity, inability to look down, and bad judgment. The dementia is similar to FTD with apathy, frontal/executive dysfunction, poor judgment, slowed thought processes, impaired verbal fluency, and difficulty with sequential actions and with shifting from one task to another. These cognitive deficits are usually evident at the time of presentation and often precede the motor syndrome.

PSP is often confused with Parkinson's disease. Dementia does occur in ~20% of Parkinson's disease patients, often secondary to DLB. Furthermore, the behavioral syndromes seen with DLB differ from those of PSP (see below). The occurrence of dementia in Parkinson's disease is more likely with increasing age, increasing severity of extrapyramidal signs, a long duration of disease, and the presence of depression. Cortical atrophy is usually present on brain imaging studies. Neuropathologically, there may be Alzheimer changes in the cortex (amyloid plaques and NFTs), neuronal Lewy body inclusions in both the substantia nigra and the cortex, or no specific microscopic changes other than gliosis and neuronal loss. →*PSP and Parkinson's disease are discussed in detail in Chap. 351.*

Cortical Basal Degeneration CBD is a slowly progressive dementing illness that typically presents with a unilateral onset with rigidity, dystonia, and apraxia of one arm and hand, sometimes called the "alien hand." Eventually the condition becomes bilateral and includes dysarthria, slow gait, action tremor, and dementia. →*CBD is discussed in detail in Chap. 351.*

DEMENTIA WITH LEWY BODIES This syndrome is characterized by visual hallucinations, parkinsonism, fluctuating alertness, and falls. Dementia can precede or follow the appearance of parkinsonism. DLB may present in a patient with longstanding Parkinson's disease without cognitive impairment who slowly develops dementia associated with visual hallucinations, parkinsonism, and fluctuating alertness. In other patients the dementia and neuropsychiatric syndrome precede the parkinsonism. DLB patients are highly susceptible to metabolic perturbations, and in some the first manifestation of illness is a delirium,

FIGURE 350-6 Voxel-based morphometry (VBM) analysis showing differing patterns of brain atrophy in the frontal variant of frontotemporal dementia (red), temporal variant of frontotemporal dementia (green), and Alzheimer's disease (blue). This technique allows comparison of MRI gray matter volumes between groups of subjects. (*Image courtesy of Marilu Gorno-Tempini, University of California at San Francisco.*)

often precipitated by an infection or other systemic disturbance. A delirium induced by L-dopa, prescribed for parkinsonian symptoms attributed to Parkinson's disease, may be the initial clue that the correct diagnosis is DLB. Even without an underlying precipitant, fluctuations can be marked in DLB patients, with the occurrence of episodic confusion admixed with lucid intervals. However, despite the fluctuating pattern, the clinical features persist over a long period of time, unlike delirium, which resolves following correction of the underlying precipitant. Cognitively, DLB patients tend to have relatively better memory, but more severe visuospatial deficits, than individuals with AD.

The key neuropathologic feature is the presence of Lewy bodies throughout the cortex, amygdala, cingulated cortex, and substantia nigra. Lewy bodies are intraneuronal cytoplasmic inclusions that stain with periodic acid–Schiff (PAS) and ubiquitin. They are composed of straight neurofilaments 7 to 20 nm long with surrounding amorphous material. They are recognized by antibodies against phosphorylated and nonphosphorylated neurofilament proteins, ubiquitin, and a presynaptic protein called α-synuclein. Lewy bodies are traditionally found in the substantia nigra of patients with idiopathic Parkinson's disease. A profound cholinergic deficit is present in many patients with DLB and may be a factor responsible for the fluctuations and visual hallucinations present in these patients. In patients without other pathologic features, the condition is referred to as *diffuse Lewy body disease*. In patients whose brains also contain excessive amounts of amyloid plaques and NFTs, the condition is called the *Lewy body variant of AD*. The quantity of Lewy bodies required to establish the diagnosis is not agreed on, but a definite diagnosis requires pathologic confirmation. At autopsy, 10 to 30% of demented patients show cortical Lewy bodies.

Due to the overlap with AD and the cholinergic deficit in DLB, anticholinesterase compounds may be helpful. Exercise programs are also helpful to maximize the motor function of these patients. Antidepressants are often necessary to treat depressive syndromes that accompany DLB. Atypical antipsychotics in low doses are sometimes needed to alleviate psychosis, although even low doses can increase extrapyramidal syndromes, which rarely may be life-threatening. As noted above, patients with DLB are extremely sensitive to dopaminergic medications, which must be carefully titrated; tolerability may be improved by concomitant use of cholinesterase inhibitors.

OTHER CAUSES OF DEMENTIA *Huntington's disease (HD)* (Chap. 351) is an autosomal dominant, degenerative brain disorder. A DNA repeat expansion (CAG repeat) of the gene encoding huntingtin on chromosome 4 forms the basis of a diagnostic blood test for the disease gene. The clinical hallmarks of the disease are chorea, behavioral disturbance, and a frontal/executive disorder. Onset is usually in the fourth or fifth decade, but there is a wide range in age of onset, from childhood to >70 years. Memory is frequently not impaired until late in the disease, but attention, judgment, awareness, and executive functions may be seriously deficient at an early stage. Depression, apathy, social withdrawal, irritability, and intermittent disinhibition are common. Delusions and obsessive-compulsive behavior may occur. The disease duration is typically about 15 years but is quite variable. There is no specific treatment, but the adventitious movements and behavioral changes may partially respond to phenothiazines, haloperidol, or benzodiazepines. Asymptomatic adult children at risk for HD should

A   **B**

FIGURE 350-7 Normal pressure hydrocephalus. *A.* Sagittal T1-weighted MR image demonstrates dilatation of the lateral ventricle and stretching of the corpus callosum (*arrows*), depression of the floor of the third ventricle (*single arrowhead*), and enlargement of the aqueduct (*double arrowheads*). Note the diffuse dilatation of the lateral, third, and fourth ventricles with a patent aqueduct, typical of communicating hydrocephalus. *B.* Axial T2-weighted MR images demonstrate dilatation of the lateral ventricles without generalized cortical atrophy. This patient underwent successful ventriculoperitoneal shunting.

receive careful genetic counseling prior to DNA testing, because a positive result may have serious emotional and social consequences.

Normal-pressure hydrocephalus (NPH) is a relatively uncommon syndrome consisting of an abnormal gait (ataxic or apractic), dementia (usually mild to moderate), and urinary incontinence. Historically, many individuals who have been treated as having NPH have suffered from other dementias, particularly AD, multi-infarct dementia, and DLB. Neuroimaging findings in NPH are those of a communicating hydrocephalus with a patent aqueduct of Sylvius (Fig. 350-7). In many cases periventricular edema is present. Lumbar puncture findings include an opening pressure in the high-normal range and normal CSF protein, sugar concentrations, and cell count. NPH is presumed to be caused by obstruction to normal flow of CSF over the cerebral convexity and delayed absorption into the venous system. The indolent nature of the process results in enlarged lateral ventricles but relatively little increase in CSF pressure. There is presumably stretching and distortion of white matter tracts in the corona radiata, but the exact physiologic cause of the clinical syndrome is unclear. Some patients have a history of conditions producing scarring of the basilar meninges (blocking upward flow of CSF) such as previous meningitis, subarachnoid hemorrhage, or head trauma. Others with longstanding but asymptomatic congenital hydrocephalus may have an adult-onset deterioration in gait or memory that is confused with NPH; in these patients, the aqueduct of Sylvius is small, in contrast to patients with NPH. Unlike in AD, the NPH patient has an early and prominent gait disturbance and no evidence of cortical or hippocampal atrophy on neuroimaging studies. A number of attempts have been made to use various special studies to improve the diagnosis of NPH and predict the success of ventricular shunting. These include radionuclide cisternography (showing a delay in CSF absorption over the convexity) and various attempts to monitor and alter CSF flow dynamics. None has proved to be specific or consistently useful. There is sometimes a transient improvement in gait or cognition following lumbar puncture (or serial punctures) with removal of ≥30 mL of CSF, but this finding is not a reliable predictor of post-shunt improvement. Approximately 30 to 50% of patients identified by careful diagnosis as having NPH will show improvement with a ventricular shunting procedure. Gait may improve more than memory. Transient, short-lasting improvement is common. Patients should be carefully selected for this operation, because subdural hematoma and infection are known complications.

Prion diseases such as CJD are rapidly progressive disorders associated with dementia, focal cortical signs, rigidity, and myoclonus. The rapidity of progression seen with CJD is uncommon in AD so that distinction between the two disorders is usually straightforward. CBD and DLB progress more rapidly than AD and are associated with prominent disorders of movement and so are more likely to be mistaken for CJD. Abnormal periodic EEG discharges and cortical and basal ganglia abnormalities on diffusion-weighted MRI are unique diagnostic features of CJD. →*Prion diseases are discussed in detail in Chap. 362.*

Dementia can accompany *chronic alcoholism* (Chap. 372). This may be a result of associated malnutrition, especially of B vitamins and particularly thiamine. However, other as yet poorly defined aspects of chronic alcohol ingestion may also produce cerebral damage. A rare syndrome of dementia and seizures with degeneration of the corpus callosum has been reported primarily in male Italian drinkers of red wine (Marchiafava-Bignami disease).

Thiamine (vitamin B₁) deficiency causes Wernicke's encephalopathy (Chap. 258). The clinical presentation is a malnourished individual (frequently but not necessarily alcoholic) with confusion, ataxia, and diplopia from ophthalmoplegia. Thiamine deficiency damages the thalamus, mammillary bodies, midline cerebellum, periaqueductal gray matter of the midbrain, and peripheral nerves. Damage to the dorsomedial thalamic regions correlates most closely with memory loss. Prompt administration of parenteral thiamine may reverse the disease if given in the first few days of symptom onset. However, prolonged untreated thiamine deficiency can result in an irreversible dementia/amnestic syndrome known as *Korsakoff's syndrome*. Here, the patient is unable to recall new information despite normal immediate memory, attention span, and level of consciousness. Memory for new events is seriously impaired, whereas memory of knowledge prior to the illness is relatively intact. Patients are easily confused, disoriented, and incapable of recalling new information for more than a brief interval. Superficially, they may be conversant, entertaining, able to perform simple tasks, and follow immediate commands. Confabulation is common, although not always present, and may result in obviously erroneous statements and elaborations. There is no specific treatment because the previous thiamine deficiency has produced irreversible damage to the medial thalamic nuclei and mammillary bodies. Mammillary body atrophy may be visible on high-resolution MRI (Fig. 258-6).

Vitamin B₁₂ deficiency, as can occur in pernicious anemia, causes a macrocytic anemia and may also damage the nervous system (Chaps. 92 and 356). Neurologically it most commonly produces a spinal cord syndrome (myelopathy) affecting the posterior columns (loss of position and vibratory sense) and corticospinal tracts (hyperactive tendon reflexes with Babinski responses); it also damages peripheral nerves, resulting in sensory loss with depressed tendon reflexes. Damage to cerebral myelinated fibers may also cause dementia. The mechanism of neurologic damage is unclear but may be related to a deficiency of S-adenosylmethionine (required for methylation of myelin phospholipids) due to reduced methionine synthase activity or accumulation of methylmalonate, homocysteine, and propionate, providing abnormal substrates for fatty acid synthesis in myelin. The neurologic signs of vitamin B₁₂ deficiency are usually associated with macrocytic anemia, but on occasion may occur in its absence. Treatment with parenteral vitamin B₁₂ stops progression of the disease if instituted promptly, but reversal of advanced nervous system damage will not occur.

Deficiency of nicotinic acid (pellagra) is associated with sun-exposed skin rash, glossitis, and angular stomatitis (Chap. 61). Severe dietary deficiency of nicotinic acid along with other B vitamins such as pyridoxine may result in spastic paraparesis, peripheral neuropathy, fatigue, irritability, and dementia. This syndrome has been seen in prisoner-of-war and concentration camps. Low serum folate levels appear to be a rough index of malnutrition, but isolated folate deficiency has not been proved to be a specific cause of dementia.

Infections of the CNS usually cause delirium and other acute neurologic syndromes (Chap. 258). However, some chronic CNS infections, particularly those associated with chronic meningitis (Chap. 361), may produce a dementing illness. The possibility of chronic infectious meningitis should be suspected in patients presenting with a dementia or behavioral syndrome who also have headache, meningismus, cranial neuropathy, and/or radiculopathy. Between 20 and 30% of patients in the advanced stages of infection with HIV become demented (Chap. 173). Cardinal features include psychomotor retardation, apathy, and impaired memory. This may result from secondary opportunistic infections but can also be caused by direct infection of CNS neurons with HIV. Neurosyphilis (Chap. 153) was a common cause of dementia in the preantibiotic era; it is now uncommon but can still be encountered in patients with multiple sex partners. Characteristic CSF changes consist of pleocytosis, increased protein, and a positive Venereal Disease Research Laboratory (VDRL) test.

Primary and metastatic neoplasms of the CNS (Chap. 358) usually produce focal neurologic findings and seizures rather than dementia. However, if tumor growth begins in the frontal or temporal lobes, the initial manifestations may be memory loss or behavioral changes. A paraneoplastic syndrome of dementia associated with occult carcinoma (often small cell lung cancer) is termed *limbic encephalitis* (Chap. 87). In this syndrome, confusion, agitation, seizures, poor memory, movement disorders, and dementia occur in association with sensory neuropathy.

A nonconvulsive seizure disorder may underlie a syndrome of confusion, clouding of consciousness, and garbled speech. Psychiatric disease is often suspected, but an EEG demonstrates the seizure discharges. If recurrent or persistent, the condition may be termed *complex partial status epilepticus*. The cognitive disturbance often responds to anticonvulsant therapy. The etiology may be previous small strokes or head trauma; some cases are idiopathic.

It is important to recognize systemic diseases that indirectly affect the brain and produce chronic confusion or dementia. Such conditions include hypothyroidism; vasculitis; and hepatic, renal, or pulmonary disease. Hepatic encephalopathy may begin with irritability and confusion and slowly progress to agitation, lethargy, and coma (Chap. 258).

Isolated vasculitis of the CNS (CNS granulomatous vasculitis) (Chaps. 306 and 349) occasionally causes a chronic encephalopathy with confusion, disorientation, and clouding of consciousness. Headache is common, and strokes and cranial neuropathies may occur. Brain imaging studies may be normal or nonspecifically abnormal. CSF studies reveal a mild pleocytosis or elevation in the protein level. Cerebral angiography often shows multifocal stenosis and narrowing of vessels. A few patients have only small-vessel disease that is not revealed on angiography. The angiographic appearance is nonspecific and may be mimicked by atherosclerosis, infection, or other causes of vascular disease. Brain or meningeal biopsy demonstrates abnormal arteries with endothelial cell proliferation and infiltrates of mononuclear cells. The prognosis is often poor; however, the disorder may remit spontaneously. Some patients respond to glucocorticoids or chemotherapy.

Chronic metal exposure may produce a dementing syndrome. The key to diagnosis is to elicit a history of exposure at work, home, or even as a consequence of a medical procedure such as dialysis. Chronic lead poisoning may present as fatigue, depression, and confusion and may be associated with episodic abdominal pain and peripheral neuropathy. Inadequately fired glazed pottery has been reported as a cause. Gray lead lines appear in the gums. There is usually an anemia with basophilic stippling of red cells. The clinical presentation can resemble that of acute intermittent porphyria, including elevated levels of urine porphyrins as a result of the inhibition of δ-aminolevulinic acid dehydrase. The treatment is chelation therapy with agents such as ethylenediamine tetraacetic acid (EDTA). Chronic mercury poisoning produces dementia, peripheral neuropathy, ataxia, and tremulousness that may progress to choreoathetosis. Chronic arsenic intoxication can produce confusion and memory loss associated with nausea, weight loss, peripheral neuropathy, pigmentation and scaling of the skin, and transverse white lines of the fingernails (Mee's lines). Treatment is chelation therapy with dimercaprol (BAL). Aluminum poisoning has been best documented with the dialysis dementia syndrome in which water used during renal dialysis was contaminated with excessive amounts of aluminum. A progressive encephalopathy ensued, associated with confusion, aphasia, memory loss, agitation, and, later, lethargy and stupor. Speech arrest and myoclonic jerks were common and associated with severe and generalized EEG changes. The condition has been eliminated by the use of deionized water for dialysis.

Recurrent head trauma in professional boxers may lead to dementia, sometimes called the "punch drunk" syndrome or *dementia pugilistica*. The symptoms can be progressive, beginning late in a boxer's career or even long after retirement. The severity of the syndrome correlates with the length of the boxing career and number of bouts. Early on, a personality change associated with social instability and sometimes paranoia and delusions occurs. Later, memory loss progresses to full dementia, often associated with parkinsonian signs and ataxia or intention tremor. At autopsy, the cerebral cortex may show changes similar to those in AD, although NFTs are usually more prominent than amyloid plaques (which are usually diffuse rather than neuritic). There may also be loss of neurons in the substantia nigra. Chronic subdural hematoma (Chap. 357) is also occasionally associated with dementia, often in the context of underlying cortical atrophy from conditions such as AD or Huntington's disease. In these latter cases, evacuation of the subdural hematoma will not alter the underlying degenerative process.

Transient global amnesia (TGA) is characterized by the sudden onset of a severe episodic memory deficit, usually occurring in persons over age 50. Often, the memory loss occurs in the setting of an emotional stimulus or physical exertion. During the attack the individual is alert and communicative, general cognition seems intact, and there are no other neurologic signs or symptoms. The patient may seem confused and repeatedly ask about present events. The ability to form new memories returns after a period of hours, and the individual returns to normal with no recall for the period of the attack. Frequently no cause is determined, but cerebrovascular disease, epilepsy (7% in one study), migraine, or cardiac arrhythmia have all been implicated. A Mayo Clinic review of 277 patients with TGA found a past history of migraine in 14% and cerebrovascular disease in 11%, but these conditions were not temporally related to the TGA episodes. Approximately one-quarter of the patients had recurrent attacks, but they were not at increased risk for subsequent stroke. Rare instances of permanent memory loss after sudden onset have been reported, usually representing ischemic infarction of the hippocampi or medial thalamic nuclei bilaterally.

The ALS/parkinsonian/dementia complex of Guam is a rare degenerative disease that has occurred in the Chamorro natives on the island of Guam. Any combination of parkinsonian features, dementia, and motor neuron disease may occur. The most characteristic pathologic features are the presence of NFTs in degenerating neurons of the cortex and substantia nigra and loss of motor neurons in the spinal cord. Epidemiologic evidence supports a possible environmental cause, such as exposure to a neurotoxin with a long latency period. One interesting but unproven candidate neurotoxin occurs in the seed of the false palm tree, which Guamanians traditionally used to make flour. The ALS syndrome is decreasing in frequency on Guam, but a dementing illness with rigidity continues to be seen.

Rarely adult-onset leukodystrophies, neuronal storage diseases, and other genetic disorders can cause dementia late in life. Adult metachromatic leukodystrophy (arylsulfatase A deficiency) can present as a dementia associated with large frontal white matter lesions. Adult presentations of adrenoleukodystrophy have been reported, and in these cases involvement of the spinal cord and posterior white matter is common. This is diagnosed with measurement of medium- and long-chain fatty acids (Chap. 356). The neuronal cerebrolipofuscinoses are a genetically heterogeneous group of disorders associated with myoclonus, seizures, and progressive dementia. Diagnosis is made by finding curvilinear inclusions within white blood cells or neuronal tissue.

Psychogenic amnesia for personally important memories is common, although whether this results from deliberate avoidance of unpleasant memories or from unconscious repression is currently unknown. The event-specific amnesia is more likely to occur after violent crimes such as homicide of a close relative or friend or sexual abuse. It may also develop in association with drug or alcohol intoxication and sometimes with schizophrenia. More prolonged psychogenic amnesia occurs in fugue states that also commonly follow severe emotional stress. The patient with a fugue state suffers from a sudden loss of personal identity and may be found wandering far from home. In contrast to organic amnesia, fugue states are associated with amnesia for personal identity and events closely associated with the personal past. At the same time, memory for other recent events and the ability to learn and use new information are preserved. The episodes usually last hours or days and occasionally weeks or months while the patient takes on a new identity. On recovery, there is a residual amnesia for the period of the fugue. Very rarely, selective loss of autobiographical information represents a focal injury in the brain areas involved with these functions.

Psychiatric diseases may mimic dementia. Severely depressed individuals may appear demented, a phenomenon called *pseudodementia*. Memory and language are usually intact when carefully tested in depressed persons, and a significant memory disturbance usually suggests an underlying dementia, even if the patient is depressed. The patient with pseudodementia may feel confused and unable to accomplish routine tasks. Vegetative symptoms are common, such as insomnia, lack of energy, poor appetite, and concern with bowel function. The onset is often abrupt, and the psychosocial milieu may suggest prominent reasons for depression. Such patients respond to treatment of the depression. Schizophrenia is usually not difficult to distinguish from dementia, but occasionally the distinction can be problematic. Schizophrenia usually has a much earlier age of onset (second and third decades) than most dementing illnesses and is associated with intact memory. The delusions and hallucinations of schizophrenia are usually more complex and bizarre than those of dementia. Some chronic schizophrenics develop an unexplained progressive dementia late in life that is not related to AD. Conversely, FTD, HD, vascular dementia, DLB, AD, or leukoencephalopathy can begin with schizophrenia-like features, leading to the misdiagnosis of a psychiatric condition. The later age of onset, presence of significant deficits on cognitive testing, and neuroimaging findings point toward a degenerative condition. Memory loss may also be part of a conversion reaction. In this situation, patients commonly complain bitterly of memory loss, but careful cognitive testing either does not confirm the deficits or demonstrates inconsistent or unusual patterns of cognitive problems. The patient's behavior and "wrong" answers to questions often indicate that he or she understands the question and knows the correct answer.

Clouding of cognition by chronic drug or medication use, often prescribed by physicians, is an important cause of dementia. Sedatives, tranquilizers, and analgesics used to treat insomnia, pain, anxiety, or agitation may cause confusion, memory loss, and lethargy, especially in the elderly. Discontinuation of the offending medication often improves mentation.

GENERAL SYMPTOMATIC TREATMENT OF THE PATIENT WITH DEMENTIA

The major goals of management are to treat any correctable causes of the dementia and to provide comfort and support to the patient and caregivers. Removal of sedating or cognition-impairing drugs and medications is often beneficial. If the patient is depressed rather than demented, the depression should be vigorously treated. Patients with degenerative diseases may also be depressed, and that portion of their condition may respond to antidepressant therapy. Antidepressants that are low in cognitive side effects, such as SSRIs (Chap. 371), are advisable when treatment is necessary. Anticonvulsants are used to control seizures.

Agitation, hallucinations, delusions, and confusion are difficult to treat. These behavioral problems represent major causes for nursing home placement and institutionalization. Before treating these behaviors with medications, a thorough search for potentially modifiable environmental or metabolic factors should be sought. Hunger, lack of exercise, toothache, constipation, urinary tract infection, or drug toxicity all represent easily correctable factors that can be treated without psychoactive drugs. Medications that may calm agitation and insomnia without worsening dementia include low-dose haloperidol (0.5 to 2 mg), trazodone, buspirone, or propranolol. The new atypical antipsychotics including risperidone, olanzapine, and quetiapine are increasingly used for patients with difficult behaviors. When patients do not respond it is usually a mistake to advance to higher doses or to use anticholinergics or sedatives (such as barbiturates or benzodiazepines). The few controlled studies comparing drugs with behavioral intervention in the treatment of agitation suggest that both approaches are effective. However, careful, daily, nondrug behavior management is often not available, rendering medication necessary. Sometimes, apathy, visual hallucinations, and other psychiatric symptoms respond to the cholinesterase inhibitors, obviating the need for other therapies.

A proactive strategy has been shown to reduce the occurrence of delirium in hospitalized patients. This includes frequent orientation, cognitive activities, sleep-enhancement measures, vision and hearing aids, and correction of dehydration.

Nondrug behavior therapy has an important place in the management of dementia. The primary goal is to make the demented patient's life comfortable, uncomplicated, and safe. Memory aids such as notebooks, lists, and posted daily reminders are frequently helpful. It is also useful to stress familiar routines, short-term tasks, walks, and simple physical exercises. For many demented patients, the memory for facts is worse than that for routine activities, and they still may be able to take part in remembered physical activities such as walking, bowling, dancing, and golf. Demented patients usually object to losing control over familiar tasks such as driving, cooking, and handling finances. Attempts to help or take over may be greeted with complaints, depression, or anger. Hostile responses on the part of the caretaker are useless and sometimes harmful. Explanation, reassurance, distraction, and calm statements are more productive responses in this setting. Eventually, tasks such as finances and driving must be assumed by others, and the patient will conform and adjust. Safety is an important issue that includes not only driving but the environment of the kitchen, bathroom, and sleeping area. These areas need to be monitored, supervised, and made as safe as possible. A move to a retirement home, assisted-living center, or nursing home can initially increase confusion and agitation. Repeated reassurance, reorientation, and careful introduction to the new personnel will help to smooth the process. Provision of activities that are known to be enjoyable to the patient can be of considerable benefit. Attention should also be paid to frustration and depression in family members and caregivers. Caregiver guilt and burn-out are common, often resulting in nursing home placement of the patient. Family members often feel overwhelmed and helpless and may vent their frustrations on the patient, each other, and health care providers. Caregivers should be encouraged to take advantage of day-care facilities and respite breaks. Education and counseling about dementia are important. Local and national support groups, such as the Alzheimer's Disease and Related Disorders Association, can be of considerable help.

FURTHER READING

BOEVE BF et al: Current management of sleep disturbances in dementia: Curr Neurol Neurosci Rep 2:169, 2002

HEJI A et al: Potentially reversible conditions in 1000 consecutive memory clinic patients. J Neurol Neurosurg Psychiatry 73:390, 2002

REISBERG B et al: Memantine in moderate to severe Alzheimer's disease. N Engl J Med 348:1333, 2003

ROSEN HJ et al: Utility of clinical criteria in differentiating frontotemporal lobar degeneration (FTLD) from AD. Neurology 58:1608, 2002

SHUMAKER SA et al: Estrogen plus progestin and the incidence of dementia and mild cognitive impairment in postmenopausal women: The Women's Health Initiative Memory Study: A randomized controlled trial. JAMA 289:2651, 2003

VERMEER SE et al: Silent brain infarcts and the risk of dementia and cognitive decline. N Engl J Med 348:1215, 2003

351 PARKINSON'S DISEASE AND OTHER MOVEMENT DISORDERS
Mahlon R. DeLong, Jorge L. Juncos

PARKINSON'S DISEASE

Parkinson's disease (PD) is the most common example of a family of neurodegenerative disorders characterized by a neuronal accumulation of the presynaptic protein α-synuclein and by variable degrees of *parkinsonism*, defined as a paucity and slowness of movement (*bradykinesia*), tremor at rest, rigidity, shuffling gait, and flexed posture. Nearly all forms of parkinsonism result from a reduction of dopaminergic transmission within the basal ganglia. Sporadic and idiopathic PD account for ~75% of all cases of parkinsonism; the remaining 25% result from genetically defined etiologies and other causes including other neurodegenerative disorders, cerebrovascular disease, and drugs.

Epidemiology PD afflicts >1 million individuals in the United States (~1% of those >55 years). Its peak age of onset is in the 60s (range is 35 to 85 years), and the course of the illness ranges between 10 and 25 years. Familial clusters of autosomal dominant and recessive forms of PD comprise ~5% of cases (Table 351-1). These are characterized by an earlier age of onset (typically before age 50 years) and a longer course than the more typical "sporadic" PD. Although most patients with PD appear to have no strong genetic determinant, epidemiologic evidence points to a complex interaction between genetic vulnerability and environmental factors (Fig. 351-1). Risk factors include a positive family history, male gender, head injury, exposure to pesticides, consumption of well water, and rural living. Factors linked to a reduced incidence of PD include coffee drinking, smoking, use of nonsteroidal anti-inflammatory drugs, and estrogen replacement in postmenopausal women.

Clinical Features A diagnosis of PD can be made with some confidence in patients who present with at least two of the three cardinal signs—rest tremor, rigidity, and bradykinesia. Tremor is particularly important, as it is present in 85% of patients with true PD; a diagnosis of PD is particularly difficult when tremor is absent. A unilateral and gradual onset of symptoms further supports the diagnosis. Masked facies, decreased eye blinking, stooped posture, and decreased arm swing complete the early picture. The onset may also be heralded by

TABLE 351-1 *Familial Parkinson's Disease*

Locus	Gene	Inheritance
PARK1	α-Synuclein	AD
PARK2	Parkin	AR
PARK4	α-Synuclein triplication	AD
PARK5	UCHL1	AD
PARK7	DJ-1	AR
PARK3,4,6,8,9	Unknown	AD and AR mutations
PARK10	Unknown	Late-onset susceptibility gene

vague feelings of weakness and fatigue, incoordination, aching, and discomfort.

Motor Features The most disabling feature of PD is bradykinesia, which interferes with all aspects of daily living such as walking, rising from a chair, turning in bed, dressing. Fine motor control is also impaired as evidenced by decreased manual dexterity and handwriting (*micrographia*). Soft speech (*hypophonia*) and sialorrhea are other troubling manifestations of (bulbar) bradykinesia. Rest tremor, at a frequency of 4 to 6 Hz, typically appears unilaterally, first distally, involving the digits and wrist where it may have a "pill-rolling" character. Tremor usually spreads proximally, ipsilaterally, and occasionally to the leg before crossing to the other side after a year or more. It may appear later in the lips, tongue, and jaw but spares the head. Rigidity is felt as a uniform resistance to passive movement about a joint throughout the full range of motion, giving rise to a characteristic "plastic" quality. Brief, regular interruptions of resistance during passive movement, corresponding to subclinical tremor, may give rise to a "cogwheeling" sensation. Dystonia involving the distal arm or leg may occur early in the disease, unrelated to treatment, especially in younger patients. It can also be provoked by antiparkinsonian drug therapy.

Gait disturbance with shuffling short steps and a tendency to turn en bloc is a prominent feature of PD. Festinating gait, a classic parkinsonian sign, results from the combination of flexed posture and loss of postural reflexes, which cause the patient to accelerate in an effort to "catch up" with the body's center of gravity. Freezing of gait, a feature of more advanced PD, occurs commonly at the onset of locomotion (start hesitation), when attempting to change direction or turn around, and upon entering a narrow space such as a doorway.

Abnormalities of balance and posture tend to increase in prominence as the disease progresses. Flexion of the head, stooping and tilting of the upper trunk, and a tendency to hold the arm in a flexed posture while walking are common, as are changes in the posture of the fingers and hands. Postural instability is one of the most disabling features of advanced PD, contributing to falls and injuries and leading to major morbidity and mortality. Significant postural instability and falls in the first years of the illness, however, strongly suggest a diagnosis other than PD.

Non-Motor Features Non-motor aspects of PD include depression and anxiety, cognitive impairment, sleep disturbances, sensory abnormalities and pain, loss of smell (*anosmia*), and disturbances of autonomic function. Together they may contribute as much to the burden of the disease as the more obvious motor abnormalities. Some of these (e.g., anosmia, depression, and sleep disorders) may be present long before the onset of motor signs. The physiologic basis of the non-motor signs and symptoms are explained in part by widespread involvement of brainstem, olfactory, thalamic, and cortical structures, as discussed below.

Sensory symptoms most often manifest as a distressing sensation of inner restlessness presumed to be a form of akathisia. Aching pain and discomfort in the extremities can be a prominent presenting symptom or develop when antiparkinson medications are wearing off. Other patients develop a subjective shortness of breath in the absence of any underlying cardiorespiratory pathology.

Sleep disorders are common in PD. Daytime drowsiness and frequent napping are typical signs of sleep disruption. Factors that disrupt sleep include nighttime reemergence of bradykinesia and rigidity, with difficulty turning in bed, as well as tremor and involuntary movements (e.g., myoclonic jerks or periodic leg movements). Restless legs and rapid eye movement–behavioral disorder (RBD) are present in considerable numbers of patients, often preceding the onset of PD. Vivid dreams and hallucinations related to dopaminomimetic therapy may

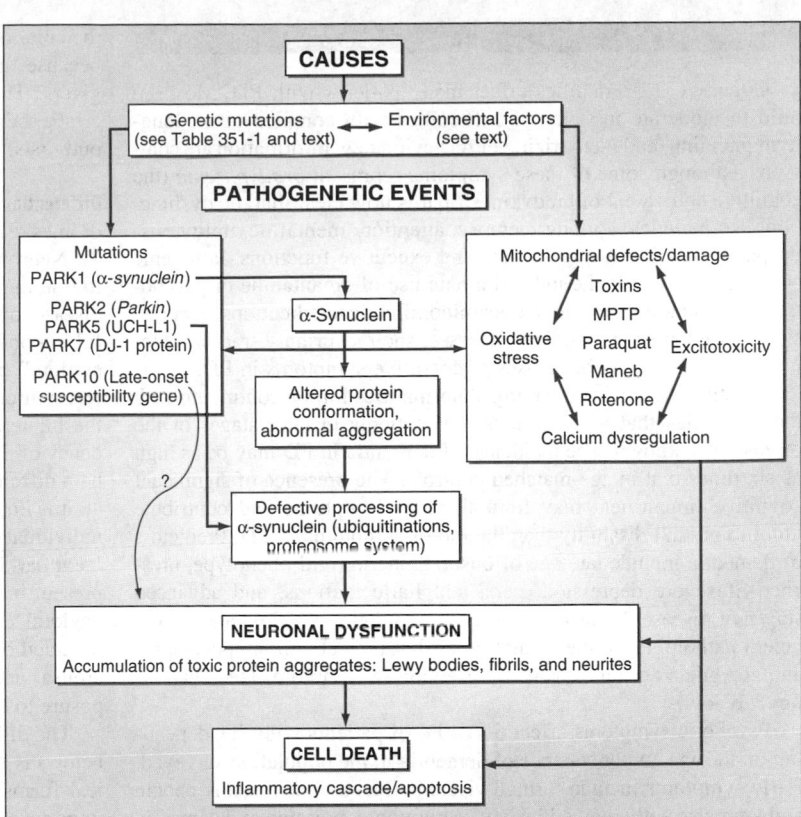

FIGURE 351-1 Possible cascade of pathogenic events leading to neuronal cell death in Parkinson's disease.

also contribute to sleep disruption. Finally, sleep apnea and other sleep disturbances can occur.

Autonomic dysfunction can produce diverse manifestations, including orthostatic hypotension, constipation, urinary urgency and frequency, excessive sweating, and seborrhea. Orthostatic hypotension is present in many patients resulting from sympathetic denervation of the heart or as a side effect of dopaminomimetic therapy. This rarely leads to syncope unless the patient has developed true autonomic failure or has an unrelated cardiac problem. Drenching sweats may occur in advanced PD, often related to wearing off of medication.

Neuropsychiatric Symptoms Changes in mood, cognition, and behavior are common accompaniments of the later stages of PD and may be the direct result of PD or its comorbid pathologies [e.g., Alzheimer's disease (AD), cortical dementia with Lewy bodies (DLB)], or occur as a side effect of its pharmacotherapy.

Depression affects approximately half of patients with PD and can occur at any phase of the illness. It is often difficult to diagnose due to the overlap between the somatic and vegetative symptoms of PD and depression. As a consequence, depression often goes unrecognized and untreated. There is compelling evidence that depression in PD is an intrinsic part of the illness and not simply a reaction to disability. Recognizing even mild depression is particularly important since it can account for otherwise unexplained worsening parkinsonian motor symptoms, new somatic symptoms, and sleep disruption. Depression can also be induced or aggravated iatrogenically by antiparkinsonian and psychotropic agents used to treat other symptoms. Finally, other causes for depressive symptoms and refractory depression should always be considered, including hypothyroidism, hypogonadism, and vitamin B_{12} deficiency.

Anxiety disorders in PD can appear in isolation or as an accompaniment of depression or progressive cognitive impairment. They can also be due to an akathisia equivalent mediated by "dopamine hunger" due to undertreatment of motor symptoms. The development of drug-induced motor fluctuations can compound the problem by precipitating fluxes in anxiety during the off periods that mimic panic attacks.

Cognitive abnormalities affect many patients with PD. Most are mild to moderate in severity. Difficulties with complex tasks, long-term planning, and memorizing or retrieving new information are common. Although some of these symptoms represent *bradyphrenia* (the cognitive equivalent of bradykinesia), it is now clear that the dysfunction also includes working memory, attention, mental flexibility, visuospatial function, word fluency, and executive functions. Iatrogenic contributors include the indiscriminate use of amantadine or psychotropic, anticholinergic, and dopaminomimetic medications. Depression and intercurrent medical illnesses, such as urinary tract or other infections, are reversible causes of cognitive symptoms in PD.

Whether these nondementing abnormalities form a continuum with the dementias that affect a subset of patients in later stages of the disease is unknown. The incidence of dementia in PD may be as high as six times that in age-matched controls. The presence of significant cognitive impairment may limit therapeutic options and contribute more to overall disability than the motor symptoms in PD. Predictors of dementia include late age of onset, akinetic rigid phenotype, presence of severe depression, persistent hallucinations, and advanced stages of disease. In most instances accumulating amyloid and α-synuclein pathologies in the frontal lobes, basal forebrain, hippocampus, and amygdala account for the progression of symptoms (see "Pathology," below).

Psychotic symptoms affect 6 to 40% of patients with PD, depending on the age and prevalence of dementia in the population surveyed. Early symptoms include formed visual hallucinations (usually people and animals) with retained insight. Although depression and dementia are the most important risk factors for psychotic symptoms in PD, the symptoms are often triggered by drug therapy and are dose-dependent. Dopaminomimetics, anticholinergics, amantadine, and selegiline are the chief offenders. Delusions are more disturbing than hallucinations because they place an even heavier burden on the family and caregivers. The prodrome to these psychotic symptoms includes subtle erratic behaviors with temperamental and sometimes unreasonable outbursts.

Differential Diagnosis   The differential diagnosis of parkinsonian syndromes requires a careful history and physical examination (Table 351-2). Neuroimaging with magnetic resonance imaging (MRI) is useful to rule out disorders such as normal pressure hydrocephalus, vascular disease, or mass lesions. Positron emission tomography (PET) is helpful in confirming suspected atypical forms (see "Corticobasal Degeneration," below). Essential tremor (ET) is sometimes confused with rest tremor in PD, but the absence of other signs of parkinsonism and the bilaterality, higher frequency (8 to 10 Hz), and postural dependency of ET plus significant relief with even a small amount of alcohol help differentiate this from the rest tremor of PD. In individuals under 40 it is important to rule out Wilson's disease (Chap. 339). In younger individuals Huntington's disease (HD) sometimes presents with prominent parkinsonian features. Although parkinsonian features are often present in AD, they are greatly outweighed by the cognitive and behavioral disturbances. In DLB, the parkinsonian features are compounded by the early appearance of hallucinations and disturbances in arousal and behavior. Parkinsonism may also develop following exposure to certain neurotoxins such as carbon monoxide or manganese.

The differentiation of sporadic PD from atypical parkinsonism (see below) is the most difficult task, since early in their course these atypical forms often meet diagnostic criteria for PD. Accordingly, it is important not to settle on a definite diagnosis at the first visit. The development of early imbalance and falls suggests progressive supranuclear palsy (PSP); early urinary incontinence, orthostatic hypotension, and dysarthria suggest multiple system atrophy (MSA). The

---

TABLE 351-2   *Differential Diagnosis of Parkinsonism*

PRIMARY PARKINSONISM	SECONDARY PARKINSONISM
I. Familial ("primary") PD (rare; see Table 351-1)	I. Repeated head trauma ("dementia pugilistica" with parkinsonian features)
II. Idiopathic ("sporadic") PD (most common form)	II. Infectious and postinfectious diseases
Phenotype may be influenced by vulnerability genes and environmental factors	A. Postencephalitic PD
III. Other neurodegenerative disorders	B. Neurosyphillis
A. Disorders associated with α-synuclein pathology	III. Metabolic conditions
1. Multiple systems atrophies (glial and neuronal inclusions)	A. Hypoparathyroidism or pseudohypoparathyroidism with basal ganglia calcifications
a. Striatonigral degeneration	B. Non-Wilsonian hepatolenticular degeneration
b. Olivopontocerebellar atrophy	IV. Drugs
c. Shy-Drager syndrome	A. Neuroleptics (typical antipsychotics)
d. Motor neuron disease with PD features	B. Selected atypical antipsychotics (see text)
2. Dementia with Lewy bodies (cortical and brainstem neuronal inclusions)	C. Antiemetics (e.g., compazine, metoclopramide)
B. Disorders associated with primary tau pathology ("tauopathies")	D. Dopamine-depleting agents (reserpine, tetrabenazine)
1. Progressive supranuclear palsy	E. ∝-Methyldopa
2. Corticobasal degeneration	F. Lithium carbonate
3. Frontotemporal dementia	G. Valproic acid
C. Disorders associated with primary amyloid pathology ("amyloidopathies")	H. Fluoxetine
1. Alzheimer's disease with parkinsonism	V. Toxins
IV. Genetically mediated disorders with occasional parkinsonian features	A. 1-Methyl-1,2,4,6 tetrahydropyridine (MPTP)
A. Wilson's disease	B. Manganese
B. Hallervorden-Spatz disease	C. Cyanide
C. Chédiak-Higashi disease	D. Methanol
D. SCA-3 spinocerebellar ataxia	E. Carbon monoxide
E. X-linked dystonia-parkinsonism (DYT3)	F. Carbon disulfide
F. Fragile X premutation associated ataxia-tremor-parkinsonism syndrome	G. *N*-hexane?
G. Huntington's disease (Westphalt variant)	
H. Prion disease	
V. Miscellaneous acquired conditions	
A. Vascular parkinsonism	
B. Normal pressure hydrocephalus	
C. Catatonia	
D. Cerebral Palsy	

Note: PD, Parkinson's disease.

early appearance of drug-induced hallucinations strongly favors the diagnosis of DLB. As a rule the different forms of atypical parkinsonism can be reliably differentiated from sporadic PD within the first 3 to 4 years.

Pathology Gross pathologic examination of the brain in PD reveals mild frontal atrophy with loss of the normal dark melanin pigment of the midbrain. Microscopically there is degeneration of the dopaminergic cells with the presence of Lewy bodies (LBs) in the remaining neurons and processes of the substantia nigra pars compacta (SNpc), other brainstem nuclei, and regions such as the medial temporal, limbic, and frontal cortices. LBs have a high concentration of α-synuclein and are the pathologic hallmark of the disorder. Mutations in the α-synuclein gene can cause familial PD by promoting the formation of α-synuclein-positive filaments that aggregate into LBs and Lewy neurites (Fig. 351-2). This pathology may begin in the anterior olfactory nuclei and lower brainstem (glossopharyngeal and vagal nerve nuclei), with ascending brainstem involvement of the locus coeruleus, n. gigantocellularis, and the raphe, before extending to the magnocellular nuclei of the basal forebrain, the central nucleus of the amygdala, and the SNpc. Involvement of these nuclei may play a role in the non-motor (e.g., autonomic, sleep, emotional, and cognitive) and refractory motor aspects (e.g., postural instability, gait, and bulbar disturbances) of PD.

The biochemical consequence of dopaminergic cell loss in the SNpc is gradual denervation of the striatum, the main target projection for the SNpc neurons. Other target regions of these neurons include the intralaminar and parafascicular nuclei of the thalamus, the globus pallidus, and the subthalamic nucleus (STN). Dopamine denervation of the striatum leads to many of the motor symptoms of PD. Symptoms develop when striatal dopamine depletion reaches 50 to 70% of normal. Pharmacologic restoration of dopamine transmission is the basis for symptomatic drug treatment of PD.

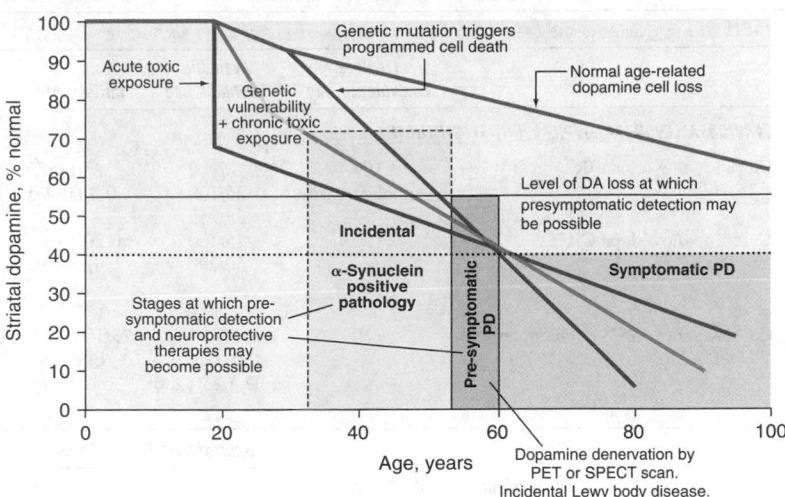

FIGURE 351-2 Proposed stages of Parkinson's disease (PD) based on extrapolations from epidemiologic field studies and on brain imaging data using PET and SPECT technology. At presymptomatic stages the patient would not meet criteria for the clinical diagnosis of PD but may instead exhibit striatal dopamine denervation on PET scan or, in familial cases, have a positive genetic test. This stage is thought to last about 5 years. The presence of incidental α-synuclein positive pathology (Lewy neurites or LBs) at autopsy may be the earliest recognizable stage of PD. PET, positron emission tomography using 18-F fluorodopa; SPECT, single proton emission computerized tomography using β-CIT, both presynaptic markers of presynaptic dopamine innervation.

Pathogenesis (Fig. 351-1) In PD dopaminergic and other cells die due to a combination of factors including: (1) genetic vulnerability, (2) oxidative stress, (3) proteosomal dysfunction, and (4) environmental factors, most of which have yet to be identified.

Oxidative stress appears to play an important role in the sporadic forms of PD. Endogenous sources of oxidative stress include the free-radicals produced by the metabolism of dopamine and melanin. Additional stress may come from defects in mitochondrial complex I of the oxidative phosphorylation chain in patients with PD. This defect has been detected in platelets and muscle and in postmortem tissue from the substantia nigra. Several toxins have been shown to cause oxidative toxicity and dopamine cell death in animal models of PD, further strengthening the above hypothesis. The most important of these are MPTP, a meperidine derivative, and rotenone, a commonly used insecticide. Both cause oxidative damage by inhibiting complex I. In vitro, oxidative stress can lead to aggregation of α-synuclein and proteosomal dysfunction. Proteosomal system abnormalities have also been described in the substantia nigra from sporadic cases of PD. The other factors of the selective dopamine neuron degeneration in PD are microglial activation, low-grade inflammation, and apoptosis, each a potential target for therapeutic intervention.

℞ TREATMENT

General Considerations The goals of therapy in PD are to maintain function and quality of life and to avoid drug-induced complications. Bradykinesia, tremor, rigidity, and abnormal posture respond well to symptomatic therapy early in the course of the illness. In contrast, cognitive symptoms, hypophonia, autonomic dysfunction, and balance difficulties respond poorly. Primary motor disability in PD is often aggravated by secondary disability resulting from physical deconditioning following a sedentary life-style. Prevention of secondary disability requires a consistent program of physical activity, thus regular activity is strongly encouraged. Remaining mentally active is probably equally important.

A current priority is to move beyond symptom control to neuroprotective therapies. Unfortunately, no such therapy is yet available, although selegiline (deprenyl) may, in addition to a mild symptomatic effect, have a neuroprotective function. High doses of coenzyme Q_{10} and intrastriatal infusion of neurotrophic factors show promise in early clinical trials. Animal studies have shown that exercise can promote neuroprotection against neurotoxins.

TABLE 351-3 *Guide to the Use of Levodopa Formulations and Dopamine Agonists in Parkinson's Disease*

		LD Dose Equivalency, mg	Available Strengths, mg	Initial Dose	Other Considerations
CARBIDOPA/LEVODOPA (TYPICAL INITIAL STRENGTH)					
Carbidopa/levodopa IR 25/100	→	100 (anchor dose)	10/100 25/100 25/250	25/100; 0.5 tab tid	Target dose = 3–6 25/100 tabs/d
Carbidopa/levodopa CR 50/200	→	150	25/100 50/200	50/200; one tab bid to tid	Increased bioavailability with food; splitting the tablet negates the CR property
Carbidopa/levodopa/entacapone 25/100/200	→	120	12.5/50/200 25/100/200 37.5/150/200	25/100/200; one tab bid to tid	Do not split tablets

	DA Equivalent to LD Anchor Dose Above, mg[a]	Available Strengths, mg	Approximate Target Doses			Other Considerations
			Initial Dose, mg	As Monotherapy, mg/d	As Adjuncts to LD, mg/d	
DOPAMINE AGONISTS						
Non-ergot alkaloids						
Ropinirole	5	0.25, 0.5, 1, 2, 3, 4, 5	0.25 tid	12–24	6–16	Hepatic metabolism; potential drug-drug interactions Occasionally associated with "sleep attacks"
Pramipexole	1	0.125, 0.25, 1, 1.5	0.125 tid	1.5–4.5	0.375–3.0	Renal metabolism; dose adjustments needed in renal insufficiency Occasionally associated with "sleep attacks"
Ergot alkaloids						
Pergolide	1	0.05, 0.25, 1.0	0.05 tid	1.5–6	0.3–3	Rare reports of valvular heart disease; fewer reports of sleep attacks compared to non-ergots
Bromocriptine	2	2.5, 5.0	1.25 bid to tid	7.5–15	3.75–7.5	Rare reports of pulmonary and retroperitoneal fibrosis Relative incidence of sleep attacks not well studied

[a] Equivalency doses are approximations based on clinical experience and may not correlate with the relative in vitro binding properties of these compounds.

Note: LD, levodopa (with carbidopa); IR, immediate release; CR, controlled release; DA, dopamine agonist. Carbidopa/levodopa/entacapone, Stalevo.

Initiation of Therapy From a practical standpoint, dopaminomimetic therapy should be initiated as soon as the patient's symptoms begin to interfere with quality of life. The ideal agent for initiation of symptomatic therapy depends on the age and cognitive status of the patient and, to a lesser extent, the patient's clinical type and finances. The choices consist of either a levodopa preparation or a dopamine agonist. Controlled studies support the view that, in early PD, dopamine agonist monotherapy is well tolerated and significantly reduces the risk of later treatment-related complications such as motor fluctuations and dyskinesias. *Motor fluctuations* are the exaggerated ebb and flow of parkinsonian signs experienced by many patients between doses of antiparkinsonian medications. *Dyskinesias* refer to choreiform and dystonic movements that can occur as a peak dose effect or at the beginning or end of the dose (diphasic dyskinesias). More than 50% of patients with PD treated over five years with levodopa will develop these complications.

Successful dopamine agonist monotherapy requires a higher dose of the agonist than is typically needed when the agonist is used to supplement levodopa (Table 351-3). In both cases titration has to be slow and cautious to avoid unnecessary side effects. Patients benefit greatly from education and support during this titration. Most patients will require the addition of levodopa or another agent within 1 to 3 years of initiating dopamine agonist monotherapy. Preclinical studies suggest that the advantages of dopamine agonist monotherapy can be maintained with agonist-dominant therapy. In this case dopamine agonists continue to provide the bulk of dopaminomimetic therapy, with levodopa playing a supplementary role.

Although dopamine agonist monotherapy is considered the initial treatment of choice for most patients with PD, the long-term benefits noted above must be balanced against a higher incidence of non-motor side effects and a slightly higher level of motor disability than with levodopa. These recommendations may need to be modified in patients with psychotic symptoms or severe daytime sleep disturbances. Older patients and those with akinetic rigid phenotypes of PD have a lower risk of motor complications and dyskinesias compared to the average PD patient and may be satisfactorily treated with levodopa.

Pharmacotherapy of Motor Symptoms The above advances in the initiation of therapy notwithstanding, levodopa remains the most effective treatment for PD. It significantly improves motor symptoms and increases quality of life and independence. The aim of all dopaminomimetic strategies is to restore dopamine transmission in the striatum. This is accomplished by stimulating postsynaptic receptors (directly with dopamine agonists), increasing dopamine precursor availability (levodopa), blocking the metabolism of levodopa in the periphery and in the brain, and blocking the catabolism of dopamine at the presynaptic terminal.

DOPAMINE AGONISTS Dopamine agonists readily cross the blood-brain barrier and act directly on postsynaptic dopamine receptors (primarily D_2 type). Compared to levodopa, they are longer acting and thus provide a more uniform stimulation of dopamine receptors. They are effective as monotherapeutic agents and as adjuncts to carbidopa/levodopa therapy. They can also be used in combination with anticholinergics and amantadine. Table 351-3 provides a guide to the doses and uses of these agents.

Available agents include two ergot alkaloids, pergolide and bromocriptine, and two non-ergot alkaloids, pramipexole and ropinirole. Apomorphine has been available for subcutaneous infusion and injection in Europe and Canada for many years and will soon become available in the United States as "rescue therapy" to help control motor fluctuations ("off" spells) in patients with moderate to advanced disease. These agents are particularly effective in treating bradykinesia and gait disturbances, but they are less effective in treating tremor. Side effects include nausea, postural hypotension, psychiatric symptoms, daytime sedation, and occasional sleep attacks. These can be managed using the above strategies and, in severe cases, through the introduction of peripheral dopamine blockers such as domperidone (not available in the United States) or short courses of trimethobenzamide or dronabinol until the symptoms subside. Patients need to be warned against the potential for sleep attacks, which can occur without warning and have resulted in traffic accidents. This phenomenon has been most often associated with agonists and less so with carbidopa/levodopa. Pergolide has recently been shown to be associated with valvular disease. When used as adjuncts to levodopa therapy these agents can aggravate dyskinesias if the doses of carbidopa/levodopa are not adjusted accordingly, and they are more expensive than carbidopa/levodopa, which is now available in generic form.

CARBIDOPA/LEVODOPA FORMULATIONS Carbidopa/levodopa is available in regular, immediate release (IR) formulations (Sinemet, Atamet and others; 10/100 mg, 25/100 mg, and 25/250 mg), controlled release (CR) formulations (Sinemet CR 25/100 mg, 50/200 mg), and more recently as Stalevo (Table 351-3). The latter combines IR carbidopa/levodopa with 200 mg of entacapone (see below). In most individuals, at least 75 mg/d of carbidopa is necessary to block peripheral levodopa decarboxylation into dopamine and thus symptoms of nausea and orthostasis often associated with the initiation of levodopa. Initial target doses of these medications are summarized in the table. Individualized and gradual escalation of these doses is recommended. Initiation of dosing at mealtimes will reduce the incidence and severity of nausea. As patients develop tolerance to nausea and other side effects, these medications can be administered on an empty stomach, which generally leads to a more brisk and predictable absorption.

LEVODOPA AUGMENTATION Selegiline is a selective and irreversible monoamine oxidase (MAO) B inhibitor with a weak symptomatic effect when used as monotherapy or as an adjunct to carbidopa/levodopa. Typically, selegiline is used as initial therapy or is added to alleviate tremor or levodopa-associated wearing-off. The usual dose is 5 mg with breakfast and lunch. At this dose there is no need for dietary restrictions, as is the case with non-selective and MAO-A inhibitors. A significant side-effect of selegiline is insomnia. Older individuals, and those with significant cardiac abnormalities, may benefit from doses as low as 2.5 mg/d. The potential role of selegiline (or desmethylselegiline) as neuroprotective therapy remains controversial.

The catechol *O*-methyltransferase (COMT) inhibitors entacapone and tolcapone offer yet another strategy to augment the effects of levodopa by blocking the enzymatic degradation of levodopa and dopamine. Entacapone is preferred to tolcapone because of the low but potentially serious incidence of hepatic and hematologic side effects of the latter. When used in conjunction with carbidopa/levodopa, these agents increase the area under the curve of plasma levodopa by >30%. They alleviate wearing-off symptoms and increase by 1 to 2 h the time a patient remains "on" (i.e., well medicated) during the day. The more common side effects are gastrointestinal and hyperdopaminergic, including increased dyskinesias that may require reductions in the dose of carbidopa/levodopa. The dose of entacapone is 200 mg coadministered with each dose of carbidopa/levodopa. The dose of tolcapone is 50 to 200 mg tid.

Anticholinergics and amantadine are appropriate adjuncts to dopaminomimetic therapy. Anticholinergics are particularly useful for controlling rest tremor and dystonia, and amantadine can reduce drug-induced dyskinesias by up to 70%. The mechanisms of action of amantadine are unknown, although there is evidence it has both anticholinergic and dopaminomimetic properties. Recently amantadine has been shown to have weak glutamate antagonist properties, a mechanism thought responsible for reducing drug-induced dyskinesias. The side-effects of amantadine are nausea, headaches, edema, erythema, and livedo reticularis. In older patients, it may aggravate confusion and psychosis. Doses need to be adjusted in patients with renal failure.

Therapy of Non-Motor Symptoms Patients with frequent nighttime awakenings due to nocturnal akinesia or tremor can be treated with supplemental doses of carbidopa/levodopa at night. A bedtime dose of dopamine agonists helps restless leg symptoms and urinary urgency. Treatment of other bladder symptoms will improve sleep for many elderly patients. Depression typically responds to antidepressants [e.g., tricyclics, selective serotonin reuptake inhibitors (SSRIs)]. The combination of SSRIs and selegiline carries an exceedingly low risk of a hyperserotonergic syndrome (delirium with myoclonus and hyperpyrexia). Electroconvulsive therapy (ECT) is highly effective in drug-refractory cases or in patients intolerant of oral antidepressants. There are several reports indicating that ECT, in addition, has short-term benefit for parkinsonian motor symptoms.

In patients with psychotic symptoms or confusion, anticholinergics and amantadine should be eliminated first. In severe cases not responding to the above approach, some dopaminomimetics may have to be reduced or eliminated. Further drug simplification and dose reductions should proceed in the following order: selegiline, nocturnal doses of dopamine agonists, Sinemet CR, daytime doses of dopamine agonists, and finally, daytime doses of carbidopa/levodopa. If the patient improves after only a modest reduction of antiparkinsonian therapy, the overall impact on the parkinsonian motor symptoms will be negligible. If in the process parkinsonian symptoms worsen, most specialists initiate treatment with an atypical antipsychotic with a low incidence of extrapyramidal side effects rather than continuing to lower dopaminomimetic therapy. Quetiapine is recommended first because, although not as well studied in PD as clozapine, it has proved to be effective in open-label studies and lacks the small risk of agranulocytosis associated with clozapine. Typical doses of quetiapine are 12.5 to 100 mg/d, and for clozapine 12.5 to 100 mg/d. Both are dosed at night to promote sleep and minimize daytime sedation and orthostasis. Other atypical antipsychotics, such as risperidone and olanzapine, are not well tolerated by most patients with PD because they are associated with dose-dependent parkinsonism. Early evidence suggests that the use of acetylcholinesterase inhibitors may be well tolerated and capable of treating hallucinations and delusions in patients with PD and dementia.

Given the complexity of the above polypharmacy, the management of non-motor symptoms is best carried out in an interdisciplinary setting, coordinated by a neurologist who specializes in PD together with a psychiatrist and the patient's primary care physician.

Neuroprotective Therapy Reducing the progression of PD through neuroprotective or restorative therapy is a major focus of research. Epidemiologic studies suggest that the chronic use of nonsteroidal anti-inflammatory agents or the use of estrogen replacement in postmenopausal women may delay or prevent the onset of PD through yet unclear mechanisms. From a pharmacologic standpoint, current strategies involve interrupting the cascade of biochemical events that leads to death of dopaminergic cells (Fig. 351-2). The first such clinical trial in PD was the large multicenter DATATOP study in which selegiline monotherapy delayed the need for levodopa therapy by 9 to 12 months in newly diagnosed patients. Most evidence indicates that this delay was due to a mild symptomatic effect of selegiline. Long-term follow-up of the DATATOP cohort revealed that patients who remained on selegiline for 7 years experienced slower motor decline compared to those who were changed to placebo after 5 years. The 7-year patient group was more likely to develop dyskinesias but less likely to develop freezing gait. Finally, the metabolite of selegiline, desmethylselegiline, has been shown in laboratory studies to have powerful neuroprotective effects, possibly through interactions of glyceraldehyde-3-phosphate dehydrogenase (GAPDH) and other cellular protective (antiapoptotic) factors. Clinical trials to test this agent are under way.

FIGURE 351-3 Schematic diagram of the basal ganglia–thalamocortical circuitry under normal conditions and in Parkinson's disease (PD). Inhibitory connections are shown as black arrows and excitatory connections as red arrows. Note that in PD, striatal dopamine denervation results in increased traffic in the indirect pathway and decreased traffic in the direct pathway. The downstream consequence of this is increased activity in striatal outflow stemming from the increased activity of STN and ultimately GPi/SNr neurons. Because striatal outflow is inhibitory to the thalamus (main neurotransmitter = γ-aminobutyric acid), there is a decrease in the ability of the thalamus to activate the frontal cortex leading to signs of parkinsonism. As discussed, changes in discharge pattern are also a major factor. D, direct pathway; I, indirect pathway; GPe, external segment of the globus pallidus; GPi, internal segment of the globus pallidus; SNr, substantia nigra, pars reticulata; SNc, substantia nigra, pars compacta; STN, subthalamic nucleus; VA/VL, ventral anterior and ventrolateral thalamus; CM, centromedian nucleus; PPN, pedunculopontine nucleus. *(Courtesy of T Wichmann, MD, Emory University School of Medicine.)*

In a recent trial, coenzyme Q_{10}, an antioxidant and a cofactor of complex I of the mitochondrial oxidative chain, appeared to delay progression of early disability in PD. Other potentially neuroprotective agents under investigation are acetyl-levo-carnitine and creatine monohydrate. A large controlled study of the antiglutamatergic agent riluzole (Chap. 353) was prematurely discontinued after a futility analysis revealed little effect on progression of symptoms. Dopamine agonists are also under investigation as putative agents to slow disease progression in PD, based on their possible antioxidant properties resulting in part from their ability in vitro to decrease dopamine turnover, scavenge free radicals, and interfere with proapoptotic cell signals. Other promising agents include nitric oxide synthetase inhibitors, anti-apoptotic agents such as Jun N-terminal kinase inhibitors, and the antibiotic minocycline. Minocycline can inhibit microglial activation in vitro and interrupt apoptosis by inhibiting caspase 1 and 3, which are involved in the enzymatic processing of α-synuclein.

Surgical Treatments Over the past decade there has been a renaissance in the surgical treatment of PD and other movement disorders. Although both pallidotomy and thalmotomy were performed widely in the 1950s, the introduction of levodopa in the 1960s led to the virtual abandonment of surgery. The resurgence in the use of surgery has been motivated by the fact that after ≥5 years of treatment, many patients develop significant drug-induced motor fluctuations and dyskinesias. Second, advances in understanding of the functional organization of the basal ganglia and the pathophysiologic basis of parkinsonism have provided a clearer rationale for the effectiveness of these procedures and guidance for targeting specific structures (Fig. 351-3). The demonstration, in animal models of PD, that ablation of the STN (subthalamotomy) resulted in a dramatic reduction in all of the cardinal features of parkinsonism was a critical finding.

The selection of suitable patients for surgery is most important, since in general patients with atypical Parkinson's do not have a favorable response. The major indications for surgery are (1) a diagnosis of idiopathic PD, (2) a clear response to levodopa, (3) significant intractable symptoms of PD, and/or (4) drug-induced dyskinesias and wearing-off. Contraindications to surgery include atypical forms of PD, cognitive impairment, major psychiatric illness, substantial medical comorbidities, and advanced age (a relative factor). Signs and symptoms not responding to levodopa, such as postural instability and falling, hypophonia, micrographia, drooling, and autonomic dysfunction, are unlikely to benefit from surgery. As a rule of thumb, the benefits from surgery are unlikely to exceed the benefits of antiparkinson medication. In general, the decision for surgery should be made by a movement disorder neurologist who is part of a team including a neurosurgeon trained in functional neurosurgery, a psychiatrist, a neuropsychologist, and trained technicians.

ABLATION VERSUS DEEP BRAIN STIMULATION (DBS) The use of ablation (e.g., pallidotomy or thalamotomy) has decreased greatly since the introduction of DBS and is generally reserved for individuals who for medical or economic reasons cannot have DBS. Major advantages of DBS are that it is somewhat less invasive and more reversible than ablation, and in addition may be adjusted to best effect following implantation. Although the choice between the STN and the internal segment of the globus pallidus for DBS has shifted toward the STN, the data to support this are lacking. Several clinical trials are now under way to compare these two targets. The available evidence suggests that both are effective for all the cardinal features of PD as well as for dyskinesias and motor fluctuations. Unilateral stimulation is appropriate for patients with asymmetric disease, although bilateral surgery is generally necessary for patients with more advanced disease and for those with significant bilateral manifestations. Reductions in drug dosages appear to be easier with STN than globus pallidus procedures.

The mechanism of action of DBS remains controversial. Since clinically it appears that ablation and stimulation of a given target have a similar effect, it has been assumed that stimulation caused a functional blockade. It is likely, however, that multiple factors are involved. The basis for improvement may be the replacement of abnormal neural activity by a more tolerable pattern of activity. Following ablation or DBS, the remaining motor systems in the brainstem, thalamus, and cortex are able to compensate more effectively for the abnormal activity associated with the parkinsonian state. Whatever the mechanism, it is clear that these approaches can offer impressive results in properly selected patients.

NEUROTRANSPLANTATION AND OTHER SURGICAL APPROACHES Despite highly encouraging open-label pilot studies of fetal cell transplantation, this approach has suffered considerable disappointment with the recent publication of the results from two large, well-controlled clinical trials. The first, using sham surgery, showed only modest benefit in patients under 60 and no benefit in those over 60. An unexpected complication in a number of patients was the development of symptomatic dyskinesias, occurring off medication. The second study has shown similar findings with regard to benefit and the development of dyskinesias. A puzzling feature of these studies is the apparent successful grafting observed by PET and autopsy. Because of these disappointing results, the considerable obstacles to obtaining sufficient fetal tissue, and opposition to the use of fetal tissue on ethical grounds, this approach is now viewed as purely investigational. It is hoped that these issues can be addressed with the development of other strategies to enhance dopaminergic cell function (e.g., carotid body cells; stem cells; encapsulated and genetically engineered cells capable of producing levodopa, dopamine, and/or trophic factors). The favorable response from direct infusion of glial cell–derived neurotrophic factor (GDNF) to the putamen in a small number of patients with PD has raised hopes that this approach, or the use of gene-transfer of trophic factors such as GDNF, will succeed. Preliminary studies in primate models of PD have been encouraging in this regard.

DEMENTIA IN PARKINSON'S DISEASE As noted above, the incidence of dementia in PD may be as high as six times that in the general non-PD population. Approximately a quarter of patients will develop dementia of the Alzheimer type simply due to the overlap of these two common age-related disorders. Pathologically, the incidence of AD-type findings in postmortem tissue from patients dying with PD is as high as 40%. Conversely, 25% of AD patients have at least mild clinical parkinsonian features such as rigidity and bradykinesia, and ≥60% have coexistent α-synuclein pathology in the cortex. Patients with PD-dementia (PDD) typically have the akinetic/rigid form of the disorder where tremor is less prominent than in idiopathic PD. The course of PDD is more rapid and the management is more difficult than in PD due to the high incidence of cognitive side effects from antiparkinsonian therapy, particularly anticholinergics and amantadine. Central dopaminomimetic toxicity can present in many ways, ranging from sleep disruption with daytime sleepiness, personality changes, depression and mental dullness, episodic confusion, hallucinations, and disruptive behaviors.

DLB is an increasingly recognized form of dementia with prominent parkinsonian features. The dementia may precede or follow the parkinsonian syndrome. In patients presenting with parkinsonian features, the dementia is often heralded by levodopa-induced sedation, myoclonus, and hallucinations. Early on, the phenotype can be indistinguishable from PD. Features that help differentiate this entity from PD include the presence of an action rather than a rest tremor, a rapidly fading response to levodopa, and rapidly fluctuating, spontaneous, and drug-induced problems with arousal. Another feature of DLB is the higher incidence of neuropsychiatric symptoms than in idiopathic PD. These symptoms include apathy, personality changes, depression, fixed delusions, and hallucinations. Finally, patients with DLB exhibit a heightened sensitivity to drug-induced parkinsonism (DIP) when exposed to any dopamine blocker. The progression of symptoms in DLB is intermediate between the PD and PD/AD overlap. →*DLB is discussed in detail in Chap. 350.*

OTHER PARKINSONIAN DISORDERS

PARKINSONIAN DISORDERS ASSOCIATED WITH ABNORMAL METABOLISM OF α-SYNUCLEIN (α-SYNUCLEINOPATHIES) ■ **Multiple System Atrophy** MSA represents a sporadic group of disorders characterized by varying degrees of parkinsonism and cerebellar, corticospinal, and autonomic dysfunction. The average age of onset is 50 years (earlier than in PD), and the median survival 6 to 9 years. The clinical presentation is highly varied and may begin with any of the above clinical signs. The unifying pathologic hallmark is the presence of α-synuclein-positive inclusions located in various brain regions.

CLINICAL PHENOTYPES With disease progression, 90% percent of patients exhibit parkinsonian signs, 80% signs of autonomic failure, and a similarly high percentage exhibit upper motor neuron signs. Tremor is common but, unlike in PD, this and other parkinsonian signs are more likely to present symmetrically. Parkinsonian symptoms are typically poorly responsive to dopaminergic therapy, although some patients may respond favorably for years. Drug-induced dyskinesias typically involve the face and neck rather than the trunk and limbs, as is the case in PD. Corticospinal signs consist of spasticity, involving the legs more than the arms, and pseudobulbar palsy. This aspect of the illness may mimic primary lateral sclerosis with lower motor neurons being occasionally involved. A few patients develop myoclonus.

Signs of autonomic failure include orthostatic hypotension, leg swelling not due to drug therapy, changes in sweating patterns, and autonomic storms with diaphoresis and flushing. Orthostatic hypotension can present with dizziness, faintness, or syncope. Once patients are successfully treated for syncope, they often develop fatigue and lassitude. This is due in part to chronic tissue hypoperfusion caused by marginal blood pressures while sitting or standing. More aggressive management of the blood pressure is warranted but not always successful. Urinary symptoms include urgency, retention, and incontinence. In men impotence is one of the earliest and most prominent signs. The autonomic dysfunction can precede or follow the development of other neurologic signs by several years. Dementia may not be as frequent as in PD.

The clinical phenotype of MSA can fall into one of three broad categories, termed *striatonigral degeneration* (SND), *olivopontocerebellar atrophy* (OPCA), and *progressive autonomic failure* (PAF), either without parkinsonism or with parkinsonism (Shy-Drager syndrome). Patients presenting with a relatively pure form of akinetic rigid parkinsonism and a limited response to levodopa are designated as SND. The diagnosis is difficult. Individuals with other signs such as ataxia, upper motor neuron and corticobulbar involvement, myoclonus, oculomotor abnormalities, peripheral neuropathy, and deafness fit into the category of OPCA. This phenotype is notably heterogeneous, with sporadic and hereditary forms. The sporadic forms are more likely to form part of the spectrum referred to in this section, with the hereditary forms usually representing one of the spinocerebellar ataxias (Chap. 352). Finally, a diagnosis of Shy-Drager syndrome is justified when the parkinsonian features are associated with prominent signs of autonomic dysfunction. Although the above categories remain clinically useful, it should be noted that as disease progresses, there tends to be more clinical and pathologic overlap than separation between these entities.

The spectrum of disease in MSA is determined by the location and density of the LB pathology. For instance, in PD the LBs are confined to neurons in the brainstem, and in DLB to the brainstem, cortex, and hippocampus. In MSA these deposits take the form of glial α-synuclein-positive intracytoplasmic inclusions in the substantia nigra, putamen, inferior olives, pontine nuclei, pigmented nuclei of the brainstem, the intermediolateral nucleus of the spinal cord, and the cerebellum. In addition in MSA there are myelin degeneration and oligodendroglia containing argyrophilic glial cytoplasmic inclusions that are immunoreactive for ubiquitin and α-synuclein. Similar inclusions can be found in neuronal cell bodies and processes.

Several diagnostic tests help differentiate MSA from PD and other parkinsonian syndromes. In OPCA, brain MRI reveals prominent atrophy of the cerebellum, pons, and olivary eminence of the medulla. In SND, prominent volume loss and T2-weighted image hyperintensity in the putamen, globus pallidus, and white matter may be present. Electrodiagnostic studies may reveal rectal sphincter abnormalities with signs of degeneration with reinnervation due to anterior horn cell loss. Commercially available genetic tests are available for many of the spinocerebellar ataxias (Chap. 352) that present with features that overlap OPCA.

℞ TREATMENT

Early in the course of the illness parkinsonian features may respond to dopaminomimetic agents. These have to be used with caution due to their tendency to provoke orthostatic hypotension.→*Treatment of orthostatic hypotension and other autonomic symptoms is discussed in Chap. 354.*

PARKINSONIAN DISORDERS ASSOCIATED WITH ABNORMALITIES OF TAU METABOLISM (TAUOPATHIES) As in the synucleopathies, the discovery that a group of familial and sporadic disorders with pathology involving the microtubule-associated protein tau has helped classify a group of disorders characterized by atypical parkinsonism and dementia. In the less common familial forms, mutations in the *tau* gene have been linked to rare forms of parkinsonism and to frontotemporal dementia, another tauopathy discussed in Chap. 350. This discussion will focus on two entities that typically present with movement disorders. The first, PSP, has not been linked to mutations in the *tau* gene but is associated with overrepresentation of the H1 *tau* gene haplotype. These and other findings support the view that abnormal processing of tau may be directly linked to the pathogenesis of sporadic and familial tauopathies.

Progressive Supranuclear Palsy This is a sporadic neurodegenerative disorder of unknown etiology associated with tau pathology. It presents in the sixth to seventh decades and progresses faster than PD, with death in 5 to 10 years. Risk factors include head trauma, vascular disease, dietary exposure to benzyl-tetrahydroisoquinolines (TIQ, reticuline), and beta-carbolines (reports from the West Indies).

PSP is characterized by akinetic rigid parkinsonism, dizziness, unsteadiness, slowness, falls, and pseudobulbar dysarthria. Tremor is distinctly uncommon. Supranuclear eye movement abnormalities affecting downgaze occur first, followed by variable limitations of upward and horizontal eye movement. Because the vestibular ocular reflex ("doll's eyes" maneuver) and the Bell's reflex (elevation and abduction of eyes on attempted lid closure) are intact, these abnormalities are termed *supranuclear*. Neurologic examination often reveals prominent stare and furrowed brow, axial (especially nuchal) and proximal distal limb rigidity and dystonia, as well as upper motor neuron and occasional cerebellar signs. Virtually all patients develop frontal-type cognitive dysfunction (Chap. 350), and a significant number may develop dementia with distinct subcortical features (e.g., abulia, mental inflexibility, and defects in memory retrieval). Brain MRI reveals midbrain atrophy (superior colliculus), and PET studies show symmetric frontal and striatal hypometabolism. Although some response may occur to levodopa and other antiparkinson medications, especially early in the course, treatment is generally not highly effective. The diagnosis is made on clinical grounds.

Pathologically, PSP is characterized by deposition of neurofibrillary tangles histochemically positive for tau (mostly 4-repeat tau) and negative for amyloid or α-synuclein. The deposits are associated with varying degrees of degeneration in the brainstem, basal ganglia, and cerebellum. There is loss of dopamine and dopamine receptors due to intrinsic striatal damage. This is thought to account for the poor response to therapy.

Corticobasal Degeneration (CBD)   CBD, another sporadic tauopathy, is less common and has a broader range of clinical presentations than PSP. As with most atypical forms of parkinsonism, it begins insidiously in the sixth to seventh decades with varying degrees of asymmetric progressive apraxia, rigidity, dystonia, bradykinesia, and myoclonic jerks with or without cortical sensory loss. Alien limb phenomena is a characteristic sign present in many cases. The disorder progresses to become bilateral over 2 to 5 years, leading to total incapacity with, ultimately, paraplegia in flexion. A significant number of cases present with frontotemporal dementia or progressive aphasia, followed by asymmetric cortical sensory signs, including abnormalities of graphesthesia and astereognosis (Chap. 350). Brain MRI reveals focal cortical loss in the contralateral superior frontal and parietal lobes with corresponding hypometabolic changes on PET scan, as well as hyperintense signal abnormalities in white matter and sometimes atrophy of the corpus callosum. Treatment is largely ineffective.

Grossly, CBD is a focal cortical degenerative process with asymmetric pathology and volume loss in the parietal and frontal regions. Most of the damage is in the dorsal peri-Rolandic, superior frontal, and superior parietal cortices, whereas cases with aphasia show abnormalities in the peri-Sylvian regions. Histologically, gliosis and swollen (ballooned) achromatic neurons and neuronal loss are present in these cortical regions as well as in the nigra, caudate, putamen, and thalamus. Recent clinicopathologic evidence indicates the syndrome can occur in the absence of basal ganglia or nigral degeneration.

SECONDARY PARKINSONISM ■ **Drug-Induced Parkinsonism**   DIP closely resembles PD except for the tremor, which is generally (but not always) less prominent. It is commonly due to neuroleptics, some atypical antipsychotics, lithium carbonate, or antiemetic agents (especially metochlopramide). Less common causes include valproic acid and, more recently, fluoxetine. DIP can be induced as well by the chronic administration of antihypertensive agents such as reserpine and alphamethyldopa. Exposure to manganese, carbon monoxide or disulfides, cyanide, and methanol can also lead to a parkinsonian state. The severity of the parkinsonian symptoms usually correlates with the dose or exposure to a medication or toxin. If due to medication, the symp-

toms tend to disappear within days to weeks after stopping the offending agent but may be permanent. Patients with permanent symptoms may have been in the process of developing parkinsonism. DIP may respond to anticholinergic agents, amantadine, and levodopa.

Vascular Parkinsonism   The concept of vascular or atherosclerotic parkinsonism remains a topic of controversy. Generally, patients with vascular parkinsonism exhibit an akinetic-rigid syndrome with short mincing steps without tremor. Most have neurologic signs distinguishable from those associated with PD, including upper motor neuron signs, pseudobulbar palsy, or dementia. A poor response to levodopa therapy is characteristic. Imaging studies are heterogeneous and may reveal basal ganglia lacunes or multiple infarcts. The hypertensive and diabetic microangiopathy and diffuse white matter disease (Chap. 349) typically present with patchy, confluent or diffuse white matter in the centrum semiovale. Other causes of microangiopathy can also rarely be a cause. The premortem diagnosis of these disorders is difficult to make with certainty, given the absence of disease markers.

TREMOR

Tremor is defined as an "approximately rhythmic and roughly sinusoidal movement of variable amplitude and frequency" (Elble and Koller). Not all tremors are abnormal; most are involuntary with occasional voluntary tremors occurring in malingerers. Individuals with conversion disorders may show partial control over their tremor symptom. Physiologic tremor is a normal high-frequency, low-amplitude tremor notable only during hyperadrenergic states. Parkinsonian rest tremor is discussed above. Cerebellar kinetic tremor is discussed in Chaps. 21 and 352. Kinetic tremors can be postural, action, or both. Postural tremor is most prominent when the arms are held in front of the chest. Action or intention tremor is most notable when reaching to a target. Most tremor disorders have a predominant tremor type and a variable representation of other tremor types.

ESSENTIAL TREMOR   ET is perhaps the most common movement disorder, affecting 5 to 10 million adults and a few children in the United States. It is characterized by a 6- to 12-Hz postural and kinetic tremor affecting the arms in almost all cases. In order of decreasing frequency, other body parts that can also be involved include the head (titubation), legs, the larynx (voice tremor), and the trunk. Diagnosis is made on clinical grounds. An autosomal dominant inheritance pattern is likely; thus a positive family history is very helpful, as is a history of partial response to alcohol consumption. Drugs that can aggravate any tremor include valproic acid, lithium, β-adrenergic agonists, methylxanthines, thyroxin, glucocorticoids, tricyclic antidepressants, and serotonin reuptake blockers. Withdrawal from drugs associated with tolerance, or medical conditions such as thyrotoxicosis and other enhanced adrenergic states, can amplify physiologic tremor, mimic pathologic tremors, or aggravate ET.

Compared to PD, symptoms of ET are generally bilateral from onset and the course slower. A small subset of patients has comorbid PD. ET can nonetheless be associated with significant disability, depending on amplitude of the tremor and the body region involved. Anxiety disorders are comorbid in a significant number of cases, and, as in all movement disorders, symptoms and signs worsen during emotional and physiologic stress. There is no consensus with respect to any pathology associated with ET, and diagnostic imaging of the brain is normal.

℞ **TREATMENT**

There is no cure for ET, but symptoms can be managed adequately with pharmacologic interventions in ~50% of cases and with surgical interventions in 80% of patients. Primidone and propranolol are the first-line treatments for ET; both have shown efficacy in double-blind, placebo-controlled studies. Primidone (50 to 750 mg/d) is often highly effective. The starting dose should be 25 mg (one-half of a 50-mg tab) at bedtime, with slowly increasing doses to minimize sedation. Propranolol (40 to 320 mg/d) is better tolerated but no more effective and is contraindicated in patients with asthma, bradycardia, and some cardiac conduction defects. Additional medications with potential efficacy (with or without the primary agents) include benzodiazepines, gabapentin, topiramate, and botulinum toxin injections to affected muscle groups. Approximately 80% of patients resistant or intolerant to pharmacotherapy respond to thalamotomy or to deep brain stimulation of the ventral intermediate nucleus of the thalamus.

HYPERKINETIC DISORDERS

Hyperkinetic movement disorders (Chap. 21) encompass a wide variety of involuntary movements, which may occur in isolation or in combination. Hyperkinesias have a wide spectrum of severity ranging from subtle restlessness to the violent movements of hemiballismus and the highly complex and emotionally laden vocal tics and coprolalia in Tourette syndrome.

HEMIBALLISMUS/HEMICHOREA Hemiballismus, a dramatic disorder, is typically acute in onset and ranges from mild chorea to the wild flinging movements of ballism. Hemiballismus may be viewed as a large-amplitude, violent form of chorea affecting the proximal more than the distal limbs. The most common cause is a lesion of the subthalamic nucleus, most often a hypertensive lacunar stroke (Fig. 351-4). Other cerebral lesions associated with hemiballismus and hemichorea include cortical, thalamic, and basal ganglia infarcts or lesions and demyelinating disease. Medical management of hemiballismus consists of supportive care to avoid injuries, exhaustion, and dehydration. The condition is difficult to treat pharmacologically but the drugs most consistently beneficial are tetrabenazine (not available in the United States), haloperidol, propranolol, phenytoin, clonazepam, and baclofen. Although hemiballismus was once thought to carry a poor prognosis, with proper treatment there is a high likelihood of survival and improvement over weeks to months. In intractable cases, pallidotomy or thalamotomy can be highly effective.

HUNTINGTON'S DISEASE HD is a fatal autosomal dominant disorder characterized by progressive motor, emotional, and cognitive dysfunction. Onset is typically between the ages of 35 and 45 years (range 3 to 70). HD occurs worldwide, with a prevalence of 10 cases per 100,000. It is caused by mutations in the Huntington's gene on the short arm of

FIGURE 351-4 Schematic diagram of the basal ganglia–thalamocortical circuitry in hemiballismus, a surrogate in this case for other hyperkinetic movement disorders. As in Fig. 351-3, inhibitory connections are shown as black arrows and excitatory connections as red arrows. In hemiballismus the sudden loss of activity in STN neurons or their connections results in the loss of the normal thalamic inhibition by basal ganglia outflow, leading to poorly modulated and excessive thalamic activation of cortex. Clinically the patient exhibits abnormal contralateral choreiform movements. Dopamine antagonists help reduce the violence of the movements by decreasing neuronal activity in the direct pathway and increasing it in the indirect pathway, elevating neuronal activity in GPi/SNr. Parodoxically, surgical lesions of GPi/SNr are also beneficial, suggesting that abnormalities in neuronal discharge patterns are a major factor as well. D, direct pathway; I, indirect pathway; GPe, external segment of the globus pallidus; GPi, internal segment of the globus pallidus; SNr, substantia nigra, pars reticulata; SNc, substantia nigra, pars compacta; STN, subthalamic nucleus; VA/VL, ventral anterior and ventrolateral thalamus; CM, centromedian nucleus; PPN, pedunculopontine nucleus. *(Courtesy of T Wichmann, MD, Emory University School of Medicine.)*

chromosome 4, specifically an expanding and unstable polyglutamine repeat (CAG) in its coding sequence. The gene encodes the highly conserved cytoplasmic protein huntingtin, which is present in all neurons.

Clinical Features A clinical diagnosis of HD can be made readily in cases with a positive family history and an insidious onset of chorea with variable degrees of dementia and emotional symptoms. The term *chorea* ("dance") refers to arrhythmic involuntary movements that are typically sudden and brief and that seem to flow from one part of the body to another. When combined with slower writhing movements or dystonic posturing, the term *choreoathetosis* is often used. Examples of other involuntary movements that may be confused with chorea include myoclonus and tics. Myoclonic jerks are lightning fast but lack the rhythmic flow of activity seen in chorea. While patients with myoclonic jerks commonly lose motor control and drop objects, this rarely happens with chorea or tics. Unlike chorea and myoclonus, motor tics can be readily suppressed voluntarily.

The clinical course of HD can last 15 to 20 years. In the early stages the chorea is focal and segmental (i.e., increased blinking, grimacing) but progresses to involve multiple body parts. The chorea typically peaks within 10 years and is gradually replaced by bradykinesia, rigidity, and dystonia. In 6 to 10% of cases HD may present with a parkinsonian syndrome rather than with chorea (Westphalt variant). The latter cases typically have an early onset (e.g., < 20 years). The behavioral and cognitive disturbances characteristic of HD most often account for the brunt of the patient's disability and most of the hardship to the family. Approximately one-third develop dysthymia or an affective disorder; one-third an intermittent explosive disorder; and the remaining third substance-abuse problems, sexual dysfunction, antisocial personality traits, or schizophreniform symptoms. Depression with suicidal tendencies is not uncommon. Even the minority who may not manifest behavioral problems ultimately succumb to dementia.

The diagnosis of HD is confirmed with genetic testing, which is also helpful in the differential diagnosis of chorea of unknown etiology and in cases of atypical dementia or psychosis. Genetic testing is also used for genetic counseling in adults but is usually not necessary in symptomatic individuals if there is genetic or pathologic confirmation of HD in other family members. Other conditions important in the differential diagnosis of HD include so-called senile chorea occurring in older individuals, benign hereditary chorea in younger individuals, and neuroacanthocytosis, a progressive autosomal recessive degeneration of the basal ganglia associated with acanthocytosis of red cells in the peripheral smear and normal plasma lipoproteins. Ancillary diagnostic measures include MRI to determine if there is caudate atrophy. Other diagnostic measures may be helpful in atypical cases without a clear family history and in cases where the genetic testing results are indeterminate. These tests include PET, which typically reveals decreased striatal metabolic activity before atrophy is apparent, and neuropsychologic testing.

Pathology and Pathophysiology The neuropathology of HD consists of widespread cerebral atrophy with prominent involvement of the striatum and cerebral cortex. Neuronal loss and gliosis are maximal in the caudate initially, with lesser involvement of the cortex and other subcortical structures. Although the mechanism of cell death in HD remains unclear, there is now experimental evidence to support the hypothesis that abnormal glutamatergic transmission with excitotoxicity of striatal cells bearing glutamate receptors plays a role.

Rx TREATMENT

Treatment should involve a multidisciplinary team that can provide social, medical, neuropsychiatric, and genetic guidance to patients and families throughout the course of the illness. Although dopamine blockers are moderately effective for chorea, they may aggravate bradykinesia and dystonia. Atypical antipsychotics such as clozapine, risperidone, and olanzapine are better tolerated but may not be as effective. The indications for treating chorea include interference with activities of daily living and social embarrassment.

Depression responds to conventional antidepressant therapy. The therapy needs to be monitored carefully since it can produce mania or precipitate suicide, a particularly serious problem in HD. Anxiety responds to benzodiazepines as well as to effective treatment of depression. Long-acting benzodiazepines are favored over short-acting ones because of the lesser potential for abuse and paradoxical excitation.

Psychosis can be treated with atypical neuroleptics clozapine (50 to 600 mg/d), quetiapine (100 to 600 mg/d), and risperidone (2 to 8 mg/d). These medications control dyskinesias as well as traditional neuroleptics but have fewer extrapyramidal side effects. When these drugs cannot be tolerated, smaller doses combined with tetrabenazine can be tried. There is currently no adequate treatment for the motor and cognitive decline of HD.

DYSTONIA ■ Clinical Features

Dystonia is a syndrome consisting of involuntary muscular contractions that result in twisting and repetitive movements and/or abnormal postures. Dystonia comprises a large and heterogeneous group of disorders. Although dystonia is one of the more common movement disorders, it is also one of the most frequently under- and misdiagnosed due to its highly variable presentations. The prevalence is not certain because of underreporting but probably exceeds 300,000 cases in the United States, a prevalence equal to that of multiple sclerosis.

Co-contraction of agonist and antagonist muscles is a fundamental feature of dystonia, distinguishing it from chorea, tics, and other dyskinesias. Also, unlike other hyperkinetic movement disorders, dystonia is characteristically present during attempted voluntary movement (so-called action dystonia). It is also associated with "overflow," the abnormal spread of activation to muscles other than those required for the intended movement. As with most movement disorders, dystonia is exacerbated by stress and fatigue. A unique feature of dystonia is that it can often be attenuated by sensory (tactile or proprioceptive) input (so-called sensory tricks). For instance, in patients with torticollis, placing a finger on the chin or the hand on the neck may reduce the twisting movements or abnormal postures. Another common feature of primary dystonia is the presence of dystonic tremor, which may appear in a form resembling essential tremor or as a succession of rapid dystonic movements.

The dystonias can be classified according to: (1) age of onset (childhood vs. adult), (2) region of the body involved, and (3) etiology. Using an etiologic scheme, similar to that used for PD, the dystonias may be divided into primary, secondary, dystonia-plus syndromes, and hereditary degenerative disorders.

PRIMARY DYSTONIA

Primary dystonia includes syndromes in which dystonia is the only clinical manifestation of the disease (other than tremor), and no pathologic changes are evident. Primary dystonia is often inherited and a number of genes have been identified. The major childhood disorder in this group is idiopathic torsion dystonia (ITD), or Oppenheim's dystonia. Sporadic adult-onset focal dystonias are the most common forms of primary dystonia.

Oppenheim's Dystonia

ITD dystonia is an autosomal dominant hereditary disorder affecting primarily Ashkenazy Jewish families (up to 90% of all cases of dystonia) but also present in non-Jewish families. The gene is located on chromosome 9q34 and results in a loss of glutamic acid in the protein Torsin A. The penetrance is about 30%. Families with ITD dystonia may exhibit either generalized or focal dystonia. The age of onset is typically in childhood for generalized and later for focal dystonia. The first signs of dystonia generally occur in the foot during walking or in the arms during voluntary movement. Dystonia later occurs at rest, leading to postural abnormalities. It usually spreads to the arm on the same side before spreading to the other side of the body. The age of onset is typically later in cases in which symptoms begin in the arm or neck. In late-onset ITD the dystonia tends to remain focal, in contrast to early-onset forms that usually become generalized.

Focal Dystonias

The most common forms of dystonia are the focal dystonias, which present primarily in adults. These may affect (1) the eyelids, causing them to close involuntarily (*blepharospasm*); (2) the neck and shoulders (*cervical dystonia*), causing the neck to twist to the side (*torticollis*), forward (*anterocollis*), or backward (*retrocollis*); (3) the lower face and jaw or a syndrome causing the jaw to move incessantly (*oromandibular dystonia*); and (4) the larynx (*spasmodic dysphonia*), causing the voice to have a strained and discontinuous quality due to involuntary closing of the vocal cords with phonation. The combination of lower facial and jaw dystonia (*Meige's syndrome*) is not uncommon. Another type of task-specific focal dystonia affects the hand and forearm in specific activities such as handwriting (writer's cramp), typing, or playing a musical instrument (musician's cramp). Dystonia can, in fact, occur in almost any situation involving repetitive activities of the hand or other body parts. The focal dystonias are still often misdiagnosed as psychiatric or orthopedic problems.

The role of hereditary and environmental factors in adult-onset focal dystonia is not well understood. There is now mounting evidence that in some cases dystonia can develop from peripheral factors such as trauma to peripheral nerves. In addition to peripheral injury, discrete cerebral lesions, typically involving the basal ganglia but also the thalamus, cortex, or brainstem, can cause unilateral dystonia. The most frequent cause is a cerebral infarction but trauma, tumor, and other lesions may be accountable. In the case of infarction, the onset of dystonia is typically delayed by weeks to months as the associated hemiparesis clears.

SECONDARY DYSTONIAS

Secondary dystonias are largely due to drugs and other environmental factors. The drug-induced phenomena include levodopa-induced dystonia as well as acute and tardive dystonia associated with dopamine receptor blockers (see "Drug-Induced Movement Disorders," below). External factors producing dystonia include cerebral palsy (athetoid form), cerebral trauma, peripheral nerve injury, cerebral hypoxia, some infectious and postinfectious states, and toxic exposure to manganese, cyanide, and 3-nitro proprionic acid.

Dystonia-Plus Syndromes

Two types of dystonia-plus syndromes deserve mention—dopamine-responsive dystonia (DRD) and myoclonic dystonia. DRD is a dominantly inherited disorder associated with mutations in the gene for cyclohydrolase I (*GTPCH*), the rate-limiting enzyme in the synthesis of the tyrosine hydroxylase cofactor tetrahydrobiopterin. Tyrosine hydroxylase is the rate-limiting enzyme for dopamine synthesis. DRD typically presents in childhood beginning in the legs and spreading to the arms. Marked diurnal fluctuations are common. In the typical case a child aged between 4 and 8 develops a stiff-legged gait that worsens as the day progresses but improves dramatically on awakening from sleep. Some patients exhibit parkinsonism and signs of spasticity. In late-onset cases the presentation may consist of parkinsonism instead of dystonia. Patients have an excellent response to levodopa and a non-progressive course. DRD may be misdiagnosed as "athetoid" cerebral palsy, "spastic" paraplegia, or parkinsonism. Although rare, DRD is so responsive to levodopa that many feel that a trial of levodopa is warranted in all cases of dystonia.

The hereditary syndrome of myoclonic dystonia (also called hereditary dystonia with lightning jerks) is not always easily distinguished from primary dystonia or heredity essential myoclonus. It is distinguished not only by its character but also by its responsiveness to alcohol.

The hereditary degenerative diseases that may manifest dystonia typically present with more prominent parkinsonian features and include Wilson's disease, HD, PD, corticobasal degeneration (CBD), progressive supranuclear palsy (PSP), the Lubag form of dystonia-parkinsonism (DYT3), Leigh's disease, and other mitochondrial encephalopathies.

Pathophysiology

There is now considerable evidence for a loss of inhibition at multiple levels in the central nervous system (CNS), including the cortex, brainstem, and spinal cord, in patients with both generalized and focal dystonia. Dystonia appears to result primarily from dysfunction within the basal ganglia. As in PD, both ablation and DBS of the internal segment of the globus pallidus are effective in ameliorating the abnormal motor signs. Experimental studies in humans and animals have demonstrated a degradation of sensorimotor representation in the cortex, suggesting a disturbance of neuroplasticity.

R℞ TREATMENT

Treatment for dystonia is for the most part symptomatic except in the rare instances such as Wilson's disease (Chap. 339) or DRD, where known mechanisms are present and specific therapies are available. The available treatments include physical and emotional support, physical therapy and neurorehabilitation, drugs, and surgery. The importance of education and supportive care must be recognized. Sensory retraining in humans with focal dystonias has resulted in a substantial recovery of function in some patients. Patients with generalized dystonia benefit from a team approach in a specialized center.

Pharmacotherapy Anticholinergic drugs are the most effective forms of treatment for generalized primary dystonia. Trihexyphenidyl is most commonly used. Doses ≥120 mg/d in children may be necessary, with a usual range of 20 to 50 mg/d. Adults can rarely tolerate these high doses. The limiting factors include constipation, dry mouth, blurred vision, and urinary retention as well as impaired short-term memory, confusion, and hallucinations. Benzodiazepines, including clonazepam or diazepam, are also effective for dystonia, alone or in combination with anticholinergics. Dosages are raised slowly until benefits are obtained or side effects, including sedation, ataxia, and confusion, prevent further escalation. Baclofen, a drug similar to the naturally occurring neurotransmitter γ-aminobutyric acid (GABA), is also effective for treating both focal and generalized dystonia. Relatively high doses are required (60 to 100 mg); however, side effects are often limiting. A baclofen pump for intrathecal infusion may be helpful for such cases. Dystonia involving the legs and trunk is most responsive to this form of therapy. Unfortunately, sustained benefits are not the rule and complications are not infrequent. Dopaminergic drugs are occasionally beneficial in both generalized and focal dystonias, but the most dramatic effects are seen in individuals with DRD, who experience a dramatic and sustained improvement with even a small dose of levodopa. Paradoxically, a fair percentage of patients with generalized dystonia (and craniocervical dystonia) respond to dopaminergic antagonists, such as haloperidol or pimozide. Sometimes the combination of tetrabenazine, pimozide, and trihexyphenidyl is effective.

Botulinum Toxin Although the focal dystonias are generally poorly responsive to drugs, they often respond dramatically to botulinum toxin injected into the affected muscle groups. Botulinum toxin can also be used in generalized dystonia for the occasional treatment of focal problems. Botulinum toxin acts by blocking the release of acetylcholine at the neuromuscular junction, resulting in dose-dependent weakness. Repeated injections are required every 2 to 5 months. Botulinum toxin serotypes A and B are now available, providing an alternative should resistance develop to either serotype.

Surgical Approaches Prior to the introduction of botulinum toxin, peripheral denervation procedures, such as dorsal or anterior cervical rhizotomy and selective peripheral denervation, were commonly performed, primarily for the treatment of cervical dystonia. These are now performed far less frequently, generally in patients with cervical dystonia who fail botulinum toxin injections. Stereotactic surgery is used primarily for severe generalized dystonia unresponsive to other treatments. In recent years following the success in PD, pallidotomy and DBS of the pallidum are being used with promising results. The best candidates for surgery appear to be individuals with primary (DYT1) dystonia. Patients with secondary forms of dystonia are less likely to benefit. Bilateral surgery is usually necessary to obtain control of axial dystonia.

TOURETTE SYNDROME

The most common disorder characterized by tics is Tourette syndrome (TS), a neurodevelopmental disorder with neurologic and behavioral manifestations. The true prevalence of TS disorders is unknown but has been estimated at 0.05%. In addition to tics, approximately half of patients develop comorbidities, specifically obsessive-compulsive disorder (OCD) and attention-deficit hyperactivity disorder (ADHD).

Clinical Features A *tic* is a brief, rapid, repetitive, and seemingly purposeless stereotyped action that may involve one or more muscle groups. Tics are divided into motor or vocal types, depending on the affected muscle group, and into simple and complex, depending on the number of muscle groups involved and the associated behaviors. They can range from the barely detectable and easily rationalized "nervous habits" such as blinking, twitching of the nose, and jerking of the neck, to the complex, emotionally laden, and sometimes offensive utterances of a minority of patients (*coprolalia*). Tics can be associated with brief focal sensory experiences termed *sensory tics* that commonly affect the face, head, and neck areas. Some tics may be difficult to distinguish from other fast "jerky" movements, such as chorea and myoclonus, but are unique in that they can be voluntarily inhibited for a brief period of time.

Developmentally, attentional problems develop before school and tics present during the first years of school. OCD symptoms develop later, just before or during adolescence. Tics and ADHD symptoms tend to stabilize with aging. The OCD symptoms have a more variable course.

The inheritance pattern of TS best fits the model of a major gene or genes with low penetrance, modifier genes, and a phenotype influenced by environmental factors. The risk of a family with one affected child of having another is 25%. No specific gene has been linked to TS, however. In PET studies using selective dopamine D_2-receptor ligands, alleles of this gene have been shown to modify symptom severity.

R℞ TREATMENT

Tic symptoms have been ascribed to an overactivity of dopaminergic circuits. Accordingly dopamine blockers have consistently improved symptoms. Tics are not the most disabling feature of the illness, and treatment is generally indicated only when tics interfere with quality of life. The typical antipsychotics, Fluphenazine, haloperidol, and pimozide, thought to be very effective at treating tics, have been associated with extrapyramidal symptoms and school phobias. More recently, selected atypical antipsychotics have been shown to control tic symptoms and to have a lower incidence of these complications compared to typical antipsychotics. Drugs in this category include risperidone (0.5 to 4 mg/d), olanzapine (5 to 30 mg/d), and ziprasidone (80 to 200 mg/d). Other treatments for tics include clonidine (0.1 to 0.4 mg/d or the equivalent as transdermal patch), guanifencine (0.5 to 2 mg/d), and clonazepam (0.5 to 4.0 mg/d). Botulinum toxin injections can be effective in controlling focal tics involving small muscle groups. In general, symptoms of anxiety and OCD should be treated first since their control may preclude the need to treat the tics (Chap. 371).

DRUG-INDUCED HYPERKINETIC DISORDERS

This important group of iatrogenic and mostly reversible movement disorders is primarily associated with drugs that directly or indirectly affect central dopaminergic transmission. CNS stimulants, levodopa, dopamine agonists, and dopamine receptor blockers are the most common offending agents. The mechanism of acute and subacute movement disorders appears to result from idiosyncratic extensions of the intended action of the compound. By contrast, the mechanism of delayed or tardive dyskinesia (TD) syndromes remains more obscure.

DRUG-INDUCED MOVEMENT DISORDERS ■ **Acute** Reactions in this category include acute dystonia in response to dopamine antagonists, which appears most frequently in a generalized form in children and in a focal form (e.g., blepharospasm, torticollis, or oromandibular dystonia) in adults. These movements can be readily treated with the parenteral administration of anticholinergics (benztropine or diphenhydramine) or benzodiazepines (lorazepam or diazepam). Other acute movement disorders include dyskinesias, stereotypic behaviors, and tics after exposure to CNS stimulants such as methylphenidate, dextroamphetamine, and pemoline.

Subacute   Probably the most common of these reactions is neuroleptic-induced akathisia, a state of motor restlessness with a feeling of restlessness and a need to move, which tends to alleviate the symptoms temporarily. Therapy consists of removing the offending agent(s). When this is not possible, symptoms can be ameliorated with benzodiazepines, anticholinergics, beta blockers, and, in some cases, dopamine agonists.

Tardive   Tardive movement disorders such as TD are primarily due to chronic exposure to central dopamine blockers. The movements are most often choreatic, affecting first the mouth, lips, and tongue and later the trunk and limbs. In a fully developed case there can be head nodding, pelvic rocking, and fine movements of the fingers and toes. The diaphragm is affected rarely, producing respiratory distress. Other tardive syndromes include tardive dystonia, which generally presents with more axial than appendicular involvement; tardive akathisia; tardive tics; and even tardive tremor.

Approximately one-third of patients with TD remit within 3 months of stopping neuroleptic therapy, and in most patients the movements will gradually remit within 5 years. Patients at risk of permanent TD include the elderly, the edentulous, and those with underlying organic cerebral dysfunction. Patients with affective illnesses appear more likely to develop TD than patients with schizophrenia. Since treatment of TD is most often unsatisfactory and frustrating for both patient and physician, it is critical that typical antipsychotics be used judiciously and that, once started, their continued need be reassessed periodically. Abrupt drug cessation may result in "withdrawal dyskinesias," which presage the development of frank TD.

℞ TREATMENT

Atypical antipsychotics (clozapine, risperidone, olanzepine, quetiapine, ziprasidone, and aripiprazole) significantly lower the risk of TD compared to typical antipsychotics. Accordingly, if withdrawal of the offending antipsychotic is not possible, replacing traditional with atypical antipsychotics should be tried. Furthermore, it appears that atypical antipsychotics can successfully block the dyskinesias themselves. Elimination of stimulants and anticholinergics will also alleviate dyskinesias. In refractory cases, choreatic TD can be treated with the catecholamine depletors reserpine and tetrabenazine. Reserpine should be started at 0.125 mg/d and escalated slowly as needed up to 6 mg/d. Tetrabenazine should be started at 12.5 mg/d and gradually increased as necessary up to 200 mg/d. The elderly are less likely to tolerate the dose-dependent sedation and orthostatic hypotension associated with these drugs. Approximately 15% of patients on catecholamine depletors develop depression with chronic use of reserpine. Another strategy employs GABAergic medications such as baclofen (40 to 80 mg/d), clonazepam (1 to 8 mg/d), or valproic acid (750 to 3,000 mg/d). The latter strategy is particularly helpful in patients with tardive dystonia, which may also benefit from anticholinergic therapy and botulinum toxin injections.

Neuroleptic Malignant Syndrome (NMS)   This serious complication of neuroleptic medications occurs in 1 to 2% of treated individuals; the mortality rate is as high as 20%. Muscle rigidity with myonecrosis; an altered mental status resembling catatonia; and autonomic dysfunction with hyperthermia, tachycardia, and a labile blood pressure constitute the principal manifestations. Symptoms typically evolve subacutely over several days and usually occur in the first few weeks following initial exposure to the drug, but can develop anytime. NMS can also be precipitated by the abrupt withdrawal of antiparkinson medications.

℞ TREATMENT

Treatment begins with immediate cessation of the offending antipsychotic drug as well as lithium and anticholinergic agents, which appear to increase the risk of NMS. Careful monitoring of body temperature, hydration, electrolytes (especially K^+), and blood pressure are essential. Specific pharmacologic agents include dopamine agonists or levodopa, amantadine, and benzodiazepines as well as dantrolene. Supportive measures include antipyretics, cooling blankets, fluids, and measures to maintain blood pressure.

FURTHER READING

AHLSKOG JE: Slowing Parkinson's disease progression: Recent dopamine agonist trials. Neurology 60:381, 2003

DAWSON TM, DAWSON VL: Molecular pathways of neurodegeneration in Parkinson's disease. Science 302:819, 2003

PAHWA R, LYONS K: Essential tremor: Differential diagnosis and current therapy. Am J Med 115:134, 2003

SIDEROWF A, STERN M: Update on Parkinson's disease. Ann Intern Med 138: 651, 2003

352   ATAXIC DISORDERS
Roger N. Rosenberg

APPROACH TO THE PATIENT

Symptoms and signs of ataxia consist of gait impairment, unclear ("scanning") speech, visual blurring due to nystagmus, hand incoordination, and tremor with movement (Chap. 21). These result from the involvement of the cerebellum and its afferent and efferent pathways, including the spinocerebellar pathways, and the frontopontocerebellar pathway originating in the rostral frontal lobe. True cerebellar ataxia must be distinguished from ataxia associated with vestibular nerve or labyrinthine disease, as the latter results in a disorder of gait associated with a significant degree of dizziness, light-headedness, or the perception of movement (Chap. 20). True cerebellar ataxia is devoid of these vertiginous complaints and is clearly an unsteady gait due to imbalance. Sensory disturbances can also on occasion simulate the imbalance of cerebellar disease; with sensory ataxia, imbalance dramatically worsens when visual input is removed (Romberg sign). Rarely, weakness of proximal leg muscles mimics cerebellar disease. In the patient who presents with ataxia, the rate and pattern of the development of cerebellar symptoms help to narrow the diagnostic possibilities (Table 352-1). A gradual and progressive increase in symptoms with bilateral and symmetric involvement suggests a biochemical, metabolic, immune, or toxic etiology. Conversely, focal, unilateral symptoms with headache and impaired level of consciousness accompanied by ipsilateral cranial nerve palsies and contralateral weakness imply a space-occupying cerebellar lesion.

Symmetric Ataxia   Progressive and symmetric ataxia can be classified with respect to onset as acute (over hours or days), subacute (weeks or months), or chronic (months to years). Acute and reversible ataxias include those caused by intoxication with alcohol, phenytoin, lithium, barbiturates, and other drugs. Intoxication caused by toluene exposure, gasoline sniffing, glue sniffing, spray painting, or exposure to methyl mercury or bismuth are additional

TABLE 352-1 Etiology of Cerebellar Ataxia

Symmetric and Progressive Signs			Focal and Ipsilateral Cerebellar Signs		
Acute (Hours to Days)	Subacute (Days to Weeks)	Chronic (Months to Years)	Acute (Hours to Days)	Subacute (Days to Weeks)	Chronic (Months to Years)
Intoxication: alcohol, lithium, diphenylhydantoin, barbiturates (positive history and toxicology screen) Acute viral cerebellitis (CSF supportive of acute viral infection) Postinfection syndrome	Intoxication: mercury, solvents, gasoline, glue; cytotoxic chemotherapeutic drugs Alcoholic-nutritional (vitamin B$_1$ and B$_{12}$ deficiency) Lyme disease	Paraneoplastic syndrome Anti-gliadin antibody syndrome Hypothyroidism Inherited diseases Tabes dorsalis (tertiary syphilis) Phenytoin toxicity	Vascular: cerebellar infarction, hemorrhage, or subdural hematoma Infectious: cerebellar abscess (positive mass lesion on MRI/CT, positive history in support of lesion)	Neoplastic: cerebellar glioma or metastatic tumor (positive for neoplasm on MRI/CT) Demyelinating: multiple sclerosis (history, CSF, and MRI are consistent) AIDS-related multifocal leukoencephalopathy (positive HIV test and CD4+ cell count for AIDS)	Stable gliosis secondary to vascular lesion or demyelinating plaque (stable lesion on MRI/CT older than several months) Congenital lesion: Chiari or Dandy-Walker malformations (malformation noted on MRI/CT)

Abbreviations: CSF, cerebrospinal fluid; CT, computed tomography; MRI, magnetic resonance imaging.

causes of acute or subacute ataxia, as is treatment with cytotoxic chemotherapeutic drugs such as fluorouracil and paclitaxel. Patients with a postinfectious syndrome (especially after varicella) may develop gait ataxia and mild dysarthria, both of which are reversible (Chap. 359). Rare infectious causes of acquired ataxia include poliovirus, coxsackievirus, echovirus, Epstein-Barr virus, toxoplasmosis, *Legionella*, and Lyme disease.

The subacute development of ataxia of gait over weeks to months (degeneration of the cerebellar vermis) may be due to the combined effects of alcoholism and malnutrition, particularly with deficiencies of vitamins B$_1$ and B$_{12}$. Hyponatremia has also been associated with ataxia. Paraneoplastic cerebellar ataxia is associated with a number of different tumors (and autoantibodies) such as breast and ovarian cancers (anti-Yo), small-cell lung cancer (anti-PQ type voltage-gated calcium channel), and Hodgkin's disease (anti-Tr) (Chap. 87). Another paraneoplastic syndrome associated with myoclonus and opsoclonus occurs with breast (anti-Ri) and lung cancers and neuroblastoma. For all of these paraneoplastic ataxias, the neurologic syndrome may be the presenting symptom of the cancer. Another immune-mediated progressive ataxia is associated with anti-gliadin (and anti-endomysium) antibodies and the HLA DQB1*0201 haplotype; in some affected patients, biopsy of the small intestine reveals villous atrophy consistent with gluten-sensitive enteropathy (Chap. 275). Finally, subacute progressive ataxia may be caused by a prion disorder, especially when an infectious etiology, such as transmission from contaminated human growth hormone, is responsible (Chap. 362).

Chronic symmetric gait ataxia suggests an inherited ataxia (discussed below), a metabolic disorder, or a chronic infection. Hypothyroidism must always be considered as a readily treatable and reversible form of gait ataxia. Infectious diseases that can present with ataxia are meningovascular syphilis and tabes dorsalis due to degeneration of the posterior columns and spinocerebellar pathways in the spinal cord.

Focal Ataxia Acute focal ataxia commonly results from cerebrovascular disease, usually ischemic infarction, or cerebellar hemorrhage. These lesions typically produce cerebellar symptoms ipsilateral to the injured cerebellum and may be associated with an impaired level of consciousness due to brainstem compression and increased intracranial pressure; ipsilateral pontine signs, including sixth and seventh nerve palsies, may be present. Focal and worsening signs of acute ataxia should also prompt consideration of a posterior fossa subdural hematoma, bacterial abscess, or primary or metastatic cerebellar tumor. Computed tomography (CT) or magnetic resonance imaging (MRI) studies will reveal clinically significant processes of this type. Many of these lesions represent

true neurologic emergencies, as sudden herniation, either rostrally through the tentorium or caudal herniation of cerebellar tonsils through the foramen magnum, can occur and is usually devastating. Acute surgical decompression may be required (Chap. 258). Lymphoma or progressive multifocal leukoencephalopathy (PML) in a patient with AIDS may present with an acute or subacute focal cerebellar syndrome. Chronic etiologies of progressive ataxia include multiple sclerosis (Chap. 359) and congenital lesions such as a Chiari malformation (Chap. 356) or a congenital cyst of the posterior fossa (Dandy-Walker syndrome).

THE INHERITED ATAXIAS

These may show autosomal dominant, autosomal recessive, or maternal (mitochondrial) modes of inheritance. A genomic classification (Table 352-2) has now largely superseded previous ones based on clinical expression alone.

Although the clinical manifestations and neuropathologic findings of cerebellar disease dominate the clinical picture, there may also be characteristic changes in the basal ganglia, brainstem, spinal cord, optic nerves, retina, and peripheral nerves. In large families with dominantly inherited ataxias, many gradations are observed from purely cerebellar manifestations to mixed cerebellar and brainstem disorders, cerebellar and basal ganglia syndromes, and spinal cord or peripheral nerve disease. Rarely, dementia is present as well. The clinical picture may be homogeneous within a family with dominantly inherited ataxia, but sometimes most affected family members show one characteristic syndrome, while one or several members have an entirely different phenotype.

AUTOSOMAL DOMINANT ATAXIAS The autosomal spinocerebellar ataxias (SCAs) include SCA type 1 through SCA22, dentatorubropallidoluysian atrophy (DRPLA), and episodic ataxia (EA) types 1 and 2 (Table 352-2). SCA1, SCA2, SCA3 [Machado-Joseph disease (MJD)], SCA6, SCA7, and SCA17 are caused by CAG triplet repeat expansions in different genes. SCA8 is due to an untranslated CTG repeat expansion, SCA12 is linked to an untranslated CAG repeat, and SCA10 is caused by an untranslated pentanucleotide repeat. The clinical phenotypes of these SCAs overlap. The genotype has become the "gold standard" for diagnosis and classification. CAG encodes glutamine, and these expanded CAG triplet repeat expansions result in expanded polyglutamine proteins, termed *ataxins*, that produce a toxic gain of function with autosomal dominant inheritance. Although the phenotype is variable for any given disease gene, a pattern of neuronal loss with gliosis is produced that is relatively unique for each ataxia. Immunohistochemical and biochemical studies have shown cytoplasmic (SCA2), neuronal (SCA1, MJD, SCA7), and nucleolar (SCA7) accumulation of the

TABLE 352-2 Genotype Classification of the Spinocerebellar Ataxias

Name	Locus	Phenotype
SCA1 (autosomal dominant type 1)	6p22-p23 with CAG repeats (exonic) Ataxin-1	Ataxia with ophthalmoparesis, pyramidal and extrapyramidal findings
SCA2 (autosomal dominant type 2)	12q23-q24.1 with CAG repeats (exonic) Ataxin-2	Ataxia with slow saccades and minimal pyramidal and extrapyramidal findings
Machado-Joseph disease/SCA3 (autosomal dominant type 3)	14q24.3-q32 with CAG repeats (exonic) MJD–ataxin-3	Ataxia with ophthalmoparesis and variable pyramidal, extrapyramidal, and amyotrophic signs
SCA4 (autosomal dominant type 4)	16q24-ter	Ataxia with normal eye movements, sensory axonal neuropathy, and pyramidal signs
SCA5 (autosomal dominant type 5)	Centromeric region of chromosome II	Ataxia and dysarthria
SCA6 (autosomal dominant type 6)	19p13.2 with CAG repeats in α_{1A}-voltage–dependent calcium channel gene (exonic)	Ataxia and dysarthria, nystagmus, mild proprioceptive sensory loss
SCA7 (autosomal dominant type 7)	3p14.1-p21.1 with CAG repeats (exonic) Ataxin-7	Ophthalmoparesis, visual loss, ataxia, dysarthria, extensor plantar response, pigmentary retinal degeneration
SCA8 (autosomal dominant type 8)	13q21 with CTG repeats; noncoding	Gait ataxia, dysarthria, nystagmus, leg spasticity, and reduced vibratory sensation
SCA10 (autosomal dominant type 10)	22q; ATTCT repeat; noncoding	Gait ataxia, dysarthria, nystagmus; partial complex and generalized motor seizures; polyneuropathy
SCA11 (autosomal dominant type 11)	15q14-q21.3 by linkage	Slowly progressive gait and extremity ataxia, dysarthria, vertical nystagmus, hyperreflexia
SCA12 (autosomal dominant type 12)	5q31-q33 by linkage; CAG repeat; protein phosphatase 2A	Tremor, decreased movement, increased reflexes, dystonia, ataxia, dysautonomia, dementia, dysarthria
SCA13 (autosomal dominant type 13)	19q13.3-q14.4	Mutation unknown
SCA14 (autosomal dominant type 14)	19q-13.4	Mutation unknown
SCA15 (autosomal dominant type 15)	Mutation unknown in 1 family; other known loci were excluded	Gait and extremity ataxia, dysarthria
SCA16 (autosomal dominant type 16)	8q22.1-24.1	Mutation unknown; pure cerebellar ataxia and head tremor, gait ataxia, and dysarthria; horizontal gaze–evoked nystagmus
SCA17 (autosomal dominant type 17)	6q27; CAG expansion in the TATA-binding protein (*TBP*) gene	Gait ataxia, dementia, parkinsonism, dystonia, chorea, seizures; MRI shows cerebral & cerebellar atrophy
SCA18 (autosomal dominant type 18)	7q22-q32	Ataxia motor/sensory neuropathy
SCA19 (autosomal dominant type 19)	1p21-q21	Ataxia, tremor, cognitive impairment, myoclonus
SCA20 (assigned but not yet published)	—	—
SCA21 (autosomal dominant type 21)	7p21.3-p15.1	Ataxia, extrapyramidal features of akinesia, rigidity, tremor, cognitive defect
SCA22 (assigned but not yet published)	—	—
Dentatorubropallidoluysian atrophy (autosomal dominant)	12p12-ter with CAG repeats (exonic) Atrophin	Ataxia, choreoathetosis, dystonia, seizures, myoclonus, dementia
Friedreich's ataxia (autosomal recessive)	9q13-q21.1 with intronic GAA repeats Frataxin	Ataxia, areflexia, extensor plantar responses, position sense deficits, cardiomyopathy, diabetes mellitus, scoliosis, foot deformities; defective iron transport from mitochondria
Friedreich's ataxia (autosomal recessive)	8q13.1-q13.3; (α-TTP deficiency)	Same as phenotype that maps to 9q but associated with vitamin E deficiency
Autosomal recessive spastic ataxia of Charlevoix-Saguenay (ARSACS)	Chromosome 13; SACS gene; loss of Sacsin peptide activity	Childhood onset of ataxia, spasticity, dysarthria, distal muscle wasting, foot deformity, retinal striations, mitral valve prolapse
Kearns-Sayre syndrome (sporadic)	mtDNA deletion and duplication mutations	Ptosis, ophthalmoplegia, pigmentary retinal degeneration, cardiomyopathy, diabetes mellitus, deafness, heart block, increased CSF protein, ataxia
Myoclonic epilepsy and ragged red fiber syndrome (MERRF) (maternal inheritance)	Mutation in mtDNA of the tRNA^{lys} at 8344; also mutation at 8356	Myoclonic epilepsy, ragged red fiber myopathy, ataxia
Mitochondrial encephalopathy, lactic acidosis, and stroke syndrome (MELAS) (maternal inheritance)	tRNA^{leu} mutation at 3243; also at 3271 and 3252	Headache, stroke, lactic acidosis, ataxia
Leigh's disease; subacute necrotizing encephalopathy (maternal inheritance or autosomal recessive)	mtDNA complex V defect (ATPase gene at 8993) or mitochondrial protein synthesis defect (both maternally inherited); or complex IV defect (autosomal recessive)	Obtundation, hypotonia, cranial nerve defects, respiratory failure, hyperintense signals on T2-weighted MRI in basal ganglia, cerebellum, or brainstem; ataxia
Episodic ataxia, type 1 (EA-1) (autosomal dominant)	12p; potassium channel gene, *KCNA1*	Episodic ataxia for minutes; provoked by startle or exercise; with facial and hand myokymia; cerebellar signs are not progressive; responds to phenytoin
Episodic ataxia, type 2 (EA-2) (autosomal dominant)	19p-13 (*CACNA1A*) (allelic with SCA6) (α_{1A}-voltage–dependent calcium channel subunit)	Episodic ataxia for days; provoked by stress, fatigue; with down-gaze nystagmus; cerebellar atrophy results; progressive cerebellar signs; responds to acetazolamide
Ataxia telangiectasia (autosomal recessive)	11q22-23; *ATM* gene for regulation of cell cycle; mitogenic signal transduction and meiotic recombination	Telangiectasia, ataxia, dysarthria, pulmonary infections, neoplasms of lymphatic system; IgA and IgG deficiencies; diabetes mellitus, breast cancer

(continued)

TABLE 352-2—(Continued)

Name	Locus	Phenotype
Infantile-onset spinocerebellar ataxia of Nikali et al (autosomal recessive)	10q23.3-q24.1	Infantile ataxia, sensory neuropathy; athetosis, hearing deficit, ophthalmoplegia, optic atrophy; primary hypogonadism in females
Hypoceruloplasminemia with ataxia and dysarthria (autosomal recessive)	Ceruloplasmin gene; 3q23-q25 (trp 858 ter)	Gait ataxia and dysarthria; hyperreflexia; cerebellar atrophy by MRI; iron deposition in cerebellum, basal ganglia, thalamus, and liver; onset in the 4th decade
Spinocerebellar ataxia with neuropathy (SCAN1) (autosomal recessive)	Tryosyl-DNA phosphodiesterase-1 (TDP-1) 14q31-q32	Onset in 2nd decade; gait ataxia, dysarthria, seizures, cerebellar vermis atrophy on MRI, dysmetria

Abbreviations: MRI, magnetic resonance imaging; CSF, cerebrospinal fluid.

specific mutant polyglutamine containing ataxin proteins. Expanded polyglutamine ataxins with more than ~40 glutamines are potentially toxic to neurons for a variety of reasons including the following: high levels of gene expression for the mutant polyglutamine ataxin in affected neurons; conformational change of the aggregated protein to a β-pleated structure; abnormal transport of the ataxin into the nucleus (SCA1, MJD, SCA7); binding to other polyglutamine proteins, including the TATA-binding transcription protein and the CREB-binding protein, impairing their functions; altering the efficiency of the ubiquitin-proteosome system of protein turnover; and inducing neuronal apoptosis. An earlier age of onset (anticipation) and more aggressive disease in subsequent generations are due to further expansion of the CAG triplet repeat and increased polyglutamine number in the mutant ataxin. The most common disorders are discussed below.

SCA1 SCA1 was previously referred to as *olivopontocerebellar atrophy*, but genomic data have shown that that entity represents several different genotypes with overlapping clinical features.

SYMPTOMS AND SIGNS SCA1 is characterized by the development in early or middle adult life of progressive cerebellar ataxia of the trunk and limbs, impairment of equilibrium and gait, slowness of voluntary movements, scanning speech, nystagmoid eye movements, and oscillatory tremor of the head and trunk. Dysarthria, dysphagia, and oculomotor and facial palsies may also occur. Extrapyramidal symptoms include rigidity, an immobile face, and parkinsonian tremor. The reflexes are usually normal, but knee and ankle jerks may be lost, and extensor plantar responses may occur. Dementia may be noted but is usually mild. Impairment of sphincter function is common, with urinary and sometimes fecal incontinence. Cerebellar and brainstem atrophy are evident on MRI (Fig. 352-1).

Marked shrinkage of the ventral half of the pons, disappearance of the olivary eminence on the ventral surface of the medulla, and atrophy of the cerebellum are evident on gross postmortem inspection of the brain. Variable loss of Purkinje cells, reduced numbers of cells in the molecular and granular layer, demyelination of the middle cerebellar peduncle and the cerebellar hemispheres, and severe loss of cells in the pontine nuclei and olives are found on histologic examination. Degenerative changes in the striatum, especially the putamen, and loss of the pigmented cells of the substantia nigra may be found in cases with extrapyramidal features. More widespread degeneration in the central nervous system (CNS), including involvement of the posterior columns and the spinocerebellar fibers, is often present.

GENETIC CONSIDERATIONS SCA1 encodes a gene product, called ataxin-1, which is a novel protein of unknown function. The mutant allele has 40 CAG repeats located within the coding region, whereas alleles from unaffected individuals have ≤36 repeats. A few patients with 38 to 40 CAG repeats have been described. There is a direct correlation between a larger number of repeats and a younger age of onset for SCA1. Juvenile patients have higher numbers of repeats, and anticipation is present in subsequent generations. Transgenic mice carrying SCA1 developed ataxia and Purkinje cell pathology. Nuclear localization, but not aggregation, of ataxin-1 appears to be required for cell death initiated by the mutant protein.

SCA2 ■ *SYMPTOMS AND SIGNS* Another clinical phenotype, SCA2, has been described in Cubans. These patients probably are descendants of a common ancestor, and the population may be the largest homogeneous group of patients with ataxia yet described. The age of onset ranges from 2 to 65 years, and there is considerable clinical variability within families. Although neuropathologic and clinical findings are compatible with a diagnosis of SCA1, including slow saccadic eye movements, ataxia, dysarthria, parkinsonian rigidity, optic disk pallor, mild spasticity, and retinal degeneration, SCA2 is a unique form of cerebellar degenerative disease.

GENETIC CONSIDERATIONS The gene in SCA2 families also contains CAG repeat expansions coding for a polyglutamine-containing protein, ataxin-2. Normal alleles contain 15 to 32 repeats; mutant alleles have 35 to 77 repeats.

Machado-Joseph Disease/SCA3 MJD was first described among the Portuguese and their descendants in New England and California. Subsequently, MJD has been found in families from Portugal, Australia, Brazil, Canada, China, England, France, India, Israel, Italy, Japan, Spain, Taiwan, and the United States. In most populations, it is the most common autosomal dominant ataxia.

SYMPTOMS AND SIGNS MJD has been classified into three clinical types. In type I MJD (amyotrophic lateral sclerosis–parkinsonism–dystonia type), neurologic deficits appear in the first two decades and involve weakness and spasticity of extremities, especially the legs, often with dystonia of the face, neck, trunk, and extremities. Patellar and ankle clonus are common, as are extensor plantar responses. The gait is slow and stiff, with a slightly broadened base and lurching from side to side; this gait results from spasticity, not true ataxia. There is no truncal

FIGURE 352-1 Sagittal MRI of the brain of a 60-year-old man with gait ataxia and dysarthria due to SCA1, illustrating cerebellar atrophy (*arrows*).

titubation. Pharyngeal weakness and spasticity cause difficulty with speech and swallowing. Of note is the prominence of horizontal and vertical nystagmus, loss of fast saccadic eye movements, hypermetric and hypometric saccades, and impairment of upward vertical gaze. Facial fasciculations, facial myokymia, lingual fasciculations without atrophy, ophthalmoparesis, and ocular prominence are common early manifestations.

In type II MJD (ataxic type), true cerebellar deficits of dysarthria and gait and extremity ataxia begin in the second to fourth decades along with corticospinal and extrapyramidal deficits of spasticity, rigidity, and dystonia. Type II is the most common form of MJD. Ophthalmoparesis, upward vertical gaze deficits, and facial and lingual fasciculations are also present. Type II MJD can be distinguished from the clinically similar disorders SCA1 and SCA2.

Type III MJD (ataxic-amyotrophic type) presents in the fifth to the seventh decades with a pancerebellar disorder that includes dysarthria and gait and extremity ataxia. Distal sensory loss involving pain, touch, vibration, and position senses and distal atrophy are prominent, indicating the presence of peripheral neuropathy. The deep tendon reflexes are depressed to absent, and there are no corticospinal or extrapyramidal findings.

The mean age of onset of symptoms in MJD is 25 years. Neurologic deficits invariably progress and lead to death from debilitation within 15 years of onset, especially in patients with types I and II disease. Usually, patients retain full intellectual function.

The major pathologic findings are variable loss of neurons and glial replacement in the corpus striatum and severe loss of neurons in the pars compacta of the substantia nigra. A moderate loss of neurons occurs in the dentate nucleus of the cerebellum and in the red nucleus. Purkinje cell loss and granule cell loss occur in the cerebellar cortex. Cell loss also occurs in the dentate nucleus and in the cranial nerve motor nuclei. Sparing of the inferior olives distinguishes MJD from other dominantly inherited ataxias.

GENETIC CONSIDERATIONS   The gene for MJD maps to 14q24.3-q32. Unstable CAG repeat expansions are present in the MJD gene coding for a polyglutamine-containing protein named ataxin-3, or MJD-ataxin. An earlier age of onset is associated with longer repeats. Alleles from normal individuals have between 12 and 37 CAG repeats, and MJD alleles have 60 to 84 CAG repeats. Polyglutamine-containing aggregates of ataxin-3 (MJD-ataxin) have been described in neuronal nuclei undergoing degeneration.

SCA6   Genomic screening for CAG repeats in other families with autosomal dominant ataxia and vibratory and proprioceptive sensory loss have yielded another locus. Of interest is that different mutations in the same gene for the α_{1A} voltage-dependent calcium channel subunit (CACNL1A4; also referred to as the *CACNA1A* gene) at 19p13 result in different clinical disorders. CAG repeat expansions (21 to 27 in patients; 4 to 16 triplets in normal individuals) result in late-onset progressive ataxia with cerebellar degeneration. Missense mutations in this gene result in familial hemiplegic migraine. Nonsense mutations resulting in termination of protein synthesis of the gene product yield hereditary paroxysmal cerebellar ataxia or EA. Some patients with familial hemiplegic migraine develop progressive ataxia and also have cerebellar atrophy.

SCA7   This disorder is distinguished from all other SCAs by the presence of retinal pigmentary degeneration. The visual abnormalities first appear as blue-yellow color blindness and proceed to frank visual loss with macular degeneration. In almost all other respects, SCA7 resembles several other SCAs in which ataxia is accompanied by various noncerebellar findings, including ophthalmoparesis and extensor plantar responses. The genetic defect is an expanded CAG repeat in the SCA7 gene. The expanded repeat size in SCA7 is highly variable. Consistent with this, the severity of clinical findings varies from

essentially asymptomatic to mild late-onset symptoms to severe, aggressive disease in childhood with rapid progression. Marked anticipation has been recorded, especially with paternal transmission. The disease protein, ataxin-7, forms aggregates in nuclei of affected neurons, as has also been described for SCA1 and SCA3/MJD.

SCA8   This form of ataxia is caused by a CTG repeat expansion in an untranslated region of a gene on chromosome 13q21. There is marked maternal bias in transmission, perhaps reflecting contractions of the repeat during spermatogenesis. The mutation is not fully penetrant. Symptoms include slowly progressive dysarthria and gait ataxia beginning at ~40 years of age with a range between 20 and 65 years. Other features include nystagmus, leg spasticity, and reduced vibratory sensation. Severely affected individuals are nonambulatory by the fourth to sixth decades. MRI shows cerebellar atrophy. The mechanism of disease may involve a dominant "toxic" effect occurring at the RNA level, as occurs in myotonic dystrophy.

Dentatorubropallidoluysian Atrophy   DRPLA has a variable presentation that may include progressive ataxia, choreoathetosis, dystonia, seizures, myoclonus, and dementia. DRPLA is due to unstable CAG triplet repeats in the open reading frame of a gene named *atrophin* located on chromosome 12p12-ter. Larger expansions are found in patients with earlier onset. The number of repeats is 49 in patients with DRPLA and ≤26 in normal individuals. Anticipation occurs in successive generations, with earlier onset of disease in association with an increasing CAG repeat number in children who inherit the disease from their father. One well-characterized family in North Carolina has a phenotypic variant known as the *Haw River syndrome*, now recognized to be due to the DRPLA mutation.

Episodic Ataxia   EA types 1 and 2 are two rare dominantly inherited disorders that have been mapped to chromosomes 12p (a potassium channel gene) for type 1 and 19p for type 2. Patients with EA-1 have brief episodes of ataxia with myokymia and nystagmus that last only minutes. Startle, sudden change in posture, and exercise can induce episodes. Acetazolamide or anticonvulsants may be therapeutic. Patients with EA-2 have episodes of ataxia with nystagmus that can last for hours or days. Stress, exercise, or excessive fatigue may be precipitants. Acetazolamide may be therapeutic and can reverse the relative intracellular alkalosis detected by magnetic resonance spectroscopy. Stop codon, nonsense mutations causing EA-2 have been found in the *CACNA1A* gene, encoding the α_{1A} voltage-dependent calcium channel subunit (see "SCA6," above).

AUTOSOMAL RECESSIVE ATAXIAS ■ **Friedreich's Ataxia**   This is the most common form of inherited ataxia, comprising one-half of all hereditary ataxias. It can occur in a classic form or in association with a genetically determined vitamin E deficiency syndrome; the two forms are clinically indistinguishable.

SYMPTOMS AND SIGNS   Friedreich's ataxia presents before 25 years of age with progressive staggering gait, frequent falling, and titubation. The lower extremities are more severely involved than the upper ones. Dysarthria occasionally is the presenting symptom; rarely, progressive scoliosis, foot deformity, nystagmus, or cardiopathy is the initial sign.

The neurologic examination reveals nystagmus, loss of fast saccadic eye movements, truncal titubation, dysarthria, dysmetria, and ataxia of trunk and limb movements. Extensor plantar responses (with normal tone in trunk and extremities), absence of deep tendon reflexes, and weakness (greater distally than proximally) are usually found. Loss of vibratory and proprioceptive sensation occurs. The median age of death is 35 years. Women have a significantly better prognosis than men.

Cardiac involvement occurs in 90% of patients. Cardiomegaly, symmetric hypertrophy, murmurs, and conduction defects are reported. Moderate mental retardation or psychiatric syndromes are present in a small percentage of patients. A high incidence of diabetes mellitus (20%) is found and is associated with insulin resistance and pancreatic β-cell dysfunction. Musculoskeletal deformities are com-

FIGURE 352-2 Sagittal MRI of the brain and spinal cord of a patient with Friedreich's ataxia, demonstrating spinal cord atrophy.

mon and include pes cavus, pes equinovarus, and scoliosis. MRI of the spinal cord shows atrophy (Fig. 352-2).

The primary sites of pathology are the spinal cord, dorsal root ganglion cells, and the peripheral nerves. Slight atrophy of the cerebellum and cerebral gyri may occur. Sclerosis and degeneration occur predominantly in the spinocerebellar tracts, lateral corticospinal tracts, and posterior columns. Degeneration of the glossopharyngeal, vagus, hypoglossal, and deep cerebellar nuclei is described. The cerebral cortex is histologically normal except for loss of Betz cells in the precentral gyri. The peripheral nerves are extensively involved, with a loss of large myelinated fibers. Cardiac pathology consists of myocytic hypertrophy and fibrosis, focal vascular fibromuscular dysplasia with subintimal or medial deposition of periodic acid–Schiff (PAS)–positive material, myocytopathy with unusual pleomorphic nuclei, and focal degeneration of nerves and cardiac ganglia.

GENETIC CONSIDERATIONS The classic form of Friedreich's ataxia has been mapped to 9q13-q21.1, and the mutant gene, *frataxin*, contains expanded GAA triplet repeats in the first intron. There is homozygosity for expanded GAA repeats in >95% of patients. Normal persons have 7 to 22 GAA repeats, and patients have 200 to 900 GAA repeats. A more varied clinical syndrome has been described in compound heterozygotes who have one copy of the GAA expansion and the other copy a point mutation in the *frataxin* gene. When the point mutation is located in the region of the gene that encodes the amino-terminal half of frataxin, the phenotype is milder, often consisting of a spastic gait, retained or exaggerated reflexes, no dysarthria, and mild or absent ataxia.

Patients with Friedreich's ataxia have undetectable or extremely low levels of *frataxin* mRNA, as compared with carriers and unrelated individuals; thus, disease appears to be caused by a loss of expression of the frataxin protein. Frataxin is a mitochondrial protein involved in iron homeostasis. Mitochondrial iron accumulation due to loss of the iron transporter coded by the mutant *frataxin* gene results in oxidized intramitochondrial iron. Excess oxidized iron results in turn in the oxidation of cellular components and irreversible cell injury.

Two forms of hereditary ataxia associated with abnormalities in the interactions of vitamin E (α-tocopherol) with very low density lipoprotein (VLDL) have been delineated. These are abetalipoproteinemia (Bassen-Kornzweig syndrome) and ataxia with vitamin E deficiency (AVED). Abetalipoproteinemia is caused by mutations in the gene coding for the larger subunit of the microsomal triglyceride transfer

protein (MTP). Defects in MTP result in impairment of formation and secretion of VLDL in liver. This defect results in a deficiency of delivery of vitamin E to tissues, including the central and peripheral nervous system, as VLDL is the transport molecule for vitamin E and other fat-soluble substitutes. AVED is due to mutations in the gene for α-tocopherol transfer protein (α-TTP). These patients have an impaired ability to bind vitamin E into the VLDL produced and secreted by the liver, resulting in a deficiency of vitamin E in peripheral tissues. Hence, either absence of VLDL (abetalipoproteinemia) or impaired binding of vitamin E to VLDL (AVED) causes an ataxic syndrome. Once again, a genotype classification has proved to be essential in sorting out the various forms of the Friedreich's disease syndrome, which may be clinically indistinguishable.

Ataxia Telangiectasia ■ *SYMPTOMS AND SIGNS* Patients with ataxia telangiectasia (AT) present in the first decade of life with progressive telangiectatic lesions associated with deficits in cerebellar function and nystagmus. The neurologic manifestations correspond to those in Friedreich's disease, which should be included in the differential diagnosis. Truncal and limb ataxia, dysarthria, extensor plantar responses, myoclonic jerks, areflexia, and distal sensory deficits may develop. There is a high incidence of recurrent pulmonary infections and neoplasms of the lymphatic and reticuloendothelial system in patients with AT. Thymic hypoplasia with cellular and humoral (IgA and IgG2) immunodeficiencies, premature aging, and endocrine disorders such as type 1 diabetes mellitus are described. There is an increased incidence of lymphomas, Hodgkin's disease, acute leukemias of the T cell type, and breast cancer.

The most striking neuropathologic changes include loss of Purkinje, granule, and basket cells in the cerebellar cortex as well as of neurons in the deep cerebellar nuclei. The inferior olives of the medulla may also have neuronal loss. There is a loss of anterior horn neurons in the spinal cord and of dorsal root ganglion cells associated with posterior column spinal cord demyelination. A poorly developed or absent thymus gland is the most consistent defect of the lymphoid system.

GENETIC CONSIDERATIONS The gene for AT (the *ATM* gene) encodes a protein that is similar to several yeast and mammalian phosphatidylinositol-3'-kinases involved in mitogenic signal transduction, meiotic recombination, and cell cycle control. Defective DNA repair in AT fibroblasts exposed to ultraviolet light has been demonstrated. The discovery of *ATM* will make possible the identification of heterozygotes who are at risk for cancer (e.g., breast cancer) and permit early diagnosis.

Mitochondrial Ataxias Spinocerebellar syndromes have been identified with mutations in mitochondrial DNA (mtDNA). Thirty pathogenic mtDNA point mutations and 60 different types of mtDNA deletions are known, several of which cause or are associated with ataxia (Chap. 368).

℞ **TREATMENT**

The most important goal in management of patients with ataxia is to identify treatable disease entities. Mass lesions must be recognized promptly and treated appropriately. Paraneoplastic disorders can often be identified by the clinical patterns of disease that they produce, measurement of specific autoantibodies, and uncovering the primary cancer; these disorders are often refractory to therapy, but some patients improve following removal of the tumor or immunotherapy (Chap. 87). Ataxia with anti-gliadin antibodies and gluten-sensitive enteropathy may improve with a gluten-free diet. Malabsorption syndromes leading to vitamin E deficiency may lead to ataxia. The vitamin E deficiency form of Friedreich's ataxia must be considered, and serum vitamin E levels measured. Vitamin E therapy is indicated for these rare patients. Vitamin B_1 and B_{12} levels in serum should be measured, and the vitamins administered to patients having deficient levels. Hypothyroidism is easily treated. The cerebrospinal fluid should be tested for a syphilitic infection in patients with progressive ataxia and other features of tabes dorsalis. Similarly, antibody titers for Lyme disease and *Legionella* should be measured, and appropriate antibiotic therapy should be instituted in antibody-positive patients. Aminoacidopathies, leukodystrophies, urea-cycle abnormalities, and mitochondrial encephalomyopathies may produce ataxia, and some dietary or metabolic therapies are available for these disorders. The deleterious effects of diphenylhydantoin and alcohol on the cerebellum are well known and these exposures should be avoided in patients with ataxia of any cause.

There is no proven therapy for any of the autosomal dominant ataxias (SCA1 to 22). There is preliminary evidence that idebenone, a free-radical scavenger, can improve myocardial hypertrophy in pa-

tients with classic Friedreich ataxia; there is no current evidence, however, that it improves neurologic function. Iron chelators and antioxidant drugs are potentially harmful in Friedreich's patients as they may increase heart muscle injury. Acetazolamide can reduce the duration of symptoms of episodic ataxia. At present, identification of an at-risk person's genotype, together with appropriate family and genetic counseling, can reduce the incidence of these cerebellar syndromes in future generations (Chap. 58).

FURTHER READING

HADJIVASSILIOU M et al: Gluten ataxia in perspective: Epidemiology, genetic susceptibility and clinical characteristics. Brain 136:685, 2003

LYNCH DR et al: Friedrich ataxia: Effects of genetic understanding on clinical evaluation and therapy. Arch Neurol 59:743, 2002

ROSENBERG RN, PAULSON HL: The inherited ataxias, in *The Molecular and Genetic Basis of Neurologic and Psychiatric Disease*, 3rd ed, RN Rosenberg et al (eds). Philadelphia, Elsevier Science, and Boston, Butterworth-Heinemann, 2003

---

353 AMYOTROPHIC LATERAL SCLEROSIS AND OTHER MOTOR NEURON DISEASES
Robert H. Brown, Jr.

AMYOTROPHIC LATERAL SCLEROSIS   Amyotrophic lateral sclerosis (ALS) is the most common form of progressive motor neuron disease. It is a prime example of a neurodegenerative disease and is arguably the most devastating of the neurodegenerative disorders.

Pathology   The pathologic hallmark of motor neuron degenerative disorders is death of lower motor neurons (consisting of anterior horn cells in the spinal cord and their brainstem homologues innervating bulbar muscles) and upper, or corticospinal, motor neurons (originating in layer five of the motor cortex and descending via the pyramidal tract to synapse with lower motor neurons, either directly or indirectly via interneurons) (Chap. 21). Although at its onset ALS may involve selective loss of function of only upper or lower motor neurons, it ultimately causes progressive loss of both categories of motor neurons. Indeed, in the absence of clear involvement of both motor neuron types, the diagnosis of ALS is questionable.

Other motor neuron diseases involve only particular subsets of motor neurons (Tables 353-1 and 353-2). Thus, in bulbar palsy and spinal muscular atrophy (SMA; also called progressive muscular atrophy), the lower motor neurons of brainstem and spinal cord, respectively, are most severely involved. By contrast, pseudobulbar palsy, primary lateral sclerosis (PLS), and familial spastic paraplegia (FSP) affect only upper motor neurons innervating the brainstem and spinal cord.

In each of these diseases, the affected motor neurons undergo shrinkage, often with accumulation of the pigmented lipid (lipofuscin) that normally develops in these cells with advancing age. In ALS, the motor neuron cytoskeleton is typically affected early in the illness. Focal enlargements are frequent in proximal motor axons; ultrastructurally, these "spheroids" are composed of accumulations of neurofilaments. Also seen is proliferation of astroglia and microglia, the inevitable accompaniment of all degenerative processes in the central nervous system (CNS).

The death of the peripheral motor neurons in the brainstem and spinal cord leads to denervation and consequent atrophy of the corresponding muscle fibers. Histochemical and electrophysiologic evidence indicates that in the early phases of the illness denervated muscle can be reinnervated by sprouting of nearby distal motor nerve terminals, although reinnervation in this disease is considerably less extensive than in most other disorders affecting motor neurons (e.g., poliomyelitis, peripheral neuropathy). As denervation progresses, muscle atrophy is readily recognized in muscle biopsies and on clinical examination. This is the basis for the term *amyotrophy*. The loss of cortical motor neurons results in thinning of the corticospinal tracts that travel via the internal capsule (Fig. 353-1) and brainstem to the lateral and anterior white matter columns of the spinal cord. The loss of fibers in the lateral columns and resulting fibrillary gliosis impart a particular firmness (*lateral sclerosis*). A remarkable feature of the disease is the selectivity of neuronal cell death. By light microscopy, the entire sensory apparatus, the regulatory mechanisms for the control and coordination of movement, and the components of the brain that are needed for cognitive processes, remain intact. However, immunostaining indicates that neurons bearing ubiquitin, a marker for degeneration, are also detected in nonmotor systems. Moreover, studies of glucose metabolism in the illness also indicate that there is neuronal dysfunction outside of the motor system. Within the motor system, there is some selectivity of involvement. Thus, motor neurons required for ocular motility remain unaffected, as do the parasympathetic neurons in the sacral spinal cord (the nucleus of Onufrowicz, or Onuf) that innervate the sphincters of the bowel and bladder.

Clinical Manifestations   The manifestations of ALS are somewhat variable depending on whether corticospinal neurons or lower motor neurons in the brainstem and spinal cord are more prominently involved. With lower motor neuron dysfunction and early denervation, typically the first evidence of the disease is insidiously developing asymmetric weakness, usually first evident distally in one of the limbs. A detailed history often discloses recent development of cramping with volitional movements, typically in the early hours of the morning (e.g., while stretching in bed). Weakness caused by denervation is associated with progressive wasting and atrophy of muscles and, particularly early in the illness, spontaneous twitching of motor units, or fasciculations. In the hands, a preponderance of extensor over flexor weakness is common. When the initial denervation involves bulbar rather than limb muscles, the problem at onset is difficulty with chewing, swallowing, and movements of the face and tongue. Early involvement of the muscles of respiration may lead to death before the disease is far advanced elsewhere. With prominent corticospinal involvement, there is hyperactivity of the muscle-stretch reflexes (tendon jerks) and, often, spastic resistance to passive movements of the affected limbs. Patients with significant reflex hyperactivity complain of muscle stiffness often out of proportion to weakness. Degeneration of the corticobulbar projections innervating the brainstem results in dysarthria and exaggeration of the motor expressions of emotion. The latter leads to involuntary excess in weeping or laughing (so-called pseudobulbar affect).

Virtually any muscle group may be the first to show signs of disease, but, as time passes, more and more muscles become involved until ultimately the disorder takes on a symmetric distribution in all regions. It is characteristic of ALS that, regardless of whether the initial disease involves upper or lower motor neurons, both will eventually be implicated. Even in the late stages of the illness, sensory, bowel

TABLE 353-1 *Etiology and Investigation of Motor Neuron Disorders*

Diagnostic Category	Investigations
Structural lesions	MRI scan of head (including
Parasagittal or foramen magnum tumors	foramen magnum), cervical spine[a]
Cervical spondylosis	
Chiari malformation or syrinx	
Spinal cord arteriovenous malformation	
Infections	CSF exam, culture[a]
Bacterial—tetanus, Lyme	Lyme antibody titer[a]
Viral—poliomyelitis, herpes zoster	Antiviral antibody titers
Retroviral myelopathy	HTLV-1 titers
Intoxications, physical agents	
Toxins—lead, aluminum, others	24-h urine for heavy metals[a]
Drugs—strychnine, phenytoin	Serum for lead level[a]
Electric shock, x-irradiation	
Immunologic mechanisms	Complete blood count[a]
Plasma cell dyscrasias	Sedimentation rate[a]
Autoimmune polyradiculoneu-ropathy	Protein immunoelectrophoresis[a]
Motor neuropathy with conduction block	Anti-GM1 antibodies[a]
Paraneoplastic	Anti-Hu antibody
Paracarcinomatous/lymphoma	MRI scan, bone marrow biopsy
Metabolic	
Hypoglycemia	Fasting blood sugar (FBS), routine chemistries including calcium[a]
Hyperparathyroidism	PTH, calcium, phosphate
Hyperthyroidism	Thyroid function[a]
Deficiency of folate, vitamin B_{12}, vitamin E	Vitamin B_{12}, vitamin E, folate levels[a]
Malabsorption	24-h stool fat, carotene, prothrombin time
Mitochondrial dysfunction	Fasting lactate, pyruvate, ammonia Consider mtDNA analysis
Hereditary biochemical disorders	
Superoxide dismutase 1 gene mutation	White blood cell DNA analysis
Androgen receptor defect (Kennedy's disease)	Abnormal CAG insert in androgen receptor gene
Hexosaminidase deficiency	Lysosomal enzyme screen
Infantile (α-glucosidase deficiency/Pompe's disease)	
Hyperlipidemia	Lipid electrophoresis
Hyperglycinuria	Urine and serum amino acids
Methylcrotonylglycinuria	CSF amino acids

[a] Denotes studies that should be obtained in all cases.
Note: CSF, cerebrospinal fluid; HTLV, human T cell lymphotropic virus; MRI, magnetic resonance imaging.

TABLE 353-2 *Sporadic Motor Neuron Diseases*

CHRONIC

  Upper and lower motor neurons
    Amyotrophic lateral sclerosis
  Predominantly upper motor neurons
    Primary lateral sclerosis
  Predominantly lower motor neurons
    Multifocal motor neuropathy with conduction block
    Motor neuropathy with paraproteinemia or cancer
    Motor-predominant peripheral neuropathies
  Other
    Associated with other degenerative disorders
    Secondary motor neuron disorders (see Table 353-1)

ACUTE

  Poliomyelitis
  Herpes zoster
  Coxsackie virus

prevalence of 3 to 5 per 100,000. Several endemic foci of higher prevalence exist in the western Pacific (e.g., in specific regions of Guam or Papua New Guinea). In the United States and Europe, males are somewhat more frequently affected than females. While ALS is overwhelmingly a sporadic disorder, some 5 to 10% of cases are inherited as an autosomal dominant trait.

Familial ALS Several forms of selective motor neuron disease are inheritable (Table 353-3). Two involve both corticospinal and lower motor neurons. The most common is familial ALS (FALS). Apart from its inheritance as an autosomal dominant trait, it is clinically indistinguishable from sporadic ALS. Genetic studies have identified mutations in the gene encoding the cytosolic, copper- and zinc-binding enzyme SOD1 as the cause of one form of FALS. However, this accounts for only 20% of inherited cases of ALS. Rare mutations in other genes are also clearly implicated in ALS-like diseases. Thus, a familial, predominantly lower motor neuron disease with bulbar predominance has been ascribed to mutations in the gene encoding the cellular motor protein dynactin. Another familial, adult-onset disorder that may mimic aspects of ALS is Kennedy's syndrome; as described below, this arises from distinctive mutations in the androgen receptor. Genetic

FIGURE 353-1 Amyotrophic lateral sclerosis. Axial T2-weighted MRI scan through the lateral ventricles of the brain reveals abnormal high signal intensity within the corticospinal tracts (*arrows*). This MRI feature represents an increase in water content in myelin tracts undergoing Wallerian degeneration secondary to cortical motor neuronal loss. This finding is commonly present in ALS, but can also be seen in AIDS-related encephalopathy, infarction, or other disease processes that produce corticospinal neuronal loss in a symmetric fashion.

and bladder, and cognitive functions are preserved. Even when there is severe brainstem disease, ocular motility is spared until the very late stages of the illness. Dementia is not a component of sporadic ALS. In some families, ALS is co-inherited with frontotemporal dementia, characterized by early behavioral abnormalities with prominent behavioral features indicative of frontal lobe dysfunction.

A committee of the World Federation of Neurology has established diagnostic guidelines for ALS. Essential for the diagnosis is simultaneous upper and lower motor neuron involvement with progressive weakness, and the exclusion of all alternative diagnoses. The disorder is ranked as "definite" ALS when three or four of the following are involved: bulbar, cervical, thoracic, and lumbosacral motor neurons. When two sites are involved, the diagnosis is "probable," and when only one site is implicated, the diagnosis is "possible." An exception is made for those who have progressive upper and lower motor neuron signs at only one site and a mutation in the gene encoding superoxide dismutase (SOD1; below).

Epidemiology The illness is relentlessly progressive, leading to death from respiratory paralysis; the median survival is from 3 to 5 years. There are very rare reports of stabilization or even regression of ALS. In most societies there is an incidence of 1 to 3 per 100,000 and a

TABLE 353-3　*Genetic Motor Neuron Diseases*

Disease	Locus	Gene
I. Upper and lower motor neurons (familial ALS)		
A. Autosomal dominant	2p	Dynactin
	21q	Superoxide dismutase
	22q	Neurofilament heavy subunit
	9q	Unknown
	16q	Unknown
	20p	Unknown
	X_{cent}	Unknown
B. Autosomal recessive (juvenile)	2q	Alsin
	15q	Unknown
C. Mitochondrial	mtDNA	Cytochrome c oxidase
II. Lower motor neurons		
A. Spinal muscular atrophies	5q	Survival motor neuron protein
B. X-linked spinobulbar muscular atrophy	Xq	Androgen receptor
C. G_{M2} gangliosidosis		
1. Adult Tay-Sach's disease	15q	Hexosaminidase A
2. Sandhoff disease	5q	Hexosaminidase B
3. AB variant	5q	G_{M2} activator protein
III. Upper motor neurons/selected FSPs		
A. Autosomal dominant	2p	Spastin
	2q	Mitochondrial heat shock protein
	12q	Kinesin heavy chain KIF5A
	14q	Unknown
B. Autosomal recessive	16q	Paraplegin
C. X-linked	Xq21	Proteolipid protein
	Xq28	L1 CAM
D. Adrenomyeloneuropathy	Xq21	Adrenoleukodystrophy protein
IV. ALS-plus syndromes		
A. ALS with frontotemporal dementia	9q	Unknown
B. Amyotrophy with behavioral disorder and parkinsonian features	17q	Tau protein

Note: ALS, amyotrophic lateral sclerosis; FSP, familial spastic paraplegia.

analyses are also beginning to illuminate the pathogenesis of some childhood-onset motor neuron diseases. For example, a slowly disabling degenerative, predominantly upper motor neuron disease that starts in the first decade is caused by mutations in a gene that expresses a novel signaling molecule with properties of a guanine-exchange factor, termed *alsin*. In other instances, chromosomal locations for motor neuron diseases, but not the causative genes themselves, have been identified. Typical FALS has been genetically mapped to chromosomes 16 and 20 in several families, and a juvenile-onset, dominantly inherited form of ALS has been mapped to the long-arm of chromosome 9.

Differential Diagnosis　Because ALS is currently untreatable, it is imperative that potentially remediable causes of motor neuron dysfunction be excluded (Table 353-1). This is particularly true in cases that are atypical by virtue of (1) restriction to either upper or lower motor neurons, (2) involvement of neurons other than motor neurons, and (3) evidence of motor neuronal conduction block on electrophysiologic testing. Compression of the cervical spinal cord or cervicomedullary junction from tumors in the cervical regions or at the foramen magnum or from cervical spondylosis with osteophytes projecting into the vertebral canal can produce weakness, wasting, and fasciculations in the upper limbs and spasticity in the legs, closely resembling ALS. The ᵃʳᵉⁿce of cranial nerve involvement may be helpful in differentiation,

although some foramen magnum lesions may compress the twelfth cranial (hypoglossal) nerve, with resulting paralysis of the tongue. Absence of pain or of sensory changes, normal bowel and bladder function, normal roentgenographic studies of the spine, and normal cerebrospinal fluid (CSF) all favor ALS. Where doubt exists, magnetic resonance imaging (MRI) scans and contrast myelography should be performed to visualize the cervical spinal cord.

Another important entity in the differential diagnosis of ALS is *multifocal motor neuropathy with conduction block* (MMCB), discussed below. A diffuse, lower motor axonal neuropathy mimicking ALS sometimes evolves in association with hematopoietic disorders such as lymphoma. In this clinical setting, the presence of an M-component in serum should prompt consideration of a bone marrow biopsy. Lyme disease (Chap. 157) may also cause an axonal, lower motor neuropathy.

Other treatable disorders that occasionally mimic ALS are chronic lead poisoning and thyrotoxicosis. These disorders may be suggested by the patient's social or occupational history or by unusual clinical features. When the family history is positive, disorders involving the genes encoding cytosolic SOD1, hexosaminidase A, or α-glucosidase deficiency must be excluded (Chap. 340). These are readily identified by appropriate laboratory tests. Benign fasciculations are occasionally a source of concern because on inspection they resemble the fascicular twitchings that accompany motor neuron degeneration. The absence of weakness, atrophy, or denervation phenomena on electrophysiologic examination usually excludes ALS or other serious neurologic disease. Patients who have recovered from poliomyelitis may experience a delayed deterioration of motor neurons that presents clinically with progressive weakness, atrophy, and fasciculations. Its cause is unknown, but it is thought to reflect sublethal prior injury to motor neurons by poliovirus (Chap. 175).

Rarely, ALS develops concurrently with features indicative of more widespread neurodegeneration. Thus, one infrequently encounters otherwise typical ALS patients with a parkinsonian movement disorder or dementia. It remains unclear whether this reflects the unlikely simultaneous occurrence of two disorders or a primary defect triggering two forms of neurodegeneration. The latter is suggested by the observation that multisystem neurodegenerative diseases may be inherited. For example, prominent amyotrophy has been described as a dominantly inherited disorder in individuals with bizarre behavior and a movement disorder suggestive of parkinsonism; many such cases have now been ascribed to mutations that alter the expression of tau protein in brain (Chap. 350). In other cases, ALS develops simultaneously with a striking frontotemporal dementia. These disorders may be dominantly co-inherited; in some families, this trait is linked to a locus on chromosome 9q, although the underlying genetic defect is not established.

Pathogenesis　The cause of sporadic ALS is not well defined. Several mechanisms that impair motor neuron viability have been elucidated in mice and rats induced to develop motor neuron disease by SOD1 transgenes with ALS-associated mutations. It is evident that excitotoxic neurotransmitters such as glutamate participate in the death of motor neurons in ALS. This may be a consequence of diminished uptake of synaptic glutamate by an astroglial glutamate transporter, EAAT2. It is striking that one cellular defense against such excitotoxicity is the enzyme SOD1, which detoxifies the free radical superoxide anion (Chap. 345). Because SOD1 is mutated in some familial cases of ALS, it may be that glutamate excitotoxicity and ALS result from free radical accumulations in motor neurons. Precisely why the SOD1 mutations are toxic to motor nerves is not established, although it is clear the effect is not simply loss of normal scavenging of the superoxide anion. The mutant protein is conformationally unstable and prone to aberrant catalytic reactions. In turn, these features lead to aggregation of SOD1 protein, impairment of axonal transport, reduced production of ATP and other perturbations of mitochondrial function, activation of cyclo-oxygenase within the ALS spinal cord, and ultimately induction of cell death via pathways that are at least partially dependent on caspases. Recent studies have raised the hypothesis that genetic variants in the vascular endothelial growth factor gene (VEGF) that reduce VEGF expression increase the risk of ALS; whether this is a consequence of spinal cord hypoxia or diminished neurotrophic influence of VEGF remains to be established.

℞ TREATMENT

No treatment arrests the underlying pathologic process in ALS. The drug riluzole (100 mg/d) was approved for ALS because it produces a modest lengthening of survival. In one trial, the survival rate at 18 months with riluzole was similar to placebo at 15 months. The mechanism of this effect is not known with certainty; riluzole may reduce excitotoxicity by diminishing glutamate release. Riluzole is generally well tolerated; nausea, dizziness, weight loss, and elevated liver enzymes occur occasionally. Several agents have failed in clinical trials in human ALS including brain-derived neurotrophic factor, glial-derived neurotrophic factor, the anti-glutamate compound topiramate, and creatine. The latter was somewhat surprising as creatine was proven to be beneficial in transgenic ALS mice, perhaps by augmenting intracellular ATP stores. Insulin-like growth factor 1 (IGF-1) produced inconsistent results in ALS patients and is undergoing further clinical trials. The finding that cyclo-oxygenase activity is enhanced in the spinal cords of ALS mice led to a preclinical study of the COX-2 inhibitor, celecoxib, which significantly increased life span in that model. As a consequence, celecoxib is currently being tested in human ALS. Analogously, because minocycline produced a modest benefit in ALS mice, presumably by inhibiting late stages of the apoptotic cascade, it is now being tested in a multicenter ALS trial.

In the absence of a primary therapy for ALS, a variety of rehabilitative aids may substantially assist ALS patients. Foot-drop splints facilitate ambulation by obviating the need for excessive hip flexion and by preventing tripping on a floppy foot. Finger extension splints can potentiate grip. Respiratory support may be life-sustaining. For patients electing against long-term ventilation by tracheostomy, positive-pressure ventilation by mouth or nose provides transient (several weeks) relief from hypercarbia and hypoxia. Also extremely beneficial for some patients is a respiratory device (In-exsufflator or Cough Assist Device) that produces an artificial cough. This is highly effective in clearing airways and preventing aspiration pneumonia. When bulbar disease prevents normal chewing and swallowing, gastrostomy is uniformly helpful, restoring normal nutrition and hydration. Fortunately, an increasing variety of speech synthesizers are now available to augment speech when there is advanced bulbar palsy. These facilitate oral communication and may be effective for telephone use.

In contrast to ALS, several of the disorders (Tables 353-1 and 353-3) that bear some clinical resemblance to ALS are treatable. For this reason, a careful search for causes of secondary motor neuron disease is warranted.

SELECTED LOWER MOTOR NEURON DISORDERS In these motor neuron diseases, the peripheral motor neurons are affected without evidence of involvement of the corticospinal motor system (Tables 353-1 to 353-3).

X-Linked Spinobulbar Muscular Atrophy (Kennedy's Disease) This is an X-linked lower motor neuron disorder in which progressive weakness and wasting of limb and bulbar muscles begins in males in mid-adult life and is conjoined with androgen insensitivity manifested by gynecomastia and reduced fertility (Chap. 325). In addition to gynecomastia, which may be subtle, two findings distinguishing this disorder from ALS are the absence of signs of pyramidal tract disease (spasticity) and the presence of a subtle sensory neuropathy in some patients. The underlying molecular defect is an expanded trinucleotide repeat (-CAG-) in the first exon of the androgen receptor gene on the X chromosome. DNA testing is available. An inverse correlation appears to exist between the number of -CAG- repeats and the age of onset of the disease.

Adult Tay-Sach's Disease Several reports have described adult-onset, predominantly lower motor neuropathies arising from deficiency of the enzyme β-hexosaminidase (hex A). These tend to be distinguishable from ALS because they are very slowly progressive; dysarthria and radiographically evident cerebellar atrophy may be prominent. In rare cases, spasticity may also be present, although it is generally absent (Chap. 340).

Spinal Muscular Atrophy The SMAs are a family of selective lower motor neuron diseases of early onset. Despite some phenotypic variability (largely in age of onset), the defect in the majority of families with SMA maps to a locus on chromosome 5 encoding a putative motor neuron survival protein (SMN, for survival motor neuron) that is important in the formation and trafficking of RNA complexes across the nuclear membrane. Neuropathologically these disorders are characterized by extensive loss of large motor neurons; muscle biopsy reveals evidence of denervation atrophy. Several clinical forms exist.

Infantile SMA (SMA I, Werdnig-Hoffmann Disease) has the earliest onset and most rapidly fatal course. In some instances it is apparent even before birth, as indicated by decreased fetal movements late in the third trimester. Though alert, afflicted infants are weak and floppy (hypotonic) and lack muscle stretch reflexes. Death generally ensues within the first year of life. *Chronic childhood SMA* (SMA II) begins later in childhood and evolves with a more slowly progressive course. *Juvenile SMA* (SMA III, Kugelberg-Welander disease) manifests during late childhood and runs a slow, indolent course. Unlike most denervating diseases, in this chronic disorder weakness is greatest in the proximal muscles; indeed, the pattern of clinical weakness can suggest a primary myopathy such as limb-girdle dystrophy. Electrophysiologic and muscle biopsy evidence of denervation distinguish SMA III from the myopathic syndromes.

Multifocal Motor Neuropathy with Conduction Block In this disorder lower motor neuron function is regionally and chronically disrupted by remarkably focal blocks in conduction. Many cases have elevated serum titers of mono- and polyclonal antibodies to ganglioside GM1; it is hypothesized that the antibodies produce selective, focal, paranodal demyelination of motor neurons. MMCB is not typically associated with corticospinal signs. In contrast with ALS, MMCB may respond dramatically to therapy such as intravenous immunoglobulin or chemotherapy; it is thus imperative that MMCB be excluded when considering a diagnosis of ALS.

Other Forms of Lower Motor Neuron Disease In individual families, other syndromes characterized by selective lower motor neuron dysfunction in an SMA-like pattern have been described. There are rare X-linked and autosomal dominant forms of apparent SMA. There is an ALS variant of juvenile onset, the Fazio-Londe syndrome, that involves mainly the musculature innervated by the brainstem. A component of lower motor neuron dysfunction is also found in degenerative disorders such as Machado-Joseph disease and the related olivopontocerebellar degenerations (Chap. 352).

SELECTED DISORDERS OF THE UPPER MOTOR NEURON ■ **Primary Lateral Sclerosis** This exceedingly rare disorder arises sporadically in adults in mid- to late life. Clinically PLS is characterized by progressive spastic weakness of the limbs, preceded or followed by spastic dysarthria and dysphagia, indicating combined involvement of the corticospinal and corticobulbar tracts. Fasciculations, amyotrophy, and sensory changes are absent; neither electromyography nor muscle biopsy shows denervation. On neuropathologic examination there is selective loss of the large pyramidal cells in the precentral gyrus and degeneration of the corticospinal and corticobulbar projections. The peripheral motor neurons and other neuronal systems are spared. The course of PLS is variable; while long-term survival is documented, the course may be as aggressive as in ALS, with ~3-year survival from onset to death. Early in its course, PLS raises the question of multiple sclerosis or other demyelinating diseases such as adrenoleukodystrophy as diagnostic considerations (Chap. 359). A myelopathy suggestive of PLS is infrequently seen with infection with the retrovirus human T cell lymphotropic virus (HTLV-I) (Chap. 356). The clinical course and laboratory testing will distinguish these possibilities.

Familial Spastic Paraplegia   In its pure form, FSP is usually transmitted as an autosomal trait; most adult-onset cases are dominantly inherited. It arises in the third or fourth decade and is characterized by progressive spastic weakness beginning in the distal lower extremities. FSP typically has a long survival, presumably because respiratory function is spared. Late in the illness there may be urinary urgency and incontinence and sometimes fecal incontinence; sexual function tends to be preserved. In pure forms of FSP, ataxia, posterior column sensory loss, and amyotrophy are absent or minimal; however, in some patients, minor sensory changes (impaired vibration and position sense) may be observed in late stages. Some family members may have spasticity without clinical symptoms. Neuropathologically, in FSP there is degeneration of the corticospinal tracts, which appear nearly normal in the brainstem but show increasing atrophy at more caudal levels in the spinal cord. It is now apparent that defects at numerous loci underlie both dominantly and recessively inherited forms of FSP (Table 353-3). An infantile-onset form of X-linked, recessive FSP arises from mutations in the gene for myelin proteolipid protein (Chap. 345). This is an example of rather striking allelic variation, as most other mutations in the same gene cause not FSP but Pelizaeus-Merzbacher disease, a widespread disorder of CNS myelin. Defects in genes encoding the proteins spastin and paraplegin have been associated respectively with dominantly and recessively inherited FSP. The latter gene is of particular interest as it has homology to metalloproteases that are important in mitochondrial function in yeast. Defects in the gene *spartin*, a protein with homology to spastin, are associated with recessively inherited spasticity and distal weakness of early childhood onset. A kinesin heavy chain protein implicated in microtubule motor function was found to be defective in a family with dominantly inherited FSP of variable onset age.

Rarely, FSP may arise concomitantly with significant involvement of other regions of the nervous system. Thus, it has been described concurrently with amyotrophy, mental retardation, mental retardation with skin thickening, optic atrophy, and sensory neuropathy. In some cases there is loss of fibers in the ascending posterior columns and the spinocerebellar tracts, features reminiscent of Friedreich's ataxia (Chap. 352). These complicated forms of FSP emphasize the challenge inherent in classifying the neurodegenerative disorders; there may be considerable overlap of the clinical phenotypes in diseases otherwise classified as distinct. Fortunately, it is likely that increasingly available genetic testing will clarify these nosologic difficulties.

WEB SITES   Several web sites provide valuable information on ALS including those offered by the Muscular Dystrophy Association (www.mdausa.org), the Amyotrophic Lateral Sclerosis Association (www.alsa.org), and the World Federation of Neurology and the Neuromuscular Unit At Washington University in St. Louis (www.neuro.wustl.edu/neuromuscular).

FURTHER READING

CLEVELAND DW, ROTHSTEIN JD: From Charcot to Lou Gehrig: Deciphering selective motor neuron death in ALS. Nat Rev Neurosci 2:806, 2001

HADANO S et al: A gene encoding a putative GTPase regulator is mutated in familial amyotrophic lateral sclerosis. Nat Genet 29:166, 2001

LAMBRECHTS D et al: VEGF is a modifier of amyotrophic lateral sclerosis in mice and humans and protects motoneurons against ischemic death. Nat Genet 34(4):384, 2003

PULS I et al: Mutant dynactin in motor neuron disease. Nat Genet 33:455, 2003

YANG Y et al: The gene encoding alsin, a protein with three guanine-nucleotide exchange factor domains, is mutated in a form of recessive amyotrophic lateral sclerosis. Nat Genet 29:160, 2001

354   DISORDERS OF THE AUTONOMIC NERVOUS SYSTEM
Phillip A. Low, John W. Engstrom

The autonomic nervous system (ANS) innervates the entire neuraxis and permeates all organ systems. It regulates blood pressure (BP), heart rate, sleep, and bladder and bowel function. It operates in the background, so that its full importance becomes recognized only when ANS function is compromised, resulting in dysautonomia. →*Hypothalamic disorders that cause disturbances in homeostasis are discussed in Chaps. 16 and 318.*

ANATOMIC ORGANIZATION   The activity of the autonomic nervous system is regulated by central neurons responsive to diverse afferent inputs. After central integration of afferent information, autonomic outflow is adjusted to permit the functioning of the major organ systems in accordance with the needs of the organism as a whole. Connections between the cerebral cortex and the autonomic centers in the brainstem coordinate autonomic outflow with higher mental functions.

The preganglionic neurons of the parasympathetic nervous system leave the central nervous system (CNS) in the third, seventh, ninth, and tenth cranial nerves as well as the second and third sacral nerves, while the preganglionic neurons of the sympathetic nervous system exit the spinal cord between the first thoracic and the second lumbar segments (Fig. 354-1). The postganglionic neurons, located in ganglia outside the CNS, give rise to the postganglionic autonomic nerves that innervate organs and tissues throughout the body. Responses to sympathetic and parasympathetic stimulation are frequently antagonistic (Table 354-1), reflecting highly coordinated interactions within the CNS; the resultant changes in parasympathetic and sympathetic activity provide more precise control of autonomic responses than could be achieved by the modulation of a single system.

Acetylcholine (ACh) is the preganglionic neurotransmitter for both divisions of the ANS as well as the postganglionic neurotransmitter of the parasympathetic neurons. Norepinephrine (NE) is the neurotransmitter of the postganglionic sympathetic neurons, except for cholinergic neurons innervating the eccrine sweat glands and perhaps some blood vessels supplying skeletal muscle.

CLINICAL EVALUATION ■ **Classification**   Disorders of the ANS may result from pathology of either the CNS or the peripheral nervous system (PNS) (Table 354-2). Signs and symptoms may result from interruption of the afferent limb, CNS processing centers, or efferent limb of reflex arcs controlling autonomic responses. For example, a lesion of the medulla produced by a posterior fossa tumor can impair BP responses to postural changes and result in orthostatic hypotension (OH). OH can also be caused by lesions of the spinal cord or peripheral vasomotor nerve fibers (e.g., diabetic autonomic neuropathy). The site of reflex interruption is usually established by the clinical context in which the dysautonomia arises, combined with judicious use of ANS testing and neuroimaging studies. Important elements of the clinical context include the presence or absence of CNS signs (pathophysiology and prognosis differ), association with sensory or motor polyneuropathy, family history, and pathologic findings. Some syndromes do not fit easily into any classification scheme.

Symptoms of Autonomic Dysfunction   Clinical manifestations result from a loss of function (e.g., impaired baroreflexes leading to OH), overactivity (e.g., hyperhidrosis, hypertension, tachycardia), or loss of regulation (e.g., autonomic storms, autonomic dysreflexia) of autonomic circuits. The disorder may be widespread or regional in distribution.

PARASYMPATHETIC   SYMPATHETIC

Parasympathetic system
from cranial nerves III, VII, IX, X
and from sacral nerves 2 and 3

Sympathetic system
from T1-L2
Preganglionic fibers — — — —
Postganglionic fibers ————

A	Ciliary ganglion	H	Superior cervical ganglion
B	Sphenopalatine (pterygopalatine) ganglion	J	Middle cervical ganglion and inferior cervical (stellate) ganglion including T1 ganglion
C	Submandibular ganglion		
D	Otic ganglion		
E	Vagal ganglion cells in heart wall	K	Coeliac and other abdominal ganglia
F	Vagal ganglion cells in bowel wall	L	Lower abdominal sympathetic ganglia
G	Pelvic ganglia		

FIGURE 354-1 Schematic representation of the autonomic nervous system. (*From M Moskowitz: Clin Endocrinol Metab 6:77, 1977.*)

An autonomic history focuses on systemic functions (BP, heart rate, sleep, thermoregulation) and individual organ systems (pupils, bowel, bladder, sexual function). More formal assessment is possible using a standardized instrument such as the autonomic symptom profile. It is also important to recognize the modulating effects of age and gender. For instance, OH commonly results in lightheadedness in the young, whereas cognitive slowing is much more important in the elderly. Specific symptoms of orthostatic intolerance are quite diverse (Table 354-3). Autonomic symptoms may vary dramatically, reflecting the dynamic nature of autonomic control over homeostatic function. For example, OH might be manifest only in the early morning, following a

TABLE 354-1 *Functional Consequences of Normal ANS Activation*

	Sympathetic	Parasympathetic
Heart rate	Increased	Decreased
Blood pressure	Increased	Mildly decreased
Bladder	Increased sphincter tone	Voiding (decreased tone)
Bowel motility	Decreased motility	Increased
Lung	Bronchodilation	Bronchoconstriction
Sweat glands	Sweating	—
Pupils	Dilation	Constriction
Adrenal glands	Catecholamine release	—
Sexual function	Ejaculation, orgasm	Erection
Lacrimal glands	—	Tearing
Parotid glands	—	Salivation

TABLE 354-2 *Classification of Clinical Autonomic Disorders*

I. Autonomic disorders with brain involvement
  A. Associated with multisystem degeneration
    1. Multisystem degeneration: autonomic failure clinically prominent
      a. Multiple system atrophy (MSA)
      b. Parkinson's disease with autonomic failure
      c. Diffuse Lewy body disease (some cases)
    2. Multisystem degeneration: autonomic failure clinically not usually prominent
      a. Parkinson's disease
      b. Other extrapyramidal disorders (inherited spinocerebellar atrophies, progressive supranuclear palsy, corticobasal degeneration, Machado-Joseph disease)
  B. Unassociated with multisystem degeneration
    1. Disorders mainly due to cerebral cortex involvement
      a. Frontal cortex lesions causing urinary/bowel incontinence
      b. Partial complex seizures
    2. Disorders of the limbic and paralimbic circuits
      a. Shapiro's syndrome (agenesis of corpus callosum, hyperhidrosis, hypothermia)
      b. Autonomic seizures
    3. Disorders of the hypothalamus
      a. Wernicke-Korsakoff syndrome
      b. Diencephalic syndrome
      c. Neuroleptic malignant syndrome
      d. Serotonin syndrome
      e. Fatal familial insomnia
      f. Antidiuretic hormone (ADH) syndromes (diabetes insipidus, inappropriate ADH)
      g. Disturbances of temperature regulation (hyperthermia, hypothermia)
      h. Disturbances of sexual function
      i. Disturbances of appetite
      j. Disturbances of BP/HR and gastric function
      k. Horner's syndrome
    4. Disorders of the brainstem and cerebellum
      a. Posterior fossa tumors
      b. Syringobulbia and Arnold-Chiari malformation
      c. Disorders of BP control (hypertension, hypotension)
      d. Cardiac arrhythmias
      e. Central sleep apnea
      f. Baroreflex failure
      g. Horner's syndrome
II. Autonomic disorders with spinal cord involvement
  A. Traumatic tetraplegia
  B. Syringomyelia
  C. Subacute combined degeneration
  D. Multiple sclerosis
  E. Amyotrophic lateral sclerosis
  F. Tetanus
  G. Stiff-man syndrome
  H. Spinal cord tumors
III. Autonomic neuropathies
  A. Acute/subacute autonomic neuropathies
    1. Subacute autoimmune autonomic neuropathy (panautonomic neuropathy, pandysautonomia)
      a. Subacute paraneoplastic autonomic neuropathy
      b. Guillain-Barré syndrome
      c. Botulism
      d. Porphyria
      e. Drug induced autonomic neuropathies
      f. Toxic autonomic neuropathies
  B. Chronic peripheral autonomic neuropathies
    1. Distal small fiber neuropathy
    2. Combined sympathetic and parasympathetic failure
      a. Amyloid
      b. Diabetic autonomic neuropathy
      c. Autoimmune autonomic neuropathy (paraneoplastic and idiopathic)
      d. Sensory neuronopathy with autonomic failure
      e. Familial dysautonomia (Riley-Day syndrome)

Note: BP, blood pressure; HR, heart rate.

TABLE 354-3 *Symptoms of Orthostatic Intolerance*

Lightheadedness (dizziness)	88%
Weakness or tiredness	72%
Cognitive difficulty (thinking/concentrating)	47%
Blurred vision	47%
Tremulousness	38%
Vertigo	37%
Pallor	31%
Anxiety	29%
Palpitations	26%
Clammy feeling	19%
Nausea	18%

Source: From Low et al.

meal, or with exercise, depending upon the regional vascular bed affected by dysautonomia.

Early symptoms may be overlooked. Impotence, although not specific for autonomic failure, often heralds autonomic failure in men and may precede other symptoms by years (Chap. 43). A decrease in the frequency of spontaneous early morning erections may occur months before loss of nocturnal penile tumescence and development of total impotence. Bladder dysfunction may appear early in men and women, particularly in those with CNS involvement. Brain and spinal cord disease above the level of the lumbar spine results first in urinary frequency and small bladder volumes, and eventually in incontinence (upper motor neuron or spastic bladder). Disease of PNS autonomic nerve fibers to and from the bladder results in large bladder volumes, urinary frequency, and overflow incontinence (lower motor neuron bladder or flaccid bladder). Measurement of bladder volume (postvoid residual) is a useful bedside test for distinguishing between upper and lower motor neuron bladder dysfunction in the early stages of dysautonomia. Gastrointestinal autonomic dysfunction typically presents as severe constipation. Diarrhea occurs occasionally (as in diabetes mellitus) due to rapid transit of contents or uncoordinated small-bowel motor activity, or on an osmotic basis from bacterial overgrowth associated with small-bowel stasis. Impaired glandular secretory function may cause difficulty with food intake due to decreased salivation or with eye irritation due to decreased lacrimation. Occasionally, temperature elevation and vasodilation can result from anhidrosis because sweating is normally important for heat dissipation (Chap. 16).

OH (also called "postural hypotension") is perhaps the most disabling feature of autonomic dysfunction. The prevalence of OH is relatively high, especially when OH associated with aging is included (Table 354-4). OH can cause a variety of symptoms including dimming or loss of vision, lightheadedness, diaphoresis, diminished hearing, pallor, and weakness. Syncope results when the drop in BP impairs cerebral perfusion. Other manifestations of impaired baroreflexes are supine hypertension, a heart rate that is fixed regardless of posture, postprandial hypotension, and an excessively high nocturnal BP. Many patients with OH have a preceding diagnosis of hypertension, reflecting the great importance of baroreflexes in maintaining postural and supine normotension. The most common causes of OH are not neurologic in origin; these must be distinguished from the neurogenic causes. →*Neurocardiogenic and cardiac syncope are considered in Chap. 20.*

APPROACH TO THE PATIENT

The first step in the evaluation of symptomatic OH is the exclusion of treatable causes. The history should include a review of medications that may cause OH (e.g., diuretics, antihypertensives, antidepressants, phenothiazines, ethanol, narcotics, insulin, barbiturates, and calcium channel blocking agents). However, the precipitation of OH by medications may also be the first sign of an underlying autonomic disorder. The history may reveal an underlying cause for symptoms (e.g., diabetes, Parkinson's disease) or specific underlying mechanisms (e.g., cardiac pump failure, re-

TABLE 354-4 *Prevalence of Orthostatic Hypotension in Different Disorders*

Disorder	Prevalence
Aging	14–20%
Diabetic neuropathy	10%
Other autonomic neuropathies	10–50 per 100,000
Multiple system atrophy	5–15 per 100,000
Pure autonomic failure	10–30 per 100,000

duced intravascular volume). The relationship of symptoms to meals (splanchnic pooling), standing on awakening in the morning (intravascular volume depletion), ambient warming (vasodilatation), or exercise (muscle arteriolar vasodilatation) should be sought.

Physical examination includes measurement of supine and standing pulse and BP. OH is defined as a sustained drop in systolic (≥20 mmHg) or diastolic (≥10 mmHg) BP within 3 min of standing up. In nonneurogenic causes of OH (such as hypovolemia), the BP drop is accompanied by a compensatory increase in heart rate of >15 beats/min. An important clinical clue that the patient has neurogenic OH is the aggravation or precipitation of OH by autonomic stressors (such as a meal, hot tub/hot bath, and exercise). Neurologic evaluation should include a mental status examination (to exclude neurodegenerative disorders), cranial nerve examination (impaired downgaze is found with progressive supranuclear palsy), abnormal pupils (Horner's or Adie's pupils), motor examination (Parkinson's disease and parkinsonian syndromes), and sensory examination (polyneuropathies). In patients without a clear initial diagnosis, follow-up neurologic examinations and repeat laboratory evaluations over 1 to 2 years may reveal an evolution of findings that enables a specific diagnosis to be made.

Disorders of autonomic function should be considered in patients with symptoms of altered sweating (hyperhidrosis or hypohidrosis), gastroparesis (bloating, nausea, vomiting of old food), constipation, impotence, or bladder dysfunction (urinary frequency, hesitancy, or incontinence).

Autonomic Testing Autonomic function tests (Table 354-5) are helpful when the history and physical examination findings are inconclusive, when detection of subclinical involvement is important to evaluate the extent and severity of abnormalities, or to follow the course of an autonomic disorder or its response to therapy.

HEART RATE VARIATION WITH DEEP BREATHING This is a test of parasympathetic influence on cardiovascular function. Results are influenced by the subject's posture, rate and depth of respiration [6 breaths per minute and a forced vital capacity (FVC) >1.5 L are optimal], age, medications, and hypocapnea. Interpretation of results requires comparison of test data with results from normal individuals collected under the same test conditions. For example, the lower limit of normal heart rate variation with deep breathing

TABLE 354-5 *Neural Pathways Underlying Some Standardized Autonomic Tests*

Test Evaluated	Procedure	Autonomic Function
HRDB	6 deep breaths/min	Cardiovagal function
Valsalva ratio	Expiratory pressure, 40 mmHg for 10–15 s	Cardiovagal function
QSART	Axon-reflex test 4 limb sites	Postganglionic sudomotor function
BP$_{BB}$ to VM	BP$_{BB}$ response to VM	Adrenergic function: baroreflex adrenergic control of vagal and vasomotor function
HUT	BP$_{BB}$ and heart rate response to HUT	Adrenergic and cardiovagal responses to HUT

Note: HRDB, heart rate response to deep breathing; BP$_{BB}$, beat-to-beat blood pressure; QSART, quantitative sudomotor axon reflex test; VM, Valsalva maneuver; HUT, head-up tilt.

in persons <20 years is >15 to 20 beats/min, but for persons over age 60 it is 5 to 8 beats/min. Heart rate variation with deep breathing (respiratory sinus arrhythmia) is abolished by the administration of atropine.

VALSALVA RESPONSE This response (Table 354-5) assesses integrity of the baroreflex control of heart rate (parasympathetic) and BP (adrenergic). The response is obtained with the subject supine. A constant expiratory pressure of 40 mmHg is maintained for 15 s while measuring changes in heart rate and beat-to-beat BP. There are four phases of BP and heart rate response to the Valsalva maneuver. Phases I and III are mechanical and related to changes in intrathoracic and intraabdominal pressure. In early phase II, reduced venous return results in a fall in stroke volume and BP, counteracted by a combination of reflex tachycardia and increased total peripheral resistance. Increased total peripheral resistance arrests the BP drop ~5 to 8 s after the onset of the maneuver. Late phase II begins with a progressive rise in BP to or above baseline. Venous return and cardiac output return to normal in phase IV. Persistent peripheral arteriolar vasoconstriction and increased cardiac adrenergic tone results in a temporary BP overshoot and phase IV bradycardia (mediated by the baroreceptor reflex).

Autonomic function during the Valsalva maneuver can be measured using beat-to-beat blood pressure or heart rate changes. The Valsalva ratio is defined as the maximum phase II tachycardia divided by the minimum phase IV bradycardia. The ratio reflects cardiovagal function.

SUDOMOTOR FUNCTION Sweating is induced by release of ACh from sympathetic postganglionic fibers. The quantitative sudomotor axon reflex test (QSART) is a measure of regional autonomic function mediated by ACh-induced sweating. A reduced or absent response indicates a lesion of the postganglionic sudomotor axon. For example, sweating may be reduced in the legs as a result of peripheral neuropathy (e.g., in diabetes) before other signs of autonomic dysfunction emerge. The thermoregulatory sweat test (TST) is a qualitative measure of regional sweat production in response to an elevation of body temperature. An indicator powder placed on the anterior body surface changes color with sweat production during temperature elevation. The pattern of color changes is a measure of regional sweat secretion. Combining TST and QSART results will determine the site of the lesion. A postganglionic lesion is present if both QSART and TST show absent sweating. In a preganglionic lesion, QSART is intact but TST shows anhidrosis. Measurement of galvanic skin responses in the limbs after an induced electrical potential is another qualitative test for detecting the presence or absence of sweating.

ORTHOSTATIC BP RECORDINGS Beat-to-beat BP measurements determined in supine, 70° tilt, and tilt-back positions are useful to quantitate orthostatic failure of BP control. It is important to allow a 20-min period of supine rest before assessing changes in BP during tilting. The BP change combined with heart rate monitoring can be useful for the evaluation of patients with suspected OH or unexplained syncope or to detect vagally mediated syncope.

PHARMACOLOGIC TESTS Pharmacologic assessments can help localize an autonomic defect to the CNS or the PNS. A useful method to evaluate the systemic adrenergic response is the measurement of plasma NE, first with the patient supine and then after standing for at least 5 min. Supine values are reduced in postganglionic disorders (such as autonomic neuropathy or pure autonomic failure) and may fail to increase in preganglionic or postganglionic disorders (e.g., multiple system atrophy).

Administration of tyramine (releases NE from postganglionic terminals) and phenylephrine (denervation supersensitivity—directly acting α_1-agonist) is often used to evaluate postganglionic adrenergic function. In a postganglionic lesion, the response to tyramine is reduced and there is an excessive response to subthreshold doses of phenylephrine. Other strategies include ganglionic blockade with trimethaphan (greater fall in resulting BP with a preganglionic lesion) or administration of arginine vasopressin (to evaluate afferent central pathways).

SPECIFIC SYNDROMES OF ANS DYSFUNCTION ■ Multiple System Atrophy

Multiple system atrophy (MSA) is an uncommon entity that comprises autonomic failure (OH and/or a neurogenic bladder are required for diagnosis) combined with either striatonigral degeneration (Shy-Drager syndrome) or sporadic olivopontocerebellar atrophy (Chap. 351). The parkinsonism is usually unassociated with rest tremor and is not responsive to levodopa. Levodopa-induced dyskinesia is also uncommon. Autonomic function tests can usually differentiate MSA from Parkinson's disease in that the severity and distribution of autonomic failure is more severe and generalized in MSA. Cardiac postganglionic adrenergic innervation, measured as labeled metaiodobenzylguanidine (MIBG) uptake on single photon emission computed tomography or fluorodopamine on positron emission tomography (PET), is markedly impaired in the dysautonomia of Parkinson's disease but is normal in MSA.

MSA generally progresses relentlessly to death 7 to 10 years after onset. Neuropathologic changes include primary neuronal degeneration with loss of neurons and gliosis in many CNS regions, including the brainstem, the cerebellum, the striatum, and the intermediolateral cell column of the thoracolumbar spinal cord.

Spinal Cord Spinal cord lesions from any cause may result in focal autonomic deficits or autonomic hyperreflexia. Spinal cord transection or hemisection may be attended by autonomic hyperreflexia affecting bowel, bladder, sexual, temperature-regulation, or cardiovascular functions. Dangerous increases or decreases in body temperature may result from inability to experience the sensory accompaniments of heat or cold exposure below the level of the injury. Quadriparetic patients exhibit both supine hypertension and OH after upward tilting. Markedly increased autonomic discharge can be elicited by bladder pressure or stimulation of the skin or muscles; suprapubic palpation of the bladder, a distended bladder, catheter insertion, catheter obstruction, or urinary infection are common and correctable precipitants. This phenomenon, termed *autonomic dysreflexia*, affects 85% of patients with a traumatic spinal cord lesion above the C6 level. In patients with supine hypertension, BP can be lowered by tilting the head upward. Vasodilator drugs may be used to treat acute elevations in BP. Clonidine is used prophylactically to reduce the hypertension resulting from bladder stimulation. Sudden, dramatic increases in BP can lead to intracranial hemorrhage and death.

Peripheral Nerve and Neuromuscular Junction Disorders Peripheral neuropathies (Chap. 363) are the most common cause of chronic autonomic insufficiency. Neuropathies that affect small myelinated and unmyelinated fibers of the sympathetic and parasympathetic nerves occur in diabetes mellitus, amyloidosis, chronic alcoholism, porphyria, and Guillain-Barré syndrome. Neuromuscular junction disorders include botulism and Lambert-Eaton syndrome.

DIABETES MELLITUS Autonomic neuropathy typically begins ~10 years after the onset of diabetes (Chap. 323) and slowly progresses. The earliest autonomic abnormalities, typically asymptomatic, consist of vagal disturbances, which can be detected as reduced heart rate variation with deep breathing, and loss of distal sudomotor function, detected by QSART. Loss of small myelinated and unmyelinated nerve fibers in the splanchnic distribution, carotid sinus, and vagus nerves is characteristic. In advanced disease, widespread enteric neuropathy can cause profound disturbances in gut motility (*gastroparesis*), nausea and vomiting, malnutrition, achlorhydria, and bowel incontinence. Other symptoms can include impotence, urinary incontinence, pupillary abnormalities, and OH. Typical symptoms and signs of hypoglycemia may fail to appear because damage to the sympathetic innervation of the adrenal gland can result in a lack of epinephrine release. Insulin increases flow through arteriovenous shunts and may also aggravate OH. Autonomic dysfunction may lengthen the QT interval, increasing the risk of sudden death due to cardiac arrhythmia. There is postganglionic cardiac denervation with some proximal segments showing increased uptake of labeled hydroxyephedrine, indicative of hyperadrenergic innervation, on PET scanning. This finding is of interest in that these areas could be potentially arrhythmogenic. Hyperglycemia appears to be a direct risk factor for autonomic involvement in diabetes. Biochemical and pharmacologic studies in diabetic neuropathy are compatible with autonomic failure localized to the PNS. Supine plasma NE levels can be reduced, and a minority of patients experience a phase of hyperadrenegic autonomic function characterized by exaggerated orthostatic pressor responsiveness.

AMYLOIDOSIS   Autonomic neuropathy occurs in both sporadic and familial forms of amyloidosis (Chap. 310). The AL (immunoglobulin light chain) type is associated with primary amyloidosis or amyloidosis secondary to multiple myeloma. The ATTR type, with transthyretin as the primary protein component, is responsible for the most common form of inherited amyloidosis. Although patients usually present with a distal painful neuropathy accompanied by sensory loss, autonomic insufficiency can precede the development of the polyneuropathy or occur in isolation. Death is usually due to cardiac or renal impairment. Postmortem studies reveal amyloid deposition in many organs, including two sites that contribute to autonomic failure: intraneural blood vessels and autonomic ganglia. Pathologic examination reveals a loss of unmyelinated and myelinated nerve fibers.

ALCOHOLIC NEUROPATHY   Abnormalities in parasympathetic vagal and efferent sympathetic function are usually mild in individuals with alcoholic neuropathy. Pathologic changes can be demonstrated in the parasympathetic (vagus) and sympathetic fibers and in ganglia. OH is usually due to brainstem involvement. Impotence is a major problem, but concurrent gonadal hormone abnormalities may obscure the parasympathetic component. Clinical symptoms of autonomic failure generally appear when the polyneuropathy is severe and there is usually coexisting Wernicke's encephalopathy (Chap. 258). Autonomic involvement may contribute to the high mortality rates associated with alcoholism (Chap. 372).

PORPHYRIA   Although each of the porphyrias can cause autonomic dysfunction, the condition is most extensively documented in the acute intermittent type (Chap. 337). Autonomic symptoms include tachycardia, sweating, urinary retention, and hypertension, or, less commonly, hypotension. Other prominent symptoms include anxiety, abdominal pain, nausea, and vomiting. Abnormal autonomic function can occur both during acute attacks and during remissions. Elevated catecholamine levels during acute attacks correlate with the degree of tachycardia and hypertension that are present.

GUILLAIN-BARRÉ SYNDROME   BP fluctuations and arrhythmias can be severe (Chap. 365). It is estimated that 2 to 10% of patients seriously ill with Guillain-Barré syndrome suffer fatal cardiovascular collapse. Gastrointestinal autonomic involvement is common. Abnormal sweating, sphincter disturbance, and pupillary dysfunction also occur. Demyelination has been described in the vagus and glossopharyngeal nerves, the sympathetic chain, and the white rami communicantes. The presence of autonomic involvement is not clearly related to the severity of motor or sensory involvement.

AUTOIMMUNE AUTONOMIC NEUROPATHY   The development of serologic testing for the ganglionic ACh receptor (A₃ AChR) autoantibody, which is a putative effector of autoimmune dysautonomia, now allows definition of the entity of autoimmune autonomic neuropathy (AAN). This disorder presents as the subacute development of autonomic failure with OH, enteric neuropathy (gastroparesis, ileus, constipation/diarrhea), and cholinergic failure; the latter consists of loss of sweating, sicca complex, and a tonic pupil. In general, the antibody titer correlates with the severity of autonomic failure. Symptoms of cholinergic failure

are also predictive of a high antibody titer. Onset of the neuropathy follows a viral infection in approximately half of cases. Some patients appear to respond to immunotherapy. The spectrum of AAN is broader than originally thought, and some antibody-positive cases have an insidious onset and slow progression with a pure autonomic failure (see below) phenotype. An experimental autonomic neuropathy has recently been produced by immunization of rabbits with this receptor.

AAN can have a paraneoplastic basis (Chap. 87). The clinical features of the autonomic neuropathy may be indistinguishable from the nonparaneoplastic form, or a coexisting paraneoplastic syndrome, such as cerebellar involvement or dementia, may be present (Tables 87-2 and 87-3). The neoplasm may be truly occult, possibly suppressed by the autoantibody.

BOTULISM   Botulinum toxin binds presynaptically to cholinergic nerve terminals and, after uptake into the cytosol, blocks ACh release. Manifestations consist of motor paralysis and autonomic disturbances that include blurred vision, dry mouth, nausea, unreactive or sluggishly reactive pupils, constipation, and urinary retention (Chap. 125).

Pure Autonomic Failure (PAF)   This sporadic syndrome consists of postural hypotension, impotence, bladder dysfunction, and defective sweating. The disorder begins in the middle decades and occurs in women more often than men. The symptoms can be disabling, but the disease does not shorten life span. The clinical and pharmacologic characteristics suggest primary involvement of postganglionic sympathetic neurons. There is a severe reduction in the density of neurons within sympathetic ganglia that results in low supine plasma NE levels and noradrenergic supersensitivity. Recent studies have questioned the specificity of PAF as a distinct clinical entity. Some cases are ganglionic antibody–positive and thus represent a type of AAN. Between 10 and 15% of cases evolve into MSA.

Postural Orthostatic Tachycardia Syndrome (POTS)   This syndrome is characterized by symptomatic orthostatic intolerance (not OH) and by either an increase in heart rate to >120 beats/min or an increase of 30 beats/min with standing that subsides on sitting or lying down. Women are affected approximately five times more often than men, and most develop the syndrome between the ages of 15 and 50 years. Approximately half of affected patients report an antecedent viral infection. Syncopal symptoms (lightheadedness, weakness, blurred vision) combined with those of autonomic overactivity (palpitations, tremulousness, nausea) are common. Recurrent unexplained episodes of dysautonomia and fatigue also occur. The pathogenesis is unclear in most cases; hypovolemia, venous pooling, impaired brainstem regulation, or β-receptor supersensitivity may play a role. In one affected individual, a mutation in the NE transporter, which resulted in impaired NE clearance from synapses, was responsible. Some cases are due to an underlying limited autonomic neuropathy. Although ~80% of patients improve, only one-quarter eventually resume their usual daily activities (including exercise and sports). Expansion of fluid volume and postural training (see "Treatment") are initial approaches to treatment. When these approaches are inadequate, midodrine, fludrocortisone, phenobarbital, beta blockers, and clonidine have been used with some success.

Inherited Disorders   There are five known hereditary sensory and autonomic neuropathies (HSAN I–V). The most important ones are HSAN I and HSAN III (Riley-Day syndrome; familial dysautonomia). HSAN I is dominantly inherited and often presents as a distal small-fiber neuropathy (burning feet syndrome). The responsible gene, on chromosome 9q, is designated *SPTLC1*. SPTLC is an important enzyme in the regulation of ceramide. Cells from HSAN I patients affected by mutation of *SPTLC1* produce higher-than-normal levels of glucosyl ceramide, perhaps triggering apoptosis.

HSAN III, an autosomal recessive disorder of infants and children that occurs among Ashkenazi Jews, is much less prevalent than HSAN I. Decreased tearing, hyperhidrosis, reduced sensitivity to pain, areflexia, absent fungiform papillae on the tongue, and labile BP may be present. Episodic abdominal crises and fever are common. Pathologic examination of nerves reveals a loss of small myelinated and unmyelinated nerve fibers. The defective gene, named *IKBKAP*, is also located on the long arm of chromosome 9. Pathogenic mutations may prevent normal transcription of important molecules in neural development.

Primary Hyperhidrosis   This syndrome presents with excess sweating of the palms of the hands and soles of the feet. The disorder affects 0.6 to 1.0% of the population; the etiology is unclear but there may be a genetic component. While not dangerous, the condition can be socially embarrassing (e.g., shaking hands) or disabling (e.g., inability to write without soiling the paper). Onset of symptoms is usually in adolescence; the condition tends to improve with age. Topical antiperspirants are occasionally helpful. More useful are potent anticholinergic drugs such as glycopyrrolate, 1 to 2 mg tid. T2 ganglionectomy or sympathectomy is successful in >90% of patients with palmar hyperhidrosis. The advent of endoscopic transaxillary T2 sympathectomy has lowered the complication rate of the procedure. The most common postoperative complication is compensatory hyperhidrosis, which improves spontaneously over months; other potential complications include recurrent hyperhidrosis (16%), Horner's syndrome (<2%), gustatory sweating, wound infection, hemothorax, and intercostal neuralgia. Local injection of botulinum toxin has also been used to block cholinergic, postganglionic sympathetic fibers to sweat glands in patients with palmar hyperhidrosis. This approach is limited by the need for repetitive injections (the effect usually lasts 4 months before waning), pain with injection, the high cost of botulinum toxin, and the possibility of temporary intrinsic hand muscle weakness. Tap water iontophoresis has been successful for some patients.

Miscellaneous   Other conditions associated with autonomic failure include infections, poisoning (organophosphates), malignancy, and aging. Disorders of the hypothalamus can affect autonomic function and produce abnormalities in temperature control, satiety, sexual function, and circadian rhythms (Chap. 318).

Reflex Sympathetic Dystrophy and Causalgia   The failure to identify a primary role of the ANS in the pathogenesis of these disorders has resulted in a change of nomenclature. Complex regional pain syndrome (CRPS) types I and II are now used in place of reflex sympathetic dystrophy (RSD) and causalgia, respectively.

CRPS type I is a regional pain syndrome that usually develops after tissue trauma. Examples of associated trauma include myocardial infarction, minor shoulder or limb injury, and stroke. *Allodynia* (the perception of a nonpainful stimulus as painful), *hyperpathia* (an exaggerated pain response to a painful stimulus), and spontaneous pain occur. The symptoms are unrelated to the severity of the initial trauma and are not confined to the distribution of a single peripheral nerve. CRPS type II is a regional pain syndrome that develops after injury to a peripheral nerve, usually a major nerve trunk. Spontaneous pain initially develops within the territory of the affected nerve but eventually may spread outside the nerve distribution.

Pain is the primary clinical feature of CRPS. Vasomotor dysfunction, sudomotor abnormalities, or focal edema may occur alone or in combination but must be present for diagnosis. Limb pain syndromes that do not meet these criteria are best classified as "limb pain—not otherwise specified." In CRPS, localized sweating (increased resting sweat output) and changes in blood flow may produce temperature differences between affected and unaffected limbs.

CRPS type I (RSD) has classically been divided into three clinical phases but is now considered to be more variable. Phase I consists of pain and swelling in the distal extremity occurring within weeks to 3 months after the precipitating event. The pain is diffuse, spontaneous, and either burning, throbbing, or aching in quality. The involved extremity is warm and edematous, and the joints are tender. Increased sweating and hair growth develop. In phase II (3 to 6 months after onset), thin, shiny, cool skin appears. After an additional 3 to 6 months (phase III), atrophy of the skin and subcutaneous tissue plus flexion contractures complete the clinical picture.

The natural history of typical CRPS may be more benign than reflected in the literature. A variety of surgical and medical treatments have been developed, with conflicting reports of efficacy. Clinical trials suggest that early mobilization with physical therapy or a brief course of glucocorticoids may be helpful for CRPS type I. Other medical treatments include the use of adrenergic blockers, nonsteroidal anti-inflammatory drugs (NSAIDs), calcium channel blockers, phenytoin, opioids, and calcitonin. Stellate ganglion blockade is a commonly used invasive therapeutic technique that often provides temporary pain relief, but the efficacy of repetitive blocks is uncertain.

Rx TREATMENT

Management of autonomic failure is aimed at specific treatment of the cause and alleviation of symptoms. Of particular importance is the removal of drugs or amelioration of underlying conditions that cause or aggravate the autonomic symptom. For instance, OH can be caused or aggravated by angiotensin-converting enzyme inhibitors, calcium channel blocking agents, tricyclic antidepressants, levodopa, alcohol, or insulin.

Patient Education   OH can be asymptomatic or symptomatic. Neurogenic OH requires treatment, but only a minority of patients require pharmacologic treatment. All patients should be taught the mechanisms of postural normotension (volume status, resistance and capacitance bed, autoregulation) and the nature of orthostatic stressors (time of day and the influence of meals, heat, standing, and exercise). Patients should learn to recognize orthostatic symptoms early in their evolution (especially subtle cognitive symptoms, weakness, and fatigue) and to modify activities that provoke episodes. Other helpful measures may include keeping a BP log, dietary education (salt/fluids), monitoring urine volume and sodium excretion, or recognizing medications and situations to avoid. Learning physical countermaneuvers that reduce standing OH, practicing postural and resistance training, and learning to manage worsening OH in specific situations and at specific times are helpful measures.

Symptomatic Treatment   Nonpharmacologic approaches are summarized in Table 354-6. Adequate intake of salt and fluids to produce a voiding volume between 1.5 to 2.5 L of urine (containing >170 meq of Na$^+$) each 24 h is essential. Sleeping with the head of the bed elevated will minimize the effects of supine nocturnal hypertension. Prolonged recumbency should be avoided when possible. Patients are advised to sit with legs dangling over the edge of the bed for several minutes before attempting to stand in the morning; other postural stresses should be similarly approached in a gradual manner. Physical countermaneuvers that can reduce OH include leg-crossing, with maintained contraction of leg muscles for 30 s. Such maneuvers compress leg veins and increase systemic resistance. Compressive garments such as compression stockings and abdominal binders may be helpful; some patients find these uncomfortable. Anemia should be corrected, if necessary, with erythropoietin, administered subcutaneously at doses of 25 to 75 U/kg three times per week. The hematocrit increases after 2 to 6 weeks. A weekly maintenance dose is usually necessary. The increased intravascular volume that accompanies the rise in hematocrit can exacerbate supine hypertension.

If these measures are not sufficient, drug treatment might be nec-

TABLE 354-6   *Initial Treatment of Orthostatic Hypotension (OH)*

Patient education: mechanisms and stressors of OH
High-salt diet (10–20 g/d)
High-fluid intake (2 L/D)
Elevate head of bed 10 cm (4 in.)
Maintain postural stimuli
Learn physical countermaneuvers
Compression garments
Correct anemia

essary. Midodrine is effective but can aggravate supine hypertension at higher doses. The drug is a directly acting α_1-agonist that does not cross the blood-brain barrier. It has a duration of action of 2 to 4 h. The usual dose is 5 to 10 mg orally tid, but some patients respond best to a decremental dose (e.g., 15 mg on awakening, 10 mg at noon, and 5 mg in the afternoon). Midodrine should not be taken after 6 P.M. Side effects include pruritus, uncomfortable piloerection, and supine hypertension. Pyridostigmine appears to improve OH without aggravating supine hypertension by enhancing ganglionic transmission (maximal when orthostatic, minimal supine). Fludrocortisone will reduce OH, but it aggravates supine hypertension. At doses between 0.1 mg/d and 0.3 mg bid orally, it enhances renal sodium conservation and increases the sensitivity of arterioles to NE. Susceptible patients may develop fluid overload, congestive heart failure, supine hypertension, or hypokalemia. Potassium supplements are often necessary with chronic administration of fludrocortisone. Sustained elevations of supine BP >180/110 mmHg should be avoided.

Postprandial OH may respond to several measures. Frequent, small, low-carbohydrate meals may diminish splanchnic shunting of blood after meals and reduce postprandial OH. Prostaglandin inhibitors (ibuprofen or indomethacin) taken with meals or midodrine (10 mg with the meal) can be helpful. The somatostatin analogue octreotide can be useful in the treatment of postprandial syncope by inhibiting the release of gastrointestinal peptides that have vasodilator and hypotensive

effects. The subcutaneous dose ranges from 25 μg bid to 100 to 200 μg tid.

The patient should be taught to self-treat transient worsening of OH. Drinking two 250-mL (8-oz) glasses of water can raise standing BP 20 to 30 mmHg for about 2 h, beginning ~20 min after the fluid load. The patient can increase intake of salt and fluids (bouillon treatment), increase use of physical countermaneuvers, temporarily resort to a full-body stocking (compression pressure 30 to 40 mmHg), or increase the dose of midodrine. Supine hypertension (>180/110 mmHg) can be self-treated by avoiding the supine position and reducing fludrocortisone. A daily glass of wine, if requested by the patient, can be taken shortly before bedtime. If these simple measures are not adequate, drugs to be considered include oral hydralazine (25 mg qhs), oral procardia (10 mg qhs), or a nitroglycerin patch.

ACKNOWLEDGMENT

In the previous edition, Lewis Landsberg and James B. Young contributed the section on the anatomic organization of the autonomic nervous system.

FURTHER READING

KLEIN CM et al: The spectrum of autoimmune autonomic neuropathies. Ann Neurol 53:752, 2003

LOW PA et al: Prospective evaluation of clinical characteristics of orthostatic hypotension. Mayo Clin Proc 70:617, 1995

SINGER W et al: Acetylcholinesterase inhibition—a novel approach in the treatment of neurogenic orthostatic hypotension. J Neurol Neurosurg Psychiatry 74:1294, 2003

355   TRIGEMINAL NEURALGIA, BELL'S PALSY, AND OTHER CRANIAL NERVE DISORDERS
M. Flint Beal, Stephen L. Hauser

Symptoms and signs of cranial nerve pathology are common in internal medicine. They often develop in the context of a widespread neurologic disturbance, and in such situations cranial nerve involvement may represent the initial manifestation of the illness. In other disorders, involvement is largely restricted to one or several cranial nerves; these distinctive disorders are reviewed in this chapter. Disorders of ocular movement are discussed in Chap. 25; disorders of smell, taste, and hearing in Chap. 26; and vertigo and disorders of vestibular function in Chap. 20.

FACIAL PAIN OR NUMBNESS

ANATOMIC CONSIDERATIONS   The trigeminal (fifth cranial) nerve supplies sensation to the skin of the face and anterior half of the head (Fig.

355-1). Its motor part innervates the masseter and pterygoid masticatory muscles.

TRIGEMINAL NEURALGIA (TIC DOULOUREUX) ■ **Clinical Manifestations**   Trigeminal neuralgia is characterized by excruciating paroxysms of pain in the lips, gums, cheek, or chin and, very rarely, in the distribution of the ophthalmic division of the fifth nerve. The pain seldom lasts more than a few seconds or a minute or two but may be so intense that the patient winces, hence the term *tic*. The paroxysms, experienced as single jabs or clusters, tend to recur frequently, both day and night, for several weeks at a time. They may occur spontaneously or with movements of affected areas evoked by speaking, chewing, or smiling. Another characteristic feature is the presence of trigger zones, typically on the face, lips, or tongue, that provoke attacks; patients may report that tactile stimuli—e.g. washing the face, brushing the teeth, or exposure to a draft of air—generate excruciating pain. *An essential feature of trigeminal neuralgia is that objective signs of sensory loss cannot be demonstrated on examination.*

Trigeminal neuralgia is relatively common, with an estimated annual incidence of 4.5 per 100,000 individuals. Middle-aged and elderly persons are affected primarily, and ~60% of cases occur in women. Onset is typically sudden, and bouts tend to persist for weeks or months before remitting spontaneously. Remissions may be longlasting, but in most patients the disorder ultimately recurs.

Pathophysiology   Symptoms result from ectopic generation of action potentials in pain-sensitive afferent fibers of the fifth cranial nerve root just before it enters the lateral surface of the pons. Compression or other pathology in the nerve leads to demyelination of large myelinated fibers that do not themselves carry pain sensation but become hyperexcitable and electrically coupled with smaller unmyelinated or poorly myelinated pain fibers in close proximity; this may explain why tactile stimuli, conveyed via the large myelinated fibers, can stimulate paroxysms of pain. Compression of the trigeminal nerve root by a blood vessel, most often the superior cerebellar artery or on occasion a tortuous vein, is the source of trigeminal neuralgia in a substantial

FIGURE 355-1   The three major sensory divisions of the trigeminal nerve consist of the ophthalmic, maxillary, and mandibular nerves.

proportion of patients. In cases of vascular compression, age-related brain sagging and increased vascular thickness and tortuosity may explain the prevalence of trigeminal neuralgia in later life.

Differential Diagnosis   Trigeminal neuralgia must be distinguished from other causes of face and head pain (Chap. 14) and from pain arising from diseases of the jaw, teeth, or sinuses. Pain from migraine or cluster headache tends to be deep seated and steady, unlike the superficial stabbing quality of trigeminal neuralgia; rarely, cluster headache is associated with trigeminal neuralgia, a syndrome known as *cluster-tic*. In temporal arteritis, superficial facial pain is present but is not typically shock-like, the patient frequently complains of myalgias and other systemic symptoms and an elevated erythrocyte sedimentation rate (ESR) is usually present (Chap. 306). When trigeminal neuralgia develops in a young adult or is bilateral, multiple sclerosis is a key consideration, and in such cases the cause is a demyelinating plaque at the root entry zone of the fifth nerve in the pons; often, evidence of facial sensory loss can be found on careful examination. Cases that are secondary to mass lesions—such as aneurysms, neurofibromas, or meningiomas—also usually produce objective signs of sensory loss in the trigeminal nerve distribution (trigeminal neuropathy, see below).

Laboratory Evaluation   An ESR is indicated if temporal arteritis is suspected. In typical cases of trigeminal neuralgia, neuroimaging studies are not necessary.

℞ TREATMENT

Drug therapy with carbamazepine is effective in ~50 to 75% of patients. Carbamazepine should be started as a single daily dose of 100 mg taken with food, and increased gradually (by 100 mg daily every 1 to 2 days) until substantial (>50%) pain relief is achieved. Most patients require a maintenance dose of 200 mg qid. Doses >1200 mg daily provide no additional benefit. Dizziness, imbalance, sedation, and rare cases of agranulocytosis are the most important side effects of carbamazepine. If treatment is effective, it is usually continued for approximately 1 month and then tapered as tolerated. If carbamazepine is not well tolerated or is ineffective, phenytoin, 300 to 400 mg daily, can be tried. Baclofen may also be administered, either alone or in combination with carbamazepine or phenytoin. The initial dose is 5 to 10 mg tid, gradually increasing as needed to 20 mg qid.

If drug treatment fails, surgical therapy should be offered. The most widely applied procedure creates a heat lesion of the trigeminal (gasserian) ganglion or nerve, a method termed *radiofrequency thermal rhizotomy*. Injection of glycerol in Meckel's cave is a method preferred by some surgeons. Either procedure produces short-term relief in >95% of patients; however, long-term studies indicate that pain recurs in a substantial percentage of treated patients. Complications are infrequent in experienced hands. These procedures result in partial numbness of the face and carry a risk of corneal denervation with secondary keratitis when used for first-division trigeminal neuralgia.

A third treatment, microvascular decompression, requires a suboccipital craniotomy. This procedure has a >70% efficacy rate and a low rate of pain recurrence in responders; in a small number of cases, there is perioperative damage to the eighth or seventh nerve. High-resolution magnetic resonance angiography may be useful preoperatively to visualize the relationships between the fifth cranial nerve root and nearby blood vessels.

TRIGEMINAL NEUROPATHY   A variety of diseases may affect the trigeminal nerve (Table 355-1). Most present with sensory loss on the face or with weakness of the jaw muscles. Deviation of the jaw on opening indicates weakness of the pterygoids on the side to which the jaw deviates. Some cases are due to Sjögren's syndrome or a collagen-vascular disease such as systemic lupus erythematosus, scleroderma, or mixed connective tissue disease. Among infectious causes, herpes zoster and leprosy should be considered. Tumors of the middle cranial fossa (meningiomas), of the trigeminal nerve (schwannomas), or of the base of the skull (metastatic tumors) may cause a combination of motor and sensory signs. Lesions in the cavernous sinus can affect the

TABLE 355-1   *Trigeminal Nerve Disorders*

Nuclear (brainstem) lesions	**Peripheral nerve lesions**
Multiple sclerosis	Nasopharyngeal carcinoma
Stroke	Trauma
Syringobulbia	Guillain-Barré syndrome
Glioma	Sjögren's syndrome
Lymphoma	Collagen-vascular diseases
Preganglionic lesions	Sarcoidosis
Acoustic neuroma	Leprosy
Meningioma	Drugs (stilbamidine, trichloroethylene)
Metastasis	Idiopathic trigeminal neuropathy
Chronic meningitis	
Cavernous carotid aneurysm	
Gasserian ganglion lesions	
Trigeminal neuroma	
Herpes zoster	
Infection (spread from otitis media or mastoiditis)	

first and second divisions of the trigeminal nerve, and lesions of the superior orbital fissure can affect the first (ophthalmic) division; the accompanying corneal anesthesia increases the risk of ulceration (neurokeratitis).

Loss of sensation over the chin (mental neuropathy) can be the only manifestation of systemic malignancy. Rarely, an idiopathic form of trigeminal neuropathy is observed. It is characterized by numbness and paresthesia, sometimes bilaterally, with loss of sensation in the territory of the trigeminal nerve but without weakness of the jaw. Gradual recovery is the rule. Tonic spasm of the masticatory muscles, known as *trismus*, is symptomatic of tetanus (Chap. 124) or may occur in patients treated with phenothiazine drugs.

FACIAL WEAKNESS

ANATOMIC CONSIDERATIONS (Fig. 355-2)   The seventh cranial nerve supplies all the muscles concerned with facial expression. The sensory component is small (the nervus intermedius); it conveys taste sensation from the anterior two-thirds of the tongue and probably cutaneous impulses from the anterior wall of the external auditory canal. The motor nucleus of the seventh nerve lies anterior and lateral to the abducens nucleus. After leaving the pons, the seventh nerve enters the internal auditory meatus with the acoustic nerve. The nerve continues its course in its own bony channel, the facial canal, and exits from the

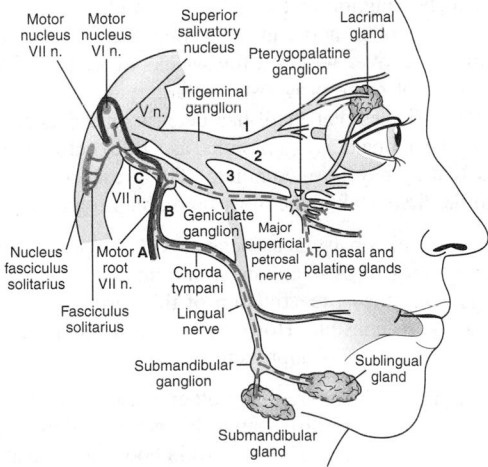

FIGURE 355-2   The facial nerve. A, B, and C denote lesions of the facial nerve at the stylomastoid foramen, distal and proximal to the geniculate ganglion, respectively. Green lines indicate the parasympathetic fibers, red line indicates motor fibers, and purple lines indicate visceral afferent fibers (taste). (*Adapted from Carpenter, 1978.*)

skull via the stylomastoid foramen. It then passes through the parotid gland and subdivides to supply the facial muscles.

A complete interruption of the facial nerve at the stylomastoid foramen paralyzes all muscles of facial expression. The corner of the mouth droops, the creases and skin folds are effaced, the forehead is unfurrowed, and the eyelids will not close. Upon attempted closure of the lids, the eye on the paralyzed side rolls upward (*Bell's phenomenon*). The lower lid sags and falls away from the conjunctiva, permitting tears to spill over the cheek. Food collects between the teeth and lips, and saliva may dribble from the corner of the mouth. The patient complains of a heaviness or numbness in the face, but sensory loss is rarely demonstrable and taste is intact.

If the lesion is in the middle ear portion, taste is lost over the anterior two-thirds of the tongue on the same side. If the nerve to the stapedius is interrupted, there is hyperacusis (sensitivity to loud sounds). Lesions in the internal auditory meatus may affect the adjacent auditory and vestibular nerves, causing deafness, tinnitus, or dizziness. Intrapontine lesions that paralyze the face usually affect the abducens nucleus as well, and often the corticospinal and sensory tracts.

If the peripheral facial paralysis has existed for some time and recovery of motor function is incomplete, a continuous diffuse contraction of facial muscles may appear. The palpebral fissure becomes narrowed, and the nasolabial fold deepens. Attempts to move one group of facial muscles may result in contraction of all (associated movements, or *synkinesis*). Facial spasms, initiated by movements of the face, may develop (*hemifacial spasm*). Anomalous regeneration of seventh nerve fibers may result in other troublesome phenomena. If fibers originally connected with the orbicularis oculi come to innervate the orbicularis oris, closure of the lids may cause a retraction of the mouth, or if fibers originally connected with muscles of the face later innervate the lacrimal gland, anomalous tearing ("crocodile tears") may occur with any activity of the facial muscles, such as eating. Another facial synkinesia is triggered by jaw opening, causing closure of the eyelids on the side of the facial palsy (jaw-winking).

BELL'S PALSY   The most common form of facial paralysis is *Bell's palsy*. The annual incidence of this idiopathic disorder is between 11 and 40 per 100,000 annually, or about 1 in 60 persons in a lifetime.

Clinical Manifestations   The onset of Bell's palsy is fairly abrupt, maximal weakness being attained by 48 h as a general rule. Pain behind the ear may precede the paralysis for a day or two. Taste sensation may be lost unilaterally, and hyperacusis may be present. In some cases there is mild cerebrospinal fluid lymphocytosis. Magnetic resonance imaging (MRI) may reveal swelling and uniform enhancement of the geniculate ganglion and facial nerve, and, in some cases, entrapment of the swollen nerve in the temporal bone. Approximately 80% of patients recover within a few weeks or months. Electromyography may be of some prognostic value; evidence of denervation after 10 days indicates that there has been axonal degeneration and that there will be a long delay (3 months, as a rule) before regeneration occurs and that it may be incomplete. The presence of incomplete paralysis in the first week is the most favorable prognostic sign.

Pathophysiology   Bell's palsy is associated with the presence of herpes simplex virus type 1 DNA in endoneurial fluid and posterior auricular muscle, suggesting that a reactivation of this virus in the geniculate ganglion may be responsible. However, a causal role for herpes simplex virus in Bell's palsy is unproven.

Differential Diagnosis   There are many other causes of facial palsy that must be considered in the differential diagnosis of Bell's palsy. Tumors that invade the temporal bone (carotid body, cholesteatoma, dermoid) may produce a facial palsy, but the onset is insidious and the course progressive. The *Ramsay Hunt syndrome*, presumably due to herpes zoster of the geniculate ganglion, consists of a severe facial palsy associated with a vesicular eruption in the pharynx, external auditory canal, and other parts of the cranial integument; often the eighth cranial nerve is affected as well. *Acoustic neuromas* frequently involve the facial nerve by local compression. Infarcts, demyelinating lesions of multiple sclerosis, and tumors are the common pontine lesions that interrupt the facial nerve fibers; other signs of brainstem involvement are usually present. Bilateral facial paralysis (facial diplegia) occurs in *Guillain-Barré syndrome* (Chap. 365) and also in a form of sarcoidosis known as *uveoparotid fever* (*Heerfordt syndrome*). Lyme disease is a frequent cause of facial palsies in endemic areas. The rare *Melkersson-Rosenthal syndrome* consists of a triad of recurrent facial paralysis, recurrent—and eventually permanent—facial (particularly labial) edema, and less constantly, plication of the tongue; its cause is unknown. Leprosy frequently involves the facial nerve, and facial neuropathy may also occur in diabetes mellitus.

All these forms of nuclear or peripheral facial palsy must be distinguished from the supranuclear type. In the latter, the frontalis and orbicularis oculi muscles are involved less than those of the lower part of the face, since the upper facial muscles are innervated by corticobulbar pathways from both motor cortices, whereas the lower facial muscles are innervated only by the opposite hemisphere. In supranuclear lesions there may be a dissociation of emotional and voluntary facial movements, and often some degree of paralysis of the arm and leg or an aphasia (in dominant hemisphere lesions) is conjoined.

Laboratory Evaluation   The diagnosis of Bell's palsy can usually be made clinically in patients with (1) a typical presentation, (2) no risk factors or preexisting symptoms for other causes of facial paralysis, (3) absence of cutaneous lesions of herpes zoster in the external ear canal, and (4) a normal neurologic examination with the exception of the facial nerve. Particular attention to the eighth cranial nerve, which courses near to the facial nerve in the pontomedullary junction and in the temporal bone, and to other cranial nerves is essential. In atypical or uncertain cases, an ESR, testing for diabetes mellitus, a Lyme titer, angiotensin-converting enzyme and chest x-ray for possible sarcoidosis, or MRI scanning may be indicated.

℞ TREATMENT

Symptomatic measures include (1) the use of paper tape to depress the upper eyelid during sleep and prevent corneal drying, and (2) massage of the weakened muscles. A course of glucocorticoids, given as prednisone 60 to 80 mg daily during the first 5 days and then tapered over the next 5 days, appears to shorten the recovery period and modestly improve the functional outcome. In one double-blind study, patients treated within 3 days of onset with both prednisone and acyclovir (400 mg five times daily for 10 days) had a better outcome than patients treated with prednisone alone.

OTHER MOTOR DISORDERS OF THE FACE   *Hemifacial spasm* consists of painless irregular involuntary contractions on one side of the face. Symptoms may develop as a sequela to Bell's palsy but may also be due to an irritative lesion of the facial nerve (e.g., an acoustic neuroma, an aberrant artery that compresses the nerve, or a basilar artery aneurysm). However, in the most common form of hemifacial spasm, the cause and pathology are unknown. Hemifacial spasm can be treated successfully with carbamazepine or, if this drug fails, with baclofen. Refractory cases due to vascular compression usually respond to surgical decompression of the facial nerve. *Blepharospasm* is an involuntary recurrent spasm of both eyelids that occurs in elderly persons as an isolated phenomenon or with varying degrees of spasm of other facial muscles. Severe, persistent cases of blepharospasm can be treated by local injection of botulinum toxin into the orbicularis oculi; the spasms are relieved for 3 to 4 months, and the injections can be repeated. *Facial myokymia* refers to a fine rippling activity of the facial muscles; it may be caused by multiple sclerosis or follow Guillain-Barré syndrome (Chap. 365).

Facial hemiatrophy occurs mainly in females and is characterized by a disappearance of fat in the dermal and subcutaneous tissues on one side of the face. It usually begins in adolescence or early adult years and is slowly progressive. In its advanced form, the affected side of the face is gaunt, and the skin is thin, wrinkled, and rather brown. The facial hair may turn white and fall out, and the sebaceous glands become atrophic. The muscles and bones are not involved as a rule. Sometimes the atrophy becomes bilateral. The condition is a form of lipodystrophy. Treatment is cosmetic, consisting of transplantation of skin and subcutaneous fat.

OTHER CRANIAL NERVE DISORDERS

GLOSSOPHARYNGEAL NEURALGIA This form of neuralgia involves the ninth (glossopharyngeal) and sometimes portions of the tenth (vagus) cranial nerves. It resembles trigeminal neuralgia in many respects but is much less common. The pain is intense and paroxysmal; it originates on one side of the throat, approximately in the tonsillar fossa. In some cases the pain is localized in the ear or may radiate from the throat to the ear because of involvement of the tympanic branch of the glossopharyngeal nerve. Spasms of pain may be initiated by swallowing or coughing. There is no demonstrable motor or sensory deficit; the glossopharyngeal nerve supplies taste sensation to the posterior third of the tongue and, together with the vagus nerve, sensation to the posterior pharynx. Cardiac symptoms—bradycardia, hypotension, and fainting—have been reported. Medical therapy is similar to that for trigeminal neuralgia, and carbamazepine is generally the first choice. If drug therapy is unsuccessful, surgical procedures, including microvascular decompression if vascular compression is evident, or rhizotomy of glossopharyngeal and vagal fibers in the jugular bulb is frequently successful.

Very rarely, herpes zoster involves the glossopharyngeal nerve. Glossopharyngeal neuropathy in conjunction with vagus and accessory nerve palsies may also occur with a tumor or aneurysm in the posterior fossa or in the jugular foramen. Hoarseness due to vocal cord paralysis, some difficulty in swallowing, deviation of the soft palate to the intact side, anesthesia of the posterior wall of the pharynx, and weakness of the upper part of the trapezius and sternocleidomastoid muscles make up the jugular foramen syndrome (Table 355-2).

DYSPHAGIA AND DYSPHONIA When the intracranial portion of one vagus (tenth cranial) nerve is interrupted, the soft palate droops ipsilaterally and does not rise in phonation. There is loss of the gag reflex on the affected side, as well as of the "curtain movement" of the lateral wall of the pharynx, whereby the faucial pillars move medially as the palate rises in saying "ah." The voice is hoarse and slightly nasal, and the vocal cord lies immobile midway between abduction and adduction. Loss of sensation at the external auditory meatus and the posterior pinna may also be present.

The pharyngeal branches of both vagal nerves may be affected in diphtheria; the voice has a nasal quality, and regurgitation of liquids through the nose occurs during the act of swallowing.

The vagus nerve may be involved at the meningeal level by neoplastic and infectious processes and within the medulla by tumors, vascular lesions (e.g., the lateral medullary syndrome), and motor neuron disease. This nerve may be involved by infection with herpes zoster virus. Polymyositis and dermatomyositis, which cause hoarseness and dysphagia by direct involvement of laryngeal and pharyngeal muscles, may be confused with diseases of the vagus nerves. Also, dysphagia is a symptom in some patients with myotonic dystrophy, →*See Chap. 33 for discussion of nonneurologic forms of dysphagia.*

The recurrent laryngeal nerves, especially the left, are most often damaged as a result of intrathoracic disease. Aneurysm of the aortic arch, an enlarged left atrium, and tumors of the mediastinum and bronchi are much more frequent causes of an isolated vocal cord palsy than are intracranial disorders. However, a substantial number of cases of recurrent laryngeal palsy remain idiopathic.

When confronted with a case of laryngeal palsy, the physician must attempt to determine the site of the lesion. If it is intramedullary, there are usually other signs, such as ipsilateral cerebellar dysfunction, loss of pain and temperature sensation over the ipsilateral face and contralateral arm and leg, and an ipsilateral Horner syndrome. If the lesion is extramedullary, the glossopharyngeal and spinal accessory nerves are frequently involved (jugular foramen syndrome). If it is extracranial in the posterior laterocondylar or retroparotid space, there may be a combination of ninth, tenth, eleventh, and twelfth cranial nerve palsies and a Horner syndrome (Table 355-2). If there is no sensory loss over the palate and pharynx and no palatal weakness or dysphagia, the lesion is below the origin of the pharyngeal branches, which leave the vagus nerve high in the cervical region; the usual site of disease is then the mediastinum.

NECK WEAKNESS Isolated involvement of the accessory (eleventh cranial) nerve can occur anywhere along its route, resulting in partial or complete paralysis of the sternocleidomastoid and trapezius muscles. More commonly, involvement occurs in combination with deficits of the ninth and tenth cranial nerves in the jugular foramen or after exit from the skull (Table 355-2). An idiopathic form of accessory neuropathy, akin to Bell's palsy, has been described, and it may be recurrent in some cases. Most but not all patients recover.

TONGUE PARALYSIS The hypoglossal (twelfth cranial) nerve supplies the ipsilateral muscles of the tongue. The nucleus of the nerve or its fibers of exit may be involved by intramedullary lesions such as tumor, poliomyelitis, or most often motor neuron disease. Lesions of the basal meninges and the occipital bones (platybasia, invagination of occipital condyles, Paget's disease) may compress the nerve in its extramedullary course or in the hypoglossal canal. Isolated lesions of unknown cause can occur. Atrophy and fasciculation of the tongue develop weeks to months after interruption of the nerve.

MULTIPLE CRANIAL NERVE PALSIES

Several cranial nerves may be affected by the same disease process. In this situation, the main clinical problem is to determine whether the lesion lies within the brainstem or outside it. Lesions that lie on the surface of the brainstem are characterized by involvement of adjacent cranial nerves (often occurring in succession) and late and rather slight involvement of the long sensory and motor pathways and segmental structures lying within the brainstem. The opposite is true of primary lesions within the brainstem. The extramedullary lesion is more likely

TABLE 355-2 *Cranial Nerve Syndromes*		
Site	**Cranial Nerves**	**Usual Cause**
Sphenoid fissure (superior orbital)	III, IV, first division V, VI	Invasive tumors of sphenoid bone; aneurysms
Lateral wall of cavernous sinus	III, IV, first division V, VI, often with proptosis	Infection, thrombosis, aneurysm, or fistula of cavernous sinus; invasive tumors from sinuses and sella turcica; benign granuloma responsive to glucocorticoids
Retrosphenoid space	II, III, IV, V, VI	Large tumors of middle cranial fossa
Apex of petrous bone	V, VI	Petrositis; tumors of petrous bone
Internal auditory meatus	VII, VIII	Tumors of petrous bone (dermoids, etc.); infectious processes; acoustic neuroma
Pontocerebellar angle	V, VII, VIII, and sometimes IX	Acoustic neuroma; meningioma
Jugular foramen	IX, X, XI	Tumors and aneurysms
Posterior laterocondylar space	IX, X, XI, XII	Tumors of parotid gland and carotid body and metastatic tumors
Posterior retroparotid space	IX, X, XI, XII and Horner syndrome	Tumors of parotid gland, carotid body, lymph nodes; metastatic tumor; tuberculous adenitis

to cause bone erosion or enlargement of the foramens of exit of cranial nerves. The intramedullary lesion involving cranial nerves often produces a crossed sensory or motor paralysis (cranial nerve signs on one side of the body and tract signs on the opposite side).

Involvement of multiple cranial nerves outside the brainstem is frequently the result of diabetes or trauma, localized infections such as herpes zoster, infectious and noninfectious (especially carcinomatous) causes of meningitis (Chap. 361), granulomatous diseases such as Wegener's granulomatosis, Behçet's disease, enlarging saccular aneurysms, or tumors. Among the tumors, nasopharyngeal cancers, lymphomas, neurofibromas, meningiomas, chordomas, cholesteatomas, carcinomas, and sarcomas have all been observed to involve a succession of lower cranial nerves. Owing to their anatomic relationships, the multiple cranial nerve palsies form a number of distinctive syndromes, listed in Table 355-2. Sarcoidosis is the cause of some cases of multiple cranial neuropathy, and chronic glandular tuberculosis the cause of a few others. Platybasia, basilar invagination of the skull, and the adult Chiari malformation are additional causes. A purely motor disorder without atrophy always raises the question of myasthenia gravis (Chap. 366). As noted above, Guillain-Barré syndrome commonly affects the facial nerves bilaterally. In the Fisher variant of the Guillain-Barré syndrome, oculomotor paresis occurs with ataxia and areflexia in the limbs (Chap. 365). Wernicke encephalopathy can cause a severe ophthalmoplegia combined with other brainstem signs.

The *cavernous sinus syndrome* (Fig. 355-3) is a distinctive and frequently life-threatening disorder. It often presents as orbital or facial pain; orbital swelling and chemosis due to occlusion of the ophthalmic veins; fever; oculomotor neuropathy affecting the third, fourth, and sixth cranial nerves; and trigeminal neuropathy affecting the ophthalmic (V_1) and occasionally the maxillary (V_2) divisions of the trigeminal nerve. Cavernous sinus thrombosis, often secondary to infection from orbital cellulitis (frequently *Staphylococcus aureus*), a cutaneous source on the face, or sinusitis (especially with mucormycosis in diabetic patients), is the most frequent cause; other etiologies include aneurysm of the carotid artery, a carotid-cavernous fistula (orbital bruit may be present), meningioma, nasopharyngeal carcinoma, other tumors, or an idiopathic granulomatous disorder (Tolosa-Hunt syndrome). The two cavernous sinuses directly communicate via intercavernous channels, thus involvement on one side may extend to become bilateral. Early diagnosis is essential, especially when due to infection, and treatment depends upon the underlying etiology. In infectious cases, prompt administration of broad-spectrum antibiotics, drainage of any abscess cavities, and identification of the offending organism is essential. Anticoagulant therapy may benefit cases of primary thrombosis. Repair or occlusion of the carotid artery may be

FIGURE 355-3 Anatomy of the cavernous sinus in coronal section, illustrating the location of the cranial nerves in relation to the vascular sinus, internal carotid artery (which loops anteriorly to the section), and surrounding structures.

required for treatment of fistulas or aneurysms. The Tolosa-Hunt syndrome generally responds to glucocorticoids.

An idiopathic form of multiple cranial nerve involvement on one or both sides of the face is occasionally seen. The syndrome consists of a subacute onset of boring facial pain, followed by paralysis of motor cranial nerves. The clinical features overlap those of the Tolosa-Hunt syndrome and appear to be due to idiopathic inflammation of the dura mater, which may be visualized by MRI. The syndrome is frequently responsive to glucocorticoids.

ACKNOWLEDGMENT

The authors acknowledge the contributions of Dr. Joseph B. Martin to this chapter in previous editions.

FURTHER READING

CARPENTER MB. *Core Text of Neuroanatomy*, 2d ed. Baltimore, Williams & Wilkins, 1978

GROGAN PM, GRONSETH GS: Practice parameter: Steroids, acyclovir, and surgery for Bell's palsy (an evidence-based review). Report of the Quality Standards Subcommittee of the American Academy of Neurology. Neurology 56:830, 2001

LOVE S, COAKHAM HB: Trigeminal neuralgia: Pathology and pathogenesis. Brain 124:2347, 2002

PATEL A et al: Microvascular decompression in the management of glossopharyngeal neuralgia: Analysis of 217 cases. Neurosurgery 50:705, 2002

SWEENEY CJ, GILDEN DH: Ramsay Hunt syndrome. J Neurol Neurosurg Psychiatry 71:149, 2001

356 | DISEASES OF THE SPINAL CORD
Stephen L. Hauser, Allan H. Ropper

Diseases of the spinal cord are frequently devastating. They can produce quadriplegia, paraplegia, and sensory deficits far beyond the damage they would inflict elsewhere in the nervous system because the spinal cord contains, in a small cross-sectional area, almost the entire motor output and sensory input of the trunk and limbs. Many spinal cord diseases are reversible if recognized and treated at an early stage (Table 356-1); thus, they are among the most critical of neurologic emergencies. The efficient use of diagnostic procedures, guided by a knowledge of the anatomy and the clinical features of common spinal ... is required for a successful outcome.

APPROACH TO THE PATIENT

SPINAL CORD ANATOMY RELEVANT TO CLINICAL SIGNS The spinal cord is a thin, tubular extension of the central nervous system contained within the bony spinal canal. It originates at the medulla and continues caudally to the conus medullaris at the lumbar level; its fibrous extension, the filum terminale, terminates at the coccyx. The adult spinal cord is ~46 cm (18 in.) long, oval or round in shape, and enlarged in the cervical and lumbar regions, where neurons that innervate the upper and lower extremities, respectively, are located. The white matter tracts containing ascending sensory and descending motor pathways are located peripherally, whereas nerve cell bodies are clustered in an inner region shaped like a four-leaf clover that surrounds the central canal (anatomically an extension

TABLE 356-1 *Some Treatable Spinal Cord Disorders*

Compressive
  Epidural, intradural, or intramedullary neoplasm
  Epidural abscess
  Epidural hemorrhage
  Cervical spondylosis
  Herniated disc
  Posttraumatic compression by fractured or displaced vertebra or
    hemorrhage
Vascular
  Arteriovenous malformation
  Antiphospholipid syndrome and other hypercoagulable states
Inflammatory
  Multiple sclerosis including neuromyelitis optica
  Transverse myelitis
  Sarcoidosis
  Vasculitis
Infectious
  Viral: VZV, HSV-1 and -2, CMV, HIV, HTLV-I, others
  Bacterial and mycobacterial: *Borrelia*, *Listeria*, syphilis, others
  Mycoplasma pneumoniae
  Parasitic: schistosomiasis, toxoplasmosis
Developmental
  Syringomyelia
  Meningomyelocoele
  Tethered cord syndrome
Metabolic
  Vitamin B_{12} deficiency (subacute combined degeneration)
  Adrenomyeloneuropathy

Note: VZV, varicella-zoster virus; HSV, herpes simplex virus; CMV, cytomegalovirus; HTLV, human T cell lymphotropic virus.

of the fourth ventricle). The membranes that cover the spinal cord—the pia, arachnoid, and dura—are continuous with those of the brainstem and cerebral hemispheres.

The spinal cord has 31 segments, each defined by an exiting ventral motor root and entering dorsal sensory root. During embryologic development, growth of the cord lags behind that of the vertebral column, and in the adult the spinal cord (conus segments) ends at approximately the first lumbar vertebral body. The lower spinal nerves take an increasingly downward course to exit via intervertebral foramina. The first seven pairs of cervical spinal nerves exit above the same-numbered vertebral bodies, whereas all the subsequent nerves exit below the same-numbered vertebral bodies; this situation is due to the presence of eight cervical spinal cord segments but only seven cervical vertebrae. The relationship between spinal cord segments and the corresponding vertebral bodies is shown in Table 356-2. These relationships assume particular importance for localization of lesions that cause spinal cord compression; a T10 spinal cord level, for example, indicates involvement of the cord adjacent to the seventh or eighth thoracic vertebral body. In addition, at every level the main ascending and descending tracts are somatotopically organized with a laminated distribution that reflects the origin or destination of nerve fibers.

Level of the Lesion (Fig. 356-1) The presence of a horizontally defined level below which sensory, motor, and/or autonomic function is impaired is a hallmark of spinal cord disease. A sensory level is sought by asking the patient to identify a pinprick or cold stimulus

TABLE 356-2 *Spinal Cord Levels Relative to the Vertebral Bodies*

Spinal Cord Level	Corresponding Vertebral Body
Upper cervical	Same as cord level
Lower cervical	1 level higher
Upper thoracic	2 levels higher
Lower thoracic	2 to 3 levels higher
Lumbar	T10-T12
Sacral	T12-L1
Coccygeal	L1

(i.e., a dry tuning fork after immersion in cold water) applied to the low back and sequentially moved up toward the neck on each side. The presence of a sensory level indicates damage to the spinothalamic tract, but the lesion is located one to two segments above the perceived level of a unilateral spinal cord lesion and at the level of the lesion when bilateral. That is the result of the ascent of second-order sensory fibers, which originate in the dorsal horn, proceed to cross anterior to the central canal, and join the opposite spinothalamic tract. Lesions that transect the descending corticospinal and other motor tracts cause paraplegia or quadriplegia, with increased muscle tone, exaggerated deep tendon reflexes, and extensor plantar signs (the upper motor neuron syndrome). Such lesions also typically produce autonomic disturbances consisting of disturbed sweating and bladder, bowel, and sexual dysfunction.

The uppermost level of a spinal cord lesion can also be localized by attention to the *segmental signs* corresponding to disturbed motor or sensory innervation by an individual cord segment. A band of altered sensation (hyperalgesia or hyperpathia) at the upper end of the sensory disturbance, fasciculations or atrophy in muscles innervated by one or several segments, or a diminished or absent deep tendon reflex may be noted. These signs also occur with focal root or peripheral nerve disorders; thus, segmental signs are most useful when they occur with signs of long tract damage. With severe and acute transverse lesions, the limbs initially may be flaccid rather than spastic. This state of "spinal shock" lasts for several days, rarely for weeks, and should not be mistaken for extensive damage to many segments of the cord or for a polyneuropathy.

The main features of transverse damage at each level of the spinal cord are summarized below.

CERVICAL CORD Extensive lesions near the junction of the cervical cord and medulla are usually fatal owing to involvement of adjacent medullary vasomotor and respiratory centers. Upper cervical cord lesions produce quadriplegia and weakness of the diaphragm. Breathing is possible only by use of accessory muscles of respiration. Lesions at C4-C5 produce quadriplegia; at C5-C6, there is loss of power and reflexes in the biceps; at C7 weakness is found in finger and wrist extensors and triceps; and at C8, finger and wrist flexion are impaired. A Horner's syndrome (miosis, ptosis, and facial hypohidrosis) may accompany a cervical cord lesion at any level.

THORACIC CORD Lesions here are localized by the sensory level on the trunk and midline back pain if it accompanies the syndrome. The sensory dermatomes of the body are shown in Fig. 22-2; useful markers are the nipples (T4) and umbilicus (T10). Leg weakness and disturbances of bladder and bowel function accompany the paralysis. Lesions at T9-T10 paralyze the lower, but not the upper, abdominal muscles, resulting in upward movement of the umbilicus when the abdominal wall contracts (Beevor's sign).

LUMBAR CORD The lumbar and sacral cord segments are small and are situated behind the T12 to L1 vertebrae. Lesions at L2-L4 paralyze flexion and adduction of the thigh, weaken leg extension at the knee, and abolish the patellar reflex. Lesions at L5-S1 paralyze movements of the foot and ankle, flexion at the knee, and extension of the thigh, and abolish the ankle jerk (S1).

SACRAL CORD/CONUS MEDULLARIS The conus medullaris is the tapered caudal termination of the spinal cord, comprising the lower sacral and single coccygeal segments. The conus syndrome is distinctive, consisting of bilateral saddle anesthesia (S3-S5), prominent bladder and bowel dysfunction (urinary retention and incontinence with lax anal tone), and impotence. The bulbocavernosus (S2-S4) and anal (S4-S5) reflexes are absent (Chap. 346). Muscle strength is largely preserved. Lesions of the conus must be distinguished from those

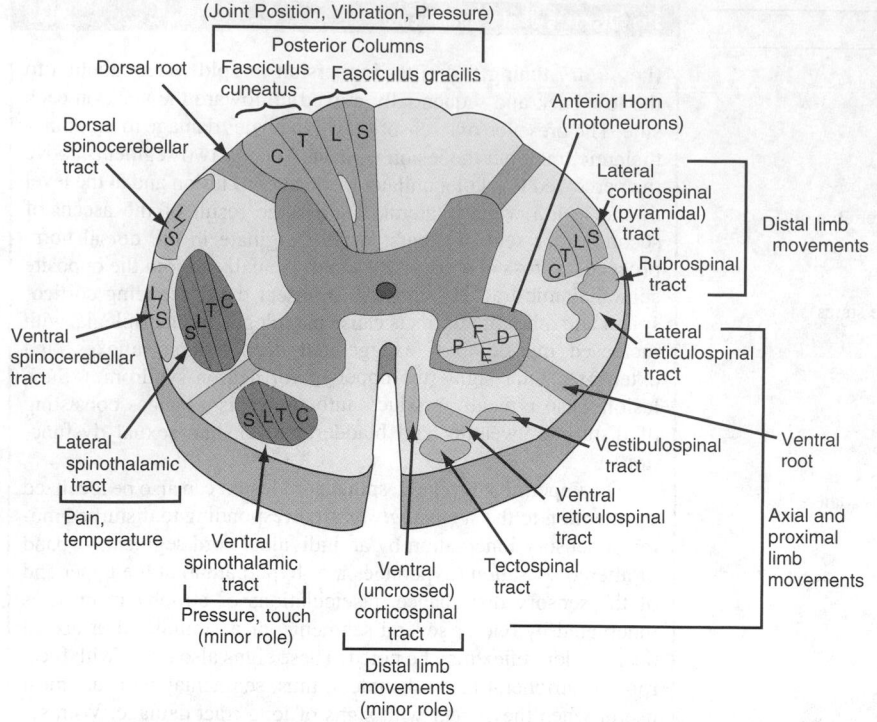

FIGURE 356-1 Transverse section through the spinal cord, composite representation, illustrating the principal ascending (*left*) and descending (*right*) pathways. The lateral and ventral spinothalamic tracts (*dark-brown*) ascend contralateral to the side of the body that is innervated. C, cervical; T, thoracic; L, lumbar; S, sacral; P, proximal; D, distal; F, flexors; E, extensors.

ANTERIOR SPINAL ARTERY SYNDROME Infarction of the cord is generally the result of occlusion or diminished flow in this artery. The result is extensive bilateral tissue destruction that spares the posterior columns. All spinal cord functions—motor, sensory, and autonomic—are lost below the level of the lesion, with the striking exception of retained vibration and position sensation.

LESIONS OF THE FORAMEN MAGNUM Partial lesions in this area interrupt decussating pyramidal tract fibers destined for the legs, which cross below those of the arms, resulting in a "crural paresis" of the lower limbs. Compressive lesions near the foramen magnum may produce weakness of the ipsilateral shoulder and arm followed by weakness of the ipsilateral leg, then the contralateral leg, and finally the contralateral arm (an "around the clock" pattern that may begin in any of the four limbs). There is typically suboccipital pain spreading to the neck and shoulders.

INTRAMEDULLARY AND EXTRAMEDULLARY SYNDROMES It is useful to differentiate intramedullary processes, arising within the substance of the cord, from extramedullary ones that compress the spinal cord or its vascular supply. The differentiating features are only relative and serve as rough guides to clinical decision making. With extramedullary lesions, radicular pain is often prominent, and there are early sacral sensory loss (lateral spinothalamic tract) and spastic weakness in the legs (corticospinal tract); this is due to the superficial location of the leg fibers in the corticospinal tract. Intramedullary lesions tend to produce poorly localized burning pain rather than radicular pain and spare sensation in the perineal and sacral areas ("sacral sparing") reflecting the laminated configuration of the spinothalamic tract with these fibers outermost; corticospinal tract signs appear later. Regarding extramedullary lesions, a further distinction is made between extradural and intradural masses, as the former are generally malignant and the latter benign (neurofibroma being the common cause); for this reason, a long duration of symptoms favors an intradural origin.

of the cauda equina, the cluster of nerve roots derived from the lower cord. Cauda equina lesions are characterized by low back or radicular pain, asymmetric leg weakness and sensory loss, variable areflexia in the lower extremities, and relative sparing of bowel and bladder function. Mass lesions in the lower spinal canal often produce a mixed clinical picture in which elements of both cauda equina and conus medullaris syndromes coexist; the typical cause is an ependymoma in that region. →*Cauda equina syndromes are discussed in Chap. 15.*

Special Patterns of Spinal Cord Disease The location of the major ascending and descending pathways of the spinal cord are shown in Fig. 356-1. Most fiber tracts—including the posterior columns and the spinocerebellar and pyramidal tracts—are situated on the side of the body they innervate. Afferent fibers mediating pain and temperature sensation ascend the spinothalamic tract contralateral to the side they supply. The anatomic relationships of these various fiber tracts produce characteristic clinical syndromes that provide clues to the underlying disease process.

BROWN-SEQUARD HEMICORD SYNDROME This consists of ipsilateral weakness (corticospinal tract) and loss of joint position and vibratory sense (posterior column), with contralateral loss of pain and temperature sense (spinothalamic tract) one or two levels below the lesion. Segmental signs, such as radicular pain, muscle atrophy, or loss of a deep tendon reflex, are unilateral. This classical syndrome is rare, and partial forms are more commonly encountered.

CENTRAL CORD SYNDROME The central cord syndrome results from damage to the gray matter nerve cells and crossing spinothalamic tracts near the central canal. In the cervical cord, the central cord syndrome produces arm weakness out of proportion to leg weakness and a "dissociated" sensory loss signifying a loss of pain and temperature sense in [a] distribution over the shoulders, lower neck, and upper trunk in [a pattern with relatively] intact light touch, joint position, and vibration sense in these [segments. Trau]ma, syringomyelia, tumors, and anterior spinal artery is[chem]ia [are the ma]in causes.

ACUTE AND SUBACUTE SPINAL CORD DISEASES

The initial symptom is often focal neck or back pain, followed by various combinations of paresthesias, sensory loss, motor weakness, and sphincter disturbance evolving over hours to several days. There may be mild sensory symptoms only or a devastating functional transection of the cord. Partial forms may selectively involve the posterior columns, anterior spinothalamic tracts, or one hemicord. Paresthesias or numbness may begin in the feet and ascend either symmetrically or asymmetrically, earlier in one leg than in the other; these symptoms may initially raise a question of Guillain-Barré syndrome, but involvement of the trunk with a sharply demarcated spinal cord level indicates the myelopathic nature of the process. In severe cases, areflexia indicating spinal shock may be present, but hyperreflexia soon supervenes; persistent areflexic paralysis indicates necrosis over multiple segments of the spinal cord.

APPROACH TO THE PATIENT

Distinguishing Compressive from Noncompressive Myelopathy The first priority is to identify a treatable mass lesion. The common causes in this category are tumor, epidural abscess or hematoma, herniated disc, or other vertebral pathology. Epidural compression due to malignancy or abscess often causes warning signs of neck or back pain, bladder disturbances, and sensory symptoms that precede the development of paralysis. Spinal subluxation, hemorrhage, and noncompressive etiologies such as infarction are more likely to produce myelopathy without antecedent symptoms. Magnetic resonance imaging (MRI) with contrast of the clinically suspected level of pathology is the initial diagnostic procedure; in some cases it is appropriate to image the entire spine (cervical through sacral regions) to search for additional, clinically silent, lesions. Once compressive lesions have been excluded, noncompressive causes of acute myelopathy that are intrinsic to the cord are considered: primarily vascular, inflammatory, and infectious etiologies.

COMPRESSIVE MYELOPATHIES ■ Neoplastic Spinal Cord Compression In adults, most neoplasms are epidural in origin, resulting from metastases to the adjacent spinal bones. The propensity of solid tumors to metastasize to the vertebral column probably reflects the high percentage of bone marrow located in the axial skeleton. Almost any malignant tumor can metastasize to the spinal column, with breast, lung, prostate, kidney, lymphoma, and plasma cell dyscrasia being particularly frequent. The thoracic cord is most commonly involved; exceptions are metastases from prostate and ovarian cancer, which occur disproportionately in the sacral and lumbar vertebrae, perhaps resulting from spread through Batson's plexus, a network of veins along the anterior epidural space. Retroperitoneal neoplasms (especially lymphomas or sarcomas) enter the spinal canal through the intervertebral foramina; they produce radicular pain and other signs of root involvement prior to cord compression.

Pain is the initial symptom; it may be either aching and localized or sharp and radiating in quality. The pain typically worsens with movement, coughing, or sneezing and characteristically awakens patients at night. A recent onset of persistent back pain, particularly if in the thoracic spine (which is uncommonly involved by spondylosis), should prompt consideration of vertebral metastasis. Rarely, pain is mild or absent. Pain typically precedes signs of cord compression by weeks or even months. However, once cord compression occurs, it usually advances rapidly. Plain radiographs of the spine and radionuclide bone scans have only a limited role in diagnosis because they do not identify 15 to 20% of metastatic vertebral lesions and fail to detect paravertebral masses that reach the epidural space through the intervertebral foramina. MRI provides excellent anatomic resolution of the site and extent of spinal tumors (Fig. 356-2); MRI has largely replaced computed tomography (CT) and myelography in the diagnosis of epidural masses. MRI can often distinguish between malignant lesions and other masses—epidural abscess, tuberculoma, or epidural hemorrhage, among others—that present in a similar fashion. Vertebral metastases are usually hypointense relative to a normal bone marrow signal on T1-weighted MRI scans; after the administration of gadolinium, contrast enhancement may "normalize" the appearance of the tumor by increasing its intensity to that of normal bone marrow. Infections of the spinal column (osteomyelitis and related disorders) are distinctive in that, unlike tumor, they may cross the disk space.

It is important to convey to the radiologist an estimate of the urgency of the imaging procedure requested. If signs of spinal cord involvement are present, imaging should be obtained promptly. If there are radicular symptoms but no evidence of myelopathy, it is usually safe, if necessary, to defer imaging for 24 to 48 h. With back or neck pain only, imaging studies may be obtained within a few days. Up to 40% of patients who present with symptomatic disease at one level are found to have asymptomatic epidural disease elsewhere; thus, the length of the spine should be imaged when epidural malignancy is in question.

℞ TREATMENT

Management includes glucocorticoids to reduce cord edema, local radiotherapy (initiated as early as possible) to the symptomatic lesion, and specific therapy for the underlying tumor type. Glucocorticoids (dexamethasone, 40 mg daily) can be administered before the imaging study if the clinical suspicion is strong and continued at a lower dose (20 mg daily in divided doses) until radiotherapy (a total of 3000 cGy administered in 15 daily fractions) is completed. Radiotherapy appears to be as effective as surgery, even for classically radioresistant metastases. Biopsy of the epidural mass is unnecessary in patients with known preexisting cancer, but the procedure may be indicated if a history of underlying cancer is lacking. Surgery, either decompression or vertebral body resection, should be considered when signs of cord compression worsen despite radiotherapy, when the maximum tolerated dose of radiotherapy has been delivered previously to the site, or when a vertebral compression fracture contributes to cord compression. A good response to radiotherapy can be expected in individuals who are ambulatory at presentation; new weakness is prevented, and some recovery of motor function occurs in approximately half of treated patients. Fixed motor deficits—paraplegia or quadriplegia—once established for >12 h, do not usually improve, and beyond 48 h the prognosis for substantial motor recovery is poor.

In contrast to tumors of the epidural space, most intradural mass lesions are slow-growing and benign. Meningiomas and neurofibromas account for most of these lesions, with occasional cases representing chordoma, lipoma, dermoid, or sarcoma (Chap. 358). Meningiomas (Fig. 356-3) are often located posterior to the thoracic cord or near the foramen magnum, although they can arise from the meninges anywhere along the spinal canal. Neurofibromas are benign tumors of the nerve sheath that typically arise near the posterior root; when multiple, neurofibromatosis is the likely etiology. Symptoms usually begin with radicular sensory symptoms followed by an asymmetric, progressive spinal cord syndrome. Therapy is by surgical resection.

Primary intramedullary tumors of the spinal cord are uncommon. They typically present as central cord or hemicord syndromes, often in the cervical region; there may be poorly localized burning pain in the extremities and sparing of sacral sensation. In adults, most of these lesions are ependymomas, hemangioblastomas, or low-grade astrocytomas (Fig. 356-4). Complete resection of an intramedullary ependymoma is often possible with microsurgical techniques. Debulking of an intramedullary astrocytoma can also be helpful, as these are often slowly growing lesions; the value of adjunctive radiotherapy is uncertain. Secondary (metastatic) intramedullary tumors are seen on most oncology services (Chap. 358).

Spinal Epidural Abscess Spinal epidural abscess presents as a clinical triad of pain, fever, and rapidly progressive weakness. Prompt recognition of this distinctive and treatable process will in most cases prevent permanent sequelae. Aching pain is almost always present, either over the spine or in a radicular pattern. The duration of pain prior to presentation is generally ≤2 weeks but may on occasion be several

FIGURE 356-2 Epidural spinal cord compression due to breast carcinoma. Sagittal T1-weighted (*A*) and T2-weighted (*B*) MRI scans through the cervicothoracic junction reveal a compression fracture of the second thoracic vertebral body with posterior displacement and compression of the upper thoracic spinal cord. The low-intensity bone marrow signal in *A* signifies replacement by tumor.

FIGURE 356-3 MRI of a thoracic meningioma. Coronal T1-weighted post-contrast image through the thoracic spinal cord demonstrates intense enhancement of a well-circumscribed extramedullary mass (*arrows*) which displaces the spinal cord to the left, widening the cistern adjacent to the mass.

FIGURE 356-5 MRI of a spinal epidural abscess due to tuberculosis. *A.* Sagittal T2-weighted free spin-echo MR sequence. A hypointense mass replaces the posterior elements of C3 and extends epidurally to compress the spinal cord (*arrows*). *B.* Sagittal T1-weighted image after contrast administration reveals a diffuse enhancement of the epidural process (*arrows*) with extension into the epidural space.

months or longer. Fever is usual, accompanied by an elevated white blood cell count and sedimentation rate. As the abscess expands, further spinal cord damage results from venous congestion and thrombosis in the epidural space. Once weakness and other signs of myelopathy appear, progression may be rapid. A more chronic granulomatous form of abscess is also known.

Risk factors include an impaired immune status (diabetes mellitus, renal failure, alcoholism, malignancy), intravenous drug abuse, and infections of the skin or other tissues. Two-thirds of epidural infections result from hematogenous spread from the skin (furunculosis), soft tissue (pharyngeal or dental abscesses), or deep viscera (bacterial endocarditis). One-third result from direct extension of a local infection to the subdural space; examples of local predisposing conditions are vertebral osteomyelitis; decubitus ulcers; or iatrogenic complications of lumbar puncture, epidural anesthesia, or spinal surgery. Most cases are due to *Staphylococcus aureus*; gram-negative bacilli, *Streptococcus*, anaerobes, and fungi can also cause epidural abscesses. Tuberculosis from an adjacent vertebral source remains an important cause in the underdeveloped world. MRI scans (Fig. 356-5) localize the abscess and exclude other causes of myelopathy. Lumbar puncture is not required but may be indicated if encephalopathy or other clinical signs raise the question of associated meningitis, a feature that is found in <25% of cases. In such situations, the level of the puncture should be planned to minimize the risk of inducing meningitis by passage of the needle through infected tissue, or herniation from decompression below an area of obstruction to the flow of cerebrospinal fluid (CSF). A high cervical tap is often the safest approach. CSF abnormalities in subdural abscess consist of pleocytosis with a preponderance of polymorphonuclear cells, an elevated protein level, and a reduced glucose level, but the responsible organism is not cultured unless there is an associated meningitis. Blood cultures are positive in <25% of cases.

℞ TREATMENT

Treatment is by decompressive laminectomy with debridement combined with long-term antibiotic treatment. Surgical evacuation prevents development of paralysis and may improve or reverse paralysis in evolution, but it is unlikely to improve deficits of more than several days duration. Antibiotics should be started empirically before surgery and then modified on the basis of culture results; medication is continued for at least 4 weeks. If surgery is contraindicated or if there is a fixed paraplegia or quadriplegia that is unlikely to improve following surgery, long-term administration of systemic and oral antibiotics can be used; in such cases, the choice of antibiotics may be guided by results of blood cultures. However, paralysis may develop or progress during antibiotic therapy; thus, initial surgical management remains the treatment of choice unless the abscess is very limited in size and causes no neurologic signs.

Epidural Hematoma   Hemorrhage into the epidural (or subdural) space causes an acute onset of focal or radicular pain followed by variable signs of a spinal cord or conus medullaris disorder. Therapeutic anticoagulation, trauma, tumor, or blood dyscrasias are predisposing conditions. Rare cases complicate lumbar puncture or epidural anesthesia, sometimes in association with use of low-molecular-weight heparin. MRI and CT confirm the clinical suspicion and can delineate the extent of the bleeding. Extrinsic spinal cord compression from any cause is an urgent condition, and appropriate treatment consists of prompt reversal of any underlying clotting disorder and surgical decompression. Surgery may be followed by substantial recovery, especially in patients with some preservation of motor function preoperatively. Because of

FIGURE 356-4   MRI of an intramedullary astrocytoma. Sagittal T1-weighted postcontrast image through the cervical spine demonstrates expansion of the upper cervical spine by a mass lesion emanating from within the spinal cord at the cervicomedullary junction. Irregular peripheral enhancement occurs within the mass (*arrows*).

the risk of hemorrhage, lumbar puncture should be avoided whenever possible in patients with thrombocytopenia or other coagulopathies.

Hematomyelia   Hemorrhage into the substance of the spinal cord is a rare result of trauma, intraparenchymal vascular malformation (see below), vasculitis due to polyarteritis nodosa or systemic lupus erythematosus (SLE), bleeding disorders, or a spinal cord neoplasm. Hematomyelia presents as an acute painful transverse myelopathy. With large lesions, extension into the subarachnoid space may occur, resulting in subarachnoid hemorrhage (Chap. 349). Diagnosis is made by MRI. Therapy is supportive, and surgical intervention is generally not useful. An exception is hematomyelia due to an underlying vascular malformation, in which selective spinal angiography may be indicated, followed by surgery to evacuate the clot and remove the underlying vascular lesion.

NONCOMPRESSIVE MYELOPATHIES   Acute transverse myelopathies (ATM) are rapidly progressive spinal cord syndromes with limb weakness, incontinence, and bilateral sensory loss accompanied by a sensory level and not due to cord compression. The time from onset to maximum symptoms is often hours or a few days, but some cases progress more slowly, over several weeks. Five general causes of ATM need to be considered: spinal cord infarction; systemic disorders including SLE and sarcoidosis; infectious (especially viral) causes; demyelinating diseases such as multiple sclerosis or neuromyelitis optica; and idiopathic transverse myelitis. The evaluation begins with a lumbar puncture and a search for systemic disease that may underlie the myelopathy (Table 356-3).

Spinal Cord Infarction   The cord is supplied by three arteries that course vertically over its surface: a single anterior spinal artery and paired posterior spinal arteries. At each segment, paired penetrating vessels branch from the anterior spinal artery to supply the anterior two-thirds of the spinal cord; the posterior spinal arteries, which often become less distinct below the midthoracic level, supply the posterior columns. Rostrally, the spinal arteries arise from the vertebral arteries. During embryogenesis, arterial feeders arise at each segmental level, but most involute before birth; generally, between three and eight major feeders remain, arising from the vertebral, subclavian, intercostal (from the aorta), iliac, and sacral arteries. In addition to the vertebral arteries, anterior spinal artery feeders arise at C6, at an upper thoracic level, and, most consistently, at T11-L2 (artery of Adamkiewicz).

Spinal cord ischemia can occur at any level; however, the presence

of the artery of Adamkiewicz creates a watershed of marginal blood flow in the upper-thoracic segments. With systemic hypotension, cord infarction occurs at the level of greatest ischemic risk, often T3-T4, and also at boundary zones between the anterior and posterior spinal artery territories. The latter may result in an acute—or more commonly progressive—syndrome of weakness and spasticity with little sensory change, superficially resembling amyotrophic lateral sclerosis (ALS).

Acute infarction in the territory of the anterior spinal artery produces paraplegia or quadriplegia, dissociated sensory loss affecting pain and temperature sense but sparing vibration and position sense, and loss of sphincter control. Onset may be sudden and dramatic but more typically is progressive over minutes or a few hours, quite unlike stroke in the cerebral hemispheres. Sharp midline or radiating back pain localized to the area of ischemia is frequent. Partial infarction of one anterior hemicord (hemiplegia or monoplegia and crossed pain and temperature loss) may also occur. Areflexia due to spinal shock is often present initially; with time, hyperreflexia and spasticity appear. Infarction in the territory of the posterior spinal arteries, resulting in loss of posterior column function, also occurs and may be underrecognized as a cause of obscure loss of position and vibration sense.

Spinal cord infarction is associated with aortic atherosclerosis, dissecting aortic aneurysm (chest or back pain with diminished pulses in legs), or hypotension from any cause. Cardiogenic emboli; vasculitis related to collagen vascular disease, particularly SLE and the antiphospholipid antibody syndrome (see below); and surgical interruption of aortic aneurysms are other causative conditions. Occasional cases develop by an unknown mechanism that leads to embolism of nucleus pulposus material into spinal vessels. In a substantial number of cases, no cause can be found, and thromboembolism in arterial feeders is suspected. The MRI may not demonstrate limited infarctions of the cord but is more often abnormal at the affected level.

Therapy is directed at treatment of any predisposing condition. In cord infarction due to presumed thromboembolism, acute anticoagulation is probably not indicated, with the exception of the unusual transient ischemic attack or incomplete infarction with a stuttering or progressive course. The antiphospholipid antibody syndrome is treated with anticoagulation, as described in Chap. 300.

Immune-Mediated Diseases   ATM occurs in ~1% of patients with SLE (Chap. 300) and may appear as the presenting manifestation of SLE. In some patients the ATM may be preceded or followed by optic neuritis (neuromyelitis optica; Chap. 359). Antiphospholipid antibodies are present in nearly two-thirds of patients with SLE-associated ATM. CSF is usually normal or shows a lymphocytic pleocytosis; oligoclonal bands are generally negative. Possible responses to glucocorticoids and/or cyclophosphamide have been reported. Other immune-mediated disorders associated with ATM include Sjögren's syndrome (Chap. 304), mixed connective tissue disease (Chap. 303), Behçet's syndrome (Chap. 307), and vasculitis with perinuclear antineutrophilic cytoplasmic (p-ANCA) antibodies (Chap. 306).

Another important consideration is sarcoid myelopathy (Chap. 309), in which a large edematous swelling of the spinal cord may mimic tumor; there is almost always enhancement of the lesion and the adjacent surface of the cord. The CSF profile consists of variable lymphocytic pleocytosis, and oligoclonal bands are present in one-third of cases. The diagnosis of sarcoid affecting the spinal cord is particularly difficult when systemic manifestations of sarcoid are meager or absent (50% of cases) or when other neurologic manifestations of the disease—such as cranial neuropathy, hypothalamic involvement, or meningeal enhancement visualized by MRI—are lacking. Whenever neurosarcoid is considered, a careful slit-lamp examination of the eye to search for uveitis, chest x-ray and CT to assess pulmonary involvement and mediastinal lymphadenopathy, serum angiotensin-converting enzyme (positive in only one-quarter of cases), serum calcium, and a gallium scan may be indicated. Initial treatment is with

---

TABLE 356-3 *Evaluation of Acute Transverse Myelopathy*

1. MRI of spinal cord with and without contrast (exclude compressive causes).
2. CSF studies: Cell count, protein, glucose, IgG index/synthesis rate, oligoclonal bands, VDRL; Gram's stain, acid-fast bacilli, and India ink stains; PCR for VZV, HSV-2, HSV-1, EBV, CMV, HHV-6, enteroviruses, HIV; antibody for HTLV-I, *B. burgdorferi, M. pneumoniae,* and *Chlamydia pneumoniae*; viral, bacterial, mycobacterial, and fungal cultures.
3. Blood studies for infection: HIV; RPR; IgG and IgM enterovirus antibody; IgM mumps, measles, rubella, group B arbovirus, *Brucella melitensis, Chlamydia psittaci, Bartonella henselae,* schistosomal antibody; cultures for *B. melitensis.* Also consider nasal/pharyngeal/anal cultures for enteroviruses; stool O&P for *Schistosoma* ova.
4. Immune-mediated disorders: ESR; ANA; ENA; dsDNA; rheumatoid factor; anti-SSA; anti-SSB, complement levels; antiphospholipid and anticardiolipin antibodies; p-ANCA; antimicrosomal and antithyroglobulin antibodies; if Sjögren syndrome suspected, Schirmer test, salivary gland scintography, and salivary/lacrimal gland biopsy.
5. Sarcoidosis: Serum angiotensin-converting enzyme; serum Ca; 24 hour urine Ca; chest x-ray; chest CT; total body gallium scan; lymph node biopsy.
6. Demyelinating disease: Brain MRI scan, evoked potentials.
7. Vascular causes: CT myelogram; spinal angiogram.

Note: VDRL, Venereal Disease Research Laboratory; PCR, polymerase chain reaction; VZV, varicella-zoster virus; HHV, human herpes virus; RPR, rapid plasma reagin (test); O&P, ova and parasites; ESR, erythrocyte sedimentation rate; ANA, antinuclear antibodies; ENA, epithelial neutrophil-activity (protein).

oral glucocorticoids; immunosuppressent drugs are used for resistant cases.

Recurrent episodes of myelitis are usually due to an immune-mediated disease such as SLE or sarcoid, a demyelinating disease, or infection with herpes simplex virus (HSV) type 2 (below).

Infectious and Parainfectious Myelitis   Many viruses have been associated with an acute myelitis that is caused by direct infection of the spinal cord. Herpes zoster is the most common viral cause of acute myelitis; HSV types 1 and 2, Epstein-Barr virus (EBV), cytomegalovirus (CMV), and rabies virus are other well-described etiologies. HSV-2 can produce a distinctive syndrome of recurrent sacral myelitis in association with outbreaks of genital herpes which mimics multiple sclerosis (MS). Poliomyelitis is the prototypic virus that produces acute infection of the spinal cord. In some cases it may be appropriate to begin specific therapy based upon the suspicion that a particular viral agent might be responsible for myelitis, pending laboratory confirmation. Herpes zoster, HSV, and EBV myelitis are treated with acyclovir (10 mg/kg tid for 10 to 14 days); CMV with ganciclovir (5 mg/kg IV bid) plus foscarnet (60 mg/kg IV tid) or with cidofovir (5 mg/kg per week for 2 weeks).

Bacterial and mycobacterial etiologies are less common than viral causes. Almost any pathogenic species may be responsible, including *Listeria monocytogenes*, *Borrelia burgdorferi* (Lyme disease), and *Treponema pallidum* (syphilis). *Mycoplasma pneumoniae* may be underrecognized as a cause of ATM.

Schistosomiasis (Chap. 203) is an important cause of parasitic myelitis in endemic areas. The myelitis is intensely inflammatory and granulomatous in nature, caused by a local response to tissue-digesting enzymes from the ova of the parasite. Toxoplasmosis (Chap. 198) can occasionally cause a focal myelopathy, and this diagnosis should be considered, particularly in patients with AIDS.

Other cases of myelitis, termed *postinfectious myelitis*, or *postvaccinial myelitis*, follow an infection or vaccination. Many infectious agents have been implicated, including influenza, measles, varicella, rubeola, and mumps. As in the related disorder, acute disseminated encephalomyelitis (Chap. 359), postinfectious transverse myelitis often begins as the patient appears to be recovering from the infection, but an infectious agent cannot be isolated from the nervous system or spinal fluid. These features suggest that the myelitis represents an autoimmune disorder triggered by infection and is not due to direct infection of the spinal cord.

Demyelinating Diseases   Multiple sclerosis (Chap. 359) may present as ATM, particularly in individuals of Asian or African ancestry. In Caucasians, MS rarely causes ATM (e.g., transverse myelitis with acute bilateral signs) but is a common cause of acute partial myelopathy. Unlike infectious and parainfectious ATM, MS-associated ATM is usually not associated with fever, rash, or other manifestations of an antecedent infection. Neuromyelitis optica (Devic's disease; Chap. 359) is a demyelinating syndrome related to MS that presents as ATM associated with optic neuritis; the optic neuritis is often bilateral and may precede or follow the myelitis by weeks or months. A neuromyelitis optica syndrome is also associated with SLE (see above) and other immune-mediated diseases, and with the antiphospholipid syndrome.

MRI findings in MS-associated ATM consist of mild swelling and edema of the cord and diffuse or multifocal areas of abnormal signal on T2-weighted sequences, often extending over several cord segments. Contrast enhancement, indicating disruption in the blood-brain barrier associated with inflammation, is present in acute cases. A brain MRI should be obtained to assess the likelihood that the myelitis represents an initial attack of MS. A normal scan indicates that the risk of evolution to MS is low—~10% over 5 years; by contrast, the finding of multiple periventricular T2-bright lesions indicates a risk of >50%. The CSF may be normal, but more often there is a mild pleocytosis, occasionally up to several hundred mononuclear cells per microliter. CSF protein

levels are normal or at most mildly elevated; oligoclonal banding is a variable finding but, when present, implicates MS.

There are no adequate trials of therapy for MS-associated ATM. Intravenous methylprednisolone (500 mg qd for 3 days) followed by oral prednisone (1 mg/kg per day for several weeks, then gradual taper) is the initial treatment of choice; a course of plasma exchange may be tried if glucocorticoids are ineffective.

Idiopathic Transverse Myelitis   In approximately one-quarter of cases of ATM, no underlying cause can be identified. Some will later manifest additional symptoms of a systemic immune-mediated disease such as SLE or a demyelinating disorder. In cases associated with inflammation (e.g., contrast enhancement of the lesion by spinal MRI or CSF pleocytosis) but not evidence of infection, glucocorticoids and plasma exchange are the first and second options, as for demyelinating causes (above).

CHRONIC MYELOPATHIES

SPONDYLITIC MYELOPATHY   Spondylitic myelopathy is one of the most common causes of gait difficulty in the elderly. Neck and shoulder pain with stiffness are early symptoms; impingement of bone and soft tissue overgrowth on nerve roots results in radicular arm pain, most often in a C5 or C6 distribution. Compression of the cervical cord produces a slowly progressive spastic paraparesis, at times asymmetric, and often accompanied by paresthesias in the feet and hands. Vibratory sense is diminished in the legs, and occasionally there is a sensory level for vibration on the upper thorax. In some cases coughing or straining produces leg weakness or radiating arm or shoulder pain. Dermatomal sensory loss in the arms, atrophy of intrinsic hand muscles, increased deep tendon reflexes in the legs, and extensor plantar responses are common. Urinary urgency or incontinence occurs in advanced cases. A tendon reflex in the arms is often diminished at some level; the biceps is most often affected (C5-C6). In individual cases, radicular, myelopathic, or combined signs may predominate. The diagnosis should be considered in cases of progressive cervical myelopathy, paresthesias of the feet and hands, or wasting of the hands.

Diagnosis is best made by MRI. Extrinsic cord compression is appreciated on axial views, and T2-weighted sequences may reveal areas of high signal intensity within the cord adjacent to the site of compression. Definitive therapy consists of surgical relief of the compression. Posterior laminectomy or an anterior approach with resection of the protruded disc material may be required. A cervical collar may be very helpful in milder cases. →*Cervical spondylosis and related degenerative diseases of the spine are discussed in Chap. 15.*

VASCULAR MALFORMATIONS   Although uncommon, vascular malformations of the cord are important lesions because they represent a treatable cause of progressive myelopathy. Arteriovenous malformations (AVMs) are most often located posteriorly, within the dura or along the surface of the cord, at or below the midthoracic level. The typical presentation is a middle-aged man with a progressive myelopathy. The myelopathy may worsen slowly or rapidly or may have periods of apparent remission with superimposed worsenings, resembling MS. Acute deterioration due to hemorrhage into the spinal cord or subarachnoid space may also occur. At presentation, most patients have sensory, motor, and bladder disturbances. The motor disorder may predominate and produce a mixture of upper and lower motor neuron signs, simulating amyotrophic lateral sclerosis (ALS). Pain, either dysesthesias or radicular pain, is also common. Other symptoms suggestive of AVM include intermittent claudication (symptoms that appear with exercise and are relieved by rest), or symptoms that change with posture, menses, or fever. A rare AVM syndrome presents as a progressive thoracic myelopathy with paraparesis developing over weeks or several months, associated with abnormally thick, hyalinized vessels (Foix-Alajouanine syndrome).

Spinal bruits are infrequent but should be sought at rest and after exercise. High-resolution MRI with contrast administration detects most AVMs (Fig. 356-6). A small number of AVMs not detected by

FIGURE 356-6 Arteriovenous malformation. Sagittal MR scans of the thoracic spinal cord: T2 fast spin-echo technique (*left*) and T1 post-contrast image (*right*). On the T2-weighted image (*left*), abnormally high signal intensity is noted in the central aspect of the spinal cord (*arrowheads*). Numerous punctate flow voids indent the dorsal and ventral spinal cord (*arrow*). These represent the abnormally dilated venous plexus supplied by a dural arteriovenous fistula. After contrast administration (*right*), multiple, serpentine, enhancing veins (*arrows*) on the ventral and dorsal aspect of the thoracic spinal cord are visualized, diagnostic of arteriovenous fistula. This patient was a 54-year-old man with a 4-year history of progressive paraparesis.

MRI may be visualized by CT myelography as enlarged vessels along the surface of the cord. Definitive diagnosis requires selective spinal angiography, which will also define the feeding vessels and the extent of the malformation. Spinal angiography should be considered when the clinical suspicion of an AVM is high, even when myelography is unrevealing. Embolization with occlusion of the major feeding vessels may stabilize a progressive neurologic deficit or produce a gradual recovery.

RETROVIRUS-ASSOCIATED MYELOPATHIES The myelopathy associated with the human T cell lymphotropic virus type I (HTLV-I), formerly called tropical spastic paraparesis, presents as a slowly progressive spastic paraparesis with variable sensory and bladder disturbance. The myelopathy typically implicates a thoracic level. Approximately half of patients have back or leg pain. The signs may be asymmetric, often lacking a well-defined sensory level; the only sign in the arms is hyperreflexia. The onset is generally insidious, and the tempo of progression is variable, but most patients are nonambulatory within 10 years of onset. This presentation may resemble primary progressive MS or a thoracic AVM. Diagnosis is made by demonstration of HTLV-I–specific antibody in serum by enzyme-linked immunosorbent assay (ELISA), confirmed by radioimmunoprecipitation or western blot analysis. There is no effective treatment, but symptomatic therapy for spasticity and bladder symptoms may be helpful. →*HTLV-I infections of the nervous system are discussed in Chap. 173.*

A progressive myelopathy may also occur in AIDS, characterized by vacuolar degeneration of the posterior and lateral tracts resembling subacute combined degeneration (see below).

SYRINGOMYELIA Syringomyelia is a developmental, slowly enlarging cavitary expansion of the cervical cord that produce progressive myelopathy. Symptoms begin insidiously in adolescence or early adulthood, progress irregularly, and may undergo spontaneous arrest for several years; most patients acquire a cervical-thoracic scoliosis. More than half of all cases are associated with Chiari type 1 malformations in which the cerebellar tonsils protrude through the foramen magnum and into the cervical spinal canal. The pathophysiology of the syrinx is controversial. Some interference with the normal flow of CSF seems likely. Acquired cavitations of the cord are also termed *syrinx cavities*; these may follow trauma, myelitis, chronic arachnoiditis due to tuberculosis and other etiologies, or necrotic spinal cord tumors.

The classic presentation is of a central cord syndrome with dissociated sensory loss and areflexic weakness in the upper limbs. The sensory deficit consists of loss of pain and temperature sensation with sparing of touch and vibration which is "suspended" over the nape of the neck, shoulders, and upper arms in a cape distribution or is in the hands. Most cases begin asymmetrically with unilateral sensory loss in the hands and unappreciated burns. Muscle wasting in the lower neck, shoulders, arms, and hands with asymmetric or absent reflexes reflects extension of the cavity to the anterior horns. As the lesion enlarges, spasticity and weakness of the legs, bladder and bowel dysfunction, and, in some cases, a Horner's syndrome appear. Thoracic kyphoscoliosis is a frequent additional finding. Some patients develop facial numbness and sensory loss from damage to the descending tract of the trigeminal nerve (C2 level or above). With Chiari malformations, cough headache, and neck, arm, or facial pain are common. Extension of the syrinx into the medulla, syringobulbia, may present as palatal or vocal cord paralysis, dysarthria, horizontal or vertical nystagmus, episodic dizziness, and/or tongue weakness.

MRI scans accurately identify developmental and acquired syrinx cavities and their associated spinal cord enlargement (Fig. 356-7). MRI scans of the brain and the entire spinal cord should be obtained to delineate the full longitudinal extent of the syrinx, assess posterior fossa structures, and determine whether hydrocephalus is present. If a Chiari malformation is not found, a contrast-enhanced MRI scan should be obtained to search for abnormal enhancement from an associated spinal cord tumor.

℞ TREATMENT

Treatment is generally unsatisfactory. Syringomyelia associated with tonsillar herniation is treated with posterior fossa decompression, generally consisting of suboccipital craniectomy, upper cervical laminectomy, and placement of a dural graft. If obstruction of fourth ventricular outflow is present, flow may be reestablished by enlargement of the opening. If the syrinx cavity is large, some surgeons recommend direct decompression of the fluid cavity, but the added benefit of this procedure is uncertain, and morbidity may occur. With Chiari malformations, shunting of hydrocephalus should generally precede any attempt to correct the syrinx. Surgery may stabilize the neurologic deficit; some patients have improvement postoperatively. Syringomyelia secondary to trauma or infection is treated with a decompression and drainage procedure in which a small shunt is inserted between the syrinx cavity and the subarachnoid space. Syringomyelia due to

FIGURE 356-7 MRI of a syringomyelia associated with a Chiari malformation. Sagittal T1-weighted image through the cervical and upper thoracic spine demonstrates descent of the cerebellar tonsils and vermis below the level of the foramen magnum (*black arrows*). Within the substance of the cervical and thoracic spinal cord, a CSF collection dilates the central canal (*white arrows*).

TABLE 356-4 *Expected Neurologic Function Following Complete Cord Lesions*

Level	Self-Care	Transfers	Maximum Mobility
High quadriplegia (C1-C4)	Dependent on others; requires respiratory support	Dependent on others	Motorized wheelchair
Low quadriplegia (C5-C8)	Partially independent with adaptive equipment	May be dependent or independent	May use manual wheelchair, drive an automobile with adaptive equipment
Paraplegia (below T1)	Independent	Independent	Ambulates short distances with aids

Source: Adapted from JF Ditunno, CS Formal: Chronic spinal cord injury. N Engl J Med 330:550, 1994; with permission.

an intramedullary spinal cord tumor is managed by resection of the tumor, if feasible; decompression of the cyst cavity may produce temporary relief, but recurrence is common.

MULTIPLE SCLEROSIS Spinal cord involvement is common in MS. It may develop acutely as an exacerbation in a patient with known MS or appear as the presenting manifestation of the disease (see above). Chronic progressive myelopathy is the most frequent cause of disability in both primary progressive and secondary progressive forms of MS. Involvement is typically asymmetric, producing motor, sensory, and bladder/bowel disturbances. Diagnosis is facilitated by identification of earlier attacks that may not be initially recalled by the patient; by MRI, CSF and evoked response testing; and by exclusion of other conditions. The diagnosis may be particularly difficult to establish in patients with primary progressive MS. Therapy with interferon β or glatiramer acetate is indicated for patients with coexisting relapses of MS. →*MS is discussed in Chap. 359.*

SUBACUTE COMBINED DEGENERATION (VITAMIN B$_{12}$ DEFICIENCY) This treatable myelopathy presents with parasthesias in the hands and feet, early loss of vibration and position sensation, and a progressive spastic and ataxic weakness. Loss of reflexes due to a superimposed peripheral neuropathy, present in many patients, is an important diagnostic clue. Optic atrophy and irritability and other mental changes may be prominent in advanced cases and on occasion are the presenting symptoms (megaloblastic madness). The myelopathy of subacute combined degeneration tends to be diffuse rather than focal; signs are generally symmetric and reflect predominant involvement of the posterior and lateral tracts, including Romberg's sign. The diagnosis is confirmed by the finding of macrocytic red cells, a low serum B$_{12}$ concentration, elevated levels of homocysteine and methylmalonic acid in uncertain cases, and a positive Schilling test (Chap. 61).

TABES DORSALIS The classic syndromes of tabes dorsalis and meningovascular syphilis of the spinal cord are rare but must be considered in the differential diagnosis of spinal cord disorders. The most common symptoms of tabes are characteristic fleeting and repetitive lancinating pains, which occur primarily in the legs and less commonly in the back, thorax, abdomen, arms, and face. Ataxia of the legs and gait due to loss of position sense occurs in half of patients. Paresthesias, bladder disturbances, and acute abdominal pain with vomiting (visceral crisis) occur in 15 to 30% of patients. The cardinal signs of tabes are loss of reflexes in the legs, impaired position and vibratory sense, Romberg's sign, and bilateral Argyll Robertson pupils, which fail to constrict to light but react with accommodation. In the modern era, diabetic polyradiculopathy simulates tabes.

FAMILIAL SPASTIC PARAPLEGIA (Chap. 353) Some cases of progressive myelopathy are genetic in origin. More than 20 different loci have been identified, including autosomal dominant, autosomal recessive, and X-linked forms. Most patients present with progressive spasticity and weakness in the legs; the syndrome is usually but not always symmetric. Sensory symptoms and signs are usually absent or mild. Sphincter disturbances may be present. In some families in which the condition is referred to as "complicated" familial spastic paraplegia, additional neurologic signs, e.g., nystagmus, ataxia, or optic atrophy,

occur. Onset may be as early as the first year of life or as late as middle adulthood. The causative mutations responsible for several forms of familial spastic paraplegia are now known (Table 353-3). No therapies are currently available.

ADRENOMYELONEUROPATHY This X-linked disorder, a variant of adrenoleukodystrophy, most commonly presents as a progressive spastic paraparesis beginning in early adulthood; some patients also have a mild peripheral neuropathy. Affected males usually have a history of adrenal insufficiency beginning in childhood. Rare heterozygous females may also present with adult-onset myelopathy. Diagnosis is usually made by demonstration of elevated levels of very long chain fatty acids in plasma and in cultured fibroblasts. The responsible gene, located at Xq17-28, encodes a protein involved in peroxysomal transport. Steroid replacement is indicated if hypoadrenalism is present, and bone marrow transplantation has been attempted for this condition, although without clear evidence of efficacy.

OTHER CHRONIC MYELOPATHIES Primary lateral sclerosis (Chap. 353) is a degenerative disorder characterized by progressive spasticity with weakness, often accompanied by dysarthria and dysphonia. Sensory function is spared. The disorder resembles ALS, but there is no evidence of a lower motor neuron disturbance. Toxic causes of spastic myelopathy include (1) lathyrism due to ingestion of chick peas containing the excitotoxin β-N-oxalylaminoalanine (BOAA) and seen primarily in the undeveloped world, and (2) nitrous oxide inhalation producing a myelopathy identical to subacute combined degeneration. SLE (Chap. 300), Sjögren's syndrome (Chap. 304), and sarcoid (Chap. 309), as mentioned above, have all been associated with progressive myelopathy, which may involve the cord even without evidence of overt systemic disease. Cancer-related causes include chronic paraneoplastic myelopathy (Chap. 87) or radiation injury (Chap. 358); metastases to the cord are probably more common than either of these. Finally, as in ATM, in some patients the etiology of a chronic myelopathy may not be determined initially. A cause can often be identified through periodic reassessment. →*Traumatic spinal cord lesions are discussed in Chap. 357.*

MEDICAL REHABILITATION OF SPINAL CORD DISORDERS

The prospects for recovery from an acute spinal cord lesion fade after ~6 months. There are currently no effective means to promote repair of injured spinal cord tissue; promising experimental approaches include the use of factors that influence reinnervation by axons of the corticospinal tract, nerve graft bridges that promote reinnervation across spinal cord lesions, and the local injection of stem cells. The disability associated with irreversible spinal cord damage is determined primarily by the level of the lesion and by whether the disturbance in function is complete or incomplete (Table 356-4). Even a complete high cervical cord lesion may be compatible with a productive life. Development of a rehabilitation plan framed by realistic expectations, and attention to the neurologic, medical, and psychological complications that commonly arise, are primary goals of treatment.

Many of the usual symptoms associated with medical illnesses, especially somatic and visceral pain, may be lacking because of the destruction of afferent pain pathways. Unexplained fever, worsening of spasticity, or deterioration in neurologic function should prompt a search for infection, thrombophlebitis, or an intraabdominal pathology; these etiologies are far more likely to be responsible than primary neurologic events such as meningitis, secondary syringomyelia, or chronic arachnoiditis. The loss of normal thermoregulation and inability to maintain normal body temperature can produce recurrent fever (*quadriplegic fever*), although most episodes of fever are due to infection of the urinary tract, lung, skin, or bone.

Bladder dysfunction generally results from loss of supraspinal innervation of the detrusor muscle of the bladder wall and the sphincter musculature. Detrusor spasticity is treated with anticholinergic drugs (oxybutinin, 2.5 to 5 mg qid) or tricyclic antidepressants with anticholinergic properties (imipramine, 25 to 200 mg/d). Failure of the sphincter muscle to relax during bladder emptying (urinary dyssynergia) may be managed with the α-adrenergic blocking agent terazosin hydrochloride (1 to 2 mg tid or qid), with intermittent catheterization, or, if that is not feasible, by use of a condom catheter in men or a permanent indwelling catheter. Surgical options include the creation of an artificial bladder by isolating a segment of intestine that can be catheterized intermittently (enterocystoplasty) or can drain continuously to an external appliance (urinary conduit). Bladder areflexia due to acute spinal shock or conus lesions is best treated by catheterization.

Bladder paralysis predisposes the patient to urinary tract infection. Bacteriuria due to asymptomatic colonization is extremely common and is generally not treated. Prophylaxis with antiseptics or antibiotics is a controversial practice. Urinary tract infections may present only as foul-smelling urine or a change in voiding pattern; the development of high fever or other systemic signs often indicates pyelonephritis. Bowel regimens and disimpaction are necessary in most patients to ensure at least biweekly evacuation and avoid colonic distention or obstruction.

High cervical cord lesions cause various degrees of mechanical respiratory failure requiring artificial ventilation. In cases of incomplete respiratory failure, chest physical therapy is useful, and a negative-pressure cuirass may alleviate atelectasis, particularly if the major lesion is below C4. With severe respiratory failure, tracheal intubation, followed by tracheotomy, provides tracheal access for ventilation and suctioning. Phrenic nerve pacing may be an option in some patients with lesions at C5 or above.

Patients with acute cord injury are at high risk for venous thrombosis and pulmonary embolism. During the first 2 weeks, use of calf-compression devices and anticoagulation with heparin (5000 U subcutaneously every 12 h) or warfarin (INR, 2 to 3) are recommended. In cases of persistent paralysis, anticoagulation should probably be continued for 3 months.

Prophylaxis against decubitus ulcers should involve frequent changes in position in a chair or bed, the use of special mattresses, and cushioning of areas where pressure sores often develop, such as the sacral prominence and heels. Early treatment of ulcers with careful cleansing, surgical or enzyme debridement of necrotic tissue, and appropriate dressing and drainage may prevent infection of adjacent soft tissue or bone.

Spasticity (Chap. 21) is aided by stretching exercises to maintain mobility of joints. Drug treatment is effective but may result in reduced function, as some patients depend upon spasticity as an aid to stand, transfer, or walk. Baclofen (15 to 240 mg/d in divided doses) is the most effective drug; it acts by facilitating GABA-mediated inhibition of motor reflex arcs. Diazepam acts by a similar mechanism and is useful for leg spasms that interrupt sleep (2 to 4 mg at bedtime). For nonambulatory patients, the direct muscle inhibitor dantrolene (25 to 100 mg qid) may be used, but it is potentially hepatotoxic. In severe cases, intrathecal baclofen administered via an implanted pump, botulinum toxin injections, or dorsal rhizotomy may be required to control spasticity.

A dramatic paroxysmal autonomic hyperreflexia may occur following lesions above the major splanchnic sympathetic outflow at T6. Headache, flushing, and diaphoresis above the level of the lesion, and hypertension with bradycardia or tachycardia, are the major symptoms. The trigger is typically a noxious stimulus—for example, bladder or bowel distention, a urinary tract infection, or a decubitus ulcer—below the level of the cord lesion. Treatment consists of removal of offending stimuli; ganglionic blocking agents (mecamylamine, 2.5 to 5 mg) or other short-acting antihypertensive drugs are useful in some patients.

Attention to these details allows longevity and a productive life for patients with myelopathy.

FURTHER READING

DE SEZE J et al: Acute myelopathies: Clinical, laboratory and outcome profiles in 79 cases. Brain 124:1509, 2001

KALB RG: Getting the spinal cord to think for itself. Arch Neurol 60:805, 2003

TRANSVERSE MYELITIS CONSORTIUM WORKING GROUP: Proposed diagnostic criteria and nosology of acute transverse myelitis. Neurology 59: 499, 2002

357 CONCUSSION AND OTHER HEAD INJURIES
Allan H. Ropper

Almost 10 million head injuries occur annually in the United States, about 20% of which are serious enough to cause brain damage. Among men under 35 years, accidents, usually motor vehicle collisions, are the chief cause of death, and >70% of these involve head injury. Furthermore, minor head injuries are so common that almost all physicians will be called upon to provide immediate care or to see patients who are suffering from various sequelae.

Medical personnel caring for head injury patients should be aware that (1) spinal injury often accompanies head injury, and care must be taken to prevent compression of the spinal cord due to instability of the spinal column; (2) intoxication is an important accompaniment of traumatic brain injury and, when appropriate, testing should be carried out for drugs and alcohol; and (3) systemic injuries, including rupture of abdominal organs, may produce vascular collapse or respiratory compromise requiring immediate attention.

TYPES OF HEAD INJURIES

CONCUSSION This refers to an immediate but transient loss of consciousness that is associated with a short period of amnesia. Patients may appear dazed or report feeling "star struck." It typically occurs after a blunt forward impact that creates a sudden deceleration of the cranium and a movement of the brain within the skull. Severe concussion may precipitate a brief convulsion or autonomic signs such as facial pallor, bradycardia, faintness with mild hypotension, or sluggish pupillary reaction, but most patients are soon neurologically normal. The mechanism of loss of consciousness in concussion is believed to be a transient electrophysiologic dysfunction of the reticular activating system in the upper midbrain caused by rotation of the cerebral hemispheres on the relatively fixed brainstem (Chap. 257).

Gross and light-microscopic changes in the brain are usually absent following concussion, but biochemical and ultrastructural changes, such as mitochondrial ATP depletion and local disruption of the blood-brain barrier, suggest that transient abnormalities occur. CT and MRI scans are usually normal; however, approximately 3% of patients will be found to have an intracranial hemorrhage of some type.

The amnesia of concussion typically occurs in individuals who have experienced at least a few moments of unresponsiveness, but on rare occasions no loss of consciousness is reported. The memory loss spans the time of, and moments before, mild impact injuries but may encompass previous weeks (rarely months) in cases of more severe trauma. In most cases, the extent of retrograde amnesia correlates with the severity of injury. Any anterograde amnesia is usually brief and disappears rapidly in alert patients. Memory is regained in an orderly way from the most distant to recent memories, with islands of amnesia occasionally remaining in severe cases. The mechanism of peritraumatic amnesia is not known. Hysterical posttraumatic amnesia is not uncommon and should be suspected when inexplicable abnormalities of behavior occur, such as recounting events that cannot be recalled

FIGURE 357-1 Traumatic cerebral contusion. Noncontrast CT scan demonstrating a hyperdense hemorrhagic region in the anterior temporal lobe.

FIGURE 357-2 Multiple small areas of hemorrhage and tissue disruption in the white matter of the frontal lobes on noncontrast CT scan. These appear to reflect an extreme type of the diffuse axonal shearing lesions that occur with closed head injury.

on later testing, a bizarre affect, forgetting one's own name, or a persistent anterograde deficit that is excessive in comparison with the degree of injury. →*For further discussion of amnesia, see Chap. 23.*

A single, uncomplicated head injury only infrequently produces permanent neurobehavioral changes in patients who are free of pre-existing psychiatric problems and substance abuse. These minor problems in memory and concentration may have an anatomic correlate in small shearing or other microscopic lesions (see below).

CONTUSION, BRAIN HEMORRHAGE, AND AXONAL SHEARING LESIONS A surface bruise of the brain, or *contusion*, consists of varying degrees of petechial hemorrhage, edema, and tissue destruction. Contusions and deeper hemorrhages result from mechanical forces that displace the hemispheres forcefully relative to the skull by deceleration of the brain against the inner skull, either under a point of impact (coup lesion) or, as the brain swings back, in the antipolar area (contrecoup lesion). Trauma sufficient to cause prolonged unconsciousness usually produces some degree of contusion. Blunt impact, as from an automobile dashboard or from falling forward while drunk, typically causes contusions on the orbital surfaces of the frontal lobes and the anterior and basal portions of the temporal lobes. With lateral forces the contusions are situated on the lateral convexity of the hemispheres. In both instances there may be contrecoup contusions on the opposite side of the impact. The clinical signs are determined by the location and size of the contusion; a hemiparesis or gaze preference is fairly typical. Large bilateral contusions produce coma with extensor posturing. Contusions limited to the frontal lobes cause an abulic-taciturn state, and those in the temporal lobe may cause an aggressive, combative, or delirious syndrome, described below.

Contusions are visible on CT and MRI scans, appearing early as inhomogeneous hyperdensities on CT and as hyperintensities on MRI; the signal changes reflect small scattered areas of cortical and subcortical blood and localized brain edema (Fig. 357-1); there is also some degree of subarachnoid bleeding, which may be detected by scans or lumbar puncture. Subacutely, contusions acquire a surrounding contrast enhancement that may be mistaken for tumor or abscess. Glial and macrophage reactions may result in scarred, hemosiderin-stained depressions on the surface (*plaques jaunes*) that are the main source of posttraumatic epilepsy.

Torsion or shearing forces in the brain can cause basal ganglial and other deep hematomas independent of surface damage. Large single hemorrhages after minor trauma may be associated with a bleeding

diathesis or cerebrovascular amyloidosis in the elderly. For unexplained reasons, deep cerebral hemorrhages may not develop until several days after severe injury. Sudden neurologic deterioration in a comatose patient or a sudden rise in intracranial pressure (ICP) should therefore prompt investigation with a CT scan.

Another type of deep white matter lesion consists of widespread acute disruption, or shearing, of axons at the time of impact. Most characteristic are small areas of tissue disruption in the corpus callosum and dorsolateral pons. The presence of widespread axonal damage of both hemispheres, a state called *diffuse axonal injury*, explains persistent coma and the vegetative state, but small ischemic-hemorrhagic lesions in the midbrain and thalamus are as often the cause. Only severe shearing lesions that contain blood are visualized by CT, usually in the corpus callosum and centrum semiovale (Fig. 357-2); however, within days of the injury, MRI scan demonstrates such lesions throughout the white matter with the use of special imaging sequences.

SKULL FRACTURES A blow to the skull causes a fracture if the elastic tolerance of the bone is exceeded. Intracranial lesions accompany two-thirds of skull fractures, and the presence of a skull fracture increases manyfold the chances of an underlying subdural or epidural hematoma. Consequently, fractures are primarily markers of the site and severity of injury. They provide pathways for entry of bacteria (meningitis) or air (pneumocephalus) to the cerebrospinal fluid (CSF) and for leakage of CSF out through the dura.

Linear fractures, which are most often associated with subdural or epidural hematomas, account for 80% of all skull fractures. They are usually oriented from the point of impact toward the base of the skull. Basilar skull fractures are often extensions of adjacent fractures over the convexity of the skull but may occur independently owing to stresses on the floor of the middle cranial fossa or occiput. They are located parallel to the petrous bone or along the sphenoid bone toward the sella turcica and ethmoidal groove. Although most are uncomplicated, basilar skull fractures can cause CSF leakage, pneumocephalus, and cavernous-carotid fistulas. Hemotympanum (blood behind the tympanic membrane), delayed ecchymosis over the mastoid process (Battle's sign), or periorbital ecchymosis ("racoon sign") all signify fracture of the base of the skull. Because routine x-ray examination may fail to disclose basilar fractures, they should be suspected if these clinical signs are present. CSF may leak through the cribriform plate or the adjacent sinus and manifest as a watery discharge from the nose (CSF rhinorrhea). Persistent rhinorrhea and recurrent meningitis are indications for surgical repair of torn dura underlying the fracture. The precise site of the leak is often difficult to determine, but useful diagnostic tests include the instillation of water-soluble contrast into the CSF followed by CT with the patient in various positions, and injection of radionuclide compounds or fluorescein into the CSF with an assessment of uptake of these compounds by absorptive nasal pledgets. The site of an intermittent leak is rarely delineated, and most resolve spontaneously. Sellar fractures, even ones associated with serious neuroendocrine dysfunction, are sometimes radiologically occult. Fractures of the dorsum sella may cause sixth or seventh nerve palsies or optic nerve damage. An air-fluid level in the sphenoid sinus suggests a fracture of the sellar floor.

Petrous bone fractures, especially those oriented along the long axis of the bone, may be associated with facial palsy, disruption of ear ossicles, and CSF otorrhea. Transverse petrous fractures are less common; they almost always damage the cochlea or labyrinths and often the facial nerve. External bleeding from the ear is usually from local abrasion of the external canal but can also result from petrous fracture.

Fractures of the frontal bone are often depressed, involving the frontal and paranasal sinuses and the orbits; permanent anosmia results if the olfactory filaments in the cribriform plate are disrupted. Depressed skull fractures are typically compound, but they are often neurologically asymptomatic because the impact energy is dissipated in breaking the bone; however, some are associated with brain contusions and focal neurologic signs caused by damage to the underlying cortical area. Prompt debridement and exploration of compound fractures are required in order to avoid infection.

CRANIAL NERVE INJURIES The cranial nerves likely to be injured with head trauma include the olfactory, optic, oculomotor, and trochlear nerves; the first and second branches of the trigeminal nerve; and the facial and auditory nerves. Anosmia and an apparent loss of taste (actually a loss of perception of aromatic flavors, with elementary tastes retained) occur in ~10% of persons with serious head injuries, particularly after falls on the back of the head. This sequela results from displacement of the brain and shearing of the olfactory nerve filaments and may occur in the absence of a fracture. Recovery is the rule, leaving residual hyposmia, but if bilateral anosmia persists for several months, the prognosis is poor. Partial optic nerve injuries from closed trauma result in blurring of vision, central or paracentral scotomas, or sector defects. Direct orbital injury may cause short-lived blurred vision for close objects and pupillary paralysis because of reversible iridoplegia. Diplopia limited to downward gaze and corrected when the head is tilted away from the affected eye indicates trochlear nerve damage. It occurs as an isolated problem after minor injury and can develop after a delay of several days. Direct facial nerve injury by a basal fracture is present immediately in 3% of severe injuries; it may also be delayed 5 to 7 days. Fractures through the petrous bone, particularly the less common transverse type, are liable to produce this injury. Delayed facial palsy, the mechanism of which is unknown, has a good prognosis. Injury to the eighth cranial nerve from a fracture of the petrous bone causes loss of hearing, vertigo, and nystagmus immediately after injury. Deafness from nerve injury must be distinguished from that due to rupture of the eardrum, blood in the middle ear, or disruption of the ossicles from fracture through the middle ear. A high-tone hearing loss occurs with direct cochlear concussion.

SEIZURES *Convulsions* are surprisingly uncommon immediately after a head injury, but a brief period of tonic extensor posturing or a few clonic movements of the limbs just after the moment of impact may occur. However, the superficial cortical scars that evolve from contusions are highly epileptogenic and may later manifest as seizures, even after many years (Chap. 348). The severity of injury determines the risk of future seizures. It has been estimated that 17% of individuals with brain contusion, subdural hematoma, or prolonged loss of consciousness will develop a seizure disorder and that this risk extends for an indefinite period of time, whereas the risk is only 2% after mild injury. The majority of convulsions in the latter group occur within 5 years of injury.

SUBDURAL AND EPIDURAL HEMATOMAS Hemorrhages beneath the dura (subdural) or between the dura and skull (epidural) may be associated with contusions and other injuries, making it difficult to determine their relative contribution to the clinical state. However, subdural and epidural hematomas as often occur as the sole manifestation of injury, and each has characteristic clinical and radiologic features. Because the mass effect and the rise in ICP caused by these hemorrhages may be life threatening, it is imperative that hemorrhages be identified immediately by CT or MRI scan and evacuated when appropriate.

Acute Subdural Hematoma These lesions become symptomatic minutes or hours after injury. Up to one-third of patients have a lucid interval before coma supervenes, but most are drowsy or comatose from the moment of injury. Direct cranial trauma is not required for acute subdural hemorrhage to occur; acceleration forces alone, as from whip-

lash, are adequate, especially in the elderly and those taking anticoagulant medications. A unilateral headache and slightly enlarged pupil on the same side are frequently but not invariably found. Stupor or coma, a hemiparesis, and unilateral pupillary enlargement are the signs of larger hematomas. In an acutely deteriorating patient with diminished alertness and with pupillary enlargement, burr (drainage) holes or an emergency craniotomy are appropriate. Small subdural hematomas may be asymptomatic and usually do not require evacuation. A subacute syndrome due to subdural hematoma occurs days to weeks after injury with drowsiness, headache, confusion, or mild hemiparesis; it is seen in alcoholics and in the elderly. Subdural hematomas appear as crescentic collections over the convexity of the hemisphere and are located over the frontotemporal region, less often in the inferior middle fossa or over the occipital poles (Fig. 357-3).

Interhemispheric, posterior fossa, or bilateral convexity hematomas are less common and are difficult to diagnose clinically, although drowsiness and the signs expected for each region can be detected (Chap. 23). Larger hematomas are primarily venous in origin, though additional arterial bleeding sites are often found; a few large hematomas, when explored surgically, have an exclusively arterial cause.

Epidural Hematoma (Fig. 357-4) These evolve more rapidly than subdural hematomas and are therefore more treacherous. They occur in up to 10% of severe head injury cases and are less often associated with underlying cortical damage than are subdural hematomas. Most patients are unconscious when first seen. A "lucid interval" of several minutes to hours before coma supervenes is most characteristic of epidural hemorrhage, but it is still uncommon, and epidural hemorrhage by no means is the only cause of this temporal sequence of events.

Chronic Subdural Hematoma A history of trauma may or may not be elicited; 20 to 30% of patients recall no head injury, particularly the elderly and those with bleeding diatheses. The causative injury may be trivial and is often forgotten because it was remote. Headache (common but not invariable), slowed thinking, change in personality, a seizure, or a mild hemiparesis emerges weeks or months afterwards. The headache may fluctuate in severity, sometimes with position changes. Many chronic subdural hematomas are bilateral and produce perplexing clinical syndromes. The initial clinical impression is of a stroke, brain tumor, drug intoxication, depression, or a dementing illness because drowsiness, inattentiveness, and incoherence of thought are more prominent than focal signs such as hemiparesis. Patients with undetected small bilateral subdural hematomas seem to have a low tolerance for surgery, anesthesia, and drugs that depress the nervous system, remaining drowsy or confused for long periods postoperatively. Occasionally a chronic hematoma causes brief episodes of hemiparesis or aphasia that are indistinguishable from transient ischemic attacks.

Skull x-rays are usually normal except for a shift of the calcified pineal body to one side or an occasional unexpected fracture. In longstanding cases the irregular calcification of membranes that surround the collection may be appreciated. CT performed soon after injury (without contrast infusion) shows a low-density mass over the convexity of the hemisphere (Fig. 357-5), but between 2 to 6 weeks after the initial bleeding the hemorrhage appears isodense compared to adjacent brain. Bilateral chronic hematomas may fail to be detected because of the absence of lateral tissue shifts; this circumstance is suggested by a "hypernormal" CT scan with fullness of the cortical sulci and small ventricles in an older patient. CT with contrast demonstrates the vascular fibrous capsule surrounding the hemorrhage. MRI reliably identifies either a subacute or chronic hematoma. Chronic subdural hematomas can expand gradually and clinically resemble tumors of the brain.

Clinical observation and serial imaging are reasonable in patients with few symptoms and small chronic subdural collections. Treatment with glucocorticoids alone is sufficient in some larger hematomas, but surgical evacuation is more often successful. The fibrous membranes

FIGURE 357-3 Acute subdural hematoma in a non-contrast CT scan. The hyperdense clot has an irregular border with the brain and causes more horizontal displacement (mass effect) than might be expected from its thickness. The disproportionate mass effect is the result of the large rostral-caudal extent of these hematomas. Compare to Fig. 357-4.

FIGURE 357-4 Acute epidural hematoma. The tightly attached dura is stripped from the inner table of the skull, producing a characteristic lenticular-shaped hemorrhage on CT scan. Epidural hematomas are usually caused by disruption of the middle meningeal artery following fracture of the temporal bone.

FIGURE 357-5 CT scan of chronic bilateral subdural hematomas of different ages. The collections began as acute hematomas and have become hypodense in comparison to the adjacent brain after a period during which they were isodense and difficult to appreciate. Some areas of resolving blood are contained on the more recently formed collection on the left (arrows).

that grow from the dura and encapsulate the region require surgical resection to prevent recurrent fluid accumulation. Small hematomas are largely resorbed, leaving only the organizing membranes.

CLINICAL SYNDROMES AND TREATMENT OF HEAD INJURY

MINOR INJURY The patient who is fully alert and attentive after head injury but who has one or more symptoms of headache, faintness, nausea, a single episode of emesis, difficulty with concentration, or slight blurring of vision has a good prognosis with little risk of subsequent deterioration. Such patients have usually sustained a concussion and are expected to have a brief amnestic period. Children and young adults are particularly prone to drowsiness, vomiting, and irritability, which is sometimes delayed for several hours after apparently minor injuries. Occasionally, vasovagal syncope follows several minutes to an hour after the injury and may cause undue concern. Constant generalized or frontal headache is common in the days following trauma; it may be migrainous (throbbing and hemicranial) in nature. After several hours of observation, patients with this category of injury may be accompanied home and observed by a family member or friend. Most patients with this syndrome do not have a skull fracture on x-ray or hemorrhage on CT. The decision to perform these tests therefore depends largely on clinical signs suggesting that the impact was severe (e.g., prolonged concussion, periorbital or mastoid hematoma, repeated vomiting, apparent fracture), on the seriousness of other bodily injuries, and on the degree of surveillance that can be anticipated at home. Persistent severe headache and repeated vomiting in the context of normal alertness and no focal neurologic signs are usually benign, but radiologic studies should be obtained and observation in the hospital is justified.

INJURY OF INTERMEDIATE SEVERITY Patients who are not comatose but who have persistent confusion, behavioral changes, subnormal alertness, extreme dizziness, or focal neurologic signs such as hemiparesis should be admitted to the hospital and soon thereafter have a CT scan. Usually a contusion or hematoma is found. The clinical syndromes most common in this group, in addition to postconcussive drowsiness, headache, dizziness, and vomiting, include (1) delirium with a disinclination to be examined or moved, expletive speech, and resistance if disturbed (anterior temporal lobe contusions); (2) a quiet, disinterested, slowed mental state (abulia) with dull facial appearance and irascibility (inferior frontal and frontopolar contusions); (3) a focal deficit such as aphasia or mild hemiparesis (due to subdural hematoma or convexity contusion, or, less often but frequently missed, carotid

artery dissection); (4) confusion with inattention, poor performance on simple mental tasks, and fluctuating or slightly erroneous orientation (associated with several types of injuries, including the first two described above as well as medial frontal contusions and interhemispheric subdural hematoma); (5) repetitive vomiting, nystagmus, drowsiness, and unsteadiness (usually from labyrinthine concussion, but occasionally due to a posterior fossa subdural hematoma or vertebral artery dissection); and (6) diabetes insipidus (damage to the median eminence or pituitary stalk). *It should be emphasized that intermediate-grade injuries are often complicated by drug or alcohol intoxication.*

Clinical observation is necessary to detect increasing drowsiness, change in respiratory pattern, or pupillary enlargement and to ensure restriction of free water (unless there is diabetes insipidus). Most patients in this category improve over several days. During the first week, the state of alertness, memory, and other cognitive functions often fluctuates, and irascibility or agitation is common. Behavioral changes are worse at night, as with many other encephalopathies, and may be treated with small doses of antipsychotic medications. Subtle abnormalities of attention, intellect, spontaneity, and memory tend to return to normal weeks or months after the injury, sometimes surprisingly abruptly; persistent problems in cognition are discussed below.

SEVERE INJURY Patients who are comatose from the onset require immediate neurologic attention and resuscitation. After intubation, with care taken to avoid deforming the cervical spine, the depth of coma, pupillary size and reactivity, limb movements, and Babinski responses are assessed. As soon as vital functions permit and cervical spine x-rays and a CT scan have been obtained, the patient should be transported to a critical care unit where ICP can be monitored, and where the systemic complications that follow severe brain injury can be treated. The finding of an epidural or subdural hematoma or large intracerebral hemorrhage is an indication for prompt surgery and intracranial decompression in otherwise salvageable patients. →*Management of raised ICP is discussed in Chap. 258.*

PROGNOSIS In severe head injury, eye opening, the best motor response of the limbs, and verbal output have been found to be roughly predictive of outcome; these are summarized using the "Glasgow Coma Scale" (Table 357-1). Over 85% of patients with aggregate scores of 3 or 4 die within 24 h. However, a number of patients with slightly higher scores and a poor initial prognosis, including a few without pupillary light responses, survive, suggesting that an initially

TABLE 357-1 *Glasgow Coma Scale for Head Injury*

Eye opening (E)		Verbal response (V)	
Spontaneous	4	Oriented	5
To loud voice	3	Confused, disoriented	4
To pain	2	Inappropriate words	3
Nil	1	Incomprehensible sounds	2
Best motor response (M)		Nil	1
Obeys	6		
Localizes	5		
Withdraws (flexion)	4		
Abnormal flexion posturing	3		
Extension posturing	2		
Nil	1		

Note: Coma score = E + M + V. Patients scoring 3 or 4 have an 85 percent chance of dying or remaining vegetative, while scores above 11 indicate only a 5 to 10 percent likelihood of death or vegetative state and 85 percent chance of moderate disability or good recovery. Intermediate scores correlate with proportional chances of recovery.

aggressive approach is justified in most patients. Patients <20 years, particularly children, may make remarkable recoveries after having grave early neurologic signs. In one large study of severe head injury, 55% of children had a good outcome at 1 year, compared with 21% of adults. Older age, increased ICP, hypoxia and hypotension, and CT scan evidence of compression of the cisterns surrounding the brainstem and shift of midline structures are all poor prognostic signs. Delayed evacuation of large intracerebral hemorrhages is associated with a poor prognosis. Carrier status for the apolipoprotein E-4 allele is also associated with poor recovery following traumatic brain injury.

POSTCONCUSSION SYNDROME

A structural basis has been sought for the posttraumatic nervous instability termed the *postconcussion syndrome*, which consists of fatigue, dizziness, headache, and difficulty in concentration after mild or moderate injury. Most instances are difficult to distinguish from asthenia and depression. Based largely on experimental models, some investigators believe that subtle axonal shearing lesions or yet undefined biochemical alterations account for the cognitive symptoms even when the findings are normal on brain imaging, evoked potentials, and electroencephalogram. In moderate and severe trauma, neuropsychological changes such as difficulty with attention, memory, and other cognitive deficits are undoubtedly present, sometimes severe, but many deficits identified in formal testing are not important for daily functioning. Test scores tend to improve rapidly during the first 6 months after injury, then more slowly for years.

Treatment of the various symptoms of the postconcussive syndrome first requires a symptomatic approach to identify and treat depression and loss of energy, sleeplessness, anxiety, persistent headache, and dizziness. Often, reassurance and treatment directed at anxious depression and sleep problems are all that are required. Care is taken to avoid prolonged use of drugs that produce dependence. Vestibular exercises (Chap. 26) and small doses of vestibular suppressants such as phenergan are helpful when dizziness is the main problem. Patients who after minor or moderate injury report difficulty with memory or with complex cognitive tasks at work may also be reassured that these problems usually improve over 6 to 12 months. It is helpful in this group to obtain focused, serial, and quantified neuropsychological testing in order to adjust the work environment to the patient's current abilities and to document improvement. Whether cognitive exercises are useful is uncertain, but patients certainly report them to be helpful. Previously energetic individuals are usually found to have the best recoveries. In patients with persistent symptoms, the possibility of malingering exists. Physicians should be aware that symptoms tend to persist when litigation regarding the injury is prolonged.

In the absence of adequate data, a common sense approach has been taken to deciding when an athlete who has suffered a concussion should resume athletic activities. Generally, it is advisable to avoid

TABLE 357-2 *Guidelines for Management of Concussion in Sports*

SEVERITY OF CONCUSSION

Grade 1: Transient confusion, no loss of consciousness (LOC), all symptoms resolve within 15 min.

Grade 2: Transient confusion, no LOC, but concussive symptoms or mental status abnormalities persist longer than 15 min.

Grade 3: Any LOC, either brief (seconds) or prolonged (minutes).

ON-SITE EVALUATION

1. Mental status testing
   a. Orientation—time, place, person, circumstances of injury
   b. Concentration—digits backward, months of year in reverse order
   c. Memory—names of teams, details of contest, recent events, recall of three words and objects at 0 and 5 min
2. Finger-nose-finger with eyes open and closed
3. Pupillary symmetry and reaction
4. Romberg and tandem gait
5. Provocative testing—40-yard sprint, 5 push ups, 5 sit ups, 5 knee bends (development of dizziness, headaches, or other symptoms is abnormal)

MANAGEMENT GUIDELINES

Grade 1: Remove from contest. Examine immediately and at 5 min intervals. May return to contest if exam clears within 15 min. A second grade 1 concussion eliminates player for 1 week, with return contingent upon normal neurologic assessment at rest and with exercise.

Grade 2: Remove from contest, cannot return for at least 1 week. Examine at frequent intervals on sideline. Formal neurologic exam the next day. If headache or other symptoms persist for 1 week or longer, CT or MRI scan is indicated. After 1 full asymptomatic week, repeat neurologic assessment at rest and with exercise before cleared to resume play. A second grade 2 concussion eliminates player for at least 2 weeks following complete resolution of symptoms.

Grade 3: Transport by ambulance to emergency department if still unconscious or worrisome signs are present; cervical spine stabilization may be indicated. Neurologic exam and, when indicated, CT or MRI scan will guide subsequent management. Hospital admission indicated when signs of pathology are present or if mental status remains abnormal. If findings are normal at the time of the initial medical evaluation, the athlete may be sent home, but daily exams as an outpatient are indicated. A brief (LOC for seconds) grade 3 concussion eliminates player for 1 week, and a prolonged (LOC for minutes) grade 3 concussion for 2 weeks, following complete resolution of symptoms. A second grade 3 concussion should eliminate player from sports for at least 1 month following resolution. Any abnormality on CT or MRI scans should result in termination of the season for the athlete, and return to play at any future time should be discouraged.

Note: CT, computed tomography; MRI, magnetic resonance imaging.
Source: Modified from Quality Standards Subcommittee of the American Academy of Neurology: *The American Academy of Neurology Practice Handbook.* The American Academy of Neurology, St. Paul, MN, 1997.

contact sports for several days at least, and for weeks after a second concussion or if there are protracted neurologic symptoms (Table 357-2). These guidelines are designed to avoid an extremely rare complication of recurrent head injury, termed the *second impact syndrome*, in which devastating cerebral swelling follows a minor head injury superimposed upon a recent concussion. There is some evidence that repeated concussions in football and soccer players are associated with mild but cumulative cognitive deficits.

FURTHER READING

LOVELL MR et al: Recovery from concussion in high school athletes. J Neurosurg 98:296, 2003

ROPPER AH (ed): *Neurological and Neurosurgical Intensive Care*, 4th ed. Philadelphia, Lippincott Williams & Wilkins, 2004

SAVOLA O, HILLBLOM M: Early predictors of post-concussion symptoms in patients with mild head injury. Eur J Neurol 10:175, 2003

Malignant primary tumors of the central nervous system (CNS) occur in ~16,500 individuals and account for an estimated 13,000 deaths in the United States annually, a mortality rate of 6 per 100,000. An approximately equal number of benign tumors of the CNS are diagnosed, with a much lower mortality rate. Glial tumors account for 50 to 60% of primary brain tumors, meningiomas for 25%, schwannomas for 10%, and all other CNS tumors for the remainder.

Brain and vertebral metastases from systemic cancer are more prevalent than primary CNS tumors. About 15% of patients who die of cancer (80,000 individuals each year in the United States) have symptomatic brain metastases; an additional 5% suffer spinal cord involvement. Brain and spinal metastases therefore pose a major problem in the management of systemic cancer.

BRAIN TUMORS

APPROACH TO THE PATIENT

Clinical Features Brain tumors usually present with one of three syndromes: (1) subacute progression of a focal neurologic deficit; (2) seizure; or (3) nonfocal neurologic disorder such as headache, dementia, personality change, or gait disorder. The presence of systemic symptoms such as malaise, weight loss, anorexia, or fever suggests a metastatic rather than a primary brain tumor.

Progressive focal neurologic deficits result from compression of neurons and white matter tracts by expanding tumor and surrounding edema. Less commonly, a brain tumor presents with a sudden stroke-like onset of a focal neurologic deficit. Although this presentation may be caused by hemorrhage into the tumor, often no hemorrhage can be demonstrated and the mechanism is obscure. Tumors frequently associated with hemorrhage include high-grade gliomas and metastatic melanoma and choriocarcinoma.

Seizures may result from disruption of cortical circuits. Tumors that invade or compress the cerebral cortex, even small meningiomas, are more likely to be associated with seizures than subcortical neoplasms. Nonfocal neurologic dysfunction usually reflects increased intracranial pressure (ICP), hydrocephalus, or diffuse tumor spread. Tumors in some areas of the brain may produce behavioral disorders; for example, frontal lobe tumors may present with personality change, dementia, or depression.

Headache may result from focal irritation or displacement of pain-sensitive structures (Chap. 14) or from a generalized increase in ICP. A headache that worsens rather than abates with recumbency is suggestive of a mass lesion. Headaches from increased ICP are usually holocephalic and episodic, occurring more than once a day. They typically develop rapidly over several minutes, persist for 20 to 40 min, and subside quickly. They may awaken the patient from a sound sleep, generally 60 to 90 min after retiring, or may be precipitated by coughing, sneezing, or straining. Vomiting may occur with severe headaches. As elevated ICP becomes sustained, the headache becomes continuous but varying in intensity. Elevated ICP may cause papilledema (Chap. 25), although it is often not present in infants or patients >55 years.

The Karnofsky performance scale is useful in assessing and following patients with brain tumors (Chap. 66). A score ≥70 indicates that the patient is ambulatory and independent in self-care activities; it is often taken as a level of function justifying aggressive therapy.

Laboratory Examination Primary brain tumors typically do not produce serologic abnormalities such as an elevated sedimentation rate or tumor-specific antigens associated with systemic cancers. In contrast, metastases to the nervous system, depending on the type and extent of the primary tumor, may be associated with systemic

signs of malignancy (Chap. 66). Lumbar puncture may precipitate brain herniation in patients with mass lesions and should be performed only in patients with suspected CNS infection or meningeal metastasis. Findings in the cerebrospinal fluid (CSF) of patients with primary and metastatic nervous system tumors may include raised opening pressure, elevated protein level, and a mild lymphocytic pleocytosis. The CSF rarely contains malignant cells, with the important exceptions of leptomeningeal metastases, primary CNS lymphoma, and primitive neuroectodermal tumors, including medulloblastoma.

Neuroimaging Computed tomography (CT) and magnetic resonance imaging (MRI) can reveal mass effect and contrast enhancement. Mass effect reflects the volume of neoplastic tissue as well as surrounding edema. Brain tumors typically produce a vasogenic pattern of edema, with accumulation of excess water in white matter. Contrast enhancement reflects a breakdown of the blood-brain barrier within the tumor, permitting leakage of contrast agent. Low-grade gliomas typically do not exhibit contrast enhancement.

Positron emission tomography (PET) and single-photon emission tomography (SPECT) have ancillary roles in the imaging of brain tumors, primarily in distinguishing tumor recurrence from tissue necrosis that can occur after irradiation (see below). Electroencephalography (EEG) has a role in the evaluation of patients with seizures. Functional imaging with PET, MRI, or magnetoencephalography may be of use in surgical or radiosurgical planning to define the anatomic relationship of the tumor to critical brain regions such as the primary motor or language cortex.

℞ TREATMENT

Symptomatic Glucocorticoids decrease the volume of edema surrounding brain tumors and improve neurologic function; dexamethasone (12 to 20 mg/d in divided doses orally or intravenously) is used because it has relatively little mineralocorticoid activity.

Tumors that involve the cerebral cortex or hippocampus may produce epilepsy. Anticonvulsants are therefore used therapeutically and prophylactically; phenytoin, carbamazepine, and valproic acid are equally effective (Chap. 348). If the tumor is subcortical in location, prophylactic anticonvulsants are unnecessary.

Gliomas and primary CNS lymphomas are associated with an increased risk for deep vein thrombosis and pulmonary embolism, probably because these tumors secrete procoagulant factors into the systemic circulation. Even though hemorrhage within gliomas is a frequent histopathologic finding, patients appear to be at no increased risk for symptomatic intracranial bleeding following treatment with an anticoagulant. Prophylaxis with low-dose subcutaneous heparin should be considered for patients with brain tumors who have lower limb immobility, which places them at risk for deep venous thrombosis.

PRIMARY BRAIN TUMORS

ETIOLOGY Exposure to ionizing radiation is the only well-documented environmental risk factor for the development of gliomas. A number of hereditary syndromes are associated with an increased risk of brain tumors (Table 358-1). Genes that contribute to the development of brain tumors, as well as other malignancies, fall into two general classes, *tumor-suppressor genes* and *proto-oncogenes* (Chap. 68). Whereas germ-line mutations of tumor-suppressor genes are rare, somatic mutations are almost invariably found in malignant tumors, including brain tumors. Likewise, the activation of proto-oncogenes occurs frequently in brain tumors. Moreover, cytogenetic analysis often reveals characteristic changes. In astrocytic tumors, DNA is commonly lost on chromosomes 10p, 17p, 13q, and 9. Oligodendrogliomas frequently have deletions of 1p and 19q. In meningiomas portions of 22q, which contains the gene for neurofibromatosis (NF) type 2, are often lost. In approximately one-third of glioblastomas, there is amplification of the *EGFR* gene.

The particular constellation of genetic alterations varies among individual gliomas, even those that are histologically indistinguishable. Moreover, gliomas are genetically unstable. Genetic abnormalities tend to accumulate with time, and these changes correspond with an increasingly malignant phenotype. There are at least two genetic routes for the development of malignant glioma (Fig. 358-1). One route involves the progression, generally over years, from a low-grade astrocytoma with deletions of chromosome 17 and inactivation of the *p53* gene to a malignant glioma with additional chromosomal alterations. The second route is characterized by the de novo appearance of a malignant glioma with amplification of the *EGFR* gene and an intact *p53* gene. In both pathways, inactivation of the *PTEN* gene as a result of the loss of chromosome 10 occurs frequently.

ASTROCYTOMAS Tumors with astrocytic cytologic features are the most common primary intracranial neoplasms (Fig. 358-2). The most widely used histologic grading system is the World Health Organization four-tiered grading system. Grade I is reserved for special histologic variants of astrocytoma that have an excellent prognosis after surgical excision. These include *juvenile pilocytic astrocytoma, subependymal giant cell astrocytoma* (which occurs in patients with tuberous sclerosis), and *pleiomorphic xanthoastrocytoma*. At the other extreme is grade IV, *glioblastoma multiforme*, a clinically aggressive tumor. *Astrocytoma* (grade II) and *anaplastic astrocytoma* (grade III) are intermediate in their histologic and clinical manifestations. The histologic features associated with higher grade are hypercellularity, nuclear and cytoplasmic atypia, endothelial proliferation, mitotic activity, and necrosis. Endothelial proliferation and necrosis are predictors of aggressive behavior.

A limitation of all grading schemes, especially when applied to a single biopsy, is that astrocytic tumors are histologically variable from region to region, and their histopathology may change with time. It is common for low-grade astrocytomas to progress over time to a higher histopathologic grade and a more aggressive clinical course.

Quantitative measures of mitotic activity also correlate with prognosis. The proliferation index can be determined by immunohistochemical staining with antibodies to the proliferating cell nuclear antigen (PCNA) or with a monoclonal antibody termed *Ki-67*, which recognizes a histone protein expressed in proliferating but not quiescent cells. These measures provide estimates of DNA synthesis and correlate with malignant clinical behavior of the tumor.

The overall prognosis is poor. In a representative Finnish population, the median survival was 93.5 months for patients with grade I or II astrocytomas, 12.4 months for patients with grade III (anaplastic astrocytoma), and 5.1 months for patients with grade IV (glioblastoma) tumors. In the United States, the median survival of patients with high-grade brain tumors is ~12 months. Clinical features that correlate with poor prognosis include age >65 and a poor functional status, as defined by the Karnofsky performance scale.

TABLE 358-1 *Hereditary Syndromes Associated with Brain Tumors*

Syndrome	Gene (Locus)	Gene Product (Function)	Nervous System Neoplasms
Neurofibromatosis type 1 (von Recklinghausen's Disease)[a]	*NF1* (17q)	Neurofibromin (GTPase activating protein)	Neuroma, schwannoma, meningioma, optic glioma
Neurofibromatosis type 2[a]	*NF2* (22q)	Merlin (cytoskeletal protein)	Schwannoma, glioma, ependymoma, meningioma
Tuberous sclerosis	*TSC1* (9q)	Hamartin (unknown function)	Astrocytoma
	TSC2 (16p)	Tuberin (GTPase activating protein)	
von Hippel-Lindau[a]	*VHL* (3p)	pVHL (modulator of cellular hypoxic response)	Hemangioblastoma of retina, cerebellum and spinal cord; pheochromocytoma
Li-Fraumeni[a]	*p53* (17p)	TP53 (cell cycle and transcriptional regulator)	Malignant glioma
Retinoblastoma[a]	*RB1* (13q)	RB (cell cycle regulator)	Retinoblastoma, pineoblastoma, malignant glioma
Turcot	*APC* (5q) (adenomatous polyposis coli)	APC (cell adhesion)	Medulloblastoma, malignant glioma
Gorlin (basal cell nevus syndrome)	*PTCH* (9q) (patched)	PTH (developmental regulator)	Medulloblastoma
Multiple endocrine neoplasia 1 (Werner syndrome)[a]	*MEN1* (11q13)	Menin (cofactor for transcription)	Pituitary adenoma, malignant schwannoma

[a] Genetic testing possible.

Low-Grade Astrocytoma Low-grade astrocytomas are more common in children than adults. Pilocytic astrocytoma, named for its characteristic spindle-shaped cells, is the most common childhood brain tumor. It frequently occurs in the cerebellum. Typically, this tumor is cystic and well demarcated from adjacent brain. Complete surgical excision usually produces long-term, disease-free survival.

The optimal management of grade II astrocytomas, termed *fibril-*

FIGURE 358-1 Model for the pathogenesis of human astrocytoma. Glioblastoma multiforme (GBM) typically presents without evidence of a precursor lesion, referred to as de novo GBM, frequently associated with amplification of the epidermal growth factor receptor (*EGFR*) gene. Less commonly, GBM arises in association with progressive genetic alterations after the diagnosis of a lower grade astrocytoma. These tumors are referred to as secondary GBM. The most widely described alterations are mutations of *p53* and *INK4a*. Other genes implicated in the development of these primary brain tumors include *CDK4*, *MDM2*, *DCC*, and *PDGFR*. LOH, loss of heterozygosity.

FIGURE 358-2 Malignant astrocytoma (glioblastoma). Coronal proton density–weighted MR scan through the temporal lobes demonstrates a heterogeneous right temporal lobe mass (*arrows*) compressing the third and lateral ventricles. The area of hypointense signal (*double arrows*) indicates either hemorrhage or calcification. Heterogeneous MR signal intensity is typical of glioblastoma.

lary astrocytomas, is controversial. For patients who are symptomatic from mass effect or poorly controlled epilepsy, surgical excision can relieve symptoms. For patients who are asymptomatic or minimally symptomatic at presentation, a diagnostic biopsy should be performed and, when surgically feasible, the tumor may be resected. The indications for postoperative radiation therapy are uncertain. In many centers, when only a biopsy or partial resection is possible, postoperative external beam radiation therapy is administered, whereas it is not used if a gross total tumor resection can be achieved. Other centers reserve radiation therapy for tumor recurrence or progression, at which time the tumor may display a more malignant phenotype. No role for chemotherapy in the management of low-grade astrocytoma has been defined.

High-Grade Astrocytoma The large majority of astrocytomas arising in adults are high grade, supratentorial, and do not have a clearly defined margin. Neoplastic cells migrate away from the main tumor mass and infiltrate adjacent brain, often tracking along white matter pathways. Imaging studies do not indicate the full extent of the tumor. These tumors are eventually fatal, although prolonged survival occurs in a few patients. Longer survival correlates with younger age, better performance status, and greater extent of surgical resection. Late in their course, gliomas, especially those located in the posterior fossa, can metastasize along CSF pathways to the spine. Metastases outside the CNS are rare.

High-grade astrocytomas are managed with glucocorticoids, surgery, radiation therapy, and chemotherapy. Dexamethasone is generally administered at the time of diagnosis and continued for the duration of radiation therapy. After completion of radiation therapy, dexamethasone is tapered to the lowest tolerated dose.

Because astrocytomas infiltrate adjacent normal brain, total surgical excision is not possible. Surgery is indicated to obtain tissue for pathologic diagnosis and to control mass effect. Moreover, retrospective studies indicate that the extent of tumor resection correlates with survival, at least in younger patients. Therefore, accessible astrocytomas are resected aggressively in patients <65 years old who are in good general medical condition.

Postoperative radiation therapy prolongs survival and improves quality of life, although the duration of benefit is only a few months. Treated with dexamethasone alone following surgery, the mean sur-

vival of patients <65 years with glioblastoma is 7 to 9 months. Survival is prolonged to 11 to 13 months with radiation therapy. Focal brain irradiation is less toxic and is as effective as whole-brain radiation for primary glial tumors. Radiation is generally administered to the tumor mass, as defined by contrast enhancement on a CT or MRI scan, plus a 3- to 4-cm margin. A total dose of 5000 to 7000 cGy is administered in 25 to 35 equal fractions, 5 days per week.

The roles of stereotaxic radiosurgery and interstitial brachytherapy in glioma treatment are uncertain. *Stereotaxic radiosurgery* is the administration of a focused high dose of radiation to a precisely defined volume of tissue in a single treatment. Stereotaxic radiosurgery can potentially achieve tumor ablation within the treated volume. A major limitation of stereotaxic radiosurgery is that it can be used for only relatively small tumors, generally <4 cm in maximum diameter. *Interstitial brachytherapy*, the implantation of radioactive material into the tumor mass, is generally reserved for tumor recurrence because of its associated toxicity—in particular, necrosis of adjacent brain tissue.

Chemotherapy is marginally effective and is often used as an adjuvant therapy following surgery and radiation therapy. Nitrosoureas, including carmustine (BCNU) and lomustine (CCNU), are the most effective available agents. Since a typical glioma infiltrates normal brain where the blood-brain barrier is relatively intact, lipid-soluble agents such as the nitrosoureas, which cross the blood-brain barrier, may reach more malignant cells than water-soluble agents. Temozolomide is an orally administered alkylating agent, has activity against gliomas, and is generally better tolerated than the nitrosoureas. Experimental approaches include intraarterial infusion of chemotherapy, the implantation of chemotherapy-releasing wafers or injection of chemotherapeutic agents into the tumor resection cavity, and administration of chemotherapy after disruption of the blood-brain barrier.

Gliomatosis cerebri is a rare form of astrocytoma in which there is diffuse infiltration of the brain by malignant astrocytes without a focal enhancing mass. It generally presents as a multifocal CNS syndrome or a more generalized disorder including dementia, personality change, or seizures. Neuroimaging studies are often nonspecific, and biopsy is required to establish the diagnosis. Gliomatosis cerebri is treated with whole-brain radiation therapy and, in selected patients, with radiation to the entire neuroaxis and systemic chemotherapy.

OLIGODENDROGLIOMAS Oligodendrogliomas, which comprise about 15% of gliomas in adults, have a more benign course and are more responsive to cytotoxic treatment than astrocytomas. Five-year survival is >50%, and 10-year survival is 25 to 34%.

Oligodendrogliomas occur chiefly in supratentorial locations; in adults, ~30% contain areas of calcification (Fig. 358-3). Many gliomas contain mixtures of cells with astrocytic and oligodendroglial features. If this mixed histology is prominent, the tumor is termed a *mixed glioma* or an *oligoastrocytoma*. The greater the oligodendroglial component, the more benign the clinical course. As a rule, oligodendrogliomas are less infiltrative than astrocytomas, permitting more complete surgical excision. Histologic features of mitoses, necrosis, and nuclear atypia are associated with a more aggressive clinical course. If these features are prominent, the tumor is termed an *anaplastic oligodendroglioma*.

Surgery, at minimum a stereotaxic biopsy, is necessary to establish a diagnosis. Many oligodendrogliomas are amenable to gross total surgical resection. In addition, oligodendrogliomas may respond dramatically to systemic combination chemotherapy with procarbazine, lomustine, and vincristine (PCV). Oligodendrogliomas with deletions of chromosome 1p always respond to PCV, but only ~25% of oligodendrogliomas lacking 1p deletion respond to chemotherapy. The simultaneous deletion of 1p and 19q predicts a durable response to chemotherapy (>31 months on average) and survival >10 years. Many centers therefore use 1p deletion as an indication for adjuvant or neo-adjuvant chemotherapy and reserve external beam irradiation for tumor recurrence.

EPENDYMOMAS In adults ependymomas are typically located in the spinal canal, especially in the lumbosacral region. They typically arise from the filum terminale of the spinal cord and have a myxopapillary histology, with a papillary arrangement of cells and mucin production. In children, ependymomas occur within the ventricles, most often the fourth ventricle, and have a different histology, typically with ependymal rosettes. Ependymomas with histologic signs of malignancy, including cellular atypia, frequent mitotic figures, or a high labeling index virtually always recur after surgical resection. Imaging with CT or MRI scans reveals ependymomas as uniformly enhancing masses that are relatively well demarcated from adjacent neural tissue. Ependymomas may metastasize via CSF pathways; brain tumor metastases that spread to the spinal cord by this means are termed *drop metastases*.

Following the gross total excision of an ependymoma, the prognosis is excellent. The 5-year disease-free survival is >80%. However, many ependymomas cannot be totally excised, and postoperative focal external beam radiation or stereotaxic radiosurgery is used. Whether focal radiation is adequate or whether the entire neuraxis needs to be irradiated is not known.

FIGURE 358-3 Oligodendroglioma. *A.* Noncontrast CT scan reveals a calcified mass involving the left temporal lobe (*arrows*) associated with mild mass effect but little edema. *B.* An MR T2-weighted image demonstrates a heterogeneous mass with hypointense signal (*black arrows*) surrounded by a zone of higher signal intensity (*white arrows*), consistent with a calcified temporal lobe mass. The tumor extends into the left medial temporal lobe and compresses the midbrain.

GERMINOMAS These tumors most commonly present during the second decade of life, generally at sites within or adjacent to the third ventricle, including the pineal region. Germinomas are the most frequent variety of *germ cell tumor*, a tumor type arising in midline structures and including *teratoma*, yolk sac tumor (*endodermal sinus tumor*), *embryonal carcinoma*, and *choriocarcinoma*. Germinomas of the CNS may be benign but are more often aggressive and invasive. Due to their location, patients frequently present with hypothalamic-pituitary dysfunction including diabetes insipidus, visual field deficits, disturbances of memory or mood, or hydrocephalus (Chap. 318). Neuroimaging demonstrates germinomas to be uniformly enhancing masses that may not have well-defined borders. The treatment of choice is complete surgical resection. For unresectable tumors, a stereotaxic biopsy is performed for diagnosis, and focal radiation is the primary therapy. When the extent of disease or very young age precludes radiotherapy as primary treatment, platinum-based chemotherapy may decrease tumor size and facilitate subsequent radiation therapy of residual disease or recurrent tumor. Prognosis depends on the histology and surgical resectability of the tumor. Germinomas are generally radiosensitive and chemosensitive. Five year survival is >85%.

MEDULLOBLASTOMAS AND PRIMITIVE NEUROECTODERMAL TUMORS (PNET) These highly cellular malignant tumors are thought to arise from neural precursor cells. Medulloblastomas of the posterior fossa are the most frequent malignant brain tumor of children. PNET is a term applied to tumors histologically indistinguishable from medulloblastoma but occurring either in adults or supratentorially in children. In adults, >50% present in the posterior fossa. These tumors frequently disseminate along CSF pathways.

If possible, these tumors should be surgically excised, although outcome is not related to the extent of surgery. In adults, surgical excision of a PNET should be followed by chemotherapy and irradiation of the entire neuraxis, with a boost in radiation dose to the primary tumor. If the tumor is not disseminated at presentation, the prognosis is generally favorable. Aggressive treatment can result in prolonged survival, although half of adult patients relapse within 5 years of treatment.

CNS LYMPHOMA ■ Primary CNS Lymphoma These are high-grade B cell malignancies that present within the neuraxis without evidence of systemic lymphoma. They occur most frequently in immunocompromised individuals, specifically organ transplant recipients or patients with AIDS (Chap. 173). In immunocompromised patients, CNS lymphomas are invariably associated with Epstein-Barr virus infection of the tumor cells.

In immunocompetent patients, neuroimaging studies most often reveal a uniformly enhancing mass lesion. In immunocompromised patients, primary CNS lymphoma is likely to be multicentric and exhibit ring enhancement or to arise in the meninges (Fig. 358-4). Stereotaxic needle biopsy can be used to establish the diagnosis. Leptomeningeal involvement is present in ~15% of patients at presentation and in 50% at some time during the course of the illness. Moreover, the disease extends to the eyes in up to 15% of patients. Therefore, a slit-lamp examination and, if indicated, anterior chamber paracentesis or vitreous biopsy is necessary to define radiation ports.

The prognosis of primary CNS lymphoma is poor compared to histologically similar lymphoma occurring outside the CNS. Many patients experience a dramatic clinical and radiographic response to glucocorticoids; however, relapse almost invariably occurs within weeks. The mainstay of definitive therapy is chemotherapy including high-dose methotrexate. This is followed in patients <60 years with whole-brain irradiation. Whole-brain irradiation is postponed as long as possible in patients >60 because of the risk of dementia as a manifestation of late-delayed radiation toxicity. Consolidation therapy is with high-dose cytarabine. Intraarterial chemotherapy with or without blood-brain barrier disruption is an alternative. Intrathecal chemotherapy with methotrexate can be added if leptomeningeal disease is present. Despite aggressive therapy, >90% of patients develop recurrent CNS disease. Historically, the survival of immunocompetent patients with CNS lymphoma has been ~18 months but is now longer with the use of systemic chemotherapy. In organ transplant recipients, reversal of the immunosuppressed state can improve outcome. Survival with AIDS-related primary CNS lymphoma is very poor, generally ≤3 months; pretreatment performance status, the degree of immunosuppression, and the extent of CNS dissemination at diagnosis all appear to influence outcome.

Secondary CNS Lymphoma Secondary CNS lymphoma is a manifestation of systemic disease and almost always occurs in adults with progressive B cell lymphoma or B cell leukemia who have tumor involvement of bone, bone marrow, testes, or the cranial sinuses. Leptomeningeal lymphoma is usually detectable with contrast-enhanced CT or gado-

FIGURE 358-4 CNS lymphoma. *A.* Proton density–weighted MR image through the temporal lobe demonstrates a low signal intensity nodule (*small arrows*) surrounded by a ring of high signal intensity edema (*larger arrows*). *B.* T1-weighted contrast-enhanced axial MRI demonstrates ring enhancement surrounded by a nonenhanced rim of edema. In this patient with AIDS, a solitary lesion of this type is consistent with either lymphoma or toxoplasmosis; the presence of multiple lesions favors toxoplasmosis. *C.* In a different patient with lymphomatous meningitis, an axial postcontrast T1-weighted MRI through the midbrain demonstrates multiple areas of abnormal enhancement in periventricular and subependymal regions (*arrows*). Lymphoma tends to spread subependymally at interfaces of CSF and brain parenchyma.

linium-enhanced MRI of the brain and spine or by CSF examination. Treatment consists of systemic chemotherapy, intrathecal chemotherapy, and CNS irradiation. It is usually possible to suppress the leptomeningeal disease effectively, although the overall prognosis is determined by the course of the systemic lymphoma.

PITUITARY ADENOMAS   See Chap. 318.

MENINGIOMAS   Meningiomas are derived from mesoderm, probably from cells giving rise to the arachnoid granulations. These tumors are usually benign and attached to the dura. They may invade the skull but only infrequently invade the brain. Meningiomas most often occur along the sagittal sinus, over the cerebral convexities, in the cerebellarpontine angle, and along the dorsum of the spinal cord. They are more frequent in women than men, with a peak incidence in middle age.

Meningiomas may be found incidentally on a CT or MRI scan or may present with a focal seizure, a slowly progressive neurologic deficit, or symptoms of raised ICP. The radiologic image of a dural-based, extraaxial mass with dense, uniform contrast enhancement is essentially diagnostic, although a dural metastasis must also be considered (Fig. 358-5). A meningioma may have a "dural tail," a streak of dural enhancement flanking the main tumor mass; however, this finding may also be present with other dural tumors.

Total surgical resection of benign meningiomas is curative. If a total resection cannot be achieved, local external beam radiotherapy or stereotaxic radiosurgery reduces the recurrence rate to <10%. For meningiomas that are not surgically accessible, targeted radiosurgery or heavy particle radiation should be considered. Small asymptomatic meningiomas incidentally discovered in older patients can safely be followed radiologically; these tumors grow at an average rate of ~0.24 cm in diameter per year and only rarely become symptomatic.

Rare meningiomas invade the brain or have histologic evidence of malignancy such as nuclear pleomorphism and cellular atypia. A high mitotic index is also predictive of aggressive behavior. *Hemangiopericytoma*, although not strictly a meningioma, is a meningeal tumor with an especially aggressive behavior. Meningiomas with features of aggressiveness and hemangiopericytomas, even if totally excised by gross inspection, frequently recur and should receive postoperative radiotherapy. Chemotherapy has no proven benefit.

SCHWANNOMAS   These tumors are also called *neuromas, neurinomas,* or *neurolemmomas.* They arise from Schwann cells of nerve roots, most frequently in the eighth cranial nerve (*vestibular schwannoma,* formerly termed *acoustic schwannoma*). The fifth cranial nerve is the second most frequent site; however, schwannomas may arise from any cranial or spinal root except the optic and olfactory nerves, which are myelinated by oligodendroglia rather than Schwann cells. NF type 2 (see below) strongly predisposes to vestibular schwannoma. Schwannomas of spinal nerve roots also occur in patients with NF type 2 as well as patients with NF type 1.

Eighth nerve schwannomas typically arise from the vestibular division of the nerve. They are densely and uniformly enhancing neoplasms on MRI (Fig. 358-6). Vestibular schwannomas enlarge the internal auditory canal, an imaging feature that helps distinguish them from other cerebellopontine angle masses. Because the vestibular system adapts to slow destruction of the eighth nerve, vestibular schwannomas characteristically present as progressive unilateral hearing loss rather than with dizziness or other vestibular symptoms. Unexplained unilateral hearing loss merits evaluation with audiometry and either brainstem auditory evoked potentials or an MRI scan (Chap. 26). As

FIGURE 358-5   Meningioma. Coronal postcontrast T1-weighted MR image demonstrates an enhancing extraaxial mass arising from the falx cerebri (*arrows*). There is a "dural tail" of contrast enhancement extending superiorly along the intrahemispheric septum.

a vestibular schwannoma grows, it can compress the cerebellum, pons, or facial nerve. With rare exceptions schwannomas are histologically and clinically benign.

Whenever possible, schwannomas should be surgically excised. When the tumors are small, it is usually possible to preserve hearing in the involved ear. In the case of large tumors, the patient is usually deaf at presentation; nonetheless, surgery is indicated to prevent further compression of posterior fossa structures. Stereotaxic radiosurgery is also effective treatment for schwannoma and has a complication rate equivalent to that of surgery.

OTHER BENIGN BRAIN TUMORS *Epidermoid tumors* are cystic tumors with proliferative epidermal cells at the periphery and more mature epidermal cells towards the center of the cyst. The mature cells desquamate into the liquid center of the cyst. Epidermoid tumors are thought to arise from embryonic epidermal rests within the cranium. They occur extraaxially near the midline, in the middle cranial fossa, the suprasellar region, or the cerebellopontine angle. These well-demarcated lesions are amenable to complete surgical excision. Postoperative radiation therapy is unnecessary.

Dermoid cysts are thought to arise from embryonic rests of skin tissue trapped within the CNS during closure of the neural tube. The most frequent locations are in the midline supratentorially or at the cerebellopontine angle. Histologically, they are composed of all elements of the dermis, including epidermis, hair follicles, and sweat glands; they frequently calcify. Treatment is surgical excision.

Craniopharyngiomas are thought to arise from remnants of Rathke's pouch, the mesodermal structure from which the anterior pituitary gland is derived (Chap. 318). Craniopharyngiomas typically present as suprasellar masses. Histologically, craniopharyngiomas resemble epidermoid tumors; they are usually cystic, and in adults 80% are calcified. Because of their location, they may present as growth failure in children, endocrine dysfunction in adults, or visual loss in either age group. Treatment is surgical excision; postoperative external beam radiation or stereotaxic radiosurgery is added if total surgical removal cannot be achieved.

Colloid cysts are benign tumors of unknown cellular origin that occur within the third ventricle and can obstruct CSF flow. *Rare benign primary brain tumors* include neurocytomas, subependymomas, and pleomorphic xanthoastrocytomas. Surgical excision of these neoplasms is the primary treatment and can be curative.

NEUROCUTANEOUS SYNDROMES

This group of genetic disorders, also known as the *phakomatoses*, produces a variety of developmental abnormalities of skin along with an increased risk of nervous system tumors (Table 358-1). These disorders are inherited as autosomal dominant conditions with variable penetrance.

NEUROFIBROMATOSIS TYPE 1 (VON RECKLINGHAUSEN'S DISEASE) NF1 is characterized by cutaneous *neurofibromas*, pigmented lesions of the skin called *café au lait spots*, freckling in non-sun-exposed areas such as the axilla, hamartomas of the iris termed *Lisch nodules*, and pseudoarthrosis of the tibia. Neurofibromas are benign peripheral nerve tumors composed of proliferating Schwann cells and fibroblasts. They present as multiple, palpable, rubbery, cutaneous tumors. They are generally asymptomatic; however, if they grow in an enclosed space, e.g., the intervertebral foramen, they may produce a compressive radiculopathy or neuropathy. Aqueductal stenosis with hydrocephalus, scoliosis, short stature, hypertension, epilepsy, and mental retardation may also occur.

Patients with NF1 are at increased risk of developing nervous system neoplasms, including plexiform neurofibromas, optic pathway gliomas, ependymomas, meningiomas, astrocytomas, and pheochro-

FIGURE 358-6 Vestibular schwannoma. *A.* Axial noncontrast MR scan through the cerebellopontine angle demonstrates an extraaxial mass that extends into a widened internal auditory canal, displacing the pons (*arrows*). *B.* Postcontrast T1-weighted image demonstrates intense enhancement of the vestibular schwannoma (*white arrow*). Abnormal enhancement of the left fifth nerve (*black arrow*) most likely represents another schwannoma in this patient with neurofibromatosis type 2.

mocytomas. Neurofibromas may undergo secondary malignant degeneration and become sarcomatous.

Mutation of the *NF1* gene on chromosome 17 causes von Recklinghausen's disease. The *NF1* gene is a tumor-suppressor gene; it encodes a protein, *neurofibromin*, which modulates signal transduction through the *ras* GTPase pathway.

NEUROFIBROMATOSIS TYPE 2 NF2 is characterized by the development of bilateral vestibular schwannomas in >90% of individuals who inherit the gene. Patients with NF2 also have a predisposition for the development of meningiomas, gliomas, and schwannomas of cranial and spinal nerves. In addition, a characteristic type of cataract, juvenile posterior subcapsular lenticular opacity, occurs in NF2. Multiple café au lait spots and peripheral neurofibromas occur rarely.

In patients with NF2, vestibular schwannomas usually present with progressive unilateral deafness early in the third decade of life. Bilateral vestibular schwannomas are generally detectable by MRI at that time (Fig. 358-6). Surgical management is designed to treat the underlying tumor and preserve hearing as long as possible.

This syndrome is caused by mutation of the *NF2* gene on chromosome 22q; *NF2* encodes a protein called *neurofibromin 2, schwannomin*, or *merlin*, with homology to a family of cytoskeletal proteins that includes moesin, ezrin, and radixin.

TUBEROUS SCLEROSIS (BOURNEVILLE'S DISEASE) Tuberous sclerosis is characterized by cutaneous lesions, seizures, and mental retardation. The cutaneous lesions include adenoma sebaceum (facial angiofibromas), ash leaf–shaped hypopigmented macules (best seen under ultraviolet illumination with a Wood's lamp), shagreen patches (yellowish thickenings of the skin over the lumbosacral region of the back), and depigmented nevi. On neuroimaging studies, the presence of subependymal nodules, which may be calcified, is characteristic. Patients inheriting the tuberous sclerosis gene are at increased risk of developing ependymomas and childhood astrocytomas, of which >90% are *subependymal giant cell astrocytomas*. These are benign neoplasms that may develop in the retina or along the border of the lateral ventricles. They may obstruct the foramen of Monro and produce hydrocephalus. Rhabdomyomas of the myocardium and angiomyomas of the kidney, liver, adrenals, and pancreas may also occur.

Treatment is symptomatic. Anticonvulsants for seizures, shunting for hydrocephalus, and behavioral and educational strategies for mental retardation are the mainstays of management. Severely affected individuals generally die before age 30.

Mutations at both 9q(*TSC-1*) and 16p(*TSC-2*) are associated with tuberous sclerosis. The mutated genes encode *tuberins*, proteins that modulate the GTPase activity of other cellular proteins.

FIGURE 358-7 Brain metastasis. *A.* Axial T2-weighted MRI through the lateral ventricles reveals two isodense masses, one in the subependymal region and one near the cortex (*arrows*). *B.* T1-weighted postcontrast image at the same level as *A* reveals enhancement of the two masses seen on the T2-weighted image as well as a third mass in the left frontal lobe (*arrows*).

VON HIPPEL–LINDAU SYNDROME

This syndrome consists of retinal, cerebellar, and spinal hemangioblastomas, which are slowly growing cystic tumors. Hypernephroma, renal cell carcinoma, pheochromocytoma, and benign cysts of the kidneys, pancreas, epididymis, or liver may also occur. Erythropoietin production by hemangioblastomas may result in polycythemia. The von Hippel–Lindau (*VHL*) gene on chromosome 3p is a tumor suppressor that encodes a protein with multiple functions, including mediating signal transduction in response to cellular hypoxia.

TUMORS METASTATIC TO BRAIN

MECHANISMS OF BRAIN METASTASES The large majority of brain metastases disseminate by hematogenous spread. The anatomic distribution of brain metastases generally parallels regional cerebral blood flow, with a predilection for the gray matter–white matter junction and for the border zone between middle cerebral and posterior cerebral artery distributions. The lung is the most common origin of brain metastases; both primary lung cancer (adenocarcinoma and small cell lung cancer) and cancers metastatic to the lung can metastasize to the brain. Breast cancer (especially ductal carcinoma) has a propensity to metastasize to the cerebellum and the posterior pituitary gland. Moreover, breast cancer that metastasizes to bone tends not to metastasize to the brain. Other common origins of brain metastases are gastrointestinal malignancies, and melanoma (Table 358-2). Certain less common tumors have a special propensity to metastasize to brain, including germ cell tumors and thyroid cancer. By contrast, prostate cancer, ovarian cancer, and Hodgkin's disease rarely metastasize to the brain.

EVALUATION OF METASTASES FROM KNOWN CANCER On MRI scans brain metastases typically appear as well-demarcated, approximately spherical lesions that are hypointense or isointense relative to brain on T1-weighted images and bright on T2-weighted images. They invariably enhance with gadolinium, reflecting extravasation of gadolinium through tumor vessels that lack a blood-tumor barrier (Fig. 358-7).

Small metastases often enhance uniformly. Larger metastases typically produce ring enhancement surrounding a central mass of nonenhancing necrotic tissue that develops as the metastasis outgrows its blood supply. Metastases are surrounded by variable amounts of edema. Blood products may also be seen, reflecting hemorrhage of abnormal tumor vessels.

The radiologic appearance of a brain metastasis is not specific. The differential diagnosis of ring-enhancement lesions includes brain abscess, radiation necrosis, toxoplasmosis, granulomas (tuberculosis, sarcoidosis), demyelinating lesions, primary brain tumors, primary CNS lymphoma, stroke, hemorrhage, and trauma. Contrast-enhanced CT scanning is less sensitive than MRI for the detection of brain metastases. Cytologic examination of the CSF is not indicated, since intraparenchymal brain metastases almost never shed cells into the CSF. Measuring CSF levels of tumor markers such as carcinoembryonic antigen (CEA) is rarely helpful in management.

BRAIN METASTASES WITHOUT A KNOWN PRIMARY TUMOR In general hospital populations, up to one-third of patients presenting with brain metastases do not have a known underlying cancer. These patients generally present with either a seizure or a progressive neurologic deficit. Neuroimaging studies demonstrate one or multiple ring-enhancement lesions. In individuals who are not immunocompromised and not at risk for brain abscesses, this radiologic pattern is most likely due to brain metastasis.

Diagnostic evaluation begins with a search for the primary tumor. Blood tests should include CEA and liver function tests. Examination of the skin for melanoma and the thyroid gland for masses should be carried out. A CT scan of the chest, abdomen, and pelvis should be obtained. If these are all negative, further imaging studies, including bone scan, other radionuclide scans, mammography, and upper and lower gastrointestinal barium studies, are unlikely to be productive. The search for a primary cancer most often discloses lung cancer, particularly small cell lung cancer, or melanoma. In 30% of patients no primary tumor can be identified, even after extensive evaluation.

A tissue diagnosis is essential. If a primary tumor is found, it will usually be more accessible to biopsy than a brain lesion. If a single brain lesion is found in a surgically accessible location, if a primary tumor is not found, or if the primary tumor is in a location difficult to biopsy, the brain metastasis should be biopsied or resected.

℞ TREATMENT

Once a systemic cancer metastasizes to the brain it is, with rare exception, incurable. Therapy is therefore palliative, designed to prevent disability and suffering and, if possible, to prolong life. Published outcome studies have focused on survival as the primary end point, leaving questions regarding quality of life unanswered. There is, however, widespread agreement that glucocorticoids, anticonvulsants, and radiation therapy improve the quality of life for many patients. The roles of surgery and chemotherapy are less well established.

General Measures Glucocorticoids frequently ameliorate symptoms of brain metastases. Improvement is often dramatic, occurs within 24 h, and is sustained with continued administration, although the toxicity of glucocorticoids is cumulative. Therefore, if possible, a more definitive therapy for metastases should be instituted to permit withdrawal of glucocorticoid therapy. One-third of patients with brain metastases have one or more seizures. Anticonvulsants are used empirically for seizure prophylaxis when supratentorial metastases are present.

Specific Measures ▪ *RADIATION THERAPY* Radiation is the primary treatment for brain metastases. Since multiple microscopic deposits of tu-

---

TABLE 358-2	Frequency of Nervous System Metastases by Common Primary Tumors		
Site of Primary Tumor	Brain Metastases, %	Leptomeningeal Metastases, %	Spinal Cord Compression, %
Lung	40	24	18
Breast	19	41	24
Melanoma	10	12	4
Gastrointestinal tract	7	13	6
Genitourinary tract	7		18
Other	17	10	30

mor cells throughout the brain are likely to be present in addition to metastases visualized by neuroimaging studies, whole-brain irradiation is usually used. Its benefit has been established in controlled studies, but no clear dose response has been shown. Usually, 30 to 37.5 Gy is administered in 10 to 15 fractions; an additional dose ("boost") of focal irradiation to a single or large metastasis may also be administered. Stereotaxic radiosurgery is of benefit in patients with four or fewer metastases demonstrable by MRI.

SURGERY Up to 40% of patients with brain metastases have only a single tumor mass identified by CT. Accessible single metastases are usually surgically excised as a palliative measure. If the systemic disease is under control, total resection of a single brain lesion has been demonstrated to improve survival and minimize disability. Survival appears to be improved if surgery is followed by whole-brain irradiation.

CHEMOTHERAPY Brain metastases of certain tumors, including breast cancer, small cell lung cancer, and germ cell tumors, are often responsive to systemic chemotherapy. Although metastases frequently do not respond as well as the primary tumor, dramatic responses to systemic chemotherapy or hormonal therapy may occur in some cases. In patients who are neurologically stable, two to four cycles of systemic chemotherapy may be administered initially to reduce tumor mass and render the residual tumor more amenable to radiation therapy. Even if a complete radiologic remission is achieved from chemotherapy, whole-brain irradiation should then be administered.

EXPERIMENTAL THERAPIES These include gene therapy, immunotherapy, intraarterial chemotherapy, and chemotherapy administered following osmotic disruption of the blood-brain barrier.

LEPTOMENINGEAL METASTASES

Leptomeningeal metastases are also called *carcinomatous meningitis, meningeal carcinomatosis*, and, in the cases of specific tumors, *leukemic meningitis* or *lymphomatous meningitis*. Clinical evidence of leptomeningeal metastases is present in 8% of patients with metastatic solid tumors; at necropsy, the prevalence is as high as 19%. Among solid tumors, adenocarcinomas of the breast, lung, and gastrointestinal tract and melanoma are the most common cause of leptomeningeal metastases (Table 358-2). In one-quarter of patients the systemic cancer is under control; thus effective control of leptomeningeal disease can improve the quality and duration of life.

Cancer usually metastasizes to the meninges via the bloodstream. Alternatively, a superficially located parenchymal brain metastasis may shed cells directly into the subarachnoid space. Some tumors, including squamous cell carcinoma of the skin and some non-Hodgkin's lymphomas, have a propensity to grow along peripheral nerves and may seed the meninges by that route.

CLINICAL FEATURES Leptomeningeal metastases present with signs and symptoms at multiple levels of the nervous system, most often in a setting of known systemic malignancy. Encephalopathy is frequent, and cranial neuropathy or spinal radiculopathy from nodular nerve root compression is characteristic. Hydrocephalus results from obstruction of CSF outflow. Focal neurologic deficits from coexisting intraparenchymal metastases may occur.

LABORATORY EVALUATION Leptomeningeal metastases are diagnosed by cytologic demonstration of malignant cells in the CSF, by MRI demonstration of nodular tumor deposits in the meninges or diffuse meningeal enhancement (Fig. 358-8), or by meningeal biopsy. CSF findings are usually those of an inflammatory meningitis, consisting of lymphocytic pleocytosis, elevated protein levels, and normal or low CSF glucose. A complete MRI examination of the neuraxis may demonstrate hydrocephalus due to obstruction of CSF pathways and identify nodular meningeal metastases.

℞ TREATMENT

In selected patients, intrathecal chemotherapy or focal external beam radiotherapy to sites of nodular leptomeningeal disease is employed.

FIGURE 358-8 Carcinomatous meningitis. Sagittal postcontrast MRI through the lower thoracic region demonstrates diffuse pial enhancement along the surface of the spinal cord (*arrows*), typical of CSF spread of neoplasm.

Although the prognosis of leptomeningeal metastases is poor, ~20% of patients treated aggressively for leptomeningeal metastases can expect a response of ≥6 months. Intrathecal therapy exposes meningeal tumor implants to high concentrations of chemotherapy with minimal systemic toxicity. Methotrexate can be safely administered intrathecally and is effective against leptomeningeal metastases from a variety of solid tumors and lymphoma; cytarabine and thiotepa are alternative agents. Intrathecal chemotherapy may be administered either by repeated lumbar puncture or through an indwelling Ommaya reservoir, which consists of a catheter in one lateral ventricle attached to a reservoir implanted under the scalp. If there is a question of patency of CSF pathways, a radionuclide flow study through the reservoir may be performed.

Large, nodular deposits of tumor on the meninges or along nerve roots are unlikely to respond to intrathecal chemotherapy, as the barrier to diffusion is too great. Therefore, external beam radiation is employed. Hydrocephalus is treated with a ventriculoperitoneal shunt, although seeding of the peritoneum by tumor is a risk.

MALIGNANT SPINAL CORD COMPRESSION

Spinal cord compression from solid tumor metastases usually results from expansion of a vertebral metastasis into the epidural space. Primary tumors that frequently metastasize to bone include lung, breast, and prostate cancer. Back pain is usually the first symptom and is prominent at presentation in 90% of patients. The pain is typically dull, aching, and may be associated with localized tenderness. If a nerve root is compressed, radicular pain is also present. The thoracic cord is most often affected. Weakness, sensory loss, and autonomic dysfunction (urinary urgency and incontinence, fecal incontinence, and sexual impotence in men) are the hallmarks of spinal cord compression. Once signs of spinal cord compression appear, they tend to progress rapidly. It is thus essential to recognize and treat this serious complication of malignancy promptly in order to prevent irreversible neurologic deficits. →*Diagnosis and management are discussed in Chap. 356.*

METASTASES TO THE PERIPHERAL NERVOUS SYSTEM

Systemic cancer may compress or invade peripheral nerves. Compression of the brachial plexus may occur by direct extension of Pancoast's tumors (cancer of the apex of the lung) or by extension of local lymph node metastases of breast or lung cancer or lymphoma. The lumbosacral plexus may be compressed by the retroperitoneal spread of prostate or ovarian cancer or lymphoma. Skull metastases may compress cranial nerve branches as they pass through the skull, and pituitary metastases may extend into the cavernous sinus. The epineurium generally provides an effective barrier to invasion of the peripheral nerves by solid tumors, but certain tumors characteristically invade and spread along peripheral nerves. Squamous cell carcinoma of the skin may spread along the trigeminal nerve and extend intracranially. Non-Hodgkin's lymphoma may be neurotrophic and cause polyradiculopathy or a syndrome resembling mononeuropathy multiplex. Focal external beam radiation may reduce pain, prevent irreversible loss of peripheral nerve function, and possibly restore function.

In patients with cancer who have brachial or lumbosacral plexopathy, it may be difficult to distinguish tumor invasion from radiation injury. High radiation dose or the presence of myokymia (rippling contractions of muscle) suggests radiation injury, whereas pain suggests tumor. Radiographic imaging studies may be equivocal, and surgical exploration is sometimes required.

COMPLICATIONS OF THERAPY

RADIATION TOXICITY   The nervous system is vulnerable to injury by therapeutic radiation. Histologically, there is demyelination, degeneration of small arterioles, and eventually brain infarction and necrosis.

Acute radiation injury occurs during or immediately after therapy. It is rarely seen with current protocols of external beam radiation but may occur after stereotaxic radiosurgery. Manifestations include headache, sleepiness, and worsening of preexisting neurologic deficits.

Early delayed radiation injury occurs within 4 months of therapy. It is associated with an increased white matter T2 signal on MRI scans. In children, the *somnolence syndrome* is a common form of early delayed radiation injury in which somnolence and ataxia develop after whole-brain irradiation. Irradiation of the cervical spine may cause Lhermitte's phenomenon, an electricity-like sensation evoked by neck flexion. Acute and early delayed radiation injury are self-limited and glucocorticoid-responsive disorders that do not appear to increase the risk of late radiation injury.

Late delayed radiation injury produces permanent damage to the nervous system. It occurs >4 months (generally 8 to 24 months) after completion of therapy; onset 15 years after therapy has been described. After whole-brain irradiation, progressive dementia can occur, sometimes accompanied by gait apraxia. White matter signal abnormalities are present on MRI studies (Fig. 358-9). Following focal brain irradiation, radiation necrosis occurs within the radiation field producing a contrast-enhancing (frequently ring-enhancing) mass. MRI or CT scans are often unable to distinguish radiation necrosis from recurrent tumor, but PET or SPECT scans may demonstrate that glucose metabolism is increased in tumor tissue but decreased in radiation necrosis. Magnetic resonance spectroscopy may demonstrate a high lactate concentration with relatively low choline concentration in areas of necrosis. Biopsy is frequently required to establish the correct diagnosis. Peripheral nerves, including the brachial and lumbosacral plexuses, may also develop late delayed radiation injury.

If untreated, radiation necrosis of the CNS may act as an expanding mass lesion, although it may resolve spontaneously or after treatment with glucocorticoids. Progressive radiation necrosis is best treated with surgical resection if the patient has a life expectancy of at least 6 months and a Karnofsky performance score >70. There are anecdotal reports that anticoagulation with heparin or warfarin may be beneficial. Radiation injury also accelerates the development of atherosclerosis in large arteries, but an increase in the risk of stroke becomes significant only years after radiation treatment.

Endocrine dysfunction frequently follows exposure of the hypothalamus or pituitary gland to therapeutic radiation. Growth hormone is the pituitary hormone most sensitive to radiation therapy, and thyroid-stimulating hormone is the least sensitive; ACTH, prolactin, and the gonadotropins have an intermediate sensitivity.

Development of a second neoplasm is another risk of therapeutic radiation that generally occurs many years after radiation exposure. Depending on the irradiated field, the risk of gliomas, meningiomas, sarcomas, and thyroid cancer is increased.

COMPLICATIONS OF CHEMOTHERAPY   Chemotherapy regimens used to treat primary brain tumors have generally included a nitrosourea and are well tolerated. Infrequently, nitrosoureas and other drugs used to treat CNS neoplasms cause altered mental states (e.g., confusion, depression), ataxia, and seizures. Chemotherapy for systemic malignancy is a more frequent cause of nervous system toxicity. Cisplatin commonly produces tinnitus and high-frequency bilateral hearing loss, especially in younger patients. At cumulative doses, >450 mg/m², cisplatin can produce a symmetric, large-fiber axonal neuropathy that is predominantly sensory; paclitaxel (Taxol) produces a similar picture. Fluorouracil and high-dose cytarabine can cause cerebellar dysfunction that resolves after discontinuation of therapy. Vincristine, which is commonly used to treat lymphoma, may cause an acute ileus and is frequently associated with development of a progressive distal, symmetric sensory-motor neuropathy with foot drop and paresthesia.

FIGURE 358-9   Radiation injury. *A.* Late-delayed radiation injury 1 year after whole-brain radiation (5500 cGy). T2-weighted MR image at the level of the temporal lobes reveals high signal intensity abnormality in periventricular white matter (*arrows*). *B* and *C.* Focal radiation necrosis 3 years after radiotherapy (7000 cGy) for carcinoma of the nasopharynx. Axial T2-weighted MRI (*B*) demonstrates a mass in the right frontal lobe with surrounding vasogenic edema. Abnormal signal changes are also present on the left. T1-weighted postcontrast MRI (*C*) reveals a heterogeneously enhancing mass in the right cingulate gyrus.

BEHIN A et al: Primary brain tumors in adults. Lancet 361:323, 2003
GLANTZ M et al: Temozolomide as an alternative to irradiation for elderly patients with newly diagnosed malignant gliomas. Cancer 97:2262, 2003

ZHU Y, PARADA LF: The molecular and genetic basis of neurological tumors. Nat Rev Cancer 2:616, 2002

359 MULTIPLE SCLEROSIS AND OTHER DEMYELINATING DISEASES
Stephen L. Hauser, Douglas S. Goodin

Demyelinating disorders are characterized by inflammation and selective destruction of central nervous system (CNS) myelin. The peripheral nervous system (PNS) is spared, and most patients have no evidence of an associated systemic illness.

MULTIPLE SCLEROSIS

Multiple sclerosis (MS) is characterized by a triad of inflammation, demyelination, and gliosis (scarring); the course can be relapsing-remitting or progressive. Lesions of MS are typically disseminated in time and location. MS affects ~350,000 Americans and 1.1 million individuals worldwide. In western societies, MS is second only to trauma as a cause of neurologic disability in early to middle adulthood. Manifestations of MS vary from a benign illness to a rapidly evolving and incapacitating disease requiring profound life-style adjustments.

PATHOGENESIS ■ Anatomy These lesions (plaques) vary in size from 1 or 2 mm to several centimeters. Acute MS lesions are characterized by perivenular cuffing with inflammatory mononuclear cells, predominantly T cells and macrophages, which also infiltrate the surrounding white matter. At sites of inflammation, the blood-brain barrier (BBB) is disrupted but, unlike vasculitis, the vessel wall is preserved. In more than half of cases, myelin-specific autoantibodies promote demyelination and stimulate macrophages and microglial cells (bone marrow—derived CNS phagocytes) that scavenge the myelin debris. As lesions evolve, astrocytes proliferate (gliosis). Surviving oligodendrocytes or those that differentiate from precursor cells may partially remyelinate the surviving naked axons, producing so-called shadow plaques. Ultrastructural studies of MS lesions suggest that fundamentally different underlying pathologies may exist in different patients. Heterogeneity has been observed in terms of: (1) whether the inflammatory cell infiltrate is associated with deposition of antibody and activation of complement, and (2) whether the target of the immunopathologic process is the myelin sheath itself or the cell body of the oligodendrocyte. Although sparing of axons is typical of MS, partial or total axonal destruction can also occur. Indirect evidence suggests that axonal loss is a major cause of irreversible neurologic disability in MS.

Physiology Nerve conduction in myelinated axons occurs in a saltatory manner, with the nerve impulse jumping from one node of Ranvier to the next without depolarization of the axonal membrane underlying the myelin sheath between nodes (Fig. 359-1). This produces considerably faster conduction velocities (~70 m/s) than the slow velocities (~1 m/s) produced by continuous propagation in unmyelinated nerves. Conduction block occurs when the nerve impulse is unable to traverse the demyelinated segment. This can happen when the resting axon membrane becomes hyperpolarized due to the exposure of voltage-dependent potassium channels that are normally buried underneath the myelin sheath. A temporary conduction block often follows a demyelinating event before the sodium channels (originally concentrated at the nodes) have had a chance to redistribute themselves along the naked axon (Fig. 359-1). This redistribution ultimately allows the continuous propagation of nerve action potentials through the demyelinated segment but, before this happens, the leakage currents are too large for the nerve impulse to jump the internode distance and conduction fails. On occasion, conduction block is incomplete, affecting, for example, high- but not low-frequency volleys of impulses. Variable conduction block can occur with raised body temperature or metabolic alterations and may explain clinical fluctuations (typical of MS) that

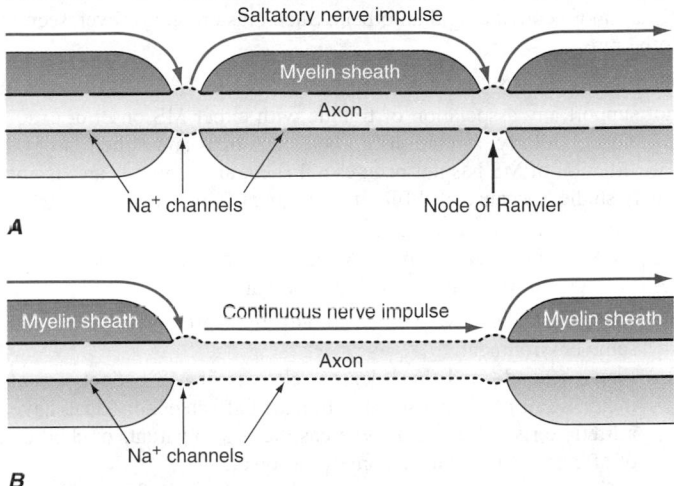

FIGURE 359-1 Nerve conduction in myelinated and demyelinated axons. *A.* Saltatory nerve conduction in myelinated axons occurs with the nerve impulse jumping from one node of Ranvier to the next. Sodium channels are concentrated at the nodes where axonal depolarization occurs. *B.* Following demyelination, the sodium channels are redistributed along the axon, thereby supporting continuous propagation of the nerve action potential in this region.

vary from hour to hour or in association with fever or exercise. Conduction slowing occurs when the demyelinated segments support only (slow) continuous nerve impulse propagation.

Epidemiology MS is approximately twice as common in women as in men. The age of onset is typically between 20 and 40 years (slightly later in men than in women). Rarely, it can begin as early as 2 years of age or as late as the eighth decade.

The highest known prevalence for MS (250 per 100,000) occurs in the Orkney islands, located north of Scotland, and similarly high rates are found throughout northern Europe, the northern United States, and Canada. By contrast, the prevalence is low in Japan (2 per 100,000), in other parts of Asia, in equatorial Africa, and in the Middle East. In general, prevalence increases with increasing distance from the equator, although certain exceptions are notable. Thus, the incidence of MS in the Eskimo population of Alaska is rare compared to the incidence in Caucasians living at similar latitudes. Similarly, native South Africans have a markedly lower prevalence compared to South Africans of European descent who live in the same geographic area. However, distinctive migration patterns of certain populations may artifactually suggest a relationship between MS and climate. Thus, when Scandanavians migrated to the United States or when the Scots migrated to New Zealand, they tended to migrate preferentially to places (e.g., the northern United States or southern New Zealand) with similar climates to their native lands. Such considerations point to potential genetic mechanisms (see below) rather than to an influence of temperate climate per se.

CHANGES IN INCIDENCE/PREVALENCE Studies from the United States, Europe, Australia, and the Middle East suggest that the prevalence of MS may be increasing, although improved methods of diagnosis may account for the apparent change. Other reports suggest that individuals who move from an area of high prevalence to one of low prevalence (or vice versa) before the age of 15 years adopt the risk of MS in their new environment, whereas if they move after this age, they retain the risk of their native land. The reliability of these observations is uncertain, although, if correct, they would suggest an environmental factor in the pathogenesis of MS.

REPORTED CLUSTERS   Clusters of MS cases are occasionally reported. Often these apparent epidemics cannot be distinguished easily from chance occurrences, although some reports (e.g., the clustering of MS cases in the Faeroe Islands after British occupation during World War II) are more convincing than others. Such clustering, however, seems to be rare.

The Relationship of MS to Trauma and Stress   The existing evidence does not support any association of trauma with either MS onset or exacerbation. Similarly, a relationship between stress and either onset or exacerbation of MS has not been established, although this area is not easily studied because of difficulties in quantifying stress.

GENETIC CONSIDERATIONS   A genetic susceptibility to MS exists, as evidenced by the following observations:

1. The prevalence of MS differs among ethnic groups residing in the same environment.
2. First-, second-, and third-degree relatives of MS patients are at increased risk for the disease. Siblings of affected individuals have a lifetime risk of 2 to 5%, whereas the risk to parents or children of affected individuals is somewhat lower.
3. Twin studies demonstrate concordance rates of 25 to 30% in monozygotic twins compared to only 2 to 5% in dizygotic twins (similar to the risk in nontwin siblings).

The inheritance of MS cannot be explained by a simple genetic model. Susceptibility is probably polygenic, with each gene contributing a relatively small amount to the overall risk. It is also likely that genetic heterogeneity (different susceptibilities among individuals) also exists. The major histocompatibility complex (MHC) on chromosome 6p21 (encoding proteins involved in presenting peptide antigens to T cells) is the most important MS susceptibility region identified to date. MS susceptibility is associated with the class II region of the MHC, specifically with the DR2 (DRB1*1501) allele and its corresponding haplotype. Other genetic regions implicated in MS susceptibility are located on chromosomal regions 19q35 and 17q13.

Immunology   An autoimmune cause for MS is supported by the laboratory model of experimental allergic encephalomyelitis (EAE) and by studies of the immune system in MS patients.

AUTOREACTIVE T LYMPHOCYTES   Myelin basic protein (MBP) is an important T cell antigen in EAE and probably also in human MS. Activated MBP-reactive T cells are often found in the blood or cerebrospinal fluid (CSF) of MS patients and, occasionally also, in MS lesions. Moreover, DR2 may influence the autoimmune response because it binds with high affinity to a fragment of MBP (spanning amino acids 89 to 96), stimulating T cell responses to this self-protein.

AUTOANTIBODIES   Autoantibodies, directed against myelin antigens such as myelin oligodendrocyte glycoprotein (MOG), probably act in concert with a pathogenic T cell response to cause the demyelinating lesions in many patients. Recent evidence suggests that the presence of anti MOG antibodies in the serum of patients with a clinically isolated syndrome (CIS) is highly predictive of the development of MS in the future. Also, evidence of an abnormal humoral immune response is present in the CSF of MS patients. Membrane attack complexes (from complement-mediated antibody damage) can be detected in CSF, and elevated CSF immunoglobulin (synthesized locally) is characteristic of MS. Oligoclonal antibody (derived from expansion of a selected group of plasma cells) is present in most cases. Oligoclonal immunoglobulin is also detected in other chronic inflammatory conditions,

including infections, and thus is not specific to MS. The pattern of banding is unique to each individual, and attempts to identify the targets of these antibodies have been unsuccessful.

CYTOKINES (Chap. 295)   The proinflammatory T_H1 cytokines such as interleukin (IL) 2, tumor necrosis factor (TNF) α, and interferon (IFN) γ are thought to be central to MS pathogenesis and some (e.g., TNF-α and IFN-γ) may directly injure oligodendrocytes or the myelin membranes. Nevertheless, the notion of an isolated T_H1 imbalance causing MS is probably simplistic. The presence of autoantibodies in MS suggests that regulatory T_H2 cytokines (including IL-4, -5, and -10) may also play a pathogenic role. Moreover, T_H1-based therapies have often proved to be unhelpful or, in the case of certain TNF-α inhibitors, harmful to patients.

TRIGGERS   Magnetic resonance imaging (MRI) has demonstrated bursts of disease activity 7 to 10 times more frequently than is clinically apparent. This finding indicates that there is a large reservoir of subclinical disease activity in MS, especially during the early stages of the disease. The triggers causing these bursts are unknown, although the fact that patients may experience relapses after nonspecific upper respiratory infections suggests that either molecular mimicry between viruses and myelin antigens or viral superantigens activating pathogenic T cells may play a role in MS pathogenesis. (Chap. 299).

Microbiology   As noted above, epidemiologic evidence supports the role of an environmental exposure in MS. MS risk also correlates with high socioeconomic status, which may reflect improved sanitation and delayed initial exposures to infectious agents. By analogy, some viral infections (e.g., poliomyelitis and measles viruses) produce neurologic sequelae more frequently when the age of initial infection is delayed. The best studied experimental model of virus-induced demyelinating disease is infection with Theiler virus, a murine coronavirus similar to measles, which produces a chronic oligodendrocyte infection with multifocal perivascular lymphocytic infiltration and demyelination, closely resembling lesions of MS.

High antibody titers against many viruses have been reported in serum and CSF of MS patients, including measles, herpes simplex, varicella, rubella, Epstein-Barr, and influenza C and some parainfluenza strains. Numerous viruses and bacteria (or their genomic sequences) have been recovered from MS tissues and fluids. Most recently human herpes virus type 6 (HHV-6) and *Chlamydia pneumoniae* have been implicated, although a causal role for any infectious agent in MS remains unproven.

CLINICAL MANIFESTATIONS   The onset of MS may be abrupt or insidious. Symptoms may be severe or seem so trivial that a patient may not seek medical attention for months or years. Indeed, at autopsy some individuals who were asymptomatic during life will be found, unexpectedly, to have MS. In other cases an MRI scan obtained for an unrelated reason may show evidence of asymptomatic MS. Symptoms of MS are extremely varied and depend upon the location of lesions within the CNS (Table 359-1). Examination generally reveals evidence of neurologic dysfunction, often in asymptomatic locations. For example, a patient may present with symptoms in one leg and signs in both.

TABLE 359-1   *Initial Symptoms of MS*

Symptom	Percent of Cases	Symptom	Percent of Cases
Sensory loss	37	Lhermitte	3
Optic neuritis	36	Pain	3
Weakness	35	Dementia	2
Paresthesias	24	Visual loss	2
Diplopia	15	Facial palsy	1
Ataxia	11	Impotence	1
Vertigo	6	Myokymia	1
Paroxysmal attacks	4	Epilepsy	1
Bladder	4	Falling	1

Source: After WD Matthews et al, *McAlpine's Multiple Sclerosis,* New York, Churchill Livingstone, 1991.

Weakness of the limbs may manifest as loss of strength or dexterity, fatigue, or a disturbance of gait. Exercise-induced weakness is a characteristic symptom of MS. The weakness is of the upper motor neuron type (Chap. 20) and is frequently accompanied by other pyramidal signs such as spasticity, hyperreflexia and Babinski signs. Occasionally, a tendon reflex may be lost (simulating a lower motor neuron lesion) if an MS lesion disrupts the afferent reflex fibers in the spinal cord.

Spasticity (Chap. 21) is often associated with spontaneous and movement-induced muscle spasms. More than 30% of MS patients have moderate to severe spasticity, especially in the legs. It is often accompanied by painful spasms and can interfere with a patient's ability to ambulate or work or with self-care. Occasionally, spasticity may provide nonvolitional support for the body weight during ambulation. In these cases, treatment of spasticity may actually do more harm than good.

Optic neuritis (ON) generally presents as diminished visual acuity, dimness, or decreased color perception (desaturation) in the central field of vision. These symptoms may be mild or may progress to severe visual loss. Rarely, there is complete loss of light perception. Visual symptoms are generally monocular but may occur bilaterally. Periorbital pain (aggravated by eye movement) often precedes or accompanies the visual loss. An afferent pupillary defect (Chap. 25) may be found. Funduscopic examination may be normal or reveal optic disc swelling (papillitis). Pallor of the optic disc (optic atrophy) commonly follows ON. Uveitis is rare and should raise the possibility of alternative diagnoses. →*ON is discussed in detail in Chap. 25.*

Visual blurring in MS may result from ON or diplopia. Visual blurring that resolves when either eye is covered is due to diplopia.

Diplopia may result from internuclear ophthalmoplegia (INO) or from palsy of the sixth cranial nerve (rarely the third or fourth). An INO consists of impaired adduction of one eye due to a lesion in the ipsilateral medial longitudinal fasciculus (Chap. 25). Prominent nystagmus is often observed in the abducting eye, along with a small skew deviation. A bilateral INO is particularly suggestive of MS. Other common gaze disturbances in MS include: (1) a horizontal gaze palsy, (2) a "one and a half" syndrome (horizontal gaze palsy plus an INO), and (3) acquired pendular nystagmus.

Sensory symptoms are varied and include both paresthesias (e.g., tingling, prickling sensations, formications, "pins and needles," or painful burning) and hypesthesia (e.g., reduced sensation, numbness or a "dead" feeling). Unpleasant sensations (e.g., feelings that body parts are swollen, wet, raw, or tightly wrapped) are also common. Sensory impairment of the trunk and legs below a horizontal line on the torso (a sensory level) suggests that the spinal cord is the origin of the sensory disturbance. It is often accompanied by a bandlike sensation of tightness around the torso. Pain is a common symptom of MS, experienced by >50% of patients. Pain can occur anywhere on the body and can change locations over time.

Ataxia usually manifests as cerebellar tremors (Chap. 21). Ataxia may also involve the head and trunk or the voice, producing a characteristic cerebellar dysarthria (scanning speech). The true extent of cerebellar involvement may be difficult to determine in an individual patient, because motor and sensory deficits can affect coordination and weakness may interfere with coordination testing.

Bladder and bowel dysfunction arise from different causes and frequently different types of dysfunction coexist. During normal reflex voiding, relaxation of the bladder sphincter (α-adrenergic innervation) is coordinated with contraction of the detrusor muscle in the bladder wall (muscarinic cholinergic innervation). Stoppage of the urinary stream is accomplished with a coordinated sphincter contraction and detrusor relaxation. Bladder-stretch (during filling) activates this reflex, which is inhibited by supraspinal (voluntary) input. Symptoms of bladder dysfunction are present in >90% of MS patients and, in a third, dysfunction results in weekly or more frequent episodes of incontinence.

Detrusor hyperreflexia, due to impairment of suprasegmental inhibition, causes urinary frequency, urgency, nocturia, and uncontrolled bladder emptying. *Detrusor sphincter dyssynergia*, due to loss of synchronization between detrusor and sphincter muscles, causes difficulty in initiating and/or stopping the urinary stream, thereby producing hesitancy. It can also lead to urinary retention, large postvoid residual volumes, overflow incontinence, and recurrent infection.

Constipation occurs in >30% of patients. Fecal urgency or *bowel incontinence* is less common (15%) but can be socially debilitating.

Cognitive dysfunction can include memory loss, impaired attention, difficulties in problem-solving, slowed information processing, and problems shifting between cognitive tasks. Euphoria (elevated mood) was once thought to be characteristic of MS but is actually uncommon, occurring in <20% of patients. Cognitive dysfunction sufficient to impair activities of daily living also occurs but is rare.

Depression, experienced by 50 to 60% of patients, can be reactive, endogenous, or part of the illness itself and can contribute to fatigue. Suicide in MS patients is 7.5-fold more common than in age-matched controls.

Fatigue is experienced by 90% of patients and is moderate or severe in half. Symptoms include generalized motor weakness, limited ability to concentrate, extreme lassitude, loss of energy, decreased endurance, and an overwhelming sense of exhaustion that requires the patient to rest or fall asleep. Fatigue (either alone or with other symptoms) is the most common reason for work-related disability in MS. Fatigue can be exacerbated by elevated temperatures, by depression, by expending exceptional effort to accomplish basic activities of daily living, or by sleep disturbances (e.g., from frequent nocturnal awakenings to urinate). MS-related fatigue may be maximum during mid-afternoon or continuous throughout the day, and it is often difficult to treat.

Sexual dysfunction is common in MS. Men report impotence, less desire, impaired genital sensation, impaired ejaculation, and inability to achieve/maintain an erection. Women report genital numbness, diminished orgasmic response, decreased libido, unpleasant sensations during intercourse, and diminished vaginal lubrication. Adductor spasticity (in women) can also interfere with intercourse, and urinary incontinence (in either men or women) can be problematic.

Facial weakness due to a lesion in the intraparenchymal pathway of the seventh cranial nerve may resemble idiopathic Bell's palsy. However, unlike Bell's palsy, facial weakness in MS is generally not associated with ipsilateral loss of taste sensation or retroauricular pain (Chap. 355).

Vertigo may appear suddenly and resemble acute labyrinthitis. A brainstem rather than end-organ origin is suggested by the presence of coexisting trigeminal or facial nerve involvement; vertical nystagmus; or nystagmus that has no latency to onset, no direction reversal, and doesn't fatigue (Chap. 20). Hearing loss may also occur in MS but is uncommon.

Ancillary Symptoms *Heat sensitivity* refers to neurologic symptoms produced by an elevation of the body's core temperature. For example, transient unilateral visual blurring or loss may occur during a hot shower or with physical exercise (*Uhthoff's symptom*). It is common for MS symptoms to worsen transiently, sometimes dramatically, during febrile illnesses (see pseudoexacerbation, below). Such heat-related symptoms probably result from transient conduction block (see above).

Lhermitte's symptom is the electric shock–like sensation (evoked by neck flexion or other movement) that radiates down the back into the legs. Rarely, it radiates into the arms. It is generally self-limited but may persist for years. Lhermitte's symptom can also occur with other disorders of the cervical spine (e.g., cervical spondylosis).

Paroxysmal symptoms are distinguished by their brief duration (30 s to 2 min), high frequency (5 to 40 episodes per day), lack of any alteration of consciousness or change in background electroencephalogram during episodes, and a self-limited course (generally lasting weeks to months). They may be precipitated by hyperventilation or movement. These syndromes include Lhermitte's symptom; tonic contractions of a limb, face, or trunk (tonic seizures); paroxysmal dysarthria/ataxia; paroxysmal sensory disturbances; and several other less well characterized syndromes. Paroxysmal symptoms probably result from spontaneous discharges, arising at the edges of demyelinated plaques, and spreading ephaptically to adjacent white matter tracts.

Trigeminal neuralgia, hemifacial spasm, and glossopharyngeal neuralgia can occur when the demyelinating lesion involves the root entry (or exit) zone of the fifth, seventh, and ninth cranial nerve, respectively. *Trigeminal neuralgia* (tic douloureux) is a very brief lancinating facial pain often triggered by an afferent input from the face or teeth. Most cases of trigeminal neuralgia are not MS-related. However, the occurrence of atypical features (Chap. 355) such as the onset before age 50 years, bilateral symptoms, objective sensory loss, or nonparoxysmal pain should raise concerns that a symptomatic cause such as MS is responsible.

Facial myokymia consists of either persistent rapid flickering contractions of the facial musculature (especially the lower portion of the orbicularis oculus) or a contraction that slowly spreads across the face. It results from lesions of the corticobulbar tracts or brainstem course of the facial nerve.

DISEASE COURSE   Four clinical types of MS have been described (Fig. 359-2):

1. *Relapsing/remitting MS* (RRMS) accounts for 85% of MS cases at onset and is characterized by discrete attacks that generally evolve over days to weeks (rarely over hours). Often, but not invariably, there is complete recovery over the ensuing weeks to months (Fig. 359-2*A*). However, when ambulation is severely impaired during an attack, approximately half will fail to improve. Between attacks, patients are neurologically stable.

2. *Secondary progressive MS* (SPMS) always begins as RRMS (Fig. 359-2*B*). At some point, however, the RRMS clinical course changes so that the patient experiences a steady deterioration in function unassociated with acute attacks (which may continue or cease during the progressive phase). SPMS produces a greater amount of fixed neurologic disability than RRMS. Approximately 50% of patients with RRMS will have developed SPMS after 15 years, and longer follow-up points indicate that the great majority of RRMS ultimately evolves into SPMS. Thus, SPMS appears to represent a late-stage of the same underlying illness as RRMS.

3. *Primary progressive MS* (PPMS) accounts for ~15% of cases. These patients do not experience attacks but only a steady functional decline from disease onset (Fig. 359-2*C*). Compared to RRMS, the

sex distribution is more even, the disease begins later in life (mean age, ~40 years), and disability develops faster. Whether PPMS is an unusual phenotype of the same underlying illness as RRMS or whether these are distinct illnesses is unknown.

4. *Progressive/relapsing MS* (PRMS) overlaps PPMS and SPMS and accounts for ~5% of MS patients. Like patients with PPMS, these patients experience a steady deterioration in their condition from disease onset. However, like SPMS patients, they experience occasional attacks superimposed upon their progressive course (Fig. 359-2*D*). The early stages of RPMS are indistinguishable from those of PPMS (i.e., until the first clinical attack).

DIAGNOSIS   There is no definitive diagnostic test for MS. Diagnostic criteria for clinically definite MS require documentation of two or more episodes of symptoms and two or more signs that reflect pathology in anatomically noncontiguous white matter tracts of the CNS (Table 359-2). Symptoms must last for >24 h and occur as distinct episodes that are separated by a month or more. At least one of the two required signs must be present on neurologic examination. The second may be documented by certain abnormal paraclinical tests such as MRI or evoked potentials (EPs). In patients who experience gradual progression of disability for ≥6 months without superimposed relapses, documentation of intrathecal IgG and visual EP testing may be used to support the diagnosis.

DIAGNOSTIC TESTS ■ **Magnetic Resonance Imaging**   MRI has revolutionized the diagnosis and management of MS (Fig. 359-3); characteristic abnormalities are found in >95% of patients. An increase in vascular permeability from a breakdown of the BBB is detected by leakage of intravenous gadolinium (Gd) into the parenchyma. Such leakage occurs early in the development of an MS lesion and serves as a useful marker of inflammation. Gd-enhancement persists for up to 3 months, and the residual MS plaque remains visible indefinitely as a focal area of hyperintensity (a lesion) on spin-echo (T2-weighted) and proton-density images. Lesions are frequently oriented perpendicular to the

TABLE 359-2   Diagnostic Criteria for MS
1. Examination must reveal *objective* abnormalities of the CNS.
2. Involvement must reflect predominantly disease of white matter long tracts, usually including (a) pyramidal pathways, (b) cerebellar pathways, (c) medial longitudinal fasciculus, (d) optic nerve, and (e) posterior columns.

3. Examination or history must implicate involvement of two or more areas of the CNS.
   a. MRI may be used to document a second lesion when only one site of abnormality has been demonstrable on examination. A confirmatory MRI must have either four lesions involving the white matter or three lesions if one is periventricular in location. Acceptable lesions must be >3 mm in diameter. For patients older than 50 years, two of the following criteria must also be met: (a) lesion size >5 mm, (b) lesions adjacent to the bodies of the lateral ventricles, and (c) lesion(s) present in the posterior fossa.
   b. Evoked response testing may be used to document a second lesion not evident on clinical examination.

4. The clinical pattern must consist of (a) two or more separate episodes of worsening involving different sites of the CNS, each lasting at least 24 h and occurring at least 1 month apart, or (b) gradual or stepwise progression over at least 6 months if accompanied by increased IgG synthesis or two or more oligoclonal bands. MRI may be used to document dissemination in time if a new T2 lesion or a Gd-enhancing lesion is seen 3 or more months after a clinically isolated syndrome.
5. The patient's neurologic condition could not better be attributed to another disease.
DIAGNOSTIC CATEGORIES
1. *Definite MS:* All five criteria fulfilled.
2. *Probable MS:* All five criteria fulfilled except (a) only one objective abnormality despite two symptomatic episodes or (b) only one symptomatic episode despite two or more objective abnormalities.
3. *At risk for MS:* Criteria 1, 2, 3, and 5 fulfilled; patient has only one symptomatic episode and one objective abnormality.

FIGURE 359-2   Clinical course of multiple sclerosis (MS). *A.* Relapsing/remitting MS. *B.* Secondary progressive MS. *C.* Primary progressive MS. *D.* Progressive/relapsing MS.

Note: CNS, central nervous system; MRI, magnetic resonance imaging; Gd, gadolinium.

ventricular surface, corresponding to the pathologic pattern of perivenous demyelination (Dawson's fingers). Lesions are multifocal within the brain, brainstem, and spinal cord. Lesions in the anterior corpus callosum are helpful diagnostically because this site is usually spared in cerebrovascular disease. Different criteria for the use of MRI in the diagnosis of MS have been proposed (Table 359-2).

The total volume of T2-weighted signal abnormality (the "burden of disease") shows a significant (albeit weak) correlation with clinical disability. Approximately one-third of T2-weighted lesions appear as hypointense lesions (black holes) on T1-weighted imaging. Black holes may be a better marker of irreversible demyelination and axonal loss than T2 hyperintensities, although even this measure depends upon the timing of the image acquisition (e.g., most acute Gd-enhancing T2 lesions are T1 dark).

Newer MRI measures such as brain atrophy, magnetization transfer ratio (MTR) imaging and proton magnetic resonance spectroscopic imaging (MRSI) may ultimately serve as surrogate markers of clinical disability. For example, MRSI can quantitate molecules such as *N*-acetyl aspartate (NAA), which is a marker of axonal integrity, and MTR may be able to distinguish demyelination from edema.

Evoked Potentials EP testing assesses function in afferent (visual, auditory, and somatosensory) or efferent (motor) CNS pathways. EPs use computer averaging to measure CNS electric potentials evoked by repetitive stimulation of selected peripheral nerves or of the brain. These tests provide the most information when the pathways studied are clinically uninvolved. For example, in a patient with a remitting and relapsing spinal cord syndrome with sensory deficits in the legs, an abnormal somatosensory EP following posterior tibial nerve stimulation provides little new information. By contrast, an abnormal visual EP in this circumstance would permit a diagnosis of clinically definite MS (Table 359-2). Abnormalities on one or more EP modalities occur in 80 to 90% of MS patients. EP abnormalities are not specific to MS, although a marked delay in the latency of a specific EP component (as opposed to a reduced amplitude) is suggestive of demyelination.

Cerebrospinal Fluid CSF abnormalities found in MS include a mononuclear cell pleocytosis and an increased level of intrathecally synthesized IgG. The total CSF protein is usually normal or slightly elevated. Various formulas distinguish intrathecally synthesized IgG from IgG that may have entered the CNS passively from the serum. One formula (the CSF IgG index) expresses the ratio of IgG to albumin in the CSF divided by the same ratio in the serum. A more complicated formula, the IgG synthesis rate, makes certain assumptions but uses the same serum and CSF IgG and albumin measurements to calculate the rate of CNS IgG synthesis. The measurement of oligoclonal banding (OCB) in the CSF also assesses intrathecal production of IgG. OCBs are detected by agarose gel electrophoresis. Two or more OCBs are

FIGURE 359-3 MRI findings in MS. *A.* Axial first-echo image from T2-weighted sequence demonstrates multiple bright signal abnormalities in white matter, typical for MS. *B.* Sagittal T2-weighted FLAIR (fluid attenuated inversion recovery) image in which the high signal of CSF has been suppressed. CSF appears dark, while areas of brain edema or demyelination appear high in signal as shown here in the corpus callosum (*arrows*). Lesions in the anterior corpus callosum are frequent in MS and rare in vascular disease. *C.* Sagittal T2-weighted fast spin echo image of the thoracic spine demonstrates a fusiform high signal intensity lesion in the mid thoracic spinal cord. *D.* Sagittal T1-weighted image obtained after the intravenous administration of gadolinium DTPA reveals focal areas of blood-brain barrier disruption, identified as high-signal-intensity regions (*arrows*).

found in 75 to 90% of patients with MS. OCBs may be absent at the onset of MS, and in individual patients the number of bands present may increase with time. It is important that paired serum samples be studied to exclude a peripheral (i.e., non-CNS) origin of any OCBs detected in the CSF.

A mild CSF pleocytosis (>5 cells/μL) is present in ~25% of cases, usually in young patients with RRMS. A pleocytosis of >75 cells/μL, the presence of polymorphonuclear leukocytes, or a protein concentration of >1.0 g/L (>100 mg/dL) in CSF should raise concern that the patient may not have MS.

DIFFERENTIAL DIAGNOSIS No single clinical sign or test is diagnostic of MS. The diagnosis is readily made in a young adult with relapsing and remitting symptoms involving different areas of CNS white matter. The possibility of an alternative diagnosis should always be considered (Table 359-3), particularly when (1) symptoms are localized exclusively to the posterior fossa, craniocervical junction, or spinal cord; (2) the patient is <15 or >60 years of age; (3) the clinical course is progressive from onset; (4) the patient has never experienced visual, sensory, or bladder symptoms; or (5) laboratory findings (e.g., MRI, CSF, or EPs) are atypical. Similarly, uncommon or rare symptoms in

TABLE 359-3 Disorders that Can Mimic MS

Acute disseminated encephalomyelitis (ADEM)
Antiphospholipid antibody syndrome
Behçet's disease
Cerebral autosomal dominant arteriopathy, subcortical infarcts, and
   leukoencephalopathy (CADASIL)
Congenital leukodystrophies (e.g., adrenoleukodystrophy, metachromatic
   leukodystrophy)
Human immunodifficiency virus (HIV) infection
Ischemic optic neuropathy (arteritic and nonarteritic)
Lyme disease
Mitochondrial encephalopathy with lactic acidosis and stroke (MELAS)
Neoplasms (e.g., lymphoma, glioma, meningioma)
Sarcoid
Sjögren's syndrome
Stroke and ischemic cerebrovascular disease
Syphilis
Systemic lupus erythematosus and related collagen vascular disorders
Tropical spastic paraparesis (HTLV I/II infection)
Vascular malformations (especially spinal dural AV fistulas)
Vasculitis (primary CNS or other)
Vitamin B_{12} deficiency

Note: HTLV, human T cell leukemia/lymphoma virus; AV, arteriovenous; CNS, central
nervous system.

MS (e.g., aphasia, parkinsonism, chorea, isolated dementia, severe muscular atrophy, peripheral neuropathy, episodic loss of consciousness, fever, headache, seizures, or coma) should increase concern about an alternative diagnosis. Diagnosis is also difficult in patients with a rapid or explosive (stroke-like) onset or with mild symptoms and a normal neurologic examination. Rarely, intense inflammation and swelling may produce a mass lesion that mimics a primary or metastatic tumor. The specific tests required to exclude alternative diagnoses will vary with each clinical situation; however, an erythrocyte sedimentation rate, serum B_{12} level, ANA, and VDRL should probably be obtained in all patients with suspected MS.

PROGNOSIS Most patients with MS experience progressive neurologic disability. Fifteen years after onset, only 20% of patients have no functional limitation; half will have progressed to SPMS and will require assistance with ambulation. Twenty-five years after onset, >80% of MS patients will have reached this level of disability. In 1998, it was estimated that the total annual economic burden of MS in the United States exceeded $6.8 billion.

However, even if the prognosis for disability is grave for the average patient, the prognosis in an individual is difficult to establish. Certain clinical features suggest a more favorable prognosis. Patients with ON or sensory symptoms at onset, patients who recover completely from early attacks, patients <40 years at onset (but not beginning in childhood), women, patients with RRMS, patients with fewer than two relapses in the first year of illness, and patients with minimal impairment after 5 years do better than patients without these clinical features. By contrast, patients with truncal ataxia, action tremor, pyramidal symptoms, or a progressive disease course are more likely to become disabled. A purely progressive disease course carries a graver outlook at all disease stages than does a disease course accompanied by occasional relapses.

Importantly, some MS patients have a benign variant of MS and never develop neurologic disability. The likelihood of having benign MS is thought to be <20%, although it may be underestimated by existing natural history studies. One recent study of patients with benign MS 15 years after onset reported that, although most patients had developed disability by 25 years, those patients with entirely normal neurologic examinations maintained their benign course.

In patients with their first demyelinating event (i.e., a clinically isolated syndrome), the brain MRI provides prognostic information. With three or more typical T2-weighted lesions, the risk of developing MS after 10 years is 70 to 80%. Conversely, with a normal brain MRI,

the likelihood of developing MS is <20%. Similarly, two or more Gd-enhancing lesions at baseline is highly predictive of future MS, as is the appearance of either new T2-weighted lesions or new Gd enhancement ≥3 months after the episode. Typical abnormalities on EP testing and CSF examination provide similar prognostic information, although these relationships are not as well characterized.

Mortality as a direct consequence of MS is uncommon, although it has been estimated that the 25-year survival is only 85% of expected. Death can occur during an acute MS attack, although this is distinctly rare. More commonly, death occurs as a complication of MS (e.g., pneumonia in a debilitated individual). Death also results from suicide.

Effect of Pregnancy Pregnant MS patients experience fewer attacks than expected during gestation (especially in the last trimester) but more attacks than expected in the first 3 months post-partum. When considering the pregnancy year as a whole (i.e., 9 months pregnancy plus 3 months post-partum), the overall disease course is unaffected. Decisions about childbearing should thus be made based upon (1) the mother's physical state, (2) her ability to care for the child, and (3) the availability of social support. Disease-modifying therapy is generally discontinued during pregnancy, although the actual risk from the interferons and glatiramer acetate (see below) appears to be quite low.

℞ TREATMENT

Current therapy for MS can be divided into several categories: (1) treatment of acute attacks as they occur; (2) treatment with disease-modifying agents that reduce the biological activity of MS, and (3) symptomatic therapy. Treatments that promote remyelination or neural repair do not currently exist but would be highly desirable.

The Kurtzke Expanded Disability Status Score (EDSS) is a measure of neurologic impairment in MS (Table 359-4). The EDSS provides a useful snapshot of the disease status of a patient at a given time and a composite picture of the disease course over time. Most patients with EDSS scores <3.5 have RRMS, walk normally, and are not disabled; by contrast, patients with EDSS scores >5.5 have progressive MS (SPMS or PPMS) and are gait-impaired and occupationally disabled.

Acute Attacks or Initial Demyelinating Episodes When patients experience an acute deterioration, it is important to consider whether this change reflects new disease activity or a "pseudoexacerbation" resulting from an increase in ambient temperature, fever, or an infection. In such instances, glucocorticoid treatment is inappropriate. Glucocorticoids are used to manage either first attacks or acute exacerbations. They provide short-term clinical benefit by reducing the severity and shortening the duration of attacks. Whether treatment provides any long-term benefit on the course of the illness is less clear. As a result, mild attacks are often not treated. Physical and occupational therapy can help with mobility and manual dexterity.

Glucocorticoid treatment is administered as intravenous methylprednisolone, 500 to 1000 mg/d for 3 to 5 days, either without a taper or followed by a course of oral prednisone beginning at a dose of 60 to 80 mg/d and gradually tapered over 2 weeks. Outpatient treatment is usually possible. If intravenous therapy is unavailable or inconvenient, oral glucocorticoids can be substituted.

Side effects of short-term glucocorticoid therapy include fluid retention, potassium loss, weight gain, gastric disturbances, acne, and emotional lability. Concurrent use of a low-salt, potassium-rich diet and avoidance of potassium-wasting diuretics is advisable. Lithium carbonate (300 mg orally bid) may help to manage emotional lability and insomnia associated with glucocorticoid therapy. Patients with a history of peptic ulcer disease may require cimetidine (400 mg bid) or ranitidine (150 mg bid).

Plasma exchange (7 exchanges: 54 mL/kg or 1.1 plasma volumes per exchange, every other day for 14 days) may benefit patients with fulminant attacks of demyelination (not only MS) that are unresponsive to glucocorticoids. However, because the cost is high, and the evidence of efficacy is preliminary, plasma exchange should be considered only in selected cases.

TABLE 359-4 *Scoring Systems for MS*

KURTZKE EXPANDED DISABILITY STATUS SCORE (EDSS)

0.0 = Normal neurologic exam [all grade 0 in functional status (FS)]	6.0 = Unilateral assistance required to walk about 100 m with or without resting
1.0 = No disability, minimal signs in one FS (i.e., grade 1)	6.5 = Constant bilateral assistance required to walk about 20 m without resting
1.5 = No disability, minimal signs in more than one FS (more than one grade 1)	7.0 = Unable to walk beyond about 5 m even with aid; essentially restricted to wheelchair; wheels self and transfers alone
2.0 = Minimal disability in one FS (one FS grade 2, others 0 or 1)	7.5 = Unable to take more than a few steps; restricted to wheelchair; may need aid to transfer
2.5 = Minimal disability in two FS (two FS grade 2, others 0 or 1)	8.0 = Essentially restricted to bed or chair or perambulated in wheelchair, but out of bed most of day; retains many self-care functions; generally has effective use of arms
3.0 = Moderate disability in one FS (one FS grade 3, others 0 or 1) or mild disability in three or four FS (three/four FS grade 2, others 0 or 1) though fully ambulatory	8.5 = Essentially restricted to bed much of the day; has some effective use of arm(s); retains some self-care functions
3.5 = Fully ambulatory but with moderate disability in one FS (one grade 3) and one or two FS grade 2; or two FS grade 3; or five FS grade 2 (others 0 or 1)	9.0 = Helpless bed patient; can communicate and eat
4.0 = Ambulatory without aid or rest for ≥ 500 m	9.5 = Totally helpless bed patient; unable to communicate or eat
4.5 = Ambulatory without aid or rest for ≥ 300 m	10.0 = Death due to MS
5.0 = Ambulatory without aid or rest for ≥ 200 m	
5.5 = Ambulatory without aid or rest for ≥ 100 m	

FUNCTIONAL STATUS (FS) SCORE

A. Pyramidal functions
 0 = Normal
 1 = Abnormal signs without disability
 2 = Minimal disability
 3 = Mild or moderate paraparesis or hemiparesis, or severe monoparesis
 4 = Marked paraparesis or hemiparesis, moderate quadriparesis, or monoplegia
 5 = Paraplegia, hemiplegia, or marked quadriparesis
 6 = Quadriplegia

B. Cerebellar functions
 0 = Normal
 1 = Abnormal signs without disability
 2 = Mild ataxia
 3 = Moderate truncal or limb ataxia
 4 = Severe ataxia all limbs
 5 = Unable to perform coordinated movements due to ataxia

C. Brainstem functions
 0 = Normal
 1 = Signs only
 2 = Moderate nystagmus or other mild disability
 3 = Severe nystagmus, marked extraocular weakness, or moderate disability of other cranial nerves
 4 = Marked dysarthria or other marked disability
 5 = Inability to swallow or speak

D. Sensory functions
 0 = Normal
 1 = Vibration or figure-writing decrease only, in 1 or 2 limbs
 2 = Mild decrease in touch or pain or position sense, and/or moderate decrease in vibration in 1 or 2 limbs, or vibratory decrease alone in 3 or 4 limbs
 3 = Moderate decrease in touch or pain or position sense, and/or essentially lost vibration in 1 or 2 limbs, or mild decrease in touch or pain, and/or moderate decrease in all proprioceptive tests in 3 or 4 limbs
 4 = Marked decrease in touch or pain or loss of proprioception, alone or combined, in 1 or 2 limbs or moderate decrease in touch or pain and/or severe proprioceptive decrease in more than 2 limbs

 5 = Loss (essentially) of sensation in 1 or 2 limbs or moderate decrease in touch or pain and/or loss of proprioception for most of the body below the head
 6 = Sensation essentially lost below the head

E. Bowel and bladder functions
 0 = Normal
 1 = Mild urinary hesitancy, urgency, or retention
 2 = Moderate hesitancy, urgency, retention of bowel or bladder, or rare urinary incontinence
 3 = Frequent urinary incontinence
 4 = In need of almost constant catheterization
 5 = Loss of bladder function
 6 = Loss of bowel and bladder function

F. Visual (or optic) functions
 0 = Normal
 1 = Scotoma with visual acuity (corrected) better than 20/30
 2 = Worse eye with scotoma with maximal visual acuity (corrected) of 20/30 to 20/59
 3 = Worse eye with large scotoma, or moderate decrease in fields, but with maximal visual acuity (corrected) of 20/60 to 20/99
 4 = Worse eye with marked decrease of fields and maximal acuity (corrected) of 20/100 to 20/200; grade 3 plus maximal acuity of better eye of 20/60 or less
 5 = Worse eye with maximal visual acuity (corrected) less than 20/200; grade 4 plus maximal acuity of better eye of 20/60 or less
 6 = Grade 5 plus maximal visual acuity of better eye of 20/60 or less

G. Cerebral (or mental) functions
 0 = Normal
 1 = Mood alteration only (does not affect EDSS score)
 2 = Mild decrease in mentation
 3 = Moderate decrease in mentation
 4 = Marked decrease in mentation
 5 = Chronic brain syndrome—severe or incompetent

Source: After JF Kurtzke, Neurology 33:1444, 1983.

Disease-Modifying Therapies for Relapsing Forms of MS (RRMS SPMS with Exacerbations) Four such agents are approved in the United States: (1) IFN-β1a (Avonex), (2) IFN-β1a (Rebif); (3) IFN-β1b (Betaseron); and (4) glatiramer acetate (Copaxone). Each of these treatments is also used in SPMS patients who still experience attacks, because SPMS can be difficult to distinguish from RRMS and the clinical trials suggest that such patients also derive therapeutic benefit. In Phase III clinical trials, recipients of IFNβ1b, IFNβ1a, and glatiramer acetate experienced ~30% fewer clinical exacerbations and fewer new MRI lesions compared to placebo recipients. Mitoxantrone (Novantrone), an immune suppressant, has also been approved in the United States, although, because of its potential toxicity, it is generally reserved for patients with progressive disability who have failed other treatments.

INTERFERON β AND GLATIRAMER ACETATE IFN-β is a class I interferon originally identified by its antiviral properties. Efficacy in MS, however,

probably results from immunomodulatory properties including: (1) downregulating expression of MHC molecules on antigen-presenting cells; (2) inhibiting proinflammatory and increasing regulatory cytokine levels; (3) inhibition of T cell proliferation; and (4) limiting the trafficking of inflammatory cells in the CNS. Glatiramer acetate is a synthetic, random polypeptide composed of four amino acids (L-glutamic acid, L-lysine, L-alanine, and L-tyrosine). Its mechanism of action may include: (1) induction of antigen-specific suppressor T cells; (2) binding to MHC molecules, thereby displacing bound MBP; or (3) altering the balance between proinflammatory and regulatory cytokines.

IFN-β reduces the attack rate (whether measured clinically or by MRI) in MS patients. It also improves disease severity measures such as EDSS progression and MRI-documented disease burden. The efficacy of IFN-β in SPMS patients is less convincing than the efficacy in RRMS patients. IFN-β should be considered in patients with either RRMS or SPMS with superimposed relapses. In patients with SPMS but without relapses, efficacy has not been established. Higher IFN-β doses appear to have slightly greater efficacy but are also more likely to induce neutralizing antibodies, which may reduce the clinical benefit (see below).

Glatiramer acetate also reduces the attack rate (whether measured clinically or by MRI) in RRMS. Glatiramer acetate may also benefit disease severity measures, although this is less well established than for the relapse rate. Therefore, glatiramer acetate should be considered in RRMS patients. However, its usefulness in progressive disease is entirely unknown.

The long-term efficacy of these treatments remains largely unknown. For the interferons, clear-cut beneficial effects in reducing the relapse rate and, more substantially, in reducing CNS inflammation inferred by MRI has not been matched by similar success in treating patients with progressive symptoms (see below). This discordance has led to a reconsideration of the MS disease process as having two separate phases: inflammatory and neurodegenerative. In this model, the former leads to attacks and the latter to progression. It is likely that a gradual loss of axons underlies progressive MS symptoms, and this process could hypothetically result from loss of trophic influences provided by intact myelin. If true, then an MS attack early in the course might lead to a progressive symptom many years later. Because of this possibility, many experts currently believe that very early treatment with a disease-modifying drug is appropriate for most MS patients. It is reasonable to delay initiating treatment in patients with (1) normal neurologic exams; (2) a single attack or a low attack frequency; and (3) a low burden of disease as assessed by brain MRI. Untreated patients need to be followed closely with periodic brain MRI scans; the need for therapy is reassessed if the scans reveal evidence of ongoing, subclinical disease.

Most treated patients with relapsing forms of MS receive IFN-β as first-line therapy. Regardless of which agent is chosen first, treatment should probably be altered in patents who continue to have frequent attacks or progressive disability (Fig. 359-4). The value of combination therapy is unknown.

IFN-β1a (Avonex), 30 μg, is administered by intramuscular injection once every week. IFN-β1a (Rebif), 44 μg, is administered by subcutaneous injection three times per week. IFN-β1b (Betaseron), 250 μg, is administered by subcutaneous injection every other day. Glatiramer acetate, 20 mg, is administered by subcutaneous injection every day. Common side effects of IFN-β therapy include flulike symptoms (e.g., fevers, chills, and myalgias) and mild abnormalities on routine laboratory evaluation (e.g., elevated liver function tests or lymphopenia). Rarely, more severe hepatotoxicity may occur. Subcutaneous IFN-β also causes reactions at the injection site (e.g., pain, redness, induration, or, rarely, skin necrosis). Side effects can usually be managed with concomitant nonsteroidal anti-inflammatory medications and with the use of an auto-injector. Depression, increased spasticity, and cognitive changes have been reported, although these symptoms can also be due to the underlying disease. In any event, side effects to IFN-β therapy usually subside with time.

Approximately 2 to 10% of IFN-β1a (Avonex) recipients, 15 to 25% of IFN-β1a (Rebif) recipients, and 30 to 40% of IFN-β1b (Betaseron) recipients develop neutralizing antibodies to IFN-β, which may disappear over time. Some evidence suggests that neutralizing antibodies reduce efficacy, especially for MRI outcomes. The current clinical data, however, are quite conflicted. Moreover, there are few situations where measurement of antibodies is necessary. Thus, for a patient doing well on therapy, the presence of antibodies should not matter. Conversely, for a patient doing poorly on therapy, alternative

A

B

FIGURE 359-4 Therapeutic decision making for MS.

treatment should be considered, even if there are no detectable antibodies.

Injection site reactions also occur with glatiramer acetate but are less severe than with IFN-β1b. Approximately 15% of patients experience one or more episodes of flushing, chest tightness, dyspnea, palpitations, and anxiety after injection. This systemic reaction is unpredictable, brief (duration <1 h), and tends not to recur.

MITOXANTRONE HYDROCHLORIDE Mitoxantrone (Novantrone), an anthracenedione, exerts its antineoplastic action by (1) intercalating into DNA and producing both strand breaks and interstrand cross-links, (2) interfering with RNA synthesis and, (3) inhibiting topoisomerase II (involved in DNA repair). The U.S. Food and Drug Administration (FDA) approved mitoxantrone on the basis of a single (relatively small) phase III clinical trial in Europe, in addition to an even smaller phase II study completed earlier. Mitoxantrone received (from the FDA) the broadest indication of any current treatment for MS. Thus, mitoxantrone is indicated for use in SPMS, in PRMS, and in patients with worsening RRMS (defined as patients whose neurologic status remains significantly abnormal between MS attacks). Despite this broad indication, however, the data supporting its efficacy are weaker than for other approved therapies.

Mitoxantrone can produce cardiac problems (e.g., cardiomyopathy, reduced left ventricular ejection fraction, and irreversible congestive heart failure). As a result, a cumulative dose >140 mg/m^2 is not recommended. At currently approved doses (12 mg/m^2 every 3 months), the maximum duration of therapy can be only 2 to 3 years. Furthermore, >40% of women will experience amenorrhea, which may be permanent. Finally, there is risk of acute leukemia, and this complication has already been reported in several mitoxantrone-treated MS patients.

Given these risks, mitoxantrone should not be used as a first-line agent in either RRMS or relapsing SPMS. It is reasonable to consider mitoxantrone in selected patients with a progressive course who have failed other approved therapies.

Disease-Modifying Therapies for SPMS without Relapses High-dose IFN-β probably has a beneficial effect in patients with SPMS who are still experiencing acute relapses. IFN-β is probably ineffective in patients with SPMS who are not having acute attacks.

Although mitoxantrone has been approved for patients with progressive MS, this is not the population studied in the pivotal trial. Therefore no evidence-based recommendation can be made with regard to its use in this setting.

PPMS No currently available therapies have shown any promise for treating PPMS at this time. A phase III clinical trial of glatiramer acetate in PPMS was recently stopped because of an apparent lack of efficacy. A trial of mitoxantrone in PPMS is in progress.

Off-Label Treatment Options for RRMS and SPMS *Azathioprine* (2 to 3 mg/kg body weight) has been used primarily in SPMS. Meta-analysis of published trials suggests that azathioprine is marginally effective at lowering relapse rates, although a benefit on disability progression has not been demonstrated.

Methotrexate (7.5 to 20 mg/wk) was shown in one study to slow the progression of upper extremity dysfunction in SPMS. Because of the possibility of developing irreversible liver damage, some experts recommend a blind liver biopsy after 2 years of therapy.

Cyclophosphamide (700 mg/m^2, every other month) may be helpful for treatment-refractory patients who are (1) otherwise in good health, (2) ambulatory, and (3) <40 years of age. Because cyclophosphamide can be used for periods in excess of 3 years, it may be preferable to mitoxantrone in these circumstances.

Intravenous immunoglobulin (IVIg), administered in monthly pulses (up to 1 g/kg) for up to 2 years, appears to reduce annual exacerbation rates. However, its use is limited because of its high cost, questions about optimal dose, and uncertainty about its effect on long-term disability outcome.

Methylprednisolone administered in one study as monthly high-dose intravenous pulses, reduced disability progression (see above).

Other Therapeutic Claims Many purported treatments for MS have never been subjected to scientific scrutiny. These include dietary therapies (e.g., the Swank diet in addition to others), megadose vitamins, calcium orotate, bee stings, cow colostrum, hyperbaric oxygen, procarin (a combination of histamine and caffeine), chelation, acupuncture, acupressure, various Chinese herbal remedies, and removal of mercury amalgam tooth fillings, among many others. Patients should avoid costly or potentially hazardous unproven treatments. Many such treatments lack biologic plausibility. For example, no reliable case of mercury poisoning resembling typical MS has ever been described.

Although potential roles for human herpes virus 6 and/or chlamydia have been suggested for MS, these reports are unconfirmed, and treatment with antiviral agents or antibiotics is not currently appropriate.

Symptomatic Therapy Potassium channel blockers (e.g., 4-aminopyridine, 10 to 40 mg/d; and 3,4-di-aminopyridine, 40 to 80 mg/d) may be helpful for *weakness*, especially for heat-sensitive symptoms. At high doses they may cause seizures. These agents are not FDA-approved but can be obtained from compounding pharmacies around the United States.

Ataxia/tremor is often intractable. Clonazepam, 1.5 to 20 mg/d; mysoline, 50 to 250 mg/d; propranolol, 40 to 200 mg/d; or ondansetron, 8 to 16 mg/d may help. Wrist-weights occasionally reduce tremor in the arm or hand. Thalamotomy or deep brain stimulation has been tried with mixed success.

Spasticity and *spasms* may improve with physical therapy, regular exercise, and stretching. Avoidance of triggers (e.g., infections, fecal impactions, bed sores) is extremely important. Effective medications include lioresal (20 to 120 mg/d), diazepam (2 to 40 mg/d), tizanidine (8 to 32 mg/d), dantroline (25 to 400 mg/d), and cyclobenzaprine hydrochloride (10 to 60 mg/d). For severe spasticity, a lioresal pump (delivering medication directly into the CSF) can provide substantial relief.

Pain is treated with anticonvulsants (carbamazepine, 100 to 1000 mg/d; phenytoin, 300 to 600 mg/d; or gabapentin, 300 to 3600 mg/d), antidepressants (amitriptyline, 25 to 150 mg/d; nortryptiline, 25 to 150 mg/d; desipramine, 100 to 300 mg/d; or venlafaxine, 75 to 225 mg/d), or antiarrhythmics (mexiletine, 300 to 900 mg/d). If these approaches fail, patients should be referred to a comprehensive pain management program.

Bladder dysfunction management is best guided by urodynamic testing. Evening fluid restriction or frequent voluntary voiding may help *detrusor hyperreflexia*. If these methods fail, propantheline bromide (10 to 15 mg/d), oxybutinin (5 to 15 mg/d), hycosamine sulfate (0.5 to 0.75 mg/d), or tolteridine tartrate (2 to 4 mg/d) may help. Coadministration of pseudoephedrine (30 to 60 mg) is sometimes beneficial.

Detrusor/sphyncter dyssynergia may respond to phenoxybenzamine (10 to 20 mg/d) or terazosin hydrochloride (1 to 20 mg/d). Loss of reflex bladder wall contraction may respond to bethanecol (30 to 150 mg/d). However, both conditions often require catheterization.

Urinary tract infections should be treated promptly. Patients with large postvoid residual urine volumes are predisposed to infections. Prevention by urine acidification (with cranberry juice or vitamin C) inhibits some bacteria. Prophylactic administration of antibiotics is sometimes necessary but may lead to colonization by resistant organisms. Intermittent catheterization may help to prevent recurrent infections.

Treatment of *constipation* includes high-fiber diets and fluids. Natural or other laxatives may help. *Fecal incontinence* may respond to a reduction in dietary fiber.

Depression should be treated. Useful drugs include the selective serotonin reuptake inhibitors (fluoxitine, 20 to 80 mg/d, or sertraline, 50 to 200 mg/d); the tricyclic antidepressants, (amitriptyline, 25 to 150 mg/d, nortryptiline, 25 to 150 mg/d, or desipramine, 100 to 300 mg/d); and the non-tricyclic antidepressants (venlafaxine, 75 to 225 mg/d).

Fatigue may improve with assistive devices, help in the home, or successful management of spasticity. Patients with frequent nocturia may benefit from anticholinergic medication at bedtime. Primary MS fatigue may respond to amantadine (200 mg/d), pemoline (37.5 to 75 mg/d), methylphenidate (5 to 25 mg/d), or modafinil (100 to 400 mg/d).

Cognitive problems may respond to the cholinesterase inhibitor donepezil hydrochloride (10 mg/d).

Paroxysmal symptoms respond dramatically to low-dose anticonvulsants (acetazolamide, 200 to 600 mg/d; carbamazepine, 50 to 400 mg/d; phenytoin, 50 to 300 mg/d; or gabapentin, 600 to 1800 mg/d).

Heat sensitivity may respond to heat-avoidance, air conditioning, or cooling garments.

Sexual dysfunction may be helped by lubricants to aid in genital stimulation and sexual arousal. Management of pain, spasticity, fatigue, and bladder/bowel dysfunction may also help. Sildenafil (50 to 100 mg) taken 1 to 2 h before sex is now the standard treatment for maintaining erections.

Promising Experimental Therapies Numerous clinical trials are currently underway. These include: (1) combination therapies; (2) higher-dose IFN-β than currently prescribed; (3) monoclonal antibodies against α_4-integrin to prevent adhesion of lymphocytes to endothelial surfaces, against CD52 to induce global lymphocyte depletion, or against CD20 to deplete B cells selectively; (4) use of statins as immunomodulators; (5) estriol to induce a pregnancy-like state; (6) bone marrow transplants; and (7) schwann cell transplants.

CLINICAL VARIANTS OF MS *Neuromyelitis optica* (NMO), or Devic's syndrome, consists of separate attacks of acute ON and myelitis. ON may be unilateral or bilateral and precede or follow an attack of myelitis by days, months, or years. In contrast to MS, patients with NMO do not experience brainstem, cerebellar, and cognitive involvement, and the brain MRI is typically normal. A focal enhancing region of swelling and cavitation, extending over three or more spinal cord segments, is typically seen on MRI. Histopathology of these lesions may reveal areas of necrosis and thickening of blood vessel walls. NMO, which is uncommon in Caucasians compared with Asians and Africans, is best understood as a syndrome with diverse causes. Some patients have a systemic autoimmune disorder, often systemic lupus erythematosus, Sjögren's syndrome, p-ANCA (perinuclear antineutrophil cytoplasmic antibody) associated vasculitis, or mixed connective tissue disease. In others, onset may be associated with acute infection with varicella-zoster virus or HIV. More frequently, however, NMO is idiopathic and probably represents an MS variant.

Occasional patients present with apparent NMO but have periventricular MRI changes indicating typical MS. Furthermore, in the MS disease model EAE, immunization with peptides of MOG can produce an NMO-like disorder. Disease-modifying therapies for MS have not been rigorously studied in NMO. Acute attacks are usually treated with high-dose glucocorticoids as for MS exacerbations (see above). Because of the possibility that NMO is antibody-mediated, plasma exchange has also been used empirically for acute episodes that fail to respond to glucocorticoids. Immunosuppressants or interferons are sometimes used in the hope that further relapses will be prevented.

Acute MS (Marburg's variant) is a fulminant demyelinating process that progresses to death within 1 to 2 years. Typically, there are no remissions. Diagnosis is established by biopsy or at autopsy, revealing widespread demyelination, axonal loss, edema, and macrophage infiltration. Discrete plaques may also be seen. Recent evidence strongly supports an antibody-mediated process in the demyelinating lesions. Marburg's variant does not seem to follow infection or vaccination, and it is unclear whether this syndrome represents an extreme form of MS or another disease altogether. No controlled trials of therapy exist; high-dose glucocorticoids, plasma exchange, and cyclophosphamide have been tried, with uncertain benefit.

ACUTE DISSEMINATED ENCEPHALOMYELITIS (ADEM)

ADEM has a monophasic course and is frequently associated with antecedent immunization (postvaccinal encephalomyelitis) or infection (postinfectious encephalomyelitis). The hallmark of ADEM is the presence of widely scattered small foci of perivenular inflammation and demyelination. In its most explosive form, acute hemorrhagic leukoencephalitis of Weston Hurst, the lesions are vasculitic and hemorrhagic, and the clinical course is devastating.

Postvaccinal encephalomyelitis may follow the administration of smallpox and certain rabies vaccines. Postinfectious encephalomyelitis is most frequently associated with the viral exanthems of childhood. Infection with measles virus is the most common antecedent (1 in 1000 cases). Worldwide, measles encephalomyelitis is still common, although use of the live measles vaccine has dramatically reduced its incidence in developed countries. An ADEM-like illness rarely follows vaccination with live measles vaccine (1 to 2 in 10^6 immunizations). ADEM is now most frequently associated with varicella (chickenpox) infections (1 in 4000 to 10,000 cases). It may also follow infection with rubella, mumps, influenza, parainfluenza, and infectious mononucleosis viruses and with *Mycoplasma*. Some patients may have a nonspecific upper respiratory infection or no known antecedent illness.

An autoimmune response to MBP can be detected in the CSF from many patients with ADEM. This response has been most clearly established after rabies vaccination and infection with measles virus. With measles infection, the induction of immune responses to a variety of CNS antigens may occur, but only the response to MBP correlates with the development of ADEM. Many cases of postvaccinal encephalomyelitis may result from sensitization with brain material that contaminates the viral vaccines. Attempts to demonstrate direct viral invasion of the CNS have been unsuccessful.

CLINICAL MANIFESTATIONS In severe cases, onset is abrupt, and progression rapid (hours to days). In postinfectious ADEM, the neurologic syndrome generally begins late in the course of the viral illness as the exanthem is fading. Fever reappears, and headache, meningismus, and lethargy progressing to coma may develop. Seizures are common. Signs of disseminated neurologic disease are consistently present (e.g., hemiparesis or quadriparesis, extensor plantar responses, lost or hyperactive tendon reflexes, sensory loss and brainstem involvement). In ADEM due to chickenpox, cerebellar involvement is often conspicuous. CSF protein is modestly elevated [0.5 to 1.5 g/L (50 to 150 mg/dL)]. Lymphocytic pleocytosis, generally 200 cells/μl, occurs in 80% of patients. Occasional patients have higher counts or a mixed polymorphonuclear-lymphocytic pattern during the initial days of the illness. Transient CSF oligoclonal banding has been reported. MRI may reveal extensive gadolinium enhancement of white matter in brain and spinal cord.

DIAGNOSIS The diagnosis is easily established when there is a history of recent vaccination or exanthematous illness. In severe cases with predominantly cerebral involvement, acute encephalitis due to infection with herpes simplex or other viruses may be difficult to exclude. The simultaneous onset of disseminated symptoms and signs is common in ADEM and rare in MS. Similarly, meningismus, drowsiness or coma, or seizures suggest ADEM rather than MS. Unlike in MS, in ADEM optic nerve involvement is generally bilateral and transverse myelopathy complete. MRI findings that may support a diagnosis of ADEM include extensive and relatively symmetric white matter abnormalities and Gd enhancement of all abnormal areas, indicating active disease and a monophasic course.

℞ TREATMENT

Initial treatment is with high-dose glucocorticoids as for exacerbations of MS (see above). Patients who fail to respond may benefit from a course of plasma exchange or intravenous immunoglobulin. The prognosis reflects the severity of the underlying acute illness. Measles encephalomyelitis is associated with a mortality rate of 5 to 20%, and most survivors have permanent neurologic sequelae. Children who recover may have persistent seizures and behavioral and learning disorders.

FURTHER READING

BERGER T et al: Antimyelin antibodies as a predictor of clinically definite multiple sclerosis after a first demyelinating event. N Engl J Med 349:139, 2003

CREE BAC et al: Neuromyelitis optica. Semin Neurol 22:105, 2002

GOODIN DS et al: Disease modifying therapies in multiple sclerosis: Report of the Therapeutics and Technology Assessment Subcommittee of the American Academy of Neurology. Neurology 58:169, 2002

OKSENBERG J et al: Mapping multiple sclerosis susceptibility to the HLA-DR locus in African Americans. Am J Hum Genet 74:160, 2004

360 MENINGITIS, ENCEPHALITIS, BRAIN ABSCESS, AND EMPYEMA
Karen L. Roos, Kenneth L. Tyler

Acute infections of the nervous system are among the most important problems in medicine because early recognition, efficient decision-making, and rapid institution of therapy can be lifesaving. These distinct clinical syndromes include acute bacterial meningitis, viral meningitis, encephalitis, focal infections such as brain abscess and subdural empyema, and infectious thrombophlebitis. Each may present with a nonspecific prodrome of fever and headache, which in a previously healthy individual may initially be thought to be benign, until (with the exception of viral meningitis) altered consciousness, focal neurologic signs, or seizures appear. Key goals of early management are to emergently distinguish between these conditions, identify the responsible pathogen, and initiate appropriate antimicrobial therapy.

APPROACH TO THE PATIENT

(Fig. 360-1) The first task is to identify whether an infection predominantly involves the subarachnoid space ("meningitis") or whether there is evidence of either generalized or focal involvement of brain tissue in the cerebral hemispheres, cerebellum, or brainstem. When brain tissue is directly injured by a viral infection the disease is referred to as "encephalitis," whereas focal bacterial, fungal, or parasitic infections involving brain tissue are classified as either "cerebritis" or "abscess," depending on the presence or absence of a capsule.

Nuchal rigidity is the pathognomonic sign of meningeal irritation and is present when the neck resists passive flexion. Kernig's and Brudzinski's signs are also classic signs of meningeal irritation. *Kernig's sign* is elicited with the patient in the supine position. The thigh is flexed on the abdomen, with the knee flexed; attempts to passively extend the knee elicit pain when meningeal irritation is present. *Brudzinski's sign* is elicited with the patient in the supine position and is positive when passive flexion of the neck results in spontaneous flexion of the hips and knees. Although commonly tested on physical examinations, the sensitivity and specificity of Kernig's and Brudzinski's signs are uncertain. Both may be absent or reduced in very young or elderly patients, immunocompromised individuals, or patients with a severely depressed mental status. The high prevalence of cervical spine disease in older individuals may result in false-positive tests for nuchal rigidity.

Initial management can be guided by several considerations: (1) Empirical therapy should be initiated promptly whenever bacterial meningitis is a significant diagnostic consideration. (2) All patients who have had recent head trauma, are immunocompromised, have known malignant lesions or central nervous system (CNS) neoplasms, or have focal neurologic findings including papilledema or a depressed level of consciousness should undergo computed tomography (CT) or magnetic resonance imaging (MRI) of the brain prior to lumbar puncture (LP). In these cases empirical antibiotic therapy should not be delayed pending test results but should be administered prior to neuroimaging and LP. (3) A significantly depressed mental status (e.g., somnolence, coma), seizures, or focal neurologic deficits only rarely occur in viral ("aseptic") meningitis; patients with these symptoms should be hospitalized for further evaluation and treated empirically for bacterial and viral meningoencephalitis. (4) Immunocompetent patients with a normal level of consciousness, no prior antimicrobial treatment, and a cerebrospinal fluid (CSF) profile consistent with viral meningitis (lymphocytic pleocytosis and a normal glucose concentration) can often be treated as outpatients, if appropriate contact and monitoring can be ensured. Failure of a patient with suspected viral meningitis to improve within 48 h should prompt a reevaluation including follow-up neurologic and general medical examination and repeat imaging and laboratory studies, often including a second LP.

ACUTE BACTERIAL MENINGITIS

DEFINITION Bacterial meningitis is an acute purulent infection within the subarachnoid space. It is associated with a CNS inflammatory reaction that may result in decreased consciousness, seizures, raised intracranial pressure (ICP), and stroke. The meninges, the subarachnoid space, and the brain parenchyma are all frequently involved in the inflammatory reaction (*meningoencephalitis*).

EPIDEMIOLOGY Bacterial meningitis is the most common form of suppurative CNS infection, with an annual incidence in the United States of >2.5 cases/100,000 population. The epidemiology of bacterial meningitis has changed significantly in recent years, reflecting a dramatic decline in the incidence of meningitis due to *Haemophilus influenzae*, and a smaller decline in that due to *Neisseria meningitidis*, following the introduction and increasingly widespread use of vaccines for both these organisms. Currently, the organisms most commonly responsible for community-acquired bacterial meningitis are *Streptococcus pneumoniae* (~50%), *N. meningitidis* (~25%), group B streptococci (~15%), and *Listeria monocytogenes* (~10%). *H. influenzae* now accounts for <10% of cases of bacterial meningitis in most series.

ETIOLOGY *S. pneumoniae* (Chap. 121) is the most common cause of meningitis in adults >20 years of age, accounting for nearly half the reported cases (1.1 per 100,000 persons per year). There are a number of predisposing conditions that increase the risk of pneumococcal meningitis, the most important of which is pneumococcal pneumonia. Additional risk factors include coexisting acute or chronic pneumococcal sinusitis or otitis media, alcoholism, diabetes, splenectomy, hypogammaglobulinemia, complement deficiency, and head trauma with basilar skull fracture and CSF rhinorrhea. Mortality remains ~20% despite antibiotic therapy.

N. meningitidis (Chap. 127) accounts for 25% of all cases of bacterial meningitis (0.6 cases per 100,000 persons per year) and for up to 60% of cases in children and young adults between the ages of 2 and 20. The presence of petechial or purpuric skin lesions can provide an important clue to the diagnosis of meningococcal infection. In some patients the disease is fulminant, progressing to death within hours of symptom onset. Infection may be initiated by nasopharyngeal colo-

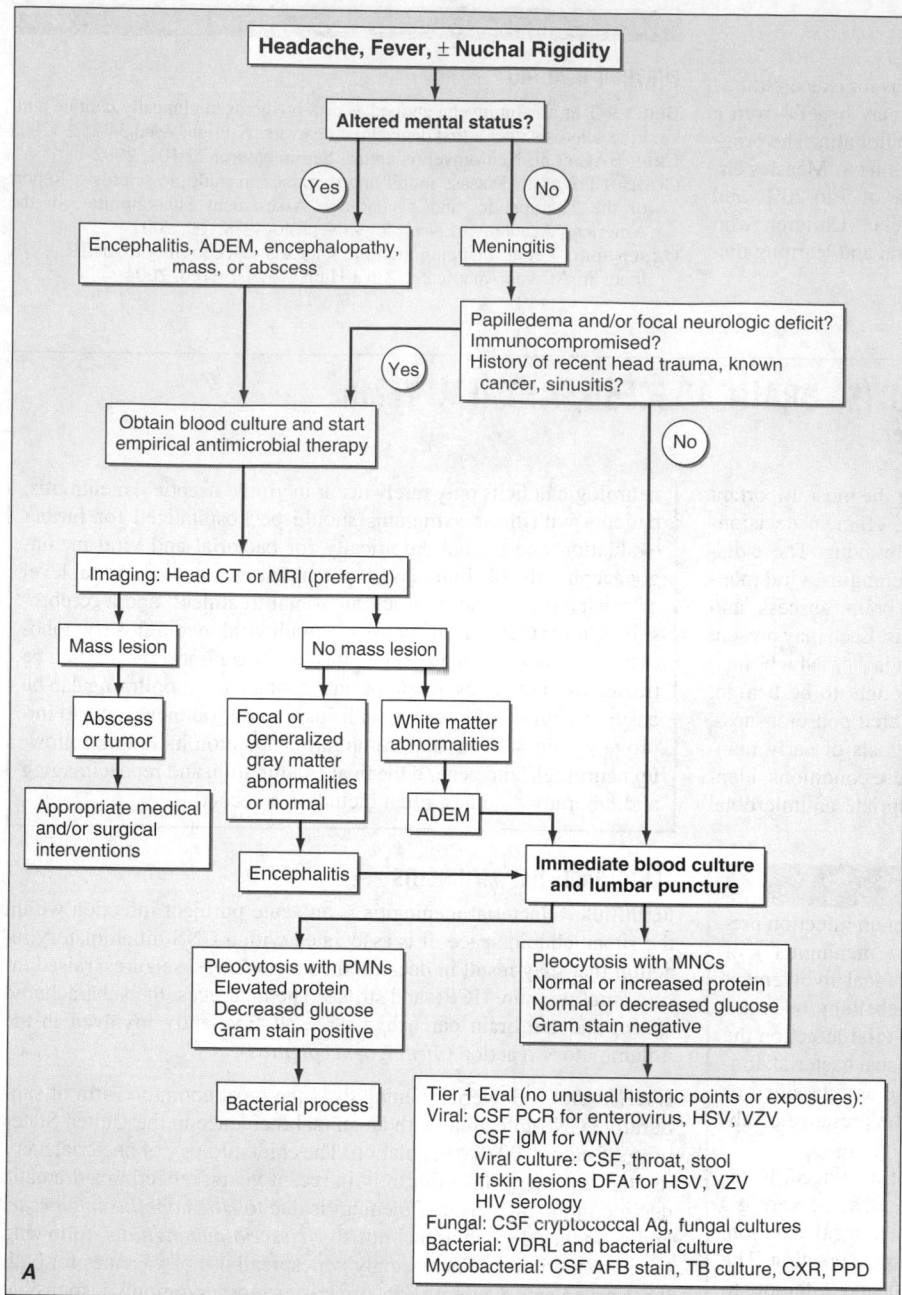

FIGURE 360-1 *A.* Algorithm for management of patients with suspected CNS infections. ADEM, acute disseminated encephalomyelitis; CT, computed tomography; MRI, magnetic resonance imaging; PMNs, polymorphonuclear leukocytes; MNCs, mononuclear cells; CSF, cerebrospinal fluid; PCR, polymerase chain reaction; HSV, herpes simplex virus; VZV, varicella-zoster virus; WNV, West Nile Virus; DFA, direct fluorescent antibody; Ag, antigen; VDRL, Venereal Disease Research Laboratory; AFB, acid-fast bacillus; TB, tuberculosis; CXR, chest x-ray; PPD, purified protein derivative; EBV, Epstein-Barr virus; CTFV, Colorado tick fever virus; HHV, human herpesvirus; LCMV, lymphocytic choriomeningitis virus.

nization, which can result in either an asymptomatic carrier state or invasive meningococcal disease. The risk of invasive disease following nasopharyngeal colonization depends on both bacterial virulence factors and host immune defense mechanisms, including the host's capacity to produce antimeningococcal antibodies and to lyse meningococci by both the classic and alternative complement pathways. Individuals with deficiencies of any of the complement components, including properdin, are highly susceptible to meningococcal infections.

Enteric gram-negative bacilli are an increasingly common cause of meningitis in individuals with chronic and debilitating diseases such as diabetes, cirrhosis, or alcoholism and in those with chronic urinary tract infections. Gram-negative meningitis can also complicate neurosurgical procedures, particularly craniotomy.

Group B streptococcus, or *S. agalactiae*, was previously responsible for meningitis predominantly in neonates, but it has been reported with increasing frequency in individuals >50 years of age, particularly those with underlying diseases.

L. monocytogenes (Chap. 123) has become an increasingly important cause of meningitis in neonates (<1 month of age), pregnant women, individuals >60 years, and immunocompromised individuals of all ages. Infection is acquired by ingesting foods contaminated by *Listeria*. Foodborne human listerial infection has been reported from contaminated coleslaw, milk, soft cheeses, and several types of "ready-to-eat" foods including delicatessen meat and uncooked hotdogs.

The frequency of *H. influenzae* type b meningitis in children has declined dramatically since the introduction of the Hib conjugate vaccine, although rare cases of Hib meningitis in vaccinated children have been reported. More frequently, *H. influenzae* causes meningitis in unvaccinated children and adults.

Staphylococcus aureus and coagulase-negative staphylococci (Chap. 120) are important causes of meningitis that follows invasive neurosurgical procedures, particularly shunting procedures for hydrocephalus, or that occurs as a complication of the use of subcutaneous Ommaya reservoirs for administration of intrathecal chemotherapy.

PATHOPHYSIOLOGY The most common bacteria that cause meningitis, *S. pneumoniae* and *N. meningitidis*, initially colonize the nasopharynx by attaching to nasopharyngeal epithelial cells. Bacteria are transported across epithelial cells in membrane-bound vacuoles to the intravascular space or invade the intravascular space by creating separations in the apical tight junctions of columnar epithelial cells. Once in the bloodstream, bacteria are able to avoid phagocytosis by neutrophils and classic complement–mediated bactericidal activity because of the presence of a polysaccharide capsule. Bloodborne bacteria can reach the intraventricular choroid plexus, directly infect choroid plexus epithelial cells, and gain access to the CSF. Some bacteria, such as *S. pneumoniae*, can adhere to cerebral capillary endothelial cells and subsequently migrate through or between these cells to reach the CSF. Bacteria are able to multiply rapidly within CSF because of the absence of effective host immune defenses. Normal CSF contains few white blood cells (WBCs) and relatively small amounts of complement proteins and immunoglobulins. The paucity of the latter two prevents effective opsonization of bacteria, an essential prerequisite for bacterial phagocytosis by neutrophils. Phagocytosis of bacteria is further impaired by the fluid nature of CSF, which is less conducive to phagocytosis than a solid tissue substrate.

A critical event in the pathogenesis of bacterial meningitis is the inflammatory reaction induced by the invading bacteria. Many of the neurologic manifestations and complications of bacterial meningitis result from the immune response to the invading pathogen rather than from direct bacteria-induced tissue injury. As a result, neurologic injury can progress even after the CSF has been sterilized by antibiotic therapy.

The lysis of bacteria with the subsequent release of cell-wall components into the subarachnoid space is the initial step in the induction of the inflammatory response and the formation of a purulent exudate in the subarachnoid space (Fig. 360-2). Bacterial cell-wall components, such as the lipopolysaccharide (LPS) molecules of gram-negative bacteria and teichoic acid and peptidoglycans of *S. pneumoniae*, induce meningeal inflammation by stimulating the production of inflammatory cytokines and chemokines by microglia, astrocytes, monocytes, microvascular endothelial cells, and CSF leukocytes. In experimental models of meningitis, cytokines including tumor necrosis factor (TNF) and interleukin (IL) 1 are present in CSF within 1 to 2 h of intracisternal inoculation of LPS. This cytokine response is quickly followed by an increase in CSF protein concentration and leukocytosis. Chemokines (cytokines that induce chemotactic migration in leukocytes) and a variety of other proinflammatory cytokines are also produced and secreted by leukocytes and tissue cells that are stimulated by IL-1 and TNF. In addition, bacteremia and the inflammatory cytokines induce the production of excitatory amino acids, reactive oxygen and nitrogen species (free oxygen radicals, nitric oxide, and peroxynitrite), and other mediators that can induce death of brain cells.

Much of the pathophysiology of bacterial meningitis is a direct consequence of elevated levels of CSF cytokines and chemokines. TNF and IL-1 act synergistically to increase the permeability of the blood-brain barrier, resulting in induction of vasogenic edema and the leakage of serum proteins into the subarachnoid space (Fig. 360-2). The subarachnoid exudate of proteinaceous material and leukocytes obstructs the flow of CSF through the ventricular system and diminishes the resorptive capacity of the arachnoid granulations in the dural sinuses, leading to obstructive and communicating hydrocephalus and concomitant interstitial edema.

Inflammatory cytokines upregulate the expression of selectins on cerebral capillary endothelial cells and leukocytes, promoting leukocyte adherence to vascular endothelial cells and subsequent migration into the CSF. The adherence of leukocytes to capillary endothelial cells increases the permeability of blood vessels, allowing for the leakage of plasma proteins into the CSF, which adds to the inflammatory exudate. Neutrophil degranulation results in the release of toxic metabolites that contribute to cytotoxic edema, cell injury, and death. Contrary to previous beliefs, CSF leukocytes probably do little to contribute to the clearance of CSF bacterial infection.

During the very early stages of meningitis there is an increase in cerebral blood flow, soon followed by a decrease in cerebral blood flow and a loss of cerebrovascular autoregulation (Chap. 258). Narrowing of the large arteries at the base of the brain due to encroachment by the purulent exudate in the subarachnoid space and infiltration of the arterial wall by inflammatory cells with intimal thickening (*vasculitis*) also occur and may result in ischemia and infarction, obstruction of branches of the middle cerebral artery by thrombosis, thrombosis of the major cerebral venous sinuses, and thrombophlebitis of the cerebral cortical veins. The combination of interstitial, vasogenic, and cytotoxic edema leads to raised ICP and coma. Cerebral herniation usually results from the effects of cerebral edema, either focal or generalized; hydrocephalus and dural sinus or cortical vein thrombosis may also play a role.

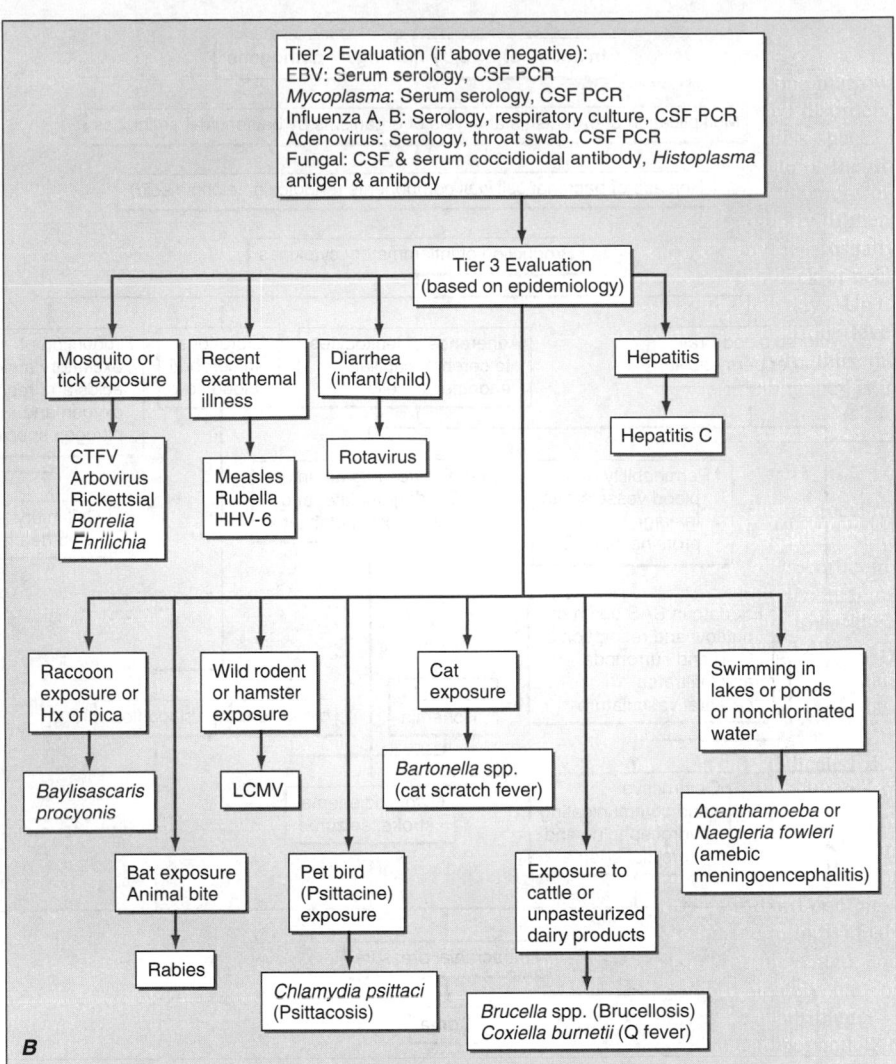

FIGURE 360-1*B*— *(Continued)*

CLINICAL PRESENTATION Meningitis can present as either an acute fulminant illness that progresses rapidly in a few hours or as a subacute infection that progressively worsens over several days. The classic clinical triad of meningitis is fever, headache, and nuchal rigidity ("stiff neck"). Each of these signs and symptoms occurs in >90% of cases. Alteration in mental status occurs in >75% of patients and can vary from lethargy to coma. Nausea, vomiting, and photophobia are also common complaints.

Seizures occur as part of the initial presentation of bacterial meningitis or during the course of the illness in 20 to 40% of patients. Focal seizures are usually due to focal arterial ischemia or infarction, cortical venous thrombosis with hemorrhage, or focal edema. Generalized seizure activity and status epilepticus may be due to hyponatremia, cerebral anoxia, or, less commonly, the toxic effects of antimicrobial agents such as high-dose penicillin.

Raised ICP is an expected complication of bacterial meningitis and is the major cause of obtundation and coma in this disease. More than 90% of patients will have a CSF opening pressure >180 mmH$_2$O, and 20% have opening pressures >400 mmH$_2$O. Signs of increased ICP include a deteriorating or reduced level of consciousness, papilledema, dilated poorly reactive pupils, sixth nerve palsies, decerebrate posturing, and the Cushing reflex (bradycardia, hypertension, and irregular respirations). The most disastrous complication of increased ICP is cerebral herniation. The incidence of herniation in patients with bacterial meningitis has been reported to occur in as few as 1% to as many as 8% of cases.

Specific clinical features may provide clues to the diagnosis of

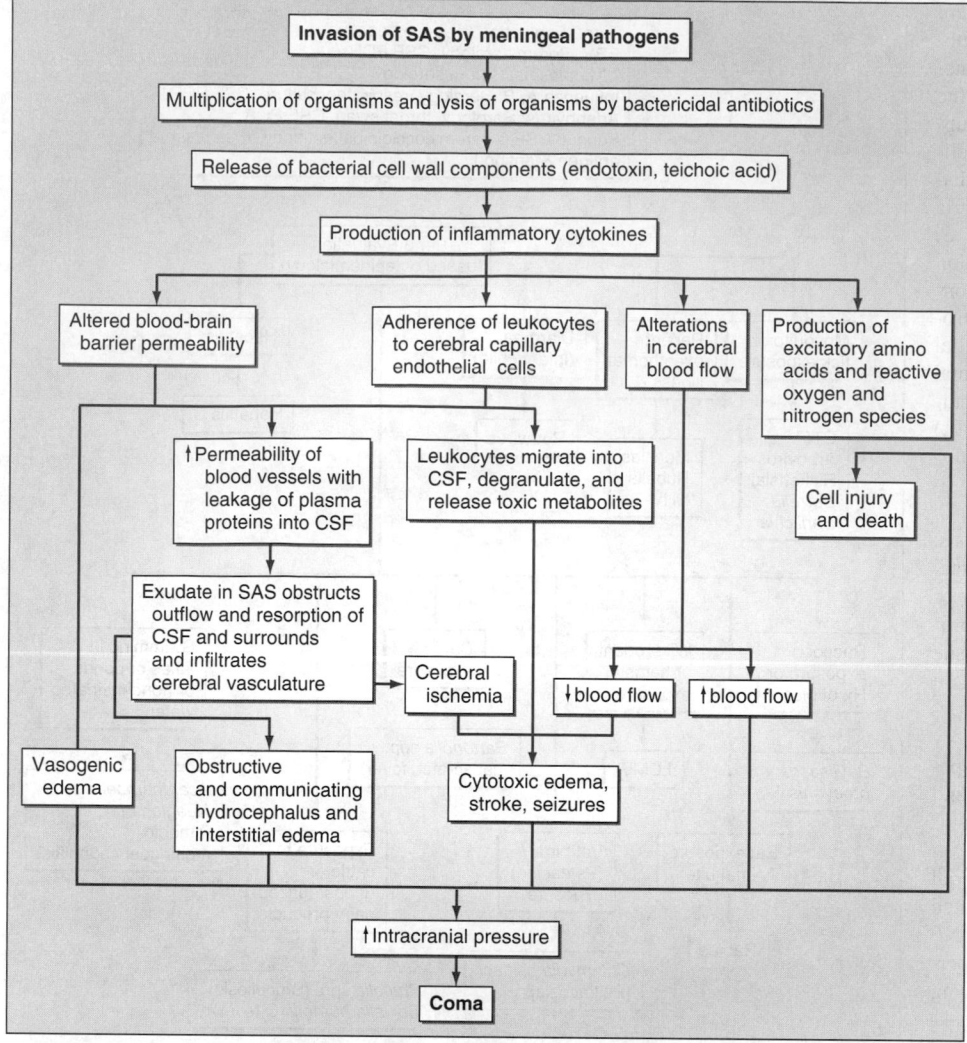

FIGURE 360-2 The pathophysiology of the neurologic complications of bacterial meningitis. SAS, subarachnoid space; CSF, cerebrospinal fluid.

individual organisms and are discussed in more detail in specific chapters devoted to individual pathogens. The most important of these clues is the rash of meningococcemia, which begins as a diffuse erythematous maculopapular rash resembling a viral exanthem, but the skin lesions of meningococcemia rapidly become petechial. Petechiae are found on the trunk and lower extremities, in the mucous membranes and conjunctiva, and occasionally on the palms and soles.

DIAGNOSIS When bacterial meningitis is suspected, blood cultures should be immediately obtained and empirical antimicrobial therapy initiated without delay. The diagnosis of bacterial meningitis is made by examination of the CSF (Table 360-1). The need to obtain neuroimaging studies (CT or MRI) prior to LP requires clinical judgment. In an immunocompetent patient with no known history of recent head trauma, a normal level of consciousness, and no evidence of papilledema or focal neurologic deficits, it is safe to perform LP without prior neuroimaging studies. If LP is delayed in order to obtain neuroimaging studies, empirical antibiotic therapy should be initiated after blood cultures are obtained. Antibiotic therapy initiated a few hours prior to LP will not significantly alter the CSF WBC count or glucose concentration, nor is it likely to prevent visualization of organisms by Gram's stain.

The classic CSF abnormalities in bacterial meningitis (Table 360-1) are (1) polymorphonuclear (PMN) leukocytosis (>100 cells/μL in 90%), (2) decreased glucose concentration [<2.2 mmol/L (<40 mg/dL) and/or CSF/serum glucose ratio of <0.4 in ~60%], (3) increased protein concentration [>0.45 g/L (>45 mg/dL) in 90%], and (4) increased opening pressure (>180 mmH₂O in 90%). CSF bacterial cul-

tures are positive in >80% of patients, and CSF Gram's stain demonstrates organisms in >60%.

CSF glucose concentrations <2.2 mmol/L (<40 mg/dL) are abnormal, and a CSF glucose concentration of zero can be seen in bacterial meningitis. Use of the CSF/serum glucose ratio corrects for hyperglycemia that may mask a relative decrease in the CSF glucose concentration. The CSF glucose concentration is low when the CSF/serum glucose ratio is <0.6. A CSF/serum glucose ratio <0.4 is highly suggestive of bacterial meningitis but may also be seen in other conditions, including fungal, tuberculous, and carcinomatous meningitis. It takes from 30 min to several hours for CSF glucose concentration to reach equilibrium with blood glucose concentrations; therefore, administration of 50 mL of 50% glucose (D50) prior to LP, as commonly occurs in emergency room settings, is unlikely to alter CSF glucose concentration significantly unless more than a few hours have elapsed between glucose administration and LP.

The latex agglutination (LA) test for the detection of bacterial antigens of *S. pneumoniae, N. meningitidis, H. influenzae* type b, group B streptococcus, and *Escherichia coli* K1 strains in the CSF is very useful for making a rapid diagnosis of bacterial meningitis, especially in patients who have been pretreated with antibiotics and in whom CSF Gram's stain and culture are negative. The CSF LA test has a *specificity* of 95 to 100% for *S. pneumoniae* and *N. meningitidis*, so a positive test is virtually diagnostic of bacterial meningitis caused by these organisms. However, the *sensitivity* of the CSF LA test is only 70 to 100% for detection of *S. pneumoniae* and 33 to 70% for detection of *N. meningitidis* antigens, so a negative test does not exclude infection by these organisms. The Limulus amebocyte lysate assay is a rapid diagnostic test for the detection of gram-negative endotoxin in CSF, and thus for making a diagnosis of gram-negative bacterial meningitis. The test has a specificity of 85 to 100% and a sensitivity approaching 100%. Thus, a positive Limulus amebocyte lysate assay occurs in virtually all patients with gram-negative bacterial meningitis, but false-positives may occur. CSF polymerase chain

TABLE 360-1 Cerebrospinal Fluid (CSF) Abnormalities in Bacterial Meningitis

Opening pressure	>180 mmH₂O
White blood cells	10/μL to 10,000/μL; neutrophils predominate
Red blood cells	Absent in nontraumatic tap
Glucose	<2.2 mmol/L (<40 mg/dL)
CSF/serum glucose	<0.4
Protein	>0.45 g/L (>45 mg/dL)
Gram's stain	Positive in >60%
Culture	Positive in >80%
Latex agglutination	May be positive in patients with meningitis due to *S. pneumoniae, N. meningitidis, H. influenzae* type b, *E. coli*, group B streptococci
Limulus lysates	Positive in cases of gram-negative meningitis
PCR for bacterial DNA	Research test

Note: PCR, polymerase chain reaction.

reaction (PCR) tests are not as useful in the diagnosis of bacterial meningitis as they are in the diagnosis of viral CNS infections. A CSF PCR test has been developed for detecting DNA from bacteria in CSF, but its sensitivity and specificity need to be better characterized before its role in diagnosis can be defined.

Almost all patients with bacterial meningitis will have neuroimaging studies performed during the course of their illness. MRI is preferred over CT because of its superiority in demonstrating areas of cerebral edema and ischemia. In patients with bacterial meningitis, diffuse meningeal enhancement is often seen after the administration of gadolinium. Meningeal enhancement is not diagnostic of meningitis but occurs in any CNS disease associated with increased blood-brain barrier permeability.

Petechial skin lesions, if present, should be biopsied. The rash of meningococcemia results from the dermal seeding of organisms with vascular endothelial damage, and biopsy may reveal the organism on Gram's stain.

DIFFERENTIAL DIAGNOSIS Viral meningoencephalitis, and particularly herpes simplex virus (HSV) encephalitis, can mimic the clinical presentation of bacterial meningitis (see "Encephalitis," below). HSV encephalitis typically presents with headache, fever, altered consciousness, focal neurologic deficits (e.g., dysphasia, hemiparesis), and focal or generalized seizures. The findings on CSF studies, neuroimaging, and electroencephalogram (EEG) distinguish HSV encephalitis from bacterial meningitis. The typical CSF profile with viral CNS infections is a lymphocytic pleocytosis with a normal glucose concentration, in contrast to PMN pleocytosis and hypoglycorrhachia characteristic of bacterial meningitis. MRI abnormalities (other than meningeal enhancement) are not seen in uncomplicated bacterial meningitis. By contrast, in HSV encephalitis parenchymal changes, especially in orbitofrontal and medial temporal lobes, are usually found. Some patients with HSV encephalitis have a distinctive periodic pattern on EEG (see below).

Rickettsial disease can resemble bacterial meningitis (Chap. 158). Rocky Mountain spotted fever (RMSF) is transmitted by a tick bite and caused by the bacteria *Rickettsia rickettsii*. The disease may present acutely with high fever, prostration, myalgia, headache, and nausea and vomiting. Most patients develop a characteristic rash within 96 h of the onset of symptoms. The rash is initially a diffuse erythematous maculopapular rash that may be difficult to distinguish from that of meningococcemia. It progresses to a petechial rash, then to a purpuric rash, and, if untreated, to skin necrosis or gangrene. The color of the lesions changes from bright red to very dark red, then yellowish-green to black. The rash typically begins in the wrist and ankles, and then spreads distally and proximally within a matter of a few hours and involves the palms and soles. Diagnosis is made by immunofluorescent staining of skin biopsy specimens.

Focal suppurative CNS infections (see below), including subdural and epidural empyema and brain abscess, should also be considered, especially when focal neurologic findings are present. MRI should be performed promptly in all patients with suspected meningitis who have focal features, both to detect the intracranial infection and to search for associated areas of infection in the sinuses or mastoid bones.

A number of noninfectious CNS disorders can mimic bacterial meningitis. Subarachnoid hemorrhage (SAH; Chap. 349) is generally the major consideration. Other possibilities include chemical meningitis due to rupture of tumor contents into the CSF (e.g., from a cystic glioma, craniopharyngioma epidermoid or dermoid cyst); drug-induced hypersensitivity meningitis; carcinomatous or lymphomatous meningitis; meningitis associated with inflammatory disorders such as sarcoid, systemic lupus erythematosus (SLE), and Behçet disease; pituitary apoplexy; and uveomeningitic syndromes (Vogt-Koyanagi-Harada syndrome).

Subacutely evolving meningitis (Chap. 361) may on occasion be considered in the differential diagnosis of acute meningitis. The principal causes include *Mycobacterium tuberculosis* (Chap. 150), *Cryptococcus neoformans* (Chap. 186), *Histoplasma capsulatum* (Chap.

183), *Coccidioides immitis* (Chap. 184), and *Treponema pallidum* (Chap. 153).

Rx TREATMENT

Empirical Antimicrobial Therapy (Table 360-2) Bacterial meningitis is a medical emergency. The goal is to begin antibiotic therapy within 60 min of a patient's arrival in the emergency room. Empirical antimicrobial therapy is initiated in patients with suspected bacterial meningitis before the results of CSF Gram's stain and culture are known. *S. pneumoniae* (Chap. 119) and *N. meningitidis* (Chap. 127) are the most common etiologic organisms of community-acquired bacterial meningitis. Due to the emergence of penicillin- and cephalosporin-resistant *S. pneumoniae*, empirical therapy of community-acquired bacterial meningitis in children and adults should include a third-generation cephalosporin (e.g., ceftriaxone or cefotaxime) and vancomycin. Ceftriaxone or cefotaxime provide good coverage for susceptible *S. pneumoniae*, group B streptococci, and *H. influenzae* and adequate coverage for *N. meningitidis*. Cefepime is a broad-spectrum fourth-generation cephalosporin with in vitro activity similar to that of cefotaxime or ceftriaxone against *S. pneumoniae* and *N. meningitidis* and greater activity against *Enterobacter* spp. and *Pseudomonas aeruginosa*. In clinical trials, cefepime has been demonstrated to be equivalent to cefotaxime in the treatment of penicillin-sensitive pneumococcal and meningococcal meningitis, but its efficacy in bacterial meningitis caused by penicillin- and cephalosporin-resistant pneumococcal organisms, *Enterobacter* spp., and *P. aeruginosa* has not been established. Ampicillin should be added to the empirical regimen for coverage of *L. monocytogenes* in individuals <3 months of age, those >55, or those with suspected impaired cell-mediated immunity because of chronic illness, organ transplantation, pregnancy, malignancies, or immunosuppressive therapy. In hospital-acquired menin-

TABLE 360-2 Antibiotics Used in Empirical Therapy of Bacterial Meningitis and Focal CNS Infections[a]

Indication	Antibiotic
Preterm infants to infants <1 month	Ampicillin + cefotaxime
Infants 1–3 mos	Ampicillin + cefotaxime or ceftriaxone
Immunocompetent children > 3 mos and adults <55	Cefotaxime or ceftriaxone + vancomycin
Adults > 55 and adults of any age with alcoholism or other debilitating illnesses	Ampicillin + cefotaxime or ceftriaxone + vancomycin
Hospital-acquired meningitis, posttraumatic or postneurosurgery meningitis, neutropenic patients, or patients with impaired cell-mediated immunity	Ampicillin + ceftazidime + vancomycin

	Total Daily Dose and Dosing Interval	
Antimicrobial Agent	Child (>1 month)	Adult
Ampicillin	200 (mg/kg)/d, q4h	12 g/d, q4h
Cefepime	150 (mg/kg)/d, q8h	6 g/d, q8h
Cefotaxime	200 (mg/kg)/d, q6h	12 g/d, q4h
Ceftriaxone	100 (mg/kg)/d, q12h	4 g/d, q12h
Ceftazidime	150 (mg/kg)/d, q8h	6 g/d, q8h
Gentamicin	7.5 (mg/kg)/d, q8h[b]	7.5 (mg/kg)/d, q8h
Meropenem	120 (mg/kg)/d, q8h	3 g/d, q8h
Metronidazole	30 (mg/kg)/d, q6h	1500–2000 mg/d, q6h
Nafcillin	100–200 (mg/kg)/d, q6h	9–12 g/d, q4h
Penicillin G	400,000 (U/kg)/d, q4h	20–24 million U/d, q4h
Vancomycin	60 (mg/kg)/d, q6h	2 g/d, q12h[b]

[a] All antibiotics are administered intravenously; doses indicated assume normal renal and hepatic function.
[b] Doses should be adjusted based on serum peak and trough levels: gentamicin therapeutic level: peak: 5–8 μg/mL; trough:<2 μg/mL; vancomycin therapeutic level: peak: 25–40 μg/mL; trough:5–15 μg/mL.

gitis, and particularly meningitis following neurosurgical procedures, staphylococci and gram-negative organisms including *P. aeruginosa* are the most common etiologic organisms. In these patients, empirical therapy should include a combination of vancomycin and ceftazidime. Ceftazidime should be substituted for ceftriaxone or cefotaxime in neurosurgical patients and in neutropenic patients, as ceftazidime is the only cephalosporin with adequate activity against CNS infection with *P. aeruginosa*. Meropenem is a carbapenem antibiotic that is highly active in vitro against *L. monocytogenes*, has been demonstrated to be effective in cases of meningitis caused by *P. aeruginosa*, and shows good activity against penicillin-resistant pneumococci. In experimental pneumococcal meningitis, meropenem was comparable to ceftriaxone and inferior to vancomycin in sterilizing CSF cultures. The number of patients with bacterial meningitis enrolled in clinical trials of meropenem has not been sufficient to definitively assess the efficacy of this antibiotic.

Specific Antimicrobial Therapy (Table 360-3) ■ *MENINGOCOCCAL MENINGITIS* Although ceftriaxone and cefotaxime provide adequate empirical coverage for *N. meningitidis*, penicillin G remains the antibiotic of choice for meningococcal meningitis caused by susceptible strains. Isolates of *N. meningitidis* with moderate resistance to penicillin have been identified, but patients infected with these strains have still been successfully treated with penicillin. CSF isolates of *N. meningitidis* should be tested for penicillin and ampicillin susceptibility, and if resistance is found, cefotaxime or ceftriaxone should be substituted for penicillin. A 7-day course of intravenous antibiotic therapy is adequate for uncomplicated meningococcal meningitis. The index case and all close contacts should receive chemoprophylaxis with a 2-day regimen of rifampin (600 mg every 12 h for 2 days in adults and 10 mg/kg every 12 h for 2 days in children >1 year). Rifampin is not recommended in pregnant women. Alternatively, adults can be treated with one dose of ciprofloxacin (750 mg), one dose of azithromycin (500 mg), or one intramuscular dose of ceftriaxone (250 mg). Close contacts are defined as those individuals who have had contact with oropharyngeal secretions either through kissing or by sharing toys, beverages, or cigarettes.

PNEUMOCOCCAL MENINGITIS Antimicrobial therapy of pneumococcal meningitis is initiated with a cephalosporin (ceftriaxone, cefotaxime, or cefepime) and vancomycin. All CSF isolates of *S. pneumoniae* should be tested for sensitivity to penicillin and the cephalosporins. Once the results of antimicrobial susceptibility tests are known, therapy can be modified accordingly (Table 360-3). For *S. pneumoniae* meningitis, an isolate of *S. pneumoniae* is considered to be susceptible to penicillin with a minimal inhibitory concentration (MIC) < 0.06 μg/mL, to have

intermediate resistance when the MIC is 0.1 to 1.0 μg/mL, and to be highly resistant when the MIC > 1.0 μg/mL. Isolates of *S. pneumoniae* that have cephalosporin MICs ≤ 0.5 μg/mL are considered sensitive to the cephalosporins (cefotaxime, ceftriaxone, cefepime). Those with MICs of 1 μg/mL are considered to have intermediate resistance, and those with MICs ≥ 2 μg/mL are considered resistant. For meningitis due to pneumococci with cefotaxime or ceftriaxone MICs ≥ 0.5 μg/mL, treatment with cefotaxime or ceftriaxone is usually adequate. If the MIC > 1 μg/mL, vancomycin is the antibiotic of choice. Rifampin can be added to vancomycin for its synergistic effect but is inadequate as monotherapy because resistance develops rapidly when it is used alone.

Patients with *S. pneumoniae* meningitis should have a repeat LP performed 24 to 36 h after the initiation of antimicrobial therapy to document sterilization of the CSF. Failure to sterilize the CSF after 24 to 36 h of antibiotic therapy should be considered presumptive evidence of antibiotic resistance. Patients with penicillin- and cephalosporin-resistant strains of *S. pneumoniae* who do not respond to intravenous vancomycin alone may benefit from the addition of intraventricular vancomycin. The intraventricular route of administration is preferred over the intrathecal route because adequate concentrations of vancomycin in the cerebral ventricles are not always achieved with intrathecal administration. A 2-week course of intravenous antimicrobial therapy is recommended for pneumococcal meningitis.

L. MONOCYTOGENES MENINGITIS Meningitis due to this organism is treated with ampicillin for at least 3 weeks (Table 360-3). Gentamicin is often added (2 mg/kg loading dose, then 5.1 mg/kg per day given every 8 h and adjusted for serum levels and renal function). The combination of trimethoprim [10 to 20 (mg/kg)/d] and sulfamethoxazole [50 to 100 (mg/kg)/d] given every 6 h may provide an alternative in penicillin-allergic patients.

STAPHYLOCOCCAL MENINGITIS Meningitis due to susceptible strains of *S. aureus* or coagulase-negative staphylococci is treated with nafcillin (Table 360-3). Vancomycin is the drug of choice for methicillin-resistant staphylococci and for patients allergic to penicillin. In these patients, the CSF should be monitored during therapy. If the CSF is not sterilized after 48 h of intravenous vancomycin therapy, then either intrathecal or intraventricular vancomycin, 20 mg once daily, can be added.

GRAM-NEGATIVE BACILLARY MENINGITIS The third-generation cephalosporins, cefotaxime, ceftriaxone, and ceftazidime, are equally efficacious for the treatment of gram-negative bacillary meningitis, with the exception of meningitis due to *P. aeruginosa*, which should be treated with ceftazidime (Table 360-3). A 3-week course of intravenous antibiotic therapy is recommended for meningitis due to gram-negative bacilli.

Adjunctive Therapy The release of bacterial cell-wall components by bactericidal antibiotics leads to the production of the inflammatory cytokines IL-1 and TNF in the subarachnoid space. Dexamethasone exerts its beneficial effect by inhibiting the synthesis of IL-1 and TNF at the level of mRNA, decreasing CSF outflow resistance, and stabilizing the blood-brain barrier. The rationale for giving dexamethasone 20 min before antibiotic therapy is that dexamethasone inhibits the production of TNF by macrophages and microglia only if it is administered before these cells are activated by endotoxin. Dexamethasone does not alter TNF production once it has been induced. The results of clinical trials of dexamethasone therapy in children, predominantly with meningitis due to *H. influenzae* and *S. pneumoniae*, have demonstrated its efficacy in decreasing meningeal inflammation and neurologic sequelae such as the incidence of sensorineural hearing loss.

A prospective European trial of adjunctive therapy for acute bacterial meningitis in 301 adults found that dexamethasone reduced the number of unfavorable outcomes (15% vs. 25%, $p = .03$) including death (7% vs. 15%, $p = .04$). The benefits were most striking in patients with pneumococcal meningitis. Dexamethasone (10 mg intra-

TABLE 360-3 *Antimicrobial Therapy of CNS Bacterial Infections Based on Pathogen*[a]

Organism	Antibiotic
Neisseria meningitides	
Penicillin-sensitive	Penicillin G or Ampicillin
Penicillin-resistant	Ceftriaxone or cefotaxime
Streptococcus pneumoniae	
Penicillin-sensitive	Penicillin G
Penicillin-intermediate	Ceftriaxone or cefotaxime
Penicillin-resistant	(Ceftriaxone or cefotaxime) + vancomycin
Gram-negative bacilli (except *Pseudomonas* spp.)	Ceftriaxone or cefotaxime
Pseudomonas aeruginosa	Ceftazidime
Staphylococci spp.	
Methicillin-sensitive	Nafcillin
Methicillin-resistant	Vancomycin
Listeria monocytogenes	Ampicillin + gentamicin
Haemophilus influenzae	Ceftriaxone or cefotaxime
Streptococcus agalactiae	Penicillin G or ampicillin
Bacteroides fragilis	Metronidazole
Fusobacterium spp.	Metronidazole

[a] Doses are as indicated in Table 360-2.

venously) was administered 15 to 20 min before the first dose of an antimicrobial agent, and the same dose was repeated every 6 h for 4 days. These results were confirmed in a second trial of dexamethasone in adults with pneumococcal meningitis. Therapy with dexamethasone should ideally be started 20 min before, or not later than concurrent with, the first dose of antibiotics. It is unlikely to be of significant benefit if started >6 h after antimicrobial therapy has been initiated. Dexamethasone may decrease the penetration of vancomycin into CSF, and it delays the sterilization of CSF in experimental models of *S. pneumoniae* meningitis. As a result, its potential benefit should be carefully weighed when vancomycin is the antibiotic of choice. Alternatively, vancomycin can be administered by the intraventricular route.

Increased Intracranial Pressure Emergency treatment of increased ICP includes elevation of the patient's head to 30 to 45°, intubation and hyperventilation (Pa_{CO_2} 25 to 30 mmHg), and mannitol. Patients with increased ICP should be managed in an intensive care unit; accurate ICP measurements are best obtained with an ICP monitoring device. →*Treatment of increased intracranial pressure is discussed in detail in Chap. 258.*

PROGNOSIS Mortality is 3 to 7% for meningitis caused by *H. influenzae*, *N. meningitidis*, or group B streptococci; 15% for that due to *L. monocytogenes*; and 20% for *S. pneumoniae*. In general, the risk of death from bacterial meningitis increases with (1) decreased level of consciousness on admission, (2) onset of seizures within 24 h of admission, (3) signs of increased ICP, (4) young age (infancy) and age >50, (5) the presence of comorbid conditions including shock and/or the need for mechanical ventilation, and (6) delay in the initiation of treatment. Decreased CSF glucose concentration [<2.2 mmol/L (<40 mg/dL)] and markedly increased CSF protein concentration [>3 g/L (>300 mg/dL)] have been predictive of increased mortality and poorer outcomes in some series. Moderate or severe sequelae occur in ~25% of survivors, although the exact incidence varies with the infecting organism. Common sequelae include decreased intellectual function, memory impairment, seizures, hearing loss and dizziness, and gait disturbances.

ACUTE VIRAL MENINGITIS

CLINICAL MANIFESTATIONS Viral meningitis presents as fever, headache, and meningeal irritation coupled with an inflammatory CSF profile (see below). Fever may be accompanied by malaise, myalgia, anorexia, nausea and vomiting, abdominal pain, and/or diarrhea. It is not uncommon to see a mild degree of lethargy or drowsiness. The presence of more profound alterations in consciousness, such as stupor, coma, or marked confusion, should prompt consideration of alternative diagnoses. Similarly, seizures or other focal neurologic signs or symptoms suggest involvement of the brain parenchyma and do not occur in uncomplicated viral meningitis. The headache associated with viral meningitis is usually frontal or retroorbital and often associated with photophobia and pain on moving the eyes. Nuchal rigidity is present in most cases but may be mild and present only near the limit of neck anteflexion. Evidence of severe meningeal irritation, such as Kernig's and Brudzinski's signs, is generally absent.

ETIOLOGY Enteroviruses account for 75 to 90% of aseptic meningitis cases in most series (Table 360-4). Viruses belonging to the *Enterovirus* genus are members of the family Picornaviridae and include the coxsackieviruses, echoviruses, polioviruses, and human enteroviruses 68 to 71. Using a variety of diagnostic techniques including CSF PCR tests, culture, and serology, a specific viral cause can be found in 75 to 90% of cases of viral meningitis. CSF cultures are positive in 30 to 70% of patients, the frequency of isolation depending on the specific viral agent. Approximately two-thirds of culture-negative cases of aseptic meningitis have a specific viral etiology identified by CSF PCR testing (see below).

EPIDEMIOLOGY The exact incidence of viral meningitis in the United States is impossible to determine since most cases go unreported to

TABLE 360-4 *Viruses Causing Acute Meningitis and Acute Encephalitis*

Common	Less Common	Rare
ACUTE MENINGITIS		
Enteroviruses	HSV-1	Adenoviruses
Arboviruses	LCMV	CMV
HIV	VZV	EBV
HSV-2		Influenza A, B, parainfluenza, mumps, rubella
ACUTE ENCEPHALITIS		
Arboviruses	CMV	Adenoviruses, CTFV, hepatitis C,
Enteroviruses	EBV	influenza A, LCMV, parainfluenza,
HSV-1	HIV	rabies, rotavirus, rubella
	Mumps	

Note: CMV, cytomegalovirus; CTFV, Colorado tick fever virus; EBV, Epstein-Barr virus; HSV, herpes simplex virus; LCMV, lymphocytic choriomeningitis virus; VZV, varicella-zoster virus

public health authorities, although a reasonable estimate would be ~75,000 cases per year. In temperate climates, there is a substantial increase in cases during the summer and early fall months, reflecting the seasonal predominance of enterovirus and arthropod-borne encephalitis virus ("arbovirus") infections, with a peak monthly incidence of about 1 reported case per 100,000 population. The dramatic seasonal predilections of some viruses causing meningitis provide a valuable clue to diagnosis (Table 360-5).

LABORATORY DIAGNOSIS ■ CSF Examination The most important laboratory test in the diagnosis of viral meningitis is examination of the CSF. The typical profile is a lymphocytic pleocytosis (25 to 500 cells/μL) a normal or slightly elevated protein concentration [0.2 to 0.8 g/L (20 to 80 mg/dL)], a normal glucose concentration, and a normal or mildly elevated opening pressure (100 to 350 mmH$_2$O). Organisms are *not* seen on Gram's or acid-fast stained smears or india ink preparations of CSF. Rarely, PMNs may predominate in the first 48 h of illness, especially in patients with infections due to echovirus 9, West Nile virus or Eastern equine encephalitis virus, or mumps. Recent studies suggest that in some patients with West Nile virus infection, PMN pleocytosis can persist for up to a week before shifting to a lymphocytic pleocytosis. Despite these exceptions, the presence of a CSF PMN pleocytosis in a patient with suspected viral meningitis should always prompt consideration of an alternative diagnosis including bacterial meningitis or parameningeal infections. The total CSF cell count in viral meningitis is typically 25 to 500/μL, although cell counts of several thousand per microliter are occasionally seen, especially with infections due to lymphocytic choriomeningitis virus (LCMV) and mumps virus. The CSF glucose concentration is typically normal in viral infections, although it may be decreased in 10 to 30% of cases due to mumps as well as in cases due to LCMV. Rare instances of decreased CSF glucose concentration occur in cases of meningitis due to echoviruses and other enteroviruses, HSV type 2, and varicella-zoster virus (VZV). As a rule, a lymphocytic pleocytosis with a low glucose concentration should suggest fungal, listerial, or tuberculous meningitis or noninfectious disorders (e.g., sarcoid, neoplastic meningitis).

A number of tests measuring levels of various CSF proteins, enzymes, and mediators, including C-reactive protein, lactic acid, lactate dehydrogenase, neopterin, quinolinate, IL-1β, IL-6, soluble IL-2 receptor, β_2-microglobulin, and TNF, have been proposed as potential

TABLE 360-5 *Seasonal Prevalence of Viruses Commonly Causing Meningitis*

Summer/Early Fall	Fall/Winter	Winter/Spring	Nonseasonal
Arboviruses	LCMV	Mumps	HSV
Enteroviruses			HIV

Note: Abbreviations are as in Table 360-4.

TABLE 360-6 Features of Selected Arbovirus Encephalitides

Feature	WNV	WEE	EEE	VEE	SLE	CE
Region	All	West, midwest	Atlantic and Gulf coasts	SW, W	All	East and NC
Age	Adults > 60	Infants, adults > 50	Children, adults > 60	Adults	Adults > 60	Children
Deaths	7%	3–15%	50–75%	1%	2–20%	<1%
Sequelae	?	Common	80%	Rare	20%	Rare
Vector	M	M	M	M	M	M
Animal reservoir	B	B	B	H, sm M	B	sm M

Note: WNV, West Nile virus; WEE, Western equine encephalitis (virus); EEE, Eastern equine encephalitis (virus); VEE, Venezuelan equine encephalitis (virus); SLE, systemic lupus erythematosus; CE, California encephalitis (virus); B, bird; H, horse; M, mosquito; NC, north central United States; sm M, small mammal; SW, southwest; W, west.

discriminators between viral and bacterial meningitis or as markers of specific types of viral infection (e.g., infection with HIV), but remain of uncertain sensitivity and specificity and are not widely used for diagnostic purposes.

Polymerase Chain Reaction Amplification of Viral Nucleic Acid Amplification of viral-specific DNA or RNA from CSF using PCR amplification has become the single most important method for diagnosing CNS viral infections. In both enteroviral and HSV infections of the CNS, PCR has become the diagnostic procedure of choice and is substantially more sensitive than viral cultures. HSV PCR is also an important diagnostic test in patients with recurrent episodes of "aseptic" meningitis, many of whom have amplifiable HSV DNA in CSF despite negative viral cultures. CSF PCR is also used routinely to diagnose CNS viral infections caused by cytomegalovirus (CMV), Epstein-Barr virus (EBV), and VZV.

CSF Culture The overall results of CSF culture for the diagnosis of viral infection are disappointing, presumably because of the generally low concentration of infectious virus present and the need to customize isolation procedures for individual viruses. For viral isolation, 2 mL of CSF should be brought promptly to the microbiology laboratory, where it should be refrigerated and processed as speedily as possible. CSF specimens for viral isolation should never be stored in a −20°C freezer since viruses are often unstable at this temperature, and most freezers have "frostfree" warm-up cycles that are detrimental to viral stability. Storage for >24 h is probably best done in a −70°C freezer.

Other Sources for Viral Isolation Viruses may also be isolated from sites and body fluids other than CSF, including throat, stool, blood, and urine. Enteroviruses and adenoviruses may be found in feces; arboviruses, some enteroviruses, and LCMV, in blood; mumps and CMV, in urine; and enteroviruses, mumps, and adenoviruses, in throat washings. During enteroviral infections, viral shedding in stool may persist for several weeks. The presence of enterovirus in stool is not diagnostic and may result from residual shedding from a previous enteroviral infection; it also occurs in some asymptomatic individuals during enteroviral epidemics.

Serologic Studies For some viruses, including many arboviruses such as West Nile virus (WNV), serologic studies remain a crucial diagnostic tool. Serum serologic studies are less useful for viruses such as HSV, VZV, CMV, and EBV for which the prevalence of antibody seropositivity in the general population is high. Diagnosis of acute viral infection can be made by documenting seroconversion between acute-phase and convalescent sera (typically obtained after 2 to 4 weeks) or by demonstrating the presence of virus-specific IgM antibodies. Documentation of intrathecal synthesis of virus-specific antibodies, as shown by an increased IgG index or the presence of IgM antibodies in CSF, is often significantly more useful than serum serology alone and can provide presumptive evidence of CNS infection. Although serum and CSF IgM antibodies generally persist for only a few months after acute infection, there are exceptions to this rule. For example, WNV IgM has been shown to persist in some patients for >1 year following acute infection. Unfortunately, the delay between onset of infection and the generation by the host of a virus-specific antibody response often means that serologic data are useful mainly for the retrospective establishment of a specific diagnosis, rather than in urgent diagnosis or management.

Agarose electrophoresis or isoelectric focusing of CSF γ-globulins may reveal the presence of oligoclonal bands. These bands have been found in association with a number of viral infections, including infections with HIV, human T cell lymphotropic virus (HTLV) type I, VZV, mumps, subacute sclerosing panencephalitis (SSPE), and progressive rubella panencephalitis. The associated antibodies are often directed against viral proteins. The finding of oligoclonal bands may be of some diagnostic utility, since typically they are not seen with arbovirus, enterovirus, or HSV infections. Oligoclonal bands are also encountered in certain noninfectious neurologic diseases (e.g., multiple sclerosis) and may be found in nonviral infections (e.g., syphilis, Lyme borreliosis).

Other Laboratory Studies All patients with suspected viral meningitis should have a complete blood count and differential; liver function tests; and measurement of the erythrocyte sedimentation rate (ESR), blood urea nitrogen (BUN), and plasma levels of electrolytes, glucose, creatinine, creatine kinase, aldolase, amylase, and lipase. Abnormalities in specific test results may suggest particular etiologic diagnoses. MRI, CT, EEG, evoked response studies, electromyography (EMG), and nerve conduction studies are not necessary in most cases. They are best used selectively when atypical presentations or unusual features present diagnostic problems.

DIFFERENTIAL DIAGNOSIS The most important issue in the differential diagnosis is the exclusion of nonviral causes that can mimic viral meningitis. The major categories of disease that should always be considered and excluded are (1) bacterial meningitis and other infectious meningitides (e.g., *Mycoplasma*, *Listeria*, *Brucella*, *Coxiella*, and *Rickettsia*); (2) parameningeal infections or partially treated bacterial meningitis; (3) nonviral infectious meningitides where cultures may be negative (e.g., fungal, tuberculous, parasitic, or syphilitic disease); (4) neoplastic meningitis; and (5) meningitis secondary to noninfectious inflammatory diseases such as sarcoid, Behçet's disease, and the uveomeningitic syndromes.

SPECIFIC VIRAL ETIOLOGIES *Enteroviruses* (Chap. 175) are the most common cause of viral meningitis (>75% of cases in which a specific etiology can be identified) and should be considered the most likely cause of viral meningitis when a typical case occurs in the summer months, especially in a child (<15 years). However, despite their summer predominance, sporadic cases of enteroviral CNS infection are seen year-round. The physical examination should include a careful search for exanthemata, hand-foot-mouth disease, herpangina, pleurodynia, myopericarditis, and hemorrhagic conjunctivitis, which may be stigmata of enterovirus infections. PCR amplification of enteroviral RNA from CSF has become the diagnostic procedure of choice for these infections.

Arbovirus infections (Chap. 180) typically occur in the summer months, may have clear circumscribed geographic localization, and occur in both endemic and epidemic form, all factors reflecting the ecology of their transmission through infected insect vectors (Fig. 360-2; Tables 360-5 and 360-6). Arboviral meningitis should be considered when clusters of meningitis cases occur in a restricted geographic region during the summer or early fall. WNV infection should be suspected when bird deaths precede clusters of human cases of meningitis or encephalitis in an area known to harbor the virus. A history of tick exposure or travel or residence in the appropriate geographic area should suggest the possibility of Colorado tick fever virus or Powassan virus infection, although nonviral diseases producing meningitis (e.g.,

Lyme disease) or headache with meningismus (e.g., RMSF) may also present this way.

HSV-2 meningitis (Chap. 163) occurs in ~25% of women and 11% of men at the time of an initial (primary) episode of genital herpes. Of these patients, 20% go on to have recurrent attacks of meningitis. In some series, HSV-2 has been the most important cause of aseptic meningitis in adults, especially women, and overall it is probably second only to enteroviruses as a cause of viral meningitis. Although HSV-2 can be cultured from CSF during a first episode of meningitis, cultures are invariably negative during recurrent episodes of HSV-2 meningitis. Diagnosis depends on amplification of HSV-2 DNA from CSF by PCR. Almost all cases of recurrent HSV meningitis are due to HSV-2, although rare cases due to HSV-1 have been reported. Most cases of benign recurrent lymphocytic meningitis, including cases previously diagnosed as "Mollaret's meningitis," appear to be due to HSV. Genital lesions may not be present, and most patients give no history of genital herpes. CSF cultures are negative, although HSV DNA can be amplified from CSF by PCR during attacks of meningitis but not during symptom-free intervals.

VZV meningitis should be suspected in the presence of concurrent chickenpox or shingles. However, it is important to recognize that in some series up to 40% of VZV meningitis cases have been reported to occur in the absence of rash. The frequency of VZV as a cause of meningitis is extremely variable, ranging from as low as 3% to as high as 20% in different series. In addition to meningitis, encephalitis (see below), and shingles (see below), VZV can also produce acute cerebellar ataxia. This typically occurs in children and presents with the abrupt onset of limb and truncal ataxia. A similar syndrome occurs less commonly in association with EBV and enteroviral infection. PCR has rapidly become a major tool in the diagnosis of VZV CNS infections. In patients with negative CSF PCR results, the diagnosis of VZV CNS infection can be made by the demonstration of VZV-specific intrathecal antibody synthesis and/or the presence of VZV CSF IgM antibodies, or by positive CSF cultures.

EBV infections may also produce aseptic meningitis, with or without accompanying evidence of the infectious mononucleosis syndrome. The diagnosis may be suggested by the finding of atypical lymphocytes in the CSF or an atypical lymphocytosis in peripheral blood. The demonstration of IgM antibody to viral capsid antigen (VCA), or antibody to the diffuse (D) component of early antigen (EA) in the absence of or preceding detectable antibody to nuclear antigen (EBNA), are indicative of acute EBV infection. EBV is almost never cultured from CSF, but EBV DNA can be amplified from CSF in some patients with EBV-associated CNS infections. HIV-infected patients with primary CNS lymphoma may have a positive CSF PCR for EBV DNA even in the absence of meningoencephalitis.

HIV meningitis should be suspected in any patient with known or identified risk factors for HIV infection. Aseptic meningitis is a common manifestation of primary exposure to HIV and occurs in 5 to 10% of cases. In some patients, seroconversion may be delayed for several months; however, detection of the presence of HIV genome by PCR or p24 protein establishes the diagnosis. HIV can be cultured from CSF in some patients. Cranial nerve palsies, most commonly involving cranial nerves V, VII, or VIII, are more common in HIV meningitis than in other viral infections. →*For further discussion of HIV infection, see Chap. 173.*

Mumps (Chap. 178) should be considered when meningitis occurs in the late winter or early spring, especially in males (male/female ratio 3:1). With the widespread use of the live attenuated mumps vaccine in the United States since 1967, the incidence of mumps meningitis has fallen by >95%. Rare cases of mumps vaccine–associated meningitis have been reported, but they are not usually seen after vaccination with the attenuated Jeryl-Lynn strain of virus used in the United States. The presence of orchitis, oophoritis, parotitis, pancreatitis, or elevations in serum lipase and amylase are suggestive but can be found with other viruses, and their absence does not exclude the diagnosis. Clinical meningitis occurs in 5% of patients with parotitis, but only 50% of patients with meningitis have associated parotitis.

Mumps infection confers lifelong immunity, so a documented history of previous infection excludes this diagnosis. The presence of hypoglycorrhachia, found in 10 to 30% of patients, may be an additional diagnostic clue, once other causes have been excluded (see above). Up to 25% of patients may have a PMN-predominant CSF pleocytosis, and CSF abnormalities may persist for months. Diagnosis is typically made by isolation of virus from CSF and/or demonstration of seroconversion between acute-phase and convalescent sera.

LCMV infection (Chap. 180) should be considered when aseptic meningitis occurs in the late fall or winter, and in individuals with a history of exposure to house mice (*Mus musculus*), pet or laboratory rodents (e.g., hamsters), or their excreta. Some patients have an associated rash, pulmonary infiltrates, alopecia, parotitis, orchitis, or myopericarditis. Laboratory clues to the diagnosis of LCMV, in addition to the clinical findings noted above, may include the presence of leukopenia, thrombocytopenia, or abnormal liver function tests. Some cases present with a marked CSF pleocytosis (>1000 cells/μL) and hypoglycorrachia (<30%).

Rx TREATMENT

In the usual case of viral meningitis, treatment is symptomatic and hospitalization is not required. Exceptions include patients with deficient humoral immunity, neonates with overwhelming infection, and patients in whom the clinical or CSF profile suggests the possibility of a bacterial or other nonviral cause of infection. Patients with suspected bacterial meningitis should receive appropriate empirical therapy pending culture results (see above). Patients usually prefer to rest undisturbed in a quiet, darkened room. Analgesics can be used to relieve headache, which is often reduced by the initial diagnostic LP. Antipyretics may help to reduce fever, which rarely exceeds 40°C. Hyponatremia may develop as a result of inappropriate vasopressin secretion [syndrome of inappropriate secretion of antidiuretic hormone (SIADH)], so fluid and electrolyte status should be monitored. Repeat LP is indicated only in patients whose fever and symptoms fail to resolve after a few days, in patients with an initial PMN pleocytosis or hypoglycorrhachia, or if there is doubt about the initial diagnosis.

Oral or intravenous acyclovir may be of benefit in patients with meningitis caused by HSV-1 or -2 and in cases of severe EBV or VZV infection. Data concerning treatment of HSV, EBV, and VZV meningitis are extremely limited. Seriously ill patients should probably receive intravenous acyclovir (30 mg/kg per day in three divided doses) for 7 days. Oral acyclovir (800 mg, five times daily), famciclovir (500 mg, tid), or valacyclovir (1000 mg, tid) for a week may be tried in less severely ill patients, although data on efficacy are lacking. Patients with HIV meningitis should receive highly active antiretroviral therapy (Chap. 173).

Patients with viral meningitis who are known to have deficient humoral immunity (e.g. X-linked agammaglobulinemia), and who are not already receiving either intramuscular γ-globulin or intravenous immunoglobulin (IVIg), should be treated with these agents. Intraventricular administration of immunoglobulin through an Ommaya reservoir has been tried in some patients with chronic enteroviral meningitis who have not responded to intramuscular or intravenous immunoglobulin.

An experimental drug, pleconaril (Viropharma Inc., VP 63843), has shown efficacy against a variety of enteroviral infections and has good oral bioavailability and excellent CNS penetration. Ongoing clinical trials in patients with enteroviral meningitis suggest that pleconaril decreases the duration of symptoms compared to placebo. Since most cases of enteroviral CNS infection are benign and self-limited, the indications for pleconaril therapy need to be better defined. Antiviral treatment might benefit patients with chronic CNS enteroviral infections in the setting of agammaglobulinemia or those who develop poliomyelitis as a complication of polio vaccine administration.

Vaccination is an effective method of preventing the development of meningitis and other neurologic complications associated with poliovirus, mumps, and measles infection. A live attenuated VZV vaccine (Varivax) is available in the United States. Clinical studies indicate an effectiveness rate of 70 to 90% for this vaccine, but a booster may be required to maintain immunity. An inactivated varicella vaccine is available for transplant recipients.

PROGNOSIS   In adults, the prognosis for full recovery from viral meningitis is excellent. Rare patients complain of persisting headache, mild mental impairment, incoordination, or generalized asthenia for weeks to months. The outcome in infants and neonates (<1 year) is less certain; intellectual impairment, learning disabilities, hearing loss, and other lasting sequelae have been reported in some studies.

VIRAL ENCEPHALITIS

DEFINITION   In contrast to viral meningitis, where the infectious process and associated inflammatory response are limited largely to the meninges, in encephalitis the brain parenchyma is also involved. Many patients with encephalitis also have evidence of associated meningitis (meningoencephalitis) and, in some cases, involvement of the spinal cord or nerve roots (encephalomyelitis, encephalomyeloradiculitis).

CLINICAL MANIFESTATIONS   In addition to the acute febrile illness with evidence of meningeal involvement characteristic of meningitis, the patient with encephalitis commonly has confusion, behavioral abnormalities, an altered level of consciousness, and evidence of either focal or diffuse neurologic signs and symptoms. Any degree of altered consciousness may occur, ranging from mild lethargy to deep coma. Patients with encephalitis may have hallucinations, agitation, personality change, behavioral disorders, and, at times, a frankly psychotic state. Focal or generalized seizures occur in many patients with severe encephalitis. Virtually every possible type of focal neurologic disturbance has been reported in viral encephalitis; the signs and symptoms reflect the sites of infection and inflammation. The most commonly encountered focal findings are aphasia, ataxia, hemiparesis (with hyperactive tendon reflexes and extensor plantar responses), involuntary movements (e.g., myoclonic jerks, tremor), and cranial nerve deficits (e.g., ocular palsies, facial weakness). Involvement of the hypothalamic-pituitary axis may result in temperature dysregulation, diabetes insipidus, or the development of SIADH. Despite the clear neuropathologic evidence that viruses differ in the regions of the CNS they injure, it is often impossible to distinguish reliably on clinical grounds alone one type of viral encephalitis (e.g., that caused by HSV) from others (see "Differential Diagnosis," below).

ETIOLOGY   In the United States, there are ~20,000 reported cases of encephalitis per year; the actual number is likely to be significantly higher. Hundreds of viruses are capable of causing encephalitis, although only a limited subset is responsible for most cases in which a specific cause is identified (Table 360-4). The same organisms responsible for aseptic meningitis are also responsible for encephalitis, although their relative frequencies differ. The most important viruses causing sporadic cases of encephalitis in immunocompetent adults are HSV-1 (Fig. 360-3), VZV and, less commonly, enteroviruses. Epidemics of encephalitis are caused by arboviruses, which belong to several different viral taxonomic groups including *Alphaviruses* (e.g. Eastern equine encephalitis virus, Western equine encephalitis virus), *Flaviviruses* (e.g., WNV, St. Louis encephalitis virus, Powassan virus), and *Bunyaviruses* (e.g., California encephalitis virus serogroup, LaCrosse virus). Historically, the largest number of cases of arbovirus encephalitis in the United States has been due to St. Louis encephalitis virus and the California encephalitis virus serogroup. However, in 2002, WNV produced the largest epidemic of encephalitis ever recorded in the United States, with 4156 cases and 284 deaths. New causes of viral encephalitis are constantly appearing, as evidenced by the recent outbreak of 257 cases of encephalitis with a 40% mortality rate in Malaysia caused by Nipah virus, a new member of the Paramyxovirus family.

FIGURE 360-3   Coronal FLAIR magnetic resonance image from a patient with herpes simplex encephalitis. Note the area of increased signal in the temporal lobe (left) confined predominantly to the gray matter. This patient had predominantly unilateral disease; bilateral lesions are more common but may be quite asymmetric in their intensity.

LABORATORY DIAGNOSIS ■ CSF Examination   CSF examination should be performed in all patients with suspected viral encephalitis unless contraindicated by the presence of severely increased ICP. The characteristic CSF profile is indistinguishable from that of viral meningitis and consists of a lymphocytic pleocytosis, a mildly elevated protein concentration, and a normal glucose concentration. A CSF pleocytosis (>5 cells/μL) occurs in >95% of patients with documented viral encephalitis. In rare cases, a pleocytosis may be absent on the initial LP but present on subsequent LPs. Patients who are severely immunocompromised by HIV infection, glucocorticoid or other immunosuppressant drugs, chemotherapy, or lymphoreticular malignancies may fail to mount a CSF inflammatory response. CSF cell counts exceed 500/μL in only about 10% of patients with encephalitis. Infections with certain arboviruses (e.g., Eastern equine encephalitis or California encephalitis viruses), mumps, and LCMV may occasionally result in cell counts >1000/μL, but this degree of pleocytosis should suggest the possibility of nonviral infections or other inflammatory processes. Atypical lymphocytes in the CSF may be seen in EBV infection and less commonly with other viruses, including CMV, HSV, and enteroviruses. The presence of substantial numbers of PMNs after the first 48 h should prompt consideration of bacterial infection, leptospirosis, amebic infection, and noninfectious processes such as acute hemorrhagic leukoencephalitis. PMN pleocytosis that can persist for up to a week has also been reported in cases of WNV encephalitis. Large numbers of CSF PMNs may be present in patients with viral encephalitis due to Eastern equine encephalitis virus, echovirus 9, and, more rarely, other enteroviruses. About 20% of patients with encephalitis will have a significant number of red blood cells (>500/μL) in the CSF in a nontraumatic tap. The pathologic correlate of this finding may be a hemorrhagic encephalitis of the type seen with HSV, Colorado tick fever virus, and occasionally California encephalitis virus. A decreased CSF glucose concentration is distinctly unusual in viral encephalitis and should suggest the possibility of bacterial, fungal, tuberculous, parasitic, leptospiral, syphilitic, sarcoid, or neoplastic meningitis. Rare patients with mumps, LCMV, or advanced HSV encephalitis may have low CSF glucose concentrations.

CSF PCR   CSF PCR has become the primary diagnostic test for CNS infections caused by CMV, EBV, VZV and enteroviruses (see "Viral Meningitis," above). The sensitivity and specificity of CSF PCRs vary with the virus being tested. Recent studies with HSV encephalitis indicate that the sensitivity (~98%) and specificity (~94%) of CSF PCR equal or exceed those of brain biopsy. It is important to recognize that CSF HSV PCR results need to be interpreted after considering the likelihood of disease in the patient being tested, the timing of the test in relationship to onset of symptoms, and the prior use of antiviral therapy. A negative HSV CSF PCR test performed in a patient with a high likelihood of HSV encephalitis based on clinical and laboratory tests significantly reduces the likelihood of HSV encephalitis but does not exclude it. There have been several recent reports of initially negative CSF HSV PCR tests that were obtained early ($\leq$72 h) following symptom onset, that became positive when repeated 1 to 3 days later. The frequency of positive CSF HSV PCRs in patients with herpes encephalitis also decreases as a function of the duration of illness, with only ~20% of cases remaining positive after $\geq$14 days. PCR results are generally not affected by $\leq$1 week of antiviral therapy. In one study 98% of CSF specimens remained PCR-positive during the first week of initiation of antiviral therapy, but the numbers fell to ~50% by 8 to 14 days and to ~21% by >15 days after initiation of therapy.

The sensitivity and specificity of CSF PCR tests for viruses other than herpes simplex have not been definitively characterized. Enteroviral CSF PCR appears to have a sensitivity and specificity of >95%. The specificity of EBV CSF PCR has not been established, and apparent false-positive results can occur in patients with CNS lymphoma and in patients with inflammatory CSF specimens. In patients with CNS infection due to VZV, CSF antibody and PCR studies should be considered complementary, as several cases with positive serologies and negative PCR studies have been reported. In the case of WNV infection, CSF PCR is considerably less sensitive (~70% sensitivity) than detection of WNV specific CSF IgM in diagnosis of WNV encephalitis.

CSF Culture Attempts to culture viruses from the CSF in cases of encephalitis are often disappointing. Cultures are invariably negative in cases of HSV-1 encephalitis.

Serologic Studies and Antigen Detection The basic approach to the serodiagnosis of viral encephalitis is identical to that discussed earlier for viral meningitis. In patients with HSV encephalitis, both antibodies to HSV-1 glycoproteins and glycoprotein antigens have been detected in the CSF. Optimal detection of both HSV antibodies and antigen typically occurs after the first week of illness, limiting the utility of these tests in acute diagnosis. Nonetheless, CSF HSV antibody testing may be of value in selected patients whose illness is >1 week in duration and who are CSF PCR-negative for HSV. Demonstration of WNV IgM antibodies is diagnostic of WNV encephalitis, as IgM antibodies do not cross the blood-brain barrier and their presence in CSF is therefore indicative of intrathecal synthesis.

MRI, CT, EEG Patients with suspected encephalitis almost invariably undergo neuroimaging studies and often EEG. These tests help identify or exclude alternative diagnoses and assist in the differentiation between a focal, as opposed to a diffuse, encephalitic process. Focal findings in a patient with encephalitis should always raise the possibility of HSV encephalitis. Examples of focal findings include: (1) areas of increased signal intensity in the frontotemporal, cingulate, or insular regions of the brain on T2-weighted, fluid-attenuated inversion recovery (FLAIR), or diffusion-weighted MRI images (Fig. 360-3); (2) temporoparietal areas of low absorption, mass effect, and contrast enhancement on CT; or (3) periodic focal temporal lobe spikes on a background of slow or low-amplitude ("flattened") activity on EEG. Approximately 10% of patients with PCR-documented HSV encephalitis will have a normal MRI, although nearly 90% will have abnormalities in the temporal lobe. CT is less sensitive than MRI and is normal in up to 33% of patients. The addition of FLAIR and diffusion-weighted images to the standard MRI sequences enhances sensitivity. EEG abnormalities occur in >90% of PCR-documented cases of HSV encephalitis; they typically involve the temporal lobes but are often nonspecific. Some patients with HSV encephalitis have a distinctive EEG pattern consisting of periodic, stereotyped, sharp-and-slow complexes originating in one or both temporal lobes and repeating at regular intervals of 2 to 3 s. The periodic complexes are typically noted

between the second and the fifteenth day of the illness and are present in two-thirds of pathologically proven cases of HSV encephalitis.

Significant MRI abnormalities are found in only ~30% of patients with WNV encephalitis, a frequency significantly less than that of HSV encephalitis. When present, abnormalities often involve deep brain structures including the thalamus, basal ganglia, and brainstem rather than the cortex. Patients with VZV encephalitis may show areas of hemorrhagic infarction reflecting the tendency of this virus to produce a CNS vasculopathy rather than a true encephalitis.

Brain Biopsy Brain biopsy is now generally reserved for patients in whom CSF PCR studies fail to lead to a specific diagnosis, who have focal abnormalities on MRI, and who continue to show progressive clinical deterioration despite treatment with acyclovir and supportive therapy. The isolation of HSV from brain tissue obtained at biopsy was once considered the "gold standard" for the diagnosis of HSV encephalitis, although with the advent of CSF PCR tests for HSV it is rarely necessary to perform brain biopsy for this purpose. The need for brain biopsy to diagnose other forms of viral encephalitis has also declined greatly with the widespread availability of CSF PCR diagnostic tests for EBV, CMV, VZV, and enteroviruses. When biopsy is performed, the tissue is cultured for virus and examined histopathologically and ultrastructurally. Tissue should be taken from a site that appears to be significantly involved on the basis of clinical and laboratory criteria. Although brain biopsy is not an innocuous procedure, the mortality rate is low (<0.2%) and serious complications occur in only 0.5 to 2.0% of cases. Potential morbidity, in addition to that related to general anesthesia, includes local bleeding and edema, the development of a seizure focus, and wound dehiscence or infection.

DIFFERENTIAL DIAGNOSIS Some of the most common illnesses masquerading as viral encephalitis, as identified in multicenter clinical trials using brain biopsy as a diagnostic standard, were vascular diseases; abscess and empyema; fungal, parasitic, rickettsial, and tuberculous infections; tumors; Reye's syndrome; toxic encephalopathy; subdural hematoma; and SLE. Acute disseminated encephalomyelitis (ADEM), limbic encephalitis, prion diseases, and Hashimoto's encephalopathy are additional considerations. Of the nonviral infections, particular attention should be paid to *Listeria*, *Mycoplasma*, *Leptospira*, *Cryptococcus*, and *Mucor* infections, as well as to toxoplasmosis and tuberculosis.

Meningoencephalitis caused by ameba can also mimic viral encephalitis. Infection caused by *Naegleria fowleri* usually causes an acute syndrome (primary amebic meningoencephalitis), whereas that caused by *Acanthamoeba* and *Balamuthia* more typically produces subacute or chronic granulomatous amebic meningoencephalitis. *Naegleria* thrive in warm iron-rich pools of water including those found in drains, canals, and both natural and man-made outdoor pools. Infection has typically occurred in immunocompetent children with a history of swimming in potentially infected water. The presentation is of an acute encephalitis, with a CSF neutrophilic pleocytosis and hypoglycorrhachia identical to that seen in bacterial meningitis. Motile trophozoites can be seen in a wet mount of warm fresh CSF. No effective treatment has been identified, and mortality approaches 100%.

There have also been several recent reports of encephalitis caused by the raccoon pinworm *Baylisascaris procyonis*. Clues to the diagnosis include a history of raccoon exposure, and especially of playing in or eating dirt potentially contaminated with raccoon feces. Most patients are children, and many have an associated eosinophilia.

Infection with *Bartonella* species, the agents of cat scratch fever, can also produce a meningoencephalitis. In some recent surveys, *Bartonella* infection has been the most common bacterial infection mimicking viral encephalitis. Infection is transmitted by the bite or scratch of a cat, with an increased risk associated with kittens and feral cats. Patients often develop regional lymphadenopathy; 2 to 4% of infected patients develop encephalopathy, retinitis, or less commonly cranial or peripheral neuropathy. CSF shows a lymphocytic pleocytosis with normal glucose in about one-third of cases, the remainder having no abnormalities or only mild protein elevation. Neuroimaging results are nonspecific, and diagnosis is based on serology. Antibiotic therapy is of uncertain value in immunocompetent hosts, although doxycycline (200 mg daily for 3 months) is often tried in patients with CNS disease.

Once nonviral causes of encephalitis have been excluded, the major diagnostic challenge is to distinguish HSV from other viruses that cause encephalitis. This distinction is particularly important because in virtually every other instance the therapy is supportive, whereas specific and effective antiviral therapy is available for HSV, and its efficacy is enhanced when it is instituted early in the course of infection. HSV encephalitis should be considered when clinical features suggesting involvement of the inferomedial frontotemporal regions of the brain are present, including prominent olfactory or gustatory hallucinations, anosmia, unusual or bizarre behavior or personality alterations, or memory disturbance. HSV encephalitis should always be suspected in patients with focal findings on clinical examination, neuroimaging studies, or EEG. The diagnostic procedure of choice in these patients is CSF PCR analysis for HSV. A positive CSF PCR establishes the diagnosis, and a negative test dramatically reduces the likelihood of HSV encephalitis (see above).

The anatomic distribution of lesions may provide an additional clue to diagnosis. Patients with rapidly progressive encephalitis and prominent brainstem signs, symptoms or neuroimaging abnormalities may be infected by flaviviruses (WNV, Japanese encephalitis virus), HSV, rabies or *L. monocytogenes*. Significant involvement of deep gray matter structures including the basal ganglia and thalamus should also suggest possible flavivirus infection. These patients may present clinically with prominent movement disorders (tremor, myoclonus) or Parkinson's disease–like features. Patients with WNV infection can also present with acute poliomyelitis-like areflexic paralysis, as can patients infected with enterovirus 71 and less commonly other enteroviruses. Despite an aggressive World Health Organization poliovirus eradication initiative, cases of wild-type poliovirus-induced poliomyelitis continue to be reported in at least seven countries worldwide: Egypt, Somalia, Niger, Nigeria, India, Pakistan, and Afghanistan. Rare cases continue to occur in the United States in nonvaccinated individuals exposed to vaccine strains of virus that have reverted to virulence. A recent outbreak of poliomyelitis on Hispaniola (the Dominican Republic and Haiti) has been attributed to vaccine strain–derived viruses that have reverted to virulence after apparently recombining with other circulating enteroviruses. Acute ascending paralysis resembling Guillain-Barré syndrome but associated with CSF pleocytosis can occur with HIV infection, rabies, and WNV infection.

Epidemiologic factors may provide important clues. Particular attention should be paid to the season of the year (Table 360-5); the age of the patient (Table 360-6); the geographic location and travel history (Table 360-6); and possible exposure to animal bites or scratches, rodents, and ticks. Although transmission from the bite of an infected dog remains the most common cause of rabies worldwide, in the United States very few cases of dog rabies occur, and the most common risk factor is exposure to bats—although a clear history of a bite or scratch is often lacking. The classic clinical presentation of encephalitic (furious) rabies is of fever and autonomic hyperactivity with fluctuating mental status. Phobic spasms of the larynx, pharynx, neck muscles, and diaphragm can be triggered by attempts to swallow water (*hydrophobia*) or by inspiration (*aerophobia*). Patients may also present with paralytic (dumb) rabies characterized by acute ascending paralysis. Patients with rabies have a CSF lymphocytic pleocytosis and may show areas of increased T2 signal abnormality in the brainstem, hippocampus, and hypothalamus. Diagnosis can be made by finding rabies virus antigen in brain tissue or in the neural innervation of hair follicles at the nape of the neck. PCR amplification of viral nucleic acid from CSF and saliva or tears may also enable diagnosis. Serology is frequently negative in both serum and CSF in the first week after onset of infection, which limits its acute diagnostic utility.

No specific therapy is available, and cases are almost invariably fatal, with isolated survivors having devastating neurologic sequelae.

Morbidity and Mortality Weekly Reports provides regular information about the prevalence of particular viruses causing encephalitis by season and region of the country. State public health authorities provide another valuable resource concerning isolation of particular agents in individual regions. Deaths in crows and other corvid birds in the local area have preceded human infection by WNV during outbreaks in the United States. Details of the occurrence of WNV in mosquitoes, birds, horses, and humans can be found on the Centers for Disease Control and Prevention (CDC) and U.S. Geological Survey (USGS) websites (and http://westnilemaps.usgs.gov/).

℞ TREATMENT

Specific antiviral therapy should be initiated when appropriate. Vital functions, including respiration and blood pressure, should be monitored continuously and supported as required. In the initial stages of encephalitis, many patients will require care in an intensive care unit. Basic management and supportive therapy should include careful monitoring of ICP, fluid restriction and avoidance of hypotonic intravenous solutions, and suppression of fever. Seizures should be treated with standard anticonvulsant regimens, and prophylactic therapy should be considered in view of the high frequency of seizures in severe cases of encephalitis. As with all seriously ill, immobilized patients with altered levels of consciousness, encephalitis patients are at risk for aspiration pneumonia, stasis ulcers and decubiti, contractures, deep venous thrombosis and its complications, and infections of indwelling lines and catheters.

Acyclovir is of benefit in the treatment of HSV and should be started empirically in patients with suspected viral encephalitis while awaiting viral diagnostic studies. Treatment should be discontinued in patients found not to have HSV encephalitis, with the possible exception of patients with severe encephalitis due to VZV or EBV. HSV, VZV, and EBV all encode an enzyme, deoxypyrimidine (thymidine) kinase, that phosphorylates acyclovir to produce acyclovir-5′-monophosphate. Host cell enzymes then phosphorylate this compound to form a triphosphate derivative. It is the triphosphate that acts as an antiviral agent by inhibiting viral DNA polymerase and by causing premature termination of nascent viral DNA chains. The specificity of action depends on the fact that uninfected cells do not phosphorylate significant amounts of acyclovir to acyclovir-5′-monophosphate. A second level of specificity is provided by the fact that the acyclovir triphosphate is a more potent inhibitor of viral DNA polymerase than of the analogous host cell enzymes.

Adults should receive a dose of 10 mg/kg of acyclovir intravenously every 8 h (30 mg/kg per day total dose) for a minimum of 14 days. Although no studies directly addressing this issue are yet available, repeating the CSF PCR after completion of acyclovir therapy should be considered. Patients with a persisting positive CSF PCR for HSV after completing a standard course of acyclovir therapy should be treated for an additional 7 days, followed by a repeat CSF PCR test. Neonatal HSV CNS infection is less responsive to acyclovir therapy than HSV encephalitis in adults; it is recommended that neonates with HSV encephalitis receive 20 mg/kg of acyclovir every 8 h (60 mg/kg per day total dose) for a minimum of 21 days.

Prior to intravenous administration, acyclovir should be diluted to a concentration ≤7 mg/mL. (A 70-kg person would receive a dose of 700 mg, which would be diluted in a volume of 100 mL.) Each dose should be infused slowly over 1 h rather than by rapid or bolus infusion, to minimize the risk of renal dysfunction. Care should be taken to avoid extravasation or intramuscular or subcutaneous administration. The alkaline pH of acyclovir can cause local inflammation and phlebitis (9%). Dose adjustment is required in patients with impaired renal glomerular filtration. Penetration into CSF is excellent, with average drug levels ~50% of serum levels. Complications of therapy include elevations in BUN and creatinine levels (5%), thrombocytopenia (6%), gastrointestinal toxicity (nausea, vomiting, diarrhea) (7%), and neurotoxicity (lethargy or obtundation, disorientation, confusion, agitation, hallucinations, tremors, seizures) (1%). Acyclovir resistance may be mediated by changes in either the viral deoxypyrimidine kinase or DNA polymerase. To date, acyclovir-resistant isolates have not been a significant clinical problem in immunocompetent individuals. However, there have been reports of clinically virulent acyclovir-resistant HSV isolates from sites outside the CNS in immunocompromised individuals, including those with AIDS.

Oral antiviral drugs with efficacy against HSV, VZV, and EBV, including acyclovir, famciclovir, and valacyclovir, have not been evaluated in the treatment of encephalitis either as primary therapy or as supplemental therapy following completion of a course of parenteral acyclovir. An NIAID/NINDS-sponsored phase III trial of supplemental oral valacyclovir therapy (2 g, tid for 3 months) following the initial 14- to 21-day course of therapy with parenteral acyclovir has recently been initiated by the Collaborative Antiviral Study Group (CASG) in patients with HSV encephalitis (CASG 204); it may help clarify the role of extended oral antiviral therapy.

Both ganciclovir and foscarnet have been shown to be effective in the treatment of CMV-related CNS infections. These drugs are often used in combination. Cidofovir (see below) may provide an alternative in patients who fail to respond to ganciclovir and foscarnet, although data concerning its use in CMV CNS infections are extremely limited.

Ganciclovir is a synthetic nucleoside analogue of 2′-deoxyguanosine. The drug is preferentially phosphorylated by virus-induced cellular kinases. Ganciclovir triphosphate acts as a competitive inhibitor of the CMV DNA polymerase, and its incorporation into nascent viral DNA results in premature chain termination. Following intravenous administration, CSF concentrations of ganciclovir are 25 to 70% of coincident plasma levels. The usual dose for treatment of severe neurologic illnesses is 5 mg/kg every 12 h given intravenously at a constant rate over 1 h. Induction therapy is followed by maintenance therapy of 5 mg/kg every day for an indefinite period. Induction therapy should be continued until patients show a decline in CSF pleocytosis and a reduction in CSF CMV DNA copy number on quantitative PCR testing (where available). Doses should be adjusted in patients with renal insufficiency. Treatment is often limited by the development of granulocytopenia and thrombocytopenia (20 to 25%), which may require reduction in or discontinuation of therapy. Gastrointestinal side effects including nausea, vomiting, diarrhea, and abdominal pain occur in ~20% of patients. Some patients treated with ganciclovir for CMV retinitis have developed retinal detachment, but the causal relationship to ganciclovir treatment is unclear.

Foscarnet is a pyrophosphate analogue that inhibits viral DNA polymerases by binding to the pyrophosphate-binding site. Following intravenous infusion, CSF concentrations range from 15 to 100% of coincident plasma levels. The usual dose for serious CMV-related neurologic illness is 60 mg/kg every 8 h administered by constant infusion over 1 h. Induction therapy for 14 to 21 days is followed by maintenance therapy (60 to 120 mg/kg per day). Induction therapy may need to be extended in patients who fail to show a decline in CSF pleocytosis and a reduction in CSF CMV DNA copy number on quantitative PCR tests (where available). Approximately one-third of patients develop renal impairment during treatment, which is reversible following discontinuation of therapy in most, but not all, cases. This is often associated with elevations in serum creatinine and proteinuria and is less frequent in patients who are adequately hydrated. Many patients experience fatigue and nausea. Reduction in serum calcium, magnesium, and potassium occur in ~15% of patients and may be associated with tetany, cardiac rhythm disturbances, or seizures.

Cidofovir is a nucleotide analogue that is effective in treating CMV retinitis and equivalent or better than ganciclovir in some experimental models of murine CMV encephalitis, although data concerning its efficacy in human CMV CNS disease are limited. The usual dose is 5 mg/kg intravenously once weekly for 2 weeks, then biweekly for 2 or more additional doses, depending on clinical response. Patients must be prehydrated with normal saline (e.g., 1 L over 1 to 2 h) prior to each dose and treated with probenecid (e.g., 1 g 3 h before cidofovir

and 1 g 2 and 8 h after cidofovir). Nephrotoxicity is common; the dose should be reduced if renal function deteriorates.

Intravenous ribavarin (15 to 25 mg/kg per day in divided doses given every 8 h) has been reported to be of benefit in isolated cases of severe encephalitis due to California encephalitis (LaCrosse) virus. Ribavarin might be of benefit for the rare patients, typically infants or young children, with severe adenovirus or rotavirus encephalitis and in patients with encephalitis due to LCMV or other arenaviruses. However, clinical trials are lacking. Hemolysis, with resulting anemia, has been the major side effect limiting therapy.

No specific antiviral therapy of proven efficacy is currently available for treatment of WNV encephalitis. Small groups of patients have been treated with interferon α, ribavarin, and IVIg preparations of non-U.S. origin containing high titer anti-WNV antibody. Evidence is insufficient to establish efficacy of any of these therapies.

SEQUELAE There is considerable variation in the incidence and severity of sequelae in patients surviving viral encephalitis. In the case of Eastern equine encephalitis virus infection, nearly 80% of survivors have severe neurologic sequelae. At the other extreme are infections due to EBV, California encephalitis virus, and Venezuelan equine encephalitis virus, where severe sequelae are unusual. For example, ~5 to 15% of children infected with LaCrosse virus have a residual seizure disorder, and 1% have persistent hemiparesis. Detailed information about sequelae in patients with HSV encephalitis treated with acyclovir are available from the NIAID-CASG trials. Of 32 acyclovir-treated patients, 26 survived (81%). Of the 26 survivors, 12 (46%) had no or only minor sequelae, 3 (12%) were moderately impaired (gainfully employed but not functioning at their previous level), and 11 (42%) were severely impaired (requiring continuous supportive care). The incidence and severity of sequelae were directly related to the age of the patient and the level of consciousness at the time of initiation of therapy. Patients with severe neurologic impairment (Glasgow coma score 6) at initiation of therapy either died or survived with severe sequelae. Young patients (<30 years) with good neurologic function at initiation of therapy did substantially better (100% survival, 62% with no or mild sequelae) compared with their older counterparts (>30 years); (64% survival, 57% no or mild sequelae). Some recent studies using quantitative CSF PCR tests for HSV indicate that clinical outcome following treatment also correlates with the amount of HSV DNA present in CSF at the time of presentation. Many patients with WNV infection have acute sequelae including cognitive impairment; weakness; and hyper- or hypo-kinetic movement disorders including tremor, myoclonus, and parkinsonism. Improvement in these symptoms may occur over the subsequent 6 to 12 months, although detailed clinical studies of the duration and severity of WNV sequelae are still lacking.

SUBACUTE MENINGITIS

CLINICAL MANIFESTATIONS Patients with subacute meningitis typically have an unrelenting headache, stiff neck, low-grade fever, and lethargy for days to several weeks before they present for evaluation. Cranial nerve abnormalities and night sweats may be present. This syndrome overlaps that of chronic meningitis discussed in detail in Chap. 361.

ETIOLOGY Common causative organisms include *M. tuberculosis*, *C. neoformans*, *H. capsulatum*, *C. immitis*, and *T. pallidum*. Initial infection with *M. tuberculosis* is acquired by inhalation of aerosolized droplet nuclei. Tuberculous meningitis in adults does not develop acutely from hematogenous spread of tubercle bacilli to the meninges. Rather, millet seed–size (miliary) tubercles form in the parenchyma of the brain during hematogenous dissemination of tubercle bacilli in the course of primary infection. These tubercles enlarge and are usually caseating. The propensity for a caseous lesion to produce meningitis is determined by its proximity to the SAS and the rate at which fibrous encapsulation develops. Subependymal caseous foci cause meningitis via discharge of bacilli and tuberculous antigens into the SAS. Mycobacterial antigens produce an intense inflammatory reaction that leads to the production of a thick exudate that fills the basilar cisterns and surrounds the cranial nerves and major blood vessels at the base of the brain.

Fungal infections are typically acquired by the inhalation of airborne fungal spores. The initial pulmonary infection may be asymptomatic or present with fever, cough, sputum production, and chest pain. The pulmonary infection is often self-limited. A localized pulmonary fungal infection can then remain dormant in the lungs until there is an abnormality in cell-mediated immunity that allows the fungus to reactivate and disseminate to the CNS. The most common pathogen causing fungal meningitis is *C. neoformans*. This fungus is found worldwide in soil and bird excreta. *H. capsulatum* is endemic to the Ohio and Mississippi River valleys of the central United States and to parts of Central and South America. *C. immitis* is endemic to the desert areas of the southwest United States, northern Mexico, and Argentina.

Syphilis is a sexually transmitted disease that is manifest by the appearance of a painless chancre at the site of inoculation. *T. pallidum* invades the CNS early in the course of syphilis. Cranial nerves VII and VIII are most frequently involved.

LABORATORY DIAGNOSIS The classic CSF abnormalities in tuberculous meningitis are as follows: (1) elevated opening pressure, (2) lymphocytic pleocytosis (10 to 500 cells/μL), (3) elevated protein concentration in the range of 1 to 5 g/L (10 to 500 mg/dL), and (4) decreased glucose concentration in the range of 1.1 to 2.2 mmol/L (20 to 40 mg/dL). *The combination of unrelenting headache, stiff neck, fatigue, night sweats, and fever with a CSF lymphocytic pleocytosis and a mildly decreased glucose concentration is highly suspicious for tuberculous meningitis.* The last tube of fluid collected at LP is the best tube to send for a smear for acid-fast bacilli (AFB). If there is a pellicle in the CSF or a cobweb-like clot on the surface of the fluid, AFB can best be demonstrated in a smear of the clot or pellicle. Positive smears are typically reported in only 10 to 40% of cases of tuberculous meningitis in adults. Cultures of CSF take 4 to 8 weeks to identify the organism and are positive in ~50% of adults. Culture remains the "gold standard" to make the diagnosis of tuberculous meningitis. PCR for the detection of *M. tuberculosis* DNA has a sensitivity of 70 to 80% but at the present time is limited by a high rate of false-positive results.

The characteristic CSF abnormalities in fungal meningitis are a mononuclear or lymphocytic pleocytosis, an increased protein concentration, and a decreased glucose concentration. There may be eosinophils in the CSF in *C. immitis* meningitis. Large volumes of CSF are often required to demonstrate the organism on India ink smear or grow the organism in culture. If spinal fluid examined by LP on two separate occasions fails to yield an organism, CSF should be obtained by high-cervical or cisternal puncture.

The cryptococcal polysaccharide antigen test is a highly sensitive and specific test for cryptococcal meningitis. A reactive CSF cryptococcal antigen test establishes the diagnosis. The detection of the *histoplasma* polysaccharide antigen in CSF establishes the diagnosis of a fungal meningitis but is not specific for meningitis due to *H. capsulatum*. It may be falsely positive in coccidioidal meningitis. The CSF complement fixation antibody test is reported to have a specificity of 100% and a sensitivity of 75% for coccidioidal meningitis.

The diagnosis of syphilitic meningitis is made when a reactive serum treponemal test [fluorescent treponemal antibody, absorbed (FTA-ABS) or microhemagglutination-*T. pallidum* (MHA-TP)] is associated with a CSF lymphocytic or mononuclear pleocytosis and an elevated protein concentration, or when the CSF VDRL is positive. A reactive CSF-FTA-ABS is not definitive evidence of neurosyphilis. The CSF-FTA-ABS can be falsely positive from blood contamination. A negative CSF VDRL does not rule out neurosyphilis. A negative CSF FTA-ABS or MHA-TP rules out neurosyphilis.

℞ TREATMENT

Empirical therapy of tuberculous meningitis is often initiated on the basis of a high index of suspicion without adequate laboratory support. Initial therapy is a combination of isoniazid (300 mg/d), rifampin (10 mg/kg per day), pyrazinamide (30 mg/kg per day in divided doses), ethambutol (15 to 25 mg/kg per day in divided doses), and pyridoxine (50 mg/d). If the clinical response is good, pyrazinamide and ethambutol can be discontinued after 8 weeks and isoniazid and rifampin continued alone for the next 6 to 12 months. A 6-month course of therapy is acceptable, but therapy should be prolonged for 9 to 12 months in patients who have an inadequate resolution of symptoms of meningitis or who have positive mycobacterial cultures of CSF during the course of therapy. Dexamethasone therapy is recommended for patients who develop hydrocephalus.

Meningitis due to *C. neoformans* is treated with amphotericin B (0.7 mg/kg per day) and flucytosine (100 mg/kg per day in four divided doses) for 2 weeks, followed by an 8- to 10-week course of fluconazole (400 to 800 mg/d). If the CSF culture is sterile after 10 weeks of acute therapy, the dose of fluconazole is decreased to 200 mg/d for 6 months to a year. Patients with HIV infection may require indefinite maintenance therapy. Meningitis due to *H. capsulatum* is treated with amphotericin B (0.7 to 1.0 mg/kg per day) for 4 to 12 weeks followed by itraconazole (400 mg/d). Therapy with amphotericin B is not discontinued until fungal cultures are sterile. After completing a course of amphotericin B, maintenance therapy with itraconazole is initiated and continued for at least 6 months to a year. *C. immitis* meningitis is treated with intravenous amphotericin B (0.5 to 0.7 mg/kg per day) for ≥4 weeks until CSF fungal cultures are negative. Intrathecal amphotericin B may be required to eradicate the infection. Lifelong therapy with fluconazole is recommended to prevent relapse. Ambisome (4 mg/kg per day) or amphotericin B lipid complex (5 mg/kg per day) can be substituted for amphotericin B in patients who have or who develop significant renal dysfunction. The most common complication of fungal meningitis is hydrocephalus. Patients who develop hydrocephalus should receive a CSF diversion device. A ventriculostomy can be used until CSF fungal cultures are sterile, at which time the ventriculostomy is replaced by a ventriculoperitoneal shunt.

Syphilitic meningitis is treated with aqueous penicillin G in a dose of 3 to 4 million units intravenously every 4 h for 10 to 14 days. An alternative regimen is 2.4 million units of procaine penicillin G intramuscularly daily with 500 mg of oral probenecid four times daily for 10 to 14 days. Either regimen is followed with 2.4 million units of benzathine penicillin G intramuscularly once a week for 3 weeks. The standard criterion for treatment success is reexamination of the CSF. The CSF should be reexamined at 6-month intervals for 2 years. The cell count is expected to normalize within 12 months, and the VDRL titer to decrease by two dilutions or revert to nonreactive within 2 years of completion of therapy. Failure of the CSF pleocytosis to resolve or an increase in the CSF VDRL titer by two or more dilutions requires re-treatment.

CHRONIC ENCEPHALITIS

PROGRESSIVE MULTIFOCAL LEUKOENCEPHALOPATHY ■ Clinical Features and Pathology Progressive multifocal leukoencephalopathy (PML) is a progressive disorder characterized pathologically by multifocal areas of demyelination of varying size distributed throughout the CNS. In addition to demyelination, there are characteristic cytologic alterations in both astrocytes and oligodendrocytes. Astrocytes are tremendously enlarged and contain hyperchromatic, deformed, and bizarre nuclei and frequent mitotic figures. Oligodendrocytes have enlarged, densely staining nuclei that contain viral inclusions formed by crystalline arrays of JC virus particles. Patients often present with visual deficits (45%), typically a homonymous hemianopia, and mental impairment (38%) (dementia, confusion, personality change). Motor weakness may not be present early but eventually occurs in 75% of cases.

Almost all patients have an underlying immunosuppressive disorder. Prior to the HIV epidemic, common associated diseases included lymphoproliferative disorders, immune deficiency states, myeloproliferative disease, and chronic infectious or granulomatous diseases. More than 60% of currently diagnosed PML cases occur in patients with AIDS. Conversely, it has been estimated that nearly 1% of AIDS patients will develop PML. The basic features of AIDS-associated and non-AIDS-associated PML are identical.

Diagnostic Studies MRI reveals multifocal asymmetric, coalescing white matter lesions located periventricularly, in the centrum semiovale, in the parietal-occipital region, and in the cerebellum. These lesions have increased T2 and decreased T1 signal, are generally nonenhancing or show only minimal peripheral enhancement, and are not associated with edema or mass effect. CT scans, which are less sensitive than MRI for the diagnosis of PML, often show hypodense nonenhancing white matter lesions.

The CSF is typically normal, although mild elevation in protein and/or IgG may be found. Pleocytosis occurs in <25% of cases, is predominantly mononuclear, and rarely exceeds 25 cells/μL. PCR amplification of JC virus DNA from CSF has become an important diagnostic tool. CSF PCR for JC virus DNA has high specificity, but sensitivity has varied among studies. Rare cases of positive CSF PCR for JC virus DNA in the absence of clinical or radiographic evidence of PML have been described in HIV-infected patients. It remains to be established whether these results are false positives or indicate preclinical PML.

A positive CSF PCR for JC virus DNA in association with typical MRI lesions in the appropriate clinical setting is diagnostic of PML. Patients with negative CSF PCR studies may require brain biopsy for definitive diagnosis; JC virus antigen and nucleic acid can be detected by immunocytochemistry, in situ hybridization, or PCR amplification. Detection of JC virus antigen or genomic material should be considered diagnostic of PML only if accompanied by characteristic pathologic changes, since both antigen and genomic material have been found in the brains of normal patients.

℞ TREATMENT

No effective therapy is available. Recent trials in HIV-associated PML failed to show benefit from either cytarabine or cidofovir. Some patients with HIV-associated PML have shown dramatic clinical improvement associated with improvement in their immune status following institution of highly active antiretroviral therapy.

SUBACUTE SCLEROSING PANENCEPHALITIS SSPE is a rare progressive demyelinating disease of the CNS associated with a chronic infection of brain tissue with measles virus. Most patients give a history of primary measles infection at an early age (2 years), which is followed after a latent interval of 6 to 8 years by the development of insidious intellectual decline and mood and personality changes. Typical signs of a CNS viral infection, including fever and headache, do not occur. Focal and/or generalized seizures, myoclonus, ataxia, and visual disturbances occur as the disease progresses. The EEG shows a characteristic periodic pattern with bursts every 3 to 8 s of high-voltage, sharp slow waves, followed by periods of attenuated ("flat") background. The CSF is acellular with a normal or mildly elevated protein level and a markedly elevated γ-globulin level (>20% of total CSF protein). CSF antimeasles antibody levels are invariably elevated, and oligoclonal antimeasles antibodies are often present. CT and MRI show evidence of multifocal white matter lesions and generalized atrophy. Measles virus can be cultured from brain tissue, and viral genome can be detected by in situ hybridization or PCR amplification. Treatment with isoprinosine (Inosiplex) (100 mg/kg per day), alone or in combination with intrathecal or intraventricular interferon, has been reported to prolong survival and produce clinical improvement in some patients but has never been subjected to a controlled clinical trial.

PROGRESSIVE RUBELLA PANENCEPHALITIS This is an extremely rare disorder that primarily affects males with congenital rubella syndrome, although isolated cases have been reported following childhood rubella. After a latent period of 8 to 19 years, patients develop progressive neurologic deterioration. The manifestations are similar to those seen in SSPE. CSF shows a mild lymphocytic pleocytosis, slightly elevated protein level, markedly increased γ-globulin, and rubella virus–specific oligoclonal bands. No therapy is available.

BRAIN ABSCESS

DEFINITION A brain abscess is a focal, suppurative infection within the brain parenchyma, typically surrounded by a vascularized capsule. The term *cerebritis* is often employed to describe a nonencapsulated brain abscess.

EPIDEMIOLOGY A bacterial brain abscess is a relatively uncommon intracranial infection, with an incidence of ~1 in 100,000 persons per year. Predisposing conditions include otitis media and mastoiditis, paranasal sinusitis, pyogenic infections in the chest or other body sites, penetrating head trauma or neurosurgical procedures, and dental infections. In most modern series, an increasing proportion of brain abscesses are not caused by classic pyogenic bacteria, but rather by fungi and parasites including *Toxoplasma gondii*, *Aspergillus* spp., *Nocardia* spp., *Mycobacteria* spp., and *C. neoformans*. These organisms are almost exclusively restricted to immunocompromised hosts with underlying HIV infection, organ transplantation, cancer, or immunosuppressive therapy. In Latin America and in immigrants from Latin America, the most common cause of brain abscess is *Taenia solium* (neurocysticercosis). In India and the Far East, mycobacterial infection (tuberculoma) remains a major cause of focal CNS mass lesions.

ETIOLOGY A brain abscess may develop (1) by direct spread from a contiguous cranial site of infection, such as paranasal sinusitis, otitis media, mastoiditis, or dental infection; (2) following head trauma or a neurosurgical procedure; or (3) as a result of hematogenous spread from a remote site of infection. In up to 25% of cases no obvious primary source of infection is apparent (cryptogenic brain abscess).

Up to one-third of brain abscesses are associated with otitis media and mastoiditis, often with an associated cholesteatoma. Otogenic abscesses occur predominantly in the temporal lobe (55 to 75%) and cerebellum (20 to 30%). In some series up to 90% of cerebellar abscesses are otogenic. Common organisms include streptococci, *Bacteroides* spp., *P. aeruginosa*, and Enterobacteriaceae. Abscesses that develop as a result of direct spread of infection from the frontal, ethmoidal, or sphenoidal sinuses and those that occur due to dental infections are usually located in the frontal lobes. Approximately 10% of brain abscesses are associated with paranasal sinusitis, and this association is particularly strong in young males in their second and third decades of life. The most common pathogens in brain abscesses associated with paranasal sinusitis are streptococci (especially *S. milleri*), *Haemophilus* spp., *Bacteroides* spp., *Pseudomonas* spp., and *S. aureus*. Dental infections are associated with ~2% of brain abscesses, although it is often suggested that many "cryptogenic" abscesses are in fact due to dental infections. The most common pathogens in this setting are streptococci, staphylococci, and *Bacteroides* and *Fusobacterium* spp.

Hematogenous abscesses account for ~25% of brain abscesses. These abscesses show a predilection for the territory of the middle cerebral artery (i.e., posterior frontal or parietal lobes). Hematogenous abscesses are often located at the junction of the gray and white matter and are often poorly encapsulated. Not surprisingly, hematogenous abscesses are often multiple, and multiple abscesses often have a hematogenous origin. The microbiology of these hematogenous abscesses is dependent on the primary source of infection. For example, brain abscesses that develop as a complication of infective endocarditis are often due to viridans streptococci or *S. aureus*. Abscesses associated with pyogenic lung infections such as lung abscess or bronchiectasis are often due to Streptococci, staphylococci, or *Bacteroides* or *Fusobacterium* spp. Enterobacteriaceae and *P. aeruginosa* are important causes of abscesses associated with urinary sepsis. Abscesses that follow penetrating head trauma or neurosurgical procedures are frequently due to staphylococci, Enterobacteriaceae, and *Pseudomonas* species. Congenital cardiac malformations that produce a right-to-left shunt (congenital cyanotic heart disease), such as tetralogy of Fallot, patent ductus arteriosus, and atrial and ventricular septal defects, allow bloodborne bacteria to bypass the pulmonary capillary bed and reach the brain. Similar phenomena can occur with pulmonary arteriovenous malformations. The decreased arterial oxygenation and saturation from the right-to-left shunt and polycythemia may cause focal areas of cerebral ischemia, thus providing a nidus for microorganisms that bypassed the pulmonary circulation to multiply and form an abscess. Streptococci are the most common pathogens in this setting.

PATHOGENESIS AND HISTOPATHOLOGY The intact brain parenchyma is relatively resistant to infection; preexisting brain ischemia, necrosis, or hypoxia appears to be a prerequisite for effective bacterial invasion. Once infection is established, brain abscess frequently evolves through a series of stages, influenced by the nature of the infecting organism and by the immunocompetence of the host. The early cerebritis stage (days 1 to 3) is characterized by a perivascular infiltration of inflammatory cells, which surround a central core of coagulative necrosis. Marked edema surrounds the lesion at this stage. In the late cerebritis stage (days 4 to 9), pus formation leads to enlargement of the necrotic center, which is surrounded at its border by an inflammatory infiltrate of macrophages and fibroblasts. A thin capsule of fibroblasts and reticular fibers gradually develops, and the surrounding area of cerebral edema becomes more distinct than in the previous stage. The third stage, early capsule formation (days 10 to 13), is characterized by the formation of a capsule that is better developed on the cortical than on the ventricular side of the lesion. This stage correlates with the appearance of a ring-enhancing capsule on neuroimaging studies. The final stage, late capsule formation (day 14 and beyond), is defined by a well-formed necrotic center surrounded by a dense collagenous capsule. The surrounding area of cerebral edema has regressed, but marked gliosis with large numbers of reactive astrocytes has developed outside the capsule. This gliotic process may contribute to the development of seizures as a sequelae of brain abscess.

CLINICAL PRESENTATION A brain abscess typically presents as an expanding intracranial mass lesion, rather than as an infectious process. Although the evolution of signs and symptoms is extremely variable, ranging from hours to weeks or even months, most patients present to the hospital 11 to 12 days following onset of symptoms. The classic clinical triad of headache, fever, and a focal neurologic deficit is present in <50% of cases. The most common symptom in patients with a brain abscess is headache, occurring in >75% of patients. The headache is often characterized as a constant, dull, aching sensation, either hemicranial or generalized, and it becomes progressively more severe and refractory to therapy. Fever is present in only 50% of patients at the time of diagnosis, and its absence should not exclude the diagnosis. The new onset of focal or generalized seizure activity is a presenting sign in 15 to 35% of patients. Focal neurologic deficits including hemiparesis, aphasia, or visual field defects are part of the initial presentation in >60% of patients.

The clinical presentation of a brain abscess depends on its location, the nature of the primary infection if present, and on the level of the ICP. Hemiparesis is the most common localizing sign of a frontal lobe abscess. A temporal lobe abscess may present with a disturbance of language (dysphasia) or an upper homonymous quadrantanopia. Nystagmus and ataxia are signs of a cerebellar abscess. Signs of raised ICP—papilledema, nausea and vomiting, and drowsiness or confusion—can be the dominant presentation of some abscesses, particularly those in the cerebellum. Meningismus is not present unless the abscess has ruptured into the ventricle or the infection has spread to the subarachnoid space.

DIAGNOSIS Diagnosis is made by neuroimaging studies. MRI (Fig. 360-4) is better than CT for demonstrating abscesses in the early (cerebritis) stages and is superior to CT for identifying abscesses in the posterior fossa. A mature brain abscess appears on CT as a focal area of hypodensity surrounded by ring enhancement. The CT and MRI appearance, particularly of the capsule, may be altered by treatment with glucocorticoids. The distinction between a brain abscess and other focal lesions such as tumors may be facilitated with diffusion-weighted imaging (DWI) sequences in which brain abscesses typically show increased signal and low apparent diffusion coefficient.

Microbiologic diagnosis of the etiologic agent is most accurately determined by Gram's stain and culture of abscess material obtained by stereotactic needle aspiration. Up to 10% of patients will also have positive blood cultures. LP should not be performed in patients with known or suspected focal intracranial infections such as abscess or empyema; CSF analysis contributes nothing to diagnosis or therapy, and LP increases the risk of herniation.

Additional laboratory studies may provide clues to the diagnosis of brain abscess in patients with a CNS mass lesion. About 50% of patients have a peripheral leukocytosis, 60% an elevated ESR, and 80% an elevated C-reactive protein.

DIFFERENTIAL DIAGNOSIS Conditions that can cause headache, fever, focal neurologic signs, and seizure activity include brain abscess, subdural empyema, bacterial meningitis, viral meningoencephalitis, superior sagittal sinus thrombosis, and acute disseminated encephalomyelitis. When fever is absent, primary and metastatic brain tumors become the major differential diagnosis. Less commonly, cerebral infarction or hematoma can have an MRI or CT appearance resembling brain abscess.

℞ TREATMENT

Optimal therapy of brain abscesses involves a combination of high-dose parenteral antibiotics and neurosurgical drainage. Empirical therapy of community-acquired brain abscess in an immunocompetent patient typically includes a third-generation cephalosporin (e.g., cefotaxime or ceftriaxone) and metronidazole (see Table 360-2 for antibiotic dosages). In patients with penetrating head trauma or recent neurosurgical procedures, treatment should include ceftazidime as the

FIGURE 360-4 Pneumococcal brain abscess. Note that the abscess wall has hyperintense signal on the axial T1-weighted image (*A*, black arrow), hypointense signal on the axial proton density images (*B*, black arrow), and enhances prominently after gadolinium administration on the coronal T1-weighted image (*C*). The abscess is surrounded by a large amount of vasogenic edema and has a small "daughter" abscess (*C*, white arrow). (*Courtesy of Joseph Lurito, MD.*)

third-generation cephalosporin to enhance coverage of *Pseudomonas* spp. and vancomycin for coverage of staphylococci. Meropenem plus vancomycin also provides good coverage in this setting.

Aspiration and drainage of the abscess under stereotaxic guidance are beneficial for both diagnosis and therapy. Empirical antibiotic coverage should be modified based on the results of Gram's stain and culture of the abscess contents. Complete excision of a bacterial abscess via craniotomy or craniectomy is generally reserved for multiloculated abscesses or those in which stereotactic aspiration is unsuccessful.

Medical therapy alone is not optimal for treatment of brain abscess and should be reserved for patients whose abscesses are neurosurgically inaccessible, for patients with small nonencapsulated abscesses (cerebritis), and patients whose condition is too tenuous to allow performance of a neurosurgical procedure. All patients should receive a minimum of 6 to 8 weeks of parenteral antibiotic therapy. The role, if any, of supplemental oral antibiotic therapy following completion of a standard course of parenteral therapy has never been adequately studied.

Patients should also receive prophylactic anticonvulsant therapy because of the high risk of seizures. Anticonvulsant therapy is continued for at least 3 months after resolution of the abscess, and decisions regarding withdrawal are then based on the EEG. If the EEG is abnormal, anticonvulsant therapy should be continued. If the EEG is normal, anticonvulsant therapy can be slowly withdrawn, with close follow-up and repeat EEG after the medication has been discontinued.

Glucocorticoids should not be given routinely to patients with brain abscesses. Intravenous dexamethasone therapy (10 mg every 6 h) is usually reserved for patients with substantial periabscess edema and associated mass effect and increased ICP. Dexamethasone should be tapered as rapidly as possible to avoid delaying the natural process of encapsulation of the abscess.

Serial MRI or CT scans should be obtained on a monthly or twice-monthly basis to document resolution of the abscess. More frequent studies (e.g., weekly) are probably warranted in the subset of patients who are receiving antibiotic therapy alone. A small amount of enhancement may remain for months after the abscess has been successfully treated.

PROGNOSIS The mortality of brain abscess has declined in parallel with the development of enhanced neuroimaging techniques, improved neurosurgical procedures for stereotactic aspiration, and improved antibiotics. In modern series the mortality is typically <15%. Significant sequelae including seizures, persisting weakness, aphasia, or mental impairment occur in ≥20% of survivors.

NONBACTERIAL CAUSES OF INFECTIOUS FOCAL CNS LESIONS

ETIOLOGY Neurocysticercosis is the most common parasitic disease of the CNS worldwide. Humans acquire cysticercosis by the ingestion of food contaminated with the eggs of the parasite *T. solium*. Eggs are contained in undercooked pork or in drinking water or other foods contaminated with human feces. *T. gondii* is a parasite that is acquired from the ingestion of undercooked meat and from handling cat feces.

CLINICAL PRESENTATION The most common manifestation of neurocysticercosis is new-onset partial seizures with or without secondary generalization. Cysticerci may develop in the brain parenchyma and cause seizures or focal neurologic deficits. When present in the subarachnoid or ventricular spaces, cysticerci can produce increased ICP by interference with CSF flow. Spinal cysticerci can mimic the presentation of intraspinal tumors. When the cysticerci first lodge in the brain, they frequently cause little in the way of an inflammatory response. As the cysticercal cyst degenerates, it elicits an inflammatory response that may present clinically as a seizure. Eventually the cyst dies, a process that may take several years, and is typically associated with resolution of the inflammatory response and often abatement of seizures.

Primary *toxoplasma* infection is often asymptomatic. However, during this phase parasites may spread to the CNS, where they become latent. Reactivation of CNS infection is almost exclusively associated with immunocompromised hosts, particularly those with HIV infection. During this phase patients present with headache, fever, seizures, and focal neurologic deficits.

DIAGNOSIS The lesions of neurocysticercosis are readily visualized by MRI or CT scans. Parenchymal brain calcifications are the most common finding. The scolex can often be visualized on MRI. A very early sign of cyst death is hypointensity of the vesicular fluid on T2-weighted images when compared with CSF. MRI findings consist of multiple lesions in the deep white matter, the thalamus, and basal ganglia and at the gray-white junction in the cerebral hemispheres. With contrast administration, the majority of the lesions enhance in a ringed, nodular, or homogeneous pattern and are surrounded by edema. In the presence of the characteristic neuroimaging abnormalities of this parasitic infection, serum anti–*T. gondii* antibodies should be obtained; if positive, the patient should be treated.

℞ TREATMENT

Anticonvulsant therapy is initiated when the patient with neurocysticercosis presents with a seizure. There is controversy about whether or not antihelminthic therapy should be given to all patients. Such therapy does not necessarily reduce the risk of seizure recurrence, but the control of seizures is easier after treatment with cysticidal drugs than when the disease is untreated. Albendazole and praziquantel are used in the treatment of neurocysticercosis. Approximately 85% of parenchymal cysts are destroyed by a single course of albendazole and ~75% are destroyed by a single course of praziquantel. The dose of albendazole is 15 mg/kg per day in two doses for 8 days. The dose of praziquantel is 50 mg/kg per day for 15 days, although a number of other dosage regimens are also frequently cited. Antiepileptic therapy can be stopped once the follow-up CT scan shows resolution of the lesion. Long-term antiepileptic therapy is recommended when seizures occur after resolution of edema and resorption or calcification of the degenerating cyst.

CNS toxoplasmosis is treated with a combination of sulfadiazine, 1.5 to 2.0 g orally qid, plus pyrimethamine, 100 mg orally to load then 75 to 100 mg orally qd, plus folinic acid, 10 to 15 mg orally qd. Folinic acid is added to the regimen to prevent megaloblastic anemia. Therapy is continued until there is no evidence of active disease on neuroimaging studies, which typically takes at least 6 weeks, and then the dose of sulfadiazine is reduced to 2 to 4 g/d and pyrimethamine to 50 mg/d. Clindamycin plus pyrimethamine is an alternative therapy for patients who cannot tolerate sulfadiazine, but the combination of pyrimethamine and sulfadiazine is more effective.

SUBDURAL EMPYEMA

A subdural empyema (SDE) is a collection of pus between the dura and arachnoid membranes (Fig. 360-5).

EPIDEMIOLOGY SDE is a rare disorder that accounts for 15 to 25% of focal suppurative CNS infections. Sinusitis is the most common predisposing condition and typically involves the frontal sinuses, either alone or in combination with the ethmoid and maxillary sinuses. Sinusitis-associated empyema has a striking predilection for young males, possibly reflecting sex-related differences in sinus anatomy and development. It has been suggested that SDE may complicate 1 to 2% of cases of frontal sinusitis severe enough to require hospitalization. As a consequence of this epidemiology, SDE shows an ~3:1 male:female predominance, with 70% of cases occurring in the second and third decades of life. SDE may also develop as a complication of head trauma or neurosurgery. Secondary infection of a subdural effusion may also result in empyema, although secondary infection of hematomas, in the absence of a prior neurosurgical procedure, is rare.

ETIOLOGY Aerobic and anaerobic streptococci, staphylococci, Enterobacteriaceae, and anaerobic bacteria are the most common causative

Subdural empyema

Thrombosed veins

S.Toal

FIGURE 360-5 Subdural empyema is a collection of pus between the dura and arachnoid membranes.

organisms of sinusitis-associated SDE. Staphylococci and gram-negative bacilli are often the etiologic organisms when SDE follows neurosurgical procedures or head trauma. Up to one-third of cases are culture-negative, possibly reflecting difficulty in obtaining adequate anaerobic cultures.

PATHOPHYSIOLOGY Sinusitis-associated SDE develops as a result of either retrograde spread of infection from septic thrombophlebitis of the mucosal veins draining the sinuses or contiguous spread of infection to the brain from osteomyelitis in the posterior wall of the frontal or other sinuses. SDE may also develop from direct introduction of bacteria into the subdural space as a complication of a neurosurgical procedure. The evolution of SDE can be extremely rapid because the subdural space is a large compartment that offers few mechanical barriers to the spread of infection. In patients with sinusitis-associated SDE, suppuration typically begins in the upper and anterior portions of one cerebral hemisphere and then extends posteriorly. SDE is often associated with other intracranial infections including epidural empyema (40%), cortical thrombophlebitis (35%), and intracranial abscess or cerebritis (>25%). Cortical venous infarction produces necrosis of underlying cerebral cortex and subcortical white matter, with focal neurologic deficits and seizures (see below).

CLINICAL PRESENTATION A patient with SDE typically presents with fever and a progressively worsening headache. The diagnosis of SDE should always be suspected in a patient with known sinusitis who presents with new CNS signs or symptoms. Patients with underlying sinusitis frequently have symptoms related to this infection. As the infection progresses, focal neurologic deficits, seizures, nuchal rigidity, and signs of increased ICP commonly occur. Headache is the most common complaint at the time of presentation; initially it is localized to the side of the subdural infection but then becomes more severe and generalized. Contralateral hemiparesis or hemiplegia is the most common focal neurologic deficit and can occur from the direct effects of the SDE on the cortex or as a consequence of venous infarction. Seizures begin as partial motor seizures that then become secondarily generalized. Seizures may be due to the direct irritative effect of the SDE on the underlying cortex or result from cortical venous infarction (see above). In untreated SDE, the increasing mass effect and increase in ICP cause progressive deterioration in consciousness, leading ultimately to coma.

DIAGNOSIS MRI (Fig. 360-6) is superior to CT in identifying SDE and any associated intracranial infections. The administration of gadolinium greatly improves diagnosis by enhancing the rim of the empyema and allowing the empyema to be clearly delineated from the underlying brain parenchyma. Cranial MRI is also extremely valuable in identifying sinusitis, other focal CNS infections, cortical venous infarction, cerebral edema, and cerebritis. CT may show a crescent-shaped hypodense lesion over one or both hemispheres or in the interhemispheric fissure. Frequently the degree of mass effect, exemplified by midline shift, ventricular compression, and sulcal effacement, is far out of proportion to the mass of the SDE.

CSF examination should be avoided in patients with known or suspected SDE as it adds no useful information and is associated with the risk of cerebral herniation.

DIFFERENTIAL DIAGNOSIS The differential diagnosis of the combination of headache, fever, focal neurologic signs, and seizure activity that progresses rapidly to an altered level of consciousness includes subdural hematoma, bacterial meningitis, viral encephalitis, brain abscess, superior sagittal sinus thrombosis, and acute disseminated encephalomyelitis. The presence of nuchal rigidity is unusual with brain abscess or epidural empyema and should suggest the possibility of SDE when associated with significant focal neurologic signs and fever. Patients with bacterial meningitis also have nuchal rigidity but do not typically have focal deficits of the severity seen with SDE.

℞ TREATMENT

SDE is a medical emergency. Emergent neurosurgical evacuation of the empyema, either through burr-hole drainage or craniotomy, is the definitive step in the management of this infection. Empirical antimicrobial therapy should include a combination of a third-generation cephalosporin (e.g., cefotaxime or ceftriaxone), vancomycin, and metronidazole (see Table 360-2 for dosages). Parenteral antibiotic therapy should be continued for a minimum of 4 weeks. Specific diagnosis of the etiologic organisms is made based on Gram's stain and culture of fluid obtained via either burr holes or craniotomy; the initial empirical antibiotic coverage can be modified accordingly.

PROGNOSIS Prognosis is influenced by the level of consciousness of the patient at the time of hospital presentation, the size of the empyema, and the speed with which therapy is instituted. Long-term neurologic sequelae, which include seizures and hemiparesis, occur in up to 50% of cases.

A B C

FIGURE 360-6 Subdural empyema. There is marked enhancement of the dura and leptomeninges (*A, B*, straight arrows) along the left medial hemisphere. The pus is hypointense on T1-weighted images (*A, B*), but markedly hyperintense on the proton density–weighted (*C*, curved arrow) image. (*Courtesy of Joseph Lurito, MD.*)

EPIDURAL ABSCESS

Cranial epidural abscess is a suppurative infection occurring in the potential space between the inner skull table and dura (Fig. 360-7).

ETIOLOGY AND PATHOPHYSIOLOGY Epidural abscess is less common than either brain abscess or SDE and accounts for <2% of focal suppurative CNS infections. A cranial epidural abscess develops as a complication of a craniotomy or compound skull fracture or as a result of spread of infection from the frontal sinuses, middle ear, mastoid, or orbit. An epidural abscess may develop contiguous to an area of osteomyelitis, when craniotomy is complicated by infection of the wound or bone flap, or as a result of direct infection of the epidural space. Infection in the frontal sinus, middle ear, mastoid, or orbit can reach the epidural space through retrograde spread of infection from septic thrombophlebitis in the emissary veins that drain these areas or by way of direct spread of infection through areas of osteomyelitis. Unlike the subdural space, the epidural space is really a potential rather than an actual compartment. The dura is normally tightly adherent to the inner skull table, and infection must dissect the dura away from the skull table as it spreads. As a result, epidural abscesses are often smaller than SDEs. Cranial epidural abscesses, unlike brain abscesses, only rarely result from hematogenous spread of infection from extracranial primary sites. The bacteriology of a cranial epidural abscess is similar to that of SDE (see above). The etiologic organisms of an epidural abscess that arises from frontal sinusitis, middle ear infections, or mastoiditis are usually streptococci or anaerobic organisms. Staphylococci or gram-negative organisms are the usual cause of an epidural abscess that develops as a complication of craniotomy or compound skull fracture.

CLINICAL PRESENTATION Patients present with fever (60%), headache (40%), nuchal rigidity (35%), seizures (10%), and focal deficits (5%). Periorbital edema and Potts puffy tumor, reflecting underlying associated frontal bone osteomyelitis, are present in ~40%. In patients with a recent neurosurgical procedure, wound infection is invariably present, but other symptoms may be subtle and can include altered mental status (45%), fever (35%), and headache (20%). The diagnosis should also be considered when fever and headache follow recent head trauma or occur in the setting of frontal sinusitis, mastoiditis, or otitis media.

DIAGNOSIS Cranial MRI is the procedure of choice to demonstrate a cranial epidural abscess. The sensitivity of CT is limited by the presence of signal artifacts arising from the bone of the inner skull table. The CT appearance of an epidural empyema is that of a lens or crescent-shaped hypodense extraaxial lesion. On MRI, an epidural empyema appears as a lentiform or crescent-shaped fluid collection that is hyperintense compared to CSF on T2-weighted images. On T1-weighted images, the fluid collection has a signal intensity that is intermediate between that of brain tissue and CSF. Following the administration of gadolinium, a significant enhancement of the dura is seen on T1-weighted images. In distinction to subdural empyema, signs of mass effect or other parenchymal abnormalities are uncommon.

FIGURE 360-7 Cranial epidural abscess is a collection of pus between the dura and the inner table of the skull.

Ⓡ TREATMENT

Immediate neurosurgical drainage is indicated. Empirical antimicrobial therapy, pending the results of Gram's stain and culture of the purulent material obtained at surgery, should include a combination of a third-generation cephalosporin, nafcillin or vancomycin, and metronidazole (Table 360-2). Ceftazidime should be substituted for ceftriaxone or cefotaxime in neurosurgical patients. Meropenem and vancomycin also provide effective empirical therapy in postneurosurgical cases. When the organism has been identified, antimicrobial therapy can be modified accordingly. Antibiotics should be continued for at least 3 weeks after surgical drainage.

PROGNOSIS Mortality is <5% in modern series, and full recovery is the rule in most survivors.

SUPPURATIVE THROMBOPHLEBITIS

DEFINITION Suppurative intracranial thrombophlebitis is septic venous thrombosis of cortical veins and sinuses. This may occur as a complication of bacterial meningitis; SDE; epidural abscess; or infection in the skin of the face, paranasal sinuses, middle ear, or mastoid.

ANATOMY AND PATHOPHYSIOLOGY The cerebral veins and venous sinuses have no valves; therefore, blood within them can flow in either direction. The superior sagittal sinus is the largest of the venous sinuses (Fig. 360-8). It receives blood from the frontal, parietal, and occipital superior cerebral veins and the diploic veins, which communicate with the meningeal veins. Bacterial meningitis is a common predisposing condition for septic thrombosis of the superior sagittal sinus. The diploic veins, which drain into the superior sagittal sinus, provide a route for the spread of infection from the meninges, especially in cases where there is purulent exudate near areas of the superior sagittal sinus. Infection can also spread to the superior sagittal sinus from nearby SDE or epidural abscess. Dehydration from vomiting, hypercoagulable states, and immunologic abnormalities, including the presence of circulating antiphospholipid antibodies, also contribute to cerebral venous sinus thrombosis. Thrombosis may extend from one sinus to another, and often at autopsy thrombi of different histologic ages can be detected in several sinuses. Thrombosis of the superior sagittal sinus is often associated with thrombosis of superior cortical veins and small parenchymal hemorrhages.

The superior sagittal sinus drains into the transverse sinuses (Fig. 360-8). The transverse sinuses also receive venous drainage from small veins from both the middle ear and mastoid cells. The transverse sinus becomes the sigmoid sinus before draining into the internal jugular vein. Septic transverse/sigmoid sinus thrombosis can be a complica-

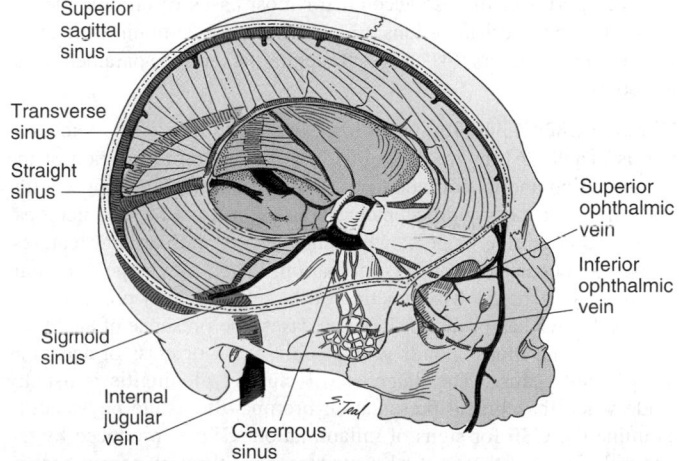

FIGURE 360-8 Anatomy of the cerebral venous sinuses.

tion of acute and chronic otitis media or mastoiditis. Infection spreads from the mastoid air cells to the transverse sinus via the emissary veins or by direct invasion. The cavernous sinuses are inferior to the superior sagittal sinus at the base of the skull. The cavernous sinuses receive blood from the facial veins via the superior and inferior ophthalmic veins. Bacteria in the facial veins enter the cavernous sinus via these veins. Bacteria in the sphenoid and ethmoid sinuses can spread to the cavernous sinuses via the small emissary veins. The sphenoid and ethmoid sinuses are the most common sites of primary infection resulting in septic cavernous sinus thrombosis.

CLINICAL MANIFESTATIONS *Septic thrombosis of the superior sagittal sinus* presents with headache, fever, nausea and vomiting, confusion, and focal or generalized seizures. There may be a rapid development of stupor and coma. Weakness of the lower extremities with bilateral Babinski signs or hemiparesis is often present. When superior sagittal sinus thrombosis occurs as a complication of bacterial meningitis, nuchal rigidity and Kernig's and Brudzinski's signs may be present.

The oculomotor nerve, the trochlear nerve, the abducens nerve, the ophthalmic and maxillary branches of the trigeminal nerve, and the internal carotid artery all pass through the cavernous sinus (Fig. 355-3). The symptoms of *septic cavernous sinus thrombosis* are fever, headache, frontal and retroorbital pain, and diplopia. The classic signs are ptosis, proptosis, chemosis, and extraocular dysmotility due to deficits of cranial nerves III, IV, and VI; hyperesthesia of the ophthalmic and maxillary divisions of the fifth cranial nerve and a decreased corneal reflex may be detected. There may be evidence of dilated, tortuous retinal veins and papilledema.

Headache and earache are the most frequent symptoms of *transverse sinus thrombosis*. A transverse sinus thrombosis may also present with otitis media, sixth nerve palsy, and retroorbital or facial pain (*Gradinego's syndrome*). Sigmoid sinus and internal jugular vein thrombosis may present with neck pain.

DIAGNOSIS The diagnosis of septic venous sinus thrombosis is suggested by an absent flow void within the affected venous sinus on MRI and confirmed by magnetic resonance venography or the venous phase of cerebral angiography. The diagnosis of thrombophlebitis of intracerebral and meningeal veins is suggested by the presence of intracerebral hemorrhage but requires cerebral angiography for definitive diagnosis.

℞ TREATMENT

Septic venous sinus thrombosis is usually treated with antibiotics and hydration. The choice of antimicrobial therapy is based on the bacteria responsible for the predisposing or associated condition. Optimal duration of therapy is unknown, but antibiotics are usually continued for 6 weeks or until there is radiographic evidence of resolution of thrombosis. Anticoagulation with dose-adjusted heparin has been reported to be beneficial in patients with aseptic venous sinus thrombosis; it is also used in the treatment of septic venous sinus thrombosis complicating bacterial meningitis in patients who are worsening despite antimicrobial therapy and intravenous fluids. The presence of a small intracerebral hemorrhage from septic thrombophlebitis is not an absolute contraindication to heparin therapy. Successful management of aseptic venous sinus thrombosis has been reported with urokinase therapy and with a combination of intrathrombus recombinant tissue plasminogen activator (rtPA) and intravenous heparin, but the efficacy of these therapies in septic venous sinus thrombosis is unknown.

FURTHER READING

DE GANS J, VAN DE BEEK D: Dexamethasone in adults with bacterial meningitis. N Engl J Med 347:1549, 2002

DWORKIN MS: A review of progressive multifocal leukoencephalopathy in persons with and without AIDS. Curr Clin Top Infect Dis 22:181, 2002

LU CH et al: Bacterial brain abscess: Microbiological features, epidemiological trends and therapeutic outcomes. Q J M ed 95:501, 2002

ROOS KL: Acute bacterial meningitis. Semin Neurol 20:293, 2000

ROSENSTEIN NE et al: Meningococcal disease. N Engl J Med 344:1378, 2001

SOLOMON T et al: West Nile encephalitis, BMJ 326:865, 2003

361 CHRONIC AND RECURRENT MENINGITIS
Walter J. Koroshetz, Morton N. Swartz

Chronic inflammation of the meninges (pia, arachnoid, and dura) can produce profound neurologic disability and may be fatal if not successfully treated. The condition is most commonly diagnosed when a characteristic neurologic syndrome exists for >4 weeks and is associated with a persistent inflammatory response in the cerebrospinal fluid (CSF) (white blood cell count >5/μL). The causes are varied, and appropriate treatment depends on identification of the etiology. Five categories of disease account for most cases of chronic meningitis: (1) meningeal infections, (2) malignancy, (3) noninfectious inflammatory disorders, (4) chemical meningitis, and (5) parameningeal infections.

CLINICAL PATHOPHYSIOLOGY Neurologic manifestations of chronic meningitis (Table 361-1) are determined by the anatomic location of the inflammation and its consequences. Persistent headache with or without stiff neck, and hydrocephalus, cranial neuropathies, radiculopathies, and cognitive or personality changes are the cardinal features. These can occur alone or in combination. When they appear in combination, widespread dissemination of the inflammatory process along CSF pathways has occurred. In some cases, the presence of an underlying systemic illness points to a specific agent or class of agents as the probable cause. The diagnosis of chronic meningitis is usually made when the clinical presentation prompts the astute physician to examine the CSF for signs of inflammation. CSF is produced by the choroid plexus of the cerebral ventricles, exits through narrow foramina into the subarachnoid space surrounding the brain and spinal cord,

TABLE 361-1 *Symptoms and Signs of Chronic Meningitis*

Symptom	Sign
Chronic headache	+/− Papilledema
Neck or back pain	Brudzinski's or Kernig's sign of meningeal irritation
Change in personality	Altered mental status—drowsiness, inattention, disorientation, memory loss, frontal release signs (grasp, suck, snout), perseveration
Facial weakness	Peripheral seventh CN palsy
Double vision	Palsy of CNs III, IV, VI
Visual loss	Papilledema, optic atrophy
Hearing loss	Eighth CN palsy
Arm or leg weakness	Myelopathy or radiculopathy
Numbness in arms or legs	Myelopathy or radiculopathy
Sphincter dysfunction	Myelopathy or radiculopathy
	Frontal lobe dysfunction
Clumsiness	Ataxia

Note: CN, cranial nerve.

circulates around the base of the brain and over the cerebral hemispheres, and is resorbed by arachnoid villi projecting into the superior sagittal sinus. CSF flow provides a pathway for rapid spread of infectious and malignant processes over the brain, spinal cord, and cranial and spinal nerve roots. Spread from the subarachnoid space into brain parenchyma may occur via the arachnoid cuffs that surround blood vessels that penetrate brain tissue (Virchow-Robin spaces).

Intracranial Meningitis Nociceptive fibers of the meninges (Chap. 14) are stimulated by the inflammatory process, resulting in headache or neck or back pain. Obstruction of CSF pathways at foramina or arachnoid villi may produce *hydrocephalus* and symptoms of raised intracranial pressure (ICP), including headache, vomiting, apathy or drowsiness, gait instability, papilledema, visual loss, impaired upgaze, or palsy of the sixth cranial nerve (CN) (Chap. 258). Cognitive and behavioral changes during the course of chronic meningitis may also result from vascular damage, which may similarly produce seizures, stroke, or myclopathy. Inflammatory deposits seeded via the CSF circulation are often prominent around the brainstem and cranial nerves and along the undersurface of the frontal and temporal lobes. Such cases, termed *basal meningitis*, often present as multiple cranial neuropathies, with visual loss (CN II), facial weakness (CN VII), hearing loss (CN VIII), diplopia (CNs III, IV, and VI), sensory or motor abnormalities of the oropharynx (CNs IX, X, and XII), decreased olfaction (CN I), or facial sensory loss and masseter weakness (CN V).

Spinal Meningitis   Injury may occur to motor and sensory roots as they traverse the subarachnoid space and penetrate the meninges. These cases present as multiple radiculopathies with combinations of radicular pain, sensory loss, motor weakness, and sphincter dysfunction. Meningeal inflammation can encircle the cord, resulting in myelopathy. Patients with slowly progressive involvement of multiple cranial nerves and/or spinal nerve roots are likely to have chronic meningitis. Electrophysiologic testing (electromyography, nerve conduction studies, and evoked response testing) may be helpful in determining whether there is involvement of cranial and spinal nerve roots.

Systemic Manifestations   In some patients, evidence of systemic disease provides clues to the underlying cause of chronic meningitis. A careful history and physical examination are essential before embarking on a diagnostic workup, which may be costly, prolonged, and associated with risk from invasive procedures. A complete history of travel, sexual practice, and exposure to infectious agents should be sought. Infectious causes are often associated with fever, malaise, anorexia, and signs of localized or disseminated infection outside the nervous system. Infectious causes are of major concern in the immunosuppressed patient, especially in patients with AIDS, in whom chronic meningitis may present without headache or fever. Noninfectious inflammatory disorders often produce systemic manifestations, but meningitis may be the initial manifestation. Carcinomatous meningitis may or may not be accompanied by clinical evidence of the primary neoplasm.

APPROACH TO THE PATIENT

The occurrence of chronic headache, hydrocephalus, cranial neuropathy, radiculopathy, and/or cognitive decline in a patient should prompt consideration of a lumbar puncture for evidence of meningeal inflammation. On occasion the diagnosis is made when an imaging study [computed tomography (CT) or magnetic resonance imaging (MRI)] shows contrast enhancement of the meninges, always abnormal with the exception of dural enhancement after lumbar puncture, neurosurgical procedures, or spontaneous CSF leakage. Once chronic meningitis is confirmed by CSF examination, effort is focused on identifying the cause (Tables 361-2 and 361-3) by (1) further analysis of the CSF, (2) diagnosis of an underlying systemic infection or noninfectious inflammatory condition, or (3) pathologic examination of meningeal biopsy specimens.

Two clinical forms of chronic meningitis exist. In the first, the symptoms are chronic and persistent, whereas in the second there are recurrent, discrete episodes of illness. In the latter group, all symptoms, signs, and CSF parameters of meningeal inflammation resolve completely between episodes without specific therapy. In such patients, the likely etiologies include infection with herpes simplex virus (HSV) type 2; chemical meningitis due to leakage into CSF of contents from an epidermoid tumor, craniopharyngioma, or cholesteatoma; primary inflammatory conditions, including Vogt-Koyanagi-Harada syndrome, Behçet's syndrome (Chap. 307), Mollaret's meningitis, and systemic lupus erythematosus (SLE; Chap. 300); and drug hypersensitivity with repeated administration of the offending agent.

The epidemiologic history is of considerable importance and may provide direction for selection of laboratory studies. Pertinent features include a history of tuberculosis or exposure to a likely case; past travel to areas endemic for fungal infections (the San Joaquin Valley in California and southwestern states for coccidioidomycosis, midwestern states for histoplasmosis, southeastern states for blastomycosis); travel to the Mediterranean region or ingestion of imported unpasteurized dairy products (*Brucella*); time spent in areas endemic for Lyme disease (e.g., Connecticut, New York, Massachusetts); exposure to sexually transmitted disease (syphilis); exposure of an immunocompromised host to pigeons and their droppings (*Cryptococcus*); gardening (*Sporothrix schenkii*); ingestion of poorly cooked meat or contact with a household cat (*Toxoplasma gondii*); residence in Thailand or Japan (*Gnathostoma spinigerum*) or the South Pacific (*Angiostrongylus cantonensis*); rural residence and raccoon exposure (*Baylisascaris procyonis*); and residence in Latin America, the Philippines, or Southeast Asia when eosinophilic meningitis is present (*Taenia solium*).

The presence of focal cerebral signs in a patient with chronic meningitis suggests the possibility of a brain abscess or other parameningeal infection; identification of a potential source of infection (chronic draining ear, sinusitis, right-to-left cardiac or pulmonary shunt, chronic pleuropulmonary infection) supports this diagnosis. In some cases, diagnosis may be established by recognition and biopsy of unusual skin lesions (Behçet's syndrome, cryptococcosis, blastomycosis, SLE, Lyme disease, intravenous drug use, sporotrichosis, trypanosomiasis) or enlarged lymph nodes (lymphoma, tuberculosis, sarcoid, infection with HIV, secondary syphilis, or Whipple's disease). A careful ophthalmologic examination may reveal uveitis [Vogt-Koyanagi-Harada syndrome, sarcoid, or central nervous system (CNS) lymphoma], keratoconjunctivitis sicca (Sjögren's syndrome), or iridocyclitis (Behçet's syndrome) and is essential to assess visual loss from hydrocephalus. Aphthous oral lesions, genital ulcers, and hypopyon suggest Behçet's syndrome. Hepatosplenomegaly suggests lymphoma, sarcoid, tuberculosis, or brucellosis. Herpetic lesions in the genital area or on the thighs suggest HSV-2 infection. A breast nodule, a suspicious pigmented skin lesion, focal bone pain, or an abdominal mass directs attention to possible carcinomatous meningitis.

Imaging   Once the clinical syndrome is recognized as a potential manifestation of chronic meningitis, proper analysis of the CSF is essential. However, if the possibility of raised ICP exists, a brain imaging study should be performed before lumbar puncture. If ICP is elevated because of a mass lesion, brain swelling, or a block in ventricular CSF outflow (obstructive hydrocephalus), then lumbar puncture carries the potential risk of brain herniation. Obstructive hydrocephalus usually requires direct ventricular drainage of CSF. In patients with open CSF flow pathways, elevated ICP can occur due to impaired resorption of CSF by arachnoid villi. In such patients, lumbar puncture is usually safe, but repetitive or continuous lumbar drainage may be necessary to prevent relatively sudden death from raised ICP. In some patients, especially with cryptococcal meningitis, life-threatening levels of ICP can occur without visible hydrocephalus on brain imaging.

Contrast-enhanced MRI or CT studies of the brain and spinal cord can identify meningeal enhancement, parameningeal infections (including brain abscess), encasement of the spinal cord (malignancy or inflammation and infection), or nodular deposits on the meninges or nerve roots (malignancy or sarcoidosis) (Fig. 361-1). Imaging studies are also useful to localize areas of meningeal disease prior to meningeal biopsy.

Cerebral angiography may be indicated in patients with chronic meningitis and stroke to identify cerebral arteritis (granulomatous angiitis, other inflammatory or infectious causes).

TABLE 361-2 *Infectious Causes of Chronic Meningitis*

Causative Agent	CSF Formula	Helpful Diagnostic Tests	Risk Factors and Systemic Manifestations
COMMON BACTERIAL CAUSES			
Partially treated suppurative meningitis	Mononuclear or mixed mononuclear-polymorphonuclear cells	CSF culture and Gram stain	History consistent with acute bacterial meningitis and incomplete treatment
Parameningeal infection	Mononuclear or mixed polymorphonuclear-mononuclear cells	Contrast-enhanced CT or MRI to detect parenchymal, subdural, epidural, or sinus infection	Otitis media, pleuropulmonary infection, right-to-left cardiopulmonary shunt for brain abscess; focal neurologic signs; neck, back, ear, or sinus tenderness
Mycobacterium tuberculosis	Mononuclear cells except polymorphonuclear cells in early infection (commonly <500 WBC/μL); low CSF glucose, high protein	Tuberculin skin test may be negative; AFB culture of CSF (sputum, urine, gastric contents if indicated); tuberculostearic acid detection in CSF; identify tubercle bacillus on acid-fast stain of CSF or protein pellicle; PCR	Exposure history; previous tuberculous illness; immunosuppressed or AIDS; young children; fever, meningismus, night sweats, miliary TB on X-ray or liver biopsy; stroke due to arteritis
Lyme disease (Bannwarth's syndrome) *Borrelia burgdorferi*	Mononuclear cells; elevated protein	Serum Lyme antibody titer; Western blot confirmation; (patients with syphilis may have false-positive Lyme titer)	History of tick bite or appropriate exposure history; erythema chronicum migrans skin rash; arthritis, radiculopathy, Bell's palsy, meningoencephalitis–multiple sclerosis-like syndrome
Syphilis (secondary, tertiary) *Treponema pallidum*	Mononuclear cells; elevated protein	CSF VDRL; serum VDRL (or RPR); fluorescent treponemal antibody-absorbed (FTA) or MHA-TP; serum VDRL may be negative in tertiary syphilis	Appropriate exposure history; HIV seropositive individuals at increased risk of aggressive infection; "dementia"; cerebral infarction due to endarteritis
UNCOMMON BACTERIAL CAUSES			
Actinomyces	Polymorphonuclear cells	Anaerobic culture	Parameningeal abscess or sinus tract (oral or dental focus); pneumonitis
Nocardia	Polymorphonuclear; occasionally mononuclear cells; often low glucose	Isolation may require weeks; weakly acid fast	Associated brain abscess may be present
Brucella	Mononuclear cells (rarely polymorphonuclear); elevated protein; often low glucose	CSF antibody detection; serum antibody detection	Intake of unpasteurized dairy products; exposure to goats, sheep, cows; fever, arthralgia, myalgia, vertebral osteomyelitis
Whipple's disease *Tropherema whippelii*	Mononuclear cells	Biopsy of small bowel or lymph node; CSF PCR for *T. whippelii*; brain and meningeal biopsy (with PAS stain and EM examination)	Diarrhea, weight loss, arthralgias, fever; dementia, ataxia, paresis, ophthalmoplegia, oculomasticatory myoclonus
RARE BACTERIAL CAUSES			
Leptospirosis (occasionally if left untreated may last 3–4 weeks)			
FUNGAL CAUSES			
Cryptococcus neoformans	Mononuclear cells; count not elevated in some patients with AIDS	India ink or fungal wet mount of CSF (budding yeast); blood and urine cultures; antigen detection in CSF	AIDS and immune suppression; pigeon exposure; skin and other organ involvement due to disseminated infection
Coccidioides immitis	Mononuclear cells (sometimes 10–20% eosinophils); often low glucose	Antibody detection in CSF and serum	Exposure history—southwestern US; increased virulence in dark-skinned races
Candida sp.	Polymorphonuclear or mononuclear	Fungal stain and culture of CSF	IV drug abuse; post surgery; prolonged intravenous therapy; disseminated candidiasis
Histoplasma capsulatum	Mononuclear cells; low glucose	Fungal stain and culture of large volumes of CSF; antigen detection in CSF, serum, and urine; antibody detection in serum, CSF	Exposure history—Ohio and central Mississippi River Valley; AIDS; mucosal lesions
Blastomyces dermatitidis	Mononuclear cells	Fungal stain and culture of CSF; biopsy and culture of skin, lung lesions; antibody detection in serum	Midwestern and Southeastern USA; usually systemic infection; abscesses, draining sinus, ulcers
Aspergillus sp.	Mononuclear or polymorphonuclear	CSF culture	Sinusitis; granulocytopenia or immunosuppression
Sporothrix schenckii	Mononuclear cells	Antibody detection in CSF and serum; CSF culture	Traumatic inoculation; IV drug use; ulcerated skin lesion
RARE FUNGAL CAUSES			
Xylohypha (formerly *Cladosporium*) *trichoides* and other dark-walled (demateaceous) fungi such as *Curvularia*, *Drechslera*; *Mucor, Pseudoallescheria boydii*			

(continued)

TABLE 361-2—(Continued)

Causative Agent	CSF Formula	Helpful Diagnostic Tests	Risk Factors and Systemic Manifestations
PROTOZOAL CAUSES			
Toxoplasma gondii	Mononuclear cells	Biopsy or response to empirical therapy in clinically appropriate context (including presence of antibody in serum)	Usually with intracerebral abscesses common in HIV seropositive patients
Trypanosomiasis *Trypanosoma gambiense T. rhodesiense*	Mononuclear cells, elevated protein	Elevated CSF IgM; identification of trypanosomes in CSF and blood smear	Endemic in Africa; chancre, lymphadenopathy; prominent sleep disorder
RARE PROTOZOAL CAUSES			
Acanthamoeba sp. causing granulomatous amebic encephalitis and meningoencephalitis in immunocompromised and debilitated individuals			
HELMINTHIC CAUSES			
Cysticercosis (infection with cysts of *Taenia solium*)	Mononuclear cells; may have eosinophils; glucose level may be low	Indirect hemagglutination assay in CSF; ELISA immunoblotting in serum	Usually with multiple cysts in basal meninges and hydrocephalus; cerebral cysts, muscle calcification
Gnathostoma spinigerum	Eosinophils, mononuclear cells	Peripheral eosinophilia	History of eating raw fish; common in Thailand and Japan; subarachnoid hemorrhage; painful radiculopathy
Angiostrongylus cantonensis	Eosinophils, mononuclear cells	Recovery of worms from CSF	History of eating raw shellfish; common in tropical Pacific regions; often benign
Baylisascaris procyonis (raccoon ascarid)	Eosinophils, mononuclear cells		Infection follows accidental ingestion of *B. procyonis* eggs from raccoon feces; fatal meningoencephalitis
RARE HELMINTHIC CAUSES			
Trichinella spiralis (trichinosis); *Echinococcus* cysts; *Schistosoma* sp. The former may produce a lymphocytic pleocytosis whereas the latter two may produce an eosinophilic response in CSF associated with cerebral cysts (*Echinococcus*) or granulomatous lesions of brain or spinal cord			
VIRAL CAUSES			
Mumps	Mononuclear cells	Antibody in serum	No prior mumps or immunization; may produce meningoencephalitis; may persist for 3–4 weeks
Lymphocytic choriomeningitis	Mononuclear cells	Antibody in serum	Contact with rodents or their excreta; may persist for 3–4 weeks
Echovirus	Mononuclear cells; may have low glucose	Virus isolation from CSF	Congenital hypogammaglobulinemia; history of recurrent meningitis
HIV (acute retroviral syndrome)	Mononuclear cells	p24 antigen in serum and CSF; high level of HIV viremia	HIV risk factors; rash, fever, lymphadenopathy; lymphopenia in peripheral blood; syndrome may persist long enough to be considered as "chronic meningitis"; or chronic meningitis may develop in later stages (AIDS) due to HIV
Herpes simplex (HSV)	Mononuclear cells	PCR for HSV DNA; CSF antibody	Recurrent meningitis due to HSV-2 (rarely HSV-1) often associated with genital recurrences

Abbreviations: AFB, acid-fast bacillus; CSF, cerebrospinal fluid; CT, computed tomography; ELISA, enzyme-linked immunosorbent assay; EM, electron microscopy; FTA, fluorescent treponemal antibody absorption test; MHA-TP, microhemagglutination assay-*T. pallidum*; MRI, magnetic resonance imaging; PAS, periodic acid–Schiff; PCR, polymerase chain reaction; RPR, rapid plasma reagin test; TB, tuberculosis; VDRL, Venereal Disease Research Laboratories test.

Cerebrospinal Fluid Analysis The CSF pressure should be measured and samples sent for bacterial culture, cell count and differential, Gram's stain, and measurement of glucose and protein. In cases without a known cause, CSF should be sent for the Venereal Disease Research Laboratories (VDRL) test, acid-fast bacillus (AFB) stain and culture, wet mount for fungus and parasites, India ink preparation and culture, culture for fastidious bacteria and fungi, assays for cryptococcal antigen and oligoclonal immunoglobulin bands, and cytology. Other specific CSF or blood tests and cultures (Tables 361-2 and 361-3) should be ordered as indicated on the basis of the history, physical examination, or preliminary CSF results (i.e., eosinophilic, mononuclear, or polymorphonuclear meningitis). Rapid diagnosis may be facilitated by serologic tests and polymerase chain reaction (PCR) testing to identify DNA sequences in the CSF that are specific for the suspected pathogen.

In most categories of chronic (not recurrent) meningitis, mononuclear cells predominate in the CSF. When neutrophils predominate after 3 weeks of illness, the principal considerations are *Nocardia asteroides*, *Actinomyces israelii*, *Brucella*, *Mycobacterium tuberculosis* (5 to 10% of early cases only), various fungi (*Blastomyces dermatitidis*, *Candida albicans*, *Histoplasma capsulatum*, *Aspergillus* species, *Pseudallescheria boydii*, *Cladophialophora bantiana*), and noninfectious causes (SLE, exogenous chemical meningitis). When eosinophils predominate or are present in limited numbers in a primarily mononuclear cell response in the CSF, the differential diagnosis includes parasitic diseases (*A. cantonensis*, *G. spinigerum*, *B. procyonis*, or *Toxocara canis* infection, cysticercosis, schistosomiasis, echinococcal disease, *T. gondii* infection), fungal infections (6 to 20% eosinophils along with a predominantly lymphocyte pleocytosis, particularly with coccidioidal meningitis), neoplastic disease (lymphoma, leukemia, metastatic carcinoma), or other inflammatory processes (sarcoidosis, hypereosinophilic syndrome).

It is often necessary to broaden the number of diagnostic tests if the initial workup does not reveal the cause. In addition, repeated samples of large volumes of CSF may be required to diagnose certain infectious and malignant causes of chronic meningitis. For instance, lymphomatous or carcinomatous meningitis may be di-

TABLE 361-3 Noninfectious Causes of Chronic Meningitis

Causative Agents	CSF Formula	Helpful Diagnostic Tests	Risk Factors and Systemic Manifestations
Malignancy	Mononuclear cells, elevated protein, low glucose	Repeated cytologic examination of large volumes of CSF; CSF exam by polarizing microscopy; clonal lymphocyte markers; deposits on nerve roots or meninges seen on myelogram or contrast-enhanced MRI; meningeal biopsy	Metastatic cancer of breast, lung, stomach, or pancreas; melanoma, lymphoma, leukemia; meningeal gliomatosis; meningeal sarcoma; cerebral dysgerminoma; meningeal melanoma or B cell lymphoma
Chemical compounds (may cause recurrent meningitis)	Mononuclear or PMNs, low glucose, elevated protein; xanthochromia from subarachnoid hemorrhage in week prior to presentation with "meningitis"	Contrast-enhanced CT scan or MRI Cerebral angiogram to detect aneurysm	History of recent injection into the subarachnoid space; history of sudden onset of headache; recent resection of acoustic neuroma or craniopharyngioma; epidermoid tumor of brain or spine, sometimes with dermoid sinus tract; pituitary apoplexy
Primary inflammation CNS sarcoidosis	Mononuclear cells; elevated protein; often low glucose	Serum and CSF angiotensin-converting enzyme levels; biopsy of extraneural affected tissues or brain lesion/meningeal biopsy	CN palsy, especially of CN VII; hypothalamic dysfunction, especially diabetes insipidus; abnormal chest radiograph; peripheral neuropathy or myopathy
Vogt-Koyanagi-Harada syndrome (recurrent meningitis)	Mononuclear cells		Recurrent meningoencephalitis with uveitis, retinal detachment, alopecia, lightening of eyebrows and lashes, dysacousia, cataracts, glaucoma
Isolated granulomatous angiitis of the nervous system	Mononuclear cells, elevated protein	Angiography or meningeal biopsy	Subacute dementia; multiple cerebral infarctions; recent zoster ophthalmicus
Systemic lupus erythematosus	Mononuclear or PMNs	Anti-DNA antibody, antinuclear antibodies	Encephalopathy; seizures; stroke; transverse myelopathy; rash; arthritis
Behçet's syndrome (recurrent meningitis)	Mononuclear or PMNs, elevated protein		Oral and genital aphthous ulcers; iridocyclitis; retinal hemorrhages; pathergic lesions at site of skin puncture
Chronic benign lymphocytic meningitis	Mononuclear cells		Recovery in 2–6 months, diagnosis by exclusion
Mollaret's meningitis (recurrent meningitis)	Large endothelial cells and PMNs in first hours, followed by mononuclear cells	PCR for herpes; MRI/CT to rule out epidermoid tumor or dural cyst	Recurrent meningitis; exclude HSV-2; rare cases due to HSV-1; occasional case associated with dural cyst
Drug hypersensitivity	PMNs; occasionally mononuclear cells or eosinophils		Exposure to ibuprofen, sulfonamides, isoniazid, tolmetin, ciprofloxacin, phenazopyridine; improvement after discontinuation of drug; recurrent episodes with recurrent exposure
Wegener's granulomatosis	Mononuclear cells	Chest and sinus radiographs; urinalysis; ANCA antibodies in serum	Associated sinus, pulmonary, or renal lesions; CN palsies; skin lesions; peripheral neuropathy

Other: multiple sclerosis, Sjögren's syndrome, neonatal onset multisystemic inflammatory disease (NOMID), and rarer forms of vasculitis (e.g., Cogan's syndrome)

Abbreviations: ANCA, anti-neutrophil cytoplasmic antibodies; CN, cranial nerve; CSF, cerebrospinal fluid; CT, computed tomography; HSV, herpes simplex virus; MRI, magnetic resonance imaging; PCR, polymerase chain reaction; PMNs, polymorphonuclear cells.

agnosed by examination of sections cut from a cell block formed by spinning down the sediment from a large volume of CSF. The diagnosis of fungal meningitis may require large volumes of CSF for culture of sediment. If standard lumbar puncture is unrewarding, a cervical cisternal tap to sample CSF near to the basal meninges may be fruitful.

Laboratory Investigation In addition to the CSF examination, an attempt should be made to uncover pertinent underlying illnesses. Tuberculin skin test, chest radiograph, urine analysis and culture, blood count and differential, renal and liver function tests, alkaline phosphatase, sedimentation rate, antinuclear antibody, anti-Ro and anti-La antibody, and serum angiotensin-converting enzyme level are often indicated. Liver or bone marrow biopsy may be diagnostic in some cases of miliary tuberculosis, disseminated fungal infection, sarcoidosis, or metastatic malignancy. Abnormalities discovered on chest radiograph or chest CT can be pursued by bronchoscopy or transthoracic needle biopsy.

Meningeal Biopsy A diagnostic meningeal biopsy should be strongly considered in patients who are severely disabled, who need chronic ventricular decompression, or whose illness is progressing rapidly. The activities of the surgeon, pathologist, microbiologist, and cytologist should be coordinated so that a large enough sample is obtained and the appropriate cultures and histologic and molecular studies, including electron microscopic and PCR studies, are performed. The diagnostic yield of meningeal biopsy can be increased by targeting regions that enhance with contrast on MRI or CT. With current microsurgical techniques, most areas of the basal meninges can be accessed for biopsy via a limited craniotomy. In a series from the Mayo Clinic reported by Cheng et al., MRI demonstrated meningeal enhancement in 47% of patients undergoing meningeal biopsy. Biopsy of an enhancing region was diagnostic in 80% of cases; biopsy of nonenhancing regions was diagnostic in only 9%; sarcoid (31%) and metastatic adenocarcinoma (25%) were the most common conditions identified.

Approach to the Enigmatic Case In approximately one-third of cases, the diagnosis is not known despite careful evaluation of CSF and potential extraneural sites of disease. A number of the organisms that cause chronic meningitis may take weeks to be identified by cultures. In enigmatic cases several options are available, determined by the extent of the clinical deficits and rate of progression. It is prudent to wait until cultures are finalized if the patient is asymptomatic or symptoms are mild and not progressive. Unfortunately, in many cases progressive neurologic deterioration occurs, and rapid treatment is required. Ventricular-peritoneal shunts may be placed to relieve hydrocephalus, but the risk of disseminating the undiagnosed inflammatory process into the abdomen must be considered.

Empirical Treatment Diagnosis of the causative agent is essential because effective therapies exist for many etiologies of chronic meningitis; if the condition is left untreated, however, progressive damage to the CNS and cranial nerves and roots is likely to occur. Occasionally, empirical therapy must be initiated when all attempts at diagnosis fail. In general, empirical therapy in the United States consists of antimycobacterial agents, amphotericin for fungal infection, or glucocorticoids for noninfectious inflammatory causes. It is important to direct empirical therapy of lymphocytic meningitis at tuberculosis, particularly if the condition is associated with hypoglycorrhachia and sixth and other CN palsies, since untreated disease is fatal in 4 to 8 weeks. In a series from the Mayo Clinic, the most useful empirical therapy was administration of glucocorticoids rather than antituberculous therapy. Carcinomatous or lymphomatous meningitis may be difficult to diagnose initially, but the diagnosis becomes evident with time.

THE IMMUNOSUPPRESSED PATIENT Chronic meningitis is not uncommon in the course of HIV infection. Pleocytosis and mild meningeal signs often occur at the onset of HIV infection, and occasionally low-grade meningitis persists. Toxoplasmosis commonly presents as intracranial abscesses and may also be associated with meningitis. Other important causes of chronic meningitis in AIDS include infection with *Cryptococcus*, *Nocardia*, *Candida*, or other fungi; syphilis; and lymphoma

FIGURE 361-1 Primary central nervous system lymphoma. A 24-year-old man, immunosuppressed due to intestinal lymphangiectasia, developed multiple cranial neuropathies. CSF findings consisted of 100 lymphocytes/μL and a protein of 250 mg/dL; cytology and cultures were negative. Gadolinium-enhanced T1 MRI revealed diffuse, multifocal meningeal enhancement surrounding the brainstem (*A*), spinal cord and cauda equina (*B*).

(Fig. 361-1). Toxoplasmosis, cryptococcosis, nocardiosis, and other fungal infections are important etiologic considerations in individuals with immunodeficiency states other than AIDS, including those due to immunosuppressive medications. Because of the increased risk of chronic meningitis and the attenuation of clinical signs of meningeal irritation in immunosuppressed individuals, CSF examination should be performed for any persistent headache or unexplained change in mental state.

FURTHER READING

LAN SH et al: Cerebral infarction in chronic meningitis: A comparison of tuberculous meningitis and cryptococcal meningitis. Q J Med. 94:247, 2001

LILIANG PC et al: Use of ventriculoperitoneal shunts to treat uncontrollable intracranial hypertension in patients who have cryptococcal meningitis without hydrocephalus. Clin Infect Dis. 34:E64, 2002

SMITH JE, AKSAMIT AJ: Outcome of chronic idiopathic meningitis. Mayo Clinic Proc 69:548, 1994

THWAITS G et al: Tuberculous meningitis. J Neurol Neurosurg Psychiatry 68: 289, 2000

---

362 PRION DISEASES
Stanley B. Prusiner, Bruce Miller

Prions are infectious proteins that cause degeneration of the central nervous system (CNS). Prion diseases are disorders of protein conformation, the most common of which in humans is called Creutzfeldt-Jakob disease (CJD). CJD typically presents with dementia and myoclonus, is relentlessly progressive, and generally causes death within a year of onset. Most CJD patients are between 50 and 75 years of age; however, patients as young as 17 years and as old as 83 years have been recorded.

In mammals, prions reproduce by binding to the normal, cellular isoform of the *pr*ion *pr*otein (PrP^C) and stimulating conversion of PrP^C into the di*s*ease-*c*ausing isoform (PrP^{Sc}). PrP^C is rich in α-helix and has little β-structure, while PrP^{Sc} has less α-helix and a high amount of β-structure (Fig. 362-1). This α-to-β structural transition in the prion protein (PrP) is the fundamental event underlying prion diseases (Table 362-1).

Four new concepts have emerged from studies of prions: (1) Prions are the only known infectious pathogens that are devoid of nucleic acid; all other infectious agents possess genomes composed of either RNA or DNA that direct the synthesis of their progeny. (2) Prion diseases may be manifest as infectious, genetic, and sporadic disorders; no other group of illnesses with a single etiology presents with such a wide spectrum of clinical manifestations. (3) Prion diseases result from the accumulation of PrP^{Sc}, the conformation of which differs substantially from that of its precursor PrP^C. (4) PrP^{Sc} can exist in a variety of different conformations, each of which seems to specify a particular disease phenotype. How a specific conformation of a PrP^{Sc} molecule is imparted to PrP^C during prion replication to produce nascent PrP^{Sc} with the same conformation is unknown. Additionally, it is

FIGURE 362-1 Structures of prion proteins. *A.* NMR structure of Syrian hamster recombinant (rec) PrP(90–231). Presumably, the structure of the α-helical form of recPrP(90–231) resembles that of PrP^C. recPrP(90–231) is viewed from the interface where PrP^{Sc} is thought to bind to PrP^C. Shown are: α-helices A (residues 144–157), B (172–193), and C (200–227). Flat ribbons depict β-strands S1 (129–131) and S2 (161–163). *(Reprinted with permission from H Lui et al: Biochemistry 38:5362, 1999.)* *B.* Theoretical structural model of PrP^{Sc}. The 90–160 region has been modeled onto a β-helical architecture while the COOH terminal helices B and C are preserved as in PrP^C. *(Image prepared by C. Govaerts.)*

unclear what factors determine where in the CNS a particular PrP^{Sc} molecule will be deposited.

SPECTRUM OF PRION DISEASES The sporadic form of CJD is the most common prion disorder in humans. Sporadic CJD (sCJD) accounts for ~85% of all cases of human prion disease, while inherited prion diseases account for 10 to 15% of all cases (Table 362-2). Familial CJD (fCJD), Gerstmann-Sträussler-Scheinker (GSS) disease, and fatal familial insomnia (FFI) are all dominantly inherited prion diseases that are caused by mutations in the PrP gene.

Although infectious prion diseases account for <1% of all cases and infection does not seem to play an important role in the natural history of these illnesses, the transmissibility of prions is an important biologic feature. *Kuru* of the Fore people of New Guinea is thought to have resulted from the consumption of brains from dead relatives during ritualistic cannibalism. With the cessation of ritualistic cannibalism in the late 1950s, kuru has nearly disappeared with the exception of a few recent patients exhibiting incubation periods of >40 years. Iatrogenic CJD (iCJD) seems to be the result of the accidental inoculation of patients with prions. Variant CJD (vCJD) in teenagers

TABLE 362-1 *Glossary of Prion Terminology*

Prion	*Pr*oteinaceous *in*fectious particle that lacks nucleic acid. Prions are composed largely, if not entirely, of PrP^{Sc} molecules. They can cause scrapie in animals and related neurodegenerative diseases of humans such as Creutzfeldt-Jakob disease (CJD).
PrP^{Sc}	Disease-causing isoform of the prion protein. This protein is the only identifiable macromolecule in purified preparations of scrapie prions.
PrP^C	Cellular isoform of the prion protein. PrP^C is the precursor of PrP^{Sc}.
PrP 27-30	A fragment of PrP^{Sc}, generated by truncation of the NH$_2$-terminus by limited digestion with proteinase K. PrP 27-30 retains prion infectivity and polymerizes into amyloid.
PRNP	PrP gene located on human chromosome 20.
Prion rod	An aggregate of prions composed largely of PrP 27-30 molecules. Created by detergent extraction and limited proteolysis of PrP^{Sc}. Morphologically and histochemically indistinguishable from many amyloids.
PrP amyloid	Amyloid containing PrP in the brains of animals or humans with prion disease; often accumulates as plaques.

TABLE 362-2 *The Prion Diseases*

Disease	Host	Mechanism of Pathogenesis
Human		
Kuru	Fore people	Infection through ritualistic cannibalism
iCJD	Humans	Infection from prion-contaminated hGH, dura mater grafts, etc.
vCJD	Humans	Infection from bovine prions
fCJD	Humans	Germ-line mutations in PRNP
GSS	Humans	Germ-line mutations in PRNP
FFI	Humans	Germ-line mutation in PRNP (D178N, M129)
sCJD	Humans	Somatic mutation or spontaneous conversion of PrP^C into PrP^{Sc}?
sFI	Humans	Somatic mutation or spontaneous conversion of PrP^C into PrP^{Sc}?
Animal		
Scrapie	Sheep	Infection in genetically susceptible sheep
BSE	Cattle	Infection with prion-contaminated MBM
TME	Mink	Infection with prions from sheep or cattle
CWD	Mule deer, elk	Unknown
FSE	Cats	Infection with prion-contaminated beef
Exotic ungulate encephalopathy	Greater kudu, nyala, or oryx	Infection with prion-contaminated MBM

Abbreviations: BSE, bovine spongiform encephalopathy; CJD, Creutzfeldt-Jakob disease; fCJD, familial Creutzfeldt-Jakob disease; iCJD, iatrogenic Creutzfeldt-Jakob disease; sCJD, sporadic Creutzfeldt-Jakob disease; vCJD, variant Creutzfeldt-Jakob disease; CWD, chronic wasting disease; FFI, fatal familial insomnia; sFI, sporadic fatal insomnia; FSE, feline spongiform encephalopathy; GSS, Gerstmann-Sträussler-Scheinker disease; hGH, human growth hormone; MBM, meat and bone meal; TME, transmissible mink encephalopathy.

and young adults in Europe is the result of exposure to tainted beef from cattle with bovine spongiform encepalopathy (BSE).

Six diseases of animals are caused by prions (Table 362-2). Scrapie of sheep and goats is the prototypic prion disease. Mink encephalopathy, BSE, feline spongiform encephalopathy, and exotic ungulate encephalopathy are all thought to occur after the consumption of prion-infected foodstuffs. The BSE epidemic emerged in Britain in the late 1980s and was shown to be due to industrial cannibalism. Whether BSE began as a sporadic case of BSE in a cow or started with scrapie in sheep is unknown. The origin of chronic wasting disease (CWD), a prion disease endemic in deer and elk in regions of North America, is uncertain.

EPIDEMIOLOGY CJD is found throughout the world. The incidence of sCJD is approximately one case per million population. Although many geographic clusters of CJD have been reported, each has been shown to segregate with a PrP gene mutation. Attempts to identify common exposure to some etiologic agent have been unsuccessful for both the sporadic and familial cases. Ingestion of scrapie-infected sheep or goat meat as a cause of CJD in humans has not been demonstrated by epidemiologic studies, although speculation about this potential route of inoculation continues. Of particular interest are deer hunters who develop CJD, because up to 90% of culled deer in some game herds have been shown to harbor CWD prions. Studies with Syrian hamsters demonstrate that oral infection with prions can occur, but the process is inefficient compared to intracerebral inoculation.

PATHOGENESIS The human prion diseases were initially classified as neurodegenerative disorders of unknown etiology on the basis of pathologic changes being confined to the CNS. With the transmission of kuru and CJD to apes, investigators began to view these diseases as infectious CNS illnesses caused by slow viruses. Even though the familial nature of a subset of CJD cases was well described, the significance of this observation became more obscure with the transmission of CJD to animals. Eventually, the meaning of heritable CJD became clear with the discovery of mutations in the *PrP* gene of these patients. The prion concept explains how a disease can manifest as a heritable as well as an infectious illness. Moreover, the hallmark of all prion diseases, whether sporadic, dominantly inherited, or acquired by infection, is that they involve the aberrant metabolism of PrP.

A major feature that distinguishes prions from viruses is the finding that both PrP isoforms are encoded by a chromosomal gene. In humans, the *PrP* gene is designated *PRNP* and is located on the short arm of chromosome 20. Limited proteolysis of PrP^{Sc} produces a smaller, protease-resistant molecule of ~142 amino acids designated PrP 27-30; PrP^C is completely hydrolyzed under the same conditions (Fig. 362-2). In the presence of detergent, PrP 27-30 polymerizes into amyloid. Prion rods formed by limited proteolysis and detergent extraction are indistinguishable from the filaments that aggregate to form PrP amyloid plaques in the CNS. Both the rods and the PrP amyloid filaments found in brain tissue exhibit similar ultrastructural morphology and green-gold birefringence after staining with Congo red dye.

Prion Strains The existence of prion strains raised the question of how heritable biologic information can be enciphered in a molecule other than nucleic acid. Various strains of prions have been defined by incubation times and the distribution of neuronal vacuolation. Subsequently, the patterns of PrP^{Sc} deposition were found to correlate with vacuolation profiles, and these patterns were also used in their characterization.

Persuasive evidence that strain-specific information is enciphered in the tertiary structure of PrP^{Sc} comes from transmission of two different inherited human prion diseases to mice expressing a chimeric human-mouse PrP transgene. In FFI, the protease-resistant fragment of PrP^{Sc} after deglycosylation has a molecular mass of 19 kDa, whereas in fCJD and most sporadic prion diseases, it is 21 kDa (Table 362-3). This difference in molecular mass was shown to be due to different sites of proteolytic cleavage at the NH$_2$ termini of the two human PrP^{Sc} molecules, reflecting different tertiary structures. These distinct conformations were not unexpected because the amino acid sequences of the PrPs differ.

Extracts from the brains of patients with FFI transmitted disease into mice expressing a chimeric human-mouse PrP transgene and induced formation of the 19-kDa PrP^{Sc}, whereas brain extracts from fCJD and sCJD patients produced the 21-kDa PrP^{Sc} in mice expressing the same transgene. On second passage, these differences were maintained, demonstrating that chimeric PrP^{Sc} can exist in two different conformations based on the sizes of the protease-resistant fragments, even though the amino acid sequence of PrP^{Sc} is invariant.

This analysis was extended when patients with sporadic fatal insomnia (sFI) were identified. Although they did not carry a *PRNP* gene mutation, the patients demonstrated a clinical and pathologic phenotype that was indistinguishable from that of patients with FFI. Furthermore, 19-kDa PrP^{Sc} was found in their brains, and on passage of prion disease to mice expressing a chimeric human-mouse PrP transgene, 19-kDa PrP^{Sc} was also found. These findings indicate that the disease phenotype is dictated by the conformation of PrP^{Sc} and not the amino acid sequence. PrP^{Sc} acts as a template for the conversion of PrP^C into nascent PrP^{Sc}. On the passage of prions into mice expressing a chimeric hamster-mouse PrP transgene, a change in the conformation of PrP^{Sc} was accompanied by the emergence of a new strain of prions.

Species Barrier Studies on the role of the primary and tertiary structures of PrP in the transmission of prion disease have given new insights into the pathogenesis of these maladies. The amino acid sequence of PrP encodes the species of the prion, and the prion derives its PrP^{Sc} sequence from the last mammal in which it was passaged. While the primary structure of PrP is likely to be the most important or even sole determinant of the tertiary structure of PrP^C, PrP^{Sc} seems to function as a template in determining the tertiary structure of nascent PrP^{Sc} mol-

A.

B.

FIGURE 362-2 *Prion protein isoforms. A. Western immunoblot of brain homogenates from uninfected (lanes 1 and 2) and prion-infected (lanes 3 and 4) Syrian hamsters. Samples in lanes 2 and 4 were digested with proteinase K. PrP^C in lanes 2 and 4 was completely hydrolyzed under these conditions, whereas in PrP^{Sc} (lane 4), ~67 amino acids were digested from the NH$_2$-terminus to generate PrP 27-30. The blot was developed with anti-PrP polyclonal rabbit antiserum. Molecular size markers (left) are in kilodaltons. B. Bar diagram of Syrian hamster PrP, which consists of 254 amino acids. After processing of the NH$_2$ and COOH termini, both PrP^C and PrP^{Sc} consist of 209 residues. After limited proteolysis, the NH$_2$ terminus of PrP^{Sc} is truncated to form PrP 27-30 composed of ~142 amino acids. [Reprinted from Les Prix Nobel T. Frängsmyr (ed), Stockholm, Norstedts Tryckeri, 1998, pp 268–323, with permission.]*

ecules as they are formed from PrP^C. In turn, prion diversity appears to be enciphered in the conformation of PrP^{Sc} and thus, prion strains seem to represent different conformers of PrP^{Sc}.

In general, transmission of prion disease from one species to another is inefficient, in that not all intracerebrally inoculated animals develop disease, and those that fall ill do so only after long incubation times that can approach the natural life span of the animal. This "spe-

TABLE 362-3 Distinct Prion Strains Generated in Humans with Inherited Prion Diseases and Transmitted to Transgenic Mice[a]

Inoculum	Host Species	Host PrP Genotype	Incubation Time [days ± SEM] (n/n$_0$)	PrP^{Sc} (kDa)
None	Human	FFI(D178N, M129)		19
FFI	Mouse	Tg(MHu2M)	206 ± 7 (7/7)	19
FFI → Tg(MHu2M)	Mouse	Tg(MHu2M)	136 ± 1 (6/6)	19
None	Human	fCJD(E200K)		21
fCJD	Mouse	Tg(MHu2M)	170 ± 2 (10/10)	21
fCJD → Tg(MHu2M)	Mouse	Tg(MHu2M)	167 ± 3 (15/15)	21

[a] Tg(MHu2M) mice express a chimeric mouse-human PrP gene.
Note: Clinicopathologic phenotype is determined by the conformation of PrP^{Sc} in accord with the results of the transmission of human prions from patients with FFI to transgenic mice. FFI, fatal familial insomnia; fCJD, familial Creutzfeldt-Jakob disease.

cics barrier" to transmission is correlated with the degree of similarity between the amino acid sequence of PrP^C in the inoculated host and of PrP^{Sc} in the prion inoculum. The importance of sequence similarity between the host and donor PrP argues that PrP^C directly interacts with PrP^{Sc} in the prion conversion process.

SPORADIC AND INHERITED PRION DISEASES

Several different scenarios might explain the initiation of sporadic prion disease: (1) A somatic mutation may be the cause and thus follow a path similar to that for germ-line mutations in inherited disease. In this situation, the mutant PrP^{Sc} must be capable of targeting wild-type PrP^C, a process known to be possible for some mutations but less likely for others. (2) The activation barrier separating wild-type PrP^C from PrP^{Sc} could be crossed on rare occasions when viewed in the context of a population. Most individuals would be spared, while presentations in the elderly with an incidence of ~1 per million would be seen. (3) PrP^{Sc} may be present at very low levels in some normal cells, where it performs some important, as yet unknown, function. The level of PrP^{Sc} in such cells is hypothesized to be sufficiently low as to be not detected by bioassay. In some altered metabolic states, the cellular mechanisms for clearing PrP^{Sc} might become compromised and the rate of PrP^{Sc} formation would then begin to exceed the capacity of the cell to clear it. The third possible mechanism is attractive since it suggests PrP^{Sc} is not simply a misfolded protein, as proposed for the first and second mechanisms, but that it is an alternatively folded molecule with a function.

More than 30 different mutations resulting in nonconservative substitutions in the human *PRNP* gene have been found to segregate with inherited human prion diseases. Missense mutations and expansions in the octapeptide repeat region of the gene are responsible for familial forms of prion disease. Five different mutations of the *PRNP* gene have been linked genetically to heritable prion disease.

Although phenotypes may vary dramatically within families, specific phenotypes tend to be observed with certain mutations. A clinical phenotype indistinguishable from typical sCJD is usually seen with substitutions at codons 180, 183, 200, 208, 210, and 232. Substitutions at codons 102, 105, 117, 198, and 217 are associated with the GSS variant of prion disease. The normal human PrP sequence contains five repeats of an eight-amino-acid sequence. Insertions from two to nine extra octarepeats frequently cause variable phenotypes ranging from a condition indistinguishable from sCJD to a slowly progressive dementing illness of many years' duration. A mutation at codon 178 resulting in substitution of asparagine for aspartic acid produces FFI if a methionine is encoded at the polymorphic 129 residue on the same allele. Typical CJD is seen if a valine is encoded at position 129 of the same allele.

Human *PRNP* Gene Polymorphisms   Polymorphisms influence the susceptibility to sporadic, inherited, and infectious forms of prion disease. The methionine/valine polymorphism at position 129 not only modulates the age of onset of some inherited prion diseases but can also determine the clinical phenotype. The finding that homozygosity at codon 129 predisposes to sCJD supports a model of prion production that favors PrP interactions between homologous proteins.

Substitution of the basic residue lysine at position 218 in mouse PrP produced dominant-negative inhibition of prion replication in transgenic mice. This same lysine at position 219 in human PrP has been found in 12% of the Japanese population, and this group appears to be resistant to prion disease. Dominant-negative inhibition of prion replication was also found with substitution of the basic residue arginine at position 171; sheep with arginine are resistant to scrapie prions but are susceptible to BSE prions that were inoculated intracerebrally.

INFECTIOUS PRION DISEASES

IATROGENIC CJD   Accidental transmission of CJD to humans appears to have occurred with corneal transplantation, contaminated electroen-cephalogram (EEG) electrode implantation, and surgical procedures. Corneas from donors with inapparent CJD have been transplanted to apparently healthy recipients who developed CJD after prolonged incubation periods. The same improperly decontaminated EEG electrodes that caused CJD in two young patients with intractable epilepsy caused CJD in a chimpanzee 18 months after their experimental implantation.

Surgical procedures may have resulted in accidental inoculation of patients with prions during their operations, presumably because some instrument or apparatus in the operating theater became contaminated when a CJD patient underwent surgery. Although the epidemiology of these studies is highly suggestive, no proof for such episodes exists.

Dura Mater Grafts   More than 120 cases of CJD after implantation of dura mater grafts have been recorded. All of the grafts were thought to have been acquired from a single manufacturer whose preparative procedures were inadequate to inactivate human prions. One case of CJD occurred after repair of an eardrum perforation with a pericardium graft.

Human Growth Hormone and Pituitary Gonadotropin Therapy   The possibility of transmission of CJD from contaminated human growth hormone (hGH) preparations derived from human pituitaries has been raised by the occurrence of fatal cerebellar disorders with dementia in >120 patients ranging in age from 10 to 41 years. These patients received injections of hGH every 2 to 4 days for 4 to 12 years. If it is assumed that these patients developed CJD from injections of prion-contaminated hGH preparations, the possible incubation periods range from 4 to 30 years. Even though several investigations argue for the efficacy of inactivating prions in hGH fractions prepared from human pituitaries with 6 *M* urea, it seems doubtful that such protocols will be used for purifying hGH because recombinant hGH is available. Four cases of CJD have occurred in women receiving human pituitary gonadotropin.

VARIANT CJD   The restricted geographic occurrence and chronology of vCJD raised the possibility that BSE prions have been transmitted to humans through the consumption of tainted beef. More than 140 cases of vCJD have occurred, with >90% of these in Britain. Because the number of vCJD cases is still small, it not possible to decide if we are at the beginning of a prion disease epidemic in Europe, similar to those seen for BSE and kuru, or if the number of vCJD cases will remain small. What is certain is that prion-tainted meat should be prevented from entering the human food supply.

The most compelling evidence that vCJD is caused by BSE prions was obtained from experiments in mice expressing the bovine PrP transgene. Both BSE and vCJD prions were efficiently transmitted to these transgenic mice and with similar incubation periods. In contrast to sCJD prions, vCJD prions did not transmit disease efficiently to mice expressing a chimeric human-mouse PrP transgene. Earlier studies with nontransgenic mice suggested that vCJD and BSE might be derived from the same source because both inocula transmitted disease with similar but very long incubation periods.

Attempts to determine the origin of BSE and vCJD prions have relied on passaging studies in mice, some of which are described above, as well as studies of the conformation and glycosylation of PrP^{Sc}. One scenario suggests that a particular conformation of bovine PrP^{Sc} was selected for heat resistance during the rendering process and was then reselected multiple times as cattle infected by ingesting prion-contaminated meat and bone meal (MBM) were slaughtered and their offal rendered into more MBM.

NEUROPATHOLOGY   Frequently, the brains of patients with CJD have no recognizable abnormalities on gross examination. Patients who survive for several years have variable degrees of cerebral atrophy.

On light microscopy, the pathologic hallmarks of CJD are spongiform degeneration and astrocytic gliosis. The lack of an inflammatory response in CJD and other prion diseases is an important pathologic feature of these degenerative disorders. Spongiform degeneration is characterized by many 1- to 5-μm vacuoles in the neuropil between nerve cell bodies. Generally, the spongiform changes occur in the cerebral cortex, putamen, caudate nucleus, thalamus, and molecular layer of the cerebellum. Astrocytic gliosis is a constant but nonspecific feature of prion diseases. Widespread proliferation of fibrous astrocytes is found throughout the gray matter of brains infected with CJD prions. Astrocytic processes filled with glial filaments form extensive networks.

Amyloid plaques have been found in ~10% of CJD cases. Purified CJD prions from humans and animals exhibit the ultrastructural and histochemical characteristics of amyloid when treated with detergents during limited proteolysis. In first passage from some human Japanese CJD cases, amyloid plaques have been found in mouse brains. These plaques stain with antisera raised against PrP.

The amyloid plaques of GSS disease are morphologically distinct from those seen in kuru or scrapie. GSS plaques consist of a central dense core of amyloid surrounded by smaller globules of amyloid. Ultrastructurally, they consist of a radiating fibrillar network of amyloid fibrils, with scant or no neuritic degeneration. The plaques can be distributed throughout the brain but are most frequently found in the cerebellum. They are often located adjacent to blood vessels. Congophilic angiopathy has been noted in some cases of GSS disease.

In vCJD, a characteristic feature is the presence of "florid plaques." These are composed of a central core of PrP amyloid, surrounded by vacuoles in a pattern suggesting petals on a flower.

CLINICAL FEATURES Nonspecific prodromal symptoms occur in about a third of patients with CJD and may include fatigue, sleep disturbance, weight loss, headache, malaise, and ill-defined pain. Most patients with CJD present with deficits in higher cortical function. These deficits almost always progress over weeks or months to a state of profound dementia characterized by memory loss, impaired judgment, and a decline in virtually all aspects of intellectual function. A few patients present with either visual impairment or cerebellar gait and coordination deficits. Frequently, the cerebellar deficits are rapidly followed by progressive dementia. Visual problems often begin with blurred vision and diminished acuity, rapidly followed by dementia.

Other symptoms and signs include extrapyramidal dysfunction manifested as rigidity, masklike facies, or choreoathetoid movements; pyramidal signs (usually mild); seizures (usually major motor) and, less commonly, hypesthesia; supranuclear gaze palsy; optic atrophy; and vegetative signs such as changes in weight, temperature, sweating, or menstruation.

Myoclonus Most patients (~90%) with CJD exhibit myoclonus that appears at various times throughout the illness. Unlike other involuntary movements, myoclonus persists during sleep. Startle myoclonus elicited by loud sounds or bright lights is frequent. It is important to stress that myoclonus is neither specific nor confined to CJD. Dementia with myoclonus can also be due to Alzheimer's disease (AD) (Chap. 350), to cryptococcal encephalitis (Chap. 186), or to the myoclonic epilepsy disorder Unverricht-Lundborg disease (Chap. 348).

Clinical Course In documented cases of accidental transmission of CJD to humans, an incubation period of 1.5 to 2.0 years preceded the development of clinical disease. In other cases, incubation periods of up to 30 years have been suggested. Most patients with CJD live 6 to 12 months after the onset of clinical signs and symptoms, whereas some live for up to 5 years.

DIAGNOSIS The constellation of dementia, myoclonus, and periodic electrical bursts in an afebrile 60-year-old patient generally indicates CJD. Clinical abnormalities in CJD are confined to the CNS. Fever, elevated sedimentation rate, leukocytosis in blood, or a pleocytosis in cerebrospinal fluid (CSF) should alert the physician to another etiology to explain the patient's CNS dysfunction.

Variations in the typical course appear in inherited and transmitted forms of the disease. fCJD has an earlier mean age of onset than sCJD. In GSS disease, ataxia is usually a prominent and presenting feature, with dementia occurring late in the disease course. GSS disease typically presents earlier than CJD (mean age, 43 years) and is typically more slowly progressive than CJD; death usually occurs within 5 years of onset. FFI is characterized by insomnia and dysautonomia; dementia occurs only in the terminal phase of the illness. Rare sporadic cases have been identified. vCJD has an unusual clinical course, with a prominent psychiatric prodrome that may include visual hallucinations and early ataxia, while frank dementia is usually a late sign of vCJD.

DIFFERENTIAL DIAGNOSIS Many conditions may mimic CJD superficially. AD is occasionally accompanied by myoclonus but is usually distinguished by its protracted course and lack of motor and visual dysfunction.

Intracranial vasculitides (Chap. 306) may produce nearly all of the symptoms and signs associated with CJD, sometimes without systemic abnormalities. Myoclonus is exceptional with cerebral vasculitis, but focal seizures may confuse the picture; furthermore, myoclonus is often absent in the early stages of CJD. Stepwise change in deficits, prominent headache, abnormal CSF, and focal magnetic resonance imaging (MRI) or angiographic abnormalities all favor vasculitis.

Neurosyphilis (Chap. 153) may present with dementia and myoclonus that progresses in a relatively rapid fashion but is easily distinguished from CJD by CSF findings, as is cryptococcal meningoencephalitis. A diffuse intracranial tumor (gliomatosis cerebri; Chap. 358) may occasionally be confused with CJD. In rare cases of CNS neoplasia, neuroimaging studies are normal and there are no signs of increased intracranial pressure; however, CSF protein is usually elevated. Adult onset leukodystrophies (ceroid lipofuscinosis; Chap. 350) and myoclonic epilepsy with Lafora bodies (Chap. 348) may be responsible for dementia, myoclonus, and ataxia; but the less acute courses and prominent seizures distinguish them from CJD. A number of diseases that may simulate CJD are easily distinguished by the clinical setting in which they occur. These diseases include anoxic encephalopathy, subacute sclerosing panencephalitis, progressive rubella panencephalitis, herpes simplex encephalitis (in immunoincompetent hosts), dialysis dementia, uremia, and hepatic encephalopathy. When CJD begins atypically, it may for a short time resemble other disorders such as Parkinson's disease, progressive supranuclear palsy (Chap. 351), or progressive multifocal leukoencephalopathy (Chap. 360).

Certain drug intoxications, particularly lithium and bismuth, may produce encephalopathy and myoclonus. The rare condition known as Hashimoto's encephalopathy, which presents with a subacute progressive encephalopathy and myoclonus with periodic triphasic complexes on the EEG, should be excluded in every case of suspected CJD. It is diagnosed by the finding of high titers of antithyroglobulin or antithyroid perioxidase (antimicrosomal) antibodies in the blood, and improves with glucocorticoid therapy. Unlike CJD, fluctuations in severity typically occur in Hashimoto's encephalopathy.

The AIDS dementia complex (Chap. 173) may occasionally imitate CJD in onset, early course, physical signs, computed tomography (CT) findings, and lack of abnormalities on routine CSF studies. The few such patients without manifestations of systemic immunodeficiency (<10%) should be questioned about risk factors and should have serum antibodies to HIV determined.

LABORATORY TESTS The only specific diagnostic tests for CJD and other human prion diseases measure PrP^{Sc}. The most widely used method involves limited proteolysis that generates PrP 27-30, which is detected by immunoassay after denaturation. The conformation-dependent immunoassay (CDI) is based on immunoreactive epitopes that are exposed in PrP^{C} but buried in PrP^{Sc}. The CDI is extremely sensitive and quantitative and is likely to find wide application in both the post- and antemortem detection of prions. In humans, the diagnosis of CJD can be established by brain biopsy if PrP^{Sc} is detected. If no attempt is made to measure PrP^{Sc}, but the constellation of pathologic changes frequently found in CJD is seen in a brain biopsy, then the diagnosis is reasonably secure (see "Neuropathology," above). Because PrP^{Sc} is not uniformly distributed throughout the CNS, the apparent absence of PrPSc in a limited sample such as a biopsy does not rule out prion disease. At autopsy, sufficient brain samples should be taken for both PrPSc immunoassay, preferably by the CDI, and immunohistochemistry of tissue sections.

Whether an antemortem test can be developed using the CDI to detect protease-sensitive forms of PrPSc in blood is uncertain. Another possibility is such a test based on PrPSc formation in muscle. PrPSc accumulation seems to be restricted to the hindlimb muscles in mice but is more widespread in hamsters. Whether muscles in humans and livestock can be identified in which PrPSc accumulates consistently remains to be established.

To establish the diagnosis of either sCJD or familial prion disease, sequencing the *PRNP* gene must be performed. Finding the wild-type *PRNP* gene sequence permits the diagnosis of sCJD if there is no history to suggest exposure to an exogenous source of prions. The identification of a mutation in the *PRNP* gene sequence that encodes a nonconservative amino acid substitution argues for familial prion disease.

CT may be normal or show cortical atrophy. The MRI scan may show a subtle increased intensity in the basal ganglia with T2- or diffusion-weighted imaging, but this finding is neither sensitive nor specific enough to make a diagnosis.

CSF is nearly always normal but may show minimal protein elevation. Although the stress protein 14-3-3 is elevated in the CSF of some patients with CJD, similar elevations of 14-3-3 are found in patients with herpes simplex virus encephalitis, multi-infarct dementia, and stroke. In AD, 14-3-3 is generally not elevated. In the serum of some patients with CJD, the S-100 protein is elevated, but as with 14-3-3, this elevation is not specific.

The EEG is often useful in the diagnosis of CJD. During the early phase of CJD, the EEG is usually normal or shows only scattered theta activity. In most advanced cases, repetitive, high-voltage, triphasic, and polyphasic sharp discharges are seen, but in many cases their presence is transient. The presence of these stereotyped periodic bursts of <200 ms duration, occurring every 1 to 2 s, makes the diagnosis of CJD very likely. These discharges are frequently but not always symmetric; there may be a one-sided predominance in amplitude. As CJD progresses, normal background rhythms become fragmentary and slower.

CARE OF CJD PATIENTS Although CJD should not be considered either a contagious or communicable disease, it is transmissible. The risk of accidental inoculation by aerosols is very small; nonetheless, procedures producing aerosols should be performed in certified biosafety cabinets. Biosafety level 2 practices, containment equipment, and facilities are recommended by the Centers for Disease Control and Prevention and the National Institutes of Health. The primary problem in caring for patients with CJD is the inadvertent infection of health care workers by needle and stab wounds. The transmission of prions through the air has never been documented. Electroencephalographic and electromyographic needles should not be reused after studies on patients with CJD have been performed.

There is no reason for pathologists or morgue dieners to resist performing autopsies on patients whose clinical diagnosis was CJD. Standard microbiologic practices outlined here, along with specific recommendations for decontamination, seem to be adequate precautions for the care of patients with CJD and the handling of infected specimens.

DECONTAMINATION OF CJD PRIONS Prions are extremely resistant to common inactivation procedures, and there is some disagreement about the optimal conditions for sterilization. Some investigators recommend treating CJD-contaminated materials once with 1 *N* NaOH at room temperature, but we believe this procedure may be inadequate for sterilization. Autoclaving at 132°C for 5 h or treatment with 2 *N* NaOH for several hours is recommended for sterilization of prions. The term "sterilization" implies complete destruction of prions; any residual infectivity can be hazardous.

PREVENTION AND THERAPEUTICS There is no known effective therapy for preventing or treating CJD. The finding that phenothiazines and acridines inhibit PrPSc formation in cultured cells led to clinical studies of quinacrine in CJD patients. Although quinacrine seems to slow the rate of decline in some CJD patients, no cure of the disease has been observed. In mice, the results of quinacrine treatment are mixed: Some investigators report treatment is ineffective, while others find that quinacrine prolongs the lives of prion-infected mice compared to untreated animals.

Like the acridines, anti-PrP antibodies have been shown to eliminate PrPSc from cultured cells. Additionally, such antibodies in mice either administered by injection or produced from a transgene have been shown to prevent prion disease when prions are introduced by a peripheral route, such as intraperitoneal inoculation. Unfortunately, the antibodies were ineffective in mice inoculated intracerebrally with prions. Several drugs delay the onset of disease in animals inoculated intracerebrally with prions if the drugs are given around the time of the inoculation.

Structure-based drug design predicated on dominant-negative inhibition of prion formation has produced several promising compounds. Modified quinacrine compounds that are more potent than the parent drug have been found. Whether improving the efficacy of such small molecules will provide general methods for developing novel therapeutics for other neurodegenerative disorders, including AD and Parkinson's disease, as well as amyotrophic lateral sclerosis (ALS), remains to be established.

Financial Disclosure: SBP has a financial interest in InPro Biotechnology, Inc.

FURTHER READING

BOSQUE PJ et al: Prions in skeletal muscle. Proc Natl Acad Sci USA 99:3812, 2002

MAY BCH et al: Potent inhibition of scrapie prion replication in cultured cells by bis-acridines. Proc Natl Acad Sci USA 100:3416, 2003

PRUSINER SB (ed): *Prion Biology and Diseases*, 2nd ed. Cold Spring Harbor, New York, Cold Spring Harbor Laboratory Press, 2004

WILL RG et al: Diagnosis of new variant Creutzfeldt-Jakob disease. Ann Neurol 47:575, 2000

Section 3   Nerve and Muscle Disorders

363 APPROACH TO THE PATIENT WITH PERIPHERAL NEUROPATHY
Arthur K. Asbury

Peripheral neuropathy is a general term indicating peripheral nerve disorders of any cause; the manifestations of neuropathy may be so diverse that it is difficult for the physician to know where to begin and how to proceed.

The clinical and electrodiagnostic (EDX) approach to evaluation and management of a neuropathic disorder is summarized in Fig. 363-1. The EDX approach consists of electrophysiologic examination of nerve and muscle, including nerve conduction studies and electromyography. It is part of the evaluation of any neuropathy and is considered to be an extension of the neurologic examination. Using this

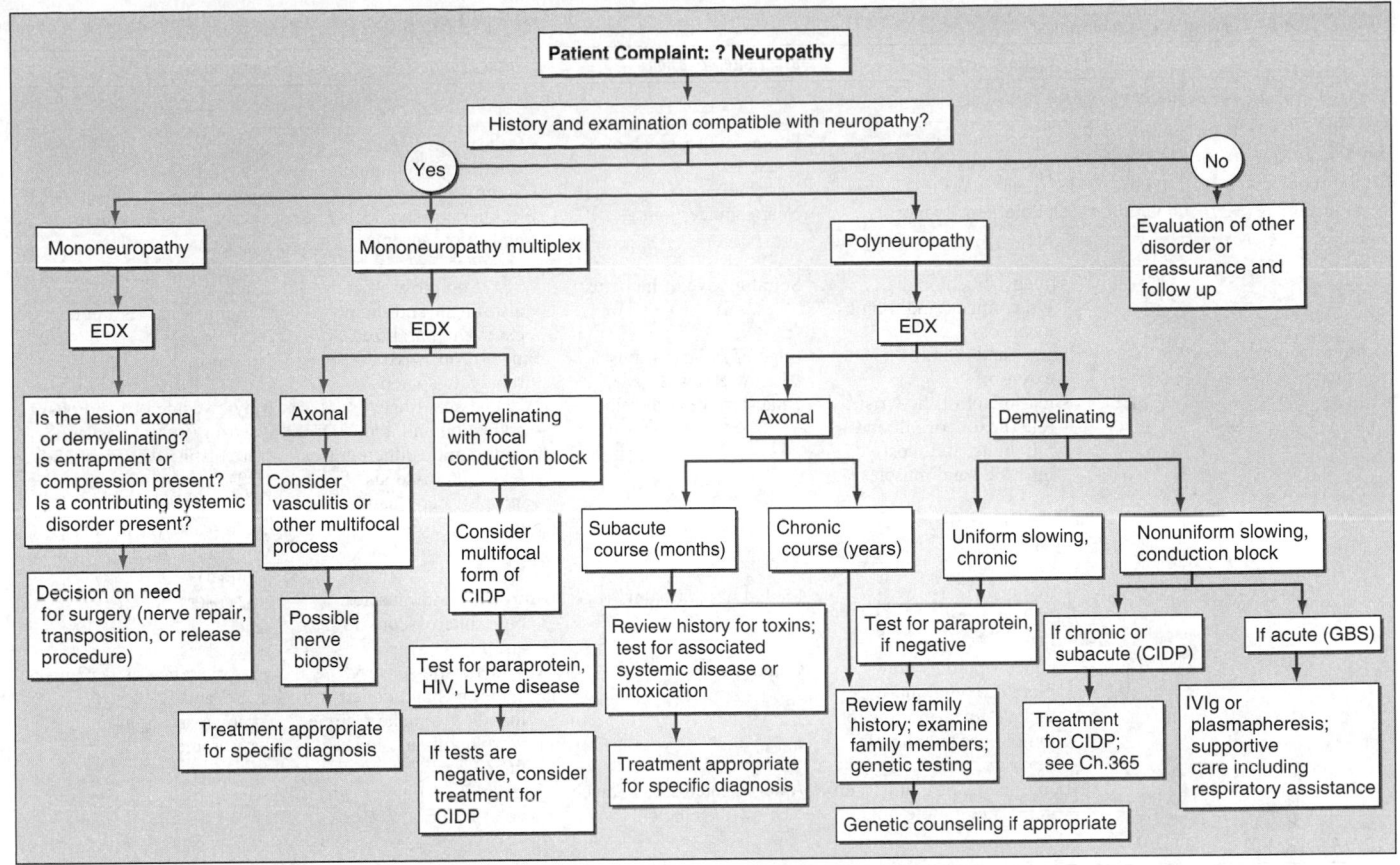

FIGURE 363-1 Approach to the evaluation of peripheral neuropathies. CIDP, chronic inflammatory demyelinating polyradiculoneuropathy; EDX, electrodiagnostic studies; GBS, Guillain-Barré syndrome; IVIg, intravenous immunoglobulin. For management and treatment considerations, see relevant sections of this chapter or of the two succeeding chapters on immune-mediated and on genetically determined neuropathies.

scheme (Fig. 363-1), the examiner determines for each patient the tempo, distribution, and severity of the neuropathy and makes a judgment as to whether the problem represents a mononeuropathy, a mononeuropathy multiplex, or a polyneuropathy. Often this distinction is obvious. With the sum of clinical and EDX information in hand, the differential diagnostic possibilities and treatment options are usually narrowed to a manageable number.

MONONEUROPATHY *Mononeuropathy* refers to focal involvement of a single nerve trunk and therefore implies a local cause. Direct trauma, compression, and entrapment are the usual causes. Ulnar neuropathies, due to lesions either at the ulnar groove or in the cubital tunnel, and median neuropathy due to compression in the carpal tunnel constitute the great majority of mononeuropathies encountered in clinical practice. These are described below, and other common mononeuropathies are listed in Table 363-1. EDX examination is part of the evaluation of mononeuropathies, mainly to judge the nature of the focal lesion (demyelinating or axonal degeneration) and, in severe mononeuropathies, to determine whether any nerve fibers remain in continuity.

In the absence of a history of trauma to the nerve trunk, factors favoring conservative management of a mononeuropathy include sudden onset, no motor deficit, few or no sensory findings (even though pain and sensory symptoms may be present), and no evidence of axonal degeneration by EDX criteria. Factors favoring active measures including surgical intervention are chronicity and worsening neurologic deficit on examination, particularly if motor and EDX evidence suggests that the lesion has produced a degree of wallerian degeneration.

Ulnar Neuropathy Complete ulnar paralysis results in a characteristic claw-hand deformity owing to wasting and weakness of many of the small hand muscles and hyperextension of the fingers at the metacarpophalangeal joints and flexion at the interphalangeal joints. The flex-

ion deformity is most pronounced in the fourth and fifth fingers. Sensory loss occurs over the fifth finger, the ulnar aspect of the fourth finger, and the ulnar border of the palm. The superficial location of the nerve at the elbow makes it a common site of pressure palsy. The ulnar nerve may also become entrapped just distal to the elbow in the cubital tunnel formed by the aponeurotic arch linking the two heads of the flexor carpi ulnaris. Also, prolonged pressure on the base of the palm, as occurs with use of hand tools or bicycle riding, may result in damage to the deep palmar branch of the ulnar nerve, causing weakness of the small hand muscles but no sensory loss (Table 363-1). Management of ulnar neuropathy depends on the timing, site, and severity of the responsible focal lesion. Entrapment of the ulnar nerve within the cubital tunnel may be released surgically, whereas ulnar nerve damage in the condylar groove is managed either conservatively, using padding to protect the nerve, or surgically by an anterior nerve transposition procedure.

Carpal Tunnel Syndrome The median nerve in the carpal tunnel lies in close quarters with nine tendons. Entrapment of the nerve at the wrist (*carpal tunnel syndrome*) is usually due to excessive use of the wrist but on occasion may be secondary to tenosynovitis with arthritis or local infiltration, e.g., by a thickening of connective tissue as in acromegaly or by deposit of amyloid or by one of the mucopolysaccharidoses. Other systemic diseases associated with carpal tunnel syndrome are hypothyroidism, rheumatoid arthritis, and diabetes mellitus, but underlying diseases account for only a small fraction of all cases. The main symptoms of carpal tunnel syndrome are nocturnal paresthesias of thumb, index, and middle fingers. With worsening, numbness occurs in that distribution and is demonstrable by pin examination. Eventually weakness and atrophy of the abductor pollicis brevis (thenar eminence) become evident. The principal treatment of carpal tunnel syndrome is surgical section of the carpal ligament to relieve entrapment.

TABLE 363-1 *Common Mononeuropathies*

Nerve	Origin[a]	Muscles Innervated	Usual Site of Lesion	Clinical Features	Comments
UPPER EXTREMITY					
Suprascapular	C5, C6	Supraspinatus Infraspinatus	Suprascapular notch of scapula	Weakness of lateral rotation of the humerus	No sensory deficit
Long thoracic	C5–C7	Serratus anterior	Variable	Winging of scapula	No sensory deficit
Axillary	C5, C6	Deltoid, teres minor	Near shoulder joint	Weakness of shoulder abduction; atrophy of shoulder	Sensory deficit similar to C5 dorsal root lesion (See Figs. 22-2 and 22-3)
Radial	C5–T1	Triceps, brachioradialis, wrist, finger, and thumb extensors	Spiral groove of humerus	Wrist drop most obvious, also finger and thumb extensors paralyzed	Saturday night palsy (acute compression) is frequent cause
Posterior interosseous branch	C7, C8	Finger and thumb extensors	Edge of supinator muscle below elbow	Finger drop; wrist relatively spared	No sensory deficit
Ulnar	C8, T1	Ulnar flexor of the wrist, long flexors of 4th and 5th digits, and most intrinsic hand muscles	Ulnar groove at the elbow	Weakness of finger adduction and abduction and thumb adduction (see text); interosseous atrophy, claw-hand	May be acute or insidious; sensory symptoms/signs are distinctive (Figs. 22-2 22-3); see also text
			Cubital tunnel	Same as above	Often pain over medial proximal forearm (cubital tunnel)
			Medial base of palm	Intrinsic hand muscles only, interosseous atrophy	No sensory deficit
Median	C6–T1	Abductor pollicis brevis; more proximal muscles include forearm pronator, long finger and thumb flexors	Carpal tunnel	Characteristic sensory symptoms and deficit and inability to make a circle with thumb and index finger	Sensory deficit as per Figs. 22-2 and 22-3 (see text); known as carpal tunnel syndrome
Anterior interosseous branch	C7–T1	Long flexors of thumb and index and middle fingers	Anterior interosseus branch below the elbow	Weakness of pinch; pain in volar forearm	No sensory deficit
LOWER EXTREMITY					
Femoral	L2–L4	Iliopsoas (hip flexor) and quadriceps femoris (knee extensor)	Proximal to inguinal ligament	Knee buckling; absent knee jerk; weak anterior thigh muscles with atrophy	Association with diabetes mellitus; sensory disturbance as per Fig. 22-2
Lateral femoral cutaneous branch	L2, L3	None	Inguinal ligament	Dysesthetic hyperpathia of lateral thigh	Known as meralgia paresthetica
Obturator	L3, L4	Thigh adductors	Intrapelvic or at pubis	Weakness of hip adduction	Sensory deficit on medial thigh
Sciatic	L4–S3	Hamstring muscles, hip abductor, and all muscles below the knee	Near sciatic notch	Severe lower leg and hamstring weakness; flail foot; severe disability	Uncommon except from war wounds; sometimes after a misdirected injection
Posterior tibial	L5–S2	Calf muscles (proximally), toe flexors, and other intrinsic foot muscles	Tarsal tunnel, near medial malleolus	Pain and numbness of sole, weak toe flexors	Known as tarsal tunnel syndrome (see text)
Peroneal	L4–S1	Dorsiflexors of toes and foot, evertors of foot	At neck of fibula	Foot drop and weakness of foot eversion	Sensory deficit is similar in distribution to L5, S1 sensory roots

[a] Spinal segments.

Tarsal Tunnel Syndrome The distal tibial nerve, along with several tendons and the posterior tibial artery, lies in the tarsal tunnel just posterior to the medial malleolus. Because of its superficial site, the distal tibial nerve is subject to compression or to direct trauma. Causes include sprain or fracture of the ankle, ill-fitting footwear, posttraumatic fibrosis, cysts or ganglia adjacent to the nerve, arthritis, and tenosynovitis. Characteristic symptoms are pain in the ankle and the sole of the foot with paresthesias, particularly while walking. On examination, the tibial nerve trunk in the tarsal tunnel is usually tender to palpation, sensory deficit should be demonstrable on the sole of the foot, and weakness of the toe plantar-flexor muscles may be noted. EDX examination and also nerve block using local anesthetic are useful in establishing the diagnosis. Definitive treatment is extensive surgical decompression of the tibial nerve in the tarsal tunnel. Tarsal tunnel syndrome, in terms of its pathophysiology and management, is similar to carpal tunnel syndrome but is much less common (Table 363-1).

Cranial Mononeuropathy Mononeuropathy affecting individual cranial nerves is a large subject and is dealt with separately in Chap. 355.

POLYNEUROPATHY The prototypical picture of polyneuropathy occurs with acquired toxic or metabolic neuropathic states. The first symptoms tend to be sensory and consist of tingling, prickling, burning, or bandlike dysesthesias in the balls of the feet or tips of the toes, or in a general distribution over the soles (Chap. 22). Symptoms and findings are usually symmetric and graded distally and often precede objective motor or sensory signs.

With progression, dysesthesias spread up the lower legs. Pansensory loss is usually found over both feet, ankle jerks are lost, and weakness of dorsiflexion of the toes, best demonstrated in the great toe, is present. In some instances, the process begins with weakness in the feet, without preceding sensory symptoms. As worsening occurs, sensory loss moves centripetally in a graded "stocking" fashion, and the patient may complain that the feet have a numb or "wooden" feeling or may say "I feel as though I'm walking on stumps." Patients have difficulty walking on their heels during examination, and their feet may slap while walking. Later, the knee jerk reflex disappears and foot drop becomes more apparent. By the time sensory disturbance has reached the upper shin, dysesthesias are usually noticed in the tips of the fingers. The degree of spontaneous pain varies but is often considerable. Light stimuli to hypesthetic areas, once perceived, may be experienced as extremely uncomfortable (*hyperpathia*). Unsteadiness of gait may be out of proportion to muscle weakness because of proprioceptive loss.

Worsening is more severe in the legs than in the arms and proceeds in a centripetal, symmetrically graded manner with pansensory loss, areflexia, and muscle atrophy; motor weakness is usually greater in the extensor muscles than in corresponding flexor groups. When the sensory disturbance reaches the elbows and mid-thighs, a tent-shaped area of hypesthesia may often be demonstrated on the lower abdomen. This area will grow broader, and its apex will extend rostrally toward the sternum as the neuropathy worsens. By this time, patients generally cannot stand or walk or hold objects in their hands.

Overall, nerve fibers are affected according to axon length, without regard to root or nerve trunk distribution—hence the aptness of the term *stocking-glove* to describe the pattern of sensory deficit. In general, the motor deficit is also graded, distal, and symmetric.

Although *polyneuropathy* connotes a widespread symmetric process, usually distal and graded, polyneuropathies are quite diverse because of the variability of tempo, severity, mix of sensory and motor features, and presence or absence of positive symptoms. For instance, a patient with a subacute, severely dysesthetic sensory polyneuropathy and alopecia who is in the early phases of thallium intoxication bears little similarity to the patient with a 40-year history of insidiously progressive clumsiness of gait whose findings are foot drop, lower leg atrophy, pes cavus, and minimal asymptomatic distal sensory deficit, all due to a hereditary polyneuropathy (Chap. 364). These two patients fall at opposite ends of the spectrum of polyneuropathy.

The classification of peripheral neuropathies has become increasingly complex as the capacity to discriminate new subgroups and identify new associations with toxins and systemic disorders improves. The important features of each major grouping of polyneuropathies are summarized in Table 363-2, and key aspects of specific polyneuropathies are given in Tables 363-3 to Table 363-6.

MONONEUROPATHY MULTIPLEX (MULTIFOCAL NEUROPATHY)

Mononeuropathy multiplex refers to simultaneous or sequential involvement of individual noncontiguous nerve trunks, either partially or completely, evolving over days to years. Since the disease process underlying mononeuropathy multiplex affects peripheral nerves in a multifocal and random fashion, progression of the disease favors the neurologic deficit becoming less patchy and multifocal and more confluent and symmetric. As a result, some patients present with what appears to be a distal symmetric neuropathy. Attention to the pattern of early symptoms is therefore important in making the judgment that a particular neuropathy is indeed a mononeuropathy multiplex and not a polyneuropathy.

ASSESSMENT AND DIAGNOSIS OF POLYNEUROPATHY AND MONONEUROPATHY MULTIPLEX

Clues to the diagnosis of these neuropathies often lie in unnoticed or forgotten events occurring weeks or months prior to the onset of symptoms. Inquiry should be made about recent viral illnesses; other systemic symptoms; institution of new medications; exposures to solvents, pesticides, or heavy metals; the occurrence of similar symptoms in family members or co-workers; habits concerning alcohol; and the presence of preexisting medical disorders. Patients should be asked if they would feel well if free of their neuropathic symptoms; answers will suggest the presence or absence of an underlying systemic illness.

How did symptoms first appear? Even with distal polyneuropathies, symptoms may appear in the sole of one foot a few days or a week before the other, but usually the patient will describe a distal graded disturbance that moves evenly and symmetrically in centripetal fashion. Symptoms that first appear in the distribution of individual digital nerves, involving only half of a digit at a time, and then gradually spread and coalesce suggest a multifocal process (mononeuropathy multiplex), as might occur with a systemic vasculitis or cryoglobulinemia.

The evolution of neuropathy ranges from rapid worsening over a few days to an indolent process lasting decades. Polyneuropathies that progress slowly, over >5 years, are most likely to be genetically determined, particularly if the major manifestations are distal atrophy and weakness with few or no positive sensory symptoms. Diabetic polyneuropathy and paraproteinemic neuropathies also progress insidiously over 5 to 10 years. Axonal degenerations of toxic or metabolic origin tend to evolve over several weeks to a year or more, and the rate of progression of demyelinating neuropathies is highly variable, ranging from a few days in Guillain-Barré syndrome (GBS; Chap. 365) to many years in others.

Major fluctuations in the course of neuropathy raise two possibilities: (1) relapsing forms of neuropathy and (2) repeated toxic exposures. Slow fluctuation in symptoms taking place over weeks or months (reflecting changes in the activity of neuropathy) should not be confused with day-to-day variation or diurnal undulation of symptoms. The latter are common to all neuropathic disorders. An example is carpal tunnel syndrome, in which dysesthesias may be prominent at night but absent during the day.

Palpation of the nerve trunk to detect enlargement is a frequently forgotten part of the neurologic examination. In mononeuropathy or mononeuropathy multiplex, the entire course of the nerve trunk in question should be explored manually for focal thickening, for the presence of neurofibroma, point tenderness, or Tinel's phenomenon (generation of a tingling sensation in the sensory territory of the nerve

---

TABLE 363-2	*Major Types of Polyneuropathy*		
Type of Polyneuropathy	**Evolution**	**Causes**	**Comments**
Axonal			
Acute	Days to weeks	Porphyria	See Table 363-3; also Chap. 337
		Massive intoxications (arsenic; inhalants)	See Table 363-4
		Guillain-Barré syndrome—axonal form	See Chap. 365
Subacute	Weeks to months	Mostly toxic or metabolic polyneuropathies; see Tables 363-3 and 363-4	Treatment involves eliminating the toxins or treating the associated systemic disorder
Chronic	Months to years	<5 years, consider toxic/metabolic causes; >5 years, consider hereditary basis, also diabetic and dysproteinemic causes	See Tables 363-3 and 363-4; also Chap. 364 on hereditary neuropathy
Demyelinating			
Acute	Days to weeks	Almost all are the common form of Guillain-Barré syndrome; see Chap. 365	Rare possibilities include diphtheritic polyneuritis or buckthorn berry intoxication
Subacute	Weeks to months	Mostly relapsing form of CIDP (see Chap. 365)	Rarely, toxins mentioned above plus aurothioglucose and taxol (see Table 363-3)
Chronic	Months to years	Many possibilities including hereditary; inflammatory-autoimmune; dysproteinemias; other metabolic and toxic neuropathies	See Chaps. 364 and 365; also Tables 363-3 and 363-4

Note: CIDP, chronic inflammatory demyelinating polyneuropathy.

TABLE 363-3 Polyneuropathy Associated with Systemic Diseases

Systemic Disease (Occurrence)	Axonal[a]			Demyelinating[a]			Sensory vs. Motor[b]	Autonomic[a]	Comment
	Acute	Subacute	Chronic	Acute	Subacute	Chronic			
Diabetes mellitus (common)	−	±	+	−	±	+	S, SM, rarely M	± to +	See Table 363-5
Uremia (sometimes)	±	+	+	−	−	−	SM	±	Controllable with proper dialysis; curable with successful renal transplant
Porphyria (3 types) (rare)	+	±	−	−	−	−	M or SM	± to +	May be proximal > distal and may have atypical proximal sensory deficits
Hypoglycemia (rare)	±	+	±	−	−	−	M	−	Usually with insulinoma; arms often > legs
Vitamin deficiency, excluding B$_{12}$ (sometimes)	−	+	+	−	−	−	SM	±	Involves thiamine, pyridoxine, folate, pantothenic acid, and probably others
Vitamin B$_{12}$ deficiency (sometimes)	−	±	+	−	−	−	S	−	Neuropathy overshadowed by myelopathy
Critical illness (sepsis) (common)	−	+	±	−	−	−	M > S	−	Sepsis patients severely ill
Chronic liver disease (sometimes)	−	−	−	−	−	+	S or SM	−	Usually mild or subclinical
Primary biliary cirrhosis (rare)	−	+	+	−	−	−	S	−	Intraneural xanthomas; dysesthesias
Primary systemic amyloidosis (rare)	−	±	+	−	−	−	SM	+	Also in amyloidosis with myeloma or macroglobulinemia
Hypothyroidism (rare)	−	−	−	−	±	+	S	−	May respond to thyroid replacement
Chronic obstructive lung disease (rare)	−	±	+	−	−	−	S or SM	−	Severe pulmonary insufficiency
Acromegaly (rare)	−	−	+	−	−	−	S	−	Carpal tunnel syndrome also frequent
Malabsorption (sprue, celiac disease) (sometimes)	−	±	+	−	−	−	S or SM	±	Basis for neuropathy unclear; deficiency?
Carcinoma (sensory) (rare)	−	+	+	−	−	−	Pure S	−	Due to ganglionitis, mostly small cell lung or breast carcinoma; paraneoplastic
Carcinoma (sensorimotor) (sometimes)	−	+	+	−	−	−	SM	±	Sensorimotor axonal neuropathy; mostly with lung cancer
Carcinoma (late) (common)	−	+	+	−	−	−	S > M	±	Mild, probably related to weight loss and wasting
Carcinoma (demyelinating) (sometimes)	−	−	−	+	+	±	SM	−	Acute or relapsing demyelinating neuropathy
HIV infection (sometimes)	−	±	+	−	−	−	S ≫ M	−	Late stages of AIDS; other neuropathies occur; see text
Lyme disease (sometimes)	−	±	+	−	−	−	S > M	−	Variable picture; see text
Lymphoma, including Hodgkin's (sometimes)	−	+	+	+	+	±	See above	±	Same as with carcinomatous types
Polycythemia vera (rare)	−	±	+	−	−	−	S	−	Also CNS manifestations; often shooting pains in limbs
Multiple myeloma, lytic type (sometimes)	−	±	+	−	−	−	S, M, or SM	±	Symptomatic neuropathy uncommon; subclinical neuropathy frequent
Multiple myeloma, osteosclerotic[c] (sometimes)	−	−	±	−	±	+	SM	−	May show severe slowing of nerve conduction velocity
MGUS[d] (sometimes):									
IgA	−	±	+	−	−	−	SM	−	IgM$_{\kappa}$ mainly; may bind to myelin-associated glycoprotein (MAG) or other glycoconjugates
IgG	−	±	+	−	−	−	SM	−	
IgM	−	−	−	−	±	+	SM or S	−	
Cryoglobulinemia (rare)	−	±	+	−	−	−	SM	−	May be mononeuropathy multiplex in presentation

[a] +, Usually; ±, sometimes; −, rare, if ever.
[b] S, sensory; M, motor; SM, sensorimotor.
[c] Some cases associated with POEMS syndrome (polyneuropathy, organomegaly, endocrinopathy, M proteins, and skin changes; see Chap. 330).
[d] Monoclonal gammopathy of undetermined significance.

TABLE 363-4 Polyneuropathy Associated with Drugs and Environmental Toxins

	Axonal[a]			Demyelinating[a]			Sensory vs. Motor[b]	Autonomic[a]	CNS[a]	Comment
	Acute	Subacute	Chronic	Acute	Subacute	Chronic				
DRUGS[c]										
Amiodarone (antiarrhythmic)	−	−	+		−	+	SM	−	−	Dose-dependent neuropathy, reversible by decreasing dose
Aurothioglucose (antirheumatic)	±	±	−	+	+	−	SM	−	−	Idiosyncratic reaction; ? immune-mediated
Cisplatin (antineoplastic)	−	+	+	−	−	−	S	−	−	Severe sensory neuropathy, also ototoxicity; dose-related
Dapsone (dermatologic agent, e.g., for leprosy)	−	±	+	−	−	−	M	−	−	Dose-related pure motor neuropathy
Disulfiram (antialcoholism agent)	±	+	+	−	−	−	SM	−	±	Usually occurs after months of treatment
Hydralazine (antihypertensive)	−	±	+	−	−	−	S > M	−	−	A pyridoxine antagonist
Isoniazid	−	±	+	−	−	−	SM	±	−	A pyridoxine antagonist, neurotoxic in slow acetylators
Metronidazole (antiprotozoal)	−	−	±	−		−	S or SM	−	+	Dose-related central-peripheral distal axonopathy
Misonidazole (radiosensitizer)	−	±	+	−	−	−	S or SM	−	+	Neurotoxicity is the limiting factor
Nitrofurantoin (urinary antiseptic)	−	±	+	−	−	−	SM	−	−	Generally total dose-related; renal failure enhances toxicity
Nucleoside analogues (ddC, ddI, d4T) (antiretroviral agents)	±	+	+	−	−	−	S ≫ M	−	?	Dose-related; painful
Phenytoin (anticonvulsant)	−	−	+	−	−	−	S > M	−	−	After 20–30 years of phenytoin use
Pyridoxine (vitamin)	−	±	+	−	−	−	S	−	−	Occurs with large intake (>300 mg/d)
Statins (HMG CoA reductase inhibitors)	−	±	+	−	−	−	S > M	−	−	Cases reported for most statins
Suramin (antineoplastic)	+	+	−	+	+	−	M > S	−	−	Related to serum levels 350 µg/mL or above
Taxol (antineoplastic)	±	+	±	±	+	±	S > M	−	−	Dose-related
Vincristine (antineoplastic)	−	+	+	−	−	−	S > M	−	−	Sensory symptoms common, hands > feet; motor signs ominous; should stop treatment
TOXINS[c]										
Acrylamide (flocculant; grouting agent)	−	±	+	−	−	−	S > M	±	+	Large-fiber neuropathy; sensory ataxia
Arsenic (herbicide; insecticide)	±	+	+	−	−	−	SM	±	±	Skin changes, Mees' lines in nails; painful; systemic effects
Diphtheria toxin	−	−	−	+	+	−	SM	−	−	Clinically very rare; can be confused with GBS
γ-Diketone hexacarbons (solvents)	−	±	+	−	−	+	SM	+	+	Neurofilamentous swelling of axons; these solvents now in restricted use
Inorganic lead	−	−	+	−	−	−	M > S or M	−	±	Selective motor neuropathy with prominent wrist drop
Organophosphates	−	±	+	−	−	−	SM	−	+	Brain and spinal cord also affected, the latter irreversibly
Thallium (rat poison)	−	+	+	−	−	−	SM	−	+	Also alopecia, Mees' lines in nails; painful

[a] +, Usually; ±, sometimes; −, rare, if ever.
[b] S, sensory; M, motor; SM, sensorimotor.
[c] The following drugs and environmental toxins are also neurotoxic, mainly to the peripheral nervous system:
Drugs: Allopurinol, amitriptyline, chloramphenicol, colchicine, ethambutol, flecainide, indomethacin, lithium, nitrous oxide, perhexiline maleate, podophyllin, sodium cyanate, thalidomide, L-tryptophan.
Environmental toxins: Allyl chloride, buckthorn berry, carbon disulfide, diglycols (either ethylene or propylene), dimethylaminoproprionitrile (DMAPN), ethylene oxide, metallic mercury, methyl bromide, polychlorinated biphenyls, styrene, trichlorethylene, vacor.
Note: CNS, central nervous system; GBS, Guillain-Barré syndrome.

TABLE 363-5   Classification of Diabetic Neuropathies

Symmetric
1. Distal, primarily sensory polyneuropathy
   a. Mainly large fibers affected
   b. Mixed[a]
   c. Mainly small fibers affected[a]
2. Autonomic neuropathy
3. Chronically evolving proximal motor neuropathy[a,b]

Asymmetric
1. Acute or subacute proximal motor neuropathy[a,b]
2. Cranial mononeuropathy[b]
3. Truncal neuropathy[a,b]
4. Entrapment neuropathy in the limbs

[a] Often painful.
[b] Recovery, partial or complete, is likely.

by tapping along the course of the nerve trunk); and for pain elicited by stretching of the nerve trunk. In leprous neuritis, fusiform thickening of nerve trunks is frequent, and beading of nerve trunks may be encountered in amyloid polyneuropathy. In genetically determined hypertrophic neuropathies, uniform thickening of all nerve trunks may occur, often to the diameter of one's little finger.

Most neuropathies involve nerve fibers of all sizes, but damage is sometimes restricted either to large or to small fibers. In a polyneuropathy affecting mainly small fibers, diminished pinprick and temperature sensation, often with painful, burning dysesthesias, will predominate, along with autonomic dysfunction, but with relative sparing of motor power, balance, and tendon jerks. Some cases of amyloid and distal diabetic polyneuropathies fall into this category. In contrast, large-fiber polyneuropathy is characterized by areflexia, sensory ataxia, relatively minor cutaneous sensory deficit (even though distal dysesthesias are common), and variable degrees of motor dysfunction, sometimes severe.

For patients with polyneuropathy or mononeuropathy multiplex, standard tests should include a complete blood count and measurement of erythrocyte sedimentation rate, urinalysis, chest x-ray or chest computed tomography (CT) scan, postprandial blood glucose determination, and serum protein electrophoresis. Further tests are dictated by the combined results of the history and the physical and EDX examination (Fig. 363-1).

Electrodiagnosis   EDX studies are an essential part of the evaluation of neuropathies and also of myopathies and neuromuscular junction disorders. Such studies indeed are critical in helping to distinguish between these three categories of disease. The EDX examination ordinarily comprises electromyography (EMG) and nerve conduction studies (NCSs). EMG involves recording for electrical potentials from a needle electrode in muscle both at rest and during voluntary contraction of the muscle. Resulting electromyographic patterns are displayed on an oscilloscope screen for analysis. EMG is generally most useful for distinguishing between and among myopathic and neuropathic disorders. Myopathic disorders are marked by small, short-duration, polyphasic muscle action potentials recruited in excessive numbers for a given degree of voluntary muscle contraction. Other patterns characteristic of specific muscle abnormalities can also be observed, such as myotonia (high-frequency discharges that wax or wane).

By contrast, EMG findings in neuropathic disorders are those of muscle denervation. Specifically, denervation features a decrease in the number of motor units[1] activated by maximal effort to contract muscle but an increase in the rate of firing of those remaining motor

units. In long-standing muscle denervation (months or years), motor unit potentials become large and polyphasic. This occurs as a result of collateral reinnervation of nearby denervated muscle fibers by axonal sprouts from surviving motor axons. In brief, when motor axons die back, their muscle fiber domains are taken over by intact neighboring axons. Other EMG features that favor denervation include fibrillations (random, unregulated firing of individual denervated muscle fibers), fasciculations (random, spontaneous firing of motor units, which in chronic states can be markedly enlarged and polyphasic), positive sharp waves, and complex repetitive discharges (Fig. 363-2).

NCSs are carried out by stimulating motor or sensory nerves electrically at two or more sites and recording from either the muscle innervated, for motor nerves (Fig. 363-3), or from yet another site on the stimulated nerve trunk, for sensory nerves. From the data recorded, the velocity of conduction and other informative characteristics of the recorded waveforms can be determined. When a disorder of the neuromuscular junction is suspected, other more specialized techniques are used, including muscle response to repetitive stimulation of nerve and single-fiber EMG. Detailed discussion of the full range of EDX techniques and their application, use, and interpretation may be found in several recent monographs listed in the references.

It is generally not possible to distinguish between axonal and demyelinating disorders by clinical examination alone; here EDX analysis is particularly useful. EDX features of demyelination are slowing of nerve conduction velocity (NCV), dispersion of evoked compound action potentials, conduction block (major decrease in amplitude of muscle compound action potentials on proximal stimulation of the nerve, as compared to distal stimulation), and marked prolongation of distal latencies. In contrast, axonal neuropathies are characterized by a reduction in amplitude of evoked compound action potentials with relative preservation of NCV. The distinction between a primarily demyelinating neuropathy and an axonal neuropathy is crucial because of the differing approaches to diagnosis and management.

EDX studies also help to determine the presence or absence of a sensory involvement when that is not clear by clinical examination alone. It provides information about the distribution of subclinical findings, thus sharpening the diagnostic focus. Other issues that may be clarified by the electrodiagnostician include:

1. The distinction between disorders primary to nerve or to muscle (neuropathy versus myopathy)
2. The distinction between root or plexus involvement and more distal nerve trunk involvement
3. The distinction between generalized polyneuropathic processes and widespread multifocal nerve trunk involvement
4. The distinction between upper and lower motor neuron weakness
5. The distinction, in a given generalized polyneuropathic process, between primary demyelinating neuropathy and primary axonal degeneration
6. The assessment, in both primary axonal and demyelinating neuropathies, of features bearing on the nature, activity, and likely prognosis of the neuropathy, particularly the extent of primary or secondary axonal degeneration
7. The assessment, in mononeuropathies, of the site of the lesion and its major effect on nerve fibers, especially the distinction between demyelinating conduction block and wallerian degeneration
8. The characterization of disorders of the neuromuscular junction
9. The identification, often in muscle of normal bulk and strength, of important features such as chronic partial denervation, fasciculations, and myotonia
10. The analysis of cramp, and its distinction from physiologic contracture

If in a particular instance of progressive polyneuropathy of subacute or chronic evolution the EDX findings are those of an axonopathy, a long list of metabolic states and exogenous toxins comes under consideration (Tables 363-3 and 363-4). If the course is protracted over several years, it raises the likelihood of a hereditary neu-

---

[1] A motor unit is, by definition, an anterior horn cell, its axon, and the motor end plates and muscle fibers it innervates. The number of muscle fibers in a normal motor unit varies widely, from as few as 20 in an extraocular muscle to over 1500 in a large leg muscle (Chap. 21, Fig. 21-2).

TABLE 363-6 *Sensory Neuropathies*

Cause or Association	Course	Nerve Fiber Size Affected Small	Large	Neuronopathy	Comment
TOXINS/DRUGS					
Cisplatin (antineoplastic)	Sub/Chr	+	++	+	Dose-related
Pyridoxine (vitamin, in megadose amounts)	Sub/Chr	+	++	+/−	Dose-related
Taxol (antineoplastic)	Acu/Sub	++	+	−	NGF may be protective
SYSTEMIC DISEASES					
Paraneoplastic	Sub	+	++	++	Most SCLC and breast
Sjögren's syndrome	Sub/Chr	+/−	+	++	Variable presentation
Dysproteinemia (mainly IgM$_\kappa$)	Chr	+	++	−	Demyelinating; may bind to MAG and other myelin glycoproteins
IDIOPATHIC					
Acute sensory neuronopathy	Acu	+/−	++	++	Poor recovery; persistent deficit
Chronic ataxic neuropathy	Chr	+/−	++	Prob.	Gradual progression
HEREDITARY					
Many varieties (see Chap. 364)	Chr	Variable		Some	Progressive

Abbreviations: ++, most; +, some; ±, occasionally; Prob, probable; Acu, acute; Sub, subacute; Chr, chronic; NGF, nerve growth factor; MAG, myelin-associated glycoprotein; SCLC, small-cell lung carcinoma.

ropathy (Chap. 364); family members must be examined and additional attention given to the family history. If the EDX findings indicate primary demyelination of nerve, the approach is entirely different. The possibilities then include acquired demyelinating neuropathy, thought to be immunologically mediated (Chap. 365), and genetically determined demyelinating neuropathies, many of which are marked by uniform and drastic slowing of nerve conduction velocities (Chap. 364).

If the clinical features indicate mononeuropathy multiplex, the EDX question is whether the process is primarily axonal or demyelinating. Almost one-third of all adults with the clinical syndrome of mononeuropathy multiplex have a clear-cut picture of a demyelinating disorder, often with foci of persistent conduction block on EDX examination. Multifocal demyelinating neuropathy may represent part of the spectrum of chronic inflammatory demyelinating polyneuropathy (CIDP) or, if multifocal and only motor, would fit into the related category of multifocal motor neuropathy. →*For further discussion of the management of multifocal motor neuropathy, see Chap. 365.*

The remaining two-thirds of patients with mononeuropathy multiplex have a picture of patchy axonal involvement by EDX examination. Although ischemia should be suspected as the basis of neuropathy in these patients, only about one-half can be shown to have

disease of the vasa nervorum, usually vasculitis. Management of those with proven vasculitis of vasa nervorum is often the same as treatment for systemic vasculitis (Chaps. 306 and 365). If the cause of mononeuropathy multiplex remains undiagnosed even on follow-up, management should be conservative. In many patients the disease will stabilize or reverse, at least partially.

Mononeuropathy multiplex syndrome may also be seen as a manifestation of leprosy, sarcoidosis, certain types of amyloidosis, hypereosinophilia syndrome, cryoglobulinemia, neuroAIDS, and multifocal types of diabetic neuropathy.

Nerve Biopsy The sural nerve at the ankle is the preferred site for cutaneous nerve biopsy. There are few indications to employ this invasive technique. The main one is in asymmetric and multifocal neu-

FIGURE 363-2 Activity recorded during EMG. *A.* Spontaneous fibrillation potentials and positive sharp waves. *B.* Complex repetitive discharges recorded in partially denervated muscle at rest. *C.* Normal triphasic motor unit action potential. *D.* Small, short-duration, polyphasic motor unit action potential such as is commonly encountered in myopathic disorders. *E.* Long-duration polyphasic motor unit action potential such as may be seen in neuropathic disorders. *(Courtesy of Prof M.J. Aminoff.)*

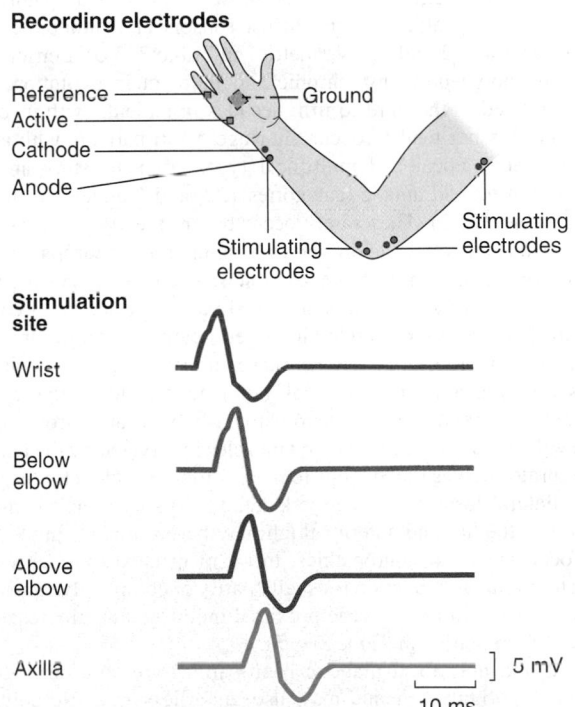

FIGURE 363-3 Arrangement for motor conduction studies of the ulnar nerve. Responses are recorded with a surface electrode from the abductor digiti minimi muscle to supramaximal stimulation of the nerve at different sites and are shown in the lower panel. *(From MJ Aminoff: Electromyography in Clinical Practice: Electrodiagnostic Aspects of Neuromuscular Disease, 3d ed. New York, Churchill Livingstone, 1998.)*

ropathic disorders producing a clinical picture of mononeuropathy multiplex, the basis of which is still unclear after other laboratory investigations are complete. Diagnostic considerations include vasculitis, multifocal demyelinating neuropathies, amyloidosis, leprosy, and occasionally sarcoidosis. Nerve biopsy is also helpful when one or more cutaneous nerves are palpably enlarged. Another clinical application is in establishing the diagnosis in some genetically determined childhood disorders such as metachromatic leukodystrophy, Krabbe's disease, giant axonal neuropathy, and infantile neuroaxonal dystrophy. In all of these recessively inherited diseases, both the central nervous system and the peripheral nervous system are affected.

There is a tendency to carry out sural nerve biopsy in distal symmetric polyneuropathies of subacute or chronic evolution. This practice is discouraged because its yield is low and not worth the risk of wound infection, poor healing, or persistent pain. Nerve biopsy in this situation may be useful as part of an approved research protocol when the biopsy will provide crucial information not otherwise obtainable.

SPECIAL CATEGORIES OF NEUROPATHY   Some neuropathies require individual description because of their importance or distinctiveness.

Diabetic Neuropathies   The neuropathies of diabetes mellitus are classified in Table 363-5. A limitation of this classification is that most patients do not fit neatly into any single category but instead have overlapping clinical features of several. For instance, many diabetic patients with distal, primarily sensory polyneuropathy can also be shown to have autonomic dysfunction, usually in the form of vasomotor disturbance in the limbs and abnormalities of sweating. Similarly, patients who develop a proximal motor syndrome often have dysautonomic features (including sexual impotence in males) and some degree of distal sensory polyneuropathy. To compound matters, such patients appear at risk of developing a cranial mononeuropathy. Pain is a frequent feature of diabetic neuropathies (Table 363-5) but is variable in incidence and degree.

Neuropathies occur in the setting of long-standing hyperglycemia, the principal manifestation of the group of metabolic disorders comprising diabetes mellitus. By far the most common neuropathies related to diabetes mellitus are the diffuse sensory and autonomic types (categories 1 and 2 under "Symmetric" in Table 363-5). Sensory and autonomic polyneuropathy, chronic and indolent in evolution, may first be noticed in the third to fifth decades in patients with juvenile-onset diabetes but tend to occur after age 50 in patients with adult-onset diabetes. Focal and multifocal types of neuropathy are less common but quite dramatic (categories 1, 2, and 3 under "Asymmetric" in Table 363-5). They rarely occur before the age of 45 and are usually subacute or acute in onset. Cranial mononeuropathies are mainly isolated sixth or third nerve palsies. The latter spares the pupil in three-fourths of cases, and some local pain or headache occurs in one-half. Truncal (thoracoabdominal) neuropathy is painful, involves one or more intercostal or lumbar nerves unilaterally, and frequently coexists with asymmetric proximal motor neuropathy in the legs. In asymmetric proximal motor neuropathy (diabetic amyotrophy), the most evident features are weakened muscles innervated by the femoral and obturator nerves (quadriceps femoris, iliopsoas, adductor magnus) and ipsilateral loss of the knee jerk reflex. Sensory deficit is minor, but pain in the hip and anterior thigh may be prominent. In all these multifocal and focal neuropathies, the pain usually subsides within weeks to a year, and function is usually partly or completely recovered. The same is true for symmetric proximal motor neuropathy (category 3 under "Symmetric" in Table 363-5).

Focal and multifocal diabetic neuropathies are considered to be ischemic in origin; ischemia may also underlie symmetric polyneuropathies, which are also thought to involve an abnormality of nerve metabolism.

Management of diabetic neuropathies is directed toward optimal glycemic control and symptomatic pain suppression. In the long-term Diabetes Control and Complications Trial, patients who controlled their diabetes meticulously showed significantly less neuropathy. The role of aldose reductase inhibitors in preventing or reversing diabetic complications, including neuropathy, remains unclear. Entrapment neuropathies are frequently amenable to surgical decompression.

Neuropathies with HIV Infection   Neuropathies are common in infection with HIV, but different types of neuropathy are seen according to the stage of the disease. GBS or CIDP (Chap. 365) are the neuropathies likely to occur following conversion to seropositivity and during the asymptomatic phase of HIV infection. Treatment is the same as for HIV-negative patients. In later, symptomatic stages, mononeuritis multiplex, axonal in nature, can occur; the course is typically subacute or chronic. In some cases, vasculitis of the vasa nervorum has been demonstrated.

A common neuropathy is a distal, symmetric, mainly sensory polyneuropathy, which evolves slowly in the late symptomatic stages of HIV infection and frequently coexists with symptomatic encephalopathy and myelopathy (Table 363-3; Chap. 173). The incidence of late-stage neurologic disorders, including sensory polyneuropathy, appears to be diminishing for HIV-positive individuals on effective highly active antiretroviral therapy (HAART) programs. Sensory polyneuropathy of late-stage HIV infection must be distinguished from toxic polyneuropathy that may result from the use of nucleoside analogue treatment (Table 363-4). At times, nucleoside analogues may precipitate a rapidly evolving, severe polyneuropathy with concurrent lactic acidemia. Clinically the neuropathy can be mistaken for GBS. Also in the late stages, a severe, destructive, subacute, asymmetric polyradiculopathy involving the cauda equina may be seen; it is caused by infection of the nerve roots with cytomegalovirus. Ganciclovir, started early, can arrest the disorder.

Neuropathies with Lyme Disease   A focal or multifocal radiculoneuropathy may occur weeks, months, or even years after primary infection by the tick-borne spirochete *Borrelia burgdorferi*. Although usually sensory and either dysesthetic or painful, the neuropathy is variable in distribution, affecting cranial nerves and spinal roots or nerves in a patchy, asymmetric fashion. Neuropathy is often chronic and persistent; cerebrospinal fluid pleocytosis is the rule. In many, improvement occurs spontaneously, but the course is shortened by treatment with antibiotics, usually intravenous ceftriaxone (Chap. 157).

Herpes Zoster   This is a sensory neuritis due to infection with varicella-zoster virus (VZV) and is characterized by acute inflammation of one or more dorsal root ganglia. Lancinating pain and hyperalgesia over the skin surface supplied by the affected roots occur for 3 to 4 days, followed by the appearance in the same segment of a herpetic eruption characterized by painful raised blisters on reddened bases. Pain usually subsides in a few weeks. If the inflammatory process spreads to involve related motor roots, segmental motor weakness and wasting appear. Paralysis of the oculomotor nerves may occur in conjunction with involvement of the ophthalmic division of the trigeminal ganglion (ophthalmoplegic zoster). Facial paralysis may occur with involvement of the geniculate ganglion and herpetic eruption on the ipsilateral tympanic membrane or external ear canal (Ramsay Hunt syndrome).

In a small proportion of patients, neuropathic pain persists in the dermatomal distribution of the affected ganglia. This pain, known as *postherpetic neuralgia*, is intense, burning, hyperpathic, and unrelenting; it often dominates the lives of those affected. Advancing age is a risk factor for this outcome. In some patients, blunting of the pain to tolerable levels is achieved by use of anticonvulsants such as carbamazepine or gabapentin or a tricyclic antidepressant such as desipramine or norpramin. Recent investigations suggest that postherpetic neuralgia reflects active persistent VZV infection of the ganglion, and that it may respond to intravenous antiviral treatment (Chap. 164).

Leprous Neuritis   This is a major worldwide cause of neuropathy. *Mycobacterium leprae* organisms readily invade Schwann cells in cutaneous nerve twigs, particularly those associated with unmyelinated nerve fibers. *M. leprae* thrives best in the coolest tissues in the body.

Two major forms of leprous neuritis are recognized, tuberculoid and lepromatous, which actually represent the ends of a spectrum of disease, the middle of which is called borderline (dimorphous) leprosy (patchy and multifocal involvement of skin and nerve). The treatment of a given case depends on where it falls in this spectrum (Chap. 151). Tuberculoid (high-resistance) leprosy consists of a single patch of hypesthetic or anesthetic skin in any location. The skin patch is frequently thickened, reddened, or hypopigmented. Few or no *M. leprae* bacilli may be demonstrated. If a superficially placed nerve trunk, typically a cutaneous nerve, courses just beneath the area of affected skin, it may be engulfed in the inflammatory reaction, resulting in an associated mononeuropathy. Such a nerve may be palpably enlarged and beaded. Lepromatous (low-resistance) leprosy is marked by immunologic tolerance; numerous bacilli; and widespread skin thickening, cutaneous anesthesia, and anhidrosis, which spare only the warmest parts of the body, notably the axilla, the groin, and beneath the scalp hair. Motor signs (focal weakness and atrophy) result from damage to mixed nerves lying close to the skin, particularly the median, ulnar, peroneal, and facial nerves.

SPECIAL NEUROPATHIC PRESENTATIONS Some disorders selectively affect the peripheral nervous system, limiting dysfunction to specific systems or sites, such as motor nerves, brachial plexus, or the autonomic nervous system.

Autonomic Neuropathy The autonomic nervous system regulates the visceral organs and vegetative functions (Chap. 354). Many pharmacologic agents modify specific autonomic functions, but autonomic neuropathy (dysautonomia) with structural changes in pre- and post-ganglionic neurons can also occur. Usually autonomic neuropathy is a manifestation of a more generalized polyneuropathy, as in diabetic neuropathy, GBS, and alcoholic polyneuropathy, but occasionally syndromes of pure pandysautonomia are encountered. Symptoms of dysautonomia are mainly negative (i.e., loss of function) and include postural hypotension with faintness or syncope, anhidrosis, hypothermia, bladder atony, obstipation, dry mouth and dry eyes from failure of salivary and lacrimal glands to secrete, blurring of vision from lack of pupillary and ciliary regulation, and sexual impotence in males. Positive phenomena (hyperfunction) may also occur and include episodic hypertension, diarrhea, hyperhidrosis, and either tachycardia or bradycardia. Management is symptomatic and also directed at the underlying cause, if it can be identified.

Pure Motor Neuropathy Disorders affecting any level of the motor unit—anterior horn cell, motor axon, or neuromuscular junction—can result in a purely lower motor syndrome without sensory disturbance. Distinguishing anterior horn cell disorders (motor neuronopathies) from motor axonopathies may be difficult clinically because they share manifestations (weakness, muscle denervation atrophy, hypo- or areflexia, fasciculations). EDX examination may also fail to localize the primary site of the lesion (neuropathic versus neuronopathic) unless the lesion is demyelinating in nature, in which case it is by definition neuropathic.

Examples of motor neuronopathies include the lower-motor form of amyotrophic lateral sclerosis, poliomyelitis, hereditary spinal muscular atrophies, and adult variant of hexosaminidase A deficiency (Chap. 353). Motor neuropathies may be seen with lead or dapsone intoxication, occasionally with porphyria, and also with multifocal motor neuropathy. The latter is a chronic asymmetric disorder of mid-life associated with persistent conduction block on EDX examination, and often high titers of antiganglioside antibodies (particularly anti-GM$_1$) (Chap. 365). Neuromuscular junction disorders (e.g., Lambert-Eaton myasthenic syndrome, tick bite paralysis, other types of toxic neuromuscular blockade) are purely motor and can be recognized and localized electrodiagnostically (Chap. 366). Some motor-sensory polyneuropathies have predominant motor symptoms and signs, such as hereditary motor-sensory neuropathies, GBS, and CIDP, but the subclinical sensory component is readily demonstrated electrodiagnostically or by quantitative sensory testing.

Pure Sensory Neuropathy Clinical presentations involving primary sensation only (Table 363-6; Chap. 22) are common. Manifestations may (1) reflect mainly large afferent fiber involvement with deficits of vibratory and proprioceptive sense, areflexia, and sensory ataxia with or without tingling dysesthesias; (2) reflect mainly small afferent fiber involvement with numbness and cutaneous hypesthesia to pin-prick and temperature stimuli, often with painful, burning dysesthesias; or (3) be pansensory, with both large- and small-fiber manifestations. The pattern of distribution, although variable, is often distal and symmetric, particularly for large-fiber neuropathies.

The most severe and widespread of these pure sensory syndromes exhibit poor or no recovery, suggesting irreversible lesions of nerve cell bodies in dorsal root and trigeminal ganglia. These are referred to as *sensory neuronopathies*. With sensory neurotoxins, moderate doses lead to potentially reversible neuropathy, but high doses appear to cause irreversible neuronopathy.

Plexopathy This term refers to disorders of either the brachial or the lumbosacral plexus. Lesions of the brachial plexus are characterized by motor and sensory signs different from those expected in either mononeuropathies of the upper limb or polyneuropathies. The usual causes are direct trauma to the plexus, idiopathic brachial neuritis (also called *neuralgic amyotrophy*; Chap. 15), cervical rib or band, infiltration by malignant tumor, or prior radiation therapy. When the upper parts of the brachial plexus, arising from cervical roots 5 through 7, are affected, weakness and atrophy of shoulder girdle and upper arm muscles occur. Injuries to the lower brachial plexus, arising from the eighth cervical and first thoracic roots, produce distal arm weakness, atrophy, and focal sensory deficit in the forearm and hand. In general, idiopathic brachial neuritis, irradiation with >60 Gy (6000 rad), and particular types of trauma (arm jerked downward) result in damage to the upper portions of the brachial plexus. In contrast, infiltration by malignant tumor, cervical rib or band, and certain other types of trauma (arm jerked upward) cause damage to the lower brachial plexus. Lumbosacral plexopathies are less common; they may be due to trauma, including intraoperative damage, retroperitoneal hemorrhage, idiopathic plexitis, or malignant tumor infiltration or may occur in association with long-standing diabetes mellitus.

Cold Effects Cold exerts direct deleterious effects on peripheral nerve, independent of ischemia. Cold injury to nerve occurs after prolonged exposure, usually of a limb, to moderately low temperatures, as with immersion of the feet in seawater; actual freezing of tissue is not required. Axonal degeneration of myelinated fibers is the pathologic expression of cold injury. Frequently, limbs affected by cold injury to nerve show sensory deficit and dysesthesias, cutaneous vasomotor instability, pain, and marked sensitivity to minimal cold exposure, which may persist for years. The pathophysiology of these phenomena is uncertain.

Trophic Changes The array of observable changes in completely denervated muscle, bone, and skin, including hair and nails, is well known, if incompletely understood. It is unclear what portion of the changes is due purely to denervation versus what is due to disuse, immobility, lack of weight bearing, and particularly recurrent, unnoticed, painless trauma. Considerable evidence favors the view that ulceration of skin, poor healing, tissue resorption, neurogenic arthropathy, and mutilation are the result of repeated unheeded injury to insensitive parts. This sequence of events is avoidable with proper attention to and care of the insensitive parts by both patient and physician.

RECOVERY FROM NEUROPATHY In contrast to axons in the central nervous system, peripheral nerve fibers have an excellent ability to regenerate under proper circumstances. The process of regeneration following axonal degeneration may take from 2 months to more than a year, depending on the severity of the neuropathy and the length of regeneration required. Regeneration can take place when the cause of the neuropathy has been eliminated, such as removal from contact with a neurotoxic substance or correction of an abnormal metabolic state. A deficit secondary to demyelination may recover rapidly, since intact axons may remyelinate in just a few weeks. For example, a patient with GBS, in whom demyelination but no secondary axonal degeneration has occurred, may recover to normal strength from bedfastness and paralysis of arms and legs in as little as 3 to 4 weeks.

PERIPHERAL NERVE TUMORS These tumors are mostly benign and can arise on any nerve trunk or twig. Although peripheral nerve tumors can occur anywhere in the body, including the spinal roots and cauda equina, many are subcutaneous in location and present as a soft swelling, sometimes with a purplish discoloration of the skin. Two major categories of peripheral nerve tumors are recognized: neurilemmoma (schwannoma) and neurofibroma. Neurilemmomas are usually solitary and grow in the nerve sheath, rendering the tumor relatively easy to dissect free. In contrast, neurofibromas tend to be multiple, grow in the endoneurial substance, which renders them difficult to dissect, may undergo malignant changes, and are the hallmark of von Recklinghausen's neurofibromatosis (NF1) (Chap. 358).

FURTHER READING

ASBURY AK, THOMAS PK: *Peripheral Nerve Disorders*, 2d ed. Oxford, Butterworth-Heinemann, 1995

BROWN WF et al (eds): *Neuromuscular Function and Disease: Basic, Clinical and Electrodiagnostic Aspects*. Philadelphia, Saunders, 2002

DYCK PJ, THOMAS PK (eds): *Diabetic Neuropathy*, 2d ed, Philadelphia, Saunders, 1999

———, ——— (eds): *Peripheral Neuropathy*, 4d ed. Philadelphia, Saunders, 2004

KATIRJI B et al (eds): *Neuromuscular Disorders in Clinical Practice*. Boston, Butterworth-Heinemann, 2002

LLEWELYN JG: The diabetic neuropathies: Types, diagnosis and management. J Neurol, Neurosurg Psychiatry 74(Suppl 2):15, 2003

MENDELL JR, SAHENK Z: Painful sensory neuropathy. N Engl J Med 348: 1243, 2003

SHAPIRO BE, PRESTON DC: Entrapment and compressive neuropathies. Med Clin North Am 87:663, 2003

STEWART JD: *Focal Peripheral Neuropathies*, 3d ed. Philadelphia, Lippincott Williams & Wilkins, 1999

WILLISON HJ, WINER JB: Clinical evaluation and investigation of neuropathy. J Neurol, Neurosurg Psychiatry 74(Suppl 2):3, 8, 2003

364 CHARCOT-MARIE-TOOTH DISEASE AND OTHER INHERITED NEUROPATHIES
Phillip F. Chance, Thomas D. Bird

CHARCOT-MARIE-TOOTH DISEASE

GENERAL CLINICAL FEATURES Charcot-Marie-Tooth (CMT) neuropathy comprises a heterogeneous group of inherited peripheral nerve diseases (Table 364-1). Transmission is most frequently autosomal dominant but may also be autosomal recessive or X-linked. An estimated 1 in 2500 persons has a form of CMT, making it one of the most frequently encountered inherited neurologic syndromes.

The neuropathy of CMT affects both motor and sensory nerves. Typical features consist of distal muscle weakness and atrophy, impaired sensation, and absent or hypoactive deep tendon reflexes. Common signs and symptoms are related to muscle weakness, initially involving the feet and legs and later progressing to the hands and forearms. A history of an abnormal high-stepped (steppage) gait with frequent tripping and falling is frequently elicited. Complaints related to foot deformity (pes cavus, or high-arched feet) result from atrophy of intrinsic muscles of the feet. Despite the involvement of sensory nerves in CMT, complaints of limb pain or sensory disturbances are unusual.

Onset is most often during the first or second decade of life, although presentation in mid-adult life is not unusual. The variation in clinical presentation is exceptionally wide, ranging from individuals whose only clinical finding is pes cavus and minimal or no distal muscle weakness to those with severe distal atrophy and marked hand and foot deformity. However, it is unusual for patients with CMT to lose ambulation. There are no therapies that can prevent the onset or delay progression of disability associated with CMT. Patients frequently benefit from physical therapy, use of ankle-foot orthoses (AFOs) to alleviate foot drop, and, in some cases, surgical procedures to the foot. Surgery should be undertaken only when pain or difficulty walking due to severe foot deformity cannot be managed by more conservative means.

CLASSIFICATION BY PHENOTYPE A widely accepted classification system distinguishes demyelinating forms of CMT (also designated as CMT type 1, or CMT1) from those due to axonal degeneration (CMT type 2, or CMT2). Individuals with CMT1 have electrophysiologic findings of reduced motor and sensory nerve conduction velocities (NCVs; typically <38 to 40 m/s) and pathologic findings of hypertrophic demyelinating neuropathy ("onion bulbs"). By contrast, in CMT2 there is relative preservation of the myelin sheath and these individuals have normal or near-normal NCVs. CMT3 refers to Déjerine-Sottas disease

TABLE 364-1 *Forms of Charcot-Marie-Tooth Disease (Hereditary Motor and Sensory Neuropathy) and Related Disorders*

	Locus	Gene	Mechanism
CHARCOT-MARIE-TOOTH TYPE 1			
(HMSNI)			
CMT1A	17p11.2-p12	*PMP22*	AD
CMT1B	1q22-q23	P_0	AD
CMT1C	16p12-p13	*SIMPLE*	AD
CMT1D	10q21-q22	*EGR2*	AD/AR
CMTX	Xq13.1	*CX32*	X-linked
CMT4A	8q13-q21	*GDAP1*	AR
CMT4B1	11q22	*MTMR2*	AR
CMT4B2	11p15	*SBF2*	AR
CMT4D (HMSN-Lom)	8q24	*NDRG1*	AR
CMT4F	19q13	*PRX*	AR
CHARCOT-MARIE-TOOTH TYPE 2			
(HMSNII)			
CMT2A	1p35-p36	*KIF1B*	AD
CMT2B	3q13-q22	*RAB7*	AD
CMT2C	12q23-q24	*Unknown*	AD
CMT2D	7p14	*GARS*	AD
CMT2E	8p21	*NEF-L*	AD
CMT2B1	11q21	*LMNA*	AR
DÉJERINE-SOTTAS			
(HMSNIII)			
DSS	17p11.2-p12	*PMP22*	AD
	1q22-p23	P_0	AD
	10q21-q22	*EGR2*	AD/AR
	19q13	*PRX*	AD
CONGENITAL HYPOMYELINATION			
CHN	1q22-23	P_0	AD
	10q21-q22	*EGR2*	AR/AD
HEREDITARY NEUROPATHY WITH PRESSURE PALSIES			
HNPP	17p11.2-p12	*PMP22*	AD

Abbreviations: *PMP22*, peripheral myelin protein 22; P_0, myelin protein zero; *SIMPLE*, small integral membrane protein of late endosome; *Cx32*, connexin32; *EGR2* (Krox-20) early growth response 2 gene; *GDAP1*, ganglioside-induced differentiation-associated protein-1; *MTMR2*, myotubularin-related protein-2; *SBF2*, SET binding factor 2; *NDRG1*, N-myc downstream regulated gene1; *PRX*, periaxin; *KIF1B*, kinesin family member 1B; *RAB7*, Ras-associated protein 7; *GARS*, Glycyl-tRNA synthetase; *NEFL*, neurofilament, light polypeptide; *LMNA*, lamin A.

(DSD; see below), CMT4 to autosomal recessive forms of CMT, and CMTX to X-linked varieties.

An alternative classification system designates these disorders as hereditary motor and sensory neuropathies (HMSN); HMSNI refers to CMT1, HMSNII to CMT2, HMSNIII to DSD, and HMSNIV to Refsum disease (see below).

APPROACH TO THE PATIENT

A clinical diagnosis of an inherited peripheral neuropathy consistent with a form of CMT (CMT1 or CMT2) should be established prior to undertaking specific genetic tests. Other causes of peripheral neuropathy (e.g., diabetes mellitus, alcoholism, heavy metal poisoning, immune neuropathies) should also be considered and, if necessary, ruled out. An environmental exposure may affect multiple family members, thereby potentially mimicking a hereditary illness. CMT is usually a chronic, slowly progressive condition. One should be suspicious of cases that seem to have a rapid course of deterioration. As noted above, the neurologic findings show great variability in patients with CMT; mild pes cavus and depressed deep tendon reflexes may be the only signs of disease.

Although symptoms related to sensory disturbances are uncommon in CMT, a careful sensory examination is nonetheless essential. In patients who have no objective signs of sensory impairment and no evidence of sensory nerve dysfunction on electrophysiologic studies, alternative diagnoses including primary motor system disorders (e.g., distal spinal muscle atrophy, juvenile amyotrophic lateral sclerosis) should be considered.

The pedigree is of paramount importance in the diagnosis of CMT. Examination of multiple family members, particularly parents, for subtle signs of neuropathy may help to establish a diagnosis. If possible, it is also important to obtain NCVs and an electromyogram (EMG) from all at-risk family members.

GENETIC CONSIDERATIONS   CMT Neuropathy Type 1A (CMT1A)   Approximately three-quarters of pedigrees with autosomal dominant CMT1 demonstrate linkage to chromosome 17p11.2-12 (CMT1A) and are associated with a tandem 1.5-megabase (Mb) DNA duplication. The duplication is usually inherited as a stable Mendelian trait; however, it may also arise as a de novo event. The de novo duplication is responsible for many sporadic cases of CMT1 and may also account for some cases previously thought to occur on the basis of an autosomal recessive mode of inheritance. When present as a de novo event, the duplication results more commonly from an error in spermatogenesis; however, ~10% of de novo cases have been found to result from an error in oogenesis.

The critical gene for CMT1A is peripheral myelin protein-22 (*PMP22*), which is expressed in Schwann cells. The *PMP22* gene encodes a 160-amino-acid protein localized to the compact portion of peripheral nerve myelin; it contains four putative transmembrane domains and is highly conserved in evolution. The level of expression of *PMP22* is crucial for proper myelination of peripheral nerves. The neuropathy in patients with the duplication results from the presence of three copies of *PMP22* leading to increased expression at this locus. In rare cases, patients homozygous for the CMT1A duplication have been identified, and in some cases these individuals exhibit a more severe phenotype than their heterozygous siblings or parents. As discussed below, monosomic underexpression of *PMP22* results in hereditary neuropathy with liability to pressure palsies (HNPP).

Rare CMT1 pedigrees that are linked to chromosome 17p11.2-p12, yet lack the duplication, may harbor missense mutations within the *PMP22* gene.

DNA testing for CMT1A (including the duplication and sequencing to detect point mutations in *PMP22*) is available and now an accepted part of the evaluation of patients with suspected hereditary neuropathies (see below).

CMT Neuropathy Type 1B (CMT1B)   CMT1B is less common than CMT1A; it results from mutations in the human myelin protein zero gene (*MPZ*,

or *P₀*), which maps to chromosome 1q22-q23. P_0 is the major structural protein component of peripheral nervous system myelin (quantitatively 50% by weight) and represents ~10% of total Schwann cell mRNA. P_0 is a member of the immunoglobulin gene superfamily of cell adhesive molecules and localizes to the compact portion of peripheral nerve myelin. P_0 protein consists of 248 amino acids and contains an intracellular and a glycosylated extracellular domain with a single transmembrane segment. Many different point mutations in the P_0 gene have been found in patients with CMT1B, and these mutations predominately map to the extracellular domain of its gene product.

At the clinical level it is not possible to differentiate patients with CMT1A from those with CMT1B. Molecular genetic testing is available.

Déjerine-Sottas Disease (CMT3)   Patients who never ambulate (or lose the ability to ambulate in infancy or childhood) are sometimes diagnosed as DSD (also called HMSNIII) or congenital hypomyelinating neuropathy (CHN). These disorders are severe, infantile- or childhood-onset, hypertrophic demyelinating polyneuropathies. NCVs are substantially slowed (typically 10 m/s), and elevations in the cerebrospinal fluid (CSF) protein level are typically present. The clinical features of DSD and CHN overlap those of severe CMT1, and for this reason the continued clinical separation of CMT1 and DSD/CHN is perhaps unwarranted. Many cases of DSD or CHN appear to be sporadic, occurring in the absence of a family history of neuropathy.

Molecular genetic studies indicate that DSD and CHN may be associated with point mutations in the P_0 or the *PMP22* genes, although pedigrees have been described that lack mutations in either the P_0, *PMP22*, or *Cx32* gene (see below). Most DSD mutations identified to date appear to function as dominant genetic traits.

Hereditary Neuropathy with Liability to Pressure Palsies   HNPP (also called *tomaculous neuropathy*) is an autosomal dominant disorder that produces an episodic, recurrent demyelinating neuropathy. HNPP typically develops during adolescence and may cause attacks of numbness, muscular weakness, and atrophy. Peroneal palsies, carpal tunnel syndrome, and other entrapment neuropathies are manifestations of HNPP. Motor and sensory NCVs are mildly reduced in affected patients as well as in asymptomatic gene carriers. Pathologic changes observed in HNPP include segmental demyelination and tomaculous, or sausage-like, formations in peripheral nerves. Due to overlap of clinical features between HNPP and CMT1, some HNPP patients may be misdiagnosed as having CMT1. Approximately 10% of patients with HNPP present with a brachial neuropathy, which is typically painless. Rare patients with HNPP have been found by magnetic resonance imaging (MRI) to have central nervous system (CNS) demyelination.

The HNPP locus maps to chromosome 17p11.2-p12 and is associated with a 1.5-Mb deletion. The duplicated CMT1A chromosome (described earlier) and the deleted HNPP chromosome are the reciprocal products of unequal crossing-over during meiosis. In the case of HNPP, loss of a copy of the *PMP22* gene and underexpression of this critical myelin gene lead to demyelination. Most HNPP patients have the associated chromosome 17 deletion; however, rare patients with HNPP have been found to have point mutations in the *PMP22* gene. Molecular genetic testing is clinically available.

Treatment for HNPP is largely supportive. Surgical decompression of nerves has been proposed but is controversial. There is some evidence that surgical repair of carpal tunnel syndrome in HNPP is of little benefit and that transposition of the ulnar nerve at the elbow may produce poor results because the nerves are especially sensitive to manipulation and minor trauma.

CMT Neuropathy Type 2   CMT2 is less common than CMT1 and, in general, has a later age of onset, produces less involvement of the intrinsic muscles of the hands, and lacks palpably enlarged nerves. Extensive demyelination with "onion bulb" formation is not present in CMT2. Motor NCVs are normal or only slightly reduced in affected persons. The CMT2A locus maps to chromosome 1p35-p36, and in one pedigree a mutation in KIF1B, an axonal motor protein, was found. Limb ulceration is a notable feature of CMT2B. CMT2B maps to chromosome 3q13-q22 and results from mutations in the *RAB7* gene, a member of the Rab family of ras-related GTPases that function in intracellular membrane trafficking. Further genetic heterogeneity within CMT2 is evidenced by the identification of kindreds with the features of axonal neuropathy, weakness of the diaphragm, and vocal cord paralysis. Such pedigrees carry the designation of CMT2C, which has been mapped to chromosome 12q23-q24. Yet another form of CMT2, designated CMT2D, maps to chromosome 7p14 and results from mutations in the glycyl tRNA synthetase gene (*GARS*). In a large Russian pedigree having an autosomal dominant axonopathy, a CMT2 gene was mapped to chromosome 8p21 (and designated CMT2E), and a mutation was found in the neurofilament-light (*NEFL*) gene.

Additionally, certain P_0 or connexin32 (*Cx32*, see below) mutations have been found to be the underlying genetic defect in a subset of patients with CMT1 or CMTX who were initially thought to have CMT2 because of only mild slowing of NCVs. With these exceptions, DNA testing is not widely available for any form of CMT2.

X-linked CMT Neuropathy   The clinical features of X-linked CMT disease (CMTX) include demyelinating neuropathy, absence of male-to-male transmission, and an earlier age of onset and faster rate of progression in males. NCVs vary widely in CMTX from nearly normal to moderately slowed. CMTX accounts for ~10% of all patients thought to have a form of demyelinating CMT (i.e., CMT1). CMTX should be suspected when the commonly associated chromosome 17 duplication is not present and there is no history of father-to-son transmission of the neuropathy.

The gene for CMTX maps to chromosome Xq13-q21 and results from point mutations in the *Cx32* gene. *Cx32* encodes a major component of gap junctions and is structurally similar to PMP22, as both of these proteins contain four putative transmembrane domains in similar orientation. Unlike PMP22 and P_0, which are present in compact myelin, Cx32 is located at uncompacted folds of Schwann cell cytoplasm around the nodes of Ranvier and at Schmidt-Lanterman incisures. This localization suggests a role for gap junctions composed of Cx32 in providing a pathway for the transfer of ions and nutrients around and across the myelin sheath of peripheral nerves. Mutations in the Cx32 protein have been suggested to alter its cellular localization and its trafficking and interfere with cell-to-cell communication. Over 200 different mutations in the *Cx32* gene have been described in patients with CMTX, and the distribution pattern of these mutations suggests that all parts of the Cx32 protein are functionally important. DNA testing is available.

Rare Forms of CMT   Mutations in the putative zinc finger domain of the early growth response 2 gene (*EGR2*, or *Krox-20*) or in the small integral membrane protein of the lyzosome/late endosome (*SIMPLE*) gene have been found in CMT1 families that were found to be negative for the CMT1A duplication, as well as for mutations in *PMP22*, P_0, or *Cx32*. EGR2 mutations have also been reported in CHN. EGR2 acts as a direct transactivator of myelination genes in differentiating Schwann cells. SIMPLE has been proposed to play a role in myelin protein degradation and turnover. Mutations have also been found in periaxin (*PRX*), an important structural myelin protein, in demyelinating forms of neuropathy clinically diagnosed as CMT1 or DSD. DNA testing is available for EGR2 and PRX.

Rare families with autosomal recessive motor and sensory neuropathy have been reported, particularly Tunisian families with parental consanguinity. Both demyelinating and axonal types of neuropathy have been described and given the designation CMT4. One form of autosomal recessive demyelinating neuropathy, CMT4A, has been mapped to chromosome 8q13-q21 and is associated with mutations in the ganglioside-induced differentiation-associated protein (GDAP1). CMT4B is characterized by focally folded myelin sheaths and maps

to chromosome 11q23. CMT4B is caused by mutations in the myotubularin-related protein-2 (*MTMR2*), which is thought to be a transcriptional regulator. Additional loci for other rare forms of CMT4 have been found, and in some cases causal genes are known (Table 364-1).

Genetic Evaluation of CMT and HNPP   An approach for evaluating a patient suspected of having an inherited peripheral neuropathy is presented in Fig. 364-1. If the proband has evidence for CMT1, determination of NCVs is a useful screening tool for parents and other at-risk family members. The *CMT1* gene is penetrant in early life, and correct disease status can probably be determined by age 5 by screening with NCVs. However, if a proband's nerve conduction is normal or only mildly prolonged, the diagnosis may be CMT2. In this case the screening examination will need to focus on determination of motor unit amplitudes and other electrical signs of denervation. Rare patients have been found to have point mutations in either P_0 or *Cx32*, resulting in very mild demyelination and misclassification as CMT2.

Most CMT1 and CMT2 pedigrees have autosomal dominant inheritance. In pedigrees lacking male-to-male transmission and whenever males are more severely affected than females and have an earlier onset, CMTX should be suspected. Determination of autosomal dominant versus X-linked CMT is important as the genetic counseling for these two modes of inheritance is different. For any form of autosomal dominant CMT, the likelihood of an affected parent (of either sex) having an affected child is 50% for each pregnancy, regardless of the sex of the child. For CMTX, all daughters of an affected father will inherit the gene, and none of the sons will be affected. For a woman with CMTX, there is a 50% likelihood that her children will be affected regardless of their sex.

Sporadic cases in males can be especially difficult to evaluate, as the neuropathy could be nongenetic or the pattern of inheritance could be autosomal dominant, X-linked, or even autosomal recessive. Sporadic cases may also represent de novo duplications (CMT1A) or de novo deletions (HNPP). False paternity is another explanation for apparent sporadic CMT or HNPP.

Molecular genetic testing is currently available for the DNA duplication (or deletion) associated with CMT1A or HNPP and for point mutations in the *PMP22*, P_0, *EGR2*, *PRX*, and *Cx32* genes associated with other forms of CMT1 and CMTX.

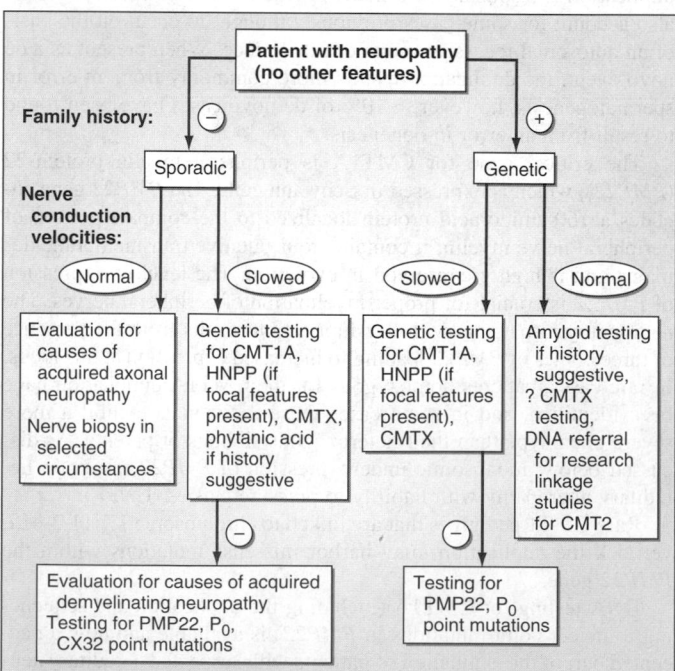

FIGURE 364-1   Evaluation of patients suspected of having an inherited peripheral neuropathy. CMT, Charcot-Marie-Tooth; HNPP, hereditary neuropathy with liability to pressure palsies. (*Modified from Lynch and Chance.*)

CHEMOTHERAPY IN PATIENTS WITH CMT
Chemotherapeutic agents known to affect peripheral nerves should be used with great caution in patients with inherited neuropathies, and in the case of vincristine, total avoidance is strongly advised. A number of reports have documented the serious consequences of vincristine treatment administered in standard oncologic dosages in patients with CMT, including CMT1A and CMT2. The complications ranged from the precipitation of severe neuropathies in clinically asymptomatic at-risk individuals, induction of marked worsening in previously symptomatic patients, and even death due to respiratory collapse.

OTHER INHERITED NEUROPATHIES

HEREDITARY SENSORY NEUROPATHIES Hereditary sensory neuropathies (HSNs) are a heterogeneous group of disorders affecting sensory neurons. The most common form of HSN, HSN type I, is an autosomal degenerative disorder of sensory and motor neurons. Phenotypically, distal sensory loss, distal muscle wasting and weakness, and variable neural deafness are observed. The disease involves progressive loss of dorsal root ganglion cells and axons in peripheral nerves. Age of onset is the second decade of life or later. The HSN-I locus maps to chromosome 9q22.1-q22.3 and results from mutations in the serine palmityl transferase (*SPTLC1*) gene. Because of the presence of muscular weakness in some patients with HSN, this disorder may be clinically confused with CMT.

FAMILIAL AMYLOID NEUROPATHY Familial amyloid polyneuropathy (FAP) is an autosomal dominant disorder that classically presents as progressive sensory peripheral neuropathy, with early involvement of the autonomic nervous system and an associated cardiomyopathy. Postmortem studies have shown extensive amyloid deposition in multiple organs throughout the body. Transthyretin (TTR) is the most common constituent amyloid fibril protein deposited in FAP. Several different point mutations in the *TTR* gene have been described in TTR-related FAP, and DNA testing for these mutations is clinically available. →*Amyloidosis is discussed in Chap. 310.*

REFSUM DISEASE This autosomal recessive disorder is characterized by a progressive sensorimotor demyelinating polyneuropathy, associated with cerebellar ataxia and retinitis pigmentosa. Neural deafness, cardiomyopathy, cataracts, and icthyosis are additional features. Onset is in late childhood or early adulthood. Patients often complain of night blindness as the earliest symptom. The CSF protein is typically elevated. Diagnosis is made by demonstration of elevated levels of phytanic acid (a 20-carbon branched-chain fatty acid) in the serum and urine. The disorder appears to be due to a deficiency of a peroxysomal enzyme, phytanic acid oxidase, responsible for alpha oxidation of phytanic acid. Therapy, consisting of avoidance of dietary sources of phytanic acid and plasmapheresis in some cases, is partially effective.

FURTHER READING

BENNETT CL, CHANCE PF: Molecular pathogenesis of hereditary motor, sensory and autonomic neuropathies. Curr Opin Neuro 14:621, 2001

CHANCE PF, SHAPIRO BE: Charcot-Marie-Tooth disease and related disorders, in B Katirji et al (eds): *Neuromuscular Disorders in Clinical Practice*. Philadelphia, Butterworth-Heinemann, pp 513–525, 2002

KAMHOLZ J et al: Charcot-Marie-Tooth disease type 1: Molecular pathogenesis to gene therapy. Brain 123:222, 2000

LYNCH D, CHANCE PF: Inherited peripheral neuropathies. Neurologist 3:277, 1997

MEULEMAN JR, CHANCE PF: Hereditary pressure palsy, in *Neurological Therapeutics: Principles and Practice*, J Noseworthy (ed). London, Martin Dunitz, 2003

SCHERER SS et al: Peripheral neuropathies, in *The Molecular and Genetic Basis of Neurological Disease*, RN Rosenberg et al (eds). Oxford, Butterworth-Heinemann, pp 435–453, 2003

365 GUILLAIN-BARRÉ SYNDROME AND OTHER IMMUNE-MEDIATED NEUROPATHIES
Stephen L. Hauser, Arthur K. Asbury

GUILLAIN-BARRÉ SYNDROME

Guillain-Barré syndrome (GBS) is an acute, frequently severe, and fulminant polyradiculoneuropathy that is autoimmune in nature. It occurs year-round at a rate of about one case per million per month, or ~3500 cases per year in the United States and Canada. Males and females are equally at risk, and in western countries adults are more frequently affected than children.

Clinical Manifestations GBS manifests as rapidly evolving areflexic motor paralysis with or without sensory disturbance. The usual pattern is an ascending paralysis that may be first noticed as rubbery legs. Weakness typically evolves over hours to a few days and is frequently accompanied by tingling dysesthesias in the extremities. The legs are usually more affected than the arms, and facial diparesis is present in 50% of affected individuals. The lower cranial nerves are also frequently involved, causing bulbar weakness and difficulty with handling secretions and maintaining an airway. Most patients require hospitalization, and almost 30% require ventilatory assistance at some time during the illness. Fever and constitutional symptoms are absent at the onset, and, if present, cast doubt on the diagnosis. Deep tendon reflexes usually disappear within the first few days of onset. Cutaneous sensory deficits, e.g., loss of pain and temperature sensation, are usually relatively mild, but functions subserved by large sensory fibers, such as deep tendon reflexes and proprioception, are more severely affected. Bladder dysfunction may occur in severe cases but is usually transient. If bladder dysfunction is a prominent feature and comes early in the course, possibilities other than GBS should be considered, particularly spinal cord disease. Once clinical worsening stops and the patient reaches a plateau, further progression is unlikely.

In severe cases of GBS requiring critical care management, autonomic involvement is common. Usual features are loss of vasomotor control with wide fluctuation in blood pressure, postural hypotension, and cardiac dysrhythmias. These features require close monitoring and management and can be fatal. Pain is another common feature of GBS; several types are encountered. Most common is deep aching pain in weakened muscles, which patients liken to having overexercised the previous day. Other pains in GBS include back pain involving the entire spine and sometimes dysesthetic pain in the extremities as a manifestation of sensory nerve fiber involvement. These pains are self-limited and should be treated with standard analgesics.

Several subtypes of GBS are now recognized, as determined primarily by electrodiagnostic and pathologic distinctions (Table 365-1). A range of limited or regional GBS syndromes may be encountered, although uncommonly. These include (1) the Miller Fisher syndrome (Table 365-1 and see "Immunopathogenesis," below); (2) pure sensory forms; (3) ophthalmoplegia with anti-GQ1b antibodies (see "Immunopathogenesis," below) as part of severe motor-sensory GBS; (4) GBS with severe bulbar and facial paralysis, sometimes associated with antecedent cytomegalovirus (CMV) infection and anti-GM2 antibodies; and (5) acute pandysautonomia.

Antecedent Events Some 75% of cases of GBS are preceded 1 to 3 weeks by an acute infectious process, usually respiratory or gastrointestinal. Culture and seroepidemiologic techniques show that 20 to 30% of all cases occurring in North America, Europe, and Australia are preceded by infection or reinfection with *Campylobacter jejuni*. A similar proportion is preceded by a human herpes virus infection, often CMV or Epstein-Barr virus. Other viruses and also *Mycoplasma pneu-*

TABLE 365-1 Subtypes of Guillain-Barré Syndrome (GBS)

Subtype	Features	Electrodiagnosis	Pathology
Acute inflammatory demyelinating polyneuropathy (AIDP)	Adults affected more than children; 90% of cases in western world; recovery rapid; anti-GM1 antibodies (<50%)	Demyelinating	First attack on Schwann cell surface; widespread myelin damage, macrophage activation, and lymphocytic infiltration; variable secondary axonal damage
Acute motor axonal neuropathy (AMAN)	Children and young adults; prevalent in China and Mexico; may be seasonal; recovery rapid; anti-GD1a antibodies	Axonal	First attack at motor nodes of Ranvier; macrophage activation, few lymphocytes, frequent periaxonal macrophages; extent of axonal damage highly variable
Acute motor sensory axonal neuropathy (AMSAN)	Mostly adults; uncommon; recovery slow, often incomplete; closely related to AMAN	Axonal	Same as AMAN, but also affects sensory nerves and roots; axonal damage usually severe
M. Fisher syndrome (MFS)	Adults and children; uncommon; ophthalmoplegia, ataxia, and areflexia; anti-GQ1b antibodies (90%)	Demyelinating	Few cases examined; resembles AIDP

moniae have been identified as agents involved in antecedent infections. Recent immunization has also been associated with GBS. The swine influenza vaccine, administered widely in the United States in 1976, is the most notable example; influenza vaccines in use from 1992 to 1994, however, resulted in only one additional case of GBS per million persons vaccinated. Older type rabies vaccine, prepared in nervous system tissue, is implicated as a trigger of GBS in developing countries where it is still used; the mechanism is presumably immunization against neural antigens. GBS also occurs more frequently than can be attributed to chance alone in patients with lymphoma, including Hodgkin's disease (Chap. 97), in HIV-seropositive individuals (Chap. 173), and in patients with systemic lupus erythematosus (Chap. 300).

Immunopathogenesis Several lines of evidence support an autoimmune basis for acute inflammatory demyelinating polyneuropathy (AIDP), the most common and best studied type of GBS; the concept extends to all of the subtypes of GBS (Table 365-1).

It is likely that both cellular and humoral immune mechanisms contribute to tissue damage in AIDP. T cell activation is suggested by the finding that elevated levels of cytokines and cytokine receptors are present in serum [interleukin (IL) 2, soluble IL-2 receptor] and in cerebrospinal fluid (CSF) (IL-6, tumor necrosis factor α, interferon-γ). AIDP is also closely analogous to an experimental T cell–mediated immunopathy designated *experimental allergic neuritis* (EAN); EAN is induced in laboratory animals by immune sensitization against protein fragments derived from peripheral nerve proteins, and in particular against the P2 protein. Based on analogy to EAN, it was initially thought that AIDP was likely to be primarily a T cell–mediated disorder; however, abundant data now suggest that autoantibodies directed against nonprotein determinants may be central to many cases.

Circumstantial evidence suggests that all GBS results from immune responses to nonself antigens (infectious agents, vaccines) that misdirect to host nerve tissue through a resemblance-of-epitope (molecular mimicry) mechanism (Fig. 365-1) (Chap. 299). The neural targets are likely to be glycoconjugates, specifically gangliosides (Table 365-2; Fig. 365-2). Gangliosides are complex glycosphingolipids that contain one or more sialic acid residues; various gangliosides participate in cell-cell interactions (including those between axons and glia), modulation of receptors, and regulation of growth. They are typically exposed on the plasma membrane of cells, rendering them susceptible to an antibody-mediated attack. Gangliosides and other glycoconjugates are present in large quantity in human nervous tissues and in key sites, such as nodes of Ranvier. Antiganglioside antibodies, most fre-

quently to GM1, are common in GBS (20 to 50% of cases), particularly in those preceded by *C. jejuni* infection. Furthermore, isolates of *C. jejuni* from stool cultures of patients with GBS have surface glycolipid structures that antigenically cross react with gangliosides, including GM1, concentrated in human nerves. Another line of evidence is derived from experience in Europe with parenteral use of purified bovine brain gangliosides for treatment of various neuropathic disorders. Between 5 and 15 days after injection some recipients developed acute motor axonal GBS with high titers of anti-GM1 antibodies that recognized epitopes at nodes of Ranvier and motor endplates.

Particularly noteworthy is the Miller Fisher syndrome (MFS), which presents as rapidly evolving ataxia and areflexia of limbs without weakness, and ophthalmoplegia often with pupillary paralysis. The MFS variant accounts for ~5% of all GBS cases. Anti-GQ1b IgG antibodies are found in >90% of patients with MFS (Tables 365-1 and 365-2; Fig. 365-2), and titers of IgG are highest early in the course. Anti-GQ1b antibodies are not found in other forms of GBS unless there is extraocular motor nerve involvement. Extraocular motor nerves are enriched in GQ1b gangli-

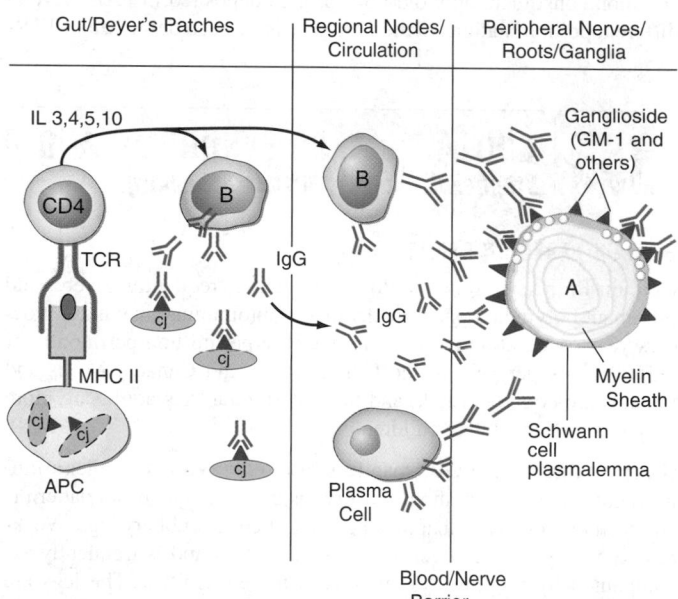

FIGURE 365-1 Postulated immunopathogenesis of GBS associated with *C. jejuni* infection. B cells recognize glycoconjugates on *C. jejuni* (Cj) (triangles) that cross-react with ganglioside present on Schwann cell surface and subjacent peripheral nerve myelin. Some B cells, activated via a T cell–independent mechanism, secrete primarily IgM (not shown). Other B cells (upper left side) are activated via a partially T cell–dependent route and secrete primarily IgG; T cell help is provided by CD4 cells activated locally by fragments of Cj proteins that are presented on the surface of antigen-presenting cells (APC). A critical event in the development of GBS is the escape of activated B cells from Peyers patches into regional lymph nodes. Activated T cells probably also function to assist in opening of the blood-nerve barrier, facilitating penetration of pathogenic autoantibodies. The earliest changes in myelin (right) consist of edema between myelin lamellae and vesicular disruption (shown as circular blebs) of the outermost myelin layers. These effects are associated with activation of the C5b-C9 membrane attack complex and probably mediated by calcium entry; it is possible that the macrophage cytokine tumor necrosis factor (TNF) also participates in myelin damage. B, B cell; MHC II, class II major histocompatibility complex molecule; TCR, T cell receptor; A, axon.

TABLE 365-2 *Principal Anti-Glycolipid Antibodies Implicated in Immune Neuropathies*

Clinical Presentation	Antibody Target	Usual Isotype
ACUTE IMMUNE NEUROPATHIES (GUILLAIN BARRÉ SYNDROMES)		
Acute inflammatory demyelinating polyneuropathy (AIDP)	No clear patterns GM1 most common	IgG (polyclonal)
Acute motor axonal neuropathy (AMAN)	GD1a, GM1, GM1b, GalNAc–GD1a (<50% for any)	IgG (polyclonal)
Miller Fisher Syndrome (MFS)	GQ1b (>90%)	IgG (polyclonal)
Acute pharyngeal cervicobrachial neuropathy (APCBN)	GT1a (? Most)	IgG (polyclonal)
CHRONIC IMMUNE NEUROPATHIES		
Chronic inflammatory demyelinating polyneuropathy CIDP (75%)	P0 in some	No clear pattern
CIDPa (MGUS associated) (25%)	Neural binding sites	IgG, IgA (monoclonal)
Chronic sensory > motor neuropathy	SPGP, SGLPG (on MAG) (50%)	IgM (monoclonal)
	Uncertain (50%)	IgM (monoclonal)
Multifocal motor neuropathy (MMN)	GM1, GalNAc–GD1a, others (25–50%)	IgM (polyclonal, monoclonal)
Chronic sensory ataxic neuropathy	GD1b, GQ1b and other b-series gangliosides	IgM (monoclonal)

Note: MGUS, monoclonal gammopathy of undertermined significance; MAG, myelin-associated glycoprotein.
Source: Modified from HJ Willison, N Yuki: Brain 125:2591, 2002.

FIGURE 365-2 Glycolipids implicated as antigens in immune-mediated neuropathies. *(Modified from HJ Willison, N Yuki: Brain 125:2591, 2002.)*

osides in comparison to limb nerves. Further, a monoclonal anti-GQ1b antibody raised against *C. jejuni* isolated from a patient with MFS blocked neuromuscular transmission experimentally.

Taken together, these observations provide strong but still inconclusive evidence that autoantibodies play an important pathogenic role in GBS. Although anti-ganglioside antibodies have been studied most intensively, other antigenic targets may also be important. One recent report identified IgG antibodies against Schwann cells and neurons (nerve growth cone region) in some GBS cases. Proof that these antibodies are pathogenic requires that they be capable of mediating disease following direct passive transfer to naïve hosts; this has not yet been demonstrated, although a case of apparent maternal-fetal transplacental transfer of GBS has been described.

Pathophysiology In the demyelinating forms of GBS, the basis for flaccid paralysis and sensory disturbance is conduction block. This finding, demonstrable electrophysiologically, implies that the axonal connections remain intact. Hence, recovery can take place rapidly as remyelination occurs. In severe cases of demyelinating GBS, secondary axonal degeneration usually occurs; its extent can be estimated electrophysiologically. More secondary axonal degeneration correlates with a slower rate of recovery and a greater degree of residual disability. When a primary axonal pattern is encountered electrophysiologically, the implication is that axons have degenerated and become disconnected from their targets, specifically the neuromuscular junctions, and must therefore regenerate for recovery to take place. In motor axonal cases in which recovery is rapid, the lesion is thought to be localized to preterminal motor branches, allowing regeneration and reinnervation to take place quickly.

Laboratory Features CSF findings are distinctive, consisting of an elevated CSF protein level [1 to 10 g/L (100 to 1000 mg/dL)] without accompanying pleocytosis. The CSF is often normal when symptoms have been present for ≤48 h; by the end of the first week the level of protein is usually elevated. A transient increase in the CSF white cell

count (10 to 100/μL) occurs on occasion in otherwise typical GBS; however, a sustained CSF pleocytosis suggests an alternative diagnosis (viral myelitis) or a concurrent diagnosis (unrecognized HIV infection; Chap. 173). Electrodiagnostic features are mild or absent in the early stages of GBS and lag behind the clinical evolution. In cases with demyelination (Table 365-1), prolonged distal latencies, conduction velocity slowing, evidence of conduction block, and temporal dispersion of compound action potential are the usual features. In cases with primary axonal pathology, the principal electrodiagnostic finding is reduced amplitude of compound action potentials without conduction slowing or prolongation of distal latencies.

Diagnosis GBS is a descriptive entity. The diagnosis is made by recognizing the pattern of rapidly evolving paralysis with areflexia, absence of fever or other systemic symptoms, and characteristic antecedent events (Table 365-3). Other disorders that may enter into the

TABLE 365-3 *Diagnostic Criteria for Guillain-Barré Syndrome*

REQUIRED

1. Progressive weakness of 2 or more limbs due to neuropathy[a]
2. Areflexia
3. Disease course <4 weeks
4. Exclusion of other causes [e.g., vasculitis (polyarteritis nodosa, systemic lupus erythematosus, Churg-Strauss syndrome), toxins (organophosphates, lead), botulism, diphtheria, porphyria, localized spinal cord or cauda equina syndrome]

SUPPORTIVE

1. Relatively symmetric weakness
2. Mild sensory involvement
3. Facial nerve or other cranial nerve involvement
4. Absence of fever
5. Typical CSF profile (acellular, increase in protein level)
6. Electrophysiologic evidence of demyelination

[a] Excluding M. Fisher and other variant syndromes.
Source: Modified from AK Asbury, DR Cornblath: Ann Neurol 27:S21, 1990.

differential diagnosis include acute myelopathies (especially with prolonged back pain and sphincter disturbances); botulism (pupillary reactivity lost early); diphtheria (early oropharyngeal disturbances); Lyme polyradiculitis and other tick-borne paralyses; porphyria (abdominal pain, seizures, psychosis); vasculitic neuropathy (check erythrocyte sedimentation rate, described below); poliomyelitis (fever and meningismus common); CMV polyradiculitis (in immunocompromised patients); critical illness neuropathy; neuromuscular disorders such as myasthenia gravis; or poisonings with organophosphates, thallium, or arsenic. Laboratory tests are helpful primarily to exclude mimics of GBS. Electrodiagnostic features may be minimal, and the CSF protein level may not rise until the end of the first week. If the diagnosis is strongly suspected, treatment should be initiated without waiting for evolution of the characteristic electrodiagnostic and CSF findings to occur. GBS patients with risk factors for HIV or with CSF pleocytosis should have a serologic test for HIV.

℞ TREATMENT

In the vast majority of patients with GBS, treatment should be initiated as soon after diagnosis as possible. Each day counts; ~2 weeks after the first motor symptoms, immunotherapy is no longer effective. Either high-dose intravenous immune globulin (IVIg) or plasmapheresis can be initiated, as they are equally effective (Table 365-4). A combination of the two therapies is not significantly better than either alone. IVIg is often the initial therapy chosen because of its ease of administration and good safety record. IVIg is administered as five daily infusions for a total dose of 2 g/kg body weight. There is some evidence that GBS autoantibodies are neutralized by anti-idiotypic antibodies present in IVIg preparations, perhaps accounting for the therapeutic effect. A course of plasmapheresis, consisting of ~40 to 50 mL/kg plasma exchange (PE) four times over a week, is usually employed. In patients who are treated early in the course of GBS and improve, relapse may occur in the second or third week. Brief retreatment with the original therapy is usually effective. Glucocorticoids have not been found to be effective in GBS. Occasional patients with very mild forms of GBS, especially those who appear to have already reached a plateau when initially seen, may be managed conservatively without IVIg or plasma exchange.

In the worsening phase of GBS, most patients require monitoring in a critical care setting, with particular attention to vital capacity, cardiovascular status, and chest physiotherapy. As noted, ~30% of patients with GBS require ventilatory assistance, sometimes for prolonged periods of time (several weeks or longer). Frequent turning and assiduous skin care are important, as are daily range-of-motion exercises to avoid joint contractures, and daily reassurance as to the generally good outlook for recovery.

Prognosis and Recovery Approximately 85% of patients with GBS achieve a full functional recovery within several months to a year, although minor findings on examination (such as areflexia) may persist. The mortality rate is <5% in optimal settings; death usually results from secondary pulmonary complications. The outlook is worst in patients with severe proximal motor and sensory axonal damage. Such axonal damage may be either primary or secondary in nature (see "Pathophysiology," above), but in either case successful regeneration cannot occur. Other factors that worsen the outlook for recovery are advanced age, a fulminant or severe attack, and a delay in the onset of treatment. Between 5 to 10% of patients with typical GBS have one or more late relapses; such cases are then classsified as chronic inflammatory demyelinating polyneuropathy (CIDP).

CHRONIC INFLAMMATORY DEMYELINATING POLYNEUROPATHY

CIDP is distinguished from GBS by its chronic course. In other respects, this neuropathy shares many features with GBS, including elevated CSF protein levels and the electrodiagnostic findings of acquired demyelination. Most cases occur in adults, and males are affected slightly more often than females. The incidence of CIDP is lower than that of GBS, but due to the protracted course the prevalence is greater.

Clinical Manifestations Onset is usually gradual, sometimes subacute; in a few, the initial attack is indistinguishable from that of GBS. Symptoms are both motor and sensory in most cases. Weakness of the limbs is usually symmetric but can be strikingly asymmetric. There is considerable variability from case to case. Some patients experience a

TABLE 365-4 *Major Clinical Trials of Treatment for Guillain-Barré Syndrome (GBS)*

Trial/Site	Reference	No. Patients (N)/ Follow Up (FU)/ Trial Arms	End Points	Results/p Value	Comment
GBS Study Group; USA/Canada (18 centers)	Neurology 35:1096, 1985	N = 245 FU = 6 months PE vs. none	1. % improved 1 grade at 4 weeks 2. Days to improve 1 grade 3. Days to reach grade 2	1. 59% (PE) vs. 39% (none) $p < .001$ 2. 19 days (PE) vs. 40 days (none) $p < .001$ 3. 53 days (PE) vs. 85 days (none) $p < .001$	First major trial showing efficacy—prior smaller trials showed conflicting results
French Coop. Group on PE in GBS; France/Switzerland (28 centers)	Ann Neurol 22:753, 1987; Ann Neurol 32:94, 1992	N = 220 FU = 1 year PE vs. none; Albumin vs. FFP in PE arm	1. Days to walk with assistance 2. Days to positive Δ score 3. Albumin vs. FFP	1. 30 days (PE) vs. 44 days (none) $p < .01$ 2. 4 days (PE) vs. 12 days (none) $p < .001$ 3. No significant difference	At 1 year, full strength recovery in 71% (PE) vs. 52% (none); $p = .007$
Dutch GB Study Group; The Netherlands (15 centers)	N Engl J Med 326: 1123, 1992	N = 150 FU = 6 months IVIg vs. PE	1. % improved 1 grade at 4 weeks 2. Days to reach grade 2	1. 53% (IVIg) vs. 34% (PE) $p = .024$ 2. 55 days (IVIg) vs. 70 days (PE) $p = .07$	Patient assignment inadvertently favored IVIg group
Plasma Exchange/ Sandoglobulin GBS Trial (38 centers in 11 countries)	Lancet 349:225, 1997	N = 329 FU = 48 weeks IVIg vs. PE vs. both (3 arms)	1. % improved 1 grade at 4 weeks 2. Secondary end points: days to reach grade 2; days to off-respirator; disability at 48 weeks	No significant difference between the 3 groups for any end points	Nonsignificant trends favoring combined therapy

Abbreviations: PE, plasma exchange; IVIg, high dose intravenous immunoglobulin; FFP, fresh-frozen plasma

Note: All studies except the French Coop. Group used the London grade scale: 0, healthy; 1, minor symptoms/signs; 2, walk 5 m unassisted; 3, walk 5 m with assistance; 4, bed/chairbound; 5, requiring assisted respiration; 6, dead.

chronic progressive course, whereas others, usually younger patients, have a relapsing and remitting course. Some have only motor findings, and a small proportion present with a relatively pure syndrome of sensory ataxia. Tremor occurs in ~10% and may become more prominent during periods of subacute worsening or improvement. A small proportion have cranial nerve findings, including external ophthalmoplegia. CIDP tends to ameliorate over time with treatment; the result is that many years after onset nearly 75% of patients have reasonable functional status. Death from CIDP is uncommon.

Diagnosis The diagnosis rests on characteristic clinical, CSF, and electrophysiologic findings. The CSF is usually acellular with an elevated protein level, sometimes several times normal. Electrodiagnostically, variable degrees of conduction slowing, prolonged distal latencies, temporal dispersion of compound action potentials, and conduction block are the principal features. In particular, the presence of conduction block is a certain sign of an acquired demyelinating process. Evidence of axonal loss, presumably secondary to demyelination, is present in >50% of patients. Serum protein electrophoresis with immunofixation is indicated to search for monoclonal gammopathy and associated conditions (see "Monoclonal Gammopathy of Undetermined Significance," below). In all patients with presumptive CIDP, it is also reasonable to exclude collagen vascular disease (especially systemic lupus erythematosus), chronic hepatitis, HIV infection, and diabetes mellitus.

Pathogenesis Although there is evidence of immune activation in CIDP, the precise mechanisms of pathogenesis are unknown. Biopsy typically reveals little inflammation and onion-bulb changes (imbricated layers of attenuated Schwann cell processes surrounding an axon) that result from recurrent demyelination and remyelination. The response to therapy suggests that CIDP is immune-mediated; interestingly, CIDP responds to glucocorticoids (see below), whereas GBS does not. Passive transfer of demyelination into experimental animals was recently accomplished using IgG purified from the serum of some patients with CIDP, lending support for a humoral autoimmune pathogenesis. Although the target antigen or antigens in CIDP have not yet been identified, one recent study implicated the myelin protein Po as a potential autoantigen in some patients. Approximately 25% of patients with clinical features of CIDP also have a monoclonal gammopathy of undetermined significance (MGUS). Cases associated with monoclonal IgA or IgG usually respond to treatment as favorably as cases without a monoclonal gammopathy. Patients with IgM monoclonal gammopathy tend to have more sensory findings, a more protracted course, and may have a less satisfactory response to treatment, although this is an area of controversy.

℞ TREATMENT

Most authorities initiate treatment for CIDP when progression is rapid or walking is compromised. If the disorder is mild, management can be expectant, awaiting spontaneous remission. Controlled studies have shown that high-dose IVIg, PE, and glucocorticoids are all more effective than placebo. Initial therapy is usually either IVIg or PE, which appear to be equally effective. IVIg is administered as 0.4 g/kg body weight daily for 5 days; most patients require periodic re-treatment at ~6-week intervals. PE is initiated at two to three treatments per week for 6 weeks; periodic re-treatment may also be required. Treatment with oral glucocorticoids is another option (60 to 80 mg prednisone daily for 1 to 2 months, followed by a gradual dose reduction of 10 mg per month as tolerated), but long-term adverse effects including bone demineralization, gastrointestinal bleeding, and cushingoid changes are problematic. Approximately one-half of patients with CIDP fail to respond adequately to the initial therapy chosen; a different treatment should then be tried. Patients who fail therapy with IVIg, PE, and glucocorticoids may benefit from treatment with immunosuppressive agents such as azathioprine, methotrexate, cyclosporine, and cyclophosphamide, either alone or as adjunctive therapy. Use of these therapies requires periodic reassessment of their risks and benefits.

MULTIFOCAL MOTOR NEUROPATHY

Multifocal motor neuropathy (MMN) is a distinctive but uncommon neuropathy that presents as a slowly progressive motor weakness and atrophy evolving over years in the distribution of selected nerve trunks, associated with sites of persistent focal motor conduction block in the same nerve trunks. Sensory fibers are relatively spared. The arms are affected more frequently than the legs, and >75% of all patients are male. Some cases have been confused with lower motor neuron forms of amyotrophic lateral sclerosis (Chap. 353). Approximately 50% of patients present with high titers of polyclonal IgM antibody to the ganglioside GM1. It is uncertain how this finding relates to the discrete foci of persistent motor conduction block, but high concentrations of GM1 gangliosides are normal constituents of nodes of Ranvier in peripheral nerve fibers. Pathology reveals demyelination and mild inflammatory changes at the sites of conduction block.

Most patients with MMN respond to high-dose IVIg (dosages as for CIDP, above) and some refractory patients have responded to cyclophosphamide. Glucocorticoids and PE are not effective.

NEUROPATHIES WITH MONOCLONAL GAMMOPATHY

MULTIPLE MYELOMA Clinically overt polyneuropathy occurs in ~5% of patients with the commonly encountered type of multiple myeloma, which exhibits either lytic or diffuse osteoporotic bone lesions. These neuropathies are sensorimotor, are usually mild but may be severe, and generally do not reverse with successful suppression of the myeloma. In most cases, electrodiagnostic and pathologic features are consistent with a process of axonal degeneration.

In contrast, myeloma with osteosclerotic features, although representing only 3% of all myelomas, is associated with polyneuropathy in one-half of cases. These neuropathies, which may also occur with solitary plasmacytoma, are distinct because they (1) are usually demyelinating in nature; (2) often respond to radiation therapy or removal of the primary lesion; (3) are associated with different monoclonal proteins and light chains (almost always lambda as opposed to primarily kappa in the lytic type of multiple myeloma); and (4) may occur in association with other systemic findings including thickening of the skin, hyperpigmentation, hypertrichosis, organomegaly, endocrinopathy, anasarca, and clubbing of fingers. These are features of the POEMS syndrome (*p*olyneuropathy, *o*rganomegaly, *e*ndocrinopathy, *M* protein, and *s*kin changes). The pathogenesis of this uncommon syndrome and the explanation for its association with lambda light chains are unknown. Treatment of the neuropathy is best directed at the osteosclerotic myeloma using surgery, radiotherapy, or chemotherapy, as indicated.

Neuropathies are also encountered in other systemic conditions with gammopathy including Waldenström's macroglobulinemia, primary systemic amyloidosis, and cryoglobulinemic states (mixed essential cryoglobulinemia, some cases of hepatitis C).

MONOCLONAL GAMMOPATHY OF UNDETERMINED SIGNIFICANCE Chronic polyneuropathies occurring in association with MGUS are usually associated with the immunoglobulin isotypes IgG, IgA, and IgM. From a clinical standpoint, many of these patients are indistinguishable from patients with CIDP without monoclonal gammopathy (see "Chronic Inflammatory Demyelinating Polyneuropathy," above), and their response to immunosuppressive agents is also similar. An exception is the syndrome of IgM kappa monoclonal gammopathy associated with an indolent, longstanding, sometimes static sensory neuropathy, frequently with tremor and sensory ataxia. Most patients are male and over age 50. In the majority, the monoclonal IgM immunoglobulin binds to a normal peripheral nerve constituent, myelin-associated glycoprotein (MAG), found in the paranodal regions of Schwann cells. Binding appears to be specific for a polysaccharide epitope that is also found in other normal peripheral nerve myelin glycoproteins, P0 and PMP22, and also in other normal nerve-related glycosphingolipids (Fig. 365-1). In the MAG-positive cases, IgM paraprotein is incorporated into the myelin sheaths of affected patients and widens the spacing of the myelin lamellae, thus producing a distinctive ultrastructural pattern. Demyelination and remyelination are the hallmarks of the lesions. The chronic demyelinating neuropathy appears to result from a destabilization of myelin metabolism rather than activation of an immune response. Therapy with chlorambucil or cyclophosphamide often results in improvement of the neuropathy associated with a prolonged reduction in the levels in the circulating paraprotein; chronic use of these alkylating agents is associated with significant risks (Chap. 70). In a small proportion of patients, MGUS will in time evolve into frankly malignant conditions, such as multiple myeloma (Chap. 98) or lymphoma (Chap. 97).

VASCULITIC NEUROPATHY

Peripheral nerve involvement is common in polyarteritis nodosa (PAN), appearing in half of all cases clinically and in 100% of cases at postmortem studies (Chap. 306). The most common pattern is multifocal (asymmetric) motor-sensory neuropathy (mononeuropathy multiplex) due to ischemic lesions of nerve trunks and roots; however, some cases of vasculitic neuropathy present as a distal, symmetric motor-sensory neuropathy. Symptoms of neuropathy are a common presenting complaint in patients with PAN. The electrodiagnostic findings are those of an axonal process. Small- to medium-sized arteries of the vasa nervorum, particularly the epineural vessels, are affected in PAN, resulting in a widespread ischemic neuropathy. A high frequency of neuropathy is also present in allergic angiitis and granulomatosis (Churg-Strauss syndrome).

Systemic vasculitis should always be considered when a subacute or chronically evolving mononeuropathy multiplex occurs in conjunction with constitutional symptoms (fever, anorexia, weight loss, loss of energy, malaise, and nonspecific pains). Diagnosis of suspected vasculitic neuropathy is made by a combined nerve and muscle biopsy, with serial section or skip-serial techniques (Chap. 363).

Approximately one-third of biopsy-proven cases of vasculitic neuropathy are "nonsystemic" in that the vasculitis appears to affect only peripheral nerve. Constitutional symptoms are absent, and the course is more indolent than that of PAN. The erythrocyte sedimentation rate may be elevated, but other tests for systemic disease are negative. Nevertheless, clinically silent involvement of other organs is likely, and vasculitis is frequently found in muscle biopsied at the same time as nerve.

Vasculitic neuropathy may also be seen as part of the vasculitis syndrome occurring in the course of other connective tissue disorders. The most frequent is rheumatoid arthritis, but ischemic neuropathy due to involvement of vasa nervorum may also occur in mixed cryoglobulinemia, Sjögren's syndrome, Wegener's granulomatosis, hypersensitivity angiitis (Chap. 306), and progressive systemic sclerosis (Chap. 303). Management of these neuropathies, including the "nonsystemic" vasculitic neuropathy, consists of treatment of the underlying condition as well as the aggressive use of glucocorticoids and other immunosuppressant drugs, usually cyclophosphamide.

ANTI-HU PARANEOPLASTIC NEUROPATHY

This uncommon immune-mediated disorder manifests as a sensory neuronopathy, i.e., selective damage to dorsal root ganglia. The onset is often asymmetric with dysesthesias and sensory loss in the limbs that soon progress to affect all limbs, the torso, and face. Marked sensory ataxia, pseudoathetosis, and inability to walk, stand, or even sit unsupported are frequent features and are secondary to the extensive deafferentation. Subacute sensory neuronopathy is often idiopathic, but ~25% of cases are paraneoplastic, primarily related to lung cancer, and most of those are small-cell lung cancer (SCLC) (Chap. 87). The target antigens are a family of RNA binding proteins (HuD, HuC, and Hel-N1) that in normal tissues are only expressed by neurons. The same proteins are usually expressed by SCLC, triggering in some patients an immune response characterized by antibodies and cytotoxic T cells that cross-react with the Hu proteins of the dorsal root ganglion neurons, resulting in immune-mediated neuronal destruction. An encephalomyelitis may accompany the sensory neuronopathy and presumably has the same pathogenesis. Neurologic symptoms usually precede, by 1 year on average, the identification of SCLC. The sensory neuronopathy runs its course in a few weeks or months and stabilizes, leaving the patient disabled. Most cases are unresponsive to treatment with glucocorticoids, IVIg, PE, or immunosuppressant drugs.

FURTHER READING

GONG Y et al: Localization of major gangliosides in the PNS: Implications for immune neuropathies. Brain 125:2491, 2002

HUGHES RAC et al: Practice parameter: Immunotherapy for Guillain-Barré syndrome. Report of the Quality Standards Subcommittee of the American Academy of Neurology. Neurology 61:736, 2003

OLNEY RK et al: Consensus criteria for the diagnosis of multifocal motor neuropathy. Muscle Nerve 27:117, 2003

WILLISON HJ, YUKI N: Peripheral neuropathies and anti-glycolipid antibodies. Brain 125:2591, 2002

366   MYASTHENIA GRAVIS AND OTHER DISEASES OF THE NEUROMUSCULAR JUNCTION
Daniel B. Drachman

Myasthenia gravis (MG) is a neuromuscular disorder characterized by weakness and fatigability of skeletal muscles. The underlying defect is a decrease in the number of available acetylcholine receptors (AChRs) at neuromuscular junctions due to an antibody-mediated autoimmune attack. Treatment now available for MG is highly effective, although a specific cure has remained elusive.

PATHOPHYSIOLOGY In the neuromuscular junction (Fig. 366-1), acetylcholine (ACh) is synthesized in the motor nerve terminal and stored in vesicles (quanta). When an action potential travels down a motor nerve and reaches the nerve terminal, ACh from 150 to 200 vesicles is released and combines with AChRs that are densely packed at the peaks of postsynaptic folds. The structure of the AChR has been fully elucidated; it consists of five subunits (2α, 1β, 1δ, and 1γ or ϵ) arranged around a central pore. When ACh combines with the binding sites on the AChR, the channel in the AChR opens, permitting the rapid entry of cations, chiefly sodium, which produces depolarization at the end-plate region of the muscle fiber. If the depolarization is sufficiently large, it initiates an action potential that is propagated along the muscle fiber, triggering muscle contraction. This process is rapidly terminated by hydrolysis of ACh by acetylcholinesterase (AChE), which is present within the synaptic folds, and by diffusion of ACh away from the receptor.

In MG, the fundamental defect is a decrease in the number of available AChRs at the postsynaptic muscle membrane. In addition, the postsynaptic folds are flattened, or "simplified." These changes result in decreased efficiency of neuromuscular transmission. Therefore, although ACh is released normally, it produces small end-plate potentials that may fail to trigger muscle action potentials. Failure of transmission at many neuromuscular junctions results in weakness of muscle contraction.

The amount of ACh released per impulse normally declines on repeated activity (termed *presynaptic rundown*). In the myasthenic patient, the decreased efficiency of neuromuscular transmission combined with the normal rundown results in the activation of fewer and fewer muscle fibers by successive nerve impulses and hence increasing weakness, or *myasthenic fatigue*. This mechanism also accounts for the decremental response to repetitive nerve stimulation seen on electrodiagnostic testing.

The neuromuscular abnormalities in MG are brought about by an autoimmune response mediated by specific anti-AChR antibodies. The anti-AChR antibodies reduce the number of available AChRs at neuromuscular junctions by three distinct mechanisms: (1) accelerated turnover of AChRs by a mechanism involving crosslinking and rapid endocytosis of the receptors; (2) blockade of the active site of the AChR, i.e., the site that normally binds ACh; and (3) damage to the postsynaptic muscle membrane by the antibody in collaboration with complement. The pathogenic antibodies are IgG and are T cell dependent. Thus, immunotherapeutic strategies directed against T cells are effective in this antibody-mediated disease.

How the autoimmune response is initiated and maintained in MG is not completely understood. However, the thymus appears to play a role in this process. The thymus is abnormal in ~75% of patients with MG; in about 65% the thymus is "hyperplastic," with the presence of active germinal centers detected histologically, though the hyperplastic thymus is not necessarily enlarged. An additional 10% of patients have thymic tumors (thymomas). Muscle-like cells within the thymus (myoid cells), which bear AChRs on their surface, may serve as a source of autoantigen and trigger the autoimmune reaction within the thymus gland.

CLINICAL FEATURES MG is not rare, having a prevalence of at least 1 in 7500. It affects individuals in all age groups, but peaks of incidence occur in women in their twenties and thirties and in men in their fifties and sixties. Overall, women are affected more frequently than men, in a ratio of ~3:2. The cardinal features are *weakness* and *fatigability* of muscles. The weakness increases during repeated use (fatigue) and may improve following rest or sleep. The course of MG is often variable. Exacerbations and remissions may occur, particularly during the first few years after the onset of the disease. Remissions are rarely complete or permanent. Unrelated infections or systemic disorders often lead to increased myasthenic weakness and may precipitate "crisis" (see below).

The distribution of muscle weakness often has a characteristic pattern. The cranial muscles, particularly the lids and extraocular muscles, are often involved early in the course of MG, and diplopia and ptosis are common initial complaints. Facial weakness produces a "snarling" expression when the patient attempts to smile. Weakness in chewing is most noticeable after prolonged effort, as in chewing meat. Speech may have a nasal timbre caused by weakness of the palate or a dysarthric "mushy" quality due to tongue weakness. Difficulty in swallowing may occur as a result of weakness of the palate, tongue, or pharynx, giving rise to nasal regurgitation or aspiration of liquids or food. In ~85% of patients, the weakness becomes generalized, affecting the limb muscles as well. The limb weakness in MG is often proximal and may be asymmetric. Despite the muscle weakness, deep tendon reflexes are preserved. If weakness of respiration becomes so severe as to require respiratory assistance, the patient is said to be in *crisis*.

DIAGNOSIS AND EVALUATION (Table 366-1) The diagnosis is suspected on the basis of weakness and fatigability in the typical distribution described above, without loss of reflexes or impairment of sensation or other neurologic function. The suspected diagnosis should always be confirmed definitively before treatment is undertaken; this is essential because (1) other treatable conditions may closely resemble MG, and (2) the treatment of MG may involve surgery and the prolonged use of drugs with adverse side effects.

Anticholinesterase Test Drugs that inhibit the enzyme AChE allow ACh to interact repeatedly with the limited number of AChRs, producing

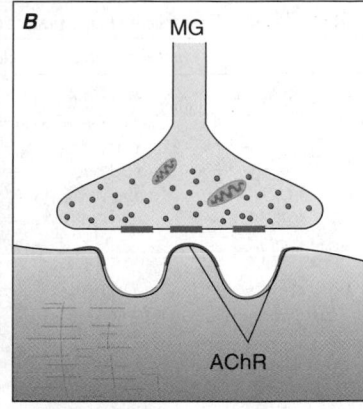

FIGURE 366-1 Diagrams of (*A*) normal and (*B*) myasthenic neuromuscular junctions. V, vesicles; M, mitochondria; AChE, acetylcholinesterase. See text for description of normal neuromuscular transmission. The MG junction shows a normal nerve terminal; a reduced number of AChRs (stippling); flattened, simplified postsynaptic folds; and a widened synaptic space.

improvement in the strength of myasthenic muscles. Edrophonium is used most commonly for diagnostic testing because of the rapid onset (30 s) and short duration (about 5 min) of its effect. An objective endpoint must be selected to evaluate the effect of edrophonium. The examiner should focus on one or more unequivocally weak muscle groups and evaluate their strength objectively. For example, weakness of extraocular muscles, impairment of speech, or the length of time that the patient can maintain the arms in forward abduction may be useful measures. An initial dose of 2 mg of edrophonium is given intravenously. If definite improvement occurs, the test is considered positive and is terminated. If there is no change, the patient is given an additional 8 mg intravenously. The dose is administered in two parts because some patients react to edrophonium with unpleasant side effects such as nausea, diarrhea, salivation, fasciculations, and rarely with severe symptoms of syncope or bradycardia. Atropine (0.6 mg) should be drawn up in a syringe, ready for intravenous administration if these symptoms become troublesome.

False-positive tests occur in occasional patients with other neurologic disorders, such as amyotrophic lateral sclerosis, and in placebo-reactors. False-negative or equivocal tests may also occur. In some cases it is helpful to use a longer-acting drug such as neostigmine (15 mg given orally), since this permits more time for detailed evaluation

TABLE 366-1   *Diagnosis of Myasthenia Gravis (MG)*

History
  Diplopia, ptosis, weakness
  Weakness in characteristic distribution
  Fluctuation and fatigue: worse with repeated activity, improved by rest
  Effects of previous treatments
Physical examination
  Ptosis, diplopia
  Motor power survey: quantitative testing of muscle strength
  Forward arm abduction time (5 min)
  Vital capacity
  Absence of other neurologic signs
Laboratory testing
  Anti-AChR radioimmunoassay: ~85% positive in generalized MG; 50% in ocular MG; definite diagnosis if positive; negative result does not exclude MG. ~40% of AChR antibody-negative patients with generalized MG have anti-MuSK antibodies.
  Edrophonium chloride (Tensilon) 2 mg + 8 mg IV; highly probable diagnosis if unequivocally positive
  Repetitive nerve stimulation; decrement of >15% at 3 Hz: highly probable
  Single-fiber electromyography: blocking and jitter, with normal fiber density; confirmatory, but not specific
  For ocular or cranial MG: exclude intracranial lesions by CT or MRI

Note: AChR, acetylcholine receptor; CT, computed tomography; MRI, magnetic resonance imaging; MuSK, muscle specific tyrosine kinase.
Source: From DB Drachman: N Engl J Med 330:1797, 1994.

TABLE 366-2 *The Congenital Myasthenic Syndromes*

Type	Clinical Features	Electrophysiology	Genetics	End-Plate Effects	Treatment
Slow channel	Most common; weak forearm extensors; onset 2d to 3d decade; variable severity	Repetitive muscle response on nerve stimulation; prolonged channel opening and MEPP duration	Autosomal dominant; α, β, ϵ AChR mutations	Excitotoxic end-plate myopathy; decreased AChRs; postsynaptic damage	Quinidine: decreases end-plate damage; made worse by anti-AChE
Low-affinity fast channel	Onset early; moderately severe; ptosis, EOM involvement; weakness and fatigue	Brief and infrequent channel openings; opposite of slow channel syndrome	Autosomal recessive; may be heteroallelic	Normal end-plate structure	3,4-DAP; anti-AChE
Severe AChR deficiencies	Early onset; variable severity; fatigue; typical MG features	Decremental response to repetitive nerve stimulation; decreased MEPP amplitudes	Autosomal recessive; ϵ mutations most common; many different mutations	Increased length of end plates; variable synaptic folds	Anti-AChE; ?3,4-DAP
AChE deficiency	Early onset; variable severity; scoliosis; may have normal EOM, absent pupillary responses	Decremental response to repetitive nerve stimulation	Mutant gene for AChE's collagen anchor	Small nerve terminals; degenerated junctional folds	Worse with anti-AChE drugs

Abbreviations: AChR, acetylcholine receptor; AChE, acetylcholinesterase; EOM, extraocular muscles; MEPP, miniature end-plate potentials; 3,4-DAP, 3-4-Diaminopyridine.

of strength. In virtually all instances, it is desirable to carry out further testing to establish the diagnosis of MG definitively.

Electrodiagnostic Testing Repetitive nerve stimulation often provides helpful diagnostic evidence of MG. Anti-AChE medication is stopped 6 to 24 h before testing. It is best to test weak muscles or proximal muscle groups. Electric shocks are delivered at a rate of two or three per second to the appropriate nerves, and action potentials are recorded from the muscles. In normal individuals, the amplitude of the evoked muscle action potentials does not change at these rates of stimulation. However, in myasthenic patients there is a rapid reduction in the amplitude of the evoked responses of >10 to 15%. As a further test, a single dose of edrophonium may be given to prevent or diminish this decremental reaction.

Antiacetylcholine Receptor Antibody As noted above, anti-AChR antibodies are detectable in the serum of ~85% of all myasthenic patients but in only about 50% of patients with weakness confined to the ocular muscles. The presence of anti-AChR antibodies is virtually diagnostic of MG, but a negative test does not exclude the disease. The measured level of anti-AChR antibody does not correspond well with the severity of MG in different patients. However, in an individual patient, a treatment-induced fall in the antibody level often correlates with clinical improvement. Recently, antibodies to muscle-specific kinase (MuSK) have been found to be present in about 40% of AChR antibody-negative patients with generalized MG, and their presence is a useful diagnostic test in these patients. MuSK antibodies are not present in AChR antibody-positive patients or in patients with MG limited to ocular muscles. The role of these antibodies in the pathogenesis of MG is as yet uncertain. However, MuSK is known to participate in clustering of AChRs at neuromuscular junctions during development.

Inherited Myasthenic Syndromes The congenital myasthenic syndromes (CMS) comprise a heterogeneous group of disorders of the neuromuscular junction that are not autoimmune but rather are due to genetic mutations in which virtually any component of the neuromuscular junction may be affected. Alterations in function of the presynaptic nerve terminal or in the various subunits of the AChR or AChE have been identified in the various forms of CMS. These disorders share many of the clinical features of autoimmune MG, including weakness and fatigability of skeletal muscles, in some cases involving extraocular muscles (EOMs), lids, and proximal muscles, similar to the distribution in autoimmune MG. CMS should be suspected when symptoms of myasthenia have begun in infancy or childhood and AChR antibody tests are consistently negative. Features of four of the most common forms of CMS are summarized in Table 366-2. Although clinical features and electrodiagnostic and pharmacologic tests may suggest the correct diagnosis, sophisticated electrophysiologic and molecular analysis are required for precise elucidation of the defect; this may lead to helpful treatment as well as genetic counseling. In the forms that involve the AChR, a wide variety of mutations have been identified in each of the subunits, but the ϵ subunit is affected in ~75% of these cases. In most of the recessively inherited forms of CMS, the mutations are heteroallelic; that is, different mutations affecting each of the two alleles are present.

Differential Diagnosis Other conditions that cause weakness of the cranial and/or somatic musculature include the nonautoimmune CMS discussed above, drug-induced myasthenia, Lambert-Eaton myasthenic syndrome (LEMS), neurasthenia, hyperthyroidism, botulism, intracranial mass lesions, and progressive external ophthalmoplegia. Treatment with penicillamine (used for scleroderma or rheumatoid arthritis) may result in true MG, but the weakness is usually mild, and recovery occurs within weeks or months after discontinuing its use. Aminoglycoside antibiotics or procainamide can cause exacerbation of weakness in myasthenic patients; very large doses can cause neuromuscular weakness in normal individuals.

LEMS is a presynaptic disorder of the neuromuscular junction that can cause weakness similar to that of MG. The proximal muscles of the lower limbs are most commonly affected, but other muscles may be involved as well. Cranial nerve findings, including ptosis of the eyelids and diplopia, occur in up to 70% of patients and resemble features of MG. However, the two conditions are readily distinguished, since patients with LEMS have depressed or absent reflexes, show autonomic changes such as dry mouth and impotence, and show incremental rather than decremental responses on repetitive nerve stimulation. LEMS is caused by autoantibodies directed against P/Q type calcium channels at the motor nerve terminals, which can be detected in ~85% of LEMS patients by radioimmunoassay. These autoantibodies result in impaired release of ACh from nerve terminals. A majority of patients with this syndrome have an associated malignancy, most commonly small-cell carcinoma of the lung, which is thought to trigger the autoimmune response. The diagnosis of LEMS may signal the presence of the tumor long before it would otherwise be detected, permitting early removal. Treatment of the neuromuscular disorder involves plasmapheresis and immunosuppression, as for MG. 3,4 Diaminopyridine (3,4-DAP) and pyridostigmine may be symptomatically

TABLE 366-3 *Disorders Associated with Myasthenia Gravis and Recommended Laboratory Tests*

Associated disorders
Disorders of the thymus: thymoma, hyperplasia
Other autoimmune disorders: Hashimoto's thyroiditis, Graves' disease, rheumatoid arthritis, lupus erythematosus, skin disorders, family history of autoimmune disorder
Disorders or circumstances that may exacerbate myasthenia gravis: hyperthyroidism or hypothyroidism, occult infection, medical treatment for other conditions (aminoglycoside antibiotics, quinine, antiarrhythmic agents)
Disorders that may interfere with therapy: tuberculosis, diabetes, peptic ulcer, gastrointestinal bleeding, renal disease, hypertension, asthma, osteoporosis, obesity
Recommended laboratory tests or procedures
CT or MRI of mediastinum
Tests for lupus erythematosus, antinuclear antibody, rheumatoid factor, antithyroid antibodies
Thyroid-function tests
PPD skin test
Chest radiography
Fasting blood glucose measurement
Pulmonary-function tests
Bone densitometry in older patients

Note: CT, computed tomography; MRI, magnetic resonance imaging; PPD, purified protein derivative.
Source: From RT Johnson, JW Griffin (eds): *Current Therapy in Neurologic Disease*, 4th ed. St. Louis, Mosby Year Book, 1993, p 379.

helpful in LEMS. 3,4-DAP acts by blocking potassium channels, which results in prolonged depolarization of the motor nerve terminals and thereby enhances ACh release. Pyridostigmine prolongs the action of ACh, allowing repeated interactions with AChRs.

Neurasthenia is the historic term for a myasthenia-like fatigue syndrome without an organic basis. These patients may present with subjective symptoms of weakness and fatigue, but muscle testing usually reveals the "jerky release" or "give-away weakness" characteristic of nonorganic disorders; the complaint of fatigue in these patients means tiredness or apathy rather than decreasing muscle power on repeated effort. Hyperthyroidism is readily diagnosed or excluded by tests of thyroid function, which should be carried out routinely in patients with suspected MG. Abnormalities of thyroid function (hyper- or hypothyroidism) may increase myasthenic weakness. Botulism can cause myasthenic-like weakness, but the pupils are often dilated, and repetitive nerve stimulation gives an incremental response. Diplopia that mimics the symptoms of MG may occasionally be due to an intracranial mass lesion that compresses nerves to the EOMs (e.g., sphenoid ridge meningioma), but magnetic resonance imaging (MRI) of the head and orbits usually reveals the lesion.

Progressive external ophthalmoplegia is a rare condition resulting in weakness of the EOMs, which may be accompanied by weakness of the proximal muscles of the limbs and other systemic features. Most patients with this condition have mitochondrial disorders that can be detected on muscle biopsy (Chap. 368).

Search for Associated Conditions (Table 366-3) Myasthenic patients have an increased incidence of several associated disorders. Thymic abnormalities occur in ~75% of patients, as noted above. Neoplastic change (thymoma) may produce enlargement of the thymus, which is detected by computed tomography (CT) or MRI scanning of the anterior mediastinum. A thymic shadow on CT scan may normally be present through young adulthood, but enlargement of the thymus in a patient >40 years old is highly suspicious of thymoma. Hyperthyroidism occurs in 3 to 8% of patients and may aggravate the myasthenic weakness. Tests of thyroid function should be obtained. Because of the association of MG with other autoimmune disorders, blood tests for rheumatoid factor and antinuclear antibodies should be carried out in all patients. Chronic infection of any kind can exacerbate MG and should be sought carefully. Finally, measurements of ventilatory function are valuable because of the frequency and seriousness of respiratory impairment in myasthenic patients.

Because of the side effects of glucocorticoids and other immunosuppressive agents used in the treatment of MG, a thorough medical investigation should be undertaken, searching specifically for evidence of chronic or latent infection (such as tuberculosis or hepatitis), hypertension, diabetes, renal impairment, and glaucoma.

℞ TREATMENT

(Fig. 366-2) The prognosis has improved strikingly as a result of advances in treatment; virtually all myasthenic patients can be returned to full productive lives with proper therapy. The most useful treatments for MG include anticholinesterase medications, immunosuppressive agents, thymectomy, and plasmapheresis or intravenous immunoglobulin (IVIg).

Anticholinesterase Medications Anticholinesterase medication produces at least partial improvement in most myasthenic patients, although improvement is complete in only a few. There is no substantial difference in efficacy among the various anticholinesterase drugs; oral pyridostigmine is the one most widely used in the United States. As a rule, the beneficial action of oral pyridostigmine begins within 15 to 30 min and lasts for 3 to 4 h, but individual responses vary. Treatment is begun with a moderate dose, e.g., 60 mg three to five times daily. The frequency and amount of the dose should be tailored to the patient's individual requirements throughout the day. For example, pa-

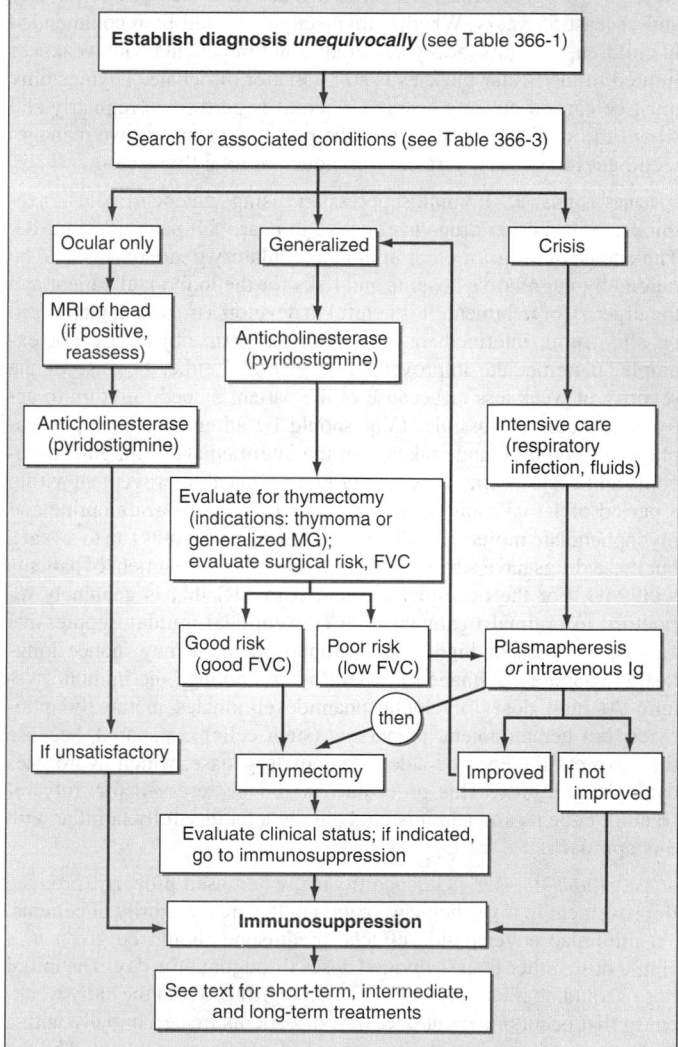

FIGURE 366-2 Algorithm for the management of myasthenia gravis. MRI, magnetic resonance imaging; FVC, forced vital capacity.

tients with weakness in chewing and swallowing may benefit by taking the medication before meals so that peak strength coincides with mealtime. Long-acting pyridostigmine may occasionally be useful to get the patient through the night but should never be used for daytime medication because of variable absorption. The maximum useful dose of pyridostigmine rarely exceeds 120 mg every 3 to 6 h during daytime. Overdosage with anticholinesterase medication may cause increased weakness and other side effects. In some patients, muscarinic side effects of the anticholinesterase medication (diarrhea, abdominal cramps, salivation, nausea) may limit the dose tolerated. Atropine/diphenoxylate or loperamide is useful for the treatment of GI symptoms.

Thymectomy Two separate issues should be distinguished: (1) surgical removal of thymoma, and (2) thymectomy as a treatment for MG. Surgical removal of a thymoma is necessary because of the possibility of local tumor spread, although most thymomas are benign. In the absence of a tumor, the available evidence suggests that up to 85% of patients experience improvement after thymectomy; of these, ~35% achieve drug-free remission. However, the improvement is typically delayed for months to years. The advantage of thymectomy is that it offers the possibility of long-term benefit, in some cases diminishing or eliminating the need for continuing medical treatment. In view of these potential benefits and of the negligible risk in skilled hands, thymectomy has gained widespread acceptance in the treatment of MG. It is the consensus that thymectomy should be carried out in all patients with generalized MG who are between the ages of puberty and at least 55 years. Whether thymectomy should be recommended in children, in adults >55 years of age, and in patients with weakness limited to the ocular muscles is still a matter of debate. Thymectomy must be carried out in a hospital where it is performed regularly and where the staff is experienced in the pre- and postoperative management, anesthesia, and surgical techniques of total thymectomy.

Immunosuppression Immunosuppression using glucocorticoids, azathioprine, and other drugs is effective in nearly all patients with MG. The choice of drugs or other immunomodulatory treatments should be guided by the relative benefits and risks for the individual patient and the urgency of treatment. It is helpful to develop a treatment plan based on short-term, intermediate-term, and long-term objectives. For example, if immediate improvement is essential either because of the severity of weakness or because of the patient's need to return to activity as soon as possible, IVIg should be administered or plasmapheresis should be undertaken. For the intermediate term, glucocorticoids and cyclosporine generally produce clinical improvement within a period of 1 to 3 months. The beneficial effects of azathioprine and mycophenolate mofetil usually begin after many months (up to a year), but these drugs have advantages for the long-term treatment of patients with MG. For the occasional patient with MG that is genuinely refractory to optimal treatment with conventional immunosuppressive agents, a course of high-dose cyclophosphamide may induce long-lasting (possibly permanent) benefit by "rebooting" the immune system. At high doses, cyclophosphamide eliminates mature lymphocytes, but hematopoietic precursors (stem cells) are spared, because they express the enzyme aldehyde dehydrogenase, which hydrolyzes cyclophosphamide. This procedure should be reserved for truly refractory patients and administered only in a facility fully familiar with this approach.

GLUCOCORTICOID THERAPY Glucocorticoids, when used properly, produce improvement in myasthenic weakness in the great majority of patients. To minimize adverse side effects, prednisone should be given in a single dose rather than in divided doses throughout the day. The initial dose should be relatively low (15 to 25 mg/d) to avoid the early weakening that occurs in about one-third of patients treated initially with a high-dose regimen. The dose is increased stepwise, as tolerated by the patient (usually by 5 mg/d at 2- to 3-day intervals), until there is marked clinical improvement or a dose of 50 to 60 mg/d is reached.

This dose is maintained for 1 to 3 months and then is gradually modified to an alternate-day regimen over the course of an additional 1 to 3 months; the goal is to reduce the dose on the "off day" to zero or to a minimal level. Generally, patients begin to improve within a few weeks after reaching the maximum dose, and improvement continues to progress for months or years. The prednisone dosage may gradually be reduced, but usually months or years may be needed to determine the minimum effective dose, and close monitoring is required. Few patients are able to do without immunosuppressive agents entirely. Patients on long-term glucocorticoid therapy must be followed carefully to prevent or treat adverse side effects. The most common errors in glucocorticoid treatment of myasthenic patients include (1) insufficient persistence—improvement may be delayed and gradual; (2) too early, too rapid, or excessive tapering of dosage; and (3) lack of attention to prevention and treatment of side effects. →*The management of patients treated with glucocorticoids is discussed in Chap. 321.*

OTHER IMMUNOSUPPRESSIVE DRUGS Azathioprine, cyclosporine, mycophenolate mofetil, or occasionally cyclophosphamide is effective in many patients, either alone or in combination with glucocorticoid therapy. Azathioprine has been the most widely used of these drugs because of its relative safety in most patients and long track record. Its therapeutic effect may add to that of glucocorticoids and/or allow the glucocorticoid dose to be reduced. However, up to 10% of patients are unable to tolerate azathioprine because of idiosyncratic reactions consisting of flulike symptoms of fever and malaise, bone marrow depression, or abnormalities of liver function. An initial dose of 50 mg/d should be used to test for adverse side effects. If this dose is tolerated, it is increased gradually until the white blood count falls to ~3000 to 4000/μL. In patients who are receiving glucocorticoids concurrently, leukocytosis precludes the use of this measure. A reduction of the lymphocyte count to <1000/μL and/or an increase of the mean corpuscular volume of red blood cells may be used as indications of adequacy of azathioprine dosage. The typical dosage range is 2 to 3 mg/kg total body weight. The beneficial effect of azathioprine takes at least 3 to 6 months to begin and even longer to peak. In patients taking azathioprine, allopurinol should never be used to treat hyperuricemia, because the two drugs share a common degradation pathway; the result may be severe bone marrow depression due to increased effects of the azathioprine.

Cyclosporine is approximately as effective as azathioprine and is being used increasingly in the management of MG. Its beneficial effect appears more rapidly than that of azathioprine. It may be used alone but is usually used as an adjunct to glucocorticoids to permit reduction of the glucocorticoid dose. The usual dose of cyclosporine is 4 to 5 mg/kg per day, given in two equally divided doses (to minimize side effects). Side effects of cyclosporine include hypertension and nephrotoxicity, which must be closely monitored. "Trough" blood levels of cyclosporine are measured 12 h after the evening dose. The therapeutic range, as measured by radioimmunoassay, is 150 to 200 ng/L.

Mycophenolate mofetil is also useful in the treatment of MG. A dose of 1 g to 1.5 g bid is recommended. Its mechanism of action involves inhibition of purine synthesis by the de novo pathway. Since lymphocytes lack the alternative salvage pathway that is present in all other cells, mycophenolate inhibits proliferation of lymphocytes but not proliferation of other cells. It does not kill or eliminate preexisting autoreactive lymphocytes, and therefore clinical improvement may be delayed for many months to a year, until the preexisting autoreactive lymphocytes die spontaneously. The advantage of mycophenolate lies in its relative lack of adverse side effects, with only occasional production of diarrhea and rare development of leukopenia. This drug may become the choice for long-term treatment of myasthenic patients. Unfortunately, the present cost of mycophenolate may be prohibitively high.

Cyclophosphamide is reserved for occasional patients refractory to the other drugs (see above for discussion of high-dose cyclophosphamide treatment).

History				
General	Normal	Good	Fair	Poor
Diplopia	None	Rare	Occasional	Constant
Ptosis	None	Rare	Occasional	Constant
Arms	Normal	Slightly limited	Some ADL impairment	Definitely limited
Legs	Normal	Walks/runs fatigues	Can walk limited distances	Minimal walking
Speech	Normal	Dysarthric	Severely dysarthric	Unintelligible
Voice	Normal	Fades	Impaired	Severely impaired
Chew	Normal	Fatigue on normal foods	Fatigue on soft foods	Feeding tube
Swallow	Normal	Normal foods	Soft foods only	Feeding tube
Respiration	Normal	Dyspnea on unusual effort	Dyspnea on any effort	Dyspnea at rest

Myasthenia Gravis Worksheet

Examination

BP _____ Pulse _____ Wt _____
Edema _____
Vital capacity _____
Cataracts? R _____ L _____
EOMS _____
Ptosis time _____
Face _____

Arm abduction time R _____ L _____
Deltoids   R _____ L _____
Biceps   R _____ L _____
Triceps   R _____ L _____
Grip   R _____ L _____
Iliopsoas   R _____ L _____
Quadriceps   R _____ L _____
Hamstrings   R _____ L _____
Other   R _____ L _____

FIGURE 366-3 Abbreviated interval assessment form for use in evaluating treatment for myasthenia gravis.

Plasmapheresis and Intravenous Immunoglobulin Plasmapheresis has been used therapeutically in MG. Plasma, which contains the pathogenic antibodies, is mechanically separated from the blood cells, which are returned to the patient. A course of five exchanges (3 to 4 L per exchange) is generally administered over a 2-week period. Plasmapheresis produces a short-term reduction in anti-AChR antibodies, with clinical improvement in many patients. It is useful as a temporary expedient in seriously affected patients or to improve the patient's condition prior to surgery (e.g., thymectomy).

The indications for the use of IVIg are the same as those for plasma exchange: to produce rapid improvement to help the patient through a difficult period of myasthenic weakness or prior to surgery. This treatment has the advantages of not requiring special equipment or large-bore venous access. The usual dose is 2 g/kg, which is typically administered over 5 days (400 mg/kg per day). If tolerated, the course of IVIg can be shortened to administer the entire dose over a 3-day period. Improvement occurs in about 70% of patients, beginning during treatment, or within 4 to 5 days thereafter, and continuing for weeks to months. The mechanism of action of IVIg is not known; the treatment has no consistent effect on the measurable amount of circulating AChR antibody. Adverse reactions are generally not serious but include headache, fluid overload, and rarely aseptic meningitis or renal shutdown. IVIg should rarely be used as a long-term treatment in place of rationally managed immunosuppressive therapy. Unfortunately, there is a growing tendency for physicians unfamiliar with immunosuppressive treatments to rely on repeated IVIg infusions, which are inconvenient, usually produce only intermittent benefit, and are costly. The intermediate and long-term treatment of myasthenic patients requires other methods of therapy outlined earlier in this chapter.

Management of Myasthenic Crisis Myasthenic crisis is defined as an exacerbation of weakness sufficient to endanger life; it usually consists of respiratory failure caused by diaphragmatic and intercostal muscle weakness. Crisis rarely occurs in properly managed patients. Treatment should be carried out in an intensive care unit staffed with physicians experienced in the management of MG, respiratory insufficiency, infectious disease, and fluid and electrolyte therapy. The possibility that the deterioration could be due to excessive anticholinesterase medication ("cholinergic crisis") is best excluded by temporarily stopping anticholinesterase drugs. The most common cause of crisis is intercurrent infection. This should be treated immediately, because the mechanical and immunologic defenses of the patient can be assumed to be compromised. The myasthenic patient with fever and early infection should be treated like other immunocompromised patients. Early and effective antibiotic therapy, respiratory assistance, and pulmonary physiotherapy are essentials of the treatment program. As discussed above, plasmapheresis or IVIg is frequently helpful in hastening recovery.

PATIENT ASSESSMENT In order to evaluate the effectiveness of treatment as well as drug-induced side effects, it is important to assess the patient's clinical status at baseline and on repeated interval examinations in a systematic manner. Because of the variability of symptoms of MG, the interval history as well as findings on examination must be taken into account. The most useful clinical tests include forward arm abduction time (up to a full 5 min), forced vital capacity, range of eye movements, and time to development of ptosis on upward gaze. Manual muscle testing or, preferably, quantitative dynamometry of limb muscles, especially proximal muscles, is also important. An interval form can provide a succinct summary of the patient's status and a guide to treatment results; an abbreviated form is shown in Fig. 366-3. A progressive reduction in the patient's AChR antibody level also provides clinically valuable confirmation of the effectiveness of treatment; conversely, a rise in AChR antibody levels during tapering of immunosuppressive medication may predict clinical exacerbation. For reliable quantitative measurement of AChR antibody levels, it is best to compare antibody levels from prior frozen serum aliquots with current serum samples in simultaneously run assays.

FURTHER READING

DRACHMAN DB et al: Treatment of refractory myasthenia gravis: "Rebooting" with high dose cyclophosphamide. Ann Neurol 53:29, 2003

KAMINSKI HJ: *Myasthenia Gravis and Related Disorders*. Totowa, NJ, Humana Press, 2003

KUPERSMITH MJ et al: Development of generalized disease at 2 years in patients with ocular myasthenia gravis. Arch Neurol 60:243, 2003

LINDSTROM JM: Acetylcholine receptors and myasthenia. Muscle Nerve 23:453, 2000

Skeletal muscle diseases, or myopathies, are disorders with structural changes or functional impairment of muscle. These conditions can be differentiated from other diseases of the motor unit (e.g., lower motor neuron or neuromuscular junction pathologies) by characteristic clinical and laboratory findings. →*Myasthenia gravis and related disorders are discussed in Chap. 366; musclar dystrophies and inherited, metabolic, and toxic myopathies in Chap. 368; inflammatory muscle diseases and inclusion body myositis in Chap. 369.*

CLINICAL FEATURES ■ Muscle Weakness Symptoms of muscle weakness can be either intermittent or persistent. Disorders causing *intermittent weakness* (Fig. 367-1) include myasthenia gravis, periodic paralyses (hypokalemic, hyperkalemic, and paramyotonia congenita), and metabolic energy deficiencies of glycolysis (especially myophosphorylase deficiency) and fatty acid utilization (carnitine palmitoyltransferase deficiency). The states of energy deficiency cause activity-related muscle breakdown accompanied by myoglobinuria, appearing as light-brown- to dark-brown-colored urine. Most muscle disorders cause *persistent weakness* (Fig. 367-2). In the majority of these, including most types of muscular dystrophy, polymyositis, and dermatomyositis, the proximal muscles are weaker than the distal, and the facial muscles are spared, a pattern referred to as *limb-girdle*. The differential diagnosis is more restricted for other patterns of weakness. Facial weakness (difficulty with eye closure and impaired smile) and scapular winging (Fig. 367-3) are characteristic of facioscapulohumeral dystrophy. Facial and distal limb weakness associated with hand grip myotonia is virtually diagnostic of myotonic dystrophy. When other cranial nerve muscles are weak, causing ptosis and extraocular muscle weakness without diplopia, the most important disorders to consider include oculopharyngeal muscular dystrophy, mitochondrial myopathies, or myotubular myopathy. A pathognomonic pattern exclusive to inclusion body myositis includes loss of strength in both proximal and distal muscles, hand grip weakness, and wasting of quadriceps muscles. Less frequently, but important diagnostically, is the presence of a dropped head syndrome indicative of selective neck extensor muscle weakness. The most common neuromuscular diseases causing this pattern of weakness include myasthenia gravis, polymyositis, and amyotrophic lateral sclerosis. A final pattern, recognized because of preferential distal extremity weakness, is typical of a unique category of muscular dystrophy, the distal myopathies (Chap. 368).

It is important to examine functional capabilities to help disclose certain patterns of weakness (Table 367-1). The Gowers' sign (Fig. 367-4) is particularly useful. Observing the gait of an individual may disclose a lordotic posture caused by combined trunk and hip weakness, frequently exaggerated by toe walking (Fig. 367-5). A waddling gait is caused by the inability of weak hip muscles to prevent hip drop or hip dip. Hyperextension of the knee (genu recurvatum or back-kneeing) is characteristic of quadriceps muscle weakness; and a steppage gait, due to footdrop, accompanies distal weakness.

Any disorder causing muscle weakness may be accompanied by *fatigue*, referring to an inability to maintain or sustain a force (pathologic fatigability). This condition must be differentiated from asthenia, a type of fatigue caused by excess tiredness or lack of energy. Associated symptoms may help differentiate asthenia and pathologic fatigability. Asthenia is often accompanied by a tendency to avoid physical activities, complaints of daytime sleepiness, necessity for frequent naps, and difficulty concentrating on activities such as reading. There may be feelings of overwhelming stress and depression. Thus, asthenia is not a myopathy. In contrast, pathologic fatigability occurs in disorders of neuromuscular transmission and in disorders altering energy production, including defects in glycolysis, lipid metabolism, or mitochondrial energy production. Pathologic fatigability also occurs in chronic myopathies because of difficulty accomplishing a task with less muscle. Pathologic fatigability is accompanied by abnormal clinical or laboratory findings. Fatigue without those supportive features almost never indicates a primary muscle disease.

Muscle Pain (Myalgias), Cramps, and Stiffness Muscle pain can be associated with cramps, spasms, contractures, and stiff or rigid muscles (Chap. 21). In distinction, true myalgia (muscle aching), which can be localized or generalized, may be accompanied by weakness, tenderness to palpation, or swelling. Certain drugs cause true myalgia (Table 367-2).

There are two painful muscle conditions of particular importance, neither of which is associated with muscle weakness. *Fibromyalgia* is a common, yet poorly understood type of myofascial pain syndrome.

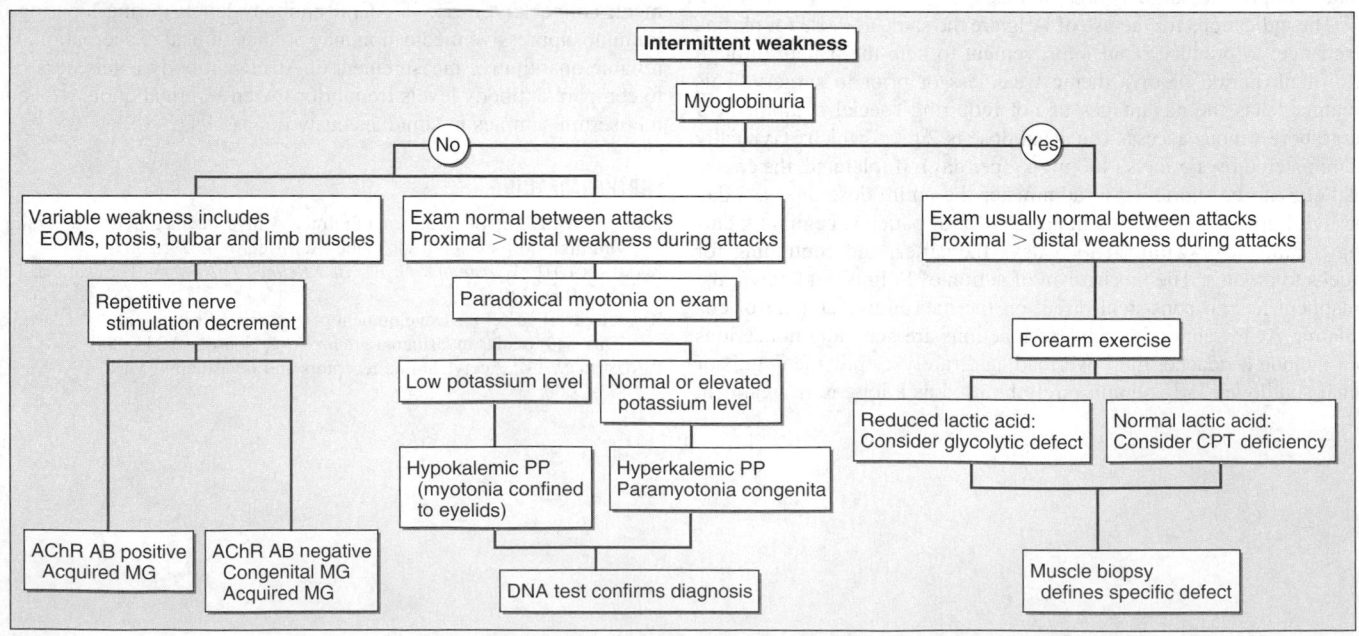

FIGURE 367-1 Diagnostic evaluation of intermittent weakness, EOMs, extraocular muscles; AChR AB, acetylcholine receptor antibody; PP, periodic paralysis; CPT, carnitine palmitoyltransferase; MG, myasthenia gravis.

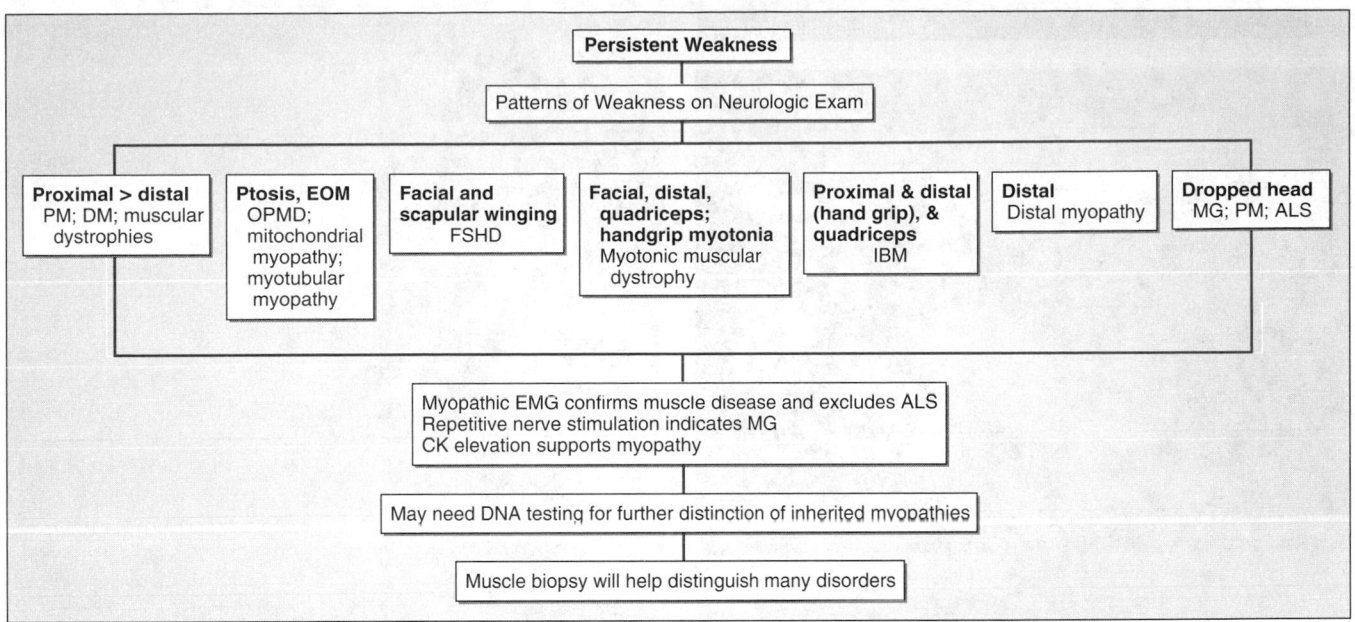

FIGURE 367-2 Diagnostic evaluation of persistent weakness. Examination reveals one of seven patterns of weakness. The pattern of weakness in combination with the laboratory evaluation leads to a diagnosis. EOM, extraocular muscle; OPMD, oculophar-yngeal muscular dystrophy; FSHD, facioscapulohumeral muscular dystrophy; IBM, inclusion body myositis; DM, dermatomyositis; PM, polymyositis; MG, myasthenia gravis; ALS, amyotrophic lateral sclerosis; CK, creatine kinase.

Patients complain of severe muscle pain and tenderness and have specific painful trigger points, sleep disturbances, and easy fatigability. Serum creatine kinase (CK) and erythrocyte sedimentation rate (ESR) are normal (Chap. 315). *Polymyalgia rheumatica* occurs mainly in patients >50 years and is characterized by stiffness and pain in the shoulders, lower back, hips, and thighs (Chap. 306). The ESR is elevated, while serum CK, electromyography (EMG), and muscle biopsy are normal. Temporal arteritis, an inflammatory disorder of medium- and large-sized arteries, usually involving one or more branches of the carotid artery, may accompany polymyalgia rheumatica. Vision is threatened due to ischemic optic neuritis. Glucocorticoids can relieve the myalgias and protect against visual loss.

Localized muscle pain is most often traumatic. A common cause of sudden abrupt-onset pain is a ruptured tendon, which leaves the muscle belly appearing rounded and shorter in appearance compared to the normal side. The biceps brachii and Achilles tendons are particularly vulnerable to rupture. Infection or neoplastic infiltration of the muscle is a rare cause of localized muscle pain.

A *muscle cramp* or *spasm* is a painful, involuntary, localized, muscle contraction with a visible or palpable hardening of the muscle. Cramps are abrupt in onset, short in duration, and may cause abnormal posturing of the joint. The EMG shows firing of motor units, reflecting an origin from spontaneous neural discharge. Muscle cramps often occur in neurogenic disorders, especially motor neuron disease (Chap. 353), radiculopathies, and polyneuropathies (Chap. 363), but are not a feature of most primary muscle diseases. Duchenne muscular dystrophy (Chap. 368) is an exception since calf muscle complaints are a common complaint. Muscle cramps are also common during pregnancy.

A *muscle contracture* is different from a muscle cramp. In both conditions, the muscle becomes hard, but a contracture is associated with energy failure in glycolytic disorders. The muscle is unable to relax after an active muscle contraction. The EMG shows electrical silence. Confusion is created because contracture also refers to a muscle that cannot be passively stretched to its proper length (fixed contracture) because of fibrosis. In some muscle disorders, especially Emery-Dreifuss muscular dystrophy and Bethlem myopathy (Chap.

FIGURE 367-3 Facioscapulohumeral dystrophy with prominent scapular winging.

TABLE 367-1 *Observations on Examination That Disclose Muscle Weakness*

Functional Impairment	Muscle Weakness
Inability to forcibly close eyes	Upper facial muscles
Impaired pucker	Lower facial muscles
Inability to raise head from prone position	Neck extensor muscles
Inability to raise head from supine position	Neck flexor muscles
Inability to raise arms above head	Proximal arm muscles (may be only scapular stabilizing muscles)
Inability to walk without hyperextending knee (backkneeing or genu recurvatum)	Knee extensor muscles
Inability to walk with heels touching the floor (toe walking)	Shortening of the Achilles tendon
Inability to lift foot while walking (steppage gait or footdrop)	Anterior compartment of leg
Inability to walk without a waddling gait	Hip muscles
Inability to get up from the floor without climbing up the extremities (Gowers' sign)	Hip muscles
Inability to get up from a chair without using arms	Hip muscles

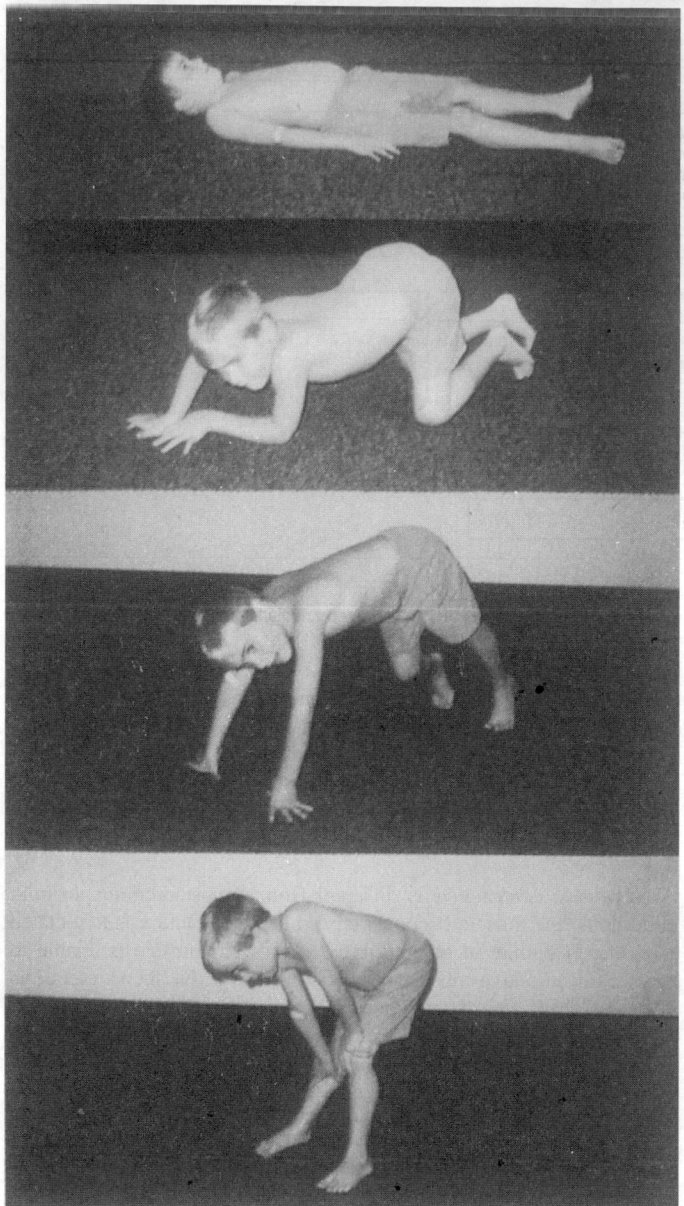

FIGURE 367-4 Gowers' sign showing a patient using arms to climb up the legs in attempting to get up from the floor.

FIGURE 367-5 Lordotic posture, exaggerated by standing on toes, associated with trunk and hip weakness.

368), fixed contractures occur early and represent distinctive features of the disease.

Muscle stiffness can refer to different phenomena. Some patients with inflammation of joints and periarticular surfaces feel stiff. This condition is different from the disorders of hyperexcitable motor nerves causing stiff or rigid muscles (Chap. 21). In *stiff-person syndrome* spontaneous discharges of the motor neurons of the spinal cord cause involuntary muscle contractions mainly involving the axial (trunk) and proximal lower extremity muscles. The gait becomes stiff and labored, with hyperlordosis of the lumbar spine. Superimposed episodic muscle spasms are precipitated by sudden movements, unexpected noises, and emotional upset. The muscles relax during sleep. Serum antiglutamic acid decarboxylase antibodies are present in approximately two-thirds of cases. In *neuromyotonia (Isaac's syndrome)* there is hyperexcitability of the peripheral nerves manifesting as continuous muscle fiber activity. *Myokymia* (continuous undulations of muscle) and impaired muscle relaxation are the result. Muscles of the leg are stiff, and the constant contractions of the muscle cause increased sweating of the extremities. This peripheral nerve hyperexcit-

ability is antibody-mediated, targeted against voltage-gated potassium channels. The site of origin of the spontaneous nerve discharges is principally in the distal portion of the motor nerves.

Myotonia is a condition of prolonged muscle contraction followed by slow muscle relaxation. It always follows muscle activation, usually voluntary, but may be elicited by mechanical stimulation (percussion myotonia) of the muscle. Myotonia typically causes difficulty in releasing objects after a firm grasp. In myotonic muscular dystrophy, weakness accompanies myotonia. Myotonia also occurs with *myotonia congenita* (a chloride channel disorder), but in this condition muscle weakness is not prominent. *Paramyotonia congenita* (a sodium channel disorder more closely aligned with hyperkalemic periodic paralysis) is named for a paradoxical phenomenon whereby the prolonged muscle contraction, with features virtually indistinguishable from myotonia, is exacerbated by repeated muscle contractions (Chap. 368). In hypokalemic periodic paralysis, myotonia of the eyelids may be present but limb muscles are usually spared.

Muscle Enlargement and Atrophy In most myopathies muscle tissue is replaced by fat and connective tissue, but the size of the muscle is usually not affected. However, in Duchenne and Becker muscular dystrophies, enlarged calf muscles are typical. In the patients with these forms of dystrophy, the enlargement represents true muscle hypertrophy; hence the term "pseudohypertrophy" should be avoided when referring to these patients. The calf muscles remain very strong even late in the course of these disorders. Muscle enlargement can also result from infiltration by sarcoid granulomas, amyloid deposits, bacterial and parasitic infections, and focal myositis.

TABLE 367-2	*Drugs That Cause True Myalgia*
Statins[a]	Emetine
Gemfibrozil	Labetalol
Vincristine	Nifedipine
Zidovudine	D-Penicillamine
Cyclosporine	L-Tryptophan
Gold	Epsilon aminocaproic acid
Danazol	Heroin
Cimetidine	Cocaine
	Methadone

[a] 3-Hydroxy-3-methylglutaryl coenzyme A reductase inhibitors.

LABORATORY EVALUATION A limited battery of tests can be used to evaluate a suspected myopathy. Nearly all patients require serum enzyme level measurements and electrodiagnostic studies as screening tools to differentiate muscle disorders from other motor unit diseases. The other tests described—DNA studies, the forearm exercise test, and muscle biopsy—are used to diagnose specific types of myopathies.

Serum Enzymes CK is the preferred muscle enzyme to measure in the evaluation of myopathies. Damage to muscle causes the CK to leak from the muscle fiber to the serum. The MM isoenzyme predominates in skeletal muscle, while CK-MB is the marker for cardiac muscle. Serum CK can be elevated in normal individuals without provocation, presumably on a genetic basis or after strenuous activity, minor trauma (including the EMG needle), a prolonged muscle cramp, or a generalized seizure. Aspartate aminotransferase (AST), alanine aminotransferase (ALT), and lactic dehydrogenase (LDH) are enzymes sharing an origin in both muscle and liver. Problems arise when the levels of these enzymes are found to be elevated in a routine screening battery, leading to the erroneous assumption that liver disease is present when in fact muscle could be the cause. An elevated gamma-glutamyl transferase (GGT) helps to establish a liver origin since this enzyme is not found in muscle. Aldolase is often thought to be a muscle-specific enzyme but is also present in liver.

Electrodiagnostic Studies EMG, repetitive nerve stimulation, and nerve conduction studies (Chap. 363) are essential methods for evaluation of the patient with suspected muscle disease. In combination they provide the information necessary to differentiate myopathies from neuropathies and neuromuscular junction diseases. Certain features of the EMG will point to an acquired, inflammatory muscle disorder (e.g., irritability on needle placement) versus a long-standing myopathic disorder (lack of irritability) that is more suggestive of a dystrophic process. Both inflammatory and noninflammatory myopathies share findings characterized by excessively recruited (too many) compound muscle action potentials for the degree of effort expended. This degree of recruitment is necessary to compensate for loss of muscle fibers related to the underlying process. The EMG can also be invaluable in helping to choose an appropriately affected muscle to sample for biopsy. The EMG can be used to fully characterize suspected involuntary activity seen during the examination, such as myokymia and myotonia.

DNA Analysis Advances in molecular diagnosis have evolved over the past decade and now serve as important tools for diagnosis. Certain muscle disorders can be definitively diagnosed by DNA analysis; these are fully discussed in Chap. 368. Nevertheless, important limitations need to be mentioned in seeking a molecular diagnosis. For example, in some disorders, such as Duchenne and Becker dystrophies, two-thirds of patients have deletion- or duplication-mutations that are easy to detect, while the remainder have point mutations that are much more difficult to find. For patients without identifiable gene defects, the muscle biopsy remains the main diagnostic tool.

Forearm Exercise Test In myopathies with intermittent symptoms, and especially those associated with myoglobinuria, there may be a defect in glycolysis. Many variations of the forearm exercise test exist. For safety, the test should not be performed under ischemic conditions to avoid an unnecessary insult to the muscle, causing rhabdomyolysis. The test is performed by placing a small indwelling catheter into an antecubital vein. A baseline blood sample is obtained for lactic acid and ammonia. The forearm muscles are exercised by asking the patient to vigorously squeeze a sphygmomanometer bulb for 1 min. Blood is then obtained at intervals of 1, 2, 4, 6, and 10 min for comparison with the baseline sample. Normal controls must be established for each laboratory. A three- to fourfold rise of lactic acid is typical. The simultaneous measurement of ammonia serves as a control, since it should also rise with exercise. In patients with myophosphorylase deficiency or other glycolytic defects (Chap. 368), the lactic acid rise will be absent or below normal, while the rise in ammonia will reach control values. If there is lack of effort, neither lactic acid nor ammonia will rise. Patients with selective failure to increase ammonia may have myoadenylate deaminase deficiency. This condition has been reported to be a cause of myoglobinuria, but deficiency of this enzyme in asymptomatic individuals makes interpretation controversial.

Muscle Biopsy Muscle biopsy analysis is an important step in establishing the final diagnosis of suspected myopathy. The microscopic evaluation uses a combination of techniques—histochemistry, immunocytochemistry with a battery of antibodies, and electron microscopy. Not all techniques need to be used on every case. A specific diagnosis can be established in many disorders. A combination of stains to identify mononuclear cells (polymyositis), complement (dermatomyositis), and amyloid (inclusion body myositis) helps to distinguish the inflammatory myopathies. Mitochondrial and metabolic (e.g., myophosphorylase and acid maltase deficiencies) myopathies demonstrate distinctive histochemical and electron-microscopic profiles. A battery of antibodies is available for the identification of missing components of the dystrophin glycoprotein complex and related proteins to help diagnose specific types of muscular dystrophies. In addition, the congenital myopathies have distinctive histologic features essential for diagnosis.

FURTHER READING

DAUBE JR: Myokymia and neuromyotonia. Muscle Nerve 24:1711, 2001

GRIGGS RC et al: Evaluation of the patient with myopathy, in *Evaluation and Treatment of Myopathies*, RC Griggs et al (eds). Philadelphia, FA Davis, 1995, pp 17–77

MEINCK HM, THOMPSON PD: Stiff man syndrome and related conditions. Mov Disord 17:853, 2002

THOMPSON PD et al: Statin-associated myopathy. JAMA 289:1681, 2003

VERNINO S, LENNON VA: Ion channel and striational antibodies define a continuum of autoimmune neuromuscular hyperexcitability. Muscle Nerve 26:70, 2002

368 MUSCULAR DYSTROPHIES AND OTHER MUSCLE DISEASES
Robert H. Brown, Jr., Jerry R. Mendell

The muscle disorders discussed in this chapter include diseases that cause acute, subacute, and chronic muscle weakness. Some cause pain in addition to or instead of weakness. →*Dermatomyositis and polymyositis are discussed in Chap. 369.*

HEREDITARY MYOPATHIES

Muscular dystrophy refers to a group of hereditary progressive diseases each with unique phenotypic and genetic features (Table 368-1).

DUCHENNE MUSCULAR DYSTROPHY This X-linked recessive disorder, sometimes also called *pseudohypertrophic muscular dystrophy*, has an incidence of ~30 per 100,000 live-born males.

Clinical Features Duchenne dystrophy is present at birth, but the disorder usually becomes apparent between ages 3 and 5. The boys fall frequently and have difficulty keeping up with friends when playing. Running, jumping, and hopping are invariably abnormal. By age 5, muscle weakness is obvious by muscle testing. On getting up from the floor, the patient uses his hands to climb up himself [Gowers' maneu

TABLE 368-1 *Progressive Muscular Dystrophies*

Type	Inheritance	Defective Gene/Protein	Onset Age	Clinical Features	Other Organ Systems Involved
Duchenne	XR	Dystrophin	Before 5 years	Progressive weakness of girdle muscles Unable to walk after age 12 Progressive kyphoscoliosis Respiratory failure in 2d or 3d decade	Cardiomyopathy Mental impairment
Becker	XR	Dystrophin	Early childhood to adult	Progressive weakness of girdle muscles Able to walk after age 15 Respiratory failure may develop by 4th decade	Cardiomyopathy
Limb-girdle	AD/AR	Several (Tables 368-2, 368-3)	Early childhood to early adult	Slow progressive weakness of shoulder and hip girdle muscles	± Cardiomyopathy
Emery-Dreifuss	XR/AD	Emerin/Lamins A/C	Childhood to adult	Elbow contractures, humeral and peroneal weakness	Cardiomyopathy
Congenital	AR	Several	At birth or within first few months	Hypotonia, contractures, delayed milestones Progression to respiratory failure in some; static course in others	CNS abnormalities (hypomyelination, malformation) Eye abnormalities
Myotonic[a] (DM1, DM2)	AD	DM1: Expansion CTG repeat DM2: Expansion CCTG repeat	Usually 2d decade May be infancy if mother affected (DM1 only)	Slowly progressive weakness of face, shoulder girdle, and foot dorsiflexion Preferential proximal weakness in DM2	Cardiac conduction defects Mental impairment Cataracts Frontal baldness Gonadal atrophy Deafness Coats' (eye) disease
Facioscapulohumeral	AD	Deletion, distal 4q	Before age 20	Slowly progressive weakness of face, shoulder girdle, and foot dorsiflexion	
Oculopharyngeal	AD	Expansion, poly-A RNA binding protein	5th to 6th decade	Slowly progressive weakness of extraocular, pharyngeal, and limb muscles	—

[a] Two forms of myotonic dystrophy, DM1 and DM2, have been identified. Many features overlap (see text).
Abbreviations: XR, X-linked recessive; AD, autosomal dominant; AR, autosomal recessive; CNS, central nervous system.

ver (Fig. 367-4)]. Contractures of the heel cords and iliotibial bands become apparent by age 6, when toe walking is associated with a lordotic posture. Loss of muscle strength is progressive, with predilection for proximal limb muscles and the neck flexors; leg involvement is more severe than arm involvement. Between ages 8 and 10 walking may require the use of braces; joint contractures and limitations of hip flexion, knee, elbow, and wrist extension are made worse by prolonged sitting. By age 12, most patients are wheelchair dependent. Contractures become fixed, and a progressive scoliosis often develops that may be associated with pain. The chest deformity with scoliosis impairs pulmonary function, which is already diminished by muscle weakness. By age 16 to 18, patients are predisposed to serious, sometimes fatal pulmonary infections. Other causes of death include aspiration of food and acute gastric dilation.

A cardiac cause of death is uncommon despite the presence of a cardiomyopathy in almost all patients. Congestive heart failure seldom occurs except with severe stress such as pneumonia. Cardiac arrhythmias are rare. The typical electrocardiogram (ECG) shows an increase net RS in lead V_1; deep, narrow Q waves in the precordial leads; and tall right precordial R waves in V_1. Intellectual impairment in Duchenne dystrophy is common; the average intelligence quotient (IQ) is approximately one standard deviation below the mean. Impairment of intellectual function appears to be nonprogressive and affects verbal ability more than performance.

Laboratory Features Serum creatine kinase (CK) levels are invariably elevated to between 20 and 100 times normal. The levels are abnormal at birth but decline late in the disease because of inactivity and loss

of muscle mass. Electromyography (EMG) demonstrates features typical of myopathy. The muscle biopsy shows muscle fibers of varying size as well as small groups of necrotic and regenerating fibers. Connective tissue and fat replace lost muscle fibers. A definitive diagnosis of Duchenne dystrophy can be established on the basis of dystrophin deficiency in a biopsy of muscle tissue or mutation analysis on peripheral blood leukocytes as discussed below.

GENETIC CONSIDERATIONS Duchenne dystrophy is caused by a mutation of the gene that encodes dystrophin, a 427-kDa protein localized to the inner surface of the sarcolemma of the muscle fiber. The dystrophin gene is >2000 kb in size and thus is one of the largest identified human genes. It is localized to the short arm of the X chromosome at Xp21. The most common gene mutation is a deletion. The size varies but does not correlate with disease severity. Deletions are not uniformly distributed over the gene but rather are most common near the beginning (5′ end) and middle of the gene. Less often, Duchenne dystrophy is caused by a gene duplication or point mutation. Identification of a specific mutation allows for an unequivocal diagnosis, makes possible accurate testing of potential carriers, and is useful for prenatal diagnosis.

A diagnosis of Duchenne dystrophy can also be made by western blot analysis of muscle biopsy specimens, revealing abnormalities on the quantity and molecular weight of dystrophin protein. In addition, immunocytochemical staining of muscle with dystrophin antibodies can be used to demonstrate absence or deficiency of dystrophin localizing to the sarcolemmal membrane. Carriers of the disease may demonstrate a mosaic pattern, but dystrophin analysis of muscle biopsy specimens for carrier detection is not reliable.

Pathogenesis Dystrophin is part of a large complex of sarcolemmal proteins and glycoproteins (Fig. 368-1). Dystrophin binds to F-actin at its amino terminus and to β-dystroglycan at the carboxyl terminus. β-Dystroglycan complexes to α-dystroglycan, which binds to laminin in the extracellular matrix (ECM). Laminin has a heterotrimeric molecular structure arranged in the shape of a cross with one heavy chain and two light chains, $\beta1$ and $\gamma1$. The laminin heavy chain of skeletal muscle is designated laminin $\alpha2$. Collagen proteins IV and VI are also found in the ECM. Like β-dystroglycan, the transmembrane sarcoglycan proteins also bind to dystrophin; these five proteins (designated α- through ε-sarcoglycan) complex tightly with each other. More recently, other membrane proteins implicated in muscular dystrophy have been found to be loosely affiliated with constituents of the dystrophin complex. These include caveolin-3, $\alpha7$ integrin, and collagen VI.

The dystrophin-glycoprotein complex appears to confer stability to the sarcolemma, although the function of each individual component of the complex is incompletely understood. Deficiency of one member of the complex may cause abnormalities in other components. For example, a primary deficiency of dystrophin (Duchenne dystrophy) may lead to secondary loss of the sarcoglycans and dystroglycan. The primary loss of a single sarcoglycan (see "Limb-Girdle Muscular Dystrophy," below) results in a secondary loss of other sarcoglycans in the membrane without uniformly affecting dystrophin. In either instance, disruption of the dystrophin-glycoprotein complexes weakens the sarcolemma, causing membrane tears and a cascade of events leading to muscle fiber necrosis. This sequence of events occurs repeatedly during the life of a patient with muscular dystrophy.

℞ TREATMENT

Glucocorticoids, administered as prednisone in a dose of 0.75 mg/kg per day, significantly slow progression of Duchenne dystrophy for up to 3 years. Some patients cannot tolerate glucocorticoid therapy; weight gain in particular represents a significant deterrent for some boys.

BECKER MUSCULAR DYSTROPHY This less severe form of X-linked recessive muscular dystrophy results from allelic defects of the same gene

FIGURE 368-1 Selected muscular dystrophy–associated proteins in the cell membrane and Golgi complex. Dystrophin localizes to the cytoplasmic face of the muscle cell membrane. It complexes with two transmembrane protein complexes, the dystroglycans and the sarcoglycans. The dystroglycans bind to the extracellular matrix protein merosin, which is also complexed with $\alpha1$ and $\alpha7$ integrins (Tables 368-1, 368-2, 368-3). Dysferlin complexes with caveolin-3 (which binds to neuronal nitric oxide synthase, or nNOS) but not with the dystrophin-associated proteins or the integrins. In each of four congenital dystrophies, there is loss of function of different Golgi-associated proteins: POMT1, POMGnT1, Fukutin, and Fukutin-related protein.

responsible for Duchenne dystrophy. Becker muscular dystrophy is approximately 10 times less frequent than Duchenne, with an incidence of about 3 per 100,000 live-born males.

Clinical Features The pattern of muscle wasting in Becker muscular dystrophy closely resembles that seen in Duchenne. Proximal muscles, especially of the lower extremities, are prominently involved. As the disease progresses, weakness becomes more generalized. Significant facial muscle weakness is not a feature. Hypertrophy of muscles, particularly in the calves, is an early and prominent finding.

Most patients with Becker dystrophy first experience difficulties between ages 5 and 15 years, although onset in the third or fourth decade or even later can occur. By definition, patients with Becker dystrophy walk beyond age 15, while patients with Duchenne dystrophy are typically in a wheelchair by the age of 12. Patients with Becker dystrophy have a reduced life expectancy, but most survive into the fourth or fifth decade.

Mental retardation may occur in Becker dystrophy, but it is not as common as in Duchenne. Cardiac involvement occurs in Becker dystrophy and may result in heart failure.

Laboratory Features Serum CK levels, results of EMG, and muscle biopsy findings closely resemble those in Duchenne dystrophy. The diagnosis of Becker muscular dystrophy requires western blot analysis of muscle biopsy samples demonstrating a reduced amount or abnormal size of dystrophin. Mutation analysis of DNA from peripheral blood leukocytes reveals deletions or duplications of the dystrophin gene in 65% of patients with Becker dystrophy, approximately the same percentage as in Duchenne dystrophy. In both Becker and Duchenne dystrophies, the size of the DNA deletion does not predict clinical severity; however, in ~95% of patients with Becker dystrophy, the DNA deletion does not alter the translational reading frame of messenger RNA. These "in-frame" mutations allow for production of some dystrophin, which accounts for the presence of altered rather than absent dystrophin on western blot analysis.

℞ TREATMENT

The use of glucocorticoids has not been adequately studied in Becker dystrophy.

LIMB-GIRDLE MUSCULAR DYSTROPHY The syndrome of limb-girdle muscular dystrophy (LGMD) represents more than one disorder. Both males and females are affected, with onset ranging from late in the first decade to the fourth decade. The LGMDs typically manifest with progressive weakness of pelvic and shoulder girdle musculature. Respiratory insufficiency from weakness of the diaphragm may occur, as may cardiomyopathy. Unlike Duchenne dystrophy, intellectual function is unaffected.

A systematic classification of LGMD is based on autosomal dominant (LGMD1) and autosomal recessive (LGMD2) inheritance. Superimposed on the backbone of LGMD1 and LGMD2, the classification employs a sequential alphabetical lettering system (LGMD1A, LGMD2A, etc.). Disorders receive letters in the order in which they are found to have chromosomal linkage. This results in an ever-expanding list of conditions. Presently there are 5 autosomal dominant and 10 autosomal recessive disorders, summarized in Tables 368-2 and 368-3. None of the conditions is as common as the dystrophinopathies; however, prevalence data for the LGMDs have not been systematically gathered for any large heterogeneous population. In referral-based clinical populations, the sarcoglycan deficiencies (LGMD2C, 2D, 2E, 2F) and dysferlinopathies (LGMD2B) have emerged as the most common disorders. Some small group analyses predict that calpain-3 deficiency (LGMD2A) and Fukutin-related protein (FKRP) deficiency (LGMD2I) may rival others for prevalence.

EMERY-DREIFUSS MUSCULAR DYSTROPHY There are two genetically distinct forms of Emery-Dreifuss muscular dystrophy (EDMD). One is

TABLE 368-2 Autosomal Dominant Limb-Girdle Muscular Dystrophies (LGMDs)

Disease	Clinical Features	Laboratory Features	Locus or Gene
LGMD1A	Onset 3d to 4th decade Muscle weakness affects distal limb muscles, vocal cords, and pharyngeal muscles	Serum CK 2 × normal EMG mixed myopathy/neuropathy NCS normal	Myotilin
LGMD1B	Onset 1st or 2d decade Proximal lower limb weakness and cardiomyopathy with conduction defects Some cases indistinguishable from Emery-Dreifuss muscular dystrophy with joint contractures	Serum CK 3–5 × normal NCS normal EMG myopathic	Lamin A/C
LGMD1C	Onset in early childhood Proximal weakness Gowers' sign, calf hypertrophy Exercise-related muscle cramps	Serum CK 4–25 × normal NCS normal EMG myopathic	Caveolin-3
LGMD1D	Onset 3d to 5th decade Proximal muscle weakness Cardiomyopathy and arrhythmias	Serum CK 2–4 × normal NCS normal EMG myopathic	Linked to chromosome 7q Gene unidentified
LGMD1E	Childhood onset Proximal muscle weakness	Serum CK usually normal NCS normal EMG myopathic	Linked to chromosome 6q23 Gene unidentified

Abbreviations: CK, creatine kinase; NCS, nerve conduction studies; EMG, electromyography.

inherited as an X-linked disorder, while the other is autosomal dominant. The latter is classified under the rubric of LGMD1B, but clinically the conditions are closely related.

Clinical Features Prominent contractures can be recognized in early childhood and teenage years, often preceding muscle weakness. The contractures persist throughout the course of the disease and are present at the elbows and neck. Muscle weakness affects humeral and peroneal muscles at first and later spreads to a limb-girdle distribution. The cardiomyopathy is potentially life threatening and may result in sudden death. A spectrum of atrial rhythm and conduction defects includes atrial fibrillation and paralysis and atrioventricular heart block. Some patients have a dilated cardiomyopathy. Female carriers of the X-linked variant may have cardiac manifestations that become clinically significant.

Laboratory Features Serum CK may be elevated two-to tenfold. EMG is myopathic. Muscle biopsy shows nonspecific dystrophic features. ECGs demonstrate atrial and atrioventricular rhythm disturbances.

GENETIC CONSIDERATIONS X-linked EDMD arises from defects in the emerin gene encoding a nuclear envelope protein. The autosomal dominant disease is caused by mutations of the *LMNA* gene on chromosome 1q21.2 encoding the lamin proteins A and C. These proteins are alternatively spliced products of the *LMNA* gene that are essential components of the filamentous network underlying the inner nuclear membrane. Loss of structural integrity of the nuclear envelope from defects in emerin or lamin A/C accounts for overlapping phenotypes.

℞ TREATMENT

Supportive care should be offered for neuromuscular disability, including ambulatory aids, if necessary. Stretching of contractures is difficult. Management of cardiomyopathy and arrhythmias can save lives.

MYOTONIC DYSTROPHY Myotonic dystrophy is also known as *dystrophia myotonica* (DM). The condition is composed of at least two clinical disorders with overlapping phenotypes and distinct molecular genetic defects: myotonic dystrophy type 1 (DM1), the classic disease originally described by Steinert, and myotonic dystrophy type 2 (DM2), also called *proximal myotonic myopathy* (PROMM).

Clinical Features The clinical expression of myotonic dystrophy varies widely and involves many systems other than muscle. Affected patients have a typical "hatchet-faced" appearance due to temporalis, masseter, and facial muscle atrophy and weakness. Frontal baldness is characteristic of men with the disease. Neck muscles, including flexors and sternocleidomastoids, and distal limb muscles are involved early. Weakness of wrist extensors, finger extensors, and intrinsic hand muscles impairs function. Ankle dorsiflexor weakness may cause footdrop. Proximal muscles remain stronger throughout the course, although preferential atrophy and weakness of quadriceps muscles occur in many patients. Palatal, pharyngeal, and tongue involvement produce a dysarthric speech, nasal voice, and swallowing problems. Some patients have diaphragm and intercostal muscle weakness, resulting in respiratory insufficiency.

Myotonia, which usually appears by age 5, is demonstrable by percussion of the thenar eminence, the tongue, and wrist extensor muscles. Myotonia causes a slow relaxation of hand grip after a forced voluntary closure. Advanced muscle wasting makes myotonia more difficult to detect.

Cardiac disturbances occur commonly in patients with DM1. ECG abnormalities include first-degree heart block and more extensive conduction system involvement. Complete heart block and sudden death can occur. Congestive heart failure occurs infrequently but may result from cor pulmonale secondary to respiratory failure. Mitral valve prolapse also occurs commonly. Other associated features include intellectual impairment, hypersomnia, posterior subcapsular cataracts, gonadal atrophy, insulin resistance, and decreased esophageal and colonic motility.

Congenital myotonic dystrophy is a more severe form of DM1 and occurs in ~25% of infants of affected mothers. It is characterized by severe facial and bulbar weakness, transient neonatal respiratory insufficiency, and mental retardation.

DM2, or PROMM, has a distinct pattern of muscle weakness affecting mainly proximal muscles. Other features of the disease overlap with DM1, including cataracts, testicular atrophy, insulin resistance, constipation, hypersomnia, and cognitive defects. Cardiac conduction defects occur but are less common, and the hatchet face and frontal baldness are less consistent features. A very striking difference is the failure to clearly identify a congenital form of DM2.

Laboratory Features The diagnosis of myotonic dystrophy can usually be made on the basis of clinical findings. Serum CK levels may be normal or mildly elevated. EMG evidence of myotonia is present in most cases. Muscle biopsy shows muscle atrophy, which selectively involves type 1 fibers in 50% of cases. Typically, increased numbers of central nuclei can be seen. Necrosis of muscle fibers and increased connective tissue, common in other muscular dystrophies, do not usually occur in myotonic dystrophy.

GENETIC CONSIDERATIONS DM1 and DM2 are both autosomal dominant disorders. New mutations do not appear to contribute to the pool of affected individuals. DM1 is transmitted by an intronic mutation consisting of an unstable expansion of a CTG trinucleotide repeat in a serine-threonine protein kinase gene (named *DMPK*) on chromosome 19q13.3. An increase in the severity of the disease phenotype in successive generations (genetic anticipation) is accompanied by an increase in the number of trinucleotide repeats. A similar type of mutation has been identified in fragile X syndrome (Chap. 56). The unstable triplet repeat in myotonic dystrophy can be used for prenatal diagnosis. Congenital disease occurs almost exclusively in infants born to affected mothers; it is possible that sperm with greatly expanded triplet repeats do not function well.

DM2 has been linked to chromosome 3q13.3-q24. At this locus, a DNA expansion mutation consists of a CCTG repeat in intron 1 of the *ZNF9* gene. The gene is believed to encode an RNA binding protein expressed in many different tissues, including skeletal and cardiac muscle.

How the DNA expansions in DM1 and DM2 impair function of muscle and other cells is not well understood. They may alter expression of an adjacent protein kinase gene (DM1), inactivate an important RNA binding protein (DM2), or influence other neighboring genes. In both DM1 and DM2, the mutant RNA appears to form intranuclear inclusions composed of aberrant RNA.

℞ TREATMENT

The myotonia in myotonic dystrophy rarely warrants treatment. Phenytoin is the preferred agent for the occasional patient who requires an antimyotonia drug; other agents, particularly quinine and procainamide, may worsen cardiac conduction. Cardiac pacemaker insertion should be considered for patients with unexplained syncope or advanced conduction system abnormalities with evidence of second-degree heart block, or trifascicular conduction disturbances with marked prolongation of the PR interval. Molded ankle-foot orthoses help prevent footdrop in patients with distal lower extremity weakness.

FACIOSCAPULOHUMERAL (FSH) MUSCULAR DYSTROPHY This form of muscular dystrophy has a prevalence of ~1 in 20,000. It is distinct from a similar disorder known as scapuloperoneal dystrophy.

Clinical Features The condition typically has an onset in childhood or young adulthood. In most cases, facial weakness is the initial manifestation, appearing as an inability to smile, whistle, or fully close the eyes. Weakness of the shoulder girdles, rather than the facial muscles, usually brings the patient to medical attention. Loss of scapular stabilizer muscles makes arm elevation difficult. Scapular winging (Fig. 367-3) becomes apparent with attempts at abduction and forward movement of the arms. Biceps and triceps muscles may be severely affected, with relative sparing of the deltoid muscles. Weakness is invariably worse for wrist extension than for wrist flexion, and weakness of the anterior compartment muscles of the legs may lead to footdrop.

In most patients, the weakness remains restricted to facial, upper extremity, and distal lower extremity muscles. In 20% of patients, weakness progresses to involve the pelvic girdle muscles, and severe functional impairment and possible wheelchair dependency result.

Characteristically, patients with FSH dystrophy do not have involvement of other organ systems, although labile hypertension is common, and there is an increased incidence of nerve deafness. *Coats' disease*, a disorder consisting of telangiectasia, exudation, and retinal detachment, also occurs.

TABLE 368-3 *Autosomal Recessive Limb-Girdle Muscular Dystrophies (LGMDs)*

Disease	Clinical Features	Laboratory Features	Locus or Gene
LGMD2A	Onset 1st or 2d decade Tight heel cords Contractures at elbows, wrists, and fingers; rigid spine in some Proximal and distal weakness	Serum CK 3–15 × normal NCS normal EMG myopathic	Calpain-3
LGMD2B	Onset 2d or 3d decade Proximal muscle weakness at onset, later distal (calf) muscles affected Miyoshi myopathy is variant of LGMD2B with calf muscles affected at onset	Serum CK 3–100 × normal NCS normal EMG myopathic Inflammation on muscle biopsy may simulate polymyositis	Dysferlin
LGMD2C–F	Onset in childhood to teenage yrs Clinical condition similar to Duchenne and Becker muscular dystrophies Cardiomyopathy uncommon Cognitive function normal	Serum CK 5–100 × normal NCS normal EMG myopathic	γ, α, β, δ sarcoglycans
LGMD2G	Onset age 10 to 15 Proximal and distal muscle weakness	Serum CK 3–17 × normal NCS normal EMG myopathic	Telethonin
LGMD2H	Onset 1st to 3d decade Proximal muscle weakness	Serum CK 2–25 × normal NCS normal EMG myopathic	TRIM32 gene
LGMD2I	Onset 1st to 3d decade Clinical condition similar to Duchenne or Becker dystrophies Cardiomyopathy (some not all) Cognitive function normal	Serum CK 10–30 × normal NCS normal EMG myopathic	Fukutin-related protein
LGMD2J[a]	Onset 1st to 3d decade Proximal lower limb weakness Mild distal weakness Progressive weakness causes loss of ambulation	Serum CK 1.5–2 × normal NCS normal EMG myopathic	Titin

[a] Tibial muscular dystrophy is a form of titin deficiency with only distal muscle weakness (see Table 368-4).
Abbreviations: CK, creatine kinase; NCS, nerve conduction studies; EMG, electromyography.

Laboratory Features The serum CK level may be normal or mildly elevated. EMG usually indicates a myopathic pattern. The muscle biopsy shows nonspecific features of a myopathy. A prominent inflammatory infiltrate, which is often multifocal in distribution, is present in some biopsy samples. The cause or significance of this finding is unknown.

⊠ **GENETIC CONSIDERATIONS** An autosomal dominant inheritance pattern with almost complete penetrance has been established, but each family member should be examined for the presence of the disease, since ~30% of those affected are unaware of involvement. FSH dystrophy is caused by deletions of tandem 3.3-kb repeats at 4q35. The deletion reduces the number of repeats to a fragment of <35 kb in most patients. This mutation results in an overexpression of upstream genes and a loss of DNA binding of a multiprotein complex mediating transcriptional repression of 4q35 genes. The mutation permits carrier detection and prenatal diagnosis. Most sporadic cases represent new mutations.

℞ TREATMENT

No specific treatment is available; ankle-foot orthoses are helpful for footdrop. Scapular stabilization procedures improve scapular winging but may not improve function.

OCULOPHARYNGEAL DYSTROPHY This form of muscular dystrophy represents one of several disorders characterized by progressive external ophthalmoplegia, which consists of slowly progressive ptosis and limitation of eye movements with sparing of pupillary reactions for light and accommodation. Patients usually do not complain of diplopia, in contrast to patients having conditions with a more acute onset of ocular muscle weakness (e.g., myasthenia gravis).

TABLE 368-4 *Distal Myopathies*

Disease	Clinical Features	Laboratory Features	Locus/Gene
Welander distal myopathy	Onset in fifth decade Weakness begins in hands Slow progression with spread to distal lower extremities Lifespan normal	Serum CK 2–3 × normal EMG myopathic NCS normal Muscle biopsy shows dystrophic features	AD inheritance Linked to chromosome 2p13
Tibial Muscular dystrophy (Markesbery/ Griggs/Udd)	Onset 4th to 8th decade Distal lower extremity weakness (tibial distribution) Upper extremities usually normal Lifespan normal	Serum CK 2–4 × normal EMG myopathic NCS normal Muscle biopsy shows dystrophic features Titin absent in M-line of muscle	AD inheritance Titin
Nonanka distal myopathy (distal myopathy with rimmed vacuoles)	Onset 2d to 3d decade Lower extremity distal weakness Mild distal upper limb weakness may be present early Progression to other muscles sparing quadriceps Ambulation may be lost in 10–15 years	Serum CK 3–10 × normal EMG myopathic NCS normal Dystrophic features on muscle biopsy plus rimmed vacuoles 15–19-nm filaments within vacuoles	AR Allelic to hereditary inclusion body myopathy GNE gene: UDP-*N*-acetylglucosamine 2-epimerase/*N*-acetylmannosamine kinase
Miyoshi myopathy	Onset 2d to 3d decade Lower extremity weakness in posterior compartment muscles Progression leads to weakness in other muscle groups Ambulation lost after 10–15 years in about one-third of cases	Serum CK 20–100 × normal EMG myopathic NCS normal Muscle biopsy shows nonspecific dystrophic features	AR Allelic to LGMD2B (see Table 368-3). Dysferlin

Abbreviations: CK, creatine kinase; AD, autosomal dominant; AR, autosomal recessive; EMG, electromyography; NCS, nerve conduction studies.

Clinical Features Oculopharyngeal muscular dystrophy has a late onset; it usually presents with ptosis and/or dysphagia in the fourth to sixth decade. The extraocular muscle impairment is less prominent in the early phase but may be severe later. The swallowing problem may become debilitating and result in pooling of secretions and repeated episodes of aspiration. Mild weakness of the neck and extremities also occurs.

Laboratory Features The serum CK level may be two to three times normal. Myopathic EMG findings are typical. On biopsy, muscle fibers are found to contain vacuoles, which by electron microscopy are shown to contain membranous whorls, accumulation of glycogen, and other nonspecific debris related to lysosomes. A distinct feature of oculopharyngeal dystrophy is the presence of tubular filaments, 8.5 nm in diameter, in muscle cell nuclei.

GENETIC CONSIDERATIONS Oculopharyngeal dystrophy has an autosomal dominant inheritance pattern with complete penetrance. The incidence is high in French-Canadians and in Spanish-American families of the southwestern United States. Large kindreds of Italian and of eastern European Jewish descent have been reported. The molecular defect in oculopharyngeal muscular dystrophy is a subtle expansion of a modest polyanine repeat tract in a poly-RNA binding protein (PABP2) in muscle.

Rx TREATMENT

Dysphagia can cause inanition, making oculopharyngeal muscular dystrophy a potentially life-threatening disease. Cricopharyngeal myotomy may improve swallowing, although it does not prevent aspiration. Eyelid crutches can improve vision in patients in whom ptosis obstructs vision; candidates for ptosis surgery must be carefully selected—those with severe facial weakness are not suitable.

DISTAL MYOPATHIES A group of muscle diseases, the distal myopathies, are notable for their preferential distal distribution of muscle weakness in contrast to most muscle conditions associated with proximal weakness. The major distal myopathies are summarized in Table 368-4.

Clinical Features Two of the conditions, *Welander distal myopathy* and *tibial muscular dystrophy*, are late-onset disorders, usually manifesting after age 40. *Nonanka distal myopathy* and *Miyoshi myopathy* are distinguished by their early onset in the late teens or twenties. Only Welander disease begins in the hands; all others start in the lower limbs. Miyoshi myopathy is unique in that gastrocnemius muscles are preferentially affected at onset. A clinical feature that makes all of these disorders confusing is that proximal muscles can be affected as the disorders progress (less so for Welander disease than others), perhaps diminishing the entire concept of the distal myopathy. In contrast to many genetic muscle diseases, the distal myopathies are for the most part limited to skeletal muscle.

Laboratory Features Serum CK is particularly helpful in diagnosing Miyoshi myopathy since it is very elevated. In the other conditions serum CK is only slightly increased. EMGs are myopathic. Muscle biopsy shows nonspecific dystrophic features. In Nonanka distal myopathy rimmed vacuoles, which contain 15- to 19-nm filaments, are common findings. Immune staining for gene product can be helpful in demonstrating titin abnormalities in tibial muscular dystrophy and reduced dysferlin in Miyoshi myopathy.

GENETIC CONSIDERATIONS Welander and tibial muscular dystrophy are inherited as autosomal dominant disorders, while Nonanka and Miyoshi myopathies are autosomal recessive conditions. The affected genes and their gene products are listed in Table 368-4. The gene for Welander disease awaits identification.

Rx TREATMENT

Occupational therapy is offered for loss of hand function; ankle-foot orthoses can support distal lower limb muscles.

CONGENITAL MYOPATHIES

These rare disorders are distinguished from muscular dystrophies by the presence of specific histochemical and structural abnormalities in muscle. Although primarily disorders of infancy or childhood, three forms that may present in adulthood are described here: central core disease, nemaline (rod) myopathy, and centronuclear (myotubular) myopathy. Other types, such as minicore myopathy (multi-minicore disease), fingerprint body myopathy, and sarcotubular myopathy, are not discussed.

CENTRAL CORE DISEASE Patients with central core disease may have decreased fetal movements and breech presentation. Hypotonia and delay in motor milestones, particularly in walking, are common. Later in childhood, patients develop problems with stair climbing, running, and getting up from the floor. On examination, there is mild facial, neck-flexor, and proximal-extremity muscle weakness. Legs are more affected than arms. Skeletal abnormalities include congenital hip dislocation, scoliosis, and pes cavus; clubbed feet also occur. Most cases are nonprogressive, but exceptions are well documented. Susceptibility to malignant hyperthermia must be considered as a potential risk factor for patients with central core disease.

The serum CK level is usually normal. Needle EMG demonstrates a myopathic pattern. Muscle biopsy shows fibers with single or multiple central or eccentric discrete zones (*cores*) devoid of oxidative enzymes. Cores occur preferentially in type 1 fibers and represent poorly aligned sarcomeres associated with Z disk streaming.

Autosomal dominant inheritance is characteristic; sporadic cases also occur. The disease is caused by point mutations of the ryanodine receptor gene on chromosome 19q, encoding the calcium-release channel of the sarcoplasmic reticulum of skeletal muscle; mutations of this gene also account for some cases of inherited malignant hyperthermia (Chap. 17). Malignant hyperthermia is an allelic condition; C-terminal mutations of the *RYR1* gene predispose to this complication.

Specific treatment is not required, but establishing a diagnosis of central core disease is extremely important, because these patients have a known predisposition to malignant hyperthermia during anesthesia.

NEMALINE MYOPATHY   The term *nemaline* refers to the distinctive presence in muscle fibers of rods or threadlike structures (Greek *nema*, "thread"). Nemaline myopathy is clinically heterogeneous. A severe neonatal form presents with hypotonia and feeding and respiratory difficulties, leading to early death. Nemaline myopathy usually presents in infancy or childhood with delayed motor milestones. The course is nonprogressive or slowly progressive. The physical appearance is striking because of the long, narrow facies, high-arched palate, and open-mouthed appearance due to a prognathous jaw. Other skeletal abnormalities include pectus excavatum, kyphoscoliosis, pes cavus, and clubfoot deformities. Facial and generalized muscle weakness, including respiratory muscle weakness, is common. An adult-onset disorder with progressive proximal weakness may be seen. Myocardial involvement is occasionally present in both the childhood and adult-onset forms. The serum CK level is usually normal or slightly elevated. The EMG demonstrates a myopathic pattern. Muscle biopsy shows clusters of small rods (nemaline bodies), which occur preferentially, but not exclusively, in type 1 muscle fibers. The muscle often shows type 1 muscle fiber predominance. Rods originate from the Z disk material of the muscle fiber.

Five genes have been associated with nemaline myopathy. All code for thin filament–associated proteins, suggesting disturbed assembly or interplay of these structures as a pivotal mechanism. Mutations of the nebulin (*NEB*) gene account for most cases, including both severe neonatal and early childhood forms, inherited as autosomal recessive disorders. Neonatal and childhood cases, inherited as predominantly autosomal dominant disorders, are caused by mutations of the skeletal muscle α-actinin (*ACTA1*) gene. In milder forms of the disease with autosomal dominant inheritance, mutations have been identified in both the slow α-tropomyosin (*TPM3*) and β-tropomyosin (*TPM2*) genes accounting for <3% of cases. Muscle troponin T (*TNNT1*) gene mutations appear to be limited to the Amish population in North America. No specific treatment is available.

MYOTUBULAR (CENTRONUCLEAR) MYOPATHY   Three distinct variants of centronuclear myopathy occur. A neonatal form, also known as *myotubular myopathy*, presents with severe hypotonia and weakness at birth. The late infancy–early childhood form presents with delayed motor milestones. Later, difficulty with running and stair climbing becomes apparent. A marfanoid, slender body habitus, long narrow face, and high-arched palate are typical. Scoliosis and clubbed feet may be present. Most patients exhibit progressive weakness, some requiring wheelchairs. Progressive external ophthalmoplegia with ptosis and varying degrees of extraocular muscle impairment are characteristic of both the neonatal and the late-infantile forms. A third variant, the late childhood–adult form, has an onset in the second or third decade. Patients have full extraocular muscle movements and rarely exhibit ptosis. There is mild, nonprogressive limb weakness and no associated skeletal abnormalities.

Normal or slightly elevated CK levels occur in each of the forms. EMG studies often give distinctive results, showing positive sharp waves and fibrillation potentials, complex and repetitive discharges, and rarely myotonic discharges. Muscle biopsy specimens in longitudinal section demonstrate rows of central nuclei, often surrounded by a halo. In transverse sections, central nuclei are found in 25 to 80% of muscle fibers.

A gene for the neonatal form of centronuclear myopathy has been localized to Xq28; this gene encodes myotubularin, a protein tyrosine phosphatase. Missense, frameshift, and splice-site mutations predict loss of myotubularin function in affected individuals. Carrier identification and prenatal diagnosis are possible. The inheritance pattern for the late infancy–early childhood disorder is probably autosomal recessive, and for the late childhood–adult form is probably autosomal dominant. No specific treatment is available.

DISORDERS OF MUSCLE ENERGY METABOLISM

There are two principal sources of energy for skeletal muscle—fatty acids and glucose. Abnormalities in either glucose or lipid utilization can be associated with distinct clinical presentations that can range from an acute, painful syndrome with rhabdomyolysis and myoglobinuria to a chronic, progressive muscle weakness simulating muscular dystrophy.

GLYCOGEN STORAGE AND GLYCOLYTIC DEFECTS ■ Disorders of Glycogen Storage Causing Progressive Weakness ■ *ACID MALTASE DEFICIENCY*   Three clinical forms of acid maltase deficiency (*type II glycogenosis*) can be distinguished. The infantile form is the most common, with onset of symptoms in the first 3 months of life. Infants develop severe muscle weakness, cardiomegaly, hepatomegaly, and respiratory insufficiency. Glycogen accumulation in motor neurons of the spinal cord and brainstem contributes to muscle weakness. Death usually occurs by 1 year of age. In the childhood form, the picture resembles muscular dystrophy. Delayed motor milestones result from proximal limb muscle weakness and involvement of respiratory muscles. The heart may be involved, but the liver and brain are unaffected. The adult form begins in the third or fourth decade. Respiratory failure and diaphragmatic weakness are often initial manifestations, heralding progressive proximal muscle weakness. The heart and liver are not involved.

In all forms of acid maltase deficiency, the serum CK level is 2 to 10 times normal. EMG examination demonstrates a myopathic pattern, but other features are especially distinctive, including myotonic discharges, trains of fibrillation and positive waves, and complex repetitive discharges. EMG discharges are very prominent in the lumbosacral paraspinal muscles. The muscle biopsy shows vacuoles containing glycogen and the lysosomal enzyme acid phosphatase. Electron microscopy reveals membrane-bound and free tissue glycogen. Definitive diagnosis is established by enzyme determination in muscle.

Acid maltase deficiency is inherited as an autosomal recessive disorder caused by mutations of the acid maltase gene. Recombinant human α-glucosidase infused intravenously is well tolerated. Clinical benefits in the infantile disease include reduced heart size, improved muscle tone, and longer life.

OTHER GLYCOGEN STORAGE DISEASES WITH PROGRESSIVE WEAKNESS   In *debranching enzyme deficiency* (*type III glycogenosis*), a slowly progressive form of muscle weakness can develop after puberty. Rarely, myoglobinuria may be seen. Patients are usually diagnosed in infancy, however, because of hypotonia and delayed motor milestones, hepatomegaly, growth retardation, and hypoglycemia. *Branching enzyme deficiency (type IV glycogenosis)* is a rare and fatal glycogen storage disease characterized by failure to thrive and hepatomegaly. Hypotonia and muscle wasting may be present, but the skeletal muscle manifestations are minor compared to liver failure.

Disorders of Glycolysis Causing Exercise Intolerance   Five glycolytic defects are associated with recurrent myoglobinuria: *myophosphorylase deficiency (type V glycogenosis), phosphofructokinase deficiency (type VII glycogenosis), phosphoglycerate kinase deficiency (type IX glycogenosis), phosphoglycerate mutase deficiency (type X glycogenosis),* and *lactate dehydrogenase deficiency (glycogenosis type XI).* Myophosphorylase deficiency, also known as *McArdle's disease,* is by far the most common of the glycolytic defects associated with exercise intolerance. These five glycolytic defects result in a common failure to support energy production at the initiation of exercise, although the exact site of energy failure remains controversial.

Clinical muscle manifestations in these five conditions usually begin in adolescence. Symptoms are precipitated by brief bursts of high-intensity exercise, such as running or lifting heavy objects. A history of myalgia and muscle stiffness usually precedes the intensely painful muscle contractures, which may be followed by myoglobinuria. Acute renal failure accompanies significant pigmenturia. Exercise tolerance can be enhanced by a slow induction phase (warm-up) or brief periods of rest, allowing for the start of the "second-wind" phenomenon (switching to utilization of fatty acids).

Certain features help distinguish some enzyme defects. Varying degrees of hemolytic anemia accompany deficiencies of both phosphofructokinase (mild) and phosphoglycerate kinase (severe). In phosphoglycerate kinase deficiency, the usual clinical presentation is a seizure disorder associated with mental retardation; exercise intolerance is an infrequent manifestation.

In all of these conditions, the serum CK levels fluctuate widely and may be elevated even during symptom-free periods. CK levels >100 times normal are expected, accompanying myoglobinuria. All patients with suspected glycolytic defects leading to exercise intolerance should undergo a forearm exercise test (Chap. 367). An impaired rise in venous lactate is highly indicative of a glycolytic defect. In lactate dehydrogenase deficiency, venous levels of lactate do not increase, but pyruvate rises to normal. A definitive diagnosis of glycolytic disease is made by muscle biopsy.

Myophosphorylase deficiency, phosphofructokinase deficiency, and phosphoglycerate mutase deficiency are inherited as autosomal recessive disorders. Phosphoglycerate kinase deficiency is X-linked recessive. Mutations can be found in the respective genes encoding the abnormal proteins in each of these disorders.

Training may enhance the second-wind phenomenon, but attempts to raise blood glucose or to modify these disorders through diet have not proved beneficial.

LIPID AS AN ENERGY SOURCE AND ASSOCIATED DEFECTS   Lipid is an important muscle energy source during rest and during prolonged, submaximal exercise. Fatty acids are derived from circulating very low density lipoprotein (VLDL) in the blood or from triglycerides stored in muscle fibers. Oxidation of fatty acids occurs in the mitochondria. To enter the mitochondria, a fatty acid must first be converted to an "activated fatty acid," acyl-CoA. The acyl-CoA must be linked with carnitine by the enzyme carnitine palmitoyltransferase (CPT) I for transport into the mitochondria. CPT I is present on the inner side of the outer mitochondrial membrane. Carnitine is removed by CPT II, an enzyme attached to the inside of the inner mitochondrial membrane, allowing transport of acyl-CoA into the mitochondrial matrix for β-oxidation.

Carnitine Palmitoyltransferase Deficiency   CPT II deficiency is the most common recognizable cause of recurrent myoglobinuria, more common than the glycolytic defects. Onset is usually in the teenage years or early twenties. Muscle pain and myoglobinuria occur after prolonged exercise. Strength is normal between attacks. Fasting predisposes to the development of symptoms. In contrast to disorders caused by defects in glycolysis, in which muscle cramps follow short, intense bursts of exercise, the muscle pain in CPT II deficiency does not occur until the limits of utilization have been exceeded and muscle breakdown has already begun. Episodes of rhabdomyolysis may produce severe weakness. In young children and newborns, CPT II deficiency can present with a very severe clinical picture including hypoketotic hypoglycemia, cardiomyopathy, liver failure, and sudden death.

Serum CK levels and EMG findings are both usually normal between episodes. A normal rise of venous lactate during forearm exercise distinguishes this condition from glycolytic defects, especially myophosphorylase deficiency. Muscle biopsy does not show lipid accumulation and is usually normal between attacks. The diagnosis requires direct measurement of muscle CPT.

CPT II deficiency is much more common in men than women (5:1); nevertheless, all evidence indicates autosomal recessive inheritance. A mutation in the gene for CPT II (chromosome 1p36) causes the disease in some individuals. It has been suggested that frequent meals and a low-fat, high-carbohydrate diet can prolong exercise tolerance. Others suggest substituting medium-chain triglycerides in the diet. Neither approach has proved beneficial.

Myoadenylate Deaminase Deficiency   The muscle enzyme myoadenylate deaminase converts adenosine 5′-monophosphate (5′-AMP) to inosine monophosphate (IMP) with liberation of ammonia. Myoadenylate deaminase may play a role in regulating adenosine triphosphate (ATP) levels in muscles. Most individuals with myoadenylate deaminase deficiency have no symptoms. There have been a few reports of patients with this disorder who have exercise-exacerbated myalgia and myoglobinuria. Many questions have been raised about the clinical effects of myoadenylate deaminase deficiency, and, specifically, its relationship to exertional myalgia and fatigability, but there is no consensus.

MITOCHONDRIAL MYOPATHIES

In 1972, Olson and colleagues recognized that muscle fibers with significant numbers of abnormal mitochondria could be highlighted with the modified trichrome stain; the term *ragged red fibers* was coined. By electron microscopy, the mitochondria in ragged red fibers are enlarged and often bizarrely shaped and have crystalline inclusions. Since that seminal observation, the understanding of these disorders of muscle and other tissues has expanded (Chap. 56).

Mitochondria play a key role in energy production. Oxidation of the major nutrients derived from carbohydrate, fat, and protein leads to the generation of reducing equivalents. The latter are transported through the respiratory chain in the process known as *oxidative phosphorylation.* The energy generated by the oxidation-reduction reactions of the respiratory chain is stored in an electrochemical gradient coupled to ATP synthesis.

A novel feature of mitochondria is their genetic composition. Each mitochondrion possesses a DNA genome that is distinct from that of the nuclear DNA. Human mitochondrial DNA (mtDNA) consists of a double-strand, circular molecule comprising 16,569 base pairs. It codes for 22 transfer RNAs, 2 ribosomal RNAs, and 13 polypeptides of the respiratory chain enzymes. The genetics of mitochondrial diseases differ from the genetics of chromosomal disorders. The DNA of mitochondria is directly inherited from the cytoplasm of the gametes, mainly from the oocyte. The sperm contributes very little of its mitochondria to the offspring at the time of fertilization. Thus, mitochondrial genes are derived almost exclusively from the mother, accounting for maternal inheritance of some mitochondrial disorders.

Patients with mitochondrial disorders have clinical manifestations that fall into three groups: chronic progressive external ophthalmoplegia (CPEO), skeletal muscle–central nervous system syndromes, and pure myopathy simulating muscular dystrophy.

PROGRESSIVE EXTERNAL OPHTHALMOPLEGIA SYNDROMES WITH RAGGED RED FIBERS   The single most common sign of a mitochondrial myopathy is CPEO, occurring in >50% of all mitochondrial myopathies. Varying degrees of ptosis and weakness of extraocular muscles are seen, usually in the absence of diplopia, a point of distinction from disorders with fluctuating eye weakness (e.g., myasthenia gravis).

KEARNS-SAYRE SYNDROME (KSS)

KSS is a widespread multiorgan system disorder with a defined triad of clinical findings: onset before age 20, CPEO, and pigmentary retinopathy plus one or more of the following features: complete heart block, cerebrospinal fluid protein > 1.0 g/L (100 mg/dL), or cerebellar ataxia. Some patients with CPEO and ragged red fibers may not fulfill all of the criteria for KSS. The cardiac disease includes syncopal attacks and cardiac arrest related to the abnormalities in the cardiac conduction system: prolonged intraventricular conduction time, bundle branch block, and complete atrioventricular block. Death attributed to heart block occurs in about 20% of the patients. Varying degrees of progressive limb muscle weakness and easy fatigability affect activities of daily living. Endocrine abnormalities are common including gonadal dysfunction in both sexes with delayed puberty, short stature, and infertility. Diabetes mellitus is a cardinal sign of mitochondrial disorders and is estimated to occur in 13% of KSS patients. Other less common endocrine disorders include thyroid disease, hyperaldosteronism, Addison's disease, and hypoparathyroidism. Both mental retardation and dementia are common accompaniments to this disorder. Serum CK levels are normal or slightly elevated. Serum lactate and pyruvate levels may be elevated. EMG is myopathic. Nerve conduction studies may be abnormal related to an associated neuropathy. Muscle biopsies reveal ragged red fibers, highlighted in oxidative enzyme stains, many showing defects in cytochrome oxidase. By electron microscopy increased numbers of mitochondria often appear enlarged with paracrystalline inclusions.

KSS is a sporadic disorder. The disease is caused by single mtDNA deletions presumed to arise spontaneously in the ovum or zygote. The most common deletion, occurring in about one-third of patients, removes 4977 bp of contiguous mtDNA. Monitoring for cardiac conduction defects is critical. Prophylactic pacemaker implantation is indicated when electrocardiograms demonstrate a bifascicular block. In KSS no benefit has been shown for supplementary therapies, including multivitamins or coenzyme Q10. Of all the proposed options, exercise might be the most applicable but must be approached cautiously because of defects in the cardiac conduction system.

AUTOSOMAL DOMINANT PROGRESSIVE EXTERNAL OPHTHALMOPLEGIA

This condition is caused by nuclear DNA mutations affecting mtDNA copy number and integrity and is thus inherited in a Mendelian fashion. Onset is usually after puberty. Fatigue, exercise intolerance, and complaints of muscle weakness are typical. Some patients notice swallowing problems. The neurologic examination confirms the ptosis and ophthalmoplegia, usually asymmetric in distribution. A sensorineural hearing loss may be encountered. Mild facial, neck flexor, and proximal weakness are typical. Rarely, respiratory muscles may be progressively affected and may be the direct cause of death. Serum CK is normal or mildly elevated. The resting lactates are normal or slightly elevated but may rise excessively after exercise. Spinal fluid protein is normal. The EMG is myopathic, and nerve conduction studies are usually normal. Ragged red fibers are prominently displayed in the muscle biopsy. Southern blots of muscle reveal a normal mtDNA band at 16.6 kb and several additional mtDNA deletion bands with genomes varying from 0.5 to 10 kb.

This autosomal dominant form of CPEO has been linked to loci on three chromosomes: 4q35, 10q24, and 15q22-26. In the chromosome 4q–related form of disease, mutations of the gene encoding the heart and skeletal muscle–specific isoform of the adenine nucleotide translocator 1 (ANT1) gene are found. This highly abundant mitochondrial protein forms a homodimeric inner mitochondrial channel through which ADP enters and ATP leaves the mitochondrial matrix. In the chromosome 10q–related disorder, mutations of the gene C10orf2 are found. Its gene product, twinkle, co-localizes with the mtDNA and is named for its punctate, starlike staining properties. The function of twinkle is presumed to be critical for lifetime maintenance of mitochondrial integrity. In the cases mapped to chromosome 15q,

a mutation affects the gene encoding mtDNA polymerase (POLG), an enzyme important in mtDNA replication.

Exercise may improve function but will depend on patients' ability to participate.

AUTOSOMAL RECESSIVE CARDIOMYOPATHY AND OPHTHALMOPLEGIA (ARCO)

ARCO is a rare mitochondrial disorder clinically important because of an associated life-threatening cardiomyopathy. CPEO is the initial manifestation, occurring between ages 8 and 10. Exercise intolerance and fatigue follow the early symptoms, accompanied by palpitations and chest pain. Examination reveals extraocular muscle weakness, ptosis, facial weakness, reduced muscle bulk, and limb weakness, greater in proximal muscles. A dilated cardiomyopathy is typical, and some patients have conduction system involvement. Death from congestive heart failure occurs as early as age 13. Serum lactate is normal at rest but increases with mild exercise. Serum CK is increased by two- to fourfold. EMG is normal or myopathic. Muscle biopsy demonstrates typical ragged red fibers. Multiple mtDNA deletions are seen on Southern blots of muscle. Echocardiograms show reduced ejection fraction. Conduction block is seen on electrocardiograms. The disease is inherited as an autosomal recessive disorder. The gene has not been identified. Heart failure may require orthotopic cardiac transplantation. Cardiac pacemakers are appropriate for patients with heart block.

mtDNA SKELETAL MUSCLE–CENTRAL NERVOUS SYSTEM SYNDROMES ■ Myoclonic Epilepsy with Ragged Red Fibers (MERRF)

The onset of MERRF is variable, ranging from late childhood to middle adult life. Characteristic features include myoclonic epilepsy, cerebellar ataxia, and progressive muscle weakness. The seizure disorder is an integral part of the disease and may be the initial symptom. Cerebellar ataxia precedes or accompanies epilepsy. It is slowly progressive, affects both trunk and limbs, and impairs gait and extremity functions. The third major feature of the disease is muscle weakness in a limb-girdle distribution. Other more variable features include dementia, peripheral neuropathy, optic atrophy, hearing loss, and diabetes mellitus.

Serum CK levels are normal or slightly increased. The serum lactate may be elevated. EMG is myopathic, and in some patients nerve conduction studies show the neuropathy. The electroencephalogram is abnormal, corroborating clinical findings of epilepsy. Typical ragged red fibers are seen on muscle biopsy. MERRF is caused by maternally inherited point mutations of mitochondrial transfer RNA (tRNA) genes. The most common mutation found in 80% of MERRF patients is an A to G substitution at nucleotide 8344 of tRNA lysine (A8344G tRNA^{lys}). Other tRNA^{lys} mutations include base-pair substitutions T8356C and G8363A. Only supportive treatment is possible, with special attention to epilepsy.

MITOCHONDRIAL MYOPATHY, ENCEPHALOPATHY, LACTIC ACIDOSIS, AND STROKE-LIKE EPISODES (MELAS)

MELAS is the most common mitochondrial encephalomyopathy. The term *stroke-like* is appropriate because the cerebral lesions do not conform to a strictly vascular distribution. The onset in the majority of patients is before age 20. Seizures, usually partial motor or generalized, are common and may represent the first clearly recognizable sign of disease. The cerebral insults that resemble strokes cause hemiparesis, hemianopia, and cortical blindness. A presumptive stroke occurring before age 40 should place this mitochondrial encephalomyopathy high in the differential diagnosis. Associated conditions include hearing loss, diabetes mellitus, hypothalamic pituitary dysfunction causing growth hormone deficiency, hypothyroidism, and absence of secondary sexual characteristics. In its full expression MELAS leads to dementia, a bedridden state, and a fatal outcome. Serum lactic acid is typically elevated. The spinal fluid protein is also increased but is usually ≤1.0 g/L (100 mg/dL). Muscle biopsies show ragged red fibers. Neuroimaging demonstrates basal ganglia calcification in a high percentage of cases. Focal lesions that mimic infarction are present predominantly in the occipital and parietal lobes. Strict vascular territories are not respected, and cerebral angiography fails to demonstrate lesions of the major cerebral blood vessels.

MELAS is caused by maternally inherited point mutations of mitochondrial tRNA genes. Most of the tRNA mutations are lethal, accounting for the paucity of multigeneration families with this syndrome. The A3243G point mutation in tRNA$^{Leu(UUR)}$ is the most common, occurring in ~80% of MELAS cases. About 10% of MELAS patients have other mutations of the tRNA$^{Leu(UUR)}$ gene including 3252G, 3256T, 3271C, and 3291C. Other tRNA gene mutations have also been reported in MELAS including G583A tRNA^{Phe}, G1642A tRNA^{Val}, G4332A tRNA^{Glu}, and T8316C tRNA^{Lys}. Mutations have also been reported in mtDNA polypeptide-coding genes. Two mutations were found in the ND5 subunit of complex I of the respiratory chain. A missense mutation has been reported at mtDNA position 9957 in the gene for subunit III of cytochrome C oxidase. No specific treatment is available. Supportive treatment is essential for the stroke-like episodes, seizures, and endocrinopathies.

PURE MYOPATHY SYNDROMES   Muscle weakness and fatigue can be the predominant manifestations of mtDNA mutations. When the condition affects exclusively muscle (pure myopathy), the disorder becomes difficult to recognize.

Mitochondrial DNA Depletion Myopathy   This disorder, clinically indistinguishable from muscular dystrophy, usually presents in the neonatal period with weakness, hypotonia, and delayed motor milestones. Some cases are rapidly fatal, with death before age 2. A milder form affects patients at a slightly later age. These patients have slowly evolving proximal muscle weakness simulating Duchenne muscular dystrophy. In some, seizures and cardiomyopathy may be present. Serum CK can reach levels of 20 to 30 times normal. Resting lactates vary from normal to mildly elevated. The EMG is myopathic, and ragged red fibers are seen on muscle biopsy. The mtDNA depletion syndrome is inherited as an autosomal recessive condition. Mutations have been identified in the *TK2* gene on chromosome 16q22 encoding thymidine kinase-2. The affected gene controls the supply of deoxyribonucleotides used for the synthesis of mtDNA. No specific treatment is available. Supportive care follows the approaches outlined for muscular dystrophy.

DISORDERS OF MUSCLE MEMBRANE EXCITABILITY

Muscle membrane excitability is affected in a group of disorders referred to as *channelopathies*. The heart may also be involved, resulting in life-threatening complications (Table 368-5).

CALCIUM CHANNEL DISORDERS OF MUSCLE ■ Hypokalemic Periodic Paralysis (HypoKPP)   Onset occurs at adolescence. Men are more often affected because of decreased penetrance in women. Episodic weakness with onset after age 25 is almost never due to periodic paralyses with the exception of thyrotoxic periodic paralysis (see below). Attacks are often provoked by meals high in carbohydrates or sodium and may accompany rest following prolonged exercise. Weakness usually affects proximal limb muscles more than distal. Ocular and bulbar muscles are less likely to be affected. Respiratory muscles are usually spared but when they are involved, the condition may prove fatal. Weakness may take as long as 24 h to resolve. Life-threatening cardiac arrhythmias related to hypokalemia may occur during attacks. Myotonia, if present, is confined to the eyelids. As a late complication, patients commonly develop severe, disabling proximal lower extremity weakness.

Attacks of thyrotoxic periodic paralysis resemble those of primary hypoKPP. Despite a higher incidence of thyrotoxicosis in women, men, particularly those of Asian descent, are more likely to manifest this complication. Attacks abate with treatment of the underlying thyroid condition.

A low serum potassium level during an attack, excluding secondary causes, establishes the diagnosis. Interattack muscle biopsies show the presence of single or multiple centrally placed vacuoles. Provocative tests with glucose and insulin to establish a diagnosis are usually not necessary and are potentially hazardous. HypoKPP is inherited as an autosomal dominant disorder with incomplete penetrance. Mutations in the voltage-sensitive, skeletal muscle calcium channel (Fig. 368-2) cause the disease.

The acute paralysis improves after the administration of potassium. Muscle strength and electrocardiogram should be monitored. Oral KCl (0.2 to 0.4 mmol/kg) should be given every 30 min. Only rarely is intravenous therapy necessary (e.g., swallowing problems or vomiting present). Administration of potassium in glucose or saline, which may further lower potassium, should be avoided. Mannitol is the preferred vehicle for administration of intravenous potassium. The long-term goal of therapy is to avoid attacks. This may reduce late-onset, fixed weakness. Patients should be made aware of the importance of a low-carbohydrate, low-sodium diet and consequences of intense exercise. Prophylactic administration of acetozolamide (125 to 1000 mg/d in divided doses) reduces or may abolish attacks. Paradoxically the potassium is lowered, but this is offset by the beneficial effect of metabolic acidosis. If attacks persist on acetozolamide, oral KCl should be added. Some patients require treatment with triamterine (25 to 100 mg/d) or spironolactone (25 to 100 mg/d).

SODIUM CHANNEL DISORDERS OF MUSCLE ■ Hyperkalemic Periodic Paralysis (HyperKPP)   The term *hyperkalemic* is misleading since patients are often normokalemic during attacks. The fact that attacks are precipitated by potassium administration best defines the disease. The onset is in the first decade. Attacks are brief and mild, usually lasting 30 min to 4 h. Weakness affects proximal muscles, sparing bulbar muscles. Attacks are precipitated by rest following exercise and fasting. In a variant of this disorder, the predominant symptom is myotonia without weakness (*potassium-aggravated myotonia*). The symptoms are aggravated by cold, and myotonia makes the muscles stiff and painful. This disorder can be confused with paramyotonia and myotonia congenita (described below).

Potassium may be slightly elevated but may also be normal during

TABLE 368-5   *Clinical Features of Periodic Paralysis and Nondystrophic Myotonias*

Feature	Calcium Channel Hypokalemic PP	Sodium Channel Hyperkalemic PP	Sodium Channel Paramyotonia Congenita	Potassium Channel Anderson's Syndrome[b]
Mode of inheritance	AD	AD	AD	AD
Age of onset	Adolescence	Early childhood	Early childhood	Early childhood
Myotonia[a]	No	Yes	Yes	No
Episodic weakness	Yes	Yes	Yes	Yes
Frequency of attacks of weakness	Daily to yearly	May be 2–3/d	With cold, usually rare	Daily to yearly
Duration of attacks of weakness	2–12 h	From 1–2 h to >1 day	2–24 h	2–24 h
Serum K⁺ level during attacks of weakness	Decreased	Increased or normal	Usually normal	Variable
Effect of K⁺ loading	No change	Increased myotonia, then weakness	Increased myotonia	No change
Effect of muscle cooling	No change	Increased myotonia	Increased myotonia, then weakness	No change
Fixed weakness	Yes	Yes	Yes	Yes

[a] May be paradoxical in paramyotonia congenita.
[b] Dysmorphic features and cardiac arrhythmias are distinguishing features (see text).

Abbreviations: AD, autosomal dominant; AR, autosomal recessive; PP, periodic paralysis.

FIGURE 368-2 Selected muscular dystrophy–associated proteins in the nuclear membrane and sarcomere. As shown in the exploded view, emerin and laminin A/C are constitutents of the inner nuclear membrane. Several dystrophy-associated proteins are represented in the sarcomere including titin, nebulin, calpain, telethonin, actinin, and myotilin. The position of the dystrophin-dystroglycan complex is also illustrated.

an attack. The EMG will often demonstrate myotonia during and between attacks. The muscle biopsy shows vacuoles that are smaller, less numerous, and more peripheral compared to the hypokalemic form. Provocative tests by administration of potassium can induce weakness but are usually not necessary to establish the diagnosis. HyperKPP and potassium-aggravated myotonia are inherited as autosomal dominant disorders. Mutations of the voltage-gated sodium channel SCN4A (Fig. 368-3) cause these conditions. For patients with frequent attacks acetozolamide (125 to 100 mg/d) is helpful.

Paramyotonia Congenita In paramyotonia congenita (PC) the attacks of weakness are cold-induced or occur spontaneously and are mild. Myotonia is a prominent feature but worsens with muscle activity (paradoxical myotonia). This is in contrast to classic myotonia in which exercise alleviates the condition. Attacks of weakness are seldom severe enough to require emergency room treatment. Over time patients develop interattack weakness as they do in other forms of periodic paralysis. PC is usually associated with normokalemia or hyperkalemia. Other features are similar to those of hyperKPP. PC is inherited as an autosomal dominant condition; voltage-gated sodium channel mutations (Fig. 368-3) are responsible. Patients with PC seldom seek treatment during attacks. Oral administration of glucose or other carbohydrates hastens recovery. Since interattack weakness may develop after repeated episodes, prophylactic treatment is usually indicated. Thiazide diuretics (e.g., chlorothiazide 250 to 1000 mg/d) and mexiletine (slowly increase dose from 450 mg/d) are reported to be helpful. Patients should be advised to increase carbohydrates in their diet.

POTASSIUM CHANNEL DISORDERS ■ Andersen's Syndrome This rare disease is characterized by episodic weakness, cardiac arrhythmias, and dysmorphic features (short stature, scoliosis, clinodactyly, hypertelorism, small or prominent low set ears, micrognathia, and broad forehead). The cardiac arrhythmias are potentially serious and life threatening. They include long QT, ventricular ectopy, bidirectional ventricular arrhythmias, and tachycardia. For many years the classification of this disorder was uncertain because episodes of weakness are associated with elevated, normal, or reduced levels of potassium during an attack. In addition, the potassium levels differ among kindreds but are consistent within a family. Inheritance is autosomal dominant, with incomplete penetrance and variable expressivity. The disease is caused by mutations of the inwardly rectifying potassium channel (*kir*) gene. The treatment is similar to that for other forms of periodic paralysis and must include cardiac monitoring. The episodes of weakness may differ between patients because of potassium variability. Acetazolamide will decrease the attack frequency and severity.

CHLORIDE CHANNEL DISORDERS Two forms of this disorder, autosomal dominant (*Thomsen's disease*) and autosomal recessive (*Becker's disease*) are related to the same gene abnormality. Symptoms are noted in infancy and early childhood. The severity lessens in the third to fourth decade. Myotonia is worsened by cold and improved by activity. The gait may appear slow and labored at first but improves with walking. In Thomsen's disease muscle strength is normal, but in Becker's, which is usually more severe, there may be muscle weakness. Muscle hypertrophy is usually present. Myotonia is prominently displayed by EMG recordings. Serum CK is normal or mildly elevated. The muscle biopsy shows hypertrophied fibers. The disease is inherited as dominant or recessive and is caused by mutations of the chloride channel gene (Fig. 368-3). Many patients will not require treatment and learn that the symptoms improve with activity. Medications that can be used to decrease myotonia include quinine, phenytoin, and mexilitene.

ENDOCRINE AND METABOLIC MYOPATHIES

Many endocrine disorders cause weakness. Muscle fatigue is more common than true weakness. The cause of weakness in these disorders is not well defined. It is not even clear that weakness results from

Sodium channel α subunit

Calcium channel α subunit

Chloride channel

FIGURE 368-3 The sodium and calcium channels are depicted here as containing four homologous domains, each with six membrane-spanning segments. The fourth segment of each domain bears positive charges and acts as the "voltage sensor" for the channel. The association of the four domains is thought to form a pore through which ions pass. Sodium channel mutations are shown along with the phenotype that they confer. HyperKPP, hyperkalemic periodic paralysis; PC, paramyotonia congenita; PAM, potassium-aggravated myotonia. See text for details.

The chloride channel is envisioned to have ten membrane-spanning domains. The positions of mutations causing dominantly and recessively inherited myotonia congenita are indicated, along with mutations that cause this disease in mice and goats.

disease of muscle as opposed to another part of the motor unit, since the serum CK level is often normal (except in hypothyroidism) and the muscle histology is characterized by atrophy rather than destruction of muscle fibers. Nearly all endocrine myopathies respond to treatment.

THYROID DISORDERS (See also Chap. 320)   Abnormalities of thyroid function can cause a wide array of muscle disorders. These conditions relate to the important role of thyroid hormones in regulating the metabolism of carbohydrates and lipids as well as the rate of protein synthesis and enzyme production. Thyroid hormones also stimulate calorigenesis in muscle, increase muscle demand for vitamins, and enhance muscle sensitivity to circulating catecholamines.

Hypothyroidism   Patients with hypothyroidism have frequent muscle complaints, and proximal muscle weakness occurs in about one-third of them. Muscle cramps, pain, and stiffness are common. Features of slow muscle contraction and relaxation occur in 25% of patients, and the relaxation phase of muscle stretch reflexes is characteristically prolonged. The serum CK level is often elevated (up to 10 times normal), even when there is minimal clinical evidence of muscle disease. *Hoffman's syndrome* results in prominent muscle enlargement and weakness with muscle stiffness. The cause of muscle enlargement has not been determined, and muscle biopsy shows no distinctive morphologic abnormalities.

Hyperthyroidism   Patients who are thyrotoxic commonly have proximal muscle weakness and atrophy on examination, but they rarely complain of the deficit. Muscle stretch reflexes are preserved and often brisk. Bulbar, respiratory, and even esophageal muscles may occasionally be affected, causing dysphagia, dysphonia, and aspiration. When bulbar involvement occurs, it is usually accompanied by chronic proximal limb weakness, but occasionally it presents in the absence of generalized thyrotoxic myopathy. Other neuromuscular disorders occur in association with hyperthyroidism, including hypokalemic, myasthenia gravis, and a progressive ocular myopathy associated with proptosis (*Graves' ophthalmopathy*). Serum CK levels are not elevated in thyrotoxic myopathy. The muscle histology usually shows only atrophy of muscle fibers.

PARATHYROID DISORDERS (See also Chap. 332) ■ **Hyperparathyroidism**   Muscle weakness is an integral part of primary and secondary hyperparathyroidism. Proximal muscle weakness, muscle wasting, and brisk muscle stretch reflexes are the main features of this endocrinopathy. Serum CK levels are usually normal or slightly elevated. Serum calcium and phosphorus levels show no correlation with the clinical neuromuscular manifestations. Muscle biopsies show only varying degrees of atrophy without muscle fiber degeneration.

Hypoparathyroidism   An overt myopathy due to hypocalcemia rarely occurs. Neuromuscular symptoms are usually related to localized or generalized tetany. Serum CK levels may be increased secondary to muscle damage from sustained tetany. Hyporeflexia or areflexia is usually present and contrasts with the hyperreflexia in hyperparathyroidism.

ADRENAL DISORDERS (See also Chap. 321)   Conditions associated with glucocorticoid excess cause a myopathy; in fact, steroid myopathy is the most commonly diagnosed endocrine muscle disease. Glucocorticoid excess, either endogenous or exogenous (see "Toxic Myopathies," below), produces various degrees of proximal limb weakness. Muscle wasting may be striking. A cushingoid appearance usually accompanies clinical signs of myopathy. Histologic sections demonstrate muscle fiber atrophy rather than degeneration or necrosis of muscle fibers. Adrenal insufficiency commonly causes muscle fatigue. The degree of weakness may be difficult to asses but is typically mild. In primary hyperaldosteronism (*Conn's syndrome*), neuromuscular complications are due to potassium depletion. The clinical picture is one of persistent muscle weakness. Long-standing hyperaldosteronism may lead to proximal limb weakness and wasting. Serum CK levels

may be elevated, and a muscle biopsy may demonstrate degenerating fibers, some with vacuoles. These changes relate to hypokalemia and are not a direct effect of aldosterone on skeletal muscle.

PITUITARY DISORDERS (See also Chap. 318)   Patients with acromegaly usually have mild proximal weakness without muscle atrophy. Muscles often appear enlarged but exhibit decreased force generation. The duration of acromegaly, rather than the serum growth hormone levels, correlates with the degree of myopathy.

DIABETES MELLITUS (See also Chap. 323)   Neuromuscular complications of diabetes mellitus are most often related to neuropathy, with cranial and peripheral nerve palsies or distal sensorimotor polyneuropathy. *Diabetic amyotrophy* is a clumsy term since the condition represents a neuropathy affecting the proximal major nerve trunks and lumbosacral plexus. More appropriate terms for this disorder include *diabetic proximal neuropathy* and *lumbosacral radiculoplexus neuropathy*.

The only notable myopathy of diabetes mellitus is ischemic infarction of thigh muscles. This condition occurs in patients with poorly controlled diabetes and presents with abrupt onset of pain, tenderness, and edema of one thigh. The area of muscle infarction is hard and indurated. The muscles most often affected include the vastus lateralis, thigh adductors, and biceps femoris. Computed tomography or magnetic resonance imaging can demonstrate focal abnormalities in the affected muscle. Diagnosis by imaging is preferable to muscle biopsy, if possible.

VITAMIN DEFICIENCY   Vitamin D deficiency (Chap. 61) due to either decreased intake, decreased absorption, or impaired vitamin D metabolism (as occurs in renal disease) may lead to chronic muscle weakness. Pain reflects the underlying bone disease (*osteomalacia*). Vitamin E deficiency may result from malabsorption. Clinical manifestations include ataxic neuropathy due to loss of proprioception and myopathy with proximal weakness. Progressive external ophthalmoplegia is a distinctive finding. It has not been established that deficiency of other vitamins causes a myopathy.

MYOPATHIES OF SYSTEMIC ILLNESS

Systemic illnesses such as chronic respiratory, cardiac, or hepatic failure are frequently associated with severe muscle wasting and complaints of weakness. Fatigue is usually a more significant problem than weakness, which is typically mild.

Myopathy may be a manifestation of chronic renal failure, independent of the better known uremic polyneuropathy. Abnormalities of calcium and phosphorus homeostasis and bone metabolism in chronic renal failure result from a reduction in 1,25-dihydroxyvitamin D, leading to decreased intestinal absorption of calcium. Hypocalcemia, further accentuated by hyperphosphatemia due to decreased renal phosphate clearance, leads to secondary hyperparathyroidism. Renal osteodystrophy results from the compensatory hyperparathyroidism, which leads to osteomalacia from reduced calcium availability and to osteitis fibrosa from the parathyroid hormone excess. The clinical picture of the myopathy of chronic renal failure is identical to that of primary hyperparathyroidism and osteomalacia. There is proximal limb weakness with bone pain.

Gangrenous calcification represents a separate, rare, and sometimes fatal complication of chronic renal failure. In this condition, widespread arterial calcification occurs and results in ischemia. Extensive skin necrosis may occur, along with painful myopathy and even myoglobinuria.

TOXIC MYOPATHIES

Toxic myopathies are relatively uncommon in clinical practice with the exception of those caused by the cholesterol-lowering agents and glucocorticoids. Others impact practice to a lesser degree but are important to consider in specific situations. Table 368-6 provides a comprehensive list of toxic myopathies with their distinguishing features.

MYOPATHY FROM LIPID-LOWERING AGENTS   All classes of lipid-lowering agents have been implicated in muscle toxicity including fibrates (clo-

TABLE 368-6 *Toxic Myopathies*

Drugs	Major Toxic Reaction

Lipid-lowering agents
  Fibric acid derivatives
  HMG-CoA reductase
    inhibitors
  Niacin (nicotinic acid)
	Drugs belonging to all three of the major classes of lipid-lowering agents can produce a spectrum of toxicity: asymptomatic serum creatine kinase elevation, myalgias, exercised-induced pain, rhabdomyolysis, and myoglobinuria.

Glucocorticoids	Acute, high-dose glucocorticoid treatment can cause acute quadriplegic myopathy. These high doses of steroids are often combined with nondepolarizing neuromuscular blocking agents but the weakness can occur without their use. Chronic steroid administration produces predominantly proximal weakness.

Nondepolarizing
  neuromuscular blocking
  agents
	Acute quadriplegic myopathy can occur with or without concomitant glucocorticoids.

Zidovudine	Mitochondrial myopathy with ragged red fibers.

Drugs of abuse
  Alcohol
  Amphetamines
  Cocaine
  Heroin
  Phencyclidine
  Meperidine
	All drugs in this group can lead to widespread muscle breakdown, rhabdomyolysis, and myoglobinuria. Local injections cause muscle necrosis, skin induration, and limb contractures.

Autoimmune toxic
  myopathy
  D-Penicillamine
	Use of this drug may cause polymyositis and myasthenia gravis.

Amphophilic cationic
  drugs
  Amiodarone
  Chloroquine
  Hydroxychloroquine
	All amphophilic drugs have the potential to produce painless, proximal weakness associated with autophagic vacuoles in the muscle biopsy.

Antimicrotubular drugs Colchicine	This drug produces painless, proximal weakness especially in the setting of renal failure. Muscle biopsy shows autophagic vacuoles.

fibrate, gemfibrozil), HMG-COA reductase inhibitors (referred to as *statins*), and niacin (nicotinic acid). Myalgia, malaise, and muscle tenderness are the most common manifestations. Muscle pain may be related to exercise. Patients may exhibit proximal weakness. Varying degrees of muscle necrosis are seen, and in severe reactions there are rhabdomyolysis and myoglobinuria. Patients improve with drug cessation. Concomitant use of statins with fibrates and cyclosporine is more likely to cause adverse reactions than use of one agent alone. Elevated serum CK is an important indication of toxicity. Muscle weakness is accompanied by a myopathic EMG, and muscle necrosis is observed by muscle biopsy. Myopathic reactions are indications for stopping the drug.

GLUCOCORTICOID-REALTED MYOPATHIES Glucocorticoid myopathy occurs with chronic treatment or as "acute quadriplegic" myopathy secondary to high-dose, intravenous glucocorticoids. Chronic administration produces proximal weakness accompanied by cushingoid manifestations, which can be quite debilitating; the chronic use of prednisone at a daily dose of ≥30 mg/d is most often associated with toxicity. Patients taking fluorinated glucocorticoids (triamcinolone, betamethasone, dexamethasone) appear to be at especially high risk for myopathy. Patients receiving high-dose, intravenous glucocorticoids for status asthmaticus, chronic obstructive pulmonary disease or other indications may develop severe generalized weakness. Involvement of the diaphragm and intercostal muscles causes respiratory failure and requires ventilatory support. In this setting, the use of glucocorticoids in combination with nondepolarizing neuromuscular blocking agents to further decrease airway resistance is particularly likely to lead to this complication. In chronic steroid myopathy the serum CK is usually normal. Serum potassium may be low. The muscle biopsy in chronic

cases shows preferential type 2 muscle fiber atrophy; this is not reflected in the EMG, which is usually normal. In acute cases with quadraplegic myopathy the muscle biopsy is abnormal, showing a distinctive loss of thick filaments by electron microscopy. By light microscopy there is focal loss of ATPase staining in central or paracentral areas of the muscle fiber. Calpain stains show diffusely reactive atrophic fibers. Withdrawal of glucocorticoids will improve the chronic myopathy. In acute quadriplegic myopathy, recovery is slow. Patients require supportive care and rehabilitation.

MYOPATHY OF NONDEPOLARIZING NEUROMUSCULAR BLOCKING AGENTS Patients may receive nondepolarizing neuromuscular blocking agents because of life-threatening airway resistance. Acute quadriplegic myopathy may result, with or without glucocorticoid use. The clinical features are identical to acute quadriplegic myopathy secondary to glucocorticoids.

DRUG INDUCED MITOCHONDRIAL MYOPATHY Zidovudine, used in the treatment of HIV infection, is a thymidine analogue that inhibits viral replication by interrupting reverse transcriptase. Myopathy is a well-established complication of this agent. Patients present with myalgias, muscle weakness, and atrophy affecting the thigh and calf muscles. The complication occurs in about 17% of patients treated with doses of 1200 mg/d for 6 months. The introduction of protease inhibitors for treatment of HIV infection has led to lower doses of zidovudine therapy and a decreased incidence of myopathy. Serum CK is elevated and EMG is myopathic. Muscle biopsy shows ragged red fibers with minimal inflammation; the lack of inflammation serves to distinguish zidovudine toxicity from HIV-related myopathy. If the myopathy is thought to be drug related the medication should be stopped or the dosage reduced.

DRUGS OF ABUSE AND RELATED MYOPATHIES Myotoxicity is a potential consequence of addiction to alcohol and illicit drugs. Ethanol is one of the most commonly abused substances with potential to damage muscle. Other potential toxins include cocaine, heroin, and amphetamines. The most deleterious reactions occur from overdosing leading to coma and seizures, causing rhabdomyolysis, myoglobinuria, and renal failure. Direct toxicity can occur from cocaine, heroin, and amphetamines causing muscle breakdown and varying degrees of weakness. The effects of alcohol are more controversial. Direct muscle damage is less certain, since toxicity usually occurs in the setting of poor nutrition and possible contributing factors such as hypokalemia and hypophosphatemia. Alcoholics are also prone to neuropathy and a variety of central nervous system disorders (Chap. 372).

Focal myopathies from self-administration of meperidine, heroin, and pentazocine can cause pain, swelling, muscle necrosis, and hemorrhage. The cause is multifactorial: needle trauma, direct toxicity of the drug or vehicle, and infection. When severe, there may be overlying skin induration and contractures with replacement of muscle by connective tissue. Elevated serum CK and myopathic EMG are characteristic of these reactions. The muscle biopsy shows widespread or focal areas of necrosis. In conditions leading to rhabdomyolysis, patients need adequate hydration to reduce serum myoglobin and protect renal function. In all of these conditions, counseling is essential to limit drug abuse.

DRUG-INDUCED AUTOIMMUNE MYOPATHIES The most consistent drug-related inflammatory or antibody-mediated myopathy is caused by D-penicillamine. This drug chelates copper and is used in the treatment of Wilson's disease. It is also used to treat other disorders including scleroderma, rheumatoid arthritis, and primary biliary cirrhosis. Adverse events include drug-induced polymyositis indistinguishable from the spontaneous disease. The incidence of this inflammatory muscle disease is about 1%. Myasthenia gravis is also induced by D-penicillamine, with a higher incidence estimated at 7%. These disorders resolve with drug withdrawal, although immunosuppressive therapy may be warranted in severe cases.

Scattered reports of other drugs causing an inflammatory myopathy are rare and include a heterogeneous group of agents: cimetidine, phenytoin, procainamide, and propylthiouracil. In most cases, a cause-and-effect relationship is uncertain. A complication of interest was related to L-tryptophan. In 1989 an epidemic of eosinophilia-myalgia syndrome (EMS) in the United States was caused by a contaminant in the product from one manufacturer. The product was withdrawn, and incidence of EMS diminished abruptly following this action.

OTHER DRUG-INDUCED MYOPATHIES Certain drugs produce painless, largely proximal, muscle weakness. These drugs include the ampho-philic cationic drugs (amiodarone, chloroquine, hydroxychloroquine) and antimicrotubular drugs (colchicine). Muscle biopsy can be useful in the identification of toxicity since autophagic vacuoles are prominent pathologic features of these toxins.

FURTHER READING

FAN X, ROULEAU GA: Progress in understanding the pathogenesis of oculo-pharyngeal muscular dystrophy. Can J Neurol Sci 30:8, 2003

FINSTERER J, STOLLBERGER C: The heart in human dystrophinopathies. Cardiology 99:1, 2003

KULLMANN DM, HANNA MG: Neurological disorders caused by inherited ion-channel mutations. Lancet Neurol 1:157, 2002

WIESER T et al: Carnitine palmitoyltransferase II deficiency: Molecular and biochemical analysis of 32 patients. Neurology 60:1351, 2003

369 POLYMYOSITIS, DERMATOMYOSITIS, AND INCLUSION BODY MYOSITIS
Marinos C. Dalakas

The inflammatory myopathies represent the largest group of acquired and potentially treatable causes of skeletal muscle weakness. They are classified into three major groups: polymyositis (PM), dermatomyositis (DM), and inclusion body myositis (IBM).

CLINICAL FEATURES The prevalence of the inflammatory myopathies is estimated at 1 in 100,000. PM as a stand-alone entity is a rare disease affecting adults. DM affects both children and adults, and women more often than men. IBM is three times more frequent in men than in women, more common in Caucasians than blacks, and is most likely to affect persons >50 years of age.

These disorders present as progressive and often symmetric muscle weakness. Patients usually report increasing difficulty with everyday tasks requiring the use of proximal muscles, such as getting up from a chair, climbing steps, stepping onto a curb, lifting objects, or combing hair. Fine-motor movements that depend on the strength of distal muscles, such as buttoning a shirt, sewing, knitting, or writing, are affected only late in the course of PM and DM, but fairly early in IBM. Falling is common in IBM because of early involvement of the quadriceps muscle with buckling of the knees. Ocular muscles are spared, even in advanced, untreated cases; if these muscles are affected, the diagnosis of inflammatory myopathy should be questioned. Facial muscles are unaffected in PM and DM, but mild facial muscle weakness is common in patients with IBM. In all forms of inflammatory myopathy, pharyngeal and neck-flexor muscles are often involved, causing dysphagia or difficulty in holding up the head (*head drop*). In advanced and rarely in acute cases, respiratory muscles may also be affected. Severe weakness, if untreated, is almost always associated with muscle wasting. Sensation remains normal. The tendon reflexes are preserved but may be absent in severely weakened or atrophied muscles, especially in IBM where atrophy of the quadriceps and the distal muscles is common. Myalgia and muscle tenderness may occur in a small number of patients, usually early in the disease, and particularly in DM associated with connective tissue disorders. Weakness in PM and DM progresses subacutely over a period of weeks or months and rarely acutely; by contrast, IBM progresses very slowly, over years, simulating a late-life muscular dystrophy (Chap. 368) or slowly progressive motor neuron disorder (Chap. 353).

SPECIFIC FEATURES (Table 369-1) ■ **Polymyositis** The actual onset of PM is often not easily determined, and patients typically delay seeking medical advice for several months. This is in contrast to DM, in which the rash facilitates early recognition (see below). PM mimics many other myopathies and is a diagnosis of exclusion. It is a subacute inflammatory myopathy affecting adults, and rarely children, who *do not have* any of the following: rash, involvement of the extraocular and facial muscles, family history of a neuromuscular disease, history of exposure to myotoxic drugs or toxins, endocrinopathy, neurogenic disease, muscular dystrophy, biochemical muscle disorder (deficiency

TABLE 369-1 *Features Associated with Inflammatory Myopathies*

Characteristic	Polymyositis	Dermatomyositis	Inclusion Body Myositis
Age at onset	>18 yr	Adulthood and childhood	>50 yr
Familial association	No	No	Yes, in some cases
Extramuscular manifestations	Yes	Yes	Yes
Associated conditions			
Connective tissue diseases	Yes[a]	Scleroderma and mixed connective tissue disease (overlap syndromes)	Yes, in up to 20% of cases[a]
Systemic auto-immune diseases[b]	Frequent	Infrequent	Infrequent
Malignancy	No	Yes, in up to 15% of cases	No
Viruses	Yes[c]	Unproven	Yes[c]
Drugs[d]	Yes	Yes, rarely	No
Parasites and bacteria[e]	Yes	No	No

[a] Systemic lupus erythematosus, rheumatoid arthritis, Sjögren's syndrome, systemic sclerosis, mixed connective tissue disease.

[b] Crohn's disease, vasculitis, sarcoidosis, primary biliary cirrhosis, adult celiac disease, chronic graft-versus-host disease, discoid lupus, ankylosing spondylitis, Behçet's syndrome, myasthenia gravis, acne fulminans, dermatitis herpetiformis, psoriasis, Hashimoto's disease, granulomatous diseases, agammaglobulinemia, monoclonal gammopathy, hypereosinophilic syndrome, Lyme disease, Kawasaki disease, autoimmune thrombocytopenia, hypergammaglobulinemic purpura, hereditary complement deficiency, IgA deficiency.

[c] HIV (human immunodeficiency virus) and HTLV-I (human T cell lymphotropic virus type I).

[d] Drugs include penicillamine (dermatomyositis and polymyositis), zidovudine (polymyositis), and contaminated tryptophan (dermatomyositis-like illness). Other myotoxic drugs may cause myopathy but not an inflammatory myopathy (see text for details).

[e] Parasites (protozoa, cestodes, nematodes), tropical and bacterial myositis (pyomyositis).

of a muscle enzyme), or IBM as excluded by muscle biopsy analysis (see below). As an isolated entity, PM is a rare (and overdiagnosed) disorder; more commonly, PM occurs in association with a systemic autoimmune or connective tissue disease, or with a known viral or bacterial infection. Drugs, especially D-penicillamine or zidovudine (AZT), may also produce an inflammatory myopathy similar to PM.

Dermatomyositis DM is a distinctive entity identified by a characteristic rash accompanying, or more often preceding, muscle weakness. The rash may consist of a blue-purple discoloration on the upper eyelids with edema (heliotrope rash; see Fig. 49-3), a flat red rash on the face and upper trunk, and erythema of the knuckles with a raised violaceous scaly eruption (*Gottron rash*; see Fig. 49-4). The erythematous rash can also occur on other body surfaces, including the knees, elbows, malleoli, neck and anterior chest (often in a *V sign*), or back and shoulders (*shawl sign*), and may worsen after sun exposure. In some patients the rash is pruritic, especially on the scalp, chest, and back. Dilated capillary loops at the base of the fingernails are also characteristic. The cuticles may be irregular, thickened, and distorted, and the lateral and palmar areas of the fingers may become rough and cracked, with irregular, "dirty" horizontal lines, resembling *mechanic's hands*. The weakness can be mild, moderate, or severe enough to lead to quadraparesis. At times, the muscle strength appears normal, hence the term *dermatomyositis sine myositis*. When muscle biopsy is performed in such cases, however, significant perivascular and perimysial inflammation is seen.

DM usually occurs alone but may overlap with scleroderma and mixed connective tissue disease. Fasciitis and thickening of the skin, similar to that seen in chronic cases of DM, have occurred in patients with the *eosinophilia-myalgia syndrome* associated with the ingestion of contaminated L-tryptophan.

Inclusion Body Myositis In patients ≥50 years of age, IBM is the most common of the inflammatory myopathies. It is often misdiagnosed as PM and suspected only later when a patient with presumed PM does not respond to therapy. Weakness and atrophy of the distal muscles, especially foot extensors and deep finger flexors, occur in almost all cases of IBM and may be a clue to early diagnosis. Some patients present with falls because their knees collapse due to early quadriceps weakness. Others present with weakness in the small muscles of the hands, especially finger flexors, and complain of inability to hold objects such as golf clubs or perform tasks such as turning keys or tying knots. On occasion, the weakness and accompanying atrophy can be asymmetric and selectively involve the quadriceps, iliopsoas, triceps, biceps, and finger flexors, resembling a lower motor neuron disease. Dysphagia is common, occurring in up to 60% of IBM patients, and may lead to episodes of choking. Sensory examination is generally normal; some patients have mildly diminished vibratory sensation at the ankles that presumably is age-related. The pattern of distal weakness, which superficially resembles motor neuron or peripheral nerve disease, results from the myopathic process affecting distal muscles selectively. Disease progression is slow but steady, and most patients require an assistive device such as cane, walker, or wheelchair within several years of onset.

In at least 20% of cases, IBM is associated with systemic autoimmune or connective tissue diseases. Familial aggregation of typical IBM may occur; such cases have been designated as *familial inflammatory IBM*. This disorder is distinct from *hereditary inclusion body myopathy* (h-IBM), which describes a heterogeneous group of recessive, and less frequently dominant, inherited syndromes; the h-IBMs are noninflammatory myopathies. A subset of h-IBM that spares the quadriceps muscles has emerged as a distinct entity. This disorder, originally described in Iranian Jews and now seen in many ethnic groups, is linked to chromosome 9p1 and results from mutations in the UDP-*N*-acetylglucosamine 2-epimerase/*N*-acetylmannosamine kinase (*GNE*) gene.

ASSOCIATED CLINICAL FINDINGS ■ Extramuscular Manifestations These may be present to a varying degree in patients with PM or DM, including:

1. *Systemic symptoms*, such as fever, malaise, weight loss, arthralgia, and Raynaud's phenomenon, especially when inflammatory myopathy is associated with a connective tissue disorder.
2. *Joint contractures*, mostly in DM and especially in children.
3. *Dysphagia and gastrointestinal symptoms*, due to involvement of oropharyngeal striated muscles and upper esophagus, especially in DM and IBM.
4. *Cardiac disturbances*, including atrioventricular conduction defects, tachyarrhythmias, dilated cardiomyopathy, and a low ejection fraction. Congestive heart failure and myocarditis may also occur, either from the disease itself or from hypertension associated with long-term use of glucocorticoids.
5. *Pulmonary dysfunction*, due to weakness of the thoracic muscles, interstitial lung disease, or drug induced pneumonitis (e.g., from methotrexate), which may cause dyspnea, nonproductive cough, and aspiration pneumonia. Interstitial lung disease may precede myopathy or occur early in the disease and develops in up to 10% of patients with PM or DM, most of whom have antibodies to t-RNA synthetases, as described below.
6. *Subcutaneous calcifications*, in DM, sometimes extruding on the skin and causing ulcerations and infections.

Association with Malignancies Although all the inflammatory myopathies can have a chance association with malignant lesions, especially in older age groups, the incidence of malignant conditions appears to be specifically increased only in patients with DM and not in PM or IBM. The most common tumors associated with DM are ovarian cancer, breast cancer, melanoma, colon cancer, and non-Hodgkin lymphoma. The extent of the search that should be conducted for an occult neoplasm in adults with DM depends on the clinical circumstances. Tumors in these patients are usually uncovered by abnormal findings in the medical history and physical examination and not through an extensive blind search. The weight of evidence argues against performing expensive, invasive, and nondirected tumor searches. A complete annual physical examination with pelvic, breast (mammogram, if indicated), and rectal examinations (with colonoscopy according to age and family history); urinalysis; complete blood count; blood chemistry tests; and a chest film should suffice in most cases. In Asians, nasopharyngeal cancer is common, and a careful examination of ears, nose, and throat is indicated.

Overlap Syndromes These describe the association of inflammatory myopathies with connective tissue diseases. A well-characterized overlap syndrome occurs in patients with DM who also have manifestations of systemic sclerosis or mixed connective tissue disease, such as sclerotic thickening of the dermis, contractures, esophageal hypomotility, microangiopathy, and calcium deposits (Table 369-1). By contrast, signs of rheumatoid arthritis, systemic lupus erythematosus, or Sjögren's syndrome are very rare in patients with DM. Patients with the overlap syndrome of DM and systemic sclerosis may have a specific antinuclear antibody, the anti-PM/Scl, directed against a nucleolar-protein complex.

PATHOGENESIS An autoimmune etiology of the inflammatory myopathies is indirectly supported by an association with other autoimmune or connective tissue diseases; the presence of various autoantibodies; an association with specific major histocompatibility complex (MHC) genes; demonstration of T cell–mediated myocytotoxicity or complement-mediated microangiopathy; and a response to immunotherapy.

Autoantibodies and Immunogenetics Various autoantibodies against nuclear antigens (antinuclear antibodies) and cytoplasmic antigens are found in up to 20% of patients with inflammatory myopathies. The antibodies to cytoplasmic antigens are directed against ribonucleoproteins involved in protein synthesis (anti-synthetases) or translational transport (anti-signal-recognition particles). The antibody directed against the histidyl-transfer RNA synthetase, called *anti-Jo-1*, accounts for 75% of all the anti-synthetases and is clinically useful because up to 80% of patients with anti-Jo-1 antibodies have interstitial lung disease. Some patients with the anti-Jo-1 antibody also have Raynaud's phenomenon, nonerosive arthritis, and the MHC molecules DR3 and DRw52. DR3 (molecular designation DRB1*0301, DQB1*0201) occurs in up to 75% of patients with PM and IBM, whereas in juvenile DM there is an increased frequency of DQA1*0501 (Chap. 296).

Immunopathologic Mechanisms In DM, humoral immune mechanisms are implicated, resulting in a microangiopathy and muscle ischemia (Fig. 369-1). Endomysial inflammatory infiltrates are composed of B cells located in proximity to CD4 T cells and macrophages; there is a relative absence of lymphocytic invasion of nonnecrotic muscle fibers. Activation of the complement C5b-9 membranolytic attack complex is thought to be a critical early event that triggers release of proinflam-

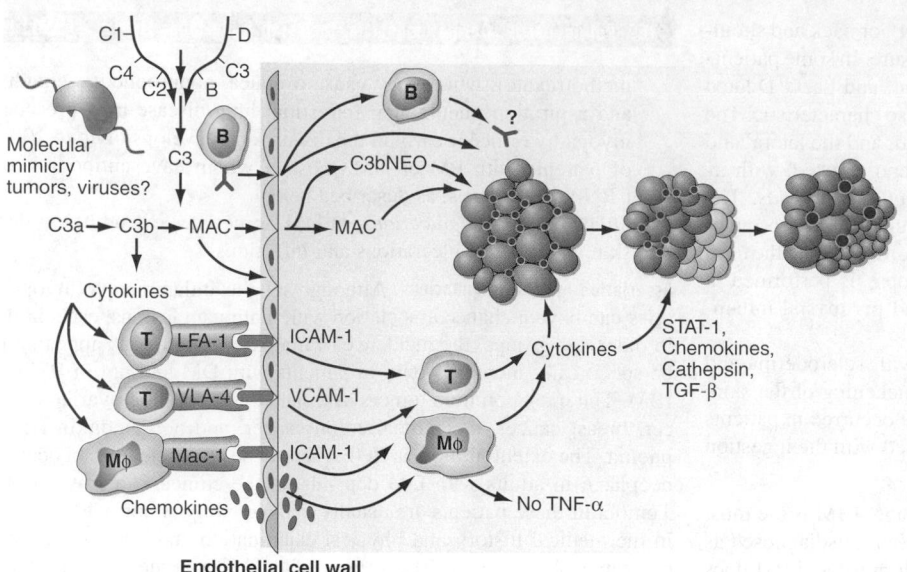

FIGURE 369-1 Immunopathogenesis of dermatomyositis. Autoantibodies (Y) possibly against endothelial cells, induce activation of complement and formation of C3 via the classic or alternative pathway. Activated C3 leads to formation of C3b, C3bNEO, and membrane attack complexes (MAC), which are deposited in and around the endothelial cell wall of the endomysial capillaries. Deposition of MAC leads to destruction of capillaries, ischemia, or microinfarcts most prominent in the periphery of the fascicles, and perifascicular atrophy. B cells, CD4 T cells, and macrophages (Mφ) traffic from the circulation to the muscle. Endothelial expression of vascular cell adhesion molecule (VCAM) and intercellular adhesion molecule (ICAM) is induced by cytokines released by the mononuclear cells. Integrins, specifically very late activation antigen (VLA)-4 and leukocyte function-associated antigen (LFA)-1, bind VCAM and ICAM and promote T cell and macrophage infiltration of muscle through the endothelial cell wall.

matory cytokines and chemokines, induces expression of vascular cell adhesion molecule (VCAM) 1 and intracellular adhesion molecule (ICAM) 1 on endothelial cells, and facilitates migration of activated lymphoid cells to the perimysial and endomysial spaces. Necrosis of the endothelial cells, reduced numbers of endomysial capillaries, ischemia, and muscle-fiber destruction resembling microinfarcts occur. The remaining capillaries often have dilated lumens in response to the ischemic process. Larger intramuscular blood vessels may also be affected in the same pattern. Residual perifascicular atrophy reflects the endofascicular hypoperfusion that is prominent in the periphery of the muscle fascicles.

By contrast, in PM and IBM a mechanism of T cell–mediated cytotoxicity is likely. CD8 T cells, along with macrophages, initially surround and eventually invade and destroy healthy, nonnecrotic muscle fibers that aberrantly express class I MHC molecules. MHC-I expression, absent from the sarcolemma of normal muscle fibers, is probably induced by cytokines secreted by activated T cells and macrophages. The CD8/MHC-I complex is characteristic of PM and IBM; its detection has now become necessary to confirm the histologic diagnosis of PM, as discussed later. The cytotoxic CD8 T cells contain perforin and granzyme granules directed towards the surface of the muscle fibers and capable of inducing myonecrosis. Analysis of T cell receptor molecules expressed by the infiltrating CD8 cells have revealed clonal expansion and conserved sequences in the antigen-binding region, both suggesting an antigen-driven T cell response. Whether the putative antigens are endogenous (e.g., muscle) or exogenous (e.g., viral) sequences is unknown. Viruses have not been identified within the muscle fibers. Key molecules involved in T cell–mediated cytotoxicity are depicted in Fig. 369-2.

The Role of Nonimmune Factors in IBM In IBM, the presence of vacuoles (almost always in fibers not invaded by T cells) together with β-amyloid deposits within the vacuolated muscle fibers and abnormal mitochondria with cytochrome oxidase–negative fibers suggest that, in addition to the autoimmune component, there is also a degenerative process. Similar to Alzheimer's disease, the amyloid deposits in IBM are immunoreactive against amyloid precursor protein (APP), chymotrypsin, apolipoprotein E, and phosphorylated tau, but it is unclear whether these deposits are directly pathogenic or represent secondary

phenomena. The same is true for the mitochondrial abnormalities, which may also be secondary to the effects of aging or a bystander effect of upregulated cytokines.

Association with Viral Infections and the Role of Retroviruses Several viruses, including coxsackieviruses, influenza, paramyxoviruses, mumps, cytomegalovirus, and Epstein-Barr virus, have been indirectly associated with myositis. For the coxsackieviruses, an autoimmune myositis triggered by molecular mimicry has been proposed because of structural homology between histidyl-transfer RNA synthetase that is the target of the Jo-1 antibody (see above) and genomic RNA of an animal picornavirus, the encephalomyocarditis virus. Sensitive polymerase chain reaction (PCR) studies, however, have repeatedly failed to confirm the presence of such viruses in muscle biopsies.

The best evidence of a viral connection in PM and IBM is with the retroviruses. Some individuals infected with HIV or with human T cell lymphotropic virus I (HTLV-1) develop PM or IBM; a similar disorder has been described in nonhuman primates infected with the simian immunodeficiency virus. The inflammatory myopathy may occur as the initial manifestation of a retroviral infection, or myositis may develop later in the disease course. Retroviral antigens have been detected only in occasional endomysial macrophages and not within the muscle fibers themselves, suggesting that persistent infection and viral replication within the muscle do not occur. Histologic findings are identical to retroviral-negative PM or IBM. This disorder should be distinguished from a toxic myopathy related to long-term therapy with AZT, characterized by fatigue, myalgia, mild muscle weakness, and mild elevation of creatine kinase (CK). AZT-induced myopathy, which generally improves when the drug is discontinued, is a mitochondrial disorder characterized histologically by "ragged-red" fibers. AZT inhibits γ-DNA polymerase, an enzyme found solely in the mitochondrial matrix.

DIFFERENTIAL DIAGNOSIS The clinical picture of the typical skin rash and proximal or diffuse muscle weakness has few causes other than DM. However, proximal muscle weakness without skin involvement can be due to many conditions other than PM or IBM.

Subacute or Chronic Progressive Muscle Weakness This may be due to denervating conditions such as the spinal muscular atrophies or amyotrophic lateral sclerosis (Chap. 353). In addition to the muscle weakness, upper motor neuron signs in the latter and signs of denervation detected by electromyography (EMG) aid in the diagnosis. The muscular dystrophies (Chap. 368) may be additional considerations; however, these disorders usually develop over years rather than weeks or months and rarely present after the age of 30. It may be difficult, even with a muscle biopsy, to distinguish chronic PM from a rapidly advancing muscular dystrophy. This is particularly true of facioscapulohumeral muscular dystrophy, dysferlin myopathy, and the dystrophinopathies where inflammatory cell infiltration is often found early in the disease. Such doubtful cases should always be given an adequate trial of glucocorticoid therapy and be screened for the respective genetic defect. Search for the MHC/CD8 lesion by immunocytochemistry is helpful to identify cases of PM as mentioned above. Some metabolic myopathies, including glycogen storage disease due to myophosphorylase or acid maltase deficiency, lipid storage myopathies due to carnitine deficiency, and mitochondrial diseases, produce weakness that is often associated with other characteristic clinical signs; diagnosis rests upon histochemical and biochemical studies of the muscle biopsy. The endocrine myopathies such as those due to hypercorticosteroidism, hyper- and hypothyroidism, and hyper- and hypoparathyroidism require the appropriate laboratory investigations for diagnosis. Muscle wasting in patients with an underlying neoplasm may be due to disuse, cachexia, or rarely to a paraneoplastic neuromyopathy (Chap. 87).

Diseases of the neuromuscular junction, including myasthenia gravis or the Lambert-Eaton myasthenic syndrome, cause fatiguing weakness that also affects the eye and cranial muscles (Chap. 366). Repetitive nerve stimulation and single-fiber EMG studies aid in diagnosis.

Acute Muscle Weakness This may be caused by an acute neuropathy such as Guillain-Barré syndrome (Chap. 365), transverse myelitis (Chap. 356), a neurotoxin (Chap. 368), or a viral infection such as poliomyelitis or West Nile virus (Chap. 360). When acute weakness is associated with painful muscle cramps, rhabdomyolysis, and myoglobinuria, it may be due to metabolic disorders including a glycogen storage disease such as myophosphorylase deficiency or carnitine palmityltransferase deficiency (Chap. 368). Acute viral infections may cause a similar syndrome. Several animal parasites, such as protozoa (*toxoplasma, trypanosoma*), cestodes (*cysticerci*), and nematodes (*trichinae*), may produce a focal or diffuse inflammatory myopathy known as *parasitic polymyositis*. *Staphylococcus aureus, Yersinia, Streptococcus,* or other anaerobic bacteria may produce a suppurative myositis, known as *tropical polymyositis*, or *pyomyositis*. Pyomyositis, previously rare in the west, is now occasionally seen in AIDS patients. Other bacteria, such as *Borrelia burgdorferi* (Lyme disease) and *Legionella pneumophila* (Legionnaire's disease) may infrequently cause myositis.

Patients with periodic paralysis develop episodes of recurrent painless acute muscle weakness, always beginning in childhood. Chronic alcoholics may develop painful myopathy with myoglobinuria after a bout of heavy drinking or present with a painless, acute hypokalemic myopathy, which is completely reversible with replacement therapy; other times they show an asymptomatic elevation of serum CK and myoglobin. Acute muscle weakness with myoglobinuria may occur with prolonged severe hypokalemia or with hypophosphatemia and hypomagnesemia, often seen in chronic alcoholics and in patients on nasogastric suction receiving parenteral hyperalimentation.

Macrophagic Myofasciitis This distinctive inflammatory muscle disorder presents as diffuse myalgias, fatigue, and mild muscle weakness. Muscle biopsy reveals pronounced infiltration of the connective tissue around the muscle by sheets of periodic acid–Schiff-positive macrophages and occasional CD8 T cells. The CK or erythrocyte sedimentation rate is variably elevated. Most patients respond to glucocorticoid therapy, and the overall prognosis seems favorable. Histologic involvement is focal and limited to sites of previous vaccinations, which may have been administered months or years earlier. This disorder, which to date has not been observed outside of France, has been linked to an aluminum-containing substrate used in vaccine preparation.

Drug-Induced Myopathies D-Penicillamine and procainamide may produce a true myositis resembling PM, and a DM-like illness had been associated with the contaminated preparations of L-tryptophan. As noted above, AZT causes a mitochondrial myopathy. Other drugs may elicit a toxic noninflammatory myopathy that is histologically different from DM, PM, or IBM. These include the cholesterol-lowering agents such as clofibrate, lovastatin, simvastatin, or provastatin, especially

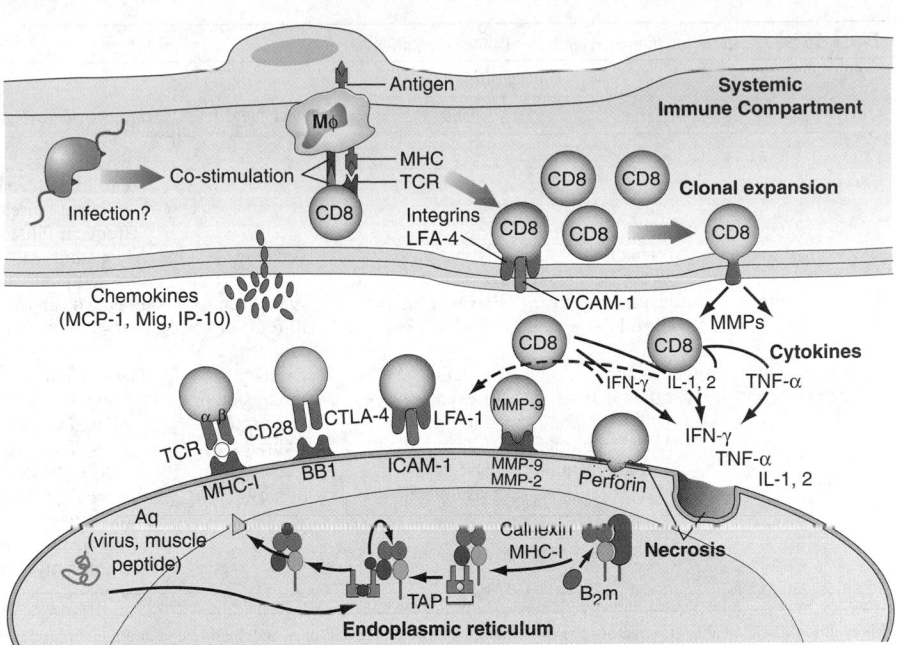

FIGURE 369-2 Cell-mediated mechanisms of muscle damage in polymyositis (PM) and inclusion body myositis (IBM). Antigen-specific CD8 cells are expanded in the periphery, cross the endothelial barrier, and bind directly to muscle fibers via T cell receptor (TCR) molecules that recognize aberrantly expressed MHC-I. Engagement of co-stimulatory molecules (BB1 and ICOSL) with their ligands (CD28, CTLA-4, and ICOS) along with ICAM-1/LFA-1, stabilize the CD8–muscle fiber interaction. Metalloproteinases (MMP) facilitate the migration of T cells and their attachment to the muscle surface. Muscle fiber necrosis occurs via perforin granules released by the autoaggressive T cells. A direct myocytotoxic effect exerted by the cytokines interferon (IFN)γ, interleukin (IL)1, or tumor necrosis factor (TNF) α may also play a role. Death of the muscle fiber is mediated by necrosis. MHC class I molecules consist of a heavy chain and a light chain [B₂ microglobulin (B₂M)] complexed with an antigenic peptide that is transported into the endoplasmic reticulum by TAP proteins (Chap. 296).

when combined with cyclosporine or gemfibrozil. Rhabdomyolysis and myoglobinuria have been rarely associated with amphotericin B, ε-aminocaproic acid, fenfluramine, heroin, and phencyclidine. The use of amiodarone, chloroquine, colchicine, carbimazole, emetine, etretinate, ipecac syrup, chronic laxative or licorice use resulting in hypokalemia, and glucocorticoids or growth hormone administration have also been associated with myopathic muscle weakness. Some neuromuscular blocking agents such as pancuronium, in combination with glucocorticoids, may cause the acute critical illness myopathy. A careful drug history is essential for diagnosis of these drug-induced myopathies, which do not require immunosuppressive therapy.

Pain on Movement and Muscle Tenderness A number of conditions including *polymyalgia rheumatica* (Chap. 306) and arthritic disorders of adjacent joints may enter into the differential diagnosis of inflammatory myopathy, even though they do not cause myositis. The muscle biopsy is either normal or discloses type II muscle fiber atrophy. Patients with *fibrositis* and *fibromyalgia* (Chap. 315) complain of focal or diffuse muscle tenderness, fatigue, and aching, which is sometimes poorly differentiated from joint pain. In other patients there may be suggestive signs of a collagen vascular disorder, such as an increased erythrocyte sedimentation rate, antinuclear antibody, or rheumatoid factor. Occasionally, there is slight but transient elevation of the serum CK. The muscle biopsy is usually normal and the prognosis favorable. Many such patients show some response to nonsteroidal anti-inflammatory agents, though most continue to have indolent complaints. *Chronic fatigue syndrome*, which may follow a viral infection, can present with debilitating fatigue, fever, sore throat, painful lymphadenopathy, myalgia, arthralgia, sleep disorder, and headache (Chap. 370). These patients do not have muscle weakness, and the muscle biopsy is normal.

DIAGNOSIS The clinically suspected diagnosis of PM, DM, or IBM is confirmed by examining the serum muscle enzymes, EMG findings, and muscle biopsy (Table 369-2).

The most sensitive enzyme is CK, which in active disease can be

TABLE 369-2 *Criteria for Diagnosis of Inflammatory Myopathies*

| Criterion | Polymyositis | | Dermatomyositis | Inclusion Body Myositis |
	Definite	Probable		
Myopathic muscle weakness[a]	Yes	Yes	Yes[b]	Yes; slow onset, early involvement of distal muscles, frequent falls
Electromyographic findings	Myopathic	Myopathic	Myopathic	Myopathic with mixed potentials
Muscle enzymes	Elevated (up to 50-fold)	Elevated (up to 50-fold)	Elevated (up to 50-fold) or normal	Elevated (up to 10-fold) or normal
Muscle biopsy findings[c]	"Primary" inflammation with the CD8/MHC-I complex and no vacuoles	Ubiquitous MCH-I expression but minimal inflammation and no vacuoles[d]	Perifascicular, perimysial, or perivascular infiltrates, perifascicular atrophy	Primary inflammation with CD8/MHC-I complex; vacuolated fibers with β-amyloid deposits; cytochrome oxygenase–negative fibers; signs of chronic myopathy[e]
Rash or calcinosis	Absent	Absent	Present[f]	Absent

[a] Myopathic muscle weakness, affecting proximal muscles more than distal ones and sparing eye and facial muscles, is characterized by a subacute onset (weeks to months) and rapid progression in patients who have no family history of neuromuscular disease, no endocrinopathy, no exposure to myotoxic drugs or toxins, and no biochemical muscle disease (excluded on the basis of muscle-biopsy findings).

[b] In some cases with the typical rash, the muscle strength is seemingly normal (dermatomyositis sine myositis); these patients often have new onset of easy fatigue and reduced endurance. Careful muscle testing may reveal mild muscle weakness.

[c] See text for details.

[d] An adequate trial of prednisone or other immunosuppressive drugs is warranted in probable cases. If, in retrospect, the disease is unresponsive to therapy, another muscle biopsy should be considered to exclude other diseases or possible evolution in inclusion body myositis.

[e] If the muscle biopsy does not contain vacuolated fibers but shows chronic myopathy with hypertrophic fibers, primary inflammation with the CD8/MHC-I complex and cytochrome oxygenase–negative fibers, the diagnosis is probable inclusion body myositis.

[f] If rash is absent but muscle biopsy findings are characteristic of dermatomyositis, the diagnosis is probable DM.

elevated as much as 50-fold. Although the CK level usually parallels disease activity, it can be normal in some patients with active IBM or DM, especially when associated with a connective tissue disease. The CK is always elevated in patients with active PM. Along with the CK, the serum glutamic-oxaloacetic and glutamate pyruvate transaminases, lactate dehydrogenase, and aldolase may be elevated.

Needle EMG shows myopathic potentials characterized by short-duration, low-amplitude polyphasic units on voluntary activation and increased spontaneous activity with fibrillations, complex repetitive discharges, and positive sharp waves. Mixed potentials (polyphasic units of short and long duration) indicating a chronic process and muscle fiber regeneration are often present in IBM. These EMG findings are not diagnostic of an inflammatory myopathy but are useful to identify the presence of active or chronic myopathy and to exclude neurogenic disorders.

Magnetic resonance imaging is not routinely used for the diagnosis of PM, DM, or IBM. However, it may guide the location of the muscle biopsy in certain clinical settings.

Muscle biopsy is the definitive test for establishing the diagnosis of inflammatory myopathy and for excluding other neuromuscular diseases. Inflammation is the histologic hallmark for these diseases; however, additional features are characteristic of each subtype.

In PM the inflammation is *primary*, a term used to indicate that T cell infiltrates, located primarily within the muscle fascicles (endomysially), surround individual, healthy muscle fibers and result in phagocytosis and necrosis. The MHC-I molecule is ubiquitously expressed on the sarcolemma, even in fibers not invaded by CD8+ cells. The CD8/MHC-I lesion is now fundamental for confirming or establishing the diagnosis and to exclude disorders with secondary, nonspecific, inflammation. When the disease is chronic, connective tissue is increased and may react positively with alkaline phosphatase.

In DM the endomysial inflammation is predominantly perivascular or in the interfascicular septae and around, rather than within, the muscle fascicles. The intramuscular blood vessels show endothelial hyperplasia with tubuloreticular profiles, fibrin thrombi, and obliteration of capillaries. The muscle fibers undergo necrosis, degeneration, and phagocytosis, often in groups involving a portion of a muscle fasciculus in a wedgelike shape or at the periphery of the fascicle, due to microinfarcts within the muscle. This results in perifascicular atrophy, characterized by 2 to 10 layers of atrophic fibers at the periphery of the fascicles. The presence of perifascicular atrophy is diagnostic of DM, *even in the absence of inflammation*.

In IBM, there is endomysial inflammation with T cells invading MHC-I-expressing nonvacuolated muscle fibers; basophilic granular deposits distributed around the edge of slitlike vacuoles (rimmed vacuoles); loss of fibers, replaced by fat and connective tissue, hypertrophic fibers, and angulated or round fibers; eosinophilic cytoplasmic inclusions; abnormal mitochondria characterized by the presence of ragged-red fibers or cytochrome oxidase–negative fibers; amyloid deposits within or next to the vacuoles; and filamentous inclusions seen by electron microscopy in the vicinity of the rimmed vacuoles.

℞ TREATMENT

The goal of therapy is to improve muscle strength, thereby improving function in activities of daily living, and ameliorate the extramuscular manifestations (rash, dysphagia, dyspnea, fever). When strength improves, the serum CK falls concurrently; however, the reverse is not always true. Unfortunately, there is a common tendency to "chase" or treat the CK level instead of the muscle weakness, a practice that has led to prolonged and unnecessary use of immunosuppressive drugs and erroneous assessment of their efficacy. It is prudent to discontinue these drugs if, after an adequate trial, there is no objective improvement in muscle strength whether or not CK levels are reduced. Agents used in the treatment of PM and DM include:

1. *Glucocorticoids*. Oral prednisone is the initial treatment of choice; the effectiveness and side effects of this therapy determine the future need for stronger immunosuppressive drugs. High-dose prednisone, at least 1 mg/kg per day, is initiated as early in the disease as possible. After 3 to 4 weeks, prednisone is tapered slowly over a period of 10 weeks to 1 mg/kg every other day. If there is evidence of efficacy and no serious side effects, the dosage is then further reduced by 5 or 10 mg every 3 to 4 weeks until the lowest possible dose that controls the disease is reached. The efficacy of prednisone is determined by an objective increase in muscle strength and activities of daily living, which almost always occur by the third month of therapy. A feeling of increased energy or a reduction of the CK level without a concomitant increase in muscle strength is not a reliable sign of improvement. If prednisone provides no objective benefit after ~3 months of high-dose therapy, the disease is probably unresponsive to the drug and tapering should be accelerated while the next-in-line immunosuppressive drug is started. Although controlled trials have not been performed, almost all patients with true PM or DM respond to glucocorticoids to *some degree and for some period of time*; in general, DM responds better than PM.

The long-term use of prednisone may cause increased weakness associated with a normal or unchanged CK level; this effect is referred to as *steroid myopathy*. In a patient who previously responded to high doses of prednisone, the development of new weakness may be related to steroid myopathy or to disease activity that either will respond to a higher dose of glucocorticoids or has become glucocorticoid-resistant. In uncertain cases, the prednisone dosage can be adjusted arbitrarily: the cause of the weakness is usually evident in 2 to 8 weeks.

2. *Other immunosuppressive drugs.* Approximately 75% of patients ultimately require additional treatment. This occurs when a patient fails to respond adequately to glucocorticoids after a 3-month trial, the patient becomes glucocorticoid-resistant, glucocorticoid-related side effects appear, attempts to lower the prednisone dose repeatedly result in a new relapse, or rapidly progressive disease with evolving severe weakness and respiratory failure develops.

The following drugs are commonly used: (1) *Azathioprine* is well tolerated, has few side effects, and appears to be as effective for long-term therapy as other drugs. The dose is up to 3 mg/kg daily. (2) *Methotrexate* has a faster onset of action than azathioprine. It is given orally starting at 7.5 mg weekly for the first 3 weeks (2.5 mg every 12 h for 3 doses), with gradual dose escalation by 2.5 mg per week to a total of 25 mg weekly. A rare side effect is methotrexate pneumonitis, which can be difficult to distinguish from the interstitial lung disease of the primary myopathy associated with Jo-1 antibodies (described above). (3) *Cyclophosphamide* (0.5 to 1 g IV monthly for 6 months) has limited success and significant toxicity. (4) *Chlorambucil* has variable results. (5) *Cyclosporine* has inconsistent and mild benefit. (6) *Mycophenolate mofetil* has recently shown some effectiveness.

3. *Immunomodulation.* In a controlled trial of patients with refractory DM, intravenous immunoglobulin (IVIg) improved not only strength and rash but also the underlying immunopathology. The benefit is often short-lived (≤8 weeks); repeated infusions every 6 to 8 weeks are generally required to maintain improvement. A dose of 2 g/kg divided over 2 to 5 days per course is recommended. Uncontrolled observations suggest that IVIg may also be beneficial for patients with PM. Neither plasmapheresis nor leukapheresis appears to be effective in PM and DM.

The following sequential empirical approach to the treatment of PM and DM is suggested: *Step 1*: high-dose prednisone; *step 2*: azathioprine or methotrexate; *step 3*: IVIg; *step 4*: a trial, with guarded optimism, of one of the following agents, chosen according to the patient's age, degree of disability, tolerance, experience with the drug, and the patient's general health: cyclosporine, chlorambucil, cyclophosphamide, mycophenolate. Patients with interstitial lung disease may benefit from aggressive treatment with cyclophosphamide.

A patient with presumed PM who has not responded to any form of immunotherapy most likely has IBM or another disease, usually a metabolic myopathy, a muscular dystrophy, a drug-induced myopathy, or an endocrinopathy. In these cases, a repeat muscle biopsy and a renewed search for another cause of the myopathy is indicated.

Calcinosis, a manifestation of DM, is difficult to treat; however, new calcium deposits may be prevented if the primary disease responds to the available therapies. Diphosphonates, aluminum hydrox-ide, probenecid, colchicine, low doses of warfarin, calcium blockers, and surgical excision have all been tried without success.

IBM is generally resistant to immunosuppressive therapies. Prednisone together with azathioprine or methotrexate is often tried for a few months in newly diagnosed patients, although results are generally disappointing. Because occasional patients may feel subjectively weaker after these drugs are discontinued, some clinicians prefer to maintain some patients on low-dose, every-other-day prednisone or weekly methotrexate in an effort to halt disease progression, even though there is no objective evidence or controlled study to support this practice. In two controlled studies of IVIg in IBM, minimal benefit in up to 30% of patients was found; the strength gains, however, were not of sufficient magnitude to justify its routine use. Another trial of IVIg combined with prednisone was ineffective. Nonetheless, many experts believe that a 2- to 3-month trial with IVIg may be reasonable for selected patients with IBM who experience rapid progression of muscle weakness or choking episodes due to worsening dysphagia.

PROGNOSIS The 5-year survival rate for treated patients with PM and DM is ~95% and the 10-year survival 84%; death is usually due to pulmonary, cardiac, or other systemic complications. Patients severely affected at presentation or treated after long delays, those with severe dysphagia or respiratory difficulties, older patients, and those with associated cancer have a worse prognosis. DM responds more favorably to therapy than PM and thus has a better prognosis. Most patients improve with therapy, and many make a full functional recovery, which is often sustained with maintenance therapy. Up to 30% may be left with some residual muscle weakness. Relapses may occur at any time.

IBM has the least favorable prognosis of the inflammatory myopathies. Most patients will require the use of an assistive device such as a cane, walker, or wheelchair within 5 to 10 years of onset. In general, the older the age of onset in IBM, the more rapidly progressive is the course.

FURTHER READING

ASKANAS V, ENGEL WK: Inclusion body myopathies: Different etiologies, possibly similar pathogenic mechanisms. Curr Opin Neurol 15:525, 2002

DALAKAS MC: The molecular and cellular pathology of inflammatory muscle diseases. Curr Opin Pharmacol 1:300, 2001

———: Understanding the immunopathogenesis of inclusion body myositis: Present and future prospects. Rev Neurol 158:948, 2002

———, HOHLFELD R: Polymyositis and dermatomyositis. Lancet. 362:971, 2003

HILTON-JONES D: Inflammatory myopathies. Curr Opin Neurol 14:591, 2001

MARIE I et al: Polymyositis and dermatomyositis: Short term and long term outcome and predictive factors of prognosis. J Rheumatol 28:2230, 2001

MASTAGLIA FL: Inflammatory myopathies: Clinical, diagnostic and therapeutic aspects. Muscle Nerve 27:407, 2003

SONTHEIMER RD: Dermatomyositis: An overview of recent progress with emphasis on dermatologic aspects. Dermatol Clin 20:387, 2002

Section 4 Chronic Fatigue Syndrome

370 CHRONIC FATIGUE SYNDROME
Stephen E. Straus

DEFINITION *Chronic fatigue syndrome* (CFS) is the current name for a disorder characterized by debilitating fatigue and several associated physical, constitutional, and neuropsychological complaints (Table 370-1). This syndrome is not new; in the past, patients diagnosed with conditions such as the vapors, neurasthenia, effort syndrome, chronic brucellosis, epidemic neuromyasthenia, myalgic encephalomyelitis, hypoglycemia, multiple chemical sensitivity syndrome, chronic candidiasis, chronic mononucleosis, chronic Epstein-Barr virus infection, and postviral fatigue syndrome may have had what is now called CFS. A subset of ill veterans of military campaigns suffer from CFS. The U.S. Centers for Disease Control and Prevention (CDC) has developed diagnostic criteria for CFS based upon symptoms and the exclusion of other illnesses (Table 370-2).

EPIDEMIOLOGY Patients with CFS are twice as likely to be women as men and are generally 25 to 45 years old, although cases in childhood and in later life have been described.

Cases are recognized in many developed countries. Most arise spo-

TABLE 370-1   *Specific Symptoms Reported by Patients with Chronic Fatigue Syndrome*

Symptom	Percentage
Fatigue	100
Difficulty concentrating	90
Headache	90
Sore throat	85
Tender lymph nodes	80
Muscle aches	80
Joint aches	75
Feverishness	75
Difficulty sleeping	70
Psychiatric problems	65
Allergies	55
Abdominal cramps	40
Weight loss	20
Rash	10
Rapid pulse	10
Weight gain	5
Chest pain	5
Night sweats	5

Source: From SE Straus: J Infect Diseases 157:405, 1988; with permission.

radically, but many clusters have also been reported. Famous outbreaks of CFS occurred in Los Angeles County Hospital in 1934; in Akureyri, Iceland, in 1948; in the Royal Free Hospital, London, in 1955; and in Incline Village, Nevada, in 1985. While these clustered cases suggest a common environmental or infectious cause, none has been identified.

Estimates of the prevalence of CFS have depended on the case definition used and the method of study. Chronic fatigue itself is a common symptom, occurring in as many as 20% of patients attending general medical clinics; CFS is far less common. Community-based studies find that 100 to 300 individuals per 100,000 population in the United States meet the current CDC case definition.

PATHOGENESIS   The diverse names for the syndrome reflect the many and controversial hypotheses about its etiology. Several common themes underlie attempts to understand the disorder: It is often postinfectious, it is associated with immunologic disturbances, and it is commonly accompanied or even preceded by neuropsychological complaints, somatic preoccupation, and/or depression.

Many studies in the 1980s and 1990s attempted to link CFS to infection with Epstein-Barr virus, a retrovirus, or an enterovirus. In many patients with chronic fatigue, titers of antibodies to several viruses are elevated. Reports that viral antigens and nucleic acids could be specifically identified in patients with CFS have not been confirmed. One study from the United Kingdom failed to detect any association between acute infections and subsequent prolonged fatigue. Another study found that chronic fatigue did not develop after typical upper respiratory infections but did in some individuals after infectious mononucleosis. Thus, while antecedent viral infections are associated with CFS, a direct viral pathogenesis is unproven and unlikely.

Changes in numerous immune parameters of uncertain functional significance have been reported in CFS. Modest elevations in titers of antinuclear antibodies, reductions in immunoglobulin subclasses, deficiencies in mitogen-driven lymphocyte proliferation, reductions in natural killer cell activity, disturbances in cytokine production, and shifts in lymphocyte subsets have been described. None of the immune findings appears in all patients, nor do any correlate with the severity of CFS. Careful comparison of affected and unaffected monozygotic twins showed no substantive immunologic differences. In theory, symptoms of CFS could result from excessive production of a cytokine, such as interleukin 1, that induces asthenia and other flulike symptoms; however, compelling data in support of this long-held hypothesis are lacking.

In some studies, patients with CFS manifest unusual sensitivity to

sustained upright tilting, resulting in hypotension and syncope, so as to suggest a form of dysautonomia.

Disturbances in the hypothalamic-pituitary-adrenal function have been identified in several controlled studies of CFS, with some evidence for normalization in patients whose fatigue abates. These neuroendocrine abnormalities could contribute to the impaired energy and depressed mood of patients.

Mild to moderate depression is present in half to two-thirds of patients. Much of this depression may be reactive, but its prevalence exceeds that seen in other chronic medical illnesses. Some propose that CFS is fundamentally a psychiatric disorder and that the various neuroendocrine and immune disturbances arise secondarily.

MANIFESTATIONS   Typically, CFS arises suddenly in a previously active individual. An otherwise unremarkable flulike illness or some other acute stress leaves unbearable exhaustion in its wake. Other symptoms, such as headache, sore throat, tender lymph nodes, muscle and joint aches, and frequent feverishness, lead to the belief that an infection persists, and medical attention is sought. Over several weeks, despite reassurances that nothing serious is wrong, the symptoms persist and other features of the syndrome become evident—disturbed sleep, difficulty in concentration, and depression (Table 370-1).

Depending on the dominant symptoms and the beliefs of the patient, additional consultations may be sought from allergists, rheumatologists, infectious disease specialists, psychiatrists, ecologic therapists, homeopaths, or other professionals, frequently with unsatisfactory results. Once the pattern of illness is established, the symptoms may fluctuate somewhat. Many patients report that diverse complaints are linked—that during periods of greatest fatigue they perceive the most pain and difficulty with concentration. Patients also commonly assert that excessive physical or emotional stress may exacerbate their symptoms.

Most patients remain capable of meeting family, work, or community obligations despite their symptoms; discretionary activities are abandoned first. Some feel unable to engage in any gainful employment. A minority of individuals require help with the activities of daily living.

Ultimately, isolation, frustration, and pathetic resignation can mark the protracted course of illness. Patients may become angry at physicians for failing to acknowledge or resolve their plight. Fortunately, CFS does not appear to progress. On the contrary, many patients experience gradual improvement, and a minority recover fully.

DIAGNOSIS   A thorough history, physical examination, and judicious use of laboratory tests are required to exclude other causes of the patient's symptoms. Prominent abnormalities argue strongly in favor of alternative diagnoses. No laboratory test, however, can diagnose this condition or measure its severity. In most cases, elaborate, expensive workups are not helpful. Early claims that magnetic resonance imaging or single photon emission computed tomography can identify

TABLE 370-2   *CDC Criteria for Diagnosis of Chronic Fatigue Syndrome*

A case of chronic fatigue syndrome is defined by the presence of:
1. Clinically evaluated, unexplained, persistent or relapsing fatigue that is of new or definite onset; is not the result of ongoing exertion; is not alleviated by rest; and results in substantial reduction of previous levels of occupational, educational, social, or personal activities; and
2. Four or more of the following symptoms that persist or recur during six or more consecutive months of illness and that do not predate the fatigue:
   - Self-reported impairment in short-term memory or concentration
   - Sore throat
   - Tender cervical or axillary nodes
   - Muscle pain
   - Multijoint pain without redness or swelling
   - Headaches of a new pattern or severity
   - Unrefreshing sleep
   - Postexertional malaise lasting $\geq$24 h

Note: CDC, U.S. Centers for Disease Control and Prevention.
Source: Adapted from K Fukuda et al: Ann Intern Med 121:953, 1994; with permission.

abnormalities in the brain of CFS patients have not withstood further study. The dilemma for patient and clinician alike is that CFS has no pathognomonic features and remains a constellation of symptoms and a diagnosis of exclusion. Often the patient presents with features that also meet criteria for other subjective disorders such as fibromyalgia and irritable bowel syndrome.

℞ TREATMENT

After other illnesses have been excluded, there are several points to address in the long-term care of a patient with chronic fatigue.

The patient should be informed about the illness and what is known of its pathogenesis; its potential impact on the physical, psychological, and social dimensions of life; and its prognosis. Patients are relieved when their complaints are taken seriously. Periodic reassessment is appropriate to identify a possible underlying process that is late in declaring itself and to address intercurrent symptoms that should not be simply dismissed as yet another subjective complaint.

Many symptoms of CFS respond to treatment. Non-steroidal anti-inflammatory drugs alleviate headache, diffuse pain, and feverishness. Allergic rhinitis and sinusitis are common; antihistamines or decongestants may be helpful. Although the patient may be averse to psychiatric diagnoses, depression and anxiety are often prominent and should be treated. Expert psychiatric assessment is sometimes advisable. Nonsedating antidepressants improve mood and disordered sleep and may attenuate the fatigue. Even modest improvements in symptoms can make an important difference in the patient's degree of self-sufficiency and ability to appreciate life's pleasures.

Practical advice should be given regarding life-style. Sleep disturbances are common; consumption of heavy meals with alcohol and caffeine at night can make sleep even more elusive, compounding fatigue. Total rest leads to further deconditioning and the self-image of being an invalid, whereas overexertion may worsen exhaustion and lead to total avoidance of exercise. A moderate, carefully graded regimen should be encouraged and has been proven to relieve symptoms and enhance exercise tolerance.

Controlled therapeutic trials have established that acyclovir, fludrocortisone, and intravenous immunoglobulin, among others, are of little or no value in CFS. Low doses of hydrocortisone provide modest benefit, but they may lead to adrenal suppression. Countless anecdotes circulate regarding other traditional and nontraditional therapies. It is important to guide patients away from those therapeutic modalities that are toxic, expensive, or unreasonable.

The physician should promote the patient's efforts to recover. Controlled trials in the United Kingdom, in Australia, and in the Netherlands showed cognitive behavioral therapy to be helpful. This approach aims to dispel misguided beliefs and fears about CFS that can contribute to inactivity and despair. For CFS, as for many other conditions, a comprehensive approach to physical, psychological, and social aspects of well-being is in order.

FURTHER READING

ALFARI N, BUCHWALD D: Chronic fatigue syndrome: A review. Am J Psychiat 160:221, 2003

WHITING P et al: Interventions for the treatment and management of chronic fatigue syndrome: A systematic review. JAMA 286:1360, 2001

Section 5   Psychiatric Disorders

371   MENTAL DISORDERS
Victor I. Reus

Mental disorders are common in medical practice and may present either as a primary disorder or as a comorbid condition. The prevalence of mental or substance use disorders in the United States is 18.5%, resulting in an annual cost of $148 billion dollars, only slightly less than the costs of cardiovascular diseases. Only 15% of these individuals are currently receiving treatment.

The revised 4th edition for use by primary care physicians of the *Diagnostic and Statistical Manual* (DSM-IV-PC) provides a useful synopsis of mental disorders most likely to be seen in primary care practice. The current system of classification is multiaxial and includes the presence or absence of a major mental disorder (axis I), any underlying personality disorder (axis II), general medical condition (axis III), psychosocial and environmental problems (axis IV), and overall rating of general psychosocial functioning (axis V).

Changes in health care delivery underscore the need for primary care physicians to assume responsibility for the initial diagnosis and treatment of the most common mental disorders. Prompt diagnosis is essential to ensure that patients have access to appropriate medical services and to maximize the clinical outcome. Validated patient-based questionnaires have been developed that systematically probe for signs and symptoms associated with the most prevalent psychiatric diagnoses and guide the clinician into targeted assessment. Prime MD (and a self-report form, the PHQ) and the Symptom-Driven Diagnostic System for Primary Care (SDDS-PC) are inventories that require only 10 min to complete and link patient responses to the formal diagnostic criteria of anxiety, mood, somatoform, and eating disorders and to alcohol abuse or dependence.

A physician who refers patients to a psychiatrist should know not only when doing so is appropriate but also how to refer, since societal misconceptions and the stigma of mental illness impede the process. Primary care physicians should base referrals to a psychiatrist on the presence of signs and symptoms of a mental disorder and not simply on the absence of a physical explanation for a patient's complaint. The physician should discuss with the patient the reasons for requesting the referral or consultation and provide reassurance that he or she will continue to provide medical care and work collaboratively with the mental health professional. Consultation with a psychiatrist or transfer of care is appropriate when physicians encounter evidence of psychotic symptoms, mania, severe depression, or anxiety; symptoms of post-traumatic stress disorder (PTSD); suicidal or homicidal preoccupation; or a failure to respond to first-order treatment.→*Eating disorders are discussed in Chap. 65.*

ANXIETY DISORDERS

Anxiety disorders, the most prevalent psychiatric illnesses in the general community, are present in 15 to 20% of medical clinic patients. Anxiety, defined as a subjective sense of unease, dread, or foreboding, can indicate a primary psychiatric condition or can be a component of, or reaction to, a primary medical disease. The primary anxiety disorders are classified according to their duration and course and the existence and nature of precipitants.

When evaluating the anxious patient, the clinician must first determine whether the anxiety antedates or postdates a medical illness or is due to a medication side effect. Approximately one-third of patients presenting with anxiety have a medical etiology for their psychiatric symptoms, but an anxiety disorder can also present with somatic symptoms in the absence of a diagnosable medical condition.

PANIC DISORDER ■ Clinical Manifestations Panic disorder is defined by the presence of recurrent and unpredictable panic attacks, which are distinct episodes of intense fear and discomfort associated with a variety of physical symptoms, including palpitations, sweating, trembling, shortness of breath, chest pain, dizziness, and a fear of impend-

TABLE 371-1 *Diagnostic Criteria for Panic Attack*

A discrete period of intense fear or discomfort, in which four or more of the
following symptoms developed abruptly and reached a peak within 10
min:
1. Palpitations, pounding heart, or accelerated heart rate
2. Sweating
3. Trembling or shaking
4. Sensations of shortness of breath or smothering
5. Feeling of choking
6. Chest pain or discomfort
7. Nausea or abdominal distress
8. Feeling dizzy, unsteady, lightheaded, or faint
9. Derealization (feelings of unreality) or depersonalization
   (being detached from oneself)
10. Fear of losing control or going crazy
11. Fear of dying
12. Paresthesias (numbness or tingling sensations)
13. Chills or hot flushes

Source: *Diagnostic and Statistical Manual of Mental Disorders,* 4th ed.

ing doom or death (Table 371-1). Paresthesias, gastrointestinal distress, and feelings of unreality are also common. Diagnostic criteria also require at least 1 month of concern or worry about the attacks or a change in behavior related to them. The lifetime prevalence of panic disorder is 1 to 3%. Panic attacks have a sudden onset, developing within 10 min and usually resolving over the course of an hour, and they occur in an unexpected fashion. The frequency and severity of panic attacks vary, ranging from once a week to clusters of attacks separated by months of well-being. The first attack is usually outside the home, and onset is typically in late adolescence to early adulthood. In some individuals, anticipatory anxiety develops over time and results in a generalized fear and a progressive avoidance of places or situations in which a panic attack might recur. *Agoraphobia*, which occurs commonly in patients with panic disorder, is an acquired irrational fear of being in places where one might feel trapped or unable to escape (Table 371-2). Typically, it leads the patient into a progressive restriction in lifestyle and, in a literal sense, in geography. Frequently, patients are embarrassed that they are housebound and dependent on the company of others to go out into the world and do not volunteer this information; thus physicians will fail to recognize the syndrome if direct questioning is not pursued.

Differential Diagnosis   A diagnosis of panic disorder is made after a medical etiology for the panic attacks has been ruled out. A variety of cardiovascular, respiratory, endocrine, and neurologic conditions can present with anxiety as the chief complaint. Patients with true panic disorder will often focus on one specific feature to the exclusion of

TABLE 371-2 *Diagnostic Criteria for Agoraphobia*

1. Anxiety about being in places or situations from which escape might be difficult (or embarrassing) or in which help may not be available in the event of having an unexpected or situationally predisposed panic attack or panic-like symptoms. Agoraphobic fears typically involve characteristic clusters of situations that include being outside the home alone; being in a crowd or standing in a line; being on a bridge; and traveling in a bus, train, or automobile.
2. The situations are avoided (e.g., travel is restricted) or else are endured with marked distress or with anxiety about having a panic attack or panic-like symptoms, or require the presence of a companion.
3. The anxiety or phobic avoidance is not better accounted for by another mental disorder, such as social phobia (e.g., avoidance limited to social situations because of fear of embarrassment), specific phobia (e.g., avoidance limited to a single situation like elevators), obsessive-compulsive disorder (e.g., avoidance of dirt in someone with an obsession about contamination), posttraumatic stress disorder (e.g., avoidance of stimuli associated with a severe stressor), or separation anxiety disorder (e.g., avoidance of leaving home or relatives).

Source: *Diagnostic and Statistical Manual of Mental Disorders,* 4th ed.

others. For example, 20% of patients who present with syncope as a primary medical complaint have a primary diagnosis of a mood, anxiety, or substance-abuse disorder, the most common being panic disorder. The differential diagnosis of panic disorder is complicated by a high rate of comorbidity with other psychiatric conditions, especially alcohol and benzodiazepine abuse, which patients initially use in an attempt at self-medication. Some 75% of panic disorder patients will also satisfy criteria for major depression at some point in their illness.

When the history is nonspecific, physical examination and focused laboratory testing must be used to rule out anxiety states resulting from medical disorders such as pheochromocytoma, thyrotoxicosis, or hypoglycemia. Electrocardiogram (ECG) and echocardiogram may detect some cardiovascular conditions associated with panic, such as paroxysmal atrial tachycardia and mitral valve prolapse. In two studies, panic disorder was the primary diagnosis in 43% of patients with chest pain who had normal coronary angiograms and was present in 9% of all outpatients referred for cardiac evaluation. Panic disorder has also been diagnosed in many patients referred for pulmonary function testing or with symptoms of irritable bowel syndrome.

Etiology and Pathophysiology   The etiology of panic disorder is unknown but appears to involve a genetic predisposition, altered autonomic responsivity, and social learning. Panic disorder shows familial aggregation; the disorder is concordant in 30 to 45% of monozygotic twins, and genome-wide screens have identified suggestive risk loci on 1q, 7p15, 10q, 11p, and 13q. Acute panic attacks appear to be associated with increased noradrenergic discharges in the locus coeruleus. Intravenous infusion of sodium lactate evokes an attack in two-thirds of panic disorder patients, as do the α_2-adrenergic antagonist yohimbine, cholecystokinin tetrapeptide (CCK-4), and carbon dioxide inhalation. It is hypothesized that each of these stimuli activates a pathway involving noradrenergic neurons in the locus coeruleus and serotonergic neurons in the dorsal raphe. Agents that block serotonin reuptake can prevent attacks. It is theorized that panic-disorder patients have a heightened sensitivity to somatic symptoms, which triggers increasing arousal, setting off the panic attack. Accordingly, therapeutic intervention involves altering the patient's cognitive interpretation of anxiety-producing experiences as well as preventing the attack itself.

℞ TREATMENT

Achievable goals of treatment are to decrease the frequency of panic attacks and to reduce their intensity. The cornerstone of drug therapy is antidepressant medication (Tables 371-3, 371-4, and 371-5). The tricyclic antidepressants (TCAs) imipramine and clomipramine benefit 75 to 90% of panic disorder patients. Low doses (e.g., 10 to 25 mg/d) are given initially to avoid transient increased anxiety associated with heightened monoamine levels. Selective serotonin reuptake inhibitors (SSRIs) are equally effective and do not have the adverse effects of TCAs. SSRIs should be started at one-third to one-half of their usual antidepressant dose (e.g., 5 to 10 mg fluoxetine, 25 to 50 mg sertraline, 10 mg paroxetine). Monoamine oxidase inhibitors (MAOIs) are also effective and may specifically benefit patients who have comorbid features of atypical depression (i.e., hypersomnia and weight gain). Insomnia, orthostatic hypotension, and the need to maintain a low-tyramine diet (avoidance of cheese and wine) have limited their use, however. Antidepressants typically take 2 to 6 weeks to become effective, and doses may need to be adjusted based upon the clinical response.

Because of anticipatory anxiety and the need for immediate relief of panic symptoms, benzodiazepines are useful early in the course of treatment and sporadically thereafter (Table 371-6). For example, alprazolam, starting at 0.5 mg qid and increasing to 4 mg/d in divided doses, is effective, but patients must be monitored closely, as some develop dependence and begin to escalate the dose of this medication. Clonazepam, at a final maintenance dose of 2 to 4 mg/d, is also helpful; its longer half-life permits twice-daily dosing, and patients appear less likely to develop dependence on this agent.

Early psychotherapeutic intervention and education aimed at symp-

TABLE 371-4 *Management of Antidepressant Side Effects*

Symptoms	Comments and Management Strategies
Gastrointestinal	
Nausea, loss of appetite	Usually short-lived and dose-related; consider temporary dose reduction or administration with food and antacids
Diarrhea	Famotidine, 20–40 mg/d
Constipation	Wait for tolerance; try diet change, stool softener, exercise; avoid laxatives
Sexual dysfunction	Consider dose reduction; drug holiday
Anorgasmia/impotence; impaired ejaculation	Bethanechol, 10–20 mg, 2 h before activity, or cyproheptadine, 4–8 mg 2 h before activity, or bupropion, 100 mg bid or amantadine, 100 mg bid/tid
Orthostasis	Tolerance unlikely; increase fluid intake, use calf exercises/support hose; fludrocortisone, 0.025 mg/d
Anticholinergic	Wait for tolerance
Dry mouth, eyes	Maintain good oral hygiene; use artificial tears, sugar-free gum
Tremor/jitteriness	Antiparkinsonian drugs not effective; use dose reduction/slow increase; lorazepam, 0.5 mg bid, or propranolol, 10–20 mg bid
Insomnia	Schedule all doses for the morning; trazodone, 50–100 mg qhs
Sedation	Caffeine; schedule all dosing for bedtime; bupropion, 75–100 mg in afternoon
Headache	Evaluate diet, stress, other drugs; try dose reduction; amitriptyline, 50 mg/d
Weight gain	Decrease carbohydrates; exercise; consider fluoxetine
Loss of therapeutic benefit over time	Related to tolerance? Increase dose or drug holiday; add amantadine, 100 mg bid, buspirone, 10 mg tid, or pindolol, 2.5 mg bid

with resultant sedation, impairment of cognition, and poor psychomotor performance. Shorter-acting compounds, such as alprazolam and oxazepam, can produce daytime anxiety, early morning insomnia, and, with discontinuation, rebound anxiety and insomnia. Although patients develop tolerance to the sedative effects of benzodiazepines, they are less likely to habituate to the adverse psychomotor effects. Withdrawal from the longer half-life benzodiazepines can be accomplished through gradual, stepwise dose reduction (by 10% every 1 to 2 weeks) over 6 to 12 weeks. It is usually more difficult to taper patients off shorter-acting benzodiazepines. Physicians may need to switch the patient to a benzodiazepine with a longer half-life or use an adjunctive medication, such as a beta blocker or carbamazepine, before attempting to discontinue the benzodiazepine. Withdrawal reactions vary in severity and duration; they can include depression,

TABLE 371-5 *Possible Drug Interactions with Selective Serotonin Reuptake Inhibitors*

Agent	Effect
Monoamine oxidase inhibitors	Serotonin syndrome—absolute contraindication
Serotonergic agonists, e.g., tryptophan, fenfluramine	Potential serotonin syndrome
Drugs that are metabolized by P450 isoenzymes: tricyclics, other SSRIs, antipsychotics, beta blockers, codeine, terfenadine, astemizole, triazolobenzodiazepines, calcium channel blockers	Delayed metabolism resulting in increased blood levels and potential toxicity—possible fatality secondary to QT prolongation with terfenadine or astemizole
Drugs that are bound tightly to plasma proteins, e.g., warfarin	Increased bleeding secondary to displacement
Drugs that inhibit the metabolism of SSRIs by P450 isoenzymes, e.g., quinidine	Increased SSRI side effects

Note: SSRI, selective serotonin reuptake inhibitor.

anxiety, delirium, lethargy, diaphoresis, tinnitus, autonomic arousal, adventitious movements, and, rarely, seizures.

Buspirone is a nonbenzodiazepine anxiolytic agent. It is nonsedating, does not produce tolerance or dependence, does not interact with benzodiazepine receptors or alcohol, and has no abuse or disinhibition potential. However, it requires several weeks to take effect and requires thrice-daily dosing. Patients who were previously responsive to a benzodiazepine are unlikely to rate buspirone as equally effective, but patients with head injury or dementia who have symptoms of anxiety and/or agitation may do well with this agent.

Administration of benzodiazepines to geriatric patients requires special care. Such patients have increased drug absorption; decreased hepatic metabolism, protein binding, and renal excretion; and an increased volume of distribution. These factors, together with the likely presence of comorbid medical illnesses and medication, dramatically increase the likelihood of toxicity. Iatrogenic psychomotor impairment can result in falls and fractures, confusional states, or motor vehicle accidents. If used, agents in this class should be started at the lowest possible dose, and effects should be monitored closely. Benzodiazepines are contraindicated during pregnancy and breast-feeding.

Anticonvulsants with GABAergic properties may also be effective against anxiety. Gabapentin, oxcarbazepine, tiagabine, pregabalin, and divalproex have all shown some degree of benefit in a variety of anxiety-related syndromes. Agents that selectively target $GABA_A$ receptor subtypes are currently under development; and it is hoped that these will lack the sedating, memory-impairing, and addicting properties of benzodiazepines.

PHOBIC DISORDERS ■ Clinical Manifestations The cardinal feature of phobic disorders is a marked and persistent fear of objects or situations, exposure to which results in an immediate anxiety reaction. The patient avoids the phobic stimulus, and this avoidance usually impairs occupational or social functioning. Panic attacks may be triggered by the phobic stimulus or may occur spontaneously. Unlike patients with other anxiety disorders, individuals with phobias usually experience anxiety only in specific situations. Common phobias include fear of closed spaces (claustrophobia), fear of blood, and fear of flying. Social phobia is distinguished by a specific fear of social or performance situations in which the individual is exposed to unfamiliar individuals or to possible examination and evaluation by others. Examples include having to converse at a party, use public restrooms, and meet strangers. In each case, the affected individual is aware that the experienced fear is excessive and unreasonable given the circumstance. The specific content of a phobia may vary across gender, ethnic, and cultural boundaries.

Phobic disorders are common, affecting ~10% of the population. Full criteria for diagnosis are usually satisfied first in early adulthood, but behavioral avoidance of unfamiliar people, situations, or objects dating from early childhood is common.

In one study of female twins, concordance rates for agoraphobia, social phobia, and animal phobia were found to be 23% for monozygotic twins and 15% for dizygotic twins. A twin study of fear conditioning, a model for the acquisition of phobias, demonstrated a heritability of 35 to 45%, and a genome-wide linkage scan has identified a risk locus on chromosome 14 in a region previously implicated in a mouse model of fear. Animal studies of fear conditioning have indicated that processing of the fear stimulus occurs through the lateral nucleus of the amygdala, extending through the central nucleus and projecting to the periaqueductal gray region, lateral hypothalamus, and paraventricular hypothalamus.

℞ TREATMENT

Beta blockers (e.g., propranolol, 20 to 40 mg orally 2 h before the event) are particularly effective in the treatment of "performance anxiety" (but not general social phobia) and appear to work by blocking the peripheral manifestations of anxiety, such as perspiration, tachycardia, palpitations, and tremor. MAOIs alleviate social phobia independently of their antidepressant activity, and SSRIs appear to be eftom control enhances the effectiveness of drug treatment. Patients can be taught breathing techniques, can be educated about physiologic changes that occur with panic, and can learn to expose themselves voluntarily to precipitating events in a treatment program spanning 12 to 15 sessions. Homework assignments and monitored compliance are important components of successful treatment. Once patients have achieved a satisfactory response, drug treatment should be maintained for 1 to 2 years to prevent relapse. Controlled trials indicate a success rate of 75 to 85%, although the likelihood of complete remission is somewhat lower.

GENERALIZED ANXIETY DISORDER ■ Clinical Manifestations Patients with generalized anxiety disorder (GAD) have persistent, excessive, and/or unrealistic worry associated with muscle tension, impaired concentration, autonomic arousal, feeling "on edge" or restless, and insomnia (Table 371-7). Onset is usually before age 20, and a history of childhood fears and social inhibition may be present. The lifetime prevalence of GAD is 5 to 6%; the risk is higher in first-degree relatives of patients with the diagnosis. Interestingly, family studies indicate that GAD and panic disorder segregate independently. Over 80% of patients with GAD also suffer from major depression, dysthymia, or social phobia. Comorbid substance abuse is common in these patients, particularly alcohol and/or sedative/hypnotic abuse. Patients with GAD worry excessively over minor matters, with life-disrupting effects; unlike in panic disorder, complaints of shortness of breath, palpitations, and tachycardia are relatively rare.

Etiology and Pathophysiology Experimental work suggests that anxiogenic agents share in common the property of altering the binding of benzodiazepines to the γ-aminobutyric acid (GABA)$_A$ receptor/chloride ion channel complex. Benzodiazepines are thought to bind two separate GABA$_A$ receptor sites: type I, which has a broad neuroanatomic distribution, and type II, which is concentrated in the hippocampus, striatum, and neocortex. The antianxiety effects of the various benzodiazepines and side effects such as sedation and memory impairment are influenced by their relative binding to type I and type II receptor sites. Serotonin [5-hydroxytryptamine (5HT)] also appears to have a role in anxiety, and buspirone, a partial 5HT$_{1A}$ receptor agonist, and certain 5HT$_{2A}$ and 5HT$_{2C}$ receptor antagonists (e.g., nefazodone) may have beneficial effects.

TABLE 371-3 Antidepressants

Name	Usual Daily Dose, mg	Side Effects	Comments
SSRIs			
Fluoxetine (Prozac)	10–80	Headache; nausea and other GI effects; jitteriness; insomnia; sexual dysfunction; can affect plasma levels of other meds (except sertraline); akathisia rare	Once daily dosing, usually in A.M.; fluoxetine has very long half-life; must not be combined with MAOIs
Sertraline (Zoloft)	50–200		
Paroxetine (Paxil)	20–60		
Fluvoxamine (Luvox)	100–300		
Citalopram (Celexa)	20–60		
Escitalopram (Lexapro)	10–30		
TCAs			
Amitriptyline (Elavil)	150–300	Anticholinergic (dry mouth, tachycardia, constipation, urinary retention, blurred vision); sweating; tremor; postural hypotension; cardiac conduction delay; sedation; weight gain	Once daily dosing, usually qhs; blood levels of most TCAs available; can be lethal in O.D. (lethal dose = 2 g); nortriptyline best tolerated, especially by elderly
Nortriptyline (Pamelor)	50–200		
Imipramine (Tofranil)	150–300		
Desipramine (Norpramin)	150–300		
Doxepin (Sinequan)	150–300		
Clomipramine (Anafranil)	150–300		
Mixed norepinephrine/ serotonin reuptake inhibitors			
Venlafaxine (Effexor)	75–375	Nausea; dizziness; dry mouth; headaches; increased blood pressure; anxiety and insomnia	Bid-tid dosing (extended release available); lower potential for drug interactions than SSRIs; contraindicated with MAOIs
Mirtazapine (Remeron)	15–45	Somnolence; weight gain; neutropenia rare	Once daily dosing
Mixed-action drugs			
Bupropion (Wellbutrin)	250–450	Jitteriness; flushing; seizures in at-risk patients; anorexia; tachycardia; psychosis	Tid dosing, but sustained release also available; fewer sexual side effects than SSRIs or TCAs; may be useful for adult ADD
Trazodone (Desyrel)	200–600	Sedation; dry mouth; ventricular irritability; postural hypotension; priapism rare	Useful in low doses for sleep because of sedating effects with no anticholinergic side effects
Nefazodone (Serzone)	300–600	Sedation; headache; dry mouth; nausea; constipation	Once daily dosing; no effect on REM sleep unlike other antidepressants
Amoxapine (Asendin)	200–600	Sexual dysfunction	Lethality in overdose; EPS possible
MAOIs			
Phenelzine (Nardil)	45–90	Insomnia; hypotension; anorgasmia; weight gain; hypertensive crisis; tyramine cheese reaction; lethal reactions with SSRIs; serious reactions with narcotics	May be more effective in patients with atypical features or treatment-refractory depression
Tranylcypromine (Parnate)	20–50		
Isocarboxazid (Marplan)	20–60		

Note: ADD, attention deficit disorder; MAOI, monoamine oxidase inhibitor; REM, rapid eye movement; SSRI, selective serotonin reuptake inhibitor; TCA, tricyclic antidepressant; EPS, extrapyramidal symptoms.

TREATMENT

A combination of pharmacologic and psychotherapeutic interventions is most effective in GAD, but complete symptomatic relief is rare. A short course of a benzodiazepine is usually indicated, preferably lorazepam, oxazepam, or temazepam. (The first two of these agents are metabolized via conjugation rather than oxidation and thus do not accumulate if hepatic function is altered.) Administration should be initiated at the lowest dose possible and prescribed on an as-needed basis as symptoms warrant. Benzodiazepines differ in their milligram per kilogram potency, half-life, lipid solubility, metabolic pathways, and presence of active metabolites. Agents that are absorbed rapidly and are lipid soluble, such as diazepam, have a rapid onset of action and a higher abuse potential. Benzodiazepines should generally not be prescribed for >4 to 6 weeks because of the development of tolerance and the risk of abuse and dependence. It is important to warn patients that concomitant use of alcohol or other sedating drugs may be neurotoxic and impair their ability to function. An optimistic approach that encourages the patient to clarify environmental precipitants, anticipate his or her reactions, and plan effective response strategies is an essential element of therapy.

Adverse effects of benzodiazepines generally parallel their relative half-lives. Longer-acting agents, such as diazepam, chlordiazepoxide, flurazepam, and clonazepam, tend to accumulate active metabolites, fective also. Benzodiazepines can be helpful in reducing fearful avoidance, but the chronic nature of phobic disorders limits their usefulness.

Behaviorally focused psychotherapy is an important component of treatment, as relapse rates are high when medication is used as the sole treatment. Cognitive-behavioral strategies are based upon the finding that distorted perceptions and interpretations of fear-producing stimuli play a major role in perpetuation of phobias. Individual and group therapy sessions teach the patient to identify specific negative thoughts associated with the anxiety-producing situation and help to reduce the patient's fear of loss of control. In desensitization therapy, hierarchies of feared situations are constructed and the patient is encouraged to pursue and master gradual exposure to the anxiety-producing stimuli.

Patients with social phobia, in particular, have a high rate of comorbid alcohol abuse, as well as of other psychiatric conditions (e.g., eating disorders), necessitating the need for parallel management of each disorder if anxiety reduction is to be achieved.

TABLE 371-6 Anxiolytics

Name	Equivalent PO dose, mg	Onset of Action	Half-life, h	Comments
Benzodiazepines				
Diazepam (Valium)	5	Fast	20–70	Active metabolites; quite sedating
Flurazepam (Dalmane)	15	Fast	30–100	Flurazepam is a pro-drug; metabolites are active; quite sedating
Triazolam (Halcion)	0.25	Intermediate	1.5–5	No active metabolites; can induce confusion and delirium, especially in elderly
Lorazepam (Ativan)	1	Intermediate	10–20	No active metabolites; direct hepatic glucuronide conjugation; quite sedating
Alprazolam (Xanax)	0.5	Intermediate	12–15	Active metabolites; not too sedating; may have specific antidepressant and antipanic activity; tolerance and dependence develop easily
Chlordiazepoxide (Librium)	10	Intermediate	5–30	Active metabolites; moderately sedating
Oxazepam (Serax)	15	Slow	5–15	No active metabolites; direct glucuronide conjugation; not too sedating
Temazepam (Restoril)	15	Slow	9–12	No active metabolites; moderately sedating
Clonazepam (Klonopin)	0.5	Slow	18–50	No active metabolites; moderately sedating
Non-benzodiazepines				
Buspirone (BuSpar)	7.5	2 weeks	2–3	Active metabolites; tid dosing—usual daily dose 10–20 mg tid; nonsedating; no additive effects with alcohol; useful for agitation in demented or brain-injured patients

STRESS DISORDERS ■ Clinical Manifestations Patients may develop anxiety after exposure to extreme traumatic events such as the threat of personal death or injury or the death of a loved one. The reaction may occur shortly after the trauma (*acute stress disorder*) or be delayed and subject to recurrence (PTSD) (Table 371-8). In both syndromes, individuals experience associated symptoms of detachment and loss of emotional responsivity. The patient may feel depersonalized and unable to recall specific aspects of the trauma, though typically it is reexperienced through intrusions in thought, dreams, or flashbacks, particularly when cues of the original event are present. Patients often actively avoid stimuli that precipitate recollections of the trauma and demonstrate a resulting increase in vigilance, arousal, and startle response. Patients with stress disorders are at risk for the development of other disorders related to anxiety, mood, and substance abuse (especially alcohol). Between 5 and 10% of Americans will at some time in their life satisfy criteria for PTSD, with women more likely to be affected than men.

Risk factors for the development of PTSD include a past psychiatric history and personality characteristics of high neuroticism and extroversion. Twin studies show a substantial influence of genetics on all symptoms associated with PTSD, with less evidence for environment effect.

Etiology and Pathophysiology It is hypothesized that in PTSD there are excessive release of norepinephrine from the locus coeruleus in response to stress and increased noradrenergic activity at projection sites in the hippocampus and amygdala. These changes theoretically facilitate the encoding of fear-based memories. Greater sympathetic responses to cues associated with the traumatic event occur in PTSD, although pituitary adrenal responses are blunted.

℞ TREATMENT

Acute stress reactions are usually self-limited, and treatment typically involves the short-term use of benzodiazepines and supportive/expressive psychotherapy. The chronic and recurrent nature of PTSD, however, requires a more complex approach employing drug and behavioral treatments. PTSD is highly correlated with peritraumatic dissociative symptoms and the development of an acute stress disorder

at the time of the trauma. TCAs such as imipramine and amitriptyline, the MAOI phenelzine, and the SSRIs (fluoxetine, sertraline, citalopram, paroxetine) can all reduce anxiety, symptoms of intrusion, and avoidance behaviors, as can prazosin, an α_1 antagonist. Trazodone, a sedating antidepressant, is frequently used at night to help with insomnia (50 to 150 mg qhs). Carbamazepine, valproic acid, or alprazolam have also independently produced improvement in uncontrolled trials. Psychotherapeutic strategies for PTSD help the patient overcome avoidance behaviors and demoralization and master fear of recurrence

TABLE 371-7 Diagnostic Criteria for Generalized Anxiety Disorder

A. Excessive anxiety and worry (apprehensive expectation), occurring more days than not for at least 6 months, about a number of events or activities (such as work or school performance).
B. The person finds it difficult to control the worry.
C. The anxiety and worry are associated with three (or more) of the following six symptoms (with at least some symptoms present for more days than not for the past 6 months): (1) restlessness or feeling keyed up or on edge; (2) being easily fatigued; (3) difficulty concentrating or mind going blank; (4) irritability; (5) muscle tension; (6) sleep disturbance (difficulty falling or staying asleep, or restless unsatisfying sleep).
D. The focus of the anxiety and worry is not confined to features of an Axis I disorder, e.g., the anxiety or worry is not about having a panic attack (as in panic disorder), being embarrassed in public (as in social phobia), being contaminated (as in obsessive-compulsive disorder), being away from home or close relatives (as in separation anxiety disorder), gaining weight (as in anorexia nervosa), having multiple physical complaints (as in somatization disorder), or having a serious illness (as in hypochondriasis), and the anxiety and worry do not occur exclusively during posttraumatic stress disorder.
E. The anxiety, worry, or physical symptoms cause clinically significant distress or impairment in social, occupational, or other important areas of functioning.
F. The disturbance is not due to the direct physiologic effects of a substance (e.g., a drug of abuse, a medication) or a general medical condition (e.g., hyperthyroidism) and does not occur exclusively during a mood disorder, a psychotic disorder, or a pervasive developmental disorder.

Source: *Diagnostic and Statistical Manual of Mental Disorders*, 4th ed.

TABLE 371-8 *Diagnostic Criteria for Posttraumatic Stress Disorder*

A. The person has been exposed to a traumatic event in which both of the following were present:
   1. The person experienced, witnessed, or was confronted with an event or events that involved actual or threatened death or serious injury, or a threat to the physical integrity of self or others.
   2. The person's response involved intense fear, helplessness, or horror.
B. The traumatic event is persistently reexperienced in one (or more) of the following ways:
   1. Recurrent and intrusive distressing recollections of the event, including images, thoughts, or perceptions.
   2. Recurrent distressing dreams of the event.
   3. Acting or feeling as if the traumatic event were recurring (includes a sense of reliving the experience, illusions, hallucinations, and dissociative flashback episodes, including those that occur on awakening or when intoxicated).
   4. Intense psychological distress at exposure to internal or external cues that symbolize or resemble an aspect of the traumatic event.
   5. Physiologic reactivity on exposure to internal or external cues that symbolize or resemble an aspect of the traumatic event.
C. Persistent avoidance of stimuli associated with the trauma and numbing of general responsiveness (not present before the trauma), as indicated by three or more of the following:
   1. Efforts to avoid thoughts, feelings, or conversations associated with the trauma
   2. Efforts to avoid activities, places, or people that arouse recollections of the trauma
   3. Inability to recall an important aspect of the trauma
   4. Markedly diminished interest or participation in significant activities
   5. Feeling of detachment or estrangement from others
   6. Restricted range of affect (e.g., unable to have loving feelings)
   7. Sense of a foreshortened future (e.g., does not expect to have a career, marriage, children, or a normal life span)
D. Persistent symptoms of increased arousal (not present before the trauma), as indicated by two (or more) of the following:
   1. Difficulty falling or staying asleep
   2. Irritability or outbursts of anger
   3. Difficulty concentrating
   4. Hypervigilance
   5. Exaggerated startle response
E. Duration of the disturbance (symptoms in criteria B, C, and D) is more than 1 month
F. The disturbance causes clinically significant distress or impairment in social, occupational, or other important areas of functioning.

Source: *Diagnostic and Statistical Manual of Mental Disorders*, 4th ed.

of the trauma; therapies that encourage the patient to dismantle avoidance behaviors through stepwise focusing on the experience of the traumatic event are the most effective.

OBSESSIVE-COMPULSIVE DISORDER ■ **Clinical Manifestations** Obsessive-compulsive disorder (OCD) is characterized by obsessive thoughts and compulsive behaviors that impair everyday functioning. Fears of contamination and germs are common, as are handwashing, counting behaviors, and having to check and recheck such actions as whether a door is locked. The degree to which the disorder is disruptive for the individual varies, but in all cases obsessive-compulsive activities take up >1 h/d and are undertaken to relieve the anxiety triggered by the core fear. Patients often conceal their symptoms, usually because they are embarrassed by the content of their thoughts or the nature of their actions. Physicians must ask specific questions regarding recurrent thoughts and behaviors, particularly if physical clues such as chafed and reddened hands or patchy hair loss (from repetitive hair pulling, or trichotillomania) are present. Comorbid conditions are common, the most frequent being depression, other anxiety disorders, eating disorders, and tics. OCD has a lifetime prevalence of 2 to 3% worldwide. Onset is usually gradual, beginning in early adulthood, but childhood onset is not rare. The disorder usually has a waxing and waning course,

but some cases may show a steady deterioration in psychosocial functioning.

Etiology and Pathophysiology A genetic contribution to OCD is suggested by twin studies. Family studies show an aggregation with Tourette's disorder. OCD is also more common in males and in first-born children.

The anatomy of obsessive-compulsive behavior is thought to involve the orbital frontal cortex, caudate nucleus, and globus pallidus. The caudate nucleus appears to be involved in the acquisition and maintenance of habit and skill learning, and interventions that are successful in reducing obsessive-compulsive behaviors also decrease metabolic activity measured in the caudate.

℞ TREATMENT

Clomipramine, fluoxetine, and fluvoxamine are approved for the treatment of OCD. Clomipramine is a TCA that is often tolerated poorly owing to anticholinergic and sedative side effects at the doses required to treat the illness (150 to 250 mg/d). Its efficacy in OCD is unrelated to its antidepressant activity. Fluoxetine (40 to 60 mg/d) and fluvoxamine (100 to 300 mg/d) are as effective as clomipramine and have a more benign side-effect profile. Only 50 to 60% of patients with OCD show adequate improvement with pharmacotherapy alone. In treatment-resistant cases, augmentation with other serotonergic agents, such as buspirone, or with a neuroleptic or benzodiazepine may be beneficial. When a therapeutic response is achieved, long-duration maintenance therapy is usually indicated.

For many individuals, particularly those with time-consuming compulsions, behavior therapy will result in as much improvement as that afforded by medication. Effective techniques include the gradual increase in exposure to stressful situations, maintenance of a diary to clarify stressors, and homework assignments that substitute new activities for compulsive behaviors.

MOOD DISORDERS

Mood disorders are characterized by a disturbance in the regulation of mood, behavior, and affect. Mood disorders are subdivided into (1) depressive disorders, (2) bipolar disorders, and (3) depression in association with medical illness or alcohol and substance abuse (Chaps. 372, 373, and 374). Depressive disorders are differentiated from bipolar disorders by the absence of a manic or hypomanic episode. The relationship between pure depressive syndromes and bipolar disorders is not well understood; depression is more frequent in families of bipolar individuals, but the reverse is not true. In the Global Burden of Disease Study conducted by the World Health Organization, unipolar major depression ranked fourth among all diseases in terms of disability-adjusted life years and was projected to rank second by year 2020. In the United States, lost productivity directly related to depression has been estimated at $44 billion per year.

DEPRESSION IN ASSOCIATION WITH MEDICAL ILLNESS Depression occurring in the context of medical illness is difficult to evaluate. Depressive symptomatology may reflect the psychological stress of coping with the disease, may be caused by the disease process itself or by the medications used to treat it, or may simply coexist in time with the medical diagnosis.

Virtually every class of *medication* includes some agent that can induce depression. Antihypertensive drugs, anticholesterolemic agents, and antiarrhythmic agents are common triggers of depressive symptoms. Among the antihypertensive agents, β-adrenergic blockers and, to a lesser extent, calcium channel blockers are the most likely to cause depressed mood. Iatrogenic depression should also be considered in patients receiving glucocorticoids, antimicrobials, systemic analgesics, antiparkinsonian medications, and anticonvulsants. To decide whether a causal relationship exists between pharmacologic therapy and a patient's change in mood, it may sometimes be necessary to undertake an empirical trial of an alternative medication.

Between 20 and 30% of cardiac patients manifest a depressive disorder; an even higher percentage experience depressive symptomatology when self-reporting scales are used. Depressive symptoms following unstable angina, myocardial infarction, or heart transplant impair rehabilitation and are associated with higher rates of mortality and medical morbidity. Depressed patients often show decreased variability in heart rate (an index of reduced parasympathetic nervous system activity), and this has been proposed as one mechanism by which depression may predispose individuals to ventricular arrhythmia and increased morbidity. Depression also appears to increase the risk of developing coronary heart disease; increased serotonin-induced platelet aggregation has been implicated as a possible cause. TCAs are contraindicated in patients with bundle branch block, and TCA-induced tachycardia is an additional concern in patients with congestive heart failure. SSRIs appear not to induce ECG changes or adverse cardiac events and thus are reasonable first-line drugs for patients at risk for TCA-related complications. SSRIs may interfere with hepatic metabolism of anticoagulants, however, causing increased anticoagulation.

In patients with cancer, the mean prevalence of depression is 25%, but depression occurs in 40 to 50% of patients with cancers of the pancreas or oropharynx. Extreme cachexia, common with some cancers, may be misinterpreted as part of the symptom complex of depression; the higher prevalence of depression in patients with pancreatic cancer nevertheless persists when compared to those with advanced gastric cancer. Initiation of antidepressant medication in cancer patients has been shown to improve quality of life as well as mood. Psychotherapeutic approaches, particularly group therapy, may have some effect on short-term depression, anxiety, and pain symptoms and, speculatively, on recurrence rates and long-term survival.

Depression occurs frequently in patients with *neurologic disorders*, particularly cerebrovascular disorders, Parkinson's disease, dementia, multiple sclerosis, and traumatic brain injury. One in five patients with left-hemisphere stroke involving the dorsal lateral frontal cortex experiences major depression. Late-onset depression in otherwise cognitively normal individuals increases the risk of a subsequent diagnosis of Alzheimer's disease. Both TCA and SSRI agents are effective against these depressions, as are stimulant compounds and, in some patients, MAOIs.

The reported prevalence of depression in patients with *diabetes mellitus* varies from 8 to 27%, with the severity of the mood state correlating with the level of hyperglycemia and the presence of diabetic complications. Treatment of depression may be complicated by effects of antidepressive agents on glycemic control. MAOIs can induce hypoglycemia and weight gain. TCAs can produce hyperglycemia and carbohydrate craving. SSRIs, like MAOIs, may reduce fasting plasma glucose, but they are easier to use and may also improve dietary and medication compliance.

Hypothyroidism is frequently associated with features of depression, most commonly depressed mood and memory impairment. Hyperthyroid states may also present in a similar fashion, usually in geriatric populations. Improvement in mood usually follows normalization of thyroid function, but adjunctive antidepressant medication is sometimes required. Patients with subclinical hypothyroidism can also experience symptoms of depression and cognitive difficulty that respond to thyroid replacement.

The lifetime prevalence of depression in HIV-positive individuals has been estimated at 22 to 45%. The relationship between depression and disease progression is multifactorial and likely to involve psychological and social factors, alterations in immune function, and central nervous system disease. Chronic hepatitis C infection is also associated with depression, which may worsen with interferon-α treatment.

Some chronic disorders of uncertain etiology, such as chronic fatigue syndrome (Chap. 370) and fibromyalgia (Chap. 315), are strongly associated with depression and anxiety and may partially benefit from antidepressant treatment, usually at lower than normal dosing.

DEPRESSIVE DISORDERS ■ Clinical Manifestations
Major depression is defined as depressed mood on a daily basis for a minimum duration

of 2 weeks (Table 371-9). An episode may be characterized by sadness, indifference, apathy, or irritability and is usually associated with: changes in sleep patterns, appetite, and weight; motor agitation or retardation; fatigue; impaired concentration and decision-making; feelings of shame or guilt; and thoughts of death or dying. Patients with depression have a profound loss of pleasure in all enjoyable activities, exhibit early morning awakening, feel that the dysphoric mood state is qualitatively different from sadness, and often notice a diurnal variation in mood (worse in morning hours).

Approximately 15% of the population experiences a major depressive episode at some point in life, and 6 to 8% of all outpatients in primary care settings satisfy diagnostic criteria for the disorder. Depression is often undiagnosed, and, even more frequently, it is treated inadequately. If a physician suspects the presence of a major depressive episode, the initial task is to determine whether it represents unipolar or bipolar depression or is one of the 10 to 15% of cases that are secondary to general medical illness or substance abuse. Physicians should also assess the risk of suicide by direct questioning, as patients are often reluctant to verbalize such thoughts without prompting. If specific plans are uncovered or if significant risk factors exist (e.g., a past history of suicide attempts, profound hopelessness, concurrent medical illness, substance abuse, or social isolation), the patient must be referred to a mental health specialist for immediate care. The physician should specifically probe each of these areas in an empathic and hopeful manner, being sensitive to denial and possible minimization of distress. The presence of anxiety, panic, or agitation significantly increases near-term suicidal risk. Approximately 4 to 5% of all de-

---

TABLE 371-9 *Criteria for Major Depressive Episode*

A. Five (or more) of the following symptoms have been present during the same 2-week period and represent a change from previous functioning; at least one of the symptoms is either (1) depressed mood or (2) loss of interest or pleasure. **Note:** Do not include symptoms that are clearly due to a general medical condition, or mood-incongruent delusions or hallucinations.
  1. Depressed mood most of the day, nearly every day, as indicated by either subjective report (e.g., feels sad or empty) or observation made by others (e.g., appears tearful)
  2. Markedly diminished interest or pleasure in all, or almost all, activities most of the day, nearly every day (as indicated by either subjective account or observation made by others)
  3. Significant weight loss when not dieting or weight gain (e.g., a change of >5% of body weight in a month), or decrease or increase in appetite nearly every day
  4. Insomnia or hypersomnia nearly every day
  5. Psychomotor agitation or retardation nearly every day (observable by others, not merely subjective feelings of restlessness or being slowed down)
  6. Fatigue or loss of energy nearly every day
  7. Feelings of worthlessness or excessive or inappropriate guilt (which may be delusional) nearly every day (not merely self-reproach or guilt about being sick)
  8. Diminished ability to think or concentrate, or indecisiveness, nearly every day (either by subjective account or as observed by others)
  9. Recurrent thoughts of death (not just fear of dying), recurrent suicidal ideation without a specific plan, or a suicide attempt or a specific plan for committing suicide
B. The symptoms do not meet criteria for a mixed episode
C. The symptoms cause clinically significant distress or impairment in social, occupational, or other important areas of functioning
D. The symptoms are not due to the direct physiologic effects of a substance (e.g., a drug of abuse, a medication) or a general medical condition (e.g., hypothyroidism)
E. The symptoms are not better accounted for by bereavement; i.e., after the loss of a loved one, the symptoms persist for >2 months or are characterized by marked functional impairment, morbid preoccupation with worthlessness, suicidal ideation, psychotic symptoms, or psychomotor retardation

Source: *Diagnostic and Statistical Manual of Mental Disorders*, 4th ed.

pressed patients will commit suicide; most will have sought help from a physician within 1 month of their death.

In some depressed patients, the mood disorder does not appear to be episodic and is not clearly associated with either psychosocial dysfunction or change from the individual's usual experience in life. *Dysthymic disorder* consists of a pattern of chronic (at least 2 years), ongoing, mild depressive symptoms that are less severe and less disabling than those found in major depression; the two conditions are sometimes difficult to separate, however, and can occur together ("double depression"). Many patients who exhibit a profile of pessimism, disinterest, and low self-esteem respond to antidepressant treatment. Dysthymic disorder exists in ~5% of primary care patients. The term *minor depression* is used for individuals who experience at least two depressive symptoms for 2 weeks, but who do not meet the full criteria for major depression. Despite its name, minor depression is associated with significant morbidity and disability and also responds to pharmacologic treatment.

Depression is approximately twice as common in women as in men, and the incidence increases with age in both sexes. Twin studies indicate that the liability to major depression in adult women is largely genetic in origin. Negative life events can precipitate and contribute to depression, but genetic factors influence the sensitivity of individuals to these stressful events. In most cases, both biologic and psychosocial factors are involved in the precipitation and unfolding of depressive episodes. The most potent stressors appear to involve death of a relative, assault, or severe marital or relationship problems.

Unipolar depressive disorders usually begin in early adulthood and recur episodically over the course of a lifetime. The best predictor of future risk is the number of past episodes; 50 to 60% of patients who have a first episode have at least one or two recurrences. Some patients experience multiple episodes that become more severe and frequent over time. The duration of an untreated episode varies greatly, ranging from a few months to ≥1 year. The pattern of recurrence and clinical progression in a developing episode are also variable. Within an individual, the nature of attacks (e.g., specific presenting symptoms, frequency and duration of episodes) may be similar over time. In a minority of patients, a severe depressive episode may progress to a psychotic state; in elderly patients, depressive symptoms may be associated with cognitive deficits mimicking dementia ("pseudodementia"). A seasonal pattern of depression, called *seasonal affective disorder*, may manifest with onset and remission of episodes at predictable times of the year. This disorder is more common in women, whose symptoms are anergy, fatigue, weight gain, hypersomnia, and episodic carbohydrate craving. The prevalence increases with distance from the equator, and improvement may occur by altering light exposure.

Etiology and Pathophysiology   Although evidence for genetic transmission of unipolar depression is not as strong as in bipolar disorder, monozygotic twins have a higher concordance rate (46%) than dizygotic siblings (20%), with little evidence for any effect of a shared family environment. A recent study indicated that a functional polymorphism in the serotonin transporter (*5-HTT*) gene may interact with stressful life events to markedly increase risk of depression and suicide. Positron emission tomography (PET) studies show decreased metabolic activity in the caudate nuclei and frontal lobes in depressed patients that returns to normal with recovery. Single-photon emission computed tomography (SPECT) studies show comparable changes in blood flow.

Postmortem examination of brains of suicide victims indicate altered noradrenergic activity, including increased binding to α_1-, α_2-, and β-adrenergic receptors in the cerebral cortex and decreased numbers of noradrenergic neurons in the locus coeruleus. Involvement of the serotonin system is suggested by findings of reduced plasma tryptophan levels, a decreased cerebrospinal fluid level of 5-hydroxyindolacetic acid (the principal metabolite of serotonin in brain), and de-

creased platelet serotonergic transporter binding. An increase in brain serotonin receptors in suicide victims and decreased expression of the cyclic AMP response element-binding (CREB) protein are also reported. Depletion of blood tryptophan, the amino acid precursor of serotonin, rapidly reverses the antidepressant benefit in depressed patients who have been successfully treated. However, a decrement in mood after tryptophan reduction is considerably less robust in untreated patients, indicating that, if presynaptic serotonergic dysfunction occurs in depression, it likely plays a contributing rather than a causal role.

Neuroendocrine abnormalities that reflect the neurovegetative signs and symptoms of depression include (1) increased cortisol and corticotropin-releasing hormone (CRH) secretion, (2) an increase in adrenal size, (3) a decreased inhibitory response of glucocorticoids to dexamethasone, and (4) a blunted response of thyroid-stimulating hormone (TSH) level to infusion of thyroid-releasing hormone (TRH). Antidepressant treatment leads to normalization of these pituitary-adrenal abnormalities. Major depression is also associated with an upregulation of proinflammatory cytokines, which normalizes with antidepressant treatment.

Diurnal variations in symptom severity and alterations in circadian rhythmicity of a number of neurochemical and neurohumoral factors suggest that biologic differences may be secondary to a primary defect in regulation of biologic rhythms. Patients with major depression show consistent findings of a decrease in rapid eye movement (REM) sleep onset (REM latency), an increase in REM density, and, in some subjects, a decrease in stage IV delta slow-wave sleep.

Although antidepressant drugs inhibit neurotransmitter uptake within hours, their therapeutic effects typically emerge over several weeks, implicating adaptive changes in second messenger systems and transcription factors as possible mechanisms of action. Antidepressant drugs have been shown to regulate neural plasticity and cell survival by increasing the expression of brain-derived neurotrophic factor (BDNF) through upregulation of the CREB protein and to alter stress responsivity through an increase in glucocorticoid receptor transcription. Secondary effects on activation of the mitogen-activated protein (MAP) kinase and phosphoinositol-3 kinase/AKT pathways and increased expression of the antiapoptotic protein, Bcl-2, are also thought to be critical to antidepressant actions.

℞ TREATMENT

Treatment planning requires coordination of short-term symptom remission with longer term maintenance strategies designed to prevent recurrence. The most effective intervention for achieving remission and preventing relapse is medication, but combined treatment, incorporating psychotherapy to help the patient cope with decreased self-esteem and demoralization, improves outcome (Fig. 371-1). About 40% of primary care patients with depression drop out of treatment and discontinue medication if symptomatic improvement is not noted within a month, unless additional support is provided. Outcome improves with (1) increased intensity and frequency of visits during the first 4 to 6 weeks of treatment, (2) supplemental educational materials, and (3) psychiatric consultation as indicated. Despite the widespread use of SSRIs, there is no convincing evidence that this class of antidepressant is more efficacious than TCAs. Between 60 and 70% of all depressed patients respond to any drug chosen, if it is given in a sufficient dose for 6 to 8 weeks. There is no ideal antidepressant; no current compound combines rapid onset of action, moderate half-life, a meaningful relationship between dose and blood level, a low side-effect profile, minimal interaction with other drugs, and safety in overdose. A rational approach to selecting which antidepressant to use involves matching the patient's preference and medical history with the metabolic and side effect profile of the drug (Tables 371-4 and 371-5). A previous response, or a family history of a positive response, to a specific antidepressant would suggest that that drug be tried first. Before initiating antidepressant therapy, the physician should evaluate the possible contribution of comorbid illnesses and consider their spe-

Determine whether there is a history of good response to a medication in the patient or a first-degree relative; if yes, begin with this agent.

↓

If not, evaluate patient characteristics and match to drug; consider health status, side effect profile, convenience, cost, patient preference, drug interaction risk, suicide potential, and medication compliance history.

↓

Begin new medication at 1/3 to 1/2 target dose if drug is a TCA, bupropion, venlafaxine or mirtazapine, or full dose, as tolerated, if drug is an SSRI.

↓

If problem side effects occur, evaluate possibility of tolerance; consider temporary decrease in dose or adjunctive treatment.

↓

If unacceptable side effects continue, taper drug over 1 week and initiate new trial; consider potential drug interactions in choice.

↓

Evaluate response after 6 weeks at target dose; if response is inadequate, increase dose in stepwise fashion as tolerated.

↓

If inadequate response after maximal dose, consider tapering and switching to a new drug vs. adjunctive treatment; if drug is a TCA, obtain plasma level to guide further treatment.

FIGURE 371-1 A guideline for the medical management of major depressive disorder. SSRI, selective serotonin reuptake inhibitor; TCA, tricyclic antidepressant.

cific treatment. In individuals with suicidal ideation, particular attention should be paid to choosing a drug with low toxicity if taken in overdose. The SSRIs and other newer antidepressant drugs are distinctly safer in this regard; nevertheless, the advantages of TCAs have not been completely superseded. The existence of generic equivalents make TCAs relatively cheap, and for several tricyclics, particularly nortriptyline, imipramine, and desipramine, well-defined relationships among dose, plasma level, and therapeutic response exist. The steady-state plasma level achieved for a given drug dose can vary more than tenfold between individuals. Plasma levels may help in interpreting apparent resistance to treatment and/or unexpected drug toxicity. The principal side effects of TCAs are antihistamine (sedation) and anticholinergic (constipation, dry mouth, urinary hesitancy, blurred vision). Cardiac toxicity due to conduction block or arrhythmias can also occur but is uncommon at therapeutic levels. TCAs are probably contraindicated in patients with serious cardiovascular risk factors. Overdoses of tricyclic agents can be lethal, with desipramine carrying the greatest risk. It is judicious to prescribe only a 10-day supply when suicide is a risk. Most patients require a daily dose of 150 to 200 mg of imipramine or amitriptyline or its equivalent to achieve a therapeutic blood level of 150 to 300 ng/mL and a satisfactory remission; some patients show a partial effect at lower doses. Geriatric patients may require a low starting dose and slow escalation. Ethnic differences in drug metabolism are significant; Hispanic, Asian, and African-American patients generally require lower doses than Caucasians to achieve a comparable blood level.

Second-generation antidepressants include amoxapine, maprotiline, trazodone, and bupropion. Amoxapine is a dibenzoxazepine derivative that blocks norepinephrine and serotonin reuptake and has a metabolite that shows a degree of dopamine blockade. Long-term use of this drug carries a risk of tardive dyskinesia. Maprotiline is a potent noradrenergic reuptake blocker that has little anticholinergic effect but may produce seizures. Bupropion is a novel antidepressant whose mechanism of action is thought to involve enhancement of noradrenergic function. It has no anticholinergic, sedating, or orthostatic side effects and has a low incidence of sexual side effects. It may, however, be associated with stimulant-like side effects, may lower seizure

threshold, and has an exceptionally short half-life, requiring frequent dosing. An extended-release preparation is available.

SSRIs such as fluoxetine, sertraline, paroxetine, citalopram, and escitalopram cause a lower frequency of anticholinergic, sedating, and cardiovascular side effects but a possibly greater incidence of gastrointestinal complaints, sleep impairment, and sexual dysfunction than do TCAs. Akathisia, involving an inner sense of restlessness and anxiety in addition to increased motor activity, may also be more common, particularly during the first week of treatment. A concern is the risk of "serotonin syndrome," thought to result from hyperstimulation of brainstem $5HT_{1A}$ receptors and characterized by myoclonus, agitation, abdominal cramping, hyperpyrexia, hypertension, and potentially death. Serotonergic agonists taken in combination should be monitored closely for this reason. Considerations such as half-life, compliance, toxicity, and drug-drug interactions may guide the choice of a particular SSRI. Fluoxetine and its principal active metabolite, norfluoxetine, for example, have a combined half-life of almost 7 days, resulting in a delay of 5 weeks before steady-state levels are achieved and a similar delay for complete drug excretion once its use is discontinued. All the SSRIs may impair sexual function, resulting in diminished libido, impotence, or difficulty in achieving orgasm. Sexual dysfunction frequently results in noncompliance and should be asked about specifically. Sexual dysfunction can sometimes be ameliorated by lowering the dose, by instituting weekend drug holidays (two or three times a month), or by treatment with amantadine (100 mg tid), bethanechol (25 mg tid) buspirone (10 mg tid), or bupropion (100–150 mg/d). Paroxetine appears to be more anticholinergic than either fluoxetine or sertraline, and sertraline carries a lower risk of producing an adverse drug interaction than the other two. Rare side effects of SSRIs include angina due to vasospasm and prolongation of the prothrombin time. Escitalopram is the most specific of currently available SSRIs and appears to have no specific inhibitory effects on the P450 system.

Venlafaxine, like imipramine, blocks the reuptake of both norepinephrine and serotonin, but it produces relatively little in the way of traditional tricyclic side effects. Unlike the SSRIs, it has a relatively linear dose-response curve. Patients should be monitored for a possible increase in diastolic blood pressure, and multiple daily dosing is required because of the drug's short half-life. An extended-release form is available and has a somewhat lower incidence of gastrointestinal side effects. Nefazadone is a selective $5HT_2$ receptor antagonist that also inhibits the presynaptic reuptake of serotonin and norepinephrine. Its side effects are similar to those of the SSRIs, and twice-daily dosing produces a steady state within 4 to 5 days. The drug is related structurally to trazodone, which is currently used more for its sedative than its antidepressant properties. Nefazadone appears to produce a lower incidence of sexual side effects than do the SSRIs. Mirtazapine is a tetracyclic antidepressant that has a unique spectrum of activity. It increases noradrenergic and serotonergic neurotransmission through a blockade of central α_2-adrenergic receptors and postsynaptic $5HT_2$ and $5HT_3$ receptors. It is also strongly antihistaminic and, as such, may produce sedation.

With the exception of citalopram and escitalopram, each of the SSRIs, as well as nefazadone, may inhibit one or more cytochrome P450 enzymes. Depending on the specific isoenzyme involved, the metabolism of a number of concomitantly administered medications can be dramatically affected. Fluoxetine and paroxetine, for example, by inhibiting 2D6, can cause dramatic increases in the blood level of type 1C antiarrhythmics, while sertraline and nefazadone, by acting on 3A4, may alter blood levels of terfenadine, carbamazepine, and astemizole. Many of these compounds have a narrow therapeutic window and can cause iatrogenic ventricular arrhythmias at toxic levels; thus, the possibility of an adverse drug interaction should always be considered.

The MAOIs are highly effective, particularly in atypical depression, but the risk of hypertensive crisis following intake of tyramine-containing food or sympathomimetic drugs makes them inappropriate as first-line agents. Common side effects include orthostatic hypotension, weight gain, insomnia, and sexual dysfunction. MAOIs should not be used concomitantly with SSRIs, because of the risk of serotonin syndrome, or with TCAs, because of possible hyperadrenergic effects.

Electroconvulsive therapy is at least as effective as medication, but its use is reserved for treatment-resistant cases and delusional depressions. Transcranial magnetic stimulation (TMS) is an investigational treatment of depression that has been shown to have efficacy in several controlled trials; it is uncertain whether the observed benefits were clinically meaningful, however. Vagus nerve stimulation (VNS) appeared to be effective in treatment-resistant depression in an initial open study, only to fail in a controlled trial.

Regardless of the treatment undertaken, the response should be evaluated after ~2 months. Three-quarters of patients show improvement by this time, but if remission is inadequate the patient should be questioned about compliance and an increase in medication dose should be considered if side effects are not troublesome. If this approach is unsuccessful, referral to a mental health specialist is advised. Strategies for treatment then include selection of an alternative drug, combinations of antidepressants, and/or adjunctive treatment with other classes of drugs, including lithium, thyroid hormone, and dopamine agonists. Patients whose response to an SSRI wanes over time may benefit from the addition of buspirone (10 mg tid) or pindolol (2.5 mg tid) or small amounts of a TCA such as desipramine (25 mg bid or tid). Once significant remission is achieved, drug treatment should be continued for at least 6 to 9 months to prevent relapse. In patients who have had two or more episodes of depression, indefinite maintenance treatment should be considered.

It is essential to educate patients both about depression and the benefits and side effects of medications they are receiving. Advice about stress reduction and cautions that alcohol may exacerbate depressive symptoms and impair drug response are helpful. Patients should be given time to describe their experience, their outlook, and the impact of the depression on them and their families. Occasional empathic silence may be as helpful for the treatment alliance as verbal reassurance. Controlled trials have shown that cognitive-behavioral and interpersonal therapies are effective in improving psychological and social adjustment and that a combined treatment approach is more successful than medication alone for many patients.

BIPOLAR DISORDER ▪ Clinical Manifestations Bipolar disorder is characterized by unpredictable swings in mood from mania (or hypomania) to depression. Some patients suffer only from recurrent attacks of *mania*, which in its pure form is associated with increased psychomotor activity; excessive social extroversion; decreased need for sleep; impulsivity and impairment in judgment; and expansive, grandiose, and sometimes irritable mood (Table 371-10). In severe mania, patients may experience delusions and paranoid thinking indistinguishable from schizophrenia. Half of patients with bipolar disorder present with a mixture of psychomotor agitation and activation with dysphoria, anxiety, and irritability. It may be difficult to distinguish *mixed mania* from *agitated depression*. In some bipolar patients (*bipolar II disorder*), the full criteria for mania are lacking, and the requisite recurrent depressions are separated by periods of mild activation and increased energy (hypomania). In *cyclothymic disorder*, there are numerous hypomanic periods, usually of relatively short duration, alternating with clusters of depressive symptoms that fail, either in severity or duration, to meet the criteria of major depression. The mood fluctuations are chronic and should be present for at least 2 years before the diagnosis is made.

Manic episodes typically emerge over a period of days to weeks, but onset within hours is possible, usually in the early morning hours. An untreated episode of either depression or mania can be as short as several weeks or last as long as 8 to 12 months, and rare patients have an unremitting chronic course. The term *rapid cycling* is used for patients who have four or more episodes of either depression or mania in a given year. This pattern occurs in 15% of all patients, almost all of whom are women. In some cases, rapid cycling is linked to an underlying thyroid dysfunction and, in others, it is iatrogenically triggered by prolonged antidepressant treatment. Approximately half of patients have sustained difficulties in work performance and psychosocial functioning.

Bipolar disorder is common, affecting ~1% of the population in the United States. Onset is typically between 20 and 30 years of age, but many individuals report premorbid symptoms in late childhood or early adolescence. The prevalence is similar for men and women; women are likely to have more depressive and men more manic episodes over a lifetime.

Differential Diagnosis The differential diagnosis of mania includes toxic effects of stimulant or sympathomimetic drugs as well as secondary mania induced by hyperthyroidism, AIDS, or neurologic disorders, such as Huntington's or Wilson's disease, or cerebrovascular accidents. Comorbidity with alcohol and substance abuse is common, either because of poor judgment and increased impulsivity or because of an attempt to self-treat the underlying mood symptoms and sleep disturbances.

Etiology and Pathophysiology Evidence for a genetic predisposition to bipolar disorder is significant. The concordance rate for monozygotic twin pairs approaches 80%, and segregation analyses are consistent with autosomal dominant transmission. Multiple genes are likely to be involved, with strongest evidence for loci on chromosomes 18p, 18q, 4p, 4q, 5q, 8p, and 21q.

The pathophysiologic mechanisms underlying the profound and recurrent mood swings of bipolar disorder remain unknown. Neuroimaging studies have documented alterations in amygdala volume as well as increases in white matter hyperintensities. Cellular models of changes in membrane Na^+- and K^+-activated ATPase and proposals of disordered signal transduction mechanisms involving the phosphoinositol system and GTP-binding proteins have received the most attention. Neurophysiologic studies suggest that patients with bipolar disorder have altered circadian rhythmicity. Lithium may exert its ther-

---

TABLE 371-10   *Criteria for a Manic Episode*

A. A distinct period of abnormally and persistently elevated, expansive, or irritable mood, lasting at least 1 week (or any duration if hospitalization is necessary)

B. During the period of mood disturbance, three (or more) of the following symptoms have persisted (four if the mood is only irritable) and have been present to a significant degree:
1. Inflated self-esteem or grandiosity
2. Decreased need for sleep (e.g., feels rested after only 3 hours of sleep)
3. More talkative than usual or pressure to keep talking
4. Flight of ideas or subjective experience that thoughts are racing
5. Distractibility (i.e., attention too easily drawn to unimportant or irrelevant external stimuli)
6. Increase in goal-directed activity (either socially, at work or school, or sexually) or psychomotor agitation
7. Excessive involvement in pleasurable activities that have a high potential for painful consequences (e.g., engaging in unrestrained buying sprees, sexual indiscretions, or foolish business investments)

C. The symptoms do not meet criteria for a mixed episode.

D. The mood disturbance is sufficiently severe to cause marked impairment in occupational functioning or in usual social activities or relationships with others, or to necessitate hospitalization to prevent harm to self or others, or there are psychotic features.

E. The symptoms are not due to the direct physiologic effects of a substance (e.g., a drug of abuse, a medication, or other treatment) or a general medical condition (e.g., hyperthyroidism).

Note: Manic-like episodes that are clearly caused by somatic antidepressant treatment (e.g., medication, electroconvulsive therapy, light therapy) should not count toward a diagnosis of bipolar I disorder.

Source: *Diagnostic and Statistical Manual of Mental Disorders*, 4th ed.

apeutic benefit through a resynchronization of intrinsic rhythms keyed to the light/dark cycle (Chap. 24).

℞ TREATMENT (Table 371-11)

Lithium carbonate is the mainstay of treatment in bipolar disorder, although sodium valproate and olanzapine are equally effective in acute mania, as is lamotrigine in the depressed phase. The response rate to lithium carbonate is 70 to 80% in acute mania, with beneficial effects appearing in 1 to 2 weeks. Lithium also has a prophylactic effect in prevention of recurrent mania and, to a lesser extent, in the prevention of recurrent depression. A simple cation, lithium is rapidly absorbed from the gastrointestinal tract and remains unbound to plasma or tissue proteins. Some 95% of a given dose is excreted unchanged through the kidneys within 24 h.

Serious side effects from lithium administration are rare, but minor complaints such as gastrointestinal discomfort, nausea, diarrhea, polyuria, weight gain, skin eruptions, alopecia, and edema are common. Over time, urine-concentrating ability may be decreased, but significant nephrotoxicity does not usually occur. Lithium exerts an antithyroid effect by interfering with the synthesis and release of thyroid hormones. More serious side effects include tremor, poor concentration and memory, ataxia, dysarthria, and incoordination. There is suggestive, but not conclusive, evidence that lithium is teratogenic, inducing cardiac malformations in the first trimester.

In the treatment of acute mania, lithium is initiated at 300 mg bid or tid, and the dose is then increased by 300 mg every 2 to 3 days to achieve blood levels of 0.8 to 1.2 meq/L. Because the therapeutic effect of lithium may not appear until after 7 to 10 days of treatment, adjunctive usage of lorazepam (1 to 2 mg every 4 h) or clonazepam (0.5 to 1 mg every 4 h) may be beneficial to control agitation. Antipsychotics are indicated in patients with severe agitation who respond only partially to benzodiazepines. Patients using lithium should be monitored closely, since the blood levels required to achieve a therapeutic benefit are close to those associated with toxicity.

Valproic acid is an alternative in patients who cannot tolerate lithium or respond poorly to it. Valproic acid may be better than lithium for patients who experience rapid cycling (i.e., more than four episodes a year) or who present with a mixed or dysphoric mania. Tremor and weight gain are the most common side effects; hepatotoxicity and pancreatitis are rare toxicities.

Carbamazepine and oxcarbazepine, although not formally approved by the U.S. Food and Drug Administration (FDA) for bipolar disorder, have clinical efficacy in the treatment of acute mania. Preliminary evidence also suggests that other anticonvulsant agents such as levtiracetam, zonisamide, and topiramate may possess some therapeutic benefit.

The recurrent nature of bipolar mood disorder necessitates maintenance treatment. A sustained blood lithium level of at least 0.8 mEq/L is important for optimal prophylaxis and has been shown to reduce risk of suicide, a finding not yet apparent for other mood stabilizers. Compliance is frequently an issue and often requires enlistment and education of concerned family members. Efforts to identify and modify psychosocial factors that may trigger episodes are important, as is an emphasis on lifestyle regularity. Antidepressant medications are sometimes required for the treatment of severe breakthrough depressions, but their use should generally be avoided during maintenance treatment because of the risk of precipitating mania or accelerating the cycle frequency. Loss of efficacy over time may be observed with any of the mood-stabilizing agents. In such situations, an alternative agent or combination therapy is usually helpful.

Consensus guidelines for the treatment of acute mania and bipolar depression are described in Table 371-12.

SOMATOFORM DISORDERS

CLINICAL MANIFESTATIONS Patients with multiple somatic complaints that cannot be explained by a known medical condition or by the effects of alcohol or of recreational or prescription drugs are com-

TABLE 371-11 *Clinical Pharmacology of Mood Stabilizers*

Agent and Dosing	Side Effects and Other Effects
Lithium Starting dose: 300 mg bid or tid Therapeutic blood level: 0.8–1.2 meq/L	*Common side effects:* Nausea/anorexia/diarrhea, fine tremor, thirst, polyuria, fatigue, weight gain, acne, folliculitis, neutrophilia, hypothyroidism Blood level is increased by thiazides, tetracyclines, and NSAIDs Blood level is decreased by bronchodilators, verapamil, and carbonic anhydrase inhibitors *Rare side effects:* Neurotoxicity, renal toxicity, hypercalcemia, ECG changes
Valproic acid Starting dose: 250 mg tid Therapeutic blood level: 50–125 µg/mL	*Common side effects:* Nausea/anorexia, weight gain, sedation, tremor, rash, alopecia Inhibits hepatic metabolism of other medications *Rare side effects:* Pancreatitis, hepatotoxicity, Stevens-Johnson syndrome
Carbamazepine/ oxcarbazepine Starting dose: 200 mg bid for carbamazepine, 150 bid for oxcarbazepine Therapeutic blood level: 4–12 µg/mL for carbamazepine	*Common side effects:* Nausea/anorexia, sedation, rash, dizziness/ataxia Carbamazepine, but not oxcarbazepine, induces hepatic metabolism of other medications *Rare side effects:* Hyponatremia, agranulocytosis, Stevens-Johnson syndrome
Lamotrigine Starting dose: 25 mg/d	*Common side effects:* Rash, dizziness, headache, tremor, sedation, nausea *Rare side effect:* Stevens-Johnson syndrome

Note: NSAID, nonsteroidal anti-inflammatory drug; ECG, electrocardiogram.

monly seen in primary care practice; one survey indicates a prevalence of such complaints of 5%. In *somatization disorder*, the patient presents with multiple physical complaints referable to different organ systems (Table 371-13). Onset is usually before age 30, and the disorder is persistent. Formal diagnostic criteria require the recording of at least four pain, two gastrointestinal, one sexual, and one pseudoneurologic symptom. Patients with somatization disorder often present with dramatic complaints, but the complaints are inconsistent. Symptoms of comorbid anxiety and mood disorder are common and may be the result of drug interactions due to regimens initiated independently by different physicians. Patients with somatization disorder may be impulsive and demanding and frequently qualify for a formal comorbid

TABLE 371-12 *Consensus Guidelines on the Drug Treatment of Acute Mania and Bipolar Depression*

Condition	Preferred Agents
Euphoric mania	Lithium
Mixed/dysphoric mania	Valproic acid
Mania with psychosis	Valproic acid with olanzapine, conventional antipsychotic, or risperidone
Hypomania	Lithium, lamotrigine, or valproic acid alone
Severe depression with psychosis	Venlafaxine, bupropion, or paroxetine *plus* lithium *plus* olanzapine, *or* risperidone; consider ECT
Severe depression without psychosis	Bupropion, paroxetine, sertraline, venlafaxine, *or* citalopram *plus* lithium
Mild to moderate depression	Lithium *or* lamotrigine alone; add bupropion if needed

Note: ECT, electroconvulsive therapy.
Source: From GS Sachs et al: Postgrad Med April, 2000.

TABLE 371-13   *Diagnostic Criteria for Somatization Disorder*

A. A history of many physical complaints beginning before age 30 years that occur over a period of several years and result in treatment being sought or significant impairment in social, occupational, or other important areas of functioning.

B. Each of the following criteria must have been met, with individual symptoms occurring at any time during the course of the disturbance:
1. *Four pain symptoms:* a history of pain related to at least four different sites or functions (e.g., head, abdomen, back, joints, extremities, chest, rectum, during menstruation, during sexual intercourse, or during urination)
2. *Two gastrointestinal symptoms:* a history of at least two gastrointestinal symptoms other than pain (e.g., nausea, bloating, vomiting other than during pregnancy, diarrhea, or intolerance of several different foods)
3. *One sexual symptom:* a history of at least one sexual or reproductive symptom other than pain (e.g., sexual indifference, erectile or ejaculatory dysfunction, irregular menses, excessive menstrual bleeding, vomiting throughout pregnancy)
4. *One pseudoneurologic symptom:* a history of at least one symptom or deficit suggesting a neurologic condition not limited to pain (conversion symptoms such as impaired coordination or balance, paralysis or localized weakness, difficulty swallowing or lump in throat, aphonia, urinary retention, hallucinations, loss of touch or pain sensation, double vision, blindness, deafness, seizures; dissociative symptoms such as amnesia; or loss of consciousness other than fainting)

C. Either of the following:
1. After appropriate investigation, each of the symptoms in criterion B cannot be fully explained by a known general medical condition or the direct effects of a substance (e.g., a drug of abuse, a medication)
2. When there is a related general medical condition, the physical complaints or resulting social or occupational impairment are in excess of what would be expected from the history, physical examination, or laboratory findings

D. The symptoms are not intentionally produced or feigned (as in factitious disorder or malingering).

Source: *Diagnostic and Statistical Manual of Mental Disorders,* 4th ed.

psychiatric diagnosis. In *conversion disorder*, the symptoms focus on deficits that involve motor or sensory function and on psychological factors that initiate or exacerbate the medical presentation. Like somatization disorder, the deficit is not intentionally produced or simulated, as is the case in factitious disorder (malingering). In *hypochondriasis*, the essential feature is a belief of serious medical illness that persists despite reassurance and appropriate medical evaluation. As with somatization disorder, patients with hypochondriasis have a history of poor relationships with physicians stemming from their sense that they have been evaluated and treated inappropriately or inadequately. Hypochondriasis can be disabling in intensity and is persistent, with waxing and waning symptomatology.

In *factitious illnesses*, the patient consciously and voluntarily produces physical symptoms of illness. The term *Munchausen's syndrome* is reserved for individuals with particularly dramatic, chronic, or severe factitious illness. In true factitious illness, the sick role itself is gratifying. A variety of signs, symptoms, and diseases have been either simulated or caused by factitious behavior, the most common including chronic diarrhea, fever of unknown origin, intestinal bleeding or hematuria, seizures, and hypoglycemia. Factitious disorder is usually not diagnosed until 5 to 10 years after its onset, and it can produce significant social and medical costs. In *malingering*, the fabrication derives from a desire for some external reward, such as a narcotic medication or disability reimbursement.

℞ TREATMENT

Patients with somatization disorders are frequently subjected to multiple diagnostic testing and exploratory surgeries in an attempt to find their "real" illness. Such an approach is doomed to failure and does not address the core issue. Successful treatment is best achieved through behavior modification, in which access to the physician is tightly regulated and adjusted to provide a sustained and predictable level of support that is less clearly contingent on the patient's level of presenting distress. Visits can be brief and should not be associated with a need for a diagnostic or treatment action. Although the literature is limited, some patients with somatization disorder may benefit from antidepressant treatment. Fluoxetine and MAOIs have both been found to be useful in reducing obsessive ruminations, dysphoria, and anxious preoccupation in patients with multiple somatic complaints.

The treatment of factitious disorder is complicated in that any attempt to confront the patient usually only creates a sense of humiliation and causes the patient to abandon treatment from that caregiver. A better strategy is to introduce psychological causation as one of a number of possible explanations and to include factitious illness as an option in the differential diagnoses that are discussed. Without directly linking psychotherapeutic intervention to the diagnosis, the patient can be offered a face-saving means by which the pathologic relationship with the health care system can be examined and alternative approaches to life stressors developed.

PERSONALITY DISORDERS

CLINICAL MANIFESTATIONS   Personality disorders are characteristic patterns of thinking, feeling, and interpersonal behavior that are relatively inflexible and cause significant functional impairment or subjective distress for the individual. The observed behaviors are not secondary to another mental disorder, nor are they precipitated by substance abuse or a general medical condition. This distinction is often difficult to make in clinical practice, as personality change may be the first sign of serious neurologic, endocrine, or other medical illness. Patients with frontal lobe tumors, for example, can present with changes in motivation and personality while the results of the neurologic examination remain within normal limits. Individuals with personality disorders are often regarded as "difficult patients" in clinical medical practice because they are seen as excessively demanding and/or unwilling to follow recommended treatment plans. Although DSM-IV portrays personality disorders as qualitatively distinct categories, there is an alternative perspective that personality characteristics vary as a continuum between normal functioning and formal mental disorder.

Personality disorders have been grouped into three overlapping clusters. *Cluster A* includes paranoid, schizoid, and schizotypal personality disorders. It includes individuals who are odd and eccentric and who maintain an emotional distance from others. Individuals have a restricted emotional range and remain socially isolated. Patients with schizotypal personality disorder frequently have unusual perceptual experiences and express magical beliefs about the external world. The essential feature of paranoid personality disorder is a pervasive mistrust and suspiciousness of others to an extent that is unjustified by available evidence. *Cluster B* disorders include antisocial, borderline, histrionic, and narcissistic types and describe individuals whose behavior is impulsive, excessively emotional, and erratic. *Cluster C* incorporates avoidant, dependent, and obsessive-compulsive personality types; enduring traits are anxiety and fear. The boundaries between cluster types are to some extent artificial, and many patients who meet criteria for one personality disorder also meet criteria for aspects of another. The risk of a comorbid major mental disorder is increased in patients who qualify for a diagnosis of personality disorder.

℞ TREATMENT

Dialectical behavior therapy (DBT) is a cognitive-behavioral approach that focuses on behavioral change while providing acceptance, compassion, and validation of the patient. Several randomized trials have demonstrated the efficacy of DBT in the treatment of personality disorders. Antidepressant medications and low-dose antipsychotic drugs have some efficacy in cluster A personality disorders, while anticonvulsant mood-stabilizing agents and MAOIs may be considered for patients with cluster B diagnoses who show marked mood reactivity, behavioral dyscontrol, and/or rejection hypersensitivity. Anxious or fearful cluster C patients often respond to medications used for axis I anxiety disorders (see above). It is important that the physician and the patient have reasonable expectations vis-à-vis the possible benefit of any medication used and its side effects. Improvement may be subtle and observable only over time.

SCHIZOPHRENIA

CLINICAL MANIFESTATIONS Schizophrenia is a heterogeneous syndrome characterized by perturbations of language, perception, thinking, social activity, affect, and volition. There are no pathognomonic features. The syndrome commonly begins in late adolescence, has an insidious (and less commonly acute) onset, and, classically, a poor outcome, progressing from social withdrawal and perceptual distortions to a state of chronic delusions and hallucinations. Patients may present with positive symptoms (such as conceptual disorganization, delusions, or hallucinations) or negative symptoms (loss of function, anhedonia, decreased emotional expression, impaired concentration, and diminished social engagement) and must have at least two of these for a 1-month period and continuous signs for at least 6 months to meet formal diagnostic criteria. "Negative" symptoms predominate in one-third of the schizophrenic population and are associated with a poor long-term outcome and a poor response to drug treatment. However, marked variability in the course and individual character of symptoms is typical.

The four main subtypes of schizophrenia are catatonic, paranoid, disorganized, and residual. Many individuals have symptoms of more than one type. *Catatonic-type* describes patients whose clinical presentation is dominated by profound changes in motor activity, negativism, and echolalia or echopraxia. *Paranoid-type* describes patients who have a prominent preoccupation with a specific delusional system and who otherwise do not qualify as having *disorganized-type* disease, in which disorganized speech and behavior are accompanied by a superficial or silly affect. In *residual-type* disease, negative symptomatology exists in the absence of delusions, hallucinations, or motor disturbance. The term *schizophreniform disorder* describes patients who meet the symptom requirements but not the duration requirements for schizophrenia, and *schizoaffective disorder* is used for those who manifest symptoms of schizophrenia and independent periods of mood disturbance. Prognosis depends not on symptom severity but on the response to antipsychotic medication. A permanent remission without recurrence does occasionally occur. About 10% of schizophrenic patients commit suicide.

Schizophrenia is present in 0.85% of individuals worldwide, with a lifetime prevalence of ~1 to 1.5%. An estimated 300,000 episodes of acute schizophrenia occur annually in the United States, resulting in direct and indirect costs estimated at >$33 billion.

DIFFERENTIAL DIAGNOSIS The diagnosis is principally one of exclusion, requiring the absence of significant associated mood symptoms, any relevant medical condition, and substance abuse. Drug reactions that cause hallucinations, paranoia, confusion, or bizarre behavior may be dose-related or idiosyncratic; β-adrenergic blockers, clonidine, cycloserine, quinacrine, and procaine derivatives are the most common prescription medications associated with these symptoms. Drug causes should be ruled out in any case of newly emergent psychosis. The general neurologic examination in patients with schizophrenia is usually normal, but motor rigidity, tremor, and dyskinesias are noted in one-quarter of untreated patients.

EPIDEMIOLOGY AND PATHOPHYSIOLOGY Epidemiologic surveys identify several risk factors for schizophrenia including genetic susceptibility, early developmental insults, winter birth, and increasing parental age. Genetic factors are involved in at least a subset of individuals who develop schizophrenia. Schizophrenia is observed in ~6.6% of all first-degree relatives of an affected proband. If both parents are affected, the risk for offspring is 40%. The concordance rate for monozygotic twins is 50%, compared to 10% for dizygotic twins. Schizophrenia-prone families are also at risk for other psychiatric disorders, including schizoaffective disorder and *schizotypal* and *schizoid personality disorders*, the latter terms designating individuals who show a lifetime pattern of social and interpersonal deficits characterized by an inability to form close interpersonal relationships, eccentric behavior, and mild perceptual distortions.

Despite evidence for a genetic causation, the results of molecular genetic linkage studies in schizophrenia are inconclusive. Major gene effects appear unlikely. Possible susceptibility genes include: neuroregulin-1 at chromosome 8p21; dysbindin at 6p22.3, proline dehydrogenase at 22q11, and G72 at 13q34. Several of these may be involved in glutamatergic regulation, increasing interest in N-methyl-D-aspartate (NMDA)-mediated glutamate signaling as a possible therapeutic target for treatment. One group has reported risk variants in the $\alpha7$ nicotinic acetycholine receptor subunit gene and linked it to a specific auditory processing deficit.

Schizophrenia is also associated with gestational and perinatal complications, including Rh factor incompatibility, fetal hypoxia, prenatal exposure to influenza during the second trimester, and prenatal nutritional deficiency. Studies of monozygotic twins discordant for schizophrenia have reported neuroanatomic differences between affected and unaffected siblings, supporting a "two-strike" etiology involving both genetic susceptibility and an environmental insult. The latter might involve localized hypoxia during critical stages of brain development.

A number of structural and functional abnormalities have been identified in schizophrenia, including (1) cortical atrophy and ventricular enlargement; (2) specific volume losses in the amygdala, hippocampus, right prefrontal cortex, fusiform gyrus, and thalamus; (3) progressive reduction in cortical volume over time; (4) reduced metabolism in the thalamus and prefrontal cortex; (5) abnormalities of the planum temporale; and (6) changes in the size, orientation, and density of cells in the hippocampus and prefrontal cortex, and decreased numbers of cortical interneurons. These observations have suggested that schizophrenia may result from a disturbance in a cortical striatal–thalamic circuit resulting in abnormalities in sensory filtering and attention.

Schizophrenic individuals are highly distractible and demonstrate deficits in perceptual-motor speed, ability to shift attention, and filtering out of background stimuli. Event-related evoked potential studies of schizophrenia have defined a specific reduction in P300 amplitude to a novel stimulus, which implicates an impairment in cognitive processing. Impaired information processing is also found in unaffected family members.

The *dopamine hypothesis* of schizophrenia is based on the discovery that agents that diminish dopaminergic activity also reduce the acute symptoms and signs of psychosis, specifically agitation, anxiety, and hallucinations. Amelioration of delusions and social withdrawal is less dramatic. Thus far, however, evidence for increased dopaminergic activity in schizophrenia is indirect, although decreased D_2 receptor occupancy by dopamine has recently been shown in drug-naïve patients. An increase in the activity of nigrostriatal and mesolimbic systems and a decrease in mesocortical tracts innervating the prefrontal cortex is hypothesized, although it is likely that other neurotransmitters, including serotonin, acetylcholine, glutamate, and GABA, also contribute to the pathophysiology of the illness. Possible involvement of excitatory amino acids is based on the genetic data cited above and finding that NMDA receptor antagonists and channel blockers, such as phencyclidine (PCP) and ketamine, produce characteristic signs of schizophrenia in normal individuals; cycloserine, an NMDA receptor agonist, can decrease the negative symptoms of psychosis.

℞ TREATMENT

Antipsychotic agents (Table 371-14) are the cornerstone of acute and maintenance treatment of schizophrenia, and are effective in the treatment of hallucinations, delusions, and thought disorders, regardless of

TABLE 371-14 *Antipsychotic Agents*

Name	Usual PO Daily Dose, mg	Side Effects	Sedation	Comments
TYPICAL ANTIPSYCHOTICS				
Low-potency				
Chlorpromazine (Thorazine)	100–600	Anticholinergic effects; orthostasis; photosensitivity; cholestasis; QT prolongation	+ + +	EPSEs usually not prominent; can cause anticholinergic delirium in elderly patients
Thioridazine (Mellaril)	100–600			
Mid-potency				
Trifluoperazine (Stelazine)	2–15	Fewer anticholinergic side effects; fewer EPSEs than with higher potency agents	+ +	Well tolerated by most patients
Perphenazine (Trilafon)	4–32		+ +	
Loxapine (Loxitane)	20–250	Frequent EPSEs	+ +	
Molindone (Moban)	50–225	Frequent EPSEs	0	Little weight gain
High potency		No anticholinergic side effects; EPSEs often prominent		Often prescribed in doses that are too high; long-acting injectable forms of haloperidol and fluphenazine available
Haloperidol (Haldol)	0.5–10		0/+	
Fluphenazine (Prolixin)	1–10	Frequent EPSEs	0/+	
Thiothixene (Navane)	2–20	Frequent EPSEs	0/+	
NOVEL ANTIPSYCHOTICS				
Clozapine (Clozaril)	200–600	Agranulocytosis (1%); weight gain; seizures; drooling; hyperthermia	+ +	Requires weekly WBC
Risperidone (Risperdal)	2–6	Orthostasis	+	Requires slow titration; EPSEs observed with doses >6 mg qd
Olanzapine (Zyprexa)	10–20	Weight gain	+ +	Mild prolactin elevation
Quetiapine (Seroquel)	350–700	Sedation; weight gain; anxiety	+ + +	Bid dosing
Ziprasidone (Geodon)	40–60	Orthostatic hypotension	+/+ +	Mimimal weight gain; increases QT interval
Aripiprazole (Abilify)	10–30	Nausea, anxiety, insomnia	0/+	Mixed agonist/antagonist

Note: EPSEs, extrapyramidal side effects; WBC, white blood count.

etiology. The mechanism of action involves, at least in part, blockade of dopamine receptors in the limbic system and basal ganglia; the clinical potencies of traditional antipsychotic drugs parallel their affinities for the D_2 receptor, and even the newer "atypical" agents exert some degree of D_2 receptor blockade. All neuroleptics induce expression of the immediate-early gene c-*fos* in the nucleus accumbens, a dopaminergic site connecting prefrontal and limbic cortices. The clinical efficacy of newer atypical neuroleptics, however, may involve D_1, D_3, and D_4 receptor blockade, α_1- and α_2-noradrenergic activity, and/or altering the relationship between $5HT_2$ and D_2 receptor activity, as well as faster dissociation of D_2 binding.

Conventional neuroleptics differ in their potency and side-effect profile. Older agents, such as chlorpromazine and thioridazine, are more sedating and anticholinergic and more likely to cause orthostatic hypotension, while higher potency antipsychotics, such as haloperidol, perphenazine, and thiothixene, are more likely to induce extrapyramidal side effects. The model atypical antipsychotic agent is *clozapine*, a dibenzodiazepine that has a greater potency in blocking the $5HT_2$ than the D_2 receptor and a much higher affinity for the D_4 than the D_2 receptor. Its principal disadvantage is a risk of blood dyscrasias. Unlike other antipsychotics, clozapine does not cause a rise in prolactin level. Approximately 30% of patients have a better response to these agents than to traditional neuroleptics, suggesting that they will increasingly displace the older-generation drugs. Clozapine appears to be the most effective member of this class and has demonstrated superiority to other atypical agents in preventing suicide; however, its side-effect profile makes it most appropriate for treatment-resistant cases. *Risperidone*, a benzisoxazole derivative, is more potent at $5HT_2$ than D_2 receptor sites, like clozapine, but it also exerts significant α_2 antagonism, a property that may contribute to its perceived ability to improve mood and increase motor activity. Risperidone is not as effective as clozapine in treatment-resistant cases but does not carry a risk of blood dyscrasias. *Olanzapine* is similar neurochemically to clozapine but has a significant risk of inducing weight gain. *Quetiapine* is distinct in having a weak D_2 effect but potent α_1 and histamine blockade. Ziprasidone causes minimal weight gain and is unlikely to increase prolactin, but may increase QT prolongation. Aripiprazole also has little risk of weight gain or prolactin increase but may increase anxiety, nausea, and insomnia as a result of its partial agonist properties.

Conventional antipsychotic agents are effective in 70% of patients presenting with a first episode. Improvement may be observed within hours or days, but full remission usually requires 6 to 8 weeks. The choice of agent depends principally on the side-effect profile and cost of treatment or on a past personal or family history of a favorable response to the drug in question. Atypical agents appear to be more effective in treating negative symptoms and improving cognitive function. An equivalent treatment response can usually be achieved with relatively low doses of any drug selected, i.e., 4 to 6 mg/d of haloperidol, 10 to 15 mg of olanzapine, or 4 to 6 mg/d of risperidone. Doses in this range result in >80% D_2 receptor blockade, and there is little evidence that higher doses increase either the rapidity or degree of response. Maintenance treatment requires careful attention to the possibility of relapse and monitoring for the development of a movement disorder. Intermittent drug treatment is less effective than regular dosing, but gradual dose reduction is likely to improve social functioning in many schizophrenic patients who have been maintained at high doses. If medications are completely discontinued, however, the relapse rate is 60% within 6 months. Long-acting injectable preparations are considered when noncompliance with oral therapy leads to relapses. In treatment-resistant patients, a transition to clozapine usually results in rapid improvement, but a prolonged delay in response in some cases necessitates a 6- to 9-month trial for maximal benefit to occur.

Antipsychotic medications can cause a broad range of side effects, including lethargy, weight gain, postural hypotension, constipation, and dry mouth. Extrapyramidal symptoms such as dystonia, akathisia, and akinesia are also frequent with traditional agents and may contribute to poor compliance if not specifically addressed. Anticholinergic and parkinsonian symptoms respond well to trihexyphenidyl, 2 mg bid, or benztropine mesylate, 1 to 2 mg bid. Akathisia may respond to beta blockers. In rare cases, more serious and occasionally life-threatening side effects may emerge, including ventricular arrhythmias, gastrointestinal obstruction, retinal pigmentation, obstructive jaundice, and neuroleptic malignant syndrome (characterized by hyperthermia, autonomic dysfunction, muscular rigidity, and elevated creatine phosphokinase levels). The most serious adverse effects of clozapine are agranulocytosis, which has an incidence of 1%, and induction of seizures, which has an incidence of 10%. Weekly white blood cell counts are required, particularly during the first 3 months of treatment.

The risk of type 2 diabetes mellitus appears to be increased in schizophrenia, and atypical agents as a group produce greater adverse effects on glucose regulation, independent of effects on obesity, than traditional agents. Clozapine, olanzapine, and quetiapine seem more likely to cause hyperglycemia, weight gain, and hypertriglyceridemia than other atypical antipsychotic drugs. Close monitoring of plasma glucose and lipid levels are indicated with the use of these agents.

A serious side effect of long-term use of the classic antipsychotic agents is *tardive dyskinesia*, characterized by repetitive, involuntary, and potentially irreversible movements of the tongue and lips (bucco-linguo-masticatory triad), and, in approximately half of cases, choreoathetosis (Chap. 21). Tardive dyskinesia has an incidence of 2 to 4% per year of exposure, and a prevalence of 20% in chronically treated patients. The prevalence increases with age, total dose, and duration of drug administration. The risk associated with the newer atypical agents appears to be much lower. The cause may involve formation of free radicals and perhaps mitochondrial energy failure. Vitamin E may reduce abnormal involuntary movements if given early in the syndrome.

Drug treatment of schizophrenia is by itself insufficient. Educational efforts directed toward families and relevant community resources have proved to be necessary to maintain stability and optimize outcome. A treatment model involving a multidisciplinary case-management team that seeks out and closely follows the patient in the community has proved particularly effective.

ASSESSMENT AND EVALUATION OF VIOLENCE

Primary care physicians may encounter situations in which family, domestic, or societal violence is discovered or suspected. Such an awareness can carry legal and moral obligations; many state laws mandate reporting of child, spousal, and elder abuse. Physicians are frequently the first point of contact for both victim and abuser. Between 1 and 2 million older Americans and 1.5 million U.S. children are thought to experience some form of physical maltreatment each year. Spousal abuse is thought to be even more prevalent. One survey of internal medicine practices found that 5.5% of all female patients had experienced domestic violence in the previous year, and that these individuals were more likely to suffer from depression, anxiety, somatization disorder, and substance abuse and to have attempted suicide. When domestic violence is suspected, direct but nonjudgmental questioning should be pursued with each party separately—"Do you feel safe at home?" and "If there's a disagreement or a conflict between the two of you, how is it worked out?" Individuals who are abused may have signs of obvious or suspected physical injury; in addition, abused individuals frequently express low self-esteem, vague somatic symptomatology, social isolation, and a passive feeling of loss of control. Although it is essential to treat these elements in the victim, the first obligation is to ensure that the perpetrator has taken responsibility for preventing any further violence. Substance abuse and/or dependence and serious mental illness in the abuser may contribute to the risk of harm and require direct intervention. Depending on the situation, law enforcement agencies, community resources such as support groups and shelters, and individual and family counseling can be appropriate components of a treatment plan. A safety plan should be formulated with the victim, in addition to providing information about abuse, its likelihood of recurrence, and its tendency to increase in severity and frequency. Antianxiety and antidepressant medications may sometimes be useful in treating the acute symptoms, but only if independent evidence for an appropriate psychiatric diagnosis exists. Antidepressants are generally not indicated when the diagnosis is linked to the social situation, such as an adjustment disorder with depressed mood. The most important element in treatment is the development of a supportive doctor-patient relationship that avoids further blame of the victim. In certain circumstances, a significant potential for societal violence may be discovered. Sympathetic, but direct, questioning about potential violent impulses, access to weapons, recreational drug use, and specific homicidal ideation is necessary and is sometimes therapeutic in its own right. The existence and possible contribution of such medical conditions as delirium and/or intoxication should be evaluated. Available disposition options for potentially violent patients include police custody, psychiatric hospitalization, and referral to home care, with involvement of family, friends, and caregivers. In deciding which treatment option is most appropriate, clinicians should endeavor to establish an empathic interaction with the patient, while avoiding interventions or stimuli that might precipitate or increase the risk of violent behavior.

MENTAL HEALTH PROBLEMS IN THE HOMELESS

There is a high prevalence of mental disorders and substance abuse among homeless and impoverished people. The total number of homeless individuals in the United States is estimated at 2 to 3 million, one-third of whom qualify as having a serious mental disorder. Poor hygiene and nutrition, substance abuse, psychiatric illness, physical trauma, and exposure to the elements combine to make the provision of medical care challenging. Only a minority of these individuals receive formal mental health care; the main points of contact are outpatient medical clinics and emergency departments. Primary care settings represent a critical site in which housing needs, treatment of substance dependence, and evaluation and treatment of psychiatric illness can most efficiently take place. Successful intervention is dependent on breaking down traditional administrative barriers to health care and recognizing the physical constraints and emotional costs imposed by homelessness. Simplifying health care instructions and follow-up, allowing frequent visits, and dispensing medications in limited amounts that require ongoing contact are possible techniques for establishing a successful therapeutic relationship.

FURTHER READING

ABLON JS, JONES EEJ: Validity of controlled clinical trials of psychotherapy: Findings from the NIMH treatment of depression collaborative research program. Am J Psychiatry 159:775, 2002

COYLE JT, DUMAN RS: Finding the intracellular signaling pathways affected by mood disorder treatments. Neuron 38:157, 2003

FISCHHOFF B, WESSELY S: Managing patients with inexplicable health problems. BMJ 326:595, 2003

KESSLER RC et al: The epidemiology of major depressive disorder: Results from the National Comorbidity Survey Replication (NCSR). JAMA 289:3095, 2003

WATHEN CN, MACMILLAN HL: Interventions for violence against women: Scientific review. JAMA 289:589, 2003

372 ALCOHOL AND ALCOHOLISM
Marc A. Schuckit

Alcohol, a drug, is consumed at some time by up to 80% of the population. At low doses alcohol can have some beneficial effects such as decreased rates of myocardial infarction, stroke, gallstones, and possibly vascular or Alzheimer's dementias, but the consumption of more than two standard drinks per day increases the risk for health problems in many organ systems. Heavy repetitive drinking, as is seen in alcohol abuse and dependence, cuts short the life span by an estimated decade in both genders, all cultural groups, and all socioeconomic strata. Even low doses of alcohol have a significant effect on many organ systems, adversely affecting most preexisting disease states and altering the effectiveness or blood levels of most over-the-counter and prescribed medications.

PHARMACOLOGY AND NUTRITIONAL IMPACT OF ETHANOL   Ethanol is a weakly charged molecule that moves easily through cell membranes, rapidly equilibrating between blood and tissues. The level of alcohol in the blood is expressed as milligrams or grams of ethanol per deciliter (e.g., 100 mg/dL or 0.10 g/dL); a level of 0.02 to 0.03 results from the ingestion of one to two typical drinks. In round figures, 340 mL (12 oz) of beer, 115 mL (4 oz) of nonfortified wine, and 43 mL (1.5 oz) (a shot) of 80-proof beverage each contain ~10 to 15 g of ethanol; 0.5 L (1 pint) of 86-proof beverage contains ~160 g (about 16 standard drinks), and 1 L of wine contains ~80 g of ethanol. Congeners found in alcoholic beverages, including low-molecular-weight alcohols (e.g., methanol and butanol), aldehydes, esters, histamine, phenols, tannins, iron, lead, and cobalt, may contribute to the adverse health consequences associated with heavy drinking.

Ethanol is a central nervous system (CNS) depressant that decreases neuronal activity, although some behavioral stimulation is observed at low blood levels. This drug has cross-tolerance with other depressants, including benzodiazepines and barbiturates, and all produce similar behavioral alterations. Alcohol is absorbed from mucous membranes of the mouth and esophagus (in small amounts), from the stomach and large bowel (in modest amounts), and from the proximal portion of the small intestine (the major site). The rate of absorption is increased by rapid gastric emptying; by the absence of proteins, fats, or carbohydrates (which interfere with absorption); by the absence of congeners; by dilution to a modest percentage of ethanol (maximum at about 20% by volume); and by carbonation (e.g., champagne).

Between 2% (at low blood alcohol concentrations) and 10% (at high blood alcohol concentrations) of ethanol is excreted directly through the lungs, urine, or sweat, but the greater part is metabolized to acetaldehyde, primarily in the liver. The most important pathway occurs in the cell cytosol where alcohol dehydrogenase (ADH) produces acetaldehyde, which is then rapidly destroyed by aldehyde dehydrogenase (ALDH) in the cytosol and mitochondria (Fig. 372-1). A second pathway in the microsomes of the smooth endoplasmic reticulum (the microsomal ethanol-oxidizing system, or MEOS), is responsible for ≥10% of ethanol oxidation at high blood alcohol concentrations.

While alcohol supplies calories (a drink contains ~300 kJ, or 70 to 100 kcal), these are devoid of nutrients such as minerals, proteins, and vitamins. Alcohol can also interfere with absorption of vitamins in the small intestine and decreases their storage in the liver with effects on folate (folacin or folic acid), pyridoxine (B_6), thiamine (B_1), nicotinic acid (niacin, B_3), and vitamin A.

An ethanol load in a fasting, healthy individual is likely to produce transient hypoglycemia within 6 to 36 h, secondary to the acute actions of ethanol on gluconeogenesis. This can result in glucose intolerance

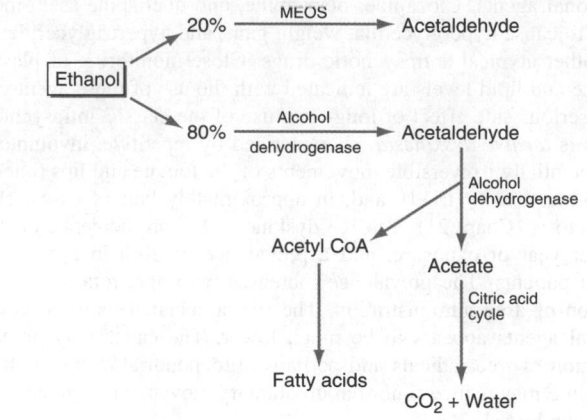

FIGURE 372-1   The metabolism of alcohol.

until the alcoholic has abstained for 2 to 4 weeks. Alcohol ketoacidosis, probably reflecting a decrease in fatty acid oxidation coupled with poor diet or recurrent vomiting, should not be misdiagnosed as diabetic ketosis. With the former, patients show an increase in serum ketones along with a mild increase in glucose but a large anion gap, a mild to moderate increase in serum lactate, and a β-hydroxybutyrate/lactate ratio of between 2:1 and 9:1 (with normal being 1:1).

BEHAVIORAL EFFECTS, TOLERANCE, AND DEPENDENCE   The effects of any drug depend on the dose, the rate of increase in plasma, the concomitant presence of other drugs, and the past experience with the agent. With alcohol, an additional factor is whether blood alcohol levels are rising or falling; the effects are more intense during the former period.

Even though "legal intoxication" requires a blood alcohol concentration of at least 80 to 100 mg/dL, behavioral, psychomotor, and cognitive changes are seen at levels as low as 20 to 30 mg/dL (i.e., after one to two drinks) (Table 372-1). Deep but disturbed sleep can be seen at twice the legal intoxication level, and death can occur with levels between 300 and 400 mg/dL. Beverage alcohol is probably responsible for more overdose deaths than any other drug.

The intoxicating effects of alcohol appear to be due to actions at a number of neurotransmitter receptors and transporters. Alcohol enhances γ-aminobutyric acid A (GABA$_A$) receptors and inhibits N-methyl-D-aspartate (NMDA) receptors. In vitro studies suggest that additional effects involve inhibition of adenosine uptake and a translocation of the cyclic AMP–dependent protein kinase catalytic subunit from the cytoplasm to the nucleus. Neurons adapt quickly to these actions, and thus different effects may be present during chronic administration and withdrawal.

At least three types of compensatory changes develop after repeated exposure to the drug, producing tolerance of higher ethanol levels. First, after 1 to 2 weeks of daily drinking, *metabolic or pharmacokinetic tolerance* can be seen, with a 30% increase in the rate of hepatic

TABLE 372-1   *Effects of Blood Alcohol Levels in the Absence of Tolerance*

Blood Level, mg/dL	Usual Effect
20	Decreased inhibitions, a slight feeling of intoxication
80	Decrease in complex cognitive functions and motor performance
200	Obvious slurred speech, motor incoordination, irritability, and poor judgment
300	Light coma and depressed vital signs
400	Death

ethanol metabolism. This alteration disappears almost as rapidly as it develops. Second, *cellular or pharmacodynamic tolerance* develops through neurochemical changes that may also contribute to physical dependence. Third, individuals can learn to adapt their behavior so that they can function better than expected under drug influence (*behavioral tolerance*).

The cellular changes caused by chronic ethanol exposure may not resolve for several weeks or longer following cessation of drinking. In the interim, the neurons require ethanol to function optimally, and the individual can be said to be physically dependent. This is distinct from psychological dependence, a concept indicating that the person is psychologically uncomfortable without the drug.

THE EFFECTS OF ETHANOL ON ORGAN SYSTEMS

Although one to two drinks per day in an otherwise healthy and non-pregnant individual can have some beneficial effects, at higher doses alcohol is toxic to most organ systems. Knowledge about the deleterious effects of alcohol helps the physician to identify alcoholic patients and provides information that can be used to help motivate them to abstain. The information offered here generally applies across ages and genders, with common sense differences (e.g., older persons carry higher health risks). It is important to remember that the typical white- or blue-collar alcoholic functions at a fairly high level for years, and that not everyone develops each problem.

CENTRAL NERVOUS SYSTEM Approximately 35% of drinkers may experience a *blackout*, an episode of temporary anterograde amnesia, in which the person forgets all or part of what occurred during a drinking evening. Another common problem, one seen after as few as several drinks, is that alcohol causes alterations between sleep stages and a deficiency in rapid eye movement and deep sleep with resulting prominent and sometimes disturbing dreams later in the night. Finally, alcohol relaxes muscles in the pharynx, which can cause snoring and exacerbate sleep apnea, with symptoms of the latter in 75% of alcoholic men over age 60. As a consequence of alcohol-related impairment in judgment and coordination, at least half of patients with physical trauma have evidence of substance-related impairment, a finding reflecting the fact that 40% of drinkers in the United States have at some time driven while intoxicated.

The effect of alcohol on the nervous system is even more pronounced among alcohol-dependent individuals. Chronic high doses cause *peripheral neuropathy* in 5 to 15% of alcoholics: patients experience bilateral limb numbness, tingling, and paresthesias, all of which are more pronounced distally. *Wernicke's syndrome* (ophthalmoparesis, ataxia, and encephalopathy) and *Korsakoff's syndrome* are seen in <10% of alcoholics as the result of thiamine deficiency, especially in persons with transketolase deficiency (Chap. 258). Approximately 1% of alcoholics develop *cerebellar degeneration*, a syndrome of progressive unsteady stance and gait often accompanied by mild nystagmus; neuroimaging studies reveal atrophy of the cerebellar vermis.

Alcoholics can manifest severe *cognitive problems* including impairment in recent and remote memory for weeks to months after an alcoholic binge. Increased size of the brain ventricles and cerebral sulci are seen in ≥50% of chronic alcoholics, but these changes are often reversible, returning toward normal within a year or so of abstinence. There is no single alcoholic dementia syndrome; rather, this label is used to describe patients who have apparently irreversible cognitive changes (possibly from diverse causes) and chronic alcoholism.

Finally, almost every psychiatric syndrome can be seen temporarily during heavy drinking or subsequent withdrawal. These include intense *sadness* lasting for days to weeks in the midst of heavy drinking in 40% of alcoholics, which is classified as an alcohol-induced mood disorder; temporary severe *anxiety* in 10 to 30% of alcoholics, often beginning during alcohol withdrawal, which can persist for many months after cessation of drinking (alcohol-induced anxiety disorder); and auditory *hallucinations* and/or paranoid delusions in a clear sensorium (*alcohol-induced psychotic disorder*) seen temporarily in 1 to

10% of alcoholics. Treatment of all forms of alcohol-induced psychopathology includes abstinence and supportive care, with the likelihood of full recovery within several days to 4 weeks. A history of alcohol intake is an important consideration in any patient with one of these psychiatric symptoms.

THE GASTROINTESTINAL SYSTEM ■ Esophagus and Stomach Acute alcohol intake can result in inflammation of the esophagus and stomach, causing epigastric distress and gastrointestinal bleeding. Chronic heavy drinking, if associated with violent vomiting, can produce a Mallory-Weiss lesion, a longitudinal tear in the mucosa at the gastroesophageal junction.

Pancreas and Liver The incidence of acute pancreatitis (~25 per 1000 per year) is almost threefold higher than in the general population, accounting for an estimated 10% or more of the cases of this disorder (Chap. 294). Alcohol impairs gluconeogenesis in the liver with a resulting fall in the amount of glucose produced from glycogen; lactate production increases; and there is a decreased oxidation of fatty acids with an increase in fat accumulation in liver cells. In the healthy individual these changes are reversible, but with repeated exposure to ethanol, more severe changes can occur, including fatty accumulation, alcohol-induced hepatitis, perivenular sclerosis, and cirrhosis, with the latter observed in an estimated 15 to 20% of alcoholics (Chap. 288).

CANCER Drinking as few as 1.5 drinks per day increases a woman's risk of breast cancer 1.4-fold. For both genders, four drinks per day increases the risk for oral and esophageal cancers approximately threefold and rectal cancers by a factor of 1.5; seven to eight or more drinks per day enhances the risks for many cancers by a factor of five.

HEMATOPOIETIC SYSTEM Ethanol causes an increase in red blood cell size [mean corpuscular volume, (MCV)], which reflects the effects on stem cells. If heavy drinking is accompanied by folic acid deficiency, there can also be hypersegmented neutrophils, reticulocytopenia, and a hyperplastic bone marrow; if malnutrition is present, sideroblastic changes can be observed. Chronic heavy drinking can decrease production of most white blood cells, decrease granulocyte mobility and adherence, and impair the delayed-hypersensitivity response to new antigens (with a possible false-negative tuberculin skin test). Finally, many alcoholics have mild thrombocytopenia, which usually resolves within a week of abstinence unless there is hepatic cirrhosis or congestive splenomegaly.

CARDIOVASCULAR SYSTEM Acutely, ethanol decreases myocardial contractility and causes peripheral vasodilation, with a resulting mild decrease in blood pressure and a compensatory increase in cardiac output. Exercise-induced increases in cardiac oxygen consumption are higher after alcohol intake. These acute effects have little clinical significance for the average healthy drinker but can be problematic in men and women with cardiac disease.

The consumption of three or more drinks per day results in a dose-dependent increase in blood pressure, which returns to normal within weeks of abstinence. Heavy drinking is an important contributor to mild to moderate hypertension. Chronic heavy drinking can cause cardiomyopathy, with symptoms ranging from unexplained arrhythmias in the presence of left ventricular impairment to heart failure with dilation of all four heart chambers and hypocontractility of heart muscle. Perhaps one-third of cases of cardiomyopathy are alcohol-induced. Mural thrombi can form in the left atrium or ventricle, while heart enlargement >25% can cause mitral regurgitation. Atrial or ventricular arrhythmias, especially paroxysmal tachycardia, can also occur after a drinking binge in individuals showing no other evidence of heart disease—a syndrome known as the "holiday heart."

Chronic intake of modest doses of alcohol can have some beneficial effects. A maximum of one to two drinks per day may decrease the risk for cardiovascular death, perhaps through an increase in high-density lipoprotein (HDL) cholesterol or changes in clotting mechanisms. In one large national study, cardiovascular mortality was reduced by 30 to 40% among individuals reporting one or more drinks daily compared to nondrinkers, with overall mortality lowest among those consuming approximately one drink per day. Recent data have also corroborated the decreased risk for ischemic, but not hemorrhagic, stroke associated with regular light drinking.

GENITOURINARY SYSTEM CHANGES, SEXUAL FUNCTIONING, AND FETAL DEVELOPMENT Acutely, modest ethanol doses (e.g., blood alcohol concentrations of ≤100 mg/dL) can both increase sexual drive and decrease erectile capacity in men. Even in the absence of liver impairment, a significant minority of chronic alcoholic men may show irreversible testicular atrophy with concomitant shrinkage of the seminiferous tubules, decreases in ejaculate volume, and a lower sperm count (Chap. 325).

The repeated ingestion of high doses of ethanol by women can result in amenorrhea, a decrease in ovarian size, absence of corpora lutea with associated infertility, and spontaneous abortions. Heavy drinking during pregnancy results in the rapid placental transfer of both ethanol and acetaldehyde, which may have serious consequences for fetal development. The *fetal alcohol syndrome* can include any of the following: facial changes with epicanthal eye folds, poorly formed concha, and small teeth with faulty enamel; cardiac atrial or ventricular septal defects; an aberrant palmar crease and limitation in joint movement; and microcephaly with mental retardation. The amount of ethanol and/or time of vulnerability during pregnancy have not been defined, making it advisable for pregnant women to abstain completely.

OTHER EFFECTS OF ETHANOL Between one-half and two-thirds of alcoholics have skeletal muscle weakness caused by acute *alcoholic myopathy*, a condition that improves but which might not disappear with abstinence. Effects of repeated heavy drinking on the *skeletal system* include alterations in calcium metabolism, lower bone density, and less growth in the epiphyses, with an increased risk for fractures and osteonecrosis of the femoral head. *Hormonal changes* include an increase in cortisol levels, which can remain elevated during heavy drinking; inhibition of vasopressin secretion at rising blood alcohol concentrations and the opposite effect at falling blood alcohol concentrations (with the final result that most alcoholics are likely to be slightly overhydrated); a modest and reversible decrease in serum thyroxine (T_4); and a more marked decrease in serum triiodothyronine (T_3).

ALCOHOLISM (ALCOHOL ABUSE OR DEPENDENCE)

Because many drinkers occasionally imbibe to excess, temporary alcohol-related pathology is common in nonalcoholics, especially those in the late teens to the late twenties. When repeated problems in multiple life areas develop, the person is likely to meet criteria for alcohol abuse or dependence.

DEFINITIONS AND EPIDEMIOLOGY *Alcohol dependence* is defined in the Fourth Diagnostic and Statistical Manual (DSM-IV) of the American Psychiatric Association as repeated alcohol-related difficulties in at least three of seven areas of functioning that cluster together over any 12-month period. A special emphasis is placed on tolerance and/or withdrawal, a condition referred to as "dependence with a physiological component," which is associated with a more severe clinical course. Dependence occurs in both men and women and in individuals from all socioeconomic strata and of all racial backgrounds. The diagnosis predicts a course of recurrent problems with the use of alcohol and the consequent shortening of the life span by a decade or more. In the absence of alcohol dependence, an individual can be given a diagnosis of *alcohol abuse* if he or she demonstrates repetitive problems with alcohol in any one of four life areas that include social, interpersonal, legal, and occupational problems, or repeated use in hazardous situations such as driving.

The lifetime risk for alcohol dependence in most western countries is about 10 to 15% for men and 5 to 8% for women. When alcohol abuse is also considered, the rates are even higher. The typical alcoholic is a blue- or white-collar worker or homemaker and not the stereotypical homeless individual.

GENETICS OF ALCOHOLISM *Alcoholism* is a complex genetically influenced disorder; genes explain about 60% of the risk. The importance of genetic influences is supported by a higher risk in the identical versus fraternal twin of an alcoholic and a fourfold increased risk in children of alcoholics even if adopted at birth and raised without knowledge of their biologic parents.

A variety of independent genetically influenced characteristics likely combine to explain the contribution of hereditary factors. For alcoholism and other substance dependencies, some families appear to carry an enhanced risk through high levels of impulsivity, as can be seen in the antisocial personality disorder. In other families the risk is associated with vulnerability for several independent psychiatric disorders such as schizophrenia and manic-depressive disease. A diminished alcoholism risk is seen in approximately half of Asian men and women; this is due to an inactive form of the enzyme ALDH, which results in higher levels of acetaldehyde following alcohol ingestion. A significant proportion of the vulnerability for alcoholism appears to relate to genes that affect the intensity of the response to alcohol. Most studies have shown that 40% of some subgroups at high risk for future alcoholism (e.g., offspring of alcoholics) require higher blood alcohol concentrations to produce the effects seen at lower blood levels in most other people. This relatively low response to alcohol predicts the risk for alcohol-related problems over the next decade, including alcohol use disorders.

NATURAL HISTORY For the "average" alcoholic, the age of first drink and first problems (e.g., an alcoholic blackout) are similar to those in the general population. However, by the early to mid-twenties, most men and women moderate their drinking (perhaps learning from minor problems), whereas difficulties for alcoholics are likely to escalate, with the first major life problem from alcohol appearing in the mid-twenties. Once established, the course of alcoholism is likely to be one of exacerbations and remissions. As a rule, there is little difficulty in stopping alcohol use when problems develop, and this step is often followed by days to months of carefully controlled drinking. Unless abstinence is maintained, these periods almost inevitably give way to escalations in alcohol intake and subsequent problems. The course is not hopeless, because between half and two-thirds of alcoholics maintain abstinence for years, and often permanently after treatment. Even without formal treatment or self-help groups there is at least a 20% chance of long-term abstinence. However, should the alcoholic continue to drink, the life span is shortened by an average of 10 years, with the leading causes of death, in decreasing order, the result of heart disease, cancer, accidents, and suicide.

IDENTIFICATION OF THE ALCOHOLIC AND INTERVENTION Physicians even in affluent areas should recognize that ~20% of patients have alcoholism. Therefore, it is important to pay attention to the alcohol-related symptoms and signs as well as laboratory tests that are likely to be abnormal in the context of regular consumption of 6 to 8 or more drinks per day. The two blood tests with between 70% and 80% sensitivity and specificity are γ-glutamyl transferase (GGT) (>30 U) and carbohydrate-deficient transferrin (CDT) (>20 U/L); the combination of the two is likely to be more accurate than either alone. Physicians should consider these tests when screening patients for high levels of alcohol intake. These serologic markers of heavy drinking can also be useful in monitoring abstinence as they are likely to return toward normal within several weeks of the cessation of drinking; thus, increases in values of as little as 10% are likely to indicate a resumption of heavy alcohol intake. Other blood tests that can be useful in identifying individuals consuming six or more standard drinks per day include high normal MCVs (>91 μm^3) and serum uric acid (>416 mol/L, or 7 mg/dL). Physical signs and symptoms that can be useful in identifying alcoholism include mild and fluctuating hypertension (e.g., 140/95), repeated infections such as pneumonia, and otherwise unexplained cardiac arrhythmias. Other disorders suggestive of dependence include cancer of the head and neck, esophagus, or stomach as well as cirrhosis, unexplained hepatitis, pancreatitis, bilateral parotid gland swelling, and peripheral neuropathy.

The clinical diagnosis of alcohol abuse or dependence ultimately rests on the documentation of a pattern of difficulties associated with alcohol use; the definition is not based on the quantity and frequency of alcohol consumption. Thus, in screening it is important to probe for life problems and then attempt to tie in use of alcohol or another substance. Information regarding marital or job problems, legal difficulties, histories of accidents, medical problems, evidence of tolerance, etc., is important. While all physicians should be able to take the time needed to gather such information, some standardized questionnaires can be helpful, including the 10-item Alcohol Use Disorder Screening Test (AUDIT). However, these are only screening tools, and a careful face-to-face interview is still required for a meaningful diagnosis. Shorter questionnaires have limited usefulness.

After alcoholism is identified, the diagnosis must be shared with the patient as part of an intervention. The presenting complaint can be used as an entrée to the alcohol problem. For instance, the patient complaining of insomnia or hypertension could be told that these are clinically important symptoms and that physical findings and laboratory tests indicate that alcohol appears to have contributed to the complaints and is increasing the risk for further medical and psychological problems. The physician should share information about the course of alcoholism and explore possible avenues of addressing the problem. This process has been codified under the names of *brief interventions* and *motivational interviewing*. The former has been shown to be effective in decreasing alcohol use and problems when instituted as two 15-min sessions 1 month apart, along with a telephone follow-up reminder. Motivational interviewing uses the clinician's level of concern and understanding of the need for patients to progress through their own stages of enhanced understanding of their problems to optimize their ability to alter their drinking behaviors.

The process of intervention is rarely accomplished in one session. For the person who refuses to stop drinking at the first intervention, a logical step is to "keep the door open," establishing future meetings so that help is available as problems escalate. In the meantime the family may benefit from counseling or referral to self-help groups such as Al-Anon (the Alcoholics Anonymous group for family members) and Alateen (for teenage children of alcoholics).

THE ALCOHOL WITHDRAWAL SYNDROME Once the brain has been repeatedly exposed to high doses of alcohol, any sudden decrease in intake can produce withdrawal symptoms, many of which are the opposite of those produced by intoxication. Features include tremor of the hands (shakes or jitters); agitation and anxiety; autonomic nervous system overactivity including an increase in pulse, respiratory rate, and body temperature; insomnia, possibly accompanied by bad dreams; and gastrointestinal upset. These withdrawal symptoms generally begin within 5 to 10 h of decreasing ethanol intake, peak in intensity on day 2 or 3, and improve by day 4 or 5. Anxiety, insomnia, and mild levels of autonomic dysfunction may persist to some degree for ≥ 6 months as a protracted abstinence syndrome, which may contribute to the tendency to return to drinking.

At some point in their lives, between 2 and 5% of alcoholics experience withdrawal seizures, often within 48 h of stopping drinking. These rare events usually involve a single generalized seizure, and electroencephalographic abnormalities generally return to normal within several days.

The term *delirium tremens* (DTs) refers to delirium (mental confusion, agitation, and fluctuating levels of consciousness) associated with a tremor and autonomic overactivity (e.g., marked increases in pulse, blood pressure, and respirations). Fortunately, this serious and potentially life-threatening complication of alcohol withdrawal is seen in <5% of alcohol-dependent individuals, with the result that the chance of DTs during any single withdrawal is <1%. DTs are most likely to develop in patients with concomitant severe medical disorders and can usually be avoided by identifying and treating medical conditions.

TREATMENT

Acute Intoxication The first priority is to be certain that the vital signs are relatively stable without evidence of respiratory depression, cardiac arrhythmia, or potentially dangerous changes in blood pressure. The possibility of intoxication with other drugs should be considered, and a blood or urine sample is indicated to screen for opioids or other CNS depressants such as benzodiazepines or barbiturates. Other medical conditions that must be evaluated include hypoglycemia, hepatic failure, or diabetic ketoacidosis.

Patients who are medically stable should be placed in a quiet environment and asked to lie on their side if fatigued in order to minimize the risk of aspiration. When the behavior indicates an increased likelihood of violence, hospital procedures should be followed, including planning for the possibility of a show of force with an intervention team. In the context of aggressiveness, patients should be clearly reminded in a nonthreatening way that it is the goal of the staff to help them to feel better and to avoid problems. If the aggressive behavior continues, relatively low doses of a short-acting benzodiazepine such as lorazepam (e.g., 1 mg orally) may be used and can be repeated as needed, but care must be taken so that the addition of this second CNS depressant does not destabilize vital signs or worsen confusion. An alternative approach is to use an antipsychotic medication (e.g., 5 mg of haloperidol), but this has the potential danger of lowering the seizure threshold. If aggression escalates, the patient might require a short-term admission to a locked ward, where medications can be used more safely and vital signs more closely monitored.

Withdrawal The first step is to perform a thorough physical examination in all alcoholics who are considering stopping drinking, including a search for evidence of liver failure, gastrointestinal bleeding, cardiac arrhythmia, and glucose or electrolyte imbalance.

The second step in treating withdrawal for even the typical well-nourished alcoholic is to offer adequate nutrition and rest. All patients should be given oral multiple B vitamins, including 50 to 100 mg of thiamine daily for a week or more. Most patients enter withdrawal with normal levels of body water or mild overhydration, and intravenous fluids should be avoided unless there is evidence of significant recent bleeding, vomiting, or diarrhea. Medications can usually be administered orally.

The third step in treatment is to recognize that most withdrawal symptoms are caused by the rapid removal of a CNS depressant. Patients can be weaned by administering any drug of this class and gradually decreasing the levels over 3 to 5 days. While many CNS depressants are effective, benzodiazepines have the highest margin of safety and lowest cost and are, therefore, the preferred class of drugs. Benzodiazepines with short half-lives (Chap. 371) are especially useful for patients with serious liver impairment or evidence of preexisting encephalopathy or brain damage, but result in rapidly changing drug blood levels and must be given every 4 h to avoid abrupt fluctuations in blood levels that may increase the risk for seizures. Therefore, most clinicians use drugs with longer half-lives, such as diazepam or chlordiazepoxide, administering enough drug on day 1 to alleviate most of the symptoms of withdrawal (e.g., the tremor and elevated pulse) and then decreasing the dose by 20% on successive days over a period of 3 to 5 days. The approach is flexible; the dose is increased if signs of withdrawal escalate, and the medication is withheld if the patient is sleeping or shows signs of increasing orthostatic hypotension. The average patient requires 25 to 50 mg of chlordiazepoxide or 10 mg of diazepam given orally every 4 to 6 h on the first day.

Treatment of the patient with DTs can be difficult, and the condition is likely to run a course of 3 to 5 days regardless of the therapy employed. The focus of care is to identify medical problems and correct them and to control behavior and prevent injuries. Many clinicians recommend the use of high doses of a benzodiazepine (as much as 800 mg/d of chlordiazepoxide have been reported), a treatment that will decrease the agitation and raise the seizure threshold but probably does little to improve the confusion. Other clinicians recommend the use of antipsychotic medications, such as haloperidol, 20 mg or more per day, an approach less likely to exacerbate confusion but which may increase the risk of seizures. Antipsychotic drugs have no place in the treatment of mild withdrawal symptoms.

Generalized withdrawal seizures rarely require aggressive pharmacologic intervention beyond that given to the usual patient undergoing withdrawal, i.e., adequate doses of benzodiazepines. There is little evidence that anticonvulsants such as phenytoin are effective in drug-withdrawal seizures, and the risk of seizures has usually passed by the time effective drug levels are reached. The rare patient with status epilepticus must be treated aggressively (Chap. 348).

While alcohol withdrawal is often treated in a hospital, efforts at reducing costs have resulted in the development of outpatient detoxification for relatively mild abstinence syndromes. This is appropriate for patients in good physical condition who demonstrate mild signs of withdrawal despite low blood alcohol concentrations and for those without prior history of DTs or withdrawal seizures. Such individuals still require a careful physical examination, evaluation of blood tests, and vitamin supplementation. Benzodiazepines can be given in a 1- to 2-day supply to be administered to the patient by a spouse or other family member four times a day. Patients are asked to return daily for evaluation of vital signs and to come to the emergency room if signs and symptoms of withdrawal escalate.

Rehabilitation of Alcoholics   After completing alcoholic rehabilitation, 60% or more of alcoholics maintain abstinence for at least a year, and many achieve lifetime abstinence. Considering the lack of evidence for the superiority of any specific treatment type, it is best to keep interventions simple.

Maneuvers in rehabilitation fall into several general categories, which are applied to all patients regardless of age or ethnic group. However, the manner in which the treatments are used should be sensitive to the practices and needs of specific populations. First are attempts to help the alcoholic achieve and maintain a high level of motivation toward abstinence. These include education about alcoholism and instructing family and/or friends to stop protecting the person from the problems caused by alcohol. The second step is to help the patient to readjust to life without alcohol and to reestablish a functional lifestyle through counseling, vocational rehabilitation, and self-help groups such as Alcoholics Anonymous. The third component, called *relapse prevention*, helps the person to identify situations in which a return to drinking is likely, formulate ways of managing these risks, and develop coping strategies that increase the chances of a return to abstinence if a slip occurs.

There is no convincing evidence that inpatient rehabilitation is always more effective than outpatient care. However, more intense interventions work better than less intensive measures, and some alcoholics do not respond to outpatient approaches. The decision to hospitalize or place into residential care can be made if (1) the patient has medical problems that are difficult to treat outside a hospital; (2) depression, confusion, or psychosis interferes with outpatient care; (3) there is a severe life crisis that makes it difficult to work in an outpatient setting; (4) outpatient treatment has failed; or (5) the patient lives far from the treatment center. The best predictors of continued abstinence include evidence of higher levels of life stability (e.g., supportive family and friends) and higher levels of functioning (e.g., job skills, higher levels of education, and absence of crimes unrelated to alcohol).

Whether the treatment begins in an inpatient or an outpatient setting, subsequent outpatient contact should be maintained for a minimum of 6 months and preferably a full year after abstinence is achieved. Counseling with an individual physician or through groups focuses on day-to-day living—emphasizing areas of improved functioning in the absence of alcohol (i.e., why it is a good idea to continue to abstain) and helping the patient to manage free time without alcohol, develop a nondrinking peer group, and handle stresses on the job.

The physician serves an important role in identifying the alcoholic, treating associated medical or psychiatric syndromes, overseeing detoxification, referring the patient to rehabilitation programs, and providing counseling. The physician is also responsible for selecting which (if any) medication might be appropriate during alcoholism rehabilitation. Patients often complain of continuing sleep problems or anxiety when acute withdrawal treatment is over, problems that may be a component of protracted withdrawal. Unfortunately, there is no place for hypnotics or antianxiety drugs in the treatment of most alcoholics after acute withdrawal has been completed. Patients should be reassured that the trouble sleeping is normal after alcohol withdrawal and will improve over the subsequent weeks and months. Patients should follow a rigid bedtime and awakening schedule and avoid any naps or the use of caffeine in the evenings. The sleep pattern will improve rapidly. Anxiety can be addressed by helping the person to gain insight into the temporary nature of the symptoms and to develop strategies to achieve relaxation as well as by using forms of cognitive therapy.

While the mainstay of alcoholic rehabilitation involves counseling, education, and cognitive approaches, several medications might be useful. The first is the opioid-antagonist drug naltrexone, 50 to 150 mg/d, which has been reported in several small-scale, short-term studies to decrease the probability of a return to drinking and to shorten periods of relapse. However, at least one longer-term large-scale trial questioned the superiority of naltrexone to placebo, and more studies are required before the cost-effectiveness of this approach can be established. A second medication, acamprosate (Campral), 2 g/d, has been tested in >5000 patients in Europe, with results that appear similar to those reported for naltrexone. Several long-term trials of naltrexone and acamprosate, used individually and in combination, are in progress, and early results are promising. A third medication, which has historically been used in the treatment of alcoholism, is the ALDH inhibitor disulfiram. In doses of 250 mg/d this drug produces an unpleasant (and potentially dangerous) reaction in the presence of alcohol, a phenomenon related to rapidly rising blood levels of the first metabolite of alcohol, acetaldehyde. However, few adequate controlled trials have demonstrated the superiority of disulfiram over placebo. Disulfiram has many side effects, and the reaction with alcohol can be dangerous, especially for patients with heart disease, stroke, diabetes mellitus, and hypertension. Thus, most clinicians reserve this medication for patients who have a clear history of longer-term abstinence associated with prior use of disulfiram and for those who might take the drug under the supervision of another individual (such as a spouse), especially during discrete periods that they have identified as representing high-risk drinking situations for them (such as the Christmas holiday).

Additional support for alcoholics and their relatives and friends is available through self-help groups such as Alcoholics Anonymous (AA). These groups, which typically consist of recovering alcoholics, offer an effective model of abstinence, provide a sober peer group, and make crisis intervention available when the urge to drink escalates. This can help patients optimize their chances for recovery, especially when incorporated into a more structured treatment milieu.

FURTHER READING

FLEMING MF et al: Brief physician advice for problem drinkers: Long-term efficacy and benefit-cost analysis. Alcohol Clin Exp Res 26:36, 2002

KIEFER F et al: Comparing and combining naltrexone and acamprosate in relapse prevention of alcoholism. Arch Gen Psychiatry 60:92, 2003

SCHUCKIT MA et al: A 5-year prospective evaluation of DSM-IV alcohol dependence with and without a physiological component. Alcohol Clin Exp Res 27:818, 2003

It is difficult to imagine modern medical practice without the use of opioid analgesics. These drugs have been part of health care since 300 B.C. Opium and codeine were isolated in the early nineteenth century, opioid-like substances produced by the body were recognized in the 1970s, and the first endogenous opioid was isolated in 1995. As important as these substances are to modern medicine, opioid drugs have many disadvantages, including overdosage and dependency; close to 1 million individuals in the United States are opioid-dependent. All opioid drugs are capable of producing a heroin-like intoxication, as well as tolerance and withdrawal.

PHARMACOLOGY The prototypic opiates, morphine and codeine (3-methoxymorphine), are derived from the milky juice of the poppy *Papaver somniferum*. The semisynthetic drugs produced from the morphine or thebane molecules include hydromorphone, diacetylmorphine (heroin), and oxycodone. The purely synthetic opioids and their cousins include meperidine, propoxyphene, diphenoxylate, fentanyl, buprenorphine, tramadol, methadone, and pentazocine.

Endogenous opioid peptides (i.e., enkephalins, endorphins, dynorphins, and others) have distinct distributions in the central nervous system (CNS) and appear to be natural ligands for opioid receptors. As summarized in (Table 373-1), the receptors with which opioid peptides interact differentially produce analgesia, respiratory depression, constipation, euphoria, and other actions. Substances capable of antagonizing one or more of these actions include nalorphine, levallorphan, cyclazocine, butorphanol, buprenorphine, and pentazocine, each of which has mixed agonist and antagonist properties, as well as naloxone, nalmefene, and naltrexone, which are pure opiate antagonists. The availability of relatively specific antagonists has helped identify at least three different receptor subtypes, including μ receptors, which influence some of the more classic opioid actions such as pain control, reinforcement, constipation, hormone levels, and respiration; κ receptors, with possible similar functions along with sedation and effects on hormones; and δ receptors, thought to relate mostly to analgesia, mood, reinforcement, and breathing. A fourth possible receptor subtype, sensitive to another endogenous peptide, is sometimes called *nociceptin* or *orphanin* and may influence pain. The major features of tolerance, dependence, and withdrawal are thought to be mediated primarily by μ receptors, and these are affected by all prescription opioids.

The most rapid and pronounced effects of opioids occur following intravenous administration, with only slightly less efficient absorption after smoking or inhaling the vapor ("chasing the dragon"). The least intense effects occur after oral consumption. Most of the metabolism of opioids occurs in the liver, primarily through conjugation with glucuronic acid, and only small amounts are excreted directly in the urine or feces. The plasma half-lives of these drugs range from 2.5 to 3 h for morphine to more than 22 h for methadone and even longer for levomethadyl acetate (LAAM).

TABLE 373-1 *Actions of Opioid Receptors*	
Receptor Type	**Actions**
Mu (μ) (e.g., morphine)	Analgesia, reinforcement euphoria, cough and appetite suppression, decreased respirations, decreased GI motility, sedation, hormone changes, dopamine and acetylcholine release
Kappa (κ) (e.g., butorphanol)	Decreased dysphoria, decreased GI motility, decreased appetite, decreased respiration, psychotic symptoms, sedation, diuresis, analgesia
Delta (δ) (e.g., etorphine)	Hormone changes, appetite suppression, dopamine release

Note: GI, gastrointestinal.

Street heroin is typically only 5 to 10% pure, mixed with sugars, quinine, powdered milk, phenacetin, caffeine, antipyrine, and strychnine. Unexpected increases in the purity of street drugs can cause unintentional lethal overdoses.

ACUTE AND CHRONIC EFFECTS OF OPIOIDS With the exception of overdose and physical dependence, most opioid effects are rapidly reversible. A major danger, however, comes through the use of contaminated needles by intravenous users, which increases the risk of hepatitis B and C, bacterial endocarditis, and infection with HIV (Chap. 173).

Effects on Organ Systems In addition to euphoria and rewarding effects of opioids due to stimulation of a dopaminergic pathway originating in the midbrain and terminating in the nucleus accumbens, CNS effects of opioid drugs include nausea and vomiting (medulla), decreased pain perception (spinal cord, thalamus, and periaqueductal gray region), and sedation (reticular activating system). The adulterants added to street drugs may contribute to nervous system damage, including peripheral neuropathy, amblyopia, myelopathy, and leukoencephalopathy. Acute opioid administration inhibits release of some hormones from the hypothalamus, including corticotropin-releasing factor (CRF) and luteinizing hormone, with a subsequent reduction in some sex hormones, actions that might contribute to the decreased sex drive and problems in handling stress. Other hormonal changes include a decrease in the release of thyrotropin and increases in prolactin and possibly growth hormone (Chap. 318).

Acute changes in the respiratory system include a CNS-mediated decrease in the cough reflex and respiratory depression, which result from a decreased response of the brainstem to carbon dioxide tension, a component of the drug overdose syndrome described below. At even low drug doses, this effect can be clinically significant for individuals with pulmonary disease. Aspiration pneumonia is an additional risk. The gastrointestinal effects of opioids can include nausea and decreased gut motility with resulting constipation and anorexia. Cardiovascular changes tend to be relatively mild, with no direct opioid effect on heart rhythm or myocardial contractility, but orthostatic hypotension can occur, probably secondary to histamine release and dilation of peripheral vessels. Bacterial endocarditis with septic emboli and stroke can occur from contaminated needles.

Opioid Toxicity and Overdosage High doses of opioids can result in a potentially lethal overdose, which may occur in >60% of opioid-dependent persons, especially with the more potent drugs such as fentanyl (80 to 100 times more powerful than morphine). The typical syndrome, which occurs immediately with intravenous overdose, includes shallow and slow respirations, pupillary miosis (with mydriasis once brain anoxia develops), bradycardia, hypothermia, and stupor or coma (Chap. 257). If not treated rapidly, respiratory depression, cardiorespiratory arrest, and death can ensue. Postmortem examination reveals few specific changes except for diffuse cerebral edema. An "allergic-like" reaction to intravenous heroin, perhaps in part related to adulterants, can also occur and is characterized by decreased alertness, frothy pulmonary edema, and an elevation in the blood eosinophil count.

The first step in managing overdose is to support vital signs, using intubation if needed. Definitive treatment is the administration of a narcotic antagonist such as 0.4 mg to 2 mg intravenous or intramuscular naloxone. A response should occur in 1 to 2 min; the dose should be repeated every 2 to 3 min up to 10 mg. Except with buprenorphene overdoses, no response after 10 mg makes an opioid toxic reaction unlikely. It is important to titrate the dose relative to the patient's symptoms to ameliorate the respiratory depression but not provoke a severe withdrawal state; the latter cannot be aggressively treated until overdose-related vital signs are relatively stable. Because the effects of naloxone diminish within 2 to 3 h, the individual must be monitored for at least 24 h after a heroin overdose and 72 h after an overdose of a longer-acting drug such as methadone. For methadone overdose, the substitution of the longer acting naltrexone should be considered. If there is little response to an opioid antagonist, the possibility of a concomitant overdose with a benzodiazepine should be considered and a challenge with intravenous flumazenil, 0.2 mg/min up to a maximum of 3 mg in an hour, might be used.

Treatment of either the typical or the "allergic" type of opioid toxic reaction often requires continued respiratory support (often with oxygen supplementation and positive-pressure breathing for the "allergic" type of overdose), intravenous fluids, pressor agents when needed to support blood pressure, and gastric lavage to remove any remaining drug. Intubation is often required to prevent aspiration in the stuporous or comatose patient. Cardiac arrhythmias and/or seizures may also be part of the opioid toxic reaction, especially with codeine, propoxyphene, or meperidine.

OPIOID ABUSE AND DEPENDENCE ■ Definition and Epidemiology The *Fourth Diagnostic and Statistical Manual* (DSM-IV) of the American Psychiatric Association defines opioid dependence as repeated use of a drug of this class to the point of causing multiple problems. The definition requires evidence of three or more problems in the same year, including tolerance, withdrawal, use of greater amounts of opiates than intended, and use despite consequences. Patients who do not have dependence but demonstrate repeated opioid-related difficulties with the law, impaired ability to meet obligations, use in hazardous situations, or continued use despite problems can be labeled as having abuse.

The use of opioids for intoxication is less prevalent than the use of alcohol, marijuana, and several other drugs. A 2002 national survey of adolescents and young adults reported that 10% of 12th graders (high school seniors) had tried an opioid outside of a doctor's prescription, including almost 2% who had used heroin. Figures for young adults and college students in 2001 were almost 12% and 2%, respectively. In all studies, prevalence rates were only slightly higher in males than females. None of the national surveys offered data regarding the prevalence of dependence, which is estimated as a lifetime risk of about 1%.

Genetics One large study of >3000 male twin pairs reported that there are genetic influences that relate uniquely to heroin dependence and also noted additional genetic factors related to an overall vulnerability toward substance-related problems. The genetic influences operate in the context of additional environmental factors that are likely to relate both to the family of upbringing and the general environment. Genetic factors might influence personality characteristics such as impulsivity and sensation-seeking or susceptibility to develop antisocial personality disorder. Genes relating to the actions of the drug on specific neurochemical systems such as dopamine are also potential candidates for an enhanced vulnerability toward developing opioid dependence.

Natural History While an opioid use disorder can develop in anyone, at least three groups are at increased risk for dependence or misuse. First, a minority of persons with chronic pain syndromes (e.g., back, joint, and muscle disorders) misuse their prescribed drugs. If physical dependence is established, any drop in opioid blood levels can then intensify the pain and promote continued drug intake. Physicians can avoid contributing to physical dependence by helping the patient to accept the goal of moderation rather than disappearance of the pain and to recognize that discomfort may not be completely eliminated (Chap. 11). Analgesic medication should be only one component of treatment and limited to the oral administration of the least potent analgesic that is able to "take the edge off" the pain (e.g., ibuprofen or, if needed, propoxyphene). Behavior-modification techniques, such as muscle relaxation and meditation, and carefully selected exercises should be used as appropriate to help increase function and decrease pain. Finally, nonmedicinal approaches, including electrical transcutaneous neurostimulation for muscle and joint disease, may be useful.

The second group at high risk are physicians, nurses, and pharmacists, primarily because of easy access to opioids. Physicians may begin use to help with sleep or to reduce stress or physical aches and pains, and then escalate doses as tolerance develops. Because of the growing awareness of these problems, programs have been developed to identify and aid substance-impaired physicians, providing peer support and education before problems escalate to the point of licensure revocation. All physicians are advised never to prescribe opioids for themselves or family members.

The third group are those who buy street drugs to get high. While some of these individuals have prior histories of severe antisocial problems, most have a relatively high level of premorbid functioning. The typical person begins using opioids occasionally, often after experimenting with tobacco, then alcohol, then marijuana, and then brain depressants or stimulants. Occasional opiate use, or "chipping," might continue for some time, and some individuals never escalate their intake to the point of developing dependence.

Opioid-dependent individuals are likely to continue to have experience with other drugs. Alcohol may be used to moderate withdrawal problems, to enhance the opioid high, and to serve as a substitute when the opioid is not available, including during methadone and other treatments. Problematic drinking, including alcohol dependence, is seen in about half of opioid-dependent persons. Cocaine appears to be taken for many of the same reasons as alcohol, and is often administered intravenously with the opioid in a mixture known as a "speedball." Another relevant class of drugs is the benzodiazepines, especially among people in methadone maintenance.

Once persistent opioid use is established, severe problems are likely to develop. At least 25% of habitual users die within 10 to 20 years (a mortality rate 15-fold higher than the general population) from suicide, homicide, accidents, or infectious diseases such as tuberculosis, hepatitis, or AIDS. The latter has become an epidemic among injection drug users, with an estimated 60% of these men and women carrying HIV (Chap. 173). Although the majority of opioid-dependent persons experience frequent exacerbations and remissions, it is important to remember that even without treatment ~35% achieve long-term, often permanent, abstinence, expecially after the age of 40. As is true with most drugs of abuse, a favorable prognosis is associated with a prior history of marital and employment stability and fewer prior criminal activities unrelated to drugs.

℞ TREATMENT

One key to diagnosis is to discard the erroneous stereotype that opioid-dependent individuals are always unemployed and homeless. Abuse or dependence is possible in any patient who demonstrates symptoms of what might be opioid withdrawal; anyone who has a chronic pain syndrome; physicians, nurses, and pharmacists or others with easy access to opioids; and all patients who repeatedly seek out prescription analgesics. Therefore, before prescribing an opioid analgesic, it is important to gather a complete history that elucidates patterns of life problems and any history of opioid use. If a problem with opioids is suspected, gathering further data from a relative or close friend can be helpful. Additionally, clinicians should search for physical stigmata of misuse (e.g., needle marks) and, when appropriate, screen blood or urine for opioids.

After identifying opioid dependence, the next step is intervention as described for alcoholism in Chap. 372. The need for continuing treatment even after the patient achieves abstinence can be presented, and the availability of help in establishing a drug-free life-style can be emphasized.

Symptoms of Withdrawal Withdrawal symptoms, generally the opposite of the acute effects of the drug, include nausea and diarrhea, coughing, lacrimation, mydriasis, rhinorrhea, profuse sweating, twitching of muscles, and piloerection (or "goose bumps") as well as mild elevations in body temperature, respiratory rate, and blood pressure. In addition, diffuse body pain, insomnia, and yawning occur, along with intense drug craving. Drugs with shorter half-lives, such as morphine or heroin, usually cause symptoms within 8 to 16 h of the last dose; intensity peaks within 36 to 72 h after discontinuation of the drug; and the acute syndrome disappears within 5 to 8 days. A protracted abstinence phase of mild moodiness, autonomic dysfunction, and changes in pain threshold and sleep patterns may persist for ≥6 months and probably contributes to relapse.

Treatment of the Withdrawal Syndrome   A thorough physical examination, including an assessment of neurologic function and a search for focal and systemic infections, especially abscesses, is mandatory. Laboratory testing includes assessment of liver function and, in intravenous users, HIV and hepatitis B and C status. Proper nutrition and rest must be initiated as soon as possible.

One treatment of withdrawal requires administration of any opioid (e.g., 10 to 25 mg of methadone bid) on day 1 to decrease symptoms. After several days of a stabilized drug dose, the opioid is then decreased by 10 to 20% of the original day's dose each day. However, detoxification with opioids is proscribed or limited in most states. Thus, pharmacologic treatments often center on relief of symptoms of diarrhea with loperamide, of "sniffles" with decongestants, and pain with nonopioid analgesics (e.g., ibuprofen). Comfort can be enhanced with administration of the α_2-adrenergic agonist clonidine in doses up to 0.3 mg given two to four times a day to decrease sympathetic nervous system overactivity. Blood pressure must be closely monitored. Some clinicians augment this regimen with low to moderate doses of benzodiazepines for 2 to 5 days to decrease agitation. An ultra-rapid detoxification procedure using deep sedation and withdrawal precipitated by naltrexone has been proposed, but has many inherent dangers and little evidence of efficacy.

A special case of opioid withdrawal is seen in the newborn made passively dependent through the mother's drug abuse during pregnancy; withdrawal consists of irritability, crying, a tremor, increased reflexes, increased respiratory rate, diarrhea, vomiting, and sneezing/ yawning/hiccuping. Treatment follows the same general steps used in the treatment of the physically dependent adult but using paregoric (0.2 mL orally every 3 to 4 h), methadone (0.1 to 0.5 mg/kg per day), phenobarbital (8 mg/kg per day), or diazepam (1 to 2 mg/kg every 8 h) in decreasing dosages for 10 to 20 days. Dependent infants of mothers on methadone maintenance also benefit by breast feeding while the mother continues to take methadone.

Rehabilitation   Despite some differences in demographics, the same general rules for rehabilitation apply to opioid-dependent persons as to alcoholics. The basic strategy includes detoxification and establishment of realistic goals, along with counseling and education to increase motivation toward abstinence. A long-term commitment by the patient to rebuilding a life-style without the substance is essential for preventing relapse.

In most programs, patients are educated about their responsibility for improving their lives, and motivation for abstinence is increased by providing information about the medical and psychological problems that can be expected if dependence continues. Patients and families are encouraged to establish an opioid-free life-style by learning to cope with chronic pain and develop realistic vocational planning (e.g., for pharmacists, physicians, and nurses). The dependent person is also advised to establish a drug-free peer group and to participate in self-help groups such as Narcotics Anonymous. Another important treatment component is relapse prevention aimed at identifying triggers for a return to drugs and developing appropriate coping strategies.

Much of this advice and counseling can be given by the physician or by referring the patients to formal drug programs, including methadone maintenance clinics, programs using narcotic antagonists, and therapeutic communities. Long-term follow-up of treated patients indicates that approximately one-third are completely drug free, and 60% no longer use opioids.

OPIOID MAINTENANCE   Maintenance programs with methadone and the longer-acting LAAM should be used only in combination with education and counseling. The goal is to provide a substitute drug that is legally accessible, safer, can be taken orally, and has a long half-life so that it can be taken once a day. This can help persons who have repeatedly failed in drug free programs to improve functioning within the family and job, to decrease legal problems, and to improve health. Individuals who stay in methadone maintenance are likely to show improvement in antisocial behavior and employment status.

Methadone is a long-acting opioid optimally dosed at 80 to 120 mg/d (a goal met through slow, careful increases over time). This level is optimally effective in blocking heroin-induced euphoria, decreasing craving, and maintaining abstinence from illegal oipoids. Over three-quarters of patients in well-supervised methadone clinics are likely to remain heroin-free for ≥6 months. Methadone is administered as an oral liquid given once a day at the program, with weekend doses taken at home. The longer-acting analogues, such as LAAM, can be given in doses up to 80 mg two or three times a week. After a period of maintenance (usually 6 months to ≥1 year), the clinician can work to slowly decrease the dose by about 5% per week.

An additional medication that has been used for maintenance treatment involves the μ opioid agonist and κ antagonist buprenorphine. Administered either as a sublingual liquid or tablet, doses of 8 to 12 mg per day (up to 32 mg in some patients) are usually given between 3 and 7 days per week. This drug has several advantages including low overdose danger, easier detoxification than is seen with methadone, and a probable ceiling effect in which higher doses do not increase euphoria. While many studies report equal effectiveness of buprenorphine and methadone, others suggest higher dropout rates or concomitant drug use with buprenorphine. As with all opioids, there is still a danger of misuse.

In the past, the British have used heroin maintenance with goals and guidelines similar to those of current methadone programs. There is no evidence that heroin maintenance has any advantages over methadone maintenance, but the heroin approach increases the risk that the drug will be sold on the streets.

OPIOID ANTAGONISTS   The opiate antagonists (e.g., naltrexone) compete with heroin and other opioids at receptors, reducing the effects of the opioid agonists. Administered over long periods with the intention of blocking the opioid "high," these drugs can be useful as part of an overall treatment approach that includes counseling and support. Naltrexone doses of 50 mg/d antagonize 15 mg of heroin for 24 h, and the possibly more effective higher doses (125 to 150 mg) block the effects of 25 mg of intravenous heroin for up to 3 days. To avoid precipitating a withdrawal syndrome, patients must be free of opioids for a minimum of 5 days before beginning treatment with naltrexone and should first be challenged with 0.4 or 0.8 mg of the shorter-acting agent naloxone to be certain they can tolerate the long-acting antagonist. A test dose of 10 mg of naltrexone is then given, which can produce withdrawal symptoms in 0.5 to 2 h. If none appear, the patient can begin with the usual dose of 40 to 150 mg three times per week.

DRUG-FREE PROGRAMS   Most opioid-dependent individuals enter treatment programs based primarily on the cognitive behavioral approaches of enhancing commitment to abstinence, helping individuals to rebuild their lives without substances, and preventing relapse. Whether carried out in inpatient or outpatient settings, patients do not receive medications.

A variation of this approach can be used for persons who are having problems maintaining a drug-free state. Here, the basic elements of treatment are incorporated into long-term (often a year or more) residence in a therapeutic community. The person begins with almost full immersion in the environment in which other individuals at various stages of recovery become the primary support group, offering advice and a drug-free atmosphere in which the opioid-dependent person progresses through ever-increasing levels of independence, including assuming a job outside the therapeutic atmosphere.

As is true for treatments of all substance-use disorders, it is likely that counseling, behavioral treatments, and relatively simple approaches to psychotherapy add significantly to a positive outcome.

Most programs focus on teaching participants to cope with stress, enhancing their understanding of personality attributes, teaching better cognitive styles, and, through the process of relapse prevention, addressing issues that might contribute to increased craving, easy access to drugs, or periods of decreased motivation. A combination of these therapies with the approaches described above appears to give the best results.

Finally, it is important to discuss prevention. Except for the terminally ill, physicians should carefully monitor opioid drug use in their patients, keeping doses as low as is practical and administering them over as short a period as the level of pain would warrant in the average person. Physicians must be vigilant regarding their own risk for opioid abuse and dependence, never prescribing these drugs for themselves. For the nonmedical intravenous drug–dependent person, all possible efforts must be made to prevent AIDS, hepatitis, bacterial endocarditis, and other consequences of contaminated needles both through methadone maintenance and by considering needle-exchange programs.

FURTHER READING

DEVRIES TJ, SHIPPENBERG TS: Neural systems underlying opiate addiction. J Neurosci 22:3321, 2002

JOHNSTON LD et al: *Monitoring the Future: National Results on Adolescent Drug Use: Overview of Key Findings*, 2002. Bethesda, MD, National Institute on Drug Abuse, 2003. NIH Publication No. 03-5374.

MATTICK RP et al: Buprenorphine versus methadone maintenance therapy: A randomized double-blind trial with 405 opioid-dependent patients. Addiction 98:441, 2003

SCHUCKIT MA et al: *Drug and Alcohol Abuse: A Clinical Guide to Diagnosis and Treatment*, 5th ed. New York, Plenum, 2000

374 COCAINE AND OTHER COMMONLY ABUSED DRUGS
Jack H. Mendelson, Nancy K. Mello

Cocaine and other psychostimulant drug abuse remains a major public health problem in the United States and throughout the world; its prevalence appears to be increasing in some metropolitan areas for both college students and adults ages 19 to 40. Drug abuse by women continues to parallel abuse of cocaine and other psychostimulant drugs by men; psychostimulant abuse among youth in the United States is a special concern.

The initiation and persistence of drug abuse are determined by a complex interaction of the pharmacologic properties and relative availability of each drug, the personality and expectations of the user, and the environmental context in which the drug is used. Polydrug abuse, the concurrent use of several drugs with different pharmacologic effects, is increasingly common among individuals from all socioeconomic strata. Particularly dangerous forms of polydrug abuse, such as the combined use of heroin and cocaine intravenously, remain a major problem in hospital emergency room settings. Drug abusers may attempt to attenuate one drug effect with another, as when heroin or alcohol is used to modulate the cocaine high. Sometimes one drug is used to enhance the effects of another, as with benzodiazepines and methadone, or cocaine plus heroin in methadone-maintained patients.

Chronic cocaine and psychostimulant abuse may cause a number of adverse health consequences, ranging from pulmonary disease to reproductive dysfunction. Preexisting disorders such as hypertension and cardiac disease may be exacerbated by drug abuse, and the combined use of two or more drugs may accentuate medical complications associated with abuse of one of them.

Drug abuse increases the risk of exposure to HIV. Cocaine and psychostimulant abuse contribute to the risk for HIV infection in part by suppression of immune function. In addition, concurrent use of cocaine and opiates (the "speedball") is frequently associated with needle-sharing by intravenous drug users. Intravenous drug abusers continue to represent the largest single group of persons with HIV infection in several major metropolitan areas in the United States as well as in urban areas in Scotland, Italy, Spain, Thailand, and China.

COCAINE Cocaine is a stimulant and local anesthetic with potent vasoconstrictor properties. The leaves of the *coca* plant (*Erythroxylon coca*) contain ~0.5 to 1% cocaine. The drug produces physiologic and behavioral effects when administered orally, intranasally, intravenously, or via inhalation following pyrolysis (smoking). Cocaine increases synaptic concentrations of the monamine neurotransmitters dopamine, norepinephrine, and serotonin by binding to transporter proteins in presynaptic neurons and blocking reuptake. The reinforcing effects of cocaine appear to be related to effects on dopaminergic neurons in the mesolimbic system.

Prevalence of Use Cocaine is widely available throughout the United States, and cocaine abuse occurs in virtually all social and economic strata of society. The prevalence of cocaine abuse in the general population has been accompanied by an increase in cocaine abuse by heroin-dependent persons, including those in methadone maintenance programs. Intravenous cocaine is often used concurrently with intravenous heroin. This combination purportedly attenuates the postcocaine "crash" and substitutes a cocaine "high" for the heroin "high" blocked by methadone.

Acute and Chronic Intoxication There has been an increase in both intravenous administration and inhalation of pyrolyzed cocaine via smoking. Following intranasal administration, changes in mood and sensation are perceived within 3 to 5 min, and peak effects occur at 10 to 20 min. The effects rarely last more than 1 h. Inhalation of pyrolyzed materials includes inhaling crack/cocaine or smoking coca paste, a product made by extracting cocaine preparations with flammable solvents, and cocaine free-base smoking. Free-base cocaine, including the free base prepared with sodium bicarbonate (crack), has become increasingly popular because of the relative high potency of the compound and its rapid onset of action (8 to 10 s following smoking).

Cocaine produces a brief, dose-related stimulation and enhancement of mood and an increase in cardiac rate and blood pressure. Body temperature usually increases following cocaine administration, and high doses of cocaine may induce lethal pyrexia or hypertension. Because cocaine inhibits reuptake of catecholamines at adrenergic nerve endings, the drug potentiates sympathetic nervous system activity. Cocaine has a short plasma half-life of ~45 to 60 min. Cocaine is metabolized by plasma esterases, and cocaine metabolites are excreted in urine. The very short duration of the euphorigenic effects of cocaine observed in chronic abusers is probably due to both acute and chronic tolerance. Frequent self-administration of the drug (two to three times per hour) is often reported by chronic cocaine abusers. Alcohol is used to modulate both the cocaine high and the dysphoria associated with the abrupt disappearance of cocaine's effects. A metabolite of cocaine, cocaethylene, has been detected in blood and urine of persons who concurrently abuse alcohol and cocaine. Cocaethylene induces changes in cardiovascular function similar to those of cocaine alone, and the pathophysiologic consequences of alcohol abuse plus cocaine abuse may be additive when both are used together.

The prevalent assumption that cocaine inhalation or intravenous administration is relatively safe is contradicted by reports of death from respiratory depression, cardiac arrhythmias, and convulsions associated with cocaine use. In addition to generalized seizures, neurologic complications may include headache, ischemic or hemorrhagic stroke, or subarachnoid hemorrhage. Disorders of cerebral blood flow and perfusion in cocaine-dependent persons have been detected with magnetic resonance spectroscopy (MRS) studies. Severe pulmonary disease may develop in individuals who inhale crack cocaine; this effect is attributed both to the direct effects of cocaine and to residual contaminants in the smoked material. Hepatic necrosis has been reported to occur following crack cocaine use.

Although men and women who abuse cocaine may report that the drug enhances libidinal drive, chronic cocaine use causes significant loss of libido and adversely affects reproductive function. Impotence and gynecomastia have been observed in male cocaine abusers, and these abnormalities often persist for long periods following cessation of drug use. Women who abuse cocaine have reported major derangements in menstrual cycle function including galactorrhea, amenorrhea, and infertility. Chronic cocaine abuse may cause persistent hyperprolactinemia as a consequence of disordered dopaminergic inhibition of prolactin secretion by the anterior pituitary. Cocaine abuse by pregnant women, particularly the smoking of crack, has been associated with both an increased risk of congenital malformations in the fetus and perinatal cardiovascular and cerebrovascular disease in the mother. However, cocaine abuse per se is probably not the sole cause of these perinatal disorders, since many problems associated with maternal cocaine abuse, including poor nutrition and health care status as well as polydrug abuse, also contribute to risk for perinatal disease.

Protracted cocaine abuse may cause paranoid ideation and visual and auditory hallucinations, a state that resembles alcoholic hallucinosis. Psychological dependence on cocaine, indicated by inability to abstain from frequent compulsive use, has also been reported. Although the occurrence of withdrawal syndromes involving psychomotor agitation and autonomic hyperactivity remains controversial, severe depression ("crashing") following cocaine intoxication may accompany drug withdrawal.

℞ TREATMENT

Treatment of cocaine overdose is a medical emergency that is usually best managed in an intensive care unit. Cocaine toxicity produces a hyperadrenergic state characterized by hypertension, tachycardia, tonic-clonic seizures, dyspnea, and ventricular arrhythmias. Intravenous diazepam in doses up to 0.5 mg/kg administered over an 8-h period has been shown to be effective for control of seizures. Ventricular arrhythmias have been managed successfully by administration of 0.5 to 1.0 mg of propranolol intravenously. Since many instances of cocaine-related mortality have been associated with concurrent use of other illicit drugs (particularly heroin), the physician must be prepared to institute effective emergency treatment for multiple drug toxicities.

Treatment of chronic cocaine abuse requires combined efforts of primary care physicians, psychiatrists, and psychosocial care providers. Early abstinence from cocaine use is often complicated by symptoms of depression and guilt, insomnia, and anorexia, which may be as severe as those observed in major affective disorders. Individual and group psychotherapy, family therapy, and peer group assistance programs are often useful for inducing prolonged remission from drug use. A number of medications used for the treatment of various medical and psychiatric disorders have been administered to reduce the duration and severity of cocaine abuse and dependence. However, no available medication is both safe and highly effective for either cocaine detoxification or maintenance of abstinence. Some psychotherapeutic interventions may be effective; however, no specific form of psychotherapy or behavioral modification is uniquely beneficial.

MARIJUANA AND CANNABIS COMPOUNDS *Cannabis sativa* contains >400 compounds in addition to the psychoactive substance, delta-9-tetrahydrocannabinol (THC). Marijuana cigarettes are prepared from the leaves and flowering tops of the plant, and a typical marijuana cigarette contains 0.5 to 1 g of plant material. Although the usual THC concentration varies between 10 and 40 mg, concentrations >100 mg per cigarette have been detected. Hashish is prepared from concentrated resin of *C. sativa* and contains a THC concentration of between 8 to 12% percent by weight. "Hash oil," a lipid-soluble plant extract, may

contain a THC concentration of 25 to 60% percent and may be added to marijuana or hashish to enhance its THC concentration. Smoking is the most common mode of marijuana or hashish use. During pyrolysis, >150 compounds in addition to THC are released in the smoke. Although most of these compounds do not have psychoactive properties, they do have potential physiologic effects.

THC is quickly absorbed from the lungs into blood and is then rapidly sequestered in tissues. It is metabolized primarily in the liver, where it is converted to 11-hydroxy-THC, a psychoactive compound, and >20 other metabolites. Many THC metabolites are excreted through the feces at a rate of clearance that is relatively slow in comparison to that of most other psychoactive drugs.

Specific cannabinoid receptors (CB_1 and CB_2) have been identified in the central nervous system, including the spinal cord, and in the peripheral nervous system. High densities of these receptors have been found in the cerebral cortex, basal ganglia, and hippocampus. B lymphocytes also appear to have cannabinoid receptors. A naturally occurring THC-like ligand has been identified in the nervous system, where it is widely distributed.

Prevalence of Use Marijuana is the most commonly used illegal drug in the United States. Use is particularly prevalent among adolescents; studies suggest that ~37% of high school students in the United States have used marijuana. Marijuana is relatively inexpensive and is often considered to be less hazardous than other controlled drugs and substances. Very potent forms of marijuana (sinsemilla) are now available in many communities, and concurrent use of marijuana with crack/cocaine and phencyclidine is increasing. Marijuana abuse by individuals from all social strata has been increasing.

Acute and Chronic Intoxication Acute intoxication from marijuana and cannabis compounds is related to both the dose of THC and the route of administration. THC is absorbed more rapidly from marijuana smoking than from orally ingested cannabis compounds. Acute marijuana intoxication usually consists of a subjective perception of relaxation and mild euphoria resembling mild to moderate alcohol intoxication. This condition is usually accompanied by some impairment in thinking, concentration, and perceptual and psychomotor function. Higher doses of cannabis may produce behavioral effects analogous to severe alcohol intoxication. Although the effects of acute marijuana intoxication are relatively benign in normal users, the drug can precipitate severe emotional disorders in individuals who have antecedent psychotic or neurotic problems. As with other psychoactive compounds, both set (user's expectations) and setting (environmental context) are important determinants of the type and severity of behavioral intoxication.

As with abuse of cocaine, opioids, and alcohol, chronic marijuana abusers may lose interest in common socially desirable goals and steadily devote more time to drug acquisition and use. However, THC does not cause a specific and unique "amotivational syndrome." The range of symptoms sometimes attributed to marijuana use is difficult to distinguish from mild to moderate depression and the maturational dysfunctions often associated with protracted adolescence. Chronic marijuana use has also been reported to increase the risk of psychotic symptoms in individuals with a past history of schizophrenia. Persons who initiate marijuana smoking before the age of 17 may subsequently develop severe cognitive and neuropsychological disorders, and may be at higher risk for later polydrug and alcohol abuse problems.

Physical Effects Conjunctival injection and tachycardia are the most frequent immediate physical concomitants of smoking marijuana. Tolerance for marijuana-induced tachycardia develops rapidly among regular users. However, marijuana smoking may precipitate angina in persons with a history of coronary insufficiency. Exercise-induced angina may be increased after marijuana use to a greater extent than after tobacco cigarette smoking. Patients with cardiac disease should be strongly advised not to smoke marijuana or use cannabis compounds.

Significant decrements in pulmonary vital capacity have been found in regular daily marijuana smokers. Because marijuana smoking typically involves deep inhalation and prolonged retention of marijuana smoke, marijuana smokers may develop chronic bronchial irritation. Impairment of single-breath carbon monoxide diffusion capacity (DL_{CO}) is greater in persons who smoke both marijuana and tobacco than in tobacco smokers.

Although marijuana has also been associated with adverse effects on a number of other systems, many of these studies await replication and confirmation. A reported correlation between chronic marijuana use and decreased testosterone levels in males has not been confirmed. Decreased sperm count and sperm motility and morphologic abnormalities of spermatozoa following marijuana use have also been reported. Prospective studies demonstrated a correlation between impaired fetal growth and development and heavy marijuana use during pregnancy. Marijuana has also been implicated in derangements of the immune system; in chromosomal abnormalities; and in inhibition of DNA, RNA, and protein synthesis; however, these findings have not been confirmed or related to any specific physiologic effect in humans.

Tolerance and Physical Dependence Habitual marijuana users rapidly develop tolerance to the psychoactive effects of marijuana and often smoke more frequently and try to secure more potent cannabis compounds. Tolerance for the physiologic effects of marijuana develops at different rates; e.g., tolerance develops rapidly for marijuana-induced tachycardia but more slowly for marijuana-induced conjunctival injection. Tolerance to both behavioral and physiologic effects of marijuana decreases rapidly upon cessation of marijuana use.

Withdrawal signs and symptoms have been reported in chronic cannabis users, with the severity of symptoms related to dosage and duration of use. These include tremor, nystagmus, sweating, nausea, vomiting, diarrhea, irritability, anorexia, and sleep disturbances. Withdrawal signs and symptoms observed in chronic marijuana users are usually relatively mild in comparison to those observed in heavy opiate or alcohol users and rarely require medical or pharmacologic intervention. More severe and protracted abstinence syndromes may occur after sustained use of high-potency cannabis compounds.

Therapeutic Use Marijuana, administered as cigarettes or as a synthetic oral cannabinoid (dronabinol), has been proposed to have a number of properties that may be clinically useful in some situations. These include antiemetic effects in chemotherapy recipients, appetite-promoting effects in AIDS, reduction of intraocular pressure in glaucoma, and reduction of spasticity in multiple sclerosis and other neurologic disorders. With the possible exception of AIDS-related cachexia, none of these attributes of marijuana compounds is clearly superior to other readily available therapies.

METHAMPHETAMINE The abuse of methamphetamine, also referred to as "meth," "speed," "crank," "chalk," "ice," "glass," or "crystal," has been declining in many metropolitan areas and communities throughout the United States. This decrease is attributed in part to drug seizures and the closures of clandestine laboratories that produce methamphetamine illegally. Prevention programs focusing upon methamphetamine abuse have also increased.

Most persons who abuse methamphetamine self-administer the drug orally, although there have been reports of methamphetamine administration by inhalation and intravenous injection. Individuals who abuse or become dependent upon methamphetamine state that use of this drug induces feelings of euphoria and decreases fatigue associated with difficult life situations. Adverse physiologic effects observed as a consequence of methamphetamine abuse include headache, difficulty concentrating, diminished appetite, abdominal pain, vomiting or diarrhea, disordered sleep, paranoid or aggressive behavior, and psychosis. Severe, life-threatening toxicity may present as hypertension, cardiac arrythmia or failure, subarachnoid hemorrhage, ischemic stroke, intracerebral hemorrhage, convulsions, or coma. Methamphetamines increase the release of monoamine neurotransmitters (dopa-

mine, norepinephrine, and serotonin) from presynaptic neurons. It is thought that the euphoric and reinforcing effects of this class of drugs are mediated through dopamine and the mesolimbic system, whereas the cardiovascular effects are related to norepinephrine. MRS studies suggest that chronic abuse may injure the frontal areas and basal ganglia of the brain.

Therapy of acute methamphetamine overdose is largely symptomatic. Ammonium chloride may be useful to acidify the urine and enhance clearance of the drug. Hypertension may respond to sodium nitroprusside or α-adrenergic antagonists. Sedatives may reduce agitation and other signs of central nervous system hyperactivity. Treatment of chronic methamphetamine dependence may be accomplished in either an inpatient or outpatient setting using strategies similar to those described above for cocaine abuse.

MDMA (3,4-methylenedioxymethamphetamine), or *Ecstasy*, is a derivative of methamphetamine. Ecstasy is usually taken orally but may be injected or inhaled. In addition to amphetamine-like effects, MDMA can induce hyperthermia and vivid hallucinations and other perceptual distortions.

During the past decade, an eighteenfold increase in MDMA-related emergency room incidents has been reported in the United States. Recent studies have revealed that MDMA induces both brain dopaminergic and serotonergic neurotoxicity. Thus, use of recreational use of MDMA by young persons may significantly increase the risk for subsequent occurrence of severe neuropsychiatric disorders.

LYSERGIC ACID DIETHYLAMIDE (LSD) The discovery of the psychedelic effects of LSD in 1947 led to an epidemic of LSD abuse during the 1960s. Imposition of stringent constraints on the manufacture and distribution of LSD (classified as a Schedule I substance by the U.S. Food and Drug Administration), as well as public recognition that psychedelic experiences induced by LSD were a health hazard, have resulted in a reduction in LSD abuse. The drug still retains some popularity among adolescents and young adults, however, and there are indications that LSD use among young persons has been increasing in some communities in the United States.

LSD is a very potent drug; oral doses as low as 20 μg may induce profound psychological and physiologic effects. Tachycardia, hypertension, pupillary dilation, tremor, and hyperpyrexia occur within minutes following oral administration of 0.5 to 2 μg/kg. A variety of bizarre and often conflicting perceptual and mood changes, including visual illusions, synesthesias, and extreme lability of mood, usually occur within 30 min after LSD intake. These effects of LSD may persist for 12 to 18 h, even though the half-life of the drug is only 3 h.

Tolerance develops rapidly for LSD-induced changes in psychological function when the drug is used one or more times per day for >4 days. Abrupt abstinence following continued use does not produce withdrawal signs or symptoms. There have been no clinical reports of death caused by the direct effects of LSD.

The most frequent acute medical emergency associated with LSD use is panic episode (the "bad trip"), which may persist up to 24 h. Management of this problem is best accomplished by supportive reassurance ("talking down") and, if necessary, administration of small doses of anxiolytic drugs. Adverse consequences of chronic LSD use include enhanced risk for schizophreniform psychosis and derangements in memory function, problem solving, and abstract thinking. Treatment of these disorders is best carried out in specialized psychiatric facilities.

PHENCYCLIDINE Phencyclidine (PCP), a cyclohexylamine derivative, is widely used in veterinary medicine to briefly immobilize large animals and is sometimes described as a dissociative anesthetic. PCP binds to ionotropic *n*-methyl-*d*-aspartate (NMDA) receptors in the nervous system, blocking ion current through these channels. PCP is easily synthesized; its abusers are primarily young people and polydrug users. It is used orally, by smoking, or by intravenous injection. It is also used as an adulterant in THC, LSD, amphetamine, or cocaine. The most common street preparation, *angel dust*, is a white granular powder that contains 50 to 100% percent of the drug. Low doses (5 mg) produce agitation, excitement, impaired motor coordination, dysarthria, and analgesia. Users may have horizontal or vertical nystagmus, flushing, diaphoresis, and hyperacusis. Behavioral changes include distortions of body image, disorganization of thinking, and feelings of estrangement. Higher doses of PCP (5 to 10 mg) may produce profuse salivation, vomiting, myoclonus, fever, stupor, or coma. PCP doses of ≥10 mg cause convulsions, opisthotonus, and decerebrate posturing, which may be followed by prolonged coma.

The diagnosis of PCP overdose is difficult because the patient's initial symptoms may suggest an acute schizophrenic reaction. Confirmation of PCP use is possible by determination of PCP levels in serum or urine. PCP assays are available at most toxicologic centers. PCP remains in urine for 1 to 5 days following high-dose intake.

PCP overdose requires life-support measures, including treatment of coma, convulsions, and respiratory depression in an intensive care unit. There is no specific antidote or antagonist for PCP. PCP excretion from the body can be enhanced by gastric lavage and acidification of urine. Death from PCP overdose may occur as a consequence of some combination of pharyngeal hypersecretion, hyperthermia, respiratory depression, severe hypertension, seizures, hypertensive encephalopathy, and intracerebral hemorrhage.

Acute psychosis associated with PCP use should be considered a psychiatric emergency since patients may be at high risk for suicide or extreme violence toward others. Phenothiazines should not be used for treatment because these drugs potentiate PCP's anticholinergic effects. Haloperidol (5 mg intramuscularly) has been administered on an hourly basis to induce suppression of psychotic behavior. PCP, like LSD and mescaline, produces vasospasm of cerebral arteries at relatively low doses. Chronic PCP use has been shown to induce insomnia, anorexia, severe social and behavioral changes, and, in some cases, chronic schizophrenia.

POLYDRUG ABUSE   Although drug abusers often report a preference for a particular drug, such as alcohol or opiates, the concurrent use of other drugs is common. Multiple drug use often involves substances that may have different pharmacologic effects from the preferred drug. Concurrent use of such dissimilar compounds as stimulants and opiates or stimulants and alcohol is not unusual. The diversity of reported drug use combinations suggests that achieving some perceptible change in state, rather than any particular direction of change (stimulation or sedation), may be the primary reinforcer in polydrug use and abuse. There is also evidence that intoxication with alcohol or opiates is associated with increased tobacco smoking. There is relatively little systematic information available about multiple drug abuse interactions.

However, the combined use of cocaine, heroin, and alcohol increases the risk for toxic effects and adverse medical consequences over risks associated with use of a single drug. One determinant of polydrug use patterns is the relative availability and cost of the drugs. There are many examples of situationally determined drug use patterns. For example, alcohol abuse, with its attendant medical complications, is one of the most serious problems encountered in former heroin addicts participating in methadone maintenance programs.

The physician must recognize that perpetuation of polydrug abuse and drug dependence is not necessarily a symptom of an underlying emotional disorder. Neither alleviation of anxiety nor reduction of depression accounts for initiation and perpetuation of polydrug abuse. Severe depression and anxiety are as frequently the consequences of polydrug abuse as they are the antecedents. There is also evidence that some of the most adverse consequences of drug use may be reinforcing and contribute to the continuation of polydrug abuse.

℞ TREATMENT

Adequate treatment of polydrug abuse, as well as other forms of drug abuse, requires innovative programs of intervention. The first step in successful treatment is detoxification, a process that may be difficult because of the abuse of several drugs with different pharmacologic actions (e.g., alcohol, opiates, and cocaine). Since patients may not recall or may deny simultaneous multiple drug use, diagnostic evaluation should always include urinalysis for qualitative detection of psychoactive substances and their metabolites. Treatment of polydrug abuse often requires hospitalization or inpatient residential care during detoxification and the initial phase of drug abstinence. When possible, specialized facilities for the care and treatment of chemically dependent persons should be used. Outpatient detoxification of polydrug abuse patients is likely to be ineffective and may be dangerous.

Polydrug abuse is a chronic disorder with an unpredictable pattern of remission and recrudescence. Definitive "cures" rarely occur. The physician should continue to assist polydrug abuse patients throughout the cyclic oscillations of this complex behavior disorder, recognizing that resumption of drug use is the rule rather than the exception.

FURTHER READING

CAMI J, FARRE M: Drug addiction. N Engl J Med 349:975, 2003

LYNSKEY MT et al: Escalation of drug use in early-onset cannabis users vs co-twin controls. JAMA 289:427, 2003

WEBER JE et al: Validation of a brief observation period for patients with cocaine-associated chest pain. N Engl J Med 348:510, 2003

375 NICOTINE ADDICTION
David M. Burns

The use of tobacco leaf to create and satisfy nicotine addiction was introduced to Columbus by Native Americans and spread rapidly to Europe. The use of tobacco as cigarettes, however, is predominantly a twentieth century phenomenon, as is the epidemic of disease caused by this form of tobacco.

Nicotine is the principal constituent of tobacco responsible for its addictive character. Addicted smokers regulate their nicotine intake and blood levels by adjusting the frequency and intensity of their tobacco use both to obtain the desired psychoactive effects and avoid withdrawal.

Unburned cured tobacco contains nicotine, carcinogens, and other toxins capable of causing gum disease and oral cancer. When tobacco is burned, the resultant smoke contains, in addition to nicotine, carbon monoxide and 4000 other compounds that result from volatilization, pyrolysis, and pyrosynthesis of tobacco and various chemical additives

used in making different tobacco products. The smoke is composed of a fine aerosol, with a particle size distribution predominantly in the range to deposit in the airways and alveolar surfaces of the lungs, and a vapor phase. The bulk of the toxicity and carcinogenicity of the smoke resides in the aerosolized particulate phase, which contains a large number of toxic constituents and carcinogenic compounds. The aggregate of particulate matter, after subtracting nicotine and moisture, is referred to as tar. The vapor phase contains carbon monoxide, respiratory irritants, and ciliotoxins as well as many of the volatile compounds responsible for the distinctive smell of cigarette smoke.

The alkaline pH of smoke from blends of tobacco utilized for pipes and cigars allows sufficient absorption of nicotine across the oral mucosa to satisfy the smoker's need for this drug. Therefore, smokers of pipes and cigars tend not to inhale the smoke into the lung, confining the toxic and carcinogenic exposure (and the increased rates of disease) largely to the upper airway for most users of these products. The acidic pH of smoke generated by the tobacco used in cigarettes dramatically reduces absorption of nicotine in the mouth, necessitating inhalation of the smoke into the larger surface of the lungs in order to absorb quantities of nicotine sufficient to satisfy the smoker's addiction. The shift to using tobacco as cigarettes, with resultant increased deposition of smoke in the lung, has created the epidemic of heart disease, lung disease, and lung cancer that dominates the current disease manifestations of tobacco use.

GENETIC CONSIDERATIONS Several genes have been associated with nicotine addiction. Some reduce the clearance of nicotine, and others have been associated with an increased likelihood of becoming dependent on tobacco and other drugs as well as a higher incidence of depression. It is unlikely that genetic factors are the principal determinants of addiction. Rates of smoking initiation among males, and corresponding rates of nicotine addiction, have dropped by almost 50% since the mid-1950s, suggesting that factors other than genetics are important. It is more likely that genetic susceptibility influences the probability that experimentation with tobacco as an adolescent will lead to addiction as an adult.

DISEASE MANIFESTATIONS OF CIGARETTE SMOKING

Over 400,000 individuals die prematurely each year in the United States from cigarette use; this represents approximately one out of every five deaths in the United States. Approximately 40% of cigarette smokers will die prematurely due to cigarette smoking unless they are able to quit.

The major diseases caused by cigarette smoking are listed in Table 375-1. The incidence of smoking-related diseases is proportionately greater in younger than in older smokers, particularly for coronary artery disease and stroke. At older ages, the background rate of disease in nonsmokers increases, diminishing the fractional contribution of smoking and the relative risk; however, absolute excess rates of disease mortality found in smokers compared to nonsmokers increase with increasing age. The organ damage caused by smoking and the number of smokers who die from smoking are both greater among the elderly, as one would expect from a process of cumulative injury.

CARDIOVASCULAR DISEASES Cigarette smokers are more likely than nonsmokers to develop large-vessel atherosclerosis as well as small-vessel disease. Approximately 90% of peripheral vascular disease in the nondiabetic population can be attributed to cigarette smoking, as can ~50% of aortic aneurysms. In contrast, 20 to 30% of coronary artery disease and ~10% of occlusive cerebrovascular disease are caused by cigarette smoking. There is a multiplicative interaction between cig-

arette smoking and other cardiac risk factors such that the increment in risk produced by smoking among individuals with hypertension or elevated serum lipids is substantially greater than the increment in risk produced by smoking for individuals without these risk factors.

In addition to its role in promoting atherosclerosis, cigarette smoking also increases the likelihood of myocardial infarction and sudden cardiac death by promoting platelet aggregation and vascular occlusion. Reversal of these effects may explain the rapid benefit of smoking cessation for a new coronary event demonstrable among those who have survived a first myocardial infarction. This effect may also explain the substantially higher rates of graft occlusion among continuing smokers following vascular bypass surgery for cardiac or peripheral vascular disease, as well as the high failure rate of angioplasty procedures among continuing smokers.

Cessation of cigarette smoking reduces the risk of a second coronary event within 6 to 12 months; rates of first myocardial infarction or death from coronary heart disease also decline within the first few years following cessation. After 15 years of cessation, the risk of a new myocardial infarction or death from coronary heart disease in former smokers is similar to that for those who have never smoked.

CANCER Tobacco smoking causes cancer of the lung, oral cavity, naso-, oro-, and hypopharynx, nasal cavity and paranasal sinuses, larynx, esophagus, stomach, pancreas, liver, kidney (body and pelvis), ureter, urinary bladder, and uterine cervix and also causes myeloid leukemia. There is evidence suggesting that cigarette smoking may play a role in increasing the risk of colorectal and possibly breast cancer. There does not appear to be a causal link between cigarette smoking and cancer of the endometrium, and there is a lower risk of uterine cancer among postmenopausal women who smoke. The risks of cancer increase with the increasing number of cigarettes smoked per day and with increasing duration of smoking, and there are synergistic interactions between cigarette smoking and alcohol use for cancer of the oral cavity, esophagus, and possibly lung. Several occupational exposures also synergistically increase lung cancer risk among cigarette smokers, most notably occupational asbestos and radon exposure.

Cessation of cigarette smoking reduces the risk of developing cancer relative to continuing smoking, but even 20 years after cessation there is a modest persistent increased risk of developing lung cancer.

RESPIRATORY DISEASE Cigarette smoking is responsible for 90% of chronic obstructive pulmonary disease. Within 1 to 2 years of beginning to smoke regularly, many young smokers will develop inflammatory changes in their small airways, although lung function measures of these changes do not predict development of chronic airflow obstruction. After 20 years of smoking, pathophysiologic changes in the lungs develop and progress proportional to smoking intensity and duration. Chronic mucous hyperplasia of the larger airways results in a chronic productive cough in as many as 80% of smokers over age 60. Chronic inflammation and narrowing of the small airways and/or enzymatic digestion of alveolar walls resulting in pulmonary emphysema can result in reduced expiratory airflow sufficient to produce clinical symptoms of respiratory limitation in ~15% of smokers.

Changes in the small airways of young smokers will reverse after 1 to 2 years of cessation. There may also be a small increase in measures of expiratory airflow among individuals who have developed chronic airflow obstruction, but the major change following cessation is a slowing of the rate of decline in lung function with advancing age rather than a return of lung function toward normal.

PREGNANCY Cigarette smoking is associated with several maternal complications of pregnancy: premature rupture of membranes, abruptio placentae, and placenta previa; there is also a small increase in the risk of spontaneous abortion among smokers. Infants of smoking mothers are more likely to experience preterm delivery, have a higher perinatal mortality, are small for their gestational age, have higher rates of infant respiratory distress syndrome, are more likely to die of sudden infant death syndrome, and appear to have a developmental lag for at least the first several years of life.

TABLE 375-1 *Relative Risks for Current Smokers of Cigarettes*

Disease or Condition	Current Smokers	
	Males	Females
Coronary heart disease		
Age 35–64	2.8	3.1
Age ≥65	1.5	1.6
Cerebrovascular lesions		
Age 35–64	3.3	4
Age ≥65	1.6	1.5
Aortic aneurysm	6.2	7.1
Chronic airways obstruction	10.6	13.1
Cancer		
Lip, oral cavity, pharynx	10.9	5.1
Esophagus	6.8	7.8
Stomach	2	1.4
Pancreas	2.3	2.3
Larynx	14.6	13
Lung	23.3	12.7
Cervix		1.6
Kidney	2.7	1.3
Bladder, other urinary organs	3.3	2.2
Sudden Infant Death syndrome		2.3
Infant respiratory distress syndrome		1.3
Low birth weight at delivery		1.8

OTHER CONDITIONS Smoking delays healing of peptic ulcers; increases the risk of osteoporosis, senile cataracts, and macular degeneration; and results in premature menopause, wrinkling of the skin, gallstones and cholecystitis in women, and male impotence.

ENVIRONMENTAL TOBACCO SMOKE Long-term exposure to environmental tobacco smoke increases the risk of lung cancer and coronary artery disease among nonsmokers. It also increases the incidence of respiratory infections, chronic otitis media, and asthma in children as well as causing exacerbation of asthma in children.

PHARMACOLOGIC INTERACTIONS

Cigarette smoking may interact with a variety of other drugs (Table 375-2). Cigarette smoking induces the cytochrome P450 system, which may alter the metabolic clearance of drugs such as theophylline. This may result in inadequate serum levels in smokers as outpatients when the dosage is established in the hospital under nonsmoking conditions. Correspondingly, serum levels may rise when smokers are hospitalized and not allowed to smoke. Smokers may also have higher first-pass clearance for drugs such as lidocaine, and the stimulant effects of nicotine may reduce the effect of benzodiazepines or beta blockers.

OTHER FORMS OF TOBACCO USE

Other major forms of tobacco use are moist snuff deposited between the cheek and gum, chewing tobacco, pipes and cigars, and recently bidi (tobacco wrapped in tendu or temburni leaf and commonly used in India) and clove cigarettes. Oral tobacco use leads to gum disease and can result in oral cancer. All forms of burned tobacco generate toxic and carcinogenic smoke similar to that of cigarette smoke. The differences in disease consequences of use relate to frequency of use and depth of inhalation. The risk of upper airway cancers is similar among cigarette and cigar smokers, while those who have smoked only cigars have a much lower risk of lung cancer, heart disease, and chronic obstructive pulmonary disease. However, cigarette smokers who switch to pipes or cigars do tend to inhale the smoke, increasing their risk; and it is likely that comparable inhalation and frequency of exposure to tobacco smoke from any of these forms of tobacco use will lead to comparable disease outcomes.

A resurgence of cigar and bidi use among adolescents of both genders has raised concerns that these older forms of tobacco use are once again causing a public health problem.

TABLE 375-2 *Interactions of Smoking and Prescription Drugs*

Drug	Interaction
Benzodiazepines	Less sedation
Beta blockers	Reduced lowering of heart rate and blood pressure
Caffeine	Faster metabolic clearance
Chlorpromazine	Decreased serum concentrations[a]
Clomipramine	Decreased serum concentrations[a]
Clozapine	Decreased serum concentrations[a]
Dextropropoxyphene	Less analgesia
Oral estrogens	Increased hepatic clearance
Flecainide	Increased first-pass clearance
Fluphenazine	Decreased serum concentrations[a]
Fluvoxamine	Decreased serum concentrations[a]
Haloperidol	Decreased serum concentrations[a]
Heparin	Faster clearance
Imipramine	Decreased serum concentrations[a]
Insulin	Delayed absorption due to skin vasoconstriction
Lidocaine	Increased first-pass clearance
Mexiletine	Increased first-pass clearance
Olanzapine	Faster clearance
Pentazocine	Less analgesia, possibly increased clearance
Propranolol	Increased first-pass clearance
Tacrine	Faster metabolic clearance
Theophylline	Faster metabolic clearance
Thiothixene	Faster metabolic clearance
Trazodone	Decreased serum concentrations[a]

[a] Clinical implication uncertain.

LOWER TAR AND NICOTINE CIGARETTES

Filtered cigarettes with lower machine-measured yields of tar and nicotine have been recommended as offering lower disease risks. However, these cigarettes commonly use ventilation holes in the filters and other engineering designs to artificially lower the machine measurements. Smokers, however, can compensate and preserve their intake of nicotine (and tar) by changing the manner in which they puff on the cigarette or the number of cigarettes smoked per day. There is no meaningful disease-reduction benefit for smokers who switch to lower-yield cigarettes, and smokers should be discouraged from thinking of low-yield cigarettes as an alternative to cessation.

CESSATION

The process of stopping smoking is often a cyclical one, with the smoker sometimes making multiple attempts to quit and failing before finally being successful. Approximately 70 to 80% of smokers would like to quit smoking, approximately one-third of current smokers attempt to quit each year, and 90% of these unassisted attempts fail. Clinician-based smoking interventions should encourage smokers to try to quit and to use different forms of cessation assistance with each new cessation attempt rather than focusing exclusively on immediate cessation at the time of the first visit.

Physician advice to quit smoking, particularly around an acute illness, is a powerful trigger for cessation attempts, with up to half of patients who are advised to quit making a cessation effort. Other triggers include the cost of cigarettes, media campaigns, and changes in rules to restrict smoking in the workplace.

PHYSICIAN INTERVENTION (Table 375-3)

All patients should be asked whether they smoke, their past experience with quitting, and whether they are currently interested in quitting. Those who are not interested in quitting should be encouraged and motivated to quit; provided a clear, strong, and personalized physician message that smoking is an important health concern; and offered assistance if they become interested in quitting in the future. There is a relationship between the amount of assistance a patient is willing to

TABLE 375-3 *Clinical Practice Guidelines*

Physician actions
 Ask: Systematically identify all tobacco users at every visit
 Advise: Strongly urge all smokers to quit
 Identify smokers willing to quit
 Assist the patient in quitting
 Arrange follow-up contact
Pharmacologic interventions—first-line therapies
 Nicotine gum (1.5)
 Nicotine 24-h patch: 21-mg patch for 4 weeks, 14-mg patch for 2 weeks, and 7-mg patch for 2 weeks (1.9)
 Nicotine nasal inhaler: one spray to each nostril 1–2 times/h for 3–6 months (2.7)
 Nicotine oral inhaler: 6–16 puffs per day for up to 6 months (2.5)
 Bupropion: 150 mg/d PO for 3 days followed by 150 mg bid for 7–12 weeks (2.1)
Pharmacologic interventions—second-line therapies
 Clonidine: Initial dose 0.1 mg bid PO, or 0.1-mg transdermal patch, increasing to 0.15–0.75 mg/d PO or 0.2-mg patch for 3–10 weeks (2.1)
 Nortriptyline: Initial dose 25 mg/d PO, increasing to 75–100 mg/d for 12 weeks (3.2)
Other interventions
 Physician or other medical personnel counseling, 10 minutes (1.3)
 Intensive smoking cessation program[a] (2.3)
 Clinic-based smoking status identification system (3.1)
 Counseling by nonclinicians and social support by family and friends
 Telephone counseling (1.2)

Note: Numerical value in parentheses is the multiple for cessation success compared to no intervention.

[a] At least four to seven sessions of 20- to 30-min duration, lasting at least 2 weeks, preferably 8 weeks.

accept and the success of the cessation attempt. A quit date should be negotiated, usually not the day of the visit but within the next few weeks, and a follow-up contact by office staff around the time of the quit date should be provided.

There are a variety of nicotine-replacement products, including over-the-counter nicotine patch and gum, as well as nicotine nasal and oral inhalers available by prescription. Recently, antidepressants such as bupropion have also been shown to be effective; some evidence supports the combined use of nicotine-replacement therapy and anti-depressants. Nicotine-replacement therapy is provided in different dosages. Clonidine or nortriptyline may be useful for patients who have failed on first-line pharmacologic treatment, or who are unable to use other therapies. Antidepressants are more effective in those with a history of depression symptoms.

Current recommendations are to offer pharmacologic treatment, usually with nicotine replacement therapy and bupropion, to all who will accept it and to provide counseling and other support as a part of the cessation attempt. Cessation advice alone by a physician or his or her staff is likely to increase success compared with no intervention; a more comprehensive approach with advice, pharmacologic assistance, and counseling can increase cessation success by almost three-fold.

In order for physicians to incorporate cessation assistance into their practice successfully, it is essential to change the infrastructure in which the physician practices. The following are simple changes: (1) including questions on smoking and interest in cessation on patient-intake questionnaires, (2) asking patients whether they smoke as part of the initial vital sign measurements made by office staff, (3) listing smoking as a problem in the medical record, and (4) automating follow-up contact with the patient on the quit date. These changes are essential to institutionalizing smoking intervention within the practice setting; without this institutionalization, the best intentions of physicians to intervene with their patients who smoke are often lost in the time crush of a busy practice.

PREVENTION

Approximately 90% of individuals who will become cigarette smokers initiate the behavior during adolescence. Factors that promote adolescent initiation are parental or older generation cigarette smoking, tobacco advertising and promotional activities, the availability of cigarettes, and the social acceptability of smoking. The need for an enhanced self-image and to imitate adult behavior is greatest for those adolescents who have the least external validation of their self-worth, which may explain in part the enormous differences in adolescent smoking prevalence by socioeconomic and school performance strata.

Prevention of smoking initiation must begin early, preferably in the elementary school years. Physicians who treat adolescents should be sensitive to the prevalence of this problem. Physicians should ask all adolescents whether they have experimented with tobacco or currently use tobacco, reinforce the facts that most adolescents and adults do not smoke, and explain that all forms of tobacco are both addictive and harmful.

FURTHER READING

INTERNATIONAL AGENCY FOR RESEARCH ON CANCER: *Tobacco Smoke and Involuntary Smoking.* IARC Monographs on the Evaluation of Carcinogenic Risks to Humans. Lyon, France, vol 83, 2003

US DEPARTMENT OF HEALTH AND HUMAN SERVICES: *The Health Consequences of Tobacco Use: A Report of the Surgeon General.* National Center for Chronic Disease Prevention and Health Promotion, Office on Smoking and Health, 2003

————: *Treating Tobacco Use and Dependence.* Clinical Practice Guideline, Public Health Service, DHHS, 2000

376 HEAVY METAL POISONING
Howard Hu

Metals pose a significant threat to health through occupational as well as environmental exposures. One indication of their importance relative to other potential hazards is their ranking by the U.S. Agency for Toxic Substances and Disease Registry, which lists all hazards present in toxic waste sites according to their prevalence and the severity of their toxicity. The first, second, third, and sixth hazards on the list are heavy metals: lead, mercury, arsenic, and cadmium, respectively. Specific information pertaining to each of these metals, including sources and metabolism, toxic effects produced, diagnosis, and the appropriate treatment for poisoning, is summarized in Table 376-1.

Metals are inhaled primarily as dusts and fumes (the latter defined as tiny particles generated by combustion). Metal poisoning can also result from exposure to vapors (e.g., mercury vapor in creating dental amalgams). When metals are ingested in contaminated food or drink or by hand-to-mouth activity (implicated especially in children), their gastrointestinal absorption varies greatly with the specific chemical form of the metal and the nutritional status of the host. Once a metal is absorbed, blood is the main medium for its transport, with the precise kinetics dependent on diffusibility, protein binding, rates of biotransformation, availability of intracellular ligands, and other factors. Some organs (e.g., bone, liver, and kidney) sequester metals in relatively high concentrations for years. Most metals are excreted through renal clearance and gastrointestinal excretion; some proportion is also excreted through salivation, perspiration, exhalation, lactation, skin exfoliation, and loss of hair and nails. The intrinsic stability of metals

TABLE 376-1 *Heavy Metals*

Metal	Main Sources	Metabolism	Toxicity	Diagnosis	Treatment
Arsenic	Smelting and microelectronics industries; wood preservatives, pesticides, herbicides, fungicides; contaminant of deep-water wells; folk remedies; and coal; incineration of these products	Organic arsenic (arsenobentaine, arsenocholine) is ingested in seafood and fish, but is nontoxic; inorganic arsenic is readily absorbed (lung and GI); sequesters in liver, spleen, kidneys, lungs, and GI tract; residues persist in skin, hair, and nails; biomethylation results in detoxification, but this process saturates.	Acute arsenic poisoning results in necrosis of intestinal mucosa with hemorrhagic gastroenteritis, fluid loss, hypotension, delayed cardiomyopathy, acute tubular necrosis, and hemolysis. Chronic arsenic exposure causes diabetes, vasospasm, peripheral vascular insufficiency and gangrene, peripheral neuropathy, and cancer of skin, lung, liver (angiosarcoma), bladder, kidney. Lethal dose: 120–200 mg (adults); 2 mg/kg (children).	Nausea, vomiting, diarrhea, abdominal pain, delirium, coma, seizures; garlicky odor on breath; hyperkeratosis, hyperpigmentation, exfoliative dermatitis, and Mees' lines (transverse white striae of the fingernails); sensory and motor polyneuritis, distal weakness. Radiopaque sign on abdominal x-ray; ECG–QRS broadening, QT prolongation, ST depression, T-wave flattening; 24-h urinary arsenic >67 μmol/d or 50 μg/d; (no seafood $\times$ 24 h); if recent exposure, serum arsenic >0.9 μmol/L (7 μg/dL). High arsenic in hair or nails.	If acute ingestion, ipecac to induce vomiting, gastric lavage, activated charcoal with a cathartic. Supportive care in ICU. Dimercaprol 3–5 mg/kg IM q4h $\times$ 2 days; q6h $\times$ 1 day, then q12h $\times$ 10 days; alternative: oral succimer.
Cadmium	Metal-plating, pigment, smelting, battery, and plastics industries; tobacco; incineration of these products; ingestion of food that concentrates cadmium (grains, cereals).	Absorbed through ingestion or inhalation; bound by metallothionein, filtered at the glomerulus, but reabsorbed by proximal tubules (thus, poorly excreted). Biological ½ life: 10–30 y. Binds cellular sulfhydryl groups, competes with zinc, calcium for binding sites. Concentrates in liver and kidneys.	Acute cadmium inhalation causes pneumonitis after 4–24 h; acute ingestion causes gastroenteritis. Chronic exposure causes anosmia, yellowing of teeth, emphysema, minor LFT elevations, microcytic hypochromic anemia unresponsive to iron therapy, proteinuria, increased urinary β_2-microglobulin, calciuria, leading to chronic renal failure, osteomalacia, and fractures.	With inhalation: pleuritic chest pain, dyspnea, cyanosis, fever, tachycardia, nausea, noncardiogenic pulmonary edema. With ingestion: nausea, vomiting, cramps, diarrhea. Bone pain, fractures with osteomalacia. If recent exposure, serum cadmium >500 nmol/L (5 μg/dL). Urinary cadmium >100 nmol/L (10 μg/g creatinine) and/or urinary β_2-microglobulin >750 μg/g creatinine (but urinary β_2-microglobulin also increased in other renal diseases such as pyelonephritis).	There is no effective treatment for cadmium poisoning (chelation not useful; dimercaprol can exacerbate nephrotoxicity). Avoidance of further exposure, supportive therapy, vitamin D for osteomalacia.

(continued)

TABLE 376-1   Heavy Metals—(Continued)

Metal	Main Sources	Metabolism	Toxicity	Diagnosis	Treatment
Lead	Manufacturing of auto batteries, lead crystal, ceramics, fishing weights, etc.; demolition or sanding of lead-painted houses, bridges; stained glass making, plumbing, soldering; environmental exposure to paint chips, house dust (in home built <1975), firing ranges (from bullet dust), food or water from improperly glazed ceramics, lead pipes; contaminated herbal remedies, candies; exposure to the combustion of leaded fuels.	Absorbed through ingestion or inhalation; organic lead (e.g., tetraethyl lead) absorbed dermally. In blood, 95–99% sequestered in RBCs—thus, must measure lead in whole blood (not serum). Distributed widely in soft tissue, with ½ life ~30 days; 15% of dose sequestered in bone with ½ life of >20 years. Excreted mostly in urine, but also appears in other fluids including breast milk. Interferes with mitochondrial oxidative phosphorylation, ATPases, calcium-dependent messengers; enhances oxidation and cell apoptosis.	Acute exposure with blood lead levels (BPb) of > 60–80 μg/dL can cause impaired neurotransmission and neuronal cell death (with central and peripheral nervous system effects); impaired hematopoiesis and renal tubular dysfunction. At higher levels of exposure (e.g., BPb > 80–120 μg/dL), acute encephalopathy with convulsions, coma, and death may occur. Subclinical exposures in children (BPb 25–60 μg/dL) are associated with anemia; mental retardation; and deficits in language, motor function, balance, hearing, behavior, and school performance. Impairment of IQ appears to occur at even lower levels of exposure with no measurable threshold above the limit of detection in most assays of 1 μg/dL. In adults, chronic subclinical exposures (BPb > 40 μg/dL) are associated with an increased risk of anemia, demyelinating peripheral neuropathy (mainly motor), impairments of reaction time, hypertension, ECG conduction delays, interstitial nephritis and chronic renal failure, diminished sperm counts, spontaneous abortions.	Abdominal pain, irritability, lethargy, anorexia, anemia, Fanconi's syndrome, pyuria, azotemia in children with blood lead level (BPb) >80 μg/dL; may also see epiphyseal plate "lead lines" on long bone x-rays. Convulsions, coma at BPb > 120 μg/dL. Noticeable neurodevelopmental delays at BPb of 40–80 μg/dL; may also see symptoms associated with higher BPb levels. In the U.S., screening of all children when they begin to crawl (~6 months) is recommended by the CDC; source identification and intervention is begun if the BPb > 10 μg/dL. In adults, acute exposure causes similar symptoms as in children as well as headaches, arthralgias, myalgias, depression, impaired short-term memory, loss of libido. Physical exam may reveal a "lead line" at the gingiva-tooth border, pallor, wrist drop, and cognitive dysfunction (e.g., declines on the mini-mental status exam); lab tests may reveal a normocytic, normochromic anemia, basophilic stippling, an elevated blood protoporphyrin level (free erythrocyte or zinc), and motor delays on nerve conduction. In the U.S., OSHA requires regular testing of lead-exposed workers with removal if BPb > 40 μg/dL.	Identification and correction of exposure sources is critical. In some U.S. states, screening and reporting to local health boards of children with BPb > 10 μg/dL and workers with BPb > 40 μg/dL is required. In the highly exposed individual with symptoms, chelation is recommended with oral DMSA (succimer); if acutely toxic, hospitalization and IV or IM chelation with edentate calcium disodium (CaEDTA) may be required, with the addition of dimercaprol to prevent worsening of encephalopathy. It is uncertain whether children with asymptomatic lead exposure (e.g., BPb 20–40 μg/dL) benefit from chelation. Correction of dietary deficiencies in iron, calcium, magnesium, and zinc will lower lead absorption and may also improve toxicity. Vitamin C is a weak but natural chelating agent.

(continued)

facilitates tracing and measurement in biologic material, although the clinical significance of the levels measured is not always clear.

Some metals, such as copper and selenium, are essential to normal metabolic function as trace elements (Chap. 61) but are toxic at high levels of exposure. Others, such as lead and mercury, are xenobiotic and theoretically are capable of exerting toxic effects at any level of exposure. Indeed, much research is currently focused on the contribution of low-level xenobiotic metal exposure to chronic diseases and to subtle changes in health that may have significant public health consequences. Research has also begun to determine how genetic factors may modify the impact of metals on health and thereby account, at least in part, for individual susceptibility to metal effects.

The most important component of treatment for metal toxicity is the termination of exposure. *Chelating agents* are used to bind metals into stable cyclic compounds with relatively low toxicity and to enhance their excretion. The principal chelating agents are dimercaprol (British Anti-Lewisite, BAL), edetate (EDTA), succimer (DMSA, dimercaptosuccinic acid), and penicillamine; their specific use depends on the metal involved and the clinical circumstances. Activated charcoal does not bind metals and thus is of limited usefulness in cases of acute metal ingestion.

In addition to the information provided in Table 376-1, several other aspects of exposure, toxicity, or management are worthy of discussion with respect to the four most hazardous toxicants (arsenic, cadmium, lead, and mercury). *Arsenic* exposure from natural contamination of shallow tube wells inserted for drinking water is a huge environmental problem for millions of residents in parts of Bangladesh and Western India. Contamination was formerly considered only a

TABLE 376-1—(Continued)

Metal	Main Sources	Metabolism	Toxicity	Diagnosis	Treatment
Mercury	Metallic, mercurous, and mercuric mercury (Hg^0, Hg^+, Hg^{2+}) exposures occur in some chemical, metal-processing, electrical-equipment, automotive industries; they are also in thermometers, dental amalgams, batteries. Mercury is dispersed by waste incineration. Environmental bacteria convert inorganic to organic mercury, which then bioconcentrates up the aquatic food chain to contaminate tuna, swordfish, and other pelagic fish.	Elemental mercury (Hg^0) is not well absorbed; however, it will volatilize into highly absorbable vapor. Inorganic mercury is absorbed through the gut and skin. Organic mercury is well absorbed through inhalation and ingestion. Elemental and organic mercury cross the blood-brain barrier and placenta. Mercury is excreted in urine and feces and has a ½ life in blood of ~60 days; however, deposits will remain in the kidney and brain for years. Exposure to mercury stimulates the kidney to produce metallothionein, which provides some detoxification benefit. Mercury binds sulfhydryl groups and interferes with a wide variety of critical enzymatic processes.	Acute inhalation of Hg^0 vapor causes pneumonitis and noncardiogenic pulmonary edema leading to death, CNS symptoms, and polyneuropathy. Chronic high exposure causes CNS toxicity (mercurial *erethism*; see diagnosis); lower exposures impair renal function, motor speed, memory, coordination. Acute ingestion of inorganic mercury causes gastroenteritis, the nephritic syndrome, or acute renal failure, hypertension, tachycardia, and cardiovascular collapse, with death at a dose of 10–42 mg/kg. Ingestion of organic mercury causes gastroenteritis, arrhythmias, and lesions in the basal ganglia, gray matter, and cerebellum at doses >1.7 mg/kg. High exposure during pregnancy causes derangement of fetal neuronal migration resulting in severe mental retardation. Mild exposures during pregnancy (from fish consumption) are associated with declines in neurobehavioral performance in offspring. Dimethylmercury, a compound only found in research labs, is "supertoxic"—a few drops of exposure via skin absorption or inhaled vapor can cause severe cerebellar degeneration and death.	Chronic exposure to metallic mercury vapor produces a characteristic intention tremor and mercurial *erethism*: excitability, memory loss, insomnia, timidity, and delirium ("mad as a hatter"). On neurobehavioral tests: decreased motor speed, visual scanning, verbal and visual memory, visuomotor coordination. Children exposed to mercury in any form may develop *acrodynia* ("pink disease"): flushing, itching, swelling, tachycardia, hypertension, excessive salivation or perspiration, irritability, weakness, morbilliform rashes, desquamation of palms and soles. Toxicity from elemental or inorganic mercury exposure begins when blood levels >180 nmol/L (3.6 μg/dL) and urine levels >0.7 μmol/L (15 μg/dL). Exposures that ended years ago may result in a >20-μg increase in 24-h urine after a 2-g dose of succimer. Organic mercury exposure is best measured by levels in blood (if recent) or hair (if chronic); CNS toxicity in children may derive from fetal exposures associated with maternal hair Hg > 30 nmol/g (6 μg/g).	Treat acute ingestion of mercuric salts with induced emesis or gastric lavage and polythiol resins (to bind mercury in the GI tract). Chelate with dimercaprol (up to 24 mg/kg per day IM in divided doses), DMSA (succimer), or penicillamine, with 5-day courses separated by several days of rest. If renal failure occurs, treat with peritoneal dialysis, hemodialysis, or extracorporeal regional complexing hemodialysis and succimer. Chronic inorganic mercury poisoning is best treated with *N*-acetyl penicillamine.

Note: GI, gastrointestinal; ECG, electrocardiogram; ICU, intensive care unit; LFT, liver function tests; RBC, red blood cell; IQ, intelligence quotient; CDC, Centers for Disease Control and Prevention; OSHA, Occupational Safety and Health Administration; CNS, central nervous system.

problem with deep wells; however, the geology of this region allows most residents only a few alternatives for potable drinking water. Serious *cadmium* poisoning from the contamination of food and water by mining effluents in Japan contributed to the 1946 outbreak of "itai-itai" ("ouch-ouch") disease, so named because of cadmium-induced bone toxicity that led to painful bone fractures. Modest exposures from environmental contamination near a smelter in Belgium were recently associated with a lower bone density, a higher incidence of fractures, and a faster decline in height in both men and women, effects that may be related to cadmium's calciuric effect on the kidney. Such research is creating concern that cadmium exposure may be contributing significantly to morbidity and mortality from osteoporosis in the general population.

Advances in our understanding of *lead* toxicity have recently benefited by the development of K-x-ray fluorescence (KXRF) instruments for making safe in vivo measurements of lead levels in bone (which, in turn, reflect cumulative exposure over many years, as opposed to blood lead levels, which mostly reflect recent exposure). High bone lead levels measured by KXRF have been linked to increased risk of hypertension in both men and women from an urban population. In addition, high maternal bone lead levels were found to predict lower birth weight, head circumference, birth length, and neurodevelopmental performance in offspring by age 2. The toxicity of low-level organic *mercury* exposure (as manifested by neurobehavioral performance) is of increasing concern based on studies of the offspring of mothers who ingested mercury-contaminated fish. However, current evidence has not supported the recent contention that ethyl mercury, used as a preservative in multiuse vaccines administered in early childhood, has played a significant role in causing neurodevelopmental problems such as autism.

Finally, a few additional metals deserve brief mention but are not covered in Table 376-1 because of the relative rarity of their being clinically encountered, or the uncertainty regarding their potential toxicities. *Aluminum* contributes to the encephalopathy in patients with severe renal disease who are undergoing dialysis (Chap. 332). High levels of aluminum are found in the neurofibrillary tangles in the cerebral cortex and hippocampus of patients with Alzheimer disease as well as in the drinking water and soil of areas with an unusually high incidence of Alzheimer disease. The experimental and epidemiologic evidence for the aluminum–Alzheimer's disease link is so far relatively weak, however, and it cannot be concluded that aluminum is a causal agent or a contributing factor in neurodegenerative disease. Hexavalent *chromium* is corrosive and sensitizing. Workers in the chromate and chrome pigment production industries have consistently had a greater risk of lung cancer. The introduction of *cobalt* chloride as a fortifier in beer led to outbreaks of fatal cardiomyopathy among heavy consumers. Occupational exposure (e.g., of miners, dry-battery manufacturers, and arc welders) to *manganese* can cause a Parkinsonian syndrome within 1 to 2 years, including gait disorders; postural instability; a masked, expressionless face; tremor; and psychiatric symptoms. With the introduction of methylcyclopentadienyl manganese tricarbonyl (MMT) as a gasoline additive, there is concern for the toxic potential of environmental manganese exposure. *Nickel* exposure induces an allergic response, and inhalation of nickel compounds with low aqueous solubility (e.g., nickel subsulfide and nickel oxide) in occupational settings is associated with an increased risk of lung cancer. Overexposure to *selenium* may cause local irritation of the respiratory system and eyes, gastrointestinal irritation, liver inflam-

mation, loss of hair, depigmentation, and peripheral nerve damage. Workers exposed to certain organic forms of *tin* (particularly trimethyl and triethyl derivatives) have developed psychomotor disturbances, including tremor, convulsions, hallucinations, and psychotic behavior.

Thallium, which is a component of some insecticides, metal alloys, and fireworks, is absorbed through the skin as well as by ingestion and inhalation. Severe poisoning follows a single ingested dose of >1 g or >8 mg/kg. Nausea and vomiting, abdominal pain, and hematemesis precede confusion, psychosis, organic brain syndrome, and coma. Thallium is radiopaque. Induced emesis or gastric lavage is indicated within 4 to 6 h of acute ingestion; Prussian blue prevents absorption and is given orally at 250 mg/kg in divided doses. Unlike other types of metal poisoning, thallium poisoning may be less severe when activated charcoal is used to interrupt its enterohepatic circulation. Other measures include forced diuresis, treatment with potassium chloride (which promotes renal excretion of thallium), and peritoneal dialysis.

FURTHER READING

ALFVÉN T et al: Low-level cadmium exposure and osteoporosis. J Bone Miner Res 15:1579, 2000

CENTENO JA et al: Pathology related to chronic arsenic exposure. Environ Health Perspect 110(Suppl 5):883, 2002

GRANDJEAN P et al: Neurotoxic risk caused by stable and variable exposure to methylmercury from seafood. Ambul Pediatr 3:18, 2003

MISRA UK: Thallium poisoning: Emphasis on early diagnosis and response to haemodialysis. Postgrad Med J 79:103, 2003

ROGAN WJ et al: The effect of chelation therapy with succimer on neuropsychological development in children exposed to lead. N Engl J Med 344: 1421, 2001

377 POISONING AND DRUG OVERDOSAGE
Christopher H. Linden, Michael J. Burns

Poisoning refers to the development of dose-related adverse effects following exposure to chemicals, drugs, or other xenobiotics. To paraphrase Paracelsus, the dose makes the poison. In excessive amounts, substances that are usually innocuous, such as oxygen and water, can cause poisoning. Conversely, in small doses, substances commonly regarded as poisons, such as arsenic and cyanide, can be consumed without ill effect. There is, however, substantial individual variability in the response to, and disposition of, a given dose. Some of this variability is genetic, and some is acquired on the basis of enzyme induction or inhibition, or because of tolerance. Poisoning may be local (e.g., skin, eyes, or lungs) or systemic depending on the chemical and physical properties of the poison, its mechanism of action, and the route of exposure. The severity and reversibility of poisoning also depend on the functional reserve of the individual or target organ, which is influenced by age and preexisting disease.

EPIDEMIOLOGY About 5 million poison exposures occur in the United States each year. Most are acute, accidental, involve a single agent, occur in the home, result in minor or no toxicity, and involve children under 6 years of age. Pharmaceuticals are involved in 47% of exposures and 84% of serious or fatal poisonings. Accidental exposures can result from the improper use of chemicals at work or play; product mislabeling; label misreading; mistaken identification of unlabeled chemicals; uninformed self-medication; and dosing errors by nurses, parents, pharmacists, physicians, and the elderly. Excluding the recreational use of ethanol, attempted suicide is the most common reason for intentional exposure. Unintended poisonings may result from the intentional use of drugs for psychotropic effects (abuse) or excessive self-dosing (misuse).

About 5% of exposures require hospitalization. They account for 5 to 10% of all ambulance transports, emergency room visits, and

intensive care unit admissions. Up to 30% of psychiatric admissions are prompted by attempted suicide via overdosage. Overall, the mortality rate is low: 0.4% of all exposures. It is much higher (1 to 2%) in hospitalized patients with nonaccidental (suicidal) overdose, who account for the majority of serious poisonings. Acetaminophen is the pharmaceutical agent most often implicated in fatal poisoning. Overall, carbon monoxide is the leading cause of death from poisoning, but this is not reflected in hospital or poison center statistics because patients with such poisoning are typically dead when discovered and are referred directly to medical examiners.

DIAGNOSIS Although poisoning can mimic other illnesses, the correct diagnosis can usually be established by the history, physical examination, routine and toxicologic laboratory evaluations, and characteristic clinical course. The *history* should include the time, route, duration, and circumstances (location, surrounding events, and intent) of exposure; the name and amount of each drug, chemical, or ingredient involved; the time of onset, nature, and severity of symptoms; the time and type of first aid measures provided; and the medical and psychiatric history.

In many cases the victim is confused, comatose, unaware of an exposure, or unable or unwilling to admit to one. Suspicious circumstances include unexplained illness in a previously healthy person; a history of psychiatric problems (particularly depression); recent changes in health, economic status, or social relationships; and onset of illness while working with chemicals or after ingesting food, drink (especially ethanol), or medications. Patients who become ill soon after arriving from a foreign country or being arrested for criminal activity should be suspected of "body packing" or "body stuffing" (ingesting or concealing illicit drugs in a body cavity). Relevant history may be available from family, friends, paramedics, police, pharmacists, physicians, and employers, who should be questioned regarding the patient's habits, hobbies, behavior changes, available medications, and antecedent events. A search of clothes, belongings, and place of discovery may reveal a suicide note or a container of drugs or chemicals. The imprint code on pills and the label on chemical products may be used to identify the ingredients and potential toxicity of a suspected poison by consulting a reference text, a computerized database, the manufacturer, or a regional poison information center.

The *physical examination* should focus initially on the vital signs, cardiopulmonary system, and neurologic status. The neurologic examination should include documentation of neuromuscular abnormalities such as dyskinesia, dystonia, fasciculations, myoclonus, rigidity, tremors. The patient should also be examined for evidence of trauma and underlying illnesses. Focal neurologic findings are uncommon in poisoning, and their presence should prompt evaluation for a structural central nervous system (CNS) lesion. Examination of the eyes (for nystagmus, pupil size and reactivity), abdomen (for bowel activity and bladder size), and skin (for burns, bullae, color, warmth, moisture, pressure sores, and puncture marks) may reveal findings of diagnostic value. When the history is unclear, all orifices should be examined for the presence of chemical burns and drug packets. The odor of breath or vomitus and the color of nails, skin, or urine may provide diagnostic clues.

The diagnosis of poisoning in cases of unknown etiology primarily relies on pattern recognition. The first step is to assess the pulse, blood pressure, respiratory rate, temperature, and neurologic status and characterize the overall physiologic state as stimulated, depressed, discordant, or normal (Table 377-1). The next step is to consider the underlying causes of the observed physiologic state and attempt to identify a pathophysiologic pattern or toxic syndrome (*toxidrome*) based on further analysis of the vital signs and neurologic status, other physical findings, and the results of ancillary diagnostic tests. Assessing the severity of physiologic derangements (Table 377-2) is useful

in this regard and also for assessing the clinical course and response to treatment. The final step is to attempt to identify the particular agent involved by looking for unique or relatively poison-specific physical or ancillary test abnormalities. This approach is summarized below.

Increased pulse, blood pressure, respiratory rate, temperature, and neuromuscular activity characterize the stimulant toxidromes: sympathetic, anticholinergic, and hallucinogen poisoning and drug withdrawal (Table 377-1). Other features are noted in Table 377-2. Mydriasis, a characteristic feature of all stimulant toxidromes, is most marked in anticholinergic poisoning. This toxidrome is distinguished by the presence of hot, dry, flushed skin; decreased bowel sounds; and urinary retention (Table 377-3). Other stimulant toxidromes increase sympathetic activity and cause diaphoresis, pallor, and increased bowel activity with varying degrees of nausea, vomiting, abnormal distress, and occasionally diarrhea. The absolute and relative degree of vital sign changes and neuromuscular hyperactivity can help distinguish among stimulant toxidromes. Since sympathetics stimulate the peripheral nervous system more directly than do hallucinogens or drug withdrawal, markedly increased vital signs and organ ischemia suggest sympathetic poisoning. Findings helpful in suggesting the particular drug or class causing physiologic stimulation include reflex bradycardia from selective α-adrenergic stimulants (e.g., decongestants), hypotension from selective β-adrenergic stimulants (e.g., asthma therapeutics), limb ischemia from ergot alkaloids, nystagmus from phencyclidine and ketamine (the only physiologic stimulants that cause this finding), and delayed cardiac conduction from high doses

---

TABLE 377-1　*Differential Diagnosis of Poisoning Based on Physiologic State*

Stimulated	Depressed	Discordant	Normal
Sympathetics	Sympatholytics	Asphyxiants	Nontoxic exposure
Sympathomimetics	α_1-Adrenergic antagonists	Cytochrome oxidase inhibitors	Psychogenic illness
Ergot alkaloids	α_2-Adrenergic agonists	Inert gases	Toxic time-bombs
Methylxanthines	ACE inhibitors	Irritant gases	Slow absorption
Monoamine oxidase inhibitors	Angiotensin receptor blockers	Methemoglobin inducers	Anticholinergics
Thyroid hormones	Antipsychotics	Oxidative phosphorylation inhibitors	Carbamazepine
Anticholinergics	β-adrenergic blockers	AGMA inducers	Concretion formers
Antihistamines	Calcium channel blockers	Alcohol (ketoacidosis)	Dilantin Kapseals
Antiparkinsonian agents	Cardiac glycosides	Ethylene glycol	Drug packets
Antipsychotics	Cyclic antidepressants	Iron	Enteric-coated pills
Antispasmodics	Cholinergics	Methanol	Lomotil
Belladonna alkaloids	Acetylcholinesterase inhibitors	Salicylate	Opioids
Cyclic antidepressants	Muscarinic agonists	Toluene	Salicylates
Muscle relaxants	Nicotinic agonists	CNS syndromes	Sustained-release pills
Mushrooms and plants	Opioids	Extrapyramidal reactions	Slow distribution
Hallucinogens	Analgesics	Hydrocarbon inhalation	Cardiac glycosides
Cannabinoids (marijuana)	GI antispasmodics	Isoniazid	Lithium
LSD and analogues	Heroin	Lithium	Metals
Mescaline and analogues	Sedative-hypnotics	Neuroleptic malignant syndrome	Salicylate
Mushrooms	Alcohols	Serotonin syndrome	Toxic metabolite
Phencyclidine and analogues	Anticonvulsants	Strychnine	Acetaminophen
Withdrawal syndromes	Barbiturates	Membrane-active agents	Carbon tetrachloride
Barbiturates	Benzodiazepines	Amantidine	Cyanogenic glycosides
Benzodiazepines	GABA precursors	Antiarrhythmics	Ethylene glycol
Ethanol	Muscle relaxants	Antihistamines	Methanol
Opioids	Other agents	Antipsychotics	Methemoglobin inducers
Sedative-hypnotics		Carbamazepine	Mushroom toxins
Sympatholytics		Cyclic antidepressants	Organophosphate insecticides
		Local anesthetics	Paraquat
		Opioids (some)	Metabolism disruptors
		Orphenadrine	Antineoplastic agents
		Quinoline antimalarials	Antiviral agents
			Colchicine
			Hypoglycemic agents
			Immunosuppressive agents
			MAO inhibitors
			Metals
			Salicylate
			Warfarins

Note: ACE, angiotensin-converting enzyme; AGMA, anion-gap metabolic alkalosis; GI, gastrointestinal; CNS, central nervous system; LSD, lysergic acid diethylamide; GABA, γ-aminobutyric acid; MAO; monoamine oxidase.

TABLE 377-2 *Severity of Physiologic Stimulation and Depression in Poisoning and Drug Withdrawal*

PHYSIOLOGIC STIMULATION

Grade 1	Anxious, irritable, tremulous; vital signs normal; diaphoresis, flushing or pallor, mydriasis, and hyperreflexia may be present
Grade 2	Agitated; may have confusion or hallucinations but is able to converse and follow commands; vital signs mildly to moderately increased
Grade 3	Delirious; unintelligible speech, uncontrollable motor hyperactivity; moderately to markedly increased vital signs; tachyarrhythmias possible
Grade 4	Coma, seizures, cardiovascular collapse

PHYSIOLOGIC DEPRESSION

Grade 1	Awake, lethargic, or sleeping but arousable by voice or tactile stimulation; able to converse and follow commands; may be confused
Grade 2	Responds to pain but not voice; can vocalize but not converse; spontaneous motor activity present; brainstem reflexes intact
Grade 3	Unresponsive to pain; spontaneous motor activity absent; brainstem reflexes depressed; motor tone, respirations, and temperature decreased
Grade 4	Unresponsive to pain; flaccid paralysis; brainstem reflexes and respirations absent; cardiovascular vital signs decreased

of cocaine and some anticholinergic agents (e.g., antihistamines, cyclic antidepressants, and antipsychotics). Seizures suggest a sympathetic etiology, an anticholinergic agent with membrane-active properties (e.g., cyclic antidepressants, orphenadrine, phenothiazines), or a withdrawal syndrome. Other manifestations of grade 4 physiologic stimulation (Table 377-2) are likely only in sympathetic poisoning.

Decreased pulse, blood pressure, respiratory rate, temperature, and neuromuscular activity are indicative of physiologic depression caused by "functional" sympatholytics (agents that decrease cardiac function and vascular tone as well as symthathetic activity), cholinergic (muscarinic and nicotinic) agents, opioids, and sedative-hypnotic [γ-aminobutyric acid (GABA)-ergic] agents (Tables 377-1 and 377-2). Miosis is also common and most pronounced in opioid and cholinergic poisoning. The latter is distinguished from other depressant toxidromes by the presence of muscarinic and nicotinic signs and symptoms (Table 377-3). Pronounced cardiovascular depression in the absence of significant CNS depression suggests a direct or peripherally acting sympatholytic. In contrast, in opioid and sedative-hypnotic poisoning, vital sign changes are secondary to depression of CNS cardiovascular and respiratory centers (or consequent hypoxemia) and significant abnormalities in these parameters do not occur until there is a marked decrease in the level of consciousness (grade 3 or 4 physiologic depression, Table 377-2). Other clues that suggest the cause of physiologic depression include cardiac arrhythmias and conduction disturbances (due to antiarrhythmics, β-adrenergic antagonists, calcium-channel blockers, digitalis glycosides, propoxyphene, and cyclic antidepressants), mydriasis (due to tricyclic antidepressants, some antiarrhythmics, meperidine, and Lomotil), nystagmus (due to sedative-hypnotics), and seizures (due to cholinergic agents, propoxyphene, cyclic antidepressants).

Discordant or mixed vital sign and neuromuscular abnormalities are characteristic of poisoning by asphyxiants, CNS syndromes, membrane-active agents, and anion-gap metabolic acidosis (AGMA) inducers (Table 377-1). In these conditions, manifestations of physiologic stimulation and physiologic depression occur together or at different times during the clinical course. For example, membrane-active agents can cause simultaneous coma, seizures, hypotension, and tachyarrhythmias. Alternatively, vital signs may be normal but the patient has altered mental status or is obviously sick or clearly symptomatic. Early, pro-

nounced vital sign and mental status changes suggest asphyxiant or membrane-active agent poisoning; the lack of such abnormalities suggests an AGMA inducer, and marked neuromuscular dysfunction without significant vital sign abnormalities suggests a CNS syndrome. As noted below, AGMA inducer poisoning can be distinguished from other causes of AGMA by the serum lactate concentration.

A normal physiologic status and physical examination may be due to a nontoxic exposure, psychogenic illness, or poisoning by "toxic time-bombs," agents that are slowly absorbed, slowly distributed to their sites of action, require metabolic activation, or disrupt metabolic processes (Table 377-1). Diagnosing a nontoxic exposure requires that the identity of the exposure agent be known or that a toxic time-bomb exposure has been excluded and that the time since exposure exceeds the longest known or predicted interval between exposure and peak toxicity. Psychogenic illness (fear of being poisoned, mass hysteria) may also occur after a nontoxic exposure and should be considered when symptoms are inconsistent with the exposure history. Anxiety reactions resulting from a nontoxic exposure can cause mild physiologic stimulation (Table 377-2) and be indistinguishable from toxicologic causes (Table 377-1) without ancillary testing or a suitable period of observation.

Laboratory assessment may be helpful in the differential diagnosis (Fig. 377-1). An increased AGMA is characteristic of advanced methanol, ethylene glycol, and salicylate intoxication but can occur with other agents (Table 377-1) and in any poisoning that results in hepatic, renal, or respiratory failure; seizures; or shock. The serum lactate concentration is low (less than the anion gap) in the former and high (nearly equal to the anion gap) in the latter. An abnormally low anion gap can be due to elevated blood levels of bromide, calcium, iodine, lithium, magnesium, or nitrate. An increased osmolal gap—a difference between the serum osmolality (measured by freezing point depression) and that calculated from the serum sodium, glucose, and blood urea nitrogen of >10 mmol/L—suggests the presence of a low-

TABLE 377-3 *Fundamentals of Poisoning Management*

SUPPORTIVE CARE

Airway protection	Treatment of seizures
Oxygenation/ventilation	Correction of temperature abnormalities
Treatment of arrhythmias	Correction of metabolic derangements
Hemodynamic support	Prevention of secondary complications

PREVENTION OF FURTHER POISON ABSORPTION

Gastrointestinal decontamination	Decontamination of other sites
Syrup of ipecac–induced emesis	Eye decontamination
	Skin decontamination
Gastric lavage	Body cavity evacuation
Activated charcoal	
Whole-bowel irrigation	
Catharsis	
Dilution	
Endoscopic/surgical removal	

ENHANCEMENT OF POISON ELIMINATION

Multiple-dose activated charcoal	Extracorporeal removal
	Peritoneal dialysis
Forced diuresis	Hemodialysis
Alteration of urinary pH	Hemoperfusion
Chelation	Hemofiltration
	Plasmapheresis
	Exchange transfusion
	Hyperbaric oxygenation

ADMINISTRATION OF ANTIDOTES

Neutralization by antibodies	Metabolic antagonism
Neutralization by chemical binding	Physiologic antagonism

PREVENTION OF REEXPOSURE

Adult education	Notification of regulatory agencies
Child-proofing	Psychiatric referral

molecular-weight solute such as acetone, an alcohol (benzyl, ethanol, isopropanol, methanol), a glycol (diethylene, ethylene, propylene), ether (ethyl, glycol), or an "unmeasured" cation (calcium, magnesium) or sugar (glycerol, mannitol, sorbitol). Ketosis suggests acetone, isopropyl alcohol, or salicylate poisoning. Hypoglycemia may be due to poisoning with β-adrenergic blockers, ethanol, insulin, oral hypoglycemic agents, quinine, and salicylates, whereas hyperglycemia can occur in poisoning with acetone, β-adrenergic agonist, caffeine, calcium channel blockers, iron, theophylline, or Vacor. Hypokalemia can be caused by barium, β-adrenergic agonists, caffeine, diuretics, theophylline, or toluene; hyperkalemia suggests poisoning with an α-adrenergic agonist, a β-adrenergic blocker, cardiac glycosides, or fluoride. Hypocalcemia may be seen in ethylene glycol, fluoride, and oxalate poisoning.

The *electrocardiogram* (ECG) can sometimes be useful for diagnostic purposes. Bradycardia and atrioventricular block may occur in patients poisoned by α-adrenergic agonists, antiarrhythmic agents, beta blockers, calcium channel blockers, cholinergic agents (carbamate and organophosphate insecticides), cardiac glycosides, lithium, magnesium, or tricyclic antidepressants. QRS- and QT-interval prolongation may be caused by hyperkalemia and by membrane-active drugs (Table 377-1). Ventricular tachyarrhythmias may be seen in poisoning with cardiac glycosides, fluorides, membrane-active drugs, methylxanthines, sympathomimetics, and agents that cause hyperkalemia or potentiate the effects of endogenous catecholamines (e.g., chloral hydrate, aliphatic and halogenated hydrocarbons).

Radiologic studies may also be useful. Pulmonary edema (adult respiratory distress syndrome, or ARDS) can be caused by poisoning with carbon monoxide, cyanide, an opioid, paraquat, phencyclidine, a sedative-hypnotic, or salicylate; by inhalation of irritant gases, fumes, or vapors (acids and alkali, ammonia, aldehydes, chlorine, hydrogen sulfide, isocyanates, metal oxides, mercury, phosgene, polymers); or by prolonged anoxia, hyperthermia, or shock. Aspiration pneumonia is common in patients with coma, seizures, and petroleum distillate ingestion. The presence of radiopaque densities on abdominal x-rays suggests the ingestion of calcium salts, chloral hydrate, chlorinated hydrocarbons, heavy metals, illicit drug packets, iodinated compounds, potassium salts, psychotherapeutic agents, lithium, phenothiazines, enteric-coated tablets, or salicylates.

Toxicologic analysis of urine and blood (and occasionally of gastric contents and chemical samples) can sometimes confirm or rule out suspected poisoning. Interpretation of laboratory data requires knowledge of the tests used for screening and confirmation (thin-layer, gas-liquid, or high-performance liquid chromatography; colorimetric and fluorometric assays; enzyme-multiplied, fluorescence polarization, and radioimmunoassays; gas chromatography; mass spectrometry), their sensitivity (limit of detection) and specificity, the preferred biologic specimen for analysis, and the optimal time of specimen sampling. Personal communication with the laboratory is essential. A negative result may mean the substance is not detectable by the test used or that its concentration is too low for detection at the time of sampling. In the latter case, repeating the test at a later time may yield a positive result.

Although rapid screening tests for a limited number of drugs of abuse are available, comprehensive screening tests require 2 to 6 h for completion, and immediate management must often be based on the history, physical examination, and routine ancillary tests. In addition, when the patient is asymptomatic, or when the clinical picture is consistent with the reported history, qualitative screening is neither clinically useful nor cost-effective. It is of greatest value in patients with severe or unexplained toxicity such as coma, seizures, cardiovascular instability, metabolic or respiratory acidosis, and non-sinus cardiac rhythms. Quantitative analysis is useful for poisoning with acetaminophen (Chap.

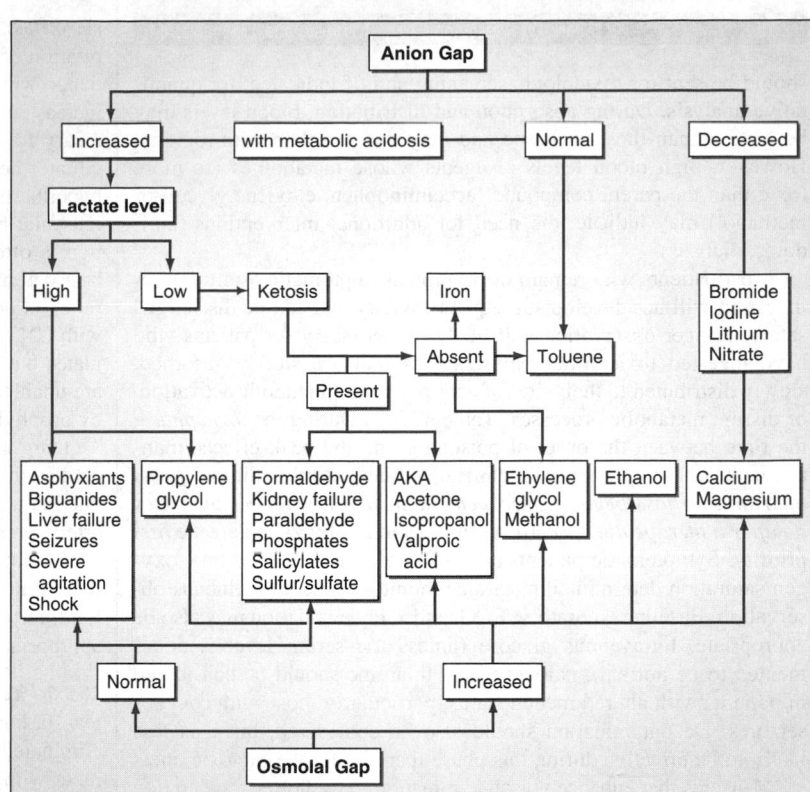

FIGURE 377-1 Differential diagnosis of poisoning based on the results of routine laboratory tests. AKA, alcoholic ketoacidosis; biguanides, metformin, phenformin.

286), acetone, alcohols (including ethylene glycol), antiarrhythmics, anticonvulsants, barbiturates, digoxin, heavy metals, lithium, paraquat, salicylate, and theophylline, as well as for carboxyhemoglobin and methemoglobin. Results can often be available within an hour.

The *response to antidotes* may be useful for diagnostic purposes. Resolution of altered mental status and abnormal vital signs within minutes of intravenous administration of dextrose, naloxone, or flumazenil is virtually diagnostic of hypoglycemia, narcotic poisoning, and benzodiazepine intoxication, respectively. The prompt reversal of dystonic (extrapyramidal) signs and symptoms following an intravenous dose of benztropine or diphenhydramine confirms a drug etiology. Although the reversal of both central and peripheral manifestations of anticholinergic poisoning by physostigmine is diagnostic of this condition, physostigmine may cause arousal in patients with CNS depression of any etiology.

℞ TREATMENT

General Principles   Treatment goals include support of vital signs, prevention of further poison absorption, enhancement of poison elimination, administration of specific antidotes, and prevention of reexposure (Table 377-3). Specific treatment depends on the identity of the poison, the route and amount of exposure, the time of presentation relative to the time of exposure, and the severity of poisoning. Knowledge of the offending agents' pharmacokinetics and pharmacodynamics is essential.

During the *pretoxic phase*, prior to the onset of poisoning, decontamination is the highest priority, and treatment is based solely on the history. The maximum potential toxicity based on the greatest possible exposure should be assumed. Since decontamination is more effective when accomplished soon after exposure, the initial history and physical examination should be focused and brief. It is also advisable to establish intravenous access and initiate cardiac monitoring, particularly in patients with potentially serious ingestions or unclear histories.

When an accurate history is not obtainable and a poison causing delayed toxicity or irreversible damage is suspected, blood and urine should be sent for toxicologic screening and, if indicated, for quantitative analysis. During absorption and distribution, blood levels may be greater than those in tissue and may not correlate with toxicity. However, high blood levels of agents whose metabolites are more toxic than the parent compound (acetaminophen, ethylene glycol, or methanol) may indicate the need for additional interventions (antidotes, dialysis).

Most patients who remain or become asymptomatic 4 to 6 h after ingestion will not develop subsequent toxicity and can be discharged safely. Longer observation will likely be necessary for patients who have ingested toxic time-bombs, agents that are slowly absorbed, slowly distributed to their sites of action, require metabolic activation, or disrupt metabolic processes (Table 377-1). During the *toxic phase*, the time between the onset of poisoning and the peak effects, management is based primarily on clinical and laboratory findings. *Effects after an overdose begin sooner, peak later, and last longer than they do after a therapeutic dose.* Resuscitation and stabilization are the first priority. Symptomatic patients should have an intravenous line, oxygen saturation determination, cardiac monitoring, and continuous observation. Baseline laboratory, ECG, and x-ray evaluation may also be appropriate. Intravenous glucose (unless the serum level is documented to be normal), naloxone, and thiamine should be considered in patients with altered mental status, particularly those with coma or seizures. Decontamination should also be considered, but it is less likely to be effective during this phase than during the pretoxic one.

Measures that enhance poison elimination may shorten the duration of toxicity and lessen its severity. However, they are not without risk, which must be weighed against the potential benefit. Diagnostic certainty (usually via laboratory confirmation) is generally a prerequisite. Intestinal dialysis with repetitive doses of activated charcoal is usually safe and can enhance the elimination of many poisons. Diuresis, urinary alkalinization, and chelation therapy enhance the elimination of a relatively small number of poisons, and their use is associated with potential complications. Extracorporeal elimination methods are effective for many poisons, but their expense and risk make their use reasonable only in patients who would otherwise have an unfavorable outcome.

During the *resolution phase* of poisoning, supportive care and monitoring should continue until clinical, laboratory, and ECG abnormalities have resolved. Since chemicals are eliminated sooner from the blood than from tissues, blood levels are usually lower than tissue levels during this phase and again may not correlate with toxicity. This is particularly true when extracorporeal elimination procedures are used. Redistribution from tissues may cause a rebound increase in the blood level after termination of these procedures. When a metabolite is responsible for toxic effects, continued treatment might be necessary in the absence of clinical toxicity.

Supportive Care The goal of supportive therapy is to maintain physiologic homeostasis until detoxification is accomplished and to prevent and treat secondary complications such as aspiration, bedsores, cerebral and pulmonary edema, pneumonia, rhabdomyolysis, renal failure, sepsis, thromboembolic disease, coagulopathy, and generalized organ dysfunction due to hypoxia or shock.

Admission to an intensive care unit is indicated for the following: patients with severe poisoning (coma, respiratory depression, hypotension, cardiac conduction abnormalities, cardiac arrhythmias, hypothermia or hyperthermia, seizures); those needing close monitoring, antidotes, or enhanced elimination therapy; those showing progressive clinical deterioration; and those with significant underlying medical problems. Patients with mild to moderate toxicity can be managed on a general medical service, intermediate care unit, or emergency department observation area, depending on the anticipated duration and level of monitoring needed (intermittent clinical observation versus continuous clinical, cardiac, and respiratory monitoring). Patients who have attempted suicide require continuous observation and measures to prevent self-injury until they are no longer suicidal.

RESPIRATORY CARE Endotracheal intubation for protection against the aspiration of gastrointestinal contents is of paramount importance in patients with CNS depression or seizures as this complication can increase morbidity and mortality. Mechanical ventilation may be necessary for patients with respiratory depression or hypoxia and to facilitate therapeutic sedation or paralysis in order to prevent or treat hyperthermia, acidosis, and rhabdomyolysis associated with neuromuscular hyperactivity. Since clinical assessment of respiratory function is often inaccurate, the need for oxygenation and ventilation is best determined by oximetry or arterial blood gas analysis. The gag reflex is not a reliable indicator of the need for intubation. A patient with CNS depression may maintain airway patency while being stimulated but not if left alone. Those who cannot respond to voice or who are unable to sit and drink fluids without assistance are best managed by prophylactic intubation.

Drug-induced pulmonary edema is usually noncardiac rather than cardiac in origin although profound CNS depression and cardiac conduction abnormalities suggest the latter. Measurement of pulmonary artery pressure may be necessary to establish the cause and direct appropriate therapy. Extracorporeal measures (membrane oxygenation, venoarterial perfusion, cardiopulmonary bypass), partial liquid (perfluorocarbon) ventilation, and hyperbaric oxygen therapy may be appropriate for severe but reversible respiratory failure.

CARDIOVASCULAR THERAPY Maintenance of normal tissue perfusion is critical for complete recovery to occur once the offending agent has been eliminated. If hypotension is unresponsive to volume expansion, treatment with norepinephrine, epinephrine, or high-dose dopamine may be necessary. Intraaortic balloon pump counterpulsation and venoarterial or cardiopulmonary perfusion techniques should be considered for severe but reversible cardiac failure. Bradyarrhythmias associated with hypotension generally should be treated as described in Chap. 213. Glucagon, calcium, and high-dose insulin with dextrose may be effective in both beta blocker and calcium channel blocker poisoning. Antibody therapy may be indicated for cardiac glycoside poisoning.

Supraventricular tachycardia associated with hypertension and CNS excitation is almost always due to agents that cause generalized physiologic excitation (Table 377-1). Most cases are mild or moderate in severity and require only observation or nonspecific sedation with a benzodiazepine. In severe cases or those associated with hemodynamic instability, chest pain, or ECG evidence of ischemia, specific therapy is indicated. When the etiology is sympathetic hyperactivity, treatment with a combined alpha and beta blocker (labetalol), a calcium channel blocker (verapamil or diltiazem), or a combination of a beta blocker and a vasodilator (esmolol and nitroprusside) is preferred. Treatment with an α-adrenergic antagonist (phentolamine) alone may sometimes be appropriate. If the cause is anticholinergic poisoning, physostigmine is the treatment of choice. Supraventricular tachycardia without hypertension is generally secondary to vasodilation or hypovolemia and responds to fluid administration.

Lidocaine and phenytoin are generally safe for ventricular tachyarrhythmias of any etiology. Beta blockers can be hazardous if the arrhythmia is due to sympathetic hyperactivity. For ventricular tachyarrhythmias due to tricyclic antidepressants and probably other membrane-active agents (Table 377-1), class IA, IC, and III antiarrhythmic agents are contraindicated (because of similar electrophysiologic effects), but sodium bicarbonate may be helpful. Magnesium sulfate and overdrive pacing (by isoproterenol or a pacemaker) may be useful in patients with torsades de pointes and prolonged QT intervals. Magnesium and anti-digoxin antibodies should be considered in patients with severe cardiac glycoside poisoning. Invasive (esophageal or intracardiac) ECG recording may be necessary to determine the origin (ventricular or supraventricular) of wide-complex tachycardias (Chap. 214). If the patient is hemodynamically stable, however, it is reasonable to simply observe them rather than to administer another potentially proarrhythmic agent. Arrhythmias may be resistant to drug therapy until underlying acid-base, electrolyte, oxygenation, and temperature derangements are corrected.

Neuromuscular hyperactivity and seizures can lead to hyperthermia, lactic acidosis, and rhabdomyolysis, with their attendant complications, and should be treated aggressively. Seizures caused by excessive stimulation of catecholamine receptors (sympathomimetic or hallucinogen poisoning and drug withdrawal), or decreased activity of GABA (isoniazid poisoning) or glycine (strychnine poisoning) receptors are best treated with agents that enhance GABA activity such as benzodiazepine or barbiturates. Since benzodiazepines and barbiturates act by slightly different mechanisms (the former increases the frequency and the latter increases the duration of chloride channel opening in response to GABA), therapy with both may be effective when neither is effective alone. Seizures caused by isoniazid, which inhibits the synthesis of GABA, may require high doses of pyridoxine (which facilitates the synthesis of GABA). Those resulting from membrane destabilization (beta blocker or cyclic antidepressant poisoning) may require a membrane-active anticonvulsant such as phenytoin as well as GABA enhancers. For poisons with central dopaminergic effects (phencyclidine), a dopamine receptor antagonist, such as haloperidol, may be useful. In anticholinergic and cyanide poisoning, specific antidotal therapy may be necessary. The treatment of seizures secondary to cerebral ischemia or edema, or to metabolic abnormalities should include correction of the underlying cause. Neuromuscular paralysis is indicated in refractory cases. Electroencephalographic monitoring and continuing treatment of seizures are necessary to prevent permanent neurologic damage.

OTHER MEASURES Temperature extremes, metabolic abnormalities, hepatic and renal dysfunction, and secondary complications should be treated by standard therapies.

Prevention of Poison Absorption ■ GASTROINTESTINAL DECONTAMINATION Whether or not to perform gastrointestinal decontamination, and which procedure to use, depends on the time since ingestion; the existing and predicted toxicity of the ingestant; the availability, efficacy, and contraindications of the procedure; and the nature, severity, and risk of complications. The efficacy of activated charcoal, gastric lavage, and syrup of ipecac decreases with time, and there are insufficient data to support or exclude a beneficial effect when they are used more than 1 h after ingestion. The average time from ingestion to presentation for treatment is >1 h for children and >3 h for adults. Most patients will recover from poisoning uneventfully with good supportive care alone, but complications of gastrointestinal decontamination, particularly aspiration, can prolong this process. Hence, gastrointestinal decontamination should be performed selectively, not routinely, in the management of overdose patients. It is clearly unnecessary when predicted toxicity is minimal or the time of expected maximal toxicity has passed without significant effect.

Activated charcoal has comparable or greater efficacy, fewer contraindications and complications, is less aversive and invasive than ipecac or gastric lavage, and thus is the preferred method of gastrointestinal decontamination in most situations. Activated charcoal suspension (in water) is given orally via a cup, straw, or small-bore nasogastric tube. The recommended dose is 1 g/kg body weight. Palatability may be increased by adding a sweetener (sorbitol) or a flavoring agent (cherry, chocolate, or cola syrup) to the suspension. Charcoal adsorbs ingested poisons within the gut lumen, allowing the charcoal-toxin complex to be evacuated with stool. The complex can also be removed from the stomach by induced emesis or lavage. In vitro, charcoal adsorbs ≥90% of most substances when given in an amount equal to 10 times the weight of the substance. Charged (ionized) chemicals such as mineral acids, alkalis, and highly dissociated salts of cyanide, fluoride, iron, lithium, and other inorganic compounds are not well adsorbed by charcoal. In animal and human volunteer studies, charcoal decreases the absorption of ingestants by an average of 73% when given within 5 min of ingestant administration, 51% when given at 30 min, and 36% at 60 min. Side effects of charcoal include nausea, vomiting, and diarrhea or constipation. Charcoal may also prevent the absorption of orally administered therapeutic agents.

Complications include mechanical obstruction of the airway, aspiration, vomiting, and bowel obstruction and infarction caused by inspissated charcoal. Charcoal is not recommended for patients who have ingested corrosives because it obscures endoscopy.

Gastric lavage is performed by sequentially administering and aspirating about 5 mL fluid per kilogram of body weight through a no. 40 French orogastric tube (no. 28 French tube for children). Except for infants, where normal saline is recommended, tap water is acceptable. The patient should be placed in Trendelenburg and left lateral decubitus positions to prevent aspiration (even if an endotracheal tube is in place). Lavage decreases ingestant absorption by an average of 52% if performed within 5 min of ingestion administration, 26% if performed at 30 min, and 16% if performed at 60 min. Its efficacy is similar to that of ipecac. Significant amounts of ingested drug are recovered in ~10% of patients. Aspiration is a common complication (occurring in up to 10% of patients), especially when lavage is performed improperly. Serious complications (esophageal and gastric perforation, tube misplacement in the trachea) occur in ~1% of patients. For this reason, the physician should personally insert the lavage tube and confirm its placement, and the patient must be cooperative or adequately restrained (with pharmacologic sedation if necessary) during the procedure. Gastric lavage is contraindicated in corrosive or petroleum distillate ingestions because of the respective risks of gastroesophageal perforation and aspiration pneumonitis. It is also contraindicated in those with a compromised unprotected airway and those at risk for hemorrhage or perforation due to esophageal or gastric pathology or recent surgery.

Syrup of ipecac can be used for the home management of patients with accidental ingestions, reliable histories, and mild predicted toxicity. It may delay the administration and decrease the effectiveness of activated charcoal, oral antidotes, and whole-bowel irrigation and is rarely appropriate for patients treated at a health care facility. It is administered orally in a dose of 30 mL for adults, 15 mL for children, and 10 mL for small infants. Clear liquids should also be given. Ipecac irritates the stomach and stimulates the central chemoreceptor trigger zone. Vomiting usually occurs about 20 min after administration. The dose may be repeated if vomiting does not occur. In animal and human volunteer studies, ipecac decreases ingestant absorption by an average of 60% if given within 5 min of ingestant administration, 32% if given at 30 min, and 30% if given at 60 min. Side effects include lethargy in children (12%) and protracted vomiting (8 to 17%). Chronic ipecac use (by patients with anorexia nervosa or bulimia) may cause electrolyte and fluid abnormalities, cardiac toxicity, and myopathy. Except for aspiration, serious complications (e.g., gastric or esophageal tears and perforations) are rare. Ipecac is contraindicated in patients with recent gastrointestinal surgery, CNS depression, or seizures, and in those who have ingested corrosives or rapidly acting CNS poisons (camphor, cyanide, tricyclic antidepressants, propoxyphene, strychnine).

Whole-bowel irrigation is performed by administering a bowel-cleansing solution containing electrolytes and polyethylene glycol (Golytely, Colyte) orally or by gastric tube at a rate of 2.0 L/h (0.5 L/h in children) until rectal effluent is clear. The patient must be in a sitting position. Although data are limited, whole-bowel irrigation appears to be as effective as other decontamination procedures. It is most appropriate for those who have ingested foreign bodies, packets of illicit drugs, slow-release or enteric-coated medications, and agents that are poorly adsorbed by charcoal (e.g., heavy metals). It is contraindicated in patients with bowel obstruction, ileus, hemodynamic instability, and compromised unprotected airways.

Cathartics are salts (disodium phosphate, magnesium citrate and sulfate, sodium sulfate) or saccharides (mannitol, sorbitol) that promote the rectal evacuation of gastrointestinal contents. The most effective cathartic is sorbitol in a dose of 1 to 2 g/kg of body weight. Alone, cathartics do not prevent ingestant absorption and should not be used as a method of gut decontamination. Their primary use is to prevent constipation following charcoal administration. Abdominal cramps, nausea, and occasional vomiting are side effects. Complications of repeated dosing include hypermagnesemia (from magnesium salts) and excessive diarrhea. Cathartics are contraindicated in patients who have ingested corrosives and in those with preexisting diarrhea. Magnesium-containing cathartics should not be used in patients with renal failure.

Dilution (i.e., drinking 5 mL/kg of body weight of water or another clear liquid) is recommended only after the ingestion of corrosives (acids, alkali). It may increase the dissolution rate (and hence absorption) of capsules, tablets, and other solid ingestants and should *not* be used in these circumstances.

Endoscopic or surgical removal of poisons may be useful in rare situations, such as ingestion of a potentially toxic foreign body that fails to transit the gastrointestinal tract, a potentially lethal amount of a heavy metal (arsenic, iron, mercury, thallium), or agents that have coalesced into gastric concretions or bezoars (barbiturates, glutethimide, heavy metals, lithium, meprobamate, salicylates, sustained-release preparations). Patients who become toxic from cocaine due to its leakage from ingested drug packets require immediate surgical intervention.

DECONTAMINATION OF OTHER SITES Immediate, copious flushing with water, saline, or another available clear, drinkable liquid is the initial treatment for topical exposures (exceptions include alkali metals, calcium oxide, phosphorus). Saline is preferred for eye irrigation. A triple wash (water, soap, water) may be best for dermal decontamination. Inhalational exposures should be treated initially with fresh air or oxygen. The removal of liquids from body cavities such as the vagina or rectum is best accomplished by irrigation. Solids (drug packets, pills) should be removed manually, preferably under direct visualization.

Enhancement of Poison Elimination Although the elimination of most poisons can be accelerated by therapeutic interventions, the pharmacokinetic efficacy (removal of drug at a rate greater than that accomplished by intrinsic elimination) and clinical benefit (shortened duration of toxicity or improved outcome) of such interventions are often more theoretical than proven. Hence, the decision to use such measures should be based on the actual or predicted toxicity and the potential efficacy, cost, and risks of therapy.

MULTIPLE-DOSE ACTIVATED CHARCOAL Repetitive oral dosing with charcoal can enhance the elimination of previously absorbed substances by binding them within the gut as they are excreted in the bile, secreted by gastrointestinal cells, or passively diffuse into the gut lumen (reverse absorption or enterocapillary exsorption). Doses of 0.5 to 1 g/kg body weight every 2 to 4 h, adjusted downward to avoid regurgitation in patients with decreased gastrointestinal motility, are generally recommended. Experimentally, this treatment enhances the elimination of nearly all substances tested. Pharmacokinetic efficacy approaches that of hemodialysis for some agents (e.g., phenobarbital, theophylline). Multiple-dose therapy is not effective in accelerating elimination of chlorpropamide, tobramycin, or agents that adsorb poorly to charcoal. Complications include intestinal obstruction, pseudoobstruction, and nonocclusive intestinal infarction in patients with decreased gut motility.

FORCED DIURESIS AND ALTERATION OF URINARY pH Diuresis and ion trapping via alteration of urine pH may prevent the renal reabsorption of poisons that undergo excretion by glomerular filtration and active tubular secretion. Since membranes are more permeable to nonionized molecules than to their ionized counterparts, acidic (low-pK_a) poisons are ionized and trapped in alkaline urine, whereas basic ones become ionized and trapped in acid urine. Saline diuresis can enhance the renal excretion of alcohols, bromide, calcium, chromium, fluoride, isoniazid, lithium, meprobamate, potassium, and thallium. Alkaline diuresis (producing a urine pH $\geq$ 7.5 and a urine output of 3 to 6 mL/kg body weight per hour by adding sodium bicarbonate to an intravenous solution) enhances the excretion of chlorphenoxyacetic acid herbicides, chlorpropamide, diflunisal, fluoride, methotrexate, phenobarbital, sulfonamides, and sa-

licylates. Contraindications include congestive heart failure, renal failure, and cerebral edema. Acid-base, fluid, and electrolyte parameters should be monitored carefully. While acid diuresis can enhance the excretion of amphetamines, chloroquine, cocaine, local anesthetics, phencyclidine, quinidine, quinine, strychnine, sympathomimetics, tricyclic antidepressants, and tocainide, such therapy is not recommended because of potential cardiovascular and renal (myoglobinuric renal failure) complications and lack of clinical efficacy.

EXTRACORPOREAL REMOVAL Peritoneal dialysis, hemodialysis, charcoal or resin hemoperfusion, hemofiltration, plasmapheresis, and exchange transfusion are capable of removing any toxin from the bloodstream. Agents most amenable to enhanced elimination by dialysis have low molecular mass (<500 Da), high water solubility, low protein binding, small volumes of distribution (<1 L/kg body weight), prolonged elimination (long half-life), and high dialysis clearance relative to total-body clearance. Molecular weight, water solubility, or protein binding do not limit the efficacy of the other forms of extracorporeal removal.

Dialysis should be considered in cases of severe poisoning due to acetone, atenolol, barbiturates, bromide, chloral hydrate, ethanol, ethylene glycol, isopropyl alcohol, lithium, methanol, procainamide, theophylline, salicylates, sotalol, and possibly heavy metals. Although hemoperfusion may be more effective in removing some of these poisons, it does not correct associated acid-base and electrolyte abnormalities. Hemoperfusion should be considered in cases of severe poisoning due to caffeine, carbamazepine, carbon tetrachloride, chloramphenicol, dapsone, disopyramide, hypnotic-sedatives (barbiturates, ethchlorvynol, glutethimide, meprobamate, methaqualone), methotrexate, mushrooms (amatoxin-containing), paraquat, phenytoin, procainamide, theophylline, and valproate. Both techniques require central venous access and systemic anticoagulation and often result in transient hypotension. Hemoperfusion may also cause hemolysis, hypocalcemia, and thrombocytopenia. Peritoneal dialysis and exchange transfusion are less effective but may be used when other procedures are either not available, contraindicated, or technically difficult (e.g., in infants). Exchange transfusion may be indicated in the treatment of severe arsine- or sodium chlorate–induced hemolysis, methemoglobinemia, and sulfhemogloginemia. Although hemofiltration can enhance elimination of aminoglycosides, vancomycin, and metal-chelate complexes, the roles of hemofiltration and plasmapheresis in the treatment of poisoning are not yet defined.

Candidates for extracorporeal removal therapies include patients with severe toxicity who deteriorate despite aggressive supportive therapy; those with potentially prolonged, irreversible, or fatal toxicity; those with dangerous blood levels of toxins; those who lack the capacity for self-detoxification because of liver or renal failure; and those with a serious underlying illness or complication that will adversely affect recovery.

OTHER TECHNIQUES The elimination of heavy metals can be enhanced by chelation, and the removal of carbon monoxide can be increased by hyperbaric oxygenation.

Administration of Antidotes Antidotes counteract the effects of poisons by neutralizing them (e.g., antibody-antigen reactions, chelation, chemical binding) or by antagonizing their physiologic effects (e.g., activation of opposing nervous system activity, provision of competitive metabolic or receptor substrate). Poisons or conditions with specific antidotes include acetaminophen, anticholinergic agents, anticoagulants, benzodiazepines, beta blockers, calcium channel blockers, carbon monoxide, cardiac glycosides, cholinergic agents, cyanide, drug-induced dystonic reactions, ethylene glycol, fluoride, heavy metals, hydrogen sulfide, hypoglycemic agents, isoniazid, membrane-active agents, methemoglobinemia, opioids, sympathomimetics, Vacor, and a variety of envenomations. Antidotes can significantly reduce morbidity and mortality, but most are potentially toxic. Since their safe use requires correct identification of a specific poisoning or syndrome, details of antidotal therapy are discussed with the conditions for which they are indicated (Table 377-4).

Physiologic Condition, Causes	Examples	Mechanism of Action	Clinical Features	Specific Treatments
STIMULATED				
Sympathetics (see also Chap. 374)				
Sympathomimetics	α_1-Adrenergic agonists (decongestants): phenylephrine, phenylpropanolamine β_2-Adrenergic agonists (bronchodilators): albuterol, terbutaline Nonspecific adrenergic agonists: amphetamines, cocaine, ephedrine	Stimulation of central and peripheral sympathetic receptors directly or indirectly (by promoting the release or inhibiting the reuptake of norepinephrine and sometimes dopamine)	Physiologic stimulation (Table 377-2); reflex bradycardia can occur with selective α_1 agonists; β agonists can cause hypotension and hypokalemia.	Phentolamine, a nonselective α_1-adrenergic receptor antagonist, for severe hypertension due to α_1-adrenergic agonists; propranolol, a nonselective β blocker, for hypotension and tachycardia due to β_2 agonists; labetalol, a β blocker with α-blocking activity, or phentolamine with esmolol, metoprolol, or other cardioselective β blocker for hypertension with tachycardia due to nonselective agents (β blockers, if used alone, can exacerbate hypertension and vasospasm due to unopposed α stimulation).
Ergot alkaloids	Ergotamine, methysergide, bromocriptine, pergolide	Stimulation and inhibition of serotonergic and α-adrenergic receptors; stimulation of dopamine receptors	Physiologic stimulation (Table 377-2); formication; vasospasm with limb (isolated or generalized), myocardial, and cerebral ischemia progressing to gangrene or infarction; hypotension, bradycardia, and involuntary movements can also occur.	Nitroprusside or nitroglycerine for severe vasospasm; prazocin (an α_1 blocker), captopril, nifedipine, and cyproheptidene (a serotonin receptor antagonist) for mild to moderate limb ischemia; dopamine receptor antagonists (antipsychotics) for hallucinations and movement disorders
Methylxanthines	Caffeine, theophylline	Inhibition of adenosine synthesis and adenosine receptor antagonism; stimulation of epinephrine and norepinephrine release; inhibition of phosphodiesterase resulting in increased intracellular cyclic adenosine and quanosine monophosphate	Physiologic stimulation (Table 377-2); pronounced gastrointestinal symptoms and β agonist effects (see above). Toxicity occurs at lower drug levels in chronic poisoning than in acute poisoning.	Propranolol, a nonselective β blocker, for tachycardia with hypotension; any β blocker for supraventricular or ventricular tachycardia without hypotension; elimination enhanced by multiple-dose charcoal, hemoperfusion, and hemodialysis; indications for hemoperfusion or hemodialysis include unstable vital signs, seizures, and a theophylline level of 80 to 100 μg/mL after acute overdose and 40 to 60 μg/mL with chronic exposure.
Monoamine oxidase inhibitors	Phenelzine, tranylcypromine, selegiline	Inhibition of monoamine oxidase resulting in impaired metabolism of endogenous catecholamines and exogenous sympathomimetic agents	Delayed or slowly progressive physiologic stimulation (Table 377-2); terminal hypotension and bradycardia in severe cases.	Short-acting agents (e.g., nitroprusside, esmolol) for severe hypertension and tachycardia; direct-acting sympathomimetics (e.g., norepinephrine, epinephrine) for hypotension and bradycardia
Anticholinergics				
Antihistamines	Diphenhydramine, doxylamine, pyrilamine	Inhibition of central and postganglionic parasympathetic muscarinic cholinergic receptors. At high doses, amantidine, diphenhydramine, orphenadrine, phenothiazines, and tricyclic antidepressants have additional nonanticholinergic activity (see below).	Physiologic stimulation (Table 377-2); dry skin and mucous membranes, decreased bowel sounds, flushing, and urinary retention; myoclonus and picking activity. Central effects may occur without significant autonomic dysfunction.	Physostigmine, an acetylcholinesterase inhibitor (see below) for delirium, hallucinations, and neuromuscular hyperactivity. Contraindications include nonanticholinergic cardiovascular toxicity (e.g., cardiac conduction abnormalities, hypotension, and ventricular arrhythmias).
Antiparkinsonian agents	Amantidine, trihexiphenydyl			
Antipsychotics	Chlorpromazine, olanzapine, quetiapine, thioridazine			
Antispasmotics	Clinidium, dicyclomine			
Belladonna alkaloids	Atropine, hyoscyamine, scopolamine			
Cyclic antidepressants	Amitriptyline, doxepin, imipramine			
Muscle relaxants	Cyclobenzaprine, orphenadrine			
Mushrooms and plants	*Amanita muscaria* and *A. pantherina*, henbane, jimson weed, nightshade			

(continued)

Physiologic Condition, Causes	Examples	Mechanism of Action	Clinical Features	Specific Treatments
DEPRESSED				
Sympatholytics α_2-Adrenergic agonists	Clonidine, guanabenz, tetra-hydrozoline and other imidazoline decongestants, tizanidine and other imidazoline muscle relaxants	Stimulation of α_2-adrenergic receptors leading to inhibition of CNS sympathetic outflow; activity at nonadrenergic imidazoline binding sites also contributes to CNS effects.	Physiologic depression (Table 377-2), miosis. Transient initial hypertension may be seen.	Dopamine and norepinephrine for hypotension. Atropine for symptomatic bradycardia. Naloxone for CNS depression (inconsistently effective).
Antipsychotics	Chlorpromazine, clozapine, haloperidol, risperidone, thioridazine	Inhibition of α-adrenergic, dopaminergic, histaminergic, muscarinic, and serotonergic receptors. Some agents also inhibit sodium, potassium, and calcium channels.	Physiologic depression (Table 377-2), miosis, anticholinergic effects (see above), extrapyramidal reactions (see below), tachycardia. Cardiac conduction delays (increased PR, QRS, JT, and QT intervals) with ventricular tachydysrhythmias, including torsades de pointes, can sometimes develop.	Sodium bicarbonate and lidocaine for ventricular tachydysrhythmias associated with QRS prolongation. Magnesium, isoproterenol, and overdrive pacing for torsades de pointes. Avoid class IA, IC, and III antiarrhythmics.
β-Adrenergic blockers	Cardioselective (β_1) blockers: atenolol, esmolol, metoprolol Nonselective (β_1 and β_2) blockers: nadolol, propranolol, timolol Partial β agonists: acebutolol, pindolol α_1 Antagonists: carvedilol, labetalol Membrane-active agents: acebutolol, propranolol, sotalol	Inhibition of β-adrenergic receptors (class II antiarrhythmic effect). Some agents have activity at additional receptors or have membrane effects (see below).	Physiologic depression (Table 377-2), atrioventricular block, hypoglycemia, hyperkalemia, seizures. Partial agonists can cause hypertension and tachycardia. Sotalol can cause increased QT interval and ventricular tachydysrhythmias. Onset may be delayed after sotalol and sustained-release formulation overdose.	Glucagon and calcium for hypotension and symptomatic bradycardia. Atropine, isoproterenol, amrinone, dopamine, dobutamine, epinephrine, and norepinephrine may sometimes be effective. High-dose insulin (with glucose and potassium to maintain euglycemia and normokalemia), electrical pacing, and mechanical cardiovascular support for refractory cases.
Calcium channel blockers	Diltiazem, nifedipine and other dihydropyridine derivatives, verapamil	Inhibition of slow (type L) cardiovascular calcium channels (class IV antiarrhythmic effect).	Physiologic depression (Table 377-2), atrioventricular block, organ ischemia and infarction, hyperglycemia, seizures. Hypotension is usually due to decreased vascular resistance rather than to decreased cardiac output. Onset may be delayed for ≥12 h after overdose of sustained-release formulations.	Calcium and glucagon for hypotension and symptomatic bradycardia. Dopamine, epinephrine, norepinephrine, atropine, and isoproterenol are less often effective but can be used adjunctively. Amrinone, high-dose insulin (with glucose and potassium to maintain euglycemia and normokalemia), electrical pacing, and mechanical cardiovascular support for refractory cases.
Cardiac glycosides	Digoxin, endogenous cardioactive steroids, foxglove and other plants, toad skin secretions (*Bufonidae* sp.)	Inhibition of cardiac Na$^+$, K$^+$-ATPase membrane pump.	Physiologic depression (Table 377-2); gastrointestinal, psychiatric, and visual symptoms; atrioventricular block with or without concomitant supraventricular tachyarrhythmia; ventricular tachyarrhythmias. Hyperkalemia in acute poisoning. Toxicity occurs at lower drug levels in chronic poisoning than in acute poisoning.	Digoxin-specific antibody fragments for hemodynamically compromising dysrhythmias, Mobitz II or third-degree atrioventricular block, hyperkalemia (>5.5 meq/L; in acute poisoning only). Temporizing measures include atropine, dopamine, epinephrine, phenytoin, and external cardiac pacing for bradydysrhythmias and magnesium, lidocaine, phenytoin, and bretylium for ventricular tachydysrhythmias. Internal cardiac pacing and cardioversion can increase ventricular irritability and should be reserved for refractory cases.

(continued)

TABLE 377-4—(Continued)

Physiologic Condition, Causes	Examples	Mechanism of Action	Clinical Features	Specific Treatments
Cyclic antidepressants	Amitriptyline, doxepin, imipramine	Inhibition of α-adrenergic dopaminergic, GABA-ergic, histaminergic, muscarinic, and serotonergic receptors; inhibition of sodium channels (see membrane-active agents); inhibition of norepinephrine and serotonin reuptake.	Physiologic depression (Table 377-2), seizures, tachycardia, cardiac conduction delays (increased PR, QRS, JT, and QT intervals; terminal QRS right axis deviation) with aberrancy and ventricular tachydysrhythmias. Anticholinergic toxidrome (see above).	Hypertonic sodium bicarbonate (or hypertonic saline) and lidocaine for ventricular tachydysrhythmias associated with QRS prolongation. Use of phenytoin is controversial. Avoid class IA, IC, and III antiarrhythmics.
Cholinergics				
Acetylcholinesterase inhibitors	Carbamate insecticides (aldicarb, carbaryl, propoxur) and medicinals (neostigmine, physostigmine, tacrine); nerve gases (sarin, soman, tabun, VX) organophosphate insecticides (diazinon, chlopyriphos, malathion)	Inhibition of acetylcholinesterase leading to increased synaptic acetylcholine at muscarinic and nicotinic cholinergic receptor sites	Physiologic depression (Table 377-2). Muscarinic signs and symptoms: seizures, excessive secretions (lacrimation, salivation, bronchorrhea and wheezing, diaphoresis), and increased bowel and bladder activity with nausea, vomiting, diarrhea, abdominal cramps, and incontinence of feces and urine. Nicotinic signs and symptoms: hypertension, tachycardia, muscle cramps, fasciculations, weakness, and paralysis. Death is usually due to respiratory failure. Cholinesterase activity in plasma and red cells <50% of normal in acetylcholinesterase inhibitor poisoning.	Atropine for muscarinic signs and symptoms. Pralidoxime (2-PAM), a cholinesterase reactivator, for nicotinic signs and symptoms due to organophosphates, nerve gases, or an unknown anticholinesterase.
Muscarinic agonists	Bethanechol, mushrooms (*Boletus, Clitocybe, Inocybe* sp.), pilocarpine	Stimulation of CNS and postganglionic parasympathetic cholinergic (muscarinic) receptors		
Nicotinic agonists	Lobeline, nicotine (tobacco)	Stimulation of preganglionic sympathetic and parasympathetic and striated muscle (neuromuscular junction) cholinergic (nicotine) receptors		
Sedative-hypnotics (see also Chap. 387)				
Anticonvulsants	Carbamazepine, ethosuximide, felbamate, gabapentin, lamotrigine, levetiracetam, oxcarbazepine, phenytoin, tiagabine, topiramate, valproate, zonisamide	Potentiation of the inhibitory effects of GABA by binding to the neuronal GABA-A chloride channel receptor complex and increasing the frequency or duration of chloride channel opening in response to GABA stimulation. Baclofen and, to some extent, GHB act at the GABA-B rector complex; meprobamate, its metabolite carisoprodol, felbamate, and orphenidrine antagonize N-methyl-D-aspartate (NDMA) excitatory receptors; ethosuximide, valproate, and zonisamide decrease conduction through T-type calcium channels; valproate decreases GABA degradation, and tiagabine blocks GABA reuptake; carbamazepine, lamotrigine, oxcarbazepine, phenytoin, topiramate, valproate, and zonisamide slow the rate of recovery of inactivated sodium channels. Some agents also have α2 agonist, anticholinergic, and sodium channel blocking activity (see above and below).	Physiologic depression (Table 377-2), nystagmus. Delayed absorption can occur with carbamazepine, phenytoin, and valproate. Myoclonus, seizures, hypertension, and tachyarrhythmias can occur with baclofen, carbamazepine, and orphenadrine. Tachyarrhythmias can also occur with chloral hydrate. AGMA, hypernatremia, hyperosmolality, hyperammonemia, chemical hepatitis, and hypoglycemia can be seen in valproate poisoning. Carbamazepine and oxcarbazepine may produce hyponatremia from SIADH. Some agents can cause anticholinergic and sodium channel (membrane) blocking effects (see above and below).	Flumazenil for benzodiazepine and zolpidem poisoning. Benzodiazepines and barbiturates for seizures. Elimination of phenobarbital and possibly other long-acting agents enhanced by multiple-dose charcoal. Hemodialysis and hemoperfusion may be indicated for severe poisoning by some agents (see "Extracorporeal Removal," in text). See above and below for treatment of anticholinergic and sodium channel (membrane) blocking effects.
Barbiturates	Short-acting: butabarbital, pentobarbital, secobarbital Long-acting: phenobarbital, primadone			
Benzodiazepines	Ultrashort-acting: estazolam, midazolam, temazapam, triazolam Short-acting: alprazolam, flunitrazepam, lorazepam, oxazepam Long-acting: chlordiazepoxide, clonazepam, diazepam, flurazepam Pharmacologically related agents: zaleplon, zolpidem			
GABA precursors	γ-Hydroxybutyrate (sodium oxybate; GHB), γ-butyrolactone (GBL), 1,4-butanediol			
Muscle relaxants	Baclofen, carisoprodol, cyclobenzaprine, etomidate, metaxalone, methocarbamol, orphenadrine, propofol, tizanidine and other imidazoline muscle relaxants.			

(continued)

Physiologic Condition, Causes	Examples	Mechanism of Action	Clinical Features	Specific Treatments
Other agents	Chloral hydrate, ethclorvynol, glutethimide, meprobamate, methaqualone, methyprylon			
DISCORDANT				
Asphyxiants				
Cytochrome oxidase inhibitors	Carbon monoxide, cyanide, hydrogen sulfide	Inhibition of mitochrondrial cytochrome oxidase, thereby blocking electron transport and oxidative metabolism. Carbon monoxide also binds to hemoglobin and myoglobin and prevents oxygen binding, transport, and tissue uptake (binding to hemoglobin shifts the oxygen dissociation curve to the left).	Signs and symptoms of hypoxia with initial physiologic stimulation and subsequent depression (Table 377-2); lactic acidosis; normal P_{O_2} and calculated oxygen saturation but decreased oxygen saturation by co-oximetry (that measured by pulse oximetry is falsely elevated but is less than normal and less than the calculated value). Headache and nausea are common with carbon monoxide. Sudden collapse may occur with cyanide and hydrogen sulfide exposure. A bitter almond breath odor may be noted with cyanide ingestion, and hydrogen sulfide smells like rotten eggs.	High-dose oxygen. Inhaled amyl nitrite and IV sodium nitrite and sodium thiosulfate (Lilly cyanide antidote kit) for coma, metabolic acidosis, and cardiovascular dysfunction in cyanide poisoning. Amyl and sodium nitrite (without thiosulfate) for similar toxicity in hydrogen sulfide poisoning. Hyperbaric oxygen for moderate to severe carbon monoxide poisoning and for cyanide or hydrogen sulfide poisoning unresponsive to other measures.
Methemoglobin inducers	Aniline derivatives, dapsone, local anesthetics, nitrates, nitrites, nitrogen oxides, nitro- and nitrosohydrocarbons, phenazopyridine, primaquine-type antimalarials, sulfonamides.	Oxidation of hemoglobin iron from ferrous (Fe^{2+}) to ferric (Fe^{3+}) state prevents oxygen binding, transport, and tissue uptake (methemoglobinemia shifts oxygen dissociation curve to the left). Oxidation of hemoglobin protein causes hemoglobin precipitation and hemolytic anemia (manifest as Heinz bodies and "bite cells" on peripheral blood smear).	Signs and symptoms of hypoxia with initial physiologic stimulation and subsequent depression (Table 377-2), gray-brown cyanosis unresponsive to oxygen at methemoglobin fractions > 15 to 20%, headache, lactic acidosis (at methemoglobin fractions > 45%), normal P_{O_2} and calculated oxygen saturation but decreased oxygen saturation and increased methehemoglobin fraction by co-oximetry (oxygen saturation by pulse oximetry may be falsely increased or decreased but is less than normal and less than the calculated value).	High-dose oxygen. Intravenous methylene blue for methemoglobin fraction > 30%, symptomatic hypoxia, or ischemia (contraindicated in G6PD deficiency). Exchange transfusion and hyperbaric oxygen for severe or refractory cases.
AGMA inducers				
	Ethylene glycol	Ethylene glycol causes CNS depression and increased serum osmolality. Metabolites (primarily glycolic acid) cause AGMA, CNS depression, and renal failure. Precipitation of oxalic acid metabolite as calcium salt in tissues and urine results in hypocalcemia, tissue edema, and crystalluria.	Initial ethanol-like intoxication, nausea, vomiting, increased osmolar gap, calcium oxalate crystalluria. Delayed AGMA, back pain, renal failure. Coma, seizures, hypotension, ARDS in severe cases.	Gastric aspiration for recent ingestions. Sodium bicarbonate to correct acidemia. Thiamine, folinic acid, magnesium, and high-dose pyridoxine to facilitate metabolism. Ethanol or fomepizole for AGMA, crytalluria or renal dysfunction, ethylene glycol level > 3 mmol/L (20 mg/dL), and for ethanol-like intoxication or increased osmolal gap if level not readily obtainable. Hemodialysis for persistent AGMA, lack of clinical improvement, and renal dysfunction. Hemodialysis also useful for enhancing ethylene glycol elimination and shortening duration of treatment when ethylene glycol level > 8 mmol/L (50 mg/dL).

(continued)

TABLE 377-4—(Continued)

Physiologic Condition, Causes	Examples	Mechanism of Action	Clinical Features	Specific Treatments
	Iron	Hydration of ferric (Fe^{3+}) ion generates H^+. Non-transferrin-bound iron catalyzes formation of free radicals that cause mitochondrial injury, lipid peroxidation, increased capillary permeability, vasodilation, and organ toxicity.	Initial nausea, vomiting, abdominal pain, diarrhea. AGMA, cardiovascular and CNS depression, hepatitis, coagulopathy, and seizures in severe cases. Radiopaque iron tablets may be seen on abdominal x-ray.	Whole-bowel irrigation for large ingestions. Endoscopy and gastrostomy if clinical toxicity and large number of tablets still visible on x-ray. IV hydration. Sodium bicarbonate for acidemia. IV deferoxamine for systemic toxicity, iron level > 90 μmol/L (500 μg/dL).
	Methanol	Methanol causes ethanol-like CNS depression and increased serum osmolality. Formic acid metabolite causes AGMA and retinal toxicity.	Initial ethanol-like intoxication, nausea, vomiting, increased osmolar gap. Delayed AGMA, visual (clouding, spots, blindness) and retinal (edema, hyperemia) abnormalities. Coma, seizures, cardiovascular depression in severe cases. Possible pancreatitis.	Gastric aspiration for recent ingestions. Sodium bicarbonate to correct acidemia. High-dose folinic acid or folate to facilitate metabolism. Ethanol or fomepizole for AGMA, visual symptoms, methanol level > 6 mmol/L (20 mg/dL), and for ethanol-like intoxication or increased osmolal gap if level not readily obtainable. Hemodialysis for persistent AGMA, lack of clinical improvement, and renal dysfunction. Hemodialysis also useful for enhancing methanol elimination and shortening duration of treatment when methanol level > 15 mmol/L (50 mg/dL).
	Salicylate	Increased sensitivity of CNS respiratory center to changes in P_{O_2} and P_{CO_2} stimulates respiration. Uncoupling of oxidative phosphorylation, inhibition of Kreb's cycle enzymes, and stimulation of carbohydrate and lipid metabolism generate unmeasured endogenous anions and cause AGMA.	Initial nausea, vomiting, hyperventilation, alkalemia, alkaluria. Subsequent alkalemia with both respiratory alkalosis and AGMA, and paradoxical aciduria. Late acidemia with CNS and respiratory depression. Cerebral and pulmonary edema in severe cases. Hypoglycemia, hypocalcemia, hypokalemia, and seizures can occur.	IV hydration and supplemental glucose. Sodium bicarbonate to correct acidemia. Alkaline diuresis for systemic toxicity. Hemodialysis for coma, cerebral edema, seizures, pulmonary edema, renal failure, progressive acid-base disturbances or clinical toxicity, salicylate level > 7 mmol/L (100 mg/dL) following acute overdose.
CNS syndromes Extrapyramidal reactions	Antipsychotics (see above), some cyclic antidepressants and antihistamines.	Decreased CNS dopaminergic activity with relative excess of cholinergic activity.	Akathisia, dystonia, parkinsonism	Oral or parenteral anticholinergic agent such as benztropine or diphenhydramine.
Isoniazid		Interference with activation and supply of pyridoxal-5-phosphate, a cofactor for glutamic acid decarboxylase, which converts glutamic acid to GABA, results in decreased levels of this inhibitory CNS neurotransmitter; complexation with and depletion of pyridoxine itself; inhibition of nicotine-adenine dinucleotide dependent lactate and hydroxybutyrate dehydrogenases resulting in substrate accumulation.	Nausea, vomiting, agitation, confusion; coma, respiratory depression, seizures, lactic and ketoacidosis in severe cases.	High-dose intravenous pyridoxine (vitamin B_6) for agitation, confusion, coma, and seizures. Diazepam or barbiturates for seizures.

(continued)

Physiologic Condition, Causes	Examples	Mechanism of Action	Clinical Features	Specific Treatments
Lithium		Interference with cell membrane ion transport, adenylate cyclase and Na$^+$, K$^+$-ATPase activity, and neurotransmitter release.	Nausea, vomiting, diarrhea, ataxia, choreoathetosis, encephalopathy, hyperreflexia, myoclonus, nystagmus, nephrogenic diabetes insipidus, falsely elevated serum chloride with low anion gap, tachycardia. Coma, seizures, arrhythmias, hyperthermia, and prolonged or permanent encephalopathy and movement disorders in severe cases. Delayed onset after acute overdose, particularly with delayed-release formations. Toxicity occurs at lower drug levels in chronic poisoning than in acute poisoning.	Whole-bowel irrigation for large ingestions. Consider endoscopic removal if high and rising drug level with progressive clinical toxicity. IV hydration. Hemodialysis for coma, seizures, severe, progressive, or persistent encephalopathy or neuromuscular dysfunction, peak lithium level > 8 meq/L (mmol/L) following acute overdose.
Serotonin syndrome	Amphetamines, cocaine, dextromethorphan, meperidine, MAO inhibitors, selective serotonin (5HT) reuptake inhibitors, tricyclic antidepressants, tramadol, triptans, tryptophan.	Promotion of serotonin release, inhibition of serotonin reuptake, or direct stimulation of CNS and peripheral serotonin receptors (primarily 5HT-1a and 5HT-2), alone or in combination.	Altered mental status (agitation, confusion, mutism, coma, seizures), neuromuscular hyperactivity (hyperreflexia, myoclonus, rigidity, tremors), and autonomic dysfunction (abdominal pain, diarrhea, diaphoresis, fever, flushing, labile hypertension, mydriasis, tearing, salivation, tachycardia). Complications include hyperthermia, lactic acidosis, rhabdomyolysis, and multisystem organ failure.	Serotonin receptor antagonist such as cyproheptadine or chlorpromazine.
Membrane-active agents	Amantidine, antiarrhythmics (class 1 and III agents; some β blockers), antipsychotics (see above), antihistamines (particularly diphenhydramine), carbamazepine, local anesthetics (including cocaine), opioids (meperidine, propoxyphene), orphenadrine, quinoline antimalarials (chloroquine, hydroxychloroquine, quinine), cyclic antidepressants (see above).	Blockade of fast sodium membrane channels prolongs phase 0 (depolarization) of the cardiac action potential, which prolong the QRS duration and promotes reentrant (monomorphic) ventricular tachycardia. Class Ia, Ic, and III antiarrhythmics also block potassium channels during phases 2 and 3 (repolarization) of the action potential, prolonging the JT interval and promoting early after-depolarizations and polymorphic (torsades de pointes) ventricular tachycardia. Similar effects on neuronal membrane channels cause CNS dysfunction. Some agents also block α-adrenergic and cholinergic receptors or have opioid effects (see above and Chap. 373).	QRS and JT prolongation (or both) with hypotension, ventricular tachyarrhythmias, CNS depression, seizures. Anticholinergic effects with amantidine, antihistamines, carbamazepine, disopyramide, antipsychotics, and cyclic antidepressants (see above). Opioid effects with meperidine and propoxyphene (see Chap. 373). Cinchonism (hearing loss, tinnitus, nausea, vomiting, vertigo, ataxia, headache, flushing, diaphoresis) and blindness with quinoline antimalarials.	Hypertonic sodium bicarbonate (or hypertonic saline) for cardiac conduction delays and monomorphic ventricular tachycardia. Lidocaine for monomorphic ventricular tachycardia (except when due to class Ib antiarrhythmics). Magnesium, isoproterenol, and overdrive pacing for polymorphic ventricular tachycardia. Physostigmine for anticholinergic effects (see above.) Naloxone for opioid effects (see Chap. 373). Extracorporeal removal for some agents (see text).

Note: AGMA, anion-gap metabolic acidosis; ARDS, adult respiratory distress syndrome; CNS, central nervous system; GABA, γ-aminobutyric acid; G6PD, glucose-6-phosphate dehydrogenase; MAO, monoamine oxidase; SIADH, syndrome of inappropriate antidiuretic hormone.

Prevention of Reexposure Poisoning is a preventable illness. Unfortunately, some adults and children are poison-prone, and recurrences are common. Adults with accidental exposures should be instructed regarding the safe use of medications and chemicals (according to labeling instructions). Confused patients may need assistance with the administration of their medications. Errors in dosing by health care providers may require educational efforts. Patients should be advised to avoid circumstances that result in chemical exposure or poisoning.

Appropriate agencies and health departments should be notified in cases of environmental or workplace exposure. The best approach with young children and patients with intentional overdose is to limit their access to poisons. In households where children live or visit, alcoholic beverages, medications, household products (automotive, cleaning, fuel, pet-care, toiletry products), nonedible plants, and vitamins should be kept out of reach or in locked or child-proof cabinets. Depressed or psychotic patients should receive psychiatric assessment, disposition, and follow-up. They should be given prescriptions for a limited supply of drugs and with a limited number of refills and be monitored for compliance and response to therapy.

SPECIFIC TOXIC SYNDROMES AND POISONINGS   Table 377-4 summarizes the pathophysiology, clinical features, and treatment of toxidromes and poisonings that are common, produce life-threatening toxicity, or require unique therapeutic interventions. In all cases, treatment should include attending to the general principles discussed above, particularly supportive care. Details regarding specific therapies can be found in the references cited here and at *harrisononline.com*. Poisonings not covered in this chapter are discussed in the referenced texts.→*Alcohol, cocaine, hallucinogen, and opioid poisoning and alcohol and opioid withdrawal are discussed in Chaps. 372 to 375; acetaminophen poisoning is discussed in Chap. 286; the neuroleptic malignant syndrome is discussed in Chap. 351; and heavy metal poisoning is discussed in Chap. 376.*

FURTHER READING

AMERICAN ACADEMY OF CLINICAL TOXICOLOGY/EUROPEAN ASSOCIATION OF POISONS CENTERS AND CLINICAL TOXICOLOGISTS: Position Statements on Gastrointestinal Decontamination: Introduction; Ipecac syrup; Gastric lavage; Single-dose activated charcoal; Cathartics; Whole bowel irrigation. Clin Toxicol 35:695, 699, 711, 721, 743, 753, 1997

————: Multi-dose activated charcoal. Clin Toxicol 37:731, 1999

BOSSE GM, MATYUNAS NJ: Delayed toxidromes. J Emerg Med 17:679, 1999

HARDMAN JG et al (eds): *Goodman and Gilman's The Pharmacologic Basis of Therapeutics*, 10th ed. New York, McGraw-Hill, 2001

KLAASSEN CD (ed): *Casarett and Doull's Toxicology: The Basic Science of Poisons*, 6th ed. New York, McGraw-Hill, 2001

LITOVITZ TL et al: 2001 Annual Report of the American Association of Poison Control Centers Toxic Exposure Surveillance System. Am J Emerg Med 20:391, 2002

378 DISORDERS CAUSED BY REPTILE BITES AND MARINE ANIMAL EXPOSURES
Paul S. Auerbach, Robert L. Norris

This chapter outlines general principles for the evaluation and management of victims of venom poisoning or intoxication by certain reptiles and marine creatures and presents a clinical approach to these emergencies. Because the incidence of serious bites and stings is relatively low in developed nations, there remains a paucity of relevant clinical research and literature, and therapeutic decision-making is often based on anecdotal information.

VENOMOUS SNAKEBITE

EPIDEMIOLOGY   The venomous snakes of the world are grouped into the families Viperidae (subfamily Viperinae: the Old World vipers; subfamily Crotalinae: the New World and Asian pit vipers), Elapidae (including the cobras, coral snakes, and all Australian venomous snakes), Hydrophiidae (the sea snakes), Atractaspididae (the burrowing asps), and Colubridae (a large group, of which the majority are nonvenomous and only a few species are dangerously toxic to humans). Bite rates are highest in temperate and tropical regions where people subsist by manual agriculture. Global estimates suggest that 30,000 to 40,000 persons die each year from venomous snakebite, but this range is likely an underestimate because of incomplete reporting.

SNAKE ANATOMY/IDENTIFICATION   The typical snake-venom apparatus consists of bilateral venom glands—one on each side of the head, below and behind the eye—connected by ducts to hollow, anterior maxillary teeth. In viperids (vipers and pit vipers), these teeth are long mobile fangs that retract against the roof of the mouth when the animal is at rest. In elapids and sea snakes, the fangs are less enlarged and are relatively fixed in an erect position. Venomous snakes can bite without injecting venom. Approximately 20% of pit viper bites and an even higher percentage of bites inflicted by some other snake families (e.g., up to 75% for sea snakes) are "dry."

Differentiation of venomous from nonvenomous snake species can be difficult. Viperids are characterized by somewhat triangular heads (a feature shared with many harmless snakes); elliptical pupils (also seen in some nonvenomous snakes, such as boas and pythons); enlarged maxillary fangs; subcaudal scalation that involves a single scale running the full width of the ventral surface of the tail for several rows just distal to the anal plate (as opposed to two scales in each subcaudal row for most nonvenomous snakes and elapids); and, in the case of pit vipers, the heat-sensing pits (foveal organs), for which they are named, located slightly inferior and anterior to the eyes on each side. Color pattern is notoriously misleading in identifying most venomous

snakes except for the coral snakes, whose other body characteristics are similar to those of harmless colubrids. The American coral snakes can be identified by red, yellow (or white), and black bands completely encircling the body; a few species have red and black bands only. North of Mexico City, the immediate contiguity of red and yellow bands is fairly reliable for distinguishing a coral snake from its many harmless mimics. Further south, differentiation by color pattern is more problematic.

In many areas of the world, such as Australia, enzyme-linked immunoassay (ELISA) kits are available to aid in determining the specific snake species involved in a bite. These kits identify venom in the victim's blood, urine, or wound aspirate. No such kit is commercially available in the United States, however.

VENOMS AND CLINICAL MANIFESTATIONS   Snake venoms are complex mixtures of enzymes, low-molecular-weight polypeptides, glycoproteins, and metal ions. Among the deleterious components are hemorrhagins that promote vascular leaking and cause both local and systemic bleeding. Various proteolytic enzymes cause local tissue necrosis, affect the coagulation pathway at various steps, and impair organ function. Myocardial depressant factors reduce cardiac output, and neurotoxins act either pre- or postsynaptically to inhibit peripheral nerve impulses. Most snake venoms have multisystem effects in their victims.

℞ TREATMENT

Field Management   Initial (prehospital) measures should focus on rapidly delivering the victim to definitive medical care while keeping him/her as inactive as possible to limit systemic spread of venom. Any other measures employed should at least do no further harm to the victim.

Although mechanical suction has been recommended in the field management of venomous snakebite for many years, there is now literature that demonstrates that this intervention is of little, if any, benefit. The amount of venom extracted from the depot site by devices purported to serve this purpose is minuscule. In addition, there is now preliminary evidence that extended use of such a device (i.e., for longer than 30 min) may actually be detrimental to local tissues.

Despite some evidence that venom can be localized to the bite site by lymph-occlusive constriction bands or by an encompassing wrap combined with splinting (pressure-immobilization), the clinical benefit of these techniques has never been demonstrated. There is concern that severely restricting venom to the bite site may, in fact, worsen local tissue necrosis. If the victim is >1 h from medical care, a constriction band or pressure-immobilization may be considered, but with the realization that one may be sacrificing tissue in order to reduce systemic toxicity. At no time should a totally occlusive arterial tourniquet be employed. Also to be avoided are incising or cooling the bite site, giving the victim an alcoholic beverage, or applying electric shocks. The bitten extremity should be splinted if possible and kept at approximately heart level.

For elapid or sea snake bites, the Australian pressure-immobilization technique, in which the entire bitten extremity is wrapped with an elastic or crepe bandage and then splinted, is highly effective. The bandage is applied with the same snugness used for a sprained ankle. This technique greatly restricts absorption and circulation of these venoms, which tend to cause more limited local tissue effects than viperid venoms.

Hospital Management   In the hospital, the victim should be closely monitored (vital signs, cardiac rhythm, and oxygen saturation) while a history is quickly obtained and a rapid but thorough physical examination is performed. The level of swelling in a bitten extremity should be marked and limb circumferences measured in several locations every 15 min until swelling has stabilized. Large-bore intravenous access in unaffected extremities should be established. Early hypotension is due to pooling of blood in the pulmonary and splanchnic vascular beds. Hours later, hemolysis and loss of intravascular volume into soft tissues may play important roles. Fluid resuscitation with normal saline or Ringer's lactate should be initiated for clinical shock. If the blood pressure response is inadequate after administration of crystalloid (20 to 40 mL/kg of body weight), then a trial of 5% albumin (10 to 20 mL/kg) is in order. If tissue perfusion fails to respond to volume resuscitation and antivenom infusion (see below), vasopressors (e.g., dopamine) should be administered. Invasive hemodynamic monitoring (central venous and/or pulmonary arterial pressures) can be helpful in such cases, although obtaining access is riskier if coagulopathy is present.

Blood should be drawn for laboratory evaluation as soon as possible. Blood typing and cross-matching procedures can be affected over time by circulating venom. Also important are a complete blood count (to evaluate the degree of hemorrhage or hemolysis and effects on platelet count), studies of renal and hepatic function, coagulation studies (to identify signs of consumptive coagulopathy), and testing of urine for blood or myoglobin. In severe cases or in the face of significant comorbidity, arterial blood gas studies, electrocardiography, and chest radiography are indicated.

Attempts to locate a source of appropriate antivenom should begin early in all cases of known venomous snakebite, regardless of symptoms. In the event that signs and symptoms progress rapidly, any delay in the administration of antivenom is dangerous. Antivenoms rarely offer cross-protection against snake species other than those used in their production unless the species are closely related. An example of good cross-protection is that of Australian tiger snake (*Notechis scutatus*) antivenom for sea snake bites (see below). The package insert accompanying a particular antivenom should be consulted for information regarding the spectrum of coverage. In the United States, assistance in finding antivenom can be obtained 24 hours a day from the University of Arizona Poison and Drug Information Center (telephone: 520-626-6016).

Progressive or severe local findings (e.g., soft tissue swelling, ecchymosis, petechiae) or manifestations of systemic toxicity (signs and symptoms or laboratory abnormalities) are indications for the administration of intravenous antivenom in cases of viperid venom poisoning. Victims of bites by elapid snakes, such as coral snakes, should be treated with an appropriate antivenom if the snake has been positively identified. In these cases, local findings are often minimal, the onset of systemic symptoms may be delayed for many hours, and progression may be difficult to halt once manifestations begin. The package insert for the appropriate antivenom should be consulted regarding the method of administration and the optimal dose. Dosing for viperid bites is guided by the severity of the bite (see Table 378-1).

Some manufacturers recommend a skin-testing procedure for potential allergy. Use of any heterologous serum product carries a risk of anaphylactic, anaphylactoid, and delayed-hypersensitivity reactions. Skin testing does not, however, reliably predict which patients will have an allergic reaction to antivenom. The newest available antivenom in the United States (CroFab, Table 378-2) is an ovine antivenom produced by techniques that yield purified Fab antibodies. This product reduces the risk of allergic sequelae, and the manufacturer does not recommend a skin test prior to its use. Table 378-2 compares the two antivenoms available for the treatment of pit viper bites in the United States: Antivenin (Crotalidae) Polyvalent (ACP) and CroFab.

If the risk of allergic reaction is deemed significant (as when a less pure antivenom is being used), the patient should receive pretreatment with appropriate loading doses of intravenous antihistamines (e.g., diphenhydramine, 1 mg/kg to a maximum of 100 mg; and cimetidine, 5 to 10 mg/kg to a maximum of 300 mg). Modest expansion of the patient's intravascular volume with crystalloids may also be beneficial in this regard. Such pretreatment is not necessary when a highly purified Fab antivenom, such as CroFab, is used. Epinephrine should always be immediately available, and the antivenom dose to be administered should be diluted in an appropriate volume of crystalloid. The antivenom should be started slowly, with the physician at the bedside to intervene in the event of an acute reaction. The rate of infusion can be increased gradually in the absence of allergic phenomena until the total starting dose has been administered (over a total period of 1 to 2 h). Further antivenom may be necessary if the patient's clinical condition fails to stabilize or worsens. After stabilization, additional doses of CroFab are recommended because this preparation contains smaller-molecular-weight Fab fragments and is more rapidly cleared from the body than ACP. Laboratory values should be rechecked hourly, particularly if abnormal, until stability is apparent.

TABLE 378-1   *Sample Grading Scale for Use in Viperid Venom Poisoning*

Severity	Local Findings	Systemic Findings		Laboratory Studies
Nonenvenomation (dry bite)	None or puncture wounds only	None	*and*	Normal
Mild	Puncture wounds Pain Soft tissue swelling confined to the bite site	None	*and*	Normal
Moderate	Swelling extending beyond the local bite site	Mild (e.g., nausea, vomiting, muscle fasciculations, paresthesias)	*or*	Mildly abnormal (e.g., mildly abnormal platelet count or fibrinogen, or elevated fibrin split products)
Severe	Generally severe pain and swelling (may be minimal swelling in deep intramuscular or intravenous poisoning)	More severe (respiratory distress, hypotension/shock, evidence of bleeding, etc.)	*or*	Very abnormal

The management of a life-threatening envenomation in a victim with an apparent allergy to antivenom requires significant expertise. Consultation with a poison specialist, an intensive care specialist, and/or an allergist is recommended. Often antivenom can still be administered in these situations under closely controlled conditions and with intensive premedication (e.g., with epinephrine, antihistamines, and glucocorticoids). Preferably, a less immunogenic product (e.g., one composed of Fab fragments) should be used.

Care of the bite wound should include application of a dry sterile dressing and splinting of the extremity with padding between the digits. Once the administration of an indicated antivenom has been initiated, the extremity should be elevated above heart level to relieve edema. Tetanus immunization should be updated as appropriate. Prophylactic antibiotics are unnecessary, as the incidence of secondary infection following venomous snakebite is quite low.

If swelling in the bitten extremity raises concern that subfascial muscle edema may be impeding tissue perfusion (muscle-compartment syndrome), intracompartmental pressures should be checked by any minimally invasive technique (e.g., a wick catheter). If pressures are elevated and remain so despite additional antivenom administration and elevation of the extremity, surgical consultation for possible fasciotomy should be obtained. This complication, fortunately, is rare after snakebites.

Whether or not antivenom is given, any patient with signs of venom poisoning should be observed in the hospital for at least 24 h. A patient with an apparently "dry" bite should be watched for at least 8 h before discharge, as significant toxicity occasionally develops after a delay of several hours. The onset of systemic symptoms is commonly delayed for a number of hours after bites by several of the elapids (including coral snakes) and sea snakes. Patients bitten by these reptiles should be observed in the hospital for 24 h. Any patient requiring antivenom treatment should be admitted to an intensive care setting.

Follow-up care should include referral for physical therapy when needed to return the patient to an optimal level of functioning. In addition, victims of viperid bite should be reevaluated for evidence of recurrent coagulopathy ~48 h after discharge and as needed thereafter. These patients should be warned to avoid any routine surgery for the first few weeks, as occult coagulopathy can recur up to 2 weeks after a viperid bite.

MORBIDITY AND MORTALITY The overall mortality rates for venomous snakebite are low in areas of the world with rapid access to medical care and appropriate antivenom. In the United States, for example, the mortality rate is <1% for victims who receive antivenom. Eastern and western diamondback rattlesnakes (*Crotalus adamanteus* and *C. atrox*, respectively) are responsible for most snakebite deaths in the United States. Snakes responsible for large numbers of deaths in other regions of the world include the cobras (*Naja* spp.) of Asia and Africa, the carpet and saw-scaled vipers (*Echis* spp.) of the Middle East and Africa, Russell's viper (*Daboia russelli*) of the Middle East and Asia, the large African vipers (*Bitis* spp.), and the lancehead pit vipers (*Bothrops* spp.) of Central and South America.

TABLE 378-2 *Comparison of Antivenoms Available for Treatment of Pit Viper Bites in the United States*

	Antivenin (Crotalidae) Polyvalent[a]	CroFab[b]
Available since	1954	2000
Origin	Equine	Ovine
Snakes used in manufacture	*Crotalus adamanteus* *C. atrox* *C. durissus terrificus* *Bothrops atrox*	*C. adamanteus* *C. atrox* *C. scutulatus* *Agkistrodon piscivorus*
Snakes covered	All North, Central, and South American and some Asian pit vipers	All North American pit vipers (and possibly some Latin American pit vipers)
Contains	IgG, equine albumin	Fab fragments
Skin testing recommended by manufacturer	Yes	No
Pretreatment with antihistamines recommended	Yes	No
Dosing		
Dry bite	None	None
Mild	0–5 vials	4–6 vials[c]
Moderately severe	10 vials	4–6 vials[c]
Severe	15–20 vials	6 vials
Repeat dosing	As needed	Repeat starting dose if patient fails to stabilize; after stabilization, 2 vials q6h for 3 more doses
Volume of diluent	1000 mL (reduce for children or in congestive heart failure)	250 mL
Administer over	2 h	1 h
Incidence of anaphylactic/-oid reaction	23–56% (some severe; some deaths)	14% (all relatively mild to date)
Incidence of delayed serum sickness	18–86% (higher with high doses)	16% (more recently, 3% with refinement of manufacturing process)

[a] Wyeth-Ayerst Laboratories, Philadelphia. There are indications that the manufacturer may soon discontinue production of this antivenom.
[b] Savage Laboratories, Melville, NY.
[c] Use of CroFab for a mild to moderate bite should be based on signs of progression of toxicity.

The incidence of morbidity—defined as permanent functional loss in a bitten extremity—is difficult to estimate but is clearly substantial. Such loss may be due to muscle, nerve, or vascular injury or to scar contracture. In the United States, such loss tends to be much more common and severe after rattlesnake bites than after bites by copperheads or water moccasins.

LIZARD BITES

Bites from the two species of venomous lizards (the gila monster, *Heloderma suspectum*, of the southwestern United States and the Mexican beaded lizard, *H. horridum*) are infrequent and usually follow attempts to capture or handle these creatures. Local findings include soft tissue trauma, significant pain, surrounding local edema, and occasionally local cyanosis and ecchymosis. Broken teeth may be embedded in the wounds. The venoms of these lizards are very similar and contain L-amino acid oxidase, phospholipases, hyaluronidase, and kallikreins. Systemic effects may include hypotension, weakness, dizziness, and diaphoresis.

Prehospital care measures for these bites should follow the guidelines listed above for viperid bites. If the biting lizard is still attached to the victim, its jaws may need to be manually pried apart for removal.

The sparseness of data on the pathophysiologic effects of helodermatid venom precludes specific recommendations regarding laboratory evaluation, but routine studies (complete blood count, coagulation studies, electrolyte analysis, blood typing and crossmatching, urinalysis, and electrocardiography) are prudent in anything other than a trivial bite. Wounds should be cleansed thoroughly and irrigated when possible. Tetanus immunization should be updated as indicated. Soft tissue radiography of the bite site and sterile probing under local anesthesia may identify retained teeth. The extremity should be splinted and elevated, but antibiotic treatment is not usually required. Systemic care is supportive (e.g., crystalloid infusion for hypotension). No antivenom exists. Pain due to local venom effects and mechanical trauma can be treated with opiates and regional nerve blocks. The mortality rate is extremely low.

MARINE ENVENOMATIONS

Management of venom poisoning by marine creatures is similar to that of venomous snakebite in that much of the treatment administered is supportive in nature. Prompt and appropriate field therapy may contribute to a successful clinical outcome. A few specific marine antivenoms can be used when appropriate.

INVERTEBRATES   *Hydroids, fire coral, jellyfish, Portuguese man-of-war*, and *sea anemones* possess specialized stinging cells called *cnidocytes*, in which reside intracytoplasmic stinging organelles called *cnidae* (including nematocysts). The venoms from these organisms are mixtures of proteins, carbohydrates, and other components. The clinical syndrome following envenomation by any of these species is similar but of variable severity. Victims usually report immediate prickling or burning, pruritus, paresthesias, and painful throbbing with radiation. The skin becomes reddened, darkened, edematous, and/or blistered. A legion of neurologic, cardiovascular, respiratory, rheumatologic, gastrointestinal, renal, and ocular symptoms have been described. Victims in unstable condition with hypotension or respiratory distress should be treated supportively. Anaphylaxis sometimes develops. During stabilization, the skin should be immediately decontaminated with a generous application of vinegar (5% acetic acid), which inactivates nematocysts. Rubbing alcohol (40 to 70% isopropyl alcohol), baking soda (sodium bicarbonate), papain (unseasoned meat tenderizer), fresh lemon or lime juice, or household ammonia may be effective, depending on the species of stinging creature. For the sting of the venomous *box-jellyfish* (*Chironex fleckeri*; Fig. 378-1), vinegar should be used. Perfume, aftershave lotion, and high-proof ethanol are less efficacious and may be detrimental. Shaving the skin helps remove remaining nematocysts. Freshwater irrigation and rubbing lead to further stinging by adherent nematocysts and should be avoided. After decontamination, application of anesthetic ointments (lidocaine, benzocaine), antihistamine creams (diphenhydramine), or steroid lotions (hydrocortisone) may be helpful. Persistent pain after decontamination may be treated with morphine or meperidine. Muscle spasms may respond to 10% calcium gluconate (5 to 10 mL) or diazepam (2 to 5 mg, titrated upwards as necessary) given intravenously. An ovine-derived antivenom is available from Commonwealth Serum Laboratories (see section on antivenom sources, below) for stings from the box-jellyfish found in Australian and Indo-Pacific waters. At the time of this writing, this antivenom has not yet been used to treat envenomation by the box-shaped jellyfish, which may be of the genus *Chiropsalmus*, recently found in Florida waters. Safe Sea, a "jellyfish-safe sun block" (www.nidaria.com) that is applied to the skin before entering the water, inactivates the recognition and discharge mechanisms of nematocysts and has been tested successfully against a number of marine stingers.

FIGURE 378-1   Skin lesions caused by *Chironex fleckeri* sting. (*Courtesy of Dr. V. Pranava Murthy.*)

Touching a *sea sponge* may result in dermatitis. If contact occurs, the skin should be gently dried and adhesive tape used to remove embedded spicules. Vinegar should be applied immediately and then for 10 to 30 min three or four times a day. Rubbing alcohol may be used if vinegar is unavailable. After spicule removal and skin decontamination, a steroid or antihistamine cream may be applied to the skin. Severe vesiculation should be treated with a 2-week course of systemic glucocorticoids.

Annelid worms (bristleworms) possess rows of soft, cactus-like spines capable of inflicting painful stings. Contact results in symptoms similar to those of nematocyst envenomation. Without treatment, pain usually subsides over several hours, but inflammation may persist for up to a week. Victims should resist the urge to scratch, since scratching may fracture retrievable spines. Visible bristles should be removed with forceps and adhesive tape or a commercial facial peel; alternatively, a thin layer of rubber cement can be used to entrap the spines. Use of vinegar, rubbing alcohol, or dilute ammonia or a brief application of unseasoned meat tenderizer (papain) may provide additional relief. Local inflammation should be treated with topical or systemic glucocorticoids.

Sea urchins possess either hollow, venom-filled, calcified spines or triple-jawed, globiferous pedicellariae with venom glands. Their venom contains several toxic components, including steroid glycosides, hemolysins, proteases, serotonin, and cholinergic substances. Contact with either venom apparatus produces immediate and intensely painful stings. The affected part should be immersed immediately in hot water (see below). Accessible embedded spines should be removed but may break off and remain lodged in the victim. Residual dye from the surface of a spine remaining after the spine's removal may mimic a retained spine but is otherwise of no consequence. Soft tissue radiography or magnetic resonance imaging (MRI) can confirm the presence of retained spines; this finding may warrant referral for attempted surgical removal if the spines are located near vital structures (e.g., joints, neurovascular bundles). Retained spines may cause the formation of granulomas that are amenable to excision or to intralesional injection with triamcinolone hexacetonide (5 mg/mL).

Cone shells are predatory, carnivorous mollusks. The most dangerous of these creatures are found in the Indian and Pacific oceans. A neurotoxic venom comprising multiple peptides is delivered through harpoon-like darts propelled from an extensible proboscis. Clinically, the sting is like that of a bee. The victim may report wound, perioral, and generalized paresthesias. Bulbar dysfunction and systemic muscular paralysis indicate severe envenomation. The sting of the geographer cone (*Conus geographus*) can cause cerebral edema, coma, and death due to respiratory or cardiac failure. Immediately after envenomation, a circumferential pressure-immobilization dressing 15 cm wide should be applied over a gauze pad measuring approximately $7 \times 7 \times 2$ cm that has been placed directly over the sting. The dressing should be applied at venous-lymphatic pressure with the preservation of distal arterial pulses. Once the victim has been transported to the nearest medical facility, the bandage can be released. Provision should be made for cardiovascular and respiratory support.

Serious envenomations and deaths have followed bites of the *Australian blue-ringed octopuses* (*Octopus maculosus* and *O. lunulata*). Although these animals rarely exceed 20 cm in length, their venom contains a potent neurotoxin (maculotoxin) that inhibits peripheral nerve transmission by blocking sodium conductance. Oral and facial numbness develop within several minutes of a serious envenomation and rapidly progress to total flaccid paralysis, including failure of respiratory muscles. If respirations are assisted, the victim may remain awake although completely paralyzed. Since there is no antidote, treatment is supportive. Immediately after envenomation, attempts should be made to limit the dispersion of venom by application of a pressure-immobilization or venous-lymphatic pressure dressing. Hot-water immersion and cryotherapy are ineffective. Artificial respiration should be provided. Even with serious envenomations, significant recovery often takes place within 4 to 10 h. Sequelae are uncommon unless related to hypoxia.

VERTEBRATES A number of marine vertebrates, including stingrays, scorpionfish, catfish, surgeonfish, and weeverfish, can envenomate humans. The management of most of these stings is similar.

A *stingray* injury is both an envenomation and a traumatic wound. The venom, which contains serotonin, 5'-nucleotidase, and phosphodiesterase, causes immediate and intense pain that may last up to 48 h. The wound often becomes ischemic in appearance and heals poorly, with adjacent soft tissue swelling and prolonged disability. Systemic effects include weakness, diaphoresis, nausea, vomiting, diarrhea, dysrhythmias, syncope, hypotension, muscle cramps, fasciculations, paralysis, and (in rare cases) death.

The designation *scorpionfish* encompasses members of the family Scorpaenidae and includes not only scorpionfish but also lionfish and stonefish. A complex venom with neuromuscular toxicity is delivered through 12 or 13 dorsal, 2 pelvic, and 3 anal spines. Pectoral spines do not contain venom. The severity of envenomation depends on the species of fish, the number of stings, and the amount of venom released. In general, the sting of a stonefish is regarded as the most serious (severe to life-threatening); that of the scorpionfish is of intermediate seriousness, and that of the lionfish is the least serious. Like that of a stingray, the sting of a scorpionfish is immediately and intensely painful. Pain from a stonefish envenomation may last for days. The systemic manifestations of scorpionfish stings are similar to those of stingray envenomations but may be more pronounced, particularly in the case of a stonefish sting. The rare deaths following stonefish envenomation usually occur within 6 to 8 h.

Two species of marine *catfish*—*Plotosus lineatus* (the oriental catfish) and *Galeichthys felis* (the common sea catfish)—as well as several species of freshwater catfish are capable of stinging humans. Venom is delivered through a single dorsal spine and two pectoral spines. Clinically, a catfish sting is comparable to that of a stingray, although marine catfish envenomations are generally more severe than those of their freshwater counterparts. *Surgeonfish* (doctorfish, tang), *weeverfish*, *ratfish*, and *horned venomous sharks* have also been implicated in human envenomations.

℞ TREATMENT

The stings of all these marine vertebrates are treated in a similar fashion. Except for stonefish and serious scorpionfish envenomations (see below), no antivenom is available. The affected part should be immersed immediately in nonscalding hot water (113°F/45°C) for 30 to 90 min or until there is significant relief of pain. This measure may inactivate heat-labile components of the venoms. Recurrent pain may respond to repeated hot-water treatment. Cryotherapy is contraindicated. Opiates will help alleviate the pain, as will local wound infiltration or regional nerve block with 1% lidocaine, 0.5% bupivacaine, and sodium bicarbonate mixed in a 5:5:1 ratio. After soaking and anesthetic administration, the wound must be explored and debrided. Radiography (in particular, MRI) may be helpful in the identification and location of foreign bodies. After exploration and debridement, the wound should be vigorously irrigated with warm sterile water, saline, or 1% povidone-iodine in solution. Bleeding can usually be controlled by sustained local pressure for 10 to 15 min. In general, wounds should be left open to heal by secondary intention or be treated by delayed primary closure. Tetanus immunization should be updated. Antibiotic treatment should be considered for serious wounds and for envenomation in immunocompromised hosts. The initial antibiotics should cover *Staphylococcus* and *Streptococcus* spp. If the victim is immunocompromised or an infection develops, antibiotic coverage should be broadened to include *Vibrio* spp.

APPROACH TO THE PATIENT

It is not uncommon for a physician to encounter a patient who has been envenomated by a marine creature that cannot be positively identified at the scene of the envenomation. Therefore, it is useful to be familiar with the local marine fauna and to recognize patterns of injury.

A large puncture wound or jagged laceration, particularly on the lower extremity, that is more painful than one would expect from the size and configuration of the wound is likely a stingray envenomation. Smaller punctures, as described above, represent the activity of a sea urchin or starfish. Stony corals cause rough abrasions and, in rare instances, lacerations or puncture wounds.

Coelenterate (marine invertebrate) stings sometimes create diagnostic skin patterns. A diffuse urticarial rash on exposed skin is often indicative of exposure to fragmented hydroids or larval anemones. A linear, whiplike print pattern appears where a jellyfish tentacle has contacted the skin. In the case of the dreaded box-jellyfish (Fig. 378-1), a cross-hatched, sometimes frosted appearance followed by the development of a dark purple coloration within a few hours of the sting heralds skin necrosis. An encounter with fire coral causes immediate pain and a swollen red skin irritation in the pattern of contact, similar to but more severe than the imprint left by exposure to an intact feather hydroid. Seabather's eruption, caused by thimble jellyfishes and larval anemones, may produce a diffuse rash that consists of clusters of erythematous macules or raised papules, accompanied by intense itching (Fig. 378-2). Toxic sponges (exposure to which usually occurs during handling) create a burning and painful red rash on exposed skin, which may blister and later desquamate. Virtually all marine stingers invoke the sequelae of inflammation, so that local erythema, swelling, and adenopathy are fairly nonspecific.

SOURCES OF ANTIVENOMS AND OTHER ASSISTANCE An antivenom for stonefish (and severe scorpionfish) envenomation, made in Australia by the Commonwealth Serum Laboratories (CSL; 45 Poplar Road, Parkville, Victoria, Australia 3052; www.csl.com.au; 61-3-389-1911; fax: 61-3-389-1434), is available in the United States through the pharmacies of Sharp Cabrillo Hospital Emergency Department, San Diego, CA, at (619) 221-3429, and Community Hospital of Monterey Peninsula (CHOMP) Emergency Department, Monterey, CA, at (408) 625-4900.

Polyvalent sea snake antivenom is available from CSL or CHOMP. If sea snake antivenom is unavailable, tiger snake (*N. scutatus*) antivenom should be used.

Divers Alert Network, a nonprofit organization designed to assist in the care of injured divers, may also help with the treatment of marine

FIGURE 378-2 Erythematous, papular rash typical of seabather's eruption caused by thimble jellyfish and larval anemones. (*Courtesy of Dr. Paul Auerbach.*)

injuries. The network can be reached on the Internet at www.diversalertnetwork.org or by telephone 24 hours a day at (919) 684-8111.

MARINE POISONINGS

CIGUATERA Ciguatera poisoning is the most common nonbacterial food poisoning associated with fish in the United States; most cases occur in Florida and Hawaii. The poisoning involves almost exclusively tropical and semitropical marine coral reef fish. Of reported cases, 75% (except in Hawaii) involve the barracuda, snapper, jack, or grouper. The ciguatera syndrome is associated with at least five polyether sodium channel activator toxins that originate in photosynthetic dinoflagellates (such as *Gambierdiscus toxicus*) and accumulate in the food chain. These toxins are unaffected by freeze-drying, heat, cold, and gastric acid. None of the toxins affects the odor, color, or taste of fish.

The onset of symptoms may come within 15 to 30 min of ingestion and typically takes place within 2 to 6 h. Symptoms then increase in severity over the ensuing 4 to 6 h. Most victims develop symptoms within 12 h of ingestion, and virtually all are afflicted within 24 h. The more than 150 symptoms reported include abdominal pain, nausea, vomiting, diarrhea, chills, paresthesias, pruritus, tongue and throat numbness or burning, sensation of "carbonation" during swallowing, odontalgia or dental dysesthesias, dysphagia, dysuria, dyspnea, weakness, fatigue, tremor, fasciculations, athetosis, meningismus, aphonia, ataxia, vertigo, pain and weakness in the lower extremities, visual blurring, transient blindness, hyporeflexia, seizures, nasal congestion and dryness, conjunctivitis, maculopapular rash, skin vesiculations, dermatographism, sialorrhea, diaphoresis, headache, arthralgias, myalgias, insomnia, bradycardia, hypotension, central respiratory failure, and coma. Death is rare.

Diarrhea, vomiting, and abdominal pain usually develop 3 to 6 h after ingestion of a ciguatoxic fish. Symptoms may persist for 48 h and then generally resolve (even without treatment). A pathognomonic symptom is the reversal of hot and cold tactile perception, which develops in some persons after 3 to 5 days and may last for months. Tachycardia and hypertension have been described, in some cases after potentially severe transient bradycardia and hypotension. More severe reactions tend to occur in persons previously stricken with the disease. Persons who have ingested parrotfish (scaritoxin) may suffer from classic ciguatera poisoning as well as a "second-phase" syndrome (after 5 to 10 days' delay) of disequilibrium with locomotor ataxia, dysmetria, and resting or kinetic tremor. This affliction may persist for 2 to 6 weeks.

The differential diagnosis of ciguatera includes paralytic shellfish poisoning, eosinophilic meningitis, type E botulism, organophosphate insecticide poisoning, tetrodotoxin poisoning, and psychogenic hyperventilation. At present, the diagnosis of ciguatera poisoning is made on clinical grounds because no routinely used laboratory test detects ciguatoxin in human blood. A ciguatoxin enzyme immunoassay or radioimmunoassay may be used to test small portions of the suspected fish, but even these tests may not detect the very small amount of toxin (0.1 ppb) necessary to render fish flesh toxic.

℞ TREATMENT

Therapy is supportive and based on symptoms. Although not of proven efficacy, a slurry of activated charcoal (100 g) in sorbitol may be of limited value if given within 3 h after ingestion. Nausea and vomiting may be controlled with an antiemetic, such as prochlorperazine (2.5 to 5 mg intravenously). Hypotension may require the administration of intravenous crystalloid and, in rare cases, a pressor drug. Bradyarrhythmias that lead to cardiac insufficiency and hypotension generally respond well to atropine (0.5 mg intravenously, up to 2 mg). Cool showers or the administration of hydroxyzine (25 mg orally every 6 to 8 h) may relieve pruritus. Amitriptyline (25 mg orally twice a day)

reportedly ameliorates pruritus and dysesthesias. In three cases unresponsive to amitriptyline, tocainide appeared to be efficacious. Nifedipine has been used to treat headache. Intravenous infusion of mannitol may be beneficial in moderate or severe cases, particularly for the relief of distressing neurologic or cardiovascular symptoms, although the efficacy of this therapy has recently been challenged. The infusion is rendered initially as 1 g/kg per day over 45 to 60 min during the acute phase (days 1 to 5). If symptoms improve, a second dose may be given within 3 to 4 h and repeated on the following day. The mechanism of the benefit against ciguatera intoxication is perhaps hyperosmotic water-drawing action, which reverses ciguatoxin-induced Schwann cell edema. Mannitol may also act in some fashion as a "hydroxyl scavenger."

During recovery from ciguatera poisoning, the victim should exclude the following from the diet: fish (fresh or preserved), fish sauces, shellfish, shellfish sauces, alcoholic beverages, and nuts and nut oils. Consumption of fish in ciguatera-endemic regions should be avoided. All oversized fish of any predacious reef species should be suspected of harboring ciguatoxin. Neither moray eels nor the viscera of tropical marine fish should ever be eaten.

PARALYTIC SHELLFISH POISONING Paralytic shellfish poisoning is induced by the ingestion of any of a variety of feral or aquacultured filter-feeding organisms, including clams, oysters, scallops, mussels, chitons, limpets, starfish, and sand crabs. The origin of their toxicity is the chemical toxin they accumulate and concentrate by feeding on various planktonic dinoflagellates and protozoan organisms. The unicellular phytoplanktonic organisms form the foundation of the food chain, and in warm summer months these organisms "bloom" in nutrient-rich coastal temperate and semitropical waters. A number of dinoflagellates produce a variety of toxins. These planktonic species can release massive amounts of toxic metabolites into the water and cause enormous mortality in bird and marine populations. The paralytic shellfish toxins are water-soluble as well as heat- and acid-stable; they cannot be destroyed by ordinary cooking. The best-characterized and most frequently identified paralytic shellfish toxin is saxitoxin, which takes its name from the Alaska butter clam *Saxidomus giganteus*. A toxin concentration of >75 µg/100 g of foodstuff is considered hazardous to humans. In the 1972 New England "red tide," the concentration of saxitoxin in blue mussels exceeded 9000 µg/100 g of foodstuff. Saxitoxin appears to block sodium conductance, inhibiting neuromuscular transmission at the axonal and muscle membrane levels.

Within minutes to a few hours after ingestion of contaminated shellfish, there is the onset of intraoral and perioral paresthesias, notably of the lips, tongue, and gums, that progress rapidly to involve the neck and distal extremities. The tingling or burning sensation later changes to numbness. Other symptoms rapidly develop and include lightheadedness, disequilibrium, incoordination, weakness, hyperreflexia, incoherence, dysarthria, sialorrhea, dysphagia, thirst, diarrhea, abdominal pain, nausea, vomiting, nystagmus, dysmetria, headache, diaphoresis, loss of vision, chest pain, and tachycardia. Flaccid paralysis and respiratory insufficiency may follow 2 to 12 h after ingestion. In the absence of hypoxia, the victim often remains alert but paralyzed.

℞ TREATMENT

Treatment is supportive and based on symptoms. Since airway loss may be rapid, induced emesis should not be attempted. If the victim comes to medical attention within the first few hours after poison ingestion, the stomach should be emptied by gastric lavage and then irrigated with 2 L (in 200-mL aliquots) of a solution of 2% sodium bicarbonate; this intervention has not been proved to be of benefit but is based on the notion that gastric acidity may enhance the potency of saxitoxin. The administration of activated charcoal (50 to 100 g) and a cathartic (sorbitol, 20 to 50 g) makes empirical sense since these shellfish toxins are believed to bind well to charcoal. Some authors advise against administration of magnesium-based solutions, such as certain cathartics, cautioning that hypermagnesemia may contribute to suppression of nerve conduction.

The most serious problem is respiratory paralysis. The victim should be closely observed in a hospital for at least 24 h for respiratory distress. With prompt recognition of ventilatory failure, endotracheal intubation and assisted ventilation prevent anoxic myocardial and brain injury.

TETRODOTOXIN FISH POISONING Tetrodotoxin is a neurotoxin that has been isolated from four different animal phyla, including puffer fish and the blue-ringed octopus. Humans ingest tetrodotoxin by eating puffer fish (toadfish, globefish, swellfish, porcupine fish) in the form of the delicacy fugu. Ingestion is intended to induce pleasurable sensations of oral tingling. The toxin is found throughout the fish, with high concentrations in the liver, viscera, gonads, and skin. It is stable to extremes of temperature. Tetrodotoxin interferes with central and peripheral neuromuscular transmission in humans via blocking effects on axonal transmission mediated by sodium conductance. In addition, the toxin causes peripheral vasodilation and hypotension, exerting these effects in a dose-dependent fashion.

Symptoms typically develop within 30 min of ingestion but may be delayed by up to 4 h. Death has occurred within 17 min of ingestion. Paresthesias of the lips and tongue are followed by sialorrhea, sweating, headache, weakness, lethargy, ataxia, incoordination, tremor, paralysis, cyanosis, aphonia, dysphagia, seizures, dyspnea, bronchorrhea, bronchospasm, respiratory failure, coma, and hypotension. Gastroenteric symptoms are often severe and include nausea, vomiting, diarrhea, and abdominal pain. Cardiac arrhythmias may precede complete respiratory failure and cardiovascular collapse.

℞ TREATMENT

Therapy is supportive and based on symptoms, with aggressive early airway management. Alpha adrenergic agonists are recommended in addition to intravenous fluids to combat hypotension. Anticholinesterase agents have been used with mixed success.

DOMOIC ACID INTOXICATION In late 1987 in eastern Canada, an outbreak of gastrointestinal and neurologic symptoms (amnestic shellfish poisoning) was documented in persons who had consumed mussels found to be contaminated with domoic acid. In 1991, an epidemic of domoic acid poisoning in the state of Washington was attributed to the consumption of razor clams. A heat-stable neuroexcitatory amino acid whose biochemical analogs are kainic acid and glutamic acid, domoic acid binds to the kainate type of glutamate receptor with three times the affinity of kainic acid and is 20 times as powerful a toxin. Shellfish can be tested for domoic acid by mouse bioassay and high-performance liquid chromatography. The regulatory limit for domoic acid in shellfish is 20 parts per million.

The abnormalities noted within 24 h of ingesting contaminated mussels (*Mytilus edulis*) include arousal, confusion, disorientation, and memory loss. The median time of onset is 5.5 h. Other prominent symptoms include severe headache, nausea, vomiting, diarrhea, abdominal cramps, hiccoughs, arrhythmias, hypotension, seizures, ophthalmoplegia, hemiparesis, mutism, grimacing, agitation, emotional lability, coma, copious bronchial secretions, and pulmonary edema. Histologic study of brain tissue taken at autopsy has shown neuronal necrosis or cell loss and astrocytosis, most prominently in the hippocampus and the amygdaloid nucleus—findings similar to those in animals poisoned with kainic acid. Several months after the primary intoxication, victims still display chronic residual memory deficits and motor neuronopathy or axonopathy. Nonneurologic illness does not persist.

℞ TREATMENT

Therapy is supportive and based on symptoms. Since kainic acid neuropathology seems to be nearly entirely seizure mediated, an emphasis

should be placed on anticonvulsive therapy, for which diazepam appears to be as effective as any other drug.

SCOMBROID Scombroid (mackerel-like) fish include the albacore, bluefin, and yellowfin tuna; mackerel; saury; needlefish; wahoo; skipjack; and bonito. Nonscombroid fish that produce scombroid poisoning include the dolphinfish (Hawaiian mahimahi, *Coryphaena hippurus*), kahawai, sardine, black marlin, pilchard, anchovy, herring, amberjack, and Australian ocean salmon. In the northeastern and mid-Atlantic United States, bluefish (*Pomatomus saltatrix*) has been linked to scombroid poisoning. Because greater numbers of nonscombroid fish are being recognized as scombrotoxic, the syndrome may more appropriately be called *pseudoallergic fish poisoning*.

Under conditions of inadequate preservation or refrigeration, the musculature of these dark- or red-fleshed fish undergoes bacterial decomposition, which includes the decarboxylation of the amino acid L-histidine to histamine, histamine phosphate, and histamine hydrochloride. Histamine levels of 20 to 50 mg/100 g are noted in toxic fish, with levels in excess of 400 mg/100 g on occasion. The toxin is heat stable and is not destroyed by domestic or commercial cooking. Affected fish typically have a sharply metallic or peppery taste; however, they may be normal in appearance, color, and flavor. Not all persons who eat a contaminated fish necessarily become ill, perhaps because of uneven distribution of decay within the fish.

Symptoms develop within 15 to 90 min of ingestion and include flushing (sharply demarcated; exacerbated by ultraviolet exposure; particularly pronounced on the face, neck, and upper trunk), a sensation of warmth without elevated core temperature, conjunctival hyperemia, pruritus, urticaria, angioneurotic edema, bronchospasm, nausea, vomiting, diarrhea, epigastric pain, abdominal cramps, dysphagia, headache, thirst, pharyngitis, burning of the gingiva, palpitations, tachycardia, dizziness, and hypotension. Without treatment, the symptoms generally resolve within 8 to 12 h. The reaction may be more severe in a person who is concurrently ingesting isoniazid because of blockade of gastrointestinal tract histaminase.

℞ TREATMENT

Therapy is directed at reversing the histamine effect with antihistamines, either H-1 or H-2. If bronchospasm is severe, an inhaled bronchodilator—or in rare, extremely severe circumstances, injected epinephrine—may be used. Glucocorticoids are of no proven benefit. Protracted nausea and vomiting, which may empty the stomach of toxin, may be controlled with a specific antiemetic, such as prochlorperazine. The persistent headache of scombroid poisoning may respond to cimetidine or a similar antihistamine if standard analgesics are not effective.

Pfiesteria In the summer of 1997, reports of adverse reactions after casual exposure to Maryland waters infested with the fish-killing dinoflagellate *Pfiesteria piscicida* prompted the Centers for Disease Control and Prevention (CDC) to undertake multistate surveillance and to establish a case definition. The route of exposure is either direct contact with the water or inhalation of aerosols. As defined by the CDC, the human disease syndrome associated with *Pfiesteria* is characterized by either of two groups of signs and symptoms: (1) memory loss, forgetfulness, or confusion *or* acute skin burning on direct contact with infested water; or (2) at least three of the following: headache, rash (flat red sores), eye irritation, upper respiratory irritation, muscle cramps, and gastrointestinal symptoms. The skin lesions—red edematous papules on the extremities and trunk—resolve within a few days to a week after exposure. Since the initial reports, cases have followed either casual exposure to infested water or laboratory work with *Pfiesteria* (which is currently conducted in biohazard III facilities).

Research on *Pfiesteria* has been complicated by a variety of factors, including the lack of a test for detection of its toxins, which have yet to be purified, and the organism's complex life cycle, which includes at least two dozen stages. In nature, the proximity of a school of fish elicits *Pfiesteria's* transformation into a flagellated zoospore that releases at least two toxins: a water-soluble, neuroactive toxin that kills fish within minutes and a fat-soluble toxin that causes epidermal delamination. Polluted environments appear to favor *Pfiesteria*.

Diagnosis is difficult because the specific toxins have not yet been identified and there is no biomarker for exposure. Detection systems using polymerase chain reaction and fluorescent markers are being developed for rapid identification of the dinoflagellate. Neurocognitive deficits appear to improve significantly within 3 to 6 months after cessation of exposure. No deaths have been reported, and most victims improve without treatment. For the treatment of persistent *Pfiesteria*-associated syndromes, one teaspoon of milk of magnesia each day followed by one scoop of cholestyramine in 8 ounces of water 4 times a day for 2 weeks has been used successfully as an empiric remedy in a limited number of cases.

FURTHER READING

AUERBACH PS (ed): *Wilderness Medicine*, 4th ed. St. Louis, Mosby, 2001

BUSH SP, HARDY DL: Immediate removal of Extractor is recommended. Ann Emerg Med 38:607, 2001

——— et al: Effects of a negative pressure venom extraction device (Extractor) on local tissue injury after artificial rattlesnake envenomation in a porcine model. Acad Emerg Med 7:495, 2000

DART RC et al: A randomized multicenter trial of Crotalinae polyvalent immune Fab (ovine) antivenom for the treatment for crotaline snakebite in the United States. Arch Intern Med 161:2030, 2001

GOLD BS et al: Bites of venomous snakes. N Engl J Med 347:347, 2002

MEIER J, WHITE J (eds): *Handbook of Clinical Toxicology of Animal Venoms and Poisons.* Boca Raton, FL, CRC Press, 1996, pp 89–176

MEYER WP et al: First clinical experiences with a new ovine Fab *Echis ocellatus* snake bite antivenom in Nigeria: Randomized comparative trial with Institute Pasteur Serum (Ipser) Africa antivenom. Am J Trop Med Hyg 56: 291, 1997

PEARN J: Neurology of ciguatera. J Neurol Neurosurg Psychiatry 70:4, 2001

379 ECTOPARASITE INFESTATIONS AND ARTHROPOD BITES AND STINGS
James H. Maguire, Richard J. Pollack, Andrew Spielman

Ectoparasites are arthropods or helminths that infest the skin of other animals, from which they derive sustenance. They may penetrate beneath the surface of the host or attach superficially by their mouthparts. These organisms damage their hosts by inflicting direct injury, by eliciting a hypersensitivity reaction, or by inoculating toxins or pathogens. The main medically important ectoparasites are arachnids (including mites and ticks), insects (including lice, fleas, and flies), pentastomes (tongue worms), and leeches. Arthropods may also harm humans through brief encounters in which they take a blood meal or attempt to defend themselves by biting, stinging, or exuding venoms. Various arachnids (spiders, scorpions), insects (including bees, hornets, wasps, ants, flies, bugs, caterpillars, and beetles), millipedes, and centipedes produce ill effects in this manner, as do certain ectoparasites of animals, including ticks, biting mites, and fleas (discussed in this chapter as biting arthropods). More people in the United States die each year as a consequence of arthropod stings than from the bites of poisonous snakes.

ECTOPARASITE INFESTATIONS

SCABIES The human itch mite, *Sarcoptes scabiei*, which infests some 300 million persons each year, is one of the most common causes of itching dermatoses throughout the world. Gravid female mites, measuring 0.3 to 0.4 mm in length, burrow superficially beneath the stratum corneum for a month, depositing two or three eggs a day. Nymphs that hatch from these eggs mature in ~2 weeks through a series of molts and then emerge as adults to the surface of the skin, where they mate and subsequently reinvade the skin of the same or another host. Transfer of newly fertilized female mites from person to person occurs by intimate contact with an infested person and is facilitated by crowding, uncleanliness, and contact with multiple sexual partners. Medical practitioners are at particular risk of infestation. Transmission via sharing of contaminated bedding or clothing is infrequent because these mites die within a day or so in the absence of host contact, depending upon ambient conditions. In the United States, scabies may account for 2 to 5% of visits to dermatologists; involved particularly often are children, immigrants from developing countries, and close household contacts. Outbreaks occur in nursing homes, mental institutions, and hospitals.

The itching and rash associated with scabies derive from a sensitization reaction directed against the excreta that the mite deposits in its burrow (Fig. 379-1). For this reason, an initial infestation remains asymptomatic for 4 to 6 weeks, and a reinfestation produces a hyper-

sensitivity reaction without delay. Scratching generally destroys the burrowing mite, but symptoms remain even in its absence. Burrows become surrounded by infiltrates of eosinophils, lymphocytes, and histiocytes, and a generalized hypersensitivity rash later develops in remote sites. By destroying these pathogens, immunity and associated scratching limit most infestations to <15 mites per person. Hyperinfestation with thousands of mites, a condition known as *crusted scabies* or *Norwegian scabies*, may result from glucocorticoid use, immunodeficiency diseases (including AIDS and infection with human T-lymphotropic virus type I), and neurologic and psychiatric illnesses that interfere with itching and scratching.

Patients with scabies report intense itching that worsens at night and after a hot shower. Typical burrows may be difficult to find because they are few in number and may be obscured by excoriations. Burrows appear as dark wavy lines in the epidermis, measure 3 to 15 mm, and end in a small pearly bleb that contains the female mite. Such lesions generally develop on the volar wrists, between the fingers, on the elbows, and on the penis. Small papules and vesicles, often accompanied by eczematous plaques, pustules, or nodules, are symmetrically distributed in these sites and in skin folds under the breasts and around the navel, axillae, belt line, buttocks, upper thighs, and scro-

FIGURE 379-1 Scabies showing typical erythematous papules and few linear burrows.

tum. Except in infants, the face, scalp, neck, palms, and soles are spared. Burrows and other typical lesions may be sparse in persons who wash frequently, and topical glucocorticoid treatment and bacterial superinfection may alter the appearance of the rash. Atypical presentations of scabies include bullous lesions, which resemble those of bullous pemphigoid, and vesicular lesions, which resemble those of dermatitis herpetiformis. Superinfection with nephritogenic strains of streptococci has led to acute glomerulonephritis. Crusted scabies resembles psoriasis in its typical widespread erythema, thick keratotic crusts, scaling, and dystrophic nails. Characteristic burrows are not seen in crusted scabies, and patients usually do not itch, although their infestations are highly contagious and have been responsible for outbreaks of classic scabies in hospitals. Bacteremia occurs frequently in AIDS patients with crusted scabies and prominent fissures. Persons with massive infestations occasionally present with diffuse pruritus and generalized papules or with minimal or no cutaneous signs.

A diagnosis of scabies should be considered in patients with pruritus and symmetric polymorphic skin lesions in characteristic locations, particularly if there is a history of household contact with a case. Burrows should be sought and unroofed with a sterile needle or scalpel blade, and the scrapings should be examined microscopically for the mite, its eggs, and its fecal pellets. A drop of mineral oil facilitates removal of the sample. Biopsies or scrapings of papulovesicular lesions may also be diagnostic. In the absence of identifiable mites or mite products, the diagnosis is based on clinical presentation and history. Diverse kinds of dermatitis due to other causes are frequently misdiagnosed as scabies. The possibility of other sexually transmitted diseases should be excluded in adults with scabies.

℞ TREATMENT

For the treatment of scabies, 5% permethrin cream is less toxic than the once commonly used 1% lindane preparations and is effective against lindane-tolerant infestations. Both scabicides are applied thinly but thoroughly behind the ears and from the neck down after bathing and are removed 8 h later with soap and water. Lindane is absorbed through the skin, and its overuse has led to seizures and aplastic anemia. It should not be applied to pregnant women or infants. Alternatives include topical crotamiton cream, benzyl benzoate, and sulfur ointments. Successful treatment of crusted scabies requires the application first of a keratolytic agent such as 6% salicylic acid (to improve the penetration of scabicides) and then of scabicides to the scalp, face, and ears (with care to avoid the eyes). Repeated treatments or the sequential use of several agents may be necessary. A single oral dose of ivermectin (200 μg/kg) effectively treats scabies in otherwise-healthy persons. Patients with crusted scabies may require two or more doses of ivermectin. Although ivermectin may become the agent of choice for treating crusted scabies, it has not yet received approval by the U.S. Food and Drug Administration (FDA) for any form of scabies. Its use should be reserved for persons who fail to respond to topical scabicides, the elderly, persons with generalized eczema, and other persons who may not tolerate topical therapy.

Although effectively treated scabies infestations become noninfectious within a day, itching and rash due to hypersensitivity frequently persist for weeks or months. Unnecessary re-treatment of the affected patients may provoke contact dermatitis. Antihistamines, salicylates, and calamine lotion relieve itching during treatment, and topical glucocorticoids are useful for the pruritus that lingers after effective treatment. An oral antibiotic may be necessary for bacterial superinfections that fail to resolve with antiscabietic therapy. Relapses of scabies may be due to infestations of the scalp when topical therapy is applied only from the neck down. To prevent reinfestations, bedding and clothing should be washed in hot water and dried in a heated dryer, and close contacts, even if asymptomatic, should be treated simultaneously.

OTHER MITE INFESTATIONS Demodectic mites infest the facial skin of virtually all people. The term *follicle mite* is applied both to *Demodex folliculorum*, which resides in hair follicles, and to *D. brevis*, which resides in sebaceous glands. These wormlike mites can be as long as

0.4 mm. They appear not to cause symptoms in humans, although they may be numerous in the skin of individuals with rosacea. Demodectic mange may be severely debilitating in certain domestic animals.

House dust mites of the genus *Dermatophagoides* infest houses throughout the world, living on furniture and rugs and feeding on shed human dander. Exposure to their allergens in the domestic environment causes asthma, rhinitis, conjunctivitis, and eczema in allergic individuals. Management includes immunotherapy with mite extracts and a variety of environmental interventions (e.g., frequent cleaning of floors and upholstered furniture, removal or acaricidal treatment of rugs in bedrooms) to reduce mite density. Although use of a high-efficiency particulate air (HEPA)–filtered vacuum may help remove mites and their food source, it may also exacerbate exposure by propelling mite allergens into the air.

PEDICULOSIS (LOUSE INFESTATION) Nymphs and adults of all three kinds of human louse feed at least once a day, and they ingest human blood exclusively. Head lice (*Pediculus capitis*) infest mainly the hair of the scalp, body lice (*P. humanus*) the clothing, and crab or pubic lice (*Pthirus pubis*) mainly the hair of the pubis. The saliva of lice produces an intensely irritating maculopapular or urticarial rash in sensitized persons. Females of head and pubic lice cement their eggs firmly to hair and body lice mainly to clothing. A nymph hatches after ~10 days of development. The empty egg (nit) may remain affixed for months or longer after the louse has hatched.

Head lice infest ~1% of elementary school–aged children in the United States and are transmitted mainly by direct person-to-person contact. The role of fomites (shared headgear and grooming implements) as a transmission vehicle seems of negligible importance. In the United States, black children are less frequently infested than other children. Excoriations of pruritic lesions on the scalp, neck, and shoulders infrequently lead to oozing, crusting, matting of hair, bacterial infections, and regional lymphadenopathy. Head lice removed from a person generally succumb to desiccation and starvation within a day. Head lice seem unimportant as natural vectors for pathogenic agents.

Body lice remain on clothing except when feeding and generally succumb within a day or two if separated from the human host. These lice mainly infest disaster victims or indigent people who are in close contact with other infested individuals and who change their clothes only infrequently. Transmission by direct contact or by sharing of clothing and bedding is enhanced under crowded conditions. The tendency of the body louse to leave febrile persons or corpses as they become cold may facilitate the transmission of louse-borne typhus, louse-borne relapsing fever, and trench fever (Chap. 158). Trench fever and endocarditis due to *Bartonella quintana* have emerged as diseases of homeless persons living in large cities of the United States and Europe. Pruritic lesions are particularly common around the neckline. Chronic infestations result in a postinflammatory hyperpigmentation and thickening of skin known as *vagabonds' disease*.

The crab or pubic louse is transmitted mainly by sexual contact but can infest eyelashes, axillary hair, and hair in other sites as well as pubic hair. Children with pubic lice generally acquire their infestations from parents rather than via sexual transmission. Polymerase chain reaction analysis of the blood meal of lice may permit identification of host DNA in cases of child abuse or rape. Intensely pruritic lesions and 2- to 3-mm blue macules (maculae ceruleae) develop at the site of bites. Blepharitis commonly accompanies infestations of the eyelashes.

Pediculosis may be suspected upon the detection of nits on hairs or in clothing. Confirmation, however, should await demonstration of a live louse. The dorsoventrally flattened adult louse measures 2 to 4 mm in length and has three pairs of legs ending in claws that enable it to grasp hair shafts or clothing. The oval nits of lice are ~0.8 mm long.

℞ TREATMENT

Generally, treatment is warranted only if live lice are discovered. The presence of nits alone does not form the basis for an active infestation.

Although some lice and their eggs may be removed mechanically by means of a fine-toothed louse or 'nit' comb, this practice often fails to eliminate infestations. Treatment of newly identified active infestations generally relies upon a 10-min application of nonprescription formulations containing 1% permethrin or pyrethrins, with a second application 10 days later. Lice persisting after this treatment may be resistant to pyrethroids. Such chronic infestations may be treated for 8 to 12 h with a prescription formulation of 0.5% malathion. Lindane seems less effective and may pose greater risk, particularly when misused.

Dead or hatched nits, which remain attached to hair sheaths and become translucent or opalescent, may falsely suggest an active infection. Although children infested by head lice are frequently isolated or excluded from school, this practice seems unjustified. Resistance of head lice to permethrin, malathion, and lindane has been reported. Ivermectin may be useful in cases of resistance to both malathion and permethrin but has not been approved for this purpose by the FDA.

Body lice can be eliminated by bathing and by applying topical pediculicides from head to foot. Clothes and bedding are effectively deloused by heat sterilization in a dryer at 65°C for 30 min or by fumigation. Emergency mass delousing of people and clothing may be warranted during periods of civil strife and after natural disasters to reduce the risk of pathogen transmission by body lice. Pubic lice infestations are treated with topical pediculicides except for eyelid infestations (*pthiriasis palpebrum*), which respond to a coating of petrolatum applied for 3 to 4 days or 1% yellow oxide of mercury ointment applied four times daily for 2 weeks.

TUNGIASIS *Tunga penetrans*, like other fleas, is a wingless, laterally flattened insect measuring 2 to 4 mm in length that feeds on blood. Also known as the chigoe flea, sand flea, or jigger, it occurs in tropical regions of Africa and the Americas. Adults live in sandy soil and burrow under the skin between toes, under nails, or on the soles of bare feet. The fleas engorge on blood and grow from pinpoint to pea size over a 2-week period. The lesions that they produce resemble a white pustule with a central black depression and may be pruritic or painful. Occasional complications include tetanus, bacterial infections, and autoamputation of toes. Tungiasis is treated by removal of the intact flea with a sterile needle or scalpel, tetanus vaccination, and topical application of antibiotics.

MYIASIS *Myiasis* refers to infestations by maggots, mainly due to the larvae produced by metallic-colored screw-worm flies or botflies. Maggots invade living or necrotic tissue or body cavities and produce different clinical syndromes, depending on the species of fly.

Furuncular Myiasis In forested parts of Central and South America, larvae of *Dermatobia hominis* (the human botfly) produce boil-like subcutaneous nodules 2 to 3 cm in diameter. The adult female captures a mosquito or other bloodsucking insect and deposits her eggs on its abdomen. When the carrier insect attacks a human or bovine host several days later, the warmth and moisture of the host's surface stimulate these eggs to hatch. The larvae promptly penetrate intact skin. After 6 to 12 weeks, the larvae mature and drop to the ground, where they pupate. The African tumbu fly, *Cordylobia anthropophaga*, produces similar lesions. Dozens of eggs are deposited on sand or drying laundry that is contaminated with urine or sweat. Larvae hatch on contact with the body, penetrate the skin, and produce boils from which they emerge 8 or 9 days later. In North America, larvae of the genus *Cuterebra* (botflies of rabbits and rodents) are an unusual cause of myiasis in persons exposed to eggs in grass or brush. A diagnosis of furuncular myiasis is suggested by uncomfortable lesions with a central breathing pore that emits bubbles when submerged in water. There is often a sensation of movement under the skin that may lead to severe emotional distress. Botfly larvae can be induced to emerge if the air pore is coated with petrolatum or another occlusive substance. Removal of *Dermatobia* larvae is facilitated by injection of a local anesthetic into the surrounding tissue, but surgical excision is often necessary because upward-pointing spines hold the larva firmly in place.

Creeping Dermal Myiasis Maggots of the horse botfly, *Gasterophilus intestinalis*, do not mature after penetrating human skin but migrate for weeks in the epidermis. The resulting pruritic and serpiginous eruption resembles cutaneous larva migrans caused by *Ancylostoma braziliense*. Horseback riders become infested when eggs deposited on the flank of the horse hatch against their bare legs. The black spines of the larvae can be identified after mineral oil is smeared over the lesion. Larvae are removed with a needle. The larvae of the cattle botfly (*Hypoderma* species) invade more deeply and produce boil-like swellings.

Wound and Body-Cavity Myiasis Certain flies are attracted to blood and pus, and their newly hatched larvae enter wounds or diseased skin. Larvae of species such as *Lucilia (Phaenicia) sericata*, the green-bottle fly, remain superficial and confined to necrotic tissue and continue to be applied on a limited basis to debride purulent wounds. Other species, including the screw-worms (*Chrysomyia bezziana* in Asia and Africa and *Cochliomyia hominivorax* in Latin America) and the flesh fly (*Wohlfahrtia vigil* in northern North America), invade more deeply into viable tissue and produce large suppurating lesions. Larvae that infest wounds also may infest body cavities such as the mouth, nose, ears, sinuses, anus, vagina, and lower urinary tract, particularly in unconscious or otherwise debilitated patients. The consequences range from harmless colonization to destruction of the nose, meningitis, and deafness. Treatment involves removal of maggots and debridement of tissue.

Other Forms of Myiasis The maggots responsible for furuncular and wound myiasis may also cause ophthalmomyiasis. Sequelae include nodules in the eyelid, retinal detachment, and destruction of the globe. In addition, the adult sheep botfly, *Oestrus ovis*, may deposit larvae in the eyes of persons tending sheep and goats, and the larvae may produce a conjunctival infestation and acute conjunctivitis. True intestinal myiasis occurs when eggs or larvae of the drone fly (*Eristalis tenax*) are ingested with contaminated food, mature in the gut, and cause enteritis. Most instances in which maggots are found in human feces are the result of larviposition by flesh flies on recently passed stools.

PENTASTOMIASIS Pentastomids, or tongue worms, are parasites with characteristics of both helminths and arthropods and generally are classified in a separate phylum. The wormlike adults inhabit the respiratory passages of reptiles and carnivorous mammals. Human infestation by *Linguatula serrata* is common in the Middle East and occurs in the Sudan following ingestion of encysted larval stages in raw liver or lymph nodes of sheep and goats, the intermediate hosts. The larvae migrate to the nasopharynx and produce an acute self-limiting syndrome known as *halzoun* (*Marrara* in the Sudan), which is characterized by pain and itching of the throat and ears, coughing, hoarseness, dysphagia, and dyspnea. Severe edema may cause obstruction and necessitate tracheostomy, and ocular invasion has been described. Diagnostic larvae measuring 5 to 10 mm in length are found in the copious nasal discharge or vomitus. Human beings become infected with *Armillifer armillatus* by ingesting eggs in contaminated food or drink or after handling the definitive host, the African python. Larvae encyst in various organs but rarely cause symptoms unless they compress vital structures or perforate an organ during migration. Cysts occasionally require surgical removal as they enlarge during molting, but they are usually encountered as an incidental finding at autopsy. There are reports of the cutaneous larva migrans syndrome due to other pentastomes (*Reighardia* and *Sebekia* species) in Southeast Asia and Central America.

LEECH INFESTATIONS Medically important leeches are annelid worms that attach to their hosts by means of chitinous cutting jaws and draw blood through muscular suckers. The medicinal leech, *Hirudo medicinalis*, is still used occasionally to reduce venous congestion in surgical flaps or replanted body parts. This practice has been complicated by wound infections, myonecrosis, and sepsis due to *Aeromonas hydrophila*, which colonizes the gullets of commercially available leeches.

Ubiquitous aquatic leeches that parasitize fish, frogs, and turtles readily attach to the skin of humans and avidly suck blood. More notorious are the land leeches (*Haemadipsa*) that live in moist vegetation of tropical rain forests. Attachment is usually painless. Hirudinin, a powerful anticoagulant secreted by the leech, causes continued bleeding after the leech has detached. Healing of the wound is slow, and bacterial infections are not uncommon. Several species of aquatic leeches in Africa, Asia, and southern Europe can enter through the mouth, nose, and genitourinary tract and attach to mucosal surfaces at sites as deep as the esophagus and trachea. Bleeding may be intense. Externally attached leeches are removed by steady gentle traction. Removal is hastened by application of alcohol, salt, vinegar, or a flame to the leech. Internally attached leeches may detach on exposure to gargled saline or may be removed by forceps.

DELUSIONAL INFESTATIONS The groundless conviction that one is infested with arthropods or other parasites is an extremely difficult disorder to treat and unfortunately is not rare. Patients report infestations of their skin, clothing, or homes and describe sensations of something moving in or on their skin. Excoriations often accompany complaints of pruritus or insect bites. Patients bring in as evidence of infestation specimens that are identified microscopically as plant-feeding or peridomestic arthropods, pieces of skin, vegetable matter, or inanimate objects. In suspected cases, it is imperative to rule out true infestations and neuropathies, environmental irritants such as fragments of fiberglass, and other causes of tingling or prickling sensations. Pharmacotherapy with pimozide, which blocks dopamine receptors, has been more helpful than psychotherapy in treating this disorder.

ARTHROPOD BITES AND STINGS

SPIDER BITES Of the more than 30,000 recognized species of spider, only about 100 defend themselves aggressively and have fangs sufficiently long to penetrate human skin. The venom that spiders use to immobilize and digest their prey can cause necrosis of skin and systemic toxicity. While the bites of most spiders are painful but not harmful, envenomations of the brown or fiddle spiders (*Loxosceles* species), widow spiders (*Latrodectus* species), and other species may be life-threatening. Identification of the offending spider should be attempted, since specific treatments exist for bites of widow and brown recluse spiders and since injuries attributed to spiders are frequently due to other causes.

Recluse Spider Bites and Necrotic Arachnidism Severe necrosis of skin and subcutaneous tissue follows envenomation by *Loxosceles reclusa*, the brown recluse spider, and by at least four other species of *Loxosceles*, mainly in the southern and midwestern United States. Other spiders that produce necrotic ulceration include the hobo spider (*Tegenaria agrestis*) in the Pacific Northwest, the sac spiders (*Chiracanthium* species) throughout the United States and abroad, the South American brown spider *Loxosceles laeta* in Central and South America, and other *Loxosceles* species in Africa and the Middle East. All these spiders measure 7 to 15 mm in body length and 2 to 4 cm in leg span. Recluse spiders are brown and have a dark violin-shaped spot on their dorsal surface; hobo spiders are brown with gray markings; and sac spiders may be pale yellow, green, or brown.

These spiders are not aggressive toward human beings and bite only if threatened or pressed against the skin. They hide under rocks and logs or in caves and animal burrows, and they emerge at night to hunt other spiders and insects. They invade homes, particularly in the fall, and seek dark and undisturbed hiding spots in closets, in folds of clothing, or under furniture and rubbish in storage rooms, garages, and attics. Bites often occur while the victim is dressing and are sustained primarily to the arms, neck, and lower abdomen.

The clear viscous venoms of these spiders contain an esterase, alkaline phosphatase, protease, and other enzymes that produce tissue necrosis and hemolysis. Sphingomyelinase B, the most important dermonecrotic factor, binds cell membranes and promotes chemotaxis of neutrophils, leading to vascular thrombosis and an Arthus-like reaction. Initially, the bite is painless or produces a stinging sensation.

Within the next few hours, the site becomes painful and pruritic, with central induration surrounded by a pale zone of ischemia and a zone of erythema. In most cases, the lesion resolves without treatment over 2 to 3 days. In severe cases, the erythema spreads, and the center of the lesion becomes hemorrhagic and necrotic with an overlying bulla. A black eschar forms and sloughs several weeks later, leaving an ulcer that may be ≥25 cm in diameter and eventually a depressed scar. Healing usually takes place within 3 to 6 months but may take as long as 3 years if adipose tissue is involved. Local complications include injury to nerves and secondary infection. Fever, chills, weakness, headache, nausea, vomiting, myalgia, arthralgia, maculopapular rash, and leukocytosis may develop within 72 h of the bite. In rare instances, acute complications such as hemolytic anemia, hemoglobinuria, and renal failure are fatal.

℞ TREATMENT

Initial management includes local cleansing, application of sterile dressings and cold compresses, and elevation and loose immobilization of the affected limb. Analgesics, antihistamines, antibiotics, and tetanus prophylaxis should be administered if indicated. Within the first 48 to 72 h, the administration of dapsone, a leukocyte inhibitor, may halt the progression of lesions that are becoming necrotic. Dapsone is given in oral doses of 50 to 100 mg twice daily after glucose-6-phosphate dehydrogenase deficiency has been ruled out. The efficacy of locally or systemically administered glucocorticoids has not been demonstrated, and a potentially useful *Loxosceles*-specific antivenin has not been approved for use in the United States. Debridement and later skin grafting may be necessary after signs of acute inflammation have subsided, but immediate surgical excision of the wound is detrimental. Patients should be monitored closely for signs of hemolysis, renal failure, and other systemic complications.

Widow Spider Bites The bite of the female widow spider is notorious for the effect of its potent neurotoxin. *Latrodectus mactans*, the black widow, has been found in every state of the United States except Alaska and is most abundant in the Southeast. It measures up to 1 cm in body length and 5 cm in leg span, is shiny black, and has a red hourglass marking on the ventral abdomen. Other dangerous North American *Latrodectus* species include *L. geometricus* (the brown widow), *L. bishopi* (the red widow), *L. variolus*, and *L. hesperus*, and there are related species in other temperate and subtropical parts of the world.

Widow spiders spin their webs under stones, logs, plants, or rock piles or in dark spaces in barns, garages, and outhouses. Bites are most common in the summer and early autumn and occur when the web is disturbed or when the spider is trapped or provoked. The buttocks or genitals are sites of bites incurred by humans while sitting in an outdoor privy. The initial bite goes unnoticed or is perceived as a sharp pinprick. Two small red marks, mild erythema, and edema develop at the fang entrance site. The oily yellow venom that is injected does not produce local necrosis, and some persons experience no other symptoms. However, α-latrotoxin, the most active component of the venom, binds irreversibly to nerves and causes release and eventual depletion of acetylcholine, norepinephrine, and other neurotransmitters from presynaptic terminals. Within 30 to 60 min, painful cramps spread from the bite site to large muscles of the extremities and the trunk. Extreme rigidity of the abdominal muscles and excruciating pain may suggest peritonitis, but the abdomen is not tender on palpation. Other features include salivation, diaphoresis, vomiting, hypertension, tachycardia, labored breathing, anxiety, headache, weakness, fasciculations, paresthesia, hyperreflexia, urinary retention, uterine contractions, and premature labor. Rhabdomyolysis and renal failure have been reported, and respiratory arrest, cerebral hemorrhage, or cardiac failure may end fatally, especially in very young, elderly, or debilitated persons. The pain begins to subside during the first 12 h but may recur during several days or weeks before resolving spontaneously.

℞ TREATMENT

Treatment consists of local cleansing, application of ice packs, and tetanus prophylaxis. Hypertension that does not respond to analgesics and antispasmodics, such as benzodiazepines or methocarbamol, requires specific antihypertensive medication. Intravenous administration of one or two vials of a widely available equine antivenin rapidly relieves pain and can be life-saving. Because of the risk of anaphylaxis and serum sickness, antivenin should be reserved for severe cases involving respiratory arrest, uncontrollable hypertension, seizures, or pregnancy.

Envenomations by Tarantulas and Other Spiders   Tarantulas are long-lived hairy spiders of which 30 species are found in the United States, mainly in the Southwest. The tarantulas that have become popular household pets are usually imported species with bright colors and a leg span of up to 25 cm. Tarantulas bite only when threatened and cause no more harm than a bee sting, but the venom occasionally provokes deep pain and swelling. Several species are covered with urticating hairs that are brushed off in the thousands when a threatened spider rubs its hind legs across its dorsal abdomen. These hairs penetrate human skin and produce pruritic papules that last for weeks. Failure to wear gloves or to wash the hands after handling the Chilean Rose tarantula, the most popular pet spider, has resulted in transfer of hairs to the eye and devastating ocular inflammation. Treatment of bites includes local washing and elevation of the bitten area, tetanus prophylaxis, and analgesic administration. Antihistamines and topical or systemic glucocorticoids are given for exposure to urticating hairs.

Atrax robustus, the Sydney funnel-web spider of Australia, and *Phoneutria* species, the South American banana spiders, are among the most dangerous spiders in the world because of their aggressive behavior and potent neurotoxins. Envenomation by *A. robustus* causes a rapidly progressive neuromotor syndrome that can be fatal within 2 h. The bite of the banana spiders causes severe local pain followed by profound systemic symptoms and respiratory paralysis that can lead to death within 2 to 6 h. Specific antivenins for envenomation by each of these spiders are available. *Lycosa* species (wolf spiders) are found throughout the world and may produce painful bites and transient local inflammation.

SCORPION STINGS   Scorpions are crablike arachnids that feed on ground-dwelling arthropods and small lizards, which they grasp with a pair of frontal pinchers and paralyze by injecting venom from a stinger on the tip of the tail. Painful but relatively harmless scorpion stings need to be distinguished from the potentially lethal envenomations that are produced by about 30 of the ~1000 known species and cause more than 5000 deaths worldwide each year. Scorpions feed at night and remain hidden during the day in crevices or burrows or under wood, loose bark, or rocks on the ground. They seek cool spots under buildings and often enter houses, where they get into shoes, clothing, or bedding or enter bathtubs and sinks in search of water. Scorpions sting human beings only when disturbed.

Scorpions of the United States   Of the 40 or so scorpion species in the United States, only the bark scorpion (*Centruroides sculpturatus* or *C. exilicauda*) produces a venom that can be lethal. Stings of the other species, such as the common striped scorpion *C. vittatus* and the large *Hadrurus arizonensis*, cause immediate sharp local pain followed by edema, ecchymosis, and a burning sensation. Symptoms typically resolve within a few hours, and skin does not slough. Allergic reactions to the venom sometimes develop.

The deadly *C. sculpturatus* of the southwestern United States and northern Mexico measures ~7 cm in length and is yellow-brown in color. Its venom contains neurotoxins that cause sodium channels to remain open and neurons to fire repetitively. In contrast to the stings of nonlethal species, *C. sculpturatus* envenomations are usually associated with little swelling, but prominent pain, paresthesia, and hy-

peresthesia can be accentuated by tapping on the affected area (the tap test). These symptoms soon spread to other locations; dysfunction of cranial nerves and hyperexcitability of skeletal muscles develop within hours. Patients present with restlessness, blurred vision, abnormal eye movements, profuse salivation, lacrimation, rhinorrhea, slurred speech, difficulty in handling secretions, diaphoresis, nausea, and vomiting. Muscle twitching, jerking, and shaking may be mistaken for a seizure. Complications include tachycardia, arrhythmias, hypertension, hyperthermia, rhabdomyolysis, and acidosis. Symptoms progress to maximal severity in ~5 h and subside within a day or two, although pain and paresthesia can last for weeks. Fatal respiratory arrest is most common among young children and the elderly.

Other Dangerous Scorpions   Envenomations by *Leiurus quinquestriatus* in the Middle East and North Africa, by *Mesobuthus tamulus* in India, by *Androctonus* species along the Mediterranean littoral and in North Africa and the Middle East, and by *Tityus serrulatus* in Brazil cause massive release of endogenous catecholamines with hypertensive crises, arrhythmias, pulmonary edema, and myocardial damage. Acute pancreatitis occurs with stings of *Tityus trinitatis* in Trinidad, and central nervous toxicity complicates stings of *Parabuthus* and *Buthotus* scorpions of South Africa. Tissue necrosis and hemolysis may follow stings of the Iranian *Hemiscorpius lepturus*.

℞ TREATMENT

Identification of the offending scorpion aids in planning therapy. Stings of nonlethal species require at most ice packs, analgesics, or antihistamines. Because most victims of dangerous envenomations (such as those produced by *C. sculpturatus*) experience only local discomfort, they can be managed at home with instructions to return to the emergency department if signs of cranial-nerve or neuromuscular dysfunction develop. Aggressive supportive care and judicious use of antivenin can reduce or eliminate deaths from more severe envenomations. Keeping the patient calm and applying pressure dressings and cold packs to the sting site decrease the absorption of venom. A continuous intravenous infusion of midazolam controls the agitation, flailing, and involuntary muscle movements produced by scorpion stings. Close monitoring during treatment with this drug and other sedatives or narcotics is necessary for persons with neuromuscular symptoms because of the risk of respiratory arrest. Hypertension and pulmonary edema respond to nifedipine, nitroprusside, hydralazine, or prazosin, and bradyarrhythmias can be controlled with atropine.

Commercially prepared antivenins are available in several countries for some of the most dangerous species. A caprine *C. sculpturatus* antivenin (not yet FDA approved) is available as an investigational drug from Arizona State University for use only in Arizona. Because of the risk of anaphylaxis or serum sickness following administration of goat serum, use of the antivenin is controversial. Intravenous administration of antivenin rapidly reverses cranial-nerve dysfunction and muscular symptoms but does not affect pain and paresthesia. The benefit of scorpion antivenin has not been established in controlled trials.

Prevention   In scorpion-infested areas, shoes, clothing, bedding, and towels should be shaken and inspected before being used. Removal of wood, stones, and debris from yards and campsites eliminates hiding places for scorpions, and household spraying of insecticides can deplete their source of food.

CHIGGERS AND OTHER BITING MITES   Chiggers are the larvae of trombiculid (harvest) mites that normally feed on mice in grassy or brush-covered sites in the tropics and subtropics and (less frequently) in temperate areas during warm months. They wait for hosts on low vegetation and attach themselves to passing animals or to people. The larva then pierces the skin of its host and deposits a tubelike structure in the dermis through which it imbibes lymph and tissue juices. This highly antigenic "stylostome" serves as the focus of an exceptionally pruritic papular, papulovesicular, or papulourticarial lesion that may be 2 cm in diameter and that develops within hours of attachment in persons previously sensitized to mite antigen. Feeding mites appear as tiny red vesicles in hair follicles. Scratching invariably destroys the body of a mite attached to a person. These lesions generally vesiculate and develop a hemorrhagic base. Itching and burning last for weeks. The rash is most common on the ankles or near tight-fitting clothes that obstruct the mites' movements. Chiggers are the vectors of scrub typhus in tropical and subtropical parts of Asia. Repellents are useful for preventing chigger bites.

Certain mesostigmatid mites that infest the nests of mice or birds feed on human beings when their usual hosts have been displaced. Intense episodes of itching dermatitis in humans, for example, may follow the removal of trash that has accumulated in a human residence or the departure of pigeons that have been nesting on a window air-conditioner. Other mites that infest grain, straw, cheese, or other animal products occasionally produce similar episodes. Persons who have close contact with dogs—and, to a lesser extent, cats—may develop a self-limited pruritic papulovesicular rash from bites of cheyletiellid mites that cause a mangelike condition in these animals. Mouse mites are the vectors of rickettsialpox in cities of the northeastern United States. Fowl and chicken mites transmit the viruses of St. Louis encephalitis and western equine encephalitis. Although sanitary measures effectively prevent rickettsialpox, removal of accumulated refuse may result in a transient period of elevated risk. Insecticidal applications applied to infested areas can eliminate mites before or while hosts and their nests are removed.

Diagnosis of mite-induced dermatitides (including those caused by chiggers) relies heavily on a history of exposure to the source of the mite, since the tiny mite may escape notice or may fall off or be scratched off the lesions. Antihistamines or topical steroids effectively reduce mite-induced pruritus.

HYMENOPTERA STINGS   Insects that sting to defend their colonies or subdue their prey belong to the order Hymenoptera, which includes apids (bees and bumblebees), vespids (wasps, hornets, and yellow jackets), and ants. Their venoms contain a wide array of amines, peptides, and enzymes that are responsible for local and systemic reactions. Although the toxic effect of multiple stings can be fatal, nearly all of the 100 or more deaths due to hymenopteran stings in the United States each year are the result of allergic reactions.

Bee and Wasp Stings   Honeybees lose their stinging apparatus and the attached venom sac in the act of stinging and subsequently die, while other bees, ants, and vespids can sting numerous times in succession. The familiar honeybees (*Apis mellifera*) and bumblebees (*Bombus* and other genera) generally attack only when a colony is disturbed. The extremely aggressive Africanized honeybees, however, respond to minimal intrusions rapidly and in large numbers. Since their introduction into Brazil in 1957, these "killer bees" have spread through South and Central America to the southern and western United States. The common vespids in the United States include the yellow jackets, notable for the yellow and black bands on their abdomens; the bald-faced hornet, with a black body and a white face; the European hornet, measuring 2.5 to 3.5 cm in length; and the paper wasps, which have variously colored elongate bodies. Vespids sting in defense of their nests, which they often build near human dwellings and suspend from eaves or shubbery, plaster onto walls, or burrow into wood or soil. All vespids feed on sugary substances and decaying meat, and certain of the yellow jackets are annoyingly abundant at recreation sites and around garbage, particularly in the late summer and fall.

Venom is produced in glands at the posterior end of the abdomen and is expelled rapidly by contraction of muscles of the venom sac, which has a capacity of up to 0.1 mL in large insects. The venoms of different species of hymenopterans are biochemically and immunologically distinct. Direct toxic effects are mediated by mixtures of low-molecular-weight compounds such as serotonin, histamine, and acetylcholine and several kinins. Polypeptide toxins in honeybee venom include mellitin, which damages cell membranes; mast cell–degranulating protein, which causes histamine release; apamin, a neurotoxin; and adolapin, which has anti-inflammatory action. Enzymes in venom include hyaluronidase, which allows the spread of other venom components, and phospholipases, which may be among the major venom allergens. There appears to be little cross-sensitization between honeybee and wasp venoms.

Uncomplicated stings cause immediate pain, a wheal-and-flare reaction, and local edema and swelling that subside in a few hours. Stings from accidentally swallowed insects may induce life-threatening edema of the upper airways. Multiple stings can lead to vomiting, diarrhea, generalized edema, dyspnea, hypotension, and collapse. Rhabdomyolysis and intravascular hemolysis may cause renal failure. Death from the direct effects of venom has followed 300 to 500 honeybee stings.

Large local reactions that spread ≥10 cm around the sting site over 24 to 48 h are not uncommon. These reactions may resemble cellulitis but are caused by hypersensitivity rather than secondary infection. Such reactions tend to recur on subsequent exposure but are seldom accompanied by anaphylaxis and are not prevented by venom immunotherapy.

An estimated 0.4 to 4.0% of the U.S. population exhibits clinical immediate-type hypersensitivity to insect stings, and 15% may have asymptomatic sensitization manifested by positive skin tests. Persons who experience severe allergic reactions are likely to have similar reactions after subsequent stings; occasionally, adults who have had mild reactions later experience serious reactions. Mild anaphylactic reactions from insect stings, as from other causes, consist of nausea, abdominal cramping, generalized urticaria, flushing, and angioedema. Serious reactions, including upper airway edema, bronchospasm, hypotension, and shock, may be rapidly fatal. Severe reactions usually begin within 10 min of the sting and only rarely develop after 5 h. Unusual complications, including serum sickness, vasculitis, neuritis, and encephalitis, develop several days or weeks after a sting.

℞ TREATMENT

Stingers from honeybees embedded in the skin should be removed as promptly as possible, using any method available, to limit the quantity of venom delivered. Previous suggestions—that the stinger be scraped or brushed off with a blade or a fingernail but not removed with forceps—simply delay removal and exacerbate the consequences. The site should be cleansed and disinfected and ice packs applied to slow the spread of venom. Elevation of the affected site and administration of analgesics, oral antihistamines, and topical calamine lotion relieve symptoms; application of meat tenderizer containing papain is of no proven value. Large local reactions may require a short course of oral therapy with glucocorticoids. Patients with numerous stings should be monitored for 24 h for evidence of renal failure or coagulopathy.

Anaphylaxis is treated with subcutaneous injection of 0.3 to 0.5 mL of epinephrine hydrochloride in a 1:1000 dilution; treatment is repeated every 20 to 30 min if necessary. Intravenous epinephrine (2 to 5 mL of a 1:10,000 solution administered by slow push) is indicated for profound shock. A tourniquet may slow the spread of venom. Parenteral antihistamines, fluid resuscitation, bronchodilators, oxygen, intubation, and vasopressors may be required. Patients should be observed for 24 h for recurrent anaphylaxis.

PREVENTION   Persons with a history of allergy to insect stings should carry a sting kit with a preloaded syringe containing epinephrine for self-administration in case of a sting. These patients should seek medical attention immediately after using the kit. To avoid stings when outdoors, individuals can wear shoes and protective clothing and avoid attracting insects with sweet foods, bright-colored clothes, perfumes, or cosmetics.

VENOM IMMUNOTHERAPY   Repeated injections of purified venom produce a blocking IgG antibody response to venom and reduce the incidence of recurrent anaphylaxis from between 50 and 60% to <5%. Honeybee, wasp, yellow jacket, and mixed vespid venoms are commercially available for desensitization and for skin testing. Adults with a history of anaphylaxis should undergo desensitization. Results of skin tests and venom-specific radioallergosorbent tests aid in the selection of patients for immunotherapy and guide the design of such treatment. The risk of a systemic reaction to a sting is ~5 to 10% after discontinuation of a ≥5-year course of immunotherapy.

Stings of Fire Ants and Other Ants All ants that are large enough can injure human beings, and some can secrete repugnant substances when handled. Stinging fire ants are an important medical problem in the United States. The imported fire ants *Solenopsis richteri* and *S. invicta* were introduced from South America into Alabama in 1918 and now infest urban and rural areas of southern states from Texas to North Carolina, with colonies in California, New Mexico, Arizona, and Virginia. They excavate open fields and yards to build tall mounds that can harbor 200,000 worker ants. Slight disturbances of the mounds have provoked massive outpourings of ants and as many as 10,000 stings on a single person. Each year fire ants sting up to 60% of the inhabitants of some cities. Waterborne ants bite on contact during times of flooding. Elderly and immobile persons are at high risk for attacks when fire ants invade dwellings.

Red-brown or brown-black fire ants attach to human skin with powerful mandibles and rotate their bodies around their heads while repeatedly injecting venom with posteriorly situated stingers. The alkaloid venom consists of cytotoxic and hemolytic piperidines and several proteins with enzymatic activity. The initial wheal-and-flare reaction, burning, and itching resolve in ~30 min, and a sterile pustule develops within 24 h. The pustule ulcerates over the next 48 h and then heals a week or 10 days later unless it becomes secondarily infected. Large areas of erythema and edema lasting several days are not uncommon and in extreme cases may compress nerves and blood vessels. Anaphylaxis occurs in ~1 to 2% of persons, and seizures and mononeuritis have been reported. Stings are treated with ice packs, topical glucocorticoids, and oral antihistamines. Covering pustules with bandages and antibiotic ointment may prevent bacterial infection. Epinephrine and supportive measures are indicated for anaphylactic reactions. Whole-body extracts are available for skin testing and immunotherapy, which appears to lower the rate of anaphylactic reactions.

The western United States is home to harvester ants (*Pogonomyrmex* species) as well as to less aggressive fire ants not yet displaced by the introduced species. The painful local reaction following harvester ant stings often extends to lymph nodes and may be accompanied by anaphylaxis. Large Australian bulldog ants and the aggressive South American *Paranopera* ants deliver extremely painful stings and may cause systemic symptoms. Velvet ants that inhabit sandy beaches in the United States and sting the bare feet of bathers are actually wingless female wasps of the genus *Dasymutilla*.

TICK BITES AND TICK PARALYSIS In the United States, hard ticks (Ixodidae) have increased in abundance since the mid-1900s to become common carriers of vector-borne disease agents. Deer ticks of the genus *Ixodes* transmit the pathogens of Lyme disease, babesiosis, and human anaplasmosis. Other ticks, such as *Dermacentor variabilis* (the dog tick), *D. andersoni* (the wood tick), and *Amblyomma americanum* (the Lone Star tick), are vectors of tularemia, Rocky Mountain spotted fever, Colorado tick fever, human monocytotropic ehrlichiosis, and ehrlichiosis ewingii. Outside the United States, hard ticks transmit pathogenic rickettsiae and arboviruses as well. Soft ticks (Argasidae) of the genus *Ornithodoros* transmit tick-borne relapsing fever (Chap. 156). Except in parts of Africa, soft ticks rarely attack human beings, and relapsing fever occurs only sporadically in the United States. Hard ticks differ from soft ticks by virtue of a dorsal scutum or plate and their preference for wooded, brushy, or weedy habitats. Soft ticks, which are nonscutate and leathery, are generally found in animal burrows and bird nests.

Ticks attach and feed painlessly; blood is their only food. Their

secretions, however, produce local reactions, a febrile illness, or paralysis. Soft ticks attach for <1 h and produce erythematous macular lesions up to 2 to 3 cm in diameter. Some species in Africa, the western United States, and Mexico produce painful hemorrhagic lesions. At the site of hard-tick bites, small areas of induration with surrounding erythema and occasionally necrotic ulcers develop. Chronic nodules, or "tick granulomas," reach several centimeters in diameter and may require surgical excision. Tick-induced fever, associated with headache, nausea, and malaise, usually resolves within 24 to 36 h after the tick is removed. Tick paralysis is an ascending flaccid paralysis believed to be caused by a toxin in tick saliva that causes neuromuscular block and decreased nerve conduction. Throughout the world, this rare complication has followed the bites of more than 40 kinds of tick—most commonly, dog and wood ticks in the United States. Children, especially girls with long hair, are most often affected. Weakness begins in the lower extremities 5 to 6 days after the tick's attachment and ascends symmetrically over several days to result in complete paralysis of the extremities and cranial nerves. Deep tendon reflexes are diminished or lacking altogether, but sensory examination and findings on lumbar puncture are typically normal. Removal of the tick generally results in improvement within a few hours and usually in complete recovery after several days. Failure to remove the tick may lead to dysarthria, dysphagia, and ultimately death from aspiration or respiratory paralysis. Diagnosis depends on finding the tick, which often is hidden beneath hair and which, when engorged, may resemble a pedunculated nevus.

An antiserum to the saliva of *Ixodes holocyclus*, the usual cause of tick paralysis in Australia, effectively reverses paralysis caused by these ticks. Ticks should be removed by firm traction with a forceps placed near their point of attachment. The site of attachment should be disinfected (e.g., with tincture of iodine). Mouthparts remaining in the skin may cause persistent irritation or lead to secondary infection. Removal of ticks during the first 48 h of attachment nearly always prevents transmission of the agents of Lyme disease, babesiosis, and erhlichiosis. Gentle handling (to avoid rupture of ticks) and use of gloves may avert accidental contamination with tick fluids containing pathogens. Protective measures against ticks include avoidance of brushy vegetation, removal of ticks from pet dogs and cats, use of protective clothing sprayed with 0.5% permethrin, and application of a repellent containing *N,N*-diethyl-*m*-toluamide (DEET). The cuffs of trousers should be tucked inside the socks. Rather than awaiting results of tick testing or patient seroconversion to Lyme disease, bites thought to be associated with deer ticks may be treated presumptively with a short course of oral antibiotics.

OTHER ARTHROPOD BITES AND ENVENOMATIONS ■ **Dipteran (Fly and Mosquito) Bites** In the process of feeding on vertebrate blood, adults of certain fly species inflict painful bites, produce local allergic reactions, or transmit pathogenic agents. Unlike insect stings, insect bites rarely cause anaphylaxis. Mosquitoes are ubiquitous pests and are the vectors of malaria, filariasis, yellow fever, dengue, and viral encephalitides. Female mosquitoes require a blood meal to produce eggs and an environment of standing water in which to deposit them. Their bite typically produces a wheal and later a pruritic papule. A similar reaction follows the bite of tiny but aggressive midges known as "no-see-ums" in the United States, which attack in swarms during warm months, or of other *Culicoides* species that transmit "nonpathogenic" filariae in tropical climates. Nodular lesions at the site of midge bites may last for months. The bite of the small humpbacked blackflies in the genus *Simulium* leaves a bleeding laceration and painful and pruritic sores that are slow to heal; regional lymphadenopathy, fever, or anaphylaxis occasionally ensues. Blackflies are common summertime nuisances in the United States and Canada and are vectors of onchocerciasis in Africa and Latin America. The widely distributed tabanids, including deerflies (*Chrysops* species) and horseflies (*Tabanus* species), are stout flies measuring 10 to 25 mm in length that attack during the day and produce large and painful bleeding punctures. Deerflies transmit loiasis in African equatorial rain forests and tularemia in the United

States and elsewhere. Tsetse flies of the genus *Glossina* transmit African trypanosomiasis in sub-Saharan Africa. Tiny phlebotomine sandflies are the vectors of leishmaniasis, bartonellosis (Carrión's disease), sandfly fever, and other arboviral infections in warm climates. *Stomoxys calcitrans*, the stable fly, which resembles a large housefly, is a fierce biter of human beings and domestic animals and a major pest in seacoast areas. Houseflies do not bite.

Rx TREATMENT

Treatment of fly bites is symptom-based. Topical application of antipruritic agents, glucocorticoids, or antiseptic lotions may relieve the itching and pain. Allergic reactions may require oral antihistamines. Antibiotics may be necessary for large bite wounds that become secondarily infected. Personal protection measures against biting flies include avoidance of infested areas, application of a DEET-containing repellent to exposed skin, and use of protective clothing and bed nets treated with permethrin. Higher concentrations of DEET provide longer-lasting protection, and 10 to 35% DEET provides adequate protection under most conditions. Repellents used on children should contain ≤10% DEET to avoid absorption of toxic levels that may provoke encephalopathy and seizures. Permethrin applied to clothing maintains its potency for at least 2 weeks, even with laundering.

Flea Bites Common human-biting fleas include the dog and cat fleas (*Ctenocephalides* species) and the rat flea (*Xenopsylla cheopis*), which inhabit the nests and resting sites of their hosts. Larval fleas feed on pellets of dried host blood that the adult fleas eject from their rectums while feeding. The high-jumping adults attack human beings or other available warm-bodied animals when the usual host abandons or is driven from its nest. The human flea (*Pulex irritans*) infests human bedding and furniture but mainly in relatively humid buildings that lack central heating. Sensitized persons develop erythematous pruritic papules, urticaria, and occasionally vesicles and bacterial superinfection at the site of the bite. Treatment consists of antihistamines and antipruritics.

Fleas transmit plague, murine typhus, a typhus-like illness due to *Rickettsia felis*, the rat and dog tapeworms, and *Bartonella henselae*. Flea infestations are eliminated by frequent cleaning of the nesting sites and bedding of the host or judicious dusting or spraying of insecticides such as pyrethrin, DDT, or malathion. Flea infestations in the home may abate if pets are treated with veterinary antiparasitic agents and insect growth regulators.

Hemipteran (True Bug) Bites Several true bugs of the family Reduviidae inflict bites that produce allergic reactions and are sometimes painful. The cone-nose bugs, so called because of their elongated heads, include the assassin and wheel bugs, which feed on other insects and bite human beings only in self-defense, and the kissing bugs, which routinely feed on vertebrate blood. Assassin and wheel bugs inhabit many parts of the world, including the United States, where they are notorious for their painful bites. The bites of the nocturnally feeding kissing bugs are painless and occur commonly in groups on the face and other exposed parts of the body. Reactions to such bites depend on prior sensitization and include tender and pruritic papules, vesicular or bullous lesions, giant urticaria, fever, lymphadenopathy, and anaphylaxis. *Triatoma infestans* and other species of kissing bug are the vectors of *Trypanosoma cruzi* in South and Central America and Mexico (causing Chagas' disease), but transmission of *T. cruzi* to humans by bugs indigenous to the United States is exceedingly rare. Bug bites are treated with topical antipruritics or oral antihistamines. Persons with anaphylactic reactions to reduviid bites should keep an epinephrine kit available. The cosmopolitan bedbug (*Cimex* species) hides in crevices in mattresses, bed frames, and other furniture and under loose wallpaper. Bedbugs are increasingly a nuisance in homes, dormitories, and even luxury hotels. The bugs hide during the day and take their blood meal at night. The bedbug's bite is painless, but sensitized persons develop erythema, itching, and wheals around a central hemorrhagic punctum. Bedbugs are not known to transmit pathogens.

Centipede Bites and Millipede Dermatitis The fangs of centipedes of the genus *Scolopendra* can penetrate human skin and deliver a venom that produces intense burning pain, swelling, erythema, and lymphangitis. Dizziness, nausea, and anxiety are occasionally described, and rhabdomyolysis and renal failure have been reported. Treatment includes washing of the site, application of cold dressings, oral analgesic administration or local lidocaine infiltration, and tetanus prophylaxis. Species of *Scolopendra*, measuring up to 25 cm, occur widely in the southern United States and other areas with warm climates worldwide. The smaller house centipede *Scutigera coleoptrata*, which is common throughout the United States, is harmless.

Millipedes, unlike centipedes, do not bite but rather secrete and in some cases eject defensive fluids that burn and discolor human skin. Affected skin turns brown overnight and may blister and exfoliate. Secretions in the eye cause intense pain and inflammation that may lead to corneal ulceration and blindness. Management includes irrigation with copious amounts of water or saline, use of analgesics, and local care of denuded skin. Millipedes are found throughout the world in leaf litter and under rocks.

Caterpillar Stings and Dermatitis The surface of caterpillars of several moth species is covered with hairs or spines that produce mechanical irritation and may contain or be coated with venom. Contact with these caterpillars causes an immediate burning sensation followed by local swelling and erythema and occasionally by regional lymphadenopathy, nausea, vomiting, and headache; shock, seizures, and coagulopathy are rare complications. In the United States, stings are most often caused by caterpillars of the io, puss, saddleback, and brown-tail moths. Contact with even detached hairs of other caterpillars, such as gypsy moth larvae (*Lymantria dispar*), can later produce a pruritic urticarial or papular rash. Spines may be deposited on tree trunks and drying laundry or may be airborne and cause irritation of the eyes and upper airways. Treatment of caterpillar stings consists of repeated application of adhesive or cellophane tape to remove the hairs, which can then be identified microscopically. Local ice packs, topical steroids, and oral antihistamines relieve symptoms.

Beetle Vesication When disturbed, blister beetles extrude cantharidin, a low-molecular-weight toxin that produces thin-walled blisters measuring up to 5 cm in diameter 2 to 5 h after contact with the beetle. The blisters are not painful or pruritic unless broken, and they resolve without treatment in a week to 10 days. Nephritis may follow unusually heavy cantharidin exposure. In the southern United States, blister beetles of several *Epicauta* species are abundant in the summer months. Contact occurs when people sit on the ground, work in the garden, or deliberately handle the beetles. In other countries, different species of beetle produce different vesicants. No treatment is necessary, although ruptured blisters should be kept clean and bandaged until healing is complete.

FURTHER READING

ARLIAN LG: Arthropod allergens and human health. Annu Rev Entomol 47: 395, 2002

AUERBACH PS (ed): *Wilderness Medicine*, 4th ed. St. Louis, Mosby, 2001

BURGESS IF: Human lice and their control. Annu Rev Entomol 49:457, 2004

FRADIN MS: Mosquitoes and mosquito repellents: A clinician's guide. Ann Intern Med 128:931, 1998

GODDARD J: *Physician's Guide to Arthropods of Medical Importance*, 4th ed. Boca Raton, FL, CRC Press, 2002

ISBISTER GK et al: Antivenom treatment in arachnidism. J Toxicol Clin Toxicol 41:291, 2003

MULLEN G, DURDEN L: *Medical and Veterinary Entomology*. Amsterdam, Academic Press, 2002

PETERS W: *A Colour Atlas of Arthropods in Clinical Medicine*. London, Wolfe, 1992

SAFDAR N et al: Autochthonous furuncular myiasis in the United States: Case report and literature review. Clin Infect Dis 36:e73, 2003

WONG HC: Importance of proper identification of stinging insects. Ann Intern Med 132:418, 2000

APPENDICES AND INDEX

APPENDICES

APPENDICES: LABORATORY VALUES OF CLINICAL IMPORTANCE
Alexander Kratz, Patrick M. Sluss, James L. Januzzi, Jr., Kent B. Lewandrowski

INTRODUCTORY COMMENTS

The following are tables of reference values for laboratory tests, special analytes, and special function tests. A variety of factors can influence reference values. Such variables include the population studied, laboratory methods and instrumentation, and even the type of container used for the collection of the specimen. Values supplied in this Appendix reflect typical reference ranges in adults. Pediatric reference ranges may vary significantly from adult values. The reference or "normal" ranges given in this appendix may therefore not be appropriate for all laboratories, and these values should only be used as general guidelines. Whenever possible, reference values provided by the laboratory performing the testing should be utilized in the interpretation of laboratory data.

In preparing the Appendix, the authors have taken into account the fact that the system of international units (SI, système international

d'unités) is used in most countries and in some medical journals. However, clinical laboratories may continue to report values in conventional units. Therefore, both systems are provided in the Appendix. The dual system is also used in the text except for (1) those instances in which the numbers remain the same but only the terminology is changed (mmol/L for meq/L or IU/L for mIU/mL), when only the SI units are given; and (2) most pressure measurements (e.g., blood and cerebrospinal fluid pressures), when the traditional units (mmHg, mmH$_2$O) are used. In all other instances in the text, the SI unit is followed by the conventional unit in parentheses.

Conversion from one system to another can be made as follows:

$$\text{mmol/L} = \frac{\text{mg/dL} \times 10}{\text{atomic weight (or molecular weight)}}$$

$$\text{mg/dL} = \frac{\text{mmol/L} \times \text{atomic weight (or molecular weight)}}{10}$$

 ## REFERENCE VALUES FOR LABORATORY TESTS

TABLE A-1 *Hematology and Coagulation*

Analyte	Specimen	SI Units	Conventional Units
Activated clotting time	WB	70–180 seconds	70–180 seconds
Activated protein C resistance (Factor V Leiden)	P	Not applicable	Ratio > 2.1
Alpha$_2$ antiplasmin	P	0.80–1.30	80–130%
Antiphospholipid antibody panel			
PTT-LA (lupus anticoagulant screen)	P	Negative	Negative
Platelet neutralization procedure	P	Negative	Negative
Dilute viper venom screen	P	Negative	Negative
Anticardiolipin antibody	S		
IgG		0–15 arbitrary units	0–15 GPL
IgM		0–15 arbitrary units	0–15 MPL
Antithrombin III	P		
Antigenic		220–390 mg/L	22–39 mg/dL
Functional		0.8–1.30 U/L	80–130%
Anti-Xa assay (Heparin assay)	P		
Unfractionated heparin		0.3–0.7 kIU/L	0.3–0.7 IU/mL
Low-molecular-weight heparin		0.5–1.0 kIU/L	0.5–1.0 IU/mL
Danaparoid (Orgaran)		0.5–0.8 kIU/L	0.5–0.8 IU/mL
Bleeding time (adult)		2–9.5 min	2–9.5 min
Bone Marrow: see Table B-3			
Carboxyhemoglobin	WB		
Nonsmoker		0–0.023	0–2.3%
Smoker		0.021–0.042	2.1–4.2%
Clot retraction	WB	0.50–1.00/2 h	50–100%/2 h
Cryofibrinogen	P	Negative	Negative
D Dimer	P	<0.5 mg/L	<0.5 μg/mL
Differential blood count	WB		
Neutrophils		0.40–0.70	40–70%
Bands		0.0–0.10	0–10%
Lymphocytes		0.22–0.44	22–44%
Monocytes		0.04–0.11	4–11%
Eosinophils		0.0–0.8	0–8%
Basophils		0.0–0.03	0–3%
Erythrocyte count	WB		
Adult males		4.50–5.90 × 10^{12}/L	4.50–5.90 × 10^6/mm^3
Adult females		4.00–5.20 × 10^{12}/L	4.00–5.20 × 10^6/mm^3
Erythrocyte lifespan	WB		
Normal survival		120 days	120 days
Chromium labeled, half life (t$_{1/2}$)		25–35 days	25–35 days
Erythrocyte sedimentation rate	WB		
Females		1–25 mm/h	1–25 mm/h
Males		0–17 mm/h	0–17 mm/h

(continued)

Analyte	Specimen	SI Units	Conventional Units
Factor II, prothrombin	P	0.60–1.40	60–140%
Factor V	P	0.60–1.40	60–140%
Factor VII	P	0.60–1.40	60–140%
Factor VIII	P	0.50–2.00	50–200%
Factor IX	P	0.60–1.40	60–140%
Factor X	P	0.60–1.40	60–140%
Factor XI	P	0.60–1.40	60–140%
Factor XII	P	0.60–1.40	60–140%
Factor XIII screen	P	Not applicable	No deficiency detected
Factor inhibitor assay	P	<0.5 Bethesda Units	<0.5 Bethesda Units
Ferritin	S		
Male		30–300 μg/L	30–300 ng/mL
Female		10–200 μg/L	10–200 ng/mL
Fibrin(ogen) degradation products	P	<2.5 mg/L	<2.5 μg/mL
Fibrinogen	P	1.50–4.00 g/L	150–400 mg/dL
Folate (folic acid)	S, P		
Normal		7.0–39.7 nmol/L	3.1–17.5 ng/mL
Borderline deficient		5.0–6.8 nmol/L	2.2–3.0 ng/mL
Deficient		<5.0 nmol/L	<2.2 ng/mL
Excess		>39.7 nmol/L	>17.5 ng/mL
Glucose-6-phosphate dehydrogenase (erythrocyte)	WB	Not applicable	No gross deficiency
Ham's test (acid serum)	WB	Negative	Negative
Haptoglobin	S	0.16–1.99 g/L	16–199 mg/dL
Hematocrit	WB		
Adult males		0.41–0.53	41.0–53.0
Adult females		0.36–0.46	36.0–46.0
Hemoglobin			
Plasma	P	0.01–0.05 g/L	1–5 mg/dL
Whole blood:	WB		
Adult males		8.4–10.9 mmol/L	13.5–17.5 g/dL
Adult females		7.4–9.9 mmol/L	12.0–16.0 g/dL
Hemoglobin electrophoresis	WB		
Hemoglobin A		0.95–0.98	95–98%
Hemoglobin A_2		0.015–0.035	1.5–3.5%
Hemoglobin F		0–0.02	0–2.0%
Hemoglobins other than A, A_2, or F		Absent	Absent
Heparin-induced thrombocytopenia antibody	P	Negative	Negative
Homocysteine	P	0–12 μmol/L	0–12 μmol/L
Iron	S	5.4–28.7 μmol/L	30–160 μg/dL
Iron binding capacity	S	40.8–76.7 μmol/L	228–428 μg/dL
Leukocytes			
Alkaline phosphatase (LAP)	WB	Not applicable	13–133/100 neutrophils
Count (WBC)	WB	4.5–11 × 10^9/L	4.5–11.0 × 10^3/mm^3
Mean corpuscular hemoglobin (MCH)	WB	26.0–34.0 pg/cell	26.0–34.0 pg/cell
Mean corpuscular hemoglobin concentration (MCHC)	WB	310–370 g/L	31.0–37.0 g/dL
Mean corpuscular volume (MCV)	WB		
Male (adult)		78–100 fl	78–100 μm^3
Female (adult)		78–102 fl	78–102 μm^3
Methemoglobin	WB		Up to 1% of total hemoglobin
Osmotic fragility of erythrocytes	WB	Not applicable	Increased hemolysis as compared to normal control
Partial thromboplastin time, activated	P	22.1–35.1 s	22.1–35.1 s
Plasminogen	P		
Antigen		84–140 mg/L	8.4–14.0 mg/dL
Functional		0.80–1.30	80–130%
Plasminogen activator inhibitor 1	P	4–43 μg/L	4–43 ng/mL
Platelet aggregation	PRP		>65% aggregation in response to adenosine diphosphate, epinephrine, collagen, ristocetin, and arachidonic acid
Platelet count	WB	150–350 × 10^9/L	150–350 × 10^3/mm^3
Platelet, mean volume	WB	6.4–11 fl	6.4–11.0 μm^3
Prekallikrein assay	P	0.60–1.40	60–140%
Prekallikrein screen	P		No deficiency detected
Protein C	P		
Total antigen		0.70–1.40	70–140%
Functional		0.70–1.40	70–140%
Protein S	P		
Total antigen		0.70–1.40	70–140%
Functional		0.70–1.40	70–140%
Free antigen		0.70–1.40	70–140%
Prothrombin gene mutation G20210A	WB	Not applicable	Not present
Prothrombin time	P	11.1–13.1 s	11.1–13.1 s
Protoporphyrin, free erythrocyte	WB	0.28–0.64 μmol/L of red blood cells	16–36 μg/dL of red blood cells
Red cell distribution width	WB	0.115–0.145	11.5–14.5%

(*continued*)

Analyte	Specimen	SI Units	Conventional Units
Reptilase time	P	16–24 s	16–24 s
Reticulocyte count	WB	0.005–0.025 red cells	0.5–2.5% red cells
Reticulocyte hemoglobin content	WB	>26 pg/cell	>26 pg/cell
Ristocetin confactor (Functional von Willebrand factor)	P		
Blood group O		0.75 mean of normal	75% mean of normal
Blood group A		1.05 mean of normal	105% mean of normal
Blood group B		1.15 mean of normal	115% mean of normal
Blood group AB		1.25 mean of normal	125% mean of normal
Schilling test, orally administered vitamin B_{12} excreted in urine	U	Not applicable	7–40%
Sickle cell test	WB	Negative	Negative
Sucrose hemolysis	WB	<0.1	<10% hemolysis
Thrombin time	P	16–24 s	16–24 s
Total eosinophils	WB	$70–140 \times 10^6$/L	70–440/mm³
Transferrin receptor	S, P	9.6–29.6 nmol/L	9.6–29.6 nmol/L
Viscosity			
Plasma	P	1.7–2.1	1.7–2.1
Serum	S	1.4–1.8	1.4–1.8
Vitamin B_{12}	S, P		
Normal		185 pmol/L	>250 pg/mL
Borderline		92–185 pmol/L	125–250 pg/mL
Deficient		<92 pmol/L	<125 pg/mL
von Willebrand factor (vWF) antigen (factor VIII:R antigen)	P		
vWF multimers	P	Normal distribution	Normal distribution
White blood cells: see *Leukocytes*			

Note: P, plasma; PRP, platelet-rich plasma; S, serum; U, urine; WB, whole blood

TABLE A-2   *Immunology*

Analyte	Specimen	SI Units	Conventional Units
Autoantibodies			
Anti-adrenal antibody	S	Not applicable	Negative at 1:10 dilution
Anti–double stranded (native) DNA	S	Not applicable	Negative at 1:10 dilution
Anti-glomerular basement membrane antibodies	S		
Qualitative		Negative	Negative
Quantitative		<5 kU/L	<5 U/mL
Anti-granulocyte antibody	S	Not applicable	Negative
Anti-Jo-1 antibody	S	Not applicable	Negative
Anti-La antibody	S	Not applicable	Negative
Anti-mitochondrial antibody	S	Not applicable	Negative
Antineutrophil cytoplasmic autoantibodies, cytoplasmic (C-ANCA)	S		
Qualitative		Negative	Negative
Quantitative (Antibodies to proteinase 3)		<2.8 kU/L	<2.8 U/mL
Antineutrophil cytoplasmic autoantibodies, perinuclear (P-ANCA)	S		
Qualitative		Negative	Negative
Quantitative (Antibodies to myeloperoxidase)		<1.4 kU/L	<1.4 U/mL
Antinuclear antibody	S	Not applicable	Negative at 1:40
Anti-parietal cell antibody	S	Not applicable	Negative at 1:20
Anti-Ro antibody	S	Not applicable	Negative
Anti-platelet antibody	S	Not applicable	Negative
Anti-RNP antibody	S	Not applicable	Negative
Anti-Scl 70 antibody	S	Not applicable	Negative
Anti-Smith antibody	S	Not applicable	Negative
Anti–smooth muscle antibody	S	Not applicable	Negative at 1:20
Anti-thyroglobulin	S	Not applicable	Negative
Anti-thyroid antibody	S	<0.3 kIU/L	<0.3 IU/mL
Bence Jones protein, serum	S	Not applicable	None detected
Bence Jones protein, urine, qualitative	U	Not applicable	None detected in 50× concentrated urine
Bence Jones Protein, urine, quantitative	U		
κ		<0.03 g/L	<2.5 mg/dL
λ		<0.05 g/L	<5.0 mg/dL
β_2-Microglobulin			
	S	<2.7 mg/L	<0.27 mg/dL
	U	<120 µg/d	<120 µg/d

(continued)

Analyte	Specimen	SI Units	Conventional Units
C-reactive protein	S		
Routine		0.08–3.1 mg/L	0.08–3.1 mg/L
High sensitivity		0.02–8.0 mg/L	0.02–8.0 mg/L
C1-esterase-inhibitor protein	S		
Antigenic		0.12–0.25 g/L	12.4–24.5 mg/dL
Functional		Present	Present
Complement			
C3 (adults)	S	0.86–1.84 g/L	86–184 mg/dL
C4 (adults)	S	0.20–0.58 g/L	20–58 mg/dL
Total complement, EIA (adult)	S	63–145 kU/L	63–145 U/L
Factor B	S	0.17–0.42 g/L	17–42 mg/dL
Cryoproteins	S	Not applicable	None detected
Immunofixation	S	Not applicable	None detected
Immunoglobulin, quantitation (adult)			
IgA	S	0.60–3.09 g/L	60–309 mg/dL
IgD	S	0–140 mg/L	0–14 mg/dL
IgE	S	24–430 μg/L	10–179 IU/mL
IgG	S	6.14–12.95 g/L	614–1295 mg/dL
IgG$_1$	S	2.7–17.4 g/L	270–1740 mg/dL
IgG$_2$	S	0.3–6.3 g/L	30–630 mg/dL
IgG$_3$	S	0.13–3.2 g/L	13–320 mg/dL
IgG$_4$	S	0.11–6.2 g/L	11–620 mg/dL
IgM	S	0.53–3.34 g/L	53–334 mg/dL
Joint fluid crystal	JF	Not applicable	No crystals seen
Joint fluid mucin	JF	Not applicable	Only type I mucin present
LE cell test	WB	Negative	Negative
Rheumatoid factor	S, JF	<30 kIU/L	<30.0 IU/mL
Serum protein electrophoresis	S	Not applicable	Normal pattern

Note: JF, joint fluid; P, plasma; S, serum; U, urine; WB, whole blood

TABLE A-3 *Clinical Chemistry*

Constituent	Specimen	SI Units	Conventional Units
Acetoacetate	P	<100 μmol/L	<1 mg/dL
Albumin	S	35–55 g/L	3.5–5.5 g/dL
Aldolase	S	0–100 nkat/L	0–6 U/L
α_1 antitrypsin	S	0.8–2.1 g/L	85–213 mg/dL
Alpha fetoprotein (adult)	S	<15 μg/L	<15 ng/mL
Aminotransferases	S		
Aspartate (AST, SGOT)		0–0.58 μkat/L	0–35 U/L
Alanine (ALT, SGPT)		0–0.58 μkat/L	0–35 U/L
Ammonia, as NH_3	P	6–47 μmol/L	10–80 μg/dL
Amylase	S	0.8–3.2 μkat/L	60–180 U/L
Angiotensin-converting enzyme (ACE)	S	<670 nkat/L	<40 U/L
Anion gap	S	7–16 mmol/L	7–16 mmol/L
Apolipoprotein A-1	S	1.2–2.4 g/L	119–240 mg/dL
Apolipoprotein B	S	0.52–1.63 g/L	52–163 mg/dL
Apo B/Apo A-1 ratio		0.35–0.98	0.35–0.98
Arterial blood gases			
[HCO_3^-]		21–28 mmol/L	21–30 meq/L
P_{CO_2}		4.7–5.9 kPa	35–45 mmHg
pH		7.38–7.44	
P_{O_2}		11–13 kPa	80–100 mmHg
β-Hydroxybutyrate	P	<300 μmol/L	<3 mg/dL
β-2-microglobulin	S	1.2–2.8 mg/L	1.2–2.8 mg/L
	U	≤200 μg/L	≤200 μg/L
Bilirubin	S		
Total		5.1–17 μmol/L	0.3–1.0 mg/dL
Direct		1.7–5.1 μmol/L	0.1–0.3 mg/dL
Indirect		3.4–12 μmol/L	0.2–0.7 mg/dL
Brain type natriuetic peptide (BNP)	P	Age and gender specific: <167 ng/L	Age and gender specific: <167 pg/mL
Calcium, ionized	WB	1.1–1.4 mmol/L	4.5–5.6 mg/dL
Calcium	S	2.2–2.6 mmol/L	9–10.5 mg/dL
CA-15-3	S	0–30 kU/L	0–30 U/mL
CA 19-9	S	0–37 kU/L	0–37 U/mL
CA 27-29	S	0–32 kU/L	0–32 U/mL
CA 125	S	0–35 kU/L	0–35 U/mL
Calcitonin	S		
Male		3–26 ng/L	3–26 pg/mL
Female		2–17 ng/L	2–17 pg/mL

(continued)

Constituent	Specimen	SI Units	Conventional Units
Carbon dioxide content (TCO$_2$)	P (sea level)	21–30 mmol/L	21–30 meq/L
Carbon dioxide tension (P$_{CO_2}$)	Arterial blood (sea level)	4.7–5.9 kPa	35–45 mmHg
Carbon monoxide content	WB	Symptoms with 20% saturation of hemoglobin	
Carcinoembryonic antigen (CEA)	S	0.0–3.4 ug/L	0.0–3.4 ng/mL
Ceruloplasmin	S	270–37 mg/L	27–37 ng/dL
Cholinesterase	S	5–12 kU/L	5–12 U/mL
Chloride	S	98–106 mmol/L	98–106 meq/L
Cholesterol: see Table A-7			
Coproporphyrins (types I and III)	U	150–460 μmol/d	100–300 μg/d
C-peptide	S	0.17–0.66 nmol/L	0.5–2.0 ng/mL
Creatine kinase (CK) (total)	S		
Females		0.67–2.50 μkat/L	40–150 U/L
Males		1.00–6.67 μkat/L	60–400 U/L
Creatine kinase-MB	S	0–7 μg/L	0–7 ng/mL
Creatine kinase relative index (ng/mL per total CK U/L) × 100	S	Method dependent	Method dependent
Creatinine	S	<133 μmol/L	<1.5 mg/dL
Erythropoietin	S	5–36 U/L	
Fatty acids, free (nonesterified)	P	0.28–0.89 mmol/L	<8–25 mg/dL
Ferritin	S		
Female		10–200 μg/L	10–200 ng/mL
Male		15–400 μg/L	15–400 ng/mL
Fibrinogen and fibrinogen split products: see Hematology and Coagulation			
Gamma glutamyltransferase	S	1–94 U/L	1–94 U/L
Glucose (fasting)	P		
Normal		4.2–6.4 mmol/L	75–115 mg/dL
Diabetes mellitus		>7.0 mmol/L	>125 mg/dL
Glucose, 2 h postprandial	P	<6.7 mmol/L	<120 mg/dL
Hemoglobin A$_{1c}$	WB	0.038–0.064 Hb fraction	3.8–6.4%
Homocysteine	P	4–12 μmol/L	4–12 μmol/L
Hydroxyproline	U, 24 hour	0–10 μmol/L	0–1.3 mg/d
Iron	S	9–27 μmol/L	50–150 μg/dL
Iron-binding capacity	S	45–66 μmol/L	250–370 μg/dL
Iron-binding capacity saturation	S	0.2–0.45	20–45%
Ketone (acetone)	S, U	Negative	Negative
Lactate dehydrogenase	S	1.7–3.2 μkat/L	100–190 U/L
Lactate	P, venous	0.6–1.7 mmol/L	5–15 mg/dL
Lactate dehydrogenase isoenzymes	S		
Fraction 1 (of total)		0.14–0.25	14–26%
Fraction 2		0.29–0.39	29–39%
Fraction 3		0.20–0.25	20–26%
Fraction 4		0.08–0.16	8–16%
Fraction 5		0.06–0.16	6–16%
Lipase	S	0–2.66 μkat/L	0–160 U/L
Lipids: see Table A-7			
Lipids, triglyceride: see Triglycerides			
Lipoprotein: see Table A-7			
Lipoprotein (a)	S	0–300 mg/L	0–30 mg/dL
Magnesium	S	0.8–1.2 mmol/L	1.8–3 mg/dL
Microalbumin urine			
24-h urine	U	<0.2 g/L or <0.031 g/24 h	<20 mg/L or <31 mg/24 h
Spot AM urine		<0.03 g albumin/g creatinine	<0.03 mg albumin/mg creatinine
Myoglobin	S		
Male		19–92 μg/L	
Female		12–76 μg/L	
5 Nucleotidase	S	0.02–0.18 ukat/L	0–11 U/L
N-telopeptide (cross linked), NTx	U	3–65 nmol/mmol creatinine	3–65 nmol/mmol creatinine
Osmolality			
	P	285–295 mmol/kg serum water	285–295 mosmol/kg serum water
	U	300–900 mmol/kg	300–900 mosmol/kg
Osteocalcin	S	3.1–14 ug/mL	3.1–14 ng/mL
Oxygen content	WB, arterial (sea level)		17–21 vol%
	WB, venous arm (sea level)		10 to 16 vol%
Oxygen percent saturation (sea level)			
	WB, arterial	0.97 mol/mol	97%
	WB, venous, arm	0.60–0.85 mol/mol	60–85%
Oxygen tension (P$_{O_2}$)	WB	11–13 kPa	80–100 mmHg
pH	WB	7.38–7.44	
Parathyroid hormone–related peptide	S	<1.3 pmol/L	<1.3 pmol/L
Phosphatase, acid	S	0.90 nkat/L	0–5.5 U/L
Phosphatase, alkaline	S	0.5–2.0 nkat/L	30–120 U/L

(continued)

TABLE A-3 Clinical Chemistry—(Continued)

Constituent	Specimen	SI Units	Conventional Units
Phosphorus, inorganic	S	1.0–1.4 mmol/L	3–4.5 mg/dL
Porphobilinogen	U	None	None
Potassium	S	3.5–5.0 mmol/L	3.5–5.0 meq/L
Prealbumin	S	195–358 mg/L	19.5–35.8 mg/dL
Prostate-specific antigen (PSA)	S		
Female		<0.5 μg/L	<0.5 ng/mL
Male			
<40 years		0.0–2.0 μg/L	0.0–2.0 ng/mL
>40 years		0.0–4.0 μg/L	0.0–4.0 ng/mL
PSA, free, in males 45–75 years, with PSA values between 4 and 20 μg/mL		>0.25 associated with benign prostatic hyperplasia (BPH)	>25% associated with BPH
Protein, total	S	55–80 g/L	5.5–8.0 g/dL
Protein fractions:	S		
Albumin		35–55 g/L	3.5–5.5 g/dL (50–60%)
Globulin		20–35 g/L	2.0–3.5 g/dL (40–50%)
Alpha$_1$		2–4 g/L	0.2–0.4 g/dL (4.2–7.2%)
Alpha$_2$		5–9 g/L	0.5–0.9 g/dL (6.8–12%)
Beta		6–11 g/L	0.6–1.1 g/dL (9.3–15%)
Gamma		7–17 g/L	0.7–1.7 g/dL (13–23%)
Pyruvate	P, venous	60–170 μmol/L	0.5–1.5 mg/dL
Sodium	S	136–145 mmol/L	136–145 meq/L
Transferrin	S	2.3–3.9 g/L	230–390 mg/dL
Triglycerides	S	<1.8 mmol/L	<160 mg/dL
Troponin I	S	0–0.4 μg/L	0–0.4 ng/mL
Troponin T	S	0–0.1 μg/L	0–0.1 ng/mL
Urea nitrogen	S	3.6–7.1 mmol/L	10–20 mg/dL
Uric acid	S		
Males		150–480 μmol/L	2.5–8.0 mg/dL
Females		90–360 μmol/L	1.5–6.0 mg/dL
Urobilinogen	U	1.7–5.9 μmol/d	1–3.5 mg/d
Vasoactive intestinal polypeptide	P	<75 ng/L	<75 pg/mL

Note: P, plasma; S, serum; U, urine; WB, blood

TABLE A-4 Metabolic and Endocrine Tests

Analyte	Specimen	SI Units	Conventional Units
Adrenocorticotropin (ACTH)	P	1.3–16.7 pmol/L	6.0–76.0 pg/mL
Aldosterone (adult)			
Supine, normal sodium diet	S, P	55–250 pmol/L	2–9 ng/dL
Upright, normal sodium diet	S, P		2- to 5-fold increase over supine value
Supine, low-sodium diet	S, P		2- to 5-fold increase over normal sodium diet level
Random, low-sodium diet	U	6.38–58.25 nmol/d	2.3–21.0 μg/24 h
Androstenedione (adult)	S	1.75–8.73 nmol/L	50–250 ng/dL
C peptide (adult)	S, P	0.17–0.66 nmol/L	0.5–2.0 ng/mL
Cortisol			
Fasting, 8 AM–Noon	S	138–690 nmol/L	5–25 μg/dL
Noon–8 PM		138–414 nmol/L	5–15 μg/dL
8 PM–8 AM		0–276 nmol/L	0–10 μg/dL
Cortisol, free	U	55–193 nmol/24 h	20–70 μg/24 h
C-peptide (insulin)	S	0.26–0.62 nmol/L	0.78–1.89 ng/mL
Dehydroepiandrosterone (DHEA) (adult)			
Male	S	6.24–41.6 nmol/L	180–1250 ng/dL
Female		4.5–34.0 nmol/L	130–980 ng/dL
DHEA sulfate	S		
Male (adult)		100–6190 μg/L	10–619 μg/dL
Female (adult, premenopausal)		120–5350 μg/L	12–535 μg/dL
Female (adult, postmenopausal)		300–2600 μg/L	30–260 μg/dL
Deoxycorticosterone (DOC) (adult)	S	61–576 nmol/L	2–19 ng/dL
11-Deoxycortisol (adult) (compound S) (8:00 AM)	S	0.34–4.56 nmol/L	12–158 ng/dL
Dihydrotestosterone			
Male	S, P	1.03–2.92 nmol/L	30–85 ng/dL
Female		0.14–0.76 nmol/L	4–22 ng/dL
Dopamine	P	<475 pmol/L	<87 pg/mL
Dopamine	U	425–2610 nmol/d	65–400 g/d
Epinepherine	P		
Supine (30 min)		<273 pmol/L	<50 pg/mL
Sitting		<328 pmol/L	<60 pg/mL
Standing (30 min)		<4914 pmol/L	<900 pg/mL

(continued)

Analyte	Specimen	SI Units	Conventional Units
Epinephrine	U	0–109 nmol/d	0–20 µg/d
Estradiol	S, P		
Female			
Menstruating			
Follicular phase		184–532 pmol/L	<20–145 pg/mL
Mid-cycle peak		411–1626 pmol/L	112–443 pg/mL
Luteal phase		184–885 pmol/L	<20–241 pg/mL
Postmenopausal		217 pmol/L	<59 pg/mL
Male		184 pmol/L	<20 pg/mL
Estrone	S, P		
Female			
Menstruating			
Follicular phase		55–555 pmol/L	1.5–15 pg/mL
Luteal phase		55–740 pmol/L	1.5–20 pg/mL
Postmenopausal		55–204 pmol/L	1.5–5.5 pg/mL
Male		55–240 pmol/L	1.5–6.5 pg/mL
Follicle-stimulating hormone (FSH)	S, P		
Female			
Menstruating			
Follicular phase		3.0–20.0 IU/L	3.0–20.0 U/L
Ovulatory phase		9.0–26.0 IU/L	9.0–26.0 U/L
Luteal phase		1.0–12.0 IU/L	1.0–12.0 U/L
Postmenopausal		18.0–153.0 IU/L	18.0–153.0 U/L
Male		1.0–12.0 IU/L	1.0–12.0 U/L
Fructosamine	S	1.61–2.68 mmol/L	1.61–2.68 mmol/L
Gastrin	S	<100 ng/L	<100 pg/mL
Glucagon	P	20–100 ng/L	20–100 pg/mL
Growth hormone (resting)	S	0.5–17.0 µg/L	0.5–17.0 ng/mL
Human chorionic gonadotropin (HCG) (nonpregnant)	S	<5 IU/L	<5 mIU/mL
17-Hydroxyprogesterone (adult)	S		
Male		0.15 nmol/L	5–250 ng/dL
Female			
Follicular phase		0.6–3.0 nmol/L	20–100 ng/dL
Midcycle peak		3–7.5 nmol/L	100–250 ng/dL
Luteal phase		3–15 nmol/L	100–500 ng/dL
Postmenopausal		≤2.1 nmol/L	≤70 ng/dL
5-Hydroindoleacetic Acid [5-HIAA]	U	10.5–36.6 µmol/d	2–7 mg/d
Insulin	S, P	14.35–143.5 pmol/L	2–20 µU/mL
17 Ketosteroids	U	10–42 µmol/d	3–12 mg/d
Luteinizing hormone (LH)	S, P		
Female			
Menstruating			
Follicular phase		2.0–15.0 U/L	2.0–15.0 U/L
Ovulatory phase		22.0–105.0 U/L	22.0–105.0 U/L
Luteal phase		0.6–19.0 U/L	0.6–19.0 U/L
Postmenopausal		16.0–64.0 U/L	16.0–64.0 U/L
Male		2.0–12.0 U/L	2.0–12.0 U/L
Metanephrine	P	Method dependent	Method dependent
Metanephrine	U	0.03–0.69 mmol/mol creatinine	0.05–1.20 µg/mg creatinine
Norepinephrine	U	89–473 nmol/d	15–80 µg/d
Norepinephrine	P		
Supine (30 min)		650–2423 pmol/L	<110–410 pg/mL
Sitting		709–4019 pmol/L	120–680 pg/mL
Standing (30 min)		739–4137 pmol/L	125–700 pg/mL
Parathyroid hormone (PTH)	S	10–60 ng/L	10–60 pg/mL
Pregnanetriol	U	Age and sex dependent	Age and sex dependent
Progesterone	S, P		
Female			
Follicular		<3.18 nmol/L	<1.0 ng/mL
Midluteal		9.54–63.6 nmol/L	3–20 ng/mL
Male		<3.18 nmol/L	<1.0 ng/mL
Prolactin	S		
Female		0–20 µg/L	1.9–25.9 ng/mL
Male		0–15 µg/L	1.6–23.0 ng/mL
Renin (adult, normal sodium diet)	P		
Supine		0.08–0.83 ng/(L·s)	0.3–3.0 ng/(mL/h)
Upright		0.28–2.5 ng/(L·s)	1–9.0 ng/(mL/h)
Serotonin	WB	0.28–1.14 µmol/L	50–200 ng/mL
Serotonin	Platelet	0.7–2.8 amol/platelet	125–500 ng/10^9 platelets
Sex hormone binding globulin (adult)	S		
Male			13–71 nmol/L
Female			18–114 nmol/L
Somatostatin	P	<25 ng/L	<25 pg/mL

(continued)

TABLE A-4 Metabolic and Endocrine Tests—(Continued)

Analyte	Specimen	SI Units	Conventional Units
Somatomedin-C (IGF-1) (adult)	S		
16–24 years		182–780 μg/L	182–780 ng/mL
25–39 years		114–492 μg/L	114–492 ng/mL
40–54 years		90–360 μg/L	90–360 ng/mL
>54 years		71–290 μg/L	71–290 ng/mL
Testosterone, total, morning sample	S		
Female		0.21–2.98 nmol/L	6–86 ng/dL
Male		9.36–37.10 nmol/L	270–1070 ng/dL
Testosterone, unbound, morning sample			
Female, adult	S	6.9–107.5 pmol/L	0.2–3.1 pg/mL
Male, adult		416–1386 pmol/L	12.0–40.0 pg/mL
Thyroglobulin	S	0–60 μg/L	0–60 ng/mL
Thyroid binding globulin	S	206–309 μg/L	16–24 μg/dL
Thyroid hormone binding index (THBI or T₃RU)	S	0.83–1.17 mol ratio	0.83–1.17
(Free) thyroxine index	S	4.2–13	4.2–13
Thyroid stimulating hormone	S	0.5–4.7 mU/L	0.5–4.7 μU/mL
Thyroxine, total (T4)	S	58–140 nmol/L	4.5–10.9 μg/dL
Triiodothyronine, total (T3)	S	0.92–2.78 nmol/L	60–181 ng/dL
Thyroxine, free (fT4)	S	10.3–35 pmol/L	0.8–2.7 ng/dL
Triiodothyronine, free (fT3)	S	0.22–6.78 pmol/L	1.4–4.4 pg/mL
Vanillylmandelic Acid (VMA)	U, 24 h	7.6–37.9 μmol/d	0.15–1.2 mg/d
Vasoactive intestinal polypeptide (VIP)	P	<75 ng/L	<75 pg/mL

Note: P, plasma; S, serum; U, urine; WB, whole blood

TABLE A-5 Toxicology and Therapeutic Drug Monitoring

Drug	Therapeutic Range Conventional Units	Therapeutic Range SI Units	Toxic Level Conventional Units	Toxic Level SI Units
Acetaminophen	10–30 μg/mL	66–199 μmol/L	>200 μg/mL	>1324 μmol/L
Amikacin				
Peak	25–35 μg/mL	43–60 μmol/L	>35 μg/mL	>60 μmol/L
Trough	4–8 μg/mL	6.8–13.7 μmol/L	>10 μg/mL	>17 μmol/L
Amitriptyline	120–250 ng/mL	433–903 nmol/L	>500 ng/mL	>1805 nmol/L
Amphetamine	20–30 ng/mL	148–222 nmol/L	>200 ng/mL	>1480 nmol/L
Antiepileptic drugs: see Table 348–8				
Barbiturates, most short-acting			>20 mg/L	>88 μmol/L
Bromide			>1250 μg/mL	>15.6 mmol/L
Carbamazepine	6–12 μg/mL	26–51 μmol/L	>15 μg/mL	>63 μmol/L
Chlordiazepoxide	700–1000 ng/mL	2.34–3.34 μmol/L	>5000 ng/mL	>16.7 μmol/L
Clonazepam	15–60 ng/mL	48–190 nmol/L	>80 ng/mL	>254 nmol/L
Clozapine	200–350 ng/mL	0.6–1 μmol/L		
Cocaine			>1000 ng/mL	>3300 nmol/L
Cyclosporine	Depends on timing after dose and transplant type with ranges of 100–400 ng/mL	Depends on timing after dose and transplant type with ranges of 83–333 nmol/L	Varies with time after dose and transplant type	Varies with time after dose and transplant type
Desipramine	75–300 ng/mL	281–1125 nmol/L	>400 ng/mL	>1500 nmol/L
Diazepam	100–1000 ng/mL	0.35–351 μmol/L	>5000 ng/mL	>17.55 μmol/L
Digoxin	0.8–2.0 ng/mL	1.0–2.6 nmol/L	>2.5 ng/mL	>3.2 μmol/L
Doxepin	30–150 ng/mL	107–537 nmol/L	>500 ng/mL	>1790 nmol/L
Ethanol			>300 mg/dL	>65 mmol/L
Behavioral changes	>20 mg/dL	>4.3 mmol/L		
Clinical intoxication	>100 mg/dL	>1 g/L		
Ethosuximide	40–100 μg/mL	283–708 μmol/L	>150 μg/mL	>1062 μmol/L
Flecainide	0.2–1.0 μg/mL	0.5–2.4 μmol/L	>1.0 μg/mL	>2.4 μmol/L
Gentamicin				
Peak	8–10 μg/mL	16.7–20.9 μmol/L	>10 μg/mL	>21 μmol/L
Trough	<2–4 μg/mL	<4.2–8.4 μmol/L	>4 μg/mL	>8.4 μmol/L
Ibuprofen	10–50 μg/mL	49–243 μmol/L	100–700 μg/mL	485–3395 μmol/L
Imipramine	125–250 ng/mL	446–893 nmol/L	>500 ng/mL	>1784 nmol/L
Lidocaine	1.5–6.0 μg/mL	6.4–26 μmol/L		26–34.2 μmol/L
CNS or Cardiovascular depression			6–8 μg/mL	>34.2 μmol/L
Seizures, obtundation, decreased cardiac output			>8 μg/mL	
Lithium	0.6–1.2 meq/L	0.6–1.2 nmol/L	>2 meq/L	>2 mmol/L
Methadone	100–400 ng/mL	0.32–1.29 μmol/L	>2000 ng/mL	>6.46 μmol/L
Methotrexate	Variable	Variable		
Low dose (1–2 weeks)			>9.1 ng/mL	>20 nmol/L
High dose (48 h)			>227 ng/mL	>0.5 μmol/L

(continued)

Drug	Therapeutic Range		Toxic Level	
	Conventional Units	SI Units	Conventional Units	SI Units
Morphine	10–80 ng/mL	35–280 μmol/L	>200 ng/mL	>700 nmol/L
Nitroprusside (as thiocyanate)	6–29 μg/mL	103–499 μmol/L		
Nortriptyline	50–170 ng/mL	190–646 nmol/L	>500 ng/mL	>1.9 μmol/L
Phenobarbital	10–40 μg/mL	43–170 μmol/L		
Slowness, ataxia, nystagmus			35–80 μg/mL	151–345 μmol/L
Coma with reflexes			65–117 μg/mL	280–504 μmol/L
Coma without reflexes			>100 μg/mL	>430 μmol/L
Phenytoin	10–20 μg/mL	40–79 μmol/L	>20 μg/mL	>79 μmol/L
Procainamide	4–10 μg/mL	17–42 μmol/L	>10–12 μg/mL	>42–51 μmol/L
Quinidine	2–5 μg/mL	6–15 μmol/L	>6 μg/mL	>18 μmol/L
Salicylates	150–300 μg/mL	1086–2172 μmol/L	>300 μg/mL	>2172 μmol/L
Theophylline	8–20 μg/mL	44–111 μmol/L	>20 μg/mL	>110 μmol/L
Thiocyanate				
After nitroprusside infusion	6–29 μg/mL	103–499 μmol/L		
Nonsmoker	1–4 μg/mL	17–69 μmol/L	>120 μg/mL	>2064 μmol/L
Smoker	3–12 μg/mL	52–206 μmol/L		
Tobramycin				
Peak	8–10 μg/mL	17–21 μmol/L	>10 μg/mL	>21 μmol/L
Trough	<4 μg/mL	<9 μmol/L	>4 μg/mL	>9 μmol/L
Valproic acid	50–150 μg/mL	347–1040 μmol/L	>150 μg/mL	>1040 μmol/L
Vancomycin				
Peak	18–26 μg/mL	12–18 μmol/L	>80–100 μg/mL	>55–69 μmol/L
Trough	5–10 μg/mL	3–7 μmol/L		

TABLE A-6 Vitamins and Selected Trace Minerals

Specimen	Analyte	SI Units	Conventional Units
Aluminum	S	<0.2 μmol/L	<5.41 μg/L
	U, random	5–30 μg/L	0.19–1.11 μmol/L
Arsenic			
	WB	0.03–0.31 μmol/L	2–23 μg/L
	U, 24 h	0.07–0.67 μmol/d	5–50 μg/d
Coenzyme Q10 (ubiquinone)	P	0.5–1.5 mg/L	0.5–1.5 μg/mL
Carotenoids	S	0.9–5.6 μmol/L	50–300 μg/dL
Copper			
	S	11–22 μmol/L	70–140 μg/dL
	U, 24 h	0.047–0.55 μmol/d	3–35 μg/d
Folic acid	RC	340–1020 nmol/L cells	150–450 ng/mL cells
Folic acid	S	7–36 nmol/L cells	3–16 ng/mL cells
Lead (adult)	S	<0.5–1 μmol/L	<10–20 μg/dL
Mercury			
	WB	3.0–294 nmol/L	0.6–59 μg/L
	U, 24 h	<99.8 nmol/L	<20 μg/L
Vitamin A	S	0.7–3.5 μmol/L	20–100 μg/dL
Vitamin B$_1$ (thiamine)	S	0–75 nmol/L	0–2 μg/dL
Vitamin B$_2$ (riboflavin)	S	106–638 nmol/L	4–24 μg/dL
Vitamin B$_6$	P	20–121 nmol/L	5–30 ng/mL
Vitamin B$_{12}$	S	148–590 pmol/L	200–800 pg/mL
Vitamin C (ascorbic acid)	S	23–57 μmol/L	0.4–1.0 mg/dL
Vitamin D$_3$, 1,25-dihydroxy	S	60–108 pmol/L	25–45 pg/mL
Vitamin D$_3$, 25-hydroxy (some labs report as a desirable level rather than a normal range)	P		
Summer		37.4–200 nmol/L	15–80 ng/mL
Winter		34.9–105 nmol/L	14–42 ng/mL
Vitamin E	S	12–42 μmol/L	5–18 μg/mL
Vitamin K	S	0.29–2.64 nmol/L	0.13–1.19 ng/mL
Zinc	S	11.5–18.5 μmol/L	75–120 μg/dL

Note: P, plasma; RC, red cells; S, serum; U, urine; WB, whole blood

TABLE A-7 Classification of LDL, Total, and HDL Cholesterol

LDL cholesterol	
<100	Optimal
100–129	Near or above normal
130–159	Borderline high
160–189	High
≥190	Very high
Total cholesterol	
<200	Desirable
200–239	Borderline high
≥240	High
HDL cholesterol	
<40	Low
≥60	High

Note: HDL, high-density lipoprotein; LDL, low-density lipoprotein
Source: Executive summary of the third report of the national cholesterol education program (NCEP) expert panel on detection, evaluation, and treatment of high blood cholesterol in adults (adult treatment panel III): JAMA 285:2486, 2001.

TABLE B-1 *Cerebrospinal Fluid[a]*

Constituent	SI Units	Conventional Units
Glucose	2.22–3.89 mmol/L	40–70 mg/dL
Lactate	1–2 mmol/L	10–20 mg/dL
Total protein		
Lumbar	0.15–0.5 g/L	15–50 mg/dL
Cisternal	0.15–0.25 g/L	15–25 mg/dL
Ventricular	0.06–0.15 g/L	6–15 mg/dL
Albumin	0.066–0.442 g/L	6.6–44.2 mg/dL
IgG	0.009–0.057 g/L	0.9–5.7 mg/dL
IgG index[b]	0.29–0.59	
Oligoclonal bands (OGB)	<2 bands not present in matched serum sample	
Ammonia	15–47 μmol/L	25–80 μg/dL
CSF pressure		50–180 mmH₂O
CSF volume (adult)	~150 mL	
Red blood cells	0	0
Leukocytes		
Total	0–5 mononuclear cells per mm³	
Differential		
Lymphocytes	60–70%	
Monocytes	30–50%	
Neutrophils	None	

[a] Since cerebrospinal fluid concentrations are equilibrium values, measurements of the same parameters in blood plasma obtained at the same time are recommended. However, there is a time lag in attainment of equilibrium, and cerebrospinal levels of plasma constituents that can fluctuate rapidly (such as plasma glucose) may not achieve stable values until after a significant lag phase.

[b] IgG index = CSF IgG(mg/dL) × serum albumin(g/dL)/Serum IgG(g/dL) × CSF albumin(mg/dL)

TABLE B-3 *Differential Nucleated Cell Counts of Bone Marrow Aspirates*

	Mean, %	Range, %	95% Confidence Intervals, %
Myeloid (total)	56.7		
Neutrophilic series (total)	53.6	49.2–65.0	33.6–73.6
Myeloblast	0.9	0.2–1.5	0.1–1.7
Promyelocyte	3.3	2.1–4.1	1.9–4.7
Myelocyte	12.7	8.2–15.7	8.5–16.9
Metamyelocyte	15.9	9.6–24.6	7.1–24.7
Band	12.4	9.5–15.3	9.4–15.4
Segmented	7.4	6.0–12.0	3.8–11.0
Eosinophilic series	3.1	1.2–5.3	1.1–5.2
Basophilic and mast cells	0.1	0–0.2	—
Erythroid (total)	25.6	18.4–33.8	15.0–36.2
Pronormoblasts	0.6	0.2–1.3	0.1–1.1
Basophilic normoblasts	1.4	0.5–2.4	0.4–2.4
Polychromatophilic normoblasts	21.6	17.9–29.2	13.1–30.1
Orthochromatic normoblasts	2.0	0.4–4.6	0.3–3.7
Lymphocytes	16.2	11.1–23.2	8.6–23.8
Plasma cells	1.3	0.4–3.9	0–3.5
Monocytes	0.3	0–0.8	0–0.6
Megakaryocytes	0.1	0–0.4	—
Reticulum cells	0.3	0–0.9	0–0.8
M:E ratio	2.3	1.5–3.3	1.1–3.5

Note: Data are from 12 healthy men.
Source: From SL Perkins: Normal blood and bone marrow values in humans, in GR Lee et al (eds): *Wintrobe's Clinical Hematology,* 10th ed, Philadelphia, Williams and Wilkins, 1999, pp 2738–2748, with permission.

TABLE B-2 *Urine Analysis*

	SI Units	Conventional Units
Acidity, titratable	20–40 mmol/d	20–40 meq/d
Ammonia	30–50 mmol/d	30–50 meq/d
Amylase		4–400 U/L
Amylase/creatinine clearance ratio [(Cl_am/Cl_cr) × 100]	1–5	1–5
Calcium (10 meq/d or 200 mg/d dietary calcium)	<7.5 mmol/d	<300 mg/d
Creatine, as creatinine		
Female	<760 μmol/d	<100 mg/d
Male	<380 μmol/d	<50 mg/d
Creatinine	8.8–14 mmol/d	1.0–1.6 g/d
Eosinophils	<100 eosinophils/mL	<100 eosinophils/mL
Glucose, true (oxidase method)	0.3–1.7 mmol/d	50–300 mg/d
5-Hydroxyindoleacetic acid (5-HIAA)	10–47 μmol/d	2–9 mg/d
"Microalbumin"	<0.02 g/L	<20 mg/L
Oxalate	228–684 μmol/d	20–60 mg/d
pH	5.0–9.0	5.0–9.0
Phosphate (phosphorus) (varies with intake)	12.9–42.0 mmol/d	400–1300 mg/d
Potassium (varies with intake)	25–100 mmol/d	25–100 meq/d
Protein	<0.15 g/d	<150 mg/d
Sediment		
Bacteria	Negative	
Bladder cells	Negative	
Broad casts	Negative	
Crystals	Negative	
Epithelial cell casts	Negative	
Granular casts	Negative	
Hyaline casts	0–5/low power field	
Red blood cell casts	Negative	
Red blood cells	0–2/high power field	
Squamous cells	Negative	
Tubular cells	Negative	
Waxy casts	Negative	
White blood cells	0–2/high power field	
White cell casts	Negative	
Sodium (varies with intake)	100–260 mmol/d	100–260 meq/d
Specific gravity	1.001–1.035	
Urea nitrogen	214–607 mmol/d	6–17 g/d
Uric acid (normal diet)	1.49–4.76 mmol/d	250–800 mg/d

TABLE B-4 *Stool Analysis*

	SI Units	Conventional Units
Bulk		
Wet weight	<197.5 (115 ± 41) g/d	<197.5 (115 ± 41) g/d
Dry weight	<66.4 (34 ± 15) g/d	<66.4 (34 ± 15) g/d
α₁ Antitrypsin	0.98 (±0.17) mg/g dry weight	0.98 (±0.17) mg/g dry weight
Coproporphyrin	600–1500 nmol/d	400–1000 μg/d
Fat		
Adult		<7 g/d
Adult on fat-free diet		<4 g/d
Fatty acid		
Free	0.01–0.10	1–10% of dry matter
Combined as soap	0.005–0.12	0.5–12% of dry matter
Nitrogen	<1.7 (1.4 ± 0.2) g/d	<1.7 (1.4 ± 0.2) g/d
Protein content	Minimal	Minimal
Urobilinogen	68–470 μmol/d	40–280 mg/d
Water	~0.65	~65%

TABLE C-1 *Renal Function Tests*

	SI Units	Conventional Units
Clearances (corrected to 1.72 m² body surface area)		
Measures of glomerular filtration rate (GFR)		
Inulin clearance (Cl)		
Males (mean ± 1 SD)	2.1 ± 0.4 mL/s	124 ± 25.8 mL/min
Females (mean ± 1 SD)	2.0 ± 0.2 mL/s	119 ± 12.8 mL/min
Endogenous creatinine clearance	1.5–2.2 mL/s	91–130 mL/min
Urea	1.0–1.7 mL/s	60–100 mL/min
Measures of effective renal plasma flow and tubular function		
p-Aminohippuric acid clearance (Cl$_{PAH}$)		
Males (mean ± 1 SD)	10.9 ± 2.7 mL/s	654 ± 163 mL/min
Females (mean ± 1 SD)	9.9 ± 1.7 mL/s	594 ± 102 mL/min
Concentration and dilution test		
Specific gravity of urine		
After 12-h fluid restriction	>1.025	>1.025
After 12-h deliberate water intake	≤1.003	≤1.003
Protein excretion, urine	<0.15 g/d	<150 mg/d
Specific gravity, maximal range	1.002–1.028	1.002–1.028
Tubular reabsorption, phosphorus	0.79–0.94 of filtered load	79–94% of filtered load

TABLE C-2 *Gastrointestinal Tests*

Test	SI Units	Conventional Units
Absorption tests		
D-Xylose: after overnight fast, 25 g xylose given in oral aqueous solution		
Urine, collected for following 5 h	33–53 mmol (or >20% of ingested dose	5–8 g (or >20% of ingested dose)
Serum, 1 h after dose	1.7–2.7 mmol/L	25–40 mg/dL
Vitamin A: a fasting blood specimen is obtained and 200,000 units of vitamin A in oil is given orally	Serum level should rise to twice fasting level in 3–5 h	Serum level should rise to twice fasting level in 3–5 h
Bentiromide test (pancreatic function): 500 mg bentiromide (chymex) orally; p-aminobenzoic acid (PABA) measured		
Plasma		>3.6 (±1.1) μg/mL at 90 min
Urine	>50% recovered in 6 h	>50% recovered in 6 h
Gastric juice		
Volume		
24 h	2–3 L	2–3 L
Nocturnal	600–700 mL	600–700 mL
Basal, fasting	30–70 mL/h	30–70 mL/h
Reaction		
pH	1.6–1.8	1.6–1.8
Titratable acidity of fasting juice	4–9 μmol/s	15–35 meq/h
Acid output		
Basal		
Females (mean ± 1 SD)	0.6 ± 0.5 μmol/s	2.0 ± 1.8 meq/h
Males (mean ± 1 SD)	0.8 ± 0.6 μmol/s	3.0 ± 2.0 meq/h
Maximal (after SC histamine acid phosphate, 0.004 mg/kg body weight, and preceded by 50 mg promethazine, or after betazole, 1.7 mg/kg body weight, or pentagastrin, 6 μg/kg body weight)		
Females (mean ± 1 SD)	4.4 ± 1.4 μmol/s	16 ± 5 meq/h
Males (mean ± 1 SD)	6.4 ± 1.4 μmol/s	23 ± 5 meq/h
Basal acid output/maximal acid output ratio	≤0.6	≤0.6
Gastrin, serum	40–200 μg/L	40–200 pg/mL
Secretin test (pancreatic exocrine function): 1 unit/kg body weight, IV		
Volume (pancreatic juice) in 80 min	>2.0 mL/kg	>2.0 mL/kg
Bicarbonate concentration	>80 mmol/L	>80 meq/L
Bicarbonate output in 30 min	>10 mmol	>10 meq

TABLE C-3 Circulatory Function Tests

Test	SI Units (Range)	Conventional Units (Range)
Arteriovenous oxygen difference	30–50 mL/L	30–50 mL/L
Cardiac output (Fick)	2.5–3.6 L/m² of body surface area per minute	2.5–3.6 L/m² of body surface area per minute
Contractility indices		
Max. left ventricular dp/dt (dp/dt)/DP when DP = 5.3 kPa (40 mmHg)	220 kPa/s (176–250 kPa/s) (37.6 ± 12.2)/s	1650 mmHg/s (1320–1880 mmHg/s) (37.6 ± 12.2)/s
Mean normalized systolic ejection rate (angiography)	3.32 ± 0.84 end-diastolic volumes per second	3.32 ± 0.84 end-diastolic volumes per second
Mean velocity of circumferential fiber shortening (angiography)	1.83 ± 0.56 circumferences per second	1.83 ± 0.56 circumferences per second
Ejection fraction; stroke volume/end diastolic volume (SV/EDV)	0.67 ± 0.08 (0.55–0.78)	0.67 ± 0.08 (0.55–0.78)
End-diastolic volume	70 ± 20.0 mL/m² (60–88 mL/m²)	70 ± 20.0 mL/m² (60–88 mL/m²)
End-systolic volume	25 ± 5.0 mL/m² (20–33 mL/m²)	25 ± 5.0 mL/m² (20–33 mL/m²)
Left ventricular work		
Stroke work index	50 ± 20.0 (g·m)/m² (30–110)	50 ± 20.0 (g·m)/m² (30–110)
Left ventricular minute work index	1.8–6.6 [(kg·m)m²]/min	1.8–6.6 [(kg·m)m²]/min
Oxygen consumption index	110–150 mL	110–150 mL
Maximum oxygen uptake	35 mL/min (20–60 mL/min)	35 mL/min (20–60 mL/min)
Pulmonary vascular resistance	2–12 (kPa·s)/L	20–130 (dyn·s)/cm⁵
Systemic vascular resistance	77–150 (kPa·s)/L	770–1600 (dyn·s)/cm⁵

Note: DP, diastolic pressure
Source: E Braunwald et al, *Heart Disease*, 6th ed. Philadelphia, Saunders, 2001, with permission

TABLE C-4 Summary of Values Useful in Pulmonary Physiology

Test	Symbol	Man Age 40, 75 kg, 175 cm Tall	Woman Age 40, 60 kg, 160 cm Tall
PULMONARY MECHANICS			
Spirometry—volume-time curves			
Forced vital capacity	FVC	4.8 L	3.3 L
Forced expiratory volume in 1 s	FEV_1	3.8 L	2.8 L
FEV_1/FVC	FEV_1%	76%	77%
Maximal midexpiratory flow	MMF (FEF 25–27)	4.8 L/s	3.6 L/s
Maximal expiratory flow rate	MEFR (FEF 200–1200)	9.4 L/s	6.1 L/s
Spirometry—flow-volume curves			
Maximal expiratory flow at 50% of expired vital capacity	V_{max} 50 (FEF 50%)	6.1 L/s	4.6 L/s
Maximal expiratory flow at 75% of expired vital capacity	V_{max} 75 (FEF 75%)	3.1 L/s	2.5 L/s
Resistance to airflow			
Pulmonary resistance	RL/(R_L)	<3.0 (cmH₂O/s)/L	
Airway resistance	Raw	<2.5 (cmH₂O/s)/L	
Specific conductance	SGaw	>0.13 cmH₂O/s	
Pulmonary compliance			
Static recoil pressure at total lung capacity	Pst TLC	25 ± 5 cmH₂O	
Compliance of lungs (static)	CL	0.2 L cmH₂O	
Compliance of lungs and thorax	C(L + T)	0.1 L cmH₂O	
Dynamic compliance of 20 breaths per minute	C dyn 20	0.25 ± 0.05 L/cmH₂O	
Maximal static respiratory pressures:			
Maximal inspiratory pressure	MIP	>90 cmH₂O	>50 cmH₂O
Maximal expiratory pressure	MEP	>150 cmH₂O	>120 cmH₂O
LUNG VOLUMES			
Total lung capacity	TLC	6.4 L	4.9 L
Functional residual capacity	FRC	2.2 L	2.6 L
Residual volume	RV	1.5 L	1.2 L
Inspiratory capacity	IC	4.8 L	3.7 L
Expiratory reserve volume	ERV	3.2 L	2.3 L
Vital capacity	VC	1.7 L	1.4 L
GAS EXCHANGE (SEA LEVEL)			
Arterial O_2 tension	Pa_{O_2}	12.7 ± 0.7 kPa (95 ± 5 mmHg)	
Arterial CO_2 tension	Pa_{CO_2}	5.3 ± 0.3 kPa (40 ± 2 mmHg)	
Arterial O_2 saturation	Sa_{O_2}	0.97 ± 0.02 (97 ± 2%)	
Arterial blood pH	pH	7.40 ± 0.02	
Arterial bicarbonate	HCO_3^-	24 + 2 meq/L	
Base excess	BE	0 ± 2 meq/L	
Diffusing capacity for carbon monoxide (single breath)	DL_{CO}	0.42 mLCO/s per mmHg (25 mL CO/min per mmHg)	
Dead space volume	V_D	2 mL/kg body wt	
Physiologic dead space; dead space-tidal volume ratio	V_D/V_T		
Rest		$\leq 35\%$ V_T	
Exercise		$\leq 20\%$ V_T	
Alveolar-arterial difference for O_2	P(A − a)$_{O_2}$	≤ 2.7 kPa ≤ 20 kPa (≤ 20 mmHg)	

TABLE C-5 *Normal Values of Doppler Echocardiographic Measurements in Adults*

	Range	Mean
RVD (cm), measured at the base in apical 4-chamber view	2.6 to 4.3	3.5 ± 0.4
LVID (cm), measured in the parasternal long axis view	3.6 to 5.4	4.7 ± 0.4
Posterior LV wall thickness (cm)	0.6 to 1.1	0.9 ± 0.4
IVS wall thickness (cm)	0.6 to 1.1	0.9 ± 0.4
Left atrial dimension (cm), anteroposterior dimension	2.3 to 3.8	3.0 ± 0.3
Aortic root dimension (cm)	2.0 to 3.5	2.4 ± 0.4
Aortic cusps separation (cm)	1.5 to 2.6	1.9 ± 0.4
Percentage of fractional shortening	34 to 44%	36%
Mitral flow (m/s)	0.6 to 1.3	0.9
Tricuspid flow (m/s)	0.3 to 0.7	0.5
Pulmonary artery (m/s)	0.6 to 0.9	0.75
Aorta (m/s)	1.0 to 1.7	1.35

Note: IVS, interventricular septum; LV, left ventricle; LVID, left ventricular internal dimension; RVD, right ventricular dimension
Source: From A Weyman: *Principles and Practice of Echocardiography,* 2d ed, Philadelphia, Lea & Febiger, with permission.

D | MISCELLANEOUS

TABLE D-1 *Body Fluids and Other Mass Data*

	Reference Range	
	SI Units	Conventional Units
Ascitic fluid: see Chap . . .		
Body fluid		
Total volume (lean) of body weight	50% (in obese) to 70%	
Intracellular	0.3–0.4 of body weight	
Extracellular	0.2–0.3 of body weight	
Blood		
Total volume		
Males	69 mL per kg body weight	
Females	65 mL per kg body weight	
Plasma volume		
Males	39 mL per kg body weight	
Females	40 mL per kg body weight	
Red blood cell volume		
Males	30 mL per kg body weight	1.15–1.21 L/m² of body surface area
Females	25 mL per kg body weight	0.95–1.00 L/m² of body surface area
Body Mass Index	18.5–24.9 kg/m²	18.5–24.9 kg/m²

TABLE D-2 *Radiation-Derived Units*

Quantity	Old Unit	SI Unit	Name for SI Unit (and Abbreviation)	Conversion
Activity	curie (Ci)	Disintegrations per second (dps)	becquerel (Bq)	1 Ci = 3.7×10^{10} Bq 1 mCi = 37 mBq 1 μCi = 0.037 MBq or 37 GBq 1 Bq = 2.703×10^{-11} Ci
Absorbed dose	rad	joule per kilogram (J/kg)	gray (Gy)	1 Gy = 100 rad 1 rad = 0.01 Gy 1 mrad = 10^{-3} cGy
Exposure	roentgen (R)	coulomb per kilogram (C/kg)	—	1 C/kg = 3876 R 1 R = 2.58×10^{-4} C/kg 1 mR = 258 pC/kg
Dose equivalent	rem	joule per kilogram (J/kg)	sievert (Sv)	1 Sv = 100 rem 1 rem = 0.01 Sv 1 mrem = 10 μSv

Bold number indicates the start of the main discussion of the topic; numbers with "f" and "t" refer to figure and table pages.